W9-BNR-886

VOLUME ONE

CANCER MEDICINE

Fourth Edition

VOLUME ONE

CANCER MEDICINE

Fourth Edition

James F. Holland
Distinguished Professor of Neoplastic Diseases
Director Emeritus, Derald H. Ruttenberg Cancer Center
Mount Sinai Medical Center
New York, New York

Robert C. Bast, Jr.
Internist and Professor of Medicine
Harry Carothers Wiess Chair for Cancer Research
Head, Division of Medicine
University of Texas M. D. Anderson Cancer Center
Houston, Texas

Donald L. Morton
Medical Director and Surgeon-in-Chief
John Wayne Cancer Institute at St. John's Hospital
Santa Monica, California
Professor and Chief, Emeritus, Surgery/Oncology
UCLA School of Medicine
Los Angeles, California

Emil Frei III
Director and Physician-in-Chief, Emeritus
Dana-Farber Cancer Institute
Richard and Susan Smith Distinguished Professor of Medicine
Harvard Medical School
Boston, Massachusetts

Donald W. Kufe
Deputy Director
Dana-Farber Cancer Center
Chief, Division of Cancer Pharmacology
Dana-Farber Cancer Institute
Professor of Medicine
Harvard Medical School
Boston, Massachusetts

Ralph R. Weichselbaum
Harold H. Hines, Jr., Professor and Chairman
Department of Radiation and Cellular Oncology
University of Chicago Hospital
Director, Chicago Tumor Institute
University of Chicago
Chicago, Illinois

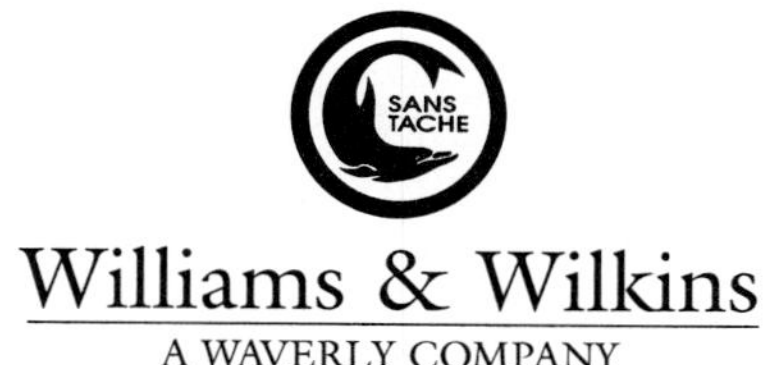

Williams & Wilkins
A WAVERLY COMPANY

BALTIMORE • PHILADELPHIA • LONDON • PARIS • BANGKOK
BUENOS AIRES • HONG KONG • MUNICH • SYDNEY • TOKYO • WROCLAW

Editor: Jonathan W. Pine, Jr.
Managing Editor: Molly Mullen
Production Coordinator: Carol Eckhart
Copy Editor: Hockett Editorial Service
Designer: Norman Och
Illustration Planner: Raymond Lowman
Cover Designer: Dan Pfisterer
Typesetter: Maryland Composition Company, Inc.
Printer and Binder: R. R. Donnelley & Sons

351 West Camden Street
Baltimore, Maryland 21201-2436 USA

Rose Tree Corporate Center
1400 North Providence Road
Building II, Suite 5025
Media, Pennsylvania 19063-2043 USA

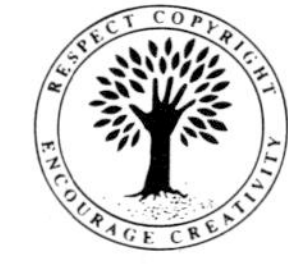

Accurate indications, adverse reactions and dosage schedules for drugs are provided in this book, but it is possible that they may change. The reader is urged to review the package information data of the manufacturers of the medications mentioned.

Printed in the United States of America

First Edition, 1973
Second Edition, 1982
Third Edition, 1993

Library of Congress Cataloging-in-Publication Data may be obtained from the Publisher.

ISBN 0-683-04095-2

The publishers have made every effort to trace the copyright holders for borrowed material. If they have inadvertently overlooked any, they will be pleased to make the necessary arrangements at the first opportunity.

To purchase additional copies of this book, call our customer service department at (800) 638-0672 or fax orders to (800) 447-8438. For other book services, including chapter reprints and large quantity sales, ask for the Special Sales department.

Canadian customers should call (800) 268-4178, or fax (905) 470-6780. For all other calls originating outside the United States, please call (410) 528-4223 or fax us at (410) 528-8550.

Visit Williams & Wilkins on the Internet: **http://www.wwilkins.com** or contact our customer service department at **custserv@wwilkins.com**. Williams & Wilkins customer service representatives are available from 8:30 am to 6:00 pm, EST, Monday through Friday, for telephone access.

97 98 99 00 01
1 2 3 4 5 6 7 8 9 10

PREFACE

This fourth edition of *Cancer Medicine* recognizes the accelerated discovery of new knowledge that must be made accessible to the clinical oncologist. Clinical chapters are written primarily by surgical, radiation, and medical oncologists to assure a multidisciplinary approach to each disease. Gynecologic, urologic, orthopedic, and otolaryngologic surgical oncologists have contributed in their specialty areas. Psycho-oncology, nursing oncology, and rehabilitation medicine are all represented. Pathology and the imaging specialties are specifically included as individual contributions and as parts of the chapters on various diseases. The editors are fortunate in having been able to attract preeminent clinicians to these tasks. This edition has greatly expanded the coverage of pediatric oncology, in large part because the editors believe that there are many lessons to be learned from these neoplasms. They are grateful to Denman Hammond, M.D., for his invaluable help with this section.

New chapters on gene therapy, minimally invasive surgery, vascular access, low-intensity electromagnetic fields, the law and cancer, outcomes assessment, and cardiac tumors have been added. Many chapters have been entirely rewritten by authors new to this volume whose selection has strengthened the book. All chapters have been brought up-to-date. The editors are grateful to their new publisher for agreeing to the introduction of many more color illustrations. These allow the oncologist a better opportunity to appreciate the characteristic appearance of patients and tissues.

Clinical oncology continues to be grounded, and now more than ever, in the fundamentals of cancer research. Understanding the science that will lead to tomorrow's diagnosis, treatment, and prevention is a necessity for the oncologist who wishes to apply the new advances. We have enjoyed the cooperation of some of the world's great scientists in this endeavor. This edition again offers the laboratory investigator an avenue to appreciate the relationship of his or her research focus to the broad perspective of cancer research and human cancer.

The editors have worked to make this the most authoritative and effective resource available for the student of cancer. If we have succeeded, it is because of the knowledge and devotion of our authors and their response to our critiques. The editors are grateful to Diane McGonnigle for her expert assistance in producing this edition. They thank their colleagues and students for provocative inquiry and advice. A companion volume has been published in a question format that serves to increase the educational value of this treatise.

The editors are grateful to their institutions and departments for the continuing support that has enabled their study of cancer. They are mindful of the forbearance and love of their families who tolerated the incursions on personal time necessary for the completion of this edition. They dedicate this book to the young scholars who will make use of it to wage battle against cancer, to the physicians and nurses who will use it on behalf of their patients, and to the patients whose participation in clinical cancer research is an indispensable component of the eventual victory.

James F. Holland
Emil Frei III
Robert Bast, Jr.
Donald Kufe
Donald Morton
Ralph Weichselbaum

CONTRIBUTORS

Stuart A. Aaronson, M.D.
Director
Derald H. Ruttenberg Cancer Center
The Mount Sinai Hospital
Mount Sinai School of Medicine
New York, New York

Arthur A. Ablin, M.D.
Professor Emeritus of Clinical Pediatrics
Past Director of Pediatric Clinical Oncology
Department of Pediatrics
University of California, San Francisco
San Francisco, California

David H. Abramson, M.D.
Clinical Professor of Ophthalmology
New York Hospital—Cornell Medical Center
New York, New York

George Acs, M.D., Ph.D.
Professor Emeritus
Department of Biochemistry
Mount Sinai School of Medicine
New York, New York

A. Leland Albright, M.D.
Associate Professor
Department of Neurological Surgery
University of Pittsburgh School of Medicine
Chief, Pediatric Neurosurgery
Children's Hospital of Pittsburgh
Pittsburgh, Pennsylvania

Nasser K. Altorki, M.D.
Associate Professor
Department of Cardiothoracic Surgery
Cornell University Medical College
Associate Attending Surgeon
Department of Cardiothoracic Surgery
The New York Hospital
New York City, New York

Edward P. Ambinder, M.D.
Associate Clinical Professor of Medicine
Mount Sinai School of Medicine
New York, New York

Kenneth C. Anderson, M.D.
Associate Professor of Medicine
Harvard Medical School
Medical Director, Blood Component Laboratory
Dana-Farber Cancer Institute
Boston, Massachusetts

Karen H. Antman, M.D.
Professor of Medicine
Chief, Division of Medical Oncology
College of Physicians and Surgeons
Columbia University
New York, New York

James B. Atkinson, M.D., F.A.C.S.
Professor of Pediatric Surgery
Department of Surgery
UCLA Medical School
Los Angeles, California

Steven D. Averbuch, M.D.
Director, Oncology
Clinical and Medical Affairs
Zeneca Pharmaceuticals
Wilmington, Delaware

Joseph S. Bailes, M.D., F.A.C.P.
Executive Vice President and National Medical Director
Physician Reliance Network, Inc.
Dallas, Texas

John Baillie, M.B., Ch.B., F.R.C.P.
Associate Professor of Medicine
Division of Gastroenterology
Duke University Medical Center
Durham, North Carolina

Erik Barquist, M.D.
Fellow in Trauma and Critical Care
Division of General Surgery
University of Miami School of Medicine
Miami, Florida

Stephen Barrett, M.D.
Consumer Advocate
Member, Board of Directors
National Council Against Health Fraud, Inc.
Allentown, Pennsylvania

Lawrence W. Bassett, M.D.
Iris Center Professor of Breast Imaging
Department of Radiological Sciences
UCLA School of Medicine
Los Angeles, California

Robert C. Bast, Jr., M.D.
Internist and Professor of Medicine
Harry Carothers Wiess Chair for Cancer Research
Head, Division of Medicine
University of Texas M.D. Anderson Cancer Center
Houston, Texas

Poonam V. Batra, M.D., F.C.C.P., F.A.C.R.
Professor
Department of Radiological Sciences
UCLA School of Medicine
Los Angeles, California

Kenneth A. Bauer, M.D.
Associate Professor
Department of Medicine
Harvard Medical School
Associate Physician
Beth Israel Hospital
Boston, Massachusetts
Chief, Hematology-Oncology Section, VA Medical Center
West Roxbury, Massachusetts

Stephen B. Baylin, M.D.
Professor of Oncology and Medicine
The Oncology Center
Johns Hopkins University School of Medicine
Baltimore, Maryland

William T. Beck, Ph.D.
Director, Cancer Center
Professor of Genetics and Pharmacology
University of Illinois College of Medicine
Chicago, Illinois
Formerly: Member
Department of Molecular Pharmacology
St. Jude's Children Research Hospital
Professor
Department of Pharmacology
University of Tennessee College of Medicine
Memphis, Tennessee

Robert S. Benjamin, M.D.
Internist, Ashbel Smith Professor of Medicine
Chairman
Department of Melanoma/Sarcoma Medical Oncology
Medical Director, Sarcoma Center
University of Texas M.D. Anderson Cancer Center
Houston, Texas

Jonathan S. Berek, M.D., F.A.C.O.G., F.A.C.S.
Professor and Vice-Chair
Chief of Gynecology and Gynecologic Oncology
Johnson Comprehensive Cancer Center
UCLA School of Medicine
Los Angeles, California

Ross S. Berkowitz, M.D.
William H. Baker Professor of Gynecology
Harvard Medical School
Director of Gynecologic Oncology
Co-Director, New England Trophoblastic Disease Center
Brigham & Women's Hospital
Boston, Massachusetts

Leslie Bernstein, Ph.D.
Professor
Department of Preventive Medicine
University of Southern California School of Medicine
Los Angeles, California

Steven H. Bernstein, M.D.
Assistant Professor of Medicine
Department of Hematological Oncology
Roswell Park Cancer Institute
Buffalo, New York

Joseph R. Bertino, M.D.
Program Chairman
Molecular Pharmacology and Therapeutics
Sloan-Kettering Institute for Cancer Research
American Cancer Society
Professor of Medicine
Memorial Sloan Kettering Cancer Center
New York, New York

William D. Bloomer, M.D.
Chairman
Department of Radiation Medicine
Evanston Hospital Corp.
Evanston, Illinois

Gerald P. Bodey, M.D.
Emeritus Professor of Medicine
Department of Medical Specialties
University of Texas M.D. Anderson Cancer Center
Houston, Texas

Gianni Bonadonna, M.D.
Director, Division of Medical Oncology
Chief, Department of Medicine
Instituto Nazionale Tumori
Milan, Italy

Ernest C. Borden, M.D.
Director, University of Maryland Cancer Center
University of Maryland
Baltimore, Maryland

Neal R. Boyd, Jr., Ed.D., M.S.P.H.
Associate Director
Tobacco Control Research
Fox Chase Cancer Center
Cheltenham, Pennsylvania

Cinda M. Boyer, Ph.D.
Assistant Research Professor
Department of Pathology
Duke University Medical Center
Durham, North Carolina

Norman E. Breslow, Ph.D.
Professor
Department of Biostatistics
University of Washington
Seattle, Washington

Edward Bresnick, Ph.D.
Vice Chancellor for Research
University of Massachusetts Medical Center
Worcester, Massachusetts

Nicholas Bruchovsky, M.D., Ph.D., F.R.C.P.
Head, Department of Cancer Endocrinology
BC Cancer Agency
Professor of Medicine
University of British Columbia
Vancouver, British Columbia, Canada
Clinical Professor, Department of Urology
University of Washington School of Medicine
Seattle, Washington

Howard W. Bruckner, M.D.
Professor of Neoplastic Diseases
Department of Medicine
Mount Sinai School of Medicine
New York, New York

Nancy J. Bunin, M.D.
Assistant Professor
Department of Pediatrics
Children's Hospital of Philadelphia
Philadelphia, Pennsylvania

Blake Cady, M.D.
Professor of Surgery
Harvard Medical School
Chief, Division of Surgical Oncology
Department of Surgery
New England Deaconess Hospital
Boston, Massachusetts

Judith Campisi, Ph.D.
Acting Department Head
Cancer Biology Department/Life Sciences Division
Berkeley National Laboratory
Berkeley, California

Robert W. Carlson, M.D.
Associate Professor of Medicine
Division of Medical Oncology
Stanford University Medical Center
Stanford, California

C. Humberto Carrasco, M.D.
Professor of Radiology
Department of Diagnostic Radiology
The University of Texas M.D. Anderson Cancer Center
Houston, Texas

Carol E. Cass, Ph.D.
Professor
Department of Biochemistry
University of Alberta
Edmonton, Alberta
CANADA

A. Philippe Chahinian, M.D.
Professor
Department of Medicine
Division of Neoplastic Diseases
Mount Sinai School of Medicine
New York, New York

Chusilp Charnsangavej, M.D.
Radiologist and Professor of Radiology
Department of Diagnostic Radiology
The University of Texas M.D. Anderson Cancer Center
Houston, Texas

George Chen, Ph.D.
Director
Medical Physics Division
University of Chicago Hospital
Chicago, Illinois

Yung-Chi Cheng, Ph.D.
Henry Bronson Professor of Pharmacology
Department of Pharmacology
Yale School of Medicine
New Haven, Connecticut

George P. Chrousos, M.D.
Chief, Section of Pediatric Endocrinology
National Institute of Child Health
National Institutes of Health
Bethesda, Maryland

John A. Cidlowski, Ph.D.
Head, Molecular Endocrinology Group
Laboratory of Integrative Biology
National Institute of Environmental Health Sciences, NIH
Research Triangle Park, North Carolina

Gary L. Clayman, D.D.S., M.D.
Associate Professor
Department of Head and Neck Surgery
University of Texas M.D. Anderson Cancer Center
Houston, Texas

James E. Cleaver, Ph.D.
Professor of Radiology
Department of Laboratory Radiology and Environmental Health
University of California
San Francisco, California

Steven K. Clinton, M.D., Ph.D.
Clinical Associate
Department of Medicine
Dana-Farber Cancer Institute
Harvard Medical School
Boston, Massachusetts

Carmel J. Cohen, M.D.
Professor of Obstetrics, Gynecology and Reproductive Science
Director, Gynecologic Services
Mount Sinai Medical Center
New York, New York

Jeffrey I. Cohen, M.D.
Senior Investigator
Laboratory of Clinical Investigation
National Institutes of Health
Bethesda, Maryland

Mervyn D. Cohen, M.B., Ch.B.
Department of Radiology
Riley Hospital for Children
Indianapolis, Indiana

O. Michael Colvin, M.D.
Director
Duke Comprehensive Cancer Center
Duke University Medical Center
Durham, North Durham

Ana Maria Comaru-Schally, M.D., M.S.
Professor of Clinical Medicine
Tulane University School of Medicine
New Orleans, Louisiana

James L. Connolly, M.D.
Director of Anatomic Pathology Division
Department of Pathology
Beth Israel Hospital
Associate Professor of Pathology
Harvard Medical School
Boston, Massachusetts

Kenneth H. Cowan, M.D., Ph.D.
Acting Chief
Medicine Branch
National Cancer Institute
Bethesda, Maryland

Carlo H. Croce, M.D.
Director
Jefferson Cancer Institute
Jefferson Cancer Center
Chairman
Department of Microbiology and Immunology
Jefferson Medical College of Thomas Jefferson University
Philadelphia, Pennsylvania

Christopher P. Crum, M.D.
Associate Professor of Pathology
Harvard Medical School
Director, Division of Women's Perinatal Pathology
Brigham and Women's Hospital
Boston, Massachusetts

Gregory A. Curt, M.D.
Clinical Director
National Cancer Institute
Bethesda, Maryland

Lisa M. DeAngelis, M.D.
Chief, Neurology Service
Memorial Sloan-Kettering Cancer Center
Associate Professor of Neurology
Cornell University Medical College
New York, New York

George D. Demetri, M.D.
Assistant Professor of Medicine
Harvard Medical School
Dana-Farber Cancer Institute
Boston, Massachusetts

Eugene R. DeSombre, Ph.D.
Professor
Ben May Institute for Cancer Research
University of Chicago
Chicago, Illinois

Ozdal Dillioglugil, M.D.
Clinical Fellow in Urological Oncology
Scott Department of Urology
Baylor College of Medicine
Houston, Texas
Assistant Professor
Department of Urology
Kocaeli University Medical School
Kocaeli, Turkey

Sarah S. Donaldson, M.D.
Professor
Department of Radiation Oncology
Stanford University School of Medicine
Stanford, California

Marguerite Donoghue, R.N., M.N.
Vice President, Research and Regulatory Affairs
Capitol Associates, Inc.
Washington, D.C.

Peter R. Dottino, M.D.
Director, Division of Gynecologic Oncology
Associate Professor
Department of Obstetrics, Gynecology and Reproductive Science
Mount Sinai Medical Center
New York, New York

Harold O. Douglass, Jr., M.D.
Professor of Surgery
State University of New York at Buffalo
Vice Chairman
Department of Surgical Oncology
Roswell Park Cancer Institute
Bufffalo, New York

Ira J. Dunkel, M.D.
Clinical Assistant
Department of Pediatrics
Memorial Sloan-Kettering Cancer Center
New York, New York

Ann M. Dvorak, M.D.
Professor of Pathology
Harvard Medical School
Senior Pathologist
Beth Israel Hospital
Boston, Massachusetts

Harold F. Dvorak, M.D.
Mallinckrodt Professor of Pathology
Harvard Medical School
Chief, Department of Pathology
Beth Israel Hospital
Boston, Massachusetts

Michael Edye, M.B., B.S.
Assistant Professor
Division of Laparoscopic Surgery
Mount Sinai Medical Center
New York, New York

Sabine Eichinger, M.D.
Assistant Professor
Department of Internal Medicine I
University of Vienna
Vienna, Austria

Lawrence H. Einhorn, M.D.
Distinguished Professor of Medicine
Indiana University
Indianapolis, Indiana

Ezekiel J. Emanuel, M.D., Ph.D.
Assistant Professor of Medicine
Division of Cancer Epidemiology & Control
Dana-Farber Cancer Institute
Boston, Massachusetts

Paul F. Engstrom, M.D.
Senior Vice President, Population Science
Fox Chase Cancer Center
Professor of Medicine
Temple University Medical School
Philadelphia, Pennsylvania

Warren E. Enker, M.D.
Vice Chaiman, Department of Surgery
Chief, Division of Colorectal Surgery
Beth Israel Medical Center
Professor of Surgery
Albert Einstein College of Medicine
New York, New York

Richard Essner, M.D.
Assistant Medical Director, Surgical Oncology
John Wayne Cancer Institute
Santa Monica, California

Michael S. Ewer, M.D., M.P.H.
Internist, Associate Professor of Medicine
Medical Specialties/Cardiology
M.D. Anderson Cancer Center
Houston, Texas

Harmon J. Eyre, M.D.
Deputy Executive Vice President for Medical Affairs and Research
American Cancer Society
Atlanta, Georgia

Jeffrey C. Faig, M.D.
Clinical Faculty
Division of Endocrinology
Harbor-UCLA Medical Center
Torrance, California

Eric R. Fearon, M.D., Ph.D.
Maisel Professor of Oncology
Associate Professor
Departments of Internal Medicine, Human Genetics and Pathology
University of Michigan Medical Center
Ann Arbor, Michigan

Paolo Fedi, M.D., Ph.D.
Assistant Professor
Derald H. Ruttenberg Cancer Center
The Mount Sinai Medical Center
New York, New York

Howard A. Fine, M.D.
Associate Professor of Medicine
Harvard Medical School
Division of Cancer Pharmacology
Dana-Farber Cancer Institute
Boston, Massachusetts

Howard J. Fingert, M.D.
Associate Professor
Tufts Medical School
Boston, Massachusetts

Bernard Fisher, M.D.
Distinguished Service Professor
Department of Surgery
University of Pittsburgh
Scientific Director
National Adjuvant Bowel and Breast Project
Pittsburgh, Pennsylvania

Thomas B. Fitzpatrick, M.D., Ph.D.
Wigglesworth, Professor of Dermatology
Harvard Medical School
Department of Dermatology
Massachusetts General Hospital
Boston, Massachusetts

Mary R. Flack, M.D.
Director
Department of Endocrine, Clinical Research
Parke-Davis Pharmaceutical Research
Ann Arbor, Michigan

Kathleen M. Foley, M.D.
Chief, Pain Service
Memorial Sloan Kettering Cancer Center
Professor of Neurology
Department of Neuroscience and Clinical Pharmacology
Cornell University Medical College
New York, New York

Judah Folkman, M.D.
Julia Dyckman Andrus Professor of Pediatric Surgery
Professor of Cell Biology
Department of Surgery
Harvard Medical School and Children's Hospital
Boston, Massachusetts

Yuman Fong, M.D.
Gastric and Mixed Tumor Service
Memorial Sloan-Kettering Cancer Center
Assistant Professor of Cell Biology and Anatomy
Cornell University Medical College
New York, New York

Charles A. Forscher, M.D.
Medical Oncologist
Department of Medical Oncology
Cedar Sinai Comprehensive Cancer Center
UCLA Medical Center
Los Angeles, California

Richard S. Foster, M.D.
Associate Professor
Department of Urology
Indiana University
Indianapolis, Indiana

Arthur Edward Frankel, M.D.
Associate Professor of Medicine
Department of Medicine
Medical University of South Carolina
Charleston, South Carolina

Arnold S. Freedman, M.D.
Associate Professor of Medicine
Harvard Medical School
Dana-Farber Cancer Institute
Boston, Massachusetts

Emil Frei III, M.D.
Director and Physician-in-Chief, Emeritus
Dana-Farber Cancer Institute
Richard and Susan Smith Distinguished Professor of Medicine
Harvard Medical School
Boston, Massachusetts

Christopher J.H. Fryer, M.D., F.R.C.P.(C)
Clinical Professor and Head
Division of Pediatric Hematology/Oncology
Department of Pediatrics
University of British Columbia
B.C. Children's Hospital
Vancouver, British Columbia
Canada

William J. Fulkerson, Jr., M.D.
Associate Professor of Medicine
Duke University Medical Center
Durham, North Carolina

John F. Gaeta, M.D.
Professor of Pathology and Urology
School of Medicine and Biomedical Sciences
State University of New York at Buffalo
Buffalo, New York

George T. Gallagher, D.M.D., D.M.Sc.
Associate Professor of Oral Pathology
Department of Oral Medicine and Diagnostic Sciences
Harvard School of Dental Medicine
Boston, Massachusetts

Paul S. Gaynon, M.D.
Professor and Clinical Director
Department of Pediatrics
University of Wisconsin
Madison, Wisconsin

Spencer Gibson, Ph.D.
Predoctoral Fellow
Department of Molecular Oncology
M.D. Anderson Cancer Center
Houston, Texas

Teresa Ann Gilewski, M.D.
Assistant Attending
Department of Medicine
Memorial Sloan Kettering Cancer Center
Assistant Professor of Medicine
Cornell University
New York, New York

Edward Giovannucci, M.D., D.P.H.
Instructor in Medicine
Harvard Medical School
Associate in Epidemiology
Department of Medicine
Brigham & Women's Hospital
Boston, Massachusetts

L. Michael Glode, M.D.
Professor of Medicine
Division of Medical Oncology
University of Colorado Health Sciences Center
Denver, Colorado

Donald P. Goldstein, M.D.
Associate Professor of Obstetrics, Gynecology and Reproductive Biology
Harvard Medical School
Co-Director, New England's Trophoblastic Disease Center
Brigham and Women's Hospital
Boston, Massachusetts

Harvey M. Golomb, M.D.
Professor of Medicine
Section Head, Hematology/Oncology
Department of Medicine
University of Chicago
Chicago, Illinois

Edward G. Grant, M.D.
Vice Chairman
Department of Radiological Sciences
UCLA School of Medicine
Chairman, Department of Radiology
VA Medical Center, West Los Angeles
Los Angeles, California

F. Anthony Greco, M.D.
Director
Sarah Cannon Cancer Center
Centennial Medical Center
Nashville, Tennessee

Daniel M. Green, M.D.
Associate Chief
Department of Pediatrics
Roswell Park Cancer Institute
Professor of Pediatrics
School of Medicine and Biomedical Sciences
State University of New York at Buffalo
Buffalo, New York

Warner C. Greene, M.D., Ph.D.
Director
Gladstone Institute of Virology & Immunology
Professor of Medicine, Microbiology and Immunology
University of California, San Francisco
San Francisco, California

Michael R. Grever, M.D.
Director
Division of Hematologic Malignancies
Johns Hopkins University
Baltimore, Maryland

Charles K. Grieshaber, Ph.D.
Acting Director
Office of Testing and Research
Center for Drug Evaluation and Research
Food and Drug Administration
Rockville, Maryland

Elizabeth A. Grimm, Ph.D.
Professor
Department of Tumor Biology and Surgical Oncology
University of Texas, M.D. Anderson Cancer Center
Houston, Texas

Paul E. Grundy, M.D.
Assistant Professor of Pediatrics
University of Alberta
Acting Director, Department of Pediatrics
Cross Center Institute
Edmonton, Alberta

Gerald M. Haase, M.D.
Clinical Professor of Surgery
Department of Pediatric Surgery
The Children's Hospital
Denver, Colorado

George M. Hahn, Ph.D.
Professor Emeritus (Active)
Department of Radiation Oncology
Division of Radiation Biology
Stanford University School of Medicine
Stanford, California

John D. Hainsworth, M.D.
Associate Director
Sarah Cannon Cancer Center
Centennial Medical Center
Nashville, Tennessee

Dennis E. Hallahan, M.D.
Assistant Professor
Department of Radiology and Cell Oncology
University of Chicago Hospital
Chicago, Illinois

Robert A. Halvorsen, Jr., M.D.
Department of Radiology
San Francisco General Hospital
San Francisco, California

G. Denman Hammond, M.D.
Associate Vice President, Health Affairs
Professor of Pediatrics
USC School of Medicine
University of Southern California
Los Angeles, California
President and Chief Executive Officer
National Childhood Cancer Foundation
Arcadia, California

Axel-R. Hanauske, M.D., Ph.D.
Professor
Abteilung Haematologie und Onkologie
I.Med. Klinik
Klinikum Rechts der Isar
München, Germany

Robert E. Handschumacher, Ph.D.
Department of Pharmacology
Yale University School of Medicine
New Haven, Connecticut

Yusuf A. Hannun, M.D.
Associate Professor of Medicine
Duke University Medical Center
Durham, North Carolina

Curtis C. Harris, M.D.
Chief of the Laboratory of Human Carcinogenesis
National Cancer Institute
Bethesda, Maryland

Harold A. Harvey, M.D.
Professor of Medicine
Hershey Medical Center
Pennsylvania State University
Hershey, Pennsylvania

Tayyaba Hasan, Ph.D.
Associate Professor of Dermatology (Biochemistry)
Harvard Medical School
Department of Dermatology
Massachusetts General Hospital
Boston, Massachusetts
Massachusetts Institute of Technology
Cambridge, Massachusetts

Randall A. Hawkins, M.D., Ph.D.
Professor of Radiology
Chief, Nuclear Medicine Program
Vice Chairman, Department of Radiology
University of California, San Francisco
San Francisco, California

Harley A. Haynes, M.D.
Director
Department of Clinical Dermatology
Brigham and Women's Hospital
Associate Professor of Dermatology
Harvard Medical School
Boston, Massachusetts

Brian E. Henderson, M.D.
Professor
Department of Preventive Medicine
University of Southern California School of Medicine
Los Angeles, California

Victor D. Herbert, M.D., J.D.
Professor of Medicine
Mount Sinai School of Medicine
Chief, Hematology and Nutrition Research Laboratory
Bronx Veterans Administration Medical Center
New York, New York

Arthur L. Herbst, M.D.
Chairman and Joseph Bolivar DeLee Distinguished Service Professor
Department of Obstetrics and Gynecology
University of Chicago
Chicago, Illinois

Andrew R. Hoffman, M.D.
Chief of Medicine, VA Medical Center
Vice Chair, Department of Medicine
Stanford University Medical Center
Palo Alto, California

John P. Hoffman, M.D.
Professor of Surgery
Temple University School of Medicine
Staff Surgeon
Department of Surgical Oncology
Fox Chase Cancer Center
Philadelphia, Pennsylvania

James F. Holland, M.D.
Distinguished Professor of Neoplastic Diseases
Director Emeritus, Derald H. Ruttenberg Cancer Center
Mount Sinai Medical Center
New York, New York

Jimmie C. Holland, M.D.
Professor of Psychiatry
Cornell University Medical College
Chief, Psychiatry Services
Wayne E. Chapman Chair in Psychiatric Oncology
Memorial Sloan-Kettering Cancer Center
New York, New York

Waun Ki Hong, M.D.
Charles A. LeMaistre Chair in Thoracic Oncology
Professor and Chairman
Department of Thoracic/Head and Neck Medical Oncology
The University of Texas M.D. Anderson Cancer Center
Houston, Texas

Antoinette F. Hood, M.D.
Professor of Pathology and Dermatology
Director of Dermatopathology
Department of Dermatology
Indiana University Medical Center
Indianapolis, Indiana

Richard T. Hoppe, M.D.
Henry S. Kaplan-Harry Lebeson Professor
Department of Cancer Biology
Chairman, Department of Radiation Oncology
Stanford University
Stanford, California

Peter J. Houghton, Ph.D.
Member
Department of Biochemistry and Clinical Pharmacology
St. Jude Children's Research Hospital
Memphis, Tennessee

Stephen B. Howell, M.D.
Professor of Medicine
University of California, San Diego
La Jolla, California

T. Scott Jennings, M.D.
Director, Division of Gynecologic Oncology
Medical University of South Carolina
Charleston, South Carolina

Elwood V. Jensen, M.D.
Professor
Institute for Hormone and Fertility Research
University of Hamburg
Hamburg, Germany

Roy B. Jones, Ph.D., M.D.
Director, Bone Marrow Transplant Program
Department of Medicine
University of Colorado Health Sciences Center
Denver, Colorado

Ralph C. Jones, Lt.Cdr., M.C., U.S.N.
Clinical Assistant Professor of Surgery
Uniformed Services University of the Health Sciences
Bethesda, Maryland
Senior Research Fellow
Department of Surgical Oncology
John Wayne Cancer Institute at St. John's Hospital
Santa Monica, California

V. Craig Jordan, Ph.D., D.Sc.
Professor of Cancer Pharmacology
Director Breast Cancer Research Program
Robert H. Lurie Cancer Center
Northwestern University Medical School
Chicago, Illinois

A. Robert Kagan, M.D.
Chief, Radiation Oncology
Kaiser Permanente
Los Angeles, California

Barton A. Kamen, M.D., Ph.D.
Professor of Pediatrics and Pharmacology
American Cancer Society Clinical Research Professor
Carl B. and Florence E. King Foundation Distinguished Chair of Pediatric Oncology Research
UT Southwestern Medical Center
Dallas, Texas

Philip W. Kantoff, M.D.
Director, Genitourinary Oncology
Department of Medicine
Dana Farber Cancer Institute
Boston, Massachusetts

Arlene F. Kantor, Dr.P.H.
Epidemiologist
Division of Cancer Epidemiology and Control
Dana-Farber Cancer Institute
Boston, Massachusetts

Lawrence D. Kaplan, M.D.
Associate Professor of Medicine
UCSF AIDS Program/Oncology Division
San Francisco General Hospital
San Francisco, California

Daniel S. Kapp, Ph.D., M.D.
Department of Radiation Oncology
Stanford University Medical Center
Stanford, California

Frederic C. Kass, M.D.
Director, Clinical Research
Cancer Foundation of Santa Barbara
Santa Barbara, California
Clinical Assistant Professor of Medicine
University of Southern California
Los Angeles, California

Peter A. Kaufman, M.D.
Assistant Professor of Medicine
Department of Hematology/Oncology
Dartmouth-Hitchcock Medical Center
Lebanon, New Hampshire

Michael J. Keating, M.D.
Professor of Medicine
Associate Head for Clinical Research
University of Texas M.D. Anderson Cancer Center
Houston, Texas

Steven M. Keller, M.D.
Associate Professor of Surgery
Albert Einstein College of Medicine
Bronx, New York

David P. Kelsen, M.D.
Chief, Gastrointestinal Oncology Service
Memorial Sloan-Kettering Cancer Center
Professor of Medicine
Cornell University Medical College
New York, New York

Karl T. Kelsey, M.D.
Associate Professor of Cancer Biology
Harvard School of Public Health
Boston, Massachusetts

Nancy Kemeny, M.D.
Professor of Medicine
Cornell University College of Medicine
Attending Physician
Department of GI Oncology
Department of Solid Tumor
Memorial Sloan-Kettering Cancer Center
New York, New York

Samuel Kenan, M.D.
Professor of Orthopedics
New York University School of Medicine
Director of Orthopedic Oncology Service
Orthopedic Institute
New York, New York

B.J. Kennedy, M.D.
Regents' Professor of Medicine, Emeritus
Masonic Professor of Oncology, Emeritus
Division of Medical Oncology
University of Minnesota Medical School
Minneapolis, Minnesota

Samir N. Khleif, M.D.
Assistant Professor of Internal Medicine
Uniformed Services University of Health Sciences
Senior Clinical Investigator
NCI-Navy Medical Oncology Branch
National Cancer Institute
Bethesda, Maryland

Youn-H. Kim, M.D.
Assistant Professor of Dermatology
Director, Residency Program
Co-Director, Mycosis-Fungoides Clinic
Stanford University School of Medicine
Stanford, California

Susan Y. Kim, M.D.
Assistant Professor
Department of Radiation Oncology
Roswell Park Cancer Institute
Buffalo, New York

John M. Kirkwood, M.D.
Professor and Chief
Division of Medical Oncology
University of Pittsburgh
Director, Melanoma Center
Pittsburgh Cancer Center
Pittsburgh, Pennsylvania

Catherine E. Klein, M.D.
Associate Professor of Medicine
Divisions of Hematology and Medical Oncology
University of Colorado Health Sciences Center
Denver Veterans Affairs Medical Center
Denver, Colorado

Elise C. Kohn, M.D.
Chief, Signal Transduction & Prevention Unit
Laboratory of Pathology
National Cancer Institute
National Institutes of Health
Bethesda, Maryland

Ritsuko Komaki, M.D., F.A.C.R.
Associate Professor of Radiotherapy
University of Texas M.D. Anderson Cancer Center
Houston, Texas

Tatsuhei Kondo, M.D.
Professor Emeritus of Surgery
Nagoya University School of Medicine
Nagoya, Japan

Ken Kondo, M.D.
Instructor in Surgery
Department of Surgery II
Nagoya University School of Medicine
Nagoya, Japan

Mark G. Kris, M.D.
Chief, Thoracic Oncology Service
Department of Medicine
Memorial Sloan-Kettering Cancer Center
Associate Professor of Medicine
Cornell University Medical College
New York, New York

Donald W. Kufe, M.D.
Deputy Director
Dana-Farber Cancer Center
Chief, Division of Cancer Pharmacology
Professor of Medicine
Harvard Medical School
Boston, Massachusetts

Joanne Kurtzberg, M.D.
Professor of Pediatrics
Duke University Medical Center
Durham, North Carolina

Beatrice C. Lampkin, M.D.
Professor Emerita of Pediatrics
Department of Pediatric Hematology-Oncology
Children's Hospital Medical Center of Cincinnati
Cincinnati, Ohio

George E. Laramore, M.D., Ph.D.
Professor and Vice-Chairman
Department of Radiation Oncology
Clinical Director, University of Washington Fast Neutron Radiotherapy Project
University of Washington
Seattle, Washington

J. Mark Lawson, M.D., F.A.C.P., F.A.C.G.
Chief, Division of Gastroenterology
Naval Medical Center
Portsmouth, Virginia
Assistant Professor of Medicine
Eastern Virginia Medical School
Norfolk, Virginia

Jin Soo Lee, M.D.
Chief, Section of Thoracic Medical Oncology
Associate Internist and Associate Professor of Medicine
Department of Thoracic/Head & Neck Medical Oncology
University of Texas M.D. Anderson Cancer Center
Houston, Texas

Bernard Levin, M.D.
Vice President for Cancer Prevention
University of Texas M.D. Anderson Cancer Center
Houston, Texas

Frederick P. Li, M.D.
Professor of Clinical Cancer Epidemiology
Harvard School of Public Health
Professor of Medicine
Harvard Medical School
Dana-Farber Cancer Institute
Boston, Massachusetts

Steven A. Lieberman, M.D.
Assistant Professor
Department of Internal Medicine
University of Texas Medical Branch
Galveston, Texas

Terry L. Lierman
President Capitol Associates, Inc.
Washington, D.C.

Lance A. Liotta, M.D., Ph.D.
Chief, Laboratory of Pathology
National Cancer Institute
National Institutes of Health
Bethesda, Maryland

Scott M. Lippman, M.D., F.A.C.P.
Associate Professor of Medicine
Department of Thoracic/Head & Neck Medical Oncology
M.D. Anderson Cancer Center
Houston, Texas

John B. Little, M.D.
James Stevens Simmons Professor of Radiobiology
Director, Laboratory of Cancer Cell Biology
Harvard School of Public Health
Lecturer on Radiation Oncology
Harvard Medical School
Boston, Massachusetts

Christopher J. Logothetis, M.D.
Chairman
Department of Genitourinary Medical Oncology
University of Texas M.D. Anderson Cancer Center
Houston, Texas

Robert Lufkin, M.D.
Professor
Department of Radiological Sciences
UCLA School of Medicine
Los Angeles, California

Cesare Maltoni, M.D.
Director
Institute di Oncologia, "F. Addarii"
Bologna, Italy

Henry J. Mankin, M.D.
Chief, Orthopaedic Service
Massachusetts General Hospital
Edith M. Ashley Professor of Orthopaedic Surgery
Harvard Medical School
Boston, Massachusetts

Andrea Manni, M.D.
Professor of Medicine
Hershey Medical Center
Pennsylvania State University
Hershey, Pennsylvania

Victor A. Marcial, M.D.
Professor and Chairman (Emeritus)
Department of Radiation Oncology
University of Puerto Rico School of Medicine
San Juan, Puerto Rico

V.A. Marcial-Vega, M.D.
Private Practice
Coconut Grove, Florida

Richard G. Margolese, M.D.
Director, Department of Oncology
Sir Mortimer B. Davis Jewish General Hospital
Herbert Black Professor
Department of Surgery
McGill University
Montreal, Quebec
Canada

Peter M. Mauch, M.D.
Associate Professor
Department of Radiation Oncology
Harvard Medical School
Boston, Massachusetts

Harold M. Maurer, M.D.
Professor of Pediatrics
University of Nebraska Medical Center
Dean
University of Nebraska College of Medicine
Omaha, Nebraska

Kenneth S. McCarty, Jr., M.D., Ph.D.
Professor of Medicine
Professor of Pathology
University of Pittsburgh Cancer Institute
Pittsburgh, Pennsylvania

Kenneth S. McCarty, Sr., Ph.D.
Professor of Biochemistry
Department of Biochemsitry
Duke University
Durham, North Carolina

Beryl McCormick, M.D.
Associate Radiation Oncologist
Department of Radiation Oncology
Memorial-Sloan Kettering Cancer Center
New York, New York

Katherine A. McGlynn, Ph.D.
Associate Member
Division of Population Science
Fox Chase Cancer Center
University of Pennsylvania
Philadelphia, Pennsylvania

Catherine M. McLachlin, M.D., F.R.C.P.C.
Pathologist
Victoria Hospital
Assistant Professor
Department of Pathology
University of Western Ontario
London, Ontario
Canada

Anna T. Meadows, M.D.
Professor of Pediatrics
University of Pennsylvania
Director of Pediatric Oncology
The Children's Hospital of Philadelphia
Philadelphia, Pennsylvania

Neal J. Meropol, M.D.
Assistant Professor of Medicine
State University of New York at Buffalo
Division of Medicine
Roswell Park Cancer Institute
Buffalo, New York

Mernin A. Merrick, M.D.
Assistant Professor of Radiation Oncology
Mount Sinai School of Medicine
New York, New York

Curtis P. Mettlin, Ph.D.
Chief of Epidemiologic Research
Roswell Park Center Institute
Buffalo, New York

Gordon B. Mills, M.D., Ph.D.
Professor and Chairman
Department of Molecular Oncology
The University of Texas M.D. Anderson Cancer Center
Houston, Texas

Franco Minardi, M.D.
Associate
European Foundation of Oncology and Environmental Sciences "Bernakdino Ramazzini"
Bologna, Italy
Thomas Mindermann, M.D.
Department of Neurosurgery
University Hospitals Basel
Basel, Switzerland
Bruce D. Minsky, M.D.
Associate Professor
Department of Radiation Oncology
Memorial Sloan-Kettering Cancer Center
New York, New York
David L. Mitchell, Ph.D.
Laboratory of Radiobiology and Environmental Health
University of California
San Francisco, California
John C. Morris, M.D.
Assistant Professor
Division of Neoplastic Diseases
Department of Medicine
Mount Sinai Medical Center
New York, New York
Visiting Scientist
Clinical Gene Therapy Branch
National Center for Human Genome Research
Bethesda, Maryland
Charles S. Morrow, M.D., Ph.D.
Assistant Professor of Biochemistry
Associate Professor of Pediatrics
Bowman Gray School of Medicine
Winston-Salem, North Carolina
Donald L. Morton, M.D.
Medical Director and Surgeon-in-Chief
John Wayne Cancer Institute at St. John's Hospital
Santa Monica, California
Professor and Chief, Emeritus, Surgery/ Oncology
UCLA School of Medicine
Los Angeles, California
Bina T. Motwani, M.D.
Formerly Assistant Clinical Professor
Division of Neoplastic Diseases
Mount Sinai Medical Center
New York, New York
Scott Murphy, M.D.
Professor of Medicine
Thomas Jefferson University
Chief Medical Officer
American Red Cross Blood Services
Penn-Jersey Region
Philadelphia, Pennsylvania
Piero Mustacchi, M.D.
Clinical Professor of Medicine and Epidemiology
Department of Epidemiology and Biostatistics
University of California, San Francisco
San Francisco, California
Charles Myers, M.D.
Director, Cancer Center
Director, Division of Hematology/Oncology
University of Virginia
Charlottesville, Virginia
Lee M. Nadler, M.D.
Professor, Harvard Medical School
Chief, Division of Hematologic Malignancies
Dana-Farber Cancer Institute
Boston, Massachusetts
Heather H. Nelson, M.P.H.
Department of Cancer Biology & Environmental Health
Harvard School of Public Health
Boston, Massachusetts
Jonathan C. Nesbitt, M.D.
Assistant Professor of Surgery
University of Texas M.D. Anderson Cancer Center
Houston, Texas
Craig R. Nichols, M.D.
Associate Professor of Medicine
Indiana University School of Medicine
Indianapolis, Indiana
Larry Norton, M.D.
Chief, Breast Cancer Medicine Service
Department of Medicine
Memorial Sloan-Kettering Cancer Center
New York, New York
Richard J. O'Reilly, M.D.
Chairman, Department of Pediatrics
Chief, Bone Marrow Transplantation Service
Memorial Sloan-Kettering Cancer Center
New York, New York
William D. Odell, M.D., Ph.D., M.A.C.P.
Professor and Chairman
Department of Internal Medicine
University of Utah Medical Center
Salt Lake City, Utah
Takao Ohnuma, M.D., Ph.D.
Professor of Neoplastic Diseases
Mount Sinai School of Medicine
Attending Physician
The Mount Sinai Hospital
New York, New York
Olufunmilayo I. Olopade, M.D.
Assistant Professor
Department of Medicine
University of Chicago
Pritzker School of Medicine
Chicago, Illinois
C. Tracy Orleans, Ph.D.
Director
Tobacco Control Research
Fox Chase Cancer Center
Cheltenham, Pennsylvania
C. Kent Osborne, M.D.
Professor of Medicine
Division of Medical Oncology, Department of Medicine
University of Texas Health Science Center at San Antonio
San Antonio, Texas
Robert F. Ozols, M.D., Ph.D.
Senior Vice President
Division of Medical Science
Fox Chase Cancer Center
Philadelphia, Pennsylvania
Roger J. Packer, M.D.
Chairman, Department of Neurology
Children's National Medical Center
Professor of Neurology and Pediatrics
George Washington University
Washington, D.C.
Esperanza B. Papadopoulos, M.D.
Assistant Professor of Medicine
Cornell University Medical College
Assistant Attending
Memorial Sloan-Kettering Cancer Center
New York, New York

Arthur B. Pardee, Ph.D.
Professor
Department of Cell Growth
Dana-Farber Cancer Institute
Boston, Massachusetts

Robert G. Parker, M.D.
Professor
Department of Radiation Oncology
University of California, Los Angeles
Los Angeles, California

David R. Parkinson, M.D.
Director, Investigational Drug Branch
Cancer Therapy Evaluation Program
National Cancer Institute
Bethesda, Maryland

John A. Parrish, M.D.
Professor and Chairman
Department of Dermatology
Harvard Medical School
Chief, Dermatology Service
Massachusetts General Hospital
Boston, Massachusetts

Roger R. Perry, M.D., F.A.C.S.
Associate Professor
Chief, Division of Surgical Oncology
Department of General Surgery
Eastern Virginia Medical School
Norfolk, Virginia

William P. Peters, M.D., Ph.D.
Director and Chief Executive Officer
Karmanos Cancer Institute
Detroit, Michigan

Barbara Pizzo, R.N., B.S.N.
Clinical Research Nurse
Memorial Sloan Kettering Cancer Center
New York, New York

Giuseppe Pizzorno, Ph.D., Pharm.D.
Assistant Professor
Departments of Internal Medicine, Pediatrics and Pharmacology
Yale University School of Medicine
New Haven, Connecticut

Elizabeth A. Platz, Sc.D., M.P.H.
Research Fellow
Departments of Epidemiology and Nutrition
Harvard School of Public Health
Boston, Massachusetts

William Plunkett, Ph.D.
Hubert L. and Olive Stringer Professor of Medical Oncology
Professor of Medicine (Pharmacology)
Division of Clinical Investigation
The University of Texas M.D. Anderson Cancer Center
Houston, Texas

Bruce A.J. Ponder, Ph.D., F.R.C.P.
Professor
CRC Human Cancer Genetics Research Group
Department of Pathology
University of Cambridge
Cambridge, United Kingdom

Jerome B. Posner, M.D.
Chairman
Department of Neurology
Memorial Sloan-Kettering Cancer Center
New York, New York

Michael D. Prados, M.D.
Associate Clinical Professor
Department of Neurosurgery
University of California, San Francisco
San Francisco, California

Antonio Puras, M.D.
Associate Professor of Urology
University of Puerto Rico School of Medicine
San Juan, Puerto Rico

Martin N. Raber, M.D.
Physician-in-Chief
M.D. Anderson Cancer Center
Houston, Texas

Kristjan T. Ragnarsson, M.D.
Dr. Lucy G. Moses Professor and Chairman
Department of Rehabilitation Medicine
Mount Sinai Medical Center
New York, New York

Kanti R. Rai, M.D.
Chief, Division of Hematology/Oncology
Long Island Jewish Medical Center
New Hyde Park, New York
Professor of Medicine
Albert Einstein College of Medicine
Bronx, New York

Mark J. Ratain, M.D.
Professor of Medicine
Chairman, Committee on Clinical Pharmacology
Department of Medicine
Section of Hematology/Oncology
University of Chicago
Chicago, Illinois

Mepur H. Ravindranath, Ph.D.
Director, Laboratory of Glycolipid Immunotherapy
John Wayne Cancer Institute at Saint John's Hospital
Santa Monica, California

Gregory H. Reaman, M.D.
Professor of Pediatrics
Department of Hematology/Oncology
The George Washington University School of Medicine
Chairman, Department of Hematology/Oncology
Children's National Medical Center
Washington, D.C.

C. Patrick Reynolds, M.D., Ph.D.
Head Developmental Therapeutics Section
Division of Hematology-Oncology
Children's Hospital Los Angeles and
University of Southern California School of Medicine
Los Angeles, California

Jerome P. Richie, M.D.
Elliott Carr Cutler Professor of Surgery
Harvard Medical School
Chairman, Harvard Program in Urology (Longwood Area)
Chief of Urology
Brigham and Women's Hospital
Boston, Massachusetts

Michael L. Ritchey, M.D.
Associate Professor of Surgery and Pediatrics
Department of Surgery
University of Texas-Houston Medical School
Houston, Texas

Arturo R. Rolla, M.D.
Assistant Clinical Professor of Medicine
Harvard Medical School
Endocrinologist
Deaconess Hospital
Boston, Massachusetts

Barrett J. Rollins, M.D., Ph.D.
Associate Professor
Department of Medicine
Dana-Farber Cancer Institute
Harvard Medical School
Boston, Massachusetts

Kenneth V.I. Rolston, M.D., F.A.C.P.
Professor of Medicine
Chief, Section of Infectious Diseases
Department of Medical Specialties
The University of Texas M.D. Anderson Cancer Center
Houston, Texas

Antonella Romanini, M.D.
Assistant Professor
Department of Medical Oncology
Santa Chiara Hospital
Pisa, Italy

Gerald Rosen, M.D.
Medical Director
Cedars-Sinai Comprehensive Cancer Center
Los Angeles, California

Warren E. Ross, M.D.
Executive Associate, Vice President for Health Affairs
Chief Executive Officer
University of Florida Health System
University of Florida
Gainesville, Florida

Ronald K. Ross, M.D.
Associate Dean
University of Florida College of Medicine
Gainesville, Florida

Elizabeth A. Rosvold, M.D.
Department of Medical Oncology
Fox Chase Cancer Center
Philadelphia, Pennsylvania

Bruce J. Roth, M.D.
Division of Hematology/Oncology
Indiana University Medical Center
Indianapolis, Indiana

Jack Alan Roth, M.D.
Professor and Chairman
Department of Thoracic and Cardiovascular Surgery
University of Texas M.D. Anderson Cancer Center
Houston, Texas

Jacob Rotmensch, M.D.
Section Chief
Professor, Department of OB/GYN
Section of Gynecology
University of Chicago
Chicago, Illinois

Leor D. Roubein, M.D.
Associate Professor of Medicine
Director, Clinical Gastroenterology
University of Kentucky
Division of Digestive Diseases and Nutrition
Department of Internal Medicine
Chandler Medical Center
Lexington, Kentucky

Janet D. Rowley, M.D., D.Sc.
Blum-Riese Distinguished Service Professor
Departments of Medicine and of Molecular Genetics and Cell Biology
University of Chicago
Chicago, Illinois

Valerie W. Rusch, M.D.
Attending Surgeon and Member
Thoracic Service, Department of Surgery
Memorial Sloan-Kettering Cancer Center
Professor of Surgery
Cornell University Medical College
New York, New York

Barry Salky, M.D., F.A.C.S.
Chief, Division of Laparoscopic Surgery
Mount Sinai Hospital
New York, New York

Peter T. Scardino, M.D.
Chairman, Department of Urology
University of Texas-Houston
Houston, Texas

Andrew V. Schally, Ph.D., D.Sci., M.D.h.c.
Professor of Medicine
Head, Section of Experimental Medicine
Tulane University Medical School
Chief, Endocrine, Polypeptide & Cancer Institute
Veterans Affairs Medical Center
New Orleans, Louisiana

Steven A. Schichman, M.D., Ph.D.
Jefferson Cancer Institute
Jefferson Cancer Center
Department of Microbiology and Immunology
Jefferson Medical College of Thomas Jefferson University
Philadelphia, Pennsylvania

Charles A. Schiffer, M.D.
Professor of Medicine & Oncology
Division of Hematologic Malignancies
University of Maryland Cancer Center
University of Maryland School of Medicine
Baltimore, Maryland

Stuart J. Schnitt, M.D.
Associate Director of Surgical Pathology
Department of Pathology
Beth Israel Hospital
Associate Professor of Pathology
Harvard Medical School
Boston, Massachusetts

Robert A. Schwartzman, Ph.D.
Post Doctoral Fellow
Department of Embryology
Carnegie Institution of Washington
Baltimore, Maryland

Leanne L. Seeger, M.D.
Associate Professor
Department of Radiological Sciences
Chief, Musculoskeletal Radiology
UCLA Center for Health Sciences
Los Angeles, California

Robert C. Seeger, M.D.
Professor of Pediatrics
Deputy Division Head for Research
Department of Hematology-Oncology
Children's Hospital of Los Angeles
Los Angeles, California

Nita L. Seibel, M.D.
Associate Professor
Department of Hematology/Oncology
Children's National Medical Center
Washington, D.C.

Michael T. Selch, M.D.
Professor
Department of Radiation Oncology
UCLA School of Medicine
Los Angeles, California

Michail Shafir, M.D.
Associate Clinical Professor
Surgery and Neoplastic Diseases
Mount Sinai School of Medicine
New York, New York

Brenda Shank, M.D., Ph.D.
Chairman and Professor of Radiation Oncology
Mount Sinai School of Medicine
Director and Attending Physician
Radiation Oncology
Mount Sinai Hospital
New York, New York

Charles L. Shapiro, M.D.
Medical Oncology
Dana-Farber Cancer Institute
Boston, Massachusetts

William U. Shipley, M.D.
Professor of Radiation Oncology
Harvard Medical School
Head, Genitourinary Oncology Unit
Department of Radiation Oncology
Massachusetts General Hospital Cancer Center
Boston, Massachusetts

Gerald Shklar, D.D.S., M.S.
Head
Department of Oral Medicine and Oral Pathology
Harvard Medical School
Boston, Massachusetts

Robert Silber, M.D.
Professor of Medicine, Emeritus
New York University Medical Center
New York, New York
Clinical Professor of Medicine
Duke University Medical Center
Durham, North Carolina

Richard T. Silver, M.D.
Clinical Professor of Medicine
Cornell University Medical College
Director, Section of Clinical Oncology Chemotherapy Research
Attending Physician
New York Hospital—Cornell Medical Center
New York, New York

Lewis R. Silverman, M.D.
Assistant Professor
Division of Neoplastic Diseases
Department of Medicine
Mount Sinai School of Medicine
New York, New York

Murray N. Silverstein, M.D., Ph.D.
Professor of Medicine
Mayo Clinic
Rochester, New York

David B. Skinner, M.D.
President/CEO
The Society of the New York Hospital
Professor of Surgery
Cornell University Medical College
Attending Surgeon
Department of Cardiothoracic Surgery
The New York Hospital-Cornell Medical Center
New York, New York

Charles R. Smart, M.D.
Retired Chief of Early Detection Branch
Division of Prevention and Control
National Cancer Institute
Salt Lake City, Utah

Joseph G. Sodroski, M.D.
Associate Professor of Pathology
Harvard Medical School
Division of Human Retrovirology
Dana-Farber Cancer Institute
Boston, Massachusetts

Morando Soffritti, M.D.
Associate
European Foundation of Oncology and Environmental Sciences "Bernardino Ramazzini"
Bologna, Italy

Stephen T. Sonis, D.M.D., D.M., Sc.
Professor of Oral Medicine
Chief, Division of Oral Medicine, Oral and Maxillofacial Surgery and Dentistry
Brigham and Women's Hospital
Boston, Massachusetts

Michael B. Sporn, M.D.
Professor of Pharmacology and Medicine
Dartmouth Medical School
Hanover, New Hampshire

Richard J. Steckel, M.D.
Chair
Department of Radiological Sciences
UCLA School of Medicine
Los Angeles, California

Charles D. Stiles, Ph.D.
Professor of Microbiology and Medical Genetics
Division of Cell and Molecular Biology
Dana-Farber Cancer Institute
Boston, Massachusetts

Richard M. Stone, M.D.
Assistant Professor of Medicine
Division of Cancer Pharmacology
Dana-Farber Cancer Institute
Boston, Massachusetts

Nelson N. Stone, M.D.
Associate Professor of Urology
Mount Sinai School of Medicine
New York, New York
Director, Department of Urology
Elmhurst Hospital Center
Elmhurst, New York

Max W. Sung, M.D.
Assistant Professor
Division of Neoplastic Diseases
Samuel Bronfman Department of Medicine
Mount Sinai School of Medicine
New York, New York

Antonella Surbone, M.D.
Associate Attending Physician
Department of Medicine
Memorial Sloan-Kettering Cancer Center
Associate Professor of Clinical Medicine
Cornell University Medical Center
New York, New York

Mario Sznol, M.D.
Head, Biologic Evaluation Section
Investigational Drug Branch
Cancer Therapy Evaluation Program
Division of Cancer Treatment
National Cancer Institute
Bethesda, Maryland

Laszlo Tabar, M.D.
Associate Professor
Department of Mammography
Falun Central Hospital
Falun, Sweden

Victor F. Tapson, M.D.
Assistant Professor of Medicine
Department of Medicine
Duke University Medical Center
Durham, North Carolina
Joseph M. Taraska, J.D.
Attorney
Taraska, Grower & Ketcham, P.A.
Orlando, Florida
Ayalew Tefferi, M.D.
Assistant Professor of Medicine
Mayo Clinic and Mayo Foundation
Rochester, Minnesota
Joel Tepper, M.D.
Professor and Chair
Department of Radiation Oncology
University of North Carolina
Chapel Hill, North Carolina
James T. Thigpen, M.D.
Professor of Medicine
University of Mississippi School of Medicine
Jackson, Mississippi
Gillian M. Thomas, M.D., F.R.C.P.C.
Head, Department of Radiation Oncology
Toronto-Sunnybrook Regional Cancer Center
North York, Ontario, Canada
Associate Professor
Departments of Radiation Oncology and Obstetrics and Gynecology
University of Toronto
Toronto, Ontario, Canada
Patrick R.M. Thomas, M.D.
Professor and Chair
Department of Radiation Oncology
Temple University Hospital
Philadelphia, Pennsylvania
Norman W. Thompson, M.D., Ph.D.
Henry King Ransom Professor of Surgery
Chief, Division of Endocrine Surgery
Department of Surgery
University of Michigan
Ann Arbor, Michigan
William M. Thompson, M.D.
Professor and Chairman
Wilhelmina and Eugene Gedguadas
Chair in Radiology
Department of Radiology
University of Minnesota Hospital and Clinic
Minneapolis, Minnesota
Swan N. Thung, M.D.
Professor of Pathology
Mount Sinai School of Medicine
New York, New York
Robert Timmerman, M.D.
Assistant Professor
Department of Radiation Oncology
Indiana University
Indianapolis, Indiana
Arthur K.F. Tong, M.D., M.B., B.S.
Dermatologist
Harvard University Health Service
Cambridge, Massachusetts
Timothy J. Triche, M.D., Ph.D.
Pathologist-in-Chief
Department of Pathology & Laboratory Medicine
Children's Hospital of Los Angeles
Professor of Pathology and Pediatrics
Department of Pathology & Laboratory Medicine
University of Southern California
Los Angeles, California
Michael E. Trigg, M.D.
Professor of Pediatrics
Director, Pediatric Bone Marrow Transplantation
University of Iowa Hospital & Clinics
Iowa City, Iowa
Steven R. Tronick, Ph.D.
Director
Research and Development
Santa Cruz Biotechnology, Inc.
Santa Cruz, California
Donald L. Trump, M.D.
Professor of Medicine and Surgery
University of Pittsburgh
Deputy Director for Clinical Investigations
Pittsburgh Cancer Institute
Pittsburgh, Pennsylvania
Fatih M. Uckun, M.D.
Professor, Director of Biotherapy Program
Departments of Therapeutic Radiology, Pediatrics, and Pharmacology
University of Minnesota
Roseville, Minnesota
John E. Ultmann, M.D.
Professor of Medicine
Section of Hematology/Oncology
Director Emeritus, University of Chicago Cancer Center
The University of Chicago
Chicago, Illinois
James Vardiman, M.D.
Department of Pathology
University of Chicago
Chicago, Illinois
Aaron I. Vinik, M.D., Ph.D., F.C.P., F.A.C.P.
Director
Diabetes Research Institute
Department of Internal Medicine
Eastern Virginia Medical School
Norfolk, Virginia
Bert Vogelstein, M.D.
Investigator
Howard Hughes Medical Institute
Professor of Oncology
Johns Hopkins School of Medicine
Baltimore, Maryland
Paul A. Volberding, M.D.
Professor of Medicine, UCSF
Director, AIDS Program
San Francisco General Hospital
San Francisco, California
Daniel D.Von Hoff, M.D., F.A.C.P.
Professor of Medicine
Department of Medicine, Oncology
University of Texas Health Science Center at San Antonio
Director, Institute for Drug Development
Cancer Therapy & Research Center
San Antonio, Texas
Sidney Wallace, M.D.
University of Texas M.D. Anderson Cancer Center
Department of Radiology
Houston, Texas

Helen H. Wang, M.D., Dr.P.H.
Medical Director of Cytopathology
Department of Pathology
Beth Israel Hospital
Assistant Professor of Pathology
Harvard Medical School
Boston, Massachusetts

William M. Wara, M.D.
Professor & Executive Vice Chairman
Department of Radiation Oncology
University of California, San Francisco
San Francisco, California

Jane Weeks, M.D., M.Sc.
Assistant Professor of Medicine
Harvard Medical School
Division of Cancer Epidemiology and Control
Dana-Farber Cancer Institute
Boston, Massachusetts

Ralph R. Weichselbaum, M.D.
Harold H. Hines, Jr., Professor and Chairman
Department of Radiation and Cellular Oncology
University of Chicago Hospital
Director, Chicago Tumor Institute
University of Chicago
Chicago, Illinois

Robert J. Wells, M.D.
Professor of Clinical Pediatrics
University of Cincinnati
Children's Hospital Medical Center
Cincinnati, Ohio

Ainsley Weston, Ph.D.
Associate Professor
Community Medicine
Mount Sinai Medical Center
New York, New York

J. Taylor Wharton, M.D.
Professor and Chairman
Department of Gynecologic Oncology
University of Texas M.D. Anderson Cancer Center
Houston, Texas

Eugene S. Wiener, M.D.
Professor of Pediatric Surgery
Department of Surgery
University of Pittsburgh School of Medicine
Children's Hospital of Pittsburgh
Pittsburgh, Pennsylvania

Charles B. Wilson, M.D.
Department of Neurosurgery
University of California, San Francisco
San Francisco, California

Kenneth Wishnow, M.D.
Associate Professor of Surgery
Department of Medicine
Dana-Farber Cancer Institute
Boston, Massachusetts

William G. Woods, M.D.
Professor and Director
Department of Pediatric Hematology-Oncology
University of Minnesota Hospital
Minneapolis, Minnesota

Antoinette J. Wozniak, M.D.
Assistant Professor of Medicine
Division of Hematology-Oncology
Wayne State University
Detroit, Michigan

Li-Teh Wu, M.D.
Clinical Assistant Professor
Department of Medicine
Division of Neoplastic Diseases
Mt Sinai School of Medicine
New York, New York

Connie Henke Yarbro, R.N., B.S.N.
Clinical Associate Professor
Division of Hematology/Oncology
University of Missouri
Columbia, Missouri

Michael R. Zalutsky, Ph.D.
Professor
Duke University Medical Center
Durham, North Carolina

Marvin Zelen, Ph.D.
Professor of Statistical Science
Harvard School of Public Health
The Dana-Farber Cancer Institute
Boston, Massachusetts

Anthony L. Zietman, M.D., F.R.C.R.
Assistant Professor
Department of Radiation Oncology
Massachusetts General Hospital
Harvard Medical School
Boston, Massachusetts

Hyman J. Zimmerman, M.D.
Professor of Medicine, Emeritus
George Washington University
Distinguished Scientist, Emeritus
Armed Forces Institute of Pathology
Washington, D.C.

Michael Zinner, M.D.
Chairman, Department of Surgery
Brigham & Women's Hospital
Moseley Professor of Surgery
Harvard Medical School
Boston, Massachusetts

CONTENTS

VOLUME ONE

SECTION I

CANCER BIOLOGY

SECTION II

TUMOR IMMUNOLOGY

SECTION III

CANCER ETIOLOGY

SECTION IV

CANCER EPIDEMIOLOGY

SECTION V

THEORY AND PRACTICE OF CLINICAL TRIALS

SECTION VI

CANCER PREVENTION

SECTION VII

CANCER SCREENING AND EARLY DETECTION

SECTION VIII

PRINCIPLES OF CANCER PATHOLOGY

SECTION IX

PRINCIPLES OF IMAGING

SECTION X

INTERVENTIONAL RADIOLOGY

SECTION XI

ENDOSCOPY

SECTION XII

PRINCIPLES OF SURGICAL ONCOLOGY

SECTION XXXIX

NEOPLASMS IN AIDS

SECTION XL

NEOPLASMS OF UNKNOWN PRIMARY SITE

SECTION XLI

NEOPLASMS IN CHILDREN

SECTION XLII

COMPLICATIONS OF CANCER AND ITS TREATMENT

SECTION XLIII

INFECTIONS IN PATIENTS WITH CANCER

SECTION XLIV

ONCOLOGIC EMERGENCIES

SECTION XLV

ONCOLOGY AND THE INFORMATION REVOLUTION

SECTION I

CANCER BIOLOGY

CHAPTER 1

Cell Proliferation and Differentiation

HOWARD J. FINGERT, JUDITH CAMPISI, AND ARTHUR B. PARDEE

Introduction

The biology of cell division and differentiation is exceedingly similar in both normal and cancer cells. The cancer cell differs from its normal counterpart in that it is aberrantly regulated. Cancer cells generally contain the full complement of biomolecules that are necessary for survival, proliferation, differentiation, and expression of many cell-type-specific functions. Failure to regulate these functions properly, however, results in an altered phenotype and cancer.

Three cellular functions tend to be inappropriately regulated in a neoplasm. First, the normal constraints on cellular proliferation are relaxed, and this is a necessary but often insufficient requirement for tumor formation. Second, differentiation can be distorted. The tumor cells may be blocked at a particular stage of differentiation, or they may differentiate into an inappropriate or abnormal cell type. Third, chromosomal and genetic organization may be destabilized such that variant cells arise with high frequency (see Chapter 7). Some variants may have an increased growth advantage, others may be resistant to killing by chemotherapeutic drugs or radiation; and others may have increased motility or enzyme production that permit invasion and metastases (see Chapters 8 and 9).

To comprehend the biology of cancer, it is necessary to understand how these three functions (i.e., growth, differentiation, and chromosome stability) are controlled in normal cells and how they become uncontrolled in cancer cells. This chapter focuses on the biology of cell proliferation and differentiation and how these functions are linked in the development of neoplasia.

Proliferation

TUMOR GROWTH AND CELL PROLIFERATION IN VIVO

In terms of population kinetics, the growth of any tissue depends on three parameters: (*a*) rate of individual cell division (Tc), (*b*) growth fraction of the cell population, and (*c*) cell loss from the growing population through differentiation, cell death, or other means (Fig. 1.1). Normal cells reach a steady state of growth that provides a balanced economy for the body as a whole. Each organ maintains tight controls over growth rate, growth fraction, and cell loss. Physiologic stimuli can alter these parameters in normal tissues, leading to increased tissue growth, but this growth will cease when the stimulus is withdrawn or a new steady state is achieved. Some normal tissues grow faster than cancers under physiologic conditions, so it is not simply rapid growth at a single time and place that distinguishes neoplasia. Biopsy samples from normal, inflammatory, and neoplastic lesions of the lung, cervix, vocal cord, or pharynx have been analyzed for the rate of cell proliferation; these studies showed that benign inflammatory lesions can grow over 20 times faster than cancer in a discrete time and place (35, 36, 126). Similarly, rapid proliferation of human lymphoid cells is induced by immunostimulants; and growth kinetics of these cells are similar to those observed in high-grade lymphomas (14). Unlike neoplastic tissues, which continue to grow over time, noncancerous neoplastic tissues cease rapid growth when healing is complete. In many ways, cancer can be thought of as a "wound that does not heal" (4).

It generally is believed that neoplastic cells multiply exponentially during the early phases of tumor cell growth, for example, 1 cell becomes 2, 2 become 4, and then 8, 16, and so on (see Chapter 52) (117). As the tumor mass increases, however, the rate of growth declines. Measuring tumor growth over time describes a curve with an exponential increase in the early period, then a flattening out of the growth rate over time (i.e., Gompertzian curve) (124). Several mechanisms have been invoked to explain this change in growth rate with larger tumors: *a*) decrease in the growth fraction, *b*) increase in cell loss (i.e., exfoliation, necrosis), (*c*) nutritional depletion of tumor cells resulting from outgrowth of available blood supply (see Chapter 10), or (*d*) lengthening of cell cycle time. Experimental tumor models suggest that cell cycle time changes only slightly when tumor growth decreases (39). Under adverse conditions, tumor cells often leave the growth fraction and enter a nongrowing state (G0 or prolonged G1) (Fig.1.2), although these same cells can reenter the division cycle when conditions improve or when stimulated by growth factors.

ANALYSIS OF CELL PROLIFERATION

Autoradiography has been a useful tool for measuring the growth rates of cell populations both in vitro and in vivo (86). This technique identifies growing cells by their uptake of radioactive precursors for DNA synthesis (e.g., tritiated thymidine). Samples of these tissues are then treated with photographic emulsion and developing agents. Black granules form over the nuclei of cells that have used the radioactive precursor and gone through DNA replication and cell division (Fig. 1.1*B*) (22, 38). A similar technique exposes cells to bromodeoxyuridine (BrdU), which is a pyrimidine analogue of thymidine selectively used by cells in DNA synthesis. Subsequently, the cell population is stained with an identifiable antibody that binds only BrdU-containing cells. This is a sensitive assay for the number of cells that are cycling through DNA synthesis (i.e., S phase).

The labeling index (LI) is a measure of cells synthesizing DNA, typically using thymidine incorporation to label S-phase cells by autoradiography. This technique provides a relatively simple method for estimating proliferative rates and growth fractions of cancerous or normal cells (5). The average time for cell division within the growing population (Tc) can be estimated by taking multiple samples over time and counting the percentage of cells that are labeled at mitosis. Timed exposure to radioactive thymidine also provides a method for estimating the length of the cell cycle and the duration of cell cycle phases (e.g., G1, S, G2, M) (86).

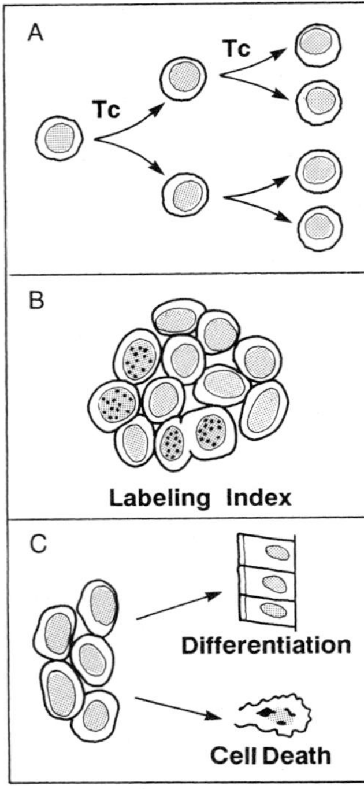

Figure 1.1. Cell proliferation and cell loss. **A.** Tc is the average time required for one cell to divide into two daughter cells. Human cancer cells exhibit a broad range, many with a Tc that is longer than rapidly dividing normal tissues such as bone marrow and intestinal mucosa (Table 1.1). **B.** Labeling index (LI) is a measure of the fraction of cells that are in the DNA synthetic phase. This is commonly measured by uptake of radioactive substrate (thymidine) for DNA synthesis. After incubation with tritiated thymidine and application of photographic emulsion, cells that incorporate thymidine are seen by the development of black dots in the photographic emulsion that overlies the nucleus. This diagram shows 4/12-33% labeling. LI also correlates with growth fraction (GF), which is the proliferating fraction of the entire cell population under study. If 4 other cells were demonstrated to be proliferating but in other phases of the cell cycle, then the GF would be 8/12-66%. **C.** Cell loss can occur by various means, including cell death and exfoliation or differentiation into nondividing cells. This diagram depicts stem cells of the gastrointestinal tract differentiating into columnar cells that line the gastrointestinal mucosa.

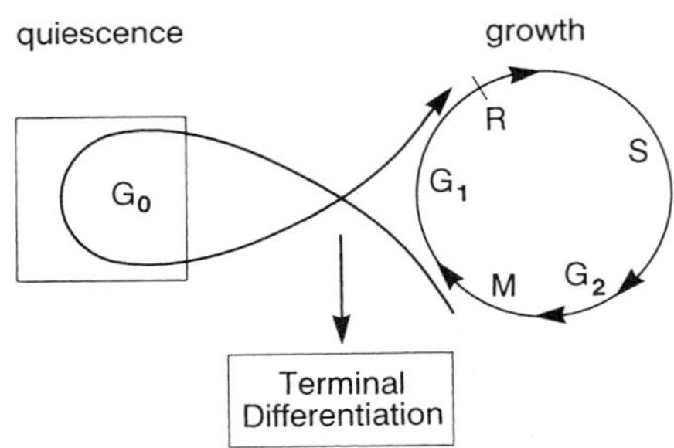

Figure 1.2. The cell cycle. When a cell is not synthesizing DNA (S phase), or completing mitosis (M phase), it is commonly termed as being in a G (gap) phase. Normal cells are capable of resting in a nondividing state, called G0. They can begin one or more cycles of cell division when there is a need to maintain or replace tissue, and they stop dividing when the necessary growth is complete. In G1, protein and RNA synthesis are active. If conditions are permissive for subsequent cell division, cells pass through the R (restriction) point and quickly move into the S (synthetic) period when new DNA is synthesized. Another gap (G2) follows when the newly duplicated chromosomes condense. In the M period, the chromosomes divide into two sets, the cell forms two nuclei, and then divides into two daughter cells. When normal cells differentiate, typically with a gain in the properties required for organ or tissue functions, they generally lose the capacity to continue cell division.

More recent studies analyzing cell proliferation have employed staining with the Ki67 mouse monoclonal antibody or quantification of DNA content by flow cytometry (85). These latter techniques can be performed with small, surgical samples of tumor. Moreover, they do not require incubation of tissues in radioactive materials or prior administration of drugs. The exact nature of the antigen bound by the antibody Ki67 is not known, but it is not appreciably expressed in quiescent (G0) cells. Expression begins in cells that have entered the cell cycle (mid-G1), and cells going through division (G2–M) are heavily positive. Thus, the ratio of Ki67-positive cells to total cells represents the percentage of cells that are cycling at any one time, which is a measure of the growth fraction (103). Monoclonal antibodies to other proliferation-related antigens also are currently under study. For example, monoclonal antibodies to "proliferation cell nuclear antigen," or PCNA, have been developed, along with methods to measure this S-phase antigen in fixed, paraffin-embedded tissues. This technique may have practical advantages in terms of clinical studies (45).

An automated technique to measure cell cycle distribution, flow cytometry, is one of the most common methods to quantify the relative number of cells in the G0–G1, S, or G2–M phases. Tissue samples are disaggregated, suspended as single cells, and stained with a fluorescent DNA dye. This sample then flows past a light source and a sensitive fluorescence detector that records the relative DNA content as measured by the amount of fluorescent signal per cell. These data are translated by computer to a histogram (Fig. 1.3), and computer programs are used to measure the relative number of cells with G0–G1, S, or G2–M DNA content. This same technique also provides a rapid method to quantify tumor ploidy (e.g., cell populations with altered chromosome number). Tumor cells with normal chromosome content (2n) are diploid, and the G0–G1 peak appears on the histogram at the same location as the G0–G1 peak from nontumor cells. The G0–G1 peak from tumor cells with abnormal (i.e., aneuploid) chromosome content, however, appears at a different position in the histogram. For example, if the aneuploid cells have more DNA in all phases of the cell cycle because of increased chromosome number, then the histogram is shifted to the right (Fig. 1.3).

Flow cytometry of DNA content has gained increasing use as a measure of proliferative activity of clinical tumor samples, because of its speed, relative simplicity with automated computer technology, and requirement of only a small tumor sample. Many investigators use the S index or S-phase fraction, computed by the relative number of cells that do not have G0–G1 or G2–M DNA content, to study proliferation of tumor cell populations. In patients with breast or ovarian cancer, a high S index was found to be an independent predictor of prognosis in patients with diploid tumors (see Chapter 36) (21, 66).

Similarly, the relative number of aneuploid tumor cells can have prognostic value, although such data often are linked to a higher S phase (21, 85). Other investigators have measured the G1 phase fraction (G1PF) to represent cells that are not in other proliferative phases and correlated a relative decrease in the G1PF with higher proliferation (72). This latter technique can be difficult, however, if the tissue sample has variable concentrations of normal cells with G0–G1 DNA content.

These techniques of measuring cell proliferation parameters provide useful information for understanding the biology of tumor growth, and they may supplement routine histology to determine diagnosis and prognosis for many cancers (103). Estimated mean values of LI and Tc for several neoplasms and some of the most rapidly proliferating normal tissues are listed in Table 1.1. These data illustrate a wide range of Tc (1–10 days) and LI (3–40%), which is similar to the wide range of growth rates observed in clinical studies of human cancers.

The LI and growth fraction (GF) are the kinetic parameters that commonly distinguish cancer from normal tissue (93). In contrast, the actual rate of cell division (Tc), is not a major determinant of the abnormal growth of neoplasms. Many cancer cells, especially those of the intestinal mucosa and bone marrow, grow at a slower Tc than normal tissues (61, 73). When comparisons have been possible between neoplastic and normal cells of the same histologic type (e.g., leukemia and normal bone marrow), it also is apparent that the Tc of cancer cells is the same as, or longer than, that of normal cells (Table 1.1). Decreased cell loss is an important parameter in many neoplasms. Cancerous tissues can increase in size faster than bone marrow or intestinal mucosa, even though the Tc and GFs predict a slower growth of the tumors compared with normal tissues (23). The normal tissues, however, balance high proliferative rates with cell loss through exfoliation or differentiation into nondividing cells.

Growth rates of individual tumors in vivo also demonstrate the importance of LI and GF (Table 1.2). Analysis of these data requires a clear distinction between the rate of cell division (Tc) and the doubling time of the tumor mass (Td). Tc refers to the time of cell division, that is, the time required for an average cell to go through one complete cell division and return to the same phase of the cell cycle. Because autora-

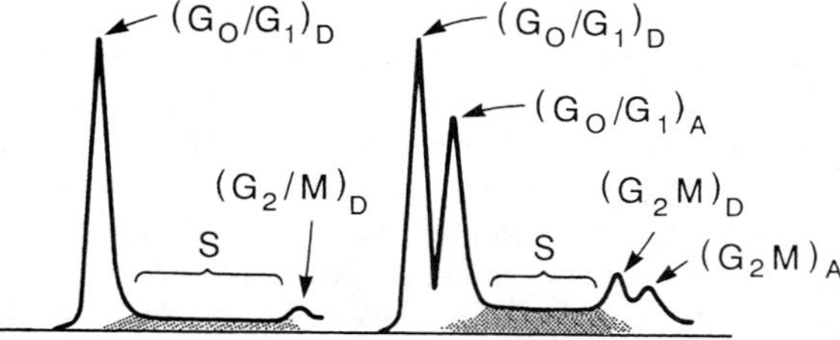

Figure 1.3. Histograms of DNA content in normal and tumor cells. Using flow cytometry, areas under the curves are measured by computer, indicating the relative number of cells in G0/G1, S, or G2/M phases of the cell cycle. **Left,** Normal cells with 2n (diploid) chromosomes. The *shaded area* represents cells in the S phase. **Right,** A clinical breast cancer removed during surgery. This tumor contains both diploid (D) and aneuploid (A) cells, and it also contains a larger number of cells in the S phase (*shaded area*).

Table 1.1. Growth Parameters of Human Neoplasms and Normal Tissues

Cell type	Labeling index (%)	Estimated cell doubling time (d)
Normal bone marrow myeloblasts	32–75	0.7–1.1
Acute myeloid leukemia	8–25	0.5–8.0
Normal B-cell lymphocytes	0–1	14–21+
High-grade lymphoma	19–29	2–3
Normal intestinal crypts	12–18	1–2
Colon adenocarcinoma	3–35	1.6–5.0
Normal epithelium/pharynx	2–3	—
Squamous cell carcinoma of the nasopharynx	5–16	2–4
Normal epithelium/bronchus	—	9–10
Epidermoid carcinoma of the lung	5–8	8–10
Normal epithelium/cervix	4–8	—
Squamous cell carcinoma of the cervix	13–40	—
Ovarian carcinoma	3–20	5–6
Benign mole of skin	0.3	—
Malignant melanoma of skin	12.8	—

Table 1.2. Correlation Between Mass Doubling Time and Growth Fraction

Tumor	Growth fraction (%)	Doubling time (d)
Experimental tumors		
L1210 (mouse)	86	0.5
B 16 (mouse)	55	1.9
LL (mouse)	38	2.9
DMBA (rat)	10	7.4
Human tumors		
Embryonal carcinoma	90	27
Lymphoma (high grade)	90	29
Squamous cell carcinoma	25	58
Adenocarcinoma	6	83

diography can identify radioactive thymidine-labeled cells as they pass through the DNA-replicative (S) phase of the cell cycle and into mitosis, Tc often is measured by the "intermitotic time" between two consecutive mitoses. In contrast, Td is the estimated time needed to double the size of an entire tumor mass using, for example, calipers or x-ray measurements. Td usually is much longer than Tc because of cell loss, change in growth rates over time, and a less than 100% GF. For example, a Tc of approximately 2 to 3 days was measured in one tumor of the head and neck, and this tumor had a Td of 21 days during the same period of measurement (12). Similarly, other human tumors have a Tc of 2 to 6 days, while the Td for the same tumor types has been in the range of 50 to 100 days. If all proliferating cells were to continue division with no cell loss, mathematic models could be employed to predict the "potential doubling time" of tumors. For example, squamous cell lung cancers may have an observed LI of approximately 7%, predicting a potential Td of 9 days; however, the observed Td typically is 1 to 2 months for these tumors, which is a difference illustrating the high level of cell loss and variable growth that occurs with these and other solid neoplasms (120).

The GF appears to correlate inversely with the overall Td of solid tumors (i.e., an increased GF corresponds to a shorter Td and a faster growth of tumor masses). This was first demonstrated in animal tumors, which can be measured more frequently than most human cancers (Table 1.2). A close correlation between increased LI and decreased Td also has been observed in studies of human cancers (126); however, methodologic differences among various laboratories present many problems for such comparisons (86, 103). A correlation between histologic grade and LI has been observed in many cancers, including lymphoma, bladder, and breast carcinomas, as well as soft-tissue sarcomas. In addition to grade or other traditional histologic criteria, several studies demonstrate that LI or the S index can be an independent determinant of prognosis, especially in breast, colon, non-small-cell lung, ovary, and primary brain neoplasms, chronic lymphocytic leukemia, and myeloma (21, 52, 84, 86).

Understanding the kinetics of tumor cell growth in vivo has provided direction for more basic investigations into the mechanisms of neoplasia at the cellular, subcellular, and molecular levels. The increased GF of cancer cells is a key property distinguishing most neoplasms from normal tissues. At the level of a single cell, the process that best determines the GF of a cell population is the initiation of cell division from a nongrowing state (i.e., the process of entering G1–S phases from a quiescent state in which DNA replication is inactive). The events leading to cell division include a complex array of biochemical and genetic signals, and many of these have been clarified using cells in culture. In addition, tumor cell proliferation in vivo is influenced by a variety of local and systemic factors, which are reviewed in later chapters.

CELLS IN CULTURE

The importance of the individual cell in cancer is clear, because a single cancer cell injected into an appropriate animal is sufficient to give rise to a tumor. Many studies, therefore, have been performed with isolated normal and tumor cells in culture. Both normal and tumor-derived mammalian cells can be grown and compared in culture, although many are not readily established in culture initially (3, 97, 98, 129). Short-term culture of human cancer cells or tissue fragments obtained from clinical biopsies can be used for evaluation of in vitro response to chemotherapies. This is a promising approach to study new anticancer agents and the mechanisms of drug action, or to predict the efficacy of clinical treatments for individual patients (44, 75). Most studies of mammalian cell biology have used fibroblasts, because this cell type is easily cultured and most likely to grow out of a tissue explant. Much has been learned from hematopoietic cells as well (26); moreover, the culture of epithelial cells has advanced considerably (105).

Cells generally are grown in a medium containing salts, amino acids, glucose, vitamins, and serum or growth factors. Plated on a plastic surface to which they may attach, normal cells can grow until they have formed a confluent monolayer, whereupon growth ceases. Growth also ceases when cells have exhausted a nutrient or a factor provided by serum or when such substances are removed by changing to a deficient medium. Thus, growth can be manipulated in culture.

Quiescence Versus Growth

Cells that have stopped growing are said to be in a G0 state, or "quiescent." Most cells in adults are in G0. They can be very active functionally and metabolically, and growth of G0 cells can be initiated by appropriately changing the cell density or the supply of nutrients. These cells then enter the cell cycle (Fig. 1.2), beginning a sequence of events that culminates in cell division. For the 3T3 murine fibroblast line, the durations of G1, S, G2, and M are approximately 6.0, 8.0, 2.0, and 0.5 hours, respectively. The duration of a cycle is relatively constant; thus, the fraction of time that a cell spends in quiescence compared with its time in cycle determines its average growth rate. The switching of cells back and forth between quiescence and cycling depends on extracellular conditions and is regulated differently in normal and tumor cells.

Molecular Events in Cell Proliferation

When a quiescent cell in culture is stimulated by the addition of serum, for example, the activated chain of events eventually leads to the formation of two cells. This requires duplication of a multitude of molecules in the original cell (10). At least three growth factors, provided in serum, have been found to act sequentially following resumption of proliferation of fibroblasts: platelet-derived growth factor (PDGF), epidermal growth factor (EGF), and insulin-like growth factor (IGF-1). Extracellular tumor growth factor-β (TGF-β) has the opposite effect. It inhibits the growth of various epithelial cells by intracellular mechanisms still being investigated (108). Paracrine production of TGF-β could limit growth of both normal and cancer cells, and experimental models suggest that it may play a role in the regression of breast cancers in response to hormonal or drug therapies (149).

Growth factor receptors are complex, large proteins that span the plasma membrane. They have a specific domain that recognizes the growth factor on the outside of the cell, and their cytoplasmic portion may have an enzymatic function, such as a protein tyrosine kinase. Binding of a growth factor or ligand to its receptor can induce transmission of a signal to the cytoplasm through activation of the kinase (31). The next step is a transduction of the cytoplasmic signal to the cell nucleus (see Chapter 4). This is accomplished by a heterogeneous group of molecules known as second messengers and include various proteins that are phosphorylated by kinases, small molecules such as inositol phosphates and cyclic AMP, and ions, including Ca^{2+}, H^{+}, and Zn^{2+}. Within the nucleus, genes are then activated in response to these second messengers. The second messengers probably modify proteins that bind to regulatory DNA sequences located near specific functional genes. "Immediate-early" genes are activated quickly and include well-known proto-oncogenes such as *jun, fos,* and *myc.* Production of new mRNAs transcribed from these genes does not require new protein synthesis, because production is not prevented by protein synthesis inhibitors. Other genes, including the *ras* and *raf* proto-oncogenes, act subsequent to the activation of immediate early genes (31).

Protein and RNA synthesis are required for cells to enter the S phase, during which DNA is synthesized, because drugs that inhibit protein or RNA synthesis also block cell passage through G1 to S (Fig. 1.4) (34, 140). Cell proliferation, particularly progression through G1, depends on molecules present in growing cells that activate quiescent cells (137). Experimental models have been developed to fuse growing and quiescent cells, and these fusions lead to rapid induction of cell division in the quiescent cells (96). These positive agents are very likely proteins induced during the latter part of G1.

A variety of proteins are produced during G1 after cells leave quiescence. Some are enzymes that expand metabolic functions lost by G0 cells, such as those providing energy, and more ribosomes are made for rapid protein synthesis as well. Others have so-called "housekeeping functions" that keep both quiescent and growing cells in metabolic balance. Only a few proteins appear to be key regulatory molecules. For example, enzymes are required for the synthesis of isoprenoids, which are necessary for activity of the *ras* oncogene, and for the synthesis of polyamines, which have many functions including ionic binding to nucleic acids. The *ras* oncogene product is synthesized as a precursor protein that requires posttranslational processing to become biologically active and capable of transforming mammalian cells. Farnesylation appears to be a critical modification of the *ras* protein, and drugs that inhibit farnesyl-protein transferase can block *ras*-dependent transformation. These agents have been proposed as a potential new class of therapy for cancer (47).

For progression through the end of the G1 period, IGF-1 appears to be the only factor necessary. Enzymes involved in the synthesis of DNA, such as thymidine kinase and DNA polymerase, as well as histones are synthesized just prior to

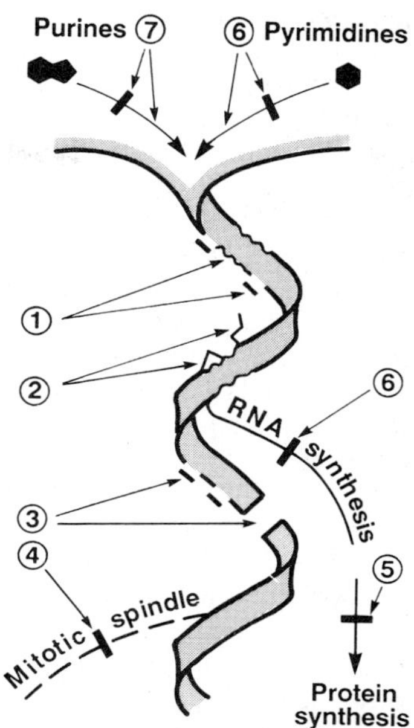

Figure 1.4. Anticancer drugs and their effects on cell proliferation. **Group 1,** Antitumor, antibiotics, and anthracyclines (doxorubicin, mitomycin, daunorubicin, mithramycin, idarubicin, dactinomycin, epirubicin, mitoxantrone). Effect: bind and disorganize DNA, prevent DNA replication and RNA synthesis. **Group 2,** Alkylating agents (mechlorethamine, cisplatin, cyclophosphamide, carboplatin, ifosfamide, nitrosoureas, thiotepa, dacarbazine). Effect: cross-link DNA, prevent DNA replication and RNA synthesis. **Group 3,** Cleaving agents (bleomycin, etoposide). Effect: cleave DNA after interaction with cellular components. **Group 4,** Tubulin binding agents (vincristine, paclitaxel, docetaxel). Effect: disrupt mitotic spindles or stabilize microtubules. **Group 5,** Protein-synthesis inhibitor (L-asparaginase). Effect: depletes extracellular asparagine, used for protein synthesis. **Group 6,** Antimetabolites (methotrexate, 5-fluorouracil, cytarabine, hydroxyurea, fludarabine). Effect: block pyrimidine or purine conversion to nucleotide, misincorporate into DNA or RNA, terminate DNA synthesis. **Group 7,** Purine analogues (6-thioguanine, 6-mercaptopurine). Effect: prevent purine ring biosynthesis, misincorporate into DNA or RNA (see Chapters 60–67).

the S phase. These enzyme molecules relocate at the beginning of DNA synthesis, moving from the cytoplasm into the nucleus. A variety of experiments show that DNA is made by a high-molecular-weight, multienzyme complex (98, 130). This complex contains many enzymes known to be involved in the process of DNA replication, but its size and other features are still a matter of debate. The onset of DNA replication has been investigated recently with in vitro systems, and these studies reveal that the synthesis of helicase enzymes, which possess DNA-unwinding ability, may provide the final factor for initiating the S phase (18). After DNA synthesis has commenced, cell growth becomes relatively independent of external controls. After completing DNA duplication, the S phase cell then goes through G2 and mitosis and finally divides to form two daughter cells. Information is rapidly accumulating regarding molecular events related to mitosis (32, 77). The daughter cells, now in the G1 phase, will then either pass through another cycle or arrest in a quiescent G0 state depending, once more, on external conditions. If these conditions are not adequate, the cell will become arrested before it reinitiates DNA synthesis.

PROLIFERATION CONTROLS

Cell growth is determined by extracellular conditions that act before the onset of DNA synthesis. The proliferation rate is initially determined by the probability of switching from the quiescent G0 to G1 phase of the cell cycle. Cells both in vivo and in culture may spend long periods of time in the G0 state depending on the cell type. Differentiated nerve and muscle cells remain quiescent permanently, and normal fibroblasts emerge to grow only when conditions are favorable and when stimulated by growth factors such as PDGF.

Two major sites of controls exist (for 3T3 cells) between G0 and S: competence and the restriction point (R). These are located approximately 12 and 2 hours before the start of the S phase, respectively. PDGF permits cells such as fibroblasts to leave G0, enter G1, and reach competence. EGF and probably insulin allow passage through mid-G1, while rapid protein synthesis and IGF-1 allow completion of G1. Once initiated, the cycle thus is not free-running; rather, it is highly regulated during the transition from G1 to the S phase (27, 98). All growth factors are dispensable a few hours before the onset of actual DNA synthesis, as is the requirement for a rapid rate of protein synthesis. This step of final regulation in G1 is the R point (98).

Much is being learned about the molecules that regulate passage through these control points. Proto-oncogenes and tumor-suppressor genes are of great interest in this regard (see Chapters 5 and 6). Some of these genes code for DNA-binding proteins such as *fos* and *jun*, which form a complex and bind to specific gene-regulatory DNA sequences during the competence process. Other proto-oncogenes code for growth factors; for example, c-*sis* codes for PDGF-β chain. Others code for growth factor receptors, such as the gene that encodes the EGF receptor. Still others, such as c-*raf*, appear to have distinct functions (e.g., coding for protein kinases that act on substrates in the cascade involved in second-messenger metabolism). Another set of gene products disappear when cells start to proliferate (112). The proteins encoded by oncogenes similarly display diverse locations, some being on the plasma membrane, others in the nucleus, and still others inside the cytoplasm (see Chapter 5) (8). Other gene products disappear in tumors, and some of these are tumor-suppressor genes, which are of increasing interest for their ability to regulate cell growth negatively (111). Several studies suggest that TGF-β blocks cell growth by blocking expression of the c-*myc* gene, possibly through interaction with the RB (retinoblastoma) protein (92).

Along with a general increase in metabolic activity during G1, changes also are observed in cell structural elements. For example, the cytoskeleton, which is composed of various filaments and microtubules, is modified. Actin, the major structural component of microfilaments, also is produced more rapidly by stimulated cells. It is not clear at present which of these changes have regulatory consequences and which are simply reorganizations of the cell to provide greater metabolic activity.

Kinetic experiments show that normal cells must synthesize proteins rapidly to reach the R point and proceed into division. The cell must make a sufficient amount of some special protein during late G1; this protein is unstable in normal cells, with a half-life of only approximately 2.5 hours in 3T3 cells. Therefore, synthesis of this protein must be quite rapid, because degradation otherwise prevents its sufficient accumulation. A protein with such properties has been identified, but its function is unknown (98).

The cyclin proteins appear to play a major role in cell cycle regulation (68). Cyclins are a family of proteins that accumulate in the G1 phase of eukaryotic cells, before the transition into the S phase (G1 cyclins), and again during late S–G2 phases before mitosis (mitotic cyclins) (77). After they reach a peak concentration, cyclin proteins are rapidly degraded. In several experimental systems, the cyclic levels of these proteins have been shown to be necessary for transition through the cell cycle (93). These proteins bind to one of several enzymes with potent kinase activity, coded by a group of "cell division cycle" genes. First discovered in yeast and sea urchin eggs, similar protein-kinase complexes have been found in various eukaryotic species, and recent studies have focused on their possible role in the regulation of neoplastic cell proliferation (68, 69). This cyclin–kinase complex becomes active to phosphorylate a variety of substrates, which trigger initiation of DNA synthesis (S phase), progression through S phase and formation of the mitotic apparatus needed for the final stage of cell division (M phase). In normal cells, the RB protein is produced throughout the cell cycle. Its phosphorylation increases at the G1/S boundary, and this inactivates the RB protein and its negative effect on cell division (80). Some studies suggest that the G1 cyclin–kinase complex phosphorylates the RB protein, thus releasing cells from G1 arrest (6).

RELAXED CONTROL IN TUMOR CELLS

The biochemistry of growth appears to be very similar qualitatively in tumor and normal cells (140). Despite numerous efforts, universal differences in biochemical machinery have not yet been discovered between normal and tumor cells (1). The fundamental difference probably lies in a relaxation of the regulation of cell growth (98). Whereas normal cells generally are quiescent at physiologic levels of growth factors, the related tumor cells are able to proliferate at these levels. In some experimental models, tumor cells proliferate in the absence of or at very low levels of growth factors. What biochemical reactions bring about this changed requirement (51)? Several general mechanisms have been proposed. One is that the limiting GFs are not needed, because the tumor cells produce their own, such as PDGF or TGF-α (Fig. 1.5) that activate their receptors (i.e., an autocrine mechanism). Alternatively, receptors may be produced in excess, as is the case for EGF receptors in numerous clinical tumors, leading to adequate stimulation at the low GF concentrations found in vivo. Moreover, mutations that alter intracellular signaling mechanisms may bypass GF dependence. Mutated forms of proto-oncogenes and inactivated tumor-suppressor genes can activate growth in these ways. Recent studies have focused on their possible role in the regulation of neoplastic cell proliferation or prognosis of epithelial or lymphoid malignancies (69). Growth inhibition of breast cancer cells in culture by antiestrogens correlates with an acute decrease

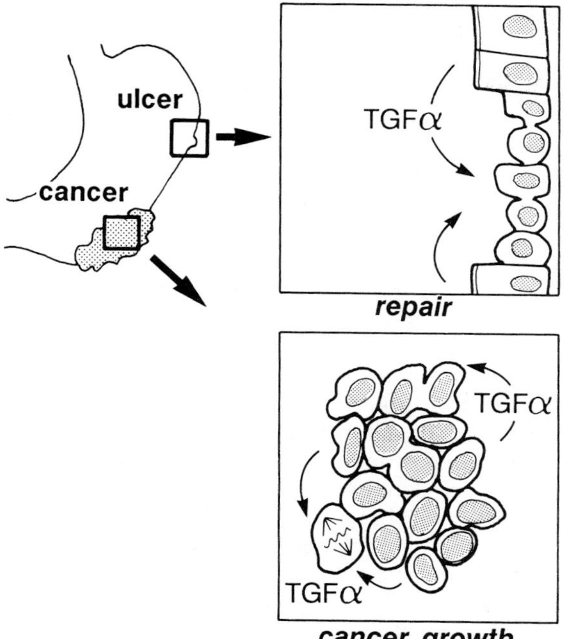

Figure 1.5. Altered regulation of growth factors. ***Top right:*** As stem cells of the normal gastric mucosa differentiate, they gain the capacity to produce TGF-α and its surface receptor (EGF receptor), both of which are presumed to help regulate normal cell growth and repair. This figure depicts a hypothetic model with release of TGF-α ***(arrows)*** in response to a gastric ulcer, thus stimulating new cell growth and repair. When the ulcer is healed, the stimulation ceases. ***Bottom right:*** In gastric neoplasms, abnormal regulation of TGF-α and/or its receptor is hypothesized to contribute to the continued growth of cancer cells (4).

in cyclin D1 expression, suggesting a possible intermediate role in response to some clinical therapies (65, 122).

Growth control can be lost as a result of transformation by a DNA virus, such as simian virus 47 (SV40) or papilloma viruses. These transformed cells are incapable of entering the G0 state. Rather, they proliferate very slowly and eventually die in vitro under conditions that cause normal cells to become quiescent, and they may bypass the normal G1 phase controls by inactivating the negative regulators p53 and pRB.

PROPERTIES OF TUMOR CELLS IN CULTURE

Cells obtained from a tumor can be distinguished from normal cells in culture by several tests. Fibroblast-derived tumor cells are less sensitive than normal cells to the presence of other cells in their immediate vicinity. Normal cells typically cease proliferation when the culture becomes confluent, but tumor cells can reach several-fold higher densities in culture. If tumor cells are plated on a dense layer of nonproliferating, homogeneous normal cells, they can continue to grow and form foci of clustered cell colonies. Such colonies show altered interactions between the tumor cells, which grow randomly, criss-crossing one another and forming clusters of viable and necrotic cells. When these cultures are fixed and stained, the number of tumor colonies is easily quantitated against the background population of normal cells. This is the basis of the commonly used "focus forming assay" for detecting transformation (e.g., the capacity of mutagens or oncogenes to produce neoplastic transformation within a population of nontumor cells).

Cells of normal solid tissue lie on a secreted extracellular matrix (ECM) that is composed of various proteins that stimulate cell growth (58). Tumor cells often are partly or completely independent of ECM for optimal growth, and they may secrete little matrix material (79). In addition, the cytoskeleton within tumor cells tends to be less well organized, and its actin filaments are less highly polymerized. Tumor cells often can be grown in the absence of a substratum, as within a semisolid medium containing agar. This formation of colonies in suspension also is used as a test of neoplastic transformation.

These properties of tumor versus normal cells are used to detect cells that have been transformed in culture. Each property provides the basis for an assay of neoplastic transformation; however, no one test is absolutely diagnostic for the ability of cells to form a tumor after implantation into a suitable animal, such as an athymic mouse. Conditions in vivo differ sufficiently from those in culture that a correlation between the two methods is essential before one can conclude that a given property of the cultured cell is typical of cancer (see Chapter 13).

GENETIC ASPECTS OF CELLS IN CULTURE

Nontumorigenic cells in culture can be transformed by a variety of agents so that they exhibit properties commonly seen in cells derived from in vivo tumors. These transformed cells can form foci on a normal cell monolayer or colonies in a semisolid medium. Often, but not always, they form tumors in experimental animals, whereas the original cells cannot.

The common thread in these modes of transformation is that they cause changes in the DNA of the cells, but the means by which this occurs differ widely. Transformation can occur spontaneously while cells continue to be cultured; this is more commonly seen in certain rodent cells and almost never in human cells. Thus, murine embryo fibroblasts spontaneously give rise to cells with altered growth control properties and changes in their karyotypes. A cause-effect relationship between chromosome rearrangements and the transformed properties is in accord with similar changes seen in cancer cells. Inheritance of constitutional chromosomal or genetic abnormalities has been linked closely to a familial susceptibility to certain cancers, including retinoblastoma, Wilms' tumor, and colon, renal, ovarian, and breast cancers. For example, familial breast cancer has been associated with the loss or mutation of a small portion of chromosome 17q21, a gene locus called "BRCA-1" (Breast Cancer-1) (88). A second breast cancer susceptibility locus, termed BRCA-2, has been reported on chromosome 13q (144), and a mutator gene, MSH2, has been associated with hereditary nonpolyposis colon cancer (40).

Radiation, which creates reactive radicals, and certain chemicals, including many of the drugs used in cancer chemotherapy, are well known to have carcinogenic activities. These agents cause defects in DNA structure through chemical reactions, creating strand breaks and producing cross-links (90). Transformation frequency has been correlated with degree of mutations, suggesting a mutational origin of carcinogenesis. However, the initiator–promoter, multistep model of carcinogenesis in vivo suggests that mutation alone is insufficient for tumorigenesis and that cell proliferation also is involved. A few compounds have been reported to be antitumorigenic, acting to alter DNA repair after cells have been damaged, probably by converting transforming reactions into lethal ones (9).

Many carcinogens induce chemical changes in DNA (43). For example, ultraviolet light creates thymine dimers, whereas x-rays produce chemical radicals within the cell that break DNA strands. Alkylating agents react with DNA bases at several sites, either on one strand or bifunctionally to cross-link DNA chains. In another mechanism, nonmethylated cytosine residues are produced by 5-azacytidine, and this change in DNA is commonly associated with transformation. Effects are sometimes more subtle, however, and some carcinogens are not reactive until they have been activated by metabolism. Oxidative enzymes of the P-450 system are found in the microsomal cell fraction of liver. They activate carcinogens such as benzo[*a*]pyrene and other aryl hydrocarbons. These changes are only the beginning of carcinogenesis. Most of the damage is eliminated by repair mechanisms that replace the damage with normal DNA components, so there is no permanent harm to the cell (57). When the chromosomes are altered by rearrangements or deletions, however, or a different base is substituted because of faulty repair, the resulting mutation can be lethal, mutagenic, or even transforming. The repair mechanisms are of several types (43); for example, in excision repair, an endonuclease cleaves the DNA strand near the site of damage, other enzymes next excise the damaged region, DNA polymerases then synthesize a replacement strand, and DNA ligase and topoisomerase(s) finally connect new and old segments. These enzymes have been identified as targets for cancer therapy (see Chapters 64 and 65) (34). Faulty DNA repair has been implicated in the pathogenesis of colon neoplasia in patients with hereditary nonpolyposis colorectal cancer (90).

Both RNA and DNA viruses can cause tumors by introducing new genetic information into cells. Retroviruses are small RNA viruses that form tumors in animals. They fall into two classes: (*a*) those that cause tumors with low efficiency, and (*b*) rare, highly oncogenic, and acutely transforming retroviruses. These latter viruses have acquired mutated sequences from mammalian cells. Such sequences have been designated as oncogenes, and when reintroduced into normal cells by the virus, they are responsible for transformation. Some of their functions have been mentioned earlier; an enormous amount of work has been performed on these oncogenes. Viral transformation appears to convert a normal cell into a tumor cell in a single step, as opposed to the multistep carcinogenesis observed with other agents. It is now evident, however, that more than one oncogene is required for transformation. The multistep progression of colonic polyps into noninvasive adenomas, and then into invasive and metastatic carcinomas, closely correlates with sequential changes in specific oncogenes (see Chapter 6) (135). Furthermore, retroviral oncogenes can destabilize other genes in the chromosomes, because of their flanking sequences, which are called long terminal repeats. These repeats can activate adjacent functional genes to cause further changes that eventually give rise to transformed phenotypes.

More recently tumor suppressor genes have been proposed and identified. Two main lines of evidence support the existence of genes that suppress tumorigenicity in normal cells. First, the loss of certain genes is seen in tumors, as in retinoblastoma and transfection of the normal RB gene has been reported to suppress the unregulated growth of these tumor cells (64). Another suppressing protein is p53, whose mutated form (or loss) can be transforming. Mutations of the p53 gene have been found in conjunction with chromosome 17p allelic deletions in tumors of the colon, brain, lung, breast, and bone (2, 123). Mutations in the p53 gene may represent the most common genetic change in human cancer (53). Similar to transfection experiments with the retinoblastoma gene, reintroduction of normal (not mutated) p53 genes into colon cancer cells inhibited tumor cell growth in vitro (2). These genes are deleted or have point mutations in their structures. Many new genes that produce their mRNAs in normal but not tumor cells also are being identified, and these are being investigated as putative tumor-suppressor genes. In normal cells, the RB protein is produced throughout the cell cycle, but its phosphorylation increases at the G1/S boundary, which inactivates the RB protein and its negative effect on cell division (80). The G1 cyclin–kinase complexes phosphorylate the RB protein, releasing cells from G1 arrest. Similarly, the p53 protein is phosphorylated by G1 cyclin–kinase enzymes, leading to release from G1 arrest in addition to phosphorylation of other substrates required for initiation of the S phase (7).

It has been reported that p53 is important in blocking entry into the S phase of cells whose DNA is damaged, thereby providing a "checkpoint" against mutations that would arise if this damaged DNA was faultily replicated (67). After normal cells are damaged, p53 increases, and its absence or mutation in many cancers could be important in permitting further genetic changes that are responsible for tumor progression.

Growth control can be lost because of transformation by a DNA virus such as SV40 or papilloma. These transformed cells are incapable of entering the G0 state; rather, they proliferate very slowly and eventually die in vitro under conditions that cause normal cells to become quiescent. They seem to bypass the normal G1 phase controls.

A widely studied DNA virus is SV40 (80). The SV40 gene coding the T antigen is responsible for the transformation of normal cells into tumor cells. Tumorigenic activity of the SV40 virus probably relates to inactivation of these tumor-suppressor genes. Both the RB and p53 proteins are bound by the T antigen and by the E6 and E7 papilloma virus gene products. Tumor cell growth is suppressed by fusion with a normal cell, suggesting that the normal cell contains tumor-suppressor genes (111). Attempts have been made to isolate such suppressor genes using the (negative) assay of inhibited tumor cell proliferation by transfected DNA, and a few have been obtained, including one that suppresses the growth of cells transformed by the *ras* oncogene (96). However, there is still much to be learned about these genes.

Differentiation

All tumor cells show abnormalities in the regulation of cell proliferation (i.e., neoplasia). In addition, most, if not all, tumor cells show abnormalities in differentiation (i.e., anaplasia). The anaplasia of tumors can provide insights into their etiology, degree of malignancy, prognosis, and sensitivity to therapeutic intervention by differentiation- or maturation-inducing agents.

WHAT IS DIFFERENTIATION?

Although somatic cells are genetically equal, it is obvious that they are not phenotypically equal. Thus, skin fibroblasts are different from T lymphocytes, muscle cells differ from gastric mucosal cells, and so on. Within an organism, however, all cells have an identical complement of DNA. Differences in phenotype arise from differences in gene expression, not in gene content.

DIFFERENTIATION AND GENE EXPRESSION

The genes expressed by a particular cell only comprise approximately 10 to 20% of the coding capacity of the genome. In humans, there are roughly 100,000 genes that code for proteins; however, an individual cell generally expresses only 10,000 to 20,000 genes. Genes expressed by a particular cell depend on its embryonic lineage, developmental stage of the organism, tissue and cellular environment, and functions that the cell must fulfill. Differential gene expression (i.e., differentiation) occurs extensively during embryogenesis, but some cell types differentiate throughout life. The mechanisms that regulate differential gene expression are incompletely understood; however, they most certainly entail the sequential action of cell-type-specific or cell-lineage-specific transcription factors that repress or activate the differentiation-specific genes. Programs of gene expression generally are instituted early in embryogenesis and sequentially altered as development proceeds (55, 65).

Some genes are expressed by many, if not all, cell types. These "housekeeping" genes generally encode proteins that participate in basic or universal cellular functions (i.e., respiration or protein synthesis). Other genes that are expressed only in specific cell types and/or stages of development, are said to be cell-type- or differentiation-specific genes. Lymphocytes, but not keratinocytes, express genes for immunoglobulins; however, keratinocytes, but not lymphocytes, express cytokeratins (i.e., intermediate filament proteins whose expression is confined to cells of epithelial origin) (91). In addition, keratinocytes express particular cytokeratin, depending on the stage of differentiation (i.e., position in the epidermis). Finally, genes that encode the cornified envelope proteins are expressed only by keratinocytes that have undergone extensive differentiation and inhabit the uppermost epidermal layers (106). Thus, the expression of specific gene products marks both the cell lineage and the stage of differentiation.

DIFFERENTIATION AND CELL PROLIFERATION

Differentiation begins shortly after the first few cell divisions that follow fertilization. Throughout development, and in adult organisms, a cell's ability to proliferate is intimately connected to its state of differentiation. Adult tissues generally express a variety of factors that act to maintain both the proliferation and the differentiation status of the cells. These include secreted molecules, transmembrane receptors, intracellular signaling molecules and transcription factors. For example, myoD (118) and c/EBP-α (132) are nuclear factors that activate the transcription of muscle- and adipocyte-specific genes, respectively; in addition, both proteins are potent inhibitors of cell proliferation.

In early embryos, cell proliferation is the primary means by which the cell mass increases. As the organism develops, however, proliferation becomes restricted. Some differentiated cells continue to proliferate, but others irreversibly lose this ability. Embryonic cells often display traits that confer on them a selective growth advantage over that of an adult cell. They proliferate vigorously, are capable of extensive migration, secrete factors that increase the local supply of blood (and, therefore, of nutrients), and produce enzymes capable of degrading basement membranes. These traits also are characteristic of tumor cells, and the malignancy of the tumor often depends on the degree to which the tumor cells express these traits. For example, the ability to increase the local blood supply (i.e., angiogenesis) is a very common feature of advanced tumors. Moreover, recent data suggest that tumor angiogenesis is an important, negative prognostic indicator for carcinomas of the prostate and breast (141, 142). Some of the machinery for angiogenesis may be similar to the processes used by tumor cells for invasion, and these are now being investigated as potential targets for cancer therapy (6). Thus, in adult organisms, mutations or conditions that activate portions of embryonic programs for gene expression or inactivate portions of the adult program can produce cells with many properties of malignant tumor cells (89).

STEM CELLS

Stem cells have the capacity for both self-renewal (i.e., proliferation without a change in phenotype) and differentiation (i.e., changing into a new phenotype). Some stem cells have already undergone considerable differentiation, so further differentiation is restricted to a single cell type or lineage (i.e., the basal keratinocytes of the epidermis or stem cells of the intestinal crypts). Other stem cells are multipotent and differentiate into a variety of cell types (i.e., hematopoietic stem cells). It has been difficult to demonstrate cells in adults that are totipotent (i.e., or capable of differentiating into most or all the cell types that comprise the organism).

In general, stem cell differentiation results in two types of changes: the expression of specialized, differentiation-specific gene products, and a partial or complete restriction of the cell's capacity for further proliferation. It then follows that another mechanism by which tumor cells might arise is through mutations that render a stem cell partly or wholly unable to differentiate.

TERMINAL DIFFERENTIATION

Some cells, particularly in adults, are terminally differentiated. These cells are irreversibly blocked in their ability to proliferate, although they may perform specialized functions for a long period of time. Some terminally differentiated cells (i.e., mature muscle and nerve cells) persist throughout much of the organism's life. Others (i.e., keratinocytes in the outer epidermal layer), die soon after terminal differentiation. Terminal differentiation is an end state, the result of a stem cell that has gone through several successive stages of differentiation.

Tumors of terminally differentiated cells are not found. Thus, tumors of mature muscle or nerve cells do not occur, although tumors of less differentiated myoblastic or neuronal stem cells do. Cell proliferation appears to be incompatible with the expression of a terminally differentiated program of gene expression. For example, cultured myoblasts or preadipocytes can be induced to differentiate terminally by modifying the culture conditions; when cells that are capable of terminal differentiation are forced to proliferate, such as by transfecting an oncogene into the cells or by providing a potent mitogen, terminal differentiation cannot be induced. In the case of adipocytes, the c-*myc* proto-oncogene appears to directly antagonize the activity of the growth-inhibitory and differentiation-specific transcription factor, c/EBP-α (42). Likewise, the protein-kinase activity stimulated by cyclin D (a G1 cyclin, discussed earlier) prevents myoblasts from arresting growth and terminally differentiating (116). When terminal differentiation is blocked, not only do cells continue to proliferate, they fail to express the characteristic gene products of the terminally differentiated state (i.e., muscle myosin or fat-metabolizing enzymes). Thus, irreversible arrest of cell division and expression of the terminally differentiated phenotype are interdependent.

In healthy tissue, whether embryonic or adult, there is always a balance between cell proliferation and cell loss through death or terminal differentiation. In many tissues, continuous proliferation is restricted to a subpopulation of cells, the stem cells, which undergo self-renewal as well as differentiation into cell types with a more restrictive proliferative potential. It then follows that mutations or conditions that interfere with the differentiation of stem cells will result in unbalanced proliferation and, thus, uncontrolled growth of the tissue. Mutations that drive proliferation are associated with an accumulation and overgrowth of less-differentiated cells in the tissue. A common feature of tumor cells is their failure to differentiate terminally under appropriate conditions either in vivo or in culture (105, 143, 148).

CELLULAR REPLICATIVE SENESCENCE

All normal, differentiated cells have a limited capacity for cell division both in vivo and in culture (82, 102). Under suitable culture conditions, cells that can proliferate in vivo will go through an initial proliferative phase, but this is invariably followed by a gradual decline in growth of the culture. This progressive decline in proliferation is termed the *finite replicative lifespan phenotype* or *cellular senescence*. For human embryonic cells, the replicative lifespan usually is approximately 50 population doublings; however, it can be much shorter for cells from older donors (13).

In cell cultures derived from several rodent species, immortal cells (i.e., cells having an infinite lifespan in culture) spontaneously arise at a low frequency. This frequency, as well as recent molecular data suggest that immortalization results from mutations that inactivate the p53 tumor-suppressor gene, and probably other genes as well. Immortal cells can be propagated indefinitely in culture and are called *cell lines*. Senescence is much more complete and irreversible with human cells cultured from normal tissues compared to rodent cells. Immortal human cell lines rarely, if ever, spontaneously occur, although radiation, carcinogenic chemicals and some viruses cause human cells to immortalize at a very low frequency (114). Whether derived from human or rodent tissues, immortal cells are much more susceptible to tumorigenic transformation than cells with a finite lifespan. Thus, escape from senescence (or immortality) permits cells to accumulate the multiple mutations that are required for tumorigenesis. Recent evidence suggests that a majority of primary human tumors contain cells that are immortal; thus, immortality may be an important step, although not necessarily an early one in tumor progression (70, 82, 111).

Once human cells senesce, it is virtually impossible to induce them to proliferate again using physiologic mitogens or normal cellular genes (13, 102). In addition, senescent cells often show an altered pattern of gene expression (13, 113). Thus, cellular senescence in some ways resembles terminal differentiation. One possibility is that the genes responsible for the loss of proliferation during terminal differentiation and those responsible for senescence are similar or have common structural or functional features.

The "finite lifespan" and the nontumorigenic phenotypes are genetically dominant. When immortal cells are fused to normal cells, the hybrid cells undergo senescence and are not immortal. Similarly, when normal and tumor cells are fused, the hybrids generally are not tumorigenic. These findings support the idea that normal cells express one or more genes that ordinarily act to restrain growth. In cell hybrids, the suppressor genes, which are expressed by the normal cell, repress the immortal and transformed phenotypes. An important step in tumorigenesis may be the loss (by mutational inactivation or deletion because of chromosomal instability) of both alleles of a tumor-suppressor gene (see Chapter 6) (147). There is evidence that some tumor-suppressor genes also function in pathways leading to cellular senescence and terminal differentiation; one example is Rb. A functional Rb protein is necessary for maintaining the senescent state (82, 114). It also is needed for the terminal differentiation of myoblasts and may interact directly with the transcription factors that regulate myogenic differentiation (54).

Studies of replicative senescence have led to a novel possibility for cancer therapy: the development of drugs or biologic molecules that inhibit the enzyme telomerase. In all cells, the DNA polymerase that replicates DNA during the S phase initiates template-dependent polymerization of nearly all of the DNA. But at each cell division, 500-200 base pairs at the 5' end of each chromosone are not replicated by this enzyme but rather, if at all, by a special enzyme named telomerase. Replicative senescence is thought to occur when the ends of the chromosomes, or telomeres, reach a critically short length. Telomeres shorten with cell division in most, if not all, somatic cells, but they do not shorten in the germ cells (and possibly in some stem cells). This is because germ cells express telomerase, which is a specialized DNA polymerase that adds telomeric sequences (which are highly repetitive) to the ends of chromosomes de novo. Recent data indicate that in most cases, the immortalization of somatic cells entails a reactivation of telomerase expression. Together with the finding that most primary tumors contain telomerase-positive immortal cells, this suggests that telomerase inhibitors may selectively target tumor cells and induce them to undergo senescence or apoptosis (70, 76, 114).

Several types of normal tissues undergo involution in response to environmental stimuli or as a terminal step in their natural lifespan. This property has been termed *programmed cell death* or *apoptosis*, and it has been studied in experimental models with cells or tissues from various mammalian species. One of these models is organ cultures of müllerian ducts from developing male embryos. These cultures undergo regression and cell death when exposed to the hormone called müllerian-inhibiting substance (MIS) (30, 136). This is similar to the growth and subsequent rapid degeneration of müllerian ducts within developing male embryos. MIS has structural similarity to TGF-β, and some studies suggest that it causes tissue regression by the inhibition of EGF-induced tyrosine phosphorylation (20, 25). Because embryonic cells that have not differentiated into müllerian ducts are not sensitive to MIS, programmed death is acquired as part of normal tissue differentiation.

Programmed cell death occurs in a variety of normal mammalian tissues in response to physiologic cues. For example, it occurs in the prostate after androgens decline, in the breast when lactation ceases, and in lymphoid cells in response to glucocorticoids. It also is involved in the pathogenesis of a variety of diseases, including autoimmunity, neurodegenerative disorders, and cancer (125, 127). Prolonged viability and growth of tumor cells may be related to inhibition of the usual apoptosis reactions. The protein coded by the *bcl*-2 oncogene is overexpressed in many human lymphoid neoplasms; *bcl*-2 is thought to prevent or interfere with apoptosis through interaction with mitochondrial and other intracellular membranes, where it appears to abrogate an oxygen-dependent apoptotic signal (59, 60). Overexpression of *bcl*-2 in transgenic mice leads to an excessive accumulation of cells in target tissues (83). *Bcl*-2 is abnormally expressed in some lung carcinomas, and its expression may have prognostic importance (101).

The molecular events leading to apoptosis are currently being defined. A large number of stimuli may induce apoptosis, including cell-type-specific ligands, ion fluxes, and DNA damage. Despite their diverse origins, however, apoptotic stimuli ultimately induce the expression of genes that actively promote cell death. Only a fraction of these genes so far have been identified in mammals (121, 146). Expression of the ICE gene of the nematode *C. elegans*, and of related genes of mammalian cells, can cause apoptosis. These genes code for proteases which that degrade proteins limiting the apoptotic process (121). Future studies may provide new approaches to cancer therapy by selective enhancement of apoptosis in neoplastic tissues (24). For example, MIS has been proposed as a potential therapeutic agent for gynecologic neoplasms, which have a müllerian duct origin and express appropriate receptors or depend on continued EGF-induced tyrosine phosphorylation (136). In experimental systems, many anticancer drugs activate the process of apoptosis, probably through an indirect mechanism after injury to DNA (17, 121, 127).

EXTRACELLULAR FACTORS THAT CONTROL DIFFERENTIATION

During embryogenesis and in a number of adult tissues, differentiation depends on external factors. These include insoluble factors such as ECM and both the proximity and type of neighboring cells as well as a growing list of soluble factors. In model systems, differentiation can be induced by a variety of biologic agents and drugs (Table 1.3). Both the ECM and differentiation-promoting soluble factors may be produced by the same cells that respond to these signals (i.e., autocrine regulation); they also may be produced by adjacent or distal cells (i.e., paracrine regulation).

Cell–cell and cell–ECM interactions are important for both the induction and maintenance of differentiation in several cell lineages. Although our understanding at a molecular level of insoluble factors is still incomplete, progress has been made in identifying key molecules and pathways through which these factors act. In the case of the ECM, specific cell surface receptors bind to particular components of the ECM (33). It now appears that the binding of an ECM component to its cellular receptor activates an intracellular signal transduction pathway that is analogous to the signalling pathways that have been identified for polypeptide GFs and growth inhibitors. Tumor cells often lose their ability to sense the ECM or neighboring cells; malignant human breast epithelial cells often can be identified by their ability to grow in an ECM gel that inhibits the growth of normal and premalignant human breast epithelial cells (100).

The soluble factors that regulate differentiation can be broadly classified into those that bind to cell surface receptors and those that freely cross the plasma membrane and bind to cytoplasmic or nuclear receptors. The first class includes molecules such as the fibroblast growth factors (FGFs)—(TGF-α and TGF-β), and hematopoietic factors such as colony-stimulating factor-1 (CSF-1), granulocyte colony-stimulating factor (G-CSF), granulocyte-macrophage colony-stimulating factor (GM-CSF), and the interleukins. These are all polypeptides and many were first identified as GFs or growth inhibitors. It now is clear, however, that these factors have a multitude of effects depending on the target cells and the cellular microenvironment. The action of these polypeptides depends on expression of cell surface receptors specific to certain cell types. For example, mononuclear

Table 1.3. Induction of Differentiation in Culture

Stem cell	Differentiation markers	Inducers
Preadipocyte	Adipocyte	Insulin, cort, cell density
Basal keratinocyte	Cornified envelope	RA deficiency, cell density
Myoblast	Myotube	GF deficiency, cell density
Squamous cell carcinoma	Cornified envelope	GF deficiency, cort
Embryonal carcinoma	Endoderm, mesoderm, ectoderm	RA, ara-C, mito, HMBA, co-culture with blastocysts
Neuroblastoma	Neuron, neurotransmitter, action potential	PI, 6TG, ara-C, MTX, dox, bleo, RA, GF deficiency
Melanoma	Dendrite, melanin, tyrosinase	PI, dox, DMSO, TPA, RA, MSH
Colon adenocarcinoma	Mucus, dome formation, CEA, columnar cell	NMF, DMSO, butyrate, low glucose, IFN, HMBA, cell density
Breast adenocarcinoma	Casein, dome formation	RA, PGE, DMSO
Bladder transitional cell carcinoma	Keratin filament, loss of surface antigen	HMBA
Erythroleukemia	Mature erythroid cell, hemoglobin	Dox, ara-C, 6TG, mito, dact, aza, hemin, DMSO, HMBA, CSF, RA, IFN
Promyelocytic	Granulocyte, macrophage	IFN, CSF, vitD, TPA, DMSO, NMF, dact, HMBA, aza, ara-C, RA
Myelocytic leukemia	Granulocyte, macrophage	CSF, RA, vitD, ara-C, dact, DMSO, TPA, cort, dox

ara-C—Cytarabine; aza—5-azacytidine; bleo—bleomycin; CEA—carcinoembryonic antigen; cort—glucocorticoids; CSF—colony stimulating factor; dact—dactinomycin; DMSO—dimethylsulfoxide; dox—doxorubicin; GF—growth factor; hemin; HMBA—hexamethylbisacetamide; IFN—alpha- or gamma-interferon; mito—mitomycin C; MSH—melanocyte-stimulating hormone; MTX—methotrexate; NMF—*N,N*-dimethylformamide; PGE—prostaglandin E; PI—phosphodiesterase inhibitor; RA—retinoic acid; TPA—12-0-tetradecanoylphorbol-13-acetate; vitD—1,25-dihydroxy vitamin D; 6TG—6-thioguanine.
Data from Cheson and colleagues (19), Reiss and colleagues (104), and Waxman and colleagues (139).

phagocytes and their precursors express high-affinity CSF-1 receptors, which are coded by the c-*fms* gene. This receptor belongs to a family of protein-tyrosine kinases. Structurally, the receptor for PDGF is similar to the CSF-1 receptor, but activation of these receptors induces different intracellular responses, such as activation of specific phosphatidylinositol kinases and changes in intracellular calcium levels (133).

Basic FGF was identified as a fibroblast mitogen in brain and pituitary extracts, but recent data suggest that FGF induces mesodermal differentiation in early embryos, is angiogenic, is a survival factor for endothelial cells (74, 107). FGF also inhibits the differentiation of some cells. Terminal differentiation into mature myotubes cannot occur unless it is withdrawn from proliferating myoblasts. Similarly, TGF-β was first identified as a stimulator of anchorage-independent growth in mesenchymal cells and later as an inhibitor of epithelial cell proliferation (109, 128). Like FGF, TGF-β stimulates the differentiation of some cells (i.e., keratinocytes or intestinal epithelial cells) but inhibits differentiation in others (i.e., myoblasts or preadipocytes). In some human tumor cells cultured in vitro or in athymic mice, TGF-β both inhibits tumor growth and promotes a more differentiated phenotype in the remaining cells. Other studies suggest that TGF-β and, probably, other growth inhibitors as well induce the expression of one or more inhibitors of cyclin-dependent protein kinases (e.g., p21, p27, p16); inhibition of these kinases in turn prevents the phosphorylation, and, thus, inactivation, of the RB protein, thereby inhibiting cell proliferation (92, 99, 115, 131).

The membrane-permeable regulators of differentiation include retinoic acid (i.e., vitamin A) and its derivatives (RA) (119). There is strong evidence that concentration gradients of RA are critical for the morphogenesis of some tissues in the early embryo (29). RA can stimulate or inhibit growth and differentiation depending on the cell type. In general, RA is required for the differentiation of many epithelial cells. It diffuses freely into cells, whereupon it binds to specific nuclear protein receptors (i.e., the retinoic acid receptors [RARs]). At least seven classes of RARs have been identified so far. Cell types vary in both the quality and quantity of RARs they express. In addition, other nuclear proteins, called RAR coregulators, have been found that interact with RARs and modulate their actions in various cell types (48). These differences may explain why specific cells and tissues differ in their responses to RA. Some differentiation-specific genes that are regulated by RA contain specific sequences to the initiation of transcription (5), to which RA–RAR complexes bind, thereby activating transcription (29, 134). The sex steroids estrogen and testosterone may regulate differentiation by similar mechanisms. Like RA, the sex steroids freely cross the plasma membrane and bind to specific nuclear receptors. The steroid receptor complexes then bind to specific sequences present in the regulatory regions of differentiation-specific genes. Whether a cell can respond to RA, or a particular steroid, depends on whether it expresses the gene for the appropriate nuclear receptor.

Tumor cells often produce factors that affect both growth and differentiation. These factors often change the growth and differentiated properties of the tumor cells themselves as well as the surrounding normal tissue. Basic FGF can confer neoplastic properties when expressed in an inappropriate cell type (e.g., a fibroblast). In addition, inappropriate expression of FGF by one cell may stimulate the growth and affect the differentiation of neighboring cell types (107).

INTRACELLULAR REGULATORS

Cellular differentiation is controlled by external factors and intrinsic programs of gene expression. In either case, the expression of differentiation-specific genes generally is under the control of a small number of master regulatory genes. Genes recently have been identified that are potential "master regulators" of developmental stages and differentiation-specific gene expression. The most globally acting master regulatory genes are known as homeotic genes, which were first identified as genetic loci that determined the developmental and spatial fates of cells in embryos of the fruit fly *Drosophila*. Similar genes have been identified in the genomes of higher organisms, including humans. Individual homeotic genes are expressed at different times during development and they also are expressed in different adult tissues. Some homeotic genes code for extracellular factors, while others code for nuclear proteins that are probably transcriptional regulatory factors. Homeotic genes regulate programs of differentiation as opposed to individual differentiation-specific genes. They appear to act by initiating cascades of gene expression that involve regulatory genes having a more restricted range of actions (46, 62). Some homeotic genes may function as tumor suppressors in normal tissues; others may promote tumorigenesis when mutated or deregulated. Mutations in homeotic genes may reactivate portions of an embryonic program of gene expression or suppress portions of an adult program of gene expression. In either case, the mutant cell may have a higher proliferative, invasive, or angiogenic potential—traits that are often shared by embryonic and tumor cells (16, 28, 82).

Some master regulatory genes appear to function only in cells of a restricted lineage and the best studied are those that regulate muscle differentiation (78). The *myoD* and *myd* genes control the differentiation of mesenchymal stem cells into myoblasts, and the myogenin gene controls the differentiation of myoblasts into mature skeletal muscle. These genes all code for transcription factors that regulate the expression of myoblast-specific or muscle-specific genes and, in the case of *myoD*, inhibit cell proliferation (118, 145). Mutations that interfere with the induction or function of *myoD, myd,* or myogenin select mesenchymal stem cells at various stages of commitment to muscle differentiation. Such cells cannot terminally differentiate and, therefore, have the potential to form a tumor.

DNA METHYLATION

In many cases, cells must go through one or more rounds of DNA replication before they can differentiate. This may be because there often is a need to modify the pattern of DNA methylation before differentiation begins. Changes in DNA methylation commonly are introduced during DNA replication. The methylation of DNA on specific cytosine residues is believed to contribute to the changes in gene expression that occur during development. Presumably, DNA methylation affects gene expression, because the transcriptional regulatory proteins that bind to methylated DNA differ from those that bind to unmethylated DNA. Many neoplastic tissues are hypomethylated relative to their normal counterparts (37, 49), and indeed, pharmacologic agents that alter the pattern of DNA methylation induce differentiation in a number of cultured cell lines. DNA methylation is probably not a universal mechanism for differentiation, however, and some cells can be induced to differentiate with either minimal or no change in the cell cycle progression (14).

DIFFERENTIATION AND CANCER THERAPY

Analysis of differentiation by tumor cells often provides valuable information for both the diagnosis and therapy of human cancers. As tumor cells grow and die, they can release glycoproteins and other products similar to those of fetal tissues, and these oncofetal products can be detected in serum or other body fluids to assist in diagnosis, follow-up, and selection of therapies. Because these markers are usually antigenic, they typically are quantified with sensitive immunologic assays. Diagnosis of male testicular carcinomas and female gestational neoplasms is greatly assisted by measuring serum levels of human chorionic gonadotropin or alpha-fetoprotein. Similarly, immunologic techniques can be used to assist the pathologist to identify the original source of tissue for metastatic neoplasms that have no obvious origin by routine studies (see Chapter 156). Examples include estrogen receptors and α-lactalbumin in breast cancer, prostate-specific antigen and prostate acid phosphatase in prostate cancers, and myoglobin and desmin in sarcomas (50).

Elevations of these markers in the serum often predict relapse of the neoplasm before any sign by routine examination or radiographic tests. In general, the specificity of such markers for a given neoplasm is poor, because minor elevations also occur with inflammatory and other benign conditions or with several types of neoplasms. Clinical studies are currently investigating serum or tissue markers of differentiation, aiming to "fine tune" the timing, type, or intensity of cancer therapy (93, 137). In carcinoma of unknown primary site, tissue markers for neuroendocrine differentiation select for a subgroup of patients with improved response to chemotherapy (56).

Some tumor cells can be induced to differentiate terminally. This has been shown most extensively in cultured cell lines (Table 1.3), but it also has been demonstrated in experimental animals (104, 131, 139). After tumor cells have been induced to undergo terminal differentiation, their ability to grow as a tumor often is stably suppressed. In contrast to most anticancer drugs, which have nonspecific toxicity to both normal and cancer cells, drug-induced differentiation can be demonstrated with agents (or drug levels) that exert minimal effects on normal cells (104). These observations have stimulated increased interest in clinical applications of differentiating agents to provide therapeutic gain with minimal toxicity (139).

A number of agents known to induce differentiation in various model systems have been used clinically (Table 1.3). Some are useful only in a particular type of tumor; for example, estrogens and androgens have been useful in treating some breast, prostate, and gynecologic tumors, providing that tumor cells express the appropriate nuclear receptor. Other differentiation-inducing drugs have been more widely studied. For example, high doses of retinoic acid, hexamethylene bisacetamide, or 5-azacytidine, which is an inhibitor of DNA methylation, can induce differentiation and inhibit the growth of several types of tumors in laboratory models (139). It also is active for myelodysprostic syndrome in humans, putatively by the same mechanism (see Chapter 141).

In fresh cultures of human promyelocytic leukemia, retinoid-induced differentiation, similar to the effects seen in passaged leukemia cell lines has been observed (11). All-*trans*-retinoic acid has been used in clinical therapy of promyelocytic leukemia with promising initial results (15, 138) and retinoids have been used in combination with interferon-α to produce responses in patients with squamous cell cancer of the skin or cervix (17). Differentiation has been observed in cultured leukemia cells exposed to mithramycin and hydroxyurea, and some investigators have proposed this mechanism to explain remissions induced in patients with the accelerated phase of chronic myelogenous leukemia (71). Because these and other proposed differentiating agents also may inhibit tumor cell growth by multiple mechanisms, it is difficult to prove specific differentiating actions of these agents when used in patients (19, 138).

Retinoids and other differentiating agents also are used in clinical trials to prevent cancer in patients with premalignant lesions or a high risk for developing cancer of the breast, cervix, colon, skin, lung, or oral cavity. Early results are encouraging, including the reversal of oral leukoplakia and prevention of second neoplasms in patients with treated squamous cell carcinoma of the head and neck (19, 63). At present, it is difficult to predict whether cells of a particular tumor (or precancerous lesion) can be induced to undergo terminal differentiation. In addition, retinoids can promote the effects of carcinogens to induce new tumors in some experimental models, although other investigators using similar models have found no such promoting effect (94). Thus, the ultimate action of these drugs may be related to the target tissue, environmental factors, experimental methods, or other unknown events. Greater knowledge about the molecular basis for the control of differentiation should lead to more accurate predictions, however, as well as a rational design of therapies for controlling tumor growth by manipulating the state of differentiation (87, 110, 139).

References

1. Ashmun RA, Look AT, Roberts WM, Roussel MF, Seremetis S, Ohtsuka M, Sherr CJ. Monoclonal antibodies to the human CSF-1 receptor detect epitopes on normal mononuclear phagocytes and on human myeloid leukemia blast cells. Blood 1989;73:827.
2. Baker SJ, Markowitz S, Fearon ER, Willson JKV, Vogelstein B. Suppression of human colorectal carcinoma cell growth by wild-type p53. Science 1990;249:912.
3. Baserga R. The Biology of Cell Reproduction. Cambridge, MA: Harvard University Press, 1985.
4. Beauchamp RD, Barnard JD, McCutchen CM, Cherner JA, Coffey RJ, Jr. Localization of transforming growth factor alpha and its receptor in gastric mucosal cells. J Clin Invest 1989;84:1017.
5. Bennington JL. Cellular kinetics of invasive squamous carcinoma of the human cervix. Cancer Res 1969;29:1082.
6. Bernstein LR, Liotta LA. Molecular mediators of interactions with extracellular matrix components in metastases and angiogenesis. Curr Opin Oncol 1994;6:106.
7. Bischoff JR, Friedman PN, Marshak DR, Prives C, Beach D. Human p53 is phosphorylated by p60-cdc2 and cyclin B-cdc2. Proc Natl Acad Sci USA 1990;87:4766.
8. Bishop JM. The molecular genetics of cancer. Science 1987;235:305.
9. Boothman DA, Schlegel R, Pardee AB. Anticarcinogenic potential of DNA-repair modulators. Mutat Res 1988;232:393.
10. Bourne HR. Signals past, present, and future. Cold Spring Harbor Symp Quant Biol 1988;LIII:1019.
11. Breitman TR, Collins SJ, Keene BR. Terminal differentiation of human promyelocytic leukemic cells in primary culture in response to retinoic acid. Blood 1981;57:1000.
12. Bresciani F, Pauluzi R, Benassi M, Nervi C, Casale C, Ziparo E. Cell kinetics and growth of squamous cell carcinomas in man. Cancer Res 1974;34:2405.
13. Campisi J, Dimri GP, Hara E. Control of replicative senescence. In Handbook of the Biology of Aging, 4th ed. Edited by E Schneider, J Rowe. New York: Academic, 1996 (in press).
14. Carlsson M, Totterman TH, Matsson P, Nilsson K. Cell cycle progression of B-chronic lymphocytic leukemia cells induced to differentiate by TPA. Blood 1988;71:415.
15. Castaigne S, Chomienne C, Daniel MT, Ballerini P, Berger R, Fenaux P, Degos L. All-*trans* retinoic acid as a differentiation therapy for acute promyelocytic leukemia. I. Clinical Results. Blood 1990;76:1704.
16. Castronovo, V, Kusaka, M, Chariot, A, Gielen, J, Sobel, M. Homeobox genes. Potential candidates for transcriptional control of the transformed and invasive phenotype. Biochem Pharmac 1994;47:137–143.
17. Chabner BA. Biologic basis for cancer treatment. Ann Intern Med 1993;118:633.
18. Challberg MD, Kelly TJ. Animal virus DNA replication. Annu Rev Biochem 1989;58: 671.
19. Cheson BD, Jasperse DM, Chun HG, Friedman MA. Differentiating agents in the treatment of human malignancies. Cancer Treat Rev 1986;13:129.
20. Cigarroa FG, Coughlin JP, Donahoe PK, White MF, Uitvlugt N, MacLaughlin DT. Recombinant human müllerian inhibiting substance inhibits epidermal growth factor receptor tyrosine kinase. Growth Factors 1989;1:179.
21. Clark GM, Dressler LG, Owens MA, Pounds G, Oldaker T, McGuire WL. Prediction of relapse or survival in patients with node-negative breast cancer by DNA flow cytometry. N Engl J Med 1989;320:627.
22. Clarkson B, Ota K, Ohkita T, O'Connor A. Kinetics of proliferation of cancer cells in neoplastic effusions in man. Cancer 1965;18:1189.
23. Coffey DS, Isaacs JT. Prostate tumor biology and cell kinetics—theory. Urology 1981;17(suppl 3):40.
24. Coffey DS, Pienta KJ. New concepts in studying the control of normal and cancer growth of the prostate. Prog Clin Biol Res 1987;239:1.
25. Coughlin JP, Donahoe PK, Budzik GP, MacLaughlin DT. Müllerian- inhibiting substance blocks autophosphorylation of the EGF receptor by inhibiting tyrosine kinase. Mol Cell Endocrinol 1987;49:75.
26. Crabtree GR. Contingent genetic regulatory events in T lymphocyte activation. Science 1989;243:355.
27. Cross F, Weintraub H, Roberts J. Simple and complex cell cycle. Annu Rev Cell Biol 1989;5:341.
28. Deschamps J, Meijlink F. Mammalian homeobox genes in normal development and neoplasia. Crit Rev Oncogenesis 1992;3:117.
29. Dolle P, Ruberte E, Kastner P, Petkovich M, Stoner CM, Gudas LJ, Chambon P. Differential expression of genes encoding alpha, beta and gamma retinoic acid receptors and CRABP in the developing limbs of the mouse. Nature 1989;342:702.
30. Donahoe PK, Cate R, MacLaughlin DT, Epstein J, Fuller AF, Takahashi M, Coughlin JP, Ninfa EG, Taylor LA. Müllerian inhibiting substance: gene structure and mechanism of action of a fetal regressor. In Recent Progress in Hormone Research, vol. 43. Edited by J.H. Clark. New York: Academic, 1987, pp 431–467.
31. Druker BJ, Mamon HJ, Roberts TM. Oncogenes, growth factors, and signal transduction. N Engl J Med 1989;321:1383.
32. Dunphy WG, Newport JW. Unraveling of mitotic control mechanisms. Cell 1988;55: 925.
33. Ekblom P, Vestweber D, Kemler R. Cell and extracellular matrix: their organization and mutual dependence. Annu Rev Cell Biol 1986;2:27.
34. Epstein RJ. Drug-induced DNA damage and tumor chemosensitivity. J Clin Oncol 1990;8:2062.
35. Fabrikant JI, Cherry J. The kinetics of cellular proliferation in normal and malignant tissues. J Surg Oncol 1969;1:23.
36. Fakuda K, Iwasaka T, Hachisuga TD, Sugimori HK, Tsugitomi H, Mutoh F. Immunocytochemical detection of S-phase cells in normal and neoplastic cervical epithelium by anti-BrdU monoclonal antibody. Anal Quant Cytol Histol 1990;12:135.
37. Feinberg AP, Vogelstein B. Hypomethylation distinguishes genes of some human cancers from their normal counterparts. Nature 1983;301:89.
38. Fettig O, Sievers R. 3H-index und mittlere Generationszeit des menschlichen Portiokarzinoms und seiner Vorstufen. Beitr Pathol 1966;133:83.
39. Fingert HJ, Campisi J, Pardee AB. Molecular Biology and Biochemistry of Cancer In Gynecologic Oncology, 2nd ed. Edited by R Knapp, R Berkowitz. New York: Macmillan, 1991, p 30.
40. Fishel R, Lescoe MK, Rao MRS, Copeland NG, Jenkins NA, Garber J, Kane M, Kolodner R. The human mutator gene homolog MSH2 and its association with hereditary nonpolyposis colon cancer. Cell 1993;75:1027.
41. Frankel SR, Eardley A, Heller G, Berman E, Miller WH, Dmitrovsky E, Warrell RP Jr. All-*trans*-retinoic acid for acute promyelocytic leukemia. Results of the New York Study. Ann Intern Med 1994;120:278.
42. Freytag SO, Geddes TJ. Reciprocal regulation of lipogenesis by *myc* and c/EBP-α. Science 1992;256:379.
43. Friedberg EC. DNA repair. New York: Freeman, 1987.
44. Fruehauf JP, Bosanquet AG. In vitro determination of drug response: a discussion of clinical applications. Princip Pract Oncol 1993;7:1.
45. Garcia RL, Coltrera MD, Gown AM. Analysis of proliferative grade using anti-PCNA/cyclin monoclonal antibodies in fixed, embedded tissues. Am J Pathol 1989;134:733.
46. Gehring WJ. Homeoboxes in the study of development. Science 1987;236:1245.
47. Gibbs JB, Oliff A, Kohl NE. Farnesyltransferase inhibitors *ras* research yields a potential cancer therapeutic. Cell 1994;77:175.
48. Glass CK, Devary OV, Rosenfeld MG. Multiple cell type-specific proteins differentially regulate target sequence recognition by the alpha retinoic acid receptor. Cell 1990;63:729.
49. Goelz SE, Vogelstein B, Hamilton SR, Feinberg AP. Hypomethylation of DNA from benign and malignant human colon neoplasms. Science 1985;228:187.
50. Gorstein F, Thor A. Tumor Markers in Diagnostic Pathology. Clinics in Laboratory Medicine, vol 10. Philadelphia: Saunders, 1990.
51. Goustin AS, Leof EB, Shipley GD, Moses HL. Growth factors and cancer. Cancer Res 1986;46:1015.
52. Graziano SL, Mazid R, Newman N, Tatum A, Oler A, Mortimer JA, Gullo JJ, DiFino SM, Scalzo AJ. The use of neuroendocrine immunoperoxidase markers to predict chemotherapy response in patients with non-small-cell lung cancer. J Clin Oncol 1989;7:1398.
53. Greenblatt MS, Bennett WP, Hollstein M, Harris CC. Mutations in the p53 tumor suppressor gene: clues to cancer etiology and molecular pathogenesis. Cancer Res 1994;54:4885.
54. Gu W, Schneider JW, Condorelli G, Kaushal S, Mahdavi V, Nadal-Ginard B. Interaction of myogenic factors and the retinoblastoma protein mediates muscle cell commitment and differentiation. Cell 1993;72:309–324.
55. Gurdon JB. Embryonic induction—molecular prospects. Development 1987;99:285.
56. Hainsworth JD, Johnson DH, Greco FA. Poorly differentiated neuroendocrine carcinoma of unknown primary site. Ann Intern Med 1988;109:364.
57. Hanawalt PC, Cooper PK, Ganesan AK, Smith CA. DNA repair in bacteria and mammalian cells. Annu Rev Biochem 1979;48:783.
58. Hawkes S, Wang JL. Extracellular Matrix. New York: Academic, 1982.
59. Hockenbery D, Nunez G, Milliman C, Schreiber RD, Korsmeyer SJ. *Bcl-2* is an inner mitochondrial membrane protein that blocks programmed cell death. Nature 1990;348:334.

60. Hockenbery D, Oltvai ZN, Yin XM, Milliman CL, Korsmeycr SJ. *Bcl-2* functions in an antioxidant pathway to prevent apoptosis. Cell 1993;75:241.
61. Hoffman RM, Connors KM, Meerson-Monosov AZ, Herrera H, Price JH. A general native-state method for determination of proliferation capacity of human normal and tumor tissues in vitro. Proc Natl Acad Sci USA 1989;86:2013.
62. Holland PWH, Hogan BLM. Expression of homeobox genes during mouse development: a review. Genes Devel 1988;2:773.
63. Hong WK, Lippman SM, Itri LM, Karp DD, Lee JS, Byers RM, Schantz SP, Kramer AM, Lotan R, Peters LJ, Dimery IW, Brown BW, Goepfert H. Prevention of second primary tumors with isotretinoin in squamous-cell carcinoma of the head and neck. N Engl J Med 1990;323:795.
64. Huang HJS, Yee JK, Shew JY, Chen PL, Bookstein R, Friedmann T, Lee EY, Lee WH. Suppression of the neoplastic phenotype by replacement of the RB gene in human cancer cells. Science 1989;242:1563.
65. Jan YN, Jan LY. HLH proteins, neurogenesis and vertebrate myogenesis. Cell 1993;75:827.
66. Kallioniemi O, Punnonen R, Mattila J, Lehtinen M, Koivula T. Prognostic significance of DNA index, multiploidy, and S-phase fraction in ovarian cancer. Cancer 1988;61:334.
67. Kastan MB, Onyekwere O, Sidransky D, Vogelstein B, Craig RW. Participation of p53 protein in the cellular response to DNA damage. Cancer Res 1991;51:6304.
68. Keyomarsi K, Pardee AB. Redundant cyclin overexpression and gene amplification in breast cancer cells. Proc Natl Acad Sci USA 1993;90:1112.
69. Keyomarsi K, O'Leary N, Molnar G, Lees E, Fingert HJ, Pardee AB. Cyclin E, a potential prognostic marker for breast cancer. Cancer Res 1994;54:380.
70. Kim NW, Platyszek M, Prowse KR, Harley CB, West MD, Ho PLC, Coviello GM, Wright WE, Weinrich SL, Shay JW. Specific association of human telomerase activity with immortal cells and cancer. Science 1994;266:2011–2015.
71. Koller CA, Miller DM. Preliminary observations on the therapy of the myeloid blast phase of chronic granulocytic leukemia with plicamycin and hydroxyurea. N Engl J Med 1986;315:1433.
72. Kroese MC, Rutgers DH, Wils IS, Van Unnik JA, Roholl PJ. The relevance of the DNA index and proliferation rate in the grading of benign and malignant soft tissue tumors. Cancer 1990;65:1782.
73. Lampkin BC. Cell kinetics as related to treatment of patients with acute nonlymphoid leukemia. Am J Pediatr Hematol Oncol 1985;7:358.
74. Lemmon SK, Riley MC, Thomas KA, Hoover GA, Maciag T, Bradshaw R. A Bovine fibroblast growth factor: comparison of brain and pituitary preparations. J Cell Biol 1982;95:162.
75. Leone LA, Meitner PA, Myers TJ, Grace WR, Gajewski WH, Fingert HJ, Rotman B. Prospective value of the fluorescent cytoprint assay (FCA): a retrospective correlation study of in vitro chemosensitivity and individual responses to chemotherapy. Cancer Invest 1991;9:491.
76. Levy MZ, Allsop RC, Futcher AB, Greider CW, Harley CB. Telomere end-replication problem and cell aging. J Molec Bio 1992;225:951–960.
77. Lewin B. Driving the cell cycle: m phase kinase, its partners, and substrates. Cell 1990;61:743.
78. Linkhart TA, Clegg CH, Hauschka SD. Control of mouse myoblast commitment to terminal differentiation by mitogens. J Supramol Struct 1980;14:483.
79. Liotta LA. Tumor invasion and metastases—role of the extracellular matrix. Cancer Res 1986;46:1.
80. Ludlow JW, De Caprio JA, Huang CM, Lee WH, Paucha E, Livingston DM. SV40 large T antigen binds preferentially to an underphosphorylated member of the retinoblastoma susceptibility gene product family. Cell 1989;56:57.
81. Maulbecker CC, Gruss P. The oncogenic potential of Pax genes. EMBO J 1993;12:2361–2367.
82. McCormick A, Campisi J. Cellular aging and senescence. Curr Opinions in Cell Bio 1991;3:230.
83. McDonnell TJ, Deane N, Platt FM, Nunez G, Jaeger U, McKearn JP, Korsmeyer SJ. *Bcl-2*-immunoglobulin transgenic mice demonstrate extended B cell survival and follicular lymphoproliferation. Cell 1989;57:79.
84. McKeever PE, Feldenzer JA, McCoy JP, Laug M, Gebarski S, Chandler WF, Greenberg HS, Junck L, D'Amato CJ, Varani J. Nuclear parameters as prognostic indicators in glioblastoma patients. J Neuropathol Exp Neurol 1990;49:71.
85. Merkel DE, McGuire WL. Ploidy, proliferative activity and prognosis. Cancer 1990;86:1194.
86. Meyer JS. Growth and cell kinetic measurements in human tumors. Pathol Ann 1981;16:53.
87. Meyskens FL Jr. Coming of age—the chemoprevention of cancer. N Engl J Med 1990;323:825.
88. Miki Y, Swenson J, Shattuck-Eidens P et al. A strong candidate for the breast and ovarian cancer susceptibility gene BRCA1. Science 1994;266:66.
89. Mintz B, Fleischman R. A Teratocarcinomas and other neoplasms as developmental defects in gene expression. Adv Cancer Res 1981;34:211.
90. Modrich P. Mismatch repair, genetic stability and cancer. Science 1994;266:1959.
91. Moll R, Francke WW, Schiller DL, Geiger B, Krepler R. The catalogue of human cytokeratins: patterns of expression in normal epithelia, tumors and cultured cells. Cell 1982;31:11.
92. Moses HL, Yang EY, Pientenpol J. A TGF-beta stimulation and inhibition of cell proliferation: new mechanistic insights. Cell 1990;63:245.
93. Murray A, Hunt T. The cell cycle; an introduction. New York: Freeman, 1993.
94. Muss HB, Thor AD, Berry DA, Kute T, Liu ET, Koemer F, Cirrincione CT, Budman DR, Wood, WC, Barcos M. C-erbB-2 expression and response to adjuvant therapy in women with node-positive early breast cancer. N Engl J Med 1994;330:1260.
95. Nauss KM, Bueche D, Newberne PM. Effect of vitamin A nutriture on experimental esophageal carcinogenesis. JNCI 1987;79:145.
96. Noda M, Kitayama H, Matsuzaki T, Sugimoto Y, Okayama H, Bassin RH, Ikawa Y. Detection of genes with a potential for suppressing the transformed phenotype associated with activated ras genes. Proc Natl Acad Sci USA 1989;86:162.
97. Pardee AB. Molecules involved in proliferation of normal and cancer cells. Cancer Res 1987;47:1488.
98. Pardee AB. G1 events and regulation of cell proliferation. Science 1989;246:603.
99. Peter M, Herskowitz I. Joining the complex: cyclin-dependent kinase inhibitory proteins and the cell cycle. Cell 79:181–184.
100. Peterson OW, Ronnov-Jessen L, Howlett AR, Bissell MJ. Interaction with basement membrane serves to rapidly distinguish growth and differentiation pattern of normal and malignant human breast epithelial cells. Proc Natl Acad Sci USA 1992;89:9064–9068.
101. Pezzella F, Turley H, Kuzu I, Tungekar MF, Dunnill MS, Pierce CB, Gatter KC, Mason DY. *Bcl-2* protein in non-small cell lung carcinoma. N Engl J Med 1993;329:690.
102. Phillips PD, Cristofalo VJ. A review of cellular aging research: regulation of cell proliferation. Rev Biol Aging Res 1985;2:339.
103. Quinn CM, Wright NA. The clinical assessment of proliferation and growth in human tumours: evaluation of methods and applications as prognostic variables. J Pathol 1990;160:93.
104. Reiss M, Gamba-Vitalo C, Sartorelli AC. Induction of tumor cell differentiation as a therapeutic approach: preclinical models for hematopoietic and solid neoplasms. Cancer Treat Rep 1986;70:201.
105. Rheinwald JG, Beckett MA. Defective terminal differentiation in culture as a consistent and selectable character of malignant human keratinocytes. Cell 1980;22:629.
106. Rice RH, Thacher SM. Involucrin. A constituent of cross-linked envelopes and marker of squamous maturation. In Biology of the Integument 2. Edited by J Bereiter-Hahn, AG Motolsky, KS Richard. New York: Springer Verlag, 1986, pp 752–761.
107. Rifkin DB, Moscatelli D. Recent developments in the cell biology of basic fibroblast growth factor. J Cell Biol 1989;109:1.
108. Rizzino A. Transforming growth factor-beta: multiple effects on cell differentiation and extracellular matrices. Dev Biol 1988;130:411.
109. Rozengurt E. Early signals in the mitogenic response. Science 1986;234:161.
110. Rowley JD, Aster JC, Sklar J. The clinical applications of new DNA diagnostic technology for the management of cancer patients. JAMA 1993;270:2331.
111. Sager R. Tumor suppressor genes: the puzzle and the promise. Science 1989;246:1406.
112. Schneider C, King RM, Phillipson L. Genes specifically expressed at growth arrest of mammalian cells. Cell 1988;54:787.
113. Seshadri T, Campisi J. Repression of c-*fos* transcription and an altered genetic program in senescent human fibroblasts. Science 1990;247:205.
114. Shay J, Wright WE. Defining the molecular mechanisms of human cell immortalization. Biochim Biophys Acta 1991;1071:1.
115. Sherr CJ. G1 phase progression: cycling on cue. Cell 1994;79:551–555.
116. Skapek SX, Rhee J, Spicer DB, Lassar AB. Inhibition of myogenic differentiation in proliferating myoblasts by cyclin D1-dependent kinase. Science 1995;267:1022–1024.
117. Skipper HE, Schabel FM Jr. Quantitative and cytokinetic studies in experimental tumor systems. In Cancer Medicine, 2nd ed. Edited by JF Holland, E Frei, III. Philadelphia: Lea & Febiger 1982, pp 663–684.
118. Sorrentino V, Pepperkok R, Davis RL, Ansorge W, Philipson L. Cell proliferation inhibited by MyoD1 independently of myogenic differentiation. Nature 1990;345:813–816.
119. Sporn MB, Roberts AB, Goodman DS. The Retinoids, vol 2. New York: Academic, 1984, p 56.
120. Steel GG. Cytokinetics of Neoplasia. In Cancer Medicine, 2nd ed. Edited by JF Holland, E Frei, III. Philadelphia: Lea & Febiger, 1982, pp 177–189.
121. Stellar H. Mechanisms and genes of cellular suicide. Science 1995;267:1445–1449.
122. Sutherland RL, Watts CK, Musgrove EA. Cyclin gene expression and growth control in normal and neoplastic human breast epithelium. J Steroid Biochem Mol 1993;47:99.
123. Takahashi T, Nau MM, Chiba I, Birrer MJ, Rosenberg RK, Vinocour M, Levitt M, Pass H, Gazdar AF, Minna JD. p53: a frequent target for genetic abnormalities in lung cancer. Science 1989;246:491.
124. Tannock I. Cell kinetics and chemotherapy: a critical review. Cancer Treat Rep 1978;62:1117.
125. Tenniswood MP, Guenette RS, Lakins J, Mooibroek M. Active cell death in hormone-dependent tissues. Cancer Metastasis Rev 1992;11:197.
126. Teodori L, Trinca ML, Goehdek W, Hemmer J, Salvatt F, Storniello G, Mauro F. Cytokinetic investigation of lung tumors using the anti-bromodeoxyuridine (BUdR) monoclonal antibody method: comparison with DNA flow cytometric data. Int J Cancer 1990;45:995.
127. Thompson C. Apoptosis in the pathogenesis and treatment of disease. Science 1995;267:1456–1462.
128. Todaro GJ, DeLarco JE, Fryling C, Johnson PA, Sporn MB. Tranforming growth factors: properties and possible mechanisms of action. J Supramol Struct Cell Biochem 1981;15:287.
129. Todaro GJ, Green H. Quantitative studies of the growth of mouse embryo cells in culture and their development into established lines. J Cell Biol 1963;17:299.
130. Tubo RA, Berezney R. Pre-replicative association of multiple replicative enzyme activities with the nuclear matrix during rat liver regeneration. J Biol Chem 1987;262:1148.
131. Twardzik DR, Ranchalis JE, McPherson JM, Ogawa Y, Gentry L, Purchio A, Plata E, Todaro GJ. Inhibition and promotion of differentiation-like phenotype of a human lung carcinoma in athymic nude mice by natural and recombinant forms of transforming growth factor-beta. JNCI 1989;81:1182.
132. Umek RM, Friedman AD, McKnight SL. CCAAT-enhancer binding protein: a component of a differentiation switch. Science 1991;251:288.
133. Varticovski L, Druker B, Morrison D, Cantley L, Roberts T. The colony stimulating factor-1 receptor associates with and activates phosphatidylinositol-3 kinase. Nature 1989;342:699.
134. Vasios GW, Gold JD, Petkovich M, Chambon P, Gudas LJ. A retinoic acid-responsive element is present in the 5″ flanking region of the laminin B1 gene. Proc Natl Acad Sci USA 1989;86:9099.
135. Vogelstein B, Kinzler KW. The multistep nature of cancer. Trends Genet 1993;9:138.
136. Wallen JW, Cate RL, Kiefer DM, Rieman MW, Martinez D, Hoffman RM, Donohoe PK, Von Hoff DD, Pepinsky B, Oliff A. Minimal antiproliferative effect of recombinant mullerian inhibiting substance on gynecological tumor cell lines and tumor explants. Cancer Res 1989;49:2005.
137. Ward AM. The value of markers in fine tuning of chemotherapy. Cancer Treat Rev 1987;14:401.
138. Warrell RP, Frankel SR, Miller WH, Scheinberg DA, Itri LM, Hittleman WN, Vyas R, Andreef M, Tafuri A, Jakubowski A, Gabrilove J, Gordon MS, Dmitrovsky E. Differentia-

tion therapy of acute promyelocytic leukemia with tretinoin (all-*trans*-retinoic acid). N Engl J Med 1991;324:1385.
139. Waxman S, Rossi GB, Takaku F. The Status of Differentiation Therapy of Cancer. New York: Raven, 1988.
140. Weber G. Biochemical strategy of cancer cells and the design of chemotherapy: G.H.A. Clowes Memorial Lecture. Cancer Res 1983;43:3466.
141. Weidner N, Carroll PR, Flax J, Blumenfeld W, Folkman J. Tumor angiogenesis correlates with metastases in invasive prostate carcinoma. Am J Pathol 1993;143:401.
142. Weidner N, Semple JP, Welch WR, Folkman J. Tumor angiogenesis and metastasis-correlation in invasive breast carcinoma. N Engl J Med. 1991;324:1.
143. Wille JJ, Maercklein PB, Scott RE. Neoplastic tranformation and defective control of cell proliferation and differentiation. Cancer Res 1982;42:5139.
144. Wooster R, Neuhausen SL, Mangion J, Quirk Y, Ford D, Collins N, Nguyen K, Seal S, Tran T, Averill D. Localization of a breast cancer susceptibility gene, BRCA2, to chromosome 13q12-13. Science 1994;265:2008.
145. Wright WE, Sasoon D, Lin VK. Myogenin, a factor regulating myogenesis, has a homologous domain to myoD. Cell 1989;56:607.
146. Wyllie AH. Apoptosis Cell death in tissue regulation. J Pathol 1987;153:313.
147. Yanishevsky RM, Stein GH. Regulation of the cell cycle in eucaryotic cells. Int Rev Cytol 1981;69:223.
148. Yuspa SH, Lichti U, Strickland J, Jaken S, Lowy D, Harper J, Roop D, Hennings H. Aberrant regulation of differentiation in epidermal carcinogenesis. In Growth Factors, Tumor Promoters and Cancer Genes. Edited by NH Colburn, HL Moses, EJ Stanbridge. New York: Liss, 1988, pp 183–189.
149. Zugmaier G, Lippman ME. Effects of TGF beta on normal and malignant mammary epithelium. Ann NY Acad Sci 1990;593:272.

CHAPTER 2

Molecular Biology

BARRETT J. ROLLINS AND CHARLES D. STILES

Cancer is a genetic disease. Abnormalities in genes that control cellular proliferation lead to the unrestrained growth that characterizes the malignant cell. Thus, to gain the initiative in cancer detection and treatment, oncologists must begin to understand the molecular roots of the disease: genes, their messenger RNAs, and the proteins they produce. In short, oncologists should be conversant with the tools of molecular biology.

This chapter is a basic survey of molecular biology and is directed toward the clinician or trainee who wants to acquire a fundamental understanding of this discipline. It is methods oriented and will serve as a frame of reference for other chapters in this section. It describes the principles that underlie procedures used most commonly by molecular biologists and provides examples of clinically relevant situations that draw on particular techniques. It will become apparent that molecular biology already plays an important role in clinical cancer medicine, from the analysis of tumors for prognostic or pathogenetic information to the production of pharmacologic agents such as the colony stimulating factors and interleukins.

We begin with an overview of genes, gene expression, and gene cloning. Our discussion of techniques will follow the flow of genetic information as we explain procedures used to analyze gene expression at the levels of DNA, RNA, and protein.

Overview—Gene Structure

GENES AND GENE EXPRESSION

The gene is the fundamental unit of inheritance and the ultimate determinant of all phenotypes. The DNA of a normal human cell contains an estimated 30,000 to 40,000 genes, but only a fraction of these are used (or expressed) in any particular cell at any given time (44, 45). For example, genes specific for erythroid cells, such as the hemoglobin genes, are not expressed in brain cells.

According to the central dogma of molecular biology, a gene exerts its effects by having its DNA transcribed into a messenger RNA (mRNA), which is in turn translated into a protein, the final effector of the gene's action. Thus molecular biologists often investigate gene expression or activation, by which is meant the process of transcribing DNA into RNA, or translating RNA into protein. The process of transcription involves creating a perfect RNA copy of the gene using the DNA of the gene as a template. Translation of mRNA into protein is a somewhat more complex process, since the structure of the gene's protein is encoded in the mRNA, and that structural message must be decoded during translation.

FUNCTIONAL COMPONENTS OF THE GENE

Every gene consists of several functional components, each involved in a different facet of the process of gene expression (Fig. 2.1). Broadly speaking, however, there are two main functional units: the promoter region and the coding region.

The promoter region controls when and in what tissue a gene is expressed. For example, the promoter of the hemoglobin gene is responsible for its expression in erythroid cells and not in brain cells. How is this tissue-specific expression achieved? In the DNA of the gene's promoter region, there are specific structural elements or nucleotide sequences (see "Structural Considerations," below) that permit the gene to be expressed only in an appropriate cell. These are the elements in the hemoglobin gene that instruct an erythroid cell to transcribe hemoglobin mRNA from that gene. These structures are often referred to as *cis*-acting elements because they reside on the same molecule of DNA as the gene. In some cases, other tissue type-specific *cis*-acting elements, called enhancers, reside on the same DNA molecule, but at great distances from the coding region of the gene (2, 52). In the appropriate cell, the *cis*-acting elements bind protein factors that are physically responsible for transcribing the gene. These proteins are often called *trans*-acting factors because they reside in the cell's nucleus separate from the DNA molecule bearing the gene. For example, brain cells would not have the right *trans*-acting factors that bind to the hemoglobin promoter, and, therefore, brain cells would not express hemoglobin. They would, however, have *trans*-acting factors that bind to neuron-specific gene promoters.

The structure of a gene's protein is specified by the gene's coding region. The coding region contains the information that directs an erythroid cell to assemble amino acids in the proper order to make the hemoglobin protein. How is this order of amino acids specified? As described in detail below, DNA is a linear polymer consisting of four distinguishable subunits called nucleotides. In the coding region of a gene, the linear sequence of nucleotides encodes the amino acid sequence of the protein. This genetic code is in triplet form,

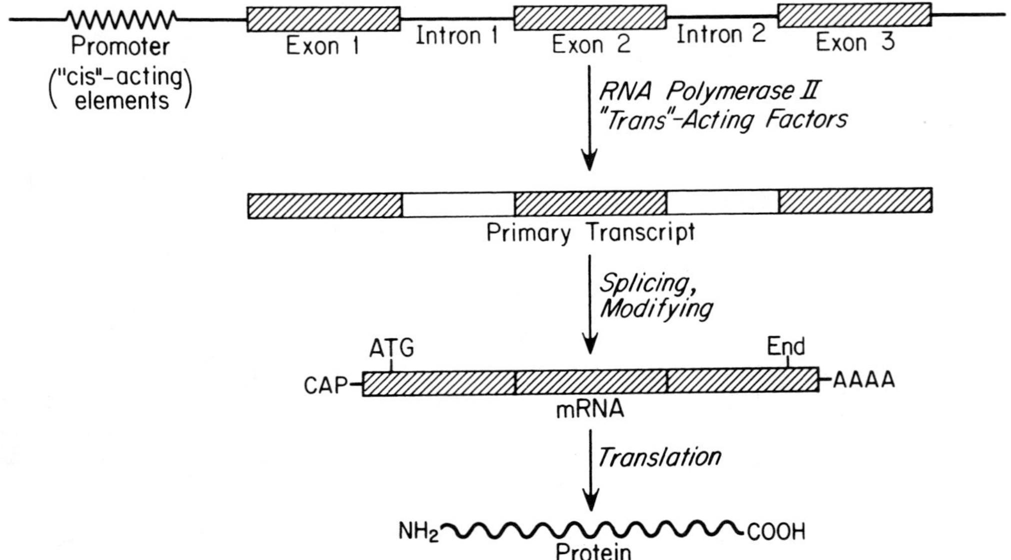

Figure 2.1. Gene expression. A gene's DNA is transcribed into mRNA, which is, in turn, translated into protein. The functional components of a gene are schematically diagrammed here. Areas of the gene destined to be represented in mature mRNA are called exons and intervening areas of DNA between exons are called introns. The portion of the gene that controls transcription, and, therefore, expression, is the promoter. This control is exerted by specific nucleotide sequences in the promoter region (so-called *cis*-acting factors) and by proteins (so-called *trans*-acting factors) that must interact with promoter DNA and/or RNA polymerase II in order for transcription to occur. The primary transcript is the RNA molecule made by RNA polymerase II that is complementary to the entire stretch of DNA containing the gene. Before leaving the nucleus, the primary transcript is modified by splicing together exons (thus removing intron sequences), adding a cap to the 5′ end, and adding a poly-A tail to the 3′ end. Once in the cytoplasm, mature mRNA undergoes translation to yield a protein.

so that every group of three nucleotides encodes a single amino acid. The number of triplets that can be formed by four nucleotides (which is 64) exceeds the number of amino acids used to make proteins (which is 20). This makes the code degenerate and allows some amino acids to be encoded by several different triplets (59). The nucleotide sequence of any gene can now be determined (see below). By translating the code, one can derive a predicted amino acid sequence for the protein encoded by a gene.

Structural Considerations

Fine Structure. The basic repeating units of the DNA polymer are nucleotides (Fig. 2.2). Nucleotides consist of an invariant portion, a five-carbon deoxyribose sugar with a phosphate group, and a variable portion, the base. Of the four bases that appear in the nucleotides of DNA, two are purines, adenine (A) and guanine (G), and two are pyrimidines, cytosine (C) and thymine (T). Nucleotides are connected to each other in the polymer through their phosphate groups, leaving the bases free to interact with each other through hydrogen bonding. This base pairing is specific, so that A interacts with T and C interacts with G. DNA is ordinarily double-stranded, that is, two linear polymers of DNA are aligned so that the bases of the two strands face each other. Base pairing makes this alignment specific, so that one DNA strand is a perfectly complementary copy of the other.

In every strand of a DNA polymer, the phosphate substitutions alternate between the 5′ and 3′ carbons of the ribose molecules. Thus, there is a directionality to DNA: the genetic code reads in the 5′ to 3′ direction. In double-stranded DNA, the strand that carries the translatable code in the 5′ to 3′ direction is called the sense strand, while its complementary partner is the antisense strand.

Gross Structure. In eukaryotes, the coding regions of most genes are not continuous. Rather they consist of areas that are transcribed into mRNA, the exons, which are interrupted by stretches of DNA that do not appear in mature mRNA, the introns (Fig. 2.1). The functions of introns are not known with certainty. A purpose of some sort is implied by their conservation in evolution. However, their overall physical structure might be more important than their specific nucleotide sequences, since the nucleotide sequences of introns diverge more rapidly in evolution than do the sequences of exons. Overall, DNA that contains genes accounts for a minor part of total DNA. Between genes, there are vast stretches of untranscribed DNA that are assumed to play an important structural role.

In the nucleus, DNA is not present as naked nucleic acid. Rather DNA is found in close association with a number of accessory proteins, such as the histones, and in this form is called chromatin (39). Although many of DNA's accessory proteins have no known specific function, they generally appear to be involved in the correct packaging of DNA. For example, DNA's double helix is ordinarily twisted on itself to form a supercoiled structure (7). This structure must unwind partially during DNA replication and transcription (86). Some of the accessory proteins (e.g., topoisomerases) are involved in regulating this process.

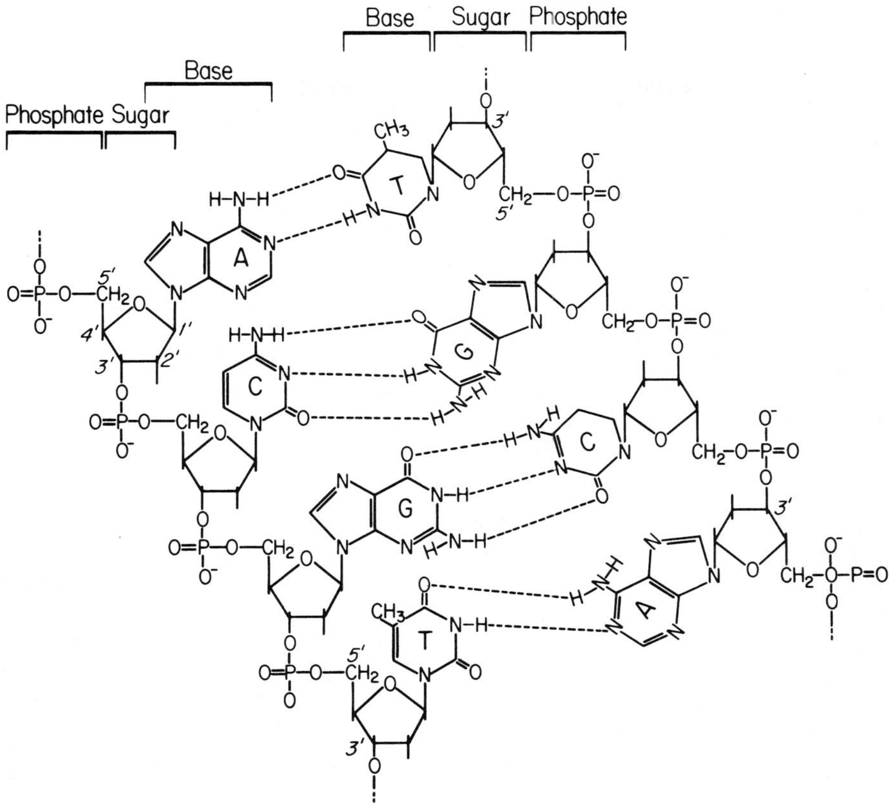

Figure 2.2. Structure of base-paired, double-stranded DNA. Each strand of DNA consists of a backbone of 5-carbon 2′-deoxyribose sugars connected to each other through phosphate bonds. Note that as one follows the sequence down the left-hand strand (A to C to G to T), one is also following the carbons of the 2′-deoxyribose ring, going from the 5′ carbon to the 3′ carbon. This is the basis for the 5′ to 3′ directionality of DNA. The 1′ carbon of each 2′-deoxyribose is substituted with a purine or pyrimidine base. In double-stranded DNA, bases face each other in the center of the molecule and base-pair via hydrogen bonds (*dotted lines*). Base pairing is specific, so that adenine pairs with thymine and guanine pairs with

SUMMARY

Genes specify the structure of proteins that are responsible for the phenotype associated with a particular gene. While the nucleus of every human cell contains 30,000 to 40,000 genes, only a fraction of them are expressed in any given cell at any given time. The promoter (with or without an enhancer) is the part of the gene that determines when and where it will be expressed. The coding region is the part of the gene that dictates the amino acid sequence of the protein encoded by the gene. DNA is a linear polymer of nucleotides. Ordinarily, the nucleotide bases of one strand of DNA interact with those of another strand (A with T, C with G) to make double-stranded DNA. In the cell's nucleus, DNA is associated with accessory proteins to make the structure called chromatin.

General Techniques

RESTRICTION ENDONUCLEASES AND RECOMBINANT DNA

In eukaryotic chromosomes, individual molecules of DNA are several million base pairs long. Because these molecules are far too large to analyze directly, scientists are usually interested in cutting DNA into fragments of manageable size. Fortunately for molecular biologists, bacteria have evolved a highly diverse set of enzymes, the restriction endonucleases, that cleave DNA internally within the polymer (77).

In nature, these enzymes have evolved to protect bacteria from invasion by foreign DNA molecules, such as phage. In order to discriminate between domestic and foreign DNA, these enzymes recognize specific nucleotide sequences. DNA without such specific sequences is left undisturbed by the enzymes. However, when a restriction endonuclease spots a recognition site, it binds to the site and cleaves both strands of the DNA to which it has bound. Individual restriction endonucleases recognize specific sequences, usually on the order of four to six bases in length, and these sequences are often palindromes; that is, the 5′ to 3′ sequence in the upper strand is identical to the 5′ to 3′ sequence in the lower strand (Fig. 2.3) (62).

While restriction endonucleases cut DNA into smaller fragments, there is a lower limit to the size of useful fragments. One would not want to cut DNA into such small pieces that the informational content of each piece is negligible. Statistically, the longer a restriction endonuclease's recognition sequence, the less frequently this sequence will occur in a stretch of DNA. Therefore, the enzymes most commonly

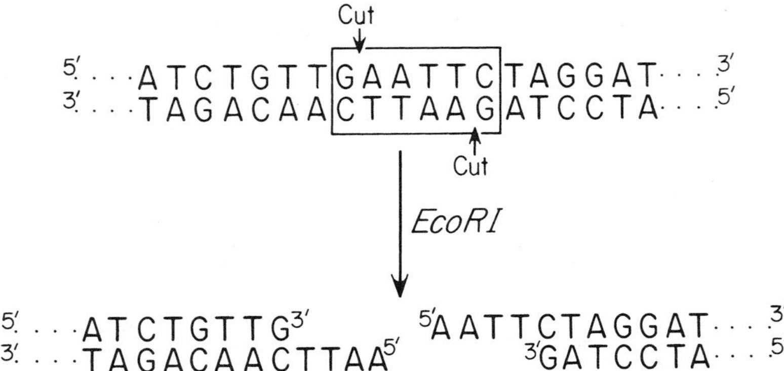

Figure 2.3. Digestion of DNA with the restriction endonuclease EcoRI. The nucleotide sequence of this stretch of DNA contains the recognition sequence for EcoRI, GAATTC (*boxed*). EcoRI cuts the DNA in both strands between the indicated nucleotides, resulting in fragments with 5´ single-stranded tails.

used to cut DNA into usefully large fragments are those that recognize a six-nucleotide recognition site (so-called six-base cutters). For example, an endonuclease isolated from *Escherichia coli*, called EcoRI, recognizes the sequence GAATTC, and wherever this occurs in double-stranded DNA, it will cleave between the G and A (Fig. 2.3). (Note that the antisense strand, which reads CTTAAG in the 3´ to 5´ direction, will also read GAATTC in the 5´ to 3´ direction. This is what is meant by a palindromic sequence.)

GENE CLONING

Mechanics. The most powerful technique available for gene analysis, and the one technique that is the cornerstone for all others, is gene cloning (Fig. 2.4). In the gene cloning process, a discrete piece of DNA is faithfully replicated in the laboratory. Cloning provides quantities of specific DNA sufficient for biochemical analysis or for any other manipulation, including joining to a foreign piece of DNA. In the early 1970s, Cohen and Boyer drew on two fundamental properties of bacteria and their viruses (phage) that made this innovation possible: plasmids and DNA ligases (18).

Plasmids are circular molecules of DNA that replicate in the cytoplasm of bacterial cells, separate from the bacteria's own DNA. In nature, plasmids often carry genetic information useful to the host bacterium, such as genes that confer resistance to antibiotics. For the purposes of gene cloning, plasmids are important because they contain all the information necessary for directing bacterial enzymes to replicate the plasmid DNA, in some cases, to many thousands of copies per bacterium.

DNA ligases are enzymes produced by bacteria (and some phage when they infect bacteria) that can link or ligate together separate pieces of DNA. The nucleotide sequence in a piece of DNA does not influence the activity of a DNA ligase, so that a DNA ligase can join two pieces of DNA that are not ordinarily connected to each other in nature.

In gene cloning, one uses a restriction endonuclease to cut open the circular plasmid DNA in a region of the plasmid not necessary for replication (Fig. 2.4). Suppose, for example, that the enzyme EcoRI cuts open the plasmid in such a nonessential area. EcoRI recognizes the sequence GAATTC, and cuts both DNA strands between the G and the A nucleotides. Protruding from the cut ends will be single-stranded DNA tails having the sequences AATT. (Note that the tail's sequence in the sense strand is the same as the sequence in the antisense strand when the nucleotides are read in the 5´ to 3´ direction.) Any other piece of DNA that has been cut with EcoRI will also have single-stranded AATT tails, and the AATT tails on this foreign piece of DNA can base-pair with the complementary TTAA tails (reading 3´ to 5´) on the cut plasmid. When this happens, the foreign DNA piece physically closes the gap in the plasmid, forming a closed circular plasmid again (which is necessary for plasmid propagation).

Although the nucleotides at the ends of the plasmid and foreign DNA now abut each other, they are not covalently connected. This is an unstable situation that the DNA ligase rectifies. DNA ligase covalently joins the plasmid and foreign DNA to create a recombinant plasmid, which still has all the information needed to be replicated in a bacterium, but which also contains a foreign DNA insert. Obviously, the EcoRI-cut ends of the plasmid can also base-pair with themselves again to reform the native plasmid, but molecular biologists have developed a number of tricks to suppress this phenomenon. It should be pointed out that single-stranded tails are not always necessary for making recombinant DNA. Under certain conditions, DNA ligase can join together two fragments of blunt-ended DNA without these tails.

When a recombinant plasmid is reintroduced into a host bacterium (by a process called transformation), the plasmid will replicate normally. Now, however, its foreign DNA insert is replicated, along with the plasmid into which it was inserted. The transformed bacteria can then be grown to large numbers in liquid culture. With each bacterial cell division, the progeny bacteria contain plasmid molecules that continue to replicate. When the bacterial culture contains the desired quantity of this plasmid (this may be milligrams of plasmid DNA in a 1-liter culture), it can be reisolated as pure DNA. The cloned foreign piece of DNA can then be cut out (with EcoRI in our example) for further analysis or manipulation. One can also use bacterial viruses (or phage) in the same manner by infecting host bacteria with recombinant phage-bearing foreign DNA sequences. In all of these ex-

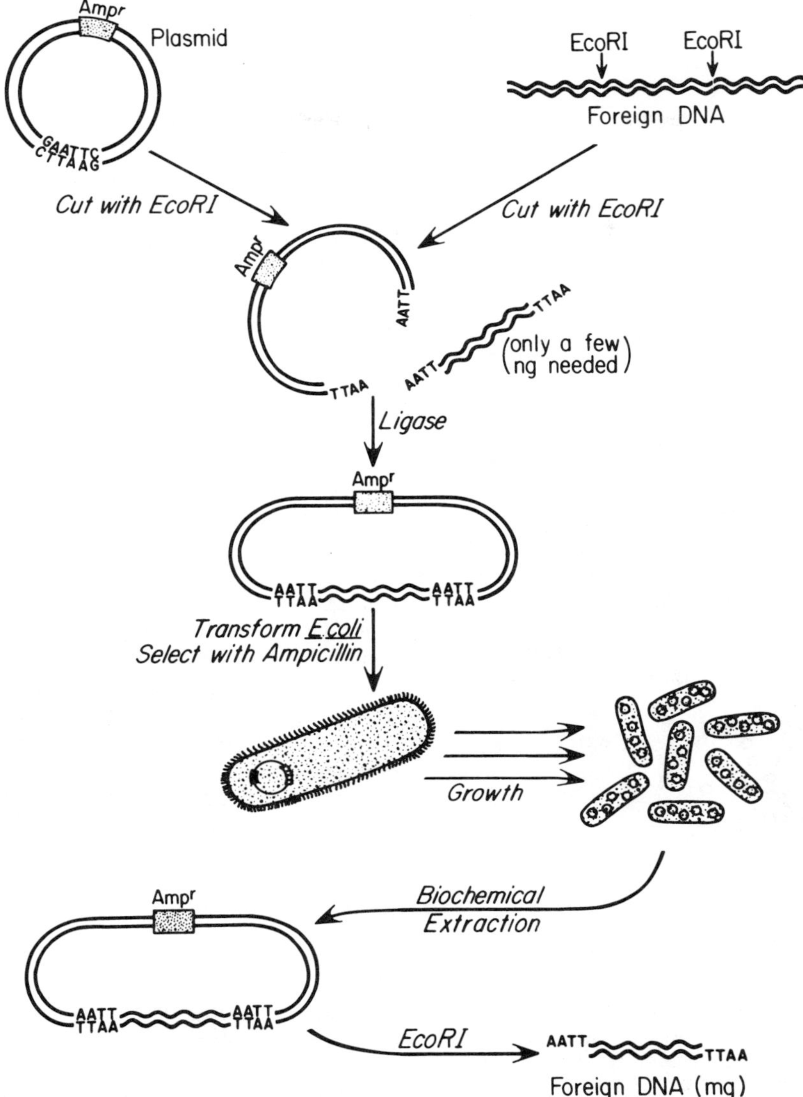

Figure 2.4. Gene cloning. In this example, a small amount of foreign DNA (a few nanograms) is digested with EcoRI. This foreign DNA can come from any source, the only requirement being that it contain the same restriction endonuclease recognition sites as the vector. Plasmid vector is also digested with EcoRI to create a linear DNA molecule. The sticky single-stranded ends of the foreign DNA can align and base-pair with the complementary sticky ends of the plasmid, after which DNA ligase covalently bonds foreign DNA to plasmid DNA. This recombinant DNA is introduced into *E. coli* by a process called transformation. Since the bacteria themselves are not resistant to ampicillin, growth in ampicillin will select only those bacteria that have taken up the plasmid DNA (which carries an ampicillin resistance gene). The plasmid contains a bacterial origin of replication, so that as the bacterial culture grows, plasmids replicate, resulting in several copies in each bacterium. When the culture has grown to sufficient size, plasmid DNA can be isolated biochemically, foreign DNA can be cut from the plasmid using EcoRI, and the resulting yield will often be milligrams of DNA, that is, greater than a 10^6-fold amplification.

periments, the plasmid or phage that houses the foreign DNA is called a vector, because it is the vehicle that directs the foreign DNA into the host bacterium.

These extraordinarily powerful tools, which are now part of the standard armamentarium of all molecular biology laboratories, have been responsible for the development of nearly all the analytic techniques described below. Several excellent manuals have been published that describe these techniques in detail (3, 9, 66).

Gene Libraries. One exceptional application of these techniques has been the construction of gene libraries (Fig. 2.5) (16, 49). A gene library contains the entire complement of DNA (and, therefore, genes) from an organism in the form of DNA fragments inserted into recombinant plasmids or phage. DNA containing an organism's genes (i.e., genomic DNA) can be isolated from a cell or tissue of interest, including human tissue, and cut into pieces of manageable size using a restriction endonuclease. These DNA fragments (several million of them, all of different lengths) can be cloned into bacterial plasmids or phage as described above so that each vector carries exactly one genomic DNA fragment. The recombinant vectors are then reintroduced into

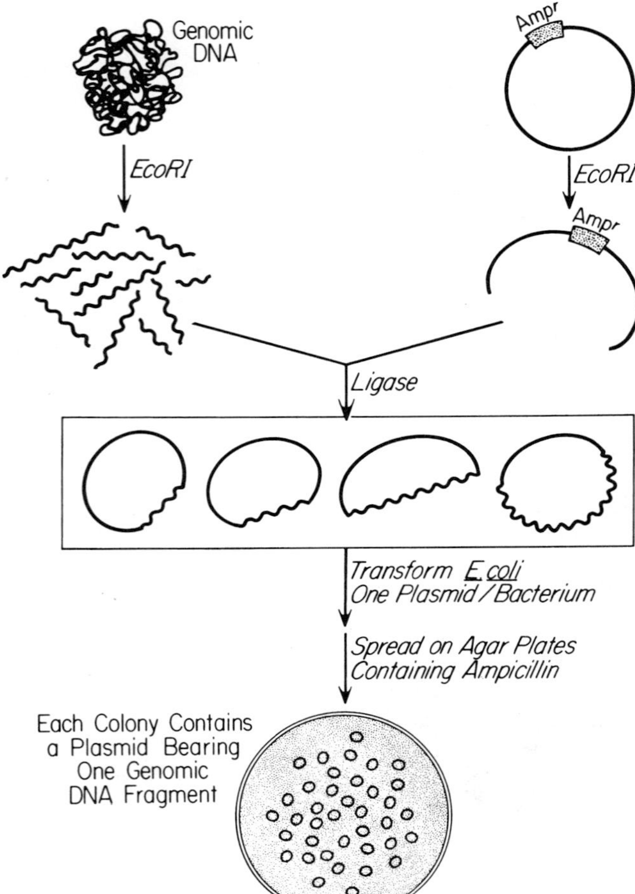

Figure 2.5. Constructing a genomic library. Genomic DNA and plasmid DNA are cut with EcoRI in preparation for cloning, as in Figure 2.4. (The vector DNA could also be bacteriophage DNA rather than plasmid DNA.) In this case, all of the variously sized EcoRI-produced genomic DNA fragments are cloned individually into the EcoRI site of the plasmid, and the recombinant DNA is introduced into *E. coli* by transformation. Transformed bacteria are selected by growth in the presence of ampicillin, as in Figure 2.4. Since each bacterium can be transformed by only one recombinant plasmid, and since each colony on the agar plate arose from a single transformed bacterium, each colony (or clone) contains amplified plasmid bearing a single genomic EcoRI fragment. Taken together, all the bacterial colonies represent the entire genetic complement of the organism from which the original genomic DNA was isolated. Taken together, all of the clones on all of the plates can be thought of as a genomic library, with each individual clone representing one volume.

bacteria, which can be plated onto agar plates and grown into individual bacterial colonies or phage plaques (areas of bacteria infected with phage). Now each bacterial colony, or each phage plaque, houses a recombinant plasmid bearing a different inserted fragment of DNA derived from the genomic DNA of the original cell or tissue. Each colony or plaque represents a different DNA clone. Specific clones containing specific genes can be identified on the basis of their nucleotide sequences (8, 32) (see below), expanded into large-scale cultures, and their recombinant DNA isolated. In this way, new genes are cloned.

GENE PROBES AND HYBRIDIZATION

We shall see in the following sections that what lies at the heart of gene analysis is the ability to identify a specific gene (or mRNA) in a complex mixture of all the DNA (or RNA) in a cell or tissue. This can be done only when one already has a cloned fragment of DNA from the gene of interest. Such fragments are usually obtained from gene libraries constructed from genomic DNA (described above) or cDNA (to be described below). These DNA fragments can be almost any size, from a fraction of the size of the gene (a few hundred nucleotides) to the size of an entire gene (several thousand nucleotides). These cloned gene fragments are called probes, because they are used to probe native DNA or RNA for the gene of interest.

To be useful, a gene probe must contain enough nucleotide sequences that it will recognize the sequences of its corresponding gene. Recognition occurs by a process called nucleic acid hybridization, in which two pieces of DNA can align themselves (or anneal) by base pairing. One can tag the probe DNA (e.g., using ^{32}P-labeled nucleotides), split apart its two strands by heating (denaturing), and add it to the DNA mixture being studied, which has usually been immobilized by sticking it to an inert flat sheet. Under appropriate reannealing conditions, wherever the probe DNA finds a complementary sequence, it will base-pair with that sequence. Any probe that has not specifically bound to its complementary DNA target can be washed away, and by exposing the flat sheet to x-ray film, the presence of the target DNA sequences can be revealed (see "Southern Blotting," below).

SUMMARY

Genes can be cut from total genomic DNA using restriction endonucleases that recognize specific nucleotide sequences. Individual genes can be captured and replicated in bulk for detailed analysis. This process is called cloning and employs bacterial plasmids and viruses (phage) as carriers for the cloned genes. Enzymes called DNA ligases join foreign DNA to plasmid or phage vectors, which can then replicate within bacterial cells to create gene libraries. Using nucleic acid hybridization, cloned genes act as probes to detect the presence of their native counterparts in complex mixtures of DNA and RNA.

Gene Analysis—DNA

SOUTHERN BLOTTING

One of the most useful techniques for analyzing a gene at the level of genomic DNA is Southern blotting, named for its originator, E.M. Southern (78). In general, it allows one to determine whether specific nucleotide sequences in a cloned probe are present in a sample of genomic DNA. The presence of these sequences usually means that the gene itself is present in the genomic DNA. Figure 2.6 diagrams the technique. Purified genomic DNA is digested with a specific restriction endonuclease, which, as described above, will produce an array of differently sized DNA fragments. Elec-

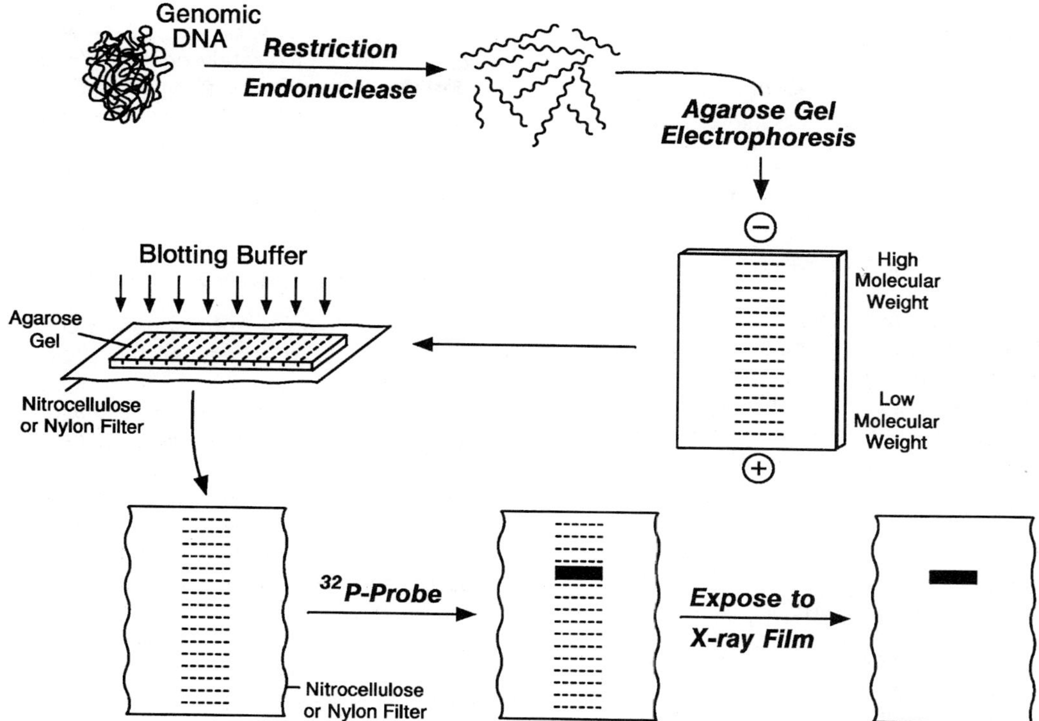

Figure 2.6. Genomic Southern blotting. Genomic DNA is digested with a single restriction endonuclease, resulting in a complex mixture of DNA fragments of different sizes (that is, molecular weights). Digested DNA is arrayed by size using electrophoresis through a semisolid agarose gel. Because DNA is negatively charged, fragments will migrate toward the anode, but their progress is variably impeded by interactions with the agarose gel. Small fragments interact less and migrate farther; large fragments interact more and migrate less. The arrayed fragments are then transferred to a sheet of nitrocellulose or nylon-based filter paper by forcing buffer through the gel as shown. The DNA fragments are carried by capillary action and can be made to bind irreversibly to the filter. Now the DNA fragments, still arrayed by size on the filter, can be probed for specific nucleotide sequences using a ^{32}P-radiolabeled nucleic acid probe. The probe will hybridize to complementary sequences in the DNA, and the position of the fragment that contains these sequences can be revealed by exposing the filter to x-ray film.

trophoresis through an agarose gel then separates these fragments according to size. (Since the phosphate groups in DNA make the molecules negatively charged, they will migrate toward the anode in an electric field. The semiporous agarose will allow molecules of DNA to pass with varying degrees of ease, at a rate inversely proportional to their size. At any time after electrophoresis begins, small molecules will be closer to the anode than large molecules.) The agarose gel is usually cast in the form of a flat rectangle a few millimeters thick.

The final goal of Southern blotting is to identify specific fragments of cut DNA using nucleic acid hybridization. Because the agarose gel used in electrophoresis is thick and the DNA fragments can move within it, DNA in the gel is not in a suitable form for further analysis. The DNA fragments must be transferred to a solid support to which they are irreversibly bound in order to carry out nucleic acid hybridization studies. Thus, after electrophoresis, a paper-thin membrane microfilter (made of nitrocellulose or nylon) is placed over the flat portion of the gel. Liquid is then forced through the agarose gel in a direction perpendicular to the direction in which the DNA moved during electrophoresis. As the liquid perfuses the gel, it carries DNA fragments with it, depositing them on the membrane filter, to which the DNA sticks. After transfer, the DNA fragments are arrayed by size on the solid support.

At this point, a fragment of cloned DNA (the probe) is radiolabeled by using any of a variety of techniques. The membrane containing the transferred DNA is then soaked in a buffer containing the radiolabeled probe. If there are any sequences in the genomic DNA that are complementary to those in the probe, the probe will hybridize to those sequences on the filter. Unbound probe can be washed away, and the remaining specifically hybridized probe can be visualized by exposing the filter to x-ray film.

What results from these studies is a pattern of one or more radiolabeled bands on x-ray film. Each band corresponds to a restriction endonuclease–generated DNA fragment containing nucleotide sequences complementary to those in the radioactive probe. For any particular gene probe, the size (i.e., length) of the band it identifies will be the same from individual to individual (although see below for a discussion of RFLPs, an important exception). Therefore, if a gene has undergone a structural rearrangement, as, for example, when the *c-abl* oncogene is translocated from chromosome 9 to 22, the pattern may change. Suppose, for example, that the c-*abl* probe ordinarily recognizes a 2,000-base EcoRI fragment in normal genomic DNA. If the translocation breakpoint in a patient with chronic myelogenous leukemia occurs within that fragment, part of the c-*abl* gene and one of its EcoRI sites will move to chromosome 22. Southern blot analysis of the patient's DNA may now detect either (*a*) a larger fragment than normal if the recipient chromosome has an EcoRI site farther away than the old EcoRI site, or (*b*) a smaller fragment if it has an EcoRI site closer than the old one. Southern blotting is thus a sensitive technique for detecting large structural rearrangements in the genome, such as those that are occasionally associated with malignancy.

Since the amount of radiolabeled probe that hybridizes to a Southern blot is proportional to the number of copies of the specific gene present in the target DNA, this technique can be used quantitatively. For example, in an analysis of primary breast cancer tissue, Southern blotting was used to determine that 30% of these samples contained multiple copies of c-*neu* oncogene DNA, that is, the gene was amplified (74).

PULSED-FIELD GEL ELECTROPHORESIS

One application for Southern blotting is the direct demonstration of physical linkage between two genes. If two different gene probes were to hybridize to the same restriction fragment in a Southern blot, this would prove that the loci of the two genes were closely linked. Unfortunately, eukaryotic genetic linkages ordinarily extend over millions of bases (megabases) of DNA, and the largest DNA fragments that can be resolved by conventional agarose gel electrophoresis are less than 100,000 bases or 100 kilobases (kb). The reason for this limitation is the tendency for all DNA molecules above a certain size to become oriented with their long axes parallel to the electric field. This prevents any appreciable interaction between the DNA molecules and the agarose gel. In the absence of such interaction, the DNA molecules are not retarded during electrophoresis, and will migrate at the same rate regardless of size. If the long axes of these large molecules are periodically reoriented perpendicular to the direction of migration, they once again interact with the agarose. Such interactions force the DNA molecules to migrate at rates inversely proportional to their lengths, and resolution by size is achieved again.

A number of ingenious techniques have been designed to accomplish this purpose: pulsed-field gel electrophoresis, in which two electrical fields are oriented perpendicularly and are alternately pulsed (68); field-inversion gel electrophoresis, in which a single field is periodically inverted (12); and contour-clamped homogeneous gel electrophoresis (CHEF), in which multiple fields of various orientations can be alternately applied (15). These techniques now allow the separation of DNA fragments that are from 2 to 5 megabases in length.

Pulsed-field gel electrophoresis has been used in the analysis of gene linkage on the long arm of chromosome 5. Genetic losses and alterations involving 5q have been associated with a variety of hematologic malignancies. The mapping of many of the genes encoding growth factors and growth factor receptors for hematologic cells on 5q has led to the suggestion that alterations in these genes are etiologic in these diseases (41). By digesting DNA with restriction endonucleases that have rarely occurring recognition sites, and performing Southern blotting experiments after pulsed-field gel electrophoresis, the genes for interleukin 3 (IL-3) and granulocyte macrophage colony-stimulating factor (GM-CSF) could be shown to lie on the same 436-kb fragment of DNA (92). Ultimately, it was demonstrated that these genes are separated by only 9 kb of DNA.

NUCLEOTIDE SEQUENCING

The nucleotide sequence of a gene's coding region encodes the amino acid sequence of its protein. This means that even in the absence of any knowledge about a gene's protein, we can predict the structure of that protein given the nucleotide sequence of the gene. How can the nucleotide sequence of a gene be determined? Two methods are used for sequencing DNA: the chemical modification method devised by Maxam and Gilbert (51), and the enzymatic chain termination method devised by Sanger and his colleagues (67). Because of its ease and wider usage, the chain termination method will be described here.

The chain termination method relies on properties of enzymes called DNA polymerases (Fig. 2.7). These are enzymes that create new DNA polymers starting from individual nucleotides. However, in order for a DNA polymerase to work, it needs a template of single-stranded DNA on which

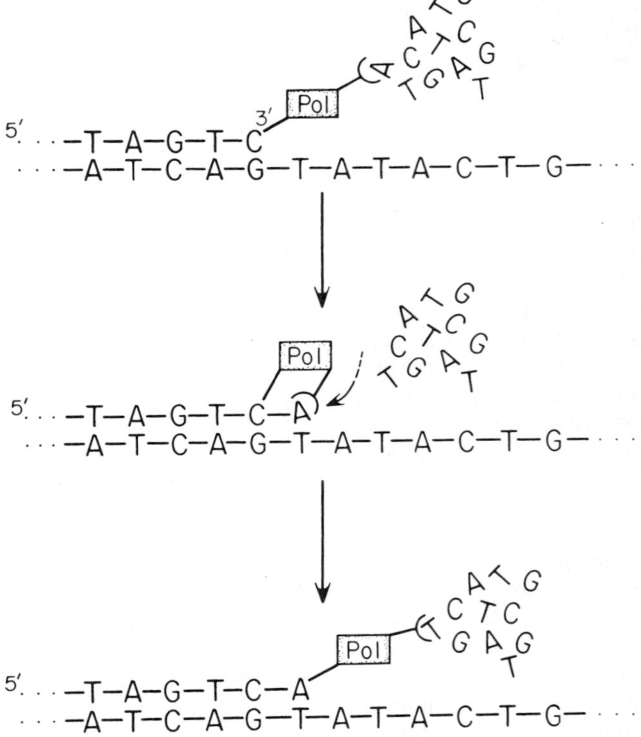

5′ . . . —T—A—G—T—C 3′ Pol
. . . —A—T—C—A—G—T—A—T—A—C—T—G— . . .

5′ . . . —T—A—G—T—C—A Pol
. . . —A—T—C—A—G—T—A—T—A—C—T—G— . . .

5′ . . . —T—A—G—T—C—A Pol
. . . —A—T—C—A—G—T—A—T—A—C—T—G— . . .

Figure 2.7. DNA polymerase. In this schematic, the enzyme DNA polymerase is creating a new DNA chain (*upper strand*) using a template (*lower strand*). Specific nucleotides are added from the 5′ to the 3′ direction as determined by the next nucleotide in the template.

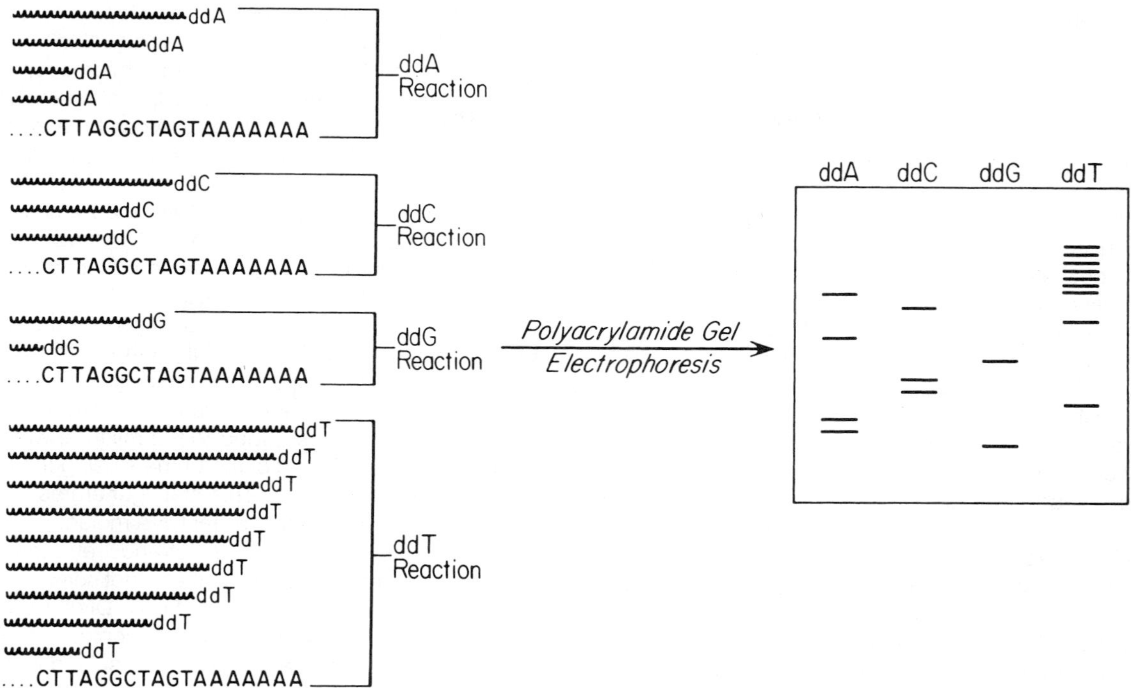

Figure 2.8. DNA sequencing using the chain termination method. In this example, DNA ending with the sequence...CTTAGGCTAGTAAAAAAA is being analyzed. Four reactions are performed, each using this DNA as a template for a DNA polymerase reaction, and each containing one of the four dideoxynucleotides (dideoxyadenosine triphosphate [ddA], dideoxycytidine triphosphate [ddC], dideoxyguanosine triphosphate [ddG], and dideoxythymidine triphosphate [ddT]). In each reaction, chain elongation will terminate when the dideoxynucleotide is incorporated at the position of its complementary nucleotide in the template. This will result in a family of chains of differing lengths that correspond to the position at which polymerization terminated. These chains can be resolved by electrophoresis through a urea-containing polyacrylamide gel in which longer chains run near the top of the gel and shorter chains near the bottom. Each new chain is radioactively labeled, and after autoradiography, the pattern of bands can be read from x-ray film. By noting the order in which bands appear, starting at the bottom of the gel, one can read the sequence of the template by substituting the complement of each dideoxynucleotide at every position. Reading from the bottom yields GAATCCGATCATTTTTTT, and substituting the complementary base at each position yields CTTAGGCTAGTAAAAAAA, the sequence of the template.

to create the new polymer. DNA polymerase adds a new nucleotide to the 3′ end of a growing DNA chain, but the base of the new nucleotide must be able to base-pair (that is, be complementary) to the base on the template over which the polymerase is positioned. After the addition of that nucleotide, the polymerase moves to the next nucleotide on the template, and adds a new nucleotide to the 3′ end of the growing chain. Again, the new nucleotide must be complementary to the next base in the template. When the process has been completed, DNA polymerase will have made a new DNA chain whose nucleotide sequence is completely complementary to the template DNA.

Nucleotide sequencing is based on the observation that when DNA polymerase adds a synthetic abnormal nucleotide to a growing chain, the polymerization stops. The synthetic terminating nucleotides used most commonly are dideoxynucleotides that have no alcohol substitutions on the 3′ carbon of their deoxyribose groups, and thus cannot be joined by a phosphate bridge to the next nucleotide (Fig. 2.2). For example, in the presence of dideoxy-adenosine triphosphate (ddATP), chain termination will occur wherever an A appears in the new DNA sequence (a T in the template) (Fig. 2.8). These reactions are performed in vitro in a test tube where millions of new DNA molecules are being made at once. If normal deoxy-ATP is mixed in the proper proportion with dideoxy-ATP, only a few of these molecules will terminate at each T in the template. This will generate a series of new DNA polymers, each one stretching from the beginning of the chain to the position of an A (i.e., a T in the template). If the newly formed DNA is radiolabeled, and the products of this reaction are separated electrophoretically in a polyacrylamide gel (see below), a ladder of radioactive bands will be generated. Each step of the ladder is a fragment of DNA that stretches from the start of the new polymer to the position of an A. Four separate reactions are performed using each of the four dideoxynucleotides. Each reaction is run in an adjacent lane on a polyacrylamide gel so that the nucleotide sequence can be read directly from the gel by reading up the steps of each ladder.

A specific application of DNA sequencing in cancer research has been the analysis of mutated sequences in the tumor suppressor gene p53. The hallmark of tumor suppressor gene involvement in cancer is loss of function of these genes. While loss of function can occur by wholesale loss of the gene, the same result can be achieved if the gene undergoes a mutation that inactivates its protein. Thus, in many types of cancers that have retained a *p53* allele as determined by Southern blotting, DNA sequencing has shown that the remaining allele has often undergone a single nucleotide, or point, mutation (58, 80).

RAPID TECHNIQUES FOR DETECTING MUTATIONS

As powerful as DNA sequencing may be, it is too cumbersome to be used as a screening tool for the identification of single mutations in patient DNA samples. A variety of clever techniques have been developed that rapidly reveal single-base mutations without resorting to DNA sequencing (19). One is denaturing gradient-gel electrophoresis (DGGE), which depends on the fact that double-stranded DNA molecules melt or denature into single strands at different temperatures or in different chemical conditions, depending on their specific sequences. For example, one can construct electrophoresis gels that contain a gradient of increasing concentrations of denaturants, such as urea or formamide, and if DNA is electrophoresed through such a gel, it will stop migrating at the position at which it has denatured. If two DNA fragments of identical length differ in their sequences at only one base pair, the concentration of denaturant at which the two fragments melt will be slightly different. Thus, electrophoresis of these two DNA fragments through a gradient of denaturant will distinguish them by the positions at which the two fragments stop migrating. One could begin with fragments isolated by the polymerase chain reaction (PCR), making this a convenient way to screen for the presence of common mutations using only a small amount of patient material.

Another, simpler technique is single-stranded conformation polymorphism (SSCP), which relies on the differences in mobility between single-stranded DNA molecules based on their secondary structures in nondenaturing gels. Single-stranded DNA molecules can fold back on themselves due to intrastrand base pairing and form unique shapes called secondary structures. Alteration of one base in a short DNA molecule, therefore, could have profound effects on secondary structure by altering the pattern of intrastrand base pairing. DNA molecules of identical length but different secondary structures will migrate at different rates in nondenaturing electrophoretic gels. Thus, DNA fragments can be isolated or synthesized by performing PCR on patient DNA samples; they can then be denatured, and individual strands allowed to reanneal to themselves rather than to their complementary strands. The products can be separated by nondenaturing electrophoresis, and fragments containing single base-pair mutations can be identified by their anomalous migration. Although technically simpler than DGGE, which can detect nearly 100% of single base-pair mutations, SSCP can only detect about 80% of such mutations (19).

POLYMERASE CHAIN REACTION

To detect gene sequences by Southern blotting, at least 1 to 2 μg of genomic DNA is required. This translates into milligram quantities of tissue that must be used fresh or freshly frozen. By amplifying specific fragments of DNA, the polymerase chain reaction (PCR) lowers the theoretical limit of detectable DNA sequences in a sample to a single molecule of DNA. With some advance knowledge of the nucleotide sequences in the DNA to be detected, microscopically small amounts of tissue, even a single cell, contain enough DNA to be amplified, and the amplified DNA can be easily analyzed. Even fixed tissue in paraffin blocks or on slides can yield sufficient DNA for analysis using PCR (91).

The concepts underlying PCR are diagrammed in Figure 2.9. Two short, single-stranded DNA fragments, called primers, have sequences complementary to those that flank the stretch of DNA to be amplified. They are added to the target DNA, the mixture is heated to dissociate the paired double strands of target DNA, and then the temperature is lowered to permit hybridization, or annealing, of the primers to their complementary sequences on the target DNA. A DNA polymerase enzyme is added to the mixture, which will add nucleotides to the 3′ end of the primers using the target DNA as a sequence template. This step generates one copy of each of the strands of one target DNA molecule. The mixture is heated again to dissociate the strands, and then cooled to allow more primers to anneal to the target sequences on both the original and new pieces of DNA. DNA polymerase is added again and now generates four copies of the target sequences. These steps are repeated, resulting in a geometrically increasing amount of target DNA—a chain reaction.

When it was first devised, this technique used a DNA polymerase from *E. coli*, which is inactivated by heating, so that fresh enzyme had to be added at every step (55, 64). With the discovery (13) and cloning (40) of the DNA polymerase from the thermophilic bacterium, *Thermus aquaticus* (the *Taq* polymerase), which retains activity after being heated to 95°C, heating and cooling steps could be carried out on the same mixture without adding new enzyme (65). This allowed the procedure to be automated. There are now automated thermal cyclers in every molecular biology laboratory, and in many clinical laboratories, that will take PCR mixtures through 20 to 50 cycles, producing large amounts of synthetic DNA for subsequent analysis.

DNA POLYMORPHISMS

A genetic polymorphism is defined as the occurrence of two or more phenotypes determined by a single genetic locus. The difference between a polymorphism and a mutation is that a polymorphism is retained in the population, that is, it occurs commonly. The usual distinction is that a gene is polymorphic when its least frequent manifestation appears in at least 1% of the population. Examples include blood types and major histocompatability complex molecules.

Polymorphisms may also occur without being associated with an obvious phenotype. For example, changes in nucleotide sequence within introns or in regions between genes would not necessarily result in altered proteins, and, therefore, would be silent. However, if these changes are polymorphic (i.e., frequent) then there is a high probability that an individual might be heterozygous for the polymorphism. In other words, it would be likely that the two chromosomes of a diploid pair would carry different versions of the polymorphism. Then, if the chromosomal position of the polymorphic change were known, it could be used as a

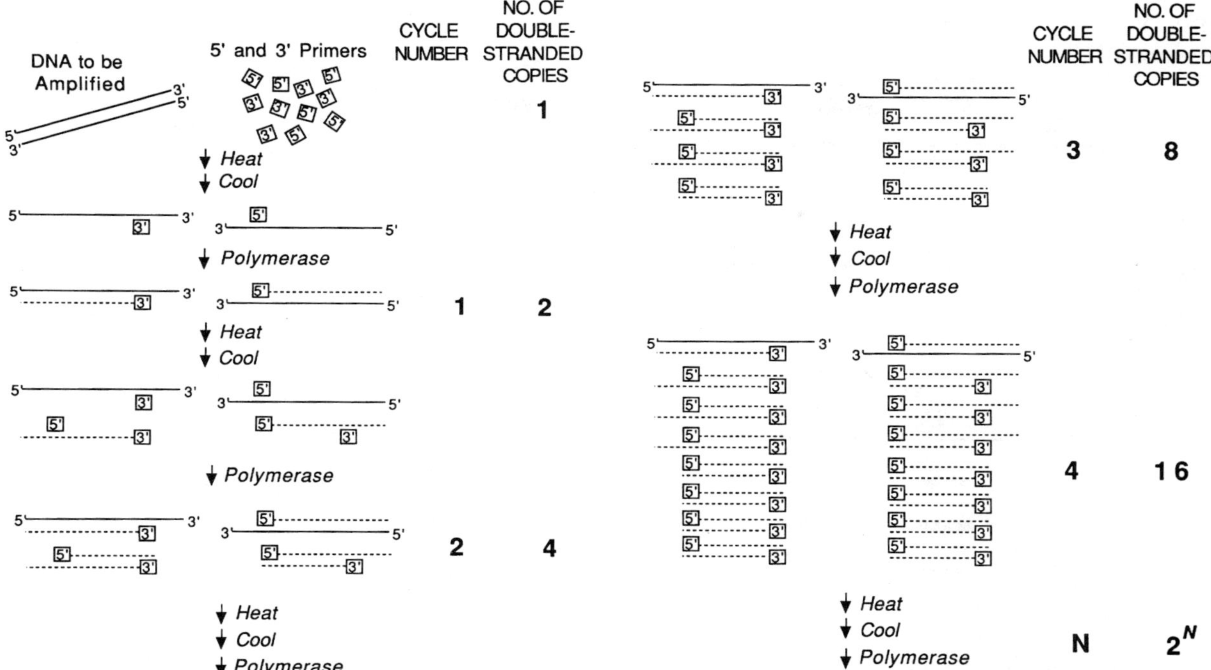

Figure 2.9. Polymerase chain reaction (PCR). DNA is mixed with short (10- to 20-base) single-stranded oligonucleotide primers that are complementary to the 5′ and 3′ ends of the sequence to be amplified. The mixture is heated to dissociate or melt all double-stranded DNA, and then cooled to permit the primers to anneal to their complementary sequences on the DNA to be amplified. Note that the 5′ primer will anneal to the lower strand, and the 3′ primer will anneal to the upper strand. A heat-resistant (thermostable) DNA polymerase (*Taq* polymerase, see text) was added to the original mixture, and it now synthesizes DNA by starting at the primers and using the strands to which the primers are annealed as a template. This results in the formation of two double-stranded DNA copies for every molecule of double-stranded DNA in the original mixture. The reaction is heated to melt double-stranded DNA and then cooled to allow reannealing, and the polymerase makes new double-stranded DNA again. There are now four double-stranded DNA copies for each original DNA molecule. This process can be repeated n times (usually 20 to 50) to result in 2^n copies of double-stranded DNA.

marker for mapping other genes. There are several varieties of DNA polymorphisms, and they provide the basis for gene mapping techniques that have identified several important cancer genes.

Restriction fragment length polymorphisms (RFLPs) appear as differences among individuals in the pattern of bands on a Southern blot probed with a single cloned DNA. There are two mechanisms whereby DNA polymorphisms are detectable by Southern blotting. First, a single nucleotide change might either create or destroy the recognition site for a restriction endonuclease. This would cause an alteration in the Southern blot pattern of that gene when the DNA is digested with a particular restriction endonuclease. For example, if a stretch of DNA with the sequence . . . AGGATTTCGA . . . in one individual contained a single nucleotide change in a second individual so that the sequence was . . . AGGAATTCGA . . ., the recognition site for EcoRI (GAATTC) would be created (Fig. 2.3). Digesting this individual's DNA with EcoRI would generate two new restriction fragments and remove one old one when compared with a nonmutated individual's DNA.

The second mechanism involves one of the more mysterious features of genomic DNA in eukaryotes, namely, that it is replete with repeated sequences of unknown function. The sequences often stretch themselves along the DNA polymer, one set of sequences after the other, in so-called tandem repeats. In humans, the best known repetitive sequence is called *alu*, and its nucleotide sequence is so specific that it can be used to identify human DNA in a mixture of DNAs from many species. There are several examples of tandemly repeated sequences in which the number of tandem repeats varies among individuals (57). One may have a DNA probe that recognizes a restriction fragment containing some tandem repeats. If the number of repeated sequences varies from one individual to the next, the size of the restriction fragment to which the probe hybridizes on a Southern blot will vary between the individuals. This will appear as an RFLP. These polymorphisms are called VNTRs for "variable number of tandem repeats."

By either mechanism, these RFLPs are stably inherited in a Mendelian fashion, which permits them to be used in gene mapping. RFLPs occur at specific positions (loci) in genomic DNA. If all the affected individuals in a family with a particular genetic disease inherit the same RFLP, this is presumptive evidence that the gene for the disease is close (or linked) to the RFLP locus. Linking a disease locus to an RFLP maps the gene for that disease and is the first step toward cloning the gene responsible for the disease. These are the tools of reverse genetics which have also led to the identifi-

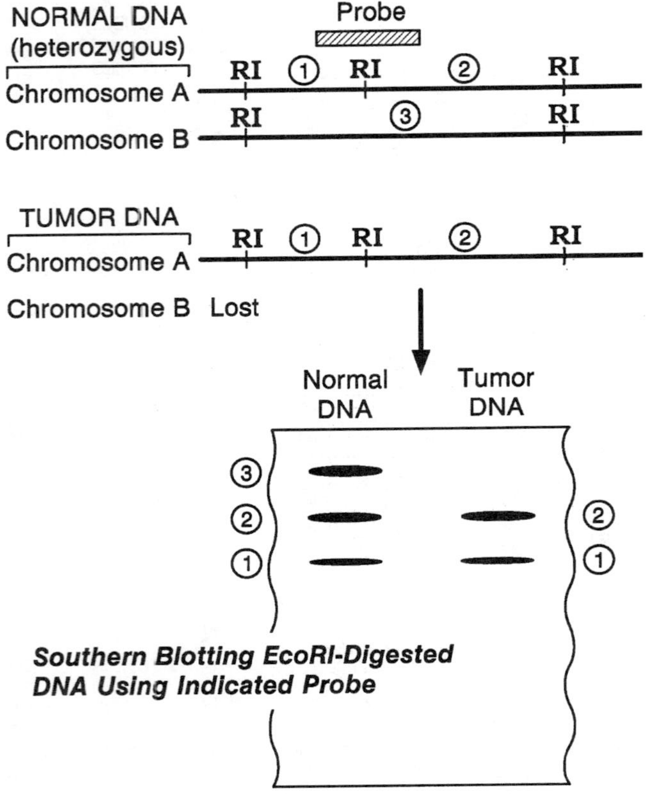

Figure 2.10. Using RFLPs and Southern blotting to detect loss of heterozygosity in tumor tissue. In this example, an individual is heterozygous for an EcoRI recognition site: the second EcoRI site on chromosome A is absent on its diploid partner chromosome B. The individual's tumor is assumed to be clonal and to have arisen from a cell that lost the region of chromosome B displayed in the figure. Southern blotting can then be performed using genomic DNA from the individual's normal DNA and tumor DNA in separate lanes of the agarose gel. Probing the DNA with the probe indicated at the top of the figure reveals a heterozygous banding pattern in normal DNA (reflecting the presence of both polymorphisms, one on each chromosome pair), and a loss of that pattern in the tumor DNA. This is one of the hallmarks of a tumor suppressor gene.

cation of some of the genes associated with malignant transformation, for example, the *BRCA1* gene on chromosome 17, whose mutations may be responsible for a significant fraction of heritable breast cancer (54).

RFLPs have also been used to demonstrate gene loss in cancer (Fig. 2.10). This approach relies on an individual's being heterozygous for an RFLP, that is, having one polymorphism on one chromosome and another polymorphism on the other. If an individual with cancer is heterozygous for a particular RFLP (termed an informative individual), his or her tumor can be analyzed by Southern blotting, using the probe that recognizes the polymorphism, and compared with normal tissue analyzed the same way. If one of the RFLPs present in the heterozygous individual's normal DNA is missing from the tumor cell DNA, the tumor is said to have undergone a reduction to homozygosity or a loss of heterozygosity. This implies a loss of genetic material from the tumor, specifically the DNA that includes the missing RFLP. This is the hallmark of a tumor suppressor gene (37). It was in this way that the involvement of the suppressor gene *p53* was found in human colon cancers (5, 85).

A particularly interesting polymorphism is known as a microsatellite. For unknown reasons, about 50,000 copies of the repetitive sequence dC-dA (tandemly repeated 10 to 60 times) are dispersed throughout the human genome (47). Because the longer tandem repeats (VNTRs) have been called minisatellite DNA, the shorter dC-dA repeats are called microsatellite DNA. (The term satellite refers to the fact that the buoyant density of repetitive DNA is different from the majority of genomic DNA. This leads to the appearance of small satellite bands distinct from the main DNA band when genomic DNA is purified by density gradient centrifugation.) The number of repeats at a particular locus varies in a polymorphic way among individuals, and because these sequences are stably inherited, they can serve as polymorphic markers. The difference in the number of repeat units between two polymorphic microsatellites can be as small as a few nucleotides. These differences cannot be detected by Southern blotting, which has a resolution of ≈100 nucleotides. However, these differences can easily be resolved using PCR: primers that flank the repeat region are used in a PCR in the presence of radiolabeled deoxynucleotides, and the products are separated on a DNA sequencing-style polyacrylamide gel. Mini- and microsatellite polymorphic markers are much more useful in gene mapping than are RFLPs because, unlike RFLPs, which usually have only two alleles, the variable number of repeats creates multiple alleles for each locus, significantly raising the likelihood that an individual will be heterozygous for the marker.

While the number of repeats in a microsatellite marker is usually stable, in some cancers, most notably colorectal cancer, the number of microsatellite repeats in the tumors differs from that in normal colorectal tissue from the same patient. Since the variability in repeat number occurs at all positions throughout the genome of the tumor, this suggests that the tumors experience overall genetic instability (1, 82). The basis of this instability is believed to be a mutation in the human homologue of a DNA proofreading gene, which, when mutated in yeast, leads to the appearance of unstable numbers of dC-dA repeats (79). This gene, which maps to chromosome 2, is probably responsible for hereditary nonpolyposis colorectal cancer (28, 42).

SUMMARY

Genomic DNA is too large to be analyzed easily in the laboratory, but it can be cut into manageable fragments using restriction endonucleases isolated from bacteria. Electrophoresis through an agarose gel can separate these fragments by size. Pulsed-field gel electrophoresis is a variation of this technique that allows the separation of extremely large DNA molecules. Fragments that carry nucleotide sequences corresponding to a gene of interest can then be detected by Southern blotting. Specific nucleotide changes (mutations) that give rise to stable genetic differences can be determined by DNA sequencing. Point mutations can be detected by anomalous migration of DNA through denaturing (DGGE) or nondenaturing (SSCP) electrophoretic gels.

PCR technology permits the detection of specific genes in extremely small amounts of tissue or in tissue that has been fixed for histologic analysis. There are polymorphic sites throughout genomic DNA; some create or destroy restriction endonuclease sites leading to RFLPs, whereas others contain a variable number of tandemly repeated sequences and are called mini- or microsatellites. Polymorphisms can be used for gene mapping or cancer diagnostics.

Gene Expression—mRNA Transcript Analysis

STRUCTURAL CONSIDERATIONS

The first step in gene expression is transcription of the genetic information in DNA into RNA. The individual building blocks of RNA, ribonucleotides, have the same structure as the deoxyribonucleotides in DNA, except that (*a*) the 2′ carbon of the ribose sugar is substituted with an OH group instead of H, and (*b*) there are no thymine bases in RNA, only uracil (demethylated thymine), which also base-pairs with adenine by hydrogen bonding. Just like the DNA polymerases described above, the enzyme RNA polymerase II uses the nucleotide sequence of the gene's DNA as a template to form a polymer of ribonucleotides with a sequence complementary to the DNA template.

In order for transcription to be correct, RNA polymerase II must (*a*) use the antisense strand of DNA as a template (*b*), begin transcription at the start of the gene, and (*c*) end transcription at the end of the gene. The signals that assure correct transcription are provided to RNA polymerase II by the DNA in the form of specific nucleotide sequences in the promoter of the gene. After reading and interpreting these signals, RNA polymerase generates a primary RNA transcript that extends from the initiation site to the termination site in a perfect complementary match to the DNA sequence used as a template. However, not all transcribed RNA is destined to arrive in the cytoplasm as mRNA. Rather, by an incompletely understood process, sequences complementary to introns (see above) are excised from the primary transcript, and the ends of exon sequences are joined together in a process termed splicing (69).

In addition to splicing, the primary transcript is further modified by the addition of a methylated GTP cap at the 5′ end (70), and the addition of a stretch of anywhere from 20 to 40 A bases at the 3′ end (11). These modifications appear to promote the translatability (27, 71) and relative stability of mRNAs, and help direct the subcellular localization of mRNAs destined for translation.

NORTHERN BLOTTING

The fundamental question in the analysis of gene expression at the RNA level is whether RNA sequences derived from a gene of interest are present in cells or tissues. Detecting specific RNA sequences can be accomplished by Northern blotting, the whimsically named analogue of Southern blotting, applied to RNA analysis. RNA can be isolated from cells in its intact form, free from significant amounts of DNA (14). Messenger RNA is much smaller than genomic DNA, so it can be analyzed by agarose gel electrophoresis without the enzymatic digestion steps that are necessary for the analysis of high-molecular-weight DNA.

RNA is single stranded and has a tendency to fold back on itself. This allows complementary bases on the same stretch of RNA to base-pair with each other and form what is termed secondary structure. Because secondary structure can lead to aberrant electrophoretic behavior, RNA is electrophoretically separated by size in the presence of a denaturing agent such as formaldehyde (43) or glyoxal/dimethyl sulfoxide (DMSO) (53). After electrophoresis through a denaturing agarose gel, the RNA is transferred to a nitrocellulose or nylon-based membrane in the same manner as DNA for Southern blotting (Fig. 2.6). Hybridization schemes and blot washing are essentially the same for Northern blotting as for Southern blotting. In this manner, specific RNA sequences corresponding to those in cloned DNA probes can easily be identified.

There is a lower limit to the sensitivity of Northern blotting, so that only moderately abundant mRNAs can be detected using this technique. One way to increase the sensitivity of Northern blotting is to enrich the RNA preparation for messenger RNA. Ordinarily, mRNA makes up less than 10% of the total RNA content of a cell or tissue. When RNA is isolated from these sources, all RNA species are being isolated—ribosomal and transfer RNA, as well as mRNA. As noted above, most mRNAs destined for the cytoplasm and translation are modified by the addition of a 3′ poly(A) tract. An RNA preparation, therefore, can be greatly enriched for mRNA species by removing all RNA molecules that lack the 3′ poly(A) tail (4). This can be done by exposing the RNA preparation to a tract of poly(U) or poly(T) bound to an immobilized support, such as a plastic bead. The poly(A) portion of mRNA will bind to the poly(U) or poly(T) material, and non–poly(A)-containing RNA can be washed away. After washing, the poly(A)-containing mRNA can be recovered from the solid support and used in Northern blot analysis. This procedure improves the sensitivity of Northern blotting by nearly two orders of magnitude.

A dramatic use of Northern blotting in cancer research has been the demonstration of oncogene expression in some human tumors. RNA was isolated from human tumor samples and analyzed by Northern blotting using cloned DNA probes derived from various oncogenes. The earliest observations included expression of c-*abl* and c-*myc* in human tumor cell lines and leukemic blasts (25, 89). Since then, however, a large number of proto-oncogenes have been shown to be transcribed in primary human tumor tissue (75).

NUCLEASE PROTECTION ASSAYS

Another technique used in the analysis of mRNA is the nuclease protection assay. This assay differs from Northern blotting in two general respects: (1) it is more sensitive than Northern blotting, and, therefore, is used for the detection of rare mRNA species; and (2) it provides detailed structural information about the mRNA being analyzed, and is thus often referred to as transcript mapping.

Nuclease protection assays (diagrammed in Fig. 2.11) use a single-stranded radioactive DNA or RNA probe. The nucleotide sequence of the probe contains at least some nu-

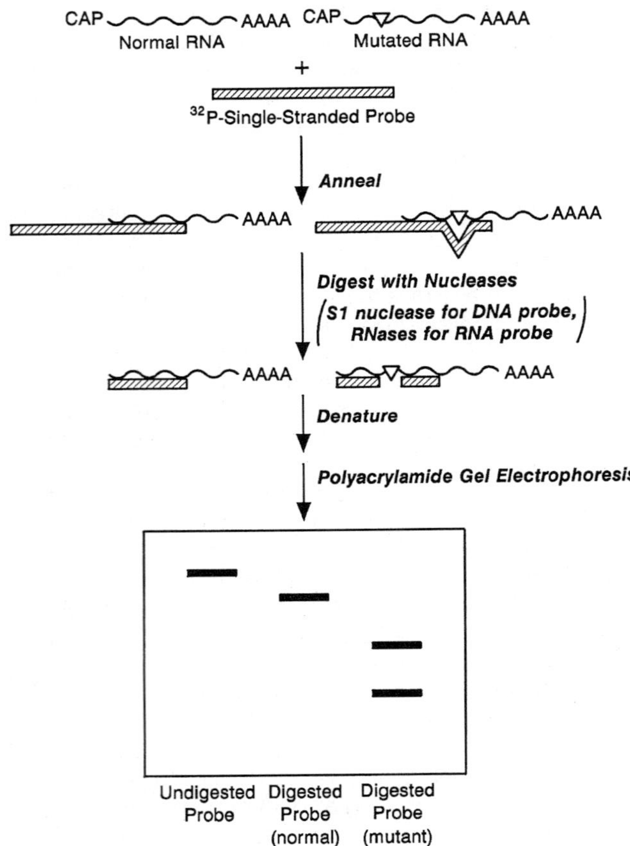

Figure 2.11. Nuclease protection assay. In this example, an mRNA containing a point mutation (indicated by the inverted triangle in the mRNA on the right) is distinguished from its normal, nonmutated counterpart (mRNA on the left). The mRNA is mixed with a single-stranded ^{32}P-labeled DNA or RNA probe that (1) has sequences perfectly complementary to the nonmutated region of interest in the mRNA, and (2) extends for some length beyond the mRNA. The mixture is heated, and then cooled to allow the probe to anneal to its complementary sequences in the mRNA. The annealed mixture is then treated with single-strand specific nucleases (S1 nuclease for a DNA probe, or RNases for an RNA probe). This results in digestion of the probe at all single-stranded areas: the extension beyond the mRNA sequences and the single base-pair mismatch overlying the mutation (*right*). The radioactive digestion products are then separated by electrophoresis through a urea-containing polyacrylamide gel. The probe that annealed to normal, nonmutated mRNA is smaller than the undigested probe (by the length of the extended region not complementary to the mRNA) and, therefore, will migrate farther than undigested probe. The probe that annealed to the mutated mRNA will have been digested into two fragments, whose summed length will equal that of the digested probe that annealed to nonmutated mRNA.

cleotides that are complementary to the mRNA being analyzed. The probe is annealed to the target mRNA by base pairing, and the regions of the probe that are complementary to the target mRNA now become double-stranded, while the noncomplementary regions of the probe remain single-stranded. The annealed mixture is then subjected to digestion with an enzyme specific for single-stranded DNA (usually S1 nuclease) (10) when using a DNA probe, or RNA (usually a mixture of RNase A and RNase T1) (48, 95) when using an RNA probe. The double-stranded annealed areas resist digestion, while all the single-stranded noncomplementary parts of the probe are digested away. In essence, areas in the probe that anneal to the mRNA are protected from digestion by the nucleases. The surviving, undigested parts of the probe can then be analyzed by electrophoresis through an agarose or polyacrylamide gel. The amount of radiolabeled probe resistant to digestion is proportional to the amount of target mRNA in the sample.

Nuclease protection assays can also provide structural information about target mRNA sequences. If there are any mismatches in the sequence of the target mRNA as compared with the probe, the areas corresponding to the mismatches will generate small single-stranded loops (Fig. 2.11). Since the nucleases that digest the annealed probe/mRNA hybrid are specific for single-stranded nucleotides, any mismatches between probe and target are susceptible to digestion. Thus, a mismatch can be detected if the nuclease-digested radiolabeled probe is smaller than would have been expected, or when the probe has been digested into multiple fragments. In fact, by careful measurement of the length of the digested probe, one can determine exactly where the mismatch has occurred in the target mRNA.

This technique has been used to detect single base mutations or small deletions in cellular mRNAs. For example, the proposed pathogenetic role of tumor suppressor genes, such as *p53*, in cancer depends on the inactivation of these genes, for example, by point mutation. A recent study used a nuclease protection assay to demonstrate the presence of point mutations in the mRNA for *p53* in several primary human lung cancer samples (80).

cDNA

The flow of genetic information usually runs from DNA to RNA to protein, following the so-called central dogma of molecular biology. There are, however, exceptions to this rule, the most prominent of which involves the life cycle of retroviruses. These viruses encode their genetic information in RNA rather than in DNA. When they invade a susceptible host cell, they direct the synthesis of a DNA intermediate that is a complementary copy of their genomic RNA. The enzyme that accomplishes this task, reverse transcriptase, is a DNA polymerase (see above) that uses RNA, rather than DNA, as a template to form a complementary DNA (cDNA) copy of the RNA (6, 81). The enzyme has been purified and can be used in vitro to make cDNA copies of any available RNA.

One important application of cDNA synthesis has been the construction of cDNA libraries (23, 63), analogues to the genomic libraries described above (Fig. 2.5). A valuable tool for the analysis of gene expression would be a gene library that consisted only of the genes that were expressed in a cell or tissue of interest. Most of the time, one is really not concerned with all the DNA in the genome, such as intron sequences, promoters, and vast regions of uninformative DNA that lie between genes. Even if one could make a library that contained only the coding regions of genes, one might still be interested only in the genes expressed by a particular cell type. For example, if one were interested in analyzing the genes expressed in a brain cell, why bother making a library that contained sequences for the hemoglobin gene? One way to construct a library comprised only of tissue-specific expressed genes would be to clone all the mRNA in a specific cell or tissue of interest. Unfortunately, there is no way to ligate single-stranded RNA to a double-stranded DNA cloning vector. However, one can use all the mRNA in a cell as a template for making double-stranded cDNA, which can then be inserted into a cloning vector.

To make a cDNA library, one isolates all the mRNA from a cell or tissue. Then, using this mRNA as a template, reverse transcriptase makes cDNA copies of each mRNA molecule in the mixture. The cDNA is ligated into plasmid or phage vectors, as described for genomic libraries, and the recombinant vectors are introduced into bacteria. After growth on agar plates, each bacterial colony or phage plaque of a cDNA library houses a unique recombinant vector containing the cDNA copy of a single mRNA. Desired clones can be detected by nucleic acid hybridization to the plaques or colonies using a radiolabeled gene probe (8, 32). Alternatively, if the vector containing the cDNA molecules can direct transcription of mRNA by host bacterial cells, mRNA will be synthesized and that mRNA will be translated. In this case, each bacterial colony or plaque will produce a different protein, and each protein will have been encoded by an mRNA from the original cell or tissue being investigated. If an antibody directed against a protein of interest is available, the cDNA clone corresponding to the mRNA that encodes that protein can be identified by binding the antibody to the colonies or plaques of the cDNA library (93). This technique, called expression cloning, often employs the bacteriophage λgt11 as the cloning vector.

cDNA libraries can be used to clone a cDNA for a known gene to discover the sequence of the mRNA it encodes. Alternatively, these libraries can be used to identify previously unknown genes. In a process called differential screening, cDNAs can be discovered that owe their existence to a particular differentiation or activation state in the cell of origin. For example, this technique has been used to identify genes whose expression is turned on by hormones or by growth factors, such as platelet-derived growth factor (PDGF) (17). A rapid modification of this technique using PCR (called differential display) is described in the next section.

PCR

Another important use of cDNA technology has allowed PCR to be applied to RNA. Since the *Taq* polymerase is a DNA polymerase, it cannot use RNA as a template. Simply adding primers and *Taq* polymerase to an RNA preparation will not result in amplification. However, if an RNA of interest could be made into DNA, then PCR would proceed as usual.

The first step in this analysis is generating a cDNA copy of the mRNA of interest using reverse transcriptase. This can be done using a primer consisting of T's (complementary to the poly(A) tail) or of a sequence complementary to some portion of the 3′ region of the mRNA. The 5′ primer can then be added along with *Taq* polymerase, and the single-stranded cDNA made in the first step will be amplified as described above (Fig. 2.10). In one of the first applications of this technique, Ph′-positive leukemias were diagnosed by identifying chimeric BCR-ABL mRNA species in clinical material using PCR. Since then, so-called RT-PCR (for reverse transcriptase PCR) has come into widespread use (36).

One inherent problem in using PCR to monitor mRNA expression is quantitation of the amplified PCR products. In Northern blotting or nuclease protection analysis, the intensity of the hybridization signal is directly proportional to the amount of target RNA in the sample. Thus, one can compare the number of RNA molecules in one sample with those in another. With PCR, a slight change in the efficiency of polymerization in an early cycle in one sample will lead to a geometrically increasing discrepancy between the amount of amplified product in that sample as compared with another sample. Fortunately, a number of techniques have been described for normalizing the products of PCR reactions to allow quantitative comparisons (33). In general, they involve amplifying an easily distinguishable control RNA template in the same reaction as the RNA of interest. Normalization of the amplified experimental PCR products to the control products then allows comparisons to be made.

One application of RT-PCR is a simple method for differential screening called differential display (46). Two cell populations to be compared are identified, and mRNA is isolated from both. Reverse transcription and PCR are performed using a poly-T primer, which will anneal to the 3′ poly-A tail of all the mRNA species, and a set of primers with random sequences, which by chance will anneal to sequences upstream of the poly-A tail in all the mRNA species. Since the upstream primer will anneal at random to different mRNA species, the lengths of the PCR products will vary for nearly every mRNA. If the amplification is performed in the presence of radiolabeled nucleotides, the products from the two reactions can be separated on a sequencing gel. Bands that are much darker in one lane as compared with another represent mRNA species that were overexpressed in one cell population compared to another. The cDNA representing this band can be recovered from the gel for further analysis and identification.

RIBOZYMES

One of the more surprising discoveries of the past decade was that some RNA molecules have enzymatic activity. These RNAs, called ribozymes, can cleave RNA at sequence-specific sites (94). They were originally discovered in *Tetrahymena* when it appeared that some of the primary RNA molecules in this species were capable of splicing out their introns without the aid of any protein enzymes. Ribozymes have also recently been described in higher organisms, and it is likely that they will be found to play a universal and important role in RNA processing. Sequence-specific ribozymes can be synthesized that will destroy specific mRNAs. One application of this technology is the introduction into malignant cells of ribozymes directed against activated oncogenes. In the laboratory, this technique can reverse the malignant phenotype of some cancer cells (34).

SUMMARY

The genetic information in DNA is copied, or transcribed, into mRNA by the enzyme RNA polymerase II. Before being transported to the cytoplasm, primary transcripts in the nucleus are modified by splicing out introns, and adding a 5′ cap and adding a 3′ poly(A) tract. Cytoplasmic mRNA can be detected by Northern blotting, nuclease protection assays, or modified PCR. Although nuclease protection assays are somewhat more demanding technically than is Northern blotting, they are more sensitive and can provide structural information about mRNA transcripts. A retroviral enzyme called reverse transcriptase can make cDNA copies of mRNA transcripts. These cDNAs can be cloned into cDNA libraries, which are useful for isolating and analyzing expressed genes. In the future, ribozymes may be useful for the selective elimination of specific mRNA species.

Gene Expression—Protein Analysis

STRUCTURAL CONSIDERATIONS

Proteins are polymeric molecules consisting of amino acids linked by peptide bonds. The sequence of amino acids in a protein is dictated by the sequence of nucleic acids in the mRNA that encodes the protein. Since amino acids are joined to each other in a linear polymer, there is a directionality to proteins, just as there is to DNA and RNA. The 5′ end of the mRNA corresponds to the amino end of its cognate protein and the 3′ end corresponds to the carboxy end (Fig. 2.1).

For many proteins, the linear polymer of amino acids must undergo a number of alterations in order to be functional. These alterations are referred to as posttranslational modifications. For example, proteins destined to be secreted from a cell initially exist as propeptides with a 20- to 30-amino-acid sequence at their amino ends. This highly hydrophobic tail, called a leader sequence, remains embedded in the membranes of the endoplasmic reticulum and secretory granule until the protein is to be secreted, at which point the leader sequence is cleaved. There are many examples of propeptides that undergo cleavage of specific amino acids before they become mature, functional proteins.

Other posttranslational modifications include the addition of various nonpeptide substituents to the side chains of amino acids. These include simple and complex carbohydrate chains, sulfate groups, and phosphate groups. Phosphorylation of intracellular proteins, usually on serine, threonine, or tyrosine residues, plays an important regulatory role in protein function. For example, many of the cell surface receptors for growth factors, such as the PDGF receptor (24) and the receptor for M-CSF (61, 72), are themselves tyrosine protein kinases. When this type of receptor binds its ligand, the receptor undergoes a conformational change that activates its kinase activity. The activated receptor then adds phosphate groups to some of its own tyrosine residues, as well as to tyrosines in other proteins. These phosphorylations are part of the signal transduction process whereby a message is sent from the cell surface receptor to the nucleus (see Chapter 4). The importance of tyrosine phosphorylation in cell growth may be reflected in the fact that tyrosine kinases form the largest functional subset of oncogenes.

SDS-PAGE

As with nucleic acids, the most common analytic technique applied to proteins is separation by size using electrophoresis. However, unlike nucleic acids, not all proteins are anionic, and they do not have a uniform charge-to-mass ratio. In the presence of an electric field, a mixture of unmodified and uncharacterized proteins would migrate in an unpredictable way, providing little or no information about their structures. This problem has been overcome by performing protein electrophoresis in the presence of the anionic detergent sodium dodecyl sulfate (SDS). SDS binds to proteins in a uniform way, approximately one molecule of SDS for every two amino acids. Thus, all proteins become polyanions in the presence of SDS, and the number of negative charges (supplied by the sulfate group in SDS) is directly proportional to the size, or molecular weight, of the protein.

Since proteins are generally smaller than the most commonly analyzed nucleic acids, electrophoresis is performed through a solid support made of polyacrylamide, which resolves low-molecular-weight molecules better than agarose. In the presence of an electric field, proteins in SDS will migrate toward the anode at a rate inversely proportional to the log of their molecular weights (38, 88). Proteins can be analyzed by SDS-polyacrylamide gel electrophoresis (SDS-PAGE) in the presence or absence of β-mercaptoethanol (β-ME), which reduces sulfhydryl groups on the sidechains of cysteines that can bind two separate protein chains together. Electrophoresis in the presence of β-ME permits the analysis of protein subunits, while electrophoresis in the absence of β-ME can reveal multimeric protein associations. SDS-PAGE is routinely employed to test the purity of a protein preparation. It is also an integral component of the techniques of immune precipitation and Western blotting.

IMMUNE PRECIPITATION

A primary goal of molecular biology is to use gene probes to detect the presence of a particular gene in a complex mixture of DNAs or RNAs. In a similar way, a specific antibody can be used as a probe to detect the presence of a particular protein in a complex mixture of proteins. An antibody directed against a protein of interest can be added to a mixture of proteins under conditions that allow the antibody to bind to its target protein (Fig. 2.12). One can then collect all the immunoglobulins (Ig's) in that mixture by adding a protein that binds to Ig's, such as anti-immunoglobulin antibodies or Staphylococcal protein A. These proteins are often bound to a solid support (e.g., polystyrene beads) that can be removed from solution by gentle centrifugation. As the beads collect at the bottom of the centrifuge tube, their attached Ig and target proteins collect there as well. When

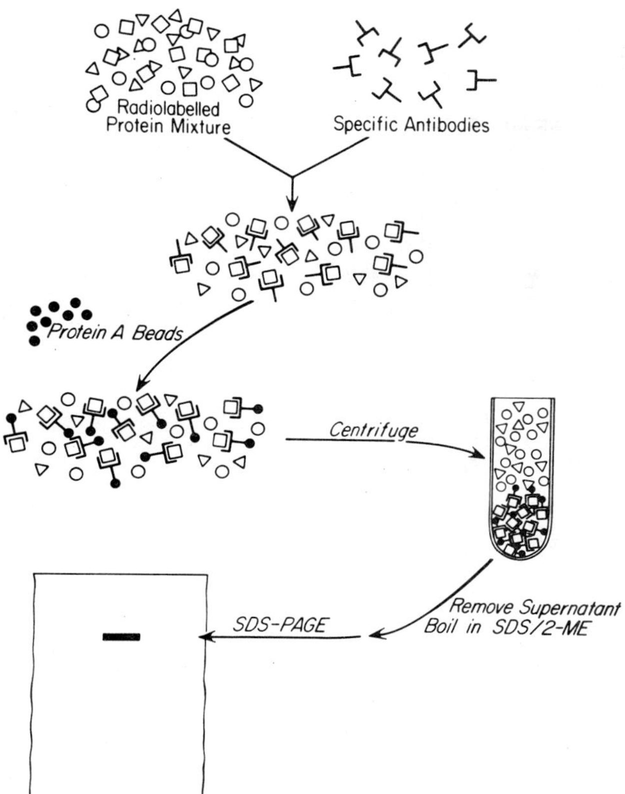

Figure 2.12. Immune precipitation. A complex mixture of radiolabeled proteins (indicated by different geometric shapes) is incubated with antibodies specific for one of those proteins (in this case, the squares). After the antibodies have bound to their protein, small polystyrene or agarose beads containing Staphylococcal protein A are added to the mixture. Protein A binds to the antibodies, and when centrifuged, the beads to which the protein A is bound will sediment to the bottom of the centrifuge tube, taking along the antibodies and the specific protein to which they have bound. The unbound proteins remain in the supernatant and can be removed. After boiling to dissociate the protein A/antibody/protein complex, specifically precipitated radiolabeled protein can be visualized by electrophoresis (SDS-PAGE) and autoradiography.

boiled in SDS and β-mercaptoethanol, the protein complexes dissociate, and they can be electrophoretically separated by SDS-PAGE. This process is called immune precipitation. To document the specificity of the antibody, a second immune precipitation is usually performed with a control antibody that does not bind the protein of interest. The two precipitations can be run side by side on SDS-PAGE, and the protein of interest identified by its presence in the experimental lane and its absence from the control lane. The proteins can be identified by staining reactions, or, if the protein preparation is radiolabeled, by autoradiography.

A recent application of this technique was the demonstration that the protein product of the retinoblastoma susceptibility gene (RB) binds to proteins encoded by DNA tumor viruses. Antibodies directed against adenovirus proteins were used in an immune precipitation of proteins from cells transformed or infected by adenovirus. In addition to the adenovirus proteins, the precipitated proteins contained another protein that proved to be the protein encoded by the retinoblastoma susceptibility gene (90). Similar experiments using antibodies directed against the large T antigen of simian virus 40 (SV40) revealed an interaction between T antigen protein and the RB protein (20). In both cases, these interactions may be central to the mechanisms whereby these viruses oncogenically transform susceptible host cells.

IMMUNOBLOTTING

Another valuable immunologic identification technique is immunoblotting (Fig. 2.13) (83). A mixture of proteins can be electrophoretically separated by SDS-PAGE, and the separated proteins can be transferred to a nitrocellulose or nylon-based filter by electrophoresis in a direction perpendicular to that of the first electrophoresis. The proteins will remain bound to the membrane support. By analogy to Southern blotting for DNA and Northern blotting for RNA, this technique for protein transfer has been called Western blotting.

The protein blot can be soaked in a solution that contains a specific antibody that binds to the protein of interest. The presence of the bound antibody on the blot can then be detected if the antibody is labeled. The label can be an enzyme that reveals its presence by catalyzing a color or light-emitting reaction, or it can be a radionuclide, such as ^{125}I, that can be detected by autoradiography. Alternatively, an unlabeled antibody can be detected by washing the blot in a solution that contains a labeled anti-immunoglobulin antibody.

This technique has been used to demonstrate overexpression of the HER-2/*neu* protein in some breast cancers in which Southern blotting revealed no gene amplification (76). Since the protein is the effector of gene function and the determinant of phenotype, overexpression of the protein can be highly significant, and is often considered to be the gold standard of overexpression.

SEQUENCING

The ultimate in protein identification is direct determination of amino acid sequence. Automated sequenators are now available that have considerably simplified this technically demanding analysis. In addition, recent advances in protein chemistry have permitted sequencing to be performed on mere picomoles of protein. In fact, Western blotting can be used to purify small amounts of protein, and the fragment of the blot containing the stained protein of interest can be used directly in an automated sequenator (50).

Direct protein sequencing was responsible for ushering in the modern era of molecular oncology. The empirically determined amino acid sequence of the B chain of human platelet-derived growth factor (PDGF) was found to be nearly identical to the protein encoded by the oncogene v-*sis*, the transforming gene of the the simian sarcoma virus (22, 87). This was the first demonstration of a connection between oncogenes and the components involved in normal cellular proliferation.

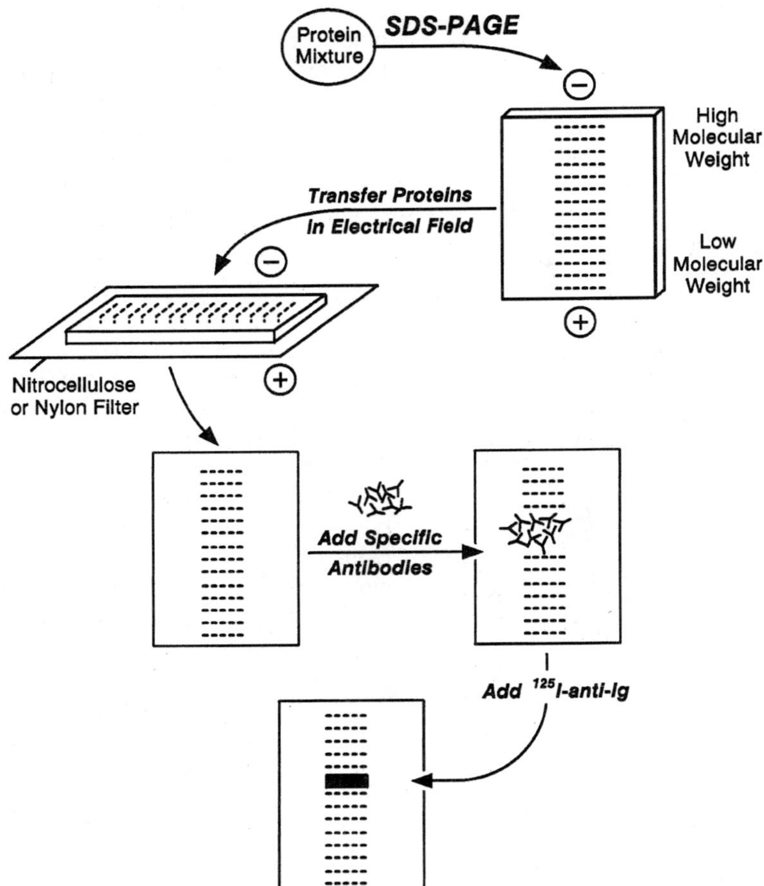

Figure 2.13. Immune (Western) blotting. A complex mixture of proteins can be separated by size using electrophoresis (SDS-PAGE). The separated proteins are then transferred to a nitrocellulose or nylon filter in an electric field, maintaining their size-specific spatial orientation on the filter. Antibodies directed against one specific protein in the original mixture are added to the filter and bind to the specific protein. Bound antibodies can be radiolabeled or enzymatically labeled themselves, or they can be visualized by incubating the filter with labeled anti-immunoglobulin antibodies.

ENGINEERED PROTEIN EXPRESSION

The final goal of many experiments in molecular biology is the use of biologic systems to synthesize the protein encoded by the gene being studied. This process, called engineered protein expression, can be an experimental end in itself. When the expressed protein synthesized by recombinant DNA methods can be shown to have all the properties of the natural protein, this is considered to be proof that the proper gene has been cloned. Alternatively, expression can be an end in itself when one wants to produce large amounts of a particular protein that might be difficult to obtain from natural sources.

In Vitro Translation. One very simple expression method is in vitro translation, in which translation occurs entirely in a test tube. All of the components necessary for translating mRNA can be obtained from cells that are highly efficient in protein synthesis, such as reticulocytes (usually from rabbits) or wheat germ. Under the appropriate conditions, and in the presence of all 20 amino acids, a synthetic or purified RNA added to such a system will be efficiently translated into protein. If a radioactive amino acid, such as [^{35}S]methionine, is included in the mix, the reaction products can be analyzed by SDS-PAGE and autoradiography. Demonstrating an appropriately sized protein or one that is recognized by a specific antibody constitutes good evidence that the mRNA in hand is the one the investigator desires.

Large-Scale Production of Recombinant Proteins. In vitro translation can only be applied at a small-scale analytic level. To produce large amounts of protein, one must turn to in vivo expression systems. One of the simplest involves cloning the cDNA for the desired protein into a bacterial plasmid or phage that contains a transcriptional promoter active in bacteria. When introduced into the appropriate bacterial host, large amounts of mRNA will be transcribed that, in turn, will be translated into protein. The recombinant protein can then be purified away from all the bacterial proteins. This is the way that some clinically available interferons (21, 31, 56) have been produced.

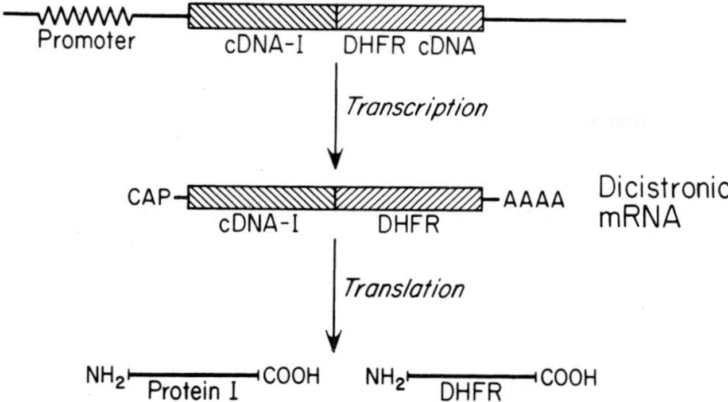

Figure 2.14. Mammalian engineered protein expression system. A cDNA encoding the protein to be produced (I) is cloned downstream (3′) of a promoter and upstream (5′) of a cDNA for dihydrofolate reductase (DHFR). After transfection into a mammalian cell, the promoter directs transcription of a dicistronic mRNA, one that contains two independent coding regions. The cDNA for I is 5′ to the cDNA for DHFR. When the mRNA is translated, two separate proteins result, the I protein and DHFR. As described in the text, the cDNA for DHFR can be amplified by methotrexate selection. This process will also result in amplification of the closely linked DNA for cDNA-I, and will ultimately lead to large amounts of dicistronic mRNA and large amounts of I protein and DHFR.

Many eukaryotic proteins require posttranslational modifications for maximal activity. Bacteria do not have the machinery required to accomplish complex modifications, such as the addition of specific carbohydrate groups. Moreover, the interior milieu of a bacterial cell is a reducing environment, so that disulfide bonds essential to the structure and function of many eukaryotic proteins cannot form. When these modifications are required, mammalian cells can be used for expression. The basic concept is the same as in bacterial systems: a cDNA is cloned into a vector having a eukaryotic transcriptional promoter and the resulting recombinant DNA is introduced into mammalian cells.

Expression systems have been modified to increase the levels of protein synthesis in number of ways. We present one particularly clever technique (diagrammed in Fig. 2.14) as an example of how observations in disparate areas of research oncology can be combined to great advantage. Here, a cDNA of interest is inserted in a plasmid downstream from a promoter sequence (in this case, one borrowed from adenovirus) and upstream from a cDNA for mouse dihydrofolate reductase (DHFR) (35). When mRNA is transcribed from this plasmid, the mRNA will be dicistronic, that is, it will contain the message sequences for two separate proteins on the same mRNA. Upstream, at the 5′ end, will be the cDNA of interest, and downstream, at the 3′ end, will be the DHFR cDNA. When the mRNA is translated, two separate proteins (not a fusion protein) will be made, since the upstream cDNA has a termination codon at the end of its coding sequences.

This recombinant plasmid is then introduced, by means of a process called transfection, into a cell line that has no endogenous DHFR gene (84). Not all the cells in the transfection experiment take up the recombinant DNA, but by growing the cells in the absence of nucleosides in the growth medium, the only cells that will survive will be those that have (*a*) taken up the DNA, (*b*) have transcribed the DHFR cDNA into mRNA, and (*c*) have translated that mRNA into DHFR protein. These surviving cells will also necessarily be expressing the protein of interest, since its cDNA was upstream from the DHFR sequences.

One can now take advantage of the fact that the major mechanism of methotrexate (MTX) resistance in mammalian cells is amplification of the DNA encoding DHFR. The expressing cells can be exposed to gradually increasing concentrations of MTX in vitro to generate resistant lines. At each level of resistance, the transfected DHFR cDNA has undergone amplification, but so has the cDNA cloned immediately upstream from DHFR. Thus, as DHFR protein expression reaches higher levels, so does the expression of the protein of interest. In this way, very high levels of several of the colony-stimulating factors have been produced for clinical use (92).

There are still significant disadvantages to the use of mammalian cells for large-scale recombinant protein production. Mammalian cells are expensive to grow in vitro because they require a medium rich in nutrients and growth factors. Yeast cells, insect cells, and even plant cells are being exploited as an attractive compromise between mammalian cell culture and bacterial culture for protein expression. These eukaryotic cells can execute most of the posttranslational modifications required by mammalian proteins, including disulfide bonding. At the same time, these cells are easier and more economical to grow in vitro. A number of expression vectors analogous to those described here for bacteria and animal cells have been developed for these alternative eukaryotic hosts.

SUMMARY

The genetic information in DNA is transcribed into RNA, and the information in RNA is ultimately translated into protein. Like DNA and RNA, proteins are directional. The amino and carboxy termini of proteins are specified by the 5′ and 3′ ends, respectively, of their cognate mRNAs. After translation, proteins may require further modification in order to be fully functional.

Proteins can be fractionated by size using electrophoresis through polyacrylamide gels in the presence of the anionic detergent, SDS (SDS-PAGE). SDS-PAGE is an integral component of the analytic techniques of immune precipitation and Western blotting. Automated analyzers are now available that can directly determine the amino acid sequence of a protein using vanishingly small amounts of material.

The mRNA that encodes a protein can be translated in vitro using cellular extracts of rabbit reticulocytes or wheat germ. The DNA that encodes a protein can be transcribed and the RNA translated in vivo by using appropriate vector and host cell combinations in culture. Bacterial cells are simple and economical vehicles for expressing foreign genes, but they cannot perform many of the posttranslational modifications required by mammalian proteins. Vectors have been designed that permit mammalian cells to express foreign proteins with great efficiency and fidelity. However, mammalian expression systems are expensive. Simpler eukaryotic expression systems using yeast cells, insect cells, or plant cells have been developed as an acceptable middle ground.

Miscellany

Molecular biologists have developed a wide variety of useful techniques that are too complex to describe in detail in this chapter. However, their increasingly common use may place them in the paths of oncologists with scientific interests. Therefore, we provide a brief description of a handful of these techniques with appropriate references.

ELECTROPHORETIC MOBILITY SHIFT ASSAYS (EMSA; GEL SHIFT ASSAYS)

This technique identifies specific DNA sequences in promoters or enhancers to which *trans*-acting factors bind. It relies on the fact that DNA bound to protein migrates more slowly in polyacrylamide gels than does naked DNA (29, 30). Radiolabeled oligonucleotides bearing candidate binding sequences are mixed with pure or crude proteins that are predicted or known to bind to specific DNA sequences. Oligonucleotides bearing the correct binding sequences will bind their appropriate proteins and have a slower electrophoretic mobility than oligonucleotides with incorrect sequences. DNase I footprinting can independently confirm that sequences identified by gel shift assays bind proteins (3).

ISOLATION OF DNA-BINDING PROTEINS (SOUTHWESTERN BLOTTING)

Major efforts are currently directed toward isolating cDNA clones that encode *trans*-acting transcription factors that bind to enhancer and promoter sequences. The approach is similar to that described for expression cloning using antibodies. In this case, however, an expression cDNA library is probed with radiolabeled oligonucleotides that will bind to clones encoding proteins that specifically recognize the oligonucleotide's DNA sequence. This can be independently confirmed by SDS-PAGE of the recombinant protein, followed by electrophoretic transfer to a nylon membrane and probing with radiolabeled oligonucleotide. Because this step mixes features of Western blotting (SDS-PAGE and protein transfer to a membrane) and Southern blotting (probing with radiolabeled DNA), it has been called Southwestern blotting (73).

TWO-HYBRID SCREEN

Protein–protein interactions are required for a variety of regulatory functions, for example, activation of cyclin-dependent kinases by interactions with cyclins (60). If one member of the protein pair is already identified, the second member can be cloned using a yeast two-hybrid screen. This technique relies on the fact that many *trans*-acting transcription factors have two separable functional domains, namely, a DNA binding domain that recognizes the appropriate promoter sequences and a transcriptional activator domain that is responsible for stimulating transcription. One of the best characterized systems is the yeast GAL4 activator. The cloning technique uses a yeast strain in which a specific promoter is linked to an indicator gene that will turn the yeast colony blue when activated. The yeasts are then transformed with a plasmid in which one of the putative interacting proteins is fused to the DNA binding domain of GAL4. They are also transformed with a cDNA library in which all the cDNA clones are fused to the transactivation domain of GAL4. If two proteins interact in the yeast, this will bring the DNA binding and transactivation domains into sufficiently close proximity to stimulate transcription of the indicator gene, turning the yeast colony blue. The cDNA responsible for interacting with the target protein can then be isolated (26).

References

1. Aaltonen LA, Peltomaki P, Leach FS, Sistonen P, Pylkkanen L, Mecklin JP, Jarvinen H, Powell SM, Jen J, Hamilton SR, Petersen GM, Kinzler KW, Vogelstein B, de la Chapelle A. Clues to the pathogenesis of familial colorectal cancer. Science 1993;260:812.
2. Atchison ML. Enhancers: mechanisms of action and cell specificity. Annu Rev Cell Biol 1988;4:127.
3. Ausubel FM, Brent R, Kingston RE, Moore DD, Seidman JG, Smith JA, Struhl K, (Editors). Current Protocols in Molecular Biology. New York: Wiley, 1993.
4. Aviv H, Leder P. Purification of biologically active globin messenger RNA by chromatography on oligothymidylic acid-cellulose. Proc Natl Acad Sci USA 1972;69:1408.
5. Baker SJ, Fearon ER, Nigro JM, Hamilton SR, Preisinger AC, Jessup JM, vanTuinen P, Ledbetter DH, Barker DF, Nakamura Y, White R, Vogelstein B. Chromosome 17 deletions and p53 gene mutations in colorectal carcinomas. Science 1989;244:217.
6. Baltimore D. RNA-dependent DNA polymerase in virions of RNA tumor viruses. Nature 1970;226:1209.
7. Bauer WR, Crick FHC, White JH. Supercoiled DNA. Sci Am 1980;243:118.
8. Benton WD, Davis RW. Screening λgt recombinant clones by hybridization to single plaques in situ. Science 1977;196:180.
9. Berger SL, Kimmel AR. Guide to molecular cloning techniques. In Methods in Enzymology, vol 152. Edited by JN Abelson, MI Simon. San Diego, CA: Academic Press, 1987.
10. Berk AJ, Sharp PA. Sizing and mapping of early adenovirus mRNAs by gel electrophoresis of S1 endonuclease-digested hybrids. Cell 1977;12:721.
11. Birnstiel ML, Busslinger M, Strub K. Transcription termination and 3′ processing: the end is in site! Cell 1985;41:349.
12. Carle GF, Frank M, Olson MV. Electrophoretic separations of large DNA molecules by periodic inversion of the electric field. Science 1986;232:65.
13. Chien A, Edgar DB, Trela JM. Deoxyribonucleic acid polymerase from the extreme thermophile *Thermus aquaticus*. J Bacteriol 1976;127:1550.
14. Chirgwin JM, Przybyla AE, MacDonald RJ, Rutter WJ. Isolation of biologically active ribonucleic acid from sources enriched in ribonuclease. Biochemistry 1979;18:5294.
15. Chu G, Vollrath D, Davis RW. Separation of large DNA molecules by contour-clamped homogeneous electric fields. Science 1986;234:1582.
16. Clarke L, Carbon J. A colony bank containing synthetic Col E1 hybrid plasmids representative of the entire *E. coli* genome. Cell 1976;9:91.
17. Cochran BH, Reffel AC, Stiles CD. Molecular cloning of gene sequences regulated by platelet-derived growth factor. Cell 1983;33:939.
18. Cohen SN, Chang ACY, Boyer HW, Helling RB. Construction of biologically functional bacterial plasmids in vitro. Proc Natl Acad Sci USA. 1973;70:3240.
19. Cotton RG. Current methods of mutation detection. Mutat Res 1993;285:125.
20. DeCaprio JA, Ludlow JW, Figge J, Shew JY, Huang CM, Lee WH, Marsilio E, Paucha E, Livingston DM. SV40 large tumor antigen forms a specific complex with the product of the retinoblastoma susceptibility gene. Cell 1988;54:275.
21. Derynck R, Remaut E, Saman E, Stanssens P, DeClercq E, Content J, Fiers W. Expression of human fibroblast interferon gene in *Escherichia coli*. Nature 1980;287:193.
22. Doolittle RF, Hunkapiller MW, Hood LE, Devare SG, Robbins KC, Aaronson SA, Antoniades HA. Simian sarcoma virus onc gene, v-*sis*, is derived from the gene (or genes) encoding a platelet-derived growth factor. Science 1983;221:275.
23. Efstradiatis A, Kafatos FC, Maniatis T. The primary structure of rabbit β-globin mRNA as determined from cloned cDNA. Cell 1977;10:571.
24. Ek B, Westermark B, Wasteson A, Heldin CH. Stimulation of tyrosine-specific phosphorylation by platelet-derived growth factor. Nature 1982;295:419.
25. Eva A, Robbins KC, Andersen PR, Srinivasan A, Tronick SR, Reddy EP, Ellmore NW, Galen AT, Lautenberger JA, Papas TS, Westin EH, Wong-Staal F, Gallo RC, Aaronson SA. Cellular genes analogous to retroviral *onc* genes are transcribed in human tumour cells. Nature 1982;295:116.
26. Fields S, Song O. A novel genetic system to detect protein-protein interactions. Nature 1989;340:245.
27. Filipowicz W. Functions of the 5′-terminal m^7G cap in eukaryotic mRNA. FEBS Lett 1978;96:1.
28. Fishel R, Lescoe MK, Rao MRS, Copland NG, Jenkins NA, Garber J, Kane M, Kolodner R. The human mutator gene homolog *MSH2* and its association with hereditary nonpolyposis colon cancer. Cell 1993;75:1027.
29. Fried M, Crothers DM. Equilibria and kinetics of *lac* repressor-operator interactions by polyacrylamide gel electrophoresis. Nucl Acids Res 1981;9:6505.
30. Garner MM, Revzin A. A gel electrophoresis method for quantifying the binding of proteins to specific DNA regions: application to components of *Escherichia coli* lactose operon regulatory system. Nucl Acids Res 1981;9:3047.

31. Goeddel DV, Yelverton E, Ullrich A, Heyneker HL, Miozzari K, Holmes W, Seeburg PH, Dull T, May L, Stebbing N, Crea R, Maeda S, McCandliss R, Sloma A, Tabor JM, Gross M, Familletti PC, Pestka S. Human leukocyte interferon produced by *E. coli* is biologically active. Nature 1980;287:411.
32. Grunstein M, Hogness DS. Colony hybridization: a method for the isolation of cloned DNAs that contain a specific gene. Proc Natl Acad Sci USA 1975;72:3961.
33. Innis MA, Gelfand DH, Sninsky JJ, White TJ. PCR Protocols. San Diego, CA: Academic, 1990.
34. Kashani SM, Funato T, Florenes VA, Fodstad O, Scanlon KJ. Suppression of the neoplastic phenotype in vivo by an anti-*ras* ribozyme. Cancer Res 1994;54:900.
35. Kaufman RJ, Murtha P, Davies M. Translational efficiency of polycistronic mRNAs and their utilization to express heterologous genes in mammalian cells. EMBO J 1987;6: 187.
36. Kawasaki ES, Clark SS, Coyne MY, Smith SD, Champlin R, Witte ON, McCormick FP. Diagnosis of chronic myeloid and acute lymphocytic leukemias by detection of leukemia-specific mRNA sequences amplified in vitro. Proc Natl Acad Sci USA 1988;85:5698.
37. Knudson AG. Hereditary cancer, oncogenes, and antioncogenes. Cancer Res 1985;45:1437.
38. Laemmli UK. Cleavage of structural proteins during the assembly of the head of bacteriophage T4. Nature 1970;227:680.
39. Laskey RA, Earnshaw WC. Nucleosome assembly. Nature 1980;286:763.
40. Lawyer FC, Stoffel S, Saiki RK, Myambo R, Drummond R, Gelfand DH. Isolation, characterization, and expression in *Escherichia coli* of the DNA polymerase gene from *Thermus aquaticus*. J Biol Chem 1989;264:6427.
41. Le Beau MM, Pettenati MJ, Lemons RS, Diaz MO, Westbrook CA, Larson RA, Sherr CJ, Rowley JD. Assignment of the GM-CSF, CSF-1, and FMS genes to human chromosome 5 provides evidence for linkage of a family of genes regulating hematopoiesis and for their involvement in the deletion (5q) in myeloid disorders. Cold Spring Harbor Sympon Quanttative Biology 1986;51:899.
42. Leach FS, Nicolaides NC, Papadopoulos N, Liu B, Jen J, Parsons R, Peltomaki P, Sistonen P, Aaltonen LA, Nystrom-Lahti M, Guan XY, Zhang J, Meltzer PS, Yu JW, Kao FT, Chen DJ, Cerosaletti KM, Fournier REK, Todd S, Lewis T, et al. Mutations of a mutS homolog in hereditary nonpolyposis colorectal cancer. Cell 1993;75:1215.
43. Lehrach H, Diamond D, Wozney JM, Boedtker H. RNA molecular weight determinations by gel electrophoresis under denaturing conditions, a critical reexamination. Biochemistry 1977;16:4743.
44. Lewin B. Gene expression, 2nd ed. New York: Wiley, 1980.
45. Lewin N. Genes IV, 4th ed. Oxford, England: Oxford University Press, 1990.
46. Liang P, Pardee AB. Differential display of eukaryotic messenger RNA by means of the polymerase chain reaction. Science 1992;257:967.
47. Litt M, Luty JA. A hypervariable microsatellite revealed by in vitro amplification of a dinucleotide repeat within the cardiac muscle actin gene. Am J Hum Genet 1989;44:397.
48. Lynn DA, Angerer LM, Bruskin AM, Klein WH, Angerer RC. Localization of a family of mRNAs in a single cell type and its precursors in sea urchin embryos. Proc Natl Acad Sci USA 1983;80:2656.
49. Maniatis T, Hardison RC, Lacy E, Lauer J, O'Connell C, Quon D, Sim GK, Efstratiadis A. The isolation of structural genes from libraries of eukaryotic DNA. Cell 1978;15:687.
50. Matsudaira P. Sequence from picomole quantities of proteins electroblotted onto polyvinylidene difluoride membranes. J Biol Chem 1987;262:10035.
51. Maxam AM, Gilbert W. A new method for sequencing DNA. Proc Natl Acad Sci USA 1977;74:560.
52. McKnight S, Tjian R. Transcriptional selectivity of viral genes in mammalian cells. Cell 1986;46:795.
53. McMaster GK, Carmichael GG. Analysis of single- and double-stranded nucleic acids on polyacrylamide and agarose gels by using glyoxal and acridine orange. Proc Natl Acad Sci USA 1977;74:4835.
54. Miki Y, Swensen J, Shattuck-Eidens D, Futreal PA, Harshman K, Tavtigian S, Liu Q, Cochran C, Bennett LM, Ding W, Bell R, Rosenthal J, Hussey C, Tran T, McClure M, Frye C, Hattier T, Phelps R, Haugen-Strano A, Katcher H, et al. A strong candidate for the breast and ovarian cancer susceptibility gene *BRCA1*. Science 1994;266:66.
55. Mullis KB, Faloona FA. Specific synthesis of DNA in vitro via a polymerase-catalyzed chain reaction. Methods Enzymol 1987;155:335.
56. Nagata S, Taira H, Hall A, Johnsrud L, Streuli M, Escodi J, Boll W, Cantell K, Weissman C. Synthesis in *E. coli* of a polypeptide with human leukocyte interferon activity. Nature 1980;284:316.
57. Nakamura Y, Leppert M, O'Connell P, Wolff R, Holm T, Culver M, Martin C, Fujimoto E, Hoff M, Kumlin E, White R. Variable number of tandem repeat (VNTR) markers for human gene mapping. Science 1987;235:1616.
58. Nigro JM, Baker SJ, Preisinger AC, Jessup JM, Hostetter R, Cleary K, Bigner SH, Davidson N, Baylin S, Devilee P, Glover T, Collins FS, Weston A, Modali R, Harris CC, Vogelstein B. Mutations in the *p53* gene occur in diverse human tumor types. Nature 1989;342:705.
59. Nirenberg MW, Leder P. RNA codewords and protein synthesis. Science 1964;145: 1399.
60. Pines J, Hunter T. Cyclin-dependent kinases: a new cell cycle motif? Trends Cell Biol 1991;1:117.
61. Rettenmier CW, Chen JH, Roussel MF, Sherr CJ. The product of the c-*fms* proto-oncogene: a glycoprotein with associated tyrosine kinase activity. Science 1985;228:320.
62. Roberts R. Restriction and modification enzymes and their recognition sequences. Nucl Acids Res 1982;10:117.
63. Rougeon F, Mach B. Stepwise biosynthesis in vitro of globin genes from globin mRNA by DNA polymerase of avian myeloblastosis virus. Proc Natl Acad Sci USA 1976;73: 3418.
64. Saiki RK, Gelfand DH, Stoffel S, Scharf SJ, Higuchi R, Horn GT, Mullis KB, Erlich HA. Primer-directed enzymatic amplification of DNA with a thermostable DNA polymerase. Science 1988;239:487.
65. Saiki RK, Scharf S, Faloona F, Mullis KB, Horn GT, Erlich HA, Arnheim N. Enzymatic amplification of β-globin genomic sequences and restriction site analysis for diagnosis of sickle cell anemia. Science 1985;230:1350.
66. Sambrook J, Fritsch EF, Maniatis T. Molecular Cloning, a Laboratory Manual, 2nd ed. Cold Spring Harbor, NY: Cold Spring Harbor Laboratory Press, 1989.
67. Sanger F, Nicklen S, Coulson AR. DNA sequencing with chain-terminating inhibitors. Proc Natl Acad Sci USA 1977;74:5463.
68. Schwartz DC, Cantor CR. Separation of yeast chromosome-sized DNAs by pulsed field gradient gel electrophoresis. Cell 1984;37:67.
69. Sharp PA. Split genes and RNA splicing. Cell 1994;77:805.
70. Shatkin AJ. Capping of eukaryotic mRNAs. Cell 1976;9:645.
71. Shatkin AJ. mRNA cap binding proteins: essential factors for initiating translation. Cell 1985;40:223.
72. Sherr CJ, Rettenmier CW, Sacca R, Roussel MF, Look AT, Stanley ER. The c-*fms* proto-oncogene product is related to the receptor for the mononuclear phagocyte growth factor, CSF-1. Cell 1985;41:665.
73. Singh H, Lebowitz JH, Baldwin AS, Sharp P. A molecular cloning of an enhancer binding protein: isolation by screening of an expression library with a recognition site DNA. Cell 1988;52:415.
74. Slamon DJ, Clark GM, Wong SG, Levin WJ, Ullrich A, McGuire WL. Human breast cancer: correlation of relapse and survival with amplification of the HER-2/*neu* oncogene. Science 1987;235:177.
75. Slamon DJ, deKernion JB, Verma IM, Cline MJ. Expression of cellular oncogenes in human malignancies. Science 1984;224:256.
76. Slamon DJ, Godolphin W, Jones LA, Holt JA, Wong SG, Keith DE, Levin WJ, Stuart SG, Udove J, Ullrich A, Press MF. Studies of the HER-2/*neu* proto-oncogene in human breast and ovarian cancers. Science 1989;244:707.
77. Smith HO. Nucleotide sequence specificity of restriction endonucleases. Science 1979;205:455.
78. Southern EM. Detection of specific sequences among DNA fragments separated by gel electrophoresis. J Molec Biol 1975;98:503.
79. Strand M, Prolla TA, Liskey RM, Petes T. Destabilization of tracts of simple repetitive DNA in yeast by mutations affecting DNA mismatch repair. Nature 1993;365:274.
80. Takahashi T, Nau MM, Chiba I, Birrer MJ, Rosenberg RK, Vinocour M, Levitt M, Pass H, Gazdar A, Minna JD. p53: a frequent target for genetic abnormalities in lung cancer. Science 1989;246:491.
81. Temin HM, Mizutani S. RNA-dependent DNA polymerase in virions of Rous sarcoma virus. Nature 1970;226:1211.
82. Thibodeau SN, Bren G, Schaid D. Microsatellite instability in cancer of the proximal colon. Science 1993;260:816.
83. Towbin H, Staehelin T, Gordon J. Electrophoretic transfer of proteins from polyacrylamide gels to nitrocellulose sheets: procedure and some applications. Proc Natl Acad Sci USA 1979;76:4350.
84. Urlaub G, Chasin LA. Isolation of Chinese hamster cell mutants deficient in dihydrofolate reductase activity. Proc Natl Acad Sci USA 1980;77:4216.
85. Vogelstein B, Fearon ER, Kern SE, Hamilton SR, Preisinger AC, Nakamura Y, White R. Allelotype of colorectal carcinomas. Science 1989;244:207.
86. Wang JC. DNA topoisomerases. Annu Rev Biochem 1985;54:665.
87. Waterfield MD, Scrace GT, Whittle N, Stroobant P, Johnsson A, Wasteson A, Westermark B, Heldin CH, Huang JS, Deuel TF. Platelet-derived growth factor is structurally related to the putative transforming protein p28^{sis} of simian sarcoma virus. Nature 1983;304:35.
88. Weber K, Osborn M. The reliability of molecular weight determinations by dodecyl sulfate-polyacrylamide gel electrophoresis. J Biol Chem 1969;244:4406.
89. Westin EH, Wong-Staal F, Gelmann EP, Dalla Favera R, Papas TS, Lautenberger JA, Eva A, Reddy EP, Tronick SR, Aaronson SA, Gallo RC. Expression of cellular homologues of retroviral *onc* genes in human hematopoietic cells. Proc Natl Acad Sci USA 1982;79:2490.
90. Whyte P, Buchkovich KJ, Horowitz JM, Friend SH, Raybuck M, Weinberg RA, Harlow E. Association between an oncogene and an anti-oncogene: the adenovirus E1A proteins bind to the retinoblastoma gene product. Nature 1988;334:124.
91. Wright DK, Manos MM. Sample preparation from paraffin-embedded tissues. In PCR Protocols: A Guide to Methods and Applications, Edited by MA Innis, et al. San Diego: Academic, 1989, p 153.
92. Yang Y-C, Ciarletta AB, Temple PA, Chung MP, Kovacic S, Witek-Giannotti JS, Leary AC, Kriz R, Donahue RE, Wong GG, Clark SC. Human IL-3 (multi-CSF).identification by expression cloning of a novel hematopoietic growth factor related to murine IL-3. Cell 1986;47:3.
93. Young RA, Davis RW. Efficient isolation of genes using antibody probes. Proc Natl Acad Sci USA 1983;80:1194.
94. Zaug AJ, Been MD, Cech TR. The Tetrahymena ribozyme acts like an RNA restriction endonuclease. Nature 1986;324:429.
95. Zinn K, DiMaio D, Maniatis T. Identification of two distinct regulatory regions adjacent to the human β-interferon gene. Cell 1983;34:865.

CHAPTER 3

Growth Factors

PAOLO FEDI, STEVEN R. TRONICK, AND STUART A. AARONSON

The evolution of multicellular organisms has involved the development of intercellular communication required for such processes as embryonic development, tissue differentiation, and systemic responses to wounds and infections. These complex signaling networks are in large part mediated by growth factors, cytokines, and hormones. Such factors can influence cell proliferation in positive or negative ways as well as inducing a series of differentiated responses in appropriate target cells. The interaction of a growth factor with its receptor by specific binding in turn activates a cascade of intracellular biochemical events that is ultimately responsible for the biologic responses observed. Cytoplasmic molecules that mediate these responses have been termed *second messengers.* The eventual transmission of biochemical signals to the nucleus leads to effects on the expression of cassettes of genes involved in mitogenic and differentiation responses.

Over the past few years it has become increasingly evident that the pathogenic expression of critical genes in growth factor-signaling pathways can contribute to altered cell growth associated with malignancy. The v-*sis* oncogene of simian sarcoma virus (SSV), which encodes a growth factor homologous to the B chain of human platelet-derived growth factor (PDGF-B), is the paradigm for such genes (70, 389). The normal counterparts of other oncogenes have been shown to encode membrane-spanning growth factor receptors (72, 331). Other genes that act early in intracellular pathways of growth factor signal transduction have been implicated as oncogenes as well. Present knowledge indicates that the constitutive activation of growth factor-signaling pathways through genetic alterations affecting these genes contributes to the development and progression of most, if not all, human cancers.

This chapter focuses on normal aspects of growth factor signaling, particularly those mediated by growth factor receptors possessing intrinsic protein tyrosine kinase activity. In addition, examples are provided where abnormalities in early steps in these pathways involving alterations in growth factor expression and/or receptor signaling have been implicated in the etiology of human malignancies. Finally, we will discuss how this knowledge may be useful in efforts to design new approaches toward therapeutic intervention with the malignant process.

The limits of space preclude a discussion of several important families of ligands and their receptors. These include the cytokines and their receptors that lack intrinsic tyrosine kinase activity but associate with cytoplasmic tyrosine kinases. Other ligand-receptor families including the tumor necrosis factor (TNF), the T-cell receptor, and the serine-threonine kinase receptor families, the last of which includes the transforming growth factor-beta (TGF-β) and activin receptors, will also not be discussed. There are excellent recent reviews concerning each of these topics (169, 241). Finally, a group of small peptides, classified as neurotransmitters, has been shown under certain conditions to stimulate proliferation (403). Their receptors, which possess seven transmembrane domains, interact with heterotrimeric G proteins. These neurotransmitters have also been the subject of review (198, 404).

Background

Hormones that act at great distances from the cells producing them have been known for many years. Hormones as signaling molecules were isolated from tissue fluids and readily characterized by their effects in vivo. In contrast, knowledge of growth factors is relatively recent. Growth factor activity capable of stimulating the growth of chicken embryonic nerve cells was found to be released by mouse sarcoma cells (191). During purification of this nerve growth factor (NGF), a second activity that promoted eyelid opening and incisor eruption in newborn mice and rats was discovered (44). Because of recognition of its effects on epithelial cells, this factor was designated epidermal growth factor (EGF). Since the early days of tissue culture, it was recognized that serum was important for growth of cell cultures. A major mitogenic activity found in serum was shown to be derived from platelets and was, therefore, designated platelet-derived growth factor (PDGF) (127, 306). Subsequent studies by several laboratories have led to detection of a series of growth factors that were often given names based on the tissue or cell of origin or the target cell initially found to be stimulated.

An important discovery concerning growth factors came from the demonstration of a unique enzymatic activity associated with binding of EGF to its receptor (28, 44). Studies of the product of the viral oncogene v-*src* had led to the demonstration of its ability to act as a protein kinase (23, 45, 139, 192). Many protein kinases had been previously identified, but these had the capacity to phosphorylate serine and/or threonine residues. Moreover, it was well-established

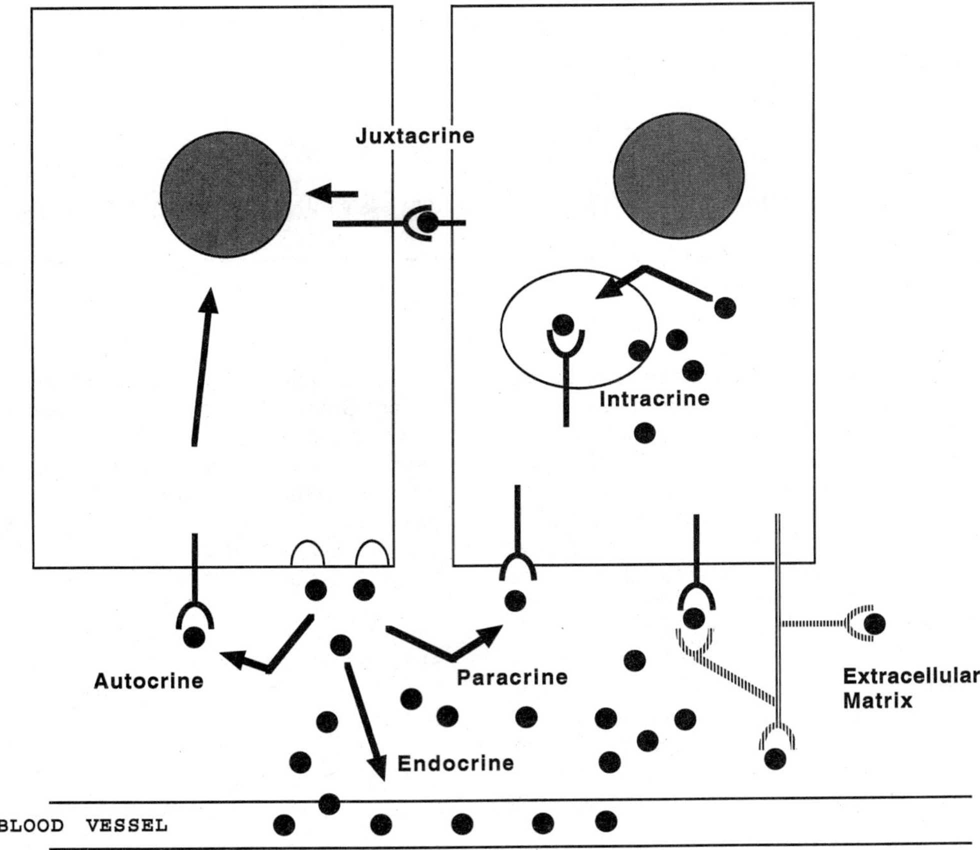

Figure 3.1. Different modes of action for growth factors (see text for specification).

that phosphorylations and dephosphorylations affected the activities of a variety of proteins. However, the *src* product was subsequently shown to have a unique specificity as a protein kinase in that it was capable of phosphorylating tyrosine residues (45, 139, 192). Cohen then showed that addition of EGF led to phosphorylation of tyrosine residues on its purified receptor (28, 44). Subsequent studies have demonstrated that the ability to perform this enzymatic function is central to the functions of a large number of mitogenic signaling molecules.

Several major modes of action for growth factors have been described. In 1980 Sporn and Todaro (346) defined *autocrine* and *paracrine* as major modes of action for growth factors, in addition to the classical means by which hormones travel great distances from their sites of production (Fig. 3.1). The autocrine mode refers to the ability of growth factor to act on the same cell releasing it. In the paracrine mode, the released growth factor from one cell acts on a nearby or adjacent cell. Certain growth factors also exist as membrane-anchored forms that can bind and activate membrane receptors only on adjacent cells. This process, considered a variant of the paracrine mode, has been termed *juxtacrine* (21, 219) and is capable of delivering spatially localized intercellular stimuli. Many researchers have observed that factors which are produced in cells but are not detectably secreted, nevertheless, can induce observable phenotypic changes in those cells. The suggestion has been made that this represents an "intracrine" mode of action, whereby the factor interacts with its receptor, for example, within the Golgi apparatus (197, 297). A sixth mode of action, in which the growth factor is bound to, and stored within, the extracellular matrix before presentation to the receptor on the cell surface, has also been demonstrated (170, 411). While this might be regarded as a separate mode, it is perhaps best thought of as a subdivision of endocrine, autocrine, and paracrine modes.

CLASSIFICATION OF GROWTH FACTORS

Platelet-Derived Growth Factor Family

PDGF is the major protein growth factor in human serum and is a markedly heat-stable, cationic protein that consists of two related but nonidentical (36.7% amino acid sequence identity) polypeptide chains designated A and B (also called PDGF-1 and PDGF-2) (70, 389). PDGF molecules exist as AA and BB homodimers as well as an AB heterodimer (127, 306). PDGF-AB is the major PDGF form found in platelets and is released into serum upon blood clotting; however, there is evidence for the natural occurrence of each of the other forms. Connective tissue and glial cells in culture are highly sensitive to the mitogenic effects of PDGF (125, 306), and it is these cells that express PDGF receptors. The α and

β PDGF receptors are encoded by distinct genes (39, 40, 222, 409), and there is evidence that they exist as receptor subunits that differentially interact with the three dimeric PDGF ligands (118, 120, 127, 222, 223). Thus, PDGF-AA can bind only the $\alpha\alpha$ receptor dimer while PDGF-BB can interact with $\alpha\alpha$, $\alpha\beta$, and $\beta\beta$ receptor dimers. The PDGF-AB heterodimer preferentially interacts with and triggers $\alpha\alpha$ and $\alpha\beta$ receptors and would bind the $\beta\beta$ receptor without, however, inducing its dimerization. This is an example of the fine degree of regulation that can evolve in the interactions of ligands with their receptors. Presumably in the case of PDGF, this relates to quantitative regulation of responses based upon differential availability in tissues of ligands and receptors, since there is evidence that the two PDGF receptors, themselves, are each capable of mediating the major known PDGF responses, including mitogenic signaling and chemotaxis (223, 400).

As noted earlier, the gene for the PDGF-B chain is the human homologue of the v-*sis* oncogene of SSV (70, 389). The transforming protein expressed by SSV shares close structural similarities with PDGF-B chain homodimers (301, 302). PDGF-B has been detected in human tumor cells that also possess PDGF receptors (41, 84, 101, 140). These findings, taken together with the demonstration that the normal PDGF-B gene can act as an oncogene when expressed at high levels (101), suggest that PDGF-B plays a role in the development of certain human cancers. The PDGF-A chain is frequently expressed by human tumor cells, and AA homodimers are produced by osteosarcoma (126), melanoma (394), and glioblastoma cells (257).

Efforts to identify factors that control angiogenesis recently led to the identification of a new growth factor that is a potent mitogen for vascular endothelial cells of small and large vessels (190). Vascular endothelial growth factor (VEGF) was initially isolated from conditioned medium of folliculostellate and bovine pituitary follicular cells using heparin-sepharose-affinity chromatography (91, 106, 288). At the same time another group reported the cloning of a transcript encoding a protein termed *vascular permeability factor* (VPF) (46, 165, 329, 330). Sequence comparisons revealed that VEGF and VPF are products of the same gene. VEGF/VPF is a glycosylated, dimeric heparin-binding protein (mol. wt. 45 kd) able to stimulate angiogenesis and to increase the permeability of capillary vessels to different macromolecules. The potent mitogenic effects of VEGF are restricted to cells of vascular endothelial origin. Even if VEGF/VPF does not show high sequence similarity to PDGF (18% overall identity with PDGF-B), they are related because each contains conserved cysteines that are the hallmark of growth factors belonging to this family (362).

VEGF 121, 165, 189, and 206 correspond in amino acid length to the four known isoforms. These arise from the alternative splicing of the primary transcriptional product. While VEGF 121 and 165 are secreted into the medium from producing cells, VEGF 189 and 206 are not efficiently secreted and seem to bind tightly to cell surface heparin-like molecules of producing cells (254). Substantial evidence indicates that the binding of VEGF 165, the best-studied form, to its receptor is dependent on cell surface-associated heparin-like molecules.

Placenta-derived growth factor (PIGF) is a member of this family whose expression appears limited to placenta (203). Two isoforms, one of which (PIGF-2) shows high-affinity binding to heparin, arise from the same gene (122). Colony-stimulating factor 1 (CSF-1) or macrophage colony-stimulating factor (MCSF) also belongs to this family (300). This molecule promotes the growth and maturation of monocytes and macrophage precursors. It also enhances the phagocytic and tumoricidal activity of human macrophage and monocytes and induces them to secrete a variety of different cytokines (115). Two active forms, one of which is secreted and the other cell associated, arise from differential splicing.

Stem-cell factor (SCF), also designated *kit ligand*, *mast cell growth factor*, *steel factor*, or *SLF*, is a hematopoietic and tissue growth factor that binds to the receptor encoded by the c-*kit* proto-oncogene (402). The naturally occurring form of this secreted molecule is a 165-amino acid polypeptide, which is heavily N- and O- glycosylated and exists as a dimer. Alternative splicing of the gene results in secreted and membrane-bound forms. The SCF/*kit* ligand is present at relatively high levels in human plasma, relative to most other cytokines. This growth factor does not stimulate hematopoietic colony formation itself but has been shown to augment proliferation in vitro of both myeloid and lymphoid hematopoietic progenitor cells in the presence of other cytokines (5, 94, 135, 215, 398, 419). It has been proposed that the SCF/*kit* ligand, produced locally in high concentrations by bone marrow stromal cells, acts as an "anchor" factor and permits stem cells to respond to physiologic concentrations of cytokines. It also promotes the activation of skin mast cells and basophils.

The cloning of a ligand for the Flt3 receptor was recently reported (201). This ligand shows similarity in the conserved cysteine residue with the *kit* ligand. This new molecule, for which several alternative splicing products have been described (202), stimulates the proliferation of a subpopulation of hematopoietic cells that are enriched for stem cells. The ligand is a transmembrane protein that undergoes proteolytic cleavage to generate a soluble factor. Both forms, soluble and bound to the cell surface, are biologically active.

Epidermal Growth Factor Family

EGF purified from mouse submaxillary glands was found to promote precocious eyelid separation by enhancing epidermal growth and keratinization while it induced early incisor eruption by enhancing the differentiation of the lips of treated animals (44). The proliferative effects of EGF on epidermal cells in organ and tissue cultures derived from avian and mammalian species were subsequently established. Some years later, the discovery was made that urogastrone (URO), a hormone with gastric antisecretory activity, was identical to EGF (44, 114). The role of EGF/URO in inhibiting gastric secretion long remained a mystery until Wright and co-workers (406) reported the induction of novel EGF/URO-secreting cells following mucosal ulceration. Although EGF/URO was known to be a potent mitogen for cells of the intestine when administered parenterally, it is not absorbed from the adult gut, nor does it have an effect when given through the gut lumen when the mucosa is intact. The new cells that form following ulceration of the human gastrointestinal tract eventually form a small gland that secretes EGF/URO whose proliferative effects stimulate ulcer healing. This is likely to be a major in vivo role of EGF/URO.

The EGF chain consists of 53 amino acids constrained by three internal disulfide bonds and is generated from a 1200-residue precursor with a remarkable structure (109, 327). That is, the sequence of the precursor includes eight units similar to EGF and a hydrophobic stretch near its carboxyl terminal such as those found in integral membrane proteins. The precursor has been detected as a glycosylated membrane protein in cells transfected with a prepro-EGF precursor and retains biologic activity similar to that of EGF (240).

Other members of this widely expressed EGF family include tumor growth factor-α (TGF-α), amphiregulin (AR), or schwannoma-derived growth factor (rat homolog of AR), heparin-binding EGF (HB-EGF), Betacellulin, the poxvirus mitogens (vaccinia [367], Shope [32], and myxoma [375] growth factors), and the Heregulin family. All of these molecules share sequence similarity, at least 28% sequence identity, and 100% conservation of the 6-cysteine residue present within the mature sequence of EGF. The EGF-like motif ($X_nCX_7CX_{2-3}GXCX_{10-13}CX\ CX_3YXGXRCX_4LX_n$) shown in each of these molecules is also present in diverse proteins found associated with the cell surface or extracellularly but that are not ligands for the EGF receptor (56). With the exception of the Heregulins, all of these proteins are able to bind to the EGF receptor and show mitogenic effects on EGF-responsive cells (303).

This class of ligands is synthesized as integral membrane precursor glycoproteins, and their extracellular domains contain an EGF-like sequence. It has been shown for EGF and TGF-α that the membrane-bound forms may interact with receptors on the surface of adjacent cells, thereby potentially contributing to cell-cell adhesion as well to cell-cell stimulation (219). Since many of these molecules bind and activate the same receptor, there appears to be substantial functional redundancy within this family. Nonetheless, quantitative differences in their biologic activities have been demonstrated. The findings that TGF-α is found in culture fluids from various oncogenically transformed cells (59, 363) gave rise to its designation as a *transforming growth factor.* TGF-α and EGF are almost indistinguishable in their ability to bind, activate, and down-modulate the EGF receptor in mammalian cells (363); however, TGF-α is more potent than EGF as an angiogenic factor in vivo (325) and in stimulating epidermal-cell colony formation in culture (13). Whereas EGF is normally expressed in kidney and submaxillary glands and is produced in response to gastrointestinal (GI) tract injury (44, 303, 406), TGF-α appears to be normally expressed by a variety of epithelial cells (61, 303).

AR is a bifunctional growth modulator that was initially purified from conditioned medium of a human breast adenocarcinoma, MCF-7, treated with phorbol 12-merystate 13-acetate (335). AR is a potent stimulator of normal keratinocytes and mammary epithelial cells (47, 336); however, it also inhibits the growth of some human carcinoma cell lines (47, 290, 335, 336). Relative to EGF, AR contains a very basic 40-amino acid stretch at its amino terminal, which is also rich in potential N- and O-linked glycosylation sites. Within this region, there are also two putative nuclear localization signals (336). In fact, AR has been detected in the nucleus as well as in the cytoplasm of treated cells (154, 155). The biologic importance of its nuclear localization is not yet understood. AR is a heparin-binding growth factor whose bioactivity can be inhibited by heparan sulfate (47). It has also been shown that extracellular heparan sulfate proteoglycans are essential for mediation of its mitogenic signal by EGFR (156).

HB-EGF, was initially purified from conditioned medium of macrophage-like U937 cells, and it is a more potent mitogen for smooth muscle cells than either EGF or TGF-α (128). It is also active on fibroblasts, but not endothelial cells. Like TGF-α and AR, HB-EGF is secreted by means of proteolytic processing of a transmembrane precursor. In some instances, this proteolytic processing does not occur with a high degree of fidelity. In fact, at least five different forms with amino terminal heterogeneity have been identified (129). Also, it has been recently demonstrated that the membrane-anchored form of HB-EGF acts as the diphtheria toxin receptor (231, 334).

Betacellulin was initially isolated from an insulinoma-derived cell line. It is a potent mitogen for retinal pigment epithelial cells and vascular smooth muscle cells (334). The relatively low-affinity of Betacellulin for the EGFR suggests that this ligand may act as a high-affinity ligand for some other related receptor.

Purification of rat and human stimulatory proteins for $p185^{neu}$, the second member of the EGF receptor family, led to the isolation of cDNAs encoding novel EGF-related proteins (17). The 44-kd rat factor, termed *Neu differentiation factor* (NDF), stimulates $p185^{neu}$ tyrosine phosphorylation and induces the production of milk components in certain breast carcinoma cell lines (280, 390). The homologous human factors, HRGs, were found to be mitogenic for certain mammary tumor cells (131, 200). At least 10 HRG isoforms have been described (391). For example, the acetylcholine receptor-inducing activity (ARIA) (85) and glial growth factors (GGF) (209) were found to represent isoforms of HRG. Multiple HRG isoforms are encoded by the same gene through alternative splicing of at least six recognizable domains: the amino terminal region, an immunoglobulin (Ig) motif, a glycosylation-rich spacer motif, an EGF-like domain, a hydrophobic transmembrane domain, and a cytoplasmic tail (391). The HRGs are classified into two groups, α and β, that differ in their EGF-like domains.

Recently, it has been discovered that two EGF receptor family members, $p180^{erbB3}$ and $p180^{erbB4}$, are the actual receptors for HRG/NDF, and the presence of one of these receptors is necessary for the HRG/NDF-stimulated tyrosine phosphorylation of $p185^{erbB2/neu}$ (368). Like TGF-α, HRGs display a wide distribution in many tissues and organs (391). Moreover, the expression patterns of some isoforms are tissue specific. For example the $\alpha 2$ isoform is the predominant form in mesenchymal tissues, while the $\beta 1$ isoform is enriched in brain tissue and spinal cord (391). Neuronal and nonneuronal tissues differ also in splicing of additional putative exons (391).

Fibroblast Growth Factor Family

Fibroblast growth factors comprise an expanding multigene family that exhibit mitogenic activity toward a wide variety of cells of mesenchymal, neuronal, and epithelial origin (15, 26). Because these proteins can bind to and have their biologic activities modulated by heparin, they have also been termed *heparin-binding growth factors* (HBGFs) (26, 170, 264). The family includes acidic FGF (aFGF, FGF-1), basic FGF (bFGF, FGF-2), *int*-2 (FGF-3), *hst*/KS3 (FGF-4), FGF-5, FGF-6, keratinocyte growth factor (FGF-7) (26, 34, 92, 211, 311, 361), androgen-induced growth factor (AIGF or FGF-8), and glia-activating factor (GAF or FGF-9). The first to be isolated, bFGF, was recognized in certain hormone preparations by its mitogenicity for fibroblasts and chondrocytes and was later purified from bovine pituitary. The factor aFGF was purified independently from acidic extracts of bovine brain (26, 34). Both acidic and basic FGF are angiogenic in vivo and are thought to function during embryogenesis. Both are single-chain polypeptides of about 17 kd and share 55% amino acid sequence identity. A striking feature of their structures, in contrast to those of other family members, is the lack of a consensus secretory signal peptide. This has generated a great deal of speculation about their mode of release from cells. It has been argued that they are liberated by lysis or escorted out of intact cells by other proteins. The presence of a nuclear translocation signal and detection of aFGF, as well as bFGF, in the nuclei of endothelial and mesenchymal cells, respectively (22, 315), have suggested that these growth factors may also act internally without requiring a secretory signal sequence (145).

Analysis of DNA of mammary tumors induced by mouse mammary tumor virus (MMTV) revealed that the viral genome frequently integrates within a genetic locus termed *int*-2 and thereby activates expression of this gene by insertional mutagenesis (343). The protein encoded by *int*-2, renamed FGF3, is predicted to be 245 amino acids long and highly similar to aFGF and bFGF. The normal expression of *int*-2 is apparently limited to embryonic tissues, and there is evidence from in vitro translation studies that it is a weak mitogen for mammary epithelial cells (69). Transgenic mouse experiments have shown that *int*-2 expression leads to mammary gland hyperplasia in female mice and benign epithelial hyperplasia in the prostate of males (242).

FGF-4 and FGF-5 were uncovered during searches for oncogenes in human tumor cells (26, 34, 361). FGF-4 was isolated independently from a human stomach tumor (*hst*) (355) and a Kaposi's sarcoma (KS3) (60). It is mitogenic for vascular endothelial cells, human melanocytes, and mouse NIH/3T3 fibroblasts (26). The FGF-5 gene was also isolated by DNA transfection, but by use of a selection system in which cell proliferation was dependent upon abrogation of growth factor requirements. Thus, DNA from a human bladder carcinoma cell line induced proliferation and morphologic transformation in the absence of added growth factors. FGF-5 was found to be activated by a DNA rearrangement that juxtaposed a retrovirus transcriptional enhancer upstream of its natural promoter. Partially purified FGF-5 preparations were found to be mitogenic for mouse fibroblasts and bovine heart endothelial cells (415).

An elegant demonstration of the critical importance of different FGF family members at specific phases of normal development derives from gene knockout experiments in mice. Such studies have shown that FGF-4 is required at a very early stage of development involving implantation of the embryo (89). The absence of FGF-5 is associated with a very different phenotype, in which affected mice develop apparently normally but show increased hair length following birth (G. Martin, personal communication).

Isolation of additional members of gene families is sometimes possible by low-stringency molecular hybridization employing probes derived from the most highly conserved sequences. FGF-6 was isolated by this approach from a cosmid library prepared from a human lymphoblastoid cell line and was shown to act as a transforming gene for NIH/3T3 cells by transfection analysis (211). Other biologic activities of FGF-6 have yet to be demonstrated.

KGF (FGF-7) was isolated from media conditioned by a human embryonic lung fibroblast cell line and was found to be a potent mitogen for epithelial cells but to lack activity on fibroblasts or endothelial cells (311). Thus, KGF is distinct in its target cell specificity, not only from other members of the FGF family but from all other known polypeptide growth factors as well. Molecular cloning and sequence analysis established KGF as a member of the FGF family, whose predicted amino acid sequence is about 38% identical to those of aFGF and bFGF (92). KGF transcripts show striking specificity of expression in stromal, but not epithelial, cells of most major epithelial tissues (92). There is also evidence that KGF plays an important role in epithelial renewal during wound repair (392) and as a stromal mediator of epithelial cell proliferation and differentiation in sex hormone-responsive tissues (3). All of these findings support the concept that this factor is important in the normal mesenchymal stimulation of epithelial cell growth.

AIGF (356) was isolated from media conditioned by a cell line derived from a testosterone-dependent mouse mammary tumor cell line. AIGF (FGF-8) is approximately equidistantly related to the other FGFs. Target cells include epithelial and fibroblast cells, and it appears to act in an autocrine fashion to stimulate the proliferation of the mammary carcinoma cells, from which it was isolated (317). It appears to be restricted to expression in the testes in the adult, and its expression during development is maximal during the period of reproductive tract development.

GAF/FGF-9 (232, 252) was purified from supernatants of a cultured human glioma cell line. It lacks an identifiable signal sequence but was found to be efficiently secreted from COS cells transfected with the cDNA. Little information is as yet available concerning its physiologic role.

Insulin Family

The diversity of metabolic effects of insulin have been studied intensively for decades (83). Its primary functions in vivo involve the regulation of rapid anabolic responses such as glucose uptake, lipogenesis, and amino acid and ion transport. In addition to its effects on metabolism, insulin stimulates DNA synthesis and cell growth. The insulin-like growth factors, IGF-1 and IGF-2, were first recognized as serum factors, antigenically distinct from insulin. These molecules are induced by growth hormone and serve as its effectors in stimulating growth of skeletal tissues (42). Subsequently, it was determined that somatomedin C is identical to IGF-1, while a polypeptide known as multiplication-stimulating factor (MSA) is homologous to IGF-2 (42).

The IGFs contribute to the insulin-like effects of serum on muscle and adipose tissue, but there are major differences between insulin and the IGFs. For example, while insulin levels fluctuate widely according to carbohydrate level, the IGFs are bound to carrier proteins and are maintained at steady concentrations in the bloodstream. The carrier proteins belong to a recently recognized class of proteins that have high affinity and specificity for the IGFs and are designated as insulin-like growth factor-binding proteins (IGFBP) (7). Five different IGFBPs have been identified in humans, and it seems that they are well conserved among mammals. The IGFBPs are involved in modulation of the proliferative and mitogenic effects of IGFs endocrine, paracrine, and autocrine levels (184).

At the structural level, IGF-1 and insulin share 48% of their amino acid sequences, and their similarity to IGF-2 is 50% (74, 371). Insulin is synthesized as a 109-amino acid precursor (preproinsulin) that is processed to a 6-kd protein consisting of two chains (A and B) linked by two disulfide bonds. The structures of IGF-1 and IGF-2 are analogous to that of proinsulin in that they consist of a single polypeptide chain.

Studies in vivo indicate that IGF-1 acts in an autocrine or paracrine mode, since infusion of IGF-1 does not give rise to its growth-promoting actions (42). Although it is not known whether overexpression of insulin family members can lead to transformation, a recent report has indicated that addition of exogenous IGF-1 or supraphysiologic levels of insulin to mouse NIH/3T3 cells overexpressing IGF-1 receptors introduced by transfection induced morphologic transformation and enabled the cells to grow in soft agar and form tumors in nude mice (159).

Hepatocyte Growth Factor

A growth factor apparently specific for hepatocytes, designated HGF, was isolated from plasma (105) or platelets (250). HGF levels were found to increase dramatically following acute liver injury, and, thus, HGF was reasoned to play an important role in liver regeneration. The biochemical and biologic properties of HGF were found to differ from those of other known growth factors (105, 250). The molecular weight of native HGF is around 90 kd and it consists of two polypeptide chains of about 70 and 34 kd linked by disulfide bonds (105, 250). Cloning of HGF cDNA showed that the growth factor is encoded as a single transcript, whose 728-amino acid product is processed by proteolytic cleavage into heavy and light chains (233, 251). Unexpectedly, the predicted amino acid sequence of HGF was found to be related to plasminogen (251). In addition to their 38% sequence identity, both molecules contain serine protease domains and disulfide bond-linked intrachain structures known as *kringles*. The latter are typical of prothrombin, tissue plasminogen activator, urokinase, and coagulation factor XII. Neither plasminogen nor plasmin has HGF-like activity, and HGF is not likely to be a protease since the histidine and serine residues in the region corresponding to the catalytic site are replaced by other amino acids.

HGF has been shown to have an expanding array of biologic activities. It is mitogenic for a variety of epithelial cells as well as endothelial cells and melanocytes. Independent studies by Stoker and co-workers led to purification of a motility factor, termed *scatter factor* (349), that is identical to HGF. HGF/scatter factor is also capable of inducing certain cell types to undergo morphogenesis when suspended in a semisolid matrix. For example, it induces tubule formation in canine epithelial cells, which undergo scattering under standard culture conditions. Thus, HGF/scatter factor is a mitogen, a motogen, and a morphogen as well (305). Recent studies have revealed that the HGF gene knockout is an embryonic lethal, leading to obvious abnormalities in liver and placenta development (322).

A ligand related to HGF, termed *HGF-like* (119) or macrophage-stimulating protein (MSP) (340, 413), is a heterodimer of a heavy chain of 53 kd (α) and a light chain of 25 kd (β). MSP shares with HGF the overall four-kringle protease domain-like structure. Liver appears to be the main source of MSP, and its major activity to date is stimulating macrophage migration.

Nerve Growth Factor Family

Substantial progress has recently been made in research on NGF and the other members of this related family of neurotrophic factors (the neurotrophins) (76, 207). Apart from NGF (192), which was discovered 40 years ago, this family includes brain-derived neurotrophic factor (BDNF), neurotrophin-3 (NT-3), neurotrophin-4 (NT-4), neurotrophin-5 (NT-5), and neurotrophin-6 (NT-6). These factors are produced in limiting amounts in their target tissues and mediate cell interactions regulating neuron survival during the period of naturally occurring neuronal death in development (76). The release of these proteins is believed to regulate not only the survival of neurons but also the extent of innervation of their target tissues (76). As well as being important in neuronal development, neurotrophic factors function in the adult nervous system.

NGF is a basic 118-amino acid protein that acts in sensory and sympathetic neurons in the peripheral nervous system (191). NGF is also present in the brain, where it serves a trophic function in the development and maintenance of cholinergic neurons of the basal forebrain (77). Brain-derived neurotrophic factor, BDNF, supports the survival of neural crest-derived embryonic sensory neurons in vitro (10, 187), and is expressed mainly in the central nervous system. NT-3 shows a strong sequence similarity to both NGF and BDNF, and displays a high degree of regional specificity. It is expressed in a subset of pyramidal and granular neurons in the hippocampus (79). NT-4 was isolated from *Xenopus* as a molecule showing the capacity to stimulate sensory neurons in culture. Soon after its isolation, another growth factor was isolated from human and rat and termed *NT-5*. However, the amino acid sequences of NT-4 and NT-5 were shown to be identical and, thus, to reflect the same gene (145). NT-6 distinguishes itself from the other known neurotrophins in that it is not found as a soluble protein in the medium of producing cells. The addition of heparin causes the release of NT-6 from the cell surface and extracellular matrix molecules (107). From studies of the recombinant neurotrophins, it is evident that, although the members of the NGF family share considerable sequence similarity, they have unique biologic activities and co-operate to support the development and maintenance of the vertebrate nervous system.

Ligands for *axl/ufo* Family

Protein S is a protease regulator that is a potent anticoagulant (54), and Gas 6 is a protein related to protein S but lacking any known function (208). These molecules have been recently shown to be the ligands for Sky and Axl, respectively, members of a previously orphan family of receptor tyrosine kinases (348, 378).

The critical role of protein S in the coagulation process is illustrated by the massive thrombotic complications suffered by infants homozygous for protein S deficiency (204, 279). It seems that protein S acts by indirectly inhibiting proteases involved in the coagulation cascade, although the precise mechanism remains unclear (54). Other functions, not directly involving coagulation, had been proposed for protein S (99, 206, 283). This 70-kd protein contains several modules, including an amino terminal region containing vitamin K-dependent γ-carboxylation sites, a thrombin-sensitive module, a series of EGF-like repeats that undergo hydroxylation modification, and a module with homology to steroid-binding globulin (54). Gas 6 was cloned as a growth arrest-specific gene (323) and shares all but the thrombin-sensitive module with protein S (208). It has been previously shown that other coagulation factors such as thrombin are able to bind and activate intracellular signaling via G protein-coupled cell surface receptors (382). It is possible to speculate that proteases and protease regulators, which activate specific cell surface receptors, may serve to integrate coagulation with associated cellular responses required for tissue repair and growth.

Ligands for *eph*-like Receptors

Four different proteins have recently been identified as ligands for the *eph*-like receptor tyrosine kinases (16, 95, 174). LERK-1, the ligand for *eph*-related kinase-1, was previously characterized as an early-response gene product (B6–1) (132) of IL-1 or TNF-treated human umbilical vein endothelial cells (68). LERK-1 is both an angiogenic factor and an endothelial chemotaxin (269). LERK-2 (or ELK-L), LERK-3/EHK1-L, and LERK-4 are three additional members of this family of cell surface-bound ligands. It has been shown that these molecules exhibit distinct but overlapping specificities for the *eph*-like kinases. They are able to function when presented in a membrane-bound form, suggesting that they require direct cell-to-cell contact to activate their receptors. Although the mechanism by which membrane attachment participates in receptor activation has not been established, the activity of clustered soluble forms of these ligands suggests that membrane attachment somehow facilitates dimerization or aggregation of these ligands (57).

Growth Factor Receptors That Possess Tyrosine Kinase Activity

Growth factors mediate their diverse biologic responses by binding to and activating cell surface receptors with intrinsic protein kinase activity (1). To date, more than 50 receptor tyrosine kinases (RTKs), which belong to at least 13 different receptor families, have been identified. All RTKs contain a large, glycosylated, extracellular ligand-binding domain, a single transmembrane region, and a cytoplasmic portion with a conserved protein tyrosine kinase domain. In addition to the catalytic domain, a juxtamembrane region and a carboxyl terminal tail can be identified in the cytoplasmic portion. Because of their configuration, RTKs can be envisioned as membrane-associated allosteric enzymes (373). In particular, RTKs have the ligand-binding domain and protein tyrosine kinase activity separated by the plasma membrane. Therefore, receptor activation due to extracellular ligand binding must be translated across the membrane barrier into activation of intracellular domain functions (reviewed in 1, 87, 124, 373). On the basis of sequence similarity and distinct structural characteristics, it is possible to classify these receptors into related groups (Fig. 3.2). Characteristic structural features of the extracellular domains of these groups include, among others, cysteine-rich motifs, immunoglobulin-like (Ig-like) repeats, fibronectin type III (FNIII) repeats, and EGF motifs that can be present singly or in different combinations.

There is substantial evidence that ligand-induced activation of the kinase domain and its signaling potential are mediated by receptor oligomerization (reviewed in 124, 373). After ligand binding, the subsequent conformational alteration of the extracellular domain induces receptor oligomerization. This event stabilizes interactions between adjacent cytoplasmic domains and leads to activation of kinase function by molecular interaction. Receptor oligomerization appears to be a universal phenomenon among growth factor receptors. Dimerization can take place between two identical receptors (homodimerization), between different members of the same receptor family, or between a receptor and an accessory protein (heterodimerization) (29, 188).

Dimerization of RTKs is responsible for activation of their intrinsic protein kinase activity and for autophosphorylation. Autophosphorylation occurs on two different classes of tyrosine residues. Autophosphorylation of certain conserved tyrosine residues within the kinase domains is commonly ob-

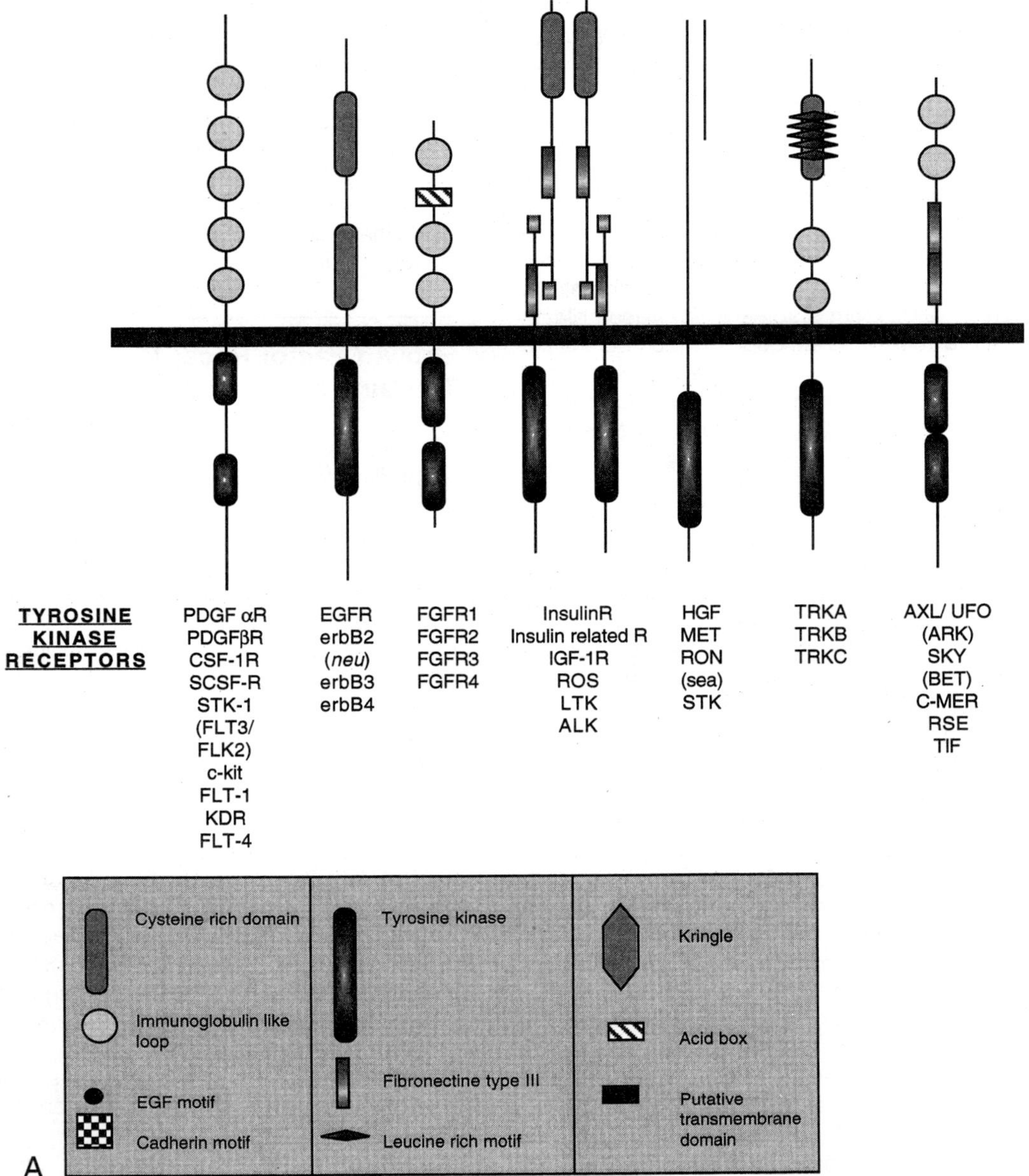

Figure 3.2. Families of receptor tyrosine kinases.

served. It is still not known how this autophosphorylation is initiated; one possibility is that the monomeric receptor has low basal kinase activity, which is sufficient to phosphorylate the companion receptor after dimerization. This would then be followed by reciprocal phosphorylation. Alternatively, the interaction between the intracellular domains of receptors in the dimer may induce a conformational change that leads to their increased kinase activity (124). The other class of autophosphorylation sites is normally localized outside the kinase domain and serves the important function of creating docking sites for downstream signal transduction molecules (see below).

Heterodimerization of RTKs has been shown to increase, on one hand, the repertoire of ligands that can be recognized by each receptor alone, and, on the other, to expand the diversity of signaling pathway that can be recruited by a given receptor. Interestingly, the insulin receptor family exists in the cell as disulfide-bonded homo- or heterodimers of receptor subunits. Thus, ligand binding does not induce receptor dimerization but presumably causes a conformational alteration in the preformed dimeric receptor that leads to receptor activation.

Most evidence indicates that the transmembrane domain does not directly influence signal transduction and is instead a passive anchor of the receptor to the membrane. Thus, the main function of the transmembrane domain would be to anchor the receptor in the plane of the plasma membrane, thereby connecting the extracellular environment with inter-

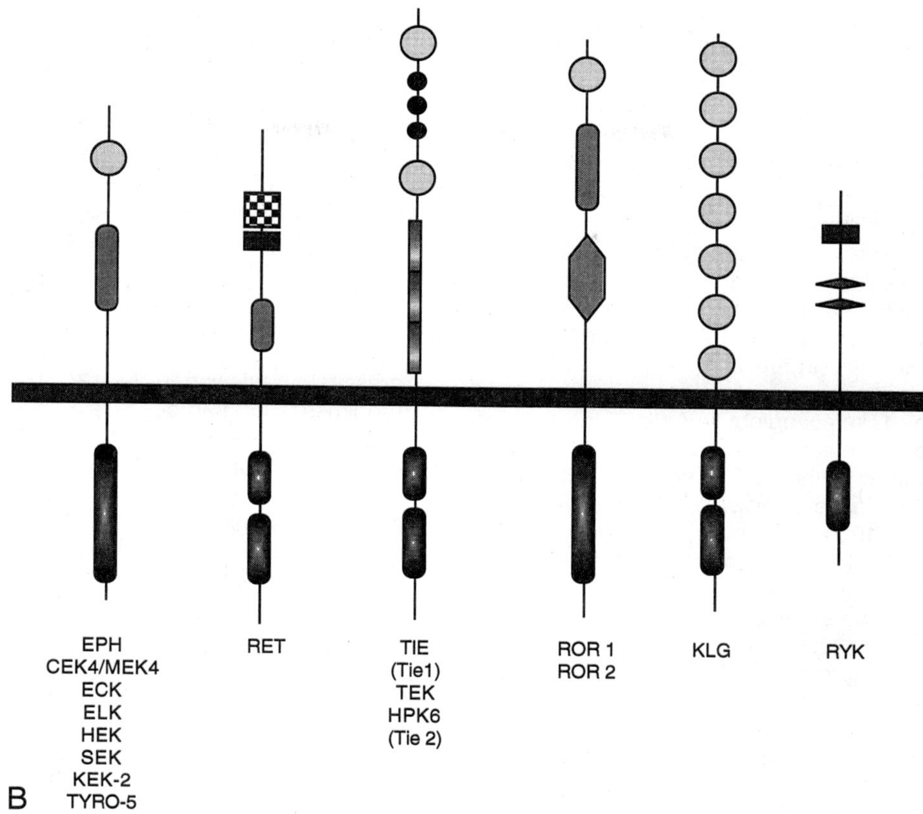

Figure 3.2. *(continued)*

nal compartments of the cell. It is important to note, however, that point mutations in the transmembrane domain of one receptor-like protein, the *neu/erb*B-2 protein, enhance its transforming properties (5). The transmembrane mutation in *neu* may have a stabilizing effect on this conformation, resulting in dimerization and constitutive activation of receptor signaling.

The juxtamembrane sequence that separates the transmembrane and cytoplasmic domains is not well conserved between different families of receptors; however, juxtamembrane sequences are very similar among members of the same family, and studies indicate that this stretch plays a role in modulation of receptor functions by heterologous stimuli, a process termed *receptor transmodulation* (373). For example, addition of PDGF to many types of cells causes a rapid decrease in high-affinity binding of EGF to its receptor. This has been shown to be a downstream effect of PDGF receptor activation in which protein kinase C, itself a serine protein kinase, is activated and, in turn, phosphorylates a site in the juxtamembrane domain of the EGF receptor (410).

The tyrosine kinase domain is the most conserved among tyrosine kinase receptors, and an intact protein tyrosine kinase domain is absolutely required for receptor signaling. For example, mutation of a single lysine in the ATP-binding site, which blocks the ability of the receptor to phosphorylate tyrosine residues, completely inactivates receptor biologic function. The kinase domain of some receptor tyrosine kinases (see Fig. 3.2) is divided into two halves by insertions of up to 100 mostly hydrophilic amino acid residues. The kinase inserts of these various receptors vary in length and show only marginal similarity. For a specific receptor, however, kinase insertion sequences are highly conserved between species, which suggests that they play an important role in receptor function. Thus, it appears that the role of the kinase insert region is to modulate receptor interactions with certain cellular substrates and effector proteins.

The carboxyl terminal tail sequences are among the most divergent between all known RTKs (410). The carboxyl terminal domain of the receptor is thought to play an important role in regulation of kinase activity. This region typically contains several tyrosine residues, which are phosphorylated by the activated kinase. In fact, the receptor itself is often the major tyrosine-phosphorylated species observed following ligand stimulation. Tyrosine phosphorylation of the carboxyl terminal domain has been postulated to modulate kinase catalytic activity, and/or the ability of the kinase to interact with substrates. Thus, mutations that alter individual tyrosine sites or deletions of the carboxyl terminal domain have the effect of attenuating kinase function in those receptors so far analyzed (410). Receptor tyrosine kinases catalyze the phosphorylation of exogenous substrates as well as tyrosine residues within their own polypeptide chains. The ability to molecularly clone related genes based upon the conserved nature of their kinase domains has led to the identification of several structurally related members of several receptor families, which are discussed next.

Platelet-Derived Growth Factor-Receptor Family

The PDGF receptor family includes PDGF-α and -β receptors, MCSF-1 receptor (MCSF-1R) also called CSF-1 receptor (CSF-1R); the SCF receptor (SCFR) or steel factor or c-*kit* receptor; and STK-1, the human homolog for the murine Flt3/Flk2 gene. One distinctive feature of these receptors is their extracellular regions, which show primary sequence characteristics and the same spacing of cysteine residues, consistent with the organization of five immunoglobulin-like domains (38). A similar organization is present in other membrane-spanning receptors without tyrosine kinase activity, including Thy 1, immunoglobulin A (IgA); the T-cell receptor, as well as interleukin 1 (IL-1) and 6 (IL-6) receptors (388). Another feature of the PDGF receptor family is the presence of a large kinase insert within the tyrosine kinase domain. These 80- to 100-amino acid stretches are highly divergent among different family members. There are reports that the kinase insert is required for interaction with certain substrates (163), and deletions in this domain impair receptor mitogenic signaling (82).

Two high-affinity receptors for VEGF have been identified. Both molecules are characterized by an extracellular region containing seven Ig-like domains and a tyrosine kinase interrupted by a large kinase insert. These receptors, termed *VEGFR-1/Flt-1* (*fms-like tyrosine* kinase-1) (67, 332) and *VEGFR-2/KDR/Flk-1* (*k*inase insert *d*omain-containing *re*ceptor/*f*etal *l*iver *k*inase-1) (220, 230, 261, 360), are expressed by vascular endothelial cells, although expression has been detected in certain hematopoietic cells, such as monocytes, as well as in melanoma cell lines. VEGFR-2 is reported as a major regulator of vasculogenesis and angiogenesis (246). VEGFR-1 is also associated with vascular development, and there is evidence that it may have a function in quiescent endothelium of mature vessels not related to cell growth. Thus, VEGF and its receptors act as a paracrine system to regulate the proliferation and differentiation of endothelial cells and neovascularization of tissues. A recent addition to this group is represented by Flt4, which is a receptor tyrosine kinase related to VEGFR that does not bind VEGF (98, 266). The extracellular domain of Flt4 is proteolytically cleaved into two disulfide-linked polypeptides (267, 268), and its expression by in situ hybridization has been detected in developing lymphatic vessels during the late stage of development (246).

EPIDERMAL GROWTH FACTOR/*erb* B-RECEPTOR FAMILY

There are four known members of the EGF-receptor family. They include (*a*) the EGF receptor (EGFR) (reviewed in 166, 293), (*b*) *erb* B-2 (also known as HER-2, for homologue of the human EGF receptor or c-*neu* for homologue of the rat proto-oncogene *neu*) (reviewed in 12, 71), (*c*) *erb* B-3 (175, 290), and (*d*) *erb* B-4 (291). The EGFR was identified and isolated by biochemical techniques, and shown to be the cellular homologue of the v-*erb* B, a retroviral oncogene (72, 408). The other members were isolated from genomic DNAs and cDNA libraries by low-stringency hybridization techniques using conserved tyrosine kinase domain probes. The extracellular domains of each of these molecules contain cysteine-rich motifs in two distinct regions and an uninterrupted tyrosine kinase domain (293).

While the EGFR and *erb* B-2 are expressed in a wide variety of cell types, the expression of *erb* B-3 is restricted to cells of epithelial or neuroectodermal origin (175). The four members of this family are normally coexpressed in various combinations in diverse tissues except in the hematopoietic system. It has been shown that they can act synergistically by heterodimer formation and can be influenced by receptor cross-talk (reviewed in 29, 124, 188). Ligand-induced heterodimerization has been demonstrated for EGFR and *erb* B-2, as well as *erb* B-2, and *erb* B-3 after exposure to EGF and HRG, respectively (4, 383). The *erb* B-3 product, p180$^{\text{erb B-3}}$, is unique among known tyrosine kinases, in that it shows a substitution in the four amino acid residues that are highly conserved or invariant in the catalytic domains of both serine/threonine and tyrosine protein kinases. This has raised the intriguing possibility that this receptor lacks, or has deficient, intrinsic tyrosine kinase activity. For this reason it has been proposed that *erb* B-3 becomes tyrosine phosphorylated after heterodimer formation with other members of this family, providing "docking sites" for proteins not recruited by autophosphorylation of kinase-active receptors (29). Gene amplification or overexpression of either the EGFR or *erb* B-2 associated with constitutive activation has been observed in a wide variety of human tumors (71, 166).

FIBROBLAST GROWTH FACTOR-RECEPTOR FAMILY

Another family of receptor proteins has the FGF receptor as its prototype (26). The receptors most closely resemble the PDGF-receptor family; instead, they contain extracellular domain variants with two or three immunoglobulin-like motifs instead of five (186). Moreover, the kinase insert within the tyrosine kinase domain of this receptor family is shorter (14 amino acids) than in members of the PDGF receptor (see Fig. 3.2). Between the first and the second Ig domain is a short domain referred to as the *acid box domain*. In FGFR1, this domain contains a core sequence of eight consecutive acidic residues. Following the TK domain is a carboxyl terminal domain of approximately 55 to 65 amino acids. Four distinct but related genes, FGFR1, FGFR2, FGFR3, and FGFR4, have been identified (well reviewed in 153, 173, 275). One FGF receptor gene is likely represented by *cek* 1 (chicken), *flg*, and N-*sam* (121) (both human). The *bek*, *cek* 3, and K-*sam* genes (121), from mouse, chicken, and human, respectively, represent another, while *cek* 2 (chicken) represents a different gene. Adding to this complexity are findings of alternatively spliced forms of FGF receptors expressed in different cell types. In the case of the FGFR1 and FGFR2 genes, multiple forms of the FGF receptor are generated via alternative splicing. Ig domain I and the acidic box are affected for FGFR1 and -2, and alternative transcripts appear to be responsible for generating three distinct carboxyl terminal domains in FGFR2. The second half of Ig domain III represents another site of alternative splicing in both FGFR1 and -2. Binding studies have shown that alternative splicing in this domain is important in determining ligand-binding specificities.

On the basis of binding studies, it has been proposed that tissues can achieve selective responsiveness to individual members of the FGF family through at least two mechanisms: tissue-specific alternative splicing in the third Ig domain, and/or tissue-specific differential gene expression. Evidence from tissue localization studies of the different receptor forms indicates that both of these mechanisms probably occur in vivo. After ligand binding, dimer formation likely occurs, but the complexity of heterodimeric interactions among different FGFR family members remains to be elucidated.

INSULIN RECEPTOR FAMILY

The insulin receptor (IR) is the prototype for a family of RTKs, whose distinctive structural feature is to function as a heterotetrameric aggregation of two α and two β subunits. The extracellular ligand-binding subunit, which contains a single cysteine-rich cluster, is disulfide linked to the transmembrane β subunit, which contains the cytoplasmic tyrosine kinase domain (78, 370, 372). The insulin receptor binds insulin with approximately 100-fold greater affinity than it does IGF-1 or IGF-2 (100 pM versus 10 nM). The IGF-1 receptor is closely related to the insulin receptor in sequence and structure but binds IGF-1 with highest affinity (100 pM), followed by IGF-2 and insulin. IGF-2 is also bound by another receptor, which has been shown to be identical to the cation-independent mannose-6-phosphate receptor. The IGF-2 receptor binds IGF-2 and IGF-1 with high affinity but does not bind insulin, and its role in IGF-2 signaling is not known (reviewed in 256, 307).

A gene encoding a third member of this family, called the *insulin receptor-related receptor* or IRR, was identified by low-stringency hybridization of Southern blots of human and guinea pig genomic DNA probed with fragments of IR cDNA (333). This new member of the IR family, unlike the genes encoding the receptors for insulin and IGF-1, has a more limited pattern of tissue expression. In situ hybridization studies revealed that IRR mRNA is most abundantly expressed in rats in sympathetic and sensory neurons and in renal distal tubule cells (298). The observed variation in expression during embryonic development suggests also that the IRR may be involved in neurogenesis. Like the other family members, the IRR is synthesized as a single polypeptide precursor that is proteolytically cleaved into α and β subunits. It has been shown that the IRR does not bind insulin or the other related molecules (158); however, the intrinsic kinase activity appears to phosphorylate endogenous proteins with a specificity very similar to that of the other two receptors of this family (416). It is possible that the IRR may form heterodimers with the IR or IGF-R. Alternatively, the IRR tyrosine kinase may be activated by an as yet unidentified ligand.

Owing to the high level of similarity of its TK domain to those of the IR and IGF-R, the c-*ros* proto-oncogene also belongs to this receptor family. The *ros* proto-oncogene is the cellular counterpart of the retroviral oncogene, v-*ros*, originally identified in the avian sarcoma virus UR2 (224, 387). The gene encodes a receptor-like PTK with an unusually large extracellular domain of nearly 2000 amino acids (20). It is closely related to the product of the sevenless gene from *Drosophila* (259, 344), which determines cellular fate during development of the compact eye. However, c-*ros* has not been, and does not appear to be, expressed in avian or mammalian eyes (344). In fact, hybridization in situ studies have indicated that c-*ros* is mainly expressed in epithelial cells of the renal collecting ducts and intestinal villi and crypts (344). A likely developmental role for c-*ros* has been implied, since expression of the proto-oncogene is detected only transiently during embryogenesis. The identification of a specific ligand should make it possible to better understand the functions of this protein.

The l*eukocyte* t*yrosine* k*inase* (*ltk*), another member of this TKR subfamily, is structurally most closely related to the c-*ros* protein (225). It has been shown that this TK receptor is expressed in B-lymphocyte precursors and forebrain neurons in the mouse (18) and in placenta and hematopoietic cells in humans (225). Recently, another member has been identified as being rearranged with the NPM nucleolar phosphoprotein gene in most anaplastic large-cell non-Hodgkin's lymphomas (236). This gene, termed a*naplastic* l*ymphoma* k*inase* (ALK), is normally expressed in the small intestine, testis, and brain, but not in normal lymphoid cells.

THE *met* RECEPTOR FAMILY

The oncogene c-*met* was initially identified as a rearranged oncogene in a human osteogenic sarcoma cell line transformed in vitro with a chemical carcinogen (48). This proto-oncogene encodes a 190-kd glycoprotein that is processed to form a heterodimer comprised of a 50-kd alpha chain and 145-kd beta chain. The extracellular, membrane, spanning, and tyrosine kinase domains are located on the beta chain. The oncogene c-*met* is expressed in a variety of tissues and cell types, but the highest levels are found in epithelial cells (30, 66, 148). The expression of HGF/SF was first detected in mesenchymal cells of various organs and in particular in stromal and non-parenchymal cells' neighboring epithelia (reviewed in 305, 379). The c-*met* receptor initiates all of known responses to HGF/SF mitogenesis including motility and morphogenesis.

The oncogene *ron* was identified and isolated as a c-*met*-related gene from cDNA libraries of human keratinocytes and a gastric carcinoma (304) by means of degenerate oligonucleotides. Its cDNA encodes a glycosylated protein that shares overall similar topology with the HGF receptor and displays 63% sequence identity in its catalytic domain as well as a similar tissue distribution. The $p185^{ron}$ product, like that of c-*met*, is synthesized as a single-chain precursor, which is converted into the mature form by proteolytic cleavage. The ligand for *ron* is the macrophage-stimulating protein (MSP) (100).

The avian erythroblastosis virus S13-encoded oncogene, v-*sea*, derives its name from the ability of the virus to cause sarcoma, erythroblastosis, and anemia (342). Its cellular homolog c-*sea* shows structural similarity to c-*met* and is expressed particularly well in peripheral white blood cell populations (137). Another member of this family was recently isolated from a murine hematopoietic stem cell and is designated STK for *s*tem cell-derived *t*yrosine *k*inase (147). STK is expressed at various stages of hematopoietic cell differentiation, but has not been detected in other adult tissues. Ligands for c-*sea* and STK remain to be identified.

NEUROTROPHIN RECEPTORS

The neurotrophins are thought to play central roles in neural development and regeneration through two distinct classes of receptors (reviewed in 76, 103, 207). One of these classes is represented by the p75/p80 LNGFR (low-affinity NGF receptor) protein (152, 295). This receptor is a glycoprotein that is highly conserved across species and is broadly expressed in neuronal and nonneuronal tissues. The extracellular region of the LNGFR contains a cysteine-rich domain (33), while the intracellular domain is not related to any known protein and has no known enzymatic function. Low-affinity binding (K_d 10^{-9} M) of all tested neurotrophins is mediated via this LNGFR, although its physiologic functions are not yet well understood (76, 207). The second class of neurotrophin receptors is encoded by the *trk* genes. As a result of efforts to isolate oncogenes from human tumor cells, *trk* or *trk*A was discovered (171). The other two members of the family, *trk* B (172) and *trk* C (183), were isolated by screening mammalian cDNA libraries with the *trk* A proto-oncogene as probe. In contrast to the LNGFR, the cytoplasmic regions of $p140^{trkA}$, $p140^{trkB}$, and $p145^{trkC}$ contain tyrosine kinase catalytic domains. Their extracellular regions contain Ig-like and FNIII domains, in addition to cysteine clusters alternated with leucine motif repeats (260, 294).

Each member of the *trk* family can bind at least one member of the neurotrophin family (76, 103, 207). While there are obvious preferences for binding of a particular neurotrophin to one of the *trk* family members, there is some promiscuity (76, 103, 207). In summary, $p140^{trkA}$ binds and becomes activated by NGF, NT-3, NT-4, and NT-5, but not BDNF. The $p140^{trkB}$ binds and is activated by BDNF, NT-3, NT-4, and NT-5, but not NGF. The *trk* C product is activated by NT-3, but not NGF or BDNF. Thus, at least three high-affinity receptors confer different but not absolute specificities for these related ligands.

Recently, a number of new RTKs (DDR/CAK/*trk* E, NEP and ptk3, TKT and tyro 10) (65, 157, 160, 182, 282, 314, 414) have been identified with several features that are unique to the *trk* family in the kinase domain; however, the extracellular domains consist of a combination of several motifs, including the constant (c1 and c2) domains of the blood coagulation Factors V and VII (150, 405) and A5, a putative retinotectal neuronal recognition protein identified in *Xenopus laevis* (357). Some members of this putative new family contain also a discoidin-1-like sequence (157). Discoidin-1 is a lectin found in *Dictyostelium discoideum*, where it is involved in cell aggregation (345).

ufo/axl RECEPTORS FAMILY

The *ufo* gene, also designated *axl* (from the Greek, *anexelekto*, "uncontrolled"), was identified and isolated independently as a transforming gene from patients with chronic myelogenous leukemia and myeloproliferative disorder, respectively, by DNA transfection-tumorigenicity analysis (149, 260). The murine homologue, *ark* (for *a*dhesion *r*elated *k*inase), was cloned on the basis of relatedness to the tyrosine kinase domain of one of the fibroblast growth factor receptors (299). The encoded *ufo/axl/ark* proteins define a new family of receptor tyrosine kinases that feature a new sequence in their cytoplasmic tyrosine kinase domains and an extracellular domain that juxtaposes two Ig-like domains and two FNIII repeats. A similar external domain topology has been observed among several neural cell adhesion molecules as well as a receptor tyrosine phosphatase (52, 350). Although the functions of the Ig-like and FNIII domains are not understood, their presence in numerous cell adhesion molecules and receptors suggests a potential function in cell-cell interactions. *ufo/axl* Expression has been detected in the majority of cell types examined (88, 149, 299). The nearly ubiquitous expression of *axl* suggests an important normal cellular function for this RTK.

In the attempt to isolate the human cellular homolog of the avian v-*sea* oncogene by means of reduced-stringency hybridization, another member of the *axl/ufo* family was identified and designated *sky* for *s*ea-related protein tyrosine *k*inase for t*y*rosine (262). The encoded protein showed around 64% amino acid identity with *axl/ufo*. Northern blot analysis further revealed that *sky* mRNA is expressed predominantly in brain (262). It has been proposed that *sky* may be involved in cell adhesion processes, particularly in the central nervous system (262). Its murine homologue has been designated *brt* for *br*ain *t*yrosine kinase (97).

Another family member was isolated from a human B-lymphoblastoid λgt11 expression library screened using antiphosphotyrosine antibodies in the attempt to identify novel B-cell *TKs* (108). Sequence comparisons showed that this gene, c-*mer*, may be the human homologue of the recently isolated chicken retroviral oncogene, v-*ryk* (renamed v-*eyk*), a truncated tyrosine kinase whose expression by retroviral infection produced sarcomas in chickens (151). Since the *ryk* designation has been used to name another tyrosine kinase (see below), the designation c-*mer* has been suggested based on its expression pattern in *m*onocytes and tissues of *e*pithelial and *r*eproductive origin. At least two other RTKs belong to this family: *rse* (for *r*eceptor *se*ctatoris) (212) and *tif* (for *t*yrosine kinase with *i*mmunoglobulin-like and *f*ibronectin III structure) (55). While *rse* is expressed at high levels in brain, *tif* shows high expression in human ovary and testis. *Tif* differs from all other members of this family in that its extracellular domain contains only one Ig loop and one FNIII structure. Recent findings that ligands for these receptors are members of a family of vitamin K-dependent proteins, involved in blood coagulation (348, 378) should help to provide insights into the physiologic roles of this family of receptors.

eph FAMILY

The *eph*-like proteins are the largest subfamily of RTKs (reviewed in 365). At least seven distinct genes that encode *eph*-like proteins have been identified, and partial cDNA sequences indicate that there may be at least five other members. These genes encode proteins of approximately 130 to 135 kd, including *eph*, *eck*, *elk*, *cek5*, *hek* (*mek4* and *cek4* appear to be murine and avian homologs, respectively), and *cek5*.

The extracellular region of these proteins contains a region with very weak similarity to an Ig-like loop, a cysteine-rich region that differs from those present in EGFR, and insulin receptor subfamilies followed by two FNIII domains (365). The presence of this last set of repeats has led to speculation that these receptors may also be involved in cell adhesion processes. The tyrosine kinase domains of the *eph*-like receptors do not contain kinase-insert sequences and are followed by a carboxyl terminal domain of approximately 90 to 100 amino acids.

While the *eph*-like receptors as a group are differentially expressed throughout the body, all members are expressed with a specific distribution in both the developing and the adult nervous system. The very recent discovery of ligands for this family should facilitate the study and the understanding of their physiologic roles (16, 95, 174).

ORPHAN RECEPTORS

The identification of new RTKs implies the existence of new growth factors as well. Several RTKs await the assignment of ligands. This group of "orphan receptors" presently includes *ret*, *tie*, *ror*, *klg*, and *ryk*.

The c-*ret* proto-oncogene (354, 358) encodes an RTK whose extracellular domain shows a unique feature, the presence of sequences similar to cadherin repeats (324). This motif is known to play an important role in Ca^{++}-dependent homophilic binding in other proteins (324). So far, only the c-*ret* protein, among all the RTKs, is known to contain this sequence. High levels of *ret* expression are detected in the peripheral nervous system (including enteric and autonomic) as well as in the excretory system during embryogenesis (265). In addition, *ret* is expressed preferentially in human tumors such as neuroblastoma, pheochromocytoma, and thyroid medullary carcinoma (142, 316). The *ret* mutations, which constitutively activate its tyrosine kinase, are carried in the germ line of families with multiple endocrine neoplasia type 2 (MEN-2) (reviewed in 289). This represents the only known example to date of a hereditary tumor caused by genetic transmission of an activated oncogene.

The *tie* (*t*yrosine kinase with *i*mmunoglobulin and *e*pidermal growth factor homology domains) family of RTKs includes two receptors that are specifically expressed in endothelial cells (75, 146, 205, 274, 318, 326, 417). The TIE (tie-1 is the murine homologue) and the HPK-6/TEK (*t*unica interna *e*ndothelial cell *k*inase) (tie-2 in the mouse) are characterized in their extracellular domains by two Ig-like loops separated by three EGF-like domains, followed by three FNIII repeats. These receptors are thought to be involved in angiogenesis and maintenance of endothelial cell function (246).

Two related genes, *Ror*-1 and *Ror*-2 (214), define another family of receptors whose extracellular domains contain Ig-like, cysteine-rich, and kringle domains. Their tyrosine kinase domains are followed by serine/threonine- and proline-rich motifs. These receptors were originally identified on the basis of the similarity of their TK domains to the *trk* family of neurotrophin receptors. Both are widely expressed and at high levels during early rat embryonic development. Dror is the corresponding gene in *Drosophila* (401), where it is expressed specifically in the developing nervous system.

The receptors *klg* and RYK represent two other distinct tyrosine kinase receptors. The *k*inase-*l*ike *g*ene, *klg*, was isolated from a cDNA library prepared from embryonic chicken tissues utilizing as a probe the v-*sea* oncogene (35). The receptor *klg* is a member of the immunoglobulin gene superfamily (24), with seven Ig-like loops in its extracellular domain. The gene *ryk* (*r*elated to t*y*rosine *k*inase) (133, 347), a ubiquitously expressed gene, encodes a protein containing two putative transmembrane segments and two leucine-rich motifs in the extracellular domain (359). The functional significance of these two genes is not known because efforts to demonstrate their tyrosine kinase activity have not yet been successful. Moreover, both genes show several unusual sequence idiosyncrasies in some of the most highly conserved elements of the conserved TK.

Growth Factor Signaling Pathways

STRINGENT REGULATION OF MITOGENIC RESPONSIVENESS TO GROWTH FACTORS

Growth factors cause cells in the resting or G_0 phase to enter and proceed through the cell cycle (1). The mitogenic response occurs in two parts; the quiescent cell must first be advanced into the G_1 phase of the cell cycle by "competence" factors, traverse the G_1 phase, and become committed to DNA synthesis under the influence of "progression" factors (286, 287) (see Chapter 1). Transition through the G_1 phase requires sustained growth factor stimulation over a period of several hours. If the signal is disrupted for a short period of time, the cell reverts to the G_0 state (393). There is also a critical period in G_1 during which simultaneous stimulation by both factors is needed to allow progression through the cell cycle (189, 190, 395). After this restriction point, only the presence of a "progression" factor, such as insulin-like growth factor 1 (IGF-1), is needed (270). Cytokines such as transforming growth factor β (TGF-β), interferon, or TNF can antagonize the proliferative effects of growth factors. In the case of TGF-β, these effects can be observed even when cells are treated with the cytokine relatively late in G_1 (238).

In some cell types, the absence of growth factor stimulation causes the rapid onset of programmed cell death or apoptosis (399, 407). Certain growth factors can also promote differentiation of a progenitor cell while they stimulate proliferation; others acting on the same cell induce only proliferation (229). Thus, there must be a specific biochemical signal responsible for differentiation that only certain factors can trigger (104, 227, 386). The action of a series of growth factors can cause a hematopoietic progenitor to move through stages to a terminally differentiated phenotype (229); however, at intermediate stages, in the absence of continued stimulation by the growth factor, this commitment may be reversible (284). Although the differentiation program of the cell governs the diversity of phenotypic responses elicited, there are some common, highly conserved biochemical pathways for mitogenic signaling. For example, transfection of cells with DNA encoding foreign receptors often allows coupling of the appropriate ligand to mitogenic signal transduction pathways inherently expressed by the cells (309, 285). The same RTK can also inhibit or cause cell proliferation when expressed in different cellular environments. For example, NGF and other neurotrophic factors elicit neuronal survival and differentiation upon activation of different members of the *trk* family of RTKs (49, 102, 196); however, NGF stimulation of the *trk* RTK induces proliferation of transfected fibroblasts (9).

GROWTH FACTOR RECEPTOR SIGNALING

Knowledge of signal transduction by RTKs has expanded dramatically over the past few years. It is not possible to cover this research topic exhaustively in this chapter. Several excellent reviews on the general events in signal transduction and on the specific signaling molecules involved have recently been published (27, 87, 124, 162, 213, 277, 278, 320, 321, 373) (see Chapter 4). It is well established that activation of intrinsic receptor kinase activity leads to tyrosine phosphorylation of a variety of intracellular substrates. The tyrosine phosphorylated RTK, or its substrates, then associate with intracellular signal enzymes that are the effectors of the RTK. These signaling molecules mediate the pleiotropic responses of cells to growth factors.

It is now clear that receptor autophosphorylation acts as a switch for the recruitment of specific substrates. The association between the tyrosine-phosphorylated regions in the RTK and the signaling proteins is mediated by a conserved region of approximately 100 amino acids termed the *src homology-2* (SH2) domain present within such molecules. These domains represent recognition motifs for specific tyrosine phosphorylated peptide sequences that direct binding of the target proteins to the receptor at specific sites of tyrosine autophosphorylation. Similarly, phosphorylation of the initial set of target proteins by the receptor allows recruitment of additional sets of proteins.

Receptor-binding proteins include a class, which, in addition to their SH2 domains, contain distinct enzyme activity. The SH2 domains of this class of signaling molecules directly mediate their interactions with the tyrosine phosphorylated receptor and other tyrosine phosphorylated proteins. These proteins include phospholipase C-γ in the protein kinase C pathway (25, 210, 228, 237, 384, 385); p91, a component of the ISGF-3 transcriptional factor in the STAT pathway (51, 96, 179, 235, 312, 313, 338, 366); p120-GAP in the Ras pathway (8, 138, 180, 364, 397); Src family cytoplasmic tyrosine kinases (51, 179, 235, 366); and phosphotyrosine phosphatases, such as Syp/SH-PTP2 (90, 164, 177, 185, 353, 381, 412). The second class of SH2-containing proteins is thought to function as adaptors or regulatory components of specific catalytic subunits. These SH2-containing proteins include the p85 regulatory component of the phosphatidylinositol 3-kinase (PI3-kinase) (272), Shc and Grb2 in the Ras pathway (199, 310), the proto-oncogene Vav product (134, 245), and Crk (221).

Recruitment to phosphorylated tyrosine residues on the receptors leads to activation of signaling molecules by several mechanisms (reviewed in 320). For example, tyrosine phosphorylation in the case of phospholipase C-γ and SH-PTP2 tyrosine phosphatase leads to enzymatic activation (381, 385). Conformational changes are induced by binding of the SH2 domain to phosphotyrosine for the PI3-kinase (50, 272). Alteration of subcellular location occurs in the case of translocation to the plasma membrane and stimulation of Ras guanine nucleotide exchange by Sos, which is recruited through interaction with Grb-2 and/or SHC adapter proteins (320). One exception to this scheme is represented by the insulin receptor. Autophosphorylation of the insulin receptor β subunit is not associated with strong binding of SH2-containing proteins. The principal insulin receptor substrate is a 165- to 185-kd protein, IRS-1. This is a docking protein that then complexes with several SH2-containing signaling molecules (248, 351, 352, 396).

It is known that growth factors can cause cytoskeletal changes, and recent evidence has shown that cytoskeleton elements can also be targets for RTKs. Sequence analysis of tensin, a protein that appears to link actin filaments to focal contact points at the membrane, has revealed the presence of an SH2 domain (58). Finally, SH2 binding to activated RTKs does not seem to be specific only for tyrosine phosphorylated residues. In fact, it has been demonstrated that, in the BCR-*abl* fusion product, which arises from a genetic translocation in CML, BCR can bind to the *abl* SH2 domain after it becomes highly phosphorylated on serine (281).

Abnormalities Associated with Growth Factors in Cancer Cells

Evidence establishing the role of growth factors in the process of transformation in vivo was provided by the demonstration that the v-*sis* oncogene encoded a protein closely related to human PDGF-B (70, 389), and that MMTV induction of mammary carcinoma in mice correlated with integration of the provirus in the region of the int-2 (FGF-3) gene (343). Moreover, the FGF-4 and FGF-5 genes were isolated by their ability to cause transformation of mouse fibroblasts in vitro (26, 34, 361). By extrapolation, it follows that the expression of any growth factor and its specific receptor by the same cell could establish an autocrine loop that contributes to tumor progression. In fact, the ability of autocrine stimulation to induce a tumorigenic phenotype in established cell lines has now been demonstrated under a variety of experimental conditions. After transfection of cDNA expression vectors encoding the specific factor and receptor, such cells overcome their growth factor dependence and become tumorigenic (43, 112, 141, 376). It should be noted however, that normal cells also have the capacity to produce growth factors under conditions that can activate autostimulatory pathways.

Autocrine transforming interactions have been identified in

a number of human malignancies. At least one PDGF chain and one of its receptors have been detected in a high fraction of sarcomas as well as in glial-derived neoplasms (127, 222, 226, 258). In tissue culture, such tumor cells exhibit evidence of a functional autocrine loop, in which chronic PDGF receptor activation can be demonstrated by the detection of tyrosine phosphorylated receptors and/or downregulation of the receptor protein. Thus, it appears that inappropriate expression of PDGF often plays an important role in such tumors.

TGF-α is often detected in carcinomas that express high levels of EGF receptors (61, 64). The role of acidic or basic FGF in tumors is less well established. Since neither of these molecules possesses a secretory signal peptide sequence, their normal route of release by cells is not the classical secretory pathway by which growth factor receptors are processed (26, 34); however, recent studies have demonstrated the expression of bFGF by human melanoma cell lines but not by normal melanocytes (116). Moreover, only the former require bFGF for proliferation in culture (117). Evidence that antagonists of FGF can inhibit growth of melanoma cells argues for a role of bFGF in the uncontrolled growth of these cells (116). Since many more ligands for tyrosine kinase receptors have recently been identified, the contribution of autocrine loops to human malignancies is probably much more extensive than is presently documented.

Small-cell lung carcinomas are thought to be of neuroectodermal origin. Cuttitta and colleagues (53) reported that secretion by such tumors (234) of bombesin-like peptides was growth stimulating. The receptor has been recently identified and is a G-protein-coupled membrane-spanning receptor (218). Antibodies to bombesin have been reported to inhibit proliferation of the small-cell carcinoma cell lines both in vitro and in vivo (244). Thus, bombesin appears to play a role as an autocrine growth factor in such tumors.

While several growth factors have been shown to induce transformation by an autocrine mode, it is also worth considering the possible role that growth factors might have in predisposing to cancer. It can be hypothesized that overexpression of growth factors by a paracrine mode might increase the proliferation of a polyclonal target cell population. This conceivably could increase the frequency of spontaneous genetic changes in the population, eventually selecting for a cancer cell. By such a model, increased production of a growth factor might act in a manner analogous to that of a tumor promoter. At the present time, this model is speculative and awaits experimental test.

Aberrations Affecting Growth Factor Receptors in Tumor Cells

While growth factor receptors can be constitutively activated by autocrine loops, a number of other mechanisms have been identified by which growth factor receptors can become transforming. Retroviral transduction of proto-oncogenes can result in mutation of the normal version of the gene. The paradigm for such alterations is v-*erb* B, the oncogenic counterpart of the EGF receptor, transduced as the viral oncogene of avian erythroblastosis virus (72, 408). The mechanism of v-*erb* B activation involved deletion of its ligand-binding domain, resulting in a truncated EGF receptor.

More subtle mutational changes are responsible for oncogenic activation of v-*fms*, whose normal homologue is the CSF-1 receptor (331). Here, a small genetic alteration affecting the external domain of the molecule was responsible for constitutive activation of this receptor as an oncogene (308). The avian v-*ros* oncogene differs from its cellular counterpart, c-*ros*, in that the entire extracellular domain is deleted with the exception of six amino acids and contains a three-amino acid insertion in the middle of the transmembrane domain (418). This results in constitutive activation of the molecule. Other examples are represented by v-*sea*, v-*sis*, and v-*kit* (see sections above). The *neu* was initially identified as an oncogene by NIH/3T3 transfection analysis (319) of cDNA from ethylnitrosourea-induced rat neuroblastomas. The transforming gene was identified as having a specific mutation in its transmembrane domain responsible for oncogenic activation (11). Recently, a novel activating mutation in the *neu* gene has been shown to be involved in induction of mammary tumors arising in transgenic mice generated with the *neu* proto-oncogene (337). The altered *neu* transcript bears in-frame deletions affecting the extracellular domain of the encoded protein.

In human malignancies, overexpression of a normal receptor, with or without the concomitant presence of the ligand, contributes to neoplastic transformation. Examples include the EGFR (63, 380), *erb* B-2 (62), the IGF-1 receptor (159), CSF-1R (309), eph (217), and *axl/ufo* (260). The most well-characterized mechanistically involve EGFR family members. Initially, *erb* B-2 was identified as an amplified gene in a primary human breast carcinoma (167) and a salivary gland tumor (328). Moreover, *erb* B-2 overexpression beyond some critical threshold level in NIH/3T3 fibroblasts was shown to be sufficient to induce the malignant phenotype (62). Clinical studies have indicated that the normal *erb* B-2 gene is frequently amplified and/or overexpressed in human breast carcinomas as well as in ovarian carcinomas (176, 253, 273, 377), and there is evidence that detection in breast carcinomas of high levels of the *erb* B-2 protein may be a prognostic indicator of poor survival (181, 341). Thus, *erb* B-2 appears to be most commonly altered in human malignancies by mechanisms leading to its overexpression.

Whereas *erb* B-2 overexpression has been observed primarily in adenocarcinomas, overexpression of an apparently normal EGF receptor has been reported frequently in squamous cell carcinomas (168) and glioblastomas (195). In many cases, the EGFR appears to be activated by autocrine stimulation by one of its ligands, most commonly TGF-α.

Genomic alterations such as mutation or rearrangement have also been shown to activate the transforming capacity of receptor tyrosine kinases in human malignancies. In some human tumors, deletions within the external domain of the EGFR receptor are associated with its constitutive activation, independent of ligand. Structural rearrangements involving *ret*, *trk*, and *met*, have also been observed. The *ret* gene is activated by rearrangement, as a somatic event, in about one third of papillary thyroid carcinomas (113); however, this is not the only mutation that activates the transforming capacity of this receptor. Germ line mutations affecting the cysteine residues in the extracellular region are responsible for multiple endocrine neoplasia (MEN) 2A (243) and for the familial medullary thyroid carcinoma (FMTC) syndrome (81), while a substitution of methionine by threonine at codon 918 in the catalytic region of the tyrosine kinase has been reported in MEN 2B (80). These mutations have been shown to up-regulate the catalytic function of this RTK in the apparent absence of a ligand, resulting in its genetic transmission as an oncogene.

The human *trk* oncogene was initially isolated from a colon carcinoma, and molecular analysis shows that the gene was a chimeric molecule in which the extracellular domain of *trk* is substituted by rearrangement with a tropomyosin sequence (216). Furthermore, the activation in vitro of the *met* oncogene by treatment of a human osteogenic sarcoma cell line with a carcinogen resulted in the fusion of two distinct loci involving *met* and a translocated promoter region (tpr) (271).

Implications for Cancer Therapy

Growth factors and their signaling pathways are potential targets for therapeutic approaches to cancer (Fig 3.3). One possible point at which to intervene is the initial interaction between the growth factor and its cognate receptor at the surface of tumor cells whose growth is dependent on autocrine or paracrine mechanisms. Specific antagonists might be developed based on knowledge of ligand-receptor binding interactions. In some cases, such molecules are produced naturally, and presumably have a physiologic role in modulating growth factor signaling (31, 73). Suramin is a highly anionic naphthalene sulfonic acid derivative (123) that interferes with certain ligand-receptor interactions (19). It has been used in clinical trials in the treatment of renal (239) and prostate carcinoma (247, 296).

A different approach is based on the production of monoclonal antibodies that specifically neutralize the activities of growth factors or interfere with ligand-receptor interactions. Monoclonal antibodies directed against receptors have also been tested in tumors in which, as discussed earlier, uncontrolled proliferation occurs as the result of receptor overexpression. For example, there are reports in experimental animal models in which administration of monoclonal receptor antibodies induced receptor down-regulation and inhibited tumor growth (6, 136, 161, 178, 249). In fact, humanized monoclonals against the EGFR, as well as *erb* B-2, are currently in phase II clinical trials (194).

Another strategy utilizes receptor monoclonals or growth factors to deliver cytotoxic agents, such as toxins or radioisotopes, to tumor cells that overexpress a particular RTK (93, 276). This approach offers the possibility that, in the normal process of signaling, the receptor is internalized. Thus, in addition to targeting an overexpressed receptor upon which tumor proliferation is dependent, this approach could provide a convenient means of targeting chemotherapeutic agents to intracellular sites within the tumor cell. As with other receptor-targeting strategies, the efficacy of this approach depends upon the specificity as well as differential magnitude of receptor expression by the tumor, as opposed to normal cells, as well as accessibility of tumor cells to the systemic administration of such agents. Other more speculative intervention strategies with tumors that overexpress cell surface receptors include specific antisense oligodeoxynucleotides or genetically engineered antisense expression vectors to block effective transcription or translation of their products. Such approaches have been successfully demonstrated in in vitro models but not as yet in vivo (36, 37, 339). Gene therapy may represent another approach with respect to tumors that exhibit overexpression of growth factor receptors. One such strategy takes advantage of the high activity in such tumors of the promoter for the receptor gene. Thus, overexpression of an introduced therapeutic gene, such as the cytokine IL-2, under the control of that promoter might specifically target the tumor cell (reviewed in 305a).

Angiogenesis is required for many physiologic processes. Neoangiogenesis can also be a limiting factor in tumor growth, and, thus, play an important role in tumor progression (246). Moreover, certain growth factors, such as VEGF, appear to be specific for endothelial cells. Recent studies have shown that administration of a neutralizing monoclonal antibody raised against VEGF inhibited the growth of human tumors in the nude mouse model (166a). Thus, intervention with endothelial cell-specific growth factor signaling could target cancer cells as an indirect consequence of inhibition of the neoangiogenesis (see Chapter 10).

Inhibition of constitutive RTK activity or the binding and activation of downstream targets represents another approach to tumor intervention. For example, protein tyrosine kinase inhibitors with rather broad specificity have been isolated from fungal extracts. Quercetin (110, 111), genistein (2), lavendustin A (263), erbstatin (144, 374), and herbimicyn A (369) have been successfully tested in vitro and are currently being used as models for the design of synthetic inhibitors (recently reviewed in 194).

A different class of compounds, the tyrphostins (to indicate a class of *tyr*osine *phos*phorylation *in*hibitors), are tyrosine analogs that act competitively to inhibit receptor substrate interactions (193). Recent evidence suggests that such analogs can exhibit specificity among different receptors and even among substrates of the same receptor under in vitro experimental conditions. Another possible approach to block interactions of the activated receptor with downstream targets has involved the generation of molecules that antagonize binding of the SH2 domains of proteins that bind the activated receptor (194).

Many of these approaches are only now being developed and tested, but they are based upon accumulating knowledge of the importance of growth factor signaling in cancer cells. Initial clinical tests combine such experimental strategies with conventional therapeutic modalities. For example, it has been shown that the combined treatment of animals bearing human tumor xenografts treated with anti-EGFR

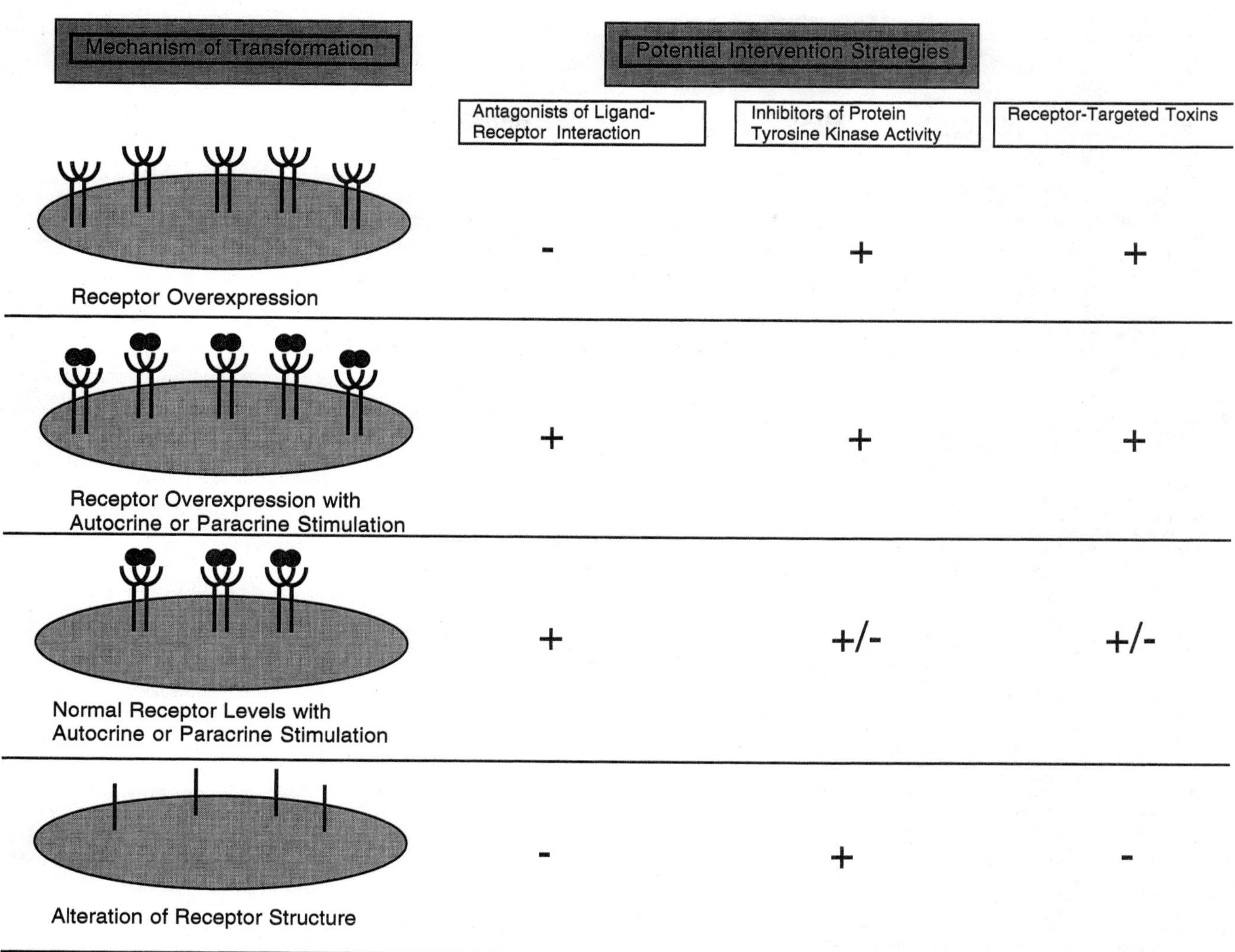

Mechanism of Transformation
Potential Intervention Strategies
Antagonists of Ligand-Receptor Interaction
Inhibitors of Protein Tyrosine Kinase Activity
Receptor-Targeted Toxins
-
+
+
Receptor Overexpression
+
+
+
Receptor Overexpression with Autocrine or Paracrine Stimulation
+
+/-
+/-
Normal Receptor Levels with Autocrine or Paracrine Stimulation
-
+
-
Alteration of Receptor Structure

Figure 3.3. Therapeutic approaches for intervening in malignant activation of growth factor-mediated proliferative pathways. Intervention strategies that might be successful are indicated by +. Treatments that could possibly affect normal cells as well as tumor cells are indicated by +/−.

monoclonal antibodies and doxorubicin or cisplatin, significantly increases the antitumor activity of these drugs (14, 86). Thus, as evidence mounts that genetic alterations in growth factor-signaling pathways underlie a major component of the malignant process, it is likely that this knowledge will lead to new approaches toward therapeutic intervention with the cancer cell.

References

1. Aaronson SA. Growth factors and cancer. Science 1991;254:1146–1153.
2. Akiyama T, Ishida J, Nakagawa S, Ogawara H, Watanabe S, Itch N, Shibuya M, Fukami Y. Genistein, a specific inhibitor or tyrosine-specific protein kinases. J Biol Chem 1987;261:5592–5595.
3. Alarid ET, Rubin JS, Young P, Chedid M, Ron D, Aaronson SA, Cunha GR. Keratinocyte growth factor functions in epithelial induction during seminal vesicle development. Proc Natl Acad Sci USA 1994;91:1074–1078.
4. Alimandi M, Romano A, Curia MC, Muraro R, Fedi P, Aaronson SA, Di Fiore PP, Kraus MH. Cooperative signaling of ErbB3 and ErbB2 in neoplastic transformation and human mammary carcinomas. Oncogene 1995;10:1813–1821.
5. Anderson DM, Lyman SD, Baird A, Wignall JM, Eisenman J, Rauch C, March CJ, Boswell HS, Gimpel SD, Cosman D. Molecular cloning of mast cell growth factor, a hematopoietin that is active in both membrane bound and soluble forms. Cell 1990;63:235–243.
6. Arteaga CL. Interference of the IGF system as a strategy to inhibit breast cancer growth. Breast Cancer Res Treat 1992;22:101–106.
7. Ballard J, Baxter R, Binoux M, Clemmons D, Hall K, Hintz R, Rechler M, Rutanen E, Schwander J. On the nomenclature of the IGF-binding proteins. Acta Endocrinol 1989;121:751–752.
8. Barbacid M. *ras* genes. Annu Rev Biochem 1987;56:779–827.
9. Barbacid M, Lamballe F, Pulido D, Klein R. The *trk* family of tyrosine protein kinase receptors. Biochim Biophys Acta 1991;1072:115–127.
10. Barde Y-A, Edgar D, Thoenen H. Purification of a new neurotrophic factor from mammalian brain. Eur Mol Biol Org J 1982;1:549–533.
11. Bargmann CI, Hung MC, Weinberg RA. Multiple independent activations of the *neu* oncogene by a point mutation altering the transmembrane domain of p185. Cell 1986;45:649–657.
12. Bargmann CI, Hung MC, Weinberg RA. The *neu* oncogene encodes an epidermal growth factor receptor-related protein. Nature 1986;319:226–230.
13. Barrandon Y, Green H. Cell migration is essential for sustained growth of keratinocyte colonies: the roles of transforming growth factor-alpha and epidermal growth factor. Cell 1987;50:1131–1137.
14. Baselga J, Norton L, Masui H, Pandiella A, Coplan K, Miller WH Jr, Mendelsohn J. Antitumor effects of doxorubicin in combination with anti-epidermal growth factor receptor monoclonal antibodies. JNCI 1993;85:1327–1333.
15. Basilico C, Moscatelli D. The FGF family of growth factors and oncogenes. Adv Cancer Res 1992;59:115–165.
16. Beckmann MP, Cerretti DP, Baum P, Vanden Bos T, James L, Farrah T, Kozlosky C, Hollingsworth T, Shilling H, Maraskovski E. Molecular characterization of a family of ligands for eph-related tyrosine kinase receptors. EMBO J 1994;13:3757–3762.
17. Ben-Buarch N, Yarder Y. Neu differentiation factors: a family of alternatively spliced neuronal and mesenchymal factors. Proc Soc Exp Biol Med 1994;206:221–227.

18. Ben-Neriah Y, Bauskin AR. Leukocytes express a novel gene encoding a putative transmembrane protein-kinase devoid of an extracellular domain. Nature 1988;333: 672–676.
19. Betsholtz C, Johnsson A, Heldin CH, Westermark B. Efficient reversion of simian sarcoma virus-transformation and inhibition of growth factor-induced mitogenesis by suramin. Proc Natl Acad Sci USA 1986;83:6440–6444.
20. Birchmeier C, O'Neill K, Riggs M, Wigler M. Characterization of ROS1 cDNA from a human glioblastoma cell line. Proc Natl Acad Sci USA 1990;87:47799–47803.
21. Bosenberg MW, Massague J. Juxtacrine cell signaling molecules. Curr Opin Cell Biol 1993;5:832–838.
22. Bouche G, Gas N, Prats H, Baldin V, Tauber JP, Teissie J, Amalric F. Basic fibroblast growth factor enters the nucleolus and stimulates the transcription of ribosomal genes in ABAE cells undergoing G0-G1 transition. Proc Natl Acad Sci USA 1987;84: 6770–6774.
23. Brugge JS, Erikson RL. Identification of a transformation-specific antigen induced by an avian sarcoma virus. Nature 1977;269:346–348.
24. Buck CA. Immunoglobulin superfamily: structure, function and relationship to other receptor molecules. Cell Biol 1992;3:179–188.
25. Burgess WH, Dionne CA, Kaplow J, Mudd R, Friesel R, Zilberstein A, Schlessinger J, Jaye M. Characterization and cDNA cloning of phospholipase C-gamma, a major substrate for heparin-binding growth factor 1 (acidic fibroblast growth factor)-activated tyrosine kinase. Mol Cell Biol 1990;10:4770–4777.
26. Burgess WH, Maciag T. The heparin-binding (fibroblast) growth factor family of proteins. Annu Rev Biochem 1989;58:575–606.
27. Cantley LC, Auger KR, Carpenter C, Duckworth B, Graziani A, Kapeller R, Soltoff S. Oncogenes and signal transduction. Cell 1991;64:281–302.
28. Carpenter G, Cohen S. Epidermal growth factor. J Biol Chem 1990;265:7709–7712.
29. Carraway KL III, Cantley LC. A *neu* acquaintance for ErbB3 and ErbB4: a role for receptor heterodimerization in growth signaling. Cell 1994;78:5–8.
30. Chan AM, King HW, Deakin EA, Tempest PR, Hilkens J, Kroezen V, Edwards DR, Wills AJ, Brookes P, Cooper CS. Characterization of the mouse *met* proto-oncogene. Oncogene 1988;2:593–599.
31. Chan AM-L, Rubin JS, Bottaro DP. Identification of a competitive HGF antagonist encoded by an alternative transcript. Science 1991;254:1382–1385.
32. Chang W, Upton C, Hu SL, Purchio AF, McFadden G. The genome of Shope fibroma virus, a tumorigenic poxvirus, contains a growth factor gene with sequence similarity to those encoding epidermal growth factor and transforming growth factor alpha. Mol Cell Biol 1987;7:535–540.
33. Chao MV. The p75 neurotrophin receptor. J Neurobiol 1994;25:1373–1385.
34. Chiu IM. Growth factor genes as oncogenes. Mol Chem Neuropathol 1989;10:37–52.
35. Chou Y-H, Hayman MJ. Characterization of a member of the immunoglobulin gene superfamily that possibly represents an additional class of growth factor receptor. Proc Natl Acad Sci USA 1991;88:4897–4901.
36. Ciardiello F, Bianco C, Normano N, Baldassarre G, Pepe S, Tortora G, Bianco AR, Salomon DS. Infection with a transforming growth factor α antisense retroviral expression vector reduces the in vitro growth and transformation of a human colon cancer cell line. Int J Cancer 1993;54:952–958.
37. Ciardiello F, Tortora G, Bianco C, Selvam MP, Basolo F, Fontanini G, Pacifico F, Normanno N, Brandt R, Persico MG, et al. Inhibition of CRIPTO expression and tumorigenicity in human colon cancer cells by antisense RNA and oligodeoxynucleotides. Oncogene 1994;9:291–298.
38. Claesson-Welsh L, Eriksson A, Moren A, Severinsson L, Ek B, Ostman A, Betsholtz C, Heldin CH. cDNA Cloning and expression of a human platelet-derived growth factor (PDGF) receptor specific for B-chain-containing PDGF molecules. Mol Cell Biol 1988;8:3476–3486.
39. Claesson-Welsh L, Eriksson A, Westermark B, Heldin CH. cDNA Cloning and expression of the human A-type platelet-derived growth factor (PDGF) receptor establishes structural similarity to the B-type PDGF receptor. Proc Natl Acad Sci USA 1989;86:4917–4921.
40. Claesson-Welsh L, Hammacher A, Westermark B, Heldin CH, Nister M. Identification and structural analysis of the A type receptor for platelet-derived growth factor. Similarities with the B type receptor. J Biol Chem 1989;264:1742–1747.
41. Clarke MF, Westin E, Schmidt D, Josephs SF, Ratner L, Wong-Staal F, Gallo RC, Reitz MS Jr. Transformation of NIH/3T3 cells by a human c-*sis* cDNA clone. Nature 1984;308:464–467.
42. Clemmons DR. Structural and functional analysis of insulin-like growth factors. Br Med Bull 1989;45:465–480.
43. Cleveland JL, Troppmair J, Packham G, Askew DS, Lloyd P, Gonzalez-Garcia M, Nunez G, Ihle JN, Rapp UR. v-raf Suppresses apoptosis and promotes growth of interleukin-3-dependent myeloid cells. Oncogene 1994;9:2217–2226.
44. Cohen S. Epidermal growth factor. Biosci Rep 1986;6:1017–1028.
45. Collett MS, Erikson RL. Protein kinase activity associated with the avian sarcoma virus *src* gene product. Proc Natl Acad Sci USA 1978;75:2021–2024.
46. Connolly DT, Olander JV, Heuvelman D, Nelson R, Monsell R, Seigel N, Haymore BL, Leimgruber R, Feder J. Human vascular permeability factor. Isolation from U937 cells. J Biol Chem 1989;264:20017–20024.
47. Cook PW, Mattox PA, Winifred KW, Pittelkow MR, Plowman GD, Shoyab M, Adelman JP, Shipley GD. A heparin sulfate-regulated human keratinocyte autocrine factor is similar or identical to amphiregulin. Mol Cell Biol 1991;11:2547–2557.
48. Cooper CS, Park, Blair DG, Oskarsson MK, Tainsky MA, Eader LA, Vande Woude GF. Molecular cloning of a new transforming gene from a chemically-transformed human cell line. Nature 1984;311:29–33.
49. Cordon-Cardo C, Tapley P, Jing S, Nanduri V, O'Rourke E, Lamballe F, Kovary K, Klein R, Jones KR, Reichardt LF, Barbacid M. The *trk* tyrosine protein kinase mediates the mitogenic properties of nerve growth factor and neurotrophin-3. Cell 1991;66:173–183.
50. Coughlin SR, Escobedo JA, Williams LT. Role of phosphatidylinositol kinase in PDGF receptor signal transduction. Science 1989;243:1191–1194.
51. Courtneidge SA, Kypta RM, Cooper JA, Kazlauskas A. PDGF receptor sequences important for kinases binding of SRC family tyrosine. Cell Growth Diff 1991;2:483–486.
52. Cunningham BA, Hemperly JJ, Murray BA, Prediger EA, Brackenbury R, Edelman GM. Neural cell adhesion molecule: structure, immunoglobulin-like domains, cell surface modulation, and alternative RNA splicing. Science 1987;236:799–806.
53. Cuttitta F, Carney DN, Mulshine J, Moody TW, Fedorko J, Fischler A, Minna JD. Bombesin-like peptides can function as autocrine growth factors in human small-cell lung cancer. Nature 1985;316:823–826.
54. Dahlback B. Protein S and C4b-binding protein: components involved in the regulation of the protein C anticoagulant system. Thromb Haemost 1991;66:49–61.
55. Dai W, Pan H, Hassanain H, Gupta SL, Murphy MJ Jr. Molecular cloning of a novel receptor tyrosine kinase, tif, highly expressed in human ovary and testis. Oncogene 1994;9:975–979.
56. Davis CG. The many faces of epidermal growth factor repeats. New Biol 1990;2: 410–419.
57. Davis S, Gale NW, Aldrich TH, Maisonpierre PC, Lhotak V, Pawson T, Goldfarb M, Yancopoulos GD. Ligands for EPH-related receptor tyrosine kinases that require membrane attachment or clustering for activity. Science 1994;266:816–819.
58. Davis S, Lu ML, Lo SH, Butler JA, Drucker BJ, Roberts TM, An Q, Chen LB. Presence of an SH2 domain in the actin-binding protein tensin. Science 1991;252:712–715.
59. de Larco JE, Todaro JG. Growth factors from murine sarcoma virus-transformed cells. Proc Natl Acad Sci USA 1978;75:4001–4005.
60. Delli Bovi P, Curatola AM, Kern FG, Greco A, Ittmann M, Basilico C. An oncogene isolated by transfection of Kaposi's sarcoma DNA encodes a growth factor that is a member of the FGF family. Cell 1987;50:729–737.
61. Derynck R. Transforming growth factor alpha. Cell 1988;54:593–595.
62. Di Fiore PP, Pierce JH, Kraus MH, Segatto O, King CR, Aaronson SA. *erb*B-2 is a potent oncogene when overexpressed in NIH/3T3 cells. Science 1987;237:178–182.
63. Di Fiore PP, Pierce JH, Fleming TP, Hazan R, Ullrich A, King CR, Schlessinger J, Aaronson SA, Antoniades HN. Overexpression of the human EGF receptor confers and EGF-dependent transformed phenotype to NIH/3T3 cells. Cell 1987;51: 1063–1070.
64. Di Marco E, Pierce JH, Fleming TP, Kraus MH, Molloy CJ, Aaronson SA, Di Fiore PP. Autocrine interaction between TGF-alpha and the EGF-receptor: quantitative requirements for induction of the malignant phenotype. Oncogene 1989;4:831–838.
65. Di Marco E, Cutuli N, Guerra L, Cancedda R, De Luca M. Molecular cloning of trkE, a novel trk-related putative tyrosine kinase receptor isolated from normal human keratinocytes and widely expressed by normal human tissues. J Biol Chem 1993;268: 24290–24295.
66. Di Renzo MF, Narsimhan RP, Olivero M, Bretti M, Giordano S, Medico E, Gaglia P, Zara P, Comoglio PM. Expression of the Met/HGF receptor in normal and neoplastic human tissues. Oncogene 1991;6:1997–2003.
67. di Vries CJ, Escobedo JA, Ueno H, Houck K, Ferrara N, Williams LT. The fms-like tyrosine kinase, a receptor for vascular endothelial growth factor. Science 1992;25: 989–991.
68. Dixit VM, Green S, Sarma V, Holzman LB, Wolf FW, O'Rourke K, Ward PA, Prochownik EV, Marks RM. Tumor necrosis factor-alpha induction of novel gene products in human endothelial cells including a macrophage-specific chemotaxin. J Biol Chem 1990;265:2973–2978.
69. Dixon M, Deed R, Acland P, Moore R, Whyte A, Peters G, Dickson C. Detection and characterization of the fibroblast growth factor-related oncoprotein INT-2. Mol Cell Biol 1989;9:4896–4902.
70. Doolittle RF, Hunkapiller MW, Hood LE, Devare SG, Robbins KC, Aaronson SA, Antoniades HN. Simian sarcoma virus *onc* gene, v-*sis*, is derived from the gene (or genes) encoding a platelet-derived growth factor. Science 1983;221:275–277.
71. Dougall WC, Qian X, Peterson NC, Miller MJ, Samanta A, Green MI. The *neu*-oncogene: signal transduction pathways, transformation mechanisms and evolving therapies. Oncogene 1994;9:2190–2223.
72. Downward J, Yarden Y, Mayes E, Scrace G, Totty N, Stockwell P, Ullrich A, Schlessinger J, Waterfield MD. Close similarity of epidermal growth factor receptor and v-*erb*B oncogene protein sequences. Nature 1984;307:521–527.
73. Duan D-SR, Werner S, Williams LT. A naturally occurring secreted form of fibroblast growth factor (FGF) receptor 1 binds basic FGF in preference over acidic FGF. J Biol Chem 1992;267:16076–16080.
74. Dull TJ, Gray A, Hayflick JS, Ullrich A. Insulin-like growth factor II precursor gene organization in relation to insulin gene family. Nature 1984;310:777–781.
75. Dumont D, Yamaguchi T, Colon R, Rossant J. *tek*, A novel tyrosine kinase gene located on mouse chromosome 4, is expressed in endothelial growth factor. Science 1992;225:989–991.
76. Ebendal T. Function and evolution in the NGF family and its receptors. J Neurosci Res 1992;32:461–470.
77. Ebendal T. NGF in CNS: experimental data and clinical implications. Progr Growth Factor Res 1989;1:143–159.
78. Ebina Y, Ellis L, Jarnagin K, Edery M, Graf L, Clauser E, Ou JH, Masiarz F, Kan YW, Goldfine ID, Roth RA, Rutter WJ. The human insulin receptor cDNA: the structural basis for hormone-activated transmembrane signalling. Cell 1985;40:747–758.
79. Enfors P, Ibanez CF, Ebendal T, Olson L, Persson H. Molecular cloning and neurotrophic activities of a protein with structural similarities to nerve growth factor: developmental and topographical expression in the brain. Proc Natl Acad Sci USA 1990;87:5454–5458.
80. Eng C, Smith DP, Muligan LM, Naigai MA, Healey CS, Ponder MA, Gardner E, Scheumann GF, Jackson CE, Tunnacliffe A, et al. Point mutation within the tyrosine kinase domain of the RET proto-oncogene in multiple endocrine neoplasia type 2B and related sporadic tumours. Hum Mol Genet 1994;3:327–241, 1994;3:686 (erratum).
81. Eng C, Smith DP, Mulligan LM, Healey CS, Zvelebil MJ, Stonehouse TJ, Ponder MA, Jackson CE, Waterfield MD, Ponder BAJ. A novel point mutation in the tyrosine kinase domain of the *ret* proto-oncogene in sporadic medullary thyroid carcinoma and in a family with FMTC. Oncogene 1995;10:509–513.
82. Escobedo JA, Williams LT. A PDGF receptor domain essential for mitogenesis but not for many other responses to PDGF. Nature 1988;335:85–87.
83. Espinal J. Mechanism of insulin action. Nature 1987;328:574–575.
84. Eva A, Robbins KC, Andersen PR, Srinivasan A, Tronick SR, Reddy EP, Ellmore NW, Galen AT, Lautenberger JA, Papas TS, Westin EH, Wong-Staal F, Gallo RC, Aaronson SA. Cellular genes analogous to retroviral *onc* genes are transcribed in human tumour cells. Nature 1982;295:116–119.
85. Falls DL, Rosen KM, Corfas G, Lane WS, Fischbach GD. ARIA, a protein that stimulates acetylcholine receptor synthesis, is a member of the *neu* ligand family. Cell 1993;72:801–815.

86. Fan Z, Baselga J, Masui H, Mendelsohn J. Antitumor effect of anti-epidermal growth factor receptor monoclonal antibodies plus *cis*-diamminedichloroplatinum on well-established A431-cell xenografts. Cancer Res 1993;53:4637–4642.
87. Fantl WJ, Johnson DE, Williams LT. Signalling by receptor tyrosine kinases. Annu Rev Biochem 1993;62:453–481.
88. Faust M, Ebensperger C, Schulz AS, Schleithoff L, Hameister H, Bartram CR, Janssen JWG. The murine *ufo* receptor: molecular cloning, chromosomal localization, and *in situ* expression analysis. Oncogene 1992;7:1287–1293.
89. Feldman B, Poueymirou W, Papaioannou VE, DeChiara TM, Goldfarb M. Requirement of FGF-4 for postimplantation mouse development. Science 1995;267:246–249.
90. Feng G-S, Hui CC, Pawson T. SH2-Containing phosphotyrosine phosphatase as a target of protein-tyrosine kinases. Science 1993;259:1607–1611.
91. Ferrara N, Henzel WJ. Pituitary follicular cells secrete a novel heparin-binding growth factor specific for vascular endothelial cells. Biochem Biophys Res Commun 1989;161:851–858.
92. Finch PW, Rubin JS, Miki T, Ron D, Aaronson SA. Human KGF is FGF-related with properties of a paracrine effector of epithelial cell growth. Science 1989;245: 752–755.
93. Fitzgerald D, Pastan I. Targeted toxin therapy for the treatment of cancer. JNCI 1989;81:1455–1463.
94. Flanagan JG, Leder P. The kit ligand: a cell surface molecule altered in steel mutant fibroblasts. Cell 1990;63:185–194.
95. Fletcher FA, Carpenter MK, Shilling H, Baum P, Ziegler SF, Gimpel S, Hollingsworth T, Vanden Bos T, James L, Hjerrild K, Davison BL, Lyman SD, Beckmann MP. LERK-2, a binding protein for the receptor-tyrosine kinase ELK, is evolutionarily conserved and expressed in a developmentally regulated pattern. Oncogene 1994;9: 3241–3247.
96. Fu X-Y, Zhang J-J. Transcription factor p91 interacts with the epidermal growth factor receptor and mediates activation of the c-*fos* gene promoter. Cell 1993;74: 1135–1145.
97. Fujimoto J, Yamamoto T. brt, A mouse gene encoding a novel receptor-type protein-tyrosine kinase, is preferentially expressed in the brain. Oncogene 1994;9:693–698.
98. Galland F, Karamysheva A, Pebusque JJ, Borg JP, Rottapel R, Dubreuil P, Rosnet O, Birnbaum D. The FLT4 gene encodes a transmembrane tyrosine kinase related to the vascular endothelial growth factor receptor. Oncogene 1993;8:1233–1240.
99. Gasic GP, Arenas CP, Gasic TB, Gasic GJ. Coagulation factors X, Xa, and protein S as potent mitogens of cultured aortic smooth muscle cells. Proc Natl Acad Sci USA 1992;89:2317–2320.
100. Gaudino G, Follenzi A, Naldini L, Collesi C, Santoro M, Gallo KA, Godowski P, Comoglio PM. Ron is a heterodimeric tyrosine kinase receptor activated by the HGF homologue MSP. EMBO J 1994;13:3524–3532.
101. Gazit A, Igarashi H, Chiu IM, Srinivasan A, Yaniv A, Tronick SR, Robbins KC, Aaronson SA. Expression of the normal human *sis*/PDGF-2 coding sequence induces cellular transformation. Cell 1984;39:89–97.
102. Glass DJ, Nye SH, Hantzopoulos P, Macchi MJ, Squinto SP, Goldfarb M, Yancopoulos GD. TrkB mediates BDNF/NT-3-dependent survival and proliferation in fibroblasts lacking the low affinity NGF receptor. Cell 1991;66:405–413.
103. Glass DJ, Yancopoulos GD. The neurotrophins and their receptors. Trends Biochem Sci 1993;3:262–268.
104. Gliniak BC, Rohrschneider LR. Expression of the M-CSF receptor is controlled post-transcriptionally by the dominant actions of GM-CSF or multi-CSF. Cell 1990;63: 1073–1083.
105. Gohda E, Tsubouchi H, Nakayama H, Hirono S, Sakiyama O, Takahashi K, Miyazaki H, Hashimoto S, Daikuhara Y. Purification and partial characterization of hepatocyte growth factor from plasma of a patient with fulminant hepatic failure. J Clin Invest 1988;81:414–419.
106. Gospodarowicz D, Abraham JA, Schilling J. Isolation and characterization of a vascular endothelial cell mitogen produced by pituitary-derived folliculo stellate cells. Proc Natl Acad Sci USA 1989;86:7311–7315.
107. Gotz R, Koster R, Winkler C, Raulf F, Lottspeich F, Schartl M, Thoenen H. Neurotrophin-6 is a new member of the nerve growth factor family. Nature 1994;372: 266–269.
108. Graham DK, Dawson TL, Mullaney DL, Snodgrass HR, Earp HS. Cloning and mRNA expression analysis of a novel human protooncogene, c-*mer*. Cell Growth Different 1994;5:647–657.
109. Gray A, Dull TJ, Ullrich A. Nucleotide sequence of epidermal growth factor cDNA predicts a 128,000-molecular weight protein precursor. Nature 1983;303:722–725.
110. Graziani Y, Chayoth R, Karny N, Feldman B, Levy J. Regulation of protein kinases activity by quercetin in Ehrlich ascites tumor cells. Biochim Biophys Acta 1982;714: 415–421.
111. Graziani Y, Erikson E, Erikson RL. The effect of quercetin on the phosphorylation activity of the Rous sarcoma virus transforming gene product in vitro and in vivo. Eur J Biochem 1983;135:583–589.
112. Greenberger JS, Eckner RJ, Sakakeeny M, Marks P, Reid D, Nabel G, Hapel A, Ihle JN, Humphries KC. Interleukin 3-dependent hematopoietic progenitor cell lines. Fed Proc 1983;42:2762–2771.
113. Grieco M, Santoro M, Berlingieri MT, Melillo RM, Donghi R, Bongarzone I, Pierotti MA, Della Porta G, Fusco A, Vecchio G. PTC is a novel rearranged form of the *ret* proto-oncogene and is frequently detected in vivo in human papillary carcinomas. Cell 1990;60:557–563.
114. Gregory H. Isolation and structure of urogastrone and its relationship to epidermal growth factor. Nature 1975;257:325–327.
115. Griffin JD. Clinical applications of colony-stimulating factors. Oncology 1988;2: 15–23.
116. Halaban R, Kwon BS, Ghosh S, Delli Bovi P, Baird A. bFGF as an autocrine growth factor for human melanomas. Oncogene Res 1988;3:177–186.
117. Halaban R, Langdon R, Birchall N, Cuono C, Baird A, Scott G, Moellmann G, McGuire J. Basic fibroblast growth factor from human keratinocytes is a natural mitogen for melanocytes. J Cell Biol 1988;107:1611–1619.
118. Hammacher A, Mellstrom K, Heldin CH, Westermark B. Isoform-specific induction of actin reorganization by platelet-derived growth factor suggests that the functionally active receptor is a dimer. EMBO J 1989;8:2489–2495.
119. Han S, Stuart LA, Degen SJ. Characterization of the DNF 15S2 locus on human chromosome 3: identification of a gene coding for four kringle domains with homology to hepatocyte growth factor. Biochemistry 1991;30:9768–9780.
120. Hart CE, Forstrom JW, Kelly JD, Seifert RA, Smith RA, Ross R, Murray MJ, Bowen-Pope DF. Two classes of PDGF receptor recognize different isoforms of PDGF. Science 1988;240:1529–1531.
121. Hattori Y, Odagiri H, Nakatani H, Miyagawa K, Naito K, Sakamoto H, Katoh O, Yoshida T, Sugimura T, Terada M. K-sam, an amplified gene in stomach cancer, is a member of the heparin-binding growth factor receptor genes. Proc Natl Acad Sci USA 1990;87:5983–5987.
122. Hauser S. A heparin-binding form of placenta growth factor (P1GF-2) is expressed in human umbilical vein endothelial cells and in placenta. Growth Factors 1993;9: 259–268.
123. Hawking F. Suramin: with special reference to onchocerciasis. Adv Pharmacol Chemother 1978;15:289–322.
124. Heldin C-H. Dimerization of cell surface receptors in signal transduction. Cell 1995;80:213–223.
125. Heldin CH, Hammacher A, Nister M, Westermark B. Structural and functional aspects of platelet-derived growth factor. Br J Cancer 1988;57:591–593.
126. Heldin CH, Johnsson A, Wennergren S, Wernstedt C, Betsholtz C, Westermark B. A human osteosarcoma cell line secretes a growth factor structurally related to a homodimer of PDGF A-chains. Nature 1986;319:511–514.
127. Heldin CH, Westermark B. Platelet-derived growth factors: a family of isoforms that bind to two distinct receptors. Br Med Bull 1989;45:453–464.
128. Higashiyama S, Abraham JA, Miller J, Fiddes JC, Klagsbrun M. A heparin-binding growth factor secreted by macrophage-like cell that is related to EGF. Science 1991;251:936–939.
129. Higashiyama S, Lau K, Besner GE, Abraham JA, Klagsbrun M. Structure of heparin-binding EGF-like growth factor. Multiple forms, primary structure, and glycosylation of the mature protein. J Biol Chem 1992;267:6205–6212.
130. Hirai H, Maru Y, Hagiwara K, Nishida J, Takaku F. A novel putative tyrosine kinase receptor encoded by the *eph* gene. Science 1987;238:1717–1720.
131. Holmes WE, Sliwkowski MX, Akita RW, Henzel WJ, Lee J, Park JW, Yansura D, Abadi N, Raab H, Lewis GD, Shepard HM, Kuang W, Wood WI, Goeddel DV, Vandlen RL. Identification of heregulin, a specific activator of $p185^{erbB2}$. Science 1992;256: 1205–1210.
132. Holzman LB, Marks RM, Dixit VM. A novel immediate-early response gene of endothelium is induced by cytokines and encodes a secreted protein. Mol Cell Biol 1990;10:5830–5838.
133. Hovens CM, Stacker SA, Andres A-C, Harpur AG, Ziemiecki A, Wilkis AF. RYK, a receptor tyrosine kinase-related molecule with unusual kinase domain motifs. Proc Natl Acad Sci USA 1992;89:11818–11822.
134. Hu P, Margolis B, Schlessinger J. Vav: a potential link between tyrosine kinases and ras-like GTPases in hematopoietic cell signaling. Bioessays 1993;15:179–183.
135. Huang E, Nocka K, Beier DR, Chu TY, Buck J, Lahm HW, Wellner D, Leder P, Besmer P. The hematopoietic growth factor KL is encoded by the S1 locus and is the ligand of the c-*kit* receptor, the gene product of the W locus. Cell 1990;63:225–233.
136. Hudziak RM, Lewis GD, Winget M. p185HER2 monoclonal antibody has antiproliferative effects in vitro and sensitized human breast tumor cells to tumor necrosis factor. Mol Cell Biol 1989;9:1165.
137. Huff JL, Jelinek MA, Borgman CA, Lansing TJ, Parsons JT. The protooncogene c-sea encodes a transmembrane protein-tyrosine kinase related to the Met/hepatocyte growth factor/scatter factor receptor. Proc Natl Acad Sci USA 1993;90:6140–6144.
138. Hunter T, Angel P, Boyle WJ, Chiu R, Freed E, Gould KL, Isacke CM, Karin M, Lindberg RA, van der Geer P. Targets for signal-transducing protein kinases. Cold Spring Harb Symp Quant Biol 1988;53:131–142.
139. Hunter T, Sefton BM. Transforming gene product of Rous sarcoma virus phosphorylates tyrosine. Proc Natl Acad Sci USA 1980;77:1311–1315.
140. Igarashi H, Rao CD, Siroff M, Leal F, Robbins KC, Aaronson SA. Detection of PDGF-2 homodimers in human tumor cells. Oncogene 1987;1:79–85.
141. Ihle JN, Askew D. Origins and properties of hematopoietic growth factor-dependent cell lines. Int J Cell Cloning 1989;7:68–91.
142. Ikeda I, Ishizaka Y, Tahira T, Suzuki T, Onda M, Siugimura T, Nagao M. Specific expression of the ret proto-oncogene in human neuroblastoma cell lines. Oncogene 1990;5:1291–1296.
143. Imamura T, Engleka K, Zhan X, Tokita Y, Forough R, Roeder D, Jackson A, Maier JAM, Hla T, Maciag T. Recovery of mitogenic activity of a growth factor mutant with a nuclear translocation sequence. Science 1990;249:1567–1570.
144. Imoto M, Umezawa K, Komuro K, Sawa T, Takeuchi T, Umezawa H. Antitumor activity of erbstatin, a tyrosine protein kinase inhibitor. Jpn J Cancer Res 1987;78: 329–332.
145. Ip NY, Ibanez CF, Nye SH, McClain J, Jones PF, Gies DR, Belluscio L, Le Beau MM, Espinosa R, Squinto SP, Persson H, Yancopoulos GD. Mammalian neutrotrophin-4 structure, chromosomal location, tissue distribution, and receptor specificity. Proc Natl Acad Sci USA 1992;89:3060–3064.
146. Iwama A, Hamaguchi I, Hashiyama M, Murayama K, Yasunaga K, Suda T. Molecular cloning and characterization of mouse TIE and TEK receptor tyrosine kinase genes and their expression in hematopoietic stem cells. Biochem Biophys Res Commun 1993;195:301–309.
147. Iwama A, Okano K, Sudo T, Matsuda Y, Suda T. Molecular cloning of a novel receptor tyrosine kinase gene, *STK*, derived from enriched hematopoietic stem cells. Blood 1994;83:3160–3169.
148. Iyer A, Kmiecik TE, Park M, Daar I, Blair D, Dunn J, Sutrave P, Ihle JN, Bodescot M, Vande Woude G. Structure, tissue-specific expression, and transforming activity of the mouse *met* protooncogene. Cell Growth Different 1990;1:87–95.
149. Janssen JW, Schulz AS, Steenvoorden AC, Schmidberger M, Strehl S, Ambros PF, Bartram CR. A novel putative tyrosine kinase receptor with oncogenic potential. Oncogene 1991;6:2113–2120.
150. Jenny RJ, Pittman R, Toole JJ, Kriz RW, Aldape RA, Hewick RM, Kaufman RJ, Mann KG. Complete cDNA and derived amino acid sequence of human factor V. Proc Natl Acad Sci USA 1987;84:4846–4850.
151. Jia R, Hanafusa H. The proto-oncogene of v-*eyk* (v-*ryk*) is a novel receptor-type protein tyrosine kinase with extracellular Ig/FN-III domains. J Biol Chem 1994;269: 1839–1844.

152. Johnson D, Lanahan A, Buck CR, Sehgal A, Morgan C, Mercer E, Bothwell M, Chao M. Expression and structure of the human NGF receptor. Cell 1986;47:545–554.
153. Johnson DE, Williams LT. Structural and functional diversity in the FGF receptor multigene family. Adv Cancer Res 1993;60:1–41.
154. Johnson GR, Saeki T, Gordon AW, Shoyab M, Salomon DS, Stromberg K. Response to and expression of amphiregulin by ovarian carcinoma and normal ovarian surface epithelial cells: nuclear localization of endogenous amphiregulin. Biochem Biophys Res Commun 1991;180:481–488.
155. Johnson GR, Saeki T, Gordon AW, Shoyab M, Salomon DS, Stromberg K. Autocrine action of amphiregulin in a colon carcinoma cell line and immunocytochemical localization of amphiregulin in human colon. J Cell Biol 1992;118:741–751.
156. Johnson GR, Wong L. Heparan sulfate is essential to amphiregulin-induced mitogenic signaling by the epidermal growth factor receptor. J Biol Chem 1994;269: 27149–27154.
157. Johnson JD, Edman JC, Rutter WJ. A receptor tyrosine kinase found in breast carcinoma cells has an extracellular discoidin I-like domain. Proc Natl Acad Sci USA 1993;90:10891.
158. Jui H-Y, Suzuki Y, Accili D, Taylor SL. Expression of a cDNA encoding the human insulin receptor-related receptor. J Biol Chem 1994;269:22446–22452.
159. Kaleko M, Rutter WJ, Miller AD. Overexpression of the human insulin-like growth factor I receptor promotes ligand-dependent neoplastic transformation. Mol Cell Biol 1990;10:464–473.
160. Karn T, Holtrich U, Brauninger A, Bohme B, Wolf G, Rubsamen-Waigmann H, Strebhardt K. Structure, expression and chromosomal mapping of TKT from man and mouse: a new subclass of receptor tyrosine kinases with a factor VIII-like domain. Oncogene 1993;8:3433–3440.
161. Kasprzyk PG, Song SU, Di Fiore PP. Therapy of an animal model of human gastric cancer using a combination of anti-erbB-2 monoclonal antibodies. Cancer Res 1992;52:2771–2776.
162. Kazlauskas A. Receptor tyrosine kinases and their targets. Curr Opin Genet Devel 1994;4:5–14.
163. Kazlauskas A, Cooper JA. Autophosphorylation of the PDGF receptor in the kinase insert region regulates interactions with cell proteins. Cell 1989;58:1121–1133.
164. Kazlauskas A, Feng G-S, Pawson T, Valius M. The 64-kDa protein that associates with the platelet-derived growth factor receptor β subunit via tyr-1009 is the SH2-containing phosphotyrosine phosphatase SYP. Proc Natl Acad Sci USA 1993;90:6939–6942.
165. Keck PJ, Hauser SD, Krivi G, Sanzo K, Warren T, Feder J, Connolly DT. Vascular permeability factor, an endothelial cell mitogen related to PDGF. Science 1989;246: 1309–1312.
166. Khazaie K, Schirrmacher V, Lichtner RB. EGF receptor in neoplasia and metastasis. Cancer Metastasis Rev 1993;12:255–274.
166a. Kim KJ, Ki B, Winer J, Armanini M, Gillett N, Phillips HS, Ferrara N. Inhibition of vascular endothelial growth factor-induced angiogenesis suppresses tumour growth in vivo. Nature 1993;362:841–844.
167. King CR, Kraus MH, Aaronson SA. Amplification of a novel v-*erb*B-related gene in a human mammary carcinoma. Science 1985;229:974–976.
168. King CR, Kraus MH, Williams LT, Merlino GT, Pastan IH, Aaronson SA. Human tumor cell lines with EGF receptor gene amplification in the absence of aberrant sized mRNAs. Nucleic Acids Res 1985;13:8477–8486.
169. Kishimoto T, Taga A, Akira S. Cytokine signal transduction. Cell 1994;76:253–262.
170. Klagsbrun M, Baird. A dual receptor system is required for basic fibroblast growth factor activity. Cell 1991;67:229–231.
171. Klein R, Jing S, Nanduri V, O'Rourke E, Barbacid M. The *trk* proto-oncogene encodes a receptor for nerve growth factor. Cell 1991;85:189–197.
172. Klein R, Parada LF, Coulier F, Barbacid M. *trk*B, a novel tyrosine protein kinase receptor expressed during mouse neural development. EMBO J 1989;8:3701–3709.
173. Korhonen J, Partanen J, Eerola E, Vainikka S, Alitalo R, Makela TP, Sandberg M, Hirvonen H, Alitalo K. Five FGF receptors with distinct expression patterns. EXS 1992;61: 91–100.
174. Kozlosky CJ, Maraskovski E, McGrew JT, VandenBos T, Teepe M, Lyman SD, Srinivasan S, Fletcher FA, Gayle RB, Cerretti DP, Beckmann MP. Ligands for the receptor tyrosine kinases hek and elk: isolation of cDNAs encoding a family of proteins. Oncogene 1995;10:299–306.
175. Kraus MH, Issing W, Miki T, Popescu NC, Aaronson SA. Isolation and characterization of *erb*B-3, a third member of the *erb*B/epidermal growth factor receptor family: evidence for overexpression in a subset of human mammary tumors. Proc Natl Acad Sci USA 1989;86:9193–9197.
176. Kraus MH, Popescu NC, Amsbaugh SC, King CR. Overexpression of the EGF receptor-related proto-oncogene *erb*B-2 in human mammary tumor cell lines by different molecular mechanisms. EMBO J 1987;6:605–610.
177. Kuhne MR, Pawson T, Lienhard GE, Feng G-S. The insulin receptor substrate 1 associates with the SH2-containing phosphotyrosine phosphatase SYP. J Biol Chem 1993;268:11479–11481.
178. Kumar R, Shepard HM, Mendelsohn J. Regulation of phosphorylation of the c-erbB-2/HER2 gene product by a monoclonal antibody and serum growth factor(s) in human mammary carcinoma cells. Mol Cell Biol 1991;11:979–986.
179. Kypta RM, Goldberg Y, Ulug ET, Courtneidge SA. Association between the PDGF receptor and members of the Src family of tyrosine kinases. Cell 1990;62:481–492.
180. Lacal JC, Tronick SR. The ras oncogene. In The Oncogene Handbook. Edited by EP Reddy, AM Skalka, T Curran. Amsterdam: Elsevier, 1988, pp 255–304.
181. Lacroix H, Iglehart JD, Skinner MA, Kraus MH. Overexpression of *erb*B-2 or EGF receptor proteins present in early stage mammary carcinoma is detected simultaneously in matched primary tumors and regional metastases. Oncogene 1989;4: 145–151.
182. Lai C, Lemke G. Structure and expression of the Tyro 10 receptor tyrosine kinase. Oncogene 1994;9:877–883.
183. Lamballe F, Klein R, Barbacid M. *trk*C, a new member of the trk family of tyrosine protein kinases, is a receptor for neurotrophin-3. Cell 1991;66:967–979.
184. Lamson G, Giudice LC, Rosenfeld RG. Insulin-like growth factor binding proteins: structural and molecular relationships. Growth Factors 1991;5:19–28.
185. Lechleider JR, Sugimoto S, Bennett AM, Kashishian SD, Cooper JA, Shoelson SE, Walsh CT, Neel BG. Activation of the SH2-containing phosphotyrosine phosphatase SH-PTP2 by its binding site, phosphotyrosine 1009, on the human platelet-derived growth factor receptor β. J Biol Chem 1993;268:21478–21481.
186. Lee PL, Johnson DE, Cousens LS, Fried VA, Williams LT. Purification and complementary DNA cloning of a receptor for basic fibroblast growth factor. Science 1989;245:57–60.
187. Leibrock J, Lottspeich F, Hohn A, Hofer M, Hengerer B, Masiakowski P, Thoenen H, Barde Y-A. Molecular cloning and expression of brain-derived neurotrophic factor. Nature 1989;341:149–152.
188. Lemmon MA, Schlessinger J. Regulation of signal transduction and signal diversity by receptor oligomerization. Trends Biochem Sci 1994;19:459–463.
189. Leof EB, Van Wyk JJ, O'Keefe EJ, Pledger WJ. Epidermal growth factor (EGF) is required only during the traverse of early G1 in PDGF stimulated density-arrested BALB/c-3T3 cells. Exp Cell Res 1983;147:202–208.
190. Leung DW, Cachianes G, Kuang WJ, Goeddel DV, Ferrara N. Vascular endothelial growth factor is a secreted angiogenic mitogen. Science 1989;246:1306–1309.
191. Levi-Montalcini R. The nerve growth factor 35 years later. Science 1987;237: 1154–1162.
192. Levinson AD, Oppermann H, Levintow L, Varmus HE, Bishop JM. Evidence that the transforming gene of avian sarcoma virus encodes a protein kinase associated with a phosphoprotein. Cell 1978;15:561–572.
193. Levitzki A. Tyrphostins: tyrosine kinase blockers as novel antiproliferative agents and dissectors of signal transduction. FASEB J 1992;6:3275–3282.
194. Levitzki A, Gazit A. Tyrosine kinase inhibition: an approach to drug development. Science 1995;267:1782–1788.
195. Libermann TA, Razon N, Bartal AD, Yarden Y, Schlessinger J, Soreq H. Expression of epidermal growth factor receptors in human brain tumors. Cancer Res 1984;44: 753–760.
196. Loeb DM, Maragos J, Martin-Zanca D, Chao MV, Parada LF, Greene LA. The *trk* proto-oncogene rescues NGF responsiveness in mutant NFG-nonresponsiveness PC12 cell lines. Cell 1991;66:961–966.
197. Logan A. Intracrine regulation at the nucleus—a further mechanism of growth factor activity? J Endocrinol 1990;125:339–343.
198. Macaulay VM, Carney DN. Neuropeptide growth factors. Cancer Invest 1991;9: 659–673.
199. Lowenstein EJ, Daly RJ, Batzer AG, Li W, Margolis B, Lammers R, Ullrich A, Bar-Sagi D, Schlessinger J. The SH2 and SH3 domain containing protein Grb2 links receptor tyrosine kinases to ras signaling. Cell 1992;70:431–442.
200. Lupu R, Colomer R, Zugmaier G, Sarup J, Shepard M, Slamon D, Lippman ME. Direct interaction of a ligand for the *erb*B2 oncogene product with the EGF receptor and p185*erb*B2. Science 1990;249:1552–1555.
201. Lyman SD, James L, Vanden Bos T, de Vries P, Brasel K, Gliniak B, Hollingsworth LT, Picha KS, McKenna HJ, Splett RR, Fletcher FA, Maraskovsky E, Farrah T, Foxworthe D, Williams DE, Beckmann MP. Molecular cloning of a ligand for the flt3/flk-2 tyrosine kinase receptor: a proliferative factor for primitive hematopoietic cells. Cell 1993;75: 1157–1167.
202. Lyman SD, James L, Escobar S, Downey H, de Vries P, Brasel K, Stocking K, Beckmann MP, Copeland NG, Cleveland LS, Jenkins NA, Belmont JW, Davison BL. Identification of soluble and membrane-bound isoforms of the murine flt3 ligand generated by alternative splicing of mRNAs. Oncogene 1995;10:149–157.
203. Maglione D, Guerriero V, Viglietto G, Delli-Bovi P, Persico MG. Isolation of a human placenta cDNA coding for a protein related to the vascular permeability factor. Proc Natl Acad Sci USA 1991;88:9267–9271.
204. Mahasandana C, Suvatte V, Chuansumrit A, Marlar RA, Manco-Johnson MJ, Jacobson LJ, Hathaway WE. Clinical and laboratory observations: homozygous protein S deficiency in an infant with purpura fulminans. J Pediatr 1990;117:750–753.
205. Maillard C, Berruyer M, Serre CM, Dechavanne M, Delmas PD. Protein-S, a vitamin K-dependent protein, is a bone matrix component synthesized and secreted by osteoblasts. Endocrinology 1992;130:1599–1604.
206. Maisonpierre PC, Goldfarb M, Yancopoulos GD, Gao G. Distinct rat genes with related profiles of expression define TIE receptor tyrosine kinase family. Oncogene 1993;8:1631–1637.
207. Maness LM, Kastin AJ, Weber JT, Banks WA, Beckman BS, Zadina JE. The neurotrophins and their receptors: structure, function, and neuropathology. Neurosci Biobehav Rev 1994;18:143–159.
208. Manfioletti G, Brancolini C, Avanzi G, Schneider C. The protein encoded by a growth arrest-specific gene (gas6) is a new member of the vitamin K-dependent proteins related to protein S, a negative coregulator in the blood coagulation cascade. Mol Cell Biol 1993;13:4976–4985.
209. Marchionni MA, Goodearl ADJ, Chen MS, Bermingham-McDonogh O, Kirk C, Hendricks M, Denehy F, Misumi D, Sundhalter J, Kobayashi K, Wroblewski D, Lynch C, Baldassare M, Hiles I, Davis JB, Hsuan JJ, Totty NF, Otsu M, McBury RN, Waterfield MD, Stoobant P, Gwynne D. Glial growth factors are alternatively spliced *erb*B-2 ligands expressed in the nervous system. Nature 1993;362:312–318.
210. Margolis B, Rhee SG, Felder S, Mervic M, Lyall R, Levitzki A, Ullrich A, Zilberstein A, Schlessinger J. EGF induces tyrosine phosphorylation of phospholipase C-II: a potential mechanism for EGF receptor signaling. Cell 1989;57:1101–1107.
211. Marics I, Adelaide J, Raybaud F, Mattei MG, Coulier F, Planche J, de Lapeyriere O, Birnbaum D. Characterization of the HST-related FGF6 gene, a new member of the fibroblast growth factor gene family. Oncogene 1989;4:335–340.
212. Mark MR, Scadden DT, Wang Z, Gu Q, Goddard A, Godowski PJ. rse, A novel receptor-type tyrosine kinase with homology to Axl/Ufo, is expressed at high levels in the brain. J Biol Chem 1994;269:10720–10728.
213. Marshall CJ. Specificity of receptor tyrosine kinase signaling: transient versus sustained extracellular signal-regulated kinase activation. Cell 1995;80:179–185.
214. Masiakowski P, Carroll RD. A novel family of cell surface receptors with tyrosine kinase-like domain. J Biol Chem 1992;267:26181–26190.
215. Martin FH, Suggs SV, Langley KE, Lu HS, Ting J, Okino KH, Morris CF, McNiece IK, Jacobsen FW, Mendiaz EA. Primary structure and functional expression of rat and human stem cell factor DNAs. Cell 1990;64:203–211.
216. Martin-Zanca D, Oskam R, Mitra G, Copeland T, Barbacid M. Molecular and biochemical characterization of the human *trk* proto-oncogene. Mol Cell Biol 1989;9: 24–33.

217. Maru Y, Hirai H, Takaku F. Overexpression confers an oncogenic potential upon the *eph* gene. Oncogene 1990;5:445–447.
218. Marx J. Bombesin receptor gene cloned. Science 1990;249:1377.
219. Massague J. Transforming growth factor-α: a model for membrane-anchored growth factors. J Biol Chem 1990;265:21393–21396.
220. Matthews W, Jorday GT, Gavin M, Jenkins N, Copeland NO, Lemischka IR. A receptor tyrosine kinase cDNA isolated from a population of enriched primitive hematopoietic cells and exhibiting close gene linkage to c-*kit*. Proc Natl Acad Sci USA 1991;88: 1026–1030.
221. Matsuda M, Mayer BJ, Fukui Y, Hanafusa H. Binding of transforming protein, P47gag-crk, to a broad range of phosphotyrosine containing proteins. Science 1990;248: 1537–1539.
222. Matsui T, Heidaran M, Miki T, Popescu N, La Rochelle W, Kraus M, Pierce J, Aaronson SA. Isolation of a novel receptor cDNA establishes the existence of two PDGF receptor genes. Science 1989;243:800–804.
223. Matsui T, Pierce JH, Fleming TP, Greenberger JS, LaRochelle WJ, Ruggiero M, Aaronson SA. Independent expression of human alpha or beta platelet-derived growth factor receptor cDNAs in a naive hematopoietic cell leads to functional coupling with mitogenic and chemotactic signaling pathways. Proc Natl Acad Sci USA 1989;86:8314–8318.
224. Matsushime H, Wang LH, Shibuya M. Human c-*ros*-1 gene homologous to the v-*ros* sequence of UR2 sarcoma virus encodes for a transmembrane receptorlike molecule. Mol Cell Biol 1986;6:3000–3004.
225. Mary Y, Hirai H, Takaku F. Human ltk: gene structure and preferential expression in human leukemic cells. Oncogene Res 1990;5:199–204.
226. Maxwell M, Naber SP, Wolfe HJ, Galanopoulos T, Hedley-Whyte ET, Black PM, Antoniades HN. Coexpression of platelet-derived growth factor (PDGF) and PDGF-receptor genes by primary human astrocytomas may contribute to their development and maintenance. J Clin Invest 1990;86:131–140.
227. McKinnon RD, Matsui T, Dubois-Dalcq M, Aaronson, SA. FGF modulates the PDGF-driven pathway of oligodendrocyte development. Neuron 1990;5:603–614.
228. Meisenhelder J, Suh PG, Rhee SG, Hunter T. Phospholipase C-gamma is a substrate for the PDGF and EGF receptor protein-tyrosine kinases *in vivo* and *in vitro*. Cell 1989;57:1109–1122.
229. Metcalf D. The molecular control of cell division, differentiation commitment and maturation in haemopoietic cells. Nature 1989;339:27–30.
230. Millauer B, Wizigmann-Voos S, Schnurch H, Martinez R, Moller NP, Risau W, Ullrich A. High affinity VEGF binding and developmental expression suggest Flk-1 as a major regulator of vasculogenesis and angiogenesis. Cell 1993;72:835–846.
231. Mitamura T, Higashiyama S, Taniguchi N, Klagsbrun M, Mekada E. Diphtheria toxin binds to the epidermal growth factor (EGF)-like domain of human heparin-binding EGF-like growth factor/diphtheria toxin receptor and inhibits specifically its mitogenic activity. J Biol Chem 1995;270:1015–1019.
232. Miyamoto M, Naruo L, Seko C, Matsumoto S, Kondo T, Kurokawa T. Molecular cloning of a novel cytokine cDNA encoding the ninth member of the fibroblast growth factor family, which has a unique secretion property. Mol Cell Biol 1993;13:4251–4259.
233. Miyazawa K, Tsubouchi H, Naka D, Takahashi K, Okigaki M, Arakaki N, Nakayama H, Hirono S, Sakiyama O, et al. Molecular cloning and sequence analysis of cDNA for human hepatocyte growth factor. Biochem Biophys Res Commun 1989;163: 967–973.
234. Moody TW, Pert CB, Gazdar AF, Carney DN, Minna JD. High levels of intracellular bombesin characterize human small-cell lung carcinoma. Science 1981;214: 1246–1248.
235. Mori S, Ronnstrand L, Yokote K, Engstrom A, Courtneidge SA, Claesson-Welsh L, Heldin C-H. Identification of two juxtamembrane autophosphorylation sites in the PDGF β-receptor; involvement in the interaction with Src family tyrosine kinases. EMBO J 1993;12:2257–2264.
236. Morris SW, Kirstein MN, Valentin MB, Dittmer KG, Shapiro DN, Saltman DL, Look AT. Fusion of a kinase gene, ALK, to a nucleolar protein gene, NPM, in non-Hodgkin's lymphoma. Science 1994;263:1281–1284.
237. Morrison DK, Kaplan DR, Rhee SG, Williams LT. Platelet-derived growth factor (PDGF)-dependent association of phospholipase C-gamma with the PDGF receptor signaling complex. Mol Cell Biol 1990;10:2359–2366.
238. Moses HL, Yang EY, Pietenpol JA. TGF-beta stimulation and inhibition of cell proliferation: new mechanistic insights. Cell 1990;63:245–247.
239. Motzer RJ, Nanus DM, O'Moore P, Scher HI, Bajorin DF, Reuter V, Tong WP, 1versen J, Louison C, Albino AP. Phase II trial of suramin in patients with advanced renal cell carcinoma: treatment results, pharmacokinetics, and tumor growth factor expression. Cancer Res 1992;52:5775–5779.
240. Mroczkowski B, Reich M, Chen K, Bell GI, Cohen S. Recombinant human epidermal growth factor precursor is a glycosylated membrane protein with biological activity. Mol Cell Biol 1989;9:2771–2778.
241. Mui AL-F, Miyajima A. Cytokine receptors and signal transduction. Prog Growth Factor Res 1994;5:15–35.
242. Muller WJ, Lee FS, Dickson C, Peters G, Pattengale P, Leder P. The *int*-2 gene product acts as an epithelial growth factor in transgenic mice. EMBO J 1990;9:907–913.
243. Mulligan LM, Kwok JBJ, Healey CS, Elsdon MJ, Eng C, Gardner E, Love DR, Mole SE, Moore JK, Papi L, Ponder MA, Telenius H, Tunnacliffe A, Ponder BAJ. Germ-line mutations of the *RET* proto-oncogene in multiple endocrine neoplasia type 2A. Nature 1993;363:458–460.
244. Mulshine JL, Avis I, Treston AM, Mobley C, Kaspryzyk P, Carrasquillo JA, Larson SM, Nakanishi Y, Merchant B, Minna JD, et al. Clinical use of a monoclonal antibody to bombesin-like peptide in patients with lung cancer. Ann NY Acad Sci 1988;547: 360–372.
245. Musacchio A, Gibson T, Rice P, Thompson J, Saraste M. The PH domain: a common piece in the structural patchwork of signaling proteins. Trends Biochem Sci 1993;18: 343–348.
246. Mustonen T, Alitalo K. Endothelial receptor tyrosine kinases involved in angiogenesis. J Cell Biol 1995;129:895–898.
247. Myers C, Cooper M, Stein C, LaRocca R, Walther MM, Weiss G, Choyke P, Dawson N, Steinberg S, Uhrich MM. Suramin: A novel growth factor antagonist with activity in hormone-refractory metastatic prostate cancer. J Clin Oncol 1992;10:881–889.
248. Myers MG Jr, Backer JM, Sun XJ, Shoelson S, Hu P, Schlessinger J, Yoakim M, Schaffhausen B, White MF. IRS-1 activates phosphatidylinositol 3′-kinase by associating with *src* homology 2 domains of p85. Proc Natl Acad Sci USA 1992;89: 10350–10354.
249. Myers JN, Drebin JA, Wada T, Greene MI. Biological effects of monoclonal antireceptor antibodies reactive with *neu* oncogene product, p185neu. Methods Enzymol 1991;198:277–290.
250. Nakamura T, Nawa K, Ichihara A, Kaise N, Nishino T. Purification and subunit structure of hepatocyte growth factor from rat platelets. FEBS Lett 1987;224:311–316.
251. Nakamura T, Nishizawa T, Hagiya M, Seki T, Shimonishi M, Sugimura A, Tashiro K, Shimizu S. Molecular cloning and expression of human hepatocyte growth factor. Nature 1989;342:440–443.
252. Naruo K, Seko C, Kuroshima K, Matsutani E, Sasada R, Kondo T, Kurokawa T. Novel secretory heparin-binding factors from human glioma cells (glia-activating factors) involved in glial cell growth. Purification and biological properties. J Biol Chem 1993;368:2857–2864.
253. Natali PG, Nicotra MR, Bigotti A, Venturo I, Slamon DJ, Fendly BM. Expression of the p185 encoded by HER2 oncogene in normal and transformed human tissues. Int J Cancer 1990;45:457–461.
254. Neufeld G, Tessler S, Gitay-Goren H, Cohen T, Levi B. Vascular endothelial growth factor and its receptors. Prog Growth Factor Res 1994;5:89–97.
255. Nichols EJ, Manger R, Hakomori SI, Rohrschneider LR. Transformation by the oncogene v-*fms*: the effects of castanospermine on transformation-related parameters. Exp Cell Res 1987;173:486–495.
256. Nissley P, Lopaczynski W. Insulin-like growth factor receptors. Growth Factors 1991;5:29–43.
257. Nister M, Hammacher A, Mellstrom K, Siegbahn A, Ronnstrand L, Westermark B, Heldin CH. A glioma-derived PDGF A chain homodimer has different functional activities from a PDGF AB heterodimer purified from human platelets. Cell 1988;52: 791–799.
258. Nister M, Libermann TA, Betsholtz C, Pettersson M, Claesson-Welsh L, Heldin CH, Schlessinger J, Westermark B. Expression of messenger RNAs for platelet-derived growth factor and transforming growth factor-alpha and their receptors in human malignant glioma cell lines. Cancer Res 1988;48:3910–3918.
259. Norton PA, Hynes RO, Rees DJ. Sevenless: seven found? Cell 1990;61:15–16.
260. O'Bryan JP, Frye RA, Cogswell PC, Neubauer A, Kitch B, Prokop C, Espinosa R III, Le Beau MM, Earp HS, Liu ET. *axl*, a transforming gene isolated from primary human myeloid leukemia cells, encodes a novel receptor tyrosine kinase. Mol Cell Biol 1991;11:5016–5031.
261. Oelrichs R, Reid HH, Bernard O, Ziemiecki A, Wilks A. NYK/FLK-1: a putative receptor tyrosine kinase isolated from E10 embryonic neuroepithelium is expressed in endothelial cells of the developing embryo. Oncogene 1992;8:11–18.
262. Ohasi K, Mizuno K, Kuma K, Miyata T, Nakamura T. Cloning of the cDNA for a novel receptor tyrosine kinase, Sky, predominantly expressed in brain. Oncogene 1994;9: 699–705.
263. Onoda T, Iinuma H, Sasaki Y, Hamada M, Isshiki K, Naganawa H, Takeuchi T, Tatsuta K, Umezawa K. Isolation of a novel tyrosine kinase inhibitor, lavendustin A, from *Streptomyces griseolavendus*. J Natl Prod 1989;52:1252–1257.
264. Ornitz DM, Yayon A, Flanagan JG, Svahn CM, Levi E, Leder P. Heparin is required for cell-free binding of basic fibroblast growth factor to a soluble receptor and for mitogenesis in whole cells. Mol Cell Biol 1992;12:240–247.
265. Pachnis V, Mankoo B, Costantini F. Expression of the c-ret proto-oncogene during mouse embryogenesis. Development 1993;119:1005–1017.
266. Pajusola K, Aprelikova O, Korhonen J, Kaipainen A, Pertovaara L, Alitalo R, Alitalo K. FLT4 receptor tyrosine kinase contains seven immunoglobulin-like loops and is expressed in multiple human tissues and cell lines. Cancer Res 1992;52:5738–5743.
267. Pajusola K, Aprelikova O, Armstrong E, Morris S, Alitalo K. Two human FLT4 receptor tyrosine kinase isoforms with distinct carboxy terminal tails are produced by alternative processing of primary transcripts. Oncogene 1993;8:2931–2937.
268. Pajusola K, Aprelikova A, Pelicci G, Welch H, Claesson-Welch KM, Alitalo BD. Signalling properties of FLT4, a proteolytically processed receptor tyrosine kinase related to two VEGF receptors. Oncogene 1994;9:3545–3555.
269. Pandy A, Shao H, Marks RM, Polverini PJ, Dixit VM. Role of B61, the ligand for the eck receptor tyrosine kinase, in TNF-α-induced angiogenesis. Science 1995;268: 567–569.
270. Pardee AB. G1 events and regulation of cell proliferation. Science 1989;246:603–608.
271. Park M, Dean M, Cooper CS, Schmidt M, O'Brien SJ, Blair DG, Vande Woude GF. Mechanism of *met* oncogene activation. Cell 1986;45:895–904.
272. Parker PJ, Waterfield MD. Phosphatidylinositol 3-kinase: a novel effector. Cell Growth Different 1992;3:747–752.
273. Parkes HC, Lillycrop K, Howell A, Craig RK. C-*erb*B-2 mRNA expression in human breast tumours: comparison with c-*erb*B-2 DNA amplification and correlation with prognosis. Br J Cancer 1990;61:39–45.
274. Partanen J, Armstrong E, Makela T, Korhonen J, Sanberg M, Renkonen R, Knuutila S, Huebner K, Alitalo K. A novel endothelial cell surface receptor tyrosine kinase with extracellular epidermal growth factor homology domains. Mol Cell Biol 1992;12: 1698–1707.
275. Partanen J, Vainikka S, Korhonen J, Armstrong E, Alitalo K. Diverse receptors for fibroblast growth factors. Prog Gowth Factor Res 1992;4:69–83.
276. Pastan I, Fitzgerald D. Recombinant toxins for cancer treatment. Science 1991;254: 1173–1177.
277. Pawson T. Tyrosine kinases and their interactions with signalling proteins. Curr Opin Genet Devel 1992;2:4–12.
278. Pazin MJ, Williams LT. Triggering signaling cascades by receptor tyrosine kinases. Trends Biochem Sci 1992;17:374–378.
279. Pegelow CH, Ledford M, Young JN, Zilleruelo G. Severe protein S deficiency in a newborn. Pediatrics 1992;89:674–676.
280. Peles E, Bacus SS, Koski RA, Lu HS, Wen D, Ogden SG, Levy RB, Yarden Y. Isolation of the Neu/HER-2 stimulatory ligand: a 44 kd glycoprotein that induces differentiation of mammary tumor cells. Cell 1992;69:205–216.
281. Pendergast AM, Muller AJ, Havlik MH, Maru Y, Witte ON. BCR sequences essential for transformation by the BCR-ABL oncogene bind to the ABL SH2 regulatory domain in a non-phosphotyrosine-dependent manner. Cell 1991;66:162–172.

282. Perez JL, Shen X, Finkernagel S, Sciorra L, Jenkins NA, Gilbert DJ, Copeland NG, Wong TW. Identification and chromosomal mapping of a receptor tyrosine kinase with a putative phospholipid binding sequence in its ectodomain. Oncogene 1994;9: 211–219.
283. Phillips DJ, Greengard JS, Fernandez JA, Ribeiro M, Evatt BL, Griffin JH, Hopper WC. Protein S, and antithrombotic factor, is synthesized and released by neural tumor cells. J Neurochem 1993;61:344–347.
284. Pierce JH, Di Marco E, Cox GW, Lombardi D, Ruggiero M, Varesio L, Wang LM, Choudhury GG, Sakaguchi AY, Di Fiore PP, et al. Macrophage-colony-stimulating factor (CSF-1) induces proliferation, chemotaxis, and reversible monocytic differentiation in myeloid progenitor cells transfected with the human c-fms/CSF-1 receptor cDNA. Proc Natl Acad Sci USA 1990;87:5613–5617.
285. Pierce JH, Ruggiero M, Fleming TP, Di Fiore PP, Greenberger JS, Varticovski L, Schlessinger J, Rovera G, Aaronson SA. Signal transduction through the EGF receptor transfected in IL-3-dependent hematopoietic cells. Science 1988;239:628–631.
286. Pledger WJ, Stiles CD, Antoniades HN, Scher CD. Induction of DNA synthesis in BALB/c 3T3 cells by serum components: reevaluation of the commitment process. Proc Natl Acad Sci USA 1977;74:4481–4485.
287. Pledger WJ, Stiles CD, Antoniades HN, Scher CD. An ordered sequence of events is required before BALB/c-3T3 cells become committed to DNA synthesis. Proc Natl Acad Sci USA 1978;75:2839–2843.
288. Plouet J, Schilling J, Gospodarowicz D. Isolation and characterization of a newly identified endothelial cell mitogen produced by AtT-20 cells. EMBO J 1989;8:3801–3806.
289. Ponder BAJ. The gene causing multiple endocrine neoplasia type 2 (MEN2) Ann Med 1994;26:199–203.
290. Plowman GD, Green JM, McDonald VL, Neubauer MG, Disteche CM, Todaro GJ, Shoyab M. The amphiregulin gene encodes a novel epidermal growth factor-related protein with tumor-inhibitory activity. Mol Cell Biol 1990;10:1969–1981.
291. Plowman GD, Culouscou J-M, Whitney GS, Green JM, Carlton GW, Foy L, Neubauer MG, Shoyab M. Ligand-specific activation of HER4/p180^{erbB4}, a fourth member of the epidermal growth factor receptor family. Proc Natl Acad Sci USA 1993;90: 1746–1750.
292. Plowman GD, Whitney GS, Neubauer MG, Green JM, McDonald VL, Todaro GJ, Shoyab M. Molecular cloning and expression of an additional epidermal growth factor receptor-related gene. Proc Natl Acad Sci USA 1990;87:4905–4909.
293. Prigent SA, Lemoine NR. The type 1 (EGFR-related) family of growth factor receptors and their ligands. Prog Growth Factor Res 1992;4:1–24.
294. Pulido D, Campuzano S, Koda T, Modoleel J, Barbacid M. Dtrk, a *Drosophila* gene related to the trk family of neurotrophin receptors, encodes a novel class of neural cell adhesion molecule. EMBO J 1992;11:391–404.
295. Radeke MJ, Misko TP, Hus C, Herzenberg LA, Shooter EM. Gene transfer and molecular cloning of the rat nerve growth factor receptor. Nature 1987;325:593–597.
296. Rapoport BL, Falkson G, Raats JI, de Wet M, Lotz BP, Potgieter HC. Suramin in combination with mitomycin C in hormone-resistant prostate cancer. A phase II clinical study. Ann Oncol 1993;4:567–573.
297. Re RN. Emerging issues in the cellular biology of the cardiovascular system. Am J Cardiol 1988;62:7G-12G.
298. Reinhardt RR, Chin E, Zhang B, Roth RA, Bondy CA. Insulin receptor-related receptor messenger ribonclelc acid is focally expressed in sympathetic and sensory neurons and renal distal tubule cells. Endocrinology 1993;133:3–10.
299. Rescigno J, Mansukhani A, Basilico C. A putative receptor tyrosine kinase with unique structural topology. Oncogene 1991;6:1903–1913.
300. Rettenmier CW, Sherr CJ. The mononuclear phagocyte colony-stimulating factor (CSF-1, M-CSF). Hematol Oncol Clin North Am 1989;3:479–493.
301. Robbins KC, Antoniades HN, Devare SG, Hunkapiller MW, Aaronson SA. Structural and immunological similarities between simian sarcoma virus gene product(s) and human platelet-derived growth factor. Nature 1983;305:605–608.
302. Robbins KC, Leal F, Pierce JH, Aaronson SA. The v-*sis*/PDGF-2 transforming gene product localizes to cell membranes but is not a secretory protein. EMBO J 1985;4: 1783–1792.
303. Roberts AB, Sporn MB. Principles of molecular cell biology of cancer: growth factors related to transformation. In Cancer: Principles and Practice of Oncology. Edited by VT DeVita Jr, S Hellman, SA Rosenberg. Philadelphia: Lippincott, 1989, pp 67–80.
304. Ronsin C, Muscatelli F, Mattei MG, Breathnach R. A novel putative receptor protein tyrosine kinase of the met family. Oncogene 1993;8:1195–1202.
305. Rosen EM, Nigam SK, Goldberg ID. Scatter factor and the c-Met receptor: a paradigm for mesenchymal/epithelial interaction. J Cell Biol 1994;127:1783–1787.
305a.Rosenberg SA. Karnotsky Memorial Lecture. The immunotherapy and gene therapy of cancer. J Clin Oncol 1992;10:180–199.
306. Ross R, Raines EW, Bowen-Pope DF. The biology of platelet-derived growth factor. Cell 1986;46:155–169.
307. Rotwein P. Structure, evolution, expression and regulation of insulin-like growth factors I and II. Growth Factors 1991;5:3–18.
308. Roussel MF, Downing JR, Rettenmier CW, Sherr CJ. A point mutation in the extracellular domain of the human CSF-1 receptor (c-*fms* proto-oncogene product) activates its transforming potential. Cell 1988;55:979–988.
309. Roussel MF, Dull TJ, Rettenmier CW, Ralph P, Ullrich A, Sherr CJ. Transforming potential of the c-*fms* proto-oncogene (CSF-1 receptor). Nature 1987;325:549–552.
310. Rozakis-Adcock M, McGlade J, Mbamalu G, Pelicci G, Daly R, Li W, Batzer A, Thomas S, Brugge J, Pelicci PG, et al. Association of the Shc and Grb2/Sem5 SH2-containing proteins is implicated in activation of the *ras* pathway by tyrosine kinases. Nature 1992;360:689–692.
311. Rubin JS, Osada H, Finch PW, Taylor WG, Rudikoff S, Aaronson, SA. Purification and characterization of a newly identified growth factor specific for epithelial cells. Proc Natl Acad Sci USA 1989;86:802–806.
312. Ruff-Jamison S, Chen K, Cohen S. Induction by EGF and interferon-γ of tyrosine phosphorylated DNA binding proteins in mouse liver nuclei. Science 1993;261: 1733–1736.
313. Sadowski HB, Shuai K, Darnell JE, Gilman MZ Jr. A common nuclear signal transduction pathway activated by growth factor and cytokine receptors. Science 1993;261:1739–1744.
314. Sanchez MP, Tapley P, Saini SS, He B, Pulido D, Barbacid M. Multiple tyrosine protein kinases in rat hippocampal neurons: isolation of Ptk-3, a receptor expressed in proliferative zones of the developing brain. Proc Natl Acad Sci USA 1994;91: 1819–1823.
315. Sano H, Forough R, Maier JA, Case JP, Jackson A, Engleka K, Maciag T, Wilder RL. Detection of high levels of heparin binding growth factor-1 (acidic fibroblast growth factor) in inflammatory arthritic joints. J Cell Biol 1990;110:1417–1426.
316. Santoro M, Rosati R, Grieco M, Berlingieri MT, D'Amato GL, de Franciscis V, Fusco A. The ret proto-oncogene is consistently expressed in human pheochromocytomas and thyroid medullary carcinomas. Oncogene 1990;5:1595–1598.
317. Sato B, Kouhara H, Koga M, Kasayama S, Saito H, Sumitani S, Hashimoto K, Kishimoto T, Tanaka A, Matsumoto L. Androgen-induced growth factor and its receptor: demonstration of the androgen-induced autocrine loop in mouse mammary carcinoma cells. J Steroid Biochem Mol Biol 1993;47:91–98.
318. Sato T, Qin Y, Kozak CA, Audus K. tie-1 and tie-2 Defined another class of putative receptor tyrosine kinase gene expressed in early embryonic vascular system. Proc Natl Acad Sci USA 1993;90:9355–9358.
319. Schechter AL, Stern DF, Vaidyanathan L, Decker SJ, Drebin JA, Greene MI, Weinberg RA. The *neu* oncogene: an *erb*B-related gene encoding a 185,000-Mr tumour antigen. Nature 1984;312:513–516.
320. Schlessinger J. SH2/SH3 signaling proteins. Curr Opin Genet Devel 1994;4:25–30.
321. Schlessinger J, Ullrich A. Growth factor signaling by receptor tyrosine kinases. Neuron 1992;9:383–391.
322. Schmidt C, Bladt F, Goedecke S, Brinkmann V, Zschiescho W, Sharpe M, Gheradi E, Birchmeir C. Scatter factor/hepatocyte growth factor is essential for liver development. Nature 1995;373:699–702.
323. Schneider C, King RM, Phillipson L. Genes specifically expressed at growth arrest of mammalian cells. Cell 1988;54:787–793.
324. Schneider R. The human protooncogene ret: a communicative cadherin? Trends Biochem Sci 1992;17:468–469.
325. Schreiber AB, Winkler ME, Derynck R. Transforming growth factor-alpha: a more potent angiogenic mediator than epidermal growth factor. Science 1986;232: 1250–1253.
326. Schnurch HA, Risau W. Expression of tie-2, a member of a novel family of receptor tyrosine kinases, in the endothelial cell linage. Development 1993;119:957–968.
327. Scott J, Urdea M, Quiroga M, Sanchez-Pescador R, Fong N, Selby M, Rutter WJ, Bell GI. Structure of a mouse submaxillary messenger RNA encoding epidermal growth factor and seven related proteins. Science 1983;221:236–240.
328. Semba K, Kamata N, Toyoshima K, Yamamoto T. A v-*erb*B-related protooncogene, c-*erb*B-2, is distinct from the c-*erb*B-1/epidermal growth factor-receptor gene and is amplified in a human salivary gland adenocarcinoma. Proc Natl Acad Sci USA 1985;82:6497–6501.
329. Senger DR, Galli SJ, Dvorak AM, Perruzzi CA, Harvey VS, Dvorak HF. Tumor cells secrete a vascular permeability factor that promotes accumulation of ascites fluid. Science 1983;219:983–985.
330. Senger DR, Perruzzi CA, Feder J, Dvorak HF. A highly conserved vascular premeability factor secreted by a human and rodent tumor cell lines. Cancer Res 1986;46: 5629–5632.
331. Sherr CJ, Rettenmier CW, Sacca R, Roussel MF, Look AT, Stanley ER. The c-*fms* proto-oncogene product is related to the receptor for the mononuclear phagocyte growth factor, CSF-1. Cell 1985;41:665–676.
332. Shibuya M, Yamaguchi S, Yamane A, Ikeda T, Tojo A, Matsushime H, Sato M. Nucleotide sequence and expression of a novel human receptor-type tyrosine kinase gene (*flt*) closely related to the *fms* family. Oncogene 1990;5:519–524.
333. Shier P, Watt VM. Primary structure of a putative receptor for a ligand of the insulin family. J Biol Chem 1989;264:14605–14608.
334. Shing Y, Christofori G, Hanahan D, Ono Y, Sasada R, Igarashi K, Folkman J. Betacellulin: a mitogen from pancreatic β cell tumors. Science 1993;259:1604–1607.
335. Shoyab M, McDonald VL, Bradley JG, Todaro GJ. Amphiregulin: a bifunctional growth-modulating glycoprotein produced by the phorbol 12-myristate 13-acetate-treated human breast adenocarcinoma cell line MCF-7. Proc Natl Acad Sci USA 1988;85:6528–6532.
336. Shoyab M, Plowman GD, McDonald VL, Bradley JG, Todaro GJ. Structure and function of human amphiregulin: a member of an epidermal growth factor family. Science 1989;14:1074–1076.
337. Siegel PM, Dankort DL, Hardy WR, Muller WJ. Novel activating mutations in the *neu* proto-oncogene involved in induction of mammary tumors. Mol Cell Biol 1994;14: 7068–7077.
338. Silvennoinen O, Schindler C, Schlessinger J, Levy DE. *ras*-independent growth factor signaling by transcription factor tyrosine phosphorylation. Science 1993;261: 1736–1739.
339. Sizeland AM, Burgess AW. Anti-sense transforming growth factor a oligonucleotides inhibit autocrine stimulated proliferation of a colon carcinoma cell line. Mol Cell Biol 1992;3:1235–1243.
340. Skeel A, Yoshimura T, Showalter SD, Tanaka S, Appella E, Leonard EJ. Macrophage stimulating protein: purification, partial amino acid sequence, and cellular activity. J Exp Med 1991;173:1227–1234.
341. Slamon DJ, Godolphin W, Jones LA, Holt JA, Wong SG, Keith DE, Levin WJ, Stuart SG, Udove J, Ullrich A, et al. Studies of the HER-2/*neu* proto-oncogene in human breast and ovarian cancer. Science 1989;244:707–712.
342. Smith DR, Vogt PK, Hayman MJ. The v-*sea* oncogene of avian erythroblastosis retrovirus S13: another member of the protein-tyrosine kinase gene family. Proc Natl Acad Sci USA 1989;86:5291–5295.
343. Smith R, Peters G, Dickson C. Multiple RNAs expressed from the *int*-2 gene in mouse embryonal carcinoma cell lines encode a protein with homology to fibroblast growth factors. EMBO J 1988;7:1013–1022.
344. Sonnenberg E, Godecke A, Walter B, Bladt F, Birchmeier C. Transient and locally restricted expression of the *ros*1 protooncogene during mouse development. EMBO J 1991;10:3693–3702.
345. Springer WR, Cooper DN, Barondes SH. Discoidin I is implicated in cell-substratum attachment and ordered cell migration of *Dictyostelium discoideum* and resembles fibronectin. Cell 1984;39:557–564.
346. Sporn MB, Todaro GJ. Autocrine secretion and malignant transformation of cells. N Engl J Med 1980;303:878–880.
347. Stacker SA, Hovens CM, Vitali A, Pritchard MA, Baker E, Sutherland GR, Wilks AF.

Molecular cloning and chromosomal localisation of the human homologue of a receptor related to tyrosine kinases (RYK). Oncogene 1993;8:1347–1356.
348. Stitt TN, Conn G, Gore M, Lai C, Bruno J, Radziejewski C, Mattsson K, Fisher J, Gles DR, Jones PF, Masiakowski P, Ryan TE, Tobkes NJ, Chen DH, DiStefano PS, Long GL, Basillico C, Goldfarb MP, Lemke G, Glass DJ, Yancopoulos GD. The anticoagulation factor protein S and its relative, gas6, are ligands for the tyro 3/*axl* family of receptor tyrosine kinases. Cell 1995;80:661–670.
349. Stoker M, Gherardi E, Perryman M, Gray J. Scatter factor is a fibroblast-derived modulator of epithelial cell mobility. Nature 1987;327:239–242.
350. Streuli M, Krueger NX, Tsai AY, Saito H. A family of receptor-linked protein tyrosine phosphatases in humans and *Drosophila*. Proc Natl Acad Sci USA 1989;86: 8698–8702.
351. Sun XJ, Miralpeix M, Myers MG Jr, Glasheen EM, Backer JM, Kahn CR, White MF. Expression and function of IRS-1 in insulin signal transmission. J Biol Chem 1992;267: 22662–22672.
352. Sun XJ, Rothenberg P, Kahn CR, Backer JM, Araki E, Wilden PA, Cahill DA, Goldstein BJ, White MF. Structure of the insulin receptor substrate IRS-1 defines a unique signal transduction protein. Nature 1991;352:73–77.
353. Sun XJ, Crimmins DL, Myers MG, Miralpeix M, White M. Pleiotropic insulin signals are engaged by multisite phosphorylation of IRS-1. Mol Cell Biol 1993;13:7418–7428.
354. Takahashi M, Buma Y, Hiai H. Isolation of *ret* proto-oncogene cDNA with an amino-terminal signal sequence. Oncogene 1989;4:805–806.
355. Taira M, Yoshida T, Miyagawa K, Sakamoto H, Terada M, Sugimura T. cDNA sequence of human transforming gene *hst* and identification of the coding sequence required for transforming activity. Proc Natl Acad Sci USA 1987;84:2980–2984.
356. Tanaka A, Miyamoto K, Minamino N, Takeda M, Sato B, Matsuo H, Matsumoto L. Cloning and characterization of an androgen-induced growth factor essential for the androgen-dependent growth of mouse mammary carcinoma cells. Proc Natl Acad Sci USA 1992;89:8928–8932.
357. Takagi S, Tsuji T, Amagai T, Takamatsu T, Fijisawa H. Specific cell surface labels in the visual centers of *Xenopus laevis* tadpole identified using monoclonal antibodies. Dev Biol 1987;122:90–100.
358. Takahashi M, Buma Y, Iwamoto T, Inaguma Y, Ikeda H, Hiai H. Cloning and expression of the *ret* proto-oncogene encoding a tyrosine kinase with two potential transmembrane domains. Oncogene 1988;3:571–578.
359. Tamagnone L, Partanen J, Armstrong E, Lasota J, Ohgami K, Tazunoki T, LaForgia S, Huebner K, Alitalo K. The human ryk cDNA sequence predicts a protein containing two putative transmembrane segments and a tyrosine kinase catalytic domain. Oncogene 1993;8:2009–2014.
360. Terman BC, Dougher-Vermazen M, Carrion ME, Dimitrov D, Amerlino D, Gospodarowicz D, Bohlen P. Identification of the KDR tyrosine kinase as a receptor for vascular endothelial growth factor. Biochem Biophys Res Commun 1992;187: 1479–1586.
361. Thomas KA. Transforming potential of fibroblast growth factor genes. Trends Biochem Sci 1988;13:327–328.
362. Tisher E, Gospodarowicz D, Mitchell R, Silva M, Schilling J, Lau K, Crisp T, Fiddes JC, Abraham JA. Vascular endothelial growth factor: a new member of the platelet-derived growth factor gene family. Biochem Biophys Res Commun 1989;165: 1198–1206.
363. Todaro GJ, Fryling C, De Larco JE. Transforming growth factors produced by certain human tumor cells: polypeptides that interact with epidermal growth factor receptors. Proc Natl Acad Sci USA 1980;77:5258–5262.
364. Trahey M, McCormick F. A cytoplasmic protein stimulates normal N-*ras* p21 GTPase, but does not affect oncogenic mutants. Science 1987;238:542–545.
365. Tuzi NL, Gullick WJ. eph, The largest known family of putative growth factor receptors. Br J Cancer 1994;69:417–421.
366. Twamley GM, Kypta RM, Hall B, Courtneidge SA. Association of fyn with the activated platelet-derived growth factor receptor: requirements for binding and phosphorylation. Oncogene 1992;7:1893–1901.
367. Twardzik ER, Brown JP, Ranchalis JE, Todaro GJ, Moss B. Vaccinia virus-infected cells release a novel polypeptide functionally related to transforming and epidermal growth factors. Proc Natl Acad Sci USA 1985;82:5300–5304.
368. Tzahar E, Levkowitz G, Karunagaran D, Yi L, Peles E, Lavi S, Chang D, Liu N, Yayon A, Wen D, Yarden Y. *Erb*B-3 and *Erb*B-4 function as the respective low and high affinity receptors of all *neu* differentiation factor/heregulin isoforms. J Biol Chem 1994;269: 25226–25233.
369. Uehara Y, Murakami Y, Suzukake-Tsuchiya K, Moriya Y, Sano H, Shibata K, Omura S. Effects of herbimycin derivatives on *src* oncogene function in relation to antitumor activity. J Antibiotics 1988;41:831–834.
370. Ullrich A, Bell JR, Chen EY, Herrera R, Petruzzelli LM, Dull TJ, Gray A, Coussens L, Liao YC, Tsubokawa M, et al. Human insulin receptor and its relationship to the tyrosine kinase family of oncogenes. Nature 1985;313:756–761.
371. Ullrich A, Berman CH, Dull TJ, Gray A, Lee JM. Isolation of the human insulin-like growth factor I gene using a single synthetic DNA probe. EMBO J 1984;3:361–364.
372. Ullrich A, Gray A, Tam AW, Yang-Feng T, Tsubokawa M, Collins C, Henzel W, Le Bon T, Kathuria S, Chen E, et al. Insulin-like growth factor I receptor primary structure: comparison with insulin receptor suggests structural determinants that define functional specificity. EMBO J 1986;5:2503–2512.
373. Ullrich A, Schlessinger J. Signal transduction by receptors with tyrosine kinase activity. Cell 1990;61:203–212.
374. Umezawa H, Imoto M, Sawa T, Isshiki K, Matsuda N, Uchida T, Iinuma H, Hamada M, Takeuchi T. Studies on a new epidermal growth factor-receptor kinase inhibitor, erbstatin, produced by MH436-hF3. J Antibiotics 1986;39:170–173.
375. Upton C, Macen JL, McFadden G. Mapping and sequencing of a gene from myxoma virus that is related to those encoding epidermal growth factor and transforming growth factor alpha. J Virol 1987;61:1271–1275.
376. Valtieri M, Tweardy DJ, Caracciolo D, Johnson K, Mavilio F, Altmann S, Santoli P, Rovera G. Cytokine-dependent granulocytic differentiation. Regulation of proliferative and differentiative responses in a murine progenitor cell line. J Immunol 1987;138: 3829–3835.
377. Van De Vijver M, Bersselaar R, Devilee P, Cornelisse C, Peterse J, Nusse R. Amplification of the neu (c-*erb*B-2) oncogene in human mammary tumors is relatively frequent and is often accompanied by amplification of the linked c-*erb*A oncogene. Mol Cell Biol 1987;7:2019–2023.
378. Varnum BC, Young C, Elliott G, Garcia A, Bartley TD, Fridell Y, Hunt RW, Trall G, Clogston C, Toso RJ, Yanaglhara D, Bennett L, Sylber M, Merewether L, Tseng A, Escobar E, Liu ET, Yamane HK. *Axl* receptor tyrosine kinase stimulated by the vitamin K-dependent protein encoded by growth arrest-specific gene 6. Nature 1995;373: 623–626.
379. Vigna E, Naldini L, Tamagnone L, Longati P, Bardelli A, Maina F, Ponzetto C, Comoglio PM. Hepatocyte growth factor and its receptor, the tyrosine kinase encoded by the c-*met* proto-oncogene. Cell Mol Biol 1994;40:597–604.
380. Velu TJ, Beguinot L, Vass WC, Willingham MC, Merlino GT, Pastan I, Lowy DR. Epidermal growth factor-dependent transformation by a human EGF receptor proto-oncogene. Science 1987;238:1408–1410.
381. Vogel W, Lammers R, Huang J, Ullrich A. Activation of a phosphotyrosine phosphatase by tyrosine phosphorylation. Science 1993;259:1611–1614.
382. Vu TK, Hung DT, Wheaton VI, Coughlin SR. Molecular cloning of a functional thrombin receptor reveals a novel proteolytic mechanism of receptor activation. Cell 1991;64:1057–1066.
383. Wata T, Qian XL, Greene MI. Intermolecular association of the p185*neu* protein and EGF receptor modulates EGF receptor function. Cell 1990;61:1339–1347.
384. Wahl MI, Daniel TO, Carpenter G. Antiphosphotyrosine recovery of phospholipase C activity after EGF treatment of A-431 cells. Science 1988;241:968–970.
385. Wahl MI, Nishibe S, Carpenter G. Growth factor signaling pathways: phosphoinositide metabolism and phosphorylation of phospholipase C. Cancer Cells 1989;1: 101–107.
386. Walker F, Nicola NA, Metcalf D, Burgess AW. Hierarchical down-modulation of hemopoietic growth factor receptors. Cell 1985;43:269–276.
387. Wang LH, Hanafusa H, Notter MF, Balduzzi PC. Genetic structure and transforming sequence of avian sarcoma virus UR2. J Virol 1982;41:833–841.
388. Waterfield MD. Growth factor receptors. Br Med Bull 1989;45:541–553.
389. Waterfield MD, Scrace GT, Whittle N, Stroobant P, Johnsson A, Wasteson A, Westermark B, Heldin CH, Huang JS, Deuel TF. Platelet-derived growth factor is structurally related to the putative transforming protein p28*sis* of simian sarcoma virus. Nature 1983;304:35–39.
390. Wen D, Peles E, Cupples R, Suggs SV, Bacus SS, Luo YI, Trail G, Hu S, Silbiger SM, Levy RB, Koski RA, Lu HS, Yarden Y. Neu differentiation factor: a transmembrane glycoprotein containing an EGF domain and an immunoglobulin homology unit. Cell 1992;69:559–572.
391. Wen D, Suggs SV, Karunagaran D, Liu N, Cupples RL, Luo Y, Janssen AM, Ben-Baruch N, Trollinger DB, Jacobsen VL, Meng S, Lu HS, Hu S, Chang D, Yang W, Yanigahara D, Koski RA, Yarden Y. Structural and functional aspects of the multiplicity of neu differentiation factors. Mol Cell Biol 1994;14:1909–1919.
392. Werner S, Smola H, Liao X, Longaker MT, Krieg T, Hofschneider PH, Williams LT. The function of KGF in morphogenesis of epithelium and reepithelialization of wounds. Science 1994;266:819–822.
393. Westermark B, Heldin CH. Similar action of platelet-derived growth factor and epidermal growth factor in the prereplicative phase of human fibroblasts suggests a common intracellular pathway. J Cell Physiol 1985;124:43–48.
394. Westermark B, Johnsson A, Paulsson Y, Betsholtz C, Heldin CH, Herlyn M, Rodeck U, Koprowski H. Human melanoma cell lines of primary and metastatic origin express the genes encoding the chains of platelet-derived growth factor (PDGF) and produce a PDGF-like growth factor. Proc Natl Acad Sci USA 1986;83:7197–7200.
395. Wexler D, Fleming TP, DiFiore PP, Aaronson SA. Unpublished data.
396. White MF, Maron R, Kahn CR. Insulin rapidly stimulates tyrosine phosphorylation of a Mr-185,000 protein in intact cells. Nature 1985;318:183–186.
397. Wigler MH. GAPS in understanding *ras*. Nature 1990;346:696–697.
398. Williams DE, Eisenman J, Baird A, Rauch C, Van Ness K, March CJ, Park LS, Martin U, Mochizuki DY, Boswell HS. Identification of a ligand for the c-*kit* proto-oncogene. Cell 1990;633:167–174.
399. Williams GT. Programmed cell death: apoptosis and oncogenesis. Cell 1991;65: 1097–1098.
400. Williams LT. Signal transduction by the platelet-derived growth factor receptor. Science 1989;243:1564–1570.
401. Wilson C, Goberdhan DC, Steller H. Dror, a potential neurotrophic receptor gene, encodes a *Drosophila* homolog of the vertebrate Ror family of Trk-related receptor tyrosine kinases. Proc Natl Acad Sci USA 1993;90:7109–7113.
402. Witte ON. Steel locus defines new multipotent growth factor. Cell 1990;63:5–6.
403. Woll PJ, Rozengurt E. Neuropeptides as growth regulators. Br Med Bull 1989;45: 492–505.
404. Woll PJ. Neuropeptide growth factors and cancer. Br J Cancer 1991;63:469–475.
405. Wood WI, Capon DJ, Simonsen CC, Eaton DL, Gitschier J, Keyt B, Seeburg PH, Smith DH, Hollingshead P, Wion KL. Expression of active human factor VIII from recombinant DNA clones. Nature 1984;312:330–337.
406. Wright NA, Pike C, Elia G. Induction of a novel epidermal growth factor-secreting cell lineage by mucosal ulceration in human gastrointestinal stem cells. Nature 1990;343: 82–85.
407. Wyllie AH, Rose KA. Rodent fibroblast tumours expressing human *myc* and *ras* genes: growth, metastasis and endogenous oncogene expression. Br J Cancer 1987;56:251–259.
408. Yamamoto T, Nishida T, Miyajima N, Kawai S, Ooi T, Toyoshima K. The *erb*B gene of avian erythroblastosis virus is a member of the *src* gene family. Cell 1983;35:71–78.
409. Yarden Y, Escobedo JA, Kuang WJ, Yang-Feng TL, Daniel TO, Tremble PM, Chen EY, Ando ME, Harkins RN, Francke U, et al. Structure of the receptor for platelet-derived growth factor helps define a family of closely related growth factor receptors. Nature 1986;323:226–232.
410. Yarden Y, Ullrich A. Growth factor receptor tyrosine kinases. Annu Rev Biochem 1988;57:443–478.
411. Yayon A, Klagsbrun M, Esko JD, Leder P, Ornitz DM. Cell surface, heparin-like molecules are required for binding of basic fibroblast growth factor to its high affinity receptor. Cell 1991;64:841–848.
412. Yi T, Ihle JN. Association of hematopoietic cell phosphatase with c-*kit* after stimulation with c-*kit* ligand. Mol Cell Biol 1993;13:3350–3358.
413. Yoshimura T, Yuhki N, Wang MH, Skeel A, Leonard EJ. Cloning, sequencing, and ex-

pression of human macrophage stimulating protein (MSP, MST1) confirms MSP as a member of the family of kringle proteins and locates the MSP gene on chromosome 3. J Biol Chem 1993;268:15461–15468.
414. Zerlin M, Julius MA, Goldfarb MD. NEP: a novel receptor-like tyrosine kinase expressed in proliferating neuroepithelia. Oncogene 1993;8:2731–2739.
415. Zhan X, Bates B, Hu XG, Goldfarb M. The human FGF-5 oncogene encodes a novel protein related to fibroblast growth factors. Mol Cell Biol 1988;8:3487–3495.
416. Zhang B, Roth RA. The insulin receptor-related receptor. Tissue expression, ligand binding specificity, and signaling capabilities. J Biol Chem 1992;267:18320–18328.
417. Ziegler SF, Bird TA, Schneringer JA, Schooley KA, Baum PR. Molecular cloning and characterization of a novel receptor protein tyrosine kinase from human placenta. Oncogene 1993;8:663–670.
418. Zong CS, Wang L-H. Modulatory effect of the transmembrane domain of the protein-tyrosine kinase encoded by oncogene *ros*: biological function and substrate interaction. Proc Natl Acad Sci USA 1994;91:10982–10986.
419. Zsebo KM, Williams DA, Geissler EN, Broudy VC, Martin FH, Atkins HL, Hsu RY, Birkett NC, Okino KH, Murdock DC. Stem cell factor is encoded at the D1 locus of the mouse and is the ligand for the c-*kit* tyrosine kinase receptor. Cell 1990;63:213–224.

CHAPTER 4

Signal Transduction in Cancer

YUSUF A. HANNUN

Introduction

The last 15 years have witnessed significant and exciting advances in understanding the mechanisms of cell regulation. This has been most notable in the area of cancer biology. The genetic and biochemical mechanisms underlying the pathogenesis of the cancerous phenotype have been yielding to the increasing sophistication and intensity of basic science approaches. In fact, it is now evident that cancer biology is amenable to investigation at a molecular level. While a complete and detailed understanding of the complex molecular pathways of cell regulation is not yet fully developed, many of the key elements responsible for control of cell growth and cell function in normal and malignant cells have been discovered and their mechanisms of action studied.

In normal cellular physiology, individual cells function in large part by responding to appropriate stimuli from their environment and by interacting with other cells. The healthy maintenance of normal physiology, therefore, demands that cells possess the ability to sense a multitude of external and internal stimuli, integrate those messages, and execute the appropriate responses (Fig. 4.1). For example, in the case of neutrophilic leukocytes, normal homeostasis requires these white blood cells to maintain an active pool of differentiated cells capable of responding to infectious agents. Similarly, the maintenance of normal epithelial tissues requires precursor cells to differentiate so as to regenerate epithelial surfaces while at the same time maintaining the precursor (stem cell) pool (Fig. 4.1). In most cases, tissues have developed mechanisms to eliminate old or damaged cells through regulated programmed cell death (or apoptosis). These examples illustrate the delicate balance that must be maintained between cellular proliferation, cell differentiation, and cell elimination (or cell death) in different body tissues.

Cancer cells, on the other hand, which are derived from normal counterparts, are characterized by their much more autonomous behavior, their nearly unchecked proliferation, and their greater resistance to elimination. Cancer cells may be afflicted by viruses, carcinogens, or endogenous mutations so that they no longer respond appropriately to their environment (Fig. 4.1). This transformation is passed on to the progeny of a cancer cell, causing an expansion of this malignant clone. Such clonal expansion results in increased susceptibility to additional mutations and consequently greater loss of growth control, increasing the potential for metastasis and growth in otherwise unfavorable environments. The pathophysiology of cancer derives from these defects which accumulate in cancer cells (whether caused by exogenous agents or spontaneous mutations).

A major hypothesis of molecular cancer biology is that such defects modify the networks that control cell proliferation, viability, or differentiation. These networks are primarily composed of signal transduction and cell regulatory pathways that normally operate to regulate tightly cellular responses to the environment. Fundamental support for this hypothesis derives from the following: (*a*) oncogenes (cancer-causing genes) encode for essential components of signal transduction and cell regulatory pathways; (*b*) transforming viruses modulate the expression and/or function of endogenous cell regulatory molecules; (*c*) spontaneous oncogenic mutations are increasingly found to result in deranged behavior of cell regulatory molecules; and (*d*) various classes of tumor promoters, which are agents that enhance cell transformation, act by interacting with basic elements of signal transduction pathways. These and other observations have begun to unify heretofore disparate fields of cancer biology. In turn, cancer biology has unified different fields of physiology, biochemistry, pharmacology and genetic research.

It is now clear that to understand cancer at a molecular level we must understand the pathways of cell regulation and signal transduction. The study of signal transduction has traditionally involved the dissection of biochemical pathways involved in the proximal events leading from external stimuli to cellular responses. As such, signal transduction is a major component of cell regulation. Advances in the study of cell regulation have merged areas of signal transduction (proximal events) with more distal events, thus blurring the demarcation of signal transduction events. The emphasis in this chapter will be predominantly on the proximal events of cell regulation—that is, on signal transduction.

This chapter reviews briefly the current state of knowledge regarding components of signal transduction, their regulation and normal operation, and their implicated roles in cancer pathogenesis. Not only is this knowledge beginning to unify our understanding of cancer biology, but it potentially identifies discrete biochemical targets for cancer therapeutics. The first section describes the general components of signaling mechanisms, while the second provides a more detailed description of individual signal transduction pathways. The third section provides a general overview of the interrelationships between different signaling pathways and describes their complexity and organization. The fourth sec-

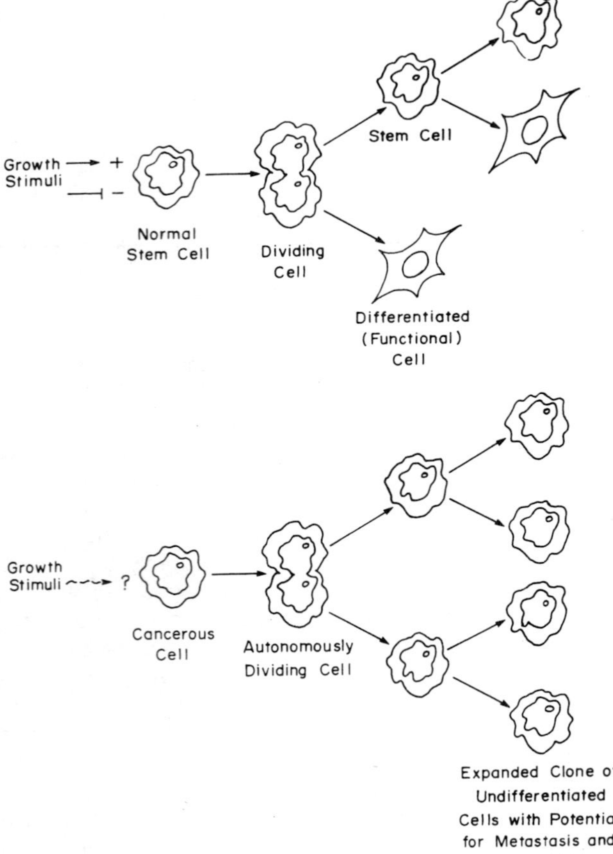

Figure 4.1. Differentiation/proliferation in normal and cancerous cells. The specialized functions of most tissues (e.g., epithelial or hematopoietic) are carried out by fully differentiated cells with little or no capacity to divide and proliferate. Therefore, normal stem cells have to divide and proliferate in order to maintain an active pool of stem cells as well as to replenish lost differentiated cells. These processes of cell proliferation and differentiation are under strict control. Cells respond to environmental signals (such as growth factors and cytokines) and execute the appropriate responses. The intra- and intercellular pathways of signal transduction and cell regulation, therefore, play essential roles in ensuring normal cell function. Breakdown of these cell regulatory processes and signal transduction mechanisms may then result in autonomously dividing cells, hyperproliferation, and an expanded clone of undifferentiated cells with poor normal function.

tion describes aberrations in signal transduction and their role in oncogenesis and tumor promotion. The fifth section outlines the therapeutic potential afforded by this increasing understanding of how cellular signaling affects cancer biology.

How Do Cells Transduce Signals?

Each cell type is capable of sensing numerous extracellular signals. Although there are extracellular agents that penetrate the plasma membrane and interact with intracellular receptors (e.g., steroids and nitric oxide), the vast majority of these agents interact with receptors in the plasma membrane (Fig. 4.2). These cell surface receptors specifically recognize and interact with a unique extracellular agent (or with a closely related set of agents). They then communicate to intracellular macromolecules the status of their receptor occupancy. This initiates flow of information through a series of signaling components and ultimately results in modulation of cell function.

EXTRACELLULAR STIMULI

The chemical composition of extracellular agents is quite diverse and includes proteins, small peptides, nucleotides, amino acid derivatives, carbohydrates, lipids, and other miscellaneous chemicals, including neurotransmitters and many xenobiotics (Fig. 4.2). With very few exceptions, each of these extracellular agents has unique structural features

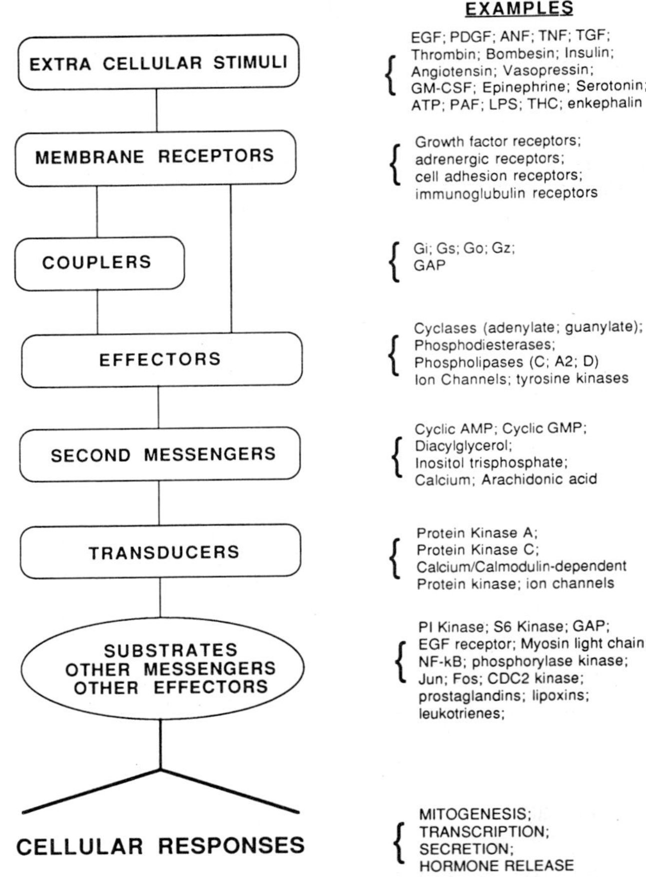

Figure 4.2. Components of signal transduction pathways. Stimuli interact with membrane receptors, which then couple effectors either directly or through couplers. Effectors usually act by generating second messengers that act on target transducers. These are usually protein kinases that modulate substrate phosphorylation. In other cases, initial signaling events lead to the activation of subsequent effectors and the generation of additional messengers. Examples of molecules belonging to each of these components are given to the right. EGF, epidermal growth factor; PDGF, platelet-derived growth factor; ANF, atrial natriuretic factor; TNF, tumor necrosis factor; TGF, transforming growth factor; GM-CSF, granulocyte-macrophage colony-stimulating factor; PAF, platelet-activating factor; LPS, lipopolysaccharide; THC, tetrahydrocannabinol; GAP, GTPase-activating protein; Gi, Gs, Go, Gz, different G proteins; PI, phosphatidylinositol; NFκB, nuclear factor κB.

that are recognized by a specific cell membrane receptor. This allows cells to recognize different stimuli accurately and to initiate the appropriate response.

Growth factors form an important subset of extracellular stimuli (see below). They play essential roles in regulating cell proliferation and growth. Most known growth factors are polypeptides or glycoproteins; these include the transforming growth factors (TGF-α and TGF-β), interleukins, hematopoietic growth factors, epidermal growth factor (EGF), and platelet-derived growth factor (PDGF). These growth factors are mitogenic (i.e., induce cell division) and, therefore, induce cell growth (30). However, a few growth factors, such as TGF-β, can also inhibit growth of many cell types (61). An important feature of growth factors is that they possess multiple functions, depending on the cell type (85). For example, TGF-β can stimulate the growth of fibroblasts but inhibits the growth of many other cell types. Thrombin is a mitogen for fibroblasts and endothelial cells (95) but also functions as a critical component of blood coagulation and platelet activation (82). Also, the action of growth factors may be dramatically influenced by the presence of other growth factors. TGF-β in the presence of PDGF stimulates the growth of fibroblasts, while the combination of TGF-β and EGF inhibits growth of these same cells (76).

MEMBRANE RECEPTORS

The currently identified membrane receptors belong to a few large subfamilies. These include growth factor receptors (64) that are predominantly membrane-spanning proteins (most receptors that have been studied are located at the plasma membrane; a few receptors have also been postulated to exist in the nuclear membrane). Receptors for growth factors are either single-chain proteins or multimers (usually homo- or heterodimers) (Fig. 4.3, Schemes I and VI). Many of the receptors in this group possess enzymatic activity in that they can phosphorylate other proteins and peptides on tyrosine residues (Fig. 4.3, Scheme I); i.e., they are tyrosine kinases (e.g., receptors for EGF, PDGF). An emerging class of membrane receptors, exemplified by the TGF-β receptor, possess serine threonine kinase activity. Other receptors, however, do not possess protein kinase activity (Fig. 4.3, Scheme V) such as those for TNF, interferon, and interleukins (1). Another major family of receptors is composed of protein molecules that appear to have seven transmembrane spanning regions (38). These receptors (as well as some of those belonging to the first group) are able to specifically interact with intracellular proteins (G proteins) that function to couple bound receptors to intracellular effector systems (Fig. 4.3, Schemes II and III). A third class of receptors is represented by the atrial natriuretic factor (ANF) receptor which has an intracytoplasmic guanylate cyclase activity (44) (Fig. 4.3, Scheme IV). A major class of receptors, the immunoglobulin-receptor superfamily (43), comprises receptors for immunoglobulins, T-cell antigens, and many cell adhesion molecules. These and related receptors for cell adhesion molecules may play important roles in cell–cell interactions, cell adhesion, and mitogenesis. However, their coupling mechanisms are poorly understood, but may involve activation of nonreceptor tyrosine protein ki-

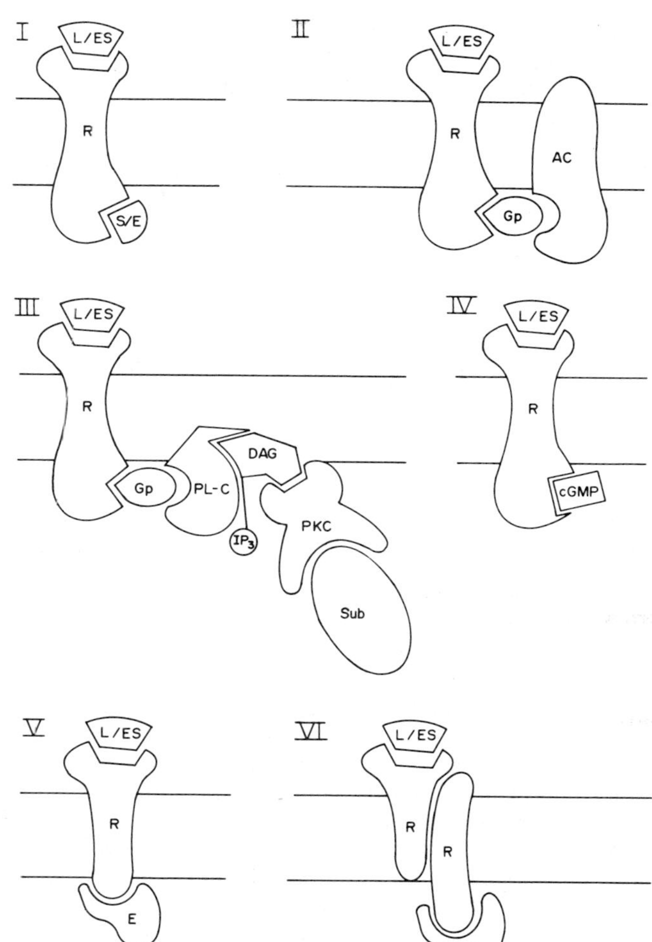

Figure 4.3. Schematic of receptor classes. Most protein receptors are transmembrane proteins with an extracellular domain that contains the ligand-binding site, an intramembranous domain, and an intracytoplasmic domain that usually harbors the site for interaction with couplers, effectors, or substrates. Many growth factor receptors are single or homodimer polypeptides with a single transmembrane domain (Scheme I and Scheme V) and an intracytoplasmic domain that has tyrosine kinase activity (Scheme I) or a short intracytoplasmic domain with no known effector function (Scheme V). A special case with the ANF receptor is the presence of guanylate cyclase activity in its intracytoplasmic domain (Scheme IV). Other receptors may exist as heterodimers with one or both components having ligand-binding sites (Scheme VI). Adrenergic and related receptors are characterized by seven transmembrane domains and an intracytoplasmic domain that couples to G proteins, which in turn couple receptors to adenylate cyclase (Scheme II) or to phospholipase C (Scheme III). Growth factor receptors may also couple to phospholipase C and the PI cycle through G proteins (Scheme III). L/ES, ligand/extracellular stimulus; R, receptors; S/E substrate/effector; Gp, G protein; PL-C, phospholipase C; DAG, diacylglycerol; IP3, inositol trisphosphate; PKC, protein kinase C; Sub, substrate.

nases. For all these receptor classes, a major question in the study of transmembrane signaling relates to the mechanism by which the binding of an extracellular agent to its membrane receptor initiates the biologic response. These are critical events that launch a series of sequential and parallel reactions in the cell. It is thought that significant changes in receptor conformation are imparted by receptor occupancy;

however, the precise nature and mechanism of these changes are unknown.

G PROTEINS (COUPLERS)

The action of many membrane receptors is transduced by a distinct class of GTP-binding proteins known as G proteins (15, 19). These proteins appear to function primarily by coupling receptors to intracellular effectors (Fig. 4.2). They, therefore, play critical regulatory functions in directing intracellular signaling traffic. Significant information has been amassed in the last decade regarding the nature, complexity, function, and roles of certain G proteins in human disease. They are known to exist as two major families. The first is a family of large G proteins that are heterotrimers composed of α, β, and γ subunits. There are multiple isoforms of these subunits that can associate in various combinations, resulting in distinct G proteins. In the resting state, the G protein exists with guanosine diphosphate (GDP) tightly bound to the α chain (Fig. 4.4). Upon receptor occupancy, an appropriate conformational change in the receptor is triggered that results in modulation of the interaction of receptors with G proteins, causing replacement of bound GPD with GTP. GTP binding is accompanied by dissociation of the α chain from the β and γ chains (19). The released GTP-liganded α chain may then interact with certain effector molecules such as adenylate cyclase and phospholipase C (Fig. 4.4), while the β and γ chains may have function on their own (such as interaction with phospholipase A_2) (15) and with phospholipase (12). Signal termination results from the ability of G proteins to hydrolyze the bound GTP, thus regenerating GDP and reassociating the α with the β and γ subunits.

Another family of G proteins consists of small molecular weight G proteins (Smgs) that share homology with the α subunit of large molecular weight G proteins. These include the proto-oncogene *ras*, and other related molecules such as *rev*, *rab*, and *rap*. Smgs are also able to bind GTP and cause its hydrolysis, i.e., they possess GTPase activity (46). GTPase-activating proteins (GAPs), which potentiate the enzymatic activity of many Smgs, have been described. The GAPs serve as substrates of tyrosine kinases and may couple receptors to Smgs and possibly serve as downstream effectors. Although the role of small molecular weight G proteins in signal transduction is not clear, mutations in some of these molecules are oncogenic (see below). They also appear to be important for other cell functions such as trafficking of macromolecules and organelle transport.

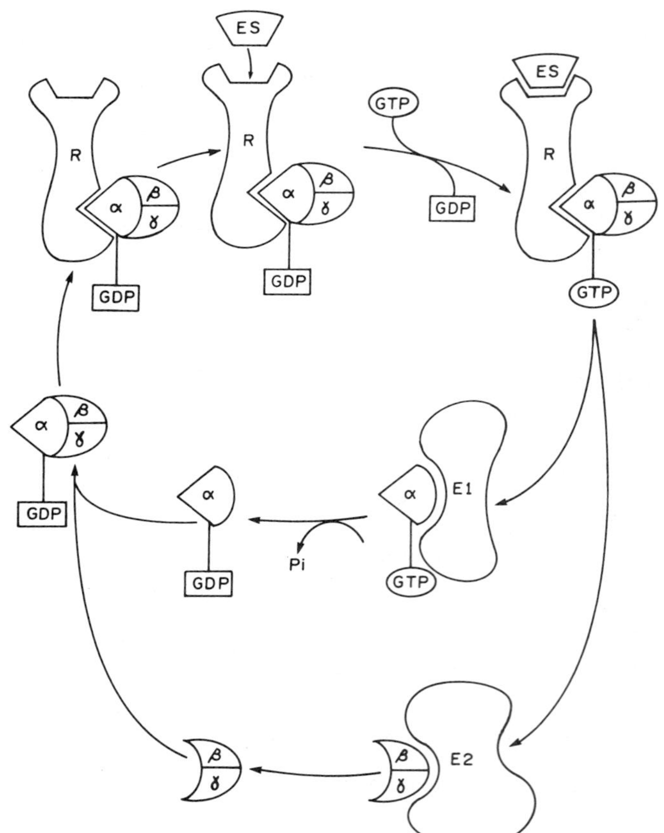

Figure 4.4. G protein cycle. Many membrane receptors may interact with G proteins, which are trimers of α, β, and γ subunits, with GDP bound to the α subunit. Upon receptor occupancy, the coupling of receptors to G proteins results in exchange of GDP for GTP. The GTP-bound α subunit then dissociates from the $\beta\gamma$ subunit and regulates either directly or indirectly effector molecules such as adenylate cyclase. The $\beta\gamma$ subunit may interact with other effector molecules such as ion channels and phospholipase A_2. The α subunit possesses GTPase activity, resulting in the release of phosphate from GTP and the generation of GDP. The GDP-bound α subunit then reassociates with the $\beta\gamma$ subunit resulting in the formation of a resting complex.

EFFECTOR MOLECULES

Effector molecules play a key role in transducing the action of extracellular agents following their interaction with their cell surface receptors. As noted above, many growth factor receptors possess intrinsic tyrosine kinase activity that is activated upon receptor occupancy (64). This enzymatic activity then serves as an effector function for this class of receptors. For receptors that are coupled to G proteins (19), however, it is these G proteins that regulate the activity of key effector enzymes (Fig. 4.2). The most notable such enzymes are adenylate cyclase and phospholipase C. Phospholipases C (57) serve to catalyze the hydrolysis of membrane phospholipids, thereby generating diacylglycerol and inositol triphosphates. Adenylate cyclase catalyzes the formation of cyclic adenosine monophosphate (AMP) from adenosine triphosphate (ATP) (49). Diacylglycerol, inositol trisphosphates, and cyclic AMP then serve as important and potent second messengers.

While the effector function of either phospholipase C or adenylate cyclase appears to be utilized by many receptors, the extent and diversity of known effector molecules are rapidly expanding (Fig. 4.2). Phospholipases C exist as a superfamily of enzymes that catalyze the hydrolysis of various membrane phospholipids (see below). Adenylate cyclase also exists as a family of related enzymes with distinct mechanisms of regulation. Other signaling effectors include guanylate cyclase, which may occur either as an intrinsic element within certain membrane receptors (44) or as a separate soluble enzyme (27). Another major effector is phospholipase A_2, which hydrolyzes membrane phospholipids such as phosphatidylcholine. The main product of phospholipase A_2 action is arachidonic acid, from which many active metabolites are derived (31, 38). Other important effectors include ion channels (16), which may be directly or indirectly regulated by transducers such as G proteins and phosphodiesterases that hydrolyze and inactivate cyclic GMP.

SECOND MESSENGERS AND MEDIATORS

The main function of effector molecules is the generation of second messengers that transduce the information generated by receptor occupancy into functional events. This function is achieved by altering the activity of key regulatory enzymes. Second messengers identified so far appear to be small molecules that are able to regulate target function specifically (Fig. 4.2). Most second messengers appear to derive from membrane lipids or intracellular nucleotides. The best studied and most ubiquitous second messengers are diacylglycerol, inositol trisphosphates, cyclic AMP, cyclic GMP, and calcium (Figs. 4.5 and 4.6). Other molecules whose status as second messengers is increasingly recognized include arachidonic acid and its metabolites, phosphatidic acid, and sphingolipid-derived molecules.

The formation of second messengers is under strict control. Their intracellular levels appear to be low in the resting state and increase, usually abruptly (Fig. 4.7), following receptor occupancy and activation of effectors such as phospholipase C or adenylate cyclase. The signal is then maintained for variable (Fig. 4.7), often short, durations (usually measured in seconds or minutes) and is terminated by metabolism of the second messenger into inactive metabolites. During this brief interval when the intracellular signal is generated, it is able to dramatically modulate the function of key target elements such as protein kinases. Obviously, deranged generation or metabolism of these second messengers could have profound effects on cell function. The magnitude of the signal is also important in determining the extent of the cellular response. In turn, this is modulated by the potency of the extracellular stimulus, the degree of receptor occupancy, the nature of the coupling mechanisms, the effectiveness of cellular enzymes in metabolizing and extinguishing the signal, and a variety of positive and negative feedback mechanisms.

IMMEDIATE TARGETS FOR SECOND MESSENGERS (TRANSDUCERS)

The targets of action of second messengers play a key role in regulating diverse cellular activities ranging from short-term effects such as hormone release and blood cell activation to long-term effects such as cell differentiation, tumor promotion, and oncogenesis. The best studied and most universal of these targets are protein kinases (25, 33) that enzymatically transfer a phosphate from cellular ATP (or GTP) to serine, threonine, or tyrosine residues on various cellular proteins. This phosphorylation event results in conformational changes in target substrates with significant functional effects such as activation/inhibition of other kinases, metabolic enzymes, and/or transcriptional factors. Other known transducers of second messenger effects include protein phosphatases, proteases, and ion channels.

Major questions in molecular cancer biology relate to the identification of physiologic targets for the action of transducers of second messenger action, linking initial events of signal transduction to the functional outcome at a molecular level and identifying mechanisms of growth suppression. At present, these remain largely elusive goals since not all components of the diverse signaling pathways have been defined and since the more distal mediators of cellular events have not yet been linked to proximal components of signaling pathways.

SUBSEQUENT MESSENGERS AND EFFECTORS

Although many second messengers go on to interact directly with enzymes that mediate their effects, a number of second messengers operate by liberating a third stage of messenger molecules. For example, inositol trisphosphate activates intracellular calcium channels, resulting in liberation of calcium from intracellular stores (9). The generation of an intracellular calcium signal activates a number of cal-

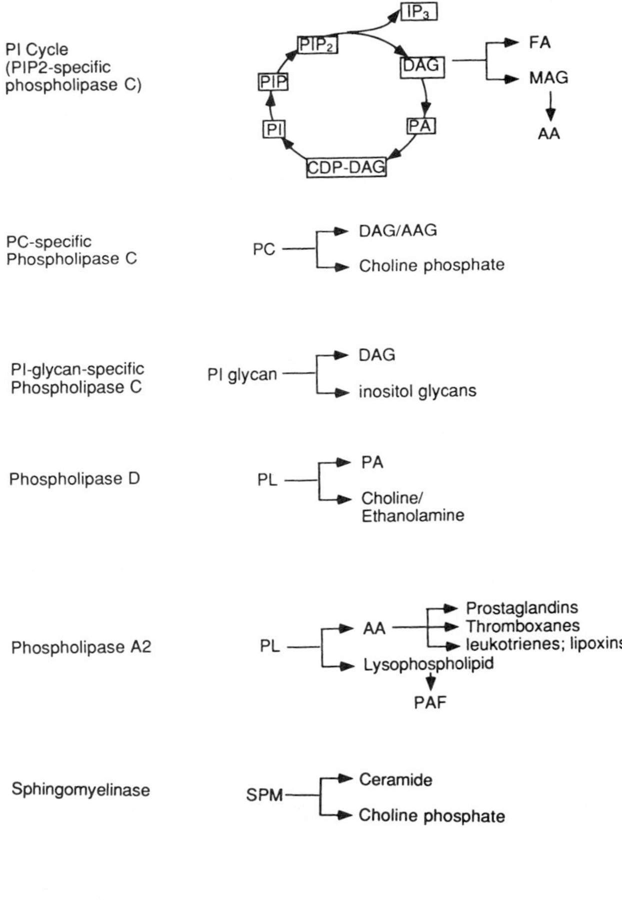

Figure 4.5. Effector/second messenger systems. The different effector systems are shown. Enzyme activities are indicated on the left side, and schematic reactions showing precursors and second messengers are indicated on the right side of the figure. For structures and explanation of abbreviations, see Figure 4.6.

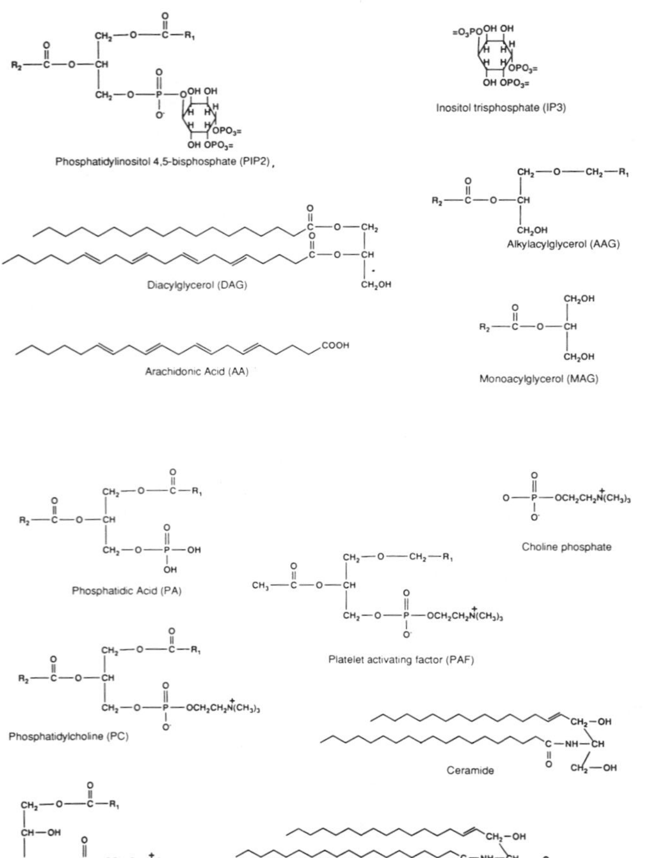

Figure 4.6. Structures of second messengers and precursors.

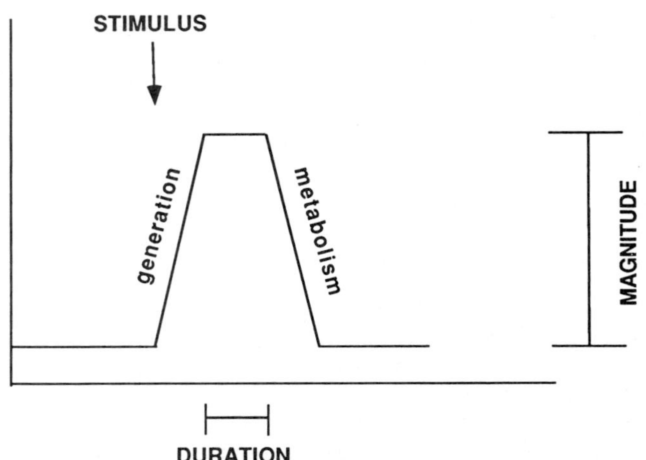

Figure 4.7. The second messenger response. The interaction of extracellular stimuli with cells leads to the activation of effector molecules with the generation of second messengers such as diacylglycerol, cyclic AMP, cyclic GMP, inositol trisphosphate, and arachidonic acid. This results in a build up of levels of those second messengers usually from very low resting levels. The magnitude of peak intracellular levels of second messengers is determined primarily by the strength of the extracellular stimulus as well as by a variety of feedback mechanisms. In most cases, the duration of the second messenger response is limited by active metabolism of second messengers to either inactive metabolites or metabolites with different spectra of activities. The duration of the response is determined by the balance between generation and metabolism and is therefore modulated by the strength of the extracellular stimulus, the presence of multiple extracellular stimuli, feedback mechanisms, and degradation.

cium-binding proteins. This is best studied in the case of arachidonic acid, which is further metabolized into active metabolites (Figs. 4.5 and 4.6) with various biologic functions (10). Diacylglycerol may be further metabolized to yield arachidonic acid and monoacylglycerol, which may have mitogenic activity (Fig. 4.5) (86). Also, cascades of protein kinases exist whereby the activation of one kinase leads to phosphorylation and activation of a subsequent kinase (Fig. 4.2) (25).

DISTAL COMPONENTS/SUBSTRATES OF PROTEIN KINASES

It appears that protein kinases play an essential role in signal transduction mechanisms. A major difficulty in understanding the mechanisms by which extracellular signals modulate discrete cellular functions relates to the identification of substrates whose phosphorylation by protein kinases results in modification of cellular responses. While many such substrates have been identified in vitro, correlating in vitro phosphorylation with an in vivo cellular response continues to be one of the most resistant problems facing investigators in this area of research.

As noted above, many of the substrates for protein kinases are protein kinases themselves. This results in signal amplification through a cascade of different protein kinases. Many of the ultimate substrates of protein kinases are (*a*) rate-limiting enzymes in metabolic cascades, a classic example being glycogen phosphorylase in the pathway of glycogen metabolism; (*b*) nuclear transcription factors; and (*c*) cytoskeletal elements that may mediate changes in cell shape, structure, and/or motility.

The pathways from protein kinases to longer term effects (Fig. 4.2) such as cell proliferation and differentiation appear to be particularly complex. At present, this trail appears to be lost in the cytoplasm, but can be picked up again in the nucleus (see above). A number of transcription regulators appear to be phosphoproteins whose activities may be significantly regulated by phosphorylation/dephosphorylation. The best studied of these factors are *myc*, *myb*, *jun*, *fos*, and nuclear factor κB, all of which have oncogenic counterparts (see below).

Signal Transduction Systems

Although signal transduction mechanisms are closely interrelated, a number of signal transduction pathways may, at a first level of approximation, be considered discrete entities. The complexities generated by cross-talk, feedback, divergence, and convergence of signal transduction mechanisms are discussed below. A brief overview of the major known signal transduction pathways with special emphasis on their role in cell regulation, mitogenesis, and possible involvement in oncogenesis follows.

RECEPTOR-REGULATED TYROSINE KINASES AND MAP KINASE PATHWAY

The receptors for many extracellular ligands possess a tyrosine kinase activity that is regulated by the status of receptor occupancy (64); ligand interaction leads to activation of the tyrosine kinase activity of the receptor. It appears that this tyrosine kinase activity plays an essential role in receptor function. Mutant receptors biochemically engineered to lack the kinase activity lose their function. Major advances in understanding signaling through receptor tyrosine kinases came with the identification of a number of regulatory and effector molecules that are substrates for these receptors. These include a form of phospholipase C that is directly phosphorylated on tyrosine by receptors for EGF and PDGF (47). This phosphorylation results in activation of phospholipase C and initiation of signaling through that pathway (see below). Another emerging target for receptor tyrosine kinases is phosphatidylinositol (PI) kinase (94). This enzyme phosphorylates inositol phospholipids at the 3 position, leading to the formation of a special class of inositol phospholipids. The role of this lipid in signaling is receiving increased attention. GTPase-activating protein (GAP) also appears to be a substrate for receptor tyrosine kinases (65), and its phosphorylation may modulate its interaction with ras-like effector molecules. A number of other cellular substrates are known to be phosphorylated on tyrosine residues, although it is not known whether this phosphorylation is due to receptor tyrosine kinases or to other nonreceptor tyrosine kinases. These substrates include the serine kinase encoded by the *CDC2* gene, which plays an important role in regulation of cell cycle (67).

Once activated, tyrosine kinase receptors not only phosphorylate key substrates, but also undergo autophosphorylation on tyrosine residues. This is a result of intramolecular interactions following receptor dimerization induced by receptor occupancy. Receptor dimerization, which usually involves homodimers or heterodimers of receptors for the same ligand, has been postulated as a key event in receptor activation. The mechanisms involved in dimerization remain, however, poorly understood. The phosphorylated tyrosines on receptors are now recognized to serve as docking sites for specific interactions with individual proteins such that a single receptor may interact with a number of molecules and substrates. Some of these molecules function as adapter proteins, forming a physical link between the receptor and key substrates and/or downstream targets. One of the best studied modular proteins is Grb-2, which interacts with tyrosine phosphorylated receptors through a motif known as src homology-2 (SH2) and serves to interact with sos, an activator of ras, through another modular domain, in this case SH3 (17, 60). In turn, activation of ras results in activation of a cascade of kinases, starting with direct activation of raf kinase and proceeding to activation of MEK (MAP kinase/Erk kinase), followed by activation of MAP kinase (for mitogen-activated protein kinase or microtubule-associated protein kinase, also known as Erk, for extracellular signal-regulated kinase) (22). MAP kinase appears to function as a major activation switch in signal transduction and especially in mitogenic pathways with important targets serving as potential substrates including Myc, phospholipase A_2, and other transcription factors. Indeed, this more or less linear signal transduction pathway from receptor tyrosine kinases to MAP kinase and its substrates is now emerging as a prototype of multiple pathways that appear to be structured similarly, including pathways that result in activation of a jun kinase (also known as stress-activated protein kinase, or SAPK). Thus, multiple trails are being identified that function to connect proximal membrane signal transduction components to nuclear events and other downstream targets.

THE PHOSPHATIDYLINOSITOL CYCLE

It has been almost four decades since investigators first observed changes in phospholipid levels following stimulation of pancreatic cells with acetylcholine (40). The changes in phospholipids were rapid and involved the incorporation of labeled phosphate into phosphatidylinositol (PI) and phosphatidic acid. This was associated with acetylcholine-induced release of amylase from pancreatic acinar cells. Since these initial observations, it has become evident that the activation of many receptors leads to degradation of inositol phospholipids, followed by resynthesis through the formation of phosphatidic acid as an intermediate (Fig. 4.5). This has come to be termed the phosphatidylinositol cycle of cell regulation or the PI cycle. The enzymes involved in PI hydrolysis, the second messengers generated from the breakdown of inositol phospholipids, and the role of this important cycle in various cellular processes are being increasingly clarified.

Phospholipase C

The first regulated enzyme in the PI cycle is a phospholipase C which has specificity toward inositol phospholipids (57). Coupling of surface receptors to phospholipase C appears to occur either through the intermediatory action of G proteins (e.g., receptors for thrombin, bombesin, and others) or through direct tyrosine phosphorylation of phospholipase C by activated receptors (e.g., receptors for EGF or PDGF) (Fig. 4.3). Phospholipase C is known to exist as a family of isoenzymes with variable tissue distribution, substrate specificity, and different requirements for calcium (75). These phospholipases share an ability to hydrolyze inositol phospholipids, especially phosphatidylinositol bisphosphate. This results in the formation of two ubiquitous and important second messengers, inositol trisphosphate and diacylglycerol (Figs. 4.5 and 4.6).

Inositol Trisphosphate

Inositol 1,4,5-trisphosphate, the released hydrophilic head group of phosphatidylinositol bisphosphate, mobilizes calcium from intracellular stores (thought to be the endoplasmic reticulum) (9). The resulting elevation in cytoplasmic calcium levels activates calcium-regulated enzymes. A critical result of calcium elevation is its binding to calmodulin, a major intracellular calcium-binding protein. The calcium/calmodulin complex then interacts with a number of enzymes (21) including calcium/calmodulin-dependent protein kinases, phosphatases, and phosphodiesterases. Calcium/calmodulin-dependent protein kinases consist of a family of related isoenzymes with wide tissue distribution (25).

There are multiple species of inositol phosphates interconnected by complex metabolic pathways (9, 57). Only inositol 1,4,5-trisphosphate has a well-defined function in endogenous release of calcium. Another close relative, inositol tetrakisphosphate, may play a role in calcium entry into the cell (63). The function of other inositol phosphates remains undetermined.

Diacylglycerol/Protein Kinase C

Diacylglycerol, the other product of phosphatidylinositol bisphosphate hydrolysis, is a neutral lipid second messenger (6) that specifically activates protein kinase C (Fig. 4.3, Scheme III). This central event in signal transduction has not only linked protein kinase C to the PI cycle but also has linked PI turnover to the field of tumor promoters (see below) (69). Protein kinase C is a calcium- and phospholipid-dependent protein kinase that is specifically activated by diacylglycerols. It is also activated by phorbol ester-type tumor promoters. Protein kinase C is now known to consist of a family of closely related isoenzymes with different tissue distribution. Activation of protein kinase C occurs whenever the PI cycle is turned on in response to various extracellular stimuli. Protein kinase C appears to have multiple roles in hormone secretion, neurotransmission, cell proliferation, and cell differentiation (69).

Protein kinase C phosphorylates a number of substrates that mediate the various physiologic responses associated with its activation. Although both the nature of these substrates and the signaling pathways leading to cellular responses remain poorly defined, certain pathways have received special attention as possible mediators of the effects of protein kinase C on mitogenesis and gene regulation (Fig. 4.8). The first involves the activation of the transcription factor NFκB. Activation of protein kinase C in lymphoid cells results in phosphorylation of IκB in cytosol, which is an inhibitor of NFκB (28). This results in liberation of NFκB and its translocation to the nucleus, where it acts by modulating the transcription of a number of genes, including those for TNF and IL-2 receptor (Fig. 4.8).

Another transcription pathway activated by protein kinase C is that involving c-fos and c-jun protein products. The phosphorylation of as yet undetermined substrates results in dimerization of these two proteins to form the AP-1 transcription factor, which modulates gene transcription (Fig. 4.8) (3). AP-1 function appears to be associated with sensitivity to tumor promotion (7). Because of the involvement of NFκB, Jun, and Fos in mitogenesis and oncogenesis, these studies implicate protein kinase C as an important regulator of these cell responses.

The discovery that protein kinase C is the predominant intracellular receptor for phorbol esters and that phorbol esters activate protein kinase C by substituting for endogenous diacylglycerol implicated protein kinase C in the process of

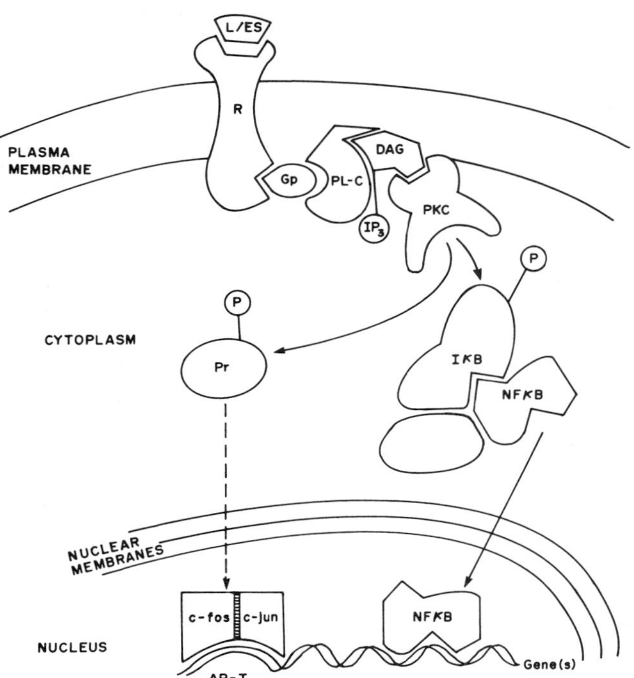

Figure 4.8. Signaling pathways and gene regulation. This scheme illustrates two potential pathways relating signal transduction to gene regulation. The generation of diacylglycerol second messengers through the operation of the PI cycle (as shown above) or from other sources (Fig. 4.5) leads to activation of protein kinase C, which in turn phosphorylates a number of proteins. Phosphorylation of IκB results in dissociation of NFκB from this inhibitory cytoplasmic complex and translocation of NFκB to the nucleus, where it is able to modulate transcription of nuclear genes as a homodimer, heterodimer, or tetramer. In another pathway, protein kinase C phosphorylation of as yet unknown substrates results in activation of AP-1 transcription factor, which is composed of a heterodimer of c-*fos* and c-*jun* that interacts with AP-1 sites on a number of genes, thus modulating gene transcription. Other pathways (not shown) involve activation of CREB nuclear factors by protein kinase C and by cAMP-dependent protein kinase.

tumor promotion and oncogenesis (69). This has been further substantiated by multiple lines of evidence. First, many non-phorbol ester tumor promoters directly activate protein kinase C. Second, overexpression of protein kinase C in fibroblasts results in altered cell growth and acquisition of a transformed phenotype (72). Third, fibroblasts containing overexpressed protein kinase C cause the formation of tumors in nude mice, a model for testing the oncogenic potential of various transformed cells (72). Finally, overproduction of protein kinase C increases the transforming potential of activated *ras* oncogenes (42). These studies suggest that protein kinase C can act as an oncogene, a predictable result given its important role in cell regulation and mitogenesis.

Increasing evidence also implicates the phospholipase C/protein kinase C pathway as a potential target for a number of oncogenes. For example, overexpression of *ras* or *sis* oncogenes results in increased levels of diacylglycerol with consequent abnormal regulation of protein kinase C (73). Prolonged elevation in intracellular diacylglycerol levels may mimic the action of tumor promoters. Thus, abnormal diacylglycerol metabolism may have oncogenic potential, and diacylglycerol may function as an endogenous tumor promoter. The exact mechanisms by which these effects are mediated and their overall contribution to the oncogenic potentials of these transforming oncogenes are yet to be determined.

OTHER LIPID-DERIVED SIGNAL TRANSDUCTION PATHWAYS

Other Phospholipase Cs

Recent investigations have demonstrated the existence of phospholipases C with specificity toward phospholipids other than inositol phospholipids (26). These appear to act primarily on phosphatidylcholine, with the resulting generation of diacylglycerol and choline phosphate (Figs. 4.5 and 4.6). The significance and regulation of this pathway have not been determined.

Other phospholipases appear to have specificity toward complex inositol phospholipids termed PI glycans (55). Hydrolysis of these lipids by a phospholipase C reaction results in the generation of diacylglycerol and inositol glycans (Figs. 4.5 and 4.6). The latter may play important roles in mediating some of the actions of insulin and nerve growth factor. The structure of these putative second messengers is complex and appears to consist of inositol linked to complex carbohydrates composed of galactose and mannose, as well as ethanolamine. The extent and significance of this signaling pathway are unclear (53).

Phospholipase D/Phosphatidic Acid Pathway

Hormone interaction with cell membrane receptor has recently been demonstrated to result in the activation of phospholipase D (11). These stimuli include epinephrine, vasopressin, EGF, PDGF, and others. The action of phospholipase D on membrane phospholipids results in a different chemical cleavage from that induced by phospholipase C. When the substrate is phosphatidylcholine, the action of phospholipase D results in the formation of choline and phosphatidic acid (Figs. 4.5 and 4.6). Phosphatidic acid may have its own cellular actions, including mitogenesis. It may also serve as a precursor for the generation of diacylglycerol. Because the plasma membrane content of phosphatidylcholine far exceeds that of inositol phospholipids (by a ratio of at least 5 : 1 or 10 : 1), induction of phosphatidylcholine hydrolysis may result in production of significantly larger quantities of diacylglycerol than observed with PI hydrolysis. This would result in prolonged elevation in diacylglycerol levels and sustained activation of protein kinase C. Therefore, the phosphatidylcholine pathway of signal transduction may be particularly relevant for mediation of mitogenic effects of cell surface receptors through the protein kinase C pathway. Although this pathway duplicates the ability of the PI cycle to generate diacylglycerol, a major distinguishing feature is the lack of concomitant generation of inositol trisphosphate with consequent elevation of intracellular calcium levels. Therefore, activation of phosphatidylcholine hydrolysis may lead to specific activation of protein kinase C independent of calcium-mediated events.

Phospholipase A_2/Arachidonic Acid Pathway

A major effect of the action of many extracellular stimuli is the activation of phospholipase A_2 (31, 88). The cytosolic form of this enzyme liberates preferentially arachidonic acid from the 2 position of membrane phospholipids. The enzyme is regulated both by calcium and by phosphorylation, especially by MAP kinase (52). Lysophospholipids (Figs. 4.5 and 4.6) generated from the action of phospholipase A_2 may have their own effects on cells, although these are not well defined. Lyso (alkyl) phosphatidylcholine may also serve as a precursor for platelet-activating factor, which has important mitogenic and cell-activating functions. Arachidonic acid, on the other hand, is known to exert effects of its own, including interaction with membrane channels, protein kinase C, and other enzymes. More important, arachidonic acid appears to serve as a precursor for major cell regulatory molecules (Figs. 4.5 and 4.6). These belong to different classes, depending on the metabolic pathways involved in their synthesis. Metabolism through the cyclooxygenase pathway results in the formation of a number of prostaglandins, prostacyclins, and thromboxanes. Alternatively, arachidonic acid may be metabolized through the lipoxygenase pathway, resulting in the formation of lipoxins and leukotrienes (78). Many of these metabolites act as intercellular stimuli/messengers. These appear to have specific cell surface receptors (90) that transduce their action by activating adenylate cyclase, phospholipase C, or other signaling mechanisms. These metabolites have pleiotropic activities including effects on smooth muscle contractility, platelet aggregation, and mitogenesis.

Sphingolipids and the Sphingomyelin Cycle

Sphingolipids are important membrane lipids that show structural diversity and complexity that far exceed that seen with glycerophospholipids. Investigations over many decades have established important roles for sphingolipids in different biologic processes, especially in cell contact, cell proliferation, and cell differentiation (32, 35). Sphingolipids serve as important tumor and differentiation markers. For example, the progression of human melanoma to more aggressive phenotypes is associated with the acquisition of novel sphingolipids. The mechanism of action of sphingolipids, however, remains poorly understood.

Recent studies have begun exploring potential roles for sphingolipids and sphingolipid-derived molecules in signal transduction and as second messengers (35). Sphingosine and related lysosphingolipids are potent inhibitors of protein kinase C. Indeed, a number of pharmacologic and cellular activities for sphingosine have been demonstrated (62). A major theme for sphingosine action seems to be directed at inhibition of activation of the DAG/protein kinase C pathway. Thus, sphingosine has been shown to activate phospholipase D, inhibit the formation of diacylglycerol from phosphatidic acid by inhibiting phosphatidic acid hydrolase, activate diacylglycerol kinase, which metabolizes diacylglycerol, and inhibit protein kinase C (54). Sphingosine has, therefore, been proposed as an endogenous long-chain amino base with important effects on signal transduction processes.

Another lysosphingolipid, sphingosine-1-phosphate, has been demonstrated to possess mitogenic activity and has been proposed as an endogenous mediator of at least certain mitogen-activated pathways (84). Sphingosine-1-phosphate appears to mobilize calcium from intracellular stores either by acting on cell membrane receptors or by acting on intracellular modulators of calcium release. *N*-methylated sphingosines have also been proposed as endogenous regulators of chemotaxis and cell migration (36). These studies are beginning to provide insight into possible functions of sphingolipid-derived products as unique second messenger molecules.

Recently, the sphingomyelin cycle (71) has emerged as an important signal transduction mechanism involved in antiproliferative pathways through the action of a novel lipid-derived second messenger, ceramide. In this pathway, the action of a number of extracellular agents (such as TNF-α, IL-1, and the fas ligand), chemotherapeutic agents, ionizing radiation, and other inducers of antiproliferation or cell stress/injury results in activation of sphingomyelinases that cause hydrolysis of membrane sphingomyelin and the release of membrane ceramide (Fig. 4.5) (34).

The product of sphingomyelin hydrolysis, ceramide (Fig. 4.6), is emerging as an important mediator of the action of these various extracellular agents, especially in mediating antiproliferative activities. Studies with cell-permeable analogues of ceramide have shown the ability of these ceramides to induce differentiation of leukemia cells and to inhibit the growth of a number of transformed and nontransformed cell lines. The inhibition of cell growth has been attributed to inhibition of cell cycle progression at the G_0/G_1 phase of the cell cycle, and evidence is pointing to a role for the product of the retinoblastoma gene product (Rb) as an important downstream target for ceramide. Indeed, Rb has been proposed as an important regulator and checkpoint for cell cycle progression, probably by interacting with key regulators of S phase such as the transcription factor E2F. These studies with ceramide suggest that the sphingomyelin/ceramide pathway may function to transduce the effects of a number of growth-inhibitory agents and signals from the cell membrane to nuclear events involving Rb and subsequent downstream targets.

In another set of studies, the cytotoxic effects of ceramide were investigated and were found to be a result of the induction of programmed cell death, or apoptosis (70). These effects of ceramide were specific in that very closely related lipids (such as dihydroceramide) were totally inactive. Moreover, these changes were reversible, such that activation of the protein kinase C pathway by diacylgylcerol prevented ceramide-induced apoptosis. Thus, the effects of ceramide appear to be specific and regulated, suggesting a specific role for endogenous ceramide in mediating the apoptotic effects of extracellular agents such as TNF-α and the Fas ligand. Because of the emerging role of apoptosis as a key event in regulation of cell growth and viability, understanding the intracellular mechanisms by which apoptosis is regulated promises to provide important insight into the regulation of this heretofore poorly understood mechanism of cell death.

Current effort is aimed at investigating the mechanisms by which ceramide transduces these important antiproliferative activities. Thus, studies have shown the ability of ceramide to regulate the activity of a number of transcription factors and nuclear proteins. For example, ceramide has been shown to down regulate the c-*myc* oncogene, activate NFkB, and activate the retinoblastoma gene product, Rb. A major pressing question in this active area of research is the determination of the most proximal target for the action of ceramide. At present a number of targets have been suggested, including serine/threonine protein phosphatases and protein kinases. The ceramide-activated phosphatase, which is inhibited by okadaic acid, has been suggested to play an important role in tumor suppressor pathways.

Overall, these recent studies are pointing to an important role for ceramide and possibly other sphingolipid-derived molecules in transmitting negative growth stimuli and apoptotic signals. It thus appears that sphingomyelin hydrolysis and ceramide generation are beginning to define a signal transduction pathway originating at the cell membrane and communicating to intranuclear factors, resulting in either apoptosis or cell cycle arrest. As a corollary, derangements in ceramide generation or action may cause significant cell growth dysregulation and may therefore contribute to the pathogenesis of the malignant phenotype. This therefore promises to be an important area of growth and development in the field of signal transduction with particular emphasis in cancer biology.

CYCLASES/CYCLIC NUCLEOTIDE SIGNAL TRANSDUCTION PATHWAYS

Adenylate Cyclase and Cyclic AMP

The first signaling mechanism to be dissected involved cyclic AMP as the second messenger. The interaction of many extracellular stimuli (e.g., adrenergic compounds, acetylcholine, serotonin) with their cell surface receptors is coupled to adenylate cyclase through the action of G proteins (19, 49). G protein–linked pathways exist for both the activation and inhibition of adenylate cyclase. This critical transmembrane enzyme catalyzes the formation of cyclic AMP from ATP (Fig. 4.5). Cyclic AMP acts as a second messenger to activate protein kinase A21 (also known as cyclic AMP-dependent protein kinase). Activation of protein kinase A results from interaction of cyclic AMP with a regulatory component of this enzyme, leading to dissociation of the catalytic subunit of the enzyme. The liberated catalytic subunit is then able to phosphorylate a number of protein substrates on serine and threonine residues, thereby modulating their activities (25). Numerous substrates for protein kinase A have been identified in vitro and in vivo, including the transcription factor(s) CREB/ATF (79).

Activation of the protein kinase A pathway of signaling has been implicated in a number of cellular processes, including neurotransmission and hormone release, as well as in mitogenesis and cell differentiation.

Guanylate Cyclases and Cyclic GMP

Signaling mechanisms involving cyclic GMP as their second messenger have come under increasing investigation as a result of two initially divergent areas of cell biology. Cell biologists had identified the existence of a factor termed EDRF (for endothelium-derived relaxing factor) that acts to cause smooth muscle relaxation. Recent evidence demonstrated that this factor is in fact nitric oxide (NO) or a closely related molecule (66). NO appears to be not only the putative EDRF but also to be the mediator of action of a number of nitroso compounds such as nitrites and nitroprusside, agents of great importance in cardiovascular pharmacology. NO also appears to mediate tumor cell killing by macrophages. A major proximal target of NO appears to be a soluble form of guanylate cyclase. NO interacts with guanylate cyclase and liberates a heme moiety. This results in activation of the enzyme (27, 66) and rapid intracellular formation of cyclic GMP. In turn, cyclic GMP is then able to activate cyclic GMP dependent protein kinase (protein kinase G).

Recent investigations have identified atrial natriuretic peptide (or factor) as an important regulator of circulating fluid volume. Studies on the structure of the cellular receptor for atrial natriuretic factor yielded the unexpected result that the intracellular domain of this receptor is a guanylate cyclase (Fig. 4.3, Scheme IV) (44). It is now established that the action of atrial natriuretic factor on its receptor results in guanylate cyclase activation and the formation of cyclic GMP as a messenger. Atrial natriuretic factor also has important mitogenic activities. These studies implicate cyclic GMP as a potentially important second messenger in the mitogenic response.

COMPLEXITY OF SIGNAL TRANSDUCTION PATHWAYS

Signaling pathways operate to transduce external stimuli to specific cellular responses. The basic structural and biochemical organization of signal transduction pathways as outlined in the previous section may, at a first level of approximation, be considered to consist of components that act in series to transduce the effect of extracellular signals. For example, growth factor interaction with cell receptors may lead to activation of phospholipase C through the coupling action of a G protein. This in turn generates a second messenger such as diacylglycerol, which activates a protein kinase. The consequent phosphorylation of key proteins would then modify cell function and lead to the desired response.

If a strict one-to-one correspondence between each two consecutive components of signal transduction pathways existed, then the action of any one extracellular agent would operate through a unique signal transduction pathway, resulting in a distinct cellular response. While such a scenario would be conceptually easy to understand and more amenable to experimental study, it does not appear to approximate reality. In fact, if cells required each unique receptor to have its own unique coupling protein and unique effector mechanisms, cells would have an enormous number of unique signaling pathways (probably measured in the hundreds). Apparently cells do not require a unique signaling mechanism for each response. This is understandable, since each unique cell type is capable of carrying only a limited repertoire of functional activities even in response to diverse extracellular agents. Also, different cells may use similar signal transduction pathways to couple unique responses to various stimuli. For example, leukocytes and blood platelets may utilize the same or similar mechanisms to couple a "killing" response to foreign organisms, on the one hand, and an aggregation response to thrombotic agents, on the other. Similar pathways may couple the mitogenic response of epithelial cells to growth factors. These features allow significant simplification of signal transduction mechanisms. Paradoxically, this introduces substantial complexity into our understanding of signaling pathways. The following section presents an overview on how signaling components may interact and how complexity is generated.

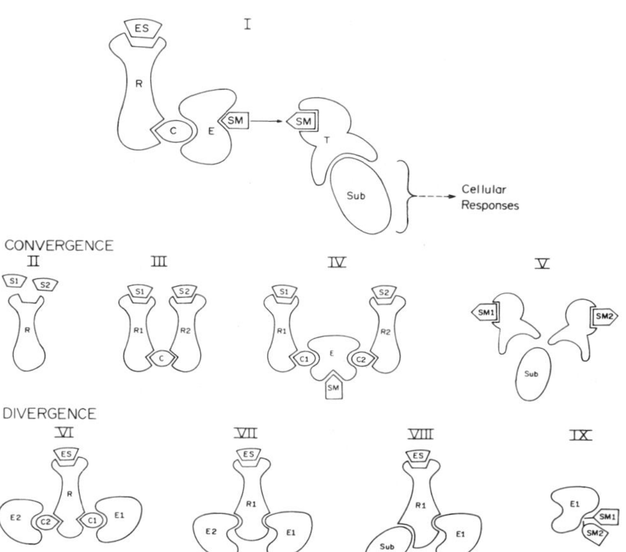

Figure 4.9. Variations of signal transduction pathways. **I.** Schematic representation of a generic signal transduction pathway involving an extracellular stimulus, receptor, G protein, effector, second messenger, and transducer, the latter usually being a protein kinase phosphorylating a substrate. Phosphorylation of one or more substrates is then translated into a cellular response. **II.** More than one extracellular substrate may interact with the same receptor, such as occurs with TGF-α and EGF. **III.** Two unique receptors may interact with the same G protein. **IV.** Two different G proteins may interact with the same effector, such as occurs with Gs and Gi acting on adenylate cyclase to stimulate and inhibit it, respectively. **V.** More distally in the signaling pathways, two protein kinases may act to phosphorylate the same substrate. **VI.** The same receptor may couple two distinct effectors via two distinct G proteins. **VII.** One receptor (such as tyrosine kinase receptors for growth factors) may phosphorylate two different effector molecules. **VIII.** A single receptor may phosphorylate one substrate and activate another effector. **IX.** A single effector may result in the generation of two distinct second messengers.

CONVERGENCE OF SIGNALING PATHWAYS

A one-to-one correspondence of signaling components requires that each extracellular stimulus (S) bind to a unique receptor (R) that interacts with a unique coupler (C), allowing it to transmit information to a unique effector (E), which then generates one second messenger (SM) which in turn activates a unique transducer (T), which in the case of a protein kinase (PK) would phosphorylate a unique substrate (Sub) (Fig. 4.9, Scheme I). Examples of deviation occur at almost each and every level, so that it is the exception where unique consecutive targets interact in series, coupling an extracellular stimulus to a cellular response. These different scenarios are illustrated in Figure 4.9.

The one-to-one correspondence is best preserved in the interaction of unique extracellular stimuli with unique cell surface molecules. There are a few isolated exceptions whereby distinct but closely related extracellular stimuli interact with the same cellular receptor. This is best illustrated in the case of TGF-α and EGF, which appear to interact with the same cellular receptor (91), the EGF receptor (Fig. 4.9, Scheme II).

Many distinct receptors appear to utilize similar coupling mechanisms. For example, many distinct receptors couple to adenylate cyclase through identical G proteins (Fig. 4.9, Scheme III) (19). Also, stimulatory and inhibitory receptors couple to stimulatory and inhibitory G proteins, respectively (19). This results in stimulation or inhibition of adenylate cyclase (Fig. 4.9, Scheme IV). Distinct signaling mechanisms may also converge at more distal components. For example, different protein kinases may phosphorylate the same substrates, resulting in similar cellular responses (Fig. 4.9, Scheme V).

DIVERGENCE OF SIGNALING

While the organization of many signaling events results in convergence of signaling pathways and induction of similar responses, signaling mechanisms also display significant divergence. A unique receptor may couple to more than one type of effector molecule (Fig. 4.9, Scheme VI). For example, certain cholinergic receptors may couple through G proteins to both adenylate cyclase and phospholipase C, thus launching these two important second messenger pathways (4). Certain tyrosine kinase receptors may directly activate phospholipase C as well as other signaling effectors (such as GTPase-activating proteins and PI kinase), which could then initiate alternate signaling mechanisms (Fig. 4.9, Scheme VII).

Further divergence of signaling pathways occurs when certain effectors result in the generation of more than one second messenger molecule. The primary example of this event is the formation of both diacylglycerol and inositol trisphosphate upon the activation of phospholipase C (Fig. 4.9, Scheme IX). Similarly, activation of phospholipase A_2 generates arachidonic acid and lysophospholipids.

REDUNDANCY

Further complexity in the organization of signal transduction mechanisms is introduced by the ability of distinct signaling pathways to mediate the same or closely related cellular responses. This is best studied in the events leading to the mitogenic response in various cell systems. It appears that activation of either the phospholipase C/protein kinase C pathway, cyclic AMP/protein kinase A pathway, tyrosine kinase pathway, or calcium mediated signaling results in mitogenesis. The level at which these pathways ultimately converge to induce a mitogenic response is not well delineated but may involve up-regulation of distinct or similar transcription factors and cell cycle regulators.

This redundancy and overlap in the action of different growth factors allows individual cells to integrate their responses. This is of paramount importance under physiologic conditions where cells receive an ever-changing input from a multitude of positive and negative growth factors and regulators.

CASCADES/AMPLIFICATION

The earliest studies on biochemical pathways of signaling established the importance of the role of cascades and signal amplification. In those studies, it was established that activation of protein kinase A by cyclic AMP results in activation of phosphorylase kinase, which in turn activates glycogen phosphorylase (25). The interpolation of additional kinases and regulatory elements ensures multiple steps of control of signaling events. It also allows for amplification of intracellular signaling in which each kinase phosphorylates many copies of its substrate kinase, which in turn amplifies the signal by phosphorylating a larger amount of the next level of substrates.

Also, as discussed previously, the MAP kinase, jun kinase, and S6 kinase pathways represent elaborate examples of linear cascades of signal transduction involving the participation of multiple serine/threonine kinases, tyrosine kinases, dual specificity kinases, and other regulator and adapter proteins such as ras and Grb-2.

FEEDBACK CONTROL

Important regulation of the propagation of signaling events is achieved by feedback mechanisms. These are of two general varieties. Positive feedback mechanisms ensure propagation and amplification of signals and second messengers. For example, inositol trisphosphate may release calcium from intracellular stores and, through yet unidentified mechanisms, may result in influx of extracellular calcium (8). This serves to maintain a longer lasting calcium signal. Similarly, activation of protein kinase C may result in further generation of diacylglycerol from membrane phospholipids through activation of phospholipase D with more prolonged activation of protein kinase C itself. More sophisticated feedback mechanisms occur when protein kinases undergo autophosphorylation and modulate their own activity. This is best illustrated with calcium/calmodulin-dependent protein kinases, which, upon autophosphorylation, become intrinsically active and independent of further calcium/calmodulin regulation (25).

On the other hand, negative feedback mechanisms operate to attenuate ongoing signals. For example, activation of protein kinase C in certain cells may result in negative feedback effects on G proteins and phospholipase C (69), thus ensuring termination of further diacylglycerol generation.

Feedback regulation also operates at the intercellular level whereby the action of some growth factors leads to the generation and secretion of additional growth factors that proceed to act on the same or proximal cells.

Although the operations of both positive and negative feedback mechanisms may appear contradictory, these mechanisms play important roles in regulating the duration and intensity of signaling events. In situations where prolonged signaling is required, such as during mitogenesis, positive feedback may predominate, while in other situations negative feedback may ensure prompt termination of signaling in response to subthreshold levels of extracellular stimuli.

CROSS-TALK BETWEEN DIFFERENT SIGNALING MECHANISMS

When different signaling mechanisms are launched independently by the action of the same or distinct extracellular stimuli, multiple interactions between those pathways ensure that they do not operate totally independently of each other. This may serve important functions in integrating cellular responses to different stimuli and in tightly regulating unique responses to the same stimulus. For example, activation of adrenergic-type receptors may lead to activation of endogenous kinases that serve to desensitize the cells to further action of the same or other stimuli (38). In regulation of mitogenesis, activation of the adenylate cyclase pathway attenuates the ras/MAP kinase pathway, possibly by direct phosphorylation of Raf with protein kinase A (22). This may explain the antimitogenic activity of cAMP in some cell types. Activation of phospholipase C may result in activation of ras (74).

SPATIAL ORGANIZATION OF SIGNAL TRANSDUCTION

The initial events of signal transduction for most classes of extracellular agents appear to localize at the plasma membrane. The propagation of signals through effectors, second messengers, and transducing targets leads to interactions in different cellular compartments. Many events occur at the plasma membrane itself, and these usually involve positive and negative feedback effects. Many other events occur in the cytosolic compartment where protein kinases may phosphorylate soluble substrates. Other events, however, may occur in specialized cellular compartments. Inositol trisphosphates may release calcium from endoplasmic reticulum, protein kinases may associate with cytoskeletal or nuclear membrane compartments, and phosphorylated substrates may migrate from cytosolic compartments to the nucleus, where they may act to modulate transcriptional events.

It is also conceivable that further complexity may be introduced by compartmentalization of signaling events. This is a particularly difficult area of research. However, the complexity of intracellular organization may impose significant limitations as to the sites of generation of second messengers, sites of their action, and the topological pathways of propagation of signaling.

TEMPORAL REGULATION OF SIGNAL TRANSDUCTION

The temporal aspects of signal transduction play critical roles in modifying cellular responses to the action of extracellular stimuli. The duration of exposure to extracellular stimuli may affect the degree and even the nature of the cellular response. Transient encounters between cells and extracellular stimuli may lead to suboptimal or aborted responses, while more prolonged or intense encounters may lead to significant changes in cell function.

The generation of internal second messengers is also subject to tight temporal control. This is achieved by the regulation of both the generation and the metabolism of these second messengers. In many situations, the formation of the second messenger is transitory, leading to immediate and specific responses. This occurs, for example, when neutrophilic leukocytes encounter extracellular organisms and mount a chemotactic and bactericidal response.

For many cellular responses such as mitogenesis, a prolonged elevation of second messenger may be required for the response. The action of a number of growth factors on cell surface receptors leads to repetitive and oscillatory elevations in intracellular calcium that serve to maintain elevated calcium levels over a prolonged duration. Similarly, prolonged elevations in diacylglycerol levels may result in persistent activation of protein kinase C, which would then result in a significant mitogenic response.

Additional temporal regulation of signal propagation is achieved by the cascade of sequential effector molecules and second messengers. While this allows for signal amplification, it may also play an important role in regulating the duration of signaling events.

These complexities of signaling mechanisms with redundancy, convergence, divergence, feedback, and cross-talk between different signaling pathways provide individual cells with sophisticated control mechanisms that ensure fidelity in signaling as well as allow fine tuning of cellular responses, depending on the nature, intensity, and duration of extracellular stimuli. For the experimentalist, this lack of a one-to-one correspondence between signaling components presents enormous problems for the dissection of physiologic pathways of signaling that mediate the effects of any one particular extracellular stimulus. If signaling operated on a one-to-one correspondence, it would be sufficient to demonstrate the effects of any one component on subsequent events to allow investigators to conclude that this component is vital for that particular cellular response. For example, demonstrating that an extracellular stimulus leads to the generation of diacylglycerol second messenger and demonstrating that diacylglycerol can cause mitogenesis would be sufficient to conclude that the mitogenic effect in response to that extracellular stimulus is mediated through phospholipase C/diacylglycerol/protein kinase C. However, the redundancy, cross-talk, and divergence of signaling mechanisms preclude such simple conclusions. Therefore, while many of the components of various signaling mechanisms are being assembled and studied, the exact relevance and contribution of each component to the overall cellular response have yet to be convincingly determined in any one situation. This is an area of active investigation with profound implications for the understanding of cell regulation and carcinogenesis.

Oncogenesis and Signal Transduction

Disturbances in signal transduction mechanisms and cell regulatory processes provide the molecular basis to explain the induction and maintenance of the cancerous phenotype. In many cases, it appears that acquisition of an overactive or poorly regulated component of a signal transduction pathway is sufficient to drive cells into unchecked proliferation. In fact, disturbances in signal transduction and cell regulatory mechanisms appear to provide a unifying basis for the molecular analysis of traditionally distinct fields of carcinogenesis (genetic, viral, and acquired). A brief overview of the role of signal transduction during various processes and stages of carcinogenesis follows.

ONCOGENES AND SIGNAL TRANSDUCTION

Oncogenes were initially identified as transforming genes carried by carcinogenic retroviruses (13). It quickly became evident, however, that these retroviral genes had cellular homologues, and that the retroviral oncogenes arose from their cellular counterparts, the proto-oncogenes. There is now ample evidence supporting the involvement of proto-oncogenes in the generation and/or the maintenance of cancer (see Chapter 5). For example, transfection (insertion of foreign DNA into cells) of cells in tissue culture with either high levels of proto-oncogenes or abnormally regulated proto-oncogenes results in cell transformation. Also, genes in retroviruses responsible for cell transformation are the viral counterparts of proto-oncogenes. When investigators searched for genes in cancer cells responsible for maintenance of the cancerous phenotype, mutated proto-oncogenes were often obtained (13). Thus, a mutation in a proto-oncogene may lead to oncogenic activation by disrupting the control and function of its protein product. Alternatively, overexpression of a proto-oncogene, as may occur following chromosomal translocation, viral insertion, or deranged activity of an essential regulator, may also result in oncogenic transformation (83).

The study of oncogenes has led to the classification of most proto-oncogene protein products as localizing to either the cytoplasm or the nucleus (13). A tantalizing realization came with the repeated finding that cytoplasmic oncoproteins (oncogenes whose protein product resides in the cytoplasm) are either actual components of signal transduction pathways or closely associated proteins. On the other hand, nuclear oncoproteins play important and critical roles in cell regulation and gene transcription, although their precise function is less well defined than those of the cytoplasmic oncoproteins. Therefore most, if not all, proto-oncogenes encode normal cellular proteins that function to regulate cell growth.

While the study of signal transduction has generally been applied to transmembrane and cytoplasmic events, an ultimate and important target of many signal transduction pathways is modulation of the function of nuclear proteins. Many of the nuclear oncoproteins are phosphoproteins and appear to be substrates for different protein kinases, thus linking them to more general signal transduction pathways. Therefore, the products of most oncogenes appear to be integral members of signal transduction pathways. An understanding of their mechanism of action must by necessity involve dissection of their impact on signal transduction during normal cell function and determining how oncogenesis is related to disruption of these processes. In the simplest formulation, it appears that when any essential component of a signal transduction pathway is rendered hyperactive or autonomous, it may acquire the ability to drive the cell into unchecked proliferation. An active area of research is aimed at determining the mechanism of action of normal proto-oncogenes and their oncogenic variants.

The intimate relationship between oncogenes and components of signal transduction pathways has been established at almost every level (Fig. 4.10). For example, the earliest observation of a proto-oncogene with effects on cell growth came from the demonstration that the c-*sis* proto-oncogene encodes for a PDGF (23). Cell transformation by an overexpressed c-*sis* oncogene then results in a mitogenic response by providing an overactive extracellular growth factor. V-*erb* B was then identified as a truncated form of the EGF receptor (24) with endogenous unchecked protein-tyrosine kinase activity. C-*fms* (81), on the other hand, encodes the homologue of the receptor for the macrophage colony-stimulating factor (M-CSF), while c-*mas* may encode an angiotensin receptor (45).

Mutated *ras* oncogenes are, so far, the most frequently detected mutated oncogenes in human cancer (92). The *ras* oncogenes belong to the family of small molecular weight GTP-binding proteins, and they play an essential role in stimulus-response coupling (see above).

Many of the other extranuclear oncoproteins appear to possess intrinsic protein-tyrosine kinase activity. These include *Src*, *Abl*, *Fes*, *Fgr*, *Yes*, *Ros*, and others (13). By analogy with receptor tyrosine kinases, these cytoplasmic or membrane-associated tyrosine kinase oncoproteins are thought to play essential roles in signal transduction mechanisms, and many of them serve as receptor-linked tyrosine kinases. Another category of extranuclear oncoproteins appears to possess protein-serine/threonine kinase activity, and these include *Raf* and *Mos* (13). Mutated G proteins have been found in pituitary and other endocrine tumors (56), while a mutated protein with homology to GAP may underlie the pathogenesis of neurofibromatosis (96).

ANTI-ONCOGENES AND CELL REGULATION

Just as increased and unchecked activity of essential components of promitogenic signaling pathways may contribute to carcinogenesis, it is becoming obvious that elimination of activity essential for inhibition of mitogenesis may also lead to increased proliferation. The existence of suppressor oncogenes (also termed recessive oncogenes, anti-oncogenes, or tumor suppressor genes) has long been postulated. A number of anti-oncogenes have recently been identified (59), including the retinoblastoma gene, the elimination of whose activity results in retinoblastoma and a num-

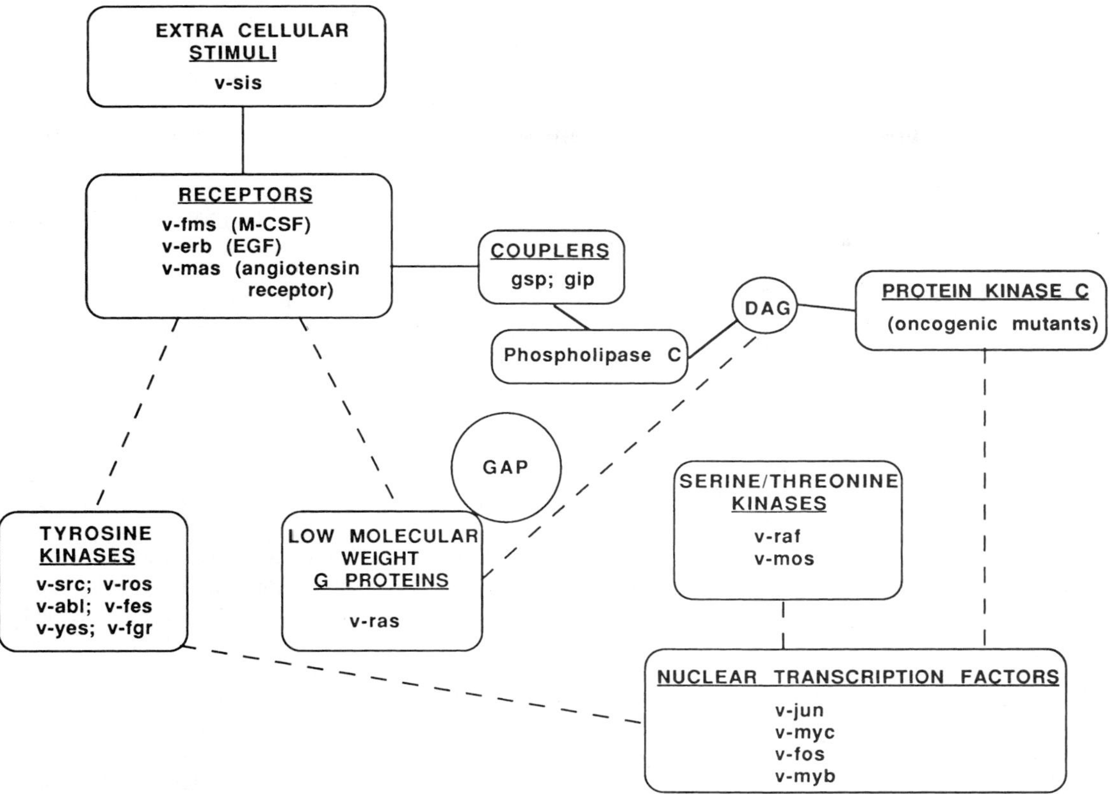

Figure 4.10. Involvement of oncogene products in signal transduction pathways. This scheme illustrates components of signal transduction pathways and the role of products of oncogenes in signal transduction. v-Sis encodes an oncogenic counterpart of platelet-derived growth factor; c-fms, c-erb, and c-mas encode for receptors for M-CSF, EGF, and angiotensin, respectively; oncogenic counterparts of G proteins have been described (gsp and gip); while other oncogenes encode for tyrosine kinases, serine-threonine kinases, and nuclear transcription factors as indicated. GAP (GTPase-activating proteins) may represent a family of proteins with possible oncogenic counterparts. *Ras* oncoproteins activate the raf-MAP kinase pathway of mitogenesis. *Solid lines* indicate established pathways of signaling, *dashed lines* indicate potential or poorly defined pathways.

ber of bladder and bone cancers (41). The cellular localization of the protein product of the retinoblastoma gene appears to be nuclear, and it functions in suppressing progression through the cell cycle (93). The study of anti-oncogenes has also led to identifying the K-*rev* (smg 21) gene as an anti-oncogene with homology to small molecular weight G proteins (48). Its function appears to be to antagonize the role of the activity of *ras* oncogenes. The neurofibromatosis gene (NF) has been cloned and found to have homology to GAP. It is hypothesized that NF acts as a tumor suppressor gene that ordinarily functions to regulate the activity of ras or ras-like proteins (96).

p53, a 53-kd nuclear protein (89), has emerged as the most frequently mutated gene in human cancers, especially in the later stages of tumor progression and transformation (68). p53 has been proposed as the guardian of DNA as well as the guardian of tissue health. Indeed, intensive investigation over the last few years has delineated important functions for p53 as a key component in mechanisms that sense DNA and intracellular damage and cause the cells to undergo either programmed cell death (apoptosis) or cell cycle arrest in order to allow for repair of cell damage (80). Therefore, normal function of p53, while not essential for cell growth and development, is critical for preventing abnormal growth and the proliferation of mutated cells. Loss of this function therefore plays an important role in providing a survival advantage for cancer cells that otherwise would have been eliminated. p53 is also involved in genetic predisposition to cancer. In the Li-Fraumeni syndrome, patients inherit a germ-line mutation in one allele of p53. This renders them highly susceptible to the development of multiple cancers, probably through the loss of function of the wild-type allele.

Additional anti-oncogenes have been identified and they also appear to be involved in mechanisms of signal transduction/cell regulation. These include RET, a receptor tyrosine kinase involved in thyroid carcinoma; and a number of transcription factors, including WT-1, which is missing in Wilms' tumor (59).

The study of tumor suppressor genes and growth suppressor mechanisms is beginning to provide an important dimension for the understanding of cancer development and progression. Thus, we may consider cancer as a multistep process that involves not only driving cells through growth, even in unfavorable environments (as in metastasis), but also the disarming of counterregulatory mechanisms that would have resulted either in repair of mutation in cancer cells or in the elimination of damaged or transformed cells. Therefore, the study of tumor suppressor mechanisms should shed important light on understanding cancer pathogenesis as well as provide a novel dimension for possible cancer therapeutics.

TUMOR PROMOTERS AND SIGNAL TRANSDUCTION

Experimental models of carcinogenesis in the mouse are consistent with a two-step carcinogenesis scheme consisting of an initiating event (step 1) followed by a tumor-promoting event (step 2). These models have allowed the identification of a number of tumor promoters over the last three decades with pleiotropic biologic effects far exceeding their role as cancer-promoting agents (14). Studies conducted in the past decade, however, generated important insights into the mechanism of action of tumor promoters and led to unification of the field of study of tumor promotion with signal transduction (Fig. 4.11).

The best studied class of tumor promoters consists of phorbol esters and related molecules. Phorbol esters were known to exert profound effects on cellular functions, including hormone release, blood cell activation, cell differentiation, mitogenesis, and tumor promotion. Insight into their mechanism of action came with the identification of protein kinase C as the main intracellular receptor for these agents (69). The interaction of phorbol esters with protein kinase C results in prolonged and unattenuated activation of this enzyme, followed by its proteolytic inactivation. This interaction appears to explain most, if not all, of the effects of phorbol

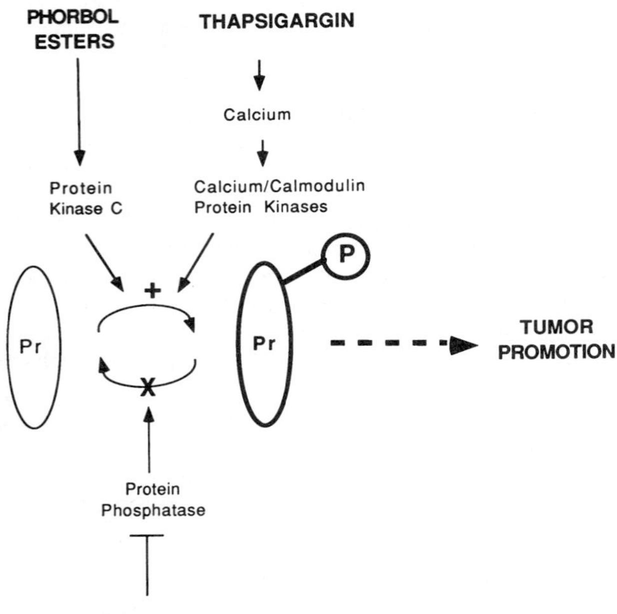

Figure 4.11. Tumor promoters and protein phosphorylation. Three classes of tumor promoters are indicated. These are phorbol esters and non-phorbol ester tumor promoters that act by activating protein kinase C; thapsigargin, which releases calcium from intracellular stores; and okadaic acid, which inhibits protein phosphatases. Phorbol esters and thapsigargin activate protein kinases that increase endogenous substrate phosphorylation, while okadaic acid inhibits protein phosphatases, thus also enhancing substrate phosphorylation. The exact nature of the phosphorylated substrates and their roles in tumor promotion are not well delineated.

esters on cell function. By extension, protein kinase C has been implicated as a main mediator of tumor promotion, (this hypothesis and the mechanisms explaining these effects are yet to be demonstrated). Protein kinase C also appears to be the target of action of other non-phorbol ester tumor promoters. These include mezerein, aplysiatoxin, and lyngbyatoxin. Arachidonic acid and its prostanoid metabolites also appear to exert tumor-promoting activity. The mechanism of action, which may or may not involve protein kinase C, is poorly understood.

More recently, two important additional links between tumor promotion and signal transduction have been established. First, it has been shown that thapsigargin, a potent tumor promoter, acts by inhibiting calcium uptake/sequestration, thereby promoting elevations in calcium levels (Fig. 4.11) (87). Okadaic acid, another tumor promoter, appears to inhibit serine-threonine protein phosphatases (39) and thus results in increased phosphorylation of protein substrates (Fig. 4.11).

It appears that activation of either protein kinase C or calcium-dependent protein kinases (and other calcium-dependent events) or inhibition of protein phosphatases results in tumor promotion. Activation of kinases or inhibition of phosphatases results in increased phosphorylation of protein substrates. In the case of tumor promoters, it appears that a common final effect is to increase phosphorylation of critical substrates on serine and threonine residues (Fig. 4.11). The nature of these substrates has not been determined, but the convergence of the action of disparate tumor promoters on specific phosphorylation of proteins on serine and threonine residues strongly implicates signal transduction processes in tumor promotion and carcinogenesis.

VIRUSES AND ONCOGENESIS

HTLV-I and hepatitis B virus are major transforming human viruses (see Chapters 23 and 146). In this context, it is sufficient to point to the role of virally encoded proteins in modifying essential components of signal transduction elements. This is especially true in the case of HTLV-I where the Tax protein drives the expression of IL-2 and IL-2 receptor, two essential components of T-lymphocyte growth and mitogenesis (5). Hepatitis B virus may activate the N-*myc* proto-oncogene.

Another important link between transforming viruses and cell regulation comes from the increasing appreciation of the direct effects of many transforming proteins of tumor viruses on cell regulatory elements (such as the interaction of large tumors of SV40 with Rb and p53 anti-oncogenes).

METASTASIS AND SIGNAL TRANSDUCTION

A crucial event in the progression of cancer is the acquisition by tumor cells of the ability to metastasize to new sites in the body (37). Although metastasis is the defining parameter of cancer lethality, it remains one of the more poorly understood manifestations of cancer at the molecular level. This may derive from the complexity of metastasis biology, including the involvement of growth, angiogenesis, invasion, and survival in an unnatural environment that would have been hostile to the development and growth of normal cells. Nevertheless, a number of hormones, angiogenesis factors, and signal transduction pathways are being examined for their involvement in invasion and metastasis. This promises to be a major frontier in the study of cancer regulation.

Recent evidence has begun to elucidate specific mechanisms involved in metastasis. A gene, nm23, has been isolated with the unique ability to suppress the ability of cancer cells to metastasize (72). Loss of its function may be one mechanism allowing tumor cells to metastasize. Therefore this gene may function as an anti-oncogene. An important link between metastasis and signal transduction came with the realization that this metastasis-suppressing gene may function as a nucleotide diphosphate kinase and that it may associate with G proteins (51).

Implications for Treatment

The detailed mapping of signaling pathways and their precise roles in cell regulation and cell transformation offers a unique advantage in the development of specific preventative and therapeutic modalities for malignant disorders. These treatments may aim at any level of the signal transduction pathways; it is expected that detailed biochemical and molecular analysis of biopsy material from individual tumors will generate insight into the cause and pathogenesis of individual tumors. This would then allow the development of specific therapeutic intervention. It is conceivable that modulation of receptors, coupling mechanisms, effectors, second messengers, protein kinases, and important substrates may also have profound therapeutic effects. For example, modifying the ability of *ras* oncogenes to function may reverse their malignant role. This may be achieved by preventing an essential biochemical step (prenylation—the covalent addition of a prenyl-derived group) that modifies *ras* in order to allow its membrane localizations (29), a necessary step in its activation (17). This example demonstrates that a highly sophisticated understanding of the biochemical and molecular mechanisms of carcinogenesis generates specific targets for cancer therapy.

Protein kinase C inhibitors are also undergoing evaluation as potential chemotherapeutic agents. Inhibitors of phospholipase A_2 and arachidonic acid metabolism have been evaluated for possible efficacy in metastasis and in tumor progression. The rational targeting and design of specific cancer therapeutics based on the evolving molecular understanding of cancer pathogenesis is in early stages of development. It is hoped that through understanding of the specific mechanisms operative in cancer pathogenesis, specific targets can be evaluated. More important, it is becoming increasingly obvious that the rational development of inhibitors of specific targets requires a thorough and detailed understanding of the biochemical regulation and mechanism of these targets. Thus, inhibitors of *ras* have only become possible after identification of farnesylation (addition of a farnesyl group) of *ras* and the purification of farnesyl transferases. The more sophisticated our understanding of these targets becomes, the more successful will rational drug design emerge.

In addition to drug design, a number of growth factors and hormones have found significant use in cancer therapy and prevention. Some, such as tumor necrosis factor, have been used for their direct toxic effect. Others, such as interleukins and interferons, have been used for their ability to modulate the body's immune response toward cancer; that is, they are biologic response modifiers. Growth factors are playing increasingly important roles as adjunctive therapy to limit the toxicity and complications of chemotherapy. For example, erythropoietin may be used to stimulate red cell production. G-CSF and GM-CSF enhance the recovery of white blood cell counts, thus allowing the use of more effective chemotherapy and curtailing the morbidity and mortality associated with prolonged decreases in white blood cell counts (see Chapter 82).

One important area of research centers on the role of signal transduction in modulating the function of the proteins (e.g., gp 170) implicated in multiple drug resistance (2). The ability to modulate the presumed pump activity of this protein may have significant therapeutic implications.

Another treatment potential arises from the observations that various tumor promoters appear to act, by different mechanisms (Fig. 4.11), to increase protein phosphorylation through elements of signal transduction pathways. Therefore, it is possible that chemopreventive treatment aimed at preventing or reversing tumor promotion may make use of agents that counteract or preempt the effects of tumor promoters on signal transduction. Such agents may include protein kinase inhibitors, protein phosphatase activators, and modulators of calcium release.

Another area of cancer prevention relating to modulation of signal transduction may make use of dietary manipulation of signaling pathways. Diet contains carcinogens and tumor promoters, as well as inhibitors of carcinogenesis and tumor promotion, although the identity of the latter remains elusive (18). Also, it is known that dietary habits may be associated with different composition of membrane lipids. Associations have been made between dietary fatty acid intake and risk of colon and breast cancer. It appears plausible that these dietary changes modulate the function of signaling pathways. For example, omega-3 fatty acids may substitute for arachidonic acids. When they are released in response to phospholipase A_2 activation, they lead to the formation of inactive metabolites instead of the powerful thromboxanes and leukotrienes (20). Clearly, the understanding of normal signaling mechanisms and the impact of dietary manipulation on these pathways may open up an area of chemoprevention through dietary manipulation.

Conclusions

Signal transduction and cell regulatory mechanisms appear to offer a unifying molecular mechanism for the pathogenesis of cancer. Rapid advances in current knowledge of the components of signaling mechanisms, their regulation, and their interrelationships have provided a major breakthrough in our understanding on how normal cell function is regulated. This has been an essential step in applying this data base toward the understanding of how abnormalities in these pathways can impact on cancer pathogenesis and progression. Further studies to define all components of signaling and regulatory pathways and their precise roles in cell regulation are clearly indicated.

Such sophisticated understanding of signaling and regulatory mechanisms is no longer an unattainable task. The achievement of this goal should open multiple avenues for novel and innovative modalities for cancer prevention and treatment, including dietary manipulation, biologic response modification, and treatments aimed at specific rectification of cancer cell behavior.

References

1. Akira S, Hirono T, Taga T, Kishimoto T. Biology of multifunctional cytokines: IL 6 and related molecules (IL 1 and TNF). FASEB J 1990;4:2860.
2. Ames G. The basis of multidrug resistance in mammalian cells: homology with bacterial transport. Cell 1986;47:323.
3. Angel P, Imagawa M, Chiu R, Stein B, Imbra RJ, Rahmsdorf HJ, Jonat C, Herrlich P, Karin M. Phorbol ester-inducible genes contain a common cis element recognized by TPA-modulated trans-acting factor. Cell 1987;49:729.
4. Ashkenazi A, Winslow JW, Peralta EG, Peterson GL, Schimerlik MI, Capon DJ, Ramachandran J. An M2 muscarinic receptor subtype coupled to both adenylyl cyclase and phosphoinositide turnover. Science 1987;238:672.
5. Ballard DW, Bohnlein E, Lowenthal JW, Wano Y, Franza BR, Greene WC. HTLV-1 Tax induces proteins that activate the kB element in the IL-2 receptor gene. Science 1988;241:1652.
6. Bell RM. Protein kinase C activation by diacylglycerol second messengers. Cell 1986;45:631.
7. Bernstein LR, Colburn NH. AP1/jun function is differentially induced in promotion-sensitive and resistant JB6 cells. Science 1989;244:566.
8. Berridge MJ. Calcium oscillations. J Biol Chem 1990;265:9583.
9. Berridge MJ, Irvine RF. Inositol phosphates and cell signalling. Nature 1989;341:197.
10. Bevan S, Wood JN. Arachidonic-acid metabolites as second messengers. Nature 1987;328:20.
11. Billah MM, Pai J-K, Mullmann TJ, Egan RW, Siegel MI. Regulation of phospholipase D in HL-60 granulocytes: activation by phorbol esters, diglyceride, and calcium ionophore via protein kinase C–independent mechanisms. J Biol Chem 1989;264:9069.
12. Birnbaumer L. Receptor-to-effector signaling through G proteins: roles for $\beta;\gamma$ dimers as well as α subunits. Cell 1992;71:1069.
13. Bishop JM. Viral oncogenes. Cell 1985;42:23.
14. Blumberg PM. In vitro studies on the mode of action of the phorbol esters, potent tumor promoters. Crit Rev Toxicol 1980;8:153.
15. Bourne HR. G-protein subunits: who carries what message? Nature 1989;337:504.
16. Brown A, Birnbaumer L. Ion channels and G proteins. Hosp Pract 1989;124:139.
17. Brown MS, Goldstein JL. Mad bet for rab. Nature 1993;366:14.
18. Carr BI. Chemical carcinogens and inhibitors of carcinogenesis in the human diet. Cancer 1985;55:218.
19. Casey PJ, Gilman AG. G protein involvement in receptor-effector coupling. J Biol Chem 1988;263:2577.
20. Cave WT. Dietary n-3 (Ω-3) polyunsaturated fatty acid effects on animal tumorigenesis. FASEB J 1991;5:2160.
21. Cheung WY. Calmodulin–An Introduction. In Calcium and Cell Function. Edited by WY Cheung. New York: Academic, 1980, pp 2–9.
22. Cook SJ, McCormick F. Inhibition by cAMP of Ras-dependent activation of Raf. Science 1993;262:1069.
23. Doolittle RF, Hunkapiller MW, Hood LE, De Vare SG, Robbins KC, Aaronson SA, Antoniades HN. Simian sarcoma virus onc gene, v-sis, is derived from the gene (or genes) encoding a platelet-derived growth factor. Science 1983;221:275.
24. Downward J, Yarden Y, Mayes E, Scrace G, Totty N, Stockwell P, Ullrich A, Schlessinger J, Waterfield MD. Close similarity of epidermal growth factor receptor and v-erb-B oncogene protein sequence. Nature 1984;307:521.
25. Edelman AM, Blumenthal DK, Krebs EG. Protein serine/threonine kinases. Annu Rev Biochem 1987;56:567.
26. Exton JH. Signaling through phosphatidylcholine breakdown. J Biol Chem 1990;265:1.
27. Gerzer R, Hofmann F, Schultz G. Purification of a soluble sodium-nitroprusside-stimulated guanylate cyclase from bovine lung. Eur J Biochem 1981;116:479.
28. Ghosh S, Baltimore D. Activation in vitro of NF-κB by phosphorylation of its inhibitor IκB. Nature 1990;344:678.
29. Gibbs JB, Oliff A, Kohl NE. Farnesyltransferase inhibitors: ras research yields a potential cancer therapeutic. Cell 1994;77:175.
30. Green AR. Peptide regulatory factors: multifunctional mediators of cellular growth and differentiation. Lancet 1989;1:705.
31. Gronich JH, Bonventre JV, Nemenoff RA. Identification and characterization of a hormonally regulated form of phospholipase A_2 in rat renal mesangial cells. J Biol Chem 1988;263:16645.
32. Hakomori S. Glycosphingolipids in cellular interaction, differentiation, and oncogenesis. Annu Rev Biochem 1981;50:733.
33. Hanks SK, Quinn AM, Hunter T. The protein kinase family: conserved features and deduced phylogeny of the catalytic domains. Science 1988;241:42.
34. Hannun YA. The sphingomyelin cycle and the second messenger function of ceramide. J Biol Chem 1994;269:3125.
35. Hannun YA, Bell RM. Functions of sphingolipids and sphingolipid breakdown products in cellular regulation. Science 1989;243:500.
36. Hannun YA, Linardic CM. Sphingolipid breakdown products: anti-proliferative and tumor-suppressor lipids. Biochim Biophys Acta 1993;00:000.
37. Hart IR, Saini A. Biology of tumour metastasis. Lancet 1992;339:1453.
38. Hausdorf WP, Caron MG, Lefkowitz RJ. Turning off the signal: desensitization of β-adrenergic receptor function. FASEB J 1990;4:2881.
39. Haystead TA, Sim AT, Carling D, Honnor RC, Tsukitani Y, Cohen P, Hardie DG. Effects of the tumour promoter okadaic acid on intracellular protein phosphorylation and metabolism. Nature 1989;337:78.
40. Hokin MR, Hokin LE. Enzyme secretion and the incorporation of ^{32}P into phospholipids of pancreas slices. J Biol Chem 1953;203:967.
41. Horowitz JM, Park S-H, Bogenmann E, Cheng J-C, Yandell DW, Kaye FJ, Minna JD, Dryja TP, Weinberg RA. Frequent inactivation of the retinoblastoma anti-oncogene is restricted to a subset of human tumor cells. Proc Natl Acad Sci USA 1990;87:2775.
42. Hsiao W-LW, Housey GM, Johnson MD, Weinstein IB. Cells that overproduce protein kinase C are more susceptible to transformation by an activated H-ras oncogene. Mol Cell Biol 1989;9:2641.
43. Hunkapillar T, Hood L. Diversity of the immunoglobulin gene superfamily. Adv Immunol 1989;4:1.
44. Inagami T. Atrial natriuretic factor. J Biol Chem 1989;264:3043.
45. Jackson TR, Blair LA, Marshall J, Goedert M, Hanley MR. The mas oncogene encodes an angiotensin receptor. Nature 1988;335:437.
46. Kawata M, Matsui, Y, Kondo J, Hishida T, Teranishi Y, Takai Y. A novel small molecular weight GTP-binding protein with the same putative effector domain as the ras proteins in bovine brain membranes. J Biol Chem 1988;263:18965.
47. Kim JW, Sim SS, Kim U-H, Nishibe S, Wahl MI, Carpenter G, Rhee SG. Tyrosine residues in bovine phospholipase C-gamma phosphorylated by the epidermal growth factor receptor in vitro. J Biol Chem 1990;265:3940.
48. Kitayama H, Sugimoto Y, Matsuzaki T, Ikawa Y, Noda M. A ras-related gene with transformation suppressor activity. Cell 1989;56:77.
49. Krupinski J, Coussen F, Bakalyar HA, Tang WJ, Feinstein PG, Orth K, Slaughter C, Reed RR, Gilman AG. Adenylyl cyclase amino acid sequence: possible channel- or transport-like structure. Science 1989;244:1558.
50. Lacal JC, Moscat J, Aaronson S. A Novel source of 1,2-diacylglycerol elevated in cells transformed by Ha-ras oncogene. Nature 1987;330:269.
51. Lacombe ML, Wallet V, Troll H, Veron M. Functional cloning of a nucleoside diphosphate kinase from *Dictyostelium discoideum*. J Biol Chem 1990;265:10012.
52. Lin L-L, Wartmann M, Lin AY, Knopf JL, Seth A, Davis RJ. cPLA2 is phosphorylated and activated by MAP kinase. Cell 1993;72:269.
53. Liscovitch M, Cantley LC. Lipid second messengers. Cell 1994;77:329.
54. Liscovitch M, Lavie Y. Sphingoid bases as endogenous cationic amphiphilic drugs. Biochem Pharmacol 1991;42:2071.
55. Low MG, Saltiel AR. Structural and functional roles of glycosyl-phosphatidylinositol in membranes. Science 1988;239:268.
56. Lyons J, Landis CA, Harsh G, Vallar L, Grunewald K, Feichtinger H, Duh QY, Clark OH, Kawasaki E, Bourne HR, McCormick F. Two G protein oncogenes in human endocrine tumors. Science 1990;249:655.
57. Majerus PW, Connolly TM, Deckmyn H, Ross TS, Bross TE, Ishii H, Bansal V, Wilson D. The metabolism of phosphoinositide-derived messenger molecules. Science 1986;234:1519.
58. Malkin D, Li FP, Stong LC, Fraumeni JF Jr, Nelson CE, Kim DH, Kassel J, Gryka MA, Bischoff FZ, Tainsky MA, Friend SH. Germ line p53 mutations in a familial syndrome of breast cancer, sarcomas, and other neoplasms. Science 1990;250:1233.
59. Marx J. Learning how to suppress cancer. Science 1993;261:1385.
60. Marx J. Two major signal pathways linked. Science 1993;262:988.
61. Massague J. The TGF-β family of growth and differentiation factors. Cell 1987;49:437.
62. Merrill AH Jr. Cell regulation by sphingosine and more complex sphingolipids. J Bioenerg Biomemb 1991;23:83.
63. Michell B. A second messenger function for inositol tetrakisphosphate. Nature 1986;324:613.
64. Michell RH. Post-receptor signalling pathways. Lancet 1989;1:765.
65. Molloy CJ, Bottaro DP, Fleming TP, Marshall MS, Gibbs JB, Aaronson SA. PDGF induction of tyrosine phosphorylation of GTPase activating protein. Nature 1989;343:711.
66. Moncada S, Palmer RMJ, Higgs EA. Biosynthesis of nitric oxide from L-arginine. A pathway for the regulation of cell function and communication. Biochem Pharmacol 1989;38:1709.
67. Morla AO, Draetta G, Beach D, Wang JYJ. Reversible tyrosine phosphorylation of cdc2: dephosphorylation accompanies activation during entry into mitosis. Cell 1989;58:193.
68. Nigro JM, Baker SJ, Preisinger AC, Jessup JM, Hostetter R, Cleary K, Bigner SH, Davidson N, Baylin S, Devilee P, Glover T, Collins FS, Weston A, Modali R, Harris CC, Vogelstein B. Mutations in the p53 gene occur in diverse human tumour types. Nature 1989;343:705.
69. Nishizuka Y. Studies and prospectives of the protein kinase C family for cellular regulation. Cancer 1989;63:1892.
70. Obeid LM, Linardic CM, Karolak LA, Hannun YA. Programmed cell death induced by ceramide. Science 1993;259:1769.
71. Okazaki T, Bell RM, Hannun YA. Sphingomyelin turnover induced by vitamin D3 in HL-60 cells: role in cell differentiation. J Biol Chem 1989;264:19076.
72. Persons DA, Wilkison WO, Bell RM, Finn OJ. Altered growth regulation and enhanced tumorigenicity of NIH 3T3 fibroblasts transfected with protein kinase C-1 cDNA. Cell 1988;52:447.
73. Preiss J, Loomis CR, Bishop WR, Stein R, Niedel JE, Bell RM. Quantitative measurement of sn-1,2-diacylglycerols present in platelets, hepatocytes, and ras- and sis-transformed normal rat kidney cells. J Biol Chem 1986;261:8597.
74. Price BD, Morris JDH, Marshall CJ, Hall A. Stimulation of phosphatidylcholine hydrolysis, diacylglycerol release, and arachidonic acid production by oncogenic ras is a consequence of protein kinase C activation. J Biol Chem 1989;264:16638.
75. Rhee SG, Suh PG, Ryu SH, Lee SY. Studies of inositol phospholipid-specific phospholipase C. Science 1989;244:546.
76. Roberts AB, Anzano MA, Wakefield LM, Roche NS, Stern DF, Sporn MB. Type β transforming growth factor: a bifunctional regulator of cellular growth. Proc Natl Acad Sci USA 1985;82:119.
77. Rosengard AM, Krutzsch HC, Shearn A, Biggs JR, Barker E, Margulies MK, King CR,

Liotta LA, Steeg PS. Reduced Mm23/Awd protein in tumour metastasis and aberrant *Drosophila* development. Nature 1989;342:177.
78. Samuelsson B, Dahlen SE, Lindgren JA, Rouzer CA, Serhan CN. Leukotrienes and lipoxins: structures, biosynthesis, and biological effects. Science 1987;237:1171.
79. Sassone-Corsi P, Ransone LJ, Verma IM. Cross-talk in signal transduction: TPA-inducible factor jun/AP-1 activates cAMP-responsive enhancer elements. Oncogene 1990;5:427.
80. Shaw P, Bovey R, Tardy S, Sahli R, Sordat B, Costa J. Induction of apoptosis by wild-type p53 in a human colon tumor-derived cell line. Proc Natl Acad Sci USA 1992;89:4495.
81. Sherr CJ, Rettenmier CW, Sacca R, Roussel MF, Look AT, Stanley ER. The c-fms proto-oncogene product is related to the receptor for the mononuclear phagocyte growth factor, CSF-1. Cell 1985;41:665.
82. Shuman MA, Greenberg CS. Platelet regulation of thrombus formation. In Biochemistry of Platelets. Edited by DR Philips, MA Shuman. Orlando, FL: Academic, 1986, pp 319–346.
83. Slamon DJ. Proto-oncogenes and human cancers. N Engl J Med 1987;317:955.
84. Spiegel S, Olivera A, Zhang H, Thompson EW, Su Y, Berger A. Sphingosine-1-phosphate, a novel second messenger involved in cell growth regulation and signal transduction, affects growth and invasiveness of human breast cancer cells. Breast Cancer Res Treat 1994;31:337.
85. Sporn MB, Roberts AB. Peptide growth factors are multifunctional. Nature 1988;332:217.
86. Takuwa N, Takuwa Y, Rasmussen H. Stimulation of mitogenesis and glucose transport by 1-monooleoylglycerol in Swiss 3T3 fibroblasts. J Biol Chem 1988;263:9738.
87. Thastrup O, Cullen PJ, Drobak BK, Hanley MR, Dawson AP. Thapsigargin, a tumor promoter, discharges intracellular Ca^{2+} stores by specific inhibition of the endoplasmic reticulum Ca^{2+}-ATPase. Proc Natl Acad Sci USA 1990;87:2466.
88. Ulevitch RJ, Watanabe Y, Sano M, Lister MD, Deems RA, Dennis EA. Solubilization, purification, and characterization of a membrane-bound phospholipase A_2 from the P388D1 macrophage-like cell line. J Biol Chem 1988;263:3079.
89. Ullrich SJ, Anderson CW, Mercer WE, Appella E. The p53 tumor suppressor protein, a modulator of cell proliferation. J Biol Chem 1992;267:15259.
90. Ushikubi F, Nakajima M, Hirata M, Okuma M, Fujiwara M, Narumiya S. Purification of the thromboxane A2-prostaglandin H2 receptor from human blood platelets. J Biol Chem 1989;264:16496.
91. Waterfield MD. Epidermal growth factor and related molecules. Lancet 1989;1:1243.
92. Weinberg RA. Ras oncogenes and the molecular mechanisms of carcinogenesis. Blood 1984;64:1143.
93. Weinberg RA. Tumor suppressor genes. Science 1991;254:1138.
94. Williams LT. Signal transduction by the platelet-derived growth factor receptor. Science 1989;243:1564.
95. Wright TM, Rangan LA, Shin HS, Raben DM. Kinetic analysis of 1,2-diacylglycerol mass levels in cultured fibroblasts. J Biol Chem 1988;263:9374.
96. Xu G, O'Connell P, Viskochil D, Cawthon R, Robertson M, Culver M, Dunn D, Stevens J, Gesteland R, White R, Weiss R. The neurofibromatosis type 1 gene encodes a protein related to GAP. Cell 1990;62:599.

CHAPTER 5

Oncogenes

STEVEN A. SCHICHMAN AND CARLO H. CROCE

Neoplasia is a multistep process that results from the accumulation of genetic changes in somatic cells. One of the major accomplishments in modern biomedical research has been the identification of many different genes that participate in the neoplastic transformation of cells. These genes fall into two broad categories, oncogenes and tumor suppressor genes (1). Oncogenes are pathologically altered versions of normal cellular genes called proto-oncogenes, that regulate cellular growth processes such as proliferation, differentiation, and programmed cell death (2). Oncogenes exert their malignant action in an autosomal dominant fashion through a gain in function mechanism. In contrast, tumor suppressor genes, which also participate in the regulation of normal cell growth, generally function in an autosomal recessive manner through a loss of function mechanism. Oncogenes were originally discovered as the transforming genes of RNA tumor viruses (3–5). Further study broadened the definition of oncogenes to include any dominantly acting gene involved in the neoplastic transformation of cells.

More than 100 different oncogenes have been discovered thus far by various methods (1). Most of these oncogenes were identified in experimental animal models of cancer (5). Only a small subset of these genes, however, seem to play a role in human cancer. A few proto-oncogenes, notably those of the *ras* and *myc* families, have been implicated repeatedly in the initiation and progression of various human tumors. Proto-oncogenes are converted into oncogenes by the genetic mechanisms of mutation, gene amplification, and chromosomal rearrangement (6). An accumulation of changes in different proto-oncogenes and tumor suppressor genes is required for full expression of the neoplastic phenotype in human tumors. Our knowledge of these gene defects is incomplete but rapidly expanding. This chapter presents an overview of current knowledge of proto-oncogene families with particular emphasis on those oncogenes involved in human cancer. First, the methods by which oncogenes were discovered will be described. Second, the various functions of cellular proto-oncogenes will be presented. Third, the genetic mechanisms of proto-oncogene activation will be summarized. Finally, the role of specific oncogenes in the initiation and progression of human tumors will be discussed.

Discovery and Identification of Oncogenes

The first oncogenes were discovered through the study of *retroviruses*, RNA tumor viruses whose genomes are reverse transcribed into DNA in infected animal cells (7). During the course of infection, retroviral DNA is inserted into the chromosomes of host cells. The integrated retroviral DNA, called the provirus, replicates along with the cellular DNA of the host (8). Transcription of the DNA provirus leads to the production of viral progeny that bud through the host cell membrane to infect other cells. Two categories of retroviruses are classified by their time course of tumor formation in experimental animals. Acutely transforming retroviruses can rapidly cause tumors within days after injection. These retroviruses can also transform cell cultures to the neoplastic phenotype. Chronic or weakly oncogenic retroviruses can cause tissue-specific tumors in susceptible strains of experimental animals after a latency period of many months. Although weakly oncogenic retroviruses can replicate in vitro, these viruses do not transform cells in culture.

Retroviral oncogenes are altered versions of host cellular proto-oncogenes that have been incorporated into the retroviral genome by recombination with host DNA, a process known as retroviral *transduction* (4). This surprising discovery was made through study of the Rous sarcoma virus (RSV). RSV is an acutely transforming retrovirus first isolated from a chicken sarcoma over 80 years ago by Payton Rous (9). Studies of RSV mutants in the early 1970s revealed that the transforming gene of RSV was not required for viral replication (10–12). Molecular hybridization studies then showed that the RSV transforming gene (designated v-*src*) was homologous to a host cellular gene (c-*src*) that was widely conserved in eukaryotic species (13). Studies of many other acutely transforming retroviruses from fowl, rodent, feline, and nonhuman primate species have led to the discovery of dozens of different retroviral oncogenes (see below and Table 5.1). In every case, these retroviral oncogenes are derived from normal cellular genes captured from the genome of the host. Viral oncogenes are responsible for the rapid tumor formation and efficient in vitro transformation activity characteristic of acutely transforming retroviruses.

In contrast to acutely transforming retroviruses, weakly oncogenic retroviruses do not carry viral oncogenes. These retroviruses, which include mouse mammary tumor virus (MMTV) and various animal leukemia viruses, induce tumors by a process called *insertional mutagenesis* (14). This process results from integration of the DNA provirus into the host genome in infected cells. In rare cells, the provirus inserts near a proto-oncogene. Expression of the proto-oncogene is then abnormally driven by the transcriptional regulatory elements contained within the long terminal repeats of

Table 5.1. Proto-oncogenes

Proto-oncogene	Function of protein product	Method of identification
Growth factors		
sis	Platelet-derived growth factor	Retroviral homologue
int-2	Growth factor	Insertional mutagenesis
Growth factor receptors		
erb B	Tyrosine kinase/EGF receptor	Retroviral homologue
erb B-2(neu/HER-2)	Tyrosine kinase	Transfection
fms	Tyrosine kinase/CSF-1 receptor	Retroviral homologue
kit	Tyrosine kinase/steel receptor	Retroviral homologue
trk	Tyrosine kinase/NGF receptor	Transfection
ret	Tyrosine kinase	Transfection
met	Tyrosine kinase/hepatocyte growth factor receptor	Transfection
sea	Tyrosine kinase	Retroviral homologue
ros	Tyrosine kinase	Retroviral homologue
mas	Angiotensin receptor	Transfection
Signal transduction		
abl	Tyrosine kinase	Retroviral homologue
fes	Tyrosine kinase	Retroviral homologue
fgr	Tyrosine kinase	Retroviral homologue
lck	Tyrosine kinase	Insertional mutagenesis
src	Tyrosine kinase	Retroviral homologue
yes	Tyrosine kinase	Retroviral homologue
raf	Serine/threonine kinase	Retroviral homologue
mos	Serine/threonine kinase	Retroviral homologue
pim	Serine/threonine kinase	Insertional mutagenesis
H-*ras*	Binds GDP/GTP	Retroviral homologue
K-*ras*	Binds GDP/GTP	Retroviral homologue
N-*ras*	Binds GDP/GTP	Transfection
gsp	G protein	Mutation
gip	G protein	Mutation
Transcription factors		
erb A	T_3 receptor/DNA binding	Retroviral homologue
ets	DNA binding	Retroviral homologue
fos	DNA binding/AP-1 complex with jun	Retroviral homologue
jun	DNA binding/AP-1 complex with fos	Retroviral homologue
myb	DNA binding	Retroviral homologue
c-*myc*	DNA binding	Retroviral homologue
L-*myc*	DNA binding	Amplification
N-*myc*	DNA binding	Amplification
rel	DNA binding	Retroviral homologue
ski	DNA binding	Retroviral homologue
Programmed cell death regulation		
bcl-2	Membrane protein/apoptosis	Chromosomal translocation

Modified with permission from Gaidano G, Dalla-Favera R. Protooncogenes and tumor suppressor genes. In *Neoplastic Hematopathology.* Edited by D Knowles. Baltimore: Williams & Wilkins, 1992, p 247.

the provirus (15, 16). In these cases, proviral integration represents a mutagenic event that activates a proto-oncogene. Activation of the proto-oncogene then results in transformation of the cell, which can grow clonally into a tumor. The long latent period of tumor formation of weakly oncogenic retroviruses is therefore due to the rarity of the provirus insertional event that leads to tumor development from a single transformed cell. Insertional mutagenesis by weakly oncogenic retroviruses, first demonstrated in bursal lymphomas of chickens, frequently involves the same oncogenes (such as *myc*, *myb*, and *erb B*) that are carried by acutely transforming retroviruses (17–20). In many cases, however, insertional mutagenesis has been used as a tool to identify new oncogenes, including *int-1*, *pim-1*, and *lck* (21).

The demonstration of activated proto-oncogenes in human tumors was first shown by the DNA-mediated transformation technique (22, 23). This technique, also called *gene transfer*, assays the ability of donor DNA from a tumor to transform a recipient strain of rodent cells called NIH 3T3, an immortalized mouse cell line (24, 25). This sensitive assay, which can detect the presence of single-copy oncogenes in a tumor sample, also enables the isolation of the transforming oncogene by molecular cloning techniques. After serial growth of the transformed NIH 3T3 cells, the human tumor oncogene can be cloned by its association with human repetitive DNA sequences. The first human oncogene isolated by the gene transfer technique was derived from a bladder carcinoma (26, 27). Overall, approximately 20% of individual human tumors have been shown to induce transformation of NIH 3T3 cells in gene transfer assays. Many of the oncogenes identified by gene transfer studies are identical or closely related to those oncogenes transduced by retroviruses. Most prominent among these are members of the *ras* family that have been repeatedly isolated from various human tumors by gene transfer (28, 29). A number of new oncogenes (such as *neu*, *met*, and *trk*) have also been identified by the gene transfer technique (30, 31). In many cases, however, oncogenes identified by gene transfer were shown to be activated by rearrangement during the experimental procedure and are not activated in the human tumors that served as the source of the donor DNA (32).

Chromosomal translocations have served as guideposts for the discovery of many new oncogenes (33, 34). Consistently recurring karyotypic abnormalities are found in many hematologic and solid tumors. These abnormalities include chromosomal rearrangements as well as the gain or loss of whole chromosomes or chromosome segments. The first consistent karyotypic abnormality identified in a human neoplasm was a characteristic small chromosome in the cells of patients with chronic myelogenous leukemia (CML) (35). Later identified as a derivative of chromosome 22, this abnormality was designated the Philadelphia chromosome after its city of discovery. The application of chromosome banding techniques in the early 1970s enabled the precise cytogenetic characterization of many chromosomal translocations in human leukemia, lymphoma, and solid tumors (36). The subsequent development of molecular cloning techniques then enabled the identification of proto-oncogenes at or near chromosomal breakpoints in various neoplasms. Some of these proto-oncogenes, such as *myc* and *abl*, had been previously identified as retroviral oncogenes. In general, however, the cloning of chromosome breakpoints has served as a rich source of discovery of new oncogenes involved in human cancer.

Functions of Proto-oncogenes

Proto-oncogenes encode proteins that are involved in the control of cell growth. Alteration of the structure and/or expression of proto-oncogenes can activate them to become oncogenes capable of transforming susceptible cells into the neoplastic phenotype. Proto-oncogenes can be classified into five groups based on the functional and biochemical properties of their protein products. These groups are (*a*) growth factors, (*b*) growth factor receptors, (*c*) signal transducers, (*d*) transcription factors, and (*e*) programmed cell death regulators. Table 5.1 lists examples of proto-oncogenes according to their functional categories.

GROWTH FACTORS

Growth factors are secreted polypeptides that function as extracellular signals to stimulate the proliferation of target cells (37, 38). Appropriate target cells must possess a specific receptor in order to respond to a specific type of growth factor. A well-characterized example is platelet-derived growth factor (PDGF), an approximately 30-kd protein consisting of two polypeptide chains (39). PDGF is released from platelets during the process of blood coagulation. PDGF stimulates the proliferation of fibroblasts, a cell growth process that plays an important role in wound healing. Other well-characterized examples of growth factors include nerve growth factor, epidermal growth factor, and fibroblast growth factor.

The link between growth factors and retroviral oncogenes was revealed by study of the *sis* oncogene of simian sarcoma virus, a retrovirus first isolated from a monkey fibrosarcoma. Sequence analysis showed that *sis* encodes the beta chain of PDGF (40). This discovery established the principle that inappropriately expressed growth factors could function as oncogenes. Experiments demonstrated that the constitutive expression of the *sis* gene product (PDGF-β) was sufficient to cause neoplastic transformation of fibroblasts, but not of cells that lacked the receptor for PDGF (41). Thus, transformation by *sis* requires interaction of the *sis* gene product with the PDGF receptor. The mechanism by which a growth factor affects the same cell that produces it is called *autocrine stimulation* (42). The constitutive expression of the *sis* gene product appears to cause neoplastic transformation by the mechanism of autocrine stimulation, resulting in self-sustained aberrant cell proliferation. Another example of a growth factor that can function as an oncogene is *int-2*, a member of the fibroblast growth factor family. *Int-2* is sometimes activated in mouse mammary carcinomas by MMTV insertional mutagenesis (43).

GROWTH FACTOR RECEPTORS

Some viral oncogenes are altered versions of normal growth factor receptors that possess intrinsic tyrosine kinase activity (44, 45). Receptor tyrosine kinases, as these growth factor receptors are collectively known, have a characteristic protein structure consisting of three principal domains: (*a*) the extracellular ligand-binding domain, (*b*) the transmembrane domain, and (*c*) the intracellular tyrosine kinase catalytic domain. Growth factor receptors are molecular machines that transmit information in a unidirectional fashion across the cell membrane. The binding of a growth factor to the extracellular ligand-binding domain of the receptor results in the activation of the intracellular tyrosine kinase catalytic domain. The recruitment and phosphorylation of specific cytoplasmic proteins by the activated receptor then trigger a series of biochemical events generally leading to cell division.

Because of the role of growth factor receptors in the regulation of normal cell growth, it is not surprising that these receptors constitute an important class of proto-oncogenes. Examples include *erb B*, *erb B-2*, *fms*, *kit*, *met*, *ret*, *ros*, and *trk*. Mutation or abnormal expression of growth factor receptors can convert them into oncogenes (46). For example, deletion of the ligand-binding domain of *erb B* (the epidermal growth factor receptor) is thought to result in constitutive activation of the receptor in the absence of ligand binding (47). Point mutation in the tyrosine kinase domain and deletion of intracellular regulatory domains can also result in the constitutive activation of receptor tyrosine kinases. Increased expression through gene amplification and abnormal expression in the wrong cell type are additional mechanisms through which growth factor receptors may be involved in neoplasia. The identification and study of altered growth factor receptors in experimental models of neoplasia have contributed much to our understanding of the normal regulation of cell proliferation.

SIGNAL TRANSDUCERS

Mitogenic signals are transmitted from growth factor receptors on the cell surface to the cell nucleus through a series of complex interlocking pathways collectively referred to as the signal transduction cascade (48). This relay of information is accomplished in part by the stepwise phosphorylation of interacting proteins in the cytosol. Signal transduction also involves guanine nucleotide-binding proteins and second messengers such as the adenylate cyclase system (49, 50). The first retroviral oncogene discovered, *src*, was subsequently shown to be involved in signal transduction.

Many proto-oncogenes are members of signal transduction pathways (51, 52). These consist of two main groups: nonreceptor protein kinases and GTP-binding proteins. The nonreceptor protein kinases are subclassified into tyrosine kinases (e.g., *abl*, *lck*, and *src*) and serine/threonine kinases (e.g., *raf-1*, *mos*, and *pim-1*). GTP-binding proteins with intrinsic GTPase activity are subdivided into monomeric and heterotrimeric groups (53). Monomeric GTP-binding proteins are members of the important *ras* family of proto-oncogenes that includes H-*ras*, K-*ras*, and N-*ras* (54). Heterotrimeric GTP-binding proteins (G proteins) implicated as proto-oncogenes currently include *gsp* and *gip*. Signal transducers are often converted to oncogenes by mutations that lead to their unregulated activity, which in turn leads to uncontrolled cellular proliferation (55).

TRANSCRIPTION FACTORS

Transcription factors are nuclear proteins that regulate the expression of target genes or gene families (56). Transcriptional regulation is mediated by protein binding to specific DNA sequences or DNA structural motifs, usually located upstream of the target gene. Transcription factors often belong to multigene families that share common DNA-binding domains such as zinc fingers. The mechanism of action of transcription factors also involves binding to other proteins, sometimes in heterodimeric complexes with specific partners. Transcription factors are the final link in the signal transduction pathway that converts extracellular signals into modulated changes in gene expression.

Many proto-oncogenes are transcription factors that were discovered through their retroviral homologues (57). Examples include *erb A*, *ets*, *fos*, *jun*, *myb*, and c-*myc*. Together, *fos* and *jun* form the AP-1 transcription factor, which positively regulates a number of target genes whose expression leads to cell division (58, 59). *Erb A* is the receptor for the T3 thyroid hormone, triiodothyronine (60, 61). Proto-oncogenes that function as transcription factors are often activated by chromosomal translocations in hematologic and solid neoplasms (62). An important example in human cancer is the c-*myc* gene, which helps to control the expression of genes leading to cell proliferation (63). As will be discussed later in this chapter, the c-*myc* gene is frequently activated by chromosomal translocations in human leukemia and lymphoma.

PROGRAMMED CELL DEATH REGULATION

Normal tissues exhibit a regulated balance between cell proliferation and cell death. Programmed cell death is an important component in the processes of normal embryogenesis and organ development. A distinctive type of programmed cell death, called apoptosis, has been described for mature tissues (64). This process is characterized morphologically by blebbing of the plasma membrane, volume contraction, condensation of the cell nucleus, and cleavage of genomic DNA by endogenous nucleases into nucleosome-sized fragments. Apoptosis can be triggered in mature cells by external stimuli such as steroids and radiation exposure. Studies of cancer cells have shown that failure to undergo programmed cell death as well as uncontrolled cell proliferation can both contribute to neoplasia.

The only proto-oncogene thus far shown to regulate programmed cell death is *bcl-2*. *Bcl-2* was discovered by the study of chromosomal translocations in human lymphoma (65, 66). Experimental studies show that *bcl-2* activation inhibits programmed cell death in lymphoid cell populations (67). The dominant mode of action of activated *bcl-2* classifies it as an oncogene. The *bcl-2* gene encodes a protein localized to the inner mitochondrial membrane, endoplasmic reticulum, and nuclear membrane. The mechanism of action of the *bcl-2* protein has not been fully elucidated, but studies indicate that it functions in part as an antioxidant that inhibits lipid peroxidation of cell membranes (68). The normal function of *bcl-2* requires interaction with other proteins, such as *bax*, also thought to be involved in the regulation of programmed cell death. It is unlikely that *bcl-2* is the only apoptosis gene involved in neoplasia, although additional proto-oncogenes await identification.

Mechanisms of Oncogene Activation

The activation of oncogenes involves genetic changes to cellular proto-oncogenes. The consequence of these genetic alterations is to confer a growth advantage to the cell. Three genetic mechanisms activate oncogenes in human neoplasms: (*a*) mutation, (*b*) gene amplification, and (*c*) chromosomal rearrangement. These mechanisms result in either an alteration of proto-oncogene structure or an increase in proto-oncogene expression. Because neoplasia is a multistep process, more than one of these mechanisms often contribute to the genesis of human tumors. Full expression of the neoplastic phenotype, including the capacity for metastasis, usually involves a combination of proto-oncogene activation and tumor suppressor gene loss or inactivation.

MUTATION

Mutations activate proto-oncogenes through structural alterations in their encoded proteins. These alterations, which usually involve critical protein regulatory regions, often lead to the uncontrolled, continuous activity of the mutated protein. Various types of mutations, such as base substitutions, deletions, and insertions, are capable of activating proto-oncogenes (69). Retroviral oncogenes, for example, often have deletions that contribute to their activation. Examples include deletions in the amino-terminal ligand-binding domains of the *erb B*, *kit*, *ros*, *met*, and *ret* oncogenes (2). In human tumors, however, most characterized oncogene muta-

Table 5.2. *Ras* Gene Mutations in Human Cancer

Tumor type	Incidence (%)	Predominant *ras* gene activated
Lung (adenocarcinoma)	30	K-*ras*
Colon (adenocarcinoma)	50	K-*ras*
Pancreas (adenocarcinoma)	90	K-*ras*
Cholangiocarcinoma	90	K-*ras*
Bladder carcinoma	6	H-*ras*
Breast	<5	K-*ras*
Cervical carcinoma	25	H-*ras*
Thyroid	>60	H-*ras*, K-*ras*, N-*ras*
Melanoma	20	N-*ras*
Seminoma	40	K-*ras*, N-*ras*
Myelodysplasia	30	N-*ras*
Acute myeloid leukemia	30	N-*ras*
Acute lymphoblastic leukemia	10	N-*ras*

Modified with permission from McCormick F. *ras* oncogenes. In *Oncogenes and the Molecular Origins of Human Cancer*. Edited by RA Weinberg. Cold Spring Harbor, NY: Cold Spring Harbor Laboratory Press, 1989, p 139.

tions are base substitutions (point mutations) that change a single amino acid within the protein.

Point mutations are frequently detected in the *ras* family of proto-oncogenes (K-*ras*, H-*ras*, and N-*ras*) (70). It has been estimated that as many as 15 to 20% of unselected human tumors may contain a *ras* mutation (Table 5.2). Mutations in K-*ras* predominate in carcinomas. Studies have found K-*ras* mutations in about 30% of lung adenocarcinomas, 50% of colon carcinomas, and 90% of carcinomas of the pancreas (71–73). N-*ras* mutations are preferentially found in hematologic malignancies, with up to a 25% incidence in acute myeloid leukemias and myelodysplastic syndromes (74, 75). The majority of thyroid carcinomas have been found to have *ras* mutations distributed among K-*ras*, H-*ras*, and N-*ras* without preference for a single *ras* family member (76). The majority of *ras* mutations involve codon 12 of the gene, with a smaller number involving other regions such as codons 13 or 61 (77). *Ras* mutations in human tumors have been linked to carcinogen exposure. The consequence of *ras* mutations is the constitutive activation of the signal transducing function of the *ras* protein.

GENE AMPLIFICATION

Gene amplification refers to the expansion in copy number of a gene within the genome of a cell. Gene amplification was first discovered as a mechanism by which some tumor cell lines can acquire resistance to growth-inhibiting drugs (78). The process of gene amplification occurs through redundant replication of genomic DNA, often giving rise to karyotypic abnormalities called double-minute chromosomes (DMs) and homogeneous staining regions (HSRs) (79). DMs are characteristic "minichromosome" structures without centromeres. HSRs are segments of chromosomes that lack the normal alternating pattern of light and dark staining bands. Both DMs and HSRs represent large regions of amplified genomic DNA containing up to several hundred copies of a gene. Amplification leads to the increased expression of genes, which in turn can confer a selective advantage for cell growth.

Table 5.3. Amplification of *myc, erb B,* and *ras* Gene Families in Human Tumors

Gene	Tumor type	Frequency of amplification (%)
c-*myc*	Breast cancer	15–23
	Colon carcinoma	3–6
	Lung—squamous cell carcinoma	12–25
N-*myc*	Neuroblastoma	10–31
c-*myc* or L-*myc*	Lung—adenocarcinoma	2–11
c-*myc*, N-*myc*, or L-*myc*	Lung—small cell carcinoma	11–23
erb B (epidermal growth factor receptor)	Breast cancer	1–4
	Gastric and esophageal carcinoma	4–8
	Head and neck squamous cell carcinoma	10
	Glioblastoma	38–50
erb B-2 (neu/HER-2)	Breast cancer	16–33
	Gastric and esophageal carcinoma	5–13
	Ovarian cancer	20–33
K-*ras*	Breast cancer	3
	Ovarian cancer	4–8
	Lung carcinoma	4

Adapted with permission from Brison O. Gene amplification and tumor progression. *Biochim Biophys Acta* 1155:26, 1993.

The frequent observation of DMs and HSRs in human tumors suggested that the amplification of specific proto-oncogenes may be a common occurrence in neoplasia (80). Studies then demonstrated that three proto-oncogene families—*myc*, *erb B*, and *ras*—are amplified in a significant number of human tumors (Table 5.3). About 10 to 20% of breast and ovarian cancers show c-*myc* amplification, and an approximately equal frequency of c-*myc* amplification is found in some types of squamous cell carcinomas (81). N-*myc* was discovered as a new member of the *myc* proto-oncogene family through its amplification in neuroblastomas (82). Amplification of N-*myc* correlates strongly with advanced tumor stage in neuroblastoma, suggesting a role for this gene in tumor progression (83). L-*myc* was discovered through its amplification in small cell carcinomas of the lung, a neuroendocrine-derived tumor (84). Amplification of *erb B*, the epidermal growth factor receptor, is found in up to 50% of glioblastomas and in 10 to 20% of squamous carcinomas of the head and neck (81). Approximately 15 to 30% of breast and ovarian cancers have amplification of the *erb B-2* (*HER-2/neu*) gene. In breast cancer, *erb B-2* amplification correlates with advanced stage and poor prognosis (85). Members of the *ras* gene family, including K-*ras* and N-*ras*, are sporadically amplified in various carcinomas.

CHROMOSOMAL REARRANGEMENTS

Recurring chromosomal rearrangements are often detected in hematologic malignancies as well as in some solid tumors (33, 86, 87). These rearrangements consist mainly of

Table 5.4A. Oncogenes Associated with Chromosomal Rearrangements in Hematologic Malignancy

A. Gene Activation

Rearrangement	Disease	Rearranged gene at breakpoint	Activated gene near breakpoint
B-cell malignancies			
t(8;14)(q24;q32)	BL, B-ALL	*IgH* (14q32)	*c-MYC* (8q24)
t(2;8)(p12;q24)	BL, B-ALL	*IgL-κ* (2p12)	*c-MYC* (8q24)
t(8;22)(q24;q11)	BL, B-ALL	*IgL-λ* (22q11)	*c-MYC* (8q24)
t(11;14)(q13;q32)	MCL	*IgH* (14q32)	*BCL1/PRAD1/cyclin D1* (11q13)
t(14;18)(q32;q21)	FL	*IgH* (14q32)	*BCL2* (18q21)
t(14;19)(q32;q13)	B-CLL	*IgH* (14q32)	*BCL3* (19p13.1)
t(3;14)(q27;q32)	DLCL	*IgH* (14q32)	*BCL6/Laz3* (3q27)
T-cell malignancies			
t(7;19)(q35;p13)	T-ALL	*TCR-β* (7q35)	*LYL1* (19p13)
t(7;9)(q35;q34)	T-ALL	*TCR-β* (7q35)	*TAL2* (9q34)
t(1;14)(p32;q11)	T-ALL	*TCR-δ* (14q11)	*TAL1/SCL/TCL5* (1p32)
t(8;14)(q24;q11)	T-ALL	*TCR-α* (14q11)	*c-MYC* (8q24)
t(10;14)(q24;q11)	T-ALL	*TCR-α* (14q11)	*HOX11* (10q24)
t(11;14)(p15;q11)	T-ALL	*TCR-δ* (14q11)	*RBTN1/Ttg1* (11p15)
inv(q11;q32)	T-CLL/T-PLL	*TCR-Cα* (14q11)	*TCL1* (14q32.1)

For abbreviations, see Table 5.4B, on page 91.

chromosomal translocations and, less frequently, chromosomal inversions. Chromosomal rearrangements can lead to hematologic malignancy by two different mechanisms: (*a*) the transcriptional activation of proto-oncogenes, or (*b*) the creation of fusion genes. Transcriptional activation, sometimes referred to as gene activation, results from chromosomal rearrangements that move a proto-oncogene close to an immunoglobulin or T-cell receptor gene. Transcription of the proto-oncogene then falls under control of regulatory elements from the immunoglobulin or T-cell receptor locus. This circumstance causes deregulation of proto-oncogene expression, which can then lead to neoplastic transformation of the cell.

Fusion genes can be created by chromosomal rearrangements when the chromosomal breakpoints fall within the loci of two different genes. The resultant juxtaposition of segments from two different genes gives rise to a composite structure consisting of the head of one gene and the tail of another gene. Fusion genes encode chimeric proteins with transforming activity. In general, both genes involved in the fusion contribute to the transforming potential of the chimeric oncoprotein. Mistakes in the physiologic rearrangement of immunoglobulin or T-cell receptor genes are thought to give rise to many of the recurring chromosomal rearrangements found in hematologic malignancy (88). Examples of chromosomal rearrangements in hematologic malignancies are given in Table 5.4. In some cases, the same proto-oncogene is involved in several different translocations.

Gene Activation. The t(8;14)(q24;q32) translocation, found in about 85% of cases of Burkitt's lymphoma, is a well-characterized example of the transcriptional activation of a proto-oncogene. This chromosomal rearrangement places the c-*myc* gene, located at chromosome band 8q24, under control of regulatory elements from the immunoglobulin heavy chain locus located at 14q32 (89). The resulting transcriptional activation of c-*myc*, which encodes a nuclear protein involved in the regulation of cell proliferation, plays a critical role in the development of Burkitt's lymphoma (90). The c-*myc* gene is also activated in some cases of Burkitt's lymphoma by translocations involving immunoglobulin light chain genes (91, 92). These "variant" translocations are t(2;8)(p12;q24), involving the κ locus located at 2p12, and t(8;22)(q24;q11), involving the λ locus at 22q11. Although the position of the chromosomal breakpoints relative to the c-*myc* gene may vary considerably in individual cases of Burkitt's lymphoma, the consequence of the translocations is the same—deregulation of c-*myc* expression, leading to uncontrolled cellular proliferation.

In some cases of T-cell acute lymphoblastic leukemia (T-ALL), the c-*myc* gene is activated by the t(8;14)(q24;q11) translocation. In these cases, transcription of c-*myc* is placed under the control of regulatory elements within the T-cell receptor α locus located at 14q11 (93). In addition to c-*myc*, several proto-oncogenes that encode nuclear proteins are activated by various chromosomal translocations in T-ALL involving the T-cell receptor α or β locus. These include *HOX11*, *TAL1*, *TAL2*, and *RBTN1/Tgt1* (94–96). The proteins encoded by these genes are thought to function as transcription factors through DNA-binding and protein–protein interactions. Over-expression or inappropriate expression of these proteins in T cells is thought to inhibit T-cell differentiation and lead to uncontrolled cellular proliferation.

A number of other proto-oncogenes are also activated by chromosomal translocations in leukemia and lymphoma. In most follicular lymphomas and some large cell lymphomas, the *bcl-2* gene (located at 18q21) is activated as a consequence of t(14;18)(q32;q21) translocations (65, 66). Over-expression of the *bcl-2* protein inhibits apoptosis, leading to an imbalance between lymphocyte proliferation and programmed cell death (67). Mantle cell lymphomas are characterized by the t(11;14)(q13;q32) translocation, which activates the *cyclin D1* (*bcl-1*) gene located at 11q13 (97, 98).

Table 5.4B.

B. Gene Fusion

Rearrangement	Disease	Fused genes at chromosomal breakpoints
t(9;22)(q34;q11)	CML/ALL	*cABL* (9q34) *BCR* (22q11)
t(1;19)(q23;p13)	pre-B-ALL	*PBX1* (1q23) *E2A* (19p13)
t(17;19)(q22;p13)	pro-B-ALL	*HLF* (17q22) *E2A* (19p13)
t(15;17)(q21;q11-22)	APL	*PML* (15q21) *RARA* (17q21)
t(11;17)(q23;q21)	APL	*PLZF* (11q23) *RARA* (17q21)
t(4;11)(q21;q23)	ALL/ANLL	*ALL1/MLL/HRX* (11q23) *AF4* (4q21)
t(6;11)(q27;q23)	ALL/ANLL	*ALL1/MLL/HRX* (11q23) *AF6* (6q27)
t(9;11)(p22;q23)	ALL/ANLL	*ALL1/MLL/HRX* (11q23) *AF9* (9p22)
t(11;19)(q23;p13.3)	ALL/ANLL	*ALL1/MLL/HRX* (11q23) *ENL* (19p13.3)
t(11;19)(q23;p13.1)	ALL/ANLL	*ALL1/MLL/HRX* (11q23) *ELL/MEN* (19p13.1)
t(11;17)(q23;q21)	ALL/ANLL	*ALL1/MLL/HRX* (11q23) *AF17* (17q21)
t(1;11)(p32;q23)	ALL/ANLL	*ALL1/MLL/HRX* (11q23) *AF1p* (1p32)
t(1;11)(q21;q23)	ALL/ANLL	*ALL1/MLL/HRX* (11q23) *AF1q* (1q21)
t(10;11)(p12;q23)	ALL/ANLL	*ALL1/MLL/HRX* (11q23) *AF10* (10p12)
t(X;11)(q13;q23)	ALL	*ALL1/MLL/HRX* (11q23) *AFX1* (Xq13)
t(8;21)(q22;q22)	AML	*AML1/CBFα* (21q22) *ETO/MTG8* (8q22)
t(3;21)(q26;q22)	CML	*AML1/CBFα* (21q22) *EVI-1* (3q26)
t(3;21)(q26;q22)	Myelodysplasia	*AML1/CBFα* (21q22) *EAP* (3q26)
t(16;21)(p11;q22)	Myeloid	*FUS* (16p11) *ERG* (21q22)
t(6;9)(p23;q34)	AML	*DEK* (6p23) *CAN* (9p34)
inv(16)(p13;q22)	AML	*Myosin MYH11* (16p13) *CBF-β* (16q22)
t(5;12)(q33;p13)	CMML	*PDGF-β* (5q33) *TEL* (12p13)
t(2;5)(p23;q35)	NHL	*NPM* (5q35) *ALK* (2p23)

Abbreviations: BL, Burkitt's lymphoma; MCL, mantle cell lymphoma; FL, follicular lymphoma; CLL, chronic lymphocytic leukemia (B- or T-cell); DLCL, diffuse large cell lymphoma; ALL, acute lymphoblastic leukemia (B- or T-cell); PLL, prolymphocytic leukemia; CML, chronic myelogenous leukemia; APL, acute promyelocytic leukemia; ANLL, acute nonlymphoblastic leukemia; AML, acute myeloid leukemia; CMML, chronic myelomonocytic leukemia; NHL, non-Hodgkin's lymphoma. Modified with permission from Schichman SA, Croce CM. Approaches to the identification and molecular cloning of chromosome breakpoints. *Methods Enzymol* 254:325, 1995; and Rabbits TH. Chromosomal translocations in human cancer. *Nature* 372:144–145, 1994, MacMillan Magazines Limited.

Cyclin D1 is a G1 cyclin involved in the normal regulation of the cell cycle. In some cases of T-cell chronic lymphocytic leukemia and prolymphocytic leukemia, the *tcl-1* gene at 14q32.1 is activated by inversion or translocation involving chromosome 14 (99). The *tcl-1* gene product is a small cytoplasmic protein whose function is not yet known.

Gene Fusion. The first example of gene fusion was discovered through the cloning of the breakpoint of the Philadelphia chromosome in CML (100). The t(9;22) (q34;q11) translocation in CML fuses the c-*abl* gene, normally located at 9q34, with the *bcr* gene at 22q11 (101). The *bcr/abl* fusion, created on the der (22) chromosome, encodes a chimeric protein of 210 kd with increased tyrosine kinase activity and abnormal cellular localization (102). The precise mechanism by which the *bcr/abl* fusion protein contributes to the expansion of the neoplastic myeloid clone is not yet known. The t(9;22) translocation is also found in up to 20% of cases of ALL. In these cases, the breakpoint in the *bcr* gene differs somewhat from that found in CML, resulting in a 185 kd bcr/abl fusion protein (103). It is unclear at this time why the slightly smaller bcr/abl fusion protein leads to such a large difference in neoplastic phenotype.

In addition to c-*abl*, two other genes encoding tyrosine kinases are involved in distinct gene fusion events in hematologic malignancy. The t(2;5)(p23;q35) translocation in anaplastic large cell lymphomas fuses the *NPM* gene (5q35) with the *ALK* gene (2p23) (104). *ALK* encodes a membrane-spanning tyrosine kinase similar to members of the insulin growth factor receptor family. The NPM protein is a nucleolar phosphoprotein involved in ribosome assembly. The *NPM/ALK* fusion creates a chimeric oncoprotein in which the ALK tyrosine kinase activity may be constitutively activated. The t(5;12)(q33;p13) translocation, characterized in a case of chronic myelomonocytic leukemia (CMML), fuses the *TEL* gene (12p13) with the tyrosine kinase domain of the platelet-derived growth factor receptor β gene (PDGFR-β at 5q33) (105). The *TEL* gene is thought to encode a nuclear DNA-binding protein similar to those of the *ets* family of proto-oncogenes.

Gene fusions sometimes lead to the formation of chimeric transcription factors (62, 87). The t(1;19)(q23;p13) translocation, found in childhood pre-B-cell ALL, fuses the *E2A* transcription factor gene (19p13) with the *PBX1* homeodomain gene (1q23) (106). The E2A/PBX1 fusion protein consists of the amino-terminal transactivation domain of the E2A protein and the DNA-binding homeodomain of the PBX1 protein. The t(15;17)(q22;q21) translocation in acute promyelocytic leukemia fuses the *PML* gene (15q22) with the *RARA* gene at 17q21 (107). The PML protein contains a zinc-binding domain called a RING finger that may be involved in protein–protein interactions (108). *RARA* encodes the retinoic acid α-receptor protein, a member of the nuclear steroid/thyroid hormone receptor superfamily. Although retinoic acid binding is retained in the fusion protein, the PML/RARA fusion protein may confer altered DNA-binding specificity to the RARA–ligand complex (109). Leukemia patients with the *PML/RARA* gene fusion respond well to retinoid treatment. In these cases, treatment with all-trans-retinoic acid induces differentiation of promyelocytic leukemia cells.

The *ALL1* gene, located at chromosome band 11q23, is involved in approximately 5 to 10% of acute leukemia cases overall in children and adults (110, 111). These include cases of ALL, AML, and leukemias of mixed cell lineage. Among leukemia genes, *ALL1* (also called *MLL* and *HRX*) is unique because it participates in fusions with a large number of different partner genes on the various chromosomes. Over 20 different reciprocal translocations involving the *ALL1* gene at 11q23 have been reported, the most common of which are those involving chromosomes 4, 6, 9, and 19 (112). In approximately 5% of cases of acute leukemia in adults, the *ALL1* gene is fused with a portion of itself (113). This special type of gene fusion is called *self-fusion* (114). Self-fusion of the *ALL1* gene, which is thought to occur through a somatic recombination mechanism, is found in high incidence in acute leukemias with trisomy 11 as a sole cytogenetic abnormality. The *ALL1* gene encodes a large protein with DNA-binding motifs, a transactivation domain, and a region with homology to the *Drosophila trithorax* protein (a regulator of homeotic gene expression) (115–117). The various partners in *ALL1* fusions encode a diverse group of proteins, some of which appear to be nuclear proteins with DNA-binding motifs (118, 119). The ALL1 fusion protein consists of the amino-terminus of ALL1 and the carboxy-terminus of one of a variety of fusion partners. It appears that the critical feature in all ALL1 fusions, including self-fusion, is the uncoupling of the ALL1 amino-terminal domains from the remainder of the ALL1 protein.

Table 5.5. Oncogenes Associated with Chromosomal Rearrangements in Solid Tumors

Rearrangement	Disease	Fused genes at chromosomal breakpoints
t(11;22)(q24;q12)	Ewing's sarcoma	*EWS* (22q12) *FLI1* (11q24)
t(21;22)(q22;q12)	Ewing's sarcoma	*EWS* (22q12) *ERG* (21q22)
t(12;22)(q13;q12)	Melanoma of soft parts	*EWS* (22q12) *ATF1* (12q13)
t(11;22)(p13;q12)	Desmoplastic small round cell tumor	*EWS* (22q12) *WT1* (11p13)
t(2;13)(q35;q14)	Alveolar rhabdomyosarcoma	*PAX3* (2q35) *FKHR* (13q14)
t(1;13)(p36;q14)	Alveolar rhabdomyosarcoma	*PAX7* (1p36) *FKHR* (13q14)
t(12;16)(q13;p11)	Myxoid liposarcoma	*FUS/TLS* (16p11) *CHOP* (12q13)
t(X;18)(p11;q11)	Synovial sarcoma	*SYT* (18q11) *SSX* (Xp11)

Modified with permission from Rabbits TH. Chromosomal translocations in human cancer. *Nature* 372;145, 1994, MacMillan Magazines Limited.

Solid tumors, especially sarcomas, sometimes have consistent chromosomal translocations that correlate with specific histologic types of tumors (Table 5.5) (120). In general, translocations in solid tumors result in gene fusions that encode chimeric oncoproteins. Studies thus far indicate that in sarcomas the majority of genes fused by translocations encode transcription factors (87). In myxoid liposarcomas, the t(12;16)(q13;p11) fuses the *FUS* (*TLS*) gene at 16p11 with the *CHOP* gene at 12q13 (121). The FUS protein contains a transactivation domain that is contributed to the FUS/CHOP fusion protein. The CHOP protein, which is a dominant inhibitor of transcription, contributes a protein-binding domain and a presumptive DNA-binding domain to the fusion. Despite knowledge of these structural features, the mechanism of action of the FUS/CHOP oncoprotein is not yet known. In Ewing's sarcoma, the t(11;22)(q24;q12) fuses the *EWS* gene at 22q12 with the *FLI1* gene at 11q24 (122). Like FUS, the EWS protein contains three glycine rich segments and an RNA-binding domain. The FLI1 protein contains an ets-like DNA-binding domain. The EWS/FLI1 fusion protein combines a transactivation domain from EWS with the DNA-binding domain of FLI1. In alveolar rhabdomyosarcoma, the t(2;13)(q35;q14) fuses the *PAX3* gene at 2q35 with the *FKHR* gene at 13q14 (123). The PAX3 protein, a transcription factor that activates genes involved in development, is a paired-box homeodomain protein with two distinct DNA-binding domains. The FKHR protein encodes a conserved DNA-binding motif (the fork head domain) similar to that first identified in the *Drosophila* fork head homeotic gene. The PAX3/FKHR fusion protein is a chimeric transcription factor containing the PAX3 DNA-binding domains, a truncated fork head domain, and the carboxy-terminal FKHR regions.

Oncogenes in the Initiation and Progression of Neoplasia

Human neoplasia is a complex, multistep process involving sequential changes in proto-oncogenes and tumor suppressor genes. Statistical analysis of the age incidence of human solid tumors indicates that five or six independent mutational events may contribute to tumor formation (124). In human leukemias, only three or four mutational events may be necessary, presumably involving different genes.

The study of chemical carcinogenesis in animals provides a foundation for our understanding the multistep nature of cancer (125). In the mouse model of skin carcinogenesis, tumor formation involves three phases, termed initiation, promotion, and progression. Initiation of skin tumors can be induced by chemical mutagens such as 7,12-dimethylbenzanthracene (DMBA). After application of DMBA, the mouse skin appears normal. If the skin is then continuously treated with a promoter, such as the phorbol ester TPA, precancerous papilomas will form. Chemical promoters such as TPA stimulate growth but are not mutagenic substances. Over a period of months of continuous application of the promoting agent, some of the papillomas will progress to skin carcinomas. Treatment with DMBA or TPA alone does not cause skin cancer. Mouse papillomas initiated with DMBA usually have H-*ras* oncogenes with a specific mutation in codon 61 of the H-*ras* gene. The mouse skin tumor model indicates that initiation of papillomas is the result of mutation of the H-*ras* gene in individual skin cells by the chemical mutagen DMBA. For papillomas to appear on the skin, however, growth of mutated cells must be continuously stimulated by a promoting agent. Additional unidentified genetic changes must then occur for papillomas to progress to carcinoma.

Although a single oncogene is sufficient to cause tumor formation by some rapidly transforming retroviruses such as RSV, transformation by a single oncogene is not usually seen in experimental models of cancer. Other rapidly transforming retroviruses carry two different oncogenes that cooperate in producing the neoplastic phenotype. One well-characterized example of this type of cooperation is the avian erythroblastosis virus, which carries the *erb A* and *erb B* oncogenes (126). Cooperation between oncogenes can also be demonstrated by in vitro transformation studies using nonimmortalized cell lines. For example, studies have shown cooperation between the nuclear myc protein and the cytoplasmic membrane-associated ras protein in the transformation of rat embryo fibroblasts (127). Collaboration between two different general categories of oncogenes (e.g., nuclear and cytoplasmic) can often be demonstrated, but is not strictly required for transformation (128). The production of transgenic mice expressing a single oncogene such as *myc* has also demonstrated that multiple genetic changes are necessary for tumor formation (129). Experimental studies with individual oncogenes generally support the multistep model of malignant transformation.

Cytogenetic studies of the clonal evolution of human hematologic malignancies have provided much insight into the multiple steps involved in the initiation and progression of human tumors (130). The evolution of CML from chronic phase to acute leukemia is characterized by an accumulation of genetic changes seen in the karyotypes of the evolving malignant clones. The early chronic phase of CML is defined by the presence of a single Philadelphia chromosome. The formation of the *bcr/abl* gene fusion as a consequence of the t(9;22) translocation is thought to be the initiating event in CML (101). The biologic progression of CML to a more malignant phenotype corresponds with the appearance of additional cytogenetic abnormalities such as a second Philadelphia chromosome, isochromosome 17, or trisomy 8 (131). These karyotypic changes are thought to reflect additional genetic changes involving an increase in oncogene dosage and loss or inactivation of tumor suppressor genes. Although the karyotypic changes in evolving CML are somewhat variable from patient to patient, the accumulation of genetic changes always correlates with progression from differentiated cells of low malignancy to undifferentiated cells of high malignancy.

The initiation and progression of human neoplasia involve the activation of oncogenes and the inactivation or loss of tumor suppressor genes. The mechanisms of oncogene activation and the time course of events, however, vary among different types of tumors. In hematologic malignancies and soft-tissue sarcomas, initiation of the malignant process predominantly involves chromosomal rearrangements that activate various oncogenes (86). Many of the chromosomal rearrangements in leukemia and lymphoma are thought to result from errors in the physiologic process of immunoglobulin or T-cell receptor gene rearrangement during normal B-cell and T-cell development. Late events in the progression of hematologic malignancies involve oncogene mutation, mainly of the *ras* family, inactivation of tumor suppressor genes such as *p53*, and sometimes additional chromosomal translocations (132).

In carcinomas such as colon and lung cancer, the initiation of neoplasia has been shown to involve oncogene and tumor suppressor gene mutations (133). These mutations are generally thought to result from chemical carcinogenesis, especially in the case of tobacco-related lung cancer. In preneoplastic adenomas of the colon, the K-*ras* gene is often mutated (29, 134). Progression of colon adenomas to invasive carcinoma frequently involves inactivation or loss of the *DCC* and *p53* tumor suppressor genes. Gene amplification is often seen in the progression of some carcinomas and other types of tumors. Amplification of the *erb B-2* oncogene may be a late event in the progression of breast cancer (85). Members of the *myc* oncogene family are frequently amplified in small cell carcinoma of the lung (84). As mentioned previously, amplification of N-*myc* strongly correlates with the progression and clinical stage of neuroblastoma (83). Although there is variability in the pathways of human tumor initiation and progression, studies of various types of malignancy have clearly confirmed the multistep nature of human cancer.

Summary and Conclusions

The initiation and progression of human neoplasia is a multistep process involving the accumulation of genetic changes in somatic cells. These genetic changes consist of the activation of oncogenes and the inactivation or loss of tumor suppressor genes. Oncogenes are altered versions of normal cellular genes called proto-oncogenes. Proto-oncogenes are a diverse group of genes involved in the regulation of cell growth. The functions of proto-oncogenes include growth factors, growth factor receptors, signal transducers, transcription factors, and regulators of programmed cell death. Proto-oncogenes may be activated by mutation, chromosomal rearrangement, or gene amplification. Chromosomal rearrangements—which include translocations and inversions—can activate proto-oncogenes by deregulation of their transcription (e.g., transcriptional activation) or by gene fusion. Tumor suppressor genes, which also participate in the regulation of normal cell growth, are usually inactivated by point mutations coupled with the loss of the normal allele.

The discovery of oncogenes represented a breakthrough for our understanding of the molecular and genetic basis of cancer. Oncogenes have also provided important knowledge concerning the regulation of normal cell proliferation, differentiation, and programmed cell death. The identification of oncogene abnormalities has provided tools for the molecular diagnosis and monitoring of cancer. Most important, oncogenes represent potential targets for new types of cancer therapies. It is hoped that a new generation of chemotherapeutic agents directed at specific oncogene targets will be developed. The goal of these new drugs will be to kill cancer cells selectively while sparing normal cells. One promising approach entails using specific oncogene targets to trigger programmed cell death. Our rapidly expanding knowledge of the molecular mechanisms of cancer holds great promise for the development of better methods of cancer therapy in the near future.

References

1. Levine AJ. The genetic origins of neoplasia. JAMA 1995;273:592.
2. Cooper GM. Oncogenes. Boston: Jones and Bartlett, 1990.
3. Bishop JM. Retroviruses and oncogenes II. In Les Prix Nobel. Stockholm: Almqvist and Wiksell, 1989, pp 220–238.
4. Varmus HE. Retroviruses and oncogenes I. In Les Prix Nobel. Stockholm: Almqvist and Wiksell, 1989, pp 194–212.
5. Varmus H. An historical overview of oncogenes. In Oncogenes and the Molecular Origins of Cancer. Edited by RA Weinberg. Cold Spring Harbor, NY: Cold Spring Harbor Laboratory Press, 1989, pp 3–44.
6. Bishop JM. Oncogenes and clinical cancer. In Oncogenes and the Molecular Origins of Cancer. Edited by RA Weinberg. Cold Spring Harbor, NY: Cold Spring Harbor Laboratory Press, 1989, pp 327–358.
7. Varmus HE. Retroviruses. Science 1988;240:1427–1435.
8. Varmus HE. Form and function of retroviral proviruses. Science 1982;216:812–820.
9. Rous P. A sarcoma of the fowl transmissible by an agent separable from the tumor. J Exp Med 1911;13:397–411.
10. Duesberg PH, Vogt PK. Differences between the ribonucleic acids of transforming and nontransforming avian tumor viruses. Proc Natl Acad Sci USA 1970;67: 1673–1680.
11. Martin GS. Rous sarcoma virus: a function required for the maintenance of the transformed state. Nature 1970;227:1021–1023.
12. Vogt PK. Spontaneous segregation of nontransforming viruses from the cloned sarcoma viruses. Virology 1971;46:939–946.
13. Stehlin D, Varmus HE, Bishop JM, Vogt PK. DNA related to the transforming gene(s) of avian sarcoma viruses is present in normal avian DNA. Nature 1976;260:170–173.
14. Nusse R, Berns KI. Cellular oncogene activation by insertion of retroviral DNA: genes identified by provirus tagging. In Cellular Oncogene Activation. Edited by G Klein. New York: Marcel Dekker, 1988, pp. 95–120.
15. Hayward WS, Neel BG, Astrin SM. Activation of a cellular onc gene by promoter insertion in ALV-induced lymphoid leukosis. Nature 1981;290:475–480.
16. Neel BG, Hayward WS, Robinson HL, Fang J, Astrin SM. Avian leukosis virus-induced tumors have common proviral integration sites and synthesize discrete new RNAs: oncogenesis by promoter insertion. Cell 1981;23:323–334.
17. Payne GS, Bishop JM, Varmus HE. Multiple arrangements of viral DNA and an activated host oncogene in bursal lymphomas. Nature 1982;295:209–214.
18. Robinson HL, Gagnon GC. Patterns of proviral insertion and deletion in avian leukosis virus-induced lymphomas. J Virol 1986;57:28–36.
19. Fung Y-KT, Lewis WG, Crittenden LB, Kung H-J. Activation of the cellular oncogene *c-erbB* by LTR insertion: molecular basis for induction of erythroblastosis by avian leukosis virus. Cell 1983;33:357–368.
20. Kanter MR, Smith RE, Hayward WS. Rapid induction of B-cell lymphomas: insertional activation of *c-myb* by avian leukosis virus. J Virol 1988;62:1423–1432.
21. Morishita K, Parker DS, Mucenski ML, Jenkins NA, Copeland NG, Ihle JN. Retroviral activation of a novel gene encoding a zinc finger protein in IL-3 dependent myeloid leukemia cell lines. Cell 1988;54:831–840.
22. Shih C, Shilo B-Z, Goldfarb MP, Dannenberg A, Weinberg RA. Passage of phenotypes of chemically transformed cells via transfection of DNA and chromatin. Proc Natl Acad Sci USA 1979;76:5714–5718.
23. Krontiris TG, Cooper GM. Transforming activity of human tumor DNAs. Proc Natl Acad Sci USA 1981;78:1181–1184.
24. Murray MJ, Shilo B-Z, Shih C, Cowing D, Hsu HW, Weinberg RA. Three different human tumor cell lines contain different oncogenes. Cell 1981;25:355–361.
25. Perucho M, Goldfarb M, Shimizu K, Lama C, Frogh J, Wigler M. Human tumor derived cell lines contain common and different transforming genes. Cell 1981;27:467–476.
26. Pulciani S, Santos E, Lauver AV, Long LK, Robbins KC, Barbacid M. Oncogenes in human tumor cell lines: molecular cloning of a transforming gene from human bladder carcinoma cells. Proc Natl Acad Sci USA 1982;79:2845–2849.
27. Parada LF, Tabin CJ, Shih C, Weinberg RA. Human EJ bladder carcinoma oncogene is homologue of Harvey sarcoma virus *ras* gene. Nature 1982;297:474–478.
28. Shimizu K, Goldfarb M, Suard Y, et al. Three human transforming genes are related to viral *ras* oncogenes. Proc Natl Acad Sci USA 1983;80:2112–2116.
29. Bos JL. *Ras* oncogenes in human cancer: a review. Cancer Res 1989;49:4682–4689.
30. Bargmann CI, Hung M-C, Weinberg RA. Multiple independent activations of the *neu* oncogene by a point mutation altering the transmembrane domain of p185. Cell 1986;45:649–657.
31. Park M, Dean M, Cooper CS, et al. Mechanism of *met* oncogene activation. Cell 1986;45:895–904.
32. Takahashi M, Ritz J, Cooper GM. Activation of a novel human transforming gene, *ret*, by DNA rearrangement. Cell 1985;42:581–588.
33. Croce CM. Role of chromosome translocations in human neoplasia. Cell 1987;49: 155–156.
34. Rowley JD. Recurring chromosome abnormalities in leukemia and lymphoma. Semin Hematol 1990;27:122–136.
35. Nowell PC, Hungerford D. A minute chromosome in human granulocytic leukemia. Science 1960;132:1497.
36. Nowell PC. Cytogenetic approaches to human cancer genes. FASEB J 1994;8: 408–413.
37. Cross M, Dexter TM. Growth factors in development, transformation, and tumorigenesis. Cell 1991;64:271–280.
38. Weinberg RA. Growth factors and oncogenes. In Oncogenes and the Molecular Origins of Cancer. Edited by RA Weinberg. Cold Spring Harbor, NY: Cold Spring Harbor Laboratory Press, 1989, pp 45–66.
39. Beckmann MP, Betsholtz C, Heldin C-H, et al. Comparison of biological properties and transforming potential of human PDGF-A and PDGF-B chains. Science 1988;241: 1346–1349.
40. Doolittle RF, Hunkapiller MW, Hood LE, et al. Simian sarcoma virus *onc* gene, *v-sis*, is derived from the gene (or genes) encoding a platelet-derived growth factor. Science 1983;221:275–277.
41. Fleming TP, Matsui T, Molloy CJ, Robbins KC, Aaronson SA. Autocrine mechanism for *v-sis* transformation requires cell surface localization of internally activated growth factor receptors. Proc Natl Acad Sci USA 1989;86:8063–8067.
42. Sporn MB, Roberts AB. Autocrine growth factors and cancer. Nature 1985;313: 745–747.
43. Peters G, Lee AE, Dickson C. Concerted action of two potential protooncogenes in carcinomas induced by mouse mammary tumor virus. Nature 1986;320:628–632.
44. Yarden Y, Ullrich A. Growth factors and receptor tyrosine kinases. Annu Rev Biochem 1988;57:443–478.
45. Gill GN. Growth factors and their receptors. In Oncogenes and the Molecular Origins of Cancer. Edited by RA Weinberg. Cold Spring Harbor, NY: Cold Spring Harbor Laboratory Press, 1989, pp. 67–96.
46. Segatto O, King CR, Pierce JH, Di Fiore PP, Aaronson SA. Different structural alterations upregulate in vitro tyrosine kinase activity and transforming potency of the *erbB-2* gene. Mol Cell Biol 1988;8:5570–5574.
47. Wells A, Bishop JM. Genetic determinants of neoplastic transformation by the retroviral oncogene *v-erbB*. Proc Natl Acad Sci USA 1988;85:7597–7601.
48. Ullrich A, Schlessinger J. Signal transduction by receptors with tyrosine kinase activity. Cell 1990;61:203–212.
49. Casey PJ, Gilman AG. G protein involvement in receptor-effector coupling. J Biol Chem 1988;236:2577–2580.
50. Gilman AG. G proteins: transducers of receptor-generated signals. Annu Rev Biochem 1987;56:615–629.
51. Cantley LC, Auger KR, Carpenter C, et al. Oncogenes and signal transduction. Cell 1991;64:281–302.
52. Bourne HR, DeFranco AL. Signal transduction and intracellular messengers. In Oncogenes and the Molecular Origins of Cancer. Edited by RA Weinberg. Cold Spring Harbor, NY: Cold Spring Harbor Laboratory Press, 1989, pp. 97–124.
53. Kaziro Y, Itoh H, Kozaso T, Nakafuku M, Satoh T. Structure and function of signal-transducing GTP-binding proteins. Annu Rev Biochem 1991;60:349–400.
54. Lowy DR, Willumsen BM. Function and regulation of *ras*. Annu Rev Biochem 1993;62: 851–891.

55. Rodrigues GA, Park M. Oncogenic activation of tyrosine kinases. Curr Opin Genet Dev 1994;4:15–24.
56. Mitchell PJ, Tjian R. Transcriptional regulation in mammalian cells by sequence-specific DNA binding proteins. Science 1989;245:371–378.
57. Lewin B. Oncogenic conversion by regulatory changes in transcription factors. Cell 1991;64:303–312.
58. Chiu R, Boyle WJ, Meek J, Smeal T, Hunter T, Karin M. The c-fos protein interacts with *c-jun*/AP-1 to stimulate transcription of AP-1 responsive genes. Cell 1988;54:541–552.
59. Angel P, Karin M. The role of jun, fos and the AP-1 complex in cell-proliferation and transformation. Biochim Biophys Acta 1991;1072:129–157.
60. Damm K, Thompson CC, Evans RM. Protein encoded by *v-erb* A functions as a thyroid-hormone receptor antagonist. Nature 1989;339:593–597.
61. Privalsky ML. *v-erb* A, nuclear hormone receptors, and oncogenesis. Biochim Biophys Acta 1992;1114:51–62.
62. Cleary ML. Oncogenic conversion of transcription factors by chromosomal translocations. Cell 1991;66:619–622.
63. Marcu KB, Bossone SA, Patel AJ. *Myc* function and regulation. Annu Rev Biochem 1992;61:809–860.
64. Wyllie AH. Apoptosis: cell death in tissue regulation. J Pathol 1987;153:313–316.
65. Tsujimoto Y, Finger LR, Yunis J, Nowell PC, Croce CM. Cloning of the chromosome breakpoint of neoplastic B cells with the t(14;18) chromosome translocation. Science 1984;226:1097–1099.
66. Cleary ML, Smith SD, Sklar J. Cloning and structural analysis of cDNAs for *bcl-2* and a hybrid *bcl-2*/immunoglobulin transcript resulting from the t(14;18) translocation. Cell 1986;47:19–28.
67. Korsmeyer SJ. Bcl-2 initiates a new category of oncogenes: regulators of cell death. Blood 1992;80:879–886.
68. Korsmeyer SJ, Shutter JR, Veis DJ, Merry DE, Oltvai ZN. Bcl-2/Bax: a rheostat that regulates anti-oxidant pathway and cell death. Semin Cancer Biol 1993;4:327–332.
69. Bishop JM. Molecular themes in oncogenesis. Cell 1991;64:235–248.
70. Rodenhuis S. *ras* and human tumors. Semin Cancer Biol 1992;3:241–247.
71. Slebos RJC, Kibbelaar RE, Dalesio O, et al. K-*ras* oncogene activation as a prognostic marker in adenocarcinoma of the lung. N Engl J Med 1990;323:561–565.
72. Forrester K, Almoguera C, Han K, Grizzle WE, Perucho M. Detection of high incidence of K-*ras* oncogenes during human colon tumorigenesis. Nature 1987;327:298–303.
73. Almoguera C, Shibata D, Forrester K, Martin J, Arnheim N, Perucho M. Most human carcinomas of the exocrine pancreas contain mutant K-*ras* genes. Cell 1988;53:549–554.
74. Liu E, Hjelle B, Morgan R, Hecht F, Bishop JM. Mutation of the Kirsten-*ras* proto-oncogene in human preleukemia. Nature 1987;330:186–188.
75. Lyons J, Janssen JWG, Bartram C, Layton M, Mufti GJ. Mutations of K-*ras* and N-*ras* oncogenes in myelodysplastic syndromes. Blood 1988;71:1707–1712.
76. Suarez HG, du Villard JA, Severino M, et al. Presence of mutations in all three *ras* genes in human thyroid tumors. Oncogene 1990;5:565–570.
77. Oudejans J, Slebos RJC, Zoetmulder FAN, Mooi WJ, Rodenhuis S. Differential activation of *ras* genes by point mutation in human colon cancer with metastases to either lung or liver. Int J Cancer 1990;49:875–879.
78. Alt FW, Kellems RE, Bertino JR, Schimke RT. Selective multiplication of dihydrofolate reductase genes in methotrexate-resistant variants of cultured mouse cells. J Biol Chem 1978;253:1357–1370.
79. Cowell JK. Double minutes and homogeneously staining regions: gene amplification in mammalian cells. Annu Rev Genet 1982;16:21–59.
80. Alitalo K, Schwab M. Oncogene amplification in tumor cells. Adv Cancer Res 1986;47:235–281.
81. Brison O. Gene amplification and tumor progression. Biochim Biophys Acta 1993;1155:25–41.
82. Schwab M, Alitalo K, Klempnauer KH, et al. Amplified DNA with limited homology to *myc* cellular oncogene is shared by human neuroblastoma cell lines and a neuroblastoma tumour. Nature 1983;305:245–248.
83. Seeger RC, Brodeur GM, Sather H, et al. Association of multiple copies of the N-*myc* oncogene with rapid progression of neuroblastomas. N Engl J Med 1985;313:1111–1116.
84. Nau MM, Brooks BJ, Battey J, et al. L-*myc*, a new *myc*-related gene amplified and expressed in human small cell lung cancer. Nature 1985;318:69–73.
85. Slamon DJ, Godolphin W, Jones LA, et al. Studies of *HER-2/neu* proto-oncogene in human breast and ovarian cancer. Science 1989;244:707–712.
86. Solomon E, Borrow J, Goddard AD. Chromosome aberrations and cancer. Science 1991;254:1153–1160.
87. Rabbits TH. Chromosomal translocations in human cancer. Nature 1994;372:143–149.
88. Haluska FG, Finver S, Tsujimoto Y, Croce CM. The t(8;14) chromosome translocation occurring in B-cell malignancies results from mistakes in V-D-J joining. Nature 1986;324:158–161.
89. Dalla Favera R, Bregni M, Erikson J, Patterson D, Gallo RC, Croce CM. Assignment of the *c-myc* oncogene to the region of chromosome 8 which is translocated in Burkitt lymphoma cells. Proc Natl Acad Sci USA 1982;79:7824–7827.
90. Nowell PC, Croce CM. Chromosome translocations and oncogenes in human lymphoid tumors. Am J Clin Pathol 1990;94:229–237.
91. Croce CM, Thierfelder W, Erikson J, et al. Transcriptional activation of an unrearranged and untranslocated *c-myc* oncogene by translocation of a Cλ locus in Burkitt lymphoma. Proc Natl Acad Sci USA 1983;80:6922–6926.
92. Emanuel BS, Selden JR, Chaganti RSK, Jhanwar S, Nowell PC, Croce CM. The 2p breakpoint of a 2;8 translocation in Burkitt's lymphoma interrupts the V κ locus. Proc Natl Acad Sci USA 1984;81:2444–2446.
93. Erikson J, Finger L, Sun L, et al. Deregulation of *c-myc* by translocation of the α-locus of the T-cell receptor in T-cell leukemias. Science 1986;232:884–886.
94. Hatano M, Roberts CWM, Minden M, Crist WM, Korsmeyer SJ. Deregulation of a homeobox gene, HOX11, by the t(10;14) in T cell leukemia. Science 1991;253:79–82.
95. Baer R. TAL1, TAL2, and LYL1: a family of basic helix-loop-helix proteins implicated in T cell acute leukemia. Semin Cancer Biol 1993;4:341–347.
96. Sanchez-Garcia I, Rabbits TH. LIM domain proteins in leukaemia and development. Semin Cancer Biol 1993;4:349–358.
97. Tsujimoto Y, Yunis J, Onorato-Showe L, Erikson J, Nowell PC, Croce CM. Molecular cloning of the chromosomal breakpoint of B-cell lymphomas and leukemias with the t(11;14) translocation. Science 1984;224:1403–1406.
98. Withers DA, Harvey RC, Faust JB, Melnyk O, Carey K, Meeker TC. Characterization of a candidate *bcl-1* gene. Mol Cell Biol 1991;11:4846–4853.
99. Virgilio L, Narducci MG, Isobe M, et al. Identification of the *TCL-1* gene involved in T-cell malignancies. Proc Natl Acad Sci USA 1994;91:12530–12534.
100. Groffen J, Stephenson JR, Heistercamp N, de Klein A, Bartram CR, Grosveld G. Philadelphia chromosomal breakpoints are clustered within a limited region, *bcr*, on chromosome 22. Cell 1984;36:93–98.
101. Shitvelman E, Lifshitz B, Gale RP, Canaani E. Fused transcript of *abl* and *bcr* genes in chronic myelogenous leukemia. Nature 1985;315:550–552.
102. Sawyers CL. The *bcr-abl* gene in chronic myelogenous leukemia. Cancer Surv 1992;15:37–51.
103. Hermans A, Heisterkamp N, von Lindern M, et al. Unique fusion of *bcr* and *c-abl* genes in Philadelphia chromosome positive acute lymphoblastic leukemia. Cell 1987;51:33–39.
104. Morris SW, Kirstein MN, Valentine MB, et al. Fusion of a kinase gene, *ALK*, to a nucleolar protein gene, *NPM*, in non-Hodgkin's lymphoma. Science 1994;263:1281–1284.
105. Golub TR, Barker GF, Lovett M, Gilliland DG. Fusion of PDGF receptor β to a novel ets-like gene, *tel*, in chronic myelomonocytic leukemia with t(5;12) chromosomal translocation. Cell 1994;77:307–316.
106. Nourse J, Mellentin JD, Galili N, et al. Chromosomal translocation t(1;19) results in synthesis of a homeobox fusion mRNA that codes for a potential chimeric transcription factor. Cell 1990;60:535–545.
107. Burrow J, Goddard AD, Sheer D, Solomon E. Molecular analysis of acute promyelocytic leukemia breakpoint cluster region on chromosome 17. Science 1990;249:1577–1580.
108. Borden KLB, Boddy MN, Lally J, et al. The solution structure of the RING finger domain from the acute promyelocytic leukaemia proto-oncoprotein PML. EMBO J 1995;14:1532–1541.
109. Gillard EF, Solomon E. Acute promyelocytic leukaemia and the t(15;17) translocation. Semin Cancer Biol 1993;4:359–367.
110. Cimino G, Moir DT, Canaani O, et al. Cloning of *ALL-1*, the locus involved in leukemias with the t(4;11)(q21;q23), t(9;11)(p22;q23), and t(11;19)(q23;p13) chromosome translocations. Cancer Res 1991;51:6712–6714.
111. Zieman-van der Poel S, McCabe NR, Gill HJ, et al. Identification of a gene, *MLL*, that spans the breakpoint in 11q23 translocations associated with human leukemias. Proc Natl Acad Sci USA 1991;88:10735–10739.
112. Thirman MJ, Gill HJ, Burnett RC, et al. Rearrangement of the *MLL* gene in acute lymphoblastic and acute myeloid leukemias with 11q23 chromosomal translocations. N Engl J Med 1993;329:909–914.
113. Schichman SA, Caligiuri MA, Gu Y, et al. *ALL-1* partial duplication in acute leukemia. Proc Natl Acad Sci USA 1994;91:6236–6239.
114. Schichman SA, Canaani E, Croce CM. Self-fusion of the *ALL-1* gene: a new genetic mechanism for acute leukemia. JAMA 1995;273:571–576.
115. Gu Y, Nakamura T, Alder H, et al. The t(4;11) chromosome translocation of human acute leukemias fuses the *ALL-1* gene, related to *Drosophila trithorax*, to the *AF-4* gene. Cell 1992;71:701–708.
116. Tkachuk DC, Kohler S, Cleary ML. Involvement of a homolog of Drosophila trithorax by 11q23 chromosomal translocations in acute leukemias. Cell 1992;71:691–700.
117. Zeleznik-Le NJ, Harden AM, Rowley JD. 11q23 translocations split the "AT-hook" cruciform DNA-binding region and the transcriptional repression domain from the activation domain of the mixed-lineage leukemia (*MLL*) gene. Proc Natl Acad Sci USA 1994;91:10610–10614.
118. Nakamura T, Alder H, Gu Y, et al. Genes on chromosomes 4, 9, and 19 involved in 11q23 abnormalities in acute leukemia share sequence homology and/or common motifs. Proc Natl Acad Sci USA 1993;90:4631–4635.
119. Prasad R, Leshkowitz D, Gu Y, et al. Leucine-zipper dimerization motif encoded by the *AF17* gene fused to *ALL-1* (*MLL*) in acute leukemia. Proc Natl Acad Sci USA 1994;91:8107–8111.
120. Sreekantaiah C, Landanyi M, Rodriguez E, Chaganti RSK. Chromosomal aberrations in soft tissue tumors: relevance to diagnosis, classification, and molecular mechanisms. Am J Pathol 1994;144:1121–1134.
121. Rabbits TH, Forster A, Larson R, Nathan P. Fusion of the dominant negative transcription regulator *CHOP* with a novel gene *FUS* by translocation t(12;16) in malignant liposarcoma. Nature Genet 1993;4:175–180.
122. Delattre O, Zucman J, Plougastel B, et al. Gene fusion with an ETS-DNA binding domain caused by chromosome translocation in human tumors. Nature 1992;359:162–165.
123. Galili N, Davis RJ, Fredericks WJ, et al. Fusion of a fork head domain gene to *PAX3* in the solid tumour alveolar rhabdomyosarcoma. Nature Genet 1993;5:230–235.
124. Peto R. Epidemiology, multistage models, and short-term mutagenicity models. Cold Spring Harbor Conf Cell Prolif 1977;4:1404–1428.
125. Weinberg RA. Oncogenes and multistep carcinogenesis. In Oncogenes and the Molecular Origins of Cancer. Edited by RA Weinberg. Cold Spring Harbor, NY: Cold Spring Harbor Laboratory Press, 1989, pp 307–326.
126. Frykberg LS, Palmieri S, Berg H, Graf T, Hayman MJ, Vennstrom B. Transforming capacities of avian erythroblastosis virus mutants deleted in *erb*A and *erb*B oncogenes. Cell 1983;32:227–238.
127. Land H, Parada LF, Weinberg RA. Tumorigenic conversion of primary embryo fibroblasts requires at least two cooperating oncogenes. Nature 1983;304:596–602.
128. Ruley HE. Transforming collaborations between *ras* and nuclear oncogenes. Cancer Cells 1990;2:258–268.
129. Stewart TA, Pattengale PK, Leder P. Spontaneous mammary adenocarcinomas in transgenic mice that carry and express MTV/*myc* fusion genes. Cell 1984;38:627–637.
130. Nowell PC. The clonal evolution of tumor cell populations. Science 1976;194:23–28.
131. Rowley JD. Chromosome abnormalities in human cancer. In Principles and Practice of Oncology. Edited by VT DeVita, S Hellman, SA Rosenberg. Philadelphia: Lippincott, 1989, pp. 81–87.
132. Feinstein E, Cimino G, Gale RP, et al. *p53* in chronic myelogenous leukemia in acute phase. Proc Natl Acad Sci USA 1991;88:6293–6297.
133. Fearon ER, Vogelstein B. A genetic model for colorectal tumorigenesis. Cell 1990;61:759–767.
134. Bos JL, Toksoz D, Marshall CJ, et al. Prevalence of *ras* gene mutations in human colorectal cancers. Nature 1987;327:293–297.

CHAPTER 6

Tumor Suppressor and DNA Repair Gene Defects in Human Cancer

ERIC R. FEARON AND BERT VOGELSTEIN

Introduction

A genetic basis for the development of cancer has been hypothesized for nearly a century, and has been supported by familial, epidemiologic, and cytogenetic studies. Only in the past 2 decades, however, has definitive evidence been obtained through molecular genetic studies that cancer is a genetic disease. A current view is that cancers arise through a multistage evolutionary process driven by inherited and somatic mutations of cellular genes and clonal selection of variant progeny with increasingly more aggressive growth properties. Three classes of genes—proto-oncogenes, tumor suppressor genes, and DNA repair genes—are targeted by the mutations. The vast majority of the mutations that contribute to the development and behavior of cancer cells are somatic and are present only in the neoplastic cells of the patient. Although only a relatively small subset of all mutations in cancer cells are present in the germ line of affected individuals, such mutations not only predispose to cancer, but can be passed on to future generations.

The identification and function of proto-oncogenes and mutant oncogenic alleles are reviewed in other chapters in this text. However, brief mention will be made here of their general properties in an effort to compare and contrast them with the tumor suppressor and DNA repair genes. Over 50 different proto-oncogenes have been identified through a variety of experimental strategies (11–13, 242, 252). In general, these genes have critical roles in a variety of growth regulatory pathways, and their protein products are distributed throughout virtually all subcellular compartments. The oncogenic variant alleles present in cancers have gain-of-function mutations resulting from point mutation, chromosomal rearrangement, or gene amplification of the proto-oncogene sequences (12, 13, 252). In the overwhelming majority of patients with cancer, mutations in the particular affected proto-oncogene arise somatically in the tumor cells, although germ-line mutations in one proto-oncogene (i.e., *RET*) have been identified in those with multiple endocrine neoplasia (241).

While oncogenic alleles harbor activating mutations, tumor suppressor genes are inactivated in human cancer (13, 122, 148, 205, 253). As will be reviewed below, a large number of tumor suppressor genes are hypothesized to exist; however, only about a dozen or so have been identified. Like proto-oncogenes, the cellular functions of the tumor suppressor genes identified thus far appear to be diverse.

Finally, DNA repair pathway gene defects have been implicated in a fairly broad spectrum of human cancers (97, 160). Like the tumor suppressor genes, the DNA repair genes are inactivated in human cancers; however, they appear to differ from the tumor suppressor genes with respect to their normal cellular functions. Specifically, while protein products of many tumor suppressor genes are likely to be directly involved in growth inhibition or differentiation, the DNA repair pathway proteins have a more passive role in regulating cell growth. Their inactivation in tumor cells results in an increased rate of mutations in other cellular genes, presumably including proto-oncogenes and tumor suppressor genes. Because of the functional differences between the DNA repair pathway genes and the tumor suppressor genes in growth suppression and differentiation, the two classes of genes will be considered separately in this chapter.

Enormous progress has been made in the identification of inherited and somatic mutations in tumor suppressor and DNA repair genes in human cancer, as well as in elucidating the means by which loss-of-function mutations in these genes may contribute to the development of cancer. It will not be possible to summarize all of these findings here. Rather, the principal aims of this chapter will be to review the following topics: the somatic cell genetic and epidemiologic studies that established the existence of tumor suppressor genes; the identification and cloning of tumor suppressor genes; selected studies that have provided insights into the function of tumor suppressor genes in growth regulation and differentiation; and recent studies implicating DNA repair gene mutations in common human cancers.

Genetic Basis for Tumor Development

That cancer in humans and other animals might be inherited has been appreciated for over a century. Broca, in 1866, described a family with a high proportion of members who developed breast or liver cancer and proposed that an inherited abnormality within the affected tissue allowed tumor development (20). Studies of differences in the rates of spontaneous mammary tumor formation among various inbred strains of mice led to the proposal by Haaland that tumorigenesis behaved in a formal sense as a Mendelian genetic trait (77). Similarly, Warthin's analysis of the pedigrees of cancer patients at the University of Michigan Hospital between 1895 and 1913 identified four multigenerational families with susceptibilities to several specific cancer types that appeared to be transmitted as autosomal dominant Mendelian traits (249; Fig. 6.1). Although these studies suggested that, in some cases, a genetic basis for cancer might exist, other explanations for familial clustering were possible, and furthermore, it was argued that most cancers arose as sporadic, isolated cases.

A role for somatic mutations in cancer was first proposed by Boveri, who noted that in sea urchin eggs fertilized by two sperm, abnormal mitotic divisions leading to the loss of chromosomes occurred in daughter cells, and atypical tissue masses could be seen in the resulting gastrula (19). He believed that these abnormal tissues appeared physically similar to the poorly differentiated tissue masses seen in tumors, and hypothesized that cancer arose from a cellular aberration that produced abnormal mitotic figures. This hypothesis apparently did not gain favor at the time, initially because of the lack of direct experimental support from studies of the karyotypes of animal and human tumors, and later because of uncertainty about whether the changes in chromosome number in tumors were a cause or an effect of the neoplastic phenotype.

A landmark observation in the identification of a genetic basis for cancer was reported by Rous in 1911, when he showed that sarcomas could be induced in chickens by cell-free filtrates of a sarcoma that arose spontaneously in a chicken (202). Although this observation furnished strong evidence that neoplasms could be virally induced, it also provided support for the proposal that cancer could be attributed to discrete genetic elements. Sixty years after Rous' initial report, the oncogenic region of the Rous sarcoma virus was identified, and further characterization and cloning of

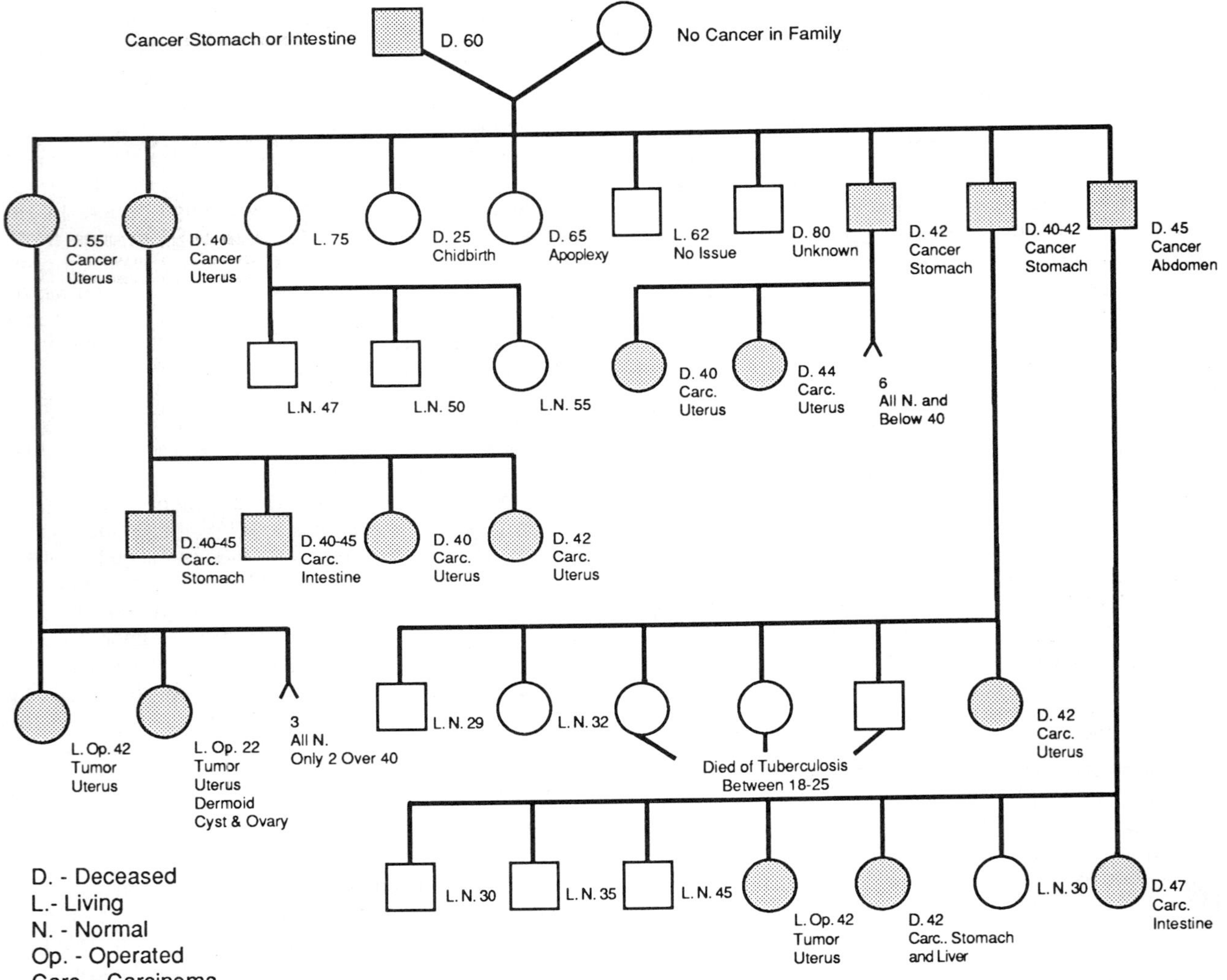

Figure 6.1. The inheritance of cancer in a family (family G). The affected members with cancer are indicated by shaded figures, as well as the type of cancer in each case. The family demonstrates a dominant inheritance pattern for the development of cancer, of either the colon, stomach, or uterus, a syndrome now referred to as hereditary nonpolyposis colorectal cancer (HNPCC). Recent studies have demonstrated that cancer predisposition in families with HNPCC results from germ-line mutation of a DNA repair gene allele (see text) (kindred described by A. S. Warthin).

this region demonstrated that the oncogenicity of the virus was dependent on v-*src*, a transduced cellular gene (11, 150, 230). Subsequently, all oncogenes of acutely transforming RNA tumor viruses have, in fact, been found to be transduced cellular genes (the proto-oncogenes; 11, 242). While the biochemical mechanisms by which most viral oncogenes cause neoplastic transformation still are not precisely defined, the viral oncogenes appear to cause transformation because they are mutated versions of cellular proto-oncogenes and/or are expressed aberrantly. In human cancers, somatic mutations generate oncogenic alleles (12, 13, 252).

Nevertheless, despite the significance of oncogenes in the genesis of many different human tumor types, many of the properties of neoplastic cells, including immortality and tumorigenicity, appear to result from the inactivation or loss of function of normal cellular genes (204, 228, 229). These cellular genes, hypothesized to regulate cellular proliferation and growth in a negative fashion, have been termed tumor suppressor genes.

Somatic Cell Genetic Studies of Tumorigenesis

While oncogenes were directly identified by their positive role in altering the growth properties of appropriate recipient cells, virtually all of the initial evidence supporting the existence of tumor suppressor genes was derived without direct identification of these genes. One of the essential difficulties in identifying tumor suppressor genes by direct selection methods is that these genes would be expected to suppress properties of tumor cells, such as their uncontrolled proliferation, unlimited life span, and tumorigenicity. Selection methods, however, for directly identifying suppressed cells in a background of transformed cells thus far have proved elusive. Nevertheless, a number of somatic cell genetic studies of tumorigenesis using both rodent and human tumor cells provided the first (albeit indirect) evidence that tumor suppressor genes must exist.

The studies of Harris and colleagues provided compelling evidence that the ability of cells to form a tumor is a recessive trait (87, 88). They observed that the growth of murine tumor cells in syngeneic animals could be suppressed when the malignant cells were fused to nonmalignant cells, although reversion to tumorigenicity often occurred when the hybrids were propagated for extended periods in culture. The reappearance of malignancy was found to be associated with chromosome losses. Their interpretation—that malignancy can be suppressed in somatic cell hybrids—was subsequently supported by additional studies of mouse, rat, and hamster intraspecies somatic cell hybrids, as well as of interspecies hybrids between rodent tumor cells and normal human cells (87, 118, 204). The karyotypic instability of the rodent–human hybrids, however, complicated the analysis of the human chromosomes involved in the suppression process. Stanbridge and his colleagues overcame this problem by studying hybrids made by fusing human tumor cell lines to normal, diploid human fibroblasts (228, 229). Their analysis confirmed that hybrids retaining both sets of parental chromosomes were suppressed, with tumorigenic segregants arising only rarely after chromosome losses in the hybrids. Moreover, it was demonstrated that the loss of specific human chromosomes, and not simply chromosome loss in general, correlated with the reversion to tumorigenicity. Tumorigenicity could be suppressed even if activated oncogenes, such as mutant *RAS* genes, were expressed in the hybrids (69).

The observation that the loss of specific chromosomes was associated with the reversion to malignancy suggested that a single chromosome (and perhaps even a single gene) might be sufficient to suppress tumorigenicity. To test this hypothesis directly, single chromosomes were transferred from normal cells to tumor cells, using the technique of microcell-mediated chromosome transfer. It was found that the transfer of a single chromosome 11 into the HeLa cervical carcinoma cell line suppressed the tumorigenic phenotype of the cells (208). Similarly, transfer of chromosome 11 into a Wilms' tumor cell line was found to suppress tumorigenicity, while the transfer of several other chromosomes had no effect (255). As shown in Table 6.1, the tumorigenic phenotype of a variety of different tumor cell lines can be suppressed by single chromosome transfer (181, 217, 228, 237).

Although the tumorigenic phenotype can often be suppressed in hybrids resulting from fusion between malignant and normal cells, other traits characteristic of the parental tumor cells (such as immortality and anchorage-independent growth) may be retained in the hybrids. This observation is consistent with the notion that most malignant tumors arise as a result of multiple genetic alterations. The suppression of tumorigenicity following cell fusion or microcell chromosome transfer thus might represent the correction of only one of the alterations. In this regard, studies using microcell-mediated chromosome transfer have demonstrated that human chromosome 1 will cause an immortal, but nontumorigenic, hamster cell line to cease cell division (232). Furthermore, these data suggest that the genes that influence the life span of normal cells may be distinct from the genes that suppress the tumorigenic phenotype. However, because each of

Table 6.1. Tumor Suppression by Single Chromosome Transfer

Tumor cell line	Chromosome transferred	
	Suppressive effect	No suppressive effect
Cervical (HeLa)	11	X
Cervical (SiHa)	11	12
Rhabdomyosarcoma (G401)	11	X, 13
Rhabdomyosarcoma (A204)	11	—
Melanoma (UACC-903, UACC-091)	6	—
Neuroblastoma (SK-N-MC)	1	11
Fibrosarcoma (HT1080)	1, 11	2, 7, 12
Endometrial (HHUA)	1, 6, 9, 11	19
Renal cell (YCR)	3	1, 11, X
Choriocarcinoma (CC1)	7	1, 2, 6, 9, 11
Colorectal cancer (CoFu)	5, 18	—
Colorectal cancer (SW480)	5, 17, 18	—

these classes of genes can suppress at least some of the phenotypic properties of tumor cells (i.e., tumorigenicity or immortality), the two classes of genes are not usually distinguished from each other, and both types are referred to as tumor suppressor genes (204).

In summary, although the somatic cell genetic studies of tumorigenesis reviewed above have not led to the direct identification of tumor suppressor genes, they did provide persuasive evidence for the existence of critical growth-regulating genes in normal cells that can suppress phenotypic traits of immortal or even fully cancerous cells.

Retinoblastoma—A Paradigm for Tumor Suppressor Gene Function

Essentially concurrent with the initial cell fusion experiments of Harris and colleagues, Knudson's analysis of the age-specific incidence of retinoblastoma led him to propose that two mutagenic events or "hits," were necessary for retinoblastoma development (119). Retinoblastoma occurs sporadically in most cases, but in some families it displays autosomal dominant inheritance. In an individual with the inherited form of the disease, Knudson proposed that the first hit is present in the germ-line, and thus, in all cells of the body. However, it was also proposed that the presence of a mutation at the susceptibility locus was insufficient for the formation of a tumor, and that a second somatic mutation was necessary for promoting tumor formation. Given the high likelihood of a somatic mutation occurring in at least one retinal cell during development, the dominant inheritance pattern of retinoblastoma in some families could be explained. In the nonhereditary form of retinoblastoma, both mutations were hypothesized to arise somatically within the same cell. Although each of the two hits could have been in different genes, subsequent studies (see below) led to the conclusion that both hits were at the same genetic locus, ultimately inactivating both alleles of the retinoblastoma (*RB1*) susceptibility gene. Knudson's hypothesis not only served to illustrate the mechanisms through which inherited and somatic genetic changes might collaborate in tumorigenesis, but it also linked the notion of recessive genetic determinants for human cancer to somatic cell genetic observations demonstrating the recessive nature of tumorigenesis.

The first clue to the location of the putative locus responsible for inherited retinoblastoma was obtained from karyotypic analyses of patients with retinoblastoma. Constitutional deletions of chromosome 13 were observed in some cases (180). Subsequent cytogenetic studies of a large number of patients with retinoblastoma revealed that detectable germ-line deletions of chromosome 13 were noted in only about 5% of the patients. However, in cases where deletions were observed, the common region of deletion was found to be centered around chromosome band 13q14 (62). Levels of esterase D, an enzyme of unknown physiologic function, were found to be reduced in patients with deletions of 13q14, as compared with karyotypically normal family members (223). This finding suggested that the *esterase D* gene might be contained within chromosome band 13q14. Indeed, analysis of the segregation patterns of esterase D isozymes and retinoblastoma development in families with inherited retinoblastoma established that the *esterase D* and *RB1* loci were very closely genetically linked (224).

Subsequently, a child with inherited retinoblastoma was found to have esterase D levels approximately one-half of normal, although no deletion of chromosome 13 was seen in karyotype studies of his blood cells and skin fibroblasts (8). Interestingly, tumor cells from this patient had a complete absence of esterase D activity, despite harboring one apparently intact copy of chromosome 13. Based on these findings, it was proposed that the copy of chromosome 13 retained in the tumor cells had a submicroscopic deletion of both the *esterase D* and *RB1* loci. Moreover, it was concluded that the initial *RB1* mutation in the child was recessive at the cellular level, that is, cells with inactivation of one *RB1* allele had a normal phenotype. The effect of the predisposing mutation, however, could be unmasked in the tumor cells by a second event, such as the loss of the chromosome 13 carrying the wild-type *RB1* allele. This proposal was entirely consistent with Knudson's two-hit hypothesis (119, 120).

To establish the generality of these observations, Cavenee, Whyte, and their colleagues undertook studies of retinoblastomas, both inherited and sporadic in nature, using DNA probes from chromosome 13. Probes detecting restriction fragment length polymorphisms (RFLPs) were used, so that the two parental copies of chromosome 13 in the cells of the patient's normal and tumor tissues could be distinguished from each other. Using such markers to compare paired normal and tumor samples from each patient, they were able to demonstrate that loss of heterozygosity (i.e., the loss of one parental set of markers) for chromosome 13 alleles had occurred during tumorigenesis in over 60% of the cases studied (26). Loss of heterozygosity (LOH) for chromosome 13, and specifically the region of chromosome 13 containing the *RB1* locus, occurred by a number of different chromosomal mechanisms (Fig. 6.2). In addition, through the study of inherited cases, it was shown that the copy of chromosome 13 retained in the tumor cells was derived from the affected parent and the chromosome carrying the wild-type *RB1* allele had been lost (27, 28). These data established that the unmasking of a predisposing mutation at the *RB1* locus, whether the initial mutation had been inherited or had arisen somatically, occurred by the same chromosomal mechanisms.

Patients with the inherited form of retinoblastoma were known to be at an increased risk for the development of second primary tumors, particularly osteosarcomas. The LOH for the chromosome 13q region containing the *RB1* locus was identified in osteosarcomas arising in patients with the inherited form of the disease, suggesting that inactivation of both *RB1* alleles was critical to the development of osteosarcomas in those with inherited retinoblastoma (83, 84). Chromosome 13q LOH was also observed in sporadic osteosarcomas. These molecular studies of retinoblastomas and osteosarcomas provided strong support for Knudson's two-hit hypothesis, and suggested that a variety of tumors might arise from the unmasking of recessive mutations at different tumor suppressor loci (83, 120, 228). In addition, the

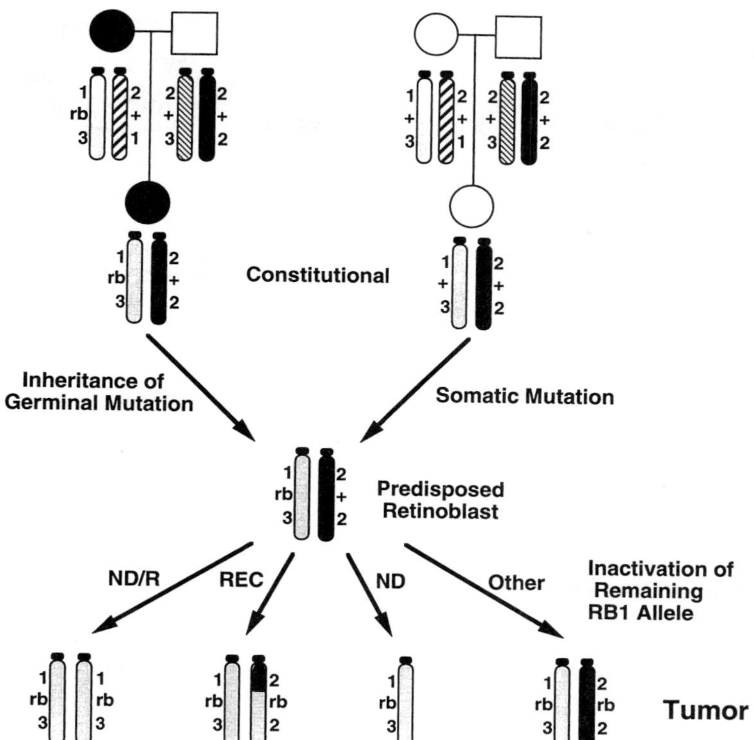

Figure 6.2. Chromosomal mechanisms which result in loss of heterozygosity for alleles at the retinoblastoma locus at chromosome band 13q14. In the inherited form of the disease, the child inherits a copy of chromosome 13 from her affected mother. This copy of chromosome 13 carries a recessive mutation at the *RB1* locus (this allele is designated *rb*). The other copy of chromosome 13 from her father has no mutation at the *RB1* locus (designated +). Thus, each of the girl's cells contains one mutated and one wild-type *RB1* allele (the genotype of the cells is *rb*/+). A retinoblastoma can arise after the loss or inactivation of the remaining wild-type retinoblastoma allele by one of the mechanisms shown. In the noninherited (sporadic) form of the disease, a recessive mutation arises somatically at one retinoblastoma allele in a developing retinal cell. Subsequently, a retinoblastoma will develop if the remaining *RB1* allele in this predisposed cell is inactivated by one of the mechanisms shown: ND/R = chromosomal nondisjunction and reduplication; REC = mitotic recombination; ND = non-disjunction; and other (e.g, localized mutation). The two parental copies of chromosome 13 present in each cell of individual can be distinguished by study of restriction fragment length polymorphisms (RFLPs) at loci flanking the *RB1* locus chromosome on 13q (the polymorphic alleles are designated "1" and 2"). (Source: Cavenee W, Krufos, Hansen M. Mut Res 1986;168:3. Modified with the permission of Elsevier Press.)

studies demonstrated that both the inherited and sporadic forms of a tumor appeared to arise as a result of similar genetic alterations. Finally, osteosarcoma, a common second primary neoplasm in patients with inherited retinoblastoma, was found to have pathogenetic mechanisms in common with retinoblastoma.

CLONING AND ANALYSIS OF THE *RB1* GENE

The isolation of the *RB1* gene was facilitated by the identification of an anonymous DNA marker from the chromosome 13q14 region that detected DNA rearrangements in retinoblastomas (43). Through the analysis of the DNA sequences flanking this DNA marker, a gene with the properties expected of *RB1* was identified (63, 66, 131). The *RB1* gene has a complex organization with 27 exons, spanning greater than 200 kilobases (kb) of DNA, spliced together to produce a messenger RNA transcript of about 4.7 kb (64). Interestingly, the *RB1* gene appears to be expressed almost ubiquitously, rather than being restricted to retinoblasts and osteoblasts in its expression.

The cloning of *RB1* allowed study of the mutations that inactivate the gene. Although gross deletions of *RB1* sequences have been observed in a small subset of retinoblastomas and osteosarcomas, most tumors appear to express full-length *RB1* transcripts and do not have detectable gene rearrangements when analyzed by Southern blots (44, 73, 251, 265). Hence, the detection of inherited and somatic mutations in the *RB1* gene in most cases has required detailed characterization of its sequence (98, 265). Mutant *RB1* alleles both from constitutional cells of individuals with the inherited form of the disease and from retinoblastomas of both the inherited and sporadic type have now been sequenced. This analysis has provided definitive molecular evidence supporting Knudson's two-hit model. As predicted, patients with inherited retinoblastoma were found to have one mutated and one normal allele in their constitutional (blood) cells. In retinoblastomas of such individuals, the remaining *RB1* allele was found to be inactivated by somatic mutation, usually by loss of the normal allele through a gross chromosomal event (see Fig. 6.2), but in some cases by point mutation. Multiple tumors arising in an individual patient with inherited retinoblastoma all were found to contain the same germ-line (initial) mutation, but had different somatic mutations affecting the remaining *RB1* allele. Finally, patients with single, sporadic retinoblastomas had two somatic mutations in their tumors and two normal alleles in their blood cells.

While the identification of mutations in both alleles of the *RB1* gene in retinoblastomas and osteosarcomas provides strong support for the proposal that the cloned gene is indeed the gene whose inactivation is a crucial step in tumor formation, additional support was provided by the demonstration that *RB1* suppressed some aspects of retinoblastoma tumorigenesis. The transfer of a cloned copy of wild-type *RB1* to retinoblastoma and osteosarcoma tumor cells in culture has been shown to affect a number of cellular properties, including morphology, growth rate in culture, and the ability of the cells to form colonies in soft agar and tumors in nude mice (18, 100).

The observation that *RB1* is ubiquitously expressed is rather puzzling, given the spectrum of tumors that develop in patients with germ-line *RB1* mutations. Patients with germ-line mutations of *RB1* are at elevated risk for the development of only a rather limited number of tumor types, including retinoblastoma in childhood, and osteosarcomas, soft tissue sarcomas, and melanomas later in life (28, 251). *RB1* germ-line mutations fail to predispose to more common cancers, despite the fact that somatic *RB1* mutations have been observed in breast, small cell lung, bladder, and prostate cancers (18, 85, 98, 133).

FUNCTION OF THE RETINOBLASTOMA PROTEIN (p105-RB)

The protein product (p105-RB) of the *RB1* gene is a nuclear phosphoprotein with a molecular weight of about 105,000 (132). The first critical insights into p105-RB function were provided by studies conducted by Harlow and colleagues. They demonstrated that p105-RB complexed with the E1A oncoprotein encoded by the murine DNA tumor virus adenovirus type 5 (258). Prior studies of E1A had established that it had many effects on cell growth, including cell immortalization and cooperation with oncogenes in neoplastic transformation. It was thus hypothesized that the functional inactivation of p105-RB through its complexing to E1A may be responsible for some of these effects. Additional support for this proposal was provided by data establishing that mutations inactivating the ability of E1A to bind to RB also inactivated the transforming ability of E1A (162, 259).

The significance of physical interaction between p105-RB and a DNA tumor virus oncoprotein was further supported by the subsequent demonstration that other DNA tumor virus oncoproteins also complexed with p105-RB, including SV40 T antigen and the E7 proteins of human papillomavirus (HPV) types 16 and 18 (38, 45; Fig. 6.3). Many of the mutations inactivating the transforming activities of these oncoproteins also inactivated their ability to complex with p105-RB. Furthermore, E7 proteins from "high risk" HPVs (i.e., those linked to cancer development), such as HPV 16 and 18, complexed more tightly with p105-RB than did E7 proteins of "low risk" viruses (e.g., HPV types 6 and 11). These studies of p105-RB provided compelling evidence that DNA tumor viruses might transform cells by inactivating tumor suppressor gene products. In addition, the studies also provided

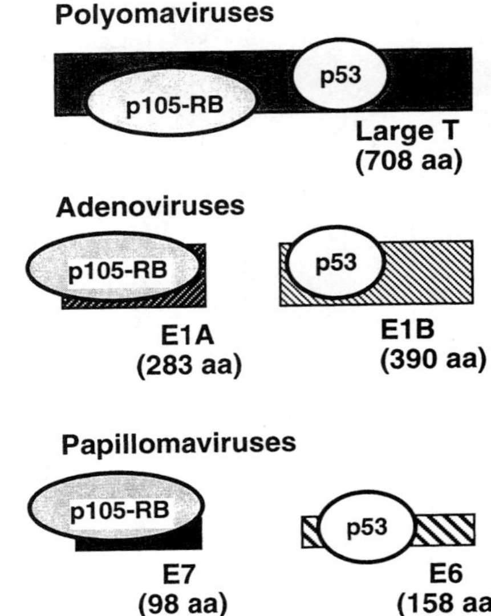

Figure 6.3. A schematic representation of the interactions between the proteins of DNA tumor viruses and tumor suppressor gene products. Large T antigen, a product of SV40 polyomavirus, interacts with both the retinoblastoma protein (p105-RB) and *p53*. In contrast, both p105-RB and *p53* bind to different adenovirus and papillomavirus transforming proteins (Source: Werness, et al. (256). Modified with permission).

support for the hypothesis that p105-RB might normally regulate cell growth by complexing cellular proteins involved in DNA replication and cell division.

At present, it appears that the function of p105-RB is regulated predominantly by phosphorylation during normal progression through the cell cycle (22, 30, 142). Indeed, p105-RB appears to be predominantly unphosphorylated or hypophosphorylated in the G_1 phase of the cell cycle and maximally phosphorylated in G_2 (Fig. 6.4). The critical phosphorylation events regulating the function of p105-RB are likely to be mediated at the boundary between the G_1 and S (DNA synthesis) phases of the cell cycle by cyclin and cyclin-dependent kinase (CDK) protein complexes (40, 52, 99, 115). Presumably, phosphorylation of p105-RB, particularly at the G_1-S boundary, inactivates its ability to interact with cellular proteins that promote entry into the S phase. For example, when it is not phosphorylated, p105-RB complexes with and inhibits E2F proteins from activating gene expression (91, 92, 109, 169, 254). However, when phosphorylated, p105-RB no longer can complex with E2Fs (Fig. 6.4). The E2F proteins when dimerized with their DP partner proteins are then capable of activating the expression of a number of genes that are likely to regulate/promote entry into the S phase, including DNA polymerase alpha, thymidine kinase, and dihydrofolate reductase (169). A number of other cellular proteins that complex with p105-RB have been identified, but their functions and the significance of their interactions with p105-RB remain less well characterized.

The retinoblastoma protein shares significant similarity with several other cellular proteins, including two proteins, known as p107 and p130, that have also been found to complex with DNA tumor virus proteins (34, 51, 82, 138). Because of their sequence similarity to 105-RB, the p107 and

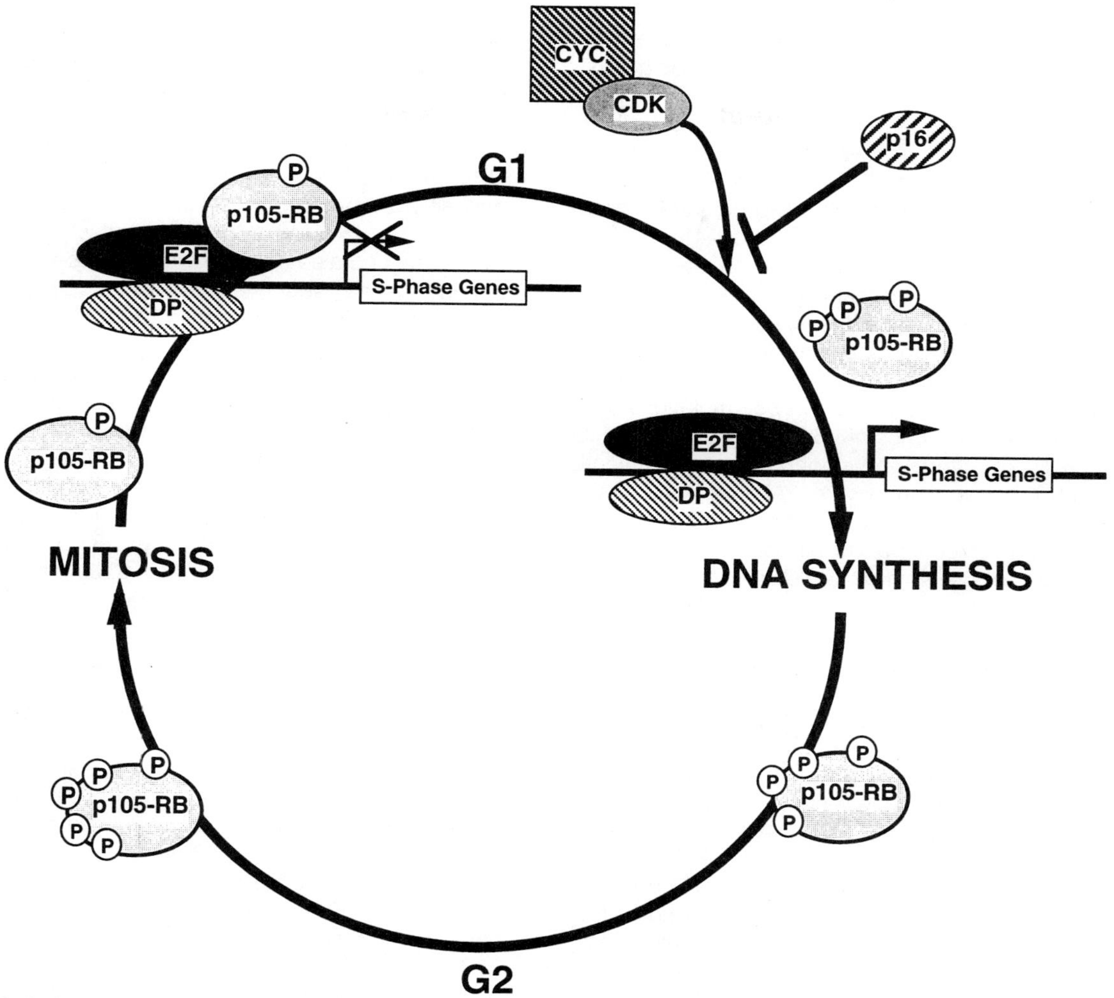

Figure 6.4. Retinoblastoma protein function is regulated during the cell cycle by phosphorylation. The retinoblastoma protein (p105-RB) is hypophosphorylated in the G_1 phase of the cell cycle, and phosphorylation (P) of specific sites appears to increase during progression through the cell cycle. One of the protein complexes that is likely to phosphorylate p105-RB prior to DNA synthesis (S phase) includes a cyclin (CYC) and a cyclin-dependent kinase (CDK) (most likely cyclin D_1 and CDK_4 or CDK_6). The protein product of the MTS1/*p16* gene (*p16*) is an inhibitor of $CYCD_1$-CDK_4 (and perhaps $CYCD_1$-CDK_6) kinase activity. Thus, *p16* acts to inhibit p105-RB phosphorylation. When p105-RB is hypophosphorylated, it can complex with E2F transcriptional regulatory proteins. E2F binds to DNA following dimerization with a DP protein and regulates the transcription of several genes involved in entry into the S phase, including DNA polymerase alpha, thymidine kinase, and dihydrofolate reductase. Other targets for regulation by p105-RB are not well defined. The p105-RB protein is dephosphorylated at or near anaphase.

p130 proteins have been termed p105-RB cousins. Although all three proteins may have closely related functions, there is no evidence yet to suggest that either inherited or somatic mutations in the *p107* or *p130* genes contribute to cancer development. Future studies will undoubtedly shed further light on the means by which loss of p105-RB function, but not that of p107 or p130, contributes to cancer development.

The *p53* Tumor Suppressor Gene

Studies in the late 1970s revealed that a cellular phosphoprotein with a relative molecular mass of about 53,000 formed a tight complex with SV40 T antigen, and hence the p53 protein was so named (126, 141). Additional studies established that p53 also complexed with other viral oncogene products, including adenovirus E1B, and that p53 was present at low levels in normal cells and at high levels in many tumors and tumor cell lines (36, 127, 206). These findings suggested that increased levels of p53 might contribute to cell transformation. Consistent with this notion, gene transfer studies provided data demonstrating that *p53* functioned as an oncogene in some in vitro experiments (48, 106, 127, 185). Other findings, however, suggested that p53 was not likely to be an oncogene. The *p53* gene was inactivated by DNA rearrangements in some viral-induced murine erythroleukemias, the HL-60 promyelocytic leukemia cell line, and some osteosarcomas (2, 127, 151, 163, 261). In addition, subsequent reexamination of the cellular transformation studies revealed that only mutant *p53* genes were capable of functioning as oncogenes and that wild-type *p53* actually inhibited transformation by oncogenes (49, 50, 57, 96).

The first evidence to suggest that *p53* might frequently be inactivated in human cancers was obtained from studies demonstrating that chromosome 17p LOH was common in a number of different tumor types, including colorectal, bladder, breast, and lung cancer (4, 54, 171, 233, 245). Analysis of the sequence of the *p53* alleles retained in cancers with 17p LOH demonstrated the remaining *p53* allele was mutated in the vast majority of such cases. Additional evidence that p53 functions as a tumor suppressor gene in human cancer has been provided by gene transfer studies (5). Based on the types of tumors in which *p53* mutations have been found and the prevalence of *p53* mutations in those tumor types, *p53* is believed to be among the most frequently mutated genes in human cancer (246). Although gross rearrangements of the *p53* gene are seen in some pediatric tumors such as osteosarcoma and rhabdomyosarcoma, and splicing mutations are seen in some SCCLs, the vast majority of the somatic mutations in *p53* are missense mutations (74, 164).

Detailed characterization of the particular base substitutions in the *p53* gene has revealed distinctly different spectra of *p53* mutations in different types of cancer (74). For example, most *p53* mutations in colorectal cancers appear to have arisen spontaneously as a result of deamination of methylated cytosine bases, leading to C → T transition mutations. By contrast, many of the *p53* mutations seen in lung cancers are transversion mutations (e.g., G → T) that may have arisen as result of direct interactions of *p53* gene sequences with carcinogens present in tobacco smoke. Furthermore, some of the most compelling data to link mutagenic and carcinogenic agents with cancer induction have come from study of the *p53* mutations seen in squamous cell cancers and hepatocellular cancers. In squamous cell cancers arising in ultraviolet light–exposed skin areas, a sizable fraction of the *p53* mutations presumably arose from the generation of pyrimidine dimer premutagenic lesions. Similar studies of the *p53* gene in hepatocellular cancers arising in individuals from geographic areas with very high exposures to aflatoxin have identified mutations that are similar to those generated by aflatoxin in in vitro studies (see Chapter 13).

Germ-line mutations in the *p53* gene have been seen in those with the Li-Fraumeni syndrome (LFS), as well as in a small subset of pediatric patients with sarcomas or osteosarcomas who do not meet the more strict criteria for diagnosis of LFS (9, 145, 227). Those with LFS are at a very elevated risk for the development of a number of tumors, including soft tissue sarcomas, osteosarcomas, brain tumors, breast cancers, and leukemias. Between one-half and two-thirds of those with LFS have been found to have germline mutations in the central core domain of the *p53* coding sequences (exons 5 to 9), resembling the somatic mutations frequently seen in *p53*. However, the remaining LFS patients have mutations outside of the *p53* coding region, and many of these mutations appear to result in the loss of transcripts from the affected *p53* allele.

In addition to somatic and inherited mutations in the gene, *p53* function can be inactivated by other mechanisms. As noted above, the majority of cervical cancers contain high-risk or cancer-associated HPV genomes (i.e., HPV type 16 or 18). The E6 gene product of high-risk, but not low-risk HPV types can mediate the degradation of *p53* (256). High-risk HPVs are present in the vast majority of cervical cancers, and only a small subset of cervical cancers have somatic mutations in *p53* (116, 209). However, when a high-risk HPV E6 protein and a somatic *p53* mutation are both present in a cervical cancer specimen, there are data to suggest that such cancers may behave more aggressively (37). A cellular p53-binding protein known as MDM-2 is overexpressed in a subset of soft tissue sarcomas as a result of gene amplification involving chromosome 12q sequences (161, 175). DNA transfection studies have shown that the *MDM2* gene will function as an oncogene in vitro when overexpressed. Presumably, one of the mechanisms by which *MDM2* overexpression may alter cell growth and promote tumorigenesis is by complexing and inactivating p53. In agreement with this proposal, sarcomas with *MDM2* amplification have not been found to harbor somatic mutations in *p53* (175, 246).

p53 FUNCTION

Although it may have other functions, the p53 protein has been shown to function as a transcriptional regulatory protein (195). The p53 protein binds to specific DNA sequences with its central core domain sequences (Fig. 6.5). The amino-terminal sequences of p53 function as a transcriptional activation domain, and its carboxy-terminal sequences appear to be critical to the ability of p53 to form dimers and tetramers with itself. p53 transcriptionally activates a number of genes that play critical roles in the control of the cell cycle, including *WAF1/CIP1/p21* (which encodes a regulator of CDK activity) and *GADD45* (a growth arrest DNA damage inducible gene) (47, 86, 113, 263). Other studies suggest that p53 may also function to repress the transcription of some genes, although the specific targets for this activity remain poorly characterized. As noted above, the vast majority of *p53* mutations in common human cancers are missense mutations (74). These missense mutations are scattered through the central domain of the *p53* coding region (exons 5 to 9). The missense mutations all appear to have marked effects on the ability of the p53 protein to bind to its cognate DNA recognition sequence through either of two mechanisms. Some of the mutations (e.g., mutations at codon 248 or 273) alter p53 sequences that are directly responsible for sequence-specific DNA binding. Other mutations (e.g., codon 175) appear to affect the folding of p53 and thus indirectly affect its ability to bind to DNA (33, 65).

The cellular function of p53 is becoming increasingly well understood (65, 195, 246). Under some circumstances, p53 acts at the G_1/S checkpoint to regulate the cell's decision to synthesize DNA. At other times, p53 appears to exert control over the cell's decision to undergo apoptosis or programmed cell death. Of interest with regard to the possible role of p53 in cancer pathogenesis is that loss of p53 function affects the ability of cells to arrest cell growth at the G_1/S checkpoint in response to DNA damage (114, 128). While

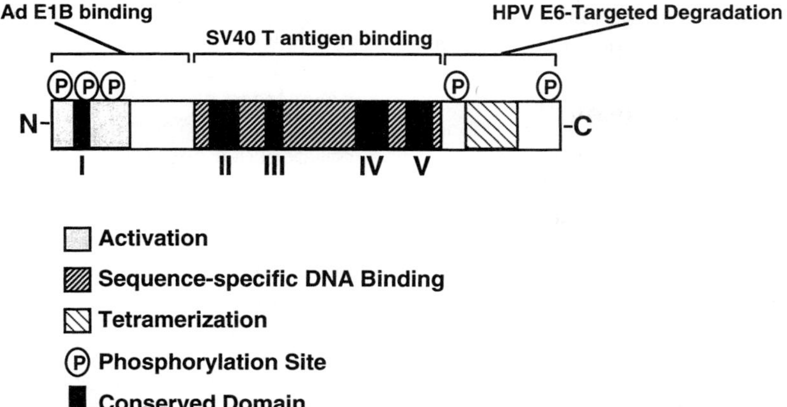

Figure 6.5. *p53* functions as a transcription factor. *p53* sequences involved in transcriptional activation, sequence-specific DNA binding, tetramerization, and binding to DNA tumor virus proteins have been characterized and are indicated. Five domains of *p53* sequence are highly conserved in all vertebrates and are indicated (I–V). Several of the *p53* regions that contain phosphorylation (P) sites are noted. Many of the *p53* mutations in human tumors are clustered in the central core region of *p53* (i.e., the DNA binding and SV40 T antigen binding regions).

many of the cells that fail to repair the DNA damage may die, a small subset may replicate damaged DNA and acquire mutations in oncogenes or tumor suppressor genes. Such mutations are presumed to promote the clonal outgrowth of affected cells with more aggressive growth properties. In this way, *p53* mutations may promote tumor progression. Furthermore, and of particular interest with regard to cancer treatment, are data from in vitro models suggesting that tumor cells lacking p53 function are less sensitive to γ-irradiation and some chemotherapeutic agents, such as cisplatin (59). Nevertheless, thus far, few studies of primary human cancers have documented a compelling relationship between *p53* mutational status and the responsiveness of the cancer to chemotherapy and/or radiation therapy.

WT1, The 11p13 Wilms' Tumor Gene

Wilms' tumor is the most common renal neoplasm of children, accounting for about 6% of all pediatric cancers (35). It is similar to retinoblastoma in a number of ways, as both tumors occur either bilaterally or unilaterally, with single or multiple foci, and in a sporadic or inherited fashion. The two-mutation model originally proposed for retinoblastoma was also proposed to be valid for Wilms' tumor: Wilms' tumor was proposed to develop from two mutational events—the first of which could arise either in the germ-line or in somatic cells, and the second of which always arose somatically (121). Hereditary cases, however, are not as common for Wilms' tumors as for retinoblastomas, and while almost all patients inheriting a mutation at the *RB1* locus develop a retinoblastoma, only about 50% of individuals inheriting the predisposition to Wilms' tumor develop the disease (35).

The first finding providing insight into an inherited genetic basis for Wilms' tumor came from a report in 1964 describing six patients with Wilms' tumor and sporadic aniridia (156). It was proposed that the simultaneous occurrence of these two very rare conditions might result from chromosomal aberrations affecting two or more loci, with mutation of one locus leading to aniridia and mutation of another leading to Wilms' tumor. This hypothesis was subsequently supported by the discovery of interstitial deletions of chromosome 11p, involving band 11p13, in peripheral blood samples from children with the WAGR syndrome of Wilms' tumor, aniridia, genitourinary abnormalities, and mental retardation (199). In addition, cytogenetic studies of the tumor tissues in a few cases of sporadic-type Wilms' tumors revealed deletions or translocations of chromosome band 11p13 (112, 221). Subsequent studies of paired samples of Wilms' tumor and normal cells from patients, using probes that detect RFLPs on chromosome 11p, revealed that 11p LOH occurred frequently in Wilms' tumors of both the inherited and sporadic type (56, 124, 179, 197).

The *WT1* gene was identified in 1990 by virtue of mutations inactivating the gene in patients with the WAGR syndrome, as well as of somatic mutations in the gene in tumors from a minority of patients with unilateral Wilms' tumor and no associated congenital malformations (16, 25, 70). *WT1* is encoded by 10 exons and its transcripts are subject to alternative splicing (78). Its mRNAs encode proteins with molecular masses of 45,000 to 49,000 and zinc finger motifs. Based on the predicted amino acid sequence, the WT1 proteins were suspected to function in transcriptional regulation. Several studies have provided evidence to support this notion (79, 196). In particular, the WT1 proteins have been found to suppress the expression of a number of growth-inducing genes; including the early growth response (EGR1), insulin like growth factor 2 (IGF-2), and platelet-derived growth factor A chain (PDGFA) genes. The ability of WT1 to regulate the expression of growth-inducing genes may account, at least in part, for the function of the *WT1* gene as a tumor suppressor gene (80). In contrast to the rather ubiquitous expression of the *RB1* and *p53* genes, high-level expression of the *WT1* gene appears to be restricted to embryonic kidney and a small subset of other tissues (79, 194, 196).

Although *WT1* inactivation clearly contributes to Wilms' tumor development in those with the WAGR syndrome, only about 10% of apparently sporadic Wilms' tumors have detectable somatic mutations in the *WT1* gene (79, 196). Furthermore, there is much evidence to suggest that Wilms' tumors may also arise through mutations in genes other than the *WT1* gene. First, the chromosome 11p allelic losses seen in Wilms' tumor frequently involve band 11p15, but not band 11p13, and the *WT1* gene (146, 198). Second, the 11p15 region harbors a gene responsible for Beckwith-Wiedemann syndrome (BWS), a congenital syndrome in which affected individuals develop hyperplasia of the kidneys, endocrine pancreas, and other internal organs; macroglossia; and hemihypertrophy (123, 188). Those affected by BWS are also at markedly increased risk for the development of embryonic tumors, such as hepatoblastoma and Wilms' tumor. Finally, linkage studies of three families with dominant inheritance of Wilms' tumor have excluded linkage of the susceptibility locus in these families to any part of chromosome 11p (76, 101). Overall, the data suggest that germ-line mutations in any one of at least three different genes (i.e., *WT1*, the *BWS* gene, and a nonchromosome *11p* gene) can predispose to Wilms' tumor. Whether a combination of inherited and somatic mutations in more than one of these genes (or even all three) is ultimately required for the transformation of a developing kidney cell to Wilms' tumor, or whether alternative genetic pathways for the development of Wilms' tumors exist, remains to be established. The genetic heterogeneity seen in Wilms' tumor development provides an important contrast to the apparently less complex genetic pathway of retinoblastoma development. The genetics of Wilms' tumor may be, therefore, more akin to the genetics of common adult cancers, such as those of the colon, lung, and breast.

The *APC* Gene

Familial adenomatous polyposis (FAP) is an autosomal dominant disorder in which thousands of benign tumors (adenomatous polyps) arise in the colon and rectum. The gene responsible for FAP (i.e., the *APC* gene, for adenomatous polyposis coli) was initially localized to chromosome 5q21 on the basis of cytogenetic studies that revealed a germ-line chromosomal deletion involving 5q21 in an unusual patient with mental retardation and polyposis (94). Subsequent linkage studies confirmed the chromosomal localization and facilitated the eventual isolation of the *APC* gene by positional cloning approaches in 1991 (14, 75, 108, 117, 135, 172). *APC* is very large, encoding a 2843 amino acid protein that is expressed in all tissues studied (75, 117, 189). The central region of the APC protein binds to β-catenin, a cytoplasmic protein that is presumed to link the cytoskeleton to E-cadherin, an adhesion molecule on the cell surface (189, 203, 231). Hence, the *APC* protein may function in relaying signals generated by cell–cell and/or cell–extracellular matrix interactions to the growth-controlling pathways within the cell.

Germ-line mutations of APC have been identified in more than two-thirds of the polyposis kindreds studied (157, 165, 166, 189, 193). Almost all of the germ-line mutations identified in FAP patients cause premature truncation of the APC protein product, as a result of either nonsense mutations or of small deletions or insertions (Fig. 6.6). This observation has led to a strategy for detecting *APC* mutations in which polymerase chain reaction (PCR)–amplified products are transcribed and translated in vitro, and the resultant APC polypeptides separated by gel electrophoresis. This assay thus is termed the in vitro synthesis of protein (IVSP) assay of the protein truncation test (PTT). In this assay, smaller-than-normal polypeptides indicate the presence of a mutant *APC* allele (193). Because of the large size of the *APC* gene, direct sequence analysis of the gene is impractical and screening tests, such as the IVSP assay, have substantial clinical value.

Several variants of FAP have been described. Gardner's syndrome is characterized by a fulminant polyposis combined with extracolonic manifestations, such as osteomas of the mandible and desmoid tumors of the skin and internal connective tissues. Patients with Gardner's syndrome have germ-line *APC* mutations that are often identical to those observed in FAP patients without extracolonic manifestations (172). The molecular basis for the predisposition to extracolonic tumors in those with Gardner's syndrome, therefore, remains undetermined. In contrast to Gardner's syndrome and other FAP patients, patients with the syndrome known as attenuated adenomatous polyposis coli (AAPC) develop only a few adenomas (136). Patients with AAPC have been found to have mutations that result in the synthesis of severely truncated APC protein products containing fewer than the first 200 amino acids (225). It thus has been hypothesized that the severely truncated proteins may be associated with a milder disease phenotype, perhaps because they fail to interact/complex with other cellular proteins, including homo-oligomerization with APC itself (95). Patients harboring a germ-line mutation in more distal regions of the *APC* gene are predisposed to the development of congenital hypertrophy of the retinal pigment epithelium (177), but the moleuclar basis for this phenotype remains to be determined. Finally, the majority of the kindreds with Turcot syndrome, in which affected individuals may exhibit brain tumors (predominantly medulloblastomas) in addition to polyposis, have been found to have germ-line *APC* mutations.

FAP is a relatively common genetic disease with a prevalence of about 1 in 7,000 individuals, and it accounts for about 0.5 to 1.0% of the annual colorectal cancer (CRC) cases in the United States. The importance of the *APC* gene, however, is not limited to FAP. Present findings suggest that virtually all colorectal cancers, whether they occur in patients with inherited predisposition to polyposis or in "sporadic" cases, harbor mutant *APC* alleles (158, 166, 189, 192). The somatic *APC* mutations arising in sporadic adenomas and carcinomas are similar in their location and nature to the germ-line *APC* mutations seen in those with FAP (189; Fig. 6.6). In FAP, one mutant *APC* allele is inherited in every colonic epithelial cell, and the first stage of colonic neoplasia is initiated when the *APC* allele from the unaffected parent is inactivated. In sporadic CRC cases, somatic mutations in both *APC* alleles arise in rare single cells within the colon. As nearly half of the adult population of the Western world

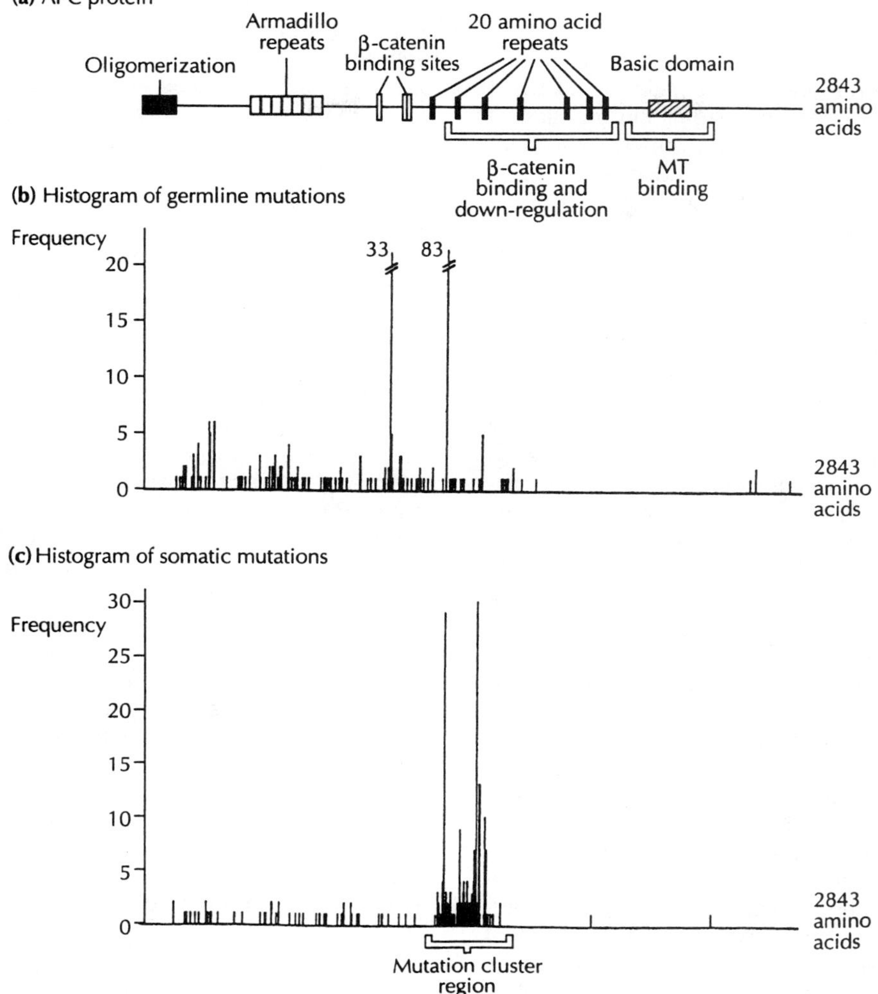

Figure 6.6. Linear representation of *APC* protein with mutational histograms. (**a**) The *APC* protein, showing the relative positions of various *APC* regions. A putative domain involved in homo-oligomerization of *APC* is located at the amino-terminus. Also noted are a series of repeats with similarity to the *Drosophila* armadillo protein, several sites known to mediate binding to *β*-catenin, and a region that appears to facilitate complexing with microtubules (MT). (**b**) germ-line mutations in the *APC* gene (predominantly chain-terminating mutations) are dispersed throughout the 5′ half of the sequence, with two apparent "hot spots" at codons 1061 and 1309. (**c**) Somatic mutations in the *APC* gene in colorectal cancer appear to cluster in a region termed the mutation cluster region, and mutations at codons 1309 and 1450 are the most common. (Source: Polakis (189).)

will develop an adenoma, and as each of these lesions is likely to harbor mutations in one or both *APC* alleles, *APC* mutations may be the most common functional genetic alterations arising in humans.

The *p16* Gene

Loss of heterozygosity affecting chromosome 9q21 has been identified in a large number of tumors, including melanomas, gliomas, bladder cancers, and leukemias (154, 178, 219, 240). A subset of such tumors was found to have homozygous deletions involving this same chromosomal region (41, 61, 105). Furthermore, linkage studies of a subset of families with inherited melanoma localized a predisposition gene to this same area of chromosome 9p (247).

In an effort to identify a tumor suppressor gene on chromosome 9p, positional cloning guided by two independent experimental approaches was undertaken. One of the approaches was to perform linkage studies in families with inherited melanoma to localize the melanoma predisposition gene on 9p. The other approach was to characterize the minimal region of 9p affected by homozygous losses in sporadic tumors of various types (176, 250). These studies delineated a small region of chromosome 9p that was presumed to contain a single tumor suppressor gene affected by both germ-line and somatic mutations. One of the genes in this region was termed *MTS1* (multiple tumor suppressor 1) (110, 173). Sequence analysis of the *MTS1* gene revealed that it was identical to a previously identified gene—*p16*. The *p16* gene was originally discovered during investigations of the cell cycle and was found to encode a protein that inhibited the cyclin-dependent kinases CDK4 and CDK6. Subsequent studies revealed that subtle mutations in one allele of the *p16* gene were present in some patients with familial melanoma (102, 111, 247), and that somatic mutations of both p16 alleles were present in a significant fraction of many different cancer types, including but not limited to, melanomas, gliomas, bladder cancers, and leukemias (17, 23, 24, 89, 226). In some of these tumors, deletions of the *p16* gene were also found to involve a nearby gene termed *p15* or *MTS2*. Of note, *p15* encodes a protein that is closely related to p16.

Perhaps unlike some of the other tumor suppressor genes discussed in this chapter, the means by which loss of *p16* function may contribute to tumorigenesis appears to be relatively more clear-cut, at least based on our present understanding of cell cycle regulation. Cyclin-dependent kinases positively regulate the cell cycle, while inhibitors, such as the p16 protein, negatively regulate the cell cycle in growth conditions that favor growth arrest rather than cell proliferation. Mutations of *p16*, therefore, presumably lead to a loss of appropriate cell cycle control with a resultant selective growth advantage for affected cells. Nevertheless, despite these insights into *p16*, many questions remain about *p16* mutations in human cancer. The *p16* gene is clearly involved in melanoma predisposition in some kindreds with inherited melanoma, but the fraction of all melanoma cases that may arise from germ-line mutation of *p16* appears to be low (247). Similarly, whether patients with germ-line mutations in *p16* are predisposed to other cancer types remains to be determined. In addition, while *p16* is mutated in a sizable percentage of some cancer types, such as gliomas and leukemias, in many other primary cancer types, such as colorectal and breast cancers, mutations of the gene apparently are infrequent (17, 110). It should also be noted that *p16* mutations are more prevalent in established cell lines than primary tumors, presumably because *p16* inactivation may provide an additional growth advantage to cultured tumor cells. Finally, although chromosome 9q LOH (and probably *p16* inactivation, as well) has been found to be an "early" event in some tumors, such as bladder cancer (178, 219), the relative timing of *p16* inactivation in other tumor types remains to be addressed.

The *NF1* and *NF2* Genes

Neurofibromatosis types 1 and 2 are diseases with autosomal dominant inheritance in which neurofibromas of the peripheral or central nervous systems, respectively, are the major neoplastic features. In addition to peripheral neurofibromas, NF1 patients also manifest café-au-lait spots on the skin and are at risk for several cancers, including pheochromocytomas, neurofibrosarcomas, gliomas, and leukemia. The *NF1* gene on chromosome 17q was identified through a positional cloning approach that was guided by linkage analysis and detailed characterization of the chromosome 17q sequences affected by chromosomal rearrangements in two unusual patients with type 1 neurofibromatosis (7, 29, 60, 137, 174, 191, 211, 243, 248). *NF1* is a large gene with over 50 exons, encoding a protein with a mass greater than 300,000 (244). Perhaps in part because of the large size and complexity of the *NF1* gene, germ-line mutations in those with type 1 neurofibromatosis have been identified in only about a third of affected families (239, 244). Nevertheless, data from linkage analyses argue that type 1 neurofibromatosis is a genetically homogeneous disease, due predominantly, if not exclusively, to germ-line mutations in the *NF1* gene (244). Inactivation of both *NF1* alleles has been demonstrated in leukemias arising in children with type 1 neurofibromatosis (216), establishing that *NF1* behaves like other tumor suppressor genes. Somatic mutations in the *NF1* gene have been seen in a few cancer types arising sporadically, including colorectal cancer, neuroblastoma, melanoma, and leukemia (107, 215, 234, 244).

The protein encoded by the *NF1* gene (termed neurofibromin) appears to function as a GTPase activating protein (GAP) for the *RAS* proto-oncogene family (6, 68, 149, 153, 264). As has been reviewed in Chapter 4, in their GTP-bound state, *RAS* proteins are active in signaling. *RAS* signaling function is inactivated by GTP hydrolysis, and the GTPase activities of the *RAS* proteins are stimulated markedly by their interaction with GAPs, such as neurofibromin (15, 236). The predominant effect of mutations inactivating NF1 function appears to be an increase in signaling through the *RAS* pathway (39, 153). The means by which increased *RAS* activity might stimulate abnormal cell growth and predispose to cancer is relatively clear-cut. However, given that *NF1* is expressed in virtually all cell types and that NF1 mutations have been identified in a fraction of common sporadic tumors (215), the molecular basis for the relatively restricted tumor spectrum seen in NF1 patients is not well understood.

NF2 patients develop schwannomas of the eighth cranial nerve, and occasionally other brain tumors, such as menin-

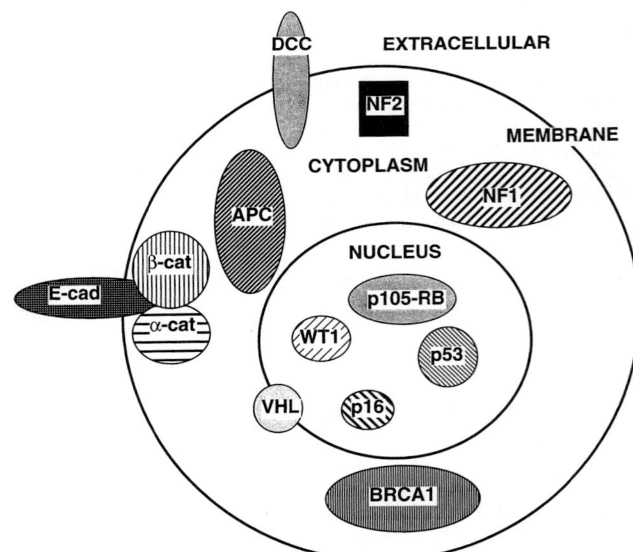

Figure 6.7. Localization of tumor suppressor protein products in various cellular compartments. The presumed localization of known and candidate (e.g., DCC, E-cadherin, α-and β-catenin) tumor suppressor protein products is indicated. The various tumor suppressor genes and proteins are described in the text. (Reprinted with permission from Fearon, E. R. Oncogenes and Tumor Suppressor Genes in Abeloff, M. D, Armitage, J. O, Lichter, A. S, Niederhuber, J. E, eds, in Clinical Oncology, Churchill Livingstone, New York. 1995, pp. 11–40.)

giomas and ependymomas. The gene responsible for NF2 was localized to chromosome 22q by linkage analyses and LOH studies in meningiomas (200, 210, 212, 213). The *NF2* gene was ultimately identified by a positional cloning approach (201). In addition to germ-line mutations in the *NF2* gene in those with central neurofibromatosis, somatic mutations of both *NF2* alleles have been identified in meningiomas and ependymomas arising sporadically (144, 201, 238). The *NF2* gene encodes a protein termed merlin (for *m*oesin-, *e*zrin-, *r*adixin-*l*ike prote*in*) or schwannomin (201, 238). Based on the similarity of its sequence to that of other proteins involved in the organization of the cell's cortical actin cytoskeleton, merlin has been hypothesized to function in transducing growth regulatory signals generated by cell–cell and cell–extracellular matrix interactions (Fig. 6.7). The NF2 protein might thereby function in a fashion somewhat similar to that of APC in the regulation of cell growth.

The *VHL* Gene

The Von Hippel-Lindau (VHL) syndrome is inherited in an autosomal dominant fashion, with affected individuals demonstrating predisposition to renal cell cancers, pheochromocytomas, hemangioblastomas of the central nervous system, retinal angiomas, and cysts of the kidney, pancreas, and epididymis (71). Linkage studies assigned the *VHL* gene to chromosome 3p and the gene was subsequently identified by positional cloning (71, 129, 214). Germline mutations in the gene have been found in the majority of those with the VHL syndrome. In addition, somatic mutations in both alleles of the *VHL* gene have been identified in the great majority of sporadic renal cell cancers of the clear cell type, but have not been seen in those of the papillary type (72, 218, 257). However, in roughly 20% of sporadic renal cell cancers of the clear cell type, no detectable mutations in the *VHL* gene have been observed. Rather, the expression of the *VHL* gene appears to be markedly decreased, perhaps as a result of abnormal methylation of the gene's upstream regulatory sequences (93). Thus, it is possible that all clear cell renal cell carcinomas, of sporadic or inherited type, are initiated by inactivation of the *VHL* gene, much like *APC* inactivation appears to initiate all colorectal tumors. Finally, while *VHL* mutations have also been seen in sporadically arising hemangioblastomas, they are infrequently, if ever, found in sporadic pheochromocytomas or common cancers, such as lung and pancreatic cancer.

Although the function of the *VHL* gene is not well known, recent studies suggest that it encodes a protein with a molecular weight of about 20,000. The VHL protein has been implicated in regulating the efficiency and processivity of the cell's transcriptional machinery. The means by which alterations in a protein product with such general function would lead to a relatively specific predisposition to renal cell cancer, rather than to cancers of many organs, is unknown. In general, the spectrum of tumors arising in patients with inherited mutations of tumor suppressor genes is mysterious, as most of these genes appear to be widely, if not ubiquitously expressed, and yet the neoplasms that develop affect only a small and specific number of cell types in each case.

The *BRCA1* and *BRCA2* Genes

Based on epidemiologic and family studies, it has been estimated that roughly 5% of breast cancer cases might be attributable in large part to a single, autosomal dominant component. As is the case in other familial cancer syndromes, women in such families not only have a markedly increased risk of breast cancer, but they often develop cancers at an earlier age. The first definitive evidence that breast cancer could be inherited as a dominant Mendelian disease was obtained through linkage studies localizing a breast cancer predisposition gene (termed *BRCA1*) to chromosome 17q21 (81). The *BRCA1* gene recently was isolated (155). It has at least 24 exons and encodes a zinc-finger protein that has been suggested to function in transcriptional regulation.

Germ-line mutations in *BRCA1* have been identified in a number of patients with premenopausal breast cancer and/or ovarian cancer, and the gene is presumed to function as a tumor suppressor gene (67, 155, 222). At present, it is estimated that about one-half of the families with apparent autosomal dominant transmission of breast and ovarian cancer susceptibility and average age of onset of less than 45 years may harbor germ-line mutations in *BRCA1* (46). Unexpectedly, the studies carried out thus far suggest that somatic mutations in the coding regions of *BRCA1* may be very infrequent in nonfamilial breast cancers and ovarian cancers (67). Another gene, termed *BRCA2*, that predisposes predominantly to premenopausal breast cancer was recently localized to chromosome 13q, but has not yet been identified (262). Together, germ-line mutations in *BRCA1* and *BRCA2* may account for the majority of cases of inherited premenopausal breast cancer. In addition, those carrying germ-line mutations of the *BRCA1* and *BRCA2* genes may be at increased risk for the development of prostate and colorectal cancer. However, further studies are needed to define more precisely the magnitude of the risk for various types of cancer in *BRCA1* and *BRCA2* mutation carriers.

Other Candidate Tumor Suppressor Genes

All of the tumor suppressor genes discussed above are noteworthy in that mutated alleles of the genes are present in individuals with specific inherited predispositions to cancer. These findings provide incontrovertible evidence of the importance of these genes in tumorigenesis. As reviewed above, other findings, such as the demonstration of LOH of one allele of a tumor suppressor gene and somatic mutation of the remaining allele in sporadic tumors, have supported a more widespread role for these genes in cancer (122, 253). Moreover, in an effort to identify novel tumor suppressor genes, investigators have sought to identify the chromosomal regions affected by LOH in sporadic cancers of various types (190).

Allelic losses affecting chromosome 18q have been noted in upward of 70% of primary colorectal cancers, and in nearly 100% of hepatic metastases arising from colorectal cancers (32, 245). The region of chromosome 18q that is affected by LOH in colorectal cancers often includes a large part of the chromosomal arm, making it difficult to localize the putative gene(s) to a small region. However, a candidate gene termed *DCC* (for deleted in colorectal cancer) was identified from the 18q region that is generally lost in this tumor type (32, 53). The *DCC* gene was discovered by virtue of recognizable somatic mutations in several colorectal cancers. These mutations included a homozygous deletion, point mutations, and insertions. In most colorectal cancers, somatic mutations in *DCC* coding regions have not yet been identified, although expression of the gene is absent or low in most cases. The *DCC* gene is enormous, spanning more than 1.3 million base pairs, which may account for some of the difficulty in identifying specific mutations that might affect its expression and function (31, 32). *DCC* encodes a protein with similarity to the immunoglobulin superfamily class of cell adhesion molecules, and accordingly the DCC protein is expressed on the cell surface (90; Fig. 6.7). Alterations of the *DCC* gene and abnormalities of its expression have been found in several other cancer types in addition to those of the colon and rectum, including breast, brain, pancreatic, and male germ cell cancers, and leukemias.

The *E-cadherin* gene on chromosome 16q encodes a protein with a critical role in epithelial cell adhesion (Fig. 6.7). Decreased expression of the E-cadherin protein has been noted in many tumor types, including those of the breast, bladder, prostate, esophagus, stomach, and liver (10). In a small subset of these tumor types, inactivating mutations in the *E-cadherin* gene have been identified by DNA sequencing studies (reviewed in 10). The region of chromosome 16q in which the *E-cadherin* gene is located is frequently affected by LOH in many cancers in which E-cadherin expression is reduced or absent, providing additional support for the proposal that *E-cadherin* might function as a tumor suppressor gene. It is interesting that E-cadherin–mediated cell adhesion, as well as its signaling function, are dependent on the ability of E-cadherin to complex with two cytosolic proteins—alpha- and beta-catenin—and that beta-catenin has been found to complex with the APC tumor suppressor gene product (189, 203, 231). Thus, these findings reinforce the notion that proper cell–cell interactions are critical in growth control. Further, mutations of the genes encoding cell components involved in either adhesion itself or in the downstream signaling mediated by cell-cell adhesion may be a common factor in the genesis of many different kinds of tumors.

DNA Repair Genes

As noted earlier in this chapter, thus far only one inherited cancer syndrome—multiple endocrine neoplasia (MEN) type 2—has been shown to result from germ-line activation of a proto-oncogene. Specifically, although it was initially hypothesized that cancer predisposition in this syndrome might result from inactivation of a normal cellular gene, the *RET* gene on chromosome 10 was found to harbor activating mutations in those with MEN type 2 (125, 152, 168, 220, 241). The remainder of the cancer syndromes for which the underlying genetic defects have been elucidated result from inactivation of normal cellular genes, either tumor suppressor genes or DNA repair genes. The tumor suppressor genes described above function directly in cell growth regulation pathways, and inactivating mutations in these genes presumably lead directly to a selective growth advantage for the affected cells. In contrast, inactivating mutations in the DNA repair genes presumably have only indirect effects on cell growth. Specifically, defects in DNA repair lead to an accelerated rate of mutations for all genes, including oncogenes and tumor suppressor genes. Thus, defective DNA repair accelerates the tumorigenic process, leading to a more rapid acquisition of the multiple mutations necessary to convert a normal cell into a malignant one.

DNA repair genes were first implicated in diseases with autosomal recessive inheritance, including xeroderma pigmentosum, ataxia telangiectasia, and Bloom syndrome. Several forms of xeroderma pigmentosum have been described, each caused by mutation in a gene participating in nucleotide excision repair. These genes are discussed more fully in Chapters 1, 8, and 137. Ataxia telangiectasia (AT) is characterized by symptoms of cerebellar dysfunction and vascular lesions of the skin. These patients are predisposed to leukemia and a variety of other tumor types. Although it was initially believed that the genetic basis of AT was heterogeneous, recent studies have suggested that a single large gene on chromosome 11q is responsible for all cases (207). Based on the similarity of its sequence to those genes regulating the response to DNA damage in simpler eukaryotic organisms, the *AT* gene may function in controlling the response to DNA damage. However, the mechanisms by which *AT* gene defects lead to the pleiotrophic clinical manifestations of the disease are as yet unclear.

DNA repair defects have been implicated more recently in cancer predisposition syndromes with autosomal dominant modes of inheritance. Hereditary nonpolyposis colorectal cancer (HNPCC) was one of the first cancer predisposition syndromes to be described. Indeed, a family with nonpolyposis colorectal cancer (illustrated in Fig. 6.1) was described by Warthin more than eighty years ago (249). Nevertheless, a number of features of HNPCC made the identification of its genetic basis particularly difficult. Unlike FAP, in which thousands of adenomatous polyps appear, HNPCC patients develop very few polyps or cancers (on average one or two). In addition, because colorectal cancers are so common in the population, affecting roughly 5% by the age of 75, and only 2 to 4% of all colorectal cancers are thought to arise in those with HNPCC, distinguishing those cases attributable to HNPCC from those merely representing chance accumulation within families can be particularly difficult. Moreover, because no physical features (e.g., intestinal polyposis) distinguish HNPCC patients from unaffected individuals, linkage studies were hindered. The diagnosis of HNPCC until recently was solely based on family history: a kindred must contain at least three affected relatives, two of whom are first degree; at least two generations must be affected; and at least one of the affected individuals must be under 50 years of age. In addition to colorectal cancer, members of HNPCC kindreds have a high risk of several other cancer types, particularly those of the endometrium and ovary in females (143).

Despite the difficulties noted, our understanding of HNPCC has advanced greatly over the past few years. Large kindreds with HNPCC were ascertained, eventually allowing a genome-wide linkage analysis that localized susceptibility genes to chromosomes 2p and 3p. As was noted for familial breast cancer and melanoma, the linkage studies of HNPCC were important not only because they represented the first step in gene identification, but also because they conclusively demonstrated that HNPCC is a Mendelian disease.

Subsequent studies allowed refinement of the chromosomal positions of HNPCC genes to chromosome 2p16 or 3p21 (140, 187). The final identification of the responsible genes was considerably facilitated by a functional approach. It was found that cancers from patients with HNPCC had characteristic changes in simple repeated sequences distributed throughout the tumor genome (1, 103, 235). Such simple repeated sequences are composed of mononucleotide, dinucleotide, trinucleotide, or tetranucleotide motifs, and are known as microsatellites. In the tumors of HNPCC patients, expansions or contractions of these repeats occur, leading to the generation of alleles not found in the normal cells of the same patients. This "microsatellite instability" was originally described in a small fraction of sporadic cancers, but was found to occur in virtually all cancers arising in HNPCC patients. The instability in microsatellite sequences was thought to reflect replication errors (RER) arising as a result of defective polymerases or repair proteins.

Investigators studying repair processes in bacteria and yeast noted that the microsatellite instability in colorectal cancers was similar to that observed in simpler organisms with "mismatch repair" gene defects. Mismatch repair is a major proofreading system through which organisms correct errors made during DNA copying (159, 160). In particular, it was found that yeast cells with mutations of the *mutS* or *mutL* classes of mismatch repair genes exhibit a microsatellite instability very similar to that observed in the colorectal tumors of HNPCC patients (160). Hence, it was hypothesized that defects in the human homologues of these genes were responsible for the predisposition to cancer in those with HNPCC. This insightful prediction was soon confirmed by biochemical studies that demonstrated that HNPCC tumors were devoid of mismatch repair activity (186). Additionally, human homologues of the *mutS* and *mutL* genes were identified and shown to be altered in the germ-lines of HNPCC patients. A human *mutS* homologue is known as *hMSH2* and maps to chromosome 2p16 (58, 130). Germ-line mutations in *hMSH2* account for the predisposition to colorectal and other tumors in about 50% of the families with HNPCC (130). One human *mutL* homologue known as *hMLH1* is located at chromosome 3p21, and germ-line mutations in this gene account for cancer predisposition in roughly a third of the HNPCC kindreds (21, 183). Three other mismatch repair genes (the *mutL* homologues *hPMS1* and *hPMS2* on chromosome 2q and 7p, respectively, and a second *mutS* homologue *GTBP* on chromosome 2p16) have also been identified (42, 170, 182, 184). Germ-line mutations in these mismatch repair genes, and perhaps others to be identified, may account for cancer predisposition in the remaining 20% or so of HNPCC families.

In normal cells of patients with HNPCC, DNA repair usually is not impaired, because the cells retain a copy of the gene inherited from the nonaffected parent. However, during tumorigenesis, inactivation of the remaining wild-type allele occurs as a result of a somatic mutation (due either to loss of a large chromosomal region containing the allele or to a subtle mutation in the allele). When this inactivation occurs, mismatch repair becomes totally deficient in the cell and mutations begin to accumulate in rapid succession. In brief, HNPCC can be thought of as a disease of tumor progression, in which a rapid acquisition of mutations leads to an accelerated transition from benign to malignant neoplasia. Indeed, in HNPCC patients, this transition may take only three to five years instead of the 20 to 40 years normally required for the development of sporadic carcinomas. As with tumor suppressor genes, the tumor type specificity associated with inherited mutations of mismatch repair genes remains enigmatic, given that these genes are expressed ubiquitously. Further studies may determine why germ-line defects in such genes predispose predominantly to cancers of the colon and endometrium, and occasionally of the ovary and hepatobiliary and urinary tracts.

Despite the enormous recent progress in characterization of DNA mismatch repair gene defects in HNPCC, much work remains in this area. As noted above, about 15% of apparently sporadic colorectal cancers demonstrate apparent alterations in mismatch repair activity. Nevertheless, neither somatic nor inherited genetic defects in the known mismatch repair genes have been identified in the vast majority of colorectal cancers arising sporadically (i.e., in those without a family history of HNPCC; 139). Furthermore, in addition to the known oncogenes and tumor suppressor genes affected in colorectal cancer (e.g., the K-*RAS* oncogene and the *p53* and *APC* tumor suppressor genes), mutations in other cellular genes that are frequently mutated in tumors with mismatch repair gene defects only now are beginning to be identified. One of the genes mutated in many of the tumors with mismatch repair deficiencies encodes a receptor for transforming growth factor beta, a small secreted polypeptide that is a powerful repressor of cell growth (147).

Finally, the spectrum of other cancer predisposition syndromes caused by defects in gene products with critical roles in replication fidelity remains to be determined. It has been shown that individuals heterozygous for ataxia telangiectasis (AT) mutations (i.e., carriers of AT) have an elevated risk of cancer, particularly cancer of the breast. These AT carriers do not show the cardinal features of AT, such as the cerebellar and skin lesions, which are only observed when both alleles of AT are mutated in the germ-line. Nevertheless, inherited mutation of one copy of the AT gene apparently can lead to cancer predisposition, perhaps in the same way as noted for DNA mismatch repair genes.

Inactivation of Multiple Tumor Suppressor Genes During Tumor Progression

Human cancers have long been hypothesized to arise from a multistep process (3). In terms of the genetic alterations underlying tumor development, colorectal tumors are one of the best understood tumor types (55). Abundant clinical and histopathologic data suggest that the malignant form of the disease (carcinoma) arises from preexisting benign tumors (adenomas). Tumors at various stages of development, from very small benign adenomas to large metastatic carcinomas, can be obtained for study. The study of LOH events in such tumors provided some of the initial evidence for the inactivation of multiple tumor suppressor genes during tumorigenesis. The multiple genetic alterations identified at different stages of colorectal tumorigenesis are outlined in Figure 6.8. Although the alterations have been found to arise in a preferred order, that order is not invariant, and the accumulation of the mutations, rather than their order with respect to one another, seems most important in promoting tumor progression (55). In addition to the mutations outlined in Figure 6.8, other alterations, including allelic losses on other chromosomes, can be observed in colorectal carcinomas. The median frequency of allelic losses in an individual colorectal carcinoma has been found to involve four to five chromosomal arms, and thus it is possible that inactivation of four to five different tumor suppressor genes may be necessary to promote the fully malignant phenotype in many colorectal tumors (55). It has been shown that patients whose primary tumors have a high frequency of allelic losses have a higher risk of developing distant metastases and dying of their cancer than do patients with a lower frequency of allelic losses in their tumors. Analysis of individual tumors for the nature and extent of tumor suppressor gene inactivation may, in the future, help to formulate prognosis more accurately.

Significant progress has also been made toward understanding the multiple genetic alterations arising in tumor suppressor genes in other human tumor types (Table 6.2). Data from epidemiologic studies of common epithelial cancers argue that multiple events are involved in the genesis of virtually all common cancers (3). Studies of somatic mutations in gliomas and bladder cancers at various stages have suggested that the progressive accumulation of alterations in tumor suppressor genes (and oncogenes) accompanies tumor progression in these tumor types (104, 134, 178, 219) much as such alterations do in colorectal tumors.

Summary

Much evidence has now been obtained to demonstrate that inactivating mutations in tumor suppressor and DNA repair pathway genes are critical in the development of many types of human tumors. However, it is important to note that only about 25 years ago the first compelling experimental evidence was obtained that tumorigenesis might result from the inactivation of normal cellular genes with essential roles in growth regulation. Additional evidence for the existence of tumor suppressor genes and their importance in tumorigenesis emerged gradually from somatic cell genetic and epidemiologic studies, as well as from studies of chromosome losses in tumor cells using cytogenetic and molecular genetic techniques. In the past decade, nearly a dozen tumor suppressor genes have been isolated by molecular cloning techniques. In some cases, these genes are lost or inactivated in the germ-line, and their inactivation predisposes to cancer. More often, tumor suppressor genes are inactivated by somatic

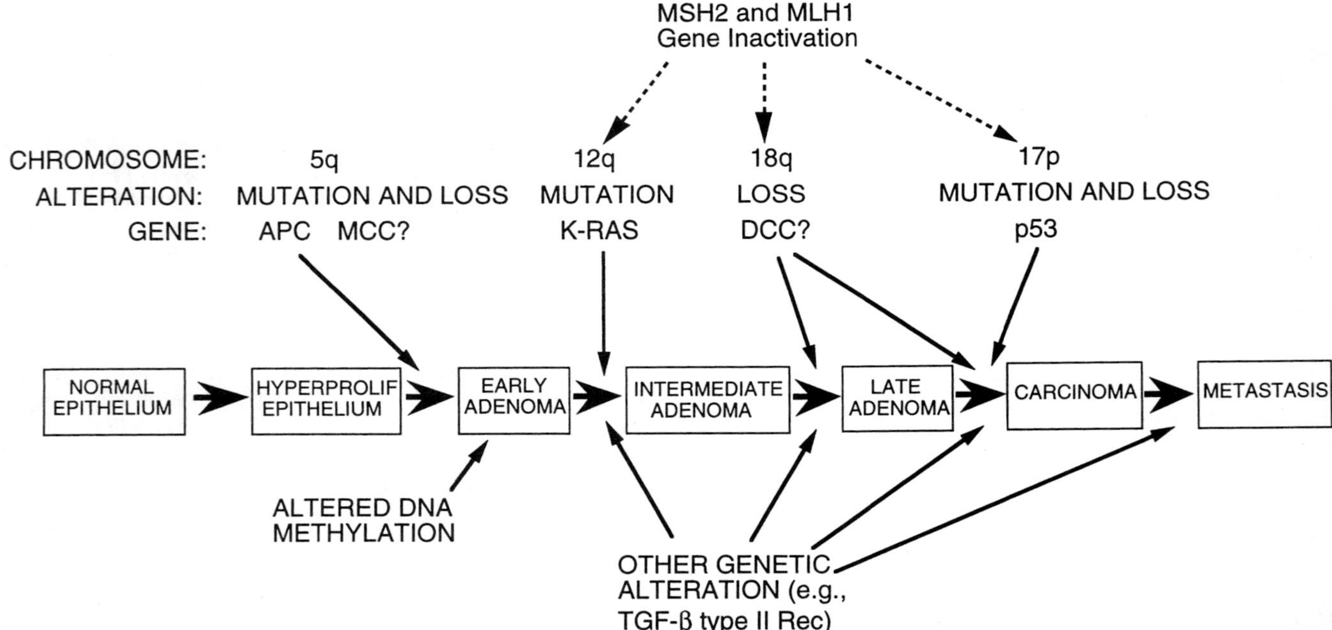

Figure 6.8. A genetic model of colorectal cancer. Evidence from clinical and histopathologic studies supports the notion that the majority of colorectal cancers arise from adenomatous polyps over a period of years, or even decades. The inherited and somatic genetic alterations found at various stages of colorectal tumorigenesis are indicated, with the specific gene affected, its chromosomal location, and the nature of the alteration in the gene noted. Many of the genetic alterations are discussed in more detail in the text. Inactivation of DNA damage repair genes (e.g., MSH2 and MLH1) in those with HNPCC may lead to more rapid acquisition of mutations in such oncogenes as *K-RAS* and in tumor suppressor genes such as *p53*, TGF-β type II receptor (TGF-β type II rec) and *DCC*. (Source: Fearon, Vogelstein (55).)

Table 6.2. Tumor Suppressor Gene Alterations in Selected Human Tumor Types or Tumor Syndromes

Tumor type/tumor syndrome	Chromosomal region	Evidence[a]
Retinoblastoma	13q14	LA, LOH, RB1 mutation
Osteosarcoma	13q14	LA, LOH, RB1 mutation
	17p13	LA, LOH, p53 mutation
Wilms' tumor	11p13	LA, LOH, WT1 mutation
	11p15	LA, LOH
	16q	LOH
	Other(s)	LA
Rhabdomyosarcoma	17p13	LA, LOH, p53 mutation
	11p15	LOH
Hepatoblastoma	11p15	LOH
Colorectal	1p	LOH
	5q21	LA, LOH, APC mutation
	8p	LOH
	17p13	LOH, p53 mutation
	18q21	LOH, DCC mutation
	Others	LOH
Breast	17p13	LA, LOH, p53 mutation
	17q	LA, LOH, BRCA1 mutation
	16q	LOH, E-cadherin mutation
	11p15	LOH
	11q	LOH
	13q	LA (BRCA2)
	13q	LOH
	13q	RB1 mutation
	Others	LOH
Lung (small cell)	3p	LOH
	13p14	LOH, RB1 mutation
	17p	LOH, p53 mutation
	Others	LOH
Lung (non-small cell)	3p	LOH
	17p13	LOH, p53 mutation
	Others	LOH
Bladder (transitional cell)	9p21	LOH, p16 (CDKN2) mutation
	9q	LOH
	11p15	LOH
	17p13	LOH
	Others	LOH
Kidney (renal cell)	3p	LA, LOH, VHL mutation
	17p13	LOH, p53 mutation
	Others	LOH
Glioblastoma	9p21	LOH, p16 (CDKN2) mutation
	10q	LOH
	17p13	LOH, p53 mutation
	Others	LOH
Melanoma	9p21	LA, LOH, p16 (CDKN2) mutation
	17q	NF1 mutation
	Others	LOH
Neurofibromatosis type 1	17q	LA, LOH, NF1 mutation
Neurofibromatosis type 2	22q	LA, LOH, NF2 mutation
Meningioma	22q	LOH, NF2 mutation

[a] LA = linkage analysis; LOH = loss of heterozygosity; the genes are described in the text.

mutations arising during tumor development. Great progress has also been made in the isolation of DNA repair pathway genes, as well as in elucidating the role of inherited and somatic mutations in these genes in tumorigenesis.

Although we have learned much about the tumor suppressor and DNA repair pathway genes, a great deal of work remains. Just as the oncogenes are involved in many different levels of growth regulation in the cell, the tumor suppressor genes are also likely to function in a wide variety of growth regulatory pathways. The products of some tumor suppressor genes may act directly to oppose the function of oncogenes, whereas others may interact only indirectly with oncogenes in pathways of growth and differentiation. In addition, the means by which loss of function mutations in the DNA repair pathway genes promotes the development of specific cancer types is not fully understood. A more complete description of tumorigenesis will undoubtedly emerge with the identification of additional tumor suppressor and DNA repair pathway genes, the detailed characterization of their normal cellular functions, and the elucidation of mutations that inactivate these genes in human tumors. These findings not only will provide new insights into cancer pathogenesis, but also should prove of critical importance in improving the management and treatment of patients with cancer.

References

1. Aaltonen LA, Peltomaki P, Leach FS, Sistonen P, Pylkkanen L, Mechklin J-P, Jarvinen H, Powell SM, Jen J, Hamilton SR, Petersen GM, Kinzler KW, Vogelstein B, de la Chapelle A. Clues to the pathogenesis of familial colorectal cancer. Science 1993;260:812.
2. Ahua H, Bar-Eli M, Advani SH, Benchimol S, Cline MJ. Alterations of the *p53* gene and the clonal evolution of the blast crises of chronic myelogenous leukemia. Proc Natl Acad Sci U.S.A. 1989;86:6783.
3. Armitage P, Doll R. The age distribution of cancer and a multi-stage theory of carcinogenesis. Br J Cancer 1954;8:1.
4. Baker SJ, Fearon ER, Nigro JM, Hamilton SR, Preisinger AC, Jessup JM, van Tuinen P, Ledbetter DH, Barker DF, Nakamura Y, White R, Vogelstein B. Chromosome 17 deletions and *p53* gene mutations in colorectal carcinomas. Science 1989;244:217.
5. Baker SJ, Markowitz S, Fearon ER, Willson JKV, Vogelstein B. Suppression of human colorectal carcinoma cell growth by wild-type *p53*. Science 1990;249:912.
6. Ballester R, Marchuk D, Boguski M, Saulino A, Letcher R, Wigler M, Collins F. The *NF1* locus encodes a protein functionally related to mammalian GAP and yeast IRA proteins. Cell 1990;63:851.
7. Barker D, Wright E, Nguyen K, Cannon L, Fain P, Goldgar D, Bishop DT, Carey J, Baty B, Kivlin J, Williard H, Waye JS, Greig G, Leinwand L, Nakamura Y, O'Connell P, Leppert M, Lalouel J-M, White R, Skolnick M. Gene for von Recklinghausen neurofibromatosis is in the pericentric region of chromosome 17. Science 1987;236:1100.
8. Benedict WF, Murphree AL, Banerjee A, Spina CA, Sparkes MC, Sparkes RS. Patient with chromosome 13 deletion: evidence that the retinoblastoma gene is a recessive cancer gene. Science 1983;219:973.
9. Birch JM, Hartley AL, Tricker KJ, Prosser J, Condie A, Kelsey AM, Harris M, Jones PHM, Binchy A, Crowther D, Craft AW, Eden OB, Gareth D, Evans R, Thompson E, Mann JR, Martin J, Mitchell ELD, Santbanez-Koref MG. Prevalence and diversity of constitutional mutations in the *p53* gene among 21 Li-Fraumeni families. Cancer Res 1994;54:1298.
10. Birchmeier W, Hulsken J, Behrens J. Adherens junction proteins in tumour progression. Cancer Surv 1995;24:129.
11. Bishop JM. Viral oncogenes. Cell 1985;42:23.
12. Bishop JM. The molecular genetics of cancer. Science 1987;235:305.
13. Bishop JM. Molecular themes in oncogenesis. Cell 1991;64:235.
14. Bodmer WF, Bailey CJ, Bodmer J, Bussey HJR, Ellis A, Gorman P, Lucibello FC, Murray VA, Rider SH, Scrambler P, Sheer D, Solomon E, Spurr NK. Localization of the gene for familial adenomatous polyposis on chromosome 5. Nature 1987;328:614.
15. Boguski MS, McCormick F. Proteins regulating *RAS* and its relatives. Nature 1993;366:643.
16. Bonetta L, Kuehn SE, Huang A, Law DJ, Kalikin LM, Koi M, Reeve AE, Brownstein BH, Yeger H, Williams BRG, Feinberg AP. Wilms' tumor locus on 11p13 defined by multiple CpG island-associated transcripts. Science 1990;250:994.
17. Bonnetta L. Tumour suppressor genes—open questions on *p16*. Nature 1994;370:180.
18. Bookstein R, Shew J-Y, Chen P-L, Scully P, Lee W-H. Suppression of tumorigenicity of human prostate carcinoma cells by replacing a mutant *RB* gene. Science 1990;247:712.
19. Boveri T. The Origin of Malignant Tumors. Baltimore: Williams & Wilkins, 1929.
20. Broca PP. Traite des Tumeurs. Paris: Asselin, 1986.
21. Bronner CE, Baker SM, Morrison PT, Warren G, Smith LG, Lescoe MK, Kane M, Earabino C, Lipford J, Lindblom A, Tannergard P, Bollag RJ, Godwin AR, Ward DC, Nordenskjold M, Fishel R, Kolodner R, Liskay RM. Mutation in the DNA mismatch repair gene homologue *hMLH1* is associated with hereditary nonpolyposis colon cancer. Nature 1994;368:258.
22. Buchkovich K, Duffy LA, Harlow E. The retinoblastoma protein is phosphorylated during specific phases of the cell cycle. Cell 1989;58:1099.
23. Cairns P, Mao L, Merlo A, Lee DJ, Schwab D, Eby Y, Tokino K, van der Riet P, Blaugrund JE, Sidransky D. Rates of *p16 (MTS1)* mutations in primary tumors with 9p loss. Science 1994;265:415.
24. Caldas C, Hahn SA, da Costa LT, Redston MS, Schutte M, Seymour AB, Weinstein CL, Hruban RH, Yeo CJ, Kern SE. Frequent somatic mutations and homozygous deletions of the *p16 (MTS1)* gene in pancreatic adenocarcinoma. Nat Genet 1994;8:27.
25. Call KM, Glaser T, Ito CY, Buckler AJ, Pelletier J, Haber DA, Rose EA, Kral A, Yager H, Lewis WH, Jones C, Housman DE. Isolation and characterization of a zinc finger polypeptide gene at the human chromosome 11 Wilms' tumor locus. Cell 1990;60:509.

26. Cavenee WK, Dryja TP, Phillips RA, Benedict WF, Godbout R, Gallie BL, Murphree AL, Strong LC, White R. Expression of recessive alleles by chromosomal mechanisms in retinoblastoma. Nature 1983;305:779.
27. Cavenee WK, Hansen MF, Koch E, Nordenskjold M, Maumenee I, Squire JA, Phillips RA, Gallie BL. Genetic origins of mutations predisposing to retinoblastoma. Science 1985;228:501.
28. Cavenee WK, Murphree AL, Shull MM, Benedict WF, Sparkes RS, Kock E, Nordenskjold M. Prediction of familial predisposition to retinoblastoma. N Engl J Med 1985;314:1201.
29. Cawthon RM, Weiss R, Xu G, Viskochil D, Culver M, Stevens J, Robertson M, Dunn D, Gesteland R, O'Connell P, White R. A major segment of the neurofibromatosis type 1 gene: cDNA sequence, genomic structure, and point mutations. Cell 1990;62:193.
30. Chen P-L, Scully P, Shew J-Y, Wang JYJ, Lee W-H. Phosphorylation of the retinoblastoma gene product is modulated during the cell cycle and cellular differentiation. Cell 1989;58:1193.
31. Cho KR, Oliner JD, Simon JW, Hedrick L, Fearon ER, Preisinger AC, Hedge P, Silverman GA, Vogelstein B. The *DCC* gene: structural analysis and mutations in colorectal carcinomas. Genomics 1994;19:525.
32. Cho KR, Fearon ER. *DCC*: linking tumor suppressor genes and altered cell surface interactions in cancer? Curr Opin Genet Dev 1995;5:72.
33. Cho Y, Gorina S, Jeffrey PD, Pavletich NP. Crystal structure of the p53 tumor suppressor–DNA complex: understanding tumorigenic mutations. Science 1994;265:346.
34. Cobrinik D, Whyte P, Peeper DS, Jacks R, Weinberg RA. Cell cycle–specific association of E2F with the p130 E1A-binding protein. Genes Dev 1993;7:2392.
35. Coppes MJ, Haber DA, Grundy PE. Genetic events in the development of Wilms' tumor. N Engl J Med 1994;331:586.
36. Crawford LV, Pim DC, Lamb P. The cellular protein *p53* in human tumors. Mol Bio Med 1984;2:261.
37. Crook T, Vousden KH. Properties of *p53* mutations detected in primary and secondary cervical cancers suggest mechanisms of metastasis and involvement of environmental carcinogens. EMBO J 1992;11:3935.
38. DeCaprio JA, Ludlow JW, Figge J, Shew J-Y, Huang C-M, Lee W-H, Marsilio E, Paucha E, Livingston DM. SV40 large tumor antigen forms a specific complex with the product of the retinoblastoma susceptibility gene. Cell 1988;54:275.
39. DeClue JE, Papageorge AG, Fletcher JA, Diehl SR, Ratner N, Vass WC, Lowy DR. Abnormal regulation of p21*ras* contributes to malignant tumor growth in von Recklinghausen (type 1) neurofibromatosis. Cell 1992;69:265.
40. Dowdy SF, Hinds PW, Louie K, Reed SI, Arnold A, Weinberg RA. Physical interaction of the retinoblastoma protein with mammalian D-type cyclins. Cell 1993;73:499.
41. Diaz MO, Rubin CM, Harden A, Ziemin S, Larson RA, Le Beau MM, Rowley JD. Deletions of interferon genes in acute lymphoblastic leukemia. N Engl J Med 1990;322:77.
42. Drummond JT, Li GM, Longley MJ, Modrich P. Isolation of an hMSH2-p160 heterodimer that restores DNA mismatch repair to tumor cells. Science 1995;268:1909.
43. Dryja TP, Rapaport JM, Joyce JM, Petersen RA. Molecular detection of deletions involving band q14 of chromosome 13 in retinoblastomas. Proc Natl Acad Sci USA 1986;83:7391.
44. Dunn JM, Phillips RA, Zhu X, Becker A, Gallie BL. Mutations in the *RB1* gene and their effects on transcription. Mol Cel Biol 1989;9:4596.
45. Dyson N, Howley PM, Munger K, Harlow E. The human papilloma virus 16 E7 oncoprotein is able to bind to the retinoblastoma gene product. Science 1989;243:934.
46. Easton DF, Bishop DT, Ford D, Crockford GP. Genetic linkage analysis in familial breast and ovarian cancer—result from 214 families. Am J Hum Genet 1993;52:678.
47. El-Deiry WS, Tokino T, Velculescu VE, Levy DB, Parsons R, Trent JM, Lin D, Mercer WE, Kinzler KW, Vogelstein B. *WAF1*, a potential mediator of *p53* tumor suppression. Cell 1993;75:817.
48. Eliyahu D, Raz A, Gruss P, Givol D, Oren M. Participation of *p53* cellular tumor antigen in transformation of normal embryonic cells. Nature 1984;312:651.
49. Eliyahu D, Goldfinger N, Pinhasi-Kimhi O, Shaulsky G, Shurnik Y, Arai N, Rotter V, Oren M. Meth A fibrosarcoma cells express two transforming mutant *p53* species. Oncogene 1988;3:313.
50. Eliyahu D, Michalovitz D, Eliyahu S, Pinhasi-Kimhi O, Oren M. Wild-type *p53* can inhibit oncogene-mediated focus formation. Proc Natl Acad Sci USA 1989;86:8763.
51. Ewen M, Xing Y, Lawrence JB, Livingston DM. Molecular cloning, chromosomal mapping, and expression of the cDNA for *p107*, a retinoblastoma gene product-related protein. Cell 1991;66;1155.
52. Ewen M, Sluss HK, Sherr CJ, Matshushime H, Kato J-Y, Livingston DM. Functional interactions of the retinoblastoma protein with mammalian D-type cyclins. Cell 1993;73:487.
53. Fearon ER, Cho KR, Nigro JM, Kern SE, Simons JW, Ruppert JM, Hamilton SR, Preisinger AC, Thomas G, Kinzler KW, Vogelstein B. Identification of a chromosome 18q gene that is altered in colorectal cancers. Science 1990;247:49.
54. Fearon ER, Hamilton SR, Vogelstein B. Clonal analysis of human colorectal tumors. Science 1987;238:193.
55. Fearon ER, Vogelstein B. A genetic model for colorectal tumorigenesis. Cell 1990;61:759.
56. Fearon ER, Vogelstein B, Feinberg AP. Somatic deletion and duplication of genes on chromosome 11 in Wilms' tumor. Nature 1984;309:176.
57. Finlay CA, Hinds PW, Levine AJ. The *p53* protooncogene can act as a suppressor of transformation. Cell 1989;57:1083.
58. Fishel R, Lescoe MK, Rao MRS, Copeland NG, Jenkins NA, Garber J, Kane M, Kolodner R. The human mutator gene homolog *MSH2* and its assocation with hereditary nonpolyposis colon cancer. Cell 1993;75:1027.
59. Fisher DE. Apopotosis in cancer therapy: crossing the threshold. Cell 1994;78:539.
60. Fountain JW, Wallace MR, Bruce MJ, Seizinger BR, Menon AG, Gusella JF, Michels VV, Schmidt MA, Dewald GW, Collins FS. Physical mapping of a translocation breakpoint in neurofibromatosis. Science 1989;244:1085.
61. Fountain JW, Karayiorgou M, Ernstoff MS, Kirkwood JM, Vlock DR, Titus-Ernstoff L, Bouchard B, Vijayasardhi S, Houghton AN, Lahti J, Kidd VJ, Housman DE, Dracopoli NC. Homozygous deletions within human chromosome band 9p21 in melanoma. Proc Natl Acad Sci USA 1992;89:10557.
62. Francke U. Retinoblastoma and chromosome 13. Cytogenet Cell Genet 1976;16:131.
63. Friend SH, Bernards R, Rogel S, Weinberg RA, Rapaport JM, Albert DM, Dryja TP. A human DNA segment with the properties of a gene that predisposes to retinoblastoma and osteosarcoma. Nature 1986;323:643.
64. Friend SH, Horowitz JM, Gerber MR, Wang XF, Bogenmann E, Li FP, Weinberg R. A Deletions of a DNA sequence in retinoblastomas and mesenchymal tumors: organization of the sequence and its encoded protein. Proc Natl Acad Sci USA 1987;84:9059.
65. Friend SH. *p53*: a glimpse at the puppet behind the shadow play. Science 1994;265:334.
66. Fung Y-KT, Murphree AL, T'Ang A, Qian J, Hinrichs SH, Benedict WF. Structural evidence for the authenticity of the human retinoblastoma gene. Science 1987;236:1657.
67. Futreal PA, Liu Q, Shattuck-Eidens D, Cochran C, Harshman K, Tavtigian S, Bennett LM, Haugen-Strano A, Swensen J, Miki Y, Eddington K, McClure M, Frye C, Weaver-Feldhaus J, Ding W, Gholami Z, Soderkvist P, Terry L, Jhanwar S, Berchuck A, Iglehart JD, Marks J, Ballinger DG, Barrett JC, Skolnick MH, Kamb A, Wiseman R. BRCA1 mutations in primary breast and ovarian carcinomas. Science 1994;266:120.
68. Gangfeng X, O'Connell P, Viskochil D, Cawthon R, Robertson M, Culver M, Dunn D, Stevens J, Gesteland R, White R, Weiss, R. The neurofibromatosis type 1 gene encodes a protein related to GAP. Cell 1990;62:599.
69. Geiser A, Der CJ, Marshall CJ, Stanbridge EJ. Suppression of tumorigenicity with continued expression of the c-Ha-*RAS* oncogene in EJ bladder carcinoma X human fibroblast hybrid cells. Proc Natl Acad Sci USA 1986;83:5029.
70. Gessler M, Poustka A, Cavenee WK, Neve RL, Orkin SH, Bruns GAP. Homozygous deletion in Wilms' tumors of a zinc-finger gene identified by chromosome jumping. Nature 1990;343:774.
71. Gnarra JR, Glenn GM, Latif F, Anglard P, Lerman MI, Zbar B, Linehan WM. Molecular genetic studies of sporadic and familial renal cell carcinoma. Urol. Clin. North Am. 1993;20:207.
72. Gnarra JR, Tory K, Weng Y, Schmidt L, Wei MW, Li H, Latif F, Liu S, Chen F, Duh F-M, Lubensky I, duan D-SR, Florence C, Pozzatti R, Walther MM, Bander NH, Grossman HB, Brauch H, Brooks JD, Isaccs WB, Lerman MI, Zbar B, Linehan WM. VHL tumor suppressor gene mutations in renal carcinoma tumorigenesis. Nat Genet. 1994;7:85.
73. Goddard AD, Balakier H, Canton M, Dunn J, Squire J, Reyes E, Becker A, Phillips RA, Gallie BL. Infrequent genomic rearrangement and normal expression of the putative RB1 gene in retinoblastoma tumors. Mol. Cell Biol. 1988;8:2082.
74. Greenblatt MS, Bennett WP, Hollstein M, Harris CC. Mutations in the *p53* tumor suppressor gene: clues to cancer etiology and molecular pathogenesis. Cancer Res. 1994;54:4855.
75. Groden J, Thlivers A, Samowitz W, Carlson M, Gelbert L, Albertsen H, Joslyn G, Stevens J, Spirio L, Robertson M, Sargeant L, Krapcho K, Wolff E, Burt R, Hughes JP, Warrington J, McPherson J, Wasmuth J, Le Paslier D, Abderrahim H, Cohen D, Leppert M, White R. Identification and characterization of the familial adenomatous polyposis coli gene. Cell 1991;66:589.
76. Grundy P, Koufos A, Morgan K, Li FP, Meadows AT, Cavenee WK. Familial predisposition to Wilms' tumor does not map to the short arm of chromosome 11. Nature 1988;336:374.
77. Haaland M. Spontaneous tumors in mice. Sci Rep Invest Imp Cancer Res Fund 1911;4:1.
78. Haber DA, Sohn RL, Buckler AJ, Pelletier J, Call K, Housman D. Alternative splicing and genomic structure of the Wilms' tumor gene *WT1*. Proc Natl Acad Sci USA 1991;88:9618.
79. Haber DA, Housman DE. The genetics of Wilms' tumor. Adv Cancer Res 1992;59:41.
80. Haber DA, Park S, Maheswaran S, Englert C, Re GG, Hazen-Martin DJ, Sens DA, Garvin AJ. *WT1*-mediated growth suppression of Wilms' tumor cells expressing a *WT1* splicing variant. Science 1993;262:2057.
81. Hall JM, Lee MK, Newman B, Morrow JE, Anderson LA, Huey B, King M-C. Linkage of early onset breast cancer to chromosome 17q21. Science 1990;250:1684.
82. Hannon GJ, Demetrick D, Beach D. Isolation of the Rb-related p130 through its interactions with CDK2 and cyclins. Genes Dev 1993;7:237.
83. Hansen MF, Cavenee WK. Genetics of cancer predisposition. Cancer Res 1987;47:5518.
84. Hansen MF, Koufos A, Gallie BL, Phillips RA, Fodstad O, Grogger A, Gedde-Dahl T, Cavenee WK. Osteosarcoma and retinoblastoma: a shared chromosomal mechanism revealing recessive predisposition. Proc Natl Acad Sci USA 1985;82:6216.
85. Harbour JW, Lai SL, Whang PJ, Gazdar AF, Minna JD, Kaye FJ. Abnormalities in structure and expression of the retinoblastoma gene in SCLC. Science 1988;241:353.
86. Harper JW, Adami GR, Wei N, Keyomarsi K, Elledge SJ. The p21 Cdk-interacting protein Cip1 is a potent inhibitor of G1 cyclin-dependent kinases. Cell 1993;75:805.
87. Harris H. The analysis of malignancy by cell fusion: the position in 1988. Cancer Res 1988;48:3302.
88. Harris H, Klein G. Malignancy of somatic cell hybrids. Nature 1969;224:1314.
89. He J, Allen JR, Collins VP, Allalunis-turner MJ, Godbout R, Day RS III, James CD. CDK4 amplification is an alternative mechanism to *p16* gene homozygous deletion in glioma cell lines. Cancer Res 1994;54:5804.
90. Hedrick L, Cho KR, Fearon ER, Wu TC, Kinzler KW, Vogelstein B. The *DCC* gene product in cellular differentiation and colorectal tumorigenesis. Genes Dev 1994;8:1174.
91. Helin K, Lees JA, Vidal M, Dyson N, Harlow E, Fattaey AA. cDNA encoding a pRB-binding protein with properties of the transcription factor E2F. Cell 1992;70:337.
92. Helin K, Wu C-L, Fattaey AR, Lees JA, Dynlact BD, Ngwu C, Harlow E. Heterodimerization of the transcription factors E2F-1 and DP-1 lead to cooperative trans-activation. Genes Dev 1993;7:1850.
93. Herman JG, Latif F, Weng Y, Lerman MI, Zbar B, Liu S, Samid D, Duan DR, Gnarra JR, Linehan WM, Baylin SB. Silencing of the VHL tumor-suppressor gene by DNA methylation in renal carcinoma. Proc Natl Acad Sci USA 1994;91:9700.
94. Herrera L, Kakati S, Gibas L, Pietrzak E, Sändberg A. Brief clinical report: Gardner syndrome in a man with an interstitial deletion of 5q. Am J Med Genet 1986;25:473.
95. Hershowitz I. Functional inactivation of genes by dominant negative mutations. Nature 1987;329:219.
96. Hinds P, Finlay C, Levine AJ. Mutation is required to activate the *p53* gene for cooperation with the *RAS* oncogene and transformation. J Virol 1989;63:739.
97. Hoeijmakers JHJ. Nucleotide excision repair. II. From yeast to mammals. Trends

Genet 1993;9:211.

98. Horowitz J, Yandell DW, Park S-H, Canning S, Whyte P, Buchkovich K, Harlow E, Weinberg RA, Dryja TP. Point mutational inactivation of the retinoblastoma antioncogene. Science 1989;243:937.
99. Hu Q, Lees JA, Buchkovich KJ, Harlow E. The retinoblastoma protein physically associates with the human cdc kinase. Mol Cell Biol 1992;12:971.
100. Huang H-JS, Yee J-K, Shew J-Y, Chen P-L, Bookstein R, Friedmann T, Lee EY-HP, Lee W-H. Suppression of the neoplastic phenotype by replacement of the *RB* gene in human cancer cells. Science 1988;242:1563.
101. Huff V, Compton DA, Chao L-Y, Strong LC, Geiser CF, Saunders GF. Lack of linkage of familial Wilms' tumor to chromosomal band 11p13. Nature 1988;336:377.
102. Hussussian CJ, Struewing JP, Goldstein AM, Higgins PAT, Ally DS, Sheahan MD, Clark WH Jr, Tucker MA, Dracopoli NC. Germ-line *p16* mutations in familial melanoma. Nat Genet 1994;8:15.
103. Ionov YM, Peinado A, Malkhosyan S, Shibata D, Perucho M. Ubiquitous somatic mutations in simple repeated sequences reveal a new mechanism for colonic carcinogenesis. Nature 1993;363:558.
104. James CD, Carlbom E, Dumanski JP, Hansen M, Nordenskjold M, Collins VP, Cavenee WK. Clonal genomic alterations in glioma malignancy stages. Cancer Res 1988;48:5546.
105. James CD, Collins VP, Allaluni-Turner MJ, Days RS. Localization of chromosome 9p homozygous deletions in glioma cell lines with markers constituting a continuous linkage map. Cancer Res 1993;53:3674.
106. Jenkins JR, Rudge K, Currie GA. Cellular immortalization by a cDNA clone encoding the transformation associated phosphoprotein *p53*. Nature 1984;312:651.
107. Johnson MR, Look AT, DeClue JE, Valentine MB, Lowy DR. Inactivation of the NF1 gene in human melanoma and neuroblastoma cell lines without impaired regulation of GTP-*RAS*. Proc Natl Acad Sci USA 1993;90:5539.
108. Joslyn G, Carlson M, Thlivers A, Albertsen H, Gelbert L, Samowitz W, Groden J, Stevens J, Spirio L, Robertson M, Sargeant L, Krapcho K, Wolff E, Burt R, Hughes JP, Warrington J, McPherson J, Wasmuth J, Le Paslier D, Abderrahim H, Cohen D, Leppert M, White R. Identification of deletion mutations and three new genes at the familial polyposis locus. Cell 1991;66:601.
109. Kaelin WG Jr, Krek W, Sellers WR, DeCaprio JA, Ajchanbaum F, Fuchs CS, Chittenden T, Li Y, Farnham PJ, Blanar MA, Livingston DM, Flemington EK. Expression cloning of a cDNA encoding a retinoblastoma-binding protein with E2F-like properties. Cell 1992;70:351.
110. Kamb A, Gruis NA, Weaver-Feldhaus J, Liu Q, Harshman K, Tavtigian SV, Stockert E, Day RS III, Johnson BE, Skolnick MH. A cell cycle regulator potentially involved in genesis of many tumor types. Science 1994;264:436.
111. Kamb A, Shattuck-Eidens D, Eeles R, Liu QQ, Gruis NA, Ding W, Hussey C, Tran T, Miki Y, Weaver-Feldhaus J, McClure M, Aitken JF, Anderson DE, Bergman W, Frants R, Goldgar DE, Green A, MacLennan R, Martin NG, Meyer LJ, Youl P, Zone JJ, Skolnick MH, Cannon-Albright LA. Analysis of the *p16* gene (CDKN2) as a candidate for the chromosome 9p melanoma susceptibility locus. Nat Genet 1994;8:22.
112. Kaneko Y, Egues MC, Rowley JD. Interstitial deletion of short arm of chromosome 11 limited to Wilms' tumor cells in a patient without aniridia. Cancer Res 1981;41:4577.
113. Kastan MB, Zhan Q, El-Deiry WS, Carrier F, Jacks T, Walsh WV, Plunkett BS, Vogelstein B, Fornace AJ Jr. A mammalian cell cycle check-point pathway utilizing *p53* and *GADD45* is defective in ataxia-telangiectasia. Cell 1992;71:587.
114. Kastan MB, Onyerkwere O, Sidransky D, Vogelstein B, Craig RW. Participation of *p53* protein in the cellular resonse to DNA damage. Cancer Res 1991;53:6304.
115. Kato J-Y, Matshushime H, Hiebert SW, Ewen ME, Sherr CJ. Direct binding of cyclin D to the retinoblastoma gene product (pRb) and pRb phosphorylation by the cyclin D-dependent knase CDK4. Genes Dev 1993;7:331.
116. Kessis TD, Slebos RJ, Han SM, Shah K, Bosch WF, Munoz N, Hedrick L, Cho KR. *p53* gene mutation and mdm-2 gene mutation are uncommon in primary carcinomas of the uterine cervix. Am J Pathol 1993;143:1398.
117. Kinzler KW, Nilbert MC, Su L-K, Vogelstein B, Bryan TM, Levy DB, Smith KJ, Presisinger AC, Hedge P, McKechnie D, Finniear R, Markham A, Groffen J, Boguski MS, Altschul SF, Horii A, Ando H, Miyoshi Y, Miki Y, Nishisho I, Nakamura Y. Identification of FAP locus genes from chromosome 5q21. Science 1991;253:661.
118. Klinger HP. Suppression of tumorigenicity. CytoGenet Cell Genet 1982;32:68.
119. Knudson AG Jr. Mutation and cancer: statistical study of retinoblastoma. Proc Natl Acad Sci USA 1971;68:820.
120. Knudson AG Jr. Hereditary cancer, oncogenes, and anti-oncogenes. Cancer Res 1985;45:1437.
121. Knudson AG Jr, Strong LC. Mutation and cancer: a model for Wilm's tumor of the kidney. J Natl Cancer Inst 1972;48:313.
122. Knudson AG Jr. Antioncogenes and human cancer. Proc Natl Acad Sci USA 1993;90:10914.
123. Koufos A, Grundy P, Morgan K, Aleck KA, Hadus T, Lampkin BC, Kalbakji A, Cavenee WK. Familial Wiedman-Beck with syndrome and a second Wilms' tumor locus both map to 11p15.5. Am J Hum Genet 1989;44:711.
124. Koufos A, Hansen MF, Lampkin BC, Workman ML, Copeland NG, Jenkins NA, Cavenee WK. Loss of alleles at loci on human chromosome 11 during genesis of Wilms' tumor. Nature 1984;309:170.
125. Landsvater RM, Mathew CGP, Smith BA, Marcu EM, Te Meerman GJ, Lips CJM, Geerdink RA, Nakamura Y, Ponder BAJ, Buys CHC. Development of multiple endocrine neoplasia type 2A does not involve substantial deletions of chromosome 10. Genomics 1989;4:246.
126. Lane DP, Crawford LV. T-antigen is bound to host protein in SV40-transformed cells. Nature 1979;278:261.
127. Lane DP, Benchimol S. *p53*: oncogene or anti-oncogene? Genes Devel 1990;4:1.
128. Lane DP. *p53*, guardian of the genome. Nature 1992;358:15.
129. Latif F, Tory K, Gnarra J, Yao M, Duh F-M, Orcutt ML, Stackhouse T, Kuzmin I, Modi W, Geil L, Schmidt L, Zhou F, Li H, Wei MH, Chen F, Glenn G, Choyke P, Walther MM, Weng Y, Duan D-SR, Dean M, Glavac D, Richards RM, Crossey PA, Ferguson-Smith MA, Le Paslier D, Chumakov I, Cchen D, Chinault C, Maher ER, Linehan WM, Zbar B, Lerman MI. Identification of the von Hippel-Lindau disease tumor suppressor gene. Science 1993;260:1317.
130. Leach FS, Nicolaides NC, Papdopoulos N, Liu B, Jen J, Parsons R, Peltomaki P, Sistonen P, Aaltonen LA, Nystrom-Lahti M, Guan X-Y, Zhang J, Melttzer PS, Yu J-W, Kao F-T, Chen DJ, Cerosaletti KM, Fournier REK, Todd S, Lewis T, Leach RJ, Naylor SL, Weissenbach J, Mecklin J-P, Jarvinen H, Petersen GM, Hamilton SR, Green J, Jass J, Watson P, Lynch HT, Trent JM, de la chapelle A, Kinzler KW, Vogelstein B. Mutations of a MutS homolog in hereditary nonpolyposis colorectal cancer. Cell 1993;75:1215.
131. Lee W-H, Bookstein R, Hong F, Young L-H, Shew J-Y, Lee EY-HP. Human retinoblastoma susceptibility gene: cloning, identification and sequence. Science 1987;235:1394.
132. Lee W-H, Shew JY, Hong FD, Sery TW, Donoso LA, Young L-J, Bookstein R, Lee EY-HP. The retinoblastoma susceptibility gene encodes a nuclear phosphoprotein associated with DNA binding activity. Nature 1987;329:642.
133. Lee EY-HP, To H, Shew J-Y, Bookstein R, Scully P, Lee W-H. Inactivation of the retinoblastoma susceptibility gene in human breast cancer. Science 1988;241:218.
134. Leon SP, Zhu J, Black P. McL Genetic aberrations in human brain tumors. Neurosurgery 1994;34:708.
135. Leppert M, Dobbs M, Scambler P, O'Connell P, Nakamura Y, Stauffer D, Woodward S, Burt R, Hughes J, Gardner E, Lathrop M, Wasmuth J, Lalouel J-M, White R. The gene for familial polyposis coli maps to the long arm of chromosome 5. Science 1987;238:1411.
136. Leppert M, Burt R, Hughes JP, Samowitz W, Nakamura Y, Woodward S, Gardner E, Lalouel J-M, White R. Genetic analysis of an inherited predisposition to colon cancer in a family with a variable number of adenomatous polyps. N Engl J Med 1990;322:904.
137. Li Y, Bollag G, Clark R, Stevens J, Conroy L, Fults D, Ward K, Friedman E, Samowitz W, Robertson M, Bradley P, McCormick F, White R, Cawthon R. Somatic mutations in the neufibromatosis 1 gene in human tumors. Cell 1992;69:275–281.
138. Li Y, Graham C, Lacy S, Duncan AMV, Whyte P. The adenovirus E1A-associated 130-kD protein is encoded by a member of the retinoblastoma gene family and physically interacts with cyclins A and E. Genes Dev 1993;7:2366.
139. Liu B, Nicolaides NC, Markowitz S, Willson JKV, Parsons RE, Jen J, Papacopolous N, Peltomaki P, de la Chapelle A, Hamilton SR, Kinzler KW, Vogelstein B. Mismatch repair gene defects in sporadic colorectal cancer with microsatellite instability. Nat Genet 1995;9:48.
140. Lindblom A, Tannergard P, Werelius B, Nordenskjold M. Genetic mapping of a second locus predisposing to hereditary nonpolyposis colorectal cancer. Nat Genet 1993;5:279.
141. Linzer DIH, Levine AJ. Characterization of a 54K dalton cellular SV40 tumor antigen present in SV40 transformed cells and uninfected embryonal carcinoma cells. Cell 1979;17:43.
142. Ludlow JW, Decaprio JA, Huang C-M, Lee W-H, Paucha E, Livingston DM. SV40 large T antigen binds preferentially to an underphosphorylated member of the retinoblastoma gene product family. Cell 1989;56:57.
143. Lynch HT, Smyrk RC, Watson P, Lanspa SJ, Lynch JF, Lynch PM, Cavalieri RJ, Boland CR. Genetics, natural history, tumor spectrum, and pathology of hereditary nonpolyposis colorectal cancer: an updated review. Gastroenterology 1993;104:1535.
144. MacCollin M, Mohney T, Trofatter J, Wertelecki W, Ramesh V, Gusella J. DNA diagnosis of neurofibromatosis 2: altered coding sequence of the merlin tumor suppressor in an extended pedigree. JAMA 1993;270:2316.
145. Malkin D, Li FP, Strong LC, Fraumeni JF, Nelson CE, Kim DH, Gryka MA, Bischoff FZ, Tainsky MA, Friend SH. germ-line *p53* mutations in a familial syndrome of breast cancer, sarcomas, and other neoplasms. Science 1990;250:1233.
146. Mannens M, Slater RM, Heytig C, Blick J, De Kraker J, Coad N, DePagter-Holthuizen P, Pearson PL. Molecular nature of genetic changes resulting in loss of heterozygosity of chromosome 11 in Wilms' tumors. Hum Genet 1988;81:41.
147. Markowitz S, Wang J, Myeroff L, Parsons R, Sun LZ, Lutterbaugh J, Zborowska E, Kinzler KW, Vogelstein B, Brattain M, Willson JKV. Inactivation of the type II TGF-beta receptor in colon cancer cells with microsatellite instability. Science 1995;268:1336.
148. Marshall CJ. Tumor suppressor genes. Cell 1991;64:313.
149. Martin GA, Viskochil D, Bollag G, McCabe PC, Crosier WJ, Haubruck H, Conroy L, Clark R, O'Connell P, Cawthon RM, Innis MA, McCormick F. The GAP-related domain of the neurofibromatosis type 1 gene product interacts with *ras* p21. Cell 1990;63:843.
150. Martin GS. Rous sarcoma virus: a function required for the maintenance of the transformed state. Nature 1970;227:1021.
151. Masuda HC, Miller C, Koeffler HP, Battifora H, Kline MJ. Rearrangement of the *p53* gene in human osteogenic sarcomas. Proc Natl Acad Sci USA 1987;84:7716.
152. Mathew CGP, Chin KS, Easton DF, Thorpe K, Carter C, Liou GI, Fong S-L, Bridges CDB, Haak H, Nieuwenhuijzen-Kruseman A, Schifterr S, Hansen HA, Telenius H, Telenius-Berg M, Ponder BAJ. A linked genetic marker for multiple endocrine neoplasia type 2A on chromosome 10. Nature 1987;328:527.
153. McCormick F. *RAS* signaling and NF1. Curr Opin Genet Devel 1995;5:51.
154. Merlo A, Gabrielson E, Askin F, Baylin S, Sidransky D. Frequent loss of chromosome 9 in human primary non-small cell lung cancer. Cancer Res 1994;54:640.
155. Miki Y, Swensen J, Shattuck-Eidens D, et al. A strong candidate for the breast and ovarian cancer susceptibility gene BRCA1. Science 1994;266:66.
156. Miller RW, Fraumeni JF Jr, Manning MD. Association of Wilms' tumor with aniridia, hemihypertrophy, and other congenital malformations. N Engl J Med 1964;270:922.
157. Miyoshi Y, Ando H, Nagase H, Nishisho I, Horii A, Miki Y, Mori T, Utsunomiya J, Baba S, Petersen G, Hamilton, Kinzler KW, Vogelstein B, Nakamura Y. Germ-line mutations of the *APC* gene in 53 adenomatous polyposis patients. Proc Natl Acad Sci USA 1992;89:4452.
158. Miyoshi Y, Nagase H, Ando H, Horii A, Ichii S, Nakatsuru S, Aoki T, Miki Y, Mori T, Nakamura Y. Somatic mutations of the *APC* gene in colorectal tumors: mutation cluster region in the *APC* gene. Hum Mol Genet 1992;1:229.
159. Modrich P. Mechanisms and biological effects of mismatch repair. Annu Rev Genet 1991;25:229.
160. Modrich P. Mismatch repair, genetic stability, and cancer. Science 1994;266:1959.
161. Momand J, Zambetti GP, Olson DC, George DL, Levine AJ. The mdm-2 oncogene product forms a complex with the *p53* protein and inhibits *p53* medicated transactivation. Cell 1992;69:1237.
162. Moran E, Matthews MB. Multiple functional domains in the adenovirus E1A gene. Cell 1987;48:177.

163. Mowat M, Cheng A, Kicumca N, Bernstein A, Benchimol S. The arrangements of the cellular *p53* gene in erythroleukemic cells transformed by Friend virus. Nature 1985;314:633.
164. Mulligan LM, Matlashewski GJ, Scrable HJ, Cavenee WK. Mechanism of *p53* loss in human sarcomas. Proc Natl Acad Sci USA 1990;87:5863.
165. Nagase H, Miyoshi Y, Horii A, Aoki T, Ogawa M, Utsunomiya J, Baba S, Sasazuki T, Nakamura Y. Correlation between the location of germ-line mutations in the APC gene and the number of colorectal polyps in familial adenomatous polyposis patients. Cancer Res 1992;52:4055.
166. Nagase H, Nakamura Y. Mutations of the *APC* (adenomatous polyposis coli) gene. Hum Mutat 1993;2:425.
167. Narod SA, Feuteun J, Lynch HT, Watson P, Conway T, Lynch J, Lenoir GM. Familial breast-ovarian cancer locus on chromosome 17q12–23. Lancet 1991;338:82.
168. Nelkin BD, Nakumura Y, White RW, deBustros AC, Herman J, Wells SA Jr, Baylin SB. Low incidence of loss of chromosome 10 in sporadic and hereditary human medullary thyroid carcinoma. Cancer Res 1989;49:4114.
169. Nevins JR. E2F: a link between the Rb tumor suppressor proteins and viral oncoproteins. Science 1992;258:424.
170. Nicolaides NC, Papadopoulos N, Liu B, et al. Mutations of two PMS homologues in hereditary nonpolyposis colon cancer. Nature 1994;371:75.
171. Nigro JM, Baker SJ, Preisinger AC, Jessup JM, Hostetter R, Cleary K, Bigner SH, Davidson N, Baylin S, Devilee P, Glover T, Collins FS, Wesxton A, Modali R, Harris CC, Vogelstein B. Mutations in the *p53* gene occur in diverse tumor types. Nature 1989;342:705.
172. Nishisho I, Nakamura Y, Miyoshi Y, Miki Y, Ando H, Horii A, Koyama K, Utsunomiya J, Baba S, Hedge P, Markham A, Krush AJ, Petersen G, Hamilton SR, Nilbert MC, Levy DB, Bryan TM, Presisinger AC, Smith KJ, Su L-K, Kinzler KW, Vogelstein B. Mutations of chromosome 5q21 genes in FAP and colorectal cancer patients. Science 1991;253:665.
173. Nobori T, Miura K, Wu DJ, Lois A, Takabayashi K, Carson DA. Deletions of the cyclin-dependent kinase-4 inhibitor gene in multiple human cancers. Nature 1994;368:753.
174. O'Connell P, Leach R, Cawthon R, Culver M, Stevens J, Viskochil D, Fournier REK, Rich D, Ledbetter D, White R. Two von Recklinghausen neurofibromatosis translocations map within a 600 kb segment of 17q11.2. Science 1989;244:1087.
175. Oliner JD, Kinzler KW, Meltzer PS, George DL, Vogelstein B. Amplification of a gene encoding a *p53*-associated protein in human sarcomas. Nature 1992;358:80.
176. Olopade OI, Bohlander SK, Pomykala H, Maltepe E, Van Melle E, Le Beau MM, Diaz MO. Mapping of the shortest region of overlap of deletions of the short arm of chromosome 9 associated with human neoplasia. Genomics 1992;14:437.
177. Olschwang S, Tiret A, Laurent-Puig P, Muleris M, Parc R, Thomas G. Restriction of ocular fundus lesions to a specific subgroup of *APC* mutations in adenomatous polyposis coli patients. Cell 1993;75:959.
178. Olumi AF, Skinner EC, Tsai YC, Jones PA. Molecular analysis of human bladder cancer. Semin Urol 1990;8:270.
179. Orkin SH, Goldman DS, Sallan SE. Development of homozygosity for chromosome 11p markers in Wilms' tumor. Nature 1984;309:172.
180. Orye E, Delbek MJ, Vandenabeele B. Retinoblastoma and long arm deletion at chromosome 13: attempts to define the deleted segment. Clin Genet 1974;5:457.
181. Oshimura M, Kugoh H, Koi M, Shimizu M, Yamada H, Satoh H, Barrett JC. Transfer of human chromosome 11 suppresses tumorigenicity of some but not all tumor cell lines. J Cell Biochem 1990;42:135.
182. Palombo R, Gallinari P, Iaccarino I, Lettieri T, Hughes M, Darrigo A, Hsuan JJ, Jiricny J. GTBP, a 160-kilodalton protein essential for mismatch-binding activity in human cells. Science 1995;268:1912.
183. Papadopoulos N, Nicolaides NC, Wei Y-F, Ruben SM, Carter KC, Rossen CA, Haseltine WA, Fleischman RD, Fraser CM, Adams MD, Venter JC, Hamilton SR, Petersen GM, Watson P, Lynch HT, Peltomaki P, Mecklin J-P, de la Chapelle A, Kinzler KW, Vogelstein B. Mutation of a *mutL* homolog in hereditary colon cancer. Science 1994;263:1625.
184. Papadopoulos N, Nicolaides NC, Liu B, Parsons R, Lengauer C, Palombo F, Darrigo A, Markowitz S, Willson JKV, Jiricny J. Mutations of GTBP in genetically unstable cells. Science 1995;268:1915.
185. Parada LF, Land H, Weinberg RA, Wolf D, Rotter V. Cooperation between gene encoding *p53* tumor antigen and *ras* in cellular transformation. Nature 1984;312:649.
186. Parsons R, Li GM, Longley MJ, Fang W-H, Papadopoulos N, Jen J, de la Chapelle A, Kinzler KW, Vogelstein B, Modrich P. Hypermutability and mismatch repair deficiency in RER$^+$ tumor cells. Cell 1993;75:1227.
187. Peltomaki P, Aaltonen LA, Sistonen P, Pylkkanen L, Mecklin J-P, Jarvinen H, Greeen JS, Jass JR, Weber JL, Leach FS, Petersen GM, Hamilton SR, de la Chapelle A, Vogelstein B. Genetic mapping of a locus predisposing to human colorectal cancer. Science 1993;260:810.
188. Ping AJ, Reeve AE, Law DJ, Young MR, Boehuke M, Feinberg AP. Genetic linkage of Beckwith-Wiedman syndrome to 11p15. Am J Hum Genet 1989;44:720.
189. Polakis P. Mutations in the *APC* gene and their implications for protein structure and function. Curr Opin Genet Devel 1995;5:66.
190. Ponder B. Gene losses in human tumors. Nature 1988;335:400.
191. Ponder B. Neurofibromatosis gene cloned. Nature 1990;346:703.
192. Powell SM, Zilz N, Beazer-Barclay Y, Bryan RM, Hamilton SR, Thibodeau SN, Vogelstein B, Kinzler KW. *APC* mutations occur early during colorectal tumorigenesis. Nature 1992;359:235.
193. Powell SM, Petersen GM, Krush AJ, Booker S, Jen J, Giardiello FM, Hamilton SR, Vogelstein B, Kinzler KW. Molecular diagnosis of familial adenomatous polyposis. N Engl J Med 1993;329:1982.
194. Pritchard-Jones K, Fleming S, Davidson D, Bickmore W, Porteous D, Gosden C, Bard J, Buckler A, Pelletier J, Housman D, van Heyningen V, Hastie N. The candidate Wilms' tumor gene is involved in genitourinary development. Nature 1990;346:194.
195. Prives C. How loops, β sheets, and α helices help us to understand *p53*. Cell 1994;78:543.
196. Rauscher FJ III. The *WT1* Wilms' tumor gene product: a developmentally regulated transcription factor in the kidney that functions as a tumor suppressor. FASEB J 1993;7:896.
197. Reeve AE, Housiaux PJ, Gardner RJM, Chewings WE, Grindley RM, Millow LJ. Loss of a Harvey *RAS* allele in sporadic Wilms' tumor. Nature 1984;309:174.
198. Reeve AE, Sih SA, Raizis AM, Feinberg AP. Loss of allelic heterozygosity at a second locus on chromosome 11 in sporadic Wilms' tumor cells. Mol Cell Biol 1989;9:1799.
199. Riccardi VM, Hittner HM, Francke U, Yunis JJ, Ledbetter D, Borges W. The aniridia-Wilms' tumor association: the clinical role of chromosome band 11p13. Cancer Genet CytoGenet 1980;2:131.
200. Rouleau GA, Wertelecki W, Haines JL, Hobbs WJ, Trofatter JA, Seizinger BR, Martuza RL, Superneau DW, Conneally PM, Gussela JF. Genetic linkage of bilateral acoustic neurofibromatosis to a DNA marker on chromosome 22. Nature 1987;329:246.
201. Rouleau GA, Merel P, Luchtman M, Sanson M, Zucman J, Marineau C, Hoang-Xuan K, Demczuk S, Cesmaze C, Plougstel B, Pulst SM, Lenoir G, Bijlsma E, Fashold R, Dumanski J, de Jong P, Parry D, Eldrige R, Aurias A, Delattere O, Thomas G. Alteration in a new gene encoding a putative membrane-organizing protein causes neurofibromatosis type 2. Nature 1993;363:515.
202. Rous P. A sarcoma of the fowl transmissible by an agent separable from the tumor cells. J Exp Med 1911;13:397.
203. Rubinfeld B, Souza B, Albert I, Muller O, Chamberlain SC, Masiarz F, Munemitsu S, Polakis P. Association of the *APC* gene product with β-catenin. Science 1993;262:1731.
204. Sager R. Genetic suppression of tumor formation: a new frontier in cancer research. Cancer Res 1986;46:1573.
205. Sager R. Tumor suppressor genes: the puzzle and the promise. Science 1989;246:1406.
206. Sarnow P, Ho YS, Williams J, Levine AJ. Adenovirus E1b-58 Kd tumor antigen and SV40 large tumor antigen are physically associated with the same 54 Kd cellular protein in transformed cells. Cell 1982;28:387.
207. Savitsky K, Barshira A, Gilad S, Rotman G, Ziv Y, Vanagaite L, Tagle DA, Smith S, Uziel T, Sfez S, Ashkenazi M, Pecker I, Frydman M, Harnik R, Patanjali SR, Simmons A, Clines GA, Sartiel A, Gatti RA, Chessa L, Sanai O, Lavin MF, Jaspers NGJ, Taylor MR, Arlett CF, Miki T, Weissman SM, Lovett M, Collins FS, Shiloh Y. A single ataxia telangiectasia gene with a product similar to PI-3 kinase. Science 1995;268:1749.
208. Saxon PJ, Srivastan ES, Stanbridge EJ. Introduction of human chromosome 11 via microcell transfer controls tumorigenic expression of HeLa cells. EMBO J. 1986;5:3461.
209. Scheffner M, Munger K, Byrne JC, Howley PM. The state of the *p53* and retinoblastoma genes in human cervical cancer cell lines. Proc Natl Acad Sci USA 1991;88:5523.
210. Seizinger BR, Martuza RL, Gusella JF. Loss of genes on chromosome 22 in tumorigenesis of human acoustic neuroma. Nature 1986;322:644.
211. Seizinger BR, Rouleau GA, Ozelius LJ, et al. Genetic linkage of von Recklinghausen neurofibromatosis to the nerve growth factor receptor gene. Cell 1987;49:589.
212. Seizinger BR, Rouleau GA, Ozelius LJ, et al. Common pathogenetic mechansim for three types in bilateral acoustic neurofibromatosis. Science 1987;236:317.
213. Seizinger BR, de la Mote S, Atkins L, Gusella JF, Martuza RL. Molecular genetic approach to human meningioma: loss of genes on chromosome 22. Proc Natl Acad Sci USA 1987;84:5419.
214. Seizinger BR, Rouleau GA, Ozelius LJ, Lane AH, Farmer GE, Lamiell JM, Haines J, Yeun JWM, Collins D, Majoor-Krakauer D, Bonner T, Matthew C, Rubenstein A, Halperin J, McConkie-Rosell A, Green JS, Trofatter JA, Ponder B, Eierman L, Bowner MI, Schmike R, Oostra B, Aronin N, Smith DI, Drabkin H, Wazari MW, Hobbs WJ, Martuza RL, Conneally PM, Hsia YE, Gusella JF. Von Hippel-Lindau disease maps to the region of chromosome 3 associated with renal cell carcinoma. Nature 1988;332:268.
215. Seizinger BR. NF1.a prevalent cause of tumorigenesis in human cancers? Nat Genet 1993;3:97.
216. Shannon KM, O'Connell P, Martin GA, Paderanga D, Olson K, Dinndorf P, McCormick F. Loss of the normal NF1 allele form the bone marrow of children with NF1 and malignant myeloid disorders. N Engl J Med 1994;330:597.
217. Shimizu M, Yokota J, Mori N, Shuin T, Shinoda M, Terada M, Oshimura M. Introduction of normal chromosome 3p modulates the tumorigenicity of a human renal cell carcinoma cell line YCR. Oncogene 1990;5:185.
218. Shuin T, Kondo K, Torigoe S, Kishida T, Kubota Y, Hosaka M, Nagashima Y, Kitamura H, Latif F, Zbar B, Lerman MI, Yao M. Frequent somatic mutations and loss of heterozygosity of the von Hippel-Lindau tumor suppressor gene in primary human renal cell carcinomas. Cancer Res 1994;54:2852.
219. Sidransky D, Messing E. Molecular genetics and biochemical mechanisms in bladder cancer: oncogenes, tumor suppressor genes, and growth factors. Urol Clin North Am 1992;19:629.
220. Simpson NE, Kidd KK, Goodfellow PJ, McDermid H, Myers S, Kidd JR, Jackson CE, Duncan AMV, Farrer LA, Brasch K, Castiglione C, Genel M, Gertner J, Greenberg CR, Gusella JF, Holden JJA, White BN. Assignment of multiple endocrine neoplasia type 2A to chromosome 10 by linkage. Nature 1987;328:528.
221. Slater RM, de Kraker J. Chromosome number 11 and Wilms' tumor. Cancer Genet CytoGenet 1982;5:237.
222. Smith SA, Easton DF, Evans DGR, Ponder BJ. Allele losses in the region 17q12-21 in familial breast and ovarian cancer involve the wild-type chromosome. Natl Genet 1991;2:128.
223. Sparkes RS, Sparkes MC, Wilson MG, Towner JW, Benedict WF, Murphree AL, Yunis JJ. Regional assignment of genes for human esterase D and retinoblastoma to chromosome 13q14. Science 1980;208:1042.
224. Sparkes RS, Murphree AL, Lingus RW, Sparkes MC, Field LL, Funderburk SJ, Benedict WF. Gene for hereditary retinoblastoma assigned to human chromosome 13 by linkage to esterase D. Science 1983;219:971.
225. Spirio L, Olschwang S, Groden J, Robertson M, Samowitz W, Joslyn G, Gelbert L, Thliveris A, Carlson M, Otterud B, Lynch H, Watson P, Lynch P, Laurent-Puig P, Burt R, Hughes JP, Thomas G, Leppert M, White R. Alleles of the *APC* gene: an attenuated form of familial polyposis. Cell 1993;75:951.
226. Spruck CHL, Gonzalez-Zulueta M, Shibata A, Simoneau AS, Lin M-F, Gonzales F, Tsai YC, Jones PA. *p16* gene in uncultured tumors. Nature 1994;370:183.
227. Srivastava S, Zou Z, Pirollo K, Blattner W, Chang EH. Germ-line transmission of a mutated *p53* gene in cancer-prone family with Li-Fraumeni syndrome. Nature 1990;348:747.
228. Stanbridge EJ, Cavenee WK. Heritable cancer and tumor suppressor genes: a tentative connection. In Oncogenes and the Molecular Origins of Cancer. Edited by RA Weinberg. Cold Spring Harbor, NY: Cold Spring Harbor Press, 1989.
229. Stanbridge EJ, Der CJ, Doerson CJ, Nighimi RY, Peehl DM, Weissman BE, Wilkinson J. Human cell hybrids: analysis of transformation and tumorigenicity. Science 1982;215:252.

230. Stehlin D, Varmus HE, Bishop JM, Vogt PK. DNA related to the transforming gene(s) of avian sarcoma viruses is present in normal avian DNA. Nature 1976;260:170.
231. Su L-K, Vogelstein B, Kinzler KW. Association of the *APC* tumor suppressor protein with catenins. Science 1993;262:1734.
232. Sugawara O, Oshimura M, Koi M, Annab LA, Barrett JC. Induction of cellular senescence in immortalized cells by human chromosome 1. Science 1990;247:707.
233. Takahashi T, Nau MM, Chibu I, Birrer MJ, Rosenberg RK, Vinocour M, Levitt M, Pass H, Gazdar AF, Minna JD. *p53*. A frequent target for genetic abnormalities in lung cancer. Science 1989;246:491.
234. The I, Murthy AE, Hannigan GE, Jacoby LB, Menon AG, Gusella JF, Bernards A. Neurofibomatosis type 1 gene mutations in neuroblastoma. Natl Genet 1993;3:62.
235. Thibodeau SN, Bren G, Schaid D. Microsatellite instability in cancer of the proximal colon. Science 1993;260:816.
236. Trahey M, McCormick F. A cytoplasmic protein stimulates normal N-*RAS* p21 GTPase, but does not affect oncogenic mutants. Science 1987;238:542.
237. Trent JM, Stanbridge EJ, McBride HL, Meese EV, Casey G, Araujo DE, Witkowski CM, Nagle RB. Tumorigenicity in human melanoma lines controlled by introduction of human chromosome 6. Science 1990;247:568.
238. Trofatter J, MacCollin M, Rutter J, Murrell JR, Duyao MP, Parry DM, Eldridge R, Kley N, Menon AG, Pulaski K, Haase VH, Abrose CM, Munroe D, Bove C, Haines JL, Martuza RL, MacDonald Seizinger BR, Short MP, Buckler AJ. A novel moesin-, ezrin-, radixin-like gene is a candidate for the neurofibromatosis 2 tumor suppressor. Cell 1993;72:791.
239. Upadhyaya M, Shen M, Cherryson A, Farnham J, Maynard J, Huson SM, Harper PS. Analysis of mutations at the neurofibromatosis 1 (*NF1*) locus. Hum Mol Genet 1992;1:735.
240. van der Riet P, Nawroz H, Hruban RH, Corio R, Tokino K, Koch W, Sidransky D. Frequent loss of chromosome 9p21–22 early in head and neck cancer progression. Cancer Res 1994;54:1156.
241. van Heyningen V. One gene—four syndromes. Nature 1994;367:319.
242. Varmus HE. The molecular genetics of cellular oncogenes. Annu Rev Genet 1984;18:553.
243. Viskochil D, Buchberg AM, Xu G, Cawthon RM, Stevens J, Wolff RK, Culver M, Carey JC, Copeland NG, Jenkins NA, White R, O'Connell P. Deletions and a translocation interrupt a cloned gene at the neurofibromatosis type 1 locus. Cell 1990;62:187.
244. Viskochil D, White R, Cawthon R. The neurofibromatosis type 1 gene. Annu Rev Neurosci 1993;16:183.
245. Vogelstein B, Fearon ER, Hamilton SR, Kern SE, Preisinger AC, Leppert M, Nakumura Y, White R, Smits AMM, Bos JL. Genetic alterations during colorectal-tumor development. N Engl J Med 1988;319:525.
246. Vogelstein B, Kinzler KW. *p53* function and dysfunction. Cell 1992;70:523.
247. Wainwright B. Familial melanoma and *p16*—a hung jury. Nat Genet 1994;8:3.
248. Wallace MR, Marchuk DA, Andersen LB, Letcher R, Odeh HM, Saulino AM, Fountain JW, Bereton A, Nicholson J, Mitchell AL, Brownstein BH, Collins FS. Type 1 neurofibromatosis gene identification of a large transcript disrupted in three NF1 patients. Science 1990;249:181.
249. Warthin AS. Heredity with reference to carcinoma: as shown by the study of the cases examined in the pathological laboratory of the University of Michigan, 1895–1913. Arch Intern Med 1913;12:546.
250. Weaver-Feldhaus J, Gruis NE, Neuhausen S, Le Paslier D, Stockert E, Skolnick MH, Kamb A. Localization of a putative tumor suppressor gene by using homozygous deletions in melanomas. Proc Natl Acad Sci USA 1994;91:7563.
251. Weichselbaum RR, Beckett M, Diamond A. Some retinoblastomas, osteosarcomas, and soft tissue sarcomas may share a common etiology. Proc Natl Acad Sci USA 1988;85:2106.
252. Weinberg RA. Oncogenes, antioncogenes, and the molecular bases of multistep carcinogenesis. Cancer Res 1989;49:3713.
253. Weinberg RA. Tumor suppressor genes. Science 1991;254:1138.
254. Weintraub SJ, Prater CA, Dean DC. Retinoblastoma protein switches the E2F site from positive to negative element. Nature 1992;358:259.
255. Weissman BE, Saxon PJ, Pasquale SR, Jones GR, Geiser AG, Stanbridge EJ. Introduction of a normal human chromosome 11 into a Wilms' tumor cell line controls its tumorigenic expression. Science 1987;236:175.
256. Werness BA, Levine AJ, Howley PM. Association of human papillomavirus types 16 and 18 E6 proteins with *p53*. Science 1990;248:76.
257. Whaley JM, Naglich J, Gelbert L, Hsia YE, Lamiell JM, Green JS, Collins D, Neumann HPH, Laidlaw J, Li FP, Klein-Szanto AJP, Seizinger BR, Kley. North Am J Hum Genet 1994;55:1092.
258. Whyte P, Buchkovich KJ, Horowitz JM, Friend SH, Raybuck J, Weinberg RA, Harlow E. Association between an oncogene and an anti-oncogene: the adenovirus E1A proteins bind to the retinoblastoma gene product. Nature 1988;334:124.
259. Whyte P, Williamson NM, Harlow E. Cellular targets for transformation by the adenovirus E1A proteins. Cell 1989;56:67.
260. Wigler MH. GAPs in understanding *ras*. Nature 1990;346:696.
261. Wolf D, Admon S, Oren M, Rotter V. Major deletions in the gene encoding the *p53* tumor antigen cause lack of *p53* expression in HL-60 cells. Proc Natl Acad Sci USA 1984;82:790.
262. Wooster R, Neuhausen SL, Mangion J, Quirk Y, Ford D, Collins N, Nguyen K, Seal S, Tran T, Averill D, Fields P, Marshall G, Narod S, Lenoir GM, Lynch HT, Feunteun J, Devilee P, Cornelisse CJ, Menko FH, Daly PA, Ormiston W, Memanus R, Pye C, Lewis CM, Cannon-Albright LA, Easton DF, et al. Localization of a breast cancer susceptibility gene, *BRCA2*, to chromosome 13q12-13. Science 1994;265:2088.
263. Xiong Y, Hannon GJ, Zhang H, Casso D, Kobayashi R, Beach D. p21 is a universal inhibitor of cyclin kinases. Science 1993;366:701.
264. Xu G, O'Connell P, Viskochil D, Cawthon R, Robertson M, Culver M, Dunn D, Stevens J, Gesteland R, White R, Weiss R. The neurofibromatosis type 1 gene encodes a protein related to GAP. Cell 1990;62:599.
265. Yandell D, Campbell TA, Dayton SH, Petersen R, Walton D, Little JB, McConkie-Rosell A, Buckley EG, Dryja TP. Oncogenic point mutations in the human retinoblastoma gene: their application to genetic counseling. N Engl J Med 1989;321:1689.

CHAPTER 7

Recurring Chromosome Rearrangements in Human Cancer

OLUFUNMILAYO I. OLOPADE AND JANET D. ROWLEY

Introduction

Over the past decade, it has become clear that acquired clonal chromosomal abnormalities are found in the malignant cells of many patients with leukemia, lymphoma, and solid tumors. Many genes involved in consistent chromosome rearrangements, notably translocations, have already been identified, and the identity of most genes affected by these aberrations likely will be determined within the next decade. Moreover, for a number of rearrangements, some of the changes in gene structure and function have been defined; therefore, some general principles that may be applicable to all chromosome rearrangements in human malignant disease are beginning to emerge. This review presents the most current data on primary chromosome rearrangements in hematologic malignancies as well as solid tumors.

Much of the detailed information regarding the relevant chromosome rearrangements is contained in a number of recent reviews, and only a general summary is presented here (75, 101, 120, 160, 174, 215). Mitelman has published five editions of his *Catalog of Chromosome Aberrations in Cancer* (119). A comparison of the number of abnormal karyotypes according to the type of neoplasia is summarized in Figure 7.1. Although carcinomas account for the greatest proportion of malignant disease, they only represent approximately 20% of the karyotypic data. From the beginning of cytogenetic analysis of human malignant disease, it has been clear that virtually all solid tumors, including the non-Hodgkin's lymphomas, have an abnormal karyotype and that some of these abnormalities are limited to a given tumor (75, 121, 169). In the 1960s and 1970s, only approximately 50% of leukemias had identifiable karyotypic abnormalities, but now over 80% have an abnormal karyotype (160). This increase has occurred because of improved culture techniques and processing methods. Certain malignant diseases, such as Hodgkin's disease or multiple myeloma, continue to show a high frequency of normal karyotypes, probably because of their low mitotic index; however, the use of fluorescence in situ hybridization is adding a new precision in chromosome identification that will have a major impact. "Painting" probes identify chromosomes that are involved in rearrangements or in marker chromosomes (163); centromere-specific probes allow enumeration of the number of chromosomes in interphase nuclei, and region-specific probes can detect deletions and translocations (163).

Different chromosome changes have been observed in neoplastic cells, and these often occur in combination, which leads to great difficulty in identifying precisely the unique abnormalities in a particular cancer. A number of international meetings over the last 25 years led to the establishment of a universally accepted system for chromosome nomenclature. The most authoritative document, *Cancer Cytogenetics, Supplement to An International System for Human Cytogenetic Nomenclature* (79), is used here. The simplest change is either a gain or a loss of a whole chromosome. Common structural alterations are translocations, which involve the exchange of material between two or more chromosomes, and deletions, which involve the loss of DNA from a chromosome and, thus, from the affected cell (Fig. 7.2). Chromosome inversions have also been observed; in this rearrangement, a single chromosome is broken in two places and the central portion inverted and rejoined to the ends of the chromosome. Each chromosome band is numbered (79). The total chromosome number is followed by the sex chromosomes, and gains and losses of whole chromosomes are identified by a "+" or a "−" before the chromosome number. A gain or loss of part of a chromosome is identified by a "+" or a "−" after the chromosome arm that is involved; "p" and "q" represent the short and the long arms, respectively. Translocations are indicated by "t" with the chromosomes involved noted in the first set of brackets and the breakpoints in the second set (Table 7.1). Other abnormalities will be defined when they are first described, and our discussion will be restricted to clonal abnormalities that are defined as at least two cells with the same extra chromosome or structural rearrangement (identified with banding) or three cells with the same missing chromosome. Banding of chromosomes is essential to cytogenetic investigations, because it allows the identification of individual chromosomes. A band is defined as a chromosome area that is distinguished from adjacent segments by appearing darker or lighter through one or more banding techniques. Various banding methods are currently used, including quinacrine-mustard (Q bands) and Giemsa stain (G bands).

Two new molecular cytogenetic techniques have proven to be particularly powerful in the identification of genetic alterations associated with hematologic malignancies and solid tumors; fluorescence in situ hybridization (FISH), and comparative genomic hybridization (CGH) (84, 148, 149, 163, 184). FISH is a technique in which the appropriate DNA

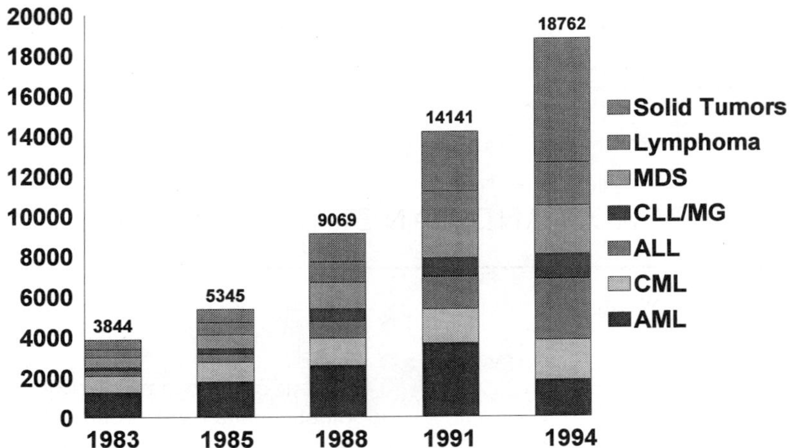

Figure 7.1. The proportion of abnormal karyotypes in the four Mitelman catalogs by disease type. The number in parentheses below the date is the total number of abnormal karyotypes in each addition. Chronic myelogenous leukemia (CML) patients with only a t(9;22) are not included. ALL, acute lymphocytic leukemia; ANLL, acute nonlymphocytic leukemia; CLL/MG, chronic lymphocytic leukemia/MG, monoclonal grammopathy; MDS, myelodysplastic syndrome.

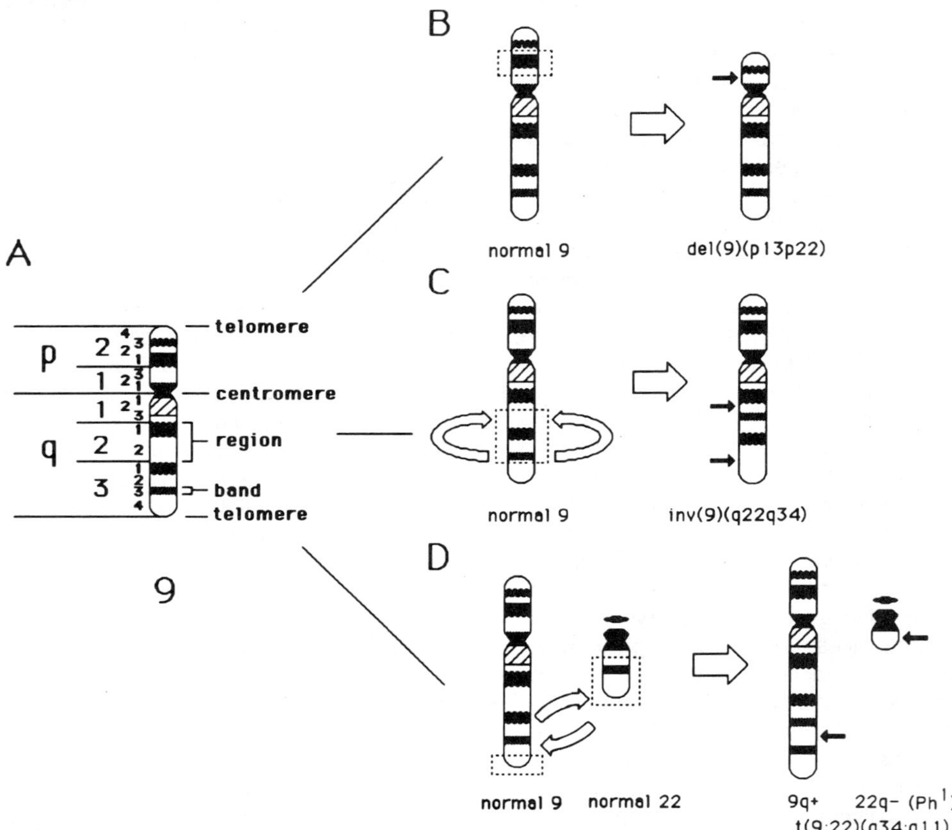

Figure 7.2. A normal chromosome and three chromosomal abnormalities observed in human neoplasms. **A.** The banding pattern of a normal chromosome 9. The chromosome arms (p, short arm; q, long arm), regions, band numbers are indicated on the left of the chromosome; specific chromosome structures are indicated on the right of the chromosome. **B.** The mechanism of an interstitial deletion of the short arm of chromosome 9, a common abnormality in acute lymphoblastic leukemia. Chromosome breaks occur in bands 9p13 and 9p22, the intervening chromosomal segment (band 9p21 and parts of bands 9p13 and 9p22) is lost [del (9)(p13p22)]. **C.** The mechanism of a paracentric inversion. Chromosome breaks occur in two bands within a single chromosome arm, in this case within 9p22 and 9q34. The intervening segment is inverted, and the chromosome breaks are repaired [inv (9)(q22q34)]. **D.** The mechanism of reciprocal translocation involving chromosomes 9 and 22, t(9;22)(q34;q11), which gives rise to the Philadelphia (Ph^1) chromosome in the malignant cells of patients with chronic myelogenous leukemia. Breaks occur in bands q34 and q11 of chromosomes 9 and 22, respectively, followed by a reciprocal exchange of chromosomal material. This rearrangement results in the translocation of the *ABL* oncogene, normally located at 9q34, adjacent to the *BCR* gene on chromosome 22, giving rise to a chimeric *BCR-ABL* gene, whose protein product plays a role in the transformation of myeloid cells. *Source*: Modified from Le Beau and Rowley (105).

Table 7.1*A*. Glossary of Cytogenetic Terminology

Centromere	The constriction along the length of the chromosome that is the site of the spindle fiber attachment. The position of the centromere determines whether chromosomes are metacentric (X-shaped, e.g., chromosomes 1, 3, 16, 19, 20) or acrocentric (inverted V-shaped, e.g., chromosomes 13–15, 21, 22, Y). During mitosis, the two exact copies of the DNA in each chromosome are separated by shortening of the spindle fibers attached to opposite sides of the dividing cell
Karyotype	Arrangement of chromosomes from a particular cell according to a well-established system such that the largest chromosomes are first and the smallest ones last. See Figure 7.5. Normal female karyotype is 46,XX; normal male karyotype is 46,XY
Translocation	A break in at least two chromosomes with exchange of material; in a reciprocal translocation, there is no obvious loss of chromosomal material. See Figure 7.5
Deletion	A segment of a chromosome is missing as the result of two breaks and loss of the intervening piece. See Figure 7.2
Inversion	Two breaks occur in the same chromosome, with rotation of the intervening segment. If both the breaks are on the same side of the centromere, it is called a paracentric inversion. If they are on opposite sides, it is called a pericentric inversion. See Figure 7.2.
Isochromosome	A chromosome that consists of identical copies of one chromosome arm with loss of the other arm. Thus, an isochromosome for the long arm of chromosome-17 [i(17q)] contains two copies of the long arm (separated by the centromere), with loss of the short arm of the chromosome
Clone	In the cytogenetic sense, this is defined as two cells with the same additional or structurally rearranged chromosome or three cells with loss of the same chromosome
Diploid	Normal chromosome number and composition of chromosomes
Hyperdiploid	Additional chromosomes; therefore, the modal number is 47 or greater
Hypodiploid	Loss of chromosomes with modal number 45 or less
Haploid	Only one-half the normal complement (i.e., 23 chromosomes)

Table 7.1*B*. Karyotype Symbols

p	Short arm
q	Long arm
+	If before the chromosome, indicates a gain of a whole chromosome (e.g., +8); if after the chromosome indicates gain of part of the chromosome (e.g., 14q+, added material at the end of the long arm of chromosome 14)
−	If before the chromosome indicates a loss of a whole chromosome (e.g., −7); if after the chromosome, indicates loss of part of the chromosome (e.q., 5q−, loss of part of the long arm of chrcmosome 5)
?	Indicates uncertainty about the identity of the chromosome or band listed just after the ?
t	Translocation
del	Deletion
inv	Inversion
i	Isochromosome

probes are labeled with various fluorochromes (e.g., rhodamine) that are detected by fluorescence microscopy. A large number of chromosome-specific centromere probes are now available that unequivocally mark a pair of chromosomes. Using these probes, gains or losses of chromosomes can be detected not only in metaphase chromosomes but also in interphase cells (Fig. 7.3). Large-size DNA probes that contain specific genes or anonymous DNA sequences (e.g., yeast artificial chromosomes P1 or cosmids) can be used to screen for recurring translocations and to identify those probes that are split by the translocation breakpoints. Currently this technique is widely used by many groups in their search for genes involved in different translocations (163). CGH is a new in situ hybridization-based procedure to detect and map relative gene copy aberrations (both gains and losses) in the tumor genome onto normal metaphase chromosomes (84). This technique is powerful, because it does not require advanced knowledge of the existence or genetic location of altered copy-number regions or cell culture, thereby eliminating the possibility of subpopulation selection during the culture. Changes in relative gene copy number detected using CGH may be associated with oncogene amplification or loss of tumor-suppressor gene function.

To be relevant to the malignant disease, chromosomes for analysis must be obtained from the tumor cells. Thus, for leukemia, bone marrow cells or peripheral blood cells processed directly or after 24- to 72-hour culture are used; lymph nodes or solid tumors are minced to yield a single cell suspension that can be harvested immediately or cultured for a short period of time. The cells are exposed to a hypotonic solution, fixed, and stained according to a variety of protocols (101, 106). Combined with a brief exposure to mitotic inhibitors such as colchicine or use of DNA-binding agents to elongate chromosomes, use of amethopterin or fluorodeoxyuridine to synchronize cells has resulted in longer chromosomes that have an increased number of bands as well as improved morphology. The addition of PHA-stimulated conditioned medium or recombinant colony-stimulating factors to the culture medium also has con-

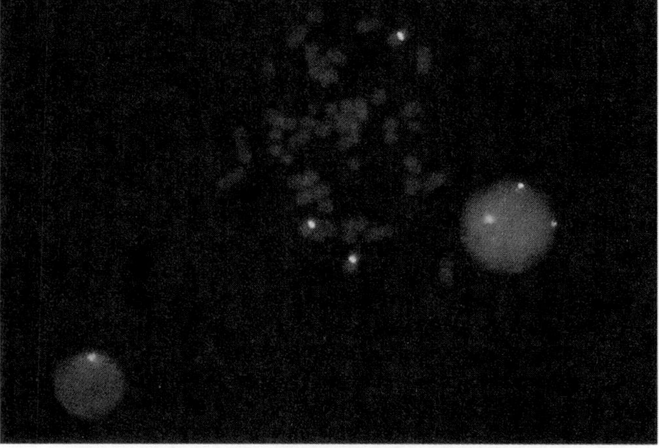

Figure 7.3. In situ hybridization with biotinylated DNA probe to chromosome 8 centromere demonstrates three copies of chromosome 8 in a metaphase and an interphase cell. The probe was detected with fluoresceinated avidin (yellow) and the cells were counterstained with propidium iodide (red). Magnification × 1,000.

tributed to the increased rate of successful cytogenetic analysis of different tumors. Cytogenetic analysis requires specimens that contain viable dividing cells; therefore, specimens should be transported without delay to the cytogenetics laboratory in a suitable culture medium at room temperature.

Myeloproliferative Disorders

CHRONIC MYELOID LEUKEMIA

The first consistent chromosome abnormality in any malignant disease was the Philadelphia or Ph^1 chromosome (now called the Ph chromosome) identified in chronic myeloid leukemia (CML) (134). This abnormality was thought to be a deletion of chromosome 22 (22q–) but was later shown to be a translocation involving chromosome 9 and 22 [t (9;22)(q34;q11)] (Fig. 7.2) (159).

The Philadelphia chromosome occurs in a pluripotential stem cell that gives rise to cells of both lymphoid and myeloid lineage. The karyotypes of many Ph+ patients with CML have been examined with banding techniques by a number of investigators. In a review of 1129 Ph+ patients, the 9;22 translocation was identified in 1036 (92%) (160). The remaining patients had variant translocations. One appeared to be a simple translocation involving chromosome 22 and some chromosome other than 9 (approximately 4% of patients), and the other was a complex translocation involving at least three or more different chromosomes, including chromosomes 9 and 22 (approximately 4%). Recent data clearly demonstrate that chromosome 9 is affected in the simple as well as the complex translocations and that its involvement in simple translocations initially had been overlooked. Virtually all chromosomes have been involved in these variant translocations, but chromosome 17 is affected more often than any other. Other studies with fluorescence markers or chromosome polymorphisms have shown that in a particular patient, the same chromosomes 9 and 22 are involved in each cell (160). The reciprocal nature of the translocation was established in 1982, when the Abelson proto-oncogene, *ABL*, which is normally on chromosome 9, was identified on the Ph chromosome (45, 46, 173). This ultimately led to cloning of the breakpoint involved in the t(9;22) (71). The site on the Ph chromosome was called *bcr*, for *b*reakpoint *c*luster *r*egion, which in the majority of translocations cluster in a small, 5.8 kb region (71). In contrast, the breaks on chromosome 9 occur over an incredible distance of more than 200 kb (167). The genetic consequences of the standard t(9;22) or the complex translocation involving at least three chromosomes is to move the *ABL* proto-oncogene on chromosome 9 next to a gene on chromosome 22, called *BCR*, whose function has recently been elucidated (Fig. 7.4) (206). The appearance of new abnormalities in the karyotype of a patient with CML often signals a change in the pace of the disease, usually to a more aggressive disorder. When patients with CML enter the terminal acute phase, approximately 10 to 20% appear to retain the chromosome 46, Ph-cell line unchanged; however, most patients show additional chromosomal abnormalities, which result in cells with modal chromosome numbers of 47 to 50 (160). During the acute phase of CML, different chromosomal abnormalities occur either singly or in combination, in a distinctly nonrandom pattern. In patients with only a single new chromosome change, this most commonly involves a second Ph chromosome, an isochromosome for the long arm of chromosome 17 [i(17q)], or a +8, in descending order of frequency. Chromosome loss is rare, but when it happens, a −7 is seen, which occurs in 3% of patients (160).

Marrow cells from some patients who appear to have CML

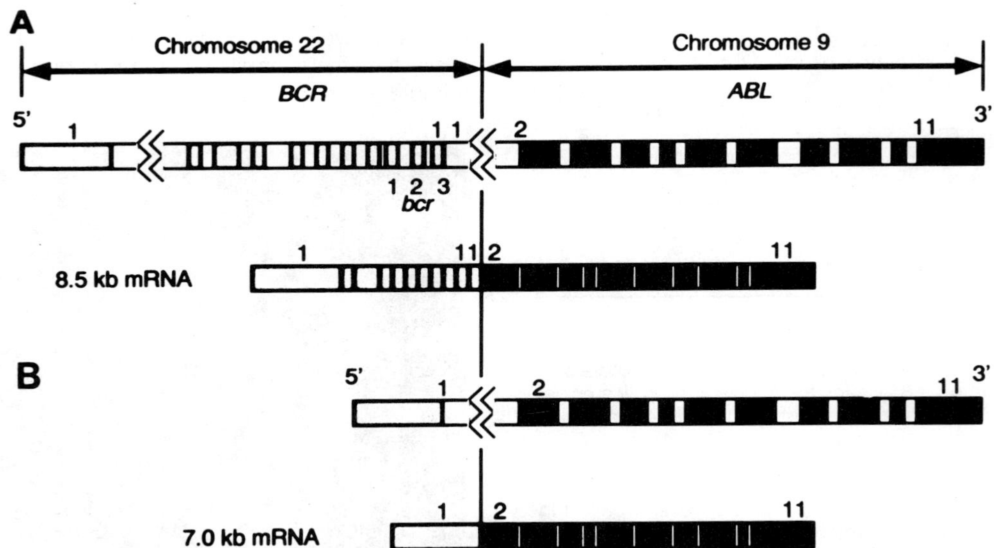

Figure 7.4. **A.** Map of the *BCR-ABL* fusion gene in chronic myeloid leukemia (CML) and in some adult acute lymphocytic leukemia (ALL) patients. In this example, the breakpoint has occurred between the third and fourth exons included in the bcr region, which are equivalent to exons 11 and 121 in the *BCR* gene. The chimeric mRNA is diagrammed below the gene. **B.** Map of the fusion gene in some patients with ALL showing the breakpoint in the first intron of *BCR*. The breakpoint in *ABL* is identical with that in CML in this example. Only one *BCR* exon is included so that the mRNA is much smaller than in CML.

on both clinical and morphologic grounds lack a Ph chromosome. Most of these patients had a normal karyotype and somewhat surprisingly, their survival was substantially shorter than those whose cells were Ph+ (203). Reviews of two series of such patients showed they did not have CML but rather some type of myelodysplasia, most commonly chronic myelomonocytic leukemia or refractory anemia with excess blasts, leading to their shorter survival (127, 150, 185). The situation has become more complex, however, because molecular analysis has shown that some patients with clinically typical CML who lack a Ph chromosome cytogenetically have evidence for the insertion of *ABL* sequences into the *BCR* gene (10, 127). Thus, it can be proposed that the sine qua non of CML is the juxtaposition of *BCR* and *ABL* with the formation of a fusion transcript *BCR-ABL* (43, 174). Several research groups are working to unravel the genetic consequences of the Ph chromosome (66, 206).

ACUTE MYELOID LEUKEMIA DE NOVO

At present, at least 80% of patients with acute myeloid leukemia (AML) have an abnormal karyotype. The most frequent abnormalities are a gain of chromosome 8 or a loss of chromosome 7, which are seen in most subtypes of AML (59, 160, 166, 169). Specific rearrangements are closely associated with particular subtypes of AML as defined by the French-American-British Cooperative Group (14) (FAB classification) (Figs. 7.5 and 7.6). The chromosomal abnormalities associated with each subtype and their frequency are summarized in Table 7.2*A* and 7.2*B*.

A translocation between chromosomes 8 and 21 [t (8;21)(q22;q22)] was first identified in 1972, and this was the first translocation to be discovered (Fig. 7.5) (161). The translocation is seen primarily in patients with AML-M2 (acute myeloblastic leukemia with maturation). Approximately 20% of all patients with AML-M2 have a t(8;21), and the t(8;21) is the most frequent abnormality in children with AML (160). Chromosomes 8 and 21 can participate in three-way rearrangements similar to those involving chromosomes 9 and 22 in CML. Moreover, the t(8;21) often is accompanied by the loss of a sex chromosome; among the cases reviewed at the Fourth International Workshop on Chromosomes in Leukemia (IWCL), 28 of 33 males (85%) were −Y and 8 of 12 females (67%) were −X. This association is particularly noteworthy, because sex chromosome abnormalities otherwise are rarely observed in AML. Recently, it has been shown that the gene for the receptor for *CSF2* (formerly *GMCSF*) is located in the pseudoautosomal region of the short arm of the X chromosome (70). It is possible that loss of this receptor is an important factor leading to the loss of an X or Y chromosome in this subtype of leukemia. The molecular consequences of this translocation have been intensely investigated, and the translocation breakpoint recently has been cloned. A novel gene *AML1* on chromosome 21 was found to be rearranged in leukemic cells of patients with a t(8;21) (126). The gene on chromosome 8 is the *ETO* or *MTG8* gene

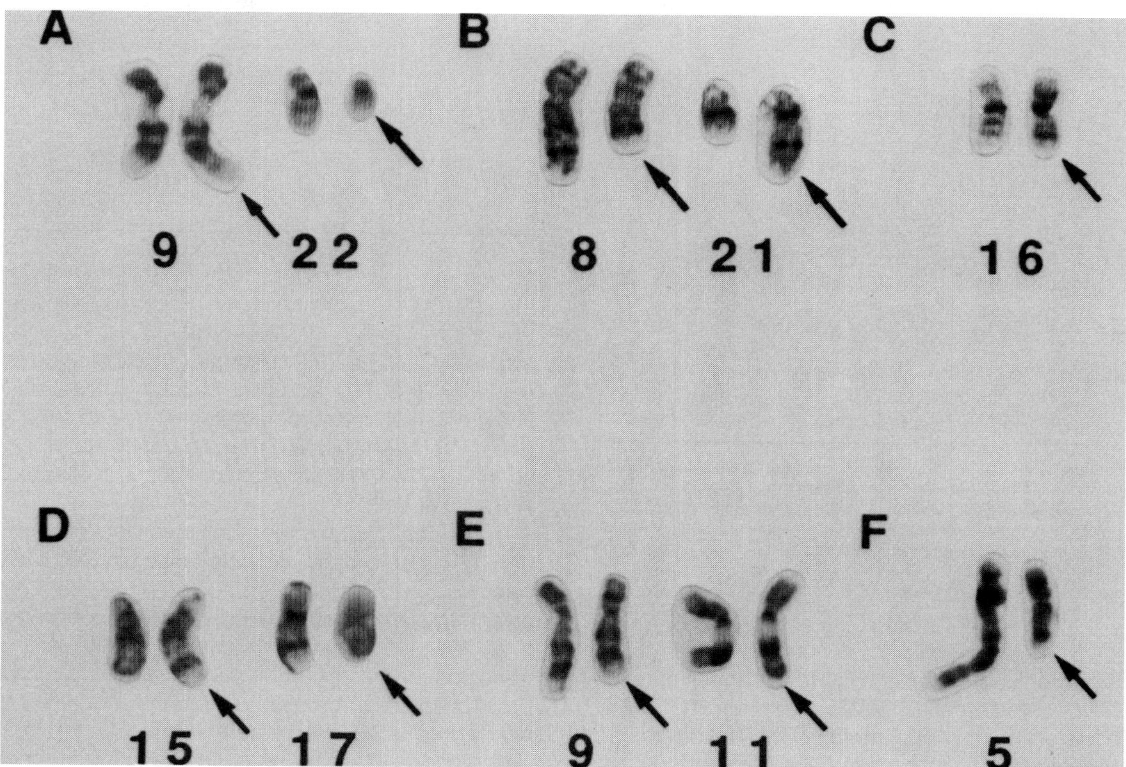

Figure 7.5. Partial karyotypes from trypsin-Giemsa-banded metaphase cells depicting nonrandom chromosomal rearrangements observed in myeloid malignant diseases. Rearranged chromosomes are identified with *arrowheads*. **A.** t(9;22)(q34;q11), chronic myelogenous leukemia. **B.** t(8;21)(q22;q22), acute myelomonocytic leukemia-M4E-M2. **C.** inv(16)(p13q22), AMMoL-M4Eo. **D.** t(15;17)(q22;q11–12), acute promyelocytic leukemia. **E.** t(9;11)(p22;q23). **F.** del(5)(q13q33), t-acute nonlymphocytic leukemia (t-ANLL).

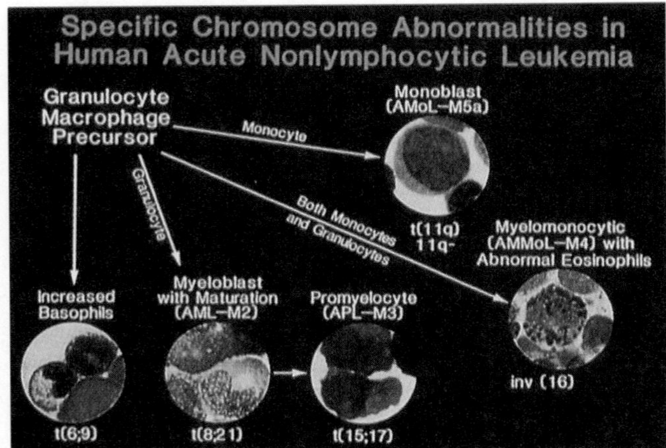

Figure 7.6. Specific chromosomal abnormalities associated with specific types of human acute nonlymphocytic leukemia.

Table 7.2A. Nonrandom Chromosomal Abnormalities in Malignant Myeloid Diseases

Disease[a]	Chromosomal abnormality[b]	Patients (%)
CML	t(9;22)(q34;q11)	~100
CML blast phase	t(9;22)(q34;q11) with +8, +Ph, +19, or i(17q)	~70
AML-M2	t(8;21)(q22;q22)	20
APL-M3,M3V	t(15;17)(q22;q11-12)	60–100
AMMoL-M4Eo	inv(16)(p13q22) or t(16;16)(p13;q22)	25 of M4
AMMo9L-M4	del(11)(q23)	35
	t(10;11)(p11-p15;q24)	
	t(11;17)(q23;q25)	
	t(11;19)(q23;p13)	
	t(11q13 or q23), del(11)(q23)	
AMoL-M5	t(9;11)(p22;q23), t(11q13 or q23)	~30
AML	+8	13
	−7	9
	−5 or del(5q)	6
M2/M4 (including basophils)	del(20q)	5
	t(12p) or del(12p)	2
	t(3;21)(q26;q22)	1
	t(6;9)(p23;q34)	2
M4 (including platelets)	t(3;3)(q21;q26) or inv(3)(q21q26)	2
Therapy-related AML	−7 or del(7q) and/or −5 or del(5q)	90
	der(1)t(1;7)(p11;p11)	2
	t(9;11)(p22;q23)	<1

[a] AML—acute myelogenous leukemia; AML-M2—acute myelogenous leukemia with maturation; AMMoL—acute myelomonocytic leukemia; AMMoL-M4Eo—acute myelomonocytic leukemia with abnormal eosinophils; AMoL—acute monoblastic leukemia; APL-M3,M3V—hypergranular (M3) and microgranular (M3V) acute promyelocytic leukemia; CML—chronic myelogenous leukemia.
[b] Literature references are given in LeBeau and Larson and Bloomfield, Trent and Van den Berghe.

Table 7.2B. Recurring Structural Rearrangements in Malignant Myeloid Diseases

Disease	Chromosomal abnormality	Involved genes
Chronic myeloid leukemia (CML)	t(9;22)(q34;q11)	*ABL-BCR*
CML blast phase	t(9;22) +8, +Ph, i(17q)	*ABL-BCR*
Chronic myelomonocytic leukemia	t(5;12)(q33;p13)	*PDGFRB-TEL*
Acute myeloid leukemia (AML)		
AML-M2	t(8;21)(q22;q22)	*ETO-AML1*
APL-M3, M3V	t(15;17)(q22;q12)	*PML-RARA*
Atypical APL	t(11;17)(q23;q12)	*PLZF-RARA*
AMMoL-M4Eo	inv(16)(p13q22) or t(16;16)(p13;q22)	*MYH11-CBFB*
AMMoL-M4/AMoL-M5	t(6;11)(q27;q23)	*AF6-MLL*
	t(9;11)(p22;q23)	*AF9-MLL*
	t(10;11)(p13;q14)	
	t(10;11)(p11-p15;q23)	*AF10-MLL*
	t(11;17)(q23;q25)	*MLL-AF17*
	t(11;19)(q23;p13.1)	*MLL-ELL*
	Other t(11q23)	*MLL*
AMegL-M7	t(1;22)(p13;q13)	
AML	t(3;3)(q21;q26) or inv(3)(q21q26)	*RPN1-EVI1*
	t(3;5)(q21;q31)	
	t(3;5)(q25;q34)	
	t(6;9)(p23;q34)	*DEK-CAN*
	t(7;11)(p15;p15)	
	t(8;16)(p11;p13)	
	t(9;12)(q34;p13)	*TEL-ABL*
	t(12;22)(p13;q13)	*TEL-NM1*
	t(16;21)(p11;q22)	*TLS(FUS)-ERG*
	−7 or del(7q)	
	−5 or del(5q)	
	del(20q)	
	del(12p)	*TEL*, ?p27^{KIP1}
Therapy-related AML	−7 or del(7q) and/or −5 or del(5q)	*IRF1?*
	t(11q23)	*MLL*
	t(3;21)(q26;q22)	*EAP/MDS1/EVI1-AML1*

(53, 125). The translocation results in the juxtaposition of 5′ *AML1* and 3′ *ETO* (also called *MTG8*), leading to a fusion gene and a fusion or chimeric protein. The critical fusion gene on the derivative (8) chromosome is transcribed from telomere to centromere. The *AML1* gene also is involved in other translocations, including the t(3;21), in which it is fused with several genes, including *EAP*, *MDSI*, and *EVI1* (135). With the availability of DNA probes and, especially, use of the reverse transcriptase-polymerase chain reaction (RT-PCR), it has been possible to detect the fusion transcript in all patients with a t(8;21) both at diagnosis and in long-term remission (135). In addition, patients whose leukemic cells show the typical morphologic features of t(8;21) cells but have a normal karyotype may be positive for the fusion transcript on RT-PCR. This situation thus is similar to Ph−, *BCR-ABL*+ CML (135).

A structural rearrangement involving chromosomes 15 and 17 in acute promyelocytic leukemia (APL) was first recognized in 1977 [t(15;17)(q22;q12)] (Fig. 7.5) (164). This rearrangement is unique to APL, or to the hypogranular variant. It is clear that all patients with APL have a t(15;17). The translocation has been cloned. In addition, the gene at the breakpoint on chromosome 17 is the α chain of the retinoic acid receptor (*RARA*), whereas that on chromosome 15 is called *PML* (48, 67). The critical junction is located on the der(15) chromosome, and it consists of the 5′ portion of *PML* fused to virtually all of the *RARA* gene (9). The fusion protein contains the DNA-binding portion of *RARA* as well as the retinoic acid response domain. It binds to a different receptor, RXR rather than RAR, and it does not respond to retinoic acid, which in normal cells leads to maturation of promyelocytes. Earlier studies from China, however, using all-*trans*-retinoic acid (ATRA) to treat patients showed that those with APL responded and entered complete remission. Even so, use of ATRA leads to remissions that may be short lived, so it needs to be combined with cytotoxic drugs. The fusion transcript can be detected with RT-PCR (67).

The close association of translocations or less often, deletions, of the long arm of chromosome 11 (11q) and acute monoblastic leukemia (M5) was first observed by Berger and colleagues (15). Abnormalities of 11q most frequently occurred in children with monoblastic leukemia and less often in adults with monoblastic leukemia. Moreover, approximately 60% of AML cases and almost 80% of ALL cases involving infants under 1 year of age with leukemia involve chromosome band 11q23 (35). The leukemias with 11q23 translocations involve both the myeloid and the lymphoid lineages. The most common translocations in AML are t(9;11), t(6;11), and t(11;19)(q23;p13.1); in ALL, they are t(4;11) and t(11;19)(q23;p13.3). These same translocations are seen in leukemias that develop in patients with a primary cancer who previously received treatment with drugs targeting topoisomerase II (162).

The gene involved in virtually all 11q23 translocations has been cloned and is called *MLL* for *m*yeloid-*l*ymphoid *l*eukemia (161). The *MLL* gene contains regions of homology to the *Drosophila trithorax* gene, especially in the zinc finger region and the most 3′ segment of the gene; consequently, it is also called *Htrx*, *HRX*, or *ALL1* (50, 73, 183). The *MLL* gene is involved with at least 25 other genes, because there are at least 25 different translocations in both myeloid and lymphoid leukemia. The breakpoint in *MLL* for virtually all patients occurs in an 8.3-kb breakpoint cluster region just 5′ of the zinc fingers; the conserved junction is on the der(11) chromosome (162, 179). Eleven translocation junctions have been cloned, and all lead to fusion genes that consist of 5′ MLL and the 3′ partner gene (162). The partner genes have different motifs, although several have serine- and proline-rich segments that are typical of activation domains. The function of neither *MLL* nor any partner gene is known at present. The clustering of the breaks in *MLL* makes it possible to use a single cDNA probe spanning the breakpoint and a single restriction-enzyme digest to detect the rearrangement on Southern blot analysis in virtually any patient (179). For the common breakpoints in which the other partner chromosome has been cloned, one can also use RT-PCR (208).

Another clinical-cytogenetic association that has been identified involves myelomonocytic leukemia with eosinophils that have unique morphologic changes (M4EO). These patients were first identified as having a del(16)(q22) and an excess of eosinophils. Knight and colleagues (88) described a series of 33 patients, most of whom had M4 leukemia with eosinophils that had large and irregular basophilic granules, a third of these patients lacked increased eosinophils, because the marrow had fewer than 5% eosinophils. Twenty-seven patients had an inversion of chromosome 16, inv(16)(p13q22), and 6 patients had a t(16;16)(p13;q22). The strong correlation between abnormal eosinophils and structural rearrangements of chromosome 16 was confirmed at the Fourth IWCL (59). In fact, the morphologic features of the eosinophils are so specific that pathologists can accurately predict which patients will have an inv(16) or a t(16;16) by examining the bone marrow aspirate. This chromosomal abnormality, which is present in approximately 25% of patients with AMMoL M4, has clinical implications as well. Among 32 patients treated by Larson and colleagues (95, 96), 78% achieved a complete remission, compared with 36% of 58 other patients with AMMoL. The median survival time was more than 65 weeks for patients with abnormal chromosome 16, compared with 29 weeks for those with a normal chromosome 16.

The recently identified gene at 16q22 is core binding factor-beta (*CBFB*), and that at 16p13 is one of the myosin heavy-chain genes (*MYH11*) (111). Both genes are transcribed from centromere to telomere. In both the inversion and translocation, the critical genetic event is the fusion of the 5′ part of *CBFB* with the 3′ part of the *MYH11* gene. It is astonishing that CBFB forms a heterodimer with CBFA, another name for the *AML1* gene involved in the t(8;21). Presumably, the CBFB protein increases the efficiency of the DNA binding of CBFA and its stability. In the inv(16), *CBFB* is fused to *MYH11*, which also has a dimerization motif. The chimeric CBFB binds to CBFA, but it has an additional dimerization partner at the C terminus, binding to *MYH11*. The breakpoints in both *CBFB* and *MYH11* are variable, but with the appropriate DNA primers, the inversion or translocation can be detected in virtually every patient using RT-PCR (36).

A unique feature of abnormalities involving the long arm of chromosome 3 [inv(3)(q21q26) or t(3;3)(q21;q26)] is the high frequency of platelet counts above 100×10^9/L (100,000/μL), and sometimes even over $1{,}000 \times 10^9$/L. A consistent finding in bone marrow is an increased number of megakaryocytes, especially micromegakaryocytes (21). This breakpoint also has been cloned, and the consequences of these rearrangements appear to differ from those of all other translocations in myeloid leukemias in that it does not result in a fusion transcript. The gene at 3q26 is *EVI1* (ecotropic viral insertion site). It is not normally expressed in myeloid cells but rather binds to the GATA1 site in the globin promoter and leads to red cell maturation. The gene at 3q21 is riboforin (*RBN1*) (176). In the translocation, *RBN1* is moved 5′ of *EVI1*, whereas in the inversion, it is 3′ of *EVI1*. In both rearrangements, the transcriptional orientation of *RBN1* is toward *EVI1* and it appears to activate transcription of *EVI1* inappropriately. This situation is similar to that in the mouse, from which *EVI1* was first cloned, because the integration of an ecotropic virus leads to *EVI1* expression and, ultimately, leukemia. Also, of note, *EVI1* inhibits the differentiation of myeloid cells.

Gains and losses of a part of or whole chromosomes frequently occur in AML, both as solitary changes usually found at diagnosis or as additions in later disease stages. Most of the structural rearrangements occur in younger patients, with a median age in the thirties, whereas some of the numeric abnormalities, such as −5 or loss of the long arm [del(5q)] or −7 or del(7q), occur in patients with a median age of over 50. Many of these latter patients have a history of working in environments that might have exposed them to mutagenic agents such as chemicals that include solvents, petroleum products, or pesticides (69, 123). Secondary chromosome changes, such as del(20q), del(9q), and i(17q), occur in AML and also are associated with other diseases, and these changes sometimes are found as the sole aberrations. Most patients with del(9q) as a secondary abnormality had a t(8;21) initially. At the Fourth IWCL (59), it was clearly shown that the type rather than the presence of a chromosomal abnormality had prognostic importance. Follow-up of 66 long-term survivors of the 711 initial Workshop patients showed that those with an inv(16) and a del(7q) as the sole anomaly had a survival rate at 11 years of 30 to 40%; those with a t(15;17), t(8 21), or a normal karyotype had a survival rate of between 10 and 20% (178).

OTHER MYELOPROLIFERATIVE DISEASES

In polycythemia vera, an abnormal clone is present in 14% of untreated patients. This number increases to 39% in treated patients (160, 169). The malignant marrow cells frequently contain additional chromosomes, +8 or +9; the two abnormalities also may occur together. In addition, del(20q) and duplication of the long arm of chromosome 1 are seen in 20 and 30% of patients, respectively. The presence of chromosomal abnormalities at diagnosis is not predictive of clinical outcome, but a change in karyotype, as with CML, is an ominous sign (160, 169). In the terminal leukemic phase, −7 (20% of patients) and del(5q) (40%) have been observed. It is not clear whether these abnormalities relate to the therapy these patients may have received.

Approximately one-third of patients with agnogenic myeloid metaplasia have clonal abnormalities, commonly −7, +8, del(11q), or del(20q) (75, 169).

ACUTE MYELOID LEUKEMIA AND MYELODYSPLASTIC SYNDROME ASSOCIATED WITH PRIOR CYTOTOXIC THERAPY

One of the most serious consequences from successful treatment of a prior malignant disease is the occurrence of treatment-related myelodysplasia (t-MDS) or acute leukemia (t-AML) (3, 102, 146, 165). These patients have two different patterns of chromosomal abnormality, which are related to the type(s) of initial cytotoxic therapy. Patients who received alkylating agents, with or without radiation, often have MDS preceding AML, which on average occurs approximately 4 years after the start of therapy, and they show loss of chromosomes 5 and/or 7 or deletion of the long arm of chromosome 5 or 7. These patients often have very abnormal karyotypes, with deletions of 12p, 17p, and 20q. The response of these patients to antileukemic therapy often is very poor. A case of therapy-related leukemia with a t(15;17) has now been reported. In contrast, with the increasing use of drugs that target topoisomerase II, such as the epipodophyllotoxins or anthracyclines, patients have balanced translocations, usually involving the *MLL* gene at 11q23 or, less often, the *AML1* gene at 21q22 (146). These leukemias may occur within less than a year of the beginning of therapy, lack an MDS phase, and often respond well to chemotherapy (146).

PRIMARY MYELODYSPLASTIC SYNDROME

Clonal chromosomal abnormalities have now been reported in more than 700 patients with MDS, 40 to 79% of whom have clonal abnormalities at diagnosis (75, 169). The common chromosomal abnormalities, +8, −5/del(5q), −7/del(7q), and del(20q), are similar to those seen in AML de novo; however in a review of 247 patients at the Sixth IWCL (63), none had t(8;21), t(15;17), t(9;22), t(9;11), or inv(16). This suggests that patients with the specific types of AML that are associated with these abnormalities exhibit a preleukemic phase of their disease only rarely. In general, unlike AML, the chromosomal changes do not show a close association with the specific subtypes of myelodysplastic syndrome; patients with complex karyotypes and abnormalities of chromosomes 5 and/or 7 have a poor prognosis (102). The exception is the "5q-" syndrome in which there is an interstitial deletion of the long arm of 5. The syndrome occurs in a subset of older patients, frequently women, with refractory macrocytic anemia, generally low blast counts, and normal or elevated platelet counts (75, 169). A number of growth factors and growth factor receptors have been localized to this region on chromosome 5q. Presumably, this region harbors a leukemia-suppressor gene, the search for which has been pioneered by members of our group (104, 105).

Malignant Lymphoproliferative Diseases

The chromosomal abnormalities in lymphoid disorders, especially in the non-Hodgkin's lymphomas have been reviewed in considerable detail elsewhere (57, 62, 90, 160, 169). A high proportion of cases of lymphoma (79%) are characterized by recurring clonal chromosomal abnormalities; many of these abnormalities correlate with histologic and immunophenotypic subtypes (Tables 7.3*A* and 7.3*B*). Chromosome band 14q32 is frequently involved in B-cell lymphoma, while T-cell lymphomas are characterized by rearrangements that involve 14q11, 7q35, or 7p15, which are the bands containing the genes for the T-cell receptor α/δ, β, or γ chains, respectively (106). This section reviews the consistent translocations seen in Burkitt's lymphoma, follicular lymphoma, chronic lymphocytic leukemia, B-cell acute lymphocytic leukemia (ALL), and in some T-cell disorders.

LYMPHOMA

In 1972, Manolov and Manolova (114) discovered that the malignant cells of patients with Burkitt's lymphoma had an additional band at the end of the long arm of one chromosome 14 (14q+). In 1976, Zech and colleagues (214) first observed that the end of one chromosome 8 was consistently absent, and they suggested that the missing part was translocated to chromosome 14 [t(8;14)(q24;q32)]. The t(8;14) also has been observed in nonendemic Burkitt's tumors from America, Europe, and Japan. Thus, it is a highly characteristic chromosome anomaly in Burkitt's lymphoma. This translocation also has been observed in other lymphomas, particularly those of the diffuse large-cell type (57).

Table 7.3*A*. Cytogenetic-Immunophenotypic Correlations in Malignant B-Lymphoid Diseases

Phenotype	Chromosome abnormality	Involved genes
Acute lymphoblastic leukemia (ALL)		
Pre-B	t(1;19)(q23;p13)	*PBX1-TCF3(E2A)*
B(SIg+)	t(8;14)(q24;q32)	*MYC-IGH*
	t(8;8)(p12;q24)	*IGK-MYC*
	t(8;22)(q24;q11)	*MYC-IGL*
B or B-myeloid	t(9;22)(q34;q11)	*ABL-BCR*
	t(4;11)(q21;q23)	*AF4-MLL*
	t(11;19)(q23;p13.3)	*MLL-ENL*
Other	50–60 chromosomes	
	t(5;14)(q31;q32)	*IL3-IGH*
	del(9p),t(9p)	*?CDKN2*(p16)
	t(9;12)(q34;p13)	*ABL-TEL*
	t(12;21)(p13;q22)	*TEL-AML1*
	del(12p)	*TEL; ?*$p27^{KIP1}$
	t(12;21)(p13;q22)	*TEL-MN1*
Non-Hodgkin's lymphoma		
Burkitt type	See SIg+ ALL	*MYC-IGH-IGK-IGL*
Follicular	t(14;18)(q32;q21)	*IGH-BCL2*
Mantle cell	t(11;14)(q13;q32)	*CCND1-IGH*
Diffuse large cell	t(3;14)(q27;q32)	*BCL6-IGH*
Chronic lymphocytic leukemia	t(11;14)(q13;q32)	*CCND1-IGH*
	t(14;19)(q32;q13)	*IGH-BCL3*
	t(2;14)(p13;q32)	*IGH*
	t(14q) and/or +12	
	del(13q14)	
Multiple myeloma	t(11;14)(q13;q32)	*CCND1-IGH*

Table 7.3*B*. Cytogenetic-Immunophenotypic Correlations in Malignant T-Lymphoid Diseases

Phenotype	Chromosome abnormality	Involved genes
Acute lymphoblastic leukemia	t(1;14)(p34;q11)	*LCK-TCRD*
	t(1;14)(p32;q11)	*TAL1-TCRA*
	—	$TAL1^{Del}$
	t(8;14)(q24;q11)	*MYC-TCRA*
	inv(14)(q11q32)	*TCRA-IGH*
	t(10;11)(p13;q14)	
	t(10;14)(q24;q11)	*HOX11-TCRA*
	t(11;14)(p15;q11)	*RBTN1-TCRA*
	t(11;14)(p13;q11)	*RBTN2-TCRA*
	t(7;9))(q35;q32)	*TCRB-TAL2*
	t(7;9)(q35;q34)	*TCRB-TAN1*
	t(7;7)(p15;q11)	*TCRG-?*
	t(14;14)(q11;q32)	*TCRA-IGH*
	t(7;14)(q35;q11)	*TCRB-TCRD*
	t(7;14)(p15;q11)	
Non-Hodgkin's lymphoma		
T	see T-cell ALL	
	t(4;16)(q26;p13.1)	*IL2-BCM*
T or B(Ki-1+)	t(2;5)(p23;q35)	*ALK-NPM1*
Chronic lymphocytic leukemia	t(8;14)(q24;q11)	*MYC-TCRA*
	inv(14)(q11q32)	*TCRA/D-IGH*
Adult T-cell leukemia	t(14;14)(q11;q32)	*TCRA-IGH*
	inv(14)(q11q32)	*TCRA/D-IGH*
	+3	

Two other related translocations were later identified in Burkitt's tumors, and all three translocations involve chromosome chromosome 8 with a break in the same band, 8q24. One variant translocation involved chromosome 2 with a break in the short arm [t(2;8)(p12;q24)], and the other involved chromosome 22 with a break in the long arm in band 22q11. All three translocations have been identified in patients with B-cell ALL as well. The translocations result in overexpression of the *MYC* gene which is located on chromosome 8 (2).

Other recurring abnormalities in B-cell lymphoma include the t(14;18)(q32;q21) and the t(11;14)(q13;q32). The t(14;18)(q32;q21) is, in fact, the most common translocation in lymphoma (Fig. 7.7). This translocation was first identified by Fukuhara and colleagues (61) in six of nine patients with poorly differentiated lymphocytic lymphoma, now called "malignant lymphoma, follicular, predominantly small cleaved cell" in the International Classification System (207). The correlation between karyotype and histology in 260 patients was reviewed at the Fifth IWCL (57). Among these patients, 15% had a normal karyotype. The karyotypic pattern varies greatly among the different subgroups. The t(14;18) is common in follicular low-grade lymphomas, whereas the t(8;14) is common in high-grade, small, non-cleaved-cell lymphomas. Occasionally, the t(14;18) is seen in lymphomas with a more aggressive, high-grade histology. Recent data suggest that patients with diffuse large-cell lymphoma and a t(14;18) likely are older and have a poorer prognosis than those without this translocation. Of 102 patients with large-cell lymphoma, 19 had a t(14;18) and a rearrangement of the *BCL2* gene located on chromosome 18. Their median disease-free survival was 33 months, while the median was not yet reached for the other patients without this rearrangement (136). Analysis of the karyotypic pattern in low-grade lymphomas also shows that certain additional chromosome changes, especially a gain of chromosome 7 or a deletion of the long arm of chromosome 6 [(del)6q] appear to correlate with a more aggressive phenotype (90). The translocation has been cloned, and breakpoints cluster in at least two sites on the *BCL2* gene. The major cluster is in the 3′ untranslated region of the third exon (190). In the lymphoma cells, expression of the normal gene is suppressed and an abnormal, chimeric *BCL2-IGH* expressed. This leads to inappropriate expression of a structurally normal protein (37). Analysis of the function of *BCL2* indicates that this gene is involved in programmed cell death (i.e., apoptosis). Its inappropriate expression because of the translocation prevents apoptosis and thus leads to a great increase in the number of B lymphocytes among tissues such as the lymph nodes and spleen (91).

Another recurrent abnormality that recently has been described is the t(2;5)(p23;q35) in Ki-1–positive, anaplastic large-cell lymphoma (20, 86, 103). Patients with this abnormality have unique clinicomorphologic characteristics and a more favorable prognosis compared to other patients with large-cell lymphoma. The genes involved in this translocation are *ALK*, a protein tyrosine kinase at 2p23, and *NPM1* (nuclear phosphoprotein or nuclearphosmin) at 5q35 (128).

More recently, the importance of several other translocations has been appreciated (75, 169). The t(11;14)(q13;q32) has been shown to be associated with 30 to 50% of B-cell lymphomas that are classified as centrocytic or low- to inter-

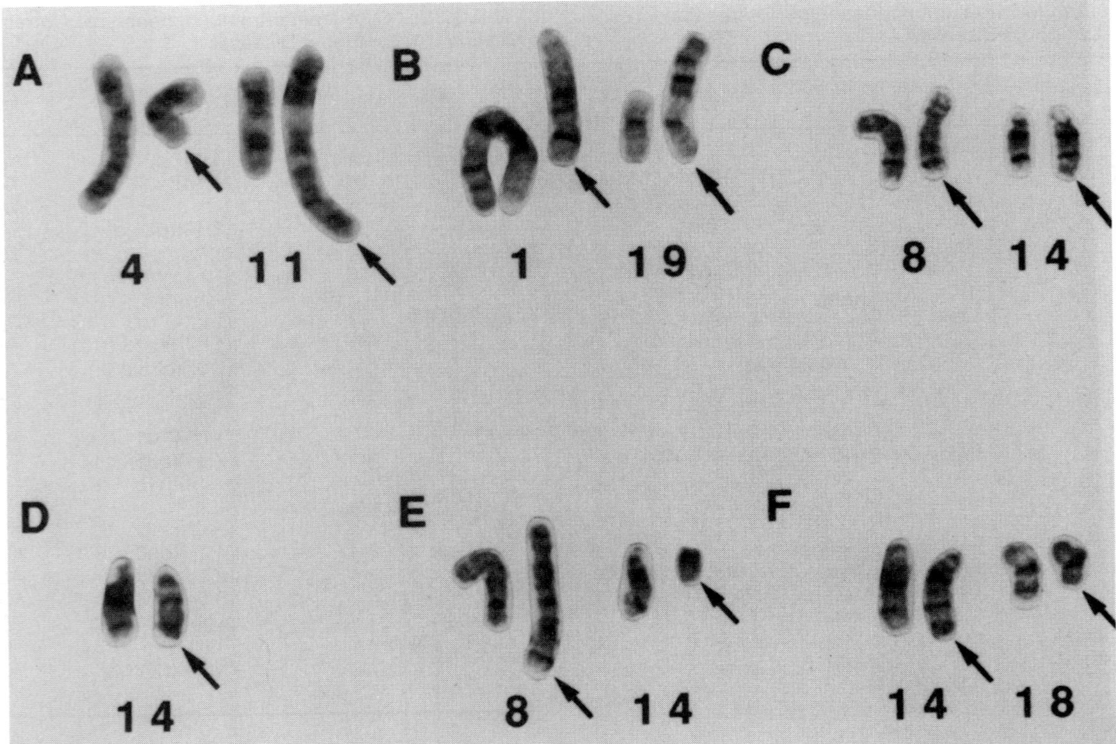

Figure 7.7. Partial karyotypes of trypsin-Giemsa-banded metaphase cells depicting nonrandom chromosomal rearrangements observed in lymphoid malignant diseases. The rearranged chromosomes are identified with *arrowheads*. **A.** t(4;11)(q21;q23), acute lymphocytic leukemia (ALL). **B.** t(1;19)(q21;p13), pre-B cell ALL. **C.** t(8;14)(q24;q32), B-cell ALL and Burkitt's lymphoma. **D.** inv(14)(9q11q32), T-cell leukemia/lymphoma. **E.** t(8;14)(q24;q11), T-cell leukemia/lymphoma. **F.** t(14;18)(q32;q21), B-cell non-Hodgkin's lymphoma. *Source:* Modified from Le Beau and Rowley (105).

mediate-grade lymphoma as well as in B-cell chronic lymphocytic leukemia (CLL) (19, 158). The breakpoint was originally cloned by Tsujimoto and colleagues (191), who called the locus at 11q13 *BCL1*. No gene was identified initially, but several other groups analyzing other genes found that one of the cyclins (*CCND1*), also called *PRAD1* because it was isolated from a parathyroid adenoma breakpoint, was a partner in the translocation (118, 158). One of the most recent breakpoints to be cloned is the t(3;14)(q27;q32) in which *IGH* and a gene called *BCL6* are involved (9). Offit, Chaganti, and their colleagues (137) used the appropriate probes to screen lymphoma samples from 102 patients with diffuse large-cell lymphoma for rearrangements of *BCL2* and *BCL6*. *BCL6* was rearranged in 23 cases, whereas *BCL2* was rearranged in 21 cases. Rearrangements of these two genes had prognostic significance, because over 80% of patients with rearranged *BCL6* and only 30% of those with rearranged *BCL2* were projected to be free of disease progression at 36 months. Thus, in the lymphomas, there are an increasing number of probes that can be used for the detection of these different translocations as well as for monitoring a patient's response to treatment.

CHRONIC LYMPHOCYTIC LEUKEMIA

The early studies of cytogenetic pattern in CLL showed a normal karyotype in most samples. As better culture and banding methods have been applied to these studies, nonrandom clonal abnormalities have been detected. These include translocations involving 14q32, such as the t(11;14)(q13;q32) and t(14;19)(q32;q13), and trisomy for chromosome 12 (19, 75, 156, 169). The gene involved in the t(11;14) is *CCND1* and that involved in the t(14;19) is the *BCL3* gene (137). This proto-oncogene plays a central role in the *NFKB* regulatory pathway (see Chapter 8). In the largest series of patients with CLL, clonal chromosomal changes were observed in 218 of 321 patients who could be examined cytogenetically (82). The most common abnormalities were trisomy 12 (67 patients) and structural abnormalities of chromosome band 13q14 encompassing the *RB1* gene (57 patients) and of chromosome 14 (41 patients). This study showed that patients with normal karyotypes had a median overall survival of more than 15 years, compared with 7.7 years for patients with clonal changes. Patients with 14q aberrations also had a poorer prognosis (82).

Acute Lymphocytic Leukemia

Whereas the correlation of cytogenetic changes with morphology in AML led to identification of the specific associations described previously, this correlation was not useful in ALL, except for the t(8;14) and its variants in L3, B-cell ALL. However, with the widespread use of precise immunophenotyping, the correlation of certain chromosome rearrangements with specific immunologic subsets of ALL has been established (Table 7.3*A*).

ALL is the most frequent leukemia in children. Patients who are between 3 and 7 years of age, with a white-blood-cell (WBC) count of less than 10,000/mL, and whose leukemic cells express the common acute lymphoblastic leukemic antigen (CALLA+ or CD10+), have the best prognosis. The systematic efforts to identify poor-risk groups and then treat them aggressively, however, has continually improved the survival rate in these patients. It was rigorously demonstrated for the first time at the Third IWCL (181) that the karyotype is an important independent prognostic factor in ALL. Of 330 patients reviewed at the Third IWCL, 112 appeared to have a normal karyotype. The largest group (39 patients) with a well-defined abnormality had a Ph chromosome. Eighteen patients had a t(4;11), 16 a t(8;14), and 15 an abnormality of chromosome 14 not involving chromosome 8. Other patients with abnormalities were classified by the modal chromosome number. These patients were reviewed again at the Sixth IWCL (63), and those data confirm both that karyotype group is an independent prognostic factor for disease-free survival in children and that karyotype in combination with presenting WBC and FAB classification can identify groups of children and adults with a markedly different prognosis.

At the Sixth IWCL (63), 29 of 172 adults with ALL (17%) and 9 of 157 children with ALL (6%) had the Ph chromosome, which is the most frequent rearrangement in adult ALL (23, 201). At the cytogenetic level, breakpoints appear to be identical to those in CML; however, recent molecular analysis indicates that the breakpoint in the *BCR* gene on chromosome 22 may be different in some patients with Ph+ALL than in those with CML (45, 160, 201). Thus, in ALL, there are two molecular subtypes of the Ph chromosome. The first is identical to that seen in CML; the translocation breakpoints are within *ABL* and bcr and the same 8.5 kb fusion mRNA and chimeric p210 protein are produced. In the second subtype, the translocation breakpoint is also in *ABL* but not within *bcr*, and the chromosome 22 breakpoint falls upstream of the *bcr*, within the first intron of the *BCR* gene (201). The transcript is a 7.0 kb fusion mRNA, and the chimeric protein is known as the $p185^{BCR\text{-}ABL}$.

Recent data suggest that a protein encoded by sequences within the first exon of *BCR* binds to the *ABL* SH2 domain. This binding is required for activation of the ABL tyrosine kinase and the transforming potential of the *BCR-ABL* chimeric protein (206). The RT-PCR technique has been applied to the diagnosis of CML and ALL. This technique is very sensitive and can detect the presence of the abnormal *BCR-ABL* message in a dilution of 1:100,000 cells. This is useful in determining whether a patient with ALL has minimal residual disease after therapy. In the Sixth IWCL (63), the children with a Ph chromosome had the second highest median leukocyte count (75,000/mL), all were non-B, non-T ALL; and they had a poor median survival of only 15 months. The Ph chromosome also carried a poor prognosis in adult ALL (201). Thus, by identifying this chromosomal abnormality or its molecular equivalent, one can detect individuals with a poor prognosis.

Of 216 patients with chromosomal abnormalities at the Third ICWL (181), 18 (8.3%) had a t(4;11)(q21;q23) rearrangement. Fifty percent of these patients were children, most of whom were less than 1 year old. The association of (4;11) with neonatal or early childhood ALL is particularly interesting in view of the low incidence of all in this age group; acute leukemias in this group usually are of the myeloid type and, as noted earlier, they usually involve the *MLL* gene (162). Children with a t(4;11) had very high leukocyte counts (median WBC, 214,000/mL), which is a poor prognostic factor. Both children and adults with this abnormality had a short median survival of 9 and 7 months, respectively; only patients with abnormalities involving 8q24 or 14q32 had shorter survivals. Although the morphology of some cells often appears to be lymphoid (L1 and L2), other features are more suggestive of a monocytic leukemia (i.e., biphenotypic leukemia). The t(4;11) has been cloned, and the *MLL* gene on 11q23, with a break in the same region as 11q23 translocations in myeloid cells, is juxtaposed to the gene on chromosome 4 called *AF4* (acute leukemia fused to chromosome 4) (73). This translocation can be detected in virtually all patients with t(4;11) by RT-PCR (208). More recently using molecular probes for *MLL* to screen cells from infant leukemias, 78% of patients screened were found to have *MLL* rearrangements, and their survival was substantially shorter than that of infants lacking an *MLL* rearrangement (35). Given the small amount of available material, molecular probes are especially useful for detecting the *MLL* rearrangement in infants.

Another recurring chromosomal abnormality is the t(1;19)(q21;p13) which has been identified in approximately 25% of patients with a pre-B phenotype (cytoplasmic Ig+ and CALLA+) (153). This breakpoint recently has been cloned using the probe for a transcription factor (*E2A*) located on chromosome 19 (119, 151). The translocation involves two genes that bind to DNA; the gene on chromosome 1 is called *PBX*. A fusion gene is formed, and thus, as in Ph+ CML and ALL, it is possible to use PCR techniques to detect abnormal cells. This technique also can be used to detect minimal residual disease following completion of therapy in patients with this translocation.

The leukemic cells of some patients with ALL are characterized by a gain of many chromosomes and fewer structural abnormalities (153, 181). Chromosome numbers usually range from 50 to 60, and a few patients have up to 65 chromosomes (i.e., hyperdiploidy). Although identical karyotypes are unusual, certain additional chromosomes commonly are seen. Among 31 patients with hyperdiploidy at the Third IWCL (14% of patients with abnormalities), +21, +6, +18, +14, +4, and +10 were seen in decreasing frequency in 10 to 33% of patients (181). It is interesting that some of these chromosomes, particularly chromosomes 10, 18, and 21, also are seen as additional chromosomes in patients with near-haploidy, with chromosome numbers of 26 to 36 (median, 28). The median age of the 22 children with a hyperdiploid karyotype was 3 years, while the median age of all 31 patients (5 years) was less than that of patients with other abnormalities. The WBC count was low (median, 6,000/mL). Thus, these patients have all of the previously recognized good prognostic factors, including age between 3 and 7 years, low WBC count, and CALLA+. In a follow-up study of these patients, the complete remission rate for children was 95%, with a median duration of remission that will be greater than 5 years. The median survival of the children with hyperdiploidy is longer than that of children with a normal karyotype; for adults, the median survival of the two groups is comparable. Chromosome losses or deletions are less frequent, and the regions involve 6q, 9p, 11q, and 12p. Deletions of 9p occur in approximately 20% of ALL cases. Homozygous deletions of DNA sequences on 9p which include the *IFN* gene cluster, methylthioadenosine phosphorylase (MTAP), CDKN2 [p16^{INK4A}, MTSI], and *CDKN2B*, have now been described in the majority of ALL cases with 9p loss (49, 51, 142). The three translocations described for Burkitt's lymphoma are seen also in B-cell ALL. Regarding karyotype and age, patients with a deletion of 6q and a modal chromosome number greater than 50 were younger, and those with a Ph chromosome or a 14q+ were older, than patients with other abnormalities. In summary, the highest remission rates were in patients with a normal karyotype and a modal number greater than 50; the lowest rates were seen in patients with a Ph chromosome, 14q+ chromosome, t(8;14), and t(4;11) (23, 63, 153).

T-CELL DISORDERS

Although fewer leukemias of T-cell origin have been studied, a distinct pattern of nonrandom karyotypic abnormalities is emerging. Rearrangements involving the proximal bands of chromosome 14 (14q11-q13) are relatively common, and those involving two regions of chromosome 7 (7q35 and 7p15) also occur in T-cell malignancies but have been observed in nonmalignant T-cell disorders as well. Breaks involving these regions are very rare in other malignant diseases (Table 7.3*B*). One recurring rearrangement in T-cell neoplasia, particularly CLL, is a paracentric inversion of chromosome 14 with a proximal breakpoint at q11 and a distal breakpoint at q32 [inv (14)(q11q32)] (196, 213). A closely related rearrangement, t(14;14)(q11;q32), is seen in T-cell neoplasia and in phytohemagglutinin-stimulated lymphocytes from patients with ataxia-telangiectasia (A-T) as well as in the leukemic cells of A-T patients in whom this disease evolved (5, 83). A number of reports from Japan have described the frequent occurrence of 14q11 breaks in adult patients with T-cell leukemia-lymphoma patients (124, 168). Williams and associates (205) have described a t(11;14)(p13;q13) in the leukemic cells of 4 of 16 patients with T-cell acute lymphoblastic leukemia; the breakpoint was later shown to be 14q11. Data confirm the observation made some time ago that the proximal region of chromosome 14 was important in T-cell neoplasia (32, 83). Analysis of these 14q11 translocations with molecular probes has shown that the T-cell receptor α- or δ-chain (*TCRA* or *D*) locus is involved (40). One of the first translocations to be cloned in T-cell leukemias was the t(8;14)(q24;q11). In this translocation the breakpoint also involves *MYC* at 8q24, but the other gene is *TCRA*. Shima and colleagues (171) have shown that the break in *MYC* is 3′ of the third exon and *MYC* remains on chromosome 8; in *TCRA*, the break is just 5′ of a Jα segment (JαD). This translocation is similar to these involving the immunoglobulin light-chain genes, in which *MYC* also remains on chromosome 8. *TCRA* also is involved with translocations affecting 14q32 and the heavy-chain gene in the inv(14).

Another translocation of special interest is the t(1;14)(p32;q11). The gene at 1p32 has several names, of which *TAL1* is the accepted one (11). The translocation juxtaposes the *TAL1* gene with the *TCRD*, and it occurs in approximately 3% of patients with T-ALL (7). Using probes for *TAL1*, several groups showed that there is a 90-kb deletion involving the 5′ region of the *TAL1* gene in up to 25% of patients (31). *TAL1* is never expressed in lymphoid cells, and the translocation or deletion results in its inappropriate expression in these cells. More recently, analysis of mRNA from T-ALL samples has revealed ectopic expression of *TAL1* in 35% of patients whose cells have neither a translocation or a deletion. Thus, *TAL1* is expressed in over 60% of patients with T-ALL, which makes it a very critical gene in this leukemia (7). More detailed analysis of rearrangements of 7q in T-cell disorders has revealed that some patients have breaks at 7q34 to 7q35, the location of the β-chain for the T-cell receptor (*TCRB*) (151, 154). Rearrangements rarely affect *TCRG* at 7p15.

Solid Tumors

Although solid tumors, carcinomas in particular, play a much larger part in human neoplasia than hematologic malignancies, much less is known about the cytogenetic abnormalities that characterize them. Among the reasons for this discrepancy is first, the difficulty of obtaining successful chromosome preparations from solid tumors because of the extensive fibrosis or necrosis that frequently is associated with these tumors. Second, until recently, many investigators questioned the relevance of the chromosome changes in malignant cells; therefore, this difficult area of research was not pursued. Third, the karyotypes of the tumor cells frequently show high modal numbers, often 60 to 90 chromosomes, with many bizarre marker chromosomes. It, therefore, is difficult to distinguish the primary change from those related to secondary evolution with progression of the malignant phenotype, because most studies have involved highly advanced, often metastatic lesions.

With newer culturing and banding techniques, patterns of relevant and consistent chromosomal rearrangements are emerging. During the last 4 years, the number of reported cytogenetic abnormalities in solid tumors has risen dramatically. A total of 5,870 chromosomal abnormalities have been reported in solid tumors (120) (Table 7.4*A*, Fig.7.1). More-

Table 7.4*A*. Solid Tumors with Chromosome Abnormalities

Epithelial	2,797 (48%)
Germ cell	254 (4%)
Mesenchymal	1,736 (30%)
Neurogenic	895 (15%)
Melanocytic	188 (3%)
Total	5,870 (100%)

Table 7.4*B*. NonRandom Chromosomal Abnormalities in Solid Tumors

Disease	Chromosomal abnormalities
Benign tumors	
Pleomorphic adenomas of the salivary glands	t(3;8)(p21;q12)
Meningioma and acoustic neuroma	Monosomy 22 or del(22q)
Lipoma	t(3;12)(q27-q28;q13-q14)
	Ring chromosome
Ovarian tumors	Trisomy 12
Leiomyoma	t(12;14)(q14-q15;q23-q24)
Adult cancers	
Breast	del(1p)
Colon	del(17p), −18
Small-cell lung carcinoma	del(3)(p14-p23)
Non-small-cell lung cancer	del(9p)
Renal carcinoma	del(3)(p11-p22)
Bladder cancer	i(5p), monosomy 9, del(19q)
Prostate	del(10)(q26)
Liposarcoma	t(12;16)(q13;p11)
Synovial sarcoma	t(X;18)(p11.2;q11.2)
Rhabdomyosarcoma (alveolar)	t(2;13)(q37;q14)
Malignant melanoma	del(1)(p11-p22), del(6)(q11q27), i(6p)
Testicular tumors	i(12p)
Glioma	−10, del(9p)
Involving embryonic cells	
Neuroblastoma	del(1)(p32 to p36)
Ewing's sarcoma/peripheral neuroepithelioma	t(11;22)(q24;q12)
Wilms' tumor	del(11)(p13)[a]
	Trisomy 1q
Retinoblastoma	del(13)(q14)[a]
	Trisomy 1q

[a] Observed as a constitutional abnormality as well as in some tumors.

over, cytogenetic analyses have demonstrated the association of specific chromosomal changes with particular types of solid tumors, most especially mesenchymal tumors (Tables 7.4*B* and 7.5*B*) Overall, the number of cytogenetically characterized solid tumors is still small compared with leukemias and lymphomas (120, 186). The number of specific chromosomal abnormalities that have been characterized by molecular studies also is quite negligible compared with translocation breakpoints in leukemia and lymphoma. The recent advances in the molecular characterization of solid tumors, however, are very encouraging (157). We are certain that the next few years will see a dramatic increase in the molecular characterization of cytogenetically detected abnormalities in solid tumors. Applications of techniques such as CGH, FISH, and molecular genetic analyses of loss of allelic heterozygosity have contributed new knowledge to our understanding of the genetic changes that characterize solid tumors (157). For this review of karyotypes in solid tumors, two broad groups of benign and malignant neoplasms are identified; each group is then divided into six categories. These are: (*a*) epithelial, (*b*) mesenchymal, (*c*) neurogenic, (*d*) germ cell, (*e*) embryonal tumors, and (*f*) tumors of unknown histogenesis.

BENIGN TUMORS

Although much of the discussion in this chapter implies that chromosomal aberrations are equivalent to a malignant phenotype, there are a number of exceptions in solid tumors. In myeloproliferative disorders, patients with clonal chromosomal abnormalities in marrow cells have been observed for up to 12 to 15 years without undergoing leukemic transformation (160). Several benign tumors have clonal abnormalities of which the meningiomas described by Mark and colleagues (116, 117) and by Zankl and Zang (211) have been studied most extensively. However, there are now several reports of clonal cytogenetic abnormalities in other benign solid tumors (129, 192).

EPITHELIAL TUMORS

There are now 363 reported chromosomal abnormalities in benign epithelial tumors (119).

Salivary Gland Tumors

Mark and associates (116) examined 100 parotid gland tumors and noted clonal chromosome abnormalities in approximately 47%. Of 47 adenomas with abnormal karyotypes, 34 had involvement of one of three particular chromosome regions; 8q12, 12q13-15, and 3p21. A t(3;8)(p21;q12) was the most common abnormality, occurring in 27% of cases. A t(11;19)(q21;13) has been described in adenolymphoma (i.e., Warthin's tumor). These abnormalities have not been reported in the few cases of malignant salivary gland tumors studied so far, and the molecular consequences of these abnormalities are unknown.

Colonic Adenomas

Trisomies for chromosomes 7, 8, 13, and 14 have been identified in a few cases reported thus far (75, 122). Trisomy 13 has been reported in 38% of cases. Other recurring abnormalities are del(1)(p36) and del(8p). By using DNA probes, loss of heterozygosity for markers on chromosome arm 5q has been reported in 20 to 50% of colorectal carcinoma and in approximately 30% of patients with sporadic colonic adenomas (174). The *APC* gene responsible for familial adenomatous polyposis was cloned from the long arm of chromosome 5 (band 5q21) (25, 87).

Benign Ovarian Tumors

Trisomy 12 has been reported as the sole abnormality in five benign ovarian tumors (thecoma or fibroma), and two other tumors had trisomy 12 in addition to other abnormalities (147). Thus, seven out of nine cytogenetically abnormal benign ovarian neoplasms are characterized by this trisomy. The high frequency of trisomy 12 in benign ovarian tumors, often as the sole abnormality, suggests that it may be a primary karyotypic event in the initiation of these tumors.

MESENCHYMAL TUMORS

Uterine Leiomyomas

More than 100 leiomyomas with karyotypic abnormalities have been reported. It appears that breaks in 14q22-24 and in 12q14-15 are the most common abnormalities (76, 133, 192). An identical translocation, t(12;14)(q13-15;q23-24), was found as the only abnormality in 4 of 34 leiomyomas (76). Other abnormalities seen in leiomyomas include rearrangements of 6p, del(7)(q21.2q31.2), and rearrangements of 1p36 (10). Endometrial polyps also have been reported with rearrangements of 6p21 and 12q13-14 (133).

Lipomas

The benign mesenchymal neoplasm that is associated with a specific chromosomal rearrangement is lipoma. Of 26 lipomas karyotyped, 70% had consistent chromosome rearrangements, and 13 of them had a reciprocal translocation involving 12q13-15 (75). This breakpoint also has been observed in liposarcomas. Analysis of 91 other cases allowed a classification of lipomas into four cytogenetic subgroups: (*a*) those with normal karyotypes, (*b*) those with hyperdiploidy with ring chromosomes, (*c*) those with pseudodiploidy and rearrangement of 12(q13-15), and (*d*) those with hypodiploid or pseudodiploid karyotypes and other aberrations (113). The region of chromosome 12 band q13-15 has now been observed to be involved in lipomas, liposarcomas, leiomyomas, and mixed salivary gland tumors. Mrozek and colleagues (129) showed that chromosome 12 breakpoints are cytogenetically different in benign and malignant tumors. The molecular mechanism involved in abnormalities of this region has been elucidated in myxoid liposarcoma, but the breakpoint in lipomas appears to be different from the liposarcomas. The t(12;16) and fusion of the *CHOP* gene at 12q13 to the *FUS* gene on chromosome 16 is characteristic of myxoid liposarcomas and is useful diagnostically in distinguishing them from lipomas (41).

NEUROGENIC TUMORS

Meningioma

This is the best characterized benign solid tumor. Zankl and colleagues (211) first described a loss of one chromosome 22 in meningioma in 1970. Monosomy 22 or del(22)(q12.3) has now been reported in approximately 70% of cases or 95% of tumors with abnormal karyotypes (115, 117). The *NF2* gene has been identified as the critical gene involved in this chromosomal region (47). Neurilemomas also have been reported to show monosomy 22 and involvement of *NF2*.

Other benign tumors with recurrent chromosomal alterations include chordoma, osteochondroma, and pulmonary hamartoma, as listed in Table 7.5*A*.

MALIGNANT TUMORS

Malignant tumors with recurrent chromosomal alterations are listed in Table 7.5*B*.

Lung Cancer

Whang-Peng and co-workers (202) first reported a specific chromosome abnormality in small cell lung cancer (SCLC). Specimens from 25 patients were successfully studied, including 1 tumor specimen, 2 pleural effusions, 8 metastatic bone marrow cells, and 16 long-term SCLC cell

Table 7.5*A*. Recurring Structural Abnormalities in Benign Solid Tumors

Tumor type	Chromosomal change	Genes involved
Lipoma	Translocations of 12q13-15 t(3;12)(q27-28;q13-15) Structural changes (t,del) of 13q Translocations of 6p	
Atypical lipoma	+r(12;?)	*MDM2?*
Lipoblastoma	der(8)(q11-13)	
Spindle cell lipoma	Loss of 16q13 → qter	
Hibernoma	Structural changes of 11q13-21	
Leiomyoma (uterus)	Structural changes of 12q13-15 t(12;14)(q13-15p;q23-24) del(7)(q21.2q31.2) Rearrangements of 6p Trisomy 12	
Fibroma (ovarian)	Trisomy 12	
Chondroma	Translocation of 12q13-15	
Osteochondroma	del(8)(q22-24)	
Hamartoma (pulmonary)	t(6;14)(p21;q24) der(12)(q13-15)	
Meningioma	−22/del(22)(q12.3)	*NF2*
Neurilemoma	−22	*NF2*

Table 7.5B. Recurring Structural Abnormalities in Malignant Solid Tumors

Tumor type	Chromosome change	Involved Genes
Liposarcoma (myxoid)	t(12;16)(q13;p11)	*CHOP;FUS*
Synovial sarcoma	t(X;18)(p11;q11)	*SSX;SYT*
Rhabdomyosarcoma (alveolar)	t(2;13)(q35;q14) t(1;13)(p36;q14)	*PAX3;FKHR*
Dermatofibrosarcoma protuberans	+r(17;?)	
Infantile fibrosarcoma	+8, +11, +17, +20	
Extraskeletal myxoid chondrosarcoma	t(9;22)(q22;q12)	?; *EWS*
Clear cell sarcoma	t(12;22)(q13;q12)	*ATF1;EWS*
Ewing's sarcoma/Askin tumor/ peripheral neuroepithelioma/ esthesioneuroblastoma	t(11;22)(q24;q12) t(21;22)(q22;q12)	*FLI1;EWS* *ERG;EWS*
Intra-abdominal desmoplastic small-cell round-cell tumor	t(11;22)(p13;q12)	*WT1;EWS*

lines. At least one chromosome 3 in all metaphases examined had a deletion of the short arm. The shortest region of overlap in all deletions was band 3p14 to p23. In their study, this abnormality was not detected in any of the non-small-cell lung cancer (NSCLC) cell lines. Other investigators have since confirmed this observation but have failed to see del(3p) in every SCLC. Moreover, Zech and associates have also reported this abnormality in all four subtypes of lung cancer (211). In addition, molecular analysis of lung cancer cells has shown that loss of heterozygosity for markers on chromosome arm 3p occurs consistently in SCLC and occasionally in NSCLC (92, 131). This region on 3p21 has been the focus of an intense search for a putative tumor-suppressor gene. The critical region has been narrowed to approximately 600 kb, spanning the smallest region of overlap of several homozygously deleted SCLC cell lines (97).

Lukeis and colleagues (112) first reported 9p abnormalities in 9 of 10 lung cancers they examined. These included five adenocarcinomas, three squamous, and two large cell carcinomas. Nonreciprocal translocations, deletions, or chromosome loss resulting in loss of material from the short arm of chromosome 9 with breakpoints in the region 9p11-p14 were observed. Thus, loss of genetic material from chromosome arm 9p also may contribute to the malignant process in these tumors. *CDKN2* ($p16^{INK4A}$), which is a gene involved in regulation of the cell cycle, recently was shown to be homozygously deleted in a significant percentage of lung cancer cell lines (85). Otterson and colleagues (142) demonstrated that only 6 of 55 SCLC samples (11%) had lost pl6 protein, and all six belonged to the rare subset of SCLC with wild-type RB expression. Conversely, of 48 SCLC samples with no or mutant RB, all showed detectable levels of p16 protein. In contrast, 23 of 33 of NSCLC samples (70%) had loss of p16. Twenty-two of 26 NSCL lines with wild-type RB had no p16, while six of seven NSCL lines with no or mutant RB had detectable p16. The inverse correlation of RB and p16 expression and the absence of p16 inactivation in RB-SCLC lines (0 of 48) confirms a common p16/RB growth suppressor pathway in human lung cancer. Whether one or several other commonly deleted genes on the short arm of chromosome 9 is involved in the malignant process in lung cancer is still unclear (139, 140, 141).

Head and Neck Cancer

Recurrent cytogenetic abnormalities in squamous cell carcinomas of the head and neck region have recently been described. The most frequent changes were deletions. Losses affecting 3p13-p24, 5q12-q23, 8p22-p23, 9p21-p24, and 18q22-q23 ranged in frequency from 40 to 60% of tumors. There was gain of 3q21-qter, 5p,7p,8q, and 11q13-q23 in 28 to 38% of tumors (197). Gain of material of 11q13 is postulated to be associated with amplification of the *CCNDI/PRADI* gene at that locus.

Renal Cell Carcinoma

A translocation between chromosomes 3 and 8 was observed in the lymphocytes of 10 affected members of a family among whom bilateral renal carcinoma segregated in an apparently autosomal dominant fashion (38, 145). Deletions or structural rearrangements of the short arm of chromosome 3 with breakpoints in bands 3p11-p21 are the changes most consistently seen in renal cell carcinoma (179). 3p Deletion also has been found as the sole abnormality in some cases, or it has been seen in 100% of cells showing clonal abnormalities (179, 200, 209). These observations suggest that del(3p) may be a primary event in the development of these tumors.

Other recurring chromosomal abnormalities that have been described in nonpapillary kidney cancer are t(3;5)(p13;q22), −4, and rearrangements of 5q22-35. Papillary carcinomas have +17 in 56% and t(X;1)(p11.2;q21) in 20% of cases (157). Mutations of the von Hippel-Lindau syndrome gene, which maps to 3p25-26, have been shown to predispose to sporadic kidney cancer as well as kidney cancer in families (98). The *VHL* gene is mutated in a high percentage of clear-cell renal carcinomas whereas it is not mutated in papillary renal cancer, thus suggesting a fundamental genetic difference between papillary and nonpapillary renal carcinoma (68).

Breast Cancer

The karyotype in a total of 332 breast tumors was reported by Mitelman (120). The two most common rearrangements are i(1q) and der(1q;16p) which were detected in approximately 40% of near diploid and hyperdiploid tumors. Further rearrangements or other derivatives from chromosome 1 also were frequently observed (i.e., approximately 20% of cases). Other recurrent abnormalities include +7, +18, and +20. Der(1;16)(q10;p10) and del(3p) are other abnormalities seen in benign fibroadenomas, fibrocystic disease, and carcinomas. In a recent study comparing chromosomal alterations in primary breast cancer to those in metastatic cancer (182, 189), random numeric changes were seen in the primary cancers while structural alterations, homogeneous-staining regions and double minutes were more commonly observed in the metastatic tumors. Chromosome 1 was significantly involved in nonrandom abnormalities in both primary and metastatic cases.

Colorectal Carcinomas

A considerable number of these tumors have been studied, but the results are difficult to interpret. The most common changes include structural rearrangements of chromosomes 1 and 17 as well as trisomy 7 and trisomy 12 (120). Loss of a chromosome 5 allele was reported by Solomon and colleagues (175).

Reports of loss of material from the short arm of chromosome 17 and long arm of chromosome 18 prompted molecular geneticists to look at these chromosomes using DNA probes. The most detailed molecular study of colorectal carcinomas was by Vogelstein and co-workers (199) who demonstrated that the progressive accumulation of genetic changes parallels the clinical progression of colorectal tumors from normal epithelium to benign tumors and, further, to the malignant stage of the disease. By molecular analysis, loss of heterozygosity for DNA sequences from chromosome regions 5q, 17p, and 18q were found to occur in a great percentage of colorectal carcinomas (55, 74, 199). Vogelstein proposed that colorectal tumorigenesis proceeds through a series of genetic alterations involving oncogenes (*RAS*) and tumor-suppressor genes *APC* on 5q, *TP53* on 17p, and *DCC* on 18q (199). Hemizygous deletions of chromosome arms 17p and 18q usually occur at a later stage of tumorigenesis than deletions of 5q or *RAS* gene mutations. Accumulation of these genetic alterations rather than the order in which they occur appears to be most important in colorectal tumorigenesis.

The *DCC* gene was identified from a segment of chromosome 18q, and it has been shown to be mutated in a few colorectal carcinomas (55). It has long been speculated that 5q deletions in colorectal carcinomas represent an inherited cancer predisposition gene, particularly in families with preceding polyposis (26). Two genes, *MCC* (mutated in colon cancer) and *APC* (adenomatosis polyposis coli), have been identified in the 5q21 chromosomal region (87). *APC* is mutated in the germline of some patients with familial adenomatous polyposis (FAP) and Gardner's syndrome.

Other chromosomal loci also have been identified as being mutated in families with nonpolyposis colon cancer (HNPCC). These loci are located on the short arm of chromosome 2 (*MSH2*), short arm of chromosome 3 (*MLH1*), and on chromosome 7 (*PMS1* and *PMS2*). These chromosomal regions are not associated with loss of material in colon cancer, but the genes are important in the repair of replication errors (25, 99, 132). Tumors arising in patients with HNPCC exhibit somatic mutations of the same genes that are involved in colorectal tumorigenesis in the general population (e.g., *RAS*, *APC*). In addition, these tumors are characterized by a marked instability of repeated sequences throughout the genome. This instability results from an absence of DNA mismatch repair, which has been traced to inactivating germline mutations in one of the four human homologues of bacterial mismatch repair genes listed earlier (143). Of families with HNPCC, 76% have been shown to have germline mutations in one (or several) of these genes.

Bladder Carcinoma

Several studies of chromosomal abnormalities in bladder cancer have reported structural rearrangements of chromosomes 1, 5, and 11 as well as numeric aberrations involving chromosomes 7 and 9 (65, 75). Monosomy 9 has been reported in 8 of 19 bladder tumors, one of which had monosomy 9 as the sole abnormality (65). Isochromosome 5p (i[5p]) has been reported in 20% of all bladder tumors, while several copies of a chromosome 5 were deleted in a few cases. This may have the same effect as an isochromosome of 5p. Thus, isochromosome 5p or del(5q) may be important in this tumor (65). The same commonly deleted region on 9p21 has been identified in bladder cancer as in other tumor types; however, it is not clear if *CDKN2* represents the only target of the chromosome 9 deletions in bladder cancer (141).

Malignant Mesenchymal Tumors

Several key advances have been made during the last few years in this group of tumors. Mesenchymal tumors are relatively rare, accounting for less than 1% of all human neoplasms. They are very heterogeneous, however, and may present diagnostic problems (42, 58, 75). Recently, cytogenetic and molecular analysis of malignant (i.e., sarcoma) and benign forms of these tumors yielded some very important clues regarding the heretofore unsuspected relationship of some of these rare neoplasms, and provided help in classifying some of the undifferentiated forms of these tumors. Moreover, that the benign and malignant forms have related karyotypic changes provides an important resource for identifying the additional genetic changes that occur in the malignant compared with the benign form. In fact, the molecular biology of soft tissue sarcomas has provided the perfect example of how cytogenetic and molecular approaches can contribute toward a clearer understanding of the development of soft-tissue sarcomas.

Sarcomas

Recurring translocations have been described in both liposarcoma and synovial sarcoma (42, 75, 193, 194). A t(12;16)(q13;p11) has been described, but only in the myxoid subgroup of liposarcomas, whereas other abnormalities, including ring chromosomes, appeared to be more frequent in well-differentiated sarcomas. As discussed previously, a breakpoint cluster region on chromosome 12q13-15 is shared by both lipomas and myxoid liposarcomas (129, 194). Mrozek and colleagues (129) recently provided evidence that the chromosome 12 breakpoints are cytogenetically different in benign and malignant lipogenic tumors. In their study, two malignant liposarcomas, one myxoid and one mixed liposarcoma, were described with t(12;16) as the sole abnormality. The breakpoints in both instances were sublocalized to bands 12q13.3 and 16p11.2. Also, in this same study, four cases of lipomas were characterized by structural rearrangements of chromosome 12. In all four cases, the chromosome 12 breakpoint could be unequivocally assigned to band q15, although the rearrangements involved different partner chromosomes.

A candidate gene called *CHOP* or human GADD153 maps to the breakpoint region at 12q13 and has been implicated in adipocyte differentiation. This gene now is known to be involved in the translocation breakpoint by fusing with *FUS*, another gene on chromosome 16 that has significant homology to the *EWS* gene on chromosome 22 (41, 152). The resultant, aberrant transcript may alter molecular pathways in adipocyte differentiation in a way that contributes to the development of myxoid liposarcomas. Benign soft-tissue tumors such as lipomas, leiomyomatas, and phleomorphic adenoma of the salivary gland with cytogenetically detectable abnormalities in the 12q13-15 region, do not demonstrate rearrangement of the *CHOP* gene. This indicates that a different breakpoint and other genes are involved in these benign tumors.

Of particular interest now are specific translocations that have been observed in distinct soft tissue sarcoma types. In leukemias and lymphomas, translocations have long been shown to be associated with the control of expression or rearrangements of particular genes. The t(2;13) associated with alveolar rhabdomyosarcomas and the t(12;16) in myeloid liposarcoma are additional recently cloned translocations. The gene on chromosome 2 that is involved in the t(2;13)(q35;q14), which occurs in approximately 50% of cases of alveolar rhabdomyosarcomas, has been identified as *PAX3* (12, 13). The *PAX* genes are a highly conserved gene family that includes nine members. This translocation results in the formation of a chimeric transcript consisting of the 5′ portion of *PAX3*, including an intact DNA-binding domain fused to the *FKHR* gene on chromosome 13. The t(1;13)(p36;q14) also seen in alveolar rhabdomyosarcomas results in the fusion of another member of the PAX family, *PAX7* to the *FKHR* gene on chromosome 13. Although detection of the chimeric transcript is a useful diagnostic tool in evaluating these tumors, it remains to be determined how this novel gene-fusion product relates to the development of rhabdomyosarcoma. The chromosomal abnormality in synovial sarcoma [t(X;18) (p11.2;q11.2)] also is of interest, because it is the first one involving a sex chromosome. This abnormality does not appear to be restricted to a particular histologic pattern (88, 110, 193).

NEUROGENIC TUMORS

Gliomas

There have been several reports on the cytogenetic abnormalities of these malignant brain tumors, covering all histologic subtypes of gliomas, including astrocytomas, oligodendroglioma, and glioblastoma multiforme. In 1971, Mark (115) demonstrated that 37 of 50 gliomas had near-diploid stem lines and that 26% contained double minute chromosomes (dmin). This study was done before the availability of banding techniques; with banding techniques, several more gliomas have been studied. Jenkins and colleagues (80) reported on 53 gliomas. No specific abnormalities were detected, but the most frequent findings were dmin, structural abnormalities of chromosome 9 [del(9p) or translocation], trisomy 7, and loss of chromosomes 10, 18, and 22 (17, 18, 76). In a report by Bigner and colleagues (17), 8 of 22 tumors contained marker chromosomes derived from chromosome 9; in 3 tumors, both chromosome 9 homologues participated in marker formation with different breakpoints for a total of 11 structural rearrangements of this chromosome. In this series, the most prevalent finding was abnormalities of chromosome 9 with breakpoints at the centromere or in 9p. A candidate tumor suppressor gene *CDKN2* ($p16^{INK4}$) recently was identified from the region on 9p (84). This gene is deleted in 70% of glioma cell lines and primary glioma tissues (51, 140). Mutations of p53, deletions of 9p and of the *CKDN2* gene, loss of chromosome 10, and *EGFR* amplification are critical genetic events in glioma progression (198).

Ewing's Sarcoma

Aurias and colleagues (6) as well as Turc-Carel and colleagues (195) independently described a t(11;22)(q24;q12) in the malignant cells of patients with Ewing's sarcoma. This translocation has now been detected in more than 90% of these tumors, and the genes involved in this translocation have been cloned. The same chromosomal translocation has been described for peripheral neuroepithelioma and Ewing's sarcoma.

Neuroepitheliomas

In 1984, Whang-Peng and colleagues (204) described a t(11;22)(q24;q12) in two cases of peripheral neuroepithelioma, which is the same translocation reported in more than 90% of Ewing's sarcoma tumors (6). Furthermore, a comparison of Ewing's sarcoma and neuroepithelioma suggests that these two tumors are histogenetically related, and it recently was shown that the neuronal phenotype of Ewing's sarcoma and neuroepithelioma is the same. This similarity has been further substantiated by molecular analysis in which identical levels of proto-oncogene expression were found in Ewing's sarcoma and neuroepithelioma (80). In both Ewing's sarcoma and neuroepithelioma (i.e., two round cell tumors of childhood), there is an association with a reciprocal t(11;22)(q24;q12). This translocation recently was demonstrated to involve the fusion of the human *FLI1* gene on chromosome 11, with coding sequence of the *EWS* gene in chromosome 22 resulting in a fusion protein (47, 195). The discovery of the same identical translocation in neuroepithelioma and Ewing's sarcoma has changed the treatment modality in neuroepithelioma. Use of therapy similar to that for Ewing's sarcoma has resulted in a marked improvement in the response of these tumors. The current thinking is that Ewing's sarcoma arises from cells of the neural crest.

Embryonic Tumors

Embryonic tumors are of particular interest to the cytogeneticist, because some occur in patients with specific constitutional chromosomal abnormalities. In all preceding sections, the karyotypic changes have been somatic mutations in malignant cells, and they have not been present in other unaffected cells except in the few cases of familial renal cell carcinoma. In contrast, some patients who are at risk of developing retinoblastoma have a variable deletion of chromosome 13 that always includes 13q14, whereas other patients with a deletion of chromosome 11 (band 11p13) are at risk of developing Wilms' tumor. In general, these sporadic deletions also are associated with various phenotypic abnormalities (60, 75, 155). Furthermore, analysis of tumor cells from patients with normal constitutional karyotypes indicate that approximately 5% of cases have tumor-specific deletions of chromosome 13, each of which includes deletions of chromosome 13, band q14. Relatively few tumors have been analyzed, however, and monosomy 13 or del(13q) are observed in less than 20% of tumor cells from some patients with retinoblastoma. These deletion cases were useful in defining the region of the genome likely to contain a locus involved in the genesis of retinoblastoma (120, 130). Further analysis of this locus using methods of molecular cloning led to the identification of the *RB1* gene (34, 53, 61, 108, 109). Suppression of tumorigenicity of human prostate carcinoma cells by replacing a mutated *RB* gene has been demonstrated (28), and the RB protein serves as an important regulatory function in controlling the cell cycle (44). The most common change that we have observed in Wilms' tumors is trisomy for the long arm of chromosome 1 (+1q), while deletions of 11p13 or unbalanced translocations occur in approximately 25% of cases (93). Recent studies suggest that three genetic loci are implicated in the development of Wilms' tumor. One locus, which is associated with the WAGR (Wilms' tumor, aniridia, genitourinary dysplasia, and mental retardation) syndrome, maps to 11p13 (27); another locus, which is associated with the Beckwith-Wiedemann syndrome, maps to 11p15; the third locus, which may be involved in familial predisposition to Wilms' tumor, was not genetically linked to any of the markers on 11p and may be on another chromosome (72, 94, 136). Two groups have independently isolated a candidate gene (*WT1*) for Wilms' tumor at 11p13, and the characterization of mutations in tumor DNA suggests that the gene product contributes to the malignant process (33, 64, 77).

Recurring chromosomal abnormalities limited to the malignant cells, also have been observed in other childhood tumors, for example, a deletion of much of the short arm of chromosome 1 [del(1p)] has been noted in neuroblastomas (29). In addition, neuroblastomas are of interest because of their proclivity to undergo gene amplification, which manifests chromosomally as hundreds or thousands of small, discrete pieces of chromosomes called double minutes or long unbanded regions on chromosomes called homogeneously staining regions or HSR (16). In some cell lines, these have been shown to represent amplification of *MYCN* (170). *MYCN* amplification also has been identified in tumor samples, and it is highly correlated with advanced stage (i.e., III and IV) and with a poor survival of these patients (30).

Germ Cell Tumors

Atkin and Baker (4) described an isochromosome for the short arm of chromosome 12 in four seminomas in 1983 [i(12p)]. The presence of this marker in various histologic types of germ cell tumors, including seminomas, teratomas, and embryonal cell carcinomas, has subsequently been confirmed in several studies (75, 187). Thus, i(12p) appears to be a highly consistent and specific cytogenetic abnormality associated with testicular germ cell tumors. Moreover, an increasing number of copies of 12p appears to be correlated with more aggressive disease and poorer survival.

Malignant Melanoma

Changes involving chromosomes 1, 6, and 7 have often been reported in the malignant cells of patients with melanoma (8). Most tumors studied have been metastatic, and there are few studies of early melanocytic lesions. Recent data from Parmiter and colleagues (144) confirm that the predominant, nonrandom abnormality in metastatic melanoma continues to be deletions and rearrangements of 1p, abnormalities of 6p and 6q, extra copies of chromosome 7, and losses of chromosome 10 (144). A translocation involving the terminal region 10q(q24-26) also was seen in some premalignant lesions, and the abnormalities of chromosome 10 were seen in both early and late lesions, suggesting that this may be a primary event in the malignant process.

Cowan and colleagues (39) described loss of one copy of chromosome 9 in two of four dysplastic nevi, and 4 of 11 melanomas. Isochromosome 1q [i(1q)] or del(1p) occur in approximately 60% of all tumors, while chromosome 6 is rearranged in more than 80% of all tumors (8, 71). Trent and colleagues (188) recently presented evidence that the insertion of a normal chromosome 6 could revert some of the malignant phenotype in malignant melanoma. *CDKN2* (p16), a gene that is involved in the cell cycle, has been shown to be frequently deleted in melanoma cell lines (85). In addition, germline mutations of this gene were recently demonstrated in cases of 9p-linked familial melanoma (78).

MOLECULAR ANALYSIS OF RECURRING CHROMOSOME ABNORMALITIES, PARTICULARLY TRANSLOCATIONS

How and When Consistent Translocations Occur

We do not know how consistent structural rearrangements occur, but there are at least two possibilities (146). Rearrangements may be random, but selection may act to eliminate the vast majority that do not provide the cell with a proliferative advantage. Alternatively, certain changes may occur preferentially, and thus, may be the ones that we see. Some tantalizing data show an association of chromosome rearrangements in tumor cells from patients with fragile sites affecting one of the chromosome bands broken in the tumor cells (99, 100, 176, 210). Much more research is required, however, to clarify the role of fragile sites as a predisposing factor to malignant transformation; no fragile site has yet been shown to be directly involved in either a translocation or a deletion breakpoint. As described by Knudson (89), the role of different mutations in cancer has been the basis of intensive research in our group.

Croce and colleagues (40) as well as Rabbitts (151) have proposed that many of the chromosome rearrangements in

B- and T-cell tumors involve sequences used in the normal recombination of the V-D-J segments of the immunoglobulin and T-cell receptor genes. The presence of heptamer and nonamer sequences in the nonimmunoglobulin gene at the site of the translocation, namely, *MYC* and *BCL2*, has been reported. However, there is no indication at present that the genes involved in the translocations in myeloid leukemias undergo similar DNA rearrangements. In fact, ALU sequences have been identified at some breakpoints (24, 170).

An equally important question is when in the multistage process of malignant transformation of a particular cell do translocations or other chromosomal aberrations occur? Some changes occur as part of the further evolution of the malignant phenotype (e.g., blast crisis of CML); therefore, they are relatively late events. However, what about the occurrence of the t(9;22) in CML, for example? Does the Ph chromosome occur in a single normal cell, which becomes the progenitor of the leukemic clone, or is there expansion of a clone, possibly a leukemic one, in which a translocation occurs in one of these already abnormal cells? Fialkow and colleagues (56) have presented detailed evidence supporting the latter proposal.

Adams and colleagues (1) have produced transgenic mice, all of whose cells have a vector containing the *myc*/*IgH* junction from a murine plasmacytoma. All cells contain this construct; however, the B-cell tumors that occur in every animal are clonal, indicating that one or more additional changes occur in one cell, resulting in clonality.

BIOLOGIC CONSEQUENCES OF CONSISTENT CHROMOSOME ABNORMALITIES

The cloning of many chromosome translocation breakpoints and identification of the involved genes have had a major impact on our understanding of at least one critical event in the transformation of a normal cell to a leukemic cell (151). Translocations in the lymphoid leukemias and lymphomas that involve the immunoglobulin genes in B-lineage tumors and the T-cell receptor genes in T-lineage tumors result in inappropriate expression of the other gene in the translocation but no alteration in its protein structure. In contrast, all of the translocations cloned to date in the myeloid leukemias (with one possible exception) result in a fusion mRNA and a chimeric protein. This same situation is true for the 1;19 translocation in pre-B ALL, and the 4;11 and 11;19 translocations in ALL (151).

Cloning of the translocation breakpoints has led to the identification of a number of new genes (140) (Table 7.6*A*). It has been pointed out repeatedly that genes cloned from the breakpoints in acute leukemia have been transcription factors. In fact, one could argue that cloning these junctions is a very effective method for identifying new transcription factors. In many instances, the translocation results in the fusion of two genes, leading to a fusion mRNA, and a fusion or chimeric protein (151, 215).

Our new sophistication regarding genetic changes in hematologic malignant disease provides us with some very

Table 7.6*A*. Functional Classification of Transforming Genes at Translocation Junctions

	Location	Translocation	Disease
SRC Family (TYR protein kinases)			
ABL	9q34	t(9;22)	CML/ALL
LCK	1p34	t(1;7)	T-ALL
ALK	2p23	t(2;5)	NHL
PDGRFRB	5q33	t(5;12)	CMMoL
Serine protein kinase			
BCR	22q11	t(9;22)	CML/ALL
Cell surface receptor			
TAN1	9q34	t(7;9)	T-ALL
Growth factor			
IL2	4q26	t(4;16)	T-NHL
IL3	5q31	t(5;14)	Pre-BALL
Mitochondrial membrane protein			
BCL2	18q21	t(14;18)	NHL
Cell cycle regulator			
CCND1 (BCL1-PRAD1)	11q13	t(11;14)	CLL/NHL
Myosin family			
MYH11	16p13	inv(16), t(16;16)	AML-M4Eo
Ribosomal protein			
EAP (L22)	3q26	t(3;21)	t-AML/CML BC
Nuclear RNA binding			
FUS (TLS)	16p11	t(16;21)	AML
Nuclear phosphoprotein			
NPM1	5q35	t(2;5)	NHL
Unknown			
DEK	6p23	t(6;9)	AML-M2/M4

ALL—Acute lymphoblastic leukemia; AML—acute myeloid leukemia; CML—chronic myeloid leukemia; CML BC—Blast crisis; CMMoL—Chronic myelomonocytic leukemia; NHL—non-Hodgkin's lymphoma; t-AML—therapy-related acute myelogenous leukemia.

Table 7.6*B*. Functional Classification of DNA Binding Factors and Transcriptional Modulators at Translocation Junctions

	Location	Translocation	Disease
DNA binding facors			
Homeobox			
PBX	1q23	t(1;19)	Pre-BALL
HOX11	10q24	t(10;14)/t(7;10)	T-ALL
Helix-loop-helix			
CAN	9q34	t(6;9)	AML
LYL1	19p13	t(7;19)	T-ALL
*MYC**	8q24	t(8;14)	B-ALL/T-ALL
TAL1(SCL)	1p32	t(1;14)	T-ALL
TAL2	9p32	t(7;9)	T-ALL
TCF3(E2A)	19p13	t(1;19)	Pre-BALL
Zinc finger			
ETO	8q24	t(8;21)	AML-M2
MLL	11q23.3	t(11q23)	ALL/AML
PLZF	11q23.1	t(11;17)	APL
PML	15q22	t(15;17)	APL
RARA	17q12	t(15;17)	APL
EVI1	3q26	inv(3), t(3;3)	AML
BCL6	3q27	t(3;14)	NHL
LIM			
RBTN1(TTG1)	11p15	t(11;14)	T-ALL
RBTN2	11p13	t(11;14)	T-ALL
Leucine zipper			
CHOP	12q13	t(12;16)	AML
Other			
AML1 (*runt* homology)	21q22	t(8;21), t(3;21)	AML-M2
LYT10 (*rel* homology)	10q24	t(10;14)	B-NHL
TEL (*ets* homology)	12p13	t(5;12)	CMMoL
ERG (*ets* homology)	21q22	t(16;21)	AML
MLL Translocation partners			
AF1p			
AF1q			
AF-4	4q21	t(4;11)	ALL
AF-6	6q27	t(6;11)	AML
AF-9	9p22	t(9;11)	AML
AF-10 Leucine zipper	10p12	t(10;11)	AML
ELL	19p13.3	t(11;19)	ALL
ENL			
Undefined			
MDS1	3q26	t(3;21)	AML
ELL	19p13.1	t(11;19)	AML
AFX	Xq24	t(X;11)	AML
Transcriptional modulators			
BCL3	19q13	t(14;19)	B-CLL
CBFB	16q22	inv(16), t(16;16)	AML-M4Eo

ALL—Acute lymphoblastic leukemia; AML—acute myelogenous leukemia; AML-M2—AML with differentiation; AML-M4Eo—AML-myelomonocytic leukemia with increased eosinophils; APL—acute promyelocytic leukemia; B-ALL—B-cell acute lymphocytic leukemia; B-CLL—B-cell chronic lymphocytic leukemia; B-NHL—B-cell non-Hodgkin's lymphoma; CMMoL—chronic myelomonocytic leukemia; NHL—non-Hodgkin's lymphoma; Pre-B ALL—Pre-B acute lymphoblastic leukemia; T-ALL—T-cell acute lymphoblastic leukemia.

critical new diagnostic tools. Standard Southern blot analysis of tumor DNA can reveal clonal rearrangements of genes using the appropriate probes. PCR can increase the sensitivity of detection of these aberrations, but the sensitivity is sometimes too great to be clinically applicable.

Our increasing precision in identifying the genetic changes in malignant cells comes at a most opportune time, because physicians will soon be in a position to use targeted therapy aimed at the specific genetic defect in the malignant cells. To use this targeted therapy effectively requires a precise genotype of the malignant cells. Although a number of genes will be involved in various genetic alterations leading to a tumor cell, those reflected in chromosomal changes may be among the easiest to monitor.

References

1. Adams JM, Harris AW, Pinkert CA, Corcoran LM, Alexander WS, Cory S, Palmiter RD, Brinster RL. The c-*myc* oncogene driven by immunoglobulin enhancers induces lymphoid malignancy in transgenic mice. Nature 1985;318:533.
2. ar-Rushdi A, Nishikura K, Erickson J, Watt R, Rovera G, Croce CM. Differential expression of the translocated and the untranslocated c-*myc* oncogene in Burkitt's lymphoma. Science 1983;222:390.
3. Arthur DC, Bloomfield CD. Banded chromosome analysis in patients with treatment-associated acute non-lymphocytic leukemia. Cancer Genet Cytogenet 1984,12:189.
4. Atkin NB, Baker MC. i:(12p): specific chromosome marker in seminoma and malignant teratoma of the testis? Cancer Genet Cytogenet 1983;10:199.
5. Aurias A. Analyse cytogenetique de 21 cas d' ataxia—telangiectasie. J Genetique Humain 1981;29:235–247.
6. Aurias A, Rimbaut C, Buffe D, Dubousset J, Mazabraud A. Chromosomal translocations in Ewing's sarcoma. N Engl J Med 1983;309:496.
7. Baer R. TAL1, TAL2, and LYL 1: a family of basic helix-loop-helix proteins implicated in T cell acute leukemia. Semin Cancer Biol 1993;4:341–347.
8. Balaban G, Herlyn M, Guerry D III, Bartolo R, Koprowski H, Clark WH, Nowell PC. Cytogenetics of human malignant melanoma and pre-malignant lesions. Cancer Genet Cytogenet 1984;11:429.

9. Baron BW, Nucifora G, McCabe N, Espinosa R II, Le Beau MM, McKeithan TW. Identification of the gene associated with the recurring translocations t(3;14)(q27;q32) and t(3;22)(q27;q11) in B cell lymphomas. Proc Natl Acad Sci USA 1993;90: 5262–5266.
10. Bartram CR. Rearrangement of the c-*abl* and *bcr* genes in pH-negative CML and pH-positive acute leukemias. Leukemia 1988;2:63.
11. Begley CG, Aplan P, Davey MP. Chromosomal translocation in a human leukemia stem cell line disrupts the T-cell antigen receptor β-chain diversity region and results in a previously unreported fusion transcript. Proc Natl Acad Sci USA 1989;86: 2031–2035.
12. Barr FG, Galili N, Holick J, Biegel JA, Rovera G, Emanuel B. Rearrangement of the PAX 3 paired box gene in the paediatric solid tumor alveolar rhabdomyosarcoma. Nature Genet 1993;3:113–117.
13. Barr FG, Holick J, Nycum L, Biegel JA, Emanuel BS. Localization of the t(2;13) breakpoint of alveolar rhabdomyosarcoma on a physical map of chromosome 2. Genomics 1992;13:1156–1163.
14. Bennett JM, Catovsky D, Daniel MT, Flandrin G, Galton DAG, Gralnick HR, Sultan C. Proposals for the classification of the acute leukemias: French-American-British (FAB) Co-operative Group. Br J Haematol 1985;51:189.
15. Berger R, Bernheim A, Sigaux F, Daniel M-T, Valensi F, Flandrin G. Acute monocytic leukemia chromosome studies. Leukemia Res 1982;6:17.
16. Biedler JL, Spengler BA. Metaphase chromosome anomaly: association with drug resistance and cell-specific products. Science 1976;191:185.
17. Bigner SH, Mark J, Bullard DE, Mahaley MS Jr, Bigner DD. Chromosomal evolution in malignant glioma starts with specific and usually numerical deviations. Cancer Genet Cytogenet 1986;22:121.
18. Bigner SH, Mark J, Burger PC, Mahaley MS Jr, Bullard DE, Muhlbaier LH, Bigner DD. Specific chromosomal abnormalities in malignant human gliomas. Cancer Res 1988;48:405.
19. Bird ML, Ueshima Y, Rowley JD, Haren JM, Vardiman JW. Chromosome abnormalities in B-cell chronic lymphocytic leukaemia and their clinical correlations. Leukemia 1989;3:182.
20. Bitter MA, Franklin WA, Larson RA, McKeithan TW, Rubin LM, LeBeau MM, Stephen JK, Vardiman JW. Morphology in Ki-1 (CD30)-positive non-Hodgkin's lymphoma is correlated with clinical features and the presence of a unique chromosomal abnormality, t(2;5)(p23;q35). Am J Surg Pathol 1990;14:305.
21. Bitter MA, Neilly ME, LeBeau MM, Pearson MG, Rowley JD. Rearrangement of chromosome 3 involving bands 3q21 and 3q26 are associated with normal or elevated platelet counts in acute nonlymphocytic leukemia. Blood 1985;66:1362.
22. Bloomfield CD, Arthur DC, Frizzera G, Levine EG, Peterson BA, Gajl-Peczalska KJ. Nonrandom chromosome abnormalities in lymphoma. Cancer Res 1983;43:2975.
23. Bloomfield CD, Goldman AI, Alimena G, Berger R, Borgstrom GH, Brandt L, Catovsky D, de la Chapelle A, Dewald GW, Garson OM, Garwicz S, Golomb HM, Hossfeld DK, Lawler SD, Mitelman F, Nilsson P, Pierre RV, Philp P, Prigogina E, Rowley JD, Sakurai M, Sandberg MAP, Secker-Walker LM, Tricot G, Vanden Berghe H, Van Orshoven A, Vupio P, Whang-Peng J. Chromosomal abnormalities identify high-risk and low-risk patients with acute lymphoblastic leukemia. Blood 1986;67:415.
24. Broeker PL, Super HG, Thirman M, Pomykala H, Yonebayashi Y, Tanabe S, Zeleznik-Le N, Rowley JD. Correlation of breakpoints in 11q23 rearrangements with topoisomerase II consensus binding sites, Alu sequences, scaffold attachment regions. Blood 1996 (In press).
25. Bronner CE, Baker SM, Morrison PT, Warren G, Smith LG, Lescoe MK, Kane M, Earabino C, Lipford J, Lindblom A, Tannergard P, Bollag RJ, Godwin AR, Ward DC, Nordenskjold M, Fishel R, Kolodner R, Liskay RM. Mutation in the DNA mismatch repair gene homologue *hMLHl* is associated with hereditary nonpolyposis colon cancer. Nature 1994;368:258–261.
26. Bodmer WF, Bailey CJ, Bodmer J, Bussey HJR, Ellis A, Gorman P, Lucibello FC, Murday VA, Rider SH, Scambler P, Sheer D, Solomon E, Spurr NK. Localization of the gene for familial adenomatous polyposis on chromosome 5. Nature 1987;328:614.
27. Bonetta L, Kuehn SE, Huang A, Law DJ, Kalikin LM, Koi M, Reeve AE, Brownstein BH, Herman Y, Williams BRG, Feinberg AP. Wilms' tumor locus on 11p13 defined by multiple CpG island-associated transcripts. Science 1990;250:994.
28. Bookstein R, Shew JY, Chen RL, Scully P, Lee WH. Suppression of tumorigenicity of human prostate carcinoma cells by replacing a mutated RB gene. Science 1990;247: 712.
29. Brodeur GM, Green AA, Hayes FA, Williams KJ, Williams DL, Tsiatis AA. Cytogenetic features of human neuroblastomas and cell lines. Cancer Res 1981;41:4678.
30. Brodeur GM, Seeger RL, Schwab M, Vermus HE, Bishop JM. Amplification of N-*myc* in untreated neuroblastoma correlates with advanced disease stage. Science 1984;224:1121.
31. Brown L, Chang J-T, Chen Q. Site specific recombination of the *tal-1* gene is a common occurrence in human T-cell leukemia. EMBO J 1990;9:3343–3351.
32. Caccia N, Bruns GA, Kirsch IR, Hollis GF, Bertness V, Mak TW. T cell receptor; gamma-chain genes are located on chromosome 14 at 14q11–14q12 in humans. J Exp Med 1985;161:1255.
33. Call KM, Glaser T, Ito CY, Buckler AJ, Pelletier J, Hasen DA, Rose EA, Kral A, Yeger H, Lewis WH. Isolation and characterization of a zinc finger polypeptide gene at the human chromosome 11 Wilms' tumor locus. Cell 1990;60:509.
34. Cavenee WK, Dryja TP, Phillips RA, Benedict WF, Godbout R, Gallie BL, Murphree AL, Strong LC, White RL. Expression of recessive alleles by chromosomal mechanisms in retinoblastoma. Nature 1983;305:779.
35. Chen C-S, Sorensen PHB, Domer PH, Reaman GH, Korsmeyer SJ, Heerema NA, Hammond GD, Kersey JH. Molecular rearrangements on chromosome 11q23 predominate in childhood acute lymphoblastic leukemia and are associated with specific biological variables and poor outcome. Blood 1993;81:2386–2393.
36. Claxton DF, Liu P, Hso HB, Mareton P, Hester J, Collins F, Deisseroth AB, Rowley JD, Siciliano MJ. Detection of fusion transcripts generated by the inversion 16 chromosome in acute myelogenous leukemia. Blood 1994;83:1750–1756.
37. Cleary ML, Smith DS, Sklar J. Cloning and structural analysis of cDNA's for *bcl-2* and a hybrid *bcl-2*/immunoglobulin transcript resulting from the t(14;18) translocation. Cell 1986;47:19.
38. Cohen AJ, Li FB, Berg S, Marchetto DJ, Tsai S, Jacobs SC, Brown RS. Hereditary renal cell carcinoma associated with a chromosomal translocation. N Engl J Med 1979;301:592.
39. Cowan JM, Halaban R, Francke U. Cytogenetic analysis of melanocytes from premalignant nevi and melanoma. JNCI 1988;80:1159.
40. Croce CM, Isobe M, Palumbo A, Puck J, Ming J, Tweardy D, Erikson J, Davis M, Rovera G. Gene for α-chain of human T-cell receptor: location on chromosome 14 region involved in T-cell neoplasms. Science 1985;227:1044.
41. Crozat A, Aman P, Mandahl N, Ron D. Fusion of CHOP as a novel RNA binding protein in human myxoid liposarcoma. Nature 1993;363:640–655.
42. Dal Cin P, Sandberg AA. Chromosome changes in soft tissue tumors: benign and malignant. Cancer Invest 1989;7:63.
43. Daley GQ, Van Etter RA, Baltimore D. Induction of chronic myelogenous leukemia in mice by p210 *bcr/abl* gene of the Philadelphia chromosome. Science 1990;247:824.
44. De Caprio JA, Ludlow JW, Lynch D, et al. The product of the retinoblastoma gene has properties of a cell cycle regulatory element. Cell 1989;58:1085.
45. De Klein A, Hagemeijer A, Bartram CR, Houwen R, Hoefsloot L, Carbonell F, Chan L, Barnett M, Greaves M, Kleihamer E, Heisterkamp N, Groffen J, Grosveld G. BCR rearrangement and translocation of the c-*abl* oncogene in Philadelphia positive acute lymphoblastic leukemia. Blood 1986;68:13184.
46. De Klein A, van Kessel AG, Grosveld G, Bartram CR, Hagemeijer A, Bootsma D, Spurr NK, Heisterkamp N, Groffen J, Stephenson JR. A cellular oncogene is translocated to the Philadelphia chromosome in chronic myelocytic leukemia. Nature 1982;300:765.
47. Delattre O, Zucman J, Plougaster B, et al. Gene fusion with an ets DNA-binding domain caused by chromosome translocation in human tumors. Nature 1992;359: 176–165.
48. De The H, Chomienne C, Lanotte M, Degos L, De Jean A. The t(15;17) translocation of acute promyelocytic leukemia fuses the retinoic acid receptor alpha gene to a novel transcribed locus. Nature 1990;347:558.
49. Diaz MO, Ziemin S, LeBeau MM, Pitha P, Smith SD, Chilcote RR, Rowley JD. Homozygous deletions of the α- and β1-interferon genes in human leukemia and derived cell lines. Proc Nat Acad Sci USA 1988;85:5259.
50. Djabali M, Selleri L, Parry P, Bower M, Young BD, Evans GA. A trithorax-like gene is interrupted by chromosome 11q23 translocations in acute leukemias. Nature Genet 1992;2:113–118.
51. Dreyling MH, Bohlander SK, Adeyanju MO, Olopade OI. Detection of CDKN2 deletions in tumor cell lines and primary glioma by interphase fluorescence in situ hybridization. Cancer Res 1995;55:984–988.
52. Dreyling M, Bohlander, S-K, LeBeeu MM, Olopade OI. Refined mapping of genomic rearrangements involving the shaft arm of chromosome 9 in acute lymphoblastic leukemias and other hematologic malignancies. Blood 86:1931-1938, 1995.
53. Dryja TP, Cavenee WK, White R, Rapaport JM, Petersen R, Albert DM, Brins GA. Homozygosity of chromosome 13 in retinoblastoma. N Engl J Med 1984;310:550.
54. Erickson PF, Robinson M, Owens G, Drabkin HA. The *ETO* portion of acute myeloid leukemia t(8;21) fusion transcript encodes a highly evolutionary conserved putative transcription factor. Cancer Res 1994;54:1782–1786.
55. Fearon ER, Cho KR, Nigro JM, Kearn SE, Simons JW, Ruppert JM, Hamilton SR, Presinger AL, Thomas G, Kinzler KW, Vogelstein B. Identification of a chromosome 18q gene that is altered in colorectal cancers. Science 1990;247:49.
56. Fialkow PJ, Singer JW, Raskind WH, Adamson JW, Jacobson RJ, Bernstein ID, Dow LW, Najfeld V, Veith R. Clonal development, differentiation, clinical remissions in acute nonlymphocytic leukemia. N Engl J Med 1987;317:468.
57. Fifth International Workshop on Chromosomes in Leukemia-Lymphoma. Correlation of chromosome abnormalities with histologic and immunologic characteristics in non-Hodgkin's lymphoma and adult T-cell leukemia-lymphoma. Blood 1987;70:1554.
58. Fletcher JA, Kozakewich HP, Hoffer FA, Lage JM, Weidner N, Tepper R, Pinkus GS, Morton CC, Corsin JM. Diagnostic relevance of clinical cytogenetic aberrations in malignant soft tissue tumors. N Engl J Med 1991;324:436–442.
59. Fourth International Workshop on Chromosomes in Leukemia. Cancer Genet Cytogenet 1984;11:249.
60. Francke U. Specific chromosome changes in the human heritable tumors retinoblastoma and nephroblastoma. In Chromosomes and Cancer. Edited by JD Rowley, JE Ultmann. Bristol-Myers Symposia Series Vol. 5. New York: Academic, 1983, p 99.
61. Friend SH, Bernards R, Rogelj S, Weinberg RA, Rapaport JM, Albert DM, Dryja TP. A human DNA segment with properties of the gene that predisposes to retinoblastoma. Nature 1986;323:643.
62. Fukuhara S, Rowley JD, Variakojis D, Golomb HM. Chromosome abnormalities in poorly differentiated lymphocytic lymphoma. Cancer Res 1979;39:3119.
63. General report of the Sixth International Workshop on Chromosomes in Leukemia. Cancer Genet Cytogenet 1989;40:149.
64. Gessler M, Poustka A, Cavene W, Neve RL, Orkin SH, Bruns GA. Homozygous deletion in Wilms' tumor of a zinc finger gene identified by chromosome jumping. Nature 1990;343:774.
65. Gibas Z, Prout G, Connoly J, Pontes JE, Sandberg AA. Nonrandom chromosomal changes in transitional cell carcinoma of the bladder. Cancer Res 1984;44:1257.
66. Gishizky ML, McLaughlin J, Pendergast AM, Witte ON. The 5′ non-coding region of the *BCR/ABL* oncogene augments its ability to stimulate the growth of immature lymphoid cells. Oncogene 1991;6:1299.
67. Gillard EF, Solomon E. Acute promyelocytic leukemia and the t(15;17) translocation. Semin Cancer Biol 1993;4:359–368.
68. Gnarra JR, Tory K, Weng Y, Schmidt L, Wei MH, Li H, Latif F, Liu S, Chen F, Duh F-M, Lubensky I, Duan R, Florence C, Pozzatti R, Walther MM, Bander NH, Grossman HB, Branch H, Pomer S, Brooks JD, Isaacs WB, Lerman MI, Zbar B, Linehan WL. Mutation of the VHL tumor suppressor gene in renal carcinoma. Nature Genet 1994;7: 85–90.
69. Golomb HM, Alimena G, Rowley JD, Vardiman JW, Testa JR, Sovik C. Correlation of occupation and karyotype in adults with acute nonlymphocytic leukemia. Blood 1982;60:404.
70. Gough NM, Geanig DP, Nicola NA, Baker E, Pritchard M, Callen DF, Sutherland GR. Localization of the human GM-GSF receptor gene to the X-Y pseudo-autosomal region. Nature 1990;345:734.

71. Groffen J, Stephenson JR, Heisterkamp N, deKlein A, Bartram CR, Grosveld G. Philadelphia chromosomal breakpoints are clustered within a limited region, *bcr*, on chromosome 22. Cell 1984;36:93.
72. Grundy P, Cavenee WK, Koufos A, Li FP, Meadows AT, Morgan K. Familial predisposition to Wilms' tumor does not map to the short arm of chromosome 11. Nature 1988;336:374.
73. Gu Y, Nakamura T, Adler H, Prasad R, Canaani O, Cimino G, Croce CM, Canaani E. The t(4;11) chromosome translocation of acute leukemia fuses the *All-1* gene related to *Drosophila trithorax*, to the *AF-4* gene. Cell 1992;71:701–708.
74. Hamilton SR. Molecular genetics of colorectal carcinoma. Cancer 1992;70:1216–1220.
75. Heim S, Mitelman F. Cancer Cytogenetics. New York: Liss, 1987.
76. Heim S, Nilbert M, Vanni R, Floderus UM, Mandahl N, Liedgren S, Lecca U, Mitelman F. A specific translocation, t(12;14)(q14–15;q23–24) characterizes a subgroup of uterine leiomyomas. Cancer Genet Cytogenet 1988;32:13.
77. Huang A, Campbell CE, Bonetta L, McAndrews-Hill MS, Chilton-MacNeill S, Coppes MJ, Law DJ, Feinberg AP, Yeger H, Williams BRG. Tissue, developmental, tumor-specific expression of divergent transcripts in Wilms' tumor. Science 1990;250:991.
78. Hussusein CJ, Struewing JP, Goldstein AM, Higgins PAT, Ally DS, Sheahan MD, Clark WH Jr, Tucker MA, Dracopoli NC. Germline p16 mutations in familial melanoma. Nature Genet 1994;8:15–20.
79. ISCN (1991). Cancer Cytogenetics. In Supplement to an International System for Human Cytogenetic Nomenclature. Edited by F Mitelman, Basel: Karger, 1991.
80. Israel MA, Helman LJ, Miser J. Patterns of proto-oncogene expression: a novel approach to the development of tumor markers. Important Adv Onc 1987; 00:87–104.
81. Jenkins RB, Kimmel DW, Moertel CA, Schultz CG, Scheithamer BW, Kelly PJ, Dewald GW. A cytogenetic study of 53 human gliomas. Cancer Genet Cytogenet 1989;39:253.
82. Juliusson G, Oscier DG, Fitchett M, Ross RM, Stockdill G, Mackie MJ, Parker AC, Castoldi GL, Guneo A, Kauutila S, et al. Prognostic subgroups in B-cell chronic lymphocytic leukemia defined by specific chromosomal abnormalities. N Engl J Med 1990;323:720.
83. Kaiser-McCaw B, Hecht F, Harnden DG, Teplitz RL. Somatic rearrangement of chromosome 14 in human lymphocytes. Proc Natl Acad Sci USA 1975;72:2071.
84. Kallionieni, A, Kallionieni OP, Sudar D, Rutovitz D, Gray JW, Waldman F, Pinkel D. Comparative genomic hybridization for molecular cytogenetic analysis of solid tumors. Science 1992;258:818–821.
85. Kamb A, Gruis NA, Weaver-Feldhaus J, Lin A, Harshmar K, Tavtigian SV, Stockert E, Day III RS, Johnson BE, Skolnick MH. A cell cycle regulator potentially involved in genesis of many tumor types. Science 1994;264:436–440.
86. Kaneko Y, Frizzera G, Edamura S. A novel translocation, t(2;5)(p23;q35) in childhood phagocytic large T-cell lymphoma mimicking malignant histiocytosis. Blood 1989;73:806–813.
87. Kinzler KW, Nilbert MC, Su L, Vogelstein B, Bryan TM, Levy DB, Smith KJ. Identification of FAP locus genes from chromosome 5q21. Science 1991;253:661–664.
88. Knight JC, Reeves BR, Kearney L, Monaco AP, Lehrach H, Cooper CS. Localization of the synovial sarcoma t(X;18)(p11.2;q11.2) breakpoint by fluorescence in situ hybridization. Human Mol Genet 1992;1:633–637.
89. Knudson AG. Mutation and cancer: statistical study of retinoblastoma. Proc Natl Acad Sci USA 1971;68:820.
90. Koduru PRK, Filippa DA, Richardson ME, Jhanwar SC, Chaganti SR, Koziner B, Clarkson BD, Lieberman PH, Chaganti RSK. Cytogenetic and histologic correlations in malignant lymphomas. Blood 1987;184:97.
91. Korsmeyer SJ. *BCL2*: an antidote to programmed cell death. Cancer Surveys 1992;15:105–118.
92. Kok K, Osinga J, Carritt B, Davis MB, Van der Hout AH, Van der Veen AY, de Leij LF, Berendsen HH, Postmus PE, Poppena S, Brys CHCM. Deletion of a DNA sequence at the chromosomal region 3p21 in all major types of lung cancer. Nature 1987;330:578.
93. Kondo K, Chilcote RR, Maurer HS, Rowley JD. Chromosome abnormalities in tumor cells from patients with sporadic Wilms' tumor. Cancer Res 1984;44:5376.
94. Koufos A, Aleck KA, Cavenee WK, Grundy P, Hadro T, Kalbakji A, Lampkin BC, Morgan K. Familial Wiedemann-Beckwith syndrome and a second Wilms' tumor locus both map to 11p15.5. Am J Hum Genet 1989;44:711.
95. Larson RA, LeBeau MM, Vardiman JW, Testa JR, Golomb HM, Rowley JD. The predictive value of initial cytogenetic studies in 148 adults with acute nonlymphocytic leukemia a 12 year study (1970–1982). Cancer Genet Cytogenet 1983;10:219.
96. Larson RA, Williams SF, LeBeau MM, Bitter MA, Vardiman JW, Rowley JD. Acute myelomonocytic leukemia with abnormal eosinophils and inv (16) or t(16;16) has a favorable prognosis. Blood 1986;68:1242.
97. Latif F, Bader S, Wei MW, Sekido Y, Duh FM, Li H, Chen JY, Geil L, Tartof, KD, Allikmet R, Dean M, Zabarovsky E, Klein G, Zbar B, Minna J, Lerman M. A 600 kb cosmid contig from 3p21.3 for isolation of candidate genes for small cell lung cancer (SCLC). Proc Am Assoc Cancer Res 1995;36:570.
98. Latif F, Tory K, Gnarra J, Yao M, Duh F-M, Orcutt ML, Stackhouse T, Kuzmin I, Modi W, Geil L, Schmidt L, Zhou F, Li H, Wei MH, Glenn G, Richards FM, Crossey PA, Ferguson-Smith MA, Le Paslier D, Chumakou I, Cohen D, Chinault C, Maher ER, Linehan WM, Zbar B, Lerman MI. Identification of the von-Hippel-Lindau disease tumor suppressor gene. Science 1993;260:1317–1320.
99. Leach FS, Nicolaides N, Papadopoulos N, Liu B, Jen J, Parsons R, Peltomaki P, Sistonen P, Aaltonen LA, Nystrom-Lahti M, Guan XY, Zhang J, Meltzer PS, Yu J, Kao FT, Chen DJ, Cerosaletti KM, Fournier REK, Todd S, Lewis T, Leach RJ, Naylor SL, Weissenbach J, Mecklin JP, Jarvinen P, Petersen H, Hamilton SR, Green J, Jass J, Watson P, Lynch HT, Trent JM, de la Chapelle A, Kinzler KW, Vogelstein B. Mutations of a muts homolog in hereditary nonpolyposis colorectal cancer. Cell 1993;75:1215–1225.
100. LeBeau MM. Chromosomal fragile sites and cancer-specific rearrangements. Blood 1986;67:849.
101. LeBeau MM. Cytogenetic analysis of hematologic malignancies. In The ACT Cytogenetics Laboratory Manual, 2nd ed. Edited by MJ Barch. New York: Raven, 1991, pp 359–449.
102. LeBeau MM, Albain KS, Larson RA, Vardiman JW, Davis EM, Blough RR, Golomb HM, Rowley JD. Clinical and cytogenetic correlations in 63 patients with therapy-related myelodysplastic syndromes and acute nonlymphocytic leukemia: further evidence for characteristic abnormalities of chromosomes 5 and 7. J Clin Oncol 1986;4:325.
103. LeBeau MM, Bitter MA, Larson RA. The t(2;5)(p23;q35): a recurring chromosomal abnormality in Ki-1 positive anaplastic large cell lymphoma. Leukemia 1989;3:866.
104. Le Beau MM, Espinosa III R, Neuman WL, Stock W, Roulston D, Larson RA, Keinanen M, Westbrook CA. Cytogenetic and molecular genetic delineation of the smallest commonly deleted region of chromosome 5. Proc Natl Acad Sci USA 1993;90:5484–5488.
105. Le Beau MM, Pettenati MJ, Lemons RS, Diaz MO, Westbrook CA, Larson RA, Sherr CJ, Rowley JD. Assignment of the GM-CSF, CSF-1, FMS genes to human chromosome 5 provides evidence for linkage of a family of genes regulating hematopoiesis and for their involvement in the deletion (5q) in myeloid disorders. Cold Spring Harbor Symp 1986;51:899.
106. LeBeau MM, Rowley JD. Cytogenetics. In Hematology 4 ed. Edited by WJ Williams, C Beutler, AJ Erslow, MA Lichtman. New York: McGraw Hill, 1989, pp 78–89.
107. Leder P, Battey J, Lenoir G, Moulding C, Murphy W, Potter H, Stewart T, Taub R. Translocations among antibody genes in human cancer. Science 1983;222:765.
108. Lee WH, Slew JY, Hong FD, Sery TW, Donoso LA, Young LJ, Bookstein R, Lee EYH-P. The retinoblastoma susceptibility gene encodes a nuclear phosphoprotein associated with DNA binding activity. Nature 1987;329:642.
109. Lee W-H, Bookstein R, Hong F, Young LT, Shew JY, Lee EYH-P. Human retinoblastoma susceptibility gene: cloning, identification, sequence. Science 1987;235:1394.
110. Leeua BD, Suijkebuijk RF, Balemans M, et al. Sublocalization of the synovial sarcoma-associated t(X;18) chromosomal translocations breakpoint in Xp11.2 using cosmid cloning and fluorescence in situ hybridization. Oncogene 1993;8:1457–1463.
111. Liu P, Tarle SA, Haira A. Fusion between transcription factor CBFb/PEBP2b and a myosin heavy chain in acute myeloid leukemia. Science 1993;261:1041–1044.
112. Lukeis R, Irving L, Garson M, Hasthorpe S. Cytogenetics of non small cell lung cancer. Analysis of consistent non-random abnormalities. Genes Chromosomes Cancer 1991;3:116.
113. Mandahl N, Heim S, Arheden K, Rydhom A, Willen H, Mitelman F. Three major cytogenetic subgroups can be identified among chromosomally abnormal solitary lipomas. Hum Genet 1988;70:203.
114. Manolov G, Manolova Y. Marker band in one chromosome 14 from Burkitt's lymphomas. Nature 1972;237:33.
115. Mark J. Chromosomal characteristic of neurogenic tumors in adults. Hereditas 1971;68:61.
116. Mark J, Dahlenfors R, Ekedahl C. Cytogenetics of the human mixed salivary gland tumor. Hereditas 1983;99:115.
117. Mark J, Levan G, Mitelman F. Identification by fluorescence of the G chromosome lost in human meningiomas. Hereditas 1972;71:163.
118. Matsushime H, Ewen ME, Strom DK, Kato J-Y, Hanks SK, Roussel FM, Sherr CJ. Identification and properties of an atypical catalytic subunit(p34 PSK-Je/cdK4) for mammalian D-type cyclins. Cell 1992;71:323–334.
119. Mellentin JD, Murre C, Donlon T, McCaw PS, Smith SD, Carroll AJ, McDonald ME, Baltimore D, Cleary ML. The gene for enhanced binding proteins E12/E47 lies at the t(1;19) breakpoint in acute leukemias. Science 1989;246:379.
120. Mitelman F. Catalog of Chromosome Aberrations in Cancer. 5th ed. Edited by F Mitelman. New York: Wiley-Liss, 1994.
121. Mitelman F, Kaneko Y, Berger R. Report of the committee on chromosome changes in neoplasia. In Human Gene Mapping 1993. 1994, pp 773–812.
122. Mitelman F, Mark J, Nilsson PL, Dencker H, Norryd C, Tranberg KG. Chromosome banding pattern in colonic polyps. Hereditas 1974;78:63.
123. Mitelman F, Nilsson PG, Brandt C, Alimena G, Gastaldi R, Dallaicola B. Chromosome pattern, occupation and clinical features in patients with acute nonlymphocytic leukemia. Cancer Genet Cytogenet 1981;4:205.
124. Miyamoto K, Tomita N, Ishii A, Miyamoto N, Nonaka H, Kondo T, Tanaka T, Tsubota T, Kitajima K. Chromosome abnormalities of leukemia cells in adult patients with T-cell leukemia. JNCI 1984;73:353.
125. Miyoshi H, Kozu T, Shimizu K, Maseki N, Kaneko Y, Ohki M. The t(8;21) translocation in acute myeloid leukemia results in production of an ANMLI-MTG transcript. EMBO J 1993:12:2715.
126. Miyoshi H, Shimizu K, Kozu T, Maseki N, Kaneko Y, Ohki M. The t(8;21) breakpoints on chromosome 21 in acute myeloid leukemia are clustered within a limited region of a single gene, AML1. Proc Natl Acad Sci USA 1991;88:10431.
127. Morris CM, Reeve AE, Fitzgerald PH, Hollings PE, Beard MEJ, Heaton DC. Genomic diversity correlates with clinical variation in Ph1-negative chronic myeloid leukemia. Nature 1986;320:281.
128. Morris SW, Kirstein MN, Valentine MB, Dittmer KG, Shapiro DN, Saltman DL, Look AT. Fusion of a kinase gene, *ALK*, to a nucleolar protein gene, *WPM*, in non-Hodgkin's lymphoma. Science 1994;263:1281–1284.
129. Mrozek K, Karakousis CP, Bloomfield CD. Chromosome 12 breakpoints are cytogenetically different in benign and malignant lipogenic tumors: locations of breakpoints in lipoma to 12q15 and in myxoid liposarcoma to 12q13.3. Cancer Res 1993;53:1670–1675.
130. Murphree AL, Benedict WF. Retinoblastoma Clues to human oncogenesis. Science 1984;219:1028.
131. Naylor SL, Johnson BE, Minna JD, Sagakuchi AY. Loss of heterozygosity of chromosome 3p markers in small cell lung cancer. Nature 1987;329:451.
132. Nicolaides NC, Papedopulos N, Liu B, Wei YF, Carter KC, Ruben SM, Rosen CA, Habertine WA, Fleischman RD, Fraser CM, et al. Mutations of the PMS homologues in hereditary non-polyposis colon cancer. Nature 1994;371:75–80.
133. Nilbert M, Heim S. Uterine leiomyoma cytogenetics. Genes Chromosomes Cancer 1990;2:3.
134. Nowell PC, Hungerford DA. A minute chromosome in human granulocytic leukemia. Science 1960;132:1497.
135. Nucifora G, Rowley JD. *AML1* and the 8;21 and 3;21 translocations in acute and chronic myeloid leukemia. Blood, in press.
136. Offit K, Hollis R, Kodurn PRK, Fillipa D, Jhanwar SC, Clarkson BC, Chaganti RSK. 18q21 rearrangement in diffuse large cell lymphoma. Incidence and clinical significance. Br J Haematol 1989;72:178.
137. Offit K, LoCoco F, Louie DC, Parsa NZ, Leung D, Portlock C, Ye BH, Lista F, Filippa DA, Rosenbaum A, Ladanyi M, Jhanwar S, Dalla-Favera R, Chaganti RSK. Rear-

rangements of the *BCL16* gene as a prognostic marker in diffuse large cell lymphoma. N Engl J Med 1994;331:74–80.

138. Ohno H, Takimoto G, McKeithan TW. The candidate proto-oncogene *bcl-3* is related to genes implicated in cell lineage determination and cell cycle control. Cell 1990;60:991.
139. Okamoto A, Dnetrick DJ, Spillare EA, Hagiwara K, Hussan SP, Bennett WP, Forrester K, Gerwin B, Serraro M, Beach DH, Harris CC. Mutations and altered expression of $p16^{INK4}$ in human cancer. Proc Natl Acad Sci USA 1994;91:11045–11049.
140. Olopade OI, Jenkins R, Cowan JM, Linnenbach AJ, Pomykala H, Rowley JD, Diaz MO. Molecular analysis of deletion of the short arm of chromosome 9 in human gliomas. Cancer Res 1992;2:2523–2529.
141. Olopade OI, Pomykala H, Sveen L, Hagos F, Gursky S, Stadler W, Dreyling M, Le Beau MM, Bohlander SK. Construction of a 2.8 megabase YAC contig and cloning of the Methylthioadenosine Phosphorylase (*MTAP*) gene from the tumor suppressor region on 9p21. Proc Natl Acad Sci USA,1995;92:6489-6493.
142. Otterson GA, Kratzker RA, Coxon A, Young WK, Kaye FJ. Absence of $p16^{INK4}$ protein is restricted to the subset of lung cancer lines that retains wildtype RB. Oncogene 1994;9:3375–3378.
143. Papadopoulus N, Nicolaides NC, Wei YF, Ruben SM, Carter KC, Rosen CA, Haseltine WA, Fleischmann RD, Fraser CM, Adams MD, Venter JC, Hamilton SR, Petersen GM, Watson P, Lynch HT, Peltomaki P, Mecklin JP, de la Chapelle A, Kinzler KW, Vogelstein B. Mutation of a mutl homolog in hereditary colon cancer. Science 1994;263:1625–1629.
144. Parmiter AH, Balaban G, Clark WH, Jr, Nowell PC. Possible involvement of the chromosome region 10q24–26 in early stages of melanocytic neoplasia. Cancer Genetics Cytogenetics 1989;30:313.
145. Pathak S, Strong LC, Ferrell RE, Trindale A. Familial renal cell carcinoma with a 3:11 chromosome translocation united to tumor cells. Science 1982;217:939.
146. Pedersen-Bjergaard J, Rowley JD. The balanced and unbalanced chromosome aberrations of acute myeloid leukemia may develop in different ways and may contribute differently to malignant transformation. Blood 1994;83:2780–2786.
147. Pejovic T, Heim S, Mandahl N, Elmfors B, Floderus UM, Furgyik S, Heim G, Willen H, Mitelman F. Trisomy 12 is a consistent chromosome aberration in benign ovarian tumors. Genes Chromosomes Cancer 1990;2:48.
148. Pinkel D, Landegent J, Collins C, Fuscoe J, Segraves R, Lucas J, Gray JW. Fluorescence in situ by hybridization with human chromosome specific libraries. Detection of trisomy 21 and translocations of chromosome 4. Proc Natl Acad Sci USA 1988;85:9138–9142.
149. Pinkel D, Straume T, Gray J. Cytogenetic analysis using quantitative high-sensitivity, fluorescence hybridization. Proc Natl Acad Sci USA 1986;83:2934–2938.
150. Pugh WC, Pearson M, Vardiman JW, Rowley JD. Philadelphia chromosome-negative chronic myelogenous leukaemia: a morphologic reassessment. Br J Haematol 1985;60:457.
151. Rabbitts TH. Chromosomal translocations in human cancer. Nature 1994;372:143–149.
152. Rabbitts TH, Forster A, Larson R, Nathan P. Fusion of the dominant negative transcription regulator CHOP with a novel gene *FUS* by translocation t(12;16) in malignant liposarcoma. Nature Genet 1993;4:175–180.
153. Raimondi SC. Current status of cytogenetic research in childhood acute lymphoblastic leukemia. Blood 1993;81:2237–2251.
154. Raimondi SD, Pui C-H, Behm FG, Williams DL. 7q32-q36 translocations in childhood T cell leukemia Cytogenetic evidence for involvement of the T cell receptor chain gene. Blood 1987;184:131.
155. Reeve AE, Sih SA, Raizis AM, Feinberg AP. Loss of allelic heterozygosity at a second locus in chromosome 11 in sporadic Wilms' tumor cells. Mol Cell Biol 1989;9:1799.
156. Robert K-H, Gahrton G, Friberg K, Zech L, Nilson B. Extra chromosome 12 and prognosis in chronic lymphocytic leukemia. Scand J Haematol 1982;28:163.
157. Rodriguez E, Sreekantaiah C, Chaganti RSK. Genetic changes in epithelial solid neoplasia. Cancer Res 1994;54:3398–3406.
158. Rosenberg CL, Wong E, Petty EM PRAD1, a candidate *BCL1* oncogene: mapping and expression in centrocytic lymphoma. Proc Natl Acad Sci USA 1991;88:9638–9642.
159. Rowley JD. A new consistent chromosomal abnormality in chronic myelogenous leukemia. Nature 1973;243:290.
160. Rowley JD. Chromosome abnormalities in leukemia and lymphoma. Semin Hematol 1990;27:122.
161. Rowley JD. Identification of translocation with quinacrine fluorescence in a patient with acute leukemia. Annal de Genet 1973;16:109.
162. Rowley JD. Rearrangements involving chromosome band 11q23 in acute leukemia. Semin Cancer Biol 1993;4:377–385.
163. Rowley JD, Diaz MO, Espinosa R III, Patel YD, Van Melle E, Ziemin S, Taillon-Miller P, Lichter P, Evans GA, Kersey JH. Mapping chromosome band 11q23 in human acute leukemia with biotinylated probes: identification of 11q23 translocation breakpoints with yeast artificial chromosome. Proc Natl Acad Sci USA 1990;87:9358.
164. Rowley JD, Golomb HM, Daugherty C. 15/17 translocation, a consistent chromosomal change in acute promyelocytic leukemia. Lancet 1977;1:549.
165. Rowley JD, Golomb HM, Vardiman JW. Nonrandom chromosome abnormalities in acute leukemia and dysmyelopoietic syndromes in patients with previously treated malignant disease. Blood 1981;58:759.
166. Rowley JD, Potter D. Chromosomal banding patterns in acute nonlymphocytic leukemia. Blood 1976;47:705.
167. Rubin CM, Carrino JJ, Dickler MN, Leibowitz D, Smith SD, Westbrook CA. Heterogeneity of genomic fusion of BCR and ABL in Philadelphia chromosome-positive acute lymphoblastic leukemia. Proc Natl Acad Sci USA 1988;85:2795.
168. Sadamori N, Nishino K, Kusano M, Tomonega Y, Tagawa M, Yao E, Sasagawa I, Nakamura H, Ichimaru M. Significance of chromosome 14 anomaly at band q11 in Japanese patients with adult T-cell leukemia. Cancer 1986;58:2244.
169. Sandburg AA. The Chromosomes in Human Cancer and Leukemia, 2nd ed. New York: Elsevier, 1990.
170. Schickman SA, Caraani E, Croce EM. Self fusion of the *ALL1* gene: a new genetic mechanism for acute leukemia. JAMA 1995;273:571–576.
171. Schwab M, Alitalo K, Klempnauer K-H, Varmuss HE, Bishop JM, Gilbert F, Brodeur G, Goldstein M, Trent J. Amplified DNA with limited homology to *myc* cellular oncogene is shared by human neuroblastoma cell lines and a neuroblastoma tumor. Nature 1983;305:245.
172. Shima EA, Le Beau MM, McKeithan TW, Minowada J, Showe LC, Mak TW, Minden MD, Rowley JD, Diaz MO. T cell receptor is moved immediately downstream of c-*myc* in a chromosomal 8;14 translocation in a cell line from a human T-cell leukemia. Proc Natl Acad Sci USA 1986;83:3439–3443.
173. Shtivelman E, Lifshitz B, Robert P, Gale RP, Canaani E. Fused transcript of *abl* and *bcr* genes in chronic myelogenous leukaemia. Nature 1985;315:550.
174. Solomon E, Borrow J, Goddard AD. Chromosome aberrations and cancer. Science 1991;254:1153–1160.
175. Solomon E, Voss R, Hall V, Bodner WF, Jass JR, Jeffreys AJ, Lucibello FC, Patel I, Rider SH. Chromosome 5 allele loss in human colorectal carcinoma. Nature 1987;328:616.
176. Sutherland GR, Hecht F. Fragile Sites on Human Chromosomes. New York: Oxford University Press, 1985.
177. Suzukawa K, Parganas E, Gajjar A, Abe T, Takahasi S, Tani K, Asano S, Asou H, Kamada N, Yokota J, Morishita K, Ihle JN. Identification of a breakpoint cluster region 3′ of the ribophorin I gene at 3q21 associated with the transcriptional activation of the *EVI1* gene in acute myelogenous leukemias with inv(3)(q21q26). Blood 1994;84:2681–2688.
178. Swansburg GJ, Lawler SD, Alemena G, Arthur D, Berger R, van den Berghe H, Bloomfield CD, de la Chappelle A, Dewald G, Garson OM, Hagemeijer A, Mitelman F, Rowley JD, Sakurai M. Long term survival in acute myelogenous leukemia: a second follow-up of the Fourth International Workshop on Chromosomes in Leukemia. Cancer Genet Cytogenet 1994;73:1–7.
179. Szucs S, Muller-Brechlin R, De Riese W, Kovacs G. Deletion 3p: the only chromosome loss in a primary renal cell carcinoma. Cancer Genet Cytogenet 1987;26:3184.
180. Thirman MJ, Gill HJ, Burnett RC, Mbangkollo D, McCabe NR, Kobayashi H, Ziemen van der Poel S, Kaneko Y, Morgan R, Sandberg AA, Chaganti RSK, Larson RA, Le Beau MM, Diaz MO, Rowley JD. Rearrangement of the *MLL* gene in acute lymphoblastic and acute myeloid leukemia with 11q23 chromosomal translocations. N Engl J Med 1993;329:909–914.
181. The Third International Workshop on Chromosomes in Leukemia. Cancer Genet Cytogenet 1981;4:95.
182. Thompson F, Emerson J, Dalton W, Yang J-M, McGee D, Villar H, Knox S, Massey K, Weinstein R, Bhattacharyya A, Trent J. Clonal chromosome abnormalities in human breast carcinomas. Twenty-eight cases with primary disease. Genes Chromosomes Cancer 1993;7:185–193.
183. Tkachuk DC, Kohler S, Cleary ML. Involvement of a homolog of *Drosophila trithorax* by 11q23 chromosomal translocations in acute leukemias. Cell 1992;71:691–700.
184. Tkachuk DC, Westbrook CA, Andreeff M, Donlon TA, Cleary ML, Suryanarayan K, Homge M, Redner A, Gray J, Pinkel D. Detection of *bcr-abl* fusion in chronic myelogenous leukemia by in situ hybridization. Science 1990;250:559–562.
185. Travis LB, Pierre RV, DeWald GW. Ph1-negative chronic granulocytic leukemia: a nonentity. Am J Clin Pathol 1986;85:186.
186. Trent JM. The Third International Workshop on Chromosomes in Solid Tumors (IWCST). Tucson, Arizona. Cancer Genet Cytogenet 1990;41:207.
187. Trent JM, Kaneko Y, Mitelman F. Report of the committee on structural chromosome changes in neoplasia. Human gene mapping 10. Cytogenet Cell Genet 1989;51:533.
188. Trent JM, Stanbridge EJ, McBride HL. Tumorigenicity in human melanoma cell lines controlled by introduction of human chromosome 6. Science 1990;247:568.
189. Trent J, Yang J-M, Emerson J, Dalton W, McGee D, Massey K, Thompson F, Villar H. Genes Chromosomes Cancer 1994;7:194–203.
190. Tsujimoto Y, Finger LR, Yunis JJ, Onorato-Showel, Nowell PC, Croce CJ. Molecular cloning of the chromosomal breakpoints of B-cell leukemias with the t(14;18) chromosomal translocation. Science 1984;226:1097.
191. Tsujimoto Y, Finger LR, Yunis JJ, Onorato-Showe L, Nowell PC, Croce CJ. Molecular cloning of the chromosome breakpoint of B-cell lymphomas and leukemias with the t(11;14) chromosome translocation. Science 1984;224:1403–1406.
192. Turc-Carel C, Dal Cin P, Boghosian L, Terk-Zakarian J, Sandberg AA. Consistent breakpoints in region 14q22-q24 in uterine leiomyoma. Cancer Genet Cytogenet 1988;32:25.
193. Turc-Carel C, Dal Cin P, Limon J, Rao U, Li FP, Corson JM, Zimmerman R, Parry DM, Cowan JM, Sandberg AA. Involvement of chromosome X in primary cytogenetic changes in human neoplasia: nonrandom translocation in synovial sarcoma. Proc Natl Acad Sci USA 1987;84:1981.
194. Turc-Carel C, Limon J, Dal Cin P, Rao U, Karakousis C, Sandberg AA. Cytogenetic studies of adipose tissue tumors. II Recurrent reciprocal translocation t(12;16)(q13;p11) in myxoid liposarcomas. Cancer Genet Cytogenet 1986;23:291.
195. Turc-Carel C, Philip I, Berger MP, Philip T, Lenoir GM. Chromosomal translocation (11;22) in cell lines of Ewing's sarcoma. CR Seances Acad Sci III 1983;296:1101.
196. Ueshima Y, Rowley JD, Variakojis D, Winter J, Gordon L. Cytogenetic studies on patients with chronic T cell leukemia/lymphoma. Blood 1984;63:1028.
197. Van Dyke DL, Worsham MJ, Benninger MS, Krause CJ, Baker SR, Wolf GT, Drumheller T, Tilley BC, Casey TE. Recurrent cytogenetic abnormalities in squamous cell carcinomas of the head and neck region. Genes Chromosomes Cancer 1994;9:192.
198. Verter DJ, Thomas DGT. Multiple sequential molecular abnormalities in the evolution of human gliomas. Br J Cancer 1991;63:753–757.
199. Vogelstein B, Fearon ER, Hamilton SR, Kern SE, Aeisinger AC, Leppert M, Nakamura Y, White R, Smits AM, Bos JL. Genetic alterations during colorectal-tumor development. N Engl J Med 1988;319:525.
200. Wang N, Perkins KL. Involvement of band 3p14 in t(3;8) hereditary renal cancer. Cancer Genet Cytogenet 1984;11:479.
201. Westbrook CA, Hooberman AL, Spino C, Bloomfield CD, Davy F, Wurster-Hill D, Sobol R. Clinical significance of the *BCR-ABL* fusion gene in adult acute lymphoblastic leukemia. Blood 1992;80:2983–2990.
202. Whang-Peng J, Bunn PA Jr, Kao-Shan CS, Lee EC, Carney DN, Gazdar A, Minna JD. A nonrandom chromosomal abnormality, del 3p(14–23), in human small cell lung cancer (SCLC). Cancer Genet Cytogenet 1982;6:119.
203. Whang-Peng J, Canellos GP, Carbone PP, Tjio JH. Clinical implications of cytogenetic variants in chronic myelocytic leukemia (CML). Blood 1968;32:755.

204. Whang-Peng J, Triche TJ, Knutsen T, Miser J, Douglass EC, Israel MA. Chromosome translocation in peripheral neuroepithelioma. N Engl J Med 1984;311:584.
205. Williams DL, Look AT, Melvin SL, Roberson PK, Dahl G, Flake T, Stass S. New chromosomal translocations correlate with specific immunophenotypes of childhood acute lymphoblastic leukemia. Cell 1984;36:101.
206. Witte O. The role of the *BCR-ABL* oncogene in human leukemia: Fifteenth Richard and Hinda Rosenthal Foundation Award Lecture. Cancer Res 1993;53:485–489.
207. Working Formulation for Clinical Usage. National Cancer Institute sponsored study of classification of non-Hodgkin's lymphomas. Cancer 1982;49:2112.
208. Yamamoto K, Seto M, Iida S, Komatsu H, Kamada N, Kajima S, Kodera Y, Nakagawa S, Saito H, Takahoshi T, Veda R. A reverse transcriptase-polymerase chain reaction detects heterogeneous chimeric mRNAs in Leukemias with 11q23 abnormalities. Blood 1994;83:2912–2921.
209. Yoshida MA, Ohyashiki K, Ochi K, Gibas A, Prout GR Jr, Pontes JE, Huben R, Sandberg AA. Rearrangement of chromosome 3 in renal cell carcinoma. Cancer Genet Cytogenet 1986;19:351.
210. Yunis JJ, Soreng AL. Constitutive fragile sites and cancer. Science 1984;226: 1199.
211. Zankl H, Zang KD. Cytological and cytogenetical studies on brain tumors. 4. Identification of the missing G chromosome in human meningiomas as no 22 by fluorescence technique. Hum Genetik 1970;14:167.
212. Zech L, Bergh J, Nilsson K. Karyotypic characterization of established cell lines and short term cultures of human lung cancer. Cancer Genet Cytogenet 1985;15:335.
213. Zech L, Gahrton G, Hammarstrom L, Juliusson G, Mallstedt H, Robert KH, Smith CI. Inversion of chromosome 14 marks human T-cell chronic lymphocytic leukemia. Nature 1984;308:858.
214. Zech L, Haglund U, Nilsson K, Klein G. Characteristic chromosomal abnormalities in biopsies and lymphoid-cell lines from patients with Burkitt and non-Burkitt lymphomas. Int J Cancer 1976;17:47.
215. Zeleznik-Le N, Nucifora G, Rowley JD. The molecular biology of myeloproliferative disorders as revealed by chromosomal abnormalities. In Seminars in Hematology. (In press)

CHAPTER 8

Biochemistry of Cancer

EDWARD BRESNICK

On Progress in Understanding the Biochemistry of the Cancer Cell

Phenomenal progress has occurred in the past 10 years, first in understanding the intricacies of communication within and between normal cells, and second in defining the biochemical differences between normal and cancer cells. Much of this progress is attributable to the discovery of oncogenes; their normal counterparts, proto-oncogenes; the mechanisms of signal transduction; and some of the details of the biochemistry of the cell cycle. Most of these topics are covered in other chapters in this section.

This chapter presents a brief historical perspective on the biochemistry of the cancer cell, concentrating on the contributions of intermediary metabolism to the development of testable hypotheses relative to cancer etiology. In addition, some of the unique aspects of the biochemistry of the cancer cell are discussed with a view to providing clues to early diagnosis of the disease in humans, depicting potential targets for therapy, and suggesting causes for the aberrancies we understand as constituting the cancer cell.

Information will be drawn from experiments with animal model systems, with cell cultures, and with humans, including both intact and in vitro systems. The central hypothesis is the universality of the mechanisms of cancer etiology and the applicability of data derived from these model systems to a discussion of the problem within the human population.

Early History of Research in Cancer Biochemistry

ENERGETICS

The biochemistry of cancer began with the work of Otto Warburg during the 1920s and 1930s (199). Warburg remained a dominant force in cancer research until 1940. Using predominantly the tissue slice technique, Warburg measured the utilization of glucose, the production of lactic acid and carbon dioxide, and the utilization of oxygen by various tumors and normal tissues. He noted a high production of lactate by tumor slices in the presence of oxygen. In contrast, in rapidly dividing normal systems, such as fetal tissue, the observed high rate of lactate production was completely abolished by the addition of oxygen.

The phenotype of elevated production of lactate in the presence of oxygen was believed by him to represent a fundamental property of cancer cells that was not found in normal tissue. Consequently, to Warburg, cancer represented a problem in intermediary metabolism. More specifically, a damage to some component of the respiratory chain was the underlying culprit.

Despite the claim by Warburg for a defect in respiration of tumor tissue, cogent arguments refuting this hypothesis were formulated, and these have been summarized by Weinhouse (201). The prevailing view currently accepts Weinhouse's analysis of the operation of both respiration and glycolysis within tumors. An excellent historical perspective on this problem can be found in the review by Shapot (170). Weinhouse pointed out that oxygen, which was consumed by neoplastic cells as effectively as by some normal cells, resulted in an inhibition of the formation of glycolytic end products. In fact, in a series of well-differentiated hepatomas, low rates of aerobic glycolysis were observed of the same magnitude as seen in normal liver with comparable rates of respiration.

The inhibition of glycolysis by oxidative phosphorylation has been called the *Pasteur effect*. Respiration is markedly dependent on the availabilities of intermediates such as adenosine diphosphate (ADP) and inorganic phosphate—that is, on respiratory control. Competition for ADP and inorganic phosphate occurs in respiration and glycolysis, resulting in an apparent inhibition of glucose utilization by oxygen due in part to a reduced availability of these cofactors for phosphorylation under aerobic conditions.

Whether or not cancers can take full advantage of energetics that are potentially derivable from both respiration and glycolysis has been a question of major concern, although the current evidence would suggest not. For example, Urbach (187) has reported a marked reduction in the partial pressure of oxygen in skin cancers as determined by inserting an oxygen electrode into the tumors as well as into the surrounding normal tissue. A very interesting confirmation and extension of these results has been provided by the experiments of Malmgren and Flanigan (114) in an animal model system. Spores of *Clostridium tetani* were implanted into normal mice as well as into several murine tumors. The normal mice survived unaffected by these spores, while the tumor-bearing mice died because the spores were able to germinate in the low pO_2 environment of the tumors. Busch and colleagues (31) have demonstrated the barely detectable level of citrate production by a tumor under in vivo conditions. Yet slices of the same tumor, when incubated in the presence of an appropriate amount of oxygen, produced citrate at a level that approximated that seen with normal liver.

All these studies strongly suggested local hypoxia as the underlying cause for the apparent deficiency in respiration of tumors; an inherent defect in respiration was not the problem. The problem of the utilization of glucose under rather unfavorable conditions by tumors, which confounded Warburg, is most probably due to the presence within tumor plasma membranes of a low K_m hexokinase that affords a "trap" mechanism for the capture of this nutrient, even when present at low concentrations in the surrounding medium (170). Indeed, a substantial body of literature (reviewed in (164)) has shown a hypoglycemic effect of large tumors as a result of this trap; this effect was not the result of ectopic hormone production. The hypoglycemic effect may in part contribute to the problems associated with cachexia in the tumor-bearing host (see later discussion).

OTHER EXAMPLES FROM INTERMEDIARY METABOLISM

Following the Warburg period, a number of technological advances enhanced the analytical capabilities of researchers by allowing for the better quantification of cofactors, enzymes, and metabolic pathways in a large number of transplantable animal tumors. Based on such measurements in a series of transplantable animal tumor models, Greenstein (70) formulated a *convergence hypothesis* to explain a number of interesting aspects of neoplasia. The convergence hypothesis was more a descriptive formulation than a mechanistic discussion of tumor etiology. Greenstein noted that cancers tended to discard certain enzymes or pathways that were not necessary for growth. This effect was particularly noted in transplanted tumors on successive rounds of transplantation. For example, the latency times before the tumors became palpable tended to decrease; i.e., a tumor of a certain size was reached within a shorter period of time after serial transplantations. Concomitant with this decrease in latency (and enhanced growth rate), the enzymatic profiles of the tumors tended to converge to a common pattern. In fact, the adoption of a similar enzymatic profile by these tumors was really a reflection of the increase in growth rate and not an inherent feature of all cancers, slow or fast growing.

Chemically induced hepatocarcinogenesis in rodents provided a number of models that could be analyzed for a number of different parameters. The Millers made several interesting observations relative to hepatocarcinogenesis induced by the administration to rats of an azo dye, *p*-dimethylaminoazobenzene (116). The azo dye tended to interact with certain proteins present in the livers of normal rats; i.e., a correlation existed between the formation of protein bound azo dye and hepatocarcinogenesis. The Millers believed that as a result of this interaction, a crucial protein(s) in the liver could have been altered in terms of function or completely deleted. This protein purportedly would be involved in the regulation of a key event in growth but would not be essential for the survival of the target cells destined to become cancer. Thus was born the *protein deletion theory of carcinogenesis*. Although the key protein or proteins have never been fully characterized, this hypothesis stimulated much research in the comparison of patterns in normal and neoplastic tissues and drove the field for a number of years.

In 1950, Potter modified the protein deletion hypothesis as a result of a number of measurements of enzymatic content of neoplastic and normal liver (145). Potter recognized the existence of alternative pathways involving common intermediates; some of these pathways favored anabolism and therefore growth, and some, catabolism. Potter further noted that competition often existed in regard to the relative amounts of the component that was subjected to either anabolism or catabolism. Based on these observations, he proposed the loss of systems of catabolism as a central feature of tumorigenesis, the *catabolic deletion hypothesis*. The beauty of this hypothesis, and in fact of much of Potter's work, was the formulation of readily testable questions. Although not providing any profound insight into the key event(s) underlying tumorigenesis, the catabolic deletion hypothesis stimulated additional correlations between the rate of tumor growth and their enzymatic composition; i.e., the more rapidly proliferating tumors were associated with the greater loss of enzymes of catabolism.

A significant blow to the catabolic deletion hypothesis as an explanation for cancer development came with the analysis of rapidly proliferating normal systems, such as regenerating and fetal liver. As pointed out by Potter in a previous edition of this text (148), a number of important enzymes that function in anabolism, such as DNA polymerase, were present in regenerating or fetal livers but were not detectable in adult liver. Conversely, catabolic enzymes, such as thymine reductase, were markedly diminished in these rapidly proliferating but normal systems when compared to adult liver. Consequently, the deletion or loss of catabolic enzymes could occur in *normal* albeit rapidly proliferating systems, as well as in tumors. The appearance of anabolic enzymes in normal, rapidly proliferating systems as well as in tumors merely reflected the rapidity of growth.

Whether or not a *specific* protein regulator, but not an enzyme, is deleted prior to oncogenesis remained to be established. Such a protein, which has been postulated by Pitot and Heidelberger (142), could function as a key in triggering a panoply of regulatory steps.

A further modification was proffered by Potter in his *minimal deviation hypothesis* in which cancer cells were noted to deviate from normal cells with regard to a number of nonessential as well as some vitally important components (146). Of great importance to this hypothesis, and subsequently to cancer research, was the development of the Morris hepatoma models. Accordingly, a brief digression on these hepatomas is germane to this discussion.

Through the selective use of a hepatocarcinogen, *N*-(2-fluorenyl)-phthalamic acid, Morris was able to develop a series of rat hepatomas that varied in growth rate, resulting in a transition from well differentiated tumors to poorly differentiated (120). These tumors were referred to as *minimal deviation hepatomas*. Subsequently, a number of these hepatomas were recruited into cell culture, which provided a further dimension to the quality of the questions that could be posed.

Potter believed that he and other investigators were now in position to reduce the important measurable differences between liver and hepatomas to only a few. The analysis of the enzymatic composition of the slow-, intermediate-, and fast-growing varieties of the Morris hepatomas could clearly show which enzymes (either by appearance or deletion) would be inextricably linked to cancer and which to growth rate. Although the minimal deviation hypothesis today appears rather simplistic, it was responsible for several important findings: (*a*) tumors of varying growth rates were analyzed as to enzyme content, and the relationship between activity and proliferation rate was further corroborated and (*b*) the hypothesis forced the realization of the lack of importance of a number of documented enzymologic changes in regard to the process of cancer development. An example of the remarkable correlation between the activity of a key enzyme in nucleotide metabolism, ribonucleotide reductase, and cell proliferation is afforded by the work of Elford et al., which is reproduced in Figure 8.1 (49).

Refinement of Potter's hypothesis came with the development of the *molecular correlation concept* by Weber (200), who noted the quantitative and qualitative variations in the

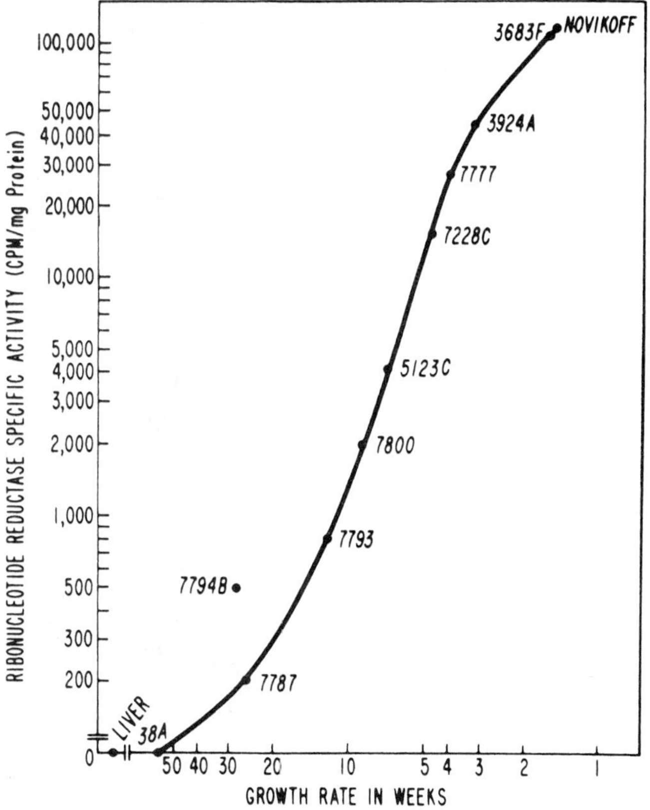

Figure 8.1. Specific activity of ribonucleotide reductase in hepatomas of varying growth rates. Rat hepatomas, indicated within the figure, were assayed for ribonucleotide reductase and the specific activity was plotted as a function of growth rate. The growth rate is expressed as the time required to reach a size that is normal for transplantation. *Source:* Elford et al. (48). Reproduced with permission.

Table 8.1. Molecular Correlation Concept and Affected Processes

Biochemical process	Alteration in cancer cells
Pyrimidine and purine synthesis	Increased
Pyrimidine and purine catabolism	Decreased
RNA and DNA syntheses	Increased
Glucose catabolism	Increased
Glucose synthesis	Decreased
Amino acid catabolism (for gluconeogenesis)	Decreased
Urea cycle	Decreased

Adapted with permission from Weber (197).

degree of neoplasia as related to the concentrations of certain regulators of key metabolic pathways. The key enzymes were defined as (*a*) regulating the rates and directions of competing (or opposing) metabolic pathways (e.g., glucokinase and glucose-6-phosphatase), (*b*) overcoming thermodynamic barriers (e.g., phosphofructokinase), (*c*) providing a common step in two or more metabolic pathways (e.g., citrate synthase), (*d*) representing the first or last step in a reaction sequence (e.g., glutamine-dependent carbamyl phosphate synthetase), (*e*) providing a target for feedback regulation of the allosteric variety (e.g., thymidine kinase), and (*f*) exhibiting isoenzymic patterns (e.g., the hexokinases).

Those metabolic pathways that contained enzymes which fulfilled one or more of these criteria are indicated in Table 8.1 along with the alteration that was observed in cancer.

One of the virtues of the molecular correlation concept is the direction of attention to control by a single regulator of metabolic pathways at multiple steps. This concept of a master regulator had previously been espoused as the *pleiotypic response hypothesis* by Tomkins and his colleagues. They proposed that under normal conditions, a constant group of metabolically unrelated steps would coordinately react in response to environmental modulation and, as a result, affect the rate of growth (82, 181). As stated by Herschko et al. (83), "the transformed phenotype itself may be the result of constant pleiotypic activation which, if true, could render transformed cells independent of growth stimulants normally required."

Therefore, a mutation in a *single* gene could affect a whole series of events that characterizes the malignant phenotype. This postulate predated and predicted the whole concept of signal transduction, which is discussed in Chapter 4.

Oncofetal Protein Expression in Cancer Cells

As indicated above, a number of the enzymatic changes that are observed in neoplastic tissues resemble those that are found in fetal systems. This observation has been responsible for the belief that neoplasia may in fact represent a dedifferentiation or retrodifferentiation of mature cells; as stated by Potter, "oncogeny is blocked ontogeny" (147). The fetal proteins that disappear as a result of maturation and are no longer expressed in adult tissues but reappear in cancerous tissues are referred to as *oncofetal proteins*. A representative list of such proteins is provided in Table 8.2.

One of the first examples of oncofetal proteins was provided by the report of Schapira et al. (165) who noted an unusual form of aldolase in primary liver cancer. Aldolase occurs in multimolecular forms of tetrameric structure, with aldolase A representing the predominant one in muscle; aldolase A is absent from normal adult liver. In fetal liver, aldolase A occurs associated with the liver-specific aldolase B. In primary hepatocellular carcinoma, only aldolase A is present.

A number of key enzymes occur as isoenzymes, with the proportions of the different forms varying as a function of ontogeny. One of the prime examples in this regard is hexokinase, i.e., glucose-ATP-phosphotransferase. This family of enzymes, which plays a vital role in the utilization of glucose, occurs in four molecular forms, types I through IV. Types I through III are referred to as hexokinases, with all possessing a low K_m for glucose. Type IV phosphotransferase is glucokinase, which is distinguished from the other hexokinases by its high K_m for glucose. The predominant forms in adult liver are types I and IV. In fetal liver, type IV glucokinase is barely detectable, while type I hexokinase is the major isoenzyme present. In hepatocarcinogenesis, a progressive reduction in the activity (and amount) of glucokinase is noted with a concomitant rise in type I hexokinase (197).

Phosphofructokinase, a key regulatory enzyme in glycolysis, also occurs in at least four molecular forms in eukaryotic systems with isozyme I found predominantly in muscle, and isozyme IV found predominantly in liver. In the normal, rapidly proliferating systems of regenerating and fetal liver, as well as in a series of hepatomas, type IV phosphofructokinase was also found, but in much higher amount than in normal liver (177). Pyruvate kinase, another key regulator of glycolysis, exists in isoenzymic forms, with type I pyruvate kinase occurring as the major type in adult liver, while representing only a minor type in fetal liver. In the latter, type III pyruvate kinase is the major form. In transplanted hepatomas, the ratio of type III to type I increases as a reflection of decreasing differentiation (174).

A considerable amount of research has been performed with the isoenzymes of alkaline phosphatase by Fishman and his colleagues (58, 59). The placental type of alkaline phosphatase, i.e., the Regan isoenzyme, was discovered in a patient with metastatic bronchogenic carcinoma. It is membrane associated, heat stable, L-phenylalanine sensitive, and neuraminidase cleavable. The Regan isoenzyme is found in the serum of one in seven cancer patients, with the highest incidence in ovarian and other gynecologic cancers.

Table 8.2. Expression of Oncofetal Proteins in Neoplasia

Fetal enzymes, e.g., hexokinase type I
Fetal antigens, e.g., α-fetoprotein
Plasminogen activator
Growth factors, e.g., platelet-derived growth factor
Polypeptide hormones, e.g., thyrocalcitonin
Cellular oncogene products, e.g., AP-1
Angiogenesis factors

TERMINAL DEOXYNUCLEOTIDYLTRANSFERASE (TdT) IN NORMAL AND LEUKEMIC CELLS

TdT has had a major impact on the biotechnology industry because of its use in a number of cloning protocols. TdT catalyzes the linear polymerization of nucleotides onto a suitable template. The substrates for this enzyme are the deoxyribonucleoside-5′-triphosphates with a polydeoxynucleotide or DNA serving as the initiator. The product is the initiator covalently linked to a polymer of deoxynucleoside monophosphates, the number of which depends on the ratio of monomer to initiator (20).

Chang was the first to describe the ontogeny of TdT in the calf thymus gland where activity appeared late during fetal development and increased during the early postnatal period (35). Subsequently, TdT was demonstrated in human and rodent bone marrow (38, 190). In normal humans, the TdT^+ cells appear exclusively in the thymus cortex and bone marrow lymphocytes. As demonstrated by Bodger et al., TdT^+ cells first appear in the lymphoid cells of the embryonic liver at the 12th to 13th week, then in fetal thymus and bone marrow at 19 to 21 and 15 to 16 weeks, respectively (19). Within the fetal thymus, TdT^+ cells constitute only 5 to 10% of the thymocytes; by 1 to 40 months of age postpartum, this number increases to 60 to 85%. In children and young adults, less than 0.02% of Ficoll-Hypaque-separated circulating lymphocytes are TdT^+.

The utility of the TdT^+ phenotype as a marker of certain leukemias arose from the observation by McCaffrey et al. of large amounts in circulating blast cells obtained from a patient with T-cell acute lymphocytic leukemia (113). Subsequently, TdT^+ cells were found in most forms of acute lymphocytic leukemia (20). Consequently, this phenotype has provided another assist in the diagnosis of the specific type of leukemia where the affected cell is of the immature lymphoid variety.

OTHER ONCOFETAL PROTEINS

Oncofetal proteins without enzyme function are also found in a variety of neoplasms. These nonenzymatic proteins are often referred to as tumor-specific antigens. A few examples will serve to illustrate this group, namely, α-fetoprotein (AFP) and carcinoembryonic antigen (CEA).

AFP is a serum protein that was first identified in human fetal cord blood but is not present in adult blood (12). AFP is produced by fetal liver, and to a lesser extent, by the yolk sac during prenatal development. It is the dominant serum protein in early extrauterine development. In many of its structural characteristics, AFP resembles albumin. However, the role of AFP has not been defined, although it does bind estrogen to some extent.

Abelev and colleagues first observed the occurrence of what later turned out to be AFP in adult mice that were bearing a transplantable hepatoma (1). Soon thereafter, elevated serum AFP levels were demonstrated in humans with hepatocellular carcinoma (181). Using the rat Morris hepatomas, Sell and Morris have determined the concentration of AFP in the serum as a function of their growth rate (168). Rats bearing poorly differentiated, rapidly growing hepatomas exhibited levels of serum AFP as high as 18×10^6 ng/mL compared with 60 ng/mL in the serum of normal rats. The serum AFP level in slow-growing, well-differentiated-hepatoma-bearing rats was close to the normal value.

That elevations in serum AFP are not restricted to tumor-bearing hosts was demonstrated in the case of toxic injury to the liver (191). Partial hepatectomy or acute liver toxicity resulted in a transient increase in serum AFP.

A second nonenzyme oncofetal protein of some import in cancer research and diagnosis is CEA, which was first reported by Gold and Freeman (68). CEA is a serum glycoprotein of molecular weight of 200 kd that is present in adenocarcinomas of the human digestive tract as well as in fetal tissues, and is shed into the blood. CEA levels are also elevated in patients with cancers of the lung and genitourinary tract. Elevated serum CEA levels may also be observed in noncancerous patients with colitis, liver cirrhosis, or alcoholic pancreatitis. CEA is one of the most thoroughly characterized tumor-associated antigens.

With the cloning of the CEA cDNA, it has been possible to define different regions of the protein molecule (131). CEA contains a 34-amino acid N-terminal sequence, followed by 107 amino acid N-terminal domain, three highly homologous repeated domains of 178 amino acids, and a 26-residue hydrophobic C-terminal domain. The three homologous regions share extensive sequence homology with the immunoglobulin gene superfamily, supporting some type of evolutionary relationship (135). The hydrophobic C-terminal region has suggested a membrane-anchoring function, which has been pursued by Hefta et al. (82) The latter investigators have demonstrated the anchoring of CEA to plasma membranes by the covalent attachment to an ethanolamine-glycosyl phosphatidylinositol moiety which is added to the protein posttranslationally. Furthermore, it has been suggested that the increased levels of CEA in the serum of patients with certain cancers may be the result of its release from the membrane by some phospholipase, or of the existence of some defect in the phosphatidylinositol complex (82).

The function of CEA has been studied by a number of investigators. Benchimol et al. have demonstrated the CEA-dependent, calcium-independent homotypic aggregation of cultured human colon adenocarcinoma cells and rodent cells that were transfected with CEA cDNA (10). CEA can facilitate the homotypic sorting of aggregating cells. It represents a new addition to the family of intercellular adhesion molecules and is structurally related to Thy-1 and neural cell adhesion molecule (138). CEA has also been demonstrated in normal tissues to be localized to epithelial cell membranes facing the lumen (10). In embryonic intestine and colonic tumors, CEA is found on the adjacent cell membranes. It has been postulated that the overproduction of CEA in colonic tumors may disrupt the normally operating intercellular adhesion forces, resulting in more cell movement, less ordered architecture, and more dedifferentiation (10). These would constitute early steps in tumorigenesis.

Although neither AFP nor CEA is specific for tumors, they do increase the diagnostic capability and, more important, allow assessment of the efficacy of therapy or the reappearance of cancer in the treated patient.

Ectopic Hormone Production by Cancer Cells

Tumors in experimental animal systems as well as in humans often exhibit "bizarre" phenotypic expressions that can have very profound effects on the host. These topics are covered in detail in Chapter 77. In 1928, Brown reported an unusual Cushing's syndrome in a patient who presented with small cell lung carcinoma (27). The symptoms included diabetes, hirsutism, hypertension, and adrenal hyperplasia. Subsequently additional cases of this lung cancer–related syndrome were observed.

In 1965, Liddle and co-workers coined the phrase, ectopic ACTH syndrome, to describe such instances in which the lung cancer elaborates an ACTH-like substance (or ACTH itself) responsible for the hypercorticosteroidism (107). It is now known that as many as 40% of patients with small cell lung carcinoma may elaborate such a polypeptide, although in a large number of these individuals, the polypeptide is either nonfunctional or possesses only a small portion of biologic activity. In the latter case, a precursor molecule, "big" ACTH (proopiomelanocortin), is often present; this substance possesses only 4% of the biologic activity of ACTH.

As indicated above, small cell lung carcinomas often display unusual phenotypic responses. They exhibit some characteristics of neuroendocrine cells in their uptake and decarboxylation of neuroactive amines (139). In this regard, very elevated levels of serotonin, antidiuretic hormone, calcitonin, and ACTH may be observed in patients with small cell lung cancer. These substances are responsible to varying degrees for the biologic syndromes seen.

Further evidence of the complications imposed on the management of cancer patients by ectopic production of a hormone by a nonendocrine tumor is afforded by the occurrence of hypercalcemia, which may be of life-threatening proportion. It was Gutman et al. who in 1936 first described an individual with hypercalcemia and hypophosphatemia as a result of a nonendocrine tumor that did not involve any osseous sites (71). Subsequently, Tashjian et al. demonstrated that extracts from nonparathyroid tumors contain a substance that is immunologically similar to parathyroid hormone (PTH) (1) (179). The ectopic secretion of PTH (or PTH-like substances) occurs in a number of nonendocrine tumors, particularly those originating in the lung and kidney. The elevated serum PTH leads to increased calcium resorption from bone and the occurrence of hypercalcemia. Hypercalcemia is relatively common in patients with disseminated cancer, occurring in approximately 10 to 20% of this population (77).

Substances in addition to hormones have been demonstrated as ectopic secretions in various human cancers. Prostaglandins, particularly of the PGE family, have been reported as ectopic substances in cancers in both experimental animal systems and in humans (124, 147). In addition, the ectopic formation of a colony-stimulating factor (CSF) has been noted in squamous cell carcinomas, resulting in hypercalcemia (79). In the latter instance, confirmation of a causal role of the carcinomas in generating hypercalcemia was provided with the nude mouse model. The squamous cell carcinomas from two patients were removed and transplanted into nude mice, and a resultant hypercalcemia was noted. On resection of these tumors, the hypercalcemia in the nude mice resolved.

Finally, osteolytic substances have been reported in other types of cancers, e.g., Burkitt's lymphoma (122). These substances were not PTH, PGE, or CSF and appeared to exert their action by directly resorbing bone independently of osteoclasts.

In summary, a number of nonendocrine cancer cells are able to manufacture and secrete ectopic substances, including hormones and growth factors, that enhance bone resorption and lead to increased levels of serum calcium (Chapter 77). The mechanisms underlying the elaboration of these substances by the cancers is not understood, although enhanced gene expression is involved.

Cancer, Cachexia, and Cachetic Factors

The growth of tumors in experimental animal systems and in humans is often accompanied by a very striking loss of weight, anorexia, asthenia, and anemia—in other words, cachexia. In several instances the cachetic response to the cancer is not directly related to the total cancer burden of the animal or patient but appears to depend more on some inherent property. Cachexia can often be the primary cause of death of the patient, with as many as 30% of patients succumbing to its effect rather than to the tumor burden (126, 192). Cachexia certainly is a major confounder in the chemotherapy of cancer. Progress in the treatment of cachetic cancer patients has been poor; wasting is predictive of a poorer survival and lower rate of response to chemotherapy. Consequently, much interest has been generated in trying to understand the mechanisms underlying the tumor-induced cachetic response so that appropriate countering measures can be instituted.

Early on, several investigators had suggested that substances released from the tumors might be directly involved in eliciting the cachectic response (reviewed in 126). Nakahara showed a marked depression in liver catalase activity in cancer patients and in tumor-bearing mice that had been treated with a water-soluble, ethanol-precipitable, and heat-stable fraction extracted from human gastric or rectal carcinomas (123). This polypeptide material was referred to as *toxohormone.* Toxohormone also caused a reduction in the concentration of iron in plasma and in the amount of liver ferritin and NAD + NADH. Toxohormone administration involuted the thymus, produced hepato- and splenomegaly, and increased hepatic protoporphyrin. Hepatic catalase activity was depressed, a phenomenon also present in humans (130). The exact mechanisms underlying these actions have never been established. However, it was clear that toxohormone played only a minor role in eliciting cachexia in the cancer patient.

A clearer picture of the cachectic response was afforded by a more detailed study of what happens in the tumor-bearing animal. In the sarcoma-bearing, noncachectic rat, an increased gluconeogenesis and an enhanced direction of glucose from peripheral tissues to the tumor are observed (30, 182). Plasma glucose levels in these rats were quite depressed and blood lactate was elevated. None of these changes were caused by alterations in insulin or glucagon levels.

Tumor-bearing rats or mice progressively lose weight and go into negative nitrogen balance as the tumor weight increases (121). Even force-feeding the host will not sustain an appropriate weight gain, although growth of the tumor is enhanced by this treatment (182). Thorough studies by Cameron and Ord (32) and by Tanaka et al. (178) using several of the Morris hepatomas and a transplantable colon adenocarcinoma model, respectively, confirmed utilization of the mechanisms of gluconeogenesis and enhanced liver glycogenolysis to sustain glucose levels for the tumor. The concept of a tumor as a "nitrogen trap" was espoused as early as 1948 by Mider and colleagues (115) who noted that rat tumors exhibited a positive nitrogen balance at the expense of the host's tissues.

The effects of tumors on the lipid status of the host were also consistent with an energy trap. Lindmark et al., using a mouse sarcoma model system, demonstrated increased fat oxidation, a decrease in body lipids, and a small but significantly elevated expenditure of energy when compared to pair-fed rats (106).

In regard to cachexia and its effects, cancer patients behave very similarly to the experimental animal models. For example, Heber et al. placed noncachectic lung cancer patients under conditions of constant calorie and nitrogen intake and then infused labeled lysine (79). They noted an increased turnover rate of total body protein and an elevation in the catabolism of muscle protein as indicated by an enhanced 3-methylhistidine/creatinine excretion rate. Although a profound increase in the rate of glucose production was observed, no changes were noted in serum ACTH, insulin, or glucagon; glucocorticoids were also normal, as indicated by a 24-hour urinary cortisol level. In the blood of a number of patients with advanced cancer, an increased concentration of alanine is apparent. This alanine, which is present as a result of increased proteolysis, participates in the Cori cycle in liver and through lactic acid is converted to glucose for utilization by the cancer (43, 54).

The above representative examples in both experimental animals and in humans dramatically demonstrate the profound effects of the tumor on intermediary metabolism in the host. The end result is to stimulate tumor growth at the expense of the host's tissue components. Furthermore, this result is accomplished by invoking very inefficient energy-producing mechanisms, i.e., glycolysis. The central question revolves about the nature of the component(s) present in tumors that is (or are) capable of directing the flow of energy from peripheral tissues to the tumor. Extensive research has shown that no shortage of willing candidates exist that are waiting to take their bows for this activity. Although interleukin 1 (IL-1) has been cast as one of the mediators of cachexia (171), a greater role falls on the shoulders of a unique polypeptide—cachectin or tumor necrosis factor (TNF).

TUMOR NECROSIS FACTOR OR CACHECTIN

The discovery of the role of TNF as a mediator in cachexia in the cancer patient drew on two independent lines of research. A group of investigators at Rockefeller University were interested in the process of cachexia that was observed in trypanosome-infected rabbits (14, 98, 157). In these rabbits, an increase in circulating triglycerides was demonstrated that was caused by a systemic suppression of lipoprotein lipase (LPL). A bacterial lipopolysaccharide-inducible serum factor was isolated from these rabbits that could suppress LPL in mice as well as the activities of other lipogenic enzymes in an adipocyte cell line. This factor was called cachectin. Chronic exposure of rabbits to cachectin led to all the signs and symptoms of cachexia seen in tumor-bearing rodents and in human cancer patients (187).

More recent work by this group has demonstrated the suppression of the expression of several mRNAs that encode essential lipogenic enzymes (e.g., glycerol-3-phosphate dehydrogenase in adipocytes) (185). That the action of cachectin is not limited to lipid metabolism was apparent with the observations of a reduction in the resting transmembrane potential, a depletion in intracellular glycogen, an increase in efflux of lactate, and an increased activity of the hexose transporters (186).

The flip side of this story began nearly a century ago with the attempts of William Coley in the late 1800s to treat cancer by administering certain bacterial toxins to cancer patients. This strategy was based on his observations of regression of some tumors in patients after a systemic bacterial infection (reviewed by Old (132)). Coley administered a mixture of killed bacteria directly into the tumor and noted some positive responses. However, with the improvement in surgical procedures and the advent of chemotherapy and radiation, the Coley treatment was abandoned.

Later, it was found that extracts of gram-negative bacteria could induce extensive hemorrhagic necrosis in mouse tumors. The active ingredient was demonstrated to contain endotoxin, a lipopolysaccharide. Indeed, the action of endotoxin appeared to be mediated through stimulation of the production of a serum factor called TNF (133). Human TNF has a molecular weight of 45,000 daltons and is dissociable into components of molecular weight 17,000.

TNF was soon demonstrated to be identical to cachectin (14). The gene has been cloned by Wang et al. (198) The role of recombinant human cachectin/TNF was determined by Oliff et al. (133), who demonstrated the severe weight loss and increased mortality of mice that bore transgenic tumors that secreted this protein.

Recently, the existence of several types of TNF has been established, with TNF-α representing the product from activated macrophages and TNF-β (lymphotoxin or LT-α) the protein from T cells (13). Both cloned products represent primary mediators of the regulation of the immune and inflammatory responses. Both TNFs require interaction with one of two distinct but homologous receptors (p75 and p55) (169). These receptors belong to a large TNF receptor subfamily consisting of at least 12 individual proteins, all of which share some commonality with regard to the extracellular region. The role of the p55 TNF receptor has been evaluated through the use of transgenic knockout mice. These mice are severely impaired with regard to their ability to clear the pathogen *Listeria monocytogenes*, die from infections, and are resistant to liposaccharide-induced septic shock. However, the lymphocyte populations appear normal, with normal T-cell development. The role of the other receptor, p75, has not yet been evaluated.

FUTILE METABOLIC CYCLES

Futile metabolic cycles can operate in carbohydrate and lipid metabolism at a number of enzymatic steps. A futile cycle may occur in a portion of a metabolic pathway where antagonistic reactions operate simultaneously. Under these conditions there is no net flux of metabolites, although a wasteful hydrolysis of ATP is observed that results in the generation of excess heat. For this reason, futile cycles have been implicated in thermogenesis (see, e.g 89, 124). A major futile cycle occurs at the level of phosphofructokinase (PFK) and fructose-1,6-diphosphatase (FDP), as indicated below:

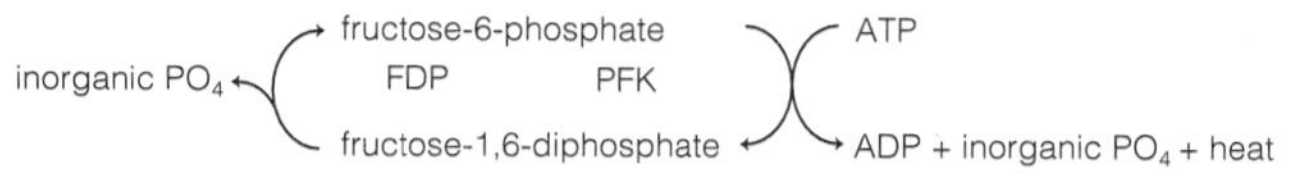

In the tumor-bearing patient, the fructose-6-phosphate/fructose-1,6-diphosphate cycle could be significantly enhanced, perhaps through the effect of TNF, with the resultant dephosphorylation of ATP and the production of heat instead of usable chemical energy. Indeed, the increased heat may contribute to the production of fever in a number of advanced cancer patients. The major source of ATP under these circumstances becomes the oxidation of fatty acids, with gluconeogenesis providing glucose for use by tissues that require this carbohydrate for energy.

In brief, TNF/cachectin is elaborated by tumors or other cells within them and binds to high-affinity receptors present in a variety of tissues, e.g., adipose tissue. The resultant complex causes the suppression of specific mRNA synthesis, which then results in major changes in intermediary metabolism, as outlined above. The end result is the feeding of the tumor at the expense of the host, i.e., cachexia.

Polyamines and Cancer

The naturally occurring polyamines putrescine, spermidine, and spermine are ubiquitously distributed throughout the eukaryotes. Although their role has not been definitively established, cell proliferation and differentiation appear to require their biosynthesis; furthermore, their generation is tightly regulated (94, 141, 176). The metabolic reactions leading to the formation of the polyamines and their biotransformation are indicated in Figure 8.2. The parent substance from which putrescine (and hence, the other

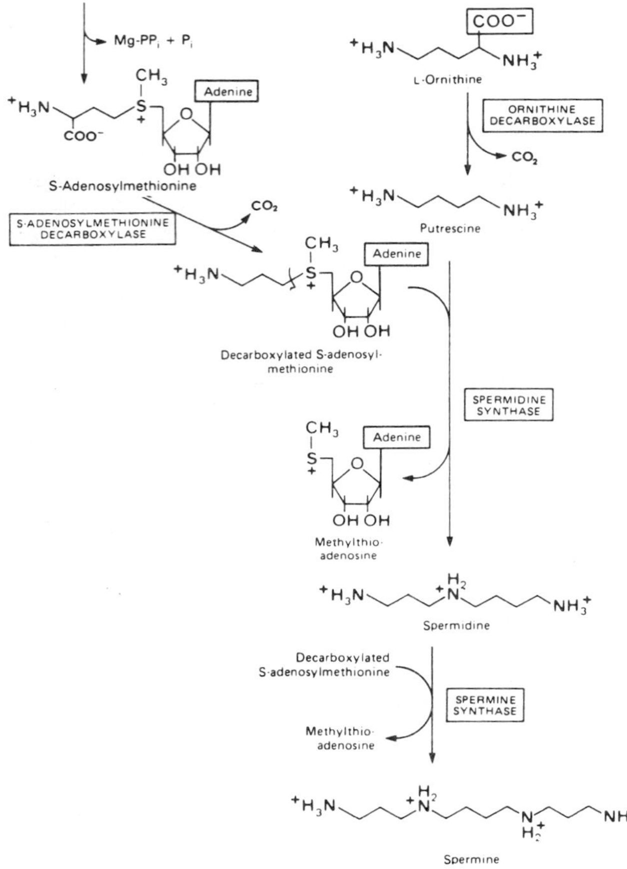

Figure 8.2. Biosynthesis of polyamines.

polyamines) is produced is ornithine in a reaction which is catalyzed by ornithine decarboxylase (ODC), the rate-limiting enzyme of this pathway (161). We will return to ODC shortly.

The formation of spermidine from putrescine and spermine from spermidine requires the addition of aminopropyl groups that are derived from decarboxylated S-adenosylmethionine. The enzymes catalyzing these steps are constitutive but are regulated by the availability of the decarboxylated substrate. S-Adenosylmethionine decarboxylase, which catalyzes the formation of the decarboxylated product, is under both positive and negative feedback control, with putrescine serving as an activator and spermidine as a repressor. The net result of this control mechanism is to regulate the supply of decarboxylated S-adenosylmethionine by the need for spermidine and the availability of putrescine (84).

The synthesis of polyamines is required for the formation of the nucleolus and for appropriate embryonic development in certain worms (80); for oocyte maturation (175); and for rodent embryogenesis (60). Some tissue hypertrophy and hyperplasia, e.g., renal and cardiac hypertrophy and regenerating liver, require polyamine synthesis (113, 140). Agents that induce terminal differentiation of the human HL60 promyelocytic leukemic cells increase putrescine and spermidine levels, suggesting a role of the polyamines in this process (88). An interesting but paradoxical requirement for polyamine synthesis in the cell cycle of normal and transformed cells has been reported. Inhibition of polyamine synthesis in Ehrlich ascites cells resulted in an accumulation of these cells in S and G_2 phases (81), while normal cells under similar conditions of blockade arrested in the G_1 phase (160).

Animal tumor models require polyamine synthesis. High polyamine levels were present in Ehrlich ascites carcinoma cells; the rate of tumor cell proliferation correlated with the increases in polyamines (94). Suppression of tumor growth has also been observed when inhibitors of polyamine synthesis were administered (see review in 82). The impact of polyamines on the growth of tumor systems has included human neoplasms. Small cell lung carcinoma cell lines were very sensitive to inhibitors of polyamine synthesis both when added in culture or administered to nude mice bearing xenografts. Other sensitive human tumors included melanoma, prostatic carcinoma, and pancreatic carcinoma cells (111).

ORNITHINE DECARBOXYLASE

As indicated above, ODC is a key regulatory enzyme in the biosynthesis of polyamines. Under normal conditions, the activity of ODC is very low in cells, although the enzyme undergoes rapid induction on their exposure to a variety of stimuli, including growth factors, hormones, and tumor promoters. These induced levels are quite ephemeral, however, as a result of the very short half-life of the protein (129, 166). ODC activity is markedly elevated in human skin tumors (164). In a mouse model system, O'Brien and colleagues have demonstrated the occurrence of a functionally altered ODC in skin tumors as compared to normal tissue; the tumor form of ODC is activated by guanosine triphosphate (GTP) (128). In a recent study from this laboratory, ODC was examined in human skin and squamous cell carcinomas and a similar altered enzyme was observed in the human skin cancers that was activated by GTP (85). O'Brien et al. have postulated that the altered protein allows the escape of the polyamine biosynthetic pathway in these tumors from normal cellular regulation.

An interesting series of experiments has been reported from the Verma laboratory relating to the localization of at least one of the human ODC genes to chromosome 2, and to further defining the role of ODC and of polyamines in tumor cell biology (44). In the normal ODC-deficient Chinese hamster ovary (CHO) cells, exogenous putrescine is required for cell growth. In CHO cells that have been transfected with the human ODC gene, the enzyme is overexpressed and the addition of putrescine is no longer required. Furthermore, in the transfected cells, considerably more G_2 + M cells are noted than in the ODC-deficient parental cell line. These studies suggest that the polyamines, and putrescine in particular, may be required for the transition from S to G_2 + M; the studies reinforce the rate-limiting nature, and hence the importance, of ODC in this pathway.

Elevated ODC activity has been reported in certain premalignant conditions in humans, e.g., in colon biopsy samples from patients with familial polyposis, a condition in which increased proliferation of the colonic mucosa is present with a high risk for the development of cancer (110). Similarly, increased ODC activity has been reported in the epithelial dysplasia associated with Barrett's esophagus, another high-risk situation for cancer development (65).

Although the exact mechanism underlying the elevation of ODC in tumor tissue is not yet understood, considerable evidence relating to the induction of this regulatory enzyme in mouse skin and in cultured keratinocytes by phorbol ester has suggested a phosphorylation-mediated gene activation. Phorbol ester is known to interact with and activate protein kinase C (see Chapter 4). The action of protein kinase C should lead to the production of certain phosphorylated trans-acting proteins. These activators may be directly responsible for enhancing the transcription of appropriate genes that contain phorbol ester–responsive elements, including ODC.

The mechanisms underlying the elevation in ODC activity in malignant and premalignant tissues are important. ODC is a protein with a very rapid turnover, i.e., minutes. Some evidence indicates that the enhanced ODC activity in these tissues may be caused in part by a posttranscriptional effect, i.e., stabilization of existing ODC molecules. The manner by which intracellular protein degradation is accomplished is just being uncovered, with at least three such mechanisms operative in mammalian cells (44): (*a*) ubiquitin-dependent, ATP-requiring proteolysis where ubiquitin forms an isopeptide linkage with the ϵ-lysine of the protein to be degraded and the targeted molecule is subjected to proteolysis by a multisubunit protease; (*b*) calcium-dependent proteases (calpains), although the role of this extralysosomal proteolytic mechanism is still unclear; and (*c*) lysosomal degradation, which is responsible for the proteolysis of many of the membranal proteins and of the long-lived cytosolic proteins.

In addition to these mechanisms, some element of structure within the amino acid sequence of the ephemeral proteins may contribute to the tagging of molecules for degradation. In this regard, the PEST hypothesis is worthy of note. Rogers et al. have examined the amino acid sequence of a number of short-lived and long-lived proteins and have noted an unusual richness of proline (P), glutamic acid (E), serine (S), and threonine (T) stretches within the primary structure of the proteins that exhibited rapid turnover rates (156). ODC is a protein with PEST sequences. It is interesting to speculate that in tumor tissues, perhaps some alteration in the PEST sequences may have occurred that would stabilize the existing ODC protein without compromising catalytic function. Indeed, Ghoda et al. (67) have noted that the removal of 37 residues from the carboxyl-terminal end of ODC resulted in a marked stabilization of the molecule; the PEST sequences are contained within this region. Whether or not alteration of the ODC gene occurs within tumors such that the PEST sequences are deleted or rendered nonfunctional, thus contributing to the increased activity of ODC, remains to be determined.

Cyclic Nucleotides as Regulators of Growth

Cyclic AMP (cAMP) may play an important role in the differentiation of certain cells. cAMP is formed from the catalytic action of adenylyl cyclase, a membrane-bound enzyme that utilizes ATP as substrate (Fig. 8.3). The

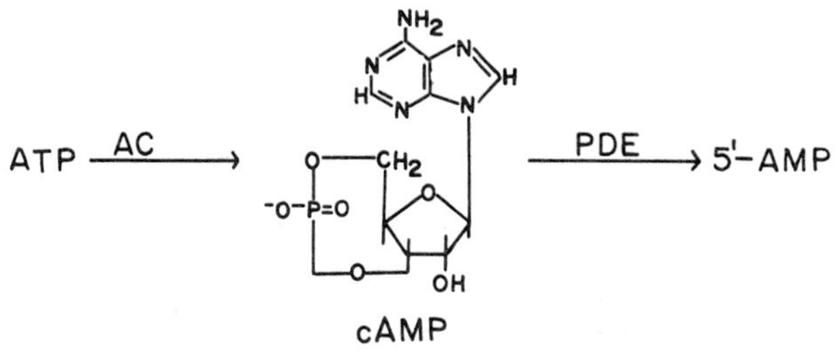

ATP —AC→ cAMP —PDE→ 5'-AMP

Figure 8.3. The biosynthesis and catabolism of cyclic AMP (cAMP). AC, adenylyl cyclase; PDE, phosphodiesterase.

intracellular level of cAMP is dependent not only on the activity of adenylyl cyclase but also on a specific phosphodiesterase. As indicated in Figure 8.3, the phosphodiesterase causes the hydrolytic cleavage of cAMP with the production of the relatively inert 5'-AMP. Although the details relative to biologic role of cAMP are discussed in some detail in Chapter 4, a brief summary of this involvement is presented below.

cAMP is involved in a number of phosphorylation reactions through the action of cAMP-dependent protein kinases, called *A-kinases*. Their dependency on cAMP is based on the existence of the A-kinases in an inactive tetrameric form consisting of two regulatory and two catalytic subunits. cAMP interacts with the regulatory subunits, releasing the catalytic oligomer for enzymatic action. The active A-kinase then catalyzes the phosphorylation of appropriate protein substrates, with ATP as the phosphorylating agent. The phosphorylated protein is responsible for eliciting a specific response relative to growth and proliferation of the cells.

cAMP levels are modulated by such external stimuli as growth factors and prostaglandins. This effect is mediated by the tight coupling that exists between the receptor for the external stimulus and the adenylyl cyclase system. An excellent review of the interplay between growth factors, oncogene products, and adenylyl cyclase is offered by Bourne and DeFranco (23).

The level of cAMP has been measured in a number of transformed cells and tumors (119). In many cases, a decrease in cAMP was observed, in others, an increase. The addition of cAMP to cultured tumor cells led to a partial reversion to a differentiated phenotype, i.e., more nearly normal. For example, neuroblastoma cells on exposure to cAMP altered their morphology with the appearance of more normal long neurites and concomitantly of enzyme profiles that were closer to normal. A similar picture has been obtained with certain glioma cells. The effect of cAMP on these cells was reversible; with its removal, the cells reverted to their previous neoplastic phenotype.

The work of Burk is also worthy of note (29). Agents that inhibit phosphodiesterase activity and, therefore, increase intracellular cAMP levels significantly depressed the growth of both normal and virally transformed baby hamster kidney cells. Furthermore, the cAMP levels increased concomitantly with the cessation of growth of nontransformed fibroblasts upon approaching confluence (162). These observations formed the basis for the belief that cAMP levels may regulate the rate of cell proliferation. It is quite clear, however, that cAMP does not play a consistent role in neoplasia, although the enzymes that are phosphorylated through the action of the A-kinases are very important determinants of proliferation.

Poly(ADP-Ribose) Polymerase and Cell Death

Poly(ADP-ribose) polymerase or synthetase is a chromatin-bound enzyme that catalyzes the formation of poly(ADP-ribose) at the expense of NAD (see reviews in 11 and 77). Poly(ADP-ribose) is capable of poly(ADP-ribosylation) of a number of proteins, thus altering their activity (e.g., DNA ligase, histones, the polymerase itself). The polymerase is involved in cell transformation, cell differentiation, and DNA repair, although the exact mechanisms in this regard have not been clearly defined. Borek and colleagues reported the inhibition of x-ray–, ultraviolet light–, and chemical carcinogen–induced malignant transformation of hamster embryo cells and mouse C3H 10T1/2 cells by administration of inhibitors of poly(ADP-ribose) polymerase, thus implicating this enzyme in that process (22).

Poly(ADP-ribosylation) is activated by DNA strand breaks, with successive transfer to nuclear proteins of the ADP-ribose moieties originating from NAD. This reaction in some manner facilitates the DNA repair process. Berger has proposed an interesting suicide response of cells with extensive DNA strand breaks that involves the poly(ADP-ribose) polymerase (11). When the damage to DNA is severe, activation of the polymerase persists, leading to depletion of the intracellular pools of both NAD and ATP. This depletion may result in rapid cell death before the DNA repair is consummated. However, some problems exist with this explanation for DNA damage-induced cell death. The depletion of NAD levels can be prevented by the administration of inhibitors of the poly(ADP-ribose) polymerase, e.g., 3-aminobenzamide. Yet these polymerase inhibitors often *potentiate* the cell toxicity of the DNA-damaging substance (33).

Ding and colleagues have investigated the effects of blocking the synthesis of poly(ADP-ribose) polymerase by antisense expression upon a variety of parameters (46). Cells in which the antisense was expressed and therefore in which synthesis of the polymerase was inhibited were delayed in their ability to initiate the repair of alkylating agent–induced DNA strand breaks. In addition, these cells depleted of the polymerase exhibited an increase in gene amplification (which requires a strand break and repair), and an alteration in chromatin structure as defined by hypersensitivity to nuclease digestion. These observations support the role of poly(ADP-ribose) polymerase in DNA repair.

APOPTOSIS AND CANCER CELL IMMORTALITY

The above discussion raises several issues in regard to damage-induced cell death and the concept of immortality, particularly as practiced in cancer cells. All normal cells are programmed for cell death, i.e., each cell has a finite lifetime. It was Wyllie's group that coined the term, *apoptosis* to describe a series of morphologic changes that result in programmed cell death (99, 203). Apoptosis occurs during differentiation, normal development, cell maturation, in immune surveillance, and following cell injury by a variety of agents. In the latter context, a number of cancer chemotherapeutic agents cause cell death by invoking the processes of apoptosis. A number of excellent reviews have recently appeared on the mechanisms of apoptosis and on the relationship to cancer etiology and therapy (48, 50, 102, 173). Although the detailed mechanisms underlying apoptosis are not yet understood, it is clear that a number of gene products are involved, including those that participate in signal transduction, in various nuclease and protease activities, and in protein phosphorylation/dephosphorylation.

Of particular interest is the apparent absence of apoptosis in cancer cells. The block in programmed cell death that occurs in cancer is related to the expression of the bcl-2 oncogene and to the relative levels of the proteins, Bcl-2 and a close relative, Bax (i.e., Bcl-2/Bcl-2, Bcl-2/Bax, Bax/Bax). Bcl-2, as discussed elsewhere in this text (Chapters 5 and 6), was first identified as a t(14;18) translocation in a human lymphoma and was expressed in hematopoietic stem cell populations. Consequently, apoptosis is negatively regulated by expression of this oncogene. Recent findings have shown that Bax as a homodimer can mediate apoptosis and that protection of cells from this type of cell death is afforded by Bcl-2 through heterodimerization with Bax or through the Bcl-2/Bcl-2 homodimer. It is evident that the expression of bcl-2 has become a focus for innovative cancer therapy.

Apoptosis is also positively regulated—induced—by expression of the tumor suppressor gene, p53. Any stimulus that affects p53 expression will therefore affect apoptosis. It is germane to mention that mutations within the p53 gene eliminate this apoptosis-inducing property.

The above discussion has raised the issue of damage-induced cell death. The rapid rate of DNA replication that is often seen in cancer cells represents the chink in the armor that has stimulated a number of approaches to cancer therapy (47). Many of the useful drugs in cancer chemotherapy are alkylating agents that interact with DNA. The binding of these agents to DNA is, however, not sufficient to explain the subsequent process of cell death. Some evidence exists that indicates that some cell cycle event(s) is or are associated with the toxicity of alkylating agents. For example, it is known that cisplatin, a useful cancer chemotherapeutic agent, is much more toxic to dividing cells, although this drug is not a cell cycle–specific substance (61). It is also known that the subsequent cell death is not related to a reduction in DNA synthesis mediated by cisplatin (172). The latter investigators have postulated some critical event in G_2 that determines the fate of treated cells.

The purpose of this discussion is to provide the reader with a framework for understanding the use of an already existing mechanism within normal and cancer cells to respond to the toxic action of a therapeutic agent. Furthermore, it is necessary to conceptualize some aberrancy in this mechanism occurring in some cancers. Thus, neoplastic cells, although exposed to an agent that can alkylate cellular DNA, may not trigger the apoptotic response, and the "resistant" cell will survive.

DNA Methylation in Cancer

A substantial body of evidence suggests a role for the methylation of DNA in the control of the expression of genes in eukaryotes. This methylation occurs exclusively in the 5-position of cytosine, and more specifically when this cytosine is part of a CpG dinucleotide. The first indications of this role came from the reports of Holliday and Pugh (86) and of Riggs (154) in 1975. A 1990 review by Jones and Buckley outlined the experimental details underlying the inverse relationship between the amount of 5-methylcytosine in DNA and the extent of gene expression (96). The conclusion from many of these studies is that hypomethylation was necessary but not sufficient for enhanced gene activity.

The dinucleotide CpG is underrepresented in vertebrates and is generally clustered in so-called CpG islands. These islands are generally defined as GC-rich regions that are hypomethylated and that do not occur with any frequency in highly tissue-specific genes (16). Methylation of these CpG islands appears associated with transcriptional inactivity. Excellent examples of this type of regulation occur with genes associated with the inactive X chromosome, e.g., hypoxanthine phosphoribosyltransferase and glucose-6-phosphate dehydrogenase. Although methylation of CpG islands within these genes is not the initial step in the inactivation, the 5-methylcytosine does stabilize the transcriptionally inactive state.

Several investigators have examined the role of DNA methylation, e.g., at CpG islands, in the production of cancer and in the maintenance of the cancerous state. This question has generally been addressed through the use of two techniques, (*a*) the sensitivity of certain restriction endonucleases to a methyl group (e.g., Msp I will cut CCGG independent of whether the middle C is methylated, while Hpa II will digest the DNA at this tetramer *only* when the middle CpG is unmethylated), and (*b*) the utilization of 5-azacytidine, an inhibitor of DNA methyltransferase, the enzyme that catalyzes the methylation of the CpG islands.

Kuo and colleagues have reported less methylation of the CpG sequences in the α-fetoprotein gene in hepatoma DNA when compared to normal liver DNA (103). On the other hand, Baylin and colleagues have noted hypermethylation of specific regions of human chromosomes in tumor cells, particularly through the use of chromosome 11 probes (9, 42). The latter studies raise the interesting possibility of increased methylation associated with the silencing of tumor suppressor genes. These studies suffer the disadvantage of using cultured tumor cells. Under these conditions, it is not known if the effects on methylation were in fact imposed by the culture per se. However, many of these types of experiments have been repeated using primary tumor samples. Gama-Sosa et al. reported a reduced level of DNA methylation in a large number of human tumors (64). Furthermore, the metastases exhibited a lower 5-methylcytosine content in their DNA than that present in benign tumors or in normal tissue. Feinberg et al. examined human colonic cells obtained from adenomas, adenocarcinomas, and normal tissue (53). They reported a hypomethylation of the DNA in the tumor with a reduction of approximately 10% in DNA 5-methylcytosine. No difference was noted in the levels of 5-methylcytosine in benign versus malignant tumors. On the other hand, a hypermethylation of the calcitonin gene has been observed in over 90% of non-Hodgkin's-type lymphoma and in 95% of the tumor cell DNA obtained from patients with acute myeloid leukemia (8).

Several groups of investigators have examined the extent of DNA methylation as a function of tumor progression. Frost and his colleagues were first to report an alteration in tumorigenicity by changing the immunogenicity of tumors after exposure to 5-azacytidine (62, 63). A reduction in DNA methylation after treatment with 5-azacytidine of clones of murine Lewis lung carcinoma cells that had been selected for their nonmetastatic potential resulted in their conversion to a metastatic phenotype (134–136). Therefore, treatment with this inhibitor of DNA methylation could result in either a loss or gain in metastatic potency, depending on the initial biologic starting material.

The methylation of DNA, principally at the CpG islands, plays a role in the tumorigenesis process and in tumor progression. However, that role is not a simple one and may be unique for each individual tumor.

Cell Cycle Control, Immortality, Genomic Instability, and Cancer

It has long been known that the transition of normal cells through the cell cycle is rather tightly controlled. Many cancer cells, however, do not exhibit the same degree of regulation of the cell cycle, and the reasons for their enhanced replication rate are slowly unfolding. Several excellent minireviews of this aspect are in print (75, 91, 127).

The transition of a normal cell from the G_1 through S, G_2, and finally M phases—i.e., the cell cycle—is controlled by both positive and negative regulators at several checkpoints, including at G_1/S, where a commitment to replication is made, and at G_2/M, where a commitment to divide is undertaken. A key event in the activation process is the association of a member of a family of cyclins with a specific cyclin-dependent kinase (CDK). The nature of the complex is constantly changing, which serves to launch the cell from one stage to another in the cycle. The resultant complex activates or inactivates various protein components by phosphorylation (catalyzed through the CDK) in this process. Almost all of the cyclins possess a short half-life, and, therefore, one is present only for a brief time for complexation to a CDK, i.e., it is present only at one stage of the cell cycle. In similar fashion, the kinase subunits also appear in successive manner during the phases of the cell cycle so that both the cyclin component and the specific CDK are constantly changing, but in a specific way. For example, the association of cyclin D with its partner CDK4 constitutes the G_1/S checkpoint. The stimulation of cell division that might normally be required would be affected through a growth factor–inducible process focused on the production of a specific cyclin. The short half-life of the cyclin would ensure only one or several rounds of cell division at most. Consequently, the cyclin-CDK system becomes a sensor for growth factors.

An additional mechanism for manifesting regulation of the cell cycle occurs by the production of cyclin-cyclin–dependent protein kinase inhibitors, e.g., p16, p15, p21, p27. These proteins all share the property of interaction with the cyclin-CDK complex and inactivating its function. For example, p16 competes with cyclin D for interaction with CDK4, and inhibits the transition of the cell through the G_1/S checkpoint.

Deregulation of the cell cycle is often observed in cancer, resulting in additional cell divisions. This loss of control which occurs at the checkpoints will also alter cancer cell growth and division by reducing the sensitivity of the cell to external stimuli, e.g., growth factors. The loss of sensitivity could result from (*a*) production of a mutant cyclin, (*b*) aberrant expression of the cyclin, or (*c*) loss of cyclin-cyclin–dependent protein kinase inhibitors. Cyclin D is overexpressed in a number of different tumors as a result of chromosomal translocation resulting in gene amplification. In this regard, the specific cyclin acts as an oncogene (see Chapter 5), and its overexpression is interpreted by the cell as a stimulus for mitosis. An increase in the steady-state level of cyclin D has also been reported to occur by stabilization of the protein through a truncation of the 3′-untranslated region of the mRNA which contributes the signal for protein degradation, i.e., is responsible for the short half-life.

While the cyclins may resemble oncogenes, the cyclin-cyclin–dependent protein kinase inhibitors are more akin to tumor suppressor genes. Thus, p16 has been mapped to a portion of chromosome 9 in the human in which a tumor suppressor gene activity is resident. The association of p21 that normally interacts with cyclin-CDK is very significantly reduced in neoplastically transformed cells. Therefore, the reduction in the cyclin-dependent protein kinase inhibitor–CDK complex in cancer cells would be accompanied by an elevated level of the active stimulus to pass through the cell cycle checkpoints, cyclin-CDK. In addition to participating in the regulation of the cell cycle at the checkpoints, p21 inhibits the replication process by interacting with and inactivating proliferating cell nuclear antigen (PCNA), an important subunit of DNA polymerase δ.

The synthesis of the cyclin-cyclin–dependent protein kinase inhibitor, p21, is itself transcriptionally activated by another tumor suppressor gene, p53. In this fashion, p53 is able to slow down cell division at the G_1/S checkpoint. In the case of damage to the DNA, such a slowdown would be required in order to facilitate repair prior to replication.

DNA DAMAGE AND THE CELL CYCLE

DNA is continuously bombarded by free radicals generated through normal cell biochemistry, e.g., through prostaglandin synthase H, or by activated toxins, mutagens, and carcinogens that may find their way into the host. These exposures lead to the production of DNA adducts such as 8-hydroxydeoxyguanosine and carcinogen-adducted bases. Most normal cells possess adequate levels of repair systems that are capable of restoring the integrity of the DNA, but the repair process must be invoked prior to replication in cell division. Were the repair process to lag, mutational events would be perpetuated by cell division. One of the mechanisms that allows a slowdown of cell division is mediated through the action of the tumor suppressor gene, p53. As indicated above, p53 transcriptionally activates the synthesis of p21, which mediates an arrest of the cell cycle at the G_1/S checkpoint by effectively competing with cyclin for CDK binding. The cell cycle arrest then allows for sufficient time for normal DNA repair processes to remove either the adducted DNA base or the alkyl group itself. p53 stimulates DNA repair by several other mechanisms: by interaction with and activation of ERCC-3, an important repair enzyme, and by transcriptionally activating the synthesis of Gadd45, another enhancer of repair.

Mutations to p53 are found in over 50% of human cancers (see Chapter 6). The mutated p53 molecules are no longer positive regulators of proteins that function in DNA repair, are not able to stimulate the production of p21, and do not arrest the cell cycle at the G_1/S checkpoint. Consequently, the mutant p53 molecules facilitate genomic instability by allowing replication to proceed before adequate repair of any adducted DNA can occur. This enhanced genomic instability undoubtedly contributes to the process of tumor progression.

DNA REPAIR ABNORMALITIES AND CANCER

A number of human genetic disorders have played a major role in establishing a relationship between a DNA repair defect and cancer development. These disorders include xeroderma pigmentosum (which actually represents a family of at least seven members), ataxia telangiectasia, Fanconi's anemia, Bloom syndrome, and Cockayne syndrome. It has long been known that individuals with xeroderma pigmentosum are very sensitive to actinic radiation-induced carcinogenesis. Cleaver subsequently established that this predisposition to skin cancer development was the result of a deficiency in nucleotide excision repair (37).

A remarkable example of the importance of postreplication DNA repair mechanisms in preserving genomic stability and serving as a component against cancer development has been reported during the past few years (26, 56, 104, 137). A connection between DNA microsatellite instability and the occurrence of reiterated dinucleotide sequences, e.g., $(CA)_n$, had been previously reported. These tandem repeats may give rise to frameshift mutations as a result of replication slippage/misalignment mediated during the DNA polymerase reaction (117). The frequency of somatic frameshift mutations in these tandem repeat regions is quite high. Ordinarily, mismatches in the tandem repeat regions such as a single base mispair, G:T, or more complex insertion-deletion loop-type mismatch nucleotides, are repaired by two families of mismatch repair genes that are conserved from bacteria to humans, *mutS* and *mutL*.

Hereditary nonpolyposis colon cancer (HNPCC) is a disease that occurs in 5 per 1,000 persons in industrialized nations. These individuals are prone to development not only of colorectal carcinoma but cancers of the female reproductive organs as well. During an analysis of genetic linkage in HNPCC families, candidate target genes were localized to chromosomes 2p and 3p. In addition, it was noted that many mono- and dinucleotide deletions and insertions occurred in the microsatellite DNA from their colon cancers and that hypervariability of this DNA appeared to be a persistent trait. Indeed, microsatellite DNA hypervariability occurs in more than 80% of HNPCC and in approximately 15% of cases of the sporadic type of colorectal cancer. Further research established the target genes on chromosomes 2p and 3p that were affected in HNPCC as *hMSH-2* and *hMSL-1*, respectively. The gene products, hMSH-2 and hMSL-1, exhibited much homology to the bacterial and yeast counterparts. These proteins functioned in postreplicative mismatch repair and maintained the integrity of regions of the chromosome in which reiterated nucleotide repeats are found, such as in microsatellites. Consequently, HNPCC and perhaps other types of cancers may result from the inability to repair these types of DNA lesions because of nonfunctional hMSH-2 and hMSL-1. It is interesting to speculate that other types of cancers may also evolve from mutations in yet other proteins that function in DNA repair.

TELOMERASE AND IMMORTALITY

One of the cardinal features of cancer cells in culture is their apparent immortality. While cultured normal cells tend either to terminally differentiate or to die off after a defined number of passages, most cancer cells continue to grow. This property of escape from senescence, i.e., immortality, has been under intense scrutiny. Recently, a striking relationship between senescence/immortality and the activity of a unique enzyme, *telomerase*, has emerged.

Telomeres, the terminal capping DNA sequences of chromosomes, play an important role in maintaining chromosomal stability (17, 71). A shortening of the telomeric ends has been observed with each round of DNA replication within normal cells. Consequently, increasing age, such as in bone marrow and epithelial cells, results in a reduction in the telomere restriction fragment length (74, 76). Indeed, the replicative capacity of human fibroblasts is correlated to the length of the telomere.

Sequence analysis of telomeric DNA in a number of eukaryotic systems has demonstrated the presence of hundreds to thousands of tandemly repeated bases, TTAGGG (18). The maximum number of these TTAGGG repeats occurs early in the gestation of a fertilized cell. With every subsequent cell division, 50 to 200 of these tandem repeats are discarded from each telomere. By the time a cultured cell has divided about 100 times, most of the telomeric TTAGGG repeats have been removed, and the cell senesces. Within a tissue, when enough cells have undergone this process over a defined normal life span, the tissue begins to "die."

Unlike normal cells, in which a continuing loss of telomeric TTAGGG repeats occurs, many neoplastic cells maintain their tandem sequences; examples include human malignant hematopoietic cells (125), ovarian carcinoma cells (37), and many others (100). The maintenance of the telomeric terminal repeats is the responsibility of a ribonucleoprotein enzyme, telomerase. This remarkable enzyme contains an RNA with a complementary sequence to the terminal repeat, thus allowing hybridization to the telomeric DNA and subsequent polymerization of deoxyribonucleotides of the TTAGGG units. In normal cells, telomerase activity appears highest in the early stages of development and is, therefore, responsible for the apparent immortalization of reproductive cells; telomerase activity diminishes with age. Cancer cells, on the other hand, maintain their levels of telomerase, which leads to continuous replenishment of the telomeric terminal repeats. The result is the immortalization of the cancer cell. The existence of the telomerase in cancer cells provides an avenue of opportunity for the development of more specific chemotherapeutic agents.

Proteases and Cancer Cells

The production and secretion of proteolytic enzymes by tumors represent very old observations. In 1925, Fischer reported that explants of virally-induced chicken tumors were able to lyse plasma clots while explants from normal connective tissue were inactive in this regard (56). Subsequently, a number of investigators observed fibrinolytic activity released by a wide variety of transformed cells (158).

Largely through the efforts of the Reich laboratory, it is clear that the fibrinolysis is the result of the secretion of plasminogen activator, which can convert the serum proteolytic zymogen, plasminogen, to an active enzyme (151, 189). Plasminogen activator is a serine protease that converts plasminogen to plasmin by cleavage of an arginine-valine bond that is present in the carboxyl portion of the zymogen. It is plasmin that subsequently dissolves the fibrin clot noted by Fischer in 1925.

Two types of plasminogen activator have been described, tissue-type (t-PA) and urokinase (u-PA). They represent different gene products and possess different enzymatic characteristics. Furthermore, at least two specific inhibitors of plasminogen activator have been reported. The plasminogen activators are involved in fibrinolysis, in tissue remodeling, and in some stages of malignancy. In particular, the plasminogen activators are participants in a number of steps of metastasis; in the initial breakdown of the basement membrane allowing the detachment of tumor cells from the primary neoplasm; in the formation of the fibrin coat on circulating tumor cells facilitating evasion of the immune response; in the proteolysis of the extracellular matrix at the site of invasion; and in angiogenesis (195).

Not only do the plasminogen activators play these roles in the malignant process, but urokinase also represents an excellent marker of malignancy. It is overexpressed in lung, colonic, breast and prostatic tumors (95).

Hyperplastic Nodules, Foci, and Biological Markers

Hepatic preneoplastic foci can be induced in rodent liver by many different carcinogens (52, 167). These nodules are characterized both histologically and biochemically and are identified long before the appearance of the hepatocellular carcinoma; i.e., they are putative precursor lesions. In these foci, alterations in specific enzymes are observed (143). The alterations in enzyme activity occurring within the liver preneoplastic foci or nodules are summarized in Table 8.3. The changes in activity represent either increases in certain enzymes or decreases. In a number of instances, the enzymatic change is the result of a reversion to a fetal-type isozyme, representing an oncofetal protein, as presented earlier above.

Of the changes in enzyme activity occurring in hepatic preneoplastic foci, three will be discussed in greater detail: γ-glutamyltranspeptidase (GGT), epoxide hydrolase, and glutathione S-transferase-P (GST-P). These represent increases in enzyme activity and, in several instances, the occurrence of a more fetal-type isozyme.

GGT

GGT has provided one of the most useful markers for preneoplasia of liver. The enzyme catalyzes the following reaction:

$$R\text{—}S\text{—}\underset{\text{Glu}}{\overset{\text{Gly}}{\text{Cys}}} \longrightarrow R\text{—}S\text{—}\underset{NH_2}{\overset{\text{Gly}}{\text{Cys}}} + \text{Glu}$$

where R = H, as in glutathione itself or an adduct:

Fiala and co-workers were the first to describe the appearance of GGT in experimental hepatomas and in preneoplastic liver (55). GGT is apparently turned on rapidly in preneoplastic nodules. Histochemistry has revealed the GGT activity within proliferating ductular cells such as bile duct and hepatic oval cells as well as in the hepatic foci. The enzyme activity shows up in both the smooth endoplasmic reticulum and the bile canaliculus (the greater activity).

Table 8.3. Marker Enzymes Found in Hepatic Preneoplastic Nodules

Enzymes with decreased activity
Specific isozymes of glucokinase, aldolase B, pyruvate kinase L
Glucose-6-phosphatase and other gluconeogenic enzymes
Liver-type glycogen phosphorylase
Tryptophan 2,3-dioxygenase
Serine dehydratase
Various cytochrome P450s and P450-dependent monooxygenases
NADPH-dependent cytochrome P450 reductase
Selenium-dependent glutathione peroxidase
Ca^{2+}, Mg^{2+}-dependent ATPase
Enzymes with increased activity
Glucose-6-phosphate dehydrogenase
Fetal-type isozymes of glycolysis
Fetal-type (type 1) UDP-glucuronosyltransferase
Epoxide hydrolase
Quinone reductase
NADP-dependent aldehyde dehydrogenase
Butyryl esterase
Glutathione transferases
γ-Glutamyltransferase
Selenium-independent glutathione peroxidase
Glutathione reductase

Modified with permission from Russell and Snyder (161).

EPOXIDE HYDROLASE

Farber and his colleagues had described the exclusive occurrence of an antigenic component of hepatic hyperplastic nodules within the endoplasmic reticulum, which they tentatively termed *PN antigen* (52). The PN antigen was purified and subsequently identified by Levin and co-workers as a microsomal form of epoxide hydrolase (105). This represented one of the first reports identifying an increased molecular form of an enzyme of biotransformation in preneoplastic nodules. The enzyme catalyzes the reaction shown below:

$$R\text{—}\underbrace{CH\text{—}CH}_{O}\text{—}R_1 + H_2O \longrightarrow R\text{—}\underset{OH}{CH}\text{—}\underset{OH}{CH}\text{—}R_1$$

GST-P

The glutathione S-transferases represent a family of isozymes that were first identified in rat liver by Booth et al. in 1961 (21). In the rat, approximately 12 molecular forms of the cytosolic enzyme involving eight different subunits have been identified; these are divided into basic, neutral, and acidic varieties (158). The generic reaction catalyzed by this family of isozymes is indicated below:

$$\text{acceptor} + \text{GSH} \longrightarrow \text{acceptor-SG}$$

The glutathione S-transferases in the human also fall into basic, neutral, and acidic categories (163). For the present discussion, the isoenzyme of interest is the acidic GT-π, which occurs in human fetal tissues as well as in adult lung, brain, and spleen. GT-π corresponds to the rat GT 7–7.

A number of laboratories have studied the changes in isoenzymic pattern for the transferases during rat liver carcinogenesis (163). Sato and co-workers first identified a form of this enzyme in rat placenta, which was later established as occurring in hepatomas but not in any appreciable amounts in normal liver (163). GT 7–7 turned out to be a good marker for preneoplastic liver foci and in fact may represent an accurate indicator of the "early" initiated cells after administration of carcinogens to rats.

Antibody to GT-π has been used in the detection of neoplasia and early preneoplastic states in a number of human organs. As reviewed by Sato, normal uterine cervical tissue was negative in response to this antibody, whereas a positive reaction was observed in cases of mild dysplasia, e.g., koilocytosis (163). Intense staining was seen in severe dysplasia and squamous cell carcinoma of the cervix. Similar positive reactions were apparent in esophageal dysplasia and carcinoma, in breast adenocarcinomas, and in colon and hepatic tumors.

In summary, GT-π may prove to be an excellent marker of certain human cancers, particularly in defining the early stages of tumorigenesis.

Cell Surface and Neoplasia

Substantial alterations to the plasma membrane of cells occurs in neoplastic transformation. In 1954, Abercrombie and Heaysman (3) reported that cultured normal cells inhibited each other by mutual contact, while many malignant cells (2) did not cease growing under similar conditions. This phenomenon of inhibition of the growth of normal cells was referred to as *contact inhibition*. For a variety of reasons, this repression of growth by contact was renamed *density-dependent inhibition of growth* by Stoker and Rubin in 1967 (174).

In culture, normal cells require a suitable surface for attachment, spreading, and proliferation, a process that is referred to as *anchorage-dependent growth*. A number of transformed cells or malignant cells can grow in suspension or in semisolid media and therefore are capable of anchorage-independent growth. The latter property has been useful in uncovering and subsequently growing malignant cells in a mixed population. Anchorage-independent growth has been closely associated with tumorigenicity (119). It is germane to mention that anchorage-independent growth, although a property of transformed rodent cells, may not be characteristic of human tumor cells.

The lack of density-dependent inhibition of growth and the presence of anchorage independence have suggested that neoplastic cells may have altered membranes as well as altered factor-mediated cell communication. Since the plasma membrane plays an important role in controlling movement and migration, in adherence to supports and to other cells, in controlling the entry of nutrients, and in the recognition of "nonself" in evoking an immune response, these alterations were pursued with some vigor.

Confirmation of a neoplasia-induced change(s) in cell membrane came with the use of a variety of lectins, each of which is capable of binding to a specific carbohydrate (70). Aub et al. were the first to report the agglutination of several transformed cells by wheat germ agglutinin (WGA) while the normal counterparts were not so affected (6). Several possibilities for this phenomenon would pertain: (*a*) transformed cells might have more plasma membrane binding sites for lectins, (*b*) surface binding sites for lectins might be more mobile, resulting in a greater concentration of these receptors by lateral movement. The latter possibility appears to be the correct one. The increased lateral mobility is undoubtedly the result of an increase in plasma membrane fluidity.

Attention was then focused on the chemistry of the cell surface and in particular on the glycoproteins and glycolipids. An excellent review of the aberrant glycosylation in malignancy has been written by Hakomori (73) who has played a major role in this research area. A more general review on alterations in neoplastic cell membrane components may be found in Ruddon (158).

In the early literature, changes in membranal sialic acid had been reported to occur in neoplasia. Later, the affected culprits were identified as glycosphingolipids and glycolipids as well as glycoproteins. The alterations were the result of (*a*) incomplete synthesis and/or processing of carbohydrate chains, resulting in marked elevations in precursor forms; (*b*) activation of glycosyltransferases that were normally absent or low in amount in normal cells; and (*c*) rearrangements in the glycolipid components of the tumor cells.

With the development and the subsequent utilization of monoclonal antibodies, it was soon recognized that these oligosaccharides were tumor-associated antigens, some of which belonged to the class of oncofetal proteins.

Among the earliest evidence that indicated aberrant glycosylation in human cancer was the observation of the incompatible expression of A antigen or the reduction of A or B determinants. A large quantity of a number of fucose-containing glycolipids were found in various adenocarcinomas (see Hakomori 73).

Cell transformation was shown to alter the gangliosides and neutral glycolipids with a number of tumor systems expressing gangliotriosylceramide (Gg3), which had not been observed in normal cells (73). The unique gangliosides found in tumors are shown in Tables 8.4 through 8.7.

The tumor-associated carbohydrate antigens fell into five classes. Class a antigens were epitope structures that were expressed in both glycosphingolipids and glycoproteins. Class b antigens were epitopes expressed only in glycosphingolipids. Class c antigens were epitopes expressed only in glycoproteins. Class d antigens were polypeptide epitopes with antigenicity expressed when single or multiple threonine or serine moieties were glycosylated, and class e antigens were poorly defined epitopes.

The class a antigens which were of the lacto series with type 1 or 2 chains, were highly expressed in tumor cells but not in progenitor cells, although a limited number were seen in some normal cells, e.g., di- or trimeric Le^x. Class b anti-

Table 8.4. Fucose-Containing Lipids and Gangliosides in Cancer

Name	Structure
Le^x	Galβ1→4GlcNAcβ1→3Galβ1→R 3 (GlcNAc) ↑ Fucα1
Le^y	Galβ1→4GlcNAcβ1→3Galβ1→R 2 (Gal) ↑ Fucα1; 3 (GlcNAc) ↑ Fucα1
Sialyl Le^x	Galβ1→4GlcNAcβ1→Galβ1→R 3 (Gal) ↑ SA2; 3 (GlcNAc) ↑ Fucα1
Trifucosyl Le^y	Galβ1→4GlcNAcβ1→3Galβ1→4GlcNAc 2 ↑ Fucα1; 3 ↑ Fucα1; 3 ↑ Fucα1
ACFH18 antigen	Galβ1→[4GlcNAcβ1→3Galβ1]$_n$→3Galβ1→4GlcNAc 6 ↑ SA2; 3 ↑ Fucα1

Abbreviations: Gal, galactose; β1→4, *β*-galactoside between 1-hydroxyl of one sugar to 4-hydroxyl of adjacent sugar; GlcNAcβ1 2-3Gal2, 1-hydroxy group of *N*-acetylglucosamine bound by *β*-linkage to the 3-hydroxyl moiety of galactose; R, residue; Fucα1, 1-hydroxy moiety of fucose linked to a group of an adjacent sugar (represented by the head of the arrow); SA2, 2-position of sialic acid covalently linked to a group in the adjacent sugar (head of the arrow).

Table 8.5. Ganglioside Series of Antigens in Cancer Cells

Name	Structure
$G\gamma_3$	GalNAc→Gal→Glc→Cer
GM_{1b}	Gal→GalNAc→Gal→Glc→Cer ↑ SA
GM_3	Gal→Glc→Cer ↑ SA
GM_2	GalNAc→Gal→Glc→Cer ↑ SA
GD_2	GalNAc→Gal→Glc→Cer ↑ SA ↑ SA
GT_2	GalNAc→Gal→Glc→Cer ↑ SA ↑ SA ↑ SA

Abbreviations: Cer, ceramide; galNAc, *N*-acetylgalactosamine. Other abbreviations are indicated in Table 8.4.

Table 8.6. Globoside Series of Antigens in Cancer Cells

Name	Structure
Forssman	GalNAcα1→3GalNAcβ1→3Galα1→4Galβ1→4Glcβ1→Cer
Antigen	
SSEA-3	Galβ1→3GalNAcβ1→3Galα1→4Galβ1→4Glcβ1→Cer
SSEA-4	NeuAcα2→3Galβ1→3GalNAcβ1→3Galα1→4Galβ1→4Glcβ1→Cer

Abbreviations: GalNAcα1, 1-hydroxyl group of *N*-acetylgalactosamine linked by α-configuration to an adjacent group of the sugar indicated at the head of the arrow; NeuAc, *N*-acetylneuraminic acid. Other abbreviations are as indicated in Tables 8.4 and 8.5.

Table 8.7. Tumor-Associated Glycoproteins in Cancer

Name	Structure
Tn	GalNAcα1-O-Ser/Thr
Sialyl Tn	NeuAcα2 ↑ 6 GalNAcα1-O-Ser/Thr

Abbreviations: O-Ser/Thr, an ester between the hydroxyl of either serine (Ser) or threonine (Thr) and a sugar. Other abbreviations are as indicated in Tables 8.4–8.6.

gens were significant components of tumor cells and were only weakly expressed in normal counterparts (e.g., GM_3). Classes c, d, and e were of the mucin-type glycoproteins, with class c exclusively located in tumor cells, e.g., incompatible blood group antigens. Examples of the unusual antigenic components are given in Tables 8.4 through 8.7.

Aberrant glycosylation has also been reported in preneoplastic cells (180). In rat liver preneoplastic nodules found in aryl amine-fed animals, fucosyl-containing carbohydrates that are absent in normal liver but highly expressed in hepatomas are also observed. These result from the significant increase in fucosyltransferase that is specific for GM_1. In humans, Le^y presence correlated with the preneoplastic state that is seen in colonic polyps. Juvenile polyps of the nonmalignant variety did not express this aberrant material (73).

A very aberrant architecture is present in hepatocellular carcinoma, which may reflect changes in the ability of the neoplastic liver cells to adhere to their neighbors and/or to support the biomatrix. These interactions are important for tissue organization and for maintenance of differentiated function in normal liver cells. The aberrant architecture of hepatoma cells has been associated with a number of biochemical changes in the cell membranes. In this regard, Walborg et al. (196) have reported the presence of a glycoprotein, dipeptidyl peptidase IV, which is related to a cell surface antigen, and is modulated as a function of the stage of malignancy. This protein, which cleaves X-proline dipeptides from the N-terminus, may be involved in the processing or binding of collagen, a major component of the biomatrix.

Extracellular Matrix

The extracellular matrix (ECM) is a complex medium that is formed from substances that are secreted by cells that make up the tissue in question. For epithelial tissues, cells from the epithelium and stroma or mesenchyme that form the base for the tissue produce the ECM components.

The ECM is important in a variety of contexts, including spreading of cells on supports, organization of cytoskeletal elements, polarization of cells, migration of cells within tissues, proliferation of cells, activation of expression of specific genes, secretion, and metastasis of cancer cells (Chapter 10). In the latter context, the ECM represents the first barrier that must be traversed so that cancer cells can invade the lymphatic or vascular systems. Consequently, it is not surprising that many cancer cells secrete proteases, glycosidases, heparanases, and type IV collagenase, enzymes that compromise the integrity of the ECM.

The proteins of the ECM, including the cell surface adhesion receptors, include a plethora of names and acronyms, which has tended to add more complexity to this field than is necessary (91). The terminology will be simplified in this discussion. As shown in Table 8.8, the cell surface adhesion receptors fall into four categories: the cadherins, integrins, immunoglobulin superfamily, and the selectins.

Table 8.8. ECM Components

Surface Adhesion Receptor	Protein Component (Examples)
Cadherins	Catenins
Integrins	Fibrinogen; fibronectin; laminin, collagens
Immunoglobulin superfamily	I-CAM, V-CAM, PECAM
Selectins	Mucins, tenascin

The *cadherins* are a family of homologous cell–cell adhesion proteins expressed by most cells; they are found in specialized contact areas such as desmosomes (67). The cadherins bind to a set of proteins called *catenins* which in turn interact with the actin-based cytoskeleton. Down-regulation of the cadherins is observed in a number of infiltrating human cancers, such as breast cancer (118), and in high-grade prostate cancer (188). The expression of decreased amount of E-cadherin appears to correlate with a poor prognosis in human bladder cancer (25). In a recent study, only E-cadherin-positive bladder carcinoma cells were found able to attach to and colonize intact urothelium. These shed cells could be responsible for attaching to other sites in this tissue, giving rise to the property of multifocality of bladder cancer on first examination (153).

The *integrins*, which represent signaling receptors, are cell–extracellular matrix receptors (92). They occur as heterodimers of two unrelated subunits, each of which is transmembrane. The integrins interact with talin and actinin and subsequently with a number of other proteins, e.g., vinculin, tensin. Tensin represents a focal adhesion-associated protein that caps actin filaments and thus anchors these filaments to focal adhesions. Tensin serves as a signal transducer, relaying the signal from the outside to the inside of the cell. Recent evidence has indicated that tensin can prevent cellular transformation as well as suppress tumorigenicity (108).

The specific receptor for fibronectin is $\alpha_V\beta_1$ integrin. High expression of this integrin normalizes many growth characteristics present in transformed cells (159). Another receptor in this category, integrin $\alpha_V\beta_3$, plays a vital role in angiogenesis. It has recently been reported that antagonists of this integrin actually promote the regression of tumors by inducing the apoptotic process in angiogenic blood vessels. The development of inhibitors of this integrin would appear to represent a high priority for cancer chemotherapy.

OTHER PROTEINS OF THE ECM

The ECM is composed of: collagen types I to V depending on the specific tissue; proteoglycans such as chondroitin sulfate, heparan sulfate, dermatan sulfate; anchorage proteins such as fibronectin and laminin that serve as attachment sites to the matrix; and sometimes elastin and entactin. The supporting structures of epithelial tissues such as in the gastrointestinal tract, mammary gland, or endocrine organs contain laminin, heparan sulfate–glycoproteins, and type IV collagen.

Fibronectin

This ECM material is a glycoprotein of MW = 450,000 that has the function of anchoring cells to the matrix. It consists of a disulfide-linked dimer that contains five N-linked oligosaccharides. Fibronectin occurs both as a cell-associated molecule and as a circulating form in the plasma (204). Fibronectin binds to a number of macromolecules such as collagen, proteoglycans, and the cell membrane itself and participates, through the interaction with a fibronectin receptor, in cell spreading, movement, and proliferation. In virally transformed cells, the cell surface fibronectin is lost as a result of increased turnover and reduced binding.

As indicated, fibronectin binds to specific receptors present on cells. The major receptor consists of a noncovalent complex of two transmembrane glycoprotein subunits. This receptor is a member of the integrin family of cell surface heterodimers. The fibronectin receptor is also referred to as VLA-5. The latter has been examined in a number of normal and transformed human cells by Yamada and colleagues (204). The fibronectin receptor in transformed cells underwent a more rapid intracellular processing mechanism, resulting in a reduction in the amount of this receptor and a more diffuse localization in the cell surface material. These events may contribute to the abnormal adhesion properties and invasiveness of the transformed human cells.

Laminin

This basement membrane protein is a glycoprotein of MW = 900,000 which contains multiple attachment points (183). It consists of two chains with attachment sites for heparan sulfate and collagenase type IV. Laminin is the first ECM protein to occur in embryonic development. It is lost from the cell surface of certain virally transformed cells (78).

TENASCIN

This ECM component is a large oligomeric glycoprotein that is synthesized during embryonic development and is found prominently in a number of tumors (79). In electron micrographs, the molecule has six long thin arms with a terminal knob on each arm, a thick distal segment, thin proximal segment, a T-junction where three arms are joined to form a trimer, and a central knob where two trimers are united into a hexamer. The connections at the T-joint and at the central knob are disulfide bonds. Tenascin is secreted by fibroblasts and glial cells in culture, with various glioma cell lines representing some of the best sources for the human protein. Tenascin binds to chondroitin sulfate–containing proteoglycans (36, 193). In contrast to fibronectin or laminin, the interaction of tenascin with the cell surface is not associated with any flattening or spreading. The cells maintain their rounded to spindle or branching morphology.

Tenascin is not seen in mammary carcinoma or squamous carcinoma cells but is prominent in the surrounding connective tissue (93, 112). The synthesis of this ECM protein occurs in the mesenchyme that surrounds a transplantable breast cancer but not in the cancer cells per se. Transformed cells increase the ability of fibroblasts of underlying connective tissue to elaborate tenascin, probably as a result of a soluble growth factor.

Tenascin is expressed in both mesenchymal tumors and carcinomas, but mostly in anaplastic tumors, e.g., in glioblastoma multiforme but not in the more differentiated astrocytomas. The presence of this substance may serve as a means for differential diagnosis of the gliomas.

Cytoskeletal Actin

Actin is one of the major components of the cytoskeleton and is ubiquitously present in eukaryotic cells (see e.g., reviews 144, 202). Actin is necessary for regulation of cell shape, motility of the cell, secretion, intracellular transport, endocytosis and exocytosis, and cell division. Actin occurs in the cytoplasm as monomers, or G-actin or as microfilaments, F-actin.

Most transformed cells exhibit marked changes in patterns of actin filaments (5, 7, 194). Cellular F-actin has been studied as a quantitative marker for transformation in relation to cell differentiation using human HL-60 cells (197). The concentration of F-actin in untransformed cells was highest during the G_1 phase of the cycle. In transformed cells, on the other hand, a major increase occurred in the G2 + M phase. Phorbol ester, which was able to differentiate the HL-60 cells, caused a large decrease in the content of F-actin. Alterations in actin may be due to point mutations in the actin gene, altered regulation of F-actin assembly, and/or changes in the actin polymerization process.

A number of actin-binding proteins occur in cells, and these may play an important role in actin skeleton rearrangements in cell motility, division, and differentiation. Among these proteins may be found gelsolin, which can bind to G-actin, cause aggregation to F-actin, and is important in the dynamic rearrangment of actin that occurs during spreading and locomotion of cells; and villin, which is related to gelsolin but is able to bundle F-actin. During the differentiation of the cytoskeleton, a 50-fold increase occurs in gelsolin synthesis (45). Villin is a component of brush border cells and is needed for the formation of microfilament bundles. It is the first actin-binding protein to appear at the site of microvilli assembly. The human colon carcinoma cell line, HT 29, can be induced to differentiate into a well-ordered brush border epithelium. Under these conditions, a marked increase in villin mRNA occurs up to levels that are found in normal intestinal mucosa (150).

Conclusions

This chapter has provided a small glimpse into the world of the neoplastic cell. Many changes are noted in the biochemistry of this cell, but a number of these changes appear to be related more to the rapid proliferation associated with some but not all human cancers. Growth-related alterations in enzyme activity or in secreted factors are adaptive mechanisms that make the cancer cell a better "machine" in regard to cell division, invasion, and ability to avoid the negative influences of its neighbors. In this context, the cancer cell is truly a magnificent creature that proves its tremendous adaptability to adversity. The cancer cell is also quite remarkable in utilizing features that are already present in the normal cell, but for reasons of ontogeny, may no longer be of value to the normal mature cell. The cancer cell, however, has resurrected these biochemical processes to be put to its own advantage. Nevertheless, these phenotypic expressions provide the Achilles heel of the cancer cell by allowing for more definitive and early diagnosis, by providing targets for potential attack with some degree of specificity, and ultimately, perhaps, for reprogramming back to normalcy. It is a challenge to the molecular and biochemical oncologist to put these phenotypic expressions to better advantage so as to rid us of this remarkable but destructive cell.

References

1. Abelev GI, Perova SD, Khamkova NI, Postnikova ZA, Irlin IS. Production of embryonal α-globulin by transplantable mouse hepatomas. Transplantation 1963;1:174.
2. Abercrombie M, Ambrose EJ. The surface properties of cancer cells: a review. Cancer Res 1962;22:525.
3. Abercrombie M, Heaysman JEM. Social behavior of cells in tissue culture II. Monolayering of fibroblasts. Exp Cell Res 1954;6:293.
4. Akiyama SK, Larjava H, Yamada KM. Differences in the biosynthesis and localization of the fibronectin receptor in normal and transformed cultured human cells. Cancer Res 1990;50:1602.
5. Antecol MH. Ontogenic potential in fibroblasts from individuals genetically predisposed to cancer. Mutation Res 1988;199:293.
6. Aub JC, Sanford BH, Cote MN. Studies on reactivity of tumor and normal cells to a wheat germ agglutinin. Proc Natl Acad Sci USA 1965;54:396.
7. Babiss LE, Liaw WS, Zimmer SG, Godman GC, Ginsberg HS, Fisher PB. Mutations in the E1a gene of adenovirus type 5 alter the tumorigenic properties of transformed cloned rat fibroblast cells. Proc Natl Acad Sci USA 1986;83:2167.
8. Baylin SB, Fearon ER, Vogelstein B, deBustros A, Sharkis SJ, Burke PJ, Staal SD, Nelkin BD. Hypermethylation of the 5′ region of the calcitonin gene is a property of human lymphoid and acute myeloid leukemia. Blood 1987;70:412.
9. Baylin SB, Hoppener JWM, deBustros A, Steenbergh PH, Lips CJM, Nelkin BD. DNA methylation patterns of the calcitonin gene in human lung cancers and lymphomas. Cancer Res 1986;46:2917.
10. Benchimol S, Fuks A, Jothy S, Beauchemin N, Shirota K, Stanners CP. Carcinoembryonic antigen, a human tumor marker, functions as an intercellular adhesion molecule. Cell 1989;57:327.
11. Berger NA. Poly(ADP-ribose) in the cellular response to DNA damage. Radiation Res 1985;101:4.
12. Bergstrand CG, Czar B. Demonstration of a new protein fraction in serum from the human fetus. Scand J Clin Lab Invest 1956;8:174.
13. Beutler B. Tumor Necrosis Factors: the Molecules and Their Emerging Role in Medicine. New York: Raven Press, 1992.
14. Beutler B, Cerami A. Cachectin and tumor necrosis factor as two sides of the same biological coin. Nature 1986;320:584.
15. Beutler B, Mahoney J, LeTrang N, Pekala P, Cerami A. Purification of cachectin, a lipoprotein lipase-suppressing hormone secreted by endotoxin-induced RAW 264.7 cells. J Exp Med 1985;161:984.
16. Bird AP. CpG-rich islands and the function of DNA methylation. Nature 1986;321:209.
17. Blackburn EH. Structure and function of telomeres. Nature 1991;350:569.
18. Blackburn EH. Telomerases. Annu. Rev. Biochem. 1992;61:113.
19. Bodger MP, Janossy G, Bollum FJ, Burford GD, Hoffbrand AV. The ontogeny of terminal deoxynucleotidyl transferase positive cells in the human fetus. Blood 1983;61:1125.
20. Bollum FJ, Chang LMS. Terminal transferase in normal and leukemic cells. Adv Cancer Res 1986;47:37.
21. Booth J, Boyland E, Sims P. An enzyme from rat liver catalysing conjugations with glutathione. Biochem J 1961;79:516.
22. Borek C, Morgan WF, Ong A, Cleaver JE. Inhibition of malignant transformation in vitro by inhibitors of poly(ADP-ribose) synthesis. Proc Natl Acad Sci USA 1984;81:243.
23. Bourne HR, DeFranco AL. Signal transduction and intracellular messengers. In Oncogenes and the Molecular Origins of Cancer. New York: Cold Spring Harbor Laboratory Press, 1989, p 97.
24. Bradstock KF, Kerr A, Bollum FJ. Antigenic phenotype of TdT-positive cells in human peripheral blood. Cell Immunol 1985;90:590.
25. Bringuier PP, Umbas R, Schaafsma HE, Karthaus HFM, DeBruyne FMJ, Schalken JA. Decreased E-cadherin correlates with poor survival in patients with bladder tumors. Cancer Res 1993;53:3241.
26. Bronner CE, Baker SM, Morrison PT, Warren G, Smith LG, Lescoe MK, Kane M, Earabino C, Lipford J, Lindblom A, Tannergard P, Bollag RJ, Godwin AR, Ward DC, Nordenskjold M, Fishel R, Kolodner R, Liskay RM. Mutation in the DNA mismatch repair gene homolog hMLH1 is associated with hereditary non-polyposis colon cancer. Nature 1994;368:258.
27. Brown NH. A case of pluriglandular syndrome-diabetes of bearded women. Lancet 1928;2:1022.
28. Brooks PC, Montgomery AMP, Rosenfeld M, Reisfeld RA, Hu T, Klier G, Cheresh DA. Integrin $\alpha_v\beta_3$ antagonists promote tumor regression by inducing apoptosis of angiogenic blood vessels. Cell 1994;79:1157.
29. Burk RR. Reduced adenyl cyclase activity in polyoma virus transformed cell line. Nature 1968;219:1272.
30. Burt ME, Lowry SF, Gorshbath C, Brennan ME. Metabolic alterations in a noncachetic animal tumor system. Cancer 1981;47:2138.
31. Busch H, Davis JR, Olle E. Citrate accumulation in slices of transplantable tumors of the rat. Cancer Res 1957;17:711.
32. Cameron IL, Ord VA. Parenteral level of glucose intake on glucose homeostasis, tumor growth, gluconeogenesis, and body consumption in normal and tumor-bearing rats. Cancer Res 1983;43:5228.
33. Carson DA, Seto S, Wasson DB, Carrera CJ. DNA strand breaks, NAD metabolism, and programmed cell death. Exp Cell Res 1986;164:273.
34. Carswell EA, Gold L, Kassel RL, Green S, Fiore N, Williamson B. An endotoxin-induced serum factor that causes necrosis of tumors. Proc Natl Acad Sci USA 1975;72:3666.
35. Chang LM. Development of terminal deoxynucleotidyl transferase activity in embryonic calf thymus gland. Biochem Biophys Res Commun 1971;44:124.
36. Chiquet M, Fambrough DM. Chick myotendinous antigen, II: a novel extracellular glycoprotein complex consisting of large disulfide-linked subunits. J Cell Biol 1984;98:1937.
37. Cleaver JE. Defective repair replication of DNA in xeroderma pigmentosum. Nature 1968;218:652.
38. Coleman MS, Hutton JJ, DeSimone P, Bollum FJ. Terminal deoxyribonucleotidyl transferase in human leukemia. Proc Natl Acad Sci USA 1974;71:4404.
39. Costa G, Holland JF. Effects of Krebs-2-carcinoma on the lipid metabolism of male Swiss mice. Cancer Res 1962;22:1081.

40. Counter CM, Hirte HW. Bacchetti S, Harley CB. Telomerase activity in human ovarian carcinoma. Proc Natl Acad Sci USA 1994;91:2900.
41. Dano K, Andreasen PA, Grondahl-Hansen J, Kristensen P, Nielsen LS, Skriver L. Plasminogen activators, tissue degradation and cancer. Adv Cancer Res 1985;44: 139.
42. deBustros A, Nelkin BD, Silverman A, Ehrlich G, Poiesz B, Baylin SB. The short arm of chromosome 11 is a "hot spot" for hypermethylation in human neoplasia. Proc Natl Acad Sci USA 1985;85:5693.
43. DeWys W. Working conference on anorexia and cachexia of neoplastic disease. Cancer Res 1970;30:2816.
44. Dice JF. Molecular determinants of protein half-lives in eukaryotic cells. FASEB J 1987;1:349.
45. Dieffenbach CW, SenGupta DN, Krause D, Sawzak D, Silverman RH. Cloning of murine gelsolin and its regulation during differentiation of embryonal carcinoma cells. J Biol Chem 1989;264:13281.
46. Ding R, Pommier Y, Kang VH, Smulson M. Depletion of poly(ADP-ribose)polymerase by antisense RNA expression: influence on genomic stability, chromatin organization and carcinogen cytotoxicity. Cancer Res 1994;54:4627.
47. Eastman A. Activation of programmed cell death by anticancer agents: cisplatin as a model system. Cancer Cells (in press).
48. Eastman A. Apoptosis. A product of programmed and unprogrammed cell death. Toxicol Appl Pharmacol 1993;121:120.
49. Elford HL, Freese M, Passamani E, Morris HP. Ribonucleotide reductase and cell proliferation: I. variations of ribonucleotide reductase activity with tumor growth rate in a series of rat hepatomas. J Biol Chem 1970;245:5228.
50. Ellis RE, Yuan JY, Horvitz HR. Mechanisms and functions of cell death. Annu Rev Cell Biol 1991;7:663.
51. Erickson HP, Bourdon MA. Tenascin: an extracellular matrix protein prominent in specialized embryonic tissues and tumors. Ann Rev Cell Biol 1989;5:71.
52. Farber E. Cellular biochemistry of the stepwise development of cancer with chemicals. Cancer Res 1984;44:5463.
53. Feinberg AP, Gehrke CW, Kuo KC, Ehrlich M. Rreduced genomic 5-methylcytosine content in human colonic neoplasia. Cancer Res 1988;48:1159.
54. Felig P, Pozefsky T, Marliss E, Cahill GE Jr. Alanine: key role in gluconeogenesis. Science 1970;167:1003.
55. Fiala S, Fiala AE, Dixon B. Gamma-glutamyl transpeptidase in transplantable, chemically induced rat hepatomas and "spontaneous" mouse hepatomas. JNCI 1972;48: 1393.
56. Fischer A. Bbetrag zur Biologie der Gewebezellen: eine vergleichend-biologische Studie der normalen und maligen Gewebezellen in vitro. Wilhelm Roux Arch Entwicklungsmech Organ 1925;104:210.
57. Fishel R, Lescoe MK, Rao MSR, Copeland NG, Jenkins NA, Garber J, Kane M, Kolodner R. The human mutator gene homolog MSH2 and its association with hereditary nonpolyposis colon cancer. Cell 1993;75:1027.
58. Fishman WH, Inglis NR, Green S. Regan isoenzyme: a carcinoplacental antigen. Cancer Res 1971;31:1054.
59. Fishman WH, Inglis NR, Green S, Anstiss CL, Ghosh NK, Reif AE, Prestigian R, Krant MJ, Stolbach LL. Immunology and biochemistry of Regan isoenzyme of alkaline phosphatase in human cancer. Nature 1968;219:697.
60. Fozard JR, Part ML, Prakash NJ, Grove J, Schechter PJ, Sjoerdsma A, Koch-Weser J. L-Ornithine decarboxylase: an essential role in early mammalian embryogenesis. Science 1980;200:505.
61. Fraval HNA, Roberts JJ. Excision repair of *cis*-diamminedichloroplatinum(II)-induced damage of Chinese hamster cells. Cancer Res 1979;39:1793.
62. Frost P, Kerbel RS. On a possible epigenetic mechanism(s) of tumor cell heterogeneity: the role of DNA methylation. Cancer Metastasis Rev 1983;2:375.
63. Frost P, Liteplo RG, Fonaghue TP, Kerbel RS. Selection of strongly immunogenic "tum-" variants from tumors at high frequency using 5-azacytidine. J Exp Med 1984;159:1491.
64. Gama-Sosa MA, Slagel VA, Trewyn RW, Oxenhandler R, Kuo K, Gehrke C, Ehrlich M. The 5-methylcytosine content of DNA from human tumours. Nucleic Acids Res 1983;11:6883.
65. Garewal HS, Gerner EW, Sampliner RE, Roe D. Ornithine decarboxylase and polyamine levels in columnar upper gastrointestinal mucosae in patients with Barrett's esophagus. Cancer Res 1988;48:3288.
66. Geiger B, Ayalon O. Cadherins. Annu Rev Cell Biol 1992;8:307.
67. Ghoda L, Wetters TV, Macrae M, Ascherman D, Coffino P. Prevention of rapid intracellular degradation of ODC by a carboxyl-terminal deficient truncation. Science 1989;243:1493.
68. Gold P, Freeman SO. Specific carcinoembryonic antigens of the human digestive system. J Exp Med 1965;122:467.
69. Goldstein IJ, Hayes CE. The lectins: carbohydrate-binding proteins of plants and animals. Adv Carbohydrate Chem Biochem 1978;35:127.
70. Greenstein JP. Some biochemical characteristics of morphologically separable cancers. Cancer Res 1956;16:641.
71. Greider CW, Telomeres. Curr Opin Cell Biol 1991;3:441.
72. Gutman AB, Tyson TL, Gutman EB. Serum calcium, inorganic phosphorus and phosphatase activity. Arch Intern Med 1936;57:379.
73. Hakomori S. Aberrant glycosylation in tumors and tumor-associated carbohydrate antigens. Adv Cancer Res 1989;52:257.
74. Harley CB, Futcher AB, Greider CW. Telomeres shorten during aging of human fibroblasts. Nature 1990;345:458.
75. Harwell LH, Kastan MB. Cell cycle control and cancer. Science 1994;266:1821.
76. Hastie ND, Dempter M, Dunlop MG, Thompson AM, Green DK, Allshire RC. Telomere reduction in human colorectalcarcinoma and with aging. Nature 1990;346:866.
77. Hayaishi O, Ueda K. Poly(ADP-ribose) and ADP-ribosylation of proteins. Annu Rev Biochem 1977;46:95.
78. Hayman EG, Engvall E, Ruoslahti E. Concomitant loss of cell surface fibronectin and laminin from transformed rat kidney cells. J Cell Biol 1981;88:352.
79. Heber D, Chlebowski RT, Ishibashi DE, Herrold JN, Block JB. Abnormalities in glucose and protein metabolism in noncachectic lung cancer patients. Cancer Res 1982;43:4815.
80. Heby O. Role of polyamines in the control of cell proliferation and differentiation. Differentiation 1981;14:1.
81. Heby O, Anderson G, Gray JW. Interference with S and G_2 phase progression by polyamine synthesis inhibitors. Exp Cell Res 1978;111:461.
82. Hefta SA, Hefta LJF, Lee TD, Paxton RJ, Shiveley JE. Carcinoembryonic antigen is anchored to membranes by covalent attachment to a glycosyl phosphatidylinositol moiety: identification of the ethanolamine linkage site. Proc Natl Acad Sci USA 1988;85: 4648.
83. Herschko A, Mamont P, Shields R, Tomkins GM. Pleiotypic responses. Nature 1971;232:206.
84. Hibasami H, Hoffman JL, Pegg AE. Decarboxylated S-adenosylmethionine in mammalian cells. J Biol Chem 1980;225:6675.
85. Hietala O, Dzubow L, Dlugosz AA, Pyle JA, Jenney F, Gilmour SK, O'Brien TG. Activation of human squamous cell carcinoma ornithine decarboxylase activity by guanosine triphosphate. Cancer Res 1988;48:1252.
86. Holliday R, Pugh JE. DNA modification mechanisms and gene activity during development. Science 1975;187:227.
87. Hsieh J-T, Denning MF, Heidel SM, Verma AK. Expression of human chromosome 2 ornithine decarboxylase gene in ornithine decarboxylase-deficient chinese hamster ovary cells. Cancer Res 1990;50:2239.
88. Huberman E, Weeks C, Herrmann A, Callahan M, Slaga T. Alterations in polyamine levels induced by phorbol diesters and other agents that promote differentiation in human promyelocytic leukemia cells. Proc Natl Acad Sci USA 1981;78:1062.
89. Hue L. The role of futile cycles in the regulation of carbohydrate metabolism in the liver. Adv Enzymol 1981;52:247.
90. Hunter T, Pines G. Cyclins and Cancer II: cyclin D and CDK inhibitors come of age. Cell 1994;79:573.
91. Hynes RO. The impact of molecular biology on models for cell adhesion. BioEssays 1994;16:663.
92. Hynes RO. Integrins: versatility, modulation and signalling cell adhesion. Cell 1992;69:11.
93. Inaguma Y, Kusakabe M, Mackie EJ, Pearson CA, Chiquet-Ehresmann R, Sakakura T. Epithelial induction of stromal tenascin in the mouse mammary gland: from embryogenesis to carcinogenesis. Dev Biol 1988;128:245.
94. Janne J, Poso H, Raina A. Polyamines in rapid growth and cancer. Biochim Biophys Acta 1978;473:241.
95. Jefferson RA, Kavanagh TA, Bevan MW. GUS fusions: beta-glucuronidase as a sensitive and versatile gene fusion marker in higher plants. EMBO J 1987;6:3901.
96. Jones PA, Buckley JD. The role of DNA methylation in cancer. Adv Cancer Res 1990;54:1.
97. Josse RG, Wilson DR, Heershe JNM, Mills JRF, Murray TM. Hypercalcemia with ovarian carcinoma: evidence of a pathological role for prostaglandins. Cancer 1981;48: 1233.
98. Kawakami M, Cerami A. Studies of endotoxin-induced decrease in lipoprotein lipase activity. J Exp Med 1981;154:631.
99. Kerr JF, Wyllie AH, Currie AR. Apoptosis: a basic biological phenomenon with wide-reaching implications in tissue kinetics. Br J Cancer 1972;26:239.
100. Kim NW, Piatyszek MA, Prowse KR, Harley CB, West MD, Ho PLC, Coviello GM, Wright WE, Weinrich SL, Shay JW. Specific association of human telomerase activity with immortal cells and cancer. Science 1994;266:2011.
101. Kondo Y, Sato K, Ohkawa H, Ueyama Y, Okabe T, Sato N, Asano S, Mori M, Ohsawa N, Kosaka K. Association of hypercalcemia with tumors producing colony-stimulating factor(s). Cancer Res 1983;43:2368.
102. Korsmeyer SJ. Bcl-2 initiates a new category of oncogenes: regulators of cell death. Blood 1992;80:879.
103. Kuo MT, Iyer B, Wu JR, Lapeyre J-N, Becker FF. Methylation of the alpha-fetoprotein gene in productive and nonproductive rat hepatocellular carcinomas. Cancer Res 1984;44:1642.
104. Leach FS, Nicolaides NC, Papadopoulos N, Liu B, Jen J, Parsons P, Peltomaki P, Sistonen P, Aaltonen LA, Nystrom-Lahti M, Guan X-Y, Zhang J, Meltzer PS, Yu J-W, Kao F-T, Chen DJ, Cersaletti KM, Fournier REK, Todd S, Lewis T, Leach RJ, Naylor SL, Weissenbach J, Mecklin J-P, Jarvinen H, Petersen GM, Hamilton SR, Green J, Jass J, Watson P, Lynch HT, Trent JM, deChapelle A, Kinzlere KW, Vogelstein B. Mutations of a *mutS* homolog in hereditary nonpolyposis colorectal cancer. Cell 1993;75:1215.
105. Levin W, Lu AYH, Thomas PE, Ryan D, Kizer DE, Griffin MJ. Identification of epoxide hydrase as the preneoplastic antigen in rat liver hyperplastic nodules. Proc Natl Acad Sci USA 1978;84:3240.
106. Lindmark L, Edstrom S, Ekman L, Karlberg I, Lundholm, K. Energy metabolism in non-growing mice with sarcoma. Cancer Res 1983;43:3649.
107. Liddle GW, Givens JR, Nicholson WE, Island DP. The ectopic ACTH syndrome. Cancer Res 1965;25:1057.
108. Lo SH, Weisberg E, Chen LB. Tensin: a potential link between the cytoskeleton and signal transduction. BioEssays 1994;16:187.
109. Luk GD. Essential role of polyamine metabolism in hepatic regeneration. Gastroenterology 1986;90:1261.
110. Luk GD, Baylin SB. ODC as a biologic marker in familial colonic polyposis. N Engl J Med 1984;311:80.
111. Luk GD, Casero RA Jr. Polyamines in normal and cancer cells. Adv Enz Regul 1987;26:91.
112. Mackie EJ, Chiquet-Ehresmann R, Pearson CA, Inaguma Y, Tayo K. Tenascin is a stromal marker for epithelial malignancy in the mammary gland. Proc Natl Acad Sci USA 1987;84:4621.
113. McCaffrey R, Smoler D, Baltimore D. Terminal deoxynucleotidyl transferase in a case of childhood acute lymphoblastic leukemia. Proc Natl Acad Sci USA 1973;70:521.
114. Malmgren RA, Flanigan CC. Localization of the vegetative form of Clostridium tetani in mouse tumors following intravenous spore administration. Cancer Res 1955;15: 473.
115. Mider GB, Tesluk H, Morton JJ. Effect of Walker carcinoma 256 on food intake, body weight and nitrogen metabolism in growing rats. Acta Un Int Cancer 1948;6:409.
116. Miller EC, Miller JA. The presence and significance of bound aminoazo dyes in the livers of rats fed p-dimethylaminoazobenzene. Cancer Res 1947;7:468.
117. Modrich P. Mechanisms and biological effects of mismatch repair. Annu Rev Genet 1991;25:229.
118. Moll R, Mitze M, Frixen UH, Birchmeier W. Differential loss of E-cadherin expression in infiltrating ductal and lobular breast carcinomas. Am J Pathol 1993;143:1731.

119. Montesano R, Drevon C, Kuroki T, Saint Vincent L, Handleman S, Sanford KK, DeFeo D, Weinstein IB. Test for malignant transformation of rat liver cells in culture: cytology, growth in soft agar, and production of plasminogen activator. JNCI 1977;59:1651.
120. Morris HP, Studies on the development, biochemistry and biology of experimental hepatomas. Adv Cancer Res 1965;9:227.
121. Morrison SD, Partition of energy expenditure between host and tumor. Cancer Res 1971;31:98.
122. Mundy GR, Luben RA, Raisz LG, Oppenhein JJ, Buell DN, Bone-resorbing activity in supernatants from lymphoid cell lines. N Engl J Med 1974;290:867.
123. Nakahara W. Toxohormone. In Methods in Cancer Research, vol. II. Edited by H Busch. New York: Academic, 1967, p 203.
124. Newsholme EA, Stanley JC. Substrate cycles: their role in control of metabolism with specific references to the liver. Diabetes Metab Rev 1987;3:295.
125. Nilsson P, Mehli C, Remes K, Roos G. Telomerase activity in vivo in human malignant hematopoietic cells. Oncogene 1994;9:3043.
126. Norton JA, Peacock JL, Morrison SD. Cancer cachexia. CRC Crit Rev Oncol Hematol 1987;7:289.
127. Nurse P. Ordering S phase and M phase in the cell cycle. Cell 1994;79:547.
128. O'Brien TG, Madara T, Pyle JA, Holmes M. Ornithine decarboxylase from mouse epidermis and epidermal papillomas: differences in enzymatic properties and structure. Proc Natl Acad Sci USA 1986;83:9448.
129. O'Brien TG, Simsiman RC, Boutwell RK. Induction of the polyamine biosynthetic enzymes in mouse epidermis by tumor-promoting agents. Cancer Res 1975;35:1662.
130. Ohnuma T, Maldia G, Holland JF. Hepatic catalase activity in advanced human cancer. Cancer Res 1966;26:1806.
131. Oikawa S, Nakazota H, Kosaki G. Primary structure of human carcinoembryonic antigen (CEA) deduced from cDNA sequences. Biochem Biophys Res Communs 1987;142:511.
132. Old LJ. Tumor necrosis factor (TNF). Science 1985;230:630.
133. Oliff A, Defeo-Jones D, Boyer M, Martinez D, Kiefer D, Vuocolo G, Wolfe A, Socher SH. Tumors secreting human TNF/cachectin induce cachexia in mice. Cell 1987;50: 555.
134. Olsson L, Behnke O, Sorenson HR. Modulating effects of 5-azacytidine, phorbol ester, and retinoic acid on the malignant phenotype of human lung cancer cells. Int J Cancer 1985;35:189.
135. Olsson L, Due C, Diamant M. Treatment of human cell lines with 5-azacytidine may result in profound alterations in clonogenicity and growth rate. J Cell Biol 1985;100: 508.
136. Olsson L, Forchhammer J. Induction of the metastatic phenotype in a mouse tumor model by 5-azacytidine and characterization of an antigen associated with metastatic activity. Proc Natl Acad Sci USA 1984;81:3389.
137. Papadopoulos N, Nicolaides NC, Wei Y-F, Ruben SM, Carter KC, Rosen CA, Haseltine WA, Fleischmann RD, Fraser CM, Adams MD, Venter JC, Hamilton SR, Petersen GM, Watson P, Lynch HT, Peltomaki P, Mecklin J-P, de la Chapelle A, Kinzler KW, Vogelstein B. Mutation in a *mutL* homolog in hereditary colon cancer. Science 1994;263: 1625.
138. Paxton RJ, Mooser G, Pande H, Lee TD, Shiveley JE. Sequence analysis of carcinoembryonic antigen: identification of glycosylation sites and homology with the immunoglobulin supergene family. Proc Natl Acad Sci USA 1987;84:920.
139. Pearse AGE. Common cytochemical and ultrastructural characteristics of cells producing polypeptide hormones (the APUD series) and their relevance to thyroid and ultimobranchial C cells and calcitonin. Proc R Soc London [Biol] 1968;170:71.
140. Pegg AE. Effect of α-difluoromethylornithine on cardiac polyamine content and hypertrophy. J Mol Cell Cardiol 1981;13:881.
141. Pegg AE, McCann PP. Polyamine metabolism and function. Am J Physiol 1982;243:c212.
142. Pitot HC, Heidelberger C. Metabolic regulatory circuits and carcinogenesis. Cancer Res 1963;23:1694.
143. Pitot HC, Sirica AE. The stages of initiation and promotion in hepatocarcinogenesis. Biochim Biophys Acta 1980;605:191.
144. Pollard T, Cooper JA. Actin and actin binding proteins: a critical evaluation of mechanisms and functions. Annu Rev Biochem 1986;55:987.
145. Potter VR. The biochemical approach to the cancer problem. Fed Proc 1958;17:691.
146. Potter VR. Transplantable animal cancer, the primary standard. Cancer Res 1961;21: 1331.
147. Potter VR. Recent trends in cancer biochemistry: the importance of studies on fetal issue. Can Cancer Conf 1969;8:9.
148. Potter VR. Biochemistry of cancer. In Cancer Medicine, 2nd ed. Edited by JJ Holland, E Frei III. Philadelphia: Lea & Febiger, 1982, p 133.
149. Prasad KN. Involvement of cyclic nucleotides in transformation. In The Transformed Cell. Edited by I Cameron, TB Pool. New York: Academic, 1981, 235.
150. Pringault E, Arpin M, Garcia A, Finidori J, Louvard D. A human villin cDNA clone to investigate the differentiation of intestinal and kidney cells in vivo and in culture. EMBO J 1986;3:119.
151. Quigley JP, Ossowski L, Reich E. Plasminogen, the serum proenzyme activated by factors from cells transformed by oncogenic viruses. J Biol Chem 1974;249:4306.
152. Rao JY, Hurst RE, Bales WD, Jones PL, Bass RA, Archer LT, Bell PB, Hemstreet GP III. Cellular F-actin levels as a marker for cellular transformation; relationship to cell division and differentiation. Cancer Res 1990;50:2215.
153. Rebel JMJ, Thijssen CDEM, Vermey M, Delouvee A, Zwarthoff EC, van der Kwast Th. E-Cadherin expression determines the mode of replacement of normal urothelium by human bladder carcinoma cells. Cancer Res 1994;54:5488.
154. Riggs AD. X-activation, differentiation and DNA methylation. Cytogenet Cell Genet 1975;14:9.
155. Robertson RP, Baylink DJ, Marini JJ, Adkinson HW. Elevated prostaglandins and suppressed parathyroid hormone associated with certain types of cancer. N Engl J Med 1975;293:1278.
156. Rogers S, Wells R, Rechsteiner M. Amino acid sequences common to rapidly degraded proteins: the PEST hypothesis. Science 1986;234:364.
157. Rouzer A, Cerami A. Hypertriglyceridemia associated with *Trypanosoma brucei* in rabbits: role of defective triglyceride removal. Mol Biochem Parasitol 1980;2:31.
158. Ruddon RW. Cancer Biology. New York: Oxford University Press, 1987.
159. Ruoslahti E, Reed JC. Anchorage dependence, integrins and apoptosis. Cell 1994;77:478.
160. Rupniak HT, Paul D. Inhibition of spermidine and spermine synthesis leads to growth arrest of rat embryo fibroblasts in G_1. J Cell Physiol 1978;94:161.
161. Russell DH, Snyder SH. Amine synthesis in rapidly growing tissues: ornithine decarboxylase in the regenerating rat liver, chick embryo, and various tumors. Proc Natl Acad Sci USA 1968;60:1420.
162. Ryan WL, Heidrick ML. Inhibition of cell growth in vitro by adenosine 3′,5′-monophosphate. Science 1968;162:1484.
163. Sato K. Glutathione transferases as markers of preneoplasia and neoplasia. Adv Cancer Res 1989;52:205.
164. Scalabrino G, Pigatto P, Ferioli ME, Modena D, Paerari M, Caru A. Levels of activity of the polyamine biosynthetic decarboxylases as indicators of the degree of malignancy of human cutaneous epitheliomas. J Invest Dermatol 1980;74:122.
165. Schapira F, Dreyfus JC, Schapira G. Aldolase in primary liver cancer. Nature 1963;200:995.
166. Seely JE, Poso H, Pegg AE. Effect of androgens on turnover of ornithine decarboxylase in mouse kidney: studies using labeling of the enzyme by reaction with [^{14}C]α-difluoromethylornithine. J Biol Chem 1982;257:7549.
167. Sell S, Hunt JM, Knoll BJ, Dunsford HA. Cellular events during hepatocarcinogenesis in rats and the question of premalignancy. Adv Cancer Res 1987;48:37.
168. Sell S, Morris HP. Relationship of rat α-fetoprotein to growth rate and chromosomal composition of Morris hepatomas. Cancer Res 1974;34:1413.
169. Smith CA, Farrah T, Goodwin RF. The TNF receptor subfamily of cellular and viral proteins: activation, costimulation, and death. Cell 1994;76:959.
170. Shapot VS. Some biochemical aspects of the relationship between the tumor and the host. Adv Cancer Res 1972;15:253.
171. Snyder DS, Unanue ER. Corticosteroids inhibit murine macrophage Ia expression and interleukin I production. J Immunol 1982;129:1803.
172. Sorenson CM, Eastman A. Influence of *cis*-diamminedichloroplatinum(II) in DNA synthesis and cell cycle progression in excision repair proficient and deficient Chinese hamster ovary cells. Cancer Res 1988;48:6703.
173. Stewart FW. Mechanisms of apoptosis: integration of genetic, biochemical, and cellular indicators. JNCI 1994;86:1286.
174. Stoker MGP, Rubin H. Density-dependent inhibition of cell growth in culture. Nature 1967;215:171.
175. Sunkara PS, Wright DA, Nishioka K. An essential role for putrescine biosynthesis during meiotic maturation of amphibian oocytes. Dev Biol 1981;87:351.
176. Tabor CW, Tabor H. Polyamines. Annu Rev Biochem 1984;53:749.
177. Tanaka T, Inamura K, Ann T, Taniuchi K. Multimolecular forms of pyruvate kinase and phosphofructokinase in normal and cancer tissues. Gann Monogr 1972;13:219.
178. Tanaka Y, Eda H, Tanaka T, Udagawa T, Ishikawa T, Horii I, Ishitsuka H, Kataoka T, Taguchi T. Experimental cancer cachexia induced by transplantable colon 26 adenocarcinoma in mice. Cancer Res 1990;50:2290.
179. Tashjian AH Jr, Levine L, Munson PL. Immunochemical identification of parathyroid hormone in non-parathyroid neoplasms associated with hypercalcemia. J Exp Med 1964;119:467.
180. Tashjian AH Jr, Voelkel EF, Levine L, Goldhaber P. Evidence that the bone ressorption-stimulating factor produced by mouse fibrosarcoma cells is prostaglandin E_2. A new model for hypercalcemia of cancer. J Exp Med 1972;136:1329.
181. Tatarinov Y. Detection of embryospecific α-globulin in the blood sera of patients with primary liver tumors. Vopr Med Khim 1964;10:90.
182. Theologides A. Pathogenesis of cachexia in cancer: a review and a hypothesis. Cancer 1972;29:484.
183. Timpl R, Engel J, Martin GR. Laminin-A multifunctional protein of basement membranes. Trends Biochem Sci 1983:207.
184. Tomkins GM, Gelehrter TD, Granner P, Martin D Jr, Samuels HH, Thompson EB. Control of specific gene expression in higher organisms. Science 1969;166:1474.
185. Torti TM, Dieckmann B, Beutler B, Cerami A, Ringold GM. A macrophage factor inhibits adipocyte gene expression: an in vitro model of cachexia. Science 1985;229: 867.
186. Tracey KJ, Lowry SF, Beutler B, Cerami A, Albert JD, Shires GT. Cachectin/tumor necrosis factor mediates changes of skeletal muscle plasma membrane potential. J Exp Med 1986;164:1368.
187. Tracey KJ, Wei H, Manogue KR, Fong Y, Hesse DG, Nguyen HT, Kuo GC, Beutler B, Cotran RS, Cerami A, Lowry SR. Cachectin/tumor necrosis factor induces cachexia, anemia and inflammation. J Exp Med 1988;167:1211.
188. Umbas R, Schalken JA, Aalders TW, Carter BS, Karthaus FM, Schaafsma HE, DeBruyne FMJ, Isaacs WB. Expression of cellular adhesion molecules: E-cadherin is reduced or absent in high grade prostate cancer. Cancer Res 1992;52:5106.
189. Unkeless J, Dano K, Kellerman GM, Reich E. Fibrinolysis associated with oncogenic transformation: partial purification and characterization of the cell factor, a plasminogen activator. J Biol Chem 1974;249:4295.
190. Urbach F. Pathophysiology of malignancy. I. Tissue oxygen tension of benign and malignant tumors of the skin. Proc Exp Biol Med 1956;92:644.
191. Uriel J. Fetal characteristics of cancer. In Cancer: A Comprehensive Treatise, vol 3. Edited by FF Becker. New York: Plenum, 1975, p 21.
192. VanEys J. Nutrition and cancer: physiological interrelationships. Ann Rev Nutr 1985;5:435.
193. Vaughan L, Huber S, Chiquet M, Winterhelter KA. A major, six-armed glycoprotein from embryonic cartilage. EMBO J 1987;6:349.
194. Verderame M, Alcorta D, Egnor M, Smith K, Pollack R. Cytoskeletal F-actin patterns quantitated with fluorescein isothiocyanate-phalloidin in normal and transformed cells. Proc Natl Acad Sci USA 1980;77:6624.
195. Vines RL, Coleman MS, Hutton JJ. Reappearance of terminal deoxynucleotidyl transferase containing cells in rat bone marrow following corticosteroid administration. Blood 1980;56:501.
196. Walborg EF Jr, Tsuchida S, Allison JP, deLourdes Ponce M, Barrick A, Weeden DS, Thomas MW, Hixson DC. Dipeptidyl peptidase IV, an enzyme shared by the hepatocyte plasma membrane and liver biomatrix altered expression in hepatocellular carcinomas. In Cell Membranes and Cancer. Edited by T Galeotti, A Cittadine, G Neri, S Pampa, LA Smits. New York: Elsevier, 1985, p 25.
197. Walker PR, Potter VR. Isozyme studies on adult, regenerating, precancerous and developing liver in relation to findings in hepatomas. Adv Enzyme Regul 1972;10:339.
198. Wang AM, Creasey AA, Ladner MB, Lin LS, Strickler J, Van Arsdell JN, Yamamoto R,

Mark DF. Molecular cloning of the complementary DNA for human tumor necrosis factor. Science 1985;228:149.
199. Warburg O. On respiratory impairment in cancer cells. Science 1956;124:269.
200. Weber G. Enzymology of cancer cells. N Engl J Med 1977;296:486, 541.
201. Weinhouse S. Oxidative metabolism of neoplastic tissues. Adv Cancer Res 1955;3: 269.
202. Wessells NK, Spooner BS, Ash JF, Bradley MO, Luduena MA, Taylor EL, Wrenn JT, Yamada KM. Microfilaments in cellular and developmental process. Science 1971;171:135.
203. Wyllie AH, Kerr JFR, Currie AR. Cell death: the significance of apoptosis. Int Rev Cytol 1980;68:251.
204. Yamada KM, Akiyama SK, Hasegawa T, Hasegawa E, Humphries MJ, Kennedy DW, Nagata K, Urishihara H, Olden K, Chen W-T. Recent advances in research on fibronectin and other cell attachment proteins. J Cell Biochem 1985;28:79.

CHAPTER 9

Invasion and Metastasis

LANCE A. LIOTTA AND ELISE C. KOHN

Invasion and metastasis are the most insidious and life-threatening aspects of cancer (9, 41, 83, 91, 142, 160). It is well accepted that most invasive epithelial cancers are derived from preexisting carcinoma in situ lesions, adenomas, or disorders of epithelial proliferation. Once the neoplasm becomes invasive, it has the capacity to disseminate via lymphatics and vascular channels. Local invasion can compromise the function of involved tissues. The most significant turning point in the disease, however, is the establishment of metastasis. At this stage, the patient no longer can be cured by local therapy alone. The patient with metastatic disease succumbs to anatomic compromise caused by cancer dissemination or to complications associated with cytotoxic therapies.

Approximately 30% of patients will have clinically detectable metastases at the time of initial diagnosis. A further 30 to 40% of the remaining patients who appear clinically free of metastases harbor occult metastases. Thus, less than one third of newly diagnosed cancer patients potentially can be cured by local therapeutic modalities alone—a number that may be optimistic. Unfortunately, most patients suffer from metastatic disease at multiple sites during the course of the disease, not all of which may present at any one time. The formation of metastatic colonies is a continuous process commencing early in the growth of the primary tumor and increasing with time. Metastases have the potential to metastasize: the presence of large identifiable metastases in a given organ is frequently accompanied by a greater number of micrometastases that may have been disseminated more recently from the primary tumor or the metastasis. The size and age variation in metastases, their dispersed anatomic locations, and their heterogeneous composition hinder complete surgical extirpation of disease and limit the effectiveness of many systemic anticancer drugs.

Tumors of comparable size and histology can have widely divergent metastatic potential, depending on their intrinsic aggressiveness. Metastatic potential can be influenced by the local tumor environment, but more significantly by the molecular phenotype, which may differ substantially between patients, and perhaps between metastases from the same primary. Thus, there is a great clinical need to (*a*) predict the aggressiveness of a patient's individual tumor, (*b*) determine methods to identify clinically occult metastatic colonies, (*c*) eradicate established metastasis and prevent further dissemination, and (*d*) develop approaches to prevent the transition from normal to malignant and from in situ to invasive neoplasm. New strategies to address these clinical goals have been provided by recent advances in our understanding of the molecular mechanisms of metastasis. We now know that the malignant phenotype is the culmination of a series of genetic changes that involve both positive and negative regulatory elements (Fig. 9.1). Investigation of the activation, regulation, mutation, or somatic deletion of genes that encode these regulatory elements is a new frontier for metastasis research.

Tumor–Host Interactions in the Metastatic Cascade

The process of metastasis is a cascade of linked sequential steps involving multiple host–tumor interactions (Table 9.1). To create a metastatic deposit successfully, a cell or group of cells must be able to leave the primary tumor, invade the local host tissue, and survive to proliferate (Fig. 9.2). This complex process requires the cells to enter into the circulation, arrest at the distant vascular bed, extravasate into the organ interstitium and parenchyma, and proliferate as a secondary colony. A large foundation of experimental work suggests that during each stage of the process, only the fittest tumor cells survive (41, 91, 142). A very small percentage (<0.01%) of circulating tumor cells ultimately initiate successful metastatic colonies. Thus, metastasis is a highly selective competition favoring the survival of a minor subpopulation of metastatic tumor cells that preexist within the primary tumor.

The distribution of metastases varies widely depending on the histologic type and anatomic location of the primary tumor. The most frequent organ location of distant metastases in many types of cancers appears to be the first capillary bed encountered by the circulating cells. Examples of this are lung metastases from sarcoma, brain metastases from primary lung carcinoma, and colorectal cancer dissemination to liver. In the gynecologic tumors, distant metastases are seen in two forms: serosal dissemination, such as liver capsule metastases from ovarian cancer; and capillary-associated dissemination, such as liver and lung parenchymal disease.

On the other hand, there are many metastatic sites that cannot be predicted on the basis of anatomic considerations alone, and can be considered examples of organ tropism. Clear cell carcinoma of the kidney often metastasizes to the thyroid, breast cancer to the ovary, and ocular melanoma to the liver. The predilection of breast and prostate cancer for bone may also reflect a degree of organ tropism. The molecular mechanisms mediating the organ distribution of metastasis have been the subject of study of a number of investigators (117). Hamilton and co-workers developed a mouse xenograft model of human ovarian cancer using the NIH: OVCAR3 cell line developed from the ascites of a patient who had progressed on primary combination chemotherapy (58). After intraperitoneal inoculation, animals develop malignant ascites—tumor masses involving ovaries and bowel serosa—and may develop liver capsular and parenchymal metastases and very late lung metastases. This pattern accurately models what is seen in women with stage III or IV ovarian cancer. Another method for studying organ tropism involves the use of organs grafted into ectopic sites. Fidler and Hart observed that the intravenously injected B16-F10 melanoma cells colonized the native lung as well as subcutaneous lung grafts (41). In order to find the ectopic site, the tumor cells must have either left the first capillary arrest site in the lungs and traveled to the ectopically implanted lung grafts, or entered the general circulation and then recognized signals from the ectopic lung to exit at that location. In control mice, ectopic kidney grafts were not colonized by the circulating tumor cells, indicating a clear organ selectivity for lung but not kidney.

There are several theoretic mechanisms for organ tropism (118). First, tumor cells disseminate equally in all organs, but preferentially grow only in specific organs. Preferential growth may be induced by local growth factors or hormones present in the target organ. For example, the insulin-like growth factors are present in liver and lung and have been shown to be important growth and motility factors for breast cancer, lung cancer, and rhabdomyosarcoma. Second, circulating tumor cells may adhere preferentially to the endothelial luminal surface only in the targeted organ. This requires that there be special recognition signals on the endothelial cells that determine the organ specificity. Last, circulating tumor cells may respond to soluble factors diffusing locally out of the target organs (78). Such factors could act in a chemotactic fashion to attract the tumor cells to extravasate. They could also cause the circulating tumor

POSITIVE
ACTIVATED ONCOGENES
GROWTH FACTORS
PROTEASES
ADHESION RECEPTORS
MOTILITY CYTOKINES
PROGRESSION
NEGATIVE
TUMOR SUPPRESSOR GENES
GROWTH INHIBITORS
METASTASIS SUPPRESSOR GENES
PROTEASE INHIBITORS

Figure 9.1. Positive and negative regulation of proliferation, invasion, and metastasis during multistep tumor progression.

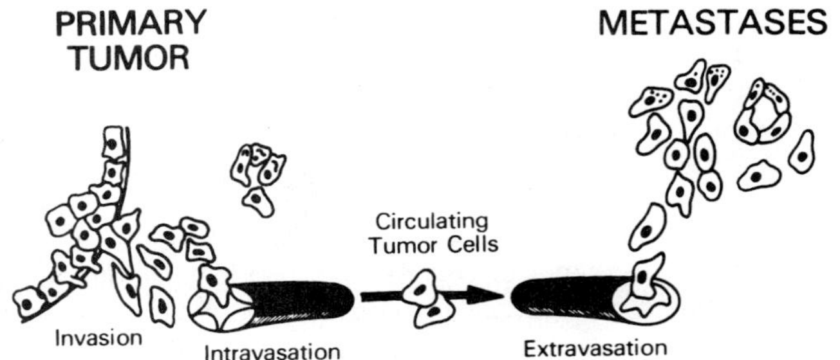

Figure 9.2. Multistep cascade of metastasis.

Table 9.1. Tumor–Host Interactions During the Metastatic Cascade

Metastatic cascade event	Potential mechanisms
1. Tumor initiation	Carcinogenic insult, oncogene activation or derepression, chromosome rearrangement
2. Promotion and progression	Karyotypic, genetic, and epigenetic instability, gene amplification; promotion-associated genes and growth factors; mutation or loss of suppressor gene products
3. Uncontrolled proliferation	Autocrine growth factors or their receptors, receptors for most hormones such as estrogen
4. Angiogenesis	Multiple angiogenesis factors including known growth factors
5. Invasion of local tissues, blood, and lymphatic vessels	Serum chemoattractants, autocrine motility factors, attachment receptors, degradative enzymes, loss of expression of proteinase inhibitors
6. Circulating tumor cell arrest and extravasation	Tumor cell homotypic or heterotypic aggregation
a. adherence to endothelium	Tumor cell interaction with fibrin, platelets, and clotting factors, adhesions to RGD-type receptors
b. retraction of endothelium	Platelet factors, tumor cell factors
c. adhesion to basement membrane	Receptors for laminin, thrombospondin and type IV collagen
d. dissolution of basement of membrane	Metalloproteinases, serine proteinases, heparinase, cathepsins
e. locomotion	Autocrine motility factors, chemotaxis factors
7. Colony formation at secondary site	Receptors for local tissue growth factors, angiogenesis factors, mutation, or loss of metastasis suppressor genes
8. Evasion of host defenses and resistance to therapy	Resistance to killing by host macrophages, natural killer cells, and activated T cells; failure to express, or blocking of tumor-specific antigens; amplification of drug-resistant genes

cells to aggregate and, therefore, embolize in the target organ. Kohn and colleagues have shown that the OVCAR3 human ovarian cancer cell line migrates in response to insulin and insulin-like growth factors, which are known to be present in many normal tissues and to be secreted by several tissues that are known metastatic target sites (78). Nicolson and colleagues have identified endothelial surface antigens that may mediate preferential adhesion of circulating tumor cells to endothelium of particular organs (117, 118). Attempts to characterize these antigens are under way.

Interaction of Metastatic Tumor Cells with the Extracellular Matrix

The mammalian organism is divided into a series of tissue compartments separated by the extracellular matrix. The basement membrane and its underlying interstitial stroma are the major connective tissue unit separating organ parenchymal compartments. During the transition from in situ to invasive carcinoma, tumor cells penetrate the epithelial basement membrane and enter the underlying interstitial stroma (8, 89). The continuous basement membrane is a dense meshwork of type IV collagen, glycoproteins, such as laminin and fibronectin, and proteoglycans and normally does not contain any pores large enough for tumor cell traversal without destructive enlargement. Therefore, invasion of the basement membrane must be an active process. Once the tumor cells enter the underlying stroma, they gain access to lymphatics and blood vessels for distant dissemination. Tumor cells must cross basement membranes to invade nerves and most organ parenchyma. During intravasation or extravasation, the tumor cells must penetrate the subendothelial basement membrane. In the distant organ where metastatic colonies are to be established, extravasated tumor cells must migrate through the perivascular interstitial stroma before tumor colony growth occurs in the organ parenchyma.

General and widespread changes occur in the organization, distribution, and quantity of the epithelial basement membrane during the transition from benign to invasive carcinoma (8). Benign proliferative disorders of the breast, such as fibrocystic disease, sclerosing adenosis, intraductal hyperplasia, fibroadenoma, and intraductal papilloma, are all characterized by disorganization of the normal epithelial stromal architecture. Extreme forms can mimic the appearance of invasive carcinoma. But regardless of the extensive nature of the architectural disorganization, these benign disorders are always characterized by a continuous basement membrane separating the epithelium from the stroma. In contrast, invasive ductal and lobular carcinomas consistently possess a defective extracellular basement membrane, with zones of basement membrane loss around the invading tumor cells in the stroma. The basement membrane is also markedly defective adjacent to tumor cells in lymph node and organ metastases. In some focal regions of well-differentiated carcinoma, partial basement membrane formation by differentiated structures can be identified. These findings have direct application to diagnostic problems in surgical pathology, such as the differentiation of tangential sections of in situ lesions from true invasion or of severe adenosis from invasive carcinoma. Loss of basement membranes in human carcinomas significantly correlates with an increased incidence of metastases and poor 5-year survivals.

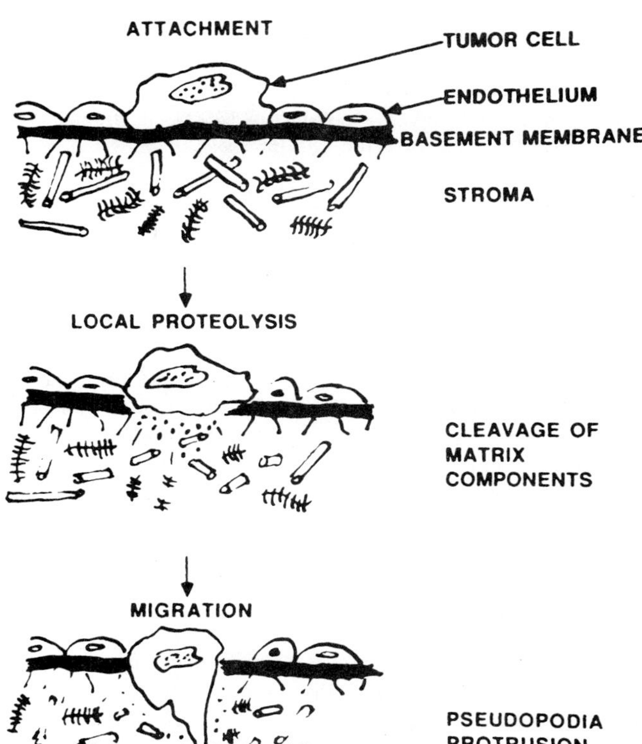

Figure 9.3. Three-step hypothesis for invasion of the extracellular matrix unit.

The general observation of defective basement membranes associated with cancer invasion and progression indicates that aggressive tumor cells may interact with basement membranes in a manner fundamentally different from that of normal cells. This provides the foundation for the investigation of molecular mechanisms of tumor cell invasion. In this regard, the interactions of the tumor cell with the basement membrane can be separated into three steps (Fig. 9.3) (64, 89, 94). For the case of a circulating tumor cell, the basement membrane is exposed by retraction of the endothelium induced by the tumor cell. The tumor cell then attaches to the basement membrane surface. This is mediated by the binding of tumor cell surface proteins to glycoproteins, such as laminin, type IV collagen, and fibronectin, in the basement membrane. Following attachment, the tumor cells must create a rent in the basement membrane. Tumor cells both secrete degradative enzymes and induce the host to secrete proteinases to degrade the matrix and its component adhesion molecules. Matrix lysis takes place in a highly localized region close to the tumor cell surface where the amount of active enzyme outbalances the natural proteinase inhibitors present in the serum or in the matrix, or that secreted by normal cells in the vicinity. The third step of invasion is translocation of the tumor cell across the basement membrane via the hole created by the local proteolysis. The direction and site of the tumor cell locomotion may by influenced by host-derived chemoattractants or tumor cell–secreted motility factors. The invasive process is a dynamic one involving cyclic repetition of these steps.

ADHESION

The first step of basement membrane invasion requires tumor cell attachment.

Laminin

An example of a major attachment protein found exclusively in the basement membrane is laminin. Laminin is a large complex cruciform glycoprotein with the ability to bind to multiple membrane components, including type IV collagen, heparan sulfate, proteoglycan, and entactin (95, 129). Laminin plays a role in cell attachment, cell spreading, mitogenesis, neurite outgrowth, morphogenesis, and cell movement. Cell surface receptors for laminin mediate these varied functions of tumor cells. A nanomolar affinity cell surface laminin receptor of 67 kd has been cloned from normal and neoplastic cells (7, 98, 104, 164). In addition, laminin may bind to heterodimeric integrins through its Arg-Gly-Asp (RGD) site (see below) or to galactins. Laminin receptors may be altered in number or degree of occupancy in human carcinomas. This may be the indirect result of defective basement membrane organization in the carcinomas (178). Breast carcinoma and colon carcinoma tissues contain a higher number of exposed, unoccupied laminin receptors as compared with benign lesions. These receptors may be amplified and distributed over the surface of the cell in contrast to the architecture of the normal cell, in which the laminin receptors are polarized at the basal surface and are occupied by the laminin in the basement membrane. There is experimental evidence to demonstrate that tumor cells exposed to the whole laminin molecule more avidly form metastases in animals. If, however, cells are treated with a fragment of laminin that cannot link the tumor cell to the basement membrane, metastases cannot be initiated.

Integrins

A second class of matrix receptors important in tumor cell attachment to the extracellular matrix is the integrins. This family of cell surface glycoproteins binds a broad array of adhesion proteins with micromolar affinity (69).The adhesion proteins that bind to integrins include fibronectin, vitronectin, fibrin, type I collagen, laminin, thrombospondin, and von Willebrand factor (60). The integrin receptor consists of a heterodimer of alpha and beta chains, which, in part, confer ligand specificity. Peptides of the Arg-Gly-Asp (RGD) group inhibit the functions of many of the integrins, a property for which the family was originally named. RGD sequences in a wide variety of proteins may serve as the recognition site for binding to the integrins. Preferential recognition of specific adhesion molecules may be conferred by ligand sequences flanking the RGD sites (137). The integrin proteins are thought to align adhesion proteins, such as fibronectin, on the cell surface with cytoskeletal components, such as talin and actin, thus altering cell shape (66). These adhesion ligands are important in the metastatic cascade. Co-injection of tumor cells with large quantities of RGD peptides inhibited metastasis formation in animal models (68). Thus, the interaction of cells and adhesion molecules of low- and high-affinity receptors is important in metastasis development. Recent data demonstrate integrin signaling through tyrosine phosphorylation and a novel tyrosine kinase, focal adhesion kinase (FAK) (70, 143). Further studies are ongoing to elucidate the downstream effectors for this signaling system and its importance in the process of cancer progression.

Cadherins

Cell–cell association is disorganized in malignant tumors. Cancer cells must disrupt their normally tight association with other cells in order to leave the primary site and metastasize. Several studies have indicated that the family of cadherin adhesion molecules plays a key role in this process (10). Cadherins are extracellular calcium-dependent cell adhesion molecules (10, 161). Three subtypes have been identified in mammals, named for their selective tissue distribution and binding specificities: epithelial (E), placental (P), and neural (N) cadherin. A role for E cadherin as an invasion suppressor molecule has been demonstrated. After treatment with anti E cadherin antibodies, nontransformed Madin-Darby canine kidney (MDCK) epithelial cells acquire an invasive phenotype in a chick heart fragment model (11). Moreover, the invasiveness of transformed MDCK cells into the chick heart fragments can be abolished by transfection and expression of E cadherin cDNA (22).

PROTEOLYSIS

The process of invasion is not a passive one due to pressure from excessive cellular proliferation alone, but is an active, dynamic process that requires protein synthesis and degradation (54, 165, 166). Inhibitors of metalloproteinases or of protein synthesis, but not of DNA synthesis, block tumor cell invasion into the matrix. Tumor cells must traverse the extracellular matrix in the process of invasion and must be able to either secrete or activate enzymes that can degrade the major components of the matrix, such as collagen types I, IV, and V, fibronectin, and proteoglycans.

Metalloproteinases

A critical proteolytic event early in the metastatic cascade appears to be the degradation of basement membrane collagen (88). Type IV collagen is a critical component of the basement membrane architectural scaffolding on which laminin, heparan sulfate, proteoglycan, and minor components of the basement membrane are assembled. Much attention has focused on the ability of metastatic tumor cells to degrade type IV collagen. Type IV collagenases are named for their ability to degrade type IV basement membrane collagen (90). They are members of the matrix metalloproteinase gene family (MMP) (Fig. 9.4). Other metalloproteases, such as stromelysin, matrilysin, and interstitial collagenases, are also important in metastases but do not proteolyze the same substrate proteins and may degrade

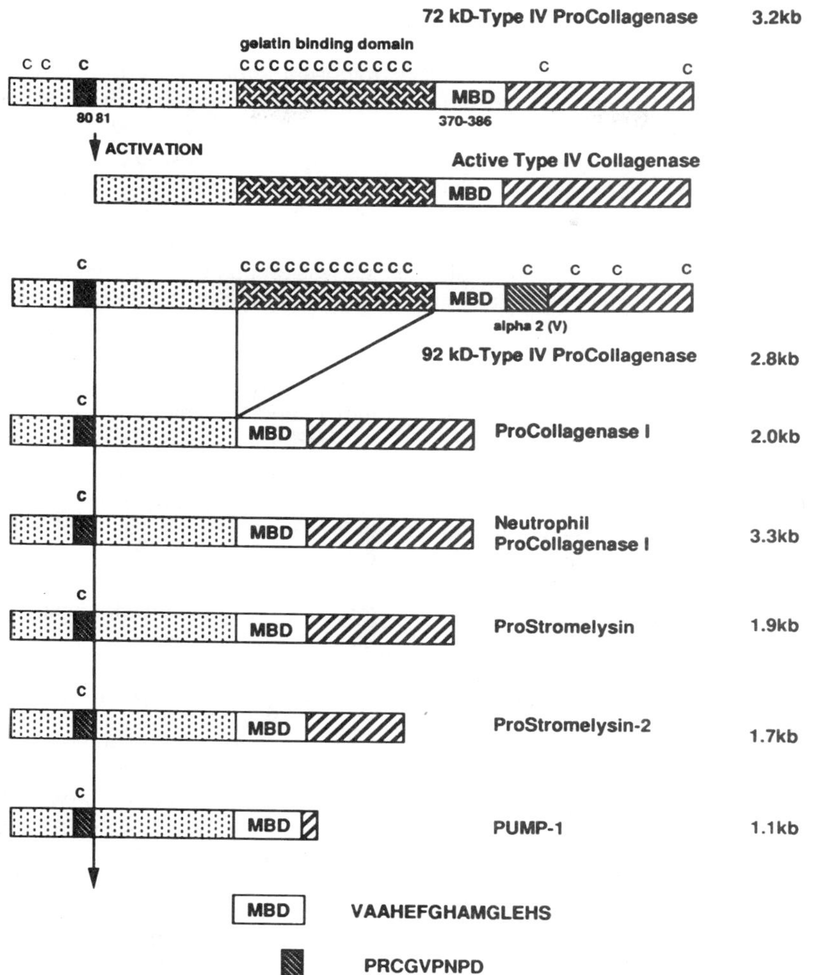

Figure 9.4. Metalloproteinase gene family. The proenzyme form of each proteinase member is shown. Activation involves cleavage of an amino terminal peptide 1–80 containing an unpaired cysteine residue. In the latent enzyme, the unpaired cysteine residue folds over and blocks the active site (MBD, metal binding domain) of the enzyme by forming a noncovalent interaction with the zinc metal atom. The type IV collagenases are distinguished by a cysteine repeat gelatin binding domain that mediates adhesion to type IV collagen. V = Val; A = Ala; H = His; E = Glu; F = Phe; G = Gly; M = Met; L = Leu; S = Ser; P = Pro; R = Arg; C = Cys; N = Asn; D = Asp; PUMP-I = putative metalloproteinase.

type IV collagen in the pepsin-sensitive nonhelical domains in a less specific fashion (102, 179).

There are at least two type IV collagenase enzymes, a 72-kd (MMP-2) and a 92-kd (MMP-9) type IV collagenase (26, 180). Both are members of the matrix metalloproteinase gene family, and share structural homologies with other members of this family (Fig. 9.4). Many earlier studies did not discriminate between the 72-kd type IV collagenase, which was originally identified and purified from a metastatic murine cell line, and the 92-kd type IV collagenase, which was originally characterized as a gelatinolytic activity from human polymorphonuclear leukocytes. MMP-2 and MMP-9 are distinguishable by immunologic, molecular, and biochemical criteria, but not by substrate specificity. Both are secreted as latent proenzymes, are activated by organomercurial compounds with the concomitant autoproteolytic removal of an amino terminal fragment, are inhibited by members of the tissue inhibitor of metalloproteinase (TIMP) family, and form specific latent proenzyme-TIMP complexes with one or the other member of the TIMP family. Both enzymes also possess potent gelatinolytic activities, for which they are also known as gelatinase A (MMP-2) and gelatinase B (MMP-9).

A positive correlation between type IV collagenase activity and tumor cell invasion has been demonstrated (50, 97, 106, 114, 131, 168). Metastatic potential has been shown to correlate in a positive fashion with type IV collagenolytic activity in murine tumor models (50, 97, 114, 168). Highly aggressive human tumors, such as carcinomas, melanomas, hepatomas, fibrosarcomas, and invasive lymphomas, all showed elevated levels of type IV collagenase activity when compared with benign controls. Immunohistochemical studies using affinity purified anti-MMP-2 antibodies have demonstrated that low levels of this enzyme are produced by normal, nontumorigenic, nonmetastatic cells, such as the myoepithelial cells of the human breast (109). Benign proliferative lesions of the breast were associated with some increase in MMP-2 immunoreactivity that was again restricted to the myoepithelial cells. With progressive severity of breast lesions from atypical hyperplasia through carcinoma in situ to frankly invasive carcinoma, there was an increase in the immunohistochemical staining for the MMP-2 that was specifically associated with the neoplastic breast epithelial cells (Fig. 9.5A) (109). Moreover, benign polyps of the colon, normal colorectal, and gastric mucosa all show negligible immunoreactivity for MMP-2 (Fig. 9.5B) (49). In contrast, almost all invasive colonic and gastric (Fig. 9.5C) adenocarcinomas were positive for this antigen. Studies have also shown a positive correlation between augmented type IV collagenase activity and the genetic induction of a metastatic phenotype (50, 168). Furthermore, use of agents that specifically inhibited type IV collagenase activity blocked invasion by tumor cells (106, 107, 131).

Measurements of MMP-2 mRNA levels and enzyme activity have shown a close correlation with the invasive and metastatic properties of c-Ha-*ras* transformed bronchial epithelial cells (168). Down regulation of type IV collagenolytic activity by retinoic acid treatment of human melanoma cells has been correlated with a loss of the invasive phenotype. Studies of the mechanism of this effect have revealed that retinoic acid treatment of human melanoma cells results in a reduction of the steady-state level of MMP-2 mRNA and loss of the invasive capacity (61). Measurements of the steady-state transcript levels for this enzyme in human colonic adenocarcinoma tissues have demonstrated a statistically significant increase over those of adjacent normal tissues, which showed consistently low levels of expression. These studies suggest that MMP-2 is a normal cell component that is dramatically overexpressed in many invasive and metastatic human cancers. Endothelial cells in culture secrete a readily detectable level of type IV collagenase activity. Antisera against MMP-2 can inhibit basic fibroblast growth factor–induced endothelial cell invasion of human amnion membrane in vitro (107). These observations suggest that MMP-2 may also function in normal physiologic processes, such as basement membrane turnover by myoepithelial cells and angiogenesis by endothelial cells.

SERINE PROTEINASES

Malignant cells have been documented as having increased amounts of plasminogen activators (29, 53, 99). In addition, oncogenic transformation of cells has been associated with increases in the extracellular release of plasminogen activators. The plasminogen activators, urokinase and tissue plasminogen activator, are independent gene products that are secreted as proenzymes. The only well-characterized physiologic substrate that is known for the plasminogen activators is plasminogen. Investigators from a number of laboratories have shown that plasminogen activator activity can be extracted from a number of human and animal tumors, and is predominantly urokinase (20, 100). Laboratory studies have indicated that matrix glycoproteins are susceptible to plasmin-mediated proteolytic degradation (71, 106, 131). Direct evidence for the role of these enzymes in invasion has been reported using an in vitro invasion assay (71). A positive correlation between plasminogen activator activity and metastatic potential has been established for the B16 murine melanoma line (173). Highly metastatic cells of the F10 generation showed high levels in the primary tumors and even higher levels in the pulmonary metastases. A recent report demonstrated a significant (six-fold) elevation of urokinase mRNA in human primary lung and breast carcinomas when compared with nonmalignant tissues (140). At present, urokinase levels are not considered sufficiently diagnostic of tumor aggressiveness to allow development as a tumor marker; however, there is a suggestion that plasminogen activator inhibitor levels may be of clinical utility.

CYSTEINE PROTEINASES

Evidence for the role of the cysteine proteinases, cathepsins B, L, and D, in cancer progression and metastasis is growing (101, 130, 145, 146). Cathepsin B is a lysosomal acid hydrolase with a broad range of endopeptidase activity against substrates, including myosin, actin, proteoglycans, fibronectin, laminin, and the nonhelical portions of type IV collagen. Cathepsin B activity has been found in association with the plasma membrane fraction of tumor cells, and in the conditioned media from tumor cell cultures (145, 146). The tumor cell–derived cathepsin B appears to be a different enzyme from that found in the lysosomes of normal cells. Studies using the B16 murine melanoma line have shown a correlation between cathepsin B activity and metastatic potential. Pietras and co-workers measured cathepsin B1 activity in the serum of patients with gynecologic malignancies and found a significant increase in cathepsin B1 activity in patients with stages III and IV squamous cell carcinoma of the uterine cervix. Minimal elevations were observed in women with lower-stage disease or dysplasia and in controls (121). They also showed that advanced-stage adenocarcinomas of the ovary and endometrium were associated with markedly elevated levels of enzyme activity up to twofold to threefold higher than seen in early-stage patients. A similarly positive correlation has been shown between cathepsin B

Figure 9.5. Type IV collagenase augmentation during human carcinoma progression. Affinity purified antisynthetic peptide antibodies were used in an immunohistochemical study of formalin-fixed, paraffin-embedded human neoplasms. The Ki67 proliferation associated marker was used as a control. Each symbol represents an individual patient's primary tumor. In each tumor, 1,000 cells were scored by three independent pathologists. **A.** Breast carcinoma. LCIS: lobular carcinoma in situ. DCIS: ductal carcinoma in situ. ILC: infiltrating lobular carcinoma. IDC: infiltrating ductal carcinoma. All invasive lesions had augmented levels of type IV collagenase (cIVase) as compared with adjacent noncancerous epithelium. **B.** Colorectal neoplasia. Duke's C cases had the highest proportion of cells positive for type IV collagenase (cIVase). Duke's A/B tumors exhibited intermediate levels, and the majority of adenomas exhibited very low type IV collagenase content. The same pattern was found when the type IV collagenase mRNA levels were compared. **C.** Gastric carcinoma. WDE: well-differentiated early (superficial). WDA: well-differentiated advanced (invading through the full thickness of the gastric wall). PDE: poorly differentiated early. PDA: poorly differentiated advanced. The advanced tumors contained the highest level of type IV collagenase.

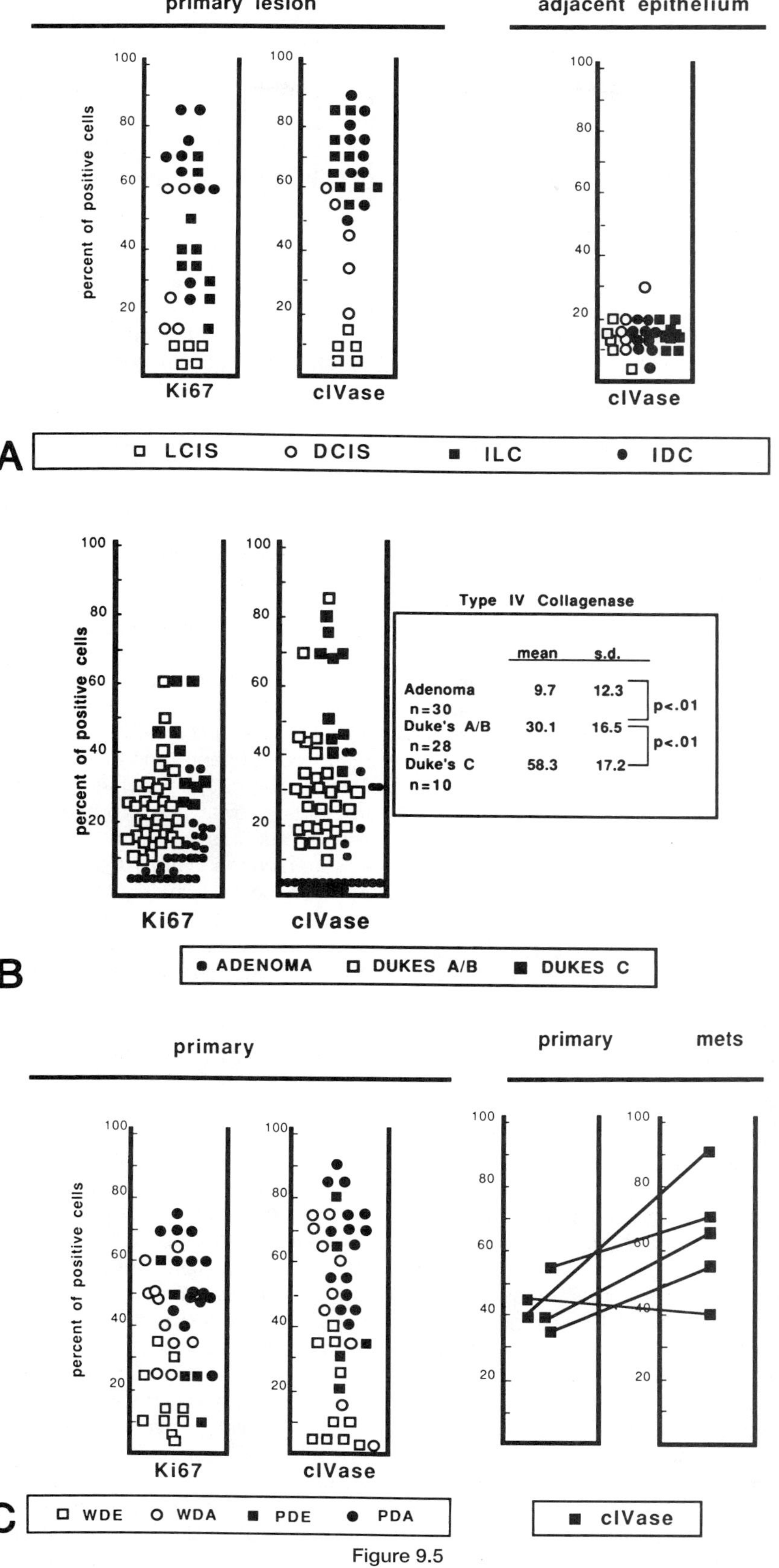
primary lesion
adjacent epithelium
percent of positive cells
Ki67
cIVase
A
LCIS
DCIS
ILC
IDC
B
Type IV Collagenase
mean s.d.
Adenoma n=30 9.7 12.3
Duke's A/B n=28 30.1 16.5
Duke's C n=10 58.3 17.2
p<.01
p<.01
ADENOMA
DUKES A/B
DUKES C
C
primary
primary
mets
WDE
WDA
PDE
PDA
cIVase

Figure 9.5

levels in other human tumors and the malignant behavior of these tumors.

Cathepsin D is also a lysosomal acid proteinase (132). It has documented mitogenic activity on estrogen-depleted MCF-7 human breast adenocarcinoma cells in culture, and its secretion is constitutive in hormone-independent breast cancer cell lines (132). This proteinase has the ability to degrade extracellular matrix components, such as proteoglycans, and is present in high levels in proliferative breast diseases, both benign and malignant, but in very low amounts in resting mammary glands (130). Two clinical studies of breast cancer patients have correlated high levels of cathepsin D with poor disease-free survival and overall survival, as an independent variable (150, 162). Cathepsin D was of most significant prognostic value in node-negative breast cancer patients. Hence, as markers of cancer invasion, cathepsin D and type IV collagenase are potential new diagnostic and prognostic markers of the aggressiveness of malignancy.

TUMOR CELL MIGRATION

An important step in the dynamic process of invasion and metastasis involves tumor cell translocation across biologic barriers. Tumor cell migration is necessary at the initiation of the metastatic cascade, at which time the tumor cells leave the primary and gain access to the circulation, as well as at the end of invasion, when the tumor cell is entering the secondary site. The movement of the cells through such biologic barriers may be driven by a number of factors (55, 103). These include tumor-derived chemotactic factors, host-derived chemoattractants, and combinations of the two. Laboratory studies of tumor cell locomotion have shown that tumor cells may respond chemotactically to growth factors, collagen peptides, matrix components and proteolytic fragments of matrix components, adhesion proteins, such as laminin and fibronectin, and tumor-derived attractants (5, 92, 103, 104, 134). These agents may stimulate both the initiation and maintenance of tumor cell motility and the directedness of that migration. Protruding pseudopodia, in response to chemoattractants, may serve multiple functions, including acting as sense organs for the migrating cell to locate directional clues, to secrete motility-stimulating factors, to provide propulsive traction for locomotion, and to induce matrix proteolysis to assist in the penetration of the matrix. The reliance on the host for migration stimulation would not favor the sustained migration seen in highly metastatic populations of tumor cells, thus emphasizing the importance of tumor-derived chemoattractants.

Investigators have demonstrated the importance of autocrine growth factors for transformed cells, leading to the hypothesis that tumor cells also secrete autocrine motility-stimulating factors (39, 78, 92). An autocrine motility factor (AMF) was originally described in the conditioned media of the A2058 human melanoma cell line. AMF-like activity has now been described in a number of systems (39, 78, 92, 93, 159). Autotaxin (ATX), the first autocrine motility factor to be isolated, purified, and cloned, is a potent motility-stimulating glycoprotein of 120 to 125 kd (93, 159). ATX has marked homology to the PC-1 protein of activated B cells and plasma cells. Both ATX and PC-1 have pyrophosphatase/type I phosphodiesterase/kinase activity and are both expressed on their respective external cell surfaces as ectokinases (159). Autotaxin is the first ectokinase to be identified in human solid tumors and opens a new field of investigation on the roles of these enzymes in normal biology and in the invasive process as motility-stimulating factors. Hepatocyte growth factor, also known as scatter factor (HGF/SF), is a paracrine motility factor that stimulates motility of epithelial and endothelial cells (156, 157). HGF/SF induces the scatter or chemokinetic locomotion of epithelial colonies, resulting in an invasive phenotype in vivo (59). HGF/SF is the preferred ligand for the c-*met* proto-oncogene product, a 190-kd transmembrane tyrosine kinase-containing receptor that is widely expressed in normal epithelial tissues (115). The transfection of a mutated *met* oncogene into the human osteosarcoma cell line, HOS, induced an invasive phenotype in vitro and tumorigenic and metastatic ability in vivo. In another experimental setting, the transfection of murine met into NIH 3T3 cells producing endogenous HGF/SF caused the cells to become highly tumorigenic and metastastic by completing the autocrine loop (133, 134). These results indicate that HGF/SF and its receptor c-*met* can play an important role during tumor progression by stimulating the growth and motility of cancer cells.

The complexity of tumor cell migration requires that more than one agent be involved in the direction, location, and magnitude of the migratory response. During the course of invasion, the tumor cell must interact with the extracellular matrix components, and be exposed to host-derived factors. Tumor cells have receptors for many of these potential attractants. Growth factors produced by normal and malignant tissues, such as the insulin-like growth factors, may also be important in the migration of tumor cells (78, 108).

These factors primarily stimulate chemotactic, or directed, motility, and may play a role in tumor cell homing to certain secondary sites. Therefore, the response of the tumor cell to autocrine motility stimulation and endocrine or paracrine stimulation by matrix components and host-derived growth factors is important in the initiation of tumor cell locomotion, its directedness, and potentially the determination of the location of the metastatic focus.

Angiogenesis

Neovascularization is a prerequisite for the local expansion of tumor colonies beyond the size restricted by oxygen and nutrient diffusion. New capillaries also provide cancer cells with conduits for entry into the circulation. Extravasated cancer cells will later require neovascularization in order to grow and form new metastatic foci. Therefore, angiogenesis is necessary at the beginning and end of the metastatic cascade. The process of blood vessel formation is functionally similar to tumor cell invasion and can be considered as a form of regulated invasion, with the independent events of adhesion, proteolysis, and migration that characterize the spreading of cancer cells also displayed by endothelial cells (80, 96). Interstitial collagenase (MMP-1), MMP-2, and urokinase have been shown to be secreted by endothelial cells in vitro and are necessary for vessel formation in vivo; inhibition of collagenolytic activity inhibits angiogenic activity (62, 76, 110). Several of these angiogenic factors may cause a pleiotropic response of enzyme production, endothelial cell migration, and/or proliferation. Basic fibroblast growth factor (FGF-2) is the most potent angiogenic factor described and is involved in many aspects of neovascularization. FGF-2 stimulates endothelial cell growth, protease secretion, and motility of endothelial cells in vitro and may be involved in the pathogenesis of a variety of human tumors (46, 141, 163).

Histologic and ultrastructural analyses of tumor vessels have revealed pronounced differences in tumor vessels as compared with normal vessels found in mature tissues. The distinction includes differences in the cellular composition of tumor vessels, the basement membrane composition and integrity, and differences in permeability (45). Due to a discontinuous basement membrane, tumor vessels are leaky and easily penetrated by cancer cells entering the circulation at high rate (millions of cells a day) (47). Recently, a positive correlation between the number of tumor microvessels in cancer specimens and patient outcome was demonstrated for a number of cancer cell types, including ovarian cancer, breast cancer, melanoma, and prostate cancers (16, 65, 151, 174, 175).

Genetic Regulation of Invasion and Metastasis

Invasion and metastasis are a very complicated multistep process. Consequently one gene product is not sufficient for metastasis. Furthermore, it is now understood that negative factors may be just as important as the positive factors discussed in the preceding sections (Fig. 9.1). In order to exhibit the metastatic phenotype, individual tumor cells must have either a deficiency in the negative factors or an augmentation in the positive factors. This is analogous to the positive and negative factors involved in tumorigenicity. Some genetic changes result in an imbalance of growth regulation, leading to uncontrolled proliferation. In terms of positive regulation, this can be due to mutational activation of oncogenes, increased production of growth factors, or a continuous activation of a growth factor signal pathway (148, 176). Uncontrolled growth can also be caused by the loss of production of growth inhibitor cytokines such as TGFβ which have their action at the cell surface, or the loss of growth suppressor gene products, such as *Rb* or *p53* which operate inside the cell (139, 140).

However, unrestrained growth does not, by itself, cause invasion and metastasis. The latter phenotype may require additional genetic changes over and above those resulting in uncontrolled proliferation. Invasion and metastasis can be facilitated by proteins that stimulate tumor cell attachment to host cellular or extracellular matrix elements, tumor cell proteolysis of host barriers to invasion, such as the basement membrane, tumor cell locomotion, and tumor cell colony formation in the target organ for metastasis (54, 95). These positive elements are counterbalanced, however, by factors that can block their production, regulation, or action. Two classes of metastasis suppressor gene products can be identified: (*a*) those that act outside the cell to block key aspects of metastasis such as proteolysis (1, 4, 15, 21, 35, 52, 62, 73, 96, 111, 112, 153, 154, 177), and (*b*) those that have their action inside the cell (12, 116, 126, 136, 167) in a regulatory pathway (12, 32, 33, 41, 85, 86, 116, 120, 126, 128, 136, 144, 152, 169).

Metastasis Suppressor Genes

The existence of tumor suppressor genes led to the hypothesis of metastasis suppressor genes (139, 147). The *ras* oncogene, which is capable of inducing the metastatic phenotype, fails to do so in all tumor cells (126, 167). C127 cells transfected with *ras* express high levels of p21 and are tumorigenic, but nonmetastatic (113). This second line of evidence indicates that the cells resistant to the induction of metastasis by *ras* may express a suppressor gene. As an extension of this finding, injection of rats with N-nitrosomethylurea-induced specific activating mutations in *ras*, resulting in mammary tumor development (152); however, only 10% of the resulting tumors were metastatic during observation periods of up to 1 year. The lack of metastatic behavior in 90% of NMU-induced tumors, despite the presence of a metastasis-inducing gene, suggested active suppression. It is, therefore, logical to postulate that highly invasive and metastatic tumor cells could be deficient in specific gene products that suppress metastasis in normal cells or in benign tumors. Given the complicated array of biologic functions involved in the metastatic process (i.e., motility, adhesiveness, proteolysis, angiogenesis, avoidance of immune recognition), any gene product that effectively stops one component of the process may block metastatic behavior, and, therefore, have suppressor activity. In addition, regulatory genes may be identified that suppress a cascade of downstream metastasis-associated genes, or suppress some aspect of cellular communication or signal transduction. Suppressor genes may also include genes that promote the stability of tumor cells, thereby reducing the genetic instability thought to fuel progression to the metastatic phenotype.

The first nonimmunologically related metastasis suppressor gene was described by Pozzatti and colleagues (126). Rat embryo fibroblasts transfected with c-Ha-*ras* were highly metastatic upon intravenous injection, but cotransfection of rat embryo fibroblasts with c-Ha-*ras* and adenovirus 2 *E1A* resulted in transformed but virtually nonmetastatic cells. The *E1A* gene, therefore, suppressed the metastasis-inducing activity of the *ras* gene. One component of the mechanism of action of *E1A* is the suppression of metalloproteinase production by the tumor cells (50). Transfection of *E1A* into malignant cells has itself abrogated the malignant phenotype, suggesting that it may also be a tumor suppressor gene (42). Other investigators attempted to identify cellular genes or homologs of viral proteins that are capable of metastasis suppression.

The first major approach to the identification of metastasis suppressor genes employed a functional analysis. A key biochemical step required for invasion and metastasis was identified and used as a target for the isolation of a cellular factor that blocked the key step. In this manner, the TIMP (tissue inhibitor of metalloproteinases) family has been proposed as a major natural inhibitor of cancer invasion. These natural inhibitor proteins, produced either by the host or by the tumor cell itself, have been shown to block the latent or the active metalloproteinases, thus functioning as metastasis suppressor proteins (35, 52, 112, 155, 177). TIMP-1, the first member of the TIMP family, is a glycoprotein with an apparent molecular size of 28.5 kd that forms a complex of 1:1 stoichiometry with activated interstitial collagenase, activated stromelysin, and the 92-kd type IV collagenase (21, 35, 62, 73).

The gene coding for TIMP-1 has been cloned, sequenced, and mapped to the X chromosome (21). The same cells that produce interstitial collagenase are capable of synthesizing and secreting TIMP-1 (62). Thus, the net collagenolytic activity for these cell types is the result of the balance between activated enzyme levels and TIMP-1 levels. Studies have shown an inverse correlation between TIMP-1 levels and the invasive potential of murine and human tumor cells. Furthermore, it has been reported that transfection of antisense RNA, which blocks TIMP-1 expression, increases the malignant phenotype (73).

Stetler-Stevenson and colleagues have isolated, purified, and cloned the second member of the TIMP family, TIMP-2, located on chromosome 17q25 (153, 154, 156). TIMP-2 is a 21-kd protein that selectively forms a complex with the latent proenzyme form of the 72-kd type IV collagenase (Fig. 9.6). TIMP-2 shows 37% identity and overall 65.6% homology to TIMP-1 at the deduced amino acid sequence level. TIMP-1 and TIMP-2 are differentially regulated at the level of mRNA expression; transforming growth factor-β reduces expression of TIMP-2 and increases TIMP-1 message (52, 153, 154). TIMP-2 inhibits the type IV collagenolytic activity and the gelatinolytic activity associated with the latent and active MMP-2 and the active forms of the other MMPs, unlike TIMP-1. Cell culture studies using cell lines that produce a variety of collagenase family enzymes, as well as both TIMP-1 and TIMP-2, suggest that TIMP-2 preferentially interacts with MMP-2. Thus, like interstitial collagenase activity, which is the balance of activated enzyme and TIMP-1, the net MMP-2 activity may depend on the balance between the levels of activated enzyme and TIMP-2 (Fig. 9.6). Further, binding of TIMP-2 to the latent form of type IV collagenase may block activation by serine proteinases, such as plasmin. Binding of TIMP-2 to the active enzyme also abolishes its activity. The binding kilodalton is in the picomolar range. In view of this stoichiometry, active proteolysis will only take place if the local number of type IV collagenase molecules is greater than the number of TIMP-2 molecules (Fig. 9.6).

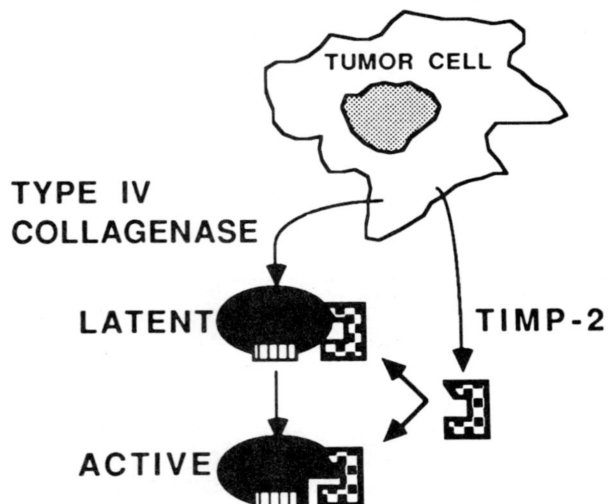

Figure 9.6. Suppressor role for TIMP-2. Tumor cells can produce both metalloproteinases and TIMPs. TIMP-2 binds in a one-to-one molar ratio with latent 72-kd type IV collagenase and blocks activation. It also binds to the activated form of the enzyme and to the activated form of all other members of the metalloproteinase family. Proteolysis via the 72-kd type IV collagenase will occur only if the local levels of the activated enzyme molecules outnumber the local number of TIMP-2 molecules. Therapeutic administration of TIMP-2 can block enzyme activation, as well as abolish the activity of the activated enzyme species.

The function of TIMP-1 and TIMP-2 may not be limited to metalloproteinase blockade. These proteins may also act as cytokines and recognize specific receptors. TIMP-2 and TIMP-1 have been cloned and sequenced from bovine endothelial cells and human fetal aorta cDNA libraries (15). TIMP-1 stimulates the proliferation of human erythroleukemia cell line K562 in vitro (4). Recently, the cartilage-derived angiogenesis inhibitor was shown to be identical to TIMP-1 (111). Furthermore, it was demonstrated that TIMP inhibited angiogenesis in vivo and both capillary endothelial cell proliferation and migration in vitro (111). These results suggest that the TIMPs may have profound biologic effects that extend well beyond their role as inhibitors of the collagenase enzymes. Natural and recombinant TIMP-1 has been shown to prevent tumor cell invasion of human amnion in vitro, and to block metastasis formation in animal models (1, 143). Thus, experimental evidence supports the concept that TIMPs may function as tumor suppressor proteins that inhibit matrix proteolysis and angiogenesis, phenomena that are necessary for tumor invasion and metastatic colony growth. It is conceivable that recombinant TIMP-2 could be considered for its therapeutic potential.

A second major method of identifying candidate metastasis suppressor genes has been the study of differentially expressed genes, that is, genes whose expression decreased as tumor cells progressed from low to high metastatic potential. The nm23 gene was identified on the basis of its reduced expression at the mRNA level in a series of seven cell lines, all derived from a single K-1735 murine melanoma. Nm23 mRNA levels were reduced 10-fold in five high metastatic potential K-1735 melanoma lines as compared with two related, low metastatic potential K-1735 melanoma lines (152). Nm23 RNA and protein levels were also examined in a small-scale prospective study of human infiltrating ductal breast carcinomas using in situ hybridization (Fig. 9.7) and immunoperoxidase staining (12, 136). At the mRNA level, all tumors from patients with evidence of metastasis to the lymph nodes at surgery contained low nm23 RNA levels. Among the patients without evidence of metastasis at surgery, nm23 RNA levels varied: approximately 75% of these tumors contained significantly greater nm23 RNA levels, in agreement with a prediction of low metastatic poten-

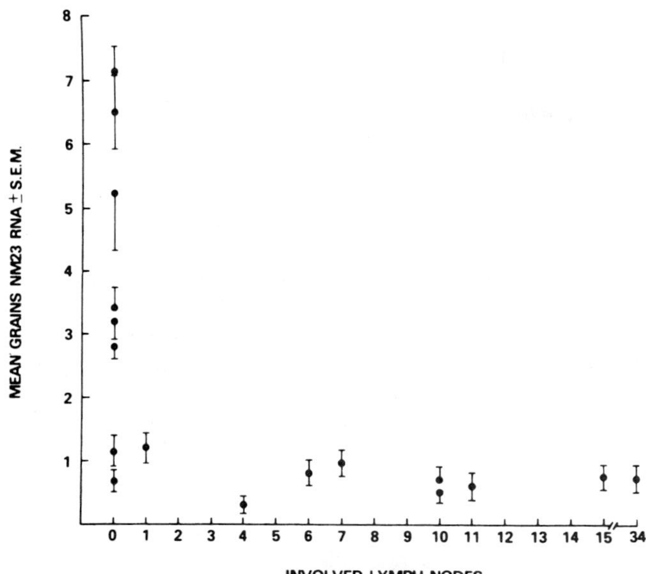

Figure 9.7. Negative correlation of nm23 mRNA levels with axillary lymph node metastasis in patients with infiltrating ductal breast carcinoma. The tumor cell nm23 mRNA levels were determined by quantitative in situ hybridization using nm23 riboprobe. The horizontal axis shows the number of lymph nodes positive for metastasis. All metastatic tumors exhibited a profound loss of nm23 expression.

tial, but 25% of the tumors contained low nm23 RNA levels. Analysis of estrogen receptor expression and histologic degree of differentiation suggested that the 25% of tumors with low nm23 RNA levels were actually of increased metastatic potential. These tumors were estrogen receptor negative and of poorly differentiated histology. Short-term (16-month) clinical follow-up data indicated that 12% of the low nm23 mRNA level patients, including one without evidence of lymph node metastases at surgery, developed disease progression, while none of the high nm23 RNA level patients did so (12).

Although the study was limited in size, the data have recently been confirmed in several other studies, again showing that nm23 RNA expression was reduced in high metastatic potential human breast tumors. This was associated with a reduction in survival, which was highly significant statistically. Of particular interest is the prognostic significance of nm23 expression in lymph node–negative breast cancer, where approximately 30% of patients will develop metastatic disease (136). Decreased nm23 expression has also been found to prognosticate short disease-free intervals in patients with carcinoma of the colon (23). Two allelic nm23 restriction fragment length polymorphisms (RFLPs), at 3 and 7 kb, respectively, were detected by Southern blots (86). In 64% of the informative (heterozygous) pairs of normal lymphocyte–breast tumor DNAs studied, deletion of one nm23 allele was observed in the tumor tissue. Thus, one mechanism of nm23 down-regulation may be its deletion from one chromosome. This characteristic stands as genetic evidence that nm23 may be a metastatic suppressor gene in breast cancer. Final proof of this function was demonstrated in transfection experiments using the K-1735 melanoma system and the MDA-231 breast cancer model (135).

What is known of the normal function of nm23? The first clue to nm23 function(s) came from its high degree of identity with the Drosophila awd gene product (136). Mutations that result in reduced awd expression or the production of a mutated protein do not significantly alter embryonic development, but do alter the development of multiple tissues after metamorphosis, when presumptive adult tissue in the wing disks begins to divide and differentiate (32, 33, 172). The second clue to nm23 function came from the study of Wallet and colleagues, who reported the identification of two developmentally regulated genes in Dictyostelium that encode NDP kinases (172). These proteins are remarkably homologous to nm23 and awd. Gip (17) was identified by screening a Dictyostelium expressing cDNA library with 35S-GTPgS. Guk 11.2 was identified in the same library by screening with an antibody to a Dictyostelium protein kinase. Compared with nm23/awd, the predicted amino acid sequences of gip 17 and guk 11.2 were 57% and 50% identical, respectively, and 70 to 75% homologous. The 17 kd size of the Dictyostelium proteins is the same as nm23/awd. Considering that Dictyostelium represents one of the lowest branches of eukaryotic evolution, this degree of amino acid identity predicts functional similarity between the Dictyostelium proteins and nm23/awd. NDP kinases make up a ubiquitous class of enzymes that catalyze the transfer of the terminal phosphate group of 5″-trisphosphate nucleotides to 5″-diphosphate nucleotides (excluding ATP) through the formation of enzyme-bound high-energy phosphate intermediates (75).

The cellular NDP kinase is an oligomer of individual NDP kinase subunits, ranging from three to six subunits, depending on the cell type. Each subunit has a size of 17 to 18 kd. NDP kinases exhibit heterogeneity in their molecular sizes and amino acid sequences, membrane versus cytoplasmic localization, the number of NDP kinase subunits, and the degree of enzyme phosphorylation. NDP kinases are known to participate in at least two major functions that could play a role in cancer and its development: microtubule assembly/disassembly, and signal transduction through G proteins (74, 75, 120). Microtubule assembly requires the exchange, or transphosphorylation without exchange, of GDP to GTP. Nickerson and Wells have isolated a microtubule-associated NDP kinase that may catalyze such transphosphorylation. Thus, changes in nm23 expression at the mRNA or protein level may be useful as a screening system for the identification of new hormones, cytokines, or synthetic compounds that may have antimetastatic activity.

Oncogene Induction of Metastasis

A long list of oncogenes has been described that, either singly or in combinations, confer anchorage-independent colony growth in soft agar, and, in many cases, tumorigenicity in animal hosts (13, 63). Since cancer cells must be tumorigenic in order to grow as a metastatic colony, oncogenes must play a basic role, at least, in the growth phase of cancer metastasis. A growing body of evidence, however, indicates that some oncogenes may also directly induce the independent phenotype of invasion and metastasis. The mechanism of this induction involves pathways separate from that which regulate growth.

The best studied oncogene capable of inducing the metastatic phenotype is H-*ras*. Mutated forms of the *ras* protein product p21 have been identified in both human and carcinogen-induced animal tumors (6). Thorgeirsson and colleagues were the first to report that acute myelogenous leukemia or bladder cancer tumor DNA-containing activated (mutated) *ras* oncogene sequences, when transfected into mouse embryo–derived fibroblasts (NIH-3T3 cells), produced numerous metastases upon intravenous injection (167). These data were confirmed by direct transfection of the cloned activated *ras* oncogene in several systems, including primary rat embryo fibroblast cultures (25, 37, 126, 167) with elevated levels of the *ras* proto-oncogene produced tumors at a rate comparable to that of cells transformed with activated *ras* (113). However, when the same cells were tested for metastatic propensity, the cells transformed by the activated *ras* were much more efficient in the production of metastases as compared with the proto-oncogene (25, 37, 170). Very high levels of normal p21 could lead to metastasis production (17, 36). Pozzatti and co-workers examined a series of diploid rat embryo fibroblasts transformed by *ras*; these clones were all highly metastatic in nude mice xenografts or experimental metastasis assays. Several genes have been associated with *ras* activity, including type IV collagenase, cathepsin L, and extracellular matrix components (50, 101, 168).

The mechanism of *ras* induction of the metastatic phenotype is under investigation. Egan and colleagues used a steroid-responsive promoter to demonstrate the importance of *ras* oncogene transcript dose on metastasis production (36). The p21 protein is associated with the inner plasma membrane, binds GTP and GDP with high affinity, and has weak GTPase activity. Based on these structural and functional properties, the *ras* p21 protein has been compared to classic G proteins, suggesting that p21 participates in the transduction of signals across the cell membrane. The transforming activity of the *ras* gene is thought to result from mutations or overexpression that causes an increase in the relative level of the p21-GTP complex. With regard to metastasis, Egan and co-workers examined the ability of two *ras* mutations to induce the metastatic phenotype: the substitution of leucine for glutamine at codon 61, which decreases GTPase activity and increases p21-GDP dissociation, resulting in a net increase in p21-GTP, and mutation in the nucleotide binding region codons 116 to 119, which also increases net p21-GTP due to the relative concentration difference of GTP and GDP pools in the cytoplasm (36, 38). Both mutations in *ras* were capable of inducing transformation and metastasis formation. Thus, the transforming and metastasis-inducing activities of p21 may involve its association with guanine nucleotides in signal transduction. The serine/threonine kinase, *raf*, has been shown to interact directly with *ras* and to propagate *ras*-related signals downstream (27, 30, 67, 169). Two observations, however, indicate that the signals used in *ras* induction of transformation and metastasis are dissimilar. The adenovirus 2 *E1A* gene has been demonstrated to suppress *ras* induction of metastatic potential without a similar effect on transformation, and the C127 cells are capable of being transformed by *ras*, but do not metastasize (113, 125, 126). Thus, it is likely that a metastasis-specific set of genes is activated by *ras*, possibly in coordinated manner, to induce metastasis formation.

However, *ras* is not the only oncogene that can induce metastatic potential. The serine/threonine kinases v-*mos*, v-*raf* and A-*raf*; tyrosine kinases v-*src*, v-*fes*, and v-*fms*; and, phosphoproteins *myc* and *p53* have all been demonstrated to induce the metastatic phenotype (38, 48, 122, 138). In addition, the *mts1* gene, encoding an S-100 calcium-binding protein, is associated with a motile and metastatic phenotype. The *mts1* gene has been found to be overexpressed in metastatic cells relative to their nonmetastatic but malignant counterparts. *Mts1* is expressed in several normal tissue types that exhibit the ability to be motile, such as T lymphocytes, activated macrophages, and trophoblasts. Metastatic mouse mammary adenocarcinoma cells (CSML-100) were shown to express *mts1* and are more motile, invasive, and metastatic than CSML-0 cells, which do not express *mts1*. In addition, transfection with *mts1* has been shown to induce the metastatic phenotype (43).

Metastasis as a Therapeutic Target

Novel targets for the treatment and prevention of cancer initiation, progression, and metastasis are needed. The cell biology of the metastatic cascade may offer new insights into therapeutic and prevention targets. The different steps of the metastatic cascade of angiogenesis, adhesion, proteolysis, motility, and proliferation, when looked at from different angles, might be both useful and novel targets. The clinical utility of this approach has been demonstrated for angiogenesis in which the inhibition of angiogenesis using interferon to inhibit angiogenic growth factor gene expression has resulted in the regression of childhood hemangiomas (42). Several antiangiogenic agents are under preclinical or clinical investigation. An important agent now in phase I clinical trial and entering phase II trials is TNP-470, a fumagillin analogue with antiangiogenic activity and direct antitumor and metastasis activity (18, 72, 181). Recently, thalidomide was shown to have antiangiogenic activity and it is now entering clinical trial (28) (see Chapter 10).

Another approach to targets for intervention in metastasis is proteolysis. While recombinant TIMPs might be a direct link between the laboratory and the clinic, this approach has not yet been developed for patient use. An analogue of the zinc binding site, BB-94, is a novel agent that has been used clinically for its inhibition of metalloproteinase activity (31). It has also been shown to be an effective inhibitor of angiogenesis. Daily administration of BB-94 has been shown to be safe and to reduce the ascitic burden of animals bearing human ovarian cancer xenografts. Clinical trials are ongoing in the United Kingdom and the United States.

Investigations into the signaling pathways underlying metastasis have suggested that calcium homeostasis, kinase activity, and *ras* activation are important signals involved in metastasis, and, therefore, may be key regulatory sites for therapeutic intervention (24, 51, 123, 124). Recent data have shown that tyrosine phosphorylation occurs in some cases of extracellular matrix proteins' binding to their related integrins (70, 143). A special tyrosine kinase, p125fak, active in cellular focal adhesion contacts, has been cloned and studied in this setting (143). Activation of p125fak is upstream to *src*-related pathways and other protein tyrosine kinases. Its specific role in promoting or preventing metastatic dissemination is as yet unknown. This tyrosine phosphorylation step might be one step through which interventions targeted against signaling events might be effective against the metastatic cascade. Many receptor tyrosine kinases have been associated with the invasive phenotype, including Met, the HGF/SF receptor FLK, the receptor for the angiogenic factor vascular endothelial cell growth factor, and the FGF family (76, 133, 163). The new class of compounds, the tyrphostins, which inhibit selective receptor tyrosine kinases, may be effective at this step (87).

Another recently developed therapeutic target in metastases is the *ras* oncoprotein signaling cascade (51). The importance of the *ras* pathway in tumorigenesis and metastasis has been discussed. Investigators have further demonstrated its utility as a therapeutic target through studies that tie *ras* to the actin cytoskeleton and its function (127). In addition, studies that suggest that p125fak activity is mediated through *src* and downstream through the *ras* signaling pathway underscore the role of this small-molecular-weight GTP-binding protein in oncogenesis. However, *ras* requires posttranslational isoprenylation to allow it to translocate and interact at the cell membrane (51). This isoprenylation can be inhibited by intervention at two points. First, interruption in the isoprenyl synthetic pathway with lovostatin, an inhibitor of HMG-coA reductase, is effective upstream of the process of farnesylation of *ras* (51). Limonene directly inhibits the isoprenylation of *ras* and has been shown to be effective in the chemoprevention of colon cancer in rat models (57). It is nontoxic and can be taken as a dietary supplement. Clinical trials are anticipated. Last, new inhibitors of farnesyltransferase, the enzyme that isoprenylates *ras* at the Cys-Ala-Ala-X carboxy terminal tail, are under development for clinical application (51).

Studies using different motility cytokines and motility-stimulating extracellular matrix proteins or tumor-derived motility factors have suggested that calcium-mediated signal transduction pathways might also be important targets. Kohn and colleagues screened for agents that would both inhibit migration in vitro and inhibit motility-requiring signaling pathways, and identified a novel inhibitor of calcium mobilization (40, 80, 82). This agent, CAI (carboxyamido-triazole), was shown to inhibit nonvoltage-gated calcium influx from receptor-operated calcium channels and ionophore-induced calcium influx, as well as to inhibit other calcium–influx dependent downstream signaling pathways, such as selected tyrosine kinase activities and the release of arachidonic acid from phospholipase A2 (40, 56, 76, 82). Studies have indicated that CAI is specific for mobilization of calcium from extracellular stores and is not directed to the internal release of calcium. These studies demonstrated a link between the calcium-mediated signaling pathways and the antiproliferative and antimetastasis effects of CAI through a structure-function analysis. Further specificity was demonstrated by the lack of activity of CAI against calcium-independent cAMP production and calcium-independent production of inositol trisphosphates through activation of phospholipase C-β (40, 56).

CAI has been show to inhibit the proliferation of a wide array of human cancer cell types in vitro (76, 77, 80, 82). In addition, CAI treatment has been shown to down regulate the expression of MMP-2, with a resultant reduction in MMP-2 activity (79). A marked inhibitory activity against neovascularization was observed with CAI in vitro and in vivo (76). Further studies showed efficacy in vivo against several human tumor xenograft models of cancer progression and metastasis using orally administered CAI (81). The blood levels in the treated animals were in the range of 1 to 10 μg/mL, which was effective in the inhibition of calcium influx and calcium-mediated signaling pathways (82). No significant toxicity was demonstrated in the animal cohorts that received daily or every-other-day CAI. These data were the basis for the now ongoing phase I clinical trials of CAI. The lack of toxicity and cytostatic effects on normal tissues with oral administration makes it a good candidate for use in adjuvant and chemopreventive approaches.

Summary

The study of invasion and metastasis, in their component parts or as a whole, offers a new approach for the development of novel therapeutics. Components of metastasis, such as angiogenesis, may also be important targets for chemoprevention or adjuvant treatments of cancer. Signal transduction therapy may alter the biology of the cell in a way that may intervene at the level of cellular transformation or at the initiation of metastatic disease. Therefore, it could be used to inhibit the initiation of cancer or to prevent the transition from in situ to invasive malignancy. Changes in the cellular and molecular biology of the cancer cell by modulation of signals thus may demonstrate that signal transduction therapy may have the potential to alter the natural history of cancer. This leads to a new paradigm of the treatment of cancer as a chronic disease by modulation of its biology.

References

1. Alvarez OA, Carmichael DF, DeClerck YA. Inhibition of collagenolytic activity and metastasis of tumor cells by a recombinant human tissue inhibitor of metalloproteinases. JNCI 1990;82:589.
2. Amstad P, Reddel RR, Pfeifer A, Malan-Shibley L, Mark GE, Harris CC. Neoplastic transformation of a human bronchial epithelial cell line by a recombinant retrovirus encoding viral Harvey *ras*. Mol Carc 1988;1:151.
3. Ananthaswamy HA, Price JE, Tainsky MA, Goldberg LH, Bales E. S. Correlation between Ha-*ras* gene amplification and spontaneous metastasis in NIH 3T3 cells transfected with genomic DNA from human skin cancers. Clin Exp Metastasis 1989;7:301.
4. Avalos B, Kaufman S, Tomonage M, Williams R, Golde D, Gasson J. K562 cells produce and respond to human erythroid potentiating activity. Blood 1988;71:1720.
5. Aznavoorian S, Stracke ML, Krutzsch H, Schiffmann E, Liotta LA. Signal transduction for chemotaxis and haptotaxis by matrix molecules in tumor cells. J Cell Biol 1990;110:1427.
6. Barbacid M. *Ras* genes. Annu Rev Biochem 1987;56:779.
7. Barsky SH, Rao CN, Williams JE, Liotta LA. Laminin molecular domains which alter metastasis in a murine model. J Clin Invest 1984;74:843.
8. Barsky SH, Siegal GP, Jannotta F, Liotta LA. Loss of basement membrane components by invasive tumors but not by their benign counterparts. Lab Invest 1983;49:140.

9. Bauer W, Igot J-P, Le Gal Y. Chronologie du cancer mammaire utilisant un modele de croissance Gompertz. Ann Anat Pathol (Paris) 1980;25:39.
10. Behrens J, Frixen U, Schipper J, et al. Cell adhesion in cancer invasion and metastasis. Semin Cancer Biol. 1992;3:169.
11. Behrens J, Mareel M, Van Roy F, Birchmeier W. Dissecting tumor cell invasion: epithelial cells aquire invasive properties after the loss of uvomorulin-mediated cell-cell adhesion. J Cell Bio 1989;108:2435.
12. Bevilacqua G, Sobel ME, Liotta LA, Steeg PS. Association of low nm23 RNA levels in human primary infiltrating ductal breast carcinomas with lymph node involvement and other histopathological indicators of high metastatic potential. Cancer Res 1989;49:5185.
13. Bishop JM. The molecular genetics of cancer. Science 1987;235:305.
14. Bondy GP, Wilson S, Chambers AF. Experimental metastatic ability of H-*ras*-transformed NIH-3T3 cells. Cancer Res 1985;45:6005.
15. Boone T, Johnson M, DeClerck Y, Langley K. CDNA cloning and expression of a metalloproteinase inhibitor related to tissue inhibitor of metalloproteinases. Proc Natl Acad Sci USA 1990;87:2800.
16. Brawer MK, Deering RE, Brown M, et al. Predictors of pathologic stage in prostatic carcinoma. Cancer 1994;73:678.
17. Bradley MO, Kraynak AR, Storer RD, Gibbs JB. Experimental metastasis in nude mice of NIH-3T3 cells containing various *ras* genes. Proc Natl Acad Sci USA 1986;83:5277.
18. Brem H, Folkman J. Analysis of experimental anti-angiogenic therapy. J Ped Surg 1993;28:445.
19. Brown PD, Levy AT, Margulies IMK, Liotta LA, Stetler-Stevenson WG. Independent expression and cellular processing of the 72-kd type IV collagenase and interstitial collagenase in human tumorigenic cell lines. Cancer Res 1990;50:6184.
20. Cajot J-F, Sordat B, Druithof EKO, Bachman F. Human primary colon carcinomas xenografted into nude mice. I. Characterization of plasminogen activators expressed by primary tumors and their xenografts. JNCI 1986;77:703.
21. Carmichael DF, Sommer A, Thomson R, Anderson DC, Smith CG, Welgus HG, Stricklin GP. Primary structure and cDNA cloning of human fibroblast collagenase inhibitor. Proc Natl Acad Sci USA 1986;83:2407.
22. Chen W, Obrink B. Cell-cell contacts mediated by E-cadherin (uvomorulin) restrict invasive behavior of L-cells. J Cell Bio 1991;144:319.
23. Cohn KH, Wang FS, DeSoto-LaPaix F, Solomon WB, Patterson LG, Arnold MR, Weimar J, Feldman JG, Levy AT, Leone A, Steeg PS. Association of nm23-H1 allelic deletions with distant metastases in colorectal carcinoma. Lancet 1991;338:722.
24. Cole KA, Kohn EC. Calcium-mediated signal transduction: biology, biochemistry, and therapy. Cancer Met Rev 1994;13:33.
25. Collard JG, Schijven JF, Roos E. Invasive and metastatic potential induced by *ras*-transfection into mouse BW5147 T-lymphoma cells. Cancer Res 1987;47:754.
26. Collier IE, Wilhelm SM, Eisen AZ, Marmer BL, Grant GA, Seltzer JL, Kronberger A, He C, Bauer EA, Goldberg GI. H-*ras* oncogene transformed human bronchial epithelial cells (TBE-1) secrete a single metalloproteinase capable of degrading basement membrane collagen. J Biol Chem 1988;263:6579.
27. Cook SJ, McCormick F. Inhibition by cAMP of *ras*-dependent activation of *raf*. Science 1993;262:1069.
28. D'Amato RJ, Loughnan MS, Flynn E, Folkman J. Thalidomide is an inhibitor of angiogenesis. Proc Natl Acad Sci USA 1994;91:4082.
29. Dano K, Andreasen PA, Grondahl-Hansen J. Plasminogen activators, tissue degradation and cancer. Adv Cancer Res 1985;44:139.
30. Daum G, Eisenmann-Tappe I, Fries H, Troppmair J, Rapp UR. The ins and outs of *raf* kinases. Trends Biol Sci 1994;19:474.
31. Davies B, Brown PD, East N, et al. A synthetic matrix metalloproteinase inhibitor decreases tumor burden and prolongs survival of mice bearing human ovarian carcinoma xenografts. Cancer Res 1993;53:2087.
32. Dearolf C, Hersperger E, Shearn A. Developmental consequences of awd, a cell-autonomous lethal mutation of Drosophilia induced by hybrid dysgenesis. Develop Biol 1988;129:159.
33. Dearolf C, Tripoulas N, Biggs J, Shearn A. Molecular consequences of awd, a cell-autonomous lethal mutation of Drosophila induced by hybrid dysgenesis. Develop Biol 1988;129:169.
34. Denhardt DT, Greenberg AH, Egan SE, Hamilton RT, Wright JA. Cysteine proteinase cathepsin L expression correlates closely with the metastatic potential of H-*ras*-transformed murine fibroblasts. Oncogene 1987;2:55.
35. Docherty AJP, Lyons A, Smith BJ, Wright EM, Stephens PE, Harris TJR, Murphy G, Reynolds JJ. Sequence of human tissue inhibitor of metalloproteinases and its identity to erythroid potentiating activity. Nature 1985;318:66.
36. Egan SE, Broere JJ, Jarolim L, Wright JA, Greenberg AH. Coregulation of metastatic and transforming activity of normal and mutant *ras* genes. Int J Cancer 1989;43:443.
37. Egan SE, McClarty GA, Jarolim L, Wright JA, Spiro I, Hager G, Greenberg AH. Expression of H-*ras* correlates with metastatic potential: evidence for direct regulation of the metastatic phenotype in lOT 1/2 and NIH-3T3 cells. Mol Cell Biol 1987;7:830.
38. Egan SE, Wright JA, Jarolim L, Yanagihara K, Bassin RH, Greenberg AH. Transformation by oncogenes encoding protein kinases induces the metastatic phenotype. Science 1987;238:202.
39. Evans CP, Walsh DS, Kohn EC. An autocrine motility factor secreted by the Dunning R-3327 rat prostatic adenocarcinoma cell subtype AT2.1. Intl J Cancer 1991;49:109.
40. Felder CC, Ma AL, Liotta LA, Kohn EC. The antiproliferative and antimetastatic compound L651582, inhibits muscarinic acetylcholine receptor-stimulated calcium influx and arachidonic acid release. J Pharmacol Exp Ther 1991;257:967.
41. Fidler IJ, Hart IR. Biologic diversity in metastatic neoplasms: origins and implications. Science, 1982;217:998.
42. Folkman J. The role of angiogenesis in tumor growth. Semin Cancer Biol 1992;3:65.
43. Ford HL, Chakravarty R, Salim M, et al. Role of the *mts1* gene and Mts1 protein in metastasis. Clin Exp Met 1994;12:30.
44. Frisch SM. Antioncogenic effect of adenovirus *E1A* in human tumor cells. Proc Natl Acad Sci USA 1991;88:9077.
45. Furcht L. Critical factors controlling angiogenesis: cell products, cell matrix, and growth factor. Lab Invest 1986;5:505.
46. Galves D. Correlation between circulating cancer cells and incidence of metastasis. Br J Cancer 1983;48:665.
47. Gajdusek CM, Luo Z, Mayberg MR. Basic fibroblast growth factor and transforming growth factor beta-1: synergistic mediators of angiogenesis in vitro. J Cell Physiol 1993;157:133.
48. Gao C, Wang L-C, Vass WC, Seth A, Chang KSS. The role of v-mos in transformation, oncogenicity and metastatic potential of mink lung cells. Oncogene 1988;3:267.
49. Garbisa S, D'Errico A, Grigioni WF, Biagini G, Caenazzo C, Fastelli G, Stetler-Stevenson WG, Liotta LA. Type IV collagenase augmentation associated with colorectal and gastric cancer progression. In Genetic Mechanisms in Carcinogenesis and Tumor Progression. Edited by CC Harris, LA Liotta. UCLA Symposia on Molecular and Cellular Biology, New Series, vol. 114. New York: Wiley-Liss, 1990, pp 203–212.
50. Garbisa S, Pozzatti R, Muschel RJ, Saffiotti U, Ballin M, Goldfarb RH, Khoury G, Liotta LA. Secretion of type IV collagenolytic protease and metastatic phenotype Induction by transfection with c-Ha-*ras* but not C-Ha-*ras* plus Ad2-*E1A*. Cancer Res 1987;47: 1523.
51. Gibbs JB, Oliff A, Kohl NE. Farnesyltransferase inhibitors: *ras* research yields a potential cancer therapeutic. Cell 1994;77:175.
52. Goldberg GI, Marmer BL, Grant GA, Eisen AZ, Wilhelm S, He C. Human 72-kd type IV collagenase forms a complex with a tissue inhibitor of metalloproteinase inhibitor. Proc Natl Acad Sci USA 1989;86:8207.
53. Goldfarb RH, Liotta LA. Proteolytic enzymes in cancer invasion and metastasis. Semin Thromb Hemost 1986;12:294.
54. Gottesman M. The role of proteases in cancer. Semin Cancer Biol 1990;1:97.
55. Grotendorst GR. Alteration of the chemotactic response of NIH/3T3 cells to PDGF by growth factors, transformation, and tumor promoters. Cell 1984;36:279.
56. Gusovsky F, Lueders JE, Kohn EC, Felder CC. Muscarinic receptor-mediated tyrosine phosphorylation of phospholipase C-gamma: an alternative mechanism for cholinergic receptor-induced phosphoinositide breakdown. J Biol Chem 1993;268: 7768.
57. Haag JD, Lindstrom MJ, Gould MN. Limonene-induced regression of mammary carcinomas. Cancer Res 1992;52:4021.
58. Hamilton TC, Young RC, Louie KG, Behrens BC, McKoy WM, Grotzinger KR, Ozols RF. Characterization of a xenograft model of human ovarian carcinoma which produces ascites and intra-abdominal carcinomatosis in mice. Cancer Res 1984;44: 5286.
59. Hartmann G, Naldini L, Weidner KM, et al. A functional domain in the heavy chain of scatter factor/hepatocyte growth factor binds the c-Met receptor and induces cell dissociation but not mitogenesis. Proc Natl Acad Sci USA 1992;89:11574.
60. Heino J, Massague J. Transforming growth factor beta switches the pattern of integrins expressed in MG-63 human osteosarcoma cells and causes a selective loss of adhesion to laminin. J Biol Chem 1989;264:21806.
61. Hendrix MJC, Wood WR, Seftor EA, Lotan D, Nakajima M, Misiorowsi RL, Seftor REB, Stetler-Stevenson WG, Bevacqua SJ, Liotta LA, Sobel ME, Raz A, Lotan R. Retinoic acid inhibition of human melanoma cell invasion through a reconstituted basement membrane and its relation to decreases in the expression of proteolytic enzymes and motility factor receptor. Cancer Res 1990;50:4121.
62. Herron GS, Banda MJ, Clark EJ, Gavrilovic J, Werb Z. Secretion of metalloproteinases by stimulated capillary endothelial cells. II. Expression of collagenase and stromelysin activities is regulated by endogenous inhibitors. J Biol Chem 1986;261: 2814.
63. Hill RP, Chambers AF, Ling V, Harris JF. Dynamic heterogeneity Rapid generation of metastatic variants in mouse B16 melanoma cells. Science 1984;224:998.
64. Hill SA, Wilson S, Chambers AF. Clonal heterogeneity experimental metastatic ability, and p21 expression in H-*ras*-transformed NIH-3T3 cells. JNCI 1988;80:484.
65. Hollingsworth HC, Kohn EC, Steinberg SM, Rothenberg ML, Merino MJ. Tumor angiogenesis in advanced stage ovarian cancer. Am J Pathol 1995. (in press)
66. Horwitz A, Duggan K, Buck C, Beckerle MC, Burridge K. Interaction of plasma membrane fibronectin receptor with talin a transmembrane linkage. Nature 1986;320:531.
67. Howe LR, Leevers SJ, Gomez N, Nakielny S, Cohen P, Marshall CJ. Activation of the MAP kinase pathway by the protein kinase raf. Cell 1992;71:335.
68. Humphries MJ, Olden K, Yamada KM. A synthetic peptide from fibronectin inhibits experimental metastasis of murine melanoma cells. Science 1986;233:467.
69. Hynes RO. Integrins. A family of cell surface receptors. Cell 1987;48:549.
70. Hynes RO. Integrins Versatility, modulation, and signaling in cell adhesion. Cell 1992;69:11.
71. Jones PA, DeClerck YA. Extracellular matrix destruction by invasive tumor cells. Cancer Metast Rev 1982;1:289.
72. Kato T, Sato K, Kakinuma H, Matsuda Y. Enhanced suppression of tumor growth by combination of angiogenesis inhibitior)-(chloroacetyl-carbamoly)fumagillol (TNP-470) and cytotoxic agents in mice. Cancer Res 1994;54:5143.
73. Khokha R, Waterhouse P, Yagel S, Lala PK, Overall CM, Norton G, Denhardt DT. Antisense RNA-induced reduction in metalloproteinase inhibitor causes mouse 3T3 cells to become tumorigenic. Science 1989;243:947.
74. Kimura N, Johnson G. Increased membrane associated nucleotide diphosphate kinase activity as a possible basis for enhanced guanine nucleotide dependent adenylate cyclase activity induced by picolinic acid treatment of simian virus 40-transformed normal rat kidney cells. J Biol Chem 1983;258:12609.
75. Kimura N, Shimada N. Membrane-associated nucleoside diphosphate kinase from rat liver. J Biol Chem 1988;263:4647.
76. Kohn EC, Alessandro R, Spoonster J, Wersto R, Liotta LA. Angiogenesis: role of calcium-mediated signal transduction. Proc Natl Acad Sci USA 1995;92:1307.
77. Kohn EC, Felder CC, Jacobs W, et al. Stucture function analysis of signal and growth inhibition by carboxyamido-triazole, CAI. Cancer Res 1994;54:935.
78. Kohn EC, Francis EA, Liotta LA, Schiffmann E. Heterogeneity of the motility responses in malignant tumor cells: a biological basis for the diversity and homing of metastatic cells. Int J Cancer 1990;46:287.
79. Kohn EC, Jacobs W, Kim YS, Alessandro R, Stetler-Stevenson WG, Liotta LA. Calcium influx modulates expression of matrix metalloproteinase-2 (72 kd type IV collagenase, gelatinase A) expression. J Biol Chem 1994;269:21505.
80. Kohn EC, Liotta LA. L651582: a novel antiproliferative and antimetastasis agent. JNCI 1990;82:54.
81. Kohn EC, Liotta LA. Molecular insights into cancer invasion: strategies for prevention and intervention. Cancer Res 1995;55:1856.

82. Kohn EC, Sandeen MA, Liotta LA. In vivo efficacy of a novel inhibitor of selected signal transduction pathways including calcium, arachidonate, and inositol phosphates. Cancer Res 1992;52:3208.
83. Koscielny S, Tubiana M, Valleron A-J. A simulation model of the natural history of human breast cancer. Br J Cancer 1985;52:515.
84. Kramer RH, Bensch KG, Wong J. Invasion of reconstituted basement membrane matrix by metastatic human tumor cells. Cancer Res 1986;46:1980.
85. Leone A, Flatow U, King CR, Sandeen MA, Liotta LA, Steeg PS. Reduced tumor incidence, metastatic potential, and cytokine responsiveness of nm23-transfected melanoma cells. Cell 1991;65:25.
86. Leone A, McBride OW, Westin A, Wang M, Anglard P, Cropp C, Linehan MW, Rees R, Callahan R, Harris C, Liotta LA, Steeg PS. Somatic allelic deletion of nm23 in human cancer. Cancer Res 1991;51:2490.
87. Levitzki A, Gilon C. Tyrphostins as molecular tools and potential antiproliferative drugs. Trends Pharmacol Sci 1991;12:171.
88. Liotta LA. Tumor invasion and metastasis—role of the basement membrane. Am J Pathol 1984;117:339.
89. Liotta LA. Tumor invasion and metastases—role of the extracellular matrix. Cancer Res 1986;46:1.
90. Liotta LA, Abe S, Robey P, Martin G. Preferential digestion of basement membrane collagen by an enzyme derived from a metastatic murine tumor. Proc Natl Acad Sci USA 1979;76:2268.
91. Liotta LA, Kleinerman J, Saidel GM. Quantitative relationships of intravascular tumor cells, tumor vessels, and pulmonary metastases following tumor implantation. Cancer Res 1974;34:997.
92. Liotta LA, Mandler R, Murano G, Katz DA, Gordon RK, Chiang PK, Schiffmann E. Tumor autocrine motility factor. Proc Natl Acad Sci USA 1986;83:3302.
93. Liotta LA, Murata J, Clair T, et al. cDNA cloning of the autocrine motility factor, autotaxin (ATX). Clin Exp Met 1994;12:3.
94. Liotta LA, Rao CN, Barsky SH. Tumor invasion and the extracellular matrix. Lab Invest 1983;49:636.
95. Liotta LA, Rao CN, Wewer UM. Biochemical interactions with the basement membranes. Annu Rev Biochem 1986;55:1037.
96. Liotta LA, Steeg PS, Stetler-Stevenson WG. Cancer metastasis and angiogenesis; an imbalance of positive and negative regulation. Cell 1991;64:327–336.
97. Liotta LA, Tryggvason K, Garbisa S, Hart I, Foltz CM, Shafie S. Metastatic potential correlates with enzymatic degradation of basement membrane collagen. Nature 1980;284:67.
98. Malinoff HL, Wicha MS. Isolation of a cell surface receptor protein for laminin from murine fibrosarcoma cells. J Cell Biol 1983;96:1475.
99. Markus G. Plasminogen activators in malignant growth. In Progress in Fibrinolysis. Edited by JF Davidson. Edinburgh: Churchill-Livingstone, 1983, p 587.
100. Markus G, Camiolo SM, Kohga S, Madeja JM, Mittelman A. Plasminogen activator secretion of human tumors in short-term organ culture, including a comparison of primary and metabolic tumors. Cancer Res 1983;43:5517.
101. Mason RW, Gal S, Gottesman MM. The identification of the major extracted protein (MEP) from a transformed mouse fibroblast cell line as a catalytically active precursor form of cathepsin L. Biochem J 1987;248:449.
102. Matrisian LM. Metalloproteinases and their inhibitors in matrix remodeling. Trends Genet 1990;6:121.
103. McCarthy JB, Basara ML, Palm SL, Sas DF, Furcht LT. The role of cell adhesion proteins—laminin and fibronectin—in the movement of malignant and metastatic cells. Cancer Met Rev 1985;4:125.
104. McCarthy JB, Skubitz APN, Palm SL, Furcht LT. Metastasis inhibition of different tumor types by purified laminin fragments and a heparin-binding fragment of fibronectin. JNCI 1988;80:108.
105. McGuire WL, Tandon AK, Allred DC, Chamness GC, Clark GM. How to use prognostic factors in axillary node-negative breast cancer patients. JNCI 1990;82:1006.
106. Mignatti P, Robbins E, Rifkin D. Tumor invasion through the human amniotic membrane: requirement for a proteinase cascade. Cell 1986;47:487.
107. Mignatti P, Tsuboi R, Robbins E, Rifkin D. In vitro angiogenesis on the human amniotic membrane: requirement for basic fibroblast growth factor-induced proteinases. J Cell Biol 1989;108:671.
108. Minniti CP, Kohn EC, Grubb JH, Sly WS, Oh Y, Muller HL, Rosenfeld RG, Helman LJ. The insulin-like growth factor II (IGF-II)/mannose 6-phosphate receptor mediates IGF-II-induced motility in human rhabdomyosarcoma cells. J Biol Chem 1992;267:9000.
109. Monteagudo C, Merino M, San-Juan J, Liotta LA, Stetler-Stevenson W. Immunohistologic distribution of type IV collagenase in normal, benign and malignant breast tissue. Am J Pathol 1990;136:585.
110. Moscatelli D, Presta M, Rifkin D. Purification of a factor from human placenta that stimulates capillary endothelial cell protease production, DNA synthesis, and migration. Proc Natl Acad Sci USA 1986;83:2091.
111. Moses MA, Sudhalter J, Langer R. Identification of an inhibitor of neovascularization from cartilage. Science 1990;248:1408.
112. Murphy G, Cawston T, Reynolds J. An inhibitor of collagenase from human amniotic fluid. Purification, characterization and action on metalloproteinases. Biochem J 1981;195:167.
113. Muschel RJ, Williams JE, Lowy DR, Liotta LA. Harvey *ras* induction of metastatic potential depends upon oncogene activation and the type of recipient cell. Am J Pathol 1985;121:1.
114. Nakajima M, Welch D, Belloni PN, Nicolson GL. Degradation of basement membrane type IV collagen and lung subendothelial matrix by rat mammary adenocarcinoma cell clones of differing metastatic potentials. Cancer Res 1987;47:4869.
115. Naldini L, Weidner KM, Vigna E, et al. Scatter factor and hepatocyte growth factor are indistinguishable ligands for the MET receptor. EMBO. 1991;10:2867.
116. Nicolson GL. Tumor cell instability, diversification and progression to the metastatic phenotype: from oncogene to oncofetal expression. Cancer Res 1987;47:1473.
117. Nicolson GL. Differential organ tissue adhesion, invasion and growth properties of metastatic rat mammary adenocarcinoma cells. Breast Cancer Res Treat 1988;12:167.
118. Nicolson GL, Dulski K, Basson C, Welch DR. Preferential organ attachment and invasion in vitro by B16 melanoma cells selected for differing metastatic colonization and invasive properties. Invas Met 1985;5:144.
119. Nigro JM, Baker SJ, Preisinger AC, Jessup JM, Hostetter R, Cleary K, Bigner SH, Davidson N, Baylin S, Devilee P, Glover T, Collins FS, Weston A, Modali R, Harris CC, Vogelstein B. Mutations in the *p53* gene occur in diverse human tumour types. Nature 1989;342:705.
120. Ohtsuki K, Ikeuchi T, Yokoyama M. Characterization of nucleoside diphosphate kinase associated guanine nucleotide binding proteins from HeLa S3 cells. Biochem Biophys Acta 1986;882:322.
121. Pietras RJ, Szego CM, Mangan CE, Seeler BJ, Burtnett MM. Elevated serum cathepsin B1-like activity in women with neoplastic disease. Gynecol Onc 1979;7:1.
122. Pohl J, Goldfinger N, Radler-Pohl A, Rotter V, Schirrmacher V. p-53 increases experimental metastatic capacity of murine carcinoma cells. Mol Cell Biol 1988;8:2078.
123. Powis G. Signaling targets for anticancer drug development. Trends in Pharmacolo Sci 1991;12:188.
124. Powis G. Drugs active against growth factor and oncogene phosphatidylinositol signaling pathways. Semin Cancer Biol 1992;3:343.
125. Pozzatti R, McCormick M, Thompson MA, Khoury G. The *E1A* gene of adenovirus type 2 reduces the metastatic potential of *ras* transformed rat embryo cells. Mol Cell Biol 1988;8:2984.
126. Pozzatti R, Muschel R, Williams J, Padmanabhan R, Howard B, Liotta LA, Khoury G. Primary rat embryo cells transformed by one or two oncogenes show different metastatic potential. Science 1986;232:223.
127. Prendergast GC, Gibbs JB. Pathways of *ras* function: connections to the actin cytoskeleton. Adv Cancer Res 1993;62:19.
128. Price JE, Polyzos A, Zhang RD, Daniels LM. Tumorigenicity and metastasis of human breast carcinoma cell lines in nude mice. Cancer Res 1990;50:717.
129. Rao CN, Margulies IMK, Tralka S, Terranova VP, Madri JA, Liotta LA. Isolation of a subunit of laminin and its role in molecular structure and tumor cell attachment. J Biol Chem 1982;257:9740.
130. Recklies AD, Poole AR, Mort JS. A cysteine proteinase secreted from human breast tumours is immunologically related to cathepsin B. Biochem J 1982;207:633.
131. Reich R, Thompson E, Iwamoto Y, Martin GR, Deason JR, Fuller GC, Miskin R. Effects of inhibitors of plasminogen activator, serine proteinases, and collagenase IV on the invasion of basement membranes by metastatic cells. Cancer Res 1988;48:3307.
132. Rochefort H, Capony F, Garcia M, Cavailles V, Freiss G, Chambon M, Morisset M, Vignon F. Estrogen-induced lysosomal proteases secreted by breast cancer cells: a role in carcinogenesis? J Cell Biochem 1987;35:17.
133. Rong S, Bodescot M, Blair D, et al. Tumorigenecity of the met proto-oncogene and the gene for hepatocyte growth factor. Mol Cell Bio 1992;12:5152.
134. Rong S, Segal S, Anver M, Resau JH, Vande Woude GF. Invasiveness and metastasis of NIH 3T3 cells induced by Met-hepatocyte growth factor/scatter factor autocrine stimulation. Proc Natl Acad Sci USA 1994;91:4731.
135. Rosengard AM, Brown P, Liotta LA, Steeg PS. Modulation of human breast carcinoma nm23 expression in vitro by transforming growth factor-beta. (personal communication).
136. Rosengard AM, Krutzsch HC, Shearn A, Biggs JR, Barker E, Margulies IMK, King CR, Liotta LA, Steeg PS. Reduced nm23/awd protein in tumor metastasis and aberrant Drosophila development. Nature 1989;342:177.
137. Ruoslahti E, Pierschbacher MD. Arg-Gly-Asp: a versatile cell recognition signal. Cell 1986;44:517.
138. Sadowski I, Pawson T, Lagarde A. v-fps protein-tyrosine kinase coordinately enhances the malignancy and growth factor responsiveness of pre-neoplastic lung fibroblasts. Oncogene 1988;2:241.
139. Sager R. Tumor suppressor genes: the puzzle and the promise. Science 1989;246:1406.
140. Sappino A-P, Busso N, Belin D, Vassali J-D. Increase of urokinase type plasminogen activator gene expression in human lung and breast carcinomas. Cancer Res 1987;47:4043.
141. Sato Y, Rifkin DB. Autocrine activities of basic fibroblast growth factor: regulation of endothelial cell movement, plasminogen activator synthesis, and DNA synthesis. J Cell Biol 1988;107:1199.
142. Schirrmacher V. Experimental approaches, theoretical concepts and impacts for treatment strategies. Adv Cancer Res 1984;43:1.
143. Schwartz MA. Signaling by integrins: implications for tumorigenesis. Cancer Res 1993;53:1503.
144. Slamon DJ, Clark GM, Wong SG, Levin WJ, Ullrich A, McGuire WL. Human breast cancer: correlation of relapse and survival with amplification of the HER-2/neu oncogene. Science 1987;235:177.
145. Sloane BR, Honn KV. Cysteine proteinases and metastasis. Cancer Metast Rev 1984;3:249.
146. Sloane BF, Rozhin J, Johnson K, Taylor H, Crissman JD, Honn KV. Cathepsin B: association with plasma membrane in metastatic tumors. Proc Natl Acad Sci USA 1986;83:2483.
147. Sobel ME. Metastasis suppressor genes. JNCI 1990;82:267.
148. Sporn M, Roberts A. Peptide growth factors: current status and therapeutic opportunities. In Important Advances in Oncology. Edited by VT DeVita Jr, S Hellman, SA Rosenberg. Philadelphia: Lippincott, 1987, pp 75–86.
149. Sporn M. Chemoprevention of cancer. Lancet 1993;342(8881):1211.
150. Spyratos F, Maudelonde T, Brouillet JP, Brunet M, Defrenne A, Andrieu C, Hacene K, Desplaces A, Rouess J, Rockefort H, Cathepsin D. An independent prognostic factor for metastasis of breast cancer. Lancet 1989;2:1115.
151. Srivastava A, Laidler P, Davies RP, et al. The prognostic significance of tumor vascularity in intermediate thickness (0.76–4.0 mm thick) skin melanoma: a quantitative histologic study. Am J Path 1988;419.
152. Steeg PS, Bevilacqua G, Kopper L, Thorgeirsson UP, Talmadge JE, Liotta LA, Sobel ME. Evidence for a novel gene associated with low tumor metastatic potential. JNCI 1988;80:200.
153. Stetler-Stevenson W, Brown P, Onisto M, Levy A, Liotta LA. Tissue inhibitor of metalloproteinase-2 (TIMP-2) mRNA expression in tumor cell lines and human tumor tissues. J Biol Chem 1990;265:13933.
154. Stetler-Stevenson WG, Krutzsch HC, Liotta LA. Tissue Inhibitor of Metalloproteinase-2 (TIMP-2), a new member of the metalloproteinase inhibitor family. J Biol Chem 1989;264:17374.
155. Stetler-Stevenson WG, Krutzsch HC, Wacher MP, Margulies IMK, Liotta LA. The activation of human type IV collagenase proenzyme. Sequence identification of the ma-

jor conversion product following organomercurial activation. J Biol Chem 1989;264: 1353.
156. Stetler-Stevenson WG, Liotta LA, Seldin MF. Linkage analysis demonstrates that the TIMP-2 locus is on mouse chromosome 11. Genomics 1992;14:828.
157. Stoker M. Effect of scatter factor on motility of epithelial cells and fibroblasts. J Cell Physiol 1989;139:565.
158. Stoker M, Gherardi E, Perryman M, et al. Scatter factor is fibroblast-derived modulator of epithelial cell motility. Nature 1987;327:239.
159. Stracke ML, Krutzsch HC, Unsworth EJ, et al. Identification, purification, and partial sequence analysis of autotaxin, a novel motility-stimulating protein. J Biol Chem 1991;267:2524.
160. Sugarbaker EV. Patterns of metastasis in human malignancies. Cancer Biol Rev 1981;2:235.
161. Takeichi M. A molecular family important in selective cell-cell adhesion. Annu Rev Biochem 1990;59:237.
162. Tandon AK, Clark GM, Chamness GC, Chirgwin I, McGuire WL. Cathepsin D and prognosis in breast cancer. N Engl J Med 1990;322:297.
163. Taylor WR, Groenberg AH, Turley EA, Wright JA. Cell motility, invasion and malignancy induced by overexpression of K-FGF or bFGF. Exp Cell Res 1993;204:295.
164. Terranova VP, Liotta LA, Russo RG, Martin GR. Role of laminin in the attachment and metastasis of murine tumor cells. Cancer Res 1982;42:2265.
165. Thorgeirsson UP, Liotta LA, Kalebic T, Margulies IMK, Thomas K, Rios-Candelore M, Russo RG. Effect of natural protease inhibitors and a chemoattractant on tumor cell invasion in vitro. JNCI 1982;69:1049.
166. Thorgeirsson UP, Turpeenniemi-Hujanen T, Neckers LM, Johnson DW, Liotta LA. Protein synthesis but not DNA synthesis is required for tumor cell invasion in vitro. Invas Met 1984;4:73.
167. Thorgeirsson UP, Turpeenniemi-Hujanen T, Williams JE, Westin E, Heilman CA, Talmadge JE, Liotta LA. NIH 3T3 cells transfected with human tumor DNA containing activated *ras* oncogenes express the metastatic phenotype in nude mice. Mol Cell Biol 1985;5:259.
168. Ura H, Bonfil RD, Reich R, Reddel R, Pfeifer A, Harris CC, Klein AJP. Expression of type IV collagenase and procollagen genes and its correlation with the tumorigenic invasive, and metastatic abilities of oncogene-transformed human bronchial epithelial cells. Cancer Res 1989;49:4615.
169. Vojtek AB, Hollenberg SM, Cooper JA. Mammalian *ras* interacts directly with the serine/threonine kinase Raf. Cell 1993;74:205.
170. Waghorne C, Kerbel RS, Breitman ML. Metastatic potential of SPI mouse mammary adenocarcinoma cells is differentially induced by activated and normal forms of c-H-*ras*. Oncogene 1987;1:149.
171. Wakefield LM, Thompson NL, Flanders KC, O'Conner-McCourt KC, Sporn MB. Transforming growth factor-beta: multifunctional regulator of cell growth and phenotype. Ann NY Acad Sci 1989;551:290.
172. Wallet V, Mutzel R, Troll H, Barzu 0, Wurster B, Vernon M, Lacombe MA. Dictyostelium nucleoside diphosphate kinase highly homologous to nm23 and awd proteins involved in mammalian tumor metastasis and Drosophila development. JNCI 1990;18: 1199.
173. Wang BS, McLoughlin GA, Richie JP, Mannick JA. Correlation of the production of plasminogen activator with tumor metastasis in B16 mouse melanoma cell lines. Cancer Res 1980;40:288.
174. Weidner N, Folkman J, Pozza F, et al. Tumor angiogenesis: a new significant and independent prognostic indicator in early-stage breast carcinoma. JNCI 1992;84:1875.
175. Weidner N, Semple J, Welch W, et al. Tumor angiogenesis and metastasis—correlation in invasive breast carcinoma. N Engl J Med 1991;324:1.
176. Weinberg RA. Oncogenes, antioncogenes and the molecular basis of multistep carcinogenesis. Cancer Res 1989;49:3713.
177. Welgus HG, Stricklin GP. Human skin fibroblast collagenase inhibitor: comparative studies in human connective tissues, serum, and amniotic fluid. J Biol Chem 1983;258:12259.
178. Wewer UM, Liotta LA, Jaye M, Ricca GA, Drohan WN, Claysmith AP, Rao CN, Wirth P, Coligan JE, Albrechtsen R, Mudryj M, Sobel ME. Altered levels of laminin receptor mRNA in various human carcinoma cells that have different abilities to bind laminin. Proc Natl Acad Sci USA 1986;83:7137.
179. Wilhelm S, Collier I, Kronberg A, Eisen A, Marmer B, Grant G, Bauer EA, Goldberg GI. Human skin fibroblast stromelysin: structure, glycosylation, substrate specificity and differential expression in normal and tumorigenic cells. Proc Natl Acad Sci USA 1987;84:6725.
180. Wilhelm SM, Collier IE, Marmer BL, Eisen AZ, Grant GA, Goldberg GI. SV40-transformed human lung fibroblasts secrete a 92-kd type-IV collagenase which is identical to that secreted by normal human macrophages. J Biol Chem 1989;264:17213.
181. Yamaoka M, Yamamoto T, Masaki T, Ikeyama S, Sudo K, Fujita T. Inhibition of tumor growth and metastasis of rodent tumors by the angiogenesis inhibitor O-(Chloroacetyl-carbamoly)fumagillol (TNP-470; AGM-1470). Cancer Res 1993;53: 4262.

CHAPTER 10

Tumor Angiogenesis

JUDAH FOLKMAN

Introduction

Angiogenesis is fundamental to reproduction, development, and repair. These processes depend mainly on brief bursts of capillary blood vessel growth that usually last only days or weeks. Such physiologic angiogenesis is tightly regulated. A variety of circulating and sequestered inhibitors ensure that for most of its existence, the vascular endothelium is out of the cell cycle. As a result, endothelial cells are among the most quiescent cells of the body. For example, turnover times of endothelial cells are measured in hundreds of days. In contrast, 5 days is the average turnover time for bone marrow cells, which divide at the rate of approximately 6×10^9 cell divisions per hour. During angiogenesis, microvascular endothelial cells proliferate as rapidly as bone marrow cells. Furthermore, endothelial proliferation is not the only event necessary for development of a new capillary blood vessel. Endothelial cells must also migrate into and invade the extracellular matrix invasion, form tubes, and connect the tips of these tubes to create loops capable of handling blood flow (12). Even in the absence of endothelial DNA synthesis in tissue that has been heavily irradiated, new capillary blood vessels and their branches still develop for a few days (284).

A hallmark of pathologic angiogenesis is persistent growth of blood vessels—that is, neovascularization out of control. Angiogenesis that continues for months or years sustains the progression of many neoplastic and nonneoplastic diseases. However, angiogenesis is almost always focal, and even pathologic angiogenesis is still spatially regulated, as is its physiologic counterpart. Neovascular suppressor mechanisms, which may be overwhelmed by local angiogenic signals from the diabetic retina or from tumors and their metastases, nevertheless manage to contain the resulting blood vessel growth and prevent it from spreading.

The vascular endothelium is a monolayer of approximately 1,000 m^2, which would cover a tennis court. An angiogenic focus appears as only a tiny fraction or a small "hot spot" of proliferating and migrating endothelial cells that originate from this expanse of resting endothelium. The fundamental objective of all antiangiogenic therapy is to return such a neovascular focus to its normal resting state or to prevent its appearance.

Historical Background

It had been observed for more than 100 years that tumors appear to be more vascular than normal tissues (336). It was long believed that simple dilation of existing host blood vessels accounted for this tumor hyperemia (50). Vasodilation was generally thought to be a side effect of tumor metabolites or of necrotic tumor products escaping from the tumor. Two reports suggested that tumor hyperemia could be related to *new* blood vessel growth—that is, to *neo*vascularization—and not to dilation. Although these observations were largely overlooked, a 1939 paper showed that while neovascularization of a wound in a transparent chamber in a rabbit ear regressed completely after the wound had healed (152), a tumor implant in the chamber was associated with accelerated growth of capillary blood vessels. The other report, which appeared in 1945, revealed that new vessels in the neighborhood of a tumor implant arose from host vessels and not from the tumor itself (3). These papers notwithstanding, debate continued in the literature for two more decades about whether tumors were supplied by pre-existing vessels or by neovascularization (58). Even among the few investigators who accepted the concept of tumor-induced neovascularization, it was generally assumed that this vascular response was an inflammatory reaction and was not necessary for tumor growth (82).

Dependence of Tumors on Angiogenesis: The Beginning of the Field of the Angiogenesis Research

A HYPOTHESIS IS ADVANCED THAT TUMOR GROWTH IS ANGIOGENESIS DEPENDENT

In 1971 I proposed a new view of the role of blood vessels in tumor growth in the form of a hypothesis that tumor growth is angiogenesis dependent (83). I suggested that tumor cells and vascular endothelial cells within a neoplasm may constitute a highly integrated ecosystem and that endothelial cells may be switched from a resting state to a rapid growth phase by a "diffusible" chemical signal from tumor cells. An additional speculation was that angiogenesis could be a relevant target for tumor therapy—i.e., antiangiogenic therapy. Because of the existing confusion between inflammation and angiogenesis, I attempted to distinguish between the two processes. The experiments that gave rise to these ideas had been carried out in the early 1960s and revealed that tumor growth in isolated perfused organs was severely restricted in association with absence of vascularization of the tumors (84–87, 91, 109).

These ideas were not accepted at the time. Although a few investigators in the early 1970s had begun to believe that tumors might induce neovascularization, this process was still widely assumed to be an inflammatory host response to necrotic tumor cells and possibly detrimental to the tumor (73). Others felt that any new vessels induced by a tumor would become "established" and thus could not undergo involution. Further, compelling evidence that tumors actually depended on neovascularization for their continued growth was lacking. The prevailing wisdom was that tumors could somehow develop around preexisting vasculature. Acceptance of the hypothesis was further hindered because the 1971 report appeared 8 years before it was possible to grow capillary endothelial cells in vitro (81), 11 years before the discovery of the first angiogenesis inhibitor (312), and 13 years before the purification of the first angiogenic protein (283).

Throughout the 1970s, laboratory studies were devoted to proving that tumor vessels were new proliferating capillaries; to elucidating the sequential steps of the angiogenic process to understand how angiogenesis might be inhibited; to developing bioassays so that angiogenesis could be quantified (88); to demonstrating that viable tumor cells released diffusible angiogenic factors that stimulated new capillary growth and endothelial mitosis in vivo (89, 90, 175), even when tumor cell proliferation had been arrested by irradiation (8); and to showing that necrotic tumor products were not angiogenic per se (for a review, see reference 92). All of these efforts were designed to provide supporting evidence that tumor growth was angiogenesis dependent. Thus, while the field of angiogenesis research began as a laboratory effort to understand tumor angiogenesis, today angiogenesis is now studied in a wide spectrum of disciplines, from developmental biology to molecular genetics, and in a variety of clinical specialties, from cardiology to ophthalmology.

EXPERIMENTAL EVIDENCE IS ASSEMBLED TO SUPPORT THE HYPOTHESIS THAT TUMOR GROWTH IS ANGIOGENESIS DEPENDENT

Indirect Evidence

By the mid-1980s, considerable indirect evidence had been assembled to support the hypothesis that tumor growth is angiogenesis dependent. By this time the idea could be stated in its simplest terms: "Once tumor take has occurred, every further increase in tumor cell population must be preceded by an increase in new capillaries which converge upon the tumor" (90). The hypothesis predicted that if angiogenesis was inhibited, tumors would become dormant at a small, possibly microscopic size (87). Thus, while neovascularization is necessary but not sufficient for expansion of a tumor, the *absence* of neovascularization prevents expansion of a primary tumor mass beyond 1 to 2 mm^3 and may restrict a metastasis to a microscopic dormant lesion. Most nonneovascularized tumors are not clinically detectable, with the exception of surface lesions on the skin or the external mucous membranes.

The indirect evidence was based on in vitro studies of tumor spheroids, in vivo studies in which a tumor mass was separated from its vascular bed, and measurements of tumors that were still in the prevascular stage of tumor progression. The following observations were made:

1. In two-dimensional flat cultures, a population of tumor cells expands indefinitely as long as fresh medium is added and unlimited cell-free surface is provided (i.e., passage of cells to a new flask). In contrast, three-dimensional spheroids of the same cells, suspended in soft agar or methylcellulose, stop enlarging at a diameter of a few millimeters, despite repeated passage of the spheroids to fresh media (98). In these "steady-state" spheroids, cell proliferation is balanced by cell death (1, 302, 303).
2. Tumors implanted into subcutaneous transparent chambers grow slowly before vascularization, and tumor volume increases linearly. After vascularization, tumor growth is rapid and tumor volume may increase exponentially (3).
3. Tumor growth in the avascular rabbit cornea proceeds slowly and at a linear rate, but switches to exponential growth after vascularization (124).
4. Tumors suspended in the aqueous fluid of the anterior chamber of the rabbit eye remain in a dormant state: viable, avascular, and limited in size (<1 mm^3). These tumors induce neovascularization of iris vessels, but the new vessels cannot reach the tumors floating in the aqueous fluid. Once a tumor spheroid is implanted contiguous to the proliferating iris vessels, the tumors can enlarge up to 16,000 times their original volume within 2 weeks (118).
5. Tumors grown in the vitreous of the rabbit eye remain viable but are restricted to diameters of less than 0.50 mm for as long as 100 days. Once such a tumor reaches the retinal surface it becomes neovascularized and within 2 weeks can undergo a 19,000-fold increase in volume over the avascular tumor (34). Cross-sectional histology of the avascular tumors reveals proliferating cells in the outer portion of the tumor and dying cells in the interior.
6. Human retinoblastomas that have metastasized to the vitreous are viable, avascular, and growth-restricted (93).
7. Within a solid tumor the H^3-thymidine labeling index of tumor cells decreases with increasing distance from the nearest open capillary. The mean labeling index for a given tumor correlates with the labeling index of the vascular endothelial cells in that tumor (311).
8. Tumors implanted into the chorioallantoic membrane of the chick embryo remain restricted in growth during the avascular phase but enlarge rapidly once they are vascularized (177).

9. Tumors implanted into the chorioallantoic membrane in successively older embryos grow at slower rates, corresponding to the reduced rates of endothelial turnover with age (177).
10. Vascular casts of metastases in the rabbit liver reveal that tumors of up to 1 mm in diameter are usually avascular, but beyond that size are vascularized (189).
11. Human ovarian carcinoma may metastasize to the peritoneal membrane as tiny avascular seeds. These implants rarely grow beyond a limited diameter of a few millimeters, until after vascularization.
12. In transgenic mice that develop carcinomas of the beta cells in the pancreatic islets, large tumors arise from a subset of preneoplastic hyperplastic islets that have become vascularized (94).
13. In another experiment, neoplastic cells injected subcutaneously develop into tumors, which become vascularized at about 0.4 mm^3. As tumor size increases, blood vessels continue to proliferate and are enveloped by encroaching tumor. The vessels eventually occupy up to 1.5% of the tumor volume. This is a 400% increase in vascular density over normal subcutaneous tissue (317). Thus, new capillary blood vessels that converge on a tumor are *enveloped* by tumor cells. Tumors are not actually penetrated by new vessels.
14. In rat colon tumors arising spontaneously after administration of a carcinogen, the vascular phase can be further divided into two distinct stages (292). In the early vascular stage (tumor diameter <3.5 mm) the tumor is temporarily supplied by preexisting host microvessels that are dilated and widened. Some of this dilation may result from proliferation and lateral migration of endothelial cells in postcapillary venules. Subsequently (tumor diameter >5.7 mm), new capillary vessels sprout and proliferate. This leads to a greater than normal microvessel density and rapid tumor growth. These studies are summarized in a recent review (95).

Direct Evidence

It was not until the late 1980s that it was possible to block angiogenesis in a tumor bed without physically separating the tumor from its vascular supply. These experiments demonstrated that tumor growth was restricted to a small volume of less than 1 to 2 mm^3 when angiogenesis was inhibited. They provided the first direct evidence that tumor growth was angiogenesis dependent. In some cases a dormant microscopic state was achieved.

1. An angiogenesis inhibitor, TNP-470 (AGM-1470), a synthetic analogue of fumagillin, potently inhibited tumor growth in vivo, but not in vitro (155). It was a selective inhibitor of proliferating endothelial cells in vitro and in vivo.
2. In another experiment, the cDNA for human basic fibroblast growth factor (bFGF) hybridized to a signal sequence was transfected into normal mouse fibroblasts (149). The transfected fibroblasts became tumorigenic, exported bFGF, and were also highly angiogenic. They formed large lethal tumors when implanted into mice. The angiogenesis was mediated solely by the bFGF released from these tumors. Furthermore, the structure of the bFGF had been modified by site-specific mutagenesis so that two serines had been substituted for cysteines. Thus, the bFGF released by the tumor could be neutralized by a specific antibody that had no effect on natural bFGF. When this antibody was administered to the tumor-bearing mice, there was dramatic reduction in neovascularization and in tumor volume.
3. In a similar experiment, a neutralizing antibody to another angiogenic protein, vascular endothelial growth factor (VEGF), was administered to mice with tumors that employed mainly VEGF as their mediator of angiogenesis (174). Tumor growth was inhibited by more than 90%. At the time of this writing, VEGF is thought to be a mitogen only for vascular endothelial cells (255).
4. The growth of a brain tumor in nude mice was significantly inhibited or prevented when tumor angiogenesis was suppressed by a strategy in which a dominant-negative mutant of the receptor (Flk-1) for the angiogenic protein VEGF was introduced into host endothelial cells (carried by a retrovirus). This signaling-defective receptor mutant formed an inactive dimer with the native Flk-1 receptor on endothelial cells and prevented the formation of new capillary blood vessels in response to VEGF released by the tumor (209).
5. Transformed cells were not tumorigenic until after they had became angiogenic (56).
6. Specific immunologic inhibition of overexpression of the integrin $\alpha_V\beta_3$ on capillary endothelial cells produced apoptosis of proliferating endothelial cells, blocked neovascularization, and caused tumor regression (36).
7. The most compelling direct evidence that tumor growth is angiogenesis dependent is based on administration of angiostatin to tumor-bearing mice (241). Angiostatin is a 38-kd internal fragment of plasminogen, which is a specific inhibitor of proliferating endothelial cells. It does not inhibit tumor cells or other nonendothelial cells in vitro. It is the most potent of the known angiogenesis inhibitors and is capable of complete blockade of angiogenesis in certain tumors and nearly complete blockade in others. When administered systemically to tumor-bearing mice, it can hold metastases in a microscopic avascular dormant state of approximately 200 μm diameter. The micrometastases form a perivascular cuff around a preexisting vessel, are unable to stimulate neovascularization, and contain proliferating tumor cells balanced by apoptotic tumor cells.

CERTAIN MISCONCEPTIONS ABOUT TUMOR ANGIOGENESIS PERSIST

As direct evidence has supported the essential role of angiogenesis in tumor growth, the angiogenic properties of tumors have become more widely understood. However, certain misconceptions have also arisen.

The presence of angiogenesis does not distinguish between a benign and a malignant tumor (265). Adrenal adenomas are benign tumors that are highly neovascularized

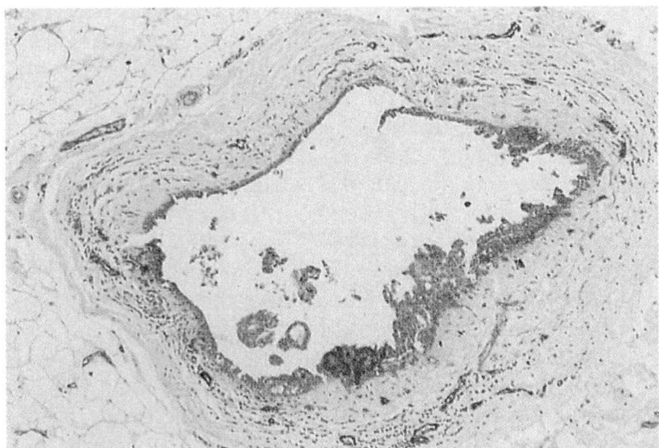

Figure 10.1. Hematoxylin-eosin–stained section with immunoperoxidase staining for Factor VIII shows cluster of endothelial cells (brown) immediately adjacent to segment of human breast duct with early carcinoma in situ. This represents the earliest switch to the angiogenic phenotype. Angiogenesis is absent near the remaining normal epithelium of the duct. *Source:* Weidner et al. (340).

but appear to lack the growth potential to take advantage of the new blood vessels they have induced. Thus, the onset of angiogenesis permits expansion of a tumor mass but does not guarantee it. In fact, the switch to the angiogenic phenotype occurs independently of other events in tumorigenesis. In most tumors, angiogenesis appears after the expression of the malignant phenotype (Fig. 10.1). However, in carcinoma of the cervix, the preneoplastic stage of dysplasia becomes neovascularized before the malignant tumor appears (294). This sequence of events also occurs in certain spontaneously arising tumors in animals (362).

Angiogenesis may not be necessary for certain tumor cells that can grow as a flat sheet between membranes, e.g., gliomatosis in the meninges.

It is still assumed by some oncologists that the blood vessels of a large tumor are "established." Proponents of this idea argue, therefore, that antiangiogenic therapy could never reduce tumor size or cause tumor regression, because "established" vessels would by definition be refractory to such treatment. Antiangiogenic therapy, however, can cause growing blood vessels to involute (72) and can bring about regression of growing tumors (37, 96, 242). Further, the replication rate of endothelial cells in tumor capillary vessels is significantly greater than in the endothelial cells of normal tissue, with the difference in rates often approaching 100-fold (60). Obviously, a few feeder vessels, usually arteries, may be observed in the midst of a histologic cross-section of a tumor and could be considered as established, but these are not the new microvessels that tumor cells induce and that bring oxygen, nutrients, and growth factors to the tumor and carry metabolites away from it.

It is commonly said that tumors outgrow their blood supply. This is as inaccurate as saying that leaves outgrow their trees. Growing tumors can gradually *compress* their blood supply because of increasing interstitial pressure. These compressed areas become ischemic, but they are not avascular. Necrosis follows. Vessel compression also interferes with the optimal delivery of therapeutic agents (162). Paradoxically, antiangiogenic therapy can decrease ischemia, apparently because of its effect of decreasing interstitial pressure.

METASTASIS IS ALSO ANGIOGENESIS DEPENDENT

Experimental and clinical evidence suggests that the process of metastasis is also angiogenesis dependent. For a tumor cell to metastasize successfully it must breach several barriers and be able to respond to specific growth factors (79, 227, 228, 347). Thus, tumor cells must gain access to the vasculature in the primary tumor, survive the circulation, arrest in the microvasculature of the target organ (226, 228), exit from this vasculature (30), grow in the target organ, and induce angiogenesis (340, 345). Therefore, angiogenesis appears to be necessary at the beginning as well as the end of the metastatic cascade.

In experimental animals, tumor cells are rarely shed into the circulation before a primary tumor is vascularized, but they can appear in the circulation continuously after neovascularization (191, 192). The number of cells shed from the primary tumor correlates with the density of tumor blood vessels as well as with the number of lung metastases observed later. Tumor cells can enter the circulation by penetrating through proliferating capillaries that have fragmented basement membranes and are leaky (64, 192). Further, angiogenic factors from tumors such as bFGF and VPF/VEGF induce increased production of plasminogen activator and collagenases in proliferating endothelial cells, thus further contributing to degradation of basement membranes (165, 217, 224). These degradative enzymes may facilitate the entry of tumor cells into the circulation. The ability of growing capillaries to liquefy extracellular matrix is clearly illustrated by the following experiment. India ink (containing carbon particles of approximately 200 Å) is injected into a rabbit cornea so that the ink is trapped in a square corneal pocket, like a tattoo, between a tumor implant and the vascular bed at the limbal edge of the cornea. As new blood vessels are attracted into the cornea by the tumor, they first encounter the India ink. India ink is dispersed only from the inferior border of the pocket, coincident with dissolution of the corneal matrix by the neovascular front. The superior border of the India ink, contiguous to the avascular tumor, remains intact. Only after the tumor has become neovascularized is it capable of invading the corneal pocket and dispersing all of the India ink. In the absence of neovascularization, India ink remains sharply demarcated in the corneal pocket for an indefinite period of time (294).

Another indication that metastasis is angiogenesis dependent is that potent angiogenesis inhibitors administered to tumor-bearing animals suppress growth of metastases. The metastases remain dormant at a microscopic size. This occurs despite the fact that angiogenesis inhibitors have no inhibitory effect on the tumor cells in vitro (172, 313). Thus, the tumor cells are "resistant" to the angiogenesis inhibitor from the beginning of therapy. Yet in these animals, the microscopic, dormant metastases are harmless and the mice appear perfectly healthy for as long as the inhibitor is administered (up to 2 months in current studies). In another animal tumor model, lung metastases remain unable to induce local angiogenesis, even after the original primary tumor has been removed. These mice appear completely healthy for as long as they have been observed (up to 1 year), or almost half the normal life span of the animals, at this writing (243). The dormant, nonangiogenic metastases can be induced to grow at any time by local trauma to the chest.

Correlative clinical data also suggest that metastatic potential may depend on the intensity of angiogenesis. Neovascularization can now be quantified in human tumors by staining histologic sections with an antibody to von Willebrand factor, an endothelial cell marker. This method also reveals a significant direct correlation between the highest density of microvessels in a histologic section of invasive breast cancer and the occurrence of future metastases (340). Microvessel counts in other tumors have also been correlated with metastatic risk and clinical outcome (see discussion under Clinical Applications of Angiogenesis, Principles in Cancer Patients, below).

Because of the clonal origin of metastases (172, 345), a primary tumor containing a high proportion of angiogenic malignant cells is more likely to generate metastases that are already angiogenic when they arrive at the target tissue.

Metastasis to lymph nodes may also depend on neovascularization of the primary tumor. Tumors are not known to induce new lymphatic vessels, and lymphatics are rarely found within tumors (162). Thus, lymph fluid that escapes from intratumoral capillaries percolates toward the tumor surface and is carried away by host lymphatics, which become engorged. Human lymph node metastases may arise from a neovascularized primary tumor, but lymph node metastasis from nonvascularized in situ carcinomas is rare. The rabbit cornea model is illuminating. India ink injected into a neovascularized cornea escapes and rapidly appears in the ipsilateral lymph nodes. In contrast, in an avascular cornea, India ink is retained indefinitely (294). Therefore, the available evidence indicates that tumor neovascularization may pump filtered plasma into the interstitial spaces of a tumor, thus increasing the flow of lymph from a tumor toward its regional lymph nodes.

ANGIOGENESIS FACILITATES INVASION

Tumor invasion may occur in the presence or absence of neovascularization. For example, in histologic sections of breast cancer with microvessels highlighted by antibody to von Willebrand factor, microinvasion may be observed in a carcinoma in situ before it has become neovascularized (340). A thin file of tumor cells breaches the basement membrane of a duct filled with tumor. However, after neovascularization has occurred, invasion into adjacent connective tissue occurs along a broad front, and tumor cords may follow the path of newly generated blood vessels (229). The experiment cited above, in which India ink escapes from a corneal pocket when the pocket is neovascularized, suggests that the proteolytic activity produced by proliferating capillary blood vessels (which presumably allows endothelial cells to invade extracellular matrix) may contribute to the invasiveness of a tumor. Thus, antiangiogenic therapy could inhibit tumor invasion; conversely, certain inhibitors of tumor proteases could also have antiangiogenic properties. An example is BB94, a metalloproteinase inhibitor, that is in clinical trial as an angiogenesis inhibitor (19, 351).

Microvascular endothelial cells under the stimulus of angiogenic proteins (e.g., bFGF or VPF/VEGF) increase their expression of proteolytic enzymes (e.g., collagenase IV), which contributes to the invasiveness of these cells during elongation of neovascular sprouts (193, 207, 217, 264). These enzymes may also enhance the invasiveness of tumor cells.

NEOVASCULAR CAPILLARY PROLIFERATION OCCURS IN SEQUENTIAL STEPS

The complexity of the angiogenic process resembles blood clotting. The generation of a new capillary blood vessel takes place in a series of sequential steps. From a therapeutic perspective, each step may be a relevant target for antiangiogenic therapy. The morphologic events of capillary growth include endothelial cell–induced degradation of the basement membrane of the parent venule, directional locomotion in concert with other endothelial cells, endothelial mitosis, lumen formation, development of sprouts and loops, generation of new basement membrane, and recruitment of pericytes (12, 212). This sequence is similar to the morphologic steps of angiogenesis in a healing wound or in a developing embryo. However, many tumors impose modifications on a new capillary bed that differ from the angiogenesis induced by nonneoplastic cells. For example, a capillary blood vessel in the normal brain usually contains one or two endothelial cells per lumen. In a brain tumor, however, 5 to 10 endothelial cells may occupy one lumen (34). Tumor-induced vessels are often dilated and saccular and may even contain tumor cells within the endothelial lining (163). Tumor microvasculature does not conform to the vasculature of normal tissues (e.g., artery to arteriole to capillary to postcapillary venule to venule to vein) (163). Tumors may contain giant capillaries, and arteriovenous shunts without intervening capillaries. Blood may even flow from one venule to another. Furthermore, organization of vessels may differ from one intratumoral location to the next (163). Capillary growth rates (i.e., the velocity of neovascularization) range from 0.23 to 0.8 mm/day, depending on the experimental system used and the type of tumor (99, 352, 355).

Although actively growing capillaries are usually pericyte-poor and do not regain their normal density of pericytes until after capillary growth has ceased, the capillaries in some tumors contain excessive numbers of pericytes (276, 327). Thus, some human tumors are pericyte-rich and others are pericyte-poor. It is not clear why these differences exist, or whether they are clinically significant. However, in a transgenic mouse model of retinoblastoma, the tumor appears to recruit an overabundance of perivascular pericytes, which themselves release a potent angiogenic factor, VEGF, thus amplifying the VEGF released from the tumor itself (39).

Many biochemical events also occur sequentially during the formation of a capillary blood vessel; however, these events have not yet been elucidated in vivo at the level of detail of the morphologic events. In the presence of an angiogenic molecule such as bFGF, there is a dramatic rise in production of plasminogen activator and collagenase by endothelial cells (133). There are changes in basement membrane components. In new capillaries growing in the chick embryo, the following observations have been made: (*a*) sulfated glycosaminoglycan synthesis is decreased (e.g., heparan sulfate) but gradually increases as the vessel matures (13); (*b*) fibronectin is one of the earliest of the basement membrane components to appear followed (within 2 days) by laminin and finally by collagen type IV as the vessels mature (111, 114); (*c*) fibrin leaks from the new vessels, undergo local degradation (224), and forms a scaffold to guide endothelial tube formation (65); (*d*) E-selectin expression also appears in new microvessels (232). Little is known about whether the production of other proteins by endothelial cells is increased in association with proliferation. These would include plasminogen activator inhibitor (PAI-1), bFGF, PDGF, HB-EGF, IL-6, and IGF-1.

Some Angiogenic Events Can Be Studied in Vitro

Because angiogenesis per se is difficult to quantify in vivo, the sequential events of capillary growth have been individually characterized by quantifiable in vitro bioassays. Capillary (81), aortic (128), and human umbilical vein endothelial cells (126, 161) are used in these systems. Locomotion in vitro is measured by chemokinetic assays that employ colloidal gold. Endothelial chemotaxis is quantified in Boyden chambers (26). Mitosis and DNA synthesis are quantified in subconfluent cultures of endothelial cells. Confluent endothelial cells, unlike fibroblasts, are generally refractory to mitogens (142). Lumen formation is studied with endothelial cells that are cultured on collagen, fibronectin, or laminin substrates (100, 132, 153, 154, 169, 198, 200, 212, 230, 231). These in vitro bioassays have been successfully used to discover and purify new angiogenic molecules (283) as well as novel angiogenesis inhibitors (155). However, whenever in vitro assays are used to guide purification of an angiogenic or an angiostatic molecule, the results must be confirmed in vivo. It is possible for a factor to be angiogenic in vivo but not mitogenic for endothelial cells in vitro (e.g., angiogenin; see below). Conversely, an endothelial mitogen in vitro may not be angiogenic in vivo (e.g., certain low-density lipoproteins) (101).

Bioassays Have Been Developed to Study Angiogenesis In Vivo

The currently available in vivo bioassays for angiogenesis are semiquantitative and have certain drawbacks. Nevertheless, they have served for the identification, purification, and characterization of almost all of the known angiogenic molecules and the inhibitors of angiogenesis. These bioassays have been extensively described and reviewed (9, 47, 101, 110). In brief, the chick embryo chorioallantoic membrane displays growth of new vessels toward an angiogenic factor implanted on the membrane in a pellet of methylcellulose or some other nonirritating vehicle. Embryos of 6 to 10 days' development are commonly used and examined 2 to 3 days later by stereomicroscopy. However, false-positive angiogenesis may be induced by any test material with abnormal osmolarity or pH which leads to cell damage. Further, angiogenesis secondary to inflammation (where infiltrating macrophages or leukocytes are the source of angiogenic activity) cannot easily be distinguished from direct angiogenic activity without detailed histologic study (270). Also, angiogenesis may be induced by fibrin degradation products that leak from embryonic vessels in response to injurious substances (66, 317). Several improvements have recently been made in the chick embryo assay (297, 309). The most quantitative method distinguishes new vessels from preexisting vessels by stimulating them to grow vertically through a collagen gel sandwiched between a top and bottom nylon mesh. The new capillary vessels that protrude through the top mesh are then counted (233).

The cornea micropocket overcomes some of the disadvantages of the chick embryo assay. A putative angiogenic factor is implanted into the cornea of the rabbit (124), mouse (223), or rat (113), usually in a polymeric sustained-release vehicle (185). The length and number of new capillaries that enter the avascular cornea can be quantified with a slit-lamp microscope or by image analysis of specimens injected with India ink (224). Vascularization of the cornea provides the most compelling evidence that new capillaries have been induced (43). This method is time-consuming and expensive in rabbits, but in mice it has become a valuable means of comparing potency among different angiogenesis inhibitors and of discovering novel endogenous inhibitors (48, 171).

Other systems include the hamster cheek pouch (278) and the subcutaneous fascia in mice (11). Recently, biodegradable and nonbiodegradable sponges (57) have been implanted into animals to study neovascularization induced by an angiogenic molecule within the sponge. These techniques facilitate histologic and immunocytochemical studies of new vessels, but neovascularization is more difficult to quantify than with other methods.

A major problem in the preclinical evaluation of antiangiogenic therapies has been the lack of an animal system that would allow quantitative comparison of the potency of different angiogenesis inhibitors administered systemically. Comparison of antitumor activity does not directly reveal "units" of antiangiogenic activity. This problem has now been solved in part by controlled release of a known quantity of bFGF or VEGF from a pellet implanted into the mouse cornea at a constant distance from the limbus. The neovascularization that appears in the next 5 days is quantified in mice given the test inhibitor or a vehicle by subcutaneous or intravenous injection (48, 171).

Human Tumors Switch to the Angiogenic Phenotype

TUMORS PROGRESS FROM A PREVASCULAR PHASE TO A VASCULAR PHASE

By the time most human tumors are detected, they are already neovascularized. However, that is not how they usually begin. Experimental and clinical data indicate that most human tumors arise without angiogenic activity, exist in situ without neovascularization for months to years, and then switch to an angiogenic phenotype (136). This phenotype is currently understood in terms of a net balance between positive and negative regulators of angiogenesis (28, 41, 176, 213, 237, 250, 254, 263). During tumor progression, one or more angiogenic factors may be overexpressed (e.g., VEGF), and/or mobilized from extracellular matrix, and/or released from macrophages recruited by the tumor. But the up-regulation of angiogenic activity may be insufficient to induce neovascularization until local tissue inhibitors of angiogenesis can be overcome (e.g., interferon alpha, beta) (290). Certain local inhibitors may be generated by tumor cells themselves as a residue from their preneoplastic parent cell. An example is thrombospondin, an angiogenesis inhibitor produced by normal human fibroblasts under the control of wild-type p53 (56). It is down-regulated by about 96% when fibroblasts from cancer-prone Li-Fraumeni patients, which already lack one allele of p53, lose or mutate the second p53 allele during progression to malignancy. Early evidence suggests that certain tumor suppressor genes may normally code for proteins that inhibit angiogenesis (326, 346).

This angiogenic "switch" has eluded analysis in experimental animals. Most transplantable animal tumors are already highly angiogenic when implanted; the prevascular phase may last only a few days. Tumor cells that are not angiogenic will not take. No take has been assumed to mean no tumor cells survived. However, stereoscopic analysis of the subcutaneous tissue at the site of implantation often reveals a viable tumor, less than 1 to 2 mm^3, that is avascular.

The switch to the angiogenic phenotype can be studied, however, in tumors that arise spontaneously. The prohibitively long time period for spontaneous tumor development can be shortened by employing transgenic mice. In transgenic mice that develop carcinomas of the beta cells of the pancreatic islets, the switch to angiogenesis occurs in a subset of hyperplastic islets before they become neoplastic. The onset of neovascularization occurs at a frequency that correlates with tumor development (94). In transgenic mice that develop fibrosarcomas, angiogenesis first appears in premalignant and then in malignant lesions. It is mediated mainly by basic fibroblast growth factor (bFGF), which can be detected as a secreted form only in vascularized tumors (166). This model is similar to certain human tumors in which the angiogenic phenotype may appear in the preneoplastic stage (362), such as cervical dysplasia or cervical intraepithelial neoplasia (CIN). For the majority of human cancers in which angiogenic activity appears after neoplasia, there are few if any suitable animal models.

THE PREVASCULAR PHASE LIMITS TUMOR ENLARGEMENT

During the prevascular phase, when angiogenic activity is absent or insufficient, tumors remain small, with volumes measured in a few cubic millimeters. Growth of the whole tumor is slow, and doubling times for the whole tumor may be years. However, this does not mean that the tumor cells are proliferating slowly. Experimental studies show that tumor cells in a prevascular neoplasm may have a ^{3}H-thymidine labeling index as high as that of a large vascularized tumor. However, the prevascular tumor has reached a steady state in which generation of new tumor cells is balanced by a high rate of tumor cell death, or apoptosis (94).

When the prevascular phase of bladder cancer (143), cervical cancer (288, 293) or cutaneous melanoma (298, 299) is first detected, these lesions are usually thin, slowly growing, stable for months to years, asymptomatic, and rarely metastatic. For the majority of tumors, however, the prevascular stage is clinically undetectable and can only be observed microscopically. For example, in breast and prostate cancer, carcinomas in situ can be observed before and after neovascularization in the same specimen (340–342).

METASTASES THAT ARE NOT NEOVASCULARIZED REMAIN DORMANT

Tumor cells that have successfully metastasized may not immediately become neovascularized after reaching the target organ. Such a metastasis lacking angiogenic activity for any of a variety of reasons may remain as a microscopic tumor of a 100 to 200 μm diameter indefinitely (102, 146, 241). In the absence of angiogenesis, the proliferation rate is balanced by a high apoptosis rate and the micrometastasis cannot expand. This prolonged dormant state has been demonstrated in mice by (*a*) treatment with angiostatin, a specific endothelial inhibitor that is also a potent angiogenesis inhibitor (241, 242), and (*b*) selection of a subclone of B-16 melanoma cells whose lung metastases are not angiogenic and have not escaped for up to 1 year at the time of this writing (244). However, simple trauma to the lungs, such as a needle puncture, is followed by rapid growth of the pulmonary metastases. This is presumably a result of wound angiogenesis.

The current dictum is that dormant metastases in patients (e.g., metastases appearing 5–10 years after removal of a breast cancer) represent tumor cells in G_0. It is quite possible, however, that dormant metastases could be based on our proposed model of blocked angiogenesis leading to balanced tumor cell proliferation and apoptosis (102, 146). This concept awaits demonstration in humans.

CLINICAL PATTERNS OF METASTASIS MAY BE GOVERNED BY ANGIOGENIC MECHANISMS

Cancer metastases may present at least four common clinical patterns (Table 10.1): (*a*) a primary tumor such as a colon carcinoma is removed, but within a few months metastases appear; (*b*) metastases are already present when the primary tumor is first detected; (*c*) metastases appear first, and the primary remains occult; (*d*) the primary is removed (or treated by other therapy), and metastases do not appear until years later (e.g., 5–10 years). A fifth and rare pattern is that metastases disappear after removal of the primary tumor (e.g., a few cases of renal cell carcinoma). These patterns of metastatic presentation are well recognized, but their biologic basis is poorly understood.

New experimental evidence suggests that the majority of the presenting patterns of metastases may be dictated by the intensity of angiogenesis in their vascular bed.

The essential role that angiogenesis plays in the metastatic cascade can be appreciated by examining ani-

Table 10.1. Common Patterns of Metastases in Cancer Patients at First Diagnosis

Pattern	Detectable (+) or not detectable (0)		Recurrence of metastases
	Primary tumor	Metastases	
1	+	0	Months
2	+	+	
3	0	+	
4	+	0	Years
5 (rare)	+	+	(Metastases regress when primary tumor is removed: e.g., some renal carcinomas)

From Folkman (102).

mal models that have been developed for each of the common presenting patterns of metastases in cancer patients.

The patient whose metastases appear within a few months after removal of the primary tumor (pattern 1 in Table 10.1) is analogous to a mouse model of Lewis lung carcinoma in which lung metastases remain microscopic while the primary is present, but grow rapidly a few days after the primary tumor is removed. In this model, the primary tumor directly inhibits angiogenesis in the bed of the lung metastases. The metastases remain unvascularized and restricted to a radius of approximately 150 μm (241). Angiogenesis in the primary tumor is mediated mainly by vascular endothelial growth factor (VEGF), which is presumably present at higher concentrations than local angiostatin. Because of up-regulation of VEGF receptors on endothelial cells in hypoxic areas (255), it is also possible that VEGF is retained in the vascular bed of the primary tumor. The half-life of VEGF in the circulation is approximately 3 minutes (N. Ferrara, pers. commun.). This rapid clearance would prevent VEGF from accumulating in the plasma. In contrast, the half-life of angiostatin is 2.5 days, and it does accumulate in the serum with increasing size of the primary tumor.

The patient whose metastases are already present when the primary tumor is first diagnosed is analogous to a mouse model of a subclone of Lewis lung carcinoma in which the primary tumor does not suppress its lung metastases and does not generate detectable levels of angiostatin in the circulation (241).

The patient who presents with metastases in the absence of a detectable primary tumor (pattern 3: occult primary) is similar to a mouse model in which metastatic cells inhibit the growth of the primary tumor (although it has not been ascertained whether the inhibition was mediated by a circulating angiostatic protein) (360). We speculate that if metastases in a patient are shed from a small primary tumor soon after it becomes neovascularized, the tumor may not be large enough to suppress angiogenesis in remote metastases. In mice with angiostatin-generating tumors, the primary tumor had to be at least 0.6 to 1.0 cm^3 before angiostatin could be detected in the circulation (241). Further, if the metastases have a slightly faster proliferation rate than the primary tumor, they could produce sufficient quantities of circulating angiogenesis inhibitor and suppress the primary tumor—an example of a secondary tumor inhibiting its primary lesion.

The patient whose metastases do not appear until years after removal of the primary tumor is analogous to a mouse model of B-16 melanoma in our laboratory in which dormant, nonangiogenic lung metastases of less than 0.1 to 0.2 mm diameter were found months after removal of the primary tumor. The mice were healthy (244). This is equivalent to 10 years of a human life span.

Although no animal model has been developed for the rare case of renal cell carcinoma in which removal of the primary tumor is followed by regression of lung metastases (pattern 5 in Table 10.1), one can speculate that the metastases may have been dependent on high production of circulating angiogenic factors and possibly other growth factors from the primary tumor (102). In renal cell carcinomas, high tissue levels of bFGF correlate with high mortality (225). In fact, in our own study of bFGF in serum and urine, 10% of a group of patients with a wide spectrum of malignancies had abnormally elevated levels of the angiogenic polypeptide bFGF in their serum and, 37% of 950 patients had abnormally elevated levels of bFGF in their urine (234).

The similarity of such animal models to human patterns of metastasis presentation does not prove that angiogenic control of metastatic growth is a central mechanism of dormancy. Nor does it mean that the human patterns are all based on angiogenic mechanisms. These models are described here because they offer a plausible general mechanism to explain the different patterns of metastasis presentation in cancer patients. The detailed experimental evidence is developed elsewhere by Holmgren et al. (146). Further attempts to uncover evidence that supports or refutes the hypothesis may be fruitful. Finally, to the extent that angiogenic processes are operating in human primary tumors and metastases, then it may be prudent to include this in thinking about the design of clinical trials of angiogenesis inhibitors.

The take-home lesson is that dormancy in all of these cases may depend on blocked angiogenesis leading to a microscopic tumor with high replication and high death rate of its tumor cells, but not necessarily cells in G_0.

THE VASCULAR PHASE PERMITS TUMOR ENLARGEMENT

Although the percentage of cycling cells in a vascularized tumor may be as high as in a nonvascularized tumor (146), the total population of replicating cells is significantly expanded by neovascularization. Human tumors that have undergone neovascularization may enter a phase of rapid growth, intensified invasion, compression of normal tissue, and increased metastatic potential. Vascularized tumors are the major cause of progressive symptoms in cancer patients. Most current conventional therapy is directed against tumors that are already well vascularized.

Neovascularization may increase metastatic potential, because the expanding tumor population increases the probability that variants of metastatic cells will arise that produce the appropriate enzymes and growth factors to penetrate a target organ and survive. The enormous enlargement of a proliferating tumor cell population may be one of the more dangerous aspects of tumor angiogenesis. Tumor cells that induce new vessels within a primary tumor are not only presented with more vascular channels in which to enter the circulation, but, upon arrival at a target organ, are already angiogenic. Thus, they have an increased chance of becoming a detectable metastasis (103).

TUMOR PERFUSION BEGINS IN THE VASCULAR PHASE

Neovascularization permits rapid tumor growth because it temporarily solves the problem of exchange of nutrients, oxygen, and wastes by a crowded three-dimensional cell population for which simple diffusion of these molecules across its outer surface has become inadequate (98, 99, 144). Blood flowing through tumor vessels may also carry survival factors and growth factors for tumor cells as well as for endothelial cells.

PARACRINE STIMULATION OF TUMOR CELLS ALSO OCCURS IN THE VASCULAR PHASE

The vascularized tumor is not only perfused, but receives paracrine stimuli from endothelial cells (103, 139, 229, 262). Endothelial cells release growth factors that stimulate tumor cells (97); these may include bFGF, PDGF, IGF-1, IGF-2 (280), and cytokines such as IL-1, IL-6 (219), IL-8 (258), and GM-CSF (363). This concept arose from experiments in which tumor cells grew preferentially along endothelial channels in vitro in the absence of blood flow (229), and from other studies (139, 262). In fact, paracrine signals within a tumor can be considered to operate in two directions: tumor cells and endothelial cells stimulate the proliferation of each other (Fig. 10.2). Further, the hypoxic conditions that arise in some areas of a tumor from vascular compression may upregulate production of specific angiogenic proteins such as VPF/VEGF (256, 285).

CLINICAL SYMPTOMS INCREASE IN THE VASCULAR PHASE

Few if any symptoms are associated with perivascular or in situ malignancies. However, the onset of neovascularization precipitates new symptoms. Blood in the urine, in the stool, in the sputum or, between menstrual periods, may signify the presence of a vascularized tumor in the bladder, colon, bronchus or, cervix. The bloody ascites associated with ovarian carcinoma indicates that the tumor has gone beyond the stage of tiny implants, which are avascular, whitish, and nearly uniform in size. The ascites is thought to be secondary to the angiogenic protein VPF/VEGF, high concentrations of which have been identified in ascites (75, 184, 192, 281).

Neovascularization is also associated with local edema,

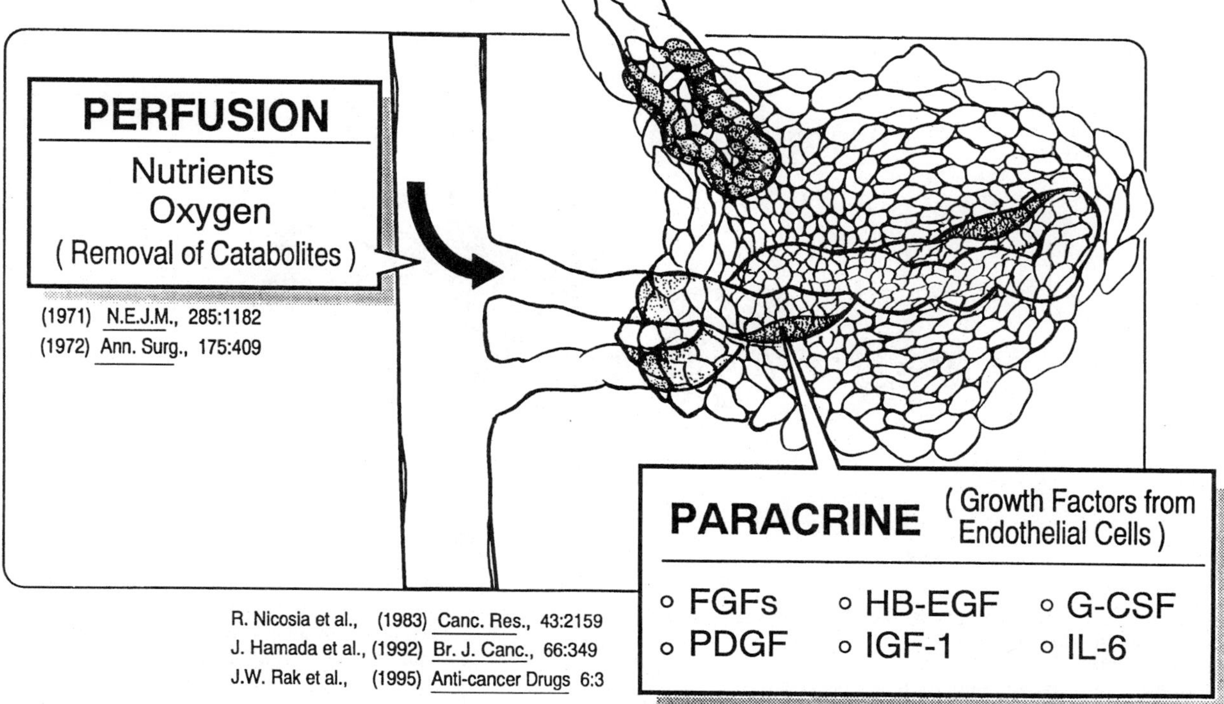

Figure 10.2. The onset of tumor neovascularization provides both a perfusion and a paracrine stimulus to tumor growth. After becoming neovascularized, a tumor is perfused, which increases the efficiency of entry of nutrients and exit of waste catabolites. In addition, growth factors produced by capillary endothelial cells stimulate tumor cells in a paracrine fashion. *Source:* Folkman (106). Reproduced with permission.

which is responsible, for example, for many of the presenting symptoms of brain tumors. Tumor rupture or hemorrhage is not uncommon when there is a large necrotic center such as in Wilms' tumor. These central areas of ischemia and necrosis are usually secondary to compression of vessels by increasing interstitial pressure.

Certain clinical signs and symptoms from tumor neovascularization are associated with specific tumor types. For example, retinoblastomas in the posterior eye induce iris neovascularization in the anterior chamber. Certain brain tumors induce angiogenesis in remote areas of the brain. Bone pain in metastatic prostate cancer may be related in part to neovascularization. A problem in the diagnosis of a primary bone tumor is that if the biopsy specimen contains only the neovascular response at the periphery of the tumor, it may be mistaken for granulation tissue or inflammation.

A variety of cancer syndromes, such as inappropriate hormonal activity, hypercoagulation, and cachexia, are secondary to the presence of biologically active peptides released into the circulation from vascularized tumors.

The angiogenesis induced by cervical cancer may be observed by colposcopy (288); the appearance of telangiectasia or "vascular spiders" in a mastectomy scar may herald local recurrence of tumor; color Doppler imaging can demonstrate neovascularization in breast cancer (170) and other tumors; bladder carcinoma is detected by cystoscopy based, in part on its vascularization; and mammography often reveals the vascularized rim of a breast tumor. In fact, a wide range of radiologic signs of cancer are based on "enhancement" of lesions by radiopaque dyes trapped in the neovasculature of a tumor. Moreover, in some tumors large central areas cannot be penetrated by radiopaque dyes because of vascular compression, a situation that is unusual in prevascular tumors.

NOT ALL TUMOR CELLS ARE ANGIOGENIC IN A VASCULARIZED TUMOR

The neovascularization of a tumor usually originates in a subset of its cells. In addition, even a highly vascularized tumor contains focal areas of high microvessel density as well as areas of low microvessel density (340). Thus, angiogenic activity is heterogeneous in many tumors. Vascularized tumors also contain a mixture of angiogenic and nonangiogenic tumor cells, as demonstrated experimentally (103) and in the following observations: (*a*) In islet cell tumors arising spontaneously in transgenic mice, only about 10% of the preneoplastic islets become angiogenic at 6 to 7 weeks of age (94). The angiogenic clusters of tumor cells then give rise to large vascularized tumors. (*b*) When multifocal fibrosarcomas arise spontaneously in transgenic mice, angiogenic activity is switched on after thin tumors have been present for a few months, but only in a subset of lesions (166). The angiogenic tumors undergo rapid expansion, while the nonangiogenic lesions remain flat and pale. (*c*) When individual tumor cells are isolated from animal tumors (such as sarcoma-180) and grown in vitro, some cells are strongly mitogenic for capillary endothelial cells, whereas other tumor cells produce little or no growth factor activity for endothelium. (*d*) In human tumors that are visible throughout their development (e.g., cutaneous melanomas), the onset of angiogenic activity appears after several years, but only in a local area of a thin, preangiogenic nevus. Neovascularization rarely envelops the entire melanoma at once. (*e*) In breast and prostate cancers, nonneovascularized as well as neovascularized carcinomas in situ can be observed in the same histologic section.

These observations further support the concept that only a subset of tumor cells acquires angiogenic activity. Based

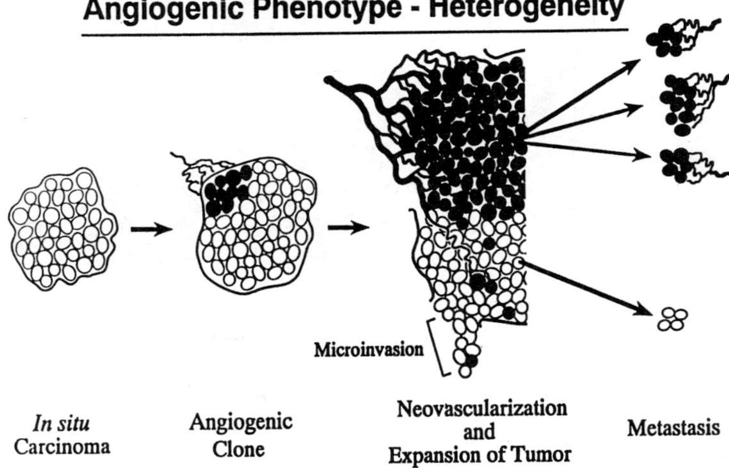

Figure 10.3. A model of how heterogeneity of the angiogenic phenotype in a primary tumor may determine whether metastases are clinically detectable. A neovascularized tumor may contain subsets of tumor cells that display the angiogenic phenotype as well as tumor cells that do not. Within a primary tumor, areas of greatest microvessel density generate greater numbers of systemically disseminated tumor cells. These metastatic cells are also more likely to express the angiogenic phenotype than tumor cells escaping from the areas with lower microvessel counts. Tumor cells that do not express the angiogenic phenotype (*open circles*) may become "dormant" micrometastases. In contrast, angiogenic tumor cells (*closed circles*) may produce rapidly growing, clinically detectable metastases. Breakdown of basement membrane and microinvasion (around a breast duct containing carcinoma) have been observed with and without neovascularization; both situations are illustrated here. *Source:* Folkman (103). Reproduced with permission.

on this model (Fig. 10.3), the vessels recruited by angiogenic tumor cells could support the growth of nonangiogenic tumor cells. Angiogenic heterogeneity among tumor cells could also provide a conceptual basis for long time periods between removal of a primary tumor and the appearance of clinically detectable metastases (e.g., 5–10 years in breast cancer).

Angiogenic Proteins Mediate Neovascularization

At least 13 positive regulators of angiogenesis have now been isolated from tumors or tissues and have been purified and sequenced (Table 10.2). Tumor angiogenesis may be mediated by one or more of these angiogenic molecules. However, basic fibroblast growth factor (bFGF) and vascular permeability factor/vascular endothelial growth factor (VPF/VEGF) have been identified in a wide spectrum of human tumors and have been studied the most extensively to date.

THE FIBROBLAST GROWTH FACTORS

Basic and acid fibroblast growth factor (bFGF and aFGF), are among the most potent of the known angiogenic proteins. They are widely distributed in normal and neoplastic tissues. Fibroblast growth factors belong to a family of related proteins for which four receptors have been identified. This is not the appropriate space for a detailed review of the biochemistry and biologic activities of the fibroblast growth factors (for a review, see Chapter 3 and reference 74).

The expression of a FGF and bFGF has been reported in a variety of different human tumors (247, 279). They lack a signal peptide and are mainly cell associated, but they are also localized in basement membranes of diverse tissues (104), where their high affinity for heparin appears to be responsible for their binding to heparan sulfate proteoglycans. An unsolved problem is how bFGF is exported from tumor cells in the absence of a signal sequence. In spontaneous tumors that arise in transgenic mice, aFGF and bFGF are exported into conditioned medium by angiogenic tumor cells, but not by preangiogenic cells in earlier stages of tumor progression (94, 166). Further, bFGF is abnormally elevated in the serum and urine of patients with many different types of cancers (see discussion under Clinical Applications of Angiogenic Principles in Cancer Patients, below). The source of these high levels of circulating and urinary bFGF is unknown. In an animal tumor transfected with a mutated bFGF that contained a signal peptide, virtually all of the urinary bFGF was exported from the tumor itself (295). However, in cancer patients, in addition to the export of bFGF from tumor cells, bFGF may also be mobilized from extracellular matrix by tumor-derived heparinases or collagenases (104, 332). As well, bFGF and other angiogenic peptides could also be released from host cells, such as macrophages, recruited into the tumor (259).

Another puzzle is why bFGF remains elevated in the serum of tumor patients when it is normally cleared within approximately 30 minutes after intravenous injection (317). The normal clearance mechanisms for bFGF (147) may be saturated or disturbed in cancer patients, but these systems remain to be studied. Circulating bFGF may be bound to soluble receptors (140). It is not known whether abnormally elevated levels of circulating bFGF maintained over prolonged periods of time may potentiate growth of dormant metastases. Endothelial cell proliferation and tumor growth were accelerated in experimental metastases when industrial strength doses of bFGF (mg/kg) were administered to the animals (134), but not when pharmacologic doses of up to 100 μg/kg were administered (243). bFGF is also abnormally elevated in the cerebrospinal fluid (CSF) of patients with different types of brain tumors (188). High bFGF levels in renal

Table 10.2. Endogenous Angiogenic Factors

Growth factor	Molecular weight	Endothelial mitogen (in vitro)[a]	Year reported	Reference[b]
Fibroblast growth factors				
Basic FGF	18,000	+	1984	283
Acidic FGF	16,400	+	1984	199
			1985	71
Angiogenin	14,100	0	1985	78
Transforming growth factor alpha	5,500	+	1986	278
Transforming growth factor beta	25,000	−	1986	267
Tumor necrosis factor alpha	17,000	−	1987	116, 187
Vascular endothelial growth factor (VPF/VEGF)	45,000	+	1983	281
			1989	51, 75, 257
Platelet-derived endothelial cell growth factor	45,000	DNA synthesis	1989	158
Granulocyte colony-stimulating factor	17,000	+	1991	44
Placental growth factor	25,000	+/0	1991	202
Interleukin 8	40,000	+	1992	178
Hepatocyte growth factor	92,000	+	1993	45, 269
Proliferin	35,000	+	1994	159

Note: TGF-β inhibits endothelial proliferation in vitro, but a focal injection in vivo stimulates angiogenesis.
[a] Symbols: + indicates stimulation; 0 indicates no effect; − indicates inhibition.
[b] The complete references may be found in Folkman (106).

carcinoma correlated with a poor outcome (225). Also, bFGF levels in the urine of children with Wilms' tumor correlated with stage of disease and tumor grade (190).

bFGF is a strong mitogen and chemotactic factor for vascular endothelial cells. It is also a mitogen for fibroblasts and smooth muscle cells and for some epithelial cells in vitro. An unresolved puzzle is that histologic sections of tumors usually reveal a predominance of capillary endothelial cell proliferation, with little fibroblast and smooth muscle proliferation. A transfected mouse sarcoma that secretes human bFGF containing a signal peptide stimulates predominantly vascular endothelial cells in vivo (149). It is not clear how such a pleiotropic growth factor as bFGF can be so relatively selective as an endothelial stimulator during tumor angiogenesis.

VASCULAR PERMEABILITY FACTOR/VASCULAR ENDOTHELIAL GROWTH FACTOR

For VPF/VEGF, the mechanism of export and the mechanism of selective stimulation of endothelial cell growth are not as problematic as for bFGF. VPF/VEGF contains a signal peptide and is secreted. At this writing it is known to be mitogenic specifically for endothelial cells in vitro, and it is angiogenic in vivo (52, 67, 76). Expression of VPF/VEGF and its receptor correlates well with blood vessel growth during embryogenesis (32, 164, 210, 253) and with angiogenesis in the female reproductive tract (286) and in tumors (40). The receptor for VPF/VEGF is restricted mainly to the endothelium of blood vessels (67, 256, 285). VPF/VEGF is also a heparin-binding protein, but, in contrast to bFGF, only two of its four forms have high heparin affinity. Of the four forms, 121, 165, 189, and 206 amino acids in length, the two higher molecular weight forms have high affinity for heparin and are not secreted. They may in fact be trapped by heparan sulfate proteoglycans on the cell surface and in the basement membrane. The two smaller forms have low heparin affinity and are secreted from tumor cells (150). The 121-amino acid form has the lowest heparin affinity and is almost completely exported as a soluble protein, whereas the 165-amino acid form of VPF/VEGF has slightly higher heparin affinity, and about 50 to 70% of it is bound to putative heparin-containing cell surface or subcellular sites in the matrix (32, 252). Thus, a signal peptide may be necessary but not sufficient for export of VPF/VEGF. The protein may also have to pass through a heparan sulfate "cage" at the cell surface. In this way, certain tumor cells that elaborate heparinases may be able to mobilize VPF/VEGF from cell surfaces and/or basement membranes. VPF/VEGF and bFGF also stimulate endothelial mitosis and chemotaxis synergistically in vitro (24, 248). Thus, tumors that export bFGF may further amplify angiogenesis by potentiating VPF/VEGF.

VPF/VEGF expression is also up-regulated by hypoxia (256, 285). Because ischemic areas usually appear during the vascular phase of tumor growth (as a result of vessel compression), the hypoxic stimulus to angiogenesis may be responsible for cyclic periods of amplified angiogenesis. Recent experimental studies suggest that a constitutive production of VPF/VEGF by tumors may be further amplified by a hypoxic stimulus in areas of ischemia (4). VPF/VEGF mRNA and protein are induced in fibroblastic and epithelial cells by transforming growth factor beta (TGF-β) (150). In contrast, mRNA for placental growth factor, an angiogenic protein related to VEGF, is not induced by TGF-β. These recent findings suggest that the angiogenic effect of TGF-β is mediated in part by its induction of VEGF in tissues. It remains to be seen whether certain human tumors will be predominantly associated with elevated levels of bFGF or VPF/VEGF (307).

ANGIOGENIN AND PLATELET-DERIVED ENDOTHELIAL CELL GROWTH FACTOR

Of interest is that two angiogenic factors, angiogenin and platelet-derived endothelial cell growth factor (PD-ECGF), are enzymes. Both are chemotactic for endothelial cells in vitro and angiogenic in vivo, but not mitogenic in vitro. Angiogenin has a unique ribonucleolytic activity that appears to be essential for its angiogenic activity (282). Angiogenin stimulates endothelial cells to form diacylglycerol (22) and to secrete prostacyclin by activating phospholipase C and phospholipase A_2, respectively (23). PD-ECGF has thymidine phosphorylase activity; 120 amino acids of human thymidine phosphorylase are identical to the sequence of PD-ECGF (119, 211). Thymidine phosphorylase and 2-deoxy-d-ribose (one of the degradation products of thymidine by thymidine phosphorylase) are both chemotactic to endothelial cells in vitro and are angiogenic in vivo (141). Angiogenin has been isolated from human colon carcinoma and from other tumors. PD-ECGF has been isolated from breast cancer and from other tumors.

Nonprotein angiogenic factors include 1-butyryl glycerol (62), the prostaglandins PGE_1 and PGE_2 (20, 112, 130) nicotinamide (183), adenosine (63), certain degradation products of hyaluronic acid (348), and the tripeptide glycine-histidine-lysine (especially when it is complexed to copper) (261).

Endogenous Inhibitors of Angiogenesis Counteract Neovascularization

It is clear that under normal conditions, vascular endothelial cells rarely proliferate and their turnover is low. However, the physiologic mechanisms that maintain this low replication rate of vascular endothelium are only now being elucidated. Regardless of how these suppressor mechanisms operate, tumors must override them in order to switch to the angiogenic phenotype. Thus, the angiogenic phenotype cannot be understood exclusively in terms of mediation by positive angiogenic factors. It represents a net balance between positive and negative regulators of angiogenesis (28, 212, 249). For this reason, many investigators are studying endothelial suppressor mechanisms. At this writing, certain components of this machinery have been elucidated, although little is known about how they integrate with each other.

Nine endothelial inhibitors are listed in Table 10.3. All except TGF-β and the soluble receptors of bFGF are known to inhibit angiogenesis as well. Some of these proteins are in the blood and others are in extracellular matrix. Several angiogenesis inhibitors are internal fragments of larger proteins, most of which themselves lack antiangiogenic activity. Four of these are generated by proteolytic cleavage. (Table 10.4).

CERTAIN ENDOTHELIAL CELL INHIBITORS CIRCULATE

Several proteins in the circulation inhibit endothelial cell proliferation and may contribute to restriction of endothelial cell growth. These include platelet factor 4 (203, 204), thrombospondin (15, 127, 222, 263, 272, 321) TGF-β, tissue inhibitors of metalloproteinases (TIMPS) (193, 201, 218), IFN-α (72, 349) and possibly a 16-kd fragment of prolactin (76). Certain angiostatic steroids, such as tetrahydrocortisol, a non-glucocorticoid, non-mineralocorticoid metabolite of cortisol, also circulate (53). Tetrahydrocortisol is lipid soluble and may be taken up by endothelial cells together with other lipids.

ENDOTHELIAL INHIBITORS ARE ALSO GENERATED BY TUMORS

In the conditioned medium of angiogenic tumor cells from transgenic mice, stimulators and inhibitors of endothelial proliferation were found together. Furthermore, a transplanted mouse tumor (Lewis lung carcinoma) was found to release the endothelial mitogen VEGF in the tumor bed, but also to release angiostatin, an inhibitor of endothelial cell proliferation, into the circulation (242). Angiostatin is not produced directly by tumor cells but appears to be cleaved from plasminogen by proteases from the tumor. Thus, our preliminary evidence suggests that the onset of angiogenesis in the tumor bed depends on an excess of positive regulators of angiogenesis in relation to negative regulators. However, in the serum, the negative regulators may accumulate in excess of positive regulators, because of the accelerated clearance of most endothelial mitogens from the circulation. We propose that in those primary tumors which

Table 10.3. Endogenous Negative Regulators of Endothelial Proliferation

Regulator	Inhibits proliferation	Inhibits chemotaxis	In circulation	In extracellular matrix	Reference
Platelet factor 4	+	+	+	−	203, 204, 312
Thrombospondin	+	+	+	+	263, 272
Tissue inhibitors of metalloproteinases (TIMP)	+/0	+	+	+	Murphy et al., 218
16-kd fragment of prolactin	+				49a
Angiostatin (38-kd fragment of plasminogen)	+	+			241
bFGF soluble receptor	+		+		140
Tranforming growth factor beta	+	+	+		267
Interferon alpha	+	+	+		287
Placental proliferin-related protein	+				159

Note: All are angiogenesis inhibitors in vivo except TGF-β. bFGF receptor has not been tested in vivo as an angiogenesis inhibitor. TIMP-2 inhibits proliferation and chemotaxis; TIMP-1 and TIMP-3 do not. TIMP-1 and TIMP-2 circulate and TIMP-3 is in the extracellular matrix.
Symbols: + indicates stimulation; 0 indicates no effect; − indicates inhibition.

Table 10.4. Endogenous Inhibitors That Are Fragments of Larger Proteins

Protein fragment	Molecular weight (kd)	Year reported	Reference[a]
Fibronectin[a]	29	1985	146a
Prolactin[a]	16	1993	49a
Thrombospondin (fragment)	140	1993	321
Angiostatin[a]	38	1994	241
SPARC fragment	4.2	1995	272a
Platelet factor 4 (fragment)[a]	7.8	1995	137
Murine EGF (fragment 33–42)	—	1995	225a

[a] Produced by proteolytic cleavage from parent protein.

suppress the growth of their metastases (260), circulating inhibitors of angiogenesis may be responsible for inhibiting metastatic growth. Indeed, when tumor cells arising from transformed hamster cells switch to the angiogenic phenotype, they may first have to down-regulate their production of thrombospondin, an angiogenesis inhibitor (28, 263).

AN ENDOTHELIAL INHIBITOR IN NORMAL TISSUES IS KNOWN TO BE UNDER THE CONTROL OF A TUMOR SUPPRESSOR GENE

Dameron et al. (Bouck) proposed that thrombospondin may normally be under the control of the p53 tumor suppressor gene (56). They studied fibroblasts from cancer-prone patients with the Li-Fraumeni syndrome. These fibroblasts contain only one allele of p53. The cells are immortal in vitro but not tumorigenic or angiogenic in vivo. After repeated passage in culture, they lose the remaining allele of p53 and become angiogenic and tumorigenic, with concomitant down-regulation of thrombospondin synthesis to approximately 4% of the parental cells. The cells could be rescued from the angiogenic phenotype by transfection with p53 or with thrombospondin. Dameron et al. concluded that wild-type p53, in addition to its many other functions (56), may negatively regulate angiogenic activity in Li-Fraumeni cells by ensuring that they produce a high level of antiangiogenic thrombospondin. In a similar study by different investigators, a glioblastoma cell line was made conditionally inducible for p53. When wild-type p53 was expressed in this cell line, it elaborated an inhibitor of angiogenesis that was not thrombospondin (325, 326). It is known that the IFN-α gene complex is deleted in certain cancers of the bladder (300), in some leukemias (61), in melanoma, and in other tumors. Because IFN-α is an angiogenesis inhibitor, it is possible that the IFN-α gene complex may be acting as an angiogenesis suppressor gene, similar to p53. Whether other tumor suppressor genes code for angiogenesis inhibitor proteins remains speculative at this time.

HOST CELLS AND EXTRACELLULAR MATRIX ALSO CONTRIBUTE TO PHYSIOLOGIC SUPPRESSION OF ENDOTHELIAL CELL GROWTH

Endothelial growth factors are sequestered. One mechanism that restricts endothelial growth is that certain endothelial mitogens such as aFGF and bFGF lack a signal peptide and remain cell associated. Endothelial mitogens are also made inaccessible to endothelial cells by being sequestered in basement membrane or on the surface of producer cells themselves. The greater the heparin affinity of an angiogenic peptide, the more likely it is to be retained in basement membrane or on the cell surface.

Endothelial Cell Shape Can Cause Unresponsiveness to Growth Factors

Endothelial cell proliferation is tightly controlled by endothelial cell shape, and this provides another mechanism of growth control (156, 157, 291). Thus, bFGF is switched from a potent mitogen for vascular endothelial cells to a nonmitogenic differentiation factor when these cells are foreshortened (to 500–700 μm^2) from a prior elongated configuration (>3,000 μm^2) in vitro. This may partly explain why early vessel dilation appears to be a prerequisite for DNA synthesis during formation of coronary collaterals, in retinal vessels of the diabetic, and in the postcapillary venules that give rise to neovascularization in a tumor bed.

Normal Host Cells Can Inhibit Endothelial Cell Proliferation

A third mechanism of endothelial growth control is inhibition by close contact with other cells. Two cell types that have been studied to date elaborate endothelial inhibitor proteins that act over short distances.

Pericytes inhibit endothelial cell proliferation in vitro by transforming growth factor beta (TGF-β). Pericytes and capillary endothelial cells in vitro release a latent form of TGF-β into the medium. However, close contact of the cells activates TGF-β, which inhibits proliferation of endothelial cells (6, 273, 274). It is not clear whether this mechanism operates in vivo. However, diabetic retinal neovascularization is often associated with pericyte dropout. Angiogenesis in some tumors is also accompanied by a paucity of pericytes, but other tumors induce capillaries rich in pericytes (277).

Fibroblasts in certain tissues appear to inhibit endothelial growth by releasing IFN-β. Singh et al. (289) showed that human renal carcinomas or colon carcinomas would grow poorly or not at all when transplanted into subcutaneous tissue of athymic mice, but would produce large tumors when transplanted into the kidney capsule or the colon wall. They discovered that these "orthotopic" tumor transplants grew well because of the relative lack of IFN-β in kidney and colon (290). In contrast, skin fibroblasts and keratinocytes produced high levels of IFN-β. They (290) further found that IFN-α and -β down-regulate mRNA and protein synthesis of aFGF and bFGF in human tumor cells and that the human colon and kidney tumors produced bFGF as an angiogenic mediator. In the subcutaneous space, these tumors were not neovascularized and their growth was inhibited. In the kidney subcapsule or in the colon these tumors were highly neovascularized. IFN-α has previously been shown to inhibit endothelial migration in vitro (38) and angiogenesis in vivo (68, 287). Thus, fibroblasts may be heterogeneous for interferon production, depending on their tissue location.

Clinical Applications of Angiogenic Principles in Cancer Patients

Both diagnostic and therapeutic studies and clinical trials in cancer patients are under way, based on applications of angiogenesis research.

INTENSITY OF TUMOR VASCULARIZATION CAN BE USED AS A PROGNOSTIC INDICATOR FOR CERTAIN TUMORS

Quantification of the intensity of angiogenesis in a biopsy specimen at the initial diagnosis of cancer may help to predict the risk of future metastases or recurrence. For example, quantitation of angiogenesis (microvessel density) in histologic specimens of invasive breast cancer provided an indicator of the risk of metastasis (340). Multivariate analysis showed that microvessel density in lymph node–negative breast cancer patients was a better predictor of metastasis than tumor grade, tumor size, estrogen receptor positivity, or other prognostic markers (341). This result has now been independently confirmed in several centers (17, 27, 114, 120, 121, 136, 148, 235, 319, 331) and by a 5-year prospective study (120). A positive association between tumor angiogenesis and risk of metastasis, tumor recurrence, or death has also been reported for a variety of other tumor types (2, 18, 31, 73, 117, 122, 131, 145, 160, 188, 196, 197, 208, 239, 271, 298, 299, 323, 329, 335, 342–344, 356); 35 published reports have demonstrated the association between angiogenesis and outcome and 5 reports have not (14a, 46, 138, 186, 324) (for a review, see Reference [343]).

Perhaps microvessel density predicts metastatic risk because areas of high microvessel density increase the vascular surface area, thus facilitating escape of tumor cells into the circulation (103, 345).

An angiogenic tumor cell shed from a primary tumor is more likely than a nonangiogenic cell to develop into a detectable metastasis. Tumor cells that are not angiogenic may become dormant micrometastases (102, 146) until they themselves eventually switch to the angiogenic phenotype (Fig. 10.3).

ANGIOGENIC PROTEINS CAN BE ACCURATELY QUANTIFIED IN BLOOD AND URINE

Quantification of angiogenic proteins in the blood and urine of cancer patients may measure progression of disease and guide therapy. Based on detection of endothelial cell stimulators in the urine of cancer patients (49), an immunoassay for bFGF (337) was developed that revealed elevated levels of the angiogenic protein in the serum of patients with renal cell carcinoma (118). High levels of bFGF were subsequently found in the serum of approximately 10% of a wide spectrum of cancer patients (338) and in the urine of more than 37% of cancer patients (234).

Biologically active bFGF was abnormally elevated in the CSF of children with brain tumors but in no children with hydrocephalus or malignant disease outside of the CNS (188). The bFGF level in CSF correlated with microvessel density in histologic sections, which itself provided a prognostic indicator of risk of mortality.

In infants with hemangiomas, urinary bFGF levels are also abnormally elevated and return toward normal with involution of the lesions. In life-threatening hemangiomas treated with IFN-α-2A (see below), quantification of urine bFGF has been a useful way of determining an effective dose and of differentiating between hemangioma and vascular malformation (Folkman et al., unpublished observations).

In some tumors, tissue levels of angiogenic proteins have correlated with severity of disease or outcome. Immunohistochemical levels of bFGF in renal carcinoma correlated with the risk of death (225). Bladder cancer expressing high levels of VEGF was found to be more invasive and more metastatic than bladder cancer expressing lower levels (236). However, it should not be a surprise if this association between tumor expression of a single angiogenic protein and disease outcome were found not to hold up for a wide variety of tumors, because tumor neovascularization and its intensity are dictated by a net balance in proteins that stimulate or inhibit microvessel growth.

ANGIOGENESIS INHIBITORS ARE UNDERGOING CLINICAL TRIALS

Antiangiogenic therapy in humans began in 1988. Of the more than 20 angiogenesis inhibitors that have been reported (10), at least 9 are currently in clinical trial. Some of these are discussed below.

IFN-α-2A for Life-Threatening or Sight-Threatening Hemangiomas

Hemangiomas consist of rapidly proliferating capillary blood vessels. They are the most common tumor of infancy, appearing in 1 to 2% of neonates (220), and in 22% of premature infants with a birth weight below 1,000 g (29). They grow rapidly for the first 8 to 12 months of life (the proliferating phase), slow down, and then gradually regress over the next 1 to 5 years (the involuting phase) (304). In over 70% of children, hemangiomas regress completely by age 7, and in the remaining children, regression continues up to age 10 to 12 years (167). Most hemangiomas do not need treatment. However, approximately 10% cause serious tissue damage, interfere with a vital organ, or are life-threatening because they obstruct the airway, produce high-output heart failure, or cause platelet-trapping thrombocytopenic coagulopathy (Kasabach-Merritt syndrome, associated with a 30–50% mortality) (69, 70). Hepatic hemangiomas have a mortality rate of 30 to 50% (70). Approximately 30% of hemangiomas respond dramatically to corticosteroid therapy and begin to regress in several days to 1 week; 40% respond equivocally; 30% do not respond at all (70); and rarely, hemangiomatous growth is accelerated. When corticosteroids fail there are no dependable, safe, and effective treatment alternatives for life-threatening hemangiomas, although there are anecdotal reports of favorable outcomes from irradiation (275), cyclophosphamide (5, 151), and embolization (7, 301). Now a new alternative treatment is under investigation—IFN-α-2A.

The discovery that IFN-α-2A was antiangiogenic (38, 68, 287) led in 1988 to its successful use in treating a life-threatening pulmonary hemangioma in a 7-year-old child (349). Results of other case studies with IFN-α were also encouraging (240, 350). In a study of infants and children with life-threatening or sight-threatening hemangiomas or large tissue–destructive hemangiomas, we found that IFN-α-2A therapy accelerated hemangioma regression in 18 of 20 patients (72). Others have reported similar results (24, 25, 195, 206, 221, 238, 266, 296, 330) and have found INF-α-2A especially useful for airway hemangiomas beyond the reach of laser therapy (238). It is unclear why some hemangiomas are unresponsive to both steroid and interferon therapy, although biopsies in some refractory cases have identified Kaposi's-like hemangiomas, and one failure of interferon therapy may have been due to insufficient dose (59). Large, endangering hemangiomas require IFN-α-2A therapy for an average of 6 to 10 months. During the first few weeks of successful IFN-α-2A therapy, hemangioma growth decreases; during the next 1 to 2 months growth stops, and during the next 9 to 14 months the lesion involutes (approximately 5–10 years before involution would occur naturally). Hemangioma regression with IFN-α-2A is less dramatic than in cases in which the lesion is highly responsive to corticosteroids.

IFN-α-2A is less toxic in infants and children than in adults, and its toxic effects are reversible. These effects include fever, transient neutropenia, anemia, and elevation of liver enzyme levels (72). Most infants taking IFN-α-2A seem to gain weight and grow normally in contrast to infants on prolonged corticosteroid therapy. A more problematic possible adverse reaction is increased motor tone of the lower extremities that has been reported in some children receiving interferon for laryngeal papillomas (330). We currently advise neurologic-developmental evaluation before beginning interferon therapy and periodic assessments during and after therapy. Combining corticosteroids and IFN-α-2A therapy has shown no advantage and may increase toxicity.

IFN-α-2B has also been used successfully (195), although one failure has been reported (316).

AGM-1470 (TNP-470)

In 1985, Donald Ingber in my laboratory discovered that a fungal contaminant, *Aspergillus fumigatus fresenius*, inhibited growth of capillary endothelial cells in culture (154). The active compound secreted by the fungus was found to be fumagillin, an old amebicide. It inhibited endothelial proliferation in vitro and angiogenesis in vivo, but was toxic. A synthetic analogue of fumagillin, angiogenesis modulator-1470 (AGM-1470), was a more potent angiogenesis inhibitor than the parent compound and was nontoxic (154, 184, 305, 306, 310). Systemic administration of AGM-1470 inhibited ocular angiogenesis in the rabbit and inhibited tumors in mice, rats, and rabbits (including human tumors in athymic mice) with little or no toxicity (354, 357–359). Picomolar concentrations of AGM-1470 specifically inhibited proliferating endothelial cells, but concentrations 100- to 10,000-fold higher were required to inhibit growth of most tumor cells. AGM-1470 apears to be rapidly cleared from the blood (80).

In 1992, phase I clinical trials commenced with AGM-1470 (also called TNP-470 [Takeda neoplastic product–470]) in patients with cancer and Kaposi's sarcoma. FDA-approved dose-escalation studies then began for AIDS-associated Kaposi's sarcoma and were extended to the treatment of metastatic carcinoma of the prostate and cervix and other solid tumors. Therapy is administered intravenously for 1 hour every other day.

Platelet Factor 4

During a study of the antiangiogenic properties of protamine, we found that platelet factor 4 inhibited angiogenesis (312). Both natural and recombinant human platelet factor 4 (184, 203, 204) inhibit endothelial proliferation in vitro and suppress angiogenesis in the chick chorioallantoic membrane. The growth of human colon cancer in nude mice and the growth of murine melanoma are inhibited significantly by intralesional administration of platelet factor 4. In contrast, these tumor cells are refractory to platelet factor 4 administered in vitro at concentrations that inhibit endothelial proliferation. Systemic administration has shown virtually no toxicity in mice. This peptide is undergoing phase I/II clinical trials for the treatment of Kaposi's sarcoma, melanoma, renal cell carcinoma, and colon cancer at four different centers in the United States. Therapeutic systemic doses, however, have not been optimized and may be higher than predicted on the basis of intralesional efficacy because the peptide is cleared from the circulation within minutes. One phase I/II study of AIDS-related Kaposi's sarcoma in which platelet factor 4 is being administered intralesionally has demonstrated safety and possible efficacy, and the agent warrants further study in an expanded population of patients. Recently a more potent fragment of platelet factor 4 was reported (137).

Carboxyaminotriazole

Carboxyaminotriazole inhibits signal transduction and blocks ligand-stimulated calcium influx (179, 180). It inhibits endothelial proliferation stimulated by bFGF, tube formation in vitro, and angiogenesis in the chick chorioallantoic membrane, and tumor growth and pulmonary metastases in mice. In a phase I clinical trial of 28 patients with pancreatic or ovarian carcinoma treated with oral carboxyaminotriazole for up to 5 to 7 months, 50% have had a cytostatic response (145).

Metalloproteinase Inhibitor BB94

BB94 (British Biotechnology 94) is a synthetic, low molecular weight inhibitor of matrix metalloproteinases. When administered by intraperitoneal injection to mice carrying a xenograft of human ovarian carcinoma, it markedly prolonged survival (351). In all treated mice, the only remaining tumor at autopsy consisted of small avascular nodules containing foci of tumor cells encapsulated by stromal tissue from the host. BB94 administered intraperitoneally is being evaluated in a phase I/II dose-escalation study of patients with malignant ascites from ovarian carcinoma (19). An oral form of this inhibitor, BB2516, is just beginning clinical trial.

Sulfated Polysaccharides

Tecogalen (DS4152), a low molecular weight peptidoglycan extracted from the bacterial wall of the bacterium *Arthrobacter*, appears to inhibit angiogenesis by interfering with binding of bFGF to endothelial cells. It is currently being evaluated in a phase I clinical trial for the treatment of refractory malignancies, including breast, lung, and head and neck cancers and, sarcoma and is administered intravenously every 21 days (322). It also is being evaluated in a phase I study for the treatment of AIDS-related Kaposi's sarcoma (162). It is administered intravenously. In addition to its antiangiogenic activity in vivo, it also has antitumor activity in vitro and in vivo.

Linomide

Quinoline-3-carboxamide (linomide) has a broad spectrum of antitumor activity against experimental solid tumors in vivo but is not cytotoxic in vitro. Its antitumor activity was initially thought to be solely by immunomodulation, but recent studies have shown that it inhibits angiogenesis in vivo (334). When administered in drinking water to mice carrying tumors in transparent skin chambers, linomide reduces capillary density by 40% and inhibits tumor growth by 60% (164). It is being used in the treatment of renal cancer and other tumors.

Thalidomide

Thalidomide, a sedative with anti-inflammatory activity, was recently discovered to inhibit angiogenesis when administered orally to rabbits (55). The antiangiogenic activity suggests a possible explanation for thalidomide's teratogenic effects in early pregnancy. Thalidomide is currently in phase II clinical trials for the treatment of recurrent brain tumors, other solid tumors, and retinal neovascularization due to macular degeneration.

Other Compounds with Possible Therapeutic Efficacy

It has recently been reported that the antibiotic minocycline is effective in arthritis (135). Minocycline is also known to inhibit angiogenesis (123, 246) and, although less potent than other inhibitors, it has a synergistic effect on other angiogenesis inhibitors and on conventional cytotoxic agents used to treat animal tumors (313). Thus, its antiangiogenic properties may contribute to its effectiveness in arthritis.

Interleukin-12. In addition to its cytotoxic properties, mediated by T-cell activation, interleukin-12 also potently inhibits angiogenesis (333). Interleukin-12 induces the up-regulation of interferon gamma, which itself up-regulates the protein IP-10 (inducible protein 10). Thus, interleukin 12 may inhibit angiogenesis through an indirect pathway that depends on a cascade of proteins.

GUIDELINES FOR ANTIANGIOGENIC THERAPY DIFFER FROM GUIDELINES FOR ANTIPROLIFERATIVE CHEMOTHERAPY

Preclinical studies in mice, rats, rabbits, and monkeys, early clinical trials of antiangiogenic therapy, and recent clinical experience with interferon treatment for hemangioma point to important principles of antiangiogenic therapy that may be useful in the future management of patients with cancer.

First, antiangiogenic therapy is directed mainly at a small focus of migrating and proliferating capillary endothelial cells. Thus, a specific angiogenesis inhibitor is not likely to cause bone marrow suppression, gastrointestinal symptoms, or hair loss. This is not to say that such drugs would have no other actions and would not produce side effects.

Second, optimal antiangiogenic therapy appears to require treatment for months to a year or more, without a break. Angiogenesis inhibitors generally down-regulate neovascularization by inhibiting endothelial cell proliferation and migration, not by a cytotoxic effect on endothelial cells. Regression or involution of a vigorously growing capillary bed is a slower process than lysis of tumor cells. Thus, in the design of clinical trials, angiogenic therapy may need to be given longer periods without a break than conventional cytotoxic agents.

Third, resistance to angiogenesis inh bitors has not been a major problem in long-term animal studies (33) or in clinical trials to date. Babies with large hemangiomas of the mediastinum or liver who were treated with INF-α2A daily for up to a year did not develop drug resistance. Of interest, antiangiogenic therapy has been proposed as a strategy to circumvent acquired resistance to anticancer agents (173).

Fourth, a combination of antiangiogenic and cytotoxic therapy may be more effective than either type alone. In tumor-bearing animals, such combinations can be curative, whereas either agent alone is only inhibitory (313–315). An angiogenesis inhibitor such as AGM1470 (TNP-470) can significantly decrease DNA synthesis in endothelial cells in a tumor bed, whereas cytotoxic agents such as Adriamycin and cisplatin do not (353). These results suggest that therapy directed against both the endothelial cell and the tumor cell compartments of a tumor is more effective than therapy directed only against tumor cells. Radiotherapy is also potentiated by antiangiogenic therapy in tumor-bearing animals, in part by decreasing tumor hypoxia (314).

The Future Use of Angiogenesis Inhibitors May Be in Combination with Conventional Anticancer Therapy

Preclinical studies suggest two potential roles for angiogenesis inhibitors in the treatment of cancer patients, independent of tumor type: angiogenesis inhibitors could be used to potentiate conventional chemotherapy and radiotherapy; and, after conventional therapy, when patients enter a remission, antiangiogenic therapy might maintain metastases in a microscopic dormant state, analogous to dormant viral infection without disease (e.g., herpes zoster). Such "dormancy therapy" has already been demonstrated in animals, who can be maintained in excellent health despite dormant micrometastases in their lungs (102, 146, 241). The long-term use of antiangiogenic therapy in humans may be similar to the paradigm for the use of low-dose methotrexate for 7 to 10 years in patients with severe psoriasis, or to the use of tamoxifen for many years to prevent recurrence of breast cancer, or to the long-term use of finasteride for benign prostatic hypertrophy.

ANTIANGIOGENIC THERAPY MAY BE ADDED TO THE TREATMENT OF CHILDHOOD LEUKEMIA

There is recent evidence that leukemias may also respond to angiogenesis inhibitors. We have found that in more than 1,000 cancer patients who have abnormal elevations of the angiogenic peptide bFGF in the urine, the leukemias have some of the highest levels (i.e., up to 200 times normal). Brunner et al. (42) showed that human hematapoietic cells express high levels of bFGF, a potent endothelial cell mitogen. Release of bFGF from bone marrow cultures has also been reported (41). Moreover, vascular endothelial cells can release G-CSF (a mitogen for marrow cells) (363). There is indirect evidence that leukemic cells stimulate bone marrow endothelium and neovascularization to support their own growth before being released into the peripheral circulation. We recently studied 61 bone marrow biopsies of 40 children with acute lymphoblastic leukemia (251). The blood vessels were highlighted by staining histologic sections with antibody to von Willebrand factor and counted according to the method described by Weidner (344). There was a statistically significant increase (>6-fold) in microvessel density (neovascularization) in all leukemic patients as compared to normal controls. Urinary bFGF was also markedly increased in all leukemic children at the time of diagnosis. Microvessel count did not correlate with relapse rate, but there were too few relapses in this study to draw statistical conclusions. Nevertheless, preliminary results such as these suggest that the growth of leukemic cells in the bone marrow may also be angiogenesis dependent. At this writing, an FDA-approved phase I clinical trial of the angiogenesis inhibitor TNP-470 (see above) has been initiated at the Dana Farber Cancer Center for children who have had a second relapse.

Summary and Future Directions

An important lesson from angiogenesis research is to think about a tumor as containing two cell compartments that stimulate each other: the endothelial cell compartment and the tumor cell compartment (Fig. 10.4). Anticancer therapy may be more efficacious if each compartment is treated by drugs that selectively target each cell type. The mutational rate is high in the tumor cell compartment and low in the endothelial cell compartment. This is the reason why it may be possible to employ antiangiogenic therapy for the long term, together with conventional chemotherapy and subsequently in the postchemotherapy period.

The field of angiogenesis research, which began as an inquiry into the mechanisms by which tumors induce a new blood supply, has now broadened to include a diverse group of disciplines. For example, the development of the vascular system itself is being explored. Genes that turn angiogenesis on or that suppress angiogenic activity are being elucidated. Angiogenic molecules are being employed to accelerate the healing of surgical wounds and peptic ulcers. Angiogenesis inhibitors intended for eventual anticancer therapy are also being studied for their potential use in ocular angiogenesis, arthritis, and other nonneoplastic diseases.

These developments in fields parallel to oncology may bring new information to bear on the problem of tumor angiogenesis. We need to understand how tumors become angiogenic, and what angiogenic molecules they employ. It will be important to know how these molecules are released, whether specific angiogenic molecules are produced by certain type of tumors, and how angiogenesis suppressor activity is downregulated during tumor progression. It is still not clear what percentage of tumor-induced angiogenesis

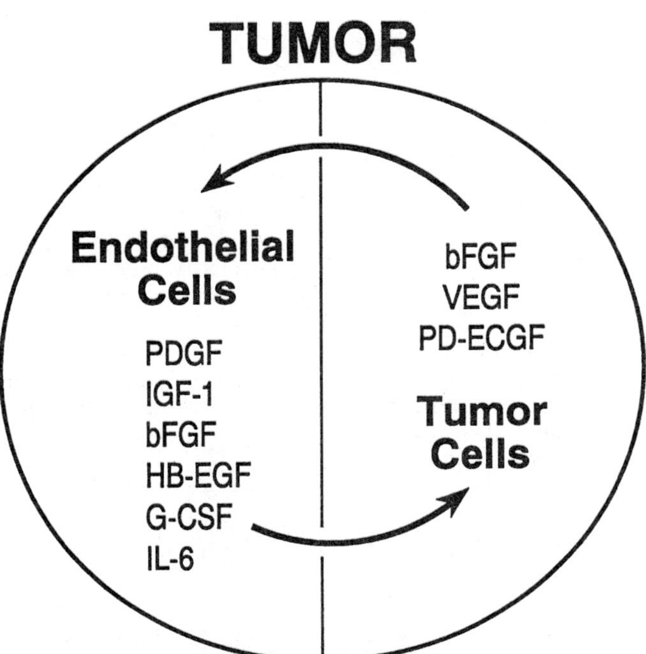

Figure 10.4. The two-cell compartment model of a tumor. Tumor cells export endothelial mitogens such as basic fibroblast growth factor (bFGF), vascular endothelial cell growth factor (VEGF), and platelet-derived endothelial cell growth factor (PD-ECGF). Endothelial cells release factors that can stimulate proliferation or motility of tumor cells. Among these factors are platelet-derived growth factor (PDGF), insulin-like growth factor 1 (IGF-1), bFGF, heparin-binding epithelial growth factor (HB-EGF), granulocyte colony-stimulating factor (G-CSF), and interleukin-6.

must be blocked before tumor growth is inhibited, nor is it known if endothelial cells can become "resistant" to angiogenesis inhibitors.

Beyond these considerations lie questions for the more distant future. Can the onset of angiogenic activity be detected in the blood or other body fluids for use in diagnosis? Can the process of angiogenesis itself be manipulated by genetic therapies, for example by administration of antisense DNA? These questions and others provide the basis for continuing excitement in the field of angiogenesis research.

Acknowledgments

I thank Wendy Foss and Pauline Breen for help with the typing and references. I thank the National Cancer Institute for many years of grant support for the studies reviewed here.

References

1. Adam JA, Maggelakis AA. Diffusion of regulated growth characteristics of a spherical prevascular carcinoma. Bull Math Biol 1990;52:549–582
2. Albo D, Granick MS, Jhala N, Atkinson B, Solomon MP. The relationship of angiogenesis to biological activity in human squamous cell carcinomas of the head and neck. Ann Plas Surg 1994;32:588–94.
3. Algire GH, Chalkely HW, Legallais FY, Park H. Vascular reactions of normal and malignant tumors in vivo: I. Vascular reactions of mice to wounds and to normal and neoplastic transplants. JNCI 1945;6:73–85.
4. Alon T, Hemo I, Itin A, Pe'er J, Stone J, Keshet E. Vascular endothelial growth factor acts as a survival factor for newly formed retinal vessels and has implications for retinopathy of prematurity. Nature Med 1995;1:1024–1028.
5. al-Rashid RA. Cyclophosphamide and radiation therapy in the treatment of hemangioendothelioma with disseminated intravascular clotting. Cancer 1971;27:364–368.
6. Antonelli-Orlidge, Saunders KB, Smith SR, D'Amore P. An activated form of transforming growth factor-β is produced by co-cultures of endothelial cells and pericytes. Proc Natl Acad Sci USA 1989;86:4544–4548.
7. Argenta LC, Bishop E, Cho KJ, Andrews AF, Coran AG. Complete resolution of life-threatening hemangioma by embolization and corticosteroids. Plas Reconstr Surg 1982;70:739–744.
8. Auerbach R, Arensman R, Kubai L, Folkman J. Tumor-induced angiogenesis: lack by irradiation. Int J Cancer 1975;15:241–245.
9. Auerbach R, Kubai L, Knighton D, Folkman J. A simple procedure for the long-term cultivation of chicken embryos. Dev Biol 1974;41:391–394
10. Auerbach W, Auerbach R. Angiogenesis inhibition: a review. Pharmacol Ther 1994;63:265–311.
11. Auerbach R. Angiogenesis-inducing factors: a review. In: Lymphokines. Edited by E Pick. London: Academic, 1981, vol 4, pp 69–88
12. Ausprunk DH, Folkman J. Migration and proliferation of endothelial cells in preformed and newly formed blood vessels during tumor angiogenesis. Microvasc Res 1977;15: 53–65.
13. Ausprunk DH. Distribution of hyaluronic acid and sulfated glycosaminoglycans during blood vessel development in the chick chorioallantoic membrane. Am J Anat 1986;177:313–331.
14. Ausprunk DH, Dethlefsen SM, Higgins ER. Distribution of fibronectin, laminin and type IV collagen during development of blood vessels in the chick chorioallantoic membrane. In The Development of the Vascular System. Edited by RN Fineberg, GK Sherer, R Averbach. Basel: S Karger, 1990, pp 93–108.

14a. Axelsson K, Ljung B-ME, Moore DH, Thor AD, Chew KL, Edgerton SM, Smith HS, Mayall BH. Tumor angiogenesis as a prognostic assay for invasive ductal breast carcinoma. JNCI 1995;87:997–1008

15. Bagavandoss P, Kaytes P, Vogeli G, Wells PA, Wilks JW. Recombinant truncated thrombospondin-1 monomer modulates endothelial cell plasminogen activator inhibitor 1 accumulation and proliferation in vitro. Biochem Biophys Res Commun 1993;192:325–332.

15a. Baird A, Durkin T. Inhibition of endothelial cell proliferation by type beta-transforming growth factor: Interactions with acidic and basic fibroblast growth factors. Biochem Biophys Res Commun 1986;138:476–482.

16. Barbareschi M, Gasparini G, Weidner N, et al. Microvessel density quantification in breast carcinomas: assessment by light microscopy vs. a computer-aided image analysis system. App Immunohistochem 1995;3:75–84.
17. Barbareschi M, Gasparini G, Morelli L, Forti S, Dalla Palma P. Novel methods for the determination of the angiogenic activity of human tumors. Breast Cancer Res Treat 1995;36:181–192.
18. Barnhill RL, Fandrey K, Levy MA, Mihm MC Jr, Hyman B. Angiogenesis and tumor progression of melanoma. Quantification of vascularity in melanocytic nevi and cutaneous malignant melanoma. Lab Invest 1992;67:332–337.
19. Beattie GJ, Young HA, Smyth JF. Phase I study of intra-peritoneal metallo-proteinase inhibitor BB94 in patients with malignant ascites. Ann Oncol 1995;5:72. Abstract.
20. Ben Ezra D. Neovasculogenic ability of prostaglandins, growth factors and synthetic chemoattractants. Am J Ophthalmol 1978;86:455–461.
21. Bevilacqua P, Barbareschi M, Verderio P, et al. Prognostic value of intratumoral microvessel density, a measure of tumor angiogenesis, in node-negative breast carcinoma: results of a multiparametric study. Breast Cancer Res Treat 1995;36:205–217.
22. Bicknell R, Vallee BL. Angiogenin activates endothelial cell phospholipase C. Proc Natl Acad Sci USA 1988;85:5961–5965.
23. Bicknell R, Vallee BL. Angiogenin stimulates endothelial cell prostacyclin secretion by activation of phospholipase A_2. Proc Natl Acad Sci USA 1989;86:1573–1577.
24. Blei F, Orlow SJ, Geronemus RG. Supraumbilical micabdominal raphe, sternal atresia, and hemangioma in an infant: response of hemangioma to laser and interferon alfa-2a. Pediatr Dermatol 1993;10:71–76.
25. Blei F, Orlow SJ, Geronemus RG. Interferon alfa-2a therapy for extensive perianal and lower extremity hemangioma. J Am Acad Dermatol 1993;23:98–99.
26. Blood CH, Zetter BR. Tumor interactions with the vasculature: angiogenesis and tumor metastasis. Biochem Biophys Acta 1990;1032:89–118.
27. Bosari S, Lee AK DeLellis RA, Wiley BD, Heatley GH, Silverman ML. Microvessel quantitation and prognosis in invasive breast carcinoma. Hum Pathol 1992;23: 755–761.
28. Bouck N. Tumor angiogenesis: The role of oncogenes and tumor suppressor genes. Cancer Cells 1990;2:179–185.
29. Bowers RE, Graham EA, Tominson KM. The natural history of the strawberry nevus. Arch Dermatol 1960;82:667–680.
30. Boxberger HJ, Paweletz N, Spiess E, Kriehuber R. An in vitro model study of BSp73 rat tumour cell invasion into endothelial monolayer. Anticancer Res 1989;9: 1777–1786.
31. Brawer MD, Keering RE, Brown M, Preston SD, Bigler SA. Predictors of pathologic stage in prostatic carcinoma. Cancer 1994;73:678–687.
32. Breier G, Albrecht U, Sterrer S, Risau W. Expression of vascular endothelial growth factor during embryonic angiogenesis and endothelial cell differentiation. Development 1992;114:521–532.
33. Brem H, Goto F, Budson A, Saunders L, Folkman J. Minimal drug resistance after prolonged antiangiogenic therapy with AGM-1470. Surg Forum 1994;45:674–677.
34. Brem S, Brem H, Folkman J, Finkelstein D, Patz A. Prolonged tumor dormancy by prevention of neovascularization in the vitreous. Cancer Res 1976;36:2807–2812.
35. Brem S, Cotran R, Folkman J. Tumor angiogenesis: a quantitative method for histologic grading. JNCI 1972;48:347–356.
36. Brooks PC, Montgomery AMP, Rosenfeld M, Reisfeld RA, Hut T, Klier G, Cheresh DA. Integrin $\alpha_v\beta_3$ antagonists promote tumor regression by inducing apoptosis of angiogenic blood vessels. Cell 1994;79:1157–1164.
37. Brooks PC, Clark RAF, Cheresh D. Requirement of vascular integrin $\alpha_v\beta_3$ for angiogenesis. Science 1994;264:569–571.
38. Brouty-Boye D, Zetter BR. Inhibition of cell motility by interferon. Science 1980;208: 516–58.
39. Browder T. Personal communication.
40. Brown LF, Berse B, Jackman RW, et al. Increased expression of vascular permeability factor (vascular endothelial growth factor) and its receptors in kidney and bladder carcinomas. Am J Pathol 1993;143:1255–1262.
41. Brunner G, Metz CN, Nguyen H, Gabrilove J, Patel SR, Davitz MA, Rifkin DB, Wilson EL. An endogenous glycosylphosphatidylinositol-specific phospholipase D releases basic fibroblast growth factor–heparan sulfate proteoglycan complexes from human bone marrow cultures. Blood 1994;83:2115–2125.
42. Brunner G, Nguyen H, Gabrilove J, Rifkin DB, Wilson EL. Basic fibroblast growth factor expression in human bone marrow and peripheral blood cells. Blood 1993;81: 631–638.
43. Burger PC, Chandler DB, Klintworth GK. Corneal neovascularization as studied by scanning electron microscopy. Lab Invest 1983;48:169–180.
44. Bussolino F, Ziche M, Wang JM, et al. In vitro and in vivo activation of endothelial cells by colony stimulating factors. J Clin Invest 1991;87:986–995.
45. Bussolino F, Di Renzo MF, Ziche M, et al. Hepatocyte growth factor is a potent angiogenic factor which stimulates endothelial cell motility and growth. J Cell Biol 1992;119:629–641.
46. Carnochan P, Briggs JC, Westbury G, Davies AJ. The vascularity of cutaneous melanoma: a quantitative histology study of lesions 0.85–1.25 mm in thickness. Br J Cancer 1991;64:102–107.
47. Castellot J, Karnovsky M, Spiegelman B. Differentiation-dependent stimulation of neovascularization and endothelial cell chemotaxis by 3T3 adipocytes. Proc Natl Acad Sci USA 1982;79:5597–5601.
48. Chen C, Parangi S, Tolentino MJ, Folkman J. A strategy to discover circulating angiogenesis inhibitors generated by human tumors. Cancer Res 1995;55:4230–4233.
49. Chodak GW, Hospelhorn V, Judge SM, Mayforth R, Koeppen H, Sasse J. Increased levels of fibroblast growth factor-like activity in urine from patients with bladder or kidney cancer. Cancer Res 1988;48:2083–2088.

49a. Clapp C, Martial JA, Guzman RC, Rentier-Delure F, Weiner RI. The 16-kilodalton *N*-terminal fragment of human prolactin is a potent inhibitor of angiogenesis. Endocrinol 1993;133:1292–1299.

50. Coman DR, Sheldon WF. The significance of hyperemia around tumor implants. Am J Pathol 1946;22:821–831.
51. Connolly DT, Heuvelman DM, Nelson R, et al. Tumor vascular permeability factor stimulates endothelial cell growth and angiogenesis. J Clin Invest 1989;84: 1470–1478.
52. Connolly DT. Vascular permeability factor: a unique regulator of blood vessel function. J Cell Biochem 1991;47:219–223.
53. Crum R, Szabo S, Folkman J. A new class of steroids inhibits angiogenesis in the presence of heparin or a heparin fragment. Science 1985;230:1375–1378.
54. Czubayko F, Schulte AM, Missner SC, Hsieh SS, Colley KJ, Wellstein A. Molecular and pharmacologic targeting of angiogenesis factors: the example of pleiotrophin. Breast Cancer Res Treat 1995;36:157–168.
55. D'Amato RJ, Loughnan MS, Flynn E, Folkman J. Thalidomide is an inhibitor of angiogenesis. Proc Natl Acad Sci USA 1994;91:4082–4085.
56. Dameron KM, Volpert OV, Tainsky MA, Bouck N. Control of angiogenesis in fibroblasts by p53 regulation of thrombospondin-1. Science 1994;265:1582–1584.
57. Davidson JM, Klagsbrun M, Hill KE, et al. Accelerated wound repair, cell proliferation, and collagen accumulation are produced by cartilage-derived growth factor. J Cell Biol 1985;100:1219–1227.
58. Day ED. Vascular relationships of tumor and host. Prog Exp Tumor Res 1964;4:57–97.
59. de Castelbajac D, Teillac D, Bodemer C, Brunelle F, Marcombes F, de Prost Y. Hemangiome cephalique tubereux d'evolution fatale: inefficacite du traitment par interferon alpha. Ann Dermatol Venereol 1990;117:821–822.

60. Denekamp J. Vascular attack as a therapeutic strategy for cancer. Cancer Metastasis Rev 1990;3:267–282.
61. Diaz MO, Rubin CM, Harden A, et al. Deletions of interferon genes in active lymphoblastic leukemia. N Engl J Med 1990;322:77–82.
62. Dobson DE, Kambe A, Block E, et al. 1 buteral glycerol: a novel angiogenesis factor secreted by differentiating adipocytes. Cell 1990;61:223–230.
63. Dusseau J, Hutchins P, Malbasa D. Stimulation of angiogenesis by adenosine on the chick chorioallantoic membrane. Circulation 1986;59:164–180.
64. Dvorak HF, Nagy JA, Dvorak JT, Dvorak AM. Identification and characterization of the blood vessels of solid tumors that are leaky to circulating macromolecules. Am J Pathol 1988;133:95–109.
65. Dvorak HF, Brown LF, Detmar M, Dvorak AM. Vascular permeability factor/vascular endothelial growth factor, microvascular hyperpermeability, and angiogenesis. Am J Pathol 1995;146:1029–1039.
66. Dvorak HF. Tumors: wounds that do not heal. Similarities between tumor stroma generation and wound healing. N Engl J Med 1986;315:1650–1659.
67. Dvorak HF, Sioussat TM, Brown LF, et al. Distribution of vascular permeability factor (vascular endothelial growth factor) in tumors: concentration in tumor blood vessels. J Exp Med 1991;174:1275–1278.
68. Dvorak HF, Gresser I. Microvascular injury in pathogenesis of interferon-induced necrosis of subcutaneous tumors in mice. JNCI 1989;81:497–502.
69. el-Dessouky M, Azmy AF, Raine PA, Young DG. Kasabach-Merritt syndrome. J Pediatr Surg 1980;23:109–111.
70. Enjolras O, Riche MC, Merland JJ, Escande JP. Management of alarming hemangiomas in infancy: a review of 25 cases. Pediatrics 1990;85:491–498.
71. Esch F, Baird A, Ling N, et al. Primary structure of bovine pituitary basic fibroblast growth factor (FGF) and comparison with the amino-terminal sequence of bovine brain acidic FGF. Proc Natl Acad Sci USA 1985;82:6507–6511.
72. Ezekowitz RA, Mulliken JB, Folkman J. Interferon alfa-2a therapy for life-threatening hemangiomas of infancy. N Engl J Med 1992;326:1456–1463 [Erratum N Engl J Med 1994;330:300].
73. Fallowfield ME, Cook MG. The vascularity of primary cutaneous melanoma. J Pathol 1991;164:241–244.
74. Fernig DG, Gallagher JT. Fibroblast growth factors and their receptors: an information network controlling tissue growth, morphogenesis and repair. Prog Growth Factor Res 1994;5:353–377.
75. Ferrara N, Henzel WJ. Pituitary follicular cells secrete a novel heparin-binding growth factor specific for vascular endothelial cells. Biochem Biophys Res Commun 1989;161:851–855.
76. Ferrara N, Houck K, Jakeman L, Leung DW. Molecular and biological properties of the vascular endothelial growth factor family of proteins. Endocr Rev 1992;13:18–32.
77. Ferrara N, Clapp C, Weiner R. The 16K fragment of prolactin specifically inhibits basal or fibroblast growth factor simulated growth of capillary endothelial cells. Endocrinology 1991;129:896–900
78. Fett JW, Strydom DJ, Lobb RR, et al. Isolation and characterization of angiogenin, an angiogenic protein, from human colon carcinoma cells. Biochemistry 1985;24: 5480–5486.
79. Fidler IJ, Gersten DM, Hart IR. The biology of cancer invasion and metastasis. Adv Cancer Res 1978;28:149–250.
80. Figg WD, Yeh HJ, Thibault A, et al. Assay of the antiangiogenic compound TNP-470, and one of its metabolites, AGM-1883, by reversed-phase high-performance liquid chromatography in plasma. J Chromatogr 1994;652:187–194.
81. Folkman J, Haudenschild CC, Zetter BR. Long-term culture of capillary endothelial cells. Proc Natl Acad Sci USA 1979;76:5217–5221.
82. Folkman J. Toward an understanding of angiogenesis: search and discovery. Perspect Biol Med 1985;29:10–36.
83. Folkman J. Tumor angiogenesis: therapeutic implications. N Engl J Med 1971;285: 1182–1186.
84. Folkman J, Long DM, Becker FF. Growth and metastasis of tumor in organ culture. Cancer 1963;16:453–467.
85. Folkman J, Cole P, Zimmerman S. Tumor behavior in isolated perfused organs: in vitro growth and metastases of biopsy material in rabbit thyroid and canine intestinal segment. Ann Surg 1966;164:491–502.
86. Folkman J Anti-angiogenesis: new concept for therapy of solid tumors. Ann Surg 1972;175:408–416.
87. Folkman J. The vascularization of tumors. Sci Am 1976;234:58–73.
88. Folkman J. Antiangiogenesis. In: Biologic Therapy of Cancer. Edited by VT DeVita Jr, S Hellman, SA Rosenberg. Philadelphia: Lippincott, 1991, pp 743–753.
89. Folkman J, Merler E, Abernathy C, Williams G. Isolation of a tumor factor responsible for angiogenesis. J Exp Med 1971;133:275–288.
90. Folkman J. Angiogenesis. In: Biology of Endothelial Cells. Edited by EA Jaffe. Boston: Nijhoff, 1984, pp 412–428.
91. Folkman J, Gimbrone MA Jr. Perfusion of the thyroid. In: Karolinska Symposia on Research Methods in Reproduction Endocrinology, 4th Symposium: Perfusion Techniques. Edited by E Diczfalusy. Stockholm, 1971, pp 237–248.
92. Folkman J, Cotran RS. Relation of vascular proliferation to tumor growth. Int Rev Exp Pathol. 1976;16:207–248
93. Folkman J. Tumor angiogenesis factor. Cancer Res 1974;34:2109–2113
94. Folkman J, Watson K, Ingber D, Hanahan D. Induction of angiogenesis during the transition from hyperplasia to neoplasia. Nature 1989;339:58–61
95. Folkman J. What is the evidence that tumors are angiogenesis dependent? JNCI 1990;82:4–6.
96. Folkman J, Langer R, Linhardt R, Haudenschild C, Taylor S. Angiogenesis inhibition and tumor regression caused by heparin or a heparin fragment in the presence of cortisone. Science 1983;221:719–725.
97. Folkman J. What is the role of angiogenesis in metastasis from cutaneous melanoma? Eur J Cancer Clin Oncol 1987;23:361–363.
98. Folkman J, Hochberg M. Self-regulation of growth in three dimensions. J Exp Med 1973;138:745–753.
99. Folkman J. Tumor angiogenesis. In Cancer: A Comprehensive Treatise, vol 3. Edited by FF Becker. New York: Plenum Press, 1975, pp 355–388.
100. Folkman J, Haudenschild CC. Angiogenesis in vitro. Nature 1980;288:551–556.
101. Folkman J, Klagsbrun M. Angiogenic factors. Science 1987;235:442–447.
102. Folkman J. Angiogenesis in cancer, vascular, rheumatoid and other disease. Nature Med 1995;1:27–31.
103. Folkman J. Angiogenesis and breast cancer. J Clin Oncol 1994;12:441–444.
104. Folkman J, Klagsbrun M, Sasse J, Wadzinski M, Ingber DE, Vlodavsky I. A heparin-binding angiogenic protein—basic fibroblast growth factor—is stored within basement membrane. Am J Pathol 1988;130:393–400.
105. Folkman J, Szabo S, Stovroff M, McNeil P, Li W, Shing Y. Duodenal ulcer: discovery of a new mechanism and development of angiogenic therapy which accelerates healing. Ann Surg 1991;214:414–427.
106. Folkman J. Tumor angiogenesis. In The Molecular Basis of Cancer. Edited by J Mendelsohn, PM Howley, MA Israel, LA Liotta. Philadelphia: Saunders, 1995, pp 206–232.
107. Folkman J. Successful treatment of an angiogenic disease. N Engl J Med 1989;320: 1211–1212.
108. Folkman J. The influence of angiogenesis research on management of patients with breast cancer. Breast Cancer Res Treat 1995;36:109–118.
109. Folkman J. The intestine as an organ culture. In Carcinoma of the Colon and Antecedent Epithelium. Edited by WJ Burdette. Springfield, IL: Thomas, 1970, pp 113–127.
110. Folkman J. Angiogenesis and its inhibitors. In Important Advances in Oncology. Edited by VT DeVita Jr, S Hellman, SA Rosenberg. Philadelphia: Lippincott, 1985, pp 42–62.
111. Form DM, Pratt BM, Madri JA. Endothelial cell proliferation during angiogenesis. In vitro modulation by basement membrane components. Lab Invest 1986;55:521–530.
112. Form DM, Auerbach R. PGE_2 and angiogenesis (41548). Proc Soc Exp Biol Med 1983;172:214–218.
113. Fournier GA, Lutty GA, Watt S, Fenselau A, Patz A. A corneal micropocket assay for angiogenesis in the rat eye. Invest Ophthalmol Visual Sci 1981;21:351–354.
114. Fox SB, Leek RD, Smith K, Hollyer J, Greenall M, Harris AL. Tumor angiogenesis in node-negative breast carcinomas: relationship with epidermal growth factor receptor, estrogen receptor, and survival. Breast Cancer Res Treat 1994;29:109–116.
115. Fox SB, Turner GDH, Leek RD, Whitehouse RM, Gatter KC, Harris AL. The prognostic value of quantitative angiogenesis in breast cancer and role of adhesion molecule expression in tumor endothelium. Breast Cancer Res Treat 1995;36:219–226.
116. Fräter-Schröder M, Risau W, Hallmann R, Gautschi P, Böhlen P. Tumor necrosis factor type a, a potent inhibitor of endothelial cell growth in vitro, is angiogenic in vivo. Proc Natl Acad Sci USA 1987;84:5277–5281.
117. Fregene TA, Khanuja PS, Noto AC, Gehani SK, Van Egmont EM, Luz DA, Pienta KJ. Tumor-associated angiogenesis in prostate cancer. Anticancer Res 1993;13: 2377–2381.
118. Fujimoto K, Ichimori Y, Kakizoe T, et al. Increased serum levels of basic fibroblast growth factor in patients with renal cell carcinoma. Biochem Biophys Res Commun 1991;180:386–392.
119. Furukawa T, Yoshimura A, Sumizawa T, Haraguchi M, Akiyama S-I. Angiogenic factor. Nature 1992;356:668.
120. Gasparini G, Weidner N, Bevilacqua P, et al. Tumor microvessel density, p53 expression, tumor size and peritumoral lymphatic invasion are relevant prognostic markers in node-negative breast carcinoma. J Clin Oncol 1994;12:454–466.
121. Gasparini G, Barbareschi M, Boracchi P, et al. Tumor angiogenesis determined by counting intratumoral microvessel density, predicts clinical outcome of node-positive breast cancer patients treated either with adjuvant hormone therapy or chemotherapy. Cancer J 1995;11:131–141.
122. Gasparini G, Weidner N, Maluta S, et al. Intratumoral microvessel density and p53 protein: correlation with metastasis in head-and-neck squamous-cell carcinoma. Int J Cancer 1993;55:739–744.
123. Gilbertson-Beadling S, Powers EA, Stamp-Cole M, et al. The tetracycline analogs minocycline and doxycycline inhibit angiogenesis in vitro by a non-metalloproteinase-dependent mechanism. Cancer Chemother Pharmacol 1995;36:418–424.
124. Gimbrone MA Jr, Cotran R, Leapman S, Folkman J. Tumor growth and neovascularization: an experimental model using rabbit cornea. JNCI 1974;52:413–427.
125. Gimbrone MA Jr, Leapman S, Cotran RS, Folkman J. Tumor dormancy in vivo by prevention of neovascularization. J Exp Med 1972;136:261–276.
126. Gimbrone MA Jr, Cotran RS, Folkman J. Endothelial regeneration and turnover. Studies with human endothelial cell cultures. Series Haematol 1973;6:453–455.
127. Good DJ, Polverini PJ, Rastinejad F, et al. A tumor suppressor-dependent inhibitor of angiogenesis is immunologically and functionally indistinguishable from a fragment of thrombospondin. Proc Natl Acad Sci USA 1990;87:6624–6628.
128. Gospodarowicz D, Moran J, Braun D, Birdwell CR. Clonal growth of bovine endothelial cells in culture: fibroblast growth factor as a survival factor. Proc Natl Acad Sci USA 1976;73:4120–4124.
129. Goto F, Goto K, Weindel K, Folkman J. Synergistic effects of vascular endothelial growth factor and basic fibroblast growth factor on the bovine capillary endothelial cells within collagen gels. Lab Invest 1993;69:508–517.
130. Graeber JE, Glaser BM, Setty BNY, Jerdan JA, Walenga RW, Stuart MJ. 15-Hydroxyeicosatetraenoic acid stimulates migration of human retinal microvessel endothelium in vitro and neovascularization. Prostaglandin 1990;39:665–673
131. Graham CH, Rivers J, Kerbel RS, Stankiewicz KS, White WL. Extent of vascularization as a prognostic indicator in thin (<0.76 mm) malignant melanomas. Am J Pathol 1994;145:510–514.
132. Grant DS, Tashiro KI, Sequi-Real B, Yamada Y, Martin GR, Kleinman HK. Two different laminin domains mediate the differentiation of human endothelial cells into capillary-like structures in vitro. Cell 1989;58:933–943
133. Gross JL, Moscatelli D, Rifkin DB. Increased capillary endothelial cell protease activity in response to angiogenic stimuli in vitro. Proc Natl Acad Sci USA 1983;80: 2623–2627.
134. Gross JL, Herblin WF, Dusak BA, Czerniak P, Diamond M, Dexter DL. Modulation of solid tumor growth in vivo by bFGF. Proc Am Assoc Cancer Res 1990;31:79. Abstract.
135. Guerin C, Laterra J, Masnyk T, Golub LM, Brem H. Selective endothelial growth inhibition by tetracyclines that inhibit collagenase. Biochem Biophys Res Comm 1992;188:740–745.
136. Guidi AJ, Fischer L, Harris JR, Schnitt SJ. Microvessel density and distribution in ductal carcinoma in situ of the breast. JNCI 1994;86:614–619.
137. Gupta SK, Hassel T, Singh JP. A potent inhibitor of endothelial cell proliferation is generated by proteolytic cleavage of the chemokine platelet factor 4. Proc Natl Acad Sci USA 1995;92:7799–7803.
138. Hall NR, Fish DE, Hunt N, Goldin RD, Guillou PJ, Monson JRT. Is the relationship between angiogenesis and metastasis in breast cancer real? Surg Oncol 1992;1: 223–229.

139. Hamada J, Cavanaugh PG, Lotan O, Nicolson GL. Separable growth and migration factors for large-cell lymphoma cells secreted by microvascular endothelial cells derived from target organs for metastasis. Br J Cancer 1992;66:349–354.
140. Hanneken A, Ying W, Ling N, Baird A. Identification of soluble forms of the fibroblast growth factor receptor in blood. Proc Natl Acad Sci USA 1994;91:9170–9174.
141. Haraguchi M, Miyadera K, Uemura K, et al. Angiogenic activity of enzymes. Nature 1994;368:198.
142. Haudenschild CC, Zahniser D, Folkman J, Klagsbrun M. Human endothelial cells in culture. Lack of response to serum growth factors. Exp Cell Res 1976;98:175–183.
143. Hicks RM, Chowaniec J. Experimental induction, histology, and ultrastructure of hyperplasia and neoplasia of the urinary bladder epithelium. Int Rev Exp Pathol 1978;18:199–280.
144. Hochberg MS, Folkman J. Mechanisms of size limitation of bacterial colonies. J Infect Dis 1972;126:629–635.
145. Hollingsworth HC, Merino M, Kohn E, Steinberg S, Rothenberg M. Tumor angiogenesis in advanced stage ovarian carcinoma. Am J Pathol 1995;147:33–41.
146. Holmgren L, O'Reilly MS, Folkman J. Dormancy of micrometastases: balanced proliferation and apoptosis in the presence of angiogenesis suppression. Nature Med 1995;1:149–153.
146a. Homandberg GA, Williams JE, Grant D, Schumacher B, Eisenstein R. Heparin-binding fragments of fibronectin are potent inhibitors of endothelial cell growth. Am J Path 1985;120:327–332.
147. Hondermarck H, Courty J, Boilly B, Thomas D. Distribution of intravenously administered acidic and basic fibroblast growth factors in the mouse. Experientia 1990;46: 973–974.
148. Horak ER, Leek R, Klenk N, et al. Angiogenesis, assessed by platelet/endothelial cell adhesion molecule antibodies, as an indicator of node metastases and survival in breast cancer. Lancet 1992;340:1120–1124.
149. Hori A, Sasada R, Matsutani E, Naito K, Sakura Y, Fujita T, Kozai Y. Suppression of solid tumor growth by immuno-neutralizing monoclonal antibody against human basic fibroblast growth factor. Cancer Res 1991;51:6180–6184.
150. Houck KA, Leung DW, Rowland AM, Winer J, Ferrara N. Dual regulation of vascular endothelial growth factor bioavailability by genetic and proteolytic mechanisms. J Biol Chem 1992;267:26031–26037.
151. Hurvitz CH, Alkalay AL, Sloninsky L, Kallus M, Pomerance J. Cyclophosphamide therapy in life-threatening vascular tumors. J Pediatr 1986;109:360–363.
152. Ide AG, Bake NH, Warren SL. Vascularization of the Brown-Pearce rabbit epithelioma transplant as seen in the transparent ear chamber. Am J Roentgenol 1939;42: 891–899.
153. Ingber DE, Madri JA, Folkman J. Endothelial growth factors and extracellular matrix regulate DNA synthesis through modulation of cell and nuclear expansion. In Vitro Cell Dev Biol 1987;23:387–394.
154. Ingber DE, Folkman J. Mechanochemical switching between growth and differentiation during fibroblast growth factor-stimulated angiogenesis in vitro: role of extracellular matrix. J Cell Biol 1989;109:317–330.
155. Ingber DM, Fujita T, Kishimoto S, Sudo K, Kanamaru T, Brem H, Folkman J. Synthetic analogues of fumagillin that inhibit angiogenesis and suppress tumour growth. Nature 1990;348:555–557.
156. Ingber DE. Fibronectin controls capillary endothelial cell growth by modulating cell shape. Proc Natl Acad Sci USA 1990;87:3579–3583.
157. Ingber DE, Folkman J. How does the extracellular matrix control capillary morphogenesis? Cell 1989;58:803–805.
158. Ishikawa F, Miyazone K, Hellman U, et al. Identification of angiogenic activity and the cloning and expression of platelet-derived endothelial cell growth factor. Nature 1989;338:557–562.
159. Jackson D, Volpert O, Bouck N, Linzer DIH. Stimulation and inhibition of angiogenesis by placental proliferin and proliferin-related protein. Science 1994;266: 1581–1584.
160. Jaeger TM, Weidner N, Chew K, et al. Tumor angiogenesis and lymph node metastases in invasive bladder carcinoma. J Urol 1994;151:348a. Abstract.
161. Jaffe EA, Nachman RL, Becker CG, Minick CR. Culture of human endothelial cells derived from umbilical veins: identification by morphologic and immunologic criteria. J Clin Invest 1972;52:2745–2756.
162. Jain RK. Delivery of novel therapeutic agents in tumors: physiological barriers and strategies. JNCI 1989;81:570–576.
163. Jain RK. Determinants of tumor blood flow. Cancer Res 1988;48:2641–2658.
164. Jakeman LB, Armanini M, Phillips HS, Ferrara N. Developmental expression of binding sites and messenger ribonucleic acid for vascular endothelial growth factor suggests a role for this protein in vasculogenesis and angiogenesis. Endocrinology 1993;133:848–859.
165. Kalebic T, Garbisa S, Glaser B, Liotta LA. Basement membrane collagen: degradation by migrating endothelial cells. Science 1983;221:281–283.
166. Kandel J, Bossy-Wetzel E, Radvanyi F, Klagsbrun M, Folkman J, Hanahan D. Neovascularization is associated with a switch to the export of bFGF in the multistep development of fibrosarcoma. Cell 1991;66:1095–1104.
167. Kasabach HH, Merritt KK. Capillary hemangiomas with extensive purpura. Am J Dis Child 1940;59:1063–1070.
168. Kato T, Sato K, Kakinuma H, Matsuda Y. Enhanced suppression of tumor growth by combination of angiogenesis inhibitor O-(chloroacetyl-carbamoyl) fumagillol (TNP-470) and cytotoxic agents in mice. Cancer Res 1994;54:5143–5147.
169. Kawasaki S, Mori M, Awai M. Capillary growth of rat aortic segments cultured in collagen gel without serum. Acta Pathol Jpn 1989;39:712–718
170. Kedar RP, Cosgrove DO, Smith IE, Mansi JL, Bamber JC. Breast carcinoma: measurement of tumor response to primary medical therapy with color doppler flow imaging. Radiology 1994;190:825–830.
171. Kenyon BM, Voest EE, Chen CC, Flynn E, Folkman J, D'Amato R. A model of angiogenesis in the mouse cornea. 1995;submitted.
172. Kerbel RS, Waghorne C, Korczak B, Lagarde A, Breitman ML. Clonal dominance of primary tumors by metastatic cells: genetic analysis and biological implications. Cancer Surv 1988;7:597–629.
173. Kerbel RS. Inhibition of tumor angiogenesis as a strategy to circumvent resistance to anti-cancer therapeutic agents. BioEssays 1991;1:31–36.
174. Kim KJ, Li B, Winer J, Armanini M, Gillett N, Phillips HS, Ferrara N. Inhibition of vascular endothelial growth factor-induced angiogenesis suppresses tumour growth in vivo. Nature 1993;362:841–844.
175. Klagsbrun M, Knighton D, Folkman J. Tumor angiogenesis activity in cell grown in tissue culture. Cancer Res 1976;36:110–114.
176. Klein S, Giancotti FG, Presta M, Albelda SM, Buck CA, Rifkin DB. Basic fibroblast growth factor modulates integrin expression in microvascular endothelial cells. Mol Biol Cell 1993;4:973–982.
177. Knighton D, Ausprunk D, Tapper D, Folkman J. Avascular and vascular phases of tumour growth in the chick embryo. Br J Cancer 1977;35:347–356.
178. Koch A, Polverini PJ, Kunkel SL, et al. Interleukin-8 as a macrophage-derived mediator of angiogenesis. Science 1992;258:1178–1801.
179. Kohn EC, Alessandro R, Spoonster J, Wersto RP, Liotta LA. Angiogenesis: role of calcium-mediated signal transduction. Proc Natl Acad Sci USA 1995;92:1307–1311.
180. Kohn EC, Liotta LA. Molecular insights into cancer invasion: strategies for prevention and intervention. Cancer Res 1995;55:1856–1862.
181. Kolber DL, Knisely TL, Maione TE. Inhibition of development of murine melanoma lung metastases by systemic administration of recombinant platelet factor 4. JNCI 1995;87:304–309.
182. Konno H, Tanaka T, Matsuda I, et al. Comparison of the inhibitory effect of the angiogenesis inhibitor, TNP-470, and mitomycin C on the growth and liver metastasis of human colon cancer. Int J Cancer 1995;61:268–271.
183. Kull FC Jr, Brent DA, Parikh I, Cuatrecasa P. Chemical identification of a tumor-derived angiogenic factor. Science 1987;236:843–845.
184. Kusaka M, Sudo K, Fujita T, Marui S, et al. Potent anti-angiogenic action of AGM-1470: comparison to the fumagillin parent. Biochem Biophys Res Commun 1991;174: 1070–1076.
185. Langer R, Folkman J. Polymers for the sustained release of proteins and other macromolecules. Nature 1976;263:797–800.
186. Leedy DA, Prune BR, Kronz JD, Weidner N, Kohen JI. Tumor angiogenesis, the p53 antigen, and cervical metastasis in squamous carcinoma of the tongue. Otolaryngol Head Neck Surg 1994;11:417–422.
187. Leibovich SJ, Polverini PJ, Shepard HM, Wiseman D, Shively V, Nuseir N. Macrophage-induced angiogenesis is mediated by tumour necrosis factor-alpha. Nature 1987;329:630–632.
188. Li VW, Folkerth RD, Watanabe H, Yu C, Rupnick M, Barnes P, Scott RM, McL Black P, Sallan S, Folkman J. Microvessel count and cerebrospinal fluid basic fibroblast growth factor in children with brain tumours. Lancet 1994;344:82–86.
189. Lien W, Ackerman NB. The blood supply of experimental liver metastases. II. A microcirculatory study of normal and tumor vessels of the liver with the use of perfused silicone rubber. Surgery 1970;68:334–340.
190. Lin RY, Argenta PA, Sullivan KM, Adzick NS. Diagnostic and prognostic role of basic fibroblast growth factor in Wilm's tumor patients. Clin Cancer Res 1995;1:327–331.
191. Liotta LA, Tryggvason K, Garbisa S, Hart I, Foltz CM, Shafie S. Metastatic potential correlates with enzymatic degradation of basement membrane collagen. Nature 1980;284:67–68.
192. Liotta LA, Saidel MG, Kleinerman J. The significance of hematogenous tumor cell clumps in the metastatic process. Cancer Res 1976;36:889–894.
193. Liotta LA, Steeg PS, Stetler-Stevenson WG. Cancer metastasis and angiogenesis: an imbalance of positive and negative regulation. Cell 1991;64:327–336.
194. Long DM. Capillary ultrastructure in human metastatic brain tumors. J Neurosurg 1979;51:53–58.
195. Loughnan MS, Elder J, Kemp A. Treatment of massive orbital capillary hemangioma with interferon alfa-2b: short term results. Arch Ophthalmol 1992;110:1366–1373.
196. Macchiarini P, Fontanini G, Hardin MJ, Squartini F, Angeletti CA. Relation of neovascularisation to metastasis of non-small-cell lung cancer. Lancet 1993;340:145–146.
197. Macchiarini P, Fontanini G, Dulmet E, de Montpreville V, Chapelier AR, Cerrin J, Le Roy Ladurie F, Dartevelle PG. Angiogenesis: an indicator of metastasis in non-small-cell lung cancer invading the thoracic inlet. Ann Thorac Surg 1994;57:1534–39.
198. Maciag T, Kadish J, Wilkins L, Stemerman MB, Weinstein R. Organization behavior of human umbilical vein endothelial cells. J Cell Biol 1982;94:511–520.
199. Maciag T, Mehlman T, Friesel R, Schreiber A. Heparin binds endothelial cell growth factor, the principal endothelial cell mitogen in bovine brain. Science 1994;25: 932–935.
200. Madri J, Williams SK. Capillary endothelial cell cultures: phenotypic modulation by matrix components. J Cell Biol 1983;97:153–165.
201. Madri JA, Sankar S, Lu T. Matrix modulation of surface molecules during angiogenesis. J Cell Biochem S118A:309. Abstract.
202. Maglione D, Guerriero V, Viglietto G, Delli-Bova P, Persico MG. Isolation of a human placenta cDNA coding for a protein related to the vascular permeability factor. Proc Natl Acad Sci USA 1991;88:9267–9271.
203. Maione TE, Sharpe RJ. Development of angiogenesis inhibitors for clinical applications. Trends Pharmacol Sci 1990;11:457–461.
204. Maione TE, Gray GS, Petro J, et al. Inhibition of angiogenesis by recombinant human platelet factor-4 and related peptides. Science 1990;247:77–79.
205. Marshall JL, Hawkins MJ. The clinical experience with antiangiogenic agents. Breast Cancer Res Treat 1995;36:253–261.
206. Mathivon F, Enjolras O, Escande JP. Hémangiomatose néonatale miliaire multiple cutanée et hépatique. Quatre observations d'évolution favorable. Ann Pediatr (Paris) 1994;41:6:337–345.
207. Mignatti P, Tsuboi R, Robbins E, Rifkin DB. In vitro angiogenesis on the human amniotic membrane: requirement for basic fibroblast growth factor-induced proteinases. J Cell Biol 1989;108:671–682.
208. Mikami Y, Tsukunda M, Mochimatsu I, Kokatsu T, Yago T, Sawaki S. Angiogenesis in head and neck tumors. Nippon Jibiinkoka Gakkai Kaiho 1991;96:645–650.
209. Millauer B, Shawver LK, Plate KH, Risau W, Ullrich A. Glioblastoma growth inhibited in vivo by a dominant-negative Flk-1 mutant. Nature 1994;367:576–579.
210. Millauer B, Wizigmann-Voos S, Schnurch H, Martinez R, Moller NPH, Risau W, Ullrich A. High affinity VEGF binding and developmental expression suggest Flk-1 as a major regulator of vasculogenesis and angiogenesis. Cell 1993;72:835–846.
211. Miyazono K, Okabe T, Urabe A, Takaku F, Heldon C. Purification and properties of an endothelial cell growth factor from human platelets. J Biol Chem 1987;262: 4098–5103.
212. Montesano R, Orci L, Vassali P. In vitro rapid organization of endothelial cells into capillary-like networks is promoted by collagen matrices. J Cell Biol 1983;97: 1648–1652.
213. Montesano R, Pepper MS, Vassalli JC, Orci L. Phorbol ester induces cultured en-

dothelial cells to invade a fibrin matrix in the presence of fibrinolytic inhibitors. J Cell Physiol 1987;132:509–516.
214. Mori S, Ueda T, Kuratsu S, Hosono N, Izawa K, Uchida A. Suppression of pulmonary metastasis by angiogenesis inhibitor TNP-470 in murine osteosarcoma. Int J Cancer 1995;6:148–152.
215. Mori S, Ueda T, Kuratsu S, Hosono N, Izawa K, Uchida A. Suppression of pulmonary metastasis by angiogenesis inhibitor TNP-470 in murine osteosarcoma. Int J Cancer 1995;61:148–152.
216. Morita T, Shinohara N, Tokue A. Antitumour effect of a synthetic analogue of fumagillin on murine renal carcinoma. Br J Urol 1994;74:416–421.
217. Moscatelli D, Gross JL, Rifkin DB. Angiogenic factors stimulate plasminogen activator and collagenase production by capillary endothelial cells [Abstract]. J Cell Biol 1981;91:201a.
218. Moses MA, Sudhalter J, Langer R. Identification of an inhibitor of neovascularization from cartilage. Science 1990;248:1408–1410.
219. Motro B, Itin A, Sachs L, Keshet E. Pattern of interleukin 6 gene expression in vivo suggests a role for this cytokine in angiogenesis. Proc Natl Acad Sci USA 1990;87: 3092–3096.
219a. Muller G, Behrens J, Nussbaumer U, Bohlen P, Birchmeier W. Inhibitory action of transforming growth factor beta on endothelial cells. PNAS USA 1987;84:5600–5604.
220. Mulliken JB, Young AE. Vascular Birthmarks: Hemangiomas and Malformations. Philadelphia: Saunders, 1988.
221. Mulliken JB, Boon LM, Takahashi K, Ohlms LA, Folkman J, Ezekowitz RAB. Pharmacologic therapy for endangering hemangioma. Curr Opin Dermatol 1995;109–113.
221a. Murphy AN, Unsworth E, Stetler-Stevenson W. Tissue inhibitor of metalloproteinase-2 (TIMP-2) inhibits bFGF-induced human microvascular endothelial cell proliferation. J Cell Physiol 1993;157:351–358.
222. Murphy-Ullrich JE, Schultz-Cherry S, Hook M. Transforming growth factor-B complexes with thrombospondin. Mol Biol Cell 1992;3:181–188.
223. Muthukkarauppan VR, Auerbach R. Angiogenesis in the mouse cornea. Science 1979;205:1416–1417.
224. Nagy JA, Brown LF, Senger DR, Lanir R, Van De Water L, Dvorak AM, Dvorak F. Pathogenesis of tumor stroma generation: a critical role for leaky blood vessels and fibrin deposition. Biochim Biophys Acta 1989;948:305–326.
225. Nanus DM, Schmitz-Drager BJ, Motzer RJ, Lee AC, Vlamis V, Cordon-Cardo C, Albino AP, Reuter VE. Expression of basic fibroblast growth factor in primary human renal tumors: correlation with poor survival. JNCI 1993;85:1597–1599.
225a. Nelson J, Allen WE, Scott WN, Bailie JR, Walker B, McFerran NV, Wilson DJ. Murine epidermal growth factor (EGF) fragment (33-42) inhibits both EGF-and laminin-dependent endothelial cell motility and angiogenesis. Cancer Res 1995;55:3772–3776.
226. Netland PA, Zetter BR. Organ-specific adhesion of metastatic tumor cells in vitro. Science 1984;224:1113–1115.
227. Nicolson GL. Cancer metastasis. Sci Am 1979;240:66–76.
228. Nicolson GL. Organ specificity of tumor metastasis: role of preferential adhesion, invasion and growth of malignant cells at specific secondary sites. Cancer Metastasis Rev 1988;7:143–188.
229. Nicosia RF, Tchao R, Leighton J. Interactions between newly formed endothelial channels and carcinoma cells in plasma clot culture. Clin Exp Metastasis 1986;4: 91–104.
230. Nicosia RF, Tchao R, Leighton J. Histiotypic angiogenesis in vitro: light microscopic, ultrastructural and radiographic studies. In Vitro 1982;18:538–549.
231. Nicosia RF, Ottinett A. Growth of microvessels in serum-free matrix culture of rat aorta: a quantitative assay of angiogenesis in vitro. Lab Invest 1990;63:115–122.
232. Nguyen M, Strubel NA, Bischoff J. A role for sialyl Lewis-X/A glycoconjugates in capillary morphogenesis. Nature 1993;365:267–269.
233. Nguyen M, Shing Y, Folkman J. Quantitation of angiogenesis and antiangiogenesis in the chick embryo chorioallantoic membrane. Microvasc Res 1994;47:31–40.
234. Nguyen M, Watanabe H, Budson AE, Richie JP, Hayes DF, Folkman J. Elevated levels of an angiogenic peptide, basic fibroblast growth factor, in the urine of patients with a wide spectrum of cancers. JNCI 1994;86:356–361.
235. Obermair A, Czerwenka K, Kurz C, Buxbaum P, Schemper M, Sevelda P. Influence of tumoral microvessel density on the recurrence-free survival in human breast cancer: preliminary results. Onkologie 1994;17:44–49.
236. O'Brien T, Cranston D, Fuggle S, Bicknell R, Harris AL. Different angiogenic pathways characterize superficial and invasive bladder cancer. Cancer Res 1995;55:510–513.
237. Odekon LE, Blasi F, Rifkin DB. Requirement for receptor-bound urokinase in plasmin-dependent cellular conversion of latent TGF-beta to active TGF-beta. J Cell Physiol 1994;158:398–407.
238. Ohlms LA, Jones DT, McGill TJI, Healy GB. Interferon alfa-2a therapy for airway hemangiomas. Ann Oto Rhinol Laryngol 1994;103:1–8.
239. Olivarez D, Ulbright T, DeRiese W, Foster R, Reister T, Einhorn L, Sledge G. Neovascularization in clinical stage A testicular germ cell tumor: prediction of metastatic disease. Cancer Res 1994;54:2800–2802.
240. Orchard PJ, Smith CH III, Woods WG, Day DL, Dehner LP, Shapiro R. Treatment of hemangioendotheliomas with alpha interferon. Lancet 1989;2:565–567.
241. O'Reilly MS, Holmgren L, Shing Y, Chen C, Rosenthal RA, Moses M, Lane WS, Cao Y, Sage EH, Folkman J. Angiostatin: a novel angiogenesis inhibitor that mediates the suppression of metastases by a Lewis lung carcinoma. Cell 1994;79:315–328.
242. O'Reilly MS, Holmgren L, Chen C, Folkman J. Suppression of angiogenesis by angiostatin produces dormancy of human primary tumors in mice. 1995;submitted.
243. O'Reilly MS, et al. Unpublished data
244. O'Reilly MS, Personal communication.
245. O'Reilly M, Rosenthal R, Sage EH, et al. The suppression of tumor metastases by a primary tumor. Surgical Forum 1993;44:474–476.
246. Paulus HE. Minocycline treatment of rheumatoid arthritis. Ann Intern Med 1995;122: 147–148.
247. Paulus W, Grothe C, Sensenbrenner M, Janet T, Bauer I, Graf M, Roggendorf W. Localization of basic fibroblast growth factor, a mitogen and angiogenic factor, in human-brain tumors. Acta Neuropathol 1990;79:418–423.
248. Pepper MS, Ferrara N, Orci L, Montesano R. Potent synergism between vascular endothelial growth factor and basic fibroblast growth factor in the induction of angiogenesis in vitro. Biochemical Biophysical Res Commun 1992;89:824–831.
249. Pepper MS, Vassalli J-D, Orci L, Montesano R. Regulation of angiogenesis in vitro: cytokine interactions and balanced extracellular proteolysis. Kidney Int 1995;47:659. Abstract.
250. Pepper MS, Montesano R. Proteolytic balance and capillary morphogenesis. Cell Different Dev 1990;32:319–328.
251. Perez-Atayde AR, Sallan SE, Tedrow U, Connors S, Folkman J. Spectrum of tumor angiogenesis in bone marrow of children with acute lymphoblastic leukemia. Lab Invest 1995;72:a141. Abstract.
252. Pertovaara L, Kaipainen A, Mustonen T, Orpana A, Ferrara N, Saksela O, Alitalo K. Vascular endothelial growth factor is induced in response to transforming growth factor-beta in fibroblastic and epithelial cells. J Biol Chem 1994;269:6271–6274.
253. Peters KG, De Vries C, Williams LT. VEGF receptor expression during embryogenesis and tissue repair suggests a role in endothelial differentiation and blood vessel growth. Proc Natl Acad Sci USA 1993;90:8915–8919.
254. Peverali FA, Mandriot SJ, Ciana P, Marelli R, Quax P, Rifkin DB, Della Valle G, Mignatti P. Tumor cells secrete an angiogenic factor that stimulates basic fibroblast growth factor and urokinase expression in vascular endothelial cells. J Cell Physiol 1994;161: 1–14.
255. Plate KH, Breier G, Millauer B, Ullrich A, Risau W. Up-regulation of vascular endothelial growth factor and its cognate receptors in a rat glioma model of tumor angiogenesis. Cancer Res 1993;53:5822–5827.
256. Plate K, Breier G, Weich HA, Risau W. Vascular endothelial growth factor is a potential tumour angiogenesis factor in human gliomas in vivo. Nature 1992;359:845–848.
257. Plouet J, Schilling J, Gospodarowicz D. Isolation and characterization of a newly identified endothelial cell mitogen produced by AT-20 cells. EMBO J 1989;8: 3801–3806.
258. Podor TJ, Jirik FR, Loskutoff DJ, Carson DA, Lotz M. Human endothelial cells produce IL-6. Lack of responses to exogenous IL-6. Ann NY Acad Sci 1989;557:374–385.
259. Polverini P, Leibovich S. Induction of neovascularization in vivo and endothelial proliferation in vitro by tumor-associated macrophages. Lab Invest 1984;51:635–642.
260. Prehn RT. The inhibition of tumor growth by tumor mass. Cancer Res 1991;51:2–4.
261. Raju KS, Alessandri G, Gullino PM. Characterization of a chemoattractant for endothelium induced by angiogenesis effectors. Cancer Res 1984;44:1579–1584.
262. Rak JW, Hegmann EJ, Lu C, Kerbel RS. Progressive loss of sensitivity to endothelium-derived growth inhibitors expressed by human melanoma cells during disease progression. J Cell Physiol 1994;159:245–255.
263. Rastinejad F, Polverini P, Bouck NP. Regulation of the activity of a new inhibitor of angiogenesis by a cancer suppressor gene. Cell 1989;56:345–355.
264. Ray JM, Stetler-Stevenson WF. The role of matrix metalloproteases and their inhibitors in tumour invasion, metastasis and angiogenesis. Eur Respir J 1994;7:2062–2072.
265. Ribatti D, Vacca A, Bertossi M, De Benedictis G, Roncali L, Dammacco F. Angiogenesis induced by B-cell non-Hodgkin's lymphomas: lack of correlation with tumor malignancy and immunologic phenotype. Anticancer Res 1990;10:401–406.
266. Ricketts RR, Hatley RM, Corden BJ, Sabio H, Howel CG Interferon-alpha-2a for the treatment of complex hemangiomas of infancy and childhood. Ann Surg 1994;219: 605–614.
267. Roberts AB, Sporn MB, Assoian RK, et al. Transforming growth factor type beta: rapid induction of fibrosis and angiogenesis in vivo and stimulation of collagen formation in vitro. Proc Natl Acad Sci USA 1986;83:4167–4171.
268. Roberts WG, Palade GE. Increased capillary permeability and endothelial fenestration induced by acute administration of vascular endothelial growth factor. Endothelium 1995;2(suppl):20. Abstract.
269. Rosen EM, Meromsky L, Setter E, Vinter DW, Goldberg ID. Purified scatter factor stimulates epithelial and vascular endothelial cell migration. Proc Soc Exp Biol Med 1990;195:34–43.
270. Ryan TJ, Stockley AT. Mechanical versus biochemical factors in angiogenesis. Microvas Res 1980;20:258–259.
271. Saclarides TJ, Speziale NJ, Drab E, Szeluga DJ, Rubin DB. Tumor angiogenesis and rectal carcinoma. Dis Colon Rectum 1994;37:921–926.
272. Sage EH, Bornstein P. Approaches for investigating matrix components produced by endothelial cells: type VIII collagen, SPARC, and thrombospondin. In Extracellular Matrix Molecules: A Practical Approach. Edited by MA Haralson, JR Hassell. Oxford: Oxford University Press, 1995.
272a. Sage EH, Bassuk JA, Yost JC, Folkman MJ, Lane TF. Inhibition of endothelial cell proliferation by SPARC is mediated through a Ca(2+)-binding EF-hand sequence. J Cell Biochem 1995;57:127–140.
273. Sato Y, Rifkin DB. Inhibition of endothelial cell movement by pericytes and smooth muscle cells: activation of a latent transforming growth factor-β1-like molecule by plasmin during co-culture. J Cell Biol 1989;109:309–315.
274. Sato Y, Tsuboi R, Lyons R, Moses H, Rifkin DB. Characterization of the activation of latent TGF-Beta by co-cultures of endothelial cells and pericytes or smooth muscle cells: a self-regulating system. J Cell Biol 1990;111:757–763.
275. Schild SE, Buskirk SJ, Frick LM, Cupps RE. Radiotherapy for large symptomatic hemangiomas. Int J Radiat Oncol Biol Phys 1991;21:729–735.
276. Schlingemann RO, Rietveld RJR, de Waal RMW, Ferrone S, Ruiter DJ. Expression of the high molecular weight melanoma-associated antigen by pericytes during angiogenesis in tumors and in healing wounds. Am J Pathol 1990;136:1393–1405.
277. Schlingemann RO, Rietveld FJ, Kwaspen F, van de Kerkhof PC, de Waal RMW, Ruiter DJ. Differential expression of markers for endothelial cells, pericytes, and basal lamina in the microvasculature of tumors and granulation tissue. Am J Pathol 1991;138: 1335–1347.
278. Schreiber AB, Winkler ME, Derynck R. Transforming growth factor-alpha: a more potent angiogenic mediator than epidermal growth factor. Science 1986;232: 1250–1253.
279. Schulze-Osthoff K, Risau W, Vollmer E, Sorg C. In situ detection of basic fibroblast growth factor by highly specific antibodies. Am J Pathol 1990;137:85–92.

280. Schweigerer L, Neufeld G, Friedman J, Abraham JA, Fiddes JC, Gospodarowicz D. Capillary endothelial cells express basic fibroblast growth factor, a mitogen that promotes their own growth. Nature 1987;325:257–259.
281. Senger DR, Galli SJ, Dvorak AM, Perruzzi CA, Harvey VS, Dvorak HF. Tumor cells secrete a vascular permeability factor that promotes accumulation of ascites fluid. Science 1983;219:983–985.
282. Shapiro R, Riordan JF, Vallee BL. Characteristic ribonucleolytic activity of human angiogenin. Biochemistry 1986;25:3527–3532.
283. Shing Y, Folkman J, Sullivan R, Butterfield C, Murray J, Klagsbrun M. Heparin affinity: purification of a tumor-derived capillary endothelial cell growth factor. Science 1984;223:1296–1298.
284. Sholley MM, Ferguson GP, Seibel HR, Montour JL, Wilson JD. Mechanisms of neovascularization: vascular sprouting can occur without proliferation of endothelial cells. Lab Invest 1984;51:624–634.
285. Shweiki D, Itin A, Soffer D, Keshet E. Vascular endothelial growth factor induced by hypoxia may mediate hypoxia-initiated angiogenesis. Nature 1992;359:843–845.
286. Shweiki D, Neeman M, Itin A, Keshet E. Induction of vascular endothelial growth factor expression by hypoxia and by glucose deficiency in multicell spheroids: implications for tumor angiogenesis. Proc Natl Acad Sci USA 1995;92:768–772.
287. Sidky YA, Borden EC. Inhibition of angiogenesis by interferons: effects on tumor- and lymphocyte-induced vascular responses. Cancer Res 1987;47:5155–5161.
288. Sillman F, Boyce J, Fruchter R. The significance of atypical vessels and neovascularization in cervical neoplasia. Am J Obstet Gynecol 1981;139:154–159.
289. Singh RK, Bucana CD, Gutman M, Fan D, Wilson MR, Fidler IJ. Organ site-dependent expression of basic fibroblast growth factor in human renal cell carcinoma cells. Am J Pathol 1994;145:365–374.
290. Singh RK, Gutman M, Bucana CD, Sanchez R, Llansa N, Fidler IJ. Interferons α and β down-regulate the expression of basic fibroblast growth factor in human carcinomas. Proc Natl Acad Sci USA 1995;92:4562–4566.
291. Singhvi R, Kumar A, Lopez GP, et al. Engineering cell shape and function. Science 1994;264:696–698.
292. Skinner SA, Tutton PJ, O'Brien PE. Microvascular architecture of experimental colon tumors in the rat. Cancer Res 1990;50:2411–2417.
293. Smith-McCune KK, Weidner N. Demonstration and characterization of the angiogenic properties of cervical dysplasia. Cancer Res 1994;54:800–804.
294. Smolin G, Hyndiuk RA. Lymphatic drainage from vascularized rabbit cornea. Am J Ophthalmol 1971;72:147–151.
295. Soutter AD, Nguyen M, Watanabe H, Folkman J. Basic fibroblast growth factor secreted by an animal tumor is detectable in urine. Cancer Res 1993;53:5297–5299.
296. Spiller JC, Sharma V, Woods GM, Hall JC, Seidel FG. Diffuse neonatal hemangiomatosis treated successfully with interferon alfa-2a. J Am Acad Derm 1992;27:102–104.
297. Splawinski J, Michna M, Palczak R, Konturek S, Splawinski B. Angiogenesis: quantitative assessment by the chick chorioallantoic membrane assay. Methods Findings Exp Clin Pharmacol 1988;10:221–226.
298. Srivastava A, Laidler P, Hughes LE, Woodcock J, Shedden EJ. Neovascularization in human cutaneous melanoma: a quantitative morphological and doppler ultrasound study. Eur J Cancer Clin Oncol 1986;22:1205–1209.
299. Srivastava A, Laidler P, Davies RP, Horfan K. The prognostic significance of tumor vascularity in intermediate-thickness (0.76–4.0 mm thick) skin melanoma. A quantitative histologic study. Am J Pathol 1988;133:419–423.
300. Stadler WM, Sherman J, Bohlander SK, et al. Homozygous deletions within chromosomal bands 9p21–22 in bladder cancer. Cancer Res 1994;54:2060–2063.
301. Stanley P, Gomperts E, Woolley MM. Kasabach-Merritt syndrome treated by therapeutic embolization with polyvinyl alcohol. Am J Pediatr Hematol Oncol 1986;8:308–311.
302. Sutherland RM. Cell and environment interactions in tumor microregions: the multicell spheroid model. Science 1988;240:177–184.
303. Sutherland RM, McCredie JA, Inch WR. Growth of multicell spheroids in tissue culture as a model of nodular carcinomas. JNCI 1971;46:113–120.
304. Takahashi K, Mulliken JB, Kozakewich HPW, Rogers RA, Folkman J, Ezekowitz RAB. Cellular markers that distinguish the phases of hemangioma during infancy and childhood. J Clin Invest 1994;93:2357–2364.
305. Takamiya Y, Brem H, Ojeifo J, Mineta T, Martuza RL. AGM-1470 inhibits the growth of human glioblastoma cells in vitro and in vivo. Neurosurgery 1994;34:869–875.
306. Takechi A. Effect of angiogenesis inhibitor TNP-470 on vascular formation in pituitary tumors induced by estrogen in rats. Neurol Med Chir 1994;34:729–733.
307. Takeshita S, Zheng LP, Brogi E, Kearney M, Pu L-Q, Bunting S, Ferrara N, Symes JF, Isner JM. Therapeutic angiogenesis: a single intra-arterial bolus of vascular endothelial growth factor augments revascularization in a rabbit ischemic hindlimb model. J Clin Invest 1994;93:662–670.
308. Takeshita S, Pu L-Q, Stein LA, et al. Intramuscular administration of vascular endothelial growth factor induces dose-dependent collateral artery augmentation in a rabbit model of chronic limb ischemia. Circulation 1994;90:II-228-II-234.
309. Tanaka NG, Sakamoto N, Tohgo A, Nishiyama Y, Ogawa H. Inhibitory effects of anti-angiogenic agents on neovascularization and growth of the chorioallantoic membrane (CAM): the possibility of a new CAM assay for angiogenesis inhibition. Exp Pathol 1986;30:143–150.
310. Tanaka T, Konno H, Matsuda I, Nakamura S, Baba S. Prevention of hepatic metastasis of human colon cancer by angiogenesis inhibitor TNP-470. Cancer Res 1995;55:836–839.
311. Tannock IF. Population kinetics of carcinoma cells, capillary endothelial cells, and fibroblasts in a transplanted mouse mammary tumor. Cancer Res 1970;30:2470–2476.
312. Taylor S, Folkman J. Protamine is an inhibitor of angiogenesis. Nature 1982;297:307–312.
313. Teicher BA, Sotomayor EA, Huang ZD. Antiangiogenic agents potentiate cytotoxic cancer therapies against primary and metastatic disease. Cancer Res 1992;52:6702–6704.
314. Teicher BA, Holden SA, Ara G, et al. Potentiation of cytotoxic cancer therapies by TNP-470 alone and with other anti-angiogenic agents. Int J Cancer 1994;57:920–925.
315. Teicher BA, Holden SA, Ara G, Northey D. Response of the FSaII fibrosarcoma to antiangiogenic modulators plus cytotoxic agents. Anticancer Res 1993;13:2101–2106.
316. Teillac-Hamel D, De Prost Y, Bodemer C, et al. Serious childhood angiomas: unsuccessful alpha-2b interferon treatment. A report of 4 cases. Br J Derm 1993;129:473–476.
317. Thompson WD, Shiach KJ, Fraser RA, Mintosh LC, Simpson JG. Tumors acquire their vasculature by vessel incorporation, not vessel ingrowth. J Pathol 1987;151:323–332.
318. Thompson RW, Whalen G, Saunders KM, Hores T, D'Amore PA. Heparin-mediated release of fibroblast growth factor-like activity into the circulation of rabbits. Growth Factors 1990;3:221–229.
319. Toi M, Kashitani J, Tominaga T. Tumor angiogenesis is a powerful prognostic indicator of primary breast carcinoma. Int J Cancer 1993;55:341–374.
320. Toi M, Inada K, Suzuki H, Tominaga T. Tumor angiogenesis in breast cancer: its importance as a prognostic indicator and the association with vascular endothelial growth factor expression. Breast Cancer Res Treat 1995;36:193–204.
321. Tolsma SS, Volpert OV, Good DJ, Frazier WA, Polverini PJ, Bouck N. Peptides derived from two separate domains of the matrix protein thrombospondin-1 have anti-angiogenic activity. J Cell Biol 1993;122:497–511.
322. Tulpule A, Snyder JC, Espina BM, et al. A Phase I study of Tecogalan, a novel angiogenesis inhibitor in the treatment of AIDS-related Kaposi's sarcoma and solid tumors. Blood 1994;84:248a. Abstract.
323. Vacca A, Ribatti D, Roncali L, Ranieri G, Serio G, Silvestris F, Dammacco F. Bone marrow angiogenesis and progression in multiple myeloma. Br J Haematol 1994;87:503–508.
324. Van Hoeff MEHM, Knox WF, Dhesi SS, Howell A, Schor AM. Assessment of tumor vascularity as a prognostic factor in lymph node negative invasive breast cancer. Eur J Cancer 1993;29A:1141–1145.
325. Van Meir EG, Polverini PJ, Chazin VR, de Tribolet N, Huang H-JS, Cavenee WK. Induction of wild type p53 expression in glioblastoma cells causes the release of an inhibitor of angiogenesis [Abstract]. Proc Am Assoc Cancer Res 1994;35:186.
326. Van Meir EG, Polverini PJ, Chazin VR, Huan H-JS, de Tribolet N, Cavenee WK. Release of an inhibitor of angiogenesis upon induction of wild type p53 expression in glioblastoma cells. Nature Genet 1994;8:171–176.
327. Verhoeven D, Buyssens N. Desmin-positive stellate cells associated with angiogenesis in a tumor and non-tumor system. Virchows Arch [B] 1988;54:263–272.
328. Vernon RB, Sage EH. Between molecules and morphology. Extracellular matrix and creation of vascular form. Am J Pathol 1995;147:873–883.
329. Vesalainen S, Lipponen P, Talja M, Alhava E, Syrjanen K. Tumor vascularity and basement membrane structure as prognostic factors in T1–2MO prostatic adenocarcinoma. Anticancer Res 1994;14:709–714.
330. Vesikari T, Nuutila A, Cantell K. Neurologic sequelae following interferon therapy of juvenile laryngeal papilloma. Acta Paediatr Scand 1988;77:619–622.
331. Visscher DW, Smilanetz S, Drozdowicz S, Wykes SM. Prognostic significance of image morphometric microvessel enumeration in breast cancer. Anal Quan Cytol Histol 1993;15:88–92.
332. Vlodavsky I, Bashkin PK, Korner G, Bar-Shavit R, Fuks Z. Extracellular matrix-resident growth factors and enzymes: relevance to angiogenesis and metastasis. Proc Annu Meet Am Assoc Cancer Res 1990;31:491–493.
333. Voest EE, Kenyon BM, O'Reilly MS, Truitt G, D'Amato RJ, Folkman J. Inhibition of angiogenesis in vivo by interleukin 12. JNCI 1995;87:581–586.
334. Vukanovic J, Passaniti A, Hirata T, Traystmann RJ, Hartley-Asp B, Isaacs JT. Antiangiogenic effects of the quinoline-3-carboxamide linomide. Cancer Res 1993;53:1833–1837.
335. Wakui S, Furusato M, Itoh T, et al. Tumour angiogenesis in prostatic carcinoma with and without bone marrow metastasis: a morphometric study. J Pathol 1992;168:257–262.
336. Warren BA. The vascular morphology of tumors. In Tumor Blood Circulation: Angiogenesis, Vascular Morphology and Blood Flow of Experimental Human Tumors. Edited by H-I Peterson. Boca Raton, FL: CRC Press, 1979, p 1–47.
337. Watanabe H, Hori A, Seno M, et al. A sensitive enzyme immunoassay for human basic fibroblast growth factor. Biochem Biophys Res Commun 1991;175:229–235.
338. Watanabe H, Nguyen M, Schizer M, et al. Basic fibroblast growth factor in human serum: a prognostic test for breast cancer. Mol Biol Cell 1992;3:324a. Abstract.
339. Watson SA, Morris TM, Robinson G, Crimmin MJ, Brown PD. Inhibition of organ invasion by the matrix metalloproteinase inhibitor batimastat (BB-94) in two human colon carcinoma metastasis models. Cancer Res 1995;55:3629–3633.
340. Weidner N, Semple JP, Welch WR, Folkman J. Tumor angiogenesis correlates with metastasis in invasive breast carcinoma. N Engl J Med 1991;324:1–8.
341. Weidner N, Folkman J, Pozza F, et al. Tumor angiogenesis: a new significant and independent prognostic indicator in early stage breast carcinoma. JNCI 1992;84:1875–1887.
342. Weidner N, Carroll PR, Flax J, Blumenfeld W, Folkman J. Tumor angiogenesis correlates with metastasis in invasive prostate carcinoma. Am J Pathol 1993;143:401–409.
343. Weidner N. Intratumoral microvessel density as a prognostic factor in cancer. Am J Pathol 1995;147:9–19.
344. Weidner N. Current pathologic methods for measuring intratumoral microvessel density within breast carcinoma and other solid tumors. Breast Cancer Res Treat 1995;36:169–180.
345. Weinstat-Saslow D, Steeg PS. Angiogenesis and colonization in the tumor metastatic process: basic and applied advances. FASEB J 1994;8:401–407.
346. Weinstat-Saslow DL, Zabrenetzky VS, VanHoutte K, Frazier WA, Roberts DD, Steeg PS. Transfection of thrombospondin 1 complementary DNA into a human breast carcinoma cell line reduces primary tumor growth, metastatic potential, and angiogenesis. Cancer Res 1994;54:6504–6511.
347. Weiss L. Biophysical aspects of the metastatic cascade. In Fundamental aspects of metastasis. Amsterdam: North-Holland, 1976, p 51–70.
348. West DC, Hampson IN, Arnold F, Kumar S. Angiogenesis induced by degradation products of hyaluronic acid. Science 1985;228:1324–1326.
349. White CW, Sondheimer HM, Crouch EC, Wilson H, Fan LL. Treatment of pulmonary

hemangiomatosis with recombinant interferon alfa-2a. N Engl J Med 1989;320: 1197–1212.

350. White CW, Wolf SJ, Korones DN, Sondheimer HM, Tosi MF, Yu A. Treatment of childhood angiomatous diseases with recombinant interferon alfa-2a. Pediatrics 1991;118:59–65.
351. Wojtowicz S, Ness E, Dickson R, Low J, Barter J, McCann P, Hawkins M. Phase I trials of batimastat (BB-94), a novel matrix metalloproteinase inhibitor in patients with advanced cancer. J Immunother 1994;16:249. Abstract.
352. Wurschmidt F, Beck-Bornboldt HP, Volger H. Radiobiology of the rhabdomyosarcoma R1H of the rat: influence of the size of irradiation field on tumor response, tumor bed effect, and neovascularization kinetics. Int J Rad Oncol Biol Phys 1990;18: 879–882.
353. Yamamoto T, Sudo K, Fujita T. Significant inhibition of endothelial cell growth in tumor vasculature by an angiogenesis inhibitor, TNP-470 (AGM-1470). Anticancer Res 1994;14:1–3.
354. Yamaoka M, Yamamoto T, Ikeyama S, Sudo K, Fujita T. Angiogenesis inhibitor TNP-470 (AGM-1470) potently inhibits the tumor growth of hormone-independent human breast and prostate carcinoma cell lines. Cancer Res 1993;53:5233–5236.
355. Yamaura H, Yamada K, Matsuzawa T. Radiation effect on the proliferating capillaries in rat transparent chamber. Int J Rad Biol 1976;30:179–187.
356. Yamazaki K, Abe S, Takekawa H, Sukoh N, et al. Tumor angiogenesis in human lung adenocarcinoma. Cancer 1994;74:2245–2250.
357. Yanai S, Okada H, Misaki M, et al. Antitumor activity of a medium-chain triglyceride solution of the angiogenesis inhibitor TNP-470 (AGM-1470) when administered via the hepatic artery to rats bearing Walker 256 carcinoma sarcoma of the liver. J Pharmacol Exp Ther 1994;271:1267–1273.
358. Yanase T, Tamura M, Fujita K, Kodama S, Tanaka K. Inhibitory effect of angiogenesis inhibitor TNP-470 on tumor growth and metastasis of human cell lines in vitro and in vivo. Cancer Res 1993;53:2566–2570.
359. Yazaki T, Takamiya Y, Costello PC, et al. Inhibition of angiogenesis and growth of human non-malignant and malignant meningiomas by TNP-470. J Neuroncol 1995;23: 23–29.
360. Yuhas JM, Pazmino NH. Inhibition of subcutaneously growing line 1 carcinoma due to metastatic spread. Cancer Res 1084; 34:2005–2010.
361. Zetter B. The cellular basis of site-specific tumor metastasis. N Engl J Med 1990;322: 605–612.
362. Ziche M, Gullino PM. Angiogenesis and neoplastic progression in vitro. JNCI 1982;69:483–487.
363. Zsebo KM, Yuschenkoff VN, Schiffer S, et al. Vascular endothelial cells and granulopoiesis: interleukin-1 stimulates release of G-CSF and GM-CSF. Blood 1988;71: 99–103.

SECTION II

TUMOR IMMUNOLOGY

CHAPTER 11

Tumor Immunology

ROBERT C. BAST, JR., GORDON B. MILLS, SPENCER GIBSON, AND CINDA M. BOYER

Introduction

Rapid expansion in our understanding of cellular and molecular mechanisms of the human immune response has better defined the concepts of host tumor immunity and signaling between lymphoreticular cells. Recognition and cloning of novel human tumor-specific antigens has demonstrated definitively that a patient's immune response can recognize and destroy tumor cells. Regardless of whether such immunity normally provides effective tumor surveillance, an individual's antitumor immunity can potentially be enhanced through genetic manipulation, tumor vaccines, cytokines, monoclonal antibodies, or the adoptive transfer of cytotoxic cells. To understand these new approaches, reviewing current models of the structure, function, and organization of the immune system is essential.

Human Immune Response

The human immune response has evolved to distinguish "self" from "nonself," permitting the detection and elimination of foreign substances and organisms. This response is mediated by different lymphoreticular cells and their products (Table 11.1). Bone marrow is the ultimate source of stem cells for both B lymphocytes, which produce antibodies, and T lymphocytes, which mediate cellular immunity (1). B and T cells are small lymphocytes that cannot be distinguished morphologically before interaction with antigen, but they bear distinct cell-surface receptors and undergo distinctive programs of differentiation. T and B cells can be identified, characterized, purified, and studied based on surface antigen expression and on their functions.

B CELLS

Mature B cells synthesize and express immunoglobulin (Ig) on their cell surface (2). After interaction with antigen and T-cell products, each clone of B cells differentiates into plasma cell(s) that produce multiple copies of a single antibody that binds noncovalently to a particular antigen. Antibodies bind to "epitopes" that are created by the three-dimensional structures of intact antigenic proteins, glycoproteins, carbohydrates, and less commonly, lipids. Epitopes can be simple linear peptides or, more frequently, arise from conformations created by the spatial apposition of multiple peptide chains or glycosyl groups. Binding depends on a precise complementarity between the antigen and the antibody's combining site. The tertiary structure of the antibody-combining site is determined by the primary amino acid sequence of each immunoglobulin. Immunoglobulin molecules consist of light (L) and heavy (H) polypeptide chains (Fig. 11.1). Each L and H chain can be divided into an amino-terminal variable (V) region and a carboxy-terminal constant region. The V region of each H chain includes three complementarity determining regions (CDRs), which contribute to the antigen-binding site and determine the specificity of the antibody (Figs. 11.2 and 11.3). The H-chain C region (C_H) determines the function and isotype of the antibody. These include IgG1, IgG2, IgG3, IgG4, IgA1, IgA2, IgM, IgD, and IgE (Table 11.2). The C_H region permits fixation of complement components, antibody-dependent cell-mediated cytotoxicity (ADCC), immunoglobulin-mediated phagocytosis, and transport of immunoglobulin across the placenta. The effector functions of immunoglobulins are particularly important for controlling viremia, bacteremia, and infection by gram-positive and encapsulated bacteria.

Antibody diversity is generated by several mechanisms, including somatic recombination of immunoglobulin gene segments, association of different H and L chains, and somatic mutation within the CDRs. Within the variable region of H-chain genes, there is recombination of segments from a library of over 100 variable (V_H), 6 joining (J_H), and 30 diversity (D_H) segments (3). To produce mature L chains, there is recombination of V_L and J_L gene segments with the L-chain genes. Some imprecision in gene-segment recombination is permitted, and additional nucleotides are added to the H-chain genes during D-region recombination by terminal deoxynucleotidyl transferase (TDT). H-chain rearrangement precedes L-chain rearrangement. Within a single B cell, only a single H and L chain associate. Following this association, hypermutable regions within the rearranged L and H chains undergo somatic mutation leading to affinity maturation. High-affinity antibody-producing cells are selected by signals transmitted following ligation of surface immunoglobulin (Ig) by the appropriate antigen, with cells expressing high Ig receptors being preferentially activated and expanded. Through these several mechanisms, more than 100,000 an-

Table 11.1. Phenotype and Functions of Human Lymphoreticular Cells

	T	B	Cell types	
			Natural killer	Monocyte/ macrophage
Phenotype				
Surface membrane immunoglobin	−	+	−	−
Fc receptors	±	+	+	+
C3 receptors	−	+	−	+
Class II MHC	±	+	±	+
TCR, CD3	+	−	−	−
Function				
Antibody formation	−	+	−	−
Antigen presentation	−	+	−	+
Tumor-cell killing	+	−	+	+
Antibody-dependent cell-mediated cytotoxicity	±[a]	−	+	+
Help to B cells	+	−	−	−
Suppression	+	−	−	+
Proliferation to				
Mitogens	+	+	−	−
Alloantigens	+	−	−	−
Soluble proteins	+	−	−	−
Cytokine production				
IL-1	−	−	±	+
IL-2	+	−	−	−
IL-3	+	−	−	−
IL-4	+	−	−	−
IL-5	+	−	−	−
IL-6	+	−	−	+
IL-8	+	−	−	+
IL-9	+	−	−	−
IL-10	+	+		−
IL-12	−	+	−	+
IL-15	+			
IFN-γ	+	−	+	−
GM-CSF	+	−	−	+
TNF-α	+	−	−	+
TGF-β	+	−	−	+

[a] Present when activated.
IL—Interleukin; MHC—major histocompatibility complex; TCR—T-cell receptors; TGF—transforming growth factor; TNF—tumor necrosis factor.
Adapted from Bast (302).

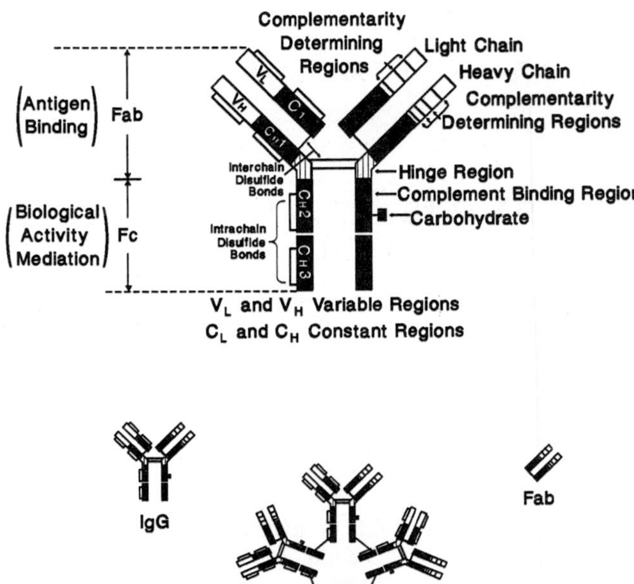

Figure 11.1. Top. Structure of an immunoglobulin monomer containing V_L, V_H, variable light- and heavy-chain regions; C_H1,2,3, constant heavy-chain regions. **Bottom.** Structure of IgG and IgM isotypes and immunoglobulin fragments. IgG consists of one immunoglobulin monomer. IgM is a pentamer consisting of five immunoglobulin monomers linked by interchain disulfide bonds. Fab fragments are generated by enzymatic cleavage with papain. Fab'$_2$ fragments are generated by enzymatic cleavage with pepsin. *Source:* Wasserman and Capra (309); Capra and Edmundson (310).

tibody specificities can be produced and specific, high-affinity antibody-producing clones selected.

Development of monoclonal antibody technology by Kohler and Milstein in 1975 (4) has resulted in the generation of reagents that have permitted precise characterization of B-cell differentiation as well as the interaction of B cells with T cells and their products. Murine monoclonal antibodies are produced by somatic cell hybridization of murine plasmacytoma cells with B cells from immune donors. Hybridomas produce essentially unlimited amounts of antibodies with defined specificity. Different monoclonal antibodies prepared against human leukocytes and tumor cells have defined "clusters of differentiation," or CD groups. Such CD groups (Table 11.3) have defined different lineages, stages of differentiation and states of activation among normal lymphoid and hematopoietic cells. In addition, CD groups have permitted classification of lymphoreticular tumors based on their similarity to normal lymphocytes of different lineages. Correlation between the phenotypes of benign and malignant cells is not always precise, because tumor cells frequently express CD determinants that are characteristic of multiple lineages, a condition described as "lineage infidelity." In defining the phenotype of tumor cells, combinations of CD epitopes often are more helpful than single determinants. CD markers not only assist in defining the phenotype of a tumor cell but also may predict prognosis and suggest appropriate therapy.

Using murine monoclonal antibodies against human B lymphocytes, several stages in differentiation have been identified (Fig. 11.4). Initial steps in the B-cell differentiation pathway are independent of antigen, but subsequent differentiation requires antigen and proceeds optimally in the presence of T-cell-derived factors. Pre-B cells initially express HLA Class II, CD9, CD19, intracellular CD22, CD34, and CD45 and, following initial steps in differentiation, CD10 and CD20. In pre-B cells, the H chain rearranges, followed by the L chain, producing cytoplasmic IgM. TDT, which

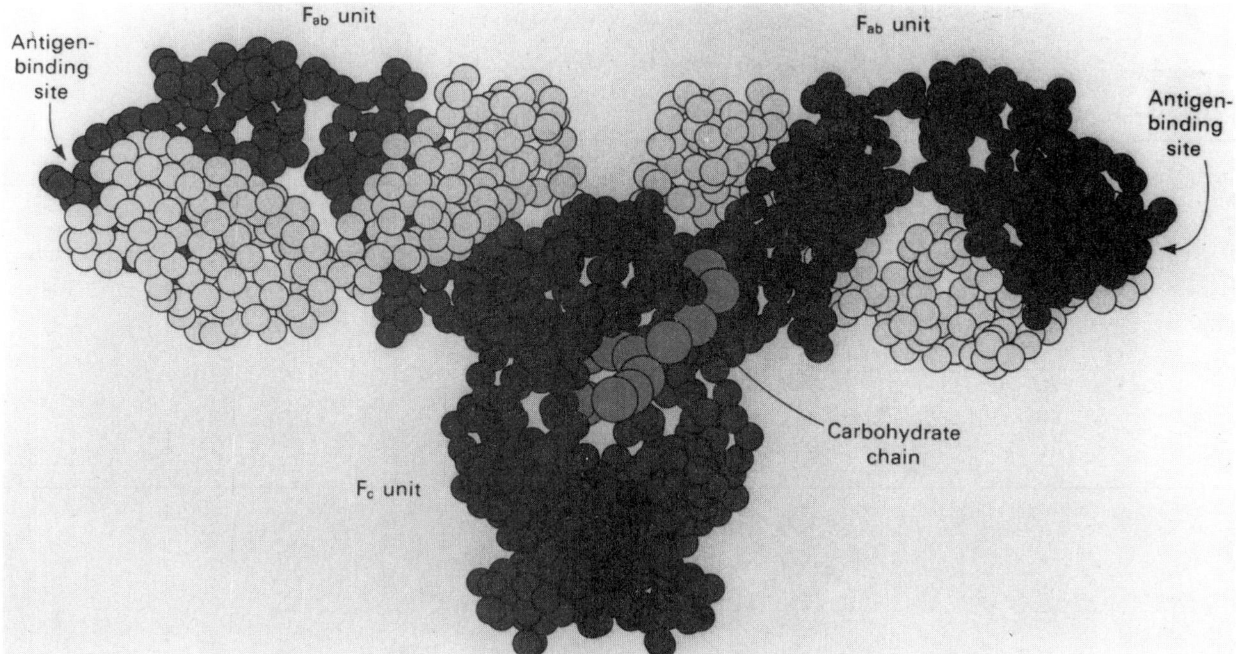

Figure 11.2. Model of an antibody molecule derived from x-ray crystallographic analysis showing the antigen-binding site along with Fab and Fc units. *Source:* Silverton and colleagues (311).

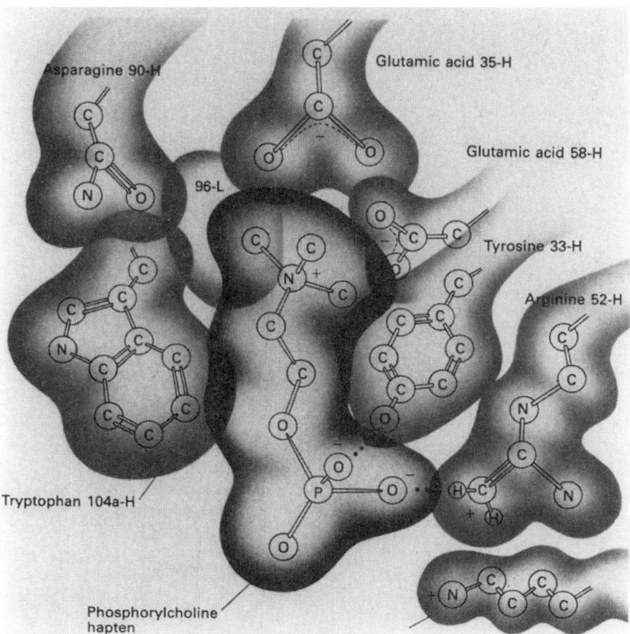

Figure 11.3. Amino acids in the complementarity-determining regions forming the antigen-binding site of an antibody molecule. Those amino acids that contact the antigen, in this case the antigen hapten phosphorylcholine, are shown. 96-L is the ninety-sixth residue of the light chain. *Source:* Capra and Edmundson (310).

adds nucleotides to the D region, is expressed in pre-B cells undergoing H-chain rearrangement. In immature B cells, monomeric IgM of a single specificity is displayed on the cell surface along with Class II major histocompatibility complex (MHC) components. CD10 and CD34 expression is lost during differentiation of pre-B to immature B cells. IgD may be co-expressed with IgM on the surface of a subpopulation of immature B cells. Survival of B-cell precursors is increased in the presence of interleukin (IL)-7 and IL-10 and potentially CD40 ligand. Mature resting B cells continue to express surface immunoglobulin, HLA Class II, CD19, CD20, surface CD22, CD23, CD40, and CD45. Mature B cells gain expression of CD21, CD35, CD44, CD11/18, CD29/49d, CD62l, and CD80 which may play roles in migration, adhesion, and cell signaling. Activated B cells express an array of new surface proteins including novel or increased expression of CD5, CD23, CD25, CD54, CD71, CD80, and CD86. Plasma cells gain expression of CD9, CD38, CD56, and PCA-1 but express lower levels or lose expression of surface immunoglobulin, Class II MHC, CD19, CD20, CD21, CD40, and CD45.

Activation of mature B cells, in contrast to that of T cells, can be triggered by antigen in the fluid phase. Cell–cell interactions between T cells and B cells can, however, provide "help" in B-cell activation and differentiation, as well as regulate sensitivity to programmed cell death through interactions between cell surface molecules such as CD40 on B cells and CD40 ligand on T cells (Fig. 11.5). When antigen binds to cell-membrane IgM in the presence of macrophage-derived factors (IL-1), T-cell factors (Il-2, IL-4, IL-5, IL-6, IL-13, and IL-14) and stromally derived survival

Table 11.2. Properties of Different Human Immunoglobulins

Antibody	Heavy chain	Serum concentration (mg/mL)	Weight (D × 10^3)	Activation of complement			
				Classical pathway	Alternate pathway	Mediation of ADCC	Molecular receptors on mast cells and basophils
IgG1	$\gamma 1$	9	150	+ +	−	−	−
IgG2	$\gamma 2$	3	150	±	−	−	−
IgG3	$\gamma 3$	1	150	+ + +	−	+	−
IgG4	$\gamma 4$	0.5	150	−	+	±	+
IgA1	$\alpha 1$	3	160	−	+	−	−
IgA2	$\alpha 2$	0.5	160	−	+	−	−
IgM	μ	1.5	950	+ + +	−	−	−
IgD	δ	0.03	175	−	+	−	−
IgE	ϵ	0.00005	190	−	−	?	+ +

ADCC—Antibody-dependent cell-mediated cytotoxicity.

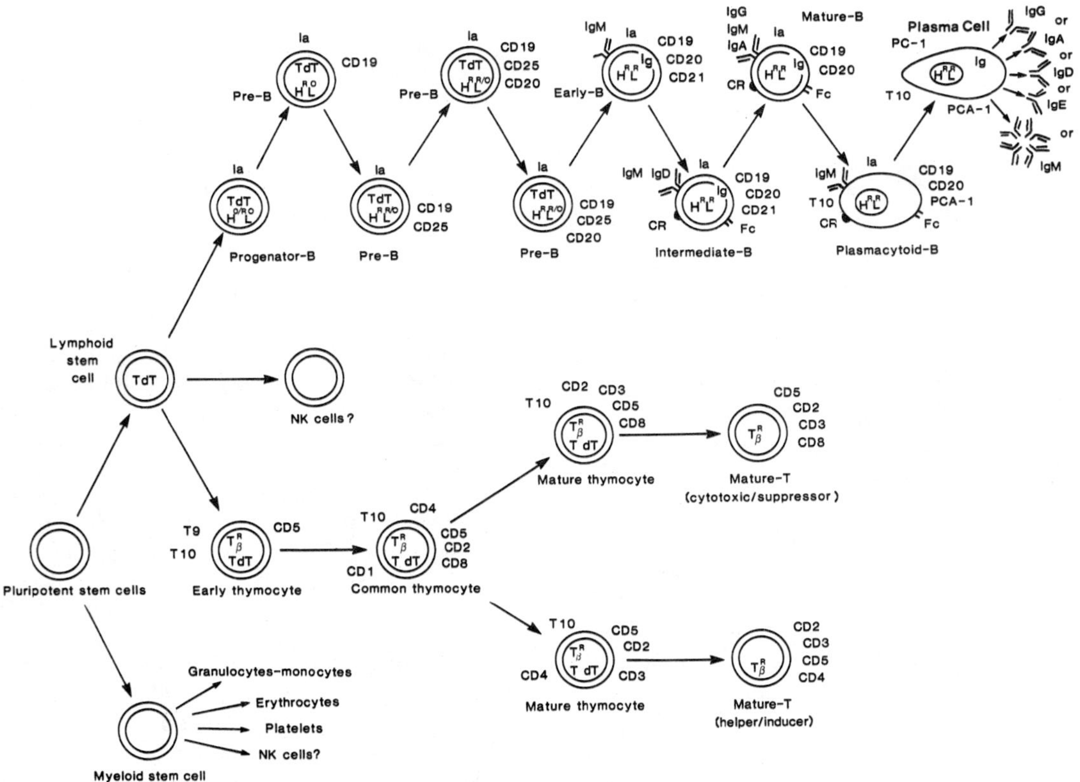

Figure 11.4. Differentiation of lymphoreticular cells from pluripotent hematopoietic stem cells. In addition, CD3 is expressed at low levels in early thymocytes and increases to high levels in common thymocytes. CD25 becomes expressed in early thymocytes and following activation of mature T lymphocytes. CR—complement receptor; γ cytoplasmic—γ heavy chain; H—heavy chain; Ia—Class II major histocompatibility complex; L—light chain; NK—natural killer; O—germ-line configuration; R—rearranged gene; $T^R\beta$—clonal rearrangement of the Tβ receptor; TdT—terminal deoxynucleotidyl transferase. *Source:* Foon and Todd (103).

Table 11.3. CD Designations

Group	Molecular weight ($x10^{-3}$D)	Cellular expression	Expression in malignancies	Function (other names)
CD1	a 49 a g5 c g3	80% of thymocytes; dendritic cells; B cell subset; Langerhans cells	Acute T lymphoblastic leukemia (<35%)	? Ligand for some $\gamma\delta$ T cells (T6)
CD2	50	70–95% thymocytes; 100% T cells, and a variable percentage of LGLs	T-cell malignancies (>70%)	Adhesion molecule (binds LFA-3); T cell activation (T11, LFA-2) (E-rosette (CD58, LFA-3) receptor)
CD3	Complex (3 chains) 16–25	20–90% thymocytes; 100% T cells	Chronic T lymphocytic leukemia (>70%) and cutaneous T-cell lymphoma (>70%), acute T lymphoblastic leukemia (<35%) and lymphoma (35%)	Signal transduction as a result of antigen recognition by T cells, associated with the T-cell antigen receptor (T3 Leu4)
CD4	59	75–80% thymocytes; 60–70% T cells ("helper/inducer" subset); MHC Class II/HIV receptor	Acute T lymphoblastic leukemia (<35%), chronic T lymphocytic leukemia (40–70%), cutaneous T-cell lymphoma (100%)	Adhesion molecule (binds to Class II MHC); signal transduction
CD5	67	10% thymocytes, most T cells, and a subset of B cells	T-cell malignancies (>70%), chronic B lymphocytic leukemia (40–70%)	? Adhesion molecule (T1)
CD6	100	Mature T cells; subset of B cells	Acute T lymphoblastic leukemia (<35%), chronic T lymphocytic leukemia (>70%) and cutaneous T-cell lymphoma (>70%), chronic B lymphocytic leukemia (40–70%)	? (T12)
CD7	40	Thymocytes; 100% T cells; some LGLs	Acute T lymphocytic leukemia (40–70%), cutaneous T-cell lymphoma (<35%)	? (T8 Leu2)
CD8	33/33	50–80% thymocytes; 35% T cells (cytotoxic/suppressor subset); MHC Class I receptor; some LGLs (low density)	Acute T lymphoblastic leukemia (<35%) and chronic T lymphocytic leukemia (<35%)	Adhesion (binds to Class I MHC); signal transduction
CD9	24	Pre-B cells; monocytes; platelets; granulocytes	Acute non-T, non-B lymphoblastic leukemia (>70%); chronic B lymphoblastic leukemia (<35%), multiple myeloma, acute myeloid leukemia	? Role in platelet activation
CD10	100	Pre-B cells; granulocytes	Acute non-T, non-B lymphoblastic leukemia (>70%)	Structurally identical to neural endopeptidase (enkephalinase); common acute lymphoblastic leukemia antigen
CD11a	180/95	Leukocytes		Adhesion (binds to ICAM-1) (LFA-1)
CD11b	165/95	Monocytes; granulocytes; LGLs	M4 (40–70%) and M5 (>70%) acute nonlymphocytic leukemia; acute lymphoblastic leukemia	Adhesion; C3Bi receptor (CR3); phagocytosis of iC3b-coated (opsonized) particles (Mac1)
CD11c	150/95	Monocytes, granulocytes, B-cell subset		Adhesion; ? phagocytosis of iC3b-coated (opsonized) particles
CD12	90–120	Monocytes, granulocytes, platelets	M4 and M5 (<35%) stages of ANLL	Phosphoprotein; no known function
CD13	150	Monocytes; granulocytes; early myeloid cells	M1 (>70%) and M4 or M5 (<35%) stages of ANLL, chronic myelogenous leukemia (40–70%)	Aminopeptidase; ? role in oxidative burst
CD14	55	70–93% monocytes; granulocytes; Langerhans cells	M4 (<35%) and M5 (40–70%) stages of acute nonlymphocytic leukemia	LPS receptor; ? role in oxidative burst (MO2)
CD15		100% monocytes; >95% mature granulocytes	Most ANLL; rare ALL; carcinoma	Sialyl form is a ligand for selectins Le^x determinant
CD16	50–65	LGLs (NK); granulocytes, monocytes, platelets		Low-affinity Fcγ receptor; ADCC, activation of NK cells; (FcγRIII)
CD17	Lactosylceramide	Granulocytes, monocytes, platelets	ANLL	?
CD18	95	T cells; B cells; LGLs; monocytes; granulocytes	ANLL	See CD11a, 11b, 11c; β chain of LFA-1 family
CD19	95	100% of pre-B cells	All non-T ALL, some ANLL, B-CLL; B-cell lymphoma	? Role in B-cell activation or regulation (B4)

(continued)

Table 11.3. *(continued)*

Group	Molecular weight ($\times 10^{-3}$D)	Cellular expression	Expression in malignancies	Function (other names)
CD20	37/32	B cells	Some non-T; ALL, B-CLL; B-cell lymphoma	? Role in B-cell activation or regulation (B1)
CD21	140	Mature B-cell subset		Receptor for C3d, Epstein-Barr virus; ? role in B-cell activation (B2)
CD22	135	B-cell subset		? Role in cell adhesion and B-cell activation
CD23	45–50	B-cell subset; activated macrophages; eosinophils	B- and T-cell lymphomas; B-CLL; Hodgkin's disease	Low-affinity Fcϵ receptor, induced by IL-4; function unknown (FcϵRIIb)
CD24	41/38	B cells; granulocytes	Non-T ALL; some ANLL; neuroblastoma	?
CD25	55	Activated T cells; B cells; monocytes; LGLs	T-ALL	Complexes with IL-2R$\beta\gamma$ high-affinity IL-2 receptor; T-cell growth (Tac)
CD26	120	Activated T and B cells; macrophages		Dipeptidyl-peptidase IV, serine peptidase; ? role in HIV infection
CD27	55 (dimer)	Thymocytes; T-cell subset	T-CLL, Sezary cells	? Role in B-cell growth; member of Fas, CD40 TNF family
CD28	44	T-cell subset		T-cell receptor for costimulatory molecule(s) B7.1, B7.2 (Tp44)
CD29	120–130	Leukocytes, platelets	ALL (T and non-T), T-CLL	Adhesion to extracellular matrix proteins, cell–cell adhesion (platelet VLAβ-chain; with IIa CD49)
CD30	105	Activated T and B cells	Reed-Sternberg cells in Hodgkin's disease	?
CD31	140	Platelets, monocytes, granulocytes, B cells		Role in leukocyte-endothelial adhesion (PECAM-1)
CD32	40	Monocytes, granulocytes, B cells		Fc receptor for aggregated IgG; role in phagocytosis, ADCC; feedback inhibition of B cells
CD33	67	Monocytes, marrow progenitors	ANLL	?
CD34	105–120	Marrow progenitors	ANLL	?
CD35	190–280	Granulocytes, B cells, monocytes, some T cells	ANLL	Binding and phagocytosis of C3b-coated particles and immune complexes
CD36	90	Monocytes, platelets, B cells	ANLL	Platelet adhesion (gpIIIb)
CD37	40–52	B cells, T cells, monocytes	B lymphomas	?
CD38	45	LGLs, B cells, activated T cells, monocytes, thymocytes, lymphoid progenitors	T-ALL, myeloma, some AML	? (T10)
CD39	70–100	B-cell subset, monocytes	Burkitt's lymphoma cells	?
CD40	44/48	B cells	B lymphomas, B-CLL, Burkitt's lymphoma; some B-ALL; carcinomas	Role in B-cell activation induced by T-cell contact
CD41	120/23	Platelets		Platelet aggregation and activation; receptor of fibrinogen, fibronectin (binds to R-G-D sequence); Platelet GPIIb-IIIa complex and GPIIb
CD42a	23	Platelets		Platelet adhesion, binding to von Willebrand factor (Platelet GPIX)
CD42b	135/25			See CD42a (Platelet GPIB)
CD43	95	T cells, granulocytes, monocytes, brain		? Role in T-cell activation
CD44	80–95	Leukocytes, brain, erythrocytes		May function as homing receptor; receptor for matrix components (e.g., hyaluronate) Pgp-1, Hermes)

(continued)

Table 11.3. *(continued)*

Group	Molecular weight ($\times 10^{-3}$D)	Cellular expression	Expression in malignancies	Function (other names)
CD45	180–220	>95% of lymphocytes; monocytes and granulocytes		Role in signal transduction, tyrosine phosphatase (T200 LCA)
CD45RA	220	T-cell subset (appears to identify suppressor/inducers); B cells; monocytes		See CD45
CD45RB	220/205/190	B cells, T-cell subset, monocytes, granulocytes		See CD45
CD45RO	180	T cells, B-cell subset, monocytes		See CD45
CD46	66/56	Leukocytes		Regulation of complement activation
CD47	47–52	Broad		?
CD48	41	Leukocytes		?
CD49b	170	Platelets, cultured T cells		Adhesion to extracellular matrix; receptor for collagen, platelet GPI, VLA-α chain
CD49c	130/25	T cells, some B-cell monocytes		Forms VLA-3 with CD29, adhesion to fibronectin, laminin
CD49d	150	Monocytes, T cells, B cells, Langerhans cells, thymocytes		Peyer's patch homing receptor, binds to VCAM-1; adhesion to fibronectin, VLA-α4 chain
CD49f	120/31/30	Platelets, T cells		Adhesion to extracellular matrix; receptor for laminin, VLA-α6 chain, platelet GPIc
CD50	148/108	Leukocytes		? GPI linked
CD51	125/25	Platelets		Adhesion: receptor for vitronectin, fibrinogen, von Willebrand factor (binds R-G-D sequence)
CD52	12–28	Leukocytes		?
CD53	32–40	Leukocytes		?
CD54	90	Broad		Adhesion; ligand for CD2 (ICAM-1)
CD55	70	Broad	LGL leukemias	Regulation of complement activation (DAF)
CD56	220/135	LGLs (NK); activated lymphocytes	LGL leukemias	Homotypic adhesion; isoform of neural cell adhesion molecule (N-CAM) (leu 19)
CD57	110	LGLs (NK); T cells; B-cell subset, brain		? (HNK1 Leu7)
CD58	40–65	LFA-3; leukocytes, epithelial cell		Dimerizes with CD51, CD41 (LFA3)
CD59	18–20	Broad		Regulation of complement (MAC) activation
CD60	NeuAc-NeuAc-Gal	T subset		?
CD61	110	Platelets		Dimerizes with CD51, CD41; integrin β3-, VNR-, β chain, platelet GPIIIa
CD62	140	Platelets		
CD62e	115	Endothelial cells		Endothelial T-cell adhesion (E-selectin ELAM-1)
CD62l	75–80	T cells		Endothelial T-cell adhesion (L-selectin LAM-1)
CD62p	130–150	Platelets, endothelial cells		Leukocyte adhesion to platelets and endothelial cells (P selectin, PADGEM)
CD63	53	Platelets, monocytes, granulocytes, T cells, B cells		?

(continued)

Table 11.3. *(continued)*

Group	Molecular weight ($x10^{-3}$D)	Cellular expression	Expression in malignancies	Function (other names)
CD64	75	Monocytes		High-affinity Fcγ receptor; role in phagocytosis, ADCC, macrophage activation
CD65	Ceramide	Granulocytes, monocytes		? Role in neutrophil activation
CD66	180–200	Granulocytes		? Role in homotypic cell–cell adhesions (carcinoembryonic antigen, or CEA, is called CD66e)
CD67	100	Granulocytes		?
CD68	110	Macrophages		?
CD69	32/28	Activated B and T cells		?
CD70	24	Activated B and T cells	Reed-Sternberg cells	?
CD71	95	Proliferating thymocytes, monocytes; activated T and B cells		Receptor for transferrin; role in iron metabolism, cell growth (T9)
CD72	43/39	B cells		Ligand for CD5; ? role in T-cell–B-cell interaction
CD73	69	B-cell subset, T-cell subset		Ecto-5′-nucleotidase, regulates nucleotide metabolism
CD74	41/35/33	B cells, monocytes		Associates with newly synthesized Class II MHC molecules
CD75	53	Mature B cells, T-cell subset		?
CD76	85/67	Mature B cells, T-cell subset		?
CD77	?	Resting B cells		Gb3
CD78	?	B cells, monocytes		?
CD79a	32–33	Mature B cells		Component of B-cell antigen receptor (Igα, Mb-1)
CD79b	37–39	Mature B cells		Component of B-cell antigen receptor (Igβ, B29)
CD80	50–60	Dendritic cells, activated B cells and macrophages		Costimulator for T-lymphocyte activation; ligand for CD28 and CTLA-4 (B7.1)
CD81	22	Broad		Association with CD19 and CD21; ? role in B-cell activation; channel complex (TAPA1)
CD82	50–53	Broad		? Co-stimulation of T cells
CD83	40–43	Some B-cell lines, Langerhans cells; others		?
CD84	73	Monocytes, lymphocytes, platelets		?
CD85	120	B cells, monocytes		?
CD86	80	B cells, monocytes		Costimulator for T-lymphocyte activation; ligand for CD28 and CTLA-4 (B7.2)
CD87	50–65	Neutrophils, monocytes, endothelial cells		?
CD88	40	Neutrophils, macrophages, mast cells, eosinophils		Receptor for complement component C5a; role in complement-induced inflammation
CD89	55–70	Neutrophils, monocytes		IgA-dependent cytotoxicity
CDw90	25–35	Thymocytes, peripheral T cells (mice), neurons (all species)		? Role in T-cell activation (Thy-1)
CD91	600	Macrophages and monocytes		α2-Macroglobulin receptor
CDw92	70	Broad		?
CD93	118–129	Neutrophils, monocytes, endothelial cells		?
CD94	43	NK cells, T-cell subset		Adhesion
CD95	42	Multiple cell types		Role in programmed cell death (Fas, Apo-1)

(continued)

Table 11.3. *(continued)*

Group	Molecular weight 10^{-3} D	Cellular expression	Expression in malignancies	Function (other names)
CD96	160/180/240	T cells	CD7+ AML	?
CD97	74/80/89	T subset, NK subset, eosinophils		?
CD98	40/80	Broad		Signaling
CD99	32	Broad		Signaling, adhesion
CD100	150	T cells, B cells, granulocytes, monocytes, NK cells		Signaling
CDw101	140	Granulocytes, monocytes		Co-expression with CD28
CD102	55–65	Endothelial cells, monocytes, other leukocytes		Ligand for LFA-1 integrin (ICAM-2)
CD103	150/25	Some T lymphocytes, other cell types		? Role in T-cell homing to mucosa (integrin subunits)
CD104	205–220	Epithelium, epithelium keratinocytes, some B cells		Adhesion, B4, integrin chain, cytoskeleton organization
CD105	95 (dimer subunits)	Endothelial cells, activated macrophages	Some B and myeloid leukemias	TGF-β III receptor (endoglin) adhesion
CD106	90–95	Endothelial cells, macrophages, follicular dendritic cells, marrow stromal cells		Receptor for VLA-4 integrin; role in cell adhesion, lymphocyte activation, hematopoiesis (VCAM-1)
CD107a	110	Platelets		Lysosomal protein of unknown function
CD107b	120	Platelets		Lysosomal protein of unknown function
CDw108	75–83	Activated T cells, some stroma		Cell activation, GPI linked
CDw109	170/150	Activated T cells, platelets, endothelium		Activation, proliferation, signaling, GPI linked
CD115	150	Monocytes, macrophages		M-CSF receptor (c-FMS)
CDw116	75–80	Myeloid cells, monocytes	Ovarian cancer, breast cancer, AML	GM-CSF receptor, α chain
CD117	145	Melanocytes, mast cells, endothelial cells	AML, breast cancer	Steel receptor (c-kit)
CDw119	90	Broad		IFN-γ receptor
CD120a	55	Broad		TNF receptor, α chain
CD120b	75	T cells, B cells, monocytes		TNF receptor, β chain
CDw121a	80	Broad		IL-1 receptor, type II
CDw121b	68	Broad		IL-7 receptor, type I
CD122	75	T cells, B cells, NK cells	Hodgkin's disease, acute leukemias	IL-2 receptor, β chain; also binds IL-15; T-cell proliferation
CDw124	140	Hematopoietic cells, fibroblasts, epithelial cells		IL-4 receptor proliferation
CD126	80	T cells, epithelium	Myeloma	IL-6 receptor α-chain signaling
CDw127	75	Hematopoietic cells		IL-7 receptor signaling
CDw128	58–67	Neutrophils, monocytes, keratinocytes	Melanoma	IL-8 receptor activation chemotaxis
CDw130	130	Broad		Common chain of IL-6, IL-11, LIF, OSM, CNTF receptors

ADCC—Antibody-dependent cell-mediated cytotoxicity; ALL—acute lymphocytic leukemia; AML—acute myelogenous leukemia; ANLL—acute nonlymphoblastic leukemia; B—B cell; CLL—chronic lymphocytic leukemia; HIV—human immunodeficiency virus; IFN—interferon; IV—intravenous; LFA—lymphocyte function antigen; LGL—large granular lymphocytes; MHC—major histocompatibility complex; NK—natural killer cell; T—T cell; TGF—transforming growth factor; TNF—tumor necrosis factor.

Data from Knapp and colleagues (303), Rosenberg and colleagues (304), Reading (305), Zola (306), and Pinto and colleagues (296).

factors (IL-11 and transforming growth factor-beta (TGF-β)), the mature virgin B cells proliferate, differentiate, and switch isotypes to IgG, IgA, or IgE. The particular array of cytokines present predisposes to the production of specific immunoglobulins. IL-2, IL-4, and IL-5 drive IgM production, whereas IL-2, IL-4, IL-6, and IFN-γ encourage IgG production; IL-5 and TGF-β promote IgA production; and IL-4 alone enhances IgE production. Signals also are transduced through the interaction of an array of accessory molecules on B cells with their cognate ligands on activated helper T cells (Fig. 11.5) (5). Following functional activation, both memory B cells and secretory plasma cells are produced.

B cells are organized in follicular aggregates within lymph nodes, spleen, and gut-associated lymphoid tissue, in proximity to T cells and antigen presenting cells. Antibody production can be augmented by T-cell help and can be down-regulated by T cells or macrophage-mediated "suppression."

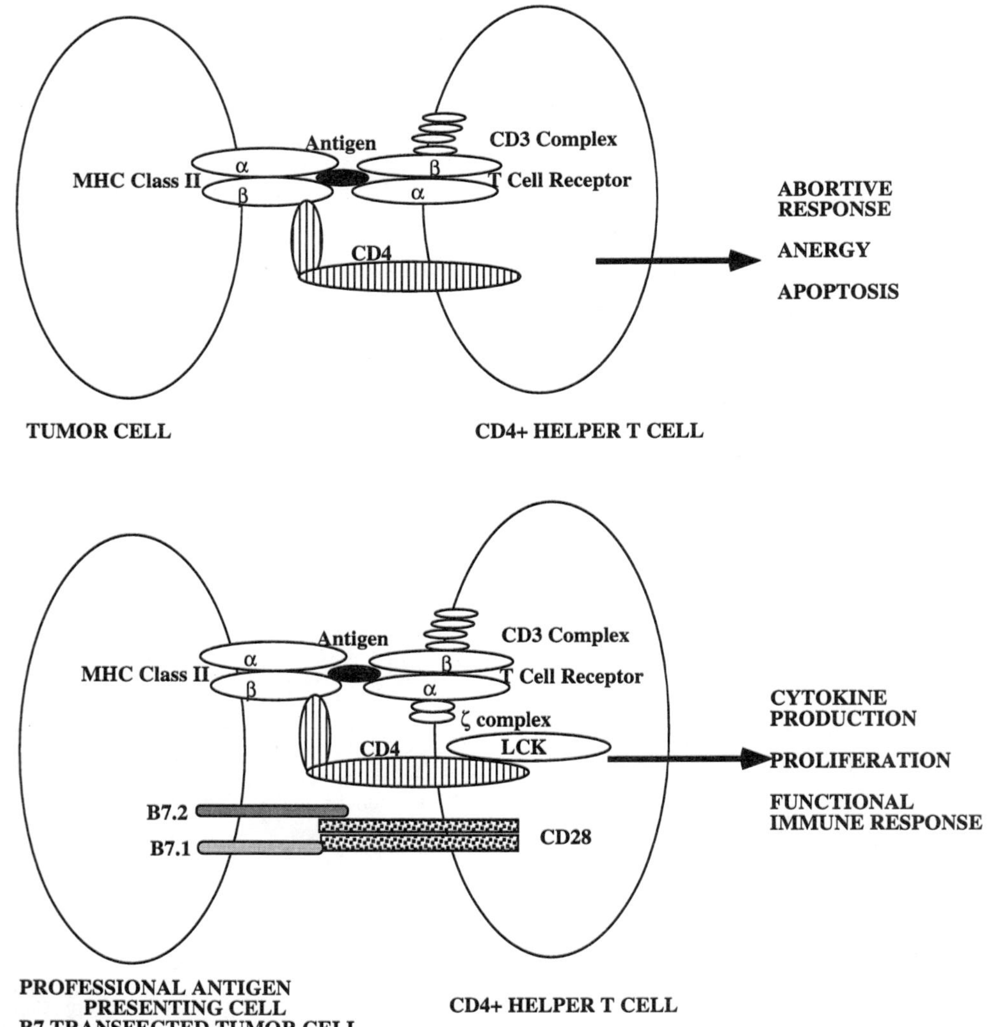

Figure 11.5. Cognate interaction between T cells and antigen-presenting cells. Adhesion and accessory molecules both increase the avidity of interactions between T cells and antigen-presenting cells as well as provide important co-stimulatory signals.

T CELLS

T lymphocytes arise in bone marrow and differentiate within the thymus (6). Over 90% of T cells, including those that recognize "self" determinants, are eliminated during thymic differentiation by apoptotic negative selection and failure to undergo positive selection. Potentially autoreactive T cells also can be rendered nonresponsive in peripheral lymphoid tissues through the induction of "anergy" or interaction with "veto" cells. Mature T cells normally traffic through the peripheral circulation and return to lymph through the venous and postcapillary venules of the skin and lymph nodes. T cells mediate the cellular immune response, including delayed hypersensitivity, graft rejection, and regulation of other T cells, B cells, monocytes, and marrow progenitors. T cells are particularly important for resistance to viruses and microbial pathogens that are destroyed by macrophages, including certain fungi, mycobacteria, *Salmonella* species, and *Listeria* monocytogenes.

The specificity of interactions with different antigens is mediated by a large family of T-cell receptors (TCR) generated by genetic recombination (7, 8). In contrast to B cells that recognize portions of intact macromolecules, the T cells generally recognize small linear peptide fragments of larger proteins only when bound to molecules of the MHC. Different clones of T cells bearing distinctive TCRs generally recognize only those antigenic peptides that are of appropriate size and sequence to permit binding to those MHC antigens inherited and expressed by the individual (Fig. 11.6).

Diversity of TCR binding sites arises through (*a*) somatic recombination of V-, D-, J-, and C-gene segments analogous to that observed during generation of Ig diversity and (*b*) addition of nucleotides during D region recombination by the action of TDT. In contrast to the process observed in B cells, somatic mutation does not play a major role in T-cell differentiation and affinity maturation thus is not a predominant process. Each TCR is an integral membrane heterodimer composed of either α/β (95%) or γ/δ (2–5%) chains. β and δ, but not α and γ, genes contain D regions. Interestingly, the δ chain in mature γ/δ T cells has tandem D

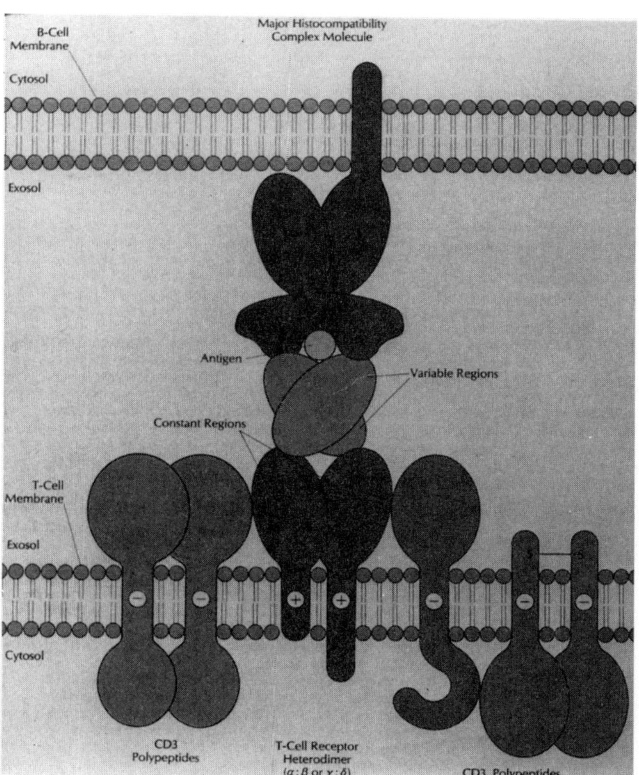

Figure 11.6. The T-cell antigen receptor CD3 complex. The T-cell receptor is a heterodimer ($\alpha\beta$ or $\gamma\delta$) with variable and constant regions found on the T-cell surface in a complex with the nonpolymorphic CD3 polypeptides. The receptor binds antigen associated with a major histocompatibility complex molecule on the surface of an antigen-presenting B cell. *Source:* Davis (312).

regions. Most γ/δ T cells are associated with the skin, lung, and intestine where they likely play a major role in resistance to parasites and mycobacteria.

Either type of TCR is found in close proximity to the CD3 and ζ peptide complexes which regulate signaling from the cell membrane to the nucleus (Fig. 11.7). Antigen-presenting cells (APC), including dendritic cells, monocytes, tissue-resident macrophages, and B cells, digest exogenous proteins in lysosomes or endosomes and display antigenic peptides of 13 to 25 amino acids at their surface in the context of Class II MHC antigens (HLA-DR, -DQ, and -DP). In addition to this exogenous pathway of antigen presentation, a recently identified endogenous pathway of antigen presentation allows the display of intracellular antigens by MHC. In this pathway, antigenic peptides of 8 to 11 amino acids produced in proteasomes from endogenous viral and cellular proteins become associated with Class I MHC antigens (HLA-A, -B, and -C) during the synthesis and expression of MHC on the cell surface, permitting immunologic recognition of changes in intracellular protein production induced by viruses, intracellular parasites, or malignant transformation. Different MHC molecules vary in their ability to bind particular antigenic peptides, resulting in a genetic limitation of the ability to present and recognize specific antigens.

In contrast to B cells, which can recognize antigen in the fluid phase, T cells are thought to recognize antigenic peptides only on the surface of APC. $CD8^+$ T cells interact with antigen bound to Class I MHC determinants, whereas $CD4^+$ T cells recognize antigen bound to Class II MHC antigens. Binding of TCR to antigen generates a "primary signal" that is transduced through the CD3-TCR- ζ complex and that activates intracellular tyrosine kinases and downstream signaling molecules, including *ras* and MAP (Fig. 11.7). Activation of tyrosine kinases and phospholipase C leads to release of intracellular calcium and activation of protein kinase C (9). Full activation of a T cell requires delivery of one or more "second signals" transmitted by an interaction between specific molecules on the surface of T cells and their cognate ligands on the surface of "professional" APCs (10, 11) (Fig. 11.8). Some of the most important costimulatory signals appear to be transduced by the interaction of CD28 homodimers on the T cell surface with B7.1 or B7.2 expressed on APCs (12, 13). In the absence of second co-stimulatory signals, the activity of T cells may be down-regulated, or T cells may be targeted to an apoptotic pathway producing tolerance or anergy to an otherwise foreign antigen (Fig. 11.8). Ligation of CD28 not only increases cytokine production through increased transcription and stabilization of mRNA but also prevents anergy and programmed cell death (12, 13). Adhesion molecules stabilize the interactions of APCs with T and B cells (Fig. 11.5). Productive activation of T cells leads to the secretion of cytokines which regulate the magnitude and duration of the subsequent immune response. Activation of mature T cells by both primary and secondary signals can trigger morphologic changes, proliferation, release of cytokines, and acquisition of cytotoxic function.

T cells mature under the influence of thymic epithelium (Fig. 11.4). Early thymocytes (Stage I), which are found in the outer cortex, express CD2, CD7, CD25, CD38, CD44, and CD71 but do not express surface T-cell receptor (TCR), CD3, CD4, or CD8, resulting in the designation of "double negative" thymocytes. Immature thymocytes (Stage II), which are found in the inner cortex, acquire CD1, low-level expression of the TCR, lose expression of CD25 and CD44, and express both CD4 and CD8, resulting in the designation of "double-positive" thymocytes. Mature thymocytes (Stage III), found in the medulla, have lost CD1 but have gained high-level expression of the TCR, CD3, CD5, and CD6. Either CD4 or CD8 is expressed, but not both, resulting in the designation of "single-positive" thymocytes. T lymphocytes that can bind to the MHC complex are positively selected, but those T cells that exhibit particularly high affinity for the MHC are eliminated through negative selection. Thus during maturation many clones that recognize "self" with high affinity are eliminated through negative selection, whereas those clones that will recognize foreign antigens in the context of MHC antigens persist through positive selection. Mature T cells constitute approximately 80% of normal peripheral blood lymphocytes, 35% of lymph node cells, and 25% of splenic lymphocytes. T cells that encounter appropriately presented and relevant antigens in the presence of stimulatory secondary signals and cytokines are expanded into functional T-cell clones. Following clearance of the foreign antigen, a population of long-lived memory T cells persists.

In general, $CD4^+$ and $CD8^+$ T cells subserve different functions, defined by the ability of CD4 to recognize Class II

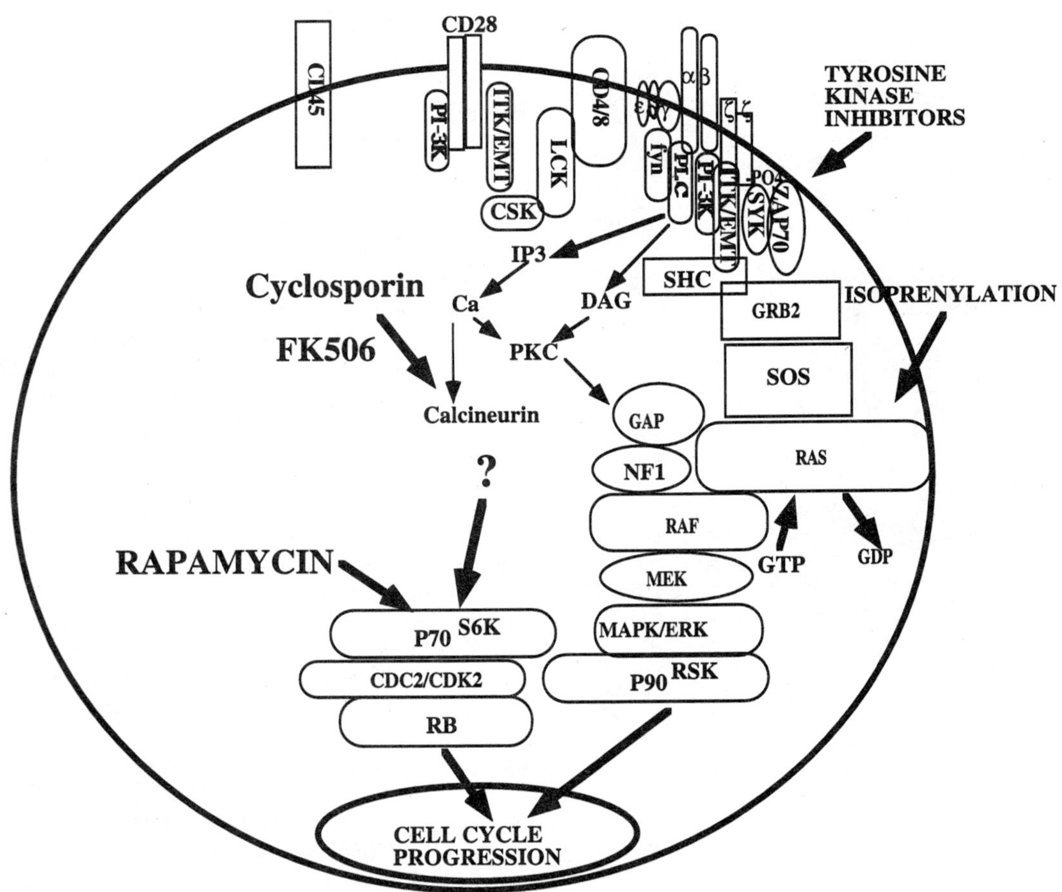

Figure 11.7. T-cell signal transduction. One of the most exciting advances made over the last decade has been the identification of a continuous signaling pathway that links cell-surface receptors, such as the T-cell receptors (TCR), to nuclear signaling events. Activation of the T-cell receptor initiates a tyrosine kinase cascade leading to activation of SOS and RAS. RAS acts as a molecular switch leading to the activation of RAF and the MAP kinase cascade. MAP kinases migrate to the nucleus, where they phosphorylate and activate transcription factors. In addition to the RAS cascade, TCR activation leads to stimulation of phospholipase C and changes intracellular calcium and activation of protein kinase C. Phosphatidylinositol 3′ kinase also is activated and, by an as-yet-poorly defined mechanism, leads to activation of P70S6 kinase. Identification of such signaling pathways may allow development of methods to specifically activate or inhibit signaling molecules: Tyrphostins by inhibiting tyrosine kinases, isoprenylation inhibitors by blocking RAS, cyclosporin by interfering with calcium-dependent signaling, FK506 by interfering with calcium-dependent signaling, and Rapamycin by blocking P70S6 kinase activation all inhibit specific intracellular signaling molecules, allowing alteration of specific pathways in T lymphocytes.

MHC and CD8 to recognize Class I MHC. $CD4^+$ T cells once were thought to be exclusively "helper/inducer" cells, but recent studies have identified populations of cytotoxic $CD4^+$ cells restricted by Class II MHC. $CD4^+$ T cells can "help" B cells, stimulate cytotoxic T cells, and activate monocytes. $CD4^+$ helper cells can be further subdivided into TH0, TH1, and TH2 cells based on their ability to produce specific cytokines. TH0, TH1, and TH2 produce TNF-α, GM-CSF, and IL-3 (Table 11.4). TH1 cells, but not TH2 cells, produce cytokines (IL-2, IFN-γ, and TNF-β), which help delayed-type hypersensitivity reactions, cytotoxic T-cell differentiation, IgG_{2a} production, NK cell maturation, macrophage activation, and cell-mediated immunity against intracellular microorganisms. TH2, but not TH1 cells, produce cytokines (IL-4, IL-5, IL-10, and IL-13), which help IgE secretion, mast cell and eosinophil production, and B cell proliferation. TH0 cells, in contrast, produce a mixture of cytokines and may be a precursor population. Suppressor T cells are predominantly $CD8^+$ and can affect B and T cells as well as hematopoietic precursors. Antigen-specific and nonspecific suppression by T cells has been documented in different systems. Nonspecific suppression of immune function also can be mediated by macrophages. Thus, the net immune response is regulated by the presence of foreign antigen, ability of antigenic peptides to be presented by the individual's MHC, presence of appropriate cytokines, and balance between the activity of helper and suppressor cells. Therefore, there are many potential sites for intervention to regulate or augment an anti-tumor immune response.

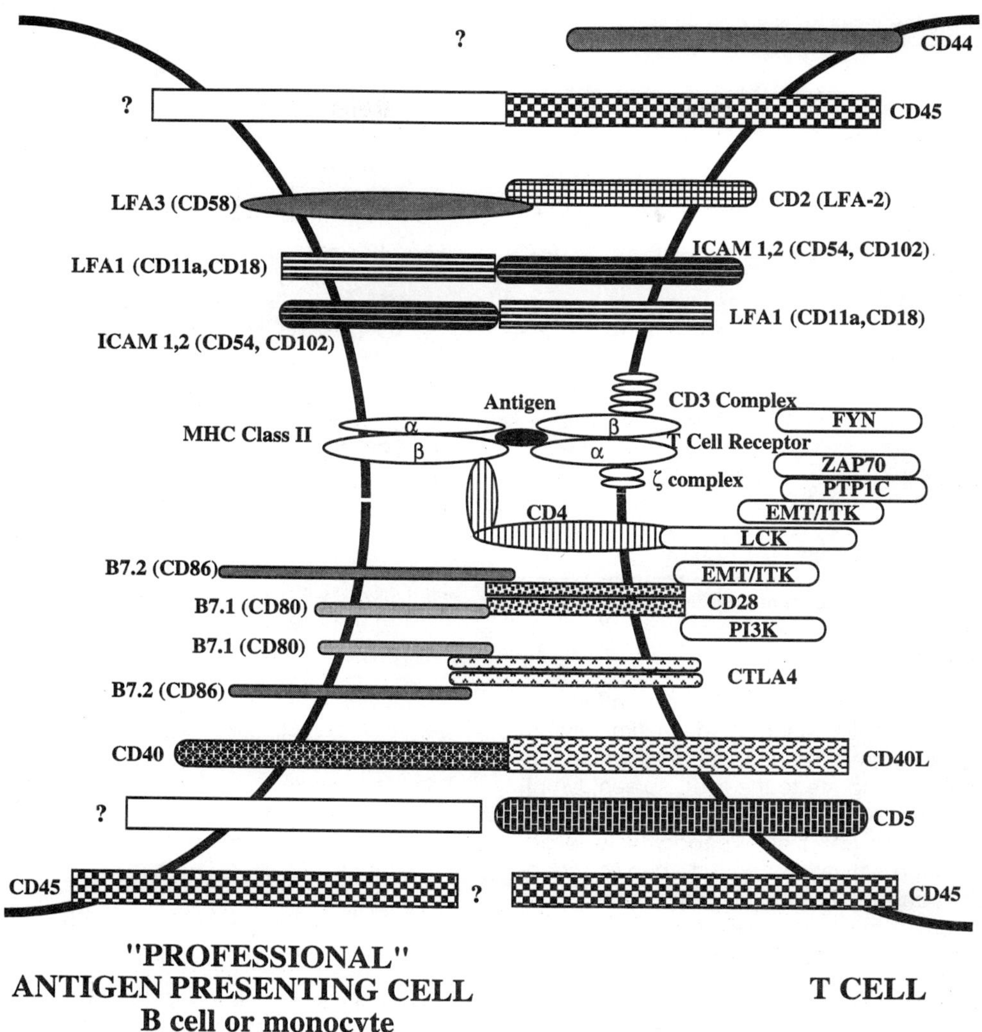

Figure 11.8. T-cell receptor (TCR) activation in the absence of appropriate co-stimulation leads to an abortive immune response. Ligation of the TCR in the absence of coligation of co-stimulatory molecules such as CD28 leads to an abortive immune response characterized by anergy or apoptosis. "Professional" antigen-presenting cells such a B cells and macrophages express B7 on their surface, resulting in activation of a functional response. Antigen presentation by interferon-activated epithelial cells or tumor cells aberrantly expressing Class II major histocompatibility complex (MHC) can lead to an abortive immune response. Transfection of B7.1 into tumor cells converts them to "functional" antigen-presenting cells, markedly increases the production of cytokines by responding T cells, and prevents the induction of anergy and apoptosis. B7.1-expressing tumor cells are capable of inducing an immune response that can clear tumors induced by the parental (non-CD28-positive) tumor.

NATURAL KILLER CELLS

A small population of lymphocytes lacks the markers associated with mature B or T cells. These express CD2, CD16, CD56, and the ζ chain (or a related chain) of the TCR complex associated with CD16. Natural killer (NK) cells express the IL-2 receptor β and γ chains, but not the α chain. This population of lymphocytes displays prominent intracytoplasmic granules that contain perforin and proteases, such as granzymes. NK cells can bind the Fc region of IgG through specific FcγR cell III surface receptors (CD16). Several potential NK receptors have been proposed, but the mechanism by which NK cells recognize targets remains obscure. NK cells can exert both ADCC and NK activity, destroying tumor cells in the presence or absence of specific IgG antibody. NK activity can be increased by IL-2, IFN-α, IFN-γ, TNF, or IL-12.

MONONUCLEAR PHAGOCYTES

In recent studies, B cells appear to be the most efficient antigen-presenting cell because of their binding, internalization and processing of specific antigen through immunoglobulin receptors as well as their display of a variety of surface co-stimulatory molecules (Fig. 11.5). Monocytes, macrophages, and dendritic cells also can present antigen to lymphocytes and, in contrast to B cells, can secrete cytokines such as IL-1, IL-6, TNF-α, interferons,

Table 11.4. CD4+ Murine T-cell Subset Functions

Effector functions	Th1	Th2	Th0
Cytokine secretion			
IL-2	+	−	+
IFN-γ	++	−	++
TNF-β	++	−	
TNF-α	++	+	
GM-CSF	++	+	+
IL-3	++	++	++
IL-4	−	++	++
IL-5	−	++	++
IL-10	−	++	++
IL-13	−	++	
IgE production	−	++	±
IgG2a production	++	+	
Eosinophil and mast cell production	−	++	
Antigen presentation	++	+	+
Macrophage activation	++	−	
Delayed-type hypersensitivity	++	−	
Parasite resistance	Live	Die	

IFN—Interferon; IL—interleukin; TNF—tumor necrosis factor.

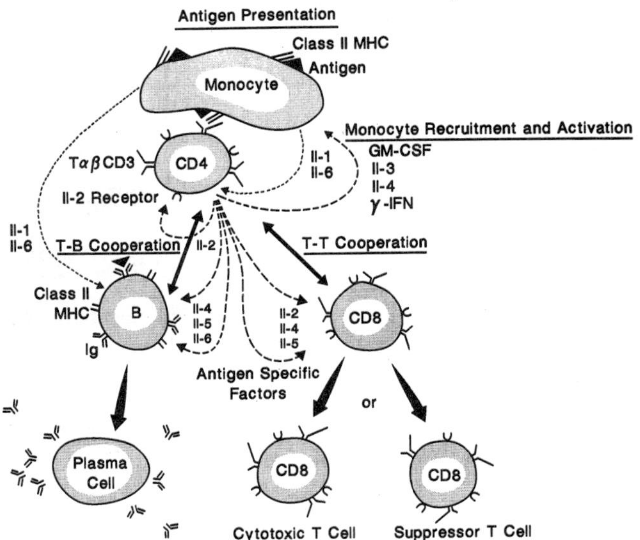

Figure 11.9. Cellular communication in the immune response via interleukins: γ-IFN; GM-CSF; IL-1 to IL-6; immunoglobulin. *Source:* Boyer and colleagues (313).

prostaglandins, and other monokines that can affect the function of both T and B cells. Macrophages ultimately are derived from promonocytes in the bone marrow, which mature into monocytes that migrate to the liver, spleen, lymph nodes, and lung. Tissue-resident macrophages can phagocytize and digest microorganisms. Phagocytosis is enhanced by macrophage activation through specific receptors for certain carbohydrates, complement, and immunoglobulin. Human monocytes express three distinct receptors for IgG (FcRI, FcRII, FcRIII) and are capable of mediating ADCC. After appropriate activation, monocytes and macrophages can inhibit tumor growth in the absence of antibody.

CYTOKINES

T cells and monocytes produce a large number of factors that mediate intercellular communication. These include the interleukins, cytokines, and hematopoietic growth factors (Table 11.5) (14). In addition, some tumors can produce one or more of these factors. Cytokines can interact synergistically and stimulate release of a cascade of secondary factors. Also, macrophages, for example, in addition to presenting antigen, can secrete IL-1. In the presence of IL-1 and antigen, T-helper cell production of IL-2 is augmented and can further activate T cells, B cells, NK cells, and monocytes. Activated T cells in turn can secrete IL-4, IL-5, IL-6, IL-10, IL-13, IL-14, and IL-15, as well as other cytokines that can stimulate the proliferation and differentiation of B lymphocytes. Activated T cells also can produce interferon-γ, which activates adjacent monocytes and modulates the proliferation of both B and T cells. Activation of monocytes and macrophages by T cells is essential for combating infection with *Salmonella*, *Listeria*, and the mycobacteria that are taken up within lysosomal vacuoles of mononuclear phagocytes (Fig. 11.9).

A number of cytokines produced by T cells, B cells, and monocytes can increase the proliferation of tumor cells and, perhaps, prevent the induction of an effective immune response. Thus, nonspecific activation of the immune system has the potential to increase as well as limit tumor growth.

Tumor-Associated Antigens

TUMOR-SPECIFIC TRANSPLANTATION ANTIGENS IN ANIMAL MODELS

One of the central concepts of contemporary tumor immunology is that cancer cells possess antigens that are not found on normal tissues and that permit the host to recognize a tumor as foreign. Evidence for the existence of tumor-associated antigens that mediate the immunologic rejection of tumor cells originally was obtained from a number of animal model systems (15–18). With the development of inbred strains of mice in the 1940s, normal tissues could be transplanted between members of a given strain without rejection. Tumors could be induced by chemical carcinogens, radiation, or tumorigenic viruses and individual cells dissociated mechanically or by digestion of the extracellular matrix with enzymes. Tumors transplanted between members of the same inbred strain would grow progressively to eventually kill the syngeneic recipient (Fig. 11.10). If tumor cells were transplanted and subsequently excised before metastasis could occur, mice would frequently reject a transplant of the same tumor that simultaneously could grow progressively in a nonimmune host (19–21). Similar immunity frequently could be induced by the injection of tumor cells that had been rendered proliferative by irradiation or treatment with cytotoxic drugs.

The specificity of tumor-specific transplantation immunity differs with the oncogenic stimulus. Mutagenic chemical carcinogens and radiation induce individually specific antigens (22–25), whereas oncogenic viruses induce antigens that

Table 11.5. **Sources, Characteristics, and Effects of Human Interleukins and Cytokines**

Factor	Source	Characteristics	Effects on other cells
IL-1	Monocyte and macrophage lines: dendritic cells; natural killer cells; B-cell lines; T-cell lines; endothelial cells; fibroblasts; astrocytes; keratinocytes	IL-1α, 15–17 kd IL-1β, 15–17 kd	Lymphokine release from activated T cells and fibroblasts Differentiation of activated B cells with IL-6 Proliferation of activated B cells with IL-5 Growth of fibroblasts, synovial cells, endothelial cells Tissue catabolism Release of PGE2, collagenase and acute phase reactants Fever Chemotaxins for neutrophils, macrophages, and lymphocytes Increase natural killer cell activity
IL-2	Activated T cells, natural killer cells (±)	15 kd	Growth of activated T cells Lymphokine production by T cells Proliferation of B cells with IL-4 or after stimulation with SAC Proliferation of CLL B cells Differentiation of B-cell lines or SAC-stimulated B cells Increases natural killer cell activity Increases LAK cell activity Increases monocyte cytotoxicity
IL-3	Activated T-cell clones, myelomonocytic cell lines (mouse)	14–28 kd	Stimulates growth of multipotential stem cells Supports growth of pre-B cell lines (mouse)
IL-4	Activated T cells	15–20 kd (mouse)	Increases B-cell proliferation Increases Fc receptor and Class II MHC antigen expression on B cells Increases IgE secretion Release of CD23 Growth factor for T cells
Il-5	T cells	45–60 kd (mouse)	Increases IgM and IgA secretion by SAC-stimulated B cells Induces eosinophil differentiation
IL-6	Monocytes; HTLV-transformed T cells; fibroblasts; carcinoma cells; sarcoma cells	34 kd	Increases growth of plasmacytomas, hybridomas Increases Ig secretion by EBV-stimulated cells Increases Class I MHC expression by fibroblasts Production of acute-phase reactants Induction of IL-2, IL-2R expression on T cells Inhibits growth and promotes differentiation of myeloid leukemia Enhances IL-3-induced colony formation by hematopoietic stem cells Induces maturation of megakaryocytes Induces mesangial cell growth Induces neural differentiation Induces keratinocyte growth
IL-7	Stromal cells isolated from the thymus	25 kd glycoprotein	Stimulates the proliferation of $CD4^-CD8^-$ thymocytes Induces proliferation of $CD4^+$ or $CD8^+$ T cells in the presence of suboptimal mitogen concentrations Acts synergistically with IL-2 to induce proliferation of $CD4^{-}$/$CD8^-$ and $CD4^+$/$CD8^+$ thymocytes
IL-8	Monocytes; keratinocytes; endothelial cells; fibroblasts; and T cells	16 kd dimer	Stimulates chemotaxis of human neutrophils in vitro Stimulates release of lactoferrin from specific granules of neutrophils Stimulates neutrophils to release superoxide anions and lysosomal enzymes I, the presence of cytochalasin Enhances the growth inhibitory activity of neutrophils to *Candida albicans* Induces MAC-1 expression on neutrophils, which promotes neutrophil adhesion to vascular endothelial cells Stimulates chemotaxis of T lymphocytes in vitro
IL-9	Activated CD4+ T cells	32–39 kd	Supports the growth of certain helper T-cell clones Stimulates growth of a human megakaryoblastic leukemia cell line Stimulates erythroid colony formation in vitro
IL-10	Activated type 2 T helper (Th2) cells, B cells	17 kd	Stimulates growth of immature and mature murine thymocytes in presence of IL-2 and/or IL-4 Stimulates differentiation of murine $CD8^+$ cytotoxic T cells Inhibits synthesis of cytokines by murine type 1 helper (Th1) cells Stimulates growth of murine cells I, presence of IL-3 or IL-4
IL-11	Primate bone marrow stroma cells	23 kd	Stimulates T-cell-dependent development of immunoglobulin-producing murine B cells

(continued)

Table 11.5. *(continued)*

Factor	Source	Characteristics	Effects on other cells
			Stimulates proliferation of IL-6-dependent murine progenitors by shortening G_0 period of stem cells Potentiates the ability of IL-3 to promote the formation of murine and human megakaryocyte colonies in vitro Supports proliferation of committed murine macrophage progenitors Inhibits adipogenesis in murine bone marrow stroma cells
IL-12	Human lymphoblastoid B cells	75 kd heterodimer	Stimulates proliferation of PHA or IL-2-activated $CD4^+$ and $CD8^+$ human T cells and $CD56^+$ natural killer cells Synergizes with low concentrations of IL-2 in the induction of cytolytic T cells and LAK cells
IL-13	Activated Th0, Th1, and Th2, CD8+ T cells	14 kd	Up-regulates monocyte/macrophage expression of CD23 and MHC class I/II antigens Inhibits expression of proinflammatory cytokines Induces proliferation and differentiation of B cells activated by CD40 ligand Induces B-cell proliferation
IL-14	T cells	17 kd	Inhibits immunoglobulin secretion
IL-15	Many cell types: mostly peripheral blood mononuclear cells, epithelial, and fibroblast cells	17 kd	Stimulates T-cell proliferation Binds to the β and γ chains of the IL-2R, but not to the α chain
IFN-α	Leukocytes, macrophages	20 kd	Antiviral activity Increases MHC class I expression Antiproliferative activity
IFN-β	Fibroblasts, epithelial cells	20 kd	Antiviral activity Increases MHC class I expression Antiproliferative activity
IFN-γ	T cells, natural killer cells, LGLs	20–25 kd	Increases proliferation of anti-Ig and SAC-stimulated B cells Increases proliferation and differentiation of CLL cells with IL-2 Increases MHC class II expression by endothelial cells, fibroblasts, myelomonocytic cells Increases antimicrobial and antitumor activity of macrophages Increases IL-4-induced proliferation of Ig-stimulated tonsillar B cells Decreases IL-4-induced activity of B-cell lines Increases natural-killer-cell activity
TNF-α	Macrophages; T cells; thymocytes; endothelial cells	17 kd (homotrimer)	Cytotoxic or cytostatic effects on certain cell lines Fever Cachexia Neutrophil chemotaxis Endothelial cell procoagulation activity Endothelial cell adhesion molecules Bone resorption Tumor necrosis
TNF-β	T cells		Cytotoxic or cytostatic for selected cell lines
G-CSF	Monocytes, fibroblasts	18–22 kd	Differentiation to granulocytes
GM-CSF	T cells, monocytes, endothelial cells, fibroblasts	22 kd	Growth and differentiation of many cell lines Differentiation of progenitors to granulocytes and mononuclear phagocytes Activation of macrophages
M-CSF	Monocytes, fibroblasts, endothelial cells, carcinoma cells	40 kd	Induces differentiation of progenitor cells to mononuclear phagocytes
EPO	Peritubular cells of the kidney, Kupffer cells	30 kd	Regulation of red blood cell production Accelerates recovery of red blood cells following hemorrhage
Angiogenin	Fibroblasts, peripheral blood lymphocytes, certain tumors	14 kd	Induces new blood vessel growth
Chemokine	Mononuclear phagocytes, endothelial cells, T cells, fibroblasts	8–10 kd 20+ related genes	Leukocyte chemotaxis and activation

CLL—Chronic lymphocytic leukemia; EBU—Epstein-Barr virus; EPO—erythropoietin; HTLV—human T-cell lymphoma virus; IFN—interferon; Ig—immunoglobulin; IL—interleukin; LAK—lymphokine-activated killer; LGL—large granular lymphocyte; MHC—major histocompatibility complex; PGE_2—prostaglandin E_2; PMA—phrobol myristate; SAC—*Staphylococcus aureus* Cowan; TNF—tumor necrosis factor.
Data from Rosenberg and colleagues (304), O'Garra and colleagues (307), and Clark and Kamen (308).

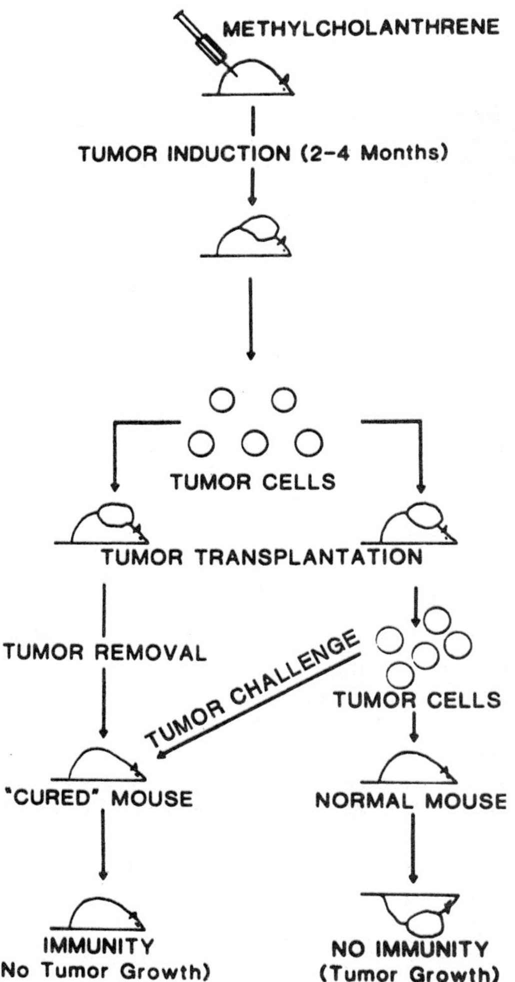

Figure 11.10. Demonstration of tumor-specific transplantation resistance. Tumors induced by an oncogenic DNA virus or a chemical carcinogen such as methylcholanthrene can be dissociated mechanically or enzymatically and transplanted to syngeneic recipients, where the tumor will grow progressively. If the blood supply of the tumor is ligated to produce necrosis or the tumor is excised before it can metastasize, the recipient will reject a second transplant of viable tumor cells that would grow progressively in a nonimmune recipient. The immune recipient would accept a graft of normal skin from the tumor donor, suggesting that the donor and recipient are indeed syngeneic and that rejection of the tumor transplant did not result from histoincompatibility of the donor and the recipient. *Source:* Bast (302).

are shared by all tumors produced by that particular virus (26–29). Shared oncofetal antigens, however, have been defined in some chemically induced tumors, and individually distinct antigens have been found in some virus-induced tumors (30, 31). Resistance to tumor transplantation is relative. A certain number of tumor cells, generally between 1 and 10,000, are required to produce a progressively growing neoplasm in mice. Immune recipients will reject several orders of magnitude more tumor cells, but a dose of tumor generally can be found that will overcome transplantation resistance. Tumor-specific immunity often can be passively transferred by T lymphocytes, but generally not by antibodies or soluble factors in immune serum. In some murine systems, $CD4^+$ T cells are required, whereas $CD8^+$ T cells have been implicated in other models (32–34). Immunity to tumors induced by oncogenic viruses and chemical carcinogens depends on the specific MHC determinants expressed by the host (i.e., are MHC restricted). Consequently, recognition of tumor-specific transplantation resistance antigen requires presentation in the context of the host's own MHC antigens. Further, because the ability to present specific antigenic peptides varies between different MHC molecules, the ability to respond to particular tumor antigens can be limited by the host's genomic complement of MHC genes.

Studies in animal model systems have demonstrated that novel expression of a normal gene, expression of mutant murine proteins, or expression of viral proteins can produce immunogenic peptide fragments that evoke transplantation resistance. Overexpression of a normal, nonmutated P1A protein renders murine mastocytomas immunogenic (35). Similarly, transplantation resistance can be induced by a murine sarcoma-associated antigen with homology to the heat-shock protein hsp90 (36–39). At least some tumors induced by mutagenic chemical carcinogens express transplantation-resistance antigens that are mutated variants of normal cellular proteins (40). In the case of virus-induced tumors, tumor-specific resistance is closely linked to peptide fragments from adenovirus E1A early genes (41–43) and from polyoma T antigen (27, 44). In both cases, intracellular viral proteins are processed and peptide fragments presented on the cell surface in the context of MHC determinants resulting in tumor rejection.

Importantly, not all animal tumors are immunogenic. Tumor-specific transplantation resistance has been observed most frequently after tumors have been induced with large doses of chemical carcinogens, ultraviolet light, or DNA viruses. Only 16% of spontaneous rat tumors evoke transplantation resistance following implantation and excision (45). Arguably, this may represent a minimal estimate of immunogenicity in that the addition of different adjuvants, administration of cytokines, or removal of suppressor cells might enhance a latent immune response to tumor-associated antigens. Mutagenic carcinogens have been used in vitro to mutate genes that can then encode immunogenic tumor-associated antigens. Rodents immunized with mutant tum^- proteins can reject tumors that bear wild type tum^+ antigen (46). Poorly immunogenic tumors have been modified by gene transfer to stimulate specific immune responses against the parental tumor and transfer of genes encoding ligands for co-stimulatory molecules (B7.1 or B7.2 activating CD28) (12, 13, 47–49), cytokines that activate T cells (IL-2 or IL-4) (47), or cytokines that enhance antigen presentation (GM-CSF or interferons) (50) have provided immunogenic vaccines in several animal models. Combinations of multiple genes have proven to be more effective than single genes alone.

Observations in murine systems have important implications for clinical immunotherapy to the extent that effective intervention depends on tumor-specific transplantation resistance. Clinically detectable human tumors have been established for long periods before presentation and often contain more than 10^9 cells at diagnosis. The tumor burden thus may exceed the capacity of even an augmented immune response. Despite the fact that different cancers arise from more than 100 tissue sites, oncogenic viruses have been implicated in the development of only a few human neoplasms, including certain T-cell leukemias, Burkitt's lymphoma, nasopharyngeal carcinoma, cervical cancer, and hepatoma. Thus, unique viral antigens likely are present only in a subset of human tumors. Many more tumors, including the frequently occurring carcinomas of lung, head and neck, bladder, and colorectum, likely are induced by chemical carcinogens. Tumor-specific transplantation antigens may be found in only a fraction of human cancers and, when present, these antigens may be individually specific, requiring modification of the patient's own tumor cells to develop effective vaccines. Further, as individually distinct antigens likely will require recognition in the context of specific MHC antigens, the appropriate MHC antigens may or may not be present in the patient's own genome. Even when tumor-associated antigens and relevant MHC components are present, appropriate mechanisms for endogenous antigen processing, transport, and presentation may not have remained intact within all tumor cells. Moreover, significant effects of immunotherapy might be seen only in patients with microscopic disease in an adjuvant setting following elimination of all clinically evident tumor with more conventional forms of treatment.

HUMAN TUMOR-SPECIFIC CELLULAR IMMUNITY

Ethical considerations preclude a formal demonstration of the presence or absence of tumor-specific transplantation-resistance antigens in humans by approaches used in animal models. Based on murine models, where T cells recognize and eliminate tumors bearing specific antigens, clinical investigators have sought to identify tumor-associated antigens that are recognized by T cells. Historically, T-cell-mediated tumor responses have been assessed in vivo by delayed cutaneous reactivity and in vitro by proliferation, cytokine production, and tumor-cell lysis. Both MHC-restricted and nonrestricted tumor-specific cytotoxic cells have been isolated from patients by co-culture of tumor cells with cytokines such as IL-2 (51, 52). Individually specific MHC-restricted cytotoxic T-cell clones have been isolated in the presence of IL-2 from patients with melanoma, sarcoma, renal cell, breast, ovarian, and head and neck carcinoma (53–57). Studies with tumor-infiltrating lymphocytes suggest that only a limited spectrum of antigens are recognized. Cytotoxic effectors most frequently are $CD3^+CD8^+CD4^-$, but $CD3^+CD8^-CD4^+$ clones have been isolated from some patients. An interesting exception to the generalization that T cells can recognize antigens only in the context of MHC molecules has been provided by the MUC-1 mucin core antigen that stimulates MHC-nonrestricted T-cell clones from patients with breast, colon, pancreatic, and ovarian cancer (58). Repeated 20 amino acid subunits in MUC-1 may provide multiple epitopes that facilitate stable association between T and tumor cells (58).

T cells are the most prevalent leukocytes infiltrating tumors of several different histologic types. Delayed cutaneous reactivity has been evoked in patients with several tumor types using autologous tumor extracts, purified proteins, and glycolipids. Lymphocyte proliferation has been produced by antigens associated with autologous tumor cells in up to 70% of patients, whereas lymphocyte-mediated cytotoxicity has been produced against autologous tumor in up to 35% of patients (11, 59, 60).

During the last 5 years, several human tumor-associated antigens that are recognized by cytotoxic human T cells have been cloned. These antigens have included peptides from normal endogenous cellular proteins and exogenous oncogenic viral proteins as well as oncogenes and tumor-suppressor genes that are mutated or overexpressed in tumor tissue (Table 11.6). Melanoma has been studied most intensively using clones of T cells isolated from patients to detect relevant antigenic peptides. Several tumor-specific antigens have been identified (*a*) by screening peptides from proteins known to be associated with melanomas, (*b*) by elution and screening of MHC-bound peptides, and (*c*) by cloning genes that restore T-cell killing after transfer to tumor-cell variants that have lost sensitivity to cytotoxic T cells. Melanoma antigens isolated to date have proven to be nonmutated cellular proteins with restricted distribution in normal tissues. MAGE-1 is expressed in testis, whereas tyrosinase, MART-1 and, gp100 are present in normal

Table 11.6. Molecules Involved in Cytolytic Function

Location	Mediator	Target	Mechanism
Secretory	Granule products		
	Perforin	Membrane	Pore formation
	Granzymes	Cytosol	Apoptosis
	Granule independent		
	lymphotoxin	LT receptor	Apoptosis
	TNF	TNF receptor	Apoptosis
	ATP	Purinergic receptor	Permeability increase
	Reactive oxygen species		Apoptosis
	Nitric oxide	Cytosol	Apoptosis
	Complement	Membrane	Apoptosis
Membrane associated	Membrane TNF	TNF receptor	Apoptosis
	FAS Ligand	FAS/Apo1	Apoptosis

LT—lymphotoxin; TNF—tumor necrosis factor.

melanocytes and retinal pigment epithelium (41, 55, 57, 61–63). Immunity to both normal and malignant melanocytes is of interest in that vitiligo has been observed during a response to immunotherapy or following spontaneous regression of melanoma. When cancers from different sites are studied, the expression of tyrosine, MART-1, and gp100 appear limited to melanoma, whereas MAGE-1, -2, and -3 are found in a variety of tumor types (41, 55, 57, 62–64). Immunologic recognition of MAGE-1, -2, and -3 is restricted by HLA-A1, whereas recognition of tyrosinase, MART-1, and gp100 is restricted by HLA-A2 (65, 66). As the HLA-A1 haplotype is expressed by 26% of whites and MAGE-1 is detected on 40% of melanomas, only approximately 10% of white patients with melanoma have the ability to respond functionally to MAGE-1. Similarly, HLA-A2 is expressed by 45% of the whites, and MART-1 is found in 80% of melanomas, suggesting that some 36% of white patients with melanoma might be able to develop an immunity to MART-1. MHC-restricted human T-cell-mediated immunity also has been demonstrated against the E6 and E7 proteins of human papilloma virus-16 (67), which is associated with development of cervical cancer, and against the Epstein-Barr virus nuclear antigen, which is associated with persistence of immunoblastic B-cell lymphoma, Burkitt's lymphoma, and nasopharyngeal carcinoma (68, 69). Human T-cell-mediated cytotoxicity also has been detected against peptides derived from mutant *ras* (70), mutant and wild-type p53 (71), bcr/c-abl (72), and c-*erb*B-2 (HER-2/*neu*) (53, 54).

Reactivity with each of these targets may be relevant to the development of vaccines. Oncogenes such as *ras* and tumor-suppressors such as p53 are mutated in a large fraction of human tumors. Mutant *ras*, p53, and fusion proteins such as the bcr/abl can provide unique antigenic determinants that can be targeted by T cells or specific antibodies. Whether these mutant peptides are expressed at sufficiently high levels and present efficiently through the endogenous antigen-processing pathway on appropriate MHC molecules remains to be ascertained.

HUMAN TUMOR-SPECIFIC HUMORAL IMMUNITY

Antibodies that bind to human tumor-associated antigens have been found in sera from patients with cancer. In up to 10% of patients with melanoma or renal cell cancer, antibodies have been isolated that bind only to the patient's own tumor cells (18). In a larger fraction of patients, antibodies can be found that bind to tumor cells of the same histologic type from other donors. Finally, antibodies that bind both to normal and tumor tissue frequently can be detected in patient sera.

Only a few tumor-associated antigens that are recognized by human antibodies have been well characterized. Individually specific, lineage-associated determinants, aberrantly glycosylated host proteins, viral proteins, antibody idiotopes, activated oncogenes, and mutated tumor-suppressor genes all can be targets for the humoral response. Approximately 10% of patients with melanoma have antibodies that bind to gp75, which is a melanosome-membrane-associated protein found both in melanomas and normal melanocytes (73). Antibodies against autologous colon cancer cells have been detected in sera from patients who have received injections of autologous colon cancer cells mixed with bacillus Calmette-Guérin (BCG) vaccine. Hybridomas have been established from the lymphocytes of these patients, and human monoclonal antibodies specific to colon cancer cells have been produced. Antibodies produced by human hybridomas developed by other investigators often have recognized glycolipids and intracellular proteins, although antibodies to unique melanoma antigens have been produced as well (74, 75). The unique idiotypic structure or idiotope created by the complementarity-determining regions for a particular antibody can serve as an antigen evoking an anti-idiotypic antibody response (Fig. 11.11). Human antibodies that are reactive with cell-surface differentiation antigens expressed by colon and ovarian cancers have

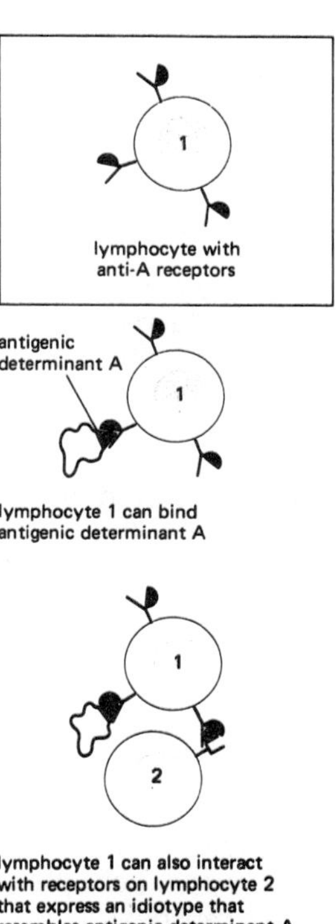

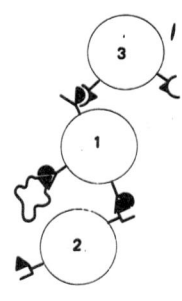

Figure 11.11. Idiotype–anti-idiotype network may play a role in the regulation of immune responses. *Source:* Alberts and colleagues (314).

been induced by the injection of murine monoclonal antibodies directed against the same tumor-associated antigens suggesting that anti-anti-idiotypic antibody had been formed (76–78). Aberrant glycosylation can produce novel antigens in human tumors (79), as, for example, antibodies against the Tn antigen (desialylated blood group Mn) are found in patients with breast cancer and titers rise following mastectomy. Antibodies also can be formed against antigens induced by human T-cell lymphoma virus type 1 (HTLV-1), Epstein-Barr virus (EBV), herpes simplex virus 2 (HSV-2), and papillomavirus (80, 81). Finally, antibodies have been detected that react with wild-type p53 in 10 to 20% of patients with breast and ovarian cancer, perhaps generated from increased stability and expression of the mutant p53 found in many patients' cells. In addition, specific antibodies have been detected in sera from patients whose tumors overexpress the HER-2/*neu* proto-oncogene. Whether humoral immunity exerts significant antitumor activity in tumor-bearing patients is not clear, but this does support the possibility that a number of antigenic targets exist for incorporation into vaccines.

MAJOR HISTOCOMPATIBILITY COMPLEX ANTIGENS

Human histocompatibility antigens are encoded on chromosome 6, and they are divided into two major classes (82). Class I antigens (HLA-A, -B, and -C) are cell-surface proteins expressed by almost all normal cells and contain a polymorphic, 42-kd peptide chain linked noncovalently to a 12-kd β_2-microglobulin molecule. Class II MHC antigens (HLA-DR, -DP, and -DQ) also are integral membrane proteins. Each is a heterodimer with an α and β chain, of approximately 33 and 29 kd, respectively. In contrast to Class I MHC molecules, the Class II MHC antigens are expressed primarily by lymphoreticular and endothelial cells and they can be detected in epithelial cells after inflammation or treatment with INF-γ.

The MHC antigens can be expressed in tumor tissue (83). Susceptibility of tumor cells to T-cell-mediated cytotoxicity depends critically on the expression of Class I determinants. Class I antigens can be down-regulated in some tumors, and this can be associated with a poor prognosis. It is uncommon, however, for Class I antigens to be lost entirely in tumor tissue. Class II MHC antigens can be expressed ectopically in malignant cells. In normal epithelium, for example, Class II antigens cannot be detected but are expressed by approximately 40% of epithelial ovarian cancers (84). Class II antigens also can be expressed in some melanoma metastases (85), but there is no consistent prognostic significance. In gestational trophoblastic neoplasia, paternal MHC antigens can be found in maternal circulating immune complexes following tumor regression (86, 87); histoincompatibility of patients and their partners does not, however, correlate with prognosis (88). Interestingly, interferons produce a highly selective induction of MHC antigens (89). To the extent that these antigens are important for recognizing tumor-associated antigens, this cytokine might affect the immunologic recognition of tumor cells.

Studies on the role of MHC in rejection within animal tumor models have provided contradictory results (83, 90, 91). Induction of MHC antigen expression by gene transfer or interferon attenuated the growth of certain animal tumors, but it did not affect other animal models (83). A role for MHC antigens in tumor recognition most often was demonstrated in virally induced tumors susceptible to MHC-restricted cytotoxic T cells. Low levels of Class I MHC antigens on both animal and human cells correlated with increased susceptibility to NK cells (92, 93). A high level of MHC Class I expression on target cells, however, is important for recognition by cytotoxic T cells. Human peripheral blood lymphocytes transformed by EBV were killed by EBV-specific MHC-restricted cytotoxic T cells, whereas EBV-positive Burkitt's lymphoma cells from the same individual expressed lower levels of MHC Class I antigens and were not killed (68, 69). The importance of MHC antigen expression for immune recognition of human tumors in vivo remains to be determined. Coexpression of class I MHC antigens with CD54 intercellular adhesion molecules appears to be important for generating a specific reaction against some human tumor cells in vitro (94). Thus, both the level and the haplotype of MHC antigens that are present in tumors may regulate the magnitude and efficacy of any antitumor immune response.

ONCOFETAL ANTIGENS

Oncofetal antigens expressed during fetal development generally are not expressed in adult tissues, but they may be reexpressed within neoplasms and in regenerating or inflamed tissues. A number of oncofetal antigens recognized by monoclonal or polyclonal reagents provide useful serum markers for monitoring the course of different neoplasms. Ideally, tumor markers are sensitive, specific, and correlate with changes in tumor burden. To affect clinical practice, it often is important that more effective or less toxic alternative therapies are available that could be used based on changes in marker levels.

Human Chorionic Gonadotrophin (HCG)

HCG is a glycoprotein heterodimer of 36.7 kd synthesized by the syncytiotrophoblast during fetal development. The α subunit is encoded on chromosome 18 and the β subunit on chromosome 19. Peak levels occur at 8 to 12 weeks of gestation during normal pregnancy. The half-life of the antigen in serum is 36 hours, assuring a rapid return of HCG to normal levels once the source of the antigen has been removed.

The major application of HCG has been in monitoring gestational trophoblastic neoplasia (95). If no metastatic disease is apparent at diagnosis, the HCG level can determine the need for chemotherapy. Failure of HCG level to fall following chemotherapy reliably indicates drug resistance. Persistent normalization of HCG level indicates cure of the disease. HCG also can be used as a marker in nongestational choriocarcinoma of the ovary and testes. These tumors are rare, and although many tumors secrete HCG, it is less reliable as a marker here than in gestational trophoblastic disease.

Alpha-fetoprotein (AFP)

AFP is a glycoprotein of 70 kd and the gene encoding AFP is linked to the serum albumin gene on chromosome 4. Peak levels during fetal development are observed at 13 weeks of gestation. The antigen is synthesized by fetal yolk sac, liver, and the upper gastrointestinal tract. AFP is immunosuppressive in high concentrations and may contribute to one of several mechanisms that protect the fetus against a maternal immune response to fetal antigens. The half-life of AFP in serum is 4 to 6 days.

In hepatoma and germ cell tumors of the ovaries and testes AFP can be a useful serum marker (96). A small subset of patients with gastric cancer also benefit from monitoring AFP concentration in that they exhibit elevated serum levels of this marker despite normal levels of carcinoembryonic antigen. Occasional patients with other cancers have elevated AFP levels. AFP levels can be elevated in benign hepatocellular disease, ataxia telangiectasia, Wiskott-Aldrich syndrome, and during pregnancy, particularly in the presence of fetal neural tube defects, thus limiting its use as a diagnostic marker for early disease.

In monitoring testicular germ cell tumors with HCG and AFP, both markers should be obtained preoperatively in all patients. Serial determinations generally are obtained monthly for the first year and every 2 months for the second. Persistently rising levels should prompt additional workup and consideration of salvage therapy. Cross-reaction between luteinizing hormone and HCG sometimes can produce false-positive elevations of HCG that decline after administration of androgens.

In monitoring ovarian germ cell tumors, AFP is particularly useful for a majority of endodermal sinus tumors and embryonal carcinomas. By contrast, HCG has greater value than AFP for nongestational choriocarcinomas. Failure to normalize is associated with persistent disease. Normal serum AFP can be associated with persistence of neoplastic elements other than endodermal sinus tumor and embryonal carcinoma. AFP is not expressed in pure dysgerminomas, but it should be measured in patients with this neoplasm in that chemotherapy is indicated for EST and embryonal carcinoma elements.

Carcinoembryonic Antigen (CEA)

CEA is a glycoprotein of 200 kd with greater than 50% carbohydrate. Analysis of its peptide core indicates that CEA is a member of the immunoglobulin supergene family (97). The marker is associated with gastrointestinal, lung, breast, gynecologic, and genitourinary tumors as well as medullary carcinomas of the thyroid (98). Studies also point to a possible role in promoting metastasis (99). Circulating levels of CEA have proven to be most useful in monitoring colon, pancreatic, stomach, and lung cancer, particularly when tumor has metastasized to the liver. Changes in CEA levels reflect both tumor burden and the ability of the liver to clear CEA (98).

Antigen levels in serum can be elevated (>2.5 ng/mL) in inflammatory bowel disease, chronic obstructive pulmonary disease, cirrhosis, and hepatobiliary disease. Levels of up to 5 ng/mL are observed in smokers without apparent cancer. Consequently, CEA has not proven to be useful in screening for occult cancer.

The primary clinical application of CEA has been in monitoring colorectal carcinoma. Preoperative CEA level should be obtained in all patients with colorectal cancer. To detect persistent disease, measurement has been repeated 1 month postoperatively in Duke's B, C, and resected Duke's D patients. The half-life of CEA is approximately 10 days (100). If the CEA level remains elevated (>5 ng/mL), values can be repeated at 2- to 4-week intervals until it is clear whether values are rising or have normalized. If CEA is not elevated, values can be repeated every 2 months for 2 years, then every 3 months for 3 additional years to assist in detecting early recurrences. CEA levels have increased 4 to 6 months before disease recurrence in two-thirds of patients (100). Persistently rising CEA levels should prompt a noninvasive work-up and, in the absence of detectable extra-abdominal disease, second-look laparotomy. Even with a negative CT scan, less than 5% of second-look operations have been negative. In one large study of 400 patients, 63% of lesions could be resected when the CEA level was less than 11 ng/mL, and 44% of these patients survived disease-free for 5 years. In patients with greater than 11 ng/mL of CEA, 5-year survival is less than 25% (101). In more than 100 patients who underwent resection of 1 to 14 liver lesions, survival at 1 and 6 years was 91 and 50%, respectively (102). A recent meta-analysis supports the impact of CEA monitoring on survival of patients with colorectal cancer.

DIFFERENTIATION AND LINEAGE-ASSOCIATED DETERMINANTS

B- and T-Cell Antigens

Antigenic determinants are expressed in normal lymphoid cells that reflect distinct stages during differentiation (103). Malignant cells can express combinations of the same antigens which may or may not correspond to the phenotypes of normal B- and T-cell precursors (Table 11.3) (104, 105). The common acute lymphoblastic leukemia antigen (CALLA; CD10), for example, is a 100-kd glycoprotein neutral endopeptidase found in 2 to 3% of normal bone marrow precursors and in approximately 50% of acute lymphoblastic leukemias (ALL), where expression of the antigen correlates with a good prognosis. ALLs that express cell-surface immunoglobulin (5%) or T-cell antigens (25 to 30%) have a relatively worse prognosis, although these differences are narrowing with improvements in therapy. Approximately 30% of ALLs lack CALLA, immunoglobulin, or T-cell markers. These "null cell" leukemias bear other B-cell determinants such as CD19 and also have a relatively poor prognosis compared with that of CALLA-positive disease.

Chronic lymphocytic leukemia more frequently is of B-cell (98%) than of T-cell (2%) origin. Cutaneous T-cell leukemia and mycosis fungoides display inducer phenotypes and express CD4. Hairy-cell leukemia expresses CD11 and the α chain of the IL-2 receptor complex (CD25). Large granular lymphocytic leukemias express CD3, CD16, CD56, and CD57.

All nodular (follicular) lymphomas and most lymphomas express B-cell antigens. A minority express T-cell antigens. The prognostic significance of these phenotypes and whether they will provide targets for therapy remains to be ascertained.

Myeloid Antigens

A number of myeloid antigens have been defined that aid in distinguishing acute myelogenous leukemia (AML) from (ALL) (104, 106). In addition, certain phenotypes may have prognostic significance within the myeloid leukemias. MY7-MY4-AML may, for example, have a more favorable prognosis than leukemias that express these markers. Leukemias of mixed myeloid and lymphcid lineage that express CD7 have a poor prognosis.

Prostate-Specific Antigen (PSA)

Lineage or tissue-specific markers also have proven useful in monitoring solid neoplasms. PSA is a glycoprotein of 33 kd that contains 7% carbohydrate (107). PSA is a serine protease that normally cleaves proteins in seminal fluid. The level of this marker is elevated in serum more frequently than that of prostatic acid phosphatase, particularly during early stages of the disease. However, low levels of PSA are found in normal serum and can be elevated in benign prostatic hypertrophy, following prostatic biopsy, and after prostatic surgery, thus limiting its use as a diagnostic marker. After total prostatectomy, values should fall to 0. Rising levels sometimes can accompany localized disease that has recurred following prostatectomy and can be treated with radiation therapy. Opinions regarding the value of PSA for early detection of prostate cancer are still mixed. A combination of PSA and digital rectal examination is more sensitive than either individual modality for the detection of early stage disease. PSA levels over 4 ng/mL generally have prompted further evaluation, including digital rectal examinations, ultrasound, and biopsy. A substantial fraction of patients will have benign prostate hypertrophy. If, however, a threshold over 10 ng/mL is chosen, a larger fraction of patients will have advanced disease that no longer can be controlled with prostatectomy or radiation therapy (108).

Increased sensitivity has been sought by evaluating the rate of PSA increase within a normal range. To increase specificity, an index has been calculated relating PSA levels to prostatic volume. The fraction of PSA bound to α-1-antichymotrypsin inhibitor may provide another useful discriminant. If all individuals aged 50 to 70 years with PSA levels over 4 ng/mL underwent diagnostic evaluation and appropriate therapy, it has been estimated that the annual cost of care for prostate cancer in the United States would increase from $255 million to $27.9 billion. Of possibly greater significance, 266,271 patients would develop impotence, some 61,618 would become incontinent, 10,563 would require colostomies, and there would be 20,563 treatment-related deaths (108). More investigation is required to identify individuals who would most benefit from PSA-based screening.

Mucins

Murine monoclonal antibodies have permitted the detection of a number of epitopes on the high-molecular-weight mucins that are associated with normal epithelium and with carcinomas of the lung, breast, ovary, and gastrointestinal tract. Mucin subunits are linked by sulfhydryl bonds, and they circulate in serum as random coiled moieties of 500 kd or greater. Mucins generally contain over 50% carbohydrate and exhibit extensive O-linked glycosylation. The protein core of each mucin contains repeating subunits of 20 amino acids, thus permitting each molecule to express multiple identical peptide as well as carbohydrate epitopes. The presence of multiple identical epitopes on each molecule has facilitated the development of double determinant "sandwich" immunoassays, in which an antibody can be used to trap antigen on a solid-phase immunoabsorbant. Radiolabeled or enzyme-conjugated antibody of exactly the same specificity can be used to detect additional free epitopes on the trapped antigen.

CA 19-9 is a sialylated Lewis blood group carbohydrate determinant that is associated both with a high-molecular-weight mucin and with cell-membrane glycolipids (109). A double determinant assay has been developed to detect CA 19-9 in serum (110). Elevated levels of CA 19-9 (>37 units/mL) are found in serum from patients with pancreatic, gastric, and colorectal carcinomas (111). CA 19-9 might supplement CEA in monitoring patients with colorectal carcinoma; among 220 patients with colorectal cancer, however, only 7 individuals had elevations of CA 19–9 without an elevated CEA. In the diagnostic workup of suspected pancreatic carcinoma, an elevated CA 19–9 level has a sensitivity of 70% and a specificity of 91%. Other mucin epitopes, such as those recognized by DUPAN-2, have been used to monitor patients with pancreatic cancer (112, 113).

A number of monoclonal and polyclonal antibodies have been prepared against mucins associated with breast cancers and normal human milk fat globule (HMFG) membranes, including HMFG1 (114), HMFG2 (114), HME-Ags (115), CA M26 (116), CA M29 (116), 115D8 (117), and DF3 (118). CA 15–3 is a heterodeterminant sandwich immunoassay that uses the 115D8 antibody as an immunoabsorbant and the DF 3 antibody as a probe (119). Elevated levels of CA 15–3 (>30 units/mL) were found in sera from patients with breast, ovarian, lung, and prostate cancers. Some 98.7% of healthy individuals have less than 30 units/mL CA 15–3, but elevated values have been found in normal pregnancy, during lactation, and in the presence of hepatitis, endometriosis, benign gynecologic tumors, and chronic pelvic inflammatory disease. CA 15–3 is more sensitive than CEA in detecting primary and metastatic breast cancer (119). Approximately 20% of patients with primary breast cancer have elevated CA 15–3 levels. Some 38% of patients with locally recurrent disease also have elevated CA 15–3 levels, as do 70% of patients with bone and liver metastases. CA 15–3 levels have correlated with disease course in up to 74% of instances studied. A combination of CEA and CA 15–3 does not appear to be superior to CA 15–3 alone, however. CA 15–3 may be valuable in monitoring selected patients who do not have readily measurable disease. Other assays for breast cancer mucins, including the Imx-BCM assay, may exhibit slightly greater sensitivity and specificity than CA 15–3 (120), but the utility of any mucin marker for managing breast cancer still remains to be defined.

CA 125

The CA 125 epitope is expressed on a high-molecular-weight glycoprotein whose smallest subunit is 220 kd (121,

122). Each antigen molecule expresses multiple CA 125 epitopes, contains less than 50% carbohydrate, and exhibits a buoyant density that sets CA 125 apart from the mucins. CA 125 is present in coelomic epithelium during embryonic development, and, it can be detected in the fetal pleura, pericardium, and peritoneum as well as in most adult tissues derived from the coelomic epithelium (123). Although CA 125 rarely is found in normal ovary, the antigen is detected in over 80% of epithelial ovarian cancers.

A double determinant radioimmunoassay has been developed for CA 125 and can be used to monitor more than 80% of patients with ovarian cancer (124). If elevated, serum CA 125 levels have correlated with disease course in 80 to 93% of instances studied (125). Recently, a second-generation assay, CA 125-II, has been developed that uses a second monoclonal antibody, M11, to trap antigen and radiolabeled OC125 antibody to detect CA125 antigen that has been trapped. Persistently rising CA 125 values are consistently associated with progressive disease. Elevation of CA 125 (>35 units/mL) at the time of a surgical surveillance procedure predicts persistence of disease with a 96% accuracy (125). The CA 125 level in a patient with primarily treated ovarian cancer, however, can return to less than 35 units/mL in response to surgery and chemotherapy before second-look surgery, and residual disease can still be found in up to 60% of patients. The serum half-life of CA 125 is approximately 4.8 days, and an apparent half-life of over 20 days during initial chemotherapy is associated with an increased number of positive second-look surgical surveillance procedures and a decreased survival rate (126, 127).

Although CA 125 levels can be elevated by adenocarcinomas that arise from a number of different sites, the marker has some value in distinguishing malignant from benign pelvic masses (128–130). In a postmenopausal patient with an adnexal mass, an elevated CA 125 level (>95 units/mL) indicates some form of malignancy with a 96% positive predictive value. Thus, preoperative determination of the CA 125 level in patients with an adnexal mass could prompt referral for surgical exploration to institutions with formal gynecologic oncology programs.

CA 125 currently is being evaluated as a marker for the early detection of ovarian cancer (131). Elevated levels can precede clinical presentation of cancer by 10 to 60 months (132, 133). CA 125 is elevated at the time of conventional diagnosis in 60% of patients with ovarian cancer and early stage disease, whereas 2% of apparently healthy postmenopausal patients have comparable levels of CA 125. False-positive values are more frequent in premenopausal patients, in whom the CA 125 level is elevated in pregnancy, endometriosis, pelvic inflammatory disease, pancreatitis, hepatic disease, renal disease, and any condition that can inflame the peritoneum, pleura, or pericardium. In prospective studies, patients with early stage ovarian cancer have been detected using CA 125 to trigger pelvic examination and transabdominal sonography (134–136). Transvaginal sonography (TVS) detects over 95% of early stage disease but is associated with an unacceptable number of false-positive determinations. Among 11,283 women screened, 486 underwent laparotomy, 7 were found to have borderline ovarian cancer, and only 6 were found to have frankly invasive ovarian neoplasms (62). Consequently, TVS is not optimally specific, and CA 125 is not optimally sensitive. The two techniques might be used together more effectively if a combination of serum markers could approach the sensitivity of TVS for detecting early stage disease. A combination of CA 125 with the novel markers OVX-1 and M-CSF detected 98% of patient with stage I ovarian cancer in a retrospective study (137); the same marker panel would have detected 11% of apparently healthy individuals in a postmenopausal population. Although this panel does not provide adequate specificity to prompt laparotomy, it could trigger more cost-effective TVS. A trial based on this design is about to begin in the United Kingdom.

Immunologic Mechanisms of Tumor-Cell Killing

T-Cell-Mediated Cytotoxicity

Tumor-specific transplantation resistance in murine systems is mediated by specific clones of T cells bearing unique receptors that are complementary to distinctive antigens associated with the tumor cell surface. Direct contact is required for specific killing, but soluble factors also can be produced. The precise mechanism of T-cell-mediated cytotoxicity is not known, but perforins, phospholipases, lymphotoxins, direct membrane interactions, and induction of apoptosis all have been proposed (138–142). Recent studies point to the importance of inducing programmed cell death through Ca^{++}-dependent granule exocytosis or Ca^{++}-independent activation of the Fas receptor by Fas ligand (141, 142).

T cells are the most prevalent lymphoreticular cells to infiltrate many solid tumors. In intraocular melanoma, the T-cell-receptor segment Vα7 was found in T lymphocytes infiltrating seven of eight tumors, which is consistent with the targeting of specific antigens by a limited repertoire of T-cell receptors (143). Both $CD4^+$ and $CD8^+$ T cells have been observed to infiltrate tumors. $CD4^+$ T cells are found at the implantation site of invasive moles and gestational trophoblastic neoplasia. Human melanomas, sarcomas, renal cell cancers, breast cancers, ovarian cancers, head and neck cancers, and HTLV-1-induced leukemias are lysed in vitro by T cells that recognize tumor-associated antigens in the context of the patient's MHC antigens. Cytotoxic T cells have been $CD3^+$, $CD4^-$, $CD8^+$ more often than $CD3^+$, $CD4^+$, and $CD8^-$. MHC nonrestricted tumor-cell killing by $CD8^+$ T-cell clones has been observed in pancreatic, colon, breast, and ovarian cancers. Mucin-like molecules may be the target insofar as killing can be blocked with monoclonal antibodies against the core protein of mucin.

Natural Killer Cells

Natural killer cells have the distinctive morphology of large granular lymphocytes (144). Granules contain a cytotoxin that is transferred to tumor targets following adhesion of the NK. NK cells are $CD5^+$, $CD56^+$, $CD16^+$ ($FcRIII^+$), TCR^-, and $CD3^-$ (145–147). Direct contact with tumor cells is required for cytotoxicity, but previous immunization is not. The cytotoxic activity of NK cells is not MHC restricted, and it is not mediated through TCR. Several candidate molecules have been identified that may be the receptors that permit NK cells to recognize and kill selectively both tumor cells and virus-infected cells (148, 149). Some, but not all, autologous, allogeneic, and xenogeneic tumor cells are more sensitive than normal cells to NK activity. Tumor cells that are deficient in Class I MHC molecules are relatively more sensitive to natural killing, which is compatible with the possibility that MHC molecules inactivate NK cells or obscure a putative NK target structure (150). Cytotoxicity can be augmented with interferons, IL-2, or TNF, and it can be inhibited by cyclic nucleotides, prostaglandins, phorbol esters, cyclophosphamide, and corticosteroids. NK cells can produce IL-1, IL-2, interferons, colony-stimulating factors, and cell growth factors in addition to cytotoxic factors.

Lymphokine-Activated Killer Cells

Lymphokine-activated killer (LAK) cells are produced from peripheral blood mononuclear cells by treatment with IL-2, lectins, or alloantigens. Continued contact with IL-2 is required for optimal cytotoxicity. Both activated NK cells and T cells can be found in LAK populations that have been generated with high concentrations of IL-2 (151). A more active adherent LAK population has been designated A-LAK. LAK, A-LAK, and cytolytic T cells contain both perforin and serine esterases (152). In the case of LAK cells mediated by T cells that are $CD3^+$ and TCR^+, it is not clear whether recognition of tumor cells depends on the TCR or some other receptor. LAK cells are selectively cytotoxic for tumor cells, and recognition is not MHC restricted. LAK cells can lyse some fresh tumor cell isolates that are resistant to NK cells. Direct contact is required between LAK cells and their targets for killing.

Tumor-infiltrating lymphocytes (TIL) have been obtained from several different human cancers. After growth in relatively low concentrations of IL-2, TIL cells have exhibited specific cytotoxicity for fresh autologous tumor in many, but not all, cases. Cytotoxic effects have been mediated more frequently by $CD3^+CD8^+$ cells than by $CD3^+CD4^+$ lymphocytes.

Macrophage-Mediated Cytotoxicity

Activated macrophages bind selectively to transformed cells and are selectively cytotoxic for them. In determining susceptibility to activated macrophages, studies with papillomavirus suggest that full transformation of cells by intact E7 protein is more important than the loss of suppressor gene function produced by mutant E7 (67). Direct contact between transformed tumor cells and macrophages is required. TNF, IL-2, a neutral protease, lysosomal hydrolases, reactive oxygen intermediates, and nitric oxide all may contribute to macrophage-mediated cytotoxicity. Perforin does not appear to be important, and destruction of different tumor cell populations may proceed by different mechanisms.

Activation of macrophages can occur in distinct stages, and it requires at least two signals (153). INF-γ and bacterial lipopolysaccharide (endotoxin) have been studied most intensively. GM-CSF and CSF-1 (M-CSF) are other macrophage activators. Complex bacterial preparations, including BCG and *Corynebacterium parvum*, can activate macrophages (154–156). Chemically defined mediators such as trehalose dimycolate and muramyl dipeptide also can activate macrophages. Activated macrophages produce prostaglandins, which down-regulate macrophages, neighboring lymphocytes, and NK cells. TGF-β also can down-regulate the activity of macrophages.

The number of macrophages in human tumors is highly variable. Tumor cells produce chemotactic factors as well as factors that inhibit chemotaxis. T cells associated with tumors can produce factors that are chemotactic for macrophages, and IL-1, IL-6, and TNF produced by macrophages can stimulate growth of a fraction of tumors. Breast and ovarian cancers can produce M-CSF that is a potent chemotactic factor for monocytes. Consequently, monocytes and macrophages may participate in the paracrine growth stimulation of some tumors.

Neutrophil-Mediated Cytotoxicity

After activation with phorbol myristate, IFN-γ, TNF-α, or TNF-β, human granulocytes can lyse tumor cells (157). Lysis by granulocytes is more protracted than lysis by T cells, which generally requires less than 8 hours. Although the mechanism of tumor-cell killing is not well understood, reactive oxygen species and lysosomal enzymes are thought to be important.

Complement-Dependent Cytotoxicity

At least nine serum complement components can participate in the lysis of tumor cells (158) and both conventional and alternative pathways for complement lysis have been described. The conventional pathway is initiated by the binding of antibody to antigen. In the conventional pathway, IgM is more potent than IgG. Nine serum proteins (C1–C9) interact sequentially to produce a "leaky patch" in the cell membrane, destroying its osmotic integrity. Many nucleated tumor cells are relatively resistant to complement-dependent cytotoxicity (159). Cell death, when it occurs, is thought to relate more often to necrosis than to apoptosis.

Antibody-Dependent Cell-Mediated Cytotoxicity

In ADCC, antibody acts as a bridge between tumor target and effector cells. Certain isotypes of IgG are effective, whereas IgM is not (Table 11.2). Activated macrophages, lymphocytes, granulocytes, and platelets all can serve as "effector" cells for ADCC that bear FcR, which binds the Fc portion of the antibody. Interaction with antibody and with tumor targets not only may provide a bridge between the effector cell and the tumor, it also may activate the effector cell, increasing its ability to kill tumor cells.

Relevanceof Different Mechanisms In Vivo

The relative importance in vivo of different mechanisms for tumor-cell killing has been difficult to assess (160). In animal models, immune serum or lymphoid cells have been transferred locally with tumor cells or injected systemically into tumor-bearing hosts. To prevent a contribution from host cells, the immune function of the recipient often has been suppressed by irradiation or through use of congenitally immunodeficient nude or SCID mice. In other studies, attempts have been made to ablate T cells, NK cells, or macrophages using thymectomy and irradiation, antisera against lymphoid antigens, or agents such as silica that are selectively toxic for phagocytic cells. In still other reports, tumor cells that have evaded host defenses in vivo have been tested for their susceptibility to different effector mechanisms in vitro and vice versa.

In studies of tumor-specific transplantation resistance, passive transfer of immunity generally has been achieved with lymphoid cells rather than with serum. T cells have been critical components of specific immunity to tumor-associated antigens. In several murine models, $CD4^+$ T cells appear to be most important, whereas in others, $CD8^+$ T cells are required as well. Antibodies against glycolipid asialo-GM1 that is expressed on NK cells can potentiate pulmonary metastases after the intravenous injection of murine tumor cells, thus arguing for a role of NK cells in controlling the growth of at least some tumors. Ultraviolet light-induced tumor cells that have evaded host defenses are resistant to killing by T cells and macrophages; however, they are susceptible to lysis by NK cells (161). Tumor cells selected for resistance to macrophage-mediated cytotoxicity in vitro were rejected by immunocompetent hosts; in contrast, tumor cells chosen for a loss of antigens recognized by T cells in vitro grew progressively in vivo (162). Infusion of cytolytic T-cell clones in the presence of exogenous IL-2 has been associated with regression of melanoma metastases in individual patients. Whether this relates to the cytolytic T cells or to infused IL-2 is difficult to resolve, however, because IL-2 alone is effective at inducing tumor regression in some patients with melanoma. Effective treatment with different immunotherapeutic agents might, of course, depend on different effector mechanisms. However, immunodeficient nude or SCID mice as well as NK-cell-deficient beige mice do not express a markedly increased propensity to develop tumors, suggesting that T, B, and NK cells may not play a major role in preventing the development of spontaneous tumors. Whether or not these cell types provide effective surveillance, it may be possible to activate them for effective therapy.

MECHANISMS BY WHICH TUMOR CELLS ESCAPE DESTRUCTION

Lack of Antigen Expression

Tumor cells may evade the immune response through a number of mechanisms. Not all tumor cells may express novel antigens; antigens may not appear at the cell surface or may not be adequately processed or presented in the context of appropriate MHC determinants. Further, the immune system can be rendered unresponsive by negative selection or peripheral tolerance through anergy or apoptosis (Fig. 11.8). Even if most cells within a tumor express potentially immunogenic antigens, a subpopulation of tumor cells may lack these antigens. Evidence for the importance of antigen-negative tumor-cell populations has been obtained in murine models and in the clinic. By using a panel of 16 murine monoclonal antibodies, distinct antigenic phenotypes were found in 16 of 18 breast cancers and in each of 16 ovarian cancers (163), suggesting that substantial heterogeneity can occur in human tumors. Similar heterogeneity has been demonstrated with polyclonal antisera and cell-mediated immunity. In some cases, heterogeneity in antigen expression relates to different phases of the cell cycle. In others, lack of antigen expression can be a stable phenotypic trait. Alternatively, cells that express a certain antigen can be grown from precursors that lack expression of that antigen, suggesting that loss of antigenic expression is not a stable phenotypic trait and may result from changes in promoter usage or methylation rather than mutational inactivation or deletion.

Antigenic Modulation and Circulating Antigen

Some antibodies are capable of inducing the modulation of antigens from the cell surface. Antigenic modulation has been observed in both murine and in human leukemias (164, 165). Not all tumor-associated antigens modulate, however. For those that do, substantial amounts of antigen can be shed into serum. This can either be in a soluble form or associated with cell-membrane vesicles. Circulating antigen can suppress cytolytic T-cell effector function and induce suppressor cells that block the generation of specific cytolytic T cells in murine melanoma models (166). For those antigens that are immunogenic in the autologous host, antigen–antibody (immune) complexes can be formed. Circulating immune complexes have been found in a number of different cancers, and in some cases, tumor-associated antigens have been detected within these complexes (86, 167, 168). To date, circulating immune complexes have not provided reliable markers for disease state or outcome of therapy.

Whether tumor-associated antigens are shed or modulate, immunoglobulin might mask epitopes on "emergence-associated tumor immunogens," thus blocking cytolytic effectors (169). IgM antibodies have apparently exerted this effect in some murine systems.

Lack of Immunologic Recognition

Potentially immunogenic tumor-associated antigens may be unable to bind to Class I or II MHC determinants from a given individual. Because many inducer T cells are of the $CD4^+$ phenotype and recognize antigens in the context of Class II determinants, whereas many cytotoxic T cells are of the $CD8^+$ phenotype and recognize antigens in the context of Class I MHC antigens, relevant epitopes from the same tumor may need to bind to both types of antigens to provide an effective cytolytic response. When T-cell clones that recognize "self" are eliminated in the thymus, whole groups of cells expressing rearranged β chain variable regions ($V\beta$) are removed from the immunologic repertoire. Thus, the ability to respond to tumors is at least in part regulated by the genomic complement of MHC antigens that are present in the individual. Consequently, clones that would recognize potentially immunogenic tumor-associated antigens may be deleted in some individuals depending on their particular complement of "self" antigens. Further, if T cells are activated in the absence of appropriate co-stimulatory molecules, they become unresponsive through the induction of anergy or apoptosis (Fig. 11.8). Anergy of the T cells apparently is reversed by the addition of exogenous IL-2.

Suppressor Cells and Factors

To the extent that tumor growth is affected by cytotoxic T lymphocytes, NK cells, and activated macrophages, cells and factors that suppress the induction or expression of immunity may be important. In recent years, the existence of antigen-specific suppression has been questioned relating to difficulties in obtaining T-cell clones with specific suppressor activity and in characterizing relevant suppressor factors (170). Substantial evidence, however, has accumulated documenting the importance of an idiotype-anti-idiotype network in regulating tumor immunity (171) as well as the role of $CD4^+$ and $CD8^+$ T-suppressor cells in well-studied animal models (172–174). Murine tumor-specific transplantation-resistance antigens can induce TS1-suppressor T cells that secrete a soluble suppressor factor that contains the α chain of the TCR and recognizes antigen by an as-yet-unknown mechanism. The TSF1-suppressor factor in turn can induce TS2-suppressor cells that bear receptors that recognize the unique idiotype expressed on TSF1 (Fig. 11.12). The TS2-suppressor cells may induce yet another generation of suppressor cells (Fig. 11.12) (175). In the case of human melanoma, $CD4^+$ T cells also have been isolated that suppress specific autologous cytotoxic responses (176–181). These suppressor cells appear to interfere with the generation of high-affinity IL-2 receptors on cytotoxic T lymphocytes.

Both humoral factors and lymphoreticular cells have been implicated in the nonspecific immunosuppression that is observed in patients with cancer that affects their T, B, or NK cell function. Cellular suppressors have included T lymphocytes, NK cells, monocytes, and macrophages in different studies. Activation of macrophages can augment their immunosuppressive activity, which is related in part to the secretion of prostaglandins. Prostaglandin E_2 levels have been increased in bronchial lavage fluid from patients with squamous cell lung cancer (182). Humoral suppressor factors may derive from tumor cells or host inflammatory cells (183). Human tumor cells produce a variety of cytokines that can affect immune effectors, including TGF-β and GM-CSF; the latter has been linked to immunosuppression in vivo in a murine mammary carcinoma model (184). Regardless of the mechanisms, defects in the ability to activate lymphocytes from tumor-bearing hosts have been detected at the level of tyrosine phosphorylation and calcium mobilization. Further, lymphocytes from tumor-bearing hosts exhibit a specific defect in expression and phosphorylation of the ζ chain of the TCR complex, which has been attributed to defective function of the $p56^{lck}$ and ZAP tyrosine kinases (185).

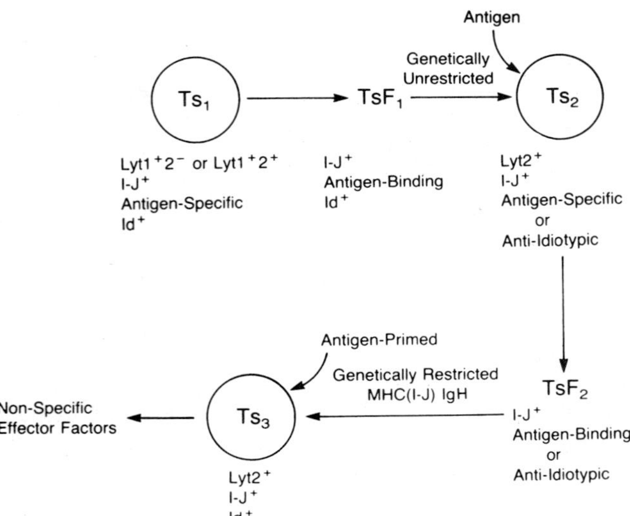

Figure 11.12. A consensus pathway of T-cell-mediated suppression. Id—idiotype; I-J—a marker for murine suppressor factors; Lyt1—the murine T-cell-differentiation antigen analogous to CD8; Ts—T suppressor cell; TsF—T suppressor factor. *Source:* Hodes (6).

IMMUNOLOGIC SURVEILLANCE

The theory of immunologic surveillance suggests that the cellular immune response has evolved to eliminate nascent clones of tumor cells before they become clinically important (186–188). In early studies, T cells were considered to be the most likely effector for surveillance, but in more recent formulations, NK cells, natural cytotoxic cells, and activated macrophages all have been proposed as candidates for maintaining surveillance (189). Evidence for immunologic surveillance has been obtained from animal models and clinical observations. Immunosuppression of mice with antithymocyte sera or thymectomy has increased their susceptibility to oncogenic DNA viruses. Greater numbers of tumors have arisen with shortened latent periods; however, this most likely results from a decreased ability to clear oncogenic viruses rather than a defect in tumor surveillance per se. Among the RNA-virus-induced tumors, thymectomy can have a paradoxic effect, particularly in the case of viruses that affect T lymphocytes. With chemically induced tumors, immunosuppression has increased oncogenesis in some studies but not in others. Finally, spontaneous tumors from most cell lineages do not appear to arise more frequently in nude mice, SCID mice, or beige mice that have defective T cells, T and B cells, or NK cells, respectively.

In patients with congenital immunodeficiency syndromes, an increased incidence of leukemias and lymphomas has been observed (190). Similarly, in patients who are immunosuppressed after the transplantation of organ allografts, large cell lymphomas of the central nervous system have occurred. In addition, squamous cell carcinomas of the skin and cervix also have been seen more frequently. Interestingly, the incidences of other solid neoplasms have not been substantially increased. In patients with AIDS, lymphomas, Kaposi's sarcoma, cervical cancer, and anal carcinomas have been observed in excess (190, 191). Whether this reflects the impact of multiple viral infections, cytokine secretion, abnormal proliferation of lymphocytes permitting pro-

Table 11.7. Immunocompetence in Different Cancers

B-cell defects
Chronic lymphocytic leukemia
Multiple myeloma
Ovarian carcinoma
T-cell defects
Hodgkin's disease
Disseminated carcinomas
Kaposi's sarcoma/AIDS
Monocyte defects
Carcinomas and sarcomas
Hodgkin's disease
Granulocyte defects
Acute lymphoblastic leukemia
Acute myeloid leukemia
Chronic myelogenous leukemia
Multiple myeloma

AIDS—Acquired immunodeficiency syndrome.

motion of tumor growth (192), or lack of immune surveillance is impossible to dissect from the current clinical data. Very high levels of soluble α chains of the IL-2 receptor are present in a significant portion of patients with solid tumors, ovarian cancer in particular (193). Because release of the soluble IL-2 receptor α chain is a highly specific marker for immune activation in solid tumor patients, this suggests that a significant number of patients with tumor have high levels of activated lymphocytes. The identity of the activating antigen and why these activated lymphocytes fail to mediate tumor clearance remain to be elucidated.

IMMUNOCOMPETENCE OF PATIENTS WITH CANCER

Immunocompetence varies inversely with tumor burden and directly with nutritional status. Protein calorie malnutrition may have a greater effect on cell-mediated immunity than on a humoral response. Phagocytic function also is impaired.

Immunocompetence and Tumor Type

The underlying cancer can also affect immunocompetence (Table 11.7). B-cell defects have been observed in chronic lymphocytic leukemia (194–197), multiple myeloma (198–200), and ovarian carcinoma (169, 201). T-cell defects are observed in advanced disseminated carcinomas (202–204), Hodgkin's disease (205–210), and Kaposi's sarcoma (190). In Hodgkin's disease, both cellular and humoral suppressors have been identified. Monocyte defects are found in carcinomas and sarcomas as well as in Hodgkin's disease. In addition to the reduced levels of granulocytes, functional defects have been identified in acute lymphocytic leukemia, acute myelogenous leukemia, chronic myelogenous leukemia, and multiple myeloma. Exaggerated delayed hypersensitivity to mosquito bites has been observed in chronic lymphocytic leukemia (211), and increased IgE levels have been observed in Hodgkin's disease (212), possibly related to a loss of T-suppressor cells.

Immunocompetence and Cancer Treatment

Surgical intervention produces a transient depression of T- and B-cell levels postoperatively (213–215). T-cell function generally recovers within 1 month. Splenectomy may predispose to a fulminant sepsis caused by *Streptococcus pneumoniae*, *Haemophilus influenzae*, or *Neisseria meningitidis* (216–218). This may relate both to loss of the spleen's phagocytic function and to decreased production of opsonizing antibodies. Whether this contributes to decreased tumor immunity remains unanswered.

Radiotherapy can depress levels of both T and B cells. B-cell function recovers over a period of months whereas certain T-cell functions can be depressed for many years, and abnormal T cells can persist for long periods (219, 220). Total nodal irradiation before antigen injection facilitates the induction of immunologic tolerance mediated by T-suppressor cells (221). Small doses of total body irradiation, however, can eliminate precursors of suppressor cells.

Intermittent chemotherapy generally is less immunosuppressive than daily treatment (222). T- and B-cell function generally rebounds between courses, although persistent defects are observed after prolonged therapy when chemotherapy and radiotherapy are combined. Most cytotoxic drugs are immunosuppressive, with the possible exception of vincristine and bleomycin. When given in conventional doses, steroids affect the recirculation as well as function of lymphocytes. T cells are affected more markedly than B cells. By contrast, cyclophosphamide has a much greater effect on B than on T cells (223). When given in relatively small doses, cyclophosphamide can deplete suppressor T cells (224). At higher doses, alkylating agents affect both B and T cells (225).

Anaphylactoid reactions can occur following the administration of a variety of chemotherapeutic agents, including L-asparaginase, cyclophosphamide, cytosine arabinoside, bleomycin, doxorubicin, methotrexate, cisplatin, dacarbazine, and L-phenylalanine mustard (226). Reactions to tartrazine dye have occurred following ingestion of hydroxyurea, and angioedema has been associated with administration of doxorubicin.

Approaches to Immunotherapy for Cancer

Over the years, two approaches have been used to provide immunotherapy for cancer. In active immunotherapy, attempts have been made to stimulate endogenous antitumor immunity within the host through the administration of bacterial products, genetic manipulation, chemically defined immunomodulators, cytokines, and vaccines. In passive immunotherapy, antibodies or lymphoreticular cells have been given to the host, providing exogenous immunity. Early attempts to treat cancers with immunotherapy were based on empiric observations. Further development of these approaches has occurred because of recent improvements in the fundamental understanding of the elements and regulation of the immune response as well as the availability of new reagents. During the last two decades, somatic cell hybridization has facilitated the production of large amounts of monoclonal antibodies, and recombinant DNA technology has provided novel cytokines and vaccines.

ACTIVE IMMUNOTHERAPY

Bacterial Immunostimulants and Contact Allergens

At the turn of the last century, William B. Coley observed tumor regression in a patient who had developed a wound infection. Subsequently, Coley treated patients with cancer using supernatants from cultures of *Streptococcus pyogenes* and *Serratia marcescens*, observing a number of responses in different types of cancers (227). More recent research suggests that the efficacy of Coley's toxins may relate to their ability to evoke the release of TNF. At least one recent randomized trial has tested the ability of Coley's toxins to augment chemotherapy for non-Hodgkin's lymphoma. Although early results suggested that patients who received chemotherapy plus toxins had a longer duration of response and survival than patients who received chemotherapy alone, differences between these groups were not maintained over time (228, 229).

Active immunotherapy with contact allergens has produced regression of cutaneous squamous and basal cell carcinomas as well as cutaneous metastases from malignant melanoma (230, 231). Cancer cells appear to be destroyed as bystanders at the site of delayed cutaneous reactions to the chemical allergens.

Cutaneous metastases of malignant melanoma also have regressed in up to 60% of patients following direct intralesional injection of viable BCG, an attenuated strain of *Mycobacterium bovis* long used as a tuberculosis vaccine (232, 233). In 10 to 15% of patients, noninjected lesions have regressed as well. Most attempts to use BCG alone for systemic therapy have failed to demonstrate an improvement in survival. The regional activity of BCG has been used to provide an advantage in the treatment of recurrent papillomas and carcinomas of the bladder; intravesical administration of BCG has delayed tumor recurrence and inhibited the development of new neoplasms. In randomized studies, BCG has proven to be superior to cytotoxic drugs such as thiotepa, mitomycin, and doxorubicin (234) and now constitutes standard therapy for superficial bladder tumors.

Other bacterial immunostimulants, including heat-killed *Corynebacterium parvum* (*Propionobacter acnes*), also have failed to consistently inhibit tumor growth following systemic administration (235). Intraperitoneal injection of *C. parvum* however, has produced regression of small ovarian cancer metastases in 30% of patients (236). Studies in animal systems generally have proven to be consistent regarding clinical experience, indicating that immunostimulants are most effective in immunocompetent hosts against small volumes of potentially immunogenic tumors growing in settings where direct contact can be achieved between cancer cells and the immunostimulant. Direct contact of immunostimulants with tumor cells optimizes not only the bystander killing by inflammatory cells but also the development of specific immunity to tumor-specific transplantation-resistance antigens. Activated macrophages, T cells, NK cells, and granulocytes all have been implicated as effectors of bystander killing in different systems. Cytokines including INF-γ, TNF, and IL-2, also may be important, but the precise mechanism(s) by which immunostimulants affect tumor growth have not yet been defined.

Chemically Defined Immunomodulators

Bacterial immunostimulants contain complex mixtures of immunomodulators. Chemically defined agents such as muramyl dipeptide and trehalose dimycolate have been used to activate macrophages and potentiate specific immunity in animal systems and in clinical trials (237–239). Despite their well-defined structure and purity, these agents exert complex effects on immunoregulation that do not consistently induce tumor regression. One of the most promising exceptions to this generalization is the use of MTP-PE to treat patients with osteogenic sarcoma (240).

Immunorestorative agents can partially correct the lack of immunocompetence that is produced by tumor growth, malnutrition, and therapy. Levamisole is a low-molecular-weight, antihelminthic drug that can affect macrophage and T-cell function. Randomized trials suggest that a combination of levamisole and 5-fluorouracil (5-FU) is significantly more effective than 5-FU alone in prolonging the survival of patients with Dukes C colon cancer treated in an adjuvant setting (241). Whether the additional activity provided by levamisole relates to immunomodulation or some other effect of the drug still remains to be determined. Levamisole in combination with 5FU, however, has become standard therapy for a subpopulation of patients with colon cancer who are at high risk for disease recurrence after primary resection.

Cytokines

Because nonspecific immunostimulants induce the release of different cytokines, purified or recombinantly derived preparations of cytokines have been evaluated individually for antitumor activity. In general, clinical protocols to evaluate cytokines have mimicked the design of trials to evaluate cytotoxic drugs; a maximally tolerated dose has been sought and used to detect antitumor activity. Optimal effects on particular immune responses may require relatively low concentrations of cytokines. Consequently, the maximally tolerated dose may not coincide with the optimal dose.

Interferon-alpha has been most thoroughly examined of these agents with regard to efficacy and toxicity (242). Lymphoreticular neoplasms have proven to be more susceptible than epithelial tumors to INF-α. Particularly impressive responses have been observed in hairy-cell leukemia (85%), chronic myelogenous leukemia (75%), and nodular non-Hodgkin's lymphoma (45%). A smaller fraction of patients with chronic lymphocytic leukemia and multiple myeloma have responded, and unlike most cytotoxic agents, INF-α has prolonged the duration of remissions in multiple myeloma. Among the solid neoplasms that respond to INF-α are Kaposi's sarcoma (33%), glioblastoma (40%), midgut carcinoids (20%), melanoma (15%), and renal cell carcinoma (15%). Recent studies suggest that INF-α prolongs disease-free and overall survival in patients with melanoma who are treated in an adjuvant setting (243). Intralesional or regional administration of interferon has produced objective tumor regression in basal cell (75%), bladder (40%), and ovarian carcinomas (45%). When all trials are considered, systemic administration of interferon produced objective responses in only 9% of 87 patients with ovarian cancer, whereas intraperitoneal administration produced responses in 45% of 11 patients (244).

Life-threatening complications rarely are observed with recombinant interferons. The patient's quality of life may not improve, however, given the side effects of optimally therapeutic doses, which include fever, chills, malaise, myalgias, headache, anorexia, nausea, weight loss, reversible neutropenia, and on occasion, abnormalities in liver function and confusion.

Interferons exert a dual effect, inhibiting tumor growth directly through interaction with tumor cells and indirectly through modulation of the immune response. Among the immunologic effects of different interferons that may be relevant are increased expression of MHC antigens, increased NK cell activity, potentiation of cytotoxic T cells, and activation of macrophages (245).

Tumor necrosis factor is a cytokine that is one of the mediators released by macrophages after exposure to endotoxin. In animal models, endotoxin produces hemorrhagic necrosis of established tumors. Serum from endotoxin-treated animals mediates the same effects. The isolated activity was named *tumor necrosis factor* and was shown to be cytotoxic or cytostatic for tumor cells in vitro (246). Administration of recombinant TNF-α to patients with cancer has been disappointing, however, with little direct antitumor activity found at dose levels having manageable toxicity (247–250). One exception to this may be intra-arterial infusion of TNF-α in combination with hyperthermia to treat melanoma that has metastasized to extremities (251).

Current studies are evaluating combinations of different cytokines as well as the use of cytokines with cytotoxic drugs. Administration of cytokines in combination may obviate very high doses of a given cytokine, which can produce untoward toxicity or exert undesirable pleiotropic effects on the immune response. Combination therapy with INF-γ and TNF-α has produced additive effects in animal models, which may have been facilitated by the ability of INF-γ to upregulate cellular receptors for TNF-α (252). Cytokines that stimulate the hematopoietic system, such as IL-3, M-CSF, G-CSF, and GM-CSF, not only can reduce the duration and degree of leukopenia but also activate immune effectors and affect the function of normal and malignant epithelial cells.

Vaccines

In animal models, tumor-specific transplantation resistance sometimes can be augmented by vaccines that present tumor-associated antigens in an immunogenic form. Different vaccines have included tumor cells from autologous or allogeneic donors, virus-infected tumor cells, purified tumor-associated antigens, and bacterial immunostimulants. Vaccines generally have been most effective against microscopic tumor burdens in immunocompetent hosts. There are few precedents for the regression of palpable tumor nodules following vaccine treatment. In clinical studies, vaccines prepared from melanoma-associated antigens and BCG or its components have evoked specific immune reactivity (253) and produced regression of clinically evident melanoma metastases in 8 to 16% of patients (254, 255).

Application of recombinant DNA technology has permitted the isolation of genes that encode immunogenic tumor-associated peptides. Several of these genes have been incorporated into vaccinia virus and other potentially immunogenic viruses (256). Pox viruses designed to deliver PSA, CEA, and other tumor-associated antigens are nearing the clinical-trial stage. Whether the local response to virally expressed human tumor antigens will potentiate antitumor immunity remains to be tested clinically. Genes for different co-stimulatory molecules such as B7 and cytokines including IL-2, IL-4, INF-γ, and GM-CSF also have been introduced directly into tumor cells, potentiating specific antitumor immunity in animal models (257–260). In these animal systems, introduction of multiple genes has been more effective than transfection of single cytokine genes. The efficacy of tumor cell vaccines likely depends on the further definition of human tumor-specific transplantation-resistance antigens, as well as a more fundamental understanding of the peptides that are actually presented to inducer and effector T cells. Future studies should better define the mechanisms that determine whether a given immunologic stimulus leads to a functional cytotoxic response or an abortive response that is characterized by anergy, tolerance, or apoptosis (Fig. 11.8). Further, given the presence of antigen-negative cells within tumor cell populations, multiple antigens may need to be incorporated into vaccines.

Even if tumor antigens are recognized, however, stimulation of the immune response may activate suppressor rather than cytotoxic effector mechanisms. Consequently, vaccines may form only one component of a program for immunoregulation that involves the inhibition of suppressor mechanisms and stimulation of local or systemic inducer function. Some suppressor cells are unusually sensitive to low concentrations of cyclophosphamide (224, 261), and to the extent that suppressor T cells exhibit a phenotype that is distinct from helper T cells, monoclonal reagents also might be used.

PASSIVE IMMUNOTHERAPY

Serotherapy

The use of antibodies as "magic bullets" was advocated by Paul Ehrlich in the early years of this century. Evaluation of polyclonal antisera for cancer treatment, however, was hampered by difficulties in producing large quantities of high-titered reagents that reacted selectively with tumor associated antigens. Clinical evaluation of serotherapy has been facilitated dramatically by the availability of monoclonal antibodies with defined specificity and high purity that can be produced in essentially unlimited amounts (4). Antibodies are capable of binding to conformational epitopes that can differ from the peptides recognized by T cells. In addition, production of antibodies in other species can further increase the repertoire of antigens that are recognized.

Monoclonal and polyclonal antibodies that are prepared in different species have defined many human tumor-associated differentiation antigens (104, 262). Even with monoclonal reagents, however, few, if any, tumor-specific epitopes have been identified. Tumor-associated antigens generally are expressed in one or more normal cell types. Distribution of some tumor-associated antigens, however, may be restricted to a small population of normal host cells that are not required for survival, limiting toxic side effects of serotherapy. Most lymphomas are monoclonal and thought to be derived from single B or T lymphocytes that bear unique cell-surface immunoglobulins or T-cell receptors. Antibodies raised against the distinctive idiotopes expressed by the monoclonal immunoglobulins that are characteristic of each human B-cell lymphoma only react with a very small fraction of the patient's nonmalignant B cells. Similar specificity should be observed with antibodies against distinctive determinants on T-cell receptors. Other tumor-associated antigens may be expressed by a larger number of host cells, but quantitative differences in antigen expression still might permit effective therapy. Oncogenes such as c-*erb*-B-2 (HER-2/*neu*) are expressed on a number of normal tissues but dramatically overexpressed in breast and ovarian cancer. In the case of those human cancers that are induced by oncogenic viruses, specific viral antigens may be recognized in transformed cells. Not all of these components, however, are accessible for antibody binding at the cell surface. The human immune response may be capable of distinguishing tumor-specific determinants from normal antigens. Human antibodies have been described that recognize antigens found only on autologous melanoma cells (235) and tumor cells with differentially glycosylated blood-group antigens (263). Production of human monoclonal antibodies recognizing tumor-associated or tumor-specific antigens, however, has proven to be technically difficult.

In contrast to T-cell-mediated therapies, serotherapy largely is directed toward cell-surface antigens. The binding of antibodies to antigens on tumor-cell surfaces generally is necessary, but not sufficient, to inhibit tumor growth. Antibodies that react with certain growth-factor receptors constitute an important exception to this generalization. Inhibition of anchorage-dependent or independent growth, and in some cases in vivo tumor growth, can be observed with some, but not all, antibodies that bind to the transferrin receptor, epidermal growth-factor receptor (EGFR), c-*erb*-B-2 (HER-2/*neu*) gene product, and the IL-2 receptor (264, 265). Moreover, antibodies against the EGFR and HER-2/*neu* have modulated resistance to cytotoxic drugs, TNF-α, and cytotoxic lymphocytes. Antibodies with appropriate isotypes can trigger complement-dependent cytotoxicity or participate in antibody-dependent cell-mediated cytotoxicity after binding to antigen. Many human tumor cells, however, are relatively resistant to lysis by human complement components. Effectors for antibody-dependent cell-mediated cytotoxicity may not be plentiful within the tumor compartment, and their function may be impaired by several factors, including the presence of endogenous antigen–antibody complexes. To compensate for deficiencies in host-effector mechanisms, antibodies may be conjugated to cytotoxic drugs, prodrugs, isotopes, or toxins, thus permitting targeted delivery of these agents.

In addition to the potency of effector mechanisms, several other factors may impede the efficacy of monoclonal antibodies, including complexing with shed antigen, failure to penetrate tissue, antigenic modulation, heterogeneity of antigen expression, and development of human antimouse antibodies (HAMA). Fortunately, not all cell-surface antigens are shed, and not all shed antigens impede the reactivity of monoclonal antibodies with tumor cells. Saturation of antigenic sites on solid-tumor nodules has proven to be difficult to achieve, although a significant fraction of sites can be occupied by monoclonal antibodies after intravenous injection. Even when antibody can gain access to a tumor nodule, a fraction of tumor cells may fail to express any given antigen. Use of multiple antibodies in combination can compensate for this heterogeneity (163). In addition, radionuclide conjugates may have the ability to kill adjacent antigen-negative tumor cells as bystanders. Although few allergic reactions been relate to HAMA, murine monoclonal antibodies are cleared more rapidly from the circulation in the presence of antimurine immunoglobulins. Human monoclonal antibodies should be less immunogenic because of a lack of the murine constant Fc region and of silencing elements potentially present in homologous antibodies, but such antibodies have been difficult to generate (266). Using recombinant technology, murine monoclonal antibodies have been "humanized" by inserting their complementarity-determining regions into the framework of human immunoglobulins (267, 268). An immune response still might be generated to idiotypic determinants in the antigen-combining region of human or chimeric antibodies.

Given the many potential limitations of serotherapy, it is remarkable that an objective response rate of 57%, with two complete remissions lasting 29 and 72 months, were observed when 14 patients with B-cell lymphomas were treated with unconjugated anti-idiotypic antibodies (269). In addition, anti-idiotypic antibodies, at least in theory, can bear the internal image of tumor-associated antigens and might be used as a vaccine (Fig. 11.11) (77, 270–272). Differentiation antigens also have provided effective targets. In lymphoreticular neoplasms, unconjugated anti-CD20 antibodies produced a 42% response rate in 37 patients with relapsed non-Hodgkin's lymphoma (273). Regression of melanoma metastases also has been produced with the systemic administration of antibodies against GD3 (274, 275) and the local injection of antibodies against GD2 (276). A prospective, randomized trial of 17–1A antibody in patients with resected Duke's C colorectal cancer yielded a 27% decrease in the recurrence rate and a 30% increase in the 5-year survival rate (277). Oncogenes have served as targets in some clinical trials, and anti-HER-2/*neu* antibodies produced a 12% response rate among patients with breast cancer whose tumors overexpressed the receptor. In preclinical studies, antibodies against the EGFR and HER-2/*neu* have potentiated the activity of cytotoxic drugs, including cisplatin

Table 11.8. Trials of Unconjugated Monoclonal Antibodies to Treat Different Malignancies

Acute lymphocytic leukemia
Acute myeloid leukemia
Chronic lymphocytic leukemia
B-cell lymphoma
T-cell lymphoma
Gastrointestinal malignancies
Lung cancer
Prostate cancer
Breast cancer
Neuroblastoma
Renal cell carcinoma

and doxorubicin. Administration of unconjugated antibodies generally has been well tolerated (Table 11.8).

Clinical trials have now been undertaken with monoclonal antibodies conjugated with cytotoxic drugs, radionuclides, or toxins. A monoclonal antibody (Br96) against Le^y has been conjugated with doxorubicin, providing promising preclinical activity (278). In phase I studies severe gastritis has been observed consistent with the known distribution of $Lewis^y$ in gastrointestinal tissue (279). Conjugates containing monoclonal antibodies and radionuclides have produced regression of lymphomas after intravenous injection (280). Intraperitoneal administration of ^{131}I linked to antibodies against HMFG protein has induced regression of small (<2 cm) ovarian cancer nodules in 36% of 24 patients treated (281). In one historically controlled study of patients with ovarian cancer but without detectable tumor, injection of ^{90}Y conjugates of anti-HMFG antibody provided a substantial survival advantage (282). Prospectively controlled studies are under way. In two independent series, (131)I conjugates with antibody against B-cell differentiation antigens produced regression of refractory lymphomas (283, 284). Bone marrow suppression occurred but could be offset by autologous stem-cell transplantation.

Several phase I trials of immunotoxins have been associated with unanticipated neurotoxicity, apparently related to the specificity of the antibody rather than the direct effect of ricin A chain or *Pseudomonas* exotoxin (285–288). Occasional responses have been observed in patients with melanoma (289, 290) and lymphoma (291). Recent preclinical studies suggest that the concurrent use of radionuclide conjugates and immunotoxins might provide additive or synergistic in vivo antitumor activity. Inhibition of protein synthesis by immunotoxins may prevent effective repair of radiation-induced DNA damage.

Monoclonal antibodies have demonstrated antitumor activity in the phase I and II studies that have been performed to date. Based on results in animal models, however, serotherapy likely will have its greatest impact on microscopic disease; critical adjuvant trials have not yet been undertaken.

Adoptive Immunotherapy

In animal tumor models, adoptive immunotherapy has been most effective when large numbers of lymphoid cells from intensely immune donors have been transferred to recipients with small tumor burdens (292). In general, micrometastatic disease has been eradicated, whereas large or established tumors have been relatively more resistant to treatment. Immunogenic tumors have been better targets than tumors with little or no demonstrable immunogenicity for adoptive immunotherapy. Recruitment of specific or nonspecific host effector cells may be important (11).

With the production of IL-2 and other cytokines by recombinant DNA technology, clinical evaluation of adoptive immunotherapy has now become feasible. Most clinical trials, however, have been performed in the setting of clinically evident metastatic disease. The immunogenicity of most human tumors has been difficult to define, and the immune response of the patients often has been compromised. LAK cells have been generated from the patient's own peripheral blood lymphocytes by incubation ex vivo with high concentrations of IL-2.

When all available studies are considered, the administration of autologous LAK cells with IL-2 has produced objective responses in 29% of patients with renal cancer, 20% with melanoma, and 16% with colorectal carcinoma (293, 294). Complete responses sometimes have been of long duration, but these occur in less than 10% of patients treated. In different trials, IL-2 alone has produced objective responses in approximately 20% of patients with renal cell carcinoma and melanoma; consequently, the precise contribution of LAK cells and IL-2 in combined therapies requires further definition. Treatment with LAK and high doses of IL-2 has been associated with fever, nausea, vomiting, diarrhea, cutaneous erythema, fluid shifts, weight gain, oliguria, increased serum creatinine, hyperbilirubinemia, hypotension, supraventricular arrhythmias, and pulmonary edema. Although intensive support has been required, toxicity generally is reversible, and few fatalities have been observed. Administration of IL-2 by continuous infusion may reduce toxicity to some extent, as may addition of *N*-methylguanine to the regimen (295). Given the relatively modest rates of complete response and the substantial morbidity observed in clinical trials, it would be useful to be able to predict which patients might respond to combination therapy with LAK cells and IL-2 (297). At present, however, there are no reliable prognostic markers for response.

Tumor-infiltrating lymphocytes can be isolated directly from tumors and cultured with IL-2 to expand the cell number (298–300). In animal models, TIL with specific antitumor reactivity have been grown in the presence of relatively low concentrations of IL-2 and are 50 to 100 times more potent than LAK cells (301). In contrast to LAK cells, TIL isolated from human tumors exhibit MHC-restricted cytotoxicity for the autologous tumor target. Treatment with TIL produced regression in 11 of 20 patients with metastatic melanoma in addition to specific antitumor reactivity (299). Based on gene-marking studies, infused TIL can be detected at tumor sites and in peripheral blood for up to 64 days (302). Phase I studies have been conducted to deliver TIL that have been transfected with TNF-α or IL-2 to achieve a high concentration of cytokine at tumor sites with acceptable systemic toxicity.

Recent studies have used gene transfer to track transferred lymphocytes. In the future, it should be possible to produce lymphocytes with specificities and functional properties that are optimal for effective adoptive transfer of tumor-rejection immunity (300). Transfer to TIL of IL-2, IL-3 receptor, and other genes has been accomplished ex vivo. Further trials may incorporate suicide genes to eliminate TIL clones that undergo autonomous proliferation. Once again, critical adjuvant trials will be required to test the efficacy of adoptive immunotherapy.

References

1. Paul WE. The immune system: an introduction. In Fundamental Immunology, 3rd ed. Edited by WE Paul. New York: Raven, 1993, p 1.
2. Kincade PW, Gimble JM. B lymphocytes. In Fundamental Immunology, 2nd ed. Edited by WE Paul. New York: Raven, 1993, p 43.
3. Rudikoff S. Principles of tumor immunity: biology of antibody-mediated response. In Biologic Therapy of Cancer. Edited by VT DeVita Jr, S Hellman, SA Rosenberg. Philadelphia: Lippincott, 1991, p 22.
4. Kohler G, Milstein C. Continuous cultures of fused cells secreting antibody of predefined specificity. Nature 1975;256:495.
5. Reth M, Hombach J, Wienands J, Campbell KS, Chien N, Justement LB, Cambier JC. The B-cell antigen receptor complex. Immunol Today 1991;12:196.
6. Hodes RJ. T-cell-mediated regulation: Help and suppression. In Fundamental Immunology, 2nd ed. Edited by WE Paul. New York: Raven, 1989, p 587.
7. Hedrick SM. T lymphocyte receptors. In Fundamental Immunology, 2nd ed. Edited by WE Paul. New York: Raven, 1989, p 291.
8. Weiss A. Structure and function of the T cell antigen receptor. J Clin Invest 1990;86: 1015.
9. Rudd CE. CD4, CD8 and the TCR-CD3 complex: a novel class of protein-tyrosine kinase receptor. Immunol Today 1990;11:400.
10. Makgoba MW, Sanders ME, Shaw S. The CD2-LFA-3 and LFA-1-ICAM pathways: relevance to T-cell recognition. Immunol Today 1989;10:417.
11. Parmiani G. An explanation of the variable clinical response to interleukin 2 and LAK cells. Immunol Today 1990;11:113.
12. Linsley PS, Ledbetter JA. The role of the CD28 receptor during T cell responses to antigen. Ann Rev Immunol 1993;11:191.
13. CD28-mediated signalling co-stimulates murine T cells and prevents induction of anergy in T-cell clones. Nature 1992;356:607.
14. Glaspy JA, Golde DW. The colony-stimulating factors: biology and clinical use. Oncology 1990;4:25.
15. Gross L. Intradermal immunization of C3H mice against a sarcoma that originated in an animal of the same line. Cancer Res 1943;3:326.
16. Herberman RB. Immunogenicity of tumor antigens. Biochim Biophys Acta 1977;473: 93.
17. Klein G. Recent trends in tumor immunology. Isr J Med Sci 1966;2:135.
18. Old LJ. Cancer immunology: the search for specificity—GHA Clowes Memorial Lecture. Cancer Res 1981;41:361.
19. Foley EJ. Antigenic properties of methylcholanthrene-induced tumors in mice of the strain of origin. Cancer Res 1953;13:835.
20. Klein G, Sjogren HO, Klein E, Hellström KE. Demonstration of resistance against methylcholanthrene-induced sarcomas in the primary autochthonous host. Cancer Res 1960;20:1561.
21. Prehn RT, Main JM. Immunity to methylcholanthrene-induced sarcomas. JNCI 1957;18:769.
22. Baldwin RW, Price MR. Neoantigen expression in chemical carcinogenesis. In Cancer, a Comprehensive Treatise Etiology: Chemical and Physical Carcinogenesis, Vol 1. Edited by FF Becker. New York: Plenum, 1975, p 353.
23. Kripke ML. Immunology of murine skin cancers. Carcinog Compr Surv 1989;11:273.
24. Old LJ, Boyse EA. Immunology of experimental tumors. Annu Rev Med 1964;15:167.
25. Schreiber H, Ward PL, Rowley DA, Stauss HJ. Unique tumor-specific antigens. Annu Rev Immunol 1988;6:465.
26. Chieco-Bianchi L, Collavo D, Biasi G. Immunologic unresponsiveness to murine leukemia virus antigens: mechanisms and role in tumor development. Adv Cancer Res 1988;51:277.
27. Dalianis T. Studies on the polyoma virus tumor-specific transplantation antigen (TSTA). Adv Cancer Res 1990;55:57.
28. Habel K. Resistance of polyoma virus immune animals to transplanted polyoma tumors. Proc Soc Exp Biol Med 1961;106:722.
29. Livingston DM, Bradley MK. The simian virus 40 large T antigen. A lot packed into a little. Mol Biol & Med 1987;4:63.
30. Morton DL, Miller GF, Wood DA. Demonstration of tumor-specific immunity against antigens unrelated to the mammary tumor virus in spontaneous mammary adenocarcinomas. JNCI 1969;42:289.
31. Vaage J. Nonvirus-associated antigens in virus-induced mouse mammary tumors. Cancer Res 1968;28:2477.
32. Greenberg PD, Cheever MA, Fefer A. Therapy of established tumors by adoptive transfer to T lymphocytes. In Basic and Clinical Tumor Immunology. Edited by RB Herberman. Boston: Martinus Nijhoff, 1983, p 301.
33. Rosenberg SA. Adoptive immunotherapy of cancer: accomplishments and prospects. Cancer Treat Rep 1984;68:233.
34. Rosenstein M, Eberlein TJ, Rosenberg SA. Adoptive immunotherapy of established syngeneic solid tumors: role of T lymphoid subpopulations. J Immunol 1984;132: 2117.
35. Van den Eynde B, Lethé B, Van Pel A, et al. The gene coding for a major tumor rejection antigen of tumor P815 is identical to the normal gene of syngeneic DBA/2 mice. J Exp Med 1991;173:1373.
36. Srivastava PK, DeLeo AB, Old LJ. Tumor rejection antigens of chemically induced sarcomas of inbred mice. Proc Natl Acad Sci USA 1986;83:3407.
37. Srivastava PK, Chen YT, Old LJ. 5′-Structural analysis of genes encoding polymorphic antigens of chemically induced tumors. Proc Natl Acad Sci USA. 1987;84:3807.
38. Srivastava PK, Old LJ. Individually distinct transplantation antigens of chemically induced mouse tumors. Immunol Today 1988;9:78.
39. Ullrich SJ, Robinson EA, Law LW, Willingham M, Appella E. A mouse tumor-specific transplantation antigen is a heat shock-related protein. Proc Natl Acad Sci USA 1986;83:3121.
40. Lurquin C, Van Pel A, Mariame B, De Plaen E, Szikora JP, Janssens C, Reddehase MJ, Lejeune J, Boon T. Structure of the gene of tum-transplantation antigen P91A: the mutated exon encodes a peptide recognized with Ld by cytolytic T cells. Cell 1989;58:293.
41. Kast WM, Offringa R, Peters PJ, Voordouw AC, Meleon RH, van der Eb AJ, Melief CJ. Eradication of adenovirus E1-induced tumors by E1A-specific cytotoxic T lymphocytes. Cell 1989;59:603.
42. Sawada Y, Urbanelli D, Raskova J, Shenk TE, Raska K Jr. Adenovirus tumor-specific transplantation antigen is a function of the E1A early region. J Exp Med 1986;163:563.
43. Urbanelli D, Sawada Y, Raskova J, Jones NC, Shenk T, Raska K Jr. C-terminal domain of the adenovirus E1A oncogene product is required for induction of cytotoxic T lymphocytes and tumor-specific transplantation immunity. Virology 1989;173:607.
44. Tanaka K, Tevethia MJ, Kalderon D, Smith AE, Tevethia SS. Clustering of antigenic sites recognized by cytotoxic T lymphocyte clones in the terminal half of SV40 T antigen. Virology 1988;162:427.
45. Baldwin RW. Specific antitumor immunity and its role in host resistance to tumors. In Basic and Clinical Tumor Immunology. Edited by RB Herberman. Boston: Martinus Nijhoff, 1983, p 107.
46. De Plaen E, Lurquin C, Van Pel A, et al. Tum-variants of mouse mastocytoma P815. IX. Immuogenic (tum)- variants of mouse tumor P815: cloning of the gene of tum-antigen P91A and identification of the tum-mutation. Proc Natl Acad Sci USA 1988;85: 2274.
47. Pardoll DM. Paracrine cytokine adjuvants in cancer immunotherapy. Ann Rev Immunol 1995;13:399.
48. Allison JP. CD28-B7 interactions in T-cell activation. Curr Opin Immunol 1994;6:144.
49. Townsend SE, Allison JP. Tumor rejection after direct costimulation of CD8+ T cells by B7-transfected melanoma cells. Science 1993;259:368.
50. Dranoff G, Jaffee E, Lazenby A, Golumbek P, Levitsky H, Brose K, Jackson V, Hamada H, Pardoll D, Mulligan RC. Vaccination with irradiated tumor cells engineered to secrete murine granulocyte-macrophage colony-stimulating factor stimulates potent, specific, and long-lasting anti-tumor immunity. Proc Natl Acad Sci USA 1993;90:3539.
51. Lotze MT, Finn OJ. Recent advances in cellular immunology: implications for immunity to cancer. Immunol Today 1990;11:190.
52. Jerome KR, Barnd DL, Boyer CM, Taylor-Papadimitriou J, McKenzie IFC, Bast RC Jr, Finn OJ. Adenocarcinoma reactive cytotoxic T lymphocytes recognize an epitope present on the protein core of epithelial mucin molecules. In Cellular Immunity and the Immunotherapy of Cancer. Edited by MT Lotze, OJ Finn. New York: Wiley-Liss, 1990, p 321.
53. Ioannides CG, Fisk B, Fan D, Biddison WE, Wharton JT, O'Brian CA. Cytotoxic T cells isolated from ovarian malignant ascites recognize a peptide derived from the HER-2/*neu* proto-oncogene. Cell Immunol 1993;151:225.
54. Yoshino I, Peoples GE, Goedegebuure PS, Maziarz R, Eberlein TJ. Association of HER2/neu expression with sensitivity to tumor-specific CTL in human ovarian cancer. J Immunol 1994;152:2393.
55. Kawakami Y, Eliyahu S, Delgaldo CH, et al. Cloning of the gene coding for a shared human melanoma antigen recognized by autologous T cells infiltrating into tumor. Proc Natl Acad Sci USA 1994;91:3515.
56. Storkus WJ, Lotze MT. Tumor antigens recognized by immune cells. In Biologic Treatment of Cancer, 2nd ed. Edited by VT De Vita, S Hellman, SA Rosenberg. Philadelphia: Lippincott, 1995, p 64.
57. Boon T, Coulir P, Marchand M, Weynants P, Wölfel T, Brichard V. Genes coding for tumor rejection antigens: perspectives for specific immunotherapy. In Important Advances in Oncology 1994. Edited by VT De Vita, S Hellman, SA Rosenberg. Philadelphia: Lippincott, 1994, p 53.
58. Barnd DL, Lan MS, Metzgar RS, Finn OJ. Specific major histocompatibility complex–unrestricted recognition of tumor-associated mucins by human cytotoxic T cells. Proc Natl Acad Sci USA 1989;86:7159.
59. Vanky F, Masucci MG, Bejarano MT, Klein E. Lysis of tumor biopsy cells by blood lymphocyte subsets of various densities. Autologous and allogeneic studies. Int J Cancer 1984;33:185.
60. Vose BM, Howell A. Cultured human antitumour T cells and their potential for therapy. In Basic and Clinical Tumor Immunology. Edited by RB Herberman. Boston: Martinus Nijhoff, 1983, p 129.
61. Kawakami Y, Eliyahu S, Jennings C, Sakaguchi K, Kang X, Southwood S, Robbins PF, Sette A, Appella E, Rosenberg SA. Recognition of multiple epitopes on the human melanoma antigen gp100 by tumor-infiltrating T lymphocytes associated with in vivo tumor regression. J Immunol 1995;154:3961.
62. Karlan BY, Platt LD. The current status of ultrasound and color Doppler imaging in screening for ovarian cancer. Gynecol Oncol 1994;55:S28.
63. Brichard V, Van Pel A, Wölfel T, et al. The tyrosinase gene codes for an antigen recognized by autologous cytolytic T lymphocytes on HLA-A2 melanomas. J Exp Med 1993;178:489.
64. Gaugler B, Van Den Eynde B, Van der Bruggen P, et al. Human gene MAGE-3 codes for an antigen recognized on a melanoma by autologous cytolytic T lymphocytes. J Exp Med 1994;179:921.
65. De Smet C, Lurquin C, Van der Bruggen P, De Plaen E, Brasseur F, Boon T. Sequence and expression pattern of the human MAGE-2 gene. Immunogenetics 1994;39:121.
66. Traversari C, van der Bruggen P, Luescher IF, et al. A non-apeptide encoded by human gene MAGE-1 is recognized on HLA-A1 by CTL directed against tumor antigen MZ2-E. J Exp Med 1992;176:1453.
67. Banks L, Moreau F, Vousden K, Pim D, Matlashewski G. Expression of the human papillomavirus E7 oncogene during cell transformation is sufficient to induce susceptibility to lysis by activated macrophages. J Immunol 1991;146:2037.
68. Masucci MG, Torsteindottir S, Colombani J, Brautbar C, Klein E, Klein G. Down-regulation of class I HLA antigens of the Epstein-Barr virus-encoded latent membrane protein in Burkitt lymphoma lines. Proc Natl Acad Sci USA 1987;84:4567.

69. Rooney CM, Rowe M, Wallace LE, Rickinson AB. Epstein-Barr virus-positive Burkitt's lymphoma cells not recognized by virus-specific T-cell surveillance. Nature 1985;317:629.
70. Jung S, Schluesener HJ. Human T lymphocytes recognize a peptide of single point-mutated, oncogenic ras protein. J Exp Med 1991;173:273.
71. Houbiers JGA, Nijman HW, van der Berg SH, Drijfhout JW, Kenemans P, van de Velde CJH, Brand A, Momberg F, Kast WM, Melief CJM. In vitro induction of human cytotoxic T lymphocyte responses against peptides of mutant and wild-type p53. Eur J Immunol 1993;23:2072.
72. Chen W, Peace DJ, Rovira DK, You S-G, Cheever MA. T-cell immunity to the joining region of p210$^{bcr\text{-}abl}$ protein. Proc Natl Acad Sci USA 1992;89:1468.
73. Vijayasaradhi S, Houghton AN. Purification of an autoantigenic 75-kDa human melanosomal glycoprotein. Int J Cancer 1991;47:298.
74. Lloyd KO, Old LJ. Human monoclonal antibodies to glycolipids and other carbohydrate antigens: dissection of the humoral immune response in cancer patients. Cancer Res 1989;49:3445.
75. Yamaguchi H, Furukawa K, Fortunato SR, Livingston PO, Lloyd KO, Oettgen HF, Old LJ. Cell-surface antigens of melanoma recognized by human monoclonal antibodies. Proc Natl Acad Sci USA 1987;84:2416.
76. Courtenay-Luck NS, Epenetos AA, Sivolapenko GB, Larche M, Barkans JR, Ritter MA. Development of anti-idiotypic antibodies against tumour antigens and autoantigens in ovarian cancer patients treated intraperitoneally with mouse monoclonal antibodies. Lancet 1988;2:894.
77. Herlyn D, Ross AH, Koprowski H. Anti-idiotypic antibodies bear the internal image of a human tumor antigen. Science 1986;232:100.
78. Loibner H, Plot R, Rot A, Werner G, Wrann M, Samonigg H, Schmid M, Stoger H, Truschnig M, Herlyn D, Koprowski H. Immunoreactivity of patients with colorectal cancer metastasis after immunisation with anti-idiotypes. Lancet 1990;335:171.
79. Hakomori S. Aberrant glycosylation in tumors and tumor-associated carbohydrate antigens. Adv Cancer Res 1989;52:257.
80. Rapp F. Herpes simplex virus type 2 and cervical cancer. Cancer 1981;6:3.
81. Yajima H, Noda T, de Villiers EM, Yajima A, Yamamoto K, Noda K, Ito Y. Isolation of a new type of human papillomavirus (HPV52B) with a transforming activity from cervical cancer tissue. Cancer Res 1988;48:7164.
82. Robinson MA, Kindt TJ. Major histo-compatibility complex antigens and genes. In Fundamental Immunology, 2nd ed. Edited by WE Paul. New York: Raven, 1989;p 489.
83. Elliott BE, Carlow DA, Rodricks AM, Wade A. Perspectives on the role of MHC antigens in normal and malignant cell development. Adv Cancer Res 1989;53:181.
84. Kabawat SE, Bast RC Jr, Welch WR, Knapp RC, Bhan AK. Expression of major histocompatibility antigens and nature of inflammatory cellular infiltrate in ovarian neoplasms. Int J Cancer 1983;32:547.b.
85. Daar AS, Fuggle SV, Ting A, Fabre JW. Anomolous expression of HLA-DR antigens on human colorectal cancer cells. J Immunol 1982;129:447.
86. Lahey SJ, Steele G Jr, Berkowitz R, Rodrick ML, Ross DS, Goldstein DP, Zamcheck N, Wilson RE, Deasy JM. Identification of material with paternal HLA antigen immunoreactivity from purported circulating immune complexes in patients with gestational trophoblastic neoplasia. JNCI 1984;72:983.
87. Rayner AA, Steele G, Rodrick ML, Harte PJ, Munroe AE, Zamcheck N, Wilson RE. Application of polyethylene glycol turbidity assay to detection of circulating immune complexes in cancer patients. Am J Surg 1981;141:460.
88. Berkowitz RS, Hornig-Rohan J, Martin-Alosco S, Klein S, Goldstein DP, Bast RC Jr, DeWolf WC. HLA antigen frequency distribution in patients with gestational choriocarcinoma and their husbands. Placenta 1981;3 (suppl):263.
89. Boyer CM, Dawson DV, Neal SE, Winchell LF, Leslie DS, Ring D, Bast RC Jr. Differential induction by interferons of major histocompatibility complex-encoded and non-major histocompatibility complex-encoded antigens in human breast and ovarian carcinoma cell lines. Cancer Res 1989;49:2928.b.
90. Gopas J, Rager-Zisman B, Bar-Eli M, Hämmerling GJ, Segal S. The relationship between MHC antigen expression and metastasis. Adv Cancer Res 1989;53:89.
91. Tanaka K, Yoshioka T, Bieberich C, Jay G. Role of the major histocompatibility complex class I antigens in tumor growth and metastasis. Annu Rev Immunol 1988;6:359.
92. Storkus WJ, Alexander J, Payne JA, Dawson JR, Cresswell P. Reversal of natural killing susceptibility in target cells expressing transfected class I HLA genes. Proc Natl Acad Sci USA 1989;86:2361.
93. Storkus WJ, Howell DN, Salter RD, Dawson JR, Cresswell P. NK susceptibility varies inversely with target cell class I HLA antigen expression. J Immunol 1987;138:1657.
94. Vanky F, Wang P, Patarroyo M, Klein E. Expression of the adhesion molecule ICAM-1 and major histocompatibility complex class I antigens on human tumor cells is required for their interaction with autologous lymphocytes in vitro. Cancer Immunol Immunother 1990;31:19.
95. Braunstein GD. Placental proteins as tumor markers. In Immunodiagnosis of Cancer, 2nd ed. Edited by RB Herberman, DW Mercer. New York: Marcel Dekker, 1990, p 673.
96. Vessella RL, Lange PH. Monitoring of patients with testicular cancer by assays for alpha-fetoprotein and human chorionic gonadotropin. In Manual of Clinical Laboratory Immunology, 3rd edition. Edited by NR Rose, H Friedman, JL Fahey. Washington, DC: American Society for Microbiology, 1986, p 810.
97. Paxton RJ, Mooser G, Pande H, Lee TD, Shively JE. Sequence analysis of carcinoembryonic antigen: identification of glycosylation sites and homology with the immunoglobulin supergene family. Proc Natl Acad Sci USA 1987;84:920.
98. Zamcheck N, Steele G, Thomas P, Mayer RJ. Use of carcinoembryonic antigen in monitoring of patients. In Manual of Clinical Laboratory Immunology, 3rd ed. Edited by NR Rose, H Friedman, JL Fahey. Washington, DC: American Society for Microbiology, 1986, p 802.
99. Jessup JM, Wagner H, Toth CA, Ford R, Thomas P. Carcinoembryonic antigen may promote metastasis by cell adhesion. Proc Am Assoc Cancer Res 1990;31:A388.
100. Begent R, Rustin GJS. Tumour markers: from carcinoembryonic antigen to products of hybridoma technology. Cancer Surv 1989;8:107.
101. Minton JP, Hoehn JL, Gerber DM, Horsley JS, Connolly DP, Salwan F, Fletcher WS, Cruz AB Jr, Gatchell FG, Oviedo M, Meyer KK, Leffall LD Jr, Berk RS, Stewart PA, Kurucz SE. Results of a 400-patient carcinoembryonic antigen second-look colorectal cancer study. Cancer 1985;55:1284.
102. Minton JP. Surgical management of recurrent colon and rectal cancers: management of recurrent colorectal carcinoma. Proceedings of the American Society of Clinical Oncology Educational Booklet, 24th Annual Meeting 1988, p 143.
103. Foon KA, Todd RF III. Immunologic classification of leukemia and lymphoma. Blood 1986;68:1.
104. Atwater SK, Borowitz MJ. Immunophenotyping of blood cells. In Practical Laboratory Hematology, 2nd ed. Edited by J Koepke. New York: Churchill Livingstone, 1991, p 193.
105. Drexler HG, Minowada J. Lymphocytic leukemia and lymphomas. In Immunodiagnosis of Cancer, 2nd ed. Edited by RB Herberman, DW Mercer. New York: Marcel Dekker, 1990, p 243.
106. Hurwitz CA, Strauss LC, Civin CI. Immunodiagnosis of acute nonlymphocytic leukemia. In Immunodiagnosis of Cancer, 2nd ed. Edited by RB Herberman, DW Mercer. New York: Marcel Dekker, 1990, p 265.
107. Chu TM. Prostate cancer-associated markers. In Immunodiagnosis of Cancer, 2nd ed. Edited by RB Herberman, DW Mercer. New York: Marcel Dekker, 1990, p 339.
108. Optenberg SA, Thompson IM. Economics of screening for carcinoma of the prostate. Urol Clin North Am 1990;17:719.
109. Magnani JL, Steplewski Z, Koprowski H, Ginsburg V. Identification of the gastrointestinal and pancreatic cancer-associated antigen detected by monoclonal antibody CA 19-9 in the sera of patients as a mucin. Cancer Res 1983;43:5489.
110. Del Villano BC, Brennan S, Brock P, Bucher C, Liu V, McClure M, Rake B, Space S, Westrick B, Schoemaker H, Zurawski VR. Radioimmunometric assay for a monoclonal antibody-defined tumor marker, CA 19-9. Clin Chem 1983;29:549.
111. Ritts RE Jr, Del Villano BC, Go VL, Herberman RB, Klug TL, Zurawski VR Jr. Initial clinical evaluation of an immunoradiometric assay for CA-19-9 using the NCI serum bank. Int J Cancer 1984;33:339.
112. Fritsche HA Jr, Gelder FB. Serum tumor markers for pancreatic cancer. In Immunodiagnosis of Cancer, 2nd ed. Edited by RB Herberman, DW Mercer. New York: Marcel Dekker, 1990, p 289.
113. Metzgar RS, Rodriguez N, Finn OJ, Lan MS, Daasch VN, Fernsten PD, Meyers WC, Sindelar WF, Sandler RS, Seigler HF. Detection of a pancreatic cancer-associated antigen (DU-PAN-2 antigen) in serum and ascites of patients with adenocarcinoma. Proc Natl Acad Sci USA 1984;81:5242.
114. Burchell J, Wang D, Taylor-Papadimitriou J. Detection of the tumour-associated antigens recognized by the monoclonal antibodies HMFG-1 and -2 in serum from patients with breast cancer. Int J Cancer 1984;34:763.
115. Ceriani RL, Rosenbaum EH. Breast epithelial antigens in the circulation of breast cancer patients. In Immunodiagnosis of Cancer, 2nd ed. Edited by RB Herberman, DW Mercer. New York: Marcel Dekker, 1990, p 223.
116. Brown JP, Linsley PS, Horn D. Breast carcinoma-associated mucins as tumor markers. In Immunodiagnosis of Cancer, 2nd ed. Edited by RB Herberman, DW Mercer. New York: Marcel Dekker, 1990, p 69.
117. Hilkens JF, Buijs J, Hilgers J. Hageman PH, Calafat J, Sonnenberg A, van der Valk M. Monoclonal antibodies against human milk-fat globule membranes detecting differentiation antigens of the mammary gland and its tumors. Int J Cancer 1984;34:197.
118. Kufe D, Inghirami G, Abe M, Hayes D, Justi-Wheeler H, Schlom J. Differential reactivity of a novel monoclonal antibody (DF3) with human malignant versus benign breast tumors. Hydridoma 1984;3:223.
119. Hayes DF, Zurawski VR Jr, Kufe DW. Comparison of circulating CA 15–3 and carcinoembryonic antigen levels in patients with breast cancer. J Clin Oncol 1986;4:1542.
120. Daly L, Ferguson J, Cram G, Haas V, Beam C, George S, McCarty K Jr, Bast R. Comparison of a new breast cancer serum marker, IMxBCM to CA15–3 and CEA. Am Soc Clin Oncol 1991;10:36.
121. Bast RC, Feeney M, Lazarus H, Nadler LM, Calvin RB, Knapp RC. Reactivity of a monoclonal antibody with human ovarian carcinoma. J Clin Invest 1981;68:1331.
122. Davis HM, Zurawski VR Jr, Bast RC Jr, Klug TL. Characterization of the CA125 antigen associated with human epithelial ovarian carcinomas. Cancer Res 1986;46:6143.
123. Kabawat SE, Bast RC Jr, Bhan AK, Welch WR, Knapp RC, Colvin RB. Tissue distribution of a coelomic-epithelium-related antigen recognized by the monoclonal antibody OC125. Int J Gynecol Pathol 1983;2:275.a.
124. Bast RC Jr, Klug TL, St. John E, Jenison E, Niloff JM, Lazarus H, Berkowitz RS, Leavitt T, Griffiths CT, Parker L, Zurawski VR Jr, Knapp RC. A radioimmunoassay using a monoclonal antibody to monitor the course of epithelial ovarian cancer. N Engl J Med 1983;309:883.a.
125. Jacobs I, Bast RC Jr. The CA125 tumour-associated antigen: a review of the literature. Hum Reprod 1989;4:1.
126. Hunter VJ, Daly L, Helms M, Soper JT, Berchuck A, Clarke-Pearson DL, Bast RC Jr. The prognostic significance of CA125 half-life in patients with ovarian cancer who have received primary chemotherapy after surgical cytoreduction. Am J Obstet Gynecol 1990;163:1164.
127. van der Burg ME, Lammes FB, van Putten WL, Stoter G. Ovarian cancer: The prognostic value of serum half-life of CA125 during induction chemotherapy. Gynecol Oncol 1988;30:307.
128. Einhorn N, Bast RC Jr, Knapp RC, Tjernberg B, Zurawski VR Jr. Preoperative evaluation of serum CA 125 levels in patients with primary epithelial ovarian cancer. Obstet Gynecol 1986;67:414.
129. Malkasian GD Jr, Knapp RC, Lavin PT, Zurawski VR Jr, Podratz KC, Stanhope CR, Mortel R, Berek JS, Bast RC Jr, Ritts RE. Preoperative evaluation of serum CA125 levels in premenopausal and postmenopausal patients with pelvic masses: discrimination of benign from malignant disease. Am J Obstet Gynecol 1988;159:341.
130. Soper JT, Hunter VJ, Daly L, Tanner M, Creasman WT, Bast RC Jr. Preoperative serum tumor-associated antigen levels in women with pelvic masses. Obstet Gynecol 1990;75:249.
131. Knapp RC, Berkowitz RS, Leavitt T Jr, Bast RC Jr. Natural history and detection of ovarian cancer. In Gynecology and Obstetrics. Edited by JW Sciarra. Philadelphia: Harper & Row, 1988, p 1.
132. Bast RC Jr, Siegal FP, Runowicz C, Klug TL, Zurawski VR Jr, Schonholz D, Cohen CJ, Knapp RC. Elevation of serum CA125 prior to diagnosis of an epithelial ovarian carcinoma. Gynecol Oncol 1985;22:115.
133. Zurawski VR Jr, Orjaseter H, Andersen A, Jellum E. Elevated serum CA 125 levels prior to diagnosis of ovarian neoplasia: relevance for early detection of ovarian cancer. Int J Cancer 1988;42:677.
134. Einhorn N, Sjovall K, Schoenfeld DA, Eklund G, Knapp RC, Bast RC Jr, Zurawski VR Jr. Early detection of ovarian cancer using the CA 125 radioimmunoassay (RIA). Proc Annu Meet Am Soc Clin Oncol 1990;9:a607.

135. Jacobs I, Stabile I, Bridges J, Kemsley P, Reynolds C, Grudzinskas J, Oram D. Multimodal approach to screening for ovarian cancer. Lancet 1988;1:268.
136. Zurawski VR Jr, Sjovall K, Schoenfeld DA, Broderick SF, Hall P, Bast RC, Jr, Eklund G, Mattsson B, Connor RJ, Eng D, Prorok PC, Knapp RC, Einhorn N. Prospective evaluation of serum CA 125 levels in a normal population, Phase I: The specificities of single and serial determinations in testing for ovarian cancer. Gynecol Oncol 1990;36: 299.
137. Woolas R, Xu FJ, Jacobs I, Oram D, Bast RC Jr. Case Report: elevated serum levels of macrophage stimulating factor and OVX1 eleven months prior to the diagnosis of stage Ic ovarian cancer. Int J Gynecol Cancer 1996.
138. Tschopp J, Nabholz M. Perforin-mediated target cell lysis by cytolytic T lymphocytes. Annu Rev Immunol 1990;8:279.
139. Young LHY, Lui C-C, Joag S, Rafii S, Young JD-E. How lymphocytes kill. Annu Rev Med 1990;41:45.
140. Nakajima H, Golstein P, Henkart PA. The target cell nucleus is not reguated for cell-mediated granzyme- or Fas-based cytotoxicity. J Exp Med 1995;181:1905.
141. El-Khatib M, Stanger BZ, Dogan H, Cui H, Ju ST. The molecular mechanism of FasL-mediated cytotoxicity by CD4+ TH1 clones. Cell Immunol 1995;163:237.
142. Podack ER. Execution and suicide: cytotoxic lymphocytes enforce Draconian laws through separate molecular pathways. Curr Opin Immunol 1995;7:11.
143. Nitta T, Oksenberg JR, Rao NA, Steinmam L. Predominant expression of T cell receptor V;ja7 in tumor-infiltrating lymphocytes of uveal melanoma. Science 1990;249: 672.
144. Trinchieri G. Biology of natural killer cells. Adv Immunol 1989;47:187.
145. Robertson MJ, Ritz J. Biology and clinical relevance of human natural killer cells. Blood 1990;76:2421.
146. Whiteside TL, Herberman RB. Short analytical review: the role of natural killer cells in human disease. Clin Immunol Immunopathol 1989;53:1.
147. Wunderlich JR, Hodes RJ. Principles of tumor immunity: biology of cellular immune response. In Biologic Therapy of Cancer. Edited by VT DeVita Jr, S Hellman, SA Rosenberg. Philadelphia: Lippincott, 1991, p 3.
148. Giorda R, Rudert WA, Vavassori C, Chambers WH, Hiserodt JC, Trucco M. NKR-P1, a signal transduction molecule on natural killer cells. Science 1990;249:1298.
149. Roder J. Immune response: killing comes naturally. Curr Biol 1991;1:242.
150. Janeway CA Jr. Immune response: to thine own self be true... Curr Biol 1991;1:239.
151. Herberman RB, Hiserodt J, Vujanovic N, Balch C, Lotzova E, Bolhuis R, Golub S, Lanier LL, Phillips JH, Riccardi C, Ritz J, Santoni A, Schmidt RE, Uchida A. Lymphokine-activated killer cell activity: characteristics of effector cells and their progenitors in blood and spleen. Immunol Today 1987;8:178.
152. Ojcius DM, Zheng LM, Sphicas EC, Zychlinsky A, Young JD. Subcellular localization of perforin and serin esterase in lymphokine-activated killer cells and cytotoxic T cells by immunogold labeling. J Immunol 1991;146:4427.
153. Johnson WJ, Somers SD, Adams DO. Expression and development of macrophage activation for tumor cytotoxicity. Contemp Topics Immunobiol 1984;13:127.
154. Adams DO, Lewis JG, Johnson WJ. Multiple modes of cellular injury by macrophages: requirement for different forms of effector activation. In Progress in Immunology V. Edited by Y Yamamura, T Tada. Tokyo: Academic, 1983, p 1009.
155. Meltzer MS, Nacy CA. Delayed-type hypersensitivity and the induction of activated, cytotoxic macrophages. In Fundamental Immunology, 2nd ed. Edited by WE Paul. New York: Raven, 1989, p 765.
156. Nathan CF, Murray HW, Cohn ZA. The macrophage as an effector cell. N Engl J Med 1980;303:622.
157. Lichtenstein A, Seelig M, Berek J, Zighelboim J. Human neutrophil-mediated lysis of ovarian cancer cells. Blood 1989;74:805.
158. Rosse WF. Mechanisms of immune destruction: complement and complement-dependent mechanisms. In Clinical Immunohematology: Basic Concepts and Clinical Applications. Boston: Blackwell, 1990, p 43.
159. Ohanian SH, Schlager SI. Humoral immune killing of nucleated cells: mechanisms of complement-mediated attack and target defense. Crit Rev Immunol 1981;1:165.
160. Schreiber H. Tumor immunology. In Fundamental Immunology, 2nd ed. Edited by WE Paul. New York: Raven, 1989, p 923.
161. Urban JL, Burton RC, Holland JM, Kripke ML, Schreiber H. Mechanisms of syngeneic tumor rejection. Susceptibility of the host-selected progressor variants to various immunological effector cells. J Exp Med 1982;155:557.
162. Urban JL, Kripke ML, Schreiber H. Stepwise immunologic selection of antigenic variants during tumor growth. J Immunol 1986;137:3036.
163. Boyer CM, Borowitz MJ, McCarty KS Jr, Kinney RB, Everitt L, Dawson DV, Ring D, Bast RC Jr. Heterogeneity of antigen expression in benign and malignant breast and ovarian epithelial cells. Int J Cancer 1989;43:55.
164. Old LJ, Stockert E, Boyse EA, Kim JH. Antigenic modulation. Loss of TL antigen from cells exposed to TL antibody. Study of the phenomenon in vitro. J Exp Med 1968;127: 523.
165. Ritz J, Pesando JM, Notis-McConarty J, Schlossman SF. Modulation of human acute lymphoblastic leukemia antigen induced by monoclonal antibody in vitro. J Immunol 1980;125:1506.
166. Takahashi K, Ono K, Hirabayashi Y, Taniguchi M. Escape mechanisms of melanoma from immune system by soluble melanoma antigen. J Immunol 1988;140:3244.
167. Theofilopoulos AN. Immune complexes in cancer. N Engl J Med 1982;307:1208.
168. Vlock DR. Immune complexes and malignancy. In Immunodiagnosis of Cancer, 2nd ed. Edited by RB Herberman, DW Mercer. New York: Marcel Dekker, 1990, p 555.
169. Mandell GL, Fisher RI, Bostick F, Young RC. Ovarian cancer: a solid tumor with evidence of normal cellular immune function but abnormal B cell function. Am J Med 1979;66:621.
170. Batchelor JR, Lombardi G, Lechler RI. Speculations on the specificity of suppression. Immunol Today 1989;10:37.
171. Schreiber H. Idiotype network interactions in tumor immunity. Adv Cancer Res 1984;41:291.
172. DiGiacomo A, North RJ. T cell suppressors of antitumor immunity. The production of Ly-1-, 2+ suppressors of delayed sensitivity precedes the production of suppressors of protective immunity. J Exp Med 1986;164:1179.
173. North RJ. Down-regulation of the antitumor immune response. Adv Cancer Res 1985;45:1.
174. North RJ, DiGiacomo A, Dye ES. Suppression of antitumor immunity. In Tumor Immunology—Mechanisms, Diagnosis, Therapy. Edited by W den Otter, EJ Ruitenberg. New York: Elsevier, 1987, p 125.
175. Germain RN, Benacerraf BA. Single major pathway of T-lymphocyte interactions in antigen-specific immune suppression. Scand J Immunol 1981;13:1.
176. Chakraborty NG, Twardzik DR, Sivanandham MT, Ergin MT, Hellstrom KE, Mukherji B. Autologous melanoma-induced activation of regulatory T cells that suppress cytotoxic response. J Immunol 1990;145:2359.
177. Mukherji B, Chakraborty NG, Sivanandham M. T-cell clones that react against autologous human tumors. Immunol Rev 1990;116:33.
178. Mukherji B, Guha A, Chakraborty NG, Sivanandham M, Nashed AL, Sporn JR, Ergin MT. Clonal analysis of cytotoxic and regulatory T cell responses against human melanoma. J Exp Med 1989;169:1961.
179. Mukherji B, Guha A, Loomis R, Ergin M. T-cell-mediated amplification and down regulation of cytotoxic immune response against autologous human cancer. J Immunol 1987;138:1987.
180. Mukherji B, Nashed AL, Guha A, Ergin MT. Regulation of cellular immune response against autologous human melanoma. II. Mechanism of induction and specificity of suppression. J Immunol 1986;136:1893.
181. Mukherji B, Wilhelm SA, Guha A, Ergin MT. Regulation of cellular immune response against autologous human melanoma. I. Evidence for cell-mediated suppression of in vitro cytotoxic immune response. J Immunol 1986;136:1888.
182. LeFever A, Funahashi A. Elevated prostaglandin E2 levels in bronchoalveolar lavage fluid of patients with bronchogenic carcinoma. Chest 1990;98:1397.
183. Bast RC Jr. Effects of cancers and their treatment on host immunity. In Cancer Medicine, 2nd ed. Edited by JF Holland, E Frei III. Philadelphia: Lea & Febiger, 1982, p 1134.
184. Lopez DM, Fu Y-X, Watson GA. Modulation of immune responses by tumor derived factors. Proc Am Assoc Cancer Res 1990;31:236.
185. Mizoguchi H, O'Shea JJ, Longo DL, Loeffler CM, McVicar DW, Ochoa AC. Alterations in signal transduction molecules in T lymphocytes from tumor-bearing mice. Science 1992;258:1732.
186. Allison AC. Immunological surveillance against tumor cells. In Cancer: A Comprehensive Treatise. Biology of Tumors: Surfaces, Immunology, and Comparative Pathology. Edited by FF Becker. New York: Plenum, 1975, p 237.
187. Bast RC, Rapp HJ. The immunology of animal tumors. In Immunological Diseases, 3rd ed. Edited by M Samter, DW Talmage, B Rose, KF Austen, JH Vaughan. Boston: Little, Brown, 1978, p 359.
188. Burnet FM. The concept of immunological surveillance. Prog Exp Tumor Res 1970;13: 1.
189. Kärre K, Ljunggren HG, Piontek G, Kiessling R. Selective rejection of H-2-deficient lymphoma variants suggests alternative immune defence strategy. Nature 1986;319: 675.
190. Penn I. Principles of tumor immunity: immunocompetence and cancer. In Biologic Therapy of Cancer. Edited by VT DeVita Jr, S Hellman, SA Rosenberg. Philadelphia: Lippincott, 1991, p 53.
191. Ioachim HL. The opportunistic tumors of immune deficiency. Adv Cancer Res 1990;54:301.
192. Prehn RT. The immune reaction as a stimulator of tumor growth. Science 1972;176: 170.
193. Hurteau J, Simon HU, Kurman C, Rubin L, Mills GB. Levels of the soluble interleukin 2 receptor alpha are elevated in epithelial ovarian cancer patients: evidence for activation of T lymphocytes and potential role in management of ovarian cancer. Am J Obstet Gynecol 1994;170:918.
194. Chiorazzi N, Fu SM, Montazeri G, Kunkel HG, Rai K, Gee T. T cell helper defect in patients with chronic lymphocytic leukemia. J Immunol 1979;122:1087.
195. Faguet GB. Mechanisms of lymphocyte activation: the role of suppressor cells in the proliferative responses of chronic lymphatic leukemia lymphocytes. J Clin Invest 1979;63:67.
196. Han T, Dadey B. In vitro functional studies of mononuclear cells in patients with CLL: evidence for functionally normal T lymphocytes and monocytes and abnormal B lymphocytes. Cancer 1979;43:109.
197. Platsoucas CD, Galinski M, Kempin S, Reich L, Clarkson B, Good R A. Abnormal T lymphocyte subpopulations in patients with chronic B cell lymphocytic leukemia: an analysis by monoclonal antibodies. J Immunol 1982;129:2305.
198. Broder S, Humphrey R, Durm M, Blackman M, Meade B, Goldman C, Strober W, Waldmann T. Impaired synthesis of polyclonal (non-paraprotein) immunoglobulins by circulating lymphocytes from patients with multiple myeloma: role of suppressor cells. N Engl J Med 1975;293:887.
199. Knapp W, Baumgartner G. Monocyte-mediated suppression of human B lymphocyte differentiation in vitro. J Immunol 1978;121:1177.
200. Platsoucas CD, Hansen HJ, Redman JR, Berenson S, Lee BJ, Clarkson BD. T-cell imbalances in patients with multiple myeloma: an analysis of monoclonal antibodies. J Clin Immunol 1983;3:227.
201. Fisher RI, DeVita VT Jr, Bostick F, Vanhaelen C, Howser DM, Hubbard SM, Young RC. Persistent immunologic abnormalities in long-term survivors of advanced Hodgkin's disease. Ann Intern Med 1980;92:595.
202. Heidenreich W, Jagla K, Schussler J, Borner P, Dehnhard F, Kalden JR, Liebold W, Peter HH, Deicher H. Immunological characterization of mononuclear cells in peripheral blood and regional lymph nodes of breast cancer patients. Cancer 1979;43: 1308.
203. Oldham RK, Wesse JL, Herberman RB, Perlin E, Mills M, Heims W, Blom J, Green D, Reid J, Bellinger S, Law I, McCoy JL, Dean JH, Cannon GB, Djeu J. Immunological monitoring and immunotherapy in carcinoma of the lung. Int J Cancer 1976;18:739.
204. Ritts RE Jr. Immune status and role of immunotherapy: overview. In Lung Cancer: Progress in Therapeutic Research and Therapy. Vol. 22. Edited by F Muggia, M Rozencweig. New York: Raven, 1979, p 457.
205. Aisenberg AC. Lymphoma, leukemia and Hodgkin's disease. In Immunological Diseases. Edited by M Samter. Boston: Little, Brown, 1978, p 530.
206. Fisher RI, Young RC. Immunologic aspects of Hodgkin's disease. In The Handbook of Cancer Immunology. Immune Status in Cancer Treatment and Prognosis. Part B, vol. 4. Edited by H Waters. New York: Garland STPM, 1978, p 1.
207. Fuks Z, Strober S, Bobrove AM, Sasazuki T, McMichael A, Kaplan HS. Long-term effects of radiation on T and B lymphocytes in peripheral blood of patients with Hodgkin's disease. J Clin Invest 1976;58:803.
208. Fuks Z, Strober S, King DP, Kaplan HS. Reversal of cell surface abnormalities of T lymphocytes in Hodgkin's disease after in vitro incubation in fetal sera. J Immunol 1976;117:1331.

209. Goodwin JS, Husby G, Williams RC. Prostaglandin E and cancer growth. Cancer Immunol Immunother 1980;8:3.
210. Twomey JJ, Rice L. Impact of Hodgkin's disease upon the immune system. Semin Oncol 1980;7:114.
211. Weed RI. Exaggerated delayed hypersensitivity to mosquito bites in chronic lymphocytic leukemia. Blood 1965;26:257.
212. Waldmann TA, Bull JM, Bruce RM, Broder S, Jost MC, Balestra ST, Suer ME. Serum immunoglobulin E levels in patients with neoplastic disease. J Immunol 1974;113: 379.
213. Berenbaum MC, Fluck PA, Hurst NP. Depression of lymphocyte responses after surgical trauma. Br J Exp Pathol 1973;54:597.
214. Jubert AV, Lee ET, Hersh EM, McBride CM. Effects of surgery, anesthesia and intraoperative blood loss on immunocompetence. J Surg Res 1973;15:399.
215. Slade MS, Simmons RL, Yunis E, Greenberg LJ. Immunodepression after major surgery in normal patients. Surgery 1975;78:363.
216. Infective hazards of splenectomy. Lancet 1976;1:1167. Editorial.
217. Eraklis AJ, Kevy SV, Diamond LK, Gross RE. Hazard of overwhelming infection after splenectomy in childhood. N Engl J Med 1967;276:1225.
218. Robinette CD, Fraumeni JF. Splenectomy and subsequent mortality in veterans of the 1939–45 war. Lancet 1977;2:127.
219. Anderson RE, Warner NL. Ionizing radiation and the immune response. Adv Immunol 1976;24:215.
220. Goh K. Radiation, cell-mediated immunity, and cancer. In The Handbook of Cancer Immunology. Basic Cancer-Related Immunology. Vol. 1. Edited by H Waters. New York: Garland STPM, 1978, p 307.
221. Slavin S, Strober S. Induction of allograft tolerance after total lymphoid irradiation (TLI): Development of suppressor cells of the mixed leukocyte reaction (MLR). J Immunol 1979;123:942.
222. Hersh EM, Gutterman JU, Mavligit G, McCredie KB, Bodey GP, Freireich EJ. Host defense, chemical immunosuppression, and the transplant recipient. Relative effects of intermittent versus continuous immunosuppressive therapy with reference to the objectives of treatment. Transplant Proc 1973;5:1191.
223. Turk JL, Parker D. The effect of cyclophosphamide on the immune response. J Immunopharmacol 1979;1:127.
224. Bast RC Jr, Reinherz EL, Maver C, Lavin P, Schlossman SF. Contrasting effects of cyclophosphamide and prednisolone on the phenotype of human peripheral blood leukocytes. Clin Immunol Immunopathol 1983;28:101.
225. Spreafico F, Anaclerio A. Immunosuppressive agents. In Immunopharmacology. Edited by JW Hadden, RG Coffey, F Spreafico. New York: Plenum, 1977, p 245.
226. Weiss RB. Hypersensitivity reactions to cancer chemotherapy. Semin Oncol 1982;9: 5.
227. Nauts HC. Beneficial effects of acute concurrent infection, inflammation, fever or immunotherapy (bacterial toxins) on ovarian and uterine cancer. Cancer Res Inst Monog 1977;17:3.
228. Kempin S, Cirrincione C, Straus DS, Gee TS, Arlin Z, Koziner B, Pinsky L, Nisce L, Myers J, Lee BJ III, Clarkson BD, Old LJ, Oettgen HF. Improved remission rate and duration in nodular non-Hodgkin's lymphoma (NNHL) with the use of mixed bacterial vaccine (MBV). Proc Am Soc Clin Oncol 1981;514.
229. Kempin S, Cirrincione C, Meyers J, Lee B III, Straus D, Koziner B, Arlin Z, Gee T, Mertelsmann R, Pinsky C, Comacho E, Nisce L, Old L, Clarkson B, Oettgen H. Combined modality therapy of advanced nodular lymphomas (NL): the role of nonspecific immunotherapy (MBV) as an important determinant of response and survival. Proc Am Soc Clin Oncol 1983;2:56.
230. Cohen M, Felix E, Jessup J, Rosenberg S. Treatment of metastatic melanoma by intralesional injection of BCG, organic chemicals, and *C. parvum*. In Neoplasm Immunity: Mechanisms. Edited by RG Crispen. Chicago: ITR, 1976, p 121.
231. Klein E. Introduction: immunotherapy of cancer in man, a reality. In Conference on the Use of BCG in Therapy of Cancer. National Cancer Institute Monograph 39. Edited by T Borsos, HJ Rapp. Washington, DC: 1973, p 139.
232. Bast RC, Zbar B, Borsos T, Rapp HJ. BCG and cancer. N Engl J Med 1974;290: 1413;1458.
233. Morton DL, Eilber FR, Malmgren RA, Wood WC. Immunological factors which influence response to immunotherapy in malignant melanoma. Surgery 1970;68:158.
234. Herr HW, Laudone VP, Badalament RA, Oettgen HF, Sogani PC, Freedman BD, Melamed MR, Whitmore WF Jr. Bacillus Calmette-Guérin therapy alters the progression of superficial bladder cancer. J Clin Oncol 1988;6:1450.
235. Oettgen HF, Old LJ. The history of cancer immunotherapy. In Biologic Therapy of Cancer. Edited by VT DeVita Jr, S Hellman, SA Rosenberg. Philadelphia: Lippincott, 1991, p 87.
236. Berek JS, Knapp RC, Hacker NF, Lichtenstein A, Jung T, Spina C, Obrist R, Griffiths CT, Berkowitz RS, Parker L, Zighelboim J, Bast RC Jr. Intraperitoneal immunotherapy of epithelial ovarian carcinoma with *Corynebacterium parvum*. Am J Obstet Gynecol 1985;152:1003.
237. Bekierkunst A, Levij IS, Yarkoni E, Vilkas E, Lederer E. Suppression of urethan-induced lung adenomas in mice treated with trehalose-6, 6-dimycolate (cord factor) and living bacillus Calmette-Guérin. Science 1971;174:1240.
238. Fidler IJ, Murray JL, Kleinerman ES. Systemic activation of macrophages in liposomes containing immunomodulators. In Biologic Therapy of Cancer. Edited by VT DeVita Jr, S Hellman, SA Rosenberg. Philadelphia: Lippincott, 1991, p 730.
239. Lederer E, Chedid L. Immunomodulation by synthetic muramyl peptides and trehalose diesters. In Immunological Aspects of Cancer Therapeutics. Edited by E Mihich. New York: Wiley, 1982, p 107.
240. Kleinerman ES, Maeda M, Jaffe N. Liposome-encapsulated muramyl tripeptide: a new biologic response modifier for the treatment of osteosarcoma. Cancer Treatment Res 1993;62:101.
241. Hamilton JM, Sznol M, Friedman MA. 5-Fluorouracil plus levamisole: effective adjuvant treatment for colon cancer. In Important Advances in Oncology 1990. Edited by VT DeVita Jr, S Hellman, SA Rosenberg. Philadelphia: Lippincott, 1990, p 115.
242. Strander H. Interferons (IFNs). Adv Cancer Res 1986;46:1.
243. Barth A, Morton DL. The role of adjuvant therapy in melanoma management. Cancer 1995;75:726.
244. Bookman MA, Bast RC Jr. The immunobiology and immunotherapy of ovarian cancer. Semin Oncol 1991;18:270.
245. Borden EC. Interferons and cancer: how the promise is being kept. Interferon 1983;5: 43.
246. Haranaka K, Satomi N. Cytotoxic activity of tumor necrosis factor (TNF) on human cancer cells in vitro. Jpn J Exp Med 1981;51:191.
247. Blick M, Sherwin SA, Rosenblum M, Gutterman J. Phase I study of recombinant tumor necrosis factor in cancer patients. Cancer Res 1987;47:2986.
248. Chapman PB, Lester TJ, Casper ES, Gabrilove JL, Wong GY, Kempin SJ, Gold PJ, Welt S, Warren RS, Starnes HF, Sherwin SA, Old LJ, Oettgen HF. Clinical pharmacology of recombinant human tumor necrosis factor in patients with advanced cancer. J Clin Oncol 1987;5:1942.
249. Jakubowski AA, Casper ES, Gabrilove JL, Templeton MA, Sherwin SA, Oettgen HF. Phase I trial of intramuscularly administered tumor necrosis factor in patients with advanced cancer. J Clin Oncol 1989;7:298.
250. Sherman ML, Spriggs DR, Arthur KA, Imamura K, Frei E, Kufe DW. Recombinant human tumor necrosis factor administered as a five-day continuous infusion in cancer patients: Phase I toxicity and effects on lipid metabolism. J Clin Oncol 1988;6:344.
251. Lejeune F, Lienard D, Eggermont A, Schraffordt-Koops H, Kroon B, Gerain J, Rosenkaimer F, Schmitz P. Clinical experience with high-dose tumor necrosis factor alpha in regional therapy of advanced melanoma. Circ Book 1994;43:191.
252. Ruddle NH. Tumor necrosis factor and related cytotoxins. Immunol Today 1987;8: 129.
253. Livingston PO, Natoli EJ, Calves MJ, Stockert E, Oettgen HF, Old LJ. Vaccines containing purified GM2 ganglioside elicit GM2 antibodies in melanoma patients. Proc Natl Acad Sci USA 1987;84:2911.
254. Berd D, Maguire HC Jr, McCue P, Mastrangelo MJ. Treatment of metastatic melanoma with an autologous tumor-cell vaccine: clinical and immunologic results in 64 patients. J Clin Oncol 1990;8:1858.
255. Mitchell MS, Harel W, Kempf RA, Hu E, Kan-Mitchell J, Boswell WD, Dean G, Stevenson L. Active-specific immunotherapy for melanoma. J Clin Oncol 1990;8:856.
256. Estin CD, Stevenson US, Plowman GD, Hu S-L, Sridhar P, Hellström I, Brown JP, Hellström KE. Recombinant vaccinia virus vaccine against the human melanoma antigen p97 for use in immunotherapy. Proc Natl Acad Sci USA 1988;85:1052.
257. Fearon ER, Pardoll DM, Itaya T, Golumbek P, Levitsky HI, Simons JW, Karasuyama H, Vogelstein B, Frost P. Interleukin-2 production by tumor cells bypasses T helper function in the generation of an antitumor response. Cell 1990;60:397.
258. Gansbacher B, Bannerji R, Daniels B, Zier K, Cronin K, Gilboa E. Retroviral vector-mediated γ-interferon gene transfer into tumor cells generates potent and long lasting antitumor immunity. Cancer Res 1990;50:7820.
259. Gansbacher B, Zier K, Daniels B, Cronin K, Bannerji R, Gilboa E. Interleukin 2 gene transfer into tumor cells abrogates tumorigenicity and induces protective immunity. J Exp Med 1990;172:1217.
260. Golumbek PT, Lazenby AJ, Levitsky HI, Jaffee LM, Karasuyama H, Baker M, Pardoll DM. Treatment of established renal cancer by tumor cells engineered to secrete interleukin-4. Science 1991;254:713.
261. Berd D, Mastrangelo MJ. Active immunotherapy of human melanoma exploiting the immunopotentiating effects of cyclophosphamide. Cancer Invest 1988;6:337.
262. Boyer CM, Lidor Y, Lottich SC, Bast RC Jr. Antigenic cell surface markers in human solid tumors. Antibody Immunocon Radiopharm 1988;1:105.
263. Kabat EA, Liao J, Shyong J, Osserman EF. A monoclonal IgM lambda macroglobulin with specificity for lacto-N-tetraose in a patient with bronchogenic carcinoma. J Immunol 1982;128:540.
264. Masui H, Moroyama T, Mendelsohn J. Mechanism of antitumor activity in mice for anti-epidermal growth factor receptor monoclonal antibodies with different isotypes. Cancer Res 1986;46:5592.
265. Taetle R, Castagnola J, Mendelsohn J. Mechanisms of growth inhibition by anti-transferrin receptor monoclonal antibodies. Cancer Res 1986;46:1759.
266. Haspel MV, McCabe RP, Pomato N, Janesch NJ, Knowlton JV, Peters LC, Hoover HC Jr, Hanna MG Jr. Generation of tumor cell reactive human mononclonal antibodies using peripheral blood lymphocytes from actively immunized colorectal carcinoma patients. Cancer Res 1985;45:3951.
267. Houghton AN. Building a better monoclonal antibody. Immunol Today 1988;9:265.
268. Morrison SL, 0I VT. Genetically engineered antibody molecules. Adv Immunol 1989;44:65.
269. Levy R, Miller RA. Therapy of lymphoma directed at idiotypes. Monogr Natl Cancer Inst 1990;10:61.
270. Mittelman A, Chen ZJ, Kageshita T, Yang T, Yamada M, Baskind P, Goldberg N, Puccio C, Ahmed T, Arlin Z, Ferrone S. Active specific immunotherapy in patients with melanoma. A clinical trial with mouse antiidiotypic monoclonal antibodies elicited with syngeneic anti-high-molecular-weight melanoma-associated antigen monoclonal antibodies. J Clin Invest 86:2136, 1990; Erratum: J Clin Invest 1991;87:757.
271. Nepom GT, Hellström KE. Anti-idiotypic antibodies and the induction of specific tumor immunity. Cancer Metastatis Rev 1987;6:489.
272. Wettendorff M, Iliopoulos D, Tempero M, Kay D, DeFreitas E, Koprowski H, Herlyn D. Idiotypic cascades in cancer patients treated with monoclonal antibody CO17–1A. Proc Natl Acad Sci USA 1989;86:3787.
273. Maloney DG, Bodkin D, Grillo-Lopez AJ, White C, Foon K, Schilder R, Neidhart J, Janakiraman N, Waldichuk C, Varns C, Royston I, Levy R. IDEC-C2B8: final report on a phase II trial in relapsed non-Hodgkin's lymphoma. Blood 1994;84:169.
274. Houghton AN, Mintzer D, Cordon-Cardo C, Welt S, Fliegel B, Vadhan S, Carswell E, Melamed MR, Oettgen HF, Old LJ. Mouse monoclonal IgG3 antibody detecting GD3 ganglioside: a phase I trial in patients with malignant melanoma. Proc Natl Acad Sci USA 1985;82:1242.
275. Vadhan-Raj S, Cordon-Cardo C, Carswell E, Mintzer D, Dantis L, Duteau C, Templeton MA, Oettgen HF, Old LJ, Houghton AN. Phase I trial of a mouse monoclonal antibody against GD3 ganglioside in patients with melanoma Induction of inflammatory responses at tumor sites. J Clin Oncol 1988;6:1636.
276. Irie RF, Morton DL. Regression of cutaneous metastatic melanoma by intralesional injection with human monoclonal antibody to ganglioside GD2. Proc Natl Acad Sci USA 1986;83:8694.
277. Reithmuller G, Schneider-Gadicke E, Schlimok G, Schmiegel W, Raab R, Hoffken K, Gruber R, Pichlmaier H, Hirche H, Pichlmayr R, et al. Randomised trial of monoclonal antibody for adjuvant therapy of resected Duke's C colorectal carcinoma.
278. Trail PA, Willner D, Lasch SJ, Henderson AJ, Hofstead S, Casazza AM, Firestone RS, Hellström I, Hellström KE. Cure of xenografted human carcinomas by Br96-doxorubicin immunoconjugates. Science 1993;261:212.
279. Sugerman S, Murray JL, Saleh M, LoBuglio AF, Jones D, Daniel C, LeBherz D, Brewer

H, Healy D, Kelley S, Hellström KE, Onetto N. A phase I study of Br96-Doxorubicin (Br96-DOX) in patients with advanced carcinoma expressing the Lewis^{Y} antigen. Am Soc Clin Oncol Edu Book 1995;14:423.

280. DeNardo SJ, DeNardo GL, O'Grady LF, Levy NB, Mills SL, Macey DJ, McGrahan JP, Miller CH, Epstein AL. Pilot studies of radiotherapy of B-cell lymphoma and leukemia using I-131 Lym-1 monoclonal antibody. Antibody Immunocon Radiopharm 1988;1: 17.
281. Epenetos AA, Munro AJ, Stewart S, Rampling R, Lambert HE, McKenzie CG, Soutter P, Rahemtulla A, Hooker G, Sivolapenko GB, Snook D, Courtenay-Luck N, Dhokia B, Krausz T, Taylor-Papadimitriou J, Durbin H, Bodmer WF. Antibody-guided irradiation of advanced ovarian cancer with intraperitoneally administered radiolabeled monoclonal antibodies. J Clin Oncol 1987;5:1890.
282. Hird V, Maraveyas A, Snook D, Dhokia B, Soutter WP, Meares C, Stewart JSW, Mason P, Lambert HE, Epenetos AA. Adjuvant therapy of ovarian cancer with radioactive monoclonal antibody. Br J Cancer 1993;68:403.
283. Press OW, Eary JF, Appelbaum FR, Martin PJ, Badger CC, Nelp WB, Glenn S, Butchki G, Fisher D, Porter B, Matthews DC, Fisher LD, Bernstein ID. Radiolabeled-antibody therapy of B-cell lymphoma with autologous bone marrow support. N Engl J Med 1993;329:1219.
284. Kaminski MS, Zasadny KR, Francis IR, Milik AW, Ross CW, Moon SD, Crawford SM, Burgess JM, Petry NA, Butchko GM, Glenn SD, Wahl RL. Radioimmunotherapy of B-cell lymphoma with (131I] anti-B anti-CD20 antibody. N Engl J Med 329:459, 1993.
285. Bookman MA, Griffin T, Godfrey S, Padavic K, Corda JP, Hamilton T, Ozols RF, Groves ES. Anti-transferrin receptor immunotoxin (IT): intraperitoneal (i.p.) phase-I trial. In Biology and Therapy of Ovarian Cancer. Marble Island Resort VT, 1990.
286. Frankel A, Borowitz M, Carter P, Hertler A, Moore JO, Brenckman W, Groves ES, Marafino B. A phase I study of continuous infusion immunotoxin for refractory metastatic breast cancer. Proc Annu Meet Am Soc Clin Oncol 1988;7:a121.
287. Pastan I, Pai L, Bookman M, Smith J, Longo D, Frankel A, Willingham M, FitzGerald DJ. OVB3-PE clinical trial. In Biology and Therapy of Ovarian Cancer. Marble Island Resort, VT, 1990.
288. Pai L, Pastan I. Immunotoxins and recombinant toxins for cancer treatment. In Important Advances in Oncology 1994. Edited by VT DeVita, S Hellman, SA Rosenberg. Philadelphia: Lippincott, 1994, p 3.
289. Oratz R, Speyer JL, Wernz JC, Hochster H, Meyers M, Mischak R, Spitler LE. Antimelanoma monoclonal antibody-ricin a chain immunoconjugate (XMMME-001-RTA) plus cyclosphamide in the treatment of metastatic malignant melanoma: results of a phase II trial. J Biol Response Mod 1990;9:345.
290. Spitler LE, del Rio M, Khentigan A, Wedel NI, Brophy NA, Miller LL, Harkonen WS, Rosendorf LL, Lee HM, Mischak RP, Kawahata RT, Stoudemire JB, Fradkin LB, Bautista EE, Scannon PJ. Therapy of patients with malignant melanoma using a monoclonal antimelanoma antibody-ricin A chain immunotoxin. Cancer Res 1987;47: 1717.
291. Nadler LM, Breitmeyer J, Coral F, Spector N, Schlossman S. Anti-B4 blocked ricin immunotherapy for patients with B cell malignancies: results of bolus and constant infusion phase I trials. Proceedings of the Second International Symposium on Immunotoxins, Orlando, 1990, p 58.
292. Sondel PM, Hank JA, Kohler PC, Sosman JA, Weil-Hillman G, Fisch P. The cellular immunotherapy of cancer: current and potential uses of interleukin-2. Crit Rev Oncol/Hematol 1989;9:125.
293. Rosenberg SA. Adoptive cellular therapy: clinical applications. In Biologic Therapy of Cancer. Edited by VT DeVita Jr, S Hellman, SA Rosenberg. Philadelphia: Lippincott, 1991, p 214.
294. Rosenberg SA, Lotze MT, Muul LM, Chang AE, Avis FP, Leitman S, Linehan WM, Robertson CN, Lee RE, Rubin JT, Seipp CA, Simpson CG, White DE. A progress report on the treatment of 157 patients with advanced cancer using lymphokine-activated killer cells and interleukin-2 or high-dose interleukin-2 alone. N Engl J Med 1987;316:889.
295. West WH, Tauer KW, Yannelli JR, Marshall GD, Orr DW, Thurman GB, Oldham RK. Constant-infusion recombinant interleukin-2 in adoptive immunotherapy of advanced cancer. N Engl J Med 1987;316:898.
296. Pinto A, Gattei V, Davide S, Parracicini C, Del Vecchio L. New molecules burst at the leukocyte surface: a comprehensive review based on the 5th International Workshop of Leukocyte Differentiation Antigens. Leukemia 1994;8:347.
297. Quirt IC, Tannock IF. Interleukin-2 for metastatic melanoma: treating polyuria with insulin? J Clin Oncol 1990;8:1125.
298. Rosenberg SA, Packard BS, Aebersold PM, Solomon D, Topalian SL, Toy ST, Simon P, Lotze MT, Yang JC, Seipp CA, Simpson C, Carter C, Bock S, Schwartzentruber D, Wei JP, White DE. Use of tumor-infiltrating lymphocytes and interleukin-2 in the immunotherapy of patients with metastatic melanoma. A preliminary report. N Engl J Med 1988;319:1676.
299. Rosenberg SA, Yannelli JR, Yang JC, Topalian SL, Schwartzentruber DJ, Weber JS, Parkinson DR, Selipp CA, Einhorn JH, White DE. Treatment of patients with metastatic melanoma with autologous tumor-infiltrating lymphocytes and interleukin 2. JNCI 1995;87:319.
300. Yang JC, Rosenberg SA. Adoptive cellular therapy: preclinical studies. In Biologic Therapy of Cancer. Edited by VT DeVita Jr, S Hellman, SA Rosenberg. Philadelphia: Lippincott, 1991, p 197.
301. Rosenberg SA, Spiess P, Lafreniere R. A new approach to the adoptive immunotherapy of cancer with tumor-infiltrating lymphocytes. Science 1986;233:1318.
302. Bast RC Jr. Principles of cancer biology: tumor immunology. In Cancer: Principles and Practice of Oncology, 2nd ed. Edited by VT DeVita Jr, S Hellman, SA Rosenberg. New York: Lippincott, 1985, p 125.
303. Knapp W, Dörken B, Gilks WR, Rieber EP, Schmidt RE, Stein H, von dem Borne AEG Jr. In Leukocyte Typing IV White Cell Differentiation Antigens. Edited by W Knapp. Oxford: Oxford University Press, 1989.
304. Rosenberg SA, Longo DL, Lotze MT. Principles and applications of biologic therapy. In Cancer Principles and Practice of Oncology. Edited by VT DeVita Jr, S Hellman, SA Rosenberg. Philadelphia: Lippincott, 1989, p 301.
305. Reading CL. Elimination of residual tumor cells from autologous bone marrow grafts using monoclonal antibodies. In Principles of Cancer Biotherapy. Edited by RK Oldham. New York: Raven, 1987, p 355.
306. Zola H. The surface antigens of human B lymphocytes. Immunol Today 1987;8:308.
307. O'Garra A, Umland S, de France T, Christiansen J. "B-cell factors" are pleiotropic. Immunol Today 1988;9:45.
308. Clark SC, Kamen R. The human hematopoietic colony-stimulating factors. Science 1987;236:1229.
309. Wasserman RL, Capra JD. Immunoglobulins. In The Glycoconjugates. Mammalian Glycoproteins and Glycolipids. Edited by MI Horowitz, W Pigman. New York: Academic, 1977, p 323.
310. Capra JD, Edmundson AB. The antibody combining site. Sci Am 1977;236:50.
311. Silverton EW, Navia MA, Davies DR. Three-dimensional structure of an intact human immunoglobulin. Proc Natl Acad Sci USA 1977;74:5140.
312. Davis MM. Molecular genetics of T cell antigen receptors. Hosp Pract 1988;23:157; 169.
313. Boyer CM, Knapp RC, Bast RC Jr. Immunology and immunotherapy. In Practical Gynecologic Oncology. Edited by JS Berek, NF Hacker. Baltimore: Williams & Wilkins, 1989, p 73.
314. Alberts B, Bray D, Lewis J, Raff M, Roberts R, Watson JD. Molecular Biology of the Cell. New York: Garland, 1983, p 988.

SECTION III

CANCER ETIOLOGY

CHAPTER 12

Genetic Predisposition to Cancer

BRUCE. PONDER

Cancer as a Genetic Disease

Several steps are necessary to turn a normal cell into a cancer cell. Most involve mutational change. Cancer, therefore, is a genetic disease at the level of the somatic cell. In some cases, cancer also may be a genetic disease at the level of the germ line. This chapter considers the inherited contribution to cancer incidence, its importance, and its investigation.

Inherited predisposition to cancer is potentially important for three reasons:

1. Predisposed individuals are a high-risk population who may benefit from prevention or from early diagnosis and treatment.
2. The existence of genetic predisposition may provide a means to study the genetic steps of carcinogenesis. Most, if not all, cancers that result from inherited predisposition have a similar nonheritable counterpart, and in the cases studied thus far, heritable and nonheritable cases are genetically similar. Study of the uncommon familial cases therefore may improve our understanding of the development of cancers in general.
3. In some cases, genetic predisposition to cancer is accompanied by abnormalities in development and control of growth, both in the tissue from which the cancer arises, and elsewhere. Many of the genes that, when mutated are cancer genes, may have important normal functions in growth and development. Cancer families are a way these genes are revealed and identified.

How Much of Cancer Depends on Inherited Predisposition?

There is no clear answer to this question. In each case, inherited predisposition, environmental exposure, and (because we are dealing with the accumulation of a series of stochastic events) chance will interact in different degrees. The question can be rephrased to ask which cases have a sufficiently strong inherited predisposition to be of practical significance for prevention or treatment (1). Perhaps fewer than 1% of cancers are "inherited cancer syndromes," and a further 5 to 10% are recognizable familial clusters of common cancers that probably have a genetic basis.

This implies that quite large numbers of individuals have an increased risk of cancer because of their family history. For example, it can be estimated from epidemiologic data that approximately 110,000 women aged from 25 to 60 years in England and Wales (total population, approximately 45 million) have a family history such that they have at least a one in six chance of developing breast cancer by age 70—approximately 2.5 times the risk in the population as a whole. Moreover, it is argued later that important inherited predisposition may exist in the absence of an obvious family history, and that "weak" predisposing genes may in fact be responsible for a greater proportion of common cancers than "strong" genes that give rise to multiple-case families.

Recognition of Inherited Predisposition

Because each heritable cancer has a histologically similar, nonheritable counterpart, it can be difficult or impossible in an individual case to know whether a cancer results from inherited predisposition (72). Until the predisposing mutations themselves can be identified, the clues to inherited predisposition are (*a*) in a few rare syndromes, a "marker phenotype" ([e.g., the multiple intestinal polyps characteristic of inherited cancer syndrome familial adenomatous polyposis (FAP]) (Fig. 12.1); and (*b*) the clinical and family history (19). Regarding the latter, if the cancer is rare, the occurrence of several cases in the family or multiple primaries in the individual is noticeable and probably significant. However, if the cancer is common (e.g., breast cancer), the significance of two or three cases in a family may be much more difficult to determine. (This point is discussed further in relation to breast and ovarian cancer in the section on familial cancers.)

A classification of inherited predisposition to cancer for practical use can be based not on biologic mechanisms (which still are largely obscure) but on the ease of recognition, using marker phenotype and family clustering. Such a classification is given in Table 12.1. The features of each group are described in the following sections.

Inherited Cancer Syndromes

GENERAL DESCRIPTION

The inherited cancer syndromes (32, 38, 59) include all cancers where a genetic effect is clearly apparent. To-

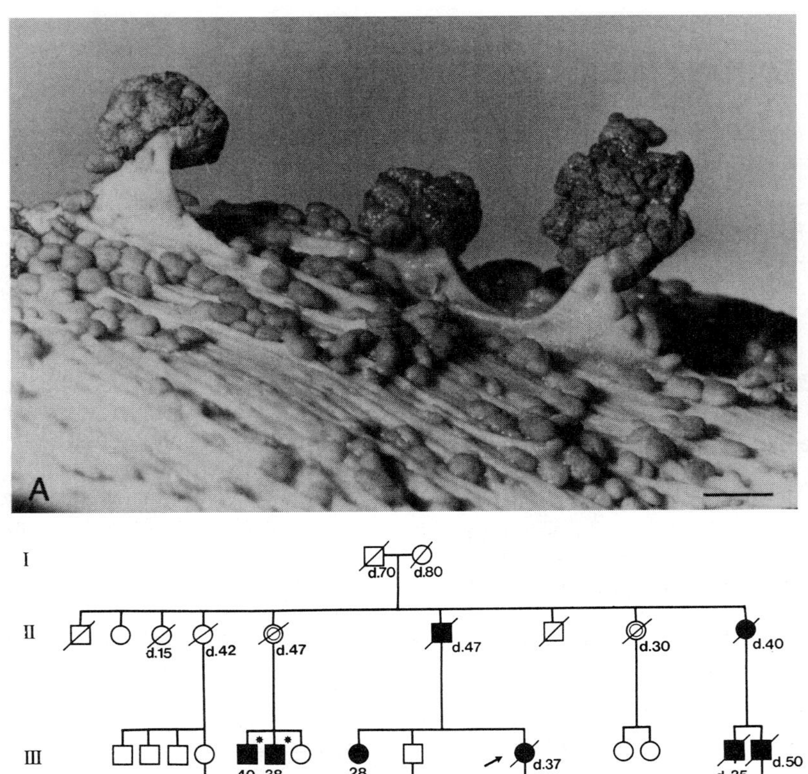

Figure 12.1. **A.** Polyps in colon of an individual with familial polyposis. Two large polyps and a smaller one are shown arising from the surface of the colonic epithelium. *Bar*, 5 mm. (Photograph provided by the ICRF Colorectal Cancer Unit, St. Mark's Hospital.) **B.** Pedigree of a family with familial polyposis of the colon (10). Family was recognized when the individual in generation III (*arrow*) presented with colonic cancer and was found to have multiple colonic polyps. Subsequently, other members have been screened by sigmoidoscopy. Three were found to already have cancer; five siblings and a cousin in generation IV had polyps and were treated by prophylactic colectomy.

Table 12.1. Classification of Genetic Predisposition to Cancer by Strength of Familial Clustering

Class	Examples
Inherited cancer syndromes	Familial polyposis Multiple endocrine neoplasia types 1 and 2 von Hippel-Lindau syndrome
Familial clusters of cancer	Breast cancer Ovarian cancer Nonpolyposis colorectal cancer
Genetic predisposition without evident familial clustering (still hypothetical)	Metabolic polymorphisms determining response to exogenous or endogenous carcinogens

gether, they probably account for less than 1% of total cancer incidence. The principal features of several of the syndromes are listed in Table 12.2.

Most cases of an inherited cancer syndrome can be recognized by a characteristic marker phenotype (Table 12.2, Fig. 12.1*A*). Of course, a striking family history (Fig. 12.1*B*) may be the first clue; but it is important to realize that such a history is lacking in many cases. This is because it has not been carefully sought, the patient has a new mutation, or the gene was not expressed in the parents (i.e., "incomplete penetrance").

In some cases (e.g., the polyps in FAP, C-cell hyperplasia in multiple endocrine neoplasia type 2 [MEN 2]), the marker phenotype results from a growth abnormality in the target tissue from which the cancer will arise, and it can be regarded as a preneoplastic lesion. In other cases (e.g., the multiple cysts of abdominal organs in Von Hippel-Lindau syndrome, the ganglioneuromatosis of the intestine in MEN 2B, the os-

Table 12.2. Examples of Inherited Cancer Syndromes

Syndrome	Tissues involved by tumor[a]	Associated phenotype[b]	
		Associated with tumor	In other tissues
Familial adenomatous polyposis (10)	Colon, small intestine, thyroid, liver	Colonic polyps	Osteomas of jaw, hypertrophy of retinal pigment epithelium (14), fibroblast proliferation of body wall (desmoid tumors), extra dentition
Multiple endocrine neoplasia type 1 (3)	Pituitary, parathyroid, pancreatic islets, adrenal cortex	Hyperplasia of target cells	—
Multiple endocrine neoplasia type 2 (91)	Thyroid C cells, adrenal medulla, parathyroid	Hyperplasia (18)[c]	Neuromas of lips, disordered autonomic ganglion plexus in viscera, skeletal abnormalities
von Hippel-Lindau syndrome (34)	Kidney, hemangioblastoma of cerebellum, adrenal medulla	—	Angiomas of retina, multiple cysts of internal organs
Basal cell nevus syndrome (32, 87)	Skin, brain (medulloblastoma)	—	Radiation sensitivity, skeletal abnormalities, plantar and palmar skin pits, jaw cysts, hamartoma of viscera
Retinoblastoma	Retina, bone (osteosarcoma), several epithelia, melanocytes (78)	—	—
Neurofibromatosis type 1 (35, 53)	Schwann cell, glia, adrenal medulla	Plexiform neurofibroma	Multiple, including: café-au-lait spots, axillary freckling, cutaneous neurofibroma, scoliosis, learning difficulties, short stature
Neurofibromatosis type 2 (53)	Schwann cells of VIII cranial n. meninges	—	Occasional cutaneous neurofibroma, café-au-lait spots

[a] Principal tumors underlined.
[b] Note that while the range of abnormalities shown may reflect the effects of mutation of a single gene, several genes may be involved in causing the phenotype in some cases.
[c] Type 2B only.

teomas of the jaw in FAP), the phenotype results from developmental defects in tissues that are remote from the cancer and presumably reflects a pleiotropic effect of the inherited mutation. The diversity of tissues and effects (Table 12.2) is puzzling, because it does not conform to current ideas of lineage or physiologic relationships in most cases.

A few cases, such as retinoblastoma, have no characteristic marker phenotype. The heritable form usually is easily recognized, because the tumor is rare. Two cases in close relatives or bilateral tumors in one individual provide strong evidence of genetic predisposition. Difficulty arises when an individual has one tumor and no family history. The majority of these is truly nonheritable, but a small number of patients will be heritable cases who by chance developed only one tumor and are new mutation cases (i.e., the start of a new family). Because the retinoblastoma gene has been cloned, it is possible to detect the germ-line mutation in some of these cases and so prove they are of the heritable type (94). In other syndromes where the gene has not been cloned, however, distinction between a truly nonheritable case and an isolated new mutation in the absence of a marker phenotype is impossible.

CHARACTERISTIC FEATURES OF INHERITED CANCER SYNDROMES

These are illustrated here mainly in reference to FAP (8–10, 29, 36, 63, 86). Similar features of other inherited cancer syndromes are summarized in Table 12.2.

Pattern of Inheritance

In FAP, as in all inherited cancer syndromes recognized thus far, the pattern of cancers in the family is that expected of an autosomal-dominant predisposing gene (Fig. 12.1*B*). In a few special cases (e.g., glomus tumors [92] and Beckwith-Wiedemann syndrome [62]), the pattern is modified according to the sex of the parent who transmitted the gene (discussed later).

Predisposition

Predisposition is not to cancers in general; rather, it is to cancers of specific sites (Table 12.2). In FAP, for example, the tumors are colorectal carcinoma, carcinoma of the ampulla of Vater, hepatoblastoma, desmoid tumors of the body wall, and thyroid tumors. It is likely that many associations are still unrecognized, and others that are claimed are disputed. For example, very large studies of retinoblastoma families have revealed a previously unsuspected association of several common epithelial cancers with this tumor (81).

VARIATIONS IN EXPRESSION OF THE SYNDROME

Variation may exist in the spectrum of tumors and other phenotypic abnormalities (i.e., "expressivity") or in the probability that each will manifest by a certain age (i.e., "penetrance"). Two possibilities can be distinguished: (*a*) clinically distinct syndromes that "breed true" in families, and so presumably result from different predisposing mutations (either at different loci or different mutant alleles at the same locus); and (*b*) variation within a family, which cannot usually result from differences in the predisposing mutation but must result from some combination of modifying genes, environment, and chance.

Clinical Variation of Familial Colorectal Cancer

Several distinct syndromes are recognized (Table 12.3) (1, 24, 49, 60). In the group that is associated with adenomatous polyps, the traditional distinction between "polyposis" and "nonpolyposis" syndromes is misleading, because the difference is in the numbers of polyps rather than their absence in the nonpolyposis group. The extent to which the different clinical syndromes are reflected in genetic differences is still unclear, however. Thus, FAP is defined genetically by mutation of the *apc* gene on chromosome 5q21 (29, 63). Some, but not all, nonpolyposis colorectal cancer families have been shown to have mutations in a family of genes that encode proteins involved in DNA repair (h-msh2, mlh-1, pms-1, and pms-2) (25, 41, 67, 68). Families carrying the *msh2* gene mutation have been found to include some with the "Muir-Torre" clinical variant of the familial colon cancer syndrome (Table 12.3). Even the distinction between familial polyposis and nonpolyposis colorectal cancer is not quite clear at the genetic level. Some families have been described with a pattern of dominantly inherited colonic cancer associated (on average), with intermediate numbers of polyps, between those typically seen in FAP and in "cancer family syndrome," which prove to have mutations in the extreme 5′ end of the *apc* gene (42, 86). Therefore, there is a spectrum of familial colorectal cancers associated with adenomatous polyps (26), and with risk of other cancers to varying degree, that result from different mutant alleles of the *apc* gene. A similar situation is seen in MEN 2 syndrome (91), where three clinically distinct varieties breed true but result from different predisposing mutations in the same gene: the proto-oncogene *ret* on chromosome 10q11 (60).

Table 12.3. Some Syndromes Associated with Inherited Risk of Colonic Cancer[a]

	Associated with adenomatous polyps	Haemartomatous
Polyposis	Familial adenomatous polyposis, Turcot syndrome (colorectal cancer, brain tumors, skin lesions)	Peutz-Jeghers Juvenile polyposis Cowden Gorlin
Nonpolyposis	Cancer family syndrome (Lynch type II: colorectal plus cancer of endometrium, breast, and ovary) Site specific colonic cancer Muir-Torre syndrome (cancer at multiple sites plus keratoacanthomas and sebaceous adenomas of face)	

[a] For reviews, see Alm and Lieznerski (1), Erbe (24), and Murday and Slack (60).

Variation in Expression Within Single Families

Some families with typical FAP (colorectal carcinoma, multiple intestinal polyps) show the additional features of pancreatic ampullary tumors, desmoid tumors, and mandibular osteomas (Table 12.2). This was originally delineated as a separate clinical variety: Gardner's syndrome (26). Families with Gardner's syndrome were found to map to the FAP locus on chromosome 5, so it seemed that FAP and Gardner's syndrome might be allelic. It now is clear that the Gardner's phenotype occurs to a greater or lesser degree in many FAP families, but especially in those with mutations in the region of the *apc* gene distal to exon 9 (12, 48, 60). Thus, Gardner's syndrome is not entirely distinct genetically from FAP, but the range of expression results from the interaction between modifying influences (as yet undefined) acting on the expression of the *apc* mutation and the precise nature of the *apc* mutant allele.

Variation in Penetrance Within and Between Families

The proportion of *apc* gene carriers who manifest colorectal polyps increases with age (60). Even by age 25, approximately 10% of carriers do not have detectable polyps (Fig. 12.2). Similarly, 10% of *MEN 2A* gene carriers still are not detected by a sensitive biochemical screening test at age 25, and 40% will not have developed clinically significant disease by age 70 (21). This variation also may result from modifying genes, environmental effects, or chance ef-

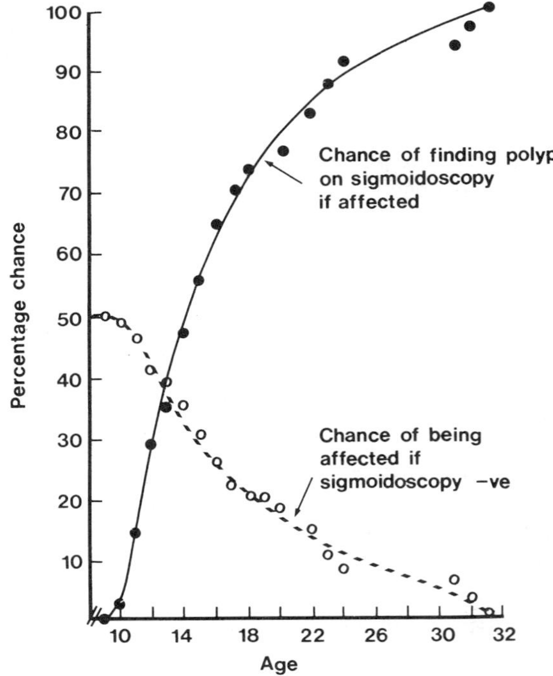

Figure 12.2. Age at detection of polyps in a family member at risk of familial adenomatous polyposis (FAP). Chance of being affected is 50% at birth because FAP is dominantly inherited. *Source:* Murday and Slack (60).

fects, and to "dissect" these factors in human families will be difficult. There is, however, a mouse equivalent of FAP resulting from mutation in the mouse homologue of the *apc* gene (called *MIN* for *m*ultiple *i*ntestinal *n*eoplasia). The number of polyps that develop in the intestine of the min mouse differs according to the genetic background of the mouse strain onto which the *min* allele is crossed. This has been exploited to demonstrate that a single background genetic modifier locus accounts for approximately 50% of the phenotypic variation seen and to map this modifier locus (MOM for *mo*difier of *m*in) to mouse chromosome 4, which is syntenic with human 1p (57, 89).

From a clinical standpoint, data about the age-related expression of marker phenotypes (or cancers) are important in family screening, because this is needed to estimate the probability that a family member with a negative screen or apparently unaffected parents at a given age may still be a gene carrier (discussed later) (76). If it were possible to predict the penetrance or expression of the predisposing gene in an individual family member, this would also have obvious application in clinical management. Unfortunately, this will not be possible until the causes of the variation are better understood and the modifier genes (where these are responsible) are identified.

Familial Cancers

GENERAL DESCRIPTION

Of greater numerical importance than the uncommon inherited cancer syndromes, this group comprises families that are at increased risk of a common cancer, such as breast, colon, or ovary (19, 37, 38, 71, 72, 88). The coincidence of several cases in a single family has been reported at some time for cancers at almost every site, thus raising two questions: (*a*) is the clustering significant and (*b*) if so, is the pattern of occurrence of the cancers in the families best explained on a genetic or some other basis? Final proof of genetic predisposition comes from demonstrating genetic linkage or the inheritance of a germ line predisposing mutation in affected families. Where this information is lacking and there is no marker phenotype comparable to those in the inherited cancer syndromes, estimates of the probability of inherited predisposition in each family must be based on the strength and pattern of the familial association in each case.

EVIDENCE THAT FAMILIAL CLUSTERING OF CANCERS IS SIGNIFICANT

Most case reports of familial clusters are clinical anecdotes. Some are very striking, but there is always the question of a chance association. Solid evidence for significant familial clustering must come from truly population-based studies (i.e., studies in which cases are initially ascertained in an unselected manner and without regard to their family history) (19).

The usual measure of familial clustering is the relative risk of cancer in family members (either all first-degree relatives or specified relatives, usually siblings) of an individual with cancer compared to the risk in the general population. This analysis may be stratified to look at groups that might be expected to have higher risk (e.g., relatives of cases diagnosed before age 50, or relatives in a family with two individuals already affected).

For most common cancers, relative risks of siblings are of the order of 2 to 3 (Table 12.4). Familial clustering of cancers therefore is real, but this does not tell us whether the clustering has a genetic origin. Nor does it tell us how the risk is distributed between individuals, because relative risk is estimated as an average over the entire population. In principle, the same overall risk might result either from a common gene that confers a slight increase in risk to many people or from a rare gene with a very strong effect in a few. These questions can be tackled by "segregation analysis."

Segregation analysis (23, 95) attempts to find the most likely explanation for an observed familial clustering of cancer by analyzing the occurrence pattern of the cancer in the families of a large series of cases ascertained without knowledge of family history. Typically, the analysis will give the relative likelihood of dominant, recessive, or polygenic genetic predisposition; environmental predisposition; or mixed models incorporating genetic and environmental components. In the case of a genetic model, an estimate will be made of the gene frequency in the population, penetrance, and risk to gene carriers versus nongene carriers.

Results from almost all analyses of the common cancers (breast, ovary, and colon) show that the most likely explanation for the observed familial clustering is dominant predisposition by an uncommon gene of strong effect that affects a small number of families (11, 15, 75, 95). This conclusion probably is broadly correct, and it is borne out by recent discoveries that many common familial cancers indeed result, at least in part, to predisposition by genes of this type. Segregation analysis alone can seldom provide conclusive evidence, however. Moreover, detailed results of segregation analysis, especially on small data sets, depend so much on the assumptions made that they should be treated with some caution. In particular, an additional contribution of a common gene that is of weaker effect may be difficult to resolve (a problem which will be discussed in detail later). Mathematic accounts of segregation analysis can be found in standard texts (23).

Table 12.4. Estimates of Relative Risks for the Same Cancer in First-Degree Relatives of Individuals Affected by Various Common Cancers

Site[a]	Relative risk
Breast (15)	2.2
Ovary (75, 84)	3.0
Endometrium (83)	2.7
Melanoma (65)	2.5
Lung (64)	2.7
Colon (45)	3.4
Stomach (50)	2.6

[a] References are mostly from the most recent substantial study; others are given in Easton and Peto (19).

Adapted from Easton and Peto (19).

CHARACTERISTIC FEATURES OF FAMILIAL CANCERS

The familial cancers resemble the inherited cancer syndromes in many of their features. Predisposition is site-specific, but there is variation between and within families. Clinical observation of pedigrees as well as population-based estimates of relative risks to siblings indicate that specific cancers are associated in familial clusters. Some of these form well-known syndromes, for example, "site-specific" colonic cancer or hereditary nonpolyposis colon cancer (HNPCC; Lynch type I) and "family cancer syndrome" (Lynch type II): colorectal, uterine, ovarian, gastric, and breast (46, 48, 49). Neither the genetic distinction between different clinically defined syndromes nor the cancers that

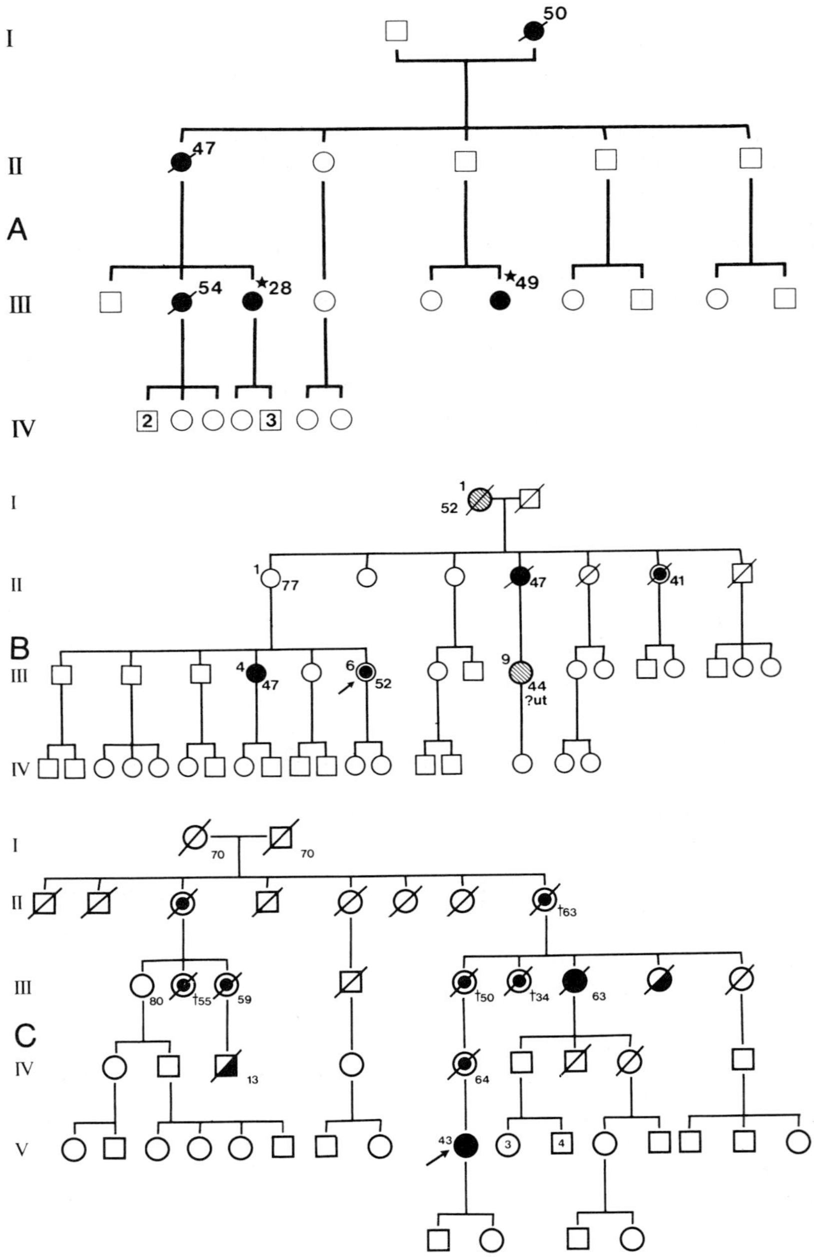

Figure 12.3. Pedigrees to illustrate different types of "breast-ovarian cancer family." Each was seen within the past 5 years in the author's familial cancer clinic. **A.** Site-specific breast cancer. Five family members have breast cancer; two of them (*stars*) have bilateral primary cancers. *Solid circle*, breast cancer, with age at diagnosis (49); *boxed numbers*, number of sons. **B.** "Breast-ovarian" family. There are two cases of breast cancer and two of ovarian cancer, all at a fairly young age. Note that II-1 (now aged 80) is an obligatory gene carrier. III-9 has probable endometrial cancer: it is difficult to know whether this is significant and what the risk of this cancer is to other family members. I-1 had probable ovarian cancer and died at age 52. *Solid circle*, breast cancer; *circled dot*, ovarian cancer, with age at diagnosis. **C.** Ovarian predominant family. There are seven cases of ovarian cancer, and two (ages 43 and 63) of breast cancer. Note the 13-year-old boy in generation IV who had a brain tumor: it is impossible to know whether this related to the presumed predisposing gene. *Double circle*, ovarian cancer; *solid circle*, breast cancer with age at diagnosis (where known) or death (†); *half-filled circle or square*, other cancer.

belong to each one are always clear, however. For example, the distinction between Lynch types I and II, or HNPCC and family cancer syndrome, is rather blurred. In fact, both clinical syndromes can almost certainly result from mutations in the same gene. Several cancers have been described as part of the "cancer family syndrome," but it is still not clear which truly are significantly associated or what the risks of cancers at each site are.

Again, breast and ovarian cancer characteristically occur together in families, but the clinical spectrum of familial disease runs from site-specific breast cancer through breast-ovarian families with each cancer in different proportions to site-specific ovarian cancer (Fig. 12.3) (47, 83). Current genetic linkage data suggest that almost all families with both young-onset breast cancer and epithelial ovarian cancer result from one of two genes: *BRCA1* on chromosome 17q21, or *BRCA2* on 13q (20, 53, 61, 98). Current unpublished data suggest that if the family has two or more cases of ovarian cancer, it is more likely to result from *BRCA1*, if there are male breast cancers in the family, it is more likely to be *BRCA2*, but neither of these distinctions is absolute. At least some site-specific breast or ovarian cancer families probably result from predisposition by other genes yet to be identified. Cancers of the colon, prostate, larynx, and possibly other sites also may form part of the *BRCA1* and *BRCA2* syndromes. The Li-Fraumeni (or SBLA—*s*arcoma, *b*reast, *l*ung, *a*drenal) syndrome (43) is easy to recognize in its most florid form, which is quite uncommon, but there are many more families in which a woman with young-onset breast cancer has a single relative with a sarcoma or a brain tumor. Are these families part of the syndrome, and what are the risks of family members? Approximately 50% of typical Li-Fraumeni pattern families have been shown to have germ-line mutations at the p53 locus (51), but many families with a similar pattern of cancers have no predisposing mutation yet identified (6).

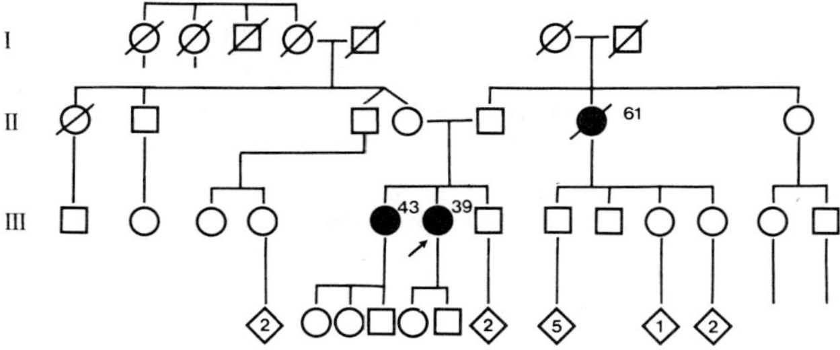

Figure 12.4. Problems of incomplete penetrance and phenocopies. There are three cases of breast cancer in the family, diagnosed at ages 39, 43, and 61. Two sisters affected at ages 39 and 43 are unlikely to be a coincidence, but if they are affected because of a dominant predisposing gene (see text), why is the family history not more extensive? A possible answer is incomplete penetrance of the gene, which would imply that other family members carry the gene but have not expressed it. A possible gene carrier is the aunt in generation II who developed breast cancer at age 61. If so, this would imply that inheritance is through the paternal side of the family, with implications for the risk to her daughters and other family members. However, it also is possible that this individual is a phenocopy—that is, she developed breast cancer independently of the predisposing gene. *Solid circle*, breast cancer; *diamonds with numbers*, number of children, sex unspecified.

Ultimately, we can expect that genetic markers will resolve the question of how syndromes should be classified. It will become clear which cancers (and associated lesions, such as benign breast disease) should be regarded as part of a syndrome, because genetic markers will make it possible to compare their incidence in known gene carriers with that in the general population. Within a single family, markers will indicate which cancers can be attributed to inherited predisposition and which are merely phenocopies (Fig. 12.4).

Inherited Predisposition Without Obvious Family Clustering

GENERAL FEATURES

So far, only cases in which inherited predisposition is strong enough to cause obvious family clustering of cancer have been considered. However, it can easily be shown that with a slight reduction in the penetrance of the predisposing gene—that is, if only a few gene carriers actually develop cancer—there can still be very significant predisposition even though enough close relatives to cause an obvious family cluster seldom are actually affected (69). Thus, a hypothetic dominant gene that results in ovarian cancer by age 55 in only 1 in 20 of female gene carriers would hardly cause any obvious multiple-case families, because the risk is only $\frac{1}{2}$ multiplied by $\frac{1}{20} = \frac{1}{40}$ by this age in each of the close female relatives and zero in the males. On average the risk is even lower in more distant relatives, who are less likely to have the gene. Even so, over a range of plausible assumptions about gene frequency, such a gene can lead to a surprising concentration of risk in a predisposed minority of the population (69). For example, if the gene is common (e.g., if 1 in 30 women carries a predisposing allele compared to the roughly 1 in 500 women who are estimated to carry a strongly predisposing allele of the *BRCA1* gene), it would result in just over 50% of all ovarian cancers below age 55 occurring in this predisposed 3% of women. A gene with these characteristics would lead to some degree of familial clustering of ovarian cancer. With the figures for frequency and relative risk quoted earlier, the relative risk of ovarian cancer in the sister of a case diagnosed before 55 years of age compared with the general population would be approximately five-fold, which in fact is roughly what is observed. However, much of the observed risk is accounted for by a minority of families who are at very high risk; those with multiple-case ovarian and breast-ovarian cancer from mutations in *BRCA1* and *BRCA2*. The question that currently is unanswered is to what extent these uncommon, high-risk families account for the observed familial clustering, or how much is left over to be explained by more common, predisposing genes of weaker effect? In lung cancer, where multiple-case families are much less common than in ovarian or breast cancer, a broadly similar relative risk for siblings is indeed presumably the result of a more even distribution of risk among the population by one or more of the more common predisposing genes of less effect. Unfortunately, epidemiologic analyses seem unlikely to resolve this problem; there is no alternative but to search for the supposed common predisposing genes and to evaluate their effects by direct measurement.

HOW CAN LOW-LEVEL PREDISPOSITION BE RECOGNIZED AND THE GENES IDENTIFIED?

The previous example suggests that multiple-case cancer families may represent only the tip of the iceberg of inherited predisposition. In public health terms, the effects of common genes of weaker effect may be much more significant. The problem is to recognize the effects and find the genes. In the inherited cancer syndromes and the familial cancers, recognition is accomplished through familial clusters and marker phenotypes. The genes can be sought empirically, with no previous knowledge of what they are, by the methods of genetic linkage, which exploit the occurrence of several cases in a family (discussed later). Without family clustering or obvious marker phenotypes, one must start with candidate genes (i.e., by guessing which genes may be involved and testing them). If sufficient pairs of affected siblings can be found, a form of genetic linkage possibly may be used, as recently was demonstrated in diabetes, for example (5, 7). More often, the approach is likely to be choosing a candidate gene, which is tested by case-control studies of a genetic variant of the candidate gene in subjects with and without cancer, or empirically, by linkage-disequilibrium-based mapping in selected populations thought to derive from a small number of founder individuals (e.g., in Finland). In such a population, most copies of the supposed predisposing gene can be expected to derive from the same ancestral copy. If so, they will be carried on the same ancestral segment of chromosome. This can possibly be identified if a number of individuals in the population with a given cancer are shown to share the same set of genetic markers across a particular chromosomal region to a greater extent than would be expected by chance.

In principle, almost any type of mechanism can be associated with a predisposing gene of low penetrance (discussed later). In practice, however, the one that has attracted most interest so far is genetic polymorphism, which might alter the interaction with potential environmental carcinogens (2, 4, 27, 28, 54, 90, 93, 96).

It is well known that individuals differ in their metabolism of exogenous chemicals used as drugs, and there seems to be no reason to expect this will be any different for chemical carcinogens. Attention therefore has focused on the genes of the cytochrome P-450 system (2, 4, 27, 28, 54, 96, 97), which is involved in the metabolism of a variety of compounds, including polycyclic hydrocarbons and both endogenous and exogenous steroid hormones, and on other enzymes involved in conjugation and detoxification that exhibit genetic variation, such as acetylating enzymes (4). There is recent evidence that variation at the locus for cytochrome P-450 *CYP1A1* may determine the risk of lung cancer in cigarette smokers (28) and that acetylator status is associated with risk of bladder cancer (4).

Heterozygotes for genetic defects of the recessive DNA repair syndromes may be another group in this category. Although still controversial, evidence from studies of the relatives of such patients is increasing that heterozygotes for the recessive disorder AT (ataxia-telangiectasia) may be at a substantially increased risk of several common cancers (90). Depending on the frequency of the *AT* gene in the population, this might account for a significant minority of these cancers at young ages. A direct test of this will be possible now that the *AT* gene has been cloned (82).

PROSPECTS

Precise definition of the contribution by this type of genetic variation to cancer incidence may never be possible, because there will be a continuum of effects, from the imperceptible to the highly significant. Identification of gene–environment interactions that result in significant levels of predisposition in a minority of individuals within the population, however, would have a significant impact on approaches to prevention and screening (4). Starting with the genes and working through them to the chemicals they interact with (i.e., a process of "reverse epidemiology") may lead to the identification of important environmental carcinogens, most of which are still unknown. The limiting factor is our knowledge of carcinogenesis and, hence, our ability to guess the relevant candidate genes.

Mechanisms of Genetic Predisposition to Cancer

GENERAL DESCRIPTION

In principle, predisposition could occur in one of three ways. The inherited mutation might (*a*) provide one of the steps in carcinogenesis ready-made in the germ line, (*b*) make one of these steps more likely to happen, or (*c*) affect the consequences of one of the steps to make the subsequent steps more likely. Most inherited cancer syndromes seem to belong to the first category. Examples of the second category are xeroderma pigmentosum, in which an inherited defect of DNA repair makes somatic mutation more likely in cells exposed to ultraviolet light, and the mutations in the *h-msh2* family of DNA repair genes, which predispose to colorectal cancer (25, 41, 67). Recent evidence (52) suggests that the type II TGF-β receptor may be one important "target" of the faulty repair in cells with the "replication error" (RER^+) defect, which results from *h-msh2* mutation. The variations in carcinogen metabolism described in the previous section also potentially fall in this group. The third group might include, for example, altered endocrine or immune effects on the nascent cancer, but as yet there are no clear examples.

INHERITED CANCER SYNDROMES

The paradigm for the mechanism of predisposition in the inherited cancer syndromes is retinoblastoma (31). Because the germ-line mutation is present in every cell of the body and not every cell becomes a tumor, it is clear that at least one further step is required. In principle, this second step might entail either loss of the remaining wild-type allele at the same locus as the inherited mutation or mutation at another locus altogether. Either way, in nonhereditary cases, both mutations must occur by chance in the same somatic cell, whereas in hereditary cases, the inheritance of one mutation in the germ line greatly increases the probability that at least one cell will acquire the second mutation and a cancer will

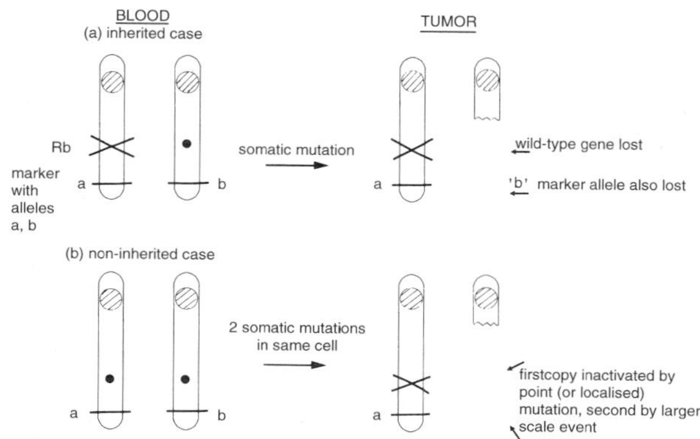

Figure 12.5. Genetic mechanism of the development of retinoblastoma and the concept of "allele loss" in tumors. Both copies of chromosome 13, which carries the retinoblastoma locus, in blood and tumor cells from (*a*) an individual with the hereditary form of the cancer and (*b*) an individual with the nonhereditary form. *Circles*, centromere of chromosome; *crossed lines*, germline mutation of one *Rb* allele in the hereditary case and somatic mutation in the nonhereditary case; *solid circle*, wild type (normal) *Rb* allele; ___ *a* and ___*b*, marker alleles further down the chromosome, detectable by restriction fragment length polymorphisms. Both alleles at the *Rb* locus must be inactivated for a tumor to develop. In inherited cases, the loss of the first allele is inherited as a germ-line mutation. In noninherited cases, both alleles must be inactivated in the same somatic cell. Usually (but not always), the first mutation is a point mutation or a small deletion within the *Rb* gene, but the second mutation may involve loss of part or all of the wild-type chromosome by various genetic mechanisms, which include nondisjunction, mitotic recombination, or chromosomal deletions (11). It is possible to infer the occurrence of such events by comparison of DNA from tumor and blood in the same individual, with the finding loss of the appropriate marker allele (here, allele b). A search for "allele losses" in tumors using probes for different marker loci is now used to search for analogous genetic events in other tumors (13, 31, 70).

result (17, 39). The model of mutations in both alleles at the same locus was confirmed in retinoblastoma, when it was shown that in a small proportion of familial cases, the first mutation involved an inherited chromosomal deletion at the Rb locus and that in the tumors, the remaining (wild-type) allele inherited from the unaffected parent also was lost (11). In nonfamilial cases, both alleles were inactivated by somatic mutation (Fig. 12.5).

Tumor-Suppressor Genes, Recessive Mutations and Dominant Pedigrees

The requirement for activity loss of both alleles of the *Rb* gene implies that the normal activity of the gene is to restrain or suppress tumorigenesis. This fits with the results from experiments in which tumor cell and normal cell hybrids are found to be nontumorigenic, again suggesting that at the cellular level, malignancy generally results from recessive mutations in a class of genes that have therefore been called *tumor-suppressor genes* (see Chapter 6) (70). The apparent paradox that familial retinoblastoma has a dominant pattern of inheritance, but the mutation is recessive at the level of the cell, is explained because in cancer (unlike other diseases), only one cell needs to acquire the genetic lesion for the phenotype to be expressed. Thus, although the inherited mutation is recessive in terms of its effect in the cell, only one retinal cell need acquire the second, somatic mutation for a tumor to develop. The number of cells at risk is such that this is very probable, and almost everyone who inherits the mutation expresses the disease. The phenotype of tumor formation therefore appears to be dominant at the level of the family pedigree.

Are Other Inherited Cancers Like Retinoblastoma?

This would imply that the germ-line mutation results in activity loss of the gene and that the wild-type allele is inactivated in tumors. In most inherited cancer syndromes, including FAP, neurofibromatosis type 1 (NF-1) and NF-2, von Hippel-Lindau syndrome, and familial breast and ovarian cancer from *BRCA1* and *BRCA2* mutations, there is evidence that this is the case (Table 12.5). MEN 2 is an exception; here, the germ-line mutations result in activation of the gene product (a membrane receptor) and are truly dominant at the level of the cell (79).

Dosage Effects

The *Rb* mutation appears to be truly recessive in that there is no discernible phenotype associated with the first mutation. The widespread phenotypic abnormalities seen in other inherited cancer syndromes suggest, however, that this is not always the case. In FAP, for example, a few patients have total germline deletions of the *apc* gene, so this first mutation, in these individuals must cause loss of activity of the gene. Yet, already in childhood, patients with FAP are reported to have a proliferative abnormality throughout their intestinal epithelium. Because every crypt is affected, this presumably is a direct expression of the germ-line mutation, without need for a somatic mutation to be superimposed. This suggests a dosage effect (i.e., that is, an effect of the level of *FAP* gene expression on phenotype). An alternative mechanism, for the large number of *apc* mutations that result in a truncated protein, is that they are "dominant negative." This is, the mutant protein interferes with the activity of the wild-type protein encoded by the remaining allele. In turn,

Table 12.5. Current Evidence of a Retinoblastoma-Like Genetic Mechanism in Other Inherited Cancer Syndromes[a]

Syndrome	Chromosomal mapping by genetic linkage	Constitutional chromosomal abnormality	Evidence of consistent allele loss in tumors
FAP	5q	Deletion	(+)
MEN 1	11q	Not found	+
MEN 2	10	Not found	Not found
von Hippel-Lindau	3p	Not found	+
NF-1	17q	Translocation	(+)
NF-2	22	Not found	+
Familial breast and ovarian cancer	17q;13a	Not found	+

[a] In rare cases. See Ponder (70) for a review.
FAP—Familial adenomatous polyposis; MEN—multiple endocrine neoplasia; NF—neurofibromatosis.

this raises the possibility that the focal lesions associated with many of the inherited cancer syndromes (e.g., the neurofibromas of NF-1, the cysts of von Hippel-Lindau syndrome, and possibly the foci of C-cell hyperplasia in MEN 2 [Table 12.2]) result from local threshold effects allowing expression of the inherited mutation rather than from second, somatic events, although this remains speculative.

Variable Expression

The concept of a dosage effect implies that loss of activity of an allele may not be "all or nothing." Different mutations in the gene may result in loss of activity to different extents or in different functional domains of the gene. In this way, different germ-line mutations may cause different expressions of the same syndrome between different families, perhaps, for example, the predominance of breast or ovarian cancer in breast-ovarian families because of different mutations in the *BRCA1* gene (Fig. 12.3).

Variation *within* a family, however, must have another cause, which might be chance, environmental effects, or genetic background effects. Some conclusions about the contribution of genetic modifiers versus environmental or chance effects to the variation in phenotype within a family can be made by observing the correlation of the phenotype between close and more distant relatives. Chance effects should result in no systematic correlation; environmental effects should result in stronger correlations among family members who have shared the same environment (e.g., within members of the same generation). The effects of modifying genes that are unlinked to the main locus of predisposition should be greatest in identical twins and become progressively weaker with an increasing distance of relationship. In other words, a hallmark of the effect of a strong modifying gene might be clustering of a particular variant of the phenotype within nuclear families in the larger pedigree. NF-1 is a good example to study, because the phenotype is not only highly variable, it also is quantifiable to the extent that the cutaneous neurofibromas and café-au-lait patches can be counted (and adjustments made for age). An analysis of the NF1 phenotype in twins and more distant family members (22) concluded that most of the observed variation could be ascribed to the effects of one or more unlinked genetic modifiers; the effect of the specific NF-1 mutation itself was relatively small. Even in this favorable situation—a common condition, quantifiable phenotype—the power to map the modifying loci in human families is likely to be very weak. Almost certainly the first clues to the identity of the modifiers will come from studies of animal models, such as the *min* mouse referred to earlier.

Genomic Imprinting

One particular type of variable expression within a family is easily identified, because it is specific to the sex of the parent from whom the gene has been inherited (77, 81). In families with dominantly inherited susceptibility to glomus tumor, for example, the phenotype is only expressed when transmitted through the male germ-line (92). After transmission through a female, the gene is almost silent until once more transmitted through a male. Similar effects are seen in families with rhabdomyosarcoma (85) and in the expression of Beckwith-Wiedemann syndrome.

Until recently, it was assumed that the paternally and maternally derived genomes were equivalent, but experiments in which mice with chromosomal translocations were bred to produce progeny in which both copies of one chromosome (or a part of one chromosome) were either of paternal or maternal origin showed this not to be so. The mice developed differently. The phenomenon affects only a minority of chromosomal regions, and transgenic mice show similar parent-of-origin-dependent expression of reporter genes such as β-galactosidase. This depends both on the chromosomal localization of the transgene and, interestingly in view of the within-family variation of expression of human genetic disorders, on the genetic background of the mouse in which the transgene is expressed.

The molecular mechanism of imprinting is unclear, but it appears to result from diminished expression of one allele, which may relate to differential methylation of genes in the male and female germ line. Its physiologic function also is unclear, but it possibly may provide a further level of control over the expression of critical genes in embryogenesis. In the transgenic systems, imprinting effects diminish as the mice age.

As inactivation of tumor-suppressor genes is an important mechanism of carcinogenesis, the possibility of epigenetic inactivation by imprinting, which moreover may be subject to genetic background influences and change over time, has potentially exciting implications (56). Only a very few cancers show imprinting defined as parent-of-origin effects in expression. Unstable epigenetic modification independent of germ-line effects might have much more general importance if it exists but unfortunately, it also is much harder to detect.

The Search for Inherited Predisposing Genes

GENERAL PRINCIPLES

The gene for hemophilia could be found because sufficient information was known about the mechanism of the disease (i.e., deficiency of clotting factor VIII) to work from the protein to the DNA sequence and, hence, the gene. Because there is no comparable understanding of the mechanisms for inherited predisposition to cancer, a different approach has been taken, starting with an empiric search for the gene by genetic linkage. Once the gene has been localized to a chromosomal region by linkage, "positional cloning" strategies lead to the construction of a physical map of the region in terms of overlapping DNA clones in yeast or other vectors, identification of coding sequences and their assembly into genes, and finally, testing of the genes as candidates by a search for mutations in affected family members. A detailed description is beyond the scope of this chapter, but an example is provided by Collins (16).

GENETIC LINKAGE

The principle of genetic linkage is simple (40, 66). The pattern of inheritance of a specific cancer through a family is taken to indicate the inheritance of the predisposing gene or, in those who are unaffected, of the corresponding wild-type allele. The cancer gene can be located by testing, in the same family, the inheritance pattern of the alleles at a "marker locus" whose chromosomal location already is known. If one allele of the marker is consistently co-inherited with the cancer (and so, by inference, with the cancer gene), the marker and the cancer gene must be adjacent on the chromosome. Otherwise, they would tend to be separated by recombination at each meiosis, and their inheritance would be independent. As the human gene map expands, the number of markers and the power of linkage approaches has increased. Current markers are mostly based on highly polymorphic "microsatellite" sequences. These are regions of the genome where the same short DNA sequence (usually a dinucleotide such as CG) is repeated many times, the precise number of repeats and, hence, the length of the repeat sequence at any given locus differing between individuals. Polymerase chain reaction (PCR) amplification across the repeat sequence using unique sequence primers flanking the repeat results in DNA segments of different lengths according to the number of repeats. These different lengths of DNA are the different marker alleles. Semiautomated methods for PCR and analysis of the alleles has led to dramatic increases in the speed with which a linkage-based search for a predisposing locus can be carried out (44).

PROBLEMS WITH LINKAGE IN CANCER FAMILIES

Phenocopies and Incomplete Penetrance

Unless there is a marker phenotype, as in some of the inherited cancer syndromes, the presence or absence of the cancer gene rather than its wild-type allele in each individual is inferred from the presence of the cancer. In the common cancers, such as breast cancer, this may be unsafe. Some individuals within a large family may have breast cancer by chance rather than predisposition: they are phenocopies (Fig. 12.4). Conversely, some individuals who do not have breast cancer still may have inherited the cancer gene but not expressed it. This will clearly be related to sex and age. With a marker phenotype, identification of gene carriers is potentially more accurate provided that good quality clinical data are available. Linkage, therefore, depends on accurate clinical data to allow the correct identification of affected and unaffected individuals which must include screening for the marker phenotype if one is available. It also depends on the assumptions made about penetrance and numbers of phenocopies.

Heterogeneity

It often is necessary to combine data from several families to achieve significant evidence for linkage. Unless the families are predisposed at the same genetic locus, however, this is a potential disaster, because positive scores from linked families will be cancelled by negative scores from unlinked families. Although mathematic procedures exist to deal with the problem of heterogeneity, the power is much reduced, and many more families must be analyzed. This is a problem, as the availability of family material usually is a limiting factor. Every effort therefore must be made to start with large families or, failing that, with families that are as homogenous as possible by clinical criteria (even though genetic homogeneity can still not be guaranteed). This problem is likely to be serious in common familial cancers, such as breast cancer (37), and less so in the inherited cancer syndromes. An example of heterogeneity in the search for the first predisposing gene for breast cancer (i.e., *BRCA1*) is detailed by Hall and colleagues (30); Wooster and colleagues (98) described the strategy that was adopted to find the locus of the second breast cancer predisposing gene (i.e., *BRCA2*) by linkage. This consisted of (*a*) excluding families that were clearly *BRCA1* carriers, (*b*) choosing the largest among the families that were left, and (*c*) using heterogeneity analysis to interpret the linkage results obtained.

Specifying the Correct Genetic Model

Most linkage analyses in familial cancers are run on the assumption of dominant inheritance, because that is what segregation analyses and clinical observation suggest. If recessive inheritance is a possibility, that model also should be run; if the familial cancer is polygenic in origin, linkage may fail.

HOW TO BEGIN LOOKING

To scan the entire genome for linkage might take a small laboratory a full year with today's resources; large laboratories can complete the task in a few weeks. Even so, it is a great deal of work, and considering whether particular genes or genome regions are especially good candidates, is worth some effort. There are four possible clues to narrow the search:

1. *Candidate genes.* Try to guess the gene that is causing the syndrome. The p53 gene in Li-Fraumeni syndrome is still the only successful example (51); however, as the genes involved in critical cellular pathways (e.g., cell cycle control) are identified, the numbers of plausible candidates will increase.
2. *Constitutional chromosomal abnormalities.* In rare cases, the germ-line mutation may be associated with cytogenetically detectable deletions or translocations. Patients in whom a young onset of cancer is associated with mental retardation or a developmental anomaly may be the best candidates, developmental problems indicating a disruption of several genes in the chromosome region. Such cases have been crucial in the mapping of several cancer genes (33), and a search for them may be well worth the effort. (10 mL) Heparinized blood should be taken for analysis by prophase banding. If positive, further blood should be taken to set up a lymphoblastoid cell line for detailed genetic mapping studies.
3. *Allele losses.* Assuming a retinoblastoma-like model, consistent regions of chromosomal loss in tumors, revealed by the loss of marker alleles (Fig. 12.5) may reflect the loss of a critical suppressor gene and, therefore, the chromosome location of a gene, the germ-line mutation of which will result in predisposition. Note, however, that it is far from clear that all the regions of allele losses that are

currently defined in fact harbor suppressor genes, nor that all suppressor-gene loci defined in this way will correspond to loci for inherited predisposition. Nevertheless, if a gene that is known to have an important and possibly relevant function is shown to map to a chromosomal region that also is affected by allele losses, that gene may become a candidate for investigation (70).

4. *Exclusion mapping*. Computer programs are available that will combine existing linkage data and generate an exclusion map, which indicates the residual probability that the gene is at any given location. This has proven to be useful in several of the inherited cancer syndromes, but if genetic heterogeneity is present, as it is with most common familial cancers, this could be seriously misleading.

PROBLEMS WITH INCOMPLETE OR SMALL FAMILIES

Classical linkage, as described earlier, is applied to families with several affected individuals in two or more generations. Often, however, real cancer families contain a small number of living, distant relatives, with all of the intervening relatives being dead. Sometimes, it will be possible to obtain archival pathology material from dead family members, and this can be analyzed for at least the smaller microsatellite marker alleles (generally <200 bp) by PCR amplification of DNA extracted from paraffin sections. In other cases (i.e., lung cancer), however, extensive families are too rare for standard linkage approaches to be practical, even with the inclusion of deceased individuals. Various modifications of linkage strategy have been developed for such situations (7, 40), and the inexperienced reader contemplating a linkage or gene-mapping study should seek expert advice at an early stage.

Investigation and Management of Cancer Families

GENERAL DESCRIPTION

In some types of familial cancers, especially the inherited cancer syndromes such as FAP, MEN 1 and 2, von Hippel-Lindau syndrome, retinoblastoma, and familial melanoma, screening and appropriate treatment of those at risk will reduce deaths and morbidity (71, 73, 88). Because the screened population is at very high risk, screening likely will be highly cost-effective where curative treatment is available. Recognition and screening of such families even in medically sophisticated countries, however, still is incomplete and often badly done.

Even when effective screening or treatment is not available, families may benefit from information and advice. Most are well aware of their history and worried by it. They often overestimate their risks and can be reassured. The fear of many doctors—that they will provoke anxiety by discussing the issues—is usually unfounded.

All of this, however, has important implications for health services. The most effective ways of informing the public and health professionals about familial cancer and methods for evaluating the costs, delivery, and results of genetic counselling for cancer families are currently the subject of much discussion. It is important that health services are not led by demand into providing costly services that are unevaluated and have uncertain benefits. Until any given procedure is proven to be beneficial and cost-effective, there is an obligation for health professionals working in this field to ensure that as far as possible, they work within a framework of research and evaluation.

WHEN IS A CANCER FAMILY CLINICALLY SIGNIFICANT?

This is the first question that confronts the family doctor or nonspecialist in a hospital clinic. Which family members merit further investigation? Putting to one side syndromes with a clearly recognizable phenotype, the question reduces to (*a*) when is a family history so striking that it is unlikely to result by chance and (*b*) what benefits are likely to follow? Unfortunately, it is impossible to provide a single, all-purpose answer. Two sisters at age 40 with breast cancer may be coincidence, but the figures for excess risk to sisters of patients of this age suggests an approximately 85% chance that such a pair is significant. Two sisters aged 70 with breast cancer, by contrast, could be significant, but it is much more likely they are not (19).

The factors that suggest genetic predisposition are listed in Table 12.6. Note, however, that the threshold at which a family history becomes "significant" and justifies further evaluation or referral for screening is a matter of opinion, and experts differ. In practice, one must take a thorough family history, evaluate these factors, and make an estimate of the cancer risks and the benefits of referral for investigation for each new family. The decision about risks often will depend critically on one or two diagnoses in family members who are now dead: if so, considerable effort may be needed to verify the information. The decision about benefits will depend on the options available for screening, prevention, or treatment. For melanoma risk in the familial dysplastic nevus syndrome, these are fairly clear; for a young woman with a family history of breast cancer or an individual in a possible Li-Fraumeni syndrome family, these are much less so.

FAMILIAL CANCER CLINIC

The purposes of a general familial cancer clinic are to (*a*) obtain as detailed a family history as possible, with confirmation of all important diagnoses; (*b*) to estimate individual risks, discuss these with family members and their doctors, and advise on the options for management; and (*c*) to main-

Table 12.6. Features Increasing the Probability that a Familial Association of Cancer Results from Genetic Susceptibility

Associated developmental or phenotypic abnormalities
Unusually early onset of cancer
Two or more close relatives on the same side of the family with the same or related cancers at a young age (e.g., <50 years)
Multiple primary cancers in one individual

tain an overview of all branches of the family (who may live at some distance from each other) to ensure that information from one branch that is relevant to the management of the other is passed on and that continuity of follow-up is maintained (74). These tasks are difficult, time consuming, and usually beyond the resources of a busy medical or surgical clinic. The purpose of the familial cancer clinic, however, is not usually to take over clinical management; screening and treatment usually remain the responsibility of local specialists who will see the family regularly.

Experience in the United Kingdom suggests that a familial cancer clinic requires, at minimum, a clinical geneticist with knowledge of cancer; one or two specially trained nurses who can obtain and confirm family information by telephone, home visits, and seeking relevant records and who can take and process blood samples; and a secretary/data manager. One clinic of this size can probably serve a population of approximately 3 million people, depending of course on local geography. Close liaison with specialist clinicians in disciplines that are relevant to assessing different syndromes (e.g., colonoscopy, ultrasonography, mammography) is helpful to ensure that advice given to families and their doctors is current. Contact with the surgeons who will be responsible for prophylactic surgery also is essential; it is important whenever possible to discuss management with the doctors who will carry it out before advising the patient. Finally, close links with a service-based molecular genetics laboratory are necessary as DNA-based diagnosis becomes possible for more familial cancers. To focus expertise and minimize the travel required of families and clinic nurses, a co-operative network of clinics has been set up throughout the United Kingdom, with clinicians in each region nominated to act as local sources of information and advice within their own speciality.

ADVISING A FAMILY

In my experience, an important first step in the clinical consultation is to establish why the individuals have come and what they hope to get from it. Some will have been sent, with little explanation, by their primary doctor and have little idea what is going on. Others will have been pressured by relatives and others will be concerned for their children. Some will want to have everything laid out for them; others will be happier to be given advice about what they should do without a detailed composition of risks. If several family members attend together, they may have different perspectives and should be given the chance to be seen individually. A preamble, during which the details of the family tree are outlined or discussed, usually will allow the clinician to "test the water" and structure the interview accordingly.

Risk Estimates

Before giving advice, the clinician must decide on the risk to the family member(s) concerned. In straightforward cases, the estimate may derive from published data on familial risk; with more complex family histories, it may require several steps (Fig. 12.6) (76). These include

1. What is the risk that the individual has inherited the predisposing gene based on a given genetic model (usually autosomal dominant) and his or her relationship to known affected individuals?
2. Might DNA testing give a more precise answer?
3. How is this risk modified by the present age of the individual (the older without signs of the disease the lower the risk), by any suggestive marker phenotype (e.g., colonic polyps), by the present age (or age at death or prophylactic surgery) of any unaffected relative through whom the gene must have been inherited, and by uncertainty that this family (or branch of the family, does in fact carry a genetic predisposition (e.g., uncertainty whether the supposed gene carrier at the head of the branch might not be a phenocopy).
4. Is there a risk of more than one type of cancer; if so, which; and are the risks different?
5. At what age does risk commence, and how is it distributed through life?
6. How is the risk affected by other known risk factors in this individual (e.g., age at menarche, parity, benign breast disease, and other factors).

Having reached an estimate, the clinician must decide how this information should be presented: in how much detail and in what form, such as a risk over a lifetime or a de-

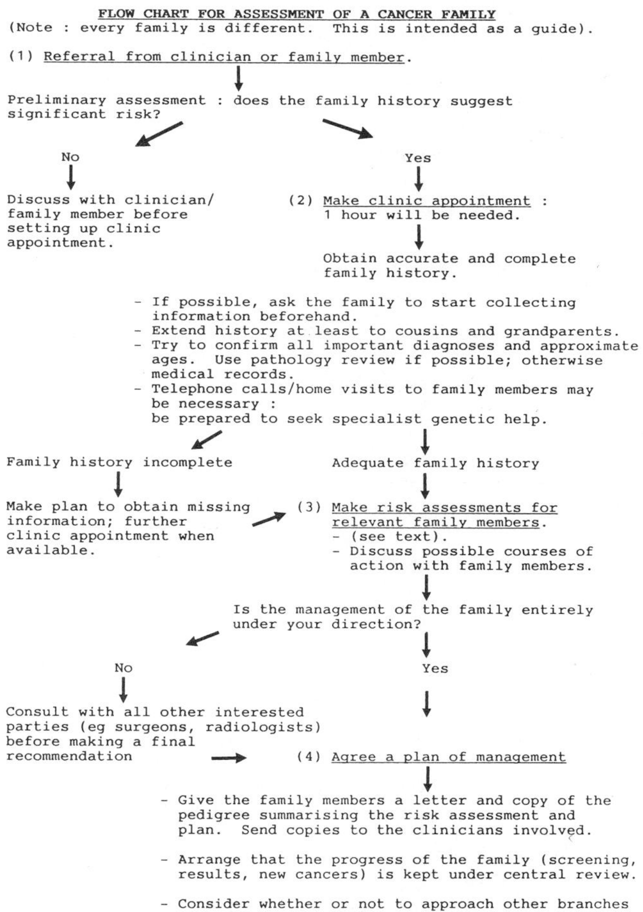

Figure 12.6. Flow chart for clinical assessment of a cancer family.

fined period (e.g., to age 50); as an absolute figure or relative to the population risk; and as percentages or betting odds. My preference generally is for betting odds and a defined period of time.

Options for Management

In general, there will be three possibilities depending on the site; do nothing, screening, and prophylactic surgery. Sensible advice about lifestyle may well be appropriate, but at present, only in a few cases (e.g., familial melanoma—keep out of the sun; breast cancer—consider enrollment in a prevention trial such as the current trial of tamoxifen) is specific advice on prevention likely to be a main option.

As a general rule, the patient or family should be helped to make their own decision rather than have it imposed on them. Of course, this rule must be adapted to the individual patient. The uncertainties of screening (e.g., for breast or ovarian cancer) and both the benefits and drawbacks of surgery must be explained in detail that is appropriate to the individual. The implications for children, even though some years away, probably will be a major source of concern. It often is helpful to provide parents with a letter detailing the family tree, the discussions you have had, and your recommendations for the children so that this can be passed on to the children for use at the appropriate time.

Other branches of the family also may be at risk. The decision to approach them will depend primarily on whether they can expect to benefit. If they are not in contact with the branch who have sought advice or are thought to be unaware of the problem, great caution is needed. Public records in the United Kingdom allow identification of the family doctor, who would be the recommended first contact in these circumstances. Family members who are enthusiastic about information should be cautioned that other relatives may respond differently.

Screening

A suggested outline of screening for some of the inherited cancer syndromes is given in Table 12.7; details must be sought elsewhere. For the common familial cancers, there is little general agreement and no present evidence of benefit; some guidelines are suggested in Table 12.8. Decisions to be made include the age to start, interval, and criteria for further investigation or surgery. Because of the generally small

Table 12.7. Current Screening Procedures for Individuals at Risk of Some Inherited Cancer Syndromes

Syndrome	Screening procedure	Starting age
Familial adenomatous polyposis	Examine for hypertrophy of retinal pigmented epithelium	Childhood
	Sigmoidoscopy for polyps	Early teens
Multiple endocrine neoplasic type 1	Plasma calcium	Teens
Multiple endocrine neoplasic type 2A	Measurement of stimulated plasma calcitonin	5 years
	Measurement of urinary catecholamines	Teens
von Hippel-Lindau	Examine for retinal angiomas urinary catecholamines	5 years
	Renal ultrasound, cranial CT/MRI, CNS clinical examination	Early twenties
	Baseline scans	20 years
Neurofibromatosis type 1	Diagnosis will usually be apparent in childhood (from CAL spots, iris nodules, other features). Once established, annual assessments for learning difficulties, visual impairment (optic glioma) and scoliosis.	—
Neurofibromatosis type 2	MRI or brain-stem auditory-evoked responses for VIII n. tumor. Clinical exam for lens opacities.	Early teens

Table 12.8. Possible Screening Policy for Individuals at High Risk in "Cancer Families"[a]

Cancer	Screen procedure	Start age[b]
Breast	Mammography (possibly ultrasound if mammography is unsatisfactory)	35 years, or 5 years earlier than earliest case in family
Ovarian	Ultrasound and serum CA-125; Doppler bloodflow scan of ovaries as "second-line"	25 years, or 5 years earlier than earliest case in family
Colorectal (not FAP)	High-risk (>2 affected first-degree relatives): colonoscopy	Repeat every 3 years if polyps; 5 years if not
	Low risk: fecal occult blood	30 years, or 5 years before first case in family
Stomach	Gastroscopy	5 years before first case in family
Endometrial	Pelvic examination, endometrial biopsy every 2 years	35 years, or 5 years before first case in family
Melanoma	Annual thorough skin examination by experienced doctor, patient/spouse education for change in nevus, excision biopsy of suspicious lesions	Childhood

[a] All screening should include a clinical examination directed to sites at risk. The procedures suggested here are not of proven effectiveness. Individual clinical judgement should always be used.
[b] Usually controversial.
FAP—Familial adenomatous polyposis.

numbers and the ethical difficulties of randomized studies using high-risk families, there are few data on which to base these decisions or prove that screening is beneficial.

DNA-BASED PREDICTION OF RISK

Once a specific, predisposing mutation is identified in a family, prediction can be based on the inheritance (or non-heritance) of this mutation in other family members. In principle, mutation-based prediction should be possible for any familial cancer in which the predisposing gene is known. In practice, however, it is important to bear in mind that even if the gene is known, in most conditions there is a proportion (ranging from a few percent in FAP and MEN 2 to the majority in NF-1) of families in whom the specific mutation cannot be identified, either for technical reasons or because it lies outside the coding region of the gene (2). Also some familial cancers are genetically heterogeneous; thus, of families with three cases of young-onset breast cancer in close relatives, perhaps one-third will result from *BRCA1* mutations, one-third to *BRCA2* mutations, and one-third to other genes yet to be identified or to chance. This means that at the time of writing, because only *BRCA1* has been identified, there is only an approximate one in three chance, at best, that such a family could be helped by mutation-based DNA prediction. It is important to point out these limitations to family members before the decision for testing is made.

For familial cancers in which the predisposing gene has been mapped but not yet cloned, or where the gene is known but the mutations cannot be identified, genetic prediction may still be possible in some cases using linked genetic markers. Care must be taken, however, to ensure there is good evidence that the familial predisposition indeed results from the linked gene, and this usually will require DNA from several affected family members. Advice from a clinical geneticist is essential as well.

The decision to have DNA predictive testing only should be made after careful explanation of the issues, usually by a clinical geneticist or genetics nurse. In conditions where the genetics are clear-cut and the information leads to a straightforward clinical decision—for example, whether to institute colonoscopic screening in a child whose parent has FAP—there may not be much controversy. In familial breast cancer, however, there are many unresolved problems. As pointed out earlier, most of smaller families will not have *BRCA1* mutations and so, at the time of this writing, cannot be helped. Even if a "mutation" is found, its significance in terms of the risk of cancer by a given age and type of cancer (e.g., breast versus ovarian) may not be clear. (The example of different *apc* mutations in FAP and its attenuated forms shows that different mutant alleles may have different significance). At the limit, some mutations may simply be neutral DNA polymorphisms, it will take time to sort this out. Finally, and most important, there is the question of how the genetic information will be used. A "negative" result implies that the individual has the same risk as the rest of the population (not no risk at all), and this might be expected to provide reassurance. However, what of a "positive" result? Unless the woman has decided that she will use this information to make a specific decision, such as whether to proceed to mastectomy, is she better off for having it? May the burden of knowledge sometimes be harmful? Clearly, these are individual matters, but the clinician who discusses DNA testing for breast cancer risk with a patient should be aware that it is not always a benign procedure and very careful discussion with an experienced counsellor likely will be needed.

How should DNA testing be organized and provided? My view is that given the need for careful counselling and support and for quality control, DNA testing for most familial cancers should only be provided through a properly set-up, clinical genetics service. "Over the counter" testing as well as that provided by well-intentioned research laboratories without professional clinical back-up are inappropriate. Much of the counselling difficulty will be resolved when there is a simple action of proven benefit that can be taken in response to a positive test.

Future Prospects

The genes that are involved in predisposition to many of the inherited cancer syndromes and some of the common familial cancers have been identified within the past 2 years. The challenges now are to devise and evaluate effective means of screening for individuals at risk, to learn how to deal with the need for education and information of the public and the health professions (especially in regard to "gene testing" for the prediction of risk), and to use knowledge of the mechanisms of action of the genes to develop new approaches to prevention and treatment.

Acknowledgments

The author is a Gibb Fellow of the Cancer Research Campaign.

References

1. Alm T, Lieznerski M. The intestinal polyposes. Clin Gastroenterol 1973;2:577.
2. Ayesh R, Idle JR, Ritchie JC, Crothers MJ, Hetzel MR. Metabolic oxidation phenotypes as markers of susceptibility to lung cancer. Nature 1984;312:169.
3. Ballard HS, Frame B, Hartsock RJ. Familial multiple endocrine adenoma-peptic ulcer complex. Medicine 1964;43:481.
4. Banbury Report 16. Genetic Variability to Chemical Exposure. Edited by GS Omenn, HV Gelboin. Cold Spring Harbor NY: Cold Spring Harbor Laboratory, 1984.
5. Bennett ST, Lucassen AM, Gough SCL, et al. Susceptibility to human type 1 diabetes at IDDM2 is determined by tandem repeat variations at the insulin gene minisatellite locus. Nature Genet 1995;9:284.
6. Birch JM, Hartley AL, Tricker KJ, et al. Prevalence and diversity of constitutional mutations in the p53 gene among 21 Li-Fraumeni families. Cancer Res 1994;54:1298.
7. Bishop DT, Williamson JA. The power of identity by state methods for linkage analysis. Am J Hum Genet 1990;46:254.
8. Bodmer WF, Bailey CJ, Bodmer J, Bussey HJR, Ellis A, Forman P, Lucibello FL, Murday VA, Rider SH, Scambler P, Sheer D, Solomon E, Spurr NK. Localization of the gene for familial adenomatous polyposis on chromosome 5. Nature 1987;328:614.
9. Bulow S. Familial polyposis coli. A clinical and epidemiologic study. Dan Med Bull 1987;34:1.
10. Bussey HJR. Familial polyposis coli. Family studies, histopathology, differential diagnosis and results of treatment. Baltimore: Johns Hopkins University Press, 1975.
11. Cannon-Albright LA, Skolnick MH, Bishop DT, Lee RG, Burt RW. Common inheritance of susceptibiity to colonic adenomatous polyps and associated colorectal cancers. N Engl J Med 1988;319:533.
12. Caspari R, Olschwang S, Friedl W, et al. Familial adenomatous polyposis: desmoid tumours and lack of ophthalmic lesions (CHRPE) associated with APC mutations beyond codon 1444. Hum Mol Genet 1995;4:337.
13. Cavenee WK, Dryja TP, Phillips RA, Benedict WF, Godbout R, Gallie BL, Murphree AL, Strong LC, White RL. Expression of recessive alleles by chromosomal mechanisms in retinoblastoma. Nature 1983;305:779.
14. Chapman PD, Church W, Burn J, Gunn A. Congenital hypertrophy of retinal pigment epithelium: a sign of familial adenomatous polyposis. Br Med J 1989;298:353.
15. Claus EB, Risch NJ, Thompson WD. Genetic analysis of breast cancer in the cancer and steroid hormone study. Am J Hum Genet 1991;42:232.
16. Collins FS. Positional cloning. Let's not call it reverse any more. Nature Genetics 1992;1:3.

17. De Mars R. In 23rd Annual Symposium on Fundamental Cancer Res M. D. Anderson Hospital 1969. Baltimore: Williams & Wilkins, 1970, p. 105.
18. Dyck PJ, Carney A, Sizemore GW, Okazaki H, Brimijoin WS, Lambert E. Multiple endocrine neoplasia type 2b: phenotype recognition. Ann Neurol 1979;6:302.
19. Easton D, Peto J. The contribution of inherited predisposition to cancer incidence. In Cancer Surveys, vol 9. Genetic Predisposition to Cancer. Edited by W Cavenee, BAJ Ponder, E Solomon. Oxford: Oxford University Press, 1991.
20. Easton DF, Ford D, Bishop DT. The Breast Cancer Linkage Consortium: breast and ovarian cancer incidence in *BRCA1*-mutation carriers. Am J Hum Genet 1995;56:265.
21. Easton DF, Ponder MA, Cummings T, Gagel RF, Hansen HH, Reichlin S, Tashjian AH, Telenius-Berg M, Ponder BAJ. The clinical and screening age-at-onset distribution for the MEN 2 syndrome. Am J Hum Genet 1989;44:208.
22. Easton DF, Ponder MA, Huson SM, Ponder BAJ. An analysis of variation in expression of neurofibromatosis type 1 : evidence for modifying genes. Am J Hum Genet 1993;53: 305.
23. Elston RC. Segregation Analysis. In Advances in Human Genetics II. Edited by H Harris, K Hirschorn. New York: Plenum, 1981, p 63.
24. Erbe RW. Inherited gastrointestinal syndromes. Ann Intern Med 1976;83:639.
25. Fishel R, Lescoe MK, Rao MRS, et al. The human mutator gene homolog MSH2 and its association with hereditary nonpolyposis colon cancer. Cell 1993;75:1027.
26. Gardner EJ. Follow-up study of a family group exhibiting dominant inheritance for a syndrome including intestinal polyps and osteomatosis. Am J Hum Genet 1962;14: 376.
27. Gonzalez FJ, Skoda RC, Kimura S, Verno M, Zanger UM, Nebert DW, Gelboin HV, Hardwick JP, Meyer UA. Characterisation of the common genetic defect in humans deficient in debrisoquin metabolism. Nature 1988;331:442.
28. Gough AC, Miles JS, Spurr NK, Moss JE, Gaedigk A, Eichelbaum M, Wolf CR. Identification of the primary gene defect at the cytochrome P450 CYP2D locus. Nature 1990;347:773.
29. Groden J, Thliveris A, Samowitz W, et al. Identification and characterization of the familial adenomatous polyposis coli gene. Cell 1991;66:589.
30. Hall JM, Lee MK, Newman B, Morrow JE, Anderson LA, Huey B, King, M-C. Linkage of early-onset familial breast cancer to chromosome 17q21. Science 1990;250:1684.
31. Hansen M. F, Cavenee W. K. Retinoblastoma and the progression of tumour genetics. Trends Genet 1988;4:125.
32. Harnden D, Morten J, Featherstone T. Dominant susceptibility to cancer in man. Adv Cancer Res 1984;41:185.
33. Herrera L, Kakati S, Gibas L, Pietrak E, Sandberg A. Gardner syndrome in a man with an interstitial deletion of 5q. Am J Med Genet 1986;25:473.
34. Horton WA, Wong V, Eldridge R. Von Hippel-Lindau disease. Arch Intern Med 1976;136:769.
35. Huson SM, Harper PS, Compston DAS. Von Recklinghausen neurofibromatosis: a clinical and population study in Southeast Wales. Brain 1988;111:1355.
36. Jagelman DG. Clinical management of familial adenomatous polyposis. Cancer Surveys 1989;8:159.
37. King, M-C. Genetic analysis of cancer in families. In Cancer Surveys, vol 9. Genetic Predisposition to Cancer. Edited by W Cavenee, BAJ Ponder, E Solomon. Oxford: Oxford University Press, 1991.
38. Knudsen AG. Hereditary cancers: clues to mechanisms of carcinogenesis. Br J Cancer 1989;59:661.
39. Knudsen AG. Mutation and cancer: statistical study of retinoblastoma. Proc Natl Acad Sci USA 1971;68:820.
40. Lander ES. Mapping complex genetic traits in humans. In Genome Analysis—A Practical Approach. Edited by KE Davies. Oxford: IRL Press, 1988, p 171.
41. Leach FS, Nicolaides NC, Papadopoulos N, et al. Mutations of a *mutS* homolog in hereditary nonpolyposis colorectal cancer. Cell 1993;75:1215.
42. Leppert M, Burt R, Hughes JP, Samowitz W, Nakamura Y, Woodward S, Gardner E, Lalouel, J-M, White R. Genetic analysis of an inherited predisposition to colon cancer in a family with a variable number of adenomatous polyps. N Engl J Med 1990;322:904.
43. Li FP, Fraumeni JF, Jr., Mulvihill JJ, Blattner WA, Dreyfus MG, Tucker MA, Miller RW. A cancer family syndrome in twenty-four kindreds. Cancer Res 1988;48:5358.
44. Livak KJ, Marmaro J, Todd JA. Towards fully automated genome-wide polymorphism screening. Nature Genet 1995;9:341.
45. Lovett E. Family studies in cancer of the colon and rectum. Br J Surg 1976;63:13.
46. Lynch HT, Kimberley W, Albano WA, Lynch JF, Biscone K, Schuelke GS, Sandberg AA, Lipkin M, Deschner EE, Mikol YB, Elston RC, Bailey-Wilson JE, Shannon Danes B. Hereditary non polyposis colonic cancer (Lynch syndrome I and II). I. Clinical description of resource. Cancer 1988;56:934.
47. Lynch HT, Lynch JF. Breast cancer genetics: clinical Nuances. In Cancer Genetics in Women, vol 1. Edited by Lynch HT, Kullander S. Boca Raton: CRC, 1987, p 49.
48. Lynch HT, Schuelke GS, Kimberling WJ, Albano WA, Lynch JE, Biscone KA, Lipkin ML, Deschner EE, Mikol YB, Sandberg AA, Elston RC, Bailey-Wilson JE, Danes BS. Hereditary nonpolyposis colorectal cancer (Lynch syndromes I and II). II. Biomarker studies. Cancer 1985;56:939.
49. Lynch HT, Smyrk TC, Watson P, et al. Genetics, natural history, tumor spectrum, and pathology of hereditary nonpolyposis colorectal cancer: an updated review. Gastroenterology 1993;104:1535.
50. Macklin MT. Inheritance of cancer of the stomach and large intestine in man. JNCI 1960;24:551.
51. Malkin D, Li FP, Strong LC, Fraumeni JF, Nelson CE, Kim DH, Kassel J, Gryka MA, Bischoff FZ, Tainsky MA, Friend SH. Germ line p53 mutations in a familial syndrome of breast cancer, sarcomas and other neoplasms. Science 1990;250:1233.
52. Markowitz Wang J, Myeroff L, Parsons R, Sun LuZhe, Lutterbaugh J, Fan RS, Zborowska E, Kinzler KW, Vogelstein B, Brattain M, Willson JKV. Inactivation of the type II TGF-β receptor in colon cancer cells with microsatellite instability. Science 1995;268:1336.
53. Martuza RL, Eldridge R. Neurofibromatosis 2. N Engl J Med 1988;318:684.
54. McLenore TL, Adelberg S, Liu M, McMahon NA, Yu SJ, Hubbard WC, Czerwincski M, Wood TG, Stoneng R, Lubet RA, Eggleston JC, Boyd MR, Hines RN. Expression of the CYP1A1 gene in patients with lung cancer. JNCI 1990;82:1333.
55. Miki Y, Swensen J, Shattuck-Eidens D, et al. A strong candidate for the breast and ovarian cancer susceptibility gene *BRCA1*. Science 1994;266:66.
56. Monk M. Variation in epigenetic inheritance. Trends Genet 1990;6:1.
57. Moser AR, Dove WF, Roth KA, Gordon JI. The *Min* (multiple intestinal neoplasia) mutation: its effect on gut epithelial cell differentiation and interaction with a modifier system. J Cell Biol 1992;116:1517.
58. Mulligan LM, Eng C, Healey CS, et al. Specific mutations of the *RET* proto-oncogene are related to disease phenotype in MEN 2A and FMTC. Nature Genet 1994;6:70.
59. Mulvihill JJ, Miller RW, Fraumeni JF. Genetics of Human Cancer Progress in Cancer Research and Therapy. New York: Raven, 1977;3.
60. Murday V, Slack J. Inherited disorders associated with colorectal cancer. Cancer Surveys 1989;8:137.
61. Narod SA, Ford D, Devilee P, et al. An evaluation of genetic heterogeneity in 145 breast-ovarian cancer families. Am J Hum Genet 1995;56:254.
62. Nikawa N, Ishikiriyama S, Takahasi S, Inagawa A, Tonoki H, Ohta Y, Hase N, Kamei T, Kajii T. The Wiedemann-Beckwith syndrome: pedigree studies on five families with evidence for autosomal dominent inheritance with variable expressivity. Am J Med Genet 1986;211:41.
63. Nishisho Y, Nakamura Y, Miyoshi Y, et al. Mutations of chromosome 5q21 genes in FAP and colorectal cancer patients. Science 1991;253:665.
64. Ooi WL, Elston RC, Chen VW, Bailey-Wilson JE, Rothschild H. Increased familial risk for lung cancer. JNCI 1986;76:217.
65. Osterlind A, Tucker MA, Hovi-Jensen K, Stone BJ, Engholm G, Jensen OM. The Danish case-control study of cutaneous malignant melanoma. I. Importance of host factors. Int J Cancer 1988;42:200.
66. Ott J. A short guide to linkage analysis. In Human Genetic Diseases: A Practical Approach. Edited by KE Davies. Oxford: IRL Press, 1986.
67. Papadopoulos N, Nicolaides NC, Wei, Y-F, et al. Mutation of a *mutL* homolog in hereditary colon cancer. Science 1994;263:1625.
68. Peltomaki P, Aaltonen LA, Sistonen P, et al. Genetic mapping of a locus predisposing to human colorectal cancer. Science 1993;260:810.
69. Peto J. Genetic predisposition to cancer. In Cancer Incidence in Defined Populations, Banbury Report 4. Edited by J Cairns, JL Lynch, MH Skolnick. Cold Spring Harbor NY: Cold Spring Harbor Laboratory, 1980, p 203.
70. Ponder BAJ. Gene losses in human tumours. Nature 1988;335:400.
71. Ponder BAJ. Genetics of malignant disease. Br Med Bull 1994;50.
72. Ponder BAJ. Inherited predisposition to cancer. Trends Genet 1990;6:213.
73. Ponder BAJ. Prospects for genetic diagnosis of inherited predisposition to cancer. Trends in Bio/Technol 1990;8:98.
74. Ponder BAJ. Setting up and running a familial cancer clinic. Br Med Bull 1994;50:732.
75. Ponder BAJ, Easton D, Peto J. Risk of ovarian cancer associated with a family history. In Ovarian Cancer. Edited by F Sharp, WD Mason, RE Leake. London: Chapman and Hall, 1990, p 3.
76. Ponder BAJ, Ponder MA, Coffey R, Pembrey ME. Gagel RF, Telenius-Berg M, Semple P, Easton D. F. Risk estimation and screening in families of patients with medullary thyroid carcinoma. Lancet 1988;i:397.
77. Reik W. Genomic imprinting and genetic disorders in man. Trends Genet 1989;5:331.
78. Riccardi VM, Eichner JE. Neurofibromatosis: phenotype, Natural History and Pathogenesis. Baltimore: Johns Hopkins University Press, 1986.
79. Santoro M, Carlomagno F, Romano A, et al. Activation of RET as a dominant transforming gene by germline mutations of MEN 2A and MEN 2B. Science 1995;267:381.
80. Sapienza C. Genome imprinting, cellular mosaicism and carcinogenesis. Mol Carcinogenesis 1990;3:118.
81. Saunders BM, Jay M, Draper GJ, Roberts GM. Non-ocular cancer in the relatives of retinoblastoma patients. Br J Cancer 1989;60:358.
82 .Savitsky K, Bar-Shira A, Gilad S, Rotman G, Ziv Y, Vanagaite L, Tagle DA, Smith S, Uziel T, Sfez S, Ashkenazi M, Pecker I, Frydman M, Harnik R, Patanjali SR, Simmons A, Clines GA, Sartiel A, Gatti RA, Chessa L, Sanal O, Lavin MF, Jaspers NGJ, Taylor AMR, Arlett CF, Miki T, Weissman SM, Lovett M, Collins FS, Shiloh Y. A single ataxia telangiectasia gene with a product similar to PI-3 kinase. Science 1995;268:1749.
83. Schildkraut JM, Risch N, Thompson WD. Evaluating genetic association among ovarian, breast and endometrial cancer: evidence for a breast ovarian relationship. Am J Hum Genet 1989;45:521.
84. Schildkraut JM, Thompson WD. Familial ovarian cancer: a population-based control study. Am J Epidemiol 1988;128:456.
85. Scrable H, Cavenee WK, Ghevimi F, Lovell M, Morgan K, Sapienza C. A model for embryonal rhabdomyosarcoma tumorigenesis that involves genomic imprinting. Proc Natl Acad Sci USA 1989;86:7480.
86. Spirio L, Olschwang S, Groden J, et al. Alleles of the APC gene: an attenuated form of familial polyposis. Cell 1993;75:951.
87. Springate JE. The nevoid basal cell carcinoma syndrome. J Pediatr Surg 1986;21:908.
88. Stoll BA. Risk Factors and Multiple Cancer–New Horizons in Oncology, vol 3. Chichester: Wiley, 1984.
89. Su L-K, Kinzler KW, Vogelstein B, et al. Multiple intestinal neoplasia caused by a mutation in the murine homolog of the APC gene. Science 1992;256:668.
90. Swift M, Reitnauer PJ, Morrell D, Chase CL. Breast and other cancers in families with ataxia-telangiectasia. N Engl J Med 1988;316:1289.
81. Thakker RV, Ponder BAJ. Multiple endocrine neoplasia. In Molecular Biology of Endocrinology (Bailliere's Clinical Endocrinology and Metabolism 2). Edited by MC Sheppard. London: Bailliere Tindall, 1988, p 1031.
92. Van der Mey AGL, Maaswinkel-Mooy PD, Cornelissa CJ, Schmidt PH, Van de Kamp JJP. Genomic imprinting in hereditary glomus tumours: evidence of new genetic theory. Lancet 1989;ii:1291.
93. Viners P, Bartschti, Caporaso N, et al. Genetically based *N*-acetyltransferase metabolic polymorphism and low level environmental exposure to carcinogens. Nature 1994;369:154.
94. Wiggs J, Nordenskj;auold M, Yandell D, Rapaport J, Grondin V, Janson M, Werelius B, Petersen R, Craft A, Riedel K, Liberfarb R, Walton D, Wilson W, Dryja TP. Prediction of the risk of hereditary retinoblastoma, using DNA polymorphisms within the retinoblastoma gene. N Engl J Med 1988;318:151.
95. Williams WR, Anderson DE. Genetic epidemiology of breast cancer: segregation analysis of 200 Danish pedigrees. Genet Epidemiol 1984;1:7.
96. Wolf CR. Cytochrome P450's.a multigene family involved in carcinogen metabolism. Trends in Genet 1986;2:209.
97. Wolf CR. Metabolic factors in cancer susceptibility. In Cancer Surveys. Edited by W Cavanee, BAS Ponder, E Solomon. Oxford: Oxford University Press, 1991.
98. Wooster R, Neuhausen SL, Mangion J, et al. Localization of a breast cancer susceptibility gene, *BRCA2*, to chromosome 13q12-13. Science 1994;265:2088.

CHAPTER 13

Chemical Carcinogenesis

AINSLEY WESTON AND CURTIS C. HARRIS

Introduction

A genetic basis for human carcinogenesis has been established through biochemical and molecular analyses of the disease (36, 179). Many different types of human cancer have been caused by occupational exposure, while others have been attributed to environmental exposure to chemical and/or viral agents (Table 13.1) (86, 158). The molecular mechanisms of human carcinogenesis are emerging through an increasing appreciation of the genetic and epigenetic changes that result from chemical–DNA interactions.

Chemical carcinogenesis is a multistage process that begins with exposure, usually to complex mixtures of chemicals that are found in the human environment. Once internalized, carcinogens frequently are subject to competing metabolic pathways of activation and detoxication, although some reactive environmental chemicals can act directly. Variations among individuals in the metabolism of carcinogens together with differences in DNA-repair capacity and response to tumor promoters govern the relative risk of an individual (64). The initial genetic change that occurs as the result of chemical–DNA interaction is termed *tumor initiation.* Thus, initiated cells are irreversibly altered and are at greater risk of malignant conversion than normal cells (177). The epigenetic effects of tumor promoters facilitate the clonal expansion of the initiated cell (192). This selective, clonal growth advantage results in the formation of a focus of preneoplastic cells. These cells are more vulnerable to progress toward tumorigenesis, because they present a larger, more rapidly proliferating target population for the further action of chemical carcinogens, oncogenic viruses, and other cofactors. Additional genetic changes occur, and consequently, the accumulation of mutations, which may activate protooncogenes and inactivate tumor-suppressor genes, leads to malignant conversion, tumor progression, and metastasis. The underlying genetic mechanisms that regulate chemical carcinogenesis are becoming increasingly well understood, and the insights generated have assisted in the development of methodologies designed to assess human cancer risk and susceptibility factors. The results of these latter studies are further intended to mold strategies for cancer prevention.

Multistage Carcinogenesis

Carcinogenesis can be divided conceptually into four steps; tumor initiation, tumor promotion, malignant conversion, and tumor progression (Fig. 13.1). The distinction between initiation and promotion was recognized through studies involving both viruses and chemical carcinogens (149, 150). This distinction was formally defined in a murine skin carcinogenesis model where mice were treated topically with a single dose of a polycyclic aromatic hydrocarbon (i.e., initiator) followed by repeated topical doses of croton oil (i.e., promoter) (16). This mechanism also has been shown to operate in a range of other rodent tissues, including bladder, colon, esophagus, liver, lung, mammary gland, stomach, and trachea (192). During the last 50 years, the sequence of events comprising chemical carcinogenesis has been systematically dissected and the model increasingly refined. It is now recognized that carcinogenesis requires the malignant conversion of hyperplastic cells from a benign or preneoplastic state and that invasion and metastasis are manifestations of further genetic and epigenetic changes (30). Study of this process in humans is necessarily indirect. Measures of age-dependent cancer incidence have shown, however, that the rate of tumor development is proportional to the sixth power of time, suggesting that four to six independent steps are necessary (134).

Tumor Initiation

Tumor initiation results from irreversible genetic damage. For mutations to accumulate, they must arise in cells that proliferate or give rise to descendants that survive the lifetime of the organism. A chemical carcinogen causes a mutation by modification of the molecular structure of DNA. Most often this is brought about by formation of an adduct between the chemical carcinogen or one of its functional groups and a nucleotide in DNA. (The process by which this occurs for the major classes of chemical carcinogens is discussed in detail under carcinogen metabolism.) In general, a positive correlation is found between the amount of carcinogen–DNA adducts that can be detected in model systems and the resulting number of tumors that develop (124, 136, 190). Thus, tumors rarely develop in tissues that do not form carcinogen–DNA adducts. Carcinogen–DNA adduct formation is central to theories of chemical carcinogenesis, and it can be considered to be a necessary, but not a sufficient, prerequisite for initiation. Some aspects of tumor initiation also can be accomplished by the activation of protooncogenes; this topic is discussed later (see Tumor Progression, Oncogenes, and Tumor-Suppressor Genes).

Table 13.1. Examples of Tumors Considered to be Induced by Chemicals[a]

Anatomical site	Subcategory	Chemical or mixture	Co-factor
External epithelia (~56% human cancer)			
Lung		Arsenic	
		Asbestos	
		Bis (chloromethyl) ether	
		Chromium	
		Hematite	
		Nickel	
	Small cell and squamous cell carcinomas	Tobacco smoke	Asbestos and radon
		Diesel exhaust	
		Coke-oven emission	
	Mesothelioma	Asbestos	
Esophagus	Squamous cell carcinoma	Tobacco smoke	Alcoholic beverages
Oral cavity	Squamous cell carcinoma	Betel nut	Calcium hydroxide
		Chewing tobacco	Alcoholic beverages
Skin	Basal cell carcinoma	Cutting oils	
		Soot	
		Coal tar	
Nasal sinuses		Nickel	
		Snuff (tobacco)	Glass powder
		Isopropyl alcohol	
Internal epithelia (~8% human cancer)			
Liver	Hepatocellular carcinoma	Aflatoxin B_1	Hepatitis virus B or C
			Alcoholic beverages
	Angioma	Vinyl chloride	
Bladder	Squamous cell carcinoma	Aromatic amines (azo-dyes)	
Sarcoma/leukemia (~8% human cancer)			
Hematologic	Acute lymphoblastic leukemia	Benzene	

[a] Information on carcinogenic risk of chemicals is found in reports by the International Agency on the Research of Cancer (86).

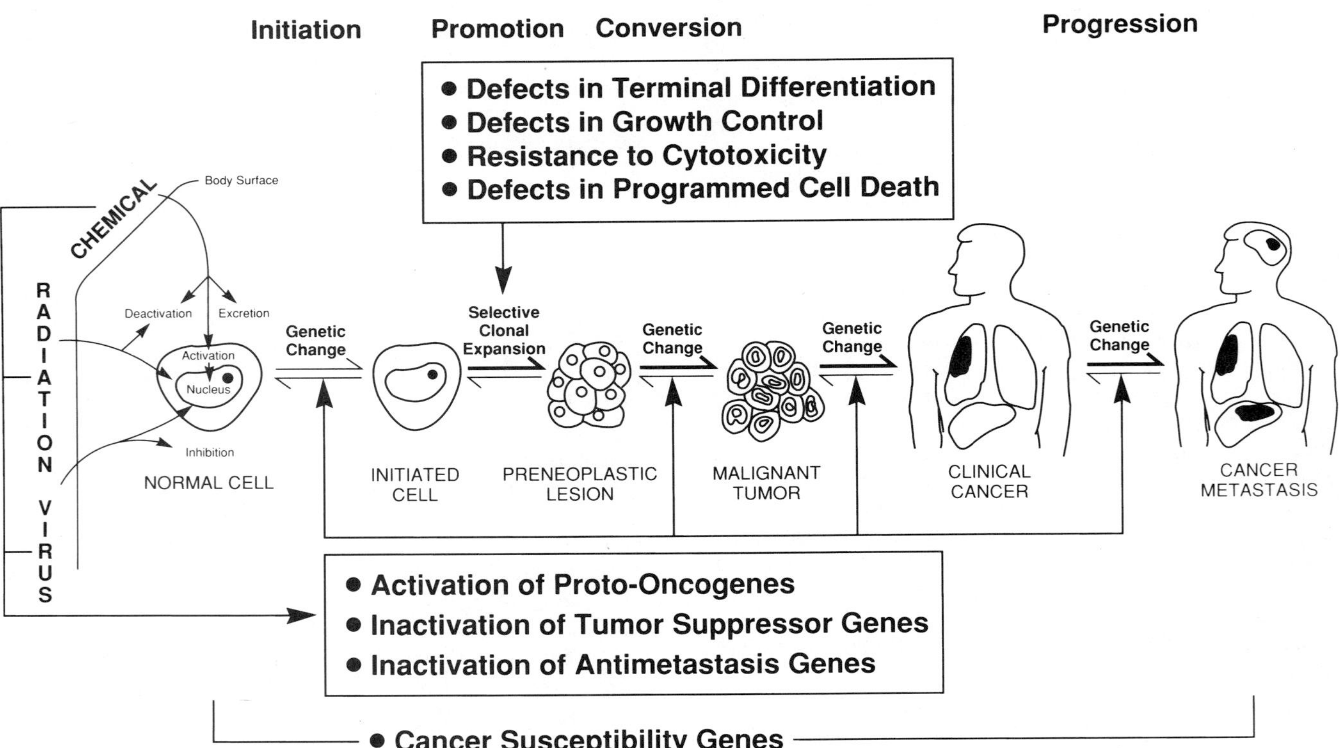

Figure 13.1. Multistage carcinogenesis. Carcinogenesis can be conceptually divided into four steps: tumor initiation, tumor promotion, malignant conversion, and tumor progression. Activation of proto oncogenes and loss of tumor-suppressor genes are genetic changes that have been found in association with carcinogenesis. The accumulation of mutations, not necessarily the order in which they occur, contributes to multistage carcinogenesis.

Tumor Promotion

Tumor promotion comprises the selective clonal expansion of initiated cells. Because the accumulation rate of mutations is proportional to the rate of cell division, or at least the rate at which stem cells are replaced, it follows that clonal expansion of initiated cells produces a larger population of cells that are at risk of further genetic changes and malignant conversion (30). Tumor promoters generally are non-mutagenic, are not carcinogenic alone, and often (but not always) are able to mediate their biologic effects without metabolic activation. These agents are characterized by their ability to reduce the latency period for tumor formation after exposure of a tissue to a tumor initiator or to increase the number of tumors formed in that tissue. In addition, they induce tumor formation in conjunction with a dose of an initiator that is too low to be carcinogenic alone. Chemicals or agents capable of both tumor initiation and promotion are known as complete carcinogens; examples are benzo-[*a*]pyrene and 4-aminobiphenyl.

Croton oil (isolated from *Croton tiglium* seeds) has been used widely as a tumor promoter in murine skin carcinogenesis, and the mechanism of action for its most potent constituent, 12-tetradecanoylphorbol-13-acetate, via activation of protein kinase C is arguably the best understood among tumor promoters (191). Protein kinase C is a calcium-phospholipid-dependent enzyme family that when activated causes phosphorylation of critical substrates and stimulates a cascade of epigenetic changes that can lead to cell growth (6, 18). Among the changes observed in cells treated with 12-O-tetradecanoylphorbol-13-acetate are altered ion flux across the cell membrane, altered hormone binding, and inhibition of cell–cell communication. With increasing recognition of redundancy in the signal transduction cascade, however, it is possible to appreciate that the effects of 12-O-tetradecanoylphorbol-13-acetate are even more diverse. Prostaglandin synthesis, which also is associated with tumor promotion, occurs because of stimulation of the arachidonic acid cascade that is mediated by protein kinase C. The cellular response to protein kinase C activation can result in the modification of differentiation or cell proliferation, and is cell-type dependent. The cell-type dependent differential response may be explained by the fact that protein kinase C is a multigene family, the members of which are differentially expressed among animal species and tissue types.

Identification of new tumor promoters in animal models has accelerated with the increasingly sophisticated development of model systems designed to assay for tumor promotion. Furthermore, ligand-binding properties also can be determined in recombinant protein kinase C isozymes that are expressed in cell cultures (42). Chemicals, complex mixtures of chemicals, or other agents that have been shown to have tumor-promoting properties include dioxin, benzoyl peroxide, macrocyclic lactones, bromomethylbenzanthracene, anthralin, phenol, saccharin, tryptophan, dichlorodiphenyltrichloroethane (DDT), phenobarbital, cigarette-smoke condensate, polychlorinated biphenyls (PCBs), teleocidins, cyclamates, estrogens and other hormones, bile acids, ultraviolet light, wounding, abrasion, and other chronic irritation (i.e., saline lavage) (192). It also has been noted that protein kinase C is activated and cellular diacylglycerol elevated in laboratory animals maintained on high-fat diets (17, 37).

Bryostatin is a macrocyclic lactone that can affect cell growth through binding to protein kinase C. Bryostatin only activates a subset of protein kinase C isozymes, but antagonizes the action of other tumor promoters (phorbol esters) by blocking protein kinase C receptors that they fail to induce (93). Bryostatin causes rapid degradation of protein kinase C, which is associated with loss of protein kinase C–regulated responses and concomitant cell proliferation (93). Staurosporine, which is a microbial alkaloid, is an anticancer agent that causes cell death and has been shown to mediate its biologic response through the protein kinase C pathway (166).

Okadaic acid is a powerful tumor promoter that is present in the marine sponge *Halichondria okadaii*. Rather than acting through modulation of protein kinase C, okadaic acid is a specific inhibitor of protein phosphatase 1 (pp1) and protein phosphatase 2A (pp2). Control of cellular processes occurs through reversible phosphorylation of pp1 and pp 2 (38). Therefore, okadaic acid actually is capable of reversing cell transformation by certain oncogenes such as c-*raf* (164). The c-*raf* gene encodes a cytoplasmic serine/threonine protein kinase that is activated through a variety of cell surface receptors, including protein kinase C (164, 168).

Malignant Conversion

Malignant conversion is the transformation of a preneoplastic cell into one that expresses the malignant phenotype. This process requires further genetic changes. The total dose of a tumor promoter is less important than frequently repeated administrations, and if the administration of a tumor promoter is discontinued before malignant conversion has occurred, premalignant or benign lesions may regress. The contribution of tumor promotion to the process of carcinogenesis is the expansion of a population of initiated cells, which will then be at risk for malignant conversion. Conversion of a fraction of these cells to malignancy will be accelerated in proportion to the rate of cell division and the quantity of dividing cells in the benign tumor or preneoplastic lesion. In part, these further genetic changes may result from infidelity of DNA synthesis (113). The relatively low probability of malignant conversion can be increased substantially by the exposure of preneoplastic cells to DNA-damaging agents (192), and it appears that this process may be mediated through the activation of protooncogenes and inactivation of tumor-suppressor genes.

Tumor Progression

Tumor progression comprises the expression of the malignant phenotype and the tendency of already malignant cells to acquire more aggressive characteristics with time. Metastasis also may involve the ability of tumor cells to secrete proteases that allow invasion beyond the immediate location of the primary tumor. A prominent characteristic of the malignant phenotype is the propensity for genomic instability and uncontrolled growth. During this process further genetic changes can occur, again including the activation of protooncogenes and the functional loss of tumor-suppressor genes. Protooncogenes frequently are activated by two major mechanisms: In the case of the *ras* gene family, point mutations are found in highly specific regions of the gene (i.e., the 12th, 13th, 59th, or 61st codons), and members of the *myc*, *raf*, *neu*, and *jun* multigene families can be overexpressed, sometimes involving amplification of chromosome segments containing these genes. Some genes are overexpressed if they are translocated and become juxtaposed to a powerful promoter (e.g., the relationship of *bcl-2* and immunoglobulin gene promoter regions in B-cell malignancies). Loss of function of tumor-suppressor genes usually occurs in a bimodal fashion, and it appears to involve point mutations in one allele and loss of the second allele by deletion, recombinational event, or chromosomal nondisjunction. These phenomena confer on the cells a growth advantage as well as the capacity for regional invasion and, ultimately distant metastatic spread. The accumulation of these mutations—and not the order or the stage of tumorigenesis in which they occur—appears to be an important determining factor (see Oncogenes and Tumor-Suppressor genes).

Interindividual Variation

Polymorphisms arise in genes through nonlethal mutations that occur during evolution. The spectrum of functional polymorphisms among humans for proteins that have, or may have, a role in chemical carcinogenesis include enzymes that metabolize (i.e., activate and detoxify) xenobiotic substances, enzymes that repair DNA damage, oncogenes, tumor-suppressor genes, and the cell surface receptors that activate the phosphorylation cascade. The cytochrome P-450 (CYP) multigene family is largely responsible for the metabolic activation and detoxication of many different chemical carcinogens in the human environment (55, 59, 60, 119, 121). Cytochrome P-450s act by adding an atom of oxygen onto the substrate; they also are inducible by polycyclic aromatic hydrocarbons and chlorinated hydrocarbons. Cytochrome P-450s are known as phase I enzymes, and the nomenclature of this enzyme family has been defined by Nelson and colleagues (123). Phase II enzymes act on oxidized substrates and also contribute to xenobiotic metabolism (40). Some phase II enzymes are methyltransferases, acetyltransferases, glutathione transferases, uridine 5′-diphosphoglucuronosyl transferases, sulfotransferases, nicotinamide-adenine dinucleotide (NAD)- and nicotinamide-adenine dinucleotide phosphate (NADP)-dependent alcohol, aldehyde and steroid dehydrogenases, quinone reductases, NADPH diaphorase, azo reductases, aldoketoreductases, transaminases, esterases and hydrolases. The pathways of activation and detoxication frequently are in competition, so the propensity of an individual to convert a procarcinogen to an ultimate metabolite that can bind covalently with DNA may vary strikingly. Moreover, differences in DNA-repair rates potentially influence the extent of carcinogen–adduct formation (i.e., biologically effective dose) and, consequently, the total amount of genetic damage that accumulates.

Carcinogen Metabolism

The chemical etiology of occupationally induced skin cancers was recognized as long ago as the eighteenth century (139). In 1933, following a 10-year research program, the first chemically pure carcinogens were isolated from coal tar pitch (40, 95). These chemicals were identified as polycyclic aromatic hydrocarbons, which are composed of variable numbers of fused benzene rings. Polycyclic aromatic hydrocarbons are formed in the incomplete combustion of fossil fuels and vegetable matter (including cooked foods and tobacco smoke), and they are common environmental contaminants. The polycyclic aromatic hydrocarbons are chemically unreactive, and it was almost 20 years before it was shown that enzymic metabolites of these compounds could bind covalently to cellular macromolecules (118).

Polycyclic aromatic hydrocarbons are activated in a multistep process involving initial epoxidation, hydration of the epoxide, and subsequent epoxidation across the remaining olefinic bond to form the ultimate carcinogenic metabolite; a diol-epoxide (22, 160). The first step in this process, formation of the arene oxide, is principally driven by cytochrome P-450, CYP1A1; the activity and inducibility of this enzyme (by exposure to polycyclic aromatic hydrocarbons) has been shown to vary among the human population (64, 87). The simple arene oxide is further metabolized to a dihydrodiol by epoxide hydrolase, the activity of which also varies among humans (40, 64). The second oxidation step, at the site of the olefinic double bond, is most extensively catalyzed by CYP3A4, which varies in activity among the population and is induced by steroids. Thus, for any individual, there can be considerable day-to-day variation in enzyme activity (59).

The molecular biology of CYP1A1 metabolism has been elucidated through cloning and sequencing of components of the signal transduction pathway that begins with ligand binding at the aryl hydrocarbon (AH) receptor and culminates in the expression of CYP1A1 (33, 122). Each component of this signal transduction cascade (the AH receptor, AH receptor nuclear translocator, dioxin-responsive elements, and CYP1A1) has been cloned and sequenced for humans and other species (33, 122). Polymorphisms in some of the components of this system give rise to different levels of activity and response (i.e., inducibility) (73, 132). Evaluation of these polymorphisms as biomarkers of susceptibility in the human population (e.g., CYP1A1) are discussed under Molecular Epidemiology.

Metabolic activation of benzo[*a*]pyrene leads to the formation of the bay-region benzo[*a*]pyrene-7,8-diol 9,10-oxide (13, 40). This vicinal diol-epoxide is asymmetric and eight stereoisomers are possible. The reactivity of each isomer is variable, and the isomers are formed in varying proportions by metabolism. Biologic response to the different enantiomers in mammalian systems suggests that the (+)anti forms are the most active mutagens and carcinogens and the (−)syn forms the least active.

The arene ring of benzo[*a*]pyrene-7,8-diol 9,10-oxide opens spontaneously at the 10 position, giving a highly reactive carbonium ion that can form a covalent addition product (i.e., adduct) with cellular macromolecules, including DNA. These adducts (an example of the structure of benzo[*a*]pyrene-7,8-diol 9,10-oxide bound to the exocyclic amino group [N2] of guanine is shown in Fig. 13.2) cause the DNA to be damaged either by their persistence and consequent interference with replication or by aberrant DNA repair. The same basic tenet holds for carcinogen–DNA adducts of other chemical classes that may be activated by different metabolic pathways.

Another class of chemical carcinogens, aromatic amines, was first linked with increased bladder cancer among dye workers in 1895 (146). A principal aromatic amine thought to be responsible for bladder cancer among workers in the rubber industry is 4-aminobiphenyl. This and many related compounds are components of cigarette smoke, diesel exhaust, and the pyrolysis of certain foods. In addition, nitrated polycyclic aromatic hydrocarbons are also environmental contaminants resulting from the incomplete combustion of vegetable matter and diesel fuel, and they are related to aromatic amines by nitroreduction.

The metabolic activation of aromatic amines is complex (13). They can be converted to an aromatic amide that is catalyzed by an acetyl coenzyme A–dependent acetylation. The acetylation phenotype varies among the population. Persons with the rapid acetylator phenotype are at higher risk of colon cancer (85, 105), whereas, those who are slow acetylators are at risk of bladder cancer (34). This latter association may result from the fact that activation of aromatic amines by *N*-oxidation is a competing pathway for aromatic amine metabolism. Also the *N*-hydroxylation products when protonated (by the acid conditions in the urinary bladder) form reactive electrophiles that bind covalently with DNA or proteins to produce macromolecular damage.

An initial activation step for both aromatic amines and amides is *N*-oxidation by CYP1A2. This cytochrome P-450 is inducible by phenobarbital, and because it is also responsible for the 3-demethylation of 1,3,7-trimethylxanthine (i.e., caffeine), the distribution of metabolic phenotypes in the population as well as the disposition of an individual with respect to CYP1A2 metabolism is relatively easy to determine (29). The reaction of *N*-hydroxy-arylamines with DNA appear to be acid catalyzed, but they can be further activated by either an acetyl coenzyme A–dependent O-acetylase or a 3′-phosphoadenosine-5′phosphosulfate-dependent O-sulfotransferase. The *N*-arylhydroxamic acids, which arise from the acetylation of *N*-hydroxy-arylamines or *N*-hydroxylation of aromatic amides, are not electrophilic; therefore, they require further activation. The predominant pathway for this occurs through acetyltransferase-catalyzed rearrangement to a reactive *N*-acetoxy-arylamine. Sulfotransferase catalysis results in the formation of *N*-sulphonyloxy arylamides. This complex pathway results in two major adduct types; amides (i.e., acetylated) and amines (i.e., non-acetylated).

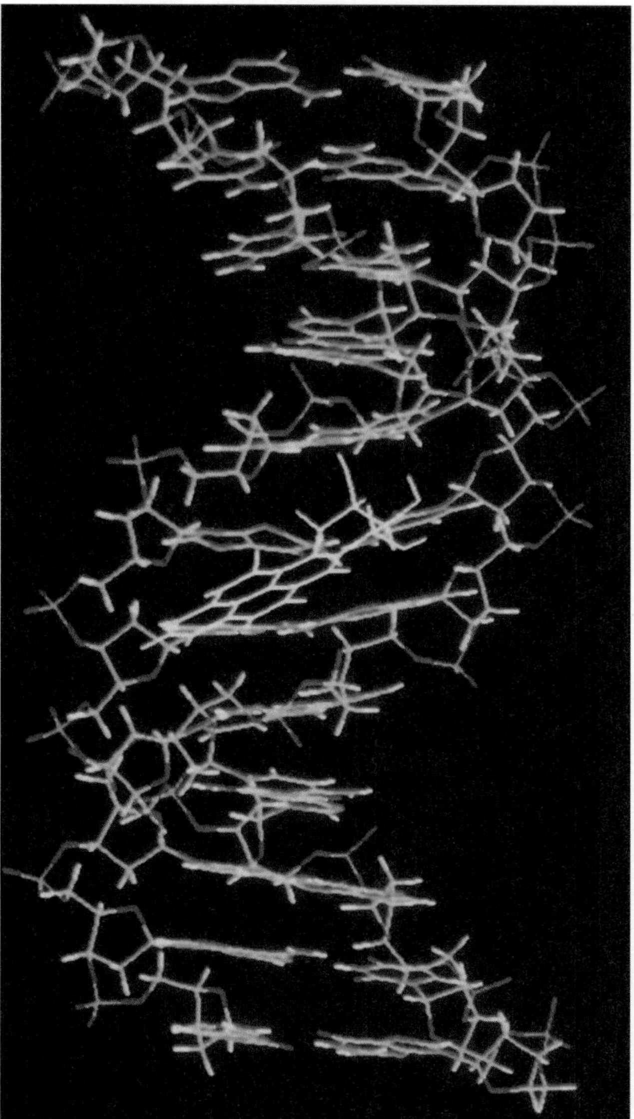

Figure 13.2. Computer-modeled image of anti-benzo[*a*]pyrene-diol epoxide deoxyguanosine adduct formed in minor groove of a 12–base pair sequence (5′-ATCggCgCggTA-3′). Structure is a half-bond color stick model: *grey*, c; *white*, H; *blue*, N; *red*, O; *green*, P; *yellow*, all atoms of the polycyclic hydrocarbon moiety.

The heterocyclic amines are formed during the preparation of cooked food, primarily from the pyrolysis (>150°C) of amino acids, creatinine, and glucose. They have been recognized as food mutagens (49, 89, 171), and they have been shown to form adducts and cause liver tumors in primates (1). Compared with other carcinogens, their metabolism is less well understood, but *N*-hydroxylation is considered to be a necessary step. Because they are similar in structure to the aromatic amines, it is not surprising that they can be activated by CYP1A2. The *N*-hydroxy metabolites of 3-amino-1-methyl-5*H*-pyrido[4,3-b]indole (Trp-P-1), 2-amino-6-

methyldipyrido[1,2-a:3′,2′-d]imidazole (Glu-P-1), and 2-amino-3-methyl-imidazo-[4,5-f]quinoline (IQ) can react directly with DNA. Unlike, however, the aromatic amines, this reaction is not facilitated by acid pH. Enzymic O-esterification of *N*-hydroxy metabolites is important in the activation of these food mutagens, and the *N*-hydroxy metabolites also are good substrates for transacetylases. This suggests a possible etiologic role for these chemicals in colorectal cancer in combination with the rapid acetylator phenotype (discussed earlier).

Aflatoxins (aflatoxin B_1, B_2, G_1, and G_2) are metabolites of *Aspergillus flavus*. They are fungal mutagens that contaminate cereals, grain, and nuts. A positive correlation exists between dietary aflatoxin exposure and incidence of liver cancer in developing countries, where grain spoilage is high. More recently, urinary levels of certain aflatoxin adducts and metabolites have been correlated with incidence of liver cancer in China (57, 58, 140, 147). It also should be noted that hepatitis B virus infection independently increases risk of liver cancer, but the effects of hepatitis B infection together with ingestion of aflatoxin are multiplicative, not additive (66, 67, 140, 147).

Aflatoxins are activated by several cytochrome P-450s, including CYP2A3, CYP2A6, and CYP3A4 (54, 60). Aflatoxin B_1 and G_1 have an olefinic double bond at the 8,9-position, and they are more mutagenic and carcinogenic than aflatoxin B_2 and G_2 which are saturated and have an ethylenic bond at this position. Along with the analysis of the DNA adducts, this implies that the olefinic 8,9-bond is the site of activation. Further support for this mechanism comes from studies of the prevalence of p53 mutations in liver cancer. In people with liver cancer from parts of China and Africa where food spoilage caused by molds is high, G:C to T:A transversions in codon 249 are frequent (2, 26, 82). This phenomenon is consistent with metabolic activation of aflatoxin B_1.

Carcinogenic *N*-nitrosamines are ubiquitous environmental contaminants and can be found in food, alcoholic beverages, cosmetics, cutting oils, hydraulic fluid, rubber, and tobacco (11). Tobacco-specific *N*-nitrosamines such as 4-(methylnitrosoamino)-1-(3-pyridyl)-1-butanone are carcinogenic in a wide range of animal species, and they may account for the carcinogenic nature of snuff and chewing tobacco (75). Endogenous nitrosation also can occur because of the reaction of an amine with nitrate alone or nitrite in the presence of acid. Thus, nitrite (used in curing meats) and L-cysteine in the presence of acetaldehyde (a metabolite of alcohol) form *N*-nitrosothiazolidine-4-carboxylic acid. The *N*-nitrosamines are activated primarily by CYP2E1. This isozyme is inducible by alcohol, but it is not known whether CYP2E1 is polymorphic (59).

N-nitrosodimethylamine undergoes α-hydroxylation to form an unstable α-hydroxynitrosamine. The breakdown products are formaldehyde and methyl diazohydroxide. The alkyl groups of compounds like methyl diazohydroxide are good leaving groups and thus are powerful methylating agents that can add a small functional group (small alkyl-adduct as opposed to the bulky aryl-adducts formed by the carcinogens discussed earlier) at more than 10 different sites in DNA. The tobacco-specific nitrosamines are not symmetric and also can form bulky adducts; 4-(methylnitrosoamino)-1-(3-pyridyl)-1-butanone metabolism gives rise to either a positively charged pyridyl-oxobutyl ion or a positively charged methyl ion, both of which are able to alkylate DNA (12, 76, 77).

DNA Damage and Repair

There are several ways in which the chemical structure of DNA can be altered by a carcinogen, including the formation of bulky aromatic-type adducts, alkylation (generally small adducts), oxidation, dimerization and deamination. Chemical carcinogens also can cause epigenetic changes, such as alteration in DNA methylation status (188). Carcinogen–DNA adducts vary in their promutagenic potential, and this is discussed later for alkyl-adducts. Figure 13.2 shows the binding of benzo[*a*]pyrene-7,8-diol 9,10-epoxide to the exocyclic (N2) amino group of deoxyguanosine. This is a bulky aromatic adduct that resides within the minor groove of the double helix, and it is typical of polycyclic aromatic hydrocarbons. Although this adduct appears to be the most common form by far of DNA damage induced by benzo[*a*]pyrene in mammalian systems, others are possible, including covalent binding of metabolites to deoxyadenosine (13, 40).

Aromatic amine adducts are more complex, not only because they have both acetylated and nonacetylated (viz. diacetylated) metabolic intermediates but also because they form covalent bonds at the C8, N2, and sometimes O6 positions of deoxyguanosine as well as deoxyadenosine. The major adducts, however, are C8-deoxyguanosine adducts, which reside predominantly in the major groove of the DNA double helix (12).

Although the evidence for activation of aflatoxins B_1 and G_1 through hydroxylation of the olefinic 8,9-position is circumstantial, the structures of the adducts are known. They are formed at the N7-position of deoxyguanosine. They are relatively unstable and have a half-life of approximately 50 hours at neutral pH, with resulting depurination. The aflatoxin B1-N7-deoxyguanosine adduct also can undergo ring opening to yield two pyrimidine adducts; alternately, aflatoxin B1-8,9-dihydrodiol could result. This latter possibility could restore the molecular structure of the DNA if hydrolysis of the original adduct occurs, but a potentially promutagenic lesion would result if formation of the 8,9-dihydrodiol results from degradation of ring-open adduct forms (Fig. 13.3) (57, 79).

Alkylation of DNA can occur at many sites either following the metabolic activation of certain *N*-nitrosamines or directly by the action of the *N*-alkylureas (*N*-methyl-*N*-nitrosourea) or the *N*-nitrosoguanidines. The protonated alkyl-functional groups that become available to form lesions in DNA generally attack the following nucleophilic centers: adenine (N1, N3, and N7), cytosine (N3), guanine (N2, O6 and N7), and thymine (O2, N3, and O4). Some of these lesions are known to be repaired (O6-methyldeoxyguanosine), while others are not (N7-methyldeoxyguanosine) (74). Furthermore, O6-methyldeoxyguanosine is a promutagenic lesion, whereas N7-methyldeoxyguanosine is not.

Oxy-radical damage can result in the modification of DNA

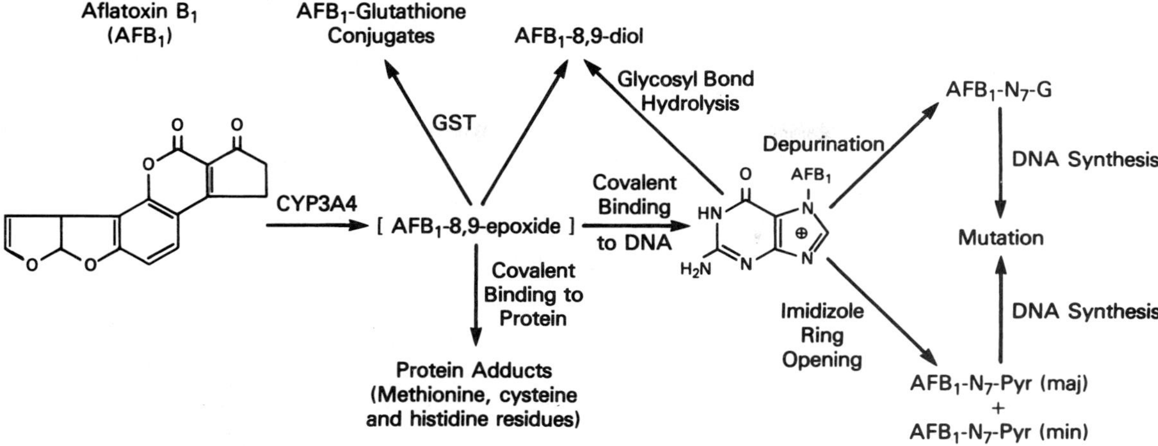

Figure 13.3. Metabolism and activation of aflatoxin B_1. The metabolic activation of aflatoxin proceeds by oxidation at the olefinic bond in the 8,9-position (CYP2A3 and CYP3A4). Aflatoxins B_2 and G_2, which do not have an 8,9-double bond, are much less carcinogenic.

to form thymine glycol or 8-hydroxydeoxyguanosine adducts. Three major pathways have been identified. Exposure to organic peroxides (catechol, hydroquinone, and 4-nitroquinoline-*N*-oxide) leads to this type of oxy-radical damage; however, oxy-radicals and hydrogen peroxide can be generated in lipid peroxidation and the catalytic cycling of some enzymes (173). Cells also can be stimulated to produce peroxisomes by treatment with certain drugs and plasticizers (145). Exposure to tumor promoters can indirectly increase oxy-radical formation, and perhaps the best-known relationship is that between the phorbol esters and inflammatory cells. In this system, mediated through protein kinase C and the subsequent activation of a membrane-localized pyridine nucleotide-dependent oxidase, oxy-radical formation is highly correlated with the relative potencies of the different phorbol esters (52). Correspondingly, promoters that do not stimulate the protein kinase C signal transduction cascade do not affect oxy-radical production.

Another potentially mutagenic cause of DNA damage is the deamination of methylated cytosine residues in DNA. 5-methylcytosine comprises approximately 3% of deoxynucleotides. In this case, deamination at a CpG dinucleotide gives rise to a TpG mismatch. Repair of this lesion most often restores the CpG; however, a mutation may be fixed by repair to TpA (172). Deamination of cytosine also can generate a C to T transition if uracil glycosylation and G-T mismatch repair are inefficient. Oxy-radicals can enhance the rate of deamination, so the activity of nitric oxide synthase could contribute to DNA damage by this mechanism (Fig. 13.4).

DNA repair enzymes act at sites of DNA damage caused by chemical carcinogens, and five major mechanisms are known; direct DNA repair, nucleotide excision repair, base excision repair, post-replication repair, and mismatch repair (19, 20, 61). These have been characterized in lower organisms, yeast, and bacteria; however, some gene homologues have been cloned from human gene libraries (e.g., *hMSH*).

Direct DNA repair is effected by suicide enzymes (i.e., alkyltransferases). These enzymes catalyze translocation of the alkyl moiety from an alkylated base (e.g., O6-methyldeoxyguanosine) to a cysteine residue at their active site in the absence of DNA strand scission. Thus, one molecule of the enzyme is capable of repairing one alkyl lesion in DNA.

In DNA-nucleotide excision repair, preincision recognition of the lesion is required. The UvrABC endonuclease complex can, for example, recognize large distortions in DNA because of the presence of adduct lesions. Removal of the lesion is achieved by the action of the endonuclease. Then using the intact strand as a template a patch is constructed by 5′ to 3′ polymerization, and ligation of the free ends then occurs. This type of transcription repair is strand specific, that is, the transcribed strand in a gene is preferentially repaired by comparison to the nontranscribed strand (19). Nucleotide excision repair is a vital mechanism in humans and lack of this function results in *Xeroderma pigmentosum.*

Base excision repair also removes a segment of DNA containing an adduct. Removal of the adducted base is, however, brought about by a glycosylase, and repair of the damaged strand is accomplished by the combined action of an exonuclease that degrades a few bases on the damaged strand and a polymerase that synthesizes a 'patch' in the 5′ to 3′ direction using the undamaged strand as a template. The patch is then ligated as in nucleotide excision repair. Generally, small alkyl-adducts (e.g., 3-methyladenine) are repaired in this way.

DNA mismatches occasionally occur because of excision repair processes and involve incorporation of unmodified or conventional, but noncomplementary, Watson-Crick bases opposite each other in the DNA helix. Transition mispairs (G-T or A-C) are repaired by the mismatch repair process more efficiently than transversion mispairs (G-G, A-A, G-A, C-C, C-T and T-T), probably because differential recognition of the mispairings. Repair efficiency of mispairings also depends on their oligonucleotide environment for the same reason. Thus, mispairings in G-C–rich regions are repaired more efficiently than those in A-T–rich regions. The mechanism for correction of mispairings essentially is the same as that for nucleotide excision repair and resynthesis described earlier,

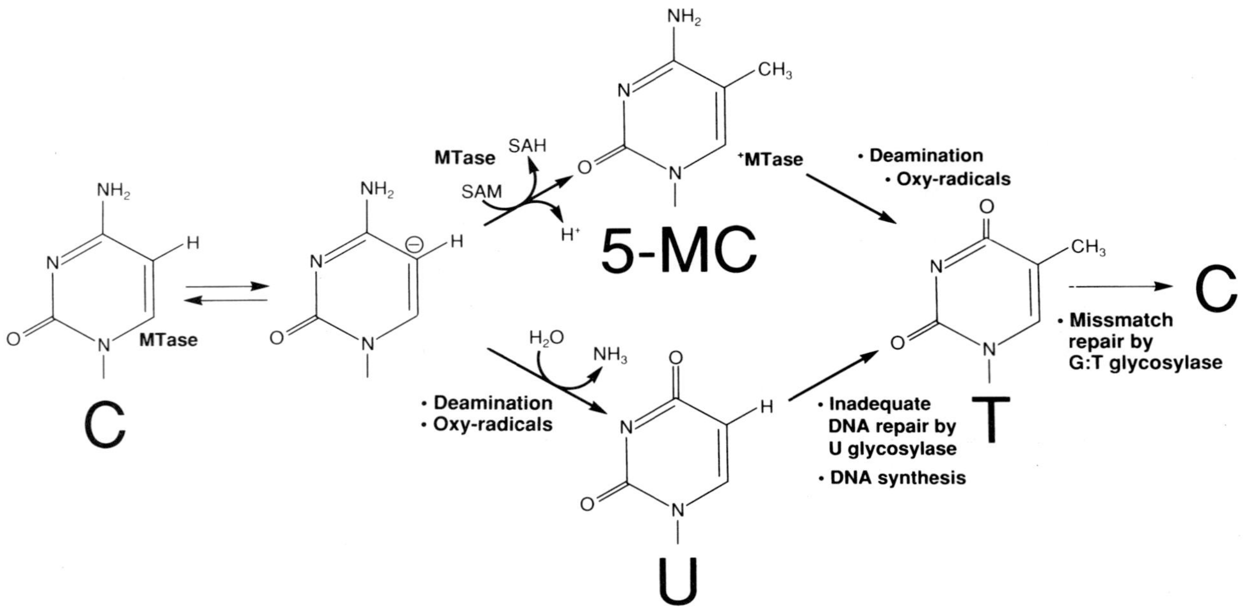

Figure 13.4. Deamination of cytosine and 5-methylcytosine is an example of endogenous mutagenesis.

but it generally involves the excision of large pieces of the DNA containing mispairings. Because the mismatch recognition protein is required to bind simultaneously the mismatch and an unmethylated adenine in a GATC recognition sequence, it removes the whole intervening DNA sequence. The parental template strand is then used by the polymerase to fill the gap.

Postreplication repair occurs by polymerase action or a recombinational mechanism in response to replication of DNA on a damaged template. The DNA polymerase stops at the replication fork when DNA damage is detected on the parental strand. Alternately, the polymerase proceeds past the lesion, leaving a gap in the newly synthesized strand. The gap is filled in one of two ways: (1) either by recombination of the homologous parent strand with the daughter strand in a process that is mediated by the RecA protein, or (2) when a single nucleotide gap remains, mammalian DNA polymerases insert an adenine residue. Consequently, this mechanism may lead to recombinational events as well as base mispairing.

The rate, but not the fidelity, of DNA repair can be measured by adduct removal or unscheduled DNA synthesis. Substantial variations among individuals have been found in these rates (64, 127, 155). Markedly reduced rates of excision repair are found in individuals with *Xeroderma pigmentosum*, and these individuals are at known risk of ultraviolet light–induced skin cancer. Among the general population, however, an approximately 5-fold variation in the rates of excision repair have been found in lymphocytes treated with carcinogens in vitro. An association also has been found between the reduced capacity of mononuclear leukocytes in vitro to repair aromatic amine adducts in individuals who have first-degree relatives with cancer. Up to 40-fold variations among humans in the activity of O6-alkylguanine-DNA alkyltransferase have been reported as well. DNA repair rates are inhibited by aldehydes, alkylating agents, and some chemotherapeutic drugs. Decreased DNA repair capacity also has been noted in the fibroblasts of patients with lung cancer compared to those patients with melanoma or noncancer controls. For benzo[*a*]pyrene-7,8-diol 9,10-epoxide–DNA adducts, a unimodal distribution of repair rates is observed in lymphocytes, but interindividual variation has been found to be substantial (155).

Among the most recent advances is the cloning of two DNA mismatch repair genes; *hMSH2*, located on chromosome 2p; and *hMSH1*, located on chromosome 3p21-23. These genes are responsible for the fidelity of DNA repair. The chromosomal regions in which these genes reside were previously found to be in linkage disequilibrium with certain forms of colon cancer (27, 51, 151, 154); subsequently, the cloning of these genes provided a biologic mechanism for the genetic defect leading to increased mutations or the mutator phenotype (113). The prevalence of mutated forms of these genes is common by comparison with other disease susceptibility genes (approximately 1 in 200 individuals), and inheritance of such gene defects accounts for early onset colon cancer. The discovery of these genes was performed through a novel combination of linkage analysis using restriction fragment length polymorphism markers that assisted localization and sequencing by positional cloning (108), and by examination of candidate DNA mismatch repair genes (51). Subsequently, two additional genes, *hPMS1* and *hPMS2*, located on chromosomes 2p and 7p, respectively, have been discovered (114).

Response to Tumor Promoters

The tumor-promoting effects of phorbol esters are reversible, and repeated doses frequently are necessary for promotion to occur (191). This suggests that tumor promotion occurs through an epigenetic mechanism based on selective clonal expansion. These effects are mediated primarily through protein kinase C activation. Resistance of initiated cells to phorbol ester–mediated terminal differentiation may relate to alteration in the expression of protein kinase C (via the initiating event). Evidence to date supports this molecular model for the differential effects of tumor promoters between normal and initiated cells.

Phorbol esters produce different effects in different cell types. This may be explained by the expression of different classes of protein kinase C receptors among cell types. In addition, multiple protein kinase C genes and mRNA species have been identified in mammalian tissues (41, 98), and different rodent strains vary in their sensitivity to promoting agents (23, 134, 163). Diversity in the elements that comprise the complex protein activation cascade likely are differentially expressed among the population, either because polymorphisms or differential exposures to environmental agents, and variation in individual response to tumor promoters could result.

Oncogenes and Tumor-Suppressor Genes

Activation of protooncogenes and loss of tumor-suppressor genes are genetic changes associated with carcinogenesis. The study of mechanisms by which chemical carcinogens cause these changes is an active area of interdisciplinary cancer research. It clearly is reasonable that chemical–DNA interactions and carcinogen–DNA adduct formation (either direct, in the case of polycyclic aromatic hydrocarbons, or indirect, in the case of oxy-radicals) lead to this type of genetic change in human cancer, because these changes have been detected in tumors with a recognized chemical etiology. Furthermore, both the recognition that carcinogen–DNA interaction is an important step in carcinogenesis and the results of short-term mutagenesis assays led to the conclusion that chemically induced DNA damage is an early step in the carcinogenic process.

Protooncogenes are normal cellular genes that control cell growth (i.e., proliferation), specialization (i.e., differentiation) and death (i.e., apoptosis). Almost all protooncogenes encode a protein component of the signal transduction cascade. This integrated, multiprocess system is responsible for the smooth, orderly, and specific transmission of extracellular signals to the nucleus, and this process regulates gene transcription with respect to replication (126). When protooncogenes are activated, they are termed *oncogenes*. Oncogenes exert a positive driving force for cell growth by their failure to desist in response to the absence of stimulation (101). The discovery of oncogenes, their role in cell transformation, and the realization that these genes arise from the activation of normal cellular genes (protooncogenes) is discussed in Chapter 5. That there are several possible mechanisms by which protooncogenes may be activated should be emphasized. These are overexpression of the gene product leading to an increased concentration of the protein (dosage hypothesis); expression of the gene at an inappropriate time or context, which could occur because of a mutation in the regulatory region of the gene (unscheduled gene expression); expression of a proto oncogene in an inappropriate cell type; and structural alteration of the gene product. The primary mechanisms by which chemicals cause oncogene activation are discussed later.

Activated *ras* genes predominate as the family of oncogenes to be isolated from solid tumors that are induced by chemicals in laboratory animals. Members of the *ras* gene family code for proteins of molecular weight 21,000 (p21); these proteins are membrane bound, have GTPase activity, and form complexes with other proteins. The *ras* genes code for small G proteins (guanine nucleotide binding) that exert a powerful proliferative response through the signal transduction cascade. They have been referred to as a molecular switch that when mutated, freezes in the "on" position. Activated *ras* binds to *raf*, a protein kinase, and through this mechanism recruits other mitogen-activated protein kinases to cause cell proliferation. Disruption of this signalling pathway holds promise for future therapeutic strategies (7, 101, 116). The first direct evidence of proto oncogene activation by a chemical carcinogen was obtained from in vitro studies (10, 115). A wild-type recombinant clone of the human *Ha-ras* gene (pEC) was modified with benzo[*a*]pyrene-diol-epoxide. The treated plasmid was then used to transfect NIH-3T3 cells, with the result that the transformed cell foci produced contained the same specific point mutations (in either codon 12 or 61) known to exist in activated ras genes isolated from human tumors including the bladder (pEJ).

In animal model systems of chemical carcinogenesis and surveys of different types of human tumors that arise from a variety of environmental exposures (Table 13.1), *ras* mutations have been found (10). In rodents, polycyclic aromatic hydrocarbons (3-methylcholanthrene, 7,12-dimethylbenz-[*a*]anthracene and benzo[*a*]pyrene)have been used repeatedly to produce both benign tumors and malignant carcinomas. A large proportion of these premalignant and malignant lesions have mutations in either the 12th or 61st codons. Similarly, treatment of rats with either 7,12-dimethylbenz[*a*]anthracene or *N*-methyl-*N*-nitrosourea resulted in the development of mammary carcinomas containing *ras* codon 12 or 61 mutations. These types of mutation also have been observed in mouse skin after initiation with 7,12-dimethylbenz[*a*]anthracene and tumor promotion with 12-O-tetradecanoylphorbol-13-acetate. Mutations in *ras* have been found in mouse liver after treatment with either vinyl carbamate, hydroxydehydroestragole or *N*-hydroxy-2-acetylaminofluorene. The same point mutations also have been found in murine thymic lymphomas after treatment with *N*-methyl-*N*-nitrosourea or γ-radiation and in other rodent skin models after treatment with either methylmethanesulphonate, *a*-propiolactone, dimethylcarbamyl chloride, or *N*-methyl-*N*′-nitro-*N*-nitrosoguanidine.

These data suggest that chemical carcinogens may produce site specific mutations based in part on nucleoside selectivity of the ultimate carcinogen. Persistence of a specific mutation, however, also depends on the amino acid substitution in that the function of the mutant protein is altered to confer on the cell a clonal growth advantage. The types of mutations that are found in chemically activated *ras* genes cause conformational changes that alter nucleotide binding to the p21 protein in such a way that the p21 GTPase activity is not reduced. Data support the hypothesis that *ras* activation is associated with malignant conversion as well as tumor initiation. Transfection of activated *ras* genes into benign papillomas that did not contain a constitutively activated *ras* gene caused malignant progression (62).

Similarly, normal human bronchial epithelial cells, or those immortalized with SV40 T antigen, have been shown to undergo malignant transformation when transfected with an activated *ras* gene (4, 142). In the immortalized cells, overexpression of *c-raf-1* and *c-myc* in combination, but not in isolation, also caused neoplastic transformation (135). In addition, *Ki-ras* gene mutations are one of a number of changes that can arise either early or late in the development of colorectal carcinoma (47). These findings suggest that the accumulation of mutations and not necessarily the order in which they occur contributes to multistage carcinogenesis. Furthermore, the stage of carcinogenesis in which each mutation occurs is not necessarily fixed. It appears that in the model for human colorectal carcinoma, *ras* mutations most often occur during malignant conversion but can be an early event (i.e., tumor initiation); in the rodent skin models, *ras* mutations appear to be primarily a tumor-initiating event. These differences may reflect type of exposure, both in terms of chemical class and chronic versus acute exposure, or they may be a function of tissue type.

Loss of the function of genes that may suppress the tumor phenotype was considered as a theoretic possibility in regard to retinoblastoma more than 20 years ago. Firm experimental evidence for the existence of tumor-suppressor genes was provided by analysis of the molecular genetics of pediatric tumors (retinoblastoma, Wilms' tumor, rhabdomyosarcoma and bilateral acoustic neurofibromatosis). Examination of DNA–restriction fragment length polymorphisms by Southern hybridization shows the loss of a restriction fragment from the tumor of a constitutive heterozygote if that genetic locus has been affected by certain mutational events (deletion, translocation, nondisjunction, mitotic recombination). This type of genetic analysis is termed loss of heterozygosity. In fact, in pediatric tumors, studies that showed loss of the normal allele and duplication of the inherited, defective allele provided the first proof of mitotic recombination in humans.

Loss of a tumor-suppressor gene is generally characterized by a mutation in one copy of the gene and loss of the homologous copy. Several genes with these characteristics have been located on specific chromosomes: the retinoblastoma gene (*Rb*) (13q14); the Wilms' tumor gene (*WT-1*) (11p13); the *p53* gene (17p13); the deleted in colon carcinoma gene (*DCC*) (18q); the mutated in colon cancer gene (*MCC*) (5q21); the nonmetastasis-23 gene (*NM23*) (17q); the von Hippel-Lindau disease gene (*VHL*) (3p25); the neurofibromatosis genes (*NF1* and *NF2*) (17q11 and 22q, respectively); the adenopolyposis coli gene (*APC*) (5q21); the protein tyrosine phosphatase gamma (*PTP-γ*) (3p), the retinoic acid receptor gene (*RAR*) (3p) and the *p16*^{ink4} gene (9p21) (9, 35, 45, 88, 97, 99, 103, 106, 109, 128, 148, 165, 167, 181). The proof that these are tumor-suppressor genes will come from experiments that test the tumor-suppressive effects of a wild-type copy reintroduced into a tumor that has only a defective copy.

Other chromosomal loci also have been identified as candidates that contain tumor-suppressor genes through loss of heterozygosity studies. Even though a model of carcinogenesis for retinoblastoma usually implies an inherited defect followed by a somatic mutation, spontaneous, nonfamilial retinoblastoma is known. Therefore, it is reasonable to suppose that chemical carcinogens may be responsible for causing genetic changes to tumor-suppressor genes. This concept has been examined in the study of a growing number of adult tumors with etiologies of implied chemical exposure (i.e., the smoking-related cancers). Frequent loss of heterozygosity has been observed in many of these tumor types (69, 117, 187). These studies have been extended to DNA sequence analysis to determine if an associated mutation has occurred in a known tumor-suppressor gene. Point mutations in the *p53* gene that give rise to amino acid changes or chain termination are observed in approximately 50% of human cancers and are frequent in lung as well as colon cancer (56, 110, 125, 174). Concerning tumor-suppressor genes, most available data are derived from studies of *p53*.

The role of tumor suppressor genes (i.e., *p53* in homeostasis) is to prevent tissue overgrowth, nullify cells with damaged genomes, and metastasis. These controlling functions, even in the presence of already severely damaged cells that are being driven by activated protooncogenes (oncogenes), may be thwarted by a fully functional p53 protein. It is of further importance to recognize that the p53 function may be compromised by viral infection (e.g., human papillomavirus). The role of p53 in the life cycle of the cell is becoming increasingly well understood, and the p53 protein has been shown to have broad functionality in cellular processes. These include cell cycle control, DNA repair, differentiation, genomic plasticity, and apoptosis (i.e., programmed cell death) (104, 110).

Molecular analysis of the *p53* may gives clues to environmental etiology of cancer. It is implicit from the preceding text (DNA damage and repair) that the covalent binding of activated carcinogens to DNA is not random. Therefore, the formation of a particular DNA lesion to some extent may be deduced from the mutation that resulted. The *p53* gene mutations in many human cancers could provide the clues. A dramatic example of this phenomenon is the previously mentioned codon 249 mutation, which is detected in almost all aflatoxin-related hepatocellular carcinomas (2, 26, 82). The striking nature of this association could arise by two distinct mechanisms. First, the third base in codon 249 (AGG) may be unusually susceptible to activated aflatoxin B_1 mutations. Indeed, it was discussed earlier that aflatoxin B_1-8,9-oxide causes a promutagenic lesion by covalent binding to the N7 position of deoxyguanosine. Alternately, cells bearing the codon 249 lesion may have a selective growth advantage. Evidence that a combination of these factors is responsible has been presented as well (138).

Another prominent example where circumstantial evidence points to specific molecular events is that of *p53* mutations indicative of pyrimidine dimer formation in ultraviolet light–related skin cancers (24). In the case of tobacco smoking and lung cancer, G:C to T:A transversions indicate formation of adducts from activated bulky carcinogens (e.g.,

Table 13.2. Mutational Spectra of *p53* in Human Cancers[a]

Carcinogen exposure	Neoplasm	Mutation
$Aflatoxin_1$	Hepatocellular carcinoma	Codon 249^{ser} mutations
Sunlight	Skin carcinoma	Dipyrimidine mutations on nontranscribed DNA strand
Cigarette smoke	Lung carcinoma	G:C to T:A mutations on nontranscribed DNA strand
Tobacco and alcohol	Head and neck carcinoma	Increase the frequency *p53* mutations
Radon	Lung cancer	Codon 249^{met} mutations
Vinyl chloride	Hepatic angiosarcomas	A:T to T:A transversions

[a] For reviews, see Greenblatt and colleagues (56) and Brennan and colleagues (25).

polycyclic aromatic hydrocarbons) (56). However, we should be cautious in our interpretation, because two major confounding factors in this approach are that different carcinogens can lead to the formation of identical mutations and that most environmental chemical carcinogens are highly complex mixtures (e.g., tobacco smoke and diesel exhaust). These and other examples (Table 13.2) of mutational spectra at the *p53* gene locus and others have been comprehensively reviewed (56, 68, 81).

The general mechanism for the loss of heterozygosity that occurs in tumors that have a familial origin may be different from that occurring in chemically induced cancer. Mitotic recombination is a common feature of pediatric neoplasms. The carcinogenic effects of the clastogens found in cigarette smoke, however, appear to be mediated in part more typically through chromosomal deletions. These deletions are primarily terminal, but they are to a lesser extent interstitial (187). Furthermore, given the complexity of tobacco smoke (a mixture of mutagens, carcinogens, and promoters), these and other mutations likely result from both direct (adduct formation) and indirect (oxy-radical formation) damage to DNA. Determination of these types of disease-associated mutational spectra, which include both oncogenes and tumor-suppressor genes, eventually may be useful in defining causal chemical exposure.

Clonal Evolution

The most extensively documented studies of sequential changes addressing the question of clonality during human tumor evolution have used cytogenetic techniques in leukemia (126) (see Chapters 7 and 142) and polymorphic gene loci in the molecular analysis of colon cancer (46, 180). With the exception of a role for benzene in the etiology of acute myeloid leukemia, however, it is not certain whether either of these malignancies have a chemical etiology. Specifically, the clonal evolution of chemically induced mouse skin tumors has been studied in chimeric or mosaic animals (144, 145).

With reference to the case of chronic myelogenous leukemia, the early disease phase is characterized by a single reciprocal translocation, t (9;22), called the Philadelphia chromosome. This genetic change activates the *c-abl* proto-oncogene through the formation of a hybrid gene of *c-abl* with the break point cluster region. The resulting gene product has elevated tyrosine kinase activity. The later stages of chronic myeloid leukemia are typified by overgrowth of one or more subclones that have additional karyotypic alterations (see Chapter 143).

In colorectal tumorigenesis, a model has been developed in which accumulated alterations include at least one dominantly acting oncogene and several tumor-suppressor genes (46). These same studies provided evidence for the progressive nature of genetic changes in carcinogenesis. Loss of heterozygosity in these and other types of tumors always results in loss of one of a pair of restriction fragments, that is, the same allele (e.g., *p53*) in all of the cells is evidence of clonality. The clonal origin of colorectal tumors in female patients with cancer has been more convincingly demonstrated by differential methylation. Inactivation of the X chromosome (by methylation) during embryogenesis is random so polyclonal female tissues develop with an approximately equal complement of inactivated maternal and paternal X chromosomes. If the tissues are monoclonal, the same inactive X chromosome should be present in all of the cells. By using a DNA–restriction fragment length polymorphism–based strategy, all of the colorectal tumors were found to be monoclonal, and 95% of all human tumors so far studied, including leukemias, have proved to be monoclonal (46, 180).

In chimeric or mosaic mice that differentially express isozymes of glucose phosphate isomerase or 3-phosphate kinase, a range of different carcinogens and initiation/promotion treatment regimes have been used to produce tumors that are monoclonal. Thus, the polyclonal tissues of the animals express more than one isotype, and the tumor tissues express a single isotype, indicating monoclonality. In a few rare cases, polyclonal tumors were observed, probably because of the coalescence of two or more neighboring primary tumors. In experiments where the isozyme type was monitored at various stages in development, the malignant phenotype was always found to contain the same isotype as the benign papillomas. When human tumors have been examined in mosaic individuals, evidence for monoclonality is most often found.

Chemical and Viral Interactions

A distinction between viral and chemical carcinogenesis was made almost 50 years ago, and these seminal studies paved the way for the multistage theory of carcinogenesis (16, 149, 150). Once inside a cell, certain viruses can integrate into the genome, and depending on their site of entry into the genome, they can potentially activate proto oncogenes and/or inactivate tumor-suppressor genes. Because viruses are able to act at every stage of carcinogenesis in this way, it is reasonable that chemicals and viruses may have interactive effects in certain forms of carcinogenesis. There now is good evidence from experiments with in vivo experimental systems that viruses and chemicals also can interact in a synergistic manner (71). The causation of cancer by purely chemical means previously has been discussed, and a number of studies clearly have demonstrated that certain forms of cancer have a viral etiology, including Burkitt's lymphoma and T-cell leukemia (see Chapters 20–23 and 147).

A number of human cancers now are considered to have both a viral and a chemical component to their etiology. These include hepatitis B virus and aflatoxin B_1 or alcoholic beverages in hepatocellular carcinoma, Epstein-Barr virus and *N*-nitrosamines in nasopharyngeal carcinoma, and human papilloma virus and tobacco smoke components in cancers of the uterine cervix, oral cavity, and larynx (66, 67, 72). These studies have provided evidence of an association between environmental agents and carcinogenesis, but association does not imply causation.

In essence chemicals can act as tumor promoters following tumor initiation by viral agents, and viruses can act as promoters following chemical initiation. Cells that are pretreated with chemical carcinogens (benzo[*a*]pyrene, 4-nitroquinoline-*N*-oxide, 3-methylcholanthrene or thymidine analogues) have been shown to be morphologically transformed more easily by SV40. Similarly, enhanced transformation by other viruses (adenovirus SA7, mutant adenovirus type 5, or herpes simplex virus type 2) also has been observed following pretreatment with several polycyclic aromatic hydrocarbons. In other cases, alkylating agents have been used (methylmethane sulphate) before infection with wild-type adenovirus 5 as a regimen to morphologically transform rat-embryo fibroblast cells in culture.

Human epithelial cells in vitro have proved to be more difficult for the study of chemical–viral interactions. Some reports exist where viruses (SV40 or Epstein-Barr) have been used first to immortalize the cells, and chemicals (3-methylcholanthrene or *N*-acetoxy-2-acetylaminofluorene) have been used to cause neoplastic transformation of the immortalized cells (96). In Epstein-Barr–immortalized B lymphocytes, however, *N*-methyl-*N*-nitrosoguanidine treatment failed to cause neoplastic transformation. Taken together, these studies may indicate that immortalization is required before malignant progression can occur and that more than one gene is involved; however, it is difficult to assess the relevance of such an immortalization step to human carcinogenesis in vivo.

Implications for Molecular Epidemiology, Risk Assessment, and Cancer Prevention

Increased understanding of the mechanisms of carcinogenesis has led to strategies for human cancer risk assessment (70, 182, 189). These studies extend to the measurement of carcinogen–macromolecular adducts present in a target organ or surrogate and of phenotypic determinants of disease disposition. The exposure of laboratory animals or cells in culture to chemical carcinogens has been shown to result in the formation of carcinogen–macromolecular adducts, and this suggests that it is reasonable to seek evidence for the presence of adducts in human tissues.

The biologically effective dose of a chemical carcinogen is governed by the amount that reaches a target tissue in a form that becomes activated in that tissue to a chemical species capable of causing lesions in DNA (130). Because chemical carcinogens in the human environment usually are not radioactive, and because humans most commonly are exposed to complex mixtures of chemicals, human carcinogen dosimetry at the molecular level requires sensitive and specific methods for carcinogen–macromolecular adduct quantitation. The low levels of adducts that are present in human DNA samples challenge the detection limits of conventional assay systems, and complex mixtures of adducted materials confound simple assay systems.

Several different methods have been developed for carcinogen–DNA dosimetry in humans. Specifically, the most commonly used techniques for adduct measurement are ^{32}P-nucleotide postlabeling, immunoassays, fluorescence spectroscopy, electrochemical conductance, and gas chromatography/mass spectroscopy. Each of these techniques currently has its own advantages and limitations, and within the framework of epidemiologic surveys, multiple corroborative end-point analyses seem to provide the most useful information. These methodologies, their application, and their limitations are reviewed extensively elsewhere (137, 182, 184, 186, 190).

Correlation of carcinogen–DNA adduct levels determined in humans with putative environmental exposure rarely has been shown in a convincing fashion. Probably the best example is the correlation of aflatoxin–DNA adducts that have been measured in urine samples from people in Africa. Aflatoxin–albumin adducts also correlated well with both exposure and 6-hydroxycortisol levels, indicating a role for CYP3A4 in aflatoxin activation (58, 140, 147). Measurements of polycyclic aromatic hydrocarbon–DNA adducts in the peripheral white blood cells of occupationally exposed people have shown that this approach to human biomonitoring is feasible. Further research and development is required, however, to establish reliable methods (159, 182). Studies to measure 4-aminobiphenyl-hemoglobin adducts have shown a dose-response relationship have shown between the extent of smoking, type of tobacco used, and adduct levels (28, 178).

Assays for human cancer risk assessment that include the use of indicator drugs are complementary to adduct studies because of the implications for biologically effective dose following exposure (137). For example, an innocuous xenobiotic that shares the same pathway of metabolism as a known or suspect carcinogen, caffeine, is an indicator of carcinogenic arylamine metabolism. Polymorphisms in xenobiotic metabolism may be determined by administration of an indicator drug and urinalysis to measure the metabolic ratio that characterizes the metabolic phenotype. Measures of metabolic ratio are the ratio between excretion of the unaltered drug to its metabolites or a ratio of excreted metabolites. Caffeine is demethylated by the action of cytochrome CYP1A2 (29, 59). The metabolites that are formed include theophylline (1,3-dimethylxanthine), paraxanthine (1,7-

dimethylxanthine), theobromine (3,7-dimethylxanthine), and 1,3,7-trimethyluric acid. The formation of paraxanthine, or demethylation of caffeine at the 3-position by CYP1A2, has been found to correlate highly with metabolic *N*-oxidation of primary arylamines (e.g., the carcinogen, 4-aminobiphenyl, that is found in cigarette smoke and food items). *N*-acetyltransferase, which leads to the acetylation of primary arylamines, is an enzyme that competes with P-450 demethylation. It also is possible to discriminate between the slow and fast acetylator phenotypes by measuring other caffeine metabolites in urine. This is achieved by the determination of the ratio of 5-acetyl-6-formylamino-3-methyluracil to 1-methylxanthine. Therefore, determination of caffeine metabolic ratios in humans may be useful in assessing the cancer risk of individuals with environmental exposures to aromatic amines in conjunction with genetic factors.

The extensive metabolizer phenotype of debrisoquine, which is an antihypertensive drug that is cleared through ring hydroxylation by the hepatic cytochrome CYP2D6, correlates with the risk of lung cancer (8, 32, 107). People who are extensive metabolizers of debrisoquine therefore appear to be at significantly greater risk of lung cancer than are poor metabolizers. There are two possible explanations for these findings, it has been hypothesized that CYP2D6 may activate a chemical carcinogen found in tobacco smoke; alternately, CYP2D6 may be in linkage disequilibrium with a lung-cancer-susceptibility gene. Even though the mechanistic basis for this association is obscure, the debrisoquine polymorphism still might prove to be a valuable tool in risk assessment. Accordingly, research efforts in this area are continuing, including further epidemiologic studies to firmly establish the association and carcinogen metabolism studies aimed at determinating a mechanistic basis for this association. With the cloning of this gene, molecular studies for the development of a genotyping test also could result in a better understanding of debrisoquine-metabolizer disposition as a risk factor in lung carcinogenesis (78, 84).

A number of other polymorphisms in carcinogen-metabolizing genes that can be detected by Southern hybridization or the polymerase chain reaction also have been described. These include polymorphisms in the *CYP1A1, CYP2E1*, glutathione-S-transferase (*GST*) and *N*-acetyltransferase (*NAT*) genes (15, 72, 131, 153, 157, 176). Several reports also claim that inheritance of specific genotypes confers susceptibility to lung, esophagus and bladder cancer, whereas others are contradictory (3, 14, 15, 21, 44, 80, 83, 90, 91, 94, 100, 119, 129, 141, 152, 193). More recently, a number of studies have correlated measures of carcinogen–DNA adduct levels with genotype; these studies are intended to more clearly elucidate the mechanistic basis for exposure–disease associations and gene–environment interactions (156).

Epidemiologic and pharmacogenetic studies have postulated the existence of an inherited predisposition for human lung and other cancers, and certain genetic polymorphisms have been suggested to be associated with risk in human lung carcinogenesis. For DNA–restriction fragment length polymorphisms at the human *HRAS-1*, *p53*, and *L-myc* loci, rare or minor restriction fragments (i.e., alleles) may either predispose to certain cancers (169, 183) or are associated with poor prognosis (92, 120). A variable, tandem repeat DNA-sequence region tightly flanked by MspI restriction sites, which is located 1.4 kb distal (3′) to the cellular *HRAS-1* structural proto-oncogene (chromosome locus 11p15.5) (31, 48), accounts for the DNA–restriction fragment length polymorphism. For *p53*, a codon 72 polymorphism in exon 4 results in either an arginine or a proline variant (5, 42). In the case of L-*myc*, the presence or absence of an EcoRI restriction site in the second intron of the gene defines a simple polymorphism. Hypotheses that rare or minor variants of these three genes might influence susceptibility to lung cancer have been tested in case-control studies (169, 175, 183, 185). Individuals with rare allelomorphs at the *HRAS-1* proto-oncogene locus have been found to be at greater risk of lung and breast cancer (53, 102, 169). No firm mechanistic basis is known for these associations, but the tandem repeat region may be sensitive to mitotic recombination and, consequently, a target for chemical carcinogens. Data for *p53* gene polymorphisms are equivocal. Some studies have suggested an increased risk of lung and colon cancer, whereas others have been negative (91, 183, 185). Most recently, studies of the *p53* locus have claimed that haplotypes rather than individual polymorphisms are more appropriate indicators of cancer risk (161, 162). No association was found with increased risk of metastasis and the L-*myc* proto-oncogene polymorphism (175). The allelic frequency distribution for all three of these polymorphisms (*HRAS-1, p53* and L-*myc*) was found to vary significantly with race (169, 183, 185).

The goal of molecular epidemiology is to identify individuals who are at increased risk of cancer by obtaining evidence of high exposure to carcinogens leading to pathobiologic lesions in target cells and/or increased susceptibility to cancer from either inherited or acquired host factors. Variation among individuals in carcinogen biodistribution, metabolism, DNA-adduct formation, DNA repair, and potential response to tumor promoters have important implications in determinating cancer risk. An increased understanding of the molecular basis of these differences among humans and their connection with critical steps in carcinogenesis may assist in future predictions of disease risk for an individual before the clinical onset of disease (65).

The two facets of molecular epidemiology of human cancer risk are the assessment of carcinogen exposure and inherited or acquired host cancer-susceptibility factors (63, 129). The interaction between these two facets determines cancer risk. When combined with carcinogen bioassays in laboratory animals and classical epidemiology, molecular epidemiology can contribute to the four traditional aspects of cancer risk assessment: (*a*) hazard identification, (*b*) dose-response assessment, (*c*) exposure assessment, and (*d*) risk characterization. Important bioethical considerations accompany the identification of high-risk individuals; these include autonomy, privacy, justice, and equity. Benefits of the knowledge of risk for the individual may be offset by specific concerns relating to that individual's responsibility to family members and pychosocial anxiety regarding the genetic testing of children. Therefore, the uncertainty of current individual risk assessments and the limited availability of genetic counseling services dictate caution. In addition, it is widely held that genetic testing should be restricted to those situations that are amenable to preventative or therapeutic intervention (111).

References

1. Adamson RH. Induction of hepatocellular carcinoma in nonhuman primates by chemical carcinogens. Cancer Detect Prev 1989;14:215.
2. Aguilar F, Hussain SP, Cerutti P. Aflatoxin B_1 induces the transversion of G→T in codon 249 of the *p53* tumor-suppressor gene in human hepatocytes. Proc Natl Acad Sci USA 1993;90:8586.
3. Alexandrie AK, Sundberg MI, Seidegard J, Tornling G, Rannug A. Genetic susceptibility to lung cancer with special emphasis on CYP1A1 and GST-M1: a study on host factors in relation to age at onset, gender and histological cancer types. Carcinogenesis 1994;15:1785.
4. Amstad P, Reddel RR, Pfeifer A, Malan-Shibley L, Mark GE, Harris CC. Neoplastic transformation of a human bronchial epithelial cell line by a recombinant retrovirus encoding viral harvey *ras*. Mol Carcinogenesis 1988;1:151.
5. Ara S, Lee PS, Hansen MF, Saya H. Codon 72 polymorphism of the TP53 gene. Nucleic Acids Res 1990;18:4961.
6. Ashendel CL. The phorbol ester receptor: a phospholipid-regulated protein kinase. Biochim Biophys Acta 1985;822:219.
7. Avruch J, Zhang XF, Kyriakis JM. *Raf* and *ras*: completing the framework of a signal transduction pathway. Trends Biochem Sci 1994;19:279.
8. Ayesh R, Idle JR, Ritchie JC, Crothers MJ, Hetzel MR. Metabolic oxidation phenotypes as markers for susceptibility to lung cancer. Nature 1984;312:169.
9. Baker SJ, Fearon ER, Nigro JM, Hamilton SR, Preisinger AC, Jessup JM, van Tuinen P, Ledbetter DH, Barker DF, Nakamura Y. Chromosome 17 deletions and *p53* gene mutations in colorectal carcinomas. Science 1989;244:217.
10. Barbacid M. Involvement of *ras* oncogenes in the initiation of carcinogen-induced tumors. Int Symp Princess Takamatsu Cancer Res Fund 1986;17:43.
11. Bartsch H, Ohshima H, Shuker DE, Pignatelli B, Calmels S. Exposure of humans to endogenous *N*-nitroso compounds: implications in cancer etiology. Mutat Res 1990;238:255.
12. Beland FA, Kadlubar FF. Formation and persistence of arylamine DNA adducts in vivo. Environ Health Perspect 1985;62:19.
13. Beland FA, Poirier MC. DNA adducts and carcinogenesis. In: Sirica AE, ed. The Pathobiology of Neoplasia. New York: Plenum, 1989:p 57.
14. Bell D, Taylor J, Paulson D, Robertson D, Mohler J, Lucier G. Genetic risk and carcinogen exposure: a common inherited defect of the carcinogen-metabolism gene glutathione-S-transferase M1 (GSTM1) that increases susceptibility to bladder cancer. JNCI 1993;85:1159.
15. Bell DA, Thompson CL, Taylor J, Miller CR, Perera F, Hsieh LL, Lucier GW. Genetic monitoring of human polymorphic cancer susceptibility genes by polymerase chain reaction: application to glutathione transferase mu. Environ Health Perspect 1992;98:113.
16. Berenblum I, Shubik P. A new quantitative approach to the study of the stages of chemical carcinogenesis in the mouse skin. Br J Cancer 1947;1:383.
17. Birt DF, Kris ES, Choe M, Pelling JC. Dietary energy and fat effects on tumor promotion. Cancer Res 1992;52:2035S.
18. Blumberg PM. In vitro studies on the mode of action of the phorbol esters, potent tumor promoters, part 2. CRC Crit Rev Toxicol 1981;8:199.
19. Bohr VA. Gene specific DNA repair. Carcinogenesis 1991;12:1983.
20. Bohr VA, Evans MK, Fornace AJ Jr. Biology of disease. DNA repair and its pathogenetic implications. Lab Invest 1989;61:143.
21. Bonney GE. Interactions of genes, environment, and life-style in lung cancer development. JNCI 1990;82:1236.
22. Borgen A, Darvey H, Castagnoli N, Crocker TT, Rasmussen RE, Wang IY. Metabolic conversion of benzo[a]pyrene by Syrian hamster liver microsomes and binding of metabolites to deoxyribonucleic acid. J Med Chem 1973;16:502.
23. Boutwell RK. Some biological aspects of skin carcinogenesis. Prog Exp Tumor Res 1964;4:207.
24. Brash DE, Rudolph JA, Simon JA, Mckenna GJ, Baden HP, Halperin AJ, Ponten J. A role for sunlight in skin cancer: UV-induced *p53* mutations in squamous cell carcinoma. Proc Natl Acad Sci USA 1991;88:10124.
25. Brennan JA, Boyle JO, Koch WM, Goodman SN, Hruban RH, Eby YJ, Couch MJ, Forastiere AA, Sidransky D. Association between cigarette smoking and mutation of the *p53* gene in squamous cell carcinoma of the head and neck. N Engl J Med 1995;332:712.
26. Bressac B, Kew M, Wands J, Ozturk M. Selective G to T mutations of *p53* hepatocellular carcinoma from southern Africa. Nature 1991;350:429.
27. Bronner CE, Baker SM, Morrison PT, et al. Mutation in the DNA mismatch repair gene homologue hMLH1 is associated with hereditary non-polyposis colon cancer. Nature 1994;368:258.
28. Bryant MS, Vineis P, Skipper PL, Tannenbaum SR. Hemoglobin adducts of aromatic amines: associations with smoking status and type of tobacco. Proc Natl Acad Sci USA 1988;85:9788.
29. Butler MA, Iwasaki M, Guengerich FP, Kadlubar FF. Human cytochrome P-450m PA (P-450IA2), the phenacetin O-deethylase, is primarily responsible for the hepatic 3-demethylation of caffeine and N-oxidation of carcinogenic arylamines. Proc Natl Acad Sci USA 1989;86:7696.
30. Cairns J. Mutation selection and the natural history of cancer. Nature 1975;255:197.
31. Capon DJ, Chen EY, Levinson AD, Seeburg PH, Goeddel DV. Complete nucleotide sequences of the T24 human bladder carcinoma oncogene and its normal homologue. Nature 1983;302:33.
32. Caporaso NE, Tucker MA, Hoover R, Hayes RB, Pickle LW, Issaq H, Muschik G, Green-Gallo L, Buivys D, Aisner S, Resau J, Trump BF, Tollerud D, Weston A, Harris CC. Lung cancer and the debrisoquine metabolic phenotype. JNCI 1990;85:1264.
33. Carrier F, Chang CY, Duh JL, Nebert DW, Puga A. Interaction of the regulatory domains of the murine CYP1A1 gene with two DNA-binding proteins in addition to the Ah receptor and the Ah receptor nuclear translocator (ARNT). Biochem Pharmocol 1994;48:1767.
34. Cartwright RA, Glashan RW, Rogers HJ, Ahmad RA, Barham-Hall D, Higgins E, Kahn MA. Role of *N*-acetyltransferase phenotypes in bladder carcinogenesis: a pharmacogenetic epidemiological approach to bladder cancer. Lancet 1982;ii:842.
35. Cavenee WK, Dryja TP, Phillips RA, Benedict WF, Godbout R, Gallie BL, Murphree AL, Strong LC, White RL. Expression of recessive alleles by chromosomal mechanisms in retinoblastoma. Nature 1983;305:779.
36. Cavenee WK, Hansen MF, Nordenskjold M, Kock E, Maumenee I, Squire JA, Phillips RA, Gallie BL. Genetic origin of mutations predisposing to retinoblastoma. Science 1985;228:501.
37. Choe M, Kris ES, Luthra R, Copenhaver J, Pelling JC, Donnelly TE, Birt DF. Protein kinase C is activated and diacylglycerol is elevated in epidemal cells from Sencar mice fed high fat diets. J Nutr 1992;122:2322.
38. Cohen P, Holmes CF, Tsukitani Y. Okadaic acid: a new probe for the study of cellular regulation. Trends Biochem Sci 1990;15:98.
39. Conney AH. Induction of microsomal enzymes by foreign chemicals and carcinogenesis by polycyclic aromatic hydrocarbons: G.H A. Clowes Memorial Lecture. Cancer Res 1982;42:4875.
40. Cooper CS, Grover PL, Sims P. The metabolism and activation of benzo[*a*]pyrene. In: Bridges JW, Chasseaud L, eds. Progress in Drug Metabolism. New York: Wiley, 1983:p 295.
41. Coussens L, Parker PJ, Rhee L, Yang-Feng TL, Chen E, Waterfield MD, Francke U, Ullrich A. Multiple, distinct forms of bovine and human protein kinase C suggest diversity in cellular signaling pathways. Science 1986;233:859.
42. de la Calle-Martin O, Fabregat V, Romero M, Soler J, Vives J, Yague J. AccII polymorphism of the *p53* gene. Nucleic Acids Res 1990;18:4963.
43. Dlugosz AA, Mischak H, Mushinski JF, Yuspa SH. Transcripts encoding protein kinase C-α, -δ, -ϵ, -ζ, and -σ are expressed in basal and differentiating mouse keratinocytes in vitro and exhibit quantitative changes in neoplastic cells. Molecular Carcinogenesis 1992;5:286.
44. Drakoulis N, Cascorbi I, Brockmoller J, gross, CR, Roots I. Polymorphisms in the human CYP1A1 gene as susceptibility factors for lung cancer: exon-7 mutation (4889 A to G), and a T to C mutation in the 3″-flanking region. Clin Invest 1994;72:240.
45. Fearon ER, Cho KR, Nigro JM, Kern SE, Simons JW, Ruppert JM, Hamilton SR, Preisinger AC, Thomas G, Kinzler KW, Vogelstein B. Identification of a chromosome 18q gene that is altered in colorectal cancers. Science 1990;247:49.
46. Fearon ER, Hamilton SR, Vogelstein B. Clonal analysis of human colorectal tumors. Science 1987;238:193.
47. Fearon ER, Vogelstein B. A genetic model for colorectal tumorigenesis. Cell 1990;61:759.
48. Feinberg AP, Vogelstein B. Hypomethylation of *ras* oncogenes in primary human cancers. Biochem Biophys Res Commun 1983;111:47.
49. Felton JS, Knize MG, Shen NH, Wu R, Becher G. Mutagenic heterocyclic imidazoamines in cooked foods. In: King CM, Romano LJ, Schuetzle D, eds. Carcinogenic and Mutagenic Responses to Aromatic Amines and Nitroarenes. New York: Elsevier, 1988:p 73.
50. Finney RE, Bishop JM. Predisposition to neoplastic transformation caused by gene replacement of *H-ras1*. Science 1993;260:1524.
51. Fishel R, Lescoe MK, Rao MR, Copeland NG, Jenkins NA, Garber J, Kane M, Kolodner R. The human mutator gene homolog MSH2 and its association with hereditary nonpolyposis colon cancer. (Erratum. Cell 1994;77:167.) Cell 1993;75:1215.
52. Floyd RA, Watson JJ, Harris J, West M, Wong PK. Formation of 8-hydroxydeoxyguanosine, hydroxyl free radical adduct of DNA in granulocytes exposed to the tumor promoter, tetradecanoylphorbolacetate. Biochem Biophys Res Commun 1986;137:841.
53. Garrett PA, Hulka BS, Kim YL, Farber RA. HRAS protooncogene polymorphism and breast cancer. Cancer Epidemiol Biomarkers Prev 1993;2:131.
54. Gonzalez FJ. The molecular biology of cytochrome P-450s. Pharmacol Rev 1988;40:243.
55. Gonzalez FJ. Molecular genetics of the P-450 superfamily. Pharmacol Ther 1990;45:1.
56. Greenblatt MS, Bennett WP, Hollstein M, Harris CC. Mutations in the *p53* tumor suppressor gene: clues to cancer etiology and molecular pathogenesis. Cancer Res 1994;54:4855.
57. Groopman JD, Donahue PR, Zhu JQ, Chen JS, Wogan GN. Aflatoxin metabolism in humans: detection of metabolites and nucleic acid adducts in urine by affinity chromatography. Proc Natl Acad Sci USA 1985;82:6492.
58. Groopman JD, Sabbioni G, Wild CP. Molecular dosimetry of human aflatoxin exposures. In: Groopman P, Skipper P, eds. Molecular Dosimetry of Human Cancer: Epidemiological, Analytical, and Social Considerations. New Jersey: Telford, 1991.
59. Guengerich FP. Characterization of human microsomal cytochrome P-450 enzymes. Annu Rev Pharmacol Toxicol 1989;29:241.
60. Guengerich FP. Metabolic activation of carcinogens. Pharm Ther 1992;54:17.
61. Hanawalt PC. Preferential DNA repair in expressed genes. Environ. Health Perspect 1987;76:9.
62. Harper JR, Roop DR, Yuspa SH. Transfection of the EJ *rasHa* gene into keratinocytes derived from carcinogen-induced mouse papillomas causes malignant progression. Mol Cell Biol 1986;6:3144.
63. Harris CC. Chemical and physical carcinogenesis: advances and perspectives. Cancer Res 1991;51:5023S.
64. Harris CC. Interindividual variation among humans in carcinogen metabolism, DNA adduct formation and DNA repair. Carcinogenesis 1989;10:1563.
65. Harris CC. Interindividual variation in human chemical carcinogenesis: implications for risk assessment. In: Moolgavkar SH, ed. Scientific Issues in Quantitative Risk Assessment. Boston: Birkhauser, 1990, p 235.
66. Harris CC. Hepatocellular carcinogenesis: recent advances and speculations. Cancer Cells 1990;2:146.
67. Harris CC. Solving the viral-chemical puzzle of human liver carcinogenesis. Cancer Epidemiol Biomarkers Prev 1994;3:1.
68. Harris CC, Hollstein M. Clinical implications of the *p53* tumor-suppressor gene. N Engl J Med 1993;329:1318.
69. Harris CC, Reddel RR, Pfeifer A, Amstad P, Mark GE, Weston A, Modali R, Iman DS, McMenamin MG, Kaighn ME, Gabrielson EW, Jones R, Trump BF. Oncogenes and tumor-suppressor genes in human lung carcinogenesis. In: Harris CC, Liotta LA, eds. Genetic Mechanisms in Carcinogenesis and Tumor Progression. New York: Wiley-Liss, 1990, p 127.

70. Harris CC, Weston A, Willey JC, Trivers GE, Mann DL. Biochemical and molecular epidemiology of human cancer: indicators of carcinogen exposure, DNA damage, and genetic predisposition. Environ Health Perspect 1987;75:109.
71. Haugen A, Harris CC. Interactive effects between viruses and chemical carcinogens. In: Cooper CS, Grover PL, eds. Carcinogenesis and Mutagenesis, Handbook of Experimental Pharmacology. London: Springer-Verlag 1990, p 249.
72. Hayashi S, Watanabe J, Kawajiri K. High susceptibility to lung cancer analyzed in terms of combined genotypes of CYP1A1 and mu-class GST genes. Jpn J Cancer Res 1992;83:866.
73. Hayashi, S-I, Watanabe J, Nakachi K, Eguchi H, Gotoh O, Kawajiri K. Interindividual difference in expression of human Ah receptor and related P-450 genes. Carcinogenesis 1994;15:801.
74. Hecht SS, Foiles PG, Carmella SG, Trushin N, Rivenson A, Hoffmann D. Recent studies on the metabolic activation of tobacco-specific nitrosamines: prospects for dosimetry in humans. In: Hoffmann D, Harris CC, eds. Banbury Report 23: Mechanisms in Tobacco Carcinogenesis. New York: Cold Spring Harbor Laboratory, 1986, p 245.
75. Hecht SS, Hoffmann D. The relevance of tobacco-specific nitrosamines to human cancer. Cancer Surv 1989;8:273.
76. Hecht SS, Hoffmann D. Tobacco-specific nitrosamines, an important group of carcinogens in tobacco and tobacco smoke. Carcinogenesis 1988;9:875.
77. Hecht SS, Trushin N, Castonguay A, Rivenson A. Comparative tumorigenicity and DNA methylation in F344 rats by 4-(methylnitrosamino)-1-(3-pyridyl)-1-butanone and *N*-nitrosodimethylamine. Cancer Res 1986;46:498.
78. Heim M, Meyer UA. Genotyping of poor metabolizers of debrisoquine by allele-specific PCR amplification. Lancet 1990;336:529.
79. Hertzog PJ, Smith JR, Garner RC. Characterisation of the imidazole ring-opened forms of *trans*-8,9-dihydro-8,9-dihydro-8-(7-guanyl)9-hydroxy aflatoxin B1. Carcinogenesis 1982;3:723.
80. Hirvonen A, Husgafvel-Pursiainen K, Karjalainen A, Antilla S, Vainio H. Point-mutational MspI and Ile-Val polymorphisms closely linked in the CYP1A1 gene: lack of association with susceptibility to lung cancer in a Finnish study population. Cancer Epidemiol Biomarkers Prev 1992;1:485.
81. Hollstein M, Sidransky D, Vogelstein B, Harris CC. *p53* mutations in human cancers. Science 1991;253:49.
82. Hsu IC, Metcalf RA, Sun T, Welsh JA, Wang NJ, Harris CC. Mutational hotspot in the p53 gene in human hepatocellular carcinomas. Nature 1991;350:427.
83. Ichiba M, Hagmar L, Rannug A, Hogstedt B, Alexandrie AK, Carstensen U, Hemminki K. Aromatic DNA adducts, micronuclei and genetic polymorphism for CYP1A1 and GST1 in chimney sweeps. Carcinogenesis 1994;15:1347.
84. Idle JR, Armstrong M, Boddy AV, Boustead C, Cholerton S, Cooper J, Daly AK, Ellis J, Gregory W, Hadidi H, et al. The pharmacogenetics of chemical carcinogenesis. Pharmacogenetics 1992;2:246.
85. Ilett KF, David BM, Detchon P, Castleden WM, Kwa R. Acetylation phenotype in colorectal carcinoma. Cancer Res 1987;47:1466.
86. International Agency for Research on Cancer. IARC Monographs on the Evaluation of Carcinogenic Risks to Humans. Overall Evaluations of Carcinogenicity: an Updating of IARC Monographs Volumes 1 to 42. Lyon: IARC, 1987.
87. Jaiswal AK, Nebert DW. Two RFLPs associated with the human P_1450 gene linked to the *MP1* locus on chromosome 15. Nucleic Acids Res 1986;14:4376.
88. Jin X, Nguyen D, Zhang, W-W, Kyritsis P, Roth J. Cell cycle arrest and inhibition of tumor cell proliferation by the $P16^{INK4}$ gene mediated by an adenovirus vector. Cancer Res 1995;55:3250.
89. Kato R. Metabolic activation of mutagenic heterocyclic aromatic amines from protein pyrolysates. Crit Rev Toxicol 1986;16:307.
90. Kato S, Shields PG, Caporaso NE, Hoover RN, Trump BF, Sugimura H, Weston A, Harris CC. Cytochrome P450IIE1 genetic polymorphisms, racial variation, and lung cancer risk. Cancer Res 1992;52:6712.
91. Kawajiri K, Nakachi K, Imai K, Watanabe J, Hayashi S. Germ line polymorphisms of *p53* and CYP1A1 genes involved in human lung cancer. Carcinogenesis 1993;14:1085.
92. Kawashima K, Shikama H, Imoto K, Izawa M, Naruke T, Okabayashi K, Nishimura S. Close correlation between restriction fragment length polymorphism of the L-MYC gene and metastasis of human lung cancer to the lymph nodes and other organs. Proc Natl Acad Sci USA 1988;85:2353.
93. Kazanietz MG, Lewin NE, Gao F, Pettit GR, Blumberg PM. Binding of [26-^{3}H]bryostatin 1 and analogs to calcium-dependent and calcium-independent protein kinase C isozymes. Mol Pharmacol 1994;46:374.
94. Kelsey KT, Wiencke JK, Spitz MR. A race-specific genetic polymorphism in the *CYP1A1* gene is not associated with lung cancer in African Americans. Carcinogenesis, 1994;15:1121.
95. Kennaway E. The identification of a carcinogenic compound in coal tar. BMJ 1955;2:749.
96. Kessler DJ, Heilman CA, Cossman J, Maguire RT, Thorgeirsson SS. Transformation of Epstein-Barr virus immortalized human B-cells by chemical carcinogens. Cancer Res 1987;47:527.
97. Kinzler KW, Nilbert MC, Vogelstein B, Bryan TM, Levy DB, Kelly JS, Pressinger AC, Hamilton SR, Hedge P, Markham A, Carlson M, Joslyn G, Groden J, White R, Miki Y, Miyoshi Y, Nishisho I, Nakamura Y. Identification of a gene located at chromosome 5q21 that is mutated in colorectal cancers. Science 1991;251:1366.
98. Knopf JL, Lee MH, Sultzman LA, Kriz RW, Loomis CR, Hewick RM, Bell RM. Cloning and expression of multiple protein kinase C cDNAs. Cell 1986;46:491.
99. Koufos A, Hansen MF, Lampkin BC, Workman ML, Copeland NG, Jenkins NA, Cavenee WK. Loss of alleles at loci on human chromosome 11 during genesis of Wilms' tumour. Nature 1984;309:170.
100. Kouri RE, McKinney CE, Slomianry DJ, et al. Positive correlation between high aryl hydrocarbon hydroxylase activity and primary lung cancer as analyzed in cryopreserved lymphocytes. Cancer Res 1982;42:5030.
101. Krontiris TG. Oncogenes. N Engl J Med 1995;333:303.
102. Krontiris TG, Devlin B, Karp DD, Robert NJ, Risch N. An association between the risk of cancer and mutations in the HRAS-1 minisatellite locus [see comments]. N Engl J Med 1993;329:517.
103. LaForgia S, Morse B, Cannizzaro LA, Li F, Nowell PC, Boghosian-Sell L, Glick J, Weston A, Harris CC, Drabkin H, Patterson D, Croce CM, Schlesinger J, Huebner K. Receptor-linker protein-tyrosine-phosphatase, PTP-γ, is a candidate tumor suppressor at human chromosome region 3p21. Proc Natl Acad Sci USA 1991;88:5036.
104. Lane DP, Benchimol S. *p53*: oncogene or anti-oncogene. Genes Dev 1990;4:1.
105. Lang NP, Chu DZ, Hunter CF, Kendall DC, Flammang TJ, Kadlubar FF. Role of aromatic amine acetyltransferase in human colorectal cancer. Arch Surg 1986;121:1259.
106. Latif F, Tory K, Gnarra J, et al. Identification of the von Hippel Lindau disease tumor suppressor gene. Science 1993;260:1317.
107. Law MR, Hetzel MR, Idle JR. Debrisoquine metabolism and genetic predisposition to lung cancer. Br J Cancer 1989;59:686.
108. Leach FS, Nicolaides NC, Papadopoulos N, Liu B, Jen J, Parsons R, Peltomaki P, Sistonen P, Aaltonen LA, et al. Mutations of a mutS homolog in hereditary nonpolyposis colorectal cancer. Cell 1993;75:1215.
109. Leone A, McBride WO, Weston A, Wang M, Anglard P, Cropp CS, Goepel JR, Lidereau R, Callahan R, Linehan WM, Rees RC, Harris CC, Liotta LA, Steeg PS. Somatic allelic deletion of nm23 in human cancer. Cancer Res 1991;51:2490.
110. Levine AJ, Momand J, Finlay CA. The *p53* tumor-suppressor gene. Nature 1991;351:453.
111. Li, FP, Garber JE, Friend SH, Strong LC, Patenaude AF, Juengst ET, Reilly PR, Correa P, Fraumeni JF. Recommendations on predictive testing for germ line p53 mutations among cancer-prone individuals. JNCI 1992;84:1156.
112. Loeb LA. Mutator phenotype may be required for multistage carcinogenesis. Cancer Res 1991;51:3075.
113. Loeb LA, Cheng KC. Errors in DNA synthesis: a source of spontaneous mutations. Mutat Res 1990;238:297.
114. Marra G, Boland CR. Hereditary nonpolyposis colorectal cancer: the syndrome, the genes and historical perspectives. JNCI 1995;87:1114.
115. Marshall CJ, Vousden KH, Phillips DH. Activation of c-Ha-*ras*-1 proto-oncogene by in vitro modification with a chemical carcinogen, benzo[*a*]pyrene diol-epoxide. Nature 1984;310:586.
116. McCormick F. *ras* GTPase activating protein: signal transmitter and signal terminator. Cell 1989;56:5.
117. McGuire WL, Naylor SL. Loss of heterozygosity in breast cancer: cause or effect [editorial; comment]. JNCI 1989;81:1764.
118. Miller JA. Carcinogenesis by chemicals: an overview—GHA Clowes memorial lecture. Cancer Res 1970;30:559.
119. Nakachi K, Imai K, Hayashi S, Watanabi J, Kawajiri K. Genetic susceptibility to squamous cell carcinoma of the lung in relation to cigarette smoking dose. Cancer Res 1991;51:5177.
120. Nau MM, Brooks BJ, Jr, Battey JF, Sausville E, Gazdar AF, Kirsch IR, McBride OW, Bertness V, Hollis GF, Minna JD. L-*myc*, a new *myc*-related gene amplified and expressed in human small cell lung cancer. Nature 1985;318:69.
121. Nebert DW, Negishi M. Multiple forms of cytochrome P-450 and the importance of molecular biology and evolution. Biochem Pharmacol 1982;31:2311.
122. Nebert DW, Puga A, Vasiliou V. Role of the Ah receptor and the dioxin inducible [Ah] gene battery in toxicity, cancer, and signal transduction. Ann NY Acad Sci 1992;698:624.
123. Nelson DR, Kamataki T, Waxman DJ, Guengerich FP, Estabrook RW, Feyereisen R, Gonzalez FJ, Coon MJ, Gunsalus IC, Gotoh O, Okuda K, Nebert DW. The P-450 superfamily: update on new sequences, gene mapping, accession numbers, early trivial names of enzymes, and nomenclature. DNA Cell Biol 1993;12:1.
124. Neumann HG. Role of extent and persistence of DNA modifications in chemical carcinogenesis by aromatic amines. Recent Results Cancer Res 1983;84:77.
125. Nigro JM, Baker SJ, Preisinger AC, Jessup JM, Hostetter R, Cleary K, Bigner SH, Davidson N, Baylin S, Devilee P, Glover T, Collins FS, Weston A, Modali R, Harris CC, Vogelstein B. Mutations in the *p53* gene occur in diverse human tumor types. Nature 1989;342:705.
126. Nowell PC, Croce CM. Chromosomal approaches to oncogenes and oncogenesis. FASEB J 1988;2:3054.
127. Oesch F, Aulmann W, Platt KL, Doerjer G. Individual differences in DNA repair capacities in man. Arch Toxicol 1987;10(suppl):172.
128. Olschwang S, Laurent-Puig P, White GR, Thomas G. Germ-line mutations in the first 14 exons of the adenomatous polyposis coli (APC) gene. Am J Hum Genet 1993;52:273.
129. Perera FP, Santella RM. Carcinogenesis. In: Schulte P, Perea FP, eds. Molecular Epidemiology: Principals and Practices. New York: Academic, p 277.
130. Perera FP, Weinstein IB. Molecular epidemiology and carcinogen-DNA adduct detection: new approaches to studies of human cancer causation. J Chronic Dis 1982;35:581.
131. Peters WHM, Wobbes T, Hennie MJR, Jansen, JBMJ. Glutathione-S-transferases in esophageal cancer. Carcinogenesis 1993;14:1377.
132. Petersen DD, McKinney CE, Ikeya K, Smith HH, Bale AE, McBride OW, Nebert DW. Human *CYP1A1* gene: cosegregation of the enzyme inducibility phenotype and an RFLP. Am J Hum Genet 1991;48:720.
133. Peto J. Genetic predisposition to cancer. In: Banbury Report No. 4. New York: Cold Spring Harbor Laboratory, 1980, p 203.
134. Peto R, Roe FJ, Lee PN, Levy L, Clack J. Cancer and ageing in mice and men. Br J Cancer 1975;32:411.
135. Pfeifer A, Mark GE, Malan-Shibley L, Graziano SL, Amstad P, Harris CC. Cooperation of c-*raf*-1 and c-*myc* proto-oncogenes in the neoplastic transformation of SV40 T-antigen immortalized human bronchial epithelial cells. Proc Natl Acad Sci USA 1989;86:10075.
136. Poirier MC, Beland FA. DNA adduct measurements and tumorincidence during chronic carcinogen exposure in animal models: implications for DNA adduct-based human cancer risk assessment. Chem Res Toxicol 1992;5:749.
137. Poirier MC, Weston A. DNA adduct determination in humans. Prog Clin Biol Res 1991;374:205.
138. Ponchel F, Puisieux A, Tabone E, Michot JP, Froschl G, Morel AP, Frebourg T, Fontaniere B, Oberhammer F, Ozturk M. Hepatocarcinoma-specific mutant p53-249ser induces mitotic activity but has no effect on transforming growth factor-β1 mediated apoptosis. Cancer Res 1994;54:2064.
139. Pott P. Chirurgical observations relative to the cancer of the scrotum. London: Hawes, Clark, and Collins, 1775.
140. Qian, G-S, Ross RK, Yu, MC, Yuan, J-M, Gao, Y-T, Henderson BE, Wogan GN, Groop-

man JD. A follow-up study of urinary markers of aflatoxin exposure and liver cancer risk in Shanghai, People's Republic of China. Cancer Epidemiol Biomarkers Prev 1994;3:3.

141. Rebbeck TR, Rosvold EA, Duggan DJ, Zhang J, Buetow KH. Genetics of CYP1A1: coamplification of specific alleles by polymerase chain reaction and association with breast cancer. Cancer Epidemiol Biomarkers Prev 1994;3:511.
142. Reddel RR, Ke, Y, Kaighn ME, Malan-Shibley L, Lechner JF, Rhim JS, Harris CC. Human bronchial epithelial cells neoplastically transformed by v-*Ki-ras*: altered response to inducers of terminal squamous differentiation. Oncogene Res 1988;3:401.
143. Reddy AL, Fialkow PJ. Multicellular origin of fibrosarcomas in mice induced by the chemical carcinogen 3-methylcholanthrene. J Exp Med 1979;150:878.
144. Reddy AL, Fialkow PJ. Papillomas induced by initiation-promotion differ from those induced by carcinogen alone. Nature 1983;304:69.
145. Reddy JK, Lalwani ND. Carcinogenesis by hepatic peroxisome proliferators: evaluation of the risk of hypolipodemic drugs and industrial plasticizers to humans. CRC Crit Rev Toxicol 1984;12:1.
146. Rehn C. Blasengeschwulste bei Fuchsinarbeitern. Arch Klin Chir 1895;50:588.
147. Ross RK, Yuan JM, Yu, MC, Wogan GN, Qian GS, Tu, JT, Groopman JD, Gao YT, Henderson BE. Urinary aflatoxin biomarkers and risk of hepatocellular carcinoma. Lancet 1992;339:943.
148. Rouleau GA, Merel P, Lutchman M, et al. Alteration in a new gene encoding a putative membrane-organizing protein causes neuro-fibromatosis type-2. Nature 1993;363:515.
149. Rous P, Friedwald WF. The effect of chemical carcinogens on virus induced rabbit carcinomas. J Exp Med 1944;79:511.
150. Rous P, Kidd JG. The carcinogenic effect of a papilloma virus on the tarred skin of rabbits. I. Description of the phenomenon. J Exp Med 1938;67:399.
151. Schaeffer L, Roy R, Humbert S, Moncollin V, Vermeulen W, Hoeijmakers JH, Chambon P, Egly JM. DNA repair helicase: a component of BTF2 (TFIIH) basic transcription factor [see comments]. Science 1993;260:58.
152. Seidegard J, Pero R, Markowitz MM, Roush G, Miller DG, Beattie EJ. Isozyme(s) of GST (class-μ) as a marker for the susceptibility to lung cancer.A follow-up study. Carcinogenesis 1990;11:33.
153. Seidegard J, Vorachek WR, Pero RW, Pearson WR. Hereditary differences in the expression of the human glutathione transferase active on trans-stilbene oxide are due to a gene deletion. Proc Natl Acad Sci USA 1988;85:7293.
154. Selby CP, Sancar A. Molecular mechanism of transcription-repair coupling [see comments]. Science 1993;260:53.
155. Setlow RB. Variations in DNA repair among humans. In: Harris CC, Autrup H (eds). Human Carcinogenesis. New York: Academic Press, 1983, p 231.
156. Shields PG, Bowman ED, Harrington AM, Doan VT, Weston A. Polycyclic aromatic hydrocarbon DNA adducts in human lung and cancer susceptibility genes. Cancer Res 1993;53:3486.
157. Shields PG, Caporaso NE, Falk RT, Sugimura H, Trivers GE, Trump BF, Hoover RN, Weston A, Harris CC. Lung cancer, race and a CYP1A1 genetic polymorphism. Cancer Epidemiol Biomarkers Prev 1993;2:481.
158. Shields PG, Harris CC. Environmental causes of cancer. Med Clin North Am 1990;74:263.
159. Shields PG, Weston A, Sugimura H, Bowman ED, Caporaso NE, Manchester DK, Trivers GE, Tamai S, Resau JH, Trump BF, Harris CC. Molecular epidemiology: dosimetry, susceptibility and cancer risk. In: Van der Laan M, ed. Immunoassays for Monitoring Human Exposure to Toxic Chemicals in Foods and the Environment. Washington DC: ACS Books, 1990, p 186.
160. Sims P, Grover PL, Swaisland A, Pal K, Hewer AJ. Metabolic activation of benzo[*a*]pyrene proceeds by a diol-epoxide. Nature 1974;252:326.
161. Själander A, Birgander R, Athlin L, Stenling R, Rutegard J, Beckman L, Beckman G. P53 germ line haplotypes associated with increased risk for colorectal cancer. Carcinogenesis 1995;16:1461.
162. Själander A, Birgander R, Kivelä A, Beckman, G. p53 polymorphisms and haplotypes in different ethnic groups. Hum Hered 1995;45:144.
163. Slaga TJ, Fischer SM, Weeks CE, Klein-Szanto AJ, Reiners JJ. Studies of mechanisms involved in multistage carcinogenesis in mouse skin. In: Harris CC, Cerutti PA, eds. Mechanisms of Chemical Carcinogenesis. New York: Liss, 1982, p 207.
164. Sozeri O, Vollmer K, Liyanage M, frith D, Kour G, Mark GE, Stabel S. Activation of the c-*raf* protein kinase by protein kinase C phosphorylation. Oncogene 1992;7:2259.
165. Spiro L, Olschwang S, Groden J, Robertson M, Samowitz W, Joslyn G, Gelbert L, Thliveris A, Carlson M, et al. Alleles of the APC gene: an attenuated form of familial polyposis. Cell 1993;75:951.
166. Strickland JE, Dlugosz AA, Hennings H, Yuspa SH. Inhibition of tumor formation from grafted murine papilloma cells by treatment of grafts with staurosporine, an inducer of squamous differentiation. Carcinogenesis 1993;14:205.
167. Su, LK, Johnson KA, Smith KJ, Hill DE, Vogelstein,B, Kinzler KW. Association between wild-type and mutant APC gene products. Cancer Res 1993;53:2728.
168. Suganuma M, Yatsunami J, Yoshizawa S, Okabe S, Fujiki H. Absence of synergistic effects on tumor promotion in CD-1 mouse skin by simultaneous applications of two different types of tumor promotors, okadaic acid and teleocidin. Cancer Res 1993;53:1012.
169. Sugimura H, Caporaso NE, Hoover RN, Modali R, Resau J, Trump BF, Lonergan JA, Krontiris TG, Mann DL, Weston A, Harris CC. Association of rare alleles of the Harvey *ras* proto-oncogene locus with lung cancer. Cancer Res 1990;50:1857.
170. Sugimura H, Suzuki J, Hamada GS, Iwase T, Takahashi T, Nagura K, Iwata H, Watanabe S, Kino I, Tsugane S. Cytochrome P-450 1A1 genotype in lung cancer patients and controls in Rio de Janeiro, Brazil. Cancer Epidemiol Biomarkers Prev 1994;3:145.
171. Sugimura T, Sato S, Wakabayashi T. Mutagens carcinogens in pyrolysates of amino acids, proteins and cooked food; heterocyclic aromatic amines. In: Woo YT, Lai DY, Arcos JT, Ardus MF, eds. Chemical Induction of Cancer. New York: Academic Press, 1988, p 681.
172. Sved J, Bird A. The expected equilibrium of the CpG dinucleotide in vertebrate genomes under a mutation model. Proc Natl Acad Sci USA 1990;87:4692.
173. Taffe BG, Kensler TW. Free radicals and signal transduction in tumor promotion. In: Colburn NH, ed. Genes and Signal Transduction in Multistage Carcinogenesis. New York: Marcel Dekker, 1989, p 391.
174. Takahashi T, Nau MM, Chiba I, Birrer MJ, Rosenberg RK, Vinocour M, Levitt M, Pass H, Gazdar AF, Minna JD. p53. A frequent target for genetic abnormalities in lung cancer. Science 1989;246:491.
175. Tamai S, Sugimura H, Caporaso NE, Resau JH, Trump BF, Weston A, Harris CC. Restriction fragment length polymorphism analysis of the L-*myc* gene locus in a case-control study of lung cancer. Int J Cancer 1990;46:411.
176. Vanden-Heuvel JP, Clark GC, Thompson CL, McCoy Z, Miller CR, Lucier GW, Bell DA. CYP1A1 mRNA levels as a human exposure biomarker: use of quantitative polymerase chain reaction to measure CYP1A1 expression in human peripheral blood lymphocytes. Carcinogenesis 1993;10:2003.
177. Verma AK, Boutwell RK. Effects of dose and duration of treatment with the tumor-promoting agent, 12-O-tetradecanoylphorbol-13-acetate on mouse skin carcinogenesis. Carcinogenesis 1980;1:271.
178. Vineis P, Caporaso N, Tannenbaum SR, Skipper PL, Glogowski J, Bartsch H, Coda M, Talaska G, Kadlubar F. Acetylation phenotype, carcinogen-hemoglobin adducts, and cigarette smoking. Cancer Res 1990;50:3002.
179. Vogelstein B, Fearon ER, Hamilton SR, Kern SE, Preisinger AC, Leppert M, Nakamura Y, White R, Smits AM, Bos JL. Genetic alterations during colorectal-tumor development. N Engl J Med 1988;319:525.
180. Vogelstein B, Fearon ER, Hamilton SR, Preisinger AC, Willard HF, Michelson AM, Riggs AD, Orkin SH. Clonal analysis using recombinant DNA probes from the X-chromosome. Cancer Res 1987;47:4806.
181. Weinberg RA. Tumor suppressor genes. Science 1991;254:1138.
182. Weston A. Physical methods for the detection of carcinogens-DNA adducts in humans. Mutat Res 1993;288:19.
183. Weston A, Ling-Cawley HM, Caporaso NE, Bowman ED, Hoover RN, Trump BF, Harris CC. Determination of the allelic frequencies of an L-*myc* and a *p53* polymorphism in human lung cancer. Carcinogenesis 1994;15:583.
184. Weston A, Manchester DK, Povey AC, Harris CC. Detection of carcinogen-macromolecular adducts in humans. J Am Coll Toxicol 1989;8:913.
185. Weston A, Perrin LS, Forrester K, Hoover RN, Trump BF, Harris CC, Caporaso NE. Allelic frequency of a p53 polymorphism in human lung cancer. Cancer Epidemiol Biomarkers Prev 1992;1:481.
186. Weston A, Poirier MC. Development of methods for chemical carcinogen-DNA adduct determination in human tissues. In: Milman HA, Weisburger EK, eds. Park Ridge NJ: Noyes, 1994, p 672.
187. Weston A, Willey JC, Modali R, Sugimura H, McDowell EM, Resau J, Light B, Haugen A, Mann DL, Trump BF, Harris CC. Differential DNA sequence deletions from chromosomes 3, 11, 13 and 17 in squamous cell carcinoma, large cell carcinoma and adenocarcinoma of the human lung. Proc Natl Acad Sci USA 1989;86:5099.
188. Wilson VL, Smith RA, Longoria J, Liotta MA, Harper CM, Harris CC. Chemical carcinogen-induced decreases in genomic 5-methyldeoxycytidine content of normal human bronchial epithelial cells. Proc Natl Acad Sci USA 1987;84:3298.
189. Wogan GN. Markers of exposure to carcinogens. Environ Health Perspect 1989;81:9.
190. Wogan GN, Gorelick NJ. Chemical and biochemical dosimetry of exposure to genotoxic chemicals. Environ Health Perspect 1985;62:5.
191. Yuspa SH. Tumor promotion. In: Fortner JG, Rhoads JE, eds. Accomplishments in Cancer Research. Philadelphia: Lippincott, 1986, p 169.
192. Yuspa SH, Poirier MC. Chemical carcinogenesis: from animal models to molecular models in one decade. Adv Cancer Res 1988;50:25.
193. Zhong S, Wyllie AH, Barnes D, Wolf CR, Spurr NK. Relationship between the GSTM1 genetic polymorphism and susceptibility to bladder breast and colon cancer. Carcinogen 1993;14:1821.

CHAPTER 14

Hormones and the Etiology of Cancer

BRIAN E. HENDERSON, LESLIE BERNSTEIN, AND RONALD K. ROSS

Introduction

A substantial and convincing body of experimental, clinical, and epidemiologic evidence indicates that hormones play a major role in the etiology of several human cancers. That hormones can increase the incidence of neoplasia was first proposed by Bittner (16), based on experimental studies of estrogens and mammary cancer in mice. This concept has been refined into epidemiologic hypotheses related to cancers of the breast, endometrium, prostate, ovary, thyroid, bone, and testis (70, 74). A key element in these hypotheses is neoplasia as the consequence of excessive hormonal stimulation of the particular target organ, the normal growth and function of which is controlled by one or more steroid or polypeptide hormones (Fig. 14.1). In this model, hormones exert an effect that will be independent of outside initiators such as chemicals or ionizing radiation.

The activation of oncogenes and inactivation of tumor-suppressor genes produce a sequence of genetic changes that leads to a malignant phenotype (Fig. 14.2). The activation of oncogenes, whether by mutation, translocation, or amplification, requires cell division. Genetic errors that precede the development of a fully malignant tumor also include the loss or inactivation during mitosis of several tumor-suppressor genes that function to control normal cellular behavior (46, 156, 161). Germline mutations have recently been described with one such gene, the *BRCA1* gene, and have been associated with susceptibility to breast and ovarian cancer in certain kindreds (111). Most of the currently favored models suggest that the first hit is inactivation by a mutational event of one allele of a tumor-suppressor gene that is present in diploid cells, followed by a reduction to homozygosity of the faulty chromosome (94). The initial mutagenic event and loss of the wild-type allele of the tumor-suppressor gene (e.g., *TP53* or *BRCA1*) both require cell division. Thus, for expression of the full malignant phenotype, cells are absolutely required to divide.

Neoplasia of hormone-responsive tissues currently accounts for more than 35% of all newly diagnosed male, and more than 40% of all newly diagnosed female, cancers in the United States. Because of the evidence that endogenous hormones affect both the risk and importance of these cancers in absolute frequency, reason for concern about the effects on cancer risk if the same or closely related hormones are administered for therapeutic purposes (e.g., contraceptives, as hormone replacement therapy, or for the prevention of miscarriage) exists (70, 74). This chapter reviews the epidemiologic and endocrinologic evidence for

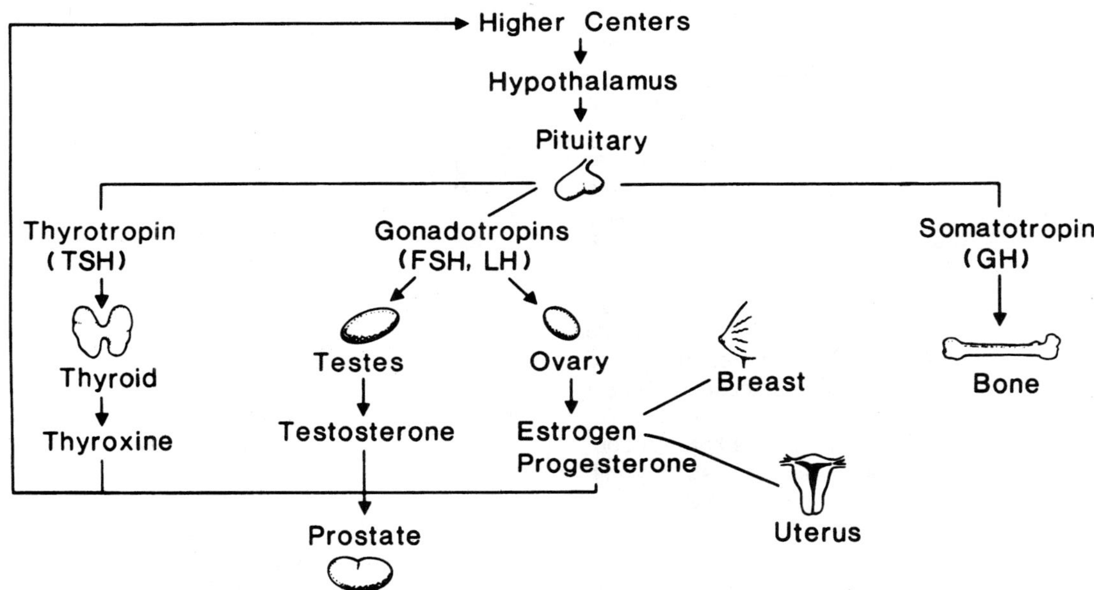

Figure 14.1. Hypothesized relationships between steroid and polypeptide hormones and human cancer.

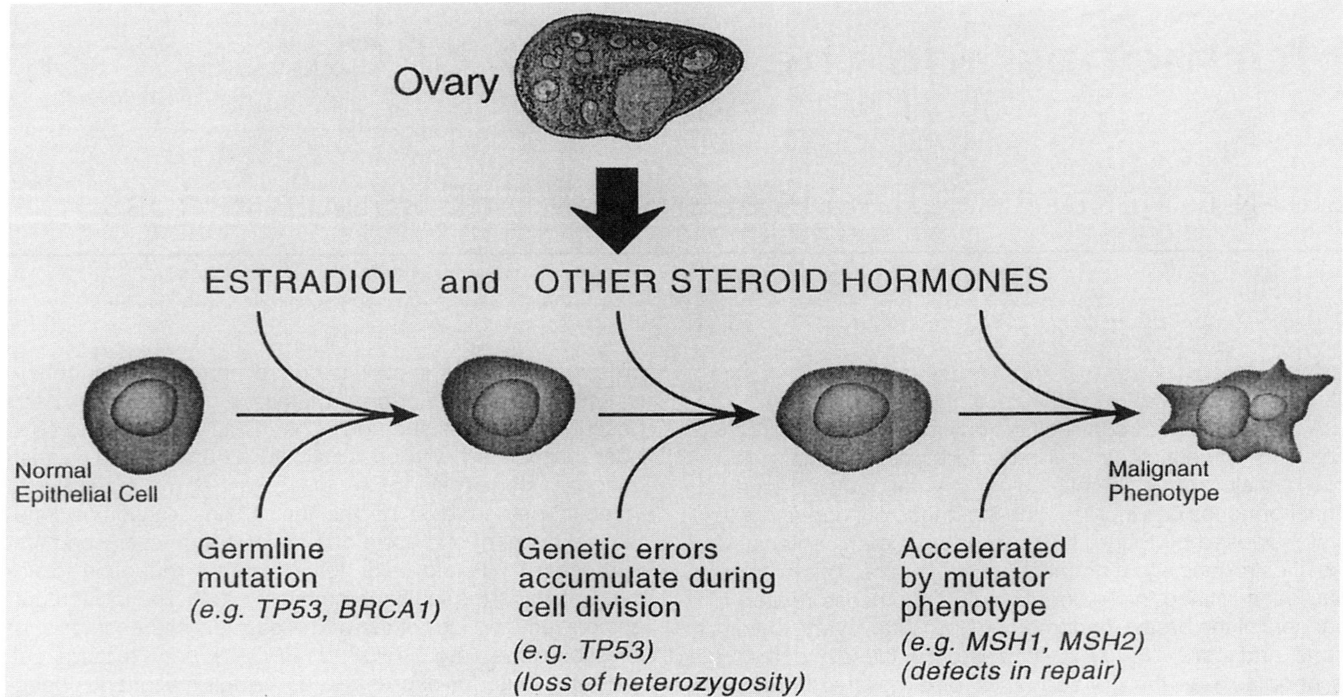

Figure 14.2. Estradiol and to a lesser degree other steroid hormones (e.g., progesterone) drive breast cell proliferation, which facilitates mutation or enhances fixation of mutations, or facilitates expression of genetic errors through loss of heterozygosity by defects in DNA repair. Germline mutations in relevant tumor-suppressor genes accelerate the transformation to the malignant phenotype.

the role of hormones in the development of specific cancers as well as the current status of the relationship between exogenous hormones and cancer of the breast, endometrium, and ovary.

Breast Cancer

Breast cancer is the most common cancer in women, and it accounted for approximately 180,000 new cancer diagnoses and 45,000 deaths in 1995 (178). Available evidence regarding the hormonal etiology of breast cancer is most consistent with the hypothesis that estrogen is the primary stimulant for breast cell proliferation (70, 74). The simultaneous presence of progesterone probably further increases the rate of proliferation (92). This latter conclusion is based largely on the fact that breast mitotic activity peaks during the luteal phase of the menstrual cycle (47).

The most consistently documented, hormonally related risk factors for breast cancer are early age at menarche, late age at menopause, late age at first full-term pregnancy, and weight (Table 14.1) (69). The age-incidence curve for breast cancer emphasizes the importance of ovulation in determining risk (73). The initial cases occur during early adulthood, and the rate of increase in incidence then rises sharply with age to the time of menopause, when it slows dramatically. The rate of increase in the postmenopausal period is only approximately one-sixth the rate of increase in the premenopausal period. This age-incidence curve appears to be shaped in a major way by the effects of ovarian activity.

REPRODUCTIVE AND RELATED LIFESTYLE FACTORS

Early age at menarche has been demonstrated to be a risk factor for breast cancer in most case-control studies (69). In general, an approximately 20% decrease in risk results from each year that menarche is delayed. In a study of young women, Henderson and colleagues (69) recorded both age at onset of menstruation and when "regular" (i.e., predictable) menstruation was first established. For a fixed age at menarche, establishment of regular menstrual cycles within 1 year of the first menstrual period more than doubled the risk of breast cancer compared to women with a 5-year or longer delay for menses to regularize. Women with early menarche (i.e., age 12 or younger) and rapid establishment of regular cycles had an almost fourfold increased risk of breast cancer compared to women with late menarche (i.e., age 13 or older) and long duration of irregular cycles.

These observations suggest that regular ovulatory cycles increase a woman's risk of breast cancer (71), and they support results from an earlier study comparing circulating hormone levels in daughters of women with breast cancer to those in age- matched daughters of controls (67). Daughters of women with breast cancer, who as a group have at least twice the risk of the general population, had higher levels of circulating estrogen and progesterone than found in controls (67).

Other evidence supporting the concept that the cumulative number of ovulatory cycles (i.e., cumulative estrogen and progesterone exposure) is a major determinant of breast cancer comes from the international studies of MacMahon and colleagues (105) who studied the frequency

Table 14.1. Established Hormonal Risk and Protective Factors for Breast Cancer

Risk factors (i.e., increased exposure to estrogen and/or progesterone)
- Early menarche
- Late menopause
- Obesity (postmenopausal women)
- Hormone replacement therapy

Protective factors (i.e., reduced exposure to estrogen and/or progesterone)
- Lactation
- Early age at full-term pregnancy
- Physical activity (exercise)

of ovulation in relation to age at and years since menarche in girls from 15–19 years of age who were selected from several populations at varying risk of breast cancer. In all of these populations, given the same number of elapsed years since menarche, women with later menarche were more likely to have anovulatory cycles than women with early menarche. Adjusting for years since menarche, the highest frequency of ovulatory cycles was observed in those populations with the highest rates of breast cancer. Apter and Vihko (4), in a longitudinal study of 200 schoolgirls, also found that those with early menarche establish ovulatory cycles more quickly than those with later onset. When followed into adult life, women with early menarche (i.e., before age 12) had higher serum estradiol concentrations during the follicular phase of the menstrual cycle (at average, age 27) than in women with later menarche (3). Furthermore, serum estradiol concentrations increased more rapidly to the midcycle peak in these women with early menarche than in those with later menarche. In addition, follicular-phase concentrations of sex-hormone binding globulin (SHBG) were approximately 30% lower in women with early menarche, which could result in higher circulating levels of bioavailable (non-SHBG-bound) estradiol.

Strenuous physical activity may delay menarche. Girls who engage in regular ballet dancing, swimming, or running experience a considerable delay in the onset of menses (49). In one study (13), ballet dancers had a mean age at menarche of 15.4 years, compared with 12.5 years for controls. Breast development also was delayed in these dancers, and they experienced intermittent amenorrhea throughout their teenage years as long as they remained active dancers. Even moderate physical activity during adolescence can lead to anovular cycles. Girls who engaged in regular, moderate physical activity (averaging at least 600 Kcal of energy expended per week) were 2.9 times more likely than girls who engaged in lesser amounts of physical activity to be anovular. More recently, Bernstein and colleagues (11) reported that adolescent and adult physical activity significantly reduces the risk of breast cancer in young women (i.e., ≤40 years of age). Risk of breast cancer among women who averaged four or more hours of exercise activity per week during their reproductive years was nearly 60% lower than that of inactive women.

In the same way that early onset of menarche and regular ovulation equate with a greater cumulative lifetime exposure to estrogen and risk of breast cancer, late occurrence of menopause and extended exposure to ovulatory cycles at the end of menstrual life also increase risk. Women whose natural menopause occurs before age 45 have only one-half the risk of breast cancer as women whose menopause occurs after age 55 (168). Artificial menopause, induced either by bilateral oophorectomy or pelvic irradiation, also markedly reduces risk of breast cancer; this effect appears to be slightly greater than that of natural menopause (168).

The relationship between body weight and risk of breast cancer is critically dependent on age. Among postmenopausal women, a 10-kg increment in body weight results in an approximately 80% increase in that person's risk of breast cancer (38). In premenopausal women, the relationship between weight and risk is less clearly established, but if anything, the situation appears to be the reverse of that in postmenopausal women (i.e., high weight appears to be associated with reduced risk) (175). This may result from the reduced prevalence of ovulation associated with high body weight.

The quantity and quality of cumulative cyclic ovarian activity among various populations of women appear to explain much of the international variation in breast cancer risk (135). The most carefully performed international studies comparing estrogen levels in populations at differing risks of breast cancer were done in the early 1970s. MacMahon and colleagues (103) conducted a series of studies on teenagers and young women to investigate whether some aspect of estrogen metabolism was responsible for the large differences in the rates of breast cancer between Asia and North America. They studied native Japanese, women who would be expected to experience low rates of breast cancer. Using overnight urine samples collected on the morning of day 21 in the menstrual cycle, they found that total urinary estrogen levels were 36% higher in the North American teenagers. In nulliparous women from age 20–24 years, total urinary estrogen levels in the North American group were 49% higher on day 21 and 38% higher on day 10 (during the follicular phase of the menstrual cycle); similar differences were found among parous women aged 30–39 years. These differences in total urinary estrogens presumably reflect both reduced frequency of ovulatory cycles and less effective corpus luteum formation during those cycles in which ovulation did occur.

Assuming that increased ovarian activity does increase the risk of breast cancer, case-control studies of breast cancer should find higher levels of circulating estradiol. Seven such studies have been undertaken, but four had insufficient numbers of subjects, producing inconclusive results (92). Bernstein and colleagues (14) recently described the results of two concurrent case-control studies in the United States (Los Angeles) and China (Shanghai). Overall, those with breast cancer had 14% higher serum estradiol concentrations, with a case-to-control excess of 17% in Chinese women and 11% in white U.S. women. Los Angeles control women had 21% greater estradiol concentrations than Shanghai control women and adjustment for body weight only accounted for 25% of this difference. These higher levels of estradiol in white U.S. women compared to Chinese women are consistent with the differences in urinary estrogen levels between these populations as described earlier.

A recent prospective study by Toniolo and colleagues (167) found a significant increase in risk of breast cancer, related to higher circulating levels of total and free estradiol.

Greater hormonal differences have been observed in comparisons of postmenopausal Asian and white U.S. women. Recently, Shimizu and colleagues (159) studied serum estrogen levels in postmenopausal women in Japan and postmenopausal white women in Los Angeles. The Japanese women were deliberately chosen from a rural, agricultural area to obtain samples representing as closely as possible the traditional Japanese "lifestyle" that gave rise to the low rates of breast cancer found in Japan. Levels of estrone and estradiol both were significantly higher (47% and 36%, respectively) in the sera of white U.S. women. Interestingly, adjustment for body weight did not account for all of this difference.

An early age at first birth (i.e., before age 20) is a protective factor, reducing the lifetime risk of breast cancer to about one-half the lifetime risk of breast cancer of nulliparous women (104). Additional completed pregnancies at any age add smaller increments of protection (184). Women who have a very late first full-term pregnancy actually are at a higher risk of breast cancer than nulliparous women (104). This paradoxic effect of a late first full-term pregnancy has been repeatedly confirmed by epidemiologic studies. Furthermore, it has been demonstrated that women who have given birth during the previous 3 years have a higher risk of breast cancer than women of the same age, parity, and age at first birth whose most recent birth occurred at least 10 years earlier (19). First-trimester abortions, whether spontaneous or induced and occurring before the first full-term pregnancy, also are associated in some studies with a higher risk of breast cancer (33, 59, 134).

Based on these results, it appears that two contradictory effects of pregnancy on risk of breast cancer are particularly notable during a first pregnancy; a short-term increase in risk, followed in the long term by a substantial reduction in risk (135). This apparent paradox has a physiologic explanation based on patterns of estrogen as well as prolactin secretion and metabolism during pregnancy. During the first trimester, the level of bioavailable estradiol rapidly rises, an effect that is more apparent during the first than in subsequent pregnancies (10). Thus, in terms of estrogen exposure to the breast, the net effect during this early part of pregnancy is an increased risk that is equivalent to the exposure from several ovulatory cycles over a relatively short period of time. In the long run, however, this negative effect of early pregnancy on risk of breast cancer can be overridden by two beneficial hormonal consequences of completing the pregnancy. It has been reported that prolactin levels are substantially lower in parous compared with nulliparous women (119, 183). In addition, parous women have been reported to have higher levels of sex-hormone binding globulin (SHBG) and lower levels of bioavailable estradiol than their nulliparous counterparts (12).

If the cumulative number of ovulatory cycles directly relates to the risk of breast cancer, a beneficial effect of long-duration lactation would be expected, because nursing substantially delays the reestablishment of ovulation following a completed pregnancy. Because only a small proportion of mothers had a large, cumulative number of nursing months, most of earlier studies were unable to assess the effects of lactation on risk of breast cancer. However, in a population-based, case-control study in China (184), a population in which long-duration nursing is the norm, risk was reduced by approximately 30% for each 5 years of nursing experience. A recent large, case-control study in the United States (121) found comparable protection from breast cancer associated with breast-feeding, but it suggested the protection may be more substantial for premenopausal disease.

DIET

Much attention has been focused on dietary differences, particularly fat consumption, to explain both the international pattern of breast cancer occurrence and changes in rates of breast cancer following migration to high-risk countries or Western nations from low-risk countries (5, 57). International breast cancer mortality rates correlate highly with per capita consumption of fat (Relative Risk RR = 0.93)(5). When international breast cancer incidence rates rather than mortality rates are considered, the magnitude of the correlation coefficient still is very high (RR = 0.84) (5). There is a wealth of evidence that nutrition profoundly influences breast cancer occurrence by modifying age at menarche and body weight, but the correlation of fat with international breast cancer mortality remains highly significant even after statistical adjustment for those factors. Hirayama (78) reported that breast cancer mortality rates in various regions of Japan are correlated highly with fat consumption.

Many case-control studies of fat consumption and breast cancer have found only small differences between cases and controls, generally no larger than the differences in total calorie consumption (126). However, Howe and colleagues (81) recently conducted a combined analysis of dietary risk factors for breast cancer drawn from 12 large, case-control studies representing populations with a wide range of dietary habits and underlying rates of breast cancer. They found a positive association between both total fat and saturated fat intake and risk of breast cancer among postmenopausal women (approximately 50% difference in risk among individuals in the highest versus the lowest quintile of intake). Nonetheless, the three cohort studies that have used food-frequency questionnaires to study the relationship of diet and breast cancer found no clear or consistent relationship with either total fat, saturated fat, or vegetable fat (80, 83, 112, 176).

High fiber diets may protect against breast cancer, perhaps because fiber may reduce the intestinal reabsorption of estrogens excreted via the biliary system (83). In one animal study (28), a high-fiber diet was associated with a reduced incidence of mammary cancer. Assessment of fiber intake in epidemiologic studies has been problematic because of a paucity of data on the fiber content of individual foods and disagreement about the most appropriate methods of biochemical analysis to determine the different types of fiber.

EXOGENOUS HORMONES

There is substantial literature on the relationship between oral contraceptive (OC) use and risk of breast cancer. As a group, these studies provide overwhelming evidence that when used during most of a woman's reproductive life, OCs do not confer protection against breast cancer as they do against ovarian and endometrial cancer (133). Several of the most recent studies, which have paid particular attention to the complex methodologic difficulties in studying this association, have provided evidence of a small but positive trend of increasing risk of breast cancer with increasing duration of OC use in women diagnosed before age 45 (with risk increasing by approximately 3.1% per year of use) but no such increase in the risk of women diagnosed over age 45.

Early epidemiologic studies that reported findings on menopausal estrogen therapy and breast cancer often were limited by small numbers, insufficient data on dose and duration of use, and inadequate attention to selecting an appropriate comparison group. More recent studies, however, which have used healthy population comparison groups and have addressed these other methodologic issues, have provided evidence for an increased risk of breast cancer in long-term users of estrogen replacement therapy (ERT). This increase is on the order of 3.1% per year for all formulations combined (73, 133). When only conjugated equine estrogen is considered, the increase in breast cancer risk is estimated to be approximately 2% per year of ERT use. The results of these population-based studies contrast with those of other recent studies using hospital patients as controls, which found no association of ERT with overall risk of breast cancer or with long duration of use. One possible explanation is that hospital controls are biased regarding HRT use because they have more contact with the health care system and therefore are more likely to use elective drugs than the population at large. Results from a recently published, population-based, prospective study in Sweden (131) are compatible with those of the population-based, case-control studies that demonstrated an approximately 70% increase in risk after 10 years of ERT use (131).

The impact on risk of breast cancer by adding progestogens to ERT is the subject of considerable debate. As indicated earlier, progestogens probably augment the mitogenic effect of estrogen on the breast. In the only study to date of combination hormone therapy, a small, increased risk of breast cancer over that reported for ERT alone was observed (131). Further observations are needed to more accurately define the potential adverse effects of progestogens on the risk of breast cancer.

GENETIC DETERMINANTS

A family history of breast cancer is associated with an increased risk of the disease. This is particularly so if the history includes a woman who was affected at an early age or had bilateral disease. Whereas a two- to three-fold increased overall risk of the disease has been observed in first-degree relatives of women with breast cancer, a nine-fold increased risk has been found in the first-degree relatives of premenopausal women with bilateral breast cancer (2). High risks (i.e., five-fold increases) also have been found in women with multiple first-degree relatives with breast cancer.

The patterns of risks observed in epidemiologic studies among the relatives of women with breast cancer are consistent with the disease having a hereditary component. More formal genetic analyses corroborate this hypothesis. The majority of segregation analyses of breast cancer pedigrees, including a recent segregation analysis of the 4,730 breast cancer cases from the Cancer and Steroid Hormone (CASH) study (15, 25, 86, 123, 177), have provided evidence for the existence of one or more rare autosomal dominant genes leading to increased susceptibility to breast cancer.

The results of segregation analyses subsequently were confirmed by linkage analyses, which provided strong evidence for a breast cancer–susceptibility gene (or genes) located on the long arm of chromosome 17 (42, 60, 61, 120). In families for whom the linkage was found, transmission of breast cancer was consistent with an autosomal dominant pattern of inheritance. Hall and colleagues (60), the first group to report the linkage of breast cancer to chromosome 17p21, found particularly strong evidence of linkage in families with an early age at onset. In 1991, Narod and colleagues (120) showed that both breast and ovarian cancer were linked to chromosome 17q12-23 by examining five families characterized by multiple cases of early onset breast and ovarian cancer. However, these authors found evidence of genetic heterogeneity as only three of the five families appeared to be linked to chromosome 17.

To confirm the aforementioned linkage results as well as to localize a breast cancer gene, designated *BRCA1*, members of the Breast Cancer Consortium (42) analyzed 214 extensive breast cancer pedigrees, including 57 families characterized by both breast and ovarian cancer. From estimates of the gene frequency in the population, the Consortium concluded that the *BRCA1* gene likely accounts for somewhat less than 5% of all breast cancers. Studies of familial breast cancer recently culminated with the characterization and identification of various mutations of *BRCA1* in some but not all breast and ovarian cancer kindreds, but not in sporadic cases of these diseases (50, 111). A second breast cancer–susceptibility locus, *BRCA2*, has been localized to chromosome 13q12–13 (179) and a third locus has also been proposed (30).

The recent finding of germline p53 mutations in the Li-Fraumeni syndrome suggests another potential mechanism of genetic susceptibility (107); breast cancer is a common feature of this syndrome. Other genes that are critical to a woman's risk of breast cancer likely are those that control the metabolism of estradiol (e.g., 17–hydroxysteroid dehydrogenase [17–HSD]) and the activity of the estrogen receptor in breast epithelial cells. In breast tissue there are at least two forms of 17–HSD (types I and II), one of which seems to favor the reductive conversion of estrone to estradiol (142). The EDH17B2 gene (which codes for 17HSH type 1)is encoded by two autosomal codominant alleles, and there is some evidence of an association between certain exon 6 polymorphisms and the risk of breast cancer in a Finnish population (108). The EDH17B2 type II is located in close proximity to *BRCA1* and the possible interrelationships of these two genes is the object of considerable research. It still is not clear if the EDH17B1 gene is a separate gene or "pseudogene." The estrogen receptor gene is a large gene (<140 kb in length) (137, 140) and several polymorphisms and mutations have been described (181, 187). Substantial polymorphism has been reported as well for a TA repeat in the upstream promoter region of the gene as well (35). The functional significance of these and presumably other yet to be described polymorphisms, needs to be clarified.

Endometrial Cancer

Among the hormone-related cancers, the best understood etiologically is endometrial cancer. All of the major demographic characteristics of the disease (as well as the major non-demographic risk factors) are explicable based on cumulative exposure of the endometrium to that fraction of estrogen unopposed by the modifying influences of progesterone (Table 14.2) (70).

MITOTIC ACTIVITY IN THE ENDOMETRIUM

Key and Pike (91) have summarized the existing data on endometrial mitotic activity during normal menstrual cycles. Mitotic rates are low during days 1 through 4 of the cycle, then increase rapidly and remain stable thereafter until day 19, after which rates drop to essentially zero for the remainder of the cycle. There appears to be a lag period of approximately 4 days before the full stimulatory effects of unopposed estrogen, or the modifying influence of progesterone on endometrial mitotic activity, are fully apparent.

The cellular basis for the antiestrogenic activity of progestogens on the endometrium is well understood (70). Progestogens reduce the concentration of estradiol receptors, and they increase the activity of the enzyme system that converts estradiol to estrone, which is a biologically less potent estrogen because of its lower affinity for cellular estrogen receptors. Luteal phase progesterone causes endometrial cells to differentiate to a secretory state, and progestogen withdrawal leads to a cyclic sloughing of endometrial tissue.

The age-incidence curve of endometrial cancer essentially consists of two straight lines of different slopes intersecting at menopause (73, 91). During the premenopausal period, the slope is steep and most likely determined by accumulation of mitotic activity in the first half of the menstrual cycle, when estrogen is unopposed by progesterone. With cessation of ovarian function at menopause, the slope of the age-incidence curve decreases dramatically, although endometrial cancer rates continue to increase during the postmenopausal period. The most likely explanation for the latter phenomenon is weight-related estrogen formation and use of ERT.

Table 14.2. Established Hormonal Risk and Protective Factors for Endometrial Cancer

Risk factors (i.e., increased exposure to "unopposed" estrogen)
Estrogen replacement therapy
Obesity
Sequential oral contraceptives
Late menopause
Protective factors (i.e., decreased exposure to "unopposed" estrogen)
Pregnancy
Oral contraceptives

Based on the concept that frequency of mitotic activity primarily determines the risk of endometrial cancer and that cumulative exposure to unopposed estrogens controls such activity, one can readily predict the most important risk factors for this disease. Pregnancies and OCs, which expose the endometrium to constant, high levels of both estrogen and progestogen, should protect against endometrial cancer development. ERT and obesity should increase risk. All of these predicted effects have been repeatedly documented in epidemiologic studies.

ESTROGEN REPLACEMENT THERAPY

Hormone replacement therapy in the form of unopposed estrogen therapy gained widespread popularity in the United States during the 1960s and 1970s. By 1974, there were nearly 30 million prescriptions of noncontraceptive estrogen being filled annually, and the most popular brand, conjugated equine estrogen, had become the fourth most frequently prescribed drug in the country (90). Concomitant with this increasing usage, incidence rates of endometrial cancer in postmenopausal women also increased rapidly, especially on the West Coast, where use of ERT was particularly common (6). By 1975, the results of epidemiologic case-control studies, demonstrating a strong overall association between ERT and risk of endometrial cancer were being published (102, 185). Although the methodologic strengths and weaknesses of these early studies were the subject of intense scrutiny and debate, it soon became apparent that this association represented a cause-and-effect relationship. Literally dozens of studies have now documented a high relative increase in the risk of endometrial cancer following ERT (73). Risk is strongly related both to dose and duration of use, but high relative increments in risk follow even moderate doses taken for moderately long periods of time. Women who use ERT for 5 years or longer have approximately a 3.5-fold increase in risk compared with that of women who have never used such therapy (Fig. 14.3*A*) (73, 180).

While use of estrogen clearly increases the incidence of aggressive endometrial cancer, the overall mortality from endometrial cancer among affected users somewhat paradoxically is much lower than among nonusers who develop endometrial cancer (24). In fact, such women have little reduction in lifespan compared with healthy women of the same age (24). The reasons for this are not completely known, but this phenomenon likely can be explained largely by the increased medical surveillance among estrogen users. Women who use ERT tend to be closely followed because the drug is known to induce vaginal bleeding. Part of this favorable survival experience also probably results from patients with estrogen-induced benign hyperplasia being misdiagnosed as endometrial cancer. While past users of ERT have a risk of endometrial cancer that is intermediate between that for current users of comparable duration and lifetime nonusers, risk in such women remains substantially elevated over baseline even after many years without treatment (129).

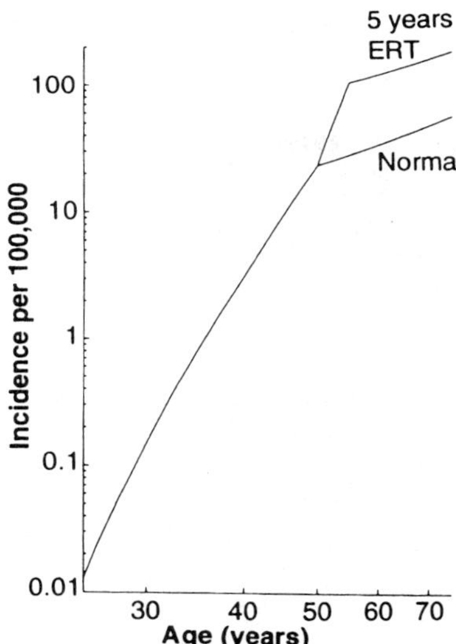

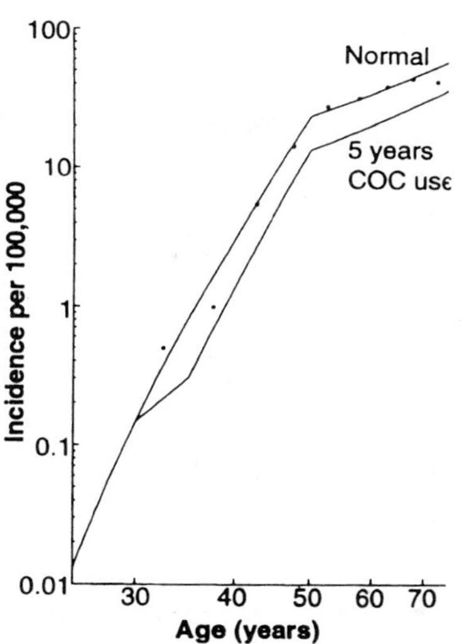

Figure 14.3. Age-specific incidence rates for cancers of the endometrium in women using estrogen replacement therapy (ERT) (**A**) and combination oral contraceptives (OCs) (**B**) for 5 years. Data are from the U.K. Birmingham Cancer Registry for the years 1968 to 1972. These data largely avoid problems arising from the high hysterectomy and oophorectomy rates in the United States, which artificially distort the age-incidence curves. *Dots*, actual incidence data; *solid lines* marked "normal," mathematic models predicting these rates from the major known risk factors for these cancers. *Source:* Pike and colleagues (135).

Tamoxifen appears to act as an estrogen agonist in the endometrium, and the risk of endometrial cancer is elevated by tamoxifen in a fashion analogous to that of ERT (170). The molecular basis of this agonist effect on the endometrium as opposed to the antagonist activity of tamoxifen on the breast, however, is not well defined.

BODY WEIGHT

High body weight leads to increased risk of endometrial cancer at all ages (44, 66, 89, 99). The three studies of postmenopausal women with the largest number of endometrial cancer cases and controls all show at least a doubling of risk between the thinnest and the heaviest women (44, 89, 99). The reason for this increased risk with increasing weight in postmenopausal women is straightforward: obese postmenopausal women have increased plasma concentrations of estradiol (186). Adipose tissue is rich in an aromatase enzyme system that converts androstenedione to estrone. In turn, estrone can be converted directly to estradiol. In addition, SHBG levels are lower in obese women, so the amount of bioavailable estradiol in such women is higher than would be expected from the peripheral conversion of androstenedione to estrone alone (186).

The explanation for the substantially increased risk of endometrial cancer with obesity in premenopausal women, as observed by Henderson and colleagues (66) and La Vecchia and colleagues (99), is less obvious. Although obesity does appear to be associated with slightly increased levels of bioavailable estradiol in premenopausal women, this alone appears to be insufficient to account for such a profound effect. The more likely explanation is that obesity in premenopausal women is associated with amenorrhea and subnormal luteal-phase progesterone levels, thus resulting in prolonged exposure of the endometrium to unopposed estrogen (148).

ORAL CONTRACEPTIVES

The role of estrogens as the principal cause of endometrial cancer is further supported by the markedly increased risk after a relatively short-duration use of sequential OCs, which deliver an unopposed estrogen during most of the monthly cycle (66). As potent as ERT and sequential OCs are in modifying the risk of endometrial cancer, these effects can be mitigated by the simultaneous administration of progestogens. A series of case- control studies have consistently demonstrated that combination OCs (the only type of OCs currently marketed), which deliver an estrogen and progestogen simultaneously during each day of use, decrease the risk of endometrial cancer by 11.7% per year (Fig. 14.3*B*) (73, 133). Two prospective studies, the Walnut Creek Contraceptive Drug Study (146) and the Royal College of General Practitioner's Oral Contraceptive Study (9), have demonstrated similar decreases in risk. In most of these studies, risk of endometrial cancer steadily decreased with increasing duration of use. In the largest case-control study, the protective effect of combination OC use persisted even for women who discontinued using OCs as much as 15 years earlier (22).

HORMONE REPLACEMENT THERAPY

The newer regimens of hormone replacement therapy typically follow a pattern not unlike that of sequential OCs; an unopposed estrogen is given early in a monthly cycle, followed by estrogen combined with a progestogen for the last 10 to 12 days. This regimen attempts to reproduce the hormonal pattern of the normal menstrual cycle, albeit at lower levels of both estrogen and progestogen. One therefore might predict that this method of hormone replacement therapy might only partially offset the increased risk of endometrial cancer that is associated with unopposed ERT.

Only one study that meets acceptable methodologic standards has reported to date the effects of combination hormone therapy on the risk of endometrial cancer. Risk in this prospective study was clearly reduced to a level below that of women using unopposed ERT, but the study did not use a sufficiently large sample to determine with confidence whether risk was reduced to baseline (130).

A continuous, combined regimen of hormone replacement therapy in which estrogen and progestogen are administered together each day, as with combination OCs, has been growing in popularity. This regimen presumably could obviate the risk of endometrial cancer but might also reduce some of the benefit from unopposed estrogen on the risk of heart disease and adversely affect the risk of breast cancer (72).

PARITY

The other major, established risk factor for endometrial cancer, low parity, also is readily explained by the unopposed estrogen hypothesis (101). The highest risk of endometrial cancer occurs in either married or unmarried nulliparous women, and an incremental decrease in risk occurs with each incremental increase in parity. Nulliparous women have a risk of endometrial cancer that is 3 to 5 times that of women with parity of greater than 3 (101). This effect is expected as no endometrial mitotic activity occurs during pregnancy, because of the persistently high progesterone levels.

Ovarian Cancer

The epidemiology of epithelial ovarian cancer, like that of breast and endometrial cancer, is well studied. However, the hormonal basis for ovarian cancer appears to differ from that of other hormone-induced cancers in that the responsible hormones, gonadotropins, act indirectly on ovarian epithelial cells. The stimulus for cell division in the etiology of ovarian cancer is not hormonal per se; rather, it follows ovulation, which is the direct result of complex hormonal changes (70). In this case, epithelial cells within the developing follicle or covering the ovarian surface have been proposed as the cells of origin for ovarian cancer. These cells replicate during or after each ovulation, thus any respite from ovulation would be protective against ovarian cancer. This hypothesis is supported by a large body of epidemiologic data that consistently demonstrates the risk of developing ovarian cancer decreases with increasing parity and with combination OC use (Table 14.3).

PARITY

Many case-control studies have been conducted since the mid-1970s in diverse populations, and parity has been consistently identified as a protective factor in most of these studies. Compared with parous women, nulliparous women have at least a 50% greater risk of ovarian cancer (174). Each pregnancy beyond the first confers additional protection. This includes both full-term and incomplete pregnancies, and it does not result from an age-at-first-pregnancy effect (122).

Table 14.3. Established Hormonal Risk and Protective Factors for Ovarian Cancer

Risk factors (i.e., increased number of ovulations)
Late menopause
Protective factors (i.e., decreased number of ovulations)
Pregnancy
Oral contraceptives

ORAL CONTRACEPTIVES

Use of combination OCs has been widely investigated and shown to be protective against ovarian cancer. On average, women who have used OCs have a 7.5% per year decreased risk compared with that of nonusers (73).

This translates into a 32% reduction in risk of ovarian cancer associated with 5 years of OC use (RR $= 1 - 0.075)^5 =$ 0.68). This is slightly less than the 45% reduction predicted from the suppression of 60 ovulatory menstrual cycles of the approximately 480 that a woman would experience during her reproductive years (135). This difference likely results from the ovarian cancer studies on which risk estimates are based including substantial numbers of premenopausal women. Among postmenopausal women, it is likely that the estimated 7.5% decline in risk of ovarian cancer per year of OC use is too conservative; the dose-response effect of OCs on risk of ovarian cancer appears to be long-lasting (i.e., 10 to 15 years after discontinuing OC use, the risk remains at a very low level) (23, 181).

ANOVULATION: A UNIFYING HYPOTHESIS

Casagrande and colleagues (21) suggested that because the protection afforded by pregnancies and OC use appears to act through a common mechanism, periods of pregnancy and OC use could be combined into a single measure of "protected time" (21). They demonstrated that the risk of ovarian cancer clearly decreased as protected time increased. Other epidemiologic studies have confirmed this observation (48, 181).

As with breast and endometrial cancer, the age-incidence curve for ovarian cancer emphasizes the importance of ovulation in determining risk. The age-incidence curve of ovarian cancer can be brought into line with the familiar linear log-log plot of other non-hormone-dependent epithelial tumors if ovarian age is considered as starting at menarche and proceeding at a reduced rate (roughly 30% of normal) during periods of anovulation, including the postmenopausal period (39, 181).

Prostate Cancer

Prostate cancer has become the most frequently diagnosed cancer among men in the United States, exceeding lung cancer. Approximately 240,000 cases were diagnosed in 1995 alone, resulting in approximately 40,000 deaths (178). The most important risk factor for prostate cancer is age. Prostate cancer is extremely rare before age 40, but thereafter, the rate of increase (i.e., the slope of the age-incidence curve) is greater than that for any other cancer (150). There is substantial international variation in incidence, with four- to five-fold difference in death rates across countries. Among those countries with reasonably reliable cancer reporting, Hong Kong and Japan have the lowest mortality rates for prostate cancer, whereas African-Americans have by far the highest rate in the world (117).

Testosterone, through metabolism to dihydrotestosterone, controls mitotic activity in the prostate although the quantitative relationship between levels of testosterone and the rate of cell proliferation in the prostate is unstudied. Free testosterone, which is the small proportion (approximately 2%) of testosterone that is not bound to either serum albumin or SHBG, diffuses into prostate cells, where it rapidly and irreversibly converts to dihydrotestosterone through the action of the type II 5α-reductase enzyme. Dihydrotestosterone is bound to the androgen receptor, and the hormone-receptor complex is translocated to the nucleus of prostate cells for DNA-binding transactivation of androgen-responsive genes (Fig. 14.4) (27).

Laboratory animals have a very low incidence of spontaneous adenocarcinomas in the prostate, and few experimental strategies are known to increase the tumor yield (147). The first and most successful experimental model was that produced by Noble (124), who demonstrated that exogenous administration of subcutaneous testosterone could, in a dose-related fashion, dramatically increase the incidence of adenocarcinoma of the prostate in Nb rats. Pollard (139) has similarly induced prostatic carcinoma in germ-free Lobund-Wistar rats through hormonal manipulation. Attempts to chemically induce prostatic adenocarcinomas other than by hormonal manipulation have been largely unsuccessful. Recently, Bosland and colleagues (17) have been able to induce invasively growing, metastasizing adenocarcinomas in the prostate of Wistar rats by a single intravenous injection of *N*-methyl-*N*-nitrosourea; hormonal priming with testosterone to induce maximal cell proliferation was required in this model for any tumor induction. In fact, all clearly established, experimental models of prostatic adenocarcinomas have an androgen requirement for tumor induction.

ENDOGENOUS HORMONE LEVELS

A number of studies have compared circulating testosterone levels measured by radioimmunoassay in cases of prostate cancer with those in controls of similar age with no known prostatic disease. The largest and best designed of these studies tend to find slightly higher levels of serum testosterone in those with cancer (150). For example, Ghanadian and colleagues (54) showed that patients with prostatic cancer had higher testosterone levels than healthy controls of similar age. Ahluwalia and colleagues (1) also found levels of serum testosterone to be significantly higher in patients with prostatic cancer than in age-matched controls in the United States, but not in African blacks. Drafta and colleagues (41) similarly found higher circulating testosterone levels among patients with prostate cancer than in "normal ambulatory controls." Others, however, have not found such differences, especially those studies that have used nonhealthy controls for comparison (82).

Three prospective studies of prostate cancer and circulating testosterone levels reported to date have produced inconsistent results. One found higher levels in patients with cancer, but the others did not (63). In a case-control study nested within a large Hawaiian prospective study, Nomura and colleagues (125) observed no difference in testosterone levels between 98 patients with prostate cancer and age- as well as hour-of-sampling-matched controls. Barrett-Connor and colleagues (8) reported results from an ongoing prospective study among a cohort of elderly residents of Rancho Bernardo, California, and they found no consistent relationship between circulatory testosterone levels and risk of subsequent prostate cancer. Rather unexpectedly, however, they also found that prostate cancer increased with increased levels of estradiol, and of the adrenal androgen, androstenedione.

The hypothesis of a hormonal etiology for prostatic cancer would predict that healthy African-American males should have higher levels of testosterone than healthy white U.S. males, who in turn should have a higher level than native Japanese and Chinese men. Because differences in the ratio of prostate cancer incidence among racial ethnic groups

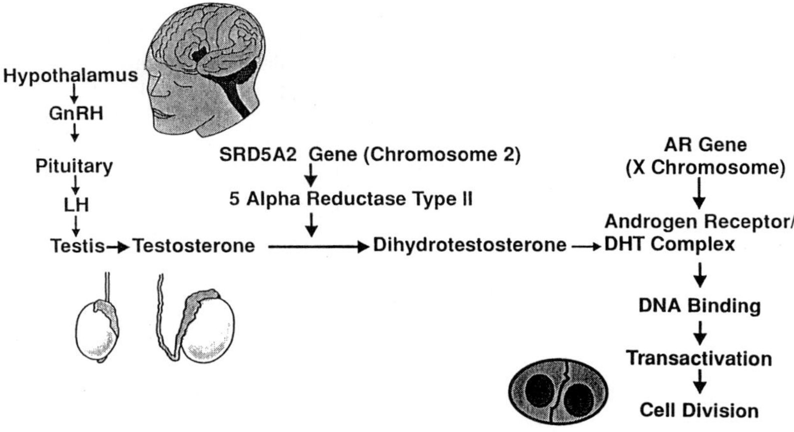

Figure 14.4. Hormonal pathway in causation of prostate cancer.

are maximal early in the age range during which prostate cancer occurs, hormonal patterns at young ages might be particularly important determinants of risk (150). Ross and colleagues (151) studied levels of circulating steroid hormone in white and black college students in Los Angeles. After adjustment for minor differences in the few known codeterminants of testosterone levels (i.e., age, alcohol use, smoking habits, time of sampling, weight), the mean testosterone level in blacks was 15% higher than in whites, and the free testosterone level was 13% higher. Although this difference is not large, it could be sufficient to explain the 1.7-fold "excess" of this disease in blacks compared to whites if such differences persist throughout adolescence and adulthood. When Ross and colleagues extended this study to include young Japanese men born and raised in rural Japan (152), a group with less than 10% of the expected lifetime risk of prostate cancer found in U.S. whites, the predicted deficit in testosterone was not found. However, these men did have levels of androstanediol and androsterone glucuronides that were some 25 to 50% less than those of U.S. whites and blacks.

These hormones are a sensitive index of 5α-reductase enzymatic activity (152). There are two distinct 5α-reductase enzymes encoded for by different genes; the type II enzyme is active primarily in the prostate and the genital skin. There is only 50% homology in the amino acid sequence between the two enzymes, and there is a clear distinction in optimal pH. The type II 5α-reductase gene (*SRD5A2*), is located on chromosome 2P and has been cloned and sequenced (97). Germline mutations of *SRD5A2* have been identified, most notably in a highly inbred community in the Dominican Republic (166). Boys with this mutated gene are phenotypically female, with a persistent vaginal pouch until puberty, at which time there is some phallic enlargement and development of some secondary sex characteristics; the prostate remains undeveloped. Davis and Russell (34) have described a polymorphism in the 3′ untranslated region of the gene, varying in the length of a TA dinucleotide repeat sequence. A subsequent small study suggests that the prevalence of variant alleles using this polymorphic marker is higher than originally described, and there may exist novel alleles of this gene that are unique to African-Americans. The significance of these to *SRD5A2* activity and, ultimately, to prostate cancer risk, however, is unknown.

ANDROGEN RECEPTOR GENE

The androgen-receptor (*AR*) gene also is potentially important in prostate carcinogenesis if the *AR* gene binds dehydrotestosterone and translocates it to the nucleus(Fig. 14.4). The gene is located on the long arm of the X chromosome (87). Within exon 1 of the *AR* gene is a highly polymorphic microsatellite, a trinucleotide (CAG) repeat sequence, of unknown function; however, abnormal expansion of this satellite is associated with X-linked spinal and bulbar muscular atrophy (i.e., Kennedy's syndrome). This syndrome is characterized by modest androgen insensitivity. Linkage analysis originally localized the gene defect for Kennedy's syndrome to the region of the *AR* gene. In investigating differences in the *AR* gene in affected compared with healthy individuals, DNA sequence variations were discovered only in exon 1, specifically in the length of the CAG repeat (98). An increased size of the repeat was absolutely associated with the disease. Normal size varies from approximately 9 to 31 repeats, whereas the mutant range associated with Kennedy's syndrome varies from 40 to 62. These mutant receptors bind androgen normally but have been shown in transfection assays to transactivate an androgen-responsive reporter gene subnormally (110).

African-Americans, U.S. whites, and Asian-Americans all show population differences in the CAG repeat polymorphism, with the entire allele frequency profile shifted toward shorter alleles in the case of African-Americans, and longer alleles in Asian-Americans, relative to U.S. whites (26, 43). Coetzee and Ross (26) have proposed that within the normal range of CAG repeats in exon 1, shorter alleles may be associated with increased transactivation of androgen-responsive genes relative to longer alleles; this hypothesis would predict the observed mean distribution of the CAG repeat polymorphism.

HORMONE MANIPULATION

Endocrine manipulation has been a mainstay for treatment of prostatic cancer for nearly 50 years. Administration of estrogens, and more recently of luteinizing hormone–releasing hormone agonists, to reduce pituitary luteinizing hormone production and thereby greatly reduce testicular testosterone production is a common strategy for treating advanced disease. Use of anti-androgens to block androgen activity at the cellular level also is growing in popularity (118).

Castration leads to an approximately 80% reduction in prostatic size. Although no systematic study of this association exists, there has never been a case report of prostatic cancer occurring in such a patient (150). A number of investigators have found evidence that factors associated with increased sexual activity also are associated with increased risk of prostate cancer, such as early age-at-first-intercourse (79), frequency of intercourse (155), number of sexual partners (162), and history of venereal disease (79, 155, 162). With the exception of the latter observation, however, results are not entirely consistent across studies (150). Findings such as these have suggested the possibility that prostate cancer may result from transmission of an infectious agent through sexual activity. However, in a cohort study of cancer mortality among Catholic priests in Los Angeles, Ross and colleagues (153) found a small but statistically nonsignificant excess of prostate cancer deaths. The absence of a marked deficit of prostate cancer mortality among such men is evidence against sexual transmission of the disease. An obvious alternative explanation is that these measures of sexual activity are indices of underlying androgen production.

DIET

The other fairly well-established risk factor for prostatic cancer relevant to a hormonal etiology is dietary fat consumption. A strong correlation exists between per capita fat consumption and prostate cancer mortality on an international basis (5). Moreover, the four largest epidemiologic case-control studies found that patients with prostate cancer tended to consume more fat than controls (56, 76, 95, 155). These studies have involved diverse target populations, including African-Americans, U.S. whites, and Asian-Americans. Studies that evaluated the risk of prostate cancer in association with an intake of specific high-fat foods (e.g., beef and pork, milk, eggs, or cheese) rather than as a specific nutrient also support the notion that fat is a risk factor.

The strongest evidence to support an association between dietary fat and prostate cancer, and the most detailed evaluation of this possible relationship, comes from two prospective studies of male health professionals conducted by investigators at Harvard (52, 55). Both studies found an association between prostate cancer and consumption of animal fat, especially from red meat, and an association with the essential fatty acid, linolenic acid. The latter association was confirmed by prediagnostic measurements of linolenic acid in blood samples. The mechanism to explain these associations is unknown, but it has been hypothesized (160, 164) that dietary fat might affect prostate cancer occurrence through an alteration in the hormonal environment. In support of this hypothesis, Hill and Wynder (77) showed in a small study a decade ago that switching from a Western diet (i.e., 40% calories from fat) to an isocaloric vegetarian, low-fat diet (i.e., 25% calories from fat) substantially reduced levels of circulating testosterone. Preliminary data from the Lobund-Wistar rat model suggest that dietary fat may enhance the effects of testosterone in inducing prostatic cancer, but isocaloric diets have not yet been evaluated in this system (138).

Adolescent and Young Adult Genital Cancer

Herbst and colleagues (75), describing the association between in utero diethylstilbestrol (DES) exposure and vaginal adenocarcinoma provided the initial suggestion that estrogen might induce anomalous development in utero which would later have neoplastic consequences in the postpubertal period (75). These neoplasms developed within a limited age range (approximately ages 15–29); and the relevant exposure nearly always occurred during the first trimester of the index pregnancy. Vaginal adenocarcinomas appear to develop from Müllerian duct remnants that are induced by DES exposure to persist beyond early fetal life. These remain dormant during childhood and are activated at puberty.

The age-specific incidence rates of malignant germ cell tumors of the testis peak in early adult life, in a pattern that is similar to that of DES-induced vaginal adenocarcinoma (154). This correspondence suggests that the etiology of testicular germ cell neoplasms may also involve in utero hormonal exposure. Risk factors for testis cancer include a history of cryptorchidism, Caucasian race and in utero exogenous estrogen exposure, and may include maternal nausea and maternal obesity as well.

Men with a cryptorchid testis have been reported to have relative risks of testis cancer ranging from 3 to 14, compared to men who experienced normal testicular descent (37, 64, 141). A persistently undescended testis is often accompanied by other structural abnormalities. The testis is smaller and tubule development and spermatogenesis are retarded. Sertoli cell development is delayed and Leydig cells are abnormal (75). It is not the abdominal location of the undescended testis that increases the risk of cancer in the undescended testis. After descent is achieved by surgical treatment, previously undescended testes retain a higher than normal risk of cancer (40, 141). Furthermore, the contralateral, normally descended testis in patients with unilateral cryptorchidism is reported to have a twofold increased risk of cancer (64, 88, 115).

Normal descent of the testis is under hormonal control. Animal experiments have shown that estrogen treatment of pregnant mice can lead to undescended and hypogenetic testes (127). Similar abnormalities have been reported in the male offspring of women exposed to DES and to OCs during pregnancy (127). Thus, it is likely that cryptorchidism is tied to estrogen levels early in pregnancy and represents another, sometimes intermediate, outcome of the pathway leading to germ cell testicular tumors.

Other potential risk factors for testis cancer may also be manifestations of excess free maternal estrogen during the critical gestation period. Excessive nausea during pregnancy of mothers of patients with testis cancer may be associated with an increased risk of testis cancer; the risk is greatest for nausea requiring medical treatment and most noticeable for sons who were the mother's first live birth (37, 64). Increased levels of bioavailable estradiol are found in the first trimester of pregnancy of women with hyperemesis gravidarum compared to controls and in the first trimester of a woman's first compared to her second pregnancy (10, 36). Since adipose tissue is a source of estrogen, and since obesity is associated with reduced levels of SHBG, the increasing risk of testis cancer observed with increased weight of the mother prior to the index pregnancy may also reflect an excess of bioavailable estrogen (100).

Three of four studies of the relationship of exogenous sex steroid exposure in pregnancy and testis cancer have shown higher risk of testis cancer in sons who experienced in utero exposure to either DES, OCs, estrogen, or the estrogen-progestin combinations used in pregnancy tests, with reported relative risks ranging from 2.8–5.3 (37, 64, 116, 157).

The rarity of testis cancer and, correspondingly, cryptorchidism, in black males, may represent a slight variation of this "estrogen excess" hypothesis (154). The substantially higher plasma testosterone as well as estrogen levels in black women compared to white women early in gestation suggest the possibility that both hormones may be important factors in the development of the testis (65). The absolute excess of testosterone in the early gestation blood of black women, by providing a "protected" environment for testicular development and descent, is one possible explanation for the subsequent lower incidence of testis cancer in black male offspring. In rats, estrogen-inhibited testicular descent can be reversed by treatment with androgens (145).

There are similarities in the epidemiology of ovarian and testicular germ-cell tumors, even though the former are comparatively rare. Ovarian tumors tend to have a peak incidence rate in the young adult age range, and as for testicular cancer, these rates have been increasing (172). Furthermore, risk of these tumors also is associated with maternal exposure to hormonal drugs during the index pregnancy (171).

Cervical Cancer

Numerous studies of the relationship between hormonal contraceptives and cervical neoplasia have been conducted; however, not much attention has been paid to the contribution of other hormonal factors to the etiology of this disease. A small study of cervical cell mitotic activity during the menstrual cycle has shown that the mitotic rate was 1.85-fold greater during the luteal phase of the cycle than in the follicular phase (96). The mitotic rate of postmenopausal women was only 33% of that in premenopausal women. These data would predict that the slope of the age-specific incidence curve for cervical cancer should decrease after menopause as it does for cancers of the breast, ovary, and endometrium. Mortality and incidence data that predate the widespread use of Pap testing suggest that this is true (29).

The relationship between OCs and risk of cervical cancer risk requires careful evaluation (9). Sexual factors such as age at first sexual intercourse and number of sexual partners, which are risk factors for cervical cancer, also may be associated with OC use. Furthermore, OC use is positively associated with the frequency of cervical Pap testing (62, 85, 163). This positive association would be expected to produce a positive association of cervical carcinoma in situ (CIS) with OC use whether or not a true etiologic association exists. It also would be expected to downwardly bias any association of OC use with invasive cervical cancer by detecting tumors at a premalignant or in situ stage. Few studies have adjusted for Pap testing and sexual history in evaluating the relationship between OC use and risk of cervical cancer risk.

Two recent case-control studies examined the issue of a possible spurious association between OC use and cervical CIS, but the studies arrived at opposite conclusions. Irwin and colleagues (85) found a higher risk of cervical CIS among OC users overall, but no increased risk was observed when they restricted analyses to subgroups of subjects for whom no association between Pap testing and OC use existed. In a study conducted by Kjaer and colleagues (93), however, OC use was associated with a higher risk of cervical CIS in women who had never had a previous Pap test as well as among those who had been tested previously.

Analytic studies involving OC use and invasive cervical cancer either have focused almost entirely on squamous cell malignancies or have not provided analyses by cell type. Results for studies that included primarily squamous cell tumors provide some evidence that OC use increases the risk of invasive cervical cancer. For example, in a case-control study conducted by Brinton and colleagues (18), the relative risk for OC users was 1.5 times that of nonusers after adjustment for possible sexual factors and Pap testing. In this study, long-term OC users (i.e., 5 or more years) had an approximately twofold higher risk than nonusers. Overall, women who had used OCs containing a high estrogen content were not at highest risk.

An increasing incidence of cervical adenocarcinoma has been reported among women under 35 years of age in Los Angeles County, California (132), and in areas served by population-based cancer registries participating in the Surveillance, Epidemiology and End Results Program (158). In these areas, however, incidence has remained essentially constant over the same period among older women. Peters and colleagues (132) hypothesized that OC use during the teenage years might account for this trend, because OCs produce morphologic changes in the endocervix that are characterized by stromal edema, excessive mucus production, and glandular hyperplasia (113). The extent of these histologic changes increases with longer continuous use of the contraceptive agents (51).

A population-based, case-control study conducted in Los Angeles County, California, that was limited to young women (born after 1935) who had been diagnosed with cervical adenocarcinoma was recently published as well (169). Based on personal interviews of 195 patients and 386 age-, race-, and neighborhood-of-residence-matched controls, the risk of cervical adenocarcinoma was statistically significantly greater among women who had used OCs than among those who had not (RR = 2.1). The highest risk was observed for OC use that exceeded 12 years (RR = 4.4). No further increased risk was suggested for early age at first use, long-term use beginning at an early age, elapsed time since first use, recent use, or particular formulations of OCs.

Thyroid Cancer

The pituitary hormone thyroid-stimulating hormone (TSH) is the principal hormone regulating the growth and function of the thyroid gland; thus, excess TSH may be of etiologic importance in the development of thyroid cancer (84). This hypothesis is supported by the observation that the growth of some thyroid cancers depends on TSH secretion, so that suppression of TSH release by administration of thyroxin often is an effective treatment for thyroid carcinomas (31). Experimental studies provide further support. Sustained elevation of TSH levels induces thyroid tumors in rodents (7, 58). The actual mechanism by which elevated TSH levels have been achieved in these studies appears to be unimportant as thyroid tumors have been produced by iodine-deficient diets, blocking thyroid hormone synthesis, administering TSH directly, and chemical goitrogens (114).

In the United States, thyroid cancer is roughly 2.5 times more common in women than in men. Incidence rates for women increase sharply from childhood to age 30 and then plateau; whereas in men, incidence rates increase gradually over the lifespan. The ratio of female-to-male incidence rates is greatest between the ages of 20 and 35, during which women have 4 to 5 times the risk of men. This ratio remains above 3 until menopause, when it begins to level off around 1.5. This suggests that sex hormones may play an important role in the development of thyroid cancer.

A history of pregnancy has been associated with elevated risk of thyroid cancer in three case-control studies (109, 143, 149). Thyroid glandular activity is increased during pregnancy, because estrogen increases thyroxine-binding globulin (TBG) concentrations (20). The level of TBG in normal females is 10 to 20% higher than in males, and during pregnancy, a 50% increase in the level of TBG globulin produces an increase in TSH of similar magnitude (53, 106, 128). It therefore also is likely that TSH levels of nonpregnant, normal females may vary and be elevated above the level of males at some point in the menstrual cycle, although not necessarily throughout the cycle.

Osteosarcoma

The age-specific incidence curve for osteosarcoma shows a distinct peak during adolescence (70). Epidemiologic findings strongly suggest that this adolescent peak is associated with the pattern of childhood skeletal growth. Osteosarcomas in adolescents most frequently occur in the epiphyses of long bones, sites of maximal bone growth, and often in conjunction with the adolescent growth spurt, when skeletal growth is maximal (144, 173). Skeletal growth results from a combination of factors, but hormonal activity is a primary stimulus.

During the preadolescent period, from approximately age 5 to age 11, girls grow faster than boys. However, their growth stops earlier, so that by the middle to late teenage years, males are considerably taller (165). The age-specific incidence curves for osteosarcoma follow this same pattern. Rates of osteosarcoma for girls up to approximately age 13 are roughly 30% higher than those for boys. In the 15- to 24-year-old age group, the male rate exceeds the female rate by some 140%. Blacks are known to have proportionately longer legs and arms than whites despite similar adult heights, and their rates of osteosarcoma under age 25 are higher than those of whites, with all excess incidence resulting from long-bone tumors (45).

Conclusion

As our understanding of the relationship between epidemiologic risk factors and the circulating levels of relevant hormones grows, avenues for primary prevention are now becoming apparent. Control of obesity has obvious implications for endometrial cancer and postmenopausal breast cancer. More information on the relationship between childhood diet and physical activity as well as the onset of puberty and the hormonal physiology of adolescence and young adulthood may provide increasing avenues for preventing breast, ovarian, and endometrial cancer in women, and perhaps even prostate cancer in men (13). Hormonal chemoprevention trials for breast cancer are currently underway based on our present understanding of the hormonal etiology of that tumor, and a national trial to prevent prostate cancer through use of finasteride, a 5α-reductase inhibitor, has just begun (32, 52, 136). Hormonal chemoprevention of ovarian and endometrial cancer is already occurring in the population at large through the widespread use of OCs and, for endometrial cancer, increasing use of combination hormone replacement therapy. Clearly, knowledge accumulated about the potential adverse impact of exogenous steroids in the form of contraceptives and hormone replacement therapy (Table 14.4) has led to continuing improvements in these products as well as in the overall balance of the health risks and benefits. A growing knowledge of the mutations and polymorphisms in genes that cause an increased risk of these cancers should lead to a better definition of individual susceptibility, and it should then be possible to focus intervention strategies on the higher-risk subgroups of the population.

Table 14.4. Established Effects of Combination Oral Contraceptives and Estrogen Replacement Therapy on Cancer Risk

	Change in risk/year (%)	Predicted relative risk	
		5 Years	10 Years
Oral contraceptives			
Ovary	−7.5	0.68	0.46
Endometrium	−11.7	0.54	0.29
Breast			
≤45 years	3.1	1.16	1.36
>45 years	0.0	1.00	1.00
Estrogen replacement therapy			
Endometrium	28.5[a]	3.50[a]	12.28[a]
Breast	3.1	1.16	1.36

[a] These estimates may be too high because of the misclassification of "hyperplasia" as "neoplasia."

References

1. Ahluwalia B, Jackson MA, Jones GW, Williams AO, Rao MS, Rajguru S. Blood hormone profiles in prostate cancer patients in high risk and low risk populations. Cancer 1981;48:2267.
2. Anderson DE. Genetic study of breast cancer: identification of a high risk group. Cancer 1974;34:1090.
3. Apter D, Reinila M, Vihko R. Some endocrine characteristics of early menarche, a risk factor for breast cancer, are preserved into adulthood. Int J Cancer 1989;44:783.
4. Apter D, Vihko R. Early menarche, a risk factor for breast cancer, indicates early onset of ovulatory cycles. J Clin Endocrinol Metab 1983;57:82.
5. Armstrong BG, Doll R. Environmental factors and cancer incidence and mortality in different countries, with special reference to dietary practices. Int J Cancer 1975;15:617.
6. Austin DF, Roe KM. Increase in cancer of the corpus uteri in the San Francisco-Oakland standard metropolitan statistical area, 1960–1975. JNCI 1979;62:13.
7. Axelrad AA, Leblond CP. Induction of thyroid tumors in rats by a low iodine diet. Cancer 1955;8:339.
8. Barrett-Connor E, Garland C, McPhillips JB, Khaw KT, Wingard DL. A prospective population-based study of androstenedione, estrogens and prostatic cancer. Cancer Res 1990;50:169.
9. Beral V, Hannaford P, Kay C. Oral contraceptive use and malignancies of the genital tract. Lancet 1988;2:1331.
10. Bernstein L, Depue RH, Ross RK, Judd HL, Pike MC, Henderson BE. Higher maternal levels of free estradiol in first compared to second pregnancy: early gestation differences. JNCI 1986;76:1035.
11. Bernstein L, Henderson BE, Hanisch, R et al. Physical exercise activity reduces the risk of breast cancer in young women. JNCI 1994;86:1403.
12. Bernstein L, Pike MC, Ross RK, Judd HL, Brown JB, Henderson BE. Estrogen and sex hormone-binding globulin levels in nulliparous and parous women. JNCI 1985;74:741.
13. Bernstein L, Ross RK, Lobo RA, Hanisch R, Krailo MD, Henderson BE. The effects of moderate physical activity on menstrual cycle patterns in adolescence: implication for breast cancer prevention. Br J Cancer 1987;55:681.
14. Bernstein L, Yuan JM, Ross RK, Pike MC, Hanisch R, Lobo R, Stanczyk F, Gao, Y-T, Henderson BE. Serum hormone levels in premenopausal Chinese women in Shang-

hai and white women in Los Angeles: results from two breast cancer case-control studies. Cancer Causes Control 1990;1:51.
15. Bishop DT, Cannon-Albright L, McLellen T,. et al. Segregation and linkage analysis of nine Utah breast cancer pedigrees. Genet Epidemiol 1988;5:151.
16. Bittner JJ. The causes and control of mammary cancer in mice. Harvey Lect 1947;42: 221.
17. Bosland MC, Prinsen MK, Kroes R. Adenocarcinomas of the prostate induced by N-nitroso-N-methylurea in rats pretreated with cyproterone acetate and testosterone. Cancer Lett 1983;18:69.
18. Brinton LA, Huggins GR, Lehman HF, Mallin K, Savitz DA, Trapido E, Rosenthal J, Hoover R. Long-term use of oral contraceptives and risk of invasive cervical cancer. Int J Cancer 1986;38:339.
19. Bruzzi P, Negri E, La Vecchia C, Decarli A, Palli D, Parazzini F, Del Turco MR. Short-term increase in risk of breast cancer after full-term pregnancy. Br Med J 1988;297: 1096.
20. Burrow GN. Thyroid function in relation to age and pregnancy. In: The Thyroid Gland. Edited by M DeVisscher. New York: Raven, 1980, p 215.
21. Casagrande JT, Louie EW, Pike MC, Roy S, Ross RK, Henderson BE. "Incessant ovulation" and ovarian cancer. Lancet 1979;2:170.
22. Centers for Disease Control: Oral contraceptive use and the risk of endometrial cancer. JAMA 1983;249:1600.
23. Centers for Disease Control: The reduction in risk of ovarian cancer associated with oral contraceptive use. N Engl J Med 1987;316:650.
24. Chu J, Schweid AI, Weiss NS. Survival among women with endometrial cancer: a comparison of estrogen users and non-users. Am J Obstet Gynecol 1982;143:569.
25. Claus EB, Risch N, Thompson WD. Genetic analysis of breast cancer in the Cancer and Steroid Hormone Study. Am J Hum Genet 1991;48:232.
26. Coetzee G, Ross R. Prostate cancer and the androgen receptor. JNCI 1994;86:872.
27. Coffey DS. Physiology of reproduction. In Androgen Excess and the Sex Accessory Tissue. Edited by E Knoble, J Neill, 1988, p 1081.
28. Cohen LA, Kendall ME, Zang E, et al. Modulation of *N*-nitrosomethylurea-induced mammary tumor promotion by dietary fiber and fat. JNCI 1991;83:496.
29. Cook GA, Draper GJ. Trends in cervical cancer and carcinoma in situ in Great Britain. Br J Cancer 1984;50:367.
30. Cornelis RS, Cornelisse CJ, Devliee P. Selection of families for predictive testing for breast cancer. Lancet 1994;344:1151.
31. Crile, G. Endocrine dependency of papillary carcinomas of the thyroid. JAMA 1966;195:721.
32. Cuzick J, Wang DY, Bulbrook RD. The prevention of breast cancer. Lancet 1986;2: 83.
33. Daling JR, Malone KE, Voigt LF, White E, Weiss NS. Risk of breast cancer among young women: relationship to induced abortion. JNCI 1994;86:1584.
34. Davis DL, Russell DW. Unusual length polymorphism in human steroid 5α-reductase type 2 gene (SRD5A2). Hum Molec Genet 1993;2:820.
35. Del Senno L, Aguiari G, Piva R. Dinucleotide repeat polymorphism in the human estrogen receptor (ESR) gene. Hum Molec Genet 1992;1:354.
36. Depue RH, Bernstein L, Ross RK, Judd HL, Henderson BE. Hyperemesis gravidarum in relation to estradiol levels, pregnancy outcome, and other maternal factors: a seroepidemiologic study. Am J Obstet Gynecol 1987;156:1137.
37. Depue RH, Pike MC, Henderson BE. Estrogen exposure during gestation and risk of testicular cancer. JNCI 1983;71:1151.
38. deWaard F, Baanders-van Halewijn EA. A prospective study in general practice on breast cancer risk in postmenopausal women. Int J Cancer 1974;14:153.
39. Doll R. The age distribution of cancer. J Stat Soc A 1977;134:133.
40. Dow JA, Mostofi FK. Testicular tumors following orchiopexy. South Med J 1967;60: 193.
41. Drafta D, Proca E, Zamfir V, Schindler AE, Neacsu E, Stroe E. Plasma steroids in benign prostatic hypertrophy and carcinoma of the prostate. J Steroid Biochem 1982;17:689.
42. Easton DF, Bishop DT, Ford D, et al. Genetic linkage analysis in familial breast and ovarian cancer: results from 214. Am J Hum Genet 1993;52:678.
43. Edwards A, Hammond, H A, Jin I, et al. Genetic variation of five trimeric and tandem repeat loci in four human population groups. Genomics 1992;12:241.
44. Elwood JM, Cole P, Rothman KJ, Kaplan SD. Epidemiology of endometrial cancer. JNCI 1977;59:1055.
45. Eveleth PB, Tunner JM. Worldwide Variation in Growth. Cambridge: Cambridge University Press, 1976.
46. Fearon E, Cho K, Nigro J, et al. Identification of a chromosome 18q gene that is altered on colorectal cancers. Science 1990;247:49.
47. Ferguson DJP, Anderson TJ. Morphological evaluation of cell turnover in relation to the menstrual cycle in the "resting" human breast. Br J Cancer 1981;44:177.
48. Franceschi S, La Vecchia C, Helmrich SP, Magnioni C, Toynoni G. Risk factors for epithelial ovarian cancer in Italy. Am J Epidemiol 1982;115:714.
49. Frisch R, Gotz-Welbergen A, McArthur J, et al. Delayed menarche and amenorrhea of college athletes in relation to age at onset of training. JAMA 1981;246:1559.
50. Futreal PA, Liu Q, Shattuck-Edens E, et al. BRCA1 mutations in primary breast and ovarian carcinomas. Science 1994;266:120.
51. Gall SA, Bourgeois CH, Maguire R. The morphologic effects of oral contraceptive agents on the cervix. JAMA 1969;202:2243.
52. Gann PH, Hennekens CH, Sacks, et al. A prospective study of plasma fatty acids and risk of prostate cancer. JNCI (in press)
53. Gershengorn MC, Glinoer D, Robbins J. Transport and metabolism of thyroid hormones. In The Thyroid Gland. Edited by M. DeVisscher. New York, Raven, 1980, p 81.
54. Ghanadian R, Puah CM, O'Donoghue EPN. Serum testosterone and dihydrotestosterone in carcinoma of the prostate. Br J Cancer 1979;39:696.
55. Giovannucci E, Rimm EB, Colditz GA, Stampfer MJ, Ascherio A, Chute CC, Willett WC. A prospective study of dietary fat and risk of prostate cancer. JNCI 1993;85: 1571.
56. Graham S, Haughey B, Marshall J, Priore R, Byers T, Rzepka T, Mettlin C, Pontes JE. Diet in the epidemiology of carcinoma of the prostate gland. JNCI 1983;70:687.
57. Gray GE, Pike MC, Henderson, BE. Breast cancer incidence and mortality rates in different countries in relation to known risk factors and dietary practices. Br J Cancer 1979;39:1.
58. Griesback WE, Kennedy TH, Purves HD. Studies on experimental goitre. III. The effect of goitrogenic diet of hypophysectomized rats. Br J Exp Pathol 1941;22:249.
59. Hadjimichael OC, Boyle CA, Meigs JW. Abortion before first live birth and risk of breast cancer. Br J Cancer 1986;53:281.
60. Hall J, Lee M, Newman B, et al. Linkage of early-onset familial breast cancer to chromosome 17q21. Science 1990;250:1684.
61. Hall JM, Friedman L, Guether C, et al. Closing in on a breast cancer gene on chromosome 17q. Am J Hum Genet 1992;50:1235.
62. Hellberg D, Valentin J, Nilsson S. Long-term use of oral contraceptives and cervical neoplasia: an association confounded by other risk factors? Contraception 1985;32: 227.
63. Henderson BE. Summary report of the sixth symposium on cancer registries in the Pacific Basin. JNCI 1990;82:1186.
64. Henderson BE, Benton B, Jing J, Yu MC, Pike MC. Risk factors for cancer of the testis in young men. Int J Cancer 1979;23:598.
65. Henderson BE, Bernstein L, Ross RK, Depue RH, Judd HL. The early *in utero* oestrogen and testosterone environment of blacks and whites. Potential effects on male offspring. Br J Cancer 1988;57:216.
66. Henderson BE, Casagrande JT, Pike MC, Mack T, Rosario I, Duke A. The epidemiology of endometrial cancer in young women. Br J Cancer 1983;47:749.
67. Henderson BE, Gerkins V, Rosario I. Elevated serum levels of estrogen and prolactin in daughters of breast cancer patients. N Engl J Med 1975;293:790.
68. Henderson BE, Pike MC, Casagrande JT. Breast cancer and the estrogen window hypothesis. Lancet 1981;2:363.
69. Henderson BE, Pike MC, Ross RK. Epidemiology and risk factors. In Breast Cancer: Diagnosis and Management. Edited by G. Bonadonna. New York, Wiley, 1984, p 15.
70. Henderson BE, Ross RK, Bernstein L. Estrogens as a cause of human cancer: The Richard and Hinda Rosenthal Foundation Award Lecture. Cancer Res 1988;48:246.
71. Henderson BE, Ross RK, Judd HL, Krailo MD, Pike MC. Do regulatory ovulatory cycles increase breast cancer risk? Cancer 1985;56:1206.
72. Henderson BE, Ross RK, Lobo RA, Pike MC, Mack TM. Reevaluating the role of progestogen therapy after the menopause. Fertility and Sterility 1988;49:98.
73. Henderson BE, Ross RK, Pike MC. Hormonal chemoprevention of cancer in women. Science 1993;259:633.
74. Henderson BE, Ross RK, Pike MC, Casagrande JT. Endogenous hormones as a major factor in human cancer. Cancer Res 1982;43:3232.
75. Herbst AL, Cole P, Norusis MJ, Welch WR, Scully RE. Epidemiologic aspects and factors related to survival in 384 registry cases of clear cell adenocarcinoma of the vagina and cervix. Am J Obstet Gynecol 1979;135:876.
76. Heshmat MY, Kaul L, Kovi J, Jackson MA, Jackson AG, Jones GW, Edson M, Enterline JP, Worrell RG, Perry SL. Nutrition and prostate cancer: a case-control study. Prostate 1985;6:7.
77. Hill PB, Wynder EL. Effect of vegetarian diet and dexamethasone on plasma prolactin, testosterone and dehydroepiandrosterone in men and women. Cancer Lett 1979;7:273.
78. Hirayama T. Epidemiology of breast cancer with special reference to the role of diet. Prev Med 1978;7:173.
79. Honda GD, Bernstein L, Ross RK, Greenland S, Gerkins V, Henderson BE. Vasectomy, cigarette smoking, age at first sexual intercourse as risk factors for prostate cancer in middle-aged men. Br J Cancer 1988;57:326.
80. Howe GR, Friederreich CM, Jain M, et al. A cohort study of fat intake and risk of breast cancer. JNCI 1991;83:336.
81. Howe GR, Hirohata T, Hislop TG, et al. Dietary factors and risk of breast cancer: combined analysis of 12 case-control studies. JNCI 1990;82:561.
82. Hulka BS, Hammond JE, DiFerdinanado G, Mickey DD, Fried FA, Checkoway H, Strumpf WE, Beckman WC, Clark DC. Serum hormone levels among patients with prostatic carcinoma or benign prostatic hyperplasia and clinic controls. Prostate 1987;11:171.
83. Hunter DJ, Willett WC. Diet, body build, and breast cancer. Annu Rev Nutr 1994;14: 393.
84. Ingbar SH, Woeber KA. The thyroid gland. In Textbook of Endocrinology. Edited by R. H. Williams. Philadelphia: Saunders, 1974, p 95.
85. Irwin KL, Rosero-Bixby L, Oberle MW, Lee NC, Whatley AS, Fortnery JA, Bonhomme MG. Oral contraceptives and cervical cancer risk in Costa Rica: detection bias or causal association? JAMA 1988;259:59.
86. Iselius L, Slack J, Littler M, et al. Genetic epidemiology of breast cancer in Britain. Ann Hum Genet 1991;55:151.
87. Jenster C, Van der Korput, HAGM, Van Vroonhoven C, et al. Domains of human androgen receptor involved in steroid binding, transcriptional activation, and subcellular localization. Molec Endocrinol 1991;5:1396.
88. Johnson DE, Woodhead DM, Pohl DR, Robison J. Cryptorchidism and testicular tumorigenesis. Surgery 1968;63:919.
89. Kelsey JL, LiVolsi VA, Holford TR, Fischer DA, Morton ED, Schwartz PE, O'Connor T, White C. A case-control study of cancer of the endometrium. Am J Epidemiol 1982;116:333.
90. Kennedy DL, Baum C, Forbes MB. Noncontraceptive estrogens and progestins: use patterns over time. Obstet Gynecol 1985;65:441.
91. Key TJA, Pike MC. The dose-effect relationship between "unopposed" estrogens and endometrial mitotic rate its central role in explaining and predicting endometrial cancer risk. Br J Cancer 1988;57:205.
92. Key TJA, Pike MC. The role of oestrogens and progestagens in the epidemiology and prevention of breast cancer. Eur J Cancer Clin Oncol 1988;24:29.
93. Kjaer SK, Engholm G, Dahl C, et al. Case-control study of risk factors for cervical squamous-cell neoplasia in Denmark. III. Role of oral contraceptive use. Cancer Causes Control 1993;4:513.
94. Knudson A. Mutation and cancer: statistical study of retinoblastoma. Proc Natl Acad Sci USA 1971;68:820.
95. Kolonel LN, Yoshizawa CN, Hankin JH. Diet and prostatic cancer: a case-control study in Hawaii. Am J Epidemiol 1988;127:999.
96. Konishi I, Fujii S, Nonogaki H, Nanbu Y, Iwai T, Mori T. Immunohistochemical analysis of estrogen receptors, progesterone receptors, Ki-67 antigen, and human papillomavirus DNA in normal and neoplastic epithelium of the uterine cervix. Cancer 1991;68:1340.
97. Labrie F, Sugimoto Y, Luu-The V, Simard J, Lachance Y, Bachvarov D, Leblanc G,

Durocher F, Paquet N. Structure of the human type II 5α-reductase gene. Endocrinology 1992;131:1571.
98. La Spada AR, Wilson EM, Lubahn DB, et al. Androgen receptor gene mutations in X-linked spinal and bulbar muscular atrophy. Nature 1991;352:77.
99. La Vecchia C, Franceschi S, Decarli A, Gallus G, Toynoni G. Risk factors for endometrial cancer at three different ages. JNCI 1984;73:667.
100. MacDonald PC, Edman CD, Hemsell DL, Porter JC, Siiteri PK. Effect of obesity on conversion of plasma androstenedione to estrone in postmenopausal women with and without endometrial cancer. Am J Obstet Gynecol 1978;130:448.
101. Mack T, Cozen W, Quinn M. Epidemiology of gynecological cancer of the endometrium, ovary, vulva, and vagina. In Gynecological Oncology, 2nd ed. Edited by M Coppleson. London: Churchill Livingston, 1991.
102. Mack TM, Pike MC, Henderson BE, Pfeffer RI, Gerkins VR, Arthur M, Brown SE. Estrogens and endometrial cancer in a retirement community. N Engl J Med 1976;294:1262.
103. MacMahon B, Cole P, Brown JB, Aoki K, Lin TM, Morgan RW, Woo, N-C. Urine estrogen profiles of Asian and North American women. Int J Cancer 1974;14:161.
104. MacMahon B, Cole P, Lin TM, Lowe CR, Mirra AP, Ravnihar B, Salber EJ, Valaoras VG, Yuasa S. Age at first birth and cancer of the breast: a summary of an international study. Bull WHO 1970;43:209.
105. MacMahon B, Trichopoulos D, Brown J, Andersen AP, Aoki K, Cole P, deWaard F, Kauraniemi T, Morgan RW, Purde M, Ravihar B, Stormby N, Westlund K, Woo, N-C. Age at menarche, probability of ovulation and breast cancer risk. Int J Cancer 1982;29:13.
106. Malkasian GD, Mayberry WE. Serum total and free thyroxine and thyrotropin in normal and pregnant women, neonates, and women receiving progestogens. Am J Obstet Gynecol 1970;108:1234.
107. Malkin D, Li FP, Strong LC, et al. Germline p53 mutations in a familial syndrome of breast cancer, sarcomas and other neoplasms. Science 1992;250:1233.
108. Mannermaa A, Peltoketo H, Winqvist R, et al. Human familial and sporadic breast cancer: analysis of the coding regions of the 17β-hydroxysteroid dehydrogenase 2 gene (EDH17B2) using a single-strand conformation polymorphism assay. Hum Genet 1994;93:319.
109. McTiernan AM, Weiss NS, Daling JR. Incidence of thyroid cancer in women in relation to reproductive and hormonal factors. Am J Epidemiol 1984;120:423.
110. Mhatte AN, Trinliro MA, Kaufman M, et al. Reduced transcriptional regulatory competence of the androgen receptor in X-linked spinal and bulbar muscular atrophy. Nature Genet 1993;5:184.
111. Miki Y, Swensen J, Shattuck-Eiders et al. A strong candidate for the breast and ovarian cancer susceptibility gene BRCA1. Science 1994;266:66.
112. Mills PK, Beeson WL, Phillips RL, et al. Dietary habits and breast cancer incidence among Seventh-Day Adventists. Cancer 1989;64:582.
113. Minteot R, Fievez CL. Endocervical changes with the use of synthetic steroids. Obstet Gynecol 1974;44:53.
114. Morris HP. Experimental thyroid tumors. Brookhaven Symp Bio 7:192;1954.
115. Morrison AS. Cryptorchidism, hernia and cancer of the testis. JNCI 1976;56:731.
116. Moss AR, Osmond D, Bacchetti P, Torti FM, Gurgin V. Hormonal risk factors in testicular cancer: a case-control study. Am J Epidemiol 1986;124:39.
117. Muir C, Waterhouse J, Mack T, Powell J, Whelan S. Cancer Incidence in Five Continents, vol 5. Lyon: IARC, 1987.
118. Murphy GP, Natarajan N, Pontes JE, Schmitz RL, Smart CR, Schmidt JD, Mettlin C. The national survey of prostate cancer in the United States by the American College of Surgeons. J Urol 1982;127:926.
119. Musey VC, Collins EC, Musey PI, Martino-Saltzman D, Preedy JR. Long-term effect of a first pregnancy on the secretion of prolactin. N Engl J Med 1987;316:229.
120. Narod SA, Feuteun J, Lynch HT, et al. Familial breast-ovarian cancer locus on chromosome 17q12-q23. Lancet 1991;338:82.
121. Newcomb PA, Storer BE, Longnecker MP, et al. Lactation and a reduced risk of premenopausal breast cancer. N Engl J Med 1994;330:81.
122. Newhouse ML, Pearson RM, Fullerton JM, Boesen EAM, Shannon HS. A case-control study of carcinoma of the ovary. Br J Prev Soc Med 1979;31:148.
123. Newman B, Austin MA, Lee M, et al. Inheritance of human breast cancer: evidence for autosomal dominant transmission in high risk families. Proc Natl Acad Sci USA 1988;85:1.
124. Noble RL. The development of prostatic adenocarcinoma in Nb rats following prolonged sex hormone administration. Cancer Res 37:1929;1977.
125. Nomura A, Heilbrun ZK, Stemmermann GN, Judd HL. Prediagnostic serum hormones and the risk of prostate cancer. Cancer Res 1988;48:3515.
126. Nomura A, Henderson BE, Lee J. Breast cancer and diet among the Japanese in Hawaii. Am J Clin Nutr 1978;31:2020.
127. Nomura T, Kanzaki T. Induction of urogenital anomalies and some tumors in the progeny of mice receiving diethylstilbestrol during pregnancy. Cancer Res 1977;37:1099.
128. Pacchiarotti A, Martino E, Bartalena L, Buratti L, Mammoli C, Strigini F, Fruzzetti F, Melis GB, Pinchera A. Serum thyrotropin by ultrasensitive immunoradiometric assay and serum free thyroid hormones in pregnancy. J Endocrinol Invest 1986;9:185.
129. Paganini-Hill A, Ross RK, Henderson BE. Endometrial cancer and patterns of use of oestrogen replacement therapy: a cohort study. Br J Cancer 1989;59:445.
130. Persson I, Adami HO, Bergkvist K, Lundgren A, Petterson B, Hoover R, Schairer C. Risk of endometrial cancer after treatment with oestrogens alone or in conjunction with progestogens: results of a prospective study. Br Med J 1989;298:147.
131. Persson I, Yuen J, Bergvist L, et al. Combined oestrogen-progestogen replacement and breast cancer risk. Lancet 1992;340:1044. (Letter)
132. Peters RK, Chao A, Mack TM, et al. Increased frequency of adenocarcinomas of the uterine cervix in young women in Los Angeles County. JNCI 1986;76:423.
133. Pike MC, Bernstein LB, Spicer V. Exogenous hormones and breast cancer risk. In Current Therapy in Oncology. Edited by J. E Niederhuber. New York: Marcel Dekker, 1993.
134. Pike MC, Henderson BE, Casagrande JT, Rosario I, Gray GE. Oral contraceptive use and early abortion as risk factors for breast cancer in young women. Br J Cancer 1981;43:72.
135. Pike MC, Krailo MC, Henderson BE, Casagrande JT, Hoel DG. "Hormonal" risk factors, "breast tissue age" and the age-incidence of breast cancer. Nature 1983;303:767.
136. Pike MC, Ross RK, Lobo RA, Key TJA, Potts M, Henderson BE. LHRH agonists and the prevention of breast and prostate cancer. Br J Cancer 1989;60:142.
137. Piva R, Gambari R, Zoratao F, et al. Analysis of upstream sequences of the human estrogen receptor gene. Biochem Biophys Res Commun 1992;183:996.
138. Pollard M, Luckert PH. Prostate cancer in a Sprague-Dawley rat. Prostate 1985;6:1.
139. Pollard M, Luckert PH, Schmidt MA. Induction of prostate adenocarcinomas in Lobund-Wistar rats by testosterone. Prostate 1982;4:563.
140. Ponglikitmongkol M, Green S, Chambon P. Genomic organization of the human oestrogen receptor gene. EMBO J 1988;7:3385.
141. Pottern LM, Brown LM, Hoover RN, Javadpour N, O'Connell KJ, Stutzman RE, Blattner WA. Testicular cancer risk among young men: role of cryptorchidism and inguinal hernia. JNCI 1985;74:377.
142. Poutanen M, Miettinen M, Vihko R. Differential estrogen substrate specificities for transiently expressed human placental 17β-hydroxysteroid dehydrogenase and an endogenous enzyme expressed in cultured COS-m6 cells. Endocrinology 1993;133:2639.
143. Preston-Martin S, Bernstein L, Pike MC, Maldonado AA, Henderson BE. Thyroid cancer among young women related to prior thyroid disease and pregnancy history. Br J Cancer 55:191;1987.
144. Price CHG. Primary bone-forming tumors and their relationship to skeletal growth. J Bone Joint Surg (Br) 1958;40:574.
145. Rajfer J, Walsh PC. Hormonal regulation of testicular descent: experimental and clinical observations. J Urol 1977;118:985.
146. Ramcharan S, Pellegrin FA, Ray R, Hsu JP. A prospective study of the side effects of oral contraceptive use. In The Walnut Creek Contraceptive Drug Study, vol 3. NIH Publ No. 81–564, Washington DC: US Government Printing Office, 1981.
147. Rivenson A, Silverman J. Prostatic cancer in laboratory animals. In Endocrinology of Cancer. Edited by D. P. Rose. Boca Raton FL: CRC, 1979, p 2.
148. Rogers J, Mitchell GW. The relation of obesity to menstrual disturbances. N Engl J Med 1952;247:53.
149. Ron E, Kleinerman RA, Boice JD, LiVolsi VA, Flannery JT, Fraumeni JF. A population-based case-control study of thyroid cancer. JNCI 1987;79:1.
150. Ross RK. Prostate cancer. In Cancer Epidemiology and Prevention, 2nd ed. Edited by D. Schottenfeld, J. Fraumeni. Philadelphia: Saunders, In press.
151. Ross RK, Bernstein L, Judd H, Hanisch R, Pike M, Henderson BE. Serum testosterone levels in young black and white men. JNCI 1986;76:45.
152. Ross RK, Bernstein L, Lobo RA, Shimizu H, Stanczyk FZ, Pike MC, Henderson BE. 5-Alpha-reductase activity and risk of prostate cancer among Japanese and U.S.white and black males. Lancet 1992;339:887.
153. Ross RK, Deapen DM, Casagrande JT, Paganini-Hill A, Henderson BE. A cohort study of mortality from cancer of the prostate in Catholic priests. Br J Cancer 1981;43:233.
154. Ross RK, McCurtis JW, Henderson BE, Menck HR, Mack TM, Martin SP. Descriptive epidemiology of testicular and prostatic cancer in Los Angeles. Br J Cancer 1979;39:284.
155. Ross RK, Shimizu H, Paganini-Hill A, Honda G, Henderson BE. Case-control studies of prostate cancer in blacks and whites in Southern California. JNCI 1987;78:869.
156. Sager R. Tumor-suppressor genes: the puzzle and the promise. Science 1989;246:1406.
157. Schottenfeld D, Warshauer ME, Sherlock S, Zauber AG, Leder M, Payne R. The epidemiology of testicular cancer in young adults. Am J Epidemiol 1980;112:232.
158. Schwartz SM, Weiss NS. Increased incidence of adenocarcinoma of the cervix in young women in the United States. Am J Epidemiol 1986;124:1045.
159. Shimizu H, Ross RK, Bernstein L, Pike MC, Henderson BE. Serum estrogen levels in postmenopausal women: comparison of U.S. whites and Japanese in Japan. Br J Cancer 1990;62:451.
160. Snowdon DA, Phillips RL, Choi W. Diet, obesity, and risk of fatal prostate cancer. Am J Epidemiol 1984;120:244.
161. Stanbridge E. Identifying tumor-suppressor genes in human colorectal cancer. Science 1990;247:12.
162. Steele R, Lees REM, Kraus AS, Rao R. Sexual factors in the epidemiology of cancer of the prostate. J Chronic Dis 1971;24:29.
163. Swan SH, Brown WL. Oral contraceptive use, sexual activity and cervical carcinoma. Am J Obstet Gynecol 1981;139:52.
164. Talamini R, La Vecchia C, Decarli A, Negri E, Franceschi S. Nutrition, social factors and prostatic cancer in a Northern Italian population. Br J Cancer 1986;53:817.
165. Tanner JM. Growth at Adolescence, 2nd ed. Oxford: Blackwell, 1962, p 1.
166. Thigpen AE, Davis DL, Milatovitch A, Mendonca BB, Imperato- Ginley J, Griffin JE, Francke U, Wilson JD, Russell DW. Molecular genetics of steroid 5α-reductase 2 deficiency. J Clin Invest 1992;90:799.
167. Toniolo PG, Levitz M, Zeleniuch-Jacquotte A, Banerjee S, Koenig KL, Shore RE, Strax P, Pasternack BS. A prospective study of endogenous estrogens and breast cancer in postmenopausal women. JNCI 87: 190;1991.
168. Trichopoulos D, MacMahon B, Cole P. The menopause and breast cancer. JNCI 1972;48:605.
169. Ursin G, Peters RK, Henderson BE, et al. Oral contraceptive use and adenocarcinoma of the cervix. Lancet 1994;344:1378.
170. van Leeuwen, FE, Benraadt J, Coeberge JWW, Kiemeney LALM, Gimrealre CHF, Otter R, Schouten LJ, Damhuis RAM, Bontenbal M, Diepenhorst FW, van den Belt-Dusebout AW, van Tinteren H. Risk of endometrial cancer after tamoxifen treatment of breast cancer. Lancet 1994;343:448.
171. Walker AH, Ross RK, Haile RWC, Henderson BE. Hormonal factors and risk of ovarian germ cell cancer in young women. Br J Cancer 1988;57:418.
172. Walker AH, Ross RK, Pike MC, Henderson BE. A possible rising incidence of malignant germ cell tumors in young women. Br J Cancer 1984;49:669.
173. Weinfeld MS, Dudley HR. Osteogenic sarcoma. J Bone Joint Surg (Am) 1962;44:269.
174. Weiss N. Ovary. In Cancer Epidemiology and Prevention. Edited by D Schottenfeld, JF Fraumeni. Philadelphia: Saunders, 1982, p 871.
175. Willett WC, Browne ML, Bain C, Lipnick RJ, Stampfer MJ, Rosner B, Colditz GA, Hennekens CH, Speizer FE. Relative weight and risk of breast cancer among premenopausal women. Am J Epidemiol 1985;122:731.
176. Willett WC, Stampfer MJ, Colditz GA, et al. Dietary fat and risk of breast cancer. N Engl J Med 1987;316:22.

177. Williams WR, Anderson DE. Genetic epidemiology of breast cancer: segregation analysis of 200 Danish pedigrees. Genet Epidemiol 1984;1:7.
178. Wingo PA, Tong T, Bolden S. Cancer statistics, 1995. CA 1995.
179. Wooster R, Neuhausen SL, Mangion J, et al. Localization of a breast cancer susceptibility gene, BRCA2, to chromosome 13q12–13. Science 1994;265:2088.
180. World Health Organization. Research on the menopause. Geneva: World Health Organization Technical Report Series 670, 1981.
181. Wu ML, Whittemore AS, Paffenbarger RS, Sarles DL, Kampert JB, Grosser S, Jung DL, Ballon S, Hendrickson M, Mohle-Boetani J. Personal and environmental characteristics related to epithelial ovarian cancer. I. Reproductive and menstrual events and oral contraceptive use. Am J Epidemiol 1988;128:1216.
182. Yaich L, Dupont W, Cavener D, et al. Analysis of the *PvuII* restriction fragment-length polymorphism and exon structure of the estrogen receptor gene in breast cancer and peripheral blood. Cancer Res 1992;52:77.
183. Yu MC, Gerkins VR, Henderson BE, Brown JB, Pike MC. Elevated levels of prolactin in nulliparous women. Br J Cancer 1981;43:826.
184. Yuan J-M, Yu MC, Ross RK, Gao YT, Henderson BE. Risk factors for breast cancer in Chinese women in Shanghai. Cancer Res 48:1949;1988.
185. Ziel HK, Finkle WD. Increased risk of endometrial carcinoma among users of conjugated estrogens. N Engl J Med 1975;293:1167.
186. Zumoff B. Relationship of obesity to blood estrogens. Cancer Res 1982;42:32898.
187. Zuppan P, Hall J, Lee M, et al. Possible linkage of the estrogen receptor gene to breast cancer in a family with late-onset disease. Am J Hum Genet 1991;48:1065.

CHAPTER 15

Ionizing Radiation

JOHN B. LITTLE

Introduction

The hazards of exposure to ionizing radiation were recognized shortly after Roentgen's discovery of the x-ray in 1895. Acute skin reactions were observed in many individuals working with early x-ray generators, and by 1902 the first radiation-induced cancer was reported arising in an ulcerated area of the skin. Within a few years, a large number of such skin cancers had been observed, and the first report of leukemia in five radiation workers appeared in 1911 (89). Indeed, Marie Curie and her daughter Irene are both thought to have died of radiation-induced leukemia. Since that time, many experimental and epidemiologic studies have confirmed the oncogenic effects of radiation in many tissues of many species.

There are a number of characteristics specific to ionizing radiation that differentiate it from chemical toxic agents or other physical carcinogens. Notable among these is its ability to penetrate cells and to deposit energy within them in a random fashion, unaffected by the usual cellular barriers presented to chemical agents. All cells in the body are thus susceptible to damage by ionizing radiation; the amount of damage incurred will be related to the physical parameters that determine the radiation dose received by the particular cells or tissue. Furthermore, the physical characteristics of ionizing radiation allow us to measure accurately very low levels of exposure, doses several orders of magnitude below those that produce measurable biologic effects in human cells.

This chapter briefly reviews the principal cellular and tissue effects of radiation, as well as what is known about cellular and molecular mechanisms for radiation carcinogenesis. The term *carcinogenesis* is used in its broad sense to include the development of all types of malignant neoplasms. A more detailed description is then presented of current knowledge concerning the induction of cancer by radiation in experimental animals and human beings. Human risk estimates are derived primarily from epidemiologic studies following relatively high-dose radiation exposures. As ionizing radiation appears in reality to be a relatively weak carcinogen and mutagen compared to many chemical agents, few reliable human data are available on its oncogenic effects in the dose range below 50 cGy.

Development of Radiation Injury

A schematic representation of the interaction of ionizing radiation with biologic tissues and the subsequent development of radiation injury is shown in Figure 15.1. Such radiation is of two major types, electromagnetic waves or ionizing particles. In either case, interaction with orbital electrons results in ionizations and excitations. The initial deposition of energy in irradiated cells thus occurs in the form of ionized and excited atoms or molecules distributed at random throughout the cells. It is the ionizations that cause most of the chemical changes in the vicinity of the event; this energy may be subsequently transferred through a chain of chemical reactions, finally producing irreversible damage to critical molecules of biologic importance to the cell. It appears that the energy that goes into producing excited molecules produces relatively few chemical reactions and is eventually dissipated in the form of heat.

The ionizing event involves the ejection of an orbital electron from a molecule, producing a positively charged or ionized molecule. These molecules are highly unstable and rapidly undergo chemical change. This change results in the production of free radicals, atoms or molecules containing unpaired electrons. These free radicals are extremely reactive and may lead to permanent damage of the affected molecule, or the energy may be transferred to another molecule. Most of the energy deposited within a cell results in the production of aqueous free radicals, since approximately 80% of the cell is water. Chemical damage may be repaired before it is irreversible by the recombination of radicals and dissipation of the associated energy, or it may be modified by agents such as molecular oxygen or sulfhydryl radioprotective compounds.

As the initial ionizing events are similar for all types of radiation, their biologic effects are also qualitatively similar. However, densely ionizing radiation such as alpha particles produce more biologic damage per unit of energy absorbed. The relative biological effectiveness (RBE) of different types of radiation relative to x-rays is thus related to their linear energy transfer (LET), a measure of the density of the ionizations produced along the radiation track. The initial critical biologic change is thought to be damage to DNA molecules in the cell. The time required for the entire chain

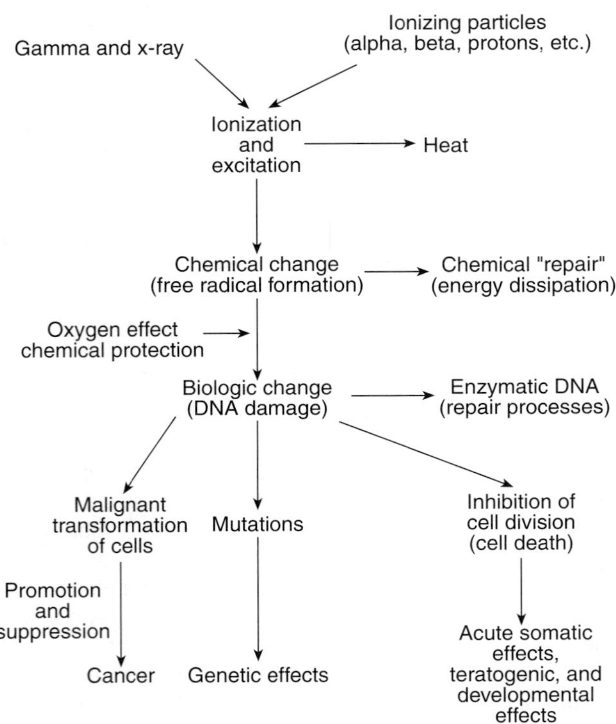

Figure 15.1. Development of radiation injury.

of physical and chemical events as shown in Figure 15.1 from the initial interaction until the production of DNA damage is of the order of a microsecond or less. The subsequent development of biochemical and physiologic changes, however, may take hours to days, whereas the induction of cancer may take many years.

Principal Cellular and Tissue Effects of Radiation

CELL KILLING

Radiation can kill cells by two distinct mechanisms. The first is apoptosis, also called programmed cell death or interphase death (47, 55). Cells undergoing apoptosis usually die in interphase within a few hours of irradiation, irrespective of and without intervening mitosis. They share distinct morphologic changes, including loss of normal nuclear structure and degradation of DNA, that can be demonstrated by a classic pattern of "laddering" on DNA blots (55). It has long been known that apoptotic cell death occurs in a few cell types, including small lymphocytes, type A spermatogonia, and oocytes, following very low doses of radiation (<50 cGy). Recently it has become evident that apoptosis may be a significant cause of death in a broader variety of cell types exposed to higher radiation doses, including lymphoid and some tumor cells. Although radiation-induced apoptosis in these cells is generally thought to depend on the functional activity of the p53 gene (55), evidence has been presented for a p53-independent pathway (79). In any case, apoptosis may be a protective mechanism by which the body gets rid of heavily radiation-damaged cells.

The second mechanism is radiation-induced reproductive failure. Radiation in sufficient doses can inhibit mitosis—the cell's ability to divide and proliferate indefinitely. The inhibition of cellular proliferation is the mechanism by which radiation kills most cells. The nature and kinetics of the cytotoxic effects of radiation in mammalian cells have been reviewed elsewhere (47). They are discussed in detail in Chapter 48 of this text, particularly as they relate to tumor cells and radiation oncology. As radiation kills cells by inhibiting their ability to divide, its effects in human beings occur primarily in tissues with high cell turnover or renewal rates characterized by a large amount of proliferative activity. These include tissues such as the bone marrow and the mucosal lining of the stomach and small intestine. Symptoms of acute exposure to whole-body irradiation in human beings are usually observed only following doses of 150 cGy or greater, whereas significant cell killing in vitro can be detected with doses as low as 50 cGy.

Another important somatic effect related to cell killing arises from irradiation of the developing embryo and fetus (6, 60). Whereas irradiation of experimental animals with doses on the order of 200 to 400 cGy during the first trimester of pregnancy has led to a variety of congenital anomalies in the offspring, no such effects were found in large populations of mice exposed to doses below 25 cGy (6). Moreover, no increase in the frequency of congenital anomalies has been observed in human beings, even following relatively high radiation doses.

Recent epidemiologic studies on the atom bomb survivors of Hiroshima and Nagasaki have focused on mental retardation and other measures of intelligence such as test scores and school performance. These are presumably more sensitive indicators of radiation effects, owing to cell depletion among the neuroblasts during development. Neuroblasts comprise by far the largest population of cells in the early fetus, and continue proliferating until the fifth or sixth month of pregnancy. The number of children with such disorders in the atom bomb survivor study is small, and the mean values for all end points are not significantly different from those in controls for the dose groups below 50 to 100 cGy. The Committee on the Biological Effects of Ionizing Radiations, of the National Search Council (BEIR V Committee) (64) concluded that for mental retardation, the best documented of the developmental abnormalities, the prevalence appeared to increase with dose in a linear manner for individuals irradiated between 8 and 15 weeks, the most sensitive time period after conception. However, the data do not exclude a threshold in the range of 20 to 40 cGy, and indeed best fit a threshold dose-response relationship with a lower bound of 12 to 20 cGy (29, 64). On the assumption of a linear, no-threshold relationship, however, the magnitude of the risk would be approximately a 4% chance of occurrence per 10 cGy for exposure at 8 to 15 weeks of gestational age, with less risk occurring for exposure at other ages.

MUTAGENESIS

The mutagenic effects of ionizing radiation were first described by Herman Muller in 1927 in his classic experiments with the fruit fly *Drosophila*. Subsequent experiments showed the dose-response relationship for such mutations to be a linear function of exposure over a wide range of radiation doses from as low as 10 to 1,000 cGy. Studies of the induction of single-gene mutations in human cells have been limited to several genetic loci. The results of these studies also suggest that the induction of mutations in human cells is a linear function of dose with doses as low as 10 and perhaps 1 cGy, and that the dose-rate effect appears to be relatively small (23, 83). DNA structural analyses have shown that the majority of radiation-induced mutations in human cells result from large-scale genetic events involving loss of the entire active gene and often extending to other loci on the same chromosome (45).

The major potential consequence of radiation-induced mutations in human populations is heritable genetic effects resulting from mutations induced in germinal cells. Such effects have been examined in several different animal systems (64). For high dose-rate exposure, the induced mutation rate per gamete generally falls in the range of 10^{-4} to 10^{-5} per cGy. The rates per locus are in the range of 10^{-7} to 10^{-8} per cGy. Protraction of exposure appears to decrease the mutation rate in rodent systems by a factor of 2 or greater. When all of the experimental data for the various genetic end points are considered, the genetic doubling dose (radiation dose necessary to double the spontaneous mutation rate) for low dose-rate exposure appears to be in the range of 100 cGy. Although significant heritable genetic effects of radiation have not yet been demonstrated in human populations, a doubling dose of 100 cGy is not inconsistent with the absence of a statistically significant increase in hereditary disease among the children of atom bomb survivors (1). Indeed, 100 cGy represents approximately the lower 95% confidence limit for the human doubling dose (64).

CHROMOSOMAL ABERRATIONS

Radiation can induce two types of chromosomal aberrations in mammalian cells. The first have been termed "aberrations" in that they are usually lethal to dividing cells. They include such changes as dicentrics, ring chromosomes, large deletions, and fragments. These types of aberrations do not allow the equal distribution of genetic material into daughter cells; in many cases, the frequency of such aberrations correlates well with the cytotoxic effects of radiation.

The second type has been termed "stable aberrations." These include changes such as small deletions, reciprocal translocations, and aneuploidy—changes that do not preclude the cell from dividing. A karyotype of a human cell showing a stable aberration is shown in Figure 15.2. Radiation-induced reciprocal translocations such as have occurred in this cell may be passed on through many generations of cell replication and emerge in clonal cell populations (31, 32).

It is well known that such deletions and translocations can result in gene mutations. It is tempting to speculate that they may play a more fundamental role in the process of carcinogenesis. Typically, cancer cells are aneuploid and contain multiple stable chromosomal aberrations. In a number of cases, specific chromosomal abnormalities have been associated with specific tumor types. This phenomenon is discussed in detail in Chapter 7. In some instances, such as the chromosome 8:14 translocation in Burkitt's lymphoma, the chromosomal change results in the activation of a specific oncogene. In others, such as the deletion of q14 of chromosome 13 found in retinoblastoma, tumor development has been ascribed to loss or inactivation of a suppressor gene.

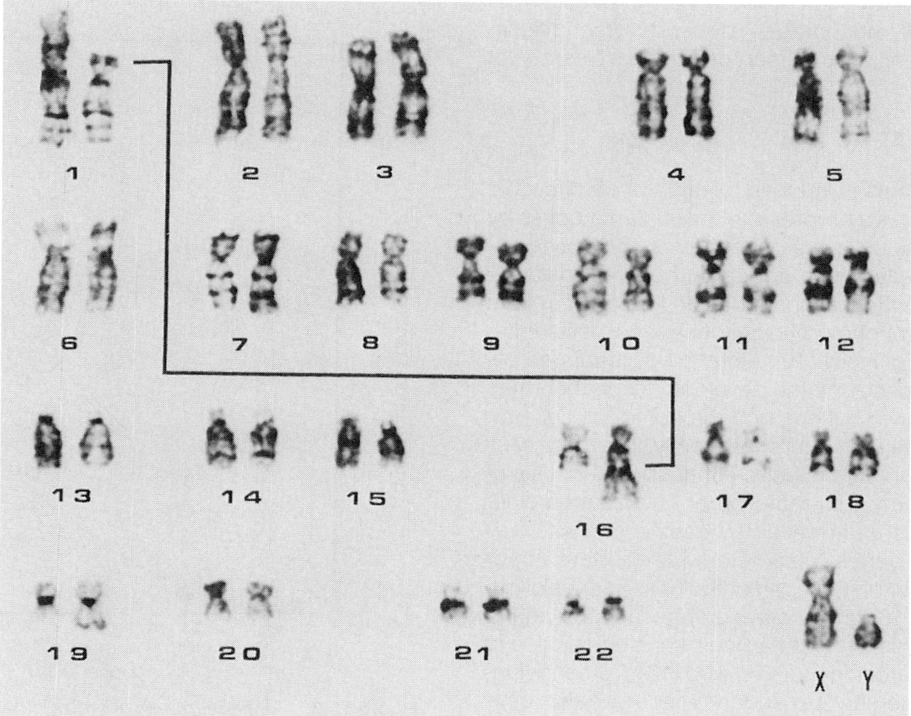

Figure 15.2. Karyotype of normal human diploid fibroblast showing stable chromosomal rearrangement (1:16 translocation) induced by radiation. The irradiated cells were serially subcultivated for 3 months (approximately 20 cell generations) before this cell was analyzed.

Further work is required, however, to define the role of such events in radiation-induced cancer in general.

NEOPLASTIC TRANSFORMATION

The final important cellular effect of radiation is neoplastic transformation, or the conversion of a normal cell to one with the phenotype of a cancer cell, including the ability to form an invasive, malignant tumor upon reinjection into syngeneic hosts. Current knowledge concerning the transformation of cells in vitro by ionizing radiation is described in the following section.

Neoplastic Transformation in Vitro by Radiation

Most human cancers have been shown to be clonal in origin. That is, all of the cells within a tumor are descendants of a single cell that has undergone neoplastic transformation. The transformation of one or more normal cells in a tissue in vivo is thought to represent the earliest step in the overall process of carcinogenesis (51). Whether or not such a transformed cell can successfully give rise to an invasive, malignant tumor depends on a number of tissue and systemic factors.

Although a number of different in vitro transformation systems involving various species and cell types are under active investigation (7), those that generate reliable quantitative data have been restricted to rodent cells, and in none of these is the entire process of malignant transformation measured. Rather, surrogate features of transformation are assayed such as changes in colony morphology, focus formation, or growth under anchorage-independent conditions. Furthermore, no quantitative human cell system has as yet been developed.

STAGES IN NEOPLASTIC TRANSFORMATION

Studies of transformation induced by radiation or chemical agents indicate that it is a progressive, multi-step process by which normal cells acquire the various phenotypic characteristics of cancer cells. There appear to be three major independent stages in the malignant transformation of cells in vitro: the development of morphologic changes, cellular immortality, and tumorigenicity (10). Morphologic changes are many and varied and include the development of abnormalities in cytology, growth pattern, and the control of cell proliferation. Immortalization occurs frequently in rodent cells but extremely rarely in human cells, either spontaneously or as a result of treatment with radiation or chemical carcinogens. It can be induced, however, by transfection with certain oncogenes or genes associated with certain tumor viruses such as the SV40 T antigen or the E6/E7 genes of human papillomavirus 16. Immortalization may thus be an important rate-limiting step in human cell transformation and perhaps in human carcinogenesis in vivo (10). Tumorigenicity also appears to be an independent phenotype that generally occurs only in previously immortalized cells. A subpopulation of such immortal cells may undergo additional genomic rearrangements that give them a selective growth advantage in vivo perhaps related to factors present in the host animal (68).

DOSE-RESPONSE RELATIONSHIPS

The observed frequency of neoplastic transformation per viable cell increases with dose up to the range of 400 to 600 cGy, reaching a plateau at higher doses. As radiation is highly cytotoxic in this higher dose range, the yield of transformants per initial cell at risk actually declines. The latter parameter, the yield of transformed cells per initial cell at risk, would be the more relevant one for the induction of cancer in vivo. The in vitro results thus predict a most effective dose for transformation in the range of 400 to 600 cGy, a phenomenon that reflects a balance between transformation and cell killing. Compared with many chemical agents, ionizing radiation is not a potent inducer of transformation. Polycyclic hydrocarbons, for example, can induce much higher frequencies of transformation at doses that produce very little cell killing (51).

Dose-response curves for the induction of transformation in two very similar mouse cell systems are shown in Figure 15.3. Although the transformation frequencies reached a similar plateau at doses above 600 rads, the shapes of the curves at lower doses differed significantly. Such findings, as well as the fact that transformation represents but an early event in the overall process of carcinogenesis, suggest that it is not relevant to predict the shape of the dose-response curve for carcinogenesis in vivo at low radiation doses from the findings with transformation in vitro. For irradiation with densely ionizing, high LET radiation, the frequency of transformation rises much more rapidly at low doses, reaching a roughly similar plateau. RBE factors in the range of 3 to 10

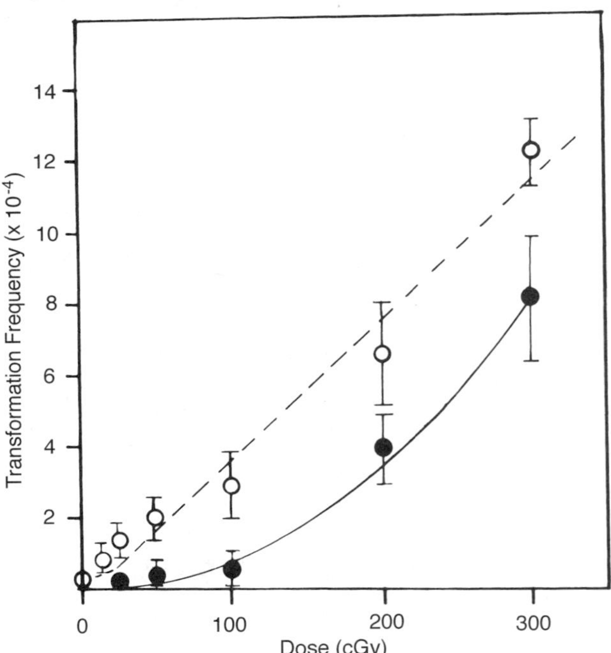

Figure 15.3. Dose-response curves for the induction of neoplastic transformation in mouse cells by x-irradiation. The upper curve is for BALB/3T3 cells and the bottom curve for C3H/10T1/2 cells.

have been calculated for high LET radiations such as fast neutrons, alpha particles, and heavy charged ions.

MODIFYING FACTORS

Incubation of cells with various agents during the 4 to 6–week postirradiation expression period can markedly modify the ultimate yield of transformed cells (50). For example, the phorbol ester compound 12–0-tetradecanoyl-phorbol-13-acetate (TPA) acts as a potent promoter of x-ray transformation if applied repeatedly beginning either immediately after irradiation or several weeks later. Indeed, these in vitro findings offered the first evidence that the initiation-promotion phenomenon was a general one and not simply limited to mouse skin. The promoting effect of TPA in vitro is shown graphically in Figure 15.4*A*.

A number of different classes of agents applied by a similar experimental protocol can suppress transformation (7, 8). These include selenium, retinoids, carotenoids, and ascorbic acid. Of particular interest are protease inhibitors (34) and the thiol radioprotective agents (27, 74), which have also shown promise as chemopreventive agents in vivo. Transformation can also be modulated by certain hormones, growth factors, and anti-inflammatory agents (8). Notable among these is thyroid hormone, specifically T^3.

Thus, it has become evident that a number of noncarcinogenic secondary factors can markedly modulate the frequency of radiation-induced transformation. As transformation can be markedly enhanced, suppressed, or completely inhibited, such factors may become the controlling ones in the overall process of transformation of cells exposed to radiation. In most cases, the effects of such agents in vitro have been predictive of those observed in experimental animal systems. It therefore seems likely that they may be of similar importance in human radiation carcinogenesis, though very few epidemiologic data to support this contention are as yet available.

The effects of dose rate on radiation transformation have proved somewhat complex. In general, protraction of exposure to low LET radiation leads to a lower frequency of trans-

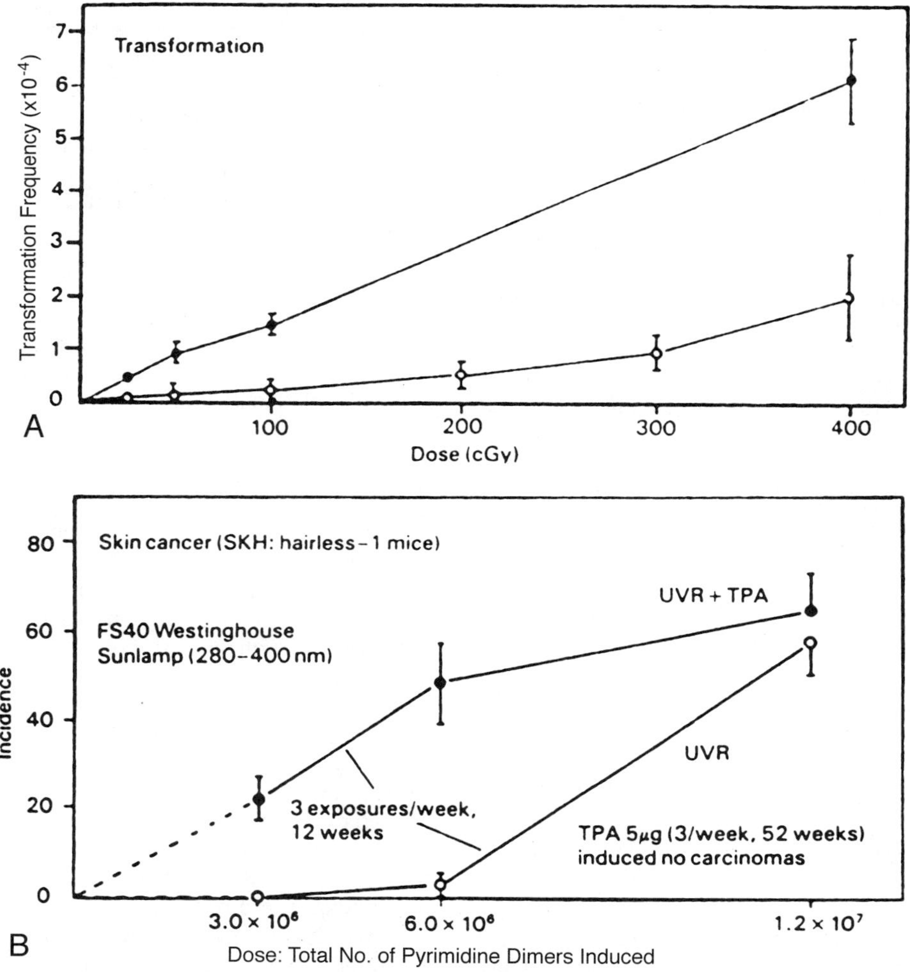

Figure 15.4. Enhancement of radiation-induced transformation in vitro and carcinogenesis in vivo by postirradiation exposure to the phorbol ester tumor-promoting agent TPA. **A.** Neoplastic transformation in mouse 10T1/2 cells. Lower curve is for cells treated with x-rays alone, whereas upper curve is for x-irradiated cells continuously incubated with TPA postirradiation. **B.** Skin tumors in mice treated with ultraviolet light irradiation. Lower curve is for mice treated with radiation alone, whereas upper curve is for irradiated mice receiving repeated applications of TPA postirradiation. *Source:* Little (51). Data in **B** are from Fry and Ley (17).

formation. However, protraction of exposure to fission spectrum neutrons at total doses of up to 100 cGy has been reported to enhance the frequency of transformation (26). The latter phenomenon has not proved to be a general finding for other high LET radiations.

INDUCED GENETIC INSTABILITY AND RADIATION TRANSFORMATION

Studies of the kinetics of radiation transformation in vitro indicate that it involves two distinct events (36, 37). The first is a frequent event that involves a large fraction of the irradiated cell population and enhances the probability of the occurrence of the second event. The second event is a low-frequency one involving the actual transformation of one or more of the progeny of the original irradiated cells after many rounds of cell division. This second step occurs with a constant frequency per cell per generation and has the characteristics of a mutagenic event (48).

This finding is in contradistinction to classic theories of carcinogenesis in which the initiating event is thought to be a rare one and likely mutagenic in nature. However, evidence from certain experimental animal systems is consistent with the hypothesis that the initiating event may indeed be a frequent one (48). Moreover, it now appears that other cellular effects of irradiation may also be delayed, appearing in the progeny of irradiated cells after many generations of replication. These include specific gene mutations in vitro (9), chromosomal aberrations in skin fibroblasts of mouse fetuses irradiated during the single-cell blastocyst stage of development (67), non-clonal cytogenetic aberrations in clonal descents of human hematopoietic stem cells exposed to alpha radiation (30), and the finding that intragenic recombinational activity persists in yeast cells for many generations of replication following exposure to ionizing radiation (15).

These findings are all consistent with the hypothesis that radiation induces a type of genetic instability in cells as a cellular response to the nonspecific DNA damage it produces. This genetic instability enhances the probability of the occurrence of malignant transformation or other cellular effects in progeny cells, sometimes after many generations of replication. The various factors modulating transformation may act on this process. Interestingly, this concept is consistent with the emerging findings in human populations which suggest that radiation-induced cancer may follow a relative risk model (see below); that is, a given dose of radiation increases the rate of occurrence of cancer at all follow-up times rather than inducing a specific cohort of new tumors.

Molecular Mechanisms

DNA DAMAGE

It is well recognized that DNA damage is central to the initiation phase of carcinogenesis induced by ionizing or ultraviolet light radiation, as well as by many chemical carcinogens (91). The cellular enzyme protein kinase C (PKC) plays a critical role in growth control and appears to be involved in the promotional phase of radiation carcinogenesis (25). PKC, activated by phorbol ester tumor promoters such as TPA, can produce a cascade of events resulting in alterations in gene expression, membrane function, and ultimately cellular differentiation and proliferation (91). The role of these factors is described in more detail in Chapters 1, 3, 4, and 5 of this text. In addition, radiation can directly induce changes in gene expression via transcriptional or posttranscriptional mechanisms (49). Given the complex multistage nature of carcinogenesis, it is reasonable to speculate that clonal evolution toward neoplasia involves a sequence of changes in gene expression driven by both genetic and epigenetic changes.

From studies of radiation-induced carcinogenesis in human populations and experimental systems, it appears that radiation acts primarily as an initiating agent by its ability to damage DNA. Radiation can induce both specific base damage and DNA strand breaks, and mammalian cells possess efficient enzymatic mechanisms for repairing these types of damage. Although it has long been assumed that unrejoined double strand breaks are the critical DNA lesions responsible for cell killing by radiation, it now appears that incorrectly rejoined DNA double strand breaks are important mutagenic and carcinogenic lesions. This DNA misrepair appears to lead to chromosomal deletions and rearrangements. DNA structural analyses of radiation-induced mutants at specific gene loci in human cells indicate that most mutations arise as a result of such large-scale genetic and chromosomal changes (45).

It is now well established that certain chromosomal rearrangements, including translocations and deletions, are associated with a wide variety of human cancers. These are described in Chapter 7. Although no consistent nonrandom chromosomal changes have as yet been associated with radiation carcinogenesis in vivo or in vitro, there is evidence to implicate specific chromosomal rearrangements in preleukemic clones in ataxia telangiectasia patients and in two types of radiation-induced murine leukemia (10).

ONCOGENES

The involvement of various oncogenes in experimental and human carcinogenesis is well established. This area is reviewed in detail in Chapter 5 of this book. The role of specific oncogene activation in radiation-induced cancer is less clear (4, 10). Activation of *ras* oncogenes occurs, though in relatively low frequencies, in mouse lymphomas induced by radiation (65), and a specific codon 146 *ras* mutation has been described in a small fraction of neutron-induced thymic lymphomas (76). Activation of c-Ki-*ras* as well as amplification of c-*myc* has been reported in some radiation-induced rat skin tumors (73), but not in mouse skin tumors (4). Amplification and rearrangement of c-*myc* has been reported in a small fraction (6–30%) of radiation-induced murine osteosarcomas (80).

If *myc* and *ras* oncogenes play a significant role in radiation carcinogenesis, activation or amplification of these genes should be found in vitro as well as in vivo. Although evidence of dominant transforming activity has been found in cells transformed by radiation in vitro, this activity has not been associated with a number of known oncogenes (39,

43). Specifically, no evidence has been found for activation or over-expression of *ras* genes. Though increased expression (but no rearrangement) of c-*myc* has been reported in some transformed cells, this appears to be a late effect occurring during the development of the transformed phenotype after the initial transforming event (43). These findings along with those of in vivo studies have led to the conclusion that distinctive, as yet unidentified transforming genes may be involved in radiation carcinogenesis.

Finally, it is not clear from such studies whether oncogene activation arose as a consequence of a direct interaction of radiation with cellular DNA or from a complex series of events initially triggered by DNA damage. The activation of *ras* oncogenes by chemical carcinogens may be either an early or a late event. In one study in which the timing of oncogene activation was studied during radiation transformation, it appeared to occur as a later event (38). As discussed above, mutations arising as a result of exposure to ionizing radiation usually involve large-scale DNA structural changes and rearrangements. As *ras* activation usually occurs by point mutations, it may not be unexpected that activation of the *ras* proto-oncogene is not an important initiating event in radiation transformation and carcinogenesis. Although the whole question of the association of oncogenes with radiation carcinogenesis needs further investigation, it is clear that the pattern of oncogene activation differs significantly for transformation and carcinogenesis induced by radiation as compared with chemical carcinogens.

TUMOR SUPPRESSOR GENES

The characteristics of tumor suppressor genes and evidence for their potential importance in human carcinogenesis are described in Chapter 6. In terms of radiation carcinogenesis, much recent interest has centered on the p53 gene, as it appears to play an important role in cell cycle control, radiosensitivity, the development of genetic instability leading to cell transformation, and perhaps in the response of human tumors to radiation or chemotherapy. p53 mutations have been found in a wide spectrum of human cancers (22) and in mouse skin tumors induced by ionizing radiation (66).

When normal human diploid fibroblasts are exposed to radiation, a significant fraction of the population remains irreversibly blocked in the G_1 phase of the cell cycle (53, 63). It has since been shown that this block is dependent on the p53 status of the cells (11, 44, 49): no radiation-induced G_1 arrest occurs in cells that lack normal p53 function. The activation of p53 by radiation damage in human tumor cells also appears to suppress the progression of G_1 cells into the DNA synthetic (S) phase of the cell cycle, as well as enhancing apoptotic cell death (40, 55). It is tempting to hypothesize that the absence of a G_1 arrest is responsible for the genetic instability that occurs in irradiated cells lacking normal p53 function; cells with extensive genetic damage progress through the cell cycle rather than becoming arrested in G_1 and undergoing apoptotic cell death or becoming senescent (24). This hypothesis, however, remains controversial (62). Whatever the mechanism, it is now evident that transgenic mice lacking p53 function are highly susceptible to radiation-induced cancer (33).

Another area of recent interest has been the role of p53 in the control of cellular radiosensitivity. The absence of normal p53 function is associated with enhanced resistance of human diploid fibroblasts to radiation-induced reproductive failure (44, 49, 81). A similar effect has been described in hematopoietic cell lineages in transgenic mice (41). For cell types that readily undergo apoptosis, the lack of an apoptotic response in p53-deficient cells renders them more resistant to radiation. The role of p53 status in the radiosensitivity of human tumor cells, however, remains unclear (5, 59). As tumor cells have undergone a number of mutagenic events in various oncogenes and tumor suppressor genes that have allowed them to escape normal growth controls, they may at the same time become refractory to the effects of p53 expression on radiosensitivity. On the other hand, preliminary results suggest that p53 status may be an important determinant of the therapeutic responsiveness of certain experimental tumors sensitive to apoptotic cell death (54). Although these results must be confirmed in other systems, it is tempting to speculate that p53 status may be a genetic marker for potential tumor response to radiation or chemotherapy. In the future, a number of such genetic markers may become available that will allow the coherent development of a predictive assay for tumor response based on a battery of molecular probes.

RB is a tumor suppressor gene that is associated with retinoblastoma, a malignant eye tumor of children. This disorder exists in both sporadic and hereditary forms. Mutations in the RB gene have in addition been associated with several other types of tumors, including osteosarcomas, soft tissue sarcomas, small cell lung cancer, and breast cancer (90). Interestingly, patients with the hereditary type of retinoblastoma appear to be at an unusually high risk for the development of radiation-induced secondary tumors, primarily osteogenic sarcomas occurring in the treatment field (14). The fact that activation of a tumor suppressor gene may result from large-scale genetic changes such as deletions, genomic rearrangements and recombinational events suggests that tumors that arise as a result of the loss of suppressor gene activity may be particularly susceptible to induction by irradiation. Although this is an intriguing hypothesis, there are at present insufficient data to establish suppressor gene inactivation as a general mechanism in radiation-induced carcinogenesis.

Experimental Radiation-Induced Carcinogenesis

GENERAL CHARACTERISTICS OF RADIATION-INDUCED CARCINOGENESIS

Ionizing radiation has been called a "universal carcinogen" in that it will induce cancer in most tissues of most species at all ages, including the fetus. It is one of the few definitely established carcinogens in human beings, and perhaps the only one for which firm dose-response data in human populations are available. It is, however, a relatively weak carcinogen and mutagen when compared to certain chemical agents. The cancers induced by radiation are of the same histologic types as occur naturally, but the distribution of types may differ. As examples, a higher percentage of small cell carcinomas of the lung occur as a result of exposure to alpha radiation in uranium miners; radiation induces follicular and papillary carcinomas of the thyroid but not anaplastic and medullary carcinomas; and chronic lymphocytic leukemia is apparently not induced by radiation, whereas other common types of leukemias are. There is a distinct latent period between exposure to radiation and the clinical appearance of a tumor.

DOSE-RESPONSE RELATIONSHIPS

It has been generally accepted that radiation carcinogenesis is a stochastic process. That is, the probability of the occurrence of the effect increases with dose, with no threshold, but the severity of the effect is not influenced by dose. This is in contradistinction to a nonstochastic or deterministic effect, for which both the probability and the severity of the effect vary with dose. There is no clear experimental evidence to suggest that the grade of malignancy, including its invasive or metastatic properties, is a function of dose; radiation-induced cancer appears to be an all-or-none effect. Stochastic effects are those that may arise from damage to a few cells or even a single cell. If this is the case, any dose, no matter how small, carries with it the finite probability of producing the effect. Studies of radiation-induced carcinogenesis in experimental animals and human populations have been designed to test this hypothesis, as most environmental exposures are in the low dose range. Unfortunately, however, it is very difficult to obtain statistically significant data in either human or animal studies at doses below 50 cGy of low LET radiation.

Many earlier studies of the effects of radiation in small animals involved its life-shortening properties. Although this effect was originally ascribed to "radiation-induced aging" in which the natural causes of death were accelerated by radiation, a critical examination of this phenomenon by use of techniques such as serial sacrifice experiments and life table analyses has shown that practically all of the life-shortening effects of radiation in experimental animals can be accounted for by the induction of cancer, except perhaps in the high, sublethal dose range (78, 84). Thus, the dose-response relationship for life shortening in animals should reflect that for cancer deaths from all types of radiation-induced tumors in that species. Such a dose-response curve is shown in Figure 15.5. A generally linear response has been observed for life shortening in a number of different studies.

The dose-response relationships for the induction of cancers in specific tissues vary with site, with sex, and with species (18, 86, 87). For low LET radiation, the frequency of induced cancers generally rises with dose in the range of 0 to 300 cGy. In some cases, tumor incidence levels off at higher doses and may even decline. This phenomenon is thought to reflect cell killing. The carcinogenic effect of low LET radiation in rodents is usually reduced with protraction of exposure. In the dose range up to 200 to 300 cGy, the dose-response curves for individual tumor types vary but generally assume a linear-quadratic to nearly linear relationship.

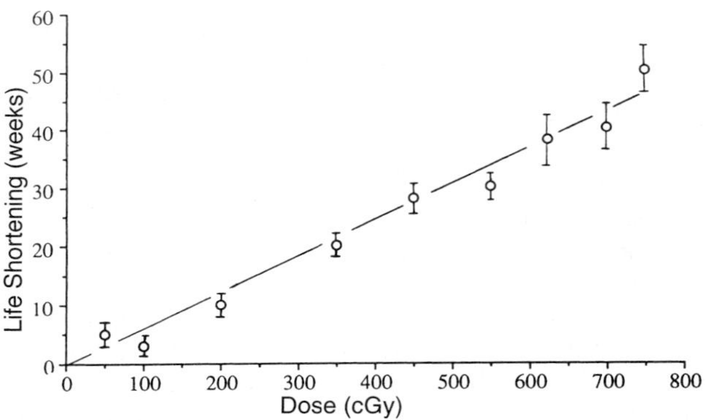

Figure 15.5. Life shortening in mice as a function of dose of ionizing radiation. The shortening of life span is ascribed to early death owing to induced cancers. *Source:* Lindop and Rotblat (46).

For high LET radiation, the rise in cancer incidence with dose is much steeper. The dose-response curves are approximately linear within the range of 0 to 20 cGy, although in some cases they bend over, reaching a plateau at higher doses (18, 85). In contradistinction to low LET radiation, significant increases in cancer and life shortening can be observed after doses as low as 10 cGy of neutrons, alpha particles, or heavy ions (18, 52, 85). RBE values in the range of 3 to 15 have been estimated for the carcinogenic effects of these radiations at low doses. There is usually no dose-rate effect for high LET radiation exposure. However, an outstanding example is the induction of mouse mammary tumors by low doses of fast neutrons, in which protraction of exposure appears to increase the carcinogenic effectiveness by a factor of 2 to 3 at doses of 2.5 to 10 cGy (85).

MODIFYING FACTORS

As in the case of neoplastic transformation, radiation-induced carcinogenesis in experimental animals can also be modulated by noncarcinogenic secondary factors. Data on the promotion by TPA of ultraviolet light–induced skin cancer in mice are shown in Figure 15.4*B*. This can be compared with the effect of this tumor promoter on neoplastic transformation in Figure 15.4*A*. A similar phenomenon has been shown for the induction of malignant squamous cell carcinoma of the skin of mice by ionizing radiation (4), and evidence is accumulating that the two-stage model of initiation and promotion generally applies to tumor induction in epithelial tissues (13).

As an illustration of the possible effects of seemingly innocuous secondary factors, eight weekly intratracheal instillations of 0.2 mL of isotonic saline given to hamsters 4 months after exposure to a relatively low dose of alpha radiation led to a 10-fold enhancement in the induction of lung cancer as compared to that occurring in animals receiving radiation alone (48). It appeared that the saline instillations, which were noncarcinogenic in themselves, had induced a transient round of cell proliferation among the target cells in the lungs of these animals, facilitating expression of the initial radiation-induced damage.

The induction of carcinogenesis in experimental animals can also be suppressed by treatment with certain agents that are known to inhibit radiation-induced transformation in vitro. These include, notably, treatment with protease inhibitors, which have been shown to suppress the induction of cancer in several different tumor systems (35). Incubation with thiol radioprotective compounds during irradiation has also been shown to protect against radiation-induced carcinogenesis and subsequent life shortening (21). In both of these cases, clinical trials are currently under way. It is well known that the hormonal environment is important in certain radiation-induced rodent cancers, particularly ovarian and mammary tumors. These and other observations again emphasize the importance of noncarcinogenic secondary factors in the induction and expression of experimental radiation-induced carcinogenesis. However, the extent to which such factors are important in radiation-induced cancer in human populations is not clear.

GENETIC SUSCEPTIBILITY TO RADIATION-INDUCED CANCER

The discovery of a number of specific genes associated with single or multiple cancer types has stimulated renewed interest in the question of genetic susceptibility to the carcinogenic effects of radiation (72). Should a fraction of the population be genetically predisposed to radiation-induced cancer, this fact could be of considerable importance in the development of protection standards. Clearly, there are marked differences in the susceptibility to radiation-induced cancer among different inbred strains of mice; in general, this susceptibility correlates with the spontaneous incidence of the particular tumor.

While there is little evidence at present to suggest that such genetic factors are involved in most human cancer, they do appear to play a role in certain rare disorders that may serve as models for radiation–genetic interactions. For example, patients with hereditary retinoblastoma whose somatic cells are heterozygous for the RB gene are at markedly increased risk for the development of radiation-induced bone sarcomas (14), whereas patients with the nevoid basal cell carcinoma syndrome are at high risk for the development of basal cell cancers in irradiated areas. Radiation has also been associated with an enhanced incidence of early-onset breast cancer, although the hereditary nature of the disease and its relation to the *BRCA1* gene remain to be clarified. Interestingly, these three disorders all involve mutations in purported tumor suppressor genes. As described earlier, transgenic mice heterozygous for the p53 tumor suppressor gene also show a markedly increased sensitivity to radiation-induced cancer (33). The involvement of tumor suppressor genes in radiation-induced carcinogenesis is not unexpected, given the fact that radiation-induced mutations involve primarily large-scale genetic events.

A rather different case is that of ataxia telangiectasia (AT). Although AT is a rare, autosomal recessive disorder, as many as 1 to 3% of people in the general population may be heterozygous for the ATM gene. It has been reported that obligate AT heterozygotes are at increased risk for the development of lymphoid and breast cancer, and that a five- to six-fold excess risk of breast cancer appeared to be associated with prior exposure to diagnostic x-rays (82). Confirmation should result from the recent cloning of the ATM gene such that heterozygous gene carriers can be identified among all breast cancer patients and in the general population. However, AT offers a model for the possible existence of a significant subpopulation with enhanced susceptibility to radiation-induced cancer.

Human Epidemiologic Studies

There is now a large body of data on radiation-induced cancer derived from epidemiologic studies in irradiated human populations, and it is largely on the basis of these data that risk estimates are derived. These data are reviewed and analyzed in detail in the latest reports from the Committee on the BEIR V (64) and the United Nations Scientific Committee on the Effects of Atomic Radiation (UNSCEAR) (88). They are derived primarily from two sources: (1) the long-term follow-up of survivors of the atomic bombings of Hiroshima and Nagasaki (56, 75), and (2) populations exposed to medical x-rays (3). Information is also available from certain occupational exposures, particularly from individuals with pulmonary and skeletal exposure to alpha radiation. The results of these studies have yielded significant dose-response data for the induction of cancer in at least five tissue sites. Such dose-response data are extremely important in ascribing radiation as the causal agent for the increased incidence of cancer, as well as for estimating the risks associated with a given exposure. Unfortunately, however, the epidemiologic studies yielding useful dose-response data all involve relatively high dose exposures (>50 cGy). Thus, risk estimates in the low-dose range must be derived from an extrapolation from the high-dose data. The shape of the dose-response relationship becomes of critical importance in making such extrapolations.

The observed dose-response curves from the human epidemiologic studies appear to be either linear or linear-quadratic in form (that is, a linear component at low doses with a quadratic component at higher doses). A linear curve implies a constant risk per cGy at all doses, whereas the linear-quadratic model implies a smaller risk per cGy in the low-dose range. The assumption of a linear model simplifies the extrapolation from high to low doses and the corresponding estimation of risks. Furthermore, it is a conservative technique; that is, if anything, it would overestimate rather than underestimate the potential risk. There is no evidence for a proportionally greater effect at low doses.

A final parameter of importance in determining the hazards of a given dose of radiation is the choice of risk models. For many years, risks were estimated on the basis of an absolute risk model. This model assumed that a specific number of excess cancers was induced by a given radiation dose. Radiation-induced cancers occurred in addition to the natural incidence. Thus, the increased risk could be expressed as the number of excess cancer cases (or cancer deaths) per 10^6 exposed people per year per cGy (the rate per year), or as the total number of excess cancers per 10^6 exposed people per cGy (the total risk or yield of cancers to be expected from a given radiation dose). The absolute risk model generally assumes a linear dose-response relationship, although with certain corrections it can be applied to the linear-quadratic situation.

An analysis of the recent data from the atomic bomb survivors suggests that some types of radiation-induced cancers more likely follow a relative risk model (64, 75). This is also true for several different tumor types in mice (78). The relative risk model implies that radiation increases the natural incidence of cancer at all ages by a dose-dependent factor. As the excess cancer risk is proportional to the natural incidence, radiation-induced cancers would occur primarily at the times when natural tumors arose, independent of the age at irradiation. Thus, the largest cohort of radiation-induced cancers would occur in older individuals. The relative risk model appears to fit the epidemiologic data for several solid tumors, although it does not appear to be valid for leukemia or bone or lung cancers.

LEUKEMIA

At one time, leukemia was thought to be the major radiation-induced cancer to arise from whole-body exposure. We now know the two reasons for this assumption: (*a*) the spontaneous occurrence of leukemia is low, and thus radiation-induced cases are more readily recognizable; and (*b*) the latency period in human beings is very short relative to the latency period of other types of cancers, so leukemias are recognized earlier. Excess leukemias begin appearing within 2 years after acute radiation exposure, reach a peak incidence within 10 years, then fall off steadily. This is in comparison to other cancers, for which the minimum latent period is 10 to 15 years and the rate of appearance of new radiation-induced tumors increases at least up to 40 years. The major sources of data for the induction of leukemia are from the 76,000 members of the life span study of the atomic bomb survivors from whom DS86 (1986) dose estimates are available, and from a study of approximately 14,000 patients in Great Britain treated with radiation for ankylosing spondylitis of the spine.

The dose-response relationship for the induction of leukemia in the atomic bomb survivors, based on the DS86 dosimetry measurements of organ-absorbed dose, is shown in Figure 15.6*A*. Various dose-response models fitted to the data are also shown on this graph. The data are best described by a linear-quadratic model with a cell killing term (dashed line), although statistically speaking the linear-quadratic fit is not significantly better than a straight linear fit (75). Based on these data, the relative risk at 100 cGy is 4.92, and the attributable risk is estimated to be 2.29 excess cancer deaths/10^6 persons exposed/yr/cGy. This latter figure is approximately fourfold higher than that estimated from the data for the British ankylosing spondylitis patients. This may be ascribed to the younger age of the atomic bomb survivors at the time of irradiation and the fact that they received a single, acute whole-body exposure (64). Children appear to be twice as sensitive as adults to the leukemogenic effects of radiation, whereas the unborn child may be about 10 times more sensitive following in utero irradiation (57).

Radiation-induced leukemia in human populations differs in several characteristics from solid tumors. These include the unusually short latent period, high relative risk (Table 15.1), and the fact that the epidemiologic data best fit a linear-quadratic dose-response relationship. This may be related to the nature of the hematopoietic system, which con-

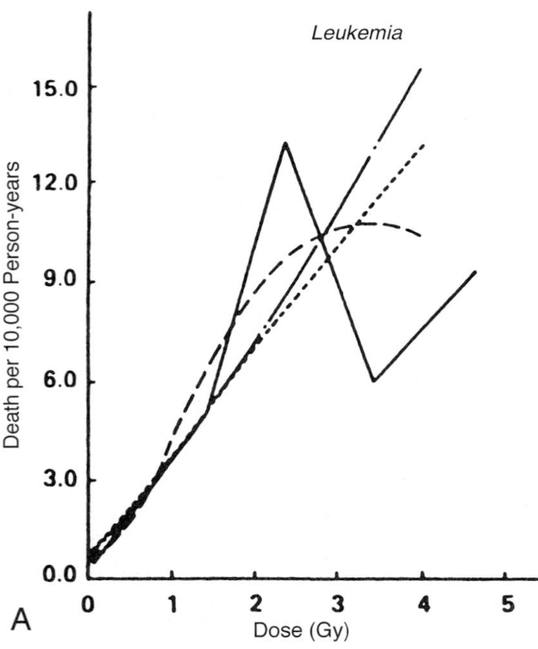

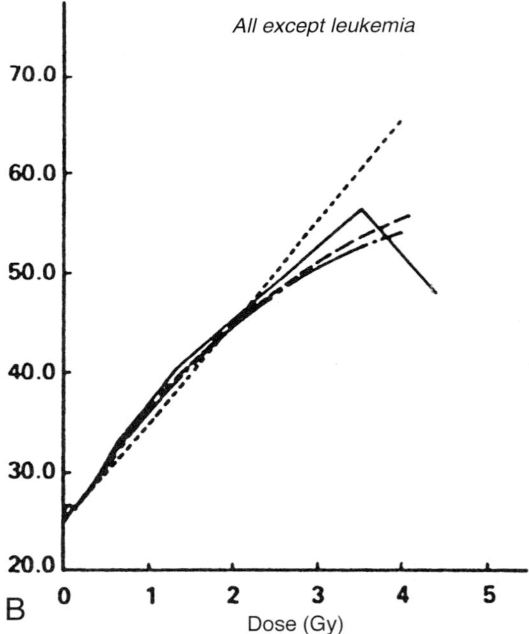

Figure 15.6. Dose-response curves for induction of cancer in human populations receiving uniform whole-body radiation exposure, derived from epidemiologic data from the atomic bomb survivors of Hiroshima and Nagasaki. **A.** Leukemia. **B.** All cancers except leukemia. *Solid lines*, actual data; *broken lines*, mathematically fitted dose-response curves based on different models: ········ linear; ——·——·—— linear-quadratic; – – – – with cell killing correction. *Source:* Shimizu et al. (75).

Table 15.1. Summary Measures of Radiation Dose-Response for Mortality at Statistically Significant Tissue Sites in Atomic Bomb Survivors of Hiroshima and Nagasaki[a]

Site of cancer	Relative risk at 100 cGy	Excess deaths (no./10^6 persons exposed/yr/cGy)	Attributable risk (%)[b]
Leukemia	4.92	2.29	55.0
All cancers (except leukemia)	1.39	7.41	7.9
Female breast	2.0	1.02	22.0
Lung	1.46	1.25	11.0
Esophagus	1.43	0.34	13.0
Stomach	1.23	2.07	6.3
Colon	1.56	0.56	15.0
Ovary	1.81	0.45	19.0
Urinary tract	2.02	0.55	23.0
Multiple myeloma	2.86	0.21	32.0

[a] Includes both sexes, all ages at exposure, 1950–1985 data. Estimates based on shielded kerma does measurements and linear extrapolation model. Data from Shimizu et al. (75).
[b] Percentage of all cancer observed that can be attributed to the radiation exposure.

tains less stroma than do most tissues. Therefore, there may be fewer constraints on cell proliferation, in essence allowing a few transformed cells to grow rapidly and be detected earlier as a clinical cancer.

OTHER TUMORS

The dose-response relationship for all cancers except leukemia is shown in Figure 15.6*B*; the data are best described by a linear model. The various risk estimates for all types of cancers in which mortality was significantly increased among the atom bomb survivors are shown in Table 15.1. These data are based on 42,000 subjects exposed to greater than 1 cGy. This group includes 144 leukemia deaths, of which 80 are ascribed to radiation exposure, and about 3,300 other cancer deaths, of which 260 are ascribed to radiation exposure. Approximately 10% of all cancer deaths in this population so far are associated with radiation, though the overall mortality rate is not significantly increased. As can be seen in Table 15.1, the relative risk at 100 cGy is considerably lower for all other cancers than it is for leukemia. The excess of cancer deaths/10^6 persons exposed/yr/cGy is approximately 10 for all cancers, ranging from 0.21 to 2.1 in individual tissues.

In addition to breast and lung cancers and leukemia, dose-response data from human epidemiologic studies are available for two other sites not shown in the atomic bomb survivor data in Table 15.1; these are the thyroid and bone. The incidence of bone cancer was not significantly elevated in the atomic bomb studies; the relative and absolute risks are low for the induction of this type of cancer by low LET radiation. The dose-response data have come from studies of persons with elevated body burdens of alpha-emitting radium isotopes as a result of occupational or medical exposures.

Thyroid cancer, on the other hand, is very efficiently induced by low LET radiation. Dose response relationships are derived from populations receiving therapeutic irradiation either for an enlarged thymus gland or tinea capitis. Relative risk estimates for the development of thyroid cancer have ranged from 7 to 69 among various age groups, ethnic origin groups, and in different studies (64). However, cancer death rates are not significantly elevated in these populations, since radiation apparently induces only papillary and follicular type tumors, which are readily curable.

In addition to the results from the atomic bomb survivors, dose-response data are available for breast cancer from several medically exposed populations (3). The results of these studies are generally consistent in terms of risk estimates. Taken as a whole, however, several other interesting findings have arisen. Radiation-induced breast cancers are similar in histopathologic types and age distribution to those arising spontaneously. Women under 20 years of age at exposure are at a higher relative risk than adults, similar to the observations for leukemia. As in the case of thyroid cancer, the development of breast cancer is profoundly dependent on hormonal status. Finally, protraction of exposure does not appear to reduce the risk of radiation-induced breast cancer.

Additional epidemiologic studies are also available for the induction of lung cancer (64). Of particular interest among the underground uranium workers on the Colorado plateau has been an apparent multiplicative interaction with cigarette smoking. This observation is consistent with certain experimental findings on alpha radiation–induced lung cancer. However, statistically significant evidence for a more than additive effect between smoking and low LET radiation on lung cancer incidence has not been observed in other epidemiologic studies. This important question needs further investigation.

RADIATION-INDUCED SECOND TUMORS

An increase in secondary tumors in the treatment field has now been observed in patients treated for several different types of cancers by radiation therapy, often in conjunction with chemotherapy. This phenomenon is described in detail in Chapter 188. In some cases the incidence of radiation-associated second tumors appears to be proportional to dose at the treatment portal, though some epidemiologic data suggest that for leukemia in particular, the tumor incidence may decline at high doses, owing to killing of the target cells (3). The extent to which genetic factors may play a general role in susceptibility to treatment-induced secondary tumors in cancer patients is unclear. Radiation alone may not be a very potent inducer of second tumors. This prediction arises from the localized nature of the exposure during clinical radiation therapy, in which the dose to normal tissues is minimized, and from the fact that ionizing radiation tends to be cytotoxic rather than mutagenic. The high radiation doses employed thus may kill potentially transformed cells in the treatment field. An exception may be Hodgkin's disease, in which lower radiation doses are delivered to a relatively large volume of tissue.

LOW-DOSE EXPOSURES

There have been a number of epidemiologic studies over the past decade that purport to show a carcinogenic effect of environmental radiation exposures in the dose range below 10 cGy. The populations involved are varied but include military personnel exposed during nuclear bomb testing, workers in various nuclear and weapons facilities, and members of the general population living near nuclear facilities or exposed to fallout.

There have been several recent reports analyzing various of these low-dose epidemiologic studies (20, 57, 61). Based on the relative and absolute risk estimates shown in Table 15.1, a significant increase in radiation-associated cancer incidence in populations of these sizes exposed to doses in the range of 10 cGy or less would imply a markedly enhanced sensitivity at low doses. That is, the dose-response curve should be concave upward at low doses, with the excess cancer incidence rising rapidly at very low doses. There are no experimental data to support such a phenomenon.

In reality, a careful analysis of nearly all of these low-dose studies indicates no significant increase in the incidence of all cancers or of cancers at specific sites. One seeming exception has been a small cluster of leukemias reported several years ago in the population surrounding the Sellafield nuclear plant in West Cumbria, Great Britain (19). The effect appeared not to correlate with irradiation of the individuals who developed leukemia, but rather with paternal irradiation of men who received doses greater than 10 cGy prior to conception. There was no experimental or epidemiologic precedent for such an effect of paternal irradiation. A wider study of nuclear facilities in England and Wales found no general increase in cancer mortality near these nuclear facilities (16), a finding that is in agreement with similar investigations in other countries. As the confidence limits in individual studies may be relatively large, owing to small numbers, they often cannot exclude a two- or threefold effect. Thus, a recent analysis examined the combined mortality data from seven cohort studies of nuclear industry workers in Canada, Great Britain, and the United States (28). The risk estimates for leukemia and all cancers derived from this population receiving protracted exposure to low-dose radiation are consistent with an extrapolation from the high-dose results and provide no evidence that the current radiation protection standards are appreciably in error. As for Sellafield, the increased cancer incidence was limited to children who lived specifically in the village of Seascale (although 5 of the 11 patients were not born there); the effect may thus be a statistical aberration or the result of other factors, such as exposure to chemicals or infective agents, that remain to be identified (12).

There has also been considerable concern about the risk of lung cancer from exposure to naturally occurring radon in the air of homes and the workplace. However, the results of several recent epidemiologic studies have been conflicting. No effect was observed in a case-control study of nonsmoking women in Missouri (2) or in a similar study carried out in Canada (42). On the other hand, a clear association between radon exposure and lung cancer was identified in a Swedish study (69); the magnitude of this effect was consistent with projections of the high-dose data from radon-exposed underground miners. A clear definition of the hazards posed by indoor radon exposure must await additional epidemiologic studies (71).

In summary, no consistent trend has emerged from a large variety of epidemiologic studies of low-dose radiation exposures such as to suggest an unexpected increase in sensitivity in the range from 0 to 10–20 cGy. The data are in general consistent with a linear extrapolation from the high-dose results. This conclusion is supported by the lack of correlation between cancer incidence and background radiation observed in several different studies. Low-dose epidemiologic studies in populations of limited size must be very carefully controlled and are often prone to bias by confounding factors.

Risk Assessment

The lifetime excess cancer risk estimates following exposure to 1 cGy as determined by the BEIR V Committee (64) are shown in Table 15.2. These estimates were derived from a composite of the epidemiologic data from the atomic bombing survivors and various medical x-ray exposures. They were derived by use of the relative risk model and assumed a linear-quadratic dose-response relationship for leukemia and a straight linear relationship for other tumors. In addition, characteristics such as the latent period, age at exposure, time after exposure, and interaction effects were taken into consideration.

The risk estimates shown in Table 15.2 are for the mean of all ages at exposure. For children under 20, excess cancer mortality per cGy is about 50% higher than the mean for all tumors, whereas it is much lower at ages over 65. The leukemia risk, on the other hand, rises quite steeply in middle and old age, where the risk is nearly four times that of young adults and twice that of children (64). The lifetime excess yield of death from all cancers, including leukemia, for acute radiation exposure as shown in Table 15.2 is approximately 800 per 10^6 exposed people per cGy; the UNSCEAR Committee (85) estimated that the yield may be 20 to 40% higher. On an individual basis, this is approximately a 1:1,250 (0.8×10^{-3}) effect per cGy. For example, a person receiving 10 cGy acute whole-body exposure would have a 0.8% chance of developing cancer as a result of this radiation exposure, whereas his or her chances of dying of can-

Table 15.2. Lifetime Excess Cancer Risk Estimates for Whole-Body Radiation Exposure to 1.0 cGy

Type of cancer	Cancer deaths per 10^6 persons exposed (excess per cGy)		
	Acute exposure[a]	Protracted exposure[b]	Normal expectation[a]
Leukemia	95	48	6,850
Non-leukemias	695	347	176,450
All cancers	790	395	183,300

[a] Estimates from BEIR V report (64). See text for discussion of these estimates. Normal expectation is the number of cancer deaths (lifetime risk) expected to occur in the general population of 10^6 people.

[b] Derived from acute exposure data by applying a dose-rate effectiveness factor of 2.

cer unrelated to radiation exposure are approximately 18%. This risk would be lower for protracted exposure (Table 15.2). It should be emphasized, however, that these risks are for uniform whole-body irradiation. For localized radiation exposures, the risks will be much lower and related to the critical tissues, including the bone marrow, included within the radiation field. For localized exposures, estimates are based on data such as those shown in Table 15.1 and the utilization of models developed for specific tissue sites as described by the BEIR V Committee (64).

It is often the perception of risk rather than the actual risk itself that is particularly important in the promotion and regulation of health and safety (77). For example, members of the League of Women Voters and a group of college students were asked to order their perception of the risk of fatality for 30 activities and technologies. Both placed nuclear power in first position, ahead of smoking, ingestion of alcoholic beverages, and riding in motor vehicles. The risk experts ranked smoking and motor vehicle accidents first (there are about 50,000 motor vehicle deaths in the United States each year, at least 50% of them involving alcohol or drug use), whereas they ranked nuclear power 20th in the same range as food coloring ingestion and the use of home appliances.

It is thus of interest to compare the risk of death from various activities associated with everyday living (58, 92). Such a comparison is shown in Table 15.3. In general, it turns out that the risk from radiation exposure is relatively small when compared with other risks associated with everyday living. Similarly, a comparison of occupational hazards shows that the risks to radiation workers are much lower than those associated with many other occupations (70). In this context, it is of interest to note the estimation that 400,000 excess deaths each year are associated with cigarette smoking in the United States (58). On the assumption that 40% of the population smokes, such an excess death rate would be comparable to that resulting from approximately 350 cGy of uniform whole-body radiation exposure.

Of concern to the clinical oncologist, however, is the risk of inducing a second malignant tumor as a result of exposure to high doses of radiation, often in conjunction with chemotherapy. This will of course depend on the particular tissue sites included in the radiation field. One could then derive risk estimates based on the type of information shown in Table 15.1. The information in Table 15.1, however, was derived from presumably normal people in the general population exposed to tens to hundreds rather than thousands of cGy. As discussed earlier, a number of factors might determine susceptibility to second tumors in cancer patients treated with high doses of radiation. One risk factor is the irradiation of large tissue volumes, as in the treatment of disorders such as Hodgkin's disease. Genetic factors would be another. It is well known, for example, that retinoblastoma patients are at very high risk for developing second tumors in the irradiated field. The extent to which genetic hypersusceptibility may be important in some of the more common cancers remains to be determined.

In most cases it would seem that a benefit-risk estimation would be positive; that is, the benefit of treatment would outweigh the risk of developing secondary tumors. However, information concerning the relative carcinogenicity of various combinations of radiation and chemotherapeutic agents is now becoming available, and it appears that certain combinations may be more carcinogenic than others. Clearly, additional knowledge is needed concerning treatment regimens that might minimize their carcinogenic effects, and thus the risk of developing secondary treatment-induced tumors, while producing an optimal therapeutic gain.

Table 15.3. Risk of Death from Various Environmental Sources (risks of 1 in 1 million)[a]

Source	Amount of Exposure	Risk
Ionizing radiation (uniform whole body)	12 μGy	Cancer
Cigarettes	1 cigarette	Cancer, heart disease
Living with cigarette smoker	2 mo	Cancer, heart disease
Wine	0.5 L	Cirrhosis of the liver
Peanut butter	10 tbsp	Liver cancer caused by aflatoxin
Miami drinking water	1 gal	Cancer caused by chloroform
Visit to Denver	1 wk	Cancer caused by cosmic rays
Jet flying	1,500 mi	Cancer caused by cosmic rays
Living near polyvinylchloride plant	20 yr	Cancer caused by vinyl chloride
In stone or brick building	1 wk	Cancer caused by radioactivity
In New York or Boston	1 d	Air pollution
In coal mine	3 h	Accident
In coal mine	1 h	Black lung disease
Canoeing	6 min	Drowning
Jet flying	2,500 mi	Accident
In automobile	50 mi	Accident
In motorcycle	5 mi	Accident

[a] Estimates derived from various sources on assumption of linear, nonthreshold response for all effects.

References

1. Abrahamson S. Risk estimates: past, present, and future. Health Phys 1990;59:99.
2. Alavanja CR, Brownson RC, Lubin JH, Berger E, Chang J, Boice JD Jr. Residential radon exposure and lung cancer among nonsmoking women. JNCI 1994;86:1829.
3. Boice JD Jr, Land CE, Preston D. Ionizing radiation. In Cancer Epidemiology and Prevention. Edited by D Schottenfeld, JF Fraumeni Jr. New York: Oxford, 1996 (in press).
4. Bowden GT, Jaffe D, Andrews, K. Biological and molecular aspects of radiation carcinogenesis in mouse skin. Radiation Res 1990;121:235.
5. Brachman DG, Beckett M, Graves D, Haraf D, Vokes E, Weichselbaum RR. p53 mutation does not correlate with radiosensitivity in 24 head and neck cancer cell lines. Cancer Res 1993;53:3667.
6. Brent RL. Radiation teratogenesis. Teratology 1980;21:281.
7. Chadwick KH, Seymour C, Barnhart B. Cell transformation and radiation-induced cancer. Edited by KH Chadwick, C Seymour, B Barnhart. New York: Hilger, 1989.
8. Chan GL, Little JB. Neoplastic transformation *in vitro*. In Radiation Carcinogenesis. Edited by AC Upton, RE Albert, FJ Burns, RE Shore. New York: Elsevier, 1986, pp 107–136.
9. Chang WP, Little JB. Persistently elevated frequency of spontaneous mutations in progeny of CHO clones surviving x-irradiation: association with delayed reproductive death phenotype. Mutat Res 1992;270:191–199.
10. Cox R, Little JB. Oncogenic cell transformation *in vitro*. In Advances in Radiation Biology, vol 15. Edited by OF Nygaard, WK Sinclair, JT Lett. New York: Academic, 1992, pp 137–158.
11. DiLeonardo AD, Linke SP, Clarkin K, Wahl GM. DNA damage triggers a prolonged p53-dependent G1 arrest and long-term induction of Cip1 in normal human fibroblasts. Genes Dev 1994;8:2540.
12. Doll R, Evans HJ, Darby SC. Paternal exposure not to blame. Nature 1994;367:678.
13. Drinkwater NR. Experimental models and biological mechanisms for tumor promotion. Cancer Cells 1990;2:8.
14. Eng C, Li FP, Abramson DH, Ellsworth RM, Wong FL, Goldman MB, Seddon J, Tarbell N, Boice JD Jr. Mortality from second tumors among long-term survivors of retinoblastoma. JNCI 1993;85:1121.
15. Fabre F. Mitotic transmission of induced recombinational ability in yeast. In Cellular Responses to DNA Damage. New York: Alan R Liss, 1983, p 379.

16. Forman D, Cook-Mozaffari P, Darby S, Davey G, Stratton I, Doll R, Pike M. Cancer near nuclear installations. Nature 1987;329:499.
17. Fry RJM, Ley RD. Ultraviolet radiation carcinogenesis. In Mechanisms of Tumor Promotion, vol II: Tumor Promotion and Skin Carcinogenesis. Edited by TJ Slaga. Boca Raton, FL: CRC, 1984, p 73.
18. Fry RJM, Storer JB. External radiation carcinogenesis. In Advances in Radiation Biology, vol 13. Edited by JT Lett. New York: Academic, 1987, p 31.
19. Gardner MJ, Snee MP, Hall AJ, Powell CA, Downes S, Terrell JD. Results of case-control study of leukemia and lymphoma among young people near Sellafield nuclear plant in West Cumbria. Br Med J 1990;300:423.
20. Gilbert ES, Omohundro E, Buchanan JA, Holter NA. Mortality of workers at the Hanford Site: 1945–1986. Health Phys 1993;64:577.
21. Gardina DJ, Carnes BA, Grahn D, Sigdestad CP. Protection against late effects of radiation by S-2-(3-aminopropylamino)-ethylphosphorothioic acid. Cancer Res 1991;51:4125–4130.
22. Greenblatt MS, Bennett WP, Hollstein M, Harris CC. Mutations in the p53 tumor suppressor gene: clues to cancer etiology and molecular pathogenesis. Cancer Res 1994;54:4855.
23. Grosovsky AJ, Little JB. Evidence for linear response for the induction of mutations in human cells by x-ray exposures below 10 rads. Proc Natl Acad Sci USA 1985;82:2092.
24. Hartwell LH, Kastan MB. Cell cycle control and cancer. Science 1994;266:1821.
25. Hei TK, Krauss R, Liu SX, Hall EJ, Weinstein IB. Effects of increased expression of protein kinase C on radiation-induced cell transformation. Carcinogenesis 1994;15:365.
26. Hill CK, Buonaguro FM, Myers CP, Han A, Elkind MM. Fission-spectrum neutrons at reduced dose rates enhance neoplastic transformation. Nature 1982;298:67.
27. Hill CK, Nagy B, Peraino C, Grdina DJ. 2-[(Aminopropyl)amino]ethanethiol (WR1065) is antineoplastic and antimutagenic when given during ^{60}Co γ-ray irradiation. Carcinogenesis 1986;7:665–668.
28. IARC Study Group on Cancer Risk Among Nuclear Industry Workers. Direct estimates of cancer mortality due to low doses of ionizing radiation: an international study. Lancet 1994;344:1039.
29. International Commission on Radiological Protection. Recommendations of the International Commission on Radiological Protection 1990. Ann ICRP 1991.
30. Kadhim MA, Lorimore SA, Hepburn MD, Goodhead DT, Buckle VJ, Wright EG. α-particle-induced chromosomal instability in human bone marrow cells. Lancet 1994;344:987.
31. Kano Y, Little JB. Persistence of x-ray-induced chromosomal rearrangements in long-term cultures of human diploid fibroblasts. Cancer Res 1984;44:3706.
32. Kano Y, Little JB. Mechanisms of human cell neoplastic transformation: x-ray-induced abnormal clone formation in long-term cultures of human diploid fibroblasts. Cancer Res 1985;45:2550.
33. Kemp CJ, Wheldon T, Balmain A. p53-deficient mice are extremely susceptible to radiation-induced tumorigenesis. Nature Gene 1994;8:66–69.
34. Kennedy AR. In vitro studies of anticarcinogenic protease inhibitors. In Protease Inhibitors as Cancer Chemopreventive Agents. Edited by W Troll, AR Kennedy. New York: Plenum Press, 1993, pp 65–91.
35. Kennedy AR. Overview. Anticarcinogenic activity of protease inhibitors. In Protease Inhibitors as Cancer Chemopreventive Agents. Edited W Troll, AR Kennedy. New York: Plenum Press, 1993, pp 9–64.
36. Kennedy AR, Fox M, Murphy G, Little JB. Relationship between x-ray exposure and malignant transformation in C3H 10T1/2 cells. Proc Natl Acad Sci USA 1980;77:7262.
37. Kennedy AR, Little JB. Evidence that a second event in x-ray induced oncogenic transformation *in vitro* occurs during cellular proliferation. Radiat Res 1984;99:228.
38. Krolewski B, Little JB. Molecular analysis of DNA isolated from the different stages of x-ray-induced transformation *in vitro*. Mol Carcinog 1989;2:27.
39. Krolewski B, Little JB. Search for oncogene mutations in x-ray-transformed mouse 10T[1/2] cells by denaturing gradient gel electrophoresis blotting. Int J Radiat Biol 1994;65:147.
40. Kuerbitz SJ, Plunkett BS, Walsh WV, Kasten MB. Wild-type p53 is a cell cycle checkpoint determinant following irradiation. Proc Natl Acad Sci USA 1992;89:7491–7495.
41. Lee JM, Bernstein A. p53 mutations increase resistance to ionizing radiation. Proc Natl Acad Sci USA 1993;90:5742.
42. Letourneau EG, Krewski D, Choi NW, Goddard MJ, McGregor RG, Zielinski JM, Du J. Case-control study of residential radon and lung cancer in Winnipeg, Manitoba, Canada. Am J Epidemiol 1994;140:310.
43. Leuthauser SWC, Thomas JE, Guernsey DL. Oncogenes in x-ray-transformed C3H 10T[1/2] mouse cells and in x-ray-induced mouse fibrosarcoma (RIF-1) cells. Int J Radiat Biol 1992;62:45.
44. Li C-Y, Nagasawa H, Tsang N-M, Little JB. Radiation-induced irreversible G (0)/G (1) block is abolished in human diploid fibroblasts transfected with the human papilloma virus E6 gene: implication of the p53-Cip1/WAF1 pathway. Int J Oncol 1995;6:233.
45. Li C-Y, Yandell DW, Little JB. Molecular mechanisms of spontaneous and induced loss of heterozygosity in human cells *in vitro*. Somat Cell Mol Genet 1992;8:77–87.
46. Lindop P, Rotblat J. Long-term effects of a single whole-body exposure of mice to ionizing radiations. I. Life-shortening. Proc R Soc Lond [Biol] 1961;154:332.
47. Little JB. Cellular effects of ionizing radiation. Parts I and II. N Engl J Med 1968;273:308,369.
48. Little JB. Low-dose radiation effects: interactions and synergism. Health Phys 1990;59:49.
49. Little JB. Characteristics of radiation-induced neoplastic transformation *in vitro*. Leuk Res 1986;10:719.
50. Little JB. Failla Memorial Lecture: changing views of cellular radiosensitivity. Radiat Res 1994;140:299.
51. Little JB. The relevance of cell transformation to carcinogenesis *in vivo*. In Low Dose Radiation: Biological Basis of Risk Assessment. Edited by KF Baverstock, JW Strather. London: Taylor & Francis, 1989, p 396.
52. Little JB, Kennedy AR, McGandy RB. Lung cancer induced in hamsters by low doses of alpha radiation from polonium-210. Science 1975;188:737.
53. Little JB, Nagasawa H. Effect of confluent holding on potentially lethal damage repair, cell cycle progression, and chromosomal aberrations in human normal and ataxia-telagiectasia fibroblasts. Radiat Res 1985;101:81.
54. Lowe SW, Bodis S, McClatchey A, Remington L, Ruley HE, Fisher DE, Housman DE, Jacks T. p53 status and the efficacy of cancer therapy *in vivo*. Science 1994;266:807.
55. Lowe SW, Schmitt EM, Smith SW, Osborne BA, Jacks T. p53 is required for radiation-induced apoptosis in mouse thymocytes. Nature 1993;362:847.
56. Mabuchi K, Thompson DE, Preston DL, Ron E, et al. Cancer incidence in atomic bomb survivors, parts I-IV. Radiat Res 1994;137(2)[suppl S1].
57. MacMahon B. Some recent issues in low-exposure radiation epidemiology. Environ Health Perspect 1989;81:131.
58. McGinnis JM, Foege WH. Actual causes of deaths in the United States. JAMA 1993;270:2207.
59. McIlwrath AJ, Vasey PA, Ross GM, Brown R. Cell cycle arrests and radiosensitivity of human tumor cell lines: dependence on wild-type p53 for radiosensitivity. Cancer Res 1994;54:3718.
60. Miller RW. Effects of prenatal exposure to ionizing radiation. Health Phys 1990;59:57.
61. Modan B. Low dose radiation carcinogenesis: issues and interpretation. Health Phys 1993;65:475.
62. Murnane JP. Cell cycle regulation in response to DNA damage in mammalian cells: a historical perspective. Cancer Metastasis Rev 1995;14:17.
63. Nagasawa H, Little JB. Comparison of kinetics of x-ray induced cell killing in normal, ataxia telangiectasia and hereditary retinoblastoma fibroblasts. Mutat Res 1983;109:297.
64. National Research Council. Health Effects of Exposure to Low Levels of Ionizing Radiation: BEIR V. Committee on the Biological Effects of Ionizing Radiations, National Research Council, Washington DC: National Academy Press, 1990.
65. Newcomb EW, Steinberg JJ, Pellicer A. Ras oncogenes and phenotypic staging in N-methylnitrosourea- and gamma-irradiation-induced thymic lymphomas in C57BL/6J mice. Cancer Res 1988;48:5514.
66. Ootsuyama A, Makino H, Nagao M, Ochiai A, Yamauchi Y, Tanooka H. Frequent p53 mutation in mouse tumors induced by repeated β-irradiation. Mol Carcinogenesis 1994;11:236.
67. Pampfer S, Streffer C. Increased chromosome aberration levels in cells from mouse fetuses after zygote x-irradiation. Int J Radiat Biol 1989;55:85.
68. Paquette B, Little JB. *In vivo* enhancement of genomic instability in minisatellite sequences of mouse C3H/10T[1/2] cells transformed *in vitro* by x-rays. Cancer Res 1994;54:3173.
69. Pershagen G, Åkerblom G, Axelson O, Clavensjö B, Damber L, Desai G, Enflo A, Langarde F, Mellander H, Svartengren M, Swedjemark GA. Residential radon exposure and lung cancer in Sweden. N Engl J Med 1994;330 159.
70. Pochin EE. Occupational and other fatality risks. Community Health Stud 1974;6:2.
71. Samet JM. Indoor radon and lung cancer: risky or not? JNCI 1994;86:1813.
72. Sankaranarayanan K, Chakraborty R. Cancer predisposition, radiosensitivity and the risk of radiation-induced cancers, I: background. Radiat Res 1995;143:121.
73. Sawey MJ, Hood AT, Burns FJ, Garte SJ. Activation of myc and ras oncogenes in primary rat tumors induced by ionizing radiation. Mol Cell Biol 1987;7:932.
74. Shigematsu N, Schwartz JL, Grdina DJ. Protection against radiation-induced mutagenesis at the hprt locus by spermine and N,N″-(dithiodi-2,1-ethanediyl)bis-1,3-propanediamine (WR-33278). Mutagenesis 1994;9:355–360.
75. Shimizu Y, Kato H, Schull WJ. Studies of the mortality of A-bomb survivors. 9. Mortality, 1950–1985: part 2. Cancer mortality based on the recently revised doses (DS86). Radiat Res 1990;121:120.
76. Sloan SR, Newcomb EW, Pellicer A. Neutron radiation can activate K-*ras* via a point mutation in codon 146 and induces a different spectrum of *ras* mutation than does gamma radiation. Mol Cell Biol 1990;10:405.
77. Slovic P. Perception of risk. Science 1987;236:280.
78. Storer JB, Mitchell TJ, Fry RJM. Extrapolation of the relative risk of radiogenic neoplasms across mouse strains and to man. Radiat Res 1988;114:331.
79. Strasser A, Harris AW, Jacks T, Cory S. DNA damage can induce apoptosis in proliferating lymphoid cells via p53-independent mechanisms inhibitable by Bcl-2. Cell 1994;79:329.
80. Sturm SA, Strauss PG, Adolph S, Hameister H, Erfle V. Amplification and rearrangement of c-*myc* in radiation-induced murine osteosarcomas. Cancer Res 1990;50:4146.
81. Su L-N, Little JB. Transformation and radiosensitivity of human diploid skin fibroblasts transfected with SV40 T-antigen mutants defective in RB and p53 binding domains. Int J Radiat Biol 1992;62:461.
82. Swift M, Morrell D, Massey RB, Chase CL. Incidence of cancer in 161 families affected by ataxia-telangiectasia. N Engl J Med 1991;325:1831.
83. Tabocchini MA, Little JB, Liber HL. Mutation induction in human lymphoblasts after protracted exposure to low doses of tritiated water. In Low Dose Radiation: Biological Basis of Risk Assessment. Edited by KF Baverstock, JW Stather. London: Taylor & Francis, 1989.
84. Thomson JF, Grahn D. Life shortening in mice exposed to fission neutrons and gamma-rays, VII: effects of 60 once-weekly exposures. Radiat Res 1988;115:347.
85. Ullrich RL. Tumor induction in BALB/c mice after fractionated or protracted exposures to fission-spectrum neutrons. Radiat Res 1984;97:587.
86. Ullrich RL, Storer JB. Influence of gamma irradiation on the development of neoplastic disease in mice, I: reticular tissue tumors. Radiat Res 1979;80:303.
87. Ullrich RL, Storer JB. Influence of gamma irradiation on the development of neoplastic disease in mice. II. Solid tumors. Radiat Res 1979;80:317.
88. United Nations Scientific Committee on the Effects of Atomic Radiation. Sources and Effects of Ionizing Radiation. United Nations Scientific Committee on the Effects of Atomic Radiation, UNSCEAR 1994 Report to the General Assembly with Scientific Annexes. New York: United Nations Press, 1994.
89. Upton AC. Historical perspectives on radiation carcinogenesis. In Radiation Carcinogenesis. Edited by AC Upton, RE Albert, FJ Burns, RE Shore. New York: Elsevier, 1986.
90. Weichselbaum RR, Beckett MA, Diamond AA. Some retinoblastomas, osteosarcomas, and soft tissue sarcomas may share a common etiology. Proc Natl Acad Sci USA 1988;85:2106.
91. Weinstein IB. The origins of human cancer: molecular mechanisms of carcinogenesis and their implications for cancer prevention and treatment. Cancer Res 1988;48:4135.
92. Wilson R, Crouch EAC. Risk assessment and comparisons: an Introduction. Science 1987;236:267.

CHAPTER 16

Ultraviolet Radiation Carcinogenesis

JAMES E. CLEAVER AND DAVID L. MITCHELL

Mad dogs and Englishmen go out in the midday sun.
—Noël Coward

Historical Perspective

Skin cancers occur in uniquely accessible sites and are caused by well-defined environmental agents; consequently, their formation illustrates numerous salient features of carcinogenesis. Skin tumors in humans account for about 30% of all new cancers reported annually (1, 2). Epidemiologic and laboratory studies provide evidence for a direct causal role of sunlight exposure in the induction of cancer (3), and the high rate of skin carcinogenesis is a direct result of the high dose rate from this causative agent. Both basal cell and squamous cell carcinomas are found on sun-exposed parts of the body (e.g., the face and trunk in men, the face and legs in women); and their incidence is correlated with cumulative sunlight exposure. Tumor incidence and mortality increase with decreasing latitude, corresponding to exposure; skin cancers are less frequent in dark-skinned populations than in lighter-skinned peoples; and tumor incidence increases with occupational exposure, such as in ranchers and fishermen. Melanoma, although also likely to be associated with sunlight exposure, shows a weaker dependence on total exposure to sunlight and a distribution over the body that is not as tightly correlated with exposed areas (4).

Exposure to direct sunlight in the mid–United States latitudes results in the accumulation of a mean lethal dose to unprotected human cells within approximately 30 minutes (5). The only other carcinogen to which we are exposed that even approaches these exposure levels would be cigarette smoke in very heavy smokers. Variations in individual susceptibility are also clearly observed in skin carcinogenesis. Human skin can be classified into types I through IV, ranging from skin that always burns and never tans to skin that tans but never burns; skin cancer susceptibility varies accordingly (6). But the most dramatic examples of variations in human susceptibility occur in the human genetic disorders that show increased responses to sunlight exposure (7). These include xeroderma pigmentosum, Cockayne syndrome, basal cell nevus syndrome, dysplastic nevus syndrome, Rothmund-Thomson syndrome, the porphyrias, and phenylketonuria. Some other disorders are associated with an acquired sun sensitivity, including polymorphous light eruption, actinic reticuloid, solar urticaria, lupus erythematosus, and Darier's disease. Less specific factors contributing to sun sensitivity include skin type, race, eye and hair color, and tendency for freckling; additional factors can include medication and immunologic status. Sunlight exposure also has a major immunosuppressive effect leading to loss of antigen-presenting Langerhans cells and the appearance of dyskeratotic keratinocytes (sunburn cells) in the upper epidermis, together with the erythemal sunburn response associated with vasodilation caused by a release of prostaglandin (8).

Epidemiology

SKIN CANCER FREQUENCY AND AGE AT ONSET

Sunlight, particularly the ultraviolet B (UVB) component, is the major environmental agent that precipitates the clinical symptoms of skin carcinogenesis. This is well established for squamous and basal cell cancers but still controversial for melanoma (9, 10). Nonmelanoma skin cancers are by far the most common cancers that occur in the United States each year (2, 11). They make up 30 to 40% of all cancers. More than 800,000 new cases were expected to occur in 1995 (12). Of these, 150,000 were expected to be squamous cell carcinomas, and 2,100 people were expected to die of nonmelanoma skin cancer in the United States in 1995. The incidence is increasing at an alarming rate (13) and may be considered a quiet 20th century epidemic. The role of the sun in inducing these cancers was suggested by a number of astute clinical observations around the turn of the 20th century and has been confirmed subsequently by epidemiologic studies. As a consequence, there is a wealth of human epidemiologic data on skin cancer risks with geographic location, skin type, and various photosensitizing, enhancing, and protective applications (13–19). Nonmelanoma skin cancer is therefore one of the few malignancies for which there is a clear evidence of the initiating agent: the UVB component of sunlight. The relationship of melanoma skin cancer to sun exposure and the possible action spectrum is less clear (9, 10) but may be related to acute burns rather than accumulated dose.

The importance of DNA as a chromophore for the shorter wavelengths is illustrated by the autosomal recessive disease xeroderma pigmentosum (XP). In this disease a failure in one cellular protective mechanism, DNA repair, is associated with a major increase in the rate of onset of squamous and basal cell carcinoma and melanoma (7). Median age at onset for skin cancer in the general U.S. population is 50 to 60 years; in XP patients carcinogenesis is accelerated and median onset is within the first decade of life (Fig. 16.1). This early onset is a direct consequence of sunlight-induced changes in the DNA of skin cells. An appreciation of the significance of these changes requires knowledge of the photochemical responses of DNA, mechanisms of DNA repair, and their mutagenic and carcinogenic consequences.

SUNLIGHT SPECTRUM AND WAVELENGTHS RESPONSIBLE FOR SKIN CANCER

The ultraviolet (UV) portion of the solar spectrum is undoubtedly the major factor in skin cancer. UV radiation is divided into three wavelength ranges on the basis of differences in photochemistry and biologic importance. UVA (320–400 nm) is photocarcinogenic and involved in photoaging but is weakly absorbed in DNA and protein. The relevant chromophores may therefore involve targets that result in production of active oxygen and free radicals, which secondarily cause damage to DNA (20, 21). Experimental studies using chronic UVA and UVB irradiation of mice indicate that the mechanism of tumor formation by UVA is different from that by UVB and may involve non-DNA absorption. UVB (290–320 nm) overlaps the upper end of the DNA and protein absorption spectra and is the range mainly responsible for skin cancer through photochemical damage to DNA. UVC (240–290 nm) is not normally present in sunlight but is readily produced by low-pressure mercury sterilizing lamps. The peak wavelength of mercury excitation (254 nm) coincides with the peak of DNA absorption (260 nm), and this wavelength has been of major importance in experimental studies. Absorption of UVC radiation by stratospheric ozone greatly attenuates these wavelengths, so that very little light shorter than 300 nm reaches the Earth's surface. Hence, although UVA and UVB light constitute a minute portion of the emitted solar wavelengths (0.0000001%), they are primarily responsible for the sun's pathological effects. The relative proportions of DNA photoproducts vary across these UV wavelengths. Physical shielding of the critical cells of the skin is achieved by melanin pigment and keratin layers; intracellular defenses depend on repair of DNA damage, antioxidant enzymes (e.g., superoxide dismutase, glutathione reductase), endogenous free radical quenchers, and inducible detoxifying enzymes and biochemical systems (20, 21). Melanin itself may play two opposite roles: not only shielding cells from direct UV damage, but also indirectly producing damaging free radicals through UV-stimulated redox reactions (22).

SUNLIGHT-INDUCED PHOTOPRODUCTS IN DNA

Action spectra for squamous cell carcinoma indicate that DNA is the target molecule; the absorption spectrum of DNA correlates well with lethality, mutation induction, and photoproduct formation (23–26). The energy absorbed by DNA produces molecular changes, some of which involve single bases (i.e., monomeric damage, single-strand breaks, and abasic sites), others resulting in interactions between adjacent bases (i.e., dimerizations) as well as between nonadjacent bases (i.e., inter- or intrastrand cross-links), and still others between DNA and its nucleosomal scaffold (i.e., DNA–protein cross-links).

Dimerizations between adjacent pyrimidines are the most prevalent photoreactions resulting from UV irradiation. The two major photoproducts induced are the cyclobutane pyrimidine dimer and, at about 25% the frequency, the pyrimidine-pyrimidone [6–4] photoproduct (Fig. 16.2). The distribution of these photoproducts in human chromatin depends on base sequence, secondary DNA structure, and DNA–protein interactions. In vivo mapping of UV photodamage at nucleotide resolution has been achieved using liga-

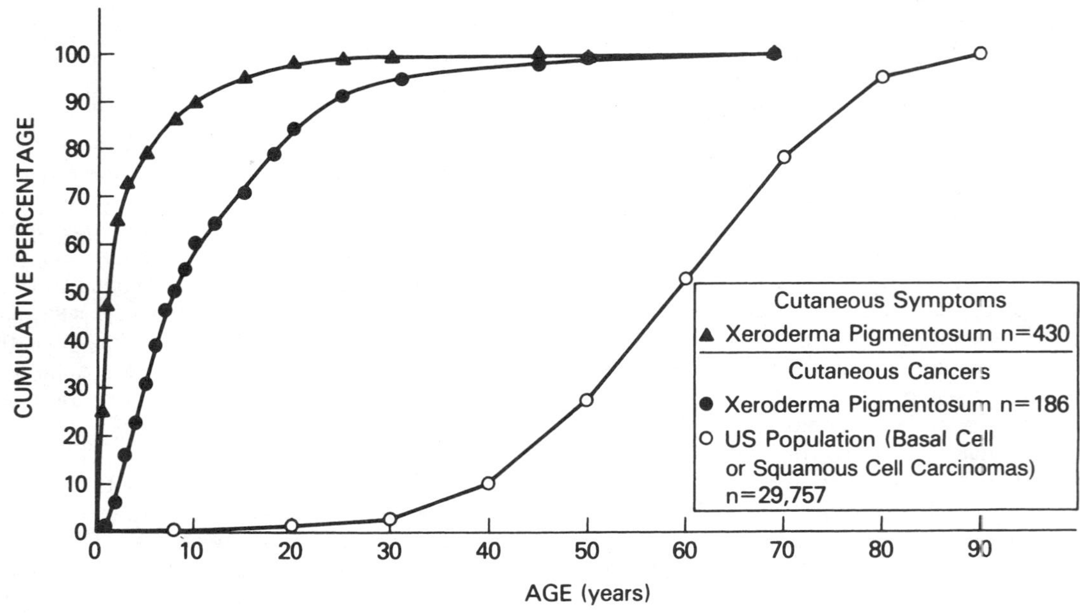

Figure 16.1. Age at onset of XP symptoms. Age at onset of cutaneous symptoms (generally sun sensitivity or pigmentation) was reported for 430 patients. Age at first skin cancer was reported for 186 patients and is compared with the age distribution of 29,757 patients with basal cell carcinoma or squamous cell carcinoma in the U.S. general population. *Source:* Kraemer et al. (119). Reproduced with permission.

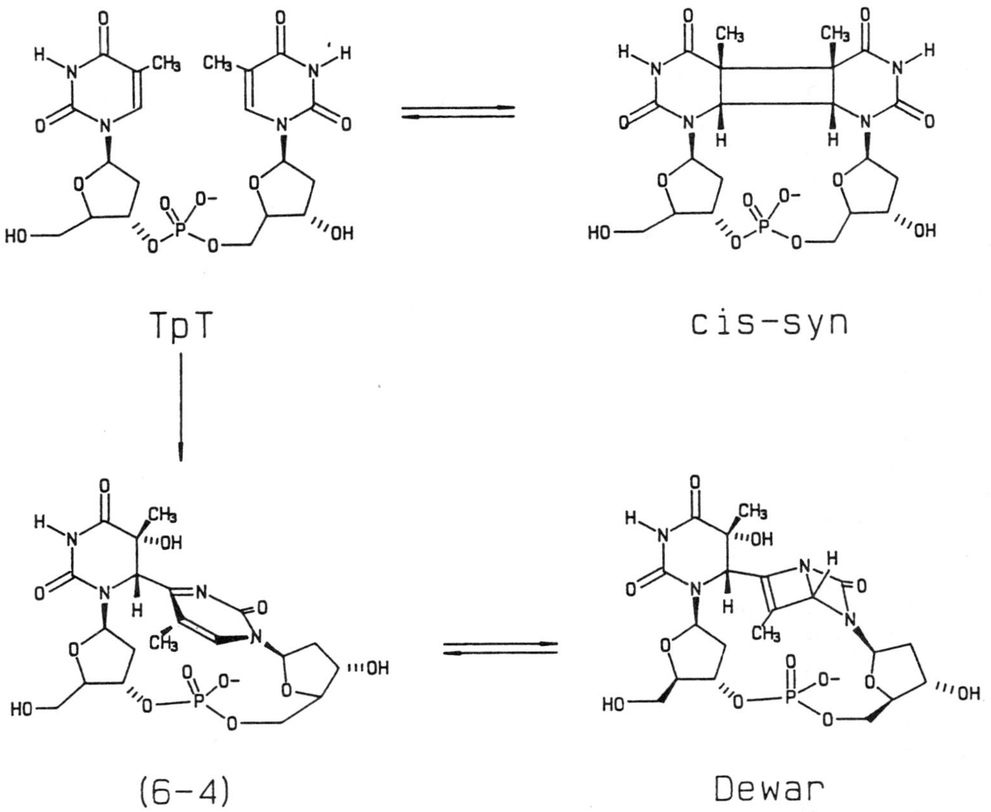

Figure 16.2. Photochemical reactions in a dipyrimidine DNA sequence leading to the formation of cyclobutane pyrimidine dimers (TpT1, TpT2) or a [cis-syn] [6–4] photoproduct (TpT4) and its photolytic derivative, the Dewar pyrimidone (TpT3). Redrawn from Taylor and Cohrs (31).

tion-mediated polymerase chain reaction (LMPCR) technology (27). With this technique, it was shown that binding of transcription factors to promoter regions can both enhance and suppress photoproduct formation at specific sites (28). The propensity of photoproduct formation for transcription factor binding sites would serve to enhance mutations in gene regulation and focus these mutations on specific tissues. The ratio of cytosine-containing cyclobutane dimers to thymine dimers increases significantly within the UVB region (29). In conjunction with [6–4] photoproducts, which are preferentially induced at thymine-cytosine dipyrimidines, cytosine-containing dimeric lesions may play a major role in UVB (solar) mutagenesis (30). The [6–4] photoproduct can further undergo a UVB-dependent conversion to its valence photoisomer, the Dewar pyrimidinone (31) (Fig. 16.2).

In addition to the major dimeric photoproducts, many other rare photoproducts can be induced in DNA, such as the 8,8-adenine dehydrodimer (32), a TA photoproduct between adjacent thymines and adenines (33), and a purine photoproduct that manifests as an enzyme-sensitive site on sequencing gels (34). Numerous monobasic pyrimidine photoproducts have also been identified, including thymine glycols (35) and a cytosine hydrate (36). Because the total yield of these photoproducts is only 3 to 4% of the yield of cyclobutane dimers, their biologic role is considered minimal; however, their importance as premutagenic lesions in specific sites cannot be excluded.

In contrast to the direct induction of DNA damage by UVB light, UVA light (wavelengths $>$ 320 nm) primarily produces damage indirectly through highly reactive chemical intermediates. UVA light generates oxygen and hydroxyl radicals, which in turn react with DNA to form monomeric damage, strand breaks, and DNA–protein cross-links. The importance of these photoproducts is not known, but evidence is accumulating to suggest that UVA light may be an important pathogenic component of sunlight. Significant levels of cell killing and mutation induction have been observed in human epidermal cells after irradiation with UVA light (23, 26). These data are consistent with earlier studies that suggested that the lethal effects of UVA (sunlight) irradiation are not mediated by dimer damage (37, 38) and that endogenous photoprotectors can mitigate the cytotoxic action of UVA light (21). The biologic importance of UVA light is perhaps best illustrated by the recent demonstration that UVA causes significant levels of tumorigenesis in hairless mice (39).

Genetic Factors in Skin Carcinogenesis

EXCISION OF UV PHOTOPRODUCTS

The idea that UV damage to DNA is an essential component of photocarcinogenesis arose from the discovery that cells from patients with the inherited disorder xeroderma pigmentosum are deficient in DNA repair (40, 41). In vivo studies measuring excision repair in the skin of these patients showed similar deficiencies (42). Since these initial studies, an abundance of data has accumulated regarding the molecular mechanisms and consequences of DNA damage and repair in XP cells, as well as cells from patients with other genetic diseases.

Two major pathways of excision repair, the nucleotide and base excision pathways, operate on different kinds of damage in DNA. The nucleotide pathway removes pyrimidine dimers and large chemical adducts to DNA and replaces the damaged site with a newly synthesized polynucleotide patch approximately 29 bases in length (Fig. 16.3) (43, 44). The base excision pathway removes DNA bases that have undergone relatively small degrees of modification, such as the monobasic UV damage to cytosines. Excision by this pathway involves glycosylases and apurinic endonucleases plus other enzymes; the patch may be smaller than that resulting from nucleotide repair. Nucleotide and base excision repair are both complex processes involving multiple gene products that interact with damaged sites in different ways according to the precise location of the damage. Adjacent bases, DNA conformation, bound proteins, transcriptional activity of the gene and strand-containing damage are among the many factors that can influence rates of repair (43).

The polymerization step of excision repair of UV damage is catalyzed predominantly by DNA polymerase α or δ, although polymerase β may also be involved to some extent, especially in base excision. The final step of repair is the sealing of the 3′, 5′ gap, a reaction catalyzed by polynucleotide ligase. Excision repair also requires a temporary relaxation of nucleosomal structure so that repaired regions are more accessible to exogenous nucleases (Fig. 16.4). The continuous excision of dimers and insertion of the bases is associated with a very low net frequency of DNA strand breaks. This suggests that during excision repair a dynamic balance is established between strand breakage and rejoining. The actual number of sites involved in excision repair at any one time is small, no more than about 1 in 2×10^8 daltons of DNA. Only about 1% of the dimers produced in DNA by a dose of 10 J/m^2 are undergoing excision at any instant. Excision must therefore be rate-limited by the enzymes involved in the early steps of repair.

There is considerable difference between cyclobutane dimers and [6–4] photoproducts in their rates of excision from the overall genome of rodent and human fibroblasts and skin (Figs. 16.5, 16.6) (45), even though the basic mechanism and patch sizes are essentially the same (46). [6–4] Photoproducts are more rapidly excised, 50% being re-

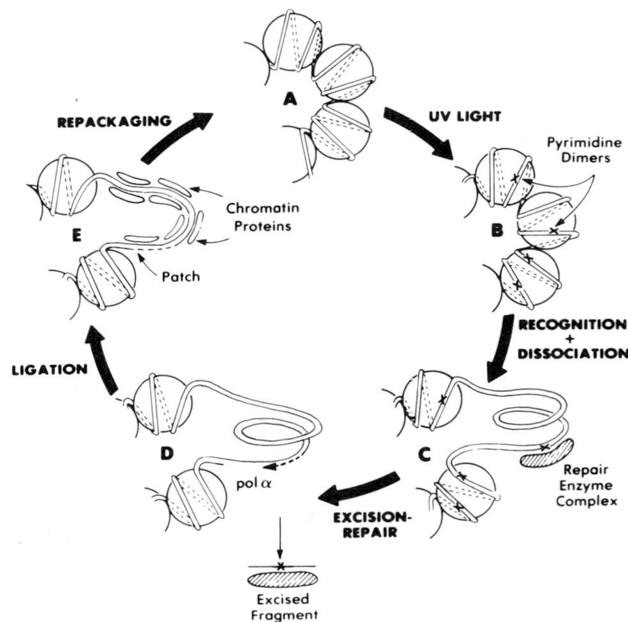

Figure 16.4. Heuristic scheme for excision repair of damaged sites on DNA in mammalian chromatin. The first step involves mechanisms that recognize damage and dissociate nucleoproteins to make the DNA accessible to repair enzymes. This is followed by sequential incision by a DNA polymerase, sealing of the patch by a polynucleotide ligase, and final reassembly and repackaging of nucleoprotein. *Source:* Cleaver and Kraemer (7). Reproduced with permission.

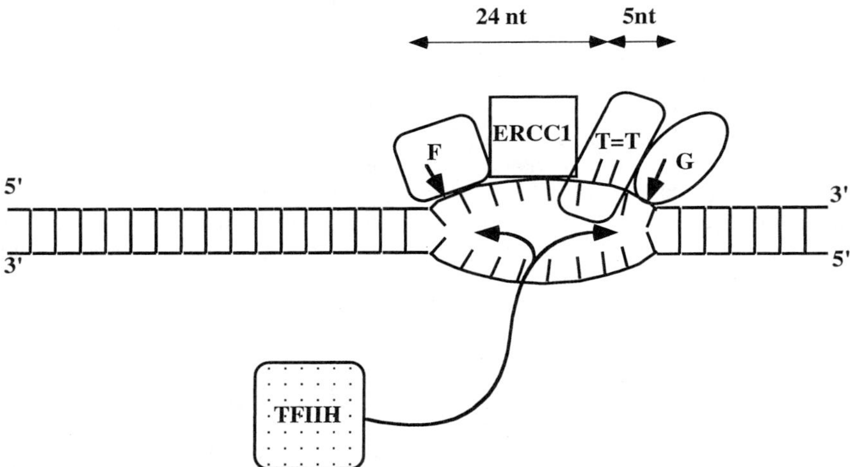

Figure 16.3. Biochemical steps for nucleotide excision repair of pyrimidine dimers in DNA prokaryotes showing biochemical details of events represented schematically in Figure 16.4. The XPA binds to photoproducts and excision occurs when UV-specific endonucleases make an incision on the 5′ and 3′ sides. Excision and subsequent polymerization releases a 29 base oligonucleotide containing the dimer.

moved from human and rodent cells in 2 to 6 hours. Cyclobutane dimers are much more slowly removed; half are removed from human cell DNA in 12 to 24 hours (47, 48), but negligible amounts are removed from rodent DNA for even longer times. There are also large variations in dimer excision between human subjects (48). The different rates of excision may reflect the fact that [6–4] photoproducts are preferentially located in internucleosomal regions of DNA, whereas dimers are distributed more randomly but with about a 10-A periodicity in the DNA wrapped around nucleosomes (49, 50). When excision is considered on an individual gene basis, additional variation exists according to transcriptional activity. Pyrimidine dimers are excised more rapidly from actively transcribed genes, especially the DNA strand used as the template for transcription (51). An increased excision rate in active genes may also occur for [6–4] photoproducts, but this is less easily resolved against the greater overall rate of excision of these photoproducts in the genome as a whole.

The differences between excision in active and inactive genes occur because a basal transcription factor, TFIIH, plays a major role in repair (52). This factor regulates basal transcription by RNA polymerase II, and most of its eight peptide components have second functions in DNA repair (53). Most of the genes that regulate this process of gene-specific repair are associated with the human disorders XP, Cockayne syndrome, and trichothiodystrophy. Two of the helicases in TFIIH correspond to the XPB and D genes of XP, and others are known to play a role from their analogues in the yeast transcription factor b (53). A detailed study of the promoter and first exons of the PGKI gene has indicated that excision is slow in regions of promoter binding but increases immediately after the ATG start site for transcription (54).

MUTAGENICITY OF UV PHOTOPRODUCTS

Two molecular mechanisms are currently considered important in the initiation of carcinogenesis: activation of proto-oncogenes and inactivation of tumor suppressor genes. Both sites of action are vulnerable to the lethal and mutagenic effects of UV light. A gene, such as the *ras* proto-oncogene, can be activated by a point mutation; p53, on the other hand, is a tumor suppressor gene commonly inactivated by point mutation in human tumors (55, 56).

The mutagenicity and tumorigenicity of a particular type of DNA damage (photoproduct) may ultimately be influenced by its lethality. This relationship has been considered in terms of a "pass/fail" rule: lesions that block DNA polymerization are lethal but nonmutagenic (55). In other words, the more cytotoxic a lesion (assuming its lethality results from termination of DNA synthesis), the less likely it will be to allow continued synthesis and mutation induction at that site.

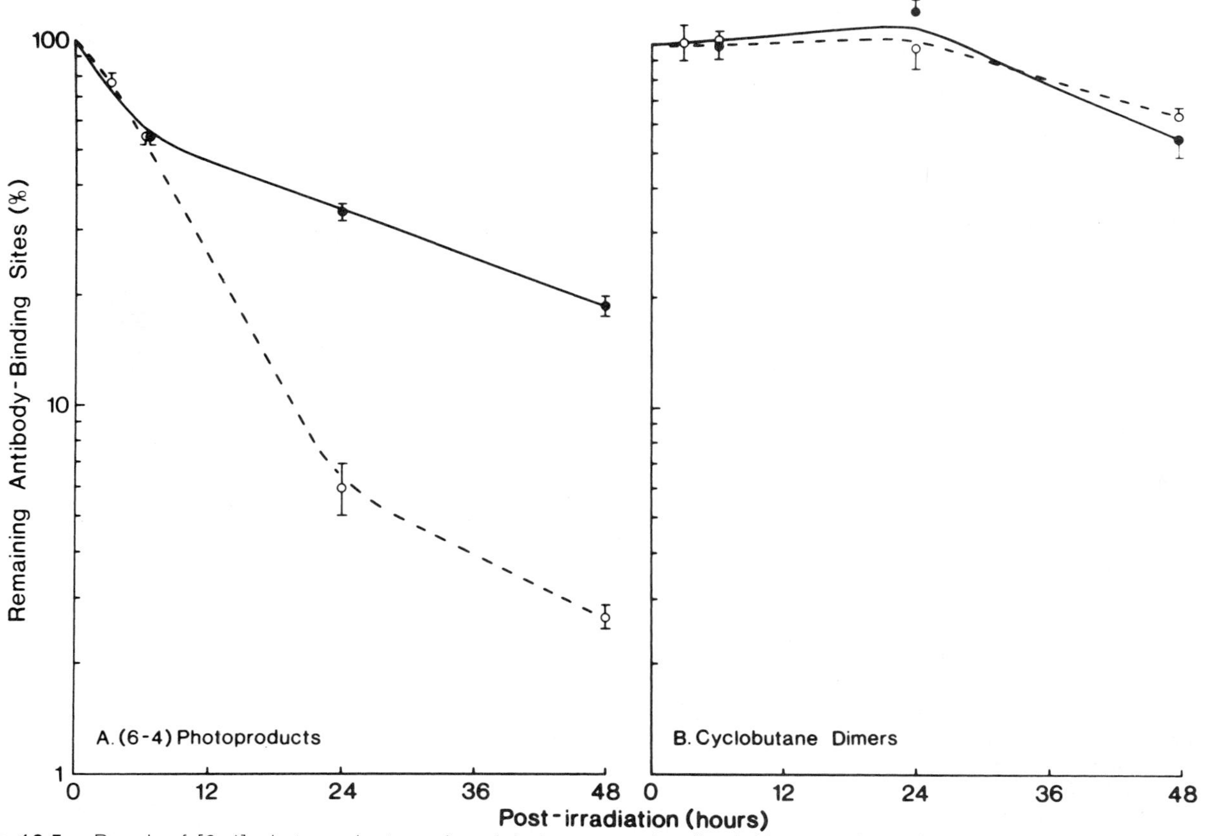

Figure 16.5. Repair of [6–4] photoproducts and cyclobutane dimers in mouse skin and cultured cells. Radioimmunoassays that specifically detect [6–4] photoproducts (**A**) or cyclobutane dimers (**B**) were used to monitor the removal of these lesions from the DNA of irradiated mouse skin (*solid lines*) and mouse cells in culture (*broken lines*). Means and standard error bars are shown for 3, 6, 24, and 48 hours after UVB irradiation of mouse skin ($n = 10$) and for 3, 4, and 24 hours after UVC irradiation of 3T3 and 10T1/2 cells ($n = 4$). *Source:* Mitchell et al. (120). Reproduced with permission.

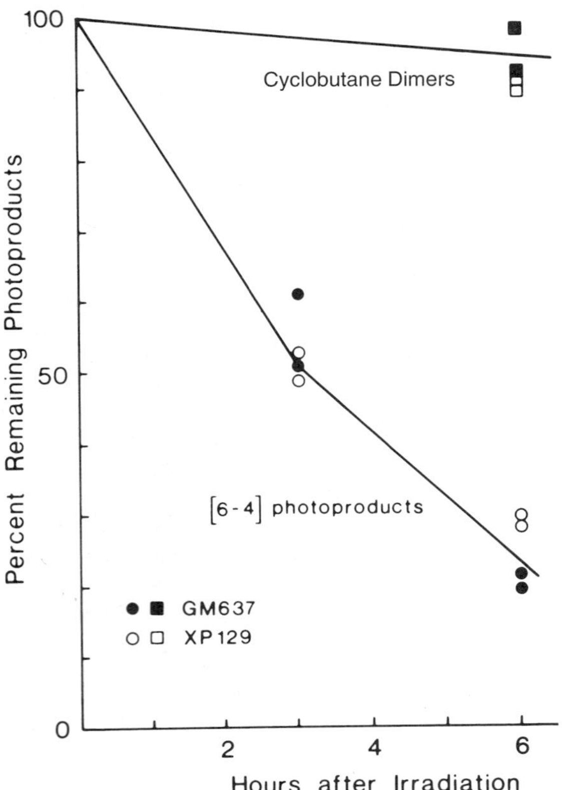

Figure 16.6. Repair of [6–4] photoproducts and cyclobutane dimers in human fibroblasts in culture. Radioimmunoassays that specifically detect [6–4] photoproducts (circles) or cyclobutane dimers (squares) were used to monitor the removal of lesions from the DNA of normal (GM637) or XP revertant (XP129) cells. *Source:* JE Cleaver, unpublished data.

In terms of this model, the mutagenicity of the major photoproducts in mammalian cells is inversely related to their cytotoxicity; their cytotoxicity is in turn modulated by repair.

Tumor progression can also be affected by UV damage in DNA. Cell death as a result of the lethal effects of UV light may enhance the clonal expansion of surviving cells that may have been mutated or initiated, increasing the probability of tumor progression (56). Thus, the interplay of UV lethality and mutagenesis in human skin cells may determine the onset and progression of UV-induced carcinogenesis, and the tumor-suppressor gene p53 plays a major role in this determination (56).

Site-specific determination of photoproduct induction in the *lacI* gene of *E. coli* suggested a correlation between UV mutation hot spots and hot spots of [6–4] photoproduct induction (57). Analysis of sites of [6–4] photoproduct induction suggested that this lesion was responsible for the major fraction of cytosine-to-thymine transition mutations in *E. coli.* Consistent with this observation, it was shown that the exclusive induction of cyclobutane dimers by acetophenone and UVB light did not increase the induction of transition mutations in lambda phage (58). A similar relationship was observed in a study of photoreactivation in *E. coli*: whereas cyclobutane dimers and [6–4] photoproducts were similarly cytotoxic, the latter were much more mutagenic (59).

The role of specific photoproducts in UV mutagenesis in human cells has been investigated with the use of shuttle vectors. In these systems UV-irradiated simian virus SV40-based plasmids are transfected into human cells, where they are replicated by the host. The plasmids are subsequently recovered, amplified in bacteria, and analyzed for mutation induction by DNA sequencing. Sites of mutations can then be compared with sites of photoproduct induction in the target sequence. The results of these studies were similar to those obtained in *E. coli*: sites of transition mutations correlated with sites of increased [6–4] photoproduct induction (Table 16.1). In particular, sites and frequencies of mutation hot spots in the *lacI* gene transfected into human cells were identical to those determined in *E. coli* (60). In a shuttle vector system in which photoproduct induction and sites of mutation were examined in the *supF* gene, transfection into SV40-transformed human fibroblasts and monkey kidney cells indicated a similar correlation (61). In the *supF* gene inserted into the mouse L cell chromosome (62) and into the endogenous *APRT* gene of Chinese hamster ovary (CHO) cells (63), most of the mutations consisted of cytosine-to-thymine transitions occurring at thymine-cytosine and cytosine-cytosine sequences. Because of the strand specificity of repair, there is a preponderance of mutations due to damage in the noncoding strand of expressed genes (64, 65). This can be more prominent in mouse cells and XP

Table 16.1. UVC-Induced Mutations Observed in Shuttle Vector pZ189 Replicated in Xeroderma Pigmentosum (XP) or Normal Human Cells[a]

Mutations	Number of plasmids with base changes[b]	
	XP	Normal
Independent plasmids sequenced[c]	61 (100%)	89 (100%)
Point mutations		
Single base substitution	47[d] (77%)	48 (53%)
Tandem base substitutions[e]	12 (20%)	16 (18%)
Multiple base substitutions[f]	1[d] (2%)	24 (28%)
Base insertions and deletions		
Single base insertion	0	2
Single or tandem base deletions	1	3
Types of single or tandem base substitutions and number of changes		
Transitions	67[d] (94%)	61 (75%)
GC to AT	66[d] (93%)	59 (73%)
AT to GC	1 (1%)	2 (2%)
Transversions	4[d] (6%)	20 (25%)
GC to TA	0[d]	8 (10%)
GC to CG	1 (1%)	5 (6%)
AT to TA	3 (4%)	6 (8%)
AT to CG	0	1 (1%)

[a] Modified with permission from Bredberg et al. (115), and previously published by Cleaver and Kraemer (7).
[b] 50 to 300 J/m^2 for XP cells, 100 to 5,000 J/m^2 for normal cells.
[c] From separate transfections or different mutations in the same transfection including all experiments.
[d] $P < .01$ versus normal.
[e] Two base substitutions zero to two bases apart, or three adjacent base substitutions.
[f] At least two base substitutions more than three bases apart.

group C cells than in normal human cells, where a high overall repair rate masks the effect.

Since the spectrum of damage induced by UVB radiation is different from that induced by UVC light, differences in the mutagenic action of these wavelengths are likely. After UVB irradiation of human cells, the ratio of ouabain-resistant mutants to thioguanine-resistant mutants is 10-fold higher than after UVC irradiation, suggesting that a unique type of premutagenic lesion is induced by the longer wavelengths (66). Mutations induced by UVB radiation have been analyzed at the sequence level in simian cells and show significant differences when compared with those induced by UVC light (67). Although GC-to-AT transition mutations still predominate from UVB, there are variations in the location of mutation hotspots, which are associated with regions of multiple base changes. In addition, UVB light induces more deletions and insertions than UVC light.

The predominance of cytosine-to-thymine transition mutations in both prokaryotic and eukaryotic cells has been explained in terms of the "A rule." This rule states that polymerases predominantly insert adenine opposite a site that lacks base coding information (68). In terms of this model, thymine-thymine cyclobutane dimers, the predominant photoproduct, would not usually be mutagenic since adenine is often correctly inserted opposite thymine. However, incorporation of adenine opposite a cytosine in a dipyrimidine photoproduct would result in a cytosine-to-thymine transition mutation. Hence, cyclobutane dimers and [6–4] photoproducts containing noninstructive cytosine base(s) are considered mutagenic, whereas thymine-thymine dimers are not.

Cyclobutane dimers and [6–4] photoproducts can both form at sequences shown to be mutation hot spots in shuttle vectors, and the identity of the mutagenic lesion has been tested by photoreactivation of the *supF* sequence in plasmids before transfection (69, 70). Enzymatic photoreversal of cyclobutane dimers reduced the mutation frequency in normal cells by 75% and in XP group A cells by 90%. Since cotransfection of monkey cells with a mixture of unirradiated *supF* plasmid and irradiated plasmid without the *supF* gene did not generate mutations, the role of an SOS-like system, as observed in *E. coli*, did not appear to be responsible for the results (70). These results are not consistent with the model developed in *E. coli* and suggest that [6–4] photoproducts may be less mutagenic in human cells. A similar analysis with photoreactivation suggested that cyclobutane dimers occurring at thymine-cytosine, cytosine-thymine, and cytosine-cytosine dipyrimidine sites were the predominant mutagenic lesions induced in human cells and that [6–4] photoproducts at these sites accounted for only about 10% of the mutations (69). However, this same study indicated that the frequencies of both cyclobutane dimers and [6–4] photoproducts at individual dipyrimidine sites did not correlate with mutation frequency, suggesting that, although UV-induced lesions are required for mutagenesis, mutation hot spots are determined by other factors.

A comparison of photoproduct yields, rates of repair, and mutations in the PGKI and p53 genes, however, has shown that regions of high UV-induced mutation can be caused by either or both high photoproduct yield and low repair (54, 71–73). A combination of initial yields and rates of repair that leave a high net persistent load of photoproducts in a particular site appears to be directly related to the mutational yield. Using LMPCR, Tormanen and Pfeifer mapped photoproduct distribution in exons 1 and 2 of three *ras* proto-oncogenes and found no correlation between photoproduct frequency and mutation induction in codon 12 of H-*ras* and K-*ras* (74). Since the initial distribution of photoproduct induction did not correlate with mutation spectra, it was possible that DNA repair may play a crucial role in the mutagenic process. Indeed, further studies with LMPCR showed that the rate of excision repair of cyclobutane dimers at specific nucleotides in the promoter and exon 1 of the PGK1 gene varied 15-fold, with much reduced repair at transcription factor–binding sites (54). DNA repair at individual nucleotides in the p53 tumor suppressor gene was highly variable and sequence dependent, with slow repair observed at seven of eight of the positions associated with mutations (72). UV-induced mutations in the p53 gene are a probable step in the formation of squamous cell carcinoma (55, 56) and may arise at DNA repair "cold spots" rather than photoproduct "hot spots."

GENETIC DISORDERS OF DNA REPAIR

The study of human sunlight-sensitive disorders and the selection of UV-sensitive hamster and mouse cells in culture have identified a large series of genetic loci that control the response of mammalian skin to damage (Table 16.2). These

Table 16.2. Complementation Groups in Xeroderma Pigmentosum (XP) and UV-Sensitive Chinese Hamster Ovary (CHO) Cells

Group	Human chromosome location	Central nervous system disorders	Relative repair (%)
Xeroderma pigmentosum			
A	9q34.1	Yes	2–5
B (Cockayne and ERCC3)[a]	2q21	Yes	3–7
C	3q25	No	5–20
D (Cockayne)[a,b]	19q13.2	Yes	25–50
E	—	No	50
F	16q13.1	No	18
G	13q32.3	Yes	<2
Variant	—	No	100
CHO (ERCC)[c]			
1	19q13.2	—	Low
2 (XPD)	19q13.2	—	Intermediate
3 (XPB)	2q21	—	Intermediate
4 (XPF)	16q13.1	—	Low
5 (XPG)	13q32.3	—	Intermediate

[a] Patients also exhibit symptoms commonly associated with Cockayne syndrome: dwarfism, cutaneous features, and mental retardation. Group B and ERCC3 represent the same complementation group as do group D and ERCC2, F and ERCC4, G and ERCC5.
[b] Some patients also have symptoms of trichothiodystrophy.
[c] Genes in the ERCC series are found in human and rodent cells, and were first identified through selection of UV-sensitive hamster cells. ERCC1 does not correspond to any XP group, but ERCC3 and XP group B are identical. There are eight or more CHO complementation groups, but the higher-numbered groups are rare and still being characterized. Relative repair in the ERCC series is classified approximately on the basis of relative sensitivity to DNA damage. We are grateful to LH Thompson for providing this summary of gene locations and group assignments.

loci are all characterized by significant increases in sensitivity to UVC or UVB radiation and include the genes associated with the following disorders: XP (approximately eight complementation groups) (7), Cockayne syndrome (CS) (approximately two complementation groups) (75, 76), trichothiodystrophy (TTD) (approximately three distinct phenotypic types) (77, 78), and basal cell nevus syndrome (BCNS) (79). Many of these genes have been defined in cell cultures as ERCC1–12 (excision repair cross complementing) (80–82).

With the exception of BCNS, all of these disorders represent increased sensitivity to UVB and UVC wavelengths due to recessive mutations. BCNS, however, exhibits a unique sensitivity to UVB wavelengths and is a dominant disorder. The recessive disorders are associated with a large family of genes that regulate human cell DNA repair. These disorders are not mutually exclusive, because CS overlaps with XP groups B, D, and G and TTD overlaps with group D. Chromosome locations are known, and the genes have been cloned for many of these loci (Table 16.2). Mutations in individual genes have pleiotropic effects on cellular sensitivity to UV light and DNA repair and are associated with a range of clinical syndromes involving skin, nervous system, and immunologic changes.

MECHANISM OF NUCLEOTIDE EXCISION REPAIR

Pyrimidine dimers and [6–4] photoproducts produced in DNA by UVC or UVB radiation are repaired by a complex multistep process involving many interacting gene products (120). In part, it is the need for interacting proteins in repair that gives rise to complex overlapping symptoms in some patients with mutations in these genes. The repair process, in principle, involves removal of a 27–29 nucleotide (nt) oligonucleotide containing the photoproduct by precisely positioned cleavages 5 nt on the 3′ side of the photoproduct, and 24 nt on the 5′ side. Once this oligonucleotide is removed, the resulting gap is filled in by DNA polymerase δ, proliferating cell nuclear antigen (PCNA), and single-strand-binding protein and ligase (43). These processes can be considered as involving sequential steps of photoproduct recognition, assembly of the excision complex, displacement of the excised fragment, and polymerization of the replacement patch.

Photoproduct recognition is achieved by specific binding of the XPA gene product, a 273-amino acid (30-kd) protein, to a photoproduct that appears to be rate-limiting for repair in human cells (83). The precise mechanism of recognition is unknown, but its greater binding coefficient for [6–4] photoproducts over dimers influences the overall rates of repair such that [6–4] photoproducts are removed much faster than dimers. Recognition may occur owing to distortions and single-strandedness in DNA from photoproducts, or the photoproducts could swing out of the DNA helix into a pocket in the protein, as occurs in some other DNA repair enzymes (84). One currently unresolved dilemma is the role of another DNA damage-binding protein in the cell, associated partially with the XPE complementation group (85). This has similar binding characteristics to the XPA protein and is present in excess, but plays a much less prominent role.

The XPA protein bound to a photoproduct acts as a site for binding two nucleases: the XPG protein that cuts 3′ to the dimer and a heterodimer of XPF and ERCC1 that cuts 5′ to the dimer (43). Interestingly, ERCC1 is a gene that is not known to be associated with a human disorder, but gene inactivation causes lethal liver failure in mice (86). This nuclease complex plus the 29–30-nt single-strand fragment is then released by the action of transcription factor TFIIH, which contains both 3′-5′ (XPB) and 5′-3′ (XPD) helicases. At least one component of TFIIH, XPB, interacts with p53 and initiates a signal cascade in damaged cells (87). This functional process requires about 100 nt of DNA along which to operate (88). This nuclease complex appears to have ready access to transcriptionally active regions of the cell, but access to nontranscribed regions requires an additional set of gene products: the XPC/HHR23B heterodimer (89, 90). PCNA, which is required for repair synthesis, also interacts with GADD45, a damage-inducible protein, which stimulates excision repair in vitro, though its in vivo function is not known (91). Many of the components of the whole excision repair machinery are the products of genes that give rise to a variety of sun-sensitive and developmental disorders. The complexity of these diseases comes not only from the specific order that gene products play in repair but also from second roles in transcription factors and signaling cascades.

XERODERMA PIGMENTOSUM

Xeroderma pigmentosum is a rare autosomal recessive disease that occurs at a frequency of about 1:250,000 in the United States (7). Affected patients (homozygotes) have sun sensitivity resulting in progressive degenerative changes of sun-exposed portions of the skin and eyes, often leading to neoplasia. Some XP patients have, in addition, progressive neurologic degeneration (119). Obligate heterozygotes (parents) are generally asymptomatic. The median age at onset is 1 to 2 years, with skin rapidly taking on the appearance of that seen in individuals with many years of sun exposure. Pigmentation is patchy, and skin shows atrophy and telangiectasia with the development of basal and squamous cell carcinomas. The frequency of cancers is 2,000 times that seen in the general population under 20 years of age, with an approximate 30-year reduction in life span.

Cells from patients with XP excise pyrimidine dimers and [6–4] photoproducts at reduced rates of 0 to 90% of normal, except for the variant group, which has near-normal rates (Table 16.3). Reduced excision is correlated with low levels of repair replication. The reductions are similar in all tissues thus far investigated, including skin in vivo, peripheral lymphocytes, fibroblasts, liver cell cultures, and tumor cells. At least seven complementation groups are known among patients who are deficient in excision repair. An eighth, the XP variant, has a defect in replication of damaged DNA (Table 16.2).

Several components of excision repair, especially the genes ERCC1 and HHR23B, have not been found among excision repair–defective complementation groups (86, 90, 92–94). Considerable genetic diversity exists within these disorders, and the capacity for excision repair correlates in many cases with the ability to survive UV irradiation. Compared with normal cells, cells from XP groups A and D are very sensitive to the lethal effects of UV light and are unable

Table 16.3. DNA Repair Characteristics of Human Cells

Phenotype	Typical cell lines	[6–4] Photoproducts repaired at 6 h (% of normal)	Incision (% of normal)	Repair synthesis (% of normal)	Cyclobutane dimer repair (% of normal)	UV resistance (% of normal)
Normal	AG1518A	100	100	100	100	100
Normal	HeLa	100	100	100	100	100
XP-A	XP12RO, XP12BE	<10	<10	<5	<5	<15
XP-A revertant	XP129	80	>80	50–90	<5	100
XP-C	XPIBE	<25	~30	<15	<10	40
XP-D	XP6BE, XP102LO	<10	15–40	25	<20	10
XP-E	XP2RO	~75		40–60	~40	70
XP variant	XP4BE, XP13BE	100	>100	70	>90	65
XP-D-like	TTD1GL	100	100	100	100	100
XP-D-like	TTD1BI	75	~50	~50	100	100
XP-D-like	TTD2GL	<25	10–40	10–40	<20	10

to excise the two major types of UV damage, the cyclobutane dimer and the [6–4] photoproduct (Table 16.3). XP group A cells also have a reduced capacity to repair the Dewar pyrimidinone, an important lesion induced with increased efficiency by UVB light (30, 95–97). XP group E cells display an intermediate phenotype, both in their UV sensitivity and in their capacity to excise UV damage, and lack a damage-specific binding protein (85, 98).

Group C is one of the largest groups and is often referred to as the common or classic form of XP. The patients show only skin disorders, which vary considerably in severity, depending on the climate. Tumors of the tongue have been observed in several patients. Cells have low but heterogeneous levels of excision repair (10–20% of normal) and are less sensitive to killing by UV light and chemical carcinogens than cells in groups A and D. One characteristic of repair unique to this group is that the reduced repair is not widespread in their genome, as it is in groups A, D, and others, but is confined to certain genomic regions (99, 100). These group C cells insert repair patches into small regions of their genome at normal rates, probably corresponding to [6–4] and cyclobutane dimer repair (99, 100), and excise thymine dimers preferentially from transcriptionally active regions (101). This raises the dilemma that high rates of cell killing, somatic mutation, and cancer from UV light in XP group C are associated with repair deficiencies in the nontranscribed regions of the genome. This in turn suggests that activating rather than silencing mutations may be important, or that mutations arise from unrepaired lesions in the nontranscribed strand of active genes.

Group E is a rare group associated with mild symptoms and residual levels of repair that are as much as 50% of normal. Some of these cells lack DNA-binding protein, but this is not seen in all cases, and the role of this protein is unclear (85).

The mechanism of UV cytotoxicity in XP variant cells does not seem to be associated with an obvious excision repair defect. These cells appear nearly normal in their ability to excise DNA damage (Table 16.3), yet show a slight but significant sensitivity to UV light. Critical regions in DNA during the S phase, such as replication forks, may be underrepaired or abnormally replicated, resulting in reduced UV resistance. The variant could, for example, be carried by mutations in a component of replication factors involved in fidelity. It is enigmatic that the genetic defect responsible for the slight reduction in UV resistance in XP variant cells is still capable of producing elevated levels of mutation and the severe clinical symptoms displayed by XP patients (7).

COCKAYNE SYNDROME

Cockayne syndrome is an autosomal recessive disease characterized by cachectic dwarfism, retinal abnormalities, microcephaly, deafness, neural defects, and retardation of growth and development after birth. Carcinomas of the skin as a result of hyperphotosensitivity are not seen in patients with CS, which sets this disease apart from XP.

Patients with CS are distributed unevenly within the complementation groups (75). Of a total of 11 patients, 2 are assigned to group A and 8 to group B. Three patients from two families are known from XP complementation group B, which also show CS symptoms (102). Symptoms of CS have also been reported in a few XPD and XPG patients. The UV sensitivity of most CS cells lies in a narrow range, with a D_{37} about half of normal, unlike XP cells, which exhibit a wide range of sensitivity. Characteristic cellular changes in CS include failure of DNA and RNA synthesis to recover to normal levels after UV irradiation (76, 103). The excision of DNA photoproducts from total genomic DNA of CS cells is normal, but repair of transcriptionally active genes is reduced (104). The CS gene products are involved in coupling excision repair to transcription, but their precise function is not yet clear.

Cockayne syndrome and XP group C therefore make an interesting contrast. CS cells repair only transcriptionally inactive genes, whereas XP group C cells repair only transcriptionally active genes. They show a similarly increased sensitivity to cell killing, indicating that all regions of the genome must be repaired for normal survival. But only XP group C shows elevated mutagenesis and carcinogenesis, indicating that defective repair of transcriptionally inactive genes is more important for these end points.

TRICHOTHIODYSTROPHY

Trichothiodystrophy is a rare autosomal recessive disorder characterized by sulfur-deficient, brittle hair, and ichthyosis. Hair shafts split longitudinally into small fibers, and this brittleness is associated with levels of cysteine or cystine in hair proteins that are 15 to 50% of those in normal individuals. The condition is also accompanied by physical and mental retardation of varying severity. The patients often have an unusual facial appearance, with protruding ears and a receding chin. Mental abilities range from low normal to severe retardation (78). Three categories of the disease can be recognized on the basis of cellular responses to UV damage: the most severe has repair deficiencies and complementation properties that place them in XP group D; intermediate cases show reduced DNA repair but normal UV sensitivity; and the third is indistinguishable in UV response from normal cells (77).

Repair profiles of three fibroblast lines derived from patients with TTD have been characterized; each displays a unique phenotype (77). One TTD cell line shows normal UV resistance and DNA repair properties; another shows an XP group D response to UV irradiation, with greatly reduced survival and repair, and is associated with mutations in the XPD gene (105, 106). Cells derived from a third patient show normal survival after UV irradiation, but the repair capacity, as evidenced by repair synthesis and repair incision, is significantly reduced. Although the excision rate of the [6–4] photoproduct in this third TTD class is slightly reduced, cyclobutane dimer repair appears normal, suggesting either that the [6–4] photoproduct is not lethal in these cells or that the observed defect in its repair is not sufficient to affect survival. Specific TTD genes (A, B) may be components of transcription factor TFIIH (53), and the symptoms of this disease indicate a role for this factor in development and hair growth.

BASAL CELL NEVUS SYNDROME

Basal cell nevus syndrome is an autosomal dominant disorder with high penetrance (>97%). The principal manifestations of this syndrome are multiple tumors (average, 50–100), primarily on sun-exposed skin, that usually appear at puberty and during the second and third decades of life (107). Other findings include palmar and plantar pitting and musculoskeletal abnormalities (scoliosis, bifurcated rib, spina bifida). The high incidence of developmental anomalies suggests that the normal allele of the BCNS gene may play a role in growth and development, in addition to accelerating sunlight-induced carcinogenesis.

The development of other tumors in BCNS, including medulloblastoma and ovarian and uterine fibromas, suggests that BCNS fits Knudson's two-mutation model for carcinogenesis (79, 107). However, the number of such mutations required to induce cancers in individuals with BCNS is unknown and could be greater than two. Nevertheless, in BCNS, one of the mutations is inherited as an autosomal dominant gene in all somatic cells, whereas the remaining mutation(s) can be induced by UV or ionizing radiation. This hypothesis is supported by the observation that presymptomatic children with BCNS who were treated with radiation for medulloblastoma developed multiple basal cell carcinomas in the area that received radiation 6 months to 3 years later.

Fibroblasts from individuals with BCNS have not shown consistent increases in sensitivity to x-rays or UVC (254-nm) radiation. They do, however, according to one report, show characteristic sensitivity to UVB, with about a fivefold reduction in the 50% survival dose (79). Although cyclobutane dimer repair is normal in these cells, excision of [6–4] photoproducts may be reduced, resembling that shown for TTD group 3 patients (108). The reduced repair of the [6–4] photoproduct may not be sufficient to affect survival after UVC irradiation. The increased sensitivity of these cells to UVB light may thus reflect an inability to excise photodamage induced with greater frequency by these wavelengths (e.g., Dewar pyrimidinones).

The dominant genetics and the lack of any sensitivity to UVC radiation make it unlikely that this disorder represents a primary deficiency in repair of the major UV photoproducts. Rather, there seems to be a specific change in some factors involved in gene expression subsequent to primary damage and repair events. In an analogy with retinoblastoma, BCNS may involve cell cycle factors and chromosome stability during progression. Alternatively, the specificity for UVB sensitivity may indicate a deficit in some products associated with melanin production or protection from UVB (22).

CARCINOGENESIS

Carcinogenesis often appears to proceed by a multi-step process, the first being an initiation event with subsequent promotional events that can often occur much later. One view of carcinogenesis would correlate initiation with the induction of somatic mutations and promotion with alterations in the expression of these mutations. Carcinogenesis appears to involve the activity of a large number of genes. These include genes for detoxifying carcinogenic chemicals, the DNA repair gene family, some 50 or more dominantly acting proto-oncogenes activated by mutation, deletion, translocation, or amplification, and tumor suppressor genes whose loss may contribute to the development of cancer (109–111).

The sequence of events seen in colorectal cancer and retinoblastoma may provide a useful model for skin carcinogenesis (110, 111). Early events may correspond to activating mutations, and various stages of tumor development occur as a result of progressive chromosome loss or conversion of heterozygosity to homozygosity. On the basis of studies with XP, early events in the skin may correspond to UV-induced mutations. Not only are major genetic defects in repair related to cancer in XP, but variations in repair among individuals also show a correlation with basal cell carcinoma. Here, however, recent studies on *ras* activation lead to a dilemma. Several investigations have led to identification of activating mutations in the Ha-*ras* and N-*ras* oncogenes at codon 61, from solar UV exposure (112–114). However, although over 75% of UV-induced mutations are cytosine-to-thymine transitions at TC or CC dimer photoproduct sites (115), Ha-*ras* and N-*ras* activation occurred in tumors at a TT site and are transversions not previously identified in model culture systems (115). Clearly, detailed investigation of oncogene activation in a number of mouse and human systems is needed to clarify the relationship between UV-induced mutations and *ras* activation. Recent studies (55, 56) have demonstrated that a large proportion of human skin tumors contain mutations in the p53 tumor suppressor gene that are caused by UV photoproducts. This demonstrates a direct causal role for UVB from sunlight in causing one of the mutagenic events in skin carcinogenesis and demonstrates that p53 mutations are early events that affect the balance of pathways of cell death versus mutation and proliferation.

Inactivation of tumor suppressor genes has been demonstrated in retinoblastoma (116), Wilms' tumor (117), and acoustic neuromas, and allelic loss resulting in conversion from heterozygosity to homozygosity appears to be a common consequence of tumor progression (111). Interestingly, chromosome 6 appears to carry a melanoma suppressor gene (118). The high levels of skin cancer in XP patients may result from increased levels of UV damage caused by defective repair, which lead to activating mutations, inactivating p53 mutations, and chromosome instability. Tumor suppressor genes could contribute to tumor advancement by incremental effects on cell growth and intercellular regulation and loss of the apototic pathway due to p53 heterozygosity (55, 56). The observation that promotion involves alterations in cell-cell communication is consistent with this interpretation. Tumor promoters may be environmental factors that mimic the effect of regulatory genes. Analysis of the various stages of skin tumor development would seem to be especially promising at this time since so many stages are accessible and the environmental causative factors are so well known.

References

1. Scotto J, Fears TR, Fraumeni JF. Incidence of nonmelanoma skin cancer in the United States. US Department of Health and Human Services, NIH Publication 83-2433, 1983.
2. Scotto J, Fraumeni JF Jr. Skin (other than melanoma). In Cancer Epidemiology and Prevention. Edited by D Schottenfeld, JF Fraumeni Jr. Philadelphia: Saunders, 1982, pp 996–1011.
3. Fitzpatrick TB, Sober AJ. Sunlight and skin cancer. N Engl J Med 1985;313:818–820.
4. Armstrong BK. Epidemiology of malignant melanoma: intermittent or total accumulated exposure to the sun? J Dermatol Surg Oncol 1988;14:835–849.
5. Trosko JE, Krause D, Isoun M. Sunlight-induced pyrimidine dimers in human cells *in vitro.* Nature 1970;228:358–359.
6. Vitaliano PP, Urbach F. The relative importance of risk factors in nonmelanoma carcinoma. Arch Dermatol 1980;116:454–456.
7. Cleaver JE, Kraemer KH. Xeroderma pigmentosum. In The Metabolic Basis of Inherited Disease, 6th ed., vol 2. Edited by CR Scriver, AL Beaudet, WS Sly, D Valle. New York: McGraw-Hill, 1989, pp 2949–2971.
8. Kripke ML. Immunological unresponsiveness induced by ultraviolet radiation. Immunol Rev 1984;80:87–102.
9. Epstein JH. Experimental models for primary melanoma. Photodermatol Photoimmunol Photomed 1992;9:91–98.
10. Kraemer KH, Lee MM, Andrews AD, Lambert WC. The role of sunlight and DNA repair in melanoma and nonmelanoma skin cancer. The xeroderma pigmentosum paradigm. Arch Dermatol 1994;130:1018–1021.
11. Serrano H, Scotto J, Shornick G, Fears TR, Greenberg ER. Incidence of nonmelanoma skin cancer in New Hampshire and Vermont. J Am Acad Dermatol 1991;24:574–579.
12. Boring CC, Squire TS, Tong T. Cancer statistics, 1993. CA 1993;43:7–26.
13. Gallagher RP, Ma D, McLean DI, Yang CP, Ho V, Carruthers JA, Warshawski LM. Trends in basal cell carcinoma, squamous carcinoma and melanoma of the skin from 1973 through 1987. J Am Acad Dermatol 1990;23:413–421.
14. Urbach F. Environmental risk factors for skin cancer. Recent Results Cancer Res 1993;128:243–262.
15. Urbach F. Man and ultraviolet radiation. In Human Exposure to Ultraviolet Radiation: Risks and Regulations. Edited by WF Passchier, BFM Boonjakovic. Amsterdam: Excerpta Medica, 1987.
16. Davies RE, Forbes PD, Urbach F. Effects of chemicals on photobiologic reactions of skin. Basic Life Sci 1990;53:127–135.
17. Robinson JK, Rademaker AW. Relative importance of prior basal cell carcinomas, containing sun exposure and circulating T lymphocytes on the development of basal cell carcinoma. J Invest Dermatol 1992;99:227–231.
18. Marks R, Staples M, Giles GG. Trends in non-melanomic skin cancer treated in Australia: the second national survey. Int J Cancer 1993;53:585–590.
19. Thompson SC. Reduction of solar keratoses by regular sunscreen use. N Engl J Med 1993;3291:1147–1151.
20. Tyrrell RM, Keyse SM. New trends in photobiology: the interaction of UVA radiation with cultured cells. J Photochem Photobiol 1990;B(4):349–361.
21. Tyrrell RM, Pidoux M. Endogenous glutathione protects human skin fibroblasts against the cytotoxic action of UVB, UVA and near-visible radiations. Photochem Photobiol 1986;44:561–564.
22. Menter JM, Willis I, Tounsel ME, Williamson GD, Moore CL. Melanin is a double-edged sword. In Photobiology: The Science and Its Applications. Edited by E Riklis. New York: Plenum 1994.
23. Jones CA, Huberman E, Cunningham ML, Peak MJ. Mutagenesis and cytotoxicity in human epithelial cells by far- and near-ultraviolet radiations: action spectra. Radiat Res 1987;110:244–254.
24. Niggli HJ, Cerutti PA. Cyclobutane-type pyrimidine photodimer formation and excision in human skin fibroblasts after irradiation with 313-nm ultraviolet light. Biochemistry 1983;22:1390–1395.
25. Peak MJ, Peak JG. Single-strand breaks induced in Bacillus subtilis DNA by ultraviolet light: action spectrum and properties. Photochem Photobiol 1982;35:675–680.
26. Tyrrell RM, Pidoux M. Action spectra for human skin cells: estimates of the relative cytotoxicity of the middle ultraviolet, near ultraviolet, and violet regions of sunlight on epidermal keratinocytes. Cancer Res 1987;47:1825–1829.
27. Pfeiffer GP, Drouin R, Riggs AD, Homquist GP. *In vivo* mapping of a DNA adduct at nucleotide resolution: detection of pyrimidine [6–4] pyrimidone photoproducts by ligation-mediated polymerase chain reaction. Proc Natl Acad Sci USA 1991;88: 1374–1378.
28. Pfeiffer GP, Drouin R, Riggs AD, Holmquist GP. Binding of transcription factors creates hot spots for UV photoproducts *in vivo.* Mol Cell Biol 1991;12:1798–1804.
29. Ellison MJ, Childs JD. Pyrimidine dimers induced in *E. coli* DNA by ultraviolet radiation present in sunlight. Photochem Photobiol 1981;34:465–469.
30. Mitchell DL, Cleaver JE. Photochemical alterations of cytosine account for most biological effects after ultraviolet irradiation. Trends Photochem Photobiol 1990;1: 107–119.
31. Taylor JS, Cohrs MP. DNA, light, and Dewar pyrimidinones: the structure and biological significance of TpT3. J Am Chem Soc 1987;109:2834–2835.
32. Gasparro FP, Fresco JR. Ultraviolet-induced 8,8-adenine dehydrodimers in oligo- and polynucleotides. Nucleic Acids Res 1986;14:4239–4251.
33. Bose SN, Kumar S, Davies RJH, Sethi SK, McCloskey JA. The photochemistry of d(T-A) in aqueous solution and in ice. Nucleic Acids Res 1984;12:7929–7947.
34. Gallagher PE, Duker NJ. Detection of UV purine photoproducts in a defined sequence of human DNA. Mol Cell Biol 1986;6:707–709.
35. Demple B, Linn S. 5,6-Saturated thymine lesions in DNA. Production by ultraviolet light or hydrogen peroxide. Nucleic Acids Res 1982;10:3781–3789.
36. Weiss RB, Gallagher PE, Brent TP, Duker NJ. Cytosine photoproduct-DNA glycosylase in *E. coli* and cultured human cells. Biochemistry 1989;28:1488–1492.
37. Elkind MM, Han A, Chiang-Liu C-M. "Sunlight"-induced mammalian cell killing. A comparative study of ultraviolet and near-ultraviolet inactivation. Photochem Photobiol 1978;27:709–715.
38. Smith PJ, Paterson MC. Abnormal responses to mid-ultraviolet light of cultured fibroblasts from patients with disorders featuring sunlight sensitivity. Cancer Res 1981;41:511–518.
39. Sterenborg HJCM, van der Leun JC. Tumorigenesis by a long wavelength UV-A source. Photochem Photobiol 1990;51:325–330.
40. Cleaver JE. Defective repair replication of DNA in xeroderma pigmentosum. Nature 1968;218:652–656.
41. Cleaver JE. Xeroderma pigmentosum: a human disease in which an initial stage of DNA repair is defective. Proc Natl Acad Sci USA 1969;63:428–435.
42. Epstein JH, Fukuyama K, Reed WB, Epstein WL. Defect in DNA synthesis in skin of patients with xeroderma pigmentosum demonstrated in vivo. Science 1970;168: 1477–1478.
43. Sancar A. Mechanisms of DNA excision repair. Science 1994;266:1954–1956.
44. Sancar A, Sancar GB. DNA repair enzymes. Annu Rev Biochem 1988;57:29–67.
45. Mitchell DL, Nairn RS. The biology of the [6–4] photoproduct. Photochem Photobiol 1989;49:805–819.
46. Cleaver JE, Jen J, Charles WC, Mitchell DL. Cyclobutane dimers and [6–4] photoproducts are mended with the same patch sizes in human cells. Photochem Photobiol 1991;54:393–402.
47. Cleaver JE. DNA damage and repair in normal, xeroderma pigmentosum and XP revertant cells analyzed by gel electrophoresis: excision of cyclobutane dimers from the whole genome is not necessary for cell survival. Carcinogenesis 1989;10: 1691–1696.
48. Freeman SE. Variations in excision repair of UVB-induced pyrimidine dimers in DNA of human skin in situ. J Invest Dermatol 1988;90:814–817.
49. Mitchell DL, Nguyen TD, Cleaver JE. Nonrandom induction of pyrimidine-pyrimidone [6–4] photoproducts in ultraviolet-irradiated human chromatin. J Biol Chem 1990;265: 5353–5356.
50. Gold JM, Smerdon MJ. UV induced [6–4] photoproducts are distributed differently than cyclobutane dimers in nucleosomes. Photochem Photobiol 1990;51:411–417.
51. Mellon I, Bohr VA, Smith CA, Hanawalt PC. Preferential DNA repair of an active gene in human cells. Proc Natl Acad Sci USA 1986;83:8878–8882.
52. Schaeffer L, Roy R, Humbert S, Moncollin V, Vermeulen W, Hoeijmakers JH, Chambon P, Egly JM. DNA repair helicase: a component of BTF2 (TFIIH) basic transcription factor. Science 1993;260:58–63.
53. Bootsma D, Hoeijmakers JH. The molecular basis of nucleotide excision repair syndromes. Mutat Res 1994;307:15–23.
54. Gao S, Drouin R, Holmquist GP. DNA repair rates mapped along the human PGK1 gene at nucleotide resolution. Science 1994;263:1438–1440.
55. Brash DE, Rudolph JA, Simon JA, Lin A, McKenna GJ, Baden HP, Halperin AJ, Ponten J. A role for sunlight in skin cancer: UV-induced p53 mutations in squamous cell carcinoma. Proc Natl Acad Sci USA 1991;88:10124.
56. Ziegler A, Jonason AS, Leffell DJ, Simon JA, Shama HW, Kimmelman J, Remington L, Jacks T, Brash DE. Sunburn and p53 in the onset of skin cancer. Nature 1994;372: 773–776.
57. Brash DE, Haseltine WA. UV-induced hotspots occur at DNA damage hotspots. Nature 1982;298:189–192.
58. Wood RD, Skopek TR, Hutchinson F. Changes in DNA base sequence induced by targeted mutagenesis of lambda phage by ultraviolet light. J Mol Biol 1984;173: 273–291.
59. Tang M-S, Hrncir J, Mitchell D, Ross J, Clarkson J. The relative cytotoxicity and mutagenicity of cyclobutane pyrimidine dimers and [6–4] photoproducts in *E. coli* cells. Mutat Res 1986;161:9–17.
60. Lebkowski JS, Clancy S, Miller JH, Calos MP. The lacI shuttle: rapid analysis of the

mutagenic specificity of ultraviolet light in human cells. Proc Natl Acad Sci USA 1985;82:8606–8610.
61. Hauser J, Seidman MM, Sidur K, Dixon K. Sequence specificity of point mutations induced during passage of a UV-irradiated shuttle vector plasmid in monkey cells. Mol Cell Biol 1986;6:277–285.
62. Glazer PM, Sarkar SN, Summers WC. Detection and analysis of UV-induced mutations in mammalian cell DNA using a lambda phage shuttle vector. Proc Natl Acad Sci USA 1986;83:1041–1044.
63. Drobetsky EA, Grosovsky AJ, Glickman BW. The specificity of UV-induced mutations at an endogenous locus in mammalian cells. Proc Natl Acad Sci USA 1987;84: 9103–9107.
64. Kress S, Sutter C, Strickland PT, Mukhtar H, Schweizer J, Schwarz M. Carcinogen-specific mutational pattern in the p53 gene in ultraviolet B radiation-induced squamous cell carcinomas of mouse skin. Cancer Res 1992;52:6400–6403.
65. Dumaz N, Drougard C, Sarasin A, Daya-Grosjean L. Specific UV-induced mutation spectrum in the p53 gene of skin tumors from DNA-repair-deficient xeroderma pigmentosum patients. Proc Natl Acad Sci USA 1993;90:10519–10533.
66. Tyrrell RM. Mutagenic action of monochromatic UV radiation in the solar range on human cells. Mutat Res 1984;129:103–110.
67. Keyse SM, Amaudruz F, Tyrrell RM. Determination of the spectrum of mutations induced by defined-wavelength solar UVB (313-nm) radiation in mammalian cells by use of a shuttle vector. Mol Cell Biol 1988;8:5425–5431.
68. Tessman I. In Abstracts of the Bacteriophage Meeting. Edited by A Bukhari, E Ljungquist. Cold Spring Harbor, NY: Cold Spring Harbor Laboratory, 1976, p 87.
69. Brash DE, Seetharam S, Kraemer KH, Seidman MM, Bredberg A. Photoproduct frequency is not the major determinant of UV base substitution hot spots or cold spots in human cells. Proc Natl Acad Sci USA 1987;84:3782–3786.
70. Protic-Sabljic M, Tuteja N, Munson PJ, Hauser J, Kraemer KH, Dixon K. UV light-induced cyclobutane pyrimidine dimers are mutagenic in mammalian cells. Mol Cell Biol 1986;6:3349–3356.
71. Tornaletti S, Rozek D, Pfeifer GP. Mapping of UV photoproducts along the human p53 gene. Ann NY Acad Sci 1994;726:324–326.
72. Tornaletti S, Pfeifer GP. Slow repair of pyrimidine dimers at p53 mutation hotspots in skin cancer. Science 1994;263:1436–1438.
73. Tornaletti S, Rozek D, Pfeifer GP. The distribution of UV photoproducts along the human p53 gene and its relation to mutations in skin cancer. Oncogene 1993;8: 2051–2057.
74. Tormanen VT, Pfeifer GP. Mapping of UV photoproducts within ras proto-oncogenes in UV irradiated cells. Correlation with mutations in human skin cancer. Oncogene 1992;7:1729–1736.
75. Lehmann AR. Three complementation groups in Cockayne syndrome. Mutat Res 1982;106:347–356.
76. Lehmann AR, Kirk-Bell S, Mayne L. Abnormal kinetics of DNA synthesis in ultraviolet light-irradiated cells from patients with Cockayne's syndrome. Cancer Res 1979;39: 4237–4241.
77. Broughton BC, Lehmann AR, Harcourt SA, Arlett CF, Sarasin A, Kleijer WJ, Beemer FA, Nairn R, Mitchell DL. Relationship between pyrimidine dimers, 6–4 photoproducts, repair synthesis and cell survival: studies using cells from patients with trichothiodystrophy. Mutat Res 1990;235:33–40.
78. Lehmann AR, Arlett CF, Broughton BC, Harcourt SA, Steingrimsdottir H, Stefanini M, Taylor AMR, Natarajan AT, Green S, King MD, Mackie RM, Stephenson JBP, Tolmie JL. Trichothiodystrophy, a human DNA repair disorder with heterogeneity in the cellular response to ultraviolet light. Cancer Res 1988;48:6090–6096.
79. Applegate LA, Goldberg LH, Ley RD, Ananthaswamy HN. Hypersensitivity of skin fibroblasts from basal cell nevus syndrome patients to killing by ultraviolet B but not by ultraviolet C radiation. Cancer Res 1990;50:637–641.
80. Busch DB, Cleaver JE, Glaser DA. Large-scale isolation of UV-sensitive clones of CHO cells. Somat Cell Genet 1980;6:407–418.
81. Busch D, Greiner C, Lewis K, Ford R, Adair G, Thompson L. Summary of complemention groups of UV-sensitive CHO cell mutants isolated by large-scale screening. Mutagenesis 1989;4:349–354.
82. Thompson LH, Rubin JS, Cleaver JE, Whitmore GF, Brookman K. A screening method for isolating DNA repair-deficient mutants of CHO cells. Somat Cell Genet 1980;6: 391–405.
83. Cleaver JE, Charles WC, McDowell ML, Mitchell DL. Overexpression of the XPA repair gene increases resistance to ultraviolet radiation in human cells. Cancer Res 1994;55:6152–6160.
84. Mol CD, Arvai AS, Shipphaug G, Kauli B, Alseth I, Krokan HE, Tarner JA. Crystal structure and mutational analysis of human uracil-DNA glycosylase: structural basis for specificity and catalysis. Cell 1995;80:869–878.
85. Patterson M, Chu G. Evidence that xeroderma pigmentosum cells from complementation group E are deficient in a homolog of yeast photolyase. Mol Cell Biol 1989;9: 5105–5112.
86. McWhir J, Selfridge J, Harrison DJ, Squires S, Melton DW. Mice with DNA repair gene (ERCC-1) deficiency have elevated levels of p53, liver nuclear abnormalities and die before weaning. Nature Genet 1993;5:217–224.
87. Greenblatt MS, Bennett WP, Hollstein M, Harris CC. Mutations in the p53 tumor suppressor gene: clues to cancer etiology and molecular pathogenesis. Cancer Res 1994;54:4855–4878.
88. Huang JC, Sancar A. Determination of minimum substrate size for human excinuclease. J Biol Chem 1994;269:19034–19044.
89. Shivji MK, Eker AP, Wood RD. DNA repair defect in xeroderma pigmentosum group C and complementing factor from HeLa cells. J Biol Chem 1994;269: 22749–22757.
90. Masutani C, Sugasawa K, Yanagisawa J, Sonoyama T, Ui M, Enomoto T, Takio K, Tanaka K, van der Spek PJ, Bootsma D, et al. Purification and cloning of a nucleotide excision repair complex involving the xeroderma pigmentosum group C protein and a human homologue of yeast RAD23. EMBO J 1994;13:1831–1843.
91. Smith ML, Chen IT, Zhan Q, Bae I, Chen CY, Gilmer TM, Kastan MB, O'Connor PM, Fornace AJ Jr. Interaction of the p53-regulated protein Gadd45 with proliferating cell nuclear antigen. Science 1994;266:1376–1380.
92. Van Duin M, de Wit J, Odijk H, Westerveld A, Yasui A, Koken MHM, Hoeijmakers JHJ, Bootsma D. Molecular characterization of the human excision repair gene ERCC-1: cDNA cloning and amino acid homology with the yeast DNA repair gene RAD10. Cell 1986;44:913–923.
93. Van Duin M, Koken MHM, van den Tol J, ten Dijke P, Odijk H, Westerveld A, Bootsma D, Hoeijmakers JHJ. Genomic characterization of the human DNA excision repair gene ERCC-1. Nucleic Acids Res 1987;15:9195–9213.
94. Van Duin M, van den Tol J, Warmerdam P, Odijk H, Meijer D, Westerveld A, Bootsma D, Hoeijmakers JHJ. Evolution and mutagenesis of the mammalian excision repair gene ERCC-1. Nucleic Acids Res 1988;16:5305–5322.
95. Mitchell DL. The induction and repair of lesions produced by the photolysis of [6–4] photoproducts in normal and UV-hypersensitive human cells. Mutat Res 1988;194: 227–237.
96. Mitchell DL, Cleaver JE, Jen J, Mullenders LH, Venema J, van Hoffen A, Simons JWIM, Zdzienicka M. The relative biological effectiveness of pyrimidine[6–4]pyrimidone photoproducts in mammalian cells. Presented at the 18th Annual Meeting of the American Society for Photobiology, Vancouver, British Columbia, June 16–20, 1990.
97. Mitchell DL, Nairn RS. The [6–4] photoproduct and human skin cancer. Photodermatol 1988;5:61–64.
98. Chu G, Chang E. Xeroderma pigmentosum group E cells lack a nuclear factor that binds to damaged DNA. Science 1988;242:564–567.
99. Cleaver JE. DNA repair in human xeroderma pigmentosum group C cells involves a different distribution of damaged sites in confluent and growing cells. Nucleic Acids Res 1986;14:8155–8165.
100. Karentz D, Cleaver JE. Excision repair in xeroderma pigmentosum group C but not group D is clustered in a small fraction of the total genome. Mutat Res 1986;165: 165–174.
101. Venema J, Van Hoffen A, Natarajan AT, van Zeeland AA, Mullenders LH. The residual repair capacity of xeroderma pigmentosum complementation group C fibroblasts is highly specific for transcriptionally active DNA. Nucleic Acids Res 1990;18: 443–448.
102. Weeda G, Reinier CA, van Ham H, Vermeulen W, Bootsma D, van der Eb AJ, Hoeijmakers JHJ. A presumed DNA helicase encoded by the excision repair gene ERCC-3 is involved in the human repair disorders xeroderma pigmentosum and Cockayne syndrome. Cell 1990;10:2570–2581.
103. Cleaver JE. Normal reconstruction of DNA supercoiling and chromatin structure in Cockayne syndrome cells during repair of damage from ultraviolet light. Am J Hum Genet 1982;34:566–575.
104. Venema J, Mullenders LHF, Natarajan AT, van Zeeland AA, Mayne LV. The genetic defect in Cockayne syndrome is associated with a defect in repair of UV-induced DNA damage in transcriptionally active DNA. Proc Natl Acad Sci USA 1990;87: 4707–4711.
105. Weber CA, Salazar EP, Stewart SA, Thompson LH. Molecular cloning and biological characterization of a human gene, ERCC2, that corrects the nucleotide excision repair defect in CHO UV5 cells. Mol Cell Biol 1988;8:1137–1146.
106. Weber CA, Salazar EP, Stewart SA, Thompson LH. ERCC2: cDNA cloning and molecular characterization of a human nucleotide excision repair gene with high homology to yeast RAD3. EMBO J 1990;9:1437–1447.
107. Gorlin RJ, Goltz RW. Multiple nevoid basal-cell epithelioma, jaw cysts and bifid rib: a syndrome. N Engl J Med 1960;262:908–912.
108. Alcalay J, Freeman SE, Goldberg LH, Wolf JE Jr. Excision repair of pyrimidine dimers induced by simulated solar radiation in the skin of patients with basal cell carcinoma. J Invest Dermatol 1990;95:506–509.
109. Sager R. Tumor suppressor genes: The puzzle and the promise. Science 1989;246: 1406–1412.
110. Stanbridge EJ. Identifying tumor suppressor genes in human colorectal cancer. Science 1990;247:12–13.
111. Vogelstein B, Fearon ER, Kern SE, Hamilton SR, Preisinger AC, Nakamura Y, White R. Allelotype of colorectal carcinomas. Science 1989;244:207–211.
112. Ananthaswamy HN, Price JE, Goldberg LH, Bales ES. Detection and identification of activated oncogenes in human skin cancers occurring on sun-exposed body sites. Cancer Res 1988;48:3341–3346.
113. Keijzer W, Mulder MP, Langeveld JC, Smit EM, Bos JL, Bootsma D, Hoeijmakers JH. Establishment and characterization of a melanoma cell line from a xeroderma pigmentosum patient: activation of N-ras at a potential pyrimidine dimer site. Cancer Res 1989;49:1229–1235.
114. Suarez HG, Daya-Grosjean L, Schlaifer D, Nardeux P, Renault G, Bos JL, Sarasin A. Activated oncogenes in human skin tumors from a repair-deficient syndrome, xeroderma pigmentosum. Cancer Res 1989;49:1223–1228.
115. Bredberg A, Kraemer KH, Seidman MM. Restricted ultraviolet mutational spectrum in a shuttle vector propagated in xeroderma pigmentosum cells. Proc Natl Acad Sci USA 1986;83:8273–8277.
116. Friend SH, Horowitz JM, Gerber MR, Wang X-F, Bogenmann E, Li FP, Weinberg RA. Deletions of a DNA sequence in retinoblastomas and mesenchymal tumors: organization of the sequence and its encoded protein. Proc Natl Acad Sci USA 1987;84: 9059–9063 [erratum Proc Natl Acad Sci USA 1988;85:2234].
117. Call KM, Glaser T, Ito CY, Buckler AJ, Pelletier J, Haber DA, Rose EA, Kral A, Yeger H, Lewis WH, Jones C, Housman DE. Isolation and characterization of a zinc finger polypeptide gene at the human chromosome 11 Wilms' tumor locus. Cell 1990;60: 509–520.
118. Trent JM, Stanbridge EJ, McBride HL, Meese EU, Casey G, Araujo DE, Witkowski CM, Nagle RB. Tumorigenicity in human melanoma cell lines controlled by introduction of human chromosome 6. Science 1990;247:568–571.
119. Kraemer KH, Lee MM, Scotto J. Xeroderma pigmentosum. Cutaneous, ocular, and neurological abnormalities in 830 published cases. Arch Dermatol 1987;123: 241–250.
120. Mitchell DL, Cleaver JE, Epstein JH. Repair of pyrimidine[6–4]-pyrimidone photoproducts in mouse skin. J Invest Dermatol 1990;95:55–59.

CHAPTER 17

Carcinogenesis from Low-Frequency Electromagnetic Fields

CESARE MALTONI AND MORANDO SOFFRITTI

Introduction

Electromagnetic fields (waves, radiation) have always been part of the natural human environment. However, their diffusion and intensity have been rapidly and greatly increasing in our century, in parallel with the growth of industrial development. Much has been known for a long time about the carcinogenic potential of short-wave/high-frequency radiation, namely the otherwise defined ionizing radiations. No scientific studies were carried out until the end of the 1970s on other electromagnetic, non-ionizing radiations.

In 1979, Wertheimer and Leeper published a case-control epidemiological study that associated extremely low-frequency electromagnetic fields (ELFEMFs) with an increase in the incidence of childhood cancer. Many well-conducted epidemiologic investigations and some laboratory studies followed up the Wertheimer and Leeper observations. They have expanded our knowledge of the carcinogenicity of ELFEMFs and have furnished cause for increasing concern about the dimensions of the carcinogenic risk from ELFEMFs and on the possible carcinogenic effects of other nonionizing radiation.

Electromagnetic Fields

GENERAL PRINCIPLES

Matter is made of particles, one of whose fundamental properties is electric charge. Electrons and protons have negative and positive charges, respectively, which are equal in magnitude. These particles seem to possess the smallest known units of electric charges.

Electrically charged particles exert forces on each other: if they are of the same sign, the force is repulsive; if they are of different signs, the force is attractive. A system of one or more electrically charged bodies produces an electric field in a given point of space.

Electric charges in physical motion produce magnetic fields. Magnetic fields, in turn, exert forces on other charges, against charges in motion. Because the most common expression of electric charge in motion is electric current, it is often said, restrictively, that magnetic fields are produced by electric currents.

Electric and magnetic fields are interrelated. However, electric fields and high-frequency magnetic fields are easily shielded by virtually all electrically conducting materials (including buildings and human bodies), whereas low-frequency magnetic fields are not. So, although interrelated, electric and magnetic fields may not be coupled. It would, therefore, be more accurate to refer to them as electric and magnetic fields instead of simply as electromagnetic fields. However, in this text, the latter terminology has been adopted because of its wide usage.

Electromagnetic fields are also defined as radiation. The term "radiation" means energy transmitted by waves. Waves are characterized by frequency and length. Frequency and length are inversely correlated. Wave frequency is expressed in hertz (Hz) (where 1 Hz corresponds to exactly one complete cycle per second) and its multiples (1,000 Hz = 1 kHz; 1,000 kHz = 1 MHz; 1,000 MHz = 1 GHz; 1,000 GHz = 1 THz; 1,000 THz = 1 PHz). Wavelength is expressed by the metric system (1,000 nm = 1 μm; 1,000 μm = 1 mm; 1,000 mm = 1 meter; 1,000 meters = 1 km).

The spectrum of electromagnetic fields, with their descriptions, sources, and characterizing effects, is presented in Table 17.1.

ELFEMFS, WITH PARTICULAR REGARD TO 50-HZ AND 60-HZ FREQUENCIES

Today, ELFEMFs are extremely diffused in the environment. They are mainly manufactured. They are generated by electric power lines and cables, industrial and domestic appliances, video display terminals, medical devices, and so on. The majority of these ELFEMFs have a 50-Hz (in Europe) or a 60-Hz (in the United States) frequency, their intensity (also intermittent) and direction (alternating) vary in time, and they induce flows of electric current in animal and human bodies.

Natural (earth) magnetic fields also have a 50–60-Hz frequency component. However, they are several orders of magnitude lower than the manufactured fields to which humans are exposed. Moreover, the main component of geomagnetic fields is static and does not induce flows of electric current in animal and human bodies.

The complete specification of a magnetic field is based on magnetic field intensity and flux density (which are almost equivalent, except in ferromagnetic materials). In the Stan-

Table 17.1. Electromagnetic Fields

Spectrum	Frequency	Wavelength	Description of band	Effects	Sources
	0 Hz		Static		Earth field magnets Direct-current (dc) supplies
			Subextremely low frequency (SELF)	Induced charge flow and molecular rotation	
Extremely low frequency	30 Hz 50 Hz 60 Hz	10,000 km 6,000 km 5,000 km	Extremely low frequency (ELF)	Induced charge flow and molecular rotation	Electric power lines and cables Domestic and industrial appliances
	300 Hz	1,000 km			
			Voice frequency (VF)	Induced charge flow and molecular rotation	Induction heaters
Radio frequency	3 kHz	100 km			
		Very low frequency (VLF)	Induced charge flow and molecular rotation	Television sets Visual display units	
	30 kHz	10 km			
			Low frequency (LF)	Induced charge flow and molecular rotation	Amplitude-modulated (AM) radio waves
	300 kHz	1 km			
			Medium frequency (MF)	Induced charge flow and molecular rotation	Induction heaters
	3 MHz	100 m			
			High frequency (HF)	Induced charge flow and molecular rotation	Radio-frequency heat sealers
	30 MHz	10 m			
			Very high frequency (VHF)	Induced charge flow and molecular rotation	Frequency-modulated (FM) radio waves
Microwave	300 MHz	1 m			
			Ultrahigh frequency (UHF)	Induced charge flow and molecular rotation	Cellular telephones, television broadcast, microwave ovens
	3 GHz	10 cm			
			Superhigh frequency (SHF)	Induced charge flow and molecular rotation	Radar Satellite links Microwave communications
	30 GHz	1 cm			
			Extra-high frequency (EHF)	Induced charge flow and molecular rotation	Point-to-point links
Infrared	300 GHz	1 mm			
				Molecular vibration	Natural Manufactured
Visible[a]	300 THz	1 μm			
				Photoactivation	Sunlight Manufactured
Ultraviolet[b]	3 PHz	100 nm			
				Covalent bond disruption	Sunlight Manufactured
X-rays	30 PHz	10 nm			
				Ionization Ionization	Manufactured Natural Manufactured
Gamma rays	3,000 PHz	0.1 nm			

[a] The wavelength range of visible radiation is 770–381 nm.
[b] The wavelength range of ultraviolet radiation is 400–200 nm.

dard International (SI) system, the magnetic field intensity is expressed in units of amperes per meter (A/m), and the flux density in teslas (T) (1 mT = 10^{-3} T; 1 μT = 1^{-3} mT). Magnetic flux density found in typical residential environments has a strength of about 0.1 μT.

Today, the diffusion of different types of electromagnetic fields is such that it is permissible to state that human beings currently live immersed in these fields.

Health problems due to ELFEMFs thus are largely, if not exclusively, related to the power industry, with all its satellite applications. More specifically, these problems mainly relate to magnetic fields, since they are not easily shielded and they are more diffuse in the environment.

The field intensity and flux intensity of the ELFEMFs depend on the flow of charge (current), which is measured in units of amperes (A). Electric charge is measured in coulombs (C). Current is simply the number of coulombs of charge that flow through a given region per second. In turn, the flow charge depends on the potential difference between opposite charges, which is expressed in units of volts (V). Magnetic field intensity and magnetic flux density decline with the distance from the source.

The dimension of manufactured ELFEMFs is expressed by the following data. In the 1980s in the United States, there were about 350,000 miles of transmission lines and about two million miles of distribution lines (26). The Computer and Business Equipment Manufacturers Association (CBEMA) calculates that the total number of personal computers in use in the United States today is over 50 million, and expects that they will increase at the rate of three million per year (3).

Carcinogenicity of ELFEMFs

BIOLOGIC DATA RELEVANT TO EVALUATION OF CARCINOGENIC RISK

Direct DNA damage from ELFEMFs has been not demonstrated. There have been reports that ELFEMF exposure may alter mRNA and protein synthesis (9, 10).

Melatonin, the principal pineal hormone, exerts a generally suppressive action on other endocrine glands. Reduced circulating concentrations of melatonin can result in increased prolactin release by the pituitary and increased estrogen and testosterone release by the gonads (29, 30). ELFEMFs have been reported to suppress melatonin production by the pineal gland (12–14, 31, 32, 46, 49). On the basis of these results it may be postulated that ELFEMFs may increase the risk of certain hormone-dependent cancers, namely, breast and prostatic carcinomas (36, 37).

EPIDEMIOLOGICAL EVIDENCE

Since the pioneering observations of Wertheimer and Leeper in 1979 (47), about 70 epidemiologic studies have been performed. These studies refer to people exposed to ELFEMFs in two different scenarios: (*a*) their dwellings were located near power-line installations, mainly high-tension electrical wires, or there were domestic sources (residential exposure); and (*b*) exposure related to their jobs and/or workplaces (occupational exposure). The studies on the risk of residential exposure deal with both children (mainly) and adults. The epidemiologic investigations include traditional case-control studies, population case-control studies, and cohort mortality studies. The epidemiological studies taken together point to the carcinogenic effect of ELFEMFs on humans.

It must be stressed, however, that the large majority of epidemiologic studies deal with the risk estimate of some specific type of neoplasia, such as leukemias (also with reference to the different types), lymphomas, neoplasms of the nervous system (with particular reference to the central nervous system, or CNS), and breast cancer in males (which, as it is infrequent, may have the value of a sentinel tumor). Only in a few instances have the epidemiologic studies considered other types of single tumors or the total number of malignancies. Therefore, at present, no studies are available on the risk estimate of all single types of neoplasms in an ELFEMF-exposed population.

The results of some of the most important epidemiologic studies on ELFEMF carcinogenic risk, following residential (of children and adults) and occupational exposure, are reported in Tables 17.2, 17.3, and 17.4. The data suggest that ELFEMFs may cause an increased risk of leukemias, lymphomas, nervous system tumors, and breast cancer in males, and also of other tumors and of total malignancies.

An increase in leukemias, in lymphomas, in tumors of the nervous system, in male breast cancer, and pituitary tumors has been found in resident children and/or in workers ex-

Table 17.2. Relevant Epidemiologic Data on Tumors Associated with Residential ELFEMF Exposure in Children

Type of study	ELFEMF source	Associated tumors	Reference
Case control	Electric power installations	Leukemias Lymphomas Nervous system tumors Other tumors	47
Case control	Electric power lines	Nervous system tumors All tumors	41
Case control	Electric power installations	Leukemias Lymphomas Brain tumors All tumors	34
Case control	Electric blanket use	Leukemias Brain tumors	33
Case control	Electric power installations	Leukemias	16
Population-based case control	Electric power lines	Leukemias	6
Population-based case control	Electric power lines	Leukemias Lymphomas Central nervous system tumors	27
Cohort	Electric power lines	Nervous system tumors (in boys)	45

Table 17.3. Relevant Epidemiologic Data on Tumors Associated with Residential ELFEMF Exposure, in Adults

Type of study	ELFEMF source	Associated tumors	Reference
Case control	Electric power installations	Lymphomas Nervous system tumors Breast cancer (females) Uterus tumors All tumors	48

Table 17.4. Relevant Epidemiologic Data on Tumors Associated with Occupational ELFEMF Exposure

Type of study	Occupation/workplace	Associated tumors	Reference
Mortality	Electrical workers	Leukemias	24
Incidence	Electrical workers	Leukemias	2
Mortality	Electrical and electronics workers	Eye cancer (largely melanoma)	39
Mortality	Electrical workers	Leukemias Non-Hodgkin's lymphomas	25
Cohort	Workers in the telecommunications industry	Melanoma	44
Cohort	Workers in the telecommunications industry	Melanoma	4
Case control	Workers employed in transportation, communication, and utilities industries	Brain tumors	35
Case control	Electrical workers	Brain tumors	17
Cohort	Several electrical jobs	Breast cancer (males)	43
Population-based case control	Several electrical jobs	Breast cancer (males)	5
Cohort	Electrical workers	Leukemias Brain tumors	42
Case control	Several electrical jobs	Leukemias Brain tumors	7
Cohort	Railway workers	Leukemias Breast cancer (males) Pituitary gland tumors	8
Population-based case control	Electrical workers	Leukemias	15
Case control	Electrical workers	Breast cancer (females)	18
Cohort case control	Electrical workers	Leukemias	40

Table 17.5. Increased Tumors Associated with Exposure to Low Flux Density of ELFEMFs[a]

Tumors	Flux density (μT)	Type of exposure	Age of exposed populations	Reference
Leukemias	≥0.2	Residential	Children	6
	≥0.4	Residential	Children	27
	4.0	Occupational	Adults	8
	0.3	Occupational	Adults	15
	≥0.2	Occupational	Adults	40
Lymphomas	≥0.4	Residential	Children	27
Nervous system tumors	≥0.4	Residential	Children	27
	≥0.4	Residential	Children	45
Male breast cancer	4.0	Occupational	Adults	8
Pituitary gland tumors	4.0	Occupational	Adults	8

[a] In this table, studies are reported in which the measurement of exposure (made in different ways) is considered adequate. There are, however, several other studies in which flux density was evaluated in a less sophisticated way, which point to the carcinogenic effect of ELFEMFs at low flux densities, that are similar to the ones listed here.

posed to ELFEMFs at the level of flux density of an order of magnitude close to that found in ordinary residential environments in industrial countries (Table 17.5).

EXPERIMENTAL ANIMAL STUDIES

Experimental animal studies on the carcinogenicity of ELFEMFs are too scanty and fragmentary, and often are inadequate, to draw definite conclusions. These studies may be divided into two categories: the first category studies the carcinogenic effects of ELFEMFs on animals not otherwise treated; the second category studies the cocarcinogenetic/promoting effects of ELFEMFs on a given anatomic site, in animals treated with chemical carcinogens that cause a known target carcinogenic effect at that site.

The main results of experimental animal studies may be summarized as follows. ELFEMFs seem to cause: (*a*) an increased incidence in malignant lymphomas and leukemias in untreated mice (23, 28) and an increased incidence of mammary tumors in rats (1); (*b*) an increase in the incidence and a decrease in the latency period, or a trend of more rapid development, of skin tumors in mice induced by 7, 12-dimethylbenz(a)anthracene (DMBA) and 12-0-tetradecanoylphorbol-13-acetate (TPA) (21, 38); and (*c*) an increase in the incidence and/or a decrease in the latency period of mammary tumors induced in rats by chemical carcinogens (DMBA and nitrosomethyl urea) (1, 19–22). However, all of these results, because of the protocol limitations of the experiments, need further confirmation.

At present, there are no experimental animal studies that may fully assess the carcinogenic potential of ELFEMFs in qualitative (types of tumor produced) and quantitative terms, also in relation to a ranking of flux intensities (including that to which humans may more often be exposed). At this time, two large, and to some extent integrated, experimental bioassays on male and female rats and mice are planned to study the carcinogenic effects of ELFEMFs of intensities ranging from 1,000 to 1 μT: one at the Cancer Research

Center of the European Ramazzini Foundation (Italy) on 5,400 Sprague-Dawley rats, and one in the framework of the U.S. National Toxicology Program (NTP) on 1,000 B6C3F1 mice and 1,000 Fisher 344 rats.

CONCLUSION

The results of the epidemiologic investigations (mainly) together with the available data from experimental carcinogenicity studies and from some basic biologic research (to a much more limited extent) converge in indicating that ELFEMFs must be considered a potential carcinogenic risk for humans. The mechanisms by which ELFEMFs exert their carcinogenetic effects are at present largely a matter of hypothesis and need-oriented research.

Perspectives

The available information suggests that ELFEMFs may cause cancer. Much research (epidemiology, animal bioassays, mechanistic studies, basic biology), however, remains to be done in order to assess the full carcinogenic potential of ELFEMFs and to evaluate, in quantitative terms, the level of risk of ELFEMF intensities of the order of magnitude to which humans are currently being exposed. Given their diffusion in the present historical scenario, ELFEMFs represent one of the priority issues of environmental and occupational carcinogenesis.

Our knowledge of the carcinogenicity of ELFEMFs leads to a wider concern about possibly similar effects of nonionizing electromagnetic radiations other than ELFEMFs. Some early experimental information, although very preliminary, has substantiated these concerns. In a long-term experimental bioassay, it was found that in male Sprague-Dawley rats, ultrahigh-frequency (namely, pulsed 2.450-GHz) radiation causes an increased incidence of pheochromocytomas of the adrenal medulla, a higher incidence of malignant tumors of the endocrine and exocrine glands, and an increased incidence of carcinomas alone and combined carcinomas and sarcomas at all sites (11).

References

1. Beniashvili DS, Bilanishvili VG, Menabde MZ. Low frequency electromagnetic radiation enhances the induction of rat mammary tumors by nitrosomethyl urea. Cancer Lett 1991;61:75.
2. Coleman M, Bell J, Skeet R. Leukaemia incidence in electrical workers. Lancet 1983;1:982.
3. Computer and Business Equipment Manufacturers Association (CBEMA): Computer and Business Equipment Marketing and Forecasting Databook. Hasbrouck Heights NJ, Hayden Books, 1985.
4. De Guire L, Thériault G, Iturra H, Provencher S, Cyr D, Case BW. Increased incidence of malignant melanoma of the skin in workers in a telecommunications industry. Br J Industr Med 1988;45:824.
5. Demers PA, Thomas DB, Rosenblatt KA, Jimenez LM, McTiernan A, Stalsberg H, Stemhagen A, Thompson WD, McCrea Curnen MG, Satariano W, Austin DF, Isacson P, Greenberg RS, Key C, Kolonel LN, West DW. Occupational exposure to electromagnetic fields and breast cancer in men. Am J Epidemiol 1991;134:340.
6. Feychting M, Ahlbom A. Magnetic fields and cancer in children residing near Swedish high-voltage power lines. Am J Epidemiol 1993;138:467.
7. Floderus B, Persson T, Stenlund C, Wennberg A, Öst Å, Knave B. Occupational exposure to electromagnetic fields in relation to leukemia and brain tumors: a case-control study in Sweden. Cancer Causes Control 1993;4:465.
8. Floderus B, Törnqvist S, Stenlund C. Incidence of selected cancers in Swedish railway workers 1961–79. Cancer Causes Control 1994;5:189.
9. Goodman R, Bassett CAL, Henderson AS. Pulsing electromagnetic fields induce cellular transcription. Science 1983;220:1283.
10. Goodman R, Shirley-Henderson A. Exposure of cells to extremely low frequency electromagnetic fields: relationship to malignancy? Cancer Cells 1990;2:355.
11. Guy AW, Chou CK, Kunz LL, Crowley J, Krupp J. Effects of Long-Term, Low-Level Radiofrequency Radiation Exposure on Rats, vol 9. Summary. Seattle: University of Washington, USAFSAM-TR-85-64, August 1985.
12. Kato M, Honma K, Shigemitsu T, Shiga Y. Effects of exposure to a circularly polarized 40-Hz magnetic field on plasma and pineal melatonin levels in rats. Bioelectromagnetics 1993;14:97.
13. Lerchl A, Nonaka KO, Reiter, RJ: Pineal gland: its apparent magnetosensitivity to static magnetic fields is a consequence of induced electric currents (eddy currents). J Pineal Res 1991;10:109.
14. Lerchl A, Nonaka KO, Stokkan KA, Reiter RJ. Marked rapid alterations in nocturnal pineal serotonin metabolism in mice and rats exposed to weak intermittent magnetic fields. Biochem Biophys Res Comm 1990;169:102.
15. London SJ, Bowman JD, Sobel E, Thomas DC, Garabrant DH, Pearce N, Bernstein L, Peters JM. Exposure to magnetic fields among electrical workers in relation to leukemia risk in Los Angeles County. Am J Industr Med 1994;26:47.
16. London SJ, Thomas DC, Bowman JD, Sobel E, Cheng TC, Peters JM. Exposure to residential electric and magnetic fields and risk of childhood leukemia. Am J Epidemiol 1991;134:923.
17. Loomis DP, Savitz DA. Mortality from brain cancer and leukaemia among electrical workers. Br J Industr Med 1990;47:633.
18. Loomis DP, Savitz DA, Ananth CV. Breast cancer mortality among female electrical workers in the United States. JNCI 1994;86:921.
19. Löscher W, Mevissen M, Lehmacher W, Stamm A. Tumor promotion in a breast cancer model by exposure to a weak alternating magnetic field. Cancer Lett 1993;71:75.
20. Löscher W, Wahnschaffe U, Mevissen M, Lerchl A, Stamm A. Effects of weak alternating magnetic fields on nocturnal melatonin production and mammary carcinogenesis in rats. Oncology 1994;51:288.
21. McLean JRN, Stuchly MA, Mitchel REJ, Wilkinson D, Yang H, Goddard M, Lecuyer DW, Schunk M, Callary E, Morrison D. Cancer promotion in a mouse-skin model by a 60-Hz magnetic field: II. Tumor development and immune response. Bioelectromagnetics 1991;12:273.
22. Mevissen M, Stamm A, Buntenkötter S, Zwingelberg R, Wahnschaffe U, Löscher W. Effects of magnetic fields on mammary tumor development induced by 7,12-Dimethylbenz(a)anthracene in rats. Bioelectromagnetics 1993;14:131.
23. Mikhail EL, Fam WZ. Development of lymphoma in third-generation mice exposed to 60-Hz magnetic field. In Abstracts of the Bioelectromagnetic Society, 13th annual meeting, Salt Lake City, UT, 1991, p 24.
24. Milham S. Mortality from leukemia in workers exposed to electrical and magnetic fields. N Engl J Med 1982;307:249.
25. Milham S. Mortality in workers exposed to electromagnetic fields. Environ Health Persp 1985;62:297.
26. Minner, D. The top 100 utilities' 1986 operating performance. Elec Light Power, August 1987.
27. Olsen JH, Nielsen A, Schulgen G. Residence near high voltage facilities and risk of cancer in children. Br Med J 1993;307:891.
28. Rannung A, Ekström T, Hansson Mild K, Holmberg B, Gimenez-Conti J, Slaga TJ. A study on skin tumour in mice with 50 Hz magnetic field exposure. Carcinogenesis 1993;14:573.
29. Reiter RJ (ed). The Pineal Gland, vols 1–3. Boca Raton, FL: CRC, 1981.
30. Reiter RJ. Effects of light and stress on pineal function. In Extremely Low Frequency Electromagnetic Fields: the Question of Cancer. Edited by BW Wilson, RG Stevens, LE Anderson. Columbus OH: Battelle Press, 1990, p 87.
31. Reiter RJ, Anderson LE, Buschbom RL, Wilson BW. Reduction of the nocturnal rise in pineal melatonin levels in rats exposed to 60-Hz electric fields in utero and for 23 days after birth. Life Sci 1988;42:2203.
32. Reuss S, Olcese J. Magnetic field effects on the rat pineal gland: role of retinal activation by light. Neurosci Lett 1986;64:97.
33. Savitz DA, John EM, Kleckner RC. Magnetic field exposure from electric appliances and childhood cancer. Am J Epidemiol 1990;131:763.
34. Savitz DA, Wachtel H, Barnes FA, John EM, Tvrdik JG. Case-control study of childhood cancer and exposure to 60-Hz magnetic fields. Am J Epidemiol 1988;128:21.
35. Speers MA, Dobbins JG, Miller VS. Occupational exposures and brain cancer mortality: a preliminary study of East Texas residents. Am J Industr Med 1988;13:629.
36. Stevens RG. Review and Commentary: electric power use and breast cancer: a hypothesis. Am J Epidemiol 1987;125:556.
37. Stevens RG. Electric power, melatonin, and breast cancer. In The Pineal Gland and Cancer. Edited by D Gupta, A Attanasio, RJ Reiter. London: Brain Research Promotion, 1988, p 233.
38. Stuchly MA, McLean JRN, Burnett R, Goddard M, Lecuyer DW, Mitchel REJ. Modification of tumor promotion in the mouse skin by exposure to an alternating magnetic field. Cancer Lett 1992;65:1.
39. Swerdlow AJ. Epidemiology of eye cancer in adults in England and Wales 1962–1977. Am J Epidemiol 1983;118:294.
40. Thériault G, Goldberg M, Miller AB, Armstrong B, Guenel P, Deadman J, Imberman E, To T, Chevalier A, Cyr D, Wall C. Cancer risk associated with occupational exposure to magnetic fields among electric utility workers in Ontario and Quebec, Canada, and France: 1970–1989. Am J Epidemiol 1994;139:550.
41. Tomenius L. 50-Hz electromagnetic environment and the incidence of childhood tumors in Stockholm County. Bioelectromagnetics 1986;7:191.
42. Törnqvist S, Knave B, Ahlbom A, Persson T. Incidence of leukaemia and brain tumours in some "electrical occupations." Br J Industr Med 1991;48:597.
43. Tynes T, Andersen A. Electromagnetic fields and male breast cancer. Lancet 1990;336:1596.
44. Vagero D, Ahlbom A, Olin R, Sahlsten S. Cancer morbidity among workers in the telecommunications industry. Br J Industr Med 1985;42:191.
45. Verkasalo PK, Pukkala E, Hongisto MY, Valjus JE, Järvinen PJ, Heikkilä KV, Koskenvuo M. Risk of cancer in Finnish children living close to power lines. Br Med J 1993;307:895.
46. Welker HA, Semm P, Willing RP, Commentz JC, Wiltschko W, Vollrath L. Effects of an artificial magnetic field on serotonin N-acetyltransferase activity and melatonin content of the rat pineal gland. Exp Brain Res 1983;50:426.
47. Wertheimer N, Leeper E. Electrical wiring configurations and childhood cancer. Am J Epidemiol 1979;109:273.
48. Wertheimer N, Leeper E. Adult cancer related to electrical wires near the home. Int J Epidemiol 1982;11:345.
49. Wilson BW, Anderson LE, Hilton DI, Phillips RD. Chronic exposure to 60-Hz electric fields: effects on pineal function in the rat. Bioelectromagnetics 1981;2:371; 1983;4:293.

CHAPTER 18

Physical Carcinogens

CESARE MALTONI AND FRANCO MINARDI

Introduction

Broadly, the term "physical carcinogens" includes a wide range of agents: electromagnetic radiations of different kinds, corpuscular (alpha and beta) radiations, low and high temperatures, mechanical traumas, and solid and gel materials. More restrictively, however, the term is currently used to define solid and gel materials, water insoluble or slightly soluble, that are capable of producing cancer. This meaning will be used in this chapter, although "solid and gel carcinogens" would be a more precise term. Both "physical carcinogens" and "solid carcinogens" are terms that have been widely used in an overly simplified manner to identify agents that produce cancer mainly if not exclusively through their physical properties and physical effects, rather than through their chemical properties and actions, as opposed to what are commonly called chemical carcinogens. Physical carcinogens include hard and soft materials, fibrous particles, nonfibrous particles, and gel materials.

The first scientific demonstration of the carcinogenic capacity of the physical agents was made by Turner, who found that Bakelite disks, implanted in rats, provoked local fibrosarcomas (43). Anecdotal cases of tumors that arose around foreign bodies (including bullets, in wartime) had been reported earlier.

The identification of physical carcinogens is based on epidemiologic and/or experimental data. The extrapolation of experimental results to humans is improved by the use of experimental models as closely equivalent to human situations as possible. The following examples illustrate this concept. Intratissue inserts of metallic alloys or plastics may well reproduce the situations in which allogenic prostheses are implanted surgically in the human body; conversely, the inhalation of particulate materials may correctly reproduce the exposure of laborers working in a dusty occupational environment. In the preamble to the Annual Reports of the U.S. National Toxicology Program (NTP), it is stated that (*a*) *known carcinogens* are "those substances for which there is sufficient evidence of carcinogenicity from studies in humans to indicate a causal relationship between the agent and human cancer," and (*b*) *substances reasonably anticipated to be carcinogens to humans* are "those substances for which there is limited evidence of carcinogenicity in humans and/or sufficient evidence of carcinogenicity in experimental animals (10).

Known Physical Carcinogens

HARD AND SOFT MATERIALS

The category of hard and soft materials includes metals and metallic alloys, synthetic products, and natural materials in the form of disks, squares, films, and foams. The studies performed in this field are nearly exclusively experimental, and the majority have been conducted on rats and have entailed intratissue implantations, mainly into the subcutaneous tissues, less frequently into other sites. The experiments of Oppenheimer and colleagues and of Nothdurft using squares and disks of metal and plastic are classic (33–36). For other studies see Hueper (11), Maltoni and Sinibaldi (28), and Maltoni et al. (29).

The most relevant available experimental data on the carcinogenicity of these materials are presented in Table 18.1. The observed tumors arise around implants and are sarcomas of different types: fibrosarcomas (Fig. 18.1), rhabdomyosarcomas (Fig. 18.2), and osteosarcomas.

Studies on the sequence of changes taking place at the site of implants, to reconstruct the histogenesis of sarcomas have shown that the implanted material induces a fibrous reaction that apparently remains unchanged for several months and may even undergo hyalinization. After several months the cells in the more internal layer of the fibrous capsule, those in direct contact with the implanted material, may start to proliferate (Fig. 18.3) and then evolve to sarcoma formation. These changes and the sequence in which they occur are independent of the nature of the implanted material (27).

Various investigators have shown that intact films of certain polymers have more potent carcinogenic effects than perforated films of the same polymer and the same shape; in fact, films are considerably more potent than powdered films. Other investigators, studying a different material, have been unable to confirm such a specific relationship between physical form and carcinogenesis. Testing vitallium in the form of intact disks, holed disks of the same diameter and thickness, and fragments (in an amount equivalent to the weight of the intact disks) confirmed the fragmentation effect but not that of holing: holed disks proved to be as carcinogenic as intact disks (Table 18.2) (29).

Surgical prostheses of metals, metallic alloys, and polymers are widely used today. To date, only a few isolated cases of human sarcomas developing around surgical implants of metal and plastic have been reported in the literature (28, 29). More information on the potential carcinogenic

Table 18.1. Hard and Soft Materials, of Different Shape and Dimension, Found to Be Carcinogenic When Implanted into Rodents

- Metals
  - Gold
  - Platinum
  - Silver
  - Steel
  - Tantalum
  - Metallic alloys
  - Vitallium (chromium, cobalt, molybdenum)
- Water-insoluble polymers
  - Hydrocarbon polymers (synthetic)
    - Polyethylene (Polythene)
    - Polymethylmethacrylate (Lucite)
    - Polyvinylbenzol (Polystyrol)
    - Cross-linked polyvinyl alcohol (Ivalon)
    - Polyester condensate of terephthalate and ethylene glycol (Dacron)
    - Phenol-formaldehyde condensate (Bakelite)
  - Halogenated hydrocarbon polymers (synthetic)
    - Polyvinyl chloride (PVC, Igelit, Vestolit, Vinnol)
    - Polyvinylidene chloride (Saran)
    - Polyfluor(chlor)-olefine (Teflon)
    - Polymethylmethacrylate chloride (Pliofilm)
    - Copolymer of vinyl chloride and acrylonitrile (Vinyon N, Dynel)
  - Aminized hydrocarbon polymers (polyamides) (synthetic)
    - Polyhexamethylene diamine adipanide (nylon)
    - Poly-e-caprolactam, polyurethane (Perlon)
  - Hydrocarbon polymers (semisynthetic and natural)
    - Processed latex gum (rubber)
    - Processed polyglucose (cellulose) (cellophane)
    - Processed cellulose (linen, parchment paper)
  - Natural organic materials (silk, keratin, ivory)
  - Silicon polymers (synthetic)
    - Processed polydimethylsiloxanes (silicone rubber) (Silastic)
- Mixture of different siloxanes (silicone gel for prostheses)

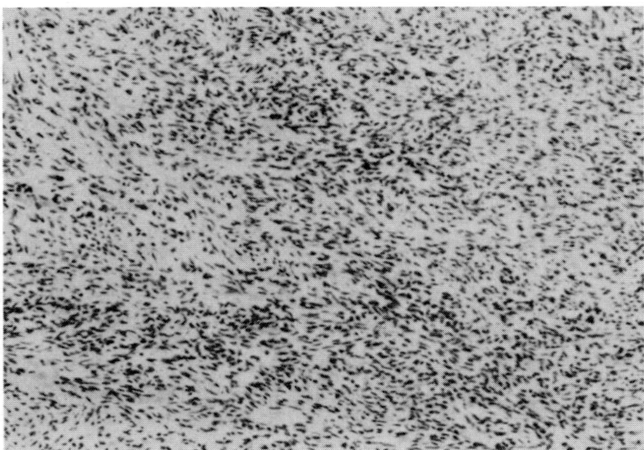

Figure 18.1. Fibrosarcoma around an implanted, holed disk of vitallium in a female Sprague-Dawley rat (hematoxylin-eosin, ×200).

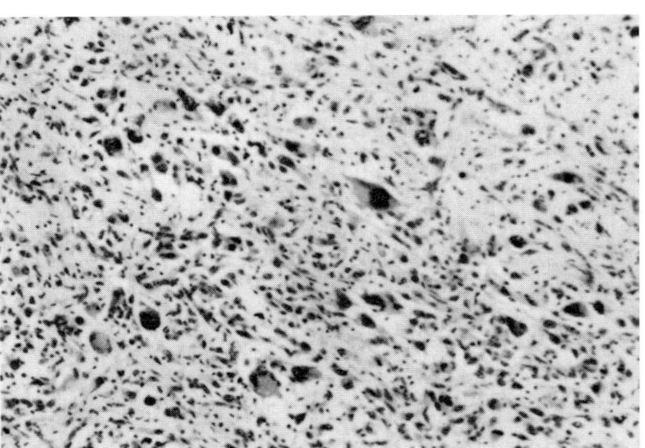

Figure 18.2. Rhabdomyosarcoma around an implanted, intact disk of vitallium in a female Sprague-Dawley rat (hematoxylin-eosin, ×200).

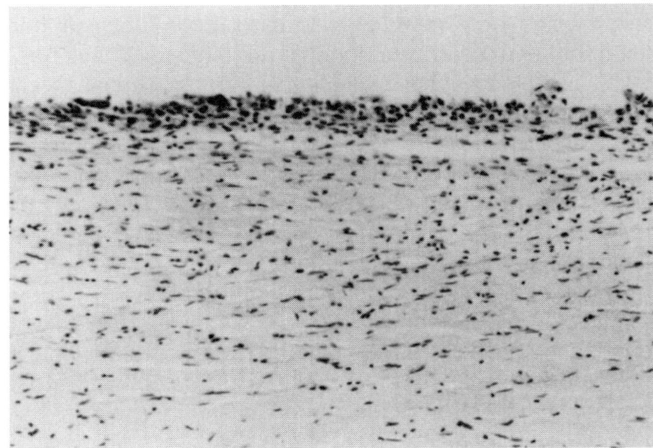

Figure 18.3. Cellular proliferation, in a fibrous capsule formed around an implant of an intact disk of vitallium, at the edge of the cavity containing the implant and therefore in direct contact with the implanted material, 15 months after the implant, in a male Sprague-Dawley rat (hematoxylin-eosin, ×200).

Table 18.2. Results of Long-term Carcinogenicity Bioassays of Vitallium, in Different Forms, Implanted into Subcutaneous Tissues of Sprague-Dawley Rats

Treatment	No. of animals	No. of animals in which sarcomas developed at site of implantation
Intact disks	30	13
Perforated disks	30	15
Fragments	30	2
None (controls)	30	0

From Maltoni et al. (29). Reproduced by permission.

risks of surgically implanted hard and soft materials could be provided by programmed long-term follow-up of patients with implants.

FIBERS

The category of fibers includes natural mineral fibers and man-made mineral fibers. The carcinogenicity of these materials has been investigated in epidemiologic and experimental studies.

Asbestos

Among the fibrous materials, asbestos has attracted the most attention because of its industrial and commercial relevance (about 3,000 uses), because of its diffusion in the occupational and general environment, and because of the early detection of its pathogenicity and carcinogenicity. Six fibrous silicates are currently characterized as asbestos: the fibrous serpentine mineral chrysotile (white asbestos) and the amphiboles actinolite, amosite, anthophyllite, crocidolite (blue asbestos), and tremolite. The most commercially important minerals of asbestos are chrysotile, amosite, and crocidolite. Chrysotile is produced in the largest amounts and is the most widely used and diffused into the environment. In the past few decades asbestos has been mined at the rate of 3 to 8 million tons per year worldwide. Asbestos is mainly used in buildings, pipes, the paper industry, maritime and railway carriers, and the clutch and brake industry. Its wide use for insulation is the major cause of environmental and occupational exposure.

Because of its great production, widespread and numerous uses, and its practical indestructibility, asbestos may be considered ubiquitous. It is present in workplaces, the general environment, and the domestic environment, where it is introduced by exposed workers who carry it on their clothes and in their hair. It is found in air, and traces of the mineral have been detected in water (including drinking water), in foods and drugs, and in a variety of consumer products. The following worker categories must be considered exposed: miners and millers of the mineral; manufacturers of asbestos products; laborers who repair, maintain, and clean structures and materials containing asbestos and those who handle waste made of or contaminated with asbestos; and workers and citizens operating in or living in an environment polluted by asbestos fibers.

Table 18.3. Tumors Related to Asbestos Exposure in Humans and Experimental Animals

Cancer type	In humans	In experimental animals
Lung cancer	+	+
Pleural mesothelioma	+	+
Peritoneal mesothelioma	+	+
Other-site mesothelioma and possibly sarcoma	+	+ (Possibly sarcomas)
Pharyngolaryngeal cancer	+	
Gastrointestinal cancer	+	
Kidney cancer	+	

The possible association between asbestos and cancer was suspected for the first time in 1935. In that year Lynch and Smith described a lung carcinoma in a patient with asbestosis (fibrosis of the lung due to the inhalation of asbestos dust) (18). The carcinogenic effect of asbestos fibers of different types on various tissues and organs, both in humans and in experimental animals, is now definitively established by a large number of clinical, epidemiologic, and experimental studies. Several comprehensive reviews on asbestos carcinogenicity are available (13, 16, 17, 38).

The major route of exposure in humans is inhalation. In animals (mainly rats, but also mice and hamsters), asbestos has been tested by inhalation; by intraperitoneal, intrapleural, and subcutaneous injection; and by ingestion. The tumors observed after an exposure to asbestos fibers in humans and experimental animals are listed in Table 18.3. Mesothelioma in different sites (mainly the pleura and peritoneum) is the tumor most specifically connected to asbestos, both in humans and in animals (Figs. 18.4 and 18.5).

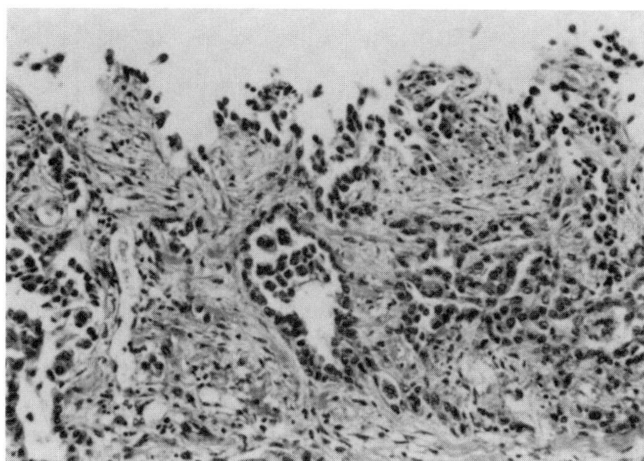

Figure 18.4. Tubular epitheliomorphic mesothelioma of the pleura in an Italian railroad machinist (hematoxylin-eosin, ×200).

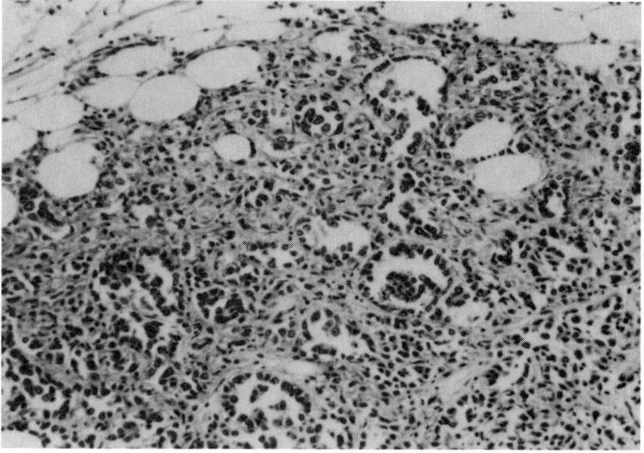

Figure 18.5. Tubular epitheliomorphic mesothelioma of the peritoneum of a male Sprague-Dawley rat injected once with 25 mg of Canadian chrysotile in 1 ml of H_2O (hematoxylin-eosin, ×200).

Table 18.4. 130 Cases of Mesothelioma in Italy due to Asbestos Used in Railroads: Distribution According to Category of Population Exposed and Site of Neoplasia

Category of population exposed	No. of cases of mesothelioma				
	Pleural	Pericardial	Peritoneal	Pleuroperitoneal	Total
Asbestos exposure due to job assignments					
Workers of the FS,[a] especially machinists	74	1	1	1	77
Rolling-stock machinists and workers engaged in the repair and demolition of the rails, of workshops not belonging to the FS	40	0	5	0	45
Subtotal	114	1	6	1	122
Asbestos exposure due to workplace pollution					
Personnel working on rolling stock, not employed by the FS	3	0	0	0	3
Asbestos exposure due to family contact					
Family members of exposed workers of the FS and of workshops not belonging to the FS	5	0	0	0	5
Total	122	1	6	1	130

[a] FS, Ferrovie dello Stato (Italian State Railroads).
From Maltoni et al. (23). Reproduced by permission.

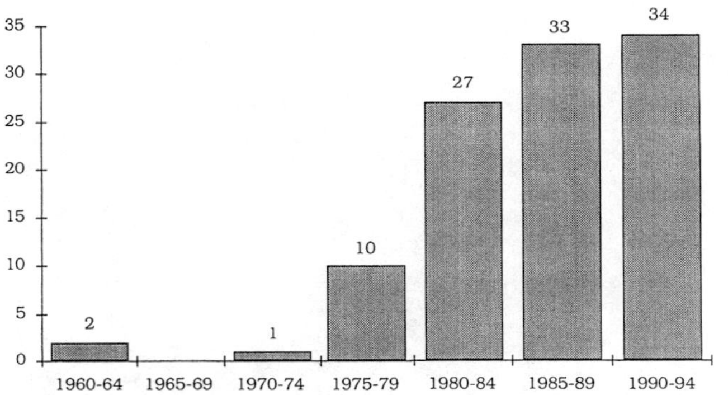

Figure 18.6. Mortality distribution by 5-year periods of 107 cases of mesothelioma in Italy following exposure to asbestos used in railroads. Note the progressive increase in mortality.

Table 18.5. 12 Cases of Mesothelioma in Italy due to Asbestos Used in Sugar Refinery Plants: Distribution According to Category of Population Exposed and Site of Neoplasia

Category of population exposed	No. of cases of mesothelioma		
	Pleural	Peritoneal	Total
Asbestos exposure due to job assignments	10	1	11
Asbestos exposure due to family contact	1	0	1
Total	11	1	12

From Maltoni et al. (26). Reproduced by permission.

Mesotheliomas in humans have been found after occupational, environmental, and family exposure.

The latency time of asbestos-correlated tumors is long. In general, tumors start to appear 20 years after the start of exposure. In people exposed to asbestos, lung carcinomas and mesotheliomas may be preceded by or associated with lung fibrosis and pleural plaques. These changes are markers of asbestos exposure, but a possible role in the natural history of these tumors has not been proved and, in fact, has been denied by several investigators.

The number of occupational groups at risk of asbestos-correlated cancer has been growing, and the incidence of asbestos-correlated tumors in some occupational categories has also been increasing in recent years. Clear examples of new risk groups whose frequency of asbestos-correlated tumors is increasing are the workers exposed to asbestos used in the railroads (Table 18.4 and Fig. 18.6) (22–24), in whom mortality due to mesothelioma is high, and sugar refinery workers exposed to the asbestos used in those factories as a heat insulator (Table 18.5) (25, 26). In consideration of the extent of the railroad network worldwide, there are good reasons to anticipate that asbestos-correlated cancer among railroad workers may become one of the most dramatic international occupational diseases.

Also increasing are the reports of asbestos mesotheliomas due to family contact (see, for example, Tables 18.4 and 18.5). Mesotheliomas due to environmental asbestos pollution may become a major problem. Three cases of mesothelioma have been recently reported in housekeepers whose houses or neighboring buildings had roofs of corrugated asbestos cement (3), which has been shown to deteriorate under atmospheric corrosion and to release asbestos fibers.

In experimental systems, the various asbestos minerals (including the serpentine chrysotile) show a similar carcinogenic potency (Table 18.6). There is evidence that each of the major non-neoplastic and neoplastic diseases associated with asbestos in humans can be produced by all of the different forms of the mineral, the amphiboles as well as the serpentine (chrysotile) (4).

The diffusion of asbestos minerals in the environment, the number of people exposed, and the high degree of carcino-

Table 18.6. Results of Long-term Carcinogenicity Bioassays on Sprague-Dawley Rats Injected Into the Peritoneal Cavity with Various Asbestos Minerals

Test material	No. of animals	No. of animals bearing peritoneal mesotheliomas
Amosite	40	36
Anthophyllite	40	33
Chrysotile (California)	40	29
Chrysotile (Canada)	40	32
Chrysotile (Rhodesia)	40	33
Crocidolite	40	39
H_2O (controls)	150	0

A single injection of 25 mg in H_2O was used.
From Maltoni and Minardi (20). Reproduced by permission.

genicity of these materials make asbestos carcinogenicity a major worldwide problem of public health.

Erionite

Erionite is a fibrous zeolite whose fibers are similar in dimension to asbestos fibers, although they are probably shorter on average. Zeolites are crystalline aluminosilicates, in which the primary building blocks are tetrahedra consisting of either silicon or aluminum atoms surrounded by four oxygen atoms. These tetrahedra combine, linked together by oxygen bridges and cations, to yield an ordered three-dimensional framework. Although there are more than 30 known natural zeolites, only four are fibrous—chabazite, clinoptilolite, erionite, and mordenite. Zeolite minerals are found as major constituents in numerous sedimentary volcanic tuffs, especially where these were deposited and have been altered by saline lake water. Many hundreds of occurrences have been recorded of zeolite deposits in over 40 countries.

Natural zeolites have many commercial uses, most of which are based on the ability of these minerals to adsorb molecules from air or liquids selectively. One such use of erionite has been documented. The exposure of humans can be occupational or environmental.

An excess of mortality due to pleural and peritoneal mesotheliomas, both in males and in females, has been reported in three remote Anatolian villages in the same area where erionite occurs. In two of these villages, the lung cancer rate also appeared to be excessive. The high rates of mesothelioma and lung cancer have been attributed to the presence of erionite in the soil, road dust, and building stones of the villages (2, 15). Asbestos is not more common in erionite villages than in control villages, where the excess of mesothelioma was not found.

It is significant that the registered increase in mesotheliomas in Sweden is partly due to cases of this neoplasia in Turkish migrant workers, who were probably exposed to erionite at an early age in their country of origin (31).

The hypothesis that erionite is the causative agent of the mesotheliomas in the Turkish workers, and therefore that it is a human carcinogen, has been supported by experimental evidence. Following inhalation exposure and intraperitoneal and intrapleural injection, erionite causes the onset of peritoneal and pleural mesotheliomas in rats and mice (15, 19–21). In rats, erionite has been shown to be the most powerful mesotheliomatogenic agent for the pleura (Table 18.7).

Table 18.7. Comparative Mesotheliomatogenic Effects on Rat Pleura of Erionite and Asbestos (Crocidolite and Chrysotile) Following Injection into the Pleural Cavity

Material	No. of animals	Animals bearing pleural mesotheliomas
Erionite	40	35
Crocidolite	40	18
Chrysotile (Canada)	40	26
H_2O (controls)	150	0

A single injection of 25 mg in H_2O was used.
From Maltoni and Minardi (20). Reproduced by permission.

The demonstration of the carcinogenic effect of erionite is also of particular relevance in light of the large amount and diffusion of natural fibrous and nonfibrous zeolites, their widespread industrial uses, which are expected to increase, and the production of man-made zeolites for several industrial applications (as detergents, and as catalysts in the petrochemical and refining industries). A systematic and integrated project of long-term carcinogenicity bioassays of natural and man-made fibrous and nonfibrous zeolites was begun several years ago at the Bologna Institute of Oncology, and the experimental data are now being processed.

Other Natural and Man-Made Mineral Fibers

Other fibers include, among the natural fibers, wollastonite (a fibrous silicate), attapulgite (a fibrous silicate), and the asbestiform fibers present in commercial talc; and among the man-made fibers, glass wool, rock wool, and slag wool (produced by blowing, centrifuging, and drawing molten rock or slag) and ceramic fibers.

Data on the carcinogenicity of natural and man-made fibers are of great public health interest because of the various industrial uses (the large majority as asbestos substitutes) of these fibers. At present more than 5 million tons of man-made mineral fibers are produced annually in more than 100 factories located throught the world. Glass fiber products account for more than 50% of the total.

Most of the carcinogenicity data come from experimental studies: only limited data are available from epidemiologic investigations. The experimental bioassays on carcinogenicity have been performed on rodents (mostly rats, but also mice and hamsters) in which the materials were administered by inhalation or (mainly) by intrapleural and intraperitoneal injection or implantation. The data on the carcinogenicity of these fibers have been extensively reviewed (12, 14–16). Results of the epidemiologic and experimental studies are shown in Table 18.8.

Fibrous glass (glass wool) carcinogenicity deserves some comments. This material was and is the most widely used substitute for asbestos. Yet, on the basis of the available information, both experimental and epidemiologic, glass wool should be reasonably anticipated to be carcinogenic for humans. As one group of investigators noted, "At least 13 stud-

Table 18.8. Results of Long-term Carcinogenicity Bioassays and Epidemiologic Investigations on Natural (Other Than Asbestos and Erionite) and Man-made Mineral Fibers

Fibrous material	Tumors in experimental animals	Tumors in humans
Wollastonite	Pleural "sarcomas"	
Attapulgite	Mesotheliomas	
Talc-containing asbestiform fibers	Mesotheliomas[a]	Lung cancer Mesotheliomas[b]
Glass wool	Lung tumors Mesotheliomas	Lung cancer
Rock wool	Mesotheliomas	
Slag wool	(Equivocal findings)	
Rock wool + slag wool		Lung cancer
Ceramic fibers	Lung tumors[b] Mesotheliomas	

[a] Studies by Minardi et al. (32).
[b] The evidence is still limited.

ies demonstrate biologically plausible and statistically significant increases in the incidence of lung cancer and mesothelioma in rats and hamsters exposed to glass wool by various routes using standard scientific methods: intrapleural injection, intrapleural implantation, intraperitoneal (i.p.) injection, and intratracheal instillation" (12). Three epidemiologic studies on workers employed in fibrous glass–manufacturing facilities—one conducted in Canada (limited to one factory) (39), one in the United States (17 factories) (7, 30), and one in Europe (13 factories) (40)—allow the conclusion that glass-wool fibers play a role in causing the excess of lung cancer risk observed among these employees (6). The production and use of fibrous glass should therefore be regulated, and prompt preventive measures should be undertaken.

NONFIBROUS PARTICULATE MATERIALS

Nonfibrous particulates include powdered metallic cobalt and nickel, and crystalline silica. Particles of pure metallic cobalt (size ranging from 3.5 × 3.5 μm to 17 × 12 μm) with large numbers of long, narrow particles on the order of 10 × 4 μm, and clumps of particles measuring up to 100 × 100 μm, when injected in the thigh muscles cause the onset of sarcomas (mainly rhabdomyosarcomas) at the site of injection (10).

After intrafemoral (marrow cavity) and subcutaneous introduction into rats, particles of pure metallic nickel, ranging in diameter from 2 to 50 μm (mean, 10–30 μm), have been shown to produce sarcomas of different histiotypes in about 28% of the animals given implants (11).

Various forms and preparations of crystalline silica (quartz, cristobalite, and tridymite) have been tested for carcinogenicity. Quartz, with particle sizes in the respirable range, administered by inhalation or by intratracheal instillation in rats, produced adenocarcinomas and squamous cell carcinomas of the lung in three of five experiments performed. When injected into the pleural and peritoneal cavities, quartz of several types with particles in the respirable range resulted in thoracic and abdominal malignant lymphomas, primarily of the histiocytic type. Cristobalite and tridymite, with particles in the respirable range, resulted in malignant lymphomas, primarily of the histiocytic type, when injected into the pleural cavity (15).

GEL MATERIALS

Two types of silicone gel used for breast prostheses have been tested by subcutaneous implantation in male and female Sprague-Dawley rats by Dow-Corning. Tumors, the large majority of which were fibrosarcomas, developed at the site of implantation in 22 to 32% of the animals in the treated groups (8). The introduction of silicone gels, used for mammary implants, in the peritoneal cavity of susceptible strains of mice caused the onset of plasmocytomas of the peritoneum (37).

The relevance of these findings for public health may be large, if one considers that silicone implants were widely used for mammary prostheses. According to the U.S. Food and Drug Administration, 130,000 silicone gel breast prostheses were implanted annually until recently, and approximately 2 million women have received implants to date. Of the breast prostheses implanted, 85% were for augmentation (cosmetic) purposes and the remainder were for breast reconstruction after mastectomy. Another use of silicone gel implants is for testicular prostheses.

Though the silicone gel is encased in a silicone envelope when used in breast prostheses, there is good evidence that silicone gel "bleeds" through the envelope and thus can get into surrounding tissues and travel to distant places in the body. The carcinogenic risk, therefore, is not only topical (at the site of injection or implantation), but also may exist at distant anatomic sites. An axillary immunoblastic lymphoma with intranodal refractile particles has been reported in a woman who received silicone prosthetic implants in the metacarpophalangeal joints of both hands (5).

Mechanisms of Carcinogenesis

It has been hypothesized that physical carcinogens produce cancer by some physical mechanisms rather than by chemical reaction. Such physical mechanisms have been regarded as the nonspecific irritative effect of hypothetical surface factors on cells that could cause cellular proliferation, the selection of spontaneously occurring transformed clones, and, finally the development of neoplasias. In favor of this view are several observations and considerations. First, the ratio of length to diameter of the fibers seems to be crucial in the carcinogenicity of asbestos and man-made mineral fibers (13, 14). For example, the incidence of pleural mesothelioma in rats following a single intrapleural implantation ranged from 0/28 to 20/29, and correlated with fiber size rather than with physicochemical properties: the most carcinogenic fibers were those > 8 μm long and < 1.5 μm in diameter (41, 42). Second, the form of implanted hard and soft materials, such as polymers and metallic alloys, also appeared to be crucial in some experiments: the carcinogenic effects of these materials were maximal when they were implanted in the form of intact disks and seemed to decrease when the disks were holed (in some experiments) or when the material was fragmented. Thus, it has been hypothesized that the fibrous reaction observed around implanted disks, squares, and films might "immunologically protect" the transformed clones formed in the core of the capsule and in contact with the implants, therefore favoring the formation of tumors. The physical hypothesis comes from the assumption that solid carcinogens are inert.

There are, however, other facts that oppose the physical hypothesis as the unique carcinogenic mechanism of physical carcinogens, and support a possible contribution of chemical mechanisms. This alternative view is based again on several observations. First, it has been observed (by several investigators, including the present authors) that many plastic polymers (the most specific example of inert material), when embedded in tissues, undergo progressive deterioration at varying rates, indicating some chemical interaction between the xenobiotic material and biologic substrates. The leaching of microquantities of soluble material from the physical carcinogens into the body may be sufficient to transform cells that are in intimate contact with the xenobiotic material. Second, the perforation effect has not been confirmed by other investigators or by us in the course of vitallium disk carcinogenesis. The discrepancy between these experimental results may be explained by the existence of different experimental conditions in various laboratories (for example, the duration of experiments), particularly when one is analyzing experiments performed many years ago, at a time when standards of good laboratory procedures may not have been uniform. Third, the fragmentation effect may be explained by the fact that fragments or powders, after insertion, usually tend to form a compact spherical mass in the body tissues, with a lesser surface of interaction with the biologic substrate than the surface area of a disk. Therefore the chemical mechanism cannot be discarded. Fourth, recent data have shown that asbestos (crocidolite and chrysotile) is mutagenic per se (T. Hei and C. Waldren, personal communication). Moreover, it has been demonstrated that chrysotile fibers have the ability to introduce plasmid DNA into cells and that this DNA can function in both replication and gene expression. The introduction of exogenous DNA into eukaryotic cells could cause mutations in several ways and thus contribute to asbestos-induced carcinogenesis (1).

The mechanisms of the action of physical carcinogens are not only scientific puzzles, but have specific practical implications. In fact, a chemical mechanism would imply a possible mutagenic effect and therefore a nonthreshold dose. It is a topic that deserves further consideration.

Conclusions

Physical carcinogenesis is an important public health, economic, and social problem because of the large-scale diffusion of particulate nonfibrous and fibrous industrial materials into the general and domestic environments and the workplace, and because of the increasing use of xenobiotic implants in plastic, orthopedic, vascular, dental, and other surgical specialties.

The dramatic carcinogenic effect of asbestos, the available data about other mineral industrial fibers, the expected introduction of new types of fibrous and nonfibrous materials into the environment, and the expanding use of alloplastic surgery all are reasons that should prompt more systematic studies of physical carcinogenesis. When such studies are positive, the consequent measures of control will be mainly preventive.

References

1. Appel JD, Fasy TM, Kohtz DS, Kohtz JD, Johnson EM. Asbestos fibers mediate transformation of monkey cells by exogenous plasmid DNA. Proc Natl Acad Sci USA 1988;85:7670.
2. Baris YI, Sahin AA, Oezesmi M, Kerse E, Oezen E, Kolacan B, Altinoers M, Goektepeli A. An outbreak of pleural mesothelioma and chronic fibrosing pleurisy in the village of Karain/Uerguep in Anatolia. Thorax 1978;33:181.
3. Chiappino G, Venerandi I. La erosione delle coperture in cemento amianto: una importante sorgente di inquinamento ambientale. Med Lav 1991;82:99.
4. Cullen MR, Lopez-Carrillo L, Alli B, Pace PE, Shalat SL, Baloyi RS. Chrysotile asbestos and health in Zimbabwe. Am J Ind Med 1991;19:161.
5. Digby JM, Wells AL. Malignant lymphoma with intranodal refractile particles after insertion of silicone prostheses. Lancet 1981;2:580.
6. Doll R. Symposium on MMMF, Copenhagen, October 1986: overview and conclusions. Ann Occup Hyg 1987;31:805.
7. Enterline PE, Marsh GM, Henderson V, Callahan C. Mortality update of a cohort of US man-made mineral fibre workers. Ann Occup Hyg 1987;31:625.
8. Analysis of Dow-Corning data regarding carcinogenicity of silicone gels. Washington DC: Food and Drug Administration, 1988.
9. Health and Human Services. Sixth Annual Report on Carcinogens. Research Triangle Park NC: National Institutes of Environmental Health Sciences, National Toxicology Program, 1991.
10. Heath JC. The production of malignant tumours by cobalt in the rat. Br J Cancer 1956;10:668.
11. Hueper WC. Experimental studies in metal carcinogenesis. IV. Cancer produced by parenterally introduced metallic nickel. JNCI 1955;16:55.
12. Infante PF, Schuman LD, Dement J, Huff J. Fibrous glass and cancer. Am J Ind Med 1994;26:559.
13. International Agency for Research on Cancer. Asbestos. IARC Monogr Eval Carcinog Risk Chem Hum, vol 14, 1977.
14. International Agency for Research on Cancer. Man-made Mineral Fibres and Radon, IARC Monogr Eval Carcinog Risk Chem Hum. vol 43, 1988.
15. International Agency for Research on Cancer. Silica and Some Silicates, IARC Monogr Eval Carcinog Risk Chem Hum. vol 42, 1987.
16. International Programme on Chemical Safety. Asbestos and Other Natural Mineral Fibres. Geneva: World Health Organization, 1986.
17. Landrigan JP, Kazemi H, eds. The Third Wave of Asbestos Disease: Exposure to Asbestos in Place. Ann NY Acad Sci 1991;special issue.
18. Lynch KM, Smith WA. Pulmonary asbestosis. III Carcinoma of lung in asbestos-silicosis. Am J Cancer 1935;24:56.
19. Maltoni C, Minardi F. The comparative potency of asbestos and erionite in producing mesothelioma, following intrapleural and intraperitoneal injection into Sprague-Dawley rats. Acta Oncol 1983;4:69.
20. Maltoni C, Minardi F. Recent results of carcinogenicity bioassays of fibres and other particulate materials. In Non-Occupational Exposure to Mineral Fibres. Edited by E Bignon, J Peto, R Saracci. Lyon: IARC Scientific Publications,1989, p 46.
21. Maltoni C, Minardi F, Morisi L. Pleural mesotheliomas in Sprague-Dawley rats by erionite: first experimental evidence. Environ Res 1982;29:238.
22. Maltoni C, Pinto C, Carnuccio R, Valenti D, Amaducci E. Mesothelioma following exposure to asbestos used in railroads: 122 Italian cases. In The Identification and Control of Environmental and Occupational Diseases: Hazards and Risks of Chemicals in the Oil Refining Industry. Edited by MA Mehlman, A Upton. Princeton, NJ: Princeton Scientific, 1994, p 635.
23. Maltoni C, Pinto C, Carnuccio R, Valenti D, Lodi P, Amaducci E. Mesotheliomas following exposure to asbestos used in railroads: 130 Italian cases. Med Lav 1995;86:461.
24. Maltoni C, Pinto C, Mobiglia A. Mesothelioma due to asbestos used in railroads in Italy. In The Third Wave of Asbestos Disease: Exposure to Asbestos in Place. Edited by PJ Landrigan, H Kazemi. Ann NY Acad Sci 1991;special issue:347.
25. Maltoni C, Pinto C, Valenti D, Carnuccio R, Amaducci E, Minardi F. Mesotheliomas following exposure to asbestos used in sugar refineries: report of the 12 Italian cases. Med Lav 1995; 86:478.
26. Maltoni C, Pinto C, Valenti D, Carnuccio R, Minardi F. Mesotheliomas following exposure to asbestos used in sugar refineries: report of the 11 Italian cases. In The Identification and Control of Environmental and Occupational Diseases: Hazards and Risk of Chemicals in the Oil Refining Industry. Edited by MA Mehlman, A Upton. Princeton NJ: Princeton Scientific, 1994, p 629.
27. Maltoni C, Santi L, Del Gaudio A. Sarcogenesi del tessuto sottocutaneo nel ratto da impianto di dischi di Teflon: sequenza delle modificazioni locali. Il Cancro 1964;17:4.
28. Maltoni C, Sinibaldi C. Carcinogenicity of acrylic resins (polymethyl methacrylate) used in dentistry. Long-term bioassays on Sprague-Dawley rats by subcutaneous implantation. Acta Oncol 1982;3:13.
29. Maltoni C, Sinibaldi C, Morisi L. Carcinogenicity of vitallium: long-term bioassays on Sprague-Dawley rats and Swiss mice by subcutaneous implantation. Acta Oncol 1980;1:11.
30. Marsh GM, Enterline PE, Stone RA, Henderson VL. Mortality among a cohort of US man-made mineral fiber workers: 1985 follow-up. J Occup Med 1990;32:594.
31. McGlashan ND, Harington JS. Unravelling cancer patterns of Southern Africa. Acta Oncol (in press).
32. Minardi F, Belpoggi F, Franch A, Maltoni C. La cancerogenesi da talco grezzo con-

taminato con amianto: primi risultati dei saggi sperimentali dell'Istituto di Oncologia di Bologna. In Recenti Progressi nelle Conoscenze e nel Controllo dei Tumori. Edited by E Triggiani, G Sammarco, G Liguori, D Carretti, C Maltoni. Bologna: Monduzzi, 1990, p 279.
33. Nothdurft H. Die experimentalle Erzeugung von Sarkomen bei Ratten und Mausen durch Implantation von Rundscheiben aus Gold, Silber, Platin oder Elfenbein. Naturwissenschaften 1955;42:75.
34. Oppenheimer BS, Oppenheimer ET, Danishefsky I, Stout AP. Carcinogenic effect of metals in rodents. Cancer Res 1956;16:439.
35. Oppenheimer BS, Oppenheimer ET, Danishefsky I, Stout AP, Eirich FR. Further studies of polymers as carcinogenic agents in animals. Cancer Res 1955;15:333.
36. Oppenheimer BS, Oppenheimer ET, Stout AP, Danishefsky I. Malignant tumours resulting from embedding plastics in rodents. Science 1953;118:305.
37. Potter M, Morrison S, Wiener F, Zang, XK, Miller FW. Induction of plasmocytomas with silicone gel in genetically susceptible strains of mice. JNCI 1994;86:1058.
38. Selikoff IJ, Lee DHK. Asbestos and disease. New York: Academic Press, 1978.
39. Shannon HS, Jamieson E, Julian JA, Muir DCF, Walsh C. Mortality experience of Ontario glass fibre workers: extended follow-up. Ann Occup Hyg 1987;31:657.
40. Simonato L, Fletcher AC, Cherrie JW, Anderson A, Bertazzi P, Charnay N, Claude J, Dodgson J, Esteve J, Frentzel-Beyme R, Gardner MJ, Jensen O, Olsen J, Teppo L, Winkelmann R, Westerholm P, Winter PD, Zocchetti C, Saracci R. The International Agency for Research on Cancer historical cohort study of MMMF production workers in seven European countries: extension of the follow-up. Ann Occup Hyg 1987;31:603.
41. Stanton MF, Layard M, Tegeris A, Miller E, May M, Morgan E, Smith A. Relation of particle dimension to carcinogenicity in amphibole asbestos and other fibrous minerals. JNCI 1981;67:965.
42. Stanton MF, Layard M, Tegaris A, MIller E, May M, Kent E. Carcinogenicity of fibrous glass: pleural response in the rat in relation to fiber dimension. JNCI 1977;58:587.
43. Turner FC. Sarcomas at sites of subcutaneous implanted Bakelite disks in rats. JNCI 1941;2:81.

CHAPTER 19

Trauma and Inflammation

JOHN F. GAETA

The normal wear and tear of life induces a multiplicity of traumas which are rarely noted or quickly forgotten until the time arises to make something out of them.

—Stewart, 1946

Introduction

The role of trauma in the causation of cancer is a subject fraught with gross exaggerations and contradictions. The literature abounds with points of view ranging from detailed descriptions of case reports of trauma followed by malignant neoplasms to others in which this relationship is minimized or flatly denied (1, 13, 26, 32, 35, 44, 47, 49).

This problem is further obscured when the medicolegal implications are brought into the picture. Compensation claims for development of a tumor ascribed to trauma are not infrequent, and although they rarely have a factual basis, some of them have been settled in favor of the injured party. Many of the causes found in the literature claiming a causal relationship between trauma and neoplasia try to fulfill a number of criteria postulated by different authors (18, 52).

Most of the conditions listed include (*a*) authenticity of trauma, (*b*) sufficient severity of the trauma, (*c*) reasonable evidence of prior integrity of the injured area, (*d*) tumor appearance at the site of trauma, and (*e*) time interval not too remote for reasonable association of trauma and tumor (41).

Additional criteria to further authenticate this possible relationship are (*a*) trauma of such magnitude that reparative proliferation of cells occurs, and (*b*) tumor of a type that might reasonably develop as a result of the regeneration and repair of specific tissues damaged during injury (52).

Unfortunately, the application of these criteria is not in itself a warranty of a scientific and objective approach to this problem. One of the main sources of disagreement between advocates and detractors of the role of trauma in the causation of cancer has been the length and significance of the time interval between the two. This factor appears to be somewhat flexible when compared to the appearance time of other neoplasms brought about by known carcinogens. The sequence of events leading to the development of leukemia following irradiation exposure is not well known, but in the case of radiation-related leukemia in Nagasaki and Hiroshima after atomic bomb exposure, we have good documentation to indicate a peak appearance time of 7.2 to 9.4 years between exposure and onset of leukemia (6). A similar time interval (8.5 years) has been demonstrated in the case of thyroid neoplasms in children following neck irradiation (54). Recent studies that correlate the appearance of some forms of vaginal adenocarcinoma in young women with mothers who received stilbestrol therapy during the gestation period indicate that the neoplasm may follow 14 to 22 years after the chemical traumatic event (22).

Mechanisms of Possible Traumatic Causation

A wide variety of malignant neoplasms have been described in the literature in association with trauma. In many cases the association is purely coincidental, judging by the lack of scientific evidence, but it emphasizes the fact that mechanical trauma may alert the patient to the presence of a preexisting neoplasm in the affected parts. Accepting the definition of trauma as a mechanical force received by the body and followed by a local reaction characteristic of injury, we exclude ionizing irradiation (see Chapter 15), chemical insults (see Chapter 13), and ultraviolet radiation (see Chapter 16) as different forms of injury discussed elsewhere in their respective relation to cancer (41). Different forms of skin cancer have been known to result from mechanical injury.

DRAINING SINUSES

In 1828, Marjolin described the development of malignant neoplastic changes in an old skin ulcer, probably the site of a draining sinus (33). In 1931, Benedict described 12 cases of cancer occurring in draining osteomyelitic sinuses and collected 52 similar cases from the literature (4). He studied 2,400 cases of osteomyelitic sinuses and found a 0.5% incidence of malignant change. The draining sinus in which cancer occurred had been present for an average of 30 years, and the subsequent neoplastic lesions were invariably slow growing. A review of all reports of cases in which metastases had occurred proved the presence of metastases in only four cases (5). Emphasizing the rarity of spread, this study postulated that some of the cases reported could have been instances of pseudoepitheliomatous hyperplasia of the skin around the sinus, mistakenly diagnosed as carcinoma.

THERMAL INJURY

Since the description by Dupuytren in 1839 of a patient treated for cancer arising in the scar of a burn caused by sulfuric acid, many cases have been described in which heat has been the initial insult that allegedly triggered the development of cancer at the site of injury and subsequent scar (16). Excellent reviews on this subject are available, concluding that the potential of a scar to undergo malignant neoplastic degeneration and the type of epithelioma resulting are related to the extent of the surface area involved and the depth of the burn (27, 46). The type of burn inflicted on the tissue is also related to the nature of the agent (tar, flame, metal), to its temperature, to the tissue's capacity for heat absorption, and to the duration of contact (1). Although most of the reported malignant lesions that follow burns correspond to epidermoid carcinomas, basal cell cancers can also originate by the same mechanism, usually when the burn is superficial and when the thermal injury results from hot solids. Based on a study of 2,465 cases of skin cancer, 2% of all epidermoid carcinomas and 0.3% of all basal cell carcinomas originate on skin subjected to thermal injury (28, 46).

Kangri Burn Cancer

The Indian kangri is an earthenware bowl heated by charcoal and worn against the skin of the thighs and abdomen. Owing to the constant application of heat, the skin in these areas becomes dry and horny and frequently shows a variable degree of chronic dermatitis. Scars resulting from previous kangri burns are frequent and apt to undergo malignant change. The average age at onset is 55 years and the average duration of life is 15 months from the recognized time of onset of the cancer. The gross lesion is variable in appearance, but microscopically it consistently shows an epidermoid type of carcinoma (36).

Kairo Burn Cancer

The kairo burn cancer in Japan relates to another system for the maintenance of body warmth, the use of a light tin box that fits snugly against the contour of the abdomen. It is generally worn for a period of at least 3 hours at a time. The continued or prolonged use of this utensil produces erythematous burns or chronic dermatitis leading to malignant neoplastic changes (46).

LUNG CANCER

A relationship between lung cancer and pulmonary scars was first noted by Friedrich and Rossle, and their association has been the subject of numerous reports (2, 9, 19, 32, 34, 39, 41, 58). The exact frequency of this association is difficult to determine from previous reports. Luders and Themel found a frequency of 28% in their study of 2,032 autopsies, whereas others report only an incidence of 14% (21, 29). These findings led to the concept of "scar cancer" as a morphologic entity embracing any inflammatory or vascular pulmonary lesion leading to the formation of scar tissue followed by the development of a local carcinoma. In most instances, the tumor arises peripherally and histologically shows the characteristics of pulmonary adenocarcinoma or bronchiolar carcinoma (9). Exact criteria have been postulated to differentiate true pulmonary scars from the dense connective tissue often encountered in lung cancer (10). Still, some believe that this association is probably much higher than suspected because of the common difficulty of convincingly demonstrating the presence of preexisting scar tissue when examining large pulmonary lesions either in surgical or in autopsy material (58).

CANCER OF THE ESOPHAGUS

This type of cancer is often related to previous injury. Studies of a substantial number of cases of stricture of the esophagus following lye ingestion indicate that at least 5.2% of the lye strictures are followed by squamous cell carcinoma (25). A number of other irritants have been implicated, such as strong alcohol, and tobacco smoking, but thermal irritation has been quoted as the most constant factor predisposing to esophageal cancer (48, 53). Some authors have stressed the frequency of this form of cancer in geographic locations where frequent ingestion of extremely hot tea is a common habit.

Cancer of the Oral Cavity

The role of these irritants is apparently reversed in relation to cancer of the oral cavity. Observations of 659 cases of carcinoma of the oral cavity emphasize the role of tobacco and alcohol in the etiology of oral cancer and diminish the significance of local trauma and dental irritation (56).

MOLES AND MALIGNANT MELANOMA

Although the exact cellular origin of malignant melanomas can still be debated, a significant number are related to preexisting nevi (moles) (30). A low percentage of nevi undergo malignant changes, but the true nature of this transformation is not well known. The fact that most malignant melanomas occur on exposed surfaces of the body, and the reported higher incidence of the disease in the sunnier parts of some countries, suggested that trauma or injury plays a part in their causation (11, 31). Another line of evidence in favor of the same hypothesis is the higher incidence of malignant melanoma in patients affected by xeroderma pigmentosum, a congenital disease characterized by failure to repair injury to DNA manifested as hypersensitivity to sunlight (27).

Evidence in favor of trauma playing a role in the development of malignant melanoma also includes reports of a significant incidence of this lesion in Sudanese patients (23). However, some studies of malignant melanoma in Australia showed that the most frequent location is the skin of the back, at least in the male, but this failed to show any direct relation to the belt area of the trunk, where the incidence of constant trauma is obviously higher (11).

Trauma and Bone Tumors

The etiologic aspect of single trauma has been repeatedly mentioned, although never elucidated, in relation to bone tumors. The preponderance of bone tumors occur in the same young age group in which the incidence of trauma is especially high. Most of the reports in the literature deal with observations of single cases. A general review of this problem in 1967 included six cases of osteogenic sarcomas following a history of trauma (36). All of them, however, presented after such a short time interval (8 days to 4 months) that their causal relationship seems highly improbable. The lack of any significant increase in the number of bone tumors following the two world wars also speaks against such a relationship (14).

OTHER TYPES OF CANCERS

Other types of cancers that have been reported occasionally in association with trauma include mammary carcinoma, brain tumors, carcinoma of the uterine cervix, meningioma, glioma, and testicular tumors, but the evidence of etiologic significance is not persuasive (3, 7, 35, 38, 43, 50).

Interactions of Trauma and Tissue Repair

There is no evidence to substantiate the production of experimental tumors by the direct action of trauma, but there are numerous studies indicating its significance as a "cocarcinogen." Since the studies of Rous and co-workers, it became apparent that, although repeated application of tar can induce tumors in rabbits under certain circumstances, a trauma can precipitate the formation of a tumor when the cells have been conditioned with previous tar treatment or by local promoters (20, 42). However, if trauma is to be considered independently as a tumor-causative factor, this could only take place as a rare event during the process of regeneration and repair. Normal regenerative process implies the restoration of lost parts by structurally and often functionally similar cells. There are some who would evoke a variety of organ-specific wound hormones liberated from the site of injury that exert a stimulating effect on homologous tissue (45). Such putative hormonal factors have been further studied more recently, and it was concluded that the hormones (chalones) liberated from the wound have a specific role as mitotic inhibitors (8). According to this view, liberation of the chalone releases cells to divide. This might also explain the mitogenic capacity of estrogens, which provide an increase in mitotic activity, possibly through neutralization of chalone substances. It is conceivable that persistent cell damage by trauma could trigger an excessive proliferative effect because of the absence of the inhibiting effect of local chalones.

Other authors have advanced the possibility of direct mutation from chronic inflammation or repair (51). This concept was chiefly based on the proposition that a sudden transformation of a gene could result from trauma leading to a change of the basic characteristics of a cell and its progeny. Because cell mutations can be brought about by different stimuli, some investigators have concluded that the effect of repeated trauma on tissues can be analogous to chemical carcinogens in their ability to induce cellular mutation (12).

Another hypothesis unrelated to a humoral factor and recently related to carcinogenesis suggests a regulatory mechanism between cytoplasmic and nuclear structures (37). Since the endoplasmic reticulum modulates DNA biosynthesis in some way, any stimulus (trauma) capable of destroying critical cytoplasmic structures or proteins could lead to a loss of a feedback mechanism, with the cell beginning actively to synthesize DNA, causing polyploidy or cell division. In this manner, differentiation of the tissue would be lost and a large increase in immature, undifferentiated cells would result from which a malignant neoplasm might emerge. Electron microscope studies corroborate the destruction of endoplasmic reticulum structures during cancerization of the liver by means of dimethylnitrosamine (17).

References

1. Abbas JS, Beecham JE. Burn wound carcinoma: case report and review of the literature. Burns Incl Therm. Inj 1988;14:222.
2. Balo J, Juhasz E, Temes J. Pulmonary infarcts and pulmonary carcinoma. Cancer 1956;9:918.
3. Barnett GH, Chou SM, Bay JW. Post-traumatic intracranial meningioma: a case report and review of the literature. Neurosurgery 1986;18:75.
4. Benedict EB. Carcinoma in osteomyelitis. Surg Gynecol Obstet 1931;53:1.
5. Bereston ES, Ney C. Squamous cell carcinoma arising in a chronic osteomyelitic sinus tract with metastasis. Arch Surg 1941;43:257.
6. Bizzozero OJ, Johnson KG, Ciocco A. Radiation-related leukemia, Hiroshima and Nagasaki, 1946–1964. I. Distribution, incidence and appearance time. N Engl J Med 1966;274:1095.
7. Boyd JT, Doll R. A study of the etiology of carcinoma uteri. Br J Cancer 1964;18:419.
8. Bullough WS. Mitotic and functional homeostasis: a speculative review. Cancer Res 1965;25:1683.
9. Carroll R. The significance of lung scars on primary lung cancer. J Pathol Bacteriol 1962;83:293.
10. Castleman B. Healed pulmonary infarcts. Arch Pathol 1940;30:130.
11. Davis NC, Herrow JJ, McLeod GR. Malignant melanoma in Queensland. Analysis of 400 skin lesions. Lancet 1966;2:407.
12. Demerec M. Mutations induced by carcinogens. Br J Cancer 1948;2:114.
13. DeNayer PP, Delloye C, Malghem J. Bone injury and late giant cell tumor occurrence: a possible relation—A case report. Orthopedics 1983;10:1279.
14. Dietrich A. Krebs Nach Kriegsverletzungen. Z Krebsforsch 1942;52:91.
15. Dolberġ DS, Hollingsworth R, Hertle M. Wounding and its role in RSV-mediated tumor formation. Science 1985;230:676.
16. Dupuytren G. Lélcons Orales de Clinique Chirurgicale. 2nd ed. Paris, 1839.
17. Emmelot E, Benedetti EL. Changes in the fine structure of rat liver brought about by dimethylnitrosamine. J Biophys Biochem Cytol 1960;7:393.
18. Ewing J. Bulkley lecture: modern attitude toward traumatic cancer. Arch Pathol 1935;10:690.
19. Friedrich G. Periphere Lungenkrebse auf dem bodem Pleuraher Narben. Virchows Arch Pathol Anat 1939;304:230.
20. Friedwald WF, Rous P. The pathogenesis of deferred cancer. J Exp Med 1950;91:459.
21. Gelzer J. Uber die peripheren Lungenkrebse in Bereich von Lungernarben. Virchows Arch Pathol Anat 1956:p. 329.
22. Herbst AL, Ulfelder H, Poskanzer DC. Adenocarcinoma of the vagina: association of maternal stilbestrol therapy with tumor appearance in young women. N Engl J Med 1971;284:878.
23. Hewer TF. Malignant melanoma in colored races: role of trauma in its causation. J Pathol Bacteriol 1935;41:473.
24. Johnson FM. The development of carcinoma in scar tissue following burns. Am Surg 1926;83:165.
25. Joske RA, Benedict EB. The role of benign esophageal obstruction in the development of carcinoma of the esophagus. Gastroenterology 1959;36:749.
26. Langer F, Pritzker KP, Gross AE, Shapiro IL. Giant cell tumor associated with trauma. Clin Orthop 1982;164:245.
27. Lever WF. Histopathology of the Skin. 4th ed. Philadelphia: Lippincott, 1967, p 63.
28. Lifeso RM, Rooney RJ, Shaker M. Post-traumatic squamous cell carcinoma. J Bone Joint Surg 1990;72:12.
29. Luders CJ, Themel KG. Die Narbenkrebse der Lungen als Beitrag zur Pathogenese des peripheren Lungencarcinoms. Virchows Arch Pathol Anat 1954;325:499.
30. McGovern JJ. Malignant Melanoma: Clinical and Histological Diagnosis. New York: Wiley, 1976, pp 47–54.
31. McKie RM, Atchison T. Severe sunburn and subsequent risk of primary cutaneous malignant melanomas in Scotland. Br J Cancer 1982;46:955.
32. Madri JA, Carter D. Scar cancers of the lung: origin and significance. Hum Pathol 1984;15:625.
33. Marjolin JN. Ulcére. Dict de méd., 2nd ed. 1846, XXX, 10. SCARS, p 22.
34. Meyer E, Liebow A. Relationship of interstitial pneumonia, honeycombing and atypical epithelial proliferation to cancer of the lung. Cancer 1965;18:322.

35. Mosinger M, Glaunes JP, Fiorentini H, Bandler H. Tumeurs et cancers post traumatiques. Ann Med Leg 1961;41:472.
36. Neve EF. Kangri Burn Cancer. Br J Med 1923;21:1255.
37. Oehlert W. The mechanism of regeneration, hyperplasia and cancerization. Acta Un Int Cancer 1963;19:605.
38. Perez-Diaz C, Cabello A, Lobato RD. Oligodendrogliomas arising in the scar of a brain contusion: report of two surgically verified cases. Surg Neurol 1985;24:581.
39. Raeburn C, Spencer H. Lung scar cancers. Brit J Tuberc 1957;51:237.
40. Rigdon RH. Trauma and cancer: a relationship based upon cell mutation. South Med J 1962;55:341.
41. Rossle R. Die Narbenkrebse der Lungen. Schweiz Med Wochenschr 1943;73:1200.
42. Rous P, Kidd JG. Conditional neoplasms and sub-threshold neoplastic states. J Exp Med 1941;73:365.
43. Stewart FW. Occupational and post-traumatic cancer. Bull NY Acad Med 1947;22:145.
44. Stoll HL, Crissey JT. Epithelioma from single trauma. NY State J Med 1962;62:496.
45. Tier H, Kiljunen A, Putkonen T. Existence of growth promoting factor in the skin of the white rat. Ann Chir Gynaecol Fenn 1951, p 40.
46. Treves N, Pack GT. The development of cancer in burn scars. Surg Gynecol Obstet 1930;51:749.
47. Troost D, Tulleken CA. Malignant glioma after bombshell injury. J Clin Neuropathol 1984;3:139.
48. Victoria CG, Munoz N, Day NE. Hot beverages and esophageal cancer in Southern Brazil: a case control study. Int J Cancer 1987;39:710.
49. Voutilainen A, Teir H, Kivivouri A. Causal relationship between trauma and malignant tumors. Ann Chir Gynaecol Fenn 1967;56(suppl 152):1.
50. Walshe F. Head injuries as a factor in the etiology of an intracranial meningioma. Lancet 1961;2:993.[ep
51. Warren S. In Pathology. Edited by WAD Anderson. St. Louis: Mosby, 1961, p 447.
52. Warren S. Minimal criteria to prove causation of traumatic or occupational neoplasms. Ann Surg 1943;117:585.
53. Watson WL, Goodner J. Carcinoma of esophagus. Am J Surg 1957;93:259.
54. Winship T, Rosvoll RV. Childhood thyroid carcinoma. Cancer 1961;14:734.
55. Wojewski A. Reticulum cell sarcoma with primary manifestation in testis. J Urol 1963;89:709.
56. Wynder EJ, Bross IJ, Feldman RM. A study of the etiological factors in cancer of the mouth. Cancer 1957;10:1300.
57. Yamamura T, Aozasa K, Honda T. Malignant fibrous histiocytoma developing in a burn scar. Br J Dermatol 1984;110:725.
58. Yokoo H, Suckow E. Peripheral lung cancers arising in scars. Cancer 1961;14:1205.

CHAPTER 20

RNA Tumor Viruses

HOWARD A. FINE AND JOSEPH SODROSKI

Introduction

The retroviruses are small single-stranded RNA containing animal viruses. The life cycle of these intracellular parasites is unique. By converting their genomic RNA into DNA and inserting it into the chromosomes of their host cells, these viruses can mutate, capture, and even transfer vital genetic information from one cell to another. The resultant effect is often an alteration in cellular growth and differentiation, leading to a wide variety of neoplastic and immunodeficient disease states in a broad range of animal hosts. The study of these viruses has led to profound insights into factors regulating the growth of normal and neoplastic cells.

The first retrovirus was identified in 1911 by Peyton Rous when he found a transmissible agent able to cause sarcomas in chickens (126). The implications of this discovery were not immediately appreciated, since most scientists believed that this phenomenon was a peculiarity specific to the avian system. Over the next 40 years, however, interest in retroviruses dramatically increased with the recognition that these agents could cause neoplasms in other animals, including mammals (14).

Although quantitative assays for these viruses were developed as early as the 1950s, our present understanding of the biology of retroviruses occurred only after discovery of the enzyme, reverse transcriptase, in 1970 (7, 146, 151). This finding significantly increased the general interest in retroviruses. However, they continued to be viewed as an enigma of nature, and their relevance to normal cellular growth and spontaneously occurring animal neoplasms remained obscure.

This all changed in 1976 when it was demonstrated that the apparent transforming genes (oncogenes) carried by these viruses were homologues of endogenous cellular genes (proto-oncogenes) (137). This discovery led to an explosion of interest in the field of retrovirology and to the identification of fewer than 60 proto-oncogenes. The impact of these discoveries has changed the way science now views how cellular genes control normal as well as neoplastic cellular growth.

This contribution to our current knowledge has alone made the study of retroviruses vitally important. Additional discoveries in the 1980s, however, made the direct relevance of these viruses to humans frightfully clear (169). These discoveries included the finding in 1980 of the first infectious human retrovirus, human T-cell lymphotropic virus type I (HTLV-1). This virus has been etiologically linked to a specific type of T-cell lymphoma/leukemia and to several degenerative neurologic diseases (see Chapter 46) (47, 114, 132, 171). It soon became clear that HTLV was not the only human pathogenic virus, for in 1984 the human immunodeficiency virus (HIV) was found to be the etiologic cause of AIDS (8, 48, 90).

With the increased understanding of how retroviruses can stably introduce and express their own genes in host cells, researchers have begun to manipulate these viruses to express heterologous genes of interest in target cells (98, 149). Thus, in a real way the study of retroviruses has brought the futuristic idea of "gene therapy" to the modern-day clinic (125).

With this as a background to the history and relevance of retrovirology, this chapter will proceed to summarize some key features concerning the classification and life cycles of retroviruses. There follows a discussion of the mechanisms by which these viruses cause neoplastic transformation and a demonstration of how our study of the life cycle of retroviruses has contributed to our understanding of cell growth regulation. The chapter concludes with a brief discussion of endogenous retroviruses and the potential for retroviral vectors to impact dramatically on the therapy of cancer and other diseases in the future.

Classification

The family of viruses known as retroviridae comprises a large group of animal viruses with roughly similar structures. The viral particles are composed of a nuclear capsid or core made up of several protein products of the gag gene (Fig. 20.1). This core is surrounded by a lipid membrane derived from the host plasma membrane and contains viral glycoprotein projections encoded by the env gene. In whole, the viral particle measures approximately 100 nm in diameter. Within the nuclear capsid reside several enzymatic proteins encoded by the pol gene. Also within the core resides the genome of the virus, consisting of two single-stranded RNA molecules.

The family of retroviruses has been subclassified using various schemas (144). Historically, they have grouped based on their apparent effects on their host cells. These three subfamilies include the spumaviruses, lentiviruses, and the oncoviruses. These subfamilies have been further broken down into different groups based on genomic structures (Table 20.1). Another somewhat dated classification

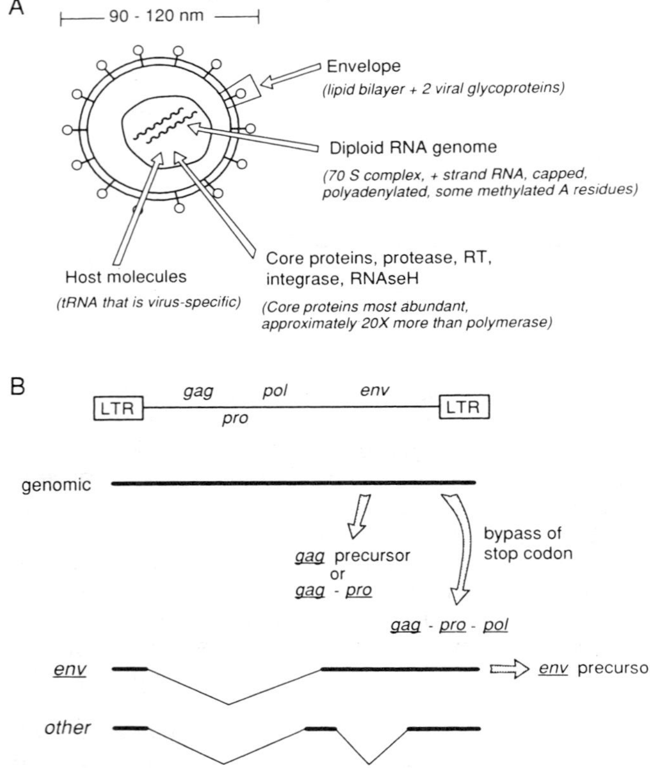

Figure 20.1. **A.** Structure of typical retrovirus virion. **B.** Structure of typical retroviral genome. All replication-competent retroviruses generate a full-length genomic RNA that encodes the gag and pol products and a singly spliced RNA that encodes the env product. Some retroviruses also generate smaller multiply-spliced messages. (pro, protease; pol, polymerase; env, envelope; gag, core proteins.)

groups retroviruses A through D based on their electron microscopic morphology (Table 20.2). Finally, retroviruses are also described as being exogenous if they only infect somatic cells, or endogenous if they are integrated into the germ line of the organism.

Structure

All replication-competent retroviral genomes contain at least three major structural genes (gag, pol, and env) and 5′ and 3′ regulatory regions known as the long terminal repeats (LTRs) (Fig. 20.1). Replication-defective retroviruses have the same general genomic structure but contain large deletions of some of the structural genes. These deleted structural genes are often replaced by oncogenes (see below). This section describes the genomic and protein components of a replication-competent retrovirus.

LONG TERMINAL REPEAT (LTR)

The LTR plays a vital role in the life cycle of the retrovirus, being not only responsible for viral gene expression, but also necessary for viral genomic integration into the host cell chromosomes. Relative to this latter function it is of interest that retroviral LTRs share structural homology with the eukaryotic transposable elements known as retrotransposons (157). The LTRs contain many regulatory signals necessary for the efficient expression and replication of the retroviral genome. Structurally, LTR is generally separated into three regions, U5, R, and U3 (Fig. 20.2). U5 is bounded by the primer binding site (see below). It is the first portion of the retroviral genome to be transcribed by the reverse transcriptase and thus becomes the 3′ LTR of the integrated provirus. This repeated structure is necessary for the reverse transcriptase process. U3 starts out adjacent to R at the 3′ portion of the end of the genomic RNA but after reverse transcription becomes the 5′ end of the viral LTR. This region,

Table 20.1. Retrovirus Groups

Oncornaviruses
- Avian leukosis-sarcoma viruses (ALSV)
- Avian reticuloendotheliosis virus
- Mammalian leukemia and sarcoma viruses (mouse/cat type C viruses)
- Mouse mammary tumor virus
- Primate type D viruses (Mason-Pfizer monkey virus/simian AIDS virus)
- Human T-cell leukemia virus/bovine leukemia virus/simian T-cell leukemia virus

Lentiviruses (including immunodeficiency viruses)
Spumaviruses

Table 20.2. Retrovirus Morphology

A-type particles
- Intracellular core formation and budding
- Intracisternal A-type particles (IAP) are products of endogenous proviruses
- Noninfectious

B-type particles (MMTV)
- Core formation occurs in the cytoplasm
- After budding at the plasma membrane, maturation to an eccentric core occurs
- Prominent surface spikes

C-type particles
- Most oncornaviruses
- Initially form electron-dense patches at the plasma membrane
- Budding at plasma membrane
- Maturation of core to yield centrally located cores
- Spikes may or may not be prominent

D-type particles
- Mason-Pfizer monkey virus, simian AIDS virus
- Intracellular nucleocapsid formation, budding at plasma membrane
- Eccentric core
- Less prominent spikes

Lentiviruses
- Visna-maidi, EIAV, CAEV, SIV, HIV, FIV, BIV
- Core formation and budding as for C-type particles
- Condensed mature core forms pyramidal shape

Spumaviruses
- IAP-like cores

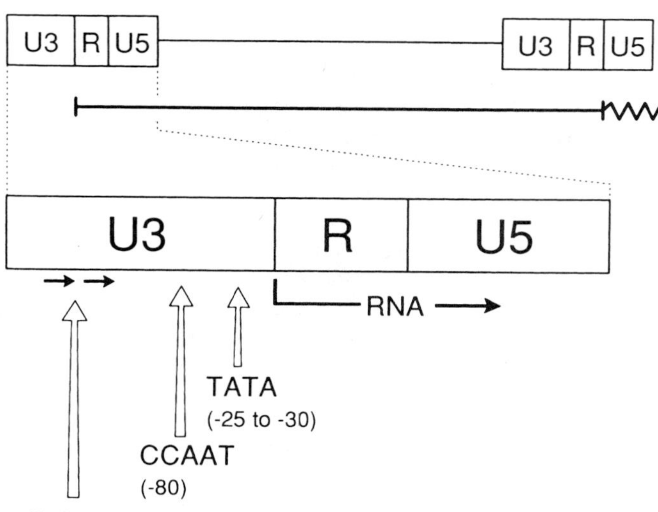

Figure 20.2. LTR structure. Replication competent retroviruses contain identical long terminal repeats (LTR) at the 5′ and 3′ ends. The U3 portion of the 5′ LTR contains all the enhancer and promoter elements necessary for efficient initiation of transcription of either retroviral or cellular genes. (MuLV, murine leukemia virus; FeLV, feline leukemia virus; MMTV, Moloney mammary tumor virus; MA, matrix protein; CA, capsid; NC, nuclear capsid; PR, protease; RT, reverse transcriptase; IN, integrase.)

therefore, contains many of the regulatory elements necessary for efficient proviral transcription. It is important to keep in mind that all primary retroviral transcripts are initiated at the 5′ portion of the LTR and are terminated at the 3′ portion of the LTR.

At the 5′ end of U3 are a series of enhancer sequences that help regulate levels of proviral gene expression. These sequences are responsive to host cell transcriptional factors. Examples of such sequences are the NFκB consensus sequence in HIV-1, the cyclic adenosine monophosphate (cAMP)-responsive elements in HTLV-I and binding sites for the glucocorticoid receptor in the mouse mammary tumor virus (MMTV) LTR (10, 52, 111, 170). It is precisely because of the dependence on these host cellular factors for efficient proviral LTR-directed transcription that the LTR ultimately plays a major role in determining the host range of the virus.

There are several other important sequences within the LTR. They include CAT and TATAAA boxes which lie downstream of the enhancer sequences and function as the promoter for RNA transcription from the proviral DNA (38, 49). At the junctions of U3 and R lies the CAP, site where RNA transcription is actually initiated (18). In the 3′ region of R exists the polyadenylation signal for the termination of transcription.

LEADER SEQUENCE

Between the 5′ LTR and the initiation codon of the gag gene lies the leader sequence. Within this short stretch of nucleotides lies three extremely important sequences. One is the primer binding site (PBS). This is the area where a specific cellular transfer RNA (tRNA) binds to its complementary sequence. The tRNA serves as the primer for the reverse transcriptase (see below) (143).

The second important structure within the leader sequences is the splice donor site for generation of subgenomic messages, usually the env transcript.

The third important function of the leader sequence is that it provides the so-called packaging sequences that allow full-length viral RNA to be recognized by gag proteins and to be incorporated into the virion particle for export out of the cell (27, 89).

GAG

The most 5′ structural gene in the genome of all retroviruses is gag. The messenger RNA (mRNA) that encodes for gag is the same size as the genomic RNA and is identical to the RNA species that encodes the pro (protease) and pol (polymerase) genes (42, 116, 117, 159). The gag protein is synthesized as a large precursor that is eventually cleaved into three to five smaller gag proteins by both cellular and virally encoded proteases. The viral protease is encoded as a carboxy extension to the gag precursor protein, as is the pol gene product.

The three major gag proteins are the nucleic acid–binding protein, the capsid protein, and the matrix protein. The nucleic acid–binding proteins are small basic proteins located in the capsid core and are associated with the RNA molecules. Their positive charges are probably vital for effective RNA packaging by neutralizing the negative charges of the RNA phosphate moieties. Another structural motif within the nuclear binding protein that allows for efficient RNA packaging is the zinc finger. This is a peptide stretch containing cysteines and histidines placed in specific positions such that a zinc atom can be incorporated. This structure is known to bind avidly to nucleic acids and is clearly necessary for the packaging of the genomic RNA into the virion (51, 130). Whether a zinc atom is actually necessary, however, remains controversial.

The capsid protein is the major structural protein of the virus and by itself forms the shell of the capsid structure. The matrix protein lies on the outside of the capsid shell and interacts with the overlying membrane of the viral particle. This hydrophobic interaction occurs via the posttranslational addition of a myristic acid to the matrix protein (131). In some viruses (e.g., HIV-1), it has been shown that the particular structure of the matrix protein is important for accommodating envelope glycoproteins with large cytoplasmic tails into virion particles (35).

PRO/POL

It is somewhat imprecise to describe pol or pro/pol as a separate gene, since, as mentioned above, these proteins are transcribed from the same RNA species as the gag proteins. In essence, they are merely carboxy terminal extensions of the gag gene. By necessity the level of production of gag protein, however, is usually greater than that of either pro or pol. How the virus regulates the level of gag production compared to the pol product varies with the specific types of virus (Fig. 20.3). In the murine leukemia virus (MuLV) there exists a stop codon at the end of the gag reading frame, thus ensuring that most transcripts encode only the gag protein. The virus, however, has the ability to periodically cause termination suppression by allowing the cellular transcription apparatus to insert a random amino acid at this codon, thus allowing for a read-through gag-pro-pol fusion precursor (172). In contrast, the Rous sarcoma virus (RSV) maintains a greater level of gag production compared to pol by having the two genes in different but overlapping reading frames. The pol product is occasionally made as a gag/pol fusion protein by virtue of a short gag sequence and resultant downstream DNA secondary structure that allows the ribosome to frameshift into the pol reading frame (70, 71, 102).

As complex as the creation of these pro-pol RNA products is, the function of their protein products is even more complex. As described above, the basic function of the protease is to cleave the gag or gag/pol fusion precursor into their individual components.

The pol gene actually encodes three different enzymes, the reverse transcriptase, a ribonuclease, and the integrase. Although reverse transcriptase was originally discovered in retroviruses, it has recently become clear that reverse transcriptase can be found in other types of viruses (Hepatitis B, Caulimoviruses) and in eukaryotic cells (67, 140). Reverse transcriptase is one of the most highly conserved parts of the retroviral genome, particularly at the amino acid level (23, 24). The major function of the reverse transcriptase is as an

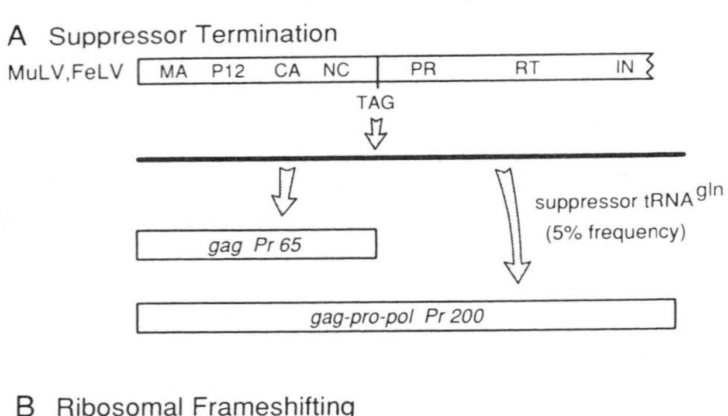

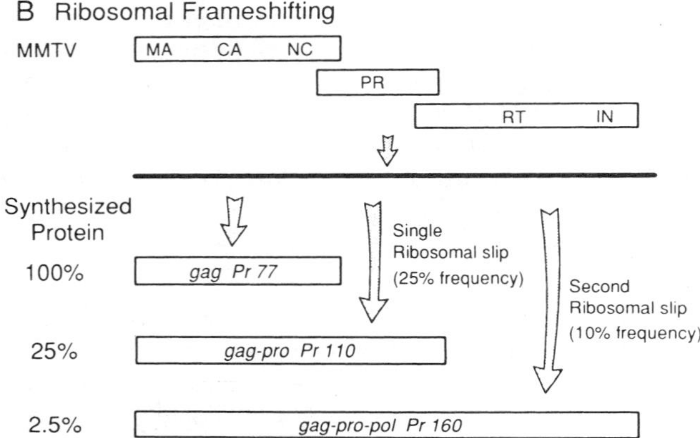

Figure 20.3. Alternative methods different retroviruses utilize to bypass the gag stop codon in order to generate the pro-pol products from the full-length genomic transcripts.

RNA-dependent DNA polymerase. However, the reverse transcriptase enzyme also has an RNase H domain located toward the carboxy terminus of the protein (73). This activity is essential for the removal of the RNA template from the reverse transcribed negative DNA strand, in order to allow synthesis of the positive DNA strand. Another unusual feature of this polymerase is its ability to utilize either RNA or DNA as a primer. As previously discussed, it is in fact a host cell tRNA that serves as the natural primer for retroviral reverse transcriptase. The structure of the HIV-1 reverse transcriptase has been solved and reveals a highly coordinated enzyme for synthesis of DNA with synchronous destruction of the RNA template (85).

Integrase is the second enzyme product of the pol gene. As its name implies, integrase is a vital component in the process of proviral integration into the host genome (see below).

ENVELOPE

The final gene that is consistently found in all replication competent retroviruses is the env gene. In contrast to the gag and pol genes, which are transcribed from a full-length proviral mRNA, the env message is the result of a single splicing event (99, 162). The cellular RNA splicing machinery utilizes the splice donor sequence localized in the leader segment and the splice acceptor sequences invariably found slightly upstream of the envelope initiation codon. Like the gag gene, env encodes a large precursor protein ranging in size from 150 to 160 kd in different viruses (31, 39, 41). This precursor is then cleaved by cellular proteases to produce a larger and smaller envelope protein. The large envelope protein is seen in electron micrographs as the spike coming out of the virion particle. This larger envelope component is glycosylated and sits outside the viral membrane (93). Its major function is to specifically bind to a host cell surface protein that serves as the receptor for that virus (30, 81). It is for this reason that the large envelope protein is generally the immunodominant portion of the virus for host neutralizing antibodies (108).

The smaller envelope component is the transmembrane protein. It is composed of three segments, the cytoplasmic, transmembrane, and external region. The external region of the transmembrane protein interacts with the larger envelope component, thus holding it onto the surface of the virion (86). The transmembrane portion of the protein is composed of hydrophobic amino acids and essentially anchors the entire envelope complex in the membrane of the virus. The function of the cytoplasmic portion of this protein remains obscure. Besides its role as an anchor of the larger envelope component, the transmembrane protein also plays a vital role in the fusion of the virion membrane with the infected cellular membrane following receptor binding (86).

VARIATIONS IN GENOMIC STRUCTURE

It should again be emphasized that the genomic composition of the retrovirus as outlined above is a generalization of the minimal amount of genetic information carried by replication-competent retroviruses. There are many retroviruses whose genomes encode other structural and/or regulatory proteins.

In particular, the lentiviruses carry many more than just the gag, pol, and env genes. HIV-1, for example, encodes at least six other regulatory or structural genes, many for which a function has not yet been ascribed (57). The HTLV-I/bovine leukemia virus (BLV) family of retroviruses also encodes at least three additional proteins in a 1- to 2-kb stretch of genome located between the env gene and U3. This region, known as the X region, has many other potential reading frames that may encode proteins that have yet to be identified. Likewise, MMTV and the spumaviruses have 3′ open reading frames, some of which, like bcl-1, encode transcriptional activators of the viral LTR.

In contrast to the complicated genomic organization of the lentiviruses are some of the acutely transforming retroviruses (i.e., RSV, A-MuLV) which are defective for replication secondary to replacement of some or all of their structural genes with host cellular sequences (i.e., oncogenes; see below).

Life Cycle

The life cycle of a retrovirus is extraordinarily complex, and the details are beyond the scope of this chapter. Nevertheless, the uniqueness of the process and the importance of understanding the general strategy the virus takes are vital to understanding the mechanism of transformation, and thus are briefly outlined below (Fig. 20.4). Although retroviral virions may nondiscriminantly attach to almost any cell membrane, actual infection is quite specific. The large exterior glycoprotein envelope functions as a specific ligand for cellular membrane–associated proteins. Thus, these proteins are effectively receptors for retroviral infection. To date, the receptors for the HIV family of viruses, the murine ecotropic retroviruses (MuLV), the Gibbon ape leukemia virus (GALV), and the amphotropic murine (A-MuLV) retroviruses have been identified (3, 92). In 1984 CD4 became the first recognized retroviral receptor with the demonstration that the large HIV exterior glycoprotein (gp120) specifically bound to it. The MuLV receptor was identified by Albritton and coworkers as a multiple membrane–spanning protein (3). Membrane-spanning proteins with phosphate transporter activity serve as the GALV and A-MuLV receptors (165).

The frequency with which a particular retroviral receptor is found in different types of cells plays a major role in the host range of that virus. The two known human retroviruses, HIV and HTLV-I, provide a dramatic contrast to this idea of receptor-mediated host range. HTLV-I has the ability to infect a broad range of cell types, including cells from nonprimate

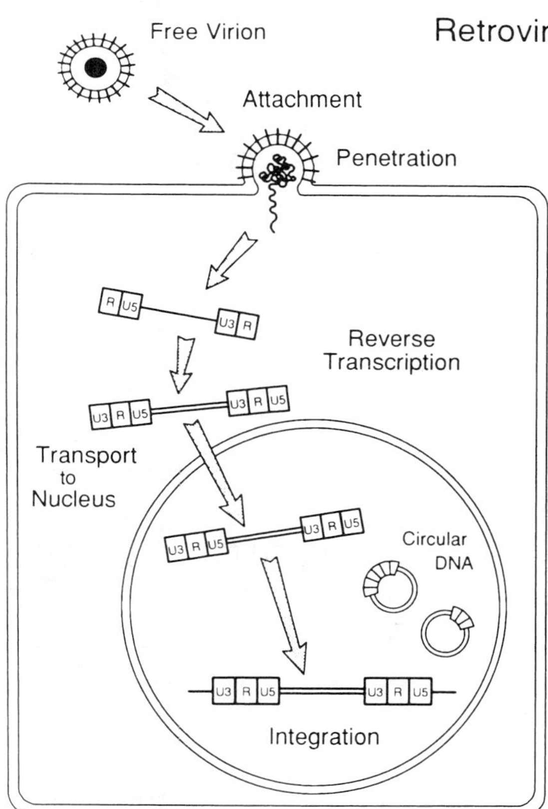

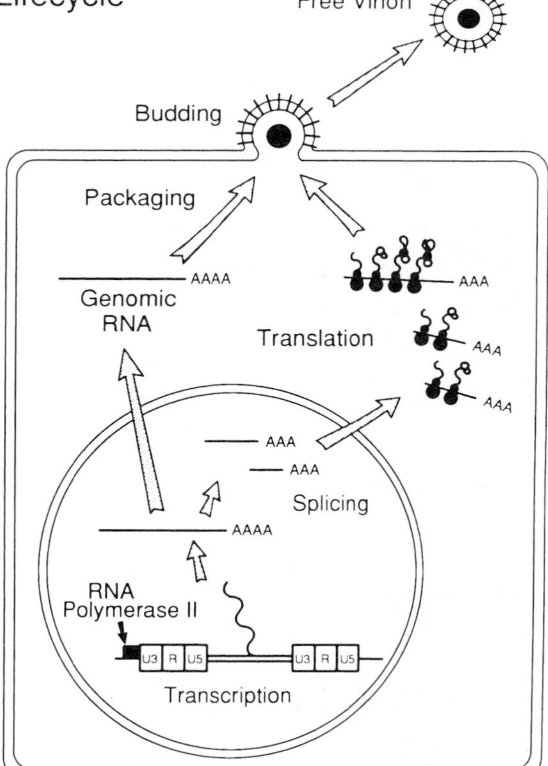

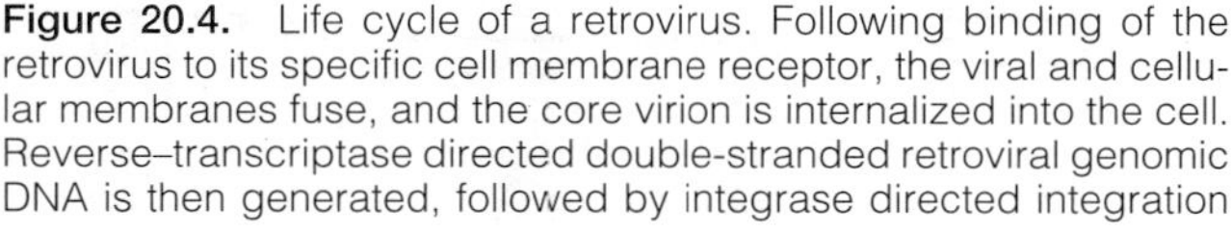

Figure 20.4. Life cycle of a retrovirus. Following binding of the retrovirus to its specific cell membrane receptor, the viral and cellular membranes fuse, and the core virion is internalized into the cell. Reverse–transcriptase directed double-stranded retroviral genomic DNA is then generated, followed by integrase directed integration into host cell DNA. Retroviral transcripts using host transcriptional machinery then proceed, with the eventual formation of new retroviral virions that bud from the cell surface, allowing a new round of infection to occur.

mammals. HIV, on the other hand, has a very restricted host range limited to CD4+ primate cells.

The frequency with which a particular retroviral receptor occurs is not, however, the only envelope property that determines retroviral host range. Following receptor binding, another envelope mediated event must occur. This is the fusion of the viral membrane with the cellular membrane. The transmembrane envelope component is thought to mediate this function (86). This reaction has apparent specificity, as demonstrated by the observation that some mouse cells transfected with and expressing human CD4 still cannot be infected with HIV. This demonstrates that infection requires more than just receptor binding.

When a retrovirus does bind to its appropriate receptor in a fusion-permissive cell, the virion particle is internalized. During the internalization process, the virion loses its membrane coat and the naked core begins to break down in the cytoplasm. At this point the process of proviral DNA generation directed by the reverse transcriptase is initiated (Fig. 20.5). This process can be summarized as follows. Using the tRNA hybridized to the PBS (located within the leader segment) as an RNA primer, the RT makes a complementary DNA in the 5 to 3′ direction, thereby creating a minus strand, U5 R LTR. This piece of DNA is known as "strong stop" (56). Utilizing the RNase activity, the RT digests the U5/R genomic RNA template. The strong stop DNA, along with the RT, thus makes the first of two "jumps" by hybridizing to the genomic RNA at the 3′ end, using the R genome as the homologous sequence. From here the remainder of the negative DNA strand is synthesized in the 5 to 3′ direction. The RNase activity now removes most of the remaining RNA genomic template except for a short stretch just 5′ to U3. This remaining small RNA piece is now used as the primer to create the second strong stop DNA, now consisting of U3, R, and U5 sequences. The 3′ PBS on the negative DNA strand is now cleaved by RNase activity, which allows the positive strong stop DNA to make the second primer "jump" and hybridize at the 5′ end of the minus DNA template, using the 5′ primer binding sequence as the homologous region. From here, the RT can complete the synthesis of the positive-strand DNA. In all, the RT reaction has taken a single strand of RNA with unique ends and created a double-stranded DNA species with duplicated LTRs.

Once this double-stranded DNA is created, it must be inserted into the host genome for successful continuation of the viral life cycle. This insertion is dependent on the virally encoded integrase protein (Fig. 20.6). At this point the integrase directs both the viral DNA and a piece of the host DNA to undergo a specific cleavage that creates staggered ends on both pieces of DNA. This reaction is accompanied by deletion of two base pairs from each end of the viral DNA and by duplication of four to six base pairs at the site of the host DNA cleavage. Following this reaction, the DNA is inserted and ligated into the chromosomal DNA. Recent stud-

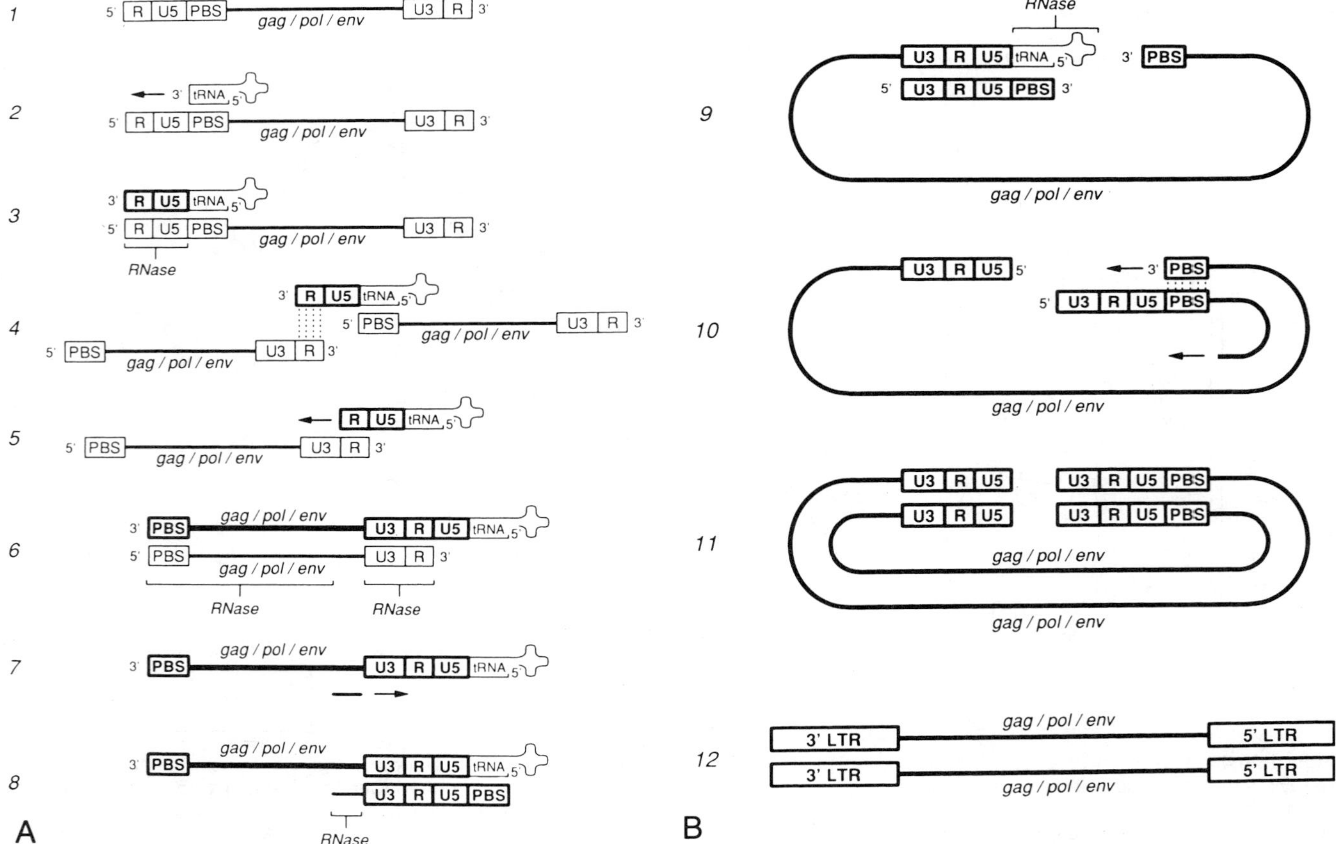

Figure 20.5. Reverse transcription. From a single stranded RNA genomic precursor, reverse transcriptase synthesizes a double-stranded DNA provirus ready for integration into host cell DNA.

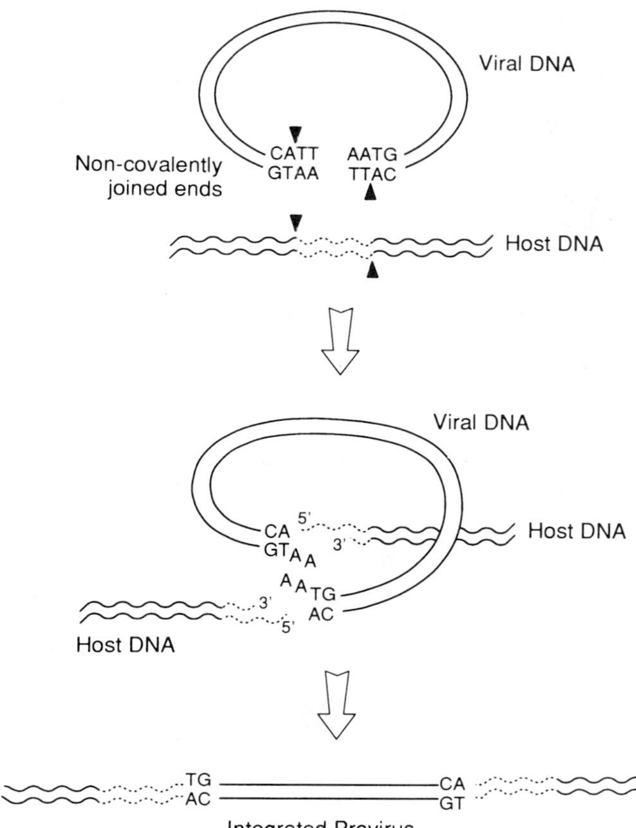

Figure 20.6. Integration. The newly reverse-transcribed double-stranded retroviral DNA genome and a piece of chromosomal DNA are specifically cleaved by the retroviral integrase protein. This is accompanied by a deletion of two base pairs from the retroviral genome and a duplication of four to six base pairs from the host DNA. Following retroviral genomic insertion into the cleaved host DNA, the DNA is relegated.

ies using purified integrase preparations have successfully demonstrated that the integrase protein is sufficient for performing all these functions (21).

Once integrated, viral transcription can proceed. As previously discussed, most retroviruses transcribe two species of mRNA. The full-length transcript can be used either as genomic RNA or as the message for the gag or gag/pol products. Factors determining how these two transcripts will be utilized have yet to be identified. The second mRNA species made by almost all retroviruses is a singly spliced message encoding the env gene. For most retroviruses the splicing reaction is dependent on host factors. Some retroviruses, such as those of the HTLV/BLV group and the lentiviruses, encode proteins that regulate the nucleus-to-cytoplasm transport of particular viral messages. The gag and the gag/pol messages are transcribed by free ribosomes and the precursor proteins localize to the cell membrane. This is directed by the fatty acid, myristic acid, which is added posttranscriptionally to the matrix protein (59, 131). At the cell surface it is the precursor gag protein that specifically interacts with and binds to the genomic RNA (168).

The envelope mRNA is transcribed by endoplasmic reticulum–associated ribosomes for eventual export to the cell surface, following extensive glycosylation in the Golgi body (123). How the gag precursor protein-reverse transcriptase complex associates with the envelope protein is still not known. The matrix protein assists in accommodating the cytoplasmic tails of the viral transmembrane envelope glycoprotein. Full processing of the gag precursors occurs at or soon after the budding of the nascent virion particle from the cell surface (173). The retrovirus can now begin a new replication cycle.

Before we leave the subject of the retroviral life cycle, several key points should be reemphasized. There is no other intracellular parasite that is so consistently efficient at integrating its entire genome into the host cell's DNA. The integration is stable and becomes a permanent genetic component of the cell and its progeny. Thus, not only are retroviruses passed down the lineage of a particular cell line, but when they infect germ cells, they become permanent genetic components of the organism. In humans, those proviruses constitute as much as 2 to 5% of the entire genome (148). Although certain DNA viruses also have the ability to integrate into host cell DNA, their persistence over a cell lineage is limited by the fact that they usually cause cell death. Retroviruses, on the contrary, are generally not cytopathic and have even developed strategies that potentiate the growth of the infected host cell line. Through these mechanisms, retroviral infection has become ubiquitous in almost all higher organisms.

Another key point to remember is that once a retrovirus has become integrated within a host cell chromosome, its transcription and replication are almost totally dependent on host cell factors. Thus, when the host cell is inactive, so is the virus. Alternately, cellular activating signals (i.e., steroid hormones in mammary tissue) will similarly activate retroviral transcription. The retrovirus has, however, evolutionarily developed some control over this process by selectively incorporating specific cellular enhancer sequences within the LTR (as previously described). This retrovirus-mediated control of transcription is taken to another level in the lentiviruses and in the HTLV/BLV group of retroviruses, where transcription is directly affected by virally encoded regulatory proteins.

The final point to be made is that retroviral integration does not always proceed without problems. Sometimes only part of the retroviral genome is incorporated into the host cell chromosome. If the incorporated segment includes the LTR and the appropriate packaging signals, a fusion transcript including both viral and cellular sequences could conceivably be made and packaged into a virion. This is exactly what occurs with the oncogene-transducing retroviruses, as will be described below.

Mechanisms of Oncogenesis

The currently accepted idea that neoplastic growth is a result of genetic alterations stems directly from the study of retroviruses (22, 82, 146) (Figure 20.7). Rous was the first to show that sarcomas in chickens could be induced by a transmissible agent (126). The concept that genetic changes were responsible for these tumors, however, was not appreciated until the isolation of mutant retroviruses that were conditionally defective (i.e., temperature sensitive) for transformation but not for replication (5, 80, 94). These viruses were uniformly found to have mutations in a 3′ extra open reading frame known as src (158). Through a series of experiments using recombinant viruses it was demonstrated that this intact src gene could act as a dominant inducer of the transformed phenotype (oncogene). Thus, for the first time it could be shown that a genetic element was directly responsible for transformation. The significance of these observations was further enhanced when it was demonstrated that the src gene hybridized with an endogenous cellular gene found in noninfected host cell DNA (137). The demonstration that normally occurring cellular genes could, in the correct context, lead to malignant transformation has shaped present-day ideas of how neoplastic growth is initiated and how it is maintained.

Since these early discoveries the study of other retroviruses has led to the identification of no fewer than 60 oncogenes (11, 12). Oncogenes are defined as genetic elements, that alone, or in cooperation with other oncogenes, transform normal cells. They are derived from their normal cellular homologues, the proto-oncogenes. Although the functions of these proto-oncogenes are quite variable, they all share the common property of being important for normal cellular growth and differentiation. It is not surprising, therefore, that either abnormal expression or mutation of these genes could result in neoplastic transformation. In the past 10 years much has been learned about the biochemistry of these proto-oncogene protein products and how they contribute to the malignant phenotype. This subject is dealt with in detail in Chapter 5. The following section of this chapter describes several different mechanisms by which retroviruses transform cells, and discusses several representative retroviruses that utilize these mechanisms.

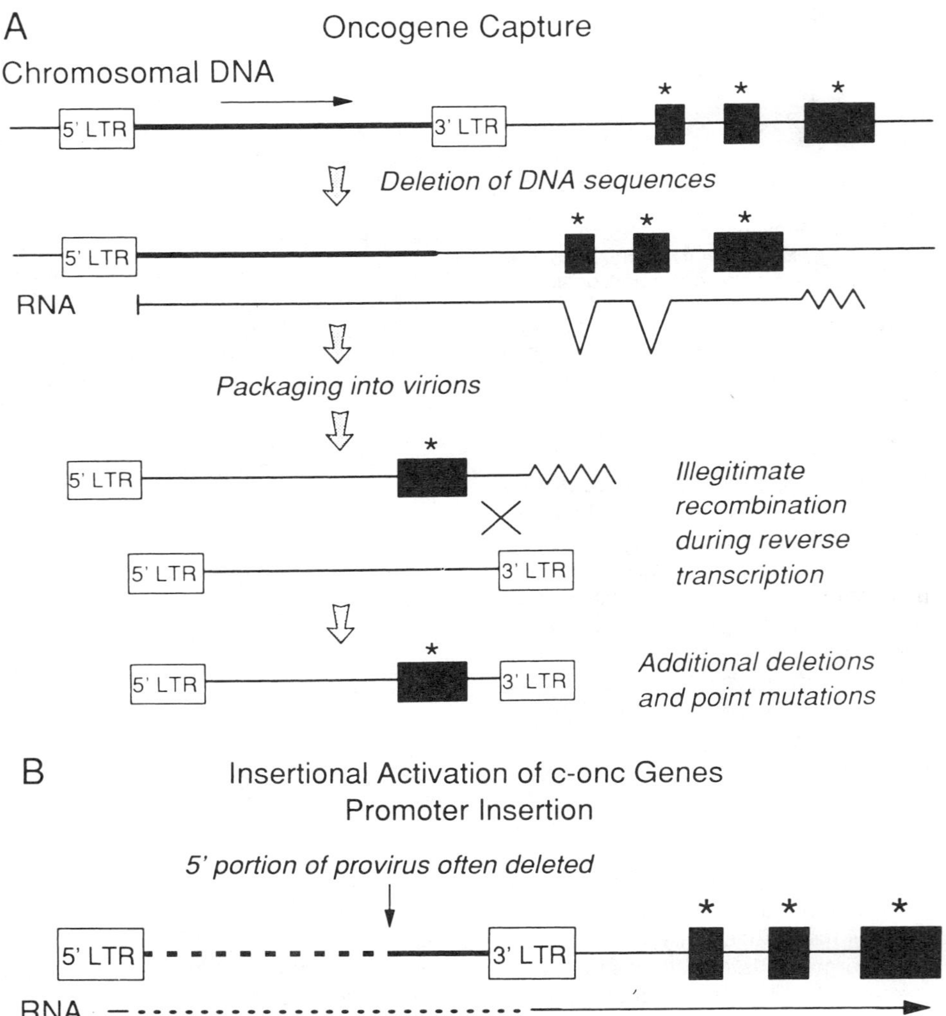

Figure 20.7. Four mechanisms of retroviral-induced oncogenesis. **A.** Oncogene capture. A mutated form of a cellular proto-oncogene (v-onc) is transferred (transduced) to a normal cell, thus inducing transformation (*c-oncogene). **B.** Insertional activation. There is a significant increase in the rate of proto-oncogene expression secondary to LTR directed transcriptional enhancement (*c-oncogene).

(figure continues on next page)

ONCOGENE TRANSDUCTION

The first oncogenic retrovirus to be described was the Rous sarcoma virus (RSV). It has become the prototypic virus representative of the group of retroviruses that transform cells by the delivery (transduction) of an oncogene (*src*, in the case of RSV) from the host cell to a target cell. These oncogene-transducing retroviruses have several common characteristics. First, these viruses are replication defective secondary to replacement of some or all of their structural genes by oncogenes (13, 64, 69). Ironically, despite RSV being the prototype of this group, it is the only member of this group that is replication competent. This is because the transduced *src* oncogene is located 3′ to the intact gag, pol, and env genes (27). Along with replication defectiveness, another common characteristic of this group of retroviruses is that they are acutely transforming. This means these viruses will produce tumors in vivo and in vitro within days to weeks of infection (37). In fact, retrovirally transduced oncogenes are the most potent carcinogens known. The final common property of this diverse group of viruses is that they cause the formation of polyclonal tumors. This probably reflects their high efficiency of transformation, so that any given tumor is made up of many different clones of cells that are the result of multiple different transformation events.

The life cycle of RSV is like that of the typical retrovirus described in the previous section. The difference, however, is that in the correct cell type, RSV induces malignant transformation. RSV induces formation of fibrosarcomas and histiocytic sarcomas when injected into young chickens (126). When these chicks (less than 1 month old) are infected, tumor formation is seen within 2 to 3 days. The tumors grow rapidly and in multiple locations (lungs, liver, spleen), and are eventually fatal. Similar tumors are seen when the same viral inoculum is used to infect adult chickens. These tumors, however, spontaneously regress if the bird's immune response is intact (9, 54).

RSV also has the capability of forming sarcomas in mammals, especially if young animals are inoculated. Tumors, however, only occasionally form, and usually only at the sites

C Growth Stimulation and Two-step Oncogenesis

RBC precursor

Step 1

Involves the interaction of a modified viral ($SFFV_p$) env product (p55) with the EPO receptor

polycythemia (neither immortal nor transformed)

SFFV

Step 2

SFFV or FrMuLV proviral integrations into Spi-1 and p53

Erythroleukemia (Immortal and transformed)

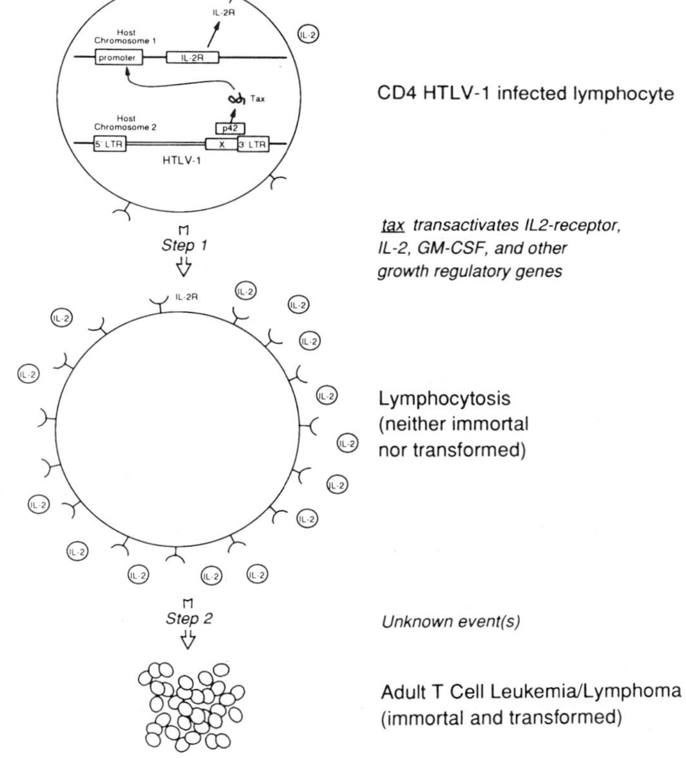

Figure 20.7. *(continued)* **C.** Growth stimulation plus two-step oncogenesis. A mutated env protein from the defective SFFV binds to the erythropoietin (EPO) receptor, causing an erythrocyte hyperplasia. This increases the susceptible target population to the actual transforming event, a retroviral insertional disruption of the Spi-I or p53 gene. (SFFV, spleen focus–forming virus; FrMuLV, Friend murine leukemia virus). **D.** Transactivation. The viral transactivating protein (tax in the case of HTLV-I) causes expansion of the potential target population through transactivation of growth regulatory genes. Some unknown second event then induces the actual transformation of a clone of these cells.

of inoculation. Furthermore, these tumors spontaneously regress as the animals grow older. This reduced oncogenic potential in mammals has been attributed to the inability of most RSV strains to replicate in mammalian cells in vivo (4, 16).

The virally encoded *src* gene (v-*src*) is expressed in all tumors and its central role in tumor induction is supported by the experimental observation that injection of the *src* DNA into young birds can induce the same tumors (45). Interestingly, these DNA-induced tumors generally regress, as is seen when the virus infects adult birds. Such regression demonstrates the importance of continued viral replication and infection of other host cells for the development of the full malignant phenotype.

Another example of an oncogene-transducing retrovirus is the Abelson murine leukemia virus (A-MuLV). The life cycle of this virus is more typical of other retroviruses that transduce oncogenes than is RSV, because A-MuLV is replication defective. A-MuLV originally arose in nude mice treated with prednisolone and the Moloney murine leukemia virus (M-MuLV) (1, 2). It was found that a transmissible agent from these animals induced lymphosarcomas in both adult and newborn nude mice (133). Unlike the well-described T-cell lymphomas induced by M-MuLV, however, these nude mice developed B-cell lymphomas. This discrepancy was finally explained by Scher and co-workers, who isolated a new retroviral strain from these mice, A-MuLV (129). A-MuLV induces a B-cell lymphoma in most strains of young mice, although adult animals seem to be resistant to tumor induction.

Molecular analysis of A-MuLV revealed a provirus almost 5,700 bp long with two open reading frames (124). The larger reading frame encodes a fusion protein consisting of the 5′ end of gag joined to the v-*abl* oncogene. One strain of A-MuLV utilizes the entire v-*abl* oncogene while another strain utilizes a v-*abl* that contains a 263 amino acid internal deletion (88). These two A-MuLV strains, therefore, respectively encode a p160 and a p120 gag-*abl* fusion oncogene respectively, both of which are transforming. Although the v-*abl* oncogene was clearly derived from the c-*abl* proto-oncogene, sequence analysis demonstrates that c-*abl* and v-*abl* differ substantially from each other (113). This demonstrates a very important principle underlying retroviral oncogene transduction. Never does the mere addition of a retroviral sequence to a cellular gene allow the creation of a transforming protein. Rather, all transduced oncogenes identified to date have exhibited some (often extensive) changes within the proto-oncogene sequence itself. Specific examples of some of these changes are noted in Table 20.3.

Another important principle highlighted by A-MuLV is that since it does not contain an intact gag, pol, or env gene it cannot replicate. A-MuLV does, however, infect and transform multiple target cells, both in vivo and in vitro. This is achieved through coinfection with a "helper virus." A helper virus is defined as a replication-competent virus that produces the structural components necessary for the packaging and infection of the defective transforming retroviral genome. In the case of A-MuLV, the helper virus is usually another murine leukemia virus, like M-MuLV. In some transformed cell lines, only defective transforming retrovirus is present. These cell lines are appropriately called "nonproducers," since no infectious virus can be made. These replication-defective transforming retroviruses can, however, be "rescued" and used to infect other target cells by the addition of a helper virus to the nonproducer cell line. The ability of retroviruses to package heterogeneous RNA genomes is a vitally important property that can be exploited in the laboratory for the creation of retroviral vectors, as will be discussed later.

Table 20.3. Differences Between v-onc and c-onc Genes

Often only a portion of the cellular oncogene is present in v-onc.

v-onc is derived from processed mRNA, which is devoid of introns and flanking sequences.

Loss of cellular control elements (promoters/repressors as well as RNA destabilizers) for some oncogenes (*myc* and *mos*) elevated level of expression in itself may be transforming.

Deletions/rearrangements may affect the structure of the protein itself:
- Loss of C-terminal Tyr-containing region of c-*src* causes loss of phosphorylation-mediated control by host cell kinases.
- v-*erb* B differs from EGF receptor by deletion of the extracellular domain.

v-onc genes are often fused to viral sequences important for transforming function:
- gag-*abl* acquires a myristilation signal → membrane localization important for transforming activity.
- v-*fms* is the CSF-1 receptor fused to the gag gene product, the latter providing a signal sequence for placement into the cell membrane.

Before we leave the subject of oncogene transduction, it is worth briefly reviewing several proposed mechanisms for how cellular sequences are incorporated into the retroviral genome. It is important to realize that the process of retroviral gene transduction has never been reproduced in the laboratory, presumably because it is such a rare event. Nevertheless, there are two leading hypotheses as to how this process may occur (Fig. 20.5*A*). In the most commonly cited hypothesis, a replication-competent retrovirus integrates into the host DNA 5′ to a particular proto-oncogene (147, 155). At some point a deletion occurs that removes the 3′ portion of the retrovirus and the 5′ portion of the proto-oncogene. This deletion leaves the remaining structural retroviral gene (usually the gag gene) in frame with the proto-oncogene. This allows the gag/proto-oncogene fusion transcript to be generated. This transcript then undergoes processing, including intron splicing, and is packaged into a virion along with a wild type retroviral genome. On subsequent infection of another cell, these two RNA species undergo RT-mediated recombination between their 3′ ends. This places a 3′ LTR onto the end of the transduced oncogene, thus allowing this defective, but oncogene-containing genome to be integrated into chromosomal DNA.

The alternative model of oncogene transduction suggests that an intact replication-competent retrovirus integrates just upstream of a proto-oncogene (Fig. 20.5*B*). On occasion, the viral genomic transcript is not appropriately terminated at the 3′ LTR termination signal but instead the RNA polymerase continues to read through into the open reading frame of the downstream proto-oncogene. This creates a full retroviral genomic RNA/proto-oncogene fusion message. At this point either a splicing event or a homologous recombination deletes the viral 3′ and proto-oncogene 5′ sequences thus creating the fusion oncogene message. This latter mechanism necessitates either areas of homology between proto-oncogene and viral sequences for recombination or appropriate splicing signals for the creation of the hybrid message. Of interest, there are extensive homologous sequences between some retroviral structural genes and proto-oncogenes. One such example is the CMII strain of the acutely transforming avian retrovirus subgroup, MC29. In this virus there is a stretch of nucleotides in the pol gene that is nearly identical to a nucleotide stretch in c-*myc*. This area corresponds directly with the junction of the gag pol/v-*myc* fusion junction in the CMII virus (161). This supports the possibility that a recombination event is responsible for the fusion protein. Alternately, Walther and co-workers have reported that the gag/v-*myc* junction in CMII corresponds to a splice acceptor site in c-*myc* (161). This site may have been used in conjunction with a potential splice donor site present in some retroviral gag sequences, thus generating the fusion message entirely by a splicing mechanism. In many other retroviruses, however, neither a splicing site nor homologous sequences can be found (74, 83). In summary, then, it seems most likely that oncogenes have been transduced by various retroviruses using either of the two mechanisms described above, and in some cases a combination of both.

INSERTIONAL ACTIVATION

The majority of transforming retroviruses are placed into the group called the leukemia viruses. (This name is actually inaccurate, since many of the acutely transforming, oncogene-transducing retroviruses also cause leukemias.) In contrast to the oncogene-transducing retroviruses, these viruses contain the entire set of structural genes and are replication competent. However, they are much less efficient at inducing in vivo transformation than are the transducing viruses and thus generally cause tumors only after long latent periods. Further, they do not induce transformation of cells in vitro. The tumors they do induce are usually monoclonal, again suggesting the rarity of the transforming event. In these virally induced tumors, the provirus is generally found within the vicinity of the proto-oncogene. It is thought that through its proximity to this gene, the proviral LTR functions as a positive enhancer of increased proto-oncogene expression. This mechanism of transformation is, therefore, often termed insertional or *cis* oncogene activation. The prototypic retrovirus in this group is the strain of avian leukosis virus (ALV) known as the lymphoid leukosis virus (LLV). LLV is passed from bird to bird by both vertical and horizontal transmission. After infection, B-cell lymphoblasts begin to accumulate in the bursa of Fabricius within 1 to 2 months (29, 106). Although most of the enlarged follicles regress with the natural involution of the bursa, some tumor nodules continue to grow. Within 6 to 8 months the chicken usually has developed a widespread metastatic lymphoma. Molecular analyses of these tumors have revealed several important points. First, although LLV appears to integrate randomly into host cell chromosomes, all tumor cells were found to have at least one provirus inserted in the vicinity of the c-*myc* gene (46, 58, 105, 151). Further, the level of c-*myc* transcription in these tumor cells was significantly elevated compared to normal cells. Another important feature of this mechanism of transformation is that once the provirus is integrated adjacent to the proto-oncogene in question (i.e., c-*myc* in the LLV example), continued transcription of viral sequences is no longer necessary to induce or maintain the malignant phenotype (105, 119). That transcription of the proto-oncogene seems to be initiated by the U3 region of the LTR is also characteristic of this mechanism of transformation. For this reason most retroviruses that act as enhancers for proto-oncogene expression are found to be oriented with the 3′ LTR upstream of the proto-oncogene (119).

The mouse mammary tumor virus (MMTV) represents another interesting example of a retrovirus that transforms cells via insertional activation of a proto-oncogene. MMTV was first detected over 50 years ago as a transmissible virus in the milk of a specific strain of inbred mice (102). These mice were known to have a very high incidence of breast carcinoma, with 90% of animals developing tumors by the age of 9 months. Animal breeding experiments showed that MMTV could be transferred horizontally or vertically as an endogenous provirus and that nearly 80% of mammary epithelium becomes infected. Although the MMTV proviral DNA has been shown to be randomly integrated in all tissue types, the breast tumor cells were consistently found to have one provirus integrated into a discrete area of chromosome 15 (110). Although examination of multiple tumors revealed that the exact integration site was always slightly different, it uniformly occurred around a discrete 30-kb sequence. In addition, the integrated provirus never interrupted this sequence (109, 154). This DNA segment has now been identified as the proto-oncogene, *int*-1 (153). It has now been established that *int*-1 is normally expressed only in the neural tube in midgestational embryos and in the testicular postmeiotic cells (72, 132). However, expression of this gene in the mammary carcinoma cells induced by MMTV suggests a role in the development of the transformed phenotype (110, 120).

The role of *int*-1 in the induction of mouse breast carcinoma was further suggested by the work of Tsukamoto and co-workers when they demonstrated that transgenic mice carrying an MMTV/*int*-1 transgene developed breast carcinoma (152). The specificity of *int*-1 expression for the development of breast tumors in transgenic mice must be questioned, however, since it has now been shown that either v-Ha-*ras*, c-*myc*, c-*neu*, or TGF-α, when driven by the MMTV promoter can induce the development of breast tumors in transgenic mice (17, 96, 134, 138). This ability of different genes to induce the same type of tumor suggests that the specificity of mammary tumor induction in these mice is a function of the viral LTR, and not the specific oncogene.

GROWTH STIMULATION AND TWO-STEP ONCOGENESIS

The defective spleen focus–forming virus (SFFV) and its helper, the Friend murine leukemia virus (Fr-MuLV), represent retroviruses with a unique mechanism of tumor induction. Infection of mice with Fr-MuLV and SFFV induces a polyclonal erythrocytosis associated with splenomegaly and hepatomegaly (55, 167). The cells, however, are neither immortal nor capable of forming tumors in nude mice. Maintenance of this erythrocytosis is dependent on continued viral replication. After a relatively long latent period one (or a few) of these proliferating clones of erythroblasts will transform into a tumorigenic clone, and the animal will develop frank erythroid leukemia. Individually, Fr-MuLV never induces the erythrocytosis stage of the disease and only rarely does it induce the erythroid leukemia when injected into nude newborn mice after a very long latent period. The defective SFFV always induces the erythrocytosis stage of the disease but this usually remits in time, because no more infectious virus is being made. Only rarely can helper-free SFFV induce progression to a full-blown erythroid leukemia (Fig. 20.5*C*).

Over the past several years, molecular analysis of these viruses has elucidated the mechanism of this two-stage oncogenic process. The erythroid hyperplasia occurs as a result of the synthesis of the one gene product of the defective SFFV, a mutant envelope protein known as gp55. Recent work has demonstrated that gp55 binds to and stimulates the erythropoietin receptor on erythroid precursors (91). It is through this mechanism that SFFV can induce erythroid hyperplasia (128). This represents a novel method by which a retrovirus stimulates cell growth. Although there are retroviruses known to transduce oncogenes that encode proteins that are homologues of normal cellular growth factors (i.e., v-*sis* and PDGF), this is the only known example of a structurally unique viral protein mimicking the function of a cellular protein.

The second component of the Fr-MuLV/SFFV transformation process can be explained by the observation that rearrangement of the cellular tumor suppressor gene, p53, occurs in a high percentage of Friend erythroleukemia cell lines (25, 103, 127). In most of these cell lines, the p53 gene disruption is secondary to SFFV (or, to a lesser extent, Fr-MuLV) proviral integration. In these tumor cells, p53 protein is either entirely absent or mutated. This concept of insertional mutagenesis of a tumor suppressor gene is another novel retroviral mechanism of transformation. These two mechanisms can be used to explain the synergistic ability of both SFFV and Fr-MuLV to induce erythroid tumors. SFFV provides a proliferation signal to expand the pool of potential target cells for transformation. Fr-MuLV, on the other hand, supplies the needed helper function for the SFFV to continue to infect new target cells. Since proviral integration tends to be a random event, the more integration events that can occur in a larger number of target cells, the greater is the likelihood of a specific disruption of the p53 locus and resultant cellular transformation.

TRANSACTIVATION

The human T-cell leukemia virus type I and II (HTLV-I and II) and BLV transform cells by an unknown but apparently unique mechanism. Like the *cis*-activation group of transforming retroviruses, HTLV-I is replication competent, carries no oncogene, and induces a monoclonal leukemia (adult T-cell leukemia, ATL) after a long latent period (15, 47, 114, 141, 171). Like the oncogene-transducing retroviruses, however, HTLV-I can immortalize lymphocytes in vitro and has no specific site of proviral integration in the transformed cell (Fig. 20.5*D*).

The transforming capability of these viruses resides in their unique 3′ genomic structure called the X region. This area is a 1- to 2-kb stretch of DNA containing several potential open reading frames. The X region has been implicated in the transformation process from the time it was first identified. This was based largely on the observation that many HTLV-I–transformed cell lines contained defective proviral genomes that encoded only the X region product. The X region of HTLV-I is known to encode at least three proteins, tax (p42), rex (p27), and p21 (33, 112, 135, 160). Although rex (a posttranscriptional regulator of viral RNA processing) and p21 (unknown function) may still be involved in the transformation process, most attention has focused on the tax protein. The role of tax in the viral life cycle is to transactivate the viral LTR, which results in a 100- to 200-fold increase in the rate of proviral transcription (135). Of even greater potential significance, however, is the ability of tax to transactivate endogenous cellular enhancers and promoters. These elements include the enhancer and promoters of the interleukine 2 (IL-2) receptor gene, the granulocyte-macrophase-colony-stimulating factor (GM-CSF) gene, the c-*fos* gene, the vimentin gene, and others (44, 68, 100, 112). It has been suggested that through transcriptional transactivation of some or all of these growth regulatory genes, tax plays a vital role in the transformation process.

In recent years three sets of experiments have added support to the idea that the X region and in particular tax is involved in oncogenesis. In the first experiment tax was shown to induce fibrosarcomas in transgenic mice when incorporated as the transgene (107). More recently, Lee Ratner and colleagues have shown that one can get leukemias of large, granular lymphocytes in transgenic mice expressing HTLV-I tax under the control of a T-cell-specific promoter (unpublished data). In the second set of experiments, tax was shown to induce soft agar colony formation when transfected into a partially transformed rat fibroblastic cell line, and to have the capability of cooperating with an activated *ras* oncogene to transform primary rat embryo cells (122, 142). These experiments clearly demonstrated the oncogenic potential of tax. The third experiment demonstrated the relevance of the X region to ATL, the in vivo disease. In this experiment the X region was inserted into a novel vector derived from the primate herpesvirus, Herpes saimiri. Infection of human bone marrow and cord blood with the H. saimiri/X region vector resulted in the immortalization of $CD4^+$ T lymphocytes that had the exact immunophenotype of ATL cells in vivo. These results provide compelling evidence that the X region, and tax in particular, is involved in the transformation process. It is probable, however, that these genes do not directly cause the development of ATL in vivo, but rather serve mainly as a proliferative stimulus to increase the number of potential transformation target cells, in much the same way that the gp55 envelope mutant of the SFFV does in the Fr-MuLV system. If this is the case, a second transforming event would be necessary for the full development of ATL. This is consistent with the observation that only a small percentage of HTLV-I–infected individuals develop lymphomas or leukemias. The search for this second event remains an active area of research in the field of human retrovirology.

Immunodeficiency

Besides neoplastic and degenerative neurologic diseases, the other major disease category associated with retroviral infection comprises immune deficiencies. The prototypic virus in this category is HIV, the etiologic agent of AIDS (8, 48). Patients with AIDS have an extraordinarily increased rate of developing high-grade lymphomas and Kaposi's sarcoma (KS). Most investigators believe that the relationship between HIV and the development of these tumors is indirect (43). Clinical experience with other types of both congenital and iatrogenically induced immune suppression has demonstrated a high rate of development of secondary tumors in these patients. These tumors are generally high-grade lymphomas, although other tumors, including KS, can be seen. The mechanism of tumor induction during immune deficiency is thought to be secondary to decreased immune surveillance resulting in inefficient destruction of early transformed cells. It has also been suggested that other viruses, particularly Epstein-Barr virus (EBV), have a direct role in tumor induction in the immune deficient state. It is of interest that many of the high-grade lymphomas in AIDS patients have been found to harbor EBV genomic DNA (53).

Some investigators, however, have suggested a more direct role for HIV in tumor induction. This is based on several studies that have demonstrated that when the tat protein of HIV (the transactivating protein) is placed into its transgenic mice, the animals develop KS-like lesions (158). In other experiments, tat protein applied directly to in vitro human endothelial cells induced a pattern of growth that morphologically resembled KS (40). The relevance of these findings to KS induction in humans with AIDS, however, remains unclear.

Before we leave the subject of immune deficiency, it is noteworthy to mention another example where tumor induction appears to be intimately related to immune deficiency. It has been known for some time that the Duplan strain of MuLV causes a severe immune deficiency disease in mice. The manifestations of this disease include a polyclonal B-cell proliferation resulting in lymphadenopathy, splenomegaly, hypergammaglobinemia, B- and T-lymphocyte functional abnormalities, increased susceptibility to infections, and malignant B-cell lymphomas (20, 84, 95, 115). In 1989 it was demonstrated that the viral stocks of the Duplan MuLV actually consisted of both a helper MuLV and a novel 4.8-kb defective retrovirus. This defective virus was shown to be the actual disease-inducing agent, since helper-free defective virus could cause the immune deficiency disease in vivo (36). Subsequent studies revealed that this defective retrovirus is oncogenic and contributes to the transformation of several B-cell clones in vivo. This transformation event results from the expression of a defective gag product (65). This oligoclonal pattern of proliferation apparently then leads to an immune deficiency state as an epiphenomenon of the leukemia or as a paraneoplastic syndrome (66). It is of interest to speculate whether other immune deficiency–inducing retroviruses may be found to be oncogenic in the future.

Endogenous Retroviruses

An important aspect in the relationship of a retrovirus to its host is that proviral DNA can become an inheritable genetic element of that organism if the retrovirus infects a germ cell. Indeed, it has now been estimated that as much as 0.5 to 1% of the mammalian genome is composed of sequences identifiable as retroviral proviruses (148). It is generally believed that these endogenous retroviruses have arisen rather late in evolution. This is based on the observation of huge variance in the type and number of endogenous retroviruses in closely related species, thus suggesting the acquisition of these viruses after divergence of closely linked species (26).

Endogenous retroviruses have several general properties. First, most of these viruses are defective, although a few endogenous retroviruses of mice and chickens can generate infectious virions. In principle, endogenous retroviruses are structurally similar to their exogenous counterparts in that they contain the gag, pol, and env genes, although they often have large deletions in their genomes, sometimes leaving only the LTRs intact. There are some endogenous retroviruses, however, that have only subtle mutations such as frameshifts or point mutations in gag and env initiation codons. Whether defective or not, it would appear that all these endogenous retroviruses were integrated into the host chromosome by the usual integrase-mediated process, as deduced from sequence analysis of their LTR–host DNA junctions.

A second property of these endogenous retroviruses is that not only are there significant differences in endogenous retroviral content between species, there are also significant variations within a given species. This suggests that endogenous retroviruses are evolutionarily unstable and thus not essential to their host. In vivo support of this hypothesis can be found by the existence of totally normal chickens and mice that were specifically bred not to contain endogenous retroviruses. It is still plausible, however, that some type of subtle evolutionary advantage is associated with the presence of specific endogenous retroviruses in a given organism (i.e., immunity against infection from certain pathogenic retroviruses). There is an example of an endogenous *env* locus in mice that protects against infection by a specific retrovirus (Cas BrE MuLV) by interfering with the receptor.

Another interesting feature of endogenous retroviruses is their variable level of expression in the host cell (156). This can span the spectrum from complete lack of transcription to production of infectious virions. There are several potential explanations for this. For example, different sites of integration within a given chromosome result in different local chromatin structure to control general levels of transcription of genes within that region. Another probable mechanism of transcriptional variation is postintegration chemical modification of the provirus. The best understood of these mechanisms is methylation of enhancer regions within the LTR, which thereby inhibits RNA polymerase transcriptional initiation (62). A third explanation for the variable expression of endogenous retroviruses probably relates to tissue tropism. Many endogenous retroviruses have been found to harbor glucocorticoid-responsive elements in their LTRs, much like the MMTV LTR. In humans, retroviral particles have been most often reported in humans in steroid-responsive tissues such as embryonic and reproductive organs. These particles have been seen in as many as 66% of all normal placentas and testicular tumors such as teratomas (6, 19, 32). It is also reasonable to speculate that other endogenous retrovirus LTRs will be found to contain additional tissue-specific enhancer sequences, thus accounting for much of the variable levels of expression seen with endogenous retroviruses.

The final general principle of endogenous retroviruses is that they are generally not pathogenic. This is not surprising, since any inherited genetic element that is deleterious to the host and that serves no vital function will be strongly selected against. MMTV is at least one exception, however, where an endogenous retrovirus can be shown to be directly responsible for disease induction. Another example of a pathogenic endogenous retrovirus can be found in the AKR mouse, a strain of animals bred specifically to select for a high rate of leukemia/lymphoma (145). It has now been demonstrated that through a complex multistage process of endogenous retroviral recombination, reinfection, and proto-oncogene *cis*-activation, most AKR mice develop a fatal T-cell lymphoma by the second year of life. Whether other examples of pathogenic endogenous retroviruses will be found, particularly in the human, is unknown. Numerous reports of retroviral particles in human tumor specimens have not been verified. For now it appears that few, if any, replication-competent human endogenous retroviruses capable of causing disease exist.

Whether or not infectious endogenous retroviral virions can be found in humans, it is clear that endogenous retroviral RNA is produced in all human cells. One specific type of human endogenous retroviral RNA accounts for .05% of the total placental RNA (79). The types of proteins encoded by these RNAs and their cellular functions remain speculative at this time. One particularly interesting endogenous retroviral transcriptional product is the RNA generated by ERV-3. The three RNA species known to be generated by this virus are 9, 7.3, and 3.5 kb in size. All three RNAs are initiated at the 5′ LTR and utilize the same splice donor site within the upstream leader sequence. The smallest RNA species is the natural subgenomic spliced env-coding RNA that is terminated in the 3′ LTR. The 9- and 7.3-kb RNA, however, extend through the 3′ LTR and are spliced into a human sequence measuring 5.5 and 3.8 kb, respectively (28, 78). The cellular function, if any, of these RNAs remains unknown. Nevertheless, the observation that all normal tissues express at least the 9.0- and 3.5-kb RNA species, while several different choriocarcinoma cell lines do not, is intriguing (78).

A final point about the potential ability of endogenous retroviruses to induce disease is notable. Up to this point we have described the potential for these viruses to encode gene products that would produce a dominant cellular phenotype. Endogenous retroviruses, however, through insertional mutagenesis could result in recessive phenotypes. Two examples of this are well described in mice, namely the D (dilute brown) and Hr (hairless) mutations. Genetic linkage mapping has placed the position of a specific endogenous murine retrovirus at the loci of these genes. Spontaneous reversions of these mutations are almost always associated with deletion of the provirus (75, 139). It is possible that some (or possibly many) variable human phenotypes are secondary to endogenous retroviral insertional mutations of a specific allele. With our growing understanding of tumor suppressor genes, like retinoblastoma and p53, it is conceivable that insertional mutagenesis of one of these alleles may eventually be identified as the recessive defect underlying some of the familial cancer syndromes.

Retroviral Vectors

As investigators begin to understand more about specific genes and their functions, the concept of gene therapy moves closer to reality (149). The problem of how to deliver a gene of interest to a target cell, however, remains a major obstacle. Traditional laboratory approaches to this problem have included inducing transient changes in the cellular membrane of a target cell, thus allowing passive influx of foreign DNA. These changes have been induced using either electrical current or chemicals (163). These methods are quite inefficient, however, allowing less than 1 in 104 to 106 cells to take up the DNA. Direct microinjection of DNA has also been used to introduce genes into target cells (136). This technique is hampered by the frequent acquisition by the target cells of multiple tandem repeats of the microinjected gene in the target cells. Furthermore, this technique is only useful for introducing foreign DNA into a few cells at a time.

Investigators have also used viruses such as the papillomavirus, adenovirus, and herpesviruses as vectors to carry the foreign gene into target cells (50, 104, 174). These vectors suffer from being large and difficult to manipulate genetically. In addition, they carry with them many of their own viral genes. Another problem with these vectors is that many of them are maintained episomally and therefore are not integrated into cellular DNA. Thus, the heterologous gene may not be subject to the same transcriptional controls active on endogenous genes.

Retroviral-based vectors can potentially overcome all these problems. Retroviruses are efficient at infecting multiple cells simultaneously and integrating a single copy of genetic information into the target cell genome. In addition, the host range of these viruses can be targeted to a particular cell type by changing the type of envelope on the virion ("pseudotyping"). Although many different types of retroviral vectors have been created, the majority have been derived from the Moloney murine leukemia virus (Mo-MuLV). The general principle underlying retroviral based vectors is that the structural components of the virion can be supplied to any given genomic RNA in *trans*, as long as the genomic

RNA contains the appropriate packaging signals. As described previously, most of these signals are contained in the nucleotide sequences in the 5′ leader segment and in the LTRs. Thus, at a minimum a retroviral vector must contain these elements. The gene of interest can then be inserted into the vector and be driven by the vector LTR or by a heterologous promoter (see Fig. 8.6).

Besides the vector itself, the other major components of this system are the genes encoding the structural proteins necessary for virion production. In most retroviral vector systems, these genes are stably introduced into cell lines ("packaging cell lines") such that these cells constitutively make viral proteins and virions. The structural genes, however, have been manipulated so that their RNAs do not contain the appropriate packaging signals, and thus the virions produced in these packaging cell lines do not contain RNA. When the vector, with the gene of interest, is introduced into these packaging cell lines, the vector RNA (which does possess the packaging signals) is incorporated into the virion. These virions then bud from the cell into the supernatant and can be collected and used to infect target cells.

The development of useful retroviral vectors has quickly progressed over the past 5 years. To date, Mo-MuLV-based vectors have been shown to efficiently infect and express heterologous genes in various cell types, including murine, canine, and human cells (61, 63, 87). Despite these early successes, the development of clinically useful retroviral vectors will have to address several key problems. One such problem is the generation of helper or wild-type viruses. This occurs through recombination between homologous areas of the vector and the structural gene expressors, such that a replication-competent genome with sufficient packaging signals for virion incorporation is generated. This problem has been largely eliminated by placing the different structural genes on different expressors, thus requiring multiple recombination events to correctly occur for the generation of wild-type virus. A second strategy to reduce the yield of helper viruses has been to minimize areas of homology between the vector and the structural gene expressor. One common method for achieving this is by replacing the native retroviral LTR of the structural gene expressor with a heterologous promoter or heterologous polyadenylation signal.

Another problem with many retroviral vectors is that in vivo gene expression does not always parallel in vitro expression. This is exemplified by a series of experiments utilizing a Mo-MuLV-based vector carrying the human adenosine deaminase (ADA) gene. Cells infected with this vector produced high levels of ADA in vitro. However, when these same cells were injected into an animal (mouse or monkey), the level of ADA production was significantly reduced (76, 77, 97, 164). The reason for this remains unexplained, but maintenance of a high level of expression of the transferred gene in vivo is a problem that must be overcome if retroviral vectors are to become clinically useful.

Another potential problem with the use of retroviral vectors is the possibility of insertional mutagenesis by the vector. With the use of helper virus–free Mo-MuLV-based vectors in primates, this concern is highly theoretical and seems quite unlikely. It is known that helper virus present in vector preparations resulted in three of seven monkeys getting lymphomas in one gene therapy study (34). Likewise, persistent viremia with replication-competent Mo-MuLV is an important factor in tumor induction in the mouse. With recent advances in the development of helper-free Mo-MuLV vectors systems, it seems unlikely that their vectors will induce tumors primates. The reason is that tumor induction is usually associated with multiple viral genomic insertions into the target cells, while retroviral vectors generally insert a single copy. Thus, Mo-MuLV vector–induced insertional mutagenesis of a primate cell leading to malignant transformation appears improbable in the absence of helper virus. Nevertheless, this theoretical problem remains a concern for vectors based on other retroviruses.

A final major problem associated with the potential clinical usefulness of retroviral vectors relates to their ability to carry only one or a few genes. These vectors, therefore, hold immediate clinical promise only for diseases caused by loss of function of a single gene, such as ADA deficiency, Lesch-Nyhan syndrome, Tay-Sachs disease, sickle cell anemia, and hemophilia. Unfortunately, most diseases, like cancer, are the result of a pathogenic process involving multiple genetic perturbations. It is unlikely, even with the discovery of tumor suppressor genes, that the addition of a single gene would completely correct the neoplastic phenotype. Thus, for cancer therapy, retroviral vectors hold most promise not for reversing the malignant phenotype but for delivering a gene that would inhibit the growth (or accelerate the destruction) of the neoplastic cells. One example of how such a strategy might work can be found in the ongoing experiments at the National Cancer Institute, where a vector carrying the tumor necrosis factor gene has been used to infect tumor infiltrating lymphocytes (TIL cells). It is hoped that these cells will then target the specific tumor they were derived from and elicit tumor cell death secondary to very high local levels of TIL-cell–produced tumor necrosis factor.

Conclusion

The study of retroviruses has contributed much to present-day knowledge in many areas of biology. Retrovirologists were the first to show that cellular transformation was the result of genetic perturbations. Through the study of these genetic changes came the discovery of oncogenes, and with it the realization that abnormal expression or mutations of a cellular gene could result in malignant transformation.

The study of the retroviral life cycle has also afforded new insights into other general concepts in molecular biology. Examples include new mechanisms of transcriptional regulation such as the glucocorticoid-responsive element in the MMTV LTR. Retroviruses have also contributed much to knowledge about the complicated mechanism of RNA splicing and factors that regulate it, such as the rev protein in HIV. Scientists have also learned novel aspects of translational control from retroviruses, such as the ribosomal frameshifting and termination suppression used to translate the polymerase protein from the gag/pol RNA. The study of gag and envelope processing and assembly has also taught us much about how macromolecules interact.

Outside of the advance in basic science knowledge, the study of retroviruses has had an even greater direct benefit. Secondary to the work in the late 1970s elucidating the basic biology underlying the life cycle of these viruses, it finally became possible to isolate two pathogenic human retroviruses, HIV and HTLV-I. In the short period since their discovery, more has been learned about HIV than about any other virus. This knowledge has already translated into the discovery of a clinically useful antiviral drug (AZT), with other drugs and vaccines in the clinical testing phase.

Finally, an important lesson learned from retrovirology has been the knowledge of how to utilize these viruses as vectors to carry heterologous genes to target cells. These vectors are uniquely equipped to deliver a single copy of the gene to multiple primary target cells, allowing integration into the host cell genome and expression of that gene at high levels. Through the use of these vectors, the age of gene therapy is at hand. It is an irony of nature that the very agents that are responsible for so many types of disease states may eventually be exploited therapeutically to eradicate these same diseases.

References

1. Abelson HT, Rabstein LS. Influence of prednisone on Moloney leukemogenic virus in BALB/c mice. Cancer Res 1970;30:2208.
2. Abelson HT, Rabstein LS. Lymphosarcoma: virus induced thymic-independent disease in mice. Cancer Res 1970;30:2213.
3. Albritton LM, Tseng L, Scadden D, Cunningham JM. A putative murine ecotropic retrovirus receptor gene encodes a multiple membrane-spanning protein and confers susceptibility to virus infection. Cell 1989;57:659.
4. Altaner C, Temin HM. Carcinogenesis by Rous sarcoma virus: XII. A qualitative study of infection of rat cells by avian sarcoma viruses. Virology 1970;40:118.
5. Bader JP. Temperature-dependent transformation of cells infected with a mutant of Bryan Rous sarcoma virus. J Virol 1972;10:267.
6. Baller K, Frank H, Lower J, Lower R, Kurth R. Structural organization of unique retrovirus-like particles budding from human terato-carcinoma cell lines. J Gen Virol 1983;64:2549.
7. Baltimore D. RNA-dependent DNA polymerase in virions of RNA tumor viruses. Nature 1970;226:1209.
8. Barré-Sinoussi F, Chermann JC, Rey F, Nugeyre MT, Chamaret S, Gruest J, Diouguet G, Axler-Blin C, Vezinet-Brun F, Rouzioux C, Rozenbaum W, Montagnier L. Isolation of a T-lymphotropic retrovirus from a patient at risk for acquired immune deficiency syndrome (AIDS). Science 1983;220:868.
9. Beard JW. Biology of oncorna viruses. In Viral Oncology. Edited by G Klein. New York: Raven Press, 1980, p 55.
10. Bielinska A, Krashow B, Nabel GJ. NF-κ B-mediated activation of the human immunodeficiency virus enhancer Site of transcription initiation is independent of the TATA box. J Virol 1989;63:4097.
11. Bishop JM. Viral oncogenes. Cell 1985;42:23.
12. Bishop JM. The molecular genetics of cancer. Science 1987;235:305.
13. Bister K, Vogt PK. Genetic analysis of the defectiveness in strain MC29 avian leukemia virus. Virology 1978;88:213.
14. Bittner JJ. Some possible effects of nursing on mammary gland tumor incidence. Science 1936;84:162.
15. Blattner WA, Kalyanaraman VS, Robert-Guroff M, Lister TA, Galton DA, Sarin PS, Crawford MH, Catovsky D, Greaves M, Gallo RC. The human type-C retrovirus, HTLV, in blacks from the Caribbean region, and relationship to adult T-cell leukemia/lymphoma. Int J Cancer 1982;30:257.
16. Boettiger D, Love DM, Weiss RA. Virus envelope markers in mammalian tropism of avian RNA tumor viruses. J Virol 1975;15:108.
17. Bouchard L, Lamore L, Tremblay PJ, Jolicoeur P. Stochastic appearance of mammary tumors in transgenic mice carrying MMTV/c-*neu* oncogene. Cell 1989;57:931.
18. Breathnach R, Chambon P. Organization and expression of eucaryotic split gene coding for proteins. Annu Rev Biochem 1981;50:349.
19. Bronson D, Saxinger W, Ritz D, Fraley E. Production of virions with retrovirus morphology by human embryonal carcinoma cells in vitro. J Gen Virol 1984;65:1043.
20. Buller RML, Yetter RA, Fredrickson TN, Morse HC III. Abrogation of resistance to severe mousepox in C47BL/6 mice infected with LP-BM5 murine leukemia viruses. J Virol 1987;61:383.
21. Bushman FD, Fujiwara T, Craigie R. Retroviral DNA integration directed by HIV integration protein in vitro. Science 1990;249:1555.
22. Cairns J. Mutation selection and the natural history of cancer. Nature 1975;255:197.
23. Chiu IM, Callahan R, Tronick SR, Schlom J, Aaronson SA. Major pol gene progenitors in the evolution of oncoviruses. Science 1984;223:364.
24. Chiu IM, Yasiv A, Dahlberg JE, Gazit A, Skuntz SF, Tronick SR, Aaronson SA. Nucleotide sequence evidence for relationship of AIDS retrovirus and lentiviruses. Nature 1985;387:364.
25. Chow V, Ben-David Y, Bernstein A, Benchimol S, Mowat M. Multistage Friend erythroleukemia: independent origin of tumor clones with normal or rearranged p53 cellular oncogenes. J Virol 1987;61:3777.
26. Coffin J. Endogenous viruses. In RNA Tumor Viruses. Edited by R Weiss, N. Teich H. Varmus, J. Coffin. Cold Spring Harbor, New York, Cold Spring Harbor Laboratory. 1984:p:1109.
27. Coffin JM. Structure of the retroviral genome. In RNA Tumor Viruses. Edited by R Weiss, N Teich, H Varmus, J Coffin. Cold Spring Harbor, New York: Cold Spring Harbor Laboratory, 1984, p 261.
28. Cohen M, Kato N, Larsson E. ERV3 human endogenous provirus mRNAs are expressed in normal and malignant tissues and cells, but not in choriocarcinoma tumor cells. J Cell Biochem 1988;36:121.
29. Cooper MD, Payne LN, Dent PB, Burmester BR, Good RA. Pathogenesis of avian lymphoid leukosis. JNCI 1968;41:373.
30. DeLarco J, Todaro GJ. Membrane receptors for murine leukemia viruses: characterization using the purified viral envelope glycoprotein, gp71. Cell 1976;8:365.
31. Dickson C, Puma JP, Nandi S. Identification of a precursor protein to the major glycoproteins of mouse mammary tumor virus. J Virol 1976;17:275
32. Dirksen E, Levy J. Virus-like particles in placentas from normal individuals and patients with systemic lupus erythematosus. JNCI 1977;59:1187.
33. Dokhelar MC, Pickford H, Sodroski J, Haseltine WA. HTLV-I p27rex regulates gag and env protein expression. J AIDS 1989;2:431.
34. Donohue RE, Kessler SW, Bodine D, McDonagh K, Dunbar C, Goodman S, Agricola B, Byrne E, Kaffeld M, Moen R, Bacher J, Zsebvo KM, Nienhuis AW. Helper virus-induced T-cell lymphoma in nonhuman primates after retroviral mediated gene transfer. J Exp Med 1992;176:1125–1135.
35. Dorfman T, Mamman F, Haseltine WA, Gottlinger HG. Role of the matrix protein in the virion association of the human immunodeficiency virus type envelope glycoprotein. J Virol 1994;68:1689–1696.
36. Douglas CA, Hanna Z, Jolicoeur P. Severe immunodeficiency cisease induced by a defective murine leukemia virus. Nature 1989;338:505.
37. Duesberg PH. Retroviral transforming genes in normal cells? Nature 1983;304:219.
38. Efstratiadle A, Posakony JW, Maniatle T, Lawn RM, O'Connell C, Spritz RA, DeRiel JR, Forget BG, Weissman SM, Slightom JL, Blachi AE, Smithiers O, Baralle FE, Shouldere CC, Proudfoot NJ. The structure and evolution of the human β-globin gene family. Cell 1980;21:653.
39. England JM, Bolognesi DP, Dietzschold B, Halpern, MS.Evidence that a precursor glycoprotein is cleaved to yield the major glycoprotein of avian tumor virus. J Virol 1977;21:810.
40. Ensoli B, Barillari G, Salahuddin SZ, Gallo RC, Wong-Staal F. Tat protein of HIV-1 stimulates growth of cells derived from Kaposi's sarcoma lesions of AIDS patients. Nature 1990;345:84.
41. Famulari NG, Buchhagen DL, Klenk HD, Fleissner E. Presence of murine leukemia virus envelope proteins gp70 and p15 (E) in a common polyprotein of infected cells. J Virol 1976;20:501.
42. Fan H, Verma IM. Size analysis and relationship of murine leukemia virus-specific mRNAs: evidence for transposition of sequences during synthesis and processing of subgenomic mRNA. J Virol 1978;26:468.
43. Fauci AS. The human immunodeficiency virus: infectivity and mechanisms of pathogenesis. Science 1988;239:617.
44. Fujii M, Sassone-Corsi P, Verma IM. c-fos promoter trans-activation by the tax1 protein of human T cell leukemia virus type 1. Proc Natl Acad Sci USA 1988;85:8526.
45. Fung YK, Crittenden LB, Fadly AM, Kung HJ. Tumor induction by direct injection of cloned v-*src* DNA into chickens. Proc Natl Acad Sci USA 1983;80:353.
46. Fung YK, Fadly AM, Crittenden LB, Kung HJ. One of the mechanisms of retrovirus-induced avian lymphoid leukosis: deletion and integration of the provirus. Proc Natl Acad Sci USA 1981;78:3418.
47. Gallo RC, Blattner WA, Reitz MB, Jr, Ito Y. HTLV. The virus of acult T-cell leukemia in Japan and elsewhere. Lancet 1982;1:683.
48. Gallo RC, Salahuddin SZ, Popovic M, Shearer GM, Kaplan M, Hayns BF, Palker TS, Redfield R, Oleske J, Safai B, White B, Fester P, Markham PD. Frequent detection and isolation of cytopathic retroviruses (HTLV-III) from patients with AIDS and at risk for AIDS. Science 1984;224:500.
49. Gannon F, O'Hare K, Perrin F, LePennec JP, Benoist C, Cochet M, Breathnach R, Royal A, Garapin A, Cami B, Chambon P. Organization and sequences at the 5′ end of a cloned complete ovalbumin gene. Nature 1979;278:428.
50. Grassman R, Dengler C, Muller-Fleckenstein I, Fleckenstein B, McGuire K, Dokhelar MC, Sodroski JG, Haseltine WA. Transformation to continuous growth of primary human T lymphocytes by human T-cell leukemia virus type I X-region genes transduced by a Herpesvirus saimiri vector. Proc Natl Acad Sci USA 1989;86:3351.
51. Green LM, Berg JM. A retroviral Cys-Xaa2-Cys-Xaa4-His-Xaa-4-Cys peptide binds metal ions: spectroscopic studies and a proposed three-dimensional structure. Proc Natl Acad Sci USA 1989;86:4047.
52. Griffin GE, Leung K, Folks TM, Kunkel S, Nabel GJ. Activation of HIV gene expression during monocyte differentiation by induction of NF-κ B. Nature 1989;339:70.
53. Groopman JE, Sullivan JL, Mulder C, Ginsburg D, Orkin SH, O Hara CJ, Falchuk K, Wong-Staal F, Gallo RC. Pathogenesis of B-cell lymphoma in a patient with AIDS Blood. 1986;87:612.
54. Gross L. The Rouse chicken sarcoma. In Oncogenic Viruses. 2nd ed. Oxford, England: Pergamon, 1970, pp 99–157.
55. Hankins WD, Kost TA, Koury MJ, Krantz, SB. Erythroid bursts produced by Friend leukemia virus in vitro. Nature 1978;276:506.
56. Haseltine WA, Kleid DG, Panet A, Rothenberg E, Baltimore, D. Ordered transcription of RNA tumor virus genomes. J Med Biol 1976;106:109.
57. Haseltine WA, Wong-Staal F. The molecular biology of the AIDS virus. Sci Am 1988;259:52.
58. Hayward WS, Neel BG, Astrin SM. Activation of a cellular on gene by promoter insertion in ALV-induced lymphoid leukosis. Nature 1981;290:475.
59. Henderson LE, Krutzsch HC, Oroszlan S. Myristyl amino-terminal acylation of murine retrovirus proteins: an unusual posttranslational protein modification. Proc Natl Acad Sci USA 1983;80:339.
60. Hidakka M, Inoue J, Yoshida M, Seiki M. Post-transcriptional regulator (rex) of HTLV-1 initiates expression of viral structural proteins but suppresses expression of regulatory proteins. EMBO J 1988;7:519.
61. Hock RA, Miller AD. Retrovirus-mediated transfer and expression of drug resistance genes in human haematopoietic progenitor cells. Nature 1986;320:275.
62. Hoffman JW, Steffer D, Gusella J, Tabin C, Bird S, Cowing D, Weinberg RW. DNA methylation affecting the expression of murine leukemia proviruses. J Virol 1982;44:144.

63. Hogge DE, Humphries RK. Gene transfer to primary normal and malignant human hemopoietic progenitors using recombinant retroviruses. Blood 1987;69:611.
64. Hu SS, Moscovici C, Vogt PK. The defectiveness of Mill Hill 2, a carcinoma-inducing avian oncovirus. Virology 1978;89:162.
65. Huan M, Jolicoeur P. Characterization of the gag/fusion protein encoded by the defective Duplan retrovirus inducing murine immunodeficiency syndrome. J Virol 1990;64:5764–5772.
66. Huang M, Simard C, Jolicoeur P. Immunodeficiency and clonal growth of target cells induced by helper-free defective retrovirus. Science 1989;246:1614.
67. Hull R, Covey SN. Does the cauliflower moseric virus replicate by reverse transcription? Trends Biochem Sci 1983;8:119.
68. Inoue J, Seiki M, Taniguchi T, Tsuru S, Yoshida M. Induction of interleukin 2 receptor gene expression by p40x encoded by human T cell leukemia virus type 1. EMBO J 1986;5:2883.
69. Ishizaki R, Langlois AJ, Chabot J, Beard JW. Component of strain MC29 avian leukosis virus with the property of defectiveness. J Virol 1971;8:821.
70. Jacks T, Varmus HE. Expression of the Rous sarcoma virus pol gene by ribosomal frameshifting. Science 1985;320:1237.
71. Jacks T, Townsley K, Varmus HE, Major J. Two efficient ribosomal frameshifting events are required for synthesis of mouse mammary tumor virus gag-related polyproteins. Proc Natl Acad Sci USA 1987;84:4298.
72. Jakobovits A, Shackleford GM, Varmus HE, Martin GR. Two proto-oncogenes implicated in mammary carcinogenesis, *int*-1 and *int*-2, are independently regulated during mouse development. Proc Natl Acad Sci USA 1986;83:7806.
73. Janese N, Goff SP. Domain structure of the Moloney murine leukemia virus reverse transcriptase: mutational analysis and separate expression of the DNA polymerase and RNAse H activities. Proc Natl Acad Sci USA 1988;85:1777.
74. Jansen HW, Bister K. Nucleotide sequence analysis of the chicken gene c-mil, the progenitor of the retroviral oncogene v-mil. Virology 1985;143:359.
75. Jenkins NA, Copeland NG, Taylor BA, Lee BK. Dilute (d) coat color mutation of DBA/2j mice is associated with the site of integration of an ecotropic MuLV genome. Nature 1981;293:370.
76. Kantoff PW, Gillio AP, McLachlin JR, Bordignon C, Eglitis MA, Kernan NA, Moen RC, Kohn DB, Yu SF, Karson E, Karlsson S, Zwiebel JA, Gilboa E, Blaese RM, Nienhuis A, O'Reilly RJ, Anderson WF. Expression of human adenosine deaminase in nonhuman primates after retrovirus-mediated gene transfer. J Exp Med 1987;166:219.
77. Kantoff PW, Kohn DB, Mitsuya H, Armentano D, Sieberg M, Zwiebel JA, Eglitis MA, McLachlin JR, Wiginton DA, Hutton JJ, Horowitz SD, Gilboa E, Blaese RM, Anderson WF. Correction of adenosine deaminase deficiency in cultured human T and B-cells by retrovirus-mediated gene transfer. Proc Natl Acad Sci USA 1986;83:6563.
78. Kato N, Larsson E, Cohen M. Absence of expression of a human endogenous retrovirus is correlated with choriocarcinoma. Int J Cancer 1988;41:380.
79. Kato N, Pfeifer-Ohlsson S, Kato M, Larsson E, Rydnert J, Ohlsson R, Cohen M. Tissue-specific expression of human provirus ERV3 mRNA in human placenta: two of the three ERV3 mRNAs contain human cellular sequences. J Virol 1987;61:2182.
80. Kawai S, Hanafusa H. The effects of reciprocal changes in the temperature on the transformed state of cells infected with a Rous sarcoma virus mutant. Virology 1971;46:470.
81. Kennel SJ, Del Villano BC, Levy R, Lesner RA. Properties of an oncornavirus glycoprotein: evidence for its presence on the surface of virions and infected cells. Virology 1973;55:464.
82. Klein G. The role of gene dosage and genetic transpositions in carcinogenesis. Nature 1981;294:313.
83. Klempnauer KH, Gonda TJ, Bishop JM. Nucleotide sequence of the retroviral leukemia gene v-myb and its cellular progenitor c-myb: the architecture of a transduced oncogene. Cell 1982;31:453.
84. Klinken SP, Fredrickson TN, Hartley JW, Yetter RA, Morse HC, 3d. Evolution of B-cell lineage lymphomas in mice with a retrovirus induced immunodeficiency syndrome, MAIDS. J Immunol 1988;140:1123.
85. Kohlstaedt LA, Wang J, Friedman JM, Rice PA, Steitz TA. Crystal structure at 2.5. A resolution of HIV-1 reverse transcriptase complexed with an inhibitor. Science 1992;256:1783–1790.
86. Kowalski M, Potz J, Basiripour L, Dorfman T, Goh WC, Terwilliger E, Dayton A, Rosen C, Haseltine W, Sodroski J. Functional regions of the envelope glycoprotein of human immunodeficiency virus type 1. Science 1987;237:1351.
87. Laneuville P, Chang W, Kamel-Reid B, Fauser AA, Dick JE. High efficiency gene transfer and expression in normal human hematopoietic cells with retrovirus vectors. Blood 1988;71:811.
88. Lee R, Paskind M, Wang JYJ, Baltimore D. Abelson (p160) murine leukemia virus (abMLV) *abl* gene. In RNA Tumor Viruses. Edited by R Weiss, N Teich, H Varmus, J Coffin. Cold Spring Harbor, New York: Cold Spring Harbor Laboratory, 1985, p 861.
89. Lever A, Gottlinger H, Haseltine W, Sodroski J. Identification of a sequence required for efficient packaging of human immunodeficiency virus type 1 RNA into virions. J Virol 1989;63:4085.
90. Levy JA, Hoffman AD, Kramer SN, Landis JA, Shimabukura JM. Isolation of lymphocytopathic retroviruses from San Francisco patients with AIDS. Science 1984;225:84.
91. Li JP, D'Andrea AD, Lodish HF, Baltimore D. Activation of cell growth by binding of Friend spleen focus-forming virus gp55 glycoprotein to the erythropoietin receptor. Nature 1990;343:762.
92. Madden PJ, Dalgleish AG, McDougal JS, Chapman PR, Weiss RA, Axel R. The TH gene encodes the AIDS virus receptor and is expressed in the immune system and the brain. Cell 1986;47:333.
93. Marguardt H, Gilden RV, Oroszlan S. Envelope glycoproteins of Rauscher murine leukemia virus: isolation and chemical characterization. Biochemistry 1977;16:710.
94. Martin GS. Rous sarcoma virus: a function required for the maintenance of the transformed state. Nature 1970;227:1021.
95. Masier DE, Yetter RA, Morse HC III. Retroviral induction of acute lymphoproliferative disease and profound immunosuppression in adult C57BL/6 mice. J Exp Med 1985;161:766.
96. Matsui Y, Halter SA, Holt JT, Hogan BL, Coffey RJ. Development of mammary hyperplasia and neoplasia in MMTV-TFGα transgenic mice. Cell 1990;61:1147.
97. McLachlin JR, Bernstein SC, Anderson WF. Separation of human from mouse and monkey adenosine deaminase by ion-exchange chromatography following retroviral-mediated gene transfer. Anal Biochem 1987;163:143.
98. McLachlin JR, Cornetta K, Eglitis MA, Anderson WF. Retroviral-mediated gene transfer. Prog Nucleic Acids Res Mol Biol 1990;38:91.
99. Mellon P, Duesberg PH. Subgenomic cellular Rous sarcoma virus RNAs contain oligonucleotides from the 3′ half and the 5′ terminus of virion RNA. Nature 1977;270:631.
100. Miyatake S, Seiki M, Yoshida M, Arai K. T-cell activation signals and human T-cell leukemia virus type 1–encoded p40x protein activate the mouse granulocyte-macrophage colony-stimulating factor gene through a common DNA element. Mol Cell Biol 1988;8:5581.
101. Moore DH, Long CA, Vaidya AD, Sheffield JB, Dion AS, Lasfargues EY. Mammary tumor viruses. Adv Cancer Res 1979;29:347.
102. Moore R, Dixon M, Smith R, Peters G, Dickson C. Complete nucleotide sequence of a milk-transmitted mouse mammary tumor virus: two frameshift suppression events are required for translation of gag and pol. J Virol 1987;61:480.
103. Mowat M, Cheng A, Kimura N, Berstein A, Berchimel S. Rearrangements of the cellular p53 gene in erythroleukemia cells transformed by Friend virus. Nature 1985;314:633.
104. Mulligan RC, Howard BH, Berg P. Synthesis of rabbit beta-globin in cultured monkey kidney cells following infection with a SV40 beta-globin recombinant genome. Nature 1979;277:108.
105. Neel BG, Hayward WS, Robinson HL, Frang J, Astrin SM. Avian leukosis virus–induced tumors have common proviral integration sites and synthetic discrete new RNAs: oncogenesis by promoter insertion. Cell 1981;23:323.
106. Neiman PE, Jordan L, Weiss RA, Payne LN. Malignant lymphoma of the bursa of Fabricius: analysis of early transformation. Cold Spring Harbor Conf Cell Proliferation 1980;7:519.
107. Nerenberg M, Hinrichs SW, Reynolds RK, Khoury G, Jay G. The tat gene of human T-lymphotropic virus type 1 induces mesenchymal tumors in transgenic mice. Science 1987;237:1324.
108. Nowinski RC, Fleissner E, Sarkar NH, Aoki T. Chromatographic separation and antigenic analysis of proteins of the oncornaviruses. J Virol 1972;9:359.
109. Nusse R, Varmus HE. Many tumors induced by mouse mammary tumor virus contain a provirus integrated in the same region of the host genome. Cell 1982;31:99.
110. Nusse RA, von Ooyen A, Cox D, Fung YK, Varmus H. Mode of proviral activation of a putative mammary oncogene (int-1) on mouse chromosome 15. Nature 1984;307:131.
111. Ohtan K, Nakamura M, Saito S, Nada T, Yoshiaki I, Sugamura K, Hinumia Y. Identification of two distinct elements in the long terminal repeat of HTLV-1 responsible for maximum gene expression. EMBO J 1987;6:389.
112. Okada M, Maeda M, Tagaya Y, Taniguchi Y, Tashigawara K, Yoshiki T, Diamantstein T, Smith KA, Uchiyama T, Honjo T, Yodoi JO. TCGF (IL 2)-receptor inducing factor(s): II. Possible role of ATL-derived factor (ADF) on constitutive IL 2 receptor expression of HTLV-1(+) T cell lines. J Immunol 1985;135:3995.
113. Opp C, Shore SC, Reddy EP. Nucleotide sequence analysis of testis-derived *c-abl* cDNAs: implications for testis-specific transcription and *abl* oncogene activation. Proc Natl Acad Sci USA 1987;84:8200.
114. Pandolfi F, Blattner WA, de Rossi B, Semenzato G, Strong DM, Gallo RC. T-cell leukemia-lymphoma virus and heterogeneity of chronic T-cell malignancies. Lancet 1982;2:1273.
115. Pattengale PK, Taylor CR, Twomey P, Hill S, Jonasson J, Beardsley T, Haas M. Immunopathology of B-cell lymphomas induced in C47BL/6 mice by dual tropic murine leukemia virus (MuLV). Am J Pathol 1982;107:362.
116. Pawson T, Harvey R, Smith AE. The size of Rous sarcoma virus mRNAs active in cell-free translation. Nature 1977;268:416.
117. Pawson T, Martin GS, Smith AE. Cell-free translation of virion RNA from nondefective and transformation-defective Rous sarcoma viruses. J Virol 1976;19:950.
118. Payne GS, Bishop JM, Varmus HE. Multiple arrangements of viral DNA and an activated host oncogene in bursal lymphomas. Nature 1982;295:209.
119. Payne GS, Courtneidge SA, Crittenden LB, Fadly AM, Bishop JM, Varmus HE. Analysis of avian leukosis virus DNA and RNA in bursal tumors: virus gene expression is not required for maintenance of the tumor state. Cell 1981;33:311.
120. Peters G, Lee A, Dickson C. Concerted activation of two potential proto-oncogenes in mouse mammary carcinomas. Nature 1986;320:628.
121. Poisz BJ, Ruscetti FW, Gazdar AD, Bunn FA, Minna JD, Gallo RC. Detection and isolation of type C retrovirus particles from fresh and cultured lymphocytes of a patient with cutaneous T-cell lymphoma. Proc Natl Acad Sci USA 1980;77:7415.
122. Pozzatti P, Vogel J, Jay G. The human T-lymphotropic virus type I tax gene can cooperate with the ras oncogene to induce neoplastic transformation of cells. Mol Cell Biol 1990;10:413.
123. Purchio AF, Jonanovich S, Erikson RL. Sites of synthesis of viral proteins in avian sarcoma virus-infected chicken cells. J Virol 1986;35:629.
124. Reddy EP, Smith MJ, Srinivason A. Nucleotide sequence of Abelson murine leukemia virus genome. Structural similarity of its transforming gene product to other onc gene products with tyrosine-specific kinase activity. Proc Natl Acad Sci USA 1983;80:3623.
125. Rosenberg SA, Asbersold P, Gornetta K, Kasid A, Morgan RA, Moen R, Karson EM, Lotze MT, Yang JC, Topalian SL, Merino MJ, Culver K, Miller AD, Blaese RM, Anderson WF. Gene transfer into humans: immunotherapy of patients with advanced melanoma using tumor-infiltrating lymphocytes modified by retroviral gene transduction. N Engl J Med 1990;323:570.
126. Rous FP. Sarcoma of the fowl transmissible by an agent separable from the tumor cells. J Exp Med 1911;13:392.
127. Rovinski B, Munroe D, Peacock J, Mowat M, Bernstein A, Benchimol S. Deletion of 5′-coding sequences of the cellular p53 gene in mouse erythroleukemia: a novel mechanism of oncogene regulation. Mol Cell Biol 1987;7:847.
128. Ruscetti SK, Janesch NJ, Chakraborti A, Sawyer ST, Hankins WD. Friend spleen focus-forming virus induces factor independence in an erythropoietin-dependent erythroleukemia cell line. J Virol 1990;64:1057.
129. Scher CD, Siegler R. Direct transformation of 3T3 cells by Abelson murine leukemia virus. Nature 1975;253:729.
130. Schiff LA, Nibert ML, Fields BN. Characterization of a zinc blotting technique: evidence that a retroviral gag protein binds zinc. Proc Natl Acad Sci USA 85:4 195;1988.
131. Schultz AM, Oroszlan S. In vivo modification of retroviral gag gene-encoded polyproteins by myristic acid. J Virol 1983;46:355.
132. Shackleford GM, Varmus HE. Expression of the proto-oncogene int-1 is restricted to

postmeiotic male germ cells and the neural tube of mid-gestational embryos. Cell 1987;50:89.

133. Siegler R, Zajdel S, Lane I. Pathogenesis of Abelson virus-induced murine leukemia. JNCI 1972;48:189.
134. Sinn E, Muller W, Pattengale P, Tepler I, Wallace R, Leder P. Co-expression of MMTV/v-Ha-ras and MMTV/c-*myc* genes in transgenic mice: synergistic action of oncogenes in vivo. Cell 1987;49:465.
135. Sodroski J, Rosen C, Goh WC, Haseltine W. A transcriptional activator protein encoded by the x-lor region of the human T-cell leukemia virus. Science 1985;228:1430.
136. Stacey DW, Allfrey VG. Microinjection studies of duck globin messenger RNA translation in human and avian cells. Cell 1976;9:725.
137. Stehelin D, Varmus HE, Bishop JM, Vogt PK. DNA related to the transforming gene of avian sarcoma virus is present in normal avian DNA. Nature 1976;260:170.
138. Stewart TA, Pattengale PK, Leder P. Spontaneous mammary adenocarcinomas in transgenic mice that carry and express MTV/c-*myc* fusion genes. Cell 1984;38:627.
139. Stoye JP, Fenner S, Greenoak GE, Moran C, Coffin JM. Role of endogenous retroviruses as mutations: the hairless mutation of mice. Cell 1988;54:383.
140. Summers J, Mason WS. Replication of the genome of a hepatitic B-like virus by reverse transcription of an RNA intermediate. Cell 1982;29:403.
141. Tajima K, Tominaga S, Suchi T, Kawagoe T, Komoda H, Hinuma Y, Oda T, Fujita K. Epidemiological analysis of the distribution of antibody to adult T-cell leukemia-virus-associated antigens: possible horizontal transmission of adult T-cell leukemia virus. Gann 1982;73:893.
142. Tanaka A, Takahashi C, Yamaoka S, Nosaka T, Maki M, Hatanaka M. Oncogenic transformation by the tax gene of human T cell leukemia virus type I in vitro. Proc Natl Acad Sci USA 1990;87:1071.
143. Taylor JM, Illmensee R. Site on the RNA of an avian sarcoma virus at which primer is bound. J Virol 1975;16:653.
144. Teich N. Taxonomy of retrovirus. In RNA Tumor Viruses. Edited by R Weiss, N Teich, H Varmus, J Coffin. Cold Spring Harbor, New York, Cold Spring Harbor Laboratory, 1984, p 509
145. Teich N, Wyke J, Mak T, Bernstein A, Hardy W. Pathogenesis of retrovirus-induced disease. In RNA Tumor Viruses. Edited by R Weiss, N Teich, H Varmus, J Coffin. Cold Spring Harbor, New York, Cold Spring Harbor Laboratory, 1984, p 785.
146. Temin HM. On the origin of the genes for neoplasia: GHA. Clowes memorial lecture. Cancer Res 1974;34:2835.
147. Temin HM. Do we understand the genetic mechanisms of oncogenesis? Keynote address for Honey Harbor meeting on cellular and molecular biology of neoplasia. J Cell Physiol Suppl 1984;3:1.
148. Temin HM. Reverse transcription in the eukaryotic genome: retroviruses, pararetroviruses, retrotransposons, and retro-transcripts. Mol Biol Eval 1985;6:455.
149. Temin HM. Retrovirus vectors: promise and reality. Science 1989;244:983.
150. Temin HM, Mizutani S. RNA-dependent DNA polymerase in virions of Rous sarcoma virus. Nature 1970;226:1211.
151. Temin HM, Rubin H. Characteristics of an assay for the Rous sarcoma virus and Rous sarcoma cells in tissue culture. Virology 1958;6:669.
152. Tsukamoto AS, Gross CR, Guzman RC, Parslow T, Varmus HE. Expression of the int-1 gene in transgenic mice is associated with mammary gland hyperplasia and adenocarcinomas in male and female mice. Cell 1988;55:619.
153. Van Ooyen A, Kwee V, Nusse R. The nucleotide sequence of the human int-1 mammary oncogene: evolutionary conservation of codon and non-codon sequences. EMBO J 1985;4:2905.
154. Van Ooyen A, Nusse R. Structure and nucleotide sequence of the putative mammary oncogene int-1; proviral insertions leave the protein-encoding-domain intact. Cell 1984;39:233.
155. Varmus HE. Form and function of retroviral proviruses. Science 1982;216:812.
156. Varmus HE. In Mobile Genetic Elements. Edited by J Shapiro. New York: Academic, 1983, p 411.
157. Vogel J, Hinrichs SH, Reynolds RK, Luciw PA, Jay G. The HIV tat gene induces dermal lesions resembling Kaposi's sarcoma in transgenic mice. Nature 1989;334:636.
158. Vogt PK. Spontaneous segregation of non-transforming viruses from cloned sarcoma viruses. Virology 1971;46:939.
159. von der Helm K, Duesberg PH. Translation of Rous sarcoma virus RNA in a cell-free system from ascites Krebs II cells. Proc Natl Acad Sci USA 1975;72:614.
160. Wachsman W, Gold DW, Temple PA, Orr EC, Clark BC, Chen IS. HTLV X-gene product: requirement for the env methionine initiation codon. Science 1985;228:1534.
161. Walther N, Lurz R, Patschinsky T, Jansen HW, Bister K. Molecular cloning of proviral DNA and structural analysis of the transduced *myc* oncogene of avian oncovirus CMII. J Virol 1985;54:576.
162. Weiss SR, Varmus HE, Bishop JM. The size and genetic composition of virus-specific RNAs in the cytoplasm of cells producing avian sarcoma-leukemia viruses. Cell 1977;12:983.
163. Wigler M, Pellicer A, Silverstein S, Axel R. Biochemical transfer of single-copy eucaryotic genes using total cellular DNA as donor. Cell 1978;14:724.
164. Williams DA, Orkin SH, Mulligan RC. Retrovirus-mediated transfer of human adenosine deaminase gene sequences into cells in culture and into murine hematopoietic cells in vivo. Proc Natl Acad Sci USA 1986;83:2566.
165. Wilson CA, Eiden MV, Anderson WB, Olah Z. The dual-function hamster receptor for amphotropic leukemia virus (MuLV), 10a1 MuLV, and Gibbon ape leukemia virus is a phosphate symporter. J Virol 1995;69:534–537.
166. Wolff JA, Yae JK, Skelly HF, Moores JC, Respess JG, Friedmann T, Leffert H. Expression of retrovirally transduced genes in primary cultures of adult rat hepatocytes. Proc Natl Acad Sci USA 1987;84:3344.
167. Wolff L, Ruscetti S. Malignant transformation of erythroid cells in vivo by introduction of a non-replicating retrovirus vector. Science 1985;228:1549.
168. Wong TC, Lewis RB, Bose HR, Kang CY. Assembly of avian reticuloendotheliosis virus: association of the core precursor polypeptide with the intracellular ribonucleoprotein complex. J Virol 1980;34:484.
169. Wong-Staal F, Gallo RC. Human T-lymphotropic retroviruses. Nature 1985;317:395.
170. Yamamoto KR. Steroid receptor regulated transcription of specific genes and gene networks. Am Rev Genet 1985;19:209.
171. Yoshida M, Miyoshi I, Hinuma Y. Isolation and characterization of retrovirus from cell lines of human adult T-cell leukemia and its implication in the disease. Proc Natl Acad Sci USA 1982;79:2031.
172. Yoshinaka Y, Katoh I, Copeland JD, Ozoszlan S. Murine leukemia protease is encoded by the gag-pol gene and is synthesized through suppression of an amber termination codon. Proc Natl Acad Sci USA 1985;82:1618.
173. Yoshinaka Y, Luftig RB. Murine leukemia virus morphogenesis: cleavage of p70 in vitro can be accompanied by a shift from a concentrically coiled internal strand ("immature") to a collapsed ("mature") form of the virus core. Proc Natl Acad Sci USA 1977;74:3446.
174. Zinn K, Mellon P, Ptashne M, Maniatis T. Regulated expression of an extrachromosomal human beta-interferon gene in mouse cells. Proc Natl Acad Sci USA 1982;79: 4897.

CHAPTER 21

Herpesviruses

JEFFREY I. COHEN

Seven herpesviruses have been isolated from humans, and an eighth herpesvirus-like DNA sequence has been identified in human tissues. Herpes simplex 1, herpes simplex 2, and varicella-zoster virus are members of the alphaherpesvirus subfamily. Cytomegalovirus, human herpesvirus 6, and human herpesvirus 7 are betaherpesviruses, and Epstein-Barr virus (EBV) is a gammaherpesvirus. A gammaherpesvirus-like sequence has been identified in tissues from AIDS patients with Kaposi's sarcoma; however, a virus has not yet been isolated. Two herpesviruses can immortalize human cells in vitro; EBV transforms human B cells and herpesvirus saimiri (a primate virus) transforms human T cells. Herpesviruses are ubiquitous in nature, and nearly every animal species is infected by at least one. The transforming animal herpesviruses include herpesvirus saimiri which induces fatal T-cell lymphomas in certain species of monkeys and rabbits, herpesvirus aeteles which causes T-cell lymphomas in tamarins and owl monkeys, gammaherpesvirus 70 which causes lymphoproliferative lesions in mice, and Marek's disease virus which induces T-cell lymphomas in birds.

Properties

Herpesviruses are enveloped virions which contain a DNA core surrounded by an icosahedral nucleocapsid and a tegument. The viral genome consists of linear, double-stranded DNA varying in size from 120 to 240 kilobase pairs, depending on the virus. The smallest herpesviruses contain approximately 70 unique open reading frames, while the largest contain about 210 open reading frames. Virions contain 30 to 35 structural proteins.

Infection of cells with herpesviruses begins with adsorption and fusion of the virion envelope with the cell membrane. The envelope glycoproteins are important mediators of adsorption and fusion. The viral capsid is released into the cytoplasm and transported to the nucleus, where the linear viral DNA circularizes. In lytic infection, immediate-early, early, and subsequently late viral genes are transcribed in the nucleus and their proteins are synthesized in the cytoplasm, while translation of host cell RNAs is inhibited. Early lytic replication is associated with irreversible cytocidal inhibition of host DNA, RNA, and protein synthesis. Virion DNA is replicated and assembled into nucleocapsids in the nucleus. Nucleocapsids undergo initial envelopment by budding through the inner lamella of the nuclear membrane. Viral proteins and glycoproteins modify the host cell's cytoplasmic membranes. Virions are released by exocytosis or by cytoplasmic deenvelopment and reenvelopment at the plasma membrane.

Herpesviruses have the capacity to establish latent infection as well as lytic infection. The capacity to establish latent infection in vivo and to reactivate from latency ensures a source of virus to infect previously uninfected persons. Herpesviruses are ubiquitous in most human populations. Almost all adults latently harbor herpes simplex 1, varicella-zoster virus, human herpesvirus 6 and 7, and EBV. Reactivation in adults results in transmission of virus to infants, children, or young adults, perpetuating nearly uniform adult infection and persistence of the virus over many generations. Reactivation from latent infection is controlled by cellular factors, although virus immediate-early genes mediate the initial reactivation from latency.

Oncogenic Features

Several features of herpesvirus replication are important for maintenance of latency and for oncogenicity. To be oncogenic, herpesviruses must be able to maintain their viral genome in the cell, avoid killing the cell, avoid destruction of the cell by the immune system, and activate appropriate cellular growth control regulatory pathways. Since EBV is the best-studied of the human herpesviruses that latently infects cells and has a strong association with human neoplasia, this virus will be used to illustrate the principles of herpesvirus infection relevant to oncogenicity (see Table 21.1).

First, viral DNA must be maintained in the cell. EBV establishes latent infection in B lymphocytes. B lymphocytes replicate so that the virus must have a way to ensure transmission to cell progeny (1). The EBV genome is usually maintained in B cells as a multicopy circular episome in the host cell, or the viral DNA can be integrated into the host genome. Episomes are formed by fusion of the direct repeat sequences, which are present at both termini of the linear genome present in virions (2). For example, the Namalwa Burkitt tumor cell line contains a complete copy of the entire EBV genome integrated into the host cell DNA and no additional episomal viral DNA. Analysis of the DNA sequence indicates that the viral genome is integrated into the host DNA at the terminal direct repeat sequence of the virus. There is no homology between the viral DNA and the cell DNA at the site of recombination (3).

Table 21.1. Diseases Associated with EBV Latent Gene Expression

Disease	EBERs	EBNA-1	EBNA-2	LMP-1	LMP-2
Burkitt's lymphoma	+	+	−	−	−
Nasopharyngeal carcinoma	+	+	−	+	+
Hodgkin's disease	+	+	−	+	+
Peripheral T-cell lymphoma	+	+	−	+	+
Lymphoproliferative disease	+	+	+	+	+

Second, a cell transformed by a virus can express only a limited number of viral genes, so as to avoid killing the cell and to avoid inciting destruction of the cell by the immune system. Replication of herpesviruses in cells results in inhibition of host cell protein synthesis and lysis of the host cell. Analysis of the EBV DNA sequence indicates nearly 100 possible gene products; however, latent infection of B cells with EBV results in expression of no more than 10 genes (reviewed in 4). This limited repertoire of gene products prevents frequent viral replication with death of the infected cell and limits the ability of the immune system to recognize a cell latently infected with the virus.

Third, specific viral genes interact with other cell proteins or directly transactivate other cell genes to provide additional functions necessary for immortalization. Proteins encoded by several DNA tumor viruses, including SV40, adenoviruses, and human papillomaviruses, have been shown to interact with cell proteins such as the retinoblastoma gene product, which appear normally to have tumor suppressor activity. In addition, proteins from these viruses also transactivate expression of cell genes that may be important to initiate or maintain neoplasia. While proteins from the EBV have not yet been shown to interact with tumor suppressor gene products, several proteins interact with cellular proteins to activate transcription of viral and cellular genes or to engage signal transduction pathways in the cell (see below).

Epstein-Barr Virus: An Oncogenic Human Herpesvirus

EFFECT ON B-CELL GROWTH IN VITRO

Infection of primary B cells with EBV in vitro results in transformation of the cells, which can then proliferate indefinitely (5). The resulting lymphoblastoid cell lines show several phenotypic changes that differentiate them from resting B cells. The lymphoblastoid cells are larger, grow in large, dense clumps (6) and secrete polyclonal immunoglobulin (7). B cell–activation antigens are also expressed on the surface of the lymphoblastoid cells, including antigens defined by monoclonal antibodies AC2, Ki-1, Ki-24 (8) and the CD23 cell surface protein (9, 10). While CD23 is expressed on the surface of EBV-transformed B cells, it is not present on normal resting B cells (11). The supernatant of EBV-transformed B cells contains a 35-kd protein thought to represent a soluble, cleaved form of CD23 (12). The soluble, cleaved form of CD23 may possess autocrine growth factor activity in EBV-transformed B cells (13). Other evidence that antibodies to CD23 can block the uptake of B-cell growth factor on the surface of the B cells suggests that CD23 could be a receptor for B-cell growth factor (14). EBV infection of Burkitt's lymphoma cells in vitro results in upregulation of a number of cellular proteins, including CD44, and two G protein–coupled peptide receptors (15).

GENE EXPRESSION IN TRANSFORMED LYMPHOCYTES

Six different EBV nuclear proteins, two membrane proteins, and two nontranslated RNAs are known to be expressed in latently infected B lymphocytes that have been growth transformed by EBV in vitro. The EBV nuclear proteins, EBNA-1, EBNA-2, EBNA-LP, EBNA-3A, EBNA-3B, and EBNA-3C make up the EBV nuclear antigen complex. EBNA-1 binds to the oriP sequence of EBV and allows the virus genome to be maintained as an episome in transformed B cells (16). Binding of EBNA-1 to oriP also has a small effect on transactivation of oriP as a *cis*-enhancer of transcription (17). Mutational analysis of EBNA-1 indicates that the carboxyl portion is required for the transactivation function (18). EBNA-1 transcripts are initiated from one of three different promoters. The Cp and Wp promoters are used to express EBNA-1 in lymphoblastoid cell lines in vitro, while the Fp promoter is used in tissues from Burkitt's lymphoma, nasopharyngeal carcinoma, and Hodgkin's disease (19–21). Transgenic mice expressing EBNA-1 develop B-cell lymphomas (22).

EBNA-2 is required for B-cell transformation by EBV. Expression of EBNA-2 in rodent fibroblasts reduces serum requirements (23). In EBV-negative Burkitt's lymphoma cells EBNA-2 causes growth in tight clumps and induces expression of two B cell– activation antigens CD23 (24) and CD21 (25). EBNA-2 also transactivates expression of the EBV genes LMP-1 (26) and LMP-2 (27), and c-*fgr* (28), a cellular gene which encodes a protein tyrosine kinase and is a member of the src gene family. EBNA-2 does not bind DNA directly but interacts with several cellular proteins. Transactivation of the CD23 promoter and the EBV Cp and LMP-1 promoters by EBNA-2 is mediated by the cellular DNA-binding protein Jκ, also referred to as CBF1 (31). This 63-kd GTG-binding protein plays a critical role in B-cell transformation by the virus (27, 32). EBNA-2 also interacts with the DNA-binding protein PU.1 to transactivate the LMP-1 promoter (33). The transactivation domain of EBNA-2 is essential for B-lymphocyte transformation (34). This domain interacts with transcription factor TFIIB and the TATA-binding protein–associated factor TAF40 (35). Recombinant viruses with EBNA-2 deletion mutants fail to transform B cells (36, 37). Mutational analysis indicates that at least four separate EBNA-2 domains are necessary for lymphocyte transformation. EBNA-2 is a major determinant of the type-specific transforming difference between the two naturally occurring types of EBV (36).

EBNA-LP is encoded by the leader sequence in EBNA-2 mRNAs (and possibly for EBNA-1 and EBNA-3 (38)). EBNA-LP localizes to the nucleus in linear arrays of granules, suggesting a possible role in RNA processing (39). EBNA-LP has DNA-binding activity (40) but has no discernible effects when expressed alone in rodent fibroblasts or B-lymphoma cells (24). Deletion of the carboxyl terminus of EBNA-LP markedly reduces the ability of the virus to transform B lymphocytes (41).

EBNA-3A, EBNA-3B, and EBNA-3C are encoded by three tandem open reading frames. These three proteins are distantly related (42, 43). EBNA-3C transactivates expression of CD21 (25), but not other B cell-activation antigens. EBNA-3A and EBNA-3C are essential for B-lymphocyte transformation in vitro (44), while EBNA-3B is dispensable (45).

Two latent membrane proteins, LMP-1 and LMP-2, are expressed in B cells that have been growth transformed by EBV. LMP-1 functions as a transforming oncogene when transfected into established rodent-cell lines (46–48). Expression of LMP-1 in EBV-negative Burkitt's lymphoma cells results in a change in morphology, and LMP-1 up-regulates expression of the B cell–activation antigen CD23, cellular adhesion molecules including ICAM-1, LFA-1, LFA-3 (49), vimentin (50), NF-κB (51, 52), and bcl-2 (52, 53). Induction of bcl-2 by LMP-1 in Burkitt's lymphoma cells protects the cells from apoptosis. LMP-1 is essential for transformation of B lymphocytes by EBV (54); the carboxyl terminus of LMP-1 provides a growth factor–like effect for transformation (55). Expression of LMP-1 in epithelial cells inhibits differentiation of the cells (56). Expression of LMP-1 in the skin of transgenic mice induces epithelial hyperplasia with increased expression of keratin 6 (57).

LMP-1 interacts with several cellular proteins. LMP-1 interacts with LAP1 and EB16, both members of the tumor necrosis factor (TNF)–receptor family (58). LAP-1 and EB16 bind to the p80 and p60 cytoplasmic domains of the TNF receptor, and LAP-1 also associates with CD40 and the lymphotoxin-β receptor. CD40, lymphotoxin-β receptor, and the TNF receptor are important components of signal transduction pathways. LMP-1 also associates with vimentin to form a patch in the cytoplasmic membrane of the B cell (59).

LMP-2 is a tyrosine-phosphorylated membrane protein that co-localizes with LMP-1 in B cells (60). Two forms of LMP-2 (LMP-2A and LMP-2B), which differ only in their first exon, are expressed in latently infected B cells. LMP-2 is expressed in latently infected peripheral blood lymphocytes in humans (61) and is dispensable for B-cell transformation by EBV in vitro (62, 63). LMP-2 is tyrosine phosphorylated and associates with the Lyn and Syk protein tyrosine kinases (64, 65). LMP-2 prevents lytic reactivation of EBV-infected primary B lymphocytes and calcium mobilization in response to cross-linking of surface immunoglobulin. This effect is mediated by the ability of LMP-2 to block protein tyrosine phosphorylation, with failure to activate the Lyn and Syk protein-tyrosine kinases (65, 66).

The two EBV-encoded RNAs, EBER 1 and EBER 2, are the two most abundant EBV RNAs in latently infected B cells; however, they have no role in latent or lytic EBV infection or cell transformation in vitro (67). These RNAs are not polyadenylated and form a complex with the nuclear antigen La (68).

Recent studies, using EBV mutants constructed with very large deletions (69, 70), indicate that only about 40% of the EBV genome is required to immortalize human B lymphocytes. These findings indicate that, except for the EBNAs and LMP1, most of the rest of the viral genome is dispensable for transformation.

EPSTEIN-BARR VIRUS GENES EXPRESSED DURING PRODUCTIVE INFECTION

Infection of epithelial cells with EBV results in productive infection with replication of virus and lysis of infected cells. Immediate-early genes encode regulators of virus gene expression, including ZEBRA, which acts as a switch to initiate lytic infection (Fig. 21.1 (71)). Early genes encode proteins that are involved in viral DNA synthesis, such as the viral

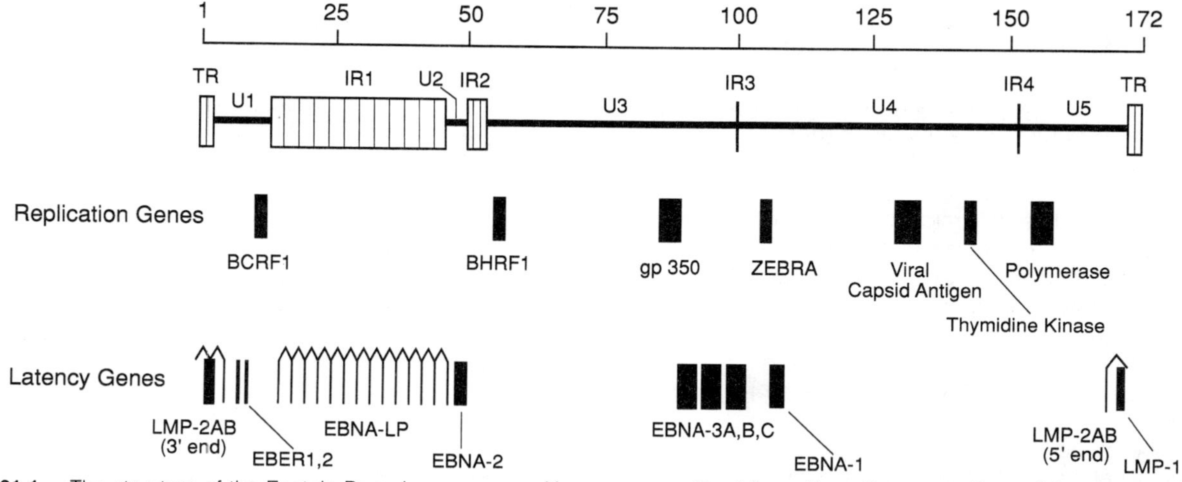

Figure 21.1. The structure of the Epstein-Barr virus genome with selected genes expressed during replication and latency. The Epstein-Barr virus genome consists of 172 kilobase pairs of DNA (*top line*) and contains unique regions (U1–5), terminal repeats (TR), and internal repeats (IR1–4) (*second line*). During replication of the viral genome about 80 genes are expressed (some of which are shown on the *third line*), while during latency only 10 genes are expressed (*fourth line*). The coding regions of EBNA-LP, LMP-1, and LMP-2AB are spliced from discontinuous portions of the genome. When the genome is circularized, LMP-2AB extends from the right end of the genome across the terminal repeats to the left end of the genome. (Adapted with permission from Cohen JI. Molecular biology of Epstein-Barr virus and its mechanism of B-cell transformation. In Epstein-Barr virus infections: biology, pathogenesis, and management. Moderated by SE Strauss. Ann Intern Med 1993:118:45–48.

DNA polymerase and thymidine kinase. Late genes encode structural proteins of the virus, including the viral capsid antigen and the major envelope glycoprotein gp350. Two viral genes that are homologues of cellular genes are expressed during productive infection and are important for survival of EBV-infected B cells.

The EBV BCRF1 protein is highly homologous to interleukin 10 and has interleukin 10 activity (72). Recombinant BCRF1 and BCRF1 secreted from EBV-infected cells inhibits release of interferon gamma from activated human peripheral blood mononuclear cells (72, 73). Since interferon gamma has been shown to inhibit outgrowth of EBV-infected B cells in vitro, expression of BCRF1 during lytic infection may prevent activation of the immune system with subsequent destruction of other latently infected cells. BCRF1 is dispensable for B-cell transformation in vitro (73).

The EBV BHRF1 protein is homologous to bcl2 (74), a cellular protein that is activated in follicular lymphomas and protects cells from apoptosis (75). BHRF1 co-localizes with bcl-2 in the cytoplasm and protects Burkitt's lymphoma cells from apoptosis (76). BHRF1 also prevents apoptosis induced by DNA-damaging agents such as cisplatin (77). BHRF1 is dispensable for B-lymphocyte transformation and virus replication (78, 79).

ANIMAL MODELS

Three types of animal models have been used to study EBV oncogenesis. In the first model, EBV-infected, growth transformed, lymphoblastoid cell lines produce B-cell tumors when inoculated intracerebrally into nude mice (80). Inoculation into subcutaneous tissue of nude mice usually is not tumorigenic; however, lymphoblastoid cell lines have induced tumors when inoculated into animals treated with antilymphocyte serum (81).

In the second model, inoculation of peripheral blood leukocytes from EBV-seropositive humans into mice with severe combined immunodeficiency results in development of B-cell lymphomas in the animals. The tumor cells are human in origin and contain EBV DNA. Inoculation of mice with peripheral blood leukocytes from EBV-seronegative humans results in engraftment of a functional human immune system, but without development of lymphomas (82). If these latter mice are subsequently inoculated with cell-free EBV, the animals develop immunoblastic lymphomas. Inoculation of lymphoblastoid cell lines into mice with severe combined immunodeficiency also results in lymphomas. These B-cell tumors contain EBV genomes and express the full complement of EBNA and LMP genes characteristic of latently infected, growth-transformed cell lines (83). This model has been useful to test the potential for agents (e.g., interleukin 2) to prevent development of EBV-associated lymphomas (84).

In the third model, cotton-top tamarins inoculated with a large dose of cell-free EBV develop multifocal large-cell lymphomas over the ensuing few weeks (85). These tumors contain EBV genomes, do not have chromosomal translocations (86), and express EBNA-1, EBNA-2, EBNA-LP, and LMP-1 (87). Tumors at different sites in an animal arise from different B-cell clones. At each site the tumors are monoclonal or oligoclonal in origin. This model has been used to test the efficacy of candidate EBV vaccines. Inoculation of cotton-top tamarins with recombinant vaccinia virus expressing EBV envelope glycoprotein 350 (88) or gp350 incorporated into immune-stimulating complexes (89) (iscoms) protects the animals from developing lymphoma when challenged with virus.

Clinical Aspects

Two types of human malignancies have been associated with EBV infection; those that occur shortly after EBV infection and those that occur long after infection. To understand the distinction it is necessary to consider normal EBV infection. EBV infection is usually spread by saliva. Virus infection is initiated in the oropharyngeal epithelium and spreads to subepithelial B lymphocytes. In the course of primary EBV infection, as many as several percent of the peripheral blood B lymphocytes are infected with EBV and have the capacity to proliferate indefinitely in vitro (reviewed in 90). The pharyngeal tonsils may be infiltrated with EBV-infected B lymphocytes. Natural killer (NK) cells (91), suppressor T-cells (92), and rapidly evolving HLA- and EBNA- (93, 94) or LMP-1 (95)-restricted cytotoxic T-cells control the latently infected B lymphocytes. T- and B-cell interactions release lymphokines and cytokines, giving rise to many of the clinical manifestations of acute infectious mononucleosis. After recovery, the fraction of B lymphocytes latently infected with EBV in the peripheral blood remains at 1 in 10^5 to 1 in 10^6. These lymphocytes or their precursors are the primary site of EBV persistence and a source of virus for persistent infection of epithelial surfaces.

B-lymphocyte tumors that occur early after EBV infection are usually lymphoproliferative processes in which latent virus infection in B lymphocytes is the principal cause of proliferation. Oral hairy leukoplakia (96) may be the epithelial counterpart. In contrast, Burkitt's lymphoma and nasopharyngeal carcinoma occur long after primary EBV infection; although etiologically related to EBV, viral gene expression may not be important to the growth of the clinically evident malignant-cells.

LYMPHOPROLIFERATIVE DISEASE

EBV is associated with B-cell lymphoproliferative disease in patients with congenital immunodeficiency. The X-linked lymphoproliferative syndrome (97) is an inherited immunodeficiency of males who have apparently normal cellular and humoral immune responses before infection with EBV (98). With primary infection, most of the patients die of fulminant hepatitis or another complication of infectious mononucleosis, one fourth develop malignant lymphoma, and a fourth, acquired hypogammaglobulinemia (97). EBV nuclear antigens and viral DNA have been detected in lesions from these patients. The mutation responsible for the X-linked lymphoproliferative syndrome has been linked to a restriction fragment length polymorphism, which may now allow prenatal diagnosis and identification of female carriers (99).

EBV has also been associated with fatal infectious mononucleosis in persons with no known underlying genetic predisposition (100, 101) and in patients with congenital immunodeficiencies (e.g., Wiskott-Aldrich syndrome and severe combined immunodeficiency (102, 103)). EBV lymphoproliferative disease occurs in patients who are immunosuppressed owing to bone marrow transplantation, solid organ transplantation, or AIDS (104). Most patients present with symptoms within 3 years of transplantation. The most common symptoms are fever, lymphadenopathy, and gastrointestinal symptoms. Lymphoproliferative lesions are most commonly in the lymph nodes, liver, lungs, kidney, bone marrow, or small intestine. Tumors in transplant patients are usually classified as lymphomas or immunoblastic sarcomas; some patients have hyperplastic lesions. The proliferating lymphocytes in these tumors generally do not have chromosomal translocations. Tumors in patients with AIDS are frequently Burkitt's or Burkitt's-type lymphomas and often have chromosomal translocations with c-*myc* rearrangements. B-cell lymphomas from immunocompromised patients generally do not contain p53 mutations unless they have the histologic features of Burkitt's lymphomas (105). The mortality rate in patients with acquired immunodeficiency and EBV lymphoproliferative disease is about 70%.

Monoclonal, oligoclonal, and polyclonal B-lymphocyte growth have been reported. Clonality can be determined by detection of immunoglobulin gene rearrangments using Southern blotting or staining of tissues for immunoglobulins. Clonality also can be assessed by analysis of the terminal repeats of the EBV genome. Monoclonal tumors are derived from a single EBV episome and have a fixed number of terminal repeats, while polyclonal tumors have varying numbers of repeats. Tissue from organ or bone marrow transplant recipients or from patients with AIDS who have EBV lymphoproliferative disease contains EBV genomes and shows expression of EBERs, EBNA-1, EBNA-2, LMP-1, CD23, ICAM-1, and LFA-3 (106, 107). The expression of these EBV genes, which are targets for cytotoxic T-cells, has important implications for therapy. Infusion of EBV-specific cytotoxic T-cells or unirradiated donor leukocytes has been effective in a few cases for treatment of EBV lymphoproliferative disease (108, 109). In one study, expression of EBER-1 in liver tissue preceded the occurrence of clinical EBV lymphoproliferative disease and provided a marker for patients at risk for this disease (110).

BURKITT'S LYMPHOMA

Burkitt's lymphoma is the most common childhood tumor in equatorial Africa and in New Guinea; in both areas the tumor is associated with holoendemic malaria. Areas with malaria control programs have a lower incidence of Burkitt's lymphoma. Burkitt's lymphoma occurs less frequently throughout the rest of the world. In Africa, most children (60%) present with tumors involving the face, while 30% have abdominal tumors; in the United States, children present at a slightly later age and 75% have abdominal tumors. Even in Africa or New Guinea, where the tumors develop at an earlier age and are closely associated with EBV infection, they occur at least several months to years after primary infection (111). Burkitt's lymphoma is classified as a high-grade malignant lymphoma with small, noncleaved cells. The cells are monoclonal B cells, which usually contain chromosome translocations. In contrast to many other childhood lymphomas, the peripheral blood and bone marrow are rarely involved with tumor.

Seroepidemiologic studies show a strong association between Burkitt's lymphoma and EBV in Africa (111). Over 90% of African Burkitt's lymphomas are associated with EBV, while only about 20% of Burkitt's lymphomas in the United States are associated with EBV. African patients with Burkitt's lymphoma often have high levels of antibody to EBV antigens (112). Antibody titers tend to correlate with the onset of tumors, an observation that is compatible with the hypothesis that virus burden is pathophysiologically linked to tumor. Tumor tissue contains EBV genomes, and virus can be recovered from the tissue (113). Burkitt's lymphoma tissues express EBERs and EBNA-1 but frequently do not express EBNA-2, EBNA-3, or LMP-1. The failure to express these latter three proteins may enhance tumor survival, since these proteins are targets for cytotoxic T-cells (94, 95). Cell lines derived from Burkitt's lymphoma that grow as individual cells express EBNA-1 but not EBNA-2, EBNA-3, EBNA-LP, or LMP-1. These cell lines do not express the B cell–activation antigen CD23 or the adhesion molecules ICAM-1 and LFA-3. However, when Burkitt's lymphoma cell lines are maintained in culture they tend to grow in tight clumps, with a lymphoblastoid cell–like morphology and express EBNA-1, EBNA-2, EBNA-3, EBNA-LP, LMP-1, CD23, and adhesion molecules (114).

Burkitt's lymphomas contain a chromosomal translocation which results in c-*myc* dysregulation. The most common chromosomal translocation is the 8/14 translocation which places a portion of the c-*myc* gene (chromosome 8) adjacent to the immunoglobulin heavy chain constant region (chromosome 14). The 8/22 translocation seen in other Burkitt's tumors places the c-*myc* oncogene (chromosome 8) at a distance from the lambda light chain constant region (chromosome 22). These latter translocations are often associated with mutations in the c-*myc* gene. The translocations result in deregulation and high constitutive c-*myc* expression. Transgenic animals that overexpress c-*myc* in breast epithelial or B-lymphoid cells develop monoclonal tumors (115, 116). Two conclusions emerge from these transgenic studies. First, c-*myc* is etiologically related to these experimental transgenic tumors. Second, dysregulated c-*myc* expression is not sufficient for malignancy.

Expression of c-*myc* (under a heterologous promoter) in EBV immortalized lymphoblastoid cell lines results in transformation of the cells with anchorage-independent growth and tumors when injected into immunodeficient mice (117). In addition, expression of c-*myc* in these cells results in down-regulation of LFA-1, an adhesion molecule, with loss of homotypic B-cell adhesion in vitro. This reduction in LFA-1 may be important for the escape of Burkitt's lymphoma cells from immunosurveillance and killing by cytotoxic T-cells, since LFA-1 is known to be involved in B-cell adhesion to NK cells and cytotoxic T-cells (118). Burkitt's lymphomas often contain p53 gene mutations (105).

EBV associated endemic Burkitt's lymphoma is thought to develop in steps (119). First, EBV infection may expand the pool of differentiating and proliferating B lymphocytes. Second, chronic holoendemic malaria may cause T-lymphocyte suppression and B-lymphocyte proliferation. Third, enhanced proliferation of differentiating B cells may favor the chance occurrence of a reciprocal c-*myc* (8/14 or 8/22) translocation placing c-*myc* partially under the control of immunoglobulin-related transcriptional enhancers with development of a monoclonal tumor.

NASOPHARYNGEAL CARCINOMA

Nasopharyngeal carcinoma is the second most common malignancy in Southern China or in emigrant Chinese from Southern China. Some northern native American populations also have a high incidence of nasopharyngeal carcinoma. North African populations have an intermediate incidence, and most Caucasian or black populations have a low incidence. The tumor presents with a metastatic lymph node in the jugular chain, with a bloody nasal discharge and nasal speech, or with unilateral secretory otitis media (secondary to compression of the eustachian tube). The third, fourth, fifth, and sixth cranial nerves may be destroyed by the tumor, which may also invade the cavernous sinus. Nasopharyngeal carcinoma frequently has a nonkeratinizing squamous cell histopathologic appearance.

The nonkeratinizing nasopharyngeal carcinomas are uniformly associated with EBV. Seroepidemiologic studies indicate that patients with nasopharyngeal carcinoma have high levels of antibodies to EBV antigens. Patients usually have elevated levels of IgA antibody to the viral capsid antigen (VCA) and early antigen (EA). EBV antibody titers are useful in screening patients for early detection of nasopharyngeal carcinoma (120). Nasopharyngeal carcinoma tissue contains EBV genomes in every cell. Biopsy tissue shows expression of EBERs, EBNA-1, LMP-1, and LMP-2 (21). EBNA-2, EBNA-3, and EBNA-LP are not expressed (121, 122). These tumors are monoclonal with regard to EBV infection, indicating that EBV infection precedes malignant-cell outgrowth at the cellular level. Unlike Burkitt's lymphoma, the association of EBV with nasopharyngeal carcinoma is uniform and universal.

HODGKIN'S DISEASE

Epidemiologic studies suggest an association of EBV with Hodgkin's disease. Patients with a history of infectious mononucleosis are at an increased risk of developing Hodgkin's disease (123). Patients with Hodgkin's disease generally have higher titers of antibody to EBV VCA than the general population (124); some patients with Hodgkin's disease have elevated antibody titers to EBV VCA and nuclear antigens before development of the disease (125). Tissues from about 40% to 60% of patients with Hodgkin's disease have EBV genomes. Cases of Hodgkin's disease from developing countries are more likely to contain EBV genomes (more than 90% of cases in some studies) than cases from industrialized countries (126,127). These lesions are usually monoclonal proliferations with the EBV genome present in Reed-Sternberg cells (128). EBV is more often associated with aggressive subtypes (nodular sclerosing, mixed cellularity) of Hodgkin's disease. Reed-Sternberg cells from tumors express EBERs, EBNA-1, LMP-1, and LMP2, but not EBNA-2 (129–131).

OTHER TUMORS ASSOCIATED WITH EBV

EBV genomes have been detected in patients with T-cell lymphomas presenting with fever, pneumonia, and numerous hematologic abnormalities. These patients have markedly elevated antibody titers to EBV VCA and early antigen (132). EBNA-1, LMP-1, and LMP-2 are expressed in peripheral T-cell lymphomas; however, EBNA-2 is not present (133). EBV DNA has also been detected in central nervous system lymphomas from patients with no underlying immunodeficiency (134), patients with carcinoma of the palatine tonsil (135), supraglottic laryngeal carcinoma (136), and angioimmunoblastic lymphadenopathy (137). EBV DNA and nuclear antigens have been detected in thymic carcinomas (138) and in T-cell lymphomas from patients with lethal midline granuloma (139).

EBV DNA has been found in leiomyosarcomas in AIDS patients (140) and viral RNA and EBNA-2 have been detected in smooth muscle tumors in organ transplant recipients (141). EBV DNA, RNA, and EBNA-1 (but not EBNA-2 or LMP-1) have been detected in 7% of primary gastric carcinomas, especially in undifferentiated lymphoepithelioma-like carcinomas (142).

Herpesvirus-like DNA in Patients with Kaposi's Sarcoma

Recently, herpesvirus-like DNA sequences were identified in Kaposi's sarcoma tissues from patients with AIDS (143). This DNA was found in nearly all of the Kaposi's sarcoma tissues examined, in 15% of lymph nodes and lymphomas from AIDS patients without Kaposi's sarcoma, but not in tissue biopsies from AIDS-free patients. This agent has been termed Kaposi's sarcoma–associated herpesvirus (KSHV), although a virus has not yet been isolated.

More recent studies have reported KSHV sequences in tissues from patients with classic Kaposi's sarcoma (elderly human immunodeficiency virus [HIV]–seronegative men with Mediterranean, Middle Eastern, or Eastern European backgrounds), African endemic Kaposi's sarcoma, and Kaposi's sarcoma in HIV-seronegative transplant recipients and HIV-seronegative homosexual men (144–147). KSHV DNA sequences were also found in uninvolved skin from many of the patients with Kaposi's sarcoma. These DNA sequences have been detected in peripheral blood mononuclear cells from patients with Kaposi's sarcoma, with or without HIV infection, but generally not in HIV–infected patients without Kaposi's sarcoma (148). KSHV sequences have also been found in association with EBV DNA in body cavity–based lymphomas of B-cell lineage (e.g., pleural, peritoneal, and pericardial lymphomas) in patients with AIDS (149). The KSHV sequences were not found, however, in other AIDS-associated lymphomas.

The KSHV DNA sequences are most closely related to herpesvirus saimiri and EBV; however, the sequences are distinct from these viruses and presumably are derived from a new member of the gammaherpesvirus subfamily. At present it is uncertain whether the DNA is present in the Kaposi's sarcoma cells or in adjacent lymphocytes and whether the virus bearing this DNA is the cause of the tumor or is colonizing the tumor.

Oncogenic Potential of Other Human Herpesviruses

Cytomegalovirus has not been shown to be oncogenic in humans. While viral antigens or viral DNA has been demonstrated in some tumors (e.g., Kaposi's sarcoma in AIDS patients, colon carcinomas, cervical carcinomas), a similar level of cytomegalovirus antigens or DNA indicative of latent infection in nontumor tissue from control patients favors the hypothesis that cytomegalovirus is not causally linked to these tumors.

While initial seroepidemiologic studies suggested a role for herpes simplex virus 2 in cervical carcinoma, there has been no convincing evidence for viral DNA or antigens in these tissues. More recent studies suggest that human papillomavirus may be a cause of cervical carcinoma and that herpes simplex virus 2 infections are seen in the same populations as are the human papillomaviruses. Herpes simplex virus 2 infection could be an adjuvant to human papillomavirus–mediated cell transformation.

Human herpesvirus 6 DNA has been detected in some lymphomas; however, it is unknown whether human herpes virus 6 is involved in the pathogenesis of these tumors or whether the virus is associated with the nonneoplastic lymphocytes.

Herpesvirus Saimiri

Herpesvirus saimiri is a member of the gammaherpesvirus subfamily that can immortalize human T cells (150). Human CD4 cells that have been immortalized with herpesvirus saimiri maintain T-cell receptors specific for various human and microbial antigens. Immortalized human CD8 cells can elicit cytotoxic T-cell responses. Transformed human T-cells express CD2, CD3, adhesion molecules, and activation markers (151).

Herpesvirus saimiri is not oncogenic in its natural host, the squirrel monkey; however, inoculation of the virus into several other species of monkeys (e.g., tamarins, owl monkeys, and marmosets) or New Zealand white rabbits results in fatal lymphoproliferative disease with T-cell leukemia, lymphoma, or lymphosarcoma. Inoculation of cotton-top marmosets with virus-free herpesvirus saimiri antigen preparations results in protection of the animals from tumors on challenge with virus (152).

References

1. Lindahl T, Adams A, Bjursell G, Bornkamm GW, Kaschka-Dierich C, Jehn U. Covalently closed circular duplex DNA of EBV in a human lymphoid cell line. J Mol Biol 1976;102:511–530.
2. Dambaugh T, Beisel C, Hummel M, King W, Fennewald S, Cheung A, Heller M, Raab-Traub N, Kieff E. Epstein-Barr virus (B95-8) DNA: molecular cloning and detailed mapping. Proc Natl Acad Sci USA 1980;77:2999–3003.
3. Matsuo T, Heller M, Petti L, O'Shiro E, Kieff E. Persistence of the entire Epstein-Barr virus genome integrated into human lymphocyte DNA. Science 1984;226: 1322–1325.
4. Kieff E, Liebowitz D. Epstein-Barr virus and its replication. In Virology. Edited by BN Fields, DM Knipe, RM Chanock, MS Hirsch, JL Melnick, TP Monath, B Roizman. New York: Raven, 1990, pp 1889–1920.
5. Henle W, Diehl B, Kohn G, zur Hausen H, Henle G. Herpes-type virus and chromosome marker in normal leukocytes after growth with irradiated Burkitt's cells. Science 1967;157:1064–1065.
6. Nilsson K, Klein G. Phenotypic and cytogenetic characteristics of human B-lymphoid cell lines and their relevance for the etiology of Burkitt's lymphoma. Adv Cancer Res 1982;37:319–380.
7. Rosen A, Gergely P, Jondal M, Klein G, Britton S. Polyclonal Ig production after Epstein-Barr virus infection of human lymphocytes in vitro. Nature 1977;267:52–54.
8. Rowe M, Rooney CM, Rickinson AB, Lenoir GM, Rupani H, Moss DJ, Stein H, Epstein MA. Distinctions between endemic and sporadic forms of Epstein-Barr virus–positive Burkitt's lymphoma. Int J Cancer 1985;35:435–441.
9. Sugden B, Metzenberg S. Characterization of an antigen whose cell surface expression is induced by infection with Epstein-Barr virus. J Virol 1983;46:800–807.
10. Thorley-Lawson DA, Nadler LM, Bhan AK, Schooley RT. BLAST-2 (EBVCS), an early cell surface marker of human B cell activation, is superinduced by Epstein-Barr virus. J Immunol 1985;134:3007–3012
11. Kinter C, Sugden B. Identification of antigenic determinants unique to the surfaces of cells transformed by Epstein-Barr virus. Nature 1981;294:458–460.
12. Thorley-Lawson DA, Swendeman SL, Edson CM. Biochemical analysis suggests distinct functional roles for the BLAST-1 and BLAST-2 antigens. J Immunol 1986;136: 1745–1751.
13. Swendeman S, Thorley-Lawson DA. The activation antigen BLAST-2, when shed, is an autocrine BCGF for normal and transformed B cells. EMBO J 1987;6:1637–1642.
14. Gordon J, Webb AJ, Walker L, Guy GR, Rowe M. Evidence for an association between CD23 and the receptor for a low molecular weight B cell growth factor. Eur J Immunol 1986;16:1627–1630.
15. Birkenbach M, Josefsen K, Yalamanchili R, Lenoir, G, Kieff E. Epstein-Barr virus induced genes: first lymphocyte-specific G protein-coupled peptide receptors. J Virol 1993;67:2209–2220.
16. Yates J, Warren N, Reisman D, Sugden, B. A *cis*-acting element from the Epstein-Barr viral genome that permits stable replication of recombinant plasmids in latently infected cells. Proc Natl Acad Sci USA 1984;81:3806–3810.
17. Reisman D, Sugden B. *Trans*-activation of an Epstein-Barr viral transcriptional enhancer by the Epstein-Barr viral nuclear antigen 1. Mol Cell Biol 1986;6:3838–3846.
18. Lupton S, Levine AJ. Mapping genetic elements of Epstein-Barr virus that facilitate extrachromosomal persistence of Epstein-Barr virus–derived plasmids in human cells. Molec Cell Biol 1985;5:2533–2542.
19. Deacon EM, Pallesen G, Niedobitek G, Crocker J, Brooks L, Rickinson AB, Young LS. Epstein-Barr virus and Hodgkin's disease: transcriptional analysis of virus latency in the malignant cells. J Exp Med 1993;177:339–349.
20. Sample J, Brooks L, Sample C, Young L, Rowe M, Gregory C, Rickinson A, Kieff E. Restricted Epstein-Barr virus protein expression in Burkitt's lymphoma is due to a different Epstein-Barr nuclear antigen 1 transcription initiation site. Proc Natl Acad Sci USA 1991;88:6343–6347.
21. Brooks, L, Yao QY, Rickinson AB, Young LS. Epstein-Barr virus latent gene transcription in nasopharyngeal carcinoma cells: coexpression of EBNA-1, LMP1, and LMP2 transcripts. J Virol 1992;66:2689–2697.
22. Wilson JB, Levine AJ. The oncogenic potential of Epstein-Barr virus nuclear antigen 1 in transgenic mice. Curr Topics Microbiol Immunol 1992;182:375–384.
23. Dambaugh T, Wang F, Hennessy K, Woodland E, Rickinson A, Kieff, E. Expression of the Epstein-Barr virus nuclear protein 2 in rodent cells. J Virol 1986;59:453–462.
24. Wang F, Gregory CD, Rowe M, Rickinson AB, Wang D, Birkenbach M, Kikutani H, Kishimoto T, Kieff, E. Epstein-Barr virus nuclear antigen 2 specifically induces expression of the B-cell activation antigen CD23. Proc Natl Acad Sci USA 1987;84: 3452–3456.
25. Wang F, Gregory C, Sample C, Rowe M, Liebowitz D, Murray R, Rickinson A, Kieff E. Epstein-Barr virus latent membrane protein (LMP-1) and nuclear proteins 2 and 3C are effectors of phenotypic changes in B lymphocytes: EBNA-2 and LMP-1 cooperatively induce CD23. J Virol 1990;64:2309–2318.
26. Wang F, Tsang SF, Kurilla MG, Cohen JI, Kieff E. Epstein-Barr virus nuclear antigen 2 transactivates latent membrane protein. J Virol 1990;64:3407–3416.
27. Zimber-Strobl U, Kremmer E, Grasser F, Marschall G, Laux G, Bornkamm GW. The Epstein-Barr virus nuclear antigen 2 interacts with an EBNA2 responsive *cis*-element of the terminal protein 1 gene promoter. EMBO J 1993;12:167–175.
28. Knutson JC. The level of c-fgr RNA is increased by EBNA-2, an Epstein-Barr virus gene required for B-cell immortalization. J Virol 1990;64:2530–2536.
29. Grossman SR, Johannsen E, Tong X, Yalamanchili R, Kieff E. The Epstein-Barr virus nuclear antigen 2 transactivator is directed to response elements by the Jκ recombination signal binding protein. Proc Natl Acad Sci USA 1994;91:7568–7572.
30. Henkel T, Ling PD, Hayward SD, Peterson MG. Mediation of Epstein-Barr virus EBNA-2 transactivation by recombination signal-binding protein Jκ. Science 1994;265: 92–95.
31. Ling PD, Rawlins DR, Hayward SD. The Epstein-Barr virus immortalizing protein EBNA-2 is targeted to DNA by a cellular enhancer-binding protein. Proc Natl Acad Sci USA 1993;90:9237–9241.
32. Yalamanchili R, Tong X, Grossman, Johannsen E, Mosialos G, Kieff E. Genetic and biochemical evidence that EBNA-2 interaction with a 63-kDa cellular GTG-binding protein is essential for B lymphocyte growth transformation by EBV. Virology 1994;204:634–641.
33. Johannsen E, Koh E, Mosialos G, Tong X, Kieff E, Grossman SR. Epstein-Barr virus nuclear protein 2 transactivation of the latent membrane protein 1 promoter is mediated by Jkappa and PU.1. J Virol 1995;69:253–262.
34. Cohen JI. A region of herpes simplex virus VP16 can substitute for a transforming domain of Epstein-Barr virus nuclear protein 2. Proc Natl Acad Sci USA 1992;89: 8030–8034.
35. Tong X, Wang F, Thut CJ, Kieff E. The Epstein-Barr virus nuclear protein 2 acidic do-

main can interact with TFIIB, TAF40, and RPA70 but not with TATA-binding protein. J Virol 1995;69:585–588.
36. Cohen JI, Wang F, Mannick J, Kieff E. Epstein-Barr virus nuclear protein 2 is a key determinant of lymphocyte transformation. Proc Natl Acad Sci USA 1989;86:9558–9562.
37. Hammerschmidt W, Sugden B. Genetic analysis of immortalizing functions of Epstein-Barr virus in human B lymphocytes. Nature 1989;340:393–397.
38. Sample J, Hummel M, Braun D, Birkenbach M, Kieff E. Nucleotide sequences of mRNAs encoding Epstein-Barr virus nuclear proteins: a probable transcriptional initiation site. Proc Natl Acad Sci USA 1986;83:5096–5100.
39. Wang F, Petti L, Braun D, Seung S, Kieff E. A bicistronic Epstein-Barr virus mRNA encodes two nuclear proteins in latently infected, growth-transformed lymphocytes. J Virol 1987;61:945–954.
40. Sauter M, Boos H, Hirsch F, Mueller-Lantzsch N. Characterization of a latent protein encoded by the large internal repeats and the BamH1 Y fragment of the Epstein-Barr virus (EBV) genome. Virology 1988;166:586–590.
41. Mannick JB, Cohen JI, Birkenbach M, Marchini A, Kieff E. The Epstein-Barr virus nuclear protein encoded by the leader of the EBNA RNAs is important in B lymphocyte transformation. J Virol 1991;65:6826–6837.
42. Petti L, Kieff E. A sixth Epstein-Barr virus nuclear protein (EBNA3B) is expressed in latently infected growth-transformed lymphocytes. J Virol 1988;62:2173–2178.
43. Petti L, Sample J, Wang F, Kieff E. A fifth Epstein-Barr virus nuclear protein (EBNA3C) is expressed in latently infected growth-transformed lymphocytes. J Virol 1988;62: 1330–1338.
44. Tomkinson B, Robertson E, Kieff E. Epstein-Barr virus nuclear proteins (EBNA) 3A and 3C are essential for B lymphocyte growth transformation. J Virol 1993;67: 2014–2025.
45. Tomkinson B, Kieff E. Use of second-site homologous recombination to demonstrate that Epstein-Barr virus nuclear protein 3B is not important for lymphocyte infection or growth transformation. J Virol 1992;66:2893–2903.
46. Baichwal VR, Sugden B. Transformation of Balb 3T3 cells by the BNLF-1 gene of Epstein-Barr virus. Oncogene 1988;2:461–467.
47. Wang D, Liebowitz D, Kieff E. An EBV membrane protein expressed in immortalized lymphocytes transforms established rodent-cells. Cell 1985;43:831–840
48. Moorthy RK, Thorley-Lawson DA. All three domains of the Epstein-Barr virus–encoded latent membrane protein LMP-1 are required for transformation of Rat-1 fibroblasts. J Virol 1993;67:1638–1646.
49. Wang D, Liebowitz D, Wang F, Gregory C, Rickinson A, Larson R, Springer T, Kieff E. Epstein-Barr virus latent membrane protein alters the human B-lymphocyte phenotype: deletion of the amino terminus abolishes activity. J Virol 1988;62:4173–4184.
50. Birkenbach M, Liebowitz D, Wang F, Sample J, Kieff E. Epstein-Barr virus latent infection membrane protein increases vimentin expression in human B-cell lines. J Virol 1989;63:4079–4084.
51. Laherty C, Hu H, Opipari A, Wang F, Dixit V. The Epstein-Barr virus LMP-1 gene product induces A20 zinc finger protein expression by activating nuclear factor, κB. J Biol Chem 1992;1267:24157–24160.
52. Rowe M, Peng-Pilon M, Huen DS, Hardy R, Croom-Carter D, Lundgren E, Rickinson, AB. Upregulation of bcl-2 by the Epstein-Barr virus latent membrane protein LMP1: a B-cell specific response that is delayed relative to NF-KB activation and to induction of cell surface markers. J Virol 1994;68:5602–5612.
53. Henderson S, Rowe M, Gregory CD, Croom-Carter D, Wang F, Longnecker R, Kieff E, Rickinson AB. Induction of bcl-2 expression by Epstein-Barr virus latent membrane protein 1 protects infected B cells from programmed cell death. Cell 1991;65: 1107–1115.
54. Kaye KM, Izumi KM, Kieff E. Epstein-Barr virus latent membrane protein 1 is essential for B-lymphocyte growth transformation. Proc Natl Acad Sci USA 1993;90: 9150–9154.
55. Kaye KM, Izumi KM, Mosialos G, Kieff, E. The Epstein-Barr virus LMP-1 cytoplasmic carboxy terminus is essential for B-lymphocyte transformation: fibroblast cocultivation complements a critical function within the terminal 155 residues. J Virol 1995;69: 675–683.
56. Dawson CW, Rickinson AB, Young LS. Epstein-Barr virus latent membrane protein inhibits human epithelial cell differentiation. Nature 1990;344:777–780.
57. Wilson JB, Weinberg W, Johnson R, Yuspa S, Levine AJ. Expression of the BNLF-1 oncogene of Epstein-Barr virus in the skin of transgenic mice induces hyperplasia and aberrant expression of keratin 6. Cell 1990;61:1315–1327.
58. Mosialos G, Birkenbach M, Yalamanchili R, VanArsdale T, Ware C, Kieff E. The Epstein-Barr virus transforming protein LMP1 engages signaling proteins for the tumor necrosis factor receptor family. Cell 1995;80:389–399.
59. Liebowitz D, Kopan R, Fuchs E, Sample J, Kieff E. An Epstein-Barr virus transforming protein associates with vimentin in lymphocytes. Molec Cell Biol 1987;7:2299–2308.
60. Longnecker R, Drucker B, Roberts TM, Kieff E. An Epstein-Barr virus protein associated with cell growth transformation interacts with a tyrosine kinase. J Virol 1991;65: 3681–3692.
61. Qu L, Rowe DT. Epstein-Barr virus latent gene expression in uncultured peripheral blood lymphocytes. J Virol 1992;66:3715–3724.
62. Kim O-J, Yates JL. Mutants of Epstein-Barr virus with a selectable marker disrupting the TP gene transform B cells and replicate normally in culture. J Virol 1993;67: 7634–7640.
63. Longnecker R, Miller CL, Tomkinson B, Miao X-Q, Kieff, E. Deletion of DNA encoding the first five transmembrane domains of Epstein-Barr virus latent membrane proteins 2A and 2B. J Virol 1993;67:5068–5074.
64. Burkhardt AL, Bolen JB, Kieff E, Longnecker R. An Epstein-Barr virus transformation–associated membrane protein interacts with src family tyrosine kinases. J Virol 1992;66:5161–5167.
65. Miller CL, Burkhardt AL, Lee JH, Stealey B, Longnecker R, Bolen JB, Kieff E. Integral membrane protein 2 of Epstein-Barr virus regulates reactivation from latency through dominant negative effects on protein-tyrosine kinases. Immunity 1995;2:155–166.
66. Miller CL, Lee JH, Kieff, E, Longnecker R. An integral membrane protein (LMP2) blocks reactivation of Epstein-Barr virus from latency following surface immunoglobulin crosslinking. Proc Natl Acad Sci USA 1994;91:772–776.
67. Swaminathan S, Tomkinson B, Kieff E. Recombinant Epstein-Barr virus with small RNA (EBER) genes deleted transforms lymphocytes and replicates in vitro. Proc Natl Acad Sci USA 1991;88:1546–1550.
68. Lerner MR, Andrews NC, Miller G, Steitz JA. Two small RNAs encoded by Epstein-Barr virus and complexed with protein are precipitated by antibodies from patients with systemic lupus erythematosus. Proc Natl Acad Sci USA 1981;78:805–809.
69. Robertson E, Kieff E. Reducing the complexity of the transforming Epstein-Barr virus genome to 64 kilobase pairs. J Virol 1995;69:983–993.
70. Kempkes B, Pich D, Zeidler R, Sugden B, Hammerschmidt W. Immortalization of human B lymphocytes by a plasmid containing 71 kilobase pairs of Epstein-Barr virus DNA. J Virol 1995;69:231–238.
71. Cohen JI. Molecular biology of Epstein-Barr virus and its mechanism of B-cell transformation. In Epstein-Barr virus infections: biology, pathogenesis, and management. Moderated by SE Strauss. Ann Intern Med 1993:118:45–48.
72. Hsu D-H, de Waal Malefyt R, Fiorentino DF, Dang M-N, Vieira P, deVries J, Spits H, Mosmann TR, Moore KW. Expression of interleukin-10 activity by Epstein-Barr virus protein BCRF1. Science 1990;250:830–832.
73. Swaminathan S, Hesselton R, Sullivan J, Kieff E. Epstein-Barr virus recombinants with specifically mutated BCRF1 genes. J Virol 1993;67:7406–7413.
74. Cleary ML, Smith SD, Sklar J. Cloning and structural analysis of cDNAs for bcl-2 and a hybrid bcl-2/immunoglobulin transcript resulting from the t(14;18) translocation. Cell 1986;47:19–28.
75. Hockenbery D, Nunex G, Milliman C, Schreiber RD, Korsmeyer SJ. Bcl2 is an inner mitochondrial membrane protein that blocks programmed cell death. Nature 1990;348:334–336.
76. Henderson S, Huen D, Rowe M, Dawson C, Johnson G, Rickinson A. Epstein-Barr virus-coded BHRF1 protein, a viral homologue of bcl-2, protects human B cells from programmed cell death. Proc Natl Acad Sci USA 1993;90:8479–8483.
77. Tarodi B, Subramanian T, Chinnadurai G. Epstein-Barr virus BHRF1 protein protects against cell death induced by DNA-damaging agents and heterologous viral infection. Virology 1994;201:404–407.
78. Marchini A, Tomkinson B, Cohen J, Kieff E. BHRF1, the Epstein-Barr virus gene with homology to bcl2, is dispensable for B-lymphocyte transformation and virus replication. J Virol 1991;65:5991–6000
79. Lee M-A, Yates JL. BHRF1 of Epstein-Barr virus, which is homologous to human proto-oncogene bcl2, is not essential for transformation of B cells or for virus replication in vitro. J Virol 1992;66:1899–1906
80. Giovanella B, Nilsson K, Zech L, Yim O, Klein G, Stehlin JS. Growth of diploid, Epstein-Barr virus–carrying human lymphoblastoid cell lines heterotransplanted into nude mice under immunologically privileged conditions. Int J Cancer 1979;24: 103–113.
81. Adams RA, Hellerstein EE, Pothier L, Foley GF, Lazarus H, Stuart A. Malignant potential of a cell line isolated from the peripheral blood in infectious mononucleosis. Cancer 1971;27:651–658.
82. Mosier DE, Gulizia RJ, Baird SM, Wilson DB. Transfer of a functional human immune system to mice with severe combined immunodeficiency. Nature 1988;335:256–259.
83. Rowe M, Young LS, Crocker J, Stokes H, Henderson S, Rickinson AB. Epstein-Barr virus (EBV)–associated lymphoproliferative disease in the SCID mouse model: implications for the pathogenesis of EBV-positive lymphomas in man. J Exp Med 1991;173:147–158.
84. Baiocchi RA, Caligiuri MA. Low-dose interleukin 2 prevents the development of Epstein-Barr virus-associated lymphoproliferative disease in scid/scid mice reconstituted i.p. with EBV-seropositive human peripheral blood lymphocytes. Proc Natl Acad Sci USA 1994;91:5577–5581.
85. Miller G, Shope T, Coope D, Waters L, Pagano J, Bornkamm GW, Henle W. Lymphoma in cotton-top marmosets after inoculation with Epstein-Barr virus: tumor incidence, histologic spectrum, antibody responses, demonstration of viral DNA, and characterization of viruses. J Exp Med 1977;145:948–967.
86. Cleary ML, Epstein MA, Finerty S, Dorfman RF, Bornkamm GW, Kirkwood JK, Morgan AJ, Sklar J. Individual tumors of multifocal EB virus–induced malignant lymphomas in tamarins arise from different B-cell clones. Science 1985;228:722–724.
87. Young LS, Finerty S, Brooks L, Scullion F, Rickinson AB, Morgan AJ. Epstein-Barr virus gene expression in malignant lymphomas induced by experimental virus infection of cottontop tamarins. J Virol 1989;63:1967–1974.
88. Morgan AJ, Mackett M, Finerty S, Arrand JR, Scullion FT, Epstein MA. Recombinant vaccinia virus expressing Epstein-Barr virus glycoprotein gp340 protects cottontop tamarins against EB virus–induced malignant lymphomas. J Med Virol 1988;25: 189–195.
89. Morgan AJ, Finerty S, Lovgren K, Scullion FT, Morein B. Prevention of Epstein-Barr (EB) virus–induced lymphoma in cottontop tamarins by vaccination with the EB virus envelope glycoprotein gp340 incorporated into immune-stimulating complexes. J Gen Virol 1988;69:2093–2096.
90. Miller G. Epstein-Barr virus. In Virology. Edited by BN Fields, DM Knipe, RM Chanock, MS Hirsch, JL Melnick, TP Monath, B Roizman. New York: Raven, 1990, pp 1921–1958.
91. Blazer B, Patarroyo M, Klein E, Klein G. Increased sensitivity of human lymphoid lines to natural killer cells after induction of the Epstein-Barr viral cycle by superinfection or sodium butyrate. J Exp Med 1980;151:614–627.
92. Tosato G, Magrath I, Koski I, Dooley N, Blase RM. Activation of suppressor T-cells during Epstein-Barr virus–induced infectious mononucleosis. N Engl J Med 1979;301:1133–1137.
93. Burrows SR, Sculley TB, Misko IS, Schmidt C, Moss DJ. An Epstein-Barr virus–specific cytotoxic T-cell epitope in EBNA 3. J Exp Med 1990;171:345–350.
94. Murray RJ, Kurilla MG, Griffin HM, Brooks JM, Mackett M, Arrand JR, Rowe M, Burrows SR, Moss DJ, Kieff E, Rickinson AB. Human cytotoxic T-cell responses against Epstein-Barr virus nuclear antigens demonstrated by using recombinant vaccinia viruses. Proc Natl Acad Sci USA 1990;87:2906–2910.
95. Murray RJ, Wang D, Young LS, Wang F, Rowe M, Kieff E, Rickinson AB. Epstein-Barr virus–specific cytotoxic T-cell recognition of transfectants expressing the virus-coded latent membrane protein LMP. J Virol 1988;62:3747–3755.
96. Greenspan JS, Greenspan D, Lennette ET, Abrams DI, Conant MA, Petersen V, Freese UK. Replication of Epstein-Barr virus within the epithelial cells of oral "hairy" leukoplakia, an AIDS-associated lesion. N Engl J Med 1985;313:1564–1571.
97. Grierson H, Purtilo DT. Epstein-Barr virus infections in males with the X-linked lymphoproliferative syndrome. Ann Intern Med 1987;106:538–545.
98. Sullivan JL, Byron KS, Brewster FE, Baker SM, Ochs HD. X-linked lymphoproliferative syndrome: natural history of the immunodeficiency. J Clin Invest 1983;71:1765–1778.
99. Skare JC, Milunsky A, Byron KS, Sullivan JL. Mapping of the X-linked lymphoproliferative syndrome. Proc Natl Acad Sci USA 1987;84:2015–2018.

100. Robinson JE, Brown N, Andiman W, Halliday K, Francke U, Robert MF, Andersson-Anvret M, Horstmann D, Miller G. Diffuse polyclonal B-cell lymphoma during primary infection with Epstein-Barr virus. N Engl J Med 1980;302:1293–1297.
101. Snydman DR, Rudders RA, Daoust P, Sullivan JL, Evan AS. Infectious mononucleosis in an adult progressing to fatal immunoblastic lymphoma. Ann Intern Med 1982;96:737–742.
102. Joncas JH, Russo P, Brochu P, Simard P, Brisebois J, Dube J, Marton D, Leclerc JM, Hume H, Rivard GE. Epstein-Barr virus polymorphic B-cell lymphoma associated with leukemia and with congenital immunodeficiencies. J Clin Oncol 1990;8: 378–384.
103. Saemundsen AK, Purtilo DT, Sakamoto K, Sullivan JL, Synnerholm AC, Hanto D, Simmons R, Anvret M, Collins R, Klein G. Documentation of Epstein-Barr virus infection in immunodeficient patients with life-threatening lymphoproliferative disease by Epstein-Barr virus complementary RNA/DNA and viral DNA/DNA hybridization. Cancer Res 1981;41:4237–4242.
104. Cohen JI. Epstein-Barr virus lymphoproliferative disease associated with acquired immunodeficiency. Medicine 1991;70:137–160.
105. Edwards RH, Raab-Traub N. Alterations of the p53 gene in Epstein-Barr virus-associated immunodeficiency-related lymphomas. J Virol 1994;68:1309–1315.
106. Thomas JA, Hotchin NA, Allday MJ, Amlot P, Rose M, Yacoub M, Crawford DH. Immunohistology of Epstein-Barr virus-associated antigens in B cell disorders from immunocompromised individuals. Transplantation 1990;49:944–953.
107. Young L, Alfieri C, Hennessy K, Evans H, O'Hara C, Anderson KC, Ritz J, Shapiro RS, Rickinson A, Kieff E, Cohen JI. Expression of Epstein-Barr virus transformation-associated genes in tissues of patients with EBV lymphoproliferative disease. N Engl J Med 1989;321:1080–1085.
108. Rooney CM, Smith CA, Ng CYC, et al. Use of gene-modified virus-specific T lymphocytes to control Epstein-Barr virus-related lymphoproliferation. Lancet 1995;345: 9–13.
109. Papadopoulos EB, Ladanyi M, Emanuel D, et al. Infusions of donor leukocytes to treat Epstein-Barr virus–associated lymphoproliferative disorders after allogeneic bone marrow transplantation. N Engl J Med 1994;330:1185–1191.
110. Randhawa PS, Jaffe R, Demetris AJ, et al. Expression of Epstein-Barr virus–encoded small RNA (by the EBER-1 gene) in liver specimens from transplant recipients with post-transplantation lymphoproliferative disease. N Engl J Med 1992;237: 1710–1714.
111. deThe G, Geser A, Day NE, Tukei PM, Williams EH, Beri DP, Smith PG, Dean AG, Bornkamm GW, Feorino P, Henle W. Epidemiological evidence for causal relationship between Epstein-Barr virus and Burkitt's's lymphoma from Ugandan prospective study. Nature 1978;274:756–761.
112. Henle G, Henle W, Clifford P, Diehl V, Kafuko GW, Kirya BG, Klein G, Morrow RH, Munube GM, Pike P, Tukei PM, Ziegler JL. Antibodies to Epstein-Barr virus in Burkitt's's lymphoma and control groups. JNCI 1969;43:1147–57.
113. Rowe M, Rowe DT, Gregory CD, Young LS, Farrell PJ, Rupani H, Rickinson AB. Differences in B cell growth phenotype reflect novel patterns of Epstein-Barr virus latent gene expression in Burkitt's's lymphoma cells. EMBO J 1987;6:2743–2751.
114. Rowe M, Gregory C. Epstein-Barr virus and Burkitt's lymphoma. Adv Viral Oncol 1989;8:237–259.
115. Adams JM, Harris AW, Pinkert CA, Corcoran LM, Alexander WS, Cory S, Palmiter RD, Brinster RL. The c-*myc* oncogene driven by immunoglobulin enhancers induces lymphoid malignancy in transgenic mice. Nature 1985;318:533–538.
116. Leder A, Pattengale PK, Kuo A, Stewart TA, Leder P. Consequences of widespread deregulation of the c-*myc* gene in transgenic mice: multiple neoplasms and normal development. Cell 1986;45:485–495.
117. Lombardi L, Newcomb EW, Dalla-Favera R. Pathogenesis of Burkitt's lymphoma: expression of an activated c-*myc* oncogene causes the tumorigenic conversion of EBV-infected human B lymphocytes. Cell 1987;49:161–170.
118. Inghirami G, Grignani F, Sternas L, Lombardi L, Knowles DM, Dalla-Favera R. Down-regulation of LFA-1 adhesion receptors by c-*myc* oncogene in human B lymphoblastoid cells. Science 1990;250:682–686.
119. Klein G. Lymphoma development in mice and humans: diversity of initiation is followed by convergent cytogenetic evolution. Proc Natl Acad Sci USA 1979;76: 2442–2446.
120. deThe G, Zeng Y. Population screening for EBV markers: toward improvement of nasopharyngeal carcinoma control. In The Epstein-Barr virus: recent advances. Edited by MA Epstein, BG Achong. New York: John Wiley, 1986, pp 237–249
121. Fahraeus R, Fu HL, Ernberg I, Finke J, Rowe M, Klein G, Falk K, Nilsson E, Yadav M, Busson P, Tursz T, Kallin B. Expression of Epstein-Barr virus-encoded proteins in nasopharyngeal carcinoma. Int J Cancer 1988;42:329–338.
122. Young LS, Dawson CW, Clark D Rupani H, Busson P, Tursz T, Johnson A, Rickinson AB. Epstein-Barr virus gene expression in nasopharyngeal carcinoma. J Gen Virol 1988;69:1051–1065.
123. Kvale G, Hoiby EA, Pedersen E Hodgkin's disease in patients with previous infectious mononucleosis. Int J Cancer 1979;23:593–597.
124. Evans AS, Gutensohn NM. A population-based case-control study of EBV and other viral antibodies among persons with Hodgkin's disease and their siblings. Int J Cancer 1984;34:149–157.
125. Mueller N, Evans A, Harris NL, Comstock G, Jellum E, Magnus K, Orentreich N, Polk BF, Vogelman J. Hodgkin's disease and Epstein-Barr virus: altered antibody pattern before diagnosis. N Engl J Med 1989;320:689–695.
126. Ambinder RF, Browning PJ, Lorenzana I, et al. Epstein-Barr virus and childhood Hodgkin's disease in Honduras and the United States. Blood 1993;81:462–467.
127. Chang KL, Albujar PF, Chen YY, Johnson RM, Weiss LM. High prevalence of Epstein-Barr virus in the Reed-Sternberg cells of Hodgkin's disease occurring in Peru. Blood 1993;81:496–501.
128. Weiss LM, Movahed LA, Warnke RA, Sklar J. Detection of Epstein-Barr viral genomes in Reed-Sternberg cells of Hodgkin's disease. N Engl J Med 1989;320:502–506.
129. Grasser FA, Murray PG, Kremmer E. Klien K, Remberger K, Felden W, Reynolds G, Niedobitek G, Young LS, Mueller-Lantzsch N. Monoclonal antibodies directed against the Epstein-Barr virus–encoded nuclear antigen 1 (EBNA1):immunohistologic detection of EBNA1 in the malignant-cells of Hodgkin's disease. Blood 1994;84: 3792–3798.
130. Herbst H, Dallenbach F, Hummel M, Niedobitek G, Pileri S, Muller-Lantzch N, Stein H. Epstein-Barr virus latent membrane protein expression in Hodgkin and Reed-Sternberg cells. Proc Natl Acad Sci USA 1991;88:4766–4770.
131. Pallesen G, Hamilton-Dutoit SJ, Rowe M, Young LS. Expression of Epstein-Barr virus latent gene products in tumour cells of Hodgkin's disease. Lancet 1991;337:320–322.
132. Jones JF, Shurin S, Abramowsky C, Tubbs RR, Sciotto CG, Wahl R, Sands J, Gottman D, Katz B, Sklar J. T-cell lymphomas containing Epstein-Barr viral DNA in patients with chronic Epstein-Barr virus infections. N Engl J Med 1988;318:733–741.
133. Chen C-L, Sadler RH, Walling DM, Su I-J, Hsieh H-C, Raab-Traub N. Epstein-Barr virus gene expression in EBV-positive T cell peripheral lymphomas. J Virol 1993;67: 6303–6308.
134. Murphy JK, Young LS, Bevan IS, Lewis FA, Dockey D, Ironside JW, O'Brien CJ, Wells M. Demonstration of Epstein-Barr virus in primary brain lymphoma by in situ DNA hybridisation in paraffin wax embedded tissue. J Clin Pathol 1990;43:220–223.
135. Brichacek B, Hirsch I, Sibl O, Vilikusova E, Vonka V. Presence of Epstein-Barr virus DNA in carcinomas of the palatine tonsil. JNCI 1984;72:809–815.
136. Brichacek B, Hirsch I, Sibl O, Vilikusova E, Vonka V. Association of some supraglottic laryngeal carcinomas with EB virus. Int J Cancer 1983;32:193–197.
137. Weiss LM, Jaffe ES, Liu X-F, Chen Y-Y, Shibata D, Medeiros LJ. Detection and localization of Epstein-Barr viral genomes in angioimmunoblastic lymphadenopathy and angioimmunoblastic lymphadenopathy-like lymphoma. Blood 1992;79:1789–1795.
138. Leyvraz S, Henle W, Chahinian AP, Perlmann C, Klein G, Gordon RE, Rosenblum M, Holland JF. Association of Epstein-Barr virus with thymic carcinoma. N Engl J Med 1985;312:1296–1299.
139. Harabuchi Y, Yamanaka N, Kataura A, Imai S, Kinoshita T, Mizuno F, Osata T. Epstein-Barr virus in nasal T-cell lymphomas in patients with lethal midline granuloma. Lancet 1990;1:128–130.
140. McClain KL, Leach CT, Jensen HB, Joshi VV, Pollock BH, Parmley RT, DiCarlo FJ, Chadwick EG, Murphy SB. Association of Epstein-Barr virus with leiomyosarcomas in young people with AIDS. N Engl J Med 1995;332:12–18.
141. Lee ES, Locker J, Nalesnik M, Reyes J, Jaffe R, Alashari M, Nour B, Tzakis A, Dickman PS. The association of Epstein-Barr virus with smooth-muscle tumors occurring after organ transplantation. N Engl J Med 1995;332:19–25.
142. Imai S, Koizumi S, Sugiura M, et al. Gastric carcinoma: monoclonal epithelial malignant-cells expressing Epstein-Barr virus latent infection protein. Proc Natl Acad Sci USA 1994:91:9131–9135.
143. Chang Y, Cesarman E, Pessin MS, Lee F, Culpepper J, Knowles DM, Moore PS. Identification of herpesvirus-like DNA sequences in AIDS-associated Kaposi's sarcoma. Science 1994;266:1865–1869.
144. Moore PS, Chang Y. Detection of herpesvirus-like DNA sequences in Kaposi's sarcoma in patients with and those without HIV infection. N Engl J Med 1995;332: 1181–1185.
145. Dupin N, Grandadam M, Calvez V, Gorin I, Aubin JT, Havard S, Lamy F, Leibowitch M, Huraux JM, Escande JP, Agut H. Herpesvirus-like DNA sequences in patients with Mediterranean Kaposi's sarcoma. Lancet 1995;345:761–762.
146. Huang YQ, Li JJ, Kaplan MH, Poiesz B, Katabira E, Zhang WC, Feiner D, Friedman-Kien AE. Human herpesvirus-like nucleic acid in various forms of Kaposi's sarcoma. Lancet 1995;345:759–761.
147. Boshoff C, Whitby D, Hatziioannou T, Fisher C, van der Walt J, Hatzakis A, Weiss R, Schulz T. Kaposi's sarcoma-associated herpesvirus in HIV-negative Kaposi's sarcoma. Lancet 1995;345:1043–1044.
148. Ambroziak JA, Blackbourn DJ, Herndier BG, Glogau RG, Gullet JH, McDonald AR, Lennette ET, Levy JA. Herpes-like sequences in HIV-infected and uninfected Kaposi's sarcoma patients. Science 1995;268:582–583.
149. Cesarman E, Chang Y, Moore PS, Said JW, Knowles DM. Kaposi's sarcoma–associated herpesvirus-like DNA sequences in AIDS-related body-cavity-based lymphomas. N Engl J Med 1995;332:1186–1191.
150. Biesinger B, Muller-Fleckenstein I, Simmer B, Lang G, Wittman S, Platzer E, Desrosiers RC, Fleckenstein B. Stable growth transformation of human T lymphocytes by herpesvirus saimiri. Proc Natl Acad Sci USA 1992;89:3116–3119.
151. Meinl E, Hohlfeld R, Wekerle H, Fleckenstein B. Immortalization of human T-cells by herpesvirus saimiri. Immunol Today 1995;16:55–58.
152. Pearson GR, Scott RE. Isolation of virus-free Herpesvirus saimiri antigen–positive plasma membrane vesicles. Proc Natl Acad Sci USA 1977;74:2546–2550.

CHAPTER 22

Papillomaviruses and Cervical Neoplasia

CATHERINE M. McLACHLIN AND CHRISTOPHER P. CRUM

In recent years, human papillomaviruses (HPVs) have become the principal focus of efforts to implicate a transmissible virus in the genesis of lower genital tract neoplasia. An explosion in technology has dictated both the tempo and direction of this research, which began with descriptive and experimental pathology, progressed to molecular biology, and finally involved molecular immunology in efforts both to implicate the virus directly in producing neoplasia and to unravel the mechanisms of host response.

Biochemical work by several laboratories has unveiled potential mechanisms by which HPV infection may produce neoplastic transformation. Studies with keratinocyte cultures, in which features of HPV-related neoplasia have been reproduced (42, 68), have put this information into morphologic perspective. Further, direct analysis of HPV nucleic acids in clinical material has identified the nature of HPV expression and provided morphologic clues as to why certain HPV types may be associated with cancer. Clinical application of this information has been attempted, based principally on the strong association between HPV and cancer. Unfortunately, the strict association between HPV nucleic acids and cervical cancer has been hampered by the discovery of latent or occult virus infection, which in turn has complicated the picture of a diagnostic molecular test that would highlight women at risk for developing cancer. Finally, the advent of molecular immunology has produced sobering observations, balancing the hope for a serologic test for HPV exposure with the reality that HPV infection (or exposure) is extremely common, whereas cervical cancer is not. This discovery has been accompanied by a shift in emphasis toward the use of immunology to prevent (by use of vaccines) rather than detect HPV-related disease. This chapter details the molecular basis for HPV-related precursor diseases of the cervix, balancing this information with the morphologic and clinical perspectives that are integral to the management of these extremely common disorders.

Definitions, Mechanisms, and Pathobiology of Genital HPV Infection

DEFINITION OF INFECTION

Genital "infections" are best defined by the presence of clinically or colposcopically identifiable flat or raised lesions that contain papillomaviral DNA, the prototype of which is genital warts. In this instance, infectious virus is likely to be identified within the epithelium (Fig. 22.1*AA*). More recently, the term infection has been expanded to include HPV-related precancerous lesions, or even cancers, infection being used loosely to denote the presence of viral DNA. However, virions are less likely to be identified in these processes (Fig. 22.1*B*) (40). As will be detailed subsequently, HPV DNA may be associated with occult viral infection, active infection, or advanced neoplasia (Table 22.1).

The hallmark of HPV infection is a morphologic transformation of the target tissue. This is not synonymous with the term transformation as classically applied to changes in cultured cells produced after introduction of HPV nucleic acids. Rather, it defines the morphologic alterations that can be most consistently associated with the presence of HPV nucleic acids. It may, depending on the host response and HPV type involved in the infection, be defined as a low- or high-grade genital precancer, either of which is distinct from normal epithelium (Figs. 22.1 and 22.2).

MECHANISM OF INFECTION

Papillomaviruses are epitheliotropic, circular, double-stranded DNA viruses that infect squamous epithelium. The interval from exposure to the development of a lesion varies from a few weeks to several months, and perhaps longer (35, 47). It is presumed that the virus gains access to the cervix or lower female genital tract through defects in the epithelium that expose basal epithelial cells to virion particles. In support of this hypothesis are the demonstration of papillomavirus DNA and RNA in basal cells and the observation that experimental infection of squamous mucosa by HPV is enhanced by disturbing the epithelial surface (and hence exposing the basal cells) prior to exposure (50). Of particular interest is the hypothesis that the viral DNA exists either in or in proximity to the epithelium for an extended interval without causing morphologic changes (73). This has been termed latent or occult infection; however, the precise definition of latency and the reservoir of latent infection remain unclear (5). As the cells containing the viral DNA approach the upper layers of the epithelium, the virus replicates and assembles into virions, which can be detected by electron microscopy or immunohistochemistry (Fig. 22.1) (76). Some of the superficial cells in the infected epithelium characteristically display enlarged, hyperchromatic nuclei, with or without cytoplasmic halos (koilocytotic atypia), and the mature virus usually concentrates in this cell population (Fig. 22.1) (31, 76). Whether koilocytosis is due exclusively to viral repli-

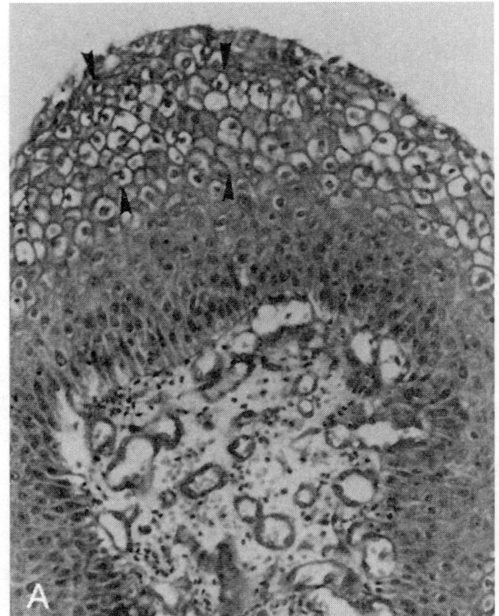

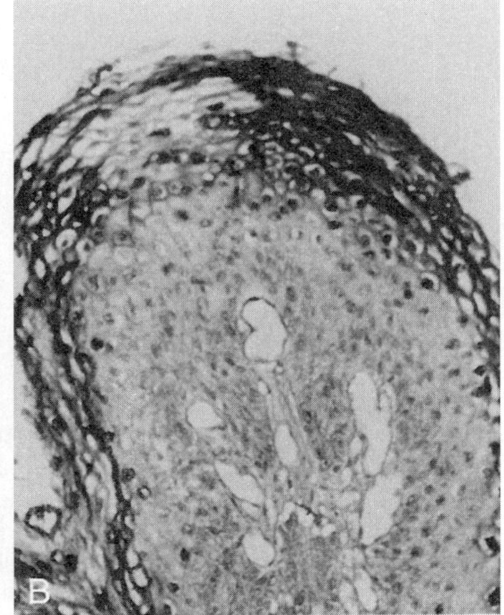

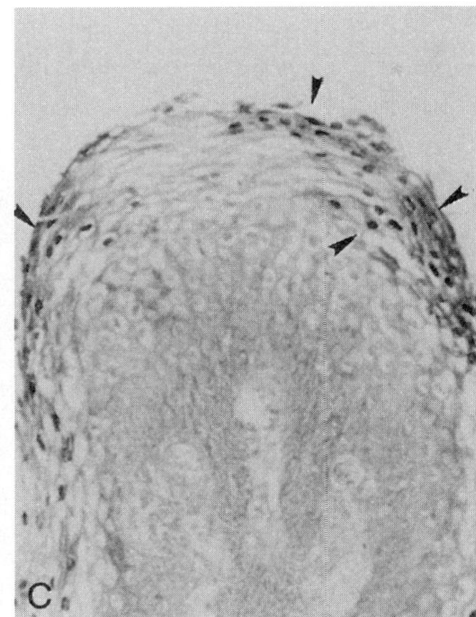

Figure 22.1. Histopathology of a classic human papillomavirus (HPV) infection (condyloma) of the cervix associated with low-risk HPV types (HPV types 6 or 11). **A.** Morphologic features of HPV infection include nuclear atypia in the superficial epithelial cells with prominent cytoplasmic halos (*arrowheads*). The lower cell layers contain minimal cytologic atypia. **B.** Appearance following in situ hybridization with a biotin-labeled mixed DNA probe containing HPV types 6 and 11 (VIRATYPE, Life Technologies, Gaithersburg, MD). The dark staining in the superficial cell nuclei and cytoplasm represent viral DNA and RNA produced during viral replication. **C.** An immunoperoxidase stain for HPV capsid proteins, highlighting several darkly staining nuclei in the superficial epithelium (*arrowheads*).

Table 22.1. Definitions

HPV	= Human papillomavirus
HPV infection	= Production of a lesion (condyloma) that contains HPV virions. Usually synonymous with condyloma or very-low-grade CIN (see Figure 22.1).
CIN	= Cervical intraepithelial neoplasia, synonymous with papillomavirus-related squamous intraepithelial lesions. Low-grade CIN (CIN I) is synonymous with flat or exophytic condyloma and exhibits nuclear atypia, principally in the upper epithelial layers. High-grade CIN (CIN II or III) is characterized by atypia in all epithelial layers.
HPV-related lesion	= Includes HPV infection, but also any lesion associated with papillomaviruses, including high-grade CIN and various invasive carcinomas.
Occult or latent HPV infection	= Presence of HPV DNA in the absence of demonstrable evidence of HPV infection (i.e., no lesion is present). Natural history is unclear.
High-risk HPV	= HPV associated with high-grade CIN and/or carcinomas.
Low-risk HPV	= HPV associated with low-grade CIN (condylomata).
Open reading frame	= Interval of DNA capable of encoding a protein of sufficient lengh to functionally justify designation as a potential "gene."

cation is controversial, principally because this cytologic phenomenon may exist in the absence of abundant capsid proteins or virions. The implication is that the nuclear hyperchromasia of koilocytotic cells signifies host DNA replication occurring in concert with viral replication (31, 76). Although genital squamous epithelium appears to be the principal site for HPV infection, there is evidence that infection may occur in germinal or undifferentiated epithelial cells that give rise to both the squamous and glandular components of the cervical mucosa. HPV nucleic acids have been isolated from neoplasms not clearly derived from squamous-committed epithelial cells, most notably adenocarcinomas and undifferentiated carcinomas (small cell carcinoma) (71, 75).

SPECIFICITY

Squamous epithelium is most susceptible to HPV infections. In particular, squamocolumnar junctions, where the glandular portion is undergoing replacement or transformation by squamous epithelium (transformation zones), are most vulnerable to the genital papillomaviruses (63). Infection with "genital types" has been demonstrated in other mucosal sites in which this process of epithelial transformation takes place, including the larynx (1), oropharyngeal mucosa (14), anus (2), esophagus (79), subungual mucosa (nail bed) (49), and conjunctiva (44). Kreider and colleagues demonstrated that some of those sites are particularly vul-

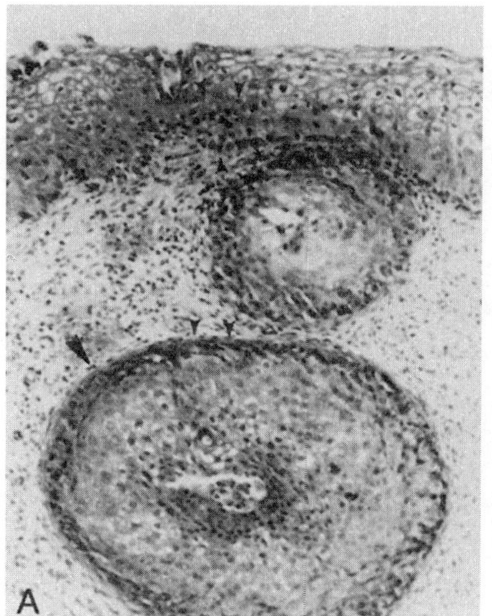

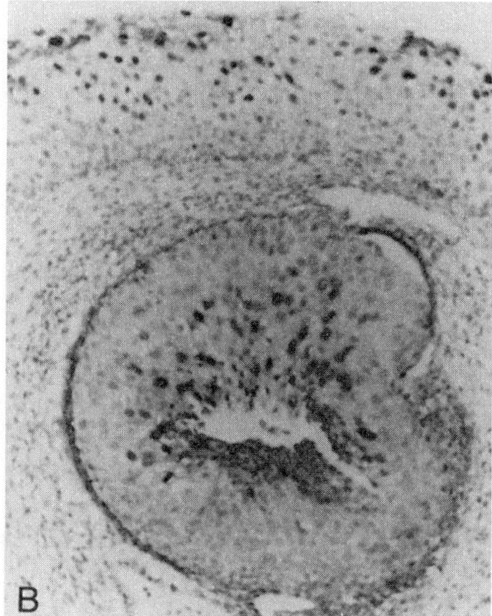

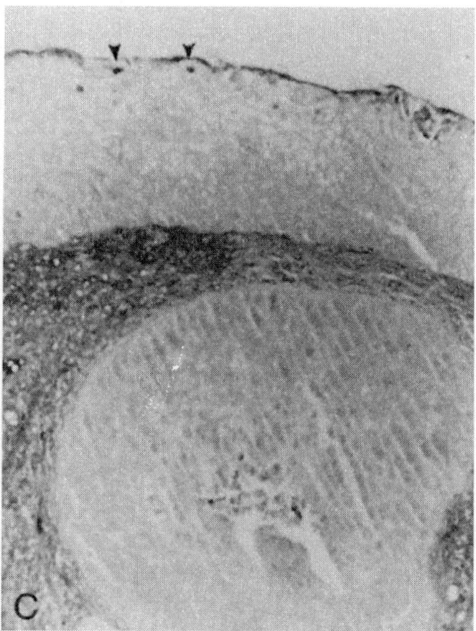

Figure 22.2. Histopathology of cervical intraepithelial neoplasm associated with high-risk HPV types (ie., 16, 31, 33, 35, and so on). **A.** Lesion involving the superficial and crypt (gland) epithelium (*large arrowhead*). Koilocytotic atypia is present (*upper right*), but in addition, nuclear atypia is conspicuous in the lower cell layers (*small arrows*). **B.** Appearance following in situ hybridization with a mixed probe containing HPV types 31, 33 and 35. Note the similar distribution of staining as in Figure 22.1*B*. In contrast to Figure 22.1*C*, capsid proteins are infrequently identified by immunostaining, with rare positive nuclei observed (*arrowheads*).

nerable to experimental infection with genital viruses (34). This indicates that genital HPV types require specific conditions provided by certain locales for infection to occur, or characteristics facilitating morphologic transformation once infection has taken place. Favoring the latter is the unusual predisposition of certain HPV types for the cervix over other genital HPVs (62).

HPV and Human Genital Neoplasia

EVOLUTION OF THE CONCEPT

Although studies with animal papillomaviruses established their potential role in the genesis of neoplasia, the most significant link between HPV and human cervical neoplasia came in the form of observations that a common cytologic feature of abnormal Papanicolaou smears, koilocytotic atypia, was a cellular marker for the presence of genital HPV infection (31, 46, 61). By virtue of its high frequency, this cytologic abnormality focused researchers on this virus and its association not only with genital warts, but also with cervical precancerous lesions (cervical intraepithelial neoplasia [CIN] or cervical dysplasia). Thus, the initial hypothesis that HPV was an oncogenic virus in the cervix was derived not only from molecular biology but also from morphologic evidence via the association between genital papillomaviruses, abnormal Papanicolaou smears, and cervical precancers (47). The cloning of genital HPVs redirected attention from the morphology of HPV infection to the molecular pathology of HPV-related diseases, in that molecular probes could identify HPV nucleic acids in the absence of viral particles or capsid proteins. Thus it became possible to identify HPV nucleic acids not only in condylomata, but also in squamous precancers and carcinomas of the female genital tract (3, 5, 18, 25). As part of this progression, the discovery of a variety of different HPV types laid the foundation for establishing that specific HPV types are associated with certain types of genital lesions (12). Currently over 60 distinct types of HPV have been identified, many of which are associated with specific clinical and pathologic characteristics (5). For example, genital warts and condylomata are associated with certain viral types (types 6, 11, and others), whereas precancerous lesions (CIN) and invasive cancer are frequently associated primarily with types 16, 18, 31, 33, 35, and others (Table 22.2) (5). In essence, the "higher grade" precancers are more likely to harbor "high-risk" HPV types, implying that, as a group, these lesions are more likely to progress to carcinoma if not treated (Fig. 22.2). The association of high-risk HPV types with both high-grade precursors and cancers has strengthened the hypothesis that infection by specific types produces specific kinds of precursor lesions that may evolve into carcinoma, depending on host factors (3, 11, 18). One interesting departure from the above concept occurs with HPV type 18, which is infrequently associated with squamous precursors and more frequently associated with invasive squamous, glandular, and undifferentiated cervical cancers (37, 71, 74, 75). However, in precursor lesions, HPV-18 is frequently identified in lesions of lower grade morphology, in contrast to the typical high-grade intraepithelial lesions associated with HPV 16 (45). The bland morphology of many HPV-18–related precursors contrasts with the high-grade morphology of HPV-18–associated cancers, but this difference cannot be linked to functional differences in sequences encoding in vitro transforming potential, transcriptional regulation, or transactivation functions.

Table 22.2. Most Common Genital HPV Types

Low-risk HPVs	
HPV-6	= Most common HPV type associated with exophytic warts; most common in vulvar condylomata, and uncommon in cervical exophytic condylomata.
HPV-11	= Second most commonly associated with exophytic warts. Uncommon in the cervix.
HPV-42	= Associated with benign genital warts.
High-risk HPVs	
HPV-16	= Most common cervical HPV, associated strongly with high-grade CIN cervical squamous carcinoma and about 30% of adenocarcinomas.
HPV-18	= Associated principally with small cell undifferentiated carcinomas, adenocarcinomas, adenocarcinomas in situ, and less than 5% of pure squamous cell carcinomas in the experience of these authors. Also associated with approximately 5% of CIN, most of which will be low grade.
HPV-31, 33, 35, 39, 51	= Additional types associated with squamous precursors and invasive cancers, less common than HPV-16. Associated with high-grade CIN, but less so than HPV-16.

Genomic Map of HPV-16

(Circular Genome)

Kb 0.0 1.0 2.0 3.0 4.0 5.0 6.0 7.0 7.9

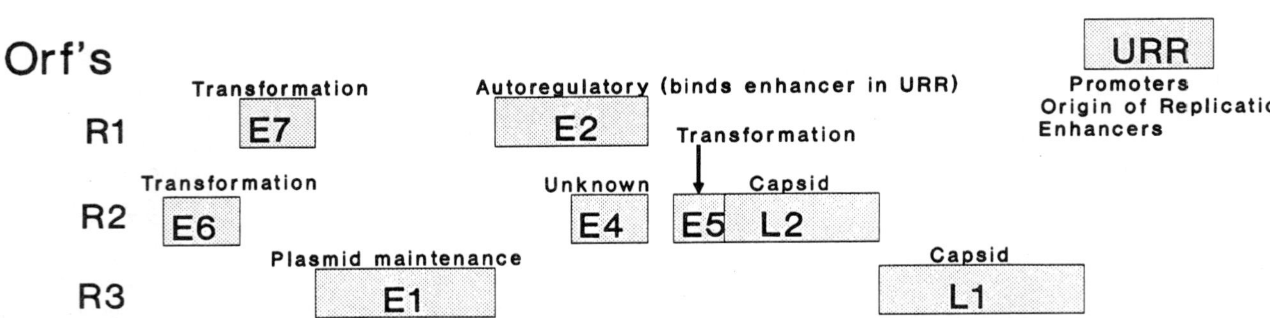

Figure 22.3. Schematic of the HPV-16 genome, outlining potential "genes" (open reading frames) and their possible functions.

MOLECULAR BASIS FOR HPV-RELATED NEOPLASIA

The molecular basis for papillomavirus effects on host squamous cells is based on and supported by the following observations.

1. Lesions associated with high-risk HPV types frequently possess morphologic and biologic characteristics that distinguish them from infection by other HPV types, suggesting that molecular events occur during infection that are unique to these virus–host relationships (11, 12, 21, 22). For example, HPV-16–related precursors produce fewer virions, are associated with greater cytologic atypia, and, by inference, frequently contain aneuploid cell populations (Fig. 22.2) (21, 22). The supposition is that some component of infection by this and similar viruses causes fundamental changes in the biology of the epithelium, which in turn increases the risk of persistence of morphologic abnormalities and, in some cases, the risk of progression to cancer.
2. HPV types associated with neoplasms (high-risk HPV types) differ from low-risk HPV types in molecular sequence and in the effects of these sequences on cells. Clues to what makes HPV-16 infection unique vis-à-vis so-called low-risk (HPV-6) infection have been forthcoming from several lines of investigation, all of which center on the viral genome itself (Fig. 22.3) (70). Mechanisms that have been studied and that may distinguish low- from high-risk viruses include (*a*) differences in the expression of so-called transforming genes, such as the E6/E7 and E5 oncoproteins; (*b*) the process of genomic integration; and (*c*) mechanisms by which the upstream regulatory region is influenced by exogenous factors such as receptor complexes. These mechanisms are summarized in Figure 22.4 (6, 19, 60, 69, 78).

Most of what is known about HPVs is derived from analogous studies with bovine papillomaviruses (BPVs). Lowy and colleagues established that 69% of the BPV genome could alter the growth characteristics of cells in culture (transformation) (41). Subsequent sequencing of this viral DNA and HPV viral DNA established that both human and animal HPVs share similar genomic organization in which the region corresponding to the transforming region of BPV is designated as the early (E) region. In contrast, the late (L) region encodes capsid proteins and does not possess transforming potential (5, 69). Studies of cell transfection and in vitro biochemical assays combined with mutational analysis have identified specific open reading frames (ORFs) that produce gene products (proteins) possessing different biologic properties (Fig. 22.3) (5). The functions of the early regions of the HPV genome and their influence on carcinogenesis have recently been delineated through structure–function analysis of these ORFs within the different viral types (59). Two genes that are actively expressed following viral integration, the E6 and E7 ORFs, are the major mediators of cellular transformation. This capability relates to their unique abilities to bind and block the function of critical cellular growth regulatory proteins. The E7 ORF encodes a 21-kd nuclear phosphoprotein that is able to cooperate with *ras* to transform primary rodent cells (28, 50, 59). Similar to the large T antigen of SV40 and the E1A protein of adenovirus, the E7 protein is able to bind the retinoblastoma gene product (RB) (50, 59). This binding capability of E7 for RB differs between the different groups of HPV in that the oncogenic viral types (HPV types 16 and 18) have a greater binding affinity for this regulatory protein than do the nononcogenic types (HPV types 6 and 11) (28). Further, the efficiency of binding correlates with the transforming capacity of these viral types (23). Binding affinity appears to be influenced by a single amino acid difference within the E7 ORF, a difference that is consistently noted between the viral types (23). Insight into the effect of this protein interaction has also been achieved. Binding of RB by E7 protein has been shown to release other cellular factors such as the E2F transcriptional factor (50, 59). Increased intracellular concentrations of free E2F may result in increased cellular proliferation, a possible mechanism for the transforming potential of HPV E7.

The product of the E6 ORF also has important functions in cellular transformation. Like E7, the E6 protein displays characteristics similar to SV40 and adenovirus by binding p53, a key cell cycle regulatory protein (47). p53 is known to block G/S-phase cell cycle progression following DNA damage, allowing repair to take place before mitosis can resume (77). Mutations in p53 that result in loss of functional protein are among the most common genetic aberrations present in solid tumors (77). However, in HPV-positive tumors, p53 mutations are uncommon and p53 levels are nearly unde-

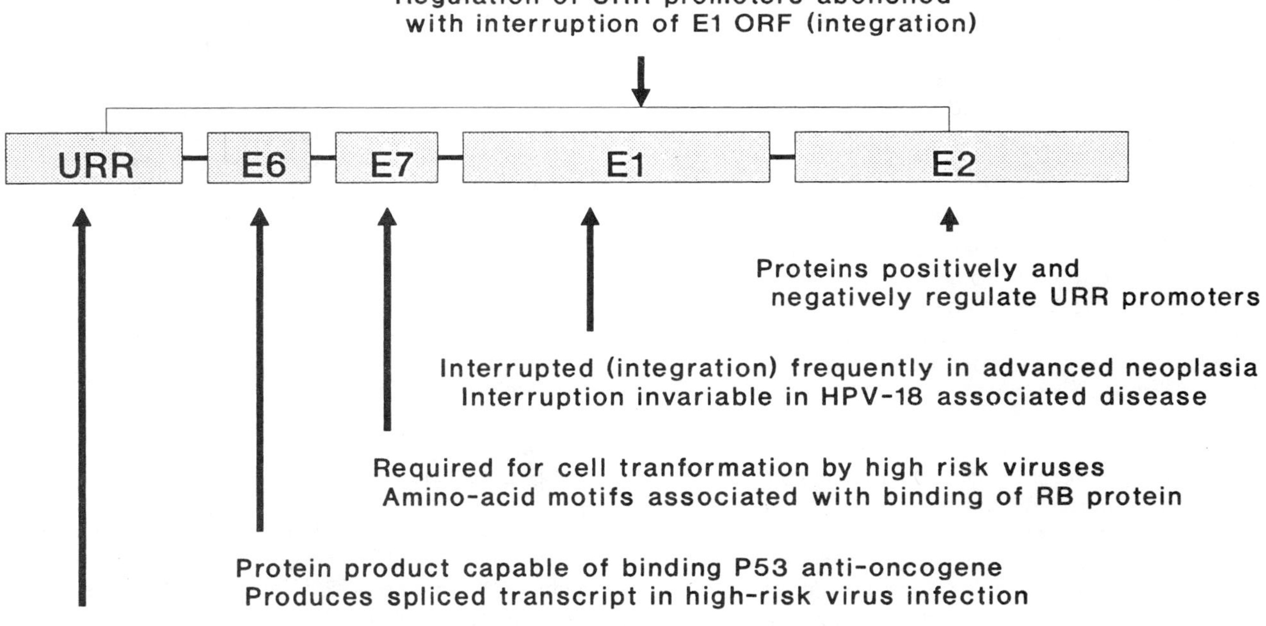

Figure 22.4. Schematic of potential mechanisms of HPV-related neoplastic transformation.

tectable (66). It appears that by binding p53, E6 is able to induce proteolysis of this protein via the ubiquitin pathway (67), effectively removing the p53-mediated block to cellular proliferation.

Another ORF with potential transforming ability is the E5 ORF, although the evidence in support of this is limited principally to the BPV system (15). The relationship of this protein to human disease is unknown. Its transforming potential relates to the ability of E5 to bind intramembrane proteins such as a 16-kd component vacuolar ATPase (8, 26) although the mechanism of this interaction is unknown. E5 also appears to modify the internalization and phosphorylation of certain growth factor receptors, EGF and CSF-1 (26). A final region that may distinguish high- from low-risk HPV is the upstream regulatory region (URR), or long control region (LCR). This enhancer within the URR activates expression of the transforming regions of the HPV genome, E6, and E7 (50, 59, 64). During viral integration into the host genome the E1 or E2 region is consistently disrupted (64). Loss of these ORFs leads to derepression of the URR enhancer, and the E6/E7 transforming proteins are expressed. Integration of the virus and interruption of E1/E2 appear to be important steps in cervical carcinogenesis. This region contains sequences that bind nuclear proteins and that contain glucocorticoid receptor sequences that will enhance transcription in a variety of HPV types when exposed to glucocorticoids. Studies by Pater and colleagues demonstrated that dexamethasone is required for oncogenic transformation of cultured cells by HPV-16 DNA and *ras* oncogene, and that this phenomenon is not reproduced with HPV-11 (58). This is of particular interest in light of epidemiologic studies associating oral contraceptive use with the risk of cervical cancer (29).

Other ORFs include those encoding capsid proteins (L1, L2) of unknown function, such as the E4 ORF (52). The latter is produced in abundance in some HPV infections (4, 11, 13, 17). In addition, the E2 ORF encodes an important product that both positively and negatively regulates the upstream regulating region (72). Finally, the intact E1 ORF is required for maintenance of the plasmid state, perhaps explaining why it is the site of interruption when genomic integration takes place (42). In recent years, the experimental infection of cervical grafts with HPV-11 has produced genital warts in nude mice (39). Moreover, transfection of human keratinocytes with HPV DNA has verified the necessity of the E7 ORF in the transformation process, and demonstrated that HPV-16 alone will produce an aneuploid cell population with many characteristics of a precursor lesion (43). Cotransfection of HPV-16 DNA with oncogenes has likewise produced similar lesions and, in some studies, neoplasms with metastatic potential (16). What has not been accomplished has been the successful completion of the life cycle of the virus in tissue culture or the production of infectious virus from cells into which DNA alone has been introduced. These remain the principal obstacles to successfully mimicking in vitro the in vivo state of the virus, as well as manipulating the viral genome to identify the critical components of infection.

Models for the putative functions of the above open reading frames in precursor and cancer development include the following: (*a*) function of the E6-E7 domain is virtually always present in tumors, via transcription of either episomal or integrated sequences; (*b*) transfection of keratinocytes with the HPV-16 E6-E7 sequences produces proliferations resembling high-grade CIN; (*c*) preservation of vegetative functions invariably segregates with low-grade CIN; (*d*) high-risk HPV types such as HPV-16 are infrequently associated with abundant vegetative functions, suggesting a lack of efficient replication and viral assembly associated with this virus; (*e*) HPV-18–associated low-grade CIN frequently produces abundant capsid proteins, much as low-risk HPV types do, implying that maintenance of vegetative functions will suppress effective expression of the HPV-18 oncogenes. In contrast, HPV-18–associated cancers invariably harbor integrated sequences. Thus, HPV-18 is a model of an HPV with powerful in vitro immortalization potential that is abrogated in vivo, provided that vegetative functions are preserved. Determining which factors influence these differences, including host functions, may provide clues to the role of host susceptibility in this disease.

OCCULT INFECTION

Considerable evidence has accumulated identifying HPV DNA in tissue or cell preparations that do not exhibit significant morphologic abnormalities. The basis for the hypothesis that clinically occult HPV infection exists has been established previously, if simply from the observation that new disease may occur in sites where previously there had been no lesion. In the first molecular analysis of this phenomenon, Steinberg and colleagues reported finding HPV DNA sequences in normal-appearing laryngeal mucosa from patients with a history of laryngeal papillomas but who were at the time in apparent remission (73). Ferenczy and colleagues linked occult infection to clinical disease in their study of patients with vulvar warts or precancers who were undergoing laser therapy. They found that grossly normal squamous epithelium adjacent to the treatment field often contained HPV DNA, and that patients with this clinically "occult" infection had a higher frequency of recurrences than those who did not (20). This finding is reinforced by observations that warts may preferentially occur at sites of trauma, emphasizing the relationship between healing and viral activation (57).

The studies described above addressed populations with documented HPV-associated lesions either concurrently or in the past. It is possible that despite appearing normal, tissue contained HPV DNA because of its proximity to tissue clinically infected by the virus or from shed cellular material (contamination) in adjacent lesions. Whatever the mechanism, the important questions to be addressed are whether it occurs in women with no history of HPV infection or abnormal Papanicolaou smears, and specifically, if it has prognostic importance.

Numerous studies have reported the detection of HPV DNA in women with no history of previous HPV-related disease (32). The detection rate of HPV in asymptomatic women varies according to age and sexual activity. HPV positivity has been correlated with lifetime number of sexual partners (38); however, other correlates include other genital infections, frequency of sexual contact, lack of use of barrier contraceptives, and number of sexual partners in the recent past. The last parameter underscores the influence of recent rather than remote sexual contact on detection of HPV DNA.

Estimates of positivity have varied according to age and the above factors. Rosenfeld et al. observed a rate as high as 39% by Southern blot analysis in young, sexually active adolescents (65). The rates in clients of sexually transmitted disease clinics are also high. In contrast, the rates in older women (ages 35–55) have been sharply reduced, measuring approximately 2 to 3% (29). In a recent study of women undergoing routine hysterectomy, we observed an index of 2.1% and a rate of high-risk types of less than 0.25% in middle-aged women (unpublished observations).

The precise location of HPV DNA sequences in normal squamous epithelium remains unknown. Numerous studies using relatively sensitive techniques such as in situ hybridization have, with rare exception, failed to localize HPV nucleic acids in normal epithelium, despite the confirmation on Southern blot hybridization (53). This does not necessarily exclude the potential importance of these sequences, in that Nuovo and colleagues found that a large proportion of HPV-related lesions contained more than one HPV type when analyzed by polymerase chain reaction, despite the fact that only one HPV type could be detected by in situ hybridization (54). This suggests that when a lesion develops from infection by a single virus type, other virus types in the vicinity are in some way inhibited from coinfecting or producing morphologic changes. In fact, the frequency of histologically demonstrable double infection is less than 5% (54). Nevertheless, Nuovo and colleagues demonstrated that recurrent lesions following ablation were frequently associated with HPV types other than the original (55). Although the role of occult infection in these recurrences is unknown, this and other findings suggest that occult infection may have clinical significance under certain circumstances.

Until recently, the predictive value of HPV DNA positives was poorly understood. Lorincz et al. did not correlate HPV DNA with a high risk of disease in the absence of clinical (or Papanicolaou) smear findings (39). However, Koutsky et al., in a study of women in a sexually transmitted disease clinic, observed that 28% of HPV-positive women developed a CIN lesion within 2 years, versus only 3% of HPV-negative women (33). Subsequent studies by Koutsky and colleagues established that many HPV infections, if followed closely, will manifest cervical abnormalities (L. Koutsky, pers communi). Based on the high incidence of abnormal Papanicolaou smears in younger women and the disproportionate number of HPV positives in this population, the model for HPV infection includes a high rate of acquisition at a young age, transient infections/lesions in many women, the development of immunity, and a low rate of lesion detection/HPV positivity in women over age 35. A proportion of high-risk HPV types will produce high-grade CIN lesions that will persist and presumably constitute a risk factor for progression to invasive carcinoma.

APPLICATIONS TO CLINICAL MEDICINE

Background

The prevention of cervical cancer is based on the Papanicolaou smear. Because the majority of cervical cancers are preceded by a cervical precursor (CIN) lesion, often by many years, the detection of these precursors is fundamental to cancer prevention. Precursor lesions are recognized clinically on colposcopy, where precursor lesions can be identified following the application of acetic acid. The use of colposcopy has maximized the targeting of lesions for biopsy, and outpatient removal is the usual approach, including cryotherapy, laser, and, recently, loop electrical excision (80). The latter procedures target the entire transformation zone, removing the lesion and replacing the process of chronic repair with a brief period of reepithelialization.

Diagnostic Classification

Because high-risk HPV types are strongly associated with squamous cell carcinomas of the cervix, efforts have been made to refine diagnostic criteria that would be most likely to identify an infection with such types. These efforts have centered on distinguishing HPV infection alone (cytopathic effect) from the more pronounced features associated with high-risk HPV types—dysplasia. In essence, cervical intraepithelial neoplasia has been redefined in practice, with CIN I corresponding to lesions closely resembling condyloma, CIN II as lesions classically called dysplasia, and CIN III as lesions previously termed carcinoma in situ (9).

Clinical Management

Because lesions in the CIN I category are least likely to progress to carcinoma, recent consensus conferences have proposed that patients whose Papanicolaou smears contain the features of condyloma or CIN I be followed by repeat smear alone (36). This is supported by the fact that 80 to 90% of smears exhibiting these features will be associated either with CIN I or with lesser changes histologically (27). Whether HPV DNA testing can be used to improve the management of these cases is less clear, and the success of this technology will depend on whether it adds information that is relevant to the management of women with low-grade cytologic abnormalities. It is generally accepted that the risk of following higher grade abnormalities (CIN II–III) is unacceptable, notwithstanding the fact that few cases will progress to carcinoma over short-term follow-up (56).

Although HPV DNA testing is an imperfect alternative to the Papanicolaou smear for preventing cancer, a significant proportion of cancer cases do develop despite screening, in addition to about one third that develop in women who have never been screened (66). More thorough health care delivery by Papanicolaou smear screening is the most effective alternative, although it is conceivable that molecular testing of certain populations with a low background index of HPV DNA (such as older women) could provide information that would augment the information from conventional Papanicolaou smear screening. However, women who do not have access to a gynecological examination will, by definition, benefit neither from a Papanicolaou smear nor from viral testing as conventionally applied.

At present, the importance of focusing on sexual transmission is unclear. Male sexual partners carry the viruses but in general, exhibit no clinical disease, or only subtle infections on the penile shaft, scrotum, and urethral meatus. Efforts to detect and eradicate disease in this group have been encouraged, but the actual impact of this approach on the cancer incidence rates is unclear, as is the importance of benign genital warts on areas less susceptible to neoplastic change, such as the vulva and vagina. The failure of high-technology therapy (laser therapy, etc.) to eradicate these infections, much less latent virus infection, has encouraged a more conservative approach to generic HPV infection and focused efforts on identifying subsets of women who are at greater risk. This group includes blacks, smokers, and individuals who have disease on the cervix as depicted by clear-cut Papanicolaou smear abnormalities (32).

Prevention

Excluding barrier methods of contraception, Papanicolaou smear screening, and HPV DNA testing, prevention of HPV-related cervical neoplasia will depend on whether these disorders can be prevented by vaccines. Concerning the immune response, the most promising studies are in the field of vaccination. Because papillomaviruses cannot be grown in culture, the study of their immunogenicity has been limited previously to serologic studies using denatured target peptides generated by recombinant technology (Fig. 22.5) (10). In contrast, the most likely targets are conformational epitopes on the surface of the capsid. Recently a number of investigators have succeeded in producing intact capsid particles by expressing the entire late region of papillomaviruses in baculovirus vectors or other eukaryotic systems. These empty capsids contain the conformational epitopes felt to be operative in generating host immunity, and their study provides the opportunity to manipulate the viral genome to produce reagents that can be used to study (or generate) host immunity (30). This avenue of investigation is, at present, the most promising because it offers the advantage of intact particles that are highly immunogenic and focuses on the capsid proteins, which are likely the first to be seen by the host immune system. Moreover, vaccination with structural components of the virus avoids the obvious concerns attendant on using proteins with known transforming potential in vitro. The major question will be whether systemic immunization will provide lasting protection to local mucosal sites such as the cervix, or whether novel delivery systems will be required.

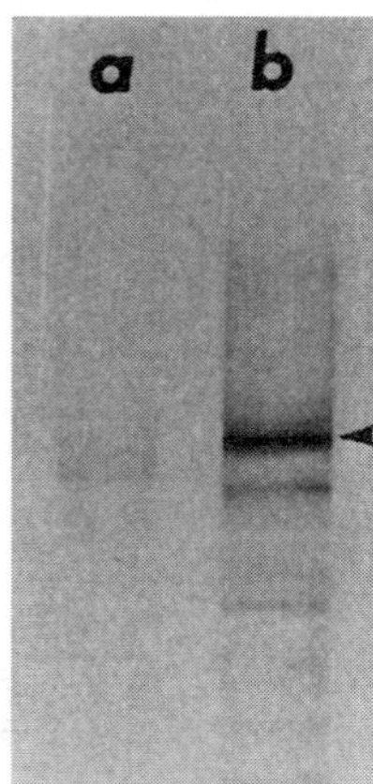

Figure 22.5. Immunoblot (Western blot) with human serum demonstrating seroreactivity to an in vitro synthesized pATH fusion protein containing HPV-16 L2 (capsid) protein. The sera react with the fusion protein (86 kd) in lane b (*arrowhead*). Lane a, containing a vector (pATH) protein alone as a control, is negative

References

1. Abramson AL, Steinberg BM, Winkler B. Laryngeal papillomatosis: clinical histopathologic and molecular studies. Laryngoscope 1987;97:678.
2. Beckmann AM, Daling JR, Sherman KJ, Miller BA, Coates RJ, Kiviat NB, Myerson D, Weiss NS, Hislop TG, Beagrie M, McDougall JK. Human papillomavirus and anal cancer. Int J Cancer 1989;43:1042.
3. Boshart M, Gissman L, Ikenberg H, Scheurlen W, zur Hausen H. A new type of papillomavirus DNA, its presence in genital cancer biopsies and in cell lines derived from cervical cancer. EMBO J 1984;3:1151.
4. Breitburd F, Croissant O, Orth G. Expression of human papillomavirus type-1 E4 gene products in warts. In Cancer Cells 5: Papillomaviruses. Edited by BM Steinberg, JL Brandsma, LB Taichman. Cold Spring Harbor, NY: Cold Spring Harbor Laboratory, 1987, p 115.
5. Broker TR, Botchan M. Papillomaviruses Retrospectives and prospectives. In Cancer Cells 4: DNA Tumor Viruses. Edited by M Botchan, T Grodzicker, PA Sharp. Cold Spring Harbor, NY: Cold Spring Harbor Laboratory, 1986, p 17.
6. Broker TR, Chow LT, Chin MT, Rhodes CR, Wolinsky SM, Whitbeck A, Stoler M. A molecular portrait of human papillomavirus carcinogenesis. In Cancer Cells 7: Molecular Diagnostics of Human Cancer. Edited by M Furth, M Greaves. Cold Spring Harbor, NY: Cold Spring Harbor Laboratory, 1989, p 197.
7. Burkett B, Peterson C, Ward BE, Nuckols M, Burch L, Brennan C, Crum CP. The relationship between contraceptives, sexual practices, and cervical human papillomavirus infection among a college population. J Clin Epidemiol 1992;45:1295.
8. Conrad M, Bubb VJ, Schlegel R. The human papillomavirus type 6 and 16 E5 proteins are membrane-associated proteins which associate with the 16 kDa pre-forming protein. J Virol 1993;67:6170.
9. Crum CP. Female Genital Tract. In Robbins Pathologic Basis of Disease. Edited by R Cotran, V Kumar, S Robbins. Philadelphia: Saunders, 1994, pp 1050–1051.
10. Crum CP, Barber S, Roche JK. Pathobiology of papillomavirus-related cervical diseases: prospects for immunodiagnosis. Clin Microbiol Rev 1991;4:270–285.
11. Crum CP, Ikenberg H, Richart R, Gissman L. Human papillomavirus type 16 and early cervical neoplasia. N Engl J Med 1984;310:380.
12. Crum CP, Mitao M, Levine RU, Silverstein S. Cervical papillomaviruses segregate within morphologicly distinct precancerous lesions. J Virol 1985;54:675.
13. Crum CP, Nuovo G, Friedman D, Silverstein SJ. Accumulation of RNA homologous to human papillomavirus type 16 open reading frames in genital precancers. J Virol 1988;62:84.
14. de Villiers EM, Weidauer H, Otto H, zur Hausen H. Papillomavirus DNA in human tongue carcinomas. Int J Cancer 1985;36:575.
15. DiMaio D, Guralski D, Schiller JT. Translation of open reading frame E5 of bovine papillomavirus is required for its transforming activity. Proc Natl Acad Sci USA 1986;83:1797.
16. DiPaolo JA, Woodworth CD, Popescu NC, Notario V, Doniger J. Induction of human cervical squamous cell carcinoma by sequential infection with human papillomavirus 16 DNA and viral Harvey ras. Oncogene 1989;4:395.
17. Doorbar J, Coneron I, Gallimore PH. Sequence divergence yet conserved characteristics among the E4 proteins of cutaneous human papillomaviruses. Virology 1989;172:51.
18. Durst M, Gissman L, Ikenberg H, zur Hausen H. A papillomavirus DNA from a cervical carcinoma and its prevalence in cancer biopsy samples from different geographic regions. Proc Natl Acad Sci USA 1983;80:3812.
19. Dyson N, Howley PM, Munger K, Harlow E. The human papillomavirus-16 E7 oncoprotein is able to bind to the retinoblastoma gene product. Science 1989;243:934.
20. Ferenczy A, Mitao M, Nagai N, Silverstein SJ, Crum CP. Latent papillomavirus and recurring genital warts. N Engl J Med 1985;313:784.
21. Fu YS, Huang I, Beaudenon S, Ionesco M, Barrasso R, de Brux J, Orth G. Correlative study of human papillomavirus DNA, histopathology, and morphometry in cervical condyloma and intraepithelial neoplasia. Int J Gynecol Pathol 1988;7:297.
22. Fu YS, Reagan JW, Richart RM. Definition of precursors. Gynecol Oncol 1981;12(suppl):220.
23. Gage JC, Meyers C, Wettstein FO. The E7 proteins of the nononcogenic human papillomavirus type 6B and of the oncogenic HPV-16 differ in retinoblastoma protein binding and other properties. J Virol 1990;64:723.
24. Genest D, Stein L, Cibas E, Sheets E, Zitz J, Crum CP. A binary (Bethesda) system for classifying cervical cancer precursors: criteria, reproducibility and viral correlates. Hum Pathol 1993;24:730–736.
25. Gissman L, De Villiers E-M, zur Hausen H. Analysis of human genital warts (condylomata acuminata) and other genital tumors for human papillomavirus type 6 DNA. Int J Cancer 1982;29:143.
26. Goldstein DJ, Schlegel R. The E5 oncoprotein of bovine human papillomavirus binds to a 16 kDa cellular protein. EMBO J 1990;9:137.
27. Hall S, Wu TC, Soudi N, Sherman ME. Low grade squamous intraepithelial lesions: cytologic predictors of biopsy confirmation. Diagn Cytopathol 1994;10:3–9.

28. Heck DV, Yee CL, Howley PM, Munger K. Efficiency of binding the retinoblastoma protein correlates with the transforming capacity of the E7 oncoproteins of the human papillomaviruses. Proc Natl Acad Sci USA 1992;89:4442.
29. Hildesheim A, Reeves WC, Brinton LA, Lavery C, Brenes M, De La Guardia ME, Godoy J, Rawls WE. Association of oral contraceptive use and human papillomavirus in invasive cervical cancers. Int J Cancer 1990;45:860.
30. Hines JF, Ghim SJ, Christensen ND, Kreider JW, Barnes WA, Schlegel R, Jenson AB. Role of conformational epitopes expressed by human papillomavirus major capsid proteins in the serologic detection of infection and prophylactic vaccination. Gynecol Oncol 1994;55:13–20.
31. Koss LG, Durfee GR. Unusual patterns of squamous epithelium of the uterine cervix: cytologic and histologic study of ko locytotic atypia. Ann NY Acad Sci 1956;63:1245.
32. Koutsky LA, Galloway DA, Holmes KK. Epidemiology of genital human papillomavirus infection. Epidemiol Rev 1988;10:122.
33. Koutsky LA, Holmes KK, Critchlow CW et al. A cohort study of the risk of cervical intraepithelial neoplasia grade 2 or 3 in relation to papillomavirus infection. N Engl J Med 1992;327:1272–1278.
34. Kreider JW, Howett MK, Stoler MH, Zaino RJ, Welsh P. Susceptibility of various human tissues to transformation in-vivo with human papillomavirus type II. Int J Cancer 1987;39:459.
35. Kreider JW, Howett MK, Wolfe SA, Bartlett GL, Zaino RJ, Sedlacek T, Mortel R. Morphologic transformation in vivo of human uterine cervix with papillomavirus from condylomata acuminata. Nature 1985;317:639.
36. Kurman RJ, Henson DE, Herbst AL, Noller KL, Schiffman MH. Interim guidelines for management of abnormal cervical cytology. JAMA 1994;271:1866–1869.
37. Kurman RJ, Shiffman RM, Lancaster WD, Reid R, Jenson AB, Temple GF, Lorincz AT. Analysis of individual human papillomavirus types in cervical neoplasia: a possible role for type 18 in rapid progression. Am J Obstet Gynecol 1988;159:1631.
38. Ley C, Bauer HM, Reingold A, Schiffman MH, Chambers JC, Tashiro CJ, Manos MM. Determinants of genital human papillomavirus infection in young women. JNCI 1991;83:997–1003.
39. Lorincz AT, Schiffman MH, Jaffurs WJ, Marlow J, Quinn AP, Temple GF. Temporal associations of human papillomavirus infection with cervical cytologic abnormalities. Am J Obstet Gynecol 1990;162:645.
40. Lorincz AT, Temple GF, Patterson JA, Jenson AB, Kurman RJ, Lancaster WD. Correlation of cellular atypia and human papillomavirus deoxyribonucleic acid sequences in exfoliated cells of the uterine cervix. Obstet Gynecol 1986;68:508.
41. Lowy DR, Dvoretzky I, Shober R, Law M-F, Engel L, Howley P. In vitro tumorigenic transformation by a defined sub-genomic fragment of bovine papillomavirus DNA. Nature 1980;287:72.
42. Lusky M, Botchan MR. Genetic analysis of bovine papillomavirus type I trans-acting replication factors. J Virol 1985;53:955.
43. McCance DJ, Kopan R, Fuchs E, Laimans LA. Human papillomavirus type 16 alters human epithelial cell differentiation in vitro. Proc Natl Acad Sci USA 1988;85:7169.
44. McDonnell JM, Mayr AJ, Martin WJ. DNA of human papillomavirus type 16 in dysplastic and malignant lesions of the conjunctiva and cornea. N Engl J Med 1989;320:1442.
45. McLachlin CM, Tate J, Zitz J, Sheets EE, Crum CP. Human papillomavirus type 18 and squamous intraepithelial lesions of the cervix. Am J Pathol 1994;1:321.
46. Meisels A, Fortin R. Condylomatous lesions of the cervix and vagina: I. Cytologic patterns. Acta Cytol 1976;20:505.
47. Meisels A, Morin C. Human papillomavirus and cancer of the uterine cervix. Gynecol Oncol 1981;12(suppl):111.
48. Melkert PWJ, Hopman E, van Den Brule AJC, Risse EKJ, van Diest PJ, Bleker OP, Helmerhorst T, Schlipper MEJ, Meijer CJ, Walboomers JMM. Prevalence of HPV in cytomorphologicly normal cervical smears as determined by polymerase chain reaction, is age-dependent. Int J Cancer 1993;53:919–923.
49. Moy RL, Eliezri YD, Nuovo GJ, Zitelli ZA, Bennett RG, Silverstein SJ. Squamous cell carcinoma of the finger is associated with human papillomavirus type 16 DNA. JAMA 1989;261:2669.
50. Munger K, Phelps WC. The human papillomavirus E7 protein as a transforming and transactivating factor. Biochim Biophys Acta 1993;115:111.
51. National Cancer Institute: Cancer control objectives for the nation: 1985–2000. Bethesda, MD, U.S. Department of Health and Human Services, Public Health Service, NIH publication No. 86-2880 (NCI Monographs No. 2), 1986.
52. Neary K, Horwitz BH, DiMaio D. Mutational analysis of open reading frame E4 of bovine papillomavirus type 1. J Virol 1987;61:1248.
53. Nuovo GJ. Correlation of histology with human papillomavirus DNA detection in the female genital tract. Gynecol Oncol 1988;31:176.
54. Nuovo GJ. Human papillomavirus (HPV) DNA in genital tract lesions histologically negative for condylomata:.analysis by in situ, Southern blot hybridization and the polymerase chain reaction. Am J Surg Pathol 1990;14[7]:643–651.
55. Nuovo GJ, Pedemonte BM. Human papillomavirus types and recurrent cervical warts. JAMA 1990;263:1223.
56. Ostör AG. Natural history of cervical intraepithelial neoplasia: a critical review. Int J Gynecol Pathol 1993;12:186–192.
57. Papay F, Wood B, Coulson M. Squamous cell papilloma at the tracheoesophageal puncture stoma. Acta Otolaryngol Head Neck Surg 1988;114:564.
58. Pater MM, Hughes GA, Hyslop DE, Nakshatri H, Pater A. Glucocorticoid-dependent oncogenic transformation by type 16 but not type 11 human papillomavirus DNA. Nature 1988;335:832.
59. Phelps WC, Muner K, Yee CL, Barnes JA, Howley PM. Structure-function analysis of the human papillomavirus type 16 E7 protein. J Virol 1992;66:2418.
60. Phelps WC, Yee CL, Munger K, Howley PM. The human papillomavirus type 16 E7 gene encodes transactivation and transformation functions similar to those of adenovirus E1A. Cell 1988;53:539.
61. Purola E, Savia E. Cytology of gynecologic condyloma acuminatum. Acta Cytol 1977;21:26.
62. Reid R, Greenberg M, Jenson AB, Husain M, Willett J, Daoud Y, Temple G, Stanhope CR, Sherman AI, Phibbs GD, Lorincz AT. Sexually transmitted papillomaviral infections: I. The anatomic distribution and pathologic grade of neoplastic lesions associated with different viral types. Am J Obstet Gynecol 1987;156:212.
63. Richart RM. Cervical intraepithelial neoplasia. In Pathology Annual. Edited by SC Sommers. New York: Appleton-Century-Crofts, 1973, p 301.
64. Romanczuk H, Howley PM. Disruption of either the E1 or the E2 regulatory gene of human papillomavirus type 16 increases the viral immortalization capacity. Proc Natl Acad Sci USA 1992;89:3159.
65. Rosenfeld WD, Vermund SH, Wentz SJ, Burk RD. High prevalence rate of human papillomavirus infection and association with abnormal Papanicolaou smears in sexually active adolescents. Am J Dis Child 1989;143:1443–1447.
66. Scheffner M, Munger K, Byrne JC, Howley PM. The state of p53 and retinoblastoma genes in human cervical cell lines. Proc Natl Acad Sci USA 1991;88:5523.
67. Scheffner M, Werness B, Huibregtse JM, Levine AJ, Howley PM. The E6 oncoprotein encoded by human papillomavirus type 16 and 18 promotes the degradation of p53. Cell 1990;63:1129.
68. Schlegel R, Phelps WC, Zhang Y-L, Barbosa M. Quantitative keratinocyte assay detects two biological activities of human papillomavirus DNA and identifies viral types associated with cervical carcinoma. EMBO J 1988;7:3181.
69. Seedorf K, Oltersdorf T, Krammer G, Rowenkamp W. Identification of early proteins of the human papillomaviruses type 16 (HPV 16) and 18 (HPV 18) in cervical carcinoma cells. EMBO J 1987;6:139.
70. Sekine H, Fuse A, Inaba N, Takamizawa H, Simizu B. Detection of the human papillomavirus 6b E2 gene product in genital condyloma and laryngeal papilloma tissues. Virology 1989;170:92.
71. Smotkin D, Berek JS, Fu YS, Hacker NF, Major FG, Wettstein FO. Human papillomavirus deoxyribonucleic acid in adenocarcinoma and adenosquamous carcinoma of the uterine cervix. Obstet Gynecol 1986;68:241.
72. Spalholz BA, Wang Y-C, Howley PM. Transactivation of a bovine papillomavirus transcriptional regulatory element by the E2 gene product. Cell 1985;42:183.
73. Steinberg BM, Topp WC, Schneider PS, Abramson AL. Laryngeal papillomavirus infection during clinical remission. N Engl J Med 1985;308:1261.
74. Stoler MH, Rhodes CR, Whitbeck A, Chow LT, Broker TR. Gene expression of HPV type 16 and 18 in cervical neoplasia. In Papillomaviruses. Edited by P Howley, T Broker. UCLA Symp Mol Biol 1990;124:1.
75. Stoler MH, Walker AN, Mills SE. Small cell neuroendocrine carcinoma of the cervix: a human papillomavirus type 18 associated cervix cancer. Lab Invest 1989;60:92A.
76. Taichman LB, Reilly SS, LaPorta RF. The role of keratinocyte differentiation in the expression of epitheliotropic viruses. J Invest Dermatol 1983;1:137.
77. Vogelstein B, Kinzler KW. p53 function and dysfunction. Cell 1992;70:523.
78. Werness BA, Levine AJ, Howley PM. Association of human papillomavirus types 16 and 18 E6 proteins with p53. Science 1990;248:76.
79. Winkler BW, Capo V, Reumann W, LaPorta R, Reilly S, Green P, Richart RM, Crum CP. Human papillomavirus infection of the esophagus: a clinicopathologic study with demonstration of papillomavirus antigen by the immunoperoxidase technique. Cancer 1985;55:149.
80. Wright TC Jr, Gagnon S, Richart RM, Ferenczy A. Treatment of CIN with the loop electrosurgical excision procedure. Obstet Gynecol 1992;79:173–178.

CHAPTER 23

Hepatitis Viruses

MAX W. SUNG, SWAN N. THUNG, AND GEORGE ACS

Introduction

Jaundice, the clinical manifestation of hepatic necroinflammation or hepatitis, was described in the Babylonian Talmud as early as the fifth century B.C. Pope Zacharias in the eighth century A.D. recognized the infectious nature of the disease when he advised the isolation of jaundiced patients. Lurman in 1885 reported an outbreak of jaundice in shipyard workers who had previously received smallpox vaccines prepared from human "lymph," proving that direct person-to-person contact was not necessary for disease transmission. The transmissible agent was subsequently found to be a "filterable" virus (1).

Epidemiologic studies have since shown that viral hepatitis can be transmitted by two routes: enteric via oral ingestion of fecal material from infected patients, and parenteral via exposure to infected bodily fluids. The viruses were not isolated until much later with the discovery of the hepatitis A and B viruses. Other infectious hepatitis cases not attributable to these two viruses were termed non-A, non-B hepatitis. Recently, three additional viruses were identified in the non-A, non-B group: the hepatitis C, D, and E viruses (2). Sensitive serologic and viral RNA tests have been developed for these viruses. However, there still exists a substantial proportion (20%) of hepatitis cases that cannot be attributed to these five viruses or to other causes of hepatitis, such as alcohol, drugs, and autoimmune disease. These cases are termed hepatitis X (2, 3). With time, additional viruses most likely will be identified. Potential candidates under investigation include the hepatitis F, G, and GB viruses.

Hepatitis A and E viruses are enterically transmitted, whereas the hepatitis B, C, and D viruses are transmitted by parenteral exposure. The enterically transmitted hepatitis viruses generally produce a self-limiting hepatitis followed by complete recovery. The parenterally transmitted hepatitis viruses, on the other hand, can persist as chronic infection with chronic hepatitis and the eventual development of cirrhosis and hepatocellular carcinoma. Other viruses, not specifically hepatotrophic, may also produce hepatic necroinflammation as part of a multisystem disease. These include cytomegalovirus, Epstein-Barr virus, human immunodeficiency virus (HIV), herpes virus, yellow fever virus, rubella, and the Ebola, Lassa, and Marburg viruses.

Hepatitis A Virus

CLINICAL PRESENTATION

Hepatitis A virus (HAV) was the first virus to be isolated from patients with enterically transmitted hepatitis. The virus is hepatotropic, and, following replication in infected hepatocytes, is excreted in the bile and feces. The virus is remarkably stable in the environment, and is most commonly transmitted by the ingestion of fecally contaminated foods and materials. Data from the Sentinel Counties study from the Centers for Disease Control and Prevention (4) showed that HAV is transmitted by person-to-person contact in a variety of settings—in households (24%), in such institutions as day care centers (18%), with male homosexual activities (11%), and during travel to endemic areas (4%). HAV can also be transmitted parenterally, since a viremic phase is seen for several weeks preceding and during clinical hepatitis. It is, therefore, not surprising that 2% of hepatitis A cases in the study occur in the setting of intravenous drug abuse, and that hepatitis A outbreaks have been reported in hemophiliacs receiving factor VIII concentrates. There still remains, however, 40% of HAV cases in the study that cannot be ascribed to known risk factors.

HAV produces a mild clinical hepatitis lasting several weeks, followed by complete recovery. Fulminant hepatitis can occur, particularly in older patients (over 50 years) and in patients with existing chronic liver disease. The fatality rate is 30 per 1,000 reported cases of hepatitis A (5). More commonly, the viral infection is effectively cleared by the host immune system with neutralizing antibodies and virus-specific cytotoxic T lymphocytes. Lifelong immunity is acquired following infection, and HAV infection is not generally associated with chronic hepatitis, cirrhosis, or hepatocellular carcinoma.

Under certain conditions, however, HAV can produce a chronic or relapsing illness. Some patients may develop persistent jaundice from cholestasis without concurrent hepatitis or active viral infection (6). Other patients may evidence disease relapse 2 or 3 months after initial presentation, but with complete resolution without permanent liver damage (7). Patients with immune dysfunction may develop chronic autoimmune hepatitis after HAV infection (8).

Table 23.1. Hepatitis Viruses

Hepatitis virus	HAV	HBV	HCV	HDV	HEV
Structure					
Family	Picornaviridae	Hepadnaviridae	Flaviviridae	Deltaviridae	Calcivir dae/togaviridae
Size (nm)	28	42	38–50	36	32
Genome	Single-stranded RNA (+) 7.5 kb	Double-stranded DNA 3.2 kb	Single-stranded RNA (+) 9.4 kb	Single-stranded RNA (+) 1.7 kb	Single-stranded RNA (+) 7.8 kb
Envelope proteins	None	Large, middle, major HBsAg	E1, E2	Yes (major HBsAg from HBV)	None
Capsid proteins	VP1, VP2, VP3	HBcAg	NS2, NS3, NS4	Small and large HDAg (p24, p27)	Two
Genomic integration	No	Yes	No	No	No
Genotypes	4	5	6 (15 subtypes)	3	3
Serotypes	1	1	?	?	1
	(Ref. 199)	(Ref. 15)	(Ref. 127)	(Ref. 174)	(Ref. 183)
Clinical					
Incubation period	30 days	75 days	50 days	75 days	40 days
Transmission	Fecal-oral	Parenteral	Parenteral	Parenteral	Fecal-oral
Tissues infected	Liver	Liver, blood mononuclear cells	Liver, blood mononuclear cells	Liver	Liver
Viral persistence	No	Yes	Yes	Yes	No
Association with HCC	No	Yes	Yes	No	No
Acute hepatitis	Yes	Yes	Yes	Yes	Yes
Chronic hepatitis	No	Yes	Yes	Yes	No
Progression to chronic hepatitis after acute infection	0%	1–10% adults, 90% neonates	50–80%	2–5% coinfection, 70–90% superinfection	0%
	(Ref. 5)	(Ref. 16)	(Ref. 143)	(Ref. 176)	(Ref. 183)
Diagnosis					
Acute	IgM anti-HAV	IgM anti-HBc, HBsAg, HBeAg, HBV-DNA	HCV-RNA, anti-HCV	IgG anti-HDAg (>1:1000), HDV-RNA	IgM anti-HEV, HEV-RNA
Chronic	NA	HBsAg, HBeAg, HBV-DNA	HCV-RNA, anti-HCV	IgG anti-HDAg (>1:1000), HDV-RNA	NA
Past infection	IgG anti-HAV*	Anti-HBs,* anti-HBc, anti-HBe	Anti-HCV	IgG anti-HDAg (<1:1000)	IgG anti-HEV
	*Also postvaccination (Ref. 5)	*Also postvaccination (Ref. 16)	(Ref. 147)	(Ref. 177)	(Ref. 186)
Treatment					
Acute	? Ribavirin (13)	? Foscarnet (55)	Interferon alpha (157)	? Foscarnet (55)	
Chronic	? Interferon beta (14)	Interferon alpha (42)	Interferon alpha, ribavirin (158)	Interferon alpha (178)	
End stage	Transplant (fulminant) (200)	Transplant + HBIG (52)	Transplant (160)	Transplant (176)	Transplant (fulminant)
Prevention					
Preexposure	HAV vaccine (11)	HBsAg vaccine (60)		HBsAg vaccine (60)	Sanitation of water supply (182)
Postexposure	Immune globulin (10)	Hepatitis B immunoglobulin + vaccine (71)			

Acute HAV infection can be diagnosed serologically by the presence of serum IgM antibody to HAV (IgM anti-HAV). The test is 99% sensitive, and the IgM antibody may persist for up to 12 months after initial presentation. IgG anti-HAV develops after resolution of the acute infection, and appears to be protective against subsequent infection.

PREVENTION AND TREATMENT

HAV hepatitis may be prevented by treatment with inactivated HAV vaccine preexposure, or with immune globulin (Ig) postexposure (9, 101).

Four genotypes of HAV have been isolated, but they are antigenically closely related, and only one serotype has been described. A whole-virus inactivated vaccine has been studied, and found to be immunogenic, with the development of IgG anti-HAV in 100% of vaccines after two or three doses. The level of antibody attained after vaccination is generally lower than that acquired after HAV infection, and more sensitive assays, such as RIFA or RIPA, are necessary for antibody detection. An anti-HAV antibody level of above 40 mIU/mL is considered protective. Efficacy trials of the inactivated HAV vaccine have shown up to 100% protection. A randomized controlled trial with 1,037 children in New York reported no HAV cases 21 to 137 days after vaccination compared with 34 cases in the placebo group (11). A randomized trial in Thailand using another strain of HAV with 40,119 children at 1 year follow-up showed two HAV cases in the vaccine group as compared with 39 cases in the control group (9).

For postexposure prophylaxis, Ig, at a dose of 0.02 mL/kg, is 90% effective when given within 2 weeks of exposure, and is protective for 2 to 3 months (10). Immune globulin is also used for preexposure prophylaxis, but most likely will be replaced by the recently developed inactivated HAV vaccine. Problems with Ig, which is derived from human serum, include the parenteral transmission of viruses. One hundred and twelve cases of acute HCV infection were recently reported following Ig administration (12). To prevent the transmission of such viruses as hepatitis C, hepatitis B, and HIV, all donors are screened for these viruses, and the Cohn-Oncley preparation technique effectively partitions out HIV and HBsAg from the Ig fractions. The combination of immunoglobulin and HAV vaccine has been used post-exposure.

Pilot studies with ribavirin and beta-interferon for the treatment of established hepatitis A infection have shown some responses (13, 14). Recommendations for use await the completion of larger randomized controlled studies.

Table 23.1 lists the characteristics of the HAV, as well as the other hepatitis viruses, discussed in this chapter.

Hepatitis B Virus

STRUCTURE AND PATHOGENICITY

The hepatitis B virus (HBV) consists of a partially double-stranded DNA genome enclosed by envelope proteins (HBsAg). The genome is packaged with a core protein (HBcAg) and a DNA polymerase. Following receptor-mediated entry into a hepatocyte, the virus enters the nucleus and may become integrated into the host genome. Protein synthesis proceeds from four open reading frames: the envelope proteins (large, middle, and major HBsAg) from the S gene, pre-S1, and pre-S2 gene sequences; the e antigen (HBeAg) and core protein (HBcAg) from the C gene and pre-C gene sequence; the DNA polymerase protein from the P gene; and the transactivator X protein from the X gene. HBeAg contains peptides from the pre-C gene sequence, which permits the protein to be secreted, in contrast to HBcAg, which lacks these peptides and remains in the cell. DNA replication proceeds via RNA intermediates in the nucleus. The virus particles are then assembled in the cytoplasm and released by the hepatocyte (15). The virus itself is not cytopathic to the host cell; viral antigens become the target of classes I and II immune responses, which, in turn, produce hepatocyte damage by virus-specific mononuclear immune cells.

In the majority of adult patients, viral infection is cleared by neutralizing antibodies and cytotoxic T lymphocytes, resulting in the disappearance of serum HBV DNA, HBeAg, and HBsAg (16). Viral infection persists chronically in up to 10% of adults and 90% of neonates following acute infection, with persistence of serum HBsAg, HBeAg, and HBV DNA (17). The frequency of viral persistence following acute infection is related to age, sex, and immune deficiency: 90% of infants under 1 year of age, 30% of children ages 1 through 5, 10% of adults; men twice as likely as women; immune-deficient individuals such as those with HIV infection (18), those with renal insufficiency requiring hemodialysis (19), and those with Down's syndrome (20). Patients exposed to large pools of potentially infected plasma, such as hemophiliacs, are also at risk for chronicity. Clearance of the virus in chronic infections may occur spontaneously, with seroconversion to negativity for HBeAg and HBsAg in 10% and 1 to 2% of cases per year, respectively (17). Chronically infected patients exhibit a wide range of pathology, from asymptomatic carriers, to a continuum of hepatic pathology from mild or severe hepatitis, to cirrhosis and/or hepatocellular carcinoma (21, 22). It is important to note that, in up to 15% of HBsAg carriers, HBeAg seroconversion may be associated with persistent high levels of HBV DNA and with high-grade histologic lesions indicative of active viral replication. These patients have been found to acquire a mutation in the pre-C region, which ablated the synthesis of HBeAg (23–25).

Hepatitis B virus is transmitted parenterally from infected patients (26), where concentrations in the blood may approach 10^{10} per milliliter (concentrations in body secretions, such as semen and saliva, are only 1/1,000 that of blood) (27). Settings where HBV may be transmitted include parenteral exposure to infected blood products, such as during transfusions (28): use of contaminated needles in intravenous drug administrations (29), sexual intercourse (30), and from mother to infant perinatally or in utero (31–34). Infants of HBeAg-positive mothers have a 70% chance of infection; following the acute infection, these infants have a 90% chance of developing chronic infection (35). Transmission has also been reported in institutions for the mentally retarded (36), day care centers (37), and family environments with close interpersonal contacts (38–40). The virus has been shown to be quite stable at ambient temperatures, and contamination of surfaces in the homes of chronically infected persons has been documented (41). The mode of transmission in intrafamilial contacts may be through inapparent percutaneous exposure, although oral spread cannot be excluded, since the accidental ingestion of HBsAg-positive human serum has been reported to result in HBV infection.

TREATMENT

Chronic HBV Infection

For the treatment of chronic HBV infection to be effective, it must eliminate viral replication, resolve hepatic necroinflammation, and prevent progression to cirrhosis and hepatocellular carcinoma. The most effective treatment to date is alpha-interferon, given at a dose of 5 million units daily or 10 million units three times a week for 12 to 24 weeks. Meta-analysis of randomized controlled trials showed that alpha-interferon produced seroconversion of HBsAg and HBeAg/HBV DNA 6% and 20%, respectively, more often than controls (42). These rates have taken into account spontaneous seroconversion rates of HBsAg and HBeAg in controls of 2% and 15% per year, respectively. For patients who clear HBeAg, 65% will also clear HBsAg at a mean follow-up of 4.3 years. For patients who clear both HBeAg and HBsAg, 50 to 100% will also clear serum HBV DNA, with improvement in hepatic necroinflammation and normalization of serum alanine aminotransferase (ALT). It should be noted that some patients may clear HBeAg but still maintain high serum levels of HBV DNA. These patients, who are HBsAg and anti-HBe positive, have acquired mutations in the pre-C sequence that ablated synthesis of HBeAg but did not affect viral replication.

Factors predicting a favorable response to alpha-interferon include high serum ALT, low serum HBV DNA, and active hepatic necroinflammation (43). Patients with normal ALT or high serum HBV DNA rarely respond to interferon. It should be noted that Oriental patients who demonstrate these favorable predictors to alpha-interferon respond as well as white and black patients (44). Patients, particularly those with more severe hepatitis, may experience a flare-up of hepatic necroinflammation with alpha-interferon treatment, but do not usually require that treatment be interrupted. Prednisone priming prior to alpha-interferon has been reported in pilot studies to be more effective than alpha-interferon alone. This has not been confirmed in large-scale studies, however, and is not used as standard treatment (45, 46).

Other drugs that have been shown to be effective and tolerated in pilot studies include lamivudine, an orally administered nucleoside analogue that inhibited HBV replication following a 1-month course of treatment. Unfortunately, patients relapsed after cessation of treatment. Of interest is a report from France that showed that HBsAg vaccine was effective in 3 of 14 patients with chronic HBV infection, with clearance of serum HBV DNA after three injections (47). 2′,3′-Dideoxynucleotides have been used to inhibit HBV replication in vitro with limited success (48). The carbocyclic analogue of 2′-deoxyguanosine, 2′-CDG, however, has been shown to produce virtual cessation of viral replication in vitro and in vivo in the duck hepatitis model. 2′-CDG can be administered orally, prolonging the antiviral effect, lasts at least 8 days after a 1 day treatment (49). Moreover, 2′-CDG was nontoxic at concentrations 200 times the minimum effective inhibitory concentration (50).

For patients with liver cirrhosis caused by chronic HBV infection, orthotopic liver transplantation may provide a benefit in long-term survival. Recurrence of HBV infection, however, occurs at a rate of 40% and 50% at 1 and 3 years following transplantation. Recurrence is particularly high in patients with positive serum HBV DNA at the time of transplantation (83% at 3 years posttransplant), compared with 58% at 3 years posttransplant in those negative for HBeAg and HBV DNA at the time of transplantation (51, 52). Long-term therapy with high-dose hepatitis B immunoglobulin (HBIG) posttransplant decreased HBV recurrence from 75% to 35%, and increased survival from 50% to 82% at 3 years posttransplant (52). These studies indicate that patients with HBV-related cirrhosis but negative HBeAg and HBV DNA may benefit from liver transplantation with HBIG treatment posttransplant.

Acute HBV Infection

Treatment of acute HBV infection ideally should shorten the clinical course, improve recovery in fulminant cases, and eliminate viral persistence. Unfortunately, alpha-interferon has not been found effective. A randomized controlled trial of alpha-interferon for acute HBV infection showed no difference when compared with placebo (53). A pilot study of alpha-interferon for fulminant HBV infection showed no improvement of mortality (80%) when compared with historic controls (54). Fulminant hepatitis was, however, effectively treated with the antiviral drug Foscarnet (trisodium phosphonoformate hexahydrate), given as a continuous intravenous infusion to maintain plasma level of 150 μg/mL for 4 to 14 days. Six of eight patients with fulminant HBV hepatitis treated with Foscarnet completely recovered, and the two nonresponders had received the drug for only 1 day (55).

PREVENTION

Preexposure Prophylaxis

Effective vaccines for prophylaxis against HBV infection were first introduced by Krugman in 1981 using inactivated human HBsAg positive serum. The HBsAg particles were subsequently purified from seropositive human sera and used in the plasma-derived vaccine. Advances in genetic engineering enabled the large-scale production of HBsAg protein product by viral expression vectors coding the S gene in Baker's yeast (56). Over 90% of patients developed adequate levels of anti-HBs (> 10 mIU/mL) following a series of three injections at 0, 1, and 6 months, and in these subjects protection from subsequent hepatitis B infection was virtually complete (57). Some patients develop "breakthrough" HBV infection despite protective levels of anti-HBs; one of these subjects has been shown to have acquired an infection with an HBsAg mutant virus, where a mutation in the S gene resulting in an amino acid substitution at position 145 rendered the virus insensitive to the neutralizing antibody raised by conventional HBsAg vaccine (58, 59).

Of vaccinated subjects, 90% and 80% retain detectable and protective levels, respectively, of anti-HBs 5 years after vaccination (60). The side effects of vaccination include mild pain at the site of injection and mild temperature elevations. There have been no reported cases of HIV transmission with either the plasma-derived or recombinant vaccines. However, 5% of the vaccinated subjects developed inadequate responses (between 2.1 and 9.9 mIU/mL), while the remaining 5% produced no anti-HBs. Lack of response may be due to immune suppression, such as in those with renal failure or HIV infection; older age (more than 60 years); or route of injection, since intramuscular is superior to subcutaneous or intradermal administration. For nonresponders or inadequate responders, an additional dose produced adequate levels of anti-HBs in 25%; an additional series of three injections produced adequate anti-HBs in 50 to 60%. For the remainder, co-administration of the vaccine with alpha-interferon, thymopentin, or interleukin-2 is being investigated for enhancement of response.

Other vaccines for preventing HBV infection are currently under investigation. HBsAg vaccines incorporating the pre-S2 polypeptide may induce responses in individuals who failed to respond to the conventional vaccine (61). A monoclonal antibody 2F10 has been raised that is an "internal image" anti-idiotype antibody capable of mimicking the group-specfic "a" determinant of HBsAg. The antibody can generate B- and T-cell responses to HBsAg when injected into mice. A 15-MER peptide from the hypervariable region of 2F10 has been isolated that is capable of generating similar immune responses as the intact antibody, and has potential for vaccine development (62). Large-scale production of immunogenic protein can be accomplished with insects or worms infected with viral vectors, or with transgenic plants (63). Recombinant HBsAg obtained from transgenic tobacco plants has been shown to elicit B- and T-cell immune responses when injected into mice (64). Tests in feeding animals with transgenic potatoes encoding recombinant HBsAg are currently in progress, and may offer a more economic program for large scale vaccinations. Vaccine administration can also be facilitated by multiple pressure/scratch techniques using vaccinia virus vectors and by oral administration using adenovirus vectors (65, 66).

Despite the development of safe and effective vaccines for HBV infection, the incidence of hepatitis B in the United States has increased. This is so in contrast to vaccination programs in Taiwan and Switzerland, where a decrease in HBV infection incidence has been demonstrated. The failure in the United States may be due to inadequate vaccination of high-risk subjects (only 10% were vaccinated) and the fact that 30 to 40% of new HBV cases did not fall into the high-risk category (67–69). The current recommendation for a universal hepatitis B vaccination program in childhood should result in the vaccination of all subjects and effectively reduce the incidence of HBV infection (70).

Postexposure Prophylaxis

For prevention after HBV exposure, such as following delivery of a neonate from an infected mother, needle-stick puncture from an infected patient, or sexual intercourse with an infected partner, administration of hepatitis B immunoglobulin (HBIG) followed by HBV vaccination has been more than 90% effective (71). Vaccination without HBIG produced only 70 to 80% anti-HBs responses.

HBV AND HEPATOCELLULAR CARCINOMA

Epidemiologic Considerations

The evidence for an epidemiologic association between chronic HBV infection and hepatocellular carcinoma (HCC) is overwhelming. Nearly 300 million people worldwide are chronic carriers of HBV and the risk of developing HCC in this population is more than 200-fold higher than in the noninfected population (72). In low endemic areas, HCC was found in about 0.4% of autopsies (73, 74), whereas in high endemic areas where HBV infection is 10-fold higher, 20 to 40% of all cancers are HCC (75–78). In the best prospective study from Taiwan, 22,707 males were tested for hepatitis B surface antigen, of whom 3,454 were positive (15.2%) (79). In the 7-year follow-up, 116 cases of HCC were diagnosed. All of them had previously tested positive for HBsAg, except for three who had serologic markers of previous HBV infection. None of the HBsAg-negative controls developed HCC. HBsAg carriers at especially high risk were those with active infection (HBeAg/HBV DNA positive) and those with cirrhosis (80). In another prospective study that of 824 native Alaskan HBsAg carriers, the annual incidence for HCC was 387 in 100,000, accounting for 57% of cancer-related deaths, compared with the noncarrier Alaskan native population, where HCC accounted for 2% of all cancer-related deaths (81). These two studies not only indicate an association between HBV and HCC, but also strongly suggest a causal relationship. It is generally accepted that carcinogenesis is a multistep process involving initiation, promotion, and progression (82). The question arises as to whether, despite this overwhelming epidemiologic evidence, HBV infection alone can be responsible for all of these processes.

There are several observations indicating that other agents alone or in combination with HBV play a role in the etiology of HCC. In industrialized countries, 68%, and in developing countries, 11% of the HCC patients do not have serologic markers of HBV infection. These data must be treated cautiously since they depend on the sensitivities of the assays for serologic markers. The numbers may change substantially by using the polymerase chain reaction, which can detect minimal amounts of HBV DNA in serum or tissue (83–85). More compelling evidence for the contribution of other factors to hepatic carcinogenesis are the following: (*a*) within one region, the prevalence of HBV infection may be relatively uniform, but HCC is not (86–89); (*b*) HCC is more frequently found in men than in women; and (*c*) in some endemic areas, variations in HCC rates have been reported according to ethnic group or place of birth (90). Besides HBV, other factors in the development of HCC may include other chronic viral hepatitis infections, such as HCV and HXV, cirrhosis of any etiology, genetic disposition, androgenic-anabolic and oral contraceptive steroids, and the role of the immune system. In addition, alcohol, cigarettes, oral contraceptives, and aflatoxin have been implicated as etiologic agents, as have α_1-antitrypsin deficiency and schistosomiasis.

Aflatoxin exposure from ingestion of aflatoxin-contaminated food has been implicated as a cause of HCC. Most of these correlation studies were done in high HBV endemic areas, and did not take into account HBV status, and were plagued by inaccurate assessments of aflatoxin exposure. A 1987 study in Swaziland addressed the relationship among aflatoxin exposure, HBV infection, and the incidence of HCC (91). In this study, HBsAg prevalence varied little from region to region, while aflatoxin exposure varied as much as fivefold. The incidence of hepatocellular carcinoma also varied up to fivefold and correlated well with aflatoxin exposure, suggesting that aflatoxin may act as an independent risk factor. Furthermore, HCC in countries where aflatoxin is highly suspect have frequent G : C to T : A transversions in codon 249 of the *p53* gene, providing a molecular epidemiologic signature by this particular mutation (92) (see Chapter 13). Alcohol consumption and cigarette smoking have also been implicated in the causation of HCC in case control and cohort studies. However, when HBV status was taken into account, alcohol consumption remained a risk factor, whereas cigarette smoking did not (93–95). The role of cirrhosis as the actual etiologic link was addressed in a cross-sectional study from France that showed that the relative risk for hepatocellular carcinoma was about twice as great in HBV-associated cirrhosis as in alcoholic cirrhosis patients (96). Of note is a study from Taiwan where up to 27% of HBV-associated hepatocellular carcinomas did not include cirrhosis

(79). Oral contraceptive use has also been recognized as a risk factor (97–99).

Mechanisms of Oncogenicity

Application of the technology of molecular biology to HBV infection gave several clues regarding the mechanisms by which HBV infection leads to HCC. A uniform mechanism, valid for every HCC, is still elusive, however. In the following sections, we review the genetic organization of HBV during infection, and the possible mechanism(s) by which it can cause HCC.

The availability of cloned HBV DNA made it possible to detect HBV DNA in hepatocellular carcinomas. The epidemiologic studies based on serologic markers were confirmed, since all the HCCs induced by HBV infection contained chromosomally integrated HBV DNA in various forms. The long latency period that elapses between infection and the development of HCC makes it very unlikely that the HBV DNA codes for a dominantly acting classic oncogene. Furthermore, during this latency period, the HBV DNA becomes fragmented and rearranged; thus, neither the HBV DNA sequences inserted nor the chromosomal sites of insertion are uniform in the various HCCs. The chromosomally integrated HBV DNA may release the growth control of hepatocytes by coding for a factor like the X protein that activates otherwise dormant genes, or activates proto-oncogenes, or silences antioncogenes; inserting of HBV DNA sequences that can also activate and influence the transcription of cellular genes; and causing chronic inflammation with cell death and hepatocyte regeneration, fibrosis, and activation of the immune system by liberating cytokines at the wrong time at the wrong place.

Role of X Protein in HCC

The X protein coded by the X gene of HBV has a transactivating activity on a number of viral and cellular genes that may be involved in the development of HCC (100–102). Its genomic localization is analogous to that of the human T-cell lymphotropic viruses (HTLV-I, II, and HIV), namely, it is at the 3′ end of the linearized genome. Interestingly, other DNA viruses with oncogenic activity also code for a transactivating activity; for example, the T antigen of SV40, the MS-EA protein of Epstein-Barr virus, the IE protein of herpes simplex, and the *tat* protein of HIV, which, despite being an RNA virus, shares some steps in its replicative cycle with HBV. The sequence coding for the X protein is well conserved among the various subtypes of HBV and in the woodchuck and ground squirrel hepatitis viruses. Despite similar genetic organizations of the hepadnaviruses, duck hepatitis virus does not contain the sequences coding for the X protein, and infection with this virus does not lead to HCC. In many HCCs, the viral DNA is inserted near or within the coding sequences of the X protein (103); thus, it is possible that expression of this protein, or of a fusion protein with cellularly coded genes, plays an important role in the development of HCC. That specific cellular proteins in concert with virally coded proteins are involved in HCC is suggested by the finding that chimpanzees infected with HBV display the classic symptoms and signs of hepatitis, as judged morphologically in liver, and by the appearance of elevated serum enzymes, together with viral antigens and the corresponding antibodies. In contrast to human disease, however, HBV infection in the chimpanzee does not lead to HCC.

Activation of Oncogenes, Growth Factors, and Receptors in HCC

Although the woodchuck hepatitis virus DNA sequences are not integrated adjacent to the coding sequences of the *myc* gene, rearrangements of the *myc* gene with a fivefold to fiftyfold higher expression were found in several HCCs. The rearrangements found in woodchuck HCCs are similar to those found in human B- and T-cell leukemias, Burkitt's lymphoma, and mouse plasmacytoma (104). Mutations and activation of the genes belonging to the *ras* family are associated with a wide variety of human cancers. Mutations in the *ras* gene(s) are not regularly found in human HCCs, but activated H-*ras* and K-*ras* genes have been detected in some HCCs (105, 106). Since, in other tissues, high expression of the *ras* genes, as well as mutated sequences, is associated with malignant transformation, the role of the *ras* gene in HCCs cannot be overlooked. Among the growth factors analyzed in HCCs, insulin-like growth factor 2 (IGF 2), originally called somatomedin A, seems to be involved in the development of HCCs. The IGF 2 RNAs are differentially spliced; the most abundant species found in fetal woodchuck liver represent the predominant species in both precancerous liver nodules and HCCs in the woodchuck. Furthermore, the pattern of IGF 2 RNAs in precancerous liver nodules is similar to that found in fully malignant HCCs. Thus, the activation of IGF 2 transcripts may contribute to the growth of precancerous nodules (107). Since the development of carcinomas can be viewed as a disturbance of the signal transducing system, it is intriguing that HBV DNA is sometimes integrated in a frame next to a liver cell sequence that bears a striking homology not only to v-*erb*-A oncogene, but also to the DNA binding domains of the human glucocorticoid receptor, estrogen receptor genes, and retinoic acid receptor. The inappropriate expression of these genes due to HBV DNA integration might be a contributory factor to the development of HCCs. The HBV DNA integration into chromosomal DNA was found to have a relationship to oncogenes, receptors, and growth factors, and, at least in one case, to a normal protein, cyclin A (107). Cyclins A and B are well conserved during evolution and play an important role in mitotic division. The finding that HBV DNA is inserted into the intron of cyclin A might influence the progression phase of HCCs. This brief and by no means complete, summation of the insertion sites of HBV DNA leads unequivocally to the conclusion that the integration of HBV DNA can be viewed only as guilt by association; the "smoking gun" has not yet been identified.

Tumor Suppressor Genes in HCC

Several lines of evidence indicate that HBV DNA insertion into chromosomes may be associated with the inactivation of a tumor suppressor gene. First, the long latency period that elapses between infection and the development of HCC and the fact that not all infections lead to HCC are compatible with the notion, as in retinoblastoma, that one allele is altered genetically while the other allele is somatically mutated. Indeed, in children with the Beckwith-Wiedemann congenital malformation syndrome, 10% of the cases are associated with mutations on chromosome 11. This leads to tumor formation, which includes hepatoblastoma, Wilms' tumor, rhabdomyosarcoma, and adrenal carcinoma (109). That chromosome 11 codes for a tumor suppressor gene was shown by Stanbridge, who found that the malignant phenotype was repressed when the normal chromosome 11 was present in somatic hybrids between tumorigenic and nontumorigenic cells (110). The loss of this chromosome led to a reversion to the malignant phenotype. The suppressor gene in retinoblastoma was mapped to chromosome 13 (111). In 45% of HCC cases, alleles from chromosome 11p are missing, and in 50% of HCCs, alleles from chromosome 13q are missing (112). In addition, HBV DNA integration was mapped to chromosome 11 in many cases. It has also been shown that the p53 gene functions as a tumor suppressor, and in many human cancers, including HCC, mutations occur in this gene, with the mutated gene subsequently acting as an oncogene (113, 114). Further, albeit circumstantial, evidence for the role of suppressor genes in HCC is furnished by transgenic mice carrying the SV40 gene coding for T antigen, the tumorigenic activity of the SV40 T antigen is associated with its ability to bind to the suppressor gene product. In transgenic mice expressing SV40 T antigen, after a long period of hyperplasia, HCC develops (115). Furthermore, mouse hepatocytes that were immortalized by T antigen were transfected with a selectable gene and HBV DNA. All the cells in which HBV replicated displayed malignant growth characteristics and were tumorigenic.

HBV-Induced Hepatocytic Hyperplasia and Necrosis in HCC

As a consequence of HBV infection leading to HCC hepatocytic nodules, ground-glass-appearing cells containing HBsAg, hyperplasia, necroinflammation, fibrosis, portal inflammation, and, in many cases, cirrhosis, can be detected in the liver (116). The causal relation between the infection and the liver cell injury has not yet been elucidated. We have only circumstantial evidence that the immune system is involved (117, 118). The availability of vaccines and the production of viral antigens by recombinant DNA technology made it possible to determine that the production of antibodies against HBsAg is T-cell dependent, while HBcAg is more immunogenic and elicits antibodies in T cell dependent and independent ways (119, 120). HBcAg-specific, functionally competent CD4+ helper and CD8+ suppressor T cells were detected in chronic infection, whereas HBsAg-specific T cells were not found (121). The T-cell clones that were HBcAg- specific were HLA-DR restricted and secreted interleukin-2, gamma-interferon, and tumor necrosis factor. For this involvement of the immune system it is obligatory that HBV enter the cells of the immune system, in order to present the antigen, and there are indications that, albeit rarely, lymphocytes and monocytes are infected with HBV in vivo. Although the involvement of the immune system could adequately explain the cascade of events that lead from infection through inflammation, necrosis, and regeneration, with subsequent genetic changes leading to HCC, the results obtained with transgenic mice indicate that HCC can develop without the contributions of the immune system. Transgenic mice carrying HBV DNA sequences have been produced in several laboratories (122–124). The livers of these animals synthesize HBsAg and secrete virus into the serum, but the immune system is tolerant. In one case, a programmed response characterized by inflammation, regenerative hyperplasia, and aneuploidy led to the development of HCC. The incidence of HCC was influenced by sex and age and was directly related to liver cell injury and nonsecreted HBsAg content of the liver cells (123).

Thus, in summation several factors, directly or indirectly, alone or in combination, can lead to HCC, but the integration of HBV DNA in one form or another is obligatory in HBV-associated hepatocarcinogenesis.

Hepatitis C Virus

STRUCTURE AND PATHOGENICITY

Hepatitis C virus (HCV) was first isolated from non-A, non-B infectious plasma in 1989 (125). HCV is a member of the family Flaviviridae, which includes yellow fever virus, dengue viruses, and Japanese encephalitis virus (126). HCV measures 30 to 60 μm and is an enveloped virus with a single-stranded, linear, positive-sense RNA genome, which is approximately 9.5 kb in length (125, 127–129). It contains one large open reading frame capable of encoding a polyprotein precursor of 3,011 amino acids. Structural proteins are encoded at the 5′ end. The 5′ noncoding region precedes the large coding sequence and represents the most highly conserved sequence among the different viral isolates. A series of three short open reading frames exist in the 5′ noncoding region (125, 128–131). The amino terminal end of the transcript is cleaved to produce the core protein, an unglycosylated, basic, 19 to 22 kd protein (p22). Two putative enveloped glycoproteins of 33 to 35 and 70 to 72 kd are designated E1 and E2. The amino terminal end of E2 contains a hypervariable region that exhibits significant variation among HCV isolates. Four nonstructural domains follow (NS2 to NS5). The NS2 region is extremely hydrophobic but its function has not been identified. The NS3 region encodes a 60 kd protein that contains a viral protease involved in polyprotein processing and a putative helicase enzyme that is probably involved in unwinding the RNA genome for replication. The NS4 region is also extremely hydrophobic and shows 50% sequence homology among the different HCV types. The function of NS4 is not known. The NS5 region encodes a 116 kd RNA-dependent RNA polymerase that replicates the RNA genome.

Phylogenetic analysis of NS5 and E1 nucleotide sequences from samples obtained worldwide led to the identification of six major genetic groups and 14 subgroups (132). The clinical consequence of the genetic heterogeneity of

HCV is not clear. Several reports have suggested correlation among these various genotypes with the severity of liver disease, the outcome of interferon treatment, and the development of hepatocellular carcinoma (133). The diversity of HCV may also explain the multiple infections and co-infections with different HCV subtypes in the same individuals (134, 135). Furthermore, this heterogeneity will make the control of HCV by vaccination difficult.

PATHOGENESIS OF LIVER DISEASE

Hepatitis C is the most common cause of nonalcoholic liver disease in the United States. More than 150,000 individuals are acutely infected with HCV annually (136). Hepatitis C is transmitted through blood and blood products. Risk factors include blood transfusion and intravenous drug abuse (4, 136–138). Sexual and perinatal transmissions are less important routes in hepatitis C. Perinatal transmission occurs more readily when the mother is co-infected with HIV (139, 140). In approximately 40% of patients with hepatitis C, there are no recognizable risk factors (141). These cases are called sporadic or community-acquired hepatitis. HCV produces a clinical picture similar to that of hepatitis B, but usually much milder. Chronic HCV infection, however, develops in up to 80% of cases and progresses to cirrhosis in 50% of them (2, 142, 143). Fulminant hepatitis is unusual in hepatitis C.

ANTI-HCV ANTIBODY AND HCV-RNA ASSAYS

The second generation of enzyme-linked immunosorbent assays (EIA-2) for the detection of anti-HCV in the serum was developed to overcome the problems of specificity and sensitivity observed with the first-generation test (EIA-1) (144–147). EIA-2 includes two additional antigens: c200 which encompasses the regions of both c100-3 (NS4 of EIA-1) and c33 (NS3) and c22-3 in the core region. A positive anti-HCV result with EIA-2 confirms HCV as the cause of the liver disease in the setting of an identifiable risk factor or clinical evidence of liver disease. In some clinical situations, confirmation of a positive antibody to HCV with recombinant immunoblot assay (RIBA) is necessary (148, 149).

The detection of HCV RNA following polymerase chain reaction (PCR) (150–152) is rarely needed to establish the diagnosis in immunocompetent patients with chronic hepatitis. In immunosuppressed patients with negative anti-HCV, however, nucleic acid assays may be necessary to establish virus presence. Quantitative methods, such as the branched DNA signal amplification assay (153) have been used to identify candidates for interferon therapy and to monitor viral load during the course of chronic infection and antiviral treatment, and prior to liver transplantation to predict recurrent infection in the allografts.

PREVENTION AND TREATMENT

Little is known about either passive or active immunity to HCV. Recent studies have shown that reinfection with HCV following a previous infection is quite common (154, 155). This finding suggests that long-lasting immunity to HCV infection is nonexistent. HCV has the ability to mutate rapidly under immune pressure and to exist simultaneously as a series of related but immunologically distinct variants, any one of which can become the predominant strain when a coexistent strain comes under immune pressure (133, 156). This coexistence of multiple mutants has been termed quasispecies. Neutralizing antibodies to HCV have been shown to develop, but they are strain specific and are ineffective against the emerging strains. Major efforts are underway to develop a vaccine that would bypass these obstacles and provide protective immunity.

Alpha-interferon-2b at a dose of 3 million units given three times a week for 6 months is the only treatment effective for chronic HCV infection (157). Three randomized trials, conducted in France and in the United States, have shown that 41% of treated patients had normalized serum ALT, and 70% of the responders had an improvement in necroinflammation of the liver on biopsy. Almost all responders lose detectable HCV RNA by the end of treatment, but responders relapse with a return of detectable HCV RNA following cessation of treatment. Favorable predictors of response to alpha-interferon-2b include the absence of advanced inflammation or cirrhosis on liver histology, low HCV RNA, and genotypes 1a and 1b. Oral ribavirin at doses of 1,000 to 1,200 mg daily produced improvement in aminotransferase activities in all 13 patients treated with the drug, but the effect was not sustained after cessation of therapy, and HCV RNA decreased only slightly during treatment (158). Other agents are currently being investigated (159).

For patients with end-stage liver cirrhosis from chronic HCV infection, orthotopic liver transplantation may prolong survival. Recurrence of HCV infection is close to 100% posttransplant, but, unlike recurrent HBV infection, the clinical course is indolent, and liver cirrhosis may not appear for years posttransplant (160). Treatment with alpha-interferon-2b posttransplant showed a 28% response with normalization of ALT, and 100% response with decrease in HCV RNA, but HCV RNA invariably returned to the pretreatment level after cessation of treatment (161).

HCV AND HEPATOCELLULAR CARCINOMA

A significant proportion of patients with HCC are infected with HCV (162–164). Patients with well-documented transfusion-related hepatitis C progressed from acute to chronic hepatitis to cirrhosis, and, finally, to HCC after 7 to 23 years. Similar observations were made in chimpanzees years after inoculation of serum with a patient with chronic non-A, non-B hepatitis (165). The epidemiologic evidence for an association of HCV with HCC is compelling. Case control studies from Japan, Italy, Spain, South Africa, and Taiwan have shown that the prevalence of anti-HCV positivity in patients with HCC is substantially higher than in the control population. Up to 60 to 70% of Japanese patients with HCC were seropositive for antibody to HCV. A similar prevalence was reported in western Europe. HCV RNA and the viral proteins can be detected in both the tumor and the surrounding cirrhotic nodules of these patients (166, 167). The role of HCV in the malignant transformation of hepatocytes, however, is not clear. While 30% of HCCs in HBV carriers developed in the absence of cirrhosis, HCC arising in chronic hepatitis C is generally associated with cirrhosis, with the exception of rare cases (168–170). These findings suggest the indirect role of HCV in hepatocarcinogenesis, probably through continuous cell regeneration (171–173) due to the chronic microinflammatory process, which predisposes hepatocytes to mutations and malignant transformation.

Hepatitis D Virus (HDV)

CLINICAL PRESENTATION

Hepatitis D virus (delta virus, or HDV) is an enveloped RNA virus whose envelope proteins are derived from proteins synthesized by the hepatitis B virus (174). It, therefore, requires the presence of HBV for infection. Acute HDV infection may occur concurrently with acute HBV infection (HDV/HBV co-infection), or may take place in the setting of an established chronic HBV infection (HDV superinfection). Acute HDV/HBV co-infection usually produces a self-limiting hepatitis, with only 2 to 5% persisting as chronic HDV infection. Acute HDV superinfection, however, persists as a chronic infection in 70 to 90% of cases, and the progression to cirrhosis is more accelerated as compared with chronic HBV infection alone (175). Generally, acute HDV superinfection presents as an acute exacerbation of chronic HBV hepatitis. However, 17% of patients with acute HDV superinfection develop fulminant hepatitis. In comparison, only 2% of patients with acute HDV/HBV co-infection develop fulminant hepatitis (176). Diagnosis of acute and chronic HDV infection is by the presence in serum of IgG anti-HDAg at titers of more than 1:1,000, HDAg, or HDV RNA (177). Serum IgG anti-HDAg may persist after resolution of HDV infection, but titers are generally less than 1:1,000.

HDV has not been associated with hepatocellular carcinoma. Patients with HBsAg-positive cirrhosis and HCC have a prevalence of chronic HDV infection similar to that of patients with HBsAg-positive cirrhosis without HCC. Chronic HDV infection, however, may accelerate the development of cirrhosis, thereby increasing the risk for hepatocellular carcinoma.

PREVENTION AND TREATMENT

Chronic HDV infection responds to alpha-interferon (178). Some 25 to 60% of treated patients have a normalization of ALT levels, with HDV RNA becoming undetectable. Time to response is generally longer (after 4 to 6 months for treatment) than with chronic HBV or HCV infection, and the doses required may be even higher than for chronic HBV infection. Relapses following cessation of therapy appear to be the rule, with 90% of patients developing increases in ALT and detectable HDV RNA 6 months after the cessation of treatment. Only those patients who clear serum HBsAg have sustained responses to interferon, with clearance even by PCR of HDV RNA from serum and liver.

Patients with HDV-related cirrhosis or fulminant hepatitis are good candidates for orthotopic liver transplantation. The risk of reinfection with HDV is lower than for HBV, and the clinical course following reinfection is more benign. The 5-year survival following liver transplant for chronic HDV infection is 88%, with a 32% risk of recurrence at 3 years (179, 180).

Transmission patterns for HDV are similar to those of HBV, namely, via parenteral exposure from contaminated blood products or intravenous drug usage. Prevention is of particular importance for patients with chronic HBV infection because of the aggressive clinical course of HDV superinfection. Current preventive measures for HDV infection include safe blood bank practices, abstinence from intravenous drug use, and vaccination against HBV. There is no commercial vaccine available for HDV. Recombinant HDAg as a vaccine has been tested in the woodchuck model and found to be immunogenic but not protective against HDV infection.

Hepatitis E Virus

CLINICAL PRESENTATION

Enterically transmitted viral hepatitis without serologic evidence for HAV infection (non-A, non-B hepatitis) was first noted in a retrospective study of an epidemic in Delhi, India, in 1956. More than 29,000 cases were reported after the water supply in the region became contaminated with sewage (181). Other epidemics involving contaminated water supplies included the 1986–1988 epidemic in Xinjiang, China, where 119, 280 people became infected over a period of 20 months (182). Hepatitis E virus (HEV) was identified as the etiology for enterically transmitted non-A, non-B hepatitis following confirmatory transmission studies in nonhuman primates (183, 184).

Like HAV, HEV is a nonenveloped RNA virus that produces a transient clinical hepatitis followed by complete recovery. Acute HEV infection in pregnant women, particularly those in the third trimester, can be fulminant and fatal in 20% of cases (185). There is no evidence for chronic hepatitis or persistent viremia following acute HEV infection. The acute infection is diagnosed by the detection of serum IgM anti-HEV antibody, which persists for up to 3 months after clinical presentation (186). HEV virus particles can also be detected in the stool by immune electronmicroscopy, and HEVAg in infected hepatocytes by immunofluorescent probes. Evidence of past infection is detected by the presence of IgG anti-HEV that arises soon after the resolution of clinical hepatitis (186).

PREVENTION

HEV hepatitis occurs primarily in developing countries in subtropical or tropical climates upon contamination of the water supply. The only reported cases in developed countries were from people who had recently returned from visits to endemic areas. Prevention of HEV hepatitis lies primarily in maintaining a sanitary water supply. Vaccine from attenuated HEV has not been prepared because of the problems of culturing HEV in vitro. A vaccine using HEV viral fusion protein trpE-C2 has been tested in cynomolgus macaques and reported to be immunogenic and protective against challenge by wild strains of HEV (187).

Hepatitis X

A sizable proportion of hepatitis cases cannot be ascribed to infection by the five known hepatitis viruses, or to other causes, such as drugs and autoimmune disease. Up to 20% of acute and chronic hepatitis cases are of unknown etiology, and are grouped under hepatitis X (2, 173, 188). Hepatitis X is of clinical importance because of its association with fulminant hepatic failure and hepatitis-associated aplastic anemia. Thirty-eight percent of fulminant hepatic failure cases are of unknown etiology (hepatitis X), and have a fatality rate of 80 to 100%. Almost all cases of hepatitis-associated aplastic anemia are of unknown etiology (hepatitis X) (189). Acute hepatitis X also progresses to chronic hepatitis in 29% of cases, and to the eventual development of cirrhosis and hepatocellular carcinoma (2).

Hepatitis X, therefore, falls into a subgroup of non-A, non-B viral hepatitis after eliminating the presence of HCV, HDV, and HEV infection. Multiple etiologies and viruses may eventually be discovered for the entity of hepatitis X. Candidates currently under study include hepatitis F, G, and G-B viruses.

Toga virus-like 60 to 70 nm enveloped particles were recovered from the hepatocytes of a number of patients transplanted for fulminant hepatic failure, which recurred within 7 days following transplantation. Since there is no evidence for hepatitis A, B, C, D, or E by PCR in the livers of these patients, these particles have been termed hepatitis F virus (190–192).

A PCR assay of a transfusion-related hepatitis virus (hepatitis G virus) has been developed that has detected the presence of the virus in 18 to 33% of groups with high risks of exposure to blood and blood products in the United States, Japan, and Europe (193, 194). There is evidence for a persistent carrier state in patients with normal transaminases that may have widespread implications for blood bank practices as the virus has been associated with acute and chronic hepatitis.

Two RNA viruses (GB virus A and GB virus B) have been isolated from a patient with acute hepatitis and successfully passaged in tamarin colonies. The GB viruses resemble agent WW-55 isolated from another jaundiced patient. WW-55 has been shown to induce hepatitis in 5 of 10 volunteers injected with the agent (195).

Clinical Significance of Viral Hepatitis to Hepatocellular Carcinoma

The epidemiologic association of chronic infection with hepatitis viruses and HCC has been well established. For patients with hepatocellular carcinoma, the presence of concurrent viral hepatitis is important because it may affect prognosis, survival, and treatment options. For patients with chronic viral hepatitis, early treatment to prevent cirrhosis and screening for HCC may be of benefit.

PROGNOSIS

Although the current UICC-TNM staging for HCC does not include liver function as a prognostic factor, other staging systems, such as that of Okuda, have included liver function because of its prognostic implications (196). Patients with advanced cirrhosis commonly succumb to complications such as encephalopathy, variceal hemorrhage, and sepsis, independently of the tumor's extent.

Treatment decisions are also based on the presence of active hepatitis or cirrhosis. Doxorubicin, the most active chemotherapy agent for HCC, is metabolized and excreted by the liver. The pharmacokinetics for doxorubicin may be changed for patients with liver dysfunction, resulting in enhanced toxicity. Hepatic resection, which is a treatment of choice for solitary HCC, can result in hepatic failure if hepatic reserve is compromised by hepatitis or cirrhosis. For patients with unresectable HCC, orthotopic liver transplantations have produced prolonged survival. Patients with stage I or II HCC have 5-year survivals following transplantation, which are comparable to those of patients transplanted for cirrhosis without HCC. This survival advantage is attenuated, however, in patients with active HBV viral replication (HBeAg or high levels of HBV DNA) because of the high incidence of severe viral reinfections of the liver allograft. Although patients with HCV infection also have a high incidence of reinfection following transplantation, the disease is indolent and eventual cirrhosis may not occur for decades.

SCREENING FOR HCC

Patients with metastatic or locally advanced HCC usually respond poorly to anticancer treatments. Early HCC is, however, effectively treated by surgical and nonsurgical modalities, with prolonged survival. It is not clear whether lead-time bias might be responsible, in part, for the survival prolongation.

Because of the high prevalence of HBV infection in certain regions of China, a screening program for hepatocellular carcinoma was instituted for adults over the age of 35 with chronic HBV infection. The screening tests used were serum alpha-fetoprotein (AFP) and liver ultrasound performed every 6 months. The AFP has a sensitivity of 70%, since up to 30% of hepatocellular carcinomas do not secrete it. The specificity of AFP depends on the threshold level chosen. For levels of more than 1,000, AFP is close to 100% specific. For levels of 20 to 200, false positivity outnumbers true positivity. Liver ultrasound has up to 70% sensitivity for the detection of HCCs that are less than 2 cm, but has poor specificity. The combination of AFP and ultrasound, however, increases both sensitivity and specificity. Of the 1.3 million people screened in this program, 500 cases of HCC were detected (197). A similar screening program was reported from Alaska, in which 1,400 HBsAg carriers were screened, and 20 cases of hepatocellular carcinoma were detected (81, 197). A randomized study demonstrating the survival benefit for the screened population as compared with controls has yet to be completed.

References

1. Zuckerman AJ. The history of viral hepatitis from antiquity to the present. In Viral Hepatitis: Laboratory and Clinical Science. Edited by F Deinhardt, J Deinhardt. New York: Marcel Dekker 1983, p 3.
2. Alter MJ, Margolis HS, Krawczynski K, et al, for the Sentinel County Chronic Non-A, Non-B Hepatitis Study Team. The natural history of community acquired hepatitis C in the United States. N Engl J Med 1992;327:1899.
3. Buti M, Jardi R, Rodriguez-Frias F, Quer J, Esteban R, Guardia J. Etiology of acute sporadic hepatitis in Spain: the role of hepatitis C and E viruses. J Hepatology 1994;20:589.
4. Francis DP, Hadler SC, Prendergast TJ, et al. Occurrence of hepatitis A, B, and non-A/non-B in the United States: CDC Sentinel County hepatitis study I. Am J Med 1984;76:69.
5. Lednar WM, Lemon SM, Kirkpatrick JW, Redfield RR, Fields ML, Kelley PW. Frequency of illness associated with epidemic hepatitis A virus infections in adults. Am J Epidemiol 1985;122:226.
6. Gordon SC, Reddy KR, Schiff L, Schiff ER. Prolonged intrahepatic cholestasis secondary to acute hepatitis A. Ann Intern Med 1984;101:635.
7. Glikson M, Galun E, Oren R, Tur-Kaspa R, Shouval D. Relapsing hepatitis A. Review of 14 cases and literature survey. Medicine 1992;71:14.
8. Vento S, Garofano T, DiPerri G, Dolci L, Concia E, Bassetti D. Identification of hepatitis A virus as a trigger for autoimmune chronic hepatitis type 1 in susceptible individuals. Lancet 1991;335:1183.
9. Innis BL, Snitbhan R, Kunasol O, et al. Protection of hepatitis A by an inactivated vaccine. JAMA 1994;271:1328.
10. Winokur PL, Stapleton JT. Immunoglobulin prophylaxis for hepatitis A. Clin Infect Dis 1992;14:580–586.
11. Werzberger A, Mensch B, Kuter B, et al. A controlled trial of a formalin inactivated hepatitis A vaccine in healthy children. N Engl J Med 1992;327:453.
12. Centers for Disease Control. Outbreak of hepatitis C associated with intravenous immunoglobulin administration—United States, October 1993–June 1994. MMWR 1994;43:505.
13. Sanchez FS, Sosa IR, Vargas GM. Treatment of type A hepatitis with ribavirin. In Clinical Applications of Ribavirin. Edited by RA Smith, V Knight, JA Smith. New York: Academic Press 1984:193.
14. Yoshiba M, Inoue K, Sekiyama K. Interferon for hepatitis A. Lancet 1994;343:288.
15. Pugh JC, Bassendine MF. Molecular biology of hepadnavirus replication. Br Med Bull 1990;46:329.
16. Hollinger FB, Dienstag JL. Hepatitis Viruses. In Manual of Clinical Microbiology, 4th ed. Edited by A Lennette, A Balrus, WH Hausler Jr, HJ Shadomy. Washington, DC: American Society of Microbiology 1985:813.
17. McMahon BL, Alward WLM, Hall DB, et al. Acute hepatitis B infection: relation of age to the clinical expression of disease and subsequent development of the carrier state. J Infect Dis 1985;151:599.
18. Taylor PZ, Stevens CE, De Cordoba SR, Rubinstein P. Hepatitis B virus and human immunodeficiency virus.possible interactions. In Viral Hepatitis and Liver Disease. Edited by AJ Zuckerman. New York: Alan Liss 1988:190.
19. Szmuness W, Prince FM, Grady GF, et al. Hepatitis B infection: a point prevalence study in 15 U.S. hemodialysis centers. JAMA 1974;227:901.
20. Hollinger FB, Goyal RK, Hersh T, Powell HC, Schulmen RJ, Melnick JL. Immune response to hepatitis virus type B in Down's syndrome and other mentally retarded patients. Am J Epidemiol 1972;95:356.
21. Desmet VJ, Gerber MA, Hoofnagle JH, Manns M, Scheuer PJ. Classification of chronic hepatitis: diagnosis, grading and staging. Hepatology 1994;19:1513.
22. Thung SN, Gerber MA, Popper H. Basic morphologic patterns of viral hepatitis A, B, non-A, non-B, and delta agent in animal and man. In Advances in Hepatitis Research. Edited by PV Chisari. New York: Masson, 1983, p 293.
23. Bonino F, Rosina F, Rizetto M, Rizzi R, Chiaberge E, Tardanico R, Callea F, Verme G. Chronic hepatitis in HBsAg carriers with serum HBV DNA and anti-HBe. Gastroenterol 1986;90:1268.
24. Brunetto M, Stemler M, Bonino F, et al. A new hepatitis B virus strain in patients with severe anti-HBe positive chronic hepatitis B. J Hepatol 1990;10:258.
25. Okamoto H, Yotsumoto S, Akahane Y, et al. Hepatitis B viruses with precore region defects prevail in persistently infected hosts along with seroconversion to the antibody against e antigen. J Virol 1990;64:1298.
26. Robinson WS, Marion PL. Biological features of hepadna viuses. In Viral hepatitis and Liver Disease. Edited by AJ Zuckerman. New York: Alan Liss, 1988, p 449.
27. Heathcote J, Cameron CH, Dane BS. Hepatitis B antigen in saliva and semen. Lancet 1974;I:71.
28. Alter HJ, Holland PV, Purcell RH. The emerging pattern of post-transfusion hepatitis. Am J Med Sci 1975;270:329.
29. Centers for Disease Control. Changing patterns of groups at high risk for hepatitis B in the United States. MMWR 1988;37:429.
30. Szmuness W, Much MI, Prince AM, Hoofnagle JH, Cherubin CE, Harley EJ, Block GH. On the role of sexual behavior in the spread and hepatitis B infection. Ann Intern Med 1975;83:489.
31. Beasley RP, Trepo C, Stevens CE, Szmuness W. The e antigen in vertical transmission of hepatitis B surface antigen. Am J Epidemiol 1977;105:94.
32. Gerety AJ, Schweitzer K. Viral hepatitis type B during pregnancy, the neonatal period, and infancy. J Pediatr 1977;90:368.
33. Schweitzer K. Vertical transmission of the hepatitis B surface antigens. Am J Med Sci 1975;270:287.
34. Schweitzer K, Dunn AEG, Peters RL, Spears RL. Viral hepatitis B in neonates and infants. Am J Med 1973;55:762.
35. Gerety RJ, Hoofnagle JH, Markenson JA, Narker LF. Exposure to hepatitis B virus and development of chronic HBsAg carrier state in children. J Pediatr 1974;84:661.
36. Szmuness W, Pick K, Prince AM. The serum hepatitis virus specific antigens (SH): a preliminary report of epidemiologic studies in an institution for the mentally retarded. Am J Epidemiol 1970;92:51.
37. Hadler SC, McFarland L. Hepatitis in day care centers: epidemiology and prevention. Rev Infect Dis 1986;8:548.
38. Heathcote J, Gateau P, Sherlock S. Role of the hepatitis-B antigen carriers in non-parenteral transmission of the hepatitis-B virus. Lancet 1974;2:370.
39. Nernier RH, Sampliner R, Gerety R, Tabor E, Hamilton F, Nathanson N. Hepatitis B infection in households of chronic carriers of hepatitis B surface antigen factors associated with prevalence of infection. Am J Epidemiol 1980;116:199.
40. Peters CJ, Purcell RH, Lander JJ, Johnson KM. Radioimmunoassay for antibody to hepatitis B surface antigen shows transmission of hepatitis B virus among household contacts. J Infect Dis 1976;134:218.
41. Bond WW, Favero MS, Petersen NJ, Gravelle CR, Ebert JW, Maynard JE. Survival and hepatitis B virus after drying and storage for one week. Lancet 1981;1:550.
42. Wong DKH, Cheung AM, O'Rourke K, Naylor CD, Detsky AS, Heathcote J. Effect of alpha-interferon treatment in patients with hepatitis B e antigen-positive chronic hepatitis B. Ann Intern Med 1993;119:312.
43. Brook MG, Karayiannis P, Thomas HC. Which patients with chronic hepatitis B virus infection will repond to alpha-interferon therapy? A statistical analysis of predictive factors. Hepatology 1989;10:761.
44. Lok AS, Wu PC, Lai CL, Lau JY, Leung EK, Wong LS, Ma OC, Lauder IJ, Ng CP, Chung HT. A controlled trial of interferon with or without prednisone priming for chronic hepatitis B. Gastroenterol 1992;102:2091.
45. Perrillo RP, Schiff ER, Davis GL, Bodenheimer HC Jr, Lindsay K, Payne J, Dienstag JL, O'Brien C, Tamburro C, Jacobson IM, Sampliner R, Feit D, Lefkowictch J, Kuhns M, Meschievitz C, Sanghvi B, Albrecht J, Gobas A, Hepatitis Interventional Therapy Group. A randomized, controlled trial of interferon alpha-2b alone and after prednisone withdrawal for the treatment of chronic hepatitis B. N Engl J Med 1990;323:295.
46. Reichen J, Bianchi L, Frei PC, Male PJ, Lavanchy D, Schmid M. Efficacy of steroid withdrawal and low dose interferon treatment in chronic active hepatitis B. Results of a randomized multicenter trial. J Hepatol 1994;20:168.
47. Pol S, Driss F, Carnot F, Michel ML, Berthelot P, Brechot C. Efficacite d'une immuinotherapie par vaccination contre le virus de l'hepatite B sur la multiplication virale B. CR Acad Sci Paris 1993;316:688–691.
48. Lee B, Luo WX, Suzuki S, Robbins MJ, Tyrrell DL. In vitro and in vivo comparison of the abilities of purine and pyrimidine 2′,3′-dideoxynucleotides to inhibit duck hepadnavirus. Antimicrob Agents Chemother 1989;33:336.
49. Fourel I, Saputelli J, Schaffer P, Mason WS. The carbocyclic analog of 2′-deoxyguanosine induces a prolonged inhibition of duck hepatitis B virus DNA synthesis in primary hepatocyte cultures and in the liver. J Virol 1994;68:1059.
50. Price PM, Banerjee R, Acs G. Inhibition of the replication of hepatitis B virus by the carbocyclic analogue of 2′-deoxyguanosine. Proc Natl Acad Sci USA 1989;86:8541.
51. Todo S, Demetris AJ, Van Thiel DH, Teperman L, Fung JJ, Starzl TE. Orthotopic liver transplantation for patients with hepatitis B virus–related liver disease. Hepatology 1991;13:619–626.
52. Samuel D, Muller R, Alexander G, Fassati L, Ducot B, Benhamou JP, Bismuth H, and the investigators of the European concerted action on viral hepatitis study. Liver transplantation in European patients with the hepatitis B surface antigen. N Engl J Med 1993;329:1942.
53. Tassopoulos NC, Hadziyannism SJ, Wright GE. Recombinant human alpha-interferon 2b in the management of acute type B hepatitis. Hepatology 1989;10:576.
54. Sanchez-Tapias JM, Mas A, Costa J, Bruguera M, Mayor A, Ballesta AM, Compernolle C, Rodes J. Recombinant 2c-interferon therapy in fulminant viral hepatitis. J Hepatol 1987;5:205.
55. Hedin G, Weiland O, Ljunggren K, Nordenfelt E, Hansson BG, Lernestedt JO, Oberg B. Treatment with Foscarnet of fulminant hepatitis B and fulminant hepatitis B and D infection, In Viral Hepatitis and Liver Disease. Edited by AJ Zuckerman. New York: Alan Liss 1988, p 947.
56. McAleer WJ, Buynak EB, Maigetter RZ, Wampler DE, Miller WJ, Hilleman MR. Human hepatitis B vaccine from recombinant yeast. Nature 1984;307:178.
57. McLean AA, Hilleman MR, McAleer WJ, Buynak EB. Summary of worldwide experience with HB-Vax (R) (B,MSD). J Infect Dis 1983;7(suppl):95.
58. Carman WF, Zanetti AR, Karayiannis P, Waters J, Manzillo G, Tanzi E, Zuckerman AJ, Thomas HC. Vaccine-induced escape mutant of hepatitis B virus. Lancet 1990;336:325.
59. Waters JA, Kennedy M, Voet P, Hauser P, Petre J, Carman W, Thomas HC. Loss of the common "a" determinant of hepatitis B surface antigen by a vaccine-induced escape mutant. J Clin Invest 1992;90:2543.
60. Hadler SC, Francis DP, Maynard JE, Thompson SE, Judson FN, Eichenberg DF, Ostrow DG, O'Malley PM, Penley KA, Altman NL, Braff E, Shipman GF, Coleman PJ, Mandel EJ. Long-term immunogenicity and efficacy of hepatitis B vaccine in homosexual men. N Engl J Med 1986;315:209.
61. Neurath AR, Kent SBH, Strick N, Stark D, Sproul P. Genetic restriction of immune responsiveness to synthetic peptides corresponding to sequences in the pre-S region of the hepatitis B virus (HBV) envelope gene. J Med Virol 1985;17:119.
62. Pride MW, Shi H, Anchin JM, Linthicum DS, LoVerde PT, Thakur A, Thanavala Y. Molecular mimicry of hepatitis B surface antigen by an anti-idiotype-derived synthetic peptide. Proc Natl Acad Sci USA 1992;89:1–1900.
63. Mason HS, Lam DM, Arntzen CJ. Expression of hepatitis B surface antigen in transgenic plants. Proc Natl Acad Sci USA 1992;89:11745.
64. Thanavala Y, Yan Y-F, Lyons P, Mason HS, Arntzen C. Immunogenicity of transgenic plant-derived hepatitis B surface antigen. Proc Natl Acad Sci USA 1995;92:3358.
65. Rutgers T, Hauser P, De Wilde M. Potential future recombinant vaccines. In Hepatitis B Vaccines in Clinical Practice. Edited by RW Ellis. New York: Marcel Dekker, 1993, p 383.
66. Lubeck MD, Davis AR, Chegavata M, Ntuk RJ, Morin JL, Molner-Kimber K, Mason BB, Bhat BM, Mizutani S, Hung PP, Purcell RH. Immunogenicity and efficacy testing in chimpanzees of an oral hepatitis B vaccine based on live recombinant adenovirus. Proc Natl Acad Sci USA 1989;86:6763.
67. Williams WW, Hickson MA, Kane MA, Kendal AP, Spika JS, Hinman AR. Immunization policies and vaccine coverage among adults The risk for missed opportunities. Ann Intern Med 1988;108:616.
68. Centers for Disease Control. Protection against viral hepatitis: recommendations of the Immunization Practices Advisory Committee (ACIP). MMWR 1990;39:1.
69. Alter MJ, Hadler SC, Margolis HS, Alexander WJ, Hu PY, Judson FN, Mares A, Niller

JK, Moyer LA. The changing epidemiology of hepatitis B in the United States: need for alternative vaccination strategies. JAMA 1990;263:1218.
70. Immunization Practices Advisory Committee. Hepatitis B virus: a comprehensive strategy for eliminating transmission in the United States through universal childhood vaccination. MMWR 1991;40(RR-13):1.
71. Stevens CE, Taylor PE, Tong MJ, et al. Yeast-recombinant hepatitis B vaccine Efficacy with hepatitis immunoglobulin in prevention of perinatal hepatitis B virus transmission. JAMA 1987;257:2612.
72. Szmuness W. Hepatocellular carcinoma and the hepatitis B virus: evidence for a causal association. Prog Med Virol 1978;24:40.
73. Hollinger FB and the North Am Regional Study Group. Controlling hepatitis B virus transmission in North America. Vaccine 1990;8(suppl):S122.
74. Yarrish RL, Werner BG, Blumberg BS. Association of hepatitis B virus infection with hepatocellular carcinoma in American patients. Int J Cancer 1980;26:711.
75. Kew MC, Desmyter J, Bradburne AF, Macnab GM. Hepatitis B virus infection in southern African blacks with hepatocellular cancer. JNCI 1979;62:517.
76. Lingao AL, Domingo EO, Nishioka K. Hepatitis B virus profile of hepatocellular carcinoma in the Philippines. Cancer 1981;48:1590.
77. Prince AM, Szmuness W, Michon J, Desmaille J, Diebolt G, Linhard J, Quenum C, Sankale M. A case-control study of the association between primary liver cancer and hepatitis B infection in Senegal. Int J Cancer 1975;16:376.
78. Sung JL and the Asian Regional Study Group. Hepatitis B virus eradication strategy for Asia. Vaccine 1990;8(suppl):S95.
79. Beasley RP, Hwang LY, Lin CC, Chien CS. Hepatocellular carcinoma and hepatitis B virus: a prospective study of 22,707 men in Taiwan. Lancet 1981;2:1129.
80. Beasley RP. Hepatitis B virus The major etiology of hepatocellular carcinoma. Cancer 1988;61:1842.
81. McMahon BJ, Alberts SR, Wainwright RB, Bulkow L, Lanier AP. Hepatitis B sequelae Prospective study in 1400 hepatitis B surface antigen-positive Alaska native carriers. Arch Intern Med 1990;150:1051.
82. Weinstein IB. Synergistic interactions between chemical carcinogens, tumor promoters, and viruses and their relevance to human liver cancer. Cancer Detect Prev 1989;14:253.
83. Brechot C. Hepatitis B virus (HBV) and hepatocellular carcinoma. HBV DNA status and its implications. J Hepatol 1987;4:269.
84. Kaneko S, Miller RH, Feinstone SM, Unoura M, Kobayashi K, Hattori N, Purcell RH. Detection of serum hepatitis B virus DNA in patients with chronic hepatitis using the polymerase chain reaction assay. Proc Natl Acad Sci USA 1989;86:312.
85. Paterlini P, Gerken G, Nakajima E, Terre S, D'Errico A, Grigiono W, Halpas B, Franco D, Wands J, Kew M, Pisi E, Tiollais P, Brechot C. Polymerase chain reaction to detect hepatitis B virus DNA and RNA sequences in primary liver cancers from patients negative for hepatitis B surface antigen. N Engl J Med 1990;323:80.
86. Peers FG, Gilman GA, Linsell CA. Dietary aflatoxins and human liver cancer. A study in Swaziland. Int J Cancer 1976;17:167.
87. Van Rensburg SJ, Cook-Mozafarri P, van Schalkwyk DJ, van der Watt JJ, Vincent TJ, Purchase IF. Hepatocellular carcinoma and dietary aflatoxin in Mozambique and Transkei. Br J Cancer 1985;51:713.
88. Yeh FS, Mo CC, Luo S, Henderson BE, Tong MJ, Tu MC. A serological case-control study of primary hepatocellular carcinoma in Guangxi, China. Cancer Res 1985;45: 872.
89. Yeh FS, Mo CC, Yen RC. Risk factors for hepatocellular carcinoma in Guangxi, People's Republic of China. Natl Cancer Inst Monog 1985;69:47.
90. Lee HP, Day NE, Shanmugaratnam K. Trends in Cancer Incidence in Singapore, 1968–1982. IARC Scientific Publications, No. 91. Lyon, France, International Agency for Research on Cancer, 1988.
91. Peers F, Bosch X, Kaldor J, Linsell A, Pluijmen M. Aflatoxin exposure, hepatitis B virus infection and liver cancer in Swaziland. Int J Cancer 1987;39:545.
92. Hsu IC, Metcalf RA, Sun T, Welsh JA. Wang NJ, Harris CC. Mutational hotspot in the p53 gene in human hepatocellular carcinogens. Nature 1991;350:427.
93. Oshima A, Tsukuma H, Hiyama T, Fujimoto I, Yamano H, Tanaka M. Follow-up study of HBsAg positive blood donors with special reference to effect of drinking and smoking on development of liver cancer. Int J Cancer 1984;34:775.
94. Trichopoulos D, Day NE, Kaklamani E, Tzonou A, Munoz N, Zavitsanos X, Koumantaki Y, Trichopoulou A. Hepatitis B virus, tobacco smoking and ethanol consumption in the etiology of hepatocellular carcinoma. Int J Cancer 1987;29:45.
95. Austin H, Delzell E, Grufferman S, Levine R, Morrison AS, Stolley PD, Cole P. A case-control study of hepatocellular carcinoma and the hepatitis B virus, cigarette smoking, and alcohol consumption. Cancer Res 1986;46:962.
96. Hadengue A, N'Dri N, Benhamou J-P. Relative risk of hepatocellular carcinoma in HBsAg positive vs. alcoholic cirrhosis. A cross-sectional study. Liver 1990;10:147.
97. Forman D, Doll R, Peto R. Trends in mortality from carcinoma of the liver and the use of oral contraceptives. Br J Cancer 1983;48:349.
98. Henderson BE, Preston-Martin S, Edmondson HA, Peters RL, Pike MC. Hepatocellular carcinoma and oral contraceptives. Br J Cancer 1983;48:437.
99. Neuberger J, Forman D, Doll R, Williams R. Oral contraceptives and hepatocellular carcinoma. Br Med J 1986;292:1355.
100. Twu JS, Schloemer RH. Transcriptional trans-activating function of hepatitis B virus. J Virol 1987;61:3448.
101. Spandau DF, Lee CH. Trans-activation of viral enhancers by the hepatitis B virus X protein. J Virol 1988;62:427.
102. Colgrove R, Simon G, Ganem D. Transcriptional activation of homologous and heterologous genes by the hepatitis B virus X gene product in cells permissive for viral replication. J Virol 1989;63:4019.
103. Wollersheim M, Debelka U, Hofscheider PH. A transactivating function encoded in the hepatitis B virus X gene is conserved in the integrated state. Oncogene 1988;3: 545.
104. Moroy T, Marchio A, Etiemble J, Trepo C, Tiollais P, Buendia MA. Rearrangement and enhanced expression of c-myc in hepatocellular carcinoma of hepatitis virus infected woodchucks. Nature 1986;324:276.
105. Ichiyada T, Fujiyama A, Fukushige S, Hatada I, Matsubara K. Molecular cloning of an oncogene from a human hepatocellular carcinoma. Proc Natl Acad Sci USA 1986;83: 4993.
106. Takada S, Koike K. Activated N-ras gene was found in human hepatoma tissue but onoy in a small fraction of the tumor cells. Oncogene 1989;4:189.
107. Yang DY, Rogler CE. Analysis of insulin-like growth factor II (IGF-II) expression in neoplastic nodules and hepatocellular carcinomas of woodchucks utilizing in situ hybridization and immunocytochemistry. Carcinogenesis 1991;12:1893.
108. Wang J, Chenivesse X, Henglein B, Brechot C. Hepatitis B virus integration in a cyclin A gene in a hepatocellular carcinoma. Nature 1990;343:555.
109. Koufos A, Hansen MF, Copeland NG, Jenkins NA, Lampkin BC, Cavenee WK. Loss of heterozygosity in three embryonla tumours suggests a common pathogenetic mechanism. Nature 1985;316:330.
110. Stanbridge EJ, Flandermeyer RR, Daniels DW, Nelson-Rees WA. Specific chromosome loss associated with the expression in tumorigenicity in human cell hybrids. Somat Cell Genet 1981;7:699.
111. Lee WH, Bookstein R, Hong F, Young LJ, Shew JY, Lee EYHP. Human retinoblastoma susceptibility gene: cloning, identification, and sequence. Science 1987;235:1394.
112. Wang HP, Rogler CE. Deletions in human chromosome arms 11p and 13q in primary hepatocellular carcinomas. Cytogenet Cell Genet 1988;48:72.
113. Bressac B, Kew M, Wands J, Ozturk M. Selective G to T mutations of p53 gene in hepatocellular carcinoma from southern Africa. Nature 1991;350:429.
114. Hsu IC, Metcalf RA, Sun T, Welsh JA, Wang NJ, Harris CC. Mutational hotspot in the p53 gene in human hepatocellular carcinomas. Nature 1991;350:427.
115. Held WA, Mullins JJ, Kuhn NJ, Gallagher JF, Gu GD, Gross KW. T antigen expression and tumorigenesis in transgenic mice containing a mouse major urinary protein/SV40 T antigen hybrid gene. EMBO J 1989;8:183.
116. Ishak KG. Light microscopic morphology of viral hepatitis. Am J Clin Pathol 1976;65: 787.
117. Montano L. Aranguibel F, Boffill M, Goodall AH, Janossy G, Thomas HC. An analysis of the composition of the inflammatory infiltrate in autoimmune and hepatitis B virus-induced chronic liver disease. Hepatology 1983;3:292.
118. Eggink HG, Houthoff HJ, Huitema S, Poppema S, Gips CH. Cellular and humoral immune reactions in chronic active liver disease: lymphocyte subsets in liver biopsies of patients with untreated idiopathic autoimmune hepatitis, chronic active hepatitis B and primary biliary cirrhosis. Clin Exp Immunol 1982;50:17.
119. Milich DR. Genetic and molecular basis for T- and B-cell recognition of hepatitis B viral antigen. Immunol Rev 1987;99:71.
120. Milich DR, McLachlan A, Moriarty A, Thornton GB. Immune response to hepatitis B virus core antigen (HNcAg): localization of T cell recognition sites within HBcAg/HBeAg. J Immunol 1987;139:1223.
121. Ferrari C, Penna A, Giuberti T, et al. Intrahepatic nucleocapsid antigen specific T cells in chronic active hepatitis B. J Immunol 1987;139:2050.
122. Chisari FV, Filippi P, Buras J, McLachlan A, Popper H, Pinkert CA, Palmiter RD, Brinster RL. Structural and pathological effects of synthesis of hepatitis B virus large envelope polypeptide in transgenic mice. Proc Natl Acad Sci USA 1987;84:6909.
123. Chisari FV, Klopchin K, Moriyama T, Pasquinelli C, Dunsford HA, Sell S, Pinkert CA, Brinster RL, Palmiter RD. Molecular pathogenesis of hepatocellular carcinoma in hepatitis B virus transgenic mice. Cell 1989;59:1145.
124. Farza H, Hadchouel M, Scotto J, Tiollais P, Babinet C, Pourcel C. Replication and gene expression of hepatitis B virus in a transgenic mouse that contains the complete viral genome. J Virol 1988;62:4144.
125. Choo QL, Kuo G, Weiner AJ, Overby LR, Bradley DW, Houghton M. Isolation of cDNA clone derived from a blood-born non-A, non-B viral hepatitis genome. Science 1989;244:359.
126. Miller RH, Purcell RH. Hepatitis C virus shares amino acid sequence similarity with pestiviruses and flaviviruses as well as members of two plant virus supergroups. Proc Natl Acad Sci USA 1990;87:2057.
127. Houghton M, Weiner A, Han JH, Kuo G, Choo QL. Molecular biology of the hepatitis C viruses: implications for diagnosis, development and control of viral disease. Hepatology 1991;14:381.
128. Kato N, Hijikata M, Ostsuyama Y, Nakagawa M, Ohkoshi S, Sugimura T, Shimotohno K. Molecular cloning of the human hepatitis C virus genome from Japanese patients with non-A, non-B hepatitis. Proc Natl Acad Sci USA 1990;87:9524.
129. Takamizawa A, Mori C, Fuke I, Manabe S, Murakami X, Fujita J, Onishi E, Andoh T, Yoshida I, Okayama H. Structure and organization of the hepatitis C virus genome isolated from human carriers. J Virol 1991;65:1105.
130. Okamoto H, Okada S, Sugiyama Y, Kurai K, Iizuka H, Machida A, Miyakawa Y, Mayumi M. Nucleotide sequence of the genomic RNA of hepatitis C virus isolated from a human carrier: comparison with reported isolates for conserved and divergent regions. J Gen. Virol 1991;72(pt 11):2697.
131. Han JH, Shyamala V, Richman KH, et al. Characterization of the terminal regions of hepatitis C viral RNA: identification of conserved sequences in the 5′ untranslated region and poly (A) tails at the 3′ end. Proc Natl Acad Sci USA 1991;88:1711.
132. Bukh J, Purcell RH, Miller RH. At least 12 genotypes of hepatitis C virus predicted by sequence analysis of the putative E1 gene of isolates collected worldwide. Proc Natl Acad Sci USA 1993;90:8234.
133. Okamoto H, Kojima M, Okada S, Yoshizawa H, Iizuka H, Tanaka T, Muchmore EE, Peterson DA, Ito Y, Mishiro S. Genetic drift of hepatitis C virus during an 8.2 year infection in a chimpanzee, variability and stability. Virology 1992;190:894.
134. Okamoto H, Sugiyama Y, Okada S, Kurai K, et al. Typing hepatitis C virus by polymerase chain reaction with type-specific primers: application to clinical surveys and tracing infectious sources. J Gen Virol 1992;73:673.
135. Tsukiyama-Kohara K, Kohara M, Tamaguchi K, Maki N, Toyoshima A, Miki K, Tanaka S, Hattori N, Nomoto A. A second group of hepatitis C virus. Virus Genes 1991;5:243.
136. Alter MJ, Sampliner RE. Hepatitis C. Miles to go before we sleep. N Engl J Med 1989;321:1538.
137. Alter MJ. Inapparent transmission of hepatitis C: footprints in the sand. Hepatology 1991;14:389.
138. Dienstag JL, Alaama A, Mosley JW, Redeker AG, Purcell RH. Etiology of sporadic hepatitis B surface antigen-negative hepatitis. Ann Intern Med 1977;87:1.
139. Thaler MM, Park CK, Landers DV, Wara DW, Houghton M, Veereman-Wauters G, Sweet RL, Han JH. Vertical transmission of hepatitis C. Lancet 1991;338:17.
140. Giovannini M, Tagger A, Ribero ML, Zuccotti G, Pogliani L, Grossi A, Ferroni P, Fiocchi A. Maternal-infant transmission of hepatitis C virus and HIV infections: a possible interaction. Lancet 1990;335:1166.
141. Alter HJ, Purcell RH, Shih JW, Melpolder JC, Houghton M, Choo QL, Kuo G. Detection of antibody to hepatitis C virus in prospectively followed transfusion recipients with acute and chronic non-A, non-B hepatitis. N Engl J Med 1989;321:1494.

142. Seeff LB, Buskell-Bales Z, Wright EC, Durako SJ, Alter HJ, Iber FL, Hollinger FB, Gitnick G, Knodell RG, Perrillo RP, Stevens CE, Hollingsworth CG, the National Heart, Lung, and Blood Institute Study Group. Long term mortality after transfusion-associated non-A, non-B hepatitis. N Engl J Med 1992;327:1906.
143. Di Bisceglie AM, Goodman ZD, Ishak KG, Hoofnagle JH, Melpolder JJ, Alter HJ. Long term clinical and histopathologic follow-up of chronic posttransfusion hepatitis. Hepatology 1991;14:969.
144. Lelie PN, Cuypers HT, Reesink HW, van der Poel CL, Winkel I, Bakker E, van Exel-Oehlers PJ, Vallari D, Allain JP, Mimms L. Patterns of serological markers in transfusion-transmitted hepatitis C virus infection using second generation HCV assays. J Med Virol 1992;37:203.
145. Li X, DeMedina M, LaRue S, Shao L, Schiff ER. Comparison of assays for HCV RNA. Lancet 1991;324:1174.
146. McHutchison JG, Person JL, Govindarajan S, Valinluck B, Gore T, Lee SR, Nelles M, Polito A, Chien D, DiNello R, Quan S, Kuo G, Redeker AG. Improved detection of hepatitis C virus antibodies in high risk population. Hepatology 1992;15:19.
147. Nakagiri I, Ichihara K, Ohmoto K, Hirokawa M, Matsuda N. Analysis of discordant test results among five second generation assays for anti-hepatitis C virus antibodies also tested by polymerase chain reaction—RNA assay and other laboratory and clinical tests for hepatitis. J Clin Microbiol 1993;31:2974.
148. Bresters D, Zaaijer HL, Cuypers HT, Reesink HW, Winkel IN. Recombinant immunoblot assay reaction patterns and hepatitis C virus RNA in blood donors and non-A, non-B hepatitis patients. Transfusion 1993;33:634.
149. Chemello L, Cavaletto D, Pontisso P, Bortolotti F, Donada C, Donadon V, Frezza M, Casarin P, Alberti A. Patterns of antibodies to hepatitis C virus in patients with chronic non-A, non-B hepatitis and their relationship to viral replication and liver disease. Hepatology 1993;17:179.
150. Lau JY, Davis GL, Kniffen J, Aian KP, Urdea MS, Chan CS, Mizokami M, Neuwald PD, Wilber JC. Significance of serum hepatitis C virus RNA levels in chronic hepatitis C. Lancet 1993;341:1501.
151. Gil B, Qian C, Riezu-Boj JI, Civeira MP, Prieto J. Hepatic and extrahepatic HCV RNA strands in chronic hepatitis C: different patterns of response to interferon treatment. Hepatology 1993;18:1050.
152. Gretch D, Lee W, Corex L. Use of aminotransferase, hepatitis C antibody, and hepatitis C polymerase chain reaction RNA assays to establish the diagnosis of hepatitis C virus infection in a diagnostic virology laboratory. J Clin Microbiol 1992;8:2145.
153. Iino S, Komata M, Kumada H, Akane T, Kiyosawa S, Hayashi N, Yoshizawa K, Tanigawa H, Yano U, Nishioka H, Suzuki H. Quantification of HCV RNA by branched DNA probe assay. J Med Pharm Sci 1993;2:327.
154. McOmish F, Chan SW, Dow BC, Gillon J, Frame WD, Crawford RJ, Yap PL, Follett EA, Simmonds P. Detection of three types of hepatitis C virus in blood donors: investigation of type of specific differences in serologic reactivity and rate of alanine aminotransferase abnormalities. Transfusion 1993;33:7.
155. Farci P, Alter HJ, Govindarajan S, Wong DC, Engle R, Lesniewski RR, Mushahwar IK, Desai SM, Miller RH, Ogata N, et al. Lack of protective immunity against reinfection with hepatitis C virus. Science 1992;258:135.
156. Ogata NR, Alter HJ, Miller RH, Purcell RH. Nucleotide sequence and mutation rate of the H strain of hepatitis C virus. Proc Natl Acad Sci USA 1991;88:3392.
157. Davis GL, Balart LA, Schiff ER, Perrillo RP, Carey W, Jacobseon IM, Payne J, Dienstag JL, VanThiel DH, Tamburro C, Lefkowitch J, Albrecht J, Mieschievitz C, Ortego TJ, Gibas A, the Hepatitis Interventional Therapy Group. Treatment of chronic hepatitis C with recombinant alpha-interferon: a multicenter randomized, controlled trial. N Engl J Med 1989;321:1501.
158. Di Bisceglie AM, Shindo M, Fong TL, Fried MW, Swain MG, Bergasa NV, Axiotis CA, Waggoner JG, Park Y, Hoofnagle JH. A pilot study of ribavirin therapy for chronic hepatitis C. Hepatology 1992;16:649.
159. Camps J, Garcia N, Roezu-Boj JI, Civiera MP, Prieto J. Ribavirin in the treatment of chronic hepatitis C unresponsive to alpha-interferon. J Hepatol 1993;19:408.
160. Wright TL, Donegan E, Hsu HH, Ferrell L, Kale JR, Kim M, Combs C, Fennessy S, Roberts JP, Ascher NL, Greenberg HB. Recurrent and acquired hepatitis C viral infection in liver transplant recipients. Gastroenterology 1992;103:317.
161. Wright TL, Combs C, Kim M, Ferrell L, Bacchetti P, Ascher N, Roberts J, Wilber J, Sheridan P, Urdea M. Interferon alpha therapy for hepatitis C virus infection following liver transplantation. Hepatology 1994;20:773.
162. Nalpas B, Driss F, Pol S, Hamelin B, Housset C, Brechot C, Berthelot P. Association between HCV and HBV infection in hepatocellular carcinoma and alcoholic liver disease. J Hepatol 1991;12:70.
163. Saito I, Miyamura T, Ohbayashi A, Harada H, Katayama T, Kikuchi S, Watanabe Y, Koi S, Onji M, Ohta Y, et al. Hepatitis C virus infection is associated with the development of hepatocellular carcinoma. Proc Natl Acad Sci USA 1990;87:6547.
164. Gerber MA. Relation of hepatitis C virus to hepatocellular carcinoma. J Hepatol 1993;17:108.
165. Muchmore E, Popper H, Peterson DA, Miller MF, Lieberman HM. Non-A, non-B hepatitis-related hepatocellular carcinoma in a chimpanzee. J Med Primatol 1988;17:235.
166. Gerber MA, Shieh YS, Shim KS, Thung SN, Demetris AJ, Schwartz M, Akyol G, Dash S. Detection of replicative hepatitis C virus sequences in hepatocellular carcinoma. Am J Pathol 1992;141:1271.
167. Haruna Y, Hayashi N, Kamada T, Hytiroglou P, Thung SN, Gerber MA. Expression of hepatitis C virus in hepatocellular carcinoma. Cancer 1994;73:2253.
168. Kew MC, Popper H. Relationship between hepatocellular carcinoma and cirrhosis. Semin Liver Dis 1984;4:136.
169. Levrero M, Tagger A, Balsano C, DeMarzio E, Avantaggiati ML, Natoli G, Diop D, Villa E, Diodati G, Alberti A. Antibodies to hepatitis C virus in patients with hepatocellular carcinoma. J Hepatol 1991;12:60.
170. Furuya K, Nakamura M, Yamamoto Y, Togei K, Otsuka H. Macroregenerative nodule of the liver: a clinicopathologic study of 345 autopsy cases of chronic liver disease. Cancer 1988;61:99.
171. Theise ND, Lapook JD, Thung SN. A macroregenerative nodule containing multiple foci of hepatocellular carcinoma in a non-cirrhotic liver. Hepatology 1993;17:993.
172. Theise ND, Schwartz M, Miller C, Thung SN. Macroregenerative nodules and hepatocellular carcinoma in 44 sequential adult liver explants with cirrhosis. Hepatology 1992;16:949.
173. Tarao K, Ohkawa S, Shimizu A, Harada M, Nakamura Y, Ito Y, Tamai S, Hoshino H, Inoue T, Kanisawa M. Significance of hepatocellular proliferation in the development of hepatocellular carcinoma from anti-hepatitis C virus–positive cirrhotic patients. Cancer 1994;73:1149.
174. Wang KS, Choo QL, Weiner AJ, Ou JH, Najarian RC, Thayer RM, Mullenbacher GT, Denniston KJ, Gerin JL, Houghton M. Structure, sequence and expression of the hepatitis delta viral genome. Nature 1986;323:508.
175. Smedile A, Rizzetto M, Gerin JL. Advances in hepatitis D virus biology and disease. Prog Liver Dis 1994;12:157.
176. Buti M, Esteban R, Allende H, Allende H, Esteban JI, Genesca J, Guardia J. Clinical and serological outcome of acute delta infection. J Hepatol 1987;5:59.
177. Di Bisceglie A, Negro F. Diagnosis of hepatitis delta virus infection. Hepatology 1989;10:1014.
178. Farci P, Mandas A, Coiana A, Lai ME, Desmet V, Van Eyken P, Gibo Y, Caruso L, Scaccabarozzi S, Criscuolo D, et al. Treatment of chronic hepatitis D with alpha-interferon-2a. N Engl J Med 1994;330:88.
179. Zignego AL, Samuel D, Gigou M, et al. Patterns of hepatitis delta reinfection after liver transplantation and their evolution during a long term follow-up. Progr Clin Biol Res 1993;382:409.
180. Ottobrelli A, Marzano A, Smedile A, Recchia S, Salizzoni M, Corni C, Lamy ME, Otte JB, DeHemptinne B, Geubel A, et al. Patterns of hepatitis delta virus reinfection and disease in transplantation. Gastroenterology 1991;101:1649.
181. Viswanathan R. Infectious hepatitis in Delhi (1955–56): a critical study. Indian J Med Res 1957;45:1.
182. Zhuang H, Cao XY, Liu CB, Wang GM. Enterically transmitted non-A, non-B hepatitis in China. In Viral Hepatitis C, D, E. Edited by T Shikata, RH Purcell, T Uchida. Amsterdam: Elsevier, 1991, p 277.
183. McCaustland KA, Bi S, Purdy MA, Bradley DW. Application of two RNA extraction methods prior to amplification of hepatitis E virus nuclei acid by the polyumerase reaction. J Virol Meth 1991;35:331.
184. Krawczynski K, Bradley DW. Enterically transmitted non-A, non-B hepatitis: identification of virus associated antigen in experimentally infected cynomolgus macaques. J Infect Dis 1989;159:1042.
185. Khuroo MS, Teli MR, Skidmore S, Sofi MA, Khuroo MI. Incidence and severity of viral hepatitis in pregnancy. Am J Med 1981;70:252.
186. Favorov MO, Fields HA, Purdy MA, Yashina TL, Alter MJ, Yarasheva DM, Bradley DW, Margolis HS. Serologic identification of hepatitis E virus infections in epidemic and endemic settings. J Med Virol 1992;36:246.
187. Purdy MA, McCaustland KA, Krawczynski K, Spelbring J, Reyes GR, Bradley DW. Preliminary evidence that a trpE-HEV fusion protein protects cynomolgus macaques against challenge with wild type hepatitis E virus (HEV). J Med Virol 1993;41:90.
188. Buti M, Jardi R, Rodriguez-Frias F, Quer J, Esteban R, Guardia J. Non-A, non-B, non-C, non-E acute hepatitis: does it really exist? In Viral Hepatitis and Liver Disease. Edited by K. Nishioka, H. Suzuki, S. Mishiro, T. Oda. Tokyo: Springer-Verlag, 1994, p 77.
189. Hibbs JR, Frickhofen N, Rosenfeld SJ, Feinstone SM, Kojima S, Bacigalupo A, Locasciulli A, Tzakis AG, Alter HJ, Young NS. Aplastic anemia and viral hepatitis. Non-A, non-B, non-C? JAMA 1992;267:2051.
190. Fagan E. A Acute liver failure of unknown pathogenesis. The hidden agenda. Hepatology 1994;19:1307.a.
191. Fagan EA, Ellis DS, Tovey GM, Lloyd G, Smith HM, Portmann B, Tan KC, Zuckerman AJ, Williams R. Toga virus-like particles in acute liver failure attributed to sporadic non-A, non-B hepatitis and recurrence after liver transplantation. J Med Virol 1992;38:71.
192. Fagan EA, Harrison TJ. Candidate hepatitis F virus in sporadic non-A, non-B acute liver failure.exclusion in liver of hepatitis viruses A to E by polymerase chain reaction. In Viral Hepatitis and Liver Disease. Edited by K Nishioka, H Suzuki, S Mishiro, T. Oda. Tokyo: Springer Verlag, 1994.
193. Kim JP, Linnen J, Wages J, et al. Hepatitis G virus (HGV), a new hepatitis virus associated with human hepatitis. J Hepatol 1995;23(suppl 1):78.
194. Hadziyannis S, Wages J, Kim JP, et al. Frequency of viraemia with a new hepatitis virus (HGV) in patients with liver disease and in groups at high risk of exposure to blood and blood products. J Hepatol 1995;23(suppl 1):78.
195. Simons JN, Pilot-Matias TJ, Leary TP, Dawson GJ, Desai SM, Schlauder GG, Muerhoff AS, Erker JC, Buuk SL, Chalmers ML, Van Sant CL, Mushahwar IS. Identification of two flavivirus-like genomes in the GB hepatitis agent. Proc Natl Acad Sci USA 1995;92:3401.
196. Okuda K, Ohtsuki T, Obata H, Tomimatsu M, Okazaki N, Hasegawa H. Natural history of hepatocellular carcinoma and prognosis in relation to treatment. Study of 850 patients. Cancer 1985;56:918.
197. Tang ZY. Subclinical hepatocellular carcinoma—historical aspects and general considerations. In Subclinical Hepatocellular Carcinoma. Edited by ZY Tang. Beijing, China: China Academic Publishers, 1985, p 1.
198. McMahon BJ, Wainwright RW, Lanier AP. The Alaska native HCC screening program: a population-based screening program for hepatocellular carcinoma. In Etiology, Pathology and Treatment of Hepatocellular Carcinoma in North America. Edited by E Tabor, AM DiBisceglie, RH Purcell. Gulf, 1991, pp 231–242.
199. Lemon SM. HAV: current concepts of the molecular virology, immunobiology and approaches to vaccine development. Rev Med Virol 1992;2:73.
200. Lidofsky SD. Liver transplantation for fulminant hepatic failure. Gastroenterol Clin North Amer Houston 1993;22:257.

CHAPTER 24

Parasites

PIERO MUSTACCHI

Intensity of parasitic infection frequently correlates with its prevalence (58). Thus, when relatively uncommon neoplasms are noted with undue frequency in countries with a high prevalence of parasitic diseases, the question of the role of the parasite arises. In this respect, the two most intriguing examples are probably the relationship of schistosomiasis to bladder cancer and that of malaria to Burkitt's lymphoma.

Schistosomiasis and Cancer of the Bladder

EPIDEMIOLOGIC ASPECTS

The data associating schistosomiasis and neoplasia are overwhelming, but explanations for this association remain speculative (16, 39). Data published so far have been retrospective and therefore have yielded only relative frequencies, with their well-known inherent limitations.

Geography

In Africa, squamous cell carcinoma of the bladder is greatly overrepresented among the fellaheen of Egypt and the Africans of Mozambique, Zimbabwe, and Zambia (formerly Rhodesia), all countries where *Schistosoma haematobium* is endemic. An age-standardized mortality rate for bladder cancer of 10.8×10^{-5} males places Egypt at the top of the list of the 54 countries providing data for the 1987 World Health Organization (WHO) data base (11). This has led to the hypothesis that infection predisposes to malignant bladder neoplasms. Observations made in Ghana are only suggestive of an association, however, but none emerges from Tanzania, Uganda, or French-speaking West Africa, where schistosomiasis is endemic but bladder cancer apparently is rare (23).

No prospective study measuring the risk of developing bladder cancer in infected and uninfected persons is yet available; thus, conflicting conclusions derived from relative frequency data remain unresolved. Although differences in relative frequencies may reflect differences in risk, the interplay of other factors, such as geopolitical variations in case finding, can result in spurious differences and erroneous associations. If the postulated association is correct, one of several conditions must obtain: the worm (*a*) produces a carcinogen, (*b*) carries a virus, or (*c*) is cocarcinogenic to some other insult. In this case, many unanswered questions must explain geographic differences in vesical cancer observed where schistosomiasis is endemic. These range from whether there is geographic uniformity in the host's reaction to infection to whether other environmental variables (such as the bright food coloring used in the candy so popular in the Nile delta) interact and are additionally responsible for vesical neoplasia.

Age and Sex

Egyptian data from the Alexandria Cancer Registry disclose a fivefold sex-linked disparity in the annual age-adjusted incidence rate of bladder cancer: 19.2×10^{-5} males and 3.6×10^{-5} females (11). Bilharzial (i.e., schistosomal) bladder cancer attacks men preferentially and seem to be especially common in those with HLA-B16 and Cw2 antigens (107). In Egyptian hospital series, their mean age is 41 years, about 5 years younger than patients with nonbilharzial bladder cancer (1, 46) and the sex ratio ranges from 5:1 to 9:1. In Ghana, 5 of 13 males with bladder cancer came to autopsy before age 36 (82). In Mozambique, too, bilharzial bladder cancer occurs earlier in life, but the sex ratio is nowhere as striking as in Egypt (M/F = 1.75:1) (86). Whether this difference from Egypt reflects greater susceptibility of females in Mozambique, a reduced risk in males, or simply a vagary resulting from underreporting remains unresolved.

Urban-Rural Distribution

In Egypt, additional support for an association with bilharzial infection can be found in the relative paucity of bladder cancer cases reported from hospitals serving the nonparasitized Italian and Greek residents of metropolitan Cairo, compared with the large number observed in hospitals attending Egyptian peasants (1).

Similarly, a survey of 624 urban and 848 rural consecutive Egyptian patients yielded 107 malignant neoplasms. Of the 33 cancers observed in urban patients, 10, or less than one third, occurred in the bladder. The fellaheen living in rural areas contributed 74 cancers, of which 45 (almost two thirds) were vesical (82).

Frequency and Severity of Infection

The association of bladder cancer with schistosomal infection seems to become stronger with longer-standing and more severe infection (38, 82). In the Nile delta, a progressively larger proportion of patients is found to have *Schistosoma* ova in the urine as the study subsets progress from bladders with cytologically benign epithelium to those with squamous metaplasia, benign tumors, and, finally, cancer.

The severity of infection tends to rise sharply with opportunities for exposure. In Egypt, it is directly related to the extent of perennial irrigation through canals, which creates constant risk of reinfection, and inversely related to control measures and availability of safe and effective therapy (74). In Ghana, where different agricultural conditions prevail, schistosomiasis is essentially a prepubertal disease, and only a small portion of the population is infested, as compared with the extent in Egypt. Comparative studies in these two countries indicate a rather good direct relationship between parasitic infection with *S. haematobium* and frequency of bladder cancer (82). Thus, the peculiar agricultural setting of the Nile Valley singles out this region for a dose-response relationship not encountered in other parts of Africa.

Variability in Diagnostic Criteria for Schistosomiasis

Many reports of schistosomal bladder cancer fail to define the diagnostic criteria for infection; moreover, there is no assurance that uniform criteria were used throughout a study. For instance, ruling out a diagnosis of schistosomiasis because of the absence of ova in the centrifuged urine specimen would be unrealistic in many cases of contracted bladder due to bilharzial fibrosis, in which the dense scar tissue precludes shedding of ova from the submucosa. Conversely, sound epidemiologic practices require that when evidence of infestation in ova-negative bilharzial patients is sought by rectal scrapings or x-ray studies, the same diagnostic refinements be used in every member of the group studied.

One such study conducted in the Nile delta concluded that only 11% of the men and 3% of the women could be considered infected, on the basis of presence of *Schistosoma* ova in the initial urinalysis. Based on this diagnostic criterion, only a suggestive association of infection and cancer of the bladder was demonstrated ($P = .04$). Conclusions based on a single specimen are notoriously unreliable. By expanding the criteria for diagnosis of schistosomiasis to include the presence of ova in any centrifuged urine sample and other evidence of infection obtained by endoscopic or radiologic procedures, the prevalence of infection was increased threefold. In either instance, after correcting for age, sex, and residence, the relative risk of developing bladder cancer among the bilharzial patients was double that in the comparison population group. By adopting the expanded definition of schistosomiasis, the association became much more probable ($P = .002$) (82).

A similar change in the force of the association emerges when the pathologist who had established a diagnosis of schistosomiasis on a surgical specimen of limited dimensions expands the anatomic substrate for infestation to a complete autopsy (46). In this situation, the P value for the association changes from .05 to less than .001.

Geographic Variability in Schistosomal Virulence

Within East Africa, a coastal strain of *S. haematobium* is more virulent than that at Lake Victoria, where infested bladders do not show severe changes. When *Schistosoma mansoni* is considered, the Brazilian and Puerto Rican strains are the most virulent, as measured by the production of liver disease in infested mice. Under the same experimental conditions, the Egyptian strain caused the least liver damage and the Tanzanian strain produced the fewest eggs (102). Variability in *S. mansoni* virulence has been cited to explain the high frequency of liver cancer in Mozambique but not in Egypt, even though schistosomal liver cirrhosis is common in both countries. This type of explanation is, at best, tentative, because other, and as yet undetected, environmental carcinogenic hazards can be at work.

Role of Urinary Tract Infection

In Egypt, but not in Mozambique, bladder calculi and incrustations of vesical ulcers are frequent complications of schistosomal infection. The experimental work linking some nitroso products of bacterial metabolism to carcinogenesis may perhaps reinvigorate the old carcinogenic hypothesis of the early Egyptian workers who implicated "alkaline urine." In fact, urinary excretion of nitrite and *N*-nitroso compounds is increased in patients with *S. haematobium* infection (98). The prevalence of urinary nitrites in symptomatic active bilharzial cystitis increases in patients who also have schistosomal bladder cancer (26). Also, in noncancerous bladders infection with *S. haematobium* increases significantly the ability of the vesical bacterial flora to reduce nitrates to the nitrite precursors of *N*-nitroso compounds (48).

Urinary tract infection has been associated with increased chromosomal breakage in the urothelium, and the frequency of micronuclei is reduced significantly after antihelminthic treatment (8). Urothelial carcinogenesis in the presence of schistosomiasis seems to proceed along pathways different from those linked to smoking, since cigarette smoking appears to have a significant impact on the mutation of the p53 gene with A:T to G:C transitions, which are not observed in bilharzial bladder cancer (43).

Pathology of Benign and Preneoplastic Schistosomal Bladder Lesions

An intense, delayed sensitivity reaction is elicited by viable *Schistosoma* eggs plugged in the vesical venules. Depending on how severe and widespread the reaction, this results in tubercules, nodules, or polyps. Thus, in bilharzial cystitis the papilloma is essentially a granuloma and not a precancerous lesion, covered as it is by one or two layers of flattened cells, which merge with the transitional epithelium at its base (86).

With recurrent inflammation and fibrosis, some transitional epithelial cells become sequestered in the vesical submucosa and acquire a globular arrangement around a central cavity. When they open in the bladder cavity, the cystic formations become pseudoglandular. These structures, as part of cystitis glandularis, are at times precancerous; an adenocarcinoma may arise from the columnar epithelium into which their lining has differentiated.

In patients with schistosomiasis (frequently termed *bilharzia* in Africa), squamous metaplasia is frequently encountered (22), because it is a common concomitant of chronic inflammation. This type of metaplasia is a nearly consistent precursor of bladder cancer, and, for this reason, leukoplakia acquires clinical importance as a precancerous condition.

SITE OF ORIGIN

In Western countries bladder cancer frequently arises in the trigone; in Egypt it usually develops in areas remote from the ureters, mostly in the anterior and posterior bladder walls. This peculiarity tends to strengthen its association with schistosomal infection, because the scanty or altogether absent submucosal tissue of the trigone discourages significant deposition of ova (Table 24.1).

HISTOLOGIC CLASSIFICATION

Table 24.2 contrasts the overrepresentation of squamous cell carcinoma of the bladder in areas like Egypt, Kuwait, Mozambique, South Africa (Bantu population) (50), and Zimbabwe, where the association with schistosomiasis is considered important, with the Ugandan and white South African experience, where the reverse applies.

Within the same country, squamous cell carcinoma of the bladder is markedly overrepresented only in areas where schistosomiasis is endemic (61, 97). Moreover, the more intense the infection, the greater is the proportion of squamous cell cancers with a concurrent decrease in the frequency of transitional cell neoplasms (Fig. 24.1) (69).

A rare, though distinct variant of squamous cell cancer is verrucous carcinoma of the bilharzial bladder (Fig. 24.2). Despite reports to the contrary, a large proportion develop into invasive squamous cell carcinoma, with which they share the same aggressive prognosis (71).

Table 24.1. Anatomic Distribution of Vesical Cancer in Egypt and the United States

Site	Egypt (%)	USA (%)
Trigone	3	21
Lateral wall	34	47
Anterior wall	22	8
Posterior wall	30	18
Vault	11	6

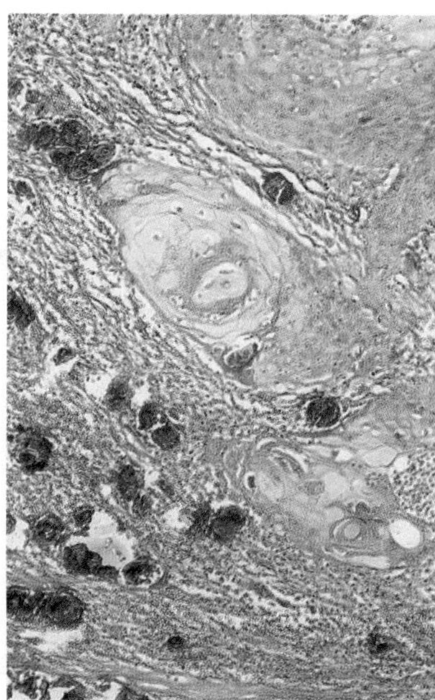

Figure 24.1. Bilharzial bladder cancer. Infiltrating well-differentiated squamous cell carcinoma with adjacent calcified *S. hematobium* eggs. (H & E × 100; Courtesy of Doctors M. R. Mahran and M. El-Baz, Mansoura University, Egypt.)

EXPERIMENTAL DATA

Half a century ago, papillomatous hyperplasia of the vesical wall was observed in African sooty monkeys within 3 months of infection with *S. haematobium.* More recently, a carcinoma of the bladder was diagnosed in a baboon killed 26 weeks after infection (41). In a number of nonhuman primates, infection with *S. haematobium* resulted in epithelial proliferation, squamous metaplasia, and transitional cell carcinoma of the urinary bladder (64). The American opossum has been found experimentally suitable for infection with *S. haematobium* (65). These experimental observations are important, because eggs of *S. haematobium*, lyophilized worms, and urine from bilharzia patients have not been found to be carcinogenic to mice (29, 93). Furthermore, *Schistosoma* ova, either dry or in the presence of 3-methylcholanthrene, lacked urothelial topical carcinogenicity or cocarcinogenicity in mice (5). However, 2-acetyl-aminofluorene appears to promote malignant and benign bladder neoplasms of mice infested with schistosomes more often than does the schistosomiasis alone or the carcinogen alone

Table 24.2. Histologic Distribution of Bladder Cancer In Africa

Type	Egypt (1,20)	Kuwait (6)	East Africa (39)	South Africa (46)		Uganda (21)	Zimbabwe (97)
				Bantus	Whites		
Squamous	232	100	58	16	11	26	207
Transitional	134	23	28	2	0	31	63
Anaplastic	2	1	13	4	129	7	7
Adenocarcinoma	20	4	0	1	0	5	20
Total	388	128	99	23	140	69	297

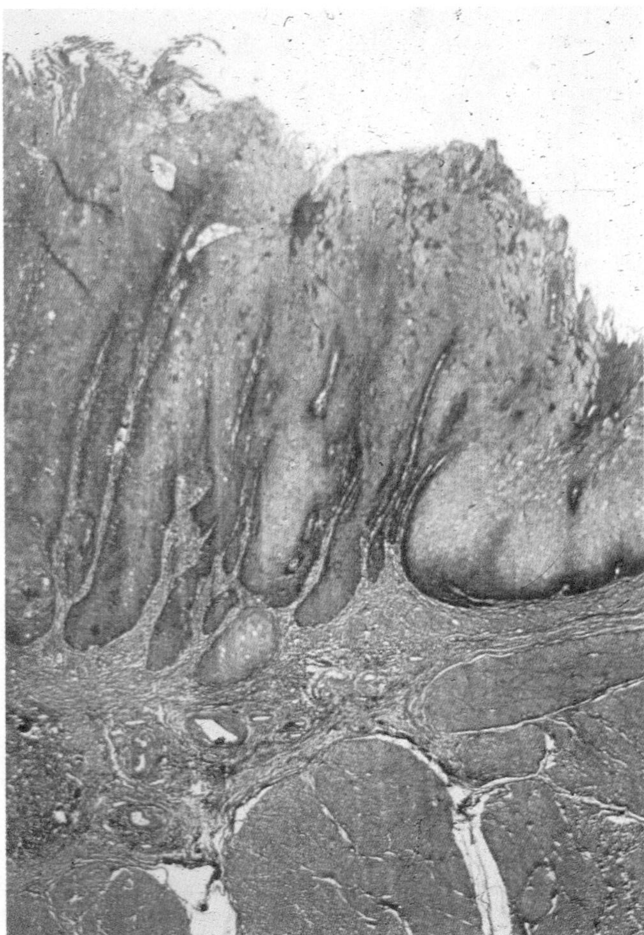

Figure 24.2. Verrucous carcinoma (noninvasive) of bladder with superficial filamentous elongated surface projections. (H & E × 40; Courtesy of Doctors M. R. Mahran and M. El-Baz, Mansoura University, Egypt.)

(45). Similarly, *N*-methyl-N-nitrosourea and *S. haematobium* caused bladder tumors in 5 of 16 hamsters, whereas, when either was given singly, no oncogenic effect was seen. Three *S. haematobium*-infected baboons treated with *N*-butyl-N-butazolnitrosamine all developed extensive bladder cancer (49).

Cancer development was thought to have been accelerated by schistosomal infection, presumably acting as a late-stage cocarcinogen by virtue of its direct proliferative effect on urothelium (47). Similarly, an increased incidence of hepatoma has been described after administration of carcinogen to mice infested with *S. mansoni* (29). This occurs even though the toxic morphologic alterations occurring in liver are fewer than those observed in noninfected mice exposed to the same hepatocarcinogen (68).

Helminthic Infestation and Viruses

No information seems to be available on the relationship between helminthic parasites and oncogenic viruses, though it is recognized that parasitic diseases exacerbate viral infection. In one of four capuchin monkeys, C-type virus particles were found in a papillary carcinoma induced by *S. haematobium* that had not been present earlier in the normal bladder tissue. Mice inoculated subcutaneously with Japanese B virus are resistant to the development of encephalitis unless they are challenged with the canine roundworm *Toxocara canis*. Also, overt disease in adult rats inoculated with encephalomyocarditis virus is promoted by concurrent trichinosis. Finally, in mice infected with *S. mansoni*, the parasitic disease may enhance the acute effect of hepatitis virus, but no evidence has yet been found that the chronic cirrhosis-like picture results therefrom (103).

Metabolic Observations During Schistosomiasis

Increased urinary excretion of free 3-hydroxykynurenine, 3-hydroxyanthranilic acid, and 2-amino-3-hydroxyacetophenone has been documented in some patients with bladder cancer. These ortho-aminophenol derivatives of tryptophan are generally excreted as conjugates of sulfuric acid or glucuronic acid. They are related to the carcinogenic metabolites of β-naphthylamine and are themselves carcinogenic to mice.

The relative resistance of the trigone to schistosomal bladder cancer would make less tenable an etiologic hypothesis predicated upon the topical action of an endogenous urinary carcinogen, were it not for the increased activity of urinary β-glucuronidase in vesical infections, including schistosomiasis. Under these circumstances the enzymatic release of the active carcinogen from its glucuronide could well become a significant biologic factor that determines the anatomic localization of the neoplasm. Thus, in the study of bilharzial cancer, the metabolism of tryptophan along the formylkynurenine pathway leading to nicotinic acid has elicited considerable interest (80). The basic justification for this interest originally stemmed from industrial oncology; however epidemiologic support is also derived from the high prevalence of classic pellagra that used to be observed in Egypt but not in other parts of Africa where squamous bladder cancer is infrequently reported despite endemic schistosomiasis. In pellagra, exaggeration of the pathway from tryptophan to nicotinic acid occurs, producing larger amounts of tryptophan intermediates along the formylkynurenine pathway.

Our understanding of the role played by *Schistosoma* infection in disturbed tryptophan metabolism is complicated by geographic variations in dietary habits. In fact, serotonin metabolites such as 5-hydroxyindoleacetic acid, which are excreted in large amounts by plantain-eating Africans, are low in Africans on other diets (36, 99). Similar differences attributable to dietary habits have been found between bilharzia patients in Mozambique and their "controls" in South Africa. Egyptian peasants are not plantain eaters but subsist mostly on beans, lentils, and rice. Those with bilharzial cancer metabolize tryptophan in a manner reminiscent of the pattern seen in many patients with spontaneous bladder cancer, because they have increased excretion of 3-hydroxyanthranilic acid, anthranilic acid, 5-hydroxyindoleacetic acid, and kynurenine. The excretion of these metabolites is enhanced by a loading dose of tryptophan.

Schistosomiasis should not be considered the only causal factor in the associated excretion of abnormal tryptophan metabolites because, with or without cancer, vesical schistosomiasis almost universally is accompanied by urinary tract infection. The bacterial flora may thus contribute to a spurious accumulation of some metabolites of tryptophan. Moreover, untreated pellagra is associated with increased urinary excretion of anthranilic acid, acetylkynurenine, and 5-hydroxyindoleacetic acid.

Potentially carcinogenic metabolites of tryptophan, which may be the true oncogenic agent in the presence of bilharzial bladder inflammation, are principally determined by hepatic metabolic patterns. Factors that bear on this are coincident infestation of the liver by *S. mansoni*, pyridoxine deficiency, and chronic protein starvation. In the presence of advanced abnormalities in any of these factors, lesser amounts of potential carcinogenic metabolites might be formed owing to lack of hepatic enzymes or cofactors; no mutagens were detected by the Ames test in the urine of patients suffering from bilharzial bladder cancer (33) or in soluble extracts of eggs and adult *Schistosoma japonicum* worms (55). A weak tumor-promoting activity was noted for *S. japonicum* soluble egg antigen, however, resulting in recovery of Epstein-Barr virus from cultured human lymphoid cells that harbored the viral genome (55).

The hepatic drug-metabolizing capacity of mice infected with *S. mansoni* is markedly reduced (15). Similarly reduced is the level of mutagen-processing potential of the *S. japonicum*–infected mouse liver (72), resulting in longer persistence of the mutagen in the animal body (3). It seems likely that the carcinogen dose is a determining factor in the aggressiveness of a bladder tumor and that a low-grade carcinoma can be converted into a high-grade one if exposed continuously to low doses of *N*-nitroso compounds (10). This would explain, at least in part, the overrepresentation of deeply invasive squamous cell cancers in the bilharzial urinary bladder (10).

A study of the frequency of active *ras* oncogenes in bilharzial bladder cancer concluded that the carcinogenic process involved in the endemic neoplasm is not associated with detectable point mutations within *ras* genes at a frequency higher than those in nonbilharzial cancer (37).

In view of its isolation from direct exposure to putative carcinogens present in the urine, a defunctionalized bilharzial bladder may seem an unlikely site for the development of neoplastic changes. Nonetheless, this has been reported in a defunctionalized bladder showing extensive metaplasia (27). Quantitative estimates of infection with *S. haematobium* have shown that its overall severity is unlikely to be the sole factor in the pathogenesis of endemic vesical cancer (28).

Schistosomiasis and Cancer of Other Sites

LARGE INTESTINE

While acknowledging the frequency of benign schistosomal polyposis (30), Egyptian data tend to discount any association of *S. mansoni* or *S. haematobium* with cancer of the large intestine (46). On the other hand, in Asia, intestinal infestation with *S. japonicum* is considered a significant contributory factor to the development of cancer of the colon and rectum. In this respect, it should be noted that *S. japonicum* lays a very large number of eggs (2,000 per day per pair of worms) while *S. mansoni*'s eggs are many fewer and, thus, cause fewer pathologic problems (56).

In one report from China, where in endemic areas the prevalence of schistosomiasis may reach 44 per 100,000 persons, 48% of colectomy specimens for colorectal carcinoma obtained from 1951 to 1974 were associated with *S. japonicum* infestation. Associated inflammatory changes, pseudopolyps, and transitional mucosal changes of schistosomal granulomatous disease progressing to mucosal atypia and to carcinoma were reminiscent of bowel carcinoma in patients with ulcerative colitis, save for the ova deposited in all layers of the bowel (18). Nonetheless, 92% were well-differentiated, as compared with 69% in the non-*Schistosoma* group. An ecologic study of 49 Chinese rural counties indicates that both schistosomal infestation and dietary factors contribute to the remarkable geographic variation of colon cancer in China (42).

In Shanghai, patients with intestinal schistosomiasis and cancer of the large intestine are, on average, 6 years younger than patients with spontaneous intestinal cancer (51, 75). However, Chinese patients whose history of schistosomiasis entailed an elevated relative risk of rectal cancer (RR = 8.3; CI = 3.1–22.6) did not show a parallel increase in their relative risk for cancer of the colon (108).

BREAST

In Egyptian hospital material, the male-to-female breast cancer ratio is substantially greater than in the West. If corroborated by incidence studies, this observation would be a valuable epidemiologic observation worthy of further investigation. Hyperestrogenism secondary to bilharzial liver fibrosis has been cited as one possible cause.

LIVER

Discordant observations on the association of schistosomiasis and hepatic cancer are difficult to reconcile without further data. In Egypt (46) and Mozambique (86) bilharzial liver cirrhosis is very common; however carcinoma of the liver is prevalent only in Mozambique, where it is the most common cancer among males. The association of cirrhosis from *S. japonicum* with hepatoma has been infrequently reported and appears invalid.

In Japan, liver cancer correlated highly with three factors: HBsAg (OR = 10.0), history of schistosomiasis (OR = 9.5), and daily intake of alcohol (OR = 3.2) with the combination of hazards acting multiplicatively or at least synergistically (54, 62). In experimental animals, infection with *S. japonicum* accelerates the occurrence of *N*-2-fluorenyl acetamide–induced liver tumors (76).

LYMPHOMA

Eight cases of solitary follicular lymphoma of the spleen were found among 863 spleens removed from patients with hepatosplenic schistosomiasis. The rarity of an isolated tumor in this site and of this type suggests a causal link, possibly mediated by cycles of follicular hyperplasia and involution occurring in the spleen in the course of advanced schistosomiasis (7). In a Nigerian series, lymphoreticular tumors were overrepresented in infected individuals (16%) as compared with uninfested ones (25).

OTHER ORGANS

Immunohistochemically confirmed invasive squamous cell carcinoma of the prostate was diagnosed in two patients with prostatic schistosomiasis coming from a population where prostatic cancer is uncommon (4). On the other hand, Egyptian cases indicate no relationship between bilharziasis and cancer of the lungs, pancreas, prostate, seminal vesicles, urethra, vulva, vagina, cervix uteri, body of the uterus, or ovaries (46). As would be expected, surgical or autopsy material in countries with high schistosomal endemicity from time to time shows the presence of schistosoma ova in various tissues, including cancerous ones. The literature contains a number of isolated reports of such coincidences. Moreover, in areas where infestation is endemic, schistosomal tissue reaction may be so intense and proliferative as to be mistaken clinically for cancer of the large intestine (81) or the cervix (91).

East Asian Distomiasis

LIVER AND PANCREAS

Clonorchis sinensis is endemic in parts of Japan, Korea, China, and Hong Kong; a similar species, *Opisthorchis viverrini*, causes distomiasis in Thailand. Liver fluke infections have been associated with multifocal intrahepatic bile duct adenocarcinoma in those areas of Asia where distomiasis is endemic: Thailand, where 70% to 90% of the population of the northeast part of the country are infected with *O. viverrini*, has the highest recorded incidence of cholangiocarcinoma in the world (59). In Indonesia, and in Taipei, Taiwan, where distomiasis is considered uncommon, cholangiocarcinoma is infrequent (40). Imported cases of distomiasis are seen in the United States, and, since the parasite can live up to 30 years, it represents a long-term hazard to infected persons (96).

Human infection results from eating raw or undercooked parasitized freshwater fish. In humans, the ingested parasites excyst in the duodenum and ascend the bile ducts and capillaries, where they mature, causing biliary epithelial hyperplasia and fibrosis. Similarities between the histopathologic responses in infected humans and experimental animals have been documented, including the development of cholangiocarcinoma in dogs and cats experimentally infected with *Clonorchis*. Hamsters infected with *Opisthorchis* and administered dimethylnitrosamine for 10 weeks all developed mucin-secreting cholangiocarcinomas, whereas noninfected animal controls failed to develop tumors, an observation in keeping with experimental evidence pointing to infection as a promoter of *N*-nitrosodimethylamine. In the Far East nitrosamines are commonly found in such traditional Chinese preserved aliments as salted fish, dried shrimp, and sausage (92).

Pancreatic ducts may also be infected with *C. sinensis*; this frequently results in squamous metaplasia and mucous gland hyperplasia. In one instance, an immigrant with *C. sinensis* in the common bile duct developed a well differentiated ductal adenocarcinoma of the pancreas (19).

Amebiasis

The association of amebiasis with neoplasms of the large intestine remains speculative, at best.

Malaria

The geographic distribution of Burkitt's lymphoma in the classic malarial belt initially suggested the possible role of an arthropod vector in oncogenesis (13, 44). The notion that drugs taken for malaria prophylaxis contribute to the development of Burkitt's lymphoma (88, 89) was considered unlikely, because no increase (and indeed a decrease) in endemic Burkitt's lymphoma (eBL) was observed in the Malagasy Republic (12) and in Imesi, West Africa (73), where intensive antimalarial prophylaxis was practiced; moreover, cases occur in Africa (53), Israel (2), and elsewhere among persons who are not receiving malaria prophylaxis.

More significant are the epidemiologic observations that have linked eBL to the combined effect of malaria and infection with the Epstein-Barr virus (EBV) (34). Regarding malaria, eBL is only found in areas where malaria is holoendemic or hyperendemic, and within these areas it is absent in pockets of no malaria such as urban centers. Within endemic areas, the peak incidence of eBL follows closely the one of severe *Plasmodium falciparum* malaria and malarial prophylaxis reduces the incidence of the lymphoma (12, 73).

Vigorous cellular and serologic responses occur during malarial infection (87). This renders very plausible the argument that the persistent reticuloendothelial stimulation experienced among malarial populations conditions the EBV-infected African patient to develop a neoplasm rather than a self-limited disease such as infectious mononucleosis (84). This view finds support in the observation that each one of the erythrocytic, exoerythrocytic, and sexual forms of the parasite is structurally differentiated and probably contains a multitude of biologically active antigenic constituents (57, 83). In this respect, it is interesting to note that in endemic malarial areas, the distribution of hyper-reactive malarial splenomegaly parallels the distribution of eBL and that the peak age incidence of eBL follows closely the peak age incidence of severe *P. falciparum* malaria (34).

One way of explaining the observation that the malaria patient harboring a multitude of parasite-derived antigens becomes a host very susceptible to eBL is the suggestion that malaria patients produce so many nonspecific and "useless" antibodies that they are unable to recognize and respond to the threat posed by a small clone of malignant lymphoid cells (104). This view is supported by experimental data. In mice, antigenic stimulation and immune suppression often result in an increased incidence of lymphomas; mice repeatedly injected with *Plasmodium berghei* sometimes develop malignant lymphoma morphologically similar to Burkitt's lymphoma, and sometimes develop persistent antigenic stimulation without significant tumorigenesis (32, 63, 95). Lymphomas are frequently induced by Moloney leukemogenic virus in mice infected with *P. berghei* but rarely occur in mice given either plasmodium or virus alone (105). Acute malaria, which increases B-cell proliferation, also impairs EBV-specific T-cell responses (44, 106). This results in a larger pool of EBV-infected cells with increased likelihood for chromosomal translocation and lymphomagenesis (70). In children, the risk of developing Burkitt's lymphoma is related to antibody titers against EBV capsid antigens (21); the clinical manifestations probably are promoted by other environmental factor(s), such as holoendemic malaria (31) and phorbol exposure (101).

Of considerable interest are studies on the frequency of sickle-cell trait in eBL patients and controls. Persons with sickle trait are not protected from being bitten by mosquitoes or from malarial infection, but they are protected against the lethal effect of overwhelming *P. falciparum* malaria in early childhood and from the intense reticuloendothelial stimulation that sometimes progresses to hyperreactive malarial splenomegaly ("big spleen" disease) (77). Sickle cells do not support the growth of parasites in vitro when exposed to low oxygen tension. A similar phenomenon may explain why children with the sickle-cell trait have a lower *P. falciparum* parasitemia. As a result, lower mortality rate, lower IgM levels, and reduced lymphoproliferation (as measured by spleen size) are found among individuals with hemoglobin AS genotype; however, most studies attempting to link eBL to AS hemoglobinopathy have failed to reach statistical significance (34). Other hemoglobinopathies (e.g., hereditary ovalocytosis) also protect against malaria. If eBL turns out to be underrepresented in populations where, as in Papua New Guinea, both ovalocytosis and malaria are prevalent (14), such information would provide strong supporting evidence for malaria as a cofactor in the genesis of eBL (34). In this event, the observation that in Uganda malarial endemicity also correlates with non-Burkitt's, non-Hodgkin's lymphoma would acquire added significance (90).

The small differences in titers of malarial antibodies observed in Burkitt's lymphoma patients and controls (78) were attributed to the fact that many in the experimental group had received several courses of antimalarial drugs, which may have lowered the level of malaria-specific antibodies (34). A probable role of malaria emerges also from the following considerations. African children with eBL develop autoantibodies, the elevated titers of which show no linear correlation with EBV titers (100) (VCA or EBNA), suggesting that a factor independent of EBV causes an immunologic imbalance and autoantibody production. The notion that this could be due to malaria is supported by the observation that Caucasians suffering from acute *P. falciparum* malaria develop autoantibodies (20, 79) and that experiments in vitro demonstrated that normal human lymphocytes will produce autoantibodies as a response to malarial antigens (60).

It has been pointed out that, in the genesis of eBL, regardless of whether one considers malaria the initiator and EBV the promoter or vice versa, neither hypothesis accounts for the fact that in vitro infection of B cells with EBV and stimulation with malaria antigens has yet to produce a cell that carries any of the chromosomal tumorigenic translocations found in both sporadic and eBL (34). Thus, it seems likely that other unidentified factors—genetic, nutritional or environmental play a significant role in this type of tumorigenesis.

AMERICAN BURKITT'S LYMPHOMA

By the early 1970s, approximately 100 cases of Burkitt's lymphoma had been confirmed by the American Burkitt's lymphoma registry (66). Space-time clustering is suggested by the American data (67, 85). Although malaria is associated with Burkitt's lymphoma in Africa, the relative rarity of the tumor in relation to the holoendemic nature of malaria indicates that a combination of genetic factors plus specific environmental factors may be operative. Host and environmental factors other than malaria are probably important in North American cases (66).

Cancer in Animals

Observations made by Fibiger (35) on gastric cancer in rats infested with a nematode are now all but discredited. A question that remains to be evaluated is whether the nematode helped localize some unidentified carcinogens in the diet (94), similar to the induction of sarcomas at the site of subcutaneous injection of sodium chloride in rats being fed 3-methylcholanthrene (52).

Sarcoma is an almost inevitable complication of infection of the liver or the subcutaneous tissues of rats with *Cysticercus fasciolaris*, the larval form of the common tapeworm of the cat, *Taenia taeniaformis*. Washed, ground-up *C. fasciolaris* produced peritoneal sarcomas in half the injected rats, the proportion reached 91% if the animals were genetically related to the parasitized host. The active agent appears to be associated with the calcium carbonate corpuscles of the parasite, but the mechanism is not clear (24). Although not directly implicated in vesical carcinogenesis, there is suggestive evidence that infestation with another nematode, *Trichosomoides crassicauda*, increases the incidence of tumors in the bladders of rats receiving 2-acetyl-aminofluorine (16).

Another nematode, *Spirocerca lupi*, has been associated with the development of esophageal sarcoma in dogs. Here, the reported association seems to be described only in the southern United States, thus adding a possible geographic dimension to the problem.

Some neoplastic responses to parasitic infestation are a kind of cecidiosis, and may represent the end of a hypothesized evolutionary sequence by which parasite secretions stimulate the host to form protective structures (cecidia) that benefit the parasite (9).

References

1. Aboul Nasr A, Gazayerli M, Fawzi RM, El-Sibai I. Epidemiology and pathology of cancer of the bladder in Egypt. Acta Unio Int Contra Cancrum 1962;18:528.
2. Aghai E, Hulu N, Virag I, Kende G, Ramot B. Childhood non-Hodgkin's lymphoma—a study of 17 cases in Israel. Cancer 1974;33:1411.
3. Aji T, Matsuoka H, Ishii A, Arimoto S, Hayatsu H. Retention of a mutagen, 3 amino-1-methyl-5 H-pyrido[4,3,6]indole (Trp P2) in the liver of mice infected with S. japonicum. Mutation Res 1994;305:265.
4. Al Adnani MS. Schistosomiasis, metaplasia and squamous cell carcinoma of the prostate: histogenesis of the squamous cells determined by localization of specific markers. Neoplasma 1985;32:613.
5. Al-Hussaini M, McDonald DF. Lack of urothelial topical tumorigenicity and cotumorigenicity of Schistosoma ova in mice. Cancer Res 1967;27:228.
6. Al-Shukry S, Alwan MH, Nayef M, Rahman AA. Bilharziasis in malignant tumors of the urinary bladder. Br J Urol 1987;59:59.
7. Andrade ZA, Abreeu WN. Follicular lymphoma of the spleen with hepatosplenic schistosomiasis mansoni. Am J Trop Med Hyg 1971;20:237.
8. Anwar WA, Rosin MP. Reduction in chromosomal damage in schistosomiasis patients after treatment with praziquantel. Mutation Res 1993;298:179.
9. Audy JR. "Hostology"—an alternative view. Trop Med Hyg News 1970;19:15.
10. Badawi AF, Mostafa MH, O'Connor PJ. Involvement of alkylating agents in schistosome-associated bladder cancer: The possible basic mechanisms of induction. Cancer Lett 1992;63:171.
11. Bedwani R, El-Khwsky F, La Vecchia C, Boffetta P, Levi F. Descriptive epidemiology of bladder cancer in Egypt. Int J Cancer 1993;55:351.
12. Bruce-Chwatt LJ. Antimalarial drugs and Burkitt's lymphoma. Lancet 1974;1:223.
13. Burchenal JH. Geographic chemotherapy—Burkitt's tumor as a stalking horse for leukemia. Presidential address. Cancer Res 1966;26:2393.
14. Castelino D, Saul A, Myler P, Kidson C, Thomas H, Cooke R. Ovalocytosis in Papua New Guinea—dominantly inherited resistance to malaria. Southeast Asian J Trop Med Public Health 1981;12:549.
15. Cha YN, Edwards R. Effects of *Schistosoma mansoni* infection on the hepatic drug-metabolizing capacity of mice. J Pharmacol Exp Ther 1976;199:432.
16. Chapman WH. The incidence of a nematode, *Trichosomoides crassicauda*, in the bladder of laboratory rats: Treatment with nitrofurantoin and preliminary report of their influence on urinary calcyli and experimental tumors. J Invest Urol 1964;2:52.
17. Cheever AW. Schistosomiasis and neoplasia. JNCI 1978;61:13.
18. Chen M-C, Chuang C-Y, Chang PY, Hu T-C. Evolution of colorectal cancer in schistosomiasis. Cancer 1980;46:1661.
19. Colquhoun BPD. Adenocarcinoma of the pancreas associated with *C. sinensis* infection. Can Med Assoc J 1987;136:153.
20. Daniel-Ribeiro CT, de Roquefeuil S, Druilhe P, Monjour L, Homberg J-C, Gentilini M. Abnormal anti-single-stranded (ss) DNA activity in sera from *Plasmodium falciparum* infected individuals. Trans R Soc Trop Med Hyg 1983;78:742.
21. de-Thé G, Geser A, Day NE, Turkey PM, Williams EH, Beri DP, Smith PG, Dean AG, Bornkamm G, Feorino P, Henle W. Epidemiological evidence for causal relationship between Epstein-Barr virus and Burkitt's lymphoma from Ugandan prospective study. Nature 1978;274:756.
22. Dimmette RM, Sproat HF, Sayegh ES. The classification of carcinoma of the urinary bladder associated with schistosomiasis and metaplasia. J Urol 1956;75:680.
23. Dodge OG. Tumors of the bladder in Uganda Africans. Acta Unio Int Contra Cancrum 1962;18:548.
24. Dunning WF, Curtis MR. Multiple peritoneal sarcoma in rats from intraperitoneal injection of washed ground Taenia larvae. Cancer Res 1946;6:668.
25. Edington GM, von Lichtenberg F, Nwabuebo I, Taylor JR, Smith JH. Pathologic effects of schistosomiasis in Ibadan, western state of Nigeria. I. Incidence and intensity of infection; distribution and severity of lesions. Am J Trop Med 1970;19:982.
26. El-Aaser AA, El-Merzabani MM, El-Bolkaini Ibrahim AS. A study on the etiological factors of bilharzial bladder cancer in Egypt: 5-Urinary nitrites in a rural population. Tumori 1980;66:400.
27. Elem B, Alam SZ. Total intestinal metaplasia with focal adenocarcinoma in a *Schistosoma*-infested defunctioned urinary bladder. Br J Urol 1984;56:331.
28. Elem B, Purohit R. Carcinoma of the urinary bladder in Zambia. A quantitative estimation of Schistosoma haematobium infection. Br J Urol 1983;55:275.
29. El-Ghaffar YA. Failure to induce bladder cancer in mice. Bladder implantation with paraffin wax pellets of lyophilized urine from bilharzial patients. Cancer 1966;19: 1225.
30. El-Masry NA, Farid Z, Bassily S, Kilpatrick ME, Watten RW. Schistosomal colonic poplyposis: Clinical, radiological and parasitological study. J Trop Med Hyg 1986;89: 13.
31. Epstein MA, Achong BG. The Epstein-Barr virus. Berlin: Springer-Verlag. 1979.
32. Evans AS. Clinical syndromes associated with EB virus infection. Adv Intern Med 1972;18:77.
33. Everson RB, Gad-el-Mawla NM, Attia MA, Chevlen EM, Thorgeirsson SS, Alexander LA, Flack PM, Staiano N, Ziegler JL. Analysis of human urine for mutagens associated with carcinoma of the bilharzial bladder by the Ames Salmonella plate assay. Interpretation employing quantitation of viable lawn bacteria. Cancer 1983;51:371.
34. Facer CA, Playfair JHL. Malaria, Epstein-Barr virus and the genesis of the lymphomas. Adv Cancer Res 1989;53:33.
35. Fibiger J. Untersuchung über eine Nematode (*Spiroptera* sp.n.) und deren Fähigkeitt, papillomatöse und karzinomatöse Geschwulstbildungen in Magen der Ratte hervorzurufen. Z Krebsforsch 1913;13:217.
36. Fripp PH. Bilharziasis and bladder cancer. Br J Cancer 1965;19:292.
37. Fujita J, Nakayama H, Onoue H, Rhim JS, El-Bolkainy MN, El-Aaser AA, Kitamura Y. Frequency of active ras oncogenes in human bladder cancers associated with schistosomiasis. Jpn J Cancer Res (Gann) 1987;78:915.
38. Gelfand M, Weinberg RW, Castle WM. Relation between carcinoma of the bladder and infestation with *Schistosoma haematobium*. Lancet 1967;1:1249.
39. Gentile JM. Schistosome related cancers: A possible role for genotoxins. Exp Mutagen 1985;7:775.
40. Gibson JB, Chan WC. Primary carcinomas of the liver in Hong Kong: Some possible aetiologic factors. Recent Results Cancer Res 1971;39:107.
41. Gillman J, Prats MD. Histologic types and histogenesis of bladder cancer in the Portuguese East African with special reference to bilharzial cystitis. Acta Unio Int Contra Cancrum 1952;18:560.
42. Guo W, Zheng W, Li JY, Chen JS, Blot WJ. Correlation of colon cancer mortality with dietary factors, markers and schistosomiasis in China. Nut Cancer 1993;20:13.
43. Habuchi T, Takahashi R, Yamada H, Ogawa O, Kakehi Y, Ogura K, Hamazaki S, Toguchida J, Ishizaki K, Fijita J, Sugiyama T, Yoshida O. Influence of cigarette smoking and schistosomiasis on p53 gene mutation in urothelial cancer. Cancer Res 1993;53:3795.
44. Haddow AJ. An improved map for the study of Burkitt's lymphoma in Africa. East Afr Med J 1963;40:429.
45. Hashem M, Boutros K. The influence of bilharzial infection on the carcinogenesis of the mouse bladder. An experimental study. J Egypt Med Assoc 1961;44:598.
46. Hashem M, Zaki SA, Hussein M. The bilharzial bladder cancer and its relation to schistosomiasis. A statistical study. J Egypt Med Assoc 1961;44:579.
47. Hicks RM. The canopic worm: Role of bilharziasis in the aetiology of human bladder cancer. J Roy Soc Med 1983;76:16.
48. Hicks RM, Ismail MM, Walters CL, Beecham PT, Rabie MF, El Alamy MA. Association of bacteriuria and urinary nitrosamine formation with *Schistosoma haematobium* infection in the Qalyub area of Egypt. Trans R Soc Trop Med Hyg 1982;76:519.
49. Hicks RM, James C, Webbe G, Nelson GS. *Schistosoma haematobium* and bladder cancer. Trans R Soc Trop Med Hyg 1977;71:288.
50. Higginson J, Oettle AG. Cancer of the bladder in the South African Bantu. Acta Unio Int Contra Cancrum 1962;18:580.
51. Huan-Wen T, Yueh-Ying Y. A pathologic study of intestinal schistosomiasis associated with cancer. Chin Med J 1958;77:244.
52. Huggins C, Grand LC. Sarcoma induced remotely in rats fed 3-methyl-cholanthrene. Cancer Res 1963;23:477.
53. Hutt MSR, Burkitt DP. Aetiology of Burkitt's lymphoma. Lancet 1973;1:439.
54. Inaba Y, Maruchi N, Matsuda M, Yoshihara N, Yamamato SA. A case-control study on liver cancer with special emphasis on the possible aetiological role of schistosomiasis. Int J Epidemiol 1984;13:408.
55. Ishii A, Matsuoka H, Aji T, Hayatsu H, Wataya Y, Arimoto S, Tokuda H. Evaluation of the mutagenicity and the tumor promoting activity of parasite extract: *Schistosoma japonicum* infection and *Clonorchis sinensis*. Mutation Res 1989;224:229.
56. Ishii A, Matsuoka H, Aji T, Ohta N, et al. Parasite infection and cancer with special emphasis on *Schistosoma japonicum* infections (*Trematoda*). A review. Mutation Res 1994;305:273.
57. Jayawardena AN. Parasitic diseases. In Immunology, vol I. Edited by JM Mansfield. New York: Dekker, 1981, pp 88–163.
58. Jordan P. Egg output in bilharziasis in relation to epidemiology, pathology, treatment and control. In *Bilharziasis*. Edited by FK Mostofi. Berlin: Springer-Verlag, 1967.
59. Juttijudata P, Chiemchaisri C, Palavatana C, et al. A high incidence of cholangiocarcinoma in patients with biliary obstructive (malignant) disease in Thailand. JNCI 1983;71:229.
60. Kataaha PK, Hacer CA, Holborow EJ. Stimulation of autoantibodies production in normal blood lymphocytes by malaria culture supernatants. Parasitol Immunol 1984;6: 481.
61. Kitinya JN, Lauren PA, Eshleman LJ, Paljarvi L, Tanaka K. The incidence of squamous and transitional cell carcinomas of the urinary bladder in northern Tanzania in areas of high and low levels of endemic *Schistosoma haematobium* infection. Trans R Soc Trop Med Hyg 1986;80:935.
62. Kojiro M, Kakizoe S, Yano H, Tsumagari J, Kenmochi K, Nakashima T. Hepatocellular carcinoma and schistosomiasis japonica. A clinicopathologic study of 59 autopsy cases of hepatocellular carcinoma associated with chronic schistosomiasis japonica. Acta Pathol Jpn 1986;36:525.
63. Kreger G, O'Conor GT. Epidemiologic and immunologic considerations on the pathogenesis of Burkitt's tumor. Recent Results Cancer Res 19712;32:211.
64. Kuntz RE, Cheever AW, Myers BJ. Proliferative epithelial lesions of the urinary bladder of nonhuman primates infested with *Schistosoma haematobium*. JNCI 1972;48: 223.
65. Kuntz RW, Myers BJ, Moore JA, Huang TC. Parasitologic aspects of *Schistosoma haematobium* (Iran) infections in the American opossum (*Didelphis marsupialis*). Int J Parasitol 1975;5:21.
66. Levine PH, Cho BR. Burkitt's lymphoma Clinical features of North American cases. Cancer Res 1974;34:1219.
67. Levine PH, Sandler SG, Komp DM, O'Conor GT, O'Conor DM. Simultaneous occurrence of "American Burkitt's lymphoma" in neighbors. N Engl J Med 1973;288:562.
68. Liu LB, Domingo EO, Stenger RJ, Warren KS, Confer DB, Johnson EA. An ultrastructural study of the toxic and carcinogenic effects of 2-amino-5-azotoluene on the livers of schistososome-infected and uninfected mice. Cancer Res 1969;29:837.
69. Lucas SB. Squamous cell carcinoma of the bladder and Schistosomiasis. East Afr Med J 1982;59:345.
70. Magrath I. The pathogenesis of Burkitt's lymphoma. Adv Cancer Res 1990;55:145.
71. Mahran MR, El-Baz M. Verrucous carcinoma of the bilharzial bladder. Scand J Urol Nephrol 1993;27:189.
72. Matsuoka H, Aji T, Ishii A, Arimoto S, Wataya Y, Hayatsu H. Reduced levels of mutagen processing potential in the *Schistosoma japonicum*-infected mouse liver. Mutation Res 1989;227:153.
73. McGucken RB. Antimalarial drugs and Burkitt's lymphoma. Lancet 1974;1:68.
74. Michelson MK, Azziz FA, Gamil FM, Wahid AA, Richards FO, Juranek DD, Habib MA, Spencer HC. Recent trends in the prevalence and distribution of schistosomiasis in the Nile delta region. Am J Trop Med Hyg 1993;49:76.
75. Ming-Chai C, Shan-Chi CW. Acute colonic obstruction in schistosomiasis japonica. A clinical study of 40 cases—14 associated with carcinoma. Chin Med J 1957;75:517.
76. Miyasato M. Experimental study on the influence of *Schistosoma japonicum* infection on carcinogenesis of mouse liver treated with *N*-2-fluorenyl acetamide (2-FAA). Jpn J Parasitol 1984;33:41.
77. Morrow RH, Sever JL, Henderson BE. Antibody levels in infectious agents other than Epstein-Barr virus in Burkitt's lymphoma patients. Cancer Res 1974;34:1212.
78. Morrow RH. Epidemiological evidence for role of falciparum Malaria. In Burkitt's Lymphoma: A Human Cancer Model. Edited by G Lenoir, G O'Conor, and C Olweny. IARC Sci Publ 1985;60:177–185.

79. Mortazavi-Milan SM, Stiele HE, Holborow EJ. Antibody to intermediate filaments of the cytoskeletons in the sera of patients with acute malaria. Clin Exp Immunol 1983;55: 177.
80. Mousa AH, Abdel Wahab AF, Mousa W, Abdel-Tawab GA, Saad AA, Kelada NL. Tryptophan metabolism in hepatosplenic bilharziasis. Trans R Soc Trop Med Hyg 1967;61:640.
81. Mustacchi PO, El-Sibai I. Advanced schistosomal proctitis simulating clinically cancer of the rectum. Gastroenterology 1951;19:137.
82. Mustacchi P, Shimkin MB. Cancer of the bladder and infestation with *Schistosoma haematobium*. JNCI 1958;20:825.
83. Neva FA, Sheagren JN, Shulman NR, Canfield CJ. Malaria: Host-defense mechanisms and complications. Ann Intern Med 1970;73:295.
84. O'Conor GT. Persistent immunologic stimulation as a factor in oncogenesis with special reference to Burkitt's tumor. Am J Med 1970;48:279.
85. Patton LL, McMillan CW, Webster WP. American Burkitt's lymphoma: A 10-year review and case study. Oral Surg Oral Med Oral Pathol 1990;69:307.
86. Prates MD, Gillman J. Carcinoma of the urinary bladder in the Portuguese East African with special reference to bilharzial cystitis and preneoplastic lesions. S Afr J Med Sci 1959;24:13.
87. Riley EM, Hviid L, Theander TG. Malaria. In Parasitic Infections and the Immune System. Edited by F Kierszenbaum. New York: Academic, 1994, pp 119–143.
88. Sadoff L. Aetiology of Burkitt's lymphoma. Lancet 1972;2:1414.
89. Sadoff L. Antimalarial drugs and Burkitt's lymphoma. Lancet 1973;2:1262.
90. Schmauz R, Mugerwa JW, Wright DH. The distribution of non-Burkitt, non-Hodgkin's lymphoma in Uganda in relation to malarial endemicity. Int J Cancer 1990;46:650.
91. Schwartz DA. Carcinoma of the uterine cervix and schisto-somiasis in West Africa. Gynecol Oncol 1984;19:365.
92. Schwartz DA. Cholangiocarcinoma associated with liver fluke infection: A preventable source of morbidity in Asian immigrants. Am J Gastroenterol 1986;81:1986.
93. Shimkin MB, Mustacchi PO, Cram EB, Wright WH. Lack of carcinogenicity of lyophilized *Schistosoma* in mice. JNCI 1955;16:471.
94. Shimkin MB, Triolo VA. History of chemical carcinogenesis: Some prospective remarks. International Symposium on Carcinogenesis and Carcinogen Testing, Boston, 1969. Prog Exp Tumor Res 1969;11:1.
95. Sizaret P, O'Conor GT, Beaumont R, Laval M. Serum protein patterns in mice following primary and challenge infection with *Plasmodium berghei*. Z Tropenmed Parasitol 1971;22:260.
96. Sun T. (ed) Chlonorchiasis and opistochiasis. In Pathology and Clinical Features of Parasitic Diseases, vol 5. New York: Masson, 1982, p 243. (Masson Monogr Diagn Pathol).
97. Thomas JE, Nassett MT, Sigola LB, Taylor P. Relationship between bladder cancer incidence, *Schistosoma haematobium* infection, and geographical region in Zimbabwe. Trans R Soc Trop Med Hyg 1990;84:551.
98. Tricker AR, Mostafa HH, Spiegelhalder P, Preussman P. Urinary nitrite and *N*-nitroso compounds in bladder cancer patients with shistosomiasis (bilharziasis). IARC Sci Publ 1991;105:178.
99. Trout GE, Gillman J, Prates MD. Bilharzial cystitis and the urinary excretion of tryptophan metabolites in the Portuguese East African. Acta Unio Int Contra Cancrum 1962;18:575.
100. Vainio E, Lenoir GM, Franklin RM. Autoantibodies in three populations of Burkitt's lymphoma patients. Clin Exp Immunol 1983;54:387.
101. Van den Bosch C, Griffin BE, Kazembe P, Dwizen C, and Kadzamira, L. Are plant factors a missing link in the evolution of endemic Burkitt's lymphoma? Br J Cancer 1993;68:1232.
102. Warren KS. A comparison of Puerto Rican, Brazilian, Egyptian, and Tanzanian strains of *Schistosoma mansoni* in mice: Penetration of cercariae, maturation of schistosomes and production of liver disease. Trans R Soc Trop Med Hyg 1967;61:795.
103. Warren KS, Rosenthal MS, Domingo EO. Mouse hepatitis virus (MHV3) infection in chronic murine Schistosomiasis mansoni. Bull NY Acad Med 1969;45:211.
104. Warrens AE. Burkitt's lymphoma and disordered immunoglobulin response. Lancet 1974;1:742.
105. Weddeburn N. Effect of concurrent malarial infection on development of virus-induced lymphoma in Balb/c mice. Lancet 1970;2:1114.
106. Whittle HC, Brown J, Marsh K, Greenwood BM, Seidelin P, Tighe H, Wedderburn L. T-cell control of Epstein-Barr virus-infected B-cells is lost during *P. falciparum* malaria. Nature 1984;312:449.
107. Wishahi M, El-Baz HG, Shaker ZA. Association between HLA-A, B, C and DR antigens and clinical manifestations of *Schistosoma haematobium* in the bladder. Eur Urol 1989;16:138.
108. Xu Z, Su D-L. *Schistosoma japonicum* and colorectal cancer: An epidemiologic study in the People's Republic of China. Int J Cancer 1984;34:315.

SECTION IV

CANCER EPIDEMIOLOGY

CHAPTER 25

Cancer Epidemiology

FREDERICK P. LI AND ARLENE F. KANTOR

Introduction

In 1995, it is estimated that newly diagnosed cancers in the United States will surpass 1.25 million, and cancer deaths will equal 547,000 for the first time (207). These figures highlight the steady rise in the occurrence of cancer and resulting deaths among Americans throughout this century. Aging and the numeric growth of the U.S. population are the major causes of these increases. At present, at least one person in three will develop cancer within a lifetime and one in five will die of cancer. The human suffering due to cancer is enormous, and the cost of care for cancer patients contributes substantially to the rising expenditures for medical services in the United States. In this era of medical cost containment, oncologists seek to develop not only better treatments for cancer but also effective programs of cancer prevention.

The prevention of cancer requires knowledge of its causes. History shows that epidemiologic studies have been the key to the control of a wide range of infectious diseases, such as tuberculosis, smallpox, cholera, and plague (107). In recent decades, epidemiologic studies have also contributed to our understanding of the origins of chronic diseases, notably heart disease and cancer (45, 50, 145, 178). This chapter describes methods used to design and conduct epidemiologic studies, and summarizes the current state of knowledge of the causes of human cancer.

Cancer epidemiology can be defined as the study of the frequencies, patterns of distribution, and determinants of tumor occurrence in humans (127). By examining who develops cancer, epidemiologists generate and test hypotheses regarding why certain individuals do so. Characterizing cancer patients helps to identify host factors in the genesis of neoplasia. The impact of environmental carcinogens is examined by determining exposures to candidate agents, and correlating these exposures with disease incidence. For most human cancers, cancer risk increases with the dose and the duration of exposure to a carcinogen. The time interval from initial oncogenic exposure to disease development is often a decade or longer, and the search for cancer causation needs to explore both the present and past histories of patients (51). In addition, the suspected carcinogen should have biologic properties that are consistent with a role in the pathogenesis of cancer. These and other tests of causal association permit the exclusion of factors that have a noncausal relation to cancer development. Identification of etiologic influences can lead to early cancer detection and prevention, particularly among populations at increased risk. Thus, scarce health care resources can be allocated to those most likely to benefit from appropriate interventions.

Design of Epidemiologic Studies

DESCRIPTIVE STUDIES

Epidemiologic studies often begin with descriptions of the patients who develop cancer. These patients are assessed to uncover demographic characteristics, medical histories, occupations, habits, and lifestyles that may predispose to cancer. The likelihood of a causal effect can be further evaluated in analytic studies.

The patterns of cancer in populations are described by several standard measures of frequency. Cancer occurrence can be expressed in terms of the number of cases, a proportion, or a rate (74). These measures can be applied to new occurrences of cancer (incidence) or cancer deaths (mortality) within a defined time interval, usually 1 year. The enumeration of cancer cases is useful, for example, in assessing levels of need for medical services. A proportion is often used to identify the fraction of total deaths that are due to cancer, or the fraction of all cancers that arise at a particular anatomic site. Rates (number of cancers per 100,000 persons) serve to standardize the measurement of disease frequency, allowing for ease of comparison among different populations. In epidemiologic studies, rates are the most useful measure of cancer incidence and mortality. Crude rates measure cancer frequency in a population without regard for its composition. Cancer rates can be specific for age, race, and sex, or adjusted to account for the influence of these factors. An age-adjusted rate is a weighted summary of age-specific rates that removes differences in age composition among populations and allows for comparisons.

Prevalence measures the proportion of the population who have cancer at a specified point or during an interval of time. Cancer prevalence reflects both the incidence of cancer and survival, and provides a measure of the cancer burden within a population (58). However, the measure includes patients who are dying of cancer, those under active treatment, those in complete remission, and long-term survivors. This heterogeneity limits the utility of prevalence as a measure of cancer frequency. Cancer incidence and mortality are better indicators in most circumstances (10).

Clinicians often need to measure the impact of therapy on survival of their patients. Absolute survival rates measure the proportion of cancer patients who survive for a specified period after diagnosis. However, survivorship from time of diagnosis can be diminished by diseases other than cancer, particularly among elderly patients. The relative survival rate is used to measure the survival of cancer patients, after eliminating the effects of deaths from other causes (26).

SOURCES OF DATA

Data on cancer incidence and mortality are obtained from several sources. Mortality data in the United States are derived primarily from death certificates. Population-based cancer registries have been established in a number of states to provide cancer incidence data. A consortium of these registries under the Surveillance, Epidemiology, and End Results (SEER) program has been the principal source of U.S. cancer rates since 1973. The SEER program, administered through the National Cancer Institute, monitors cancer incidence, mortality, and survival in approximately 10% of the U.S. population. SEER data are not representative of this population, but do encompass diverse geographic, ethnic, and racial groups. The quality of cancer frequency data available outside the United States is variable. Several European countries have established nationwide cancer incidence registries of high quality; registration of cancer incidence and mortality is more limited in developing nations. The available data are summarized and updated periodically in *Cancer Incidence in Five Continents* (31).

The quality and completeness of data may vary among cancer registries, which can employ different methods of case ascertainment. Diagnostic practice and classification of cancers differ among geographic areas and change over time. Ascertainment is usually less complete among elderly patients and those with limited access to medical care. Treatable cancers (such as skin cancers) may not be identified by the surveillance mechanisms of cancer registries, whereas cancer deaths are more likely to be recorded. Comparability of data must be considered in analyses of incidence and mortality figures from different cancer registries (80).

Cancer Incidence and Mortality

Table 25.1 shows the estimates of the annual numbers of new cancers and cancer deaths in 1995 in the United States. Cancers of the breast, lung, colon, and rectum account for nearly 40% of the more than one million incident cases. Cancers of the prostate, oral cavity, pancreas, endometrium, and bladder are also commonly diagnosed. Data for over 500,000 cancer deaths show the same general patterns. Lung cancer is, by far, the leading cause of cancer death, accounting for approximately 30% of the total. Mortality also approximates incidence for multiple myeloma, brain tumors, and cancers of the esophagus and pancreas. By comparison, survival is better for colorectal and breast cancers, with reported mortality equaling 25 to 40% of incidence.

Table 25.2 shows age-adjusted U.S. mortality and incidence rates, by sex, 1987–1991. The mortality rate in males for all sites combined is more than 50% higher than that in fe-

Table 25.1. Estimated Numbers of New Cancer Cases and Cancer Deaths in the United States, 1995

Tumor type	New cases (thousands)	Deaths (thousands)
Oral cavity	28.2	8.4
Esophagus	12.1	10.9
Stomach	22.8	14.7
Colon and rectum	138.2	55.3
Liver and biliary	18.5	14.2
Pancreas	24.0	27.0
Larynx	11.6	4.1
Lung	169.9	157.4
Breast	183.4	46.2
Cervix	15.8	4.8
Endometrium	32.8	5.9
Ovary	26.6	14.5
Prostate	244.0	40.4
Melanoma	34.1	7.2
Bladder	50.5	11.2
Kidney	28.8	11.7
Thyroid	13.9	1.1
Leukemias	25.7	20.4
Hodgkin's disease	7.8	1.5
Non-Hodgkin's lymphoma	50.9	22.7
Multiple myeloma	12.5	10.3
Brain	17.2	13.3
Other sites	82.7	43.8
All cancers	1252.0	547.0

Excluded are all in situ cancers and carcinomas of the skin (189).

Table 25.2. Age-Adjusted Incidence and Mortality Rates per 100,000 Population, United States. All Races, by Sex, 1987–1991

Tumor type	Incidence rate		Mortality rate	
	Males	Females	Males	Females
Oral cavity	16.4	6.2	4.6	1.7
Esophagus	6.4	1.9	6.0	1.5
Stomach	11.6	5.0	7.0	3.1
Colon and rectum	58.9	40.4	23.6	16.0
Liver	4.2	1.4	3.5	1.5
Pancreas	10.4	7.9	10.0	7.2
Larynx	7.9	1.7	2.5	0.5
Lung	82.1	40.4	74.9	30.5
Breast	0.9	109.5	0.2	27.2
Cervix	—	8.6	—	3.0
Uterus	—	21.2	—	3.5
Ovary	—	14.8	—	7.8
Prostate	123.0	—	25.6	—
Testis	4.5	—	0.3	—
Melanoma	13.1	9.7	3.1	1.5
Bladder	29.9	7.4	5.7	1.7
Kidney	12.1	5.9	5.0	2.3
Thyroid	2.5	6.4	0.3	0.4
Leukemias	13.1	7.7	8.3	4.9
Multiple myeloma	5.5	3.6	3.7	2.4
Brain	7.0	5.0	5.0	3.4
Hodgkin's disease	3.3	2.5	0.7	0.4
Non-Hodgkin's lymphoma	17.9	11.5	7.6	5.0
Other sites	35.0	23.8	22.8	15.6
All cancers	465.7	342.5	220.2	141.1

Rates are age-adjusted to the 1970 U.S. standard population.
SEER program (147).

males. At present, lung cancer is the leading cause of cancer deaths both in men and women in the United States. The lung cancer mortality rate in women recently surpassed that for breast cancer, but is much lower than the lung cancer rate in men. Mortality rates are also at least twice as high in men for cancers of the oral cavity, esophagus, stomach, liver, larynx, bladder, and kidney. Cancers of the male reproductive organs (prostate and testis) account for approximately 11% of all cancer deaths in men, whereas cancer of the breast and female reproductive organs account for nearly 30% of cancer deaths in women. Cancer incidence data reiterate these patterns, and will be described in subsequent discussions only when noteworthy divergences from mortality data are found.

Cancer Patterns by Age

Cancer is rare in childhood, rises in frequency throughout adulthood, and occurs most often in the elderly. The high frequency of cancer in the elderly is consistent with the multistage nature of carcinogenesis; cancer usually requires decades to develop following exposures to etiologic agents (51). Approximately 20% of the U.S. population is 55 years of age or older, but more than 80% of invasive cancers occur in this age group. At these ages, the leading causes of cancer mortality include cancer of the lung, colon, and pancreas (Fig. 25.1). Prostate cancer in men and cancers of the breast and ovary in women are also common in elderly patients.

Patterns of cancer differ between the elderly and persons aged 15 to 54. In young adults, the leading cause of cancer mortality is breast cancer in women and lung cancer in men. Brain tumors, leukemias, lymphomas, and melanoma also account for a substantial proportion of deaths in young adults. Mortality from cancers of the colon and ovary start to rise after the age of 37.

Childhood cancers make up less than 1% of all incident cancers. However, cancer accounts for more than 10% of mortality from all causes in children under 15 years of age (210). Cancer mortality rates in children have decreased almost 50% in the last few decades as a result of the improved treatment of many childhood cancers (206). Leukemia accounts for approximately one third of all cancer mortality in children 0 to 14 and remains one of the most common causes of cancer death in young adults. From childhood onward, more males develop cancer than do females, a trend that continues into adulthood.

Time Trends

Heart disease mortality, the leading cause of death in the United States, has declined in frequency in recent years. More people live to die of cancer, which now accounts for more than 20% of deaths from all causes. Overall, age-adjusted cancer mortality rates have risen approximately 10% since 1950. Lung cancer mortality is a major contributor to this increase (2).

Rates of certain cancers in the United States have changed substantially in recent decades, suggesting effects of the introduction of or disappearance of environmental oncogenic factors (Fig. 25.2*A*). Lung cancer mortality has risen sharply over the past several decades due to the increase in tobacco use by men dating to World War I and by women during World War II (51). The sex-specific mortality curves depicted in Figures 25.2*B* and 25.2*C* show sharper rises in lung cancer mortality after 1940 in men and after 1960 in women. The lag time between the start of habitual tobacco use and lung cancer development typifies the long latency of most carcinogens. In recent years, tobacco consumption has declined, and lung cancer rates in men have plateaued, although rates in women continue to rise unabated. Reported mortality rates for cancers of the stomach have decreased dramatically since 1950. Among women, mortality rates for uterine cancers, particularly cancers of the uterine cervix, have declined steadily, primarily due to the decreased incidence of invasive lesions. Breast cancer mortality has not changed in any apparent way since 1950, despite an increase in reported incidence. Colorectal cancer mortality has fallen slightly in recent decades, whereas prostate cancer mortality rates have increased slightly. These trends reflect changes in disease incidence, diagnostic practices, screening, and treatment effects (199). While incidence rates for most cancers have been increasing, mortality rates have been generally level.

Racial, Ethnic, and International Variation

In the United States, overall cancer incidence is reportedly 6% higher in blacks than in whites, while cancer mortality for blacks is approximately 30% higher. Socioeconomic status and access to health care appear to account for part of this differential (3, 12, 35, 132). Compared with whites in the United States, blacks currently have higher mortality rates for multiple myeloma and cancers of the esophagus, cervix, prostate, larynx, stomach, oropharynx, liver, corpus uteri, pancreas, and lung (Fig. 25.3). Blacks tend to smoke more than other groups in the United States, which likely accounts for their higher rates of cancers of the lung and several other sites (67).

Other ethnic groups in the United States also differ from United States whites with regard to certain site-specific cancer rates (31). Relative to whites, age-adjusted incidence and mortality rates among Mexican-Americans (Hispanics) are higher for gallbladder, stomach, and cervical cancers. In addition, increased rates have been reported for gallbladder, stomach, and cervical cancers among Native Americans; stomach cancer among Japanese Americans; nasopharyngeal and liver cancers in Chinese Americans; lung, stomach, and cervical cancers among Hawaiians; and liver cancer among Filipino-Americans.

Cancer incidence rates differ throughout the world, and migrant studies have helped elucidate environmental factors in cancer development. Migrants to the United States tend to acquire the patterns of cancer rates of United States whites. For example, the low incidence rates of breast and colon cancers in Japan have increased in those who migrate to the United States, while the high stomach cancer rates have fallen (73).

Worldwide, developed countries generally have higher reported incidence rates for cancers of the breast (North America, Europe), lung (British Isles), and prostate (United

Reported Deaths for the Five Leading Cancer Sites for Males by Age, United States, 1991

All Ages	Under 15	15-34	35-54	55-74	75+
All Cancer 272,380	All Cancer 982	All Cancer 3,699	All Cancer 27,529	All Cancer 142,089	All Cancer 98,067
Lung 91,690	Leukemia 350	Leukemia 661	Lung 8,741	Lung 55,890	Lung 26,896
Prostate 33,564	Brain & CNS 252	Non-Hodgkin's Lymphomas 501	Colon & Rectum 2,393	Colon & Rectum 13,888	Prostate 20,909
Colon & Rectum 28,178	Endocrine 111	Brain & CNS 414	Non-Hodgkin's Lymphomas 1,726	Prostate 12,306	Colon & Rectum 11,686
Pancreas 12,375	Non-Hodgkin's Lymphomas 64	Skin 298	Brain & CNS 1,577	Pancreas 6,730	Pancreas 4,299
Leukemia 10,194	Connective Tissue 46	Hodgkin's Disease 233	Pancreas 1,298	Esophagus 4,600	Bladder 3,698

Source: Vital Statistics of the United States.[6]

Reported Deaths for the Five Leading Cancer Sites for Females by Age, United States, 1991

All Ages	Under 15	15-34	35-54	55-74	75+
All Cancer 242,277	All Cancer 727	All Cancer 3,434	All Cancer 29,302	All Cancer 111,419	All Cancer 97,388
Lung 52,068	Leukemia 260	Breast 660	Breast 9,188	Lung 30,154	Lung 16,400
Breast 43,583	Brain & CNS 220	Leukemia 432	Lung 5,372	Breast 19,900	Colon & Rectum 15,727
Colon & Rectum 29,017	Endocrine 69	Uterus 343	Colon & Rectum 1,999	Colon & Rectum 11,117	Breast 13,834
Ovary 13,247	Connective Tissue 33	Brain & CNS 328	Uterus 1,978	Ovary 6,720	Pancreas 6,637
Pancreas 13,161	Bone 28	Non-Hodgkin's Lymphomas 209	Ovary 1,779	Pancreas 5,669	Ovary 4,601

Source: Vital Statistics of the United States.

Figure 25.1. Cancer deaths for the five leading cancer sites, by sex and age, United States 1991. *Source:* American Cancer Society (1). Reproduced with permission.

States blacks, Scandinavia). Elevated rates have been reported for cancer of the stomach in Japan and China, nasopharyngeal cancer in southern China, colon cancer in Denmark and New Zealand, cervical cancer in Brazil, liver cancer in parts of China and sub-Saharan Africa, and melanoma in Australia. Investigations of the exceptionally high rates of esophageal cancers in parts of China and the Caspian littoral have shown associations with vitamin and other dietary deficiencies (100). Data for developing countries are more difficult to evaluate because of underreporting. In these countries, cancers of the cervix uteri, liver, stomach, and esophagus often occur more frequently (31).

ANALYTIC STUDIES

Case-Control Studies

Descriptive epidemiologic findings and observations at the bedside can be further assessed in analytic studies of suspected risk factors. A case-control method is usually em-

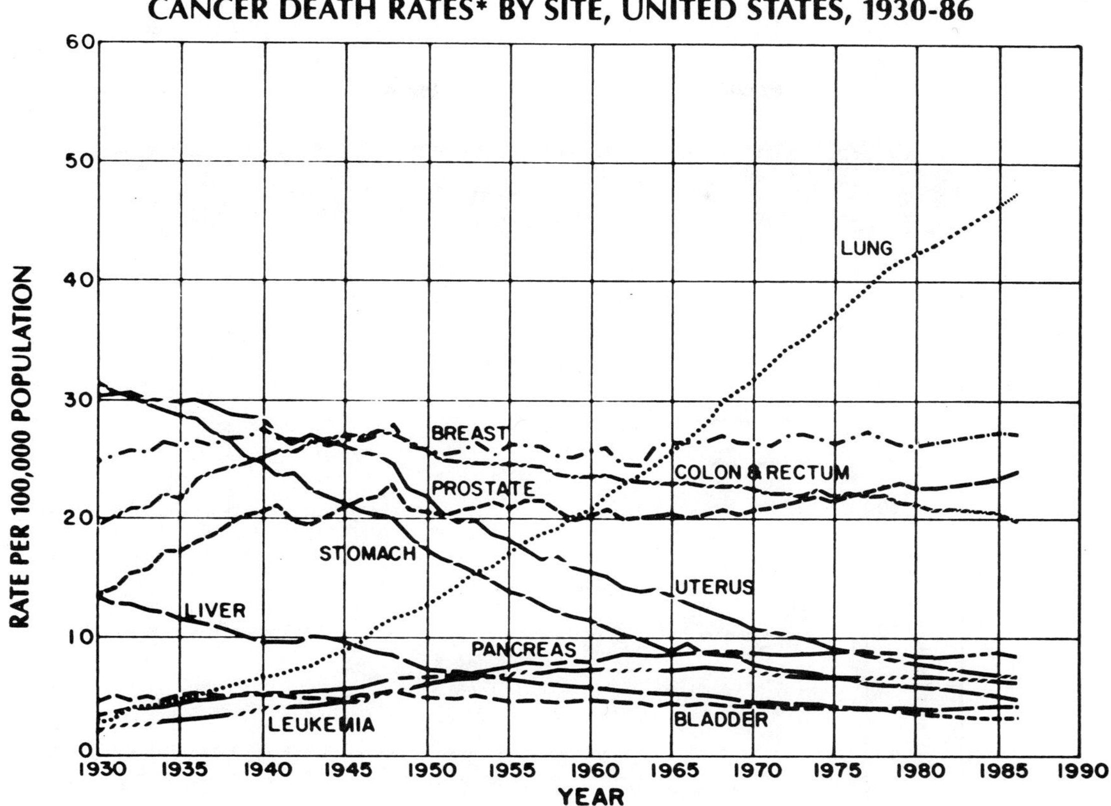

Figure 25.2A. Trends in age-adjusted cancer mortality rates per 100,000 population, by site, both sexes, United States 1930–1986. *Source:* American Cancer Society (1). Reproduced with permission.

ployed, which both can test specific etiologic hypotheses and generate new hypotheses for further examination (168). These studies compare a group of cancer patients (cases) with a group of individuals who are free of cancer (controls). Cases can be chosen, for example, from among cancer patients diagnosed during a defined period in a geographic area or hospital. Controls can be drawn from the same region or hospital as the cases, or from other appropriate sources. The case-control method has been useful, for instance, in clarifying aspects of the relation between vaginal adenocarcinoma and in utero exposure to diethylstilbestrol (82, 83).

At the outset of a case-control study, the investigators may know of certain characteristics, such as sex, race, and age that are strongly related to the distribution of the cancer. To account for these influences, a decision is often made to match controls individually to cases on these variables, or to obtain the same frequency or proportion of subgroups in both series (frequency matching). Additionally, a control series that is larger than the case series has statistic advantages in certain situations.

Information for cases and controls on oncogenic exposures and risk factors can be obtained by various means. Clinical data are usually obtained from medical records and pathology reports. In-person or telephone interviews of cases and controls are conducted in a similar manner. The data may be supplemented by employment records and other relevant documents. For deceased patients, interviews of next of kin may be conducted. Mailed questionnaires are used less often than direct interviews because the quality of information and the response rate tend to be inferior.

Case-control studies are well suited to and practical for the evaluation of uncommon diseases, such as cancer. The sizes of the case and control series are defined at the outset, and results from a case-control study are achieved relatively quickly. Ideally, the case series should be a representative sample of all cases in a population or demographic subgroup. A control series must also be carefully chosen. In a population-based case-control study, an unbiased sample of cases from a roster of all patients diagnosed in a geographic area is compared with a series of controls randomly selected from the general nondiseased population in the same area. If this is not practical, as with a hospital-based case series, the use of more than one type of control group is helpful in searching for consistent findings across all comparisons.

The case-control design is vulnerable to bias. Information on past events obtained in records or by personal recall may

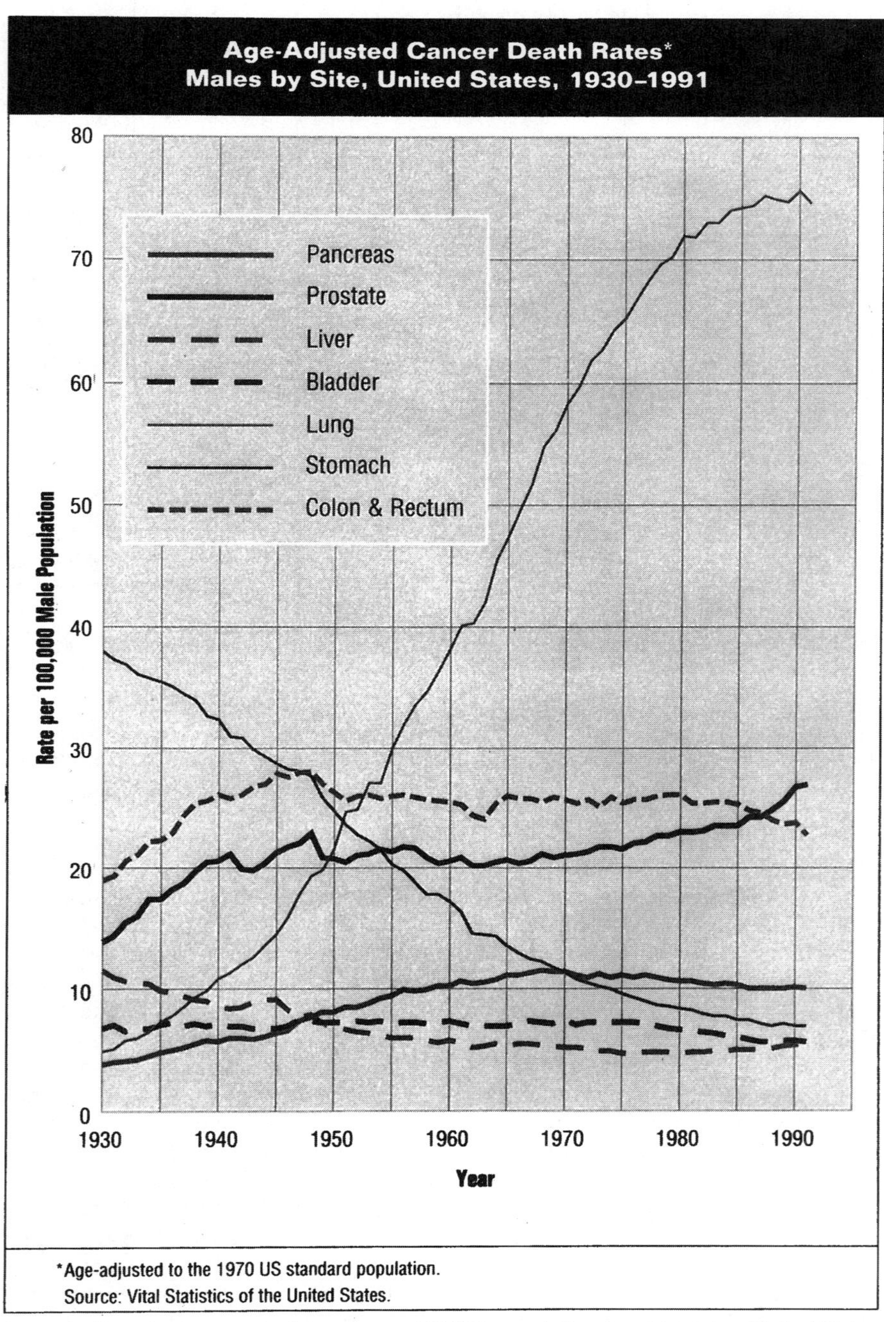

Figure 25.2B. Trends in age-adjusted cancer mortality rates per 100,000 population, by site, males, United States 1930–1991. *Source:* American Cancer Society (1). Reproduced with permission.

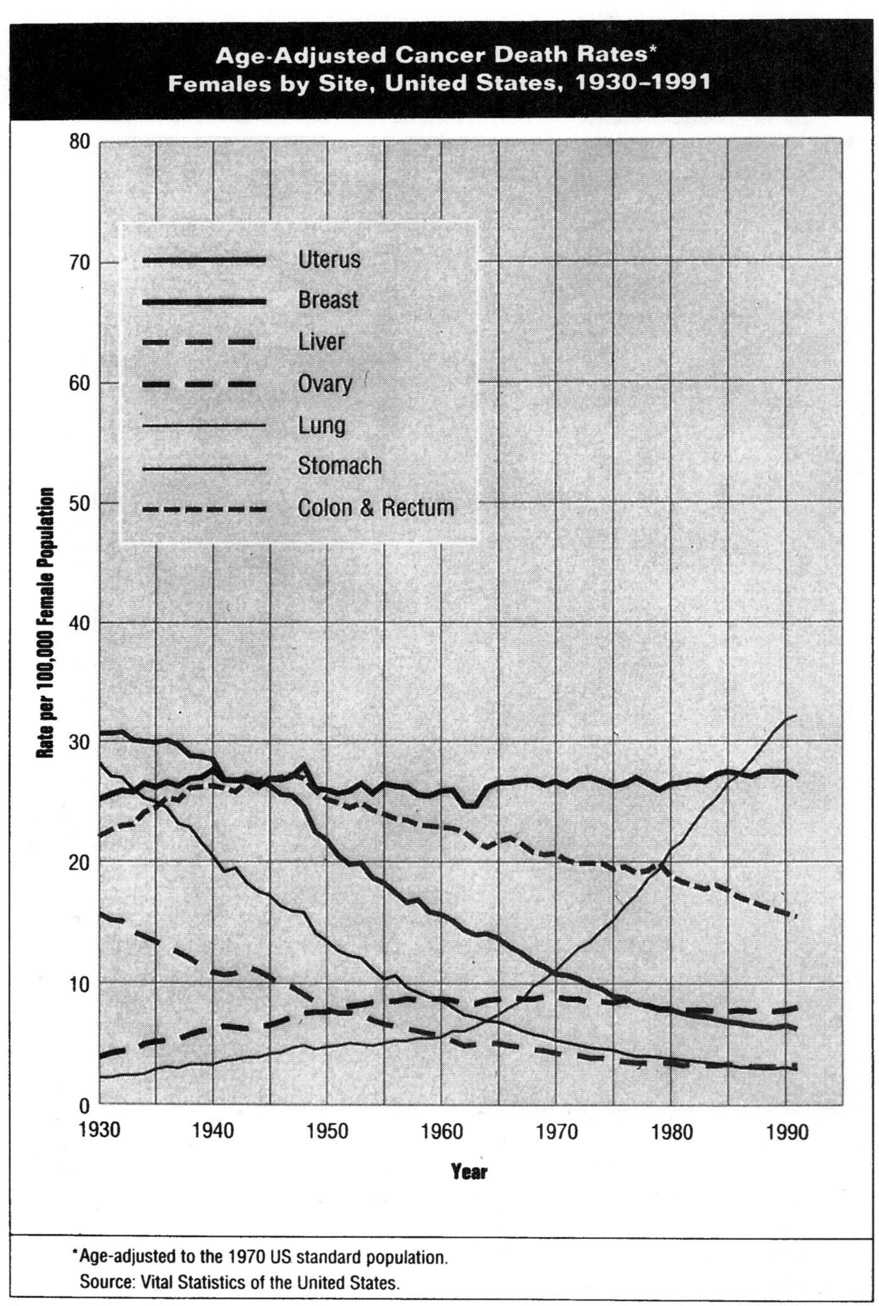

Figure 25.2C. Trends in age-adjusted cancer mortality rates per 100,000 population, by site, females, United States 1930–1991. *Source:* American Cancer Society (1). Reproduced with permission.

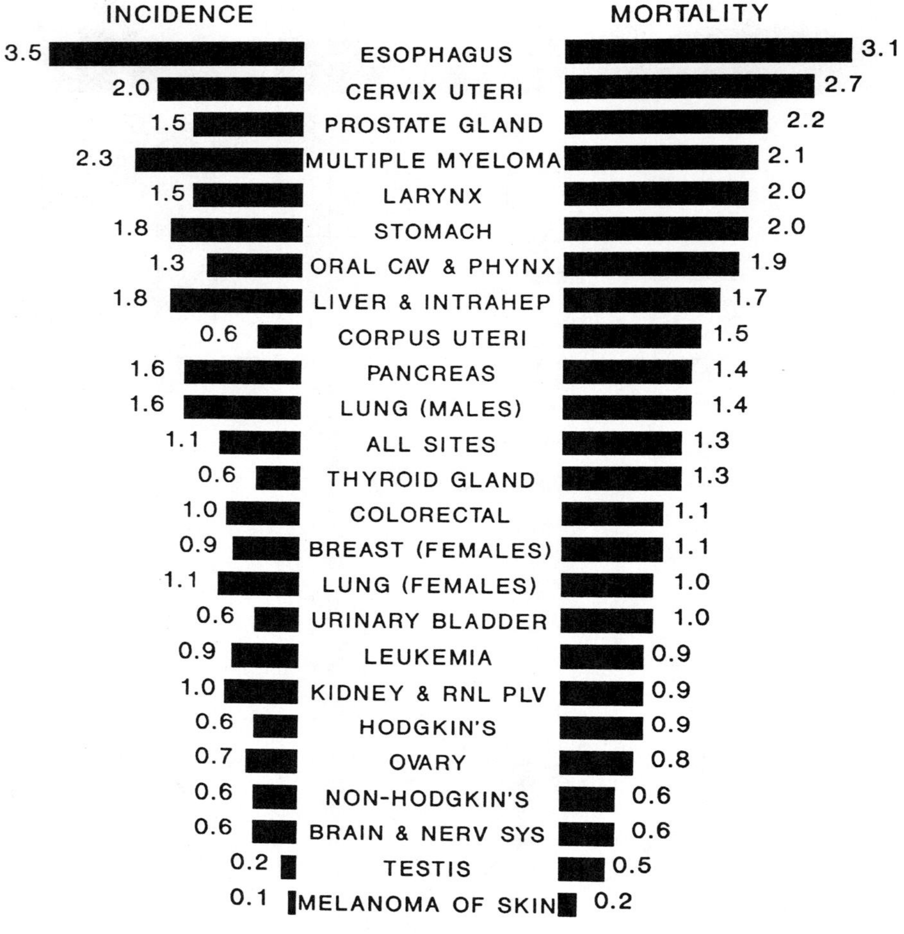

Figure 25.3. Ratios of cancer incidence and mortality rates for blacks and whites, by site, all ages, United States 1983–1987. *Source:* Doll and Peto (51).

be flawed or incomplete. Moreover, cases and controls may interpret and respond differently to questions. The choice of a control group can be the most vexing aspect of this type of study. The population-based case-control study theoretically avoids such selection bias, but it is not used in the majority of situations because of logistic problems and the expense. Hospital- or practice-based studies are more common, but also more hazardous when controls are selected from the same patient population. Selection bias for admission may not be similar for different diagnoses, or the controls may suffer from a condition that is also related to the exposure under study. Health plan enrollees, relatives, friends, and neighbors of the patients have also been used as controls. Recently, random-digit dialing has begun to be used to select controls by telephone. Once a study is underway, an additional bias in an interview study is a suboptimal response rate, particularly among controls as compared with cases.

Cohort Studies

In contrast to the case-control method, a study can be conducted in which a group (cohort) of cancer-free individuals is observed for disease development over time. After adequate numbers of years or cancers have been accrued, tumor occurrence is examined in relation to level of exposure to the risk factor under investigation (137). Thus, cohort studies compare the rates of cancer in exposed and nonexposed individuals. In a prospective cohort study, exposed and nonexposed persons will be followed over a period of years for the development of cancer. A retrospective cohort study analyzes exposure and cancer occurrence data for events that have already taken place. The cohort method has been useful, for example, in the follow-up of atomic bomb survivors for carcinogenic effects of radiation (39).

Cohort studies are useful in evaluating etiologic hypotheses and confirming leads from case-control studies. Prospective cohort studies accurately categorize exposure to the study factor at the start of follow-up, and the quality of this information is usually unaffected by subsequent disease status. Surrogates for exposure dose, such as DNA adducts in tissues of cancer patients, may facilitate the classification of exposure levels and the quantitation of risk estimates (149, 150). Cohort studies can also provide incidence rates associated with various levels of exposure to carcinogens. However, a large cohort study often involves thousands of subjects. A long period of time must elapse in order to yield a sufficient number of persons with cancer. For these reasons, cohort studies are expensive. The retrospective cohort design is less costly, and is more often used in cancer epidemiology. However, it poses some difficulties in categorizing exposure based on historic data. Both types suffer from losses to follow-up and to changes in the diagnostic criteria for the tumor under study.

A newer approach to examining causes of cancer is the intervention study. These are clinical trials in which the effect of an intervention, designed to reduce or eliminate exposure to a known or suspected carcinogen, is evaluated for its capacity to reduce or delay cancer development. A finding of no effect among the group receiving treatment might be due to insufficient study sample size (which should be addressed in the design phase of the study), poor compliance, losses to follow-up, or a period of observation that is too short to detect a beneficial effect. Random allocation of subjects in intervention trials reduces the likelihood of false-positive results. Harm from the intervention should not outweigh its potential benefits.

Intervention trials in the area of cancer prevention are limited by the long latent period between the initiation of an intervention (such as a vaccine or a change in diet or lifestyle) and a resultant reduction in cancer occurrence. The role of the hepatitis B virus (HBV) in the etiology of hepatocellular carcinoma is being assessed in clinical trials of a HBV vaccine in areas where liver cancer is endemic (21). The role of nutrients and micronutrients in cancer prevention and etiology is being explored, but there are few definitive data regarding beneficial effects. Biologic markers of intermediate end points are being sought that indicate retardation or reversal of the oncogenic process as a result of nutritional or other interventions. For example, recent biomarker studies have shown a possible reduction of oral leukoplakia, the premalignant lesions of oral cancer, by 13-*cis*-retinoic acid. Additional uses of such biomarkers in epidemiologic studies and intervention studies are being developed (118).

Analysis of Results

In assessing the degree of the association between a risk factor and a disease, a standard concept for comparison is the relative risk. Relative risk is defined as the ratio of the disease rate (usually incidence rate) among those exposed to the disease rate among those not exposed. Thus, the relative risk can only be obtained from a cohort study. However, it can be estimated from a case-control study through a figure called the odds ratio (ratio of the odds of the factor among cases to the odds of the factor among controls). The odds ratio is easily calculated from a fourfold table, as shown in Table 25.3. The odds ratio would be $(a/b)/(c/d)$, or ad/bc. The odds ratio is considered an adequate approximation of the relative risk when the disease is relatively uncommon (as is the case with cancer).

Table 25.3. Odds Ratio Calculation Table

	Cases	Controls
Exposed	*a*	*b*
Not exposed	*c*	*d*

The validity of a study may be enhanced by controlling for confounding factors. These are extraneous independent factors that are associated with both the exposure factor of interest and the disease under study. Common confounding variables are sex, age, race, and socioeconomic status. These can be handled through stratification in the analysis (or alternatively, through matching during the study's design) (61). Analysis may also include multivariate techniques, in particular, multiple regression (27).

Since valid associations may suggest prevention strategies, it is important to evaluate causal plausibility versus spurious association. If an association is not statistically significant, it may be disregarded, or alternatively, pursued in a larger study group. However, in order to demonstrate causation, several additional criteria beyond statistic significance must be met. Evidence to support a causative role for the exposure includes the following: strength of association (i.e., larger relative risks, dose–response effects are more likely to indicate a causal relationship); consistency of the association across appropriate subgroups in the study, as well as across studies of various populations and methods; temporality (a reasonable induction period has elapsed from time of exposure to disease); and biologic plausibility.

Cancer epidemiology research has produced a number of conflicting reports of an association. In evaluating these reports, appropriate questions would include not only standard statistical considerations, but also the following: (*a*) Did the conflicting studies use different designs, for example, case control versus cohort? (*b*) Was the exposure rare, so that the number of cases was not sufficiently large to detect an association? (*c*) Were so many "fishing expedition" (a posteriori) comparisons made that a few showed a statistically significant association by chance alone? (*d*) If a case-control interview design was used, was the response rate suboptimal, particularly among controls? (*e*) If a cohort was used, was the follow-up rate sufficiently high?

Established and Suspected Environmental Carcinogens in Humans

In this era of powerful computer technologies, multiple possible associations can be explored in the analysis of an epidemiologic study. Statistically significant results can be found that, in fact, are noncausal associations.

The literature on cancer epidemiology is voluminous, and often is difficult for clinicians to evaluate (211). Some reports have failed to distinguish unproved etiologic hypotheses from established oncogenic effects of such agents as tobacco and ionizing radiation. The lay press has added to this confusion by touting preliminary reports of suspected environmental carcinogens as proven fact. Carcinogens that account for many thousands of deaths annually in the United States have, on occasion, received less attention than agents that are responsible for only rare cases of cancer, such as diethylstilbestrol (82). In the following discussion, an effort is made to distinguish commonly encountered carcinogens from exposures limited to small subgroups and suspected hazards (Table 25.4).

Table 25.4. Established Environmental Causes of Human Cancer[a]

Carcinogen	Cancer site
Industrial chemicals and fibers	
Arsenicals	Skin, lung
Asbestos	Lung, pleura, peritoneum, pericardium
Benzene	Acute myleocytic leukemia
Bis(chloromethyl) ether	Lung
Chromium	Lung
Isopropyl alcohol production	Nasal sinuses
Mustard gas	Lung, larynx, nasal sinuses
Nickel dust	Lung, nasal sinuses
Polycyclic hydrocarbons	Lung, scrotum, skin (squamous carcinoma)
Vinyl chloride	Liver (angiosarcoma)
Drugs	
Epipodophyllotoxins (Etoposide, teniposide)	Acute myelocytic leukemia
Alkylating agents (melphalan, cyclophosphamide, chlorambucil, nitrosoureas)	Acute myelocytic leukemia, (also bladder, osteosarcoma for cyclophosphamide)
Androgenic steroids	Liver
Diethylstilbestrol (prenatal exposure)	Vagina (adenocarcinoma)
Immunosuppressive drugs (azathioprine, cyclosporine)	Non-Hodgkin's lymphoma
Phenacetin	Renal pelvis, bladder
Synthetic estrogens	Endometrium
Radiation	
Ionizing radiation	Almost all organs
Sunlight (ultraviolet)	Skin, intraocular melanoma
Personal habits	
Alcoholic beverages	Liver, esophagus, mouth, pharynx, larynx
Tobacco	Lung, mouth, pharynx, larynx, esophagus, pancreas, bladder, kidney, renal pelvis
Viruses	
Chronic hepatitis B infection	Liver
HTLV-I	Adult T-cell leukemia
HIV	AIDS-associated lymphomas
Human papillomavirus (HPV)	Cervical neoplasia

[a] Only well-established carcinogens in humans are listed.

TOBACCO

Cigarette smoking is the most important cause of preventable morbidity and mortality in the United States (13, 59, 126). More than 350,000 excess deaths from cigarette smoking occur annually nationwide. The majority of these deaths are due to cardiac and pulmonary diseases, but one third (130,000 deaths) are attributable cancer. Cigarette smoking is the predominant cause of lung cancer and a major cause of cancers of the larynx, oral cavity, and bladder (185). Smoking has also been linked to development of cancers of the esophagus, pancreas, and kidney (178). The annual cost of smoking-related illness and lost productivity in the United States is many billions of dollars. Carcinomas of the lung, due largely to smoking, have been the leading cause of cancer death in the United States for more than 2 decades (178). One cancer death in three among American men is the result of lung cancer, which has also surpassed breast cancer as the leading cause of neoplastic disease mortality among women. Smoking is associated primarily with squamous and small cell carcinomas of the lung, but also increases the risk of adenocarcinoma. Elimination of tobacco use is the major method of cancer prevention available (71).

The oncogenic effect of cigarette smoking on humans is beyond doubt. Data show that increased tobacco consumption in the United States and elsewhere was followed several decades later by a rise in lung cancer rates. A series of reports of the United States Surgeon General have summarized the data from diverse epidemiologic studies (178). At least nine large prospective cohort studies of up to a million subjects each and 50 case-control studies worldwide have consistently shown that cigarette smoking increases the risk of lung cancer. The cancer risk is correlated with the amount of smoke exposure as measured by years of tobacco use, number of cigarettes consumed daily, their tar and nicotine content, and depth of inhalation of the smoke. The risk declines with smoking cessation, but the lapse of a decade is required for the lung cancer risk in former smokers to approximate the low risk of nonsmokers. These findings indicate that early cessation is important among current smokers, and that adolescents need to be strongly discouraged from starting the habit (194, 195) (see Chapter 27). Recent studies using biomarkers of carcinogens in tobacco smoke further support epidemiologic data that incriminate tobacco products as a major cause of human cancer. These biomarkers of carcinogen exposure are found not only in active smokers but also in adults and children in physical proximity to active smokers (41, 77, 177).

Cigarette smoking and alternative methods of tobacco use also increase the risk of cancer (28, 57, 177). Pipe and cigar smokers develop relatively fewer lung cancers but are at particularly high risk of oral cancers, including lip cancer in pipe users, and buccal cancers in snuff dippers. Recent evidence suggests oncogenic effects in nonsmokers who inhale the smoke of nearby cigarette smokers. Although the risk to individual "passive smokers" appears relatively small, the aggregate oncogenic effect on the population appears to be substantial (19, 41, 198). Pregnant women who smoke can harm the developing fetus, and young parents who smoke increase the frequency of respiratory diseases in their young children. The increased risk of oral cancer among users of snuff and chewing tobacco is of concern in view of their growing popularity among youth (130, 208).

Clinicians are familiar with the difficulties of convincing patients to cease smoking, but they need to persevere (185). Nevertheless, per capita cigarette sales for adults in the United States have declined steadily in recent years (196). Historically, the decline in tobacco use appeared first in physicians and dentists, who knew of its hazards (56). Lung cancer death rates among physicians in the United States and England have declined steadily as a consequence of smoking cessation. Other health-conscious segments of society have also reduced tobacco consumption. The poor and the undereducated in the United States and the peoples of the third world may gradually become the remnant population who smoke frequently. Many smokers have quit on the advice of their physicians, who are well situated to influence the lifestyles of their patients (4, 185). Additional strategies to reduce tobacco consumption include smoking restriction in workplaces and public areas, enforcement of the prohibition of tobacco sales to minors, elimination of tobacco subsidies, and tobacco taxes that can be used for public education programs. In addition, limitations on advertising of tobacco products as well as increases in tobacco prices through taxation, have contributed to a reduction in smoking (44, 126). With time, the reduction in smoking in the population will inevitably result in a decline in tobacco-induced cancers (108, 194) (see Chapter 27).

ALCOHOL

Tobacco and alcohol consumption combine to multiply the risk of cancers of the upper aerodigestive tract, including the mouth, tongue, esophagus, pharynx, and larynx (52, 131). Epidemiologic studies in humans strongly implicate alcohol as a causal factor in these neoplasms, though ethanol rarely induces cancers in laboratory animals. Cancer might be due to other ingredients in alcoholic beverages or to oral mucosal injury by alcohol, which magnifies the oncogenic effects of tobacco products (139). Heavy drinkers also tend to have poor oral hygiene and poor diet, which may contribute to cancer development (128). Cancers of the esophagus and liver often occur among chronic alcoholics in the United States (25). In addition, recent data have raised the possibility that moderate alcohol ingestion elevates the risk of breast cancer, although other studies have failed to find an association (133, 164, 166, 204). Excessive alcohol consumption often starts in adolescence under the same social and psychologic influences that promote cigarette smoking. Prevention of addiction to drugs and alcohol is beginning to receive more attention from educational, social, and legal agencies (54, 112).

RADIATION

The oncogenic effects of ionizing radiation have been identified in studies of nuclear bomb survivors, occupationally irradiated workers, and patients treated for cancer and other diseases (39). Data have been gathered on types of radiation-induced tumors, time from exposure to tumor development (latency), radiation dose effects, and the influence of sex and age at exposure (63). Assessment of risk for humans is often hindered by incomplete radiation dose data, the paucity of large study populations, and the diversity of conditions of exposure. Nevertheless, the aggregate data show that, under certain conditions, ionizing radiation induces many types of leukemia, as well as cancers of the thyroid, breast, respiratory system, digestive system, skin, bone, soft tissues, and other sites (22). An apparent exception is chronic lymphocytic leukemia, which has not developed excessively among large study populations, such as atomic bomb survivors and patients irradiated for ankylosing spondylitis.

Data on radiation carcinogenesis have been gleaned primarily from studies of persons exposed to doses of tens to hundreds of centigray (cGy; rem). The radiation was delivered as either whole-body exposure or partial-body radiotherapy for diverse diseases (23, 155). Among atom bomb survivors, excess leukemias developed within 3 years of exposure, with a peak rate at 5 to 8 years after irradiation (155). Acute lymphocytic leukemia has been observed primarily in those who were children at the time of the bombing. Myelogenous leukemias developed in both exposed children and adults. Chronic myelogenous leukemia tended to develop sooner following radiation exposure than did acute myelogenous leukemia, which continues to occur excessively 4 decades after the bombing. The time to diagnosis of solid tumors has been longer than a decade from radiation exposure. Brain tumors, carcinomas, and sarcomas have occurred excessively among atom bomb survivors and patients irradiated for tinea capitis, thymic enlargement in infancy, metropathia hemorrhagica, postpartum mastitis, and follow-up of pneumothorax therapy for pulmonary tuberculosis (22). In patients who received partial-body radiation, the excess cancers have developed in tissues within or adjacent to the radiation portal.

Malignant tumors have been induced by radiotherapy in doses of thousands of centigray for childhood cancers, Hodgkin's disease, and carcinoma of diverse sites. Second neoplasms after childhood cancer include a high proportion of sarcomas, but also leukemias, lymphomas, and carcinomas of the skin, breast, and lung (18, 23). It has been difficult to separate the role of radiotherapy in these patients from the effects of host susceptibility. Among patients irradiated for carcinoma of the cervix, a small excess of leukemia and solid tumors has been observed in several large studies (23). The failure to detect a continuing rise in cancer risk with higher doses of radiotherapy might be due to dominance of the cell-killing effects over the transforming effects of the exposure.

The oncogenic effects in humans of low-dose radiation (less than 20 cGy) cannot be quantified with precision (78). Estimates of risk have been based on extrapolation from effects detected at higher doses. Recently the BEIR (Biological Effects of Ionizing Radiation) Committee of the National Research Council issued its fifth report, "Health Effects of Exposure to Low Levels of Ionizing Radiation (BEIR-V)" (39, 78). After reviewing relevant epidemiologic and laboratory data on radiation carcinogenesis, the report concluded that children are more susceptible than are adults to the oncogenic effects of ionizing radiation. For doses up to several hundred centigray, excess cancer mortality (excluding leukemia) increases in a direct linear relationship to dose (doubling the dose doubles the cancer risk). The slope of the line suggests no more than 1,000 excess cancer deaths over the lifetime of 100,000 persons exposed to 10 rem, a dose approximating the lifetime dose from background irradiation. The figure is a small fraction of the 23,000 cancer deaths from all causes expected in a United States population of 100,000. Nevertheless, the excess radiation-induced cancer mortality is higher than prior BEIR estimates by severalfold (63). The upward revision is due in part to accumulation of data favoring the relative-risk model for radiation effects. According to this model, a given dose of radiation increases cancer frequency by a fraction of the underlying cancer risk, which rises sharply with age. This model is consistent with the finding, for example, that breast irradiation is much more hazardous to females who have a higher underlying risk of the cancer. Radiogenic breast cancers also arise more frequently in older women, who have higher underlying breast cancer rates as compared with younger women. However, considerable uncertainty exists in present dose–risk estimates for humans, particularly with regard to lifetime effects (90). Additionally, the issue of threshold dose for tumor induction is unresolved, and is not readily measured in human populations (158). For purposes of protecting radiation workers and the public, it is assumed that oncogenic effects of ionizing radiation do not have a threshold. A minute radiation dose is presumed to have a small oncogenic potential.

Studies of the oncogenic effects of radionuclides have focused primarily on occupationally exposed workers, such as underground miners and radium dial painters, and on patients injected with thorium dioxide (Thorotrast) (43). However, concern has been raised recently about the development of lung cancer, and perhaps acute myelogenous leukemias, after inhalation of radon gases in dwellings (20, 81). Some studies have raised the possibility of thousands of lung cancers annually in the United States as a consequence of radon exposure, but additional studies are needed (20). The availability of biomarkers of radiation damage, as measured in somatic mutations within oncogenes and tumor suppressor genes, has strengthened the evidence for ionizing radiation carcinogenesis (183, 184). If validated, these biomarkers of radiation exposure might be particularly useful in assessing the carcinogenic effects of low-dose exposure.

In the past decade, concerns have been raised by the finding of increased cancers among individuals exposed to electric or magnetic fields (162, 187). Public attention has been further aroused by the lay press (94). Definitive data are not available, in part because of difficulties in assessing exposure, the paucity of supporting laboratory data, and discordant results from epidemiologic studies (92, 94, 162, 187).

SUNLIGHT

Excessive exposure to sunlight increases the risk of several forms of skin cancer in exposed surfaces. These include basal and squamous cell carcinomas and, to a lesser extent, melanoma (99, 170). The risk of cancer is higher among Caucasian populations residing in tropical areas as compared with those in more temperate climates. A particularly high risk of sun-induced skin cancer has been found among fair-skinned individuals of Celtic origin and in groups with ultraviolet light sensitivity, such as patients with xeroderma pigmentosum and dysplastic nevus syndrome (11, 161). The increase in popularity of sunbathing and outdoor activities among adolescents and young adults has heightened exposure to ultraviolet radiation. Molecular genetic evidence of sunburn-induced damage to cancer-associated genes further supports epidemiologic data on skin cancer development among light-skinned populations (212). Education regarding the protective effects of clothing and topical sunscreens can be an effective method of reducing sunlight exposure, particularly among sensitive individuals.

ASBESTOS FIBERS

Asbestos is an important cause of cancers of the respiratory tract, notably lung cancer and mesothelioma of both pleura and peritoneum (40). The oncogenic hazards of asbestos exposure were recognized after lung cancers were found in patients with asbestosis. In 1960, Wagner and coworkers reported 33 cases of mesothelioma in workers and residents near an asbestos mine in South Africa (193). Subsequent studies have reported mesothelioma in other asbestos workers and exposed populations.

Asbestos is a useful thermal insulator that has been mined in large quantities over the past century. The material is a family of fibrous silicates that are widely distributed geographically (40). Oncogenic asbestos fibers are the rodlike amphiboles (crocidolite, amosite, anthophyllite, tremolite, and actinolyte). The oncogenic effect of asbestos appears to be a consequence of its physical properties rather than of its chemical structure. Linear fibers of narrow diameter are more likely to induce tumors in laboratory animals. The widespread presence of asbestos in urban industrialized environments is illustrated by its use in fire-retardant ceiling materials in nearly 10% of United States schools (180). No cancers have yet been linked to attendance in these schools, but pleural and peritoneal mesotheliomas have been reported to develop after a single exposure to asbestos. In contrast, lung cancer develops chiefly among heavily exposed workers, such as pipe fitters and shipyard employees. Lung cancer risk in asbestos workers is multiplied severalfold by cigarette smoking, and the combination of these exposures is particularly hazardous (139).

Asbestos is estimated to be a causal factor in thousands of cancers, primarily lung cancers, each year in the United States. The number may increase in the future because the latency for asbestos-associated cancers is 3 to 4 decades. The incidence of asbestos-induced mesothelioma is difficult to assess (179). The neoplasm is not easy to diagnose, and death certificate data are unreliable. A reasonable estimate is that 2,000 new cases of mesothelioma occur annually in the United States (179). Projections of future incidence suggest that the number of mesothelioma cases will rise moderately early in the next century, and then decline when the benefits of environmental protection regulations of the 1970s and beyond are realized.

The deterioration of asbestos-containing products over time can cause the release of asbestos fibers into the environment (40). The demolition and repair of structures with friable asbestos also pose health hazards. The proper handling of these materials can be difficult and costly. Removal of the asbestos is a permanent solution. However, removal is expensive and requires the installation of effective barrier systems to avoid asbestos dissemination. Encapsulation of friable asbestos is another option, but the solution is not permanent because encapsulating materials can deteriorate. The cost of dealing with asbestos in schools alone is billions of dollars, and homes, factories, offices, and public buildings are also contaminated (139).

DIETARY FACTORS

Available experimental and epidemiologic data implicate diet as a factor in the etiology of cancers of the digestive tract and other sites (143). Diet alters the risk of tumors in certain laboratory animals. In addition, migrant studies and international comparisons of cancer rates have provided evidence that dietary factors can modify the risk of cancers of the esophagus, stomach, colon, rectum, breast, endometrium, and prostate (203). However, epidemiologic investigations of specific dietary constituents have often yielded inconsistent results.

Precise dietary causes of cancers in humans remain uncertain despite extensive investigations (146). The lengthy list of suspected oncogenic influences include the basic nutritional components of foods (fats, total calories, and low fiber content), food additives (dyes), flavoring agents (saccharin), contaminants (aflatoxin), preservatives (salt curing, pickling), and cooking methods (smoking, charcoal broiling) (143, 146, 203, 204). Animal and human studies of obesity and cancer are complicated by the difficulty of separating the effects of calories, fat, and body weight (165, 201). Moreover, some animal studies suggest that a marked restriction of total caloric intake is needed to reduce the incidence of cancer. Epidemiologic studies have noted a correlation between diets low in fiber, folate, or other constitutents and an increased risk for colon cancer, but results are not fully consistent (7, 65, 201, 202). Work in progress is examining the effects of different types of fiber on cancer occurrence. Other reports raise the possibility of protective factors in the diet, such as calcium, selenium, and vitamins A, C, D, E, and β-carotenes (143). A lower risk of carcinomas of the oral cavity, bladder, stomach, ovary, and lung have been reported with the ingestion of higher levels of vitamin A, carotenoids, or fruits and vegetables (134, 143, 174, 209). However, the possibility exists that the protection originates from other constitutents of fruits and vegetables or from other differences in lifestyle. Dietary intervention studies are difficult to perform because of the requirements for accurate reporting, a large patient series, problems with long-term compliance, and the lapse of years required to detect reductions in cancer occurrence (134). Intermediate biochemical markers of the effects of diet modification are being developed. In rare instances, a discernible reduction in cancer occurrence has been reported in small series of patients (143).

Controversy remains regarding the appropriate recommendations to the public regarding diet modification in cancer prevention (143, 146). Dietary studies of the Seventh-Day Adventists, who are often vegetarians and nonsmokers, show lower rates of cancers of the lung and digestive tract (151). For the general American population, some have advocated cancer control through major public education programs that encourage consumption of a balanced diet adequate in protein and other needed nutrients, with energy content sufficient to maintain a stable and normal body weight. These measures include reducing caloric and alcohol intake, decreasing fats to less than 30% of total calories, and increasing the consumption of fresh fruits and vegetables (203). While research continues, these recommendations seem prudent. Recent cohort studies reveal an increased risk of colon cancer among those who consume more meat and animal fat (206). Even if benefits in terms of prevention of breast, colon, prostate, and other cancers were small, these measures are likely to provide protection against cardiovascular diseases, the leading cause of death nationally (see Chapter 28).

VIRUSES AND OTHER INFECTIOUS AGENTS

Viruses have long been invoked as causes of human cancers (70). Both DNA and RNA viruses have been demonstrated to induce cancers in experimental animals. With the recent advances in molecular biology, the role of viruses in human cancer development is now under intensive study. Results to date show the presence of diverse viruses in cancer patients, but their contributions to the oncogenic process often remains uncertain (79). Some viruses appear to be etiologic agents; others might enhance the oncogenic process by stimulating cellular proliferation or suppressing immunity; and the remainder are found in association with cancer but have no apparent causal role. A better understanding of the molecular mechanisms of oncogenesis should help distinguish etiologic agents from secondary changes. Studies of the oncogenic RNA viruses have unexpectedly shown that transforming virogenes originate from cellular genes acquired during the intracellular phase of the viral life cycle. These cellular genes (proto-oncogenes) gain tumorigenic potential when incorporated into the viral genome. Additional studies have shown that proto-oncogenes have been strictly conserved through evolution, suggesting that they produce proteins vital to the function and survival of the organism. Some proto-oncogenes have now been shown to encode proteins that are growth factors or growth factor receptors. Qualitative or quantitative changes (activation) of these genes can confer certain behavioral characteristics of neoplasia. Oncogenes that are involved in the development of many human cancers are usually activated by mechanisms unrelated to viral infection.

Squamous cell carcinoma of the uterine cervix and its precursor lesions are associated with viral infections that may be acquired through sexual intercourse (167, 192). The incidence of the neoplasm is increased in prostitutes and in women who have had multiple sexual partners, had first coitus at an early age, and have a history of venereal diseases (79, 192). Cervical carcinoma has also been reported to occur excessively in women whose partners have carcinoma of the penis (173). Other studies show that these male partners tend to have a history of multiple sexual partners, suggesting that an infectious oncogenic agent is transmitted by males (173). Genital infections, particularly with papillomavirus types 16 and 18, are suspected as etiologic factors (150, 213) (see Chapter 21). Temporal trends show that the mortality rates for cervix cancer have declined substantially over the last several decades in the United States (48). The decline may be due to both screening for cervix cancer with the Papanicolaou smear and a lower disease incidence attributable to reduced exposure to risk factors. A worrisome exception is a recently reported increase in cervical cancer in young women (6).

Human T-cell leukemia/lymphoma virus I (HTLV-I) has been linked to the development of a rare aggressive form of leukemia in young adults (17). The disease has an unusual geographic distribution, with clusters in parts of Japan and the Caribbean. Human immunodeficiency disease virus (HIV; HTLV-III), the cause of AIDS, is associated with a markedly increased risk of Kaposi's sarcoma, non-Hodgkin's lymphoma, and perhaps other cancers in early adulthood (89) (see Chapter 139). Non-Hodgkin's lymphoma in AIDS patients might be, in part, the consequence of the profound immunosuppression that accompanies the infection. Recently, high levels of HIV p24 expression were found in the lymphoma cells of AIDS patients. The identification of a common clonal HIV integration site raises the possibility that the virus can participate directly in the genesis of certain lymphomas (172). In other studies, the detection of herpesvirus-like DNA sequences in patients with Kaposi's sarcoma suggests that the organism might be a causal factor in the neoplasm (138). Evidence of the infectious agent has been found not only in AIDS-associated Kaposi's sarcoma, but also in the classic and other forms of Kaposi's sarcoma (138).

Other viruses have been implicated in human oncogenesis. Epstein-Barr virus (EBV) is a suspected oncogenic virus that is associated with the development of non-Hodgkin's lymphoma, Burkitt's lymphoma, and nasopharyngeal carcinoma (72) (see Chapter 20). A recent study of EBV antibody titers in Hodgkin's disease patients revealed that elevations of certain titers often preceded the neoplasm by several years. The finding suggests that enhanced activation of EBV might be involved in the pathogenesis of Hodgkin's disease, or serve as a marker of altered immune control of the infection (125). Recently, EBV has been linked to the development of sarcomas in immunosuppressed children.

Cancer of the liver is a relatively rare disease in the United States and occurs largely among patients with alcoholic cirrhosis (24, 98). Worldwide, primary liver cancer is a leading cause of cancer death in developing nations, particularly in Africa and Asia. The major risk factor in these patients is chronic hepatitis B infection acquired initially in infancy (9) (see Chapter 23). Risk of primary liver cancer is increased up to 200-fold among carriers of hepatitis B virus. Hepatitis B vaccination decreases the risk of infection and holds the promise of reducing the incidence of liver cancer; trials are in progress in several endemic areas. In areas endemic for liver cancer, the contamination of food by aflatoxins and other mycotoxins might be an additional etiologic factor (8, 87). Evidence for an oncogenic role of hepatitis C virus is emerging (95, 168).

Recent studies have linked *Helicobacter pylori* infections with the development of gastric cancer and gastric duodenal ulcers (16, 148, 182). Early age of the infection may be an important factor for gastric cancer development (16). However, it remains uncertain whether *H. pylori* is the cause of gastric cancer. The use of nonsteroidal anti-inflammatory drugs (NSAIDs) has been known to heal *H. pylori*–associated gastric ulcers and to reduce the risk of their recurrence (182). Studies of NSAIDs for chemopreventive effects in gastric cancer will require many years to complete.

CANCER CLUSTERS

In recent decades, much public attention has focused on reports of localized temporal–geographic clusters of cancer, which may indicate the action of a point exposure to carcinogens (29). Many clusters have involved childhood cancers, notably leukemia, occurring within a short time in a small geographic area. Investigations of most suspected clusters have failed to identify an etiologic agent. Moreover, application of appropriate statistic methods to analyze such aggregates have shown that these "clusters" were probably explainable on the basis of chance (66). An exception is a study of Woburn, Massachusetts, showing that childhood leukemia rates were double the expected frequency between 1969 and 1979 (105, 106). Prospective observation of the community has revealed that childhood leukemias have continued to develop excessively. The explanation is unknown, and extensive efforts are in progress to identify the cause. Many other reports of cancer clusters have involved residents near chemical dumps such as in Love Canal, New York (93). In most instances, no excess cancers have been shown to be caused by ambient pollutants (46). However, the latent period for carcinogenesis is long, and cleanup of these toxic sites needs to proceed. In other studies, the clustering of childhood leukemia near nuclear power plants has led to a hypothesis regarding an infectious etiology (99). The development of molecular footprints in biomarkers of infectious exposures might be applicable to analyses of these and other cancer clusters (87).

Another pattern of clustering is based on linking cancer patients who have a history of personal contact with each other, despite dissimilar times and geographic locations at diagnosis of cancer (72). This model postulates person-to-person transmission of a hypothetic infectious agent, perhaps an oncogenic virus. Clustering of cancer by personal contact has been most often examined in connection with Hodgkin's disease in young adults, but the results are inconsistent (73).

CHEMICAL EXPOSURES IN THE WORKPLACE

Among hundreds of chemicals examined in some detail for oncogenic effects, approximately 20 have been determined to be oncogenic in humans (158). These compounds are shown, in Table 25.4 along with the cancers that occur as a result of exposure. Most chemical carcinogens induce carcinomas of the lung and upper airway; others cause acute leukemia and carcinomas of the bladder, liver, skin, and other organs. Additional chemicals have been found to induce cancer in laboratory animals, but the relevant data for humans are insufficient or inconsistent and additional research is needed. Oncogenic chemical exposures often occur in the workplace, and these are estimated to account for approximately 5% of all cancers in the United States (51). Lung cancer has developed excessively among workers exposed to chromium, arsenic, mustard gas, polycyclic hydrocarbons, and *bis*(chloromethyl)ether. Bladder cancer develops excessively after exposure to certain aromatic amines in tanners and in workers with dyes, rubber, and organic chemicals. Liver damage by vinyl chloride predisposes to angiosarcomas of the liver. Acute myelogenous leukemia occurs excessively in benzene workers. There is uncertainty as to whether atmospheric pollution resulting from the release of industrial chemicals causes a small portion of lung and other cancers (51). However, other ill effects of these pollutants are well documented, and control measures should be instituted.

Preliminary data suggest that dioxins might increase the risk of soft-tissue sarcomas among forestry workers, but additional data are needed. Dioxins are an ingredient in the defoliant Agent Orange, and its effects on exposed Vietnam-era veterans remains the subject of intense scientific and political debate. Studies of these veterans are reported to show no overall excess of cancers, but non-Hodgkin's lymphoma rates are elevated. It has been difficult to relate cancer occurrence in these veterans to their exposure to defoliants. Herbicides have been linked to non-Hodgkin's lymphoma in several groups of farmers in the United States, Canada, and elsewhere (84). The oncogenic herbicide has not been identified with certainty, although phenoxyacetic acids, particularly 2,4-D, are suspected to be causal agents (15, 84, 200). Recently, DDT, a common household and industrial pesticide, was linked to the development of breast cancer in women. Subsequent studies have yielded inconsistent results, and the carcinogenic effects of DDT on humans remain uncertain (89).

MEDICATIONS

Drugs are routinely tested for oncogenic activity in animals prior to their approval for clinical use in humans (169). The few medications strongly implicated as carcinogens in humans are listed in Table 25.4 (169). The risk of cancer associated with most of these drugs is small, and for some diseases, better treatment alternatives are not available. Alkylating agents, alone or in combination with other therapies, are the treatment of choice for certain cancers and immunologic diseases, even though a few patients may subsequently develop acute myelogenous leukemia (34, 68, 103, 156). All alkylating agents appear to have leukemogenic potential, including cyclophosphamide, melphalan, mechlorethamine, procarbazine, and nitrosoureas (34). Recent data have established the role of the epipodophyllotoxins, teniposide and etoposide, in the development of secondary acute myelogenous leukemia in patients treated for childhood acute lymphocytic leukemia and other cancers (156, 157, 176). Bladder cancers have also been reported after cyclophosphamide-associated cystitis (186). Bladder cancer after the administration of chlornaphazine, an alkylating agent that is no longer in use, may be the result of its biotransformation to the bladder carcinogen β-naphthylamine. Recently, secondary osteosarcoma was reported to occur in association with alkylating agent therapy among a series of survivors of childhood cancer, but confirmation is needed (189). Drugs and diagnostic agents used for nonneoplastic diseases, such as hormones, radionuclides, and immunosuppressants, have also been linked to the development of malignant tumors (36, 152, 169). Some of these drugs, such as inorganic arsenicals and thorium dioxide (Thorotrast), are no longer in use, but continue to produce cancers because their latency period extends for decades.

Organ transplant recipients are at high risk of non-Hodgkin's lymphoma, Kaposi's sarcoma, and skin cancer (82). The lymphomas may appear within several weeks after renal or cardiac transplantation, and differ from most environmental cancers, which arise many years after exposure to carcinogens. Molecular analyses reveal the lymphoproliferative diseases in transplant recipients to be monoclonal, oligoclonal, or polyclonal (38). The transplant-associated lymphomas have a predilection for the central nervous system. Immunosuppressive therapy with azathioprine and cyclosporin has been implicated as a risk factor in transplant recipients, although the transplanted organ may also have an oncogenic influence. Among leukemic patients who received bone marrow transplants, leukemia was found to recur occasionally in the transplanted donor cells.

Hormonal factors, both endogenous and exogenous, have been implicated in the development of cancers of the breast, ovary, endometrium, and other sites (88, 145, 171). The evidence appears strongest for the proliferative effects of conjugated estrogens on the endometrium, which produce a form of endometrial carcinoma with an excellent prognosis. Data are less consistent regarding the increased risk of breast cancer after prolonged use of oral contraceptives starting in early adulthood (36). In other studies, however, hormonal agents are being followed in chemoprevention trials (142). In particular, tamoxifen is useful not only in the treatment of hormone-responsive breast cancer, but also to reduce the risk of cancer in the opposite breast. Several trials are in progress to study whether tamoxifen can reduce cancer incidence in high-risk women. Pilot studies indicate that tamoxifen therapy might preserve bone density and lower the serum risk profile for cardiovascular disease, but at the cost of a slightly increased risk of endometrial carcinoma. The issue of breast cancer prevention using tamoxifen remains unanswered (119, 120).

HOST SUSCEPTIBILITY FACTORS

Inherited susceptibility to cancer often becomes manifest by the occurrence of the same neoplasm among multiple blood relatives. These neoplasms tend to occur at earlier ages than usual, bilaterally in paired organs, and in multiple primary foci within the predisposed organ. Familial aggregation has been reported for virtually every form of cancer in humans. In general, close relatives of a cancer patient appear to have a twofold to threefold increase in risk for that tumor. Among cancer families, however, the level of excess risk is heterogeneous and ranges up to 10,000-fold, as in carriers of the retinoblastoma gene (101). Survivors of hereditary retinoblastoma are prone to second cancers, particularly osteosarcoma and soft-tissue sarcomas (55). Clinicians are often asked by patients about the clinical implications of a family history of cancer. To provide an informative response, data are needed on the sex of affected family member(s), the relationship to the patient, age(s) at diagnosis, primary site and histology of each tumor, and disease outcome. A pedigree can be used as a concise record of cancer occurrence in multiple members of a family. In families of particular interest, confirmation of the medical history of family members should be sought through examinations of pathology reports, medical records, and death certificates. If indicated, available family members should be examined for physical evidence of inherited disorders that predispose to cancer (147). It is noteworthy that cancer is a common disease over a lifetime in the United States, occurring in one of every three persons (132). Therefore, a family history of cancer is the rule, and not the exception. Seemingly striking family aggregates of cancer can occur solely on the basis of chance (115). However, cancers in childhood are rare, and their occurrence in families is much less likely to be due to chance association (147). Estimates vary on the proportion of human cancers that are due to hereditary influences (113). Cancers of the colon, breast and other common sites of involvement demonstrate a familial tendency (109, 116). On the other hand, few cancers consistently follow a strictly Mendelian (autosomal dominant, autosomal recessive, or X-linked) pattern, or occur excessively in association with an underlying single-gene disorder, such as hereditary retinoblastoma. When the retinoblastoma gene was cloned, however, it was found to be altered in a wide spectrum of cancers, including sarcomas and carcinomas of the lung, breast, and other sites. In addition, genetic factors can play a role in the development of cancers triggered by environmental factors, through inherited mechanisms that influence the metabolism of carcinogens (96, 102, 154).

An inherited susceptibility to certain cancers can be recognized by the presence of a predisposing syndrome (Table 25.5). More than 200 single-gene traits are known to be associated with the development of neoplasia (101, 123). The frequency of tumors differs markedly among these inherited disorders. Benign and malignant tumors are the sole manifestation of some disorders, but are rarely featured in others. Hereditary cancers can present as multiple primary tumors in organs that share the same embryologic origins, as in the multiple endocrine neoplasia (MEN) syndromes (101). In addition, neoplasia occurs as a feature of diverse inherited diseases, such as neurofibromatosis types 1 and 2, which predispose to tumors of peripheral nerves and brain (86). A list of some important predisposing conditions is shown in Table 25.5. In addition, families have been reported with cancer syndromes that affect diverse anatomic sites and tissues. These families generally have no characteristic clinical features, and they are identified primarily on the basis of statistical association. A syndrome of multiple primary adenocarcinomas of the colon, endometrium, breast, and other sites has been described (125) (Lynch syndrome 2), but was difficult to diagnose (121, 122). Another syndrome of breast cancer in young women, childhood sarcomas, and other neoplasms (the Li-Fraumeni syndrome) has been extensively studied (101). Prospective study of these families has shown a marked excess of the component neoplasms during follow-up observation.

The syndrome of breast cancer and childhood neoplasms has also been identified in population-based series of children with sarcomas and in segregation analysis of families with a case of childhood sarcoma (76, 181). A tumor suppressor gene, p53, has been implicated in tumor development in sporadic and familial cases of diverse tumors, including those of the Li-Fraumeni syndrome (144). Germ-line p53 mutations have been found in approximately 50% of Li-Fraumeni families (14, 62). As somatic alterations, characteristic mutations in p53 are caused by several carcinogens. For example, aflatoxin B1 exposure is correlated with a mutation in the third base of codon 249 in the p53 gene in hepatocellular carcinoma. Lung cancer associated with cigarette smoking is frequently characterized by a transversion of G:C to T:A in the p53 gene. The type and frequency of p53 mutations may thus serve to identify the carcinogenic exposure, and contribute to the molecular epidemiology of human cancer risk (75).

Family aggregation of cancer can be due to both hereditary influences and shared exposure to environmental carcinogens (110). Dietary factors may modify the frequency of colonic tumors in patients with familial adenomatous polyposis. Recent studies show that a reduction in dietary fat intake, grain fiber supplementation, or the use of sulindac can inhibit the development of new rectal polyps in small series of polyposis patients (47). Carcinomas of the skin and malignant melanomas are, for example, often considered neoplasms induced by environmental factors, particularly sunlight and other sources of ultraviolet radiation. However, skin cancers differ markedly in frequency among the races. They are most common among fair-skinned Caucasians but are rare among blacks. The finding indicates that genetically determined skin pigmentation is also an important etiologic factor. Furthermore, in several rare hereditary disorders of DNA repair, such as xeroderma pigmentosum (XP), an exceptionally high risk of skin cancers has been found (160). In vitro studies of cells of XP patients show reduced repair of ultraviolet radiation damage, which normally involves a multistep process of incision near the damaged strand, excision of the dimer, repair of the DNA, and rejoining (53). At least nine distinct mutations (complementation groups) along this enzymatic pathway have been identified. A second disease featuring increased sensitivity to ionizing radiation is ataxia telangiectasia (AT) (64). Patients with AT are at very high risk of lymphoid neoplasms that, when treated with standard doses of radiotherapy, can produce fatal toxicity.

Knowledge that a family history of cancer is a consistent risk factor for neoplasia can be used to enhance the primary and secondary prevention of cancer (147, 197). In families with a known predisposing gene, the risk of cancer can often be estimated and used in genetic counseling. Inherited precursor lesions of cancer can be useful in early diagnosis and surveillance, as illustrated in families with dysplastic nevus syndrome and susceptibility to melanoma (11, 69).

Table 25.5. Single-Gene Traits Associated with Cancers of Internal Organs[a]

Organ system	Predisposing genetic disorder[b] (inheritance; names of cloned genes)	Type of cancer
Digestive and respiratory	Polyposis coli (AD; APC)	Carcinoma of colon and rectum
	Gardner's syndrome (AD; APC)	
	Hereditary colorectal cancer (AD; MSH2, MLH1, etc.)	
	Hereditary hemochromatosis (AD); and tyrosinemia (AR)	Primary liver cancer
	Palmar-plantar hyperkeratosis (tylosis) (AD)	Esophageal carcinoma
	Hereditary pancreatitis (AD; VHL)	Pancreatic carcinoma
	Fibrocystic pulmonary dysplasia (AD)	Carcinoma of lung
Genitourinary organs	Gonadal dysgenesis (AR)	Dysgerminoma of ovary
	Von Hippel-Lindau (AD; VHL)	Renal carcinoma (also retinal tumor)
	Wilms' tumor (AD; WT1)	Wilms' tumor
Brain and endocrine	Neurofibromatosis (AD; NF1, NF2), and tuberous sclerosis (AD)	Tumors of brain and peripheral nerves
	Multiple endocrine neoplasia type 1 (AD)	Parathyroid, pituitary, pancreatic islet tumors
	Nevoid basal cell carcinoma (AD)	Medulloblastoma (and other tumors)
	Multiple endocrine neoplasia types II, III (AD; RET)	Medullary thyroid carcinoma, pheochromocytoma
	Multiple hamartoma syndrome (Cowden's disease) (AD)	Thyroid and breast cancer (also colon and other)
Female reproductive organs	Hereditary breast/ovarian cancer (AD; BRCA1)	Breast, ovary, other
Hematologic system	Agammaglobulinemia (XL, AR), Wiskott-Aldrich syndrome (XL) ataxia-telangiectasia (AR), and X-linked lymphoproliferative syndrome (XL)	Lymphoma
	Bloom's syndrome (AR) and Fanconi's anemia (AR)	Leukemia
Musculoskeletal system and other	Li-Fraumeni syndrome (AD; p53)	Sarcoma, breast, other
	Multiple exostosis (AD) Paget's disease (AD) and multiple enchondromatosis (AD)	Osteogenic sarcoma
	Werner's syndrome (adult progeria) (AR)	Sarcoma, melanoma

[a] Excluding familial site-specific cancers and cancer syndromes.
[b] AD = autosomal dominant, AR = autosomal recessive, XL = X-linked; name of gene, if cloned.

These kindreds can be identified by obtaining a complete family history and performing a thorough skin examination of all blood relatives. Suspicious pigmented lesions should be excised and submitted for histopathologic examination (70). High-risk individuals should be taught to recognize changes in size, color, and shape of lesions that might indicate early melanoma. Since ultraviolet radiation is an etiologic factor in melanoma, avoidance of exposure is particularly important in predisposed families. In addition, early cancer detection can be undertaken in susceptible families that have no discernible precursor lesions and biomarkers of a carrier state. In breast cancer, early detection has been demonstrated to reduce mortality rates, and a family history of breast cancer is known to elevate a woman's risk of the neoplasm. The magnitude of the effect of a family history of breast cancer is determined by the number of affected relatives (163). Breast cancer in these families tends to occur in younger women, and studies in progress should help quantify the benefits of directed screening of women in high-risk families (5, 37). A similar rationale argues for the early detection of colorectal carcinomas in predisposed families, particularly in light of new evidence that inherited factors contribute to the development of a high proportion of colonic adenomas and carcinomas (32). Recently, germ-line mutations in several genes for DNA mismatch repair (MSH2, MLH1, PMS1 and 2) have been identified in hereditary colorectal cancers (also called Lynch syndrome) (29, 60). Likewise, BRCA1 mutations were found to account for a substantial fraction of hereditary breast/ovarian cancers (135). The challenge to clinicians is to define optimal approaches to using genetic data to reduce cancer mortality and morbidity, while ensuring minimal psychologic, social, and economic risk (114, 116, 124, 141).

References

1. American Cancer Society. Ca—A Cancer Journal for Clinicians. Edited by Al Holleb. New York: H&W, 1995.
2. American Cancer Society. Cancer Facts and Figures—1990. Atlanta, GA.
3. American Cancer Society. Special report on cancer in the socioeconomically disadvantaged. American Cancer Society Subcommittee on Cancer in the Economically Disadvantaged, 1986.
4. Anda RF, Remington PL, Sienko DG, Davis RM. Are physicians advising smokers to quit? The patient's perspective. JAMA 1987;257:1916.
5. Anderson DE, Badzioch MD. Risk of familial breast cancer. Cancer 1985;56:383.
6. Anello C, Lao C. U.S. trends in mortality from carcinoma of cervix. Lancet 1979;i:1038.
7. Ausman LM. Fiber and colon cancer: Does the current evidence justify a preventive policy? Nutr Rev 1993;52:57–63.
8. Ayoola EA. Synergism between hepatitis B virus and aflatoxin in hepatocellular carcinoma. IARC Sci Publ 1984;63:167.
9. Arthur MJP, Hall AJ, Wright R. Hepatitis B, hepatocellular carcinoma, and strategies for prevention. Lancet 1984;i:607.
10. Bailar JC, Smith EM. Progress against cancer? N Engl J Med 1986;314:1226.
11. Bale SJ, Dracopoli NC, Tucker MA, Clark WH, Fraser MC, Stanger BZ, Green P, Donis-Keller H, Housman DE, Greene MH. Mapping the gene for hereditary cutaneous malignant melanoma-dysplastic nevus to chromosome 1p. N Engl J Med 1989;320:1367.
12. Baquet CR, Ringen K. Cancer Among Blacks and Other Minorities. Publication 86-2785. U.S. Department of Health and Human Services, Public Health Service, National Institutes of Health, March 1986.
13. Bartecchi CE, MacKenzie TD, Schrier RW. The human costs of tobacco use (1). N Engl J Med 1994;330:907–912.
14. Birch JM, Hartley AL, Tricker KJ, Prosser J, Condle A, Kelsey AM, Harris M, Morris-Jones PH, Binchy A, Crowther D, Craft AW, Eden OB, Evans GR, Thompson E, Mann JR, Martin J, Mitchell EL, Santibanez-Koref MF. Prevalence and diversity of constitutional mutations in the p53 gene among 21 Li-Fraumeni families. Cancer Res 1994;54:1298–1304.
15. Blair A. Herbicides and non-Hodgkin's lymphoma: New evidence from a study of Saskatchewan farmers. JNCI 1990;82:544.
16. Blaser MJ, Chyou PH, Nomura A. Age at establishment of *Helicobacter pylori* infection and gastric carcinoma, gastric ulcer, and duodenal ulcer risk. Cancer Res 1995;55:562–565.
17. Blattner WA, Nomura A, Clark JW, Ho, G. Y, Nakao Y, Gallo R, Robert-Guroff M.

Modes of transmission and evidence for viral latency from studies of human T-cell lymphotrophic virus type I in Japanese migrant populations in Hawaii. Proc Natl Acad Sci USA 1986;83:4895.

18. Blayney DW, Longo DL, Young RC, Greene MH, Hubbard SM, Postal MG, Duffey PL, DeVita VT Jr. Decreasing risk of leukemia with prolonged follow-up after chemotherapy and radiotherapy for Hodgkin's disease. N Engl J Med 1987;316:710.
19. Blot WJ, Fraumeni JF Jr. Passive smoking and lung cancer (editorial). JNCI 1986;77:993.
20. Blot WJ, Xu ZY, Boice JD Jr, Zhao DZ, Stone BJ, Sun J, Jing LB, Fraumeni JF Jr. Indoor radon and lung cancer in China. JNCI 1990;82:1025.
21. Blumberg BS, London WT. Hepatitis B virus and the prevention of primary cancer of the liver. JNCI 1985;74:267.
22. Boice JD Jr, Fraumeni JF. Radiation carcinogenesis. Epidemiology and biological significance. In Progress in Cancer Research and Therapy, vol 26. New York: Raven, 1984.
23. Boice JD Jr, Blettner M, Kleinerman RA, Stovall M, Moloney WC, Engholm G, Austin DF, Bosch A, Cookfair DL, Krementz ET, Latourette HB, Peters LJ, Schulz MD, Lundell M, Pettersson F, Storm HH, Bell CMJ, Coleman MP, Fraser P, Palmer M, Prior P, Choi NW, Hislop TG, Koch M, Robb D, Robson D, Spengler RF, von Fournier D, Frischkorn R, Lochm;auuller, H, Pompe-Kirn V, Rimpela A, Kjitorstad K, Pejovic MH, Sigurdsson K, Pisani P, Kucera H, Hutchison GB. Radiation dose and leukemia risk in patients treated for cancer of the cervix. JNCI 1987;79:1295.
24. Boutron MC, Faivre J, Milan C, Bedenne L, Hillon P, Klepping C. Primary liver cancer in Côte D'Or (France). Int J Epidemiol 1988;17:21.
25. Brechot C, Nalpas B, Courouce A, Duhamel G, Callard P, Carnot F, Tiollais P, Berthelot P. Evidence that hepatitis B virus has a role in liver-cell carcinoma in alcoholic liver disease. N Engl J Med 1982;306:1384.
26. Breslow L, Bailar JC, III, Brown BW Jr, Brown HG, Darity WA, Defendi V, Fisher B, Goodman RL, Mosteller F, Shapiro S. Measurement of progress against cancer. JNCI 1990;82:825.
27. Breslow NE, Day NE. Statistical methods in cancer research. The analysis of case-control studies. IARC Sci Publ 1981:1.
28. Brinton LA, Schairer C, Haenszel W, Stolley R, Lehman HF, Levine R, Savitz D. A. Cigarette smoking and invasive cervical cancer. JAMA 1986;255:3265.
29. Bronner CE, Baker SM, Morrison PT, Warren G, Smith LG, Lescoe MK, Kane M, Earabino C, Lipford J, Lindblom A, Tannergard P, Bollag RJ, Godwin AR, Ward DC, Nordenskjold M, Fishel R, Kolodner R, Liskay RM. Mutation in the DNA mismatch repair gene homologue hMLH1 is associated with hereditary nonpolyposis colon cancer. Nature 1994;368:258–261.
30. Caldwell GC, Heath CW. Case clustering in cancer. South. Med. J 1976;69:1598.
31. Muir C, Waterhouse J, Mack T, et al. Cancer incidence in five continents. IARC Sci Publ 1987:5.
32. Cannon-Albright LA, Skolnick MH, Bishop DT, Lee RG, Burt RW. Common inheritance of susceptibility to colonic adenomatous polyps and associated colorectal cancers. N Engl J Med 1988;319:533.
33. Caporaso NE, Tucker MA, Hoover RN, Hayes RB, Pickle LW, Issaq HJ, Muschik GM, Green-Gallo L, Buivys D, Aisner S, Resau JH, Trump BF, Tollerud D, Weston A, Harris CC. Lung cancer and the debrisoquine metabolic phenotype. JNCI 1990;82:1264.
34. Casciato DA, Scott JL. Acute leukemia following prolonged cytotoxic agent therapy. Medicine 1979;58:32.
35. Centers for Disease Control. Black-white differences in cervical cancer mortality—United States 1980–1987. MMWR 1990;39:245.
36. Chilvers C, McPherson K, Peto J, Pike MC, Vessey MP. Oral contraceptive use and breast cancer risk in young women. Lancet 1989;i:973.
37. Claus EB, Risch N, Thompson WD. Genetic analysis of breast cancer in the cancer and steroid hormone study. Am J Hum Genet 1991;48:232–242.
38. Cleary ML, Sklar J. Lymphoproliferative disorders in cardiac transplant recipients are multiclonal lymphomas. Lancet 1984;ii:489.
39. Committee on the Biological Effects of Ionizing Radiations. Health Effects of Exposure to Low Levels of Ionizing Radiation. BEIR-V. Washington DC: National Academy Press, 1990.
40. Craighead JE, Mossman BT. The pathogenesis of asbestos-associated diseases. N Engl J Med 1982;306:1446.
41. Crawford FG, Mayer J, Santella RM, Cooper TB, Ottman R, Tsai WY, Simon-Cereijido G, Wang M, Tang D, Perera, F.P. Biomarkers of environmental tobacco smoke in preschool children and their mothers. JNCI 1994;86:1398–1402.
42. Cremer KJ, Spring SB, Gruber J. Role of human immunodeficiency virus type 1 and other viruses in malignancies associated with acquired immunodeficiency disease syndrome. JNCI 1990;82:1016.
43. Darby SC, Whitley E, Howe GR, Hutchings SJ, Kusiak RA, Lubin JH, Morrison HI, Tirmarche M, Tomasek L, Radford EP, Roscoe RJ, Samet JM, Yao, S.X. Radon and cancers other than lung cancer in undeground miners: a collaborative analysis of 11 studies. JNCI 1995;87:378–384.
44. Davis RM. Current trends in cigarette advertising and marketing. N Engl J Med 1987;316:725.
45. Dawber TR. The Framingham Study: The Epidemiology of Atherosclerotic Disease. Cambridge MA: Harvard University Press, 1980.
46. Day R, Ware JH, Wartenberg D, Zelen M. An investigation of a reported cancer cluster in Randolph, Massachusetts. J Clin Epidemiol 1989;42:137.
47. DeCosse JJ, Miller HH, Lesser ML. Effect of wheat fiber and vitamins C and E on rectal polyps in patients with familial adenomatous polyposis. JNCI 1989;81:1291.
48. Devesa SS. Descriptive epidemiology of cancer of the uterine cervix. J Am College Obstet Gynecol 1984;63:605.
49. Devesa SS, Blot WJ, Stone BJ, Miller BA, Tarone RE, Fraumeni JF Jr. Recent cancer trends in the U.S. JNCI 1995;87:175–182.
50. Doll R, Hill AB. Lung cancer and other causes of death in relation to smoking: A second report on the mortality of British doctors. Br Med J 1965;10:1071.
51. Doll R, Peto R. The causes of cancer: Quantitative estimates of avoidable risks of cancer in the United States today. JNCI 1981;66:1193.
52. Editorial: Alcohol and Cancer. Lancet 1990;335:634.
53. Editorial: Sunlight, DNA repair, and skin cancer. Lancet 1989;i:1362.
54. Ellickson PL, Bell R. M. Drug prevention in junior high: A multi-site longitudinal test. Science 1990;247:1299.
55. Eng C, Li, FP, Abramson DH, Ellsworth RM, Wong FL, Goldman MB, Seddon J, Tarbell N, Boice JD. Mortality from second tumors among long-term survivors of retinoblastoma. JNCI 1993;85:1121–1128.
56. Enstrom JE. Trends in mortality among California physicians after giving up smoking: 1950–79. Br Med J 1983;286:1101.
57. Ernster VL, Grady DG, Greene JC, Walsh M, Robertson P, Daniels TE, Benowitz N, Siegel D, Gerbert B, Hauck W. W. Smokeless tobacco use and health effects among baseball players. JAMA 1990;264:218.
58. Feldman AR, Kessler L, Myers MH, Naughton MD. The prevalence of cancer: Estimates based on the Connecticut Tumor Registry. N Engl J Med 1986;315:1394.
59. Fielding JE. Smoking: Health effects and control. N Engl J Med 1985;313:491.
60. Fishel R, Lescoe MK, Rao RS, Copland N, Jenkins N, Garber J, Kane M, Kolodner R. The human mutator gene homolog MSH2 and its association with hereditary nonpolyposis colon cancer. Cell 1993;75:1027–1038.
61. Fleiss JL. Statistical Methods for Rates and Proportions. New York: John Wiley and Sons, 1981.
62. Frebourg T, Barbier N, Yan Y, Garber JE, Dreyfus M, Fraumeni JF, Li, FP, Friend SH. Germline p53 mutations in 15 families with Li-Fraumeni syndrome. Am J Hum Genet 51995;6:608–615.
63. Fry RJ, Sinclair WK. New dosimetry of atomic bomb radiations. Lancet 1987;ii:845.
64. Gatti RA, Berkel I, Boder E, Braedt G, Charmley P, Concannon P, Ersoy F, Foroud T, Jaspers NG, Lange K, et al. Localization of an ataxia-telangiectasia gene to chromosome 11q22–23. Nature 1988;336:577.
65. Giovanucci E, Rimm EB, Ascherio A, Stampfer MJ, Colditz GA, Willett WC. Alcohol, low-methionine-low-folate diets, and risk of colon cancer in men. JNCI 1995;87:265–273.
66. Glass AG, Mantel N. Lack of time-space clustering of childhood leukemia in Los Angeles County 1960–1964. Cancer Res 1969;29:1995.
67. Gloeckler Ries LA, Hankey BF, Edwards BK. Cancer Statistics Review 1973–1987. Department of Health and Human Services, NIH Publication 90-2789, 1989.
68. Greene MH, Boice JD, Greer BE, Blessing JA, Dembo AJ. Acute nonlymphocytic leukemia after therapy with alkylating agents for ovarian cancer. N Engl J Med 1982;307:1416.
69. Greene MH, Clark WH Jr, Tucker MA, Kraemer KH, Elder DE, Fraser MC. High risk of malignant melanoma in melanoma-prone families with dysplastic nevi. Ann Intern Med 1985;102:458.
70. Greene MH, Clark WH Jr, Tucker MA, Elder DE, Kraemer KH, Guerry D, IV, Witmer WK, Thompson J, Matozzo I, Fraser, M.C. Acquired precursors of cutaneous malignant melanoma. N Engl J Med 1985;312:91.
71. Gritz ER. Paving the road from basic research to policy: Cigarette smoking as a prototype issue for cancer control science. Cancer Epidemiol Biomarkers Prev, Vol 1992;1:427–434.
72. Grufferman S, Raab-Traub N, Marvin K, Borowitz MJ, Pagano JS. Burkitt's and other non-Hodgkin's lymphomas in adults exposed to a visitor from Africa. N Engl J Med 1985;313:1525.
73. Gutensohn N, Cole P. Childhood social environment and Hodgkin's disease. N Engl J Med 1981;304:135.
74. Haenszel W. Migrant Studies. In Cancer Epidemiology and Prevention. Edited by D Schottenfeld, JF Fraumeni. Philadelphia: Saunders, 1982, p 194.
75. Harris CC. p53: At the crossroads of molecular carcinogenesis and risk assessment. Science 1993;262:1980.
76. Hartley AL, Birch JM, Marsden HB, Harris M. Breast cancer risk in mothers of children with osteosarcoma and chondrosarcoma. Br J Cancer 1986;54:819.
77. Hecht SS, Carmella SG, Murphy SE, Akerkar S, Brunnemann KD, Hoffmann, D: A tobacco-specific lung carcinogen in the urine of men exposed to cigarette smoke. N Engl J Med 1993;329:1543–1546.
78. Hendee WR. Estimation of radiation risks. JAMA 1992;268:621–624.
79. Henderson BE. Establishment of an association between a virus and a human cancer. JNCI 1989;81:320.
80. Hennekens CH, Buring JE. In Epidemiology in Medicine. Edited by SL Mayrent. Boston: Little, Brown, 1987.
81. Henshaw DL, Eatough JP, Richardson RB. Radon as a causative factor induction of myeloid leukemia and other cancers. Lancet 1990;335:1008.
82. Herbst AL, Ulfelder J, Poskanzer DC. Adenocarcinoma of the vagina: Association of maternal stilbestrol therapy with tumor appearance in young women. N Engl J Med 1971;284:878.
83. Herbst AL, Anderson S, Hubby MM, Haenszel WM, Kaufman RH, Noller KL. Risk factors for the development of diethylstilbestrol-associated clear-cell adenocarcinoma: a case-control study. Am J Obstet Gynecol 1986;154:814.
84. Hoar SK, Blair A, Holmes FF, Boysen CD, Robel RJ, Hoover R, Fraumeni JF, Jr. Agricultural herbicide use and risk of lymphoma and soft-tissue sarcoma. JAMA 1986;256:1141.
85. Hoover R, Fraumeni JF, Jr. Risk of cancer in renal-transplant recipients. Lancet 1973;ii:55.
86. Hope DG, Mulvihill JJ. Malignancy in neurofibromatosis. In Neurofibromatosis: Genetics, Cell Biology, and Biochemistry. Edited by VM Riccardi and JJ Mulvihill. New York: Raven, 1981, p 33.
87. Hsu IC, Metcalf RA, Sun T, Welsh JA, Wang NJ, Harris CC. Mutational hotspot in the p53 gene in human hepatocellular carcinomas. Nature 1991;350:427–428.
88. Hulka BS, Chambless LE, Kaufman DG, Fowler WC, Greenberg BG. Protection against endometrial carcinoma by combination-product oral contraceptives. JAMA 1982;247:475.
89. Hunter DJ, Kelsey KT. Pesticide residues and breast cancer: The harvest of a silent spring. JNCI 1993;85:598–599.
90. IARC Study Group on Cancer Risk Among Nuclear Industry Workers. Direct estimates of cancer mortality due to low doses of ionising radiation: An international study. Lancet 1994;344:1039–1043.
91. Iglehart JK. The campaign against smoking gains momentum. N Engl J Med 1986;314:1059.
92. Jackson JD. Are the stray 60-Hz electromagnetic fields associated with the distribution and use of electric power a significant cause of cancer. Proc Natl USA 89:3508–3510, 1992.
93. Janerich DT, Burnett WS, Feck G, Hoff M, Nasca P, Polednak AP, Greenwald P, Vianna N. Cancer incidence in the Love Canal area. Science 1981;212:1404.

94. Jauchem JR. Epidemiologic studies of electric and magnetic fields and cancer: A case study of distortions by the media. J Clin Epidemiol 1992;45:1137–1142.
95. Johnson PJ, Williams R. Hepatitis C antibodies and hepato-cellular carcinoma: New clues or a false trail? JNCI 1990;82:986.
96. Kaisary A, Smith P, Jacqz E, McAllister CB, Wilkinson GR, Ray, W.A, Branch R. A. Genetic predisposition to bladder cancer: Ability to hydroxylate debrisoquine and mephenytoin as risk factors. Cancer Res 1987;47:5488.
97. Kaplan MH, Susin M, Pahwa SG, Fetten J, Allen SL, Lichtman S, Sarngadharon MG, Gallo R. C. Neoplastic complications of HTLVIII infection: Lymphomas and solid tumors. Am J Med 1987;82:389.
98. Keller AZ. Alcohol, tobacco and age factors in the relative frequency of cancer among males with and without liver cirrhosis. Am J Epidemiol 1977;106:194.
99. Kinlen LJ, Hudson CM, Stiller CA. Contacts between adults as evidence for an infective origin of childhood leukemia: An explanation for the excess near nuclear establishments in West Berkshire? Br J Cancer 1991:64:549–554.
100. Kmet J, Mahboubi E. Esophageal cancer in the Caspian littoral of Iran: Initial studies. Science 1972;175:846.
101. Knudson AG, Jr. Hereditary cancers disclose a class of cancer genes. Cancer 1989;63:1888.
102. Knudson AG, Jr. All in the (cancer) family. Nature Genet 1993;5:103–104.
103. Kraemer KH, DiGiovanna JJ, Moshell AN, Tarone RE, Peck G. L. Prevention of skin cancer in xeroderma pigmentosum with the use of oral isotretinoin. N Engl J Med 1988;318:1633.
104. Kripke ML, Sass ER. International Conference on Ultraviolet Carcinogenesis. Department of Health, Education and Welfare Publication (NIH) 78-1532. Washington DC: U.S. Government Printing Office, 1977.
105. Deleted in proof.
106. Lagakos SW, Wessen BJ, et al. An analysis of contaminated well water and health effects in Woburn, Massachusetts. J Am Stat Assoc 1986;81:583.
107. Langmuir AD. The surveillance of communicable diseases of national importance. N Engl J Med 1963;268:182.
108. Lee L, Gilpin EA, Pierce JP. Changes in the patterns of initiation of cigarette smoking in the United States: 1950 1965, and 1980. Cancer Epidemiol Biomarkers Prev 1993;2:593–597.
109. Leppert M, Burt R, Hughes JP, Samowitz W, Nakamura Y, Woodward S, Gardner E, Lalouel JM, White R. Genetic analysis of an inherited predisposition to colon cancer in a family with a variable number of adenomatous polyps. N Engl J Med 1990;322: 904.
110. Li FP. Cancer epidemiology and prevention. Sci Am 1978;10:12.
111. Li FP, Fraumeni JF Jr, Mulvihill JJ, Blattner WA, Dreyfus MG, Tucker MA, Miller RW. A cancer family syndrome in twenty-four kindreds. Cancer Res 1988;48:5358.
112. Li FP, Mulvihill JJ. Preventative pediatric oncology: the childhood origins of adult cancer. In Principles and Practices of Pediatric Oncology. Edited by PA Pizzo, DG Poplack. Philadelphia: Lippincott, 1988, p 1075.
113. Li FP. Familial cancer syndromes and clusters. Curr Probl Cancer 1990;14:75–106.
114. Li FP, Fraumeni JF Jr. Predictive testing for inherited mutations in cancer-susceptibility genes. J Clin Oncol 1992;10:1203–1204.
115. Li FP. Molecular epidemiology of familial cancers. Br J Cancer 1993;68:217–219.
116. Li FP. Translational research on hereditary colon, breast and ovarian cancers. NCI Monogr 1995;17:1–4.
117. Liebowitz D. Epstein-Barr virus—an old dog with new tricks. N Engl J Med 1995;332: 55–57.
118. Lippman SM, Lee JS, Lotan R, Hittelman W, Wargovich MJ, Hong WK. Biomarkers as intermediate end points in chemoprevention trials. JNCI 1990;82:555.
119. Love R, Mazess RB, Barden HS, Epstein S, Newcomb PA, Jordan C, Carbone PP, DeMets, D.L. Effects of tamoxifen on bone mineral density in postmenopausal women with breast cancer. N Engl J Med 1992;326:852–856.
120. Love R, Wiebe DA, Feyzi JM, Newcomb PA, Chappell RJ. Effects of tamoxifen on cardiovascular risk factors in postmenopausal women after 5 years of treatment. JNCI 1994;86:1534–1539.
121. Lynch HT, Krush AJ. Cancer family "G" revisited: 1895–1970. Cancer 1971;27:1505.
122. Lynch HT, Lynch PM. Hereditary and gastrointestinal tract cancer. In Gastrointestinal Tract Cancer. Edited by M Lipkin, RA Good. New York: Plenum, 1980, p 259.
123. Lynch HT, Hirayama T. Genetic Epidemiology of Cancer. Boca Raton: CRC Press, 1989.
124. Lynch HT, Lynch JF. Familial predisposition and cancer management. Contempory Oncol 1993:12–25.
125. Lynch HT, Smyrk TC, Watson P. Genetics, natural history, tumor spectrum, and pathology of hereditary nonpolyposis colorectal cancer: An updated review. Gastroenterology 1993;104:1535–1549.
126. MacKenzie TD, Bartecchi CE, Schrier RW. The human costs of tobacco use (2): N Engl J Med 1994;330:975–980.
127. MacMahon B, Pugh TF. Epidemiology: Principles and Methods. Boston: Little, Brown, 1970.
128. Mahboubi E, Sayed GM. Oral Cavity and Pharynx. In Cancer Epidemiology and Prevention. Edited by D Schottenfeld, JF Fraumeni. Philadelphia: Saunders, 1982, p 583.
129. Malkin D, Li, FP, Strong LC, Fraumeni JF Jr, Nelson CE, Kim DH, Kassel J, Gryka MA, Bischoff FZ, Tainsky MA, Friend SH. Germ line p53 mutations in a familial syndrome of breast cancer, sarcomas, and other neoplasms. Science 1990;250:1233.
130. Mattson ME, Winn DM. Smokeless tobacco: Association with increased cancer risk. NCI Monogr 1989;8:13.
131. McMichael AJ. Increases in laryngeal cancer in Britain and Australia in relation to alcohol and tobacco consumption trends. Lancet 1978;ii:1244.
132. McWhorter WP, Schatzkin AG, Horm JW, Brown CC. Contribution of socioeconomic status to black/white differences in cancer incidence. Cancer 1989;63:982.
133. Meara J, McPherson K, Roberts M, Jones L, Vessey M. Alcohol, cigarette smoking, and breast cancer. Br J Cancer 1989;60:70.
134. Menkes MS, Comstock GW, Vuilleumier JP, Helsing KJ, Rider AA, Brookmeyer R. Serum beta-carotene, vitamins A and E, selenium, and the risk of lung cancer. N Engl J Med 1986;315:1250.
135. Miki Y, Swensen J, Shattuck-Eldens D, Futreal PA, Harshman K, et al. Isolation of BRCA1, the 17q-linked breast and ovarian cancer susceptibility gene. Science 1994;266:61–71.
136. Mills JL. Data torturing. N Engl J Med 1993;329:1196–1199.
137. Monson RR. Occupational Epidemiology. Boca Raton, FL: CRC Press, 1980.
138. Moore PS. and Chang Y. Detection of herpesvirus-like DNA sequences in Kaposi's sarcoma in patients with and those without HIV infection. N Engl J Med 1995;332: 1181–1185.
139. Mossman BT, Gee JBL. Asbestos-related diseases. N Engl J Med 1989;320:1721.
140. Mueller N, Evans A, Harris NL, Comstock GW, Jellum E, Magnus K, Orentreich N, Polk BF, Vogelman, J Hodgkin's disease and Epstein-Barr virus. N Engl J Med 1989;320: 689.
141. National Advisory Council of the Human Genome Program. Statement on use of DNA testing for presymptomatic identification of cancer risk. JAMA 1994;271:785.
142. Nayfield SG, Karp JE, Ford LG. Potential role of tamoxifen in prevention of breast cancer. JNCI 1991;83:1450–1459.
143. Nestle M, Bailar J. The Surgeon General's Report on Nutrition and Health. DHHS Publication 88-50210. Washington, DC: U.S. Government Printing Office, 1988.
144. Nigro JM, Baker SJ, Preisinger AC, Jessup JM, Hostetter R, Cleary K, Bignerm SH, Davidson N, Baylin S, Devilee P, Glover T, Collins FS, Weston A, Modali R, Harris CC, Vogelstein B. A tumor suppressor gene, p53, has been implicated in tumor development in sporadic and familial cases of diverse tumors, including those of the Li-Fraumeni syndrome. Nature 1989;342:705.
145. Cancer and Steroid Hormone Study of the Centers for Disease Control and the National Institute of Child Health and Human Development. Oral-contraceptive use and the risk of breast cancer. N Engl J Med 1986;315:405.
146. Pariza MW. A perspective on diet, nutrition, and cancer. JAMA 1984;251:455.
147. Parry DM, Mulvihill JJ, Miller RW, Berg K, Carter CL. Strategies for controlling cancer through genetics. Cancer Res 1987;47:6814.
148. Parsonnet J, Friedman GD, Vandersteen DP, Chang Y, Vogelman JH, Orentreich N, Sibley RK. *Helicobacter pylori* infection and the risk of gastric carcinoma. N Engl J Med 1991;325:1127–1131.
149. Perera F, Mayer J, Jaretzki A, Hearne S, Brenner D, Young TL, Fischman HK, Grimes M, Grantham S, Tang MX, Tsai, W.-Y, Santella R. M. Comparison of DNA adducts and sister chromatid exchange in lung cancer cases and controls. Cancer Res 1989;49: 4446.
150. Perera FP, Weinstein IB. Molecular epidemiology and carcinogen-DNA adduct detection: new approaches to studies of human cancer causation. J Chron Dis 1982;35: 581.
151. Phillips RL. Role of life-style and dietary habits in risk of cancer among Seventh-Day Adventists. Cancer Res 1975;35:3513.
152. Piper JM, Tonascia J, Matanoski GM. Heavy phenacetin use and bladder cancer in women aged 20 to 49 years. N Engl J Med 1985;313:292.
153. Pollack ES, Nomura AMY, Heilbrun LK, Stemmerman GN, Green SB. Prospective study of alcohol consumption and cancer. N Engl J Med 1984;310:617.
154. Potter JD. Reconciling the epidemiology, physiology, molecular biology of colon cancer. JAMA 1992;268:1573–1577.
155. Preston DL, Kato H, Kopecky KJ, Fujita S. Studies of the mortality of A-bomb survivors. Radiat Res 1987;111:151.
156. Pui CH, Behm FG, Raimondi SC, Dodge RK, George SL, Rivera GK, Mirro J Jr, Kalwinsky DK, Dahl GV, Murphy SB. Secondary acute myeloid leukemia in children treated for acute lymphoid leukemia. N Engl J Med 1989;321:136.
157. Pui CH, Ribeiro RC, Hancock ML, Rivera GK, Evans WE, Raimondi SC, Head DR, Behm FG, Mahmoud MH, Sandlund JT, Crist WM. Acute myeloid luekemia in children treated with epipodophyllotoxins for acute lymphoblastic leukemia. N Engl J Med 1991;325:1682–1687.
158. Report of an IARC Working Group: An evaluation of chemicals and industrial processes associated with cancer in humans based on human and animal data. IARC monographs vol 1–20. Cancer Res 1980;40:12.
159. Ries LAG, Miller BA, Hankey BF, Kosary CL, Harras A, Edwards BK (editors). SEER Cancer Statistics Review 1973–1991: Tables and Graphs, National Cancer Institute. NIH Publ 94-2789. Bethesda, MD, 1994.
160. Robbins JH. Xeroderma pigmentosum. Defective DNA repair causes skin cancer and neurodegeneration. JAMA 1988;260:384.
161. Rosen S. Xeroderma pigmentosum. Defective DNA repair causes skin cancer and neurodegeneration. JAMA 1988;260:384.
162. Sagan LA. Epidemiological and laboratory studies of power frequency electric and magnetic fields. JAMA 1992;268:625–629.
163. Sattin RW, Rubin GL, Webster LA, Huezo CM, Wingo PA, Ory HW, Layde PM. Family history and the risk of breast cancer. JAMA 1985;253:1908.
164. Schatzkin A, Carter CL, Green SB, Kreger BE, Splansky GL, Anderson KM, Helsel WE, Kannel WB. Is alcohol consumption related to breast cancer? Results from the Framingham heart study. JNCI 1989;81:31.
165. Schatzkin A, Greenwald P, Byar DP, Clifford CK. The dietary fat-breast cancer hypothesis is alive. JAMA 1989;261:3284.
166. Schatzkin A, Jones DY, Hoover RN, Taylor PR, Brinton LA, Ziegler RG, Harvey EB, Carter CL, Licitra LN, Dufour MC, Larson DB. Alcohol consumption and breast cancer in the epidemiologic follow-up study of the first National Health and Nutrition Examination Survey. N Engl J Med 1987;316:1169.
167. Schiffman MH, Bauer HM, Hoover RN, Glass AG, Cadell DM, Rush BB, Scott DR, Sherman ME, Kurman RJ, Wacholder S, Stanton CK, Manos MM. Epidemiologic evidence showing that human papillomavirus infection causes most cervical intraepithelial neoplasia. JNCI 1993;85:958–964.
168. Schlesselman JJ. Case-Control Studies: Design, Conduct, Analysis. New York: Oxford University Press, 1982.
169. Schmahl D, Thomas C, Auer R. Iatrongenic Carcinogenesis. Berlin: Springer-Verlag, 1977.
170. Sellers TA, Bailey-Wilson JE, Elston RC, Wilson AF, Elston GZ, Ooi WL, Rothschild H. Evidence for Mendelian inheritance in the pathogenesis of lung cancer. JNCI 1990;82:1272.
171. Shapiro S, Kelly JP, Rosenberg L, Kaufman DW, Helmrich SP, Rosenshein NB, Lewis JL Jr, Knapp RC, Stolley PD, Schottenfeld D. Risk of localized and widespread endometrial cancer in relation to recent and discontinued use of conjugated estrogens. N Engl J Med 1985;313:969.
172. Shiramizu B, Herndier BG, McGrath MS. Identification of a common clonal human immunodeficiency virum integration site in human immunodeficiency virus-associated lymphomas. Cancer Res 1994;54:2069–2072.
173. Skegg DC, Corwin PA, Paul C, Doll R. Importance of the male factor in cancer of the cervix. Lancet 1982;ii:581.
174. Slattery ML, Schuman KL, West DW, French TK, Robison LM. Nutrient intake and ovarian cancer. Am J Epidemiol 1989;130:497.

175. Smith PG, Kinlen LJ, White GC, Adelstein AM, Fox AJ. Mortality of wives of men dying with cancer of the penis. Br J Cancer 1980;41:422.
176. Smith MA, Rubinstein L, Cazenave L, Ungerleider RS, Maurer HM, Heyn R, Khan FM, Gehan E. Report of the cancer therapy evaluation program monitoring plan for secondary acute myeloid leukemia following treatment with epipodophyllotoxins. JNCI 1993;85:554–558.
177. Smokeless Tobacco or Health: An International Perspective (Monograph 2). U.S. Department of Health and Human Services, National Cancer Institute, NIH Publication 93-3461, 1993.
178. Smoking and Health: A report of the Surgeon General. U.S. Department of Health, Education, and Welfare, DHEW Publication (PHS) 79-50066. Washington, DC: U.S. Government Printing Office, 1979.
179. Spirtas R, Beebe GW, Connelly RR, Wright WE, Peters JM, Sherwin RP, Henderson BE, Stark A, Kovasznay BM, Davies JN. Recent trends in mesothelioma incidence in the United States. Am J Med 1986;9:397.
180. Sponner CM. Asbestos in schools: A public health problem. N Engl J Med 1979;301:782.
181. Strong LC, Stine M, Norsted TL. Cancer in survivors of childhood soft tissue sarcoma and their relatives. JNCI 1987;79:1213.
182. Sung JJY, Chung S, Ling TKW, Yung MY, Leung VKS, Ng, EKW, Li, MKK, Cheng AFB, Li, AKC. Antibacterial treatment of gastric ulcers associated with *Helicobacter pylori.* N Engl J Med 1995;332:139–142.
183. Takeshima Y, Seyama T, Bennett WP, Akiyama M, Tokuoka S, Inai K, Mabuchi K, Land CE, Harris, C.C. P53 mutations in lung cancers from non-smoking atomic-bomb survivors. Lancet 1993;342:1520–1521.
184. Taylor JA, Watson MA, Devereux TR, Michels RY, Saccomanno G, Anderson M. P53 mutation hotspot in radon-associated lung cancer. Lancet 1994;343:86–87.
185. Tobacco and the Clinician: Interventions for Medical and Dental Practice (Monograph 5), Edited by DM Burns. U.S. Department of Health and Human Services; National Cancer Institute, NIH Publication 94-3693, 1994.
186. Travis LB, Curtis RE, Boice JD Jr, Fraumeni JF, Jr. Bladder cancer after chemotherapy for non-Hodgkin's lymphoma. N Engl J Med 1989;321:544.
187. Trichopoulos D. Are electric or magnetic fields affecting mortality from breast cancer in women? JNCI 1994;86:885–886.
188. Tsukuma H, Hiyama T, Tanaka S, Nakao M, Yabuuchi T, Kitamura T, Nakanishi K, Fujimoto I, Inoue A, Yamazaki H, Kawashima T. Risk factors for hepatocellular carcinoma among patients with chronic liver disease. N Engl J Med 1993;328:1797–1801.
189. Tucker MA, D'Angio GJ, Boice JD Jr, Strong LC, Li, FP, Stovall M, Stone BJ, Green DM, Lombardi F, Newton W. Bone sarcomas linked to radiotherapy and chemotherapy in children. N Engl J Med 1987;312:588.
190. Tucker MA, Shields JA, Hartge P, Augsburger J, Hoover RN, Fraumeni JF, Jr. Sunlight exposure as risk factor for intraocular malignant melanoma. N Engl J Med 1985;313:789.
191. Upton AC. oncogenic effects of low-level ionizing radiation. JNCI 1990;82:448.
192. Villa LL, Franco EL. Epidemiologic correlates of cervical neoplasia and risk of human papillomavirus infection in asymptomatic women in Brazil. JNCI 1989;81:332.
193. Wagner JC, Sleggs CA, Marchang P. Diffuse pleural mesothelioma and asbestos exposure in the North Western Cape Province. Br J Ind Med 1960;17:260.
194. Walker WJ, Brin BN. U.S. lung cancer mortality and declining cigarette tobacco consumption. J Clin Epidemiol 1988;41:179.
195. Walter HJ, Vaughan RD, Wynder EL. Primary prevention of cancer among children: Changes in cigarette smoking and diet after six years of intervention. JNCI 1989;81:995.
196. Warner KE. Cigarette smoking in the 1970's: The impact of the antismoking campaign on consumption. Science 1981;211:729.
197. Wattenberg LW. Prevention-therapy basic science and the resolution of the cancer problem. Cancer Res 1993;53:5890–5896.
198. White JR, Froeb HF. Small-airways dysfunction in nonsmokers chronically exposed to tobacco smoke. N Engl J Med 1980;302:720.
199. White E, Lee CY, Kristal AR. Evaluation of the increase in breast cancer incidence in relation to mammography use. JNCI 1990;82:1546.
200. Wigle DT, Semenciw RM, Wilkins K, Riedel D, Ritter L, Morrison HI, Mao Y. Mortality study of Canadian male farm operators: Non-Hodgkin's lymphoma mortality and agricultural practices in Saskatchewan. JNCI 1990;82:575.
201. Willett W. The search for the causes of breast and colon cancer. Nature 1989;338:389.
202. Willett WC, Hunter DJ, Stampfer MJ, Colditz G, Manson JE, Spiegelman D, Rosner B, Hennekens CH, Speizer FE. Dietary fat and fiber in relation to risk of breast cancer. JAMA 1992;268:2037–2044.
203. Willett WC, MacMahon B. Diet and cancer—an overview (pt. 1). N Engl J Med 1984;310:633.
204. Willett WC, Stampfer MJ, Colditz GA, Rosner BA, Hennekens C. H, Speizer F. E. Moderate alcohol consumption and the risk of breast cancer. N Engl J Med 1987;316:1174.
205. Willett WC, Stampfer MJ, Colditz GA, Rosner BA, Hennekens CH, Speizer F. E. Dietary fat and the risk of breast cancer. N Engl J Med 1987;316:22.
206. Willett WC, Stampfer MJ, Colditz GA, Rosner BA, Speizer FE. Relation of meat, fat, fiber intake to the risk of colon cancer in a prospective study among women. N Engl J Med 1990;323:1664.
207. Wingo PA, Tong T, Bolden S. Cancer statistics 1995. Ca—A Cancer J Clinic 1995;45:8–30.
208. Winn DM, Blot WJ, Shy CM, Pickle LW, Toledo A, Fraumeni JF, Jr. Snuff dipping and oral cancer among women in the southern United States. N Engl J Med 1981;304:745.
209. You WC, Blot WJ, Chang YS, Ershow AG, Yang ZT, An, Q, Henderson B, Xu, G. W, Fraumeni JF Jr, Wang TG. Diet and high risk of stomach cancer in Shandong, China. Cancer Res 1988;48:3518.
210. Young JL, Gloekler Ries L, Silverberg E, Horm JW, Miller RW. Cancer incidence, survival, and mortality for children younger than age 15 years. Cancer 1986;58:598.
211. Zeckhauser RJ, Viscusi WK. Risk within reason. Science 1990;248:559.
212. Ziegler A, Jonason AS, Leffell DJ, Kimmelman J, Remington L, Jacks T, Brash DE. Sunburn and p53 in the onset of skin cancer. Nature 1994;372:773–776.
213. Zur Hausen H. Papillomaviruses in anogenital cancer as a model to understand the role of viruses in human cancers. Cancer Res 1989;49:4677.

SECTION V

THEORY AND PRACTICE OF CLINICAL TRIALS

CHAPTER 26

Theory and Practice of Clinical Trials

MARVIN ZELEN

Introduction

The modern era of therapeutics in cancer is dominated by clinical data arising from cancer clinical trials. This reliance on clinical trial methodology to generate scientific data on the value of therapies not only has been adopted by the oncology community but is true for those working with all chronic diseases. The U.S. effort to find AIDS therapies is principally relying on clinical trials. Applications for drug approval to the U.S. Food and Drug Administration (FDA) can only be made on the basis of scientific evidence generated by clinical trials. The development and widespread acceptance of clinical trials is one of the major conceptual advances in experimental therapeutics made during the latter half of the twentieth century.

A clinical trial is defined as an experiment on humans being carried out in order to evaluate one or more potentially beneficial therapies. The clinical investigator is assumed to have control of both the therapies being evaluated and the patient population to which these therapies are administered.

The basic ideas that are associated with clinical trials have been discussed for at least 150 years. An important intellectual landmark is the treatise *Essays in Clinical Instruction*, written by French physician P.C.A. Louis in 1834 (9). He advocated the use of the "numerical method" to study the benefits of therapy. His view was that only with "counting" is it possible to learn about the scientific basis of medicine; however, counting is not easy. It is necessary to account for the different circumstances of age, sex, temperament, physical condition, natural history of the disease, and errors in giving therapy. Louis wrote, "The only reproach which can be made to the Numerical Method is that it offers real difficulties in its execution . . . this method requires much more labor and time than the most distinguished members of our profession can dedicate to it." Dr. Louis' comments are as appropriate today as when he wrote them.

Types of Clinical Trials

Ordinarily clinical trials are characterized by three phases, which are referred to as phase I, II, or III trials. The characterization of these trials has arisen from drug trials, but the language has been used for radiotherapy and surgical trials as well.

A phase I trial refers to a new treatment (usually a drug) that is to be tried on humans for the first time. The aim is to find an acceptable dose and schedule with respect to toxicity. Use of the term *acceptable* is particularly important. Therapies for life-threatening illnesses generally will allow for greater risks of serious side effects than those targeted at less serious illnesses. In cancer, patients who are refractory to therapies that are believed to be beneficial usually are the patients who are entered in phase I trials. As a result, evaluation of side effects in this population with very advanced disease may not necessarily be the same for patients who ultimately receive the therapy for an evaluation of its benefit.

Phase II cancer trials are initiated after the completion of phase I trials. The goal is to determine if the therapy has any beneficial effect. The patient population in phase II trials sometimes is composed of newly diagnosed patients with advanced cancer. Entering such patients may be justified in non-small-cell lung cancer trials, but it may not be appropriate for cancer sites for which therapies with proven benefit do exist. As a result, most patients entering phase II trials are those who no longer benefit from therapies that are believed to be beneficial. The dilemma of phase II trials is that the trial may not be a satisfactory test of an experimental therapy if a patient population is used that has failed or been found to be unresponsive to therapies with proven benefit. Another criticism is that some trials are designed to investigate a single dose and schedule while others test combinations of drugs. The particular dose-schedule combination of a drug may be far from optimal. Scientific considerations dictate that tests of drugs in phase II trials should include a spectrum of doses and schedules that still have acceptable toxicity. In some circumstances it may be appropriate to combine phase I and II trials into a single phase I–II trial.

Phase III studies always are comparative trials: one or more experimental therapies are compared with the best standard therapy or competitive therapies. They tend to have many more patients than phase II trials, and they often require patients from many co-operating hospitals.

RANDOMIZED VS. NONRANDOMIZED CLINICAL TRIALS

The fundamental scientific principle underlying the comparison of patient groups receiving different therapies is that these groups must be alike in all important aspects and differ only in the treatment that each receives. Otherwise, differences between groups may not be caused by the treatments under study but may be attributed to the particular characteristics of the group. In clinical experimentation, patients may vary widely in their ability to respond to therapy. Furthermore, therapies cannot be reproduced exactly from occasion to occasion, in contrast to the physical sciences, in which the treatments applied to experimental units are exactly reproducible and the experimental units homogeneous. Variability in clinical experimentation arises from the heterogeneity of the patient populations and the lack of exact reproducibility of the treatment, whereas in the physical sciences, variability often is a secondary factor and arises from slight changes in the ambient environment and the variability of the measuring instrument.

The use of randomization refers to the process used to generate comparable patient groups. The term *randomization* refers to allocating the treatments to patients using a chance mechanism; it is equivalent to tossing a coin to assign therapies when only two treatments are under investigation. Classic randomized clinical trials require that neither the physician nor patient knows in advance the treatment to be given before entering a trial. Randomization makes the treatment groups "alike on the average" with respect to all factors that are likely to affect the principal end points of a trial. Randomization ensures that each patient has the same opportunity of being assigned to any of the therapies in the trial. In actual practice, a randomization schedule is generated by a computer or from a table of random numbers (16).

Randomized clinical trials (often designated as RCTs) are regarded by many investigators as the "ideal" scientific standard for comparing therapies. Randomization creates balanced patient subgroups with the same average baseline characteristics. This "balance" not only applies to known but to unknown prognostic factors as well, and randomization eliminates both physician and patient selection biases. The former refers to the physician creating a bias by only putting a special class of patients in one of the treatment arms (e.g., assigning patients in the poorest physical condition to the least toxic treatment). The patient selection bias refers to a comparable bias but is induced by the patient.

Another implicit advantage of an RCT is that the experimental therapy is compared with a concurrent control group. Hence, every group in the trial will have the same criteria for diagnosing and staging of disease, patient management, supportive care, and the same data quality and methods of evaluation.

Despite widespread acceptance of the scientific merits of randomization, many physicians are reluctant to participate in RCTs (14). The principal reason for nonparticipation is that physicians feel that the patient–physician relationship is compromised if the physician must explain to the patient that the treatment for their cancer would be chosen by a "coin toss" or "computer." The U.S. Code of Federal Regulations governing human experimentation has been interpreted to imply that a physician must tell the patient about the use of randomization. Thus, as a result of the nonparticipation by subpopulations with disease, results of an RCT may not necessarily apply to the entire patient population. Caution must be exercised when extrapolating the inference from a clinical trial to the entire population with disease.

An interesting example of biases that arise in physician and patient selection is illustrated in the trial reported by Antman and colleagues (2). An RCT was carried out jointly by the Dana Farber Cancer Institute and the Massachusetts General Hospital for the treatment of sarcoma (intermediate, high grade). The trial compared Adriamycin against observation (i.e., no active treatment). Over a period of time, there were 84 eligible patients seen among both institutions, of whom only 36 were entered in the RCT. Among the 48 patients who did not go in the trial, patient or physician refusal each accounted for 50%. Of these 48 patients, 29 did not receive any active treatment and for all practical purposes received the same treatment as the control treatment of the RCT. Thus, the control arm and a portion of the patient population (nonrandomized) can be compared. The 20-month disease-free survival for the control patients in the RCT was 64% compared with 16% for the nonrandomized patients receiving no treatment; the 30-month survival was 68% for the RCT controls, compared with 29% for the nonrandomized "controls." Even after adjustment for differences in prognostic factors, the differences still persisted. This example illustrates the need for concurrent control groups.

Because of the unpopularity of RCTs with many physicians, many nonrandomized trials aim to make conclusions about the value of an experimental treatment. Generally, data on an experimental treatment is generated prospectively and compared with a historic "control" group of patients. Of course, if the value of the treatment is overwhelmingly beneficial, no comparison may be necessary. For example, if patients with pancreatic cancer are living long periods of time (e.g., 5 years) without evidence of disease, no formal comparison is necessary, because we know that the prognosis of this disease is uniformly dismal. Unfortunately, the available therapies for cancer are not likely to result in dramatic benefits. Consequently, the benefit of an active therapy is likely to be of moderate magnitude, requiring care in its evaluation. Moderate benefits are, however, of real clinical importance (e.g., increasing the cure rate of breast cancer by 10–20%, will result in saving thousands of lives).

The use of historical controls for evaluating the benefits of an experimental therapy is fraught with many problems. There are ample opportunities for serious biases to distort the conclusions, and even when known biases are considered, there may be other unknown biases that can distort the conclusions of a clinical trial. Nevertheless, nonrandomized trials may be important as part of the overall scientific process in evaluating an experimental treatment. They have a role in pilot and exploratory studies as well as in phase II trials. Consider a phase II study to identify an active drug or drug combination. Good scientific strategy would dictate that the study be carried out in the most desirable conditions possible to identify an active therapy (e.g., selection of patient population). Comparison of the magnitude of the effect with other available therapies, however, is best done with an RCT.

The reporting of a nonrandomized trial requires special care, especially when claims are made about efficacy. Reporting should address the potential biases that could affect the conclusions, such as the six discussed below that arise in all nonrandomized trials which employ a comparison with a historical control group:

1. *Physician Selection Bias*. Selection of patients for the experimental treatment may be biased; this is not true in RCTs.

2. *Patient Selection Bias*. Patients self-select themselves for the experimental treatment. There is no self-selection in the historical control group, and this leads to potential biases in comparing outcome with a historical control group. RCTs have patient self-selection only for those who enter the trial. However, because the assignment to treatment is randomized, the self-selection does not bias comparisons between therapies within the same trial.
3. *Diagnosis and Staging*. Methods of diagnosis and staging must be the same for the experimental therapy and the historical groups. If methods have improved during recent years, this may not be reflected in the historical control group. For example, a significant number of newly diagnosed cases of breast cancer are found by mammography. This precludes using a historical group for comparisons of adjuvant treatment unless one accounts for the method of diagnosis. This problem does not exist with a concurrent control group.
4. *Patient Management and Supportive Care*. This must be the same for both groups.
5. *Evaluation Methods*. This factor reflects on the quality of data. If the historical control group has significant missing or unknown data for important variables, then unbiased comparisons may be impossible.
6. *Prognostic Factors*. The key prognostic factors must be the same for both groups. Statistical adjustments often can be used to make the groups comparable when the prognostic factors are known. It is not possible to adjust when data are missing or if there are unknown prognostic factors.

Some investigators have suggested that complex staging is a strong argument against the use of historical controls. For example, at one time, metastatic colon cancer was considered to be incurable. Early stages had variable prognoses with a high death rate. When adjuvant therapy became available through clinical trials, staging was pursued much more vigorously. As a result, more lymph nodes are now examined, multiple step sections made, and liver biopsies carried out. Consequently, a higher proportion of more recent patients may be in a better prognostic state than controls, even though they may both be classified in the same stage. Because they have better prognoses, their survival will be greater than the historical controls.

Use of consecutive patients for generating data on the new treatment and use of "matched" controls are two common methods for investigating new treatments without resorting to randomization. Both have drawbacks. Entering consecutive patients in a study eliminates the opportunity for physician bias that is associated with the selection of patients. If patient consent is necessary, however, a patient selection bias will still be present. If the mix of patients has not changed over time, the prognostic variables associated with each group may be comparable; however, issues such as patient bias, diagnosis and staging, patient management and supportive care, and different methods of evaluation still must be considered. The consecutive patient experimental design is targeted mainly at eliminating bias arising from physician selection of patients.

Employment of matched controls is another method often used to compare a new treatment with a historical control. This involves forming a group of one or more control patients for each patient receiving the new treatment. Patients are selected from the historical group so that they are comparable to the new treatment group on a patient-by-patient basis for known prognostic variables. This method is limited in that only a few key variables can be matched on any practical basis. For example, in matching, one would perhaps aim to have patients who are comparable with respect to anatomic staging, pathology, performance status, and extra disease characteristics such as demographic factors, prior treatment history, and so forth.

Statistical modeling is a generalization of matching that enables one to adjust for several factors simultaneously. This method also has limitations, however, because the statistical adjustment for bias introduces additional variability in the analysis from the "uncertainty" of the adjustment. Such adjustments can be made only for known prognostic factors. Patient and physician self-selection cannot be factored into the adjustments; neither can questions about different criteria for diagnosis and staging, different methods of patient support and management, and different methods of evaluation.

In summary, the nonrandomized methods for the evaluation of new therapies are useful for exploratory and pilot studies. They are not to be relied on for generating credible conclusions, unless the issues of potential biases are carefully discussed or the therapy outcome is so dramatic that it could not be credited to the aggregate effect of the potential biases.

Another type of nonrandomized study that will likely gain more popularity in the future is the study attempting to correlate disease markers with survival. The simplest example is to relate tumor response for measurable disease with eventual survival. The logic is that patients enter a trial with a positive disease marker (e.g., tumor), receive treatment, and the tumor becomes smaller or disappears. Survival comparisons are made between patient groups with positive marker vs. negative marker (i.e., tumor has significant reduction in volume or disappears). A straightforward comparison as described is invalid (1), the reason being that the longer a patient lives, the greater the opportunity to observe a change in disease marker status. This means that even if a change in marker status is not related to increased survival, a direct comparison of survival data on negative vs. positive disease markers will show a positive relationship. This relationship is spurious; however, new statistical techniques of analysis are being developed that can overcome this problem (8). It is expected that the new techniques will strengthen phase II studies in that they will enable inferences to be made relating a change in marker status to survival (or any other appropriate time metric). Inference, however, will only be able to answer the question, "Is a change in disease marker positively related to survival for the patients under study?"

MULTICENTER VS. SINGLE-CENTER TRIALS

The available experimental therapies for cancer are likely to have only moderate benefit. Nevertheless, a moderate benefit can be important. For example, the number of cases

Table 26.1. Characterization of Clinical Trials

Phase	Single center		Multicenter	
	Randomized	Nonrandomized	Randomized	Nonrandomized
I	Never	Yes	Never	Rare
II	Rare	Yes	Yes	Yes
III	Yes	Use of historical controls	Yes	Use of historical controls

of breast cancer diagnosed in a year is estimated to be more than 190,000 in the United States. Approximately 50% of these new cases have positive axillary nodal involvement. If the cure rate were increased by 10%, then at least 9,000 more women would be cured every year.

The end points for nearly all definitive phase III studies are survival or the disease-free period. Furthermore, the clinical course of the disease is complicated and highly variable. As a consequence of both the need for making an inference on survival and the variability of data, it is necessary to have a relatively long follow-up time with a large number of patients. Because few hospitals have enough patients to meet this need, it is necessary to carry out these phase III trials using many co-operating hospitals. Consequently, nearly all phase III trials are multicenter trials in which patients are pooled into a common study. Carrying out a multicenter trial results in increased administrative difficulties and quality assurance problems; it is one of the most difficult and complicated experiments in science.

Multicenter studies are not only used in phase III clinical trials but in phase II trials as well. The use of multicenters enables patient-accrual goals to be achieved much more rapidly. Table 26.1 is a summary of current practice regarding multicenter studies and their use in phase I, II, and III trials.

Planning Clinical Trials

OVERALL CONSIDERATIONS

The overall planning for a clinical trial depends critically on whether the trial is an "exploratory" or a "management" trial. A management trial seeks to determine whether a therapy is beneficial under conditions as close to clinical circumstances as possible. (Sometimes the term *demonstration trial* is used to describe a management trial.) A management trial should be carried out by a large number of hospitals; when the trial is collecting data from many representative hospitals, it will be possible to determine if a therapy is beneficial. An exploratory trial seeks to determine whether a therapy is efficacious under ideal or restricted circumstances, which may not necessarily correspond to a practical clinical situation.

Objectives in clinical trials may vary greatly. Possible objectives are (*a*) to find the best overall treatment, (*b*) to find the best treatment by prognostic subgroup, (*c*) to determine the relationship between the natural history of disease and treatment, (*d*) to identify an active treatment, and (*e*) to evaluate the effects of augmenting a beneficial therapy.

The choice of the eligible patient population in a trial is crucial to reaching accrual goals in a reasonable time. It is necessary to decide whether to have narrow eligibility requirements, so that patients are relatively homogeneous with regard to baseline prognostic variables, or to have broad eligibility requirements that will accelerate accrual. The pros and cons about this choice of the population depend on whether it is a management or exploratory trial. If the trial is exploratory, then having a relatively homogeneous patient population will result in less variability in the end points of the trial and make the trial more sensitive at showing real differences among treatments. Alternatively, if the trial is management, there is some advantage in having broad eligibility criteria, because one will be able to explore how therapy benefit varies among subgroups of patients; using post-hoc stratification and statistical modeling in the analysis will reduce the statistical fluctuations generated from having heterogeneous patient groups. An operational problem with defining narrow eligibility criteria is that accrual may take a long time.

Another basic decision in the choice of population is to determine if the patient population should be newly diagnosed patients or should include those who have been shown to be refractory to beneficial therapies. A newly diagnosed patient represents the most promising "patient material" for study. On the other hand, it is necessary to consider the ethics of withholding therapies of proven benefit in favor of an experimental treatment of unknown benefit. If one chooses to use a patient population that is refractory to beneficial therapies, then it may not be possible to evaluate the experimental therapy suitably. This decision on choice of patient population must balance the ethics of denying a patient a beneficial (but still noncurative) therapy with the opportunity of a patient receiving an experimental therapy with the potential of significantly better benefit.

Another consideration in planning a study is to determine the treatment plan if a patient has failed or does not appear to benefit from the treatment. Does one not change the treatment, or should a new therapy plan be prescribed? If the end point is survival, then introducing a new therapy may complicate interpretation of the survival data. If the protocol does not specify what to do after failure, however, the attending physicians may introduce a large number of new therapies, which will complicate the interpretation of the survival data even further.

It generally is accepted that phase III trials should be randomized. However, should phase II trials be randomized? Because the object of a phase II trial is to determine if there is any activity against the disease rather than to make comparisons with other therapies, most are nonrandomized. One reason for evaluating several therapies in the same phase II trial, however, is to evaluate them simultaneously with the same clinical trial process and for the same patient population. Another strategy is to include a treatment with proven benefit but which has not yet been used on the phase II patient population as one of the therapies. If the proven therapy cannot demonstrate benefit, then the phase II trial may not have a suitable patient population to permit the evaluation of experimental therapies. Thus, if several therapies are to be evaluated in the same phase II trial, randomization should be used for the treatment assignment.

What endpoints should be chosen to evaluate the therapies? There is widespread agreement that adjuvant trials should use survival as an end point; however, patients with recurrent disease will receive additional or alternate therapies. This will certainly be true for placebo or no-treatment control patients. Those on therapy also will receive alternate therapies on recurrence. Thus, survival data may not be clear-cut. Other end points could be the disease-free period and time to "progression" (progression must be carefully defined). Phase II trials often use tumor response or other disease markers. In practice, there will be a number of end points in any trial.

During the past few years, use of surrogate markers as the major end point of phase III studies has increased. Some disease markers have a high correlation with survival. The idea is that conclusions about treatment benefit can be made in a shorter time frame. For example, many phase III trials in AIDS use the CD4+ counts as the major end point. In cancer, complete responses may have a high correlation with survival. One problem with using a gross measurement like complete response in cancer vs. a survival end point is that in many cancers, the anticipated frequency of complete responses still is too low to provide meaningful comparisons.

Quality of life issues are being widely recognized as important end points in cancer (see Chapter 20). A patient cured of leukemia by bone marrow transplantation but who has chronic graft-vs.-host disease has a severely compromised quality of life. The paper by Goldhirsch and colleagues (6) discusses new methods for objectively evaluating quality of life and represents an important advance. They call their method Q-TWiST (Quality-adjusted Time Without Symptoms and Toxicity of treatment).

STATISTICAL TESTS AND PROBABILITIES OF REACHING INCORRECT CONCLUSIONS

Almost all clinical trials are analyzed using statistical procedures that are based on the frequency theory of probability. This simply means that if, for example, an outcome has a probability of happening of 10% in an experiment, then in an infinite number of repetitions of that experiment, one would observe the outcome 10% of the time. It will be assumed in the following discussion that probability statements refer to the relative frequency notion of probability.

Consider a trial in which two treatments are being evaluated. After the trial is completed and an analysis made, the two main conclusions are that (*a*) the treatments are equivalent, or (*b*) the treatments differ. These conclusions are referred to as the null and alternate hypotheses, respectively. The statistical procedures (called tests) chosen for analysis enable the specification of the error probabilities:

α: probability of concluding treatments are different when they are actually the same

β: probability of concluding treatments are the same when they are actually different.

The two probabilities often are referred to as type I and II errors, respectively. These error probabilities are the false-positive and false-negative rates, respectively (i.e., calling a result positive when it should be negative, and calling a result negative when it should be positive).

The practical application of these tests is that using observed data from the trial, one calculates a probability or significance level. This is the probability of observing the same or more extreme differences among therapies than those observed if the two treatments actually are equivalent. The reasoning behind the probability calculations is that if the investigator is willing to accept the differences observed in the trial as being scientific evidence in favor of a difference between the two treatments, then the scientific evidence would be stronger if the differences were larger than those observed. This probability is called a tail area, significance level, or simply the *P* value. If the *P* value is less than .05, then the practice is to accept the hypothesis that the treatments differ. Thus, if the treatments truly are equivalent, the probability would be less than 5% that the observed differences could have arisen from statistical fluctuations in the data.

The power or sensitivity of a test is equal to $1 - \beta$ and denotes the probability that the clinical trial will be able to detect differences among the treatments when in fact the differences are real. The power is fundamental in planning all clinical trials. It depends on the significance level chosen, the number of patients in the trial, and the magnitude of the difference between the treatments. Large numbers of patients and large differences between treatments increase the power. For studies in which survival is an end point, longer follow-up time also increases the power. When a trial concludes with "no difference between the treatments" or the result is not "statistically significant," it may be because either (*a*) there is no difference between the treatments or (*b*) the power of the trial was so low that the trial could not detect a difference.

We illustrate here the concept of power and its relation to sample size in a phase I trial. Suppose that a phase I trial is being conducted to determine the probability of life-threatening toxicity from an experimental drug. Suppose that if no life-threatening toxicity is observed, the drug will be declared to be "free of life-threatening toxicity." Table 26.2 shows the relationship between true toxicity rate, number of patients, and the power (i.e., probability of observing at least one life-threatening toxic event). For example, if only five patients are in the trial and the true toxicity rate is 10%, there is only a 41% probability of observing one or more toxic reactions. As the sample size increases, this probability goes to unity. Similarly, if the true toxic rate is high, it is easy to show that the power is increased (e.g., if the toxic rate is 40% and only five patients are in the trial, the power is 0.92). This

Table 26.2. Probability of Observing at Least One Toxic Event as a Function of True Rate and Number of Patients in Trial[a]

True toxicity (%)	Patients (n)			
	5	10	20	30
10	.41	.65	.88	.96
20	.67	.89	.99	.999
30	.89	.97	.999	1.0
40	.92	.994	1.0	1.0
50	.97	.999	1.0	1.0

[a] If true toxicity is 10% and observations are made on 10 patients, there is a probability of .65 that at least one of the patients will show toxicity.

Table 26.3. Number of Patients Per Treatment Required to Detect Differences Between Proportions for Different Values of Power[a]

Proportion comparisons	Power				
	0.3	0.5	0.7	0.8	0.9
55 vs. 60%	406	752	1,202	1,530	2,050
50 vs. 60%	103	190	304	390	520
40 vs. 60%	27	48	77	97	130
30 vs. 60%	12	22	34	44	56

[a] The test assumes a two-sided, false-positive rate of 5%.

same table also can be used to determine the probability of observing one or more responses or solutions to any problem in which events are being observed.

As another example of the use of power in a clinical trial, consider a trial in which the proportion of recurrences is the principal end point of interest. Suppose that one desires to calculate the sample size necessary to detect a difference between two groups when one has a recurrence rate of 60% and another may have a possible recurrence rate within the range 30 to 55%. Table 26.3 shows the number of patients per treatment for different levels of power comparing the two recurrence rates. For example, one needs more than 2,000 patients for each treatment group to have a power of 0.9 to detect a difference between 55% vs. 60%. However, the sample size is reduced to 130 patients per group to test 40% vs. 60% for the same power (0.9). It is clear that increasing the number of patients results in an increase in power. Also, as the differences between groups become large, a high level of power can be attained for the same sample size.

In practice, one does not know the recurrence rates to compare. Therefore, a range of comparisons is chosen based on past data that are of clinical interest, and a sample size is then chosen that will give high power. Generally, a power less than 0.8 for clinically important differences is unacceptable in planning a trial.

DATA COLLECTION AND FORMS DESIGN

There is a great deal of misunderstanding over the amount of data required to evaluate a clinical trial properly. Ordinarily, clinical trials performed by the pharmaceutical industry with the intent of submitting the trial to the FDA for drug ap-

Table 26.4. Characteristics of Data Collection Forms in Cancer Clinical Trials

Form identification	Data items
On study	Identification, demographic characteristics, disease presentation, prior treatment history, special tests, protocol treatment
Flow sheet(s)	Record of each visit, treatment given, tests, disease assessment, intercurrent medications, toxicity, psychologic assessment, other events
Evaluation (at end of every step in study)	Summary of outcome, toxicity, medications received, confounding events
Follow-up (periodic)	Patient status
Death form	Cause of death, autopsy results if available
Final evaluation	Summary of relevant patient information
Special forms	Surgery, pathology, radiation therapy, psychological assessments (self or observer), special diagnostic tests

proval collect very large amounts of data. A great deal of these data may be unnecessary and it is not uncommon to have data forms exceeding 100 pages for each patient. One reason motivating the large collection of data items is the "antagonistic" relationship between the FDA and industry. Essentially, industry-sponsored data-collection plans have the theme "to leave no stone unturned." Another motivating factor is that many trials are planned to show that two treatments are equivalent ("me too trials"). Usually, a new drug is compared with a competitor's drug that already has received FDA approval. Large amounts of data are collected in these trials to answer unanticipated questions that might be raised by the FDA.

Disregarding the special problems between the FDA and industry, data chosen for collection in a clinical trial must supply information to determine (*a*) eligibility of the patient, (*b*) whether the protocol was followed, and (*c*) objective measures of the study end points. In general, the more data collected, the greater the opportunity for data degradation. A nonrandomized study attempting to make treatment comparisons ordinarily would require a greater amount of data to check for biases than a randomized study would. A randomized study, by definition, has comparable patient groups that differ only in the treatment assigned to those groups.

In general, a cancer clinical trial is likely to have six different types of forms for collecting data as well as special forms. The data forms and types of information collected are outlined in Table 26.4.

Data forms should be designed so they are self-coding. As much as possible, boxes should only need to be checked to supply information. Care should be taken to prevent the person filling in the form from making interpretive decisions (e.g., calling a toxicity life-threatening). Space should be provided to allow the physician to note or comment on special features of the patient that were not collected by the data form or that require further comment.

EXPERIMENTAL DESIGN

This section briefly discusses experimental designs for randomized studies. Generally, phase III cancer clinical trials have two to four treatment groups. The reason for keeping the number of treatments small is that the patient-consent process requires the physician to discuss all treatment options with the patient. Having more than four treatment programs likely will confuse the patient. The logistics of having a large number of treatments in a multicenter trial also may be overwhelming.

Clinical trials ordinarily are designed using stratified randomization (16). After a patient is found to be eligible for a trial, he or she may be classified into two or more subgroups or strata that are defined by available data at the time of registering a patient into the trial. The subgroup should be defined so that patients in the same stratum have a more common prognosis than those from different strata. For example, a study for advanced breast cancer may have eight strata defined by: (*a*) performance status (0, 1 vs. 2, 3), (*b*) number of recurrent sites (two or less vs. more than two), and (*c*) disease-free interval (1 year vs. more than 1 year). All possible combinations of these three factors result in eight distinct strata. In each stratum, the treatments are assigned at random. Stratification tends to balance the treatment assignments so that treatment groups are equally balanced among the different strata. This is especially important in the early stages of a study, in which only a small number of patients have been registered. If unexpected events are observed (e.g., unusual toxicities) within a treatment group, one would be able to analyze whether the events arose from an aggregate of prognostic factors in one treatment group that was not present in other groups. As the number of patients becomes large, the patient groups tend to be comparable on the average, and the need for stratification diminishes or even disappears. Relatively small clinical trials always should be stratified, however.

There are obvious practical limits to the number of strata that can be used. If there is a large number of strata relative to the number of patients, then many of the strata will not have any patients. Having empty strata does not cause a loss of efficiency. If the number of patients in a single stratum is less than the number of treatments, there will be a loss of efficiency. For example, if there are two treatments, then all strata containing only one patient will not contribute to the analysis unless additional modeling assumptions are made.

Table 26.5. Experimental Designs for Phase III Randomized Trials[a]

Name	Design	Comment
Simple two treatment	[R] — A; — B	Compare A vs. B
Adjuvant treatment	[R] — A; — A + B	Does addition of B to A result in greater benefit?
Combination	[R] — A; — B; — A + B	Is A + B superior to each alone?
New treatment after event (event may be failure, response, or a fixed period of time)	[R] — A, — B → [E] — C	Compare treatment programs A or B followed by C
Common initial treatment	A — [E] — [R] — B; — C	Compare treatment program A followed by B or C
Cross-over	[R] — A — [E] — B; — B — [E] — A	Compare A vs. B both before and after event
Two randomizations	[R] — A, — B → [E] — [R] — C; — D	Compare A vs. B Compare C vs. D after event

[a]E—event; R—randomize.

In practice, the maximum number of patient/disease variables in a trial is approximately 12 to 15 for trials involving several hundred patients. A rough "rule of thumb" is

$$(\text{number of patients per treatment})/(\text{number of strata}) \geq 4.$$

Table 26.5 shows a variety of experimental designs that are useful in phase III trials. It is assumed that the only patients who are randomized are those who have given consent. As the designs become more complicated, the statistical methods for analysis also become more complex.

Another design that should be used more often is the factorial experiment. Suppose that the class of therapies can be characterized by two factors, which will be designated as A and B (e.g., A might refer to drug A and B to drug B). Suppose that drugs A and B are given at two doses, A_0, A_1 for drug A and B_0 and B_1 for drug B. Then, there will be four drug combinations, given by A_0B_0, A_0B_1, A_1B_0, and A_1B_1. If the clinical trial is carried out with these four groups, then one can determine: (*a*) if a low dose is different from a higher dose of A or B, and (*b*) if there is an interaction (i.e., synergy) between A and B. In general, the factors may refer to different modalities of treatment or to dose or schedule. The advantage of a factorial design is that it enables two questions to be answered for the same patient. Factorial experiments need not be restricted to two factors, however, and the number of conditions for each factor need not be two. Even so, because of the need to keep the number of treatment groups small, the factorial design with two factors each under two different conditions appears to be the most practical in clinical trials.

In some instances, it may be possible to investigate simultaneously three factors, each at two conditions, by having only four treatments. Consider the case where an investigation is planned to explore three drugs (denoted by A, B, and C) each at two different doses. All possible combinations result in eight distinct treatments; however, by choosing a special set of four treatments, it is possible to investigate the contribution to outcome for each drug by changing the dose. There are two sets of four treatments that can be chosen for this purpose. If the dose levels are designated by (A_0, A_1), (B_0, B_1), and (C_0, C_1), then any treatment combination will be made up of three letters where the subscript 0 or 1 denotes the dose. The two sets of four treatment combinations, each of which is suitable for a trial, are

$$\text{Set I: } A_0B_0C_0,\ A_0B_1C_1,\ A_1B_0C_1,\ A_1B_1C_0$$

$$\text{Set II: } A_0B_0C_1,\ A_0B_1C_0,\ A_1B_0C_0,\ A_1B_1C_1.$$

Note that the two sets together comprise the eight possible treatment combinations. This experimental design is called a Latin square or, equivalently, a "$\frac{1}{2}$ replicate of a 2^3 factorial design."

Some care must be exercised in making these comparisons. If it was necessary to change the doses of A and B when C is added, then the comparison of $A_1B_1C_1$ with $A_1B_1C_0$ may not properly reflect the change in outcome with the addition of C. In other words, the two drugs A and B have different doses when combined with C compared to the two-drug combination A and B without C.

ROLE OF COMPLIANCE

One of the key problems in interpreting results of a clinical trial is the effect of compliance on the conclusions. If the conclusions of a trial result in no difference between the therapies under investigation, it may be caused by a lack of compliance. The effect of noncompliance is to lower the sensitivity of a trial at finding differences as well as to create possible biases.

As an example of the potential for bias, consider a randomized clinical trial comparing two treatment programs for head and neck cancer. One therapy is radiation followed by surgery; the other is surgery followed by radiation. Patients in whom the disease has disappeared after radiation may refuse surgery; whereas patients doing poorly after surgery may refuse radiation. For the first treatment program, the better prognosis patients do not comply, while in the other, the poorer prognosis patients do not comply.

To understand more fully the role of bias and loss of efficiency, we use a simple mathematical model. Consider a trial comparing two treatments A and B. Let the proportion of noncompliers be P_a and P_b for the two treatments, respectively. Also let the outcome for each treatment be m_a and m_b for compliers and m_a' and m_b' for noncompliers. (The outcome could be the proportion of responders, the median survival, or whatever is appropriate.) Then, the average outcome for each treatment group will consist of a mixture of outcomes of compliers and noncompliers. Define M_a and M_b as the aggregate outcome for each group. We can write M_a and M_b as

$$M_a = (1 - P_a)m_a + P_a m_a'$$
$$M_b = (1 - P_b)\, m_b + P_b m_b'$$

Note that the effect of noncompliance is to dilute the outcomes for each group. The comparison ($M_a - M_b$), which compares treatment A with treatment B, is

$$M_a - M_b = (m_a - m_b) + P_a(m_a' - m_a) - P_b(m_b' - m_b). \quad (1)$$

Now consider a case in which there is no difference between treatments for compliers ($m_a = m_b = m$) and noncompliers ($m'_a = m'_b = m'$). Then, the value of ($M_a - M_b$) is

$$M_a - M_b = (P_a - P_b)\,(m' - m).$$

which will result in a bias if the noncompliance rates P_a, P_b are different and if $m \neq m'$. As a result, the analysis could show a difference between treatments when in truth there is none.

As another example, suppose that treatment A is an observation group having complete compliance ($P_a = 0$). Suppose that treatment B is an experimental therapy and noncompliance is simply not taking the medication. Then, the noncompliers on the intervention arm are likely to have the same outcome as the compliers on the observation treatment arm ($m_b' = m_a$). Hence, substituting $P_a = 0$ and $m_b' = m_a$ in Equation 1 gives

$$M_a - M_b = (1 - P_b)\,(m_a - m_b).$$

Thus, the effect of noncompliance is to make the treatment difference smaller. (The multiplier ($1 - P_b$) is always less than 1 unless $P_b = 0$, in which case it is unity.) The net

Table 26.6. Proportion Not Complying vs. Statistical Efficiency (One Treatment Group Is an Observational Group)

Proportion not complying	Statistical efficiency
0.0	1.0
0.10	0.81
0.25	0.56
0.50	0.25

Table 26.7 Average Compliance vs. Statistical Efficiency Trials (Noncompliance Refers to Receiving Intervention Treatment of Other Group)

$P = (P_a + P_b)/2$	Statistical efficiency
0.0	1.0
0.10	0.64
0.25	0.25
0.40	0.04

effect of noncompliance for patients assigned to B is to lower the statistical efficiency. The statistical efficiency is $(1 - P_b)^2$. Table 26.6 is instructive about statistical efficiencies for various values of P_b. The statistical efficiency means that if, for example, the proportion not complying is 10%, it is equivalent to using effectively only 81% of the accrual. In other words, 100 patients having a 10% noncompliance rate is equivalent to having 81 patients who completely comply.

Compliance issues are fundamentally important in cancer prevention trials. Consider a clinical trial in which A is an observation arm and B an intervention aimed at preventing cancer. Contemplated interventions may be to reduce smoking, reduce intake of dietary fats, or similar activity. However, it is quite possible that individuals in the control group will not comply because they eliminated smoking or changed their diet. In this case, $m'_a = m_b$ and $m'_b = m_a$. (Those in the control group who adopt the intervention are noncompliers but will have the same expected outcome as compliers in the intervention group; similarly, those in the intervention group who do not comply will have the same outcome as the compliers in the control groups.) Substituting $m'_a = m_b$ and $m'_b = m_a$ in Equation 1 results in

$$M_a - M_b = (1 - P_a - P_b)\,(m_a - m_b).$$

Note that it is necessary for the sum of the two noncompliance rates to be less than unity ($P_a + P_b < 1$), otherwise the multiplier will be negative. Also, even though $(m_a - m_b)$ may be positive, $M_a - M_b$ will be negative. Thus, trials with very large noncompliance rates will be worthless. The statistical efficiency in this case is $(1 - P_a - P_b)^2$. Table 26.7 shows how the statistical efficiency changes with the average compliance rate $P = (P_a + P_b)/2$. Thus, a trial with a 10% noncompliance rate is only 64% efficient and is losing approximately one-third of its effective number of patients.

As an example of the reality of noncompliance, one can use the experience of the Multiple Risk Factor Intervention Trial, often referred to as the MRFIT Trial (10). The intervention consisted of an educational program to change the lifestyle habits thought to be risk factors for coronary heart disease. Smoking was the most important factor and it is interesting to note that 30% of the control group gave up smoking compared with 46% of the intervention group. Thus, $P_a = 0.30$ and $P_b = 0.54$. Hence, the statistical efficiency of this trial is $(1 - 0.30 - 0.54)^2 = 0.0256$. The study enrolled 12,866 men. Therefore, with a statistical efficiency of 2.56%, this trial was equivalent to having $(0.0256) \times (12{,}866) = 320$ men who complied 100%.

INTERIM ANALYSES, MULTIPLE LOOKS AT DATA, AND EARLY STOPPING

Nearly all ongoing clinical trials are monitored at periodic intervals both in the accrual and follow-up phases. A common time period for such monitoring is every 6 months. At these times, an interim analysis is performed to review the toxicity and end point data. If the toxicity is unexpectedly high, the trial is likely to be modified. Also, if one treatment appears to be significantly superior or inferior to the other under investigation, ethical considerations would dictate that the trial be terminated or modified. Results of these interim analyses are reviewed by the principals who are responsible for carrying out the trial (Study Chair, Study Statistician, Key Investigators); in many instances, there may be a disinterested, formal monitoring committee charged with reviewing interim analyses. In a multicenter trial, detailed interim analyses ordinarily are not made available to all trial participants unless the outcome information is blinded with respect to treatment identification. The reason for masking treatment identification with respect to end point data is to avoid accrual to a study being influenced by statistical fluctuations in the end point data. Toxicity information usually is identified, but even this can influence the subsequent conduct of a trial.

The decision to terminate a trial early because of the apparent inferiority or superiority of one or more therapies is a difficult problem. The difficulty arises because the false-positive rate (i.e., the probability of concluding a therapy is beneficial when it is not) increases as the number of interim analyses increases. For example, if a clinical trial is planned to have a false-positive rate of 5% at every interim analysis, then that rate would be changed to 14% if there were five interim analyses. The false-positive rate is changed because the more occasions the data are reviewed, the greater the opportunity that a large statistical fluctuation may be mistaken for a real effect. Table 26.8 shows how the false-positive rate changes with a varying number of multiple "looks" at the data.

In recent years, new statistical techniques have been developed to aid decision making on the early stopping of clinical trials. The idea behind these methods is that one specifies not only the overall false-positive and false-negative rates, as in conventional clinical trials, but also the number of "looks" at data and the maximal sample size of the trial. This results in objective rules for early stopping. These methods are called "sequential methods," and they are modifications of concepts from the era of World War II, when sequential methods were developed for the acceptance sampling of

Table 26.8. Multiple "Looks" at Data vs. False-Positive Rate[a]

Number of "looks"	False-positive rate
1	.05
2	.08
3	.11
4	.13
5	.14
10	.19

[a] The larger the number of interim analyses ("looks"), the greater the chance of finding false-positive effects. This same table can be used to determine the overall false-positive rate of an experiment when the analysis "looks" at several subgroups separately. For example, if there are five subgroups in a study, where each is analyzed separately with a 5% false-positive rate, then the overall false-positive rate is 14%.

equipment. Essentially, these sequential methods are derived so that at each interim analysis, the trial may be stopped if the significance level of the statistical tests comparing the treatments is very low. For example, an early stopping rule for a trial with five interim analyses may stop the trial if the first analysis was significant at the $P = .00001$ level; stopping at the second analysis would be done if the results were significant at the $P = .001$ level, with subsequent stopping rules if the significance levels were $P = .008$, $P = .023$, and $P = .041$ for the third, fourth, and fifth interim analyses, respectively. This set of rules preserves an overall 5% false-positive rate for the trial. In essence, the trial results would have to be very dramatic to result in early stopping of the trial.

In practice, these rules should only serve as a guide to aid investigators. It is especially important in using these rules that the data are current, recently reviewed, and that prognostic subgroups are comparable between the various treatments being compared.

If sequential method trials continue to the last interim analysis, it generally results in an approximately 5 to 20% increase in sample size compared with a study design with a preassigned, fixed number of patients. The potential gain in using sequential methods is to have the option of terminating the trial in the accrual phase of the study. This option may be realized in trials in which the end point is the proportion of responders, but it is not likely to happen when the end point is survival. An experiment carried out by Rosner and Tsiatis (12) is particularly instructive. They reviewed 72 completed studies from the Eastern Cooperative Oncology Group in which survival or some other time metric was an end point. Various sequential experimental plans were superimposed to determine what would have happened if the studies had been originally designed to have early stopping. They found that among the 72 studies, 66 (92%) would have terminated earlier using the best sequential plan. (They simulated four different sequential plans.) Among these, 26 (36%) would have been terminated in the accrual phase. It is particularly important to note that all conclusions made from the sequential analysis simulation agreed with those made by the clinical investigators using the full data set. This study shows that the use of sequential methods in clinical trials can result in a positive gain. A fuller discussion of sequential methods in the context of cancer trials can be found in Geller (5).

STRATEGY OF EXPERIMENTATION

There are a very large number of cancer clinical trials being carried on throughout the world and a positive outcome is likely to affect clinical practice. One question that arises is: what proportion of these trials reporting beneficial results is true? The answer is important in deciding when a practicing physician should adopt a new therapy.

To discuss this problem, it is necessary to understand how conclusions from a trial are made. All analyses of clinical trials use statistical methods that are based on concepts of the probabilities of making incorrect decisions. The previous section discussed statistical tests and the role of false-positive and false-negative rates (i.e., the false positive rate refers to the probability of concluding positive benefit when there is no benefit, the false-negative rate is the probability of concluding there is no benefit when a treatment is beneficial). In addition to these concepts, we need another, which is the "prior probability of success." This depends on the level of clinical innovation and basic science that motivates the trial. Prior probability of success is subjective and cannot be measured objectively; however, it increases with knowledge of successful exploratory or pilot studies. Phase III studies should only be initiated based on successful exploratory and phase II studies; alternatively, if a trial tests a drug combination in which each individual drug is without benefit, the prior probability of success will be low. What values of the prior probability of success should one adapt for cancer trials? Because the concept is subjective, it is difficult to be precise, but prior probabilities in the range of 5 to 15% seem to be reasonable for most cancer trials.

Define α, β, and θ to be:

α—false positive rate,
β—false negative rate, and
θ—prior probability of success.

Let us adopt the values $\alpha = .05$, $\beta = .7$, and $\theta = .10$. The value of $\alpha = .05$ is commonly chosen as a false positive rate in most studies; a false negative rate of $\beta = .7$ arises if one has 50 patients in each of two groups and is attempting to determine if there is a 50% difference in the median survivals of the two groups. Figure 26.1 illustrates this process for 1,000 trials. Because the false negative rate is $\beta = .7$, the true-positive rate is $1 - \beta = 0.30$. With $\theta = .10$, one can expect 100 true-positive trials; however, only 30% of these will be reported as positive. In addition, among the true-negative trials, 5% or 45 trials will be reported as false positives. Thus, there will be a total of 75 reported positive trials from among the 1,000 trials. The true-positive trials are indistinguishable from the false positive trials. Thus, the proportion of true positives among the reported 75 positives is $30/75 = .40$. Hence, with these parameters, we would expect (on the average) 4 among every 10 reported positive therapies to be true positives.

If the trials had very large patient numbers, the false-negative rate β would be close to zero. If $\beta = 0$, then all 100 true-positive trials will be reported to be positive, and the proportion of true positives would be $100/145 = .69$ (i.e., approximately 7 of 10 reported positive trials are true positives). Thus, we have shown that with a prior probability of

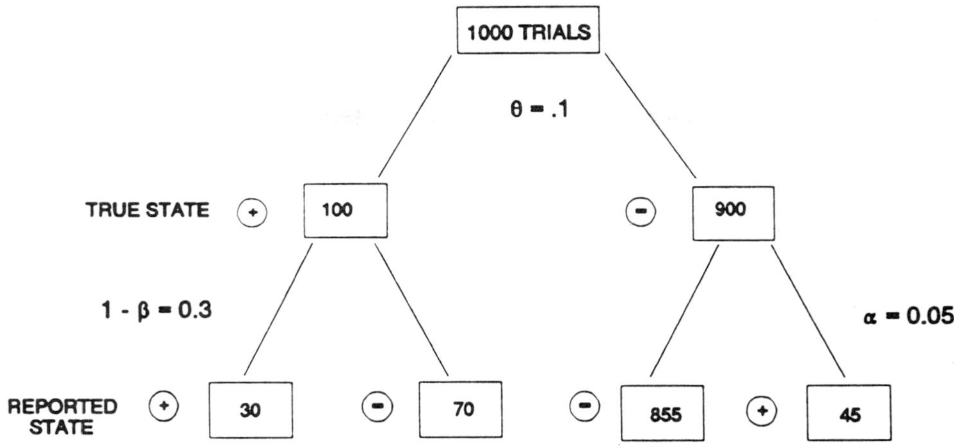

Figure 26.1. The clinical trial process θ—prior probability of success; α—false-positive probability; β—false-negative probability.

Table 26.9. Probability that a Reported Positive Treatment Is a True Positive (False-Positive Probability Fixed at 5%)[a]

θ	β		
	.7	.4	.1
.1	.40	.57	.67
.2	.60	.75	.82
.4	.80	.89	.92
.6	.90	.95	.96

[a] β—false-negative probability; θ—prior probability of success.

success of .10, the probability that a treatment reported to be beneficial is in truth beneficial may range from .40 to .69.

If $P(+)$ denotes the probability that a reported positive trial is a true positive, then we can write

$$P(+) = 1/\left[1 + \frac{1-\theta}{\theta}\frac{\alpha}{1-\beta}\right].$$

which shows that $P(+)$ depends on θ, α, and β. If θ is close to unity, then $P(+)$ is close to unity.

Table 26.9 is a summary of $P(+)$ for various values of θ and β with $\alpha = .05$. Note that as θ goes toward unity, $P(+)$ will approach unity. These considerations indicate that in assessing the conclusions of a trial reported to be positive, it is necessary to review the prior scientific evidence that led up to the trial. Also, one should avoid initiating phase III trials that are not preceded by positive pilot and phase II studies.

Reporting of Clinical Trials

The practicing oncologist must rely heavily on the published literature to help make decisions about therapy. Unfortunately, there are too many cancer sites and the current views on the systemic treatment of disease may appear to be moving too quickly for most oncologists to have personal experience with the "latest treatments." This section outlines the guidelines for assessing the quality of reporting for a clinical trial. These guidelines should be useful both to readers of the literature and authors of clinical trial manuscripts (16).

GENERAL GUIDELINES

Population Under Study

There should be clear statements describing the population under study. Major subgroups of patients who are excluded should be mentioned (e.g., "patients over age 65 were not eligible for the study").

Therapy

Reporting of the protocol therapy (especially chemotherapy) should be outlined in sufficient detail so that the therapy can be duplicated by another physician. Not only the contents of the written protocol but the therapy actually received by patients must be stated. This is especially important for chemotherapy, for which full doses as written in a protocol often may not have been given to patients. Summary measures, such as average dose per course, proportion of patients receiving incomplete courses, proportion of patients receiving full doses, and average number of courses, should be provided as well, and their effect on outcome analyzed. If the written protocol provided for a deescalation or escalation of dose(s) as a function of toxicity, details should be given. In addition, information should be given on the extent to which changes in dose followed protocol criteria.

Study Design

The study design should be outlined. A schema, which is a pictorial display of the study design, is helpful to the reader. If the study is randomized, it is not sufficient simply to state that it was a randomized study; a statement should indicate how the randomization was carried out (e.g., central randomization, closed envelope, or other methods). The actual randomization scheme should be described. Occasionally, a randomization schedule or procedure may be changed during the course of the study. If so, details should be given regarding the reasons for the change. If there is institutional balancing or other kinds of stratification, this should be stated as well.

Patient Accounting

There should be a detailed accounting of all patients registered for the study, and registration should be carefully defined. How is a patient officially registered? Are all patients officially registered before the first day of treatment or after treatment has begun? It is disappointing to learn that in many single-institution, nonrandomized studies, registration may take place months after the first day of treatment. This leaves open the possibility that not all patients on a protocol are registered. In a randomized study, patients are registered from the moment of randomization. Nonrandomized studies should have similarly precise rules for registration.

The number of patients who are classified as "canceled" or "evaluable" should be given by treatment received. A canceled patient is defined as a registered patient who withdrew from the study before the first day of treatment. An unevaluable patient may be one who has incomplete information. Some studies classify an unevaluable patient as one who has major deviations from the protocol. If the reasons for patients being classified as canceled or unevaluable relate to the treatment assignment, then it is mandatory that all patients be included in the treatment comparisons. Otherwise, the selective inclusion of patients may result in wrong conclusions being drawn from the study.

Follow-Up

The follow-up period for patients should be given separately for each treatment. Statistics should be included on the average follow-up time, the number followed for each time period (1 year, 2 years), and maximum and minimum follow-up times. The number of patients lost to follow-up and the reasons why should be reported for each treatment. If a relatively large number of patients is lost to follow-up (i.e., 10%), then statements about long-term effects may not be correct.

Data Quality

There should be a discussion of the quality control methods used for the data. Was there "Second-Party Review?" A Second-Party Review is defined as a patient data review by individuals other than the investigator who generated the patient record. This could be carried out by the Study Chair or a special committee. If there was central data management, it should be mentioned. The review should be centered on answering three major questions for each patient: (*a*) was the patient eligible? (*b*) was the protocol followed? and (*c*) was there objective documentation of the major end points? There should be statements about the quality control of radiotherapy and surgery if these treatment modalities were involved in the study, and similar remarks hold for pathology quality control.

End Points and Censored Data

Trials in which the end point for evaluating therapy is a time metric, such as survival or disease-free survival, often may have patients with incomplete data. This happens if patients are still alive or in the disease-free state at the time of analysis. Such observations are called censored observations. Several situations arise in defining censored observations that could seriously skew results. We mention only two here which are in widespread use and could lead to incorrect conclusions.

The first occurs when a patient dies from a cause other than cancer (e.g., cardiovascular disease, suicide, and so on). Appreciable numbers of patients dying from competing causes of death could seriously alter the conclusions of the study if these patients were treated as censored observations. The cancer may have been an important contributing factor in the death.

The other reporting problem arises when a patient is taken off the protocol treatment because of lack of response or progression of disease and receives some other therapy that may be more beneficial. If the survival time is classified as censored (still alive) at the time the patient ceased to be on protocol therapy, then the statistical analysis will be biased (being purged of an imminent death). This will bias a poor therapy to make it appear to be better. It is unfortunate that such practices are widespread. For this reason, the report of a clinical trial should indicate the reasons for classifying patients as censored when the classification arises, other than the usual situation where not enough follow-up time has elapsed to have a complete observation.

Statistical Analysis

The report on therapeutic benefit should be presented so there is no ambiguity if a treatment difference refers to the entire patient population or special subgroups of patients. It is necessary that the analysis consider all known major prognostic factors that can affect the outcome. Otherwise, there may be disappointment when the therapy is applied in practice. The comparison of response proportions and disease-free and survival curves must be made using objective statistical procedures. If a complicated statistical model is used, it should be described in the paper itself or an appendix. The description of the statistical methods must be adequate for another statistician to reproduce the analysis if the source data were available.

The outcome of statistical tests depends both on the existence of a true difference and the number of patients in the study. If the number of patients is small, then the study will have low sensitivity (i.e., power) to detect small or moderate treatment differences. Failure to find statistical significance may result from small numbers, rather than lack of benefit. For this reason, every paper reporting a null effect should have a discussion of statistical power and how it can influence the conclusions of the paper.

The analysis also should contain a discussion relating to ending patient entry to the study. For example, was the trial (or part of the trial) stopped because of an unusual outcome associated with a treatment (i.e., a very good or poor result)? Was patient accrual terminated after a predetermined number of patients entered the trial? Was an early stopping rule used? All of these affect the reader's interpretation of the study conclusions.

STATISTICAL TECHNIQUES

The most common end points in cancer clinical trials are: "success" (defined in the context of the trial), response (complete, partial, or both), toxicity (lethal, life-threatening, severe, moderate, or mild), survival, disease-free survival, and duration of response. These end points fall into two general classes, which often are called categorical data (success, response, toxicity) and time metric or survival data (survival, disease-free survival, and duration of response). Categorical data are characterized by having outcomes that belong in a category and can be counted (e.g., number of successes or failures) or other events. The *survival data* (this is the term most often used to describe time metric data, even though the data may not actually refer to survival) are characterized by two events (beginning and end); the time between these two events is the time measurement.

CATEGORICAL DATA

Suppose a trial evaluating objective tumor response observed 20 complete or partial responses in 100 patients. The reported response rate is 20%. The statistical model for this study envisions a true or theoretical response rate that could only be calculated if the experiment enrolled the entire population of patients with the particular disease characteristics. Theoretically, this number would be very large. The clinical trial enrolling 100 patients is a sample from this population. The proportion of 20% is only an estimate of the true proportion as it is based on a sample of patients. How close is the reported value to the true value? To judge how close the reported or sample value is to the true value, one uses a statistical technique called a confidence interval. The formula for the confidence interval is

$$\hat{p} \pm 2\sqrt{\hat{p}(1-\hat{p})/n} \qquad (2)$$

where n is the sample size and $\hat{p}$ = (number of successes)/(sample size). The caret (ˆ) often is used to remind one that the proportion is based on a sample of observations; the true value would be designated by p. More correctly, the formula given by Equation 2 is an approximate 95% confidence limit. The confidence interval for our example is calculated to be 0.20 ± 0.08. The operational interpretation of the confidence interval is that the true value of response is within the interval (12%, 28%). The reason it is referred to as a 95% confidence interval is that on average, 95% of such confidence intervals will be correct (i.e., the true value of response will be within the interval). It is possible to raise the "confidence" to 99% or even higher at the expense of widening the interval, but in practice, most scientists use 95%.

Another common statistical problem arising in the analysis of a clinical trial is comparing two proportions. The comparison can be made by calculating a confidence interval between two proportions or carrying out a statistical test of significance. To illustrate the problem, suppose that outcome is measured by success and failure and the proportion of successes for two treatments, designated as A and B, are $\hat{p}_a$ = 50/90 = .56 and $\hat{p}_b$ = 40/100 = .40, respectively. The formula for calculating an approximate 95% confidence interval for the (true) difference ($p_a - p_b$) is

$$(\hat{p}_a - \hat{p}_b) \pm 2\sqrt{\frac{\hat{p}_a(1-\hat{p}_a)}{n_a} + \frac{\hat{p}_b(1-\hat{p}_b)}{n_b}} \qquad (3)$$

where n_a *and* n_b are the respective sample sizes. Carrying out the calculations results in 0.16 ± 0.14. The interpretation is that the true value of the difference can be as low as 0.02 or as high as 0.30. The interval (0.02, 0.30) is referred to as a 95% confidence interval for the difference between two proportions. The formula in Equation 3 is only an approximation for the 95% confidence interval, but it is accurate enough for sample sizes above 20. The interpretation of the 95% confidence intervals is that on average, 95 of every 100 intervals so calculated will have the true difference within the interval. In this particular example, we conclude there is a real difference between the success proportions, because a difference of 0 is not a possible value of the true difference.

Another common way to compare proportions is to carry out a statistical test of significance. Usually the data are put in the form of a 2 × 2 table, as shown in Table 26.10.

The statistical test calculates the probability of obtaining a result that was observed as well as more extreme outcomes if there actually is no difference between the treatments. The calculation is based on the following reasoning: if the outcome is regarded as scientific evidence in favor of a treatment difference, then outcomes having a greater difference would constitute even stronger evidence of a real difference between treatments. Essentially, the probabilities of all the more extreme tables are calculated where the totals in the margins are kept constant. The probabilities are then summed to form a P value. For example, a more extreme table is depicted in Table 26.11, and those data would be even stronger evidence in favor of a difference.

Table 26.10. Statistical Test of Significance (2 × 2 Table)

Group	Success	Failure	Total
A	50	40	90
B	40	60	100
Total	90	100	190

Table 26.11. Statistical Test of Significance (More Extreme 2 × 2 Table)

Group	Success	Failure	Total
A	51	39	90
B	39	61	100
Total	90	100	190

If the P value is small, then the probability of the observed table, or more extreme tables, arising by chance (i.e., no difference between treatments) is unlikely. Hence, we would conclude that the premise on which the calculation is made (i.e., no treatment difference) is incorrect and the treatments differ. Usually, a P value of less than .05 is declared to be "significant," resulting in a conclusion that treatments differ.

The statistical test is based on a hypothesis, called the null hypothesis, in which the true values are equal. This is usually designated as H_0: $p_a = p_b$. The alternative hypothesis is that the true proportions are different (e.g., usually specified by H_1: $p_a \neq p_b$). This alternative hypothesis is called a two-sided alternative, because it refers either to $p_a < p_b$, or $p_a > p_b$. Occasionally the alternative hypothesis would be a one-sided hypothesis (e.g., H_1: $p_a > p_b$). As a working rule, one should routinely use two-sided alternative hypotheses. A one-sided hypothesis is used when one treatment can never have a less beneficial effect than the other treatment. In some instances, investigators have reasoned that in comparing a potentially beneficial treatment against a control or observation group, a one-sided test would be suitable (i.e., therapy will be no different from having no treatment or will be better). This excludes the possibility that the active treatment may adversely affect the patient; there have been instances when one-sided tests have been used to evaluate the outcome of clinical trials in which, on further follow-up, the active treatment was found to be detrimental.

The statistical test for calculating the test of significance is often referred to as Fisher's exact test after R. A. Fisher, the statistician who derived it. The numeric procedure for the test is complicated; however, it is available in almost all computer software programs for statistical analyses. The statistical test for computing Fisher's exact test comparing the two proportions

$$\hat{p}_a = \frac{50}{90} = .56 \text{ vs. } \hat{p}_b = \frac{20}{100} = .20$$

resulted in a P value of .0415.

Because any value less than .05 is significant, we would conclude that the proportions differ. An approximate test for comparing the two proportions can be carried out by calculating the chi-square test for comparing two proportions. That formula is

$$\chi^2 = (\hat{p}_a - \hat{p}_b)^2 / \left[\frac{\hat{p}_a(1-\hat{p}_a)}{n_a} + \frac{\hat{p}_b(1-\hat{p}_b)}{n_b}\right] \tag{4}$$

and then comparing the calculated values from a table of the chi-square distribution. Large values of χ^2 reflect evidence of a treatment difference. Table 26.12 is a short table of the chi-square distribution. Note that if $\chi^2 > 3.8$, the P value is certainly less than .05. Using the same data from which Fisher's exact test was carried out results in a value of $\chi^2 =$ 4.97; this gives a P value of .03. If the sample sizes are of moderate size (i.e., at least 20 for each group), the chi-square test will give an answer that is quite close to that of Fisher's exact test.

The difference between the confidence interval approach and the test of significance is that the significance test does not indicate the magnitude of the difference between two proportions. The significance test refers to the probability of observing the given difference, or larger differences, between the two observed proportions if the two theoretical proportions actually are the same. In other words, it calculates the probability of these differences arising from chance fluctuations.

Table 26.12. Key Values of the Chi-Square Distribution and Their Associated Probabilities (One Degree of Freedom)

P	χ^2	P	χ^2
.50	0.46	.04	4.20
.40	0.71	.03	4.71
.30	1.08	.02	5.43
.20	1.64	.01	6.56
.10	2.69	.001	10.82
.05	3.84		

SURVIVAL DATA

A characteristic of survival data is that at the time of analysis, some patients may still be alive. These observations are called censored observations and represent incomplete data; however, they do contain important information by providing a lower bound on survival. Both complete and censored observations must be included in any analysis of survival-type data. Censored data arise from a variety of different circumstances. The two chief reasons for observing a censored observation are: (*a*) the period of follow-up is short, and (*b*) the patient may have been lost to follow-up. The first reason for censoring is referred to as "noninformative censoring" because apart from providing a lower bound on survival, the fact that the patient is censored conveys no further information about the treatment. Patients who are lost to follow-up may arise because the patient has moved, leaving no trace, or may have died without the investigator being aware of it. In some cases, loss of contact may have arisen because the treatment was unsuccessful or too toxic. Alternatively, the loss to follow-up may be unrelated to the patient's progress. The latter represents noninformative censoring; however, the other reasons contain information about the treatment and may be informative. Because information on the reasons for patients being lost to follow-up is not generally available, clinical trials with a significant number of such patients could be seriously biased. A rule of thumb is that if more than 10% of the patients are lost to follow-up, then care must be taken in the interpretation of data. One way to assess the importance of these patients is to carry out the analysis in two separate ways: (*a*) regarding all the lost patients as censored, and (*b*) assuming the observations on the lost patients are complete and represent the survival time. If the general conclusions of both analyses are the same, then these patients do not constitute a source of bias.

A theoretical survival distribution exists for any defined population of patients, and it may be altered by treatment. The theoretical survival distribution is the probability distribution of the different survival times if a (conceptually) infinite number of patients has received the same therapy. Figure 26.2 plots a theoretical survival function. (It is a plot of a probability vs. time.) Denoting the survival function by $S(t)$ it represents the proportion of patients who will have a longer survival than time t. For example, if t_m is the time for which the survival time is exceeded by half of the patients, then $S(t_m) = \frac{1}{2}$. The quantity t_m is called the median survival, and the median survival in figure 26.2 is $t_m = 2$ years. In general, one can define the survival time t_p such that $S(t_p) = p$. The survival time t_p represents that point on the theoretical survival curve such that a proportion p of patients will have longer survival time. For example, if $p = .25$, then 25% of the patients are expected to have longer survival times than $t.25$. The value t_p is called the pth percentile or upper pth percentile.

The theoretical survival distribution is never really known. Instead, as in any real-life situation, we have a limited amount of data, which can be used to estimate the theoretical survival distribution. The estimate of the theoretical survival distribution can be considered as being a summary or condensation of the data.

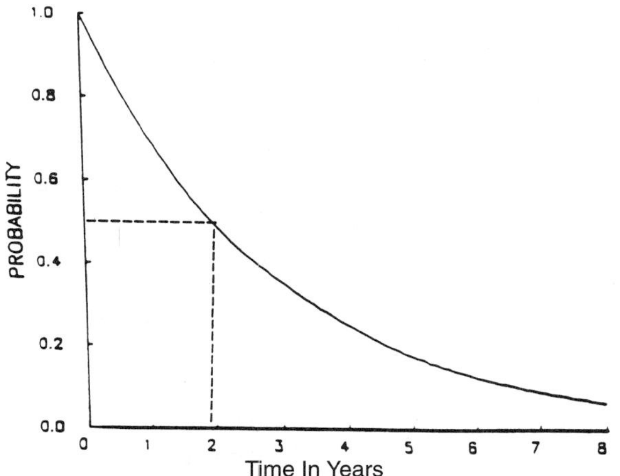

Figure 26.2. Plot of theoretical survival distribution. The median is 2 years and corresponds to the time for which half of the patients survive a longer time.

There are two principal ways of estimating the survival curve from actual data. These are called the life-table method and the Kaplan-Meier or maximum likelihood method. The life table method generally is used with a large number of observations, whereas the maximum likelihood method is used with a small number of observations. There are many different computer programs that automatically calculate these estimates. We illustrate the calculations for the life table method here as this is the more common method. Calculations for data on $n = 118$ patients with advanced adenocarcinoma of the lung are outlined in Table 26.13. The starting point for the calculations is to select a time interval to summarize the survival times. In Table 26.13, this interval is 1 month. A summary of the data is given in columns 2 to 4; the calculations in this table are self-explanatory. Figure 26.3 plots the survival function; note that it

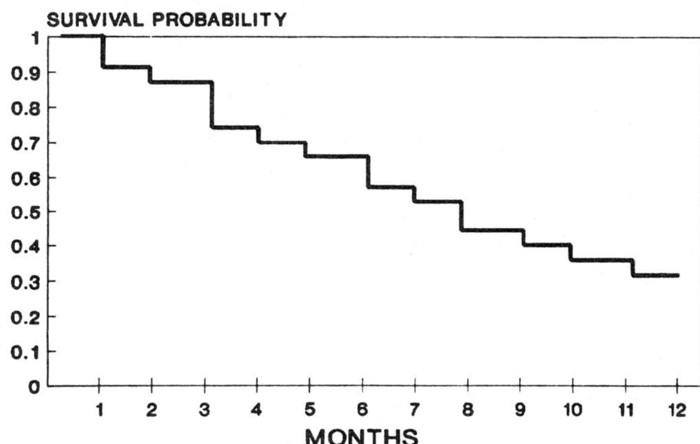

Figure 26.3. Survival for patients with adenocarcinoma of the lung ($n = 118$), plotted as a step function.

Table 26.13. Estimating the Survival Function for Patient with Advanced Carcinoma of the the Lung ($n = 118$)

Interval no.	Interval (month)	No. censored (a)	No. deaths (b)	No. alive at beginning of interval (c)[a]	No. at risk (d = c − a/2)	Probability of surviving (e = 1 − b/d)	Survival[b]
1	0–1	3	12	118	116.5	.897	.897
2	1–2	3	10	103	101.5	.901	.809
3	2–3	5	13	90	88	.852	.689
4	3–4	9	8	72	67.5	.881	.607
5	4–5	6	6	55	52	.885	.537
6	5–6	2	5	43	42	.881	.473
7	6–7	6	5	36	33	.848	.402
8	7–8	1	5	25	24.5	.796	.320
9	8–9	1	3	19	18.5	.838	.268
10	9–10	3	2	15	13.5	.852	.228
11	10–11	3	1	10	8.5	.882	.201
12	11–12	1	2	6	5.5	.636	.128
13	12+	3	0	3	3		

[a] The number of patients alive at the beginning of each interval is calculated by setting $c_1 = 118$ (the sample size of the study) for interval 1. The calculation for c_2, c_3, and so on proceeds by using the formula $c_i = c_{i-1} - (a_{i-1} + b_{i-1})$. For example, $c_2 = c_1 - (a_1 + b_1) = 118 - (3 + 12) = 103$.
[b] The last column gives the survival probabilities. The formulas for these entries are $f_1 = e_1$, $f_2 = e_2 f_1$, $f_3 = e_3 f_2$, . . . $f_i = e_i f_{i-1}$. For example, $f_2 = (.901)(.897) = .809$.

is plotted as a step function. The last column of Table 26.13 refers to the survival probability. For example, the probability is .897 of surviving 1 month and .809 of surviving 2 months. The number at risk within any interval is the number of patients who are "candidates" for dying within that interval. For example, for the first interval, 118 patients were alive at the beginning, but 3 were censored within the interval. The number at risk is calculated by assuming that three censored patients are equivalent to half the number who would be available for a potential death. Hence, the number at risk is calculated as $118 - 3/2 = 116.5$. The larger the number of patients at risk, the greater the reliability of the survival probability. As a result, survival probabilities in the "tails" of the distribution do not have the same reliability as those in the beginning of the distribution.

TEST OF SIGNIFICANCE FOR COMPARING TWO SURVIVAL DISTRIBUTIONS

There are several ways to perform a statistical test of significance for comparing two survival distributions. The most widely used test is the "log rank test." The calculation of the test is relatively complicated; however, it is widely available on computer systems. The key assumption in using the log rank test is that if the two survival distributions are denoted by $S_1(t)$ and $S_2(t)$, then the ratio of their logarithms is always a constant, i.e., $\log S_1(t)/\log S_2(t) = \beta$ (constant independent of time). The log rank procedure tests the null hypothesis that $\beta = 0$. If the assumption is that the ratio of the logarithms of the survival function is not constant, then the log rank test would be inappropriate to use for comparing two survival distributions. This assumption sometimes is referred to as the "proportional hazard" assumption. (See the section on Statistical Models for a discussion of hazard functions.) One situation in which this assumption does not hold is when the two survival distributions are observed to cross or intersect; this corresponds to the case in which one therapy appears to be better during early follow-up but, as time progresses, a higher proportion of patients on the other therapy live for longer periods of time.

Statistical Models

Evaluation of any therapy in a clinical trial should consider all factors that influence outcome. In addition to a potential for the therapy under investigation to influence outcome, features associated with the natural history of the disease also influence outcome. For example, it is well known that the probability of observing a response for advanced lung cancer depends both on performance status and weight loss. Another example is that the survival of women participating in adjuvant breast cancer trials is affected by menopausal status, nodal involvement, tumor size, and ER status. Incorporation of these baseline variables into the statistical analysis ordinarily results in a more precise analysis.

The way in which these co-variates are incorporated into a statistical analysis is through statistical models. General statistical models have been developed for both categorical and survival data; the models commonly used for these two kinds of end points are referred to as logistic and proportional hazards models, respectively. Very often, the proportional hazards models are called "Cox models" in honor of D. R. Cox, who first proposed them. The computations for using these models are extensive and ordinarily would be impossible to carry out on a hand calculator; however, calculations for both types of models are widely available in many statistical software analysis packages. Therefore, it is only appropriate to give the basic concepts here.

The basic idea of models are presented as if one had two therapies that are being compared and a single covariates. The generalization of these ideas to many covariates is straightforward.

LOGISTIC MODELS

Suppose there are two therapies (labeled A and B) having theoretical response probabilities p_a and p_b, which are unknown. The odds of response for each therapy is defined as the ratio of the probability of a response to the probability of no response, i.e., p_a/q_a and p_b/q_b where $q_a = 1 - p_q$ and $q_b = 1 - q_b$. The model for comparing two therapies would be to write the logarithm of the odds ratio as

$$\log(p_a/q_a) = \alpha, \qquad \log(p_b/q_b) = \alpha + \beta$$

The quantities α and β are unknown parameters in the model. If $\beta = 0$, then the two treatments are the same. This formulation of the modeling is equivalent to writing

$$p_a = e^{\alpha}/1 + e^{\alpha},\ q_a = 1/1 + e^{\alpha}$$
$$p_b = e^{\alpha+\beta}/1 + e^{\alpha+\beta},\ q_b = 1/1 + e^{\alpha+\beta}$$

The quantities p_a and p_b are expressed in terms of parameters (α, β), respectively. The functional form is the logistic function; hence, the name logistic models. Often, the logarithms of the odds ratios $\log(p_a/q_a)$ and $\log(p_b/q_b)$ are called logits.

Now suppose that the response is affected by gender. This is incorporated into the model by writing the logit for response as

Treatment A:	$\log(p_a/q_a) = \alpha + \gamma$	for males
	$\log(p_a/q_a) = \alpha$	for females
Treatment B:	$\log(p_b/q_b) = \alpha + \beta + \gamma$	for males
	$\log(p_b/q_b) = \alpha + \beta$	for females

where the parameters (α, β, γ) are unknown. This model assumes that the effect of gender is additive and independent of treatment. A more complex model would be to allow the effect of treatment to depend on gender. This can be done by defining a new parameter δ and writing the model for males receiving treatment B as $\log(p_b/q_b) = \alpha + \beta + \gamma + \delta$. The quantity δ is called an interaction term. The parameters for the logit model with interaction can be summarized as in Table 26.14.

Table 26.14. Summary of Logit Model

	Female	Male
Treatment A	α	$\alpha + \gamma$
Treatment B	$\alpha + \beta$	$\alpha + \beta + \gamma + \delta$
Difference in logits	β	$\beta + \delta$

Table 26.15. Model Interpretation

Parameter values	Interpretation
$\delta = 0$	Gender does not affect response differently for each treatment
$\delta \neq 0$	Treatments differ, but difference depends on gender
$\delta = 0, \beta = 0$	No difference between treatments
$\delta \neq 0, \beta = 0$	No difference in treatment for females, but difference in treatment for males
$\beta = -\delta \neq 0$	No difference in treatment for males, but difference in treatment for females
$\delta = 0, \gamma = 0$	Gender does not influence outcome
$\delta \neq 0, \gamma = 0$	Gender only influences outcome for treatment B

Statistical methods also exist for finding the numeric values of the parameters and for making tests of significance. The numeric calculations are readily carried out on computers. The model is very flexible and gives an organized way to interpret the data. Table 26.15 summarizes the various possibilities for drawing conclusions from this data set. The extension to many more covariates can be made as well.

In using a statistical model to analyze data, there are many opportunities to draw incorrect conclusions because the model was incorrect. For example, if the interaction term (δ) was omitted in the model and the effect of treatment depended on gender, then conclusions from the analysis might be wrong. Unfortunately, details of the "goodness of fit" of mathematic models often are omitted from scientific papers so that it is difficult even for the most experienced reader to verify the adequacy of a given model.

PROPORTIONAL HAZARD MODELS FOR SURVIVAL (COX SURVIVAL MODELS)

Modeling of survival data to account for other factors than influence survival is carried out by modeling the "hazard function" or "failure rate." To illustrate these ideas, consider the survival (years) of 10 patients: 0.2+, 0.5+, 0.5, 1.2+, 1.2, 1.8, 2.0, 2.1, 3.5, 5.0+, where + denotes a censored observation. Out of 10 observations, there are 6 deaths. Hence, the proportion of deaths is $p = 6/10 = 0.6$. The proportion of deaths, however, depends on the length of the follow-up time. The longer the follow-up time, the greater the proportion of deaths. (Total follow-up time is the sum of all observations. In this example, it is 18 years.) A more useful summary of the data is provided by the ratio of the proportion of deaths to the average follow-up time. This results in an expression that has units of "deaths per unit follow-up time" or, equivalently, "proportion of failures per average follow-up time." This quantity is called the "failure rate" (FR) and is calculated by

$$\text{FR} = \text{observed proportion of deaths/average follow-up time}$$
$$= \frac{6/10}{18/10} = \tfrac{1}{3} \text{ deaths per patient per year.}$$

Sometimes, it is convenient to report the deaths as per 100 or 1,000 patients. In our example, the failure rate could be reported as 1 death per 3 patients per year, 33 deaths per 100 patients per year, or 333 deaths per 1,000 patients per year.

Table 26.16. Calculation of Interval Failure Rates

Time interval	Proportion of failures	Average follow-up time	FR
First year	1/3	1.2/3 = 0.4	0.82
Second year	2/3	4.2/3 = 1.4	0.48
Third year and beyond	3/4	12.6/4 = 3.15	0.24

Alternatively, the time units may be changed to be deaths per month, in which case the death rate would be 2.75 deaths per 100 patients per month. The FR = 0.333 represents an average failure rate over the entire set of data. One could have calculated separate failure rates for the first year, second year, and so on, and these calculations are shown in Table 26.16.

Clearly, the failure rate keeps dropping with time, and the FR = 0.33 is an average failure rate. With a very large number of patients, the failure rate can be calculated for smaller and smaller time intervals (e.g., monthly, weekly, daily). One can envision an interval of time that gets progressively smaller as the interval shrinks to a point. With each of these smaller and smaller intervals, a failure rate can be calculated, provided that the number of patients is very large (theoretically infinite). This limiting process defines the "instantaneous failure rate" or the "hazard function, which is directly related to the survival function. If one knows the hazard function, then the survival function is completely defined, and vice versa. Letting $S(t)$ define the survival function and $h(t)$ the hazard function, the relationship between the two is given by

$$h(t) = -\frac{d}{dt} \log S(t)$$

or

$$S(t) = \exp\left[-\int_0^t h(x)dx\right].$$

Suppose that a clinical trial is comparing two treatments denoted by A and B. The proportional hazards model for making the comparison is to specify that $h_B(t) = e^{\beta}h_A(t)$ where $h_A(t)$, $h_B(t)$ are the hazard functions for the two treatments and β is an unknown constant. Clearly, if $\beta = 0$, the two treatments have the same hazard function and consequently the same survival functions. A more formal way of writing this model is

$$h_A(t) = h_0(t)$$
$$h_B(t) = h_0(t)e^{\beta}$$

Thus, the hazard function of treatment B is proportional to the hazard function of treatment A. This model leads to the log rank test, which has been discussed earlier. Note that

$$S_A(t) = \exp\left[-\int_0^t h_0(x)dx\right]$$

and

$$S_B(t) = \exp\left[-e^{\beta}\int_0^t h_0(x)dx\right].$$

Therefore, $\log S_B(t)/\log S_A(t) = \beta$, which is the assumption for the log rank test discussed earlier.

Now suppose that survival not only depends on the treatment but on gender. The hazard function then can be modeled in a way similar to the logistic function. Explicitly, we can model the hazard function for each treatment by

$$\begin{aligned} \log h_A(t) &= \log h_0(t) && \text{for treatment A, females} \\ \log h_B(t) &= \log h_0(t) + \beta && \text{for treatment B, females} \\ \log h_A(t) &= \log h_0(t) + \gamma && \text{for treatment A, males} \\ \log h_B(t) &= \log h_0(t) + \beta + \gamma + \delta && \text{for treatment B, males} \end{aligned}$$

The quantities β, γ, δ can be estimated from the data, and statistical tests are available for making inferences on these parameters. Note that this is a parallel model to the logistic regression model. The only difference is that $h_0(t)$, which is the baseline hazard rate, replaces α in the logistic model. The inferences from this proportional hazard model regarding the parameters are the same as in the logistic model (Table 26.15).

Many applications of this type of model fail to verify whether the proportional hazards assumption is correct. Furthermore, it is rare that an interaction term is included in the model. Investigators should be wary of presenting a statistical analysis that does not address issues of the inclusion of interaction terms to determine if the treatment effect depends on one or more prognostic or other baseline factors as well as the correctness of the proportional hazard assumption. To illustrate further how modeling for proportional hazard models is carried out, a detailed example is presented in order.

The Eastern Cooperative Oncology Group (ECOG) performed a randomized clinical trial on recurrent head and neck cancer with three treatment groups: (*a*) low-dose (40 mg/m^2) methotrexate (M), (*b*) high-dose (240 mg/m^2) methotrexate plus leucovorin rescue (ML), and (*c*) high-dose (240 mg/m^2) methotrexate plus leucovorin rescue plus cyclophosphamide (500 mg/M^2) plus cytosine arabinoside (300 mg/M^2) (MLCC). It is known that survival depends on performance status, time since first symptoms, disease site, and weight loss. The trial registered 237 patients, and Table 26.17 summarizes the medians.

Table 26.17. Summary of Median Survival by Treatment and Prognostic Factors: Head and Neck Trial ECOG[a]

	Sample size	Median survival (weeks)
Treatment		
M	81	22
ML	80	19
MLCC	76	14
Total	237	
Performance status		
Ambulatory	144	24
Nonambulatory	93	10
Weight loss		
None	93	24
<5%	61	14
5–10%	39	14
>10%	44	16
Disease site		
Tongue	45	21
Larynx	42	21
Hypopharynx	19	17
Oral mesopharynx	33	14
Floor of mouth	30	16
Other (mouth)	16	9
Other	34	22

[a] ECOG—Eastern Cooperative Oncology Group; M—methotrexate; ML—methotrexate plus leucovorin rescue; MLCC—methotrexate plus leucovorin rescue plus cyclophosphamide plus cytosine arabinoside.

It is clear that this trial is complex and a candidate for statistical modeling. The particular variables chosen for modeling and their associated levels are summarized in Table 26.18.

Table 26.18 represents a condensation of the data because performance status is measured on a five-point scale (0, 1, 2, 3, 4). An ambulatory patient is someone with a performance status of 2 or less. Similarly, the time from first symptoms has been condensed to three levels. Even with this condensation, however, the number of possible combinations is $3 \times 2 \times 3 \times 4 \times 4 = 288$. The entire trial only registered 237 patients, so there are more experimental combinations than patients.

In setting up the statistical model, each variable will generate parameters in the model. Ordinarily, the number of parameters is one less than the number of levels. For example, treatment will have two parameters because it has three groups. This can be modeled by using the parameters β_1 and β_2, that is, $h(M) = h_0(t)$, $h(ML) = h_0(t)e^{\beta_1}$, $h(MLCC) = h_0(t)e^{\beta_2}$. Because $h(ML)/h(M) = e^{\beta_1}$, positive values of β_1 imply that treatment ML has a higher failure rate than treatment M. A similar interpretation holds for $h(MLCC)/h(M) = e^{\beta_2}$. The comparisons of ML to MLCC results in $h(MLCC)/h(ML) = e^{\beta_2 - \beta_1}$. Hence, if $\beta_2 > \beta_1$, then MLCC has a higher failure rate than ML. The same scheme is set up for the other variables.

Table 26.19 summarizes the elements of this model. Note that weight loss is only one parameter (δ), even though there are four levels. This variable has been modeled as a continuous variable, where a new variable x is introduced that takes on values (0, 2, 3, 4) corresponding to increasing levels of weight loss. The estimates β_1 and β_2 are significantly greater than zero. Hence, M (low-dose methotrexate) has better survival (smaller hazard function) than the other two treatments. To compare the hazard ratios of h(ML) to

Table 26.18. Factors for Modeling[a]

Variable	Levels	No. of levels
Treatment	M, ML, MLCC	3
Performance status	Ambulatory, nonambulatory	2
Time since first symptoms	<1 year, 1–2 years, >2 years	3
Site	Other, tongue, hypopharynx, larynx	4
Weight loss	None, <5%, 5–10%, >10%	4

[a] M—Methotrexate; ML—methotrexate plus leucovorin rescue; MLCC—methotrexate plus leucovorin rescue plus cyclophosphamide plus cytosine arabinoside.

Table 26.19. Elements of Proportional Hazard Model[a]

Variable	Level	Model	Estimates of parameters[b]
Performance status	Ambulatory	1	
	Nonambulatory	e^{α}	$\hat{\alpha} = .66 \pm 16$
Treatment	M	1	
	ML	e^{β_1}	$\hat{\beta}_1 = .36 \pm .17$
	MLCC	e^{β_2}	$\hat{\beta}_x = .49 \pm .18$
Site	Other	1	
	Tongue	e^{γ_1}	$\hat{\gamma}_1 = .26 \pm .26$
	Hypopharynx	e^{γ_2}	$\hat{\gamma}_2 = .18 \pm .32$
	Larynx	e^{γ_3}	$\hat{\gamma}_3 = .45 \pm .26$
Weight loss	None ($x = 0$)	1	
	<5% ($x = 2$)	$e^{2\delta}$	
		$e^{\delta x}$	$\hat{\delta} = .14 \pm .05$
	5–10% ($x = 3$)	$e^{3\delta}$	
	>10% ($x = 4$)	$e^{4\delta}$	

[a] M—Methotrexate; ML—methotrexate plus leucovorin rescue; MLCC—methotrexate plus leucovorin rescue plus cyclophosphamide plus cytosine arabinoside.
[b] ±figures respresent 95% confidence intervals.

h(MLCC), we have h(ML)/h(MLCC) = $e^{\beta_1 - \beta_2}$. Making the comparison, we have $(\hat{\beta}_1 - \hat{\beta}_2) = -0.13 \pm .25$. Because zero is a possible value of $(\hat{\beta}_1 - \hat{\beta}_2)$, we would conclude that the two high-dose methotrexate arms have the same survival. Reviewing other parameters, we note that performance status, time since first symptoms, weight loss, and disease sites are all significant.

This model is an example of an additive model. There are no interaction terms with treatment. It concludes that low-dose methotrexate is superior, but it does not explore, for example, how this superiority relates to ambulatory status (i.e., does the superiority hold in the same way for both ambulatory and nonambulatory patients?). Similar remarks can be made about the other prognostic factors. Another potential criticism is that the way in which the weight loss is modeled requires further documentation.

Meta-Analysis

The last decade has seen increasing use of the statistical technique termed *meta-analysis*, which refers to the use of formal statistical techniques to sum up a collection of separate studies attempting to investigate the same hypothesis. Its purpose is the same as the scientific review of independent studies aimed at studying the same hypothesis. The difference between meta-analysis and an ordinary scientific review is that a scientific review tends to be somewhat personal, reflecting the views of the reviewer. Meta-analysis, however, attempts to synthesize data in a quantitative way, and the end product is a numeric estimate of a quantity that usually reflects the advantage of a treatment or a method.

The impetus for carrying out meta-analyses of cancer clinical trials is that the trials may be too small to find small but important therapeutic effects. For example, there are approximately 40,000 annual deaths from breast cancer every year in the United States. If the cure rate was increased by 10%, then one would expect 4,000 fewer deaths. A clinical trial to compare a treatment with a very low cure rate, in the neighborhood of 10 to 20%, with one that caused a 10% increase would require approximately 10,000 to 25,000 patients in a clinical trial. No breast cancer trials have ever been designed with this large a sample size.

Meta-analytic methods have been used in a wide variety of fields. They have been applied to observational as well as randomized studies. The initial applications were made in education research, but these ideas now are being applied to a large number of scientific fields. Although performing a meta-analysis is relatively straightforward, carrying out a good analysis is difficult.

The principal difficulties in applying meta-analysis to clinical trials are: (*a*) the therapies may be different, (*b*) the patient populations may be different, (*c*) the follow-up times may vary, and (*d*) the quality of the studies may vary. To illustrate these ideas, suppose that a meta-analysis is to be performed to determine if adjuvant chemotherapy prolongs survival for patients with breast cancer. In fact, a recent meta-analysis of this kind has been carried out: the Early Breast Cancer Trialists' Collaborative Group (3). Which trials should be included in this analysis? Trials exist that are both randomized and nonrandomized. To include nonrandomized studies would introduce all of the well-known biases that are associated with nonrandomized trials; hence, the meta-analysis should be restricted to randomized studies only. Among the randomized trials, some exist comparing a chemotherapy vs. placebo or observation group, whereas others may be comparing chemotherapy plus postoperative radiation vs. postoperative radiation. Should the latter trials be included in a meta-analysis? Hypothetically, if the radiation therapy is of no benefit, then such trials should be included. Alternatively, if the radiation therapy does improve survival, then it will ameliorate the effect of chemotherapy to improve survival. Among the randomized chemotherapy trials, there are a variety of treatment regimens. Some have used tamoxifen, cyclophosphamide, combination therapy [cyclophosphamide, methotrexate, 5-fluorouracil (CMF)], CMF with prednisone, or melphalan. The schedules have ranged from short intensive courses to long courses of therapy. Doses also may have differed among the studies. Some studies have been made on node-negative patients only, and some have been on node-positive patients. Still others have included both. The eligibility requirements for the trials may differ in substantial ways as well.

Should the meta-analysis be restricted to published studies only, or should it include both published and unpublished studies? Published studies tend to be positive, whereas unpublished studies tend to be negative. The data quality of unpublished studies may not be the same as for published studies. How does one find unpublished studies? Finally, the methods used to carry out the meta-analysis give more weight to studies with larger sample sizes and do not give any weight to the quality of a study. Nevertheless, proponents of meta-analysis believe that despite these problems, meta-analysis is worthwhile.

To discuss the basic issues, the meta-analysis performed by the Early Breast Cancer Trialists' Collaborative Group of cytotoxic therapy for patients with early breast cancer will be reviewed (3). The meta-analysis includes almost all randomized clinical trials (both published and unpublished) that were made available for analysis. The only exclusions were trials in Japan and the former Soviet Union. The number of trials in the analysis totalled 35, which were divided into four major subgroups: (*a*) trials of CMF or CMF and prednisone (CMFP); (*b*) trials of CMF and extra cytotoxic agents; (*c*) trials of combination therapy that include some C, M, or F; and (*d*) trials of single agents. The analysis was divided into two sets, corresponding to women younger than 50 years of age at entry to the trial and those 50 or older. We only consider here the analysis for the younger women.

The essential summary of the analysis has been put in graphic form by the authors and appears as Figure 26.4. The columns are self-explanatory, except for the last two. The authors have calculated the difference between the observed number of deaths (O) and the expected number of deaths (E) for the treatment, assuming there is no difference between treatment and control. This difference is written as O − E and the results are given for each trial. A negative value reflects that the treatment group had fewer deaths than expected. The value of O − E is given for each trial. The graphic portion of the figure plots the ratio of treatment to control mortality rates with a 99% confidence interval for each trial. A value of less than unity indicates that mortality is less for the treatment than control group. The diamond symbol is centered on the average ratio of mortality rates; its length represents a 95% confidence interval. The figure contains the average mortality ratios for each of the four subgroups of trials as well as an overall ratio, which appears at the bottom. The overall conclusions are that: (*a*) trials including CMF (group a) have a significant reduction in the annual mortality rate (37 ± 9%); (*b*) none of the other three clinical trial groups indicates a significant reduction in mortality; and (*c*) all four groups combined together share a 22 ± 6% reduction in overall mortality. This last conclusion mainly reflects the inclusion of CMF trials in the overall average.

If we examine the CMF (group a) trials, 3 among the 11 trials listed had fewer than five patients per treatment group and did not warrant inclusion. Of the remaining 8 trials, all had a no-treatment control group except Glasgow, which had a control group receiving radiotherapy. Both the ECOG

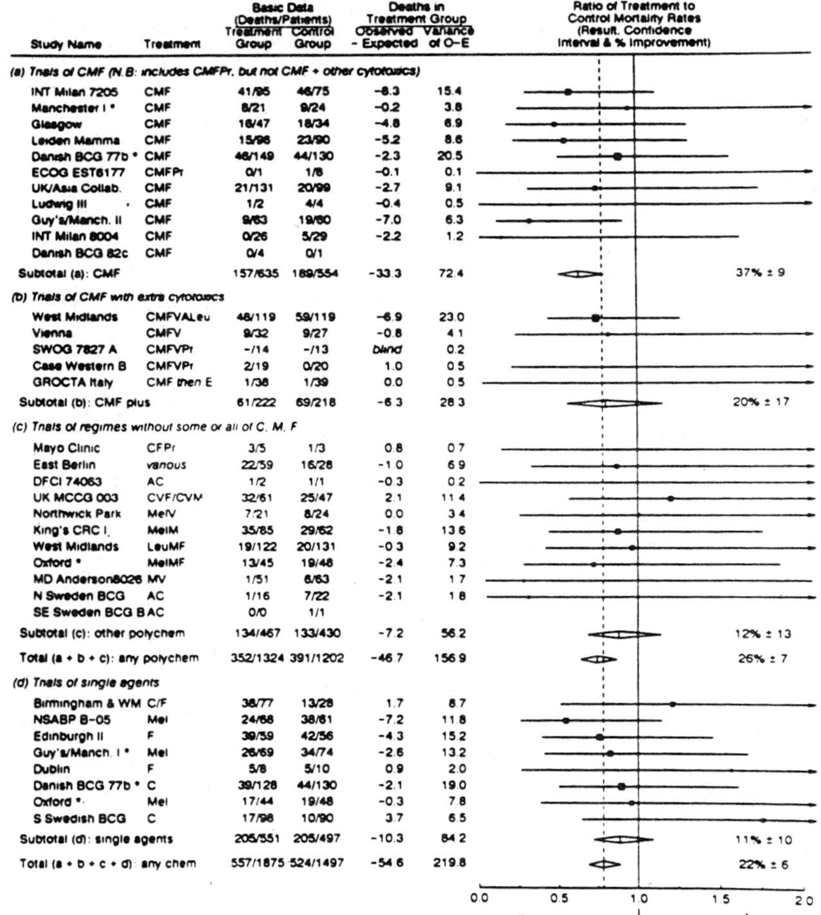

Figure 26.4. Results of meta-analysis of clinical trials evaluating cytotoxic drugs as adjuvant treatment for breast cancer: women aged <50 years at entry. From Early Breast Cancer Trialists' Collaborative Group (3).

(6177) and the Ludwig III trials added prednisone to the CMF, with the Ludwig trial also adding tamoxifen. With the exception of the Leiden and UK/Asia trials, all had a 12-month course of therapy, with the former having a 24-month course of therapy. Thus, the trials were not all comparable, but they were reasonably close with respect to therapy. It is questionable whether the Glasgow study should be included, because it does not have a no-treatment control group. In any event, excluding trials with small numbers, all of the remaining 8 trials produced a negative O − E, which indicates an excess of deaths in the control group. The chance of this happening if treatment is not beneficial is the same as tossing a fair coin eight times and observing all heads or all tails. This probability is $P = .016$ and is unlikely to have happened by chance. Hence, one could have readily concluded that the aggregate of trials having CMF as their therapy reduces mortality. Among the 8 mature trials, 5 are individually significant at the .05 level (i.e., INT Milan 7205, Glasgow, Leiden, Guys/Manch II, INT Milan 8004). Thus, it is no surprise that the meta-analysis reached a similar conclusion. The use of a 99% confidence interval for the individual trials obscures those trials significant at the conventional 5% level. It is not clear why this was done.

The overall value of O − E essentially gives more weight to trials with larger numbers of patients. There is no attempt to weight or judge the quality of these studies. However, one clue to quality is that there should be equal numbers of patients in each treatment group for every trial, except for chance fluctuations. Note that the total number of patients in the treatment and control groups are 635 and 554, respectively, in the group a analysis. The probability that such a split could arise by chance is $P = .02$; in other words, the split is not random and probably reflects differential quality among these trials. The major contributors to this imbalance are INT Milan 7205, Glasgow, and UK/Asia. These trials represent 40% of the total number of patients in group a. Additional trials have been analyzed in a recent report of the Early Breast Cancer Trialists (4).

It is not at all certain that many poor trials, considered as a constellation in a meta-analysis, will shed more light than two good trials that reach similar conclusions. The strength of meta-analysis is numbers, but the weakness is failure to consider the inherent quality of the research design and execution by better investigators. Babe Ruth and Hank Aaron could doubtless teach more about home run hitting than their 16 additional teammates combined.

Falsification of Data

The veracity of cancer clinical trials was seriously questioned when it was discovered in 1994 that false patient data were submitted by at least two participating hospitals in the breast cancer clinical trials carried out by the National Surgical Adjuvant Breast and Bowel Project (NSABP) (11). The NSABP is a multicenter-clinical-trials group mainly performing trials in breast cancer. The public announcement of the data falsification not only became a political issue, but raised questions about the way that cancer clinical trials are being carried out. Among the issues raised were: (*a*) why the falsification had not been discovered earlier, and (*b*) the effect of the false data on conclusions drawn from these clinical trials. This section discusses these two issues.

Quality control of data from cancer clinical trials usually is carried out by a combination of data managers, automated computer data checks, and record reviews by Study Chairmen and possibly other senior physicians. This program is supplemented by periodic audits at each clinical site. These involve either a full audit, an audit of all significant events, or drawing a random sample of hospital records for patients entered in trials. The audit consists of comparing the hospital record data with that submitted to the data coordinating center for the trial.

One of the NSABP clinical investigators had been submitting falsified data over a period of 15 years. A complete review audit of this investigator resulted in the discovery of 99 patients with discrepancies from among 1,511 patients. All but one of these discrepancies involved eligibility rather than toxicity or relapse. The falsified data included changing the dates of surgeries performed before patients enrolled in studies, altering dates of biopsies, changing or fabricating estrogen-receptor values, altering dates of chemotherapy, and lack of appropriate informed consent. The nature of these falsifications could only be discovered at an audit of the records in the hospital. Actually, the NSABP audit process did discover that the investigator had submitted some false data; however questions were raised by the U.S. Congress and National Cancer Institute officials as to why the data discrepancies had not been uncovered earlier by the NSABP.

It should be noted that an audit on a random sample of patient records can only assess the quality control system that is in place at the hospital. It cannot certify that all submitted data are correct. One point of view is that data fraud is at the end of a road marked by a careless and sloppy data collection system. Demands have been made to increase the frequency and scope of data audits in order to have a better chance of detecting data falsification. However, one must be realistic in proposing such a program. Our experience is that data falsification is relatively rare among clinical investigators.

It is unfortunate that this much publicized case of data fabrication only led to punitive actions rather than an investigation of why it occurred and how to reduce the incentives for such behavior. The motivation for submitting false data may arise from a variety of reasons. Among these are: (*a*) the eligibility criteria may appear to be arbitrary (e.g., patient must be entered onto the study within 28 days of surgery); (*b*) laboratory tests may be required that are non-routine, expensive, too frequent or inconvenient to the patient, and are to be used in an ancillary study but are not necessary for patient care, or (*c*) investigators receive funds on a per patient basis (which may result in additional income if the physician is in private practice).

The other issue to be addressed is the effect of data fabrication on the principal conclusions of a study. Clearly, if the amount of falsified data is relatively small compared to patient accrual, it will unlikely alter previous conclusions. It also is necessary to account for the nature of the data fabrication. All but one of the known discrepancies in the NSABP con-

Table 26.20. Loss of Power as a Function of Dropping a Percentage of the Original Number of Patients[a]

Patients dropped (%)	Reduction of Power (%)
0	0
1	0.5
5	2.5
10	5
20	11
30	19
40	28
50	36

[a] Original power of 80% with a two-sided significance level of 5%.

sisted of altered eligibility criteria. Furthermore, all of these trials were randomized. As a result, these ineligible patients were randomly assigned to the treatment groups; so each of the treatments under study had the same opportunity to be tested on these ineligible patients. Consequently, the comparisons among treatments will still be unbiased, even though the inclusion of these patients may require a modified interpretation of the conclusions of the study because of the altered patient population. The randomization process ensures that unknown factors (e.g., data ineligibility) affect all treatment groups the same way (on average). On the other hand, if the data fabrication affected the principal end points, there could be serious biases in the data.

In any event, discovery of falsified data submitted by an investigator is a serious matter. The prevailing view is that all data from that investigator (as well as his or her hospital) should be expunged from the database of the clinical trial. This will result in reduced power to detect real differences among therapies in a trial. Table 26.20 shows the loss of power relative to the percentage of data expunged from the database when a trial is designed to have 80% power at a 5% level of significance. For example, if 10% of the patients are dropped, it will result in a 5% loss of power. Hence, the power changes from 0.80 to 0.76. A rule of thumb is that there is a loss of 0.5% power for every 1% removal of patients when less than 20% of the patients are dropped.

Our general conclusion is that if the original trial showed a statistical difference between treatments, then a removal of fewer than 10% of patients from the original analysis is unlikely to change the conclusions with a re-analysis. Also, submission of fraudulent eligibility data does not affect the unbiasedness of a randomized trial.

References

1. Anderson JR, Cain KC, Gelber RD. Analysis of survival by tumor response. J Clin Oncol 1983;1:710.
2. Antman K, Amato D, Wood W, et al. Selection bias in clinical trials. J Clin Oncol 1985;3:1142.
3. Early Breast Cancer Trialists' Collaborative Group. Effects of adjuvant tamoxifen and of cytotoxic therapy on mortality in early breast cancer. N Engl J Med 1988;319:1687.
4. Early Breast Cancer Trialists' Collaborative Group. Systemic treatment of early breast cancer by hormonal, cytotoxic, or immune therapy. One hundred thirty-three randomized trials involving 31,000 recurrences and 24,000 deaths among 75,000 women. Lancet 1992;339:1(Part 1),85(Part 2).
5. Geller NL. Planned interim analysis and its role in cancer clinical trials. J Clin Oncol 1987;5:1485.
6. Goldhirsch A, Gelber RD, Simes RJ, et al. Costs and benefits of adjuvant therapy in breast cancer: a quality adjusted survival analysis. J Clin Oncol 7:36, 1989.
7. Hill AB: Principles of Medical Statistics, 5th ed. London: Lancet, 1956.
8. Lefkopoulou M, Zelen M. Intermediate clinical events, surrogate markers and survival. Lifetime Data Analysis. 1:73–85, 1995.
9. Louis PCA. Essays in Clinical Instruction. London: P. Martin, 1834.
10. Neaton JD, Brose S, Fishman EL, et al. The Multiple Risk Factor Interventions Trial (MR-FIT). VII. A comparison of risk factor changes between two study groups. Prev Med 1981;10:519.
11. Nowak R. Problems in clinical trials go far beyond misconduct. Science 1994;264:1538–1541.
12. Rosner GL, Tsiatis AA. The impact that group sequential tests would have made on ECOG clinical trials. Stat Med 1989;8:505.
13. Simes RJ, Zelen M. Exploratory data analysis and the use of the hazard function for interpreting survival data: an investigator's primer. J Clin Oncol 1985;3:1418.
14. Taylor KM, Margolese RG, Saskolne CL. Physicians' reasons for not entering eligible patients in a randomized clinical trial of surgery for breast cancer. N Engl J Med 1984;310:1363.
15. Zelen M. Guidelines for publishing papers on cancer clinical trials: responsibilities of editors and authors. J Clin Oncol 1983;1:1614.
16. Zelen M. The randomization and stratification of patients to clinical trials. J Chron Dis 1974;27:365.

ADDITIONAL READINGS

A good overall book on general features of clinical trials is Pocock SJ. Clinical Trials: A Practical Approach. Chichester: Wiley, 1983. There are a number of books devoted to clinical trials in which individual authors have written chapters on specialized topics. Among those that contain expository chapters on statistical methods are: Miké V, Stanley KE, eds. Statistics in Medical Research. New York: Wiley, 1982; and Shapiro SH, Louis TA, eds. Clinical Trials. New York: Marcel Dekker, 1983. A more general compilation that stresses the practical problems of performing cancer clinical trials is: Buyse ME, Staquet MJ, Sylvester RJ, eds., Cancer Clinical Trials. Oxford: Oxford University Press, 1984. A compilation of chapters targeted at early breast cancer trials is found in Baum M, Kay R, Scheurlen H, eds. Clinical Trials In Early Breast Cancer: Second Heidelberg Symposium. Basel: Birkhaeuser-Verlag, 1982.

There are a number of papers that provide charts or extensive tables for making sample size calculations. Among these are: Feigl P. A graphical aid for determining sample size when comparing two independent proportions. Biometrics 1978;34:111; Freedman LS. Tables of the number of patients required in clinical trials using the logrank test. Stat Med 1982;1:121; Schoenfeld DA, Richter JR. Nomograms for calculating the number of patients needed for a clinical trial with survival as an endpoint. Biometrics 1982;38:163.

Meta-analysis of clinical trials will continue to be a source of debate in medical research. A popular, but not dispassionate, account of this topic, is Mann C. Meta-analysis in the breech. Science 1990;249:476. Another overview of breast cancer adjuvant trials that uses hazard functions is Zelen M, Gelman R. Assessment of adjuvant trials in breast cancer. NCI Monograph. Adjuvant Chemotherapy and Endocrine Therapy for Breast Cancer. Washington, D.C.: U.S. Government Printing Office, 1986.

The planning of sequential trials requires complex calculations and specialized software that is not widely available. A software package that is suitable for personal computers and easy to use is called EAST and is available from Cytel Inc. (Cambridge, MA).

SECTION VI

CANCER PREVENTION

CHAPTER 27

Prevention of Tobacco-Related Cancers

PAUL F. ENGSTROM, ELIZABETH A. ROSVOLD, NEAL R. BOYD, JR., AND C. TRACY ORLEANS

Introduction

In the United States, approximately 46.3 million people smoke, and nearly 400,000 people die prematurely each year from tobacco-related diseases. This includes 151,000 deaths from cancer, 179,800 from cardiovascular diseases, and 84,500 deaths from respiratory diseases. Cigarette smoking remains the greatest cause of preventable mortality in the United States (12).

Americans have dramatically altered their smoking behavior since the first Surgeon General's report on tobacco was released in 1964. At that time, approximately 40% of the U.S. population smoked; in 1987, it was 29%. The smoking rate is higher among men (32%) than among women (27%); it also is higher among African Americans (34%) than among whites (29%). Smoking is inversely related to level of education: 36% of those without a high school diploma, 33% with a high school diploma, 26% with some college, and 16% of college graduates smoke (233). There also is a similar pattern of higher smoking rates among blue-collar and service workers compared with white-collar workers. Tobacco use is influenced heavily by the tobacco industry's $2 billion annual advertising and marketing campaigns. Women, minorities, blue-collar workers, adolescents, and even children are bombarded by clever and often insidious marketing and advertising gimmicks.

Richard Peto (174) estimates that worldwide, 3 million deaths will be attributed to smoking in 1995, and in 2025, there will be approximately 10 million such deaths, 7 million of which will occur in the developing world. For instance, more than 70% of men age 25 and older in China, smoke cigarettes. At current smoking rates, there will eventually be approximately 2 million deaths per year directly related to smoking. Worldwide cigarette smoking is the largest single cause of premature death.

This chapter reviews the pathogenesis and epidemiology of smoking-related cancer. It also discusses addiction, prevention, and cessation of tobacco use.

Physicochemical Composition of Tobacco Smoke

More than 4000 known compounds are estimated to be present in tobacco smoke. These occur as volatile constituents forming a vapor phase and, in particulate form, suspended in the vapor phase. The majority of carcinogens and mutagens are found in the particulate phase. Currently, 43 carcinogens have been identified in tobacco smoke, including polynuclear aromatic hydrocarbons (PAH), nitrosamines, heterocyclic hydrocarbons, benzene, and radioactive polonium-210 (233). Tobacco-specific nitrosamines (TSNAs) are the carcinogens that are present in the highest concentration; they occur in even higher concentrations in smokeless tobacco. For risk assessment, tobacco smoke is classified as either mainstream smoke (MS) or sidestream smoke (SS). The MS represents smoke that is directly inhaled through the butt end of the cigarette, while the SS is continuously emitted from the burning end into the environment. Most of the components that have been identified in tobacco smoke occur in both MS and SS, but the concentrations of many toxic and tumorigenic agents (e.g., nitrosamines) are higher in SS (102).

Nicotine is the pharmacologic agent that is responsible for the addictive properties of tobacco, and it also is a major source of TSNA through *N*-nitrosation reactions (102). It is present in both MS and SS and is rapidly absorbed from the small airways and alveoli of the lung. Nicotine from smokeless tobacco is absorbed through the oral mucous membranes. Once in the blood, nicotine is transported to specific receptor sites on the brain, and interaction with these receptor sites is believed to be the basis for producing a chemical dependence on tobacco. The liver is the primary site of nicotine metabolism, with cotinine as the major metabolite (236).

Carcinogenesis Bioassays and Markers of Genotoxicity

Tobacco smoke and smokeless tobacco both contain compounds that function as tumor initiators, promoters, or cocarcinogens. Tumor initiators are mutagens that bond covalently to cellular DNA; their effects generally are irreversible and may require only a single exposure. Promoters are compounds that stimulate excessive proliferation of initiated cells; they produce reversible effects that result in cancer after prolonged application. Cocarcinogens enhance the effects of carcinogens; however, they are not essential to the carcinogenic process and may have little or no direct carcinogenic activity (23).

Experimental simulation of human smoking has been performed by Auerbach and colleagues (9) using dogs. The dogs were exposed to a maximum of 14 months of tobacco smoke via tracheostoma. Although no tumors developed, bronchial epithelial sections exhibited atypical nuclei, loss of ciliated columnar cells with squamous replacement, and hyperplasia. These changes are similar to those seen in tissue specimens from patients with lung cancer and were almost absent in sections from tobacco-unexposed dogs. Only limited success has been achieved at inducing respiratory cancers in animals in response to tobacco-smoke inhalation, both because of acute toxic effects and the animals' resistance to deep inhalation of such smoke. In these studies, animals are placed in exposure chambers and exposed to alternating, short periods of tobacco smoke, diluted with air, and followed by air alone. An excess incidence of respiratory tumors has been demonstrated in mice, rats, dogs, and hamsters (the latter develop laryngeal tumors only) compared with unexposed controls. Overall incidence has been low, however, and dominated by adenomas and alveologenic adenocarcinomas (102, 235).

The majority of carcinogenesis bioassays in animals have used direct application of tobacco-smoke condensates (i.e., tars) or subfractions of the particulate phase. Tumor initiation and cocarcinogenesis primarily have been associated with the neutral subfractions that are rich in PAH, while promoters are found in the weakly acidic subfractions (102). Intrapulmonary administration of tobacco-smoke condensates or fractions have produced lung carcinomas and adenomas in rats and hamsters, respectively (102, 235). The TSNAs are potent carcinogens. 4-(Methylnitrosamino)-1-(3-pyridyl)-1-butanone (NNK) and *N'*-nitrosonornicotine (NNN) are the strongest carcinogens. The dose of TSNA to which smokers and snuff-dippers are exposed is comparable to that which is carcinogenic in animals (96). Subcutaneous injection of TSNA causes tumors of the nasal cavity, trachea, and lung in hamsters and of the nasal cavity, esophagus, lung, and liver in mice (96). Tumors of the nasal cavity, lung, liver, and esophagus have been produced in rats by intraperitoneal administration of TNSA (97). Application of TSNA into the rat oral cavity produces tumors of the cheek, tongue, hard palate, and lung (85). The carcinogenicity of NNK appears to be organ specific for the lung, regardless of the route of administration or the animal model used (84). Skin-painting of cigarette-smoke condensates has consistently produced papillomas and carcinomas in over 40% of mice, compared with a near-zero incidence in control animals. Condensates from pipes and cigars also have produced a high incidence of tumor in animal bioassays. Application of cigarette-smoke condensates in vivo to xenotransplanted, human bronchial epithelial cells has produced invasive neoplasms (117).

A large number of in vitro studies have been conducted with tobacco smoke (MS and SS) as well as condensates. Mutagenicity has been demonstrated for smoke and condensates in *Salmonella typhimurium* (the Ames test) (6), and urine from smokers also has been shown to be mutagenic in this system, with some evidence of a dose response. In mammalian tissue-culture systems, condensates, fresh tobacco smoke, and the gas phase of smoke have induced sister chromatid exchange and other mutations, cell transformation, and the inhibition of both DNA repair and intercellular communication (102).

Several markers of genetic damage occur in those who are exposed to tobacco products. An excess prevalence of sister chromatid exchanges and micronuclei has been observed in the peripheral blood lymphocytes and bone marrow of smokers compared with nonsmokers. Many of these studies have demonstrated dose-response trends with number of cigarettes or durations of smoking (102). DNA adducts are complexes that are formed by the covalent bonding of carcinogens with DNA, and they serve as a marker of initiation (78, 168, 181). Adducts may be formed by the interaction of carcinogens with DNA; those formed by PAH are detected in the lung, bronchus, and larynx of smokers but at much lower levels, or even absent, in nonsmokers. Levels correlate with the dose and duration of smoking. Levels decrease in a time-dependent fashion in former smokers. Adducts also are found in the kidney, bladder, esophagus, liver, and aorta of smokers (14). Bronchial tissue levels are potentiated by the use of alcohol (47), and the levels of PAH adducts are not reliably isolated from the oral mucosa of those using oral tobacco products (14). The adducts formed by TSNA take several forms. The 7-methylguanine adducts in peripheral white blood cells (142) and bronchial tissue (143) are found at higher levels in smokers than in nonsmokers. Levels of O_6-methyldeoxyguanosine adducts are similar in the peripheral lung tissue of smokers and nonsmokers (246). A third form of adduct is specific for nicotine exposure and is found complexed with DNA and hemoglobin. It is more frequent in smokers than in nonsmokers, and it also is detected in snuff users (60). In addition, an aromatic amine adduct has been found at higher levels in the urinary bladder tissue of smokers compared with nonsmokers, thus providing a possible link between smoking and bladder cancer (217).

The predictive value of DNA adducts and sister chromatid exchange as markers of cancer risk has not yet been determined (166–168). Studies to date that have examined the levels of DNA adducts and sister chromatid exchange in relation to cancer susceptibility have been small and their results mixed. Sister chromatid exchange frequency correlates with smoking, but it does not seem to correlate with lung cancer (166). PAH adduct levels in peripheral blood cells are higher for lung cancer cases than controls, but only when stratified by smoking status (166). Likewise, adduct levels in bronchial tissues are not associated with lung cancer independent of smoking (47). Adduct levels in bladder cells also are not different in controls versus bladder cancer cases independent of smoking intensity (218). Interpretation of these results must be tempered by the small numbers of subjects, potential confounding factors, significant interindividual variation in DNA binding, multiple sources of PAH exposure, and the fact that the assay is relatively crude (i.e., does not discern between different but structurally related PAHs) (166). Heterogeneity is seen in the level of TSNA adducts in tobacco-exposed individuals not due to level of exposure (60). This heterogeneity may reflect individual differences in the ability to activate TSNA, but other factors, (e.g., DNA repair mechanisms) may affect adduct levels. At present, both adducts and sister chromatid exchanges should be considered to be important, chiefly as markers of carcinogen-induced genetic damage, because the significance of this initiating step regarding cancer risk or susceptibility is not clear.

Genetic Variation in Susceptibility

Susceptibility to the carcinogenic effects of tobacco smoke appears to be genetically determined. A number of epidemiologic studies have observed an apparent familial aggregation of lung cancer risk, with one (151) demonstrating possible synergism between familial risk and cigarette smoking (62, 151, 221). Segregation analysis has provided evidence that such familial clustering is strongly consistent with mendelian codominant inheritance of a two-allele autosomal gene, with age of onset dependent on genotype (193). This analysis suggested that the joint effect of the gene and cigarette smoking could be responsible for 42% of lung cancer cases at age 50, 34% at age 60, and 13% at age 70. In contrast, the corresponding percentages that are attributable to smoking alone were 27% at age 50, 49% at age 60, and 72% at age 70 (193).

Several enzyme systems involved in the metabolism of xenobiotics exhibit distinct genetic polymorphisms that may be associated with differential susceptibility. This raises the possibility that certain phenotypes can serve as markers to identify individuals who are at increased risk. Enzymes that have received the most study include the P450 enzyme involved in debrisoquine metabolism; the *N*-acetyltransferases, which acetylate aryl amines in the liver; aryl hydrocarbon hydroxylase (AHH), which catalyzes monooxygenation of aromatic hydrocarbons; and the glutathione S-transferases which conjugate reactive intermediates of carcinogen metabolism.

The cytochrome P450 superfamily of genes encodes a system of enzymes that is responsible for the oxidative metabolism of endogenous compounds (e.g., fatty acids, prostaglandins) as well as drugs and other xenobiotics. Because enzymatic oxidation produces highly reactive intermediates, it is thought that metabolism by P450 enzymes activates carcinogens such as PAH, and genetic variation in P450 enzymes may alter the capacity to metabolically activate certain carcinogens, thus influencing cancer risk. The metabolism of debrisoquine (a β-blocker used as an antihypertensive agent) involves a P450 enzyme encoded by the gene *CYP2D6*. It is hypothesized that the *CYP2D6* enzyme also may be involved in metabolism of the carcinogenic compounds found in cigarette smoke. Polymorphisms of this gene are manifested by variations in the extent of metabolism, with phenotypes categorized as extensive, intermediate, or poor metabolizers (91). The extensive and poor metabolizer phenotypes occur in 20 to 30% and 5 to 10% of whites respectively; the former is an autosomal dominant trait (31, 134). Initial studies demonstrated that individuals who exhibit the extensive metabolizer phenotype (as determined by the ratio of unchanged debrisoquine to 4-hydroxydebrisoquine in the urine) have an increased risk of lung cancer compared with intermediate or poor metabolizers (10, 31, 32, 126), with one study showing that risk associated with the extensive metabolizer phenotype was higher in whites (odds ratio, 10.2) than in blacks (odds ratio, 4.5) after controlling for age, gender, and smoking (32).

Other studies of susceptibility based on metabolic phenotype have been performed with equivocal or negative results (17, 46, 185, 206). The molecular basis for the deficient metabolism of debrisoquine has been determined, and the responsible polymorphisms are detectable by restriction fragment length polymorphism (RFLP) or polymerase chain reaction techniques (87). Numerous studies have examined the metabolic phenotype, genetic polymorphism(s), or both in relation to lung cancer susceptibility. Their results remain controversial, however, with several studies supporting (71, 91, 213) but others failing to support such an association (196, 219, 249). No consistent findings have been shown regarding histologic subtype of lung cancer and phenotype/genotype, although one study did reveal an increased risk for squamous and small-cell carcinomas but not adenocarcinomas (32). The *CYP2D6* polymorphism has been studied with respect to bladder cancer susceptibility, yet these results also are not conclusive, with both positive (16, 34, 71, 108) and negative findings (108). One study has shown an association of aggressive tumor grade with EM phenotype; increased recurrence risk also has been associated with EM phenotype independent of tumor grade (59).

Acetylation rates are under genetic control at a single locus, with two different phenotypes that are categorized as "rapid" and "slow." The latter is autosomal recessive and occurs in approximately 50 to 60% of Western populations, compared with 10% among Asian populations (149). Slow acetylators are less efficient at detoxifying aryl amines, which are potent bladder carcinogens (33, 81, 131, 141). Several studies have examined the association of acetylation status and bladder cancer. Data combined from 12 such studies with varying results revealed a significant relative risk for bladder cancer for slow versus rapid acetylators (odds ratio, 1.5) (88). A more recent study failed to show any increased risk in slow acetylators (80). When considering those cases developing in individuals with occupational exposure to aryl amines, the relative risk of slow acetylators is increased, with an odds ratio of 2.2 (88). One recent study from Poland has confirmed this association (80), although in a Chinese population, no increased risk was found (83). Aryl amines are present in tobacco smoke, but studies have not shown any association between acetylator status and smoking (33, 81, 88, 141). Several studies have shown that adducts between tobacco-related aryl amines and hemoglobin are found at higher levels in slow acetylators relative to rapid acetylators, and that adduct levels increase with the number of cigarettes smoked per day (241, 251). This may help to explain the association of acetylator phenotype and bladder cancer. A study of acetylation status in larynx cancer showed an increased risk in slow acetylators (45), but one of lung cancer failed to demonstrate any difference in risk based on acetylation rate (125). Neither of these studies has not been confirmed.

Aryl hydrocarbon hydroxylase is a P450-dependent monooxygenase that can be induced to a variable degree by exposure to aromatic compounds such as benzpyrene. Considerable disagreement exists as to whether this trait is associated with variation in lung cancer susceptibility (165). Kouri and colleagues (120) found significantly higher AHH-inducibility in lymphocytes from patients with lung cancer compared with controls having other pulmonary disease and matched for age, sex, and cigarette smoking. Another study that examined inducibility in lung tissue from patients with lung cancer, and lymphocytes from smoking and nonsmoking controls as well as patients, found no evidence of excess risk associated with high inducibility (109). Levels of *CYP1A1*, the gene responsible for AHH activity, have been found to be expressed in both normal and malignant lung tissue in smokers, with little expression in nonsmokers (136). Another study showed that high AHH activity in lung correlated with the level of DNA adducts, and that high lung expression of *CYP1A1* is associated with risk of lung cancer in smokers (13).

Two polymorphisms in the *CYP1A1* gene have been studied extensively for association with lung cancer. Initial reports in Japanese patients revealed that an *Msp*I RFLP was associated with lung cancer, with a relative risk of 3.21 for squamous cell cancers (112, 113). There also appeared to be a cigarette dose effect in that those with the susceptible genotype had a relative risk of 7.31 at low cigarette doses compared with those with other genotypes (112). The polymorphic allele is felt to be associated with high AHH inducibility (144). Further studies in Japanese populations have confirmed the association of the *Msp*I polymorphism with increased lung cancer risk (144, 145). This polymorphism has been examined in white populations, and no association with lung cancer has been noted (44, 92, 93, 95, 199, 200, 220). Furthermore, no association was seen in various ethnic groups in a Brazilian study (214). A polymorphism in exon 7, which results in an amino acid substitution, also has been shown in Japanese patients to be associated with lung cancer; two studies have shown this, again with a cigarette dose effect (144) and higher risk for squamous cell cancers in susceptible genotypes (82). One study in a German population revealed a twofold higher frequency of the susceptible genotype in patients with lung cancer, with an odds ratio of 2.51 for squamous cell cancer in those who were susceptible (44), although a Finnish study revealed no association for this polymorphism with lung cancer (95). A third polymorphism in *CYP1A1* has been found and is thought to be specific for blacks, but this polymorphism has shown no association with risk for lung cancer in this population (114). The *Msp*I polymorphism is 10 times less common in white than Japanese populations (144). The frequency of the polymorphic allele in exon 7 was 0.007 in one white population and 0.019 in a Japanese population (144). Differential ethnic frequencies in these polymorphisms may account for their differing contribution to lung cancer susceptibility.

The P450IIE1 enzyme has been found to catalyze oxidation and DNA adduct formation of nitrosamines and other carcinogens (110). A polymorphism in this enzyme's gene has been associated with lung cancer in Japanese populations (224–226) with a cigarette dose effect noted in one (224). This association has not been replicated in whites (92, 173). Other polymorphisms have been described as well. No increased susceptibility for lung cancer has been noted (110), although one polymorphism may relate to decreased risk (173).

The glutathione S-transferases (GSTs) are a family of enzymes that catalyze the conjugation of PAHs and other toxic intermediates with glutathione, thus making them more easily excreted. The mu form of the enzyme family is not expressed in approximately 50% of white populations (22). In 1986, Seidegard and colleagues (192) found that the lack of GST mu activity was associated with an increased risk for lung cancer in smokers. Many studies using metabolic assays, genetic assays, or both also have examined this association in lung and other smoking-related cancers. In lung cancer, there appears to be a positive association of increased risk and lack of GST mu activity in both white populations (94, 147, 191), and in Japanese populations (82, 115, 116, 144), although not all studies support this association (24, 86, 253). The overall increased risk is approximately twofold in both populations. Several studies also demonstrate an increased risk for the development of squamous cell and small-cell cancers in smokers compared with the risk for adenocarcinoma (82, 94, 115, 116, 191, 253), although one study does demonstrate the opposite association (189). A dose effect of smoking has been demonstrated as well, particularly for the development of squamous cell cancers. The proportion of the null genotype in this cancer subtype increased with increasing cigarette exposure (115). Null individuals were found to develop squamous cell cancers at lower cigarette doses than GST-positive individuals (144). This effect was even more pronounced when susceptible genotypes for GST and *CYP1A1* were combined, with odds ratios reaching as high as 41 (144).

The GST mu phenotype and/or genotype also has been examined for an association with bladder cancer. Four studies show an increased risk for bladder cancer in those lacking GST mu activity (15, 25, 42, 122), with odds ratios ranging from 1.40 to 3.80. The increased risk was only found in those who were smokers in one study (15), although no effect of smoking was seen in two others (25, 42). No association with tumor grade was seen (25). Two studies do not support an association with bladder cancer susceptibility (129, 254). One study has reported an association of GST mu null activity in laryngeal cancer, demonstrating an increased risk of approximately twofold for smokers lacking activity (122).

In addition to the enzyme systems described previously, a number of oncogenes have been identified in tobacco-related cancers (51, 63, 121, 202, 212, 216). Mutations in the p53 tumor-suppressor gene have been described in tobacco-related cancers, including those of the lung, head and neck, esophagus, and bladder (73). In lung cancers, the most frequent mutations are G:C $\rightarrow$ T:A transversions, which are seen after experimental exposure to carcinogens from tobacco (184). This mutation has been shown to correlate with cigarette consumption (186, 215). Mutations of p53 also are seen more frequently in smoking-related forms of lung cancer, such as small-cell as opposed to adenocarcinomas (77 vs. 33%, respectively) (73). Such mutations are seen in 34% of laryngeal and pharyngeal cancers, with a spectrum of mutations similar to that for lung cancer. In oral cancers, mutations are seen in 81% of tumors, and the mutations differ from those in the other head and neck cancers. These differences may reflect exposure to different carcinogens in tobacco (73). Approximately 34% of bladder cancers also have p53 mutations, again with a different spectrum compared to lung cancer (73). There is some evidence for a dose effect of smoking (252), although the mutations are similar in both smokers and nonsmokers (208). Mutations in the *ras* oncogene family also have been observed in tobacco-related cancers. Approximately 20% of non-small-cell lung cancers have a mutation in one of the three *ras* genes (105), with the highest frequency seen in adenocarcinomas (101). A relationship between smoking status and K-*ras* mutation has been observed as well (105), and the frequency of *ras* mutations in head and neck cancers ranges from approximately 2 (198) to 50% (8). Eighteen percent of bladder cancers were found to have H-*ras* mutations in one recent study, although no relationship with tumor grade or stage was seen (30). How mutations in these oncogenes and others relate to susceptibility for tobacco carcinogenesis is still unclear, although determining the relationship between exposures and mutational spectra may provide clues.

Cancers Associated with Tobacco Use

The 1989 Surgeon General's report on smoking and health characterizes specific cancers as to whether tobacco smoke plays a causal role, acts as a contributory factor, or is merely associated with the cancer (233). Cancers in each of these categories are listed in Table 27.1, which also summarizes data on mortality and attributable risk from the 1989 report (233).

Table 27.1. Tobacco Smoke and Risks of Specific Cancers in Western Countries

Cancer site	Mortality ratio	Attributable risk (%)[a]
Causal role of tobacco		
Lung and bronchus	7.0–15.9	90 (M), 79 (F)
Larynx	6.1–13.1	81 (M), 87 (F)
Oral cavity[b]	1.0–12.5	92 (M), 61 (F)
Esophagus	1.7–6.6	78 (M), 75 (F)
Contributory role of tobacco		
Bladder	0.7–3.0	47 (M), 37 (F)
Kidney	1.1–1.6	48 (M), 12 (F)
Pancreas	1.6–6.0	29 (M), 34 (F)
Association with tobacco		
Stomach	0.9–2.3	NA
Cervix (invasive)	0.7–2.9[c]	NA

[a] Percent risk attributable to tobacco.
[b] Buccal cavity and pharynx.
[c] Estimated relative risk. (F)—Females; (M)—males; NA—data not availiable. Data from U.S. Department of Health and Human Services (233) and International Association for Research in Cancer (102).

All cancer sites listed in Table 27.1 exhibit a dose response with the level of cigarette smoking (e.g., number of cigarettes per day). Lung, larynx, oral, esophageal, and bladder cancers also exhibit a dose response with duration of smoking; duration effects have been less widely studied for other cancer sites (235). In addition, pipe and cigar smoking are associated with increased risk of cancers of the lung, oral cavity, larynx, and esophagus; for all but the former, excess risk is similar to that for cigarettes. Cessation of smoking is associated with a gradual decline in that person's risk relative to a nonsmoker (233). Patients with oral cancer who quit smoking also have approximately 50% of the risk of second primaries as do patients who continue to smoke (201).

Smoking cessation has had the largest effect on lung cancer mortality rates among white males. From 1973 to 1986, lung cancer mortality increased by 15.9% in white males (from 62.4 to 72.3 per 100,000), compared with 28.7% in black males (from 76.3 to 98.2 per 100,000). The corresponding figures for females were a 96.2% increase among whites (from 13.8 to 27.1 per 100,000) and 87.4% among blacks (from 13.8 to 25.9 per 100,000). Black males also exhibit higher mortality rates and less favorable mortality trends for cancers of the larynx, esophagus, oral cavity, and pancreas (227).

Cancer Related to Environmental Tobacco Smoke

Many investigations of the risk of cancer resulting from environmental tobacco smoke (ETS, also known as passive or involuntary smoke) have been performed since the early 1970s. Most studies have addressed the risk of lung cancer in the nonsmoking spouse of a smoker, and most have demonstrated small increases in risk (50, 64, 107, 207). Exposure to ETS in the workplace also has been linked to excess cancer risk in nonsmokers (111, 207, 250). Studies such as these led the U.S. Surgeon General and the National Research Council to conclude in 1986 that the risk of lung cancer was increased from exposure to ETS by approximately 30% in nonsmokers (146, 234). In 1992, the Environmental Protection Agency reviewed 30 epidemiologic studies of ETS and lung cancer and concluded that ETS is a human carcinogen, is causally associated with lung cancer in adults, and results in 2500 to 3000 deaths from lung cancer annually (238).

Three large studies have been published since the EPA analysis. One is an update on a study included in the EPA analysis, confirming the 30% excess risk of lung cancer in nonsmoking spouses of smokers, with an increase in relative risk associated with increasing pack-years of exposure (61). A second study revealed an increased risk (relative risk, 1.3) for lung cancer only in those exposed to over 40 pack-years of exposure (27). A third demonstrated a relative risk of 1.6 for lung cancer in those who have ever been exposed to ETS and of 2.4 for those with 40 or more years of exposure (211).

Several studies also have addressed the risk for lung cancer in adults exposed to ETS as children. One demonstrated a doubling of adult lung cancer risk associated with heavy exposure during childhood and adolescence among nonsmokers and ex-smokers (103). Another showed an increased risk of lung cancer in females who were exposed to household smoke as children, the odds ratio increasing with the amount of passive smoke exposure (243). In addition, adducts of tobacco-associated carcinogens have been found in the cord blood of newborns with both smoking and nonsmoking mothers, thus indicating that such carcinogens can cross the placenta (36); adduct levels were higher in the fetuses of smoking compared with nonsmoking mothers. Cotinine and PAH-albumin adduct levels also have been demonstrated to be higher in children whose mothers smoked compared with the children of nonsmoking mothers (39). These studies have implications for both the monitoring and risk assessment of ETS exposure, and not only for the development of cancer but for other diseases as well, such as respiratory infections and asthma.

There have been limited reports of ETS association with other cancers. Bladder cancer has not been associated with ETS in two studies (29, 106). Several studies have examined the risk of cervical cancer in those exposed to ETS, and in one, a twofold risk for cervical cancer was seen in nonsmokers (188). Another demonstrated a similar risk but did not control for the personal smoking habits of the women (28). ETS exposure was shown in another study to result in an increased risk of cervical cancer in both smokers and nonsmokers. The risk in nonsmokers increased with the number of hours per day they were exposed to ETS, and it remained elevated after adjustment for sexual practices and other potential confounding factors (203). Increased risk for cancers of the nasal sinus, maxillary sinus, and the brain have been reported (222), as has an increased risk for cancer of the breast, especially in premenopausal women (188). However, one recent study did not confirm this effect (204).

Factors Modifying Tobacco-Related Cancer Risk

Several factors strongly potentiate the carcinogenic effects of tobacco smoke. The strongest synergistic effects have been seen with asbestos and radon, and several studies have found evidence suggesting that the effects of asbestos and cigarette smoking are multiplicative, particularly for insulation workers exposed to high levels of asbestos dust (79, 90, 102, 189). In one very large cohort of insulation workers, the mortality ratio for the combined exposure was 53.2 compared with unexposed nonsmokers (79).

Most data concerning radon exposure are based on studies of uranium miners, which have produced widely varying estimates of the combined risk. Some studies also have been based on small numbers. Nevertheless, the combined effect likely is more than additive, and it may be multiplicative. Relative risks exceeding 10 have been observed for the combined exposure in several studies (102, 187, 190).

The applicability of these results to residential radon exposure has been questioned. Several large case-control studies have examined the risk of lung cancer from radon exposure, but the results are inconsistent. Two studies showed no association (21, 128), and one showed a trend only for adenocarcinoma (2). Four others found positive associations (132, 171, 172, 190) and a trend for increased risk with increasing exposure has been demonstrated in three of these four studies (171, 172, 190). The combined effect of smoking and radon exposure has not been well studied, but a trend was seen for heavy smokers in one study (172) but not in another even though the number of heavy smokers with high radon exposure was small. One study demonstrated no trend with analysis by smoking history (171).

Synergistic effects of alcohol have been observed in many studies of oral, laryngeal, and esophageal cancers, with relative risks as high as 10 to 20 for heavy smoking and drinking (48, 89, 150). In most studies, the combined effect of alcohol and tobacco appeared to be multiplicative, that is, the risk associated with the combined exposure was approximately equal to the product of the risks associated with the individual exposures (102). In animals, alcohol increases the carcinogenicity of PAH and potentiates the activity of microsomal enzyme systems (235). Further evidence for synergism comes from a study that observed significantly elevated levels of micronucleated cells in buccal mucosa from persons with heavy smoking and drinking habits but no elevation in subjects with exposure to only alcohol or tobacco (209).

In contrast to the agents just described, many studies suggest that high intake of dietary β-carotene reduces the risk of cancer among smokers (98, 244, 255). There are sufficient data from both retrospective and prospective studies to support an inverse correlation between dietary β-carotene intake and lung cancer. In most studies, risk reductions on the order of 30 to 60% have been observed. Effects have been strongest for squamous cell and small-cell cancers, thus suggesting inhibition of tobacco-related carcinogenesis. In contrast to studies on β-carotene or total carotenoids, these studies specifically addressing dietary intake of preformed vitamin A do not support a protective effect for lung cancer (244). Studies examining serum levels of retinol have produced inconsistent results (242, 244, 245), possibly because serum vitamin A levels tend to be tightly regulated, and although carotenoid levels more accurately reflect dietary intake, measurement is more difficult technically (255).

Protective effects of β-carotene also have been observed for other cancers associated with smoking, such as head and neck (197), oral cavity (135, 248), larynx (133), esophagus (26), bladder (72, 163), and cervical (72). The synthetic retinoid isotretinoin (13-*cis*-retinoic acid) has been evaluated for the prevention of second primary cancers of the head and neck. A persistent decreased incidence of second primary cancers in those patients initially rendered disease free by surgery and/or radiation therapy has been demonstrated (18), and treatment of premalignant oral lesions (i.e., leukoplakia) with isotretinoin and β-carotene also has been successful, with isotretinoin appearing to be more effective (98). One study showed reduction in second tumors with the administration of a vitamin A preparation for those patients with a history of lung cancer (164). A large, randomized, double-blind, placebo-controlled primary prevention trial examining the use of daily supplementation with β-carotene in those at high risk for lung cancer has recently been reported; in the Alpha-Tocopherol, Beta Carotene (ATBC) Lung Cancer Prevention Study, over 29,000 male smokers from Finland aged 50 to 69 years received β-carotene and/or α-tocopherol (vitamin E) or placebo daily (7). After at least 5 years of follow-up, there was an unexpected 18% increase in the incidence of lung cancer among those receiving β-carotene, thus raising the question of whether supplementation may actually be harmful. β-Carotene had no effect on the incidence of other cancers. Several trials examining the use of vitamin A preparations and β-carotene in the primary prevention of head and neck as well as lung cancer, and the prevention of second primary tumors at these sites, are currently in progress.

Vitamin E intake has been suggested as being protective against cancer. In several longitudinal studies examining serum vitamin E levels, individuals with cancer (all sites) had approximately 3% lower levels than found in controls (118). Significant associations have not been seen for lung cancer, however, except in one study (138), and no association was seen in a combined group of smoking-related cancers (118). The use of vitamin E supplementation has been associated with a decrease in oral cancer in one study (11); however, in the ATBC study (7), no effect on the incidence of lung cancer was observed with supplementation.

The effect of intake of vitamin C or fruits and vegetables that are high in vitamin C has been investigated in many studies (20). Most support an increased risk of approximately 1.5- to 2.0-fold in those with the lowest amounts of vitamin C intake. This effect has been seen for oral, laryngeal, esophageal, lung, stomach, and cervical cancers.

Strategies for Cessation

Whether smokers quit on their own or in a formal treatment program, they are more likely to succeed if they expect many health and other benefits from quitting, use a variety of active methods to stay off cigarettes and cope with withdrawal (e.g., avoiding smoking places and people, thinking "positive," finding alternative ways to cope with stress) and have social support for their efforts to quit and remain smoke free (40, 151).

The Transtheoretic Model of behavioral change, introduced by Prochaska colleagues (176, 177) provides a critical framework for understanding how smokers quit on their own (Fig. 27.1). According to this model, smokers achieve long-term quitting success by advancing through a sequence of five motivational and behavioral stages of change, often "recycling" through these stages over repeated quit attempts: *precontemplation*, or not thinking about quitting smoking; *contemplation*, or seriously planning to quit in the next six months; *determination or preparation*, or planning to quit in the next month with at least one attempt in the last year; *action*, or active efforts to stop smoking and remain smoke free; and *maintenance*, which begins 6 months after quitting and involves efforts to resist relapse and remain smoke free permanently.

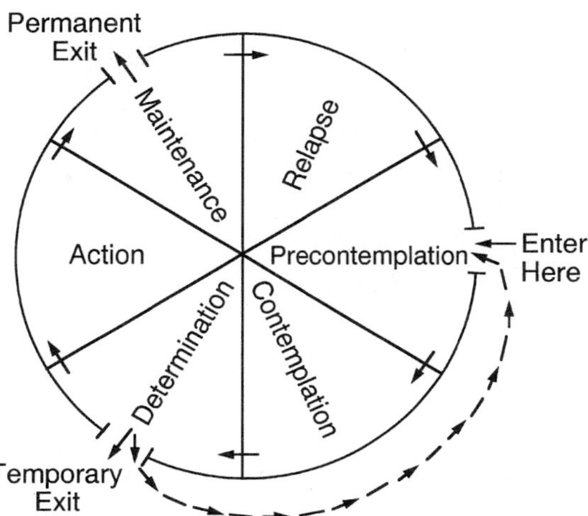

Figure 27.1. A stage model of the process of change. *Source:* Prochaska and DiClemente (176).

Cross-sectional and longitudinal studies supporting the stage model have found that different motivational and behavioral self-change processes are important in different stages of quitting (177). Accordingly, the stage model has fueled new interest in motivational treatments—including those involving personal biofeedback of smoking-related harms (127) and motivational interviewing techniques (139)—of high-risk patients to move early stage smokers (precontemplators and contemplators) into stages of greater readiness for change. Recent interventional studies have shown that stage-matched treatments produce greater accrual and quit rates than stage-mismatched treatments (178). In general, accrual is defined as the proportion of the total number of smokers in a population who are recruited into treatment. Quit rates typically are defined as the proportion of all treated smokers who report tobacco abstinence for 1 week or more at 6- and/or 12-month follow-up. Although self-reports of quitting appear to be reasonably accurate, smoking status can be verified through cotinine assays or alveolar carbon monoxide monitoring (240).

SELF-HELP METHODS

Most smokers prefer "do it yourself" and minimal contact strategies over formal treatment programs, and in fact, 90% of U.S. ex-smokers have quit on their own without the benefit of any formal treatment program (54). The 8 to 15% 1-year quit rates that are typically achieved by smokers without formal assistance (54) or with self-help materials and aids (37) are quite respectable compared with the 20 to 25% 1-year quit rates of most formal treatment programs.

Self-help programs that are designed to equip smokers with needed motivations, skills, and support and to help them progress through these stages of change can boost the success rate of self-quit efforts. In 1991, the National Cancer Institute (NCI) published a practical guide to self-help quitting programs entitled *Guided Strategies for Smoking Cessation: A Program Planner's Guide* (67). This guide presents five basic strategies for self-help programs, including (*a*) implementing policy and motivational strategies to motivate more smokers to try to quit on their own, (*b*) targeting self-change programs to all the stages of smoking cessation, (*c*) including critical cessation information and quitting methods in self-guide programs, (*d*) using adjuncts proven to boost self-quitting success rates, and (*e*) targeting programs to specific populations.

This guide also reviews a wide spectrum of low-cost, generic quitting guides, like the NCI's *Calling it Quits*, the American Cancer Society's *Smart Move,* and the American Lung Association's *Freedom from Smoking for You and Your Family*, as well as newer, population-tailored quitting guides, including those designed especially for Latino, black, and women smokers, pregnant smokers, and older adults. Three adjunctive treatment strategies are singled out as raising self-help treatment success: personalized, computer-generated feedback (41, 178); brief, personalized telephone counseling (159, 162); and nicotine replacement therapy (99). Increasingly, state-of-the-art medical and commercial self-help quit smoking programs include these adjuncts.

FORMAL QUIT SMOKING CLINICS

Smoking cessation clinics provide help beyond that of self-help programs, and they tend to attract smokers seeking extra help. In fact, formal clinics might be seen as providing quitters with the motivations, skills, and supports they otherwise lack for a *self*-quit attempt. Formal quit smoking clinics in the United States are sponsored by voluntary organizations (e.g., American Cancer Society, American Lung Association), proprietary organizations (SmokeLess, Smoke Stoppers), hospitals, managed-care organizations and health plans, health departments, and other groups. Regional American Cancer Society, American Lung Association, and Cancer Information Servicer (1-800-4-CANCER) offices can supply details on local programs.

Over the years, formal clinic programs have become increasingly similar. Most use accepted, state-of-the-art cognitive behavioral treatment techniques to help smokers get ready to quit (e.g., brand switching, motivational techniques), quit (e.g., abrupt quit date quitting, aversive smoking), cope with withdrawal symptoms and cravings, and both resist and recover from relapse. Most programs of this nature achieve similar 20 to 25% 1-year quit rates, although some programs produce 1-year quit rates as high as 40 to 50% (124, 233). Promising results have been reported for behavioral quit smoking clinics that include nicotine replacement therapy, especially transdermal nicotine. These approaches can double the quit rates achieved with cognitive behavioral techniques alone (55, 99).

PHYSICIAN-BASED INTERVENTIONS

An estimated 70% of all U.S. smokers see a physician on an annual basis, and most do so more than once (43). Glynn and Manley (70) projected that if only *half* of U.S. physicians delivered even a brief "quitting" message to their patients who smoked and were successful with only 1 in 10, this would yield 1.75 million new ex-smokers every year—more than double the national annual quit rate (54). Using conservative estimates, over 5 million U.S. smokers could be reached through hospital-based programs each year (157). In all medical settings, given physicians' very limited time for preventive interventions, nonphysician health care providers (e.g., nurses, physician assistants, respiratory therapists) play a critical role as change agents (156).

Numerous controlled trials have demonstrated the efficacy of so-called "minimal contact," office-based interventions employing techniques that can be easily integrated into routine care and delivered on a population basis to *all* smokers in the practice regardless of their motivation or readiness to quit. Glynn (66), for instance, reviewed 28 physician-based trials and found that advice or counseling alone produced 6- to 12-month quit rates of approximately 5 to 10%; more intensive physician-based interventions resulted in 20 to 25% quit rates. Similarly, five randomized, controlled, clinical trials funded by the NCI and involving over 30,000 patients and over 1000 providers (e.g., primary care physicians, some dentists) showed that patients in intervention groups had long-term quit rates two to six times higher than those of patients receiving "usual care" (69).

The core elements of these effective primary care interventions included a brief (i.e., 3 to 5 minute) but strong physician quit smoking message; self-help materials presenting state-of-the-art motivational, behavioral, and relapse prevention strategies; prescription of nicotine replacement, if appropriate; brief cessation counseling, including setting a quit date (usually provided by a nonphysician health professional); and follow-up support (119, 148). Kottke and colleagues (119) found that the most effective interventions involved more than one modality (e.g., face-to-face advice/counseling, nicotine replacement therapy), involvement of both physician *and* nonphysician counselors, and a greater number of smoking-related contact and follow-up visits.

Glynn and Manley (69) distilled these core elements into a four-step treatment algorithm that could be applied in a variety of health care settings by a variety of providers. This algorithm was first presented in *How to Help Your Patients Stop Smoking: A National Cancer Institute Manual for Physicians* (69) and since has been widely applied by physicians (5), nurses (230), respiratory care practitioners (229), and the oral health care team (e.g., dentists, hygienists) (137), and covers counseling not only of smokers, but of smokeless-tobacco users as well. The algorithm is (*a*) *ask* about smoking (tobacco use) at every opportunity; (*b*) *advise* all smokers/smokeless tobacco users to quit; (*c*) *assist* smokers/smokeless tobacco users to quit using self-help materials and, when appropriate, nicotine replacement therapy; and (*d*) *arrange* follow-up contacts or visits.

Most recently, the NCI's four-step treatment algorithm has been incorporated into the American Medical Association's stage-based model for the treatment of nicotine addiction (5, 153). This stepped-care model is outlined in Figure 27.2. This wider model starts with a practice environment that encourages nonsmoking and minimizes operational barriers to smoking cessation interventions (69), and it includes routine

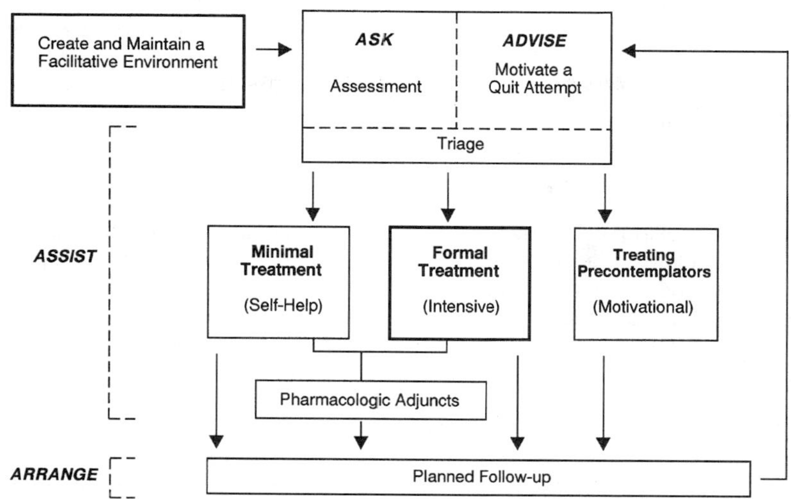

Figure 27.2. Minimal-contact treatments in a stepped-care model. *Source:* Orleans et al. (156).

surveillance or assessment of smoking status, preferably through adoption of tobacco use as a "vital sign" (52). All smokers receive a personal quitting message that is tailored to their particular health risks and includes clear advice to *quit* (versus cutting down). Then, they are triaged either to *smoking cessation* treatment (either minimal or intensive) or a *motivational* treatment depending on their answer to the question: "If we can give you some help to quit, are you willing to give it a try?" (156).

For most of those smokers who answer "yes" to this question, self-help strategies represent the best starting point. They are the easiest to deliver, the most preferred by smokers, and the most cost-effective. For smokers who have tried and repeatedly failed using self-help strategies, prefer more intensive treatments, or present with co-morbidity requiring special assistance or urgent behavior change (e.g., smokers with other chemical dependencies, those who have had a myocardial infarction, early stage cancer patients, pregnant smokers), however, triage to more intensive treatment is the best initial step. Follow-up is required for smokers who are triaged to any treatment path, and it includes a therapeutic mix of support, surveillance, quitting assistance, and remotivation delivered over return health visits. Past trials of physician quit smoking advice have shown that quitting and maintenance are related to the frequency and intensity of follow-up contacts after the initial advice or intervention (119).

PHARMACOLOGIC TREATMENTS

Pharmacologic treatments are reserved as adjuncts for smokers in active cessation programs and never offered as treatments on their own. Nicotine replacement therapy via nicotine gum or transdermal patches is the most effective pharmacologic aid to smoking cessation, and it should be considered for regular smokers who have had difficulty with nicotine withdrawal effects in past attempts and have no medical contraindications (e.g., heart attack in the past 3 months, certain severe arrhythmias, pregnancy). However, research suggests that nicotine replacement has little benefit when used on its own (55, 99, 156). To date, no other pharmacologic interventions have proven to be as consistently effective as nicotine gum or transdermal nicotine (104).

Nicotine gum helps to alleviate nicotine withdrawal—especially irritability, restlessness, anxiety, and difficulty in concentrating—and significantly boosts the quit rates of minimal contact and intensive treatments, especially with highly dependent smokers (i.e., one pack or more per day, those who smoke within 30 minutes of awakening) (99, 223). However, unless it is chewed properly (e.g., chewed slowly and then "parked" between the cheek and gum to release nicotine before further chewing), the gum often causes unpleasant side effects (e.g., burning sensation in throat, nausea, gas) that deter adherence to recommended daily regimens. For this reason, nicotine gum has *not* consistently proven to be effective in the context of brief medical advice, which may not allow for adequate instruction in appropriate use of the gum (99, 100, 123). The 4-mg gum likely is to be more effective than the 2-mg gum, but problems with side effects and appropriate use are not avoided with the stronger dose. In addition, possible problems of long-term dependence on the gum by smokers who do, and do not, quit indicate the need for careful follow-up to monitor use and weaning (76).

A meta-analysis by Fiore and colleagues (55) showed more promising results for transdermal nicotine patches in the context of routine provider intervention. Existing studies suggest that while the benefits of nicotine gum are greatest for smokers with the highest levels of nicotine dependence, transdermal nicotine appears to equally benefit smokers at all levels of dependence, with quit rates being two to three times higher than those for brief medical advice alone. The authors attributed the higher efficacy of the patch to its greater ease of adherence (relative to the gum) and a more positive side-effect profile (e.g., skin rash). A recent large-scale study of "real world" patch users, however, showed that provider instruction is still important for optimal benefit (158). Only 54% of patients in this study said they had received *any* advice on patch use or quitting from their physician or pharmacist, yet the amount of provider instruction was significantly related to higher quit rates and lower rates of concomitant smoking (i.e., smoking while using the patch). Dosing and weaning schedules for transdermal nicotine have not been systematically studied, but a lower initial patch dose (e.g., 14 mg vs. 21 mg) is recommended for patients weighing less than 100 lbs and for those with cardiovascular disease (53).

TAILORING FOR SPECIAL POPULATIONS

Considerable evidence demonstrates that interventions are most effective when they are based on the needs of the specific target population. Interventions that are personalized, relevant, and reflect the health concerns and conditions of the intended recipients have greater success rates than interventions not meeting these criteria (210). Tailoring treatment for high-risk subgroups is likely to add the treatment's efficacy and appeal. Tailoring can occur based on sociodemographic and ethnic/cultural group membership, related psychosocial and smoking habit variables, and on factors related to a smoker's unique medical/psychiatric comorbidity.

Minority Smokers

Disproportionately high rates of smoking and disease caused by smoking, including cancer, within the U.S.' adult racial/ethnic minority groups, combined with poor access to mainstream quit smoking programs and services, have made efforts to reach minority populations a national priority (3, 35). To date, progress has been greatest in clarifying the smoking patterns and quitting needs of African American and Hispanic smokers, with growing attention being paid to the special needs of Native-American and Asian-American smokers (180).

Tailored treatments have not yet been systematically compared with "generic" treatments in any of these populations. However, formative research conducted with African American and Hispanic smokers has confirmed that culturally sensitive self-help quitting guides are more likely to be read and recalled—and are rated more highly—than generic guides, even when generic guides are multiracial (160, 170). Because tailored guides address unique smoking patterns, quitting barriers, and motives, they may prove to be more effective as well. Research currently underway will shed light on these issues and help to clarify the most important channels for reaching smokers in varied U.S. racial/ethnic groups (35, 169, 180).

Women Smokers

Today, lung cancer claims more lives among U.S. women than breast cancer (3). As the U.S. population has aged and tobacco industry advertising helped make smoking an "equal opportunity addiction," there are increasingly fewer differences in the smoking or quitting habits of male and female smokers (205, 230, 231). Important gender differences remain, however, in the health consequences of smoking and in related quitting motives and barriers. Therefore, women frequently have been the target of efforts to tailor quit smoking treatments.

Solomon and Flynn (205) identified several concerns that merit special attention in treatments aimed at women. These include helping women to replace smoking as a palliative coping technique, to elicit better social support for quitting, and to cope better with fears of weight gain following quitting. Because depression is more common among women than men, helping women to cope with depression both during and after quitting also may improve the effectiveness of treatment (77); however, no studies to date confirm the benefits of tailoring on either these or related dimensions. Efforts to combine weight management and smoking cessation treatments for weight-worried women have not proven to be beneficial, but this may be a result of overburdening the quitter with too many demands for behavioral change (175).

The single area in which tailoring has proven to be effective for women quitters is during pregnancy (75). Windsor and colleagues (247) found that pregnancy-tailored quitting guides were more effective than generic guides when used as part of a brief, public health maternity-clinic intervention to help pregnant smokers quit.

Adolescents

The 1994 Surgeon General's report (231) includes the strong recommendation to develop and evaluate effective, youth-tailored programs and materials. Young smokers and smokeless-tobacco users possess a strong "optimistic bias" about the safety and benefits of smoking as well as about the ease of quitting (58, 129, 195). Moreover, sensitivity to the adolescent "culture" and appropriate "channel selection" is required for materials and programs targeted toward younger smokers and smokeless-tobacco users.

Older Smokers

Smokers at the other end of the age continuum are equally likely to benefit from tailoring and corrective messages about the actual (versus perceived) harms and benefits of smoking (e.g., "It's never too late to quit."). Relative to younger adult smokers (i.e., aged 21 to 49), older U.S. smokers (i.e., aged 50 to 74) are likely to underestimate the "cons" of smoking, especially the personal and general health risks of smoking, and to overestimate the "pros," such as viewing smoking as useful to control stress and as a weight control tactic (183). This "age gap" in adult perceptions of the health risks and benefits of smoking likely reflects the fact that today's older smokers came of age in an era when smoking was widely promoted as safe and desirable (182).

Fisher and Hill (57) stress the need for brief, physician-initiated interventions aimed at older smokers. "Remembering not to underestimate the benefits of quitting among older smokers, even the busiest specialist should view such interventions as worth the small amount of time they consume" (57). One program specifically developed for older smokers, the *Clear Horizons* program, addresses unique quitting benefits and barriers of such smokers, and recommends quitting activities tailored to the capabilities, resources, and lifestyles of older Americans. Results of a relevant, large clinical trial showed higher-than-expected recruitment rates (a single short announcement in the magazine of the American Association of Retired People elicited 10,000 inquiries), greater use and more favorable ratings of the tailored *Clear Horizons* quitting guide compared with a comparable generic guide, and better 3- and 12-month results (183).

Cancer Patients

Especially for patients with early stage cancer, smoking cessation confers enormous benefits. Whether or not the diagnosed cancer is smoking related, quitting smoking can lower the patient's risks for future smoking-caused tumors, optimize immune response, and prevent smoking-caused exacerbations of unpleasant radiation and chemotherapy side effects (75). Even so, Eriksen and Kondo (49), found that while 40 to 75% of patients with diagnosed cancer stopped smoking right after their diagnosis and initial treatment, most returned to cigarettes once the immediate crisis had passed.

To promote lasting cessation when treatment outcome expectancies are positive, the four-step NCI physician advice-model outlined earlier can be followed. Medical advice should emphasize the benefits of smoking cessation and offer solace to smokers with smoking-caused malignancies, including the explanation that most people began to smoke before the harms were widely known or understood and continued through a strong nicotine addiction. Gritz and colleagues (74, 75) recently reported the results of a physician-initiated quit smoking program for smokers with a primary squamous cell carcinoma of the upper aerodigestive tract. Smoking-cessation guides were developed for this intervention that were tailored to the lifestyles and treatment regimens of these newly diagnosed patients. Quit smoking advice and assistance were initiated immediately after surgery, or before radiation for nonsurgical patients, and continued during regular medical contacts over a 6-month period. All members of the health care team were involved. High continuous abstinence rates (70%) were observed at 6-month follow-up both for intervention-group subjects and for smokers receiving physician advice only, thus suggesting that physician advice alone may be relatively more effective in the presence of life-threatening disease. Predictors of cessation included stage of change, intensity of medical treatment, and level of nicotine dependence.

Smokeless Tobacco

At the outset of the twentieth century, cigarette smoking was relatively nonexistent (140). Less than 3% of the U.S. public's tobacco consumption was in the form of cigarettes; tobacco use was mainly in the form of pipes, cigars, and smokeless tobacco (i.e., chewing tobacco and snuff). In fact, chewing tobacco itself made up over 50% of all tobacco consumed. However, in 1913, the marketing of a milder and blended smoking tobacco in cigarettes (238), which could be inhaled and allowed for quicker nicotine absorption, led to a greater acceptance of the product and, eventually, to the decline of smokeless tobacco as the most preferred form. By 1950, smokeless tobacco made up only a very small percentage of U.S. tobacco consumption (140).

Beginning in the 1970s, smokeless tobacco regained some of its previous popularity. With the announcement by the U.S. Surgeon General in 1964 that cigarette smoking was a primary cause of lung cancer (179), smokers sought safe alternatives to cigarettes. Many erroneously assumed that the industry marketing ploy of moist snuff and chewing tobacco as "smokeless products" implied that these products posed no dangers (195). This new wave of users preferred moist snuff, whereas chewing tobacco was the primary form of smokeless tobacco earlier in the century (195).

While the prevalence of smoking cigarettes has been regularly assessed, use of smokeless tobacco has not. Based on several adult surveys conducted since 1970 (152), use of snuff and chewing tobacco has doubled over the last 25 years. According to the latest surveys, use among men 18 years of age and older indicate that 3.2% use snuff and 4.1% use chewing tobacco (152). Except for African American females in the U.S., smokeless tobacco use among adult females is approximately 1%. Current, overall smokeless tobacco use is 6% (195). Prevalence data are not available for U.S. youth (195). Current estimates indicate that approximately 20% of the white high-school males use smokeless tobacco daily, while less than 1% of young females use smokeless tobacco (231).

The chemical composition of smokeless tobacco includes four classes of carcinogens: (*a*) certain volatile aldehydes, (*b*) radioactive polonium-210, (*c*) polycyclic aromatic hydrocarbons, and (*d*) *N*-nitrosamines (237). The leading carcinogenic constituents in smokeless tobacco are the TSNAs NNN and NNK, which are both mutagenic and carcinogenic. Although these elements are present in the product, it is thought that they also form in the mouth from a reaction of saliva nitrates with the nicotine present in tobacco. NNN and NNK are present in amounts from 10 to 1400 times greater than that allowable in food and beverages (195).

Smokeless-tobacco users appear to suffer from nicotine addiction as much as smokers (19). Other health effects are halitosis and a range of oral problems, including tooth decay and periodontal gum disease (65). One of the more serious complications of using smokeless tobacco is a precancerous condition known as leukoplakia, which is a small white patch in the oral cavity that can transform into squamous cell carcinoma if left untreated. It is estimated that over 50% of the regular smokeless-tobacco users have at least a degree I or early stage leukoplakia lesion (195). Using smokeless tobacco, especially moist snuff, has causal relationship with cancers of the mouth, tongue, gum, pharynx, larynx, esophagus, nasal cavity, stomach, kidney, bladder, and pancreas (237). In addition, the synergistic effects of smokeless tobacco with both smoking and alcohol increase the risk of oral cancer. Cancer risk increases with the length of smokeless tobacco use.

There is tremendous potential for smokeless-tobacco cessation (4). Dentists and dental hygienists have an excellent opportunity to increase users' awareness of the health effects of smokeless tobacco as well as to advocate cessation. Pointing out lesions found during an examination that relate to smokeless tobacco use is a "teachable moment," when users are more apt to respond to a quitting message. A survey of male users revealed that over two-thirds of snuff users reported that they had tried to quit (195); the most frequently cited withdrawal symptoms were irritability, tension, and hunger. The urge to quit has been so compelling that some smokeless quitters have started smoking to assist their quitting efforts (195). Many smokeless-tobacco users report that their motivation to quit would be greater in the event of a smokeless tobacco-related health problem (195). Although interest in quitting exists, little research has focused on minimal-contact, self-help, and formal treatment programs. While cessation materials have been developed for major-league baseball players (154), athletic trainers and coaches (161), and young athletes (155), few self-help materials targeted at the general public are available. Two worthy exceptions are available through the American Cancer Society (3) and a comprehensive self-help cessation manual developed by Severson (194). Formal treatment programs for smokeless tobacco have adapted standard, cognitive behavioral smoking-cessation strategies for smokeless users (195); however, little research has been conducted with these formal programs. The most urgent need is to determine how smokeless cessation differs from the well-documented smoking-cessation process.

Youths

Youths represent the nation's greatest natural resource, yet as more adults are quitting smoking, an increasing number of youths are just beginning to smoke. Approximately 3000 U.S. youths start smoking daily (68). Of these 3000, around 750 will eventually die from a smoking-related disease (68). It is now estimated that over 3 million U.S. youths between 12 and 18 years of age are current smokers (i.e., smoking during the last 30 days) (231). Recent estimates concerning high-school seniors suggest that over 25% are current smokers; however, these figures are conservative given that smoking prevalence among school dropouts likely is much higher (231). Surveys among this group in one urban area indicate that at least 75% smoke daily (175). When high-school senior smoking rates are combined with those of high-school dropouts, the smoking prevalence among teenagers is comparable to that of adults (68). Also, equal numbers of young males and females now smoke cigarettes, and white youths are more likely to smoke than black or Hispanic youths (231).

Young smokers report similar levels of nicotine addiction and withdrawal as adult smokers (59). Smoking by young people also increases their risk for significant health problems during childhood and adolescence, and it places them at increased risk for health complications associated with smoking as adults (231). Significant, smoking-related childhood health problems include (*a*) coughing, (*b*) wheezing, (*c*) shortness of breath, (*d*) increased risk of respiratory diseases, (*e*) retardation of lung growth, and (*f*) reduced lung function and corresponding reduction in physical ability (231). Also, youth smoking has been observed to (*a*) increase low-density lipoprotein, (*b*) increase triglycerides, and (*c*) reduce high-density lipoproteins (38). Of course, the majority of young smokers who continue smoking as adults have increased risks for heart disease, lung cancer, chronic obstructive pulmonary disease, and other serious smoking-related diseases (231).

Tobacco use has been identified as a "gateway" drug (68), increasing the risks for experimentation/use of alcohol, marijuana, and hard drugs such as cocaine. Experimenting with smoking does not cause youth to try other drugs. Tobacco is usually the first drug that youth try, however, and such use increases the risk that other drugs also will be tried.

Most young smokers have indicated that they would like to quit smoking, and 95% say they expect to quit sometime in the future (68). Even so, few ever succeed in becoming ex-smokers (68). Little research has focused on smoking cessation among youth. Of the studies that do exist, most are anecdotal and descriptive in nature, offering little insight regarding the process of quitting among youth (231). School cessation programs have had difficulty enrolling and retaining young smokers in formal quit programs, and available data suggest there is virtually no response to treatment strategies among youth (231). With the absence of interventions, young smokers are very likely to become adult smokers. The 1994 Surgeon General's report on the prevention of tobacco use among youths concluded that effective treatment programs as well as enforcement of laws limiting tobacco sales to minors are needed (231). (Refer to the section on prevention for additional information on prevention activities for youth.)

Tobacco Addiction

In the 1964 Surgeon General's report (239), smoking was described as an habituation. In 1988, the U.S. Department of Health and Human Services (230) identified tobacco use for the first time as nicotine addiction, concluding that "cigarettes and other forms of tobacco are addictive. Nicotine is the drug in tobacco that causes addiction. Moreover, the processes that determine nicotine addiction are similar to those that determine addiction to drugs such as heroin and cocaine" (230). Drug dependence involves the repeated administration of a substance that contains a psychoactive chemical. Like other drug dependencies, nicotine dependence is a progressive, chronic, relapsing disorder that is characterized by (*a*) stereotypic patterns of use, (*b*) use despite harmful effects, and (*c*) relapse following abstinence and recurrent drug cravings. Dependence-producing drugs often produce tolerance, physical dependence, and pleasant effects (236).

The intensity of nicotine's effects relates to the dose given, time since last dose, and level of preexisting or acquired tolerance (236). An interplay exists between the addictive nature of cigarettes and their behaviorally reinforced properties. Over time, smoking becomes associated with a number of cues that reinforce the behavior (56). It is this combination of physiologic and psychologic dependence that makes cessation such a challenge.

Prevention of Tobacco Use

With tobacco use (smoking and smokeless) beginning earlier than ever, the best strategy is to prevent such use from ever starting. Recent surveys indicate that both U.S. smokers and nonsmokers strongly favor policies to prevent use of tobacco by youths (68). Such policies include (*a*) mandated public-school education on tobacco, (*b*) an absolute ban of smoking in the school environment by students and all staff, (*c*) increased restrictions on tobacco advertising and promotion, (*d*) enforcement of laws banning tobacco sales to minors, and (*e*) increases in tobacco taxes. School programs are crucial to the success of prevention efforts. Such prevention programs, which teach students to identify social influences that encourage smoking and train them in skills to resist those influences, have significantly reduced smoking prevalence among youths; however, these effects have lasted from 1 to 3 years only (231). School programs to prevent use of smokeless tobacco, based on methods comparable to the smoking prevention model, have had similar limited success (231). School programs, however, are only part of the solution. Evidence suggests that school-based prevention curricula are enhanced when they are combined with community programs that include (*a*) involvement of parents, (*b*) mass media, (*c*) counteradvertising, (*d*) community organizations, and (*e*) other segments of the school-aged child's environment (68, 231).

The American Academy of Pediatrics (AAP) has recommended that children have a minimum of 20 physician visits from birth to age 21. Such visits provide medical personnel with a teachable moment, because children consider health professionals to be important and credible sources of health information (231). Thus, children may be more likely to follow a health practitioner's advice about tobacco use than what is said by their parents. Success in preventing tobacco use depends on the physician's knowledge of risk factors leading to tobacco use, ability to recognize potentially vulnerable children, and ability to apply an appropriate intervention strategy (231).

Health care providers need to be skilled in advocating tobacco abstinence (231). Tobacco education should be a part of every clinic visit that children and their parents have. Every opportunity should be used to advise parents who smoke to quit and to relate the hazards of environmental tobacco smoke to infant health problems, and the NCI and AAP have developed recommendations for assisting health professionals' attempts to prevent tobacco use among youths. This five-step program includes (*a*) *anticipate* the risks of tobacco use that are associated with the child's stage of development, (*b*) *ask* both the child and parents about tobacco exposure and use at each visit, (*c*) *advise* users to stop tobacco use, (*d*) *assist* users to stop tobacco use by providing a choice of quitting methods, and (*e*) *arrange* for follow-up visits to provide further intervention and assessment as needed (231).

Summary

Reducing tobacco use as well as the morbidity and mortality of smoking-related diseases have been national public health priorities since publication of the first Surgeon General's report on tobacco and health in 1964 (239). As a result, tobacco control has been a major focus of the U.S. Department of Health and Human Services' "Objectives for the Nation" for the year 1990 (232) and the year 2000 (228). Specific objectives attack tobacco use and tobacco-related diseases among targeted populations using multiple methods and channels, including (*a*) education, (*b*) health services, (*c*) legislation, and (*d*) research. Never before in the history of the United States has there been such a comprehensive effort.

During the last 30 years, considerable progress has been made. The adult smoking prevalence has been reduced by approximately 35% (228), and attitudes about tobacco use have changed. Most people now believe that tobacco use is a health hazard. Many organizations and businesses ban indoor smoking, and legislation to curb tobacco use is considerably more widespread. Limitations on tobacco advertising and promotion have become more stringent. State tobacco excise taxes also have been increased, and support for additional levies has been embraced by the public and lawmakers (228).

Although there has been considerable success, much work still remains. Tobacco kills over 400,000 Americans each year, primarily from heart disease, cancer, and respiratory diseases (228). Current estimates indicate that tobacco will have killed approximately 4.5 million Americans from 1990 to 2000. Considering only health care costs and lost productivity, tobacco use amounts to $65 billion per year (68). In addition, the alarming increase in tobacco use among youths gives little cause for hope.

As the number of people who smoke decreases and our ability to help quitting smokers succeed increases, the greater the likelihood of our nation achieving the smoke-free society as advocated by the Surgeon General in 1989 (233). No single approach exists that will achieve such an outcome. A multifaceted model that includes education, mass media, legislation, and community organization provides the optimal channels to prevent tobacco use (231). Widespread availability of cessation programs, both minimal-contact and formal treatment programs, through all public health agencies, worksite health promotion/wellness programs, health maintenance organizations, and private medical and dental practices increases the probability that all tobacco users will have sufficient access to the appropriate treatment that will lead to cessation (153).

References

1. Agundez JAG, Martinez C, Ladero JM, et al, MC Ramos JM, Martin R, Rodriguez A, et al. Debrisoquin oxidation genotype and susceptibility to lung cancer. Clin Pharmacol Ther 1994;55:10–14.
2. Alavanja CRM, Brownson RC, Lubin JH, Berger E, Chang J, and Boice JD Jr. Residential radon exposure and lung cancer among nonsmoking women. JNCI 1994;86:1829–1837.
3. American Cancer Society. Cancer Facts and Figures. Atlanta GA: American Cancer Society, 1994.
4. American Cancer Society. Smokeless Tobacco, Check It Out, Think It Out, Throw It Out, Snuff It Out, Keep It Out (91-10M-2090) 1991. Atlanta GA: American Cancer Society, 1991.
5. American Medical Association. How to Help Patients Stop Smoking. Chicago: American Medical Association, 1993.
6. Ames BN, Durston WE, Yamasaki E, Lee FD. Carcinogens are mutagens: a simple test system combining liver homogenates for activation and bacteria for detection. Proc Natl Acad Sci USA 1973;70:2281.
7. Anonymous. The effect of vitamin E and beta carotene on the incidence of lung cancer and other cancers in male smokers. The Alpha-Tocopherol, Beta Carotene Cancer Prevention Study Group. N Eng J Med 1994;330:1029–1035.
8. Anwar K, Nakakuki K, Naiki H, Inuzuka, M. *Ras* Gene mutations and HPV infection are common in human laryngeal carcinoma. Int J Cancer 1993;53:22–28.
9. Auerbach O, Hammond EC, Kirman D, Garfinkel L, Stout AP. Histologic changes in bronchial tubes of cigarette-smoking dogs. Cancer 1967;20:2055.
10. Ayesh R, Idle JR, Ritchie JC, Crothers MJ, Hetzel MR. Metabolic oxidation phenotypes as markers for susceptibility to lung cancer. Nature 1984;312:169–170.
11. Barone J, Taioli E, Hebert JR, Wynder EL. Vitamin supplement use and risk of oral and esophageal cancer. Nutr Cancer 1992;18:31–41.
12. Bartecchi CE, MacKenzie TD, Schreir RW. The human costs of tobacco use. N Eng J Med 1994;330:907–912.
13. Bartsch H, Castegnaro M, Rojas M, Camus AM, Alexandrov K, Lang M. Expression of pulmonary cytochrome P4501A1 and carcinogen DNA adduct formation in high risk subjects for tobacco-related cancer. Toxicol Lett 1992;64–65: 477–483.
14. Beach AC, Gupta RC. Human biomonitoring and the ^{32}P-postlabeling assay. Carcinogenesis 1992;13:1053–1074.
15. Bell DA, Taylor JA, Paulson DF, Robertson CN, Mohler JL, Lucier GW. Genetic risk and carcinogen exposure: a common inherited defect of the carcinogen-metabolism gene glutathione S-transferase M1 (GSTM1) that increases susceptibility to bladder cancer. JNCI 1993;85:1159–1164.
16. Benitez J, Ladero JM, Fernandez-Gundin MJ, et al. Polymorphic oxidation of debrisoquine in bladder cancer. Ann Med 1990;22:157–160.
17. Benitez J, Ladero JM, Jara C, Carrillo JA, et al. Polymorphic oxidation of debrisoquine in lung cancer patients. Eur J Cancer 1991;27:158–161.
18. Benner SE, Pajak TF, Lippman SM, Early C, Hong WK. Prevention of second primary tumors with isotretinoin in inpatients with squamous cell carcinoma of the head and neck: long-term follow-up. JNCI 1994;86:140–141.
19. Benowitz NL. Nicotine and smokeless tobacco. CA 1988;38:244–247.
20. Block G. Vitamin C and cancer prevention: the epidemiologic evidence. Am J Clin Nutr 1991;53:270S–282S.
21. Blot WJ, Xu Z-Y, Boice JD, et al. Indoor radon and lung cancer in China. JNCI 1990;82:1025–1030.
22. Board PG. Biochemical genetics of glutathione-S-transferase in man. Am J Hum Genet 1981;33:36–43.
23. Boutwell RK. On the role of tumor promotion in chemical carcinogenesis. In Models, Mechanisms, and Etiology of Tumour Promotion. Edited by M Borzsonyi, NE Day. Lyon: IARC, 1984, p 3.
24. Brockmoller J, Kerb R, Drakoulis N, Nitz M, Roots I. Genotype and phenotype of glutathione S-transferase class μ isoenzymes μ in lung cancer patients and controls. Cancer Res 1993;53:1004–1011.
25. Brockmoller J, Kerb R, Drakoulis N, Staffeldt B, Roots I. Glutathione-*S*-transferase M1 and its variants A and B as host factors of bladder cancer susceptibility: a case-control study. Cancer Res 1994;54:4103–4111.
26. Brown LM, Blot WJ, Schuman SH, et al: Environmental factors and high risk of esophageal cancer among men in coastal South Carolina. JNCI 1988;80:1620.
27. Brownson RC, Alavanja MCR, Hock ET, Loy TS. Passive smoking and lung cancer in nonsmoking women. Am J Public Health 1992;82:1525–1530.
28. Buckley JD, Harris RWC, Doll R, Vessey MP, Williams PT. Case-control study of the husbands of women with dysplasia or carcinoma of the cervix uteri. Lancet 1981;ii:1010–1015.
29. Burch JD, Rohan TE, Howe GR, et al. Risk of bladder cancer by source and type of tobacco exposure: a case-control study. Int J Cancer 1989;44:622–628.
30. Burchill SA, Neal DE, Lunec J. Frequency of H-*ras* mutations in human bladder cancer detected by direct sequencing. Br J Urol 1994;73:516–521.
31. Caporaso N, Hayes R, Dosemeci M, et al. Lung cancer risk, occupational exposure, and the debrisoquine metabolic phenotype. Cancer Res 1989;49:3675.
32. Caporaso NE, Tucker MA, Hoover RN, et al: Lung cancer and the debrisoquine metabolic phenotype. JNCI 1990;82:1264.
33. Cartwright RA, Glashan RW, Rogers HJ, et al. Role of *N*-acetyltransferase phenotypes in bladder carcinogenesis: a pharmacogenetic epidemiological approach to bladder cancer. Lancet 1982;16:842.
34. Cartwright RA, Philip PA, Rogers HJ, Glashan RW. Genetically determined debrisoquine oxidation capacity in bladder cancer. Carcinogenesis 1984;5:1191–1192.
35. Centers for Disease Control and Prevention. Chronic Disease in Minority Populations. Atlanta: Centers for Disease Control and Prevention, 1994.
36. Coghlin J, Gann PH, Hammond SK, et al. 4-aminobiphenyl hemoglobin adducts in fetuses exposed to the tobacco smoke carcinogen in utero. JNCI 1991;83:2374–2380.
37. Cohen S, Lichtenstein E, Prochaska J, et al. Debunking myths about self-quitting. Am Psychol 1989;44:1335–1365.
38. Craig WY, Palomaki GE, Johnson AM, Haddow JE. Cigarette smoking-associated changes in blood lipid and lipoprotein levels in the 8- to 19-year-old age group. Pediatrics 1990;85:155–158.
39. Crawford FG, Mayer J, Santella RM, et al. Biomarkers of environmental tobacco smoke in preschool children and their mothers. JNCI 1994;86:1398–1402.
40. Curry S. Self-help interventions for smoking cessation. J Consult Clin Psychol 1993;61:790–803.
41. Curry SJ, Wagner EH, Grothaus LC. Evaluation of intrinsic and extrinsic motivation interventions with self-help smoking cessation program. J Consult Clin Psychol 1991;59:318–324.
42. Daly AK, Thomas DJ, Cooper J, Pearson WR, Neal DE, Idle JR. Homozygous deletion of gene for glutathione S-transferase M1 in bladder cancer. Br Med J 1993;307:481–482.
43. Davis RM. Uniting physicians against smoking: the need for a coordinated national strategy. JAMA 1988;259:2900–2901.
44. Drakoulis N, Cascorbi I, Brockmoller J, Gross CR, Roots I. Polymorphisms in the human *CYP1A1* gene as susceptibility factors for lung cancer: exon-7 mutation (4889 A to G), and a T to C mutation in the 3′-flanking region. Clin Investigator 1994;72:240–248.
45. Drozdz M, Gierel T, Jendryczko A, Pilch J, Piekarska J. *N*-acetyltransferase phenotype of patients with cancer of the larynx. Neoplasma 1987;34:481–484.
46. Duche JC, Joanne C, Barre J, et al. Lack of a relationship between the polymorphism of debrisoquine oxidation and lung cancer. Br J Clin Pharmacol 1991;31:533–536.
47. Dunn BP, Vedal S, San RHC, et al. DNA adducts in bronchial biopsies. Int J Cancer 1991;48:485–492.
48. Elwood JM, Pearson JCG, Skippen DH, Jackson SM. Alcohol, smoking, social, and occupational factors in the aetiology of cancer of the oral cavity, pharynx and larynx. Int J Cancer 1984;34:603.
49. Eriksen MP, Kondo AT. Smoking cessation for cancer patients: rationale and approaches. Health Ed Res 1989;4:489–494.
50. Eriksen MP, Lemaistre CA, Newell GR. Health hazards of passive smoking. Ann Rev Public Health 1988;9:47.
51. Field JK, Spandidos DA. Expression of oncogenes in human tumours with special reference to the head and neck region. Oral Pathol 1987;16:97.
52. Fiore M. The new vital sign: assessing and documenting smoking status. JAMA 1991;22:751–760.
53. Fiore M, Jorneby DE, Baker TB, Kenford SL. Tobacco dependence and the nicotine patch: clinical guidelines for effective use. JAMA 1992;268:2687–2694.
54. Fiore M, Novotny T, Pierce J, et al. Methods used to quit smoking in the United States: do cessation programs help? JAMA 1990;268:2687–2694.
55. Fiore M, Smith SS, Jorneby DE, Baker TB. The effectiveness of the nicotine patch for smoking cessation: a meta-analysis. JAMA 1994:1940–1947.
56. Fisher EB, Bishop DB, Goldmuntz J, Jacobs A. Implications for the practicing physician of the psychosocial dimension of smoking. Chest 1988;93:69S.
57. Fisher EB, Hill RD. Perspectives on older smokers. Chest 1990;97:517–518.
58. Flay BR. Youth tobacco use: risks, patterns and control. In Nicotine Addiction: Principles and Management. Edited by CT Orleans, J Slade. New York: Oxford University Press, 1993, pp 365–385.
59. Fleming CM, Kaisery A, Wilkinson GR, Smith P, Branch RA. The ability to 4-hydroxylate debrisoquine is related to recurrence of bladder cancer. Pharmacogenetics 1992;2:128–134.
60. Foiles PG, Murphy SE, Peterson LA, Carmella SG, Hecht SS. DNA and hemoglobin adducts as markers of metabolic activation of tobacco-specific carcinogens. Cancer Res 1992;52:2698S–2701S.
61. Fontham ETH, Correa P, Reynolds P, et al. Environmental tobacco smoke and lung cancer in nonsmoking women. JAMA 1994;271:1752–1759.
62. Fraumeni JF Jr, Wertelecki W, Blattner WA, Jensen RD, Leventhal BG. Varied manifestations of a familial lymphoproliferative disorder. Am J Med 1975;59:145.
63. Gallick GE, Sacks PG, Maxwell SA, Steck PA, Gutterman JU. Head and neck squamous cell carcinoma lines as a model system for the study of oncogene expression during tumor progression and metastasis. Prog Clin Biol Res 1986;212:97.
64. Garfinkel L. Time trends in lung cancer mortality among nonsmokers and a note on passive smoking. JNCI 1981;66:1061.
65. Glover ED, Schroeder KL, Henningfield JE, Severson HH, Charksten AG. An interpretative review of smokeless tobacco research in the United States: Part I. Drug Ed 1988;18:305–330.
66. Glynn TJ. Relative effectiveness of physician-initiated smoking cessation programs. Cancer Bull 1988;40:359–364.
67. Glynn TJ, Boyd G, Gruman J. Self-Guided Strategies for Smoking Cessation. A Program Planner's Guide. NIH publication No 91-3104. Washington DC: National Cancer Institute, 1991.
68. Glynn TJ, Greenwald P, Mills SM, Manley MW. Youth tobacco use in the United States: problems, progress, goals, and potential solutions. Prev Med 1993;22:560–575.
69. Glynn TJ, Manley M. How to Help Your Patients Stop Smoking: A National Cancer Institute Manual for Physicians. NIH publication No 89-3064. Washington DC: National Cancer Institute, 1989.
70. Glynn TJ, Manley MW. Physicians, cancer control and the treatment of nicotine dependence: defining success. Health Ed Res 1989;4:479–487.
71. Gough AC, Miles JS, Spurr NK, et al. Identification of the primary gene defect at the cytochrome P450 CYP2D locus. Nature 1990;347:773–776.
72. Graham S. Epidemiology of retinoids and cancer. JNCI 1984;73:1423.
73. Greenblatt MS, Bennett WP, Hollstein M, Harris CC. Mutations in the p53 tumor suppressor gene: clues to cancer etiology and molecular pathogenesis. Cancer Res 1994;54:4855–4878.
74. Gritz ER, Carr CR, Rapkin DA, Abemayor E, et al. Predictors of long-term smoking cessation in head and neck cancer patients. Cancer Epidemiol Biomarkers Prev 1993;2:261–270.
75. Gritz ER, Kristeller J, Burns DMN. Treating nicotine addiction in high-risk groups and patients with medical comorbidity. In Nicotine Addiction: Principles and Management. Edited by CT Orleans, J Slade. New York: Oxford University Press, 1993, pp 279–310.
76. Hajek P, Jackson P, Belcher M. Long-term use of nicotine chewing gum. JAMA 1988;260:1593–1596.
77. Hall SM, Munoz RF, Reus VI, Sees KI. Nicotine, negative affect and depression. J Consult Clin Psychol 1993;61:761–767.

78. Hammond EC, Garfinkel L, Lew EA. Longevity, selective mortality, and competitive risks in relation to chemical carcinogenesis. Environ Res 1978;16:153.
79. Hammond EC, Selikoff IJ, Seidman H. Asbestos exposure, cigarette smoking and death rates. Ann NY Acad Sci 1979;330:473.
80. Hanke J, Krajewska B. Acetylation phenotypes and bladder cancer. J Occupational Med 1990;32:917–918.
81. Hanssen HP, Agarwal DP, Goedde HW, et al. Association of *N*-acetyltransferase polymorphism and environmental factors with bladder carcinogenesis. Study in a North German population. Eur Urol 1985;11:263.
82. Hayashi S, Watanabe J, Kawajir K. High susceptibility to lung cancer analyzed in terms of combined genotypes of P450IA1 and mu-class glutathione S-transferase genes. Jpn J Cancer Res 1992;83:866–870.
83. Hayes RB, Bi W, Rothman N, Broly F, et al. *N*-acetylation phenotype and genotype and risk of bladder cancer in benzidine-exposed workers. Carcinogenesis 1993;14:675–678.
84. Hecht SS, Hoffman D. Tobacco-specific nitrosamines: an important group of carcionogens in tobacco and tobacco smoke. Carcinogenesis 1988;9:875–884.
85. Hecht SS, Rivenson A, Braley J, DiBello J, Adams JD, Hoffman D. Induction of oral cavity tumors in F344 rats by tobacco-specific nitrosamines and snuff. Cancer Res 1986;46:4162–4166.
86. Heckbert SR, Weiss NS, Hornung SK, Eaton DL, Motulsky AG. Glutathione S-transferase and epoxide hydrolase activity in human leukocytes in relation to risk of lung cancer and other smoking-related cancers. JNCI 1992;84:414–422.
87. Heim M, Meyer UA. Genotyping of poor metabolisers of debrisoquine by allele-specific PCR amplification. Lancet 1990;336:529–532.
88. Hein DW. Acetylator genotype and arylamine-induced carcinogenesis. Biochim Biophys Acta 1988;948:37–66.
89. Herity B, Moriarty M, Daly L, Dunn J, Bourke GJ. The role of tobacco and alcohol in the aetiology of lung and larynx cancer. Br J Cancer 1982;46:961.
90. Hilt B, Langard S, Andersen A, Rosenberg J. Asbestos exposure, smoking habits, and cancer incidence among production and maintenance workers in an electrochemical plant. Am J Ind Med 1985;8:565.
91. Hirvonen A, Husgafvel-Pursiainen K, Anttila S, Karjalainen A, Pelkonen O, Vainio H. PCR-based CYP2D6 genotyping for Finnish lung cancer patients. Pharmacogenetics 1993;3:319–327.
92. Hirvonen A, Husgafvel-Pursiainen K, Anttila S, Karjalainen A, Sorsa M, Vainio H. Metabolic cytochrome P450 genotypes and assessment of individual susceptibility to lung cancer. Pharmacogenetics 1992;2:259–263.
93. Hirvonen A, Husgafvel-Pursiainen K, Anttila S, Karjalainen A, Vainio H. Polymorphism in CYP1A1 and CYP2D6 genes: possible association with susceptibility to lung cancer. Environment Health Perspect 1993;101(suppl 3):109–112.
94. Hirvonen A, Husgafvel-Pursiainen K, Anttila S, Vainio H. The GSTM1 null genotype as a potential risk modifier for squamous cell carcinoma of the lung. Carcinogenesis 1993;14:1479–1481.
95. Hirvonen A, Husgafvel-Pursiainen K, Karjalainen A, Anttila S, Vainio H. Point mutational MspI and Ile-Val polymorphisms closely linked in the CYP1A1 gene: lack of association with susceptibility to lung cancer in a Finnish study population. Cancer Epidemiol Biomarkers Prev 1992;1:485–489.
96. Hoffman D, Hecht SS. Nicotine-derived *N*-nitrosamines and tobacco related cancer: current status and future directions. Cancer Res 1985;45:935–944.
97. Hoffman D, Melikian A, Adams JD, Brunnemann KD, Haley N. New aspects of tobacco carcinogenesis. Carcinogenesis 1985;8:239.
98. Huber MH, Hong WK. Biology and chemoprevention of head and neck cancer. Curr Probl Cancer 1994;18:81–140.
99. Hughes JR. Pharmacotherapy for smoking cessation: unvalidated assumptions, anomalies and suggestions for future research. J Consult Clin Psychol 1993;61:751–760.
100. Hughes JR, Gust SW, Keenan RM, Fenwick JW, Healey ML. Nicotine vs. placebo gum in general medical practice. JAMA 1989;261:1300–1305.
101. Husgafvel-Pursiainen K, Ridanpaa M, Hackman P, et al. Detection of *ras* gene mutations in human lung cancer: comparison of two screening assays based on the polymerase chain reaction. Environment Health Perspect 1992;98:183–185.
102. International Association for Research in Cancer. IARC Monographs on the Evaluation of the Carcinogenic Risk of Chemicals to Humans, Vol. 38. Tobacco Smoking. Lyon: IARC, 1986.
103. Janerich DT, Thompson W. Douglas, Varela LR, et al. Lung cancer and exposure to tobacco smoke in the household. N Engl J Med 1990;323:632.
104. Jarvik M, Henningfield J. Pharmacological adjuncts for the treatment of tobacco dependence. In Nicotine Addiction: Principles and Management. Edited by CT Orleans, J Slade. New York: Oxford University Press, 1993, pp 245–262.
105. Johnson BE, Kelley MJ. Overview of genetic and molecular events in the pathogenesis of lung cancer. Chest 1993;103:1S–3S.
106. Kabat GC, Dieck GS, Wynder EL. Bladder cancer in nonsmokers. Cancer 1986;57:362–367.
107. Kabat GC, Wynder EL. Lung cancer in nonsmokers. Cancer 1984;53:1214.
108. Kaisary A, Smith P, Jaczq E, et al. Genetic predisposition to bladder cancer: ability to hydroxylate debrisoquine and mephenytoin as risk factors. Cancer Res 1987;47:5488–5493.
109. Karki NT, Pokela R, Nuutinen L, Pelkonen O. Aryl hydrocarbon hydroxylase in lymphocytes and lung tissue from lung cancer patients and controls. Int J Cancer 1987;39:565.
110. Kato S, Shields PG, Caporaso NE, et al. Cytochrome P450IIE1 genetic polymorphisms, racial variation, and lung cancer risk. Cancer Res 1992;52:6712–6715.
111. Kawachi I, Pearce NE, Jackson RT. Deaths from lung cancer and ischaemic heart disease due to passive smoking in New Zealand. N Engl Med J 1989;102:337.
112. Kawajiri K, Nakachi K, Imai K, Hayashi S, Watanabe J. Individual differences in lung cancer susceptibility in relation to polymorphisms of P-450IA1 gene and cigarette dose. Int Symp Princess Takamatsu Cancer Res Fund 1990;21:55–61.
113. Kawajiri K, Nakachi K, Imai K, Yoshii A, Shinoda N, Watanabe J. Identification of genetically high risk individuals to lung cancer by DNA polymorphisms of the cytochrome P450IA1 gene. FEBS Lett 1990;263:131–133.
114. Kelsey KT, Wiencke JK, Spitz MR. A race-specific genetic polymorphism in the *CYP1A1* gene is not associated with lung cancer in African-Americans. Carcinogenesis 1994;15:1121–1124.
115. Kihara M, Kihara M, and Noda K. Lung cancer risk of GSTM1 null genotype is dependent on the extent of tobacco smoke exposure. Carcinogenesis 1994;15:415–418.
116. Kihara M, Kihara M, Noda K, Okamoto N. Increased risk of lung cancer in Japanese smokers with class mu glutathione S-transferase gene deficiency. Cancer Lett 1993;71:151–155.
117. Klein-Szanto AJP, Iizasa T, Momiki S, et al. A tobacco-specific *N*-nitrosamine or cigarette smoke condensate causes neoplastic transformation of xenotransplanted human bronchial epithelial cells. Proc Natl Acad Sci USA 1992;89:6693–6697.
118. Knekt P, Aromaa A, Maatela J, et al. Vitamin E and cancer prevention. Am J Clin Nutr 1991;53:283S–286S.
119. Kottke TE, Battista RN, DeFriese G, Brekke ML. Attributes of successful smoking cessation interventions in medical practice: a meta-analysis of 39 trials. JAMA 1988;259:2883–2889.
120. Kouri RE, McKinney CE, Slomiany DJ, Snodgrass DR, Wray NP, McLemore TL. Positive correlation between high aryl hydrocarbon hydroxylase activity and primary lung cancer as analyzed in cryopreserved lymphocytes. Cancer Res 1982;42:5030.
121. Krontiris TG, DiMartino NA, Mitcheson HD, Lonergan JA, Begg C, Parkinson DR. Human hypervariable sequences in risk assessment: rare Ha-*ras* alleles in cancer patients. Environ Health Perspect 1987;76:147.
122. Lafuente A, Pujol F, Carretero P, Villa JP, Cuchi A. Human glutathione S-transferase mu (GST mu) deficiency as a marker for the susceptibility to bladder and larynx cancer among smokers. Cancer Letters 1993;68:49–54.
123. Lam W, Sze PC, Sacks HS, Chalmers TC. Meta-analysis of randomized controlled trials of nicotine chewing gum. Lancet 1987;2:27–29.
124. Lando H. Formal quit smoking treatments. In Nicotine Addiction: Principles and Management. Edited by CT Orleans, J Slade. New York: Oxford University Press, 1993, pp 221–244.
125. Laredo Quesada JM. Jara Sanchez C, Benitez Rodriguez J, et al. Acetylation polymorphism in lung cancer. Ann Med Int 1991;8:66–68.
126. Law MR, Hetzel MR, Idle JR. Debrisoquine metabolism and genetic predisposition to lung cancer. Br J Cancer 1989;59:686–687.
127. Lerman CL, Orleans CT, Engstrom PF. Biological markers in smoking cessation treatment. Semin Oncol 1993;4:359–367.
128. Letourneau EG, Krewski D, Choi NW, et al. Case-control study of residential radon and lung cancer in Winnipeg, Manitoba, Canada. Am J Epidemiol 1994;140:310–322.
129. Leventhal H, Glynn K, Fleming R. Is the smoking decision an "informed choice?" Effect of smoking risk factors on smoking. JAMA 1987;257:3373–3376.
130. Lin HJ, Han CY, Bernstein DA, Hsiao W, Lin BK, Hardy S. Ethnic distribution of the glutathione transferase Mu 1-1 (GSTM1) null genotype in 1473 individuals and application to bladder cancer susceptibility. Carcinogenesis 1994;15:1077–1081.
131. Lower GM, Nilsson T, Nelson CE, Wolf H, Gamsky TE, Bryan GT. *N*-acetyltransferase phenotype and risk in urinary bladder cancer: approaches in molecular epidemiology. Preliminary results in Sweden and Denmark. Environ Health Perspect 1979;29:71.
132. Lubin JH. Invited commentary: lung cancer and exposure to residential radon. Am J Epidemiol 1994;140:323–332.
133. Mackerras D, Buffler PA, Randall DE, Nichaman MZ, Pickle LW, Mason TJ. Carotene intake and the risk of laryngeal cancer in coastal Texas. Am J Epidemiol 1988;128:980.
134. Manus ME, Boobis AR, Minchin RF, et al. Relationship between oxidative metabolism of 2-acetylaminofluorene, debrisoquine, bufuralol, and aldrin in human liver microsomes. Cancer Res 1984;44:5692.
135. Marshall J, Graham S, Mettlin C, Sheed D, Swanson, M. Diet in the epidemiology of oral cancer. Nutr Cancer 1982;3:145.
136. McLemore TL, Adelberg S, Liu MC, et al. Expression of CYP1A1 gene in patients with lung cancer: Evidence for cigarette smoke-induced gene expression in normal lung tissue and for altered gene regulation in primary pulmonary carcinomas. JNCI 1990;82:1333.
137. Mecklenburg RE, Christen AG, Gerbert B, et al. How to Help Your Patients Stop Using Tobacco: A National Institute Manual for the Oral Health Team. NIH publication 91-3191. Washington DC: Department of Health and Human Services, 1991.
138. Menkes MS, Comstock GW, Vuilleumier JP, Helsing KJ, Rider AA, Brookmeyer R. Serum beta-carotene, vitamins A and E, selenium, and the risk of lung cancer. N Engl J Med 1986;315:1250–1254.
139. Miller WR, Rollnick S. Motivational Interviewing. New York: Guilford, 1991.
140. Milmore BK, Conover AG. Tobacco consumption in the United States, 1880–1955. In Tobacco Smoking Patterns in the United States. Edited by W Haenszel, MB Shimkin, HP Miller. Washington DC: Government Printing Office, 1956, pp 107–111.
141. Mommsen S, Agaard J. Susceptibility in urinary bladder cancer: acetyltransferase phenotypes and related risk factors. Cancer Lett 1986;32:199.
142. Mustonen R, Hemminki K. 7-Methylguanine levels in DNA of smokers' and nonsmokers' total white blood cells, granulocytes and lymphocytes. Carcinogenesis 1992;13:1951–1955.
143. Mustonen R, Schoket B, Hemminki K. Smoking-related DNA adducts: ^{32}P-postlabeling analysis of 7-methylguanine in human bronchial and lymphocyte DNA. Carcinogenesis 1993;14:151–154.
144. Nakachi K, Imai K, Hayashi S, Kawajiri K. Polymorphisms of the CYP1A1 and glutathione S-transferase genes associated with susceptibility to lung cancer in relation to cigarette dose in a Japanese population. Cancer Res 1993;53:2994–2999.
145. Nakachi K, Imai K, Hayashi S, Watanabe J, Kawajiri K. Genetic susceptibility to squamous cell carcinoma of the lung in relation to cigarette smoking dose. Cancer Res 1991;51:5177–5180.
146. National Research Council: Environmental Tobacco Smoke. Measuring Exposures and Assessing Health Effects. Washington DC: National Academy Press, 1986.
147. Nazer-Stewart V, Motulsky AG, Eaton DL, et al. The glutathione S transferase mu polymorphism as a marker for susceptibility to lung carcinoma. Cancer Res 1993;53:2313–2318.
148. Ockene JK. Clinical perspectives: Physician-delivered interventions for smoking cessation: strategies for increasing effectiveness. Prev Med 1987;16:723–737.

149. Office of Technology Assessment: The Role of Genetic Testing in The Prevention of Occupational Disease. Washington DC: Office of Technology Assessment, 1983, p 95.
150. Olsen J, Sabroe S, Fasting, U. Interaction of alcohol and tobacco as risk factors in cancer of the laryngeal region. J Epidemiol Commun Health 1985;39:165.
151. Ooi WL, Elston RC, Chen VW, Bailey-Wilson JE, Rothschild H. Increased familial risk for lung cancer. JNCI 1986;76:217.
152. Orlandi MA, Boyd GM. Smokeless tobacco use among adolescents: a theoretical overview. Natl Cancer Inst Monogr 1989;8:6.
153. Orleans CT. Treating nicotine dependence in medical settings: a stepped care model. In Nicotine Addiction: Principles and Management. Edited by CT Orleans, J Slade. New York: Oxford University Press, 1993, pp 145–161.
154. Orleans CT, Connolly G, Workman S. Beat the Smokeless Habit. Philadelphia: Fox Chase Cancer Center, 1991.
155. Orleans CT, Cooper J, Telepchak J, Masny A, Benincasa T. Spitting into the Wind. Philadelphia: Fox Chase Cancer Center, 1993.
156. Orleans CT, Glynn TJ, Manley MW, Slade J. Minimal contact quit smoking strategies for medical settings. In Nicotine Addiction: Principles and Management. Edited by CT Orleans, J Slade. New York: Oxford University Press, 1993, pp 181–120.
157. Orleans CT, Kristeller JL, Gritz ER. Helping hospitalized smokers quit: New directions for treatment and research. J Consult Clin Psychol 1993;61:778–789.
158. Orleans CT, Resch N, Noll E, et al. Use of transdermal nicotine in a state-wide prescription plan for the elderly: a first look at "real world" patch users. JAMA 1994;271: 601–607.
159. Orleans CT, Schoenbach VJ, Wagner E. et al. Self-help quit smoking interventions: Effects of self-help materials, social support instructions and telephone counseling. J Consult Clin Psychol 1991;59:439–448.
160. Orleans CT, Sutton C, Noll EL, Resch N, James D, Blais LM, Corcoran RD, Robinson R. A formative evaluation of "pathways to freedom": a tobacco control guide for the African American community 1995 (unpublished).
161. Orleans CT, Telepchak J, Masny A, Benincasa T, Cooper J. Quitting Spit. Philadelphia: Fox Chase Cancer Center, 1993.
162. Ossip-Klein DJ, Giovino G, Megahed N. et al. Effects of a smokers' hotline: results of a 10-county self-help trial. J Consult Clin Psychol 1991;59:325–332.
163. Paganini-Hill A, Chao A, Ross RK, Henderson BE. Vitamin A, beta-carotene, and the risk of cancer: a prospective study. JNCI 1987;79:443–448.
164. Pastorino U, Infante M, Maioli M, et al. Adjuvant treatment of stage I lung cancer with high-dose vitamin A. J Clin Oncol 1993;11:1216–1222.
165. Pelkonen O, Karki NT, Sotaniemi EA. Determination of carcinogen activating enzymes in the monitoring of high-risk groups. In Human Cancer. Its Characterization and Treatment. Edited by W Davis, KR Harrap, G Stathopoulos. Amsterdam: Excerpta Medica, 1980, pp.48–57.
166. Perera F, Mayer J, Jaretzki A, et al. Comparison of DNA adducts and sister chromatid exchange in lung cancer cases and controls. Cancer Res 1989;49:4446.
167. Perera FP, Poirier MC, Yuspa SH, et al. A pilot project in molecular cancer epidemiology: determination of benzo(a)pyrene-DNA adducts in animal and human tissues by immunoassays. Carcinogenesis 1982;3:1405.
168. Perera FP, Santella RM, Brenner D, et al. DNA adducts, protein adducts, and sister chromatid exchange in cigarette smokers and nonsmokers. JNCI 1987;79:449.
169. Perez-Stable EJ, Marin B, Marin G. A comprehensive smoking cessation program for the San Francisco Bay area Latino community: programa latino para dejar defumar. Ann J Health Promo 1993;7:430–442, 475.
170. Perez-Stable EJ, Sabogal F, Marin BV, Otero-Sabogal R. Evaluation of "Guia para Dejar de fumar," a self-guide in Spanish to quit smoking. Public Health Rep 1991;87: 564–570.
171. Pershagen G, Akerblom G, Axelson O, et al. Residential radon exposure and lung cancer in Sweden. N Engl J Med 1994;330:159–164.
172. Pershagen G, Liang ZH, Hrubec Z, Swensson C, Boice JD Jr. Residential radon exposure and lung cancer in Swedish women. Health Physics 1992;63:179–186.
173. Persson I, Johansson I, Bergling H, et al. Genetic polymorphism of cytochrome P4502E1 in a Swedish population. FEBS Lett 1993;319:207–211.
174. Peto R. Smoking and death: the past 40 years and the next 40. Br Med J 1994;309: 937–939.
175. Pirie PL, Murray DM, Luepker RV. Smoking prevalence in a cohort of adolescents including absentees, dropouts, and transfers. Am J Public Health 1988;78:176–178.
176. Prochaska JO, DiClemente CC. Stages and processes of self-change of smoking: toward an integrative model. J Consult Clin Psychol 1983;51:390–395.
177. Prochaska JO, DiClemente CC, Norcross J. In search of how people change: applications to addictive behavior. Am Psychol 1992;47:1102–1114.
178. Prochaska JO, DiClemente CC, Velicer WF, Rossi JS. Standardized, individualized, interactive and personalized self-help programs for smoking cessation. Health Psychol 1993;12:399–405.
179. Public Health Service. Smoking and Health: Report of the Advisory Committee to the Surgeon General of the Public Health Service. Washington DC: U.S. Public Health Service, 1964.
180. Ramirez AG, Gallion KJ. Nicotine dependence among blacks and Hispanics. In Nicotine Addiction: Principles and Management. Edited by CT Orleans, J Slade. New York: Oxford University Press, 1993.
181. Randerath E, Miller RH, Mittal D, Avitts TA, Dunsford HA, Randerath K. Covalent DNA damage in tissues of cigarette smokers as determined by 32P-postlabeling assay. JNCI 1989;81:341.
182. Rimer B, Orleans CT, Keintz MK, Cristinzio S, Fleisher L. The older smoker: status, challenges and opportunities for intervention. Chest 1990;97:547–553.
183. Rimer BK, Orleans CT, Fleisher L, Cristinzio S, Telepchak J, Keintz MK. Does tailoring matter? The impact of a tailored guide on ratings and short-term smoking related outcomes for older smokers. Health Ed Res 1994;9:69–84.
184. Ronai ZA, Gradia S, Peterson LA, Hecht SS. G to A transitions and G to T transversions in codon 12 of the Ki-*ras* oncogene isolated from mouse lung tumors induced by 4-(methylnitrosamino)-1-(3-pyridyl)-1-butanone (NNK) and related DNA methylating and pyridoxobutylating agents. Carcinogenesis 1993;14:2419–2422.
185. Roots I, Drakoulis N, Ploch M, et al. Debrisoquine hydroxylation phenotype, acetylation phenotype, and ABO blood groups as genetic host factors of lung cancer risk. Klin Wochenschr 1988;66 (suppl XI):87–97.
186. Ryberg D, Kure E, Lystad S, et al. p53 Mutations in lung tumors: relationship to putative susceptibility markers for cancer. Cancer Res 1994;54:1551–1555.
187. Saccomanno G. The contribution of uranium miners to lung cancer histogenesis. Recent results. Cancer Res 1982;82:43.
188. Sandler DP, Everson RB, Wilcox AJ. Passive smoking in adulthood and cancer risk. Am J Epidemiol 1985;121:37–48.
189. Saracci R. Asbestos and lung cancer: An analysis of the epidemiological evidence on the asbestos-smoking interaction. Int J Cancer 1977;20:323.
190. Schoenberg JB, Klotz JB, Wilcox HB, et al. Case-control study of residential radon and lung cancer among New Jersey women. Cancer Res 1990;50:6520–6524.
191. Seidegard J, Pero RW, Markowitz MM, Roush G, Miller DG, Beattie EJ. Isoenzyme(s) of glutathione transferase (class Mu) as a marker for the susceptibility to lung cancer: a follow up study. Carcinogenesis 1990;11:33–36.
192. Seidegard J, Pero RW, Miller DG, Beattie EJ. A glutathione transferase in human leukocytes as a marker for the susceptibility to lung cancer. Carcinogenesis 1986;7: 751–753.
193. Sellers TA, Bailey-Wilson JE, Elston RC, et al. Evidence for Mendelian inheritance in the pathogenesis of lung cancer. JNCI 1990;82:1272.
194. Severson HH. Enough Snuff: A Manual for Quitting Smokeless Tobacco on Your Own. Eugene OR: Rainbow Productions, 1992.
195. Severson HH. Smokeless tobacco: Risks, epidemiology, and cessation. In Nicotine Addiction: Principles and Management. Edited by CT Orleans, J Slade. New York: Oxford University Press, 1993.
196. Shaw GL, Falk RT, Tucker MA, et al. Debrisoquine metabolism and lung cancer risk. Proc Am Assoc Cancer Res 1994;35:294. Abstract.
197. Shekelle RB, Lepper M, Liu S, et al. Dietary vitamin A and risk of cancer in the Western Electric Study. Lancet 1981;ii:1185–1190.
198. Shidara K, Suzuki T, Hara F, Nakajima T. Lack of synergistic association between human papillomavirus and *ras* gene point mutation in laryngeal carcinomas. Laryngoscope 1994;104:1008–1012.
199. Shields PG, Caporaso NE, Falk RT, et al. Lung cancer, race, and a CYP1A1 genetic polymorphism. Cancer Epidemiol Biomarkers Prev 1993;2:481–485.
200. Shields PG, Sugimura H, Caporaso NE, et al. Polycyclic aromatic hydrocarbon-DNA adducts and the CYP1A1 restriction fragment length polymorphism. Environment Health Perspect 1992;98:191–194.
201. Silverman S, Gorsky M, Greenspan D. Tobacco usage in patients with head and neck carcinomas: A follow-up study on habit changes and second primary oral/oropharyngeal cancers. J Am Dent Assoc 1983;106:33.
202. Slamon DJ, deKernion JB, Verma IM, Cline MJ. Expression of cellular oncogenes in human malignancies. Science 1984;224:256.
203. Slattery ML, Robison LM, Schuman KL, et al. Cigarette smoking and exposure to passive smoke are risk factors for cervical cancer. JAMA 1989;261:1593.
204. Smith SJ, Deacon JM, Chilvers CE. Alcohol, smoking, passive smoking and caffeine in relation to breast cancer risk in young women. UK National Case-Control Study Group. Br J Cancer 1994;70:112–119.
205. Solomon LJ, Flynn BS. Women who smoke. In Nicotine Addiction: Principles and Management. Edited by CT Orleans, J Slade. New York: Oxford University Press, 1993, pp 339–349.
206. Spiers CJ, Murray S, Davies DS, Biola-Mabadeije AF, Boobis AR. Debrisoquine oxidation phenotype and susceptibility to lung cancer. Br J Clin Pharmacol 1990;29: 101–109.
207. Spitzer WO, Lawrence V, Dales R, et al. Links between passive smoking and disease: A best evidence synthesis. A report of the Working Group on Passive Smoking. Clin Invest Med 1990;13:17.
208. Spruck CH, Rideout WM, Olumi AF, et al. Distinct patterns of p53 mutations in bladder cancer: relationship to tobacco usage. Cancer Res 1993;53:1162–1166.
209. Stich HF, Rosin MP. Quantitating the synergistic effect of smoking and alcohol consumption with the micronucleus test on human buccal mucosa cells. Int J Cancer 1983;31:305.
210. Stockwell HG, Goldman AL, Lyman GH, et al. Environmental tobacco smoke and lung cancer risk in nonsmoking women. JNCI 1992;84:1417–1422.
211. Strecher VJ, Rimer BK, Monaco KD. Development of a new self-help guide—freedom from smoking for you and your family. Health Ed Q 1990;16:101–112.
212. Sugimura H, Caporaso NE, Modali RV, et al. Association of rare alleles of the Harvey *ras* protooncogene locus with lung cancer. Cancer Res 1990;50:1857.
213. Sugimura H, Caporaso NE, Shaw GL, et al. Human debrisoquine hydroxylase gene polymorphisms in cancer patients and controls. Carcinogenesis 1990;11:1527–1530.
214. Sugimura H, Suzuki I, Hamada GS, et al. Cytochrome P-450 1A1 genotype in lung cancer patients and controls in Rio de Janeiro, Brazil. Cancer Epidemiol Biomarkers Prev 1994;3:145–148.
215. Suzuki H, Takahashi T, Kuroishi T, Suyama M, Ariyoshi Y, Ueda R. p53 Mutations in non-small cell lung cancer in Japan: association between mutations and smoking. Cancer Res 1992;52:734–736.
216. Tabin CJ, Bradley SM, Bargmann CI, et al. Mechanism of activation of a human oncogene. Nature 1982;300:143.
217. Talaska G, Al-Juburi AZSS, Kadlubar FF. Smoking related carcinogen-DNA adducts in biopsy samples of human urinary bladder: identification of *N*-(deoxyguanosin-8-yl)-4-aminobiphenyl as a major adduct. Proc Natl Acad Sci USA 1991;88:5350–5354.
218. Talaska G, Schamer M, Casetta G, Tizzani A, Vineis P. Carcinogen-DNA adducts in bladder biopsies and urothelial cells: a risk assessment exercise. Cancer Lett 1994;84:93–97.
219. Tefre T, Daly AK, Armstrong M, et al. Genotyping of the CYP2D6 gene in Norwegian lung cancer patients and controls. Pharmacogenetics 1994;4:47–57.
220. Tefre T, Ryberg D, Haugen A, et al. Human CYP1A1 (cytochrome P(1)450) gene: lack of association between the MspI restriction fragment length polymorphism and incidence of lung cancer in a Norwegian population. Pharmacogenetics 1991;1:20–25.
221. Tokuhata GK, Lilienfeld AM. Familial aggregation of lung cancer in humans. JNCI 1963;30:289.
222. Tredaniel J, Boffetta P, Saracci R, Hirsch A. Environmental tobacco smoke and the risk of cancer in adults. Eur J Cancer 1993;29A;2058–2068.
223. Tonnesen P. Dose and nicotine dependence as determinants of nicotine gum efficacy. In Nicotine Replacement: A Critical Evaluation. Edited by OF Pomerleau, CS Pomerleau. New York: Liss, 1988, pp 129–144.

224. Uematsu F, Ikawa S, Kikuchi H, et al. Restriction fragment length polymorphism of the human CYP2E1 (cytochrome P450IIE1) gene and susceptibility to lung cancer: possible relevance to low smoking exposure. Pharmacogenetics 1994;4:58–63.
225. Uematsu F, Kikuchi H, Motomiya M, et al. Association between restriction fragment length polymorphism of the human cytochrome P450IIE1 gene and susceptibility to lung cancer. Jpn J Cancer Res 1991;82:254–256.
226. Uematsu F, Kikuchi H, Motomiya M, et al. Human cytochrome P450IIE1 gene: Dral polymorphism and susceptibility to cancer. Tohoku J Exp Med 1992;168:113–117.
227. U.S. Department of Health and Human Services: Cancer Statistics Review 1973–1986. NIH publication 89-2789. Bethesda MD: U.S. Public Health Service, 1989.
228. U.S. Department of Health and Human Services. Healthy People 2000: National Health Promotion and Disease Prevention Objectives. Washington DC: Government Printing Office, Public Health Service, 1991.
229. U.S. Department of Health and Human Services. How you can help patients stop smoking: Opportunities for respiratory care practitioners. DHHS publication 89-2961. Washington DC: National Heart, Lung, and Blood Institute, 1989.
230. U.S. Department of Health and Human Services. Nurses: Help Your Patients Stop Smoking. DHHS publication 90-2962. Washington DC: National Heart, Lung, and Blood Institute, 1990.
231. U.S. Department of Health and Human Services. Preventing Tobacco Use Among Young People: A Report of the Surgeon General. Washington DC: Public Health Service, 1994.
232. U.S. Department of Health and Human Services. Promoting Health/Preventing Disease: Objectives for the Nation. Washington DC: Public Health Service, 1980.
233. U.S. Department of Health and Human Services. Reducing the Health Consequences of Smoking: 25 Years of Progress—A Report of the Surgeon General. DHHS publication (CDC) 89-8411. Washington DC: Government Printing Office, 1989.
234. U.S. Department of Health and Human Services: The Health Consequences of Involuntary Smoking. A Report of the Surgeon General. DHHS publication (CDC) 87-8398. Washington DC: U.S. Department of Health and Human Services, Public Health Service, Centers for Disease Control. 1986.
235. U.S. Department of Health and Human Services. The Health Consequences of Smoking: Cancer. A Report of the Surgeon General. Washington DC: U.S. Department of Health and Human Services, 1982.
236. U.S. Department of Health and Human Services. The Health Consequences of Smoking: Nicotine Addiction. A Report to the Surgeon General. Washington DC: Public Health Service, 1988.
237. U.S. Department of Health and Human Services. The Health Consequences of Using Smokeless Tobacco. A Report to the Advisory Committee to the Surgeon General. Washington DC: Public Health Service, 1986.
238. U.S. Environmental Protection Agency (USEPA). Respiratory Health Effects of Passive Smoking: Lung Cancer and Other Disorders. EPA/600/6-90/006F. Washington DC: Office of Research and Development, 1992.
239. U.S. Public Health Service: Smoking and Health. Report of the Advisory Committee to the Surgeon General of the Public Health Service. PHS publication 1103. Washington DC: U.S. Department of Health, Education, and Welfare, Public Health Service, Center for Disease Control, 1964.
240. Velicer WF, Prochaska JO, Rossi JS, Snow, M.G. Assessing outcome in smoking cessation studies. Psychol Bull 1992;111:23–41.
241. Vineis P. Epidemiological models of carcinogenesis: the example of bladder cancer. Cancer Epidemiol Biomarkers Prev 1992;1:149–153.
242. Wald N, Idle M, Boreham, J. Low serum vitamin-A and subsequent risk of cancer. Lancet 1980;ii:813.
243. Wang FL, Love EJ, Liu N, Dai, X.D. Childhood and adolescent passive smoking and the risk of female lung cancer. Int J Epidemiol 1994;23:223–230.
244. Willett, W.C. Vitamin A and lung cancer. Nutr Rev 1990;48:201–211.
245. Willett WC, Polk BF, Underwood BA, et al. Relation of serum vitamins A and E and carotenoids to the risk of cancer. N Engl J Med 1984;310:430.
246. Wilson VL, Weston A, Manchester DK, et al. Alkyl and aryl carcinogen adducts detected in human peripheral lung. Carcinogenesis 1989;10:2149–2153.
247. Windsor RA, Cutter G, Morris J, Reese Y, Adams B, Bartlett E. Effectiveness of self-help smoking cessation intervention for pregnant women in public health maternity clinics. Am J Public Health 1985;76:1389–1392.
248. Winn DM, Ziegler KG, Pickle LW. Diet in the etiology of oral and pharyngeal cancer among women from the southern United States. Cancer Res 1984;44:1216.
249. Wolf CR, Smith CAD, Gough AC, et al. Relationship between the debrisoquine hydroxylase polymorphism and cancer susceptibility. Carcinogenesis 1992;13:1035–1038.
250. Wu AH, Henderson BE, Pike MC, Yu MC. Smoking and other risk factors for lung cancer in women. JNCI 1985;74:747.
251. Yu, MC, Skipper PL, Taghizadeh K, Tannenbaum SR, Chan KK, Henderson, BE, Ross, RK. Acetylator phenotype, aminobiphenyl-hemoglobin adduct levels, and bladder cancer risk in white, black, and Asian men in Los Angeles, California. JNCI 1994;86:712–716.
252. Zhang ZF, Sarkis AS, Cordon-Cardo C, et al. Cancer epidemiology biomarkers and prevention. 1994;3:19–24.
253. Zhong S, Howie AF, Ketterer B, et al. Glutathione S-transferase mu locus: use of genotyping and phenotyping assays to assess association with lung cancer susceptibility. Carcinogenesis 1991;12:1533–1537.
254. Zhong S, Wyllie AH, Barnes D, Wolf CR, Spurr NK. Relationship between the GSTM1 genetic polymorphism and susceptibility to bladder, breast and colon cancer. Carcinogenesis 1993;14:1821–1824.
255. Ziegler RG. Vegetables, fruits, and carotenoids and the risk of cancer. Am J Clin Nutr 1991;53:251S–259S.

CHAPTER 28

Nutrition in the Etiology and Prevention of Cancer

STEVEN K. CLINTON AND EDWARD L. GIOVANNUCCI

Introduction

Throughout human evolution, the often precarious food supply was typically low in fat and high in complex carbohydrates and fiber. Over the last two centuries, improvements in food production, processing, storage, and distribution have led to major changes in diet composition within the industrialized nations. During this period, life expectancy also dramatically increased in economically developed countries because of a combination of factors including public health measures, improved occupational safety, and major reductions in nutrient deficiency syndromes. As the population has aged, we have seen a shift in the major causes of morbidity and mortality towards chronic diseases such as cancer and cardiovascular disease. These changes have been associated with an increasingly overweight and sedentary population. Although nutritional deficiencies still plague subpopulations in industrial nations, such as the poor, the aged, alcoholics, and the chronically ill, we now recognize the "affluent" diet contributing to the pathogenesis of chronic diseases that afflict the vast majority of the population. Efforts to understand the etiologies of the cancers have led to epidemiologic and laboratory studies that strongly implicate certain dietary patterns and specific nutrients.

The diet not only is a source of nutrients, it serves as a vehicle for many other substances that may participate in promoting or inhibiting carcinogenesis. Although frequently implicated by the lay press and public, food additives such as dyes, artificial sweeteners, and flavoring agents appear to contribute very little to the overall cancer burden (302, 303). The potential risks of man-made contaminants such as pesticides, herbicides, and industrial wastes that enter the food chain have not yet been clearly defined. Many natural carcinogens that are produced by plants or fungi (e.g., aflatoxins in moldy grains) probably play a role in the etiology of some human cancers. Increasing evidence also implicates food processing or cooking methods (e.g., salt-pickling, charcoal-broiling) as sources of carcinogens or tumor-promoting substances (302, 303). A rapidly expanding area of research focuses upon the identification of natural substances in foods, such as phytochemicals, which are not nutrients but have anticarcinogenic properties that ultimately may be used in chemoprevention programs (25, 135, 136, 302, 303).

This review is devoted to the role of nutrients and foods in the etiology of cancer. Laboratory studies have proven that nutritional status has a major influence on host susceptibility to oncogenic events. Nutrients are classified into six main categories: protein, carbohydrate, fat, vitamins, minerals, and water. The only components providing energy are protein, carbohydrates, and fat, at approximately 4, 4, and 9 kilocalories per gram, respectively. Vitamins and minerals provide no energy but function as structural components or co-factors in numerous vital metabolic processes. Dietary fiber has not been considered as an essential nutrient category, although considerable efforts have been devoted to understanding its complexities and role in human health and disease. Alcohol also has been a component of the human diet throughout recorded history and has numerous metabolic and physiologic effects in addition to its contribution to energy intake (7 kcal/g). The potential complex interactions among the dozens of established nutrients and the genetic as well as environmental factors participating in human carcinogenesis have precluded precise quantification of the risks and benefits associated with any single nutrient. Recent publications have provided comprehensive overviews of the nutrition and cancer field (6, 36, 90, 280, 302, 303, 348, 359). Rather than detailing here the complex, often incomplete, and occasionally contradictory literature concerning the role of nutrients in the etiology of human cancer, this chapter is a general guide to this rapidly expanding discipline, emphasizing the major emerging concepts in the area.

Methodologic Issues in Diet, Nutrition, and Cancer Studies

Several approaches are used by epidemiologists and laboratory-based scientists to study the effects of diet and nutrion on the development of cancer. Each type of study has its strengths and limitations that need to be understood in order to interpret individual studies within the context of a large body of data. Nutritional epidemiology poses some unique obstacles in that food is an exposure that is universal, which is in stark contrast to other cancer causing environmental exposures such as cigarette smoke (69, 102, 169, 188). The unbiased detection and quantification of risks that are associated with variations in nutrient intake would ideally be achieved through randomized, prospective trials. Unfortunately, the enormous costs of long-term nutrition studies and the scientific difficulties in controlling or measuring nutrient intake limit feasibility. Current nutritional guidelines for disease prevention and future refinements therefore will be based upon the integration of information derived from a variety of different epidemiologic approaches and laboratory investigations. The etiologies of most chronic diseases, including cancer, are multifactorial. Human cancers show striking variations based on factors such as age, sex, race, socioeconomic status, genetics, and many occupational and lifestyle factors. The potential for complex interactions between these factors and nutrients is enormous, and this emphasizes the difficulties in demonstrating causal associations with the same clarity as is demonstrable for high-risk environmental exposures such as cigarette smoking.

ASSESSMENT OF THE HUMAN DIET

The critical limiting feature of most human studies designed to examine the role of nutrients in cancer is the imprecision of quantifying nutrient intake. Estimating the usual intake of foods or nutrients as well as accounting for intraindividual variation over time is a critical area of research (35, 278). An estimate of human nutrient intake is derived from a two-step process. First, the amounts and types of foods that are consumed must be determined by interviews, questionnaires, or food diaries. This information can then be used to calculate nutrient intake if an accurate data-base has been established that quantifies the amount of each nutrient contained in the foods that are consumed by the population under investigation. Each step can be associated with significant error and makes nutrient–cancer associations difficult to detect.

There are four basic methodologies for assessing intake: dietary recalls, food records, diet histories, and food-frequency questionnaires. Dietary recalls and food records focus upon current intake, whereas diet histories and food-frequency questionnaires focus on usual intake over a period of time. For recall studies, participants are contacted and asked to list all foods they have ingested over a defined period of time, usually 24 hours; multiple 24-hour recalls collected over a period of time for different days of the week will more fully assess current intake. The food-record method requires that subjects record their intake as they consume their meals over a period of time, such as a week or month. This methodology may incorporate the estimation or measurement of portion size and the method of food preparation. Diet histories are obtained by interview using open-ended questions regarding usual intake, which may include portion size using food models as an aid. A number of food-frequency questionnaires have been developed that vary in length and complexity. Subjects record the frequency of intake for each item on the list, typically using a format that allows for rapid coding into computerized databases. Self-administered food-frequency questionnaires typically are used in large cohort or case-control studies.

There are several potential advantages and disadvantages to each diet-assessment technique. A very active and critical area of research involves improving the design and subsequent validation of dietary questionnaires and interview techniques to measure both long- and short-term dietary intake (69, 102). Several issues must be addressed by investigators in this field. The human diet is a complex array of foods that exhibits significant day-to-day and seasonal variation. The complexity of diet also differs widely among populations, cultures, and geographic areas. This often requires the development of different assessment methods for each population. For example, food variety in specific counties within the People's Republic of China is very homogeneous and may be limited to less than 25 items produced locally (191). In contrast, 90% (by weight) of the U.S. diet is derived from over 500 different food items (325). An efficient and accurate assessment tool that was designed for China would be useless in the United States. Within a nation or geographic area, food selections among individuals also show significant variation with age, gender, ethnicity, and social and economic status; specific assessment tools may be necessary for certain subgroups within a population. Most human cancers have a long latency period, and the methodologic difficulties associated with estimating the intake of foods or nutrients consumed many years before the diagnosis are a major concern for retrospective studies (465).

Once an estimate of food choices has been obtained, estimation of nutrient intake depends on a database that defines the nutrient composition of the chosen foods. The U.S. Department of Agriculture handbooks provide an estimate of the nutrient composition of most foods consumed in North America (439). However, the nutrient content of foods in many underdeveloped nations has not been as precisely defined. The content of some nutrients in a food may be relatively constant and even regulated by law in some nations (e.g., the amount of fat in whole milk); however, the contents of other nutrients in food items may be highly variable. For example, the selenium concentration in grains and vegetables will vary greatly depending on the soil selenium content. In nations where foods are shipped large distances, an estimate of selenium intake may require direct measurement of its content in food samples from the study population. A very important area of research also concerns how to accurately measure energy intake in the participants of the studies (447).

In many studies, the consumption of certain foods that account for the greatest variance in the nutrient of interest serves as a surrogate indicator of nutrient intake. For example, many investigators present an analysis of meat intake relative to the risk of certain cancers as a surrogate indicator of saturated fat intake. Similarly, the consumption of certain vegetables and citrus fruits often is used as an estimate of β-carotene or vitamin C intake. Studies using surrogate measures for nutrient intake, however, can greatly underestimate or fail to detect a real association between a nutrient and cancer because of imperfect exposure data. In addition, most foods are a source of more than one potentially active nutrient; for example, many fruits and vegetables are not only sources of vitamin C but also contribute significantly to carotenoid, and fiber intake. Caution should be used in making assumptions concerning the role of specific nutrients when investigators use food items or groups as the primary focus of the analysis.

BIOCHEMICAL ASSESSMENT OF NUTRIENT INTAKE

Future progress will depend in part upon innovative epidemiologic strategies employing accurate biochemical and molecular indicators for the intake of many nutrients (69, 319). Identifying biomarkers of nutrient exposure offers the promise of improved precison in epidemiologic studies because of reduced misclassification of participants according to intake estimates. An additional application will be in the measurement of compliance with dietary regimens during prospective intervention trials. For some nutritional factors, such as total fat intake, we have no useful screening test that can be applied to a large population. For others, such as cholesterol consumption, the measurement of serum cholesterol only provides a crude indictor of intake and is modulated by many other genetic and dietary factors. Serum retinol as a measure of vitamin A status is buffered by tissue stores and reflects nutrient status only at the extremes of deficiency or excess (452). In contrast, measuring the selenium content of hair or toenail clippings provides an integrated measure of selenium intake over an extended period of time and can be used in epidemiologic studies (296). Because the presence of a disease may alter dietary intake and the metabolism of specific nutrients, the biochemical or molecular assessment of nutrient intake will be less useful in retrospective and case-control studies; they will be most informative in prospective and cohort studies, geographic correlational investigations, and studies of migrant populations.

CORRELATION AND ECOLOGIC STUDIES

In correlation and ecologic studies, the unit of observation is a group of people. Cancer incidence or mortality among groups is compared with estimates of the average group intake of foods or nutrients. Often quoted examples are the studies showing a relationship between dietary fat intake and breast cancer (14, 53). Armstrong and Doll (14) reported a correlation of 0.89 between the estimated average per-capita fat intakes and breast cancer mortality rates in nations around the world. Ecologic studies also can be conducted within a single country. One example is a study in China based on an analysis of data from 65 Chinese counties (267). Per capita fat intake varied from 6 to 45% of energy and was positively, but weakly, associated with risk of breast cancer. These two examples illustrate that researchers must be particularly careful in making strong or quantitative conclusions based on correlations between cancer rates and single nutrients. Nations showing large differences in cancer incidence often exhibit dietary patterns so dramatically different that conclusions concerning the contribution of individual dietary components or nutrients are impossible. For example, the Chinese exhibit an overall age-adjusted breast cancer mortality rate that is approximately 10 to 20% of that found in the United States, and they consume a diet that is lower in total fat, animal protein, refined carbohydrates, vitamin A, and calcium but higher in carotenoids, starches, and fiber (Table 28.1) (191). In addition to variations in dietary content, populations also exhibit significant differences in food processing and preparation that are associated with the shift from an agrarian to industrial society. Inaccuracies in the available data on food consumption also may limit these studies. In many nations, data are crude and based on food-disappearence information of varing accuracy. Furthermore, food-disappearence data may be affected by spoilage or waste.

Table 28.1. Estimated Average Intake of Several Dietary and Nutritional Factors in the People's Republic of China and United States

Dietary intake	China	United States
Plant protein (% of total)	89	30
Starch (g/d)	371	120
Fat (% of calories)	14	39
Vitamin A (retinol equivalents/d)	28	990
Total carotinoids (retinol equivalents/d)	836	429
Vitamin C (mg/d)	140	73
Total fiber (g/d)	33	11

From Junshi and colleagues (191).

The major strength of international correlational studies is that the contrast in a dietary variable is much larger than likely will be found within geographically restricted populations. For example, dietary fat intake varies over a wide range between nations, but it is relatively homogeneous within a nation such as the United States. Despite the inherent difficulties in interpretation, ecologic studies also will continue to provide a very important resource for the generation of nutrition and cancer hypotheses.

CASE-CONTROL STUDIES

Many weaknesses of correlational studies are potentially avoidable in case-control investigations, in which information about previous diet is obtained from patients with disease and compared to that from subjects without the disease. Because the populations tend to be more homogeneous in various ways than those in international studies and detailed information on a variety of potentially confounding factors such as smoking can be obtained, positive results from these studies may provide more convincing evidence regarding a particular nutrient and cancer. These studies can be conducted over a relatively short period of time, and they are particularly useful in studying relatively rare cancers if a mechanism for identifying cases in a large geographic area is established.

These studies have been useful in many situations, but they have some limitations when studying diet and cancer. This is particularly true if serum markers of nutrient intake are being evaluated. For example, if blood β-carotene concentrations are different between subjects with and without lung cancer, it is difficult to know whether the difference reflects a true variation in intake or a change that is related to the disease. In addition, the possibility of selection or recall bias must be considered in evaluating case control studies. Selection bias occurs if a nonrepresentative control group is selected or if some of the cases or controls refuse to participate and have characteristics that may bias the results. Recall bias could occur if subjects having a specific cancer remember and report their diet differently from controls. The magnitude of this source of bias has been examined in two studies. One was conducted among members of the Nurses' Health Study cohort (118), and among participants in 1986 who prospectively completed food-frequency questionnaires, 398 were subsequently diagnosed with breast cancer in the following 2 years. The investigators attempted to contact these women and 798 age-matched controls, and they asked responders to complete a second food-frequency questionnaire inquiring about their diet in 1985 (before the diagnosis of breast cancer) to mimic a case-control study. Using the prospective data, no appreciable association was seen between total fat intake and risk of breast cancer, but a 43% higher risk was observed using the questionnaires completed after diagnosis.

A similar study that focused on recall bias (105), however, found no significant differential error in the recall of past diet by patients with cancer and controls. Recall bias is more likely in situations where participants may be familiar with a particular hypothesis, such as fat and breast cancer. Another limitation is that only dietary factors that are etiologically relevant relatively shortly before the diagnosis of cancer can be studied. Whereas many studies indicate that diet within the past few years can be recalled with reasonable accuracy, it is less likely that diet in past decades can be assessed with any degree of precision. In addition, study populations in case-control investigations may be very homogeneous relative to the intake of certain nutrients, and differences between patients with cancer and matched controls may not be demonstrable using current assessment techniques. Case-control studies may prove to be most useful in migrant populations moving to areas that exhibit dramatic differences in dietary content (e.g., migrants from countries exhibiting a low-risk of colon cancer, such as China, moving to high-risk areas, such as the United States) (445). Cases and controls can then be evaluated according to the degree of adaptation to the high-risk U.S. diet.

PROSPECTIVE OR COHORT STUDIES

The prospective approach defines a study population and monitors the incidence of disease over time as well as exposure to potential risk factors. These studies avoid some of the inaccuracies of estimating dietary intake retrospectively and the recall bias typically found in case-control studies because a description of dietary exposures can be obtained before the development of the disease. A disadvantage is the enormous costs that are associated with a large number of participants and long periods of follow-up, and a potential problem that investigators must address is the loss of participants over time because of inefficient follow-up. If disease incidence or specific dietary exposures are related to a loss to follow-up, then estimates of risk are biased or may not be detected. An additional consideration for some cancers (e.g., breast) is that nutrients acting during childhood and adolescence may be very crucial, and a prospective study initiated in adult women may not accurately identify critical dietary risk factors. One important advantage is that dietary intake can be updated periodically so that long-term intake can be more precisely estimated. For example, in the Nurses' Health Study of approximately 88,000 women (450), dietary intake was assessed in 1980, 1984, 1986, 1990, and 1994. Recent technologic advances such as self-administered, computer-scannable dietary questionnaires allow these studies to become more efficient and cost-effective. There are currently at least six large dietary cohort studies underway, ranging in size from 17,000 to over 89,000 women.

Prospective studies are especially useful when evaluating biochemical markers for nutrient intake using samples of blood, urine, feces, or tissue that may ultimately correlate with cancer risk. One approach, referred to as a nested case-control study, requires that biologic specimens be collected from all members of the cohort. Because it may not be cost-effective to measure nutrient markers in samples from all individuals, the experiment can be limited to those who develop a specific cancer and matched controls from the cohort. For example, several studies have used this technique to examine the relationship between serum β-carotene and risk of lung cancer (279). Prospectively collected sera from those developing lung cancer were analyzed and compared with controls matched by age, sex, time of serum collection, and smoking history. In each study, serum β-carotene was observed to be lower among individuals who subsequently developed lung cancer compared with controls.

RANDOMIZED TRIALS AND INTERVENTION STUDIES

Oncologists routinely use randomized trials to assess the utility of therapeutic interventions in the treatment of cancer or the prevention of relapse. Despite the scientific advantages, this method is difficult to implement for the evaluation of many nutrition and cancer hypotheses. Experiments in otherwise healthy individuals can only be justified when considerable observational data have been collected and supported by studies from the laboratory. It is critical that the potential benefits be well defined and that adverse outcomes unlikely. Because of the length of the induction period for most cancers, intervention trials will require large numbers of particiants and many years of follow-up to detect the effects of most dietary interventions. Use of individuals who are at high risk of cancer from a genetic marker or premalignant condition (i.e., colonic polyps) may increase the frequency with which an outcome of interest occurs over time.

For some nutritional variables, compliance may be an issue. It may be difficult to ensure that a large population adheres to a strict diet, such as a low-fat regimen, over a long period of time. The biochemical methodology to assess compliance with a low-fat diet does not currently exist. Trials of dietary change cannot be blinded. The control group may change nutrient intake over time based on societal adaptation to currently publicized recommendations or dietary fads, thus limiting the power of the study. Randomized trials will be most useful in the testing of potential cancer inhibitors, such as certain vitamins, minerals, and other chemopreventive agents that can be incorporated into pills or capsules and provided in a double-blind fashion over a period of years (440).

Because the length of time between a dietary intervention and a measureable effect on cancer may be years or decades, an intermediate end point may be used as an earlier indicator of efficacy. For example, the ability of supplemental wheat bran to decrease colon mucosal cell proliferative rates (5) and reduce polyp formation (83) in patients who are at high risk for colon cancer have been completed. However, intermediate end points may not completely predict cancer risk. Efforts to define intermediate markers for common cancers that can be used in prospective studies is of major importance to the nutrition and cancer field.

The manipulation of single dietary components in large-scale intervention studies is difficult. For example, increasing fruit and vegetable intake or reducing the proportion of calories from fat alters the intake of many food items and a number of nutrients. Although these studies may provide useful information regarding public health recommendations, interpretation of the precise role a specific nutrient plays may be problematic. Even when scientifically and ethically feasible, the large costs of randomized trials limit their implementation. In addition, negative results in intervention studies often are difficult to interpret. They could be explained by a lack of treatment effect, inappropriate dose of supplement, dietary intervention of ineffective magnitude, failure of participants to comply with the intervention, or insufficient duration of treatment and follow-up.

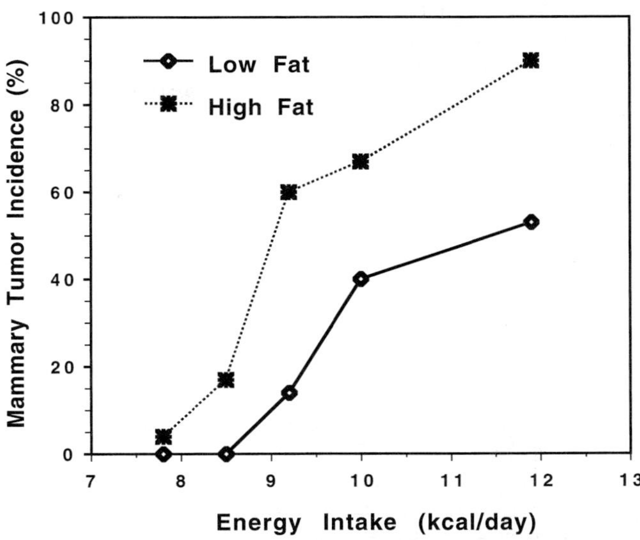

Figure 28.1. The effects of low- and high-fat diets at different levels of caloric intake on spontaneous mammary tumorigenesis in C3H female mice. *Source:* Tannenbaum (410).

LABORATORY ANIMAL MODELS

The effects of nutrients and their interactions on carcinogenesis can be rigorously tested in animal models. Although the information derived from animal models must be extrapolated to humans with caution, it does provide important evidence for the biologic plausibility of relationships suggested by epidemiologic studies. The nutrient requirements of most laboratory animals have been precisely defined, and purified ingredients can be used to formulate diets for cancer studies (10, 11, 305, 312). Unfortunately, many published studies do not provide useful information because of the investigators' failure to appreciate two critical observations derived from decades of experimentation (359). The first is the strong, positive correlation between energy intake and the incidence or growth of tumors in virtually every animal model system (1, 12, 60, 64, 100, 302, 303, 359, 368, 409). The second issue is the frequent observation that animals fed nutritionally complete diets that are composed of unrefined foods, usually referred to as chow, often exhibit a reduction in tumorigenesis compared to those fed a complete diet derived from purified nutrients (302, 359, 440).

Because energy intake has a major influence on tumorigenesis (Fig. 28.1), recording food consumption and body weight is an essential aspect of all rodent studies (410). Unfortunately, failure to document the effects of dietary treatments on feed (i.e., energy) intake frequently limits the interpretation of published experiments. Nutritional deficiencies, imbalances, or excesses can significantly alter energy intake. For example, vitamin A deficiency, or supplementation of the diet with selenium at high concentrations, can inhibit carcinogenesis through an indirect effect on energy intake. Readers of nutrition and carcinogenesis literature must carefully evaluate dietary treatments, identify the variables that are present, and determine if energy intake has confounded interpretation of the data. In some cases, pair-feeding and other methods of compensating for treatment-induced differences in energy intake can be used.

Another problem frequently found in the literature is the inappropriate use of cereal-based commercial laboratory chows. Some investigators use these products as the control or "normal" diet for comparison against synthetic diets with a different concentration of a specific nutrient. Although commercial laboratory chows provide excellent nutrition, they vary over time and between companies in the sources of natural ingredients. Chow diets contain varying concentrations of cereals, vegetables, legumes, fish meal, and milk products that are a function of local market availability and cost. Although the nutrient content of these diets satisfies the established minimum requirements for mice and rats, the concentrations of individual nutrients may vary substantially. For example, the vitamin A and β-carotene content of different batches of the NIH-07 chow diet varied over 6- and 20-fold, respectively (346). In addition, detectable levels of aflatoxins, nitrosamines, antioxidants, pesticides, herbicides and heavy metals are observed (346). Many undefined substances found in grains and vegetables are thought to have anticarcinogenic activity and contribute to the tumor-preventive properties that are associated with chow diets. In general, natural-ingredient diets are inconsistent and therefore inadequate for use in experiments to quantify the subtle effects of specific nutrients on carcinogenesis. Diets must be precisely defined in publications and confounding variables eliminated whenever possible.

Nutrition and the Etiology of Common Cancers

It is unlikely that any food, nutrient, or dietary pattern will influence all cancers uniformly (47). In reviewing the relationships between nutrition and cancer, it is convenient to examine the data for each tissue or organ separately; however, this approach will ultimately prove to be inadequate. A key feature of human cancer is interindividual heterogeneity in biologic characteristics and response to treatment. Clearly, cancer of the breast, colon, or any tissue represents a family of diseases. As laboratory methodology improves, we will be able to subclassify cancers according to molecular, biochemical, genetic, and biologic characteristics. Coupled with future improvements in nutritional assessment, the more precise classification of human cancers will allow a more accurate quantification of the relationship between nutrients and specific neoplasms.

LUNG

In affluent nations, lung cancer is the leading cause of cancer-related death (37). Cigarette smoking accounts for the vast majority of cases (87). Certain occupational exposures, such as to asbestos or radiation, may act synergistically with cigarette smoking to increase risk (87), but potential interactions between smoking and nutritional status have not been adequately assessed. The inverse relationship between the greater intake of fruits and vegetables and lower risk of lung cancer has been one of the most consistent findings in human nutritional epidemiology (36, 398–400). The active agents in a diet rich in these food items remains to be determined. Many have hypothesized that carotenoids, particularly β-carotene, or vitamin A may be important (25, 48, 68, 151, 155, 256, 270, 302, 303, 370, 388). A series of studies from Norway (31, 221), Japan (155), England (137), and the United States (139) have reported inverse associations between estimated intakes of vitamin A and risk of lung cancer (466). For example, Bjelke's prospective study in Norway (31) involved over 8,000 men responding to a mailed food-frequency questionnaire that was designed to assess dietary vitamin A intake. The relative risk for lung cancer was increased by over twofold for smokers in the low–vitamin A group compared with those in the high–vitamin A group. Prospective studies also have compared serum β-carotene levels in individuals subsequently developing lung cancer to matched controls and have found them to be correlated inversely with risk (279). Similar inverse correlations with serum vitamin A, however, have not been consistently observed (101, 279, 324, 369, 435, 436). Studies in rodent models occasionally have observed protective effects of vitamin A or analogues against respiratory tract carcinogenesis induced by a variety of polycyclic aromatic hydrocarbons, which are found in cigarette smoke, or nitrosamines (12).

Several ongoing intervention trials may help to determine if β-carotene supplementation has anticancer properties. A recent evaluation of a Finnish study (7) found no reduction, and perhaps an increase, in the incidence of lung cancer among male smokers after 5 to 8 years of supplementation with β-carotene at 20 mg/day. This report emphasizes the importance of considering other components of a diet rich in vegetables and fruit as contributors to lower risk. A number of other nutrients, such as low-vitamin C (48, 151, 221), high total fat (48, 461), and cholesterol (150), have been investigated relative to modulating the risk of lung cancer in human or rodent studies (302, 303, 359); however, their roles remain obscure. Overall, elimination of cigarette smoking and occupational risk factors will have the greatest impact on decreasing the incidence of lung cancer. Among high-risk individuals, the frequent consumption of a diverse array of fruits and vegetables may provide some degree of protection against lung cancer.

ORAL CAVITY, LARYNX, AND OROPHARYNX

Like lung cancer, cancers of the oral cavity and the larynx are strongly related to the use of tobacco products (15, 261, 269, 358, 418). Case-control studies completed over several decades also have documented associations between the consumption of alcoholic beverages and cancers of these tissues (125, 199, 201, 268, 385, 462). A dose-response relationship of alcohol and oral cancer, independent of tobacco usage, has been observed in a number of studies (Fig. 28.2) (45, 95, 147, 318, 365, 460). Additional evidence is derived from studies of populations, such as alcoholics who exhibit increased risk and Seventh-Day Adventists and Mormons in the United States who abstain from alcohol and have lower risk (85, 251). It is of interest that feeding pure alcohol as part of a nutritionally sound diet does not produce oral cancers in experimental animals (358). The extent that this represents biochemical differences between man and rodents, the lack of a direct carcinogenic effect of ethanol, the presence of carcinogens in alcoholic beverages consumed by man, the passive inhalation of ambient tobacco smoke in the places where ethanol is consumed, or the importance of other interacting carcinogens and nutritional deficits must be further evaluated.

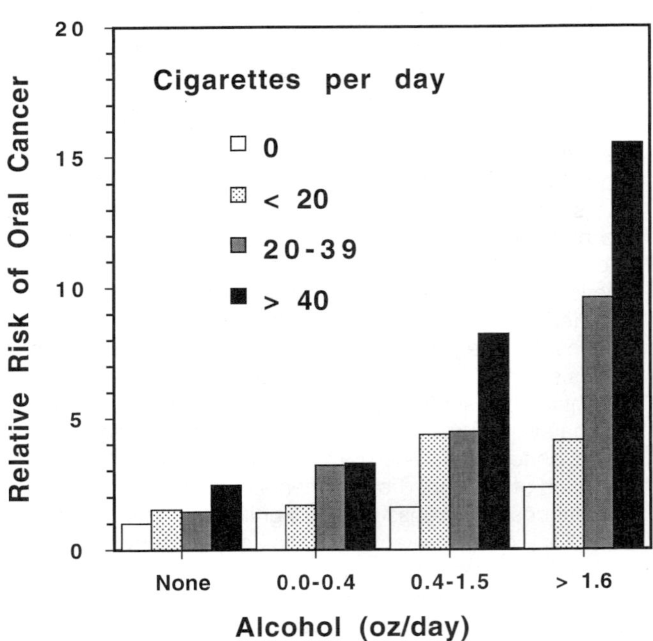

Figure 28.2. The interactions between alcohol intake and cigarette smoking on the relative risk of oral cancer. *Source:* Rothman and Keller (365).

Table 28.2. The Effects of 13-*cis*-Retinoic Acid on the Incidence of Primary Treatment Failure and of Second Primary Tumors in Squamous Cell Carcinoma of the Head and Neck

Type of failure	13-*cis*-Retinoic acid (%)[a]	Placebo (%)[b]	*P* value
Disease progression[c]	31%	33%	.772
Local	8%	14%	.373
Regional	16%	14%	.719
Distant	14%	10%	.490
Second primary tumor	4%	24%	.005

[a] $n = 49$.
[b] $n = 51$.
[c] Retinoid treatment had no effect on progression of the primary tumor but significantly reduced the incidence of second primary cancers (See Chapter 105).
From Hong and colleagues (165).

Both epidemiologic and laboratory studies support a role of vitamin A as a modulator of carcinogenesis of the oral and respiratory epithelia. Vitamin A deficiency leads to squamous metaplasia of these tissues that is corrected by treatment with vitamin A and a number of related retinoids. The metaplasia that is associated with vitamin A deficiency is similar histologically to the premalignant changes that are observed following exposure of the oral mucosa to chemical carcinogens. Several animal studies have suggested that vitamin A, carotenoids, or synthetic retinoids may retard carcinogenesis of the oral cavity, and case-control studies occasionally have reported increased risk associated with lower estimated vitamin A intake (266). A number of chemoprevention trials have been undertaken using leukoplakia, a premalignant condition of the oral mucosa, as the surrogate end point. In a randomized trial, Stich and colleagues (404) treated patients having leukoplakia with β-carotene, β-carotene plus vitamin A, or placebo for 6 months. On follow-up evaluation, the complete remission rates were 15, 28, and 3%, respectively. A subsequent study reported a 57% complete remission rate in a group treated with vitamin A at 200,000 IU/wk compared to only 3% in the placebo group (404). Several nonrandomized studies using synthetic retinoids also have suggested dramatic reversals in oral leukoplakia. Subsequent randomized studies using 13-*cis*-retinoic acid also showed significantly lower relapse rates in the treated groups (164).

The beneficial effects of vitamin A and synthetic retinoids in preventing premalignant changes of the oral mucosa led to a landmark clinical chemoprevention trial designed to determine its effectiveness in preventing second primary tumors of the aerodigestive tract (165). Second cancers occur at a rate of 3 to 4% per year in patients who have received potentially curative treatment of their initial, early stage cancer. Patients rendered disease-free after primary treatment of their head and neck cancer were randomized to placebo or 13-*cis*-retinoic acid. There were no significant differences in the local, regional, or distant recurrences of the primary cancers (Table 28.2). However, the treated group had significantly fewer second primary tumors compared with placebo controls, at 4 vs. 24%, respectively, after 32 months (see Chapter 105) (165). This study suggests that vitamin A or retinoids influence early stages in carcinogenesis and that these compounds probably have little utility for the treatment of established cancers of the oral pharynx. Frequent consumption of fruits and vegetables has been suggested to be beneficial by a number of studies (36, 266, 302, 303), and among the many factors in fruits and vegetables that may be active in preventing cancers are the carotenoids, some of which are precursors to vitamin A.

ESOPHAGUS

Cancer of the esophagus varies several-hundred-fold between nations and regions within nations (37). The incidence is particularly high in an area extending from the southern border of the Caspian Sea in Iran across central Asia to China. Within nations, such as China or Iran, there frequently are large differences in risk between different locations and population groups (260). For example, age-adjusted annual mortality in the Caspian region of Iran is 165 and 195 per 100,000 for males and females, respectively, but it is 10- and 20-fold lower in other areas of the country (260). The incidence of esophageal cancer in the United States is relatively low, at less than 7 per 100,000 (37).

In most affluent nations, correlational analyses and case-control studies indicate that the major risk factors are ethanol and cigarette smoking (302, 303, 358, 459). Risk increases in proportion to the amount of alcohol consumed (268, 417, 418, 422, 460). A number of studies have shown an alcohol dose-response relationship after controlling for cigarette smoking, although the two factors may show a significant additive effect (198, 268, 422). In the United States, mortality from esophageal cancer in the white population has decreased gradually over recent decades whereas the mortality has doubled for black men in the last 25 years (381, 382). It has been postulated that the threefold greater risk in blacks compared to whites may result from differences in alcohol intake, tobacco smoking, and undefined dietary or nutritional factors (337, 382, 467). Increasing consumption of alcohol generally is associated with the marginal intake of many nutrients, which is thought to predispose individuals to greater risk (34, 70). For example, alcohol may interact with folate, vitamin B_{12}, and methyl group metabolism to modulate risk. One study (184) found significantly lower concentrations of B_{12} and folic acid in the blood of patients with cytologic dysplasia or malignancy of the esophagus; there also was a reduction in DNA methylation of nucleated blood cells of individuals whose esophagus displayed signs of folic acid-related deficiency. As has been suggested for lung cancer, a number of studies have reported an inverse relationship between risk of esophageal cancer and the consumption of fresh fruits and vegetables (36, 129, 282). For example, the relative risk was increased 4.5-fold among Americans eating less than 40 servings of fruits and vegetables per month compared with those eating over 80 servings (282).

Alcohol consumption does not explain the high risk for esophageal cancer in certain parts of Asia (302). Populations in these areas frequently consume diets that are marginal or deficient in a number of nutrients (73, 167, 426, 463). Low intakes of fresh fruits, vegetables, and animal products are noted, and the estimated intakes of vitamin A, vitamin C, riboflavin, zinc, and several trace elements such as molybdenum frequently are cited as being low as well (70, 71, 73, 167, 463). It has been postulated that dietary deficiencies may alter susceptibility to carcinogens that are indigenous to these populations. Although not firmly established, a role for *N*-nitroso compounds in pickled foods and mycotoxins from moldy grains has been postulated (73, 167, 265, 463). In some areas, associations have been found with the intake of foods that are at high temperatures when consumed (73, 84, 463).

Several nutrient hypotheses have been evaluated in animal models using nitrosamine-induced esophageal cancer (12, 389). Overall, vitamin A and several synthetic analogues have shown little effect on risk in these models (307, 429). Some, but not all, studies with supplemental selenium (308, 429), or molybdenum (248, 429) have reduced tumorigenesis. A role for zinc has been proposed based on the prevalence of zinc deficiency in many high-risk areas of the world (298, 302, 303). Some animal studies have observed increased risk with zinc deficiency and a reduction in carcinogenesis with supplementation, although a number of experiments have found no significant effect (18, 96, 97, 107, 427–429).

In summary, cigarette smoking and alcohol consumption are the most important etiologic factors in affluent nations. The possibility that marginal intakes of one or more nutrients, secondary to the infrequent consumption of fruits and vegetables, may contribute to risk in affluent populations has been suggested but not firmly established. In some areas of the world, such as the high-risk area between Iran and China, micronutrient deficiencies coupled with the exposure to carcinogenic substances associated with intake of salt-pickled vegetables or moldy foods may be contributing factors.

STOMACH

A dramatic decrease in the incidence of stomach cancer in many affluent nations has been observed over the last 50 years. In the United States, the current rate is among the lowest in the world, whereas in 1930, gastric cancer was the most frequently diagnosed cancer in Americans (119). Gastric cancer remains a major worldwide problem (Fig. 28.3) (37). The incidence varies dramatically among countries and is highest in parts of Asia (e.g., Japan) and South America. In addition, subpopulations within a nation can show risks several-fold greater than other groups (77, 141). Studies of Japanese migrants to Hawaii or North America show that risk is significantly reduced in the second- and third-generation after migration (139, 141, 142, 207).

Although general agreement exists that diet plays a role in gastric carcinogenesis, the mechanisms that account for the geographic and temporal incidence patterns have not been firmly established (77, 302, 305). Efforts to define the causes of stomach cancer have proceeded in several directions: (a) the identification of natural carcinogens or precursors found in the food, (b) the production of carcinogens during food processing or cooking, (c) the synthesis of carcinogens from dietary precursors in the stomach, (d) the identification of dietary protective factors that may be consumed in inadequate quantities by high-risk groups, (e) the identification of nutrients that increase risk for initiation by carcinogens or act directly as promoters, and (f) the role of infectious agents.

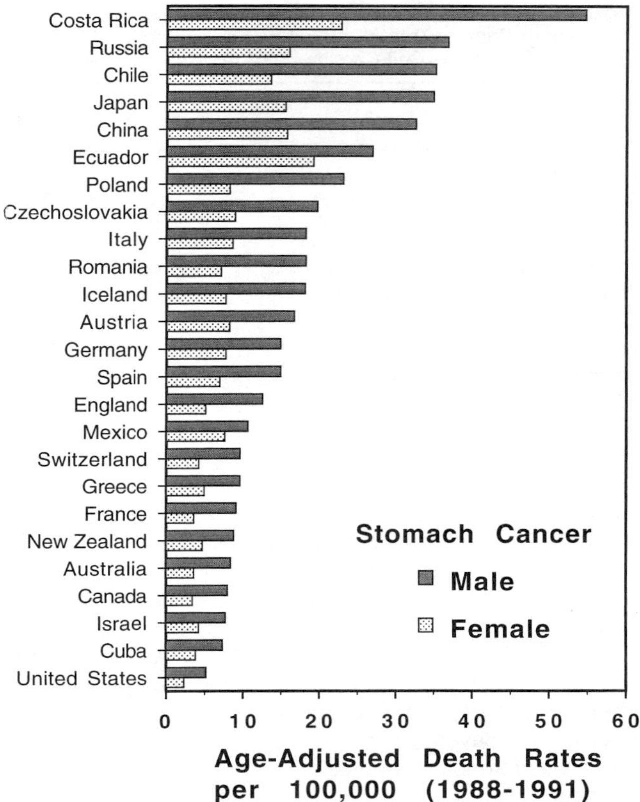

Figure 28.3. Age-adjusted death rates per 100,000 population from gastric cancer in selected countries. *Source:* Koring and colleagues (37).

The polycyclic aromatic hydrocarbons are a heterogeneous class of lipophilic compounds, many of which are carcinogenic and mutagenic. When administered orally, several have been reported to produce forestomach tumors in mice and hamsters (57, 353). These compounds are produced during the heating of foods to high temperatures or incorporated into foods that are cooked over a flame or smoked. They are found in high quantities in grilled, charbroiled, and smoke-cured meats (168, 230, 236). For example, the quantity of polycyclic aromatic hydrocarbons in a large, well-done charbroiled steak is equivalent to that found in the smoke of 600 cigarettes (230). Hot-air drying and roasting of grains and coffee also produces polycyclic aromatic hydrocarbons (106). Subpopulations at high risk for gastric cancer in Iceland, Hungary, and Latvia were found to have greater exposure to polycyclic aromatic hydrocarbons in smoked meats (56, 91, 397, 434). Overall, dietary exposure to polycyclic aromatic hydrocarbons has not been fully evaluated in large populations that differ in gastric cancer risk (302).

It has been postulated that nitrosamines found in food or produced in the stomach from precursors may play a role in gastric carcinogenesis (77, 294, 302, 380). Many nitrosamines are potent mutagens and stomach carcinogens in experimental animals, and several studies have suggested an association between increased levels of nitrate in the diet or drinking water and risk of gastric cancer (78, 302). Nitrate itself is not carcinogenic, however. Dietary nitrate first must undergo reduction to nitrite, which in turn nitrosates other compounds in the stomach contents, thus producing nitrosamines (320, 371). Factors that modulate the conversion of dietary nitrate to nitrite probably are more important than the amount of nitrate in the diet (77). One hypothesis suggests that disruption of the gastric mucosa by surgery, dietary irritants, or nutritional deficits produces focal areas of gastritis or atrophy, leading to colonization by bacteria that are known to produce nitrate reductases (143). These changes are thought to promote increased formation of nitrosamines and to initiate the malignant cascade. For example, pernicious anemia is a well-known metabolic disease of nutrient metabolism that leads to atrophic gastritis and increased risk of carcinoma (367). A number of food items and drugs have been found to yield mutagens after nitrosation; for example, nitrosation of a substance in fish consumed in Japan yields a carcinogen for the stomach of rats (442). A compound in fava beans, which are consumed by high-risk populations in Colombia, also yields a potent mutagen after nitrosation (331). Bile acids can be nitrosated and may contribute to carcinoma at the anastomotic site following partial gastrectomy (222). Laboratory studies suggest that vitamins C or E and other antioxidants may protect against the formation of nitrosamines (193, 245).

Continuing efforts are directed toward the identification of dietary factors that may accentuate the endogenous production of mutagens, alter mucosal cell susceptibility to transformation, or act as promoters. Epidemiologic studies have consistently identified an increased risk that is associated with the intake of excessive salt, which is used in many cultures as a preservative of dried meats and pickled vegetables (78, 141, 142, 157, 190, 300, 354, 420). Salt-cured foods induce gastric irritation in humans and rodents (254, 374, 375), and although salt alone will not induce stomach tumors in experimental models, increased intake potentiates tumorigenesis induced by other agents (379, 405).

Populations consuming abundant quantities of fresh fruits and vegetables generally have a lower risk of stomach cancer (36, 77, 132, 140, 142, 149, 153, 323, 354), and efforts to identify components of these foods that have protective properties are underway. Several possibilities have been proposed, including vitamin A, carotenoids, tocopherols, and vitamin C (77, 193, 245). Other studies have suggested a protective effect of dairy products, better refrigeration and sanitation, and the increased use of antioxidants by the food industry (77, 157).

Infection of the gastric mucosa with *Helicobacter pylori* (previously known as *Campylobacter pylori*) has been strongly associated with chronic atrophic gastritis and gastric carcinoma (314, 322). The vast majority of infected individuals, however, do not develop gastric cancer. The dietary and environmental factors that interact with *H. pylori* infection to modulate risk are a critical and very active area of investigation.

Although risk of gastric cancer has been associated with several dietary variables, it is not possible at this time to quantitate the contribution of these components or their mechanisms of action. In general, the diet of high-risk populations is low in animal products, high in complex carbohydrates derived from grains, high in salt-preserved and pickled foods, and low in fresh fruits and leafy green vegetables (36, 77, 302, 303). In some populations additional risk may derive from diets high in smoked foods or nitrates.

LIVER

Primary hepatocellular carcinoma is very rare in the United States and Northern Europe (37). In contrast, it is one of the most frequent types of cancer in sub-Saharan Africa, China, and Southeast Asia (37). Hepatitis B infection appears to be the major etiologic factor in many high-risk areas, where the carrier state imparts a relative risk of approximately 200-fold (19). Contamination of foods with carcinogenic fungal products, such as certain aflatoxins, also may contribute to risk in some populations (13, 231, 302, 303, 454). Aflatoxins are found in geographic areas where food processing and storage are not optimal. Some aflatoxins induce hepatocellular carcinoma in rodent models at the concentrations found in the diet of high-risk populations (456). Quantifying the contribution of aflatoxins to the incidence of hepatocellular carcinoma in many nations is limited by the difficulties of accurately assessing aflatoxin intake and the actual incidence of cancer in these populations. In addition, groups with high aflatoxin exposure often have high rates of hepatitis B infection, parasitic infections, and nutritional deficiencies, which may interact to determine risk.

In low-risk nations, it has been proposed that alcohol intake may be an important dietary factor in the pathogenesis of liver cancer (14, 16, 345, 358, 417). The data are inconsistent, however (152, 249, 250, 414), and other co-factors may act in an additive or synergistic fashion (40, 464). It has been hypothesized that liver cancer primarily occurs in those whose cumulative experiences with ethanol, viral hepatitis, and toxin exposure lead to cirrhosis. The cellular and molecular events that are associated with cirrhosis and regenerative nodules that may participate in the initiation and progression to cancer are under investigation. Additional evidence suggests that vinyl chloride, oral contraceptives, and androgenic-anabolic steroids also may participate in liver carcinogenesis in susceptible individuals.

Animal studies have shown that a number of dietary factors modulate experimental liver carcinogenesis using various carcinogens, including aflatoxin. Diets that are high in protein, energy, or lipid or deficient in lipotropes generally enhance hepatocarcinogenesis (9, 302, 303, 359). The role of these and other nutrients in modulating hepatocellular carcinoma in humans, however, has not been defined.

PANCREAS

The association between increased risk of pancreatic cancer and cigarette smoking has been firmly established. The relative risk of smoking at least a pack per day is approximately fourfold compared with that of nonsmokers (458). The important roles for nutrients in regulating normal pancreatic growth and function suggest that diet and nutrition may contribute to the pathogenesis of pancreatic cancer (242). The exocrine pancreas, which is the origin for 90% of pancreatic cancers, readily alters the pattern of digestive enzyme secretion in response to the nutrient content of the diet (396). Dietary restriction produces acinar cell atrophy, reduces DNA synthesis (311), and inhibits experimental pancreatic carcinogenesis (356). Pancreatic cell replication and differentiation are modulated by a number of gastrointestinal hormones, such as cholecystokinin and gastrin, and many dietary factors are potent mediators of gastrointestinal hormone secretion (242). Nonnutritive components such as trypsin inhibitors, frequently found in certain vegetables and legumes, have dramatic stimulatory effects on pancreatic cell DNA synthesis, induce hyperplasia and hypertrophy, and enhance pancreatic carcinogenesis in laboratory studies (242). The strong evidence supporting a role for dietary and nutritional factors in modulating pancreatic cell replication and differentiation suggests that diet may be important in pancreatic carcinogenesis.

The descriptive epidemiology of pancreatic cancer is complicated by the fact that estimates of incidence depend on conventions of medical care that vary in different geographic areas and socioeconomic conditions (255). The symptoms of pancreatic cancer often are vague, and significant cost and risk is associated with obtaining tissue for histologic diagnosis in many nations. Errors in clinical impressions and the difficulty of accurately reporting clinical diagnoses from medical records by cancer registries suggest that extreme caution should be used when comparing rates from populations with different standards of medical care or living in different times and places. Meaningful clues from epidemiologic studies concerning diet and nutrition in the pathogenesis of pancreatic cancer likely will be obscured by inconsistencies in diagnosis among different geographic and socioeconomic population groups. Overall, reports have suggested a higher incidence in affluent populations of North America and Northern Europe (37). Descriptive studies have suggested associations between an increased risk for pancreatic cancer and a number of components that are characteristic of the affluent diet, such as meat, fat, protein, eggs, milk and alcohol (14, 242, 255, 257, 302, 303). In contrast, however, the majority of epidemiologic studies suggest that the frequent consumption of fruits and vegetables may reduce the risk of pancreatic cancer (36).

Several animal models for pancreatic cancer have been characterized and used to examine the roles of dietary and nutritional components in modulating carcinogenesis under precisely controlled conditions (12, 238, 341). Diet and energy restriction dramatically reduces the number of pancreatic cancers in rodent models (12, 356), which is consistent with many studies showing a strong inhibitory effect of diet or energy restriction on carcinogenesis in other tissues (12, 368). High-fat diets, in the range of those consumed in affluent nations, enhance azaserine- and *N*-nitrosobis (2-oxopropyl)amine-induced pancreatic carcinogenesis (12, 27, 29, 357). The effects of protein quantity and quality on pancreatic carcinogenesis have not yet been clearly defined, but protein or amino acid deficiency and lower protein quality lead to pancreatic atrophy that is reversible on improvement of the diet (390, 391, 441). Roebuck and colleagues observed no effect of increasing protein on azaserine-induced cancer in rats (356), whereas others (29, 338, 340) have reported a reduced incidence of *N*-nitrosobis (2-oxopropyl)amine-induced pancreatic carcinoma in hamsters with severe protein deficiency. A potential interaction between fat and protein has been reported in the hamster model (29, 339). Those fed diets high in both fat and protein develop more pancreatic neoplasms than those fed diets that are low in both components.

Among the vitamins, studies suggest that vitamin A and synthetic retinoids may modulate experimental pancreatic carcinogenesis (12, 242). Several retinoids inhibit azaserine-induced pancreatic cancer in rats (239–241), but results using the hamster model have been less conclusive (26, 28, 239, 240). Other studies have observed stimulatory effects of vitamin A and retinoids (12). The effects of retinoid supplementation appear to depend on the dose, the baseline vitamin A status, and a number of host factors. Additional efforts to define synthetic retinoids that can be used as chemopreventive or therapeutic agents should be encouraged, although findings based on the pharmacologic doses of compounds not naturally found in foods may have little relevance to the role of dietary vitamin A status and pancreatic cancer risk.

Laboratory studies suggest that the pancreas is sensitive to dietary selenium intake. Selenium deficiency has been observed to produce pancreatic atrophy and fibrosis that is reversed with selenium supplementation (242, 316); however, supplemental selenium has not significantly altered experimental pancreatic carcinogenesis in several studies (12, 316).

Trypsin inhibitors found in many legumes and vegetables may contribute to the pathogenesis of pancreatic cancer (242). The heat-labile trypsin inhibitors are thought to be the factors responsible for pancreatic acinar hyperplasia and the spontaneous carcinomas that are observed in rats fed diets containing raw soy flour (272, 274, 275). Diets containing trypsin inhibitors also enhance the progression of pancreatic carcinomas that are induced by carcinogens such as azaserine (238, 275, 295). The ability of trypsin inhibitors to enhance pancreatic carcinogenesis probably is closely related to an increased production of trophic hormones and growth factors that contribute to acinar cell hyperplasia. It is unlikely, however, that the average cooked human diet that is characteristic of high-risk nations contains significant concentrations of active trypsin inhibitors. Additional information concerning the risk associated with various amounts and durations of exposure to the wide variety of different trypsin inhibitors is necessary.

A role for alcohol intake remains speculative (242). Ethanol does produce toxic injury to pancreatic cells, and the recurrent injury and regeneration may enhance risk in a fashion similar to partial pancreatectomy (86) and other chemical injuries (273); however, laboratory (340, 424) and epidemiologic studies (242, 255, 257) remain inconclusive.

In summary, laboratory studies clearly indicate that pancreatic carcinogenesis is sensitive to a number of dietary and nutritional components. For some nutrients, the limited data from laboratory and epidemiologic studies are in agreement. The most consistent epidemiologic data have been generated concerning reduced risk with diets rich in fruit and vegetables (36). However, additional investigations designed to define more clearly the associations identified and the mechanisms involved must be completed to develop dietary recommendations that will significantly decrease the risk of this devastating cancer.

COLON AND RECTUM

Colorectal cancer is a major public health problem in affluent westernized cultures (37). In the United States and Western Europe, up to 5% of the population may develop cancer of the large bowel by the age of 75 years (438). The international variation in large bowel cancer is large (Fig. 28.4), and although diagnostic differences may account for some of the international variation, it is unlikely to account for the greater than 10-fold variations that are observed between many nations (37). The lower rates in Japan suggest that cultural and lifestyle factors rather than industrialization are the critical factors (37). The geographic incidence patterns for colon and rectal cancer also generally vary in concert, suggesting that some similarity in etiology exists (186, 437). Studies in immigrant populations, such as Chinese migrants to the United States (445), clearly indicate that international variations primarily result from environmental influences rather than genetic background (139, 185, 277).

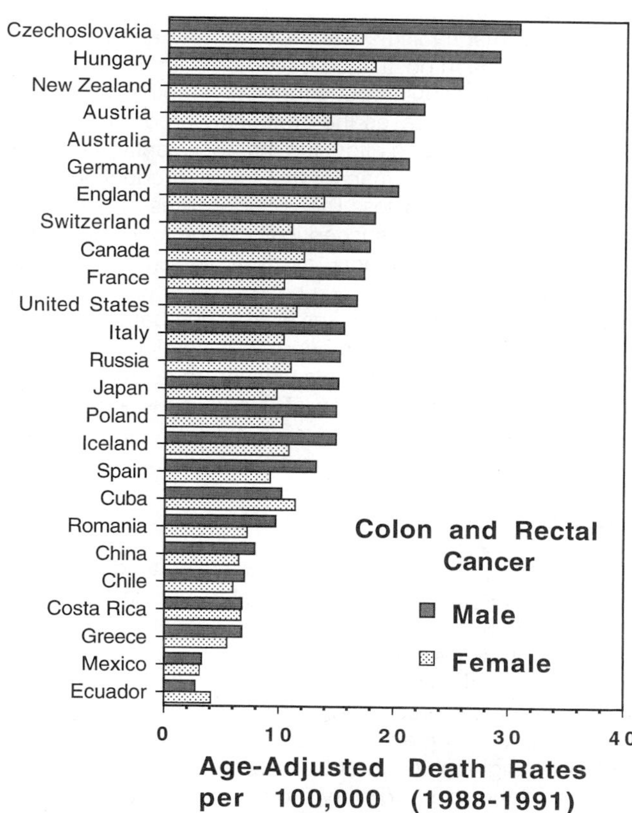

Figure 28.4. Age-adjusted death rates per 100,000 population from colon and rectal cancer in selected countries. *Source:* Koring and colleagues (37).

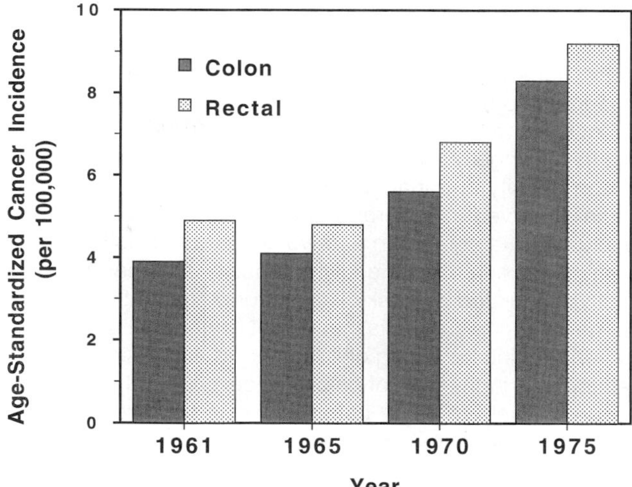

Figure 28.5. Age-standardized colon and rectal cancer incidence per 100,000 men in Japan from 1960 through 1977.

Japanese migrants to the United States also show a definite shift towards the colorectal cancer rates of the adopted country within the first generation (139). Examination of time trends in colorectal cancer incidence also suggests major contributions from environmental and lifestyle factors (185). Increases in the rate of large bowel cancer have been particularly striking within Japan in recent decades (Fig. 28.5) (139, 219). The desire to understand these variations in incidence and to institute preventive measures has prompted efforts to identify specific substances that are initiators or promoters of colon cancer (154). The role of diet and nutrition in the production of initiators and promoters or in modulating the sensitivity of the host to these agents has led to the generation of a number of hypotheses (33).

The diets most frequently associated with increased risk of colorectal cancer have several characteristics: rich in total fat, rich in total protein, rich in meat products, a high proportion of saturated fats, low in fruits and vegetables, and low in estimated fiber (36, 139, 288, 302, 303, 347). In addition, excessive caloric intake, sedentary lifestyle, and obesity have been implicated in some, but not all, studies (228, 444). The relative contribution of each variable alone as well as the potential interactions among them are currently under investigation in both human and laboratory studies.

Energy Balance

Energy intake, metabolic efficiency, physical activity, and various measures of body size or mass are intimately interrelated. It is difficult to quantitate or ascertain the role of each component in cancer risk without considering them as a group. An inverse association between physical activity and risk of colon cancer has been observed in studies limited to occupational activity (42, 98, 99, 109, 113, 321, 326, 431, 432) and those examining both job-related and recreational activity (2, 17, 112, 114, 195, 225, 334, 392, 445, 457). In addition, many studies have found an association between body mass index and elevated risk of colon cancer in men, although this relation is weaker among women (38, 110, 130,

202, 224, 229, 277, 299, 330). The association with a sedentary lifestyle appears stronger but is not limited to the distal colon. One study indicated that waist or waist-to-hip ratio and indicators of central or abdominal obesity are strongly associated with risk of colon cancer (115), perhaps explaining the stronger association in men. These associations between obesity and inactivity with risk of colon cancer have been observed in several countries (U.S., China, Sweden, and Japan), among men and women, and for both occupational and recreational activity. Obesity also has been directly associated with risk of colon adenoma (115, 234, 309). Some evidence suggests that height (perhaps a proxy of the net energy intake during childhood and adolesence) also is related to a higher risk of colon cancer (3, 4, 58). Studies in rodent models of colon carcinogenesis have reported enhanced tumorigenesis with greater ad libitum intake (65) and reduced risk with restricted intake (203, 213, 351).

Fat

Food consumption data from geographically defined populations have shown striking correlations between estimated fat intake, especially saturated fat, and colorectal cancer incidence (14, 53, 361). Many (41, 121, 130, 182, 214, 217, 218, 252, 327, 336, 373, 392, 445, 448) but not all (21, 185, 259, 271, 284, 359, 403, 421) report a positive association between dietary fat and risk of colon cancer. Most of these studies also show a direct association between total energy intake and risk of colon cancer, which is not surprising given the high correlation between fat and energy intake. Moreover, at least some of the studies indicate that nonlipid sources of energy contribute to the association between energy intake and colon cancer, which raises the question of the relative contribution of total energy consumed or of the fat composition of the diet that is etiologically relevant. For most of the studies, the investigators have not attempted to separate the influence of dietary fat from that of total energy intake.

A population-based, case-control study suggests that dietary fat accounts for 60% of colorectal cancer risk among Chinese migrants to the United States (Fig. 28.6). The relative risk of a high-fat diet, however, depends on the level of physical activity and on sex. Several other cohort studies report that fat from red meats, rather than total fat, may be more important. A recent prospective study in a cohort of 88,000 U.S. nurses supports a role for animal fat in colon cancer (451). An increased relative risk of 1.89 (95% confidence interval, 1.13 to 3.15) was observed for the highest quintile (>65 g/d) compared with the lowest quintile (<39 g/d) of animal fat intake. Other cohort studies have supported a positive association with red meat, particularly processed meats, but not with total fat, animal fat, or saturated fat (32, 38, 121, 123, 329).

Most studies in carcinogen-induced rodent models for colon cancer have observed increased tumor incidence and multiplicity in rats fed diets containing fat concentrations similar to those observed in the high-risk human diet (12, 211, 347). A promotional effect has been observed for both saturated and unsaturated fats (12); however, several well-controlled rodent studies have failed to document an in-

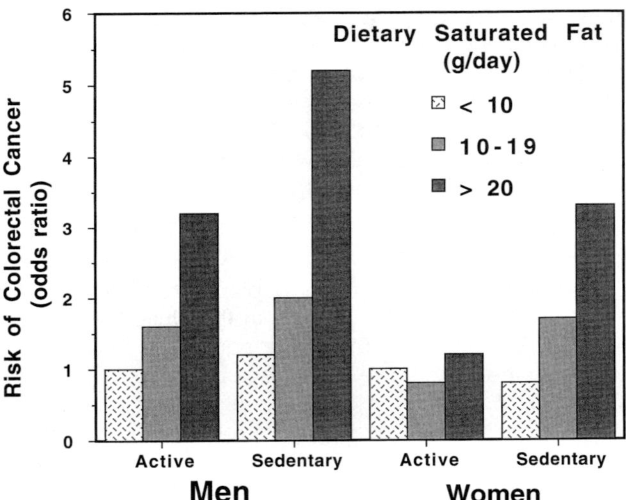

Figure 28.6. The risk of colorectal cancer in Chinese migrants to the United States according to dietary fat intake and level of physical activity. *Source:* Whittemore and colleagues (445).

creased tumor incidence with greater dietary fat (65, 313) suggesting that the effect of fat may not be a simple direct relationship and may depend on other variables not yet clearly defined, such as the timing of carcinogen exposure relative to dietary intervention, type of carcinogen and its mechanism of action, and consumption of other interacting nutrients.

Potential mechanisms whereby fat may enhance colon cancer have been postulated based on both human and rodent studies. A popular, but unproven, hypothesis suggests that dietary fat increases the concentration of bile acids in the colon contents and alters the metabolic activity of the intestinal microflora in a manner that favors production of certain bile-acid metabolites. These metabolites may be weak carcinogens, increase susceptibility of the mucosa to other carcinogens, or act directly as promoters (347). Low-risk populations in Asia and Africa have lower concentrations of bile acids and their metabolites in stool compared with high-risk populations in North America (347). Similar results have been observed in rats fed diets that vary in fat content (347). The intrarectal administration of bile-acid metabolites also has been reported to increase carcinogen-induced colon cancer in some studies (347) but not in others (62).

Protein

A role for dietary protein or specific amino acid patterns in colorectal cancer has been postulated but not yet established (302, 303, 413, 433). The international variation in total protein intake is much less than for fat. The source of protein does vary significantly, however, and is primarily derived from vegetable sources among low-risk populations in many nations and from meat and dairy products in those areas exhibiting high-risk (302, 303). Few rodent studies have investigated the role of dietary protein in colon carcinogenesis. Increasing protein intake enhanced 1,2-dimethylhydrazine-induced intestinal carcinogenesis in rats, whereas no effect of protein source was observed (63, 413).

It has been proposed that high-protein diets may enhance colon carcinogenesis via increasing colonic ammonia concentrations (62). It is interesting that in several prospective cohort studies of colon cancer and in studies of adenomatous polyps, protein intake has been associated with a reduced risk of colon cancer. This is even more remarkable given that red meat, which is a good source of protein, has been associated with an increased risk. A protective effect of dietary protein may relate to increased consumption of the amino acid methionine, which is required for normal methyl group metabolism and DNA methylation (72). Aberrant DNA methylation may be one step in the cascade of genetic defects associated with colon cancer development and progression (93, 122, 161, 163, 262).

Fiber

Burkitt and Trowell (46) popularized the hypothesis that low dietary fiber intake may be a critical variable enhancing risk of colon cancer. Trowell (416) provided a useful definition of fiber as components of plant cells that resist digestion by secretions of the human gastrointestinal tract; however, the precise definition continues to be debated and refined among nutritional scientists (302, 303). In general, dietary fiber is a complex collection of substances, including cellulose, hemicelluloses, pectin, lignin, gums, some polysaccharides, and mucilages. It is possible to expand the definition to include indigestible substances that are not derived from plant sources, such as chitins from fungi and crustaceans, aminopolysaccharides from animals, or nonenzymatic browning products that form during food processing. The chemistry of dietary fiber is exceptionally complex, and standardization of analytic techniques is a dynamic and evolving field of nutritional science. The different fiber components have widely varying physical and chemical properties, such as water-holding capacity or ion-exhange characteristics. At present, our limited understanding of these physical and chemical characteristics has not allowed adequate insight into the biologic properties of high-fiber foods, which makes it particularly difficult to understand their roles in diseases such as colon cancer (302, 303).

Studies of several populations consuming diets similar in fat but differing in total fiber intake suggest a protective role for fiber (186, 263, 349, 415); however, most international and intracountry studies have provided little insight (14, 23, 235, 253). This should not be surprising, because there is a lack of complete analytic data concerning the content of fiber components in foods consumed by many populations. Superimposed on the analytic difficulties, the epidemiologic methodology for estimating fiber intake exhibits tremendous imprecision. Inverse associations between total fiber intake and risk of colon cancer have been observed in some, but not all, case-control studies (80, 175, 178, 182, 214, 218, 252, 336, 451). A meta-analysis of case-control studies of colon cancer found a combined odds ratio of 0.58 between the highest and lowest quintiles based on fiber intake but an even stronger odds ratio of 0.48 based on vegetable consumption (415). Prospective data regarding fiber intake and risk of colon cancer generally have been less convincing, with only one study (411) showing a clear inverse association, but others are suggestive (38, 145, 398). Among the case-control and cohort studies that examined sources of fiber separately, intake of fruits or vegetables generally is protective, whereas grain fiber or cereal intake either is unrelated or positively associated with risk of colon cancer. Studies of colorectal adenomas also tend to more consistently support a beneficial effect of fruit and vegetable fiber and, possibly, cereal fiber (20, 117, 233, 258, 310, 372). Others have pointed out that of 13 analytic studies reporting an association between sucrose and colon neoplasia, 11 have reported a positive association (with significant or nearly significant findings in 6), 1 reported a null association, and 1 found a nonsignificant inverse association (22, 38, 328, 332). Overall, epidemiologic data suggest that some component of dietary fiber, or a factor associated with diets rich in fiber, may reduce risk. In addition, some characteristic of highly refined, fiber-depleted foods may enhance the risk for colon cancer.

The chemical complexity of fiber suggests that estimated total fiber intake may not be an adequate measure for epidemiologic studies attempting to determine its role in colon cancer, thus emphasizing the need for standardized analytic techniques in fiber chemistry. A number of case-control studies have not attempted to calculate fiber intake per se; rather they use the frequency of consumption of high-fiber foods as an indirect indicator. In general, these studies suggest a protective effect of fiber-rich diets and especially vegetable consumption (30, 80, 126, 258, 264, 293, 415). Intervention trials with dietary fiber are now beginning to yield results relative to the risk of colon cancer. For example, a recent double-blind, placebo-controlled study showed that a daily supplement of 22.5 g of wheat bran significantly reduced the number of adenomatous polyps in the sigmoid colon and rectum of patients with familial polyposis (83). A subsequent, single-arm study reported a reduction in rectal mucosal cell DNA synthesis rates in patients with a history of resected colon or rectal cancer who were fed wheat-bran fiber (5). Future randomized studies will determine if supplements of wheat-bran fiber prevent the development of colon cancer in a high-risk population. Studies to determine the validity of colon cell proliferative rates as a marker of carcinogenic risk also are needed. An intermediate marker will be especially useful for rapid assessment of the chemopreventative effects of various types of dietary fiber.

Animal studies have reinforced the concept that fiber nutrition may play a role in colon carcinogenesis but that the relationship is not simple (179, 180, 210, 302, 303). Studies have observed no effect, increased, and decreased tumorigenesis depending on the amount, type, and source of fiber, its particle size, the amount of other nutrients, type of carcinogen, timing of fiber feeding relative to carcinogen administration, and the strain and species of animal. The results of rodent studies reflect the complexities of fiber nutrition and emphasize the importance of avoiding strong conclusions based on single laboratory or epidemiologic studies. Among the fiber sources evaluated, wheat bran has shown a relatively consistent ability to inhibit experimental colon carcinogenesis (210, 302, 303).

A number of mechanisms may contribute to the protective effect of dietary fiber against colon cancer (210, 302, 303).

Fiber may increase fecal bulk and reduce the concentration of colon mutagens or promoters. Many high-fiber diets decrease transit time, thus providing another mechanism to reduce exposure of the colon to genotoxic agents or tumor promoters in the fecal stream. Many fibers also may bind carcinogens in the diet, further limiting exposure (67). Most fibers are metabolized to varying degrees by the bacterial flora which may lead to the production of metabolites that can either increase or decrease risk. In summary, each type of fiber has unique properties which may modulate carcinogenesis by different mechanisms. Evidence suggests that diets containing foods that have varying amounts and sources of fiber probably influence risk of colon cancer, although the details of this relationship remain to be defined.

Alcohol

An association between alcohol intake and risk of colon cancer is consistent with many ecologic (216) cohort (32, 54, 81, 154, 202, 335, 402, 453, 457) and population-based, case-control studies (104, 192, 215, 243, 335, 418). As further evidence, alcohol is consistently related to higher risk of colorectal adenoma (58, 74, 166, 200, 209, 215, 372, 401). A recent extensive review (216) concluded that a positive association between alcohol intake and colorectal cancer was found in 5 of 7 correlational studies, in 9 of 10 studies using community controls, but in only 5 of 17 studies that used hospital-based controls. These authors suggested that some of the hospital-based studies may be biased, because alcohol intake is related to many conditions requiring hospitalization (162), which could cause an overestimate of intake among controls. They also found that of 14 cohort studies, an association with alcohol was found in 10, while in 3 of the 4 cohort studies not demonstrating an association, the alcohol data collected were limited. Studies suggest that the elevated risk associated with alcohol occurs predominantly in the rectum or distal colon (216), whereas fewer studies report an elevated risk associated with proximal colon cancer. Recent studies indicate that high intakes of folate or methionine, both of which are crucial for normal methyl groupmetabolism and, particularly, DNA methylation, appeared to mitigate the influence of alcohol. The risk of colorectal adenoma and cancer was elevated in individuals with high intakes of alcohol and low intakes of methionine and folate, and the excess risk was particularly high among those with deleterious combinations such as high alcohol–low folate intake (116, 119). This suggests that alcohol, which has a well-known, adverse effect on methyl group metabolism, increases the risk of colorectal cancer via this mechanism (94).

Colon Carcinogens

The recent characterization of a series of very specific mutational events in human colon cancer ultimately must be linked with etiologic agents that participate in the accumulation of genotoxic events. At present, no definitive data implicate specific ingested carcinogens for human large bowel cancer; however, the potential for the production of initiators or promoters during cooking and food processing has not been thoroughly investigated (43). Food preparation varies among different cultures and could be a critical factor contributing to the large geographic differences in cancer incidence. For example, in China, many foods are prepared with steam, whereas similar foods more frequently are fried by Chinese migrants to the United States. These differences in food preparation may lead to a different pattern or concentration of pyrolysis products in food. A number of mutagenic pyrolysis products are produced during cooking, and several have been found to be carcinogenic in laboratory animals, even if very few have been found to be specific for the colon (43, 377, 378). Short-term studies that examine nuclear aberrations and microadenoma formation in the colonic mucosa have been used as an indirect measure of carcinogenic potential (43), and rodents fed diets containing cooked food items such as fried bacon or hamburger show a higher frequency of nuclear aberrations in the colon mucosa than do controls (43, 76).

Other investigations have focused on the production of mutagens within the digestive tract as a result of bacterial metabolism (43). Human feces contain substances that are mutagenic in bacterial test systems (43), and correlational studies have indicated that fecal mutagenicity is greater in populations that are at high risk for colorectal cancer (92, 297). For example, the concentration of stool mutagens in rural black South Africans at low risk of colon cancer was lower than in urban blacks and whites who experience greater risk (92). Human subjects fed a high-risk diet rich in protein, fat, energy, and animal products showed greater concentrations of fecal mutagens than those fed a low-risk diet (212).

One class of mutagenic compounds, known as fecapentaenes, was characterized and found to be produced by the colonic bacteria (90, 138, 430). However, fecapentaenes have not yet been proven to be carcinogenic for the colon, and their role in tumorigenesis remains speculative (205, 437). The concentrations of these compounds have been reported to decrease in individuals whose diet is supplemented with ascorbic acid and alpha-tocopherol (88), or dietary fiber (350). However, a randomized study on polyp recurrence found no beneficial effect of these supplements (43). Another large study found no significant differences in the content of stool fecapentaenes between 68 patients with colon cancer and 114 controls (377, 378). Although fecapentaenes may have some role in colon cancer, it does not appear that they are the major, or only, initiator. Metabolites, such as the ketosteroids, that are produced by bacteria or during food processing from cholesterol or bile acids also have genotoxic and cytotoxic properties (29). The concentration of these compounds in the fecal contents varies widely, and the dietary factors that modulate their formation remain to be defined.

In summary, increased risk of colorectal cancer is strongly associated with an affluent diet, which is rich in high-fat foods (especially from animal products) and low in fruits, grains, and vegetables. The individual contributions of alcohol, energy balance and exercise, folate, methionine, and specific fiber components are undergoing further investigation. The potential interactions among these components are numerous. At present, it is prudent to consider the impact of the total diet when making recommendations rather than focusing on a single nutrient.

BREAST

Cancer of the breast is frequent in the affluent nations of North America and Western Europe and much less common in many parts of Asia and Africa (37). Migrants from low-risk nations show increasing risk after moving to a high-risk nation (44, 139, 302, 303, 359). The increase in breast cancer risk among Japanese immigrants to the United States is most noticeable over several generations, in contrast to colon cancer risk, which increases significantly over the lifespan of the original migrant population (446). This observation suggests that nutritional or other environmental factors that are active during youth and adolescence may have a long-term and major impact on subsequent risk of breast cancer (360). These findings are consistent with the hypothesis that some dietary patterns established early in life are associated with increased height and weight, leading to a hormonal environment contributing to an earlier age of menarche, which in turn is associated with an increased risk of breast cancer (134).

A number of dietary and nutritional factors have been proposed to enhance or protect against breast cancer. Geographic studies have identified associations between national breast cancer rates and diets high in fat, protein, milk, eggs, refined sugar, and animal products (14, 53, 124, 287, 291, 302, 303). All of these components are characteristic of the Western diet, and the individual contribution of each factor to breast cancer risk cannot be determined by correlational studies alone. Case-control studies frequently have supported associations between breast cancer and components of the affluent diet, but results have not been uniform (131, 158, 159, 160, 169, 247, 289, 407, 412).

Energy Balance, Weight, and Obesity

The role of energy intake as a stimulator of mammary carcinogenesis has been well established by rodent studies using diet or energy restriction (410) or by regression analysis of ad libitum feeding (60, 64). Higher body weight or body mass index in women has been associated with greater risk (1); furthermore, adult weight gain is associated independently of body weight with enhanced risk of postmenopausal breast cancer (226, 237). However, the precise relationships between energy intake, energy expenditure, anthropometrics, and risk of breast cancer must be examined for different critical periods in a woman's life cycle. The effects of these factors may vary during adolescence, the reproductive years, and the postmenopausal period.

Fat

The controversy concerning the contribution of dietary fat to risk of breast cancer can best be appreciated through examination of the representative data presented in Fig. 28.7 and Tables 28.3 and 28.4. Geographic studies show strong correlations between national rates of breast cancer and the estimated per-capita fat consumption (52, 53, 342). There are wide international variations in breast cancer rates as well as per-capita fat consumption or the percentage of calories derived from fat. In general, the relationship between estimated dietary fat and risk of breast cancer appears to be linear, and correlation coefficients range between 0.75 and 0.90 (52, 53, 342). Breast cancer rates also have been observed to increase significantly in populations migrating from low-risk areas such as Japan, where diets are low in fat, to high-risk areas such as the United States, where populations consume diets high in fat (44, 139, 303, 303, 359). Time-trend studies also support the fat–breast cancer association. Within Japan, estimates of per-capita daily fat intake rose from 23 to 52 g/d over the 15-year period before 1973 (156). During this period, breast cancer mortality increased in Japan by over 30% (219). Not all ecologic studies support a strong effect of dietary fat, however. A study from 65 Chinese counties showed only a weakly positive association between fat intake and breast cancer mortality, despite a striking variation in fat intake from 6 to 45% of energy (191). Correlation does not prove cause and effect, and many investigators argue that fat intake may be an indicator of some other unidentified combination of diet and environmental components that are the truly critical risk factors. The strong correlations observed may indicate the overall effect of many dietary factors that change simultaneously.

The relationship between fat intake and risk of breast cancer has been examined in many case-control studies. Although these are too numerous to examine here, a recent meta-analysis of 17 such studies that included 6,831 cases and 7,105 controls found only 4 (of 17) showing a statistically significant, positive association between fat intake and breast cancer (39). When all 17 studies were combined, however, a modest but statistically significant, 21% increase in risk was found comparing the highest to the lowest level of intake from each study. It is of interest that no association between fat intake and risk of breast cancer was seen in a case-control study in Japan (159), where the lower-fat-consumption groups were likely to have consumed less than 20% of energy from fat.

Data from cohort studies assessing the relation between dietary fat intake and breast cancer have become available in recent years. Ten prospective studies have not provided compelling evidence for the high dietary fat–breast cancer association (49, 133, 170, 189, 204, 220, 291, 425, 448, 449). In the largest cohort study, the Nurses' Health Study (448), 1,439 cases of breast cancer were documented among 89,494 women followed for 8 years. The relative risk comparing the highest and lowest deciles of fat intake as a percent of energy intake at baseline was 0.86 (95% confidence interval, 0.67–1.08). The estimated range of total fat intake expressed as percent of calories from fat was 29 to over 49% in this population. In contrast, a cohort study of Canadian women (183) reported an increased risk of dying from breast cancer associated with a greater saturated fat intake but not with total fat.

Almost all case-control and cohort investigations have related the influence of current dietary intake of adults to short-term breast cancer risk (of approximately 10 years). It remains possible that dietary fat intake during childhood and adolescence may affect breast cancer risk decades later. Also, it may take even greater reductions in fat intake (e.g., to less than 20% of calories from fat) to reduce risk. Most

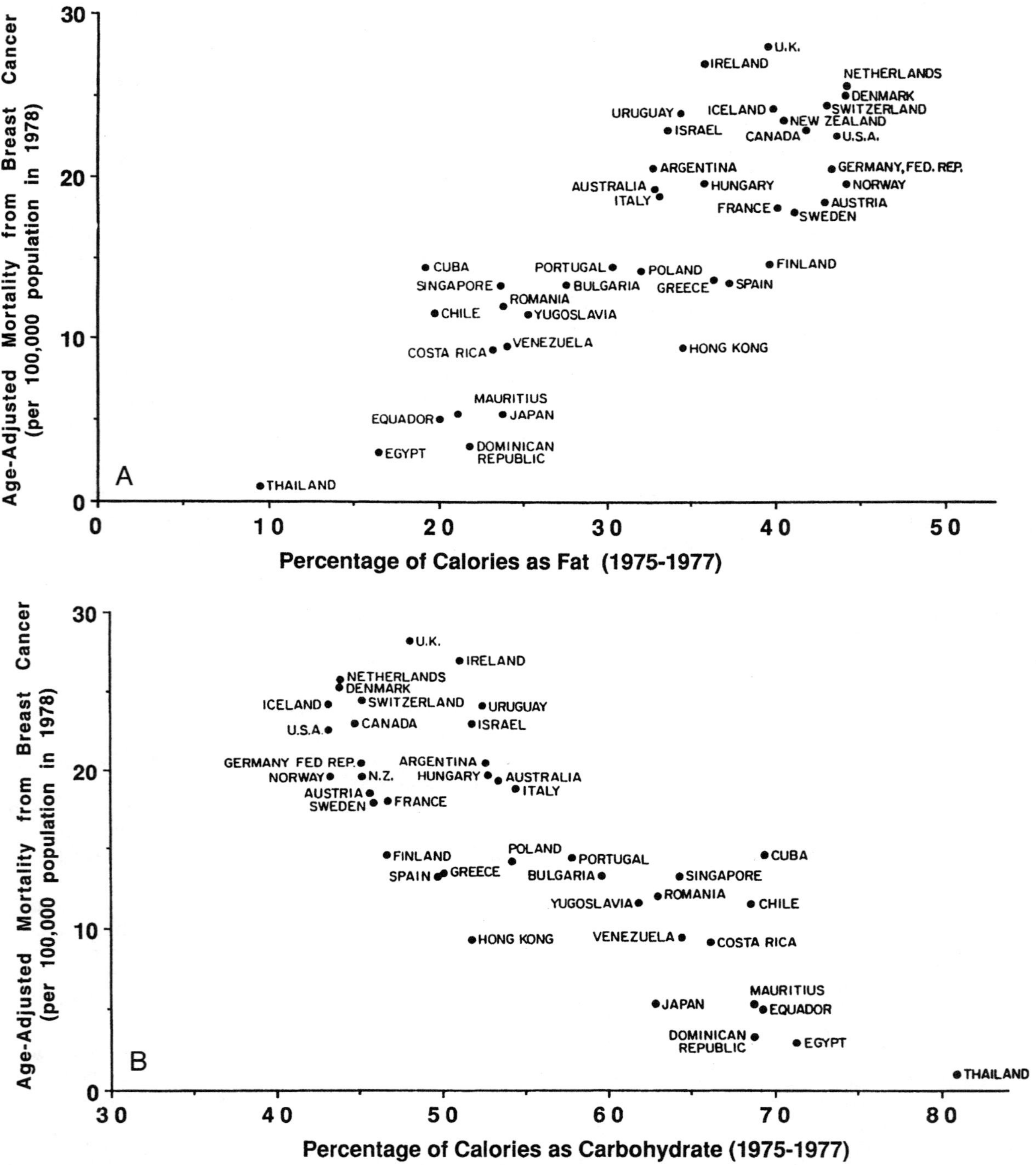

Figure 28.7. International correlation of (A) estimated dietary fat intake (percentage of calories as fat and (B) estimated carbohydrate intake (percentage of calories as carbohydrate) and age-adjusted breast cancer mortality. *Source:* Carroll (51).

case-control and cohort studies do not have significant numbers of participants with energy intakes of 20% or less.

Although the epidemiologic data have not provided definitive results concerning dietary fat and breast cancer, accumulated evidence from over 100 animal studies using chemical carcinogens, hormones, irradiation, or viruses to induce breast cancer indicate that as a single variable, fat enhances mammary carcinogenesis (100). For example, a large study in rats using diets containing fat concentrations ranging from 12 to 48% of calories clearly indicates a strong enhancement of mammary carcinogenesis over the range of fat intake observed in human populations (60, 61, 64). Well-controlled rodent studies also have shown that dietary fat enhances the risk of breast cancer independently of caloric intake (Fig. 28.1) (60, 64, 409). In addition, both saturated or polyunsaturated fats will similarly enhance mammary carcinogenesis

Table 28.3. Dietary Fat and Risk of Breast Cancer in 89,538 U.S. Nurses Aged 34 to 59 Years at Initial Evaluation in 1980[a]

Measurement	Quintile				
	1	2	3	4	5
Total fat					
Mean calorie adjusted (g/d)	56	64	69	72	78
Mean % of calories	32	36	39	41	44
Multivariate relative risk	1.00	0.80	0.88	0.80	0.82
Saturated fat					
Mean calorie adjusted (g/d)	19	22	24	26	30
Mean % of calories	11	13	14	15	17
Multivariate relative risk	1.00	0.80	0.91	0.77	0.84
Cholesterol					
Mean calorie adjusted (mg/d)	216	268	301	337	423
Multivariate relative risk	1.00	1.06	1.02	1.07	0.91

[a] During 4 years of follow-up, 601 cases of breast cancer were diagnosed among participants. The multivariate age-adjusted relative risk of breast cancer is expressed according to the quintile estimates of calorie-adjusted total fat, saturated fat, and cholesterol intake.
From Willet and colleagues (448).

Table 28.4. Effects of Dietary Fat Intake (12, 24, 48% of Calories) on 7,12-Dimethylbenz[a]anthracene (DMBA)-Induced Mammary Carcinogenesis in Female Rats[a]

Dietary fat (% kcal)	Rats (n)	Daily energy intake (kcal/d)	Final body weight (g)	Adenocarcinoma incidence (%)	Cancers (n)
12	120	46	263	19	34
24	120	47	262	35	53
48	120	47	260	62	125

[a] Rats were fed diets with corn oil providing 12, 24, or 48% of total energy from 4 weeks of age for a period of 30 weeks. DMBA was given as a single dose (2.0 mg per 100 g body weight) after 4 weeks of feeding. Each doubling of energy intake from fat multiplied the odds of developing an adenocarcinoma by 2.7 ($P < .001$).
From Clinton and colleagues (64).

once minimal amounts of essential fatty acids have been provided (52). The possibility that omega-3 fatty acids have a unique ability to reduce breast carcinogenesis or growth rates requires additional investigation.

Overall, the large body of data from animal investigations and human geographic epidemiologic studies supports the hypothesis that dietary fat may be one component of an affluent diet that contributes to an increased risk of breast cancer. The negative findings from recent analytic epidemiologic studies, however, have led many to revise hypotheses. Perhaps the effect of fat is most important early in life, when breast development is most pronounced (343, 376). Additional efforts should be directed toward defining how dietary fat interacts with other nutrients to modulate breast development and risk of initiating the carcinogenic cascade. The possibility that achievable reductions in fat intake during adulthood will cause an appreciable reduction in breast cancer risk remains uncertain; several intervention trials are underway to evaluate low-fat dietary patterns on breast cancer risk.

Protein

Dietary protein has a major impact on the early growth and development of humans and laboratory animals. Marginal intakes of protein and energy may be factors contributing to the later onset of menarche in many populations in developing nations exhibiting lower risk of breast cancer. In general, geographic correlational and case-control studies have not shown strong or consistent associations. Laboratory studies show no major influence on breast cancer when protein is varied over a wide range after rats have reached sexual maturity (61, 64). In contrast, a stimulatory effect of protein has been observed in a two-generation model (144). High-protein diets fed to dams throughout mating and lactation, and then fed to female offspring, accelerated sexual maturation and increased the incidence of chemically induced mammary cancer (144). The role of protein nutrition during childhood and adolescence as a risk factor for breast cancer later in life has not been clearly ascertained.

Alcohol

Recent reviews of the accumulated evidence concerning alcohol intake and risk of breast cancer suggest a positive association (146, 244, 362). Overall, it was estimated that 13 to 14% of all breast cancer in the United States may be attributed to alcohol alone (244, 450). The relative risk from the consumption of one typical serving of beer, wine, or liquor (approximately 12 g of ethanol) per day was estimated to be 1.4, whereas three drinks per day would approximately double the risk. Most investigators have not concluded that the association is definitely causal, however, because of the possibility of residual confounding given that the causes of breast cancer are poorly understood. Nonetheless, that the association has been observed in the United States, Spain, France, Greece, Italy, Australia, Denmark, Holland, and New Zealand, even after controlling for known or suspected risk factors, argues against residual confounding. It appears to be unlikely that the hypothetic factor would have the same pattern for all types of alcoholic beverages over all these countries. Recent data showing that two to three drinks could result in significant changes in both plasma and urinary estrogens suggest hormonal changes as one plausible mechanism (352).

Vitamins

There are no prospective cohort studies, retrospective case-control studies, or nested case-control studies using serum samples of vitamin concentrations that support a strong relationship between a specific vitamin and risk of breast cancer. Based on the accumulated evidence, the most suggestive data concerns vitamin A and provitamin A carotenoids. Some studies suggest an inverse correlation between breast cancer risk and estimated intakes of vitamin A (176, 280, 302, 303, 359). The majority of rodent experimentation also suggests a protective effect of vitamin A and related compounds (12). Vitamins E and C frequently have been investigated relative to breast cancer risk, but no major role for these or other vitamins has been firmly established.

Minerals

Selenium has been most extensively studied relative to breast cancer risk, primarily in animal models (12, 302, 303). It is difficult to assess human selenium intake by dietary questionnaires, because plants are very sensitive to the soil selenium content, thus leading to tremendous variation in the selenium content of foods. Although questionnaires are of little utility, tissue samples can be used to estimate recent intake. This approach will be useful only if evaluated prospectively, however, because the presence of a cancer may alter the results obtained (296, 303). A recent prospective analysis among women revealed that greater toenail selenium as a marker of intake was not associated with reduced risk of breast cancer or other malignancies (111). Because of the difficulties in assessment, human studies have not provided strong evidence for increased risk with low intakes. Animal studies have suggested that elevated selenium intake may inhibit mammary carcinogenesis under some conditions (12, 59, 303); however, it is apparent that the protective effect of selenium depends on other nutritional factors, such as the amount and source of fat and protein in the diet and, possibly, vitamin E and antioxidants. Because the role of selenium in human cancer is uncertain and it has potential for significant toxicity, individuals should be discouraged from consuming selenium as a supplement (12, 302, 303).

In summary, geographic epidemiologic data, studies of migrant populations, and rodent experiments strongly suggest that diet may have a significant impact on risk of breast cancer. However, the contribution of individual components of the diet and the time period during a woman's life when they may be most active are not well understood. In addition to the possible risk associated with the affluent diet, alcohol consumption may play a role in mammary cancer and warrants further study.

PROSTATE

Cancer of the prostate has become one of the most frequently diagnosed malignancies in U.S. men, and it is especially common among the U.S. black population (55, 333, 364). Prostate cancer is a disease of aging men and is rare under the age of 45 years. The international distribution of prostate cancer is similar to that of colon and breast cancer; therefore, it correlates with Western culture and affluent diets (37). The role of nutrition in prostate cancer has not been widely investigated. Increased body weight or obesity has been associated with risk of prostate cancer in some (229, 395, 408), but not all (208) studies. More detailed investigations of diet, adolescent growth and development, adult energy balance, and prostate cancer risk clearly are needed.

International and intracountry correlational studies have suggested associations between prostate cancer mortality and the per capita intake of total fat (14, 34, 172, 361). Similarly, several analytic epidemiologic studies have reported associations between total fat or the consumption of high-fat foods and prostate cancer (128, 148, 208, 383, 395). For example, a correlational analysis based on diet history data conducted within Hawaii showed that both animal and saturated fat intake had a high correlation with prostate cancer incidence (208). Within Italy, strong positive correlations exist between prostate cancer mortality and the consumption of foods rich in fat, such as milk and cheese (82, 285). The majority (127, 148, 208, 292, 328, 364, 366, 383, 393, 406, 408, 443), but not all (197, 283, 317), of the case-control studies support an association between some component of diets rich in fat, particulary saturated or animal fats, and risk of prostate cancer. Several of the earlier prospective or cohort studies have been inconsistent regarding fat intake and prostate cancer risk. Some of this variation may relate to the design of the studies. Several of the null studies had a very long time interval between dietary assessment and diagnosis of cancer, a limited dietary assessment, or were conducted in Japan, which has a low fat-consumption level (174, 386). Studies of Seventh-Day Adventists provide suggestive evidence that animal fat consumption increases the risk of prostate cancer, particularly fatal cancers (291, 395). Several recent cohort studies found similar positive associations between prostate cancer and red meat consumption, total animal fat consumption, and intake of fatty animal foods (108, 120, 227). The recent studies assessed dietary intake over a relatively short period before diagnosis (mostly within 5 years). Thus, excluding the studies from Japan, where the overall intake of animal fat is quite low, most cohort studies have supported a positive association between some component of dietary fat, especially animal fat, and risk of prostate cancer.

Few rodent models of prostate cancer have been characterized and used to investigate nutritional hypotheses derived from epidemiologic studies. Even so, essential fatty acid deficiency was found to inhibit the growth rate of a transplantable prostate adenocarcinoma, whereas dietary fat concentrations over the wide range of intake observed in human populations had no significant effect (66). This observation does not preclude the possibility of significant effects of dietary fat on earlier stages in the carcinogenic process, which cannot be evaluated in a transplantable tumor model.

Evidence suggests a complex role for vitamin A, provitamin A carotenoids, or synthetic retinoids in prostate carcinogenesis. In a series of studies, estimates of vitamin A intake have been reported to have no relationship or to be associated with increased or decreased risk of prostate cancer (128, 148, 208, 361, 364, 388). Clearly, the relationship between vitamin A status, ranging from deficiency to excess, and prostate cancer has not been defined. The high intake of foods rich in carotenoids, which have biologic activities in addition to their contribution to vitamin A status, has been associated with decreased risk in some studies (36, 363, 383).

Recent studies have established a hypothesis that a dysregulation of the vitamin D metabolism may relate to risk of prostate cancer (75). In a large, prospective, case-control study, mean serum 1,25-dihydroxyvitamin D levels were lower in cases than in matched controls. Further epidemiologic and laboratory-based studies are needed to determine which components of vitamin D intake, metabolism, and biologic action in the prostate may relate to prostate cancer risk.

In summary, a role for diet in prostate cancer has been suggested by epidemiologic studies and a limited number of laboratory investigations. Rates of prostate cancer are higher in nations consuming an affluent diet, although the contribution of specific components such as fat and energy intake have not been well defined. The biologic plausibility is further enhanced by the knowledge that many nutrients modulate the secretion of or tissue sensitivity to hormones such as testosterone, which are thought to participate in prostate carcinogenesis.

ENDOMETRIUM

In general, endometrial cancer shows an international distribution similar to that of other cancers of affluence, such as breast, colon, and prostate (37). An association between endometrial cancer and excess weight often has been reported (302, 306, 359). One established risk factor is the use of exogenous estrogens at high dosages (302, 306). It has been postulated, although the evidence is minimal, that dietary factors contributing to obesity may influence risk though changes in the hormonal environment. The potential interactions between dietary components and supplemental estrogens should be investigated.

OVARY

There are considerable international and geographic variations in the incidence and mortality rates of ovarian cancer. The disease is more common in nations exhibiting Western culture, especially among the higher socioeconomic groups (37, 223, 302, 306, 359). Although some of the geographic variation may result from reproductive variables, there also are suggestive relationships to dietary components (302, 303, 359). Several studies have implicated fat, particularly from animal sources (79, 223, 355). In contrast, the consumption of vegetables and grain products was associated with lower risk (223). At present, no conclusive role for dietary components in the pathogenesis of ovarian cancer has been established, but additional studies are needed.

BLADDER

Bladder cancer is more frequent in industrialized nations, especially among those in urban areas and of lower socioeconomic status (37). Bladder cancer is associated with cigarette smoking, occupational exposures to certain industrial chemicals, and parasitic bladder infections. There so far have been very limited efforts to investigate the role of diet and nutrition in bladder cancer etiology (14, 36, 302, 303, 359). The majority of epidemiologic studies suggest that the frequent consumption of fruits and vegetables may reduce risk (36). Laboratory studies have found that the nonnutritive sweeteners, cyclamates and saccharine, may be weak initiators or promoters of bladder carcinogenesis in rodents (344), but their contribution to human cancer probably is very small (302–304). Although some studies have suggested an association between coffee consumption and bladder cancer (3, 81, 394), most do not support a significant relationship (181, 187, 303).

Summary of Research Efforts Concerning Nutrients and Cancer

ENERGY BALANCE

Striking and consistent inhibitory effects of reduced energy intake on most types of cancer have been observed in rodent studies (12, 60, 64, 65, 100, 302, 303, 359, 368). An understanding of the diverse mechanisms underlying these observations should be relevant to human cancer prevention. Experimental evidence suggests that energy intake modulates a range of metabolic, endocrinologic, and immunologic processes that influence cellular proliferative rates, proto-oncogene expression, and DNA repair capabilities (368).

Because of the complex interrelations among total energy consumption, energy expenditure and genetic differences in energy metabolism, and limitations of current assessment methodologies, the associations between energy balance and cancer are not easily interpretable in human studies (171). Accurate measures of energy intake are difficult to obtain with current food-frequency questionnaires. Variation in energy expenditure among individuals within a population can be attributed to three general sources; physical activity, body size, and metabolic efficiency (447). The balance between energy intake and expenditure will determine whether an individual gains or loses weight; even small differences between intake and expenditure over time can lead to appreciable differences in body weight. Surrogate measures, such as the development of obesity or weight change in adulthood may reflect an imbalance between energy intake and expenditure. In human studies, obesity is associated with endometrial cancer, cancer of the biliary system, and colon cancer, particularly in men. More modest associations are evident for breast and renal cell cancer. Attained adult height, which is another surrogate marker of energy balance, may reflect in part dietary patterns during in utero development, childhood, and adolescence. In some industrialized countries, however, there may be a paucity of individuals who were sufficiently energy restricted during development to have experienced a failure to obtain their full potential for height. Mean national heights, perhaps as an index of energy balance during development, have a strong correlation with international rates of breast cancer (177, 286). Similar associations with height have been observed for colon and, possibly, prostate cancer. Greater physical activity, the other component of the equation, has been consistently related to lower risk of colon cancer and possibly breast cancer. Overall, the epidemiologic evidence supports animal studies that an imbalance of energy consumption versus requirements could be an important risk factor for a variety of cancers.

PROTEIN

Like energy intake, dietary protein has dramatic effects on many physiologic and biochemical processes that may participate in carcinogenesis (433). The Western diet typically is greatly in excess of the recommended protein requirement. The major change in protein intake as nations develop economically is a shift from plant to animal products as the major source of protein. At this time, it is not possible to precisely delineate the specific contribution of protein quality and quantity to human cancer risk. Laboratory studies generally have found minimal effects of dietary protein content, except at the extremes of feeding (302, 359, 433). Experimental studies of the breast (144), colon (62, 413), and liver (302, 303) have provided some evidence for an increased risk of carcinogenesis with greater protein intake.

LIPIDS

Defining the contribution of dietary fat in the etiology of many cancers, especially those of the breast, colon, pancreas, endometrium, and prostate, is an active area of investigation (211, 302, 303, 359). Improved epidemiologic and biochemical methods are needed to assess accurately past and current lipid intake in humans. Many previous studies lack the sensitivity and specificity that are necessary to quantify the risk associated with high-fat diets. Although human studies at this time are not totally consistent, precisely controlled laboratory studies in rodent models support a contribution of dietary fat concentration and source in the pathogenesis of several malignant neoplasms, such as breast and colon cancer. Dietary fat modulates many metabolic and endocrine processes that may alter tissue susceptibility to transformation and tumor progression. In addition, dietary lipids influence the lipid composition of cell membranes and thereby may modulate the cellular response of many growth-stimulating and -inhibitory pathways by altering ligand-receptor binding and signal transduction.

CHOLESTEROL

Dietary cholesterol derives from meat and dairy products and therefore is correlated with cancers that are frequent in affluent nations. The close association of cholesterol with other nutrients such as fat has made it difficult to establish a contribution to the risk of breast, colon, or prostate cancer (158, 196, 271, 302, 303, 336, 359). Several long-term prospective studies originally designed to evaluate cardiovascular disease have reported an inverse relationship between overall cancer risk and serum cholesterol levels at the start of the study (276). These observations have created a potentially difficult problem for those concerned with public health and dietary guidelines. At present, however, it is not clear if the information relative to a preexisting low serum cholesterol level can be extrapolated to a population with deliberately lowered serum levels to reduce risk of cardiovascular disease. Overall, the relationship between dietary cholesterol, serum cholesterol, and cancer risk in humans is far from clear.

CARBOHYDRATES

Very few studies have examined the relationship between carbohydrates and cancer (51, 302, 303, 359). The few laboratory studies have suggested that carcinogenesis in some models can be modulated to a limited degree by the source of carbohydrate, although the mechanisms remain obscure.

FIBER

The complexities of dietary fiber chemistry and in vivo physiologic effects have made it impossible to define the overall contribution of total fiber intake or specific fractions to cancer risk (210, 302, 303). However, recent data concerning the inhibition of colon polyp formation by specific fiber supplements suggests potential benefits for high-risk individuals. This is a rapidly expanding area of nutrition research, and significant improvements in our understanding of dietary fiber in health and disease should be forthcoming.

FRUITS AND VEGETABLES

Several hundred studies have examined the relationship between fruit and vegetable intake and cancer risk (36, 302, 303, 399). The vast majority suggest a significant protective effect of diets rich in fruits and vegetables relative to cancer risk at many sites. How these associations are mediated have not been clearly established, however, but it may involve many interacting factors. For example, the protective effect of fruits and vegetables may relate in part to an associated reduction in the consumption of risk-enhancing foods and nutrients, such as fat or energy. Perhaps the increased dietary fiber derived from fruits and vegetables contributes to reduced risk of some cancers; however, specific fruits and vegetables likely will prove to have unique protective effects for certain cancers. The critical task for investigators is to identify the specific foods and the chemical constituents that may have potential to inhibit carcinogenesis in specific organs. This information will allow us to target more precisely high-risk individuals with specific fruits and vegetables, food extracts, or even purified chemical components in rational, preventive studies.

VITAMINS

The public perceives vitamin supplements as an important form of self-therapy for the prevention and treatment of many ailments, including cancer (280). Vitamin supplements are inexpensive, easy to consume, relatively free of side effects when taken at the recommended dosages, and can be obtained without a prescription. A particularly attractive aspect of vitamin supplementation is the belief that these nutrients may counteract the adverse effects of diet or lifestyle that are much more difficult to change (315). These issues emphasize the importance of scientifically sound studies to define the risks and benefits of vitamin nutrition in the origins of human cancer. It is important to stress that major organizations providing dietary guidelines emphasize the importance of obtaining proper vitamin nutrition through the consumption of vitamin-rich foods rather than the use of supplements. Caution is advisable, because vitamin supplementation may not be uniformly beneficial and enhanced tumor promotion may occur in some situations.

The role of vitamin A in the normal growth and development of epithelial tissues has been known for decades. Vitamin A is provided in the diet as retinol and its esters, primarily from milk and organ meats, and as β-carotene and a few other carotenoids in yellow and leafy green vegetables. Interest in vitamin A and related compounds in the etiology, prevention, and treatment of cancer is rapidly expanding. A protective effect of consuming foods rich in vitamin A has been suggested for several types of cancer (36, 280, 302, 303, 359); however, at this time, there is no clear evidence that vitamin A supplementation will decrease the risk of cancer in populations consuming a typical diet. Although many studies in laboratory models indicate that vitamin A deficiency increases the susceptibility of many tissues to chemical carcinogenesis, these observations should not suggest that supplements may reduce this risk in those with adequate vitamin A status. The role of vitamin A excess has not been frequently assessed in rodent models. The use of vitamin A and synthetic retinoids as pharmacologic agents in chemoprevention trials to determine their efficacy in specific high risk populations is an important area of research (135, 136). Although evidence is lacking to support the use of vitamin A supplements, the consumption of foods that are rich in provitamin A carotenoids is supported by a large body of data (36).

Very few studies have investigated the role of vitamin D in human cancer (280, 303), but several studies have suggested a relationship between lower vitamin D intake and colon cancer (208, 303). Cancer cells derived from many human tumors have been shown to express the receptor for 1,25-dihydroxyvitamin D_3 and respond to this agent in vitro, but the pathophysiologic significance in human cancer remains to be determined (280). The development of vitamin D analogues that do not have hypercalcemic effects but continue to interact with receptors on many epithelial tissues may lead to the development of novel chemopreventive or therapeutic agents.

Vitamin E is a family of eight compounds that collectively are referred to as tocopherols. Vegetable oil, eggs, and whole grains are the major sources of dietary vitamin E. The antioxidant and free radical scavenger properties of vitamin E have suggested a possible role as an antineoplastic vitamin (280); however, few rodent or epidemiologic studies have provided strong evidence to support the consumption of vitamin E supplements to prevent cancer.

Vitamin C, which includes ascorbic acid and dehydroascorbic acid, functions as a general antioxidant and a component of several enzymatic reactions in intermediary metabolism (280). Citrus fruits, leafy vegetables, tomatoes, and potatoes are rich sources of vitamin C. Despite the large volume of publications in the last decade, very little evidence supports a critical role of vitamin C in the etiology of most human cancers (280, 302, 303). Some provocative evidence concerns the ability of vitamin C to inhibit the formation of carcinogenic nitrosamines, which ultimately may reduce the incidence of cancers that are thought to be associated with nitrosamines, such as gastric cancer. At present, there is no evidence to suggest that consumption of vitamin C supplements at levels higher than can be achieved in a well-balanced diet containing ample fresh fruits and vegetables is useful in the prevention or treatment of human cancer.

Folate is essential for the normal metabolism of amino acids, methyl groups, and nucleotides, and folate plays a role in the methylation of DNA, which may be critical for the normal regulation of gene expression and tissue differentiation. Epidemiologic and laboratory studies are beginning to accumulate suggesting that insufficient folate may relate to the risk of several malignancies, particularly colon cancer (103, 119). Folate primarily is derived from fruit and vegetables and may be one component contributing to the reduced risk of cancer associated with the consumption of these foods. Unlike many other nutrients, mild to moderate folate deficiency is relatively prevalent in the U.S. population.

MINERALS

A number of minerals are required for normal structural development of the skeleton and soft tissue and for numerous biochemical and physiologic reactions. Those that are required in large amounts, such as calcium, phosphorus, and magnesium, are to be considered macrominerals. The trace elements are needed in much smaller amounts and include zinc, selenium, fluoride, iron, copper, iodine, manganese, and molybdenum. The contributions of variations in the dietary intake of minerals to carcinogenesis have not been clearly defined (280, 302, 303, 359), and specific recommendations concerning supplemental intake should be avoided. Among the minerals, roles for selenium and calcium in human cancer have been actively investigated.

Recent evidence suggests a role for calcium in colon carcinogenesis. A prospective, cohort study in the United States found that those who develop colon cancer had a significantly lower intake of calcium and vitamin D (110); however, case-control studies have been inconsistent. Calcium supplementation of 1.2 g/d reduced the proliferative rate of colonic cells in patients who are considered to be at an increased risk of colon cancer (232). Laboratory studies have reported that calcium reduces the loss of superficial epithelial cells and the proliferation of basal crypt cells (50). Clinical trials to determine the effects of calcium supplementation on polyp formation are currently underway.

Selenium is an essential constituent of glutathione peroxidase, and it participates in the destruction of hydrogen peroxide and organic hydroperoxides using reducing equivalent from glutathione. Selenium therefore participates in cellular and tissue defense against oxidative damage. Marginal selenium intake does not produce major physiologic changes, but it may predispose to injury by other agents, such as chemical carcinogens. A major obstacle for epidemiologic studies is that estimates of dietary selenium intake are unreliable, especially in industrialized nations where foods are extensively processed and shipped large distances, since food content is very sensitive to soil concentrations. An inverse association between the selenium levels in forage crops and mortality rates from certain cancers in different geographic areas has been suggested (59, 303). Other studies have compared blood selenium levels in patients with cancer and controls (303). Although these studies frequently are small and do not control for other risk factors, many have observed lower selenium levels in patients with cancer. Prospective studies, where serum has been obtained before the onset of disease, have provided inconsistent results (303). A recent prospective analysis among women indicated no protection against cancer and perhaps an increase in risk with greater toenail selenium as a marker of intake (111). Animal studies also have provided contradictory results concerning the effects of excess selenium or selenium deficiency and carcinogenesis (303). Overall, conclusions concerning a role for selenium in human cancer cannot be justified, and dietary supplementation with a mineral that has a significant risk of toxicity cannot be supported. However, further studies are warranted to define the degree to which risk may be modulated and the conditions under which adjustments of selenium intake may be beneficial.

ETHANOL

Chronic consumption of alcohol is strongly associated with cancers of the oropharynx, larynx, and esophagus (303, 358). Tobacco smoking acts synergistically with alcohol in the pathogenesis of these cancers. Ethanol beverages probably contribute to liver cancer, and they may have a role in gastric, pancreatic, colon, and breast cancer. Even so, additional studies are necessary to firmly establish and quantify risk for the latter tissues. The risks associated with moderate alcohol intake and cancer are not well established but have been suggested in some studies (303, 358). Ethanol itself probably is not a carcinogen, and a number of mechanisms are under investigation whereby ethanol may modulate carcinogenesis (358). Ethanol may have direct effects on the target tissue, altering cell turnover, permeability to carcinogens, or carcinogen metabolism. Ethanol may alter nutrient requirements of the target tissue, thereby disrupting the normal structure and function and altering carcinogenic risk. Some alcoholic beverages may contain chemical substances that are carcinogens or tumor promoters. The systemic effects of alcohol on hepatic carcinogen or hormone metabolism may indirectly alter the risk of cancer in many tissues. Ethanol may contribute to malnutrition with regard to a number of nutrients by altering absorption and metabolism or through the poor dietary habits that are associated with excessive consumption of alcoholic beverages.

Dietary and Nutritional Recommendations

Considerable controversy exists within the lay public, scientific community, food industry, and government regulatory agencies concerning the establishment of dietary guidelines to prevent cancer. Some argue that dietary changes should not be recommended until scientific uncertainties have been resolved. Others believe that the associations observed justify instituting changes in the diet while more definitive data are obtained. Because cancer ranks as the second-leading cause of death in affluent nations, there is a large public demand for nutritional remedies to prevent cancer. Without sound guidelines, the public will overinterpret inconclusive studies and pursue dietary habits, including supplements that are useless and even harmful. Unfortunately, absolute proof for many diet and cancer hypotheses will be difficult to obtain because of the expense that is required to support long-term studies with large numbers of subjects. The decision to formulate recommendations must take into account several factors, including strength of the evidence, potential benefits to society if the disease could be avoided, likelihood and severity of an adverse effect, and the feasibility of reducing exposure to the risk factor. In addition, economic issues relative to the food and agricultural industry are factors that may influence the decisions of committees to define nutritional guidelines. Although much remains to be learned before the impact of proposed recommendations on health can be precisely quantified, most experts agree that a number of recommendations can be made with a reasonable degree of certainty, with the likelihood of minimal risk, and the potential for significant public health benefits (301, 303, 455).

In general, there are two different, but complementary, approaches to reducing dietary risk factors for cancer and other chronic diseases. One focuses on the individuals or groups and is aimed at identifying those who are at high risk and providing dietary intervention. A second addresses the population as a whole and is the public health approach. For some cases, we can, with a very high degree of certainty, identify individuals who will develop a specific cancer and institute preventive measures. For example, those with familial polyposis have a very high incidence of colon cancer, and a prophylactic colectomy frequently is performed before the age at which tumor risk increases. Most future patients with cancer, however, cannot be identified with a similar degree of certainty before the onset of their disease. The eventual application of sophisticated, individually based nutritional or chemopreventative interventions will be greatly facilitated by the identification of susceptible genotypes and additional environmental risk factors.

The public health approach is a preventive strategy to decrease the overall disease incidence by reducing the adverse dietary habits of the entire population. Implementation of dietary recommendations requires cooperation among the media, food industry, nutritional scientists, public health personnel, medical practitioners, educators, and the government (303). To achieve success, dietary recommendations must be simple and feasible to implement and have minimal risk, low cost to society, and the potential to benefit many people (303). Past efforts have been successful in the area of nutrition. For example, iron fortification of cereals benefits a large number of children and adult women, while risk is limited to a small number of individuals with hemochromatosis.

Tables 28.5 and 28.6 present population-based dietary recommendations published over the last decade by several organizations to lower the risk from chronic diseases (8, 9, 302, 303). Most groups recommend reducing total fat intake to 30% or less of calories, with saturated fats reduced to less than 10% of calories and cholesterol limited to less than 300 mg/d. Although the roles of fat level, saturation, and cholesterol in cancer have not been precisely quantified, a large body of evidence supports a contribution of these dietary factors to cardiovascular diseases. These goals can be accomplished by substituting fish, poultry without skin, lean meats, and low- or nonfat dairy products for fatty meats and whole-milk dairy products, and by selecting more fruits, vegetables, cereals, and legumes in conjunction with limiting fats and oils in cooking, spreads, and dressings (303). With a decrease in lipid calories, carbohydrates should increase to approximately 55% of total energy through increased consumption of green and yellow vegetables, citrus fruits, and whole-grain cereals and breads, which typically are low in fat and rich in many vitamins, minerals, and fiber. Most groups suggest moderation in protein intake. Protein is an essential nutrient, but in many affluent nations, intake is in twofold excess of the established recommended daily allowance (RDA). The contribution of protein to the risk of cancer and other major diseases is less clear than for lipid intake. The National Academy of Sciences has recommended protein intake at levels lower than twice the RDA for all age groups. Consumption of meat frequently is associated with certain cancers and cardiovascular disease; however, at this time, it is not possible to implicate meat per se other than through its contribution to high total or saturated fat and cholesterol intake. Lean meats can remain a component of a low-fat diet.

Excess weight has been associated with increased morbidity and mortality from a number of diseases, including diabetes, hypertension, cardiovascular disease, and some forms of cancer (8, 9, 302, 303). Laboratory studies indicate a strong relationship between energy intake and carcinogenesis, but the relevance of these studies, which frequently use severely restricted diets, to the human situation is unknown. The increasingly sedentary populations of many affluent nations exhibit higher average body weight or other indices of body mass even while total energy intake is slightly decreasing. It is recommended that food intake and physical activity be balanced to maintain an appropriate body weight.

Table 28.5. A Comparison of Dietary Recommendations to Lower Cancer Risk in the United States

Organization	Maintain appropriate body weight	Limit or reduce total fat (% of kcal)	Ratio of saturated to unsaturated dietary fats	Fruit and vegetable intake	Complex carbohydrate intake	Sodium intake	Food preparation and processing	Food additives and contaminants	Alcohol	Other
National Research Council, National Academy of Sciences, 1982	No Comment	<30	Not defined	Increase citrus fruits and green, yellow, and cruciferous vegetables	Increase whole-grain products	Indirectly	Reduce cured, pickled, and smoked foods	Continue to monitor, test, and reduce exposure	Drink less, if at all	Monitor and test for mutagens
American Cancer Society, 1984	Yes	<30	Not defined	Especially those with vitamin A and C, cruciferous vegetables	Whole-grain foods and high-fiber foods	Not defined	Reduce cured, pickled, and smoked foods	No comment	Drink less, if at all	—
National Cancer Institute, 1987	Yes	<30	Not defined	Citrus fruits, cruciferous vegetables, vitamin A–rich green and yellow vegetables	Whole-grain products, eat 20–30 g fiber per day	Not defined	Reduce cured, pickled, and smoked foods. Avoid frying and high temperature cooking	No comment	Drink less, if at all	Varied and balanced diet
National Research Council, National Academy of Sciences, 1989	Yes	<30	Reduce saturated fat to <10% of energy, reduce cholesterol intake to <300 mg/d	Eat 5 or more servings of green and yellow vegetables and citrus fruits per day	Eat 6 or more servings of breads, cereals, and legumes per day	Limit salt intake to ≤6 g per day	Highly processed salty, salt-preserved, and salt-pickled foods should be consumed sparingly	No comment	Limit pure alcohol intake to 1 oz per day, if at all	Avoid taking dietary supplements in excess of the RDA in any one day

Table 28.6. Population Nutrient Goals Established by the World Health Organization to Prevent Diet-Related Chronic Diseases

	Lower limit	Upper limit
Total fat	15% of energy	30% of energy[a]
Saturated fats	0% of energy	10% of energy
Polyunsaturated fats	3% of energy	7% of energy
Dietary cholesterol	0 mg/d	300 mg/d
Total carbohydrate	55% of energy	75% of energy
Complex carbohydrates[b]	50% of energy	70% of energy
Dietary fiber[c] as nonstarch polysaccharides	16 g/d	24 g/d
Total dietary fiber	27 g/d	40 g/d
Free sugars[d]	0% of energy	10% of energy
Protein	10% of energy	15% of energy
Salt	Not defined	6 g/d
Total energy	Energy intake must be sufficient to allow for normal childhood growth, the needs of pregnancy and lactation, work and desirable physical activities, and to maintain appropriate body reserves of energy in children and adults. Adult populations on average should have a body mass index (BMI) of 20–22.[e]	

[a] An interim goal for nations with high fat intakes: further benefits would be expected by reducing fat intake toward 15% of total energy.
[b] A daily minimum intake of 400 g of vegetables and fruits, including at least 30 g of pulses, nuts, and seeds, should contribute to this component.
[c] Dietary fiber includes the nonstarch polysaccharides (NSP), the goals for which are based on NSP obtained from mixed food sources. Because the definition and measurement of dietary fiber remain uncertain, the goals for total dietary fiber have been estimated from the NSP values.
[d] These sugars include monosaccharides, disaccharides, and other short-chain sugars extracted from carbohydrates by refining. These refined or purified sugars do not include the natural sugars consumed when eating fruits and vegetables or drinking milk.
[e] Body mass index = [body mass in kg]/[height in m]^2.

Most expert committees do not recommend alcohol consumption based on its role in cancer, other diseases, accidents, and birth defects. For those who drink, the National Academy of Sciences has suggested limiting intake to less than 1 ounce of alcohol per day, which is equivalent to two cans of beer or small glasses of wine (303). Salt intake should be limited to less than 6 g/d, primarily by reducing its use in cooking and at the table (303). The evidence linking salt intake to hypertension is strong. The consumption of salt-preserved or -pickled foods should be limited based on the frequent association with stomach cancer, although the causative agents in these foods have not been identified. The National Academy of Sciences does not recommend calcium intake above the current RDA (303). Benefits of intake above these levels to prevent osteoporosis, hypertension, or colon cancer have not been adequately documented. It is recommended that fluoride intake be optimized especially during the years of tooth formation (303). There is no substantial evidence linking fluoride intake to cancer risk.

An increasing proportion of the U.S. population consumes some type of self-prescribed nutritional supplement on a daily basis. The benefits of nutrient supplements that are in great excess of the RDA have not been proven, although significant risks are well known. The appropriate mechanism to obtain the recommended concentrations of nutrients is through a diverse and varied diet. It is important to view these guidelines as reflecting an overall dietary pattern rather than individual recommendations. Most of the evidence suggests that a major impact on cancer incidence would require the combination of changes recommended in these guidelines.

References

1. Albanes D. Caloric intake, body weight and cancer. A review. Nutr Cancer 1987;9: 199.
2. Albanes D, Blair A, Taylor PR. Physical activity and risk of cancer in the NHANES I population. Am J Public Health 1989;79:744.
3. Albanes D, Jones DY, Schatzkin A, Micozzi M, Taylor P. Adult stature and risk of cancer. Cancer Res 1988;48:1658.
4. Albanes D, Taylor PR. International differences in body height and weight and their relationship to cancer incidence. Nutr Cancer 1990;14:69.
5. Alberts DS, Einspahr J, Rees-McGee S, Ramanujam P, Buller MK, Clark L, Ritenbaugh C, Atwood J, Pethigal P, Earnest D, Villar H, Phelps J, Lipkin M, Wargovich M, Meyskens FL Jr. Effects of dietary wheat bran fiber on rectal epithelial cell proliferation in patients with resection for colorectal cancers. JNCI 1990;82:1280.
6. Alfin-Slater RB, Kritchevsky D. In Human Nutrition: A Comprehensive Treatise, vol 7; Cancer and Nutrition. New York: Plenum, 1991.
7. Alpha-Tocopherol, Beta-Carotene Cancer Prevention Study Group. The effect of vitamin E and beta carotene on the incidence of lung cancer and other cancers in male smokers. N Engl J Med 1994;330:1029–1035.
8. American Cancer Society. Guidelines on diet, nutrition, and cancer. CA 1991;41:334.
9. American Cancer Society. Nutrition and Cancer: Cause and Prevention. American Cancer Society Special Report, New York, 1984.
10. American Institute of Nutrition. Report of the AIN ad hoc committee on standards for nutritional studies. J Nutr 1977;110:1340.
11. American Institute of Nutrition Second report of the AIN ad hoc committee on standards for nutritional studies. J Nutr 1980;110:1726.
12. Angres G, Beth M. Effects of dietary constituents on carcinogenesis in different tumor models: an overview from 1975 to 1988. In Human Nutrition: A Comprehensive Treatise, vol 7; Cancer and Nutrition. Edited by RB Alfin-Slater, D Kritchevsky. New York: Plenum, 1991, p 51.
13. Anthony PP. Cancer of the liver: pathogenesis and recent aetiological factors. Trans R Soc Trop Med Hyg 1977;71:466.
14. Armstrong B, Doll R. Environmental factors and cancer incidence and mortality in different countries, with special reference to dietary practices. Int J Cancer 1975;15: 617.
15. Austin DF. Larynx. In Cancer Epidemiology and Prevention. Edited by D Schottenfeld, JF Fraumeni Jr. Philadelphia: Saunders, 1982, p 554.
16. Austin H, Delzell E, Grufferman S, Levine R, Morrison A, Stolley PD, Cole P. A case control study of hepatocellular carcinoma and the hepatitis B virus, cigarette smoking, and alcohol consumption. Cancer Res 1986;46:962.
17. Ballard-Barbash R, Schatzkin A, Albanes D, Schiffman M, Kreger B, Kannel W, Anderson K, Helsel W. Physical activity and risk of large bowel cancer in the Framingham Study. Cancer Res 1990;50:3610.
18. Barch DH, Kuemmerle SC, Hollenberg PF, Iannaccone PM. Esophageal microsomal metabolism of N-nitrosomethylbenzylamine in the zinc-deficient rat. Cancer Res 1984;44:5629.
19. Beasley RP, Lin CC, Hwan LY, Chien CS. Hepatocellular carcinoma and hepatitis B virus: a prospective study of 22, 707 men in Taiwan. Lancet 1981;ii:1129.

20. Benito E, Cabeza E, Moreno V, Obrador A, Bosch FX. Diet and colorectal adenomas: a case-control study in Majorca. Int J Cancer 1993;55:213.
21. Berta JL, Coste T, Rautureau J, Guilloud-Bataille M, Pequignot G. Diet and rectocolonic cancers. Results of a case-control study. Gastroenterol Clin Biol 1985;9:348.
22. Bidoli E, Franceschi S, Talamini R, Barra S, La Vecchia C. Food consumption and cancer of the colon and rectum in north-eastern Italy. Int J Cancer 1992;50:223.
23. Bingham SA, Williams DRR, Cummings JH. Dietary fiber consumption in Britain: new estimates and their relation to large bowel cancer mortality. Br J Cancer 1985;52:399.
24. Birt D, Julius A, White L, Pour P. Enhancement of pancreatic carcinogenesis in hamsters fed a high-fat diet ad libitum and at a controlled calorie intake. Cancer Res 1989;49:5848.
25. Birt DF, Bresnick E. Chemoprevention by nonutrient components of vegetables and fruits. In Human Nutrition: A Comprehensive Treatise, vol 7; Cancer and Nutrition. Edited by RB Alfin-Slater, D Kritchevsky. New York: Plenum, 1991, p 221.
26. Birt DF, Davies MH, Pour PM, Salmasi S. Lack of inhibition by retinoids of bis (2-oxopropyl)nitrosamine-induced carcinogenesis in Syrian hamsters. Carcinogenesis 1983;4:1216.
27. Birt DF, Salmasi S, Pour PM. Enhancement of experimental pancreatic cancer in Syrian golden hamsters by dietary fat. JNCI 1981;67:1327.
28. Birt DF, Sayed S, Davies MH, Pour PM. Sex differences in the effects of retinoids on carcinogenesis by *N*-nitrosobis (2-oxopropyl)amine in Syrian hamsters. Cancer Lett 1981;14:13.
29. Birt DF, Stepan KR, Pour PM. Interaction of dietary fat and protein on pancreatic carcinogenesis in Syrian golden hamsters. JNCI 1983;71:355.
30. Bjelke E. Dietary factors and the epidemiology of cancer of the stomach and large bowel. Aktuel Ernaehrungs Med Klin Prax 1978;2(Suppl):10.
31. Bjelke E. Dietary vitamin A and human lung cancer. Int J Cancer 1975;15:561.
32. Bjelke E. Epidemiologic studies of cancer of the stomach, colon and rectum. Scand J Gastroenterol 1974;9(Suppl 1):1.
33. Bjelke E. Epidemiology of colorectal cancer, with emphasis on diet. In Human Cancer. Its Characterization and Treatment. Edited by W Davis, KR Harrup, G Stathopoulos. Amsterdam: Exerpta-Medica, 1980, p 158.
34. Blair A, Fraumeni JF Jr. Geographic patterns of prostate cancer in the United States. JNCI 1978;61:1379.
35. Block G. A review of validations of dietary assessment methods. Am J Epidemiol 115: 492.
36. Block G, Patterson B, Subar A. Fruit, vegetables, and cancer prevention: a review of the epidemiological evidence. Nutr Cancer 1992;18:1.
37. Boring CC, Squires TS, Tong T, Montgomery S. Cancer statistics, 1994. CA 1994;44: 7.
38. Bostick RM, Potter JD, Kushi LH Sellers TA, Steinmetz KA, McKenzie DR, Gapstur SM, Folsom AR. Sugar, meat, and fat intake, and non-dietary risk facotrs for colon cancer incidence in Iowa women (United States). Cancer Causes Control 1994;5:38.
39. Boyd NF, Martin LJ, Noffel MM, Lockwood GA, Tritchler DL. A meta-analysis of studies of dietary fat and breast cancer risk. Br J Cancer 1993;68:627.
40. Brechot C, Nalpas B, Courouce A, Duhamel G, Callard P, Carnot F, Tiollais P, Berthelot P. Evidence that hepatitis B virus has a role in liver-cell carcinoma in alcoholic liver disease. N Engl J Med 1982;306:1384.
41. Bristol JB, Emmett PM, Heaton KW, Williamson RC. Sugar, fat, and the risk of colorectal cancer. BMJ 1985;291:1467.
42. Brownson RC, Zahm SH, Chang JC, Blair A. Occupational risk of colon cancer. An analysis by anatomic subsite. Am J Epidemiol 1989;130:675.
43. Bruce W. R Recent hypotheses for the origin of colon cancer. Cancer Res 1987;47: 4237.
44. Buell P. Changing incidence of breast cancer in Japanese-American women. JNCI 1973;51:1479.
45. Burch JD, Howe GR, Miller AB, Semenciw R. Tobacco, alcohol, asbestos, and nickel in the etiology of cancer of the larynx: a case-control study. JNCI 1981;67:1219.
46. Burkitt DP, Trowell HC. Refined Carbohydrate Foods and Disease: Some Implications of Dietary Fibre. London: Academic, 1975.
47. Byers TE, Graham S. The epidemiology of diet and cancer. Adv Cancer Res 1984;41:1.
48. Byers TE, Graham S, Haughey BP, Marshall JR, Swanson MK. Diet and lung cancer risk: findings from the Western New York Diet Study. Am J Epidemiol 1987;125:351.
49. Byrne C, Ursin G, Ziegler R. Dietary fat and breast cancer in NHANES I continued follow-up. Am J Epidemiol 1992;136:1024.
50. Caderni G, Stuart EW, Bruce WR. Dietary factors affecting the proliferation of epithelial cells in the mouse colon. Nutr Cancer 1988;11:147.
51. Carroll KK. Carbohydrate and cancer. In Human Nutrition. A Comprehensive Treatise, vol 7; Cancer and Nutrition. Edited by RB Alfin-Slater, D Kritchevsky. New York: Plenum, 1991, p 97.
52. Carroll KK, Hopkins GJ. Dietary polyunsaturated fat versus saturated fat in relation to mammary carcinogenesis. Lipids 1979;14:155.
53. Carroll KK, Khor HT. Dietary fat in relation to tumorigenesis. Prog Biochem Pharmacol 1975;10:308.
54. Carstensen JM, Bygren LO, Hatschek T. Cancer incidence among Swedish brewery workers. Int J Cancer 1990;45:393.
55. Chiarodo A. National Cancer Institute roundtable on prostate cancer: future research directions. Cancer Res 1991;51:2498.
56. Choi NW, Entwistle DW, Michaluk W, Nelson N. Gastric cancer in Icelanders in Manitoba. Isr J Med Sci 1971;7:1500.
57. Chu EW, Malmgren RA. An inhibitory effect of vitamin A on the induction of tumors for forestomach and cervix in the Syrian hamster by carcinogenic polycyclic hydrocarbons. Cancer Res 1965;25:884.
58. Chute CG, Willett WC, Colditz GA, Stampfer MJ, Baron JA, Rosner B, Speizer FE. A prospective study of body mass, height, and smoking on the risk of colorectal cancer in women. Cancer Causes Control 1991;2:117.
59. Clark LC. The epidemiology of selenium and cancer. Fed Proc 1985;44:2584.
60. Clinton SK, Alster JM, Imrey PB, Nandkumar S, Truex CR, Visek WJ. Effects of dietary protein, fat and energy intake during an initiation phase study of 7, 12-dimethylbenz[a]anthracene-induced breast cancer in rats. J Nutr 1986;116:2290.
61. Clinton SK, Alster JM, Imrey PB, Simon J, Visek WJ. The combined effects of dietary protein and fat intake during the promotion phase of 7, 12-dimethylbenz[a]anthracene-induced breast cancer in rats. J Nutr 1988;118:1577.
62. Clinton SK, Bostwick DG, Olson LM, Mangian HJH, Visek WJ. Effects of ammonium acetate and sodium cholate on *N*-methyl-*N*-nitrosoquanidine-induced colon carcinogenesis on rats. Cancer Res 1988;48:3035.
63. Clinton SK, Destree R, Anderson DB, Truex CR, Imrey PB, Visek WJ. 1,2-dimethylhydrazine-induced colon cancer in rats fed beef or vegetable protein. Nutr Reports Int 1979;20:335.
64. Clinton SK, Imrey PB, Alster JM, Simon J, Truex CR, Visek WJ. The combined effects of dietary protein and fat on 7,12-dimethylbenz(a)anthracene-induced breast cancer in rats. J Nutr 1984;114:1213.
65. Clinton SK, Imrey PB, Mangian HJ, Nandkumar S, Visek WJ. The combined effects of dietary fat, protein, and energy intake on azoxymethane-induced intestinal and renal carcinogenesis. Cancer Res 1992;52:857–865.
66. Clinton SK, Palmer SS, Spriggs CE, Visek WJ. The growth of Dunning transplantable prostate adenocarcinomas in rats fed diets varying in fat content. J Nutr 1988;118: 1577.
67. Clinton SK, Visek WJ. Wheat bran and the induction of intestinal benzo(a)pyrene-hydroxylase by dietary benzo(a)pyrene. J Nutr 1989;119:395.
68. Colditz GA, Stampfer MJ, Willett WC. Diet and lung cancer. A review of the epidemiologic evidence in humans. Arch Intern Med 1987;147:157.
69. Colditz GA, Willet WC. Epidemiologic approaches to the study of diet and cancer. In Human Nutrition: A Comprehensive Treatise, vol 7; Cancer and Nutrition. Edited by RB Alfin-Slater, D Kritchevsky. New York: Plenum, 1991, p 51.
70. Cook-Mozaffari P. The epidemiology of cancer of the oesophagus. Nutr Cancer 1979;1:51.
71. Cook-Mozaffari PJ, Azordegan F, Day WE, Ressicaud A, Sabai C, Aramesh B. Oesophageal cancer studies in the Caspian littoral of Iran: results of a case-control study. Br J Cancer 1979;39:293.
72. Cooper AJL. Biochemistry of sulfur-containing amino acids. Annu Rev Biochem 1983;52:187.
73. Coordinating Group for Research on Etiology of Esophageal Cancer in North China. The epidemiology and etiology of esophageal cancer in North China. A preliminary report. Chin Med J (Peking, Engl Ed) 1975;1:167.
74. Cope GF, Wyatt JI, Pinder IF, Lee PN, Heatley RV, Kelleher J. Alcohol consumption in patients with colorectal adenomatous polyps. Gut 1991;32:70.
75. Corder EH, Guess HA, Hulka BS, Friedman GD, Sadler, M, Vollmer RT, Lobaugh B, Drezner KMK, Vogelman JH, Orenteich N. Vitmain D and prostate cancer: a prediagnostic study with stored sera. Cancer Epidemiol Biomarkers Prevention 1993;2: 467–472.
76. Corpet CE, Stamp D, Medline A, Minkin S, Archer M, Bruce W. Promotion of colonic microadenoma growth in mice and rats fed cooked sugar or cooked casein and fat. Cancer Res 1990;50:6955.
77. Correa P. The new era of cancer epidemiology. Can Epidemiol Control 1991;1:5.
78. Correa P, Cuello C, Fajardo LF, Haenszel W, Bolanos O, deRamirez, B Diet and gastric cancer: nutrition survey of a high-risk area. JNCI 1983;70:673.
79. Cramer DW, Welch WR, Hutchinson GB, Willett W, Scully RE. Dietary animal fat in relation to ovarian cancer risk. Obstet Gynecol 1984;63:833.
80. Dales LG, Friedman GD, Ury HK, Grossman S, Williams SR. A case-control study of relationships of diet and other traits to colorectal cancer in American blacks. Am J Epidemiol 1979;109:132.
81. Dean G, MacLennan R, McLoughlin H, Shelley E. Causes of death of blue collar workers at a Dublin brewery 1954–73. Br J Cancer 1979;40:581.
82. Decarli A, La Vecchia C. Environmental factors and cancer mortality in Italy: correlational exercise. Oncology 1986;43:116.
83. DeCosse JJ, Miller HH, Lesser ML. Effect of wheat fiber and vitamins C and E on rectal polyps in patients with familial adenomatous polyposis. JNCI 1989;81:1290.
84. de Jong UW, Breslow N, Hong JGE, Sridharan M, Shanmugaratnam K. Aetiological factors in oesophageal cancer in Singapore Chinese. Int J Cancer 1974;13:291.
85. DeLint J, Levinson T. Mortality among patients treated for alcoholism: a 5-year follow-up. Can Med Assoc J 1975;113:385.
86. Denda A, Inui S, Sunagawa M, Takahashi S, Konishi Y. Enhancing effect of partial pancreatectomy and ethionine-induced pancreatic regeneration on the tumorigenesis of azaserine in rats. Gann 1978;69:633.
87. Department of Health, Education, and Welfare (DHEW). Smoking and Health: A Report of the Surgeon General. DHEW Publ. No. (PHS) 79-50066. Rockville, MD: Office on Smoking and Health, Office of the Assistant Secretary for Health, Public Health Service, U. S. Department of Health, Education and Welfare, 1979, p 1164.
88. Dion P, Bruce WR. Mutagenicity of different fractions of extracts of human feces. Mutation Res 1983;119:151.
89. Dion PW, Bright-See EB, Smith CC, Bruce WR. The effect of dietary ascorbic acid and alpha-tocoperhol on fecal mutagenicity. Mutation Res 1982;102:27.
90. Doll R, Peto R. Quantitative estimates of avoidable risks of cancer in the United States today. JNCI 191;66:1;1981.
91. Dungal N. The special problem of stomach cancer in Iceland. With particular reference to dietary factors. JAMA 1961;176:789.
92. Ehrich M, Aswell JE. Van Tassell RL, Wilkins TD. Mutagens in the feces of 3 South African populations at different levels of risk for colon cancer. Mutation Res 1979;64: 231.
93. Feinberg AP, Vogelstein B. Hypomethylation distinguishes genes of some human cancers from their normal counterparts. Nature 1983;301:89.
94. Finkelstein JD, Cello JP, Kyle WE. Ethanol-induced changes in methionine metabolism in rat livers. Biochem Biophys Res Commun 1974;61:525.
95. Flanders WD, Rothman KJ. Occupational risk for laryngeal cancer. Am J Public Health 1982;72:369.
96. Fong LYY, Lee JSK, Chan WC, Newberne PM. Zinc deficiency and the development of esophageal and forestomach tumors in Sprague-Dawley rats fed precursors of N-nitro-N-benzylmethylamine. JNCI 1984;72:419.
97. Fong LYY, Sivak A, Newberne PM. Zinc deficiency and methylbenzylnitrosamine-induced esophageal cancer in rats. JNCI 1978;61:145.
98. Fraser G, Pearce N. Occupational physical activity and risk of cancer of the colon and rectum in New Zealand males. Cancer Causes Control 1993;4:45.

99. Fredriksson M, Bengtsson NO, Hardell L, Axelson O. Colon cancer, physical activity, and occupational exposures. A case-control study. Cancer 1989;63:1838.
100. Freedman LS, Clifford C, Messina M. Analysis of dietary fat, calories, body weight, and the development of mammary tumors in rats and mice: a` review. Cancer Res 1990;50:5710.
101. Freidman GD, Blaner WS, Goodman DS, Vogelman JH, Brind JL, Hoover R, Fireman BH, Orentreich N. Serum retinol and retinol-binding protein levels do not predict subsequent lung cancer. Am J Epidemiol 1986;123:781.
102. Freudenheim JL. A review of study designs and methods of dietary assessment in nutritional epidemiology of chronic disease. J Nutr 1993;123:401–405.
103. Freudenheim JL, Graham S, Marshall JR, Haughey BP, Cholewinski S, Wilkinson G. Folate intake and carcinogenesis of the colon and rectum. Int J Epidemiol 1991;20: 368.
104. Freudenheim JL, Graham S, Marshall JR, Haughey BP, Wilkinson G. Lifetime alcohol intake and risk of rectal cancer in Western New York. Nutr Cancer 1990;3:101.
105. Friedenreich CM, Howe GR, Miller AB. An investigation of recall bias in the reporting of past food intake among breast cancer cases and controls. Ann Epidemiol 1991;1: 439.
106. Fritz W, Zum Losungsverhalten der Polyaromaten beim Kochen von Kaffee-Ersatzstoffen und Bohnenkaffee. Dtsh Lebensm Rundsch 1969;65:83.
107. Gabrial GN, Schrager TF, Newberne PM. Zinc deficiency, alcohol, and a retinoid: association with esophageal cancer in rats. JNCI 1982;68:785.
108. Gann PH, Hennekens CH, Sacks FM, Grodstein F, Giovannucci E, Stampfer MJ. A prospective study of plasma fatty acids and risk of prostate cancer. JNCI 1994;86: 281.
109. Garabrant DH, Peters JM, Mack TM, Bernstein L. Job activity and colon cancer risk. Am J Epidemiol 1984;119:1005.
110. Garland C, Shekelle RB, Barrett-Connor E, Criqui MH, Rossof AH, Paul O. Dietary vitamin D and calcium and risk of colorectal cancer: a 19-year prospective study in men. Lancet 1985;i:307.
111. Garland M, Morris S, Stampfer MJ, Colditz GA, Spate VL, Baskett CK, Rosner B, Speizer FE, Willett WC, Hunter DJ. Prospective study of toenail selenium levels and cancer among women. JNCI 1995;87:497.
112. Gerhardsson M, Floderus B, Norell SE. Physical activity and colon cancer risk. Int J Epidemiol 1988;7:743.
113. Gerhardsson M, Norell SE, Kiviranta H, Pedersen NL, Ahlbom A. Sedentary jobs and colon cancer risk. Am J Epidemiol 1986;123:775.
114. Gerhardsson de Verdier M, Steineck G, Hagman U, Rieger A, Norell S. Physical activity and colon cancer: a case-referent study in Stockholm. Int J Cancer 1990;46:985.
115. Giovannucci E, Ascherio A, Rimm EB, Colditz GA, Stampfer MJ, Willett WC. Physical activity, obesity and risk for colon cancer and adenoma in men. Ann Intern Med 1995;122:327.
116. Giovannucci E, Ascherio A, Rimm EB, Stampfer MJ, Colditz GA, Willett WC. Intake of alcohol, folate amd methionine and risk of colon cancer in men. JNCI 1995;87:265.
117. Giovannucci E, Stampfer MJ, Colditz G, Rimm EB, Willett WC. Relationship of diet to risk of colorectal adenoma in men. JNCI 1992;84:91.
118. Giovannucci E, Stampfer MJ, Colditz GA, Manson JE, Rosner BA, Longnecker M, Speizer FE, Willett WC. A comparison of prospective and retrospective assessments of diet in the study of breast cancer. Am J Epidemiol 1993;137:502.
119. Giovannucci E, Stampfer MJ, Colditz GA, Rimm E, Trichopoulos D, Rosner B, Speizer F, Willett W. Folate, methionine, and alcohol intake and risk of colorectal adenoma. JNCI 1993;85:875.
120. Giovannucci E, Rimm EB, Colditz GA, Ascherio A, Chute C, Willett W. A prospective study of dietary fat and risk of prostate cancer. JNCI 1993;85:1571.
121. Giovannucci E, Rimm EB, Stampfer MJ, Colditz GT, Ascherio A, Willett W. Intake of fat, meat and fiber in relation to risk of colon cancer in men. Cancer Res 1994;54: 2390.
122. Goelz SE, Vogelstein B, Hamilton SR, Feinberg AP. Hypomethylation of DNA from benign and malignant human colon neoplasms. Science 1985;228:187.
123. Goldbohm RA, van den Brandt PA, van't Veer P, Brants HAM, Dorant E, Sturmans F, Hermus RJJ. A prospective cohort study on the relation between meat consumption and the risk of colon cancer. Cancer Res 1994;54:718.
124. Goodwin PJ, Boyd NF. Critical appraisal of the evidence that dietary fat intake is related to breast cancer risk in humans. JNCI 1987;79:473.
125. Graham S, Dayal H, Rohrer T, Swanson M, Sultz H, Shedd D, Fischman, S Dentition, diet, tobacco, and alcohol in the epidemiology of oral cancer. JNCI 1977:59:1611.
126. Graham S, Dayal H, Swanson M, Mittelman A, Wilkinson G. Diet in the epidemiology of cancer of the colon and rectum. JNCI 1978;61:709.
127. Graham S, Haughey B, Marshall J, Priore R, Byers T, Rzepka T, Mettlin C, Pontes J. Diet in the epidemiology of carcinoma of the prostate gland. JNCI 1983;70:687.
128. Graham S, Haughey B, Marshall J, Priore R, Byers T, Rzepka T, Mettlin C, Pontes JE. Diet in the epidemiology of carcinoma of the prostate gland. JNCI 1983;70:687.
129. Graham S, Marshall J, Haughey B, Brasure J, Freudenheim J, Zielezny M, Wilkinson G, Nolan J. Nutritional epidemiology of cancer of the esophagus. Am J Epidemiol 1990;131:454.
130. Graham S, Marshall J, Haughey B, Mittelman A, Swanson M, Zielezny M, Byers T, Wilkinson G, West D. Dietary epidemiology of cancer of the colon in western New York. Am J Epidemiol 1988;128:490.
131. Graham S, Marshall J, Mettlin C, Rzepka T, Nemoto T, Byers T. Diet in the epidemiology of breast cancer. Am J Epidemiol 1982;116:68.
132. Graham S, Schotz W, Martino P. Alimentary factors in the epidemiology of gastric cancer. Cancer 1972;30:927.
133. Graham S, Zielezny M, Marshall J, Priore R, Freudenheim J, Brasure J, Haughey B, Nasca P, Zdeb M. Diet in the epidemiology of postmenopausal breast cancer in a New York State cohort. Am J Epidemiol 1992;36:1327.
134. Gray GE, Pike MC, Henderson BE. Breast cancer incidence and mortality rates in different countries in relation to known risk factors and dietary practices. Br J Cancer 1979;39:1.
135. Greenwald P, Nixon DW, Malone WF, Kelloff GJ, Stern HR, Witkin KM. Concepts in cancer chemoprevention research. Cancer 1990;65:1483.
136. Greenwald P, Sondik E, Lynch B. S Diet and chemoprevention in NCIs research strategy to achieve national cancer control objectives. Ann Prev Public Health 1986;7: 267.
137. Gregor A, Lee PN, Roe FJC, Wilson MJ, Melton A. Comparison of dietary histories in lung cancer cases and controls with special reference to vitamin A. Nutr Cancer 1980;2:93.
138. Gupta I, Suzuki K, Bruce WR, Krepinsky JJ, Yates PA. A model study of fecapentaenes: mutagens of bacterial origin with alkylating properties. Science 1984;255: 521.
139. Haenszel W. Cancer mortality among the foreign-born in the United States. JNCI 1961;26:37.
140. Haenszel W. Variation in the incidence of and mortality from stomach cancer, with particular reference to the United States. JNCI 1958;21:213.
141. Haenszel W, Kurihara M, Locke FB, Shimuzu K, Segi M. Stomach cancer in Japan. JNCI 1976;56:265.
142. Haenszel W, Kurihara M, Segi M, Lee RKC. Stomach cancer among Japanese in Hawaii. JNCI 1972;49:969.
143. Hawksworth G, Hill MJ, Gordillo G, Cuello C. Possible relationship between nitrates, nitrosamines and gastric cancer in southwest Colombia, in *N*-nitroso compounds in the environment. IARC Sci Publ 1975;9:229.
144. Hawrylewicz EJ, Huang HH, Kissane JQ, Drab EA. Enhancement of 7, 12-dimethylbenz(a)anthracene (DMBA) mammary tumorigenesis by high protein in rats. Nutr Reports Int 1982;26:793.
145. Heilbrun LK, Nomura A, Hankin JH, Stemmermann G.Diet and colorectal cancer with special reference to fiber intake. Int J Cancer 1989;44:1.
146. Henderson IC. What can a woman do about her risk of dying of breast cancer? Curr Probl Cancer 1990;14:163.
147. Herity B, Moriarty M, Daly L, Dunn J, Bourke GJ. The role of tobacco and alcohol in the aetiology of lung and larynx cancer. Br J Cancer 1982;46:961.
148. Heshmat MY, Kaul L, Kovi J, Jackson MA, Jackson AG, Jones GW, Edson M, Enterline JP, Worrell RG, Perry SL. Nutrition and prostate cancer: a case-control study. Prostate 1985;6:7.
149. Higginson J. Etiological factors in gastro-intestinal cancer in man. JNCI 1966;37:527.
150. Hinds MW, Kolonel LN, Hankin JH, Lee J. Dietary cholesterol and lung cancer risk in a multiethnic population in Hawaii. Int J Cancer 1983;32:727.
151. Hinds MW, Kolonel LN, Hankin JH, Lee J. Dietary vitamin A, carotene, vitamin C and risk of lung cancer in Hawaii. Am J Epidemiol 1984;119:227.
152. Hinds MW, Kolonel LN, Lee J, Hirohata T. Associations between cancer incidence and alcohol/cigarette consumption among five ethnic groups in Hawaii. Br J Cancer 1980;41:929.
153. Hirayama T. A study of the epidemiology of stomach cancer, with special reference to the effect of diet factor. Bull Inst Publ Health 1963;12:85.
154. Hirayama T. Association between alcohol consumption and cancer of the sigmoid colon: observations from a Japanese cohort study. Lancet 1989:2:725.
155. Hirayama T. Diet and cancer. Nutr Cancer 1979;1:67.
156. Hirayama T. Epidemiology of breast cancer with special reference to the role of diet. Prev Med 1978;7:173.
157. Hirayama T. The epidemiology of cancer of the stomach in Japan, with special reference to the role of diet. Gann Monogr 1968;3:15.
158. Hirohata T, Nomura AM, Hankin JH, Kolonel LN, Lee J. An epidemiologic study on the association between diet and breast cancer. JNCI 1987;78:595.
159. Hirohata T, Shigematsu T, Nomura AM, Nomura Y, Horie A, Hirohata I. Occurrence of breast cancer in relation to diet and reproductive history: a case-control study in Fukuoka, Japan. Natl Cancer Inst Monogr 1985;69:187.
160. Hislop TG, Coldman AJ, Elwood JM, Brauer G, Kan L. Childhood and recent eating patterns and risk of breast cancer. Cancer Detect Prev 1986;9:47.
161. Hoffman RM. Altered methionine metabolism, DNA methylation and oncogene expression in carcinogenesis. Biochim Biophys Acta 1984;738:49.
162. Holden C. Alcoholism and the medical cost crunch. Science 1987;235:1132.
163. Holliday R. The inheritance of epigenetic defects. Science 1987;38:163.
164. Hong WK, Endicott J, Itri LM, Doos W, Batsakis JG, Bell R, Fofonoff S, Byers R, Atkinson EN, Vaughan C, Toth B, Kramer A, Dimery I, Skipper P, Strong S. 13 *cis*-Retinoic acid in the treatment of oral leukoplakia. N Engl J Med 1986;315:1501.
165. Hong WK, Lippman SM, Itri LM, Karp DD, Lee JS, Byers RM, Schantz SP, Kramer AM, Lotan R, Peters LJ, Dimery IW, Brown BW, Goepfert H. Prevention of second primary tumors with isotretinoin in squamous-cell carcinoma of the head and neck. N Engl J Med 1990;323:1278.
166. Honjo S, Kono S, Shinchi K, Imanishi K, Hirohata T. Cigarette smoking, alcohol use and adenomatous polyps of the sigmoid colon. Jpn J Cancer Res 1992;83:806.
167. Hormozdiari H, Day NE, Aramesh B, Mahboubi E. Dietary factors and esophageal cancer in the Caspian littoral of Iran. Cancer Res 1975;35:3493.
168. Howard JW, Fazio T. Review of polycyclic aromatic hydrocarbons in foods. Analytical methodology and reported findings of polycyclic aromatic hydrocarbons in foods. J Assoc Off Anal Chem 1980;63:1077.
169. Howe G. R.The use of polytomous dual response data to increase power in case-control studies: an application to the association between dietary fat and breast cancer. J Chronic Dis 1985;38:663.
170. Howe GR, Friedenreich CM, Jain M, Miller AB. A cohort study of fat intake and risk of breast cancer. JNCI 1991;83:336.
171. Howe GR, Miller AB, Jain M. Re: "total energy intake: implications for epidemiologic analyses." Am J Epidemiol 1986;124:157.
172. Howell MA. Factor analysis of international cancer mortality data and per capita food consumption. Br J Cancer 1974;29:328.
173. Howson CP, Hiryama T, Wynder EL. The decline in gastric cancer: epidemiology of an unplanned triumph. Epidemiol Rev 1986;8:1.
174. Hsing AW, Mclaughlin JK, Schuman LM. Diet, tobacco use and fatal prostate cancer: results from the Lutheran brotherhood cohort study. Cancer Res 1990;50:6836.
175. Hu, J, Liu Y, Yu, Y, Zhao T, Liu S, Wong Q. Diet and cancer of the colon and rectum: a case-control study in China. Int J Epidemiol 1991;20:362.
176. Hunter DJ, Manson JE, Colditz GA, Stampfer MJ, Rosner B, Hennekens CH, Speizer FE, Willett WC. A prospective study of consumption of vitamins C, E and A and breast cancer risk. N Engl J Med 1993;3329:234.
177. Hunter DJ, Willett WC. Diet, body size, and breast cancer. Epidemiol Rev 1993;15: 110.
178. Iscovich JM, L'Abbe KA, Castelleto R, Calzona A, Bernedo A, Chopita NA, Jmelnitzsk AC, Kaldor J, Howe G. Colon cancer in Argentina. II. Risk from fiber, fat and nutrients. Int J Cancer 1992;858.
179. Jacobs LR. Dietary fiber and cancer. J Nutr 1987;117:1319.

180. Jacobs LR. Relationship between dietary fiber and cancer: metabolic, physiologic and cellular mechanisms. Proc Soc Exp Biol Med 1986;183:290.
181. Jacobsen BK, Bjelke E, Kvale G, Heuch I. Coffee drinking, mortality and cancer incidence: results from a Norweigan prospective study. JNCI 1986;76:823.
182. Jain M, Cook GM, Davis FG, Grace MG, Howe GR, Miller AB. A case-control study of diet and colo-rectal cancer. Int J Cancer 1980;26:757.
183. Jain M, Miller AB, To T. Premaorbid diet and the prognosis of women with breast cancer. JNCI 1994;86:1390.
184. Jaskiewicz K, Marasas WFO, Lazarus C, Beyers AD, van Helden PD. Association of esophageal cytological abnormalities with vitamin and liporope deficiencies in populations at risk for esophageal cancer. Anticancer Res 1988;8:711.
185. Jensen OM. The epidemiology of large bowel cancer. In Diet, Nutrition, and Cancer: A Critical Evaluation, vol 1; Macronutrients and Cancer. Edited by BS Reddy, LA Cohen. Boca Raton, FL: CRC, 1986, p 27.
186. Jensen OM, Maclennan R, Wahrendorf J. Diet, bowel function, fecal characteristics and large bowel cancer in Denmark and Finland. Nutr Cancer 1982;4:5.
187. Jensen OM, Wahrendorf J, Knudsen JB, Sorenson BL. The Copenhagen case-control study of bladder cancer. II. The effect of coffee and other beverages. Int J Cancer 1986;37:651.
188. Johansen HL, Neutel CI. Epidemiological studies in nutrition: utility and limitations. J Nutr 1988;118:137.
189. Jones DY, Schatzkin A, Green SB, Block G, Brinton L, Ziegler R, Hoover R, Taylor P. Dietary fat and breast cancer in the National Health and Nutrition Examination Survey I epidemiologic follow-up study. JNCI 1987;79:465.
190. Joosens JV, Geboers J. Dietary salt and risks to health. Am J Clin Nutr 1987;45:1277.
191. Junshi C, Campbell TC, Junyao L, Peto R. Diet, Life-style, and mortality in China. Oxford: Oxford University Press, 1990.
192. Kabat CC, Howson CP, Wynder EL. Beer consumption and rectal cancer. Int J Epidemiol 1986;15:494.
192a. Karmali RA, Marsh J, Fuchs C. Effects of omega-3 fatty acids on growth of a rat mammary tumor. JNCI 1984;73:457–461.
193. Kamiyama S, Ohshima H, Shimada A, Saito N, Bourgade M, Ziegler P, Bartsch H. Urinary excretion of *N*-nitrosamino acids and nitrate by inhabitants in high- and low-risk areas for stomach cancer in northern Japan. IARC Sci Publ 1987;84:497.
194. Deleted in proof.
195. Kato I, Tominaga S, Matsuura A, Yoshii Y, Shirai M, Kobayashi SA. comparative case-control study of colorectal cancer and adenoma. Jpn J Cancer Res 1990;81:1101.
196. Katsouyanni K, Willett W, Trichopoulos D, Boyle P, Trichopoulou A, Vasilaros S, Papadiamanits J, MacMahon B. Risk of breast cancer among Greek women in relation to nutrient intake. Cancer 1988;61:181.
197. Kaul L, Heshmat M, Kovi J, Jackson M, Jackson A, Jones,G, Edson M, Enterline J, Worrell R, Perry S. The role of diet in prostate cancer. Nutr Cancer 1987;9:123.
198. Keller AZ. The epidemiology of esophageal cancer in the west. Prev Med 1980;9:607.
199. Keller AZ, Terris M. The association of alcohol and tobacco with cancer of the mouth and pharynx. Am J Public Health 1965;55:1578.
200. Kikendall JW, Bowen PE, Burgess MB, Magnetti C, Woodward J, Langenberg P. Cigarettes and alcohol as independent risk factors for colonic adenomas. Gastroenterol 1989;97:660.
201. Kirchner JA, Malkin JS. Cancer of larynx: 30-Year survey at New Haven Hospital. Arch Otolaryngol 1953;58:19.
202. Klatsky AL, Armstrong MA, Friecman GD, Hiatt RA. The relations of alcoholic beverage use to colon and rectal cancer. Am J Epidemiol 1988;128:1007.
203. Klurfeld DM, Weber MM, Kritchevsky D. Inhibition of chemically induced mammary and colon tumor promotion by caloric restriction in rats fed increased dietary fat. Cancer Res 1987;47:2759–2762.
204. Knekt P, Albanes D, Seppanen R, Aromaa A, Jarvinen R, Hyvonen L, Teppo L, Pukkala E. Dietary fat and risk of breast cancer. Am J Clin Nutr 51990;2:903.
205. Kok T, Pachen D, van Iersel S, Baeten C, Engels L, tenHoor,F, Lleinjans J. Case control study on fecapentaene excretion and adenomatous polyps in the colon and rectum JNCI 1993;85:1241–1244.
206. Kolonel LN, Hankin JH, Lee J, Chu SY, Nomura AM, Hinds MW. Nutrient intakes in relation to cancer incidence in Hawaii. Br J Cancer 1981;44:332.
207. Kolonel LN, Hinds MW, Hankin JH. Cancer patterns among migrant and native-born Japanese in Hawaii in relation to smoking, drinking, dietary habits. In *Genetic and Environmental Factors in Experimental and Human Cancer*. Edited by HV Gelboin, M MacMahon, T Matsushima, T Sugimura, S Takayama, H Takebe. Tokyo: Japan Scientific, 1980, pp 327.
208. Kolonel LN, Yoshizawa CN, Hankin JH. Diet and prostatic cancer: a case-study control in Hawaii. Am J Epidemiol 1988;127:999.
209. Kono S, Ikedu N, Yanai F, Shinchi K, Imanishi K. Alcoholic beverages and adenomatous polyps of the sigmoid colon: a study of male self-defence officials in Japan. Int J Epidemiol 1990;9:848.
210. Kritchevsky D, Klurfeld DM. Dietary fiber and cancer. In Human Nutrition: A Comprehensive Treatise, vol 7; Cancer and Nutrition. Edited by RB Alfin-Slater, D Kritchevsky. New York: Plenum, 1991, p 211.
211. Kritchevsky D, Klurfeld DM. Fat and cancer. In Human Nutrition: A Comprehensive Treatise, vol 7; Cancer and Nutrition. Edited by RB Alfin-Slater, D Kritchevsky. New York: Plenum, 1991, p 51.
212. Kuhnlein H, Kuhnlein U, Bell PA. The effect of short-term dietary modification on human fecal mutagenic activity. Mutation Res 1983;113:1.
213. Kumar SP, Roy SJ, Todumo K, Reddy BS. Effect of different levels of calorie restriction on azoxymethane-incuced colon carcinogenesis in male F344 rats. Cancer Res 1990;50:5761.
214. Kune GA, Kune S. The nutritional causes of colorectal cancer: an introduction to the Melbourne study. Nutr Cancer 1987;9:1.
215. Kune GA, Kune S, Read A, MacGowan K, Penfold C, Watson LF. Colorectal polyps, diet, alcohol, and family history of colorectal cancer: a case-control study. Nutr Cancer 1991;16:25.
216. Kune GA, Vitetta L. Alcohol consumption and the etiology of colorectal cancer: a review of the scientific evidence from 1957 to 1991. Nutr Cancer 1992;18:97.
217. Kune S, Kune GA, Watson LF. Case-control study of alcoholic beverages as etiologic factors: the Melbourne colorectal cancer study. Nutr Cancer 1987;9:43.
218. Kune S, Kune GA, Watson LF. Case-control study of dietary etiological factors: the Melbourne Colorectal Cancer Study. Nutr Cancer 1987;9:21.
219. Kurihara M, Aoki K, Tominaga S. Cancer Mortality Statistics in the World. Nagoya: University of Nagoya Press, 1984.
220. Kushi LH, Sellers TA, Potter JD, Nelson C, Munger R, Kaye S, Folsom A. Dietary fat and postmenopausal breast cancer. JNCI 1992;84:1092.
221. Kvale G, Bjelke E, Gart JJ. Dietary habits and lung cancer risk. Int J Cancer 1983;31: 397.
222. Langhans P, Heger RA, Hoberstein J, Bunte H. Operation-sequel carcinoma. An experimental study. Hepato-Gastroenterology 1981;28:34.
223. La Vecchia C, Decarli A, Negri E, Parazzini F, Gentile A, Cecchetti G, Fasoli M, Franceschi S. Dietary factors and the risk of epithelial ovarian cancer. JNCI 1987;79: 663.
224. Lee IM, Paffenbarger RS. Quetelet's index and risk of colon cancer in college alumni. JNCI 1992;84:1326.
225. Lee IM, Paffenbarger RS, Hsieh CC. Physical activity and risk of developing colorectal cancer among college alumni. JNCI 1991;83:1324.
226. Le Marchand L, Kolonnel, Earle ME, et al. Body size at different periods of life and breast cancer risk. Am J Epidemiol 1988;128:137.
227. Le Marchand L, Kolonel LN, Wilkins LR, Myers BC, Hirohata T. Animal fat consumption and prostate cancer: a prospective study in Hawaii. Epidemiology 1994;5:276.
228. Le Marchand L, Wilkins LR, Mi, MP. Obesity in youth and middle age and risk of colorectal cancer in men. Cancer Causes Control 1992;3:349.
229. Lew EA, Garfinkel L. Variations in mortality by weight among 750,000 men and women. J Chronic Dis 1979;32:563.
230. Lijinsky W, Shubik P. Benzo(a)pyrene and other polynuclear hydrocarbons in charcoal-broiled meat. Science 1964;145:53.
231. Linsell CA, Peers FG. Aflatoxin and liver cell cancer. Trans R Soc Trop Med Hyg 1977;71:471.
232. Lipkin M. Calcium modulation of intermediate biomarkers in the gastrointestinal tract. In Calcium, Vitamin D and Cancer. Edited by M Lipkin, G Kelloff, H Newmark. Boca Raton, FL: CRC, 1991.
233. Little J, Logan RFA, Hawtin PG, Hardcastle JD, Turner ID. Colorectal adenomas and diet: a case-control study of subjects participating in the Nottingham faecal occult blood screening programme. Br J Cancer 1993;67:177.
234. Little J, Logan RFA, Hawtin PG, Hardcastle JD, Turner ID. Colorectal adenomas and energy intake, body size and physical activity: a case-control study of subjects participating in the Nottingham faecal occult blood screening programme. Br J Cancer 1993;67:172.
235. Liu K, Stamler J, Moss D, Garside D, Persky V, Soltero I. Dietary cholesterol, fat, and fibre, and colon-cancer mortality. Lancet 1979;ii:782.
236. Lo M-T, Sandi E. Polycyclic aromatic hydrocarbons (polynuclears) in foods. Residue Rev 1978;69:35.
237. London SJ, Colditz GA, Stampfer MJ, Prospective study of relative weight, height and risk of breast cancer JAMA 1989;262:2853.
238. Longnecker DS, Roebuck BD, Yager JD Jr, Lilja HS, Siegmund BT. Pancreatic carcinoma in azaserine-treated rats: induction, classification, and dietary modulation of incidence. Cancer 1981;47:1562.
239. Longnecker DS, Kuhlmann ET, Curphey TJ. Divergent effects of retinoids on pancreatic and liver carcinogenesis in azaserine-treated rats. Cancer Res 1983;43:3219.
240. Longnecker DS, Kuhlmann ET, Curphey TJ. Effects of four retinoids in *N*-nitrosobis (2-oxopropyl)amine-treated hamsters. Cancer Res 1983;43:3226.
241. Longnecker DS, Curphey TJ, Kuhlmann ET, Roebuck BD. Inhibition of pancreatic carcinogenesis by retinoids in azaserine-treated rats. Cancer Res 1982;42:19.
242. Longnecker DS, Morgan RGH. Diet and cancer of the pancreas: epidemiological and experimental evidence. In Diet, Nutrition, and Cancer: A Critical Evaluation, vol 1; Macronutrients and Cancer. Edited by BS Reddy, LA Cohen. Boca Raton, FL: CRC, 1986, p 11.
243. Longnecker MP. A case-control study of alcoholic beverage consumption in relation to risk of cancer of the right colon and rectum in men. Cancer Causes Control 1990;1:5.
244. Longnecker MP, Berlin JA, Orza MJ, Chlmers TC. A metaanalysis of alcohol consumption in relation to risk of breast cancer. JAMA 1988;260:652.
245. Lu, S, Ohshima H, Fu, H, Tian Y, Li, F, Blettner M, Wahrendorf J, Bartsch H. Urinary excretion of *N*-nitrosoamino acids and nitrate by inhabitants of high- and low-risk areas for esophageal cancer in northern China: endogenous formation of nitrosoproline and its inhibition by vitamin C. Cancer Res 1986;46:1485.
246. Deleted in proof.
247. Lubin JH, Burns PE, Blot WJ, Ziegler RG, Lees AW, Fraumeni JF Jr. Dietary factors and breast cancer risk. Int J Cancer 1981;28:685.
248. Lubin F, Ruder AM, Wax Y, Lemarchand L. Overweight and changes in weight throughout adult life in breast cancer etiology: a case-control study. Am J Epidemiol 1988;128:137–152.
248a. Luo XM, Wei HJ, Yang SP. Inhibitory effect of molybdenum on esophageal and forestomach carcinogenesis in rats. JNCI 1983;71:75.
249. Lyon JL, Gardner JW, West DW. Cancer risk and lifestyle: cancer among Mormons (1967–1975). In Genetic Environmental Factors in Experimental and Human Cancer. Edited by HV Gelboin, B MacMahon, T Matsushima, T Sugimura, S Takayama, H Takebe. Tokyo: Japan Scientific, 1980, p 273.
250. Lyon JL, Gardner JW, West DW. Cancer risk and lifestyle: cancer among Mormons (1967–1975). In Cancer Incidence in Defined Populations. Banbury Report 4. Edited by J Cairns, JL Lyon, M Skolnick. Cold Spring Harbor, NY: Cold Spring Harbor Laboratory, 1980, p 3.
251. Lyon JL, Klauber MR, Gardner JW, Smart CR. Cancer incidence in Mormons and non-Mormons in Utah 1966–1970. N Engl J Med 1976;294:129.
252. Lyon JL, Mahoney AW, West DW, Gardner JW, Smith KR, Sorenson AW, Stanish W. Energy intake Its relationship to colon cancer risk. JNCI 1987;78:853.
253. Lyon JL, Sorenson AW. Colon cancer in a low-risk population. Am J Clin Nutr 1978;31:s227.
254. MacDonald WE, Anderson FH, Hashimoto S. Histological effect of certain pickles on the human gastric mucosa. Can Med Assoc J 1967;96:1521.
255. Mack TM. Pancreas. In Cancer Epidemiology and Prevention. Edited by D Schottenfeld, EF Fraumeni Jr. Philadelphia: Saunders, 1982, p 638.
256. MacLennan R, DaCosta J, Day NE, Law CH, Ng YK, Shanmugaratnam K. Risk factors for lung cancer in Singapore Chinese, a population with high female incidence rates. Int J Cancer 1977;20:854.

257. MacMahon B. Risk factors for cancer of the pancreas. Cancer 1982;50:2676.
258. Macquart-Moulin G, Riboli E, Cornee J, Charnay B, Berthezene P, Day N. Case-control study on colorectal cancer and diet in Marseilles. Int J Cancer 1986;38:183.
259. Macquart-Moulin G, Riboli E, Cornee J, Kaaks R, Berthezene P. Colorectal polyps and diet: a case-control study in Marseilles. Int J Cancer 1987;40:179.
260. Mahboubi E, Kmet J, Cook PJ, Day NE, Ghadirian P, Salmasizadeh S. Oesophageal cancer studies in the Caspian Littoral of Iran: the Caspian cancer registry. Br J Cancer 1973;28:197.
261. Mahboudi E, Sayed GM. Oral cavity and pharynx. In Cancer Epidemiology and Prevention. Edited by D Schottenfeld, JF Fraumeni Jr. Philadelphia: Saunders, 1982, p 583.
262. Makos M, Nelkin BD, Lerman MI, Latif F, Zbar B, Baylin S. Distinct hypermethylation patterns occur at altered chromosome loci in human lung and colon cancer. Proc Natl Acad Sci USA 1992;89:1929.
263. Malhotra SL. Dietary factors in a study of colon cancer from cancer registry, with special reference to the role of saliva, milk and fermented milk products and vegetable fibre. Med Hypotheses 1977;3:122.
264. Manousos O, Day NE, Trichopoulos D, Gerovassilis F, Tzonou A, Polychronopoulou A. Diet and colorectal cancer: a case-control study in Greece. Int J Cancer 1983;32:1.
265. Marasas WFO, van Rensburg SJ, Mirocha CJ. Incidence of *Fusarium* species and the mycotoxins, deoxynivalenol and zearalenone, in corn produced in esophageal cancer areas in Transkei. J Agric Food Chem 1979;27:1108.
266. Marshall J, Graham S, Mettlin C. Diet in the epidemiology of oral cancer. Nutr Cancer 1982;3:145.
267. Marshall JR, Yinsheng Q, Junshi C, Parpia B, Campbell TC. Additional ecological evidence: lipids and breast cancer mortality among women aged 55 and over in China. Eur J Cancer 1992;28A:1720.
268. Martinez I. Factors associated with cancer of the esophagus, mouth and pharynx in Puerto Rico. JNCI 1969;42:1069.
269. Mashberg A, Garfinkel L, Harris S. Alcohol as a primary risk factor in oral squamous carcinoma. CA 1981;31:146.
270. Mayne S, Janerich D, Greenwald P, Chorost S, Tucci C, Zaman M, Melamed M, Kiely M, McKneally M. Dietary beta carotene and lung cancer risk in U.S. nonsmokers. JNCI 1994;86:33.
271. McGee D, Reed D, Stemmermann G, Rhoads G, Yano K, Feinleib M. The relationship of dietary fat and cholesterol to mortality in 10 years: the Honolulu Heart Program. Int J Epidemiol 1985;14:97.
272. McGuinness EE, Hopwood D, Wormsley KG. Further studies of the effects of raw soya flour on the rat pancreas. Scand J Gastroenterol 1982;17:273.
273. McGuinness EE, Hopwood D, Wormsley KG. Potentiation of pancreatic carcinogenesis in the rat by DL-ethionine-induced pancreatitis. Scand J Gastroenterol 1983;18:189.
274. McGuinness EE, Morgan RGH, Levison DA, Frape DL, Hopwood D, Wormsley KG. The effects of long-term feeding of soya flour on the rat pancreas. Scand J Gastroenterol 1980;15:497.
275. McGuinness EE, Morgan RGH, Levison DA, Hopwood D, Wormsley KG. Interaction of azaserine and raw soya flour on the rat pancreas. Scand J Gastroenterol 1981;16:49.
276. McMichael AJ. Serum cholesterol and human cancer. In Human Nutrition: A Comprehensive Treatise, vol 7; Cancer and Nutrition. Edited by RB Alfin-Slater, D Kritchevsky. New York: Plenum, 1991, p 141.
277. McMichael AJ, McCall MG, Hartshome JM, Woodlings TL. Patterns of intestinal cancer in European migrants to Australia: the role of dietary change. Int J Cancer 1980;25:431.
278. Medlin C, Skinner JD. Individual dietary intake methodology: a 50-year review of progress. J Am Diet Assoc 1988;88:1250.
279. Menkes MS, Comstock GW, Vuilleumier JP, Helsing KJ, Rider AA, Brookmeyer R. Serum beta-carotene, vitamins A and E, selenium, and the risk of lung cancer. N Engl J Med 1986;315:1250.
280. Merrill AH, Foltz AT, McCormick DB. Vitamins and cancer. In Human Nutrition: A Comprehensive Treatise, vol 7; Cancer and Nutrition. Edited by RB Alfin-Slater, D Kritchevsky. New York: Plenum, 1991, p 262.
281. Mettlin C, Graham S. Dietary risk factors in human bladder cancer. Am J Epidemiol 1979;110:255.
282. Mettlin C, Graham S, Priore R, Marshall J, Swanson, M. Diet and cancer of the esophagus. Nutr Cancer 1980;2:143.
283. Mettlin C, Selenskas S, Natarajan MS, Huben R. Beta-carotene and animal fats and their relationship to prostate cancer risk. Cancer 1989;64:605.
284. Meyer F, White E. Alcohol and nutrients in relation to colon cancer in middle-aged adults. Am J Epidemiol 1993;138:225.
285. Mezzanotte G, Cislaghi C, Decarli A, La Vecchia C. Cancer mortality in broad Italian geographical areas 1975–1977. Tumori 1986;72:145.
286. Micozzi MS. Nutrition, body size, and breast cancer. Yearbook Phys Anthropol 1985;28:175.
287. Miller AB. Nutrition and the epidemiology of breast cancer. In Diet Nutrition, and Cancer: A Critical Evaluation, vol 1, Macronutrients and Cancer. Edited by BS Reddy, LA Cohen. Boca Raton, FL: CRC, 1986.
288. Miller AB, Howe GR, Jain M, Craib KJP, Harrison L. Food items and food groups as risk factors in a case-control study of diet and colo-rectal cancer. Int J Cancer 1983;32:155.
289. Miller AB, Kelly A, Choi NW, Matthews V, Morgan RW, Munan L, Burch JD, Feather J, Howe GR, Jain M. A study of diet and breast cancer. Am J Epidemiol 1978;107:499.
290. Mills PK, Beeson WL, Phillips RL, Fraser GE. Cohort study of diet, lifestyle and prostate cancer in Adventist men. Cancer 1989;64:598.
291. Mills PK, Beeson WL, Phillips RL, Fraser GE. Dietary habits and breast cancer incidence among Seventh-Day Adventists. Cancer 1989;64:582.
292. Mishina T, Watanabe H, Araki H, Nakao M. Epidemiological study of prostatic cancer by matched-pair analysis. Prostate 1985;6:423.
293. Modan B, Barell V, Lubin F, Modan M, Greenberg RA, Graham S. Low-fiber intake as an etiologic factor in cancer of the colon. JNCI 1975;55:15.
294. Montes G, Cuello C, Gordillo G, Pelon W, Johnson W, Correa P. Mutagenic activity of gastric juice. Cancer Lett 1979;7:307.
295. Morgan RGH, Levinson DA, Hopwood D, Saunders JHB, Wormsley KG. Potentiation of the action of azaserine on the rat pancreas by raw soya bean flour. Cancer Lett 1977;3:87.
296. Morris JSI, Stampfer JJ, Willet WC. Dietary selenium in humans. Toenails as an indicator. Biol Trace Element Res 1983;5:529.
297. Mower HF, Ichinotsubo D, Wang LW, Mandel M, Stemmermann G, Nomura A, Heilbrun L, Kamiyama S, Shimada A. Fecal mutagens in two Japanese populations with different colon cancer risks. Cancer Res 1982;42:1164.
298. Munoz N, Wahrendorf J, Lu JB, Crespi M, Day NE, Thurnham DI, Zhang CY, Zheng HJ, Li B, Li WY, Lin GL, Lan XZ, Correa P, Grassi A, O'Connor GT, Bosch FX. No effect of riboflavine, retinol, and zinc on precancerous lesions of the oesophagus: a randomized double-blind intervention study in a high-risk population in China. Lancet 1985;ii:111.
299. Must A, Jacques PF, Dallal GE, Bajema CJ, Dietz WH. Long-term morbidity and mortality of overweight adolescents. A follow-up of the Harvard Growth Study of 1922 to 1935. N Engl J Med 1992;37:1350.
300. Nagai M, Hashimoto T, Yanagawa H, Yokoyama H, Minowa M. Relationship of diet to the incidence of esophageal and stomach cancer in Japan. Nutr Cancer 1982;3:257.
301. National Academy of Sciences. Toward Healthful Diets. Washington, DC: National Academy Press, 1978.
302. National Academy of Sciences. Committee on Diet, Nutrition, and Cancer. In Diet, Nutrition, and Cancer. Washington, DC: National Academy Press, 1982.
303. National Academy of Sciences, Committee on Diet and Health, Food and Nutrition Board, Commission on Life Sciences, National Research Council. In Diet and Health: Implications for Reducing Chronic Disease Risk. Washington, DC: National Academy Press, 1989.
304. National Academy of Sciences, National Research Council. Evaluation of Cyclamate for Carcinogenicity. Report of Committee on the Evaluation of Cyclamate for Carcinogenicity, Commission of Life Sciences. Washington, DC: National Academy Press, 1985.
305. National Academy of Sciences, National Research Council. Nutrient Requirements of Laboratory Animals, No. 10. Washington, DC: National Academy Press, 1978.
306. National Cancer Institute. Diet, Nutrition, and Cancer Prevention: A Guide to Food Choices. NIH Pub. No. 87-28-78. Washington, DC: National Institutes of Health, Public Health Service, U.S. Dept. Health and Human Services, U.S. Government Printing Office, 1987.
307. Nauss KM, Bueche D, Newberne PM. Effect of vitamin A nutriture on experimental esophageal carcinogenesis. JNCI 1987;79:145.
308. Nauss KM, Bueche D, Soule N, Fu P, Yew K, Newberne PM. Effect of dietary selenium levels on methylbenzylnitrosamine-induced esophageal cancer in rats. Cancer Lett 1986;33:107.
309. Neugut AI, Garbowski GC, Lee WC, Murray T, Nieves JW, Forde KA, Treat MR, Waye JD, Fenoglio-Preiser C. Dietary risk factors for the incidence and recurrence of colorectal adenomatous polyps. A case-control study. Ann Intern Med 1993;11:91.
310. Neugut AI, Lee WC, Garbowski GC, Waye JD, Forde KA, Treat MR, Wayne J, Forde K, Treat M, Fenoglio-Preiser C. Obesity and colorectal adenomatous polyps. JNCI 1991;83:359.
311. Nevalainen TJ, Janigan DT. Degeneration of mouse pancreatic acinar cells during fasting. Virchows Arch B 1974;15:107.
312. Newberne PM, Bieri JG, Briggs GM, Nesheim MC. Control of diets in laboratory animal experimentation. ILAR News 1978;21:A3.
313. Newberne PM, Nauss KM. Dietary fat and colon cancer: variable results in animal models. Prog Clin Biol Res 1986;222:311.
314. Nomura A, Stemmermann G, Chyou P, Kato I, Perez-Perez G, Blaser M. *Helicobacter pylori* infection and gastric carcinoma among Japanese Americans in Hawaii. N Engl J Med 1991;325:1132.
315. Nomura AM, Stemmermann GN, Heilbrun LK, Salkeld RM, Vuilleumier JP. Serum vitamin levels and the risk of cancer of specific sites to men of Japanese ancestry in Hawaii. Cancer Res 1985;45:2369.
316. O'Connor TP, Youngman LD, Campbell TC. Effect of selenium on development of L-azaserine induced preneoplastic abnormal acinar cell nodules in rat pancreas. Fed Proc 1983;42:670.
317. Ohno Y, Yoshida O, Oishi K, Okada K, Yamabe H, Schroeder F. Dietary beta-carotene and cancer of the prostate: a case-control study in Kyoto, Japan. Cancer Res 1988;48:1331.
318. Olsen J, Sabreo S, Fasting U. Interaction of alcohol and tobacco risk factors in cancer of the laryngeal region. J Epidemiol Community Health 1985;39:165.
319. Olson JA. Nutrition monitoring and nutrition status assessment: an overview. J Nutr 1990;120:1431–1432.
320. Oshima H, Bartsch H. Quantitative estimation of endogenous nitrosation in humans by monitoring *N*-nitrosoproline excreted in the urine. Cancer Res 1981;41:3568.
321. Paffenbarger RS Jr, Hyde RT, Wing AL. Physical activity and incidence of cancer in diverse populations: a preliminary report. Am J Clin Nutr 1987;45:312.
322. Parsonnet J, Friedman G, Vandersteen D, Chang Y, Vogelman J, Orentreich N, Sibley R. *Helicobacter pylori* infection and the risk of gastric carcinoma. N Engl J Med 1991;325:1127.
323. Paymaster JC, Sanghvi LD, Gangadharan P. Cancer in the gastrointestinal tract in Western India. Epidemiologic study. Cancer 1968;21:279.
324. Peleg I, Heyden A, Knowles M, Hames CG. Serum retinol and risk of subsequent cancer: extension of the Evans County, Georgia, study. JNCI 1984;73:1455.
325. Pennington JAT. Revision of the total diet study food list and diets. J Am Dietetic Assoc 1983;82:166.
326. Peters RK, Garabrant DH, Yu MC, Mack T. A case-control study of occupational and dietary factors in colorectal cancer in young men by subsite. Cancer Res 1989;49:5459.
327. Peters RK, Pike MC, Garabrandt D, Mack TM. Diet and colon cancer in Los Angeles County, California. Cancer Causes Control 1992;3:457.
328. Phillips R. Role of life-style and dietary habits in risk of cancer among Seventh-Day Adventists. Cancer Res 1975;35:3513.
329. Phillips RL, Snowdon DA. Association of meat and coffee use with cancers of the large bowel, breast, and prostate among Seventh-Day Adventists: preliminary results. Cancer Res 1983;43(Suppl):2403.
330. Phillips RL, Snowden DA. Dietary relationships with fatal colorectal cancer among Seventh-Day Adventists. JNCI 1985;74:307.
331. Piacek-Llanes B, Tannenbaum SR. Formation of an activated *N*-nitroso compound in nitrite-treated fava beans (*Vicia faba*). Carcinogenesis 1982;3:1379.

332. Pickle LW, Greene MH, Ziegler RG, Toledo A, Hoover R, Lynch H, Fraumeni J. Colorectal cancer in rural Nebraska. Cancer Res 1984;44:363.
333. Pienta KJ, Espar PS. Risk factors for prostate cancer. Annals of Int Med 1993;118:793.
334. Polednak AP. College athletics, body size, and cancer mortality. Cancer 1976;38:382.
335. Pollack ES, Nomura AMY, Heilbrun LK, Stemmermann G, Green S. Prospective study of alcohol consumption and cancer. N Engl J Med 1984;310:617.
336. Potter JD, McMichael AJ. Diet and cancer of the colon and rectum: a case-control study. JNCI 1986;76:557.
337. Pottern LM, Morris LE, Blot WJ, Ziegler RG, Fraumeni JF. Esophageal cancer among black men in Washington, D.C. I. Alcohol, tobacco and other risk factors. JNCI 1984;67:777.
338. Pour PM, Birt DF. Modifying factors in pancreatic carcinogenesis in the hamster model. IV. Effects of dietary protein. JNCI 1983;71:347.
339. Pour PM, Birt DF, Salmasi SZ, Gotz U. Modifying factors in pancreatic carcinogenesis in the hamster model. I. Effect of protein-free diet fed during the early stages of carcinogenesis. JNCI 1983;70:141.
340. Pour PM, Reber HA, Stepan K. Modification of pancreatic carcinogenesis in the hamster model. XII. Dose-related effect of ethanol. JNCI 1983;71:1085.
341. Pour PM, Runge RG, Birt D, Gingell R, Lawson T, Nagel D, Wallacave L, Salmasi SZ. Current knowledge of pancreatic carcinogenesis in the hamster and its relevance to the human disease. Cancer 1981;47:1573.
342. Prentice RL, Kakar F, Hursting S, Sheppard L, Klein R, Kushi LH. Aspects of the rationale for the Women's Health Trial. JNCI 1988;80:802.
343. Prentice RL, Pepe M, Self SG. Dietary fat and breast cancer: a quantitative assessment of the epidemiological literature and a discussion of methodological issues. Cancer Res 1989;49:3147.
344. Price JM, Biava CG, Oser BL, Vogin EE, Steinfeld J, Ley HL. Bladder tumors in rats fed cyclohexamine or high doses of a mixture of cyclamate and saccharin. Science 1970;167:1131.
345. Purtilo DT, Gottlieb LS. Cirrhosis and hepatoma occurring at Boston City Hospital (1917–1968). Cancer 1973;32:458.
346. Rao GN, Knapka JJ. Contaminant and nutrient concentrations of natural ingredient rat and mouse diet used in chemical toxicology studies. Fund Appl Toxicol 1987;9:329.
347. Reddy BS. Diet and colon cancer: evidence from human and animal model studies. In Diet, Nutrition, and Cancer: A Critical Evaluation, vol 1; Macronutrients and Cancer. Edited by BS Reddy, LA Cohen. Boca Raton, FL: CRC, 1986, p 47.
348. Reddy BS, Cohen LA. Diet, Nutrition and Cancer. A Critical Evaluation, vol 1; Macronutrients and Cancer. Boca Raton, FL: CRC, 1986.
349. Reddy BS, Hedges AR, Laakso K, Wynder EL. Metabolic epidemiology of large bowel cancer: fecal bulk and constituents of high-risk North Am and low-risk Finnish population. Cancer 1978;42:2832.
350. Reddy BS, Sharma C, Simi B, Engle A, Laakso K, Puska P, Korpela R. Metabolic epidemiology of colon cancer: effect of dietary fiber on fecal mutagens and bile acids in healthy subjects. Cancer Res 1987;47:644.
351. Reddy BS, Wang, C-X, Maruyama H. Effect of restricted caloric intake on azoxymethane-induced colon tumor incidence in male F344 rats. Cancer Res 1987;47:1226.
352. Reichman ME, Judd JT, Longcope C, Schatzkin A, Clevidence BA, Nair PP, Campbell WS, Taylor PR. Effects of alcohol consumption on plasma and urinary hormone concentrations in premenopausal women. JNCI 1993;85:722.
353. Rigdon RH, Neal J. Relationship of leukemia to lung and stomach tumors in mice fed benzo(a)pyrene. Proc Soc Exp Biol Med 1969;130:146.
354. Risch HA, Jain M, Choi NW, Fodor JG, Pfeiffer CJ, Howe GR, Harrison LW, Craib KJ, Miller AB. Dietary factors and the incidence of cancer of the stomach. Am J Epidemiol 1985;122:947.
355. Risch HA, Jain M, Marrett LD, Howe GR. Dietary fat intake and risk of epithelial ovarian cancer. JNCI 1994;86:1409.
356. Roebuck BD, Yager JD Jr, Longnecker DS. Dietary modulation of azaserine-induced pancreatic carcinogenesis in the rat. Cancer Res 1981;41:888.
357. Roebuck BD, Yager JD Jr, Longnecker DS, Wilpone SA. Promotion by unsaturated fat of azaserine-induced pancreatic carcinogenesis in the rat. Cancer Res 1981;41:3961.
358. Rogers AE, Conner MW. Interrelationships of alcohol and cancer. In Human Nutrition: A Comprehensive Treatise, vol 7; Cancer and Nutrition. Edited by RB Alfin-Slater, D Kritchevsky. New York: Plenum, 1991, p 51.
359. Rogers AE, Longnecker MP. Biology of disease. Dietary and nutritional influences on cancer: a review of epidemiological and experimental data. Lab Invest 1988;59:729.
360. Rohan TEI, Bain CJ. Diet in the etiology of breast cancer. Epidemiol Rev 1987;9:120.
361. Rose DP, Boyar AP, Wynder EL. International comparisons of mortality rates for cancer of the breast, ovary, prostate, and colon, and per capita food consumption. Cancer 1986;58:2363.
362. Rosenberg L, Metzger LS, Palmer JR. Alcohol consumption and risk of breast cancer: a review of the epidemiologic evidence. Epidemiol Rev 1993;5:133.
363. Ross RK, Paganini-Hill A, Henderson BE. The etiology of prostate cancer: what does the epidemiology suggest? Prostate 1983;4:333.
364. Ross RK, Shimizu H, Paganini-Hill A, Honda G, Henderson BE. Case-control studies of prostate cancer in blacks and whites in Southern California. JNCI 1987;78:869.
365. Rothman K, Keller A. The effect of joint exposure to alcohol and tobacco on risk of cancer of the mouth and pharynx. J Chronic Dis 1972;25:711.
366. Rotkin ID. Studies in the epidemiology of prostatic cancer: expanded sampling. Cancer Treat Rep 1977;61:173.
367. Ruddell WSJ, Bone ES, Hill MJ, Walters CL. Pathogenesis of gastric cancer in pernicious anaemia. Lancet 1978;i:521.
368. Ruggeri B. The effects of caloric restriction on neoplasia and age-related degenerative processes. In Human Nutrition: A Comprehensive Treatise, vol 7; Cancer and Nutrition. Edited by RB Alfin-Slater, D Kritchevsky. New York: Plenum, 1991, p 187.
369. Salonen JT, Salonen R, Lappetelainen R, Maenpaa PH, Alfthan G, Puska P. Risk of cancer in relation to serum concentrations of selenium and vitamins A and E: matched case-control analysis of prospective data. Br Med J 1985;290:417.
370. Samet JM, Skipper BJ, Humble CG, Pathak DR. Lung cancer risk and vitamin A consumption in New Mexico. Am Rev Respir Dis 1985;131:198.
371. Sander J, Burkle G, Schweinsberg F. Induktion malignen tumoren bei ratten durch gleichzeitge verfutterung von nitrit und sek underen aminen. Z Krebsforsch 1969;73:54.
372. Sandler RS, Lyles CM, McAuliff C, Woosley JT, Kupper LL. Cigarette smoking, alcohol, and the risk of colorectal adenomas. Gastroenterol 1993;104:1445.
373. Sandler RS, Lyles CM, Peipins LA, McAuliffe CA, Woosley JT, Kupper LL. Diet and the risk of colorectal adenomas: macronutrients, cholesterol and fiber. JNCI 1993;85:875.
374. Sato T, Fukuyama T, Susuki T, Takayanagi J. The relationship between gastric cancer mortality rate and salted food intake in several places in Japan. Bull Inst Publ Health 1959;8:187.
375. Sato T, Fukuyama T, Urata G, Suzuki T. Bleeding in the glandular stomach of mice by feeding highly salted foods and a comment on salted foods in Japan. Bull Inst Publ Health 1959;8:10.
376. Schatzkin A, Greenwald P, Byer D, Clifford C. The dietary fat-breast cancer hypothesis is alive. JAMA 1989;261:3284.
377. Schiffman MH, Andrews AW, Van Tassell RL, Smith L, Daniel J, Robinson A, Hoover RN, Rosenthal J, Weil R, Nair PP, Schwartz S, Pettigrew H, Batist G, Shaw R, Wilkins TD. Case control study of colorectal cancer and fecal mutagenicity. Cancer Res 1989;49:3420.
378. Schiffman MH, Felton JS. Re: "Fried foods and the risk of colon cancer." Am J Epidemiol 1990;131:376.
379. Schirai T, Imaida K, Fukushima S, Hasegawa R, Tatematsu M, Ito N. Effects of NaCl, Tween 60 and a low dose of *N*-ethyl-*N'*-nitro-*N*-nitrosoguanidine on gastric carcinogenesis of rats given a single dose of *N*-methyl-*N'*-nitro-*N*-nitrosoguanidine. Carcinogenesis 1982;12:1419.
380. Schlag P, Ulrich H, Merkle P, Bockler R, Peter M, Herfarth C. Are nitrite and *N*-nitroso compounds in gastric juices risk factors for carcinoma of the operated stomach? Lancet 1980;i:727.
381. Schoenberg B, Bailar JC, Fraumeni JF. Certain mortality patterns of esophageal cancer in the United States 1930–1967. JNCI 1971;46:63.
382. Schottenfeld D. Epidemiology of cancer of the esophagus. Semin Oncol 1984;11:92.
383. Schuman LM, Mandel JS, Radke A, Seal U, Halberg F. Some selected features of the epidemiology of prostatic cancer: Minneapolis-St. Paul, Minnesota case-control study 1976–1979. In Trends in Cancer Incidence: Causes and Practical Implications. Edited by K Magnus. Washington, DC: Hemisphere, 1982, p 345.
384. Schwartz GG. Letter to the editor. Correspondence re: E.H. Corder et al. Vitamin D and prostate cancer: a prediagnostic study with stored sera. Cancer Epidemiol Biomarkers Prevention 1977;3:183.
385. Schwartz D, Lellouch J, Flamant R, Denoix PF. Alcohol and cancer. Results of a retrospective investigation. Rev Fr Etud Clin Biol 1962;7:590.
386. Severson RK, Nomura AMY, Grove JS, Stemmermann GN. A prospective analysis of physical activity and cancer. Am J Epidemiol 1989;130:522.
387. Severson RK, Nomura AMY, Grove JS, Stemmermann GN. A prospective study of demographics, diet, and prostate cancer among men of Japanese ancestry in Hawaii. Cancer Res 1989;49:1857.
388. Shekelle RB, Lepper M, Liu S, Maliza C, Raynor WJ Jr, Rossof AH, Paul O, Shryock AM, Stamler J. Dietary vitamin A and risk of cancer in the Western Electric study. Lancet 1981;ii:1186.
389. Shuker DEG, Tannenbaum SR, Wishnok JS. *N*-nitroso bile acid conjugates. I. Synthesis, chemical reactivity and mutagenic activity. J Org Chem 1981;46:2092.
390. Sidransky H. Chemical and cellular pathology of experimental acute amino acid deficiency. Methods Achiev Exp Pathol 1972;6:1.
391. Sidransky H. Chemical pathology of nutritional deficiency induced by certain plant proteins. J Nutr 1960;71:387.
392. Slattery ML, Schumacher MC, Smith KR, West DW, Abd-Elghany N. Physical activity, diet, and risk of colon cancer in Utah. Am J Epidemiol 1988;128:989.
393. Slattery ML, Schumacher MC, West DW, Robison LM, French TK. Food-consumption trends between adolescent and adult years and subsequent risk of prostate cancer. Am J Clin Nutr 1990;52:752.
394. Snowdon DA, Phillips RL. Coffee consumption and risk of fatal cancers. Am J Public Health 1984;74:820.
395. Snowdon DA, Phillips RL, Choi W. Diet, obesity and risk of fatal prostate cancer. Am J Epidemiol 1984;120:244.
396. Solomon TE. Regulation of exocrine pancreatic cell proliferation and enzyme synthesis. In Physiology of the Gastrointestinal Tract, vol 2. Edited by LR Johnson. New York: Raven, 1981, p 873.
397. Soos K. The occurrence of carcinogenic polycyclic hydrocarbons in foodstuffs in Hungary. Arch Toxicol suppl 1980;4:446.
398. Steinmetz KA, Kushi LH, Bostick RM, Folsom AR, Potter JD. Vegetables, fruit, and colon cancer in the Iowa Women's Study. Am J Epidemiol 1994;139:1.
399. Steinmetz KA, Potter JD. Vegetables, fruit, and cancer. I. Epidemiology. Cancer Causes Control 1991 2:325.
400. Steinmetz KA, Potter JD, Folsom AR. Vegetables, fruit, and lung cancer in the Iowa Women's Health Study. Cancer Res 1993;53:536.
401. Stemmermann GN, Heilbrun LK, Nomura AMY. Association of diet and other factors with adenomatous polyps of the large bowel: a prospective autopsy study. Am J Clin Nutr 1988;47:312.
402. Stemmermann GN, Nomura AMY, Chyou PH, Yoshizawa C. Prospective study of alcohol intake and large bowel cancer. Dig Dis Sci 1990;35:1414.
403. Stemmermann GN, Nomura AMY, Heilbrun KL. Dietary fat and the risk of colorectal cancer. Cancer Res 1984;44:4633.
404. Stich HF, Rosin MP, Hornby AP, Mathew B, Sankaranarayanan R, and Nair MK. Remission or oral leukoplakias and micronuclei in tobacco/betel quid chewers treated with beta-carotene and with beta-carotene plus vitamin A. Int J Cancer 1988;42:195.
405. Takahashi M, Kokuho T, Furukawa F, Kurokawa Y, Tatematsu M, Hayashi Y. Effect of high salt diet on rat gastric carcinogenesis induced by MNNG. Gann Monogr 1983;74:28.
406. Talamini R, Franceschi S, La Vecchia C, Serraino D, Barra S, Negri E. Diet and prostatic cancer: a case-control study in Northern Italy. Nutr Cancer 1992;18:277.
407. Talamini R, LaVecchia C, Decarli A, Francechi S, Grattoni E, Grigoletto E, Liberati A, Tognoni G. Social factors, diet and breast cancer in Northern Italian population. Br J Cancer 1984;49:723.
408. Talamini R, LaVecchia C, Decarli A, Negri E, Francechi S. Nutrition, social factors and prostatic cancer in Northern Italian population. Br J Cancer 1986;53:817.

409. Tannenbaum A. Nutrition and cancer. In The Physiopathology of Cancer. Edited by F Homburger. New York: Hoeber-Harper, 1959.
410. Tannenbaum A. The dependence of tumor formation on the composition of the calorie-restricted diet as well as on the degree of restriction. Cancer Res 1945;5:616.
411. Thun MJ, Calle EE, Namboodiri MM, Flanders W, Coates R, Byers T, Boffetta P, Garfinkel L, Heath C. Risk factors for fatal cancer in a large prospective study. JNCI 1992;84:1491.
412. Toniolo P, Riboli E, Protta F, Charrel M, Cappa APM. Calorie-providing nutrients and risk of breast cancer. JNCI 1989;81:278.
413. Topping DC, Visek WJ. Nitrogen intake and tumorigenesis in rats injected with 1,2-dimethylhydrazine. J Nutr 1976;106:1583.
414. Trichopoulos D, Day NE, Kaklamani E, Tzonou A, Munoz N, Zavitsanos X, Koumantaki Y, Trichopoulou A. Hepatitis B virus, tobacco smoking, and ethanol consumption in the etiology of hepatocellular carcinoma. Int J Cancer 1987;39:45.
415. Trock B, Ianza E, Greenwald P. Dietary fiber, vegetables, and colon cancer: critical review and meta-analysis of the epidemiologic evidence. JNCI 1990;82:650.
416. Trowell H. Definition of dietary fiber and hypotheses that it is a protective factor in certain diseases. Am J Clin Nutr 1976;29:417.
417. Tuyns A. Alcool et Cancer. Lyon: International Agency for Research on Cancer, 1978.
418. Tuyns AJ. Alcohol. In Cancer Epidemiology and Prevention. Edited by D Schottenfeld, JF Fraumeni Jr. Philadelphia: Saunders, 1982, p 293.
419. Tuyns AJ. Oesophageal cancer in non-smoking drinkers and in non-drinking smokers. Int J Cancer 1983;32:433.
420. Tuyns AJ. Sodium chloride and cancer of the digestive tract. Nutr Cancer 1983;4:198.
421. Tuyns AJ, Haelterman M, Kaaks R. Colorectal cancer and the intake of nutrients: oligosaccharides are a risk factor, fats are not: a case-control study in Belgium. Nutr Cancer 1987;10:181.
422. Tuyns AJ, Pequignot G, Abbatucci JS. Oesophageal cancer and alcohol consumption: importance of type of beverage. Int J Cancer 1979;23:443.
423. Tuyns AJ, Pequignot G, Gignoux M, Valla A. Cancers of the digestive tract, alcohol and tobacco. Int J Cancer 1982;30:9.
424. Tweedie JH, Reber HA, Pour PM, Pounder DM. Protective effect of ethanol on the development of pancreatic cancer. Surg Forum 1981;32:222.
425. Van den Brandt PA, Van't Veer P, Goldbohm RA, Dorant E, Volovics A, Hermus R, Sturmans F. A prospective cohort study on dietary fat and the risk of postmenopausal breast cancer. Cancer Res 1993;53:75.
426. van Rensburg SJ. Epidemiologic and dietary evidence for a specific nutritional predisposition to esophageal cancer. JNCI 1981;67:243.
427. van Rensburg SJ, du Bruyn DB, van Schalkwyk DJ. Promotion of methylbenzylnitosamine-induced esophageal cancer in rats by subclinical zinc deficiency. Nutr Reports Int 1980;22:891.
428. van Rensburg SJ, Hall JM, du Bruyn DB. Effects of various dietary staples on esophageal carcinogenesis induced in rats by subcutaneously administered *N*-nitrosomethylbenzylsamine. JNCI 1985;75:561.
429. van Rensburg SJ, Hall JM, Gathercole PS. Inhibition of esophageal carcinogenesis in corn-fed rats by riboflavin, nicotinic acid, selenium, molybdenum, zinc, and magnesium. Nutr Cancer 1986;8:163.
430. Van Tassell RL, Schram RM, Wilkins TD. Microbial biosynthesis of fecapentaenes. In Genetic Toxicology of the Diet. Edited by I Knudson. New York: Liss, 1986, p 199.
431. Vena JE, Graham S, Zielezny M, Swanson MK, Barnes RE, Nolan J. Lifetime occupational exercise and colon cancer. Am J Epidemiol 1985;122:357.
432. Vena JE, Graham S, Zielezny M, Swanson MK, Barnes RE, Nolan J. Occupational exercise and risk of cancer. Am J Clin Nutr 1987;45:318.
433. Visek WJ, Clinton SK. Dietary Protein and Cancer. In Human Nutrition: A Comprehensive Treatise, vol 7; Cancer and Nutrition. Edited by RB Alfin-Slater, D Kritchevsky. New York: Plenum, 1991, p 103.
434. Voitalovich EA, Deekoon PP, Deemarsky LU, Shabad LM. Comparative study of malignant tumor frequency in Tookoom District of the Latvian SSR. Vopr Onkol 1957;3:351.
435. Wald N, Boreham J, Bailey A. Serum retinol and subsequent risk of cancer. Br J Cancer 1986;54:957.
436. Wald N, Idle M, Boreham J, Bailey A. Low serum-vitamin-A and subsequent risk of cancer. Preliminary results of a prospective study. Lancet 1980;ii:813.
437. Ward JM, Anjo T, Ohannesian L, Keefer LK, Devor DE, Donovan PJ, Smith GT, Henneman JR, Streeter AJ, Konishi N, Rehm S, Reist EJ, Bradford WW, Rice JM. Inactivity of fecapentaene-12 as a rodent carcinogen or tumor initiator and guidelines for its use in biological studies. Cancer Lett 1988;42:49.
438. Waterhouse J, Muir CS, Shanmugaratnam K, Powell J. Incidence in Five Continents IARC Sci Publ 1982;4:no.42.
439. Watt BK, Merrill AL. Composition of Foods. Agriculture Handbook, No. 8. Washington, DC: U.S. Department of Agriculture, 1975.
440. Wattenberg LW. Inhibitors of chemical carcinogens. In Cancer: Achievements, Challenges, and Prospects for the 1980s, vol 1. Edited by JH Burchenal, HF Oettgen. New York: Grune and Stratton 1981, p 517.
441. Weisblum B, Herman L, Fitzgerald PJ. Changes in pancreatic acinar cells during protein deprivation. J Cell Biol 1962;12:313.
442. Weisburger JH, Marquardt H, Hirota N, Mori H, Williams GM. Induction of cancer of the glandular stomach in rats by extract of nitrite-treated fish. JNCI 1980;64:163.
443. West DW, Slattery MI, Robison LM, French TK, Mahoney AW. Adult dietary intake and prostate cancer risk in Utah: a case-control study with special emphasis on aggressive tumors. Cancer Causes Control 1991;2:85.
444. West DW, Slattery ML, Robison LM, Schuman KL, Ford MH, Mahoney AW, Lyon JL, Sorensen AW. Dietary intake and colon cancer: sex and anatomic site-specific associations. Am J Epidemiol 1989;130:883.
445. Whittemore AS, Wu-Williams AH, Lee M, Shu Z, Gallagher RP, Deng-as J, Lun Z, Xianghui W, Kun C, Jung D, Teh C-Z, Chengde L, Yao XJ, Paffenbarger RS Jr, Henderson BE. Diet, physical activity, and colorectal cancer among Chinese in North America and China. JNCI 1990;82:915.
446. Willett W. The search for the causes of breast and colon cancer. Nature 1989;338: 389.
447. Willett W, Stampfer MJ. Total energy intake: implications for epidemiologic analyses. Am J Epidemiol 11986;24:17.
448. Willett WC, Hunter DJ, Stampfer MJ, Colditz G, Manson J, Spiegelman D, Rosner B, Hennekens C, Speizer F. Dietary fat and fiber in relation to risk of breast cancer: an eight year follow-up. JAMA 1992;268:2037.
449. Willett WC, Stampfer MJ, Colditz GA, Rosner BA, Hennekens CH, Speizer FE. Dietary fat and the risk of breast cancer. N Engl J Med 1987;316:22.
450. Willett WC, Stampfer MJ, Colditz GA, Rosner BA, Hennekens CH, Speizer FE. Moderate alcohol consumption and the risk of breast cancer. N Engl J Med 1987;316: 1174.
451. Willett WC, Stampfer MJ, Colditz GA, Rosner BA, Speizer FE. Relation of meat, fat, and fiber intake to the risk of colon cancer in a prospective study among women. N Engl J Med 1990;323:1664.
452. Willett WC, Stampfer MJ, Underwood BA, Sampson LA, Hennekens CH, Wallingford JC, Cooper LC, Hsieh CC, Speizer FE. Vitamin A supplementation and plasma retinol levels. A randomized trial among women. JNCI 1984;73:1445.
453. Williams RR, Horm JW. Association of cancer sites with tobacco and alcohol consumption and socioeconomic status of patients: interview study from the Third National Cancer Survey. JNCI 1977;58:525.
454. Wogan GN. Dietary factors and special epidemiological situations of liver cancer in Thailand and Africa. Cancer Res 1975;35:3499.
455. World Health Organization. Diet, Nutrition and the Prevention of Chronic Diseases. Technical Report Series, No. 797. Geneva: WHO, 1990.
456. World Health Organization. Environmental Health Criteria 11. Mycotoxins. Geneva: WHO, 1979.
457. Wu AH, Paganini-Hill A, Ross RK, Henderson BE. Alcohol, physical activity and other risk factors for colorectal cancer: a prospective study. Br J Cancer 1987;55:687.
458. Wynder EL. An epidemiological evaluation of the causes of cancer of the pancreas. Cancer Res 1975;35:2228.
459. Wynder EL, Bross IJ. A study of etiological factors in cancer of the esophagus. Cancer 1961;14:389.
460. Wynder EL, Bross IJ, Feldmann RM. A study of the etiological factors in cancer of the mouth. Cancer 1957;10:1300.
461. Wynder EL, Hebert JR, Kabat GC. Association of dietary fat and lung cancer. JNCI 1987;79:631.
462. Wynder EL, Hultberg S, Jacobson F, Bross IJ. Environmental factors in cancer of the upper alimentary tract: a Swedish study with special reference to Plummer-Vinson (Paterson-Kelly) syndrome. Cancer 1957;10:470.
463. Yang CS. Research on esophageal cancer in China: a review. Cancer Res 1980;40: 2633.
464. Yu MC, Mack T, Hanisch R, Peters RL, Henderson BE, Pike MC. Hepatitis, alcohol consumption, cigarette smoking, and hepatocellular carcinoma in Los Angeles. Cancer Res 1983;43:6077.
465. Zaridze DG, Muir CS, McMichael AJ. Diet and cancer: value of different types of epidemiological studies. In Diet and Human Carcinogenesis. Edited by JV Joossens, MJ Hill, J Geboers. New York: Excerpta Medica, 1985, p 221.
466. Ziegler RG, Mason TJ, Stemhagen A, Hoover R, Schoenberg JB, Gridley G, Virgo PW, Altman R, Fraumeni JF Jr. Dietary carotene and vitamin A and risk of lung cancer among white men in New Jersey. JNCI 1984;73:1429.
467. Ziegler RG, Morris LE, Blot WJ, Pottern LM, Hoover R, Fraumeni JF Jr. Esophageal cancer among black men in Washington DC. II. Role of nutrition. JNCI 1981;67: 1199.

CHAPTER 29

Chemoprevention of Cancer

MICHAEL B. SPORN AND SCOTT M. LIPPMAN

Introduction

There are two general approaches to the problem of control of cancer. The classic approach, which has been followed for more than a hundred years, has been to deal with the disease once it has manifested itself in its terminal stages, which are characterized by clinical symptoms or laboratory findings related to the phenomena of invasiveness or metastasis. Invasion and metastasis have long been considered the "true" hallmarks of cancer. Once patients have been diagnosed with "cancer," as defined by the above criteria, they have then been treated with the various modalities of surgery, radiation therapy, chemotherapy, immunotherapy, or other treatments directed at the eradication of detectable lesions. Despite some spectacular successes in the treatment of relatively rare cancers, this approach has not yet led to a significant decrease in cancer mortality resulting from the common forms of many metastatic epithelial cancers, such as carcinoma of the lung, breast, colon, prostate, pancreas, and other sites (1).

An alternative approach to the problem of control of cancer is one that attempts first, to provide new understanding of the fundamental nature of the chronic disease process which eventually leads to invasive and metastatic carcinoma, and second, to develop new pharmacologic agents that arrest or reverse this chronic disease process in its earliest stages before it reaches its terminal invasive and metastatic phase (2, 3). This alternative approach is known as *chemoprevention* (2, 4). It is based on the concept that the very term "cancer," widely used by clinicians, laboratory scientists, and laypersons alike, is a misnomer, in that it is inadequate to describe the pathogenesis of the disease process as it actually occurs in the patient. The term "cancer" denotes a static circumstance, whereas the disease in reality is an evolving chronic molecular and cellular process—that is, "carcinogenesis." By focusing on end-stage invasive and metastatic disease, we lose the opportunity to intervene in the disease process at earlier stages, when it may be more amenable to the use of pharmacologic agents for its prevention. Since 20 years or more may elapse between the original mutagenic initiation of the carcinogenic process and the subsequent development of invasive or metastatic cells (5, 6), there is a long window of opportunity in which to use preventive agents. Indeed, since there is only a stochastic probability that an early stage of carcinogenesis will progress to a later one, the intrinsic biology of the carcinogenic process suggests that preventive agents can be developed and successfully used (5, 6). Perhaps the most significant aspect of carcinogenesis as a process is that most people do *not* develop invasive and metastatic carcinoma during their lifetime, despite their endogenous and exogenous mutational burden, and often despite the presence of significant preinvasive neoplastic lesions in their various epithelia.

The natural history of the disease process of carcinogenesis thus convincingly indicates that there are intrinsic biologic mechanisms that protect the organism against the development of clones of malignant cells (7, 8). It would therefore seem reasonable to utilize these mechanisms to design strategies for prevention of cancer. It is paradoxical that the phenomenon that not all dysplastic, preinvasive lesions progress to invasiveness has been used as an argument against the clinical use of chemopreventive agents, with the false premise that since a patient may not yet have an invasive lesion (does not yet have "cancer"), the patient is therefore "healthy" (9). In this regard the oncology community lags far behind the cardiovascular community in recognizing and accepting the importance of early precursor lesions as antecedents of clinically symptomatic and life-threatening disease. In cardiovascular medicine it is well accepted that precursor lesions, such as fatty streaking and arterial plaques, have an important causal relationship to the end-stage clinical outcomes of myocardial infarction and stroke (10), and great advances have been made in the development of new drugs, such as agents that can lower cholesterol levels, and that have had major impact on lowering mortality from cardiovascular disease (11). Moreover, the fact that not all arterial precursor lesions progress to a thrombotic or embolic state has not been used as an argument against interventive chemoprevention, and it is generally accepted that patients with extensive precursor lesions in their arterial tree may be at high risk for serious, life-threatening events. There is widespread acceptance of the concepts that patients with such lesions are *not* healthy from a cardiovascular perspective, even though they may not be symptomatic, and that it is appropriate to use pharmacologic agents to prevent further progression of early arterial lesions.

Rather than dismissing precursor lesions of invasive cancer as biologically insignificant on the ground that not all of these lesions progress to invasiveness, it would seem more reasonable to attempt to understand the intrinsic mechanisms in epithelia that prevent progression of these lesions, and then design new pharmacologic agents that could enhance the activity of such mechanisms. These concepts provide the basis for the ultimate use of chemoprevention to control cancer death rates.

Agents for Chemoprevention and Their Mechanism of Action

TYPES OF CHEMOPREVENTIVE AGENTS

In the broadest sense, agents for chemoprevention of cancer fall into two principal categories (4): (*a*) those that prevent the mutagenic initiation of the carcinogenic process ("blocking" agents) and (*b*) those that prevent the further promotion or progression of lesions that have already been established ("suppressing" agents). Since mutation continues as part of the entire chronic process of carcinogenesis, the distinction between the two categories, at least in the dimension of time, is artifactual; however useful the concept of two-stage carcinogenesis (initiation followed by promotion) was in the past to describe relatively simple experimental systems in laboratory rodents, it can no longer be accepted as a valid model for the process of carcinogenesis in human subjects, in whom mutation, with its consequent continuation of the initiation of new molecular lesions, plays an ongoing role throughout the life span of the individual. Particularly as extensive information is now available on the ability of cells such as neutrophils and macrophages to generate potent agents such as superoxide, hydrogen peroxide, hydroxyl radical, and nitric oxide, all of which can damage DNA, it is clear that endogenous metabolism, as well as exposure to exogenous agents, can have a major influence on the process of carcinogenesis (12).

In this chapter, we discuss both types of agents, since both have found clinical application. Although various dietary constituents, such as calcium, and vitamins, such as ascorbic acid, β-carotene, folic acid, and α-tocopherol (vitamin E), have been the subject of many clinical trials to prevent cancer (reviewed in the last part of this chapter), for the most part the results with vitamins and other nutrients have been disappointing. It should be clear by now that if chemoprevention is truly to have a practical impact on the control of cancer, it will be necessary to develop a fundamentally pharmacologic approach to the problem. In the face of the intense mutagenic pressure that drives the process of carcinogenesis, it will be necessary to use agents that either are potent antimutagens or can significantly alter patterns of gene expression.

RETINOIDS

The set of molecules that has been most intensively studied for chemoprevention of carcinogenesis are the retinoids, which are defined as natural and synthetic analogues of retinol (vitamin A) (2, 13). More than a thousand such molecules have been made by synthetic chemistry (14), and as knowledge of the receptors that mediate their mechanism of action increases, so also does the number of new agents that are ligands for these receptors. Of particular importance to retinoid studies has been the unification in molecular and cell biology that has occurred with the discovery of the steroid receptor superfamily (15, 16). This has been a major advance in the attempt to develop new agents for the chemoprevention of carcinogenesis, since it is now apparent that the intracellular receptors for the retinoids, vitamin D, and thyroid hormone, as well as those for the classic steroids such as estrogens, progestogens, androgens, and glucocorticoids, all belong to a superfamily involved in the selective regulation of transcription of specific genes that control cell differentiation and proliferation (15–17). Studies on the mechanism of action of the above ligands with their respective receptors now provide the basis for rational design, development, and testing of new agents for the chemoprevention of carcinogenesis.

The impact of this new knowledge has been especially important in studies of retinoids. Many years ago Wolbach and Howe demonstrated that the normal function of retinoids was essential for the proper regulation of the differentiation and proliferation of all the epithelia that are the common sites of carcinogenesis in men and women (18). They clearly recognized that during retinoid deficiency there was a failure of stem cells to mature into appropriate differentiated cells; this was accompanied by enhanced cellular proliferation, with the formation of lesions resembling those found in malignant or premalignant tissues. It is now known that retinoids are required to maintain normal differentiation and proliferation of almost all cells, including nonepithelial cells of mesenchymal origin, during both embryogenesis and adult life (19).

Further advances related to the chemoprevention of carcinogenesis came from organ culture and cell culture studies. It was shown that retinoids could reverse the premalignant lesions induced in mouse prostate organ cultures by carcinogenic hydrocarbons such as 3-methylcholanthrene (20) and that retinoids could act directly on cells previously treated with such carcinogens to suppress the appearance of the malignant phenotype (21). The latter cell culture studies were particularly important, because they emphasized that the continuing presence of the retinoid was essential for the suppression of malignancy; removal of the retinoids from the cultures allowed the expression of the transformed state in cells that had previously been exposed to carcinogen. This phenomenon of a continued requirement for a retinoid to suppress carcinogenesis has also been seen repeatedly in many studies in intact animals and undoubtedly is clinically relevant. However, there are also some situations in which retinoids can alter the differentiation of invasive neoplastic cells and induce terminal differentiation. The most striking examples of this phenomenon are the induction of terminal differentiation in many types of teratocarcinoma and leukemia cells, of both animal and human origin (22–24).

Several synthetic retinoids have been successfully used in a large number of studies for the prevention of carcinogenesis in experimental animals. Among those that have potential for clinical application are the following: all-*trans*-retinoic acid (tretinoin), 4-hydroxyphenyl all-*trans*-retinoic acid amide (4-HPR, fenretinide), 13-*cis*-retinoic acid (isotretinoin), and 9-*cis*-retinoic acid. There are six known retinoic acid receptors (RAR) that mediate the actions of these retinoids. The first receptors to be cloned, RAR-α, RAR-β, and RAR-γ, bind all-*trans*-retinoic acid and 9-*cis*-retinoic acid with high affinity (25, 26), but bind neither 4-HPR nor 13-*cis*-retinoic acid. These latter two retinoids are presumably prodrugs: the isomerization of 13-*cis*- to all-*trans*-retinoic acid occurs readily; however, the enzymatic hydrolysis of 4-HPR to the free acid has yet to be shown, either in cell culture or in vivo.

More recently three new retinoid receptors, known as RXR-α, RXR-β, and RXR-γ, have been cloned (27); these RXRs bind only 9-*cis*-retinoic acid (25, 26), and do not bind any of the other three retinoids just mentioned above. However, since all-*trans*-retinoic acid can be metabolized to the 9-*cis* derivative, it is ultimately a potential ligand for the RXRs in vivo. The importance of the RXRs is emphasized by their ability to form heterodimers with many other members of the steroid receptor superfamily, including RARs, the vitamin D receptor, and the thyroid hormone receptor. RXRs and their ligands are thus permissive systems that can modulate the activity of other ligands and receptors in the steroid receptor superfamily; with the recent demonstration that terpenoid molecules other than 9-*cis*-retinoic acid can act as ligands for RXRs, the functional domain of this system now appears to be even broader than anticipated.

There is an extensive literature on the use of retinoids to arrest or reverse the process of carcinogenesis and to prevent the development of invasive carcinoma in experimental animals (28). Of particular importance are the many studies that have shown efficacy of retinoids when they are administered after animals have been treated with carcinogen; this experimental design is highly relevant to human populations. Significant activity has been shown for all-*trans*-retinoic acid, 13-*cis*-retinoic acid, 9-*cis*-retinoic acid (29), 4-HPR, and many other retinoids, as reviewed by Moon et al. (28). The epithelial sites studied include breast, skin, lung, bladder, pancreas, liver, oropharynx, esophagus, stomach, and prostate. In addition to efficacy as single agents, retinoids have been particularly effective when used in combination with other preventive agents, especially tamoxifen.

TAMOXIFEN

Tamoxifen is a nonsteroidal triphenylethylene derivative that binds to the estrogen receptor (30). It has both estrogenic and antiestrogenic actions, depending on the target tissue. Thus, it is strongly antiestrogenic on mammary epithelium (which provides the basis for its use in both the prevention and treatment of breast cancer), while it is proestrogenic on uterine epithelium (which provides the basis for the current controversy regarding the safety of the use of tamoxifen for cancer prevention (9); an increased incidence of endometrial carcinoma has been found in women treated chronically with tamoxifen (30)). It is therefore inappropriate to refer to tamoxifen simply as an antiestrogen. The term "estrogen response modifier" is perhaps more appropriate.

Tamoxifen was originally screened in a drug development program oriented toward discovering new contraceptive agents. Although it was effective in rats, it was not a useful drug for control of fertility in women, and it was not until the early 1970s that it was shown to be useful for clinical palliation of advanced breast cancer. Subsequently, animal studies performed in rats, using both dimethylbenzanthracene (DMBA) and nitrosomethylurea (NMU) as carcinogens, showed that tamoxifen was highly effective in preventing the development of experimental breast cancer (31, 32); these results have also been confirmed in the mouse model in which mammary tumor virus (MMTV) is the carcinogen.

The mechanism of action of tamoxifen is complex. Clearly, its principal mechanism of action is mediated by its binding to the estrogen receptor and the blocking of the proliferative actions of estrogen on mammary epithelium. One mechanism that has been suggested for this antiproliferative action is the induction by tamoxifen of the synthesis of the cytokine, transforming growth factor-beta (TGF-β), which acts as a negative autocrine regulatory molecule (33). However, it has also been shown that tamoxifen can induce synthesis of TGF-β in estrogen receptor–negative cells, such as fetal fibroblasts (34). Moreover, immunohistochemical studies have shown that tamoxifen induces the synthesis of TGF-β in the stromal (mesenchymal) compartment of breast cancers, suggesting a paracrine, as well as autocrine, mechanism of action, independent of an interaction with the estrogen receptor (35). Reports of some clinical efficacy of tamoxifen in the treatment of women with estrogen receptor-negative breast carcinomas would appear to be in accord with these mechanistic conclusions (36). Other studies that are in accord with these observations are the findings that tamoxifen can lower the circulating levels of insulin-like growth factor 1 (IGF-1) in breast cancer patients (37, 38). IGF-1 is a potent mitogen for breast cancer cells and may act by endocrine, paracrine, and autocrine routes to stimulate their growth.

RALOXIFENE

Although the risks are actually quite small, there is major concern at the present time about the safety of the use of tamoxifen as a chemopreventive agent for the prophylaxis of breast cancer, because of its estrogenic effect on uterine epithelium and the attendant increased risk for development of uterine cancer. Thus, there has been a search for new agents that would resemble tamoxifen in their overall mechanism of action but would be inhibitory to the growth of uterine epithelium. One such molecule is raloxifene, the chemical structure of which is totally different from that of tamoxifen; tamoxifen is a triphenylethylene derivative, while raloxifene is a benzothiophene. Like tamoxifen, raloxifene binds to the estrogen receptor and has both estrogenic and antiestrogenic actions; it is another "estrogen response modifier." It has been shown to have both therapeutic and preventive activity on breast tumors induced in rats by chemical carcinogens (32). Most notably, in contrast to tamoxifen, raloxifene does not act as an estrogen agonist in the uterus and does not stimulate the growth of uterine epithelium in ovariectomized rats (39). However, raloxifene is strongly estrogenic in its positive actions on bone and serum lipids; it is a potent agent for prevention of bone loss in the ovariectomized rat (39). Because of this unusual spectrum of pharmacologic activity, raloxifene is an attractive agent for the prevention of bone loss in osteoporotic, postmenopausal women, which is its primary therapeutic application at the present time. If large numbers of women are treated chronically with raloxifene for the prevention of osteoporosis, this therapy may also provide a clinical trial of the efficacy of this agent for prevention of breast cancer.

DELTANOIDS (VITAMIN D AND ITS SYNTHETIC ANALOGUES)

Another important ligand of the steroid receptor superfamily is 1,25-dihydroxycholecalciferol (1,25-D_3), the active metabolite of dietary vitamin D. 1,25-D_3 has potent actions in controlling the expression of many genes and can induce differentiation in many tumor cells, particularly those of myeloid lineage (40, 41). However, because of its marked hypercalcemic activity, it is not a suitable agent for clinical chemoprevention. A large number of synthetic analogues of 1,25-D_3 have been made, with the goal of increasing differentiative activity and decreasing calcemic actions (42); we have suggested the term "deltanoids," analogous to "retinoids," for the entire family of natural and synthetic molecules related to 1,25-D_3 (43). Many of the new analogues are markedly less calcemic and more active in inducing differentiation, and some have been shown to be active in the prevention of breast cancer in animal experiments (43, 44). The clinical potential for the use of these agents is still unrealized.

FINASTERIDE (PROSCAR)

Prostate carcinogenesis in both experimental animals and humans is driven by androgen, in much the same way that mammary carcinogenesis is driven by estrogen. The testosterone metabolite, 5-α-dihydrotestosterone (DHT), has higher binding affinity for the androgen receptor than testosterone and is believed to play a critical role in the development of the prostate gland. DHT is formed from testosterone by the action of the enzyme, 5 α-reductase, and several androgen analogues have been developed as antagonists of this enzyme. One of these analogues, finasteride (Proscar), is now in widespread use to treat benign prostatic hypertrophy (BPH) (45).

Although there are essentially no published studies on the use of finasteride to prevent prostate cancer in experimental animals, because of its known molecular mechanism of action and its known clinical efficacy in the treatment of BPH, this agent is now being evaluated for chemoprevention of prostate carcinogenesis in a large clinical trial.

DIFLUOROMETHYLORNITHINE

Agents that can suppress cell proliferation are obvious candidates for chemoprevention, if they have sufficient selectivity. One such molecule is difluoromethylornithine (DFMO), a potent irreversible inhibitor of the enzyme ornithine decarboxylase (ODC), that catalyzes the formation of putrescine, a polyamine involved in DNA synthesis (46). There is a very extensive literature on the use of DFMO to prevent carcinogenesis in animal models of colon, bladder, breast, liver, skin, and stomach cancer (47). The National Cancer Institute (NCI) has conducted extensive preclinical and clinical toxicologic evaluations of this drug, and further clinical trials are planned.

NONSTEROIDAL ANTI-INFLAMMATORY DRUGS

A large number of anti-inflammatory agents have shown potent chemopreventive activity in many test systems. Among the NSAIDs that have been studied at length are aspirin, ibuprofen, sulindac, and piroxicam. All of these molecules are cyclooxygenase inhibitors that block prostaglandin synthesis, and they are in widespread clinical use for the chronic treatment of various inflammatory diseases, most notably osteoarthritis or rheumatoid arthritis. There is therefore an abundance of information about the safe dosage for their long-term administration that would be required for a chemoprevention trial. All of these inhibitors of prostaglandin synthesis have been shown to be active in a multiplicity of animal models for the suppression of carcinogenesis, with particular efficacy in preventing experimental colon carcinogenesis (48). Based on these results, a number of clinical trials have been designed.

N-ACETYLCYSTEINE AND OLTIPRAZ

Glutathione in its reduced form (GSH) is a critical molecule in the chemical deactivation of many carcinogens. Since glutathione itself is not a practical agent for chemoprevention, a great deal of effort has been devoted to the development of exogenous agents that would elevate intracellular GSH levels. This principle, termed electrophile counterattack (49), has been the basis of extensive investigation. *N*-acetylcysteine and oltipraz are two of the most important such molecules that act by this mechanism. Both of these agents can block the mutagenic activity of a variety of carcinogens by preventing their binding to DNA; a substantial decrease in DNA adducts has been seen if either *N*-acetylcysteine or oltipraz is given to animals when they are treated with carcinogens such as aflatoxin, benzo(*a*)pyrene, or acetylaminofluorene (50, 51). Both agents are active in animal test systems for the prevention of cancer, and both are in clinical trial.

Chemoprevention Trials

Approximately 60 randomized chemoprevention trials have been reported to date (Table 29.1). These include premalignancy (Phase II) studies in the head and neck, lung, colon, skin, esophagus, bladder, and cervix, and cancer incidence (Phase III) trials for cancer of the head and neck, lung, colon, skin, breast, esophagus, and stomach. Although chemoprevention has yet to enter the realm of standard clinical practice, several ongoing Phase II and Phase III trials may bring this approach closer to standard practice in certain settings (52, 53).

HEAD AND NECK

Oral Premalignancy

Oral leukoplakia is a premalignant lesion that manifests with a white patch unclassifiable as any other disorder (54). Current therapy is excisional. Chemoprevention may become standard systemic therapy in certain cases, such as

Table 29.1. Randomized Chemoprevention Trials*

Author (Year)	Study Setting	Design	Number	Intervention	Outcome
Head and Neck					
Hong et al. (1986) (60)	Oral leukoplakia	Phase II	44	Isotretinoin (1–2 mg/kg/d)	Positive
Stich et al. (1988) (62)	Oral leukoplakia	Phase II	65	Vitamin A (200,000 IU/wk)	Positive
Han et al. (1990) (63)	Oral leukoplakia	Phase II	61	Retinamide (40 mg/d)	Positive
Lippman et al. (1993) (61)	Oral leukoplakia	Phase II maintenance	70	Isotretinoin (0.5 mg/kg/d)	Positive
Chiesa et al. (1993) (64)	Oral leukoplakia	Phase II maintenance	80	Fenretinide (200 mg/d)	Positive
Epstein et al. (1994) (65)	Oral leukoplakia	Phase II	22	Topical bleomycin (1%)	Positive
Hong et al. (1990) (72)	Prior SCC	Phase III	103	Isotretinoin (50–100) mg/ m^2/d)	Positive (SPT)
Bolla et al. (1994) (75)	Prior SCC	Phase III	316	Etretinate (50, 25 mg/d)	Negative
Lung					
Heimburger et al. (1988) (79)	Metaplasia (sputum)	Phase II	73	Vitamin B_{12} (500 μg/d), folic acid (10 mg/d)	Positive (atypia)
Arnold et al. (1992) (77)	Metaplasia (sputum)	Phase II	150	Etretinate (25 mg/d)	Negative
Van Poppel et al. (1992) (80)	Micronuclei (sputum)	Phase II	114	β-Carotene (20 mg/d)	Positive
Lee et al. (1994) (78)	Metaplasia (biopsy)	Phase II	87	Isotretinoin (1 mg/kg/d)	Negative
Van Poppel et al. (1995) (81)	8-oxoDG	Phase II	122	β-Carotene (20 mg/d)	Negative
McLarty et al. (1995) (82)	Metaplasia (sputum)	Phase II	755	β-Carotene (50 mg/d), retinol (25,000 IU q.o.d.)	Negative
ATBC (1994) (83)	Lung cancer	Phase III	29,133	β-Carotene (20 mg/d); α-tocopherol (50 mg/d)	Negative
Pastorino et al. (1993) (85)	Prior NSCLC	Phase III	307	Retinyl palmitate (300,000 IU/d)	Positive (SPT)
Colon					
Bussey et al. (1982) (104)	FAP	Phase II	36	Vitamin C (3 g/d)	Positive (polyp)
McKeown-Eyssen et al. (1988) (105)	Resected adenoma	Phase II	137	Vitamins C (400 mg/d) and E (400 mg/d)	Negative
DeCosse et al. (1989) (106)	FAP	Phase II	58	Vitamins C (4 g/d), E (400 mg/d), and fiber (22.5 g/d)	Positive (polyp)
Gregoire et al. (1989) (96)	Prior colon cancer	Phase II	30	Calcium (1,200 mg/d)	Negative (LI)
Stern et al. (1990) (95)	Prior FAP	Phase II	31	Calcium (1,200 mg/d)	Negative (LI)
Labayle et al. (1991) (90)	FAP	Phase II	10	Sulindac (300 mg/d)	Positive (polyps)
Kikendall et al. (1991) (102)	Resected adenoma	Phase II	257	β-carotene (15 mg/d)	Negative
Barsoum et al. (1992) (97)	Adenoma	Phase II	14	Calcium (1.25 g/d)	Positive (LI)
Wargovich et al. (1992) (94)	Resected adenoma	Phase II	20	Calcium (2,000 mg/d)	Positive (LI)
Paganelli et al. (1992) (111)	Resected adenoma	Phase II	41	Vitamins A (30,000 IU/d), E (70 mg/d), C (1 g/d)	Negative (LI)
Alberts et al. (1992) (107)	Resected adenoma	Phase II	100	WBF (2.0 or 13.5 g/d), calcium (250 or 1,500 mg/d)	Negative (LI)
Giardiello et al. (1993) (91)	FAP	Phase II	22	Sulindac (300 mg/d)	Positive (polyps)
MacLennan et al. (1995) (109)	Resected adenoma	Phase II	395	Fat (≤25% of calories), WBF (11 g/d), β-Carotene (20 mg/d)	Negative (polyps)
Bostick et al. (1993) (98)	Resected adenoma	Phase II	21	Calcium (1,200 mg/d)	Negative (LI)
Roncucci et al. (1993) (112)	Resected adenoma	Phase II	209	Vitamins A (30,000 IU/d), C (1 g/d), E (70 mg/d); lactulose (20 g/d)	Positive (Vitamins > lactulose)
Gann et al. (1993) (92)	U.S. male physicians	Phase III	22,071	Aspirin (325 mg q.o.d.)	Negative
Greenberg et al. (1994) (113)	Resected adenoma	Phase II	751	β-Carotene (25 mg/d); vitamins E (400 mg/d), C (1 g/d)	Negative
Cats et al. (1995) (99)	HNPCC families	Phase II	30	Calcium (1,500 mg/d)	Negative (LI)
Baron et al. (1995) (100)	Resected adenoma	Phase II	333	Calcium (3,000 mg/d)	Negative (LI)

(continued)

Table 29.1. *(continued)*

Author (Year)	Study Setting	Design	Number	Intervention	Outcome
Skin					
Moriarty et al. (1982) (115)	Actinic keratoses	Phase II	50	Etretinate (75 mg/d)	Positive
Watson (1986) (116)	Actinic keratoses	Phase II	15	Etretinate (75 mg/d)	Positive
Kligman & Thorne (1991) (114)	Actinic keratoses	Phase II	527	Topical tretinoin (0.05%)	Negative
Kligman & Thorne (1991) (114)	Actinic keratoses	Phase II	455	Topical tretinoin (0.10%)	Positive
Moon et al. (1993) (121)	Prior BCC/SCC	Phase III	524	Isotretinoin (5–10 mg/d); retinol (25,000 IU/d)	Negative
Greenberg et al. (1990) (119)	Prior BCC/SCC	Phase III	1,805	β-Carotene (50 mg/d)	Negative
Tangrea et al. (1992) (120)	Prior BCC	Phase III	981	Isotretinoin (10 mg/d)	Negative
Moon et al. (1993) (121)	Prior actinic keratoses	Phase III	2,298	Retinol (25,000 IU/d)	Positive
Bouwes Bavinck et al. (1995) (118)	Renal transplant recipients	Phase III	38	Acitretin (30 mg/d)	Positive
Breast					
De Palo (1995) (123)	Breast cancer	Phase III	2,849	Fenretinide (200 mg/d)	Positive (ovarian cancer); breast cancer (pending)
Esophagus/Stomach					
Munoz et al. (1985) (126,127)	Geographic high risk (Huixian)	Phase II	610	Retinol (50,000 IU/wk), riboflavin (200 mg/wk), zinc (50 mg/wk)	Negative (dysplasia); Positive (micronuclei)
Zaridze et al. (1993) (129)	Geographic high risk (Uzbekistan) (oral leukoplakia and/or chronic esophagitis)	Phase II	532	Riboflavin (80 mg/wk); vitamins A (100,000 IU/wk), E (80 mg/wk), β-Carotene (40 mg/d)	Negative
Blot et al. (1993) (130)	Geographic high risk (Linxian)	Phase III	29,584	Multiple vitamins/minerals	Positive (stomach)
Li et al. (1993) (131)	Geographic high risk (Linxian)	Phase III	3,318	Multiple vitamins/minerals	Negative (dysplasia)
Buiatti et al. (1994) (132)	Geographic high risk (Venezuela)	Phase II	222	Bismuth (120 mg q.i.d.), Amoxicillin (500 mg q.i.d.)	Negative (*H. pylori*)
Bladder					
Alfthan et al. (1983) (134)	Superficial tumors (resected)	Phase II	32	Etretinate (25–50 mg/d)	Positive
Pederson et al. (1984) (135)	Superficial tumors (resected)	Phase II	73	Etretinate (50 mg/d)	Negative
Studer et al. (1984) (136)	Superficial tumors (resected)	Phase II	86	Etretinate (25–50 mg/d)	Positive
Lamm et al. (1994) (137)	Superficial tumors (resected)	Phase II	65	Megadose vitamins	Positive
Cervix					
Byrne et al. (1986) (139)	Dysplasia (CIN 2, 3)	Phase II	26	HLI (0.8×10^6 IU/wk)	Negative
Yliskoski et al. (1990) (140)	Dysplasia (CIN 1, 2)	Phase II	20	HLI (9×10^6 IU/d)	Negative
Frost et al. (1990) (141)	Dysplasia (CIN 2)	Phase II	10	IFN-α2b (4×10^6 IU/wk)	Negative
Dunham et al. (1990) (142)	Dysplasia (CIN 1–3)	Phase II	14	IFN-α2b (6×10^6 IU/wk)	Negative
de Vet et al. (1991) (145)	Dysplasia (CIN 1–3)	Phase II	278	β-Carotene (10 mg/d)	Negative
Butterworth et al. (1992) (143)	Dysplasia (CIN 1, 2)	Phase II	235	Folic acid (10 mg/d)	Negative
Meyskens et al. (1994) (146)	Dysplasia (CIN 2, 3)	Phase II	301	Topical tretinoin (0.372%)	Positive (CIN 2)
Childers et al. (1995) (144)	Dysplasia (CIN 1, 2)	Phase II	331	Folic acid (5 mg/d)	Negative

Abbreviations: SCC, squamous cell carcinoma; SPT, second primary tumors; NSCLC, non-small cell carcinoma; FAP, familial adenomatous polyposis; LI, labeling index; WBF, wheat bran fiber; q.o.d., every other day; BCC, basal cell carcinoma; CIN, cervical intraepithelial neoplasia; CIN 1, mild dysplasia; CIN 2, moderate dysplasia; CIN 3, severe dysplasia; HLI, human leukocyte interferon; IFN; interferon.

* Modified and updated from Table 2 of Lippman et al. (52)

those involving extensive multiple lesions or field carcinogenesis, that is, carcinogenic exposure of the field extending from the oral cavity to the lungs (55). These cases cannot be controlled by local therapy.

Oral leukoplakia is an excellent model system for clinical testing of chemopreventive agents with potential activity throughout the aerodigestive tract. This lesion is related to tobacco use and associated with squamous cell carcinoma; is easily monitored clinically, cytologically, and histologically; and is related to carcinogenesis in other aerodigestive tract sites (54, 55). The oral leukoplakia system has been used for clinical laboratory translational studies of agent effects on histopathologic and other intermediate end point biomarkers of carcinogenesis (56, 57).

Systemic retinoid, β-carotene, vitamin E, and selenium intervention have been active in uncontrolled chemoprevention trials in oral leukoplakia (54–59). Only the retinoids have had their preliminary activity confirmed in randomized trials (60–64). In the only other randomized drug intervention trial significant activity was reported with topical bleomycin (65). Although interesting, the potential value of this local approach is limited by its inability to treat the diffuse aerodigestive epithelial field at risk.

Five randomized retinoid trials in oral premalignancy have been reported. The first of these, reported in 1986, was a short-term, placebo-controlled, double-blind study of high-dose isotretinoin (60). Forty-four subjects received either 3 months of 1 to 2 mg/kg/d of isotretinoin or placebo. Major clinical responses occurred in 67% (16/24) of isotretinoin recipients and in 10% (2/20) of placebo recipients ($P = .0002$). Histologic major responses (reversal of atypia) occurred in 54% (13/24) of isotretinoin recipients and 10% (2/20) of placebo recipients ($P = .01$). Although isotretinoin was active, over half of responders recurred or developed new lesions within 3 months of stopping it. Also, the high-dose isotretinoin regimen was unacceptably toxic for long-term use.

A second randomized trial was conducted to solve the toxicity and relapse problems encountered in the first (61). In an induction phase, 70 patients received high-dose isotretinoin therapy (1.5 mg/kg/d for 3 months). In a subsequent maintenance phase, stable and responding patients were randomized to 9 months of low-dose isotretinoin (0.5 mg/kg/d) or β-carotene (30 mg/d). Fifty-three subjects qualified for full evaluation. Treatment failure (disease progression or new lesion development) during or after maintenance therapy was 8% (2/24) and 55% (16/29) in the isotretinoin and β-carotene groups, respectively ($P < .001$). The toxic effects of low-dose isotretinoin therapy were generally mild, although significantly greater than those of β-carotene. The maintenance isotretinoin dose produced tolerable and reversible mucocutaneous dryness and hypertriglyceridemia.

The three other randomized trials reported significant retinoid activity in oral premalignancy. Natural vitamin A had significant activity in a 6-month placebo-controlled trial in 54 Asian betel nut chewers (62). The synthetic retinamide, *N*-4-(hydroxycarbophenyl) retinamide had significant activity in a 4-month placebo-controlled trial (63). A maintenance trial of fenretinide versus no treatment in preventing relapse or new lesion development after complete laser resection of premalignant oral lesions is ongoing (64). Parallelling results in the earlier low-dose isotretinoin maintenance trial (61), recent interim results on 137 randomized patients who received no treatment or fenretinide at a dose of 200 mg/d for 52 weeks and with 1-year follow-up, indicate a significantly lower failure rate in the retinoid arm. There were 11 treatment failures (9 recurrences, 2 new premalignant oral lesions, 0 cancers) in the fenretinide arm and 21 treatment failures (8 recurrences, 12 new lesions, and 1 cancer) in the no-treatment control arm (64).

Adjunctive laboratory studies of retinoic acid receptors and p53 have been integrated into recent clinical retinoid trials in oral premalignancy. Earlier in vitro and in vivo studies show that expression of the RAR-β mRNA is sequentially lost with carcinogenic progression to dysplasia and cancer in the head and neck, and that RAR-β expression can be up-regulated by retinoic acid in vitro in cancer cell lines. In a recent prospective isotretinoin trial, RAR-β mRNA was detected via in situ hybridization with antisense RNA in only 21 (40%) of 52 premalignant oral lesions ($P = 0.003$) (66). RAR-β mRNA expression increased significantly in response to high-dose isotretinoin (from 40% to 90%, $P < .001$), in direct association with clinical response ($P = .04$). These translational data conform with strong preclinical data indicating that RAR-β is the nuclear receptor most highly regulated by retinoids. These prospective results in human specimens also support the earlier evidence of loss of RAR-β expression in the development of head and neck cancer, and of up-regulation of RAR-β involvement in retinoid chemopreventive activity in the head and neck.

Studies of p53 are another major area of translational research within head and neck cancer chemoprevention trials. Frequent alterations of the p53 gene and its protein product occur in head and neck cancer and in adjacent normal-appearing and premalignant tissue (67, 68). Also, retinoids appear to modulate p53 mRNA and p53 protein levels associated with carcinogenesis in certain in vitro systems. Based on these findings, a study of p53 was conducted in the retinoid–oral premalignancy model (69). With the use of a very sensitive microwave technique, a wide range of p53 protein levels was detected in 40 (89%) of 45 lesions but not in any of eight oral cavity specimens from seven healthy nonsmoking controls. The level of protein accumulation was directly related to histologic severity ($P < .001$) that resembles recent findings in lung (70) and esophageal (71) premalignant lesions. The pattern of p53 expression also varied according to histologic grade. Expression of p53 in the parabasal layer increased in direct association with increasing histologic severity. This prospective study also revealed a lack of p53 modulation by isotretinoin, and a significant correlation between lesion resistance to isotretinoin and levels of p53 accumulation ($P = .006$). The mechanism of this resistance is not clear. It may involve a lesser up-regulation of RAR-β, also observed in nonresponding lesions. Other genetic alterations are associated with altered p53 function and may contribute to retinoid resistance.

Prevention of Second Primary Tumors

Compelling factors support the testing of retinoids in the adjuvant setting of second primary tumor prevention after definitive therapy of primary head and neck cancer (54–56). Oral premalignancy, which is linked to second primary tumor development through field carcinogenesis and other shared etiologic and biologic features, responds to retinoids. Second primary tumors occur in a diffuse pattern throughout the aerodigestive tract and bladder, making them beyond the control of local therapies. Second primary tumors are a major cause of death following "cure" of head and neck cancer and are the leading cancer-related cause of death after resection of early-stage disease. Second primary tumors develop at a constant rate of approximately 6% per year (52).

The first phase III adjuvant trial to prevent these second primary tumors involved high-dose isotretinoin (72). Following definitive local therapy of primary head and neck tumors, 103 patients received either isotretinoin (100 $mg/m^2/d$) or placebo for 1 year. This isotretinoin regimen was intolerable, and protocol doses were reduced after the first 44 enrolled patients to start at 50 $mg/m^2/d$. At a median follow-up for all patients of 32 months, the rate of second primary tumors was significantly lower in the retinoid group (4%) than in the placebo group (24%) ($P = .005$). The retinoid, however, had no significant effect on disease recurrence, disease-free survival, or overall survival.

A follow-up analysis of this trial after a median of 55 months was recently reported (73). Isotretinoin's protective effect against all second primary tumors had decreased since the 32-month follow-up but remained statistically significant ($P = .04$). In the subset of only tobacco-related second primary tumors, the retinoid's protective effect remained at a similar level of statistical significance ($P = .008$). Reversible retinoid effects in all second primary tumors and other carcinogenic settings are the norm. The strong long-term retinoid effect, absent treatment, against these tobacco-related second primary tumors is unprecedented.

Stringent prospective methods employed to effect surgical salvage of second primary tumor patients (most of whom came from the placebo group) may have masked the retinoid's ability to improve survival. The study population included a large percentage of patients with stages III and IV disease, who frequently experience early treatment failure and death from primary disease recurrence. Therefore, this trial could not indicate whether isotretinoin can improve survival in patients with early-stage disease.

Isotretinoin's significant activity in this initial second primary tumor prevention trial led to a multicenter, phase III trial of isotretinoin that was designed to prevent second primary tumors associated with stage I and II head and neck cancer. This trial's design called for low-dose isotretinoin to solve the toxicity problems encountered in the first trial. An interim report of this ongoing trial, which included 268 total patients (divided into two arms), 64% of whom were treated for at least 6 months and 26% for at least 1 year, indicates that the low-dose regimen is well tolerated (74). These toxicity data confirm the results from the smaller oral premalignancy maintenance trial that included 58 evaluable patients (26 on low-dose isotretinoin) who had completed at least 1 month of the planned 9-month maintenance therapy (61).

Investigators in France recently assessed the efficacy of the synthetic retinoid etretinate in preventing second primary tumors following definitive therapy of stage I-III squamous cell carcinomas of the oral cavity and oral pharynx (75). By random assignment, patients received either etretinate or placebo at doses of 50 mg/d for 1 month, followed by 25 mg/d for 2 years. Second primary tumor rates in the two study arms did not differ significantly. Interpretation of this trial was clouded by insufficient details on study compliance and second primary tumor diagnostic criteria. Still, certain valuable data were reported. The French trial confirmed earlier prospective data on the high rate of second primary tumors associated with head and neck cancer. After 41 months' median follow-up, 24% of placebo recipients had developed second primary tumors. Also, data from this trial support the field carcinogenesis theory concerning aerodigestive tract cancers: approximately 80% of second primary tumors developed in the head and neck, lungs, or esophagus.

LUNG

Premalignancy

Premalignant conditions of the lung have been the arena for several chemoprevention trials. The early report of an uncontrolled trial of etretinate (25 mg/d) for 6 months in heavy smokers raised enthusiasm for this approach in the lung (76). Metaplasia was assessed in bronchoscopic biopsy specimens. Twenty-nine of 40 participants experienced a reduction in metaplasia index, the mean reduction being from 35% before treatment to 27% after. It appeared that the retinoid had effectively reversed squamous metaplasia. Two randomized trials of retinoids in smokers with metaplasia soon followed.

The first of these trials was a placebo-controlled trial of etretinate for the reversal of metaplasia appearing in sputum samples (77). Therapy lasted 6 months. Metaplasia was reversed in the sputum of 32% of etretinate subjects and 30% of placebo subjects. The second trial was a placebo-controlled trial of isotretinoin (78). As in the uncontrolled French trial, this trial evaluated metaplasia in bronchial biopsy specimens. By random assignment, 87 subjects received either placebo or isotretinoin for 6 months. Both study groups experienced a substantial reduction in metaplasia index: 54% in the isotretinoin arm and 60% in the placebo arm. Smoking cessation was closely correlated with a significant reduction in the index of metaplasia. These two randomized trials strongly suggest that the French study's conclusion of retinoid activity (76) was invalid. They emphasize the necessity of confirming preliminary, single-arm trial results with placebo-controlled testing.

Another randomized, placebo-controlled trial in metaplasia, involving the combination of folic acid and vitamin B_{12} for 4 months in 73 smokers, has been completed (79). The folic acid–vitamin B_{12} treatment group reportedly had a significant improvement in atypia over the placebo group ($P = .02$). This result is questionable, however. The sample size was small, substantial spontaneous and interobserver variability occurred in regard to atypia assessed in subjects' sputum, and complex and nonstandard statistical methods were used to analyze results. When subjected to standard statistical analysis, this study's sputum cytology results showed no significant difference in atypia between the placebo and treatment groups (52).

A placebo-controlled trial of β-carotene in smokers used biomarker changes—sputum micronuclei frequency and urinary 8-oxo-7,8-dihydro-2′-deoxyguanosine (8-oxodG)—rather than metaplasia, dysplasia, or cancer as study end points. The nonspecific marker of DNA damage, micronuclei frequency, was reduced significantly (80), and the marker of oxidative DNA damage, 8-oxodG, was unchanged (81) in the β-carotene arm. There was no correlation between these two markers of DNA damage ($r = +.035$) and these results were not compared with any clinical or histologic endpoints.

The most recently reported intermediate end point trial in the lung was a randomized, placebo-controlled trial of β-carotene (50 mg/d) plus retinol (25,000 IU every other day) in 755 asbestos workers (82). The study was designed to test whether the natural agent combination could reduce the incidence and prevalence of atypical cells in the sputum. With a mean follow-up of 58 months, there was no significant reduction in the prevalence of sputum atypia or in progression to more severe degrees of atypia.

Metaplasia and dysplasia in sputum or bronchial biopsy specimens are the most studied intermediate end points in the lung. They frequently improve spontaneously. This has led to positive results in noncomparison trials, that have not held up in randomized placebo-controlled trials. Fluorescent localization techniques might make metaplasia and dysplasia more useful intermediate end points because of more precise monitoring of these otherwise grossly invisible lesions. New and more specific intermediate end point biomarkers are also needed for chemoprevention trials in the lung.

PREVENTION OF PRIMARY LUNG CANCER

A recent NCI-sponsored phase III trial of α-tocopherol and β-carotene to prevent primary lung cancer involved 29,133 male smokers between 50 and 69 years of age who had smoked an average of one pack of cigarettes per day for approximately 36 years (83). This trial's 2 × 2 factorial design called for α-tocopherol (50 mg/d) and β-carotene (20 mg/d) to be given in a randomized, double-blind, placebo-controlled fashion. The factorial design allowed the study scientists to assess the individual effects of each agent. Significant increases in lung cancer incidence (18% increase, $P = .01$) and total mortality (8%, $P = .02$) occurred in the β-carotene-treated subjects after 6.1 years' median follow-up. α-Tocopherol had no significant impact on the lung cancer mortality rate, and there was no evidence of an interaction between α-tocopherol and β-carotene. The β-carotene results from this large-scale phase III trial are consistent with experimental lung carcinogenesis studies (84). These laboratory data and definitive clinical results contradict the epidemiologic data on β-carotene and underscore the need to confirm data of this type before public health recommendations are made.

The other major NCI phase III lung cancer chemoprevention trial is ongoing. This placebo-controlled trial is testing the combination of β-carotene (30 mg/d) plus retinyl palmitate (25,000 IU/d) in 17,000 smokers and asbestos workers (52, 53). This trial, called CARET (β-Carotene and Retinol Efficacy Trial), has provided detailed data on the long-term tolerability of this natural agent combination.

PREVENTION OF SECOND PRIMARY TUMORS

Second primary tumors in lung cancer are related to those associated with head and neck cancer through etiology, region, and biology. An adjuvant trial of the natural vitamin A ester retinyl palmitate achieved a significant reduction in lung second primary tumors (85). Patients were randomly assigned to receive either 300,000 IU of retinyl palmitate daily (150 patients) or no treatment (157 patients) for 12 months following complete resection of stage I non-small cell lung cancer. Compliance was over 80%, and toxic effects were minimal.

At a median follow-up of 46 months, second primary tumors occurred in 29 (48%) of control patients and in 18 (39%) of retinyl palmitate recipients. Thirteen patients in the retinoid group and 25 in the control group developed tobacco-related second primary tumors. The time to development of tobacco-related second primary tumors was significantly shorter in the control arm than in the retinoid arm ($P = .045$). Recurrence rates were not significantly different in the two study arms. The 5-year estimated disease-free and overall survival rates were not significantly different between the retinoid (64% and 62%, respectively) and placebo (51% and 54%, respectively) groups ($P = .054$ and .44, respectively). The survival impact of retinyl palmitate in this trial may have been blunted by surgical salvage of second primary tumors.

These encouraging results with second primary tumors and retinoid activity in related carcinogenic systems led to two large-scale, ongoing phase III retinoid trials in the setting of second primary tumor prevention, one in Europe and the other in the United States (52, 53). The European trial, called Euroscan, is a multicenter trial of retinyl palmitate and *N*-acetylcysteine (in a 2 × 2 factorial design) to prevent second primary tumors following definitive therapy of early-stage head and neck and lung cancer. The U.S. multicenter trial (intergroup NCI I 91–0001) involves low-dose isotretinoin to prevent second primary tumors after definitive therapy of stage I non-small cell lung cancer. Several other phase III trials in this setting are in the design phase.

There is a great need for chemoprevention study in small cell lung cancer (86). Patients cured of small cell lung cancer develop second primary tumors at an alarmingly high rate (approximately twofold higher than the rate of second primary tumors related to head and neck cancer), which actually increases over time. Second primary tumors are the most common cause of cancer death 4 or more years after definitive primary therapy for small cell lung cancer. Second primary tumors related to small cell lung cancer occur most frequently in tobacco-exposed sites, with non-small cell lung cancer being the most common. The non-small cell lung cancer that develops in this setting is usually unresectable, further indicating the pressing need for chemoprevention.

COLON AND RECTUM

Colorectal trial designs have primarily employed the intermediate end points of adenomatous polyp development and response and hyperproliferation markers. Several NSAIDs, calcium salts, and vitamins-micronutrient combinations have been studied in the prevention of colon cancer.

Inhibition of colon carcinogenesis in laboratory models by drugs in the NSAID class may perhaps be due to local suppression of prostaglandin synthesis. Aspirin's ability to inhibit colon carcinogenesis is suggested by epidemiologic studies of colon cancer and adenomas (87). Piroxicam, reported to suppress rectal mucosal prostaglandin E_2 levels (but not cell proliferation) in an uncontrolled study, is currently being studied in a randomized trial (88).

Sulindac data in familial polyposis are the most promising chemoprevention results in the colon to date. Trials of this agent have focused on polyp response. Sulindac has produced reversible responses of polyps in patients with Gardner's syndrome and familial polyposis in uncontrolled trials (89). Two subsequent randomized trials of sulindac in patients with familial adenomatous polyposis have been reported that confirm the earlier favorable indications (90, 91).

The only cancer incidence trial data in the colon come from the low-dose aspirin arm of the U.S. Physicians' Health Study. No significant aspirin effect on the incidence of colon polyps or cancer was detected (92). A highly significant reduction in myocardial infarction among aspirin recipients, however, led to early closure of this arm after 5 years' average follow-up. This eliminated the possibility of detecting a potential long-term effect of aspirin on cancer development in the colon.

Early uncontrolled clinical trials of calcium in the colon were based on positive data from preclinical studies and epidemiologic surveys. Although positive (93), these early trials had a major methodologic limitation in their designs. Subjects with very high proliferative rates were selected, and it is not certain that the decrease in cell proliferation observed after calcium administration in certain patients was caused by calcium rather than by a statistical regression to the mean.

Seven randomized chemoprevention trials of calcium were based on the positive uncontrolled results (94–100). These randomized trials employed response of overall cell proliferation rates (e.g., determined by tritiated thymidine labeling index and proliferating cell nuclear antigen) within the crypts of colonic mucosa as their end points.

Results of the randomized calcium trials have been mostly negative. The two positive trials, which reported marginally significant suppression of epithelial cell proliferation in adenoma polyp patients, included one trial that enrolled only 14 total patients. The other, a 20-patient trial, was flawed by a single-blind design and analysis of only study adherers (94, 97). None of the other five studies, including a trial of over 300 patients, found that calcium significantly suppressed overall cell proliferation. In two studies, a nearly significant (P = .06) increase in cell proliferation occurred in the calcium arm compared to the placebo arm.

Epidemiologic data consistently show that diets high in fat and low in fruits, vegetables, and fiber are associated with an increased risk of colon cancer (101). Randomized trials of dietary interventions are now under way (102–112). One such trial is of wheat bran, which unlike oat bran fiber, has been shown to reduce fecal mutagen activity (103).

Trials of vitamins alone in the colon have achieved largely negative results (Table 29.1). The largest randomized trial of β-carotene or combined vitamins C and E given in a placebo-controlled, 2 × 2 factorial fashion was recently completed (113). Lasting 4 years, this study included 864 patients with at least one histologically confirmed colorectal adenoma within 3 months of study entry, and excluded patients with familial polyposis or a history of colorectal cancer. Neither β-carotene nor the vitamin combination was active.

Current phase I–II trials in the colon are evaluating new agents (such as DFMO and oltipraz) and agent combinations, such as calcium plus fiber and calcium plus NSAIDs.

SKIN

Chemoprevention trials in reversing premalignant skin lesions (e.g., actinic keratoses) and in preventing skin cancer have been conducted. Topical application of the retinoid tretinoin has exhibited dose-related activity against actinic keratoses in nonrandomized and randomized trials (114). Systemic retinoid therapy has achieved significant activity against actinic keratoses in two placebo-controlled trials (115, 116).

The NCI has sponsored a series of small trials of isotretinoin that achieved reductions in skin tumor incidence. One of these trials was conducted in five xeroderma pigmentosum patients at extremely high risk for developing nonmelanoma skin cancer (117). This trial achieved a significant reduction in the number of skin cancers during the 2 years of high-dose isotretinoin (2 mg/kg/d) treatment (P = .02). Subsequent studies from these investigators have shown that this chemopreventive effect was dose related. The beneficial effect of this approach was lost after cessation of treatment. A randomized placebo-controlled trial of the retinoid acitretin in 38 renal transplant recipients was recently reported (118). This study showed significant reductions in premalignant lesions and skin cancers. The chemopreventive effects were reversible after the 6-month retinoid intervention.

Four large-scale, long-term phase III chemoprevention trials have been conducted in subjects at much lower risk of developing skin cancer (119–121). Only one of these trials was positive. In this trial, retinol (25,000 IU/d) significantly reduced the incidence of primary squamous cell (but not basal cell) skin cancer in patients with actinic keratosis (121). The other three trials, all negative, involved β-carotene (119), retinol (121), and very low-dose isotretinoin (120, 121) in patients with previous skin cancers. The contrast between the one positive and three negative trials raises several issues to be considered in future skin cancer chemoprevention trials, including retinoid dose, biologic timing of intervention, and histopathology (squamous cell versus basal cell). These studies and others suggest that current chemoprevention approaches are most active in early phases of carcinogenesis, i.e., activity in the setting of premalignancy but not in the setting of previous cancer.

The NCI has also sponsored an ongoing U.S. trial of selenium to prevent skin cancer in regions with low endogenous levels. This trial is based on case-control and prospective cohort epidemiologic studies showing an association between low selenium and an increased risk of skin cancer (53).

BREAST

The retinoid fenretinide has exhibited potent chemopreventive activity in breast carcinogenesis models and a favorable clinical toxicity profile. These data led to a large-scale, placebo-controlled Italian trial of fenretinide to prevent contralateral breast cancer (second primary tumors) in approximately 3,000 women who had previously undergone resection for early-stage (node-negative) breast cancer (122). Contralateral breast cancers in this setting occur at a rate of approximately 0.8% per year. The intervention will last 5 years and consists of 200 mg of fenretinide per day, with monthly 3-day drug holidays to avoid ocular toxicity (reduced night vision) associated with fenretinide-induced reductions in plasma retinol levels. Preliminary data indicate significant 4-HPR activity in preventing contralateral breast cancer in premenopausal (but not postmenopausal) women. (A. Costa, personal communication, November 1995). In a recent interim analysis after over 60,000 person-months' follow-up on each study arm, fenretinide had achieved a secondary study end point of suppressing ovarian cancer (123): six new cases of ovarian cancer developed in the control group, versus no new cases in the fenretinide group ($P =$ .016). This trial has also provided important information on the long-term tolerability of this promising synthetic retinoid.

Tamoxifen is the other major chemoprevention agent studied thus far in the breast. Pooled data from over 30,000 women in 40 randomized adjuvant trials (124) show a highly significant 39% reduction in overall contralateral second primary tumor rates within the tamoxifen treatment groups over non-tamoxifen-treated groups ($P <$ .00001). Tamoxifen's significant preventive effects required long-term treatment and were most significant in postmenopausal women. Tamoxifen has several major potential favorable and adverse effects, discussed elsewhere (52, 53) (see Chapter 73), which have greatly affected breast chemoprevention designs.

The efficacy of single-agent tamoxifen in preventing breast cancer in high-risk women will be determined by large-scale trials, now under way throughout the world. The National Surgical Adjuvant Breast and Bowel Project (NSABP) is conducting one of these trials, which will enroll 16,000 women at twofold greater than average risk of developing breast cancer. The trial will also systematically evaluate tamoxifen's potential beneficial effects on women's cardiovascular and skeletal systems.

In vivo laboratory studies have shown that the combination of fenretinide and tamoxifen is significantly more active than either agent alone in suppressing mammary carcinogenesis. This combination was also active in a recent phase I study in patients with advanced breast cancer; the regimen was well tolerated and produced a substantial reduction in plasma IGF-I levels (125). A recently designed phase III U.S. breast cancer chemoprevention trial will study the combination in high-risk women.

ESOPHAGUS AND STOMACH

In the United States, esophageal carcinoma is strongly associated with tobacco and alcohol abuse. Causes of this cancer in other parts of the world, such as China, however, appear to include nutritional deficiencies and exposure to carcinogens, such as N-nitroso compounds.

Five large placebo-controlled chemoprevention trials against esophageal/gastric carcinogenesis have been conducted. Three were Phase IIb trials and two were Phase III trials. Subjects for these trials came from geographic regions with established high risks of esophageal/gastric cancers. Four trials were of multiple natural compounds. The applicability of the findings in developing countries to esophageal cancer in the United States and other developed countries with different epidemiologic risk profiles is not clear.

The first placebo-controlled, randomized trial to reverse esophageal carcinogenesis was conducted in Huixian, China (126). This trial was based on several factors, including epidemiologic and endoscopic studies in high-risk geographic areas. Subjects received a combination of retinol, riboflavin, and zinc for 13.5 months. The intervention achieved no overall reduction in the occurrence of premalignant lesions (126). Two subset analyses revealed that (1) micronuclei frequency in the esophagus, but not in the oral cavity, decreased significantly in association with the chemopreventive regimen (127) and (2) increased plasma micronutrient levels (primarily retinol) were associated with a reduction in dysplastic lesions, regardless of treatment arm (128). This trial also illustrated an issue of concern to many investigators studying vitamins, minerals, and micronutrients. Plasma micronutrient levels in the Huixian trial increased substantially in about 50% of placebo recipients. Evidently these control subjects obtained readily available trial compounds via their diet or in over-the-counter preparations of vitamins and minerals. Poor study compliance, either in the form of drop-ins or dropouts, can greatly reduce the statistical power of a randomized trial.

The second phase IIb trial was conducted in Uzbekistan. Retinol, β-carotene, and vitamin E with or without riboflavin were given in a factorial design to high-risk subjects with oral leukoplakia and/or chronic esophagitis (129). As in the Huixian study, none of the vitamin regimens had a significant effect on esophageal premalignancy.

Two NCI placebo-controlled phase III trials of multiple vitamins and minerals were conducted in the high-risk area of Linxian, China. One trial employed a complex modified factorial design to test four different vitamin-mineral combinations given to 29,584 subjects for 5 years at doses of one to two times the U.S. RDA (130). The combination of β-carotene, α-tocopherol, and selenium was associated with 4% and 21% reductions in the esophageal cancer and gastric cancer mortality rates, respectively. The gastric cancer mortality reduction was significant ($P <$ .05). In the other phase III trial, only higher risk subjects with esophageal dysplasia received either 26 vitamins and minerals (including β-carotene, α-tocopherol, and selenium, at two to three times the U.S. RDA) or placebo in a straightforward two-arm design (131). This intervention was associated with two non-significant changes: an 18% increase in the mortality from gastric cancer and a 16% reduction in the mortality from esophageal cancer. Interpretation of these two contrasting studies is made difficult by the many different interventions and end points.

A recent placebo-controlled study of 220 subjects from Venezuela reported no significant effect of bismuth and amoxicillin on *Helicobacter pylori* eradication rates (132). The bacterium *H. pylori* has been implicated in the etiology of gastric carcinogenesis.

BLADDER

In vivo animal model, in vitro, and epidemiologic studies have shown that retinoids are active against bladder carcinogenesis (133). The retinoid etretinate has been tested in three randomized clinical trials in patients following resection of superficial bladder tumors (134–136). Two of these trials employed prolonged low-dose etretinate, that appeared to be effective (134, 136). Results of the two positive trials require confirmation, however, because of these trials' limited patient numbers and follow-up. A fourth randomized trial compared a multivitamin preparation at recommended dietary allowance (RDA) levels alone or supplemented with 40,000 IU retinol, 100 mg pyridoxine, 2,000 mg ascorbic acid, 400 units of alpha-tocopherol and 90 mg zinc. The estimated 5-year tumor recurrence rate was 91% in the RDA arm versus 41% in the megadose arm (p=0.0014) (137).

Fenretinide is a leading candidate for new trials in bladder cancer chemoprevention. This retinoid has a high therapeutic index against rodent bladder carcinogenesis and has produced encouraging clinical results in a phase IIa trial (138).

CERVIX

The characteristic multistep histologic evolution of cervical carcinogenesis, the well-documented rates of progression and spontaneous regression within each histopathologic grade (CIN 1, 2, and 3), and ease in monitoring make cervical carcinogenesis an excellent human model for studying chemoprevention agents.

Cervical dysplasia has been studied in eight randomized trials. Four of these trials involved locally applied interferon and were negative (139–142). Two involved folic acid and were negative (143, 144). One involved β-carotene and was negative (145). Only one of the several trials was positive, and it involved the retinoid tretinoin (146).

The positive, randomized tretinoin trial proceeded from years of extensive phase I–IIa study of topical tretinoin in cervical dysplasia. The previous phase IIa trial employed a 0.372% solution of tretinoin delivered by an inert collagen sponge in a cervical cap for a period of 1 year. The initial protocol called for giving the drug for 4 days. Subsequently the dose was given for 2 days every 3 months. Complete responses occurred in 50% of cases (147). The positive placebo-controlled phase IIb trial was completed recently (146). Also using an intermittent schedule of locally applied tretinoin, this trial was conducted in 301 subjects—141 with biopsy-proved moderate (CIN 2) cervical dysplasia and 160 with severe (CIN 3) dysplasia. Compared to placebo, tretinoin had significant activity in moderate dysplasia (complete regression rates of 43% vs 27%, $P = .04$) but not severe dysplasia. This tretinoin delivery system was associated with some toxic effects, primarily mild vaginal inflammation, that occurred in fewer than 5% of participants. Problems with study adherence have cast a shadow over the positive aspect of this trial.

CHEMOPREVENTION AND OVERALL CANCER INCIDENCE

Two important large trials are under way to test the ability of chemoprevention to reduce overall cancer incidence. The Physicians' Health Study was begun in the United States in 1982. In this trial, β-carotene and aspirin are being given in a 2 × 2 factorial design to prevent cancer and cardiovascular disease in 22,071 male physicians (148). This trial's β-carotene results have yet to be reported. The Women's Health Study was begun more recently in the United States. This trial will determine the impact of β-carotene, vitamin E, and aspirin on cancer incidence and cardiovascular disease incidence in over 40,000 female nurses (149). These two enormous primary chemoprevention trials will require long-term follow-up to assess results because of the subjects' low cancer risks. These trial designs are extremely expensive and fraught with logistic difficulties, but may eventually have a major impact on public health.

References

1. Devesa SS, Blot WJ, Stone BJ, Miller BA, Tarone RE, Fraumeni JF Jr. Recent cancer trends in the United States. JNCI 1995;87:175–182.
2. Sporn MB, Dunlop NM, Newton DL, Smith JM. Prevention of chemical carcinogenesis by vitamin A and its synthetic analogues (retinoids). Fed Proc 1976;35:1332–1338.
3. Sporn MB. Carcinogenesis and cancer: different perspectives on the same disease. Cancer Res 1991;51:6215–6218.
4. Wattenberg LW. Chemoprevention of cancer. Cancer Res 1985;45:1–8.
5. Symposium on early lesions and the development of epithelial cancer. Cancer Res 1976;36:2475–2706.
6. Boone CW, Kelloff GJ, Steele VE. Natural history of intraepithelial neoplasia in humans with implications for cancer chemoprevention strategy. Cancer Res 1992;52:1651–59.
7. Cairns J. Mutation selection and the natural history of cancer. Nature 1975;255:197–200.
8. Sporn MB. Approaches to prevention of epithelial cancer during the preneoplastic period. Cancer Res 1976;36:2699–2702.
9. Fugh-Berman A, Epstein S. Tamoxifen: disease prevention or disease substitution? Lancet 1992;340:1143–1145.
10. Ross R. The pathogenesis of atherosclerosis: a perspective for the 1990s. Nature 1993;362:801–809.
11. Manson JE, Tosteson H, Ridker PM, et al. The primary prevention of myocardial infarction. N Engl J Med 1992;326:1406–1416.
12. Ames BN, Shigenaga MK, Hagen TM. Oxidants, antioxidants, and the degenerative diseases of aging. Proc Natl Acad Sci USA 1993;90:7915–7922.
13. Sporn MB, Roberts AB, Goodman DS, eds. The retinoids. 2nd ed. New York: Raven Press, 1994, 679 pp.
14. Dawson MI, Hobbs PD. The synthetic chemistry of retinoids. In The Retinoids, 2nd ed. Edited by MB Sporn, AB Roberts, DS Goodman. New York: Raven Press, 1994, pp 5–178.
15. Green S, Chambon P. A superfamily of potentially oncogenic hormone receptors. Nature 1986;324:615–617.
16. Evans RM. The steroid and thyroid hormone receptor super-family. Science 1988;240:889–895.
17. O'Malley B. The steroid receptor superfamily: more excitement predicted for the future. Mol Endocrinol 1990;4:363–69.
18. Wolbach SB, Howe PR. Tissue changes following deprivation of fat soluble A vitamin. J Exp Med 1925;42:753–777.
19. Sporn MB, Roberts AB. Role of retinoids in differentiation and carcinogenesis. Cancer Res 1983;43:3034–3040.
20. Lasnitzki I. The influence of A hypervitaminosis on the effect of 20-methylcholanthrene on mouse prostate glands grown in vitro. Br J Cancer 1955;9:434–441.
21. Merriman RL, Bertram JS. Reversible inhibition by retinoids of 3-methylcholanthrene-induced neoplastic transformation in C3H/10T1/2 CL8 cells. Cancer Res 1979;39:1661–1666.
22. Strickland S, Mahdavi V. The induction of differentiation in teratocarcinoma stem cells by retinoic acid. Cell 1978;15:393–403.
23. Breitman TR, Selonick SE, Collins SJ. Induction of differentiation of the human promyelocytic leukemia cell line (HL-60) by retinoic acid. Proc Natl Acad Sci USA 1980;77:2936–2940.
24. Gudas LJ, Sporn MB, Roberts AB. Cellular biology and biochemistry of the retinoids. In The Retinoids, 2nd ed. Edited by MB Sporn, AB Roberts, DS Goodman. New York; Raven Press, 1994, pp 443–520.
25. Allegretto EA, McClurg MR, Lazarchik SB, et al. Transactivation properties of retinoic acid and retinoid X receptors in mammalian cells and yeast. J Biol Chem 1993;268:26625–26633.
26. Allenby G, Janoch R, Kazmer S, Speck J, Grippo JF, Levin AA. Binding of 9-cis-retinoic acid and all-trans-retinoic acid to retinoic acid receptors α, β, and γ. J Biol Chem 1994;269:16689–16695.
27. Mangelsdorf DJ, Umesono K, Evans RM. The retinoid receptors. In The Retinoids, 2nd ed. Edited by MB Sporn, AB Roberts, DS Goodman. New York: Raven Press, 1994, pp 319–349.

28. Moon RC, Mehta RG, Rao KV. Retinoids and cancer in experimental animals. In The Retinoids, 2nd ed. Edited by MB Sporn, AB Roberts, DS Goodman. New York: Raven Press, 1994, pp 573–596.
29. Anzano MA, Byers SW, Smith JM, et al. Prevention of breast cancer in the rat with 9-cis-retinoic acid as a single agent and in combination with tamoxifen. Cancer Res 1994;54:4614–4617.
30. Jordan VC, ed. Long-Term Tamoxifen Treatment for Breast Cancer. Madison: University of Wisconsin Press, 1994, pp 289.
31. Jordan VC, Allen KE, Dix CJ. Pharmacology of tamoxifen in laboratory animals. Cancer Treat Rep 1980;64:745–749.
32. Gottardis MM, Jordan VC. Antitumor actions of keoxifene and tamoxifen in the N-nitrosomethylurea-induced rat mammary carcinoma model. Cancer Res 1987;47:4020–4024.
33. Knabbe C, Lippman ME, Wakefield LM, et al. Evidence that TGF-β is a hormonally regulated negative growth factor in human breast cancer cells. Cell 1987;48:417–428.
34. Colletta AA, Wakefield LM, Howell LM, et al. Antioestrogens induce the secretion of active TGF-β from human fetal fibroblasts. Br J Cancer 1990;62:405–409.
35. Butta A, MacLennan K, Flanders KC, et al. Induction of transforming growth factor β1 in human breast cancer in vivo following tamoxifen treatment. Cancer Res 1992;52:4261–4264.
36. Nolvadex Adjuvant Trial Organization Controlled trial of tamoxifen as a single adjuvant agent in the management of early breast cancer. Br J Cancer 1988;57:608–611.
37. Colletti RB, Roberts JD, Devlin JT, Copeland KC. Effect of tamoxifen on plasma insulin-like growth factor I in patients with breast cancer. Cancer Res 1989;49:1882–1884.
38. Pollak MJ, Costantino C, Polychronakos SA, et al. Effect of tamoxifen on serum insulin-like growth factor I levels in stage I breast cancer patients. JNCI 1990;82:1693–1697.
39. Black LJ, Sato M, Rowley ER, et al. Raloxifene (LY139481 HCl) prevents bone loss and reduces serum cholesterol without causing uterine hypertrophy in ovariectomized rats. J Clin Invest 1994;93:63–69.
40. Lowe KE, Maiyar AC, Norman AW. Vitamin D–mediated gene expression. Crit Rev Eukaryot Gene Expr 1992;2:65–109.
41. Studzinski GP, McLane JA, Uskokovic MR. Signalling pathways for vitamin D-induced differentiation: implications for therapy of proliferative and neoplastic diseases. Crit Rev Eukaryot Gene Expr 1993;3:279–312.
42. Ikekawa N, Ishizuka S. Molecular structure and biological activity of vitamin D metabolites and their analogues. In Molecular Structure and Biological Activity of Steroids. Edited by M Bol, WL Daux. Boca Raton: CRC Press, 1992, pp 293–316.
43. Anzano MA, Smith JM, Uskokovic MR, et al. 1α,25-Dihydroxy-16-ene-23-yne-26,27-hexafluorocholecalciferol (Ro24-5531), a new deltanoid (vitamin D analogue) for prevention of breast cancer in the rat. Cancer Res 1994;54:1653–1656.
44. Colston KW, Mackay AG, James SY, Binderup L, Chander S, Coombes RC. EB1089: a new vitamin D analogue that inhibits the growth of breast cancer cells in vivo and in vitro. Biochem Pharmacol 1992;44:2273–2280.
45. Stoner E. The clinical effects of a 5α-reductase inhibitor, finasteride, on benign prostatic hyperplasia. The Finasteride Study Group. J Urol 1992;147:1298–1302.
46. Pegg AE. Polyamine metabolism and its importance in neoplastic growth and as a target for chemotherapy. Cancer Res 1988;48:759–774.
47. Ratko TA, Detrisac CJ, Rao KV, Thomas CF, Kelloff GJ, Moon RC. Interspecies analysis of the chemopreventive efficacy of dietary α-difluoromethylornithine. Anticancer Res 1990;10:67–72.
48. Reddy BS. Inhibitors of the arachidonic acid cascade and their chemoprevention of colon carcinogenesis. In Cancer Chemoprevention. Edited by L Wattenberg, M Lipkin, CW Boone, GJ Kelloff. Boca Raton: CRC Press, 1992, pp 153–164.
49. Prestera T, Zhang Y, Spencer SR, Wilczak CA, Talalay P. The electrophile counterattack response: protection against neoplasia and toxicity. Adv Enzyme Regul 1993;33:281–296.
50. DeFlora S, Izzotti A, D'Agostini F, Balansky R, Cesarone CF. Chemopreventive properties of *N*-acetylcysteine and other thiols. In Cancer Chemoprevention. Edited by L Wattenberg, M Lipkin, CW Boone, GJ Kelloff. Boca Raton: CRC Press, 1992, pp 183–194.
51. Kensler TW, Egner PA, Trush MA, Bueding E, Groopman JD, Roebuck BD. Mechanisms of protection against aflatoxin tumorigenicity in rats fed 5-(2-pyrazinyl)-4-methyl-1,2-dithiol-3-thione (oltipraz) and related 1,2-dithiol-3-thiones and 1,2-dithiol-3-ones. Cancer Res 1987;47:4271–4277.
52. Lippman SM, Benner SE, Hong WK. Cancer chemoprevention. J Clin Oncol 1994;12:851–873.
53. Lippman SM, Benner SE, Hong WK. The chemoprevention of cancer. In Cancer Prevention and Control. Edited by P Greenwald P, BS Kramer, DL Weed. New York: Marcel Dekker, 1995, pp 329–352.
54. Vokes EE, Weichselbaum RR, Lippman SM, et al. Head and neck cancer. N Engl J Med 1993;328:184–194.
55. Lippman SM, Hong WK. Retinoid chemoprevention of upper aerodigestive tract carcinogenesis. In Important Advances in Oncology. Edited by VT DeVita, SA Hellman, SA Rosenberg. Philadelphia: Lippincott, 1992, pp 93–109.
56. Hong WK, Lippman SM, Wolf GT. Recent advances in head and neck cancer: larynx preservation and cancer chemoprevention. Cancer Res 1994;53:5113–5120.
57. Lippman SM, Lee JS, Lotan R, et al. Biomarkers as intermediate end points in chemoprevention trials. JNCI 1990;82:555–560.
58. Stich HF, Rosin MP, Hornby AP, et al. Remission of oral leukoplakia and micronuclei in tobacco/betel quid chewers treated with β-carotene and with β-carotene plus vitamin A. Int J Cancer 1988;42:195–199.
59. Benner SE, Winn RJ, Lippman SM, et al. Regression of oral leukoplakia with α-tocopherol: a community clinical oncology program chemoprevention study. JNCI 1993;85:44–47.
60. Hong WK, Endicott J, Itri LM, et al. 13-cis-retinoic acid in the treatment of oral leukoplakia. N Engl J Med 1986;315:1501–1505.
61. Lippman SM, Batsakis JG, Toth BB, et al. Comparison of low-dose isotretinoin with β-carotene to prevent oral carcinogenesis. N Engl J Med 1993;328:15–20.
62. Stich HF, Hornby AP, Mathew B, et al. Response of oral leukoplakias to the administration of vitamin A. Cancer Lett 1988;40:93–101.
63. Han J, Lu Y, Sun Z, et al. Evaluation of N-4-(hydroxycarbophenyl) retinamide as a cancer prevention agent and as a cancer chemotherapeutic agent. In Vivo 1990;4:153–160.
64. Chiesa F, Tradati N, Marazza M, Rossi N, Boracchi P, Mariani L, Formelli F, Giardini R, Costa A, DePalo G, Veronesi U. Fenretinide (4-HPR) in chemoprevention of oral leukoplakia. J Cell Biochem 1993;17F:255–261.
65. Epstein JB, Wong FLW, Millner A, Le ND. Topical bleomycin treatment of oral leukoplakia: a randomized double-blind clinical trial. Head Neck 1994;16:539–544.
66. Lotan R, Xu X-C, Lippman SM, Ro JY, Lee JS, Lee JJ, Hong WK. Suppression of retinoic acid receptor β in premalignant oral lesions and its upregulation by isotretinoin. N Engl J Med, 1995;332:1405–1410.
67. Shin DM, Kim J, Ro JY, et al. Activation of p53 gene expression in premalignant lesions during head and neck tumorigenesis. Cancer Res 1994;54:321–326.
68. Brennan JA, Boyle JO, Koch WM, et al. Association between cigarette smoking and mutation of the p53 gene in squamous-cell carcinoma of the head and neck. N Engl J Med 1995;332:712–717.
69. Lippman SM, Shin DM, Lee JJ, et al. p53 and retinoid chemoprevention of oral carcinogenesis. Cancer Res 1995;55:16–19.
70. Bennett WP, Colby TV, Travis WD, et al. p53 protein accumulates frequently in early bronchial neoplasia. Cancer Res 1993;53:4817–4822.
71. Gao H, Wang LD, Zhou Q, Hong JY, Huang TY, Yang CS. p53 tumor suppressor gene mutation in early esophageal precancerous lesions and carcinoma among high-risk populations in Henan, China. Cancer Res 1994;54:4342–4346.
72. Hong WK, Lippman SM, Itri LM, et al. Prevention of second primary tumors with isotretinoin in squamous-cell carcinoma of the head and neck. N Engl J Med 1990;323:795–801.
73. Benner SE, Pajak TF, Lippman SM, et al. Prevention of second primary tumors with isotretinoin in squamous cell carcinoma of the head and neck: long term follow-up. JNCI 1994;86:140–141.
74. Benner SE, Pajak TF, Lippman SM, et al. Toxicity of isotretinoin in a chemoprevention trial to prevent second primary tumors following head and neck cancer. JNCI 1994;86:1799–1801.
75. Bolla M, Lefur R, Ton Van J, et al. Prevention of second primary tumours with etretinate in squamous cell carcinoma of the oral cavity and oropharynx: results of a multicentric double-blind randomized study. Eur J Cancer 1994;30A:767–772.
76. Gouveia J, Mathe G, Hercend T, et al. Degree of bronchial metaplasia in heavy smokers and its regression after treatment with a retinoid. Lancet 1983;1:710–712.
77. Arnold AM, Browman GP, Levine MN, et al. The effect of the synthetic retinoid etretinate on sputum cytology: results from a randomized trial. Br J Cancer 1992;65:737–743.
78. Lee JS, Lippman SM, Benner SE, et al. A randomized placebo-controlled trial of isotretinoin in chemoprevention of bronchial squamous metaplasia. J Clin Oncol 1994;12:937–945.
79. Heimburger DC, Alexander B, Birch R, et al. Improvement in bronchial squamous metaplasia in smokers treated with folate and vitamin B_{12}: report of a preliminary randomized, double-blind intervention trial. JAMA 1988;259:1525–1530.
80. van Poppel G, Kok FJ, Hermus RJJ. Beta-carotene supplementation in smokers reduces the frequency of micronuclei in sputum. Br J Cancer 1992;66:1164–1168.
81. van Poppel G, Poulsen H, Loft, Verhagen H. No influence of β-carotene on oxidative DNA damage in male smokers. JNCI 1995;87:310–311.
82. McLarty J, Holiday DB, Dirard WM, Yanagihara RH, Kummet RD, Greenberg SD. Beta-carotene, vitamin A and lung cancer chemoprevention: results of an intermediate endpoint study. Presented at the Second International Conference on Antioxidant Vitamins and Beta-Carotene in Disease Prevention, Berlin, October 1994. Proceedings to be published as a supplement to the Am J Nutr, 1995.
83. The Alpha-Tocopherol, Beta-Carotene Cancer Prevention Study Group. The effect of vitamin E and beta-carotene on the incidence of lung cancer and other cancers in male smokers. N Engl J Med 1994;330:1029–1035.
84. Murakoshi M, Nishino H, Satomi Y, Takayasu J, Hasegawa T, Tokunda H, Iwashima A, Okuzumi J, Okabe H, Kitano H, Iwasaki R. Potent preventive action of α-carotene against carcinogenesis: spontaneous liver carcinogenesis and promoting stage of lung and skin carcinogenesis in mice are suppressed more effectively by α-carotene than by β-carotene. Cancer Res 1992;52:6583–6587.
85. Pastorino U, Infante M, Maioli M, et al. Adjuvant treatment of stage I lung cancer with high-dose vitamin A. J Clin Oncol 1993;11:1216–1222.
86. Heyne K, Lippman SM, Lee JJ, et al. The incidence of second primary tumors in long-term survivors of small cell lung cancer. J Clin Oncol 1992;10:1519–1524.
87. Greenberg ER, Baron JA, Freeman Jr DH, et al. Reduced risk of large-bowel adenomas among aspirin users. JNCI 1993;85:912–916.
88. Earnest DL, Hixson LJ, Fennerty MB, et al. Inhibition of prostaglandin synthesis: potential for chemoprevention of human colon cancer. Cancer Bull 1991;43:561–568.
89. Rigau J, Pique JM, Rubio E, et al. Effects of long-term sulindac therapy on colonic polyposis. Ann Intern Med 1991;115:952–954.
90. Labayle D, Fischer D, Vielh P, et al. Sulindac causes regression of rectal polyps in familial adenomatous polyposis. Gastroenterology 1991;101:635–639.
91. Giardiello FM, Hamilton SR, Krush AJ, et al. Treatment of colonic and rectal adenomas with sulindac in familial adenomatous polyposis. N Engl J Med 1993;328:1313–1316.
92. Gann PH, Manson JE, Glynn RJ, et al. Low-dose aspirin and incidence of colorectal tumors in a randomized trial. JNCI 1993;85:1220–1224.
93. Lipkin M, Newmark H. Effects of dietary calcium on colonic epithelial cell proliferation in subjects at high risk for familial colonic cancer. N Engl J Med 1985;313:1381–1384.
94. Wargovich MJ, Isbell G, Shabot M, et al. Calcium supplementation decreases rectal epithelial cell proliferation in subjects with sporadic adenoma. Gastroenterology 1992;103:92–97.
95. Stern HS, Gregorie RC, Koshtan H. Long-term effects of dietary calcium on risk markers for colon cancer in patients with familial polyposis. Surgery 1990:108:528–533.
96. Gregoire RC, Stern HS, Yeung KS, et al. Effect of calcium supplementation on mucosal cell proliferation in high risk patients for colon cancer. Gut 1989;30:376–382.
97. Barsoum GH, Hendrickse C, Winslet MC, et al. Reduction of mucosal crypt cell proliferation in patients with colorectal adenomatous polyps by dietary calcium supplementation. Br J Surg 1992;79:581–583.
98. Bostick RM, Potter JD, Fosdick L, et al. Calcium and colorectal epithelial cell proliferation: a preliminary randomized, double-blinded, placebo-controlled clinical trial. JNCI 1993;85:132–141.

99. Cats A, Kleibeuker JH, van der Meer R, et al. Randomized, double-blind, placebo-controlled intervention study with supplemental calcium in families with hereditary nonpolyposis colorectal cancer. JNCI 1995;87:598–603.
100. Baron JA, Tosteson TD, Wargovich MJ, et al. Calcium supplementation and rectal mucosal proliferation: a randomized controlled trial . JNCI 1995;87:1303–1307.
101. Schatzkin A, Freedman LS, Lanza E, Tangrea J. Diet and Colorectal Cancer: Still an open question. JNCI 1995;87:1733–1735.
102. Kikendall JW, Mobarhan S, Nelson R, Burgess M, Bowen PE. Oral beta carotene does not reduce the recurrence of colorectal adenomas [Abstract]. Am J Gastroenterol 1991;36:1356.
103. Reddy BS, England A, Katsifis S, et al. Biochemical epidemiology of colon cancer: effect of types of dietary fiber on fecal mutagens, acid, and neutral sterols in healthy subjects. Cancer Res 1990;82:1280–1285.
104. Bussey HJR, DeCosse JJ, Deschner EE, et al. A randomized trial of ascorbic acid in polyposis coli. Cancer 1982;50:1434–1439.
105. McKeown-Eyssen G, Holloway C, Jazmaji V, et al. A randomized trial of vitamins C and E in the prevention of recurrence of colorectal polyps. Cancer Res 1988;48:4701–4705.
106. DeCosse JJ, Miller HH, Lesser ML. Effect of wheat fiber and vitamins C and E on rectal polyps in patients with familial adenomatous polyposis. JNCI 1989;81:1290–1297.
107. Alberts D, Rees-McGee S, Einspahr J, et al. Effects of dietary fiber on rectal epithelial cell proliferation in patients with resection for colorectal cancers. JNCI 1990;82:1280–1285.
108. McKeown-Eyssen G, Bright-See E, Bruce WR. Recurrence of colorectal polyps: a randomized trial of a low fat high fibre diet. Presented at the 24th meeting of the Society for Epidemiologic Research 1991;215.
109. MacLennan R, Macrae F, Bain C, et al. Randomized trial of intake of fat, fiber, and beta carotene to prevent colorectal adenomas. J Natl Cancer Inst 1995;87:1760–1766.
110. Alberts D, Rees-McGee S, Einspahr J, et al Double-blind, placebo controlled study of wheat bran fiber (WBF) vs. calcium carbonate (CALC) in patients with resected adenomatous polyps. Proc Am Assoc Cancer Res 1992;33:207.
111. Paganelli GM, Biasco G, Brandi G, et al. Effect of vitamins A, C, and E supplementation on rectal cell proliferation in patients with colorectal adenomas. JNCI 1992;84:47–51.
112. Roncucci L, Donato PD, Carati L, et al. Antioxidant vitamins or lactulose for the prevention of the recurrence of colorectal adenomas. Dis Colon Rectum 1993;36:227–234.
113. Greenberg ER, Baron JA, Tosteson TD, et al. A clinical trial of antioxidant vitamins to prevent colorectal adenoma. N Engl J Med 1994;331:141–147.
114. Kligman AM, Thorne EG. Topical therapy of actinic keratosis with tretinoin. In Retinoids in Cutaneous Malignancy. Edited by R Marks. Cambridge, MA: Blackwell Scientific Publications, 1991, pp 66–73.
115. Moriarity M, Dunn J, Darragh A, et al. Etretinate in treatment of actinic keratosis: a double blind crossover study. Lancet 1982;1:364–365.
116. Watson AB. Preventative effect of etretinate therapy on multiple actinic keratoses. Cancer Detect Prev 1986;9:161–165.
117. Kraemer KH, DiGiovanna JJ, Moshell AN, et al. Prevention of skin cancer in xeroderma pigmentosum with the use of oral isotretinoin. N Engl J Med 1988;318:1633–1637.
118. Bouwes Bavinck JN, Tiben LM, Van Der Woude FJ, et al. Prevention of skin cancer and reduction of keratotic skin lesions during acitretin therapy in renal transplant recipients: a double-blind, placebo-controlled study. J Clin Oncol 1995;13: 1933–1938.
119. Greenberg ER, Baron JA, Stukel TA, et al. A clinical trial of β-carotene to prevent basal-cell and squamous-cell cancers of the skin. N Engl J Med 1990;323:789–795.
120. Tangrea JA, Edwards BK, Taylor PR, et al Long-term therapy with low-dose isotretinoin for prevention of basal cell carcinoma: a multicenter clinical trial. JNCI 1992;84:328–332.
121. Moon TE, Cartmel B, Levine N, et al. The Arizona Skin Cancer Study Group. Chemoprevention and etiology of non-melanoma skin cancers. In Program and Abstracts, 17th Annual Meeting of the American Society of Preventive Oncology, March, 1993.
122. Costa A, Formelli F, Chiesa F, et al. Prospects of chemoprevention of human cancers with the synthetic retinoid fenretinide. Cancer Res 1994;54:2032s–2037s.
123. De Palo G, Veronesi U, Camerini T, Formelli F, et al. Can Fenretinide protect women against ovarian cancer? JNCI 1995;87:146–147.
124. Early Breast Cancer Trialists' Collaborative Group Systemic treatment of early breast cancer by hormonal, cytotoxic, or immune therapy. Lancet 1992;339:1–15, 71–85.
125. Cobleigh MA, Oleske DM, Nickerson T, Pollak M. Serum IGF-I levels in stage IV breast cancer treated with tamoxifen and fenretinide. Proc Am Assoc Cancer Res 1995;36:245.
126. Munoz N, Bang LJ, Day NE, et al. No effect of riboflavin, retinol, and zinc on prevalence of precancerous lesions of oesophagus: randomized double-blind intervention study in high-risk population of China. Lancet 1985;2:111–114.
127. Munoz N, Hayashi M, Bang LJ, et al. Effect of riboflavin, retinol and zinc on micronuclei of buccal mucosa and of the esophagus: a randomized double-blind intervention study in China. JNCI 1987;79:687–691.
128. Wahrendorf J, Munoz N, Jian-Bang L, et al. Blood, retinol and zinc riboflavin status in relation to precancerous lesions of the esophagus: findings from a vitamin intervention trial in the People's Republic of China. Cancer Res 1988:48:2280–2283.
129. Zaridze D, Evstifeeva T, Boyle P. Chemoprevention of oral leukoplakia and chronic esophagitis in an area of high incidence of oral and esophageal cancer. Ann Epidemiol 1993;3:225–234.
130. Blot WJ, Li Jy, Taylor PR, et al. Linxian nutrition intervention trials: supplementation with specific vitamin/mineral combinations, cancer incidence, and disease-specific mortality in the general population. JNCI 1993;85:1483–1492.
131. Li J-Y, Taylor PR, Li B, et al. Linxian nutrition intervention trials: multiple vitamin/mineral supplementation, cancer incidence, and disease-specific mortality among adults with esophageal dysplasia. JNCI 1993;85:1492–1498.
132. Buiatti E, Munoz N, Vivas J, Cano E, et al. Difficulty in eradicating *Helicobacter pylori* in a population at high risk for stomach cancer in Venezuela. Cancer Causes and Control 1994;5:249–254.
133. Sporn MB, Squire RA, Brown CC, et al. 13-cis-retinoic acid Inhibition of bladder carcinogenesis in the rat. Science 1977;195:487–489.
134. Alfthan O, Tarkkanen J, Grohn P, et al. Tigason (etretinate) in prevention of recurrence of superficial bladder tumors. Eur Urol 1983;9:6–9.
135. Pederson H, Wolf H, Jensen SK, et al. Administration of a retinoid as prophylaxis of recurrent noninvasive bladder tumors. Scand J Urol Nephrol 1994;18:121–123.
136. Studer UE, Biedermann C, Chollet D, et al. Prevention of recurrent superficial bladder tumors by oral etretinate: preliminary results of a randomized, double-blind, multicenter trial in Switzerland. J Urol 1984;131:1469–1472.
137. Lamm DL, Riggs DR, Shrivers JS, vanGilder PF, Rach JF, DeHaven JI. Megadose vitamins in bladder cancer: a double-blind clinical trial. J Urol 1994;151:21–26.
138. Decensi A, Bruno S, Costantini M, et al. Phase IIa study of fenretinide in superficial bladder cancer, using DNA flow cytometry as an intermediate end point. JNCI 1994;86:138–141.
139. Byrne MA, Moller BR, Taylor-Robinson D, et al. The effect of interferon on human papillomaviruses associated with cervical intraepithelial neoplasia. Br J Obstet Gynacol 1986;93:1136–1144.
140. Yliskoski M, Cantell K, Syrjanen K, et al. Topical treatment with human leukocyte interferon of HPV 16 infections associated with cervical and vaginal intraepithelial neoplasias. Gynecol Oncol 1990;36:353–357.
141. Frost L, Skajaa K, Hvidman LE, et al. No effect of intralesional injection of interferon on moderate cervical intraepithelial neoplasia. Br J Obstet Gynaecol 1990;97:626–630.
142. Dunham AM, McCartney JC, McCance DJ, et al. Effect of perilesional injection of alpha-interferon on cervical intraepithelial neoplasia and associated human papillomavirus infection. J R Soc Med 1990;83:490–492.
143. Butterworth CE, Hatch KD, Soong S-J, et al. Oral folic acid supplementation for cervical dysplasia: a clinical intervention trial. Am J Obstet Gynecol 1992;166:803–809.
144. Childers, JM, Chu J, Voigt LF, et al. Chemoprevention of cervical cancer with folic acid: a phase III Southwest Oncology Group intergroup study. Cancer Epidemiol Biom Prev 1995;4:155–159.
145. De Vet HCW, Knipschild PG, Willebrand D, et al. The effect of beta-carotene on the regression and progression of cervical dysplasia: a clinical experiment. J Clin Epidemiol 1991;44:273–283.
146. Meyskens FL, Surwit E, Moon TE, et al. Enhancement of regression of cervical intraepithelial neoplasia II (moderate dysplasia) with topically applied all-trans-retinoic acid: a randomized trial. JNCI 1994;86:539–543.
147. Graham V, Surwit ES, Weiner S, et al. Phase II trial of beta-all-trans-retinoic acid for cervical intraepithelial neoplasia delivered via a collagen sponge and cervical cap. West J Med 1986;145:192–195.
148. Hennekens CH. Issues in the design and conduct of clinical trials. JNCI 1984;73:1473–1476.
149. Buring JE, Hennekens CH. The Women's Health Study: summary of the study design. J Myocard Ischemia 1992;4:27–29.

SECTION VII

CANCER SCREENING AND EARLY DETECTION

CHAPTER 30

Cancer Screening and Early Detection

CHARLES R. SMART, CURTIS P. METTLIN, LASZLO TABAR, AND HARMON J. EYRE

Introduction

Cancer screening and early detection have major importance in the survival of patients with cancer. For virtually every site, statistics show far better survival rates for early cancers than for advanced cancers. The success of treatment is largely determined by the extent of disease at the time of diagnosis with the exception of the leukemias and lymphomas. Treatment of advanced cancers, using any known modalities, is seldom curative. The objective of early detection and screening is to shift the extent of disease at diagnosis from advanced to early through the systematic examination of asymptomatic and symptomatic people. The examinations vary from self-examination and routine physical examinations by primary care deliverers, to using endoscopy, ultrasound, x-rays, and laboratory tests. A screening test is intended to distinguish those most likely to have a neoplastic disease from those least likely. Those detected then undergo diagnostic tests to confirm the presence or absence and type of cancer. Since the incidence of cancer increases with age and may vary by sex, race, habits, and geographic areas, the type and frequency of examinations vary from site to site.

In the 1960s, behavioral scientists focused on goals, objectives, procedures, and the evaluation of resultant behavior. In 1963, the first randomized cancer screening trial (RCT) using mortality from breast cancer as the endpoint was initiated in the Health Insurance Plan of Greater New York (HIP) study. In the 1970s similar studies were initiated in the United States for lung and colorectal cancers.

RCTs have the advantage of minimizing selection bias. Using a mortality endpoint minimizes any possible lead time bias or length bias. In screening asymptomatic individuals, we hope to detect cancer several years earlier than if we were to wait for symptoms to bring the individual to the doctor. This difference is called lead time. If earlier treatment results in a cure, then there is no bias. If the person eventually dies of the disease, then the increased survival time from diagnosis to death may have been only apparent, a bias, since life may not have been extended. In screening, length bias is the detection of more indolent cancers or cancers which may never have surfaced in life, which when added to clinically aggressive cancers, increases the percentages of early cases and increases overall survival percentages. In screening, a decrease in the rate (not percentage) of cases of advanced disease is one of the best predictors of a future decrease in mortality.

While theoretically ideal, RCTs of screening with a mortality endpoint are impractical for most cancer sites because of sample size, the necessary 10- to 20-year follow-up, and the need to determine cause of death in all cases. In addition, the problems of compliance in the study group, contamination of the control group, and the dependence upon the sensitivity of the screening test all greatly affect the outcome.

In 1979, the Canadian Task Force on the Periodic Health Examination evaluated the literature using strict experimental trial criteria to determine the efficacy of various procedures. One of the weaknesses of this approach is that procedures in common use, which may be highly effective, frequently have not been evaluated in an experimental trial published in the medical literature. In 1984, a similar organization using nearly identical criteria, the U.S. Preventative Services Task Force (USPSTF) was appointed by the assistant secretary of the Department of Health and Human Services (HHS). In 1980, the American Cancer Society (ACS) published Guidelines for the Cancer-Related Checkup: Recommendations and Rationale (1). In 1987, the National Cancer Institute (NCI), another division of HHS, with consultation from the ACS and representatives of medical professional organizations, developed seven early detection guidelines based upon best available evidence. In 1989, the USPSTF published their recommendations, which were at great variance with those adopted by the NCI (2).

In late 1992, after the publication of results of the Canadian National Breast Screening Study (NBSS) (3), which at 7-year follow-up showed no benefit to the study group offered screening mammography, both the NCI and ACS initiated a review of their guidelines. In February 1993, the ACS and the NCI held separate meetings to analyze existing data on screening mammography, particularly screening in women 40 to 49 years of age. While the ACS concluded that there were insufficient new data to change the consensus guideline (4), the NCI's International Workshop on Screening for Breast Cancer laid the groundwork for NCI's withdrawal of support for the consensus guidelines (5).

In December 1993, NCI dropped their endorsement of routine mammography screening for women aged 40 to 49, in spite of a near unanimous (14 to 1) recommendation of its National Cancer Advisory Board (NCAB) not to do so. In the tumult that followed changing the guidelines for women 40 to 49, NCI decided to drop the screening guidelines for all sites. These changes were triggered by a shift in leadership and in viewpoint toward recognizing only experimental trial evidence for setting public health policy.

The third edition of this book presented the early detection and screening guidelines of the NCI. NCI has since abandoned all guidelines. New information has become available on screening for breast, colorectal, and prostate cancers. The guidelines of the ACS and of most professional medical societies have been based upon "best available evidence," which will be the focus of this chapter.

Breast Cancer

SIGNIFICANCE

In 1995, it is estimated that 182,000 women will be diagnosed as having breast cancer and 46,000 will die of the disease (Fig. 30.1) (6). Breast cancer is the leading cause of death in women aged 40 to 44, and thereafter becomes even more important (Fig. 30.2). Mortality rates are based on age at death rather than age at diagnosis and thus do not truly reflect the importance of breast cancer in younger women. A second factor relates to disparities in population age groups. Age-specific incidence and mortality curves (Fig. 30.3) are slightly different from frequency distributions of actual cases diagnosed and women who later die. The latter reflects more women developing breast cancer under age 50, because of the expanded population of "baby boomers" born after World War II.

The population-based Surveillance Epidemiology and End Results (SEER) program of the NCI, which monitors cancer in nine geographic areas and covers approximately 10% of the U.S. population, registered 194,829 women with breast cancer between 1973 and 1989 with 1990 follow-up (Table 30.1). The median relative survival time was 17 years. The proportion of deaths from breast cancer in women diagnosed when they were under 50 years of age depended heavily upon the length of follow-up (Table 30.2). For the women diagnosed in 1974 after 16-year follow-up, 27% of all women who died of breast cancer were diagnosed when they were under 50 years of age.

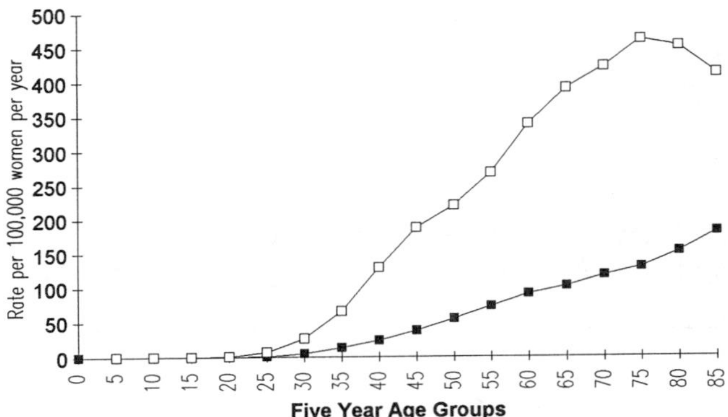

Figure 30.2. Breast cancer: age-specific incidence (*open boxes*) and mortality (*black boxes*). (SEER data 1984–1988.)

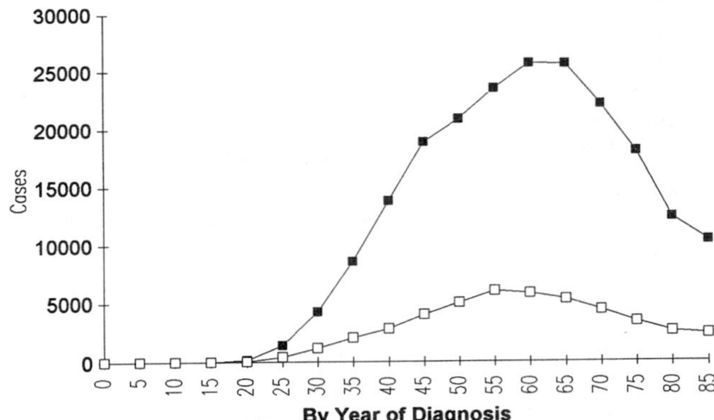

Figure 30.3. 194,829 Female breast cancers (*black boxes*) in SEER 1973–1989 with deaths from breast cancer (*open boxes*) by age at diagnosis.

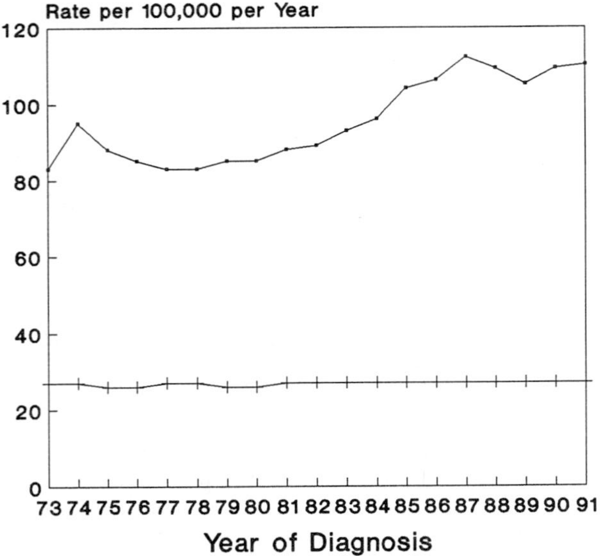

Figure 30.1. Breast cancer trends: incidence (●) and mortality (+). (SEER Cancer Statistics Review, 1971–1991. National Cancer Institute, NIH publication no. 94-2789.)

While there have been numerous reports regarding the poorer prognosis of women diagnosed under age 50, SEER data show a higher proportion of deaths from breast cancer in women diagnosed under age 40 but not for women 40 to 49. The latter group appeared to have a lower percentage of deaths from breast cancer than older women, based on death certificates (Fig. 30.1).

The 13-year relative survival rates for women with positive lymph nodes were 50% for women in their forties, 36% for women in their twenties, and 43% for the others (Fig. 30.4). Survival rates were similar for those with localized disease by age groups, as well as for those with distant disease by age groups. This was also the finding in the Breast Cancer Detection Demonstration Project (BCDDP), where women whose disease was detected in their 40s had relatively fewer lymph nodes involved than women 50 to 59 or 60 to 69 years

Table 30.1. Female Breast Cancers Diagnosed in SEER 1973–1989

Age groups (yr)	Cancers diagnosed	Patient deaths	
		No.	(%)
0	3	1	
5	0	0	
10	2	0	0
15	25	6	24
20	188	55	29
25	1,438	430	30
30	4,246	1,179	28
35	8,558	2,042	24
40	13,784	2,799	20
45	18,815	4,003	21
50	20,822	4,977	24
55	23,430	5,969	25
60	25,583	5,774	23
65	25,550	5,280	21
70	22,065	4,366	20
75	17,989	3,362	19
80	12,331	2,552	21
85	10,356	2,353	23
ALL	194,829	45,148	23

Table 30.2. SEER Data on Breast Cancer Deaths[a]

Deaths from breast cancer in women diagnosed 1973–1989 followed up in 1990			Deaths from breast cancer in women diagnosed in 1974 followed up in 1990		
Age group	**Number**	**Percentage**	**Age group**	**Number**	**Percentage**
Under 30	489	1	Under 30	27	1
30–39	3202	6	30–39	228	7
40–49	6753	13	40–49	619	19
50–59	19886	37	50–59	918	28
60–69	10996	20	60–69	812	25
70–79	7695	14	70–79	559	17
80 Plus	4887	9	80 Plus	126	4
All	53908	100	All	3289	100%

[a] The percentage of deaths in women under 50 depends upon the cohort examined. In this analysis all women diagnosed with breast cancer from 1973–1989 were analyzed; 20% of the deaths were in women under 50 years of age.

If one were to analyze those with longer follow-up, such as only women diagnosed in 1974, the percentage increases to 27%; women 40–49 take longer to die of breast cancer.

of age (7). This may be one reason why it requires more years of follow-up to evaluate breast cancer deaths in women 40 to 49 years of age in RCTs than for older women.

EVIDENCE OF BENEFIT

There is nearly unanimous agreement, based upon RCTs, that screening women 50 to 69 years of age with mammography decreases mortality by about 30%. The first randomized trial (HIP study with 18 years follow-up) showed an early decrease in mortality for the study group over age 50 starting 3 to 5 years after entry into the trial, while for women 40 to 49 years of age the decrease was delayed and did not

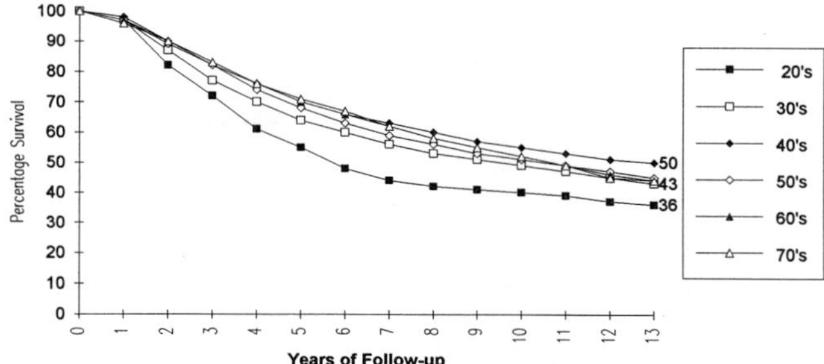

Figure 30.4. SEER breast cancer relative survival 1973–1988 among 50,480 women with regional disease by age groups.

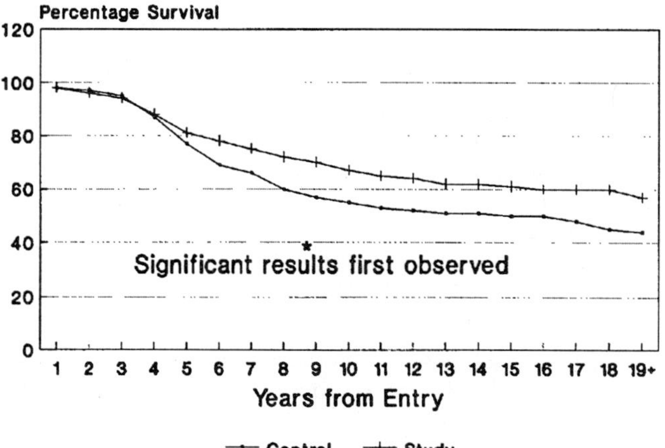

Figure 30.5. Breast cancer survival in women 40 to 49 years of age upon entry to HIP screening study. Significant difference was first attained at 9 years (8).

reach statistical significance until 9 years after entry (Fig. 30.5) (8).

The Swedish Two-County study with 13-year follow-up began in Kopparberg county in 1977 and in Östergötland county in 1978. The study had 78,085 women in the study group and 56,782 in the control group. The study group were offered single-view mammography without physical examination at average intervals of 24 months for women aged 40 to 49 years and at average intervals of 33 months for women aged 50 to 74. Compliance was 89.2% in the first round and 83.3% in the second. By the end of 1984 there was a 31% reduction in breast cancer mortality in the study group (P= .013, two-sided test). There was a highly significant reduction (P = .001) in the rate of stage II and more advanced breast cancers (25%) (9). Both of these differences began to emerge some 4 years after randomization and subsequently increased in magnitude. As of 1995, the two-county study is the only randomized controlled trial using mammography as the only screening modality that has demonstrated a significant decrease in the mortality from breast cancer (10). Based on the natural history of breast cancer and the interval breast cancer rates provided by this trial, the data strongly suggest that the periodicity of mammograms in women under 50 years of age should be every 12 months whereas for older women it might be every two years (11–16).

Some of the reasons for the delayed reduction in mortality in RCTs for women 40 to 49 years of age are these:

1. Breast cancer incidence and mortality rates are lower in women aged 40 to 49 than n women 50 and over. In the combined eight trials, less than a third of the total number of women were under 50 years of age. Therefore, statistical significance required more years of follow-up.
2. On average, the lead time cf mammography is shorter in women 40 to 49 than in women 50 and over (i.e., the prevalence screen yields comparatively fewer cases in the screened group in the overall analysis).
3. Women aged 40 to 49 years have a slight survival advantage and delayed mortality because of fewer involved regional lymph nodes than women 50 to 59 and 60 to 69 years of age in the data of the BCDDP (7) and in the population-based SEER program.
4. The sensitivity of mammography appears to be lower in women aged 40 to 49 than in women 50 and over.
5. The higher relative rates of ductal carcinoma in situ (DCIS) found in women 40 to 49 progress slowly from DCIS to invasive carcinoma and thus require a longer time to manifest a mortality difference between screen-detected DCIS in the study group and the control group.

These factors make it more difficult to detect differences between study and control groups in women 40 to 49, as compared with women 50 and older in the first 7 years of follow-up. Thus, more time is needed to manifest a statistically significant mortality reduction in women aged 40 to 49.

Recognition of the limited statistical power in individual RCTs, especially among women aged 40 to 49, has led some investigators to perform meta-analyses of RCT results (17–20). Meta-analyses benefit by combining results from different studies, thereby increasing the total number of deaths and woman-years of follow-up in the collective study and control groups. Meta-analyses, however, are blind to potential differences among studies in design, conduct, quality, and completeness of data.

RCTs are designed to study the efficacy of mammography, and they do so indirectly by comparing mortality in groups invited to screening with that in the group not invited to screening. The failure to achieve a statistically significant difference in mortality between the two groups may be due to a true lack of benefit from screening women in this age group. Alternatively, it could be due to an ineffective screening protocol, to inadequate numbers of women enrolled, or to inadequate years of follow-up.

Table 30.3 summarizes all of the breast cancer RCTs. Only the HIP and Kopparberg trials have demonstrated a statistically significant mortality reduction over their designed age ranges (8, 18, 21, 22). Table 30.4 summarizes the published subgroup data for women 40 to 49 years of age from each trial, including the number of women entering each arm. Table 30.5 summarizes the number of woman-years and breast cancer deaths used in a meta-analysis of the eight trials (10).

Figure 30.6 best depicts the results of RCTs of mammography in women aged 40 to 49 at current follow-up, with and without including the NBSS-1 trial designed to study women aged 40 to 49 (3). Five of the eight trials suggest benefit, although no single trial using standard statistical methods showed statistically significant benefit at the 95% confidence level. Including the NBSS-1 trial, the meta-analysis of

Table 30.3. Randomized Controlled Trials of Mammography

Trial (dates)	Age at entry (yr)	Screening regimen frequency		F/U (yr)	Subjects (no.)		RR 95% CI
					Invited	Control	
HIP (1963–1969)	40–64	2V, MM, CBE	Annually, 4 rounds	18	30,131	30,565	0.77[a] 0.61–0.97
Malmö (1976–1986)	45–69	1 or 2V, MM	18–24 mo, 5 rounds	12	20,695	20,783	0.81 0.62–1.07
Kopparberg (1977–1985)	40–74	1V, MM	24–33 mo, 4 rounds	13	38,562	18,478	0.60 0.46–0.79
Östergötland (1977–1985)	40–74	1V, MM	24–33 mo, 4 rounds	13	38,405	37,145	0.78 0.60–1.01
Edinburgh (1979–1988)	45–64	1 or 2V, MM	24 mo, 4 rounds	10	23,226	21,904	0.84[b] 0.63–1.12
Stockholm (1981–1985)	40–64	1V, MM	28 mo, 2 rounds	8	38,525	20,651	0.80 0.53–1.22
Gothenburg (1982–1988)	40–59	2V, MM	18 mo, 4 rounds	7	20,724	28,809	0.86 0.54–1.37
NBSS-1 (1980–1987)	40–49	2V, MM, CBE	Annually, 5 rounds	7	25,214	25,216	1.36 0.84–2.21
NBSS-2 (1980–1987)	50–59	2V, MM, CBE vs. CBE	Annually, 5 rounds	7	19,711	19,694	0.97 0.62–1.52

Key: RR, relative risk of breast cancer mortality; 95% CI, 95% confidence interval; MM, mammography; CBE, clinical breast exam; F/U, follow-up.
[a] From References 3 and 11 (for 18 years of follow-up). Other sources report slightly different results for this trial. For example, Reference 8 reports RR = 0.79 (0.62–0.99) at 18-year follow-up.
[b] From Reference 3. Reference 8 reports RR = 0.85 (0.65–1.12).

Table 30.4. Summary of Randomized Controlled Trials: Results for Women Aged 40 to 49

Study (dates)	Screening		F/U (yr)	Subjects (no.)		RR 95% CI
	Regimen	Frequency		Invited	Control	
HIP Study (11) (1963–1969)	2V, MM, CBE	Annually, 4 rounds	18	14,432	14,701	0.77[a] 0.53–1.11
Malmö (6) (1976–1986)	1 or 2V, MM	18–24 mo, 5 rounds	12	3,658[b]	3,679[b]	0.51[b] 0.22–1.17
Kopparberg (6) (1977–1985)	1V, MM	24 mo, 4 rounds	13	9,582	5,031	0.73 0.37–1.41
Östergötland (6) (1977–1985)	1V, MM	24 mo, 4 rounds	13	10,262	10,573	1.02 0.52–1.99
Edinburgh (7) (1979–1988)	1 or 2V, MM	24 mo, 4 rounds	11	5,913	5,810	0.78 0.46–1.51
Stockholm (6) (1981–1985)	1V, MM	28 mo, 2 rounds	8	14,375	7,103	1.04[c] 0.53–2.05
Gothenburg (6) (1982–1988)	2V, MM	18 mo, 4 rounds	7	10,600	12,800	0.73[d] 0.27–1.97
NBSS-1 (1) (1980–1987)	2V, MM, CBE	12 mo, 5 rounds	7	25,214	25,216	1.36 0.84–2.21

[a] From reference 11. Reference 8 reported RR = 0.78 (0.52–1.18).
[b] Includes only women aged 45–49 at entry.
[c] Use of the raw data on deaths and on woman-years of follow-up in each group results in a slightly different RR and 95% CI than that published in Reference 6 and listed above: 1.00 (0.49–2.05).
[d] This RR and 95% CI corresponds to 7 years' follow-up. At 10 years' follow-up, the RR and 95% CI are estimated to be 0.60 (0.34–1.08).
V, views, 1 or 2; MM, mammography; CBE, clinical breast exam; F/U, follow-up.

Table 30.5. Data Used in Meta-Analyses of Women Aged 40–49

Screening study	Woman-Years		Breast cancer deaths (no.)	
	Invited	Control	Invited	Control
HIP	248,454	253,085	49	65
Malmö[a]	46,000	47,000	8	16
Kopparberg	119,775	62,888	22	16
Östergötland	128,275	132,163	23	23
Edinburgh[a]	56,750	54,588	17	21
Stockholm	107,000	64,000	20	12
Gothenburg—A	64,000	77,000	6	10
Gothenburg—B	90,753	109,179	17	34
NBSS-1	173,474	173,488	38	28

[a] Includes only women aged 45–49 at entry.

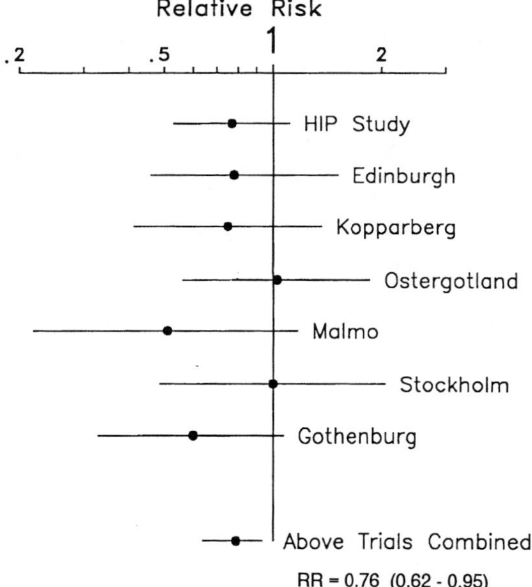

Figure 30.6. Meta-analysis of all randomized controlled trials (Tables 30.4 and 30.5) of the effect of screening women aged 40 to 49 for breast cancer on their relative risk of breast cancer mortality.

all currently available RCT results for women aged 40 to 49 suggests an insignificant 16% reduction in mortality in the group invited to screening, as compared with women assigned to an unscreened control group. Exclusion of the NBSS-1 trial results in a 24% statistically significant reduction in mortality from breast cancer in women aged 40 to 49.

The NBSS-1 trial suggests detriment from mammography, with 36% more deaths among those assigned to the study group than among women assigned to the control group. The NBSS-1 trial has a wide 95% confidence interval, ranging from 0.84 to 2.21. The NBSS-1 trial was different from all other trials in that it was the only trial that recruited volunteers rather than randomizing participants from a defined population and it was the only trial that prescreened women in both the study and control groups with a clinical breast examination. The fact that so many more advanced cancers were detected clinically in the initial screen that were randomized to the mammography plus clinical breast examination arm suggests a flaw not found in other RCTs. This is presently being reexamined by the Canadian government. It has also been suggested that future use of the NBSS-1 trial data should ignore the initial (prevalence) year (23).

Because of the delayed benefit of screening mammography in women aged 40 to 49, some have suggested that the benefit of mammography in RCTs may result from screening at or after age 50, even though the women were under 50 when they entered the trials (20). Beginning screening at 50 entirely misses the leading cause of death in women 40 to 44 years of age and the 19% of breast cancer deaths that occur in women diagnosed when 40 to 49 years of age (Table 30.1).

The true benefit of mammography today is likely to exceed the benefit demonstrated in RCTs for at least two reasons. First, RCTs test the efficacy of the *offer* of mammography to a predefined study group as compared with a predefined control group. In RCTs screening compliance rates for obtaining a first screening mammogram ranged from 61% to 89%. The true benefit for women who receive regular screening mammography will be higher than the benefit demonstrated among women who were offered only mammography in the RCTs. Second, the technology of mammography has improved considerably since the time of even the most recent RCTs (24). Women receiving regular, high-quality mammography today are more likely to have their cancers detected at smaller sizes and at earlier stages than women who participated in the eight RCTs (24–26).

Evidence from the 14-year follow-up (7, 27, 28) of the nonrandomized breast cancer detection demonstration project with 98% compliance with annual two-view mammography plus a clinical breast examination yielded equally good results for the 1004 women aged 40 to 49 whose breast cancer was detected as in the 1560 women aged 50 to 59 and the 1001 women aged 60 to 69. The initial (prevalence) screening detected progressively more cases per 1000 examinations with increasing age 40 through 70, but in the second screening, the detection rate varied little from age 45 to 70. After the initial screen, the yield and cost should not be much different for women 45 through 70 years of age (Fig. 30.7).

In both the HIP and the BCDDP the screening interval was 1 year. In the Swedish two-county trial, women 40 to 49 years of age were screened with only single-view mammography every 2 years, and women over 50 every 3 years. The Swedish analysis of interval cases (those occurring between screenings after a negative mammogram) is very informative. In the women aged 40 to 49, the interval cases for the first and second year were 38 and 68%, respectively, of the control incidence rate, as compared with 13 and 29% observed in women aged 50 to 69. This is consistent with the shorter lead time (sojourn time) observed in younger women, suggesting the need for 1-year screening intervals for women of 40 to 49. Longer intervals may be acceptable for older women (11, 12, 29–31).

In light of the new evidence of benefit for 40- to 49-year-old women, derived from meta-analysis of RCTs with longer follow-up, it would appear that the recommendation of the ACS to screen women from age 40 to 49 every 1 to 2 years, and annually after age 50, should be reconsidered and perhaps reversed (see Chapter 136).

SUGGESTION

Women should be encouraged to do monthly breast self-examination; a clinical breast examination should be included in the routine physical examination; and, beginning at age 40, mammography should be encouraged every year. After age 50 the interval might be lengthened to 2 years. Special attention should be given women with a personal history of breast cancer or atypical ductal hyperplasia or with a history of breast cancer in a mother or sister.

Colorectal Cancer

SIGNIFICANCE

Colorectal cancer is the second leading cause of death from cancer in the United States, where it is estimated that there will be 138,200 new cases and 55,300 deaths in 1995 (6). The incidence and the mortality rates are both decreasing (Fig. 30.8). The incidence is higher in men than in women (Fig. 30.9); 58.9 versus 40.4 per 100,000 per year. Age-specific incidence and mortality rates show that nearly all cases are diagnosed after 50 years of age (32).

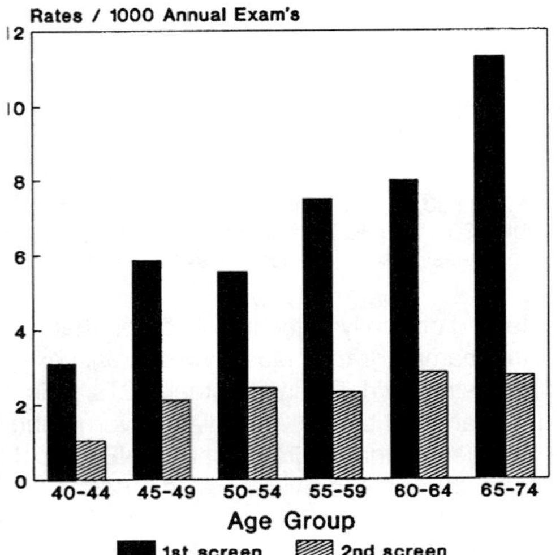

Figure 30.7. BCDDP breast cancer detection rate by 1st and 2nd screenings and age group. From JNCI 1979; 62(3):665

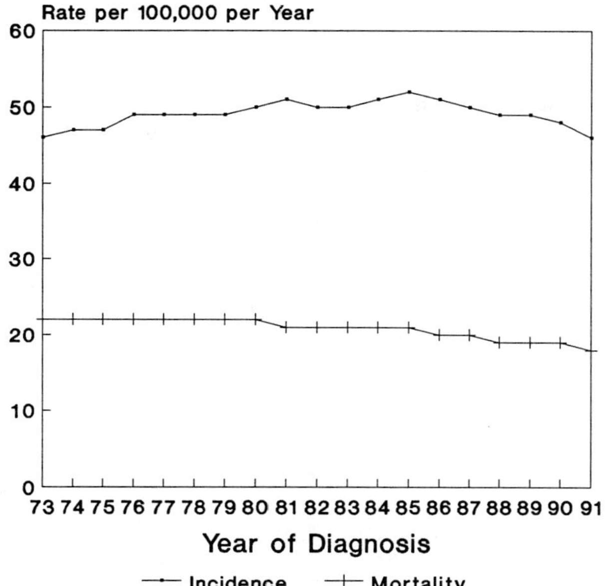

Figure 30.8. Colorectal cancer trends: incidence and mortality. (SEER Cancer Statistics Review, 1973–1991.)

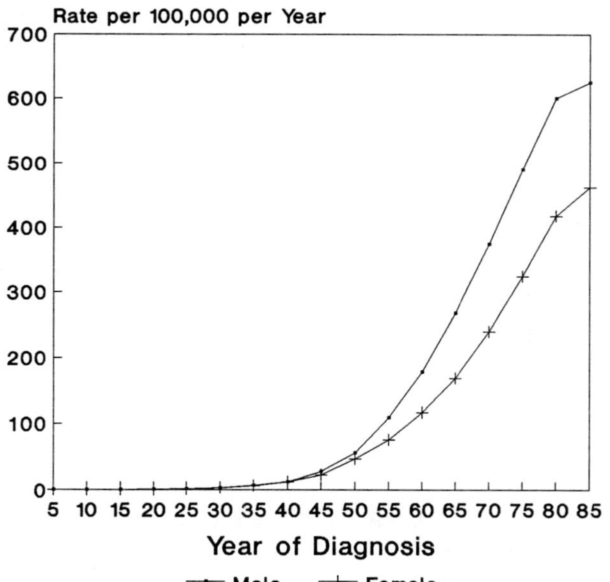

Figure 30.9. Colorectal cancer trend: age-specific rates by sex. (SEER Cancer Statistics Review, 1973–1991.)

Most patients (57%) present with regional or distant disease (Fig. 30.10). The overall 5-year relative survival rate was 60% (case-fatality rate 40%). For localized disease, the 5-year survival rate approaches 91%, for regional 61%, and for distant disease 7% (Fig. 30.11) (6).

There are groups that have a high incidence of colorectal cancer. These include those with hereditary conditions, such as familial polyposis, nonpolyposis syndromes, the cancer family syndrome (autosomal-dominant) (see Chapter 121), hereditary site-specific colon cancer, and ulcerative colitis. Together, they account for 6% of colorectal cancers. More common conditions associated with increased risk include a personal history of colorectal cancer or adenomas, first-degree family history of colorectal cancer or adenomas, and a personal history of ovarian, endometrial, or breast cancer (33). These high-risk groups account for only 23% of all colorectal cancers. Limiting screening or early cancer detection to only these high-risk groups would miss the majority of colorectal cancers (34).

A large percentage of early cancers can be detected by screening asymptomatic individuals over 50 years of age with a digital rectal examination, fecal occult blood testing, and sigmoidoscopy. The removal of premalignant polyps should decrease mortality. The discovery of polyps in the distal colon or rectum or the presence of occult blood mandates colonoscopy or a barium enema to search the entire colon.

EVIDENCE OF BENEFIT

Virtually all screening studies using any of these modalities have demonstrated an increase in the proportion of early cases and a corresponding increase in survival compared with cases diagnosed in a nonscreening environment (35). The Memorial-Strang Clinic sigmoidoscopy study (36) was conducted between 1946 and 1954 with 26,124 patients. The survival rate in the 58 patients discovered with cancer was 90% after a follow-up period of 15 years. The Gilbertsen study, conducted over a 25-year period, subjected 18,158 patients to periodic rigid sigmoidoscopy. It showed a significant reduction in the incidence of cancer in the rectosigmoid colon when compared with statewide data (37). There were 14 rectal cancers in the study group, which was only 15% of those expected in that state.

The Kaiser-Permanente Multiphasic Health Checkup was a randomized study of 10,713 health plan members between age 35 and 54 years. After 16 years, the study reported more favorable stage distribution and survival rates and reduced mortality for the study group (12 deaths versus 29 for controls), which was statistically significant. However in a recent reevaluation considering only those cancers within reach of the sigmoidoscope, no statistical difference could be demonstrated (38).

Two case-control studies have been reported that evaluate the efficacy of screening sigmoidoscopy in preventing colorectal cancer mortality (39, 40). Both were conducted in prepaid health plans. Rigid sigmoidoscopy was used during the period evaluated by Selby and co-workers. Rigid and flexible sigmoidoscopy were used during the period evaluated by Newcomb and associates. Both studies suggested a significantly decreased risk (60 to 80%) of fatal cancer of the distal colon or rectum among individuals with a history of one or more sigmoidoscopic examinations compared with unscreened patients (39, 40).

Five controlled clinical trials have been completed or are in progress to evaluate the efficacy of screening utilizing the fecal occult blood test. The Memorial Sloan-Kettering Cancer Center–Strang Clinic (MSKCC) trial, completed in 1985, was an evaluation of the fecal occult blood test as a supplement to annual rigid sigmoidoscopy (41). The patient and

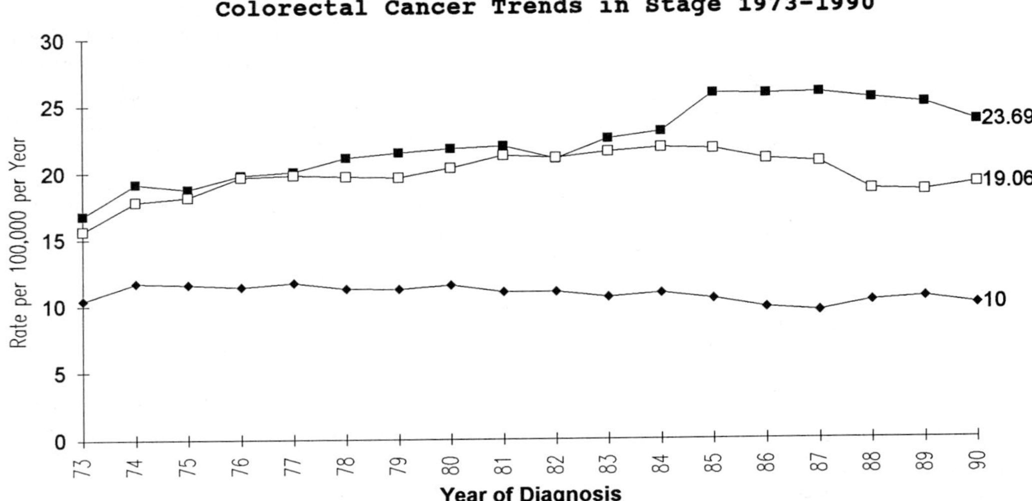

Figure 30.10. Colorectal cancer trends in stage 1973–1990. *Black boxes*, in situ or localized tumor; *open boxes*, regional metastasis; *diamonds*, distant metastasis.

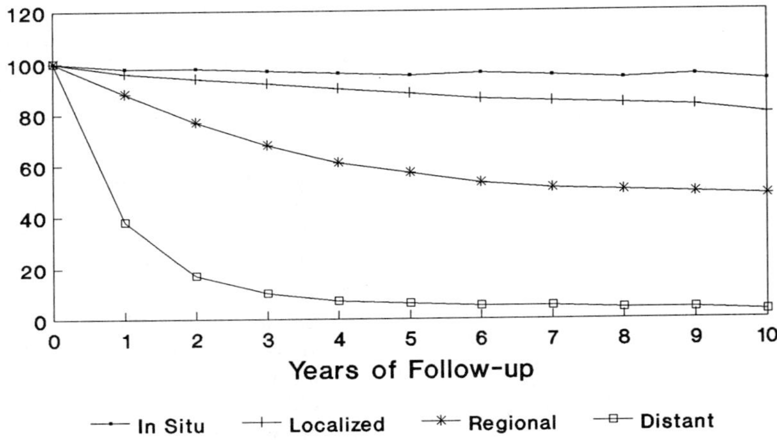

Figure 30.11. Colorectal cancer: relative survival by stage. (SEER Statistics Review, 1973–1991.)

control groups were selected by calendar periods. In the MSKCC trial, two different groups of patients were studied. Group I had a history of periodic check-ups at the Strang Clinic, whereas Group II were new patients at the Clinic. Group II had different characteristics than Group I. They reported more symptoms (8 to 9%), the rate of positivity was higher, and more findings were present on the initial proctosigmoidoscopy than in Group I. The preliminary analysis of survival indicates a significant difference between Groups I and II. At this time, comparison of the two groups suggests a difference in colorectal cancer mortality of borderline statistical significance.

The Minnesota trial demonstrated that annual fecal occult blood testing using hydrated samples decreased mortality from colorectal cancer by 33% (42). The Swedish trial is a targeted study for the 60- to 64-year age group (43). The English program selects candidates from lists of family practitioners (44). The Danish trial offers screening to a population between 45 and 75 years of age allocated at random to a control and a study group (45, 46).

In general, on initial (prevalence) examinations, some 1 to 5% of unselected persons tested with fecal occult blood tests have positive test results. Of those with positive test results, approximately 10% have cancer and approximately 20 to 30% have adenomas (47, 48). The positivity and predictive value for neoplastic lesions (both cancers and adenomas) is as follows: All trials have shown a consistent improvement in the stage of disease in the screened population. Recent data from the Danish trial indicate a high percentage of Dukes' A and B lesions compared with the control groups (Table 30.6).

Mathematical models have been constructed to estimate outcome and costs of screening strategies for average-risk and high-risk groups. These models project a significant re-

Table 30.6. Colorectal Cancer Screening Trials

Trial	Study population	Positivity (%)	Predictive value (%)	Dukes' A & B (%)	
				Screened	Control
MSKCC[41]	22,000	1.4 (Group I)	36	60	50
		2.6 (Group II)[a]	*	60	50
Sweden[43]	27,000	1.9	22	65	33
England[44]	150,000	2.1	40	90	40
Minnesota[42]	48,000	2.4	31	78	35
Denmark[45,46]	62,000	1.0	58	71	55

[a] Averages of prevalence and incidence cases in groups I and II.

duction in colorectal cancer mortality using currently available screening methods. For example, using the most accurate available information, an annual fecal occult blood test might result in a mortality reduction of 30%. An annual fecal occult blood test and flexible sigmoidoscopy every 5 years might reduce mortality by 40% (47, 49).

National trends show an increase in earlier-stage (in situ and localized) disease, from 32% in 1973 to 43% in 1987. In addition, there has been an increase in survival and a decrease in mortality from colorectal cancer (see Chapter 121).

SUGGESTION

A rectal examination should be included in routine periodic check-ups. Beginning at age 50, annual fecal occult blood testing should be included with a sigmoidoscopy every 3 to 5 years. Special attention should be given to patients with a personal history of adenomas or colon cancer or a strong family history of colon cancer or inflammatory bowel disease.

Prostate Cancer

SIGNIFICANCE

Prostate cancer is the most frequent major cancer in men in the United States (an estimated 244,000 new cases and 40,400 deaths in 1995) (6). In the last decade, prostate cancer has increased more rapidly than any other cancer. From 1973 to 1991, prostate cancer incidence increased by 126.3% with 60% occurring from 1986 to 1991 (Fig. 30.12). Although prostate cancer mortality has not increased at the same rate, in 1995 prostate cancer is estimated to be second only to lung cancer as a cause of cancer deaths (6, 32). The increase in incidence which was evident across all age groups between 40 and 80 years of age (Fig. 30.13) was the product mainly of an increase in the detection of localized disease (Fig. 30.14). The increase also was greatest for moderately differentiated cancer (Gleason grades 5 to 7) as opposed to the less aggressive Gleason grades 1 to 4 (Figs. 30.14 and 30.15).

An impression exists among some physicians that prostate cancer is a relatively benign disease that is infrequently a cause of death. It is true that competing causes of death play major roles because of the older age of prostate cancer patients, but SEER data demonstrate that prostate cancer is a killing disease that does not abate with increasing age. Ninety-eight percent of prostate cancers occurred in men over 50 years of age (Fig. 30.13). The average age at diagnosis is 72 years, the same as the present life expectancy of men in the United States. In the population-based SEER program, 146,707 prostate cancers were registered over an 18-year period (1973–1990), and in the 1990 follow-up of all cases, based on death certificate, 37% of all deaths were from prostate cancer (Table 30.7). The cause of death correlated with advancing age. As age increased, death from other causes increased; at 40 to 49 years of age nearly 60% of the deaths were from prostate cancer while at 80 years it was only 28% (Table 30.8). To compare across age groups and to correct for death from other causes relative survival rates were used. Overall, this method estimated the 10-year relative death rate from prostate cancer to be 42%. Men diagnosed in their 40s did not survive as well as men aged 50 to 79 although better than men in their 80s (Fig. 30.16). Of men in their 40s, 22% had distant disease at diagnosis compared with 16% for men 50 to 59 and 14% for men 60 to 69 years of age. Men with less distant stage disease benefited, with fewer dying of prostate cancer.

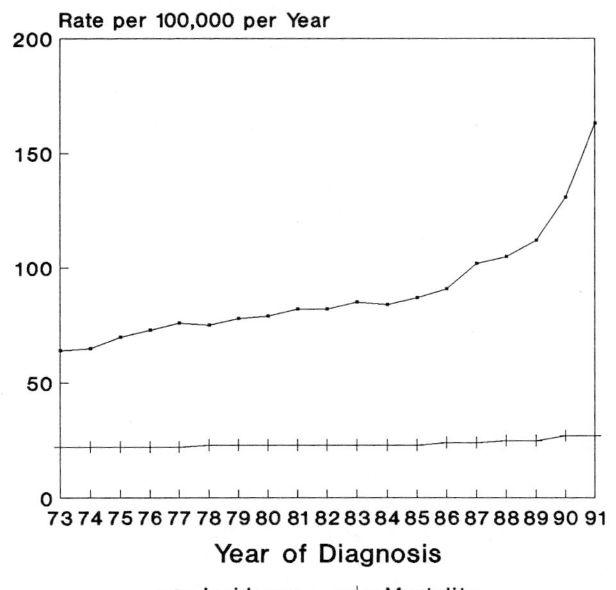

Figure 30.12. Cancer of the prostate: trends in incidence and mortality. (SEER Cancer Statistics Review, 1973–1991.)

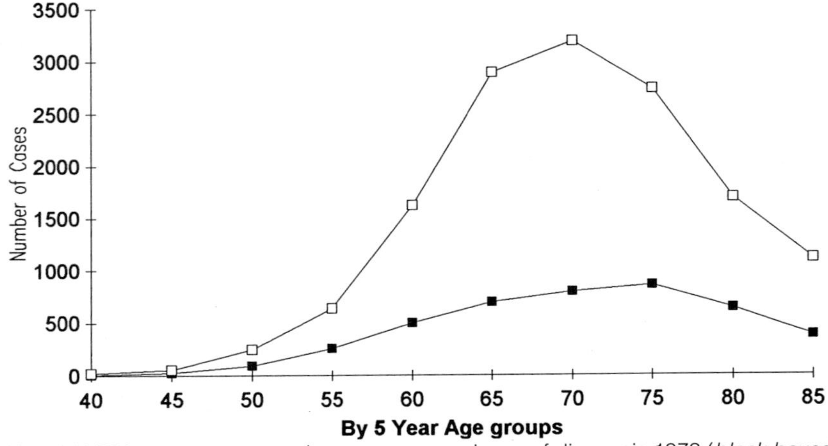

Figure 30.13. 146,709 prostate cancers by age group and year of diagnosis 1973 (*black boxes*) and 1990 (*open boxes*).

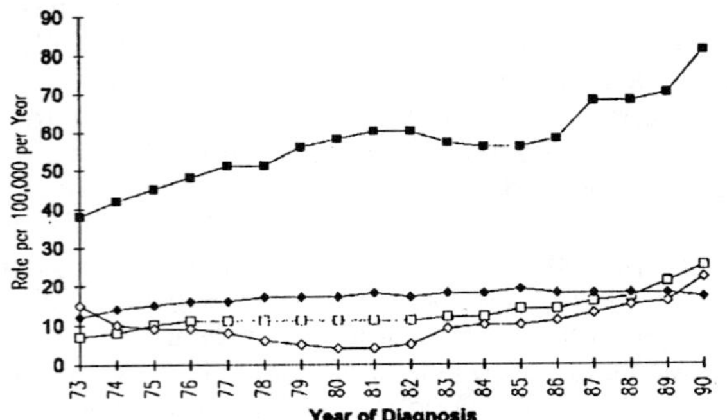

Figure 30.14. Prostate cancer incidence by stage and years: SEER registry 146,709 cases. *Black boxes*, localized; *open boxes*, regional; *black diamonds*, distant; *diamonds*, unknown.

Black men had an overall one-third higher incidence rate, 128.2 per 100,000 per year versus 84.4 for white men, and a mortality rate of 44.6 versus 22.6 per 100,000, respectively (Fig. 30.17). Among black men, more were detected with distant stage disease (26% of black men and 17% of white men), resulting in a lower 5-year relative survival rate for black men—63.4% compared with 79.3% for white men (death rates of 36.6% versus 20.7%, respectively). Again, men with less distant stage disease benefited, as fewer died of prostate cancer.

TRENDS IN DETECTION AND TREATMENT

The results of repeated national surveys on patterns of prostate cancer detection and management in the United States have been published (50, 51) and are summarized (Table 30.9). The data show trends of increasing attention given to histologic grading and Gleason scoring, as well as greater use of bone scanning and computed tomography (CT) to detect the presence of distant metastases and more accurately to stage the disease. In 1974, the most common methods of diagnosis of prostate cancer were transurethral resection (TURP) and the digital rectal examination (DRE). In the mid-1980s transrectal ultrasound (TRUS) and the biopsy gun for automatic transrectal biopsy enhanced earlier detection compared with the DRE, with a two- to threefold increase in sensitivity. The biopsy gun allowed multiple transrectal biopsies under ultrasound guidance as an office procedure without anesthesia and little discomfort, and with greater accuracy.

In the 1987–1988 era, prostate-specific antigen (PSA) was evaluated in urologic practice as a screening test in symptomatic or asymptomatic men (6, 52, 53), frequently in conjunction with TRUS. PSA was not only elevated in patients with prostate cancer but was elevated in many patients with benign prostatic hypertrophy. PSA testing was negative in some patients with cancer of the prostate as well. The use of PSA increased from 5.8% in 1983 to 68.4% in 1990. Despite its limitations, PSA enhanced the detection of many localized prostate cancers (51, 54). The increase in incidence has been generally attributed to widespread PSA screening. With increased screening and increased numbers of patients whose disease is localized to the prostate, the percentage of patients treated by radical prostatectomy increased from 8.9% in 1984 to 21.4% in 1990 (51).

In 1991, the American Urologic Association (AUA) recommended that all men over 50 years of age be screened annually by DRE and PSA. In 1992, a similar guideline was made by the ACS (5, 55, 56).

Recent reports indicate that men with localized untreated prostate cancer have survival similar to men treated by radical prostatectomy (57–59). It has also been estimated that 30% of men over 50 years of age have occult prostate cancer (found at autopsy) which rarely has been causal in their deaths (60). In view of this, plus the lack of randomized controlled trials, considerable concern exists that some of the cancers being detected may be being treated unnecessarily (61, 62).

EVIDENCE OF BENEFIT

In the ACS National Prostate Cancer Detection Project (ACS-NPCDP) (6, 63) initiated in 1987, 2,999 asymptomatic men were screened multiple times using TRUS, PSA, and DRE and subsequently were followed. The clinical and pathologic characteristics of the prostate cancers detected have been reported (64). Only 5% of cancers detected were

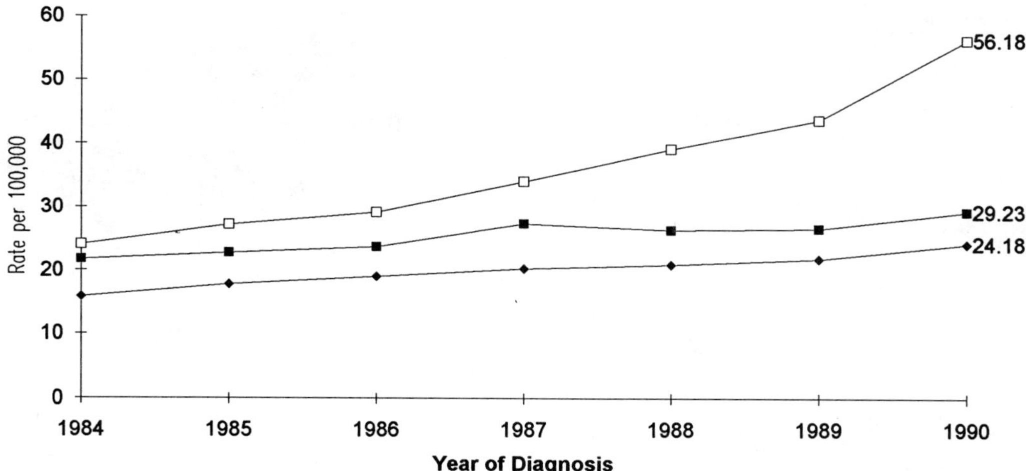

Figure 30.15. Prostate cancer: trends in Gleason scores. *Black boxes*, Gleason 2–4; *open boxes*, 5–7; *diamonds*, 8–10.

Table 30.7. 146,710 Prostate Cancers Over an 18-year Period, and their Lethality

Year	Cases (no.)	Status as of 1990 Alive (%)	Dead (%)	Prostate cancer deaths (%)
73	4,231	7	93	41
74	5,021	7	93	40
75	5,795	10	90	39
76	6,147	11	89	39
77	6,498	14	86	37
78	6,542	16	84	38
79	6,934	18	82	37
80	7,245	20	80	36
81	7,606	24	76	37
82	7,790	28	72	38
83	8,189	32	68	37
84	8,318	37	63	37
85	8,845	43	57	39
86	9,335	50	50	38
87	10,722	59	41	39
88	11,227	67	33	36
89	12,066	75	25	36
90	14,199	85	15	33
Total	146,710	40	60	37

Table 30.8. Age at Diagnosis (1973–1989) of 86,644 Prostate Cancer Patients Known Dead (SEER Data)

Age at diagnosis (yr)	Cases (No.)	Cause of death: Prostate cancer (%)	Other (%)	Unknown (%)	Total (%)
40–49	363	59	33	7	100
50–59	4,697	50	41	9	100
60–69	21,194	39	52	9	100
70–79	34,965	32	59	8	100
80+	25,391	28	65	7	100
All	86,644	34	58	8	100

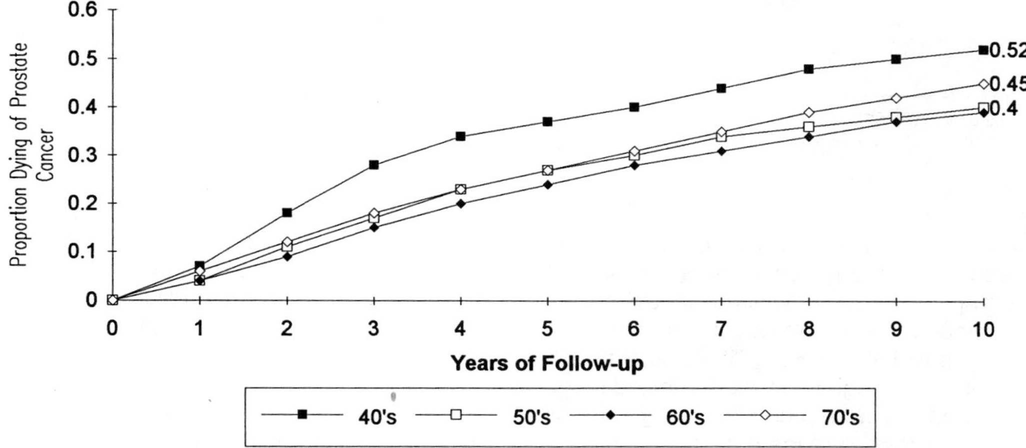

Figure 30.16. Death potential from prostate cancer by age groups in 105,705 patients.

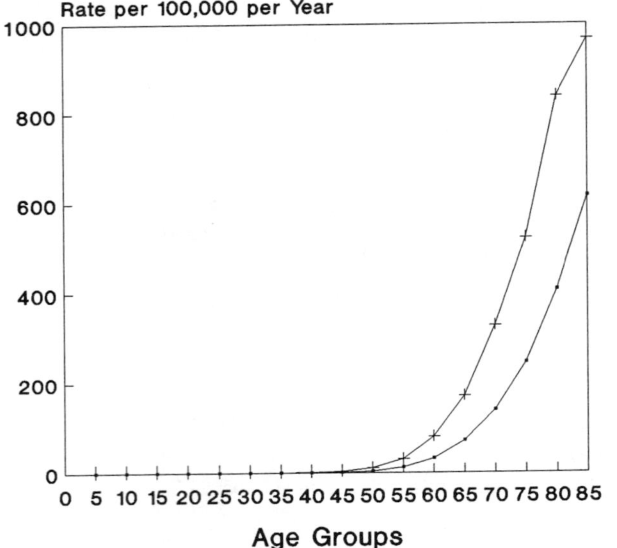

Figure 30.17. Prostate cancer: age-specific incidence by race (black (+) and white (•)). (SEER Cancer Statistics Review, 1973–1988.)

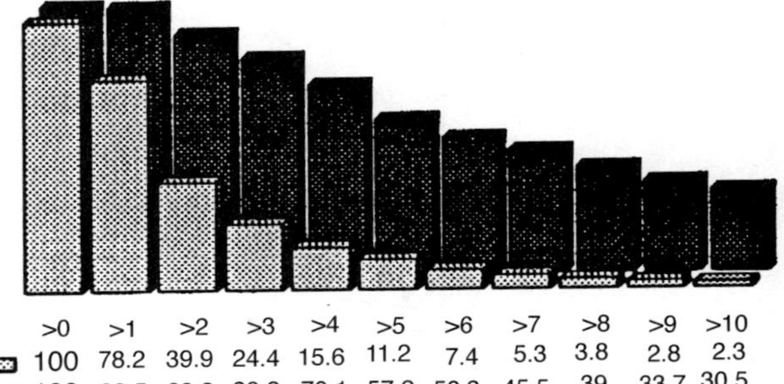

Figure 30.18. Distribution of PSA levels in 1974 cancers and 2,805 normal men.

Table 30.9. Commission on Cancer Patient Care Evaluation

	Years of survey			
	1974	1979	1983	1990
Total patients (no.)	20166	14079	17511	23183
Mode of detection				
DRE	30	45	54.3	54
TRUS			10.2	19.7
PSA			5.8	68.4
TURP	54.5	57.8	56	40.8
Needle aspiration	16.6	17.4	18.1	
Perineal biopsy	13.3	12.7	12.4	5.1
Transrectal biopsy	7	10.1	10.2	19.7
Staging procedures				
Bone survey	23.1	13.6	12.2	
Bone scan	21.5	59.3	68.9	73
CT			20.3	34.6
Acid phosphatase	65.9	72.4	72.4	68.4
Initial treatment				
None			36.1	28.9
TURP	23.6	33.2	36	
Prostatectomy	16.4	14.5	8.9	21.4
Radiation	16.4	14.5	22.8	22.6
Hormone	49.4	34.2	24	14

Key: DRE, digital rectal exam; TRUS, transrectal ultrasound; PSA, prostatic-specific antigen; TURP, transurethral resection of prostate.

at advanced clinical stage at time of diagnosis. This compares very favorably with the national pattern of 40% of prostate cancers diagnosed at an advanced stage. Cancers detected by DRE tended to be more advanced than those found on the basis of only TRUS or PSA. The tumors discovered in this early detection program showed a limited range of aggressiveness. Cancers were predominantly graded as Gleason score 4 or 5 across all of the detection modalities studied. Data from the American College of Surgeons surveys show, in contrast, that before the era of PSA screening in 1987, 7 was the Gleason score most often assigned (65).

Figure 30.18 shows the pattern of PSA observed in men found to have cancer and in men with no detected prostate cancer. These data reveal that only 15% of men without cancer exhibited PSA levels greater than 4.0 ng/ml. In contrast, more than 70% of men subsequently found to have cancer had PSA levels greater than 4.0 ng/ml.

Different indices that may enhance the early detection capability of PSA have been studied. In addition to those relating to the standard level of normal, PSA level relative to prostate gland volume (PSA density), age-referenced PSA level, and PSA change have been proposed as potentially useful indices (66, 67). To assess the performance of these different measures, specificity was studied in 2,011 ACS-NPCDP men without prostate cancer; sensitivity was determined for 171 men with prostate cancer (68). PSA change showed the highest specificity (96.4%) and PSA density the lowest (85.3%).

PSA density was the most sensitive index, positive for 74.7% of the 171 known cancers. PSA change of more than 0.75 ng/ml per year was least sensitive (54.8%). Sensitivity and specificity varied in a narrow range. Improved performance in specificity was achieved only with the loss of sensitivity. None of the alternative indexes commonly used in general early detection practice demonstrated particular advantage compared with normal PSA (defined as no greater than 4.0 ng/ml).

The cost effectiveness of DRE, TRUS, and PSA has been addressed using ACS-NPCDP results (69). Prostate cancer early detection was observed to be comparable to breast cancer screening in reducing treatment costs. The savings achieved by the lower cost of cancer treatment for early-detected cases were compared with the high costs for the treatment of more advanced cancers typically diagnosed in the United States. The procedure that appears least expensive, the DRE, can involve higher costs in a program of periodic screening. This is largely the result of the lower sensitivity of the DRE to early cancer after an initial normal examination.

While in this study it is not possible to evaluate reduction in mortality related to screening, there is evidence that, after an initial screen, the rate of detecting cancers at an advanced stage was decreased. Of the six advanced cancers, five were detected at the initial screen and only one in the second; thereafter, no advanced cancers were detected (63).

A randomized Canadian PSA screening trial using PSA in 7,350 unscreened males aged 45 to 80 was reported (54). PSA used as a prescreening test (a positive test being a value above 3.0 ng/ml) detected 88%; an additional 12% were detected by adding the DRE on the initial screen, but only 3% on follow-up screens. Four hundred seven cancers were detected. After the initial screen, no more cases of advanced cancer were detected over six screening periods.

GENERALIZED PSA SCREENING IN THE UNITED STATES

The dynamics gleaned from RCTs suggest that successful screening trials should demonstrate the following findings for the study compared with the control group: (*a*) in the initial (prevalence) screen, many more cases should be detected; (*b*) in the study group there should be more early cases—a shift in stage; (*c*) in subsequent (incidence) screenings, there should be a marked decrease in the number of cases detected; (*d*) in subsequent screenings, there should be a reduction in the number of advanced cases; (*e*) with years of follow-up, there should be a reduction in the number of deaths due to prostate cancer.

The first indication of a successful screening program is observing a detection rate that is two to three times greater than the expected incidence rate (as seen in Fig. 30.12). Cases detected at a first screening ordinarily might not have been detected for several years. Second, the increase was largely in localized (Fig. 30.14) and Gleason grade 5 to 7 cancers (see Fig. 30.15), which suggests that the increase in detected cancers was clinically important and that they were of a type that might be benefited by treatment, rather than the indolent occult type which should not be treated. Third, after the majority of men have been screened a first time and the prevalent cancers detected, one should see the incidence rate decrease. In 1993 the incidence rate decreased in two SEER registries, Utah and Seattle. Fourth, in the Utah registry there has also been a decrease in the rate of distant disease. A decrease in advanced disease should be an intermediate indicator, suggesting future decreases in mortality. Fifth, no decrease in mortality should be expected for several years. The present national trends are encouraging, and, hopefully, will lead to a decrease in the mortality rate from prostate cancer (see Chapter 126).

SUGGESTION

The present recommendation of the ACS and the AUA that men over 50 years of age have annual screening by DRE and PSA has a scientific basis suggesting greater possible benefit than harm. Screening should continue to determine its ultimate effect on mortality. Further studies and follow-up are important in assessing the ultimate value for PSA screenings. Special attention should be given those at higher risk, namely, black males and men with a family history of prostate cancer.

Oral Cancer

SIGNIFICANCE

An estimated 28,150 new cases of oral cancer will be diagnosed in the United States and 8,370 deaths will occur in 1995 (6). The disease will affect approximately 19,800 men and 9,700 women. Oral cancer accounts for about 4% of cancers in men and 2% in women. It occurs more frequently in blacks than in whites. More than 90% of all oral cancers occur in patients over the age of 45. Incidence increases steadily with age until about age 65, when the rate levels off at 45 to 50 cases per 100,000 population (Fig. 30.19) (3, 32). Trends over the past 11 years show no change in incidence and a slight decrease in mortality rate (Fig. 30.20).

The primary risk factors in American men and women are

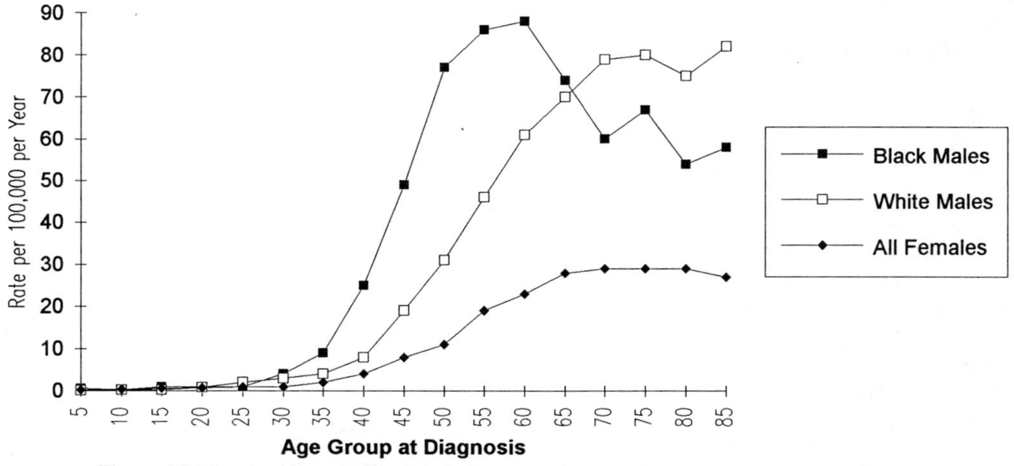

Figure 30.19. Incidence of oral and pharyngeal cancer by age group, sex, and race.

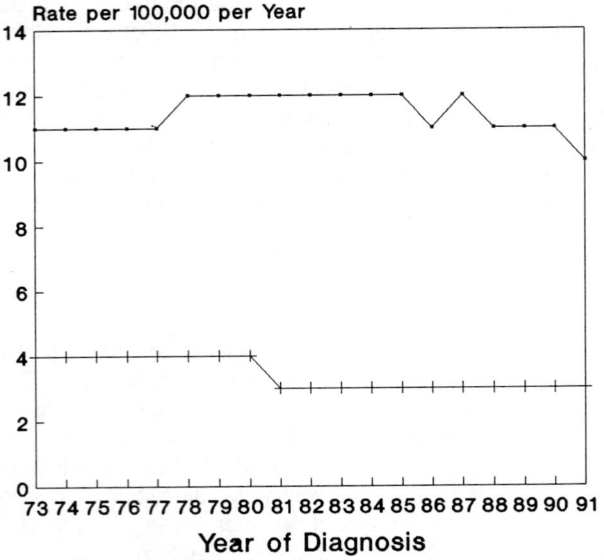

Figure 30.20. Oropharyngeal cancer: trends in incidence (•) and mortality (+). (SEER Cancer Statistics Review, 1973–1991.)

tobacco (including smokeless tobacco) and alcohol use, lower socioeconomic status, poor oral hygiene, and decayed teeth (70). Oral cancer occurs in a region of the body that is generally accessible to physical examination by the patient, the dentist, and the physician. Screening can be made more efficient by inspecting the high-risk sites where 90% of all squamous cell cancers arise: the floor of the mouth, the ventrolateral aspect of the tongue, and the soft palate complex (71). Leukoplakia and erythroplastic lesions are the earliest and most serious signs of squamous cell carcinoma (72). It has been pointed out that high-risk persons visit their medical doctors more frequently than they visit their dentists. An inspection of the oral cavity should be part of every physical examination in a dentist's or physician's office (73).

Although easily detected and often cured in its early stages, most oral cancers are moderately advanced (regional stage) at the time of diagnosis. Unfortunately, this trend has not changed. The overall survival rate has increased slightly (see Chapter 105).

EVIDENCE OF BENEFIT

Routine examination of asymptomatic patients results in the detection of earlier-stage cancers as well as premalignant lesions. In 1982, routine oral examinations were performed on 672,000 veteran patients examined on their initial visit, with the detection of 814 oral squamous cell cancers. In high-risk heavy smokers and drinkers over 40 years of age, the detection rate can be as high as one cancer in every 200 to 250 individuals examined (71).

In a regional oral cancer detection program in the Boston area, early-stage disease increased from 20 to 33% over a 3-year period when investigators stressed the importance of the routine oral examination (74). It did not require an intricate, time-consuming procedure, just an examination. In Sri Lanka, primary health care workers were trained in the oral examination, and they sent to a referral center 660 persons with suspected cancers, of which only 10% had no lesion and 58% were confirmed as having oral cancer (75).

Early oral carcinomas are amenable to treatment. The effect of stage of disease at diagnosis on survival in oral cancer is demonstrated in Figures 30.21 and 30.22, showing a difference in stage at presentation between white and black males and a corresponding difference in survival.

Although no randomized clinical trials show the efficacy of early detection, as measured by improvement in survival or decrease in mortality, until proven otherwise, it must be assumed that early detection and treatment will prevent deaths from oral cancer.

SUGGESTION

Visual oral examination, including palpation of the tongue, floor of the mouth, salivary glands, and lymph nodes of the neck, should be a routine part of the physical examination. Special attention should be given those at high risk due to tobacco and alcohol use.

Testicular Cancer

SIGNIFICANCE

It is estimated that 7,100 new cases of testicular cancer will be diagnosed, and 370 men will die of the disease in 1995 (6). Testicular cancer accounts for only 1% of all cancers in men. Despite a slow apparent increase in incidence, there has been a dramatic decrease in the mortality as a result of recent new treatments (Fig. 30.23) (32).

Unlike most other cancers, this disease is generally found in young men (Fig. 30.24) (6, 32). In white men, it is the most common cancer between 20 and 34 years of age, the second most common from 35 to 39 years of age, and the third most common from age 15 to 19 years. This type of cancer is 4.5 times more common among white men than blacks, with intermediate incidence rates for Hispanics, Native Americans, and Asians. High-risk groups exist. Males with cryptorchidism have 3 to 17 times the average risk; this means that, for every 10 patients with the condition, one will develop testicular cancer. There is also an increased risk in males with gonadal dysgenesis and Klinefelter's syndrome (76), as well as in the sons of women who took diethylstilbestrol (DES) to minimize spontaneous abortion.

Most testicular cancers are discovered by patients themselves, by accident or by self-examination. Approximately 60% are localized, 24% regional, and 14% distant stage at diagnosis (6).

In 1974, cisplatin and multidrug combination chemotherapy and radical retroperitoneal lymph node dissections were introduced for the treatment of advanced-stage disease. Excellent results are now achieved for regional as well as localized disease. There is, however, still a 30% case fatality rate for patients diagnosed with disseminated nonsemi-

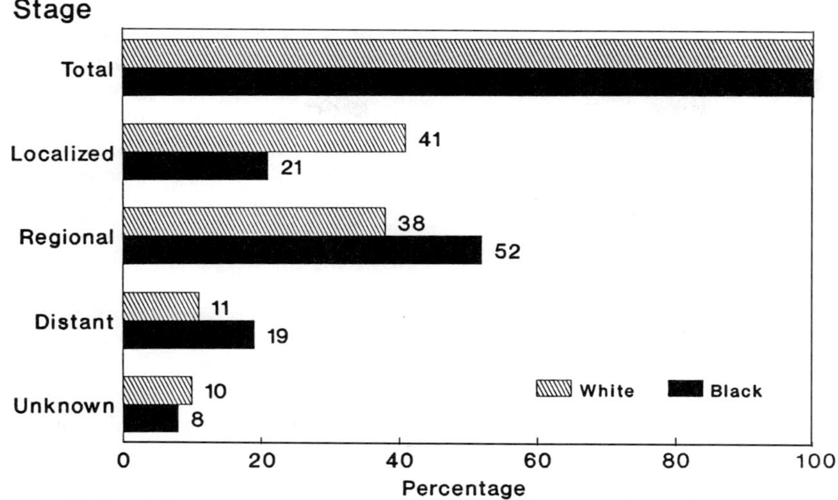

Figure 30.21. Oral and pharyngeal cancer in males, stage at diagnosis by race. (SEER Data 1974–1986, 1990 Report.)

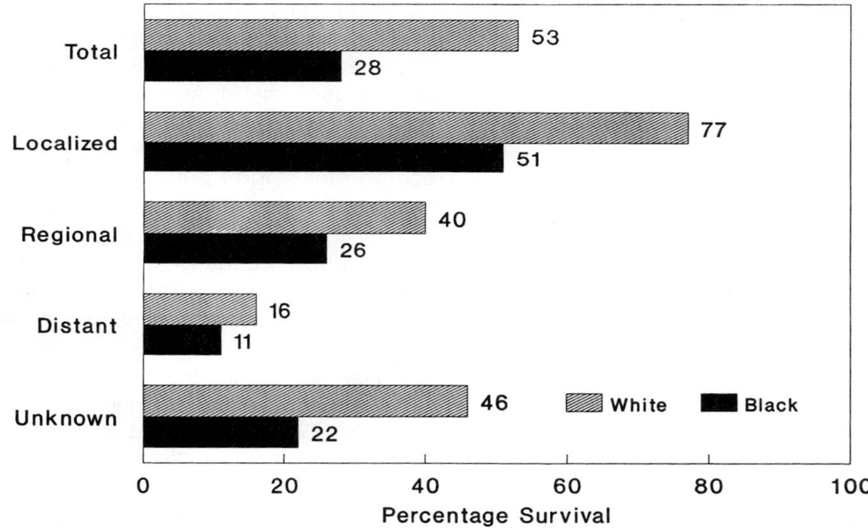

Figure 30.22. Oral and pharyngeal cancer in males, 5-year relative survival by race. (SEER Data 1973–1986.)

nomatous testicular cancer, including a 5% death rate from the toxicity of chemotherapeutic regimens (77). In Einhorn's initial experience with platinum-based multiagent chemotherapy, 93 to 96% of patients with minimal pulmonary or minimal pulmonary plus minimal abdominal disease, respectively, attained complete response following treatment. In contrast, only 65% of patients with advanced or bulky abdominal disease responded completely. Complete response usually means cure, while partial response is followed by relapse and death. Nevertheless, the majority of patients with regional and early advanced disease benefited from the new treatment, resulting in a marked increase in overall survival. There has also been a 60% decrease in mortality, without any appreciable change in the stage distribution at diagnosis (see Chapter 138).

EVIDENCE OF BENEFIT

Most testicular cancers are first detected by the patient by accident or by self-examination. Some are discovered by routine physical examination. Both detection methods entail little cost or morbidity. Delayed diagnosis leading to advanced disease has detrimental effects beyond a decrease in patient survival. The amount of treatment required, in terms of courses of chemotherapy and extent of surgery, is greater and carries higher morbidity and cost than for patients diagnosed early with a low-stage tumor.

SUGGESTION

Education in testicular self-examination should be encouraged, and clinical testicular examination should be part of

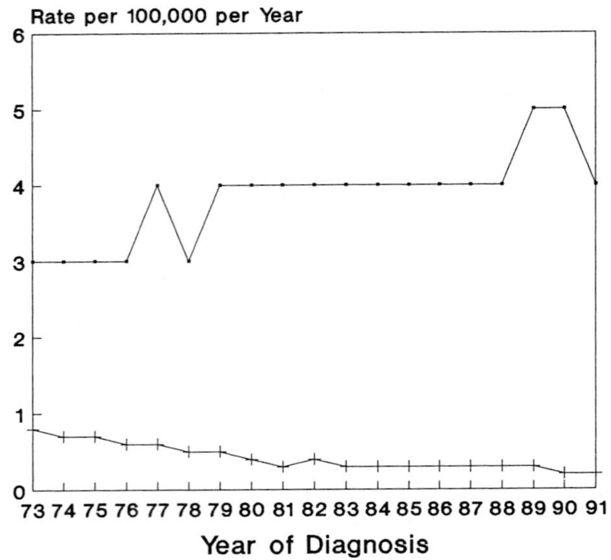

Figure 30.23. Testicular cancer: trends in incidence (●) and mortality (+). (SEER Cancer Statistics Review, 1973–1991.)

the routine physical examination. Special attention should be given men at high risk, individuals with a history of cryptorchidism, gonadal dysgenesis, and Klinefelter's syndrome.

Skin Cancer

SIGNIFICANCE

Skin cancer, the most common cancer in the United States, affects some 600,000 white Americans every year. It accounts for 1% of all cancer deaths (6). Nearly all skin cancers occur in fair-skinned individuals who have been exposed to the sun, x-rays, or ultraviolet light for prolonged periods (see Chapter 137). There are three main types: basal cell, squamous cell (the most prevalent), and malignant melanoma. Basal and squamous cell cancers have an excellent prognosis, but persons with nonmelanoma skin cancer are at high risk for developing additional skin cancers (78). They are easily detected clinically and are often cured by excisional biopsy. When neglected, they can be very deforming and can cause death.

In 1995, about 34,100 individuals are expected to develop melanoma and almost 7,200 will die from it (6). Melanoma, the rarest but most virulent form of skin cancer, is responsible for 75% of all deaths from skin cancer and will be the focus of this discussion. The incidence of melanoma rises rapidly in Caucasians after age 20 (Fig. 30.25). In recent years, the mortality from melanoma has increased (Fig. 30.26), especially in white males (79, 80), possibly as a result of increased recreational exposure to sunlight. Incidence increased nearly 80% between 1973 and 1991, at a rate of approximately 4% per year (32). Fair-skinned individuals exposed to the sun are at higher risk. The best defense against skin cancer is protection from the sun and ultraviolet light. Patients should be counseled to avoid excessive and continuous sun exposure and to use protective clothing and sunscreens (81). Individuals with certain types of pigmented lesions (sporadic dysplastic nevi, congenital nevus, lentigo maligna) and those with familial dysplastic nevus syndrome are at higher risk for developing melanoma (82). Patients who have a history of melanoma are at greater risk for developing a second melanoma (83).

EVIDENCE OF BENEFIT

Progress can be measured in overall survival rates. The 5-year rate has continued to increase over time. In 1973, the 5-year survival rate was 71.9%, whereas in 1986 it had increased to 87.0%. Over 90% of melanomas that arise in the skin can be recognized with the naked eye. Very often, there is a prolonged horizontal growth phase during which time the tumor expands centrifugally beneath the epidermis but does not invade the underlying dermis. This horizontal growth phase provides lead time for early detection. Melanoma is 100% curable if treated prior to the onset of the vertical growth phase with its metastatic potential (78). Two countries, Australia and Scotland, have had vigorous public and professional education programs, resulting in a shift to earlier-stage disease detection and improved survival. In Queensland, Australia, which has the highest incidence of melanoma in the world, the overall survival rate for 1,187 patients was greater than 82%. No deaths were recorded for stage I patients, and stage II patients had a 10-year survival of 90% (84). A similar program in Scotland also led to the detection of early-stage disease (85). Following a public education program in Scotland, the proportion of patients with primary melanomas categorized as "thin, good prognosis" had risen from 38 to 62%. The proportion of tumors categorized as "thick, poor prognosis" had fallen from 34 to 15%.

The probability of tumor recurrence in 10 years is less than 10% with tumors less than 1.4 mm thick. For patients with tumors less than 0.76 mm thick, the likelihood of recurrence is less than 1% in 10 years (86).

An important additional advantage of early detection is a reduction in the need for admission to the hospital and, thus, decreased hospital costs. A high proportion of patients with thin melanoma require only local excision, which can be performed on an outpatient basis. The treatment of early lesions is less morbid than the treatment of advanced lesions. A recent retrospective analysis suggests that early detection of melanoma decreases mortality from the disease (87).

SUGGESTION

Education in the dangers of excessive sun and ultraviolet light exposure, especially for fair-skinned individuals, should continue as should awareness of the importance of investigating changing skin lesion, with particular attention to those that are black or multicolored. An examination of the skin should be a part of the routine physical examination. Special attention should be given those with a personal or family history of melanoma or dysplastic nevi.

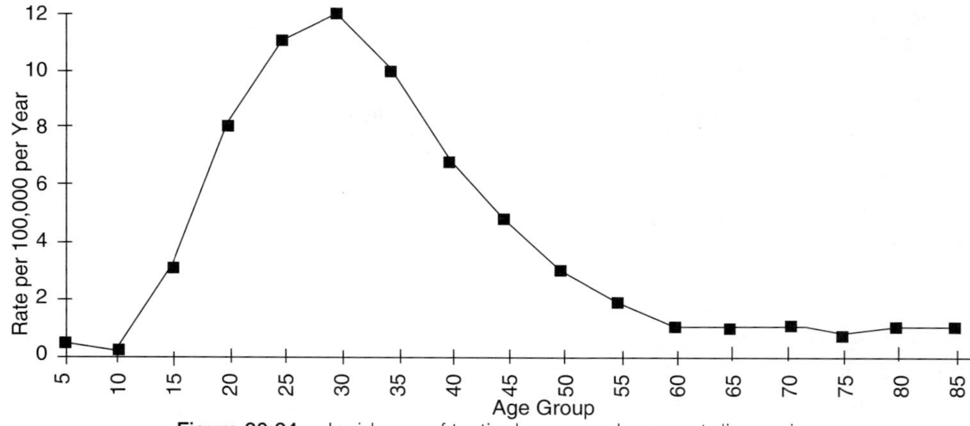

Figure 30.24. Incidence of testicular cancer by age at diagnosis.

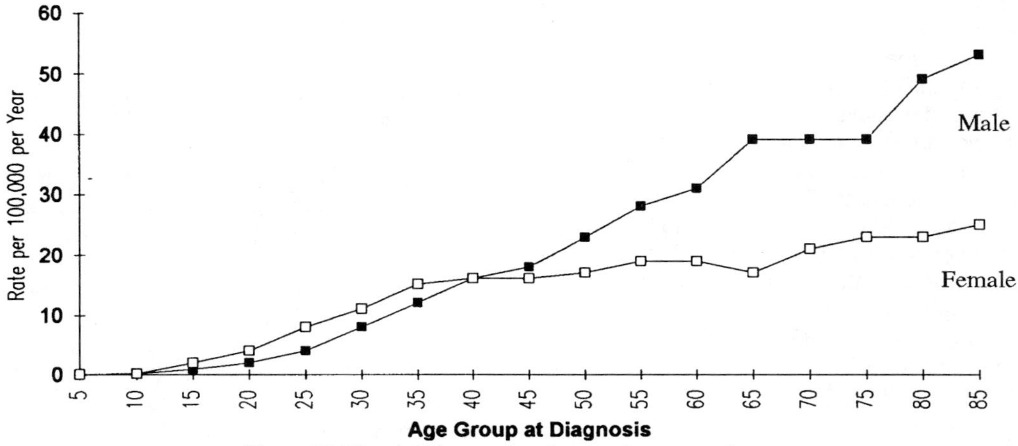

Figure 30.25. Incidence of melanoma by age and sex.

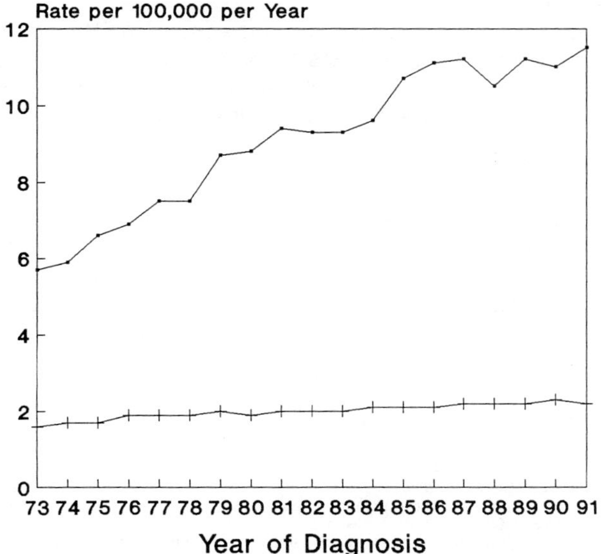

Figure 30.26. Melanoma skin cancer: trends in incidence (•) and mortality (+). (SEER Cancer Statistics Review, 1973–1991.)

Cervical Cancer

SIGNIFICANCE

In 1995, more than 15,800 cases of invasive cervical cancer are expected to occur, with about 4,800 women dying from this disease (6). From 1950 to 1970, the incidence and mortality rates for invasive cervical cancer fell impressively, by more than 70% (88). Since the early 1980s, however, the rates for incidence and mortality appear to be decreasing more slowly (Fig. 30.27). According to incidence and mortality rates, screening for cervical cancer should start in the late teens, when these rates begin their upward trend (Fig. 30.28). Rates for carcinoma in situ reach peak for both black and white women between 20 and 30 years of age. After age 25, however, the incidence of invasive cancer in black women increases rapidly with age, while in white women the incidence rises more slowly. Mortality also increases with advancing age, with dramatic differences between black and white women. Extra effort is warranted to reach older women who have not been screened. More than 25% of all invasive cervical cancers occur in women older than 65, and 40 to 50% of all women who die from cervical cancer are over 65 years of age (89, 90). A large proportion of women, particularly elderly black women and middle-aged poor women, do not get regular Pap smears (91). In some areas, as many as 75% of women over 65 have not had a Pap smear within the previous 5 years (92). These patterns underscore the importance of special screening efforts targeted to reach women who do not receive regular screening (see Chapter 130).

EVIDENCE OF BENEFIT

The widespread acceptance of the Pap smear makes the possibility of testing the efficacy of cervical cytology by randomized trials remote. Nevertheless, substantial evidence from observational studies indicates that mortality from cervical cancer can be reduced by screening.

Mortality from cervical cancer has decreased in several large populations following the introduction of well-run screening programs (93, 94). Data from several large Scandinavian studies show sharp reductions in incidence and mortality following the initiation of organized screening programs. Iceland reduced mortality rate by 80% over 20 years, and Finland and Sweden reduced their mortality rate 50 and 34%, respectively (93). Similar reductions have been found in large populations in the United States and Canada.

Reductions in incidence and mortality seem to be proportional to the intensity of screening efforts. The Scandinavian countries with the highest rates of screening activity reported greater reductions in mortality than those countries with lower rates of screening (93, 95). Mortality in the Canadian provinces was reduced most remarkably in British Columbia, which had screening rates two to five times those of the other provinces (96).

Case-control studies have found that the risk of developing invasive cervical cancer is three to ten times greater in women who have not been screened (97, 98). Risk also increases with longer duration following the last normal Pap smear, or similarly, with decreasing frequency of screening (99, 100). Screening every 2 to 3 years, however, has not been found to increase significantly the risk of finding invasive cervical cancer above the risk expected with annual screening (100, 101).

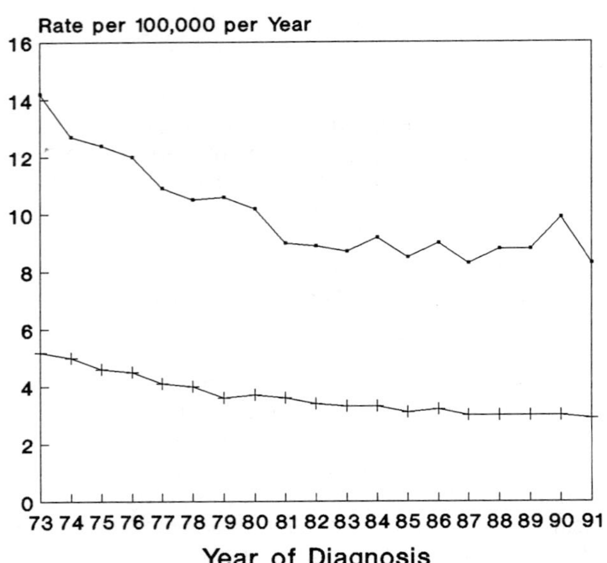

Figure 30.27. Cancer of the cervix: trends in incidence (•) and mortality (+). (SEER Cancer Statistics Review, 1973–1991.)

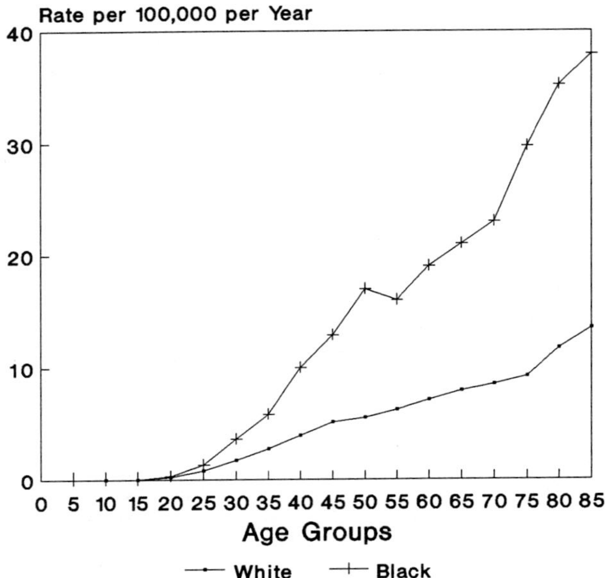

Figure 30.28. Cancer of the cervix: age-specific incidence. (SEER Cancer Statistics Review, 1973–1988.)

The analysis of survival data shows that survival appears to be directly related to the stage of disease at diagnosis. The 5-year relative survival rate for cervical cancer is 91% for women with an initial diagnosis of localized disease. For those initially diagnosed with distant disease, survival is only 12% (6). Early detection, using cervical cytology, is currently the only practical means of detecting cervical cancer in localized or premalignant stages.

Evidence strongly suggests a decrease in mortality from regular screening with Pap tests in women who are sexually active or who have reached 18 years of age. The upper age limit at which to cease screening is unknown.

SUGGESTION

An annual Pap smear and pelvic examination should be done on all women who are, or have been sexually active or are at least 18 years of age. After a woman has had three or more consecutive satisfactory normal annual examinations, the Pap test may be performed less frequently, at the discretion of her physician.

References

1. American Cancer Society Guidelines for the cancer-related checkup: recommendations and rationale. CA 1980;30:194–240.
2. Smart CR. The impact of the U.S. Preventive Services Task Force guidelines on cancer screening: perspective from the National Cancer Institute. J Gen Intern Med 1990;5:S28–S33.
3. Miller AB, Baines CJ, To T, Wall C. Canadian National Breast Screening Study: 1. Breast cancer detection and death rates among women aged 40 to 49 years. Can Med Assoc J 1992;147:1459–1476.
4. Mettlin C, Smart CR. Breast cancer detection guidelines for women aged 40 to 49 years: rationale for the American Cancer Society reaffirmation of recommendations. American Cancer Society. CA 1994;44:248–255.

5. Fletcher SW, Black W, Harris R, Rimer BK, Shapiro S. Report of the International Workshop on Screening for Breast Cancer. JNCI 1993;85:1644–1656.
6. Wingo PA, Tong T, Bolden S. Cancer statistics 1995. CA 1995;45:8–30.
7. Byrne C, Smart CR, Chu KC, Hartmann WH. Survival advantage differences by age. Evaluation of the extended follow-up of the Breast Cancer Detection Demonstration Project. Cancer 1994;74:301–310.
8. Chu KC, Smart CR, Tarone RE. Analysis of breast cancer mortality and stage-distribution by age for the Health Insurance Plan Study: a randomized trial with breast cancer screening. JNCI 1988;80:1125–1132.
9. Tabar L, Fagerberg CJ, Gad A, Baldetorp L, Holmberg LH, Grontoft O, Ljungquist U, Lundstrom B, Manson JC, Eklund G. Reduction in mortality from breast cancer after mass screening with mammography. Randomised trial from the Breast Cancer Screening Working Group of the Swedish National Board of Health and Welfare. Lancet 1985;1:829–832.
10. Smart CR, Hendrick RE, Rutledge JH Jr, Smith RA. Benefit of mammography screening in women aged 40–49: current evidence from randomized controlled trials. Cancer 1995;75:1619–1626.
11. Tabar L, Fagerberg G, Chan HH, Duffy SW, Smart CR, Gad A, Smith RA. Efficacy of breast cancer screening by age: new results from the Swedish Two-County Trial. Cancer 1995;75:2507–2517.
12. Duffy SW, Tabar L, Fagerberg G, Gad A, Gröntoft O, South MC, Day NE. Breast screening, prognostic factors and survival—results from the Swedish two county study. Br J Cancer 1991;64:1133–1138.
13. Tabar L, Duffy SW, Burhenne LW. New Swedish breast cancer detection results for women aged 40–49. Cancer 1993;72:1437–1448.
14. Tabar L, Duffy SW, Krusemo UB. Detection method, tumour size and node metastases in breast cancers diagnosed during a trial of breast cancer screening. Eur J Cancer Clin Oncol 1987;23:959–962.
15. Tabar L, Dean PB. The control of breast cancer through mammography screening. What is the evidence? Radiol Clin North Am 1987;25:993–1005.
16. Tabar L, Faberberg G, Day NE, Holmberg L. What is the optimum interval between mammographic screening examinations? An analysis based on the latest results of the Swedish two-county breast cancer screening trial. Br J Cancer 1987;55:547–551.
17. Elwood JM, Cox B, Richardson AK. The effectiveness of breast cancer screening by mammography in younger women. Online. J Curr Clin Trials 1993;1:32–227.
18. Nyström L, Rutqvist LE, Wall S, Lindgren A, Lindqvist M, Ryden S, et al. Breast cancer screening with mammography: overview of the Swedish randomized trials. Lancet 1993;341:973–978.
19. Wald N, Chamberlain F, Hackshaw A. Report of the European Society for Mastology: Breast Cancer Screening Evaluation Committee (1993). Breast 1993;2:206–216.
20. Kerlikowske K, Grady D, Rubin SM, Sandrock C, Ernster VL. Efficacy of screening mammography: a meta-analysis. JAMA 1995;273:149–154.
21. Shapiro S, Venet W, Strax P, Venet L. Periodic Screening for Breast Cancer: The Health Insurance Plan Project and Its Sequelae. 1963–1986. Baltimore: Johns Hopkins, 1988.
22. Tabár L, Fagerberg CJG, Gad A, Baldertorp L, Holmberg LH, Grontoft O, et al. Reduction in mortality from breast cancer after mass screening with mammography: randomized trial from the Breast Cancer Screening Working Group of the Swedish National Board of Health and Welfare. Lancet 1985;1:829–832.
23. Tarone RE. The excess of patients with advanced breast cancer in young women screened with mammography in the Canadian National Breast Screening Study. Cancer 1995;75:997–1003.
24. Sickles EA, Kopans DB. Deficiencies in the analysis of breast cancer data. JNCI 1993;85:1621–1624.
25. Kopans DB, Feig SA. The Canadian National Breast Screening Study: a critical review. AJR 1993;161:755–760.
26. Curpen BN, Sickles EA, Sollitto RA, Ominsky SH, Galvin HB, Frankel SD. The comparative value of mammographic screening for women 40–49 years old versus women 50–64 years old. Am J Roentgenol 1995;164:1099–1103.
27. Smart CR, Hartmann WH, Beahrs OH, Garfinkel L. Insights into breast cancer screening of younger women. Evidence from the 14-year follow-up of the Breast Cancer Detection Demonstration Project. Cancer 1993;72:1449–1456.
28. Smart CR. Highlights of the evidence of benefit for women aged 40–49 years from the 14-year follow-up of the Breast Cancer Detection Demonstration Project. Cancer 1995;74:296–300.
29. Kopans DB. Breast screening in women under 50 (letter). Lancet 1991;338:447.
30. Moskowitz M. Guidelines for screening for breast cancer. Is a revision in order? Radiol Clin North Am 1992;30:221–233.
31. Moskowitz M. Overview of guidelines for screening. Cancer 1992;69:1932–1937.
32. Ries LAG, Miller BA, Hankey BF, Kosary CL, Harras A, Edwards BK. SEER Cancer Statistics Review 1973–1991: Tables and Graphs. NIH publication no. 94-2789, 1994.
33. Ransohoff DF, Lang C. Screening for colorectal cancer. N Engl J Med 1991;325: 37–41.
34. Winawer SJ. Screening for colorectal cancer. Cancer Prin Pract Oncol Updates 1987;2:1–16.
35. Smart CR. Screening and early diagnosis. Cancer 1992;70:1246–1251.
36. Hertz RE, Deddish MR, Day Z. Value of periodic examinations in detecting cancer of the rectum and colon. Postgrad Med 1960;27:290–294.
37. Gilbertsen VA. Proctosigmoidoscopy and polypectomey in reducing the incidence of rectal cancer. Cancer 1974;34(suppl 3):936–939.
38. Friedman GD, Collen MF, Fireman BH. Multiphasic health checkup evaluation: a 16-year follow-up. J Chronic Dis 1986;39:453–463.
39. Selby JR, Friedman GD, Quesenberry CP. A case-controlled study of screening sigmoidoscopy and mortality from colorectal cancer. N Engl J Med 1992;326:653–657.
40. Newcomb PA, Norfleet RG, Storer BE. Screening sigmoidoscopy and colorectal cancer mortality. JNCI 1992;84:1572–1575.
41. Winawer SJ, Flehinger BJ, Schottenfeld D. Screening for colorectal cancer with fecal occult blood testing and sigmoidoscopy. JNCI 1993;85:1311–1318.
42. Mandel JS, Bond JH, Church TR. Reducing mortality from colorectal cancer by screening for fecal occult blood. N Engl J Med 1993;328:1365–1371.
43. Kewenter J, Bjork S, Haglind Z. Screening and rescreening for colorectal cancer: a controlled trial of fecal occult blood testing in 27,700 subjects. Cancer 1988;62: 645–651.
44. Hardcastle JD, Thomas WM, Chamberlain J. Randomised, controlled trial of faecal occult blood screening for colorectal cancer. Lancet 1989;1:1160–1164.
45. Kronborg O, Fenger C, Snergaard O. Initial mass screening for colorectal cancer with fecal occult blood test. Scand J Gastroenterol 1987;22:677–686.
46. Kronborg O, Fenger C, Olsen J. Repeated screening for colorectal cancer with fecal occult blood test. A prospective. Scand J Gastroenterol 1989;24:599–606.
47. Eddy D. Screening for colorectal cancer. Ann Intern Med 1990;113:373–384.
48. Allison JE, Feldman R, Takawa IS. Hemoccult screening in detecting colorectal neoplasms: sensitivity and specificity. Ann Intern Med 1990;112:328–333.
49. Eddy D, Nugent FW, Eddy JF. Screening for colorectal cancer in a high-risk population: results of a mathematical model. Gastroenterology 1987;682–692.
50. Murphy GP, Natarajan N, Pontes JE, Schmitz RL, Smart CR, Schmidt JD, Mettlin C. The national survey of prostate cancer in the United States by the American College of Surgeons. J Urol 1982;127:928–934.
51. Mettlin C, Murphy GP, Menck H. Trends in treatment of localized prostate cancer by radical prostatectomy: observations Cancer (in press).
52. Cooner WH, Mosley Br, Rutherford CL Jr, Beard JH, Pond HS, Terry WJ, Igel TC, Kidd DD. Prostate cancer detection in a clinical urological practice by ultrasonography, digital rectal examination and prostate-specific antigen. J Urol 1990;143:1146–52.
53. Richie JP, Catalona WJ, Ahmann FR, Hudson MA, Scardino PT, Flanigan RC, deKernion JB, Ratliff TL, Kavoussi LR, Dalkin BL. Effect of patient age on early detection of prostate cancer with serum prostate-specific antigen and digital rectal examination. Urology 1993;42:365–374.
54. Labrie F, Dupont A, Suburu R, Cusan L, Gomez JL, Koutsilieris M, Diamond P, Emond J, Lemay M, Candas B. Optimized strategy for detection of early stage, curable prostate cancer: role of prescreening with prostate-specific antigen. Clin Invest Med 1993;16:425–439.
55. Mettlin C, Dodd GD. The American Cancer Society Guidelines for the cancer-related checkup: an update. CA 1991;41:279–282.
56. Mettlin C, Jones G, Averette H, Gusberg SB, Murphy GP. Defining and updating the American Cancer Society guidelines for the cancer-related checkup: an update. CA 1993;43:42–46.
57. Johansson FE, Adami HO, Andersson SO, Bergstrom R, Holmberg L, Krusemo UB. High 10-year survival rate in patients with early, untreated prostatic cancer. JAMA 1993;267:2191–2196.
58. Chisholm GD, Rana A. Is the outcome of conservative management for localized prostate cancer acceptable? An overview. Eur Urol 1993;24(suppl 2):64–66.
59. Chodak GW, Thisted RA, Gerber GS, Johansson JE, Adolfsson J, Jones GW, Chisholm GD, Moskovitz B, Livne PM, Warner J. Results of conservative management of clinically localized prostate. N Engl J Med 1994;330:242–248.
60. Franks LM. Etiology, epidemiology and pathology of prostatic cancer. Cancer 1973;32:1092–1095.
61. Kramer BS, Brown ML, Prorok PC, Potosky AL, Gohagan JK. Prostate cancer screening: what we know and what we need to know. Ann Intern Med 1993;119:914–923.
62. Gerber GS, Chodak GW. Value of prostate cancer screening. Eur Urol 1993;24: 161–165.
63. Mettlin C, Murphy GP, Ray P, Shanberg A, Toi A, Chesley A, Babaian R, Badalament R, Kane RA, Lee F. American Cancer Society—National Prostate Cancer Detection Project. Results from multiple examinations using transrectal ultrasound, digital rectal examination, prostate specific antigen. Cancer 1993;71:891–898.
64. Mettlin C, Murphy GP, Lee F, Littrup PJ, Chesley A, Babain R, Badalament R, Kane RA, Mostofi FK. Characteristics of prostate cancers detected in a multimodality early detection program. Cancer 1993;72:1701–1706.
65. Mettlin C, Jones GW, Murphy GP. Trends in prostate cancer care in the United States 1974–1990: observations from the patient care evaluation studies of the American College of Surgeons Commission on Cancer. CA 1993;43:83–91.
66. Oesterling JE, Jacobsen SJ, Chute CG, Guess HA, Girman CJ, Panse LA, et al. Serum prostate-specific antigen in a community-based population of healthy men. Establishment of age-specific reference ranges. JAMA 1993;270:860–864.
67. Carter HB, Pearson JD, Metter EJ, Brant LJ, Chan DW, Andres R, et al. Longitudinal evaluation of prostate-specific antigen levels in men with and without prostate disease. JAMA 1992;267:2215–2220.
68. Mettlin C, Littrup PJ, Kane RA, Murphy GP, Lee F, Chesley A, Badalament R, Mostofi FK. Relative sensitivity and specificity of serum PSA level compared to age-referenced PSA, PSA density and PSA change: data from the American Cancer Society National Prostate Cancer Detection Project. Cancer 1994;74:1615–1620.
69. Littrup PJ, Goodman AC, Mettlin CJ. The benefit and cost of prostate cancer early detection. CA 1993;43:134–149.
70. Elwood JM, Gallagher RP. Factors influencing early diagnosis of cancer of the oral cavity. Can Med Assoc J 1985;133:651–655.
71. Mashberg A, Barsa P. Screening for oral and oropharyngeal squamous carcinomas. CA 1995;34:262–268.
72. Chiodo GT, Eigner T, Rosenstein DI. Oral cancer detection: the importance of routine screening for prolongation of survival. Postgrad Med 1986;80:231–236.
73. Smart CR. Screening for cancer of the aerodigestive tract. Cancer 1993;72: 1061–1065.
74. Prout M. Follow-up studies on head and neck screening. Unpublished 1990.
75. Warnakulasuriya S, Pindborg JJ. Reliability of oral precancer screening by primary health care workers in Sri Lanka. Commun Dent Health 1990;7:73–79.
76. Henderson BE, Benton B, Jing J. Risk factors for cancer of the testis in young men. Int J Cancer 1979;23:598–602.
77. Morse MJ, Whitmore WF. Neoplasms of the Testis. Campbell's Urology, 5th ed. Edited by PW Walsh. 1986.
78. Friedman RJ, Rigel DS, Kopf AW. Early detection of malignant melanoma: the role of physician examination and self-examination. CA 1985;35:130–151.
79. National Cancer Institute. 1986 Annual Cancer Review. Bethesda: National Institutes of Health, 1989.
80. Morbidity and Mortality Report Centers for Disease Control Atlanta. Death rates of malignant melanoma among white men—United States 1973–1988. Arch Dermatol 1992;128:451–452.
81. Drolet BA, Connor MJ. Sunscreens and the prevention of ultraviolet radiation-induced skin cancer. J Dermatol Surg Oncol 1992;18:571–576.
82. Mihm MC, Barnhill RL, Sober AJ. Precursor lesions of melanoma: do they exist? Semin Surg Oncol 1992;8:358–365.

83. Karagas MR, Stukel TA, Greenberg ER. Risk of subsequent basal cell carcinoma and squamous cell carcinoma. JAMA 1992;267:3305–3310.
84. Holman CD, James IR, Gattey PH. An analysis of trends in mortality from malignant melanoma of the skin in Australia. Int J Cancer 1980;26:703–709.
85. Doherty VR, MacKie M. Reasons for poor prognosis in British patients with cutaneous malignant melanoma. Br Med J 1986;292:987–989.
86. Blois MS, Sagebiel RW, Abarbanel RM. Malignant melanoma of the skin: I. the association of tumor depth and type. Cancer 1983;52:1330–1341.
87. Cristofolini M, Bianchi R, Boi S. Analysis of the cost-effectiveness ratio of the health campaign for the early diagnosis of cutaneous melanoma in Trentino, Italy. Cancer 1993;71:370–374.
88. National Cancer Institute. Cancer Statistics Review 1973–1987. NIH publication no. 90-2789, 1990.
89. Surveillance Program. Division of Cancer Prevention and Control, National Cancer Institute, 1990 (unpublished data).
90. Remington P, Lantz P, Phillips JL. Cervical cancer deaths among older women: implications for prevention. Wisc Med J 1990;89:30, 32–34.
91. Makuc DM, Freid VM, Kleinman JC. National trends in the use of preventive health care by women. Am J Public Health 1989;79:21–26.
92. Mandelblatt J, Gopaui I, Wistreich M. Gynecological care of elderly women: another look at Papanicolaou smear testing. JAMA 1986;256:367–371.
93. Laara E, Day NE, Hakama M. Trends in mortality from cervical cancer in the Nordic countries: association with organised screening programmes. Lancet 1987;1: 1247–1249.
94. Johannesson G, Geirsson G, Day N. The effect of mass screening in Iceland, 1965–1974, on the incidence and mortality of cervical carcinoma. Int J Cancer 1978;21:418–425.
95. Sigurdsson K. Effect of organized screening on the risk of cervical cancer: evaluation of screening activity in Iceland. Int J Cancer 1993;54:563–570.
96. Benedet JL, Anderson MB, Matisic JP. A comprehensive program for cervical cancer detection and management. J Obstet Gynecol 1992;166:1254–1259.
97. Aristizabal N, Cuello C, Correa P. The impact of vaginal cytology on cervical cancer risks in Calf, Colombia. Int J Cancer 1984;34:5–9.
98. Herrero R, Brinton LA, Reeves WC. Screening for cervical cancer in Latin America: a case-control study. Int J Epidemiol 1992;21:1050–1056.
99. Celentano DD, Klassen AC, Weisman CS. Duration of relative protection of screening for cervical cancer. Prevent Med 1989;18:411–422.
100. International Agency for Research on Cancer Working Group on. Screening for squamous cervical cancer: duration of low risk after negative results of cervical cytology and its implication for screening policies. Br Med J 1986;293:659–664.
101. Kleinman JC, Kopstein A. Who is being screened for cervical cancer? Am J Public Health 1981;71:73–76.

SECTION VIII

PRINCIPLES OF CANCER PATHOLOGY

CHAPTER 31

Principles of Cancer Pathology

JAMES L. CONNOLLY, STUART J. SCHNITT, HELEN H. WANG, ANN M. DVORAK, AND HAROLD F. DVORAK

Introduction

Pathologists are physicians who are concerned primarily with the study of disease in all of its aspects—causation, diagnosis, pathogenesis, mechanisms, natural history, anatomic and biochemical features, progression, and prognosis. There is a great deal of truth in the old adage that pathologists are "doctors' doctors," consultants with specialized knowledge that can be helpful to the clinician who is caring directly for the patient. Nowhere in medicine is this adage truer than in the care of patients with cancer.

Pathologists engage in three major types of activity: anatomic pathology, which includes surgical pathology, cytology, and autopsy pathology; clinical pathology, also known as laboratory medicine, that is, the direction of clinical laboratories; and experimental pathology or basic investigations of the pathogenesis of disease. While oncologists are apt to interact most closely, most consistently, and on a more personal level with anatomic pathologists in the course of their practice, they need to be aware of the roles played by pathologists of all three types if they are to provide optimal patient care. This is particularly true now that the distinctions differentiating the several traditional types of pathologists have become blurred as advances in technology have moved from the research laboratory into the clinic—immunohistochemistry, flow cytometry, molecular biologic approaches to cancer diagnosis, and so on.

This chapter reviews some of the basic principles of pathology as they apply to neoplastic disease. Primary emphasis is on solid tumors, although much of what is said also applies to tumors of other types, such as lymphomas and leukemias. The goal is to provide for oncologists a better feeling for what pathologists do; how they arrive at diagnoses, what tools, and especially what modern tools, they have at their disposal, and how the oncologist can interact most productively with the pathologist to achieve the greatest benefit for the patient.

Solid Tumor Structure and Tumor Stroma Generation

STRUCTURE OF SOLID TUMORS

What is a tumor? Although physicians know very well what they mean when they use the term, the question is not a simple one that can be answered in a concise and comprehensive manner. The word "tumor" is of Latin origin and means "swelling." But not all swellings (e.g., the swellings of inflammation and repair) are tumors in the modern sense of the term. The distinguished pathologist Sir Rupert Willis has offered what is widely considered the best definition of a tumor: "A neoplasm (tumor) is an abnormal mass of tissue, the growth of which exceeds and is uncoordinated with that of the normal tissues and persists in the same excessive manner after cessation of the stimuli which evoked the change" (196). To this definition have been added three other properties (35): tumors are apparently purposeless, they prey on the host, and they are virtually autonomous. Rowlatt has modernized the definition as follows: "A neoplasm is a mass of tissue generated by cells capable of division which have acquired either permanent expressible heritable change or stable epigenetic change so that the same or other cells no longer respond appropriately to one or more normal tissue organizing stimuli, chemical or physical, intracellular or extracellular, in the organism in which it occurs" (155). However, even these rather cumbersome definitions are not perfectly satisfactory in that they fail to consider tumors that do not form discrete masses, such as leukemias and ascites tumors. Also, they do not take into consideration the fact that many neoplasms change in character as the result of tumor progression and acquire the ability to metastasize; that is, to form new tumors at sites discontinuous with the primary tumor.

Solid tumors do have a distinct structure that mimics that of normal tissues (35, 52, 53, 56). At all but perhaps their earliest stage of development, they form a mass that is composed of two distinct but interdependent compartments: the parenchyma (neoplastic cells) and the stroma that the neoplastic cells induce and in which they are dispersed. In many tumors, including those of epithelial cell origin, a basal lamina generally separates clumps of tumor cells from the stroma. However, the basal lamina is often incomplete, especially at points of tumor invasion.

The stroma is interposed between malignant cells and normal host tissues and is essential for tumor growth. It is largely a product of the host and is induced as the result of tumor cell–host interactions. Thus, it is composed of nonmalignant supporting tissue and includes connective tissue, blood vessels, and very often inflammatory cells. The stroma has as one of its components the vascular supply that tumors require for obtaining nutrients and for gas exchange and waste disposal. Most tumors, and certainly all solid tumors, regardless of their type or cellular origin, require stroma if they are to grow beyond a minimal size of 1 to 2 mm (68). On the other hand, the stroma may also limit the influx of inflammatory cells, or, alternatively, may limit the egress of tumor cells (invasion). The stroma, therefore, at once provides a lifeline that is necessary for tumor growth and imposes a barrier that inhibits and may regulate interchange of fluids, gases, and cells with the host.

The singular importance of new blood vessel formation to tumor survival and growth has rightly led to an emphasis on angiogenesis; however, this emphasis has been accompanied by an unfortunate tendency to undervalue other tumor stromal components. Blood vessels are only one component of tumor stroma. In fact, in many tumors, the bulk of the stroma is made up of interstitial connective tissue, and blood vessels are only a minor component of stromal mass. For the most part, tumor stroma is formed by elements that are derived from the circulating blood and from adjacent host connective tissues (199). Plasma components include water and plasma proteins, together with various types and numbers of inflammatory cells. Almost any element found in normal connective tissues may be represented in tumor stroma, even including bone and cartilage. Generally speaking, the major components of tumor stroma include, in addition to new blood vessels, leaked plasma and plasma proteins; proteoglycans and glycosaminoglycans; interstitial collagens (types I, III, and, to a lesser extent, V); fibrin (Fig. 31.1); fibronectin; and cells of two general types, fixed tissue cells, such as fibroblasts, that reside in normal connective tissue and inflammatory cells that are derived from the blood (199).

Although the same basic building blocks make up all tumor stroma, pathologists have long recognized that tumors differ markedly from one another in stromal content. Sometimes these differences are primarily quantitative. At one extreme are desmoplastic tumors, such as many carcinomas of the breast, stomach, and pancreas, in which up to 90% or more of the total tumor mass consists of stroma. At the other extreme are such tumors as medullary carcinomas of the breast and many lymphomas in which only minimal stroma is deposited.

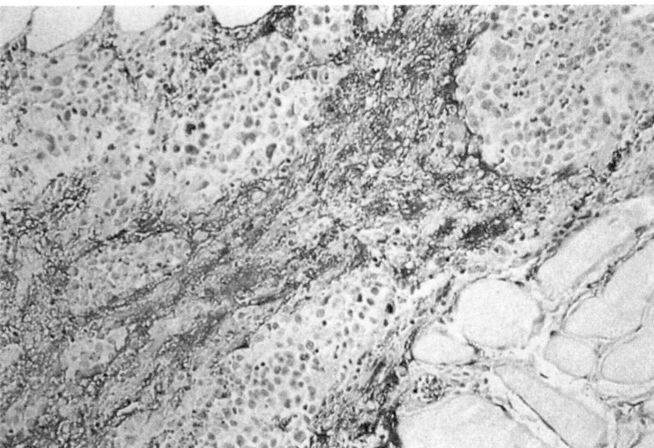

Figure 31.1. Immunoperoxidase staining reaction of line 10 guinea pig undifferentiated bile duct carcinoma exposed to a monoclonal antibody specific for fibrin (supplied by Dr. Gary Matsueda). Tumor comprises nests of malignant cells interspersed in a stroma that stains heavily for fibrin. Immunoperoxidase; magnification: ×50.

In other cases, differences in stromal content among different tumors are largely qualitative. For example, some carcinomas of the breast provoke the deposition of abundant elastic tissue along with collagen, whereas others (e.g., medullary carcinoma of the breast) induce an extensive lymphocytic infiltrate and little else in the way of stroma. Even within a single tumor there may be significant variations in stromal composition from one area to another. This stromal heterogeneity should not be surprising in view of the well-recognized heterogeneity of parenchymal cells present in individual tumors.

TUMOR STROMA GENERATION

Stroma Generation in Animal Tumors

Studies of transplantable tumors have revealed important new information concerning the pathogenesis of tumor stroma generation (Fig. 31.2) (52, 53, 199). The initial event in this process, commonly evident within an hour or less of tumor transplant, is locally increased vascular permeability to circulating macromolecules. This permeability increase cannot be accounted for by mast cell release of mediators, such as histamine, or by an immune or inflammatory response on the part of the host. Rather, it is attributable to a

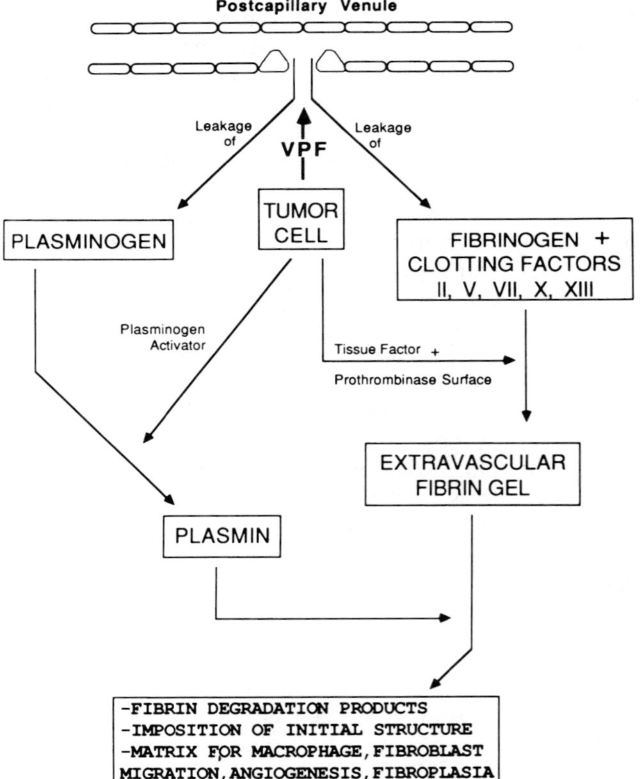

Figure 31.2. Pathogenesis of tumor stroma generation. VPF, vascular permeability factor.

protein, vascular permeability factor (VPF), that has been found to be synthesized and secreted by the great majority of tumors thus far studied. The VPF renders the microvasculature hyperpermeable to plasma and plasma proteins with a potency some 50,000 times that of histamine and ranks among the most powerful vascular permeabilizing substances known (Fig. 31.3) (53, 54, 57, 163, 164, 199). VPF has been purified to homogeneity and its cDNA has been cloned (101, 114, 162). It possesses several isoforms that result from alternative splicing of a single gene that is highly conserved in species as diverse as mice and humans (97). When injected into skin or other normal tissues, VPF, like mediators of inflammation, such as histamine, provokes the extravasation of a protein-rich plasma exudate; like histamine, the primary target of VPF action is postcapillary venules and small veins.

Local VPF-induced microvascular hyperpermeability is now thought to be an initial step in tumor angiogenesis and stroma generation (53). An important and almost immediate consequence of VPF action is plasma protein leakage with coagulation and cross-linking of fibrinogen to form an extravascular fibrin gel (52–54, 57). Fibrinogen extravasates, along with other plasma proteins, from leaky blood vessels, and is rapidly clotted by thrombin to form fibrin monomers that polymerize spontaneously and subsequently are covalently cross-linked by clotting factor XIII, a plasma protein transglutaminase that also extravasates from leaky vessels and is itself activated by thrombin. Thrombin is generated from prothrombin by activation of the extrinsic clotting pathway, primarily through the agency of tissue factor, a phospholipoprotein that is associated with tumor cells and also with various host inflammatory and connective tissue cells. In addition to tissue factor, several extravasated plasma clotting factors (i.e., clotting factors V and VII in addition to prothrombin) and a suitable surface are required for prothrombinase assembly and thrombin generation. The overall result is that within hours of transplant tumor cells have induced host blood vessels to become leaky and, as a result, have become enmeshed in a fibrin gel "cocoon" (Fig. 31.2).

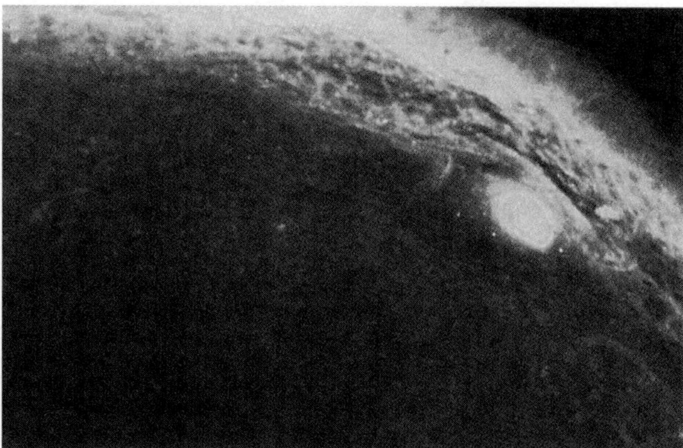

Figure 31.3. Lewis lung carcinoma growing in flank of a syngeneic C57Bl/6 mouse that had received a macromolecular tracer, 70 kD fluoresceinated dextran, 15 minutes previously. Bright-staining apple-green fluorescence forming a rim around the tumor represents extensive extravasation of tracer into surrounding normal connective tissue from leaky blood vessels at tumor-host interface. Tumor itself is virtually unstained, appearing as a "black hole," because tracer at its periphery diffuses poorly into tumor. Fluorescence microscopy; magnification: ×15.

The importance of fibrin deposits is that they provide initial structure and a provisional matrix that favors and apparently stimulates inward migration of host mesenchymal cells (25, 53). Indeed, when fibrin deposits are implanted in animals, they rapidly induce the invasion of new blood vessels and fibroblasts, resulting in a vascularized connective tissue that is not dissimilar in appearance or composition from tumor stroma (54, 55). Other plasma proteins (e.g., plasma fibronectin), as well as locally synthesized structural proteins (e.g., cellular fibronectins, tenascin) and the glycosaminoglycan hyaluronan, likely also contribute to this new tissue. In any event, by inducing microvascular hyperpermeability and initiating the leakage of fibrinogen and other plasma proteins, VPF has triggered a cascade of events that leads to both angiogenesis and mature stroma generation. More recently, VPF has been shown to have a second role in promoting angiogenesis, that of a selective endothelial cell mitogen (32, 65, 86). Discovery of this second activity has led to a second name for VPF, vascular endothelial growth factor (VEGF), and has reinforced its importance as a tumor angiogenesis factor (104).

As implied above, the fibrin gel deposited by tumors is modulated by proteases (Fig. 31.1) and is gradually replaced by the ingrowth of fibroblasts and new blood vessels that give rise to loose connective tissue, similar to the granulation tissue of healing wounds. After an additional period, this granulation tissue is further transformed into the poorly vascularized, densely collagenous scarlike connective tissue characteristic of tumor desmoplasia. Simultaneously, of course, other tumor cells have broken away from the original tumor site and have begun to recapitulate at nearby sites, and particularly at the tumor's growing edge, the same sequence of events—increased vascular permeability and new fibrin deposition. Thus, at any one time, growing desmoplastic tumors consist of older, generally more centrally placed portions composed of tumor cell units that are encased in poorly vascularized, dense collagenous stroma and a more active, newer, fibrin-rich peripheral zone that interfaces with the surrounding host tissue.

From this description, it is apparent that the events of stroma generation in transplantable tumors closely resemble those of wound healing (52). This similarity has been strengthened by the finding that VPF/VEGF expression is strikingly up-regulated in cutaneous wound healing (26), as well as in a variety of analogous pathologic and physiologic processes that involve new blood vessel and stroma formation; these include rheumatoid arthritis, psoriasis, delayed hypersensitivity, diabetic retinopathy, and corpus luteum formation (53). In all of these processes, the initial event is a local increase in vascular permeability, followed, in turn, by extravascular clotting, fibrin deposition, and the infiltration of new blood vessels and connective tissue cells, leading to the development of granulation tissue and, finally, of dense fibrous connective tissue (termed desmoplasia in tumors and scars or fibroplasia in the other entities). It would seem, therefore, that tumors have preempted and subverted for their own purposes a fundamental host mechanism, the wound healing response, as the means to acquire the stroma they need to grow and spread (52). Of course, there are some differences. Platelets, which play several critical roles in wound healing, seem not to participate in tumor stroma generation; apparently, platelet functions are subsumed by tumor cells that make similar or analogous cytokines and growth factors. Tumors differ from healing wounds in another important respect. At wound sites, vascular hyperpermeability is self-limited and returns to normal within a few days (26); in contrast, vascular hyperpermeability persists indefinitely in tumors. Thus, tumors behave in some sense as wounds that do not heal (52).

The analogy between wound healing and tumor stroma generation may be taken one step farther. Except in lower vertebrates (capable of regenerating normal tissues), wound healing does not recapitulate ontogeny, but, instead, replaces injured parenchyma and stroma with connective tissue whose functional capacities fall short of the original normal tissue. In the same manner, tumor stroma, especially that of poorly differentiated malignant tumors, is generally a disorganized and poorly supportive parody of normal connective tissue. The vascular supply is often marginal. Tumor blood vessels are generally poorly differentiated, unevenly spaced, and often unequal to the task of supporting the growth, and even the life, of rapidly metabolizing tumor cells (182). The result is irregular blood flow, uneven perfusion, shifting zones of anoxia, low pH and, commonly, coagulative necrosis—a necrosis resulting from vascular insufficiency (177). In fact, the presence of necrosis may sometimes be helpful to the pathologist in distinguishing malignant tumors from their benign counterparts and certain nonneoplastic processes.

Stroma Generation in Autochthonous Human Tumors

Detailed, interventional studies of the type required to elucidate the pathogenesis of tumor stroma generation in animal tumors are not ethically feasible in patients. Nonetheless, there is good reason to believe that similar mechanisms are involved in human malignancy. First, VPF/VEGF is overexpressed at both the mRNA and protein levels in the great majority of primary and metastatic human tumors that have been studied thus far; these include carcinomas arising in the gastrointestinal tract, pancreas, stomach, breast, kidney, and bladder (22–24, 58), as well as glioblastomas (150). Second, both specific, high-affinity receptors for VPF/VEGF are also overexpressed in the microvascular endothelial cells supplying tumors that overexpress VPF/VEGF (22–24, 150). Finally, many human tumors exhibit evidence of vascular hyperpermeability to plasma proteins, including spillage of fibrinogen with deposition of cross-linked extravascular fibrin as observed in animal tumors (34, 52, 200). Taken together, there is strong evidence that the pathogenesis of stroma formation in human tumors closely follows that in animal tumors, although allowance must be made for species differences and for the generally slower growth rate of autochthonous human tumors.

THE ROLE OF THE SURGICAL PATHOLOGIST IN THE DIAGNOSIS AND MANAGEMENT OF THE CANCER PATIENT

Surgical pathologists have the definitive role in tumor diagnosis. No matter how high the index of clinical suspicion, the diagnosis of cancer is not conclusively established or safely assumed in the absence of a tissue diagnosis. With very few exceptions, definitive therapy for cancer should not be undertaken in the absence of a tissue diagnosis. Policies supporting this practice are written into the bylaws of most hospitals and are regularly monitored by hospital tissue committees and by accrediting agencies.

It is the task of the surgical pathologist to provide an accurate, specific, and sufficiently comprehensive diagnosis to enable the clinician to develop an optimal plan of treatment and, to the extent possible, estimate prognosis. There was a time not many years ago when the simple designation "benign" or "malignant" gave the clinician all of the information necessary to provide appropriate care for the patient. This is no longer the case. Cancer is not a single disease. There are more than 300 distinct varieties of tumors, each with a characteristic biology. Moreover, tumors have a course of historic development and progression; in an individual patient, they may be first recognized at any stage along that course. The tremendous advances in all fields of oncology necessitate obtaining a great deal of additional information, and nearly every case requires a fuller understanding of the patient's particular tumor to allow the most appropriate classification for purposes of research, prognosis, and therapeutic intervention. Details of the type and origin of the tumor, its differentiation and its level of invasion, the numbers of lymph nodes with and without metastatic tumor, and their architecture, the presence or absence of hormone receptors, the activity of specific enzymes, ploidy, frequency of mitosis, and cells in the S phase may all be relevant in the pathologic assessment of neoplasia. Molecular pathology, for example, using nucleic acid probes with or without amplification by the polymerase chain reaction to detect the expression of specific tumor genes or gene mutations, has not yet reached standard practice, but promises to introduce a golden age for pathology within the next decade.

Surgical pathologists deal primarily with structure. Careful gross examination of excised tissue with the naked eye or with the help of a dissecting microscope is followed by a more detailed examination of tissue sections in the compound light microscope. Preliminary examination may make use of frozen tissue sections, but, in most instances, pathologists rely on the better preservation of structure afforded by permanent tissue sections stained with hematoxylin and eosin (H&E) and occasionally other dyes. Histochemistry, immunohistochemistry, and electron microscopy are helpful or necessary supplements to diagnosis in 10 to 15% of solid tumors. In addition, surgical pathologists collaborate closely with cytopathologists in diagnoses involving exfoliated cells or needle aspirates and with clinical pathologists who make use of other techniques, such as culture for microorganisms, flow cytometry, and specialized laboratory tests of a biochemical, immunologic, or molecular nature. In order to perform most of these supplementary studies, the specimen must be specially processed while it is still fresh; that is, prior to routine fixation. It is a responsibility of the surgical pathologist to coordinate these various activities and to synthesize the information they provide into a comprehensive diagnosis that is maximally informative to the clinician who is caring for the patient.

METHODS FOR OBTAINING SPECIMENS

Tissue may be obtained in a number of ways, each with its appropriate place and uses depending on the clinical circumstances. Cytologic examination of exfoliated, scraped, or brushed cells can be a rapid, efficient, and low-risk technique for establishing an accurate diagnosis. This approach, along with the related technique of fine-needle aspiration, is discussed in greater detail later; for obvious reasons, these approaches do not always reveal the primary tumor site or the extent of disease. Cutting needle biopsies, core needle biopsies, and drill biopsies obtain tissue cores for histologic examinations or special studies that permit evaluation of architectural structure, but may result in tissue distortion and pose a greater risk of bleeding and patient discomfort than the use of fine needles. Incisional biopsy (along with fine-needle aspiration) is often the method of choice for lesions that are inoperable or are too large for ready excision, or when excision could lead to functional or cosmetic impairment. Care must be taken that incisional biopsies are performed in a fashion that will not compromise definitive therapy; that is, the tissue excised should be confined to an area that will be encompassed by subsequent treatment. Excisional biopsy is often favored because it provides generous amounts of tissue for diagnosis and may itself afford sufficient surgical therapy for some tumors, such as small- to medium-sized breast cancers.

There are many potential pitfalls in biopsy interpretation. These include inadequate tissue sampling and artifacts induced by the procedure itself, such as thermal damage caused by an electrocautery or laser. Except for excisional biopsies, negative findings do not exclude the possibility that a tumor or other significant pathologic condition is present but was not included in the tissue submitted for examination. Thus, for procedures short of complete excision, the clinician must be prepared to perform a second, often more extensive, procedure if the first does not yield sufficient diagnostic information.

GROSS HANDLING OF SPECIMENS

The pathologist must regard (and, therefore, properly triage) biopsies, and particularly excisional biopsies, as the definitive surgical specimen. To do this well, the pathologist must be informed about the clinical history, differential diagnosis, relevant laboratory results, gross tissue examination, and frozen section findings, if any, since they may individually or together dictate whether special studies are required. Specimens should be marked with clips or sutures to provide anatomic orientation, and these should be described on the pathology submission sheet. Often, tissue arrives in the pathology lab in formalin or other fixatives. At that stage, it is already too late to perform many special studies (e.g., microbiologic cultures, certain types of immunohistochemistry, and optimal electron microscopy) that may prove to be critical for diagnosis. This fact emphasizes the importance of consulting the pathologist in advance in order to avoid the need for rebiopsy. Frequently, the goal of biopsy is to determine whether the lesion is benign or malignant, with the expectation of performing additional surgery if it proves to be malignant. In this case, supplementary tests may properly be deferred to subsequent, more definitive surgery, at which time larger amounts of tissue become available.

The gross specimen should be described with regard to its appearance and characteristics, taking care to measure in three dimensions the size of the specimen and, if visible, the lesion itself, along with the distances between the lesion edges and the excision (resection) margins. Excision margins should be identified and marked with ink prior to any dissection, thus permitting accurate measurement of these distances microscopically. Depending on the type of specimen and the clinical circumstances, margins can be evaluated by analysis of frozen sections. All lymph nodes associated with the specimen need to be dissected out; described, along with their location; and processed for histology.

A still more careful examination is required for certain biopsies, for example, those of the breast, where no lesion may be visible to the naked eye. In addition, breast specimens with calcification often require specimen radiography. Ideally, therefore, a radiograph should be made of the intact specimen, following which the margins should be inked, the specimen "bread-loafed," and radiographs taken of each slice. Sections should then be coded, processed individually for histology, and correlated with the corresponding radiographs (33, 141).

PREPARATION OF MICROSCOPIC SECTIONS

Microscopic examination requires that tissues be cut with a microtome into thin sections that can be stained with such dyes as H&E, toluidine blue, and other special stains for specific tissue components, such as mucus, glycogen, cytoplasmic granules, collagen, bacteria, and fungi. Two types of sections are most commonly used: frozen sections and paraffin-embedded or permanent sections. Frozen sections can be prepared rapidly (within minutes) during the course of surgery while the patient is still under anesthesia, and so are of the greatest practical value in situations requiring an immediate answer to an important clinical question. At one time, frozen sections were commonly obtained intraoperatively in patients with suspected breast cancer with the expectation that definitive radical surgery would follow immediately if cancer were found. With the less aggressive surgical therapy now common for the treatment of breast cancer, this practice has precipitously declined.

However, frozen sections continue to have many important applications. First, they are useful for determining whether a lesion is a neoplasm, and, if so, whether it is benign or malignant. Second, they can provide information as to the extent of regional tumor metastases, which may govern decisions concerning further surgery; for example, mediastinal lymph node involvement in primary carcinoma of the lung or peripancreatic lymph node involvement by carcinoma of the pancreas. Third, they allow the pathologist to determine whether the resection margins are adequate following definitive cancer surgery, such as resection of skin, gut, or pulmonary lesions. If resection margins are inadequate, additional tissue can be removed immediately, without the need for a subsequent operation. Some tumors, such as those arising in soft tissues or the breast, are best evaluated in permanent sections, however. Finally, perhaps the most common current use of frozen sections is to determine the appropriate additional workup necessary for a particular tissue specimen while it is still fresh; for example, if the metastatic tumor found in a lymph node is recognized as a poorly differentiated carcinoma, electron microscopy and hormone receptor studies may be required for proper diagnosis. On the other hand, if the tumor is a lymphoma, an entirely different set of studies may be required, such as those for cell surface antigen markers and gene rearrangement.

In contrast to frozen sections, permanent sections are prepared from tissues that have been fixed, dehydrated, and embedded in paraffin wax as a supporting medium prior to sectioning. Although they require more time for preparation (generally 12 to 24 hours), permanent sections offer a number of important advantages over frozen tissue sections. Sections are generally thinner (typically 5 μm) and, by avoiding freezing artifacts, are of better overall quality and thus permit greater certainty of interpretation. A broader repertoire of stains is also available for permanent sections. Certain tissues, such as those containing fat or bone, cut poorly as frozen sections but may be satisfactorily studied in permanent sections. As a general rule, if insufficient tissue is available for both frozen and permanent sections, only permanent sections should be prepared. But while these opinions certainly represent a majority view, some excellent pathology departments routinely diagnose tumors on the basis of frozen sections and prepare permanent sections primarily for archival purposes.

MICROSCOPIC INTERPRETATION OF TISSUE SECTIONS

In cases of suspected cancer, the first task of the surgical pathologist is to decide whether a neoplasm is present. As noted earlier in this chapter, the word "tumor" is Latin for "swelling," and various types of swelling can masquerade as neoplasms. These include inflammatory lesions, repair, hypertrophy, hyperplasia (e.g., keloids), choristomas (ectopic rests), and hamartomas (masses of mature cells that are appropriate to a given site but are arranged in a disorganized fashion as the result of aberrant differentiation). This initial distinction is often made easily; for example, hyperplastic polyps of the colon, nasal polyps, and skin tags are not likely to be confused with true neoplasms. Sometimes, however, the task is less straightforward. Tumors not infrequently generate an extensive inflammatory response, and it is not unusual (as in endoscopic biopsies of gastric carcinomas) to find after a prolonged search rare individual cancer cells "buried" in an extensive inflammatory cell infiltrate. Healing ulcerations of the gastrointestinal or cervical mucosae may sometimes closely resemble the carcinomas or premalignant lesions (e.g., squamous intraepithelial lesions, low or high grade) that arise in those tissues. Finally, atypical hyperplasia can be very difficult to distinguish from in situ carcinoma, and even when no evidence of tumor is found, may represent an important diagnostic finding. For instance, patients whose breast biopsies show atypical hyperplasia and who have a positive family history for breast cancer have a ninefold increased risk for developing breast cancer at a later time (43).

Having decided that a neoplasm is present on the basis of such criteria as cellular abnormalities or invasion (see below), the pathologist's next task is to classify it. A number of classification schemes are possible, but the most important of these is based on the tumor's histogenetic or cytogenetic origin. Histogenetic/cytogenetic classification is often supplemented by other useful descriptors, such as those provided by the tumor's gross or microscopic appearance (e.g., polypoid, papillomatous), the degree of cellular differentiation (e.g., well or poorly differentiated [Fig. 31.4]), and, perhaps most important, by the expected biologic behavior (benign versus malignant). Broadly speaking, tumors of epithelial cell origin are termed adenomas or papillomas when benign and carcinomas when malignant. Carcinomas account for approximately 80% of all malignant tumors. Their classification is often further qualified on the basis of the type of epithelium present; for example, glandular (adenocarcinoma; Fig. 31.5), squamous (squamous cell carcinoma; Fig. 31.6), and transitional cell (transitional cell carcinoma). Addition of the suffix *-oma* to the cell of origin also describes benign tumors of mesenchymal origin (e.g., lipomas, fibromas, leiomyomas). Malignant tumors of mesenchymal origin are designated sarcomas (e.g., liposarcomas, fibrosarcomas, leiomyosarcomas). Most tumors are composed of a single type of neoplastic cell. However, a few tumors contain neoplastic cells of more than a single type, such as Wilms' tumors. Even rarer are tumors containing neoplastic cells that derive from more than a single germ layer, such as teratomas (dermoid cysts). Certain tumors have long been identified with trivial names that do not follow any well or-

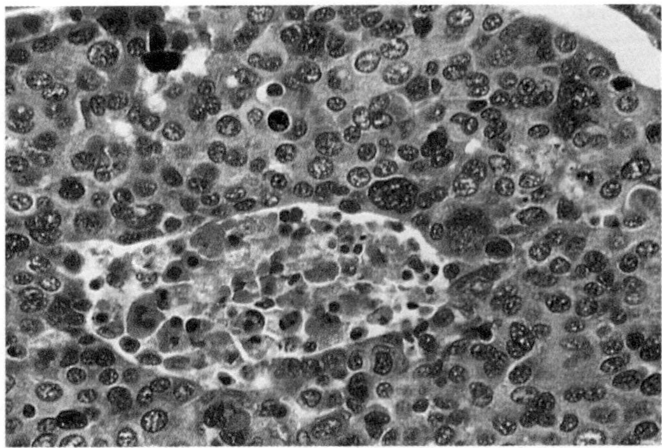

Figure 31.4. Undifferentiated carcinoma of lung. Tumor is composed of irregularly arranged pleomorphic tumor cells with large nuclei and prominent nucleoli. A central necrotic zone, typical of this type of tumor, is present. There is little stroma. H&E; magnification: ×100.

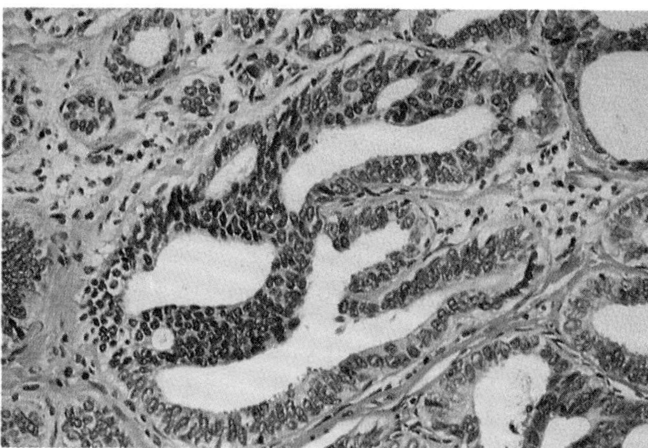

Figure 31.5. Adenocarcinoma of breast. Tumor is arranged in the form of fairly well-differentiated glands separated by a fibrous connective tissue stroma. Moderate numbers of inflammatory cells, mostly lymphocytes, are present in stroma. H&E; magnification: ×65.

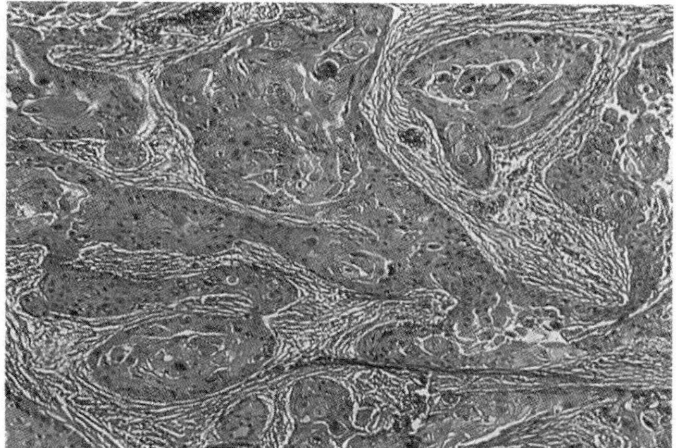

Figure 31.6. Squamous cell carcinoma of the skin of the face. Tumor consists of island of well-differentiated squamous epithelium separated by fibrous connective tissue stroma. Note that epithelium forms "keratin pearls." H&H; magnification: ×60.

dered classification scheme. Examples include seminomas (for carcinomas of testicular epithelial cell origin), hypernephromas (for renal cell carcinomas), and melanomas (for melanocarcinomas) (Fig. 31.7). Other tumors, due to prolonged use, continue to bear eponyms (e.g., Hodgkin's disease, Ewing's sarcoma, Kaposi's sarcoma).

The pathologist must carry classification further still. Even within a single organ and within a single type of epithelium, several different types of tumors may arise, each with its own special characteristics, prognosis, and response to therapy. In the breast, for example, the two most common types of malignant tumor are infiltrating ductal carcinoma (sometimes designated as carcinoma not otherwise specified or NOS), which accounts for approximately 78% of infiltrating breast cancers, and infiltrating lobular carcinomas, which account for an additional 9% or so of breast cancers. These two tumors, together accounting for nearly 90% of breast cancers,

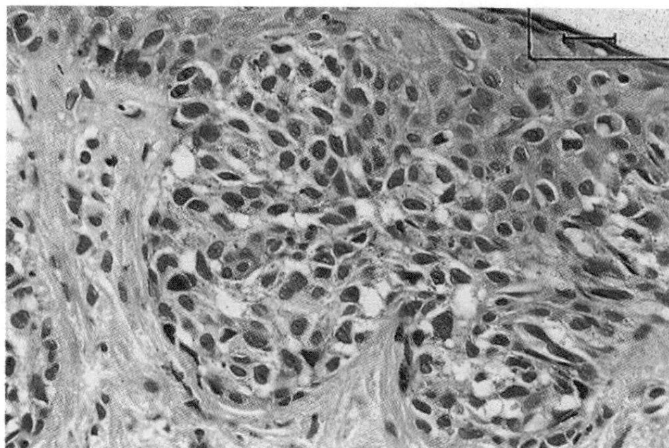

Figure 31.7. Malignant melanoma arising in skin. Tumor is composed of large, irregular cells with large nuclei, prominent nucleoli, and abundant, clear cytoplasm, peppered with dots and larger accumulations of melanin pigment. H&E; magnification: ×100.

have similar prognoses that are less favorable than those of the other, less common types of breast carcinoma (i.e., tubular, mucinous or colloid, medullary, papillary, and adenoid cystic carcinomas) (123).

One of the most important distinctions the surgical pathologist can make is that between benign or malignant tumors. In general, benign tumors share certain properties. The neoplastic cells making up the tumor are usually well differentiated, closely resembling the corresponding cells of normal tissue. Benign tumors tend to expand uniformly in all directions unless impeded from doing so by surrounding structures; for example, compression by the bony skull often causes meningiomas to take on a flattened appearance. As expansile masses, benign tumors cause compression atrophy of surrounding normal tissues that results in the formation of a thin rim of fibrous connective tissue; this enveloping connective tissue rim may serve as a capsule that renders benign tumors discrete, readily palpable, and easily movable. Not all benign tumors have capsules, however, including leiomyomas of the uterus, hemangiomas, and tubular adenomas (adenomatous polyps) of the large intestine.

Malignant tumors, or cancers, are characterized primarily by the abnormality of their neoplastic cells. These cellular abnormalities are of two general types, those involving intercellular relationships and those affecting individual neoplastic cells. With regard to the former, malignant tumors commonly exhibit increased cell number and altered orientation of both neoplastic cells and stroma that may be best described as helter-skelter or disorganized. Although carcinomas of the skin may comprise squamous cells that differentiate and mature fairly normally, the cells are commonly organized into nests in which the least differentiated cells are situated peripherally and the most differentiated cells are positioned centrally, where they form keratin pearls. Further, these tumor cell nests are surrounded by disorganized stroma. Disturbed intercellular arrangements such as these are of great help to the pathologist when reading a tissue section; much of tumor diagnosis depends on the pathologist's ability to recognize altered microscopic tissue patterns.

Abnormalities of individual neoplastic cells may also be helpful in diagnosis, particularly increased numbers of mitoses and cytologic features relating to the state of tumor cell differentiation. Cytologic features of malignancy include altered polarity, tumor cell enlargement, increased ratio of nuclear to cytoplasmic area (it may approach 1:1 instead of the normal 1:4 or 1:6, although exceptions exist), pleomorphism (variation in size and shape) of tumor cells and their nuclei, clumping of nuclear chromatin and distribution of chromatin along the nuclear membrane, enlarged nucleoli, atypical or bizarre mitoses (e.g., tripolar), and tumor giant cells with one or more nuclei. Some malignant tumors, however, are so well differentiated that their malignant cells cannot be distinguished from those of benign tumors, or even from normal cells, by any available diagnostic method. In such instances, the recognition of abnormal cellular relationships becomes especially important for correct diagnosis.

Anaplasia (Greek for "to form backwards") is the term pathologists commonly use to describe the degree of tumor cell differentiation, or, more correctly, the lack thereof. Although it is well entrenched, the term is an unfortunate one. It implies that tumors arise from mature, differentiated cells by a process of dedifferentiation (i.e., differentiation in reverse). Few pathologists hold that view today. Mammalian cells, once differentiated, generally lack the capacity to reverse that process. Also, there is strong and growing evidence for the alternative explanation, namely, that tumors arise from populations of undifferentiated "stem" or "reserve" cells that are present in many, perhaps in all, organs capable of cell renewal (108, 147, 176). Stem cells compose a minority cell population that lacks differentiation markers, making them difficult to identify. However, positive recognition of stem cells has been achieved in several organs, including bone marrow, epidermis, liver, and gastrointestinal tract mucosa (153). Stem cells have a high capacity for cell proliferation, but, unless stimulated, may divide infrequently. Stem cells alone have the capacity to regenerate normal tissues and, by extension, tumor cell populations. Oncologists, of course, are well aware that stem cells are the critically important target of cancer therapy. Destruction of differentiated tumor cells, without simultaneous killing of tumor stem cells, will not lead to permanent tumor eradication.

Malignant tumors invariably lack a capsule. Instead, they extend crablike projections into the surrounding host tissues without respect for normal anatomic boundaries. This behavior is referred to as invasion. Malignant tumor cells often invade lymphatics and veins and are transported by lymph or blood flow to distant sites, opening the possibility of metastasis (see Chapter 9). Invasion is not a property confined to malignant tumor cells; many proliferations in fetal life, placental trophoblasts, and inflammatory cells also have the capacity to invade tissues. However, cancers need not be invasive at the time of removal, either because they have been caught before they have had time to invade, or because they have not yet progressed to the point where they have acquired the capacity to invade. Epithelial tumors with all other properties of malignancy that have not extended through the underlying basement membrane at the time of diagnosis are described as in situ carcinomas and almost certainly can be cured by complete excision (161).

ANCILLARY STAINING AND ANALYTICAL METHODS

Special stains are commonly employed to aid in tumor differential diagnosis and classification. Examples include the van Gieson's solution or the Masson trichrome method for distinguishing collagen and muscle, Weigert's stain for elastic tissue, silver stains for reticulin fibers, and special stains for mucins, amyloid, lipids, myelin, and glycogen—all substances whose identification may aid in the diagnosis of one or another type of tumor. In other instances, enzyme histochemistry may be essential for defining cell lineage, as in certain types of leukemia; for example, chloroacetate esterase or endogenous peroxidase staining for cells of myelomonocytic lineage, μ-naphthyl butyrate esterase (so-called nonspecific esterase) staining for monocytes and macrophages.

Other techniques that may occasionally aid the surgical pathologist in tumor diagnosis are specimen x-ray (for localizing and analyzing crystalline material, such as calcium, in breast biopsies) and morphometry.

EXCISION MARGINS

An important concern for the pathologist is the adequacy of tumor excision. Depending on the tissue, this decision can be made on either frozen or permanent sections. If the tumor forms a discrete mass and the margins of the specimen are clearly recognizable, determination of excision margins is usually straightforward. Examples of tumors whose excision is likely to give clearly defined margins include those arising in the gastrointestinal tract, lung, and skin. On the other hand, the margins of tumors arising in soft tissues (e.g., many sarcomas and breast carcinomas) and diffusely infiltrating tumors (e.g., infiltrating lobular carcinoma of the breast, signet ring tumors of the gastrointestinal tract; nerve-invading tumors, such as adenoid cystic carcinomas of the salivary glands; gliomas; and glioblastomas) may be much more difficult to define. With at least certain histologic patterns of breast carcinoma, such factors as the extent of intraductal growth may be more reliable predictors of residual tumor than are adequate excision margins (96, 160). In patients treated with excision and radiotherapy for invasive breast cancer, the evaluation of excision margins in the context of an extensive intraductal component provides more prognostic information than does the evaluation of margins alone (159).

TUMOR GRADING, STAGING, AND PROGNOSIS

Finally, pathologists are often called on to grade tumors or to participate in their staging in order to estimate tumor prognosis. Tumor staging (e.g., the well-known TNM system) has proved to be of great value in estimating prognosis. Staging attempts to measure the extent of spread of a cancer in a patient based on such parameters as the size of the primary tumor, the degree of lymph node involvement, and the presence of metastases. It is obvious that objective determinations made by the pathologist on resected tumor specimens have a critical impact on accurate tumor staging. With perhaps only one exception (papillary carcinoma of the thyroid), the most important risk factor in determining tumor progno-

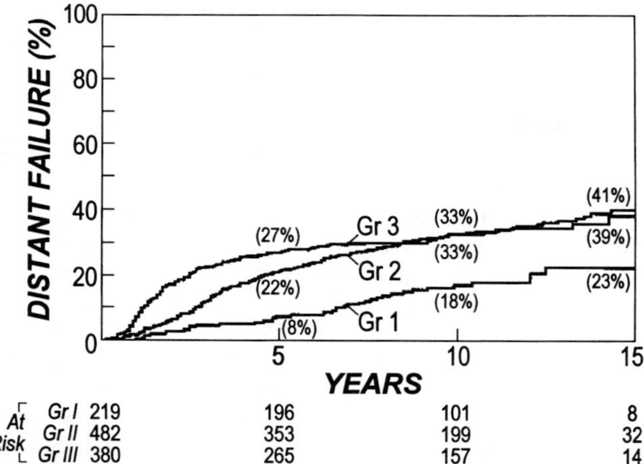

Figure 31.8. Actuarial rates of distant failure for 1,081 patients with invasive breast cancer related to histologic grade of tumor. Grading was performed using Elston's modification of the Bloom and Richardson grading system, which takes into consideration architectural pattern, nuclear grade, and mitotic activity (J. Connolly and S. Schnitt, unpublished data).

sis is the presence of metastases to regional lymph nodes. Therefore, the pathologist must search diligently to find, examine, and prepare histologic sections from all lymph nodes included in resected tissue.

Tumor grading has traditionally referred to a pathologist's judgment as to a tumor's degree of differentiation and growth rate, often on a scale of I to III, where III represents the least differentiated, fastest dividing tumors (i.e., those tumors presumed to have the worst prognosis). Formal grading systems have improved in recent years with stricter standardization of criteria (61) (Fig. 31.8). Tumor grading does, however, have shortcomings. First, a different scale is required for each type of tumor, and scoring is subjective and not always reproducible. Second, tumors are typically heterogeneous so that areas differing significantly in differentiation and mitotic activity exist side by side, with the attendant risk of sampling error. Because prognosis is invariably linked to the most malignant portions of a tumor, it follows that, for accurate diagnosis and grading, sufficient tissue and microscopic sections must be sampled so that the most malignant areas are found. Moreover, a regular (although not invariant) feature of malignant tumors is progression (69, 95), the property by which tumors become more and more malignant over time. Tumor progression is thought to result from genomic instability (135) that leads to specific mutations of oncogenes and tumor suppressor genes; from other genetic alterations, such as gene amplification; and from epigenetic changes that result in altered patterns of gene expression. Overt carcinogens, environmental promoters, and local factors, such as hypoxia and nutrient deprivation, may all contribute to these changes and, therefore, to tumor progression. Finally, the correlation between histologic appearance and biologic behavior is seldom perfect.

Of course, pathologists are continually on the lookout for more useful tumor-specific features that may be important independent predictors of tumor prognosis. Recent attempts to identify such predictors have borne fruit in certain specific cancers. Thus, carcinomas of the prostate may be usefully graded on the basis of tissue architecture and neoplastic cell pattern (84). A number of different criteria, including nuclear differentiation, degree of gland or tubule formation, and mitotic activity, have been usefully combined to grade breast carcinomas (15, 61, 158). Two common and much-studied solid tumors, cutaneous melanomas and carcinoma of the breast, illustrate other tumor-specific factors that affect prognosis in important ways.

Histologic Grading and Prognosis of Cutaneous Melanomas

Cutaneous melanomas (Fig. 31.7) are subclassified clinically as being of the nodular (NM), superficial spreading (SSM), and lentigo maligna (LMM) types. LMMs generally have the best prognosis and NMs the worst (30, 31, 80, 111, 124, 126, 127, 195). In addition to clinical subtype, many additional factors affect the prognosis of patients bearing these tumors, including tumor ulceration, thickness, cell type (i.e., spindle, epithelioid, etc.), mitotic activity, lymphocytic reaction, the presence or absence of pigment, vascular invasion and anatomic site of the primary tumor, sex of the patient, and histologic regression (125).

Recently, a model incorporating 23 separate tumor characteristics was developed (30). By multivariate analysis, six of these characteristics were found to be independent prognosticators: (*a*) mitotic rate, (*b*) presence of tumor-infiltrating lymphocytes, (*c*) tumor thickness, (*d*) anatomic site, (*e*) sex of the patient, and (*f*) evidence of histologic regression (30). One of the most useful prognostic factors was the extent (i.e., the depth) of vertical invasion into the skin. Two widely regarded systems have been developed to classify melanomas using this criterion. Clark and colleagues (31) originally categorized melanoma invasion as follows: Level 1, tumor confined to the epidermis (in situ); Level 2, tumor invasion into the papillary dermis; Level 3, tumor extends through the papillary dermis and abuts on, but does not actually invade, the reticular dermis; Level 4, tumor invades the reticular dermis; and Level 5, tumor extends through the reticular dermis and invades the subcutaneous fat. Utilizing this system, Level 1 tumors were found not to metastasize and Level 2 tumors rarely did so. However, tumors scored as Levels 3 to 5 commonly metastasized and yielded progressively worse survival rates (31).

One confounding limitation to the Clark system is that dermal anatomy varies significantly in different parts of the body. Breslow (21), therefore, developed an alternative scoring method, measuring with an ocular micrometer the vertical dimension of tumor invasion from the top of the granular cell layer of the epidermis. Patients whose tumors were 0.75 mm or less in vertical dimension rarely developed metastases, whereas patients with thicker lesions had an increasingly worse prognosis. The Breslow system of measurement also has its limitations, as when pseudoepitheliomatous hyperplasia or tumor ulceration is present.

Using measurement schemes such as these, the supposed differences in prognosis between SSM and NM tend to blur, because NMs have generally extended deeper into the dermis at the time of diagnosis than have SSMs (63,

125–127). LMM, however, continues to be an exception, maintaining its more favorable prognosis even when tumor thickness is taken into consideration (112). For this reason, it is important to determine if a melanoma has arisen in the context of lentigo maligna.

Factors Important in Predicting Risk for Breast Cancer

Separate consideration must be given to the risks of local recurrence of cancer in the breast and distant metastases; the factors that affect them are not identical.

Local Recurrence. In patients treated for infiltrating ductal carcinoma with breast-conserving surgery and radiation therapy, the factors predictive of local recurrence are not clearly related to known factors that predict for the development of distant metastasis. A recent large study on a total of 584 patients with clinical stage I or II infiltrating ductal carcinomas of the breast makes this point (93). Treatment consisted of complete surgical excision of the primary tumor without microscopic margin evaluation, followed by radiation therapy totaling at least 60 Gy to the primary site. Of 34 separate tumor characteristics that were subjected to multivariate analysis, the only factor that was found to be associated with an increased risk of local breast recurrence was the presence of an extensive intraductal component (EIC positive). EIC positivity was identified in two distinct groups of tumors: tumors that were predominantly ductal carcinomas in situ with areas of focal invasion and primarily invasive tumors in which (*a*) the ducts and lobules were not obliterated, (*b*) virtually all preserved ducts were involved by ductal carcinoma in situ, and (*c*) ductal carcinoma in situ was present adjacent to the invasive tumor.

Twenty-eight percent of all cases fell into the EIC-positive group and 26% of such patients developed local tumor recurrence as compared with only 7% of patients with EIC-negative tumors ($p = .001$) (89). A number of other investigators have now confirmed the finding that the presence of EIC is associated with a higher risk for breast recurrence after local excision and radiation therapy (99, 145).

There seem to be two likely explanations for the increased risk of local recurrence in patients with EIC-positive tumors. One is that the residual tumor in this group of patients is less radiosensitive than in patients with EIC-negative tumors. The second is that the subclinical residual tumor burden following excision is consistently larger in EIC-positive than in EIC-negative patients, and may be too large to have been eradicated by the cosmetically acceptable doses of radiation therapy that were delivered. While both of these explanations are possible, it has been found that the residual tumor burden is consistently larger in EIC-positive than in EIC-negative patients (96).

Distant Metastases. As with many other tumors, the most important factor predicting for the systemic spread of breast cancer is involvement of the regional lymph nodes. Unless treated, most patients with involved axillary lymph nodes will ultimately die of metastatic spread of their disease. Since the natural history of breast cancer is often protracted, clinically evident metastases may not appear for many years, perhaps 10 to 20 years or more after the primary tumor and axillary lymph nodes have been removed. The greater the number of involved axillary lymph nodes, the greater is the likelihood that tumor cells have spread elsewhere in the body to indeterminate locations, only to become clinically manifest at a later time. Thus, in one large series, 87% of the patients with 13 or more involved axillary lymph nodes developed metastatic spread within 10 years, whereas only 20% of node-negative patients did so (67).

Given the important prognostic significance of positive lymph nodes and recent evidence that patient survival improves with adjuvant therapy, criteria are now urgently needed for identifying the 20 to 30% of lymph-node–negative patients who nonetheless will develop metastatic disease after primary breast treatment. Factors worthy of consideration include the degree of tumor differentiation and the mitotic index as discussed above. In addition, other, more specific factors may play a role. One likely candidate is the capacity of tumor cells to find their way into vascular spaces, such as lymphatics or small blood vessels (62, 113, 154, 180).

Newer Criteria for Assessing Breast Carcinomas. Several scoring systems have been used to grade breast cancers. Generally speaking, most include the degree of nuclear differentiation, the degree to which the tumor is able to form glands, and some attempt to estimate tumor growth rate by measuring mitotic activity. Using such criteria, the survival rates at 5 years in one series of node-negative patients with grade I through grade III tumors varied from 86% through 64%, and at 15 years, from 49% through 25% (14).

One approach for assessing tumor differentiation involves the use of flow cytometry. Tumors with normal diploid or tetraploid DNA content have been repeatedly shown to have a better prognosis than aneuploid tumors (29, 64, 184). However, not all workers agree with this conclusion as it applies to node-negative patients (133, 151).

Tumor growth rate may be measured in a number of ways, including standard counts of mitotic figures per 10 high-power fields, the percentage of cells in S phase as determined by flow cytometry, and [^{3}H]-thymidine labeling index (15, 61, 158). In a large study of DNA ploidy and S-phase fraction in lymph-node–negative patients with breast cancer, no correlation was found between S-phase fraction and survival among patients with aneuploid tumors (29). These aneuploid tumors constituted two thirds of the cases studied. Among diploid tumors, however, the S-phase fraction was highly predictive for the risk of recurrence (29).

One of the most intensively studied and widely used measures of evaluating breast cancers is their expression of estrogen (ER) and progesterone hormone receptors (PR). These are, in fact, the only measures for which standardized quality control is currently available. Most studies have shown that lymph-node–negative patients with ER-positive tumors have a significantly better disease-free survival, and, in some cases, better overall survival, than patients whose tumors are ER negative (66). The difference between the survival rates of patients with ER-positive tumors and those with ER-negative tumors decreases with time, and some studies have suggested that the survival curves will eventually merge (20). Taken together, these observations suggest that tumors expressing estrogen and progesterone receptors tend to proliferate more slowly than do tumors lacking such receptors. Thus, ER measurements may not represent an independent prognostic factor per se, but may instead provide yet another method of assessing tumor growth rate or differentiation.

Another criterion for assessing breast cancer prognosis has come into prominence recently, that of measuring microvascular density. As noted earlier, tumors must induce new blood vessels if they are to grow beyond minimal size. Therefore, intratumor microvascularity, taken as a measure of tumor angiogenesis, might be expected to provide a useful index of tumor aggressiveness. Investigating this possibility, Weidner and colleagues (189, 190) performed counts of blood vessel frequency on breast cancer tissue sections. Immunostaining sections with antifactor VIII–related antigen to ensure detection of all microvessels, they found that, as with other tumor properties, such as mitotic index, individual breast cancers were heterogeneous with respect to microvessel density. They thus selected zones that exhibited the highest blood vessel density (hot spots) and found that hot spots in cancers of patients with metastases had mean vessel counts of 101 ± 49 per 200× field, significantly higher than the value of 45 ± 21 for patients without metastases. Multivariate analysis of the data revealed that intratumor microvascular density provided an independent prognostic indicator of lymph node metastasis and of both relapse-free and overall patient survival. The majority of follow-up studies have confirmed these findings (discussed by Gasporiai and Harris [77]). Unfortunately, measurements of tumor microvascular density are laborious and subject to interobserver variability, and for these reasons are unlikely to be used routinely outside of research settings. Nonetheless, Weidner's studies emphasize the importance of angiogenesis in human tumor biology and support the principle that angiogenesis may be a worthy target in biologic approaches to breast cancer therapy. Recent studies suggest that measurements of microvessel density may also provide useful prognostic information for carcinomas arising in organs other than the breast, including the head and neck (78), lung (118, 197), and prostate (185).

A large number of studies are now in progress attempting to identify other factors that may predict for risk in node-negative patients. These include evaluation of Ki-67 (76), epidermal growth factor receptors (16, 142, 157), insulin-like growth factors (18, 105), transforming growth factor-alpha (5, 188), cathepsin D (175), and various oncogenes and their products. For a recent review of prognostic factors in breast cancer, see Mansour and co-workers (119).

REPORT ISSUED BY SURGICAL PATHOLOGIST

The findings should be presented descriptively and comprehensively in terms that are understandable to both the pathologist and the clinicians caring for the patient. The report should provide enough information so that the clinician caring for the patient can follow the thought processes of the pathologist, much as though viewing the case with the pathologist at a double-headed microscope. The report should contain all the information to which the pathologist has access (i.e., tumor size, grade, and nodal status) that is necessary to stage a patient with cancer. This information varies with tumor origin, its type, and its staging system employed. The report should include the results of all specialized tests performed, their interpretation, and the synthesis and coordination of all clinically useful information available to the pathologist that may be of aid in diagnosis and management. Finally, reports should be issued in a timely manner so that they are available to the clinician within a few days of tissue submission. Failure to report results promptly may delay patient care (thus uselessly adding to the cost of medical care), lead to error and confusion, and, at the very least, prolong anxiety in patients who are often already distraught.

Role of Cytopathologist

Cytology is used for both the screening and diagnosis of lesions that may represent cancer or its precursors. Cytology is particularly useful for the definitive diagnosis of those malignancies that either are inoperable or do not require surgery for treatment, such as metastatic carcinomas and malignant lymphomas. Specific benefits include cost-effectiveness, rapid turnaround time, and tissue diagnosis with minimal patient risk. Since cytologic specimens usually consist of a small sample of cells or tissue fragments, an optimal technique for both specimen collection and preparation is crucial. Diagnosis should be attempted only by experienced personnel on well-fixed, appropriately stained materials. Moreover, as in all areas of pathology, cytologic diagnosis should never be made "in a vacuum"; pertinent clinical data and communication between the cytopathologist and clinician are essential, and will facilitate rapid, accurate, and definitive cytologic diagnoses.

METHODS FOR OBTAINING SPECIMENS

Two categories of methods are involved in obtaining cells for microscopic examination. The first is to obtain the medium that contains naturally exfoliated cells, such as urine, sputum, and body cavity fluids. The second is specifically to obtain the cells of interest for examination with an instrument, such as a brush or a needle. Diagnostic cells contained in the specimens of the first category tend to be degenerated and few in number, whereas diagnostic cells in the specimens of the second category are often well preserved and numerous.

PREPARATION OF CYTOLOGIC SPECIMENS FOR MICROSCOPIC EXAMINATION

The preparation of cytologic specimens depends on the types of specimens. Cells collected with an instrument can be either rinsed into a preservative solution, such as Saccomanno's, 50% ethanol, a balanced electrolyte solution, or other preservatives, or simply spread directly onto slides (2, 37, 41, 193). When the cells are collected in a medium, whether natural or artificial, the specimen needs to go through a process in order to separate the medium from the cells. This can be done with centrifugation, cytocentrifugation, filtering, or processing through a machine that spreads a monolayer of cells on the slides. The goal of these processes is to separate the cells from the medium and then to spread the concentrated cells evenly and thinly on slides. Cells thinly spread on a slide dry out very easily; therefore, the slides spread with unpreserved cells need to be fixed (either in 95% ethanol or with commercially available spray fixatives) immediately and then stained with Papanicolaou or H&E stain. These slides can also be left to air dry and then stained with a Romanowsky-type stain.

MICROSCOPIC INTERPRETATION OF CYTOLOGIC SPECIMENS

In contrast with surgical pathologists, cytopathologists deal primarily with cells without regard to stroma. Although some architectural features are maintained in cytologic specimens, many are lost in the process of specimen collection and preparation. Therefore, cytopathologists rely mainly on the cytologic features of malignancy described earlier and residual structural features, such as cohesion versus dyshesion, to determine the benign versus malignant nature of the lesion. Cytopathologists usually report the result in one of four categories: positive, suspicious, atypical, or negative. A positive cytology report should indicate that the pathologist is sufficiently confident of the malignant nature of the lesion that he or she is prepared to have the patient undergo definitive treatment, such as surgical resection or chemotherapy, based on that diagnosis alone. Where there is any doubt, the report should be less definitive and in the "suspicious" category. Other diagnostic tests, such as a repeat cytology sample or biopsy, should be done to determine with certainty the nature of the lesion before the patient undergoes definitive therapy. Occasionally, other signs of malignancy, such as clinical or radiologic evidence, are so strong that clinicians feel confident in implementing definitive therapy with a suspicious diagnosis. That should be the decision of the responsible clinician. When cellular abnormalities are present whose clinical significance is not known, the report should be in the "atypical" category. Other diagnostic tests may be in order, depending on the clinical situation. Definitive therapy should never be initiated solely on the basis of "atypia." A "negative" cytology means that no abnormal cells were found in the sample examined. It is important for all to realize that this does not necessarily indicate absence of malignancy in the patient. False negative cytologies are often the result of sampling error. However, laboratory error may result in both false-negative and false-positive results.

EXFOLIATIVE CYTOLOGY

Exfoliated cytology involves microscopic examination of cells exfoliated from the female genital (Pap smear), respiratory (sputum), and urinary (urine) tracts. The use of the Pap smear to screen for cervical cancer and its precursors in the general asymptomatic population has been instrumental in lowering the mortality rate from cervical cancer over the last four decades (28, 36, 88, 102, 131, 132). A problem inherent in all screening tests is the need to balance sensitivity and specificity. Lowering the threshold for diagnosis of atypia means that fewer cases of neoplasia will be missed. However, the trade-off is that more patients without neoplastic disease will require additional, expensive studies, such as colposcopy, to rule out the presence of cancer or its precursors. The importance of proper sample collection and preparation needs to be emphasized. Failure to fix samples immediately, thick smears, and the presence of significant amounts of blood may all result in specimens that are inadequate or suboptimal for diagnosis. Sensitivity can be increased by using a cytobrush because of its ability to sample a broad area (19, 79). Pap smears obtained through colposcopy with a brush are, in fact, similar to endoscopic cytology.

Cytologic examinations of sputum and urine are not currently used to screen the general population, but instead to detect cancers in high-risk patients who either have had exposures that increase their risk of developing cancers or already have symptoms that may be caused by cancers in the lung or urinary bladder. Cytology is more sensitive for diagnosing larger and higher-grade lesions arising in the urinary and respiratory tracts and cervix than for smaller, lower-grade lesions; indeed, detection of low-grade lesions may require multiple samplings. In patients with symptoms or other clinical evidence of disease, the economic and noninvasive advantages of cytology are largely lost after collection of three indeterminate specimens, and more invasive procedures, such as bronchoscopy, cystoscopy, and colposcopy, are called for to collect cells or tissue for cytologic and/or histologic examination.

ENDOSCOPIC CYTOLOGY

In areas amenable to endoscopy, such as the bronchial tree and gastrointestinal and urinary tracts, cytologic specimens obtained with brushing and washing techniques may serve a screening function, and, in fact, not uncommonly permit a definitive diagnosis. The brush can be rolled on slides to make direct smears or can be immersed in a preservative, such as CytoLyt, for subsequent preparation of slides by machine. Specimens collected by washing are processed like those collected with medium. Paired cytology and biopsy can improve the likelihood of diagnosing malignancy in a single procedure (12, 187). Because brush samples cover a wide area, they provide greater diagnostic sensitivity, particularly for the diagnosis of early lesions that are not obvious on gross examination. However, endoscopic biopsies generally provide more information, particularly in determining tumor type and the presence of invasion.

CYTOLOGY OF BODY CAVITY AND CEREBROSPINAL FLUIDS

Fluids are removed from body cavities not only for the purpose of diagnosis, but also as a form of therapy (e.g., to relieve pressure on vital organs). Although immediate fixation is not necessary, fluids do need to be refrigerated promptly, and also require anticoagulation (heparin, 1 unit per 100 mL) if the fluid is bloody. Certain morphologic clues may allow the cytopathologist to suggest the site of primary tumor origin. For example, three-dimensional clusters of adenocarcinoma cells present in effusions collected from female pa-

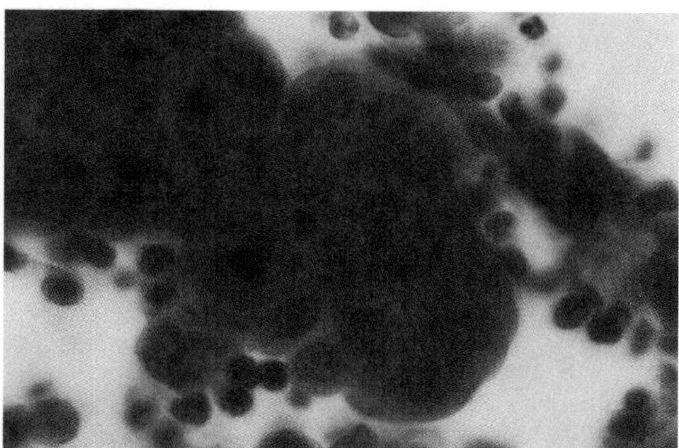

Figure 31.9. Ovarian papillary serous adenocarcinoma in ascitic fluid. Cells are present in three-dimensional clusters with nuclear molding and irregular hyperchromatic nuclei. Papanicolaou; magnification: ×250.

tients are likely derived from tumors arising in breast, ovary, or lung (Fig. 31.9). In men, adenocarcinoma cells in effusions are most likely to be of pulmonary or gastrointestinal tract origin. If consistent with the clinical findings and results from other studies, a positive cytologic diagnosis can lead directly to treatment without the need for additional biopsies or other diagnostic procedures. As always, current cytology specimens should be compared with previous cytology or histology specimens, if available.

Reactive mesothelial cells share certain characteristics with carcinoma cells, including large nuclei with nucleoli and even mitotic figures, and should always be considered in the differential diagnosis. Such features as cellular aggregates with smooth outlines, nuclear molding and irregularity, and lack of intercytoplasmic spaces or windows help to distinguish carcinoma cells from reactive mesothelial cells. Panels of immunocytochemical stains may also prove useful (see below). Unfortunately, there are no available antibodies that distinguish benign from malignant mesothelial cells, and very few that reliably identify the site of origin of metastatic cancers (42, 121). Mesothelial cells survive and multiply when exfoliated into effusions.

Sometimes (e.g., mesotheliomas) tumor growth may be confined to the surfaces lining body cavities without significant exfoliation of malignant cells. Under these circumstances, examination of effusions for exfoliated cells may be fruitless, requiring a biopsy of the cavity wall. An alternative approach for future investigation may be to analyze tumor cell-free effusions for secreted products of malignant cells or other tumor cell markers. One successful, although preliminary, application of this approach has been the finding of high levels of the angiogenic factor VPF/VEGF in effusions by immunoassay (198).

ASPIRATION CYTOLOGY

The earliest work on aspiration cytology was reported from the Memorial Hospital in New York in the 1930s (120). Subsequently, the impetus for this technique shifted to Europe and was not "rediscovered" in the United States until the 1970s (115). Prior to aspiration, the skin is prepared with alcohol; local anesthetic may be administered, but often is not necessary. A 22- to 25-gauge needle is inserted into the center of palpable lesions, and 5 to 20 cc of suction is applied to the syringe. The needle may be moved rapidly from side to side within the lesion to sample multiple foci. Suction is then released completely, and the needle is withdrawn. The needle should always be withdrawn immediately if any blood enters its hub; however, cysts need to be drained completely with reaspiration if any mass remains. In highly vascular tissues, such as thyroid, it is often useful to start with a smaller-gauge needle (e.g., 25 gauge) and to move to a larger-size needle only if the initial aspirate does not yield diagnostic material.

Considerable controversy exists over who is best qualified to perform fine-needle aspirates (FNA). At present, cytopathologists, surgeons, and other clinicians successfully perform such aspirations (72). In fact, the most critical and technically demanding step in aspiration cytology is generally not the aspiration itself, but the preparation of adequate slides after the sample has been obtained (70, 116, 139). Smears can be made directly, or the needle can be rinsed with a preservative solution as described above (37). For preparation of smears, the needle is detached from the syringe, and the syringe is filled with air, reattached, and its contents expelled onto glass slides, where they are spread in much the same manner as a blood smear, using a second slide or cover slip. Such preparations can be air dried for staining with Romanowsky-type stains or can be fixed and stained with the Papanicolaou or H&E stains.

In the case of nonpalpable lesions, aspiration is performed by a radiologist under computed tomography (CT), ultrasound, or fluoroscopic guidance. Such deep aspiration procedures are expensive, time-consuming, and invasive. For these reasons, it is desirable that a cytotechnologist or cytopathologist attend the procedure to ensure specimen adequacy and optimal slide preparation. A further advantage of this attendance is the ability of experienced personnel to triage material effectively for special studies, such as immunocytochemistry, electron microscopy, flow cytometry, and tissue culture.

Definitive aspiration cytology diagnoses, rendered by an experienced cytopathologist, can provide the basis for definitive therapy. However, such diagnoses need to be viewed in the context of all other laboratory studies and clinical findings. Specific problems and pitfalls that attend aspirations of various sites are briefly discussed in the following sections.

Thyroid

Fine-needle aspiration permits the accurate diagnosis of papillary, medullary, and anaplastic carcinomas but is less useful in the diagnosis of follicular nodules. There are cytologic features that help to distinguish among the various types of follicular lesions (75, 103), but a definitive diagnosis may not be possible by FNA, particularly the distinction between follicular adenomas and carcinoma. Thus, in some instances, FNA will serve only to distinguish patients needing immediate surgery for thyroid disease from those who may be safely followed with or without hormonal suppression (70, 90, 91). However, even this limited information can eliminate much unnecessary surgery.

Breast

The diagnostic specificity of breast aspiration is very high in the hands of an experienced cytopathologist, and a positive diagnosis may safely lead to mastectomy or other definitive treatment (70, 71, 106). Of course, atypical and suspicious cases will require a further workup. Aspiration cytology of the breast may also be performed on nonpalpable lesions under the guidance of conventional or stereotaxic mammography or ultrasound (3, 13, 39, 92, 117), but the ultimate value of this new technique is not yet clear. Inherent problems for breast cytology include the inability to distinguish infiltrating from in situ ductal carcinoma (186), and the lesser degree of accuracy, in comparison with biopsies, in correctly categorizing premalignant and benign lesions of the breast (e.g., lobular carcinoma in situ, atypical ductal hyperplasia, ductal hyperplasia, and intraductal papilloma) (1, 59, 169–171, 186).

Lung

Aspiration cytology of the lung may lead to the diagnosis of both primary and metastatic tumors and nonneoplastic lesions, such as tuberculosis and fungal infections (70, 139, 178). As with histologic tissue sections, it is not always possible to distinguish primary from metastatic carcinomas.

Abdomen

Aspiration cytology is particularly useful in diagnosing malignancies in the liver, pancreas, kidney, and retroperitoneum prior to treatment (139). A diagnosis of metastatic tumor or lymphoma spares the patient major surgery, and provides the basis for definitive therapy. Poorly differentiated tumors may be difficult to type, but the use of adjunct techniques is often helpful in establishing a definitive diagnosis (see Fig. 31.10).

Lymph Nodes

Many cytopathologists believe that aspiration cytology has only a limited role in the diagnosis of lymph node lesions. However, FNA can provide useful information to obviate the need for surgery in cases of suspected metastatic carcinoma to palpable lymph nodes with a known primary. Lymph node aspirates may also be useful for diagnosing lymphoproliferative diseases and infections (72, 73).

APPLICATION OF ANCILLARY STUDIES TO CYTOLOGIC MATERIALS

Virtually all ancillary studies, such as those involving immunohistochemistry, electron microscopy, flow cytometry, and molecular biology, can be applied to cytologic materials (see below for details).

Few diagnostic tests have been introduced into medicine that have actually lowered the cost of high-quality patient care. Cytopathology is such a test. It offers the advantages of low morbidity, rapid turnaround time, and outstanding cost-effectiveness. The problems with and pitfalls of cytology should not detract from its usefulness. All procedures have limitations, and the oncologist needs to be informed as to both the benefits of this approach and its pitfalls.

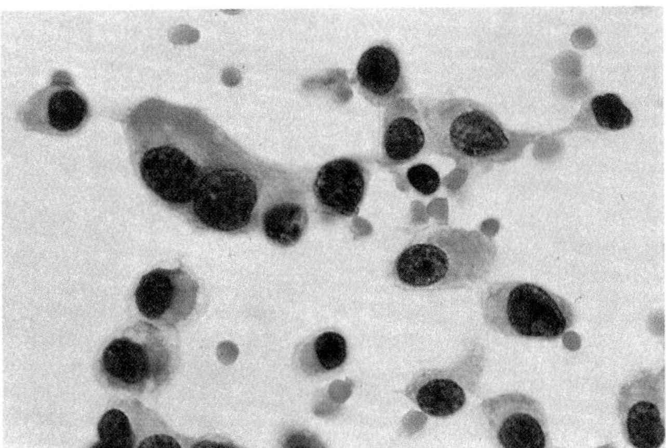

Figure 31.10. Metastatic neuroendocrine tumor as seen in a fine-needle aspiration of liver. Note eccentric nuclei with "salt and pepper" chromatin and abundant granular cytoplasm. Immunocytochemical stains confirmed the diagnosis. Papanicolaou; magnification: ×250.

Role of Immunohistochemist

Immunohistochemistry has become an important adjunct in the evaluation of human neoplasms. A detailed discussion of the technical aspects of immunohistochemistry is beyond the scope of this chapter, and the interested reader is referred to several review articles and monographs (98, 166, 172, 179). The commercial availability of a broad range of reagents (including prediluted reagents in kit form) has made it possible for high-quality immunohistochemistry to be performed in most pathology laboratories. The most commonly employed immunohistochemical techniques are those in which such enzymes as horseradish peroxidase or alkaline phosphatase are used in conjunction with specific antibodies (to provide color reactions at sites of antigen-antibody interactions). Such methods as the peroxidase-antiperoxidase (PAP) technique and the avidin-biotin complex (ABC) technique are the most widely utilized in current practice. In the PAP technique, antigen-containing tissues or cells are sequentially incubated with (*a*) an unlabeled specific rabbit antibody directed against the antigen of interest (primary antibody), (*b*) a secondary (bridging) reagent consisting, for example, of swine antibodies directed against rabbit immunoglobulin if the primary antibody was prepared in rabbits, and (*c*) a tertiary reagent consisting of peroxidase-rabbit-antiperoxidase complexes. The second (swine) antirabbit immunoglobulin antibody serves as a bridge that links the primary antibody with peroxidase-antiperoxidase complexes. The ABC procedure also requires three sequential steps: an unlabeled primary antibody, a biotin-labeled anti-immunoglobulin secondary antibody, and, finally, preformed avidin-biotin-peroxidase complexes. One variation of the ABC method employs streptavidin, which has greater sensitivity than avidin and exhibits less nonspecific binding (27). Although both the PAP and avidin-biotin methods provide satisfactory staining results, the latter is often somewhat more sensitive (167). It should be noted that the sensitivity of any immunohistochemical procedure is, in large part, related to the reagents and detailed procedures employed. As a consequence it is difficult to compare the results of immunohistochemical studies from different institutions that employ different reagents and methods.

Virtually any type of pathologic specimen may be suitable for immunohistochemical staining, including fresh frozen tissue, fixed tissue, and cytologic preparations. Unfortunately, however, not all antigens are equally well preserved after these various treatments, and the approach taken for immunohistochemical staining must depend on the antigen(s) of interest. For example, while a large number of cytoplasmic antigens are detectable in fixed, paraffin-embedded tissue, other antigens, such as many cell surface–associated antigens, are destroyed or masked by common fixatives and may be demonstrable only in fresh frozen tissue or in cytologic preparations. Antigen retrieval methods, such as pretreatment with proteolytic enzymes or heating in a microwave oven, may permit the identification of otherwise undemonstrable antigens in fixed, paraffin-embedded tissue sections (11). Finally, not all fixatives are equivalent with regard to antigen preservation. While cross-linking fixatives, such as formaldehyde, are often suitable, they are suboptimal for detecting certain antigens of diagnostic importance, such as those located on intermediate filaments, which are best demonstrated in fresh-frozen or alcohol-fixed tissue (7, 134, 149).

APPLICATIONS

Immunohistochemistry has widespread applicability in the evaluation of human tumors. Some of the more common applications are listed in Table 31.1 and are discussed below.

Table 31.1. Common Applications of Immunohistochemistry in the Evaluation of Human Tumors

- Categorization of "undifferentiated" malignant tumors
- Determination of site of origin of metastatic tumors
- Subclassification of tumors in various organ systems and tissue compartments (e.g., central nervous system tumors, germ cell tumors, sarcomas)
- Distinction between carcinomas and malignant mesotheliomas
- Categorization of leukemias and lymphomas
- Detection of antigens of potential prognostic or therapeutic importance:
  - Estrogen and progesterone receptors
  - Oncogene products
  - Markers of proliferative activity
  - P-glycoprotein

CATEGORIZATION OF "UNDIFFERENTIATED" MALIGNANT TUMORS

Not infrequently, a pathologist examining routine H&E-stained paraffin sections recognizes the presence of a malignant tumor but is unable to characterize it further. This is understandable in that undifferentiated tumors often lack characteristics that would permit more accurate classification. Yet, further classification is often important in making clinical decisions related to appropriate therapy and prognosis. Immunohistochemistry may be helpful in such situations (Fig. 31.11). Before performing immunohistochemistry, however, the pathologist must first develop a differential diagnosis, and this will depend on the tumor's histologic appearance, its anatomic location, and the clinical setting. Only then is he or she in a position to select antibodies that will permit a more definitive diagnosis.

One common problem in tumor diagnosis, that of undifferentiated tumors composed of large cells with an epithelioid appearance, will serve as an example. The differential diagnosis in such cases typically includes undifferentiated carcinoma, lymphoma, and melanoma. Distinction among these tumor types can often be made using a panel of antibodies, as illustrated in Table 31.2. Unfortunately, this table presents

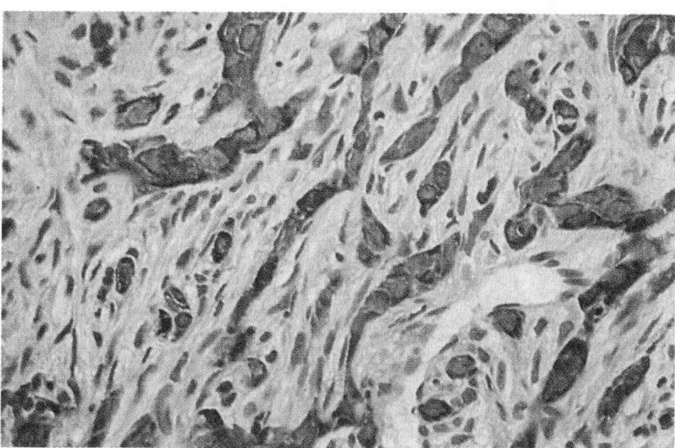

Figure 31.11. Immunoperoxidase staining of a monoclonal antibody specific for keratin in a poorly differentiated squamous cell carcinoma of skin. This "spindle cell" form of the tumor mimics tumors of connective tissue origin, and its true nature can often be determined only by immunohistochemistry. Immunoperoxidase; magnification: ×100.

Table 31.2. Idealized Immunohistochemical Evaluation of the "Undifferentiated" Malignant Tumor in Which the Differential Diagnosis Includes Carcinoma, Lymphoma, and Melanoma

Antibody to	Tumor type		
	Carcinoma	Lymphoma	Melanoma
Keratin	+	−	−
Epithelial membrane antigen	+	−	−
Vimentin	−	+ or −	+
Leukocyte common antigen	−	+	−
S-100 protein	−	−	+
Melanoma-associated antigen	−	−	+

an ideal result that is not always achieved in practice. Some carcinomas show staining for vimentin (4, 87) or S100 protein (40), some lymphomas express epithelial membrane antigen (148), and some melanomas show immunoreactivity for keratin (201). Such results emphasize the need to use a panel of antibodies, rather than a single antibody, when evaluating tumors.

Determination of Site of Origin of Metastatic Tumors

On routine microscopic examination, tumors may be classifiable with regard to general type (e.g., carcinoma) but not with regard to site of origin. It would be highly desirable to have available antibodies specific for tumors arising in different sites. At present, however, very few organ- or tissue-specific antigens have been identified, thus limiting the ability of immunohistochemistry to resolve such problems in every instance. A number of useful antigens are listed in Table 31.3. It should be noted that antigens specific for some of the more common tumors such as carcinomas of the lung, colon, endometrium, and pancreas, are not currently available. Furthermore, some of the antigens listed in Table 31.3 have now been demonstrated in neoplasms other than those for which they were initially thought to be "specific." For example, the melanoma-associated antigen detected by one widely used antibody (HMB-45) has been found in some breast carcinomas (17).

SUBCLASSIFICATION OF TUMORS IN VARIOUS ORGAN SYSTEMS

In some organs and tissue compartments, it may be difficult to subclassify certain tumors based solely on histologic grounds because of overlapping features. Some of these distinctions are (at least at present) only of academic interest (e.g., determining whether a high-grade spindle cell sarcoma shows neural, myogenous, or fibrohistiocytic differentiation), but others have therapeutic and prognostic significance. For example, in some cases, it may be difficult or impossible to distinguish with certainty an anaplastic seminoma from an embryonal carcinoma of the testis by routine microscopic examination, a distinction with both therapeutic and prognostic implications. However, immunostaining for the intermediate filament keratin is often useful in making this distinction, because seminomas are typically keratin negative whereas embryonal carcinomas are usually keratin positive (8, 130). Similar situations are encountered in other organ systems and tissue compartments.

Distinction Between Carcinomas and Malignant Mesotheliomas

A common problem encountered by the surgical pathologist is distinguishing between metastatic adenocarcinoma and malignant mesothelioma involving the pleura or peritoneum (138, 140, 165, 194). Immunohistochemical staining using a panel of antibodies may be useful in assisting the pathologist in making this distinction (Table 31.4).

CATEGORIZATION OF LEUKEMIAS AND LYMPHOMAS

One of the most common uses for immunohistochemistry is in correctly diagnosing and classifying leukemias and lymphomas. A detailed discussion of this subject is beyond the scope of this chapter, and the interested reader is referred to several recent articles and reviews (10, 38, 107, 143, 146). In brief, immunohistochemistry, in conjunction with morphology and histochemistry, is a useful adjunct in making the distinction between acute leukemias of the lymphoid and nonlymphoid types and in distinguishing hairy cell leukemia from other types of leukemic infiltrates in the bone marrow and at other sites. In addition, this technique is useful for subclassifying non-Hodgkin's lymphomas and Hodgkin's disease and in distinguishing them from each other in problematic cases.

Detection of Antigens of Potential Prognostic or Therapeutic Significance

A variety of antigens of possible prognostic and therapeutic importance can be detected using immunohistochemistry, including estrogen and progesterone receptors in breast cancers (6, 144, 173), protein products of oncogenes (such as HER-2/*neu* in breast cancers) (168, 181); antigens associated with tumor cell proliferation, such as Ki-67 and PCNA/cyclin (74, 82); and the P-glycoprotein product of the multiple-drug resistance (MDR) gene (191). Ki-67 is of particular interest (81). It is a nuclear antigen present in all proliferating cells; that is, it is present in the G_1, S, G_2, and M phases of the cell cycle, but absent from G_0 cells. Therefore, by staining for this antigen, it is possible to measure the tumor growth fraction directly and in a simpler manner that is

Table 31.3. Antigens with Highly Restricted Specificity

Antigen	Tumor specificity
Factor VIII–related antigen	Vascular tumors
Gross cystic disease fluid protein	Breast carcinomas; cutaneous tumors with apocrine differentiation
Melanoma-associated antigen	Melanoma
Muscle-specific actin	Smooth muscle and skeletal muscle tumors
Myoglobin	Skeletal muscle tumors
Prostate specific antigen	Prostatic carcinomas
Thyroglobulin	Thyroid follicular cell tumors

Table 31.4. Immunohistochemical Distinction Between Metastatic Adenocarcinoma and Malignant Mesothelioma Involving the Pleura or Peritoneum

	Adenocarcinoma	Mesothelioma
Keratin	+	+
Vimentin	+ or −	+ or −
Carcinoembryonic antigen	+ or −	−
Leu M1	+ or −	−
B72.3	+ or −	−
Ber-EP4	+ or −	−

more readily applicable to clinical specimens than are radioactive labeling methods using [^{3}H]-thymidine. Ki-67 staining also yields results that are more reproducible than those obtained by counting mitotic figures. Recently, a number of antibodies have become available to identify the Ki-67 antigen in formalin-fixed, paraffin-embedded tissue sections (122).

LIMITATIONS

An appreciation of the limitations of immunohistochemistry in tumor diagnosis is as important as is an understanding of its many useful applications. Potential limitations in the immunohistochemical evaluation of solid tumors can be broadly characterized as technical and interpretive.

Technical Limitations

Because the demonstration of different types of antigens by immunostaining requires appropriate tissue preparation, advance planning for immunohistochemistry is essential so that the specimen may be handled appropriately. For example, if a lymph node excised on clinical grounds or at intraoperative examination (i.e., frozen section or tissue imprint) conveys features suspicious for a lymphoma, a portion of the specimen should be snap-frozen to permit reliable demonstration of lymphocyte surface markers since these are not well demonstrated in fixed, paraffin-embedded tissue. In cases of suspected carcinoma, in which the demonstration of intermediate filament proteins is likely to be important, fixation of a portion of the tumor in an alcohol-based fixative is advisable.

As with any laboratory procedure, the use of appropriate positive and negative controls is mandatory in immunohistochemistry and serves as a check on the technical adequacy of the procedure. Results of immunostaining must always be viewed with caution if the appropriate controls are omitted or suboptimal.

Interpretive Limitations

The correct interpretation of immunohistochemical stains performed on tumor specimens depends not only on the technical adequacy of the procedure, but on interpretive factors as well. In most situations, it is more useful to employ a panel of antibodies than a single antibody. The antibodies making up the panel must be selected thoughtfully, based on a carefully prepared differential diagnosis. A "shotgun" approach to immunostaining is strongly discouraged, and may only serve to compound diagnostic confusion.

Accurate interpretation of staining also requires familiarity with the characteristics of true-positive, false-positive, true-negative, and false-negative staining. Negative reactions are more difficult to interpret than are positive reactions. Even with the use of other controls, it is difficult to be certain that a reaction is a "true negative" unless the section in question stains positively for a complementary antigen. For example, in the analysis of an undifferentiated malignant tumor in which the differential diagnosis includes lymphoma and carcinoma, a negative reaction for keratin (the intermediate filament characteristic of many carcinomas) does not by itself rule out the possibility of carcinoma. However, if a negative keratin stain is accompanied by positive staining for leukocyte common antigen (a marker present in most lymphomas), the likelihood of lymphoma is greatly enhanced.

Some antibodies are of great diagnostic value in terms of both sensitivity and specificity (e.g., antibodies to prostate specific antigen), whereas others are of limited diagnostic value even when used as part of a panel (e.g., antibodies to the intermediate filament vimentin). Pathologists who use immunohistochemistry must be experienced and aware of the limitations of a methodology that is evolving at a rapid pace. An antigenic profile suitable today for diagnosing a particular type of tumor tomorrow may be shown to be suboptimal or less specific than was originally thought. Immunohistochemistry is a valuable tool for aiding in the diagnosis of difficult tumors. However, it is only an adjunct to diagnosis, and the results must be interpreted in the context of other findings, particularly routine histologic sections and the clinical setting.

Role of Electron Microscopist

Although making use of radically different technology, electron microscopy seeks the same type of information as that gleaned from immunohistochemistry; that is, detection of differentiation markers that permit more accurate tumor identification and classification. Electron microscopy (EM) is generally not useful in determining whether individual cells are malignant or benign (but see McNutt and colleagues [128] for an exception). It is a powerful tool for recognizing subcellular structures that are not detectable by light microscopy, but which, when present, allow confident identification of cells as, for example, of epithelial or melanocyte origin. Although advances in immunohistochemistry have somewhat reduced the need for EM in tumor diagnosis, they by no means have eliminated this need altogether, and EM remains at present a powerful but generally underutilized approach to tumor diagnosis (49–51, 83, 94). Moreover, validation of new immunohistochemical reagents is often best accomplished by ultrastructural study of replicate tissue samples.

TECHNICAL CONSIDERATIONS

Appropriate tissue handling, fixation, and processing are of even greater importance in EM than they were for immunohistochemistry (44). Advanced planning and consultation among the clinician, surgical pathologist, and electron microscopist thus are important. In many cases, it is advantageous to have a pathologist or knowledgeable technician in the operating room or at the bedside at the time of biopsy in order that tissue may be fixed immediately and trimmed appropriately. Tissues must be cut into small pieces because chemical fixatives penetrate tissues slowly (over minutes to hours) and the electron microscope glaringly exposes artifacts in poorly fixed tissues that are not detectable at the lower resolution afforded by light microscopy. In at least one dimension, tissues must be no thicker than 1 mm, and to achieve this small size, further trimming may be necessary after brief preliminary fixation. Mixtures of glutaraldehyde and paraformaldehyde (e.g., Karnovsky's fixative) provide optimal fixation (44). Although these reagents are best when freshly prepared, it is also possible to freeze vials of fixative beforehand that may be thawed immediately before use. Tissues fixed in formalin or in other "routine" fixatives designed for light microscopy give inadequate tissue preservation for electron microscopy. Once tissues are fixed inappropriately, they generally cannot be recovered for adequate electron microscopy, and rebiopsy becomes the best option. Peripheral blood, bone marrow, and cell-containing fluids (e.g., pleural effusions, spinal or synovial fluids) are handled somewhat differently from samples of solid tissue and require a member of the electron microscopy staff to be present as the sample is obtained (44).

APPLICATIONS

The great strength of EM lies in its exquisite resolution, which permits the recognition of intracellular structures, organelles, or products that are undetectable by light microscopy.

Electron microscopy is often helpful in the diagnosis of "undifferentiated" malignant tumors and in determining the origin of metastatic tumors of unknown primary site (Figs. 31.12 and 31.13) (47). The recognition of cytoplasmic premelanosomes within tumor cells permits the distinction of amelanotic malignant melanomas from undifferentiated carcinomas and lymphomas with which they can be confused. Other ultrastructural features whose recognition may permit definitive diagnosis are the cytoplasmic granules characteristic of carcinoid tumors; the norepinephrine- and epinephrine-containing granules found in pheochromocytomas; "terminal webs" characteristic of primary gastrointestinal carcinomas of absorptive epithelial cell origin (46); lamellar (surfactant) bodies found only in type II pneumocytes, and, therefore, diagnostic of alveolar cell carcinomas of the lung (48); tonofilaments and desmosomes found in mesothelial cells and squamous cells; and cytoplasmic glycogen aggregates and calligraphic nucleoli typical of germinomas. The presence of intercellular junctions permits

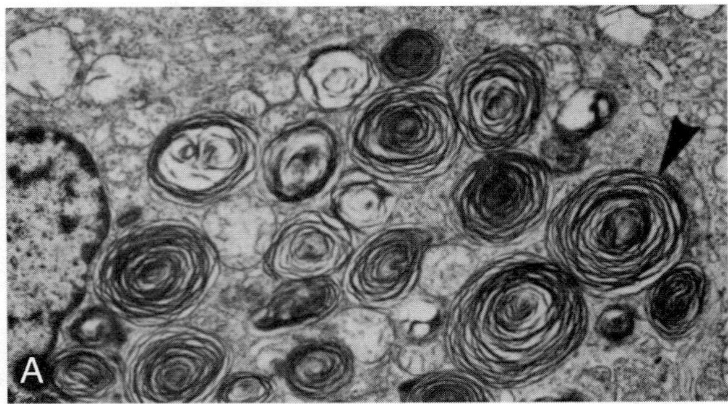

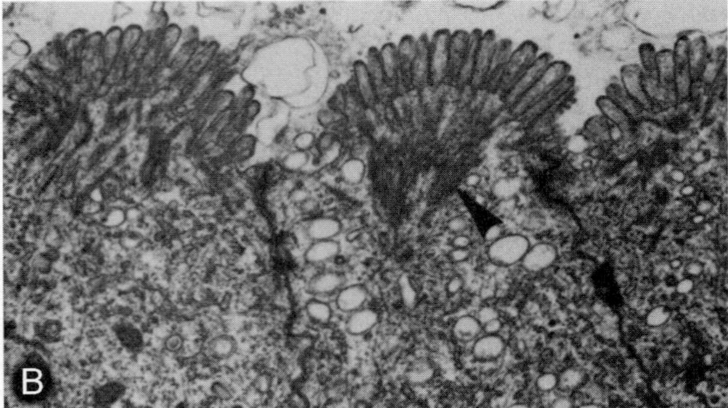

Figure 31.12. **A.** Electron micrograph from lung mass shows typical surfactant-containing lamellar bodies (surfactant bodies) (*arrowhead*) that fill cytoplasm of a tumor cell, allowing specific diagnosis of primary alveolar cell carcinoma of the lung to be made. Magnification: ×12,500. **B.** Electron micrograph from lung mass shows apical cytoplasm of three tumor cells at high magnification. Note short, blunt surface microvilli and dense terminal web (*arrowhead*) of cytoskeletal filaments that traverse apical cytoplasm to enter individual microvilli. Tumor cells are joined by epithelial junctions and contain numerous apical cytoplasmic vesicles. Identification of differentiated organelle, the terminal web, allows specific diagnosis to be made of metastatic adenocarcinoma of gut absorptive epithelial cell origin. Magnification: ×19,000.

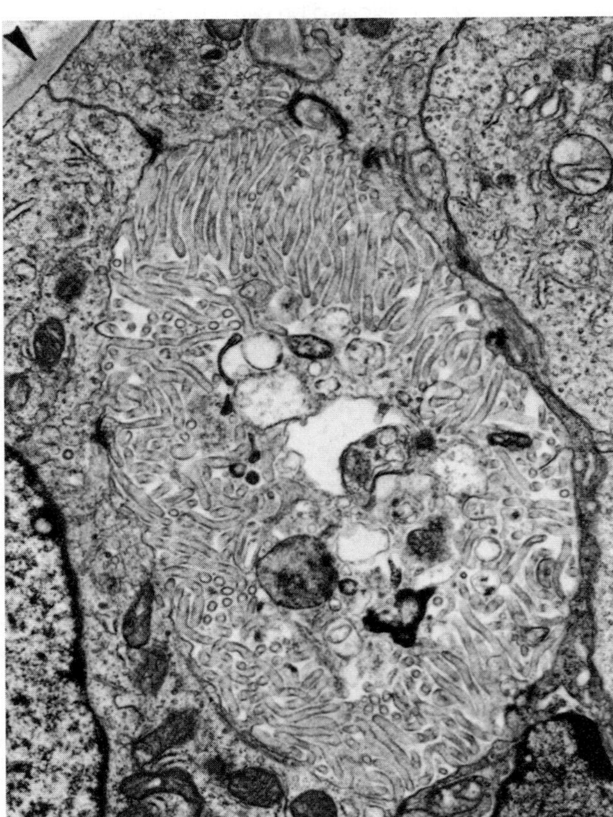

Figure 31.13. High-magnification electron micrograph of pleural tumor shows three typical features of mesothelial cells: numerous elongated, thick-surface microvilli that do not display evidence of terminal web differentiation; desmosomes that connect individual cells surrounding the extracellular acinar space; and basal lamina (*arrowhead*). Another diagnostic feature of mesothelial cells, dense bundles of tonofilaments, is not seen in this high-magnification image. These four ultrastructural findings in concert allow the ultrastructural diagnosis of mesothelioma to be made in the presence of light microscopic evidence of a malignant tumor proliferation of the pleura. Magnification: ×22,000.

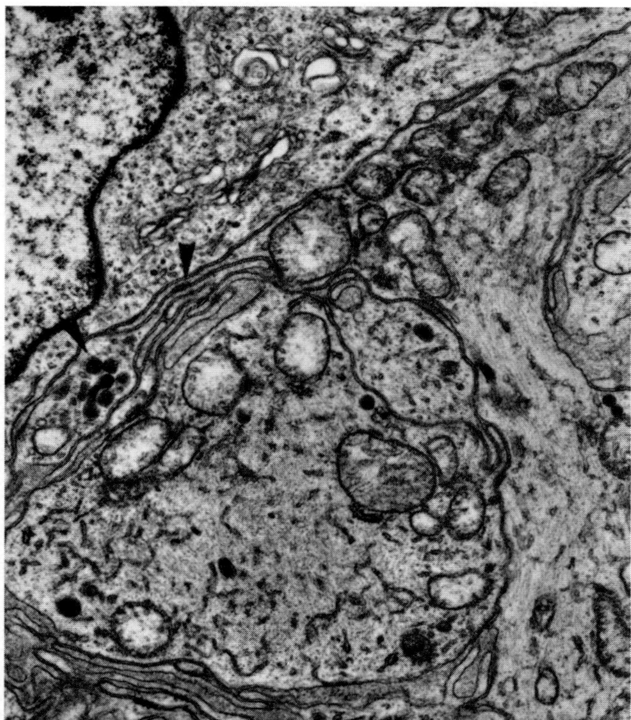

Figure 31.14. High-magnification micrograph of a gastric tumor shows tumor cells diagnostic for the newly delineated entity, the gastrointestinal autonomic nerve tumor (GAN tumor). Elongated tumor cells are neurites that contain numerous mitochondria and neurofilaments; small numbers of dense core granules are present in larger cell processes adjacent to tumor plasma membranes and in Golgi areas (not shown). Number of dense core granules increases in smaller axons with synaptic connections to adjacent neurites (*arrowheads*). Basal lamina is absent from these cells, thus ruling out its origin from Schwann cells. Magnification: ×19,000.

the distinction of carcinomas from lymphomas, even if the carcinoma's primary site cannot be determined. Other examples include some thyroid carcinomas that may be identified by the polarized nature of their cells, which often contain small apical vesicles filled with colloid at one pole and a basal lamina underlying the opposite pole. Large numbers of mitochondria characterize oncocytomas whether they originate in the thyroid or elsewhere. Electron microscopy combined with morphometric analysis to calculate a nuclear contour index may be required for the diagnosis of mycosis fungoides (128). Also, at times, EM may correct faulty impressions derived from light microscopy. For example, a mistaken diagnosis of poorly differentiated adenocarcinoma may result from the misinterpretation of vascular spaces as tumor cell acini.

Electron microscopy is helpful, as well, in subclassifying tumors, an exercise that may have important therapeutic implications. The use of ultrastructural cytochemistry for endogenous peroxidase may allow the important distinction of acute myeloblastic leukemia from acute lymphoblastic leukemia. Histiocytosis X may be diagnosed by the identification of Birbek bodies characteristic of Langerhans cells and EM may also permit accurate diagnosis of lysosomal storage diseases and of bacterial, fungal, and viral infections.

Finally, EM is important in recognizing the histogenesis of newly recognized neoplasms. A recent example (Fig. 31.14) is the recognition that certain spindle cell tumors of the gastrointestinal tract, previously thought to be of smooth muscle origin, in fact arise from autonomic neurons (gastrointestinal tract autonomic nerve tumors or GAN tumors) (45).

LIMITATIONS

As with immunohistochemistry, the limitations are both technical and interpretive. We have already alluded to certain technical limitations (those involving tissue handling, prompt and appropriate fixation, and suitable processing). Another is sampling error, attributable to the very small size of a specimen that can be studied on an EM grid. One other limitation that deserves mention is expense. Whereas the availability of commercial reagents, defined protocols, and relatively simple interpretation have permitted immunohistochemistry to be established in almost any hospital pathology laboratory, the same cannot be said for diagnostic electron microscopy. The costly electron microscope and its fairly elaborate support equipment and the need for experienced technical and professional personnel have limited the application of this methodology to large secondary and tertiary care centers, mostly at academic institutions. Of particular importance is the need for a pathologist who is well trained in both surgical pathology and electron microscopy. The widely employed practice of asking a basic science-oriented electron microscopist or an electron microscopy technician to take a few pictures of a tumor specimen is a prescription for almost certain failure and must be deplored.

Role of Clinical Pathologist

The role of the clinical pathologist or "laboratorian" is obvious and familiar to the oncologist and requires only brief mention here. Clinical pathologists direct hospital laboratories, and, thus, in addition to routine laboratory testing of cancer patients, are interested in measurements on body fluids that could lead to the early detection and monitoring of cancer. There has been a great deal of interest in the field of tumor antigens and tumor markers, and some of these are discussed elsewhere in this text. At least in theory, tumor-specific antigens circulating in the plasma could be of utility in tumor diagnosis and prognosis, assessment of tumor burden, prediction of recurrence, and guidance for treatment. Properties of an ideal tumor marker include great sensitivity, specificity, and accuracy in reflecting total tumor burden. A tumor marker should also be prognostic of outcome and predictive of tumor recurrence. Unfortunately, none of the tumor markers discovered to date fulfill all of these criteria. In fact, none of the markers are uniquely produced by tumor cells. Normal cells of one sort or another produce all of the tumor markers thus far recognized, and plasma or serum levels in tumor patients differ only quantitatively, not qualitatively, from those of normal controls or patients with other diseases.

The role of the clinical pathologist, however, has expanded into other areas of oncology. Particularly important is the molecular biologic diagnosis of tumors, for example, T-cell lymphomas, by the detection of gene rearrangements (100, 192). Demonstration of such rearrangements may be especially important as a supplement to the work of the surgical pathologist and immunohistochemist in distinguishing clonal, and so presumably malignant, lesions from benign but highly reactive lymph nodes. There is increasing interest in the clinical laboratory in the assessment of solid tumor clonality in understanding tumorigenesis and as an aid to the diagnosis and estimation of prognosis. In recent years, the cytogenetics laboratory has enjoyed a renaissance of activity in recognizing consistent chromosome abnormalities in a growing list of leukemias, lymphomas, and solid tumors. At present, specific chromosomal abnormalities are of greatest clinical importance in only a few tumors, primarily lymphomas and leukemias (109, 137); for example, in acute and chronic myeloid leukemia and in acute lymphocytic leukemia. However, it is now clear that nonrandom chromosomal changes are to be found in a variety of solid tumors, and it is likely that cytogenetic information will become increasingly useful in defining tumor progression and prognosis (136, 152, 156, 176, 183). In a similar vein, there has been increasing interest in recent years in the use of flow cytometric analysis of tumor cell suspensions for the determination of tumor ploidy and the fraction of replicating cells (see above). Early results indicate that such information is of use in defining the prognosis of renal, breast, and certain other types of tumors (29, 60, 64, 133, 176).

Role of Autopsy Pathologist

Autopsies do not receive the respect that was at one time accorded them, and the autopsy rate has declined throughout the United States from approximately 90% of hospital deaths in some teaching hospitals in the late 1960s to the current average rate of only 15% (9, 85, 100, 110, 129, 174). One widely voiced but erroneous reason for this change in attitude and practice is the belief that autopsies no longer yield much in the way of useful information because they have been preempted by new technologies, such as magnetic resonance imaging and other pathologic and biochemical tests performed on the patient during life. Another is the fear of malpractice suits by clinicians who are said to be afraid of litigation that might result from new findings revealed at autopsy that had not been diagnosed during life. Still another reason is the fact that the Joint Commission for the Accreditation of Health Care Organizations has greatly reduced its emphasis on the hospital autopsy rate for accreditation purposes. Psychologic factors may also play a negative role. Because of the significant side effects that accompany the longer survivals achieved with modern cancer therapy, the deceased's family may feel that the patient has "suffered enough." Also, the autopsy serves as a symbol of failure, reminding the clinician that he or she was unable to cure the patient. Finally, there is a negative economic incentive for performing autopsies. Neither the pathologist, the hospital, nor the oncologist is reimbursed for the cost in time, effort, and materials involved in performing an autopsy or in persuading a reluctant family to permit an autopsy.

Despite these objections, the autopsy continues to play an important role in patient care. In fact, advances in technology have done little to change the incidence of unexpected, clinically significant findings at autopsy. In our experience, it is most unusual for an unexpected autopsy finding to lead to litigation, and if an egregious error in patient management has occurred, is it not the responsibility of the medical profession to discover this?

The autopsy has an important part in evaluating the care of the cancer patient who has succumbed to the illness. While the autopsy obviously will not offer direct benefit to the dead patient, it may be essential for supporting or refuting clinical impressions, determining the extent of residual disease and the adequacy of therapy, evaluating new therapies, identifying the ultimate and proximate causes of death, and revealing unexpected findings that affected patient care. As a means of advancing knowledge, clinicians should regard autopsy permission as the final contribution they can make to science and that the deceased patient can make to an understanding of the disease to which the patient succumbed. The usefulness of the autopsy is greatly enhanced if the clinician takes the time to ask the pathologist specific questions that he or she would like answered at postmortem examination, if the clinician makes it a point to view the dissected organs, and if the pathologist issues a timely and clinician-friendly report that contains a minimum of jargon and that attempts to integrate the anatomic findings into the clinical picture.

Summary and Conclusions

Perhaps the most important theme of this chapter has been its emphasis on the role of the pathologist as a member of the medical team caring for the patient with cancer. The importance of close communication among the oncologist, surgeon, radiotherapist, other clinicians, and the pathologist cannot be overemphasized. Patient care will be optimized if the pathologist is consulted in advance of procedures designed to obtain tissue samples for definitive diagnosis. There may be only a single opportunity to obtain tissue that will make a complete diagnosis possible, and it is unfortunate if that opportunity is lost because portions of the specimen were not appropriately triaged for immunohistochemistry, electron microscopy, flow cytometry, culture, or other special procedures. Implementation of a high level of communication and cooperation between pathologists and clinicians has led to important contributions to the treatment and care of patients with malignant melanoma and breast cancer, among other examples. These examples should serve as useful models for the study of other types of cancers.

Acknowledgments

This work was supported by United States Public Health Service Grants, CA-50453, CA-58845, and AI-33372; by the

Beth Israel Hospital Pathology Foundation, Inc.; and under terms of a contract from the National Foundation for Cancer Research. The authors thank Peter K. Gardner for his expertise in compiling this manuscript.

References

1. Abendroth CS, Wang HH, Ducatman BS. Comparative features of carcinoma in situ and atypical ductal hyperplasia of the breast on fine-needle aspiration biopsy specimens. Am J Clin Pathol 1991;96:654.
2. Atkinson BF. Carbowax fixation of needle aspirates. Diagn Cytopathol 1986;2:231.
3. Azavedo E, Svane G, Auer, G Stereotactic fine-needle biopsy in 2594 mammographically detected non-palpable lesions. Lancet 1989;1:1033.
4. Azumi N, Battifora H. The distribution of vimentin and keratin in epithelial and nonepithelial neoplasms. A comprehensive immunohistochemical study on formalin- and alcohol-fixed tumors. Am J Clin Pathol 1987;88:286.
5. Barrett-Lee P, Travers M, Luqmani Y, Coombes RC. Transcripts for transforming growth factors in human breast cancer: clinical correlates. Br J Cancer 1990;61:612.
6. Battifora H. Immunocytochemistry of hormone receptors in routinely processed tissues. The new gold standard. Appl Immunohistochem 1994;2:143.
7. Battifora H, Kopinski M. The influence of protease digestion and duration of fixation on the immunostaining of keratins. A comparison of formalin and ethanol fixation. J Histochem Cytochem 1986;34:1095.
8. Battifora H, Sheibani K, Tubbs RR, Kopinski MI, Sun T-T. Antikeratin antibodies in tumor diagnosis. Distinction between seminoma and embryonal carcinoma. Cancer 1984;54:843.
9. Battle RM, Pathak D, Humble CG, Key CR, Vanatta PR, Hill RB, Anderson RE. Factors influencing discrepancies between premortem and postmortem diagnoses. JAMA 1987;258:339.
10. Beckstead JH. An approach to practical problems in the diagnosis of lymphoproliferative disorders using cytochemistry and immunocytochemistry. Clin Lab Med 1988;8:211.
11. Beckstead JH. Improved antigen retrieval in formalin-fixed, paraffin-embedded tissues. Appl Immunohistochem 1994;2:274.
12. Behmard S, Sadeghi A, Bagheri SA. Diagnostic accuracy of endoscopy with brushing cytology and biopsy in upper gastrointestinal lesions. Acta Cytol 1978;22:153.
13. Bibbo M, Scheiber M, Cajulis R, Keebler CM, Wied GL, Dowlatshahi K. Stereotaxic fine needle aspiration cytology of clinically occult malignant and premalignant breast lesions. Acta Cytol 1988;32:193.
14. Bloom HJ, Field JR. Impact of tumor grade and host resistance on survival of women with breast cancer. Cancer 1971;28:1580.
15. Bloom HJG, Richardson WW. Histological grading and prognosis in breast cancer. Br J Cancer 1957;11:359.
16. Bolla M, Chedin M, Souvignet C, Arnould C, Marron J, Chambaz EM. Prognostic value of epidermal growth factor receptor (EGFR) in breast carcinoma. Proceedings ECCO5, London, 1989.
17. Bonetti F, Colombari R, Manfrin E, Zamboni G, Martignoni G, Mombello A, Chilosi M. Breast carcinoma with positive results for melanoma marker (HMB-45). HMB-45 immunoreactivity in normal and neoplastic breast. Am J Clin Pathol 1989;92:491.
18. Bonneterre J, Peyrat JP, Beuscart R, Lefebvre J, Demaille A. Prognostic significance of IGF1 receptors (IGF1-R) in human breast cancer. Breast Cancer Res Treat 1989;14:166.
19. Boon ME, Alons-van Kordelaar JJ, Rietveld-Scheffers PE. Consequences of the introduction of combined spatula and Cytobrush sampling for cervical cytology. Improvements in smear quality and detection rates. Acta Cytol 1986;30:264.
20. Boyages J, Recht A, Connolly J, Schnitt S, Rose MA, Silver B, Harris JR. Factors associated with local recurrence as a first site of failure following the conservative treatment of early breast cancer. Recent Results Cancer Res 1989;115:92.
21. Breslow A. Thickness, cross-sectional areas and depth of invasion in the prognosis of cutaneous melanoma. Ann Surg 1970;172:902.
22. Brown LF, Berse B, Jackman RW, Tognazzi K, Guidi AJ, Dvorak HF, Senger DR, Connolly JL, Schnitt SJ. Expression of vascular permeability factor (vascular endothelial growth factor) and its receptors in breast cancer. Hum Pathol 1995;26:86.
23. Brown LF, Berse B, Jackman RW, Tognazzi K, Manseau EJ, Dvorak HF, Senger DR. Vascular permeability factor (vascular endothelial growth factor) and its receptors in kidney and bladder carcinomas. Am J Pathol 1993;143:1255.
24. Brown LF, Berse B, Jackman RW, Tognazzi K, Manseau EJ, Senger DR, Dvorak HF. Expression of vascular permeability factor (vascular endothelial growth factor) and its receptors in adenocarcinomas of the gastrointestinal tract. Cancer Res 1993;53:4727.
25. Brown LF, Lanir N, McDonagh J, Czarnecki K, Estrella P, Dvorak AM, Dvorak HF. Fibroblast migration in fibrin gel matrices. Am J Pathol 1993;142:273.
26. Brown LF, Yeo KT, Berse B, Yeo TK, Senger DR, Dvorak HF, Van De Water L. Expression of vascular permeability factor (vascular endothelial growth factor) by epidermal keratinocytes during wound healing. J Exp Med 1992;176:1375.
27. Cartun RW, Pedersen CA. An immunocytochemical technique offering increased sensitivity and lowered cost with a streptavidin-horseradish peroxidase conjugate. J Histotechnol 1989;12:273.
28. Christopherson WM. Mass population screening for cervix cancer. Tumori 1976;62:297.
29. Clark GM, Dressler LG, Owens MA, Pounds G, Oldaker T, McGuire WL. Prediction of relapse or survival in patients with node-negative breast cancer by DNA flow cytometry. N Engl J Med 1989;320:627.
30. Clark WH Jr, Elder DE, Guerry DT, Braitman LE, Trock BJ, Schultz D, Synnestvedt M, Halpern AC, Guerry D. Model predicting survival in stage I melanoma based on tumor progression. JNCI 1989;81:1893.
31. Clark WH Jr, From L, Bernardino EA, Mihm MC. The histogenesis and biologic behavior of primary human malignant melanomas of the skin. Cancer Res 1969;29:705.
32. Connolly DT, Heuvelman DM, Nelson R, Olander JV, Eppley BL, Delfino JJ, Siegel NR, Leimgruber RM, Feder J. Tumor vascular permeability factor stimulates endothelial cell growth and angiogenesis. J Clin Invest 1989;84:1470.
33. Connolly JL, Schnitt SJ. Evaluation of breast biopsy specimens in patients considered for treatment by conservative surgery and radiation therapy for early breast cancer. Pathol Annu 1988;23(Pt.I):1.
34. Costantini V, Zacharski LR, Memoli VA, Kisiel W, Kudryk BJ, Rousseau SM. Fibrinogen deposition without thrombin generation in primary human breast cancer tissue. Cancer Res 1991;51:349.
35. Cotran RS, Kumar V, Robbins SL, eds. Robbins Pathologic Basis of Disease, 5th ed. Philadelphia: Saunders, 1994.
36. Craemer DW. The role of cervical cytology in the declining morbidity and mortality of cervical cancer. Cancer 1974;34:2018.
37. Crystal BS, Wang HH, Ducatman BS. Comparison of different preparation techniques for fine needle aspiration specimens. A semiquantitative and statistical analysis. Acta Cytol 1993;37:24.
38. Davey FR, Elghetany MT, Kurec AS. Immunophenotyping of hematologic neoplasms in paraffin-embedded tissue sections. Am J Clin Pathol 1990;93(suppl 1):S17.
39. Dowlatshahi K, Gent HJ, Schmidt R, Jokich PM, Bibbo M, Sprenger E. Nonpalpable breast tumors: diagnosis with stereotaxic localization and fine-needle aspiration. Radiology 1989;170:427.
40. Drier JK, Swanson PE, Cherwitz DL, Wick MR. S100 protein immunoreactivity in poorly differentiated carcinomas. Immunohistochemical comparison with malignant melanoma. Arch Pathol Lab Med 1987;111:447.
41. Ducatman BS, Hogan CL, Wang HH. A triage system for processing fine needle aspiration cytology specimens. Acta Cytol 1989;33:797.
42. Duggan MA, Masters CB, Alexander F. Immunohistochemical differentiation of malignant mesothelioma, mesothelial hyperplasia and metastatic adenocarcinoma in serous effusions, utilizing staining for carcinoembryonic antigen, keratin and vimentin. Acta Cytol 1987;31:807.
43. Dupont WD, Page DL. Risk factors for breast cancer in women with proliferative breast disease. N Engl J Med 1985;312:146.
44. Dvorak AM. Monograph—procedural guide to specimen handling for the ultrastructural pathology service laboratory. J Electron Microsc Technol 1987;6:255.
45. Dvorak AM. Gut autonomic nerve (GAN) tumors. In Digestive Disease Pathology, vol 2. Edited by S Watanabe, M Wolff, SC Sommers. Philadelphia: Field & Wood, 1989, p 49.
46. Dvorak AM. Metastatic intestinal adenocarcinomas identified by ultrastructural analysis of a site-specific organelle—the terminal web. In Digestive Disease Pathology, vol 2. Edited by S Watanabe, M Wolff, SC Sommers. Philadelphia: Field & Wood, 1989, p 39.
47. Dvorak AM, Monahan RA. Metastatic adenocarcinoma of unknown primary site. Diagnostic electron microscopy to determine the site of tumor origin. Arch Pathol Lab Med 1982;106:21.
48. Dvorak AM, Monahan-Earley RA. Neurological findings and loss of consciousness in a previously well forty seven year old woman: alveolar cell carcinoma of the lung, metastatic to the brain. Norelco Reporter 1985;32:29.
49. Dvorak AM, Monahan-Earley RA. Diagnostic Ultrastructural Pathology. I. A Text-Atlas of Case Studies Illustrating the Correlative Clinical-Ultrastructural Pathologic Approach to Diagnosis. Boca Raton, FL: CRC Press, 1992.
50. Dvorak AM, Monahan-Earley RA. Diagnostic Ultrastructural Pathology. II. A Text-Atlas of Case Studies with Emphasis on Respiratory and Nervous Systems Illustrating the Correlative Clinical-Ultrastructural Pathologic Approach to Diagnosis. Boca Raton, FL: CRC Press, 1995.
51. Dvorak AM, Monahan-Earley RA. Diagnostic Ultrastructural Pathology. III. A Text-Atlas of Case Studies with Emphasis on Endocrine and Hematopoietic Systems Illustrating the Correlative Clinical-Ultrastructural Pathologic Approach to Diagnosis. Boca Raton, FL: CRC Press, 1995.
52. Dvorak HF. Tumors: wounds that do not heal. Similarities between tumor stroma generation and wound healing. N Engl J Med 1986;315:1650.
53. Dvorak HF, Brown LF, Detmar M, Dvorak AM. Vascular permeability factor/vascular endothelial growth factor, microvascular hyperpermeability, and angiogenesis. Am J Pathol 1995;146:1.
54. Dvorak HF, Dvorak AM, Manseau EJ, Wiberg L, Churchill WH. Fibrin-gel investment associated with line 1 and line 10 solid tumor growth, angiogenesis, and fibroplasia in guinea pigs. Role of cellular immunity, myofibroblasts, microvascular damage, and infarction in line 1 tumor regression. JNCI 1979;62:1459.
55. Dvorak HF, Harvey VS, Estrella P, Brown LF, McDonagh J, Dvorak AM. Fibrin containing gels induce angiogenesis. Implications for tumor stroma generation and wound healing. Lab Invest 1987;57:673.
56. Dvorak HF, Nagy JA, Dvorak AM. Structure of solid tumors and their vasculature: implications for therapy with monoclonal antibodies. Cancer Cells 1991;3:77.
57. Dvorak HF, Orenstein NS, Carvalho AC, Churchill WH, Dvorak AM, Galli SJ, Feder J, Bitzer AM, Rypysc J, Giovinco P. Induction of a fibrin-gel investment: an early event in line 10 hepatocarcinoma growth mediated by tumor-secreted products. J Immunol 1979;122:166.
58. Dvorak HF, Sioussat TM, Brown LF, Nagy JA, Sotrel A, Manseau E, Van De Water L, Senger DR. Distribution of vascular permeability factor (vascular endothelial growth factor) in tumors: concentration in tumor blood vessels. J Exp Med 1991;174:1275.
59. Dziura BR, Bonfiglio TA. Needle cytology of the breast. A quantitative and qualitative study of the cells of benign and malignant ductal neoplasia. Acta Cytol 1979;23:332.
60. El-Naggar AK, Batsakis JG, Teague K, Giacco G, Guinee VF, Swanson D. Acridine orange flow cytometric analysis of renal cell carcinoma. Clinicopathologic implications of RNA content. Am J Pathol 1990;137:275.
61. Elston CW. The assessment of histological differentiation in breast cancer. Aust NZ J Surg 1984;54:11.
62. Epstein AH, Connolly JL, Gelman R, Schnitt SJ, Silver B, Boyages J, Rose MA, Recht A, Harris JR. The predictors of distant relapse following conservative surgery and radiotherapy for early breast cancer are similar to those following mastectomy. Int J Radiat Oncol Biol Phys 1989;17:755.
63. Everall JD, Dowd PM. Diagnosis, prognosis, and treatment of melanoma. Lancet 1979;2:286.
64. Fallenius AG, Franzen SA, Auer GU. Predictive value of nuclear DNA content in breast cancer in relation to clinical morphologic factors. A retrospective study of 227 consecutive cases. Cancer 1988;62:521.
65. Ferrara N, Henzel WJ. Pituitary follicular cells secrete a novel heparin-binding growth factor specific for vascular endothelial cells. Biochem Biophys Res Commun 1989;161:851.

66. Fisher B, Redmond C, Fisher ER, Caplan R. Relative worth of estrogen or progesterone receptor and pathologic characteristics of differentiation as indicators of prognosis in node negative breast cancer patients: findings from National Surgical Adjuvant Breast and Bowel Project Protocol B-06. J Clin Oncol 1988;6:1076.
67. Fisher ER, Sass R, Fisher B. Pathologic findings from the National Surgical Adjuvant Project for Breast Cancers (protocol no. 4). X. Discriminants for tenth year treatment failure. Cancer 1984;53(3 suppl):712.
68. Folkman J, Shing Y. Angiogenesis. J Biol Chem 1992;267:10931.
69. Foulds L. The experimental study of tumor progression: a review. Cancer Res 1954;14:327.
70. Frable WJ. Thin-needle aspiration biopsy. In Major Problems in Pathology, vol 14. Edited by JL Bennington. Philadelphia: Saunders, 1983, p 7.
71. Frable WJ. Needle aspiration of the breast. Cancer 1984;53(3 suppl):671.
72. Frable WJ. Needle aspiration biopsy: past, present, and future. Hum Pathol 1989;20: 504.
73. Frable WJ, Kardos TF. Fine needle aspiration biopsy. Applications in the diagnosis of lymphoproliferative diseases. Am J Surg Pathol 1988;12(suppl 1):62.
74. Garcia RL, Coltrera MD, Gown AM. Analysis of proliferative grade using anti-PCNA/cyclin monoclonal antibodies in fixed, embedded tissues. Comparison with flow cytometric analysis. Am J Pathol 1989;134:733.
75. Gardner HA, Ducatman BS, Wang HH. Predictive value of fine-needle aspiration of the thyroid in the classification of follicular lesions. Cancer 1993;71:2598.
76. Gasparini G, Dal Fior S, Pozza F, Bevilacqua P. Correlation of growth fraction by Ki-67 immunohistochemistry with histologic factors and hormone receptors in operable breast carcinoma. Breast Cancer Res Treat 1989;14:329.
77. Gasparini G, Harris AL. Clinical importance of the determination of tumor angiogenesis in breast carcinoma: much more than a new prognostic tool. J Clin Oncol 1995;13:765.
78. Gasparini G, Weidner N, Bevilacqua P, Maluta S, Boracchi P, Testolin A, Pozza F, Folkman J. Intratumoral microvessel density and p53 protein: correlation with metastasis in head-and-neck squamous-cell carcinoma. Int J Cancer 1993;55:739.
79. Gay JD, Donaldson LD, Goellner JR. False-negative results in cervical cytologic studies. Acta Cytol 1985;29:1043.
80. Geelhoed GW, Breslow A, McCune WS. Malignant melanoma correlation of long-term follow-up with clinical staging, level of invasion and thickness of the primary tumor. Ann Surg 1977;43:77.
81. Gerdes J. Ki-67 and other proliferation markers useful for immunohistological diagnostic and prognostic evaluations in human malignancies. Semin Cancer Bio 1990;1: 199.
82. Gerdes J, Lelle RJ, Pickartz H, Heidenreich W, Schwarting R, Kurtsiefer L, Stauch G, Stein H. Growth fractions in breast cancers determined in situ with monoclonal antibody Ki-67. J Clin Pathol 1986;39:977.
83. Ghadially FN. Diagnostic Electron Microscopy of Tumours. London: Butterworths, 1980.
84. Gleason DF. Histologic grade, clinical stage, and patient age in prostate cancer. NCI Monogr 1988;7:15.
85. Goldman L, Sayson R, Robbins S, Cohn LH, Bettmann M, Weisberg M. The value of the autopsy in three medical eras. N Engl J Med 1983;308:1000.
86. Gospodarowicz D, Abraham JA, Schilling J. Isolation and characterization of a vascular endothelial cell mitogen produced by pituitary-derived folliculo stellate cells. Proc Natl Acad Sci USA 1989;86:7311.
87. Gould VE. The coexpression of distinct classes of intermediate filaments in human neoplasms. Arch Pathol Lab Med 1985;109:984.
88. Greenberg RS, Chow WH, Liff JM. Recent trends in the epidemiology of cervical neoplasia. Acta Cytol 1989;33:463.
89. Hahnel R, Woodings T, Vivian AB. Prognostic value of estrogen receptors in primary breast cancer. Cancer 1979;44:671.
90. Hamberger B, Gharib H, Melton LJ, IIIrd, Goellner JR, Zinsmeister AR. Fine-needle aspiration biopsy of thyroid nodules. Impact on thyroid practice and cost of care. Am J Med 1982;73:381.
91. Hamburger JI. Consistency of sequential needle biopsy findings for thyroid nodules. Management implications. Arch Intern Med 1987;147:97.
92. Hann L, Ducatman BS, Wang HH, Fein V, McIntire JM. Nonpalpable breast lesions: evaluation by means of fine-needle aspiration cytology. Radiology 1989;171:373.
93. Harris JR, Hellman S, Henderson IC, Kinne DW, eds. Breast Diseases, 2nd ed. Philadelphia: Lippincott, 1991.
94. Henderson DW, Papadimitriou JM. Ultrastructural Appearances of Tumours. A Diagnostic Atlas. Edinburgh: Churchill Livingstone, 1982.
95. Hill RP. Tumor progression: potential role of unstable genomic changes. Cancer Metastasis Rev 1990;9:137.
96. Holland R, Connolly JL, Gelman R, Mravunac M, Hendriks JH, Verbeek AL, Schnitt SJ, Silver B, Boyages J, Harris JR. The presence of an extensive intraductal component (EIC) following a limited excision correlates with prominent residual disease in the remainder of the breast. J Clin Oncol 1990;8:113.
97. Houck KA, Ferrara N, Winer J, Cachianes G, Li B, Leung DW. The vascular endothelial growth factor family: identification of a fourth molecular species and characterization of alternative splicing of RNA. Mol Endocrinol 1991;5:1806.
98. Hsu SM, Raine L. The use of avidin-biotin-peroxidase complex (ABC) in diagnostic and research pathology. In Advances in Immunohistochemistry. Edited by RA DeLellis. New York: Masson, 1984, p 31.
99. Jacquemier J, Kurtz J, Amalric R, Brandone H, Ayme Y, Spitalier JM. An assessment of extensive intraductal component as a risk factor for local recurrence after breast-conserving therapy. Br J Cancer 1990;61:873.
100. Kadin ME, Said J. T-cell lymphomas and leukemias of post-thymic differentiation. Clin Lab Med 1988;8:135.
101. Keck PJ, Hauser SD, Krivi G, Sanzo K, Warren T, Feder J, Connolly DT. Vascular permeability factor, an endothelial cell mitogen related to PDGF. Science 1989;246: 1309.
102. Kim K, Rigal RD, Patrick JR, Walters JK, Bennett A, Nordin W, Claybrook JR, Parekh RR. The changing trends of uterine cancer and cytology: a study of morbidity and mortality trends over a twenty year period. Cancer 1978;42:2439.
103. Kini SR, Miller JM, Hamburger JI, Smith-Purslow MJ. Cytopathology of follicular lesions of the thyroid gland. Diagn Cytopathol 1985;1:123.
104. Klagsbrun M, Soker S. VEGF/VPF. The angiogenesis factor found? Curr Biol 1993;3: 699.
105. Klijn JG, Portengen H, van Putten WL, Trapman AM, Reubi JC, Alexieva-Figusch J, Foekens JA. The prognostic value of receptors for somatostatin (SS-R), insulin-like growth factor-1 (IGF-1-R) and epidermal growth factor (EGF-R) in human breast cancer. Proc Annu Meet Am Soc Clin Oncol 1989;8:A78.
106. Kline TS, Kline IK. Breast. In Guides to Clinical Aspiration Cytology. Edited by TS Kline. New York/Tokyo: Igaku-Shoin, 1989, p 1.
107. Knowles DM. Lymphoid cell markers. Their distribution and usefulness in the immunophenotypic analysis of lymphoid neoplasms. Am J Surg Pathol 1985;9(suppl):85.
108. Knudson AG. Stem cell regulation, tissue ontogeny, and oncogenic events. Semin Cancer Biol 1992;3:99.
109. Kurzrock R, Gutterman JU, Talpaz M. The molecular genetics of Philadelphia: chromosome-positive leukemias. N Engl J Med 1988;319:990.
110. Landefeld CS, Chren MM, Myers A, Geller R, Robbins S, Goldman L. Diagnostic yield of the autopsy in a university hospital and a community hospital. N Engl J Med 1988;318:1249.
111. Larsen TE, Grude TH. A retrospective histological study of 669 cases of primary cutaneous malignant melanoma in clinical stage I. I. Histological classification, sex and age of the patients, localization of tumour and prognosis. Acta Pathol Microbiol Scand [A], 1978;86:437.
112. Larsen TE, Grude TH. A retrospective histological study of 669 cases of primary cutaneous malignant melanoma in clinical stage I. V. The consequences of reclassification of the original group of lentigo maligna melanomas. Acta Pathol Microbiol Scand [A], 1979;87:255.
113. Lee AK, DeLellis RA, Wolfe HJ. Intramammary lymphatic invasion in breast carcinomas. Evaluation using ABH isoantigens as endothelial markers. Am J Surg Pathol 1986;10:589.
114. Leung DW, Cachianes G, Kuang WJ, Goeddel DV, Ferrara N. Vascular endothelial growth factor is a secreted angiogenic mitogen. Science 1989;246:1306.
115. Linsk JA. Aspiration cytology in Sweden: the Karolinska group. Diagn Cytopathol 1985;1:332.
116. Linsk JA, Franzen S. Clinical Aspiration Cytology. Philadelphia: Lippincott, 1983.
117. Löfgren M, Andersson I, Bondeson L, Lindholm K. X-ray guided fine-needle aspiration for the cytologic diagnosis of nonpalpable breast lesions. Cancer 1988;61:1032.
118. Macchiarini P, Fontanini G, Hardin MJ, Hardin MJ, Squartini F, Angeletti CA. Relation of neovasculature to metastasis of non-small-cell lung cancer. Lancet 1992;340:145.
119. Mansour EG, Ravdin PM, Dressler L. Prognostic factors in early breast carcinoma. Cancer 1994;74(suppl):381.
120. Martin HE, Ellis EB. Biopsy by needle puncture and aspiration. Ann Surg 1930;92: 169.
121. Mason M, Bedrossian CWM. Value of immunocytochemistry in the study of malignant effusions. Acta Cytol 1986;30:569.
122. Mauri FA, Girlando S, Dalla Palma P, Buffa G, Perrone G, Doglioni C, Kreipe H, Barbareschi M. Ki-67 antibodies (Ki-S5, MIB-1, and Ki-67) in breast carcinomas. A brief quantitative comparison. Appl Immunohistochem 1994;2:171.
123. McDivitt RW, Stewart FW, Berg JW. Tumors of the Breast. Bethesda, MD: Armed Forces Institute of Pathology, 1968.
124. McGovern VJ. The classification of melanoma and its relationship with prognosis. Pathology 1970;2:85.
125. McGovern VJ. Melanoma histological diagnosis and prognosis. In Biopsy Interpretation Series. New York: Raven Press, 1983, p 158.
126. McGovern VJ, Shaw HM, Milton GW, Farago GA. Prognostic significance of the histological features of malignant melanoma. Histopathology 1979;3:385.
127. McGovern VJ, Shaw HM, Milton GW, Farago GA. Is malignant melanoma arising in a Hutchinson's melanotic freckle a separate disease entity? Histopathology 1980;4: 235.
128. McNutt NS, Heilbron DC, Crain WR. Mycosis fungoides: diagnostic criteria based on quantitative electron microscopy. Lab Invest 1981;44:466.
129. McPhee SJ, Bottles K. Autopsy: moribund art or vital science? Am J Med 1985;78: 107.
130. Miettinen M, Virtanen I, Talerman A. Intermediate filament proteins in human testis and testicular germ-cell tumors. Am J Pathol 1985;120:402.
131. Miller AB. Evaluation of screening for carcinoma of the cervix. Mod Med Canada 1973;28:1067.
132. Miller AB, Lindsay J, Hill GB. Mortality from cancer of the uterus in Canada and its relationship to screening for cancer of the cervix. Int J Cancer 1976;17:602.
133. Muss HB, Kute TE, Case LD, Smith LR, Booher C, Long R, Kammire L, Gregory B, Brockschmidt JK. The relation of flow cytometry to clinical and biologic characteristics in women with node negative primary breast cancer. Cancer 1989;64:1894.
134. Nagle RB. Intermediate filaments: efficacy in surgical pathology diagnosis. Am J Clin Pathol 1989;91(4 suppl 1):S14.
135. Nowell PC. Mechanisms of tumor progression. Cancer Res 1986;46:2203.
136. Nowell PC. Cytogenetic approaches to human cancer genes. FASEB J 1994;8:408.
137. Nowell PC, Croce CM. Chromosomal approaches to oncogenes and oncogenesis. FASEB J 1988;2(15):3054.
138. Ordonez NG. The immunohistochemical diagnosis of mesothelioma. Differentiation of mesothelioma and lung adenocarcinoma. Am J Surg Pathol 1989;13:276.
139. Orell S, Sterrett GF, Walters MNI, Whitaker D. Manual and Atlas of Fine Needle Aspiration Cytology. New York: Churchill Livingstone, 1986.
140. Otis CN, Carter D, Cole S, Battifora H. Immunohistochemical evaluation of pleural mesothelioma and pulmonary adenocarcinoma. A bi-institutional study of 47 cases. Am J Surg Pathol 1987;11:445.
141. Owings D, Hann L, Schnitt SJ. How thoroughly should needle localization breast biopsies be sampled for microscopic examination? A prospective mammographic-pathologic correlative study. Am J Surg Pathol 1990;14:578.
142. Perez R, Pascual M, Macias A, Lage A. Epidermal growth factor receptors in human breast cancer. Breast Cancer Res Treat 1984;4:189.
143. Perkins SL, Kjeldsberg CR. Immunophenotyping of lymphomas and leukemias in paraffin-embedded tissues. Am J Clin Pathol 1993;99:362.
144. Pertschuk LP, Feldman JG, Eisenberg KB, Carter AC, Thelmo WL, Cruz WP, Thorpe SM, Christensen IJ, Rasmussen BB, Rose C, Greene GL. Immunocytochemical detection of progesterone receptor in breast cancer with monoclonal antibody. Relation to biochemical assay, disease-free survival, and clinical endocrine response. Cancer 1988;62:342.

145. Peterse JL, van Dongen JA, Bartelink H. Recurrence of breast carcinoma after breast conserving treatment. Eur J Surg Oncol 1988;14:123.
146. Picker LJ, Weiss LM, Medeiros LJ, Wood GS, Warnke RA. Immunophenotypic criteria for the diagnosis of non-Hodgkin's lymphoma. Am J Pathol 1987;128:181.
147. Pierce GB. The cancer cell and its control by the embryo. Rous-Whipple Award lecture. Am J Pathol 1983;113:117.
148. Pinkus GS, Kurtin PJ. Epithelial membrane antigen—a diagnostic discriminant in surgical pathology: immunohistochemical profile in epithelial, mesenchymal, and hematopoietic neoplasms using paraffin sections and monoclonal antibodies. Hum Pathol 1985;16:929.
149. Pinkus GS, O'Connor EM, Etheridge CL, Corson JM. Optimal immunoreactivity of keratin proteins in formalin-fixed, paraffin-embedded tissue requires preliminary trypsinization. An immunoperoxidase study of various tumours using polyclonal and monoclonal antibodies. J Histochem Cytochem 1985;33:465.
150. Plate KH, Breier G, Weich HA, Risau W. Vascular endothelial growth factor is a potential tumour angiogenesis factor in human gliomas in vivo. Nature 1992;359:845.
151. Powles TJ, Hardy JR, Ashley SE, Cosgrove D, Davey JB, Dowsett M, McKinna A, Nash AG, Rundle SK, Sinnett HD, Tillyer CR, Treleaven JG. Chemoprevention of breast cancer. Breast Cancer Res Treat 1989;14:23.
152. Rabbitts TH. Chromosomal translocations in human cancer. Nature 1994;372:143.
153. Reid LM. Stem cell biology, hormone/matrix synergies and liver differentiation. Curr Opin Cell Biol 1990;2:121.
154. Rosen PP, Groshen S. Factors influencing survival and prognosis in early breast carcinoma (T1N0M0-T1N1M0). Assessment of 644 patients with median follow-up of 18 years. Surg Clin North Am 1990;70:937.
155. Rowlatt C. Tissue organization and neoplasms. In The Functional Integration of Cells into Animal Tissues. Cambridge: Cambridge University Press, 1982, p 319.
156. Rowley JD. Molecular cytogenetics Rosetta stone for understanding cancer—twenty-ninth G.H.A. Clowes Memorial Award lecture. Cancer Res 1990;50:3816.
157. Sainsbury JR, Farndon JR, Needham GK, Harris AL, Malcolm AJ. Epidermal-growth-factor receptor status as predictor of early recurrence of and death from breast cancer. Lancet 1987;1:1398.
158. Scharf ERW, Hadley RS. Prognosis in carcinoma of the breast. Lancet 1938;2:582.
159. Schnitt SJ, Abner A, Gelman R, Connolly JL, Recht A, Duda RB, Eberlein TJ, Mayzel K, Silver B, Harris JR. The relationship between microscopic margins of resection and the risk of local recurrence in patients with breast cancer treated with breast-conserving surgery and radiation therapy. Cancer 1994;74:1746.
160. Schnitt SJ, Connolly JL, Khettry U, Mazoujian G, Brenner M, Silver B, Recht A, Beadle G, Harris JR. Pathologic findings on re-excision of the primary site in breast cancer patients considered for treatment by primary radiation therapy. Cancer 1987;59: 675.
161. Schnitt SJ, Silen W, Sadowsky NL, Connolly JL, Harris JR. Ductal carcinoma in situ (intraductal carcinoma) of the breast. N Engl J Med 1988;318:898.
162. Senger DR, Connolly DT, Van De Water L, Feder J, Dvorak HF. Purification and NH_2-terminal amino acid sequence of guinea pig tumor-secreted vascular permeability factor. Cancer Res 1990;50:1774.
163. Senger DR, Galli SJ, Dvorak AM, Perruzzi CA, Harvey VS, Dvorak HF. Tumor cells secrete a vascular permeability factor that promotes accumulation of ascites fluid. Science 1983;3219:983.
164. Senger DR, Van De Water L, Brown LF, Nagy JA, Yeo KT, Yeo TK, Berse B, Jackman RW, Dvorak AM, Dvorak HF. Vascular permeability factor (VPF, VEGF) in tumor biology. Cancer Met Rev 1993;12:303.
165. Sheibani K. Immunopathology of malignant mesothelioma. Hum Pathol 1994;25:219.
166. Sheibani K, Tubbs RR. Enzyme immunohistochemistry: technical aspects. Semin Diagn Pathol 1984;1:235.
167. Shi ZR, Itzkowitz SH, Kim YS. A comparison of three immunoperoxidase techniques for antigen detection in colorectal carcinoma tissues. J Histochem Cytochem 1988;36:317.
168. Slamon DJ, Godolphin W, Jones LA, Holt JA, Wong SG, Keith DE, Levin WJ, Stuart SG, Udove J, Ullrich A, Press MF. Studies of the HER-2/neu proto-oncogene in human breast and ovarian cancer. Science 1989;244 (4905):707.
169. Sneige N, Staerkel GA. Fine-needle aspiration cytology of ductal hyperplasia with and without atypia and ductal carcinoma in situ. Hum Pathol 1994;25:485.
170. Sneige N, White VA, Katz RL, Troncoso P, Libshitz HI, Hortobagyi GN. Ductal carcinoma-in-situ of the breast: fine-needle aspiration cytology of 12 cases. Diagn Cytopathol 1989;5:371.
171. Stanley MW, Henry-Stanley MJ, Zera R. Atypia in breast fine-needle aspiration smears correlates poorly with the presence of a prognostically significant proliferative lesion of ductal epithelium. Hum Pathol 1993;24:630.
172. Sternberger LA. Immunocytochemistry, 3rd ed. New York: Wiley, 1986.
173. Symposium on Estrogen Receptor Determination with Monoclonal Antibodies. Cancer Res 1986;46:4231S.
174. Symposium on the Autopsy. A Professional Obligation Dissected. Hum Pathol 1990;21:127.
175. Tandon AK, Clark GM, Chamness GC, Chirgwin JM, McGuire WL. Cathepsin D and prognosis in breast cancer. N Engl J Med 1990;322:297.
176. Tannock IF, Hill RP, eds. The Basic Science of Oncology, 2nd ed. New York: McGraw-Hill, 1992.
177. Tannock IF, Rotin D. Acid pH in tumors and its potential for therapeutic exploitation. Cancer Res 1989;49:4373.
178. Tao LC. Lung, pleura, and mediastinum. In Guides to Clinical Aspiration Biopsy. Edited by TS Kline. New York/Tokyo: Igaku-Shoin, 1988, p 1.
179. Taylor CR. Immunomicroscopy. A Diagnostic Tool for the Surgical Pathologist. Philadelphia: Saunders, 1986.
180. Toikkanen S, Joensuu H, Klemi P. Nuclear DNA content as a prognostic factor in T1–2N0 breast cancer. Am J Clin Pathol 1990;93:471.
181. van de Vijver MJ, Peterse JL, Mooi WJ, Wisman P, Lomans J, Dalesio O, Nusse R. Neu-protein overexpression in breast cancer. Association with comedo-type ductal carcinoma in situ and limited prognostic value in stage II breast cancer. N Engl J Med 1988;319:1239.
182. Vaupel P, Kallinowski F, Okunieff P. Blood flow, oxygen and nutrient supply, and metabolic microenvironment of human tumors: a review. Cancer Res 1989;49:6449.
183. Vogelstein B, Fearon ER, Hamilton SR, Kern SE, Preisinger AC, Leppert M, Nakamura Y, White R, Smits AM, Bos JL. Genetic alterations during colorectal-tumor development. N Engl J Med 1988;319:525.
184. von Rosen A, Rutqvist LE, Carstensen J, Fallenius A, Skoog L, Auer G. Prognostic value of nuclear DNA content in breast cancer in relation to tumor size, nodal status, and estrogen receptor content. Breast Cancer Res Treat 1989;13:23.
185. Wakui S, Furusato M, Itoh T, Sasaki H, Akiyama A, Kinoshita I, Asano K, Tokuda T, Aizawa S, Ushigome S. Tumor angiogenesis in prostatic carcinoma with and without bone marrow metastasis: a morphometric study. J Pathol 1992;168:257.
186. Wang HH, Ducatman BS, Eick D. Comparative features of ductal carcinoma in situ and infiltrating ductal carcinoma of the breast on fine-needle aspiration biopsy. Am J Clin Pathol 1989;92:736.
187. Wang HH, Jonasson JG, Ducatman BS. Brushing cytology of the upper gastrointestinal tract. Obsolete or not? Acta Cytol 1991;35:195.
188. Watson P, Barrett J, Pantazis C, Guthrie T. Color video analysis of transforming growth factor alpha expression in female breast cancer. Proceedings American Society Clinical Oncology, vol 7, 1988, p A138.
189. Weidner N, Folkman J, Pozza F, Bevilacqua P, Allred EN, Moore DH, Meli S, Gasparini G. Tumor angiogenesis: a new significant and independent prognostic indicator in early-stage breast carcinoma. JNCI 1992;84:1875.
190. Weidner N, Semple JP, Welch WR, Folkman J. Tumor angiogenesis and metastasis—correlation in invasive breast carcinoma. N Engl J Med 1991;324:1.
191. Weinstein RS, Kuszak JR, Kluskens LF, Coon JS. P-glycoproteins in pathology: the multidrug resistance gene family in humans. Hum Pathol 1990;21:34.
192. Weiss LM, Hu, E, Wood GS, Moulds C, Cleary ML, Warnke R, Sklar J. Clonal rearrangements of T-cell receptor genes in mycosis fungoides and dermatopathic lymphadenopathy. N Engl J Med 1985;313:539.
193. Werneke S, Sovie S, Trawinski G, Garcia L, Abu-Jawdeh G, Upton MP, Wang HH. ThinPrep processing of endoscopic brushing specimens. Acta Cytol 1994;38:842 [abstract].
194. Wick MR, Loy T, Mills SE, Legier JF, Manivel JC. Malignant epithelioid pleural mesothelioma versus peripheral pulmonary adenocarcinoma: a histochemical, ultrastructural, and immunohistologic study of 103 cases. Hum Pathol 1990;21:759.
195. Williams WJ, Davies K, Jones WM, Roberts MM. Malignant melanoma of the skin: prognostic value of histology in 89 cases. Br J Cancer 1968;22:452.
196. Willis RA. The Spread of Tumors in the Human Body. London: Butterworths, 1952.
197. Yamazaki K, Abe S, Takekawa H, Sukoh N, Watanabe N, Ogura S, Nakajima I, Isobe H, Inoue K, Kawakami Y. Tumor angiogenesis in human lung adenocarcinoma. Cancer 1994;74:2245.
198. Yeo KT, Wang HH, Nagy JA, Sioussat TM, Ledbetter SR, Hoogewerf AJ, Zhou Y, Masse EM, Senger DR, Dvorak HF, Yeo T-K. Vascular permeability factor (vascular endothelial growth factor) in guinea pig and human tumor and inflammatory effusions. Cancer Res 1993;53:2912.
199. Yeo TK, Dvorak HF. Tumor stroma. In Diagnostic Immunopathology. 2nd ed. Edited by RB Colvin, AK Bhan, RT McCluskey. New York: Raven Press, 1995, p 685.
200. Zacharski LR, Memoli VA, Ornstein DL, Rousseau SM, Kisiel W, Kudryk BJ. Tumor cell procoagulant and urokinase expression in carcinoma of the ovary. JNCI 1993;85: 1225.
201. Zarbo RJ, Gown AM, Nagle RB, Visscher DW, Crissman JD. Anomalous cytokeratin expression in malignant melanoma: one- and two-dimensional western blot analysis and immunohistochemical survey of 100 melanomas. Mod Pathol 1990;3:494.

SECTION IX

PRINCIPLES OF IMAGING

CHAPTER 32

Introduction

RICHARD J. STECKEL

Introduction

The technological revolution that is being fueled by the development of increasingly powerful computers and rapid telecommunications is currently affecting all branches of medicine, but none more than diagnostic imaging. Malignant tumors often alter the normal spatial relationships in tissues, and radiologic imaging is critical not only for diagnosing cancer but also for staging tumors and following patients after they have received treatment. In the future it is expected that technological advances related to imaging may assist clinicians in evaluating functional parameters in tumors and in assessing the effects of treatment (2, 3, 6, 8). Among the imaging studies undergoing rapid development are magnetic resonance (MR) spectroscopy and brain activation analyses, rapid computed tomographic (CT) volume acquisitions, positron emission tomography (PET) with new metabolic agents, and MR blood flow and diffusion studies.

It may be appropriate to review briefly some of the technical similarities, as well as salient differences, between three cross-sectional imaging techniques that are used frequently to study cancer patients: CT, MRI, and PET. These techniques offer computerized image reconstructions of two-dimensional sections of the body in different viewing planes. Three-dimensional volume or surface images are also possible, as well as "see-through" or projectional images. To perform CT, an external radiation source and a detector are required on opposite sides of the body, as in other radiographic imaging techniques. On the other hand, MRI uses powerful magnetic fields and radiofrequency waves to create images of the head or body without the need for ionizing radiation (see below). PET entails the injection of trace amounts of short-lived radionuclides that have been produced in a cyclotron and that concentrate in tumors and various organs. The small amounts of radiation emitted by these radionuclides can be picked up by external radiation detectors positioned on opposite sides of the body, and then used to create planar or volume images. The radionuclides first emit subatomic particles called positrons. Each positron quickly combines with an electron inside the body to produce two x-ray photons, which leave the body in opposite directions and can be detected. The radiation doses delivered to tissues in PET are less than those in ordinary radiographic studies.

With CT, the tissue densities depicted on cross-sectional images have the same significance as the densities produced on ordinary x-ray radiographs. These densities correspond to the relative amounts of diagnostic radiation absorbed by each tissue that is depicted in the image, but CT is much more sensitive to minor differences in tissue absorption (i.e., exhibits greater tissue contrast) than ordinary roentgenography. In addition, CT can "peel away" superimposed layers of tissue that may obscure detail on ordinary radiographs of the head, chest, abdomen, and extremities, revealing the anatomy of a single layer or section of tissue. An external ionizing radiation source is required, and the x-ray doses to tissues are similar to those delivered during ordinary chest, abdomen, bone, and skull radiography.

With MRI, a powerful unidirectional magnetic field is used to orient or polarize hydrogen atoms within tissue in the direction of the field. Short pulses of radiowaves are then sent into the body at a frequency that is resonant with the polarized hydrogen atoms. The polarized hydrogen atoms are deflected momentarily from their axes by these radiowave pulses, and subsequently they emit radiowaves at their resonant frequency. These emissions can be picked up by an external radiowave detector. With a powerful computer, the radiowave emission patterns from the resonant hydrogen atoms can then be used to synthesize a three-dimensional volume image (or multiple adjacent planar images) of the specific region of the head or body that is under study. MR images therefore represent a computer-generated map of the hydrogen atom radiowave emitters in a single body region. The MR emissions from these hydrogen atoms are referred to as echoes. The TE or "echo delay time" for a given MR image is the split-second delay that occurs between the excitation of hydrogen atoms in the tissues by the external pulsed radiowaves and the detection of radiowave "echoes" from the same atoms by an external detector. The interval between each successive radiowave pulse emitted by the MRI machine (which, like the echo delay time, can be selected by the MRI machine operator) is called the TR, or "repetition time." Depending on the TE and TR settings (measured in milliseconds [ms]) used for each clinical MRI examination, the operator can produce an image that is characterized as a T1-weighted image or a T2-weighted image. With the most commonly used MRI technique, known as spin echo imaging, T1-weighted images can be produced by using relatively *short* TE and TR settings (e.g., a TE of 40 ms and a TR of 200 ms), whereas T2-weighted images require *longer* settings (e.g., a TE of 120 ms and a TR of 2,000 ms). Tumors may appear relatively dark on T1-weighted MR images, but they often appear bright on T2-weighted images. Anatomic detail is shown more clearly on T1-weighted images, but tumors (and the edema and reactive tissue that may surround them) often stand out in better contrast to adjacent normal tissues on T2-weighted studies.

It is also worthy of note that (*a*) MR images can be generated easily in *any* plane (not just the axial plane, as with ordinary CT images); (*b*) the contrast between soft tissues of different types (e.g., tumor and adjacent muscle) is better with MRI than with CT; and (*c*), one can discern flowing blood in vessels on MRI without necessarily injecting contrast material into the bloodstream (parenthetically, Doppler ultrasound (US) methods can also demonstrate flow in tumor vessels noninvasively, and may have future applications in clinical cancer diagnosis). Among the limitations of MRI, small amounts of calcium cannot be detected easily with MRI, whereas CT is quite sensitive to calcium deposits in tissues. Most MR scans also take longer to obtain than CT scans; they may require several minutes rather than a few seconds to perform. Body motion therefore remains a potential problem with some MRI studies. The physical confines of MRI machines are usually quite restrictive for patients, and up to 10 to 15% of patients may experience claustrophobic reactions in the "tunnel" of the machine that preclude their undergoing the studies. Because of limited physical access to the patient in position in the scanner, very ill patients who are on life support systems are also difficult to study with most MRI machines. These limitations in MRI equipment may be less of a problem in the future, as faster MRI studies become feasible and as specialized open field units with easy access to patients become available for certain clinical applications.

It is also possible to do semiquantitative spectroscopic analyses of metabolites within living tissues using MR, and MR images can be used to pinpoint the regions of interest for spectroscopic analyses. MR spectroscopy might be used in the future to improve diagnostic specificity or to assess early responses of tumors to therapy. These ideas are still undergoing investigation.

PET, like MR spectroscopy, may also be capable of providing unique information on the metabolism of human tumors, including early changes that may result from treatment. The short-lived positron-emitting radionuclides that are used in PET can serve as "tags" on certain metabolites (e.g., radioactive fluorine-labeled glucose analogues). The metabolites are injected intravenously prior to scanning, and the rate of accumulation of the metabolites is then determined to assess tumor metabolism and the alterations caused by treatment. Unsuspected deposits of metastatic tumor can also be detected in some instances with PET because of their metabolic activity. With its ability to sample the metabolism of targeted volumes of tissue in situ, PET therefore may offer a powerful new tool for studying tumors in the laboratory as well as in selected clinical situations.

The technological advances that have led to transmission (CT) and positron emission (PET) computed tomography, as well as to MR imaging or spectroscopy and modern US methods, have also led to fundamental innovations in our ability to visualize tumors and to assess their metabolism. Although the traditional radiologic imaging techniques that are still used throughout the world (e.g., radiography of the chest, skeleton, and abdomen; gastrointestinal (GI) barium studies; radionuclide scintigraphy of bone) may demonstrate tumors directly (e.g., show tumor nodules in the lung) *or* indirectly (e.g., demonstrate widening of the duodenal loop on a GI series by a pancreatic mass), cross-sectional imaging techniques, often with contrast materials, are capable of producing direct images of tumors anywhere in the head or body. In addition to showing the internal structure or "texture" of an individual tumor, these techniques can accurately delineate the tumor's margins and demonstrate its effects on adjacent structures. Some tumors may become more visible ("enhance") after vascular contrast materials are infused during CT or MRI, or when certain MRI sequences are used (e.g., T2-weighted images). The ability to image deep tumors directly as well as to show their effects upon surrounding organs in vivo, and the corresponding ability of cross-sectional imaging techniques to strip away overlying structures that may obscure tumor masses, constitute fundamental advances for managing cancer patients that have come about in the last two decades with these imaging techniques (7, 9, 12).

Even with the availability of these new diagnostic imaging techniques, it is important to emphasize that the radiologist cannot make tissue diagnoses; relevant clinical information is always needed to make the best use of our diagnostic images. Furthermore, US, CT, and MRI have not replaced standard radiologic techniques, which have been at the core of the diagnostic armamentarium of clinicians for almost a century. The newer imaging methods are powerful complements to these techniques. Cross-sectional imaging methods have made cancer diagnosis, tumor staging, and patient follow-up more accurate (particularly with regard to diagnostic sensitivity), more rapid and less invasive than ever before. Despite their relatively high cost, particularly for CT and MRI, the impact of these techniques on the net costs of cancer care may not be self-evident. A good argument can be made that cross-sectional techniques decrease the overall costs of patient care in several important ways (5). First, planar imaging methods have lessened the need for invasive diagnostic techniques such as angiography and standard myelography, and they have eliminated painful and hazardous studies like pneumoencephalography. They have also expedited the diagnosis of cancer (as well as our efforts to rule it out), and they may obviate unnecessary surgery in patients who are shown to have metastatic or locally extensive disease. The newer imaging methods are also invaluable for directing percutaneous aspirations or needle biopsies and for planning open biopsies and surgical resections when necessary, and they have lessened the requirements for hospitalization by facilitating diagnosis and tumor staging on an outpatient basis. For these reasons and many others, modern diagnostic imaging techniques have not only improved care and decreased patient suffering, they may also have reduced overall medical expenditures and losses of income to patients by simplifying diagnostic procedures, shortening the time to diagnosis, decreasing the need for hospitalization, and helping to tailor therapeutic approaches to individual patient needs.

In contrast to modern radiology's impact on diagnosis, staging, and cancer patient follow-up, only one imaging technique has had a significant impact on screening asymptomatic individuals for cancer: low-dose mammography. Breast cancer mortality in a defined population of women can be reduced by up to one-third through regular screening mammography in accordance with nationally published guidelines (1, 4).

Physicians are also cautioned that, although cross-sectional imaging techniques may have increased sensitivity for detecting tumor masses and delineating their extent, the specificity of these same techniques in diagnosing cancer may not have improved to the same degree (11). Both the clinician and the diagnostic radiologist should exercise restraint in interpreting positive radiologic findings in patients with established or suspected cancer diagnoses, particularly findings that suggest metastases or extensive local disease for the first time. Many conditions besides metastases can present as lung nodules on CT, or as "hot spots" on skeletal radionuclide scintigraphy. As always, careful correlation of the abnormalities seen on an imaging study with a patient's clinical, laboratory, and other imaging findings is essential. Comparing serial images that have been obtained over days, weeks, or months will improve diagnostic specificity when certain kinds of abnormalities have been noted: tumor masses in the lungs cannot be expected to double in size over a few days; conversely, primary tumor masses or metastatic lesions ordinarily do not remain unchanged for many months or years. Comparing a new study with a baseline imaging study obtained 6 months or a year previously can sometimes be the critical step in reaching a correct diagnosis. Correlating findings on different types of imaging studies from the same patient (e.g., comparing focal radionuclide bone scan abnormalities with radiographs of precisely the same areas in patients who have suspected breast cancer metastases) may also be extremely helpful.

Finally, much research still needs to be done on the most appropriate applications of diagnostic imaging techniques for cancer management. It is entirely possible that the divergent results reported in different cancer therapy trials might be caused in part by inaccurate stratification of patients (12). A heterogeneous group of cancer patients who are improperly stratified in a trial of therapy may have stages of disease different from those reported in another trial. The applications of imaging techniques to oncology practice, and in particular, to clinical research studies, are still less than optimal, and some reported patient trials may in fact be mixing apples and oranges (10). The more judicious use of radiologic techniques in clinical trial protocols may have much to offer here.

An area for continuing research is the appropriate type of radiologic studies to use and the appropriate intervals between radiologic examinations for following cancer patients after they have been treated. The clinical questions inherent in this area of concern must be subjected to carefully controlled trials. Whether or not to use imaging examinations at all for the posttreatment surveillance of cancer patients should depend on whether effective palliative or salvage methods (second- or third-line treatments) are currently available. Equally germane to following cancer patients who have received definitive treatment is whether or not a second- or third-line therapy is more effective when a recurrence has been detected early as opposed to late: some treatments for recurrent disease may be just as effective (or just as ineffective) when a recurrence has become manifest through new symptoms or physical findings, rather than through regular surveillance with laboratory studies and/or imaging examinations. It is likely that some diagnostic imaging techniques are currently being used in inappropriate ways to follow treated patients at treatment centers as well as in community practice, in the absence of reliable data from controlled trials to determine what the actual effects of periodic imaging studies are on patient outcomes.

The basic principles of diagnostic imaging and their current applications to cancer management, as described in this section, are the informed recommendations of several contributing experts. While their recommendations must suffice for now, additional clinical studies and more corroborative data will be needed if recent advances in diagnostic imaging are to be applied optimally to the care of cancer patients.

References

1. Cady B. New diagnostic, staging and therapeutic aspects of early breast cancer. Cancer 1990;65(suppl 3):634.
2. Carrasquillo JA, Bunn PA, Keenan AM, Reynolds JC, Schroff RW, Foon KA, Su MH, Gazdar AF, Mulshine JL, Oldham RK, Perentesis P, Horowitz M, Eddy J, James P, Larson SM. Radioimmunodetection of cutaneous T-cell lymphoma with ^{111}In-labelled T101 monoclonal antibody. N Engl J Med 1986;315:673.
3. Dodd GD. Advances in cancer diagnosis. Cancer 1990;65(suppl 3):595.
4. Henson DE, Ries LA. Progress in early breast cancer detection. Cancer 1990;65(suppl 9):2155.
5. Kuhns LR, Thornbury JR, Tryback D. Decision Making in Imaging. Chicago: Year Book, 1989.
6. Larson SM. Positron emission tomography in oncology and allied diseases. In Principles and Practice of Oncology Updates. Edited by V DeVite, S Hillman, S Rosenberg. Philadelphia: Lippincott, 1989, p 1.
7. Platt JF, Glazer GM, Gross BH, Quint LE, Francis IR, Orringer MB. CT evaluation of mediastinal lymph nodes in lung cancer: influence of lobar site of the primary neoplasm. AJR 1987;149:683.
8. Schlom J. Innovations in monoclonal antibody tumors targeting: diagnostic and therapeutic implications. JAMA 1989;261:744.
9. Siegelman SS, Khouri NF, Leo FP, Fishman EK, Braverman RM, Zerhouni EA. Solitary pulmonary nodules: CT assessment. Radiology 1986;160:307.
10. Simon R. The importance of prognostic factors in clinical trials. Cancer Treat Rev 1984;68:185.
11. Steckel RJ, Kagan AR. Pitfalls in the diagnosis of metastatic disease or local tumor extension with modern imaging techniques. Invest Radiol 1990;25:818.
12. Zerhouni GA, Stitik FP, Siegelman SS, Naidich DP, Sagel SS, Proto AV, Muhm JR, Walsh JW, Martinez CR, Heelan RT. CT of the pulmonary nodule: a cooperative study. Radiology 1986;160:319.

CHAPTER 33

Imaging Cancer of Unknown Primary Site

A. ROBERT KAGAN AND RICHARD J. STECKEL

Oncologists may perceive that the more they know about an individual patient, the better they can treat the patient. Unfortunately, when this perception leads to the uncritical use of imaging examinations in a patient with disseminated cancer and an unknown primary, errant clinical judgments may sometimes be made.

Unknown primary tumors are far from rare. In a large radiation oncology referral practice, we see about one new patient per week with metastatic disease and an unknown primary. One study described 255 patients with unknown primary tumors; autopsy results were available in 34 (9). The primary site could be identified at autopsy in only 14 of the 34 patients; it was in the lung (*not* small cell lung cancer) in 7 cases, in the pancreas in 2 cases, in the kidney, bladder, biliary ducts, and mediastinum, in 1 case each, and there was 1 case of visceral Kaposi's sarcoma. In none of the 14 tumors that were identified at autopsy would prior knowledge of the primary site have affected the patient's course. In patients presenting with metastatic disease and unknown primaries, the most common primary tumors identified later in the patient's course or at autopsy are in the lung or pancreas; these are incurable when they have spread beyond the primary site, and in most cases there is still no effective palliation available. On the other hand, palliation is attainable with some disseminated carcinomas of the breast, prostate, endometrium, thyroid, and ovary, and identification of a primary could be helpful. Curative treatments might also be undertaken for certain disseminated cancers, including lymphomas (8), testicular germ cell tumors, and gestational choriocarcinomas. However, treatable conditions still represent only a small fraction (<10%) of disseminated cancers presenting with unknown primaries.

Patients with unknown primaries that are metastatic to cervical lymph nodes are often referred to an otolaryngologist, but those with isolated axillary or inguinal lymph node metastases may be referred directly to a medical oncologist (3, 6, 15). The differential diagnosis when a patient presents initially with lymph node metastases includes lymphoma, germ cell tumor, thyroid or an upper airway tumor (with cervical node metastases), carcinoma from another site, or melanoma. A final diagnosis can often be made by biopsy using histochemical, immunohistologic, or electron microscopic techniques (see Chapter 156), not by performing extensive imaging studies or laboratory tests. Isolated lymph node metastases that first present in the supraclavicular fossa usually originate from primary tumors below the clavicle (1, 13). However, many patients who present with masses that are confined to the supraclavicular area and a biopsy diagnosis of undifferentiated carcinoma are still being referred for computed tomography (CT) and/or magnetic resonance imaging (MRI) of the head and neck. Many are also subjected to triple endoscopy with blind biopsies of the nasopharynx, tonsil, base of tongue, piriform sinus, or esophagus in a fruitless search for an upper aerodigestive tract lesion.

In a review of 57 consecutive patients with an initial diagnosis of metastatic carcinoma, primary undetermined, the histologic findings ultimately revealed that most responders to treatment had non-Hodgkin's lymphomas (5). A diagnosis of lymphoma may be missed if the tissue is poorly fixed, sparse, or weakly stained. Granulomatous infections can yield biopsy material that consists of large numbers of plasma cells or small lymphocytes, which can simulate myeloma or lymphoma, respectively. "Infectious" plasma cells are polyclonal, whereas myelomatous cells are monoclonal.

It has been suggested that patients presenting with *non*-lymphomatous anterior mediastinal masses on chest radiographs but with undifferentiated histology be managed as if they had a germ cell neoplasm, whether or not they have elevated serum levels of human chorionic gonadotropin and/or α-fetoprotein (7). A similar approach has been recommended for patients who present initially with infradiaphragmatic adenopathy and no identifiable primary. However, Abeloff was not able to corroborate these recommendations (2).

With the exception of breast cancer, malignant ascites or malignant pleural effusions often arise from primary tumors that are within the cavity containing the fluid (16). However, effective palliative measures are only available for cancer of the ovary, small cell carcinoma of the lung, or lymphoma. These primary tumor types can usually be diagnosed by cytology or by a serosal biopsy and concurrent clinical findings, not through the extensive use of imaging. There may be clinical pitfalls when serum tumor markers are slightly elevated but are still in the low range. Ascites in a woman with a moderate CA 125 elevation may suggest ovarian carcinoma, but when the liver is small the clinician should suspect cirrhosis instead. A man with widespread bony metastases, a lung lesion, a hard prostate, and a moderately elevated prostate-specific antigen level (PSA) is more likely to have disseminated lung cancer than disseminated adenocarcinoma of the prostate. Increases in serum α-fetoprotein levels are more likely to occur with metastases to the liver in pa-

Table 33.1. Diagnostic Imaging Recommendations for Patients with Metastatic Carcinoma and an Occult Primary

Presenting site of metastatic disease	Imaging studies to consider initially (chest radiography is always indicated)
Abdominal mass/hepatomegaly	Abdominal CT or MRI Consider barium enema/Upper GI series
Biliary tract (painless jaundice)	Percutaneous and/or endoscopic cholangiopancreatography Abdominal CT or MRI
Malignant ascites	Abdominal CT or MRI Consider barium enema/upper GI series
Malignant pleural effusion	Mammography for women Consider chest CT
Upper cervical lymph nodes	MRI or CT of upper airways if endoscopy is negative Consider thyroid scan
Lower cervical lymph nodes	CT of chest/abdomen Consider mammography in women
Axillary lymph nodes (undifferentiated cancer)	Mammography in women Consider chest CT
Brain (diagnosed on CT or MRI)	Chest/abdominal CT (if chest radiographs are nondiagnostic)
Spinal epidural space (on myelogram, contrast CT, or MRI)	Chest CT (if radiographs are nondiagnostic)
Bone	Radionuclide bone scan survey, with correlative radiographs of selected areas CT of chest/abdomen (if chest radiographs are nondiagnostic) Consider ultrasound of prostate (men) or mammography (women)
Lungs (multiple nodules)	CT or MRI of abdomen/pelvis Consider barium enema/upper GI

Adapted with permission from Kagan and Steckel (10).

tients who have non-germ cell primaries than in patients with gonadal tumors.

The imaging examinations that can be justified in initial attempts to establish a site of origin for an unknown primary tumor are relatively few (Table 33.1). In one clinical series, 65 consecutive patients with a diagnosis of unknown primary were subjected to extensive imaging studies (10, 18). In only 18 of the 65 patients was a diagnostic imaging procedure later identified as having been helpful: chest roentgenography in 9, barium enema examination in 4, transhepatic cholangiography in 3, and renal arteriography and xeromammography in 1 patient each. In other series, chest imaging was identified as the most fruitful diagnostic study (17), but contributory results occasionally came from imaging other anatomic sites as well (4).

Some clinicians may use the shotgun approach and perform multiple imaging examinations on patients with unknown primaries, in part to deflect peer criticism by covering all clinical possibilities and avoiding diagnostic pitfalls. However, clinicians are not the only ones who use this approach. After careful microscopic analysis of a solitary brain metastasis in a patient with an unknown primary and a normal chest roentgenogram, a pathologist may suggest the ovary, thyroid, breast, or gastrointestinal tract as possible primary sources for the patient's tumor. This diffuse opinion may lead, in turn, to a further exhaustive search for the primary tumor—a search that is often fruitless (11). Diagnostic radiologists may also contribute to the shotgun approach by suggesting that gastrointestinal imaging studies be repeated following optimal bowel preparation, that questionable CT findings be confirmed with MRI or vice versa, or that angiography or endoscopy be performed to confirm possible abnormalities that were suggested on other diagnostic studies.

In conclusion, extended diagnostic workups that are performed for metastatic disease with a persistently unknown primary site frequently do not identify the primary tumor (12, 14). Furthermore, even if the primary tumor is eventually found, exhaustive studies, including multiple imaging examinations, often do not provide information that contributes to the length or quality of the patient's life. Therefore, except in carefully defined clinical circumstances the use of multiple imaging examinations to evaluate patients who have a disseminated cancer, with the purpose of uncovering a stubbornly occult primary tumor, may yield little information of direct benefit to the afflicted patient.

References

1. Abbruzzese JL, Abbruzzese MC, Hess KR, Raber MN, Lenzi R, Frost P. Unknown primary carcinoma: natural history and prognostic factors in 657 consecutive patients. J Clin Oncol 1994;12:1272–1280.
2. Abeloff MD. Adenocarcinoma of Unknown Primary. John Hopkins Medical Grand Rounds, vol XII, Program 2, Presentation 4, 1985.
3. Anderson PJ, Kagan AR, Smith DE, Peddada AV, Rao AR. Squamous cell carcinoma of undetermined primary in the head and neck region: indications for Radiotherapy. Laryngoscope (in press).
4. Daugaard G. Unknown primary tumours. Cancer Treat Rev 1994;20:119–147.
5. de Campos ES, Menasce LP, Radford J, Harris M, Thatcher N. Metastatic carcinoma of uncertain primary site: a retrospective review of 57 patients treated with vincristine, doxorubicin, cyclophosphamide (VAC) or VAC alternating with cisplatin and etoposide (VAC/PE). Cancer 1994;73:470–475.
6. Guarischi A, Keane TJ, Elhakim T. Metastatic inguinal nodes from an unknown primary neoplasm. Cancer 1987;59:572–577.
7. Hainsworth JD, Greco FA. Treatment of patients with cancer of an unknown primary site. N Engl J Med 1993;329:257–263.
8. Horning SJ, Carrier EK, Rouse RV, Warnke RA, Michie SA Lymphomas presenting as histologically unclassified neoplasms: characteristics and response to treatment. J Clin Oncol 1989;7:1281–1287.
9. Kagan AR, Steckel RJ. Diagnosis of metastatic cancer with an unknown primary site. In Cancer Diagnosis: New Concepts and Techniques. Edited by RJ Steckel, AR Kagan. New York: Grune and Stratton, 1982, pp 289–296.
10. Kagan AR, Steckel RJ. Diagnostic imaging in clinical cancer management of metastases from unknown primary tumors. Invest Radiol 1988;23:545–547.

11. LeChevalier T, Smith FP, Caille P, Costans JP, Rouesse JG. Sites of primary malignancies in patients presenting with cerebral metastases. Cancer 1985;56:880–882.
12. Lee NK, Byers RM, Abbruzzese JL, Wolf P. Metastatic adenocarcinoma to the neck from an unknown primary source. Am J Surg 1991;162:306–309.
13. Lefebvre J-L, Coche-Dequ`eant B, Van JT, Buisset E, Adenis A. Cervical lymph nodes from an unknown primary tumor in 190 patients. Am J Surg 1990;160:443–446.
14. Nystrom JS, VanEgmond EM, Leonard RJ. Appropriate therapy for metastatic cancer of unknown primary origin. Adv Oncol 1989;5:27–30.
15. Patel J, Nemoto T, Rosner D, Dao TL, Pickren JW. Axillary lymph node metastasis from an occult breast cancer. Cancer 1981;47:2923–2927.
16. Ringenberg QS, Doll DC, Loy TS, Yarbro JW. Malignant ascites of unknown origin. Cancer 1989;64:753–755.
17. Rougraff BT, Kneisl JS, Simon MA. Skeletal metastases of unknown origin. J Bone Joint Surg 1993;75A:1276–1281.
18. Steckel RJ, Kagan AR. Metastatic tumors of unknown origin. Cancer 1991;67:1242–1244.

CHAPTER 34

Imaging Neoplasms of the Head and Neck and Central Nervous System

ROBERT LUFKIN

Magnetic resonance imaging (MRI) has come to dominate diagnostic imaging of extracranial head and neck structures and the central nervous system (CNS) in the few years since its introduction. Whereas it has reduced the need for computed tomography (CT), myelography, and diagnostic angiography, there are still situations where MRI does not provide sufficient diagnostic information and a more invasive study is indicated. To appreciate their relative roles in imaging cancer of the head and neck and CNS, it is particularly important to consider the strengths and weaknesses of MRI as it compares with CT.

MRI

ADVANTAGES

No Ionizing Radiation

The fact that the MR images are produced using only magnetism and radio waves is an advantage over other studies that require ionizing radiation. This is particularly important for individuals who require many serial examinations, for pediatric patients, and for pregnant women.

Sensitivity to Flow

The exquisite sensitivity of MRI to flow is based on the fact that any change in location of protons due to arterial, venous, or cerebrospinal fluid pulsations during MR imaging results in a change in signal. This obviates intravenous contrast materials (as with x-ray CT) to demonstrate vascular structures. In fact, most experts agree that, in most clinical situations, MR without contrast is superior to x-ray CT with contrast for the definition of vascular anatomy. Intravenous contrast material may also be valuable with MRI in the CNS to show blood-brain barrier disruption, but it is not necessary for the simple demonstration of flowing blood. The inherent sensitivity of MRI to flow is now exploited to perform projection images of flowing blood in patients using a new technique referred to as "MR angiography."

Multiplanar Capabilities

With x-ray CT the scan plane is defined by the x-ray tube-detector axis through the gantry. In most patients this means that scanning is limited to the axial—and, in some cases, the coronal—plane. With MRI the scan plane is defined instead by the selection of radio frequencies (RF) and magnetic field gradients, which can be varied and are under electronic, rather than physical, control.

Iron Sensitivity

Because of the paramagnetic and ferromagnetic properties of many forms of iron (with their unpaired electrons) these substances have special effects on MR images. Many types of iron result in subtle alterations in the local magnetic field environment of tissue protons; this, in turn, causes relaxation enhancement or shortening of T1 or T2 relaxation times. The type and amount of shortening reflect the form and quantity of the iron compounds. As a result of the high sensitivity of MR to iron it has been said that iron is to MR as calcium is to CT.

The accumulation of "nonheme" iron in the form of ferritin that occurs with normal aging has been demonstrated in the brain by MR (2). Ferritin iron results in a loss of MR signal owing to preferential T2 shortening. It is found most commonly in the globus pallidus, red nucleus, and substantia nigra.

Heme iron has a characteristic appearance on MR because of the changes it undergoes as hemoglobin passes through several breakdown stages. While the iron in normal oxyhemoglobin does not result in any significant relaxation enhancement, the reversible transformation to deoxyhemoglobin results in preferential T2 shortening on MR images. After 72 to 90 hours the deoxyhemoglobin in extravasated blood is irreversibly converted to methemoglobin which has a characteristic high signal intensity on T1-weighted images because of its T1-shortening effect. Gradually, this breakdown product is converted to hemosiderin, which will show up as a low intensity MR signal because of T2 shortening. While CT is sensitive to acute hemorrhage because of the protein content of blood within brain tissue, MR is far more sensitive to the later phases of a hematoma (more than 72 hours) when much of the protein has broken down.

High Soft-Tissue Contrast Resolution

The great sensitivity of MRI to variations in tissue proton density and in T1 and T2 relaxation times is extremely valuable for imaging CNS lesions. All forms of cerebral edema are generally shown better with MRI than with CT. The lack of beam-hardening artifact from bone, a common problem with CT, results in superior MRI of the vertex, posterior fossa, floor of the middle fossa, skull base, and spinal contents.

DISADVANTAGES

Low Calcium Sensitivity

MRI is inferior to CT for detecting calcification in masses and/or in association with hyperostosis. In some cases this lower sensitivity to calcium is more than offset by the superior soft tissue resolution of MRI. Newer types of pulse sequences, that have greater T2 sensitivity may improve the ability of MRI to detect calcium.

Acute Hemorrhage

While MRI is clearly superior to CT for the evaluation of subacute (more than 72 hours) and chronic hemorrhage (see above), the high sensitivity of CT to blood protein in acute CNS hemorrhage has made it the study of choice for recent bleeding. Other pulse sequences with high T2 sensitivity are under investigation for the evaluation of acute hemorrhage with MRI.

CONTRAINDICATIONS

Despite the noninvasive nature of MRI, exposures to magnetic fields and radiofrequencies (RF) may be contraindicated in certain patients. These patients are best studied with other techniques, such as CT. The operation of cardiac and other forms of pacemakers may be adversely affected by MRI, so patients with these devices are generally excluded from examination. Some types of ferromagnetic clips for intracranial aneurysms may develop torque from changing magnetic fields and may actually twist off vessels, so these patients are also excluded from MRI. New nonferromagnetic clips which are unaffected by magnetic fields are now available for aneurysm clipping (2). MRI study of patients with skull plates, wires, surgical clips that have been in place for a long time, or even large metallic implants may produce some image artifacts but is safe to perform. These appliances are well-fixed in the tissues and are resistant to magnetic field torques; thus, these do not represent contraindications to MRI.

Slow Image Acquisition

Conventional MRI is generally slower than a comparable CT study. This means that patients who are too ill to be placed within the MR magnet for scan times in excess of 10 minutes are best studied with techniques other than MRI. The problem of slow data acquisition with MR may be overcome in the near future, as newer pulse sequence strategies are developed. These may allow scan times comparable to or shorter than those for CT, and several investigators are even considering MR fluoroscopy.

Cost

MRI studies generally are more expensive than CT. This is a relative disadvantage for MRI in situations where CT and MRI can provide similar information. With the introduction of lower-cost MR scanners, it is anticipated that the cost per MR examination will decrease in the near future. As a result, the cancer-imaging applications of MR will continue to increase.

Specific Applications

EXTRACRANIAL HEAD AND NECK CANCER

MRI has replaced CT as the study of choice for many extracranial lesions of the head and neck. The notable exceptions where CT is still essential are lesions in which subtle bone destruction or new bone formation (e.g., osteomas of the sinuses) must be recognized. MRI easily surpasses CT in its ability to differentiate subtle differences in soft-tissue boundaries and local extensions of tumors of the head and neck. The use of intravenous gadolinium chelates in MRI of the head and neck is valuable for certain clinical indications (24). Studies indicate that, while tumor enhancement occurs with contrast infusions, little clinically relevant information is added in many cases. When intracranial tumor extension is present, however, the gadolinium contrast can improve the detection of blood-brain barrier and leptomeningeal abnormalities (e.g., cerebral edema and tumor involvement).

SALIVARY GLANDS

MRI has replaced CT for the imaging evaluation of most masses in the major salivary glands (3, 19, 21, 23, 28, 29). Since MRI can rarely suggest the histology of tumors, its value in most cases (like that of CT) is to define the tumor outline. While poor tumor margination may be a clue to malignancy, it is certainly not a pathognomonic finding in MRI or in CT studies. Deep parapharyngeal space involvement may be demonstrated with CT; however, MRI provides much better soft tissue contrast. The real advantage of MRI in evaluating masses in the parotid area is its ability to define more accurately the extent of a mass, to localize a tumor as extraparotid or intraparotid, and to determine whether an intraparotid tumor is in the superficial or deep lobes of the gland.

PARANASAL SINUSES

While CT remains the study of choice for inflammatory sinus disease, MRI is extremely valuable for evaluating masses of the paranasal sinuses. It allows excellent delineation of soft tissue masses that are surrounded by secretions in the sinuses. Erosions of the bony walls can also be demonstrated on MR by the absence of the signal void that is normally present with cortical bone. For tumor extensions outside the bony sinuses, MRI is clearly the study of choice because it can differentiate normal skeletal muscle from deep tumor extension, which can sometimes be difficult on CT studies. In cases where there is a question of extension into the anterior or middle cranial fossa, MRI with gadolinium enhancement is now the study of choice.

NASOPHARYNX

The relative lack of motion and the abundant fascial planes of the nasopharynx result in high-quality MRI (10, 30). Retropharyngeal adenopathy, tumor infiltration beyond the pharyngobasilar fascia, and hypertrophic lymphoid tissue are all identified more easily with MRI than CT (31). In particular, direct coronal and sagittal MR scans can be valuable to assess the craniocaudal extent of a tumor and possible intracranial involvement. While CT scanning is unquestionably more accurate in detecting small amounts of calcification or losses of bone, MR examinations are quite adequate to evaluate skull base invasion. Abnormalities of the skull base are detected on MRI by replacement of the normal low-signal cortical bone with the higher-intensity signal of a neoplasm. The capability for multiplanar imaging and the far superior soft tissue resolution of MRI thus make it the imaging study of choice to evaluate the nasopharynx.

TONGUE AND OROPHARYNX

In general, MRI produces soft tissue detail superior to CTs for evaluating the tongue and oropharynx (Fig. 34.1). Therefore, MRI is also considered the study of choice for cancer in

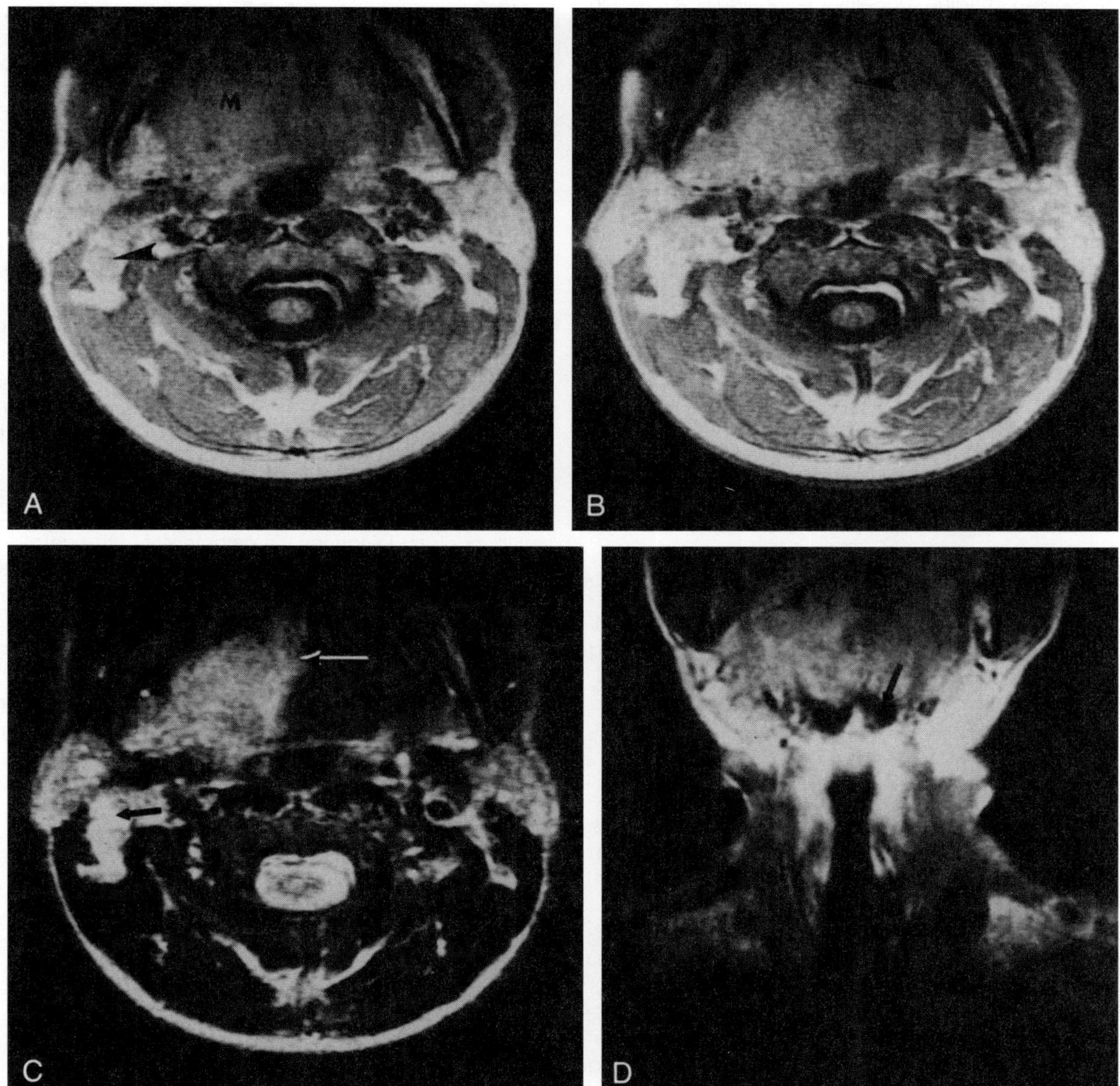

Figure 34.1. Squamous carcinoma of the tongue base imaged with MR, and without gadolinium contrast. **A.** Axial T1-weighted image (Se/800/30) through the tongue base reveals mass effect (M) on the right and associated adenopathy (*arrowhead*). The spinal cord is well-demonstrated with this pulse sequence (note central gray matter and low-signal CSF surrounding the cord). Bone cortices in the mandible and vertebral bodies appear as areas of low signal (*black*). CT scanning is generally more sensitive than MRI for detecting small calcifications or subtle bone erosions. **B.** MR image at level similar to (**A**), with same pulse sequence, after administration of gadolinium DTPA. Mild enhancement of the tongue mass is noted (*arrowhead*), with slight decrease in visibility of the abnormal lymph node. **C.** T2-weighted image (SE/2000/85) without gadolinium reveals high signal in the tongue mass (*white arrowhead*) and increased signal in the area of adenopathy (*arrow*), somewhat similar to appearance with gadolinium on T1-weighted images (**B**). **D.** Coronal T1-weighted image is useful for defining the extent of the mass (*arrowhead*) and showing that there is no extension to the supraglottic larynx. The vallecula is free of tumor (*arrow*).

this area. Lack of artifacts from dental amalgam and beam-hardening artifacts from the mandible on MRI also eliminates two major shortcomings of CT in examining the area. Finally, the ability of MRI to obtain direct coronal and sagittal scan planes is a distinct advantage in evaluating the intrinsic tongue musculature and assessing tumor volume for treatment planning (18, 32).

LARYNX AND HYPOPHARYNX

Rarely does an imaging modality play a significant role in making the primary diagnosis of malignancy in the larynx or hypopharynx. These regions are so accessible to clinical examination that the combination of visual inspection and cytology/biopsy usually suffices to confirm a diagnosis of cancer. Therefore, the role of MRI is the same as that of CT for cancer in this area: to define the extent of disease. While laryngoscopy can show normal mucosal surfaces and masses involving the airway, deep tumor extensions are difficult to detect from clinical examination alone. In several areas these extensions may have profound implications for the management and control of disease. CT, and now MR to an even greater degree, can define this critically important deep anatomy (2, 7, 8, 13–15, 20, 26, 27).

As compared with CT, MRI provides superior soft-tissue definition. Direct coronal and sagittal scanning planes allow the visualization of intrinsic laryngeal musculature and better define cranial-caudal tumor extensions. Thus, MRI is now the imaging study of choice to evaluate tumor stage within the larynx and hypopharynx.

THYROID

Ultrasound and nuclear medicine techniques are generally more cost effective than MRI for imaging malignancies of the thyroid. However, the latter is valuable for demonstrating extensions of thyroid tumors into the mediastinum where ultrasound is a less effective modality.

CENTRAL NERVOUS SYSTEM CANCER

It is difficult to generalize about the role of MRI in brain tumor imaging, because there is such variability in the results for different tumors and for different locations (22, 33). In general, MRI is effective for detecting intracranial tumors, because it is so sensitive to the cerebral edema which accompanies most tumors. Therefore, MRI is particularly advantageous for detecting small lesions such as metastases, which are found in greater numbers by MRI than by CT (12).

Bleeding into a CNS tumor may also be appreciated better by MRI than by CT, both because the abnormal signal from blood persists longer on MRI and because there is no problem in distinguishing hemorrhage from calcification. Cysts associated with tumors are visible with MRI, as they are with CT, but considerable information may be available from MRI regarding the contents of the cysts, since the signal intensity of fluid varies greatly with protein content.

MRI also has disadvantages for detecting and defining CNS tumors. Tumors may frequently be obscured by the high signal from surrounding brain edema. The use of a variety of MRI sequences may allow the tumor to be seen in such cases. MRI also benefits from the use of intravenous paramagnetic contrast media that pass into CNS regions lacking an effective blood-brain barrier, thus highlighting some tumors. Gadolinium-enhanced MRI therefore results in clear MRI demonstration of most neoplasms (6, 9).

Initially, it was hoped that it might be possible to perform tissue characterization in brain tumors by determining T1 and T2 values; however, there appears to be such wide overlap in these values that neither tumor type nor the degree of malignancy can be predicted (10). The inability of MRI to demonstrate calcification is also a disadvantage in characterizing some intracranial brain tumors. MRI probably gives a better representation than CT of the extent of a primary brain tumor. It is known that primary CNS tumors often extend beyond the apparent outlines of a mass, as demonstrated by either CT or MRI, and it may be safer to consider that a brain tumor has spread throughout the surrounding zone of visible edema, which is better delineated by MRI (25).

While it appears, at present, that both MRI and CT are quite effective in demonstrating brain tumors, MRI has the advantage of greater sensitivity for detecting edema as well as the potential for demonstrating lesions in several different planes or projections. With the use of intravenous gadolinium chelates, MRI is better able to show meningiomas and can help to characterize brain neoplasms better. While tumor boundaries may be obscured with either CT or MRI by extensive brain edema, contrast enhancement may be valuable for delineating blood-brain barrier abnormalities and subarachnoid tumor spread (11). Standard arteriography with contrast injections via catheters into the carotid or vertebrobasilar system is required relatively rarely to characterize CNS neoplasms in the era of CT and MRI. Its remaining applications for studying space-occupying lesions lie principally in the realm of arteriovenous malformations and aneurysms.

A solitary brain metastasis may be difficult to differentiate from a glioma; however, multiplicity of lesions strongly suggests metastatic disease. MRI is particularly valuable for evaluating the common complication of bleeding into brain metastases that may be seen with melanoma, choriocarcinoma, and oat-cell carcinoma of the lung.

CT scanning can better define tumor calcifications and the associated hyperostosis of a meningioma; however, both CT and MRI can easily demonstrate meningeal lesions with intravenous contrast enhancement. MRI consistently demonstrates small acoustic angle tumors with greater detail than CT. This eliminates the need for injecting intrathecal air or other contrast materials. Acoustic neuromas show striking intravenous contrast enhancement with both CT and MRI, however.

CT- and MRI-Guided Aspiration Cytology

The use of guided aspiration cytology for deep or impalpable lesions has contributed to the evaluation of many patients with extracranial head and neck and CNS tumors (16, 17). With this technique, aspiration of cells through fine nee-

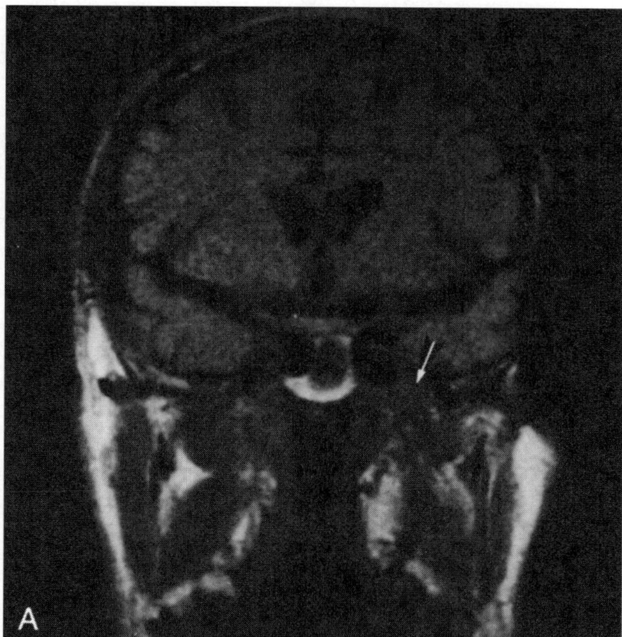

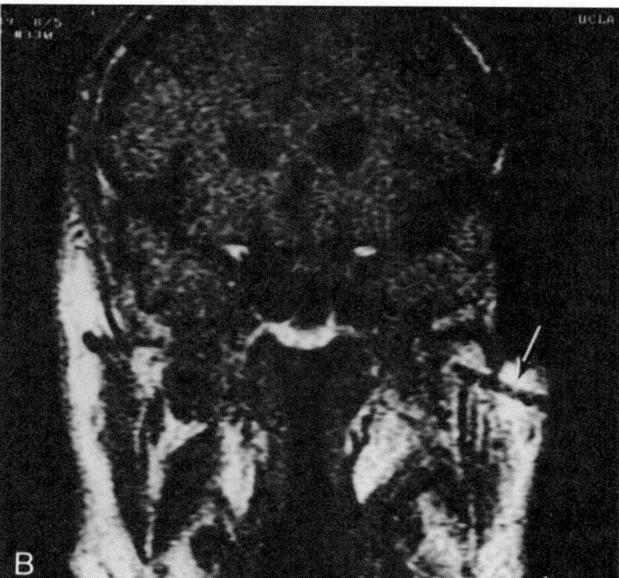

Figure 34.2. Diagnosis made by MRI-guided aspiration cytology, of recurrent squamous carcinoma in the parapharyngeal space extending to the skull base. **A.** Coronal image (SE/700/30) shows mass high in the infratemporal fossa (*arrow*). **B.** Gradient echo image after needle placement. Although image quality is less with newer rapid scanning techniques, the needle is well visualized (*arrow*) and scan time is reduced to 48 seconds (SE/480/30/60° flip angle).

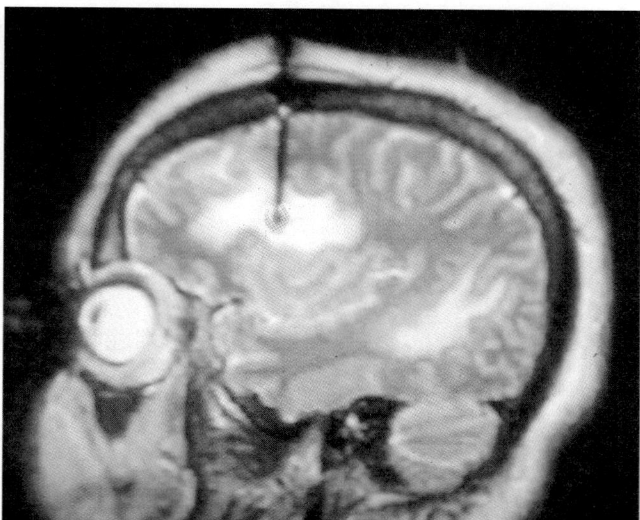

Figure 34.3. Sagittal MRI demonstrating MRI-guided thermal ablation of a metastatic tumor. The treatment electrode is shown as a low-signal line, and tissue coagulation necrosis following heat application is visible at the tip.

dles allows a diagnosis by cytology rather than by histology, which requires a larger specimen and a formal biopsy. While the aspiration technique has long been used with ultrasound and CT guidance, there are a number of areas such as the skull base where beam-hardening artifacts limit the effectiveness of CT to guide this procedure.

At our institution, MRI has been the modality of choice for guiding aspiration cytology procedures in the head and neck over the last 3 years (Fig. 34.2). In addition to the lack of beam-hardening artifacts and the availability of high soft tissue contrast and flow sensitivity, the ability to do multiplanar imaging with MRI is particularly advantageous in complex cases. Recent studies have even suggested the possibility of MR-guided ablation of brain tumors in a new application of "interventional MRI" (Fig. 34.3) (34).

References

1. Brothers M, Fox AJ, Lee DH, et al. MR imaging after surgery for vertebrobasilar aneurysm. Am J Neuroradiol 1990;11:49.
2. Castelijns JA, Gerritsen GJ, Kaiser, MC, Valk J, Jansen W, Meyer CJ, Snow, GB. MRI of normal or cancerous laryngeal cartilages: histopathologic correlation. Laryngoscope 1987;97:1085.
3. Casselman JW, Mancuso, AA. Major salivary gland masses: comparison of MR imaging and CT. Radiology 1987;165:183.
4. Dillon WP, Mills CM, Kjos B, Degroot J, Brant-Zawadzki M. Magnetic resonance imaging of the nasopharynx. Radiology 1984;152:731.
5. Drayer B, Burger P, Darwin R, Riederer, S, Herfkens R, Johnson GA. MRI of brain iron. AJR 1986;147:103.
6. Felix R, Schnorner W, Laniado M, Niendorf HP, Claussen C, Flieger W, Speck U. Brain tumors. MR imaging with gadolinium-DTPA. Radiology 1985;156:681.
7. Glazer HS, Niemeyer JH, Balfe D, Devieni VR, Emami B, Hayden RE, Aronberg DJ, Levitt RG, Ward MP, Sagel SS, Lee JK. Neck neoplasms: MR imaging. Part I. Initial evaluation. Radiology 1986;160:343.
8. Glazer HS, Niemeyer JH, Balfe D, Hayden RE, Emami B, Devineni VR, Levitt R G, Aronberg DJ, Ward MP, Lee JK, Sagel SS. Neck neoplasms: MR imaging. Part II. Post treatment evaluation. Radiology 1986;160:349.
9. Graif M, Bydder G, Steiner R, Niendord P, Thomas DG, Young IR: Contrast-enhanced MR imaging of malignant brain tumors. Am J Neuroradiol 1985;6:855.
10. Komiyama M, Yaguro H, Baba M, Yasui T, Hakuba A, Nishimura S, Inoue Y. MR imaging: possibility of tissue characterization of brain tumors using T1 and T2 values. Am J Neuroradiol 1987;8:65.
11. Krol G, Sze G, Malkin M, Walker R. MR of cranial and spinal meningeal carcinomatosis; comparison with CT and myelography. AJR 1988;151:583.
12. Lee B, Kneeland J, Cahill P, Deck M. MR recognition of supratentorial tumors. Am J Neuroradiol 1985;6:871.
13. Lufkin RB, Hanafee WN. Application of surface coils to MR anatomy of the larynx. AJR 1985;145:483.
14. Lufkin R, Hanafee W, Wortham D, Hoover L. MRI of the larynx and hypopharynx using surface coils. Radiology 1986;158:747.
15. Lufkin R, Larsson S, Hanafee W. NMR anatomy of the larynx and tongue. Radiology 1983;148:173.
16. Lufkin R, Teresi L, Chiu L, Hanafee W. A technique for MR guided needle placement in the head and neck. AJR 1988;151:193.

17. Lufkin R, Teresi L, Hanafee W. New needle for MRI guided aspiration cytology. AJR 1987;149:380.
18. Lufkin RB, Wortham DG, Dietrich RB, Hoover LA, Larsson SG, Kangarloo H, Hanafee WN. Tongue and oropharynx: findings on MR imaging. Radiology 1986;161:69.
19. Mandelblatt SM, Braun IF, Davis PC, Fry SM, Jacobs LH, Hoffman JC Jr. Parotid masses: MR Imaging. Radiology 1987;163:411.
20. McArdle CB, Bailey BJ, Amparo EG. Surface coil magnetic resonance imaging of the normal larynx. Arch Otolaryngol Head Neck Surg 1986;112:616.
21. Mirich DR, McArdle CB, Kulkarni MV. Benign pleomorphic adenomas of the salivary glands: surface coil MR imaging versus CT. J Comput Assist Tomogr 1987;11:620.
22. Muller-Forell W, Schroth G, Egan PJ. MR imaging in tumors of the pineal region. Neuroradiology 1988;30:224.
23. Rice DH, Becker T. Magnetic resonance imaging of the salivary glands. Arch Otolaryngol Head Neck Surg 1987;113:78.
24. Robinson JD, Crawford S, Teresi L, Schiller VL, Lufkin RB, Harnsberger, HR, Dietrich RB, Crim JR, Duckwiler GR, Spickler E, Hanafee W. Extracranial lesions of the head and neck: preliminary experience with Gd-DTPA–enhanced MR imaging. Radiology 1989;172:165–170.
25. Shuman W, Griffin B, Haynor D, Jones DC, Johnson DS, Cromwell LD, Laramore GE. The utility of MR in planning the radiation therapy of oligodendroglioma. Am J Neuroradiol 1988;151:583.
26. Stark DD, Moss AA, Gamsu G, Glark OH, Gooding GW, Webb WR. Magnetic resonance imaging of the neck. Part 1. Normal anatomy. Radiology 1984;150:447.
27. Stark DD, Moss AA, Gamsu G, Clark OH, Gooding GW, Webb WR. Magnetic resonance imaging of the neck. Part 2. Pathologic findings. Radiology 1984;150:455.
28. Teresi L, Lufkin R, Kolin E, Hanafee W. MRI of the intraparotid facial nerve. Am J Neuroradio 1987;8:253.
29. Teresi L, Lufkin R, Wortham D, Abemayor E, Hanafee W. Parotid masses: magnetic resonance imaging. Radiology 1987;163:405.
30. Teresi LM, Lufkin RB, Vinuela F, Dietrich RB, Wilson GH, Bentson JR, Hanafee WN. MR imaging of the nasopharynx and floor of the middle crania fossa. Part I. Normal anatomy. Radiology 1987;164:811.
31. Teresi LM, Lufkin RB, Vinuela F, Dietrich RB, Wilson GH, Bentson JR, Hanafee WN. MR imaging of the nasopharynx and floor of the middle crania fossa. Part II. Malignant tumors. Radiology 1987;164:817.
32. Unger JM. The oral cavity and tongue: magnetic resonance imaging. Radiology 1985;155:151.
33. Yuh WT, Barloon TJ, Jacoby CG, Schultz DH. MR of fourth-ventricular epidermoid tumors. Am J Neuroradiol 1988;9:794.
34. Anzai Y, Lufkin RB, DeSalles A, Hamilton DR, Farahani K, Black K. Initial Clinical Experience with MR-Guided Thermal Ablation of Brain Tumor. Am J Neuroradiol 1995;16:39–48.

CHAPTER 35

Imaging Neoplasms of the Thorax

POONAM V. BATRA

Lung Cancer

Conventional posteroanterior and lateral chest radiographs obtained with high-kilovoltage (kVp) technique represent the most valuable and cost effective imaging examination for lung cancer. Oblique or over penetrated views may be obtained in selected cases to evaluate equivocal findings on the chest radiographs, and fluoroscopy may be used to verify the presence or absence of a suspected lung lesion. In the case of a solitary pulmonary nodule, a comparison with previous chest radiographs should be performed. If there is no change in the dimensions of the nodule on serial chest radiographs for 2 or more years, then the nodule can certainly be considered benign (1). If no prior chest radiographs are available, then a radiograph obtained with low-kVp technique or fluoroscopy may show a benign pattern of calcification and obviate further study. An obvious exception may be a "scar cancer," in which a calcific focus may be present in an eccentric location and the nodule spiculated or irregular in appearance. Fluoroscopy may also be used to guide a percutaneous biopsy of a lesion in the lung, mediastinum, or pleura.

Computer tomography (CT), by virtue of its cross-sectional display of anatomy and its superior contrast resolution, has become the principal radiographic technique to supplement chest radiographic findings. The morphology of a lung lesion, including its size, margins, and presence or absence of calcification, can be demonstrated well by CT. In general, a lung lesion less than 3 cm in size, with clearly defined margins and a high attenuation value suggesting that it might contain calcium (Hounsfield numbers greater than 164) can be considered as benign (2). A lung lesion with an irregular spiculated border and a diameter greater than 3 cm may be regarded as particularly suspicious for cancer. CT can depict the segmental and subsegmental bronchial anatomy and can, therefore, help to determine the exact location of endobronchial cancers (3). Furthermore, it can assess the extraluminal component of an endobronchial cancer, which is not visible to the bronchoscopist. Because of its relatively low signal-to-noise ratio and respiratory motion problems, magnetic resonance imaging (MRI) is not generally as useful as CT for imaging lung cancer (4). Difficulty in recognizing calcification is also a limitation in evaluating primary lung lesions with MRI. However, coronal or sagittal MR images can be particularly useful for detecting the superior extent of tumors at the lung apex (Fig. 35.1) or assessing involvement of the subclavian artery or brachial plexus.

Recently, positron emission tomography (PET) using fluorine-18 fluorodeoxy glucose (FDG) has been shown to be helpful in differentiating benign from malignant solitary pulmonary nodules (5).

Accurate preoperative staging of non-small-cell lung cancer is essential when selecting patients with localized disease for curative surgery and those with widespread neoplasms for palliative therapy (6). CT is clearly superior to conventional radiography in demonstrating the extent of the primary lesion, invasion of the hilum or mediastinum, and the presence of enlarged lymph nodes (7). Most potential surgical candidates with non-small-cell lung cancer should have a preoperative chest CT scan, but the role of CT when a small peripheral lesion is the only radiographic abnormality is controversial. Some investigators believe that a patient with a peripheral nodule less than 3 cm in size and a normal hilum and mediastinum on plain chest radiographs (presumed T1, NO, MO) does not require a CT scan, because the likelihood of detecting mediastinal lymphadenopathy is low (8). Others maintain that CT scanning is indicated in those patients, because of the high prevalence (21%) of lymph node metastases (9). In patients with an enlarged hilum, it may be difficult on plain films to distinguish between hilar adenopathy and a prominent pulmonary artery. Both CT and MRI can be used to make this distinction; however, it may be somewhat easier with MRI, particularly in those patients who cannot receive intravenous contrast agents during CT. While both contrast enhanced CT and MRI are highly sensitive in detecting hilar adenopathy, specificity for tumor is low (66% for CT, and 50% for MRI) (10). CT is reported to have a sensitivity of 44 to 79% in diagnosis of mediastinal adenopathy. The specificity is low (62 to 65%), however, because some enlarged nodes may be tumor-free (11, 12). Patients with enlarged mediastinal nodes that are demonstrated by CT must have biopsy of the nodes. While it was originally hoped that MRI could differentiate benign from malignant nodes on the basis of their signal intensities on T1- and T2-weighted images, no significant difference in T1 or T2 values has been noted between inflammatory and malignant nodes (13). MRI and CT have proved to be comparable for detecting abnormal mediastinal lymph nodes, but MRI appears to be more accurate than CT in diagnosing mediastinal invasion (14). While some normal-sized nodes may harbor microscopic metastases, the predictive value of a negative CT scan is good. It has been stated that patients who have a completely normal mediastinum on a CT scan can proceed directly to thoracotomy without prior medi-

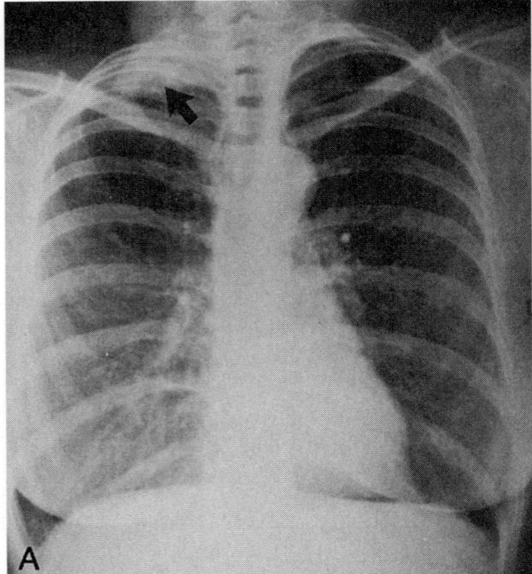

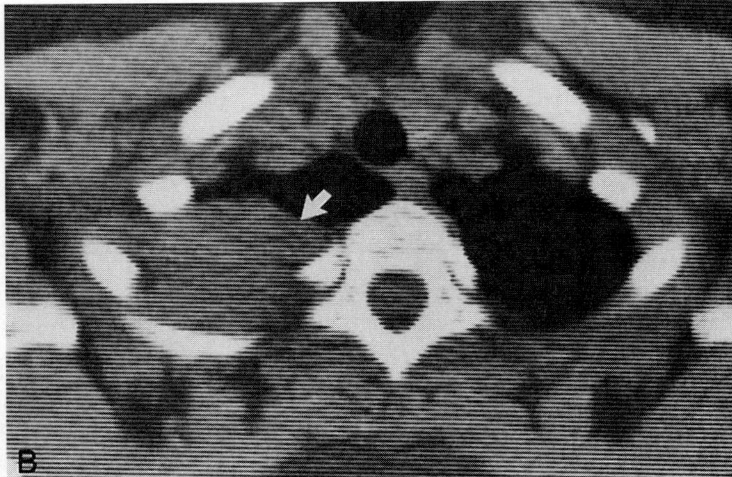

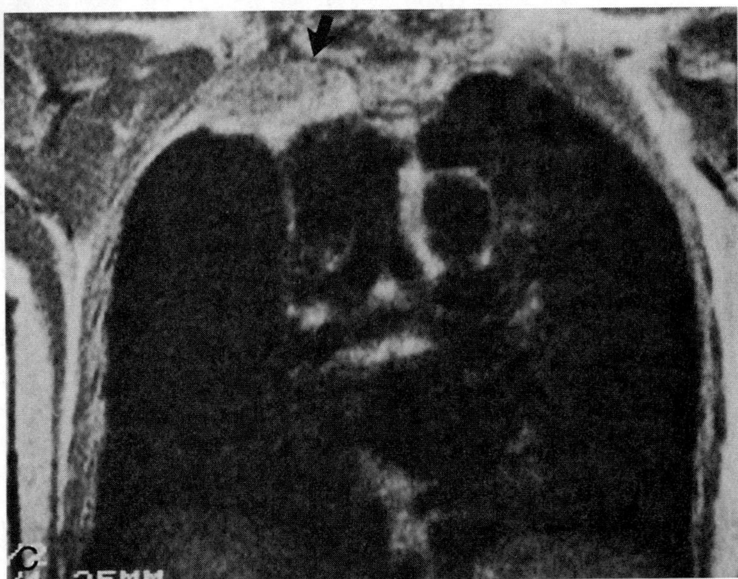

Figure 35.1. Superior sulcus lung cancer in a 46-year-old woman. **A.** Posteroanterior chest radiograph reveals a soft-tissue density at right lung apex (*arrow*); ribs are intact. **B.** CT scan shows lung mass at right apex (*arrow*). **C.** MRI coronal image (T1-weighted spin-echo image obtained with a TE of 28 msec, and TR gated to heart rate) clearly demonstrates cephalad extent of tumor (*arrow*).

astinoscopy (15). On the other hand, patients who have unequivocal mediastinal adenopathy on plain chest radiographs usually do not require CT for staging purposes. Nevertheless, CT may still be valuable in such cases for biopsy or for radiation therapy planning. Preliminary data indicate that PET with FDG imaging may be more accurate than CT in detecting mediastinal node metastases in patients with lung cancer (16).

Conventional radiographic examination and CT scanning can detect chest wall invasion when rib destruction is seen. However, in the absence of rib destruction or a definite mass within the chest wall, CT may be inaccurate in assessing chest wall invasion by a peripheral lung cancer (17). Recently, it has been shown that MRI can detect chest wall invasion in some patients with lung cancer when the CT findings are equivocal (18). MRI has also offered a slight advantage over CT in evaluating superior sulcus tumor invasion into the lower neck (19). Ultrasound examination has been reported to have a high sensitivity (100%) and specificity (98%) in demonstrating chest wall invasion in lung cancer (20).

Thoracic CT scanning should include the upper abdomen in patients with lung cancer, given the frequency of metastases to the adrenals, liver, and upper abdominal lymph nodes. Nevertheless, a small adrenal nodule in a patient with lung cancer is more likely to represent an adenoma than a metastasis, and needle biopsy is currently required to make an absolute diagnosis (21). In the future, MR may have a role in helping to distinguish adrenal metastases from benign adrenal lesions (22).

Mediastinal Masses

Close to half of the patients with mediastinal tumors are asymptomatic. Posteroanterior and lateral chest radiographs continue to be the most valuable imaging modality for detecting primary mediastinal tumors. Oblique views or fluoroscopy may assist in evaluating patients with equivocal chest radiographic abnormalities. In most institutions, CT has now replaced conventional tomography as the most useful technique for evaluating mediastinal abnormalities after they have been identified or suspected on plain chest radiographs, or when clinical findings suggest the possibility of disease in this region (23). As an example, CT examination is indicated in patients with myasthenia gravis to search for an occult thymoma, even when the chest radiographs are normal. CT can also serve as an important adjunct to plain chest radiographs in planning radiotherapy, and it can suggest the best approach for biopsy or resection of a mediastinal mass. The superior contrast of CT allows differentiation of mediastinal tumors from lymph nodes, opacified vessels and airways. When required, intravenous contrast material can help to distinguish between vascular and nonvascular abnormalities. CT delineates the morphology of a mass as well as its size, extent, and relationships to adjacent mediastinal structures (24) (Fig. 35.2). Calcifications, fat or fluid components within the mass can be demonstrated, but a reliable distinction between benign and malignant lesions is not always possible. Demonstration by CT of invasion into adjacent pleura, pericardium or lung, with encasement or narrowing of vessels and bronchi, may point to the malignant nature of a mass.

More recently, MRI has been shown to be equivalent to CT in detection of enlarged mediastinal lymph nodes and masses (25). While MRI is no more specific than CT in differentiating benign from malignant masses for purposes of primary diagnosis, there is evidence to suggest that it may be helpful in distinguishing postradiation fibrosis from residual or recurrent mediastinal or lung tumors (26). Invasion or encasement of cardiovascular structures by tumor may also be demonstrated better with MRI than CT, without the need for contrast injections. Furthermore, MRI can be used as the primary examination for imaging posterior mediastinal masses, including neurogenic tumors and paravertebral masses, as the sagittal and coronal planes facil-

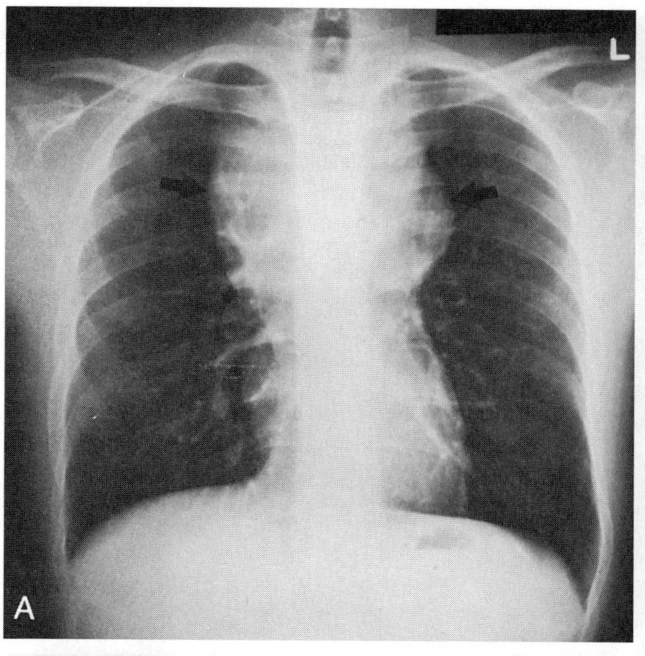

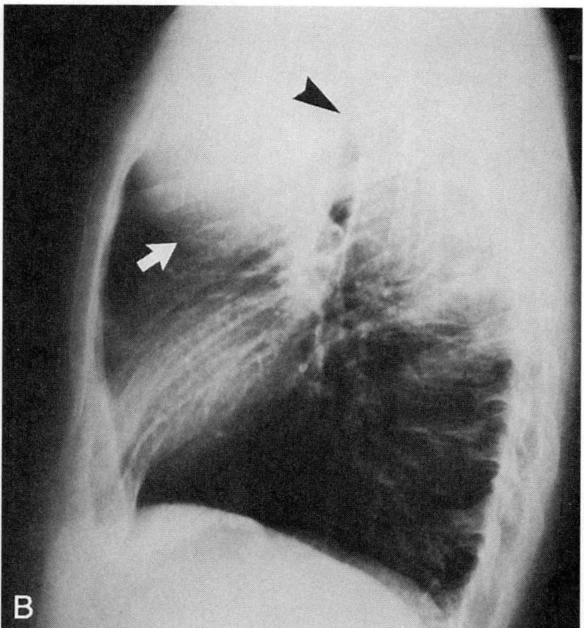

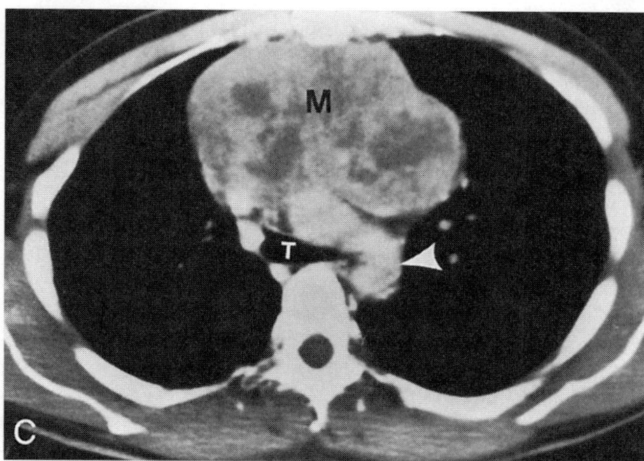

Figure 35.2. Nonseminoma germ cell tumor in a 25-year-old man. Posteroanterior (**A**) and lateral (**B**) chest radiographs reveal a large, well-defined mass in anterior mediastinum (*arrows*). Note marked narrowing of tracheal air column (*arrowhead*). CT scan (**C**) 1 cm above level of carina shows a large anterior mediastinal mass (M) containing low-density regions of fat or necrosis. Mass has displaced aortic arch (*arrowhead*) posteriorly, which in turn has compressed the anterolateral aspect of the trachea (T).

itate accurate assessment of tumor extension into the spinal canal (27).

Pleural Cancers

Extensive pleural involvement from a malignant mesothelioma can be demonstrated easily on plain chest radiographs. While the distinction between some pleural masses and loculated pleural effusions may be difficult with chest radiographs alone, it can be accomplished easily with a CT examination (Fig. 35.3). A malignant mesothelioma frequently appears to be more extensive on a CT scan than on plain chest radiographs. Invasion of pleural tumor into the mediastinum, diaphragm, retroperitoneum, or chest wall and involvement of mediastinal lymph nodes can also be suggested by CT (28). The CT appearance of malignant mesothelioma is not specific, however, and a similar radiographic appearance may occur with metastatic disease to the pleura (29). At present, MRI does not play a significant role in evaluating pleural cancer, but it may be used in the coronal or sagittal plane to clarify CT findings (30, 31).

Metastatic Disease in the Thorax

While the focus of this chapter has been on primary malignancies occurring within the chest, a word may be in order on the use of imaging techniques to detect and evaluate thoracic metastases. Bone metastases are covered in Chap-

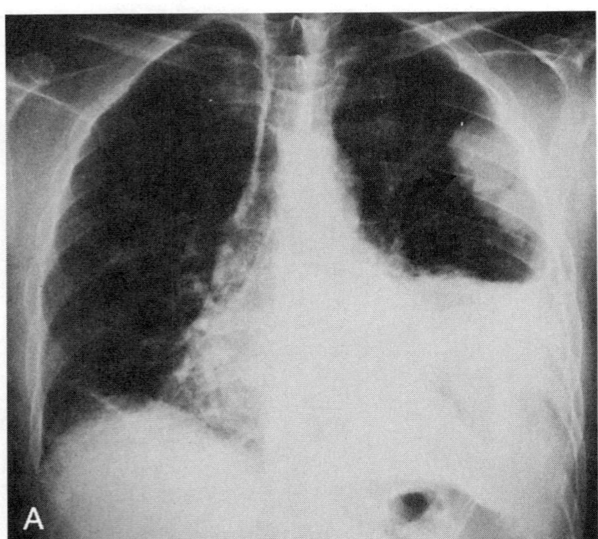

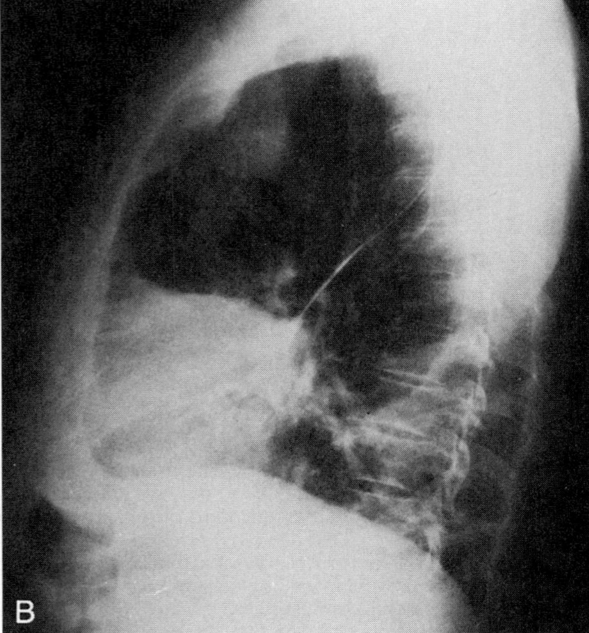

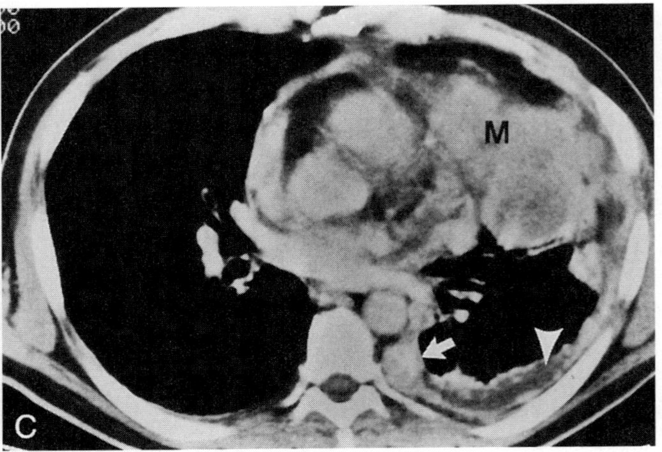

Figure 35.3. Malignant mesothelioma in a 55-year-old man. Posteroanterior (**A**) and lateral (**B**) chest radiographs show a pleural effusion associated with a lobulated mass in lateral and anterior portion of the left hemithorax (*arrows*). CT scan with intravenous contrast material (**C**) reveals enhanced pleural neoplasm (*arrow*) and nonenhanced pleural effusion (*arrowhead*). inhomogenous mass (M) is seen to invade anterior mediastinal fat. Circumferential involvement of left hemithorax is well demonstrated.

ter 40 on radionuclide imaging. Plain radiographs may be used to clarify abnormalities that have been detected by bone scans and/or clinical symptoms, or by CT and/or MRI imaging techniques in the case of mediastinal or hilar enlargement. However, CT has been most useful in detecting small lung metastases (32). Recently, a new technique known as spiral CT has been shown to be capable of detecting a greater number of pulmonary nodular metastases than conventional CT. This is related to the ability of spiral CT to image the entire thorax during a single breath-hold, thus eliminating gaps in coverage from respiratory motion that may be associated with conventional CT (33). In some geographic areas, benign lung nodules (healed granulomas) are relatively common, and the clinical context in which positive CT findings occur must therefore be taken carefully into account. CT can also be used to guide percutaneous needle biopsies of suspected metastatic lesions.

Conclusion

Conventional posteroanterior and lateral chest radiographs continue to be most useful for the detection and initial evaluation of cancer in the chest. CT, by virtue of its cross-sectional imaging display which allows thoracic structures to be visualized without superimposition, is now the imaging modality of choice to supplement the chest radiographic findings. MRI, because of its inferior spatial resolution, its longer data acquisition times leading to motion unsharpness, and its inability to display calcifications, still has a limited role to play in evaluating intrathoracic cancers. Furthermore, MRI is not suitable for critically ill patients who require close monitoring, or for those with implanted pacemakers. Accordingly, MRI is currently used as a "problem solving" modality to clarify complex findings on other studies, by virtue of its direct coronal or sagittal imaging capability. MRI can also be used to define mediastinal or hilar masses which may be difficult to distinguish from vessels on CT, to depict mediastinal and cardiovascular invasion, to confirm chest wall invasion (particularly in superior sulcus tumors), to evaluate the causes of adrenal nodules, or to distinguish recurrent tumor from postradiation fibrosis. Recently, PET imaging with FDG has shown promise in detecting and diagnosing malignant lung nodules and mediastinal lymph nodes.

References

1. Nathan MH. Management of solitary pulmonary nodules. An organized approach based on growth rate and statistics. JAMA 1974;227:1141.
2. Siegelman SS, Khouri NF, Leo FP, Fishman EK, Braverman RM, Zerhouni EA. Solitary pulmonary nodules: CT assessment. Radiology 1986;160:307.
3. Mayr B, Heywang SH, Ingrisch H, Huber RM, Haussinger K, Lissner J. Comparison of CT with MR imaging of endobronchial tumors. J Comput Assist Tomogr 1987;11:43.
4. Batra P, Brown K, Collins JD, Ovenfors CO, Steckel RJ. Evaluation of intrathoracic extent of lung cancer by plain chest radiography, computed tomography, and magnetic resonance imaging. Am Rev Respir Dis 1988;137:1456.
5. Gupta NC, Frank AR, Dewan NA, Redepenning LS, Rothberg ML, Mailliard JA, Phalen JJ, Sunderland JJ, Frick MP. Solitary pulmonary nodules: detection of malignancy with PET with 2-(F-18)-fluoro-2-deoxy-D-glucose. Radiology 1992;184:441.
6. Batra P, Brown K, Steckel R. Diagnostic imaging techniques in lung carcinoma. Am J Surg 1987;153:517.
7. Libshitz HI. Computed tomography in bronchogenic carcinoma. Semin Roentgenol 1990;25:64.
8. Bragg DG. The diagnosis and staging of primary lung cancer. Radiol Clin North Am 1994;32:1.
9. Seely JM, Mayo JR, Miller RR, Muller NL. T1 lung cancer: prevalence of mediastinal nodal metastases and diagnostic accuracy of CT. Radiology 1993;186:129.
10. Gefter WB. Magnetic resonance imaging in lung cancer. Semin Roentgenol 1990;25:73.
11. McLoud TC, Bourgouin PM, Greenberg RW, Kosiuk JP, Templeton PA, Shepard JO, Moore EH, Wain JC, Mathisen DJ, Grillo HE. Bronchogenic carcinoma: analysis of staging in the mediastinum with CT by correlative lymph node mapping and sampling. Radiology 1992;182:319.
12. Staples CA, Muller NL, Miller RR, Evans KG, Nelems B. Mediastinal nodes in bronchogenic carcinoma: comparison between CT and mediastinoscopy. Radiology 1988;167:367.
13. Glazer GM, Orringer MB, Chenevert TL, Borrello JA, Penner MW, Quint LE, Li KC, and Aisen AM. Mediastinal lymph nodes: relaxation time/pathologic correlation and implications in staging of lung cancer with MR imaging. Radiology 1988;168:429.
14. Webb WR, Gatsonis C, Zerhouni EA, Heelan RT, Glazer GM, Francis IR, McNeil BJ. CT and MR imaging in staging non-small cell bronchogenic carcinoma: report of the radiologic diagnostic oncology group. Radiology 1991;178:705.
15. Rea HH, Shevland JE, House AJS. Accuracy of computed tomographic scanning in assessment of the mediastinum in bronchial carcinoma. J Thorac Cardiovasc Surg 1981;81:825.
16. Wahl RL, Quint LE, Greenough RL, Meyer CR, White RI, Orringer MB. Staging of mediastinal non-small cell lung cancer with FDG PET, CT, and fusion images: preliminary prospective evaluation. Radiology 1994;191:371.
17. Pennes DR, Glazer GM, Wimbish KJ, Gross BH, Long RW, Orringer MB. Chest wall invasion by lung cancer: limitations of CT evaluation. AJR 1985;144:507.
18. Padovani B, Mouroux J, Seksik L, Chanalet S, Sedat J, Rotomondo C, Richelme H, Serres JJ. Chest wall invasion by bronchogenic carcinoma: evaluation with MR imaging. Radiology 1993;187:33.
19. Heelan RT, Demas BE, Caravelli JF, Martini N, Bains MS, McCormack PM, Burt M, Panicek DM, Mitzner A. Superior sulcus tumors: CT and MR imaging. Radiology 1989;170:637.
20. Suzuki N, Saitoh T, Kitamura S. Tumor invasion of the chest wall in lung cancer: diagnosis with US. Radiology 1993;187:39.
21. Oliver TW, Bernardino ME, Miller JI, Mansour K, Greene D, Davis WA. Isolated adrenal masses in nonsmall-cell bronchogenic carcinoma. Radiology 1984;153:217.
22. Krestin GP, Steinbrich W, Friedmann G. Adrenal masses: evaluation with fast gradient-echo MR imaging and Gd-DTPA-enhanced dynamic studies. Radiology 1989;171:675.
23. Batra P, Brown K, Steckel R. Diagnostic imaging techniques in mediastinal malignancies. Am J Surg 1988;156:4.
24. Tecce PM, Fishman EK, Kuhlman JE. CT evaluation of the anterior mediastinum: spectrum of disease. RadioGraphics 1994;14:973.
25. Batra P, Brown K, Collins JD, Holmes EC, Steckel RJ, Shapiro BJ. Mediastinal masses: magnetic resonance imaging in comparison with computed tomography. J Natl Med Assoc 1991;83:969.
26. Glazer HS, Levitt RG, Lee JK, Emami B, Gronemeyer S, Murphy WA. Differentiation of radiation fibrosis from recurrent pulmonary neoplasm by magnetic resonance imaging. AJR 1984;143:729.
27. Webb WR, Sostman HD. MR imaging of thoracic disease: clinical uses. Radiology 1992;182:621.
28. Kawashima A, Lipshitz MI. Malignant pleural mesothelioma: CT manifestations in 50 cases. AJR 1990;155:965.
29. Leung AN, Muller NL, Miller RR. CT in differential diagnosis of diffuse pleural disease. AJR 1990;154:487.
30. Patz EF, Shaffer K, Piwnica-Worms DR, Jochelson M, Sarin M, Sugarbaker DJ, Pugatch RD. Malignant pleural mesothelioma: value of CT and MR imaging in predicting resectability. AJR 1992;159:961.
31. Dynes MC, White EM, Fry WA, Ghabremani GG. Imaging manifestations of pleural tumors. RadioGraphics 1992;12:1191.
32. Davis SD. CT evaluation for pulmonary metastases in patients with extrathoracic malignancy. Radiology 1991;180:1.
33. Remy-Jardin M, Remy J, Giraud F, Marquette CH. Pulmonary nodules: detection with thick-section spiral CT versus conventional CT. Radiology 1993;187:513,

CHAPTER 36

Imaging Neoplasms of the Abdomen and Pelvis

ROBERT A. HALVORSEN, JR. AND WILLIAM M. THOMPSON

With recent technologic innovations, computed tomography (CT), magnetic resonance imaging (MRI), and endoluminal sonography are now able to provide much more accurate delineation of tumors, improving the ability to diagnose, stage, and follow neoplasms of the abdomen and pelvis.

The choice of whether to use CT, MRI, or sonography to evaluate abdominopelvic abnormalities depends on the organ system being studied and the patient's condition. CT has the advantages of lower cost, greater availability, and the ability to evaluate a number of organ systems during one diagnostic study (see below, and Table 36.1). Disadvantages of CT include ionizing radiation and the potential for allergic reactions to intravenous contrast media. Advantages of MRI include absence of ionizing radiation and the ability to obtain direct sagittal and coronal images, which can be especially helpful in the pelvis. Early studies have suggested that the use of intravenous gadolinium diethylene triamine pentacetic acid (Gd-DTPA) may further increase the accuracy of MRI in the abdomen and pelvis. Disadvantages of MRI include scan times (generally 3 to 9 minutes) too long for breath holding. High-quality studies can be obtained only if the patient is capable of remaining immobile for such scan times. MRI studies also cover only a limited anatomic area. For example, a thorough MRI study of the liver may require several pulse sequences and images of the upper abdomen only, taking up to an hour to complete. To also evaluate the pelvis with MRI, additional scanning periods may be required; this could double the cost. Since some patients with claustrophobia, severe illnesses that require continuous monitoring, intracerebral surgical clips, other metallic foreign bodies, or cardiac pacemakers are not candidates for MRI in the immediate future, CT is likely to remain the primary modality for staging and following cancers of the abdomen and pelvis.

Diagnosis

Visualization of the mucosal surfaces is essential to diagnose early lesions in the hollow organs of the gastrointestinal tract. The conventional upper gastrointestinal (UGI) series, small bowel follow-through, and barium enema (or endoscopic evaluation of the upper and lower tracts) are superior to either CT or MRI for detecting mucosal lesions (Table 36.2). On the other hand, CT, MRI, and sonography are superior to barium studies for evaluating the wall and extramural portions of the GI tract for tumor involvement, and are useful in detecting distant metastases (1–4).

Both CT and MRI can detect neoplasms of the solid organs in the abdomen and pelvis. CT plays the dominant role in pretreatment evaluation, and CT-guided biopsy of masses is extremely useful (Fig. 36.1). In conjunction with endoscopic retrograde cholangiopancreatography (ERCP), CT is now used in the evaluation of most patients with potential pancreatic neoplasms.

With current third- and fourth-generation CT scanners, scan times have been reduced to 1 to 2 seconds per image; this eliminates most motion artifacts. MRI technology is advancing rapidly, as well. The initial enthusiasm for MRI was due not only to the absence of ionizing radiation, but, more important, to the potential for improved tissue characterization. When MRI was introduced, it was hoped that differences in the signal intensities of abnormal tissues would enable examiners to differentiate benign masses from malignant ones. Unfortunately, tissue characterization has not proved to be as reliable as we hoped, and, in the abdomen and pelvis, the only tumor that has a relatively "pathognomonic" appearance is adrenal pheochromocytoma. All other tumors (and inflammatory processes) signal characteristics overlap.

The standard pulse sequence used in MRI has been spin echo (5). T1-weighted spin echo images provide better spatial resolution than T2-weighted images and, therefore, provide more helpful anatomic information. T2-weighted images more clearly show contrast differences between normal and abnormal tissues. In general, pathologic lesions appear relatively dark (low–signal intensity) on T1-weighted images and bright (high-signal) on T2-weighted ones. Unfortunately, many different pathologic processes (not just tumors) can produce this "dark-bright" appearance (6, 7). For instance, edema adjacent to a tumor, as well as the tumor itself, may look similar under some circumstances. A simple cyst may also be "dark-bright" on T1- and T2-weighted images, as do abscesses and some benign tumors. Therefore, while MRI may be quite sensitive for detecting an abnormality, absolute characterization of the abnormality usually is not possible.

Recently, new pulse sequences have been developed

that allow MRI imaging data to be acquired in 20 seconds or less, during one breathhold (8). This eliminates respiratory motion artifacts. In general, breath-holding MRI techniques produce images with poorer spatial resolution than do standard spin-echo techniques. Therefore, they are useful as problem-solving tools but have not yet replaced standard MRI techniques for tumor detection and staging.

Table 36.1. Imaging Abdomen and Pelvis: CT vs. MRI

Variable	CT	MRI
Cost[a]	$1034.	$2144.
Availability	Generally available	Limited in some areas
Detectability of tumor	Good	Superior
Spatial resolution	Excellent	Excellent (w/co-operative patient)
Scan planes	Axial only	Multiple planes
Ionizing radiation	Yes	No
IV contrast required	Yes	Helpful
Body areas covered	Large	Smaller

[a] Cost at University of Minnesota, 1994.

Table 36.2. Imaging Techniques for Diagnosis

Organ/system	Barium	IVU	US	CT	MRI
GI tract	+ +	—	—	—	—
Liver	—	—	+	+ +	+ +
Pancreas	—	—	+	+ +	—
Kidneys	—	+	+	+ +	+
Uterus/ovaries	—	—	+ +	+	+ +
Prostate	—	+	+ +	—	—

Key: + +, superior; +, helpful; —, not useful; Barium, intraluminal contrast; IVU, intravenous urography; US, ultrasonography; CT, computed tomography; MRI, magnetic resonance imaging.

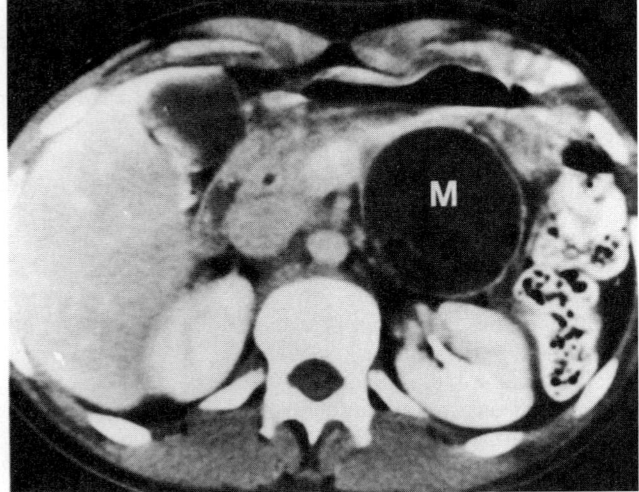

Figure 36.1. Cystic pancreatic mass. Contrast enhanced CT image of upper abdomen demonstrates large cystic mass (M) in tail of pancreas, anterior to left kidney and posterior to stomach. Operative specimen was diagnosed as pancreatic cystadenoma.

Intravenous contrast is used routinely with CT. Initially, no contrast injection was thought to be necessary with MRI, but Gd-DTPA and other agents have proven useful as intravenous contrast agents especially during T1-weighted pulse sequences. The role of these MR intravenous contrast agents during abdominal and pelvic MRI is still being evaluated. Like conventional iodinated contrast agents, MRI contrast media diffuse rapidly from the blood into the interstitial space. Therefore, MRI scanning of the liver should be performed during—not following—intravenous administration of these contrast media. Fast scanning techniques may be required to maximize the effectiveness of MRI with intravascular contrast materials. The combination of fast MRI scanning and intravenous contrast has great promise and may eventually replace CT with contrast as the standard imaging technique for solid organs in the abdomen and pelvis.

Staging

After a malignant lesion has been diagnosed in the abdomen or pelvis, imaging techniques can be helpful for tumor staging (Table 36.3). With certain limitations, the cross-sectional imaging abilities of both CT and MRI are helpful in detecting extramural spread of tumor from the GI tract (9). For instance, either CT or MRI can detect abnormal tissue infiltrating the fat that surrounds the rectum, but neither may be able to differentiate inflammatory strands from neoplastic invasion. Another limitation of both CT and MRI is their inability to detect tumor in normal-sized lymph nodes. CT is more successful in detecting lymph node involvement with cancers such as seminoma and lymphoma, which produce considerable lymph node enlargement, than with GI tract carcinomas, which often replace regional lymph nodes rather than enlarging them. Neither CT nor MRI can determine the depth of invasion of a mucosal or submucosal tumor in the wall of the GI tract. Therefore, the major role of CT and MRI in staging abdominopelvic malignancies is the detection of distant metastases.

Posttreatment Surveillance

CT is now the standard imaging technique in most institutions for following cancers of the abdomen and pelvis (10,

Table 36.3. Imaging Techniques for Staging/Follow-Up

	Barium	IVU	US	CT	MRI
GI tract	+	—	+	+ +	+
Liver	—	—	+	+ +	+ +
Pancreas	—	—	—	+ +	+
Uterus/ovaries	—	—	+ +	+	+ +
Prostate	—	—	+ +	+	+

Key: + +, superior; +, helpful; —, not useful; Barium, intraluminal contrast; IVU, intravenous urography; US, ultrasonography; CT, computed tomography; MRI, magnetic resonance imaging.

11). It is also used routinely for detecting liver metastases. While MRI now approaches or equals CT in the ability to depict liver metastases, its sensitivity for detecting extrahepatic metastatic disease in the abdomen is relatively limited. Therefore, a CT examination of the upper abdomen can potentially detect more metastatic lesions than an MRI study. The higher cost and limited availability of MRI have also permitted CT to maintain its role as the primary abdominal imaging modality for posttreatment surveillance of cancer patients.

Gastrointestinal Tract: Hollow Organs

While evaluation of the mucosal surfaces with barium studies and endoscopy still plays a primary role in diagnosis of cancers of the stomach, small bowel, and colon, CT is widely used as the first imaging test in the staging and follow-up of these tumors (4, 10, 12). CT is somewhat limited in its ability to detect mesenteric lesions because of the difficulty of differentiating unopacified loops of bowel from tumor masses, but it is useful for detecting metastases to solid organs and retroperitoneal lymph nodes (see above). MRI has achieved only limited use in the upper abdomen until now because of the lack of a suitable oral contrast medium and the prolonged imaging times. As described in Chapter 39, endoscopic ultrasound techniques, especially transrectal sonography, represent an evolving technology which has promise for evaluating wall invasion by tumors in the GI tract (2, 3, 13, 14). Endoscopic sonography is limited by its inability to depict lesions further than 5 cm from the GI lumen, however, and by problems of access to the ultrasound probe. Tumors that prevent passage of the probe because of obstruction or severe narrowing cannot be evaluated adequately by endosonography. The role of nuclear medicine in the diagnosis, staging, and follow-up of GI tract cancers has declined with the introduction of newer imaging modalities. CT, MRI, and ultrasound, all are more sensitive and reliable techniques for demonstrating liver metastases than is radionuclide scanning.

Liver Metastases

The diagnosis, staging, and follow-up of primary and metastatic liver lesions can now be attained with multiple imaging modalities. CT is the most widely used technique in the United States for ascertaining liver involvement by cancer. In Europe, many institutions use hepatic ultrasound first and use CT or MRI as a second study only in problem cases. Sonography is limited in its ability to detect smaller hepatic lesions: reported sensitivity is only 20% for lesions less than 1 cm in diameter, as compared with 31% for MRI and 49% for CT (15). With the development of fast scanning techniques and new contrast media, MRI has the potential for replacing CT and ultrasound as the primary diagnostic tool for liver disease; currently CT and MRI of the liver should be considered complementary procedures (Fig. 36.2) (6, 7). Neither study is perfect, and not infrequently lesions that are missed by CT are detected by MRI, or vice versa. Therefore, when it is important to detect all metastatic lesions in the liver before hepatic resection, both CT and MRI may be indicated.

Helical CT, which allows continuous scanning while the patient is moved slowly through the scanner, is now possible with recently developed equipment. While no large series are yet available, initial reports suggest that helical scanning may be superior to other CT techniques for detection and characterization of abdominal neoplasms. Currently, the most widely used technique for CT examination of the liver is dynamic bolus–enhanced CT (DBCT), which requires slow continuous infusion of intravenous contrast media during the examination. Unenhanced CT is less sensitive than DBCT for liver lesions. CT scans obtained following, rather than during administration of intravenous contrast are even less sensitive, since the contrast material may diffuse into a liver tumor and make it indistinguishable from the normal liver. DBCT not only can detect more lesions than other CT techniques, but it can also help to characterize some masses. Cavernous hemangioma, the most frequent benign hepatic mass, may appear on DBCT as a liver mass with well-defined margins and occasionally demonstrates "globular enhancement." Globular enhancement describes the CT findings of a small area of parenchymal enhancement on the rim of the mass, similar in degree to vessels at the same level. This finding is highly suggestive of cavernous hemangioma. When the CT findings are suggestive, but not characteristic, of a hemangioma, MRI can also be useful. The characteristic MRI appearance of a liver hemangioma is a well-defined, low–signal intensity mass on T1-weighted images and a "light bulb" or high–signal intensity mass on T2-weighted pulse sequences (6–8, 16, 17). Unfortunately, this MRI appearance can sometimes be encountered also with necrotic neoplasms or with metastases from hypervascular primary tumors such as islet cell carcinomas.

A radionuclide scan procedure performed with technetium-99m–labeled red blood cells (Tc-RBC) can also be used to make a specific diagnosis of hemangioma of the liver. The diagnosis is made when there is diminished radionuclide activity in a liver lesion during the early (vascular) phase of a labeled red cell infusion, and increased activity (a hot spot) on delayed or blood-pool scan images. While this "flip-flop" in the appearance of a liver mass on such a scan is diagnostic of a hemangioma, the Tc-RBC study is limited in its ability to detect hemangiomas that are smaller than 2 cm in diameter.

Both CT and ultrasound can also be helpful in guiding fine-needle biopsies of liver lesions. While sonographically guided biopsies require more technical expertise than biopsies monitored with CT, the ability to image the needle tip with sonography while advancing the needle into a lesion is a definite advantage over CT. The performance of a CT-guided biopsy can be considered as partially "blind," since the needle tip cannot be visualized while it is being advanced inside the liver. Sonographic biopsies are also less expensive than CT-directed biopsies in most institutions.

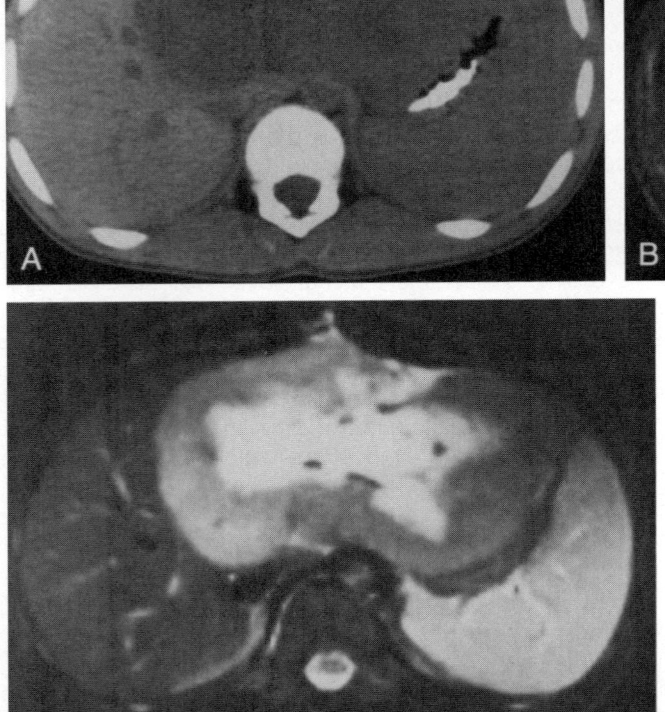

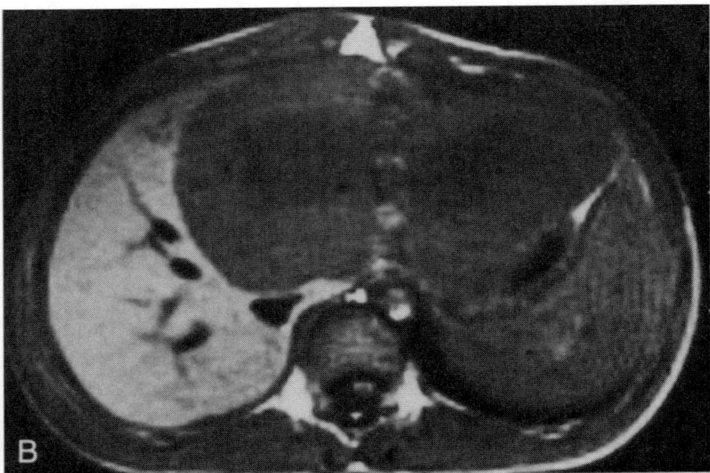

Figure 36.2. Hepatic embryonal cell sarcoma. **A.** CT demonstrates large lesion with a central low-density area occupying the entire left lobe and probably extending into right lobe of liver. **B.** Liver MRI. A T1-weighted image demonstrates more clearly than CT the interface between normal liver and mass. **C.** T2-weighted image demonstrates central area of high signal consistent with necrosis. (Reprinted with permission: Halvorsen RA Jr, Letourneau JG. Malignant liver disease. In *CT and MRI of the Liver and Biliary System*. Edited by PM Silverman, RK Zeman. New York: Churchill Livingstone, 1990.)

Pancreas

CT and sonography both play important roles in evaluating the jaundiced cancer patient. Sonographic studies are quite accurate in diagnosing bile duct dilatation and in helping to determine whether "medical" or "surgical" jaundice is present. CT can then be used to confirm the presence of ductal dilatation, and it is usually superior to sonography in determining the cause of obstruction, because of CT's ability to image the extrahepatic biliary tree and to visualize the actual obstructing lesion (e.g., a pancreatic mass).

CT has also become the primary imaging modality to evaluate suspected pancreatic disease (18). Pancreatic CT, using a bolus of intravenous contrast material and thin collimation, can detect a majority of pancreatic adenocarcinomas and islet cell tumors, and CT-guided biopsy can confirm the diagnosis (see Fig. 36.1). Ultrasound has been used to evaluate the pancreas but, in general, its application is limited by interposed bowel gas, which makes evaluation of the entire pancreas difficult for most patients. MRI is still limited in evaluating the pancreas, because of the difficulty in differentiating pancreatic tissue from adjacent bowel (19). Once ade-

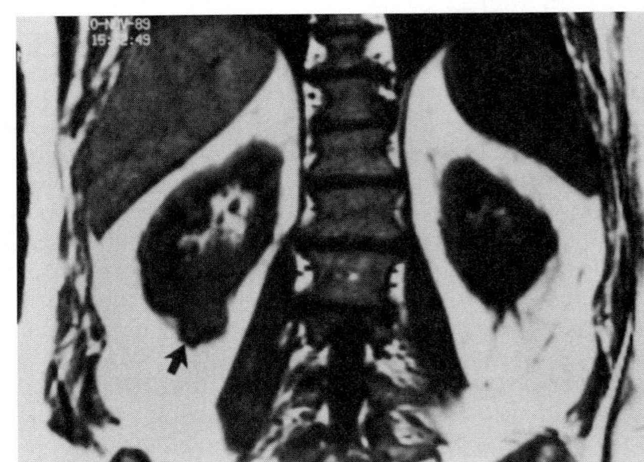

Figure 36.3. Renal cell carcinoma. Coronal T1-weighted MRI demonstrates exophytic mass (*arrow*) extending from lower pole of right kidney. Note that signal intensities of tumor and normal kidney are identical.

quate oral contrast agents become available for use with MRI, the role of MRI in pancreatic imaging will increase.

Angiography of the pancreas has declined in popularity since the advent of CT, but it still can be helpful as a complementary problem-solving tool in certain circumstances.

Kidney

Standard intravenous urography (IVU) remains a prime screening tool for suspected stone disease of the urinary tract in adult patients, but is used less frequently in the work-up of patients with a suspected renal neoplasm. While ultrasound is the preferred test for detecting hydronephrosis, CT, without and then with intravenous contrast, is the primary study whenever a solid mass in the kidney is suspected. CT can differentiate certain benign tumors from malignant lesions. For instance, a renal mass that contains fat and no calcification is presumed to be angiomyolipoma, since no renal carcinoma has been reported that contains only fat without calcification that was detectable by CT. CT is useful in staging renal carcinomas (reported accuracy, 91% [20]). MRI also has considerable potential for staging renal tumors, especially with the use of Gd-DTPA (Fig. 36.3). Two major advantages of MRI for tumor staging, as compared to CT, are better detection of tumor thrombus in renal veins and superior ability to distinguish collateral vessels in the renal hilus from renal hilar lymph nodes. In two studies comparing CT to MRI for staging renal cell carcinoma, CT's staging accuracy was 70 to 78%, compared with 92 to 96% for MRI (21, 22).

Tumors of the Female Reproductive Tract

Sonography remains the primary screening tool for pelvic lesions. Transvaginal sonographic examinations can now

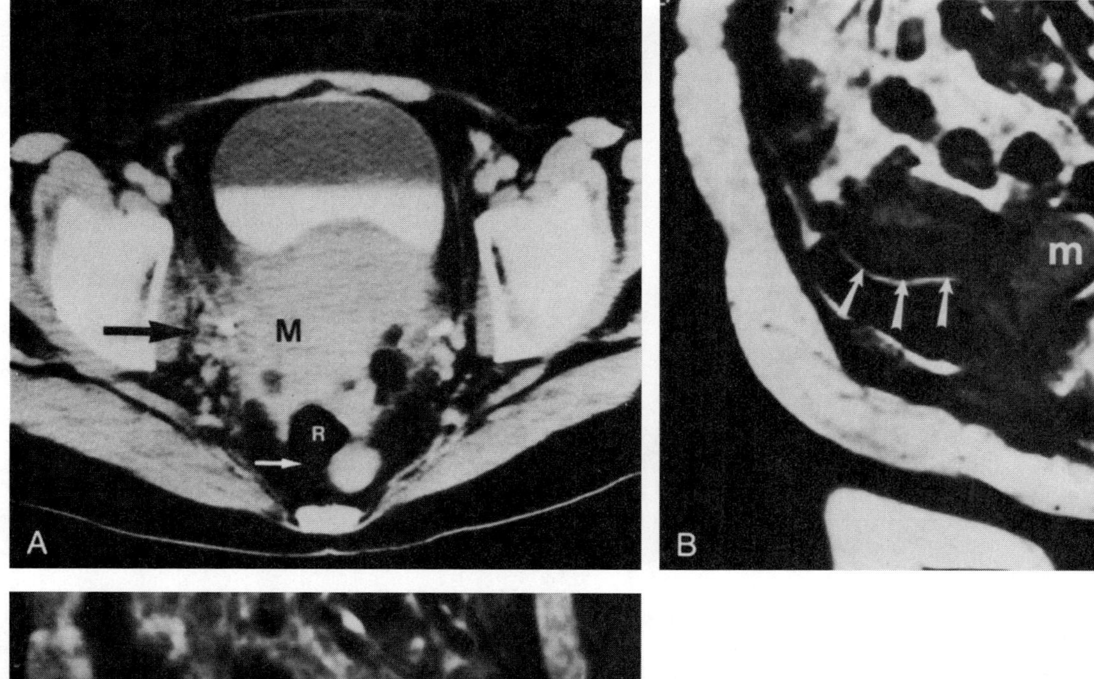

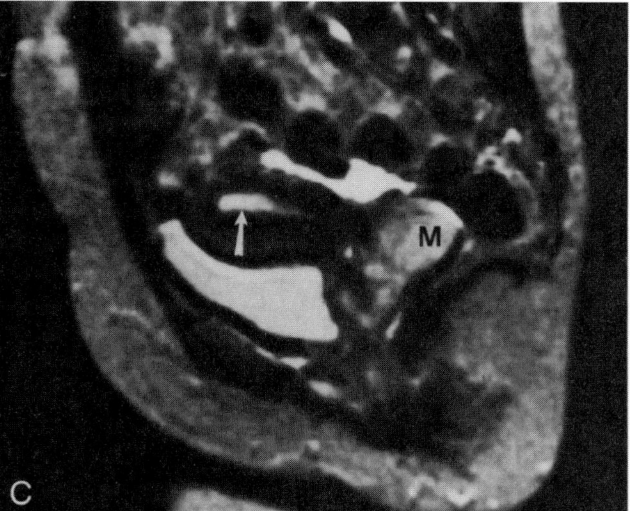

Figure 36.4. Lymphoma of uterine cervix. **A.** CT demonstrates ill-defined mass (M) between the bladder (containing layered urine and contrast material) and the rectum (R). Note that mass extends lateral to the right ureter (*arrow*) and is inseparable from body of uterus. **B.** Sagittal MRI. T1-weighted sequence demonstrates cervical tumor mass (M), which is clearly distinguishable from body of uterus (*arrows*). **C.** T2-weighted image at same level shows higher signal intensity in tumor mass (M) than normal myometrium, which is to the left. Note fluid in endometrial canal, which produces high signal (*arrow*). Bright fluid is also present in space between uterus and rectosigmoid, as well as in bladder lumen.

provide excellent visualization of lower pelvic structures (see Chapter 39). Combined with transabdominal sonography, which uses the distended bladder as an acoustic window, transvaginal sonography is usually performed as the initial examination when a pelvic mass is suspected. Sonography is ideally suited to differentiating between cystic masses and solid ones. When further evaluation is warranted, MRI can be extremely helpful in the pelvis (Fig. 36.4). Because of the relative lack of motion in this body area, the MRI is more useful in the pelvis than in the upper abdomen. The ability of MRI to obtain coronal, sagittal, and oblique images, rather than just the axial views available with CT, may be particularly useful in depicting uterine and adnexal masses (23). In a study of such masses, Mitchell and coworkers found that MRI provided additional information or increased diagnostic confidence in 25 of 35 patients who had also undergone ultrasonography or CT (24). MRI can depict the level of myometrial invasion by uterine carcinomas and is helpful in detecting extramural spread of the disease (25).

Prostate

After physical examination, transrectal sonography is the most helpful technique for detecting nodules in the prostate. While sonography has not been established as an efficacious method for screening asymptomatic men for prostate cancer, sonographically guided biopsy of suspicious lesions can provide a diagnosis of malignant neoplasms. The role of sonography in staging prostatic cancer is still uncertain, and CT is not particularly helpful in assessing the extent of local disease. With its multiplanar capability, MRI is probably the most accurate imaging modality now available for staging prostate cancer. In a study of 46 patients with prostatic carcinoma who subsequently underwent radical prostatectomy, CT staging had an accuracy rate of 65%; with MRI staging, accuracy increased to 83% (26).

Conclusion

Conventional imaging techniques, including barium studies and intravenous urography, remain the primary diagnostic tools of the radiologist for evaluating the luminal portions of the gastrointestinal and the genitourinary tracts. Diagnosis of tumors of the solid organs usually requires a cross-sectional imaging method such as CT, MRI or, occasionally, sonography, often followed by guided biopsy. CT has now replaced conventional radiographic studies for staging and following abdominopelvic malignancies; in the future, MRI may have comparable applications.

References

1. Butch RJ, Stark DD, Wittenberg J, Tepper JE, Saini S, Simeone JF, et al. Staging rectal cancer by MR and CT. AJR 1986;146:1155.
2. Hulsmans, F JJ. Staging of rectal CA: US and CT. Radiology 1989;170:319.
3. Hulsmans, F JJH, Tio TL, Fockens P, Bosma A, Tytgat GNJ. Assessment of tumor infiltration depth in rectal cancer with transrectal sonography: caution is necessary. Radiology 1994;190:715.
4. Thompson WM, Halvorsen RA, Foster WL Jr., Roberts L, Gibbons R. Preoperative and postoperative CT staging of rectosigmoid carcinoma. AJR 1986;146:703.
5. Turnbull LW, Kean DM. Tumour identification using magnetic resonance imaging. Cancer Surv 1987;6:343.
6. Li KC, Glazer GM, Quint LE, Francis IR, Aisen AM, Ensminger WD, et al. Distinction of hepatic cavernous hemangioma from hepatic metastases with MR imaging. Radiology 1988;169:409.
7. Wittenberg J, Stark DD, Forman BH, Hahn PF, Saini S, Weissleder R, et al. Differentiation of hepatic metastases from hepatic hemangiomas and cysts by using MR imaging. AJR 1988;171:79
8. Glazer GM. MR imaging of the liver, kidneys and adrenal glands. Radiology 1988;166:303.
9. Thompson WM, Halvorsen RA Jr. Computed tomographic staging of the gastrointestinal malignancies. Part II. The small bowel, colon and rectum. Invest Radiol 1987;22:96.
10. Charnsangavej C. New imaging modalities for follow-up of colorectal carcinoma. Cancer 1993;71:4236.
11. De Lange EE, Fechner RE, Wanebo HJ. Suspected recurrent rectosigmoid carcinoma after abdominoperineal resection: MR imaging and histopathologic findings. Radiology 1989;170:323.
12. Sussman SK, Halvorsen RA Jr., Illescas FF, Cohan RH, Saeed M, Liverman PM, et al. Gastric adenocarcinoma: CT versus surgical staging. Radiology 1988;167:335.
13. Carroll BA. US of the gastrointestinal tact. Radiology 1989;172:605.
14. Rifkin MD, Ehrlich SM, Marks G. Staging of rectal carcinoma: prospective comparison of endorectal US and CT. Radiology 1989;170:319.
15. Wernecke K, Rummeny E, Bongarte G, Vassallop, Kivelitz D, Weismann W, et al. Detection of hepatic metastases in patients with carcinoma: comparative sensitivities of sonography, CT and MR imaging. AJR 1991 157:731
16. Yamashita Y, Hatanaka Y, Yamamoto H, Arakawa A, Matsukawa T, Miyazaki T, Takahasi M. Differential diagnosis of focal liver lesions: role of spin echo and contrast-enhanced dynamic MR imaging. Radiology 1994;193:59.
17. McFarland EG, Mayo-Smith WW, Saini S, Hahn PF, Goldberg MA, Lee MJ. Hepatic hemangiomas and malignant tumors: improved differentiation with heavily T2-weighted conventional spin-echo MR imaging. Radiology 1994;193:43.
18. Freeny PC, Traverso LW, Ryan JA. Diagnosis and staging of pancreatic adenocarcinoma with dynamic computed tomography. Am J Surg 1993:165:600.
19. Vellet AD, Romano W, Bach DB, Passi RB, Taves DH, Munk PL. Adenocarcinoma of the pancreatic ducts: comparative evaluation with CT and MR imaging at 1.5 T. Radiology 1992;183:87.
20. Johnson CD, Dunnick NR, Cohan RH, Illescas FF. Renal adenocarcinoma: CT staging of 100 tumors. AJR 1987;148:59.
21. Hricak H, Demas BE, Williams RD, McNamara MT, Kedgcock MW, Amparo EG, et al. Magnetic resonance imaging in the diagnosis and staging of renal and perirenal neoplasms. Radiology 1985;154:709.
22. Semelka RC, Shoenat JP, Magro CM, Krocker MA, MacMahon R, Greenberg HM. Renal cancer staging: comparison of contrast-enhanced CT and gadolinium-enhanced fat-suppressed spin-echo and gradient-echo MR imaging. J Magn Reson Imaging 1993;3:597.
23. Lee MJ, Munk PL, Poon PY, Hassell P. Ovarian cancer: computed tomography findings. Can Assoc Radiol J 1995;45:185.
24. Mitchell DG, Mintz, MC Spritzer CE, Gussman D, Arger PH, Coleman BG, et al. MR imaging observations at 1.5 T, with US and CT correlation and pulse sequence optimization. Radiology 1988;169:359.
25. Hricak H, Stern JL, Fisher MR, Shapeero LG, Winkler ML, Lacy CG. Endometrial carcinoma staging by MR imaging. Radiology 1987;162:297.
26. Hricak H, Dooms GC, Jeffrey RB, Avallone A, Jacobs D, Benton WK, et al. Prostatic carcinoma: staging by clinical assessment, CT, and MR imaging. Radiology 1987;162:331.

CHAPTER 37

Cross-Sectional Imaging of Musculoskeletal Neoplasms

LEANNE L. SEEGER

Introduction

Since the advent of cross-sectional scanning techniques, the evaluation of the patient with a primary musculoskeletal cancer has changed dramatically. Choosing the imaging modality best suited to a particular problem can be complex and depends on several factors.

A diagnosis of a musculoskeletal tumor can often be suspected clinically and may be supported by the findings on plain radiographs. Radionuclide scans may be used to screen for additional lesions that lie within or are invading bone, and the tissue diagnosis is confirmed by biopsy. In this situation, the role of magnetic resonance imaging (MRI) and computed tomography (CT) is not to obtain a diagnosis but rather to supply additional information about the location and extent of the tumor (2, 9).

If one is attempting initially to determine the presence or absence of a lesion (e.g., bone pain, with negative or equivocal radiographic findings), MRI is now generally considered the modality of choice. Because of the inherently high contrast between normal and abnormal marrow and soft tissues on MRI, it is a highly sensitive means of documenting or ruling our disease. However, findings on MR are often nonspecific, and malignant and benign tumors, infection, and trauma may look similar (4, 7, 10).

When a bone lesion is known to exist and additional information is needed for a differential diagnosis, CT is usually the preferred imaging modality. This reflects not only the nonspecificity of MRI abnormalities but also the fact that MRI may be relatively insensitive to tumor mineralization and to the presence of subtle cortical or periosteal abnormalities (see below). MRI is usually the preferred cross-sectional modality to evaluate soft tissue masses which are clinically evident (6).

When obtaining cross-sectional images in patients with a known primary neoplasm in an extremity, the information of greatest interest includes a determination of the extent of the tumor in the marrow and soft tissues, a definition of the tumor's relationship to major neural and vascular structures, and evaluation of adjacent joints for intra-articular or synovial infiltration. If amputation or limb salvage is anticipated, MRI and CT can also be used to provide accurate measurements of tumor size and distance to adjacent joints. These measurements may be used to manufacture endoprostheses or for surgical planning. For primary pelvic tumors involving the ilium or sacrum, preoperative imaging must be capable of identifying infiltration into pelvic soft tissues or the epidural space and defining the relationships of tumor to sacral and sciatic nerves, major vessels, and the hip and sacroiliac joints.

Either MRI or CT can answer many of these questions during the preoperative evaluation, and one of the two studies usually suffice (Fig. 37.1); however, there are some advantages to each modality, and the study that is chosen depends largely on the experience of the referring physician and the radiologist. Several studies have compared MRI and CT for the evaluation of primary bone tumors (1, 3, 5, 8, 12). Since these studies address many different facets in tumor evaluation, it is difficult to determine from the reports if one modality is superior overall. There is, however, fairly uniform agreement that MRI is superior to CT for delineating the margins of a tumor with respect to adjacent normal muscle and that CT is superior in evaluating subtle cortical abnormalities. Under most circumstances, MRI and CT are comparable in their ability to determine the extent of intramedullary tumor involvement to a level of accuracy that is clinically important. This is especially true if CT scans are acquired with the help of intravenous contrast medium, and if thin-section images are obtained through the tumor margins.

Using conventional spin echo techniques for MRI, a determination of tumor extent and the relationships to major neurovascular structures and to adjacent joints is done by comparing T1- and T2-weighted images. Intravenous contrast administration generally does not add significant information (11). With CT, optimal visualization of the extraosseous (soft tissue) and intramedullary extent of a tumor usually requires administration of intravenous contrast medium. In the case of pelvic tumors, when preliminary radiographs reveal little or no calcified tumor matrix in the soft tissues, ingested contrast material to opacify pelvic bowel loops may also be helpful for determining the presence or absence of intrapelvic soft-tissue invasion. If an extraosseous pelvic tumor mass is highly mineralized, however, it may be difficult to differentiate osteoblastic tumor from contrast-filled loops of bowel on CT. All CT images should be evaluated with bone- as well as soft-tissue window settings. Bone windows best display calcified tumor matrix and cortical involvement. Soft-tissue window settings are needed to evaluate the marrow space for tumor invasion (which appears as loss of normal low-density fat in the mar-

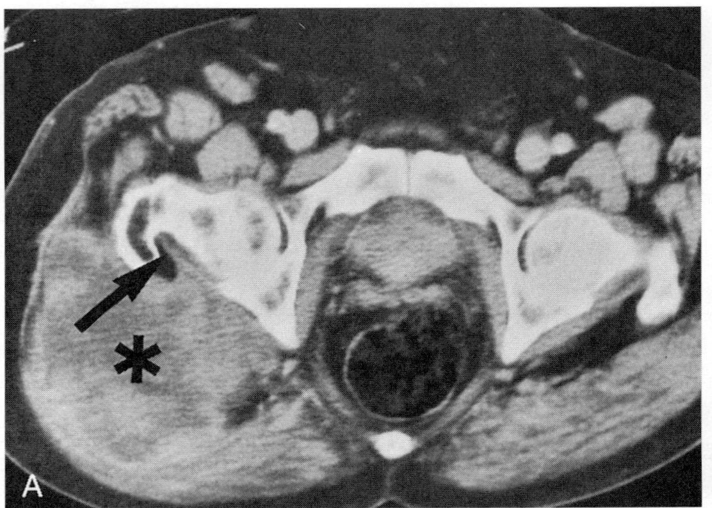

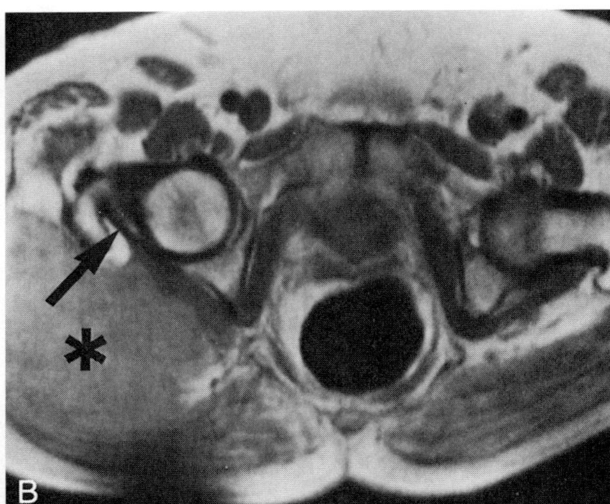

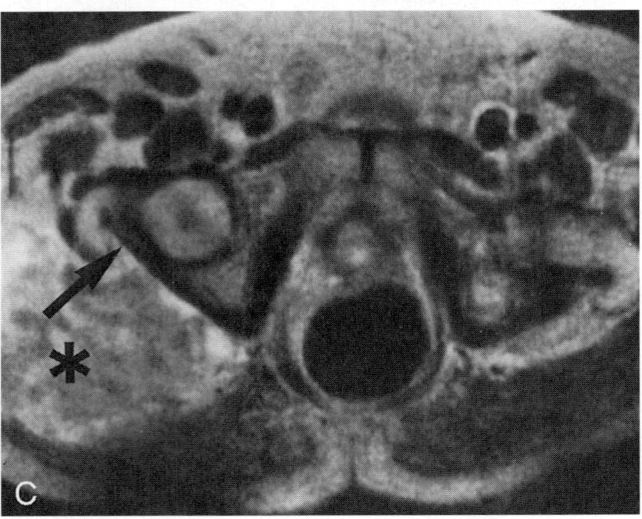

Figure 37.1. MRI vs. CT: 69-year-old male with liposarcoma of the right buttock (*). Both imaging modalities clearly show tumor extent. Tumor extends to the hip joint posteriorly, but the capsule is not invaded (*arrow*). **A.** Contrast-enhanced CT scan, soft tissue window. **B.** Axial T1-weighted MR scan (SE 22/700). **C.** Axial T2-weighted MR scan (SE 85/2000).

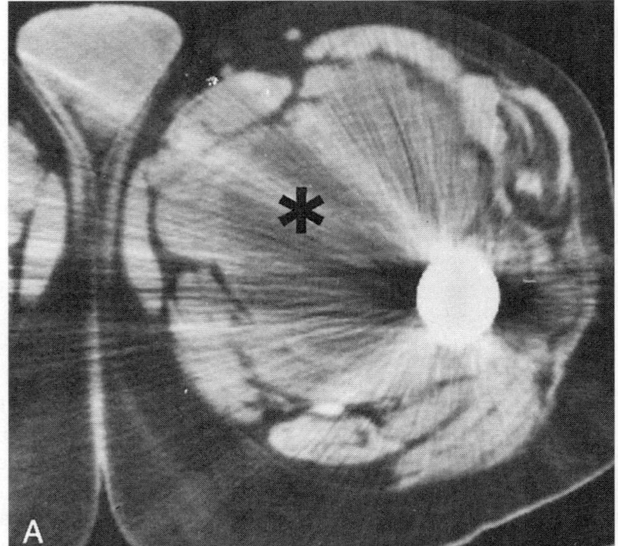

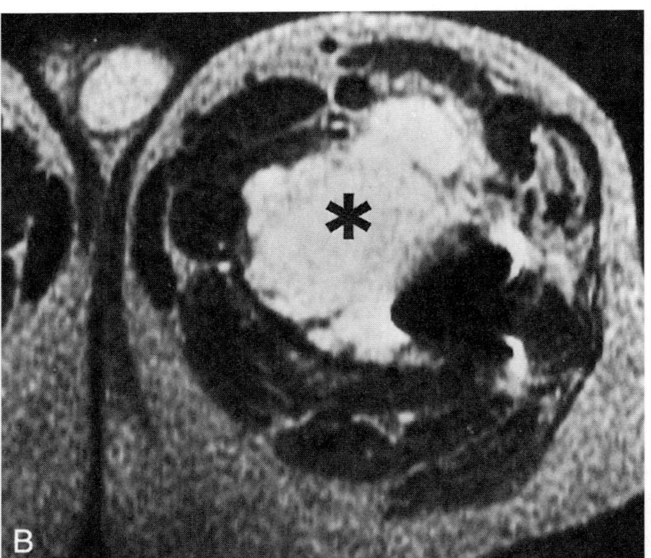

Figure 37.2. MRI vs. CT: 71-year-old male with recurrent chondrosarcoma (*) after proximal femoral limb salvage with custom endoprosthesis (titanium alloy). **A.** Contrast-enhanced CT scan (soft-tissue window). Despite significant artifact, recurrent tumor is readily evident. **B.** Axial T2-weighted MR scan (SE 85/2000) obtained on a 0.3 Tesla MR system. Titanium causes minimal artifact with low- to moderate-field–strength magnets. Recurrent tumor is evident as a high–signal intensity mass surrounding the prosthesis.

row cavity), the soft-tissue extent of the tumor, and the relationships of the tumor to major neurovascular structures (with the assistance of intravenous contrast material).

Either MRI or CT may be used for postoperative evaluation of patients who have undergone amputation, hemipelvectomy, or local tumor excision. Cross-sectional studies may be useful for identifying recurrent tumor in patients who have undergone limb salvage with a custom endoprosthesis (Fig. 37.2), especially if the region of concern lies proximal or distal to the endoprosthesis. With both MRI and CT, metal-induced artifacts may sometimes be a problem. The severity of an artifact will be determined, in part, by the type of metal used for endoprosthesis manufacture (e.g., ferrous metals degrade MR images). For MRI, the field strength of the imaging system is also important; low-field magnets induce the least amount of artifact.

For limb salvage, methylmethacrylate bone cement is frequently used to anchor the endoprosthesis. The cement appears as well-defined areas of high density on CT images and as a signal void on MRI, and it should not be mistaken for residual or recurrent osteoblastic tumor. Confusion can be avoided by correlating the MR or CT images with radiographs.

References

1. Aisen AM, Martel, Braunstein EM, McMillan KI, Phillips WA, Kling TF. MRI and CT evaluation of primary bone and soft-tissue tumors. AJR 1986;146:749.
2. Berquist TH. Magnetic resonance imaging of primary skeletal neoplasms. Radiol Clin North Am 1993;31:411.
3. Bloem JL, Taminiau AHM, Eulderink F, Hermans J, Pauwels EK. Radiologic staging of primary bone sarcoma: MR imaging, scintigraphy, angiography and CT correlated with pathologic examination. Radiology 1988;169:805.
4. Crim JR, Seeger LL, Yao L, Chandnani V, Eckardt JJ. Diagnosis of soft-tissue masses with MR imaging: can benign masses be differentiated from malignant ones? Radiology 1992;185:581.
5. Gillespy T III, Manfrini M, Ruggieri P, Spanier SS, Pettersson H, Springfield DS. Staging of intraosseous extent of osteosarcoma: correlation of preoperative CT and MR imaging with pathologic macroslides. Radiology 1988;167:765.
6. Kransdorf MJ, Jelinek JS, Moser RP. Imaging of soft tissue tumors. Radiol Clin North Am 1993;31:359.
7. Ma LD, Frassica FJ, Scott FJ, Fishman EK, Zerhouni EA. Differentiation of benign and malignant musculoskeletal tumors: potential pitfalls with MR imaging. Radiographics 1995;15:349.
8. Pettersson H, Gillespy T III, Hamlin DJ, Enneking WF, Springfield DS, Andrew ER, Spanier S, Slone R. Primary musculoskeletal tumors: examination with MR imaging compared with conventional modalities. Radiology 1987;164:237.
9. Seeger LL, Eckardt JJ, Bassett LW. Cross-sectional imaging in the evaluation of osteogenic sarcoma: MRI and CT. Semin Roentgenol 1989;24:174.
10. Seeger LL, Dungan DH, Eckardt JJ, Bassett LW, Gold RH. Nonspecific findings on MRI: the importance of correlative studies and clinical information. Clin Orthop 1991;270:306.
11. Seeger LL, Widoff BE, Bassett LW, Rosen G, Eckardt JJ. Preoperative evaluation of osteosarcoma: value of gadopentetate dimeglumine-enhanced MR imaging. AJR 1991;157:347–351.
12. Zimmer WD, Berquist TH, McLeod RA, Sim FH, Pritchard DJ, Shives TC, Wold LE, May G. Bone tumors: magnetic resonance imaging versus computed tomography. Radiology 1995;155:709.

CHAPTER 38

Imaging the Breast

LAWRENCE W. BASSETT

Introduction

It is estimated that 183,400 new cases of breast cancer were diagnosed in 1995 and that 46,240 women died from this disease (1). The risk of breast cancer is greatest for women older than 40 years, and risk increases with age. Although some women are known to be at higher risk, 75% of women who develop breast cancer have no known special risk factors (2). The best hope for improved survival still is early detection by screening, and the most effective method of breast cancer screening is mammography (3). Mammography also is an important diagnostic tool for women with breast symptoms, because it can define the nature of breast abnormalities and identify unexpected malignancy, including multifocal disease, which can have implications for therapy.

Indications for Mammography

There are two types of mammography: screening mammography and diagnostic mammography (4).

SCREENING MAMMOGRAPHY

Screening mammography is indicated for asymptomatic women to detect clinically occult breast cancer (5). While debate exists over the effectiveness of screening mammography for women aged 40 to 49 years, there is general agreement that it reduces mortality from breast cancer in women over 50 (6). Citing the lack of evidence for benefit from a review of randomized controlled studies, the National Cancer Institute (NCI) withdrew its support for mammographic screening of women aged 40 to 49; however, this change in policy was not supported by the NCI's National Cancer Advisory Board. A congressional review committee also was not convinced that the evidence against screening women aged 40 to 49 was conclusive, and it was concerned that the change in guidelines confused women (7). Furthermore, based on evidence of benefit from some randomized controlled studies, recognized flaws in others, and encouraging results in nonrandomized clinical trials, the American Cancer Society as well as professional medical societies continue to recommend mammographic screening for women aged 40 to 49 years (8).

DIAGNOSTIC MAMMOGRAPHY

Also called consultative or problem-solving mammography, diagnostic mammography is indicated when there are clinical findings such as a palpable lump or an abnormal screening mammogram that require additional imaging. The diagnostic examination involves a complete work-up that is tailored to the individual symptomatic patient or the woman with an abnormal screening examination (9) and often includes additional views of the abnormal breast using spot compression and magnification devices, correlative breast examination, and breast ultrasonography. With few exceptions, the radiologist should be on-site while diagnostic mammography is performed. Diagnostic mammography should be performed even when a biopsy is being planned on a woman over 30 years of age; the purpose of mammography before a planned biopsy is to define better the nature of the mass and to find unexpected (i.e., nonpalpable) lesions, including multifocal carcinomas or intraductal extensions of invasive carcinomas.

Performing the Examination

Although xeromammography has been advocated in the past, today, mammography is performed with the film-screen method, involving use of an x-ray–sensitive screen combined with a high-contrast film. With continuing advances in technology, film-screen mammography provides more information than was possible in the past. The examination must be performed with x-ray equipment specifically designed for breast radiography. Among other features, these dedicated mammography units have an x-ray source that is designed for soft-tissue imaging and a built-in breast compression device. Continuous improvements have been and are being made in dedicated mammography units, and equipment should be updated periodically.

The importance of proper breast compression for mammography cannot be overemphasized. Compression holds the breast still and thereby prevents motion unsharpness, brings objects closer to the film and reduces blur, separates overlapping tissues that might prevent the detection of lesions, and decreases the x-ray dose by making the breast less thick. While breast compression may be uncomfortable, it is rarely painful if properly performed (10). Surveys show that women rarely avoid having mammograms because of the discomfort of compression (11), and several strategies are used to minimize this discomfort. Because a leading factor predisposing to pain may be the expectation of pain, education and reassurance are paramount (12). Also, experienced radiologic technologists accomplish more compression with less patient discomfort, because they have learned to inform the woman before instituting compression, apply the compression in gradations rather than all at once, and get input from the woman so that she has control over the amount of compression that is finally applied (4).

SCREENING MAMMOGRAPHY

To have the greatest possible impact, screening mammography must be widely available. Therefore, screening should be done as efficiently as possible and at the lowest possible cost. It has been recommended that mammographic screening be done in a high-volume setting, where the radiologic technologist performs as many examinations as can be done properly each day and the interpreting physician reads all of the films at one sitting later in the day (5, 13). For screening, it is not necessary for the radiologist to be on-site during the actual performance of examinations. Strategies such as storing films in a light-tight box after exposures and batch processing the films at the end of the day rather than after each examination also have been used to increase both efficiency and volume. Interestingly, the U.S. General Accounting Office has studied costs and quality in mammography and concluded that high-volume performance sites are more likely to provide lower-cost as well as higher quality examinations (14). Many facilities still do not differentiate screening from diagnostic mammography, however, and this reluctance to change the way that screening is performed undoubtedly has limited access for women of lower socioeconomic groups (15).

Only mediolateral oblique (MLO) and craniocaudal (CC) views of each breast (i.e., the "standard views") are done for screening. The MLO is the most effective single view, because it includes the most breast tissue and is the only whole-breast view to include the upper-outer quadrant and the axillary tail (Fig. 38.1) (16). It has been argued that screening should be done with a single view to reduce radiation exposure, cost and time (17, 18); however, some experienced radiologists have found that the sensitivity for cancer detection decreases when only the MLO view is performed. While it does not include as much breast tissue overall, the CC view better depicts the medial aspect of the breast and often gives sharper, higher-contrast images because better compression can be achieved (19). Furthermore, because of the lower specificity of single view screening, more patients need to be called back for additional views before a definitive interpretation (20, 21); therefore, two-view screening actually may be more cost-effective.

DIAGNOSTIC MAMMOGRAPHY

If the standard MLO and CC views have not been done as part of a recent screening examination, the diagnostic examination should begin with them. In addition to the standard views, a variety of additional views often are employed in diagnostic mammography. Exaggerated CC positioning to improve visualization of the lateral or medial aspects of the breast, magnification, and spot compression over an area of interest are examples of methods that are used to localize or define a lesion better.

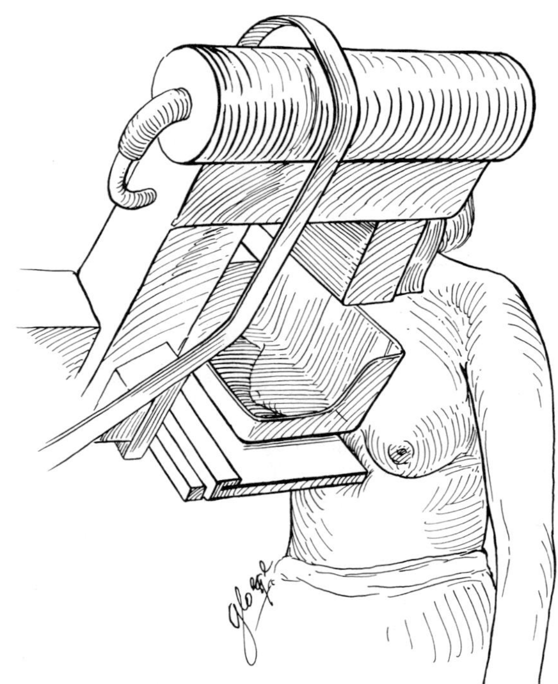

Figure 38.1. Positioning of the breast for mediolateral oblique projection. The film is placed under the breast and parallel to the plane of the pectoral muscle. The x-ray beam is directed from superomedial to inferolateral and perpendicular to the plane of the muscle. This view provides the most complete visualization of the breast and, in particular, the best depiction of the upper-outer quadrant and axillary tail of the breast.

It is important that the mammography facility be informed of any palpable mass at the time the mammogram is scheduled. At many facilities, a correlative physical examination is done on women with palpable masses to verify the location of the mass for purposes of positioning and interpretation. Once the location of the palpable mass is verified by an experienced radiologic technologist or the radiologist, a radiopaque lead shot (BB) is placed directly over the mass. The BB is used by the radiologic technologist during positioning to be certain that the lesion is included on the image, and the radiologist uses the visible BB to correlate mammographic findings with known clinical abnormalities while interpreting the examination. If the films show a circumscribed mass or the palpable mass cannot be seen because of overlying dense tissue, ultrasonography usually is performed.

Standardized Mammography Terminology and Reporting

Development of a standardized lexicon and report organization system is an important, recent advance in mammography. The American College of Radiology Breast Imaging

Data and Reporting System (BI-RADS™) was devised to standardize mammographic terminology, reduce confusing interpretations, and facilitate outcome monitoring (22). Terminology used to describe mammographic findings has evolved over many years, and lack of uniformity led to a great deal of confusion about the meanings of the terms used in reports. Confusing terms and equivocal reports also have been an impediment to assessing the impact of mammography on screened populations (23).

Once adopted nationwide, it is hoped that standardized reporting will eliminate confusing interpretations. In the standardized system, each descriptor used to describe abnormalities indicates a probability of malignancy. For example, the descriptors for the shape of a mass, listed in ascending order of probability of malignancy, are "round," "oval," "lobulated," or "irregular." The margins of a mass are described, in order of increasing likelihood of malignancy, as "circumscribed," "microlobulated," "obscured," "indistinct," or "spiculated."

The conclusion of the standardized mammography report always includes an overall, final assessment that indicates the probability of malignancy stated as one of five categories (Table 38.1). This scheme eliminates the possibility of equivocation or misunderstanding, identifies a specific management recommendation, and facilitates the follow-up and tracking of abnormal cases.

Normal Mammogram

The mammographic appearance of the normal breast can be quite variable. Appearance is based on the amount and distribution of fat and fibroglandular tissue. Fat is radiolucent (i.e., black) on mammograms and fibroglandular tissue is radiodense (i.e., white). Radiolucent fat provides a background in which small cancers can be detected more readily, which increases the accuracy of mammography (Fig. 38.2). Because dense tissue can obscure lesions, mammography is less accurate in women with dense breasts. Because more fibroglandular tissue is present in younger women, their breasts tend to be more "dense" (i.e., radiopaque, or white, on the mammogram) than the breasts of older women (Fig. 38.3). There is a wide variation in patterns, however. Dense tissue may be present in the mammograms of some older women, and some younger women may have fatty breasts. Nonetheless, the fibroglandular tissue tends to be replaced by fat as women age and have more children. This process is reversed during pregnancy, when the breasts become more dense, and an increase in density also has been associated with exogenous hormone therapy in postmenopausal women.

Abnormal Mammogram

Mammographic manifestations of malignancy can be divided into primary, secondary, and subtle or indirect signs. Primary signs include a mass and calcifications (Fig. 38.4). Secondary signs, such as skin thickening and retraction, usually are evident on clinical breast examination; when seen on mammograms, they usually are associated with an advanced cancer. Subtle or indirect signs include distortion of the "architecture" of the fibroglandular tissue, appearance of a new or evolving density in the breast, or asymmetry of the breast tissue.

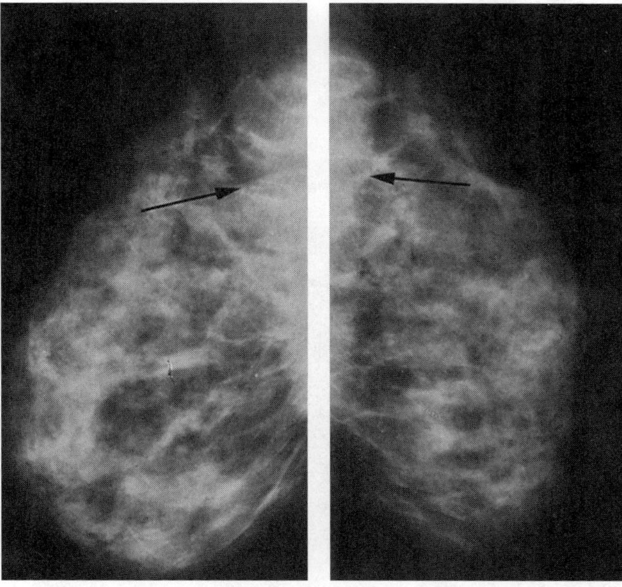

Figure 38.2. Bilateral mediolateral oblique views in a 45-year-old woman. These breasts are a mixture of dense fibroglandular tissue (*white*) and radiolucent fat (*dark gray*). The pectoral muscles (*arrows*) are seen at the posterior aspect of the breast. A small carcinoma could easily be obscured within one of the dense tissue areas.

Table 38.1. Mammography Final Assessment Categories

Category	Assessment	Description
1	Negative	—
2	Benign finding	A definitely benign finding is described
3	Probably benign finding	Very high probability of being benign. Short-term follow-up recommended to establish stability.
4	Suspicious abnormality	Not characteristic, but has reasonable probability of being malignant. Biopsy should be considered.
5	Highly suggestive of malignancy	High probability of being cancer. Appropiate action should be taken.

Adapted from American College of Radiology (22).

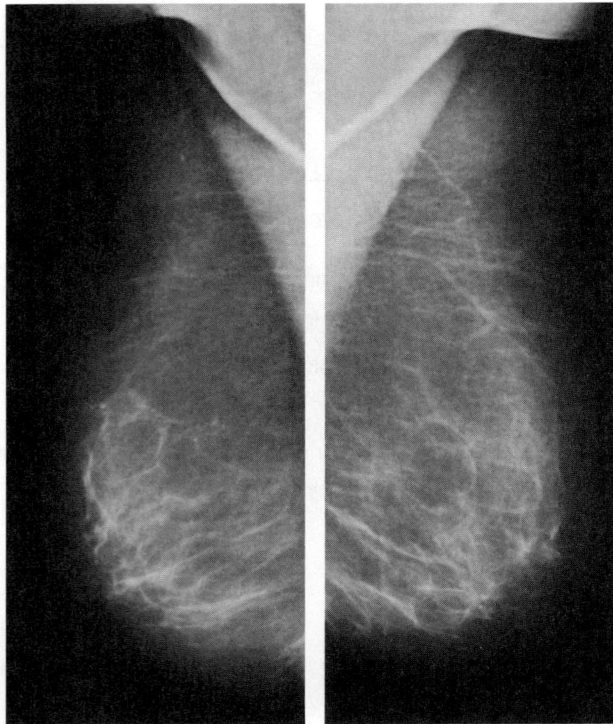

Figure 38.3. Bilateral mediolateral oblique views of a 65-year-old woman. Almost all fibroglandular tissue has been replaced by radiolucent fat. A small tumor would be visible at any location in this breast, unless it were not positioned properly over the film.

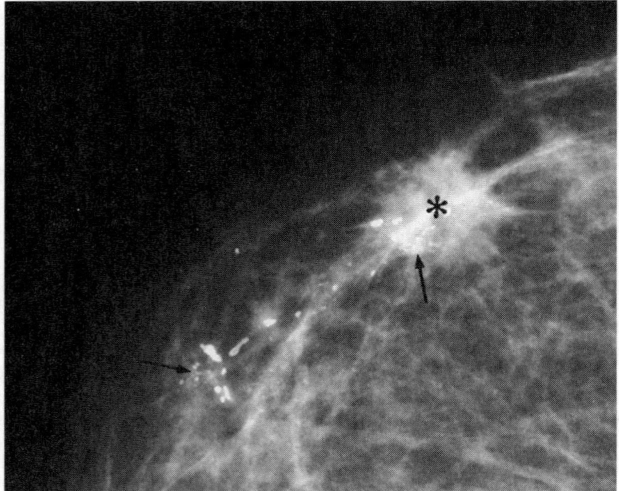

Figure 38.4. Ductal carcinoma manifested by a spiculated mass (*) and clusters of fine, malignant calcifications (*arrows*) both within and outside the tumor. The mass was an invasive carcinoma, with the calcifications representing extensive intraductal extension. The interpretation was "Highly suggestive of malignancy."

MALIGNANT MASSES

An irregular shape and ill-defined or spiculated margins are characteristic features indicating that a mass is malignant. The more highly infiltrative the lesion, the more spiculated the margin will appear on the mammogram (Fig. 38.4) (24).

MALIGNANT CALCIFICATIONS

Malignant calcifications may occur with or without an apparent mass (25). Calcifications typically are numerous, clustered, heterogeneous in size and shape, and linear and/or branching (Fig. 38.4). Calcifications often are the only evidence of an intraductal carcinoma (26), and the etiology of the calcifications of ductal carcinoma in situ (DCIS) is of interest. In comedo DCIS, the typical linear, branching calcifications form in the necrotic debris at the center of ducts filled with tumor cells. In noncomedo DCIS, the tiny calcifications of varying size and shape may result from an active, secretory process that produces aggregates of calcifications lodged within cribriform spaces or tumor excrescences within the duct.

SUBTLE OR INDIRECT SIGNS

Subtle signs have been reported to be the only findings in up to 20% of mammographically detected cancers (27). To recognize these signs, it is important to compare the right and left breasts and to have any previous mammograms available for comparison. Furthermore, a biopsy often can be avoided when the current findings are stable in comparison with those of previous mammograms.

The two breasts tend to be quite symmetrical with each other in their distribution of fibroglandular tissue. For this reason mammograms should be viewed so that the right and left breasts can be compared back to back on the viewbox. A minor asymmetry in fibroglandular tissue usually is a normal variant, but marked asymmetry should be worked up further. Our approach to the work-up of marked asymmetry on mammography begins with a correlative physical breast examination (i.e., palpation directed to the area of concern). Depending on the degree of suspicion, the next steps may be spot compression, ultrasonography, or 6-month follow-up mammography. When asymmetry is associated with architectural distortion, the probability of malignancy is greater and a biopsy should be considered.

BENIGN MASSES

The majority of benign masses (e.g., cysts, intramammary lymph nodes, fibroadenomas) have round or oval shapes. A circumscribed margin is the hallmark of a benign mass (Fig. 38.5) (24).

BENIGN CALCIFICATIONS

Compared with malignant calcifications, benign calcifications are more likely to be round, uniform, and coarse (Fig. 38.5). Calcifications that are widely scattered in both breasts are more likely to be benign.

PITFALLS IN MAMMOGRAPHIC INTERPRETATION

While masses with ill-defined or spiculated margins have a high probability of being malignant, a similar appearance occasionally may be seen with benign radial scars, sclerosing adenosis, posttraumatic fat necrosis, or biopsy scars (Fig. 38.6). With some cancers, the margins may only be slightly ill-defined, or even circumscribed. Occasionally, a

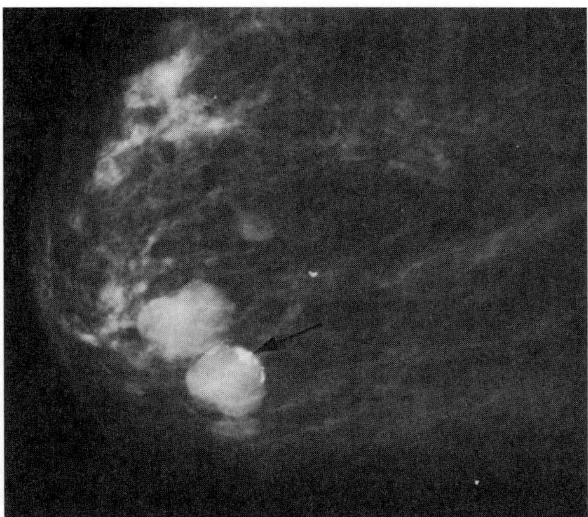

Figure 38.5. Benign lobulated masses in a 42-year-old woman. A combination of multiple masses with circumscribed margins and coarse calcifications (*arrow*) in the wall of one mass all point to benignity. Accordingly, biopsy was not done. The interpretation was "Benign findings: multiple fibroadenomas."

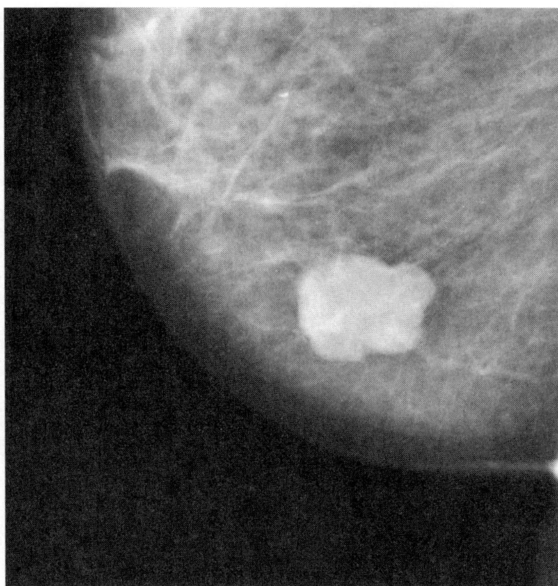

Figure 38.7. Circumscribed cancer in a 55-year-old woman. Ultrasonography revealed a solid mass. Because of its size and the woman's age, this solitary mass was of concern, even though the margins were circumscribed. The interpretation was "Suspicious abnormality. Biopsy should be considered." Biopsy revealed medullary carcinoma.

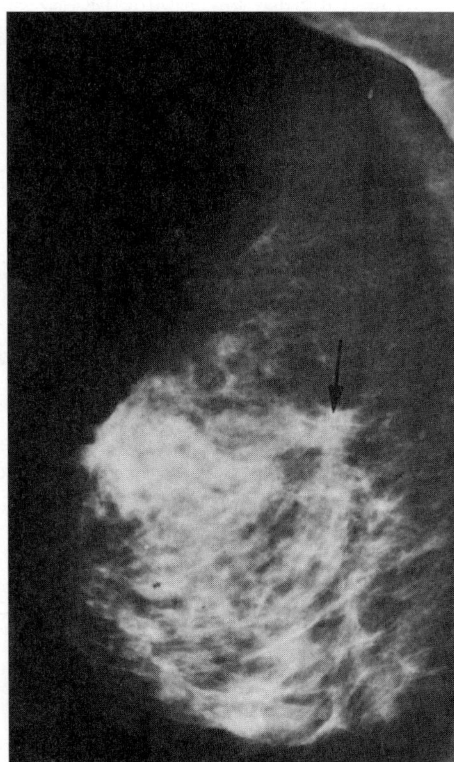

Figure 38.6. Biopsy scar mimicking malignancy. Routine mammography 6 months after surgery shows architectural distortion (*arrow*) where a fibroadenoma had been excised. The history of recent surgery at this location and the absence of a palpable mass are consistent with the radiologic interpretation of "Benign findings; post-surgical scar." Mammograms 1 year later revealed a decrease in the size of the scar.

carcinoma is so well circumscribed that it appears identical to a benign lesion (Fig. 38.7). Papillary, medullary, and colloid carcinomas are particularly likely to have circumscribed margins; however, because of their overall frequency, ductal carcinomas make up the largest percentage of circumscribed cancers.

Calcifications that are associated with sclerosing adenosis, fat necrosis, hyperplasia, or fibroadenoma sometimes can mimic those seen in malignancy, thus leading to false-positive mammograms. Therefore, clustered microcalcifications should be considered to be a sensitive, but not a specific, sign of breast cancer.

Imaging-Guided Needle Biopsy of the Breast

The positive predictive value for biopsies that are generated by mammographic abnormalities (i.e., the number of cancers detected divided by the number of biopsies done) is reported to be in the range of 10 to 40% (28). The costs of the nonproductive excisional biopsies generated by screening mammography therefore may exceed the costs of the screening mammograms, with the majority of biopsies yielding benign results (29). False-positive screening that lead to excisional biopsy also may lead to unnecessary morbidity and anxiety and have been reported to be a barrier that keeps women from participating in screening projects (30).

Needle biopsy is an attractive alternative to excisional biopsy. It is less expensive, is associated with less morbidity, and leaves no scar. At some institutions, particularly in Europe, fine-needle aspiration cytology (FNAC) has replaced excisional biopsies for mammographic abnormalities, thus reducing the overall costs of screening programs (31). Barriers to the wide acceptance of FNAC for mammographically detected abnormalities in the United States have included inadequate numbers of skilled cytopathologists to promote and validate the procedure, variability in the reported accuracy from one institution to another, high rates of insufficient samples, the requirement for extremely accurate needle placement, and the difficult U.S. medicolegal environment (32). The reported sensitivity for FNAC is in the range of 68 to 100%, specificity is from 82 to 100%, and rates of insufficient specimens from 2 to 36% (33). Even if adequate specimens are obtained, however, a definitive diagnosis is not always possible. Furthermore, infiltrating carcinoma cannot be differentiated from in situ carcinoma on FNAC.

Core needle biopsy (CNB) of the breast, which uses a large-bore, 14- or 16-gauge needle, is replacing FNAC for evaluating mammographic abnormalities at some institutions. Several investigators believe that CNB is superior to FNAC because (*a*) the interpretation can be rendered by surgical pathologists without special training in cytology, (*b*) insufficient specimens are less frequent, (*c*) CNB usually can differentiate in situ from invasive carcinoma, and (*d*) CNB can characterize lesions more completely (34). CNB of the breast for nonpalpable lesions can be guided by mammography or ultrasonography, but special stereotactic equipment is necessary to achieve the accuracy needed for mammographically guided core biopsy. Ultrasonography is gaining in popularity for the guidance of needle biopsies, partly because it does not require the purchase of new imaging equipment (35).

A range of sensitivities and specificities for core biopsy have been reported. In general, better results have been obtained with 14-gauge needles than with smaller-bore needles. One recent investigation showed that five specimens per lesion obtained with a 14-gauge needle achieved a 99% accuracy for breast masses (36); however, more than five specimens may be needed when the only mammographic abnormality is calcifications.

Several strategies will improve the results of CNB. Correlation of biopsy results with the mammographic findings is particularly important. If the results of mammography and CNB are discordant, consideration should be given to excisional biopsy, or at least to very close follow-up. Atypical ductal hyperplasia (ADH) is difficult to differentiate from ductal carcinoma in situ by CNB (37). Therefore, it is recommended that an excisional biopsy be performed when ADH has been diagnosed by CNB.

Prebiopsy Needle Localization

Imaging-guided needle localization is indicated before surgical excision of any nonpalpable mammographic lesion. The purpose of needle localization is to ensure the removal of a clinically occult lesion with the smallest possible breast deformity. Some variations on this method include (*a*) a direct needle approach, where the tip of a hypodermic needle is inserted as close as possible to the mammographic abnormality and left in place when the patient goes to surgery; (*b*) a "spot" method, which involves injecting methylene blue dye (0.1 mL) into the breast tissue through a needle that is positioned near the mammographic abnormality before the needle is removed; and (*c*) use of a needle to introduce a malleable wire with a barbed or round end, which is positioned at the site of the abnormality before open biopsy (38–41). Specimen radiography should be performed to verify that a nonpalpable lesion has been removed (42). If the abnormality (e.g., suspicious calcifications) is not identified in the specimen radiograph, removal of more tissue usually is indicated.

Postsurgical Breast

Postsurgical changes on mammograms may include skin thickening or retraction, architectural distortion (Fig. 38.6), asymmetry, calcification, and fat necrosis (43). Any of these changes can mimic carcinoma, and knowing the location of previous breast surgeries is important when interpreting mammograms. If patients have undergone breast-conserving surgery for carcinoma, it is particularly useful to know the location of the scar and to compare the current study with previous baseline studies when interpreting the mammograms. We routinely place a wire over a previous surgical site so that it can be recognized on the mammogram. When breast-conservation therapy is performed for extensive, intraductal carcinoma manifested by calcifications, we perform magnification mammography directly over the surgical site before radiotherapy to identify any residual malignant calcifications (44).

Mammography for Staging

In addition to clinical examination and diagnostic blood work, the pretreatment staging protocol for breast cancer should include chest radiography and bilateral mammography. Mammography before biopsy of a palpable abnormality is used to exclude bilateral and multifocal lesions; however, mammography is not performed preoperatively to evaluate the axillary nodes. While normal-sized or enlarged axillary nodes can be visualized in MLO views, there are no mammographic criteria that can exclude nodal involvement (45). Therefore, histologic assessment is essential when staging invasive carcinomas.

Other Breast Imaging Methods

DIGITAL MAMMOGRAPHY

Digital mammography records the image electronically in a digital format rather than primarily on film. The digital image can be displayed on a fluorescent monitor and stored in a computer database. Potential uses of digital studies are image manipulation to bring out areas of interest, computer-aided diagnosis, and teleradiography. Hopefully, digital mammography eventually will overcome some of the problems that are inherent in film mammography, such as limited resolution, film-storage space requirements, and the possibility of films being lost. The ability to send digital images almost instantaneously over long distances also opens the possibility for greater access to studies and consultations with experts (46). The technology required to make whole-breast digital images of the quality obtained with film-screen combinations is not yet available, however, but it is possible to make excellent digital images of small areas within the breast. Because film processing is eliminated, digital images can be viewed within seconds; as a result, digital imaging already is useful for stereotactic guidance of needle biopsies.

ULTRASONOGRAPHY

While ultrasonography is not reliable for screening, breast sonography is an important adjunct to mammography for diagnostic examinations (47). It frequently is used to characterize palpable abnormalities and to clarify ambiguous mammographic findings. Ultrasonography also is used to guide many interventional procedures, including cyst aspiration and needle biopsy (35). Its most important use, however, is in the evaluation of circumscribed masses to determine whether they are cystic or solid (Fig. 38.8), especially when the masses are seen mammographically but are not palpable (48). The sonographic features of a solid mass also contribute evidence as to the probability of malignancy (Fig. 38.9). In addition, ultrasonography also can be used to evaluate the integrity of breast implants, but it is not as accurate as magnetic resonance imaging (MRI) for detecting implant ruptures (49).

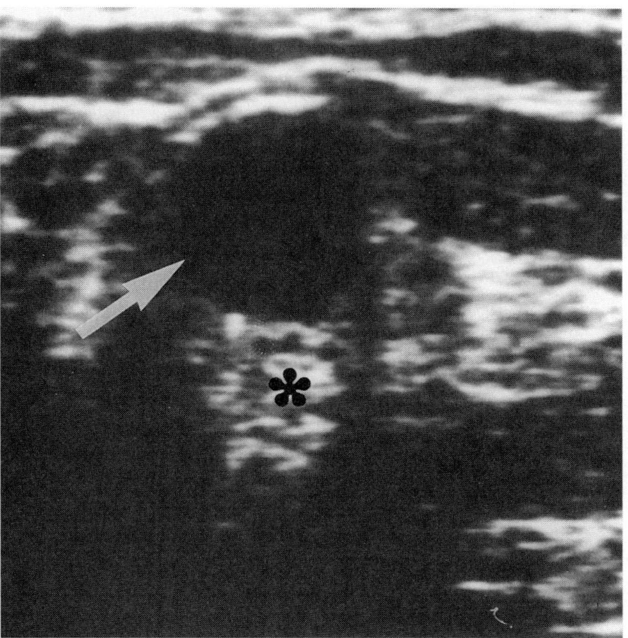

Figure 38.8. Ultrasonogram of a palpable mass in a 45-year-old woman. Mammograms with a BB placed over the site of the palpable finding showed dense tissue but no mass. At ultrasonography, the mass (*arrow*) had no internal echoes and showed enhanced sound transmission (*) distal to the mass, indicating a typical cyst. The interpretation of the diagnostic examination was "Benign findings. Ultrasound revealed a cyst at the site of the palpable mass."

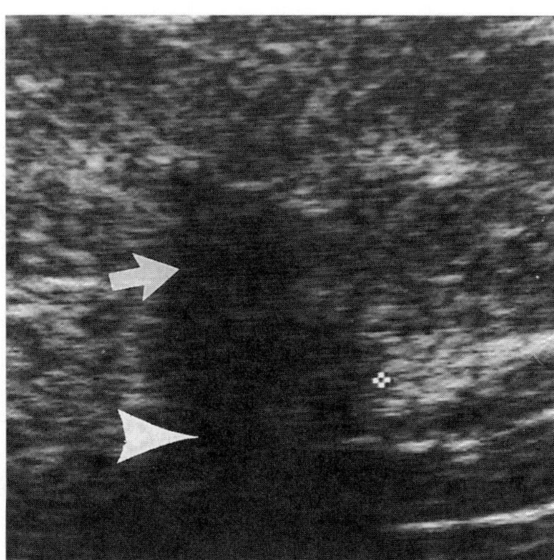

Figure 38.9. Ultrasonogram of a palpable mass in a 32-year-old woman revealing a mass (*arrow*) with an irregular shape, heterogeneous low-level echoes, and attenuation of distal echoes (*arrowhead*). These signs are associated with malignancy, but subsequent mammography revealed only dense fibroglandular tissue. The interpretation of the diagnostic examination was "Suspicious abnormality. Ultrasound reveals irregular mass at the site of the palpable abnormality."

MAGNETIC RESONANCE IMAGING OF THE BREAST

Magnetic resonance imaging has been applied successfully to the evaluation of silicone breast implants for intracapsular and extracapsular rupture; in fact, it is the most sensitive method to detect ruptures (50). Initial studies were conducted in the 1980s to determine the potential value of MRI for detecting breast cancer (51), and these early studies failed to identify a potential role for MRI. Recent investigations, however, using newer technology and intravenous magnetic resonance contrast injections show promise (52–55). When used with contrast agents, MRI has a high sensitivity for the detection of breast cancers; however, both high cost and the requirement for an intravenous injection currently prohibit its use as a screening tool. In addition, many benign lesions show contrast enhancement on MRI. Another limitation is that MRI does not identify malignant calcifications reliably. Nonetheless, there are several potential roles for MRI of the breast including (*a*) determining the size and extent of invasive cancers (i.e., staging), (*b*) imaging the extremely dense breast, (*c*) identifying recurrence of cancer in the conservatively treated breast, and (*d*) preoperative evaluation of suspicious mammographic abnormalities. Further investigation is needed before the exact role of MRI in the evaluation of breast cancer can be determined.

OTHER MODALITIES

Another area of active investigation involves radionuclide scanning of the breast after the injection of radionuclide-labelled substances that concentrate in breast tumors. For example, tumor uptake has been identified on positron emission tomography after the injection of fluorine-18 2-deoxy-2-fluoro-D-glucose (56). This agent also accumulates in axillary nodes which could potentially provide information about nodal status without surgery. Other investigators are scanning the breasts after the injection of technetium-99m sestamibi (2-methoxy isobutyl isonitral) (57). These methods will require additional studies to determine sensitivity and specificity in clinical populations as well as their cost-effectiveness.

References

1. Wingo PA, Tong T, Bolden S. Cancer Statistics, 1995. CA 1995;45:8–30.
2. Seidman H, Stellman SD, Mushinski MH. A different perspective on breast cancer risk factors: some implications for the nonattributable risk. CA 1982;32:301.
3. Tabár L, Fagerberg CJ, Gad A, Baldetorp L, Holmberg LH, Grontoft O, Ljungquist U, Lundstrom B, Manson JC, Eklund G, Day NE, Pettersson F. Reduction in mortality from breast cancer after mass screening with mammography. Randomized trial from the Breast Cancer Screening Working Group of the Swedish National Board of Health and Welfare. Lancet 1985;1:829.
4. Bassett LW, Hendrick RE, Bassford TL, Butler PF, Carter D, DeBor M, D'Orsi CJ, Garlinghouse CJ, Jones RF, Langer AS, Lichtenfeld JL, Osuch JR, Reynolds LN, de Paredes ES, Williams RE. Quality Determinants of Mammography. Clinical Practice Guideline, No. 13. AHCPR Publication No. 95-0632. Rockville, MD: Agency for Health Care Policy and Research, Public Health Service, U.S. Department of Health and Human Services, 1994.
5. American College of Radiology (ACR) Standards for the performance of screening mammography [Adopted by the ACR Council 1990; Revised 1994]. In ACR Digest of Official Actions. Reston, VA: ACR, 1994.
6. Fletcher SW, Black W, Harris R, Rimer BK, Shapiro S. Report of the international workshop on screening for breast cancer. JNCI 1993;85:1644.
7. Committee on Government Relations. Misused science: the National Cancer Institute's elimination of mammography guidelines for women in their forties. Washington, DC: U.S. Government Printing Office, 1994.
8. Mettlin C, Smart CR. Breast cancer detection guidelines for women aged 40 to 49 years: rationale for the American Cancer Society reaffirmation of recommendations. CA 1994;44:248.
9. American College of Radiology (ACR). Standards for the performance of diagnostic mammography and problem-solving breast evaluation [Adopted by the ACR Council 1994]. In ACR Digest of Official Actions. Reston, VA: ACR, 1994.
10. Jackson VP, Lex AM, Smith DJ. Patient discomfort during screen-film mammography. Radiology 1988;168:421.
11. Stomper PC, Kopans DB, Sadowsky NL, Sonnenfeld MR, Swann CA, Gelman RS, Meyer JE, Jochelson MS, Hunt MS, Allen PD. Is mammography painful: a multicenter patient study. Arch Intern Med 1988;148:521.
12. Brew MD, Billings JD, Chisholm RJ. Mammography and breast pain. Australas Radiol 1989;33:335.
13. Sickles EA, Weber WN, Galvin HB, Ominsky SH, Sollitto RA. Mammographic screening: how to operate successfully at low cost. Radiology 1986;160:95.
14. U.S. General Accounting Office. Screening Mammography: Low Cost Services Do Not Compromise Quality. General Accounting Office Report HRD-90-92. Washington, D.C.: General Accounting Office, 1990.
15. Houn F, Brown ML. Current practice of screening mammography in the United States: Data from the National Survey of Mammography Facilities. Radiology 1994;190:290.
16. Bassett LW, Gold RH. Breast radiography using the oblique projection. Radiology 1983;149:585.
17. Lundgren B, Jakobsson. Single view mammography: a simple and efficient approach to breast cancer screening. Cancer 1976;38:1124.
18. Moskowitz M, Libshitz H. Mammographic screening for breast cancer by lateral view only: is it practical? J Can Assoc Radiol 1977;28:259.
19. Helvie MA, Chang H-P, Adler DD, Boyd PG. Breast thickness on routine mammograms: effect on image quality and radiation dose. AJR 1994;163:1371.
20. Bassett LW, Bunnell DHR, Gold RH, Arndt RD, Linsman J. Breast cancer detection: one versus two views. Radiology 1987;165:95.
21. Sickles EA, Weber WN, Galvin HB, Ominsky SH, Sollitto RA. Baseline screening mammography: one versus two views per breast. AJR 1986;147:1149.
22. American College of Radiology (ACR). Breast Imaging Reporting and Data System (BI-RADS). Reston, VA: ACR, 1992.
23. Farria DM, Anderson L, Rawson TK, Smith RA, Bassett LW, Mund DF, Maxwell JR. Mammography reports: are they really a problem? Radiology 1994;193(P):217.
24. Gold RH, Montgomery CK, ON. Significance of margination of benign and malignant infiltrative mammary lesions: roentgenographic-pathological correlation. AJR 1973;118:881.
25. Egan RL, McSweeney MB, Sewell C. Intramammary calcifications without an associated mass in benign and malignant diseases. Radiology 1980;137:1.
26. Stomper PC, Connelly JL, Meyer JE, Harris JR. Clinically occult ductal carcinoma in situ detected with mammography: analysis of 100 cases with radiologic-pathologic correlation. Radiology 1989;172:235.
27. Sickles EA. Mammographic features of 300 consecutive nonpalpable breast cancers. AJR 1986;146:661.
28. Bassett LW, Liu T-H, Giuliano AE, Gold RH. The prevalence of carcinoma in palpable vs impalpable mammographically detected lesions. AJR 1991;157:21.
29. Cyrlak D. Induced costs of low-cost screening mammography. Radiology 1988;168:661.
30. Howard J. Using mammography for cancer control: an unrealized potential. CA 1987;37:33.
31. Assayed E, Sane G, Auer G. Stereotactic fine needle biopsy in 2594 mammographically-detected nonpalpable lesions. Lancet 1989;1:1033.
32. Jackson VP, Bassett LW. Stereotactic fine-needle aspiration biopsy for nonpalpable breast lesions. AJR 196;154:1;1990.
33. Masood S. Occult breast lesions and aspiration biopsy: a new challenge. Diagnostic Cytopathol 1993;9:613.
34. Parker SH, Lovin JD, Jobe WE, Burke FJ, Hopper KD, Yakes WF. Nonpalpable breast lesions: stereotactic automated large-core biopsies. Radiology 1991;180:403.
35. Fornage BD, Coan JD, David CL. Ultrasound-guided needle biopsy of the breast and other interventional procedures. Radiol Clin North Am 1992;30:167.
36. Liberman L, Dershaw DD, Rosen PP, Abramson AF, Deutch BM, Hann LE. Stereotaxic 14-gauge breast biopsy: how many core biopsy specimens are needed? Radiology 1994;192:793.
37. Jackman RJ, Nowels KW, Shepard MJ, Finkelstein SI, Marzoni FA Jr. Stereotaxic large-core needle biopsy of 450 nonpalpable breast lesions with surgical correlation in lesions with cancer or atypical hyperplasia. Radiology 1994;193:91.
38. Egan JF, Sayler CB, Goodman MJ. A technique for localizing occult breast lesions. CA 1976;26:32.
39. Homer MJ. Nonpalpable breast lesion localization using a curved-end retractable wire. Radiology 1985;157:259.
40. Kopans DB, Meyer JE. Versatile spring hookwire breast lesion localizer. AJR 1982;138:586.
41. Threatt B, Appelman H, Dow R, O'Rourke T. Percutaneous needle localization of clustered mammary microcalcifications prior to biopsy. Am J Roentgenol Radium Ther Nucl Med 1974;121:839.
42. Snyder RE. Specimen radiography and preoperative localization of nonpalpable breast cancer. Cancer 1980;46:950.
43. Sickles EA, Herzog KA. Mammography of the postsurgical breast. AJR 1981;136:585.
44. Mendelson EB. Evaluation of the postoperative breast. Radiol Clin North Am 1992;30:107.
45. Kalisher L, Chu AM, Peyster RG. Clinicopathological correlations of xeroradiography in determining involvement of metastatic axillary nodes in female breast cancer. Radiology 1976;121:333.
46. Shtern F. Digital mammography and related technologies: a perspective from the National Cancer Institute. Radiology 1992;183:629.
47. Bassett LW, Kimme-Smith C, Sutherland LK, Gold RH, Sarti D, King W III. Automatic and hand-held breast US: effect on patient management. Radiology 1987;165:130.
48. Hilton SV, Leopold GR, Olson LK, Willson SA. Real-time breast sonography: application in 300 consecutive patients. AJR 1986;147:479.
49. DeBruhl ND, Gorczyca DP, Ahn CY, Shaw WW, Bassett LW. Silicone breast implants: US evaluation. Radiology 1993;189:95.
50. Gorczyca DP, Sinha S, Ahn CY, DeBruhl ND, Hayes MK, Gausche VR, Shaw WW, Bassett LW. Silicone breast implants *in vivo*: MR imaging. Radiology 1992;185:407.
51. El Yousef SJ, O'Connell DM, Duchesneau RH, Smith MJ, Hubay CA, Guyton SP. Benign and malignant breast disease: magnetic resonance and radiofrequency pulse sequences. AJR 1985;145:1.
52. Harms SE, Flamig DP, Evans WP, Harries SA, Bown S. MR imaging of the breast: current status and future potential. AJR 1994;163:1039.
53. Heywang SH, Wolf A, Pruss E, Hilbertz T, Eiermann W, Permanetter W. MR imaging of the breast with Gd-DTPA: use and limitations. Radiology 1989;171:95.
54. Heywang-Kobrunner SH, Schlegel A, Beck R, Wendt T, Kellner W, Lommatzsch B, Untch M, Nathrath WB. Contrast-enhanced MRI of the breast after limited surgery and radiation therapy. J Comput Assist Tomogr 1993;17:891.
55. Orel SG, Schnall MD, LiVolsi VA, Troupin RH. Suspicious breast lesions: MR imaging with radiographic-pathologic correlation. Radiology 1994;190:485.
56. Adler LP, Crowe JP, Al-Kaisi NK, Sunshine JL. Evaluation of breast masses and axillary lymph nodes with (F-18) 2-deoxy-2-fluoro-D-glucose PET. Radiology 1993;187:743.
57. Khalkhali I, Mena I, Jouanne E, Diggles L, Venegas R, Block J, Alle K, Klein S. Prone scintimammography in patients with suspicion of carcinoma of the breast. J Am Coll Surg 1994;178:491.

CHAPTER 39

Ultrasound in Cancer Medicine

EDWARD G. GRANT

Sonography has been used for more than 30 years for the simple differentiation of cystic and solid lesions. Although variations in this application continue to have some clinical value, advances in technology now enable ultrasonography (US) to be used for an increasing number of applications that appear to be far removed from its original purpose. Technical breakthroughs in US equipment have led, in particular, to improvements in spatial resolution and tissue contrast. US imaging is also performed in real time (like fluoroscopic imaging). The incorporation of Doppler (both duplex and color) technology permits the noninvasive evaluation of vascular abnormalities, including some that may be associated with tumors.

Despite these technological advancements, some basic limitations of US imaging persist, particularly the inability of sound waves to penetrate bone or gas. Therefore, US is infrequently used in the evaluation of the central nervous system (CNS) or the parenchyma of the lung.

Central Nervous System Ultrasonography

There is one notable exception in the CNS, however, and that is the use of US during intracranial surgery. In this procedure, a sheathed US transducer is placed directly on the exposed brain to facilitate the approach to a known lesion and minimize damage to surrounding normal brain (Fig. 39.1) (12). In addition, US can be used to ensure that a resection has been complete. Intraoperative US can also be used to assist in the resection of spinal masses (19), including tumors and arteriovenous malformations (24).

Head and Neck Ultrasonography

Although the role of US imaging inside the skull is limited, the soft tissues of the head and neck are readily accessible to high-resolution US. US has been used to differentiate cystic from solid thyroid nodules, and it can readily depict small thyroid masses. In this regard, US has better resolution than either nuclear scintigraphy or computed tomography (CT). The ability to identify small lesions can be of particular value in differentiating solitary from multiple nodules, and it makes US an excellent method of evaluating and following patients with a history of thyroid irradiation early in life. In addition, the ability to identify small thyroid masses and to guide biopsies makes US the preferred method for finding an occult thyroid cancer in a patient who presents with metastatic disease that is compatible with a thyroid origin (28). US can also distinguish adenopathy involving anterior cervical nodes from thyroid masses. Gooding and colleagues also showed that US is uniquely capable of demonstrating whether or not there is carotid involvement by cervical adenopathy (9).

Although US is less commonly used in the United States for this purpose than in Europe, a number of studies indicate that it may be useful for staging patients with cancer of the floor of the mouth (8, 11). The relative lack of enthusiasm in the United States for using US to evaluate oral neoplasms probably reflects the ready availability of CT and magnetic resonance imaging (MRI). US does have the advantage of being a real-time examination, however, and, therefore, may be of special value in identifying fixation when a tumor invades the tongue, vocal cords, or other normally mobile structures. Other uses for US in the head and neck include the identification of enlarged parathyroid glands in patients with hypercalcemia (Fig. 39.2) and the evaluation of parotid masses (24, 31).

Thoracic Ultrasonography

In the thorax, the use of US is usually limited to localizing or evaluating pleural opacities that have been identified previously on radiographs. The ultrasonographer should be capable of differentiating between free and loculated effusions, determining which are amenable to thoracentesis (an effusion with numerous internal septa or locules may require thoracotomy), and finding the optimum site for puncture. Tube insertion for pleural drainage or drug administration and other interventional procedures can also be performed under US guidance (17). Within the effusion itself, US can also demonstrate collapsed lung and differentiate it from consolidation without atelectasis.

Color Doppler imaging can be used to evaluate vessels in the neck, upper thorax, and arms. Thrombosed vessels can be readily differentiated from normal ones or those compressed by extraluminal masses. The ability to depict venous flow may be of particular value in the cancer patient who presents with acute or chronic arm swelling, and color Doppler US should be highly accurate for evaluating thromboses in the jugular, subclavian, and axillary veins (Fig. 39.3) (10, 13). The proximal subclavian and innominate veins may be difficult to image with US, however, and may require MRI

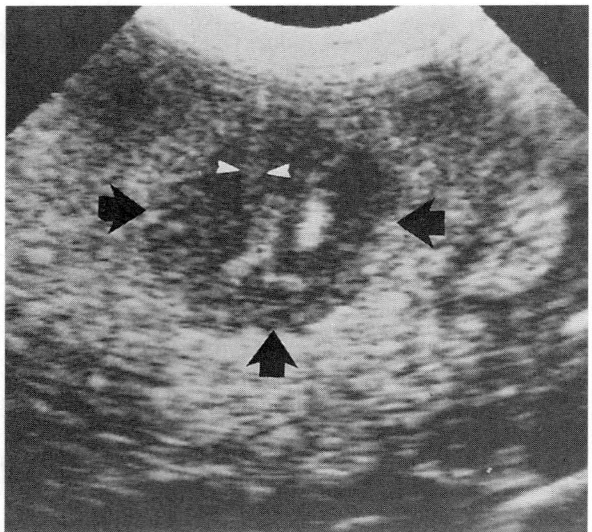

Figure 39.1. Intraoperative sonogram of a patient with a history of melanoma who was found to have a small superficial mass in the right frontal lobe on CT. At surgery the lesion was not palpable, and US was used to guide biopsy and resection. Note well-defined hypoechoic mass (*arrows*) and biopsy needle within the metastasis (*arrowheads*).

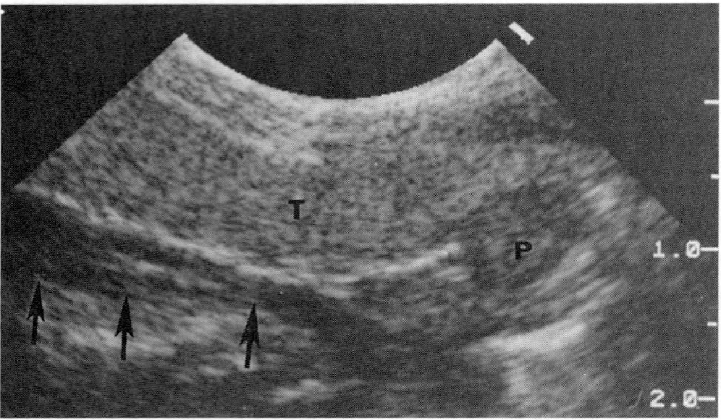

Figure 39.2. Parathyroid adenoma: US study on patient with metastatic breast carcinoma and elevated calcium levels. On a longitudinal (sagittal) section through left thyroid gland (T), note well-defined hypoechoic mass inferior to the thyroid, which is typical of parathyroid adenoma (P). *Arrows*, longus colli muscle (head of patient is to the left; foot is to the right; skin of anterior neck is at top).

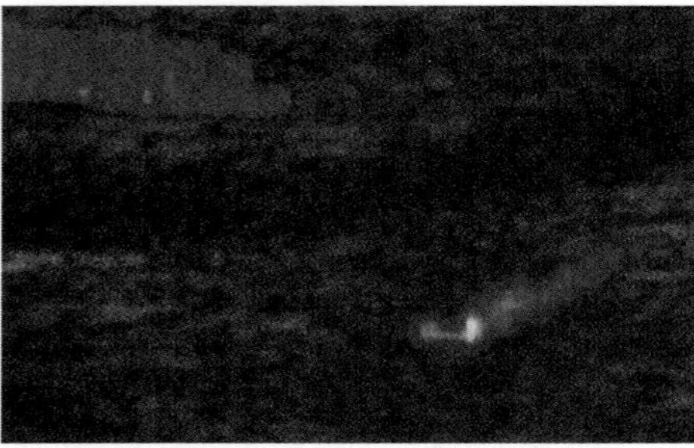

Figure 39.3. After a left mastectomy and subsequent irradiation, a 55-year-old woman presented with acute onset of severe left arm swelling. Color Doppler imaging revealed extensive thrombosis of left subclavian/brachial venous system. Note arterial flow (*red*) adjacent to vein (*no color*), which shows no flow and is filled with low-level echoes representing a blood clot.

or contrast venography. The potential of color Doppler imaging for evaluating patients with the superior vena cava syndrome remains to be investigated.

Endoscopic US is a relatively new adaptation of sonography. This technique requires the incorporation of a minute transducer into the tip of an endoscope and enables the operator to see tissues that are deep to mucosal surfaces. This technique is being used increasingly, and it is an excellent method for assessing the depth of penetration of esophageal and gastric neoplasms, identifying nodal involvement, and defining the internal characteristics of submucosal masses, both benign and malignant (Fig. 39.4) (29). Endoscopic US may eventually prove to be an essential component in evaluating the mediastinum of patients who have potential nodal spread to that area, since neither CT nor MRI has proved to be as accurate as once hoped.

Breast Ultrasonography

Outside the pleural cavity, the main application of thoracic US is in breast imaging. It is typically used to differentiate solid from cystic masses. Some investigators have attempted to use US Doppler analysis to differentiate benign from malignant breast masses, but the technique is not yet sufficiently developed to obviate the need for biopsy (26). Another recent application of US in breast cancer has been to detect adenopathy in the internal mammary lymph node

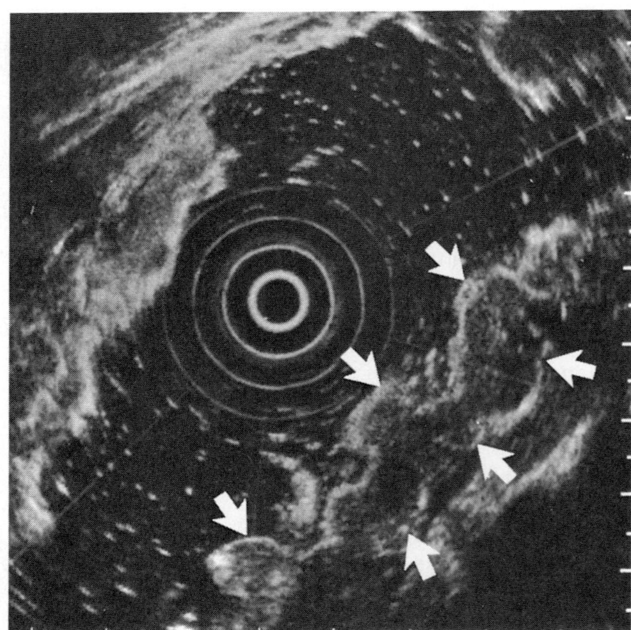

Figure 39.4. Endoscopic sonogram of a patient with weight loss. Thickened gastric folds were noted on an upper GI study. Endoscopic US is suggestive of lymphoma. Note marked thickening of wall of stomach (*arrows*), with preservation of mucosa. Central ring-like structure is a combination of the endoscopic US scanner itself and reverberation artifact. Dark, speckled area is water (with small air bubbles) that has been instilled into the stomach for better imaging of the wall. No perigastric lymph nodes were identified.

chain (24). The addition of color Doppler imaging will facilitate identification of the internal mammary vessels as they course beneath the upper ribs, and therefore help to define adjacent adenopathy.

Abdominal Ultrasonography

US is often considered to be an adjunctive imaging technique for evaluating the abdomen in the cancer patient. Screening for metastatic liver disease, for example, is better done with CT. However, US can be of use in many situations, such as in the differentiation of cystic and solid lesions in the liver. Brick and colleagues found US to be of particular value when further characterization was necessary for small indeterminate lesions identified on CT scan (2). US is also an excellent method for following measurable abdominal disease in patients who are on treatment protocols. The spatial resolution of US is currently comparable to that of CT, the study is far less expensive (usually one-third to one-half the cost of CT), it requires no contrast agent injection, and it may be more readily available at some institutions.

Although CT is generally preferred now for evaluating metastatic liver disease, US has been applied widely as the primary screening modality for asymptomatic patients who are at risk for hepatocellular carcinoma (3). Yearly US studies are recommended in people with chronic active hepatitis and some forms of cirrhosis. In patients with hepatocellular carcinoma, US has also been used to monitor the placement of needles for percutaneous ethanol ablation (15). US remains an excellent and cost-efficient method for guiding percutaneous biopsy of any hepatic (Fig. 39.5) or other abdominal mass, and it has also been used to guide the placement of radiation trocars in patients with metastatic liver disease (6).

US is the primary imaging modality in the initial evaluation of patients with jaundice and can demonstrate intrahepatic ductal dilation quite accurately. Although the actual identification of an obstructing lesion may not always be possible (strictures and stones may be particularly difficult to image), pancreatic masses or adenopathy should be visualized in the majority of patients and can then be biopsied under US guidance (14). Once biliary obstruction is identified, color Doppler imaging can be used to differentiate dilated biliary radicals from adjacent portal veins. This can be of practical import when percutaneous biliary drainage is being considered, since US can be used to guide the needle into a nonvascular lumen.

Although most of the uses for conventional US in the liver are now well established, color Doppler imaging has opened up several new windows of opportunity. In particular, this technique provides a noninvasive method for evaluating the hepatic vasculature. Portal vein thrombosis or compression by external masses is readily depicted with color Doppler imaging (5). Color Doppler imaging is also an excellent method for evaluating a suspected Budd-Chiari syndrome, and it is capable of differentiating venous compression by tumor from thrombosis of the hepatic veins or inferior vena cava (Fig. 39.6) (8). A unique group of cancer patients at risk for hepatic veno-occlusive disease are those who have undergone certain regimens of intensive chemotherapy and bone marrow transplantation. Unlike most patients with Budd-Chiari syndrome, who have gross thrombosis or tumor involvement of the major hepatic veins, patients with the syndrome who have undergone chemotherapy and bone mar-

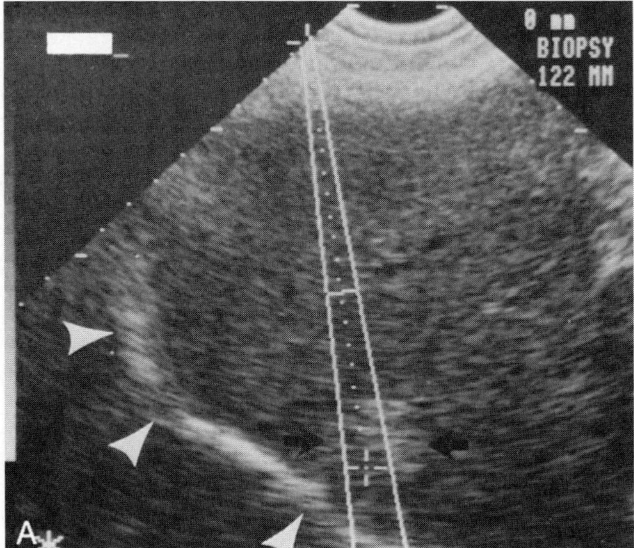

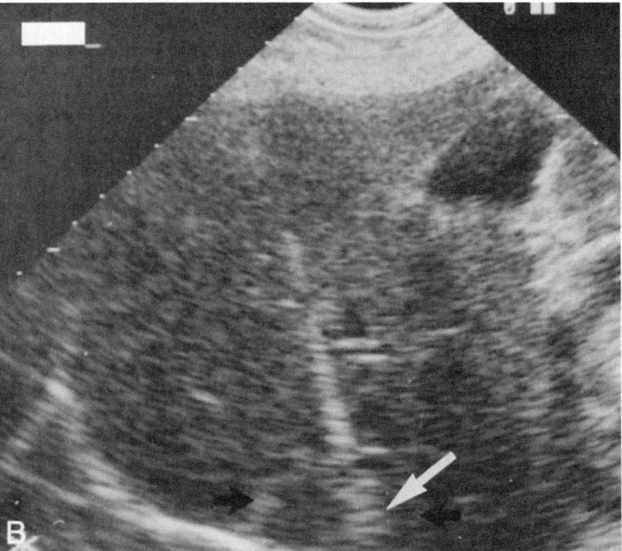

Figure 39.5. US-guided biopsy, sagittal scans. An echogenic mass was identified in posterior right lobe of the liver in a patient with a history of ovarian carcinoma. **A.** *Arrows*, demarcate liver mass adjacent to diaphragm (*arrowheads*). A needle guide was placed on the US transducer, and the expected path of the biopsy needle through the liver was displayed electronically (*white lines*) on the US monitor. Depth of the lesion can also be determined. **B.** Repeat scan obtained during biopsy confirmed proper position of needle (*white arrow*). Head of patient is toward left on both scans; foot is toward the right. Anterior abdominal wall is at top.

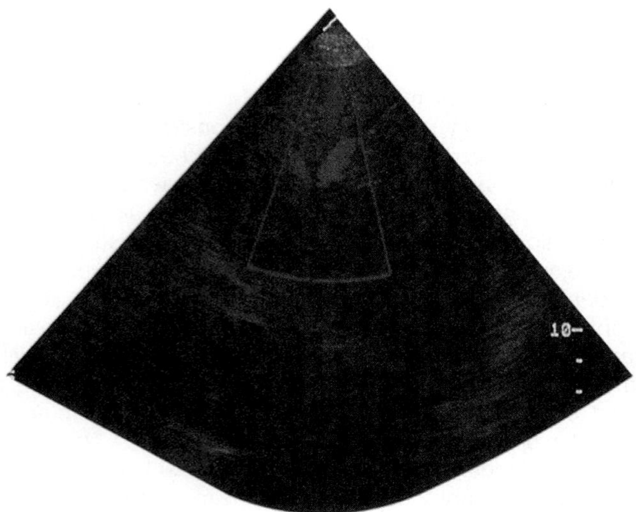

Figure 39.6. Color flow Doppler reveals normally directed flow in one hepatic vein branch (*blue, lower left*) and reversed flow in an adjacent branch (*red*). This finding is diagnostic of Budd-Chiari syndrome.

row transplantation have obstruction at the level of the hepatic venules. The major hepatic veins remain patent, and contrast venography may be normal. However, Doppler imaging may indicate the correct diagnosis by showing reversal of portal vein flow (1). Although Doppler imaging can be of assistance in evaluating the hepatic veins and the portal vein, it has not led to increased specificity in characterizing hepatic masses. Color Doppler imaging can assist in determining if a mass is relatively vascular or nonvascular, but so far it seems incapable of distinguishing among primary cancers, metastases and benign lesions, particularly hemangiomas.

Intraoperative Ultrasonography

A recent adaptation of conventional US that has direct application to the cancer patient is its intraoperative use in patients undergoing hepatic resection for hepatoma or metastatic disease. In this situation, US has both diagnostic and therapeutic potential. Several authors have shown that intraoperative US is more accurate at identifying hepatic masses than are any of the routinely used noninvasive techniques, including CT and MRI (4). The finding of previously unknown masses during intraoperative US has serious implications. Small or deep tumors may not be obvious to the surgeon and could be left behind. Additionally, new masses may be found in a separate segment or lobe of the liver, requiring a change in surgical approach (18). In some cases, depending on the location of the newly found lesions, resection may not be indicated at all, saving the patient a major surgical procedure that would have had little or no benefit. Finally, intraoperative US can be used to guide the surgeon to hepatic (or other abdominal) tumors when such tumors are difficult to palpate.

Retroperitonal Ultrasonography

In the retroperitoneum, the primary uses for US include assessments of kidney size, contour, and internal echo characteristics; the detection of hydronephrosis; and the characterization of cystic or solid masses. Although several authors have reported specific Doppler signal patterns in renal carcinomas, this is probably of little practical significance, since surgery or biopsy must still be performed on all solid renal masses (26). However, color Doppler imaging can be used to identify renal vein thrombosis (with or without tumor) and the level of extension of a thrombus into the inferior vena cava. In fact, inferior vena caval obstruction of any type can be assessed using color Doppler, and iliofemoral thromboses also may now be assessed using duplex or color Doppler imaging.

Although US can readily demonstrate vessels in the retroperitoneum, the presence or absence of adenopathy is usually better determined with CT. A notable exception may be patients with testicular tumors (27). However, the improved accuracy of US for identifying para-aortic adenopathy in this disease may be the result of the thinner body habitus of many young patients with testicular cancer, and it is probably not inherent in the pathology. In general, US may be an excellent alternative to CT for evaluating the retroperitoneum in thin patients.

Pelvic and Endovaginal Ultrasonography

In pelvic neoplastic diseases, current staging procedures now rely primarily on CT for definitive imaging information. However, the preliminary evaluation of most pelvic masses continues to be done with US. US has been quite successful in separating lesions that are gynecologic from those that are not, and in helping to characterize lesions of the uterus and ovaries. A new variation in US technique is endovaginal US. The proximity of the endovaginal transducer to the uterus and ovaries produces images that are far superior to those obtained with transabdominal scanning methods. The endovaginal technique is readily accepted by most women (including postmenopausal women) and does not require a full bladder.

In examining the uterus, thickening of the endometrial lining is exquisitely depicted by endovaginal US (Fig. 39.7A), as are small submucosal leiomyomas. In particular, small leiomyomas that may be sources of vaginal bleeding often are not seen with conventional transabdominal scanning techniques. In a patient with a known or suspected adnexal mass, endovaginal US can define the lesion's internal characteristics far better than conventional US and can provide a more definitive diagnosis in many cases (Fig. 39.7B). The improved resolution of this technique also may facilitate differentiation of a large ovary from a true mass. A recent potential application of endovaginal US is to screen asymptomatic women for ovarian carcinoma, since the technique is capable of demonstrating ovarian lesions before they cause a palpable mass. Unfortunately, unlike mammographic

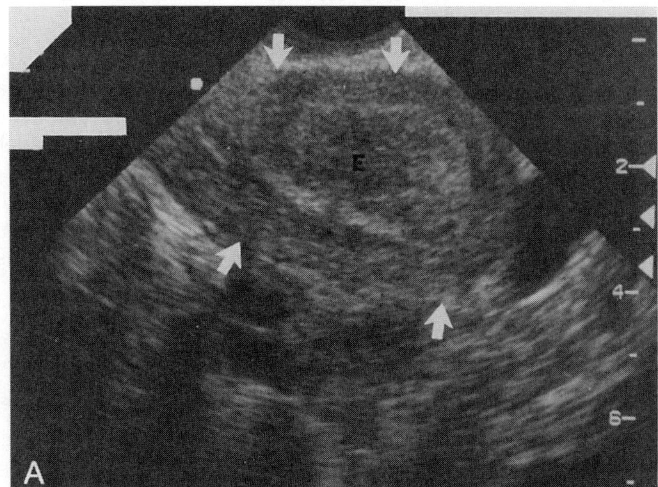

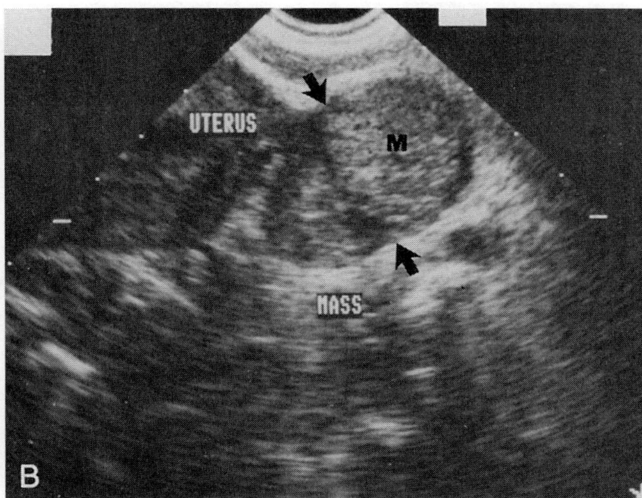

Figure 39.7. Transvaginal US. **A.** Longitudinal US scan through uterus of a 66-year-old woman with vaginal bleeding. Uterus (*arrows*) is enlarged for a postmenopausal patient, measuring 4.2 cm. Endometrium (E) is markedly thickened, a finding suggestive of endometrial carcinoma. **B.** In a postmenopausal patient with vague pelvic pain, endovaginal US scan through left adnexal area revealed a normal-sized ovary containing a 1-cm echogenic mass (M). Lesion proved to be a benign ovarian fibroma. Upper limit of both scans represents US transducer within the vagina.

screening, endovaginal US in its present form would probably not be cost-effective as a screening technique if it were applied to the general population. Selected patients who are at higher risk but not symptomatic (women who have a strong family history of ovarian cancer or a personal history of breast cancer, or middle-aged women who are nulliparous) may benefit from its application (30).

Prostatic and Transrectal Ultrasonography

A minor adaptation of the endovaginal probe allows it to be inserted into the rectum, thereby affording excellent images of the prostate and seminal vesicles. Again, its utility as a screening procedure for prostate cancer remains in question. At this point relatively little is known about the natural history of small asymptomatic prostatic nodules, which are quite common. The transrectal technique is also nonspecific with regard to differentiating from benign malignant nodules (22). Transrectal US can be an excellent guidance method for biopsying prostate nodules, and it is widely used to guide biopsies into various quadrants of the gland in patients with elevated prostate-specific antigen levels.

Another use for transrectal US is in evaluation of the rectal mucosa. Not all transrectal probes are optimally designed for this purpose, however. Only those having transducers oriented at 90 degrees to the shaft of the probe will suffice. "End-fire" probes are not optimal because the sound beam/transducer cannot be oriented perpendicular to the rectal mucosa. Because of excellent near-field resolution, various layers of the normal mucosa can be delineated clearly; depth of invasion can be depicted readily and with considerable accuracy. Additionally, submucosal lesions and local adenopathy can be identified. Several recent publications have found transrectal US to be superior to CT and other imaging modalities for both preoperative staging and follow-up of rectal cancer (32).

Testicular Ultrasonography

High-resolution US remains the primary imaging modality for testicular masses. Intratesticular masses may be differentiated from those that arise outside the gland (Fig. 39.8) and lesions rendered impalpable by overlying pathologic processes (e.g., a hydrocele or varicocele) should be easily identifiable. In this connection, patients who present with metastatic nodes in the retroperitoneum or mediastinum and whose histology is compatible with a testicular origin should undergo testicular US to identify a possible occult primary. In patients with lymphoma or leukemia, US may also define residual disease in the testis that may not be palpable.

Venous Ultrasonography

US has become the primary examination for the evaluation of deep venous thrombosis of the legs. This noninvasive technique should replace contrast venography in almost all cases. A particular advantage of US over contrast venography in cancer patients is its ability to differentiate true thromboses from a neoplasm compressing or invading the vessel.

The sonographic examination for deep venous thrombosis of the leg is usually a combination of several techniques, including gray-scale, duplex, and color flow imaging. Gray-scale US provides high-resolution anatomic images of the veins but must include a thorough compression examination. Compression US is necessary because fresh thrombus may be totally anechoic and, as such, indistinguishable from a patent vessel. Compression, however, will clearly differen-

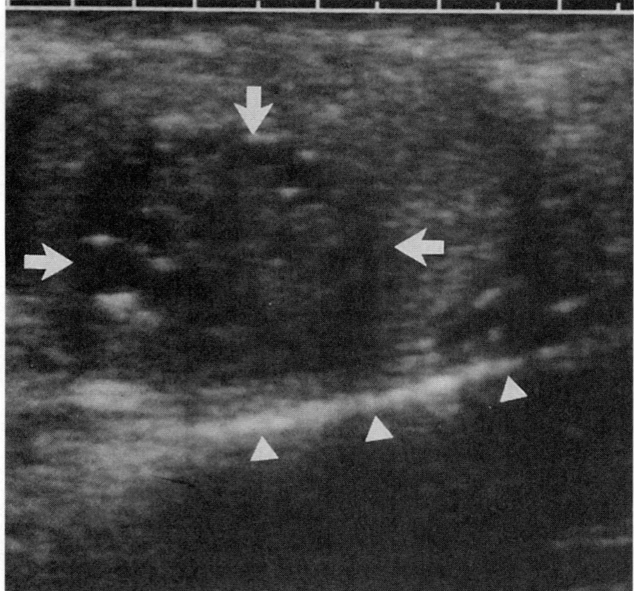

Figure 39.8. Testicular sonogram, longitudinal section through right side of scrotum in a 20-year-old man with painless enlargement of the testis. A well-defined hypoechoic mass is seen posteriorly (*arrows*). Mass contained multiple cystic spaces; other sections revealed internal calcifications. Although the sonographic appearance is not usually specific for cell type, calcifications are typical of teratocarcinoma. Diagnosis was confirmed at surgery. *Arrowheads* outline anterior scrotal wall. Epididymis is not visible in this particular section.

tiate normal from abnormal, as vessels containing thrombus will not collapse completely when pressure is applied. Duplex sonography is used to identify secondary signs of vessel compromise such as the decrease in normal respiratory variation seen with iliac vein thrombosis. Finally, color Doppler technology allows real-time imaging of the blood flow itself. This technique helps demonstrate veins that may be otherwise difficult to see and even outlines nonocclusive clot.

Subcutaneous Ultrasonography

The fine resolution of high-frequency transducers also makes US an ideal method for the evaluation of nonspecific subcutaneous masses. The differential diagnostic possibilities are several, and many of these masses have sufficiently specific appearances to obviate the need for further workup. Masses arising from unrecognized trauma, for example, should produce a mixed cystic/solid appearance, while metastatic lesions tend to produce well-defined nodules with parenchymal echo patterns. Fatty tumors, such as lipomas, are brightly echogenic with definable borders, while lobular fat is poorly defined and blends imperceptibility with the surrounding soft tissues. US can also serve to optimally direct a biopsy needle into any superficial mass when the diagnosis remains uncertain.

Summary

Modern US is an extemely versatile tool with applications to cancer management in many areas of the body. The uses for conventional (B-mode or real-time) techniques are well established and are known to most clinicians. The newer adaptations of US (color Doppler intraoperative and endoluminal scanning, in particular) provide incremental advantages that support their inclusion in the imaging techniques available to modern cancer medicine.

References

1. Abu-Yousef MM, Brown BP, Gingrich RD, LaBrecque DR. Duplex doppler sonography in the diagnosis of veno-occlusive disease. J Ultrasound Med 1990;9:S1.
2. Brick SH, Hill MC, Lande IM. Mistaken or indeterminate CT diagnosis of hepatic metastases: the value of sonography. AJR 1987;148:723.
3. Choi BI, Kim CW, Han MC, Kim CY, Lee HS, Kim ST, Kim YI. Sonographic characteristics of small hepatocellular carcinoma. Gastrointest. Radiology 1989;14:255.
4. Clarke MP, Kane RA, Steele Jr G, Hamilton ES, Ravikumar TS, Onik G, Clouse ME. Prospective comparison of preoperative imaging and intraoperative ultrasonography in the detection of liver tumors. Surgery 1989;106:849.
5. Dodd GD, Carr BI. Percutaneous biopsy of portal vein thrombus: a new staging technique for hepatocellular carcinoma. AJR 1993;161:229.
6. Dritschilo A, Grant EG, Harter KW, Holt RW, Rustgi SN, Rodgers JE. Interstitial radiation therapy for hepatic metastases: sonographic guidance for applicator placement. AJR 1986;147:275.
7. Foley WD, Middleton WD, Lawson TL, Erickson S, Quiroz FA, Macrander S. Color Doppler ultrasound imaging of lower-extremity venous disease. AJR 1989;152:371.
8. Fruehwald F, Salomonowitz E, Neuhold A, Pavelka R, Mailath G. Tongue cancer: sonographic assessment of tumor stage. J Ultrasound Med 1987;6:121.
9. Gooding GAW, Langman AW, Dillon WP, Kaplan MJ. Malignant carotid artery invasion: sonographic detection. Radiology 1989;171:435.
10. Grassi CJ, Polak JF. Axillary and subclavian venous thrombosis: follow-up evaluation with color Doppler flow US and venography. Radiology 1990;175:651.
11. Gritzmann N, Traxler M, Grasl M, Pavelka R. Advanced laryngeal cancer: sonographic assessment. Radiology 1989;171:171.
12. Hatfield MK, Rubin JM, Gebarski SS, Silbergleit R. Intraoperative sonography in low-grade gliomas. J Ultrasound Med 1989;8:131.
13. Knudson GJ, Wiedmeyer DA, Erickson SJ, Foley WD, Lawson TL, Mewissen MW, Lipchik EO. Color Doppler sonographic imaging in the assessment of upper-extremity deep venous thrombosis. AJR 154:399.
14. Laing FC, Jeffrey RB Jr, Wing VW, Nyberg D. A Biliary dilatation: defining the level and cause by real-time US. Radiology 1986;160:39.
15. Livraghi T, Salmi A, Bolondi L, Marin G, Arienti V, Monti F, Vettori C. Small hepatocellular carcinoma: percutaneous alcohol injection. Results in 23 patients. Radiology 1988;168:313.
16. Millener P, Grant EG, Rose S, Duerinckx A, Tessler FN, Perrella RR, Ragavendra N. Color Doppler imaging findings in patients with Budd-Chiari syndrome: correlation with venographic findings. AJR 1993;161:307.
17. O'Moore PV, Mueller PR, Simeone JF, Saini S, Butch RJ, Hahn PF, Steiner E, Stark DD, Ferruchi JT, Jr. Sonographic guidance in diagnostic and therapeutic interventions in the pleural space. AJR 1987;149:1.
18. Parker GA, Lawrence W Jr, Horsley S, Neifeld JP, Cook D, Walsh J, Brewer W, Koretz MJ. Intraoperative ultrasound of the liver affects operative decision making. Ann Surg 1989;209:569.
19. Raghavendra N, Epstein FJ, McCleary L. Intramedullary spinal cord tumors in children: localization with intraoperative sonography. AJNR 1984;5:395.
20. Ramos IM, Taylor KJW, Kier R, Burns PN, Snower DP, Carter D. Tumor vascular signals in renal masses: detection with Doppler US. Radiology 1988;168:633.
21. Reading CC, Charboneau JW, James EM, Karsell PR, Purnell DC, Grant CS, Van Heerden J. A High resolution parathyroid sonography. AJR 1982;139:539.
22. Rifkin MD. Endorectal sonography of the prostate: clinical implications. AJR 1987;148:1137.
23. Rose SC, Zwiebel WJ, Nelson BD, Preist DL, Knighton RA, Brown JW, Lawrence PF, Stults BM, Reading JC, Miller FJ. Symptomatic lower extremity deep venous thrombosis: accuracy, limitations, and role of color duplex flow imaging in diagnosis. Radiology 1990;175:639.
24. Rubin JM, Hatfield MK, Chandler WF, Black KL, Dipietro MA. Intracerebral arteriovenous malformations: intraoperative color Doppler flow imaging. Radiology 1989;170:219.
25. Scatarige JC, Hamper UM, Sheth S, Allen HA III. Parasternal sonography of the internal mammary vessels: technique, normal anatomy, and lymphadenopathy. Radiology 1989;172:453.
26. Schoenberger SG, Sutherland CM, Robinson AE. Breast neoplasms: duplex sonographic imaging as an adjunct in diagnosis. Radiology 1988;168:665.
27. Schwerk WB, Schwerk WN, Rodeck G. Testicular tumors: prospective analysis of real-time US patterns and abdominal staging. Radiology 1987;164:369.
28. Simeone JF, Daniels GH, Mueller PR. High-resolution real-time sonography of the parathyroid. Radiology 1982;145:431.
29. Tio TL, Coene PPLO, Schouwink MH, Tytgat GNJ. Esophagogastric carcinoma: preoperative TNM classification with endosonography. Radiology 1989;173:411.
30. Van Nagell JR, Higgins RV, Donaldson ES, Gallion HH, Powell DE, Pavlik EJ, Woods CH, Thompson EA. Transvaginal sonography as a screening method for ovarian cancer. Cancer 1990;65:573.
31. Whyte AM, Byrne JV. Comparison of computed tomography and ultrasound in the assessment of parotid masses. Clin Radiol 1987;38:339.
32. Wong WD, Orrom WJ, Jensen LL. Preoperative staging of rectal cancer with endorectal ultrasonography. Perspect Colon Rectal Surg 1990;3:315.

CHAPTER 40

Radionuclide Imaging in Cancer Medicine

RANDALL A. HAWKINS

Radionuclide evaluations of cancer have been a major emphasis of nuclear medicine practice and research for decades. While methods, techniques, and applications have changed dramatically over the years, the fundamental goals of applying radionuclide methods to cancer detection and diagnosis, staging, and treatment monitoring, in addition to some direct therapeutic applications, have continued to guide research and clinical practice with these techniques.

While primarily a diagnostic modality, radionuclide methods are also used therapeutically. Except for in vitro methods such as radioimmunoassay (RIA), radionuclide applications in cancer involve the administration (usually intravenously) of a labeled compound of biological interest. The label is an isotope with a decay scheme that facilitates detection and imaging with gamma camera systems, or the more specialized technique of positron emission tomography (PET).

Some of the first radionuclide applications in cancer, including the use of iodine isotopes for diagnosis and treatment of thyroid carcinomas and other thyroid abnormalities, remain important parts of radionuclide cancer applications today, even though the diagnostic environment in which these methods are now employed is quite different from the one that existed when the methods were first developed.

Advances in radionuclide methods in cancer medicine have occurred along two parallel paths: (*a*) radiochemistry developments and (*b*) new imaging methods. While new imaging developments including software and hardware applications related to standard gamma camera imaging, single photon emission computed tomography (SPECT), and PET have fundamentally altered and improved radionuclide approaches to cancer detection and treatment, the direction of basic and clinical research in this field, including hardware design, has been determined largely by advances in radiochemistry.

It is convenient to divide radiochemistry and hardware methods in radionuclide imaging into two categories: (*a*) "single photon" methods based on commonly used isotopes including Tc-99m, I-131, Tl-201, and others that produce a variety of detectable decay products (primarily gamma photons in the energy range of about 75–300 KeV); and (*b*) "dual photon" techniques employing positron emitting isotopes (e.g., F-18, N-13, C-11, and O-15).

Positron producing isotopes emit a positively charged electron (e^+), which, after traveling a short distance through tissue, undergoes annihilation with a negatively charged electron (e^-) resulting in the emission of two oppositely directed 511-KeV photons. These two antiparallel 511-KeV photons can be detected external to the body by PET systems. PET units consist of rings of solid-state detectors designed to detect the annihilation photons more or less "simultaneously" or, in some systems, to use small differences in arrival times at the detectors in the image reconstruction process ("time-of-flight devices").

For simplicity, in the remainder of this section these two different approaches to radionuclide imaging will be referred to as (*a*) "gamma camera methods" (including the gamma camera method known as SPECT) and (*b*) PET methods.

In addition to research and development in radiopharmaceuticals and imaging devices, another feature in the development of radionuclide applications for cancer medicine is the evolution of a better understanding of relationships between radionuclide methods and cancer biology (e.g., studies of the relationships between in vivo cancer metabolism, as defined by imaging techniques, and in vitro indicators of malignant potential such as cellular oncogene expression). Modern image-processing methods have also made possible the systematic combination of other imaging modalities [such as projectional radiologic images or "plain films," ultrasound, computed tomography (CT) and magnetic resonance imaging (MRI)] with radionuclide methods through computer-based (digital) techniques that produce three-dimensional images to reflect physiology and biochemistry (by radionuclide methods) as well as anatomy (by CT, MRI, and other methods). It is now possible, therefore, to visualize function as well as anatomy of cancer in vivo with a level of precision not previously imagined before the advent of modern digital imaging methods.

Gamma Camera Methods Including SPECT

Standard nuclear medicine techniques, as practiced at virtually every major hospital in the United States, continue to comprise the bulk of cancer-related radionuclide applications. Space does not permit an encyclopedic review of these applications, but some issues of current and future relevance are identified in the following sections.

BONE SCANNING

Radionuclide evaluation of the skeletal system (bone scanning) remains one of the most useful diagnostic methods in cancer medicine (1). The radiopharmaceutical in widest use (Tc-99m methyelenediphosphonate, or MDP), can be produced easily in nuclear medicine laboratories, and focal MDP uptake is related to skeletal osteoblastic activity. While its molecular mechanism of binding to bone is not as clearly defined as that of the positron emitter F-18 (fluoride) ion, which exchanges with hydroxyl ions in the hydroxyapatite crystal, MDP is a sensitive indicator of bone metabolic activity and continues to be used extensively in planar and SPECT-imaging studies of the skeletal system, particularly for radionuclide metastatic surveys.

The relatively widespread availability now of SPECT systems makes it possible to generate tomographic (transverse, coronal, and sagittal) images of skeletal structures within the field of view of the gamma camera (i.e., approximately 14–17 inches in diameter). Whole body skeletal surveys are still performed usually in a planar, nontomographic mode. Since SPECT requires additional imaging time for equal volumes of tissue as compared to planar radionuclide techniques, routine whole body SPECT surveys would be too time-consuming with currently available systems.

It has been recognized for decades that MDP bone scans are very sensitive but not highly specific indicators of altered bone metabolism. Approximately 50% of the local bone mass must be lost before lesions can be seen on plain radiographs, and bone scans are abnormal long before that. However, abnormal uptake on a bone scan can occur in disease processes besides cancer, including inflammatory, traumatic, and metabolic conditions. Therefore, plain films are used routinely during the initial reviews of bone scans to increase the specificity of the results. Additional imaging methods (CT, MRI, etc.) can be used as needed to better define the conditions underlying abnormalities that are seen on bone scans.

The development of more sophisticated biochemical methods for cancer detection/diagnosis has also had an impact on in vivo imaging methods. It is now known, for example, that the likelihood of an abnormal bone scan is low in a patient with prostatic carcinoma when the prostate-specific antigen (PSA) is under 10 μg/L (2, 3). Therefore, bone scanning can now be used more selectively in patients with prostate cancer. At the same time, the better definition and anatomic precision of SPECT may help identify patients with critically located metastases, such as those who are at risk for developing pathologic fractures.

In addition to radionuclide bone scanning and plain radiographs, other skeletal-imaging methods, particularly CT and MRI, are very useful for evaluating the skeletal system (see Chapter 37). The resolution of CT and its sensitivity to calcium density within tissues makes it particularly useful for identifying cortical bone abnormalities. MRI is similarly useful for detecting metastases in the marrow cavity as well as selected cortical and trabecular bone abnormalities. Some studies have indicated that MRI has a higher sensitivity, overall, than radionuclide scans for detecting bone metastases (4, 5, 6). Nevertheless, properly performed radionuclide bone scans remain useful because of their relatively low cost and because they offer options for whole body surveys and SPECT imaging (see above).

An important therapeutic application of radionuclides in the skeletal system is the use of β-emitting radiopharmaceuticals for pain relief in patients with widespread skeletal metastases. Strontium-89 was approved relatively recently by the Food and Drug Administration (FDA) for use in this context, and several other bone-seeking radiopharmaceuticals that emit β particles are also under evaluation for radiation therapy of skeletal metastases (7, 8, 9). Two of these agents, rhenium-186 HEDP and samarium-153 EDTMP (both now in phase III trials) also emit gamma photons in an energy range that is suitable for gamma camera imaging, which helps to ascertain the distribution of the administered pharmaceutical.

While this approach to treatment will not help patients who have pathologic fractures, it can be useful for pain relief in patients with otherwise uncomplicated bone metastases. Bone scanning with MDP can also be a useful method for identifying appropriate patients for this form of therapy. Studies have shown that, while life expectancy does not appear to be lengthened significantly by the treatment, the therapeutic radionuclides can lessen skeletal pain considerably in patients with end-stage skeletal involvement by cancer. To date, these agents have been used most widely in patients with widespread prostate cancer metastases, but they have also been applied to patients with skeletal metastases from cancers of the breast, lung, and other organ systems. Clinical monitoring of the platelet and leukocyte counts during and after therapy is necessary, as well as adherence to standard dosimetry protocols for administration of the radioactive agents (7, 8, 9).

THYROID

The treatment of remnants of functioning tissue within the thyroid bed with oral I-131 following total thyroidectomy for thyroid cancer, as well as the treatment of disease recurrence and metastases with I-131, remain standard approaches in this disease. The requirements of I-131 treatment include histologic and/or imaging evidence that the tumor actually metabolizes I-131 (as do most papillary or follicular carcinomas of the thyroid, whereas medullary carcinomas of the thyroid do not) (10).

The non-β-emitting isotope of iodine, I-123, is the agent of choice for simple diagnostic evaluations of iodine uptake by the thyroid. In thyroid cancer patients, however, I-131 is still widely used as a diagnostic scanning agent. The long physical half-life of 8 days makes it possible to image patients several days after the compound is administered, permitting clearance of the agent and resulting in better contrast of tumor as compared to background tissues.

As with PSA determinations in prostate cancer patients, evaluating serum thyroglubulin concentrations (11) may be a useful indicator of the presence of cancerous thyroid tissue in the body. I-131 imaging is used primarily to guide I-131 treatment. In the absence of abnormal uptake of I-131 on diagnostic scans, the likelihood of a good treatment response to I-131 is lower.

GALLIUM, THALLIUM, AND OTHER NONSPECIFIC TUMOR TRACERS

Gallium-67 citrate and thallium-201 chloride are two well-known single photon radiopharmaceuticals that have been used traditionally for locating neoplastic or inflammatory foci (gallium) and for myocardial perfusion imaging (thallium). Gallium-67 citrate remains a useful tumor localization agent, particularly for lymphomas, but its use has been somewhat limited by its relatively complex biodistribution pattern. The radiopharmaceutical has an affinity for iron-binding proteins (ferritin, lactoferrin, bacterial siderophores, and others), is actively excreted through the mucosa of the gastrointestinal tract, undergoes urinary excretion as well, and has a significant amount of normal marrow uptake. As a result, it is often necessary to image gallium distribution 24 to 72 hours after administration; this makes it a relatively time-consuming but still useful test (12).

Thallium has demonstrated utility as a myocardial perfusion agent. It has also attracted attention recently as a useful biochemical marker for the presence of viable tumor tissue with several neoplasms, including brain tumors, breast cancer, and others (13, 14, 15). Thallium, in addition to being taken up by tissues in proportion to their blood perfusion, is also concentrated by the (Na^+–K^+)-adenosine triphosphatase (ATPase) pump and is an indicator of tumor viability. Black et al. (13) have shown that SPECT brain imaging of astrocytomas with thallium-201 produces results that correlate with the histologic grade of lesions. They report that the method can identify tumor recurrences, complementing the information available from contrast-enhanced CT or MRI scans. While PET imaging with the glucose analog 2-[F-18]fluoro-2-deoxy-D-glucose (FDG) is a more precise method for this application (see below), thallium-201 SPECT can produce useful studies when PET is not available.

Both thallium-201 and another agent that is used for myocardial perfusion imaging, Tc-99m sestamibi, have been employed to identify primary lesions and nodal metastases from breast cancer (14, 16). Tc-99m sestamibi has also been demonstrated to be a substrate for the P-glycoprotein *mdr* gene transporter (17).

RECEPTOR-TARGETED IMAGING METHODS

A particularly appealing approach to radionuclide applications in cancer medicine is the design of radiolabeled macromolecules that are targeted to specific receptors on cancer cells. These approaches have both diagnostic and therapeutic potential, and they can be used potentially with gamma camera (including SPECT) and with PET imaging.

Imaging and therapy with monoclonal antibodies (MAb) were made possible with the development of the hybridoma technique by Kohler and Milstein (18). While research on the use of MAb for the diagnosis and treatment of cancer has grown enormously since their discovery, early expectations that the field would yield "magic bullets" analogous to I-131 for the treatment of thyroid cancer have remained largely unrealized for two reasons (19): (*a*) most available MAb's are currently of murine origin, resulting in the production of human antimouse antibodies (HAMA) by patients who are treated with repeated administrations of the monoclonals. This produces lower plasma concentrations of the MAb than might be necessary to achieve a therapeutic effect; and (*b*) the cellular heterogeneity of cancer cells results in variable recognition of the cells by a given MAb. Partial solutions to the former problem have been pursued by developing immunogenic Fab fragments and "humanized" MAb (20, 21).

The MAb used in imaging have been labeled primarily with iodine-131, indium-111, iodine-123, and technetium-99m. As discussed by Goldenberg (22), three "generations" of labeled MAb have been studied, including: (*a*) first generation whole IgG molecules labeled with I-131; (*b*) second generation whole IgG molecules labeled with In-111; and (*c*) third generation Tc-99m labeled antibody fragments (bivalent $F(ab')_2$ and monovalent Fab′ and Fab fragments). These third generation products are less immunogenic, resulting in a decreased HAMA response. They are also cleared from the general circulation more quickly; higher ratios of tumor to background can therefore be reached earlier following injection than with first and second generation agents, thus facilitating tumor detection with imaging. Additional physical advantages are the wide availability and relatively low cost of Tc-99m as a label (virtually all hospitals have access to Tc-99m generators) and the better gamma camera-imaging characteristics of Tc-99m (greater number of photons for external detection and lower absorbed radiation dose), as compared to the other isotopes listed above.

Several excellent reviews of the clinical experience with MAb imaging for cancer detection are available (22, 23). These agents have shown good potential in a variety of published series, including their ability to identify primary tumors and metastases that have not been found with anatomic imaging techniques (CT and MRI). Nevertheless, labeled MAb have not yet achieved routine clinical use status.

Reports of clinical experience with MAb imaging in a wide variety of cancers are available, including cancers of the colon, ovary, prostate, breast, lung, and liver, as well as trophoblastic and germ cell tumors, lymphomas, melanoma, and neuroblastoma (23). Goldenberg estimates that approximately 60 to 90% of identified lesions in the published studies have been pinpointed correctly by MAb imaging (termed "RAID" for radioimmuno-detection). The largest clinical experience to date has been acquired with colorectal and ovarian cancers (22).

In addition to imaging, cancer therapy (radioimmunotherapy or "RAIT") has also shown promise with MAb (22–26). The studies of therapeutic applications have used MAb conjugated with drugs (chemotherapeutic agents), toxins, or β-emitting radiopharmaceuticals (22, 23). The difficult challenge faced by RAIT remains achieving a high enough local concentration of labeled MAb to deliver effective levels of therapeutic radiation. Isotopes emitting β particles (electrons) are potentially well-suited for this task. Depending on their energy, the path lengths of these ionizing particles may be relatively short (e.g., less than 1 mm for the β particle from I-131).

In addition to the physical characteristics of a given isotope, other critical factors affecting tumor dosimetry from RAIT include the residence time of the labeled antibody at its target, the relative affinity of the antibody for tumor cells (taking into account the immunological heterogeneity of many tumors, as mentioned above), and the rate of clearance from normal tissues (which affects the therapeutic ratio, or the dose delivered to the tumor as compared to the dose delivered to normal tissues).

Stanley Order and his colleagues (25) were the first to use a form of RAIT (I-131 antiferritin antibodies for hepatocellular cancer patients); recent work has indicated that lymphomas and leukemias may be the most suitable tumor systems for RAIT (22, 26).

OTHER RECEPTOR-TARGETED AGENTS

Receptor-targeted imaging with other agents besides monoclonals is another exciting developmental application for radionuclides in cancer medicine. This area of research also has potential relevance to treatment as well as to diagnosis because of the increasing sophistication of radiolabeling procedures, along with advances in our understanding of the molecular biology of cancer (27). MAb technology makes it possible to target specific tumor receptors such as the epidermal growth factor receptor (EGF) with MAb (28), and parallel progress with non-MAb methods is now occurring. Metabolite and receptor-targeted imaging with PET has already achieved clinically significant results (see below).

Examples of non-MAb receptor-targeted methods are the imaging and treatment of tumors that express somatostatin receptors using the somatostatin analogue octreotide (Sandoz, Inc.) (29). A variety of neuroendocrine tumors have somatostatin receptors, including insulinomas, carcinoids, vasoactive intestinal peptide-secreting tumors, glucagonomas, and gastrinomas. Octreotide is more resistant to enzymatic degradation than is somatostatin and, therefore, has a longer plasma half-life than somatostatin itself. Octreotide has been evaluated both as a potential therapeutic agent for gastrointestinal endocrine tumors (30) and (using a modified form of octreotide in which the phenylalanine at position 3 is replaced by tyrosine) as an imaging agent (30, 31).

Kvols et al. (31) found that 22 of 28 patients with carcinoids and islet cell tumors had positive uptake of I-123 octreotide. In a larger series of neuroendocrine and nonneuroendocrine tumors that had somatostatin receptors, the same research group demonstrated the effectiveness of octreotide for imaging; they also reported a positive correlation between the scans and subsequent responses to treatment with radiolabeled octreotide in some patients (32).

These promising results with octreotide explain the current widespread interest in developing other peptide agents as diagnostic tools for oncology. These agents again have potential utility not just for cancer detection but also for monitoring of therapy and for new therapeutic strategies based on receptor-binding characteristics.

Positron Emission Tomography (PET)

PET, which was initially developed and applied primarily for neurological and cardiac applications (33), has now become used widely as both an investigative and a clinical tool in cancer medicine (34). While PET differs from gamma camera radionuclide methods in terms of the detector systems and the radiopharmaceuticals used (see above), it shares with gamma camera methods the fundamental approach of quantifying and mapping the distribution in vivo of administered radiopharmaceuticals. Table 40.1 is a partial list of some of the positron-emitting radiopharmaceuticals that have been used for investigative and clinical applications with PET in oncology.

Table 40.1. Radiopharmaceuticals Used for PET Studies of Cancer

Process	Radiopharmaceutical
General biochemical and physiological processes	
Glucose metabolism (glycolysis)	FDG
Perfusion	[^{13}N]Ammonia ($^{13}NH_3$)
	[^{15}O]Water ($H_2{}^{15}O$)
Oxygen metabolism	[^{15}O]Oxygen ($^{15}O_2$)
Amino acid uptake and protein synthesis	[^{11}C]Methionine
	[^{11}C]Leucine
	[^{13}N]Glutamate
Nucleic acid metabolism (DNA replication)	[^{11}C]Thymidine
Polyamine metabolism	[^{11}C]Putrescine
Glucosamine uptake	[^{18}F]Fluoroacetyl-D-glucosamine
Organ-specific or other specialized biochemical and physiological processes	
Blood-brain barrier permeability	^{82}Rb ion
	[^{68}Ga]EDTA
Receptor-specific ligands	[^{18}F]Fluoroestradiol
Monoclonal antibodies	[^{124}I]HMFG1 (epithelial neoplasms)
	[^{124}I]3F8 (neuroblastoma, astrocytoma)
Hypoxic cell agents	[^{18}F]Fluoromisonidazole
Chemotherapeutic agents	^{18}F UdR
	[^{18}F]Tamoxifen
Skeletal metabolic (osteoblastic activity)	[^{18}]Fluoride ion

Adapted from 34.

PET applications in cancer medicine have been focused on three clinical goals: (*a*) cancer detection and diagnosis; (*b*) cancer staging; and (*c*) cancer treatment monitoring. Paralleling these clinical goals, basic investigations are being pursued to develop better PET methods that are specific for cancer and, more fundamentally, to use PET as a tool for achieving a better understanding of cancer biology.

The observation by Otto Warburg in 1930 that malignant transformation of cells is associated with an increased glycolytic rate (even in the presence of oxygen) (35, 36) has stimulated many of the current PET studies. FDG, a metabolite analogue that was initially developed in the form of C-14 deoxyglucose to evaluate cerebral glucose metabolism by Sokoloff and colleagues (37–41), has been used widely to image and quantify glucose metabolic rates in the brain, heart (33) and other organ systems, as well as to detect and map the distribution of cancer deposits in the body. FDG, like glucose, is transported from plasma into tissues via carrier-facilitated diffusion and is then phosphorylated to FDG-6-PO4 by hexokinase (the same enzyme that catalyzes the phosphorylation of glucose to glucose-6-PO4). However, FDG-6-PO4 does not serve as a substrate for further metabolism, and it does not diffuse across cell membranes.

Therefore, clinical PET FDG images, usually acquired about 1 hour after intravenous administration of the compound, actually delineate closely the tissue distribution of glucose-6-PO4 as a metabolite of exogenous glucose. Mathematical modeling techniques make it possible to measure the rate of glucose metabolism using PET FDG images coupled with measurements of plasma F-18 and glucose concentrations (see references 37–41 for details). While rigorous quantification of glucose metabolism (or other physiologic or biochemical processes) with PET requires careful attention to the biochemical assumptions and the mathematical and imaging methods employed (41, 42), PET FDG images are proving to be useful for cancer detection and mapping because the pattern of uptake of FDG on images correlates directly with local glucose (glycolytic) metabolic rates.

BRAIN TUMORS

Di Chiro and his colleagues (43, 44) were the first to use the PET FDG method in a clinical oncologic environment. They found that elevated uptakes of FDG in astrocytomas were related directly to the histology of these lesions (grade III and IV astrocytomas have higher glucose metabolic rates than grade I and II lesions), and that the method can distinguish reliably between radiation necrosis of the brain and tumor recurrences in treated patients. Since FDG uptake requires the presence of hexokinase, PET FDG localization indicates where active metabolism is occurring. Vascular contrast enhancement on CT or MRI images of the brain indicates the presence of increased permeability through the blood-brain barrier, but it does not necessarily indicate that the tissue is viable.

Since the original work by Di Chiro et al. (43, 44), many other investigators have demonstrated that PET FDG imaging is useful for characterizing the biochemical activity of brain tumors and for detecting tumor recurrences (Fig. 40.1). Recent studies have also indicated that glucose consumption (as indicated by FDG uptake) in astrocytomas correlates with tumor cell density, and it is by this means that FDG uptake correlates with histologic grade. Other metabolic signals such as elevated choline levels in local brain regions measured by magnetic resonance spectroscopy (MRS) can also signify viable tumor as opposed to encephalomalacia (46). Investigations to compare the relative utility and the possible complementarity of PET and MRS for brain tumor characterization are currently in progress.

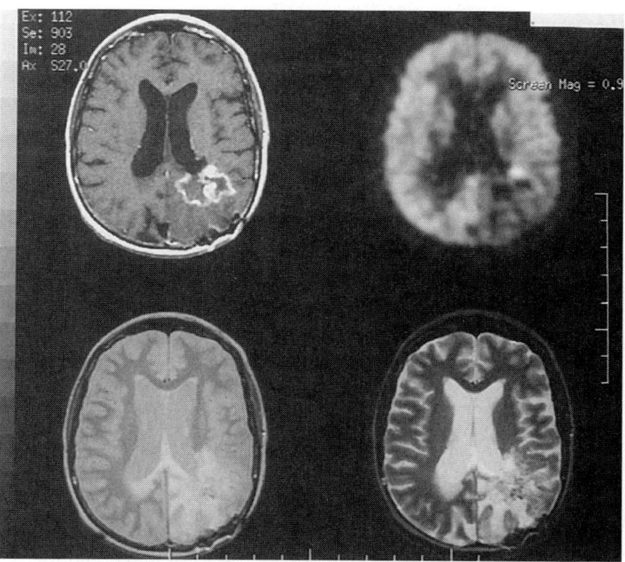

Figure 40.1. High grade astrocytoma: registered MRI and PET images. Contrast-enhanced spin echo T1 MRI (*upper left*), registered PET FDG (*upper right*), and two T2-weighted MRI images [less T2-weighting Te = 30 ms, TR = 2,500 ms (*lower left*); more T2-weighting (Te = 80 ms, tR = 2,500 ms) (*lower right*)] in a patient with a recurrent high-grade astrocytoma. Note irregular zone of contrast enhancement on contrast-enhanced T1 MRI image adjacent to posterior margin of lateral ventricle. PET FDG image was registered and aligned to correspond to the level and angle of the MRI images. Note zone of increased uptake of FDG, indicating viable tumor, best seen on anterior margin of lesion. Central zone of decreased FDG uptake and low signal on contrast-enhanced MRI within the lesion is consistent with central necrosis of the lesion. Also note diminished FDG uptake in overlying occipital cortex, corresponding in distribution to edema evident on T2 images (*lower row*).

HEAD AND NECK AND OTHER TUMORS

Outside the central nervous system, other tumors that have been studied with FDG include those of the head and neck, lung, breast, colon, pancreas, musculoskeletal system, and ovary, as well as disseminated tumors such as metastatic melanoma and the lymphomas (34).

The resolution of modern PET systems makes it possible to use PET FDG imaging to detect relatively small lesions. For example, Jabour et al (47), reported a series of 12 patients with primary squamous cell carcinomas of the head and neck in which all of the primary lesions were identified (CT and MRI missed one), and metastatic disease was detected in one lymph node that was anatomically normal by MRI criteria. Because of the structural complexity of the head and neck region, both the anatomic precision of MRI and the biochemical information yielded by PET can be helpful in staging cancers, particularly in identifying lymph node metastases. Following treatment (surgery and/or radiation therapy), PET FDG imaging can also help to detect residual or recurrent disease, even when MRI scans are equivocal.

While PET FDG imaging can be useful in detecting subclinical tumor deposits and depicting their distribution throughout the body using whole body PET-imaging methods (34), it is also important to remember that glucose utilization is ubiquitous throughout the body. Accordingly, normal glucose utilization patterns and other (nonmalignant) causes of elevated local tissue glucose utilization rates must also be considered when interpreting PET FDG images.

For example, tissue inflammation can lead to increased glucose utilization rates and increased FDG uptake on PET images (48). Nonmalignant reactive changes in lymph nodes may also produce increased FDG uptake on PET images (49) in patients with cancer. Because of the quantitative precision of PET, it may be possible eventually to differentiate benign from malignant levels of glucose utilization (50). Additional clinical experience and controlled studies are needed, however, to define the specificity of various numerical thresholds for differentiating benign from malignant disease. In addition to quantitative methods, the localizing information provided by PET images and the appropriate use of clinical data in context will often facilitate the correct interpretation of PET scans.

BREAST CANCER

Breast cancer is another focus of current PET FDG-imaging research. While mammography is an excellent screening tool, it may be falsely negative in up to 10% of women with cancer because of radiographically dense breast tissue. Moreover, mammography and other imaging methods, including MRI, cannot detect lymph node involvement accurately. Studies have shown that PET FDG imaging can detect primary breast lesions as well as axillary and other metastases in some patients when studies with other imaging modalities have been normal (51–53).

At this time, it appears that the most likely clinical role for PET in breast cancer will be in staging the disease. Because many, if not most, women currently have axillary dissections for staging purposes, staging with PET could potentially spare some women this invasive procedure. Ongoing studies have been designed to collect enough clinical information to make meaningful sensitivity and specificity calculations that may be applicable to larger groups of patients, but initial results in smaller series of patients have already been promising.

Investigators at Washington University have developed a fluorinated form of estrogen [16α-F[18]fluoroestradiol-17β (FES)] and have shown that it is possible to estimate estrogen receptor density noninvasively with PET FES imaging. This form of receptor-targeted imaging also suggests another potential application of radionuclide methods in breast cancer management: combinations of FDG and FES imaging in breast cancer patients may yield insights into which patients may benefit most from antiestrogen therapy with tamoxifen (54, 55).

LUNG CANCER

Another tumor type for which a significant amount of clinical experience with PET has accumulated is lung cancer. Benign nodules can be distinguished from malignant ones based on FDG uptake, and PET with FDG has also contributed to accurate staging of mediastinal involvement in patients who have undergone combined CT and PET FDG imaging. The best results have been obtained by registering (matching with the use of computer methods) the CT and PET FDG images, so that individual lymph nodes and other structures shown on CT can be characterized biochemically with PET FDG (56).

In addition to FDG studies, initial evaluations of cancer patients with other agents listed in Table 40.1 will illustrate that the field of biochemical characterization of cancers with in vivo imaging methods is currently in its initial phase. Beyond the biochemically based approaches with PET, such as measuring glucose utilization, receptor-targeted methods promise to further facilitate detection, staging, and treatment monitoring. As an example, the hypoxic cell marker F-18 fluoromisonidazole now makes it possible to image viable but hypoxic cells. This method is not only capable of yielding insights into mechanisms of radioresistance in different tumors based on hypoxic cell fractions, but it may also become a useful predictor of treatment responsiveness in individual patients.

Conclusion

Radionuclide evaluations in cancer medicine remain a mix of standard, but still evolving techniques that are based on gamma camera methods for whole body tumor surveys and new methods that are being driven by striking advances in radiochemistry and instrumentation. The future should see continued growth in quantitative receptor-targeted imaging approaches with SPECT and PET that will facilitate cancer detection, staging, and treatment monitoring.

References

1. Pomeranz SJ, Pretorius HT, Ramsingh PS. Bone scintigraphy and multimodality imaging in bone neoplasia: strategies for imaging in the new health care climate. Semin Nucl Med 1994;24:188–207.
2. Oesterling JE, Martin SK, Bergstralh EJ, Lowe FC. The use of prostate-specific antigen in staging patients with newly diagnosed prostate cancer. JAMA 1993;269:57–60.
3. Oesterling JE. Prostate specific antigen: a critical assessment of the most useful tumor marker for adenocarcinoma of the prostate. J Urol 1991;145:907–928.
4. Gosfield E, Alavi A, Kneeland B. Comparison of radionuclide bone scans and magnetic resonance imaging in detecting spinal metastases. J Nucl Med 1993;34: 2191–2198.
5. Avrahami E, Tadmor R, Dally O, Hadar H. Early MR demonstration of spinal metastases in patients with normal radiographs and CT and radionuclide bone scans. J Comput Assist Tomogr 1989;13:598–602.
6. Froelich JW. Is the whole really the sum of the parts? J Nucl Med 1993;34:2198–2200. (Editorial)
7. Robinson RG, Preston DF, Spicer JA, Baxter KG. Radionuclide therapy of intractable bone pain: emphasis on strontium-89. Semin Nucl Med 1992;22:28–32.
8. Silberstein EB. The treatment of painful osseous metastases with phosphorous-32-labeled phosphates. Semin Oncol 1993;20(suppl 2):10–21.
9. Silberstein EB. The treatment of painful osteoblastic metastases: what can we expect from nuclear oncology? J Nucl Med 1994;35:1994–1995.
10. Werner. The thyroid: A Fundamental and Clinical Text. 5th ed. Edited by SH Ingbar, Braverman LE. Philadelphia: Lippincott, 1986.
11. Vanherle AJ, Uller RP, Matthews NL, Brown J. Radioimmunoassay for measurement of thryglobulin in human serum. J Clin Invest 1973;52:1320–1327.
12. Uchiyama M, Kantoff PW, Kaplan WE. Gallium-67-citrate imaging in estragonadal and gonadal seminomas: relationship to radiologic findings. J Nucl Med 1994;35: 1624–1630.
13. Black KL, Emerick T, Hoh C, Hawkins RA, Mazziotta J, Becker DP. Thallium-201 SPECT and positron emission tomography equal predictors of glioma grade and recurrence. Neurol Res 1994;16:93–96.
14. Waxman AD, Ramanna L, Memsic LD, Foster CE, et al. Thallium scintigraphy in the evaluation of mass abnormalities of the breast. J Nucl Med 1993;34:18–23.
15. Matsuno S, Tanabe M, Kawasaki Y, Satoh K, et al. Effectiveness of planar image and single photon emission tomography of thallium-201 compared with gallium-67 in patients with primary lung cancer. Eur J Nucl Med 1992;19:86–95.
16. Khalkhali I, Mena I, Diggles L. Review of imaging techniques for the diagnosis of breast cancer: a new role of prone scintimammography using technetium-99m sestamibi. Eur J Nucl Med 1994;21:357–362.
17. Piwnica-Worms D, Chiu ML, Budding M, et al. Functional imaging of multidrug-resistant P-glycoprotein with an organotechnetium complex. Cancer Res 1993;53:1–8.
18. Kohler G, Milstein C. Continuous cultures of fused secreting antibody of redefined specificity. Nature 1975;256:495–497.
19. Leon JA, Goldstein NI, Fisher PB. New approaches for the development and application of monoclonal antibodies for the diagnosis and therapy of human cancer. Pharmacol Ther 1994;61:237–278.
20. Larson SM. Radioimmunology: imaging and therapy. Cancer (suppl) 1991;67: 1253–1260.
21. LoBuglio AF, Wheeler RH, Trang J, et al. Mouse/human chimeric monoclonal antibody in man: kinetics and immune response. Proc Natl Acad Sci USA 1989;86:4220–4224.
22. Goldenberg DM. Monoclonal antibodies in cancer detection and therapy. Am J Med 1993;94:297–312.
23. Goldenberg DM, Larson SM. Radioimmunodetection in cancer identification. J Nucl Med 1992;33:803–814.
24. Wahl RL. Experimental radioimmunotherapy. A brief overview. Cancer 1994;73(suppl):989–992.
25. Order SE, Stillwagon GB, Klein JL, et al. I-131 antiferritin: a new treatment modality in hepatoma: a Radiation Therapy Oncology Group study. J Clin Oncol 1985;3: 1573–1582.
26. Kaminski MS, Zasadny KR, Francis IR, Milik AW, Ross CW, Moon SD, et al. Radioimmunotherapy of B-cell lymphoma with [I-131]abtu-B1 (anti-CD20) antibody. N Engl J Med 1993;329:459–465.
27. Kerr DJ, Workman P, eds. New Molecular Targets for Cancer Chemotherapy. Boca Raton, FL: CRC, 1994.

28. Divgi CR, Welt C, Kris M, et al. Phase I and imaging trial of indium-111 labeled anti-EGF receptor monoclonal antibody 225 in patients with squamous cell lung carcinoma. JNCI 1991;83:97–104.
29. O'Dorisio TM. Rational and clinical applications of neuropeptide congeners for diagnosis and therapy of neuroendocrine tumors. Regul Pept Lett 1994;5:52–55.
30. Lamberts SWJ, Hofland LF, Van Koetsveld PM, et al. Parallel in vivo and in vitro detection of functional somatostatin receptors in human endocrine pancreatic tumors: consequences with regard to diagnosis, localization and therapy. J Clin Endocrinol Metab 1990;761:566–574.
31. Kvols LK, Brown ML, O'Connor MK, Hung JC, Hayostek RJ, Reubi JC, Lamberts SWJ. Evaluation of a radiolabeled somatostatin analog (I-123 octreotide) in the detection and localization of carcinoid and islet cell tumors. Radiology 1993;187: 129–133.
32. Krenning EP, Kwekkeboom DJ, Bakker WH, Breeman WAP, Kooij PPM, Oei HY, et al. Somatostatin receptor scintigraphy with [^{111}In-DTPA-D-Phe^{1}]- and [^{123}I-Tyr^{3}]-octreotide: the Rotterdam experience with more than 1000 patients. Eur J Nucl Med 1993;20:716–731.
33. Phelps ME, Mazziotta JC, Schelbert HR, eds. Positron Emission Tomography and Autoradiography. Principles and Applications for the Brain and Heart. New York: Raven, 1986.
34. Hawkins RA, Hoh C, Glaspy J, Choi Y, et al. The role of positron emission tomography in oncology and other whole-body applications. Semin Nucl Med 1992;22:268–284.
35. Warburg O. The Metabolism of Tumors. London, England: Constabel, 1930.
36. Warburg O. On the origin of cancer cells. Science 1956;123:309–314.
37. Sokoloff L, Reivich M, Kennedy C, et al. The (11C)-deoxyglucose method for the measurement of local cerebral glucose utilization: theory, procedure and normal values in the conscious and anesthetized albino rat. J Neurochem 1977;28:897–916.
38. Reivich M, Kuhl DE, Wolf A, et al. The (18F)flurodeoxyglucose method for the measurement of local cerebral glucose utilization in man. Circ Res 1979;44:127–137.
39. Phelps ME, Huang SC, Hoffman EJ, et al. Tomographic measurement of local cerebral glucose metabolic rate in humans with (f-18)-2-deoxy-D-glucose: validation of method. Ann Neurol 1979;6:371–388.
40. Huang SC, Phelps ME, Hoffman EJ, et al. Noninvasive determination of local cerebral metabolic rate of glucose in man. Am J Physiol 1980;238:E69–E82.
41. Hawkins RA, Phelps ME, Huang SC. Effects of temporal sampling, glucose metabolic rates and disruptions of the blood brain barrier (BBB) on the FDG model with and without a vascular compartment: studies in human brain tumors with PET. J Cereb Blood Flow Metab 1986;6:170–183.
42. Sorenson J, Phelps ME. Physics of Nuclear Medicine. New York: Raven, 1986.
43. Di Chiro G. Positron emission tomography using [18F]fluorodeoxyglucose in brain tumors. Invest Radiol 1987;22:360–371.
44. Di Chiro G, Oldfield E, Wright DC, et al. Cerebral necrosis after radiotherapy and/or intra-arterial chemotherapy for brain tumors: PET and neuropathologic studies. AJR 1988;150:189–197.
45. Herholz K, Pietrzyk U, Voges J, et al. Correlation of glucose consumption and tumor cell density in astrocytomas. J Neurosurg 1993;79:853–858.
46. Barker PB, Glickson JD, Bryan RN. In vivo magnetic resonance spectroscopy of human brain tumors. Top Magn Reson Imaging 1993;5:32–45.
47. Jabour BA, Choi Y, Hoh CK, Rege SD, Soong JC, Lufkin RB, Hanafee WN, Maddahi J, Chaiken L. Bailet J. Phelps ME, Hawkins RA. PET imaging of the extra cranial head and neck using 2-[F-18]fluoro-2-deoxy-D-glucose (FDG) with MRI correlation. Radiology 1993;186:27–35.
48. Kubota R, Yamada S. Kubota K. Ishiwata K, Tamahashi N, Ido T. Intratumoral distribution of fluorine-18-fluorodeoxyglucose in vivo: high accumulation in macrophages and granulation tissues studied by microautoradiology. J Nucl Med 1992;33:1972–1980.
49. Wahl RL, Kaminski MS, Ethier Sp, et al. The potential of 2-deoxy-2[^{18}F]fluoro-d-glucose (FDG) for the detection of tumor involvement in lymph nodes. J Nucl Med 1990;31: 1831–1835.
50. Hawkins RA, Choi Y, Huang SC, et al. Quantitating tumor glucose metabolism with FDG and PET. J Nucl Med 1992;33:339–344.
51. Wahl RL, Cody RL, Hutchins GD, et al. Primary and metastatic breast carcinoma: initial clinical evaluation with PET with the radiolabeled glucose analogue 2-[F-18]fluoro-2-deoxy-D-glucose (FDG). Radiology 1991;179:765–770.
52. Tse N, Hoh CK, Hawkins RA, et al. Application of positron emission tomography with 2-[F-18]fluoro-2-deoxy-D-glucose (FDG) to the evaluation of breast disease. Ann Surg 1992;216:27–34.
53. Adler DD, Wahl RL. New methods for imaging the breast: techniques, findings, and potential. AJR 1995;164:19–30.
54. McGuire A, Dehdashti F, Siegel B, Lyss A, Brodack J, Mathias C, Mintun M, Katzenellenbogen J, Welch M. Positron tomographic assessment of 16a[^{18}F]fluoro-17b-estradiol uptake in metastatic breast carcinoma. J Nucl Med 1991;32:1526–1531.
55. Mintun M, Welch M, Siegel B, Matthias C, Brodack J, McGuire A, Katzenellenbogen J. Breast Cancer: PET imaging of estrogen receptors. Radiology 1988;169:45–48.
56. Wahl RL, Quint LE, Greenough RL, Meyer CR, et al. Staging of mediastinal nonsmall cell lung cancer with FDG PET, CT and fusion images: preliminary prospective evaluation. Radiology 1994;191:371–377.

CHAPTER 41

Perspectives in Imaging

RICHARD J. STECKEL

A number of recent developments in diagnostic imaging that have potential import for the detection, diagnosis, staging, and follow-up of cancer patients have been described in the preceding sections. They include rapid magnetic resonance imaging (MRI) sequences that will mitigate the problem of motion during MRI examinations, new scanning agents, endoluminal (e.g., endovaginal, endorectal, endoesophageal and endobronchial) ultrasound scanning techniques, and other improvements in existing radiologic modalities. Developments in positron emission tomography (PET) include new compounds to evaluate tumor metabolism and total body imaging methods for detecting asymptomatic metastases (Fig. 41.1, *A* and *B*. Scanning agents are under development that have greater specificity for certain tumors, including "designer compounds" which attach to epitopes on the surfaces of tumor cells. The in vivo imaging capability of a radioactive ligand for benzodiazepine receptors is also being studied for possible applications to the diagnosis and staging of brain tumors (Fig. 41.2).

Over the next several years, there is a need for more concerted evaluations of existing diagnostic imaging methods and their appropriate applications to cancer management. We now have available to us a plethora of imaging techniques, without sufficient data to use them in the most efficient manner to detect and diagnose cancer, to guide treatment and follow-up care, and to prevent morbidity. Accelerating medical costs and the growth of managed care will compel us to evaluate imaging methods more systematically for their contributions to cancer management and clinical outcomes.

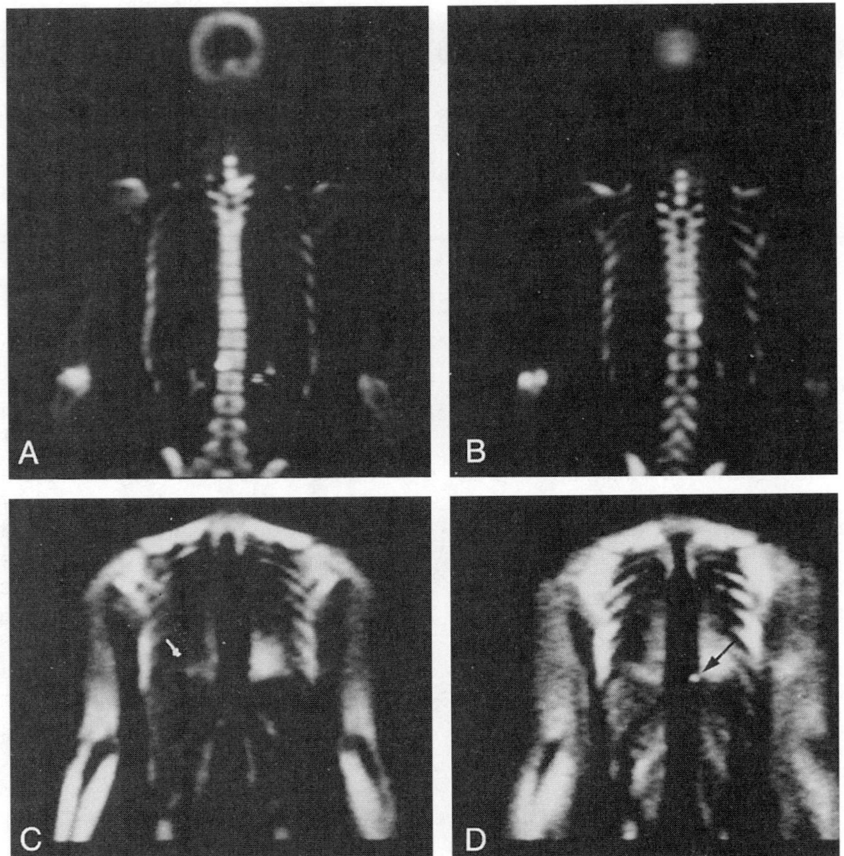

Figure 41.1. **A** and **B.** Anterior coronal images of a fluorine-18 PET bone scan in a patient with breast cancer demonstrating focal activity at several levels of the spine. **A.** Focal osteoblastic activity is evident in metastatic lesions at T-1 and T-12 levels. **B.** On a slightly more posterior "cut," focal uptake is seen at T-10 level. On both images, a "hot" area is noted in right antecubital fossa at radionuclide injection site. **C** and **D.** Posterior coronal images of 18-fluoro-deoxyglucose scan of the same patient. **C.** Focal increase in metabolic activity is confirmed at site of metastatic lesion in pedicle and transverse process of T-10 (*arrow*). **D.** A similar increase in metabolic activity is seen in T-12 vertebra (*arrow*). (Courtesy of Randall Hawkins, M.D., University of California, San Francisco School of Medicine.)

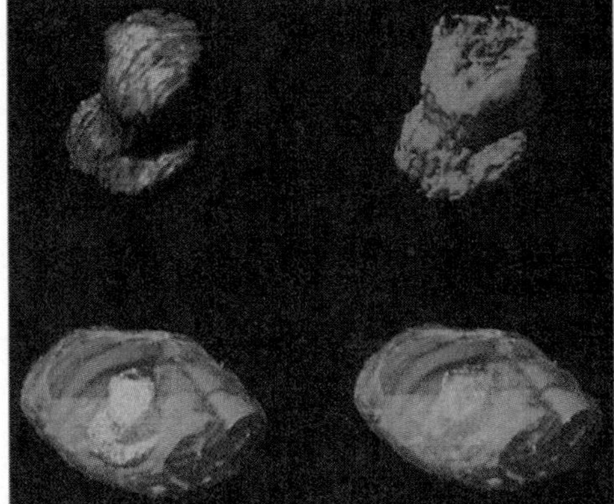

Figure 41.2. Three-dimensional model of a rat brain tumor (*brown*) was constructed of thionine-stained histologic sections and corresponds almost exactly with *green* three-dimensional tumor model constructed from autoradiograms. Autoradiograms were made using tritiated ligand, which binds to peripheral benzodiazepine receptors on tumor. *Blue*, tumor models within transparent rat brain. (Courtesy of KL Black, MD, Division of Neurosurgery, University of California Los Angeles School of Medicine.)

SECTION X

INTERVENTIONAL RADIOLOGY

CHAPTER 42

Interventional Radiology

SIDNEY WALLACE, CHUSILP CHARNSANGAVEJ, AND C. HUMBERTO CARRASCO

Introduction

Utilizing imaging that best defines the target organ, the interventional radiologist applies percutaneous procedures for a more aggressive and invasive approach to the diagnosis and management of the patient with cancer. Both percutaneous vascular and nonvascular interventional radiologic techniques, adapted from established surgical procedures, are done rapidly and efficiently. At the University of Texas M. D. Anderson Cancer Center (MDACC), more than 3,500 interventional radiologic procedures are performed each year. These procedures include biopsy and drainage; intra-arterial infusion, embolization, and chemoembolization; repositioning of central venous catheters; placement of long-term venous access devices, metallic stents, and inferior vena caval filters; and intravascular foreign body retrieval and thrombolysis.

Biopsy

Almost all tissues, including the myocardium, are accessible to percutaneous biopsy. The success of biopsy depends on the expertise and interest of the radiologist and the cytopathologist. A variety of needles (14 to 25 gauge) as well as biopsy forceps are efficient in obtaining representative specimens. Superficial palpable masses are biopsied by the cytopathologist, while others requiring imaging techniques—fluoroscopy, ultrasonography (US), computed tomography (CT), and magnetic resonance imaging (MRI)—are sampled by the radiologist (54, 79). Most biopsies of lesions in adults are scheduled electively on an outpatient basis. Prothrombin time, partial thromboplastin time, and platelet counts are determined and any correctable coagulopathies are remedied. Intravenous (IV) sedation and local analgesia are usually adequate, while general anesthesia is reserved for children. After the biopsy, the patient is observed for approximately 1 hour before discharge from the radiology department.

THORAX

Guidance by fluoroscopy or CT is usually adequate for biopsy of the lung or mediastinum. The reported accuracy (sensitivity) of percutaneous transthoracic needle biopsy of patients with lung cancer and pulmonary metastases is 90 to 98% (68, 80), while the diagnostic yield by percutaneous biopsy for focal pulmonary infection in immunocompromised patients is reported to be 73% (17). Positive cytology is disclosed in 72% of attempted biopsies of mediastinal masses, with a 9% incidence of complications (64). The major complication of lung biopsy is pneumothorax, which occurs in 10 to 50% of cases; in 2 to 50% of these a thoracic tube must be placed, usually by the interventional radiologist (42).

BREAST

The combination of the clinical examination, mammography, and histologic evaluation of core biopsy or aspiration cytology specimens establishes a correct diagnosis of malignancy in 95 to 98% of breast lesions (24, 39). At MDACC, cytology, especially if performed under sonographic (US) guidance, yields positive results in 75 to 80% of suspicious lesions (24). Localization of small lesions, less than 1 cm in diameter, for surgical excision is frequently accomplished by mammography.

In a multi-institutional study of core biopsies in 6,152 breast lesions, including 1,637 with microcalcifications and 984 malignancies (78.2%, 15 mm or smaller), it was concluded that percutaneous automated large-core breast biopsy with stereotactic or US guidance is a reproducible and reliable alternative to surgical biopsy (55). The core biopsy miss rate of 1.2% compares well with the miss rate of surgical excisional biopsy of 0.2 to 20%. However, the cost of percutaneous core biopsy is one-fourth to one-half that of surgical biopsy. The technique is well tolerated by patients, with no adverse cosmetic results and no time lost from work (55).

ABDOMEN

Guided by fluoroscopy, US, CT, and more recently, MRI, 84 to 93% of biopsies yielded adequate diagnostic material for cytologic analysis. When a 20- to 23-gauge needle is used, biopsies of the liver, pancreas, kidney, adrenal, spleen, and ovary, among other organs, are performed with a sensitivity of 86.6%, a specificity of 98.6%, and an accuracy of 90% (Fig. 42.1*A*). The overall complication rate in another study of 63,180 biopsies was 0.16%. Seeding of malignant cells along the needle tract was 0.05%.

LYMPH NODES

Metastatic lymphadenopathy from carcinoma can be detected with a high degree of accuracy—83 to 95%—by fine-needle aspiration (FNA) directed by fluoroscopy of lymph nodes that opacified on lymphography, CT, or US (Figs. 42.1*B* and *C*) (87). At MDACC the accuracy of needle biopsy of lymph nodes involved by lymphoma is now 80% with the help of immunocytochemical cell markers, DNA flow cytometry, cytogenetics, molecular studies, and cytospin and cell block techniques for cytology (15).

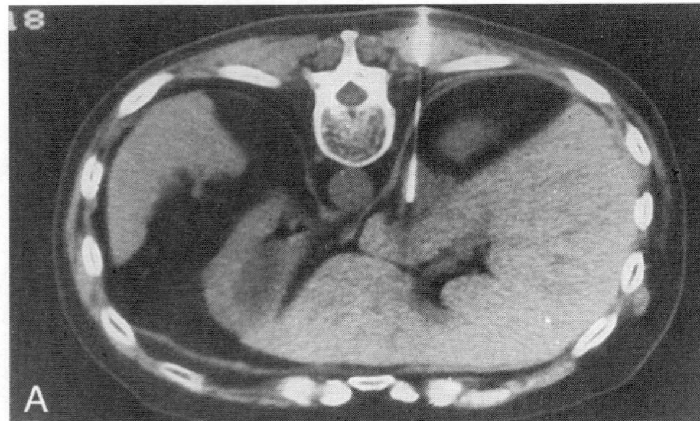

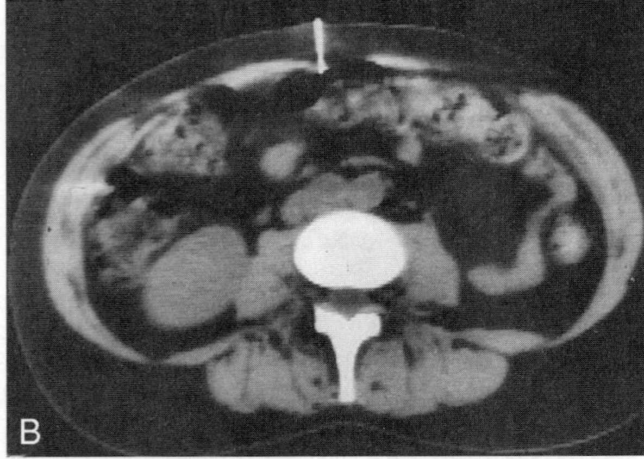

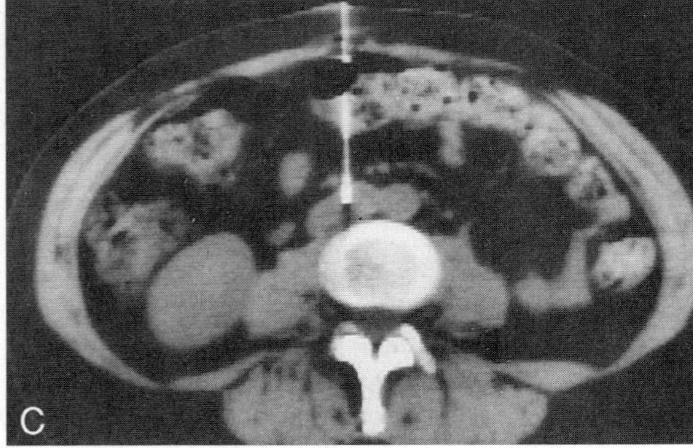

Figure 42.1. Percutaneous biopsy. **A.** Metastatic melanoma of the right adrenal. The patient is prone. Tip of needle is in the right adrenal. **B and C.** Metastatic ovarian carcinoma to the aorticocaval node. The patient is supine. Tip of needle is in the metastatic node.

MUSCULOSKELETAL

The diagnostic accuracy of percutaneous skeletal biopsy is 80% (range, 50–94%) (11). At MDACC an overall diagnostic accuracy of 78.6% was reported in a series of 178 patients with primary skeletal tumors who underwent percutaneous needle biopsy. The procedure was more accurate for malignant neoplasms (83%) than benign tumors (64.2%) (5). In unsuspected infectious diseases the frequency of positive bacterial cultures has been low (11, 70).

Drainage Procedures

Percutaneous catheter drainage of obstructed urinary, biliary, and gastrointestinal (GI) tracts as well as abnormal fluid collections such as abscesses, empyemas, bilomas, urinomas, and lymphocysts can be accomplished under radiologic guidance utilizing the Seldinger technique with needle, wire, and catheter.

NEPHROSTOMY

In cancer patients, urinary tract obstruction usually develops as the result of compression or direct extension of primary or metastatic neoplasms in the pelvis or retroperitoneum. Less frequently, obstruction in these patients is caused by calculi or benign strictures. Percutaneous nephrostomy is the primary procedure performed to improve renal function and to decrease blood pressure, to treat sepsis in cases of pyonephrosis, and to divert flow away from a urinary fistula. It is particularly important in patients whose therapy will include agents that depend on renal excretion and are also potentially nephrotoxic. The decision to perform a nephrostomy takes into consideration the patient's expected survival and the available therapeutic options. The mortality rate for percutaneous nephrostomy is less than 0.2%. The 0.7% incidence of complications immediately following the nephrostomy procedure consists of hemorrhage, septicemia, and endotoxic shock (32). Although clinically detectable retroperitoneal hemorrhage is unusual, CT demonstrated its presence in 13% of patients (32).

Percutaneous nephrostomy is usually performed under fluoroscopic guidance following antegrade nephrostography or under US guidance. A pigtail catheter can be placed into the renal pelvis through a posterior calyx and a loop is formed in the renal pelvis to minimize dislodgement. Twenty-four to 48 hours later, nephrostography should be performed to determine the cause of obstruction and to plan for further manipulation, including ureteral stenting or placement of an internal-external or indwelling catheter. We prefer a percutaneous approach as our primary procedure because of the high success rate and because it provides immediate relief of urinary obstruction, regardless of cause.

Ureteral stents, whether internal-external or indwelling, offer a more comfortable alternative to nephrostomy for long-term urinary tract decompression. Nephrostomy and ureteral stenting provide adequate palliation for ureteral obstruction by malignant neoplasms. In cancer patients, benign fibrotic ureteral strictures may occur after pelvic surgery, at ureteral anastomotic sites, and, less frequently, after radiation therapy. In a series of 44 patients with benign ureteral strictures, immediately successful dilation was accomplished in 48% of the patients (7). The best results are achieved in patients with relatively recent strictures, whereas balloon dilation of long-standing, severely fibrotic strictures is more likely to fail. Other endourologic methods of treating strictures include endoscopic incision and electrolysis.

BILIARY DRAINAGE

Percutaneous drainage of an obstructed biliary system is achieved by inserting a catheter through the hepatic parenchyma into a dilated bile duct. The endoscopic approach through the ampulla of Vater is employed as the procedure of choice, however, when that access is available.

Three types of biliary drainage are performed percutaneously: external, combined external-internal, and drainage through indwelling stents. Percutaneous drainage is an important adjunct to the palliative treatment of patients with inoperable cancer, in whom it is performed to improve metabolic and nutritional status, relieve pruritus, and allow the administration of chemotherapeutic agents that require unimpeded biliary excretion. In addition, percutaneous drainage is used to treat acute suppurative cholangitis, in failed biliary enteric bypass, and for diversion of bile flow in treating bile leaks and fistulas.

In 131 patients at MDACC with cancer, the overall median survival from the time of percutaneous drainage until death was only 57 days (16). The short survival time reflects the terminal nature of these patients with biliary obstruction, who frequently undergo the procedure before starting chemotherapy for their neoplasms. Patients who underwent subsequent biliary bypass had a better median survival time (172 days), suggesting the better clinical status of the surgical candidates.

The acute complications of biliary drainage are related to the procedure, whereas delayed complications are related to chronic catheter drainage. The incidence of acute complications is low; a review of 200 patients showed sepsis in 7, hemorrhage in 6, and death in 3. Fever and hemobilia occurred in 21 and 18 patients, respectively (48). Cholangitis, the most frequent complication in chronic drainage, was experienced by 47% of 161 patients. This often happened during periods of myelosuppression (16). In a randomized trial after endoscopic stenting, the combination of the choleretic ursodeoxycholic acid and the antibiotic norfloxacin produced significant improvement compared with conservative management alone. Median patency was 38 weeks versus 7 weeks for controls. Median survival was 67 weeks versus 18 weeks; furthermore the mean hospital stay was significantly shorter (8). Dislodgement of the catheter was noted in 18%, and in 14% the catheter became occluded (16). Intrahepatic vascular lesions, including pseudoaneurysms and arterioportal fistulas, have been reported in 26 to 33% but are usually asymptomatic. Pleural empyema, hemothorax, pneumothorax, and bilious pleural effusion may occur in 1 to 2.5% of patients (48, 53). A cholerrhagic state with bile output of 7 L/day was seen in 5% of our patients (16). It is usually temporary, but it creates severe fluid and electrolyte loss with hypotension and hyponatremia requiring aggressive replacement therapy.

Because external drainage can be associated with the cholerrhagic state, fluid and electrolyte imbalance, and catheter dislodgement, it is preferable to convert the external drainage catheter to an external-internal drainage catheter. Through the tract created by the external drainage catheter, a guidewire can be manipulated past the obstruction site and advanced into the duodenum. A catheter with multiple side holes can then be placed into the bile duct with the tip advanced into the duodenum, leaving the side holes above and below the obstruction site. This would allow external drainage of the bile and would also allow the bile to drain down into the duodenum. One of the disadvantages of this catheter is that a portion of the catheter still remains outside the patient and may cause pain and discomfort as well as become a psychological burden. Another alternative is to replace the whole catheter with an internal drain only. However, this technique may be painful and result in more discomfort than endoscopic placement of an internal drainage catheter.

The adequacy of catheter drainage depends on the physical properties of the catheter material, its luminal diameter, its length, and the total area of its inflow and outflow side holes, as well as the pressure gradient and the type of fluid being drained. Although stents larger than 8 to 10 F are best for internal drainage, their transhepatic insertion is painful and requires a well-established tract. Expandable metallic stents may be placed by the transhepatic or endoscopic approach, but thus far, mucosal hypertrophy and tumor ingrowth through interstices limit their usefulness and long-term patency.

PERCUTANEOUS GASTROSTOMY

Percutaneous gastrostomy offers a useful route for providing nutritional support to patients with esophageal and head and neck neoplasms that compromise swallowing function. Patients with chronic intestinal obstruction caused by unresectable neoplasms and those who have multiple enteric strictures secondary to irradiation should undergo decompressive gastrostomy. Although previously considered exclusively a surgical procedure, gastrostomy can be done by a percutaneous approach with a needle, wire, and catheter placed under fluoroscopic guidance or through an endoscope (59, 60, 65).

Percutaneous gastrostomy was performed under fluoroscopy in 100 cancer patients at MDACC (52). A nasogastric tube was placed into the stomach and the stomach was distended by air insufflation. The distended stomach was then punctured percutaneously through the abdominal wall under fluoroscopic guidance, and the guidewire and catheter were placed using a modified Seldinger technique. In 67 patients with bowel obstruction the procedure was done for gastric drainage, with 24 to 28 F Malecot catheters inserted in one sitting. The remaining 33 patients had supragastric obstructions or fistulas and required 10 to 14 F pigtail catheters for feeding purposes. The average postgastrostomy hospitalization was 3.6 days. Drainage gastrostomies were ready for use immediately after the procedure, whereas the use of feeding gastrostomies started an average of 2 days after tube insertion. There were no major complications or deaths related to the procedure. Percutaneous gastrostomy is a simple, safe technique even when large-caliber catheters are used, and it does not require gastric fixation to the abdominal wall to prevent spillage into the peritoneum, since the inflammatory response around the tube isolates the channel.

ABSCESS DRAINAGE

In patients with cancer, an intra-abdominal abscess may be life-threatening. It is usually caused by perforation of a hollow viscus affected by a neoplasm or by a postoperative complication. A septic episode is often accompanied by renal, pulmonary, or cardiovascular failure, and when untreated has a mortality rate of nearly 100%. Thirty-six percent of intra-abdominal abscesses are located intraperitoneally, 38% retroperitoneally, and 26% viscerally (2).

CT and US are used to diagnose and localize abscesses. The radiologic features are nonspecific, and an abscess must be differentiated from biloma, urinoma, lymphocele, seroma, pancreatic pseudocyst, hematoma, neoplasm, and a fluid-filled viscus. Cross-sectional scans are used to determine the depth, the cutaneous entry site, and the angle through which the collection is best approached (27).

A diagnostic fine-needle (21–22 gauge) puncture is made and a sample is taken for Gram stain and culture. If the Gram stain is negative, the remaining fluid is aspirated for bacterial culture and cytologic assay and the needle is withdrawn. A catheter may be left in place until the results of the culture are known, but no longer than 48 hours to avoid infecting a sterile collection. A drainage catheter is inserted if infection has been confirmed.

Selection of a safe route for diagnostic puncture and drainage is the most crucial aspect of the procedure. Nonviscous collections are drained adequately by 6 to 10 F catheters, which are also used to drain renal and hepatic parenchymal abscesses. For viscous nonparenchymal collections, 12 to 14 F sump catheters are employed. Irrigating drainage catheters with saline, chemical, or antibiotic solutions is usually not necessary and may disseminate the infection. If the exudate is viscous, gentle irrigation with 5 to 10 mL of physiologic solution may be necessary to maintain catheter patency. Drainage of simple abscesses usually ceases by the 5th to 10th day. With an associated fistula, drainage may persist for weeks (73).

Successful percutaneous drainage was accomplished in 83.6% of 250 abdominal abscesses and fluid collections, with 21 failures and 20 recurrences (73). The overall complication rate was 10% (3% severe and 7% minor). Complications included septicemia, infection of a previously sterile cavity, bowel perforation, and one death. Transvaginal US-guided drainage is effective treatment for pelvic abscess, being either completely curative or temporizing in 78% of patients (23). Transrectal US-guided aspiration-lavage was successful in treating 28 (85%) of 33 pelvic abscesses in 21 (88%) of the 24 patients. This offers a one-step method that does not require catheter placement or prolonged drainage (38). Treatment failures occurred with multiloculated abscesses and with cellulitis associated with fistulas, viscous hematomas, or organized collections. Similar parameters can be used for the percutaneous approach to treatment of empyema.

Intra-arterial Therapy

Intra-arterial management of neoplasms by the percutaneous transcatheter approach necessitates the participation of chemotherapist, surgeon, radiotherapist, and interventional radiologist in the infusion of chemotherapeutic agents, embolization, and chemoembolization. Intra-arterial management is rarely used in widely disseminated cancers since multiple circulatory beds are seldom treated.

INFUSION

Most cytotoxic agents have a steep dose-response curve; that is, the higher the concentration, the greater the tumor effect (26). Intra-arterial infusion exposes the neoplasm to a higher local concentration of chemotherapy with no increase in systemic toxicity but frequently an increase in local side effects (31). The pharmacokinetics of regional chemotherapy are discussed in detail in Chapter 55. Those agents most effective when delivered systemically should be the initial choice for intra-arterial therapy. Neoplasms refractory to IV chemotherapy may respond to the intra-arterial infusion of the same drugs at the same dose rate. Those drugs tolerated by the local tissues can be administered intra-arterially, while others can be delivered IV at the same time or sequentially. Doxorubicin and the vinca alkaloids are local irritants that cause endarteritis and are better tolerated by the liver than the extremities. Intra-arterial delivery, however, can be accomplished even with these agents by decreasing the dose per unit of time and extending the infusion over a longer period.

Hypervascular neoplasms act as a sump to draw the blood and chemotherapeutic agents almost exclusively to the tumor. Intra-arterial delivery is even more essential for hypovascular neoplasms to increase the drug concentration, which may be associated with a higher incidence of local complications.

The delivery of chemotherapeutic agents requires selective arterial catheterization, which is accomplished by tailoring the catheter configuration to the vascular anatomy. Coaxial systems with 2 to 3 F catheters have facilitated the technical challenge. A nonthrombogenic environment is created by systemic heparinization (15,000–25,000 units of aqueous heparin over each 24 hours) injected intra-arterially or IV to maintain the clotting parameters at 1.5 to 2 times normal (77). Heparin and doxorubicin are incompatible and must be infused through different catheters; one is IV and the other is intra-arterial.

Occlusion for Infusion

Temporary or permanent occlusion of branch vessels using Gelfoam segments and/or stainless steel coils can minimize the exposure of normal tissues and maximize the infusion of the tumor. This is especially helpful in the pelvis, where the superior and inferior gluteal arteries are occluded to decrease the chemodermatitis of the buttocks and to increase the concentration to neoplasms of pelvic viscera (82). Occlusion of the superficial temporal and middle meningeal arteries directs flow into the internal maxillary artery in treating neoplasms of the maxillary sinuses. The gastroduodenal artery may be occluded at its junction with the common hepatic artery to lessen gastric, duodenal, and pancreatic complications. Selective occlusion is not associated with ischemia because of adequate collateral circulation.

Redistribution of the vascular supply can be achieved by the selective occlusion of most of the vessels contributing to the neoplasm so that a single artery (through collateral circulation) will supply the entire organ and neoplasm. This is especially effective in converting multiple arteries supplying the liver to a single artery to be infused through a single catheter.

Pulsatile Flow

The conventional flow rate for intra-arterial infusion is 50 to 200 mL/h, delivered at constant pump pressure. This slow rate results in laminar flow or streaming and unequal distribution of the chemotherapeutic agents. A pulsatile pump can be attached to the constant infusion pump to create turbulence at the tip of the catheter, thereby dispersing the infusate. This can improve the infusate distribution in 20% of patients treated by hepatic arterial infusion and control chemodermatitis in 90% of the patients with osteosarcoma of an extremity treated intra-arterially.

Flow Studies

Radionuclide flow studies are used routinely to evaluate the distribution following catheter placement for intra-arterial chemotherapy infusion (34), as follows: 37 to 185 MBq (1–5 mCi) of technetium-99m macroaggregated albumin (MAA) in a volume of 0.5 to 1 mL is delivered by a mechanical pump at a rate similar to that of the chemotherapy infusion. Scintigraphy of the area of interest is performed; flow distribution is evaluated as to tumor uptake, normal adjacent organ uptake, and systemic escape. This information assists in the prediction of tumor response, the possibility of complications, and dose adjustment.

Therapeutic Agents for Intra-arterial Delivery

The cytotoxic agents delivered by the intra-arterial route include acridinyl anisidide (AMSA); actinomycin D; aziridinylbenzoquinone (AZQ); bleomycin; carboplatin; carmustine (BCNU); cisdiamminedichloroplatinum (cisplatin, CDDP); cyclophosphamide (Cytoxan); dimethyltriazenoimidazole carboxamide (DTIC); doxorubicin (Adriamycin); etoposide (epipodophyllotoxin, VP 16-213); 5-fluorouracil (5-FU); floxuridine (FUDR); ifosfamide (Ifex); methotrexate (MTX); mitomycin C (MMC); mitoxantrone (Novantrone); nitrogen mustard (mechlorethamine); phenylalanine mustard (melphalan, PAM, Alkeran); streptozocin; vinblastine (VLB, Velban); vincristine (VCR, Oncovin); and vindesine. Immunomodifiers that have been administered intra-arterially include Bacille Calmette-Guérin (BCG), *corynebacterium parvum*, interferon (IFN), interleukin-2 (IL-2), platelet factor 4, and tumor necrosis factor (TNF). Almost all water-soluble antibiotics can be delivered intra-arterially. Corticosteroids (Solucortef, Decadron) have also been administered by this route. Before the use of a new agent intra-arterially, laboratory trials are necessary to determine the dose tolerated by the patient, the organ, and the artery infused.

EMBOLIZATION

Embolization is the occlusion of the arterial supply of the tumor to create ischemia and tumor necrosis and to arrest tumor growth by the intra-arterial delivery of particulate materials, sclerosing solutions, and substances introduced in the liquid state that eventually solidify. Interruption of a vessel at its origin has an effect similar to that of surgical ligation. Collateral circulation is available immediately; the more central the occlusion, the more abundant the collateral circulation. The closer the occlusion is to the tumor, the smaller is the opportunity for collateral circulation.

Embolic Agents for Intra-arterial Delivery

The materials available for embolization include autologous clot and tissue, clot modified by thrombin, ϵ-aminocaproic acid (Amicar), and heat; absorbable gelatin sponge (Gelfoam); oxidized cellulose (Oxycel); polyvinyl alcohol foam (Ivalon); cyanoacrylates; Ethibloc; microfibrillar collagen hemostat (Avitene, Angiostat); sclerosing solutions (absolute ethanol and sodium tetradecyl sulfate [Sotradecol]); balloon catheters and detachable balloons; metallic brushes and stainless steel coils.

In general, at MDACC, peripheral embolization is accomplished with absorbable gelatin sponge particles and powder (Gelfoam) or polyvinyl alcohol foam (Ivalon) granules, and central occlusion is achieved with gelatin sponge segments or stainless steel coils.

The indications for transcatheter embolization of neoplasms are (*a*) to control hemorrhage, particularly GI hemorrhage from ulcerated tumors in patients who are not operative candidates; (*b*) preoperatively, to facilitate surgical resection by decreasing blood loss and operating time, particularly for vertebral and other axial skeletal neoplasms; (*c*) to inhibit tumor growth; and (*d*) to relieve pain by decreasing tumor bulk.

The complications of embolization were analyzed by Hemingway and Allison (30) over a 10-year period in 284 patients who underwent 410 embolizations. Minor complications occurred in 16%, serious complications (ischemia, hemorrhage, and others) in 6.6%, and death in 2%. The postembolization syndrome (fever, elevated white blood cell count, and discomfort) was encountered after 42.7% of the procedures. The underlying abnormality usually determined the nature of the complication.

CHEMOEMBOLIZATION

This technique as proposed by Kato et al. is the combination of intra-arterial infusion of chemotherapeutic agents and arterial embolization of the vascular supply to the neoplasm (36). In addition to the direct effect of ischemia on the neoplasm by occlusion, the emboli prolong the transit time through the tumor vascular bed, theoretically increasing the contact time between the chemotherapeutic agent and the neoplastic cell. The increased local drug concentration is enhanced by the increased tissue permeability caused by anoxia. The overall effect is cytotoxic not only to the neoplasm but to the vessels embolized and infused, compounding the vasculitis and occlusion. The systemic toxic effect may be reduced by metabolism of the drug on its first passage through the infused organ, thereby confining the higher concentration to the target organ.

Kato et al. incorporated mitomycin C in ethylcellulose microcapsules (225 μm in diameter) for gradual and sustained release (36). Aronsen et al. (4) and Dakhil et al. (21) injected starch microspheres (40 μm in diameter), degraded by the blood serum amylase, prior to the intra-arterial infusion of chemotherapy to slow flow and increase contact time. In Japan, management of hepatocellular carcinoma and, to a lesser extent, hepatic metastases includes the intra-arterial delivery of Gelfoam, Lipiodol ultra-fluid (Ethiodol), and the chemotherapeutic agents mitomycin C, doxorubicin, actinomycin D, cisplatin, or neocarcinostatin (18). Ethibloc, a solution of prolamine in alcohol, has also been used in Europe in combination with pulverized lyophilized cytotoxic drugs, such as mitomycin C, doxorubicin, and/or cisplatin. At MDACC, cisplatin, mitomycin C, doxorubicin, floxuridine, actinomycin D, streptozocin, and other drugs are mixed with Ivalon, Gelfoam particles, or Gelfoam powder for intra-arterial administration. These combinations frequently increase the tumor response but also increase local toxicity. Microencapsulation of most chemotherapeutic agents with a variety of polymers (particles of 100 μm and less in diameter) have been formulated in our laboratory (78, 87). Liposomes of less than 5 μm in diameter are also available for chemoembolization. Hepatic uptake of liposomes delivered IV was 50%, compared to 70% when injected into the hepatic artery (83).

MUSCULOSKELETAL APPLICATIONS

Osteosarcoma

The rationale for the preoperative intra-arterial infusion of osteosarcoma is to control the local primary tumor, to facilitate local resection with limb salvage rather than amputation, and to identify effective chemotherapy for adjuvant treatment based on the degree of tumor necrosis observed in the resected specimen (9). The treatment regimen at MDACC consists of cisplatin (120–200 mg/m^2) delivered intra-arterially over 2 to 24 hours, preceded by doxorubicin (90 mg/m^2) administered IV over 96 hours. Limb salvage surgery is now possible in 80% of skeletally mature patients. Patients treated between 1983 and 1988 had a 68% complete response rate, a 27% partial response rate, and a 76% 3-year continuous disease-free survival (9). This compares well with our historical control of 20% in patients treated by surgery alone or by surgery plus radiation therapy. Similar survival rates have been reported with the IV delivery of multiple drugs (81).

The intra-arterial approach starts with cisplatin and doxorubicin delivered IV; only in the face of failure are other drugs added, including methotrexate, ifosfamide, bleomycin, and others. The long-term implications of the multiple drugs are yet to be determined.

Giant Cell Tumors and Aneurysmal Bone Cysts

At MDACC, most of the giant cell tumors in a group of 21 patients were located in the sacrum, ilium, and thoracolumbar spine and had not responded to other forms of therapy. Sequential embolization resulted in complete control of pain and radiographic healing of the tumors in 48% of the patients. Partial relief of symptoms was observed in an additional 19% of patients, for a total response rate of 67% (12). After embolization, seven patients received chemotherapy or radiation therapy. One patient underwent subsequent surgery for an iliac tumor that responded to embolization. Ischemic neuropathy and a single unexplained death were major complications seen after extensive arterial embolization.

Similar results have been reported in patients with aneurysmal bone cysts not amenable to surgical management that were treated by embolization (37).

Metastatic Skeletal Neoplasms

Embolization of skeletal neoplasms was initially performed as an adjunct to surgical resection of hypervascular tumors to decrease operative blood loss. Subsequently, this technique was used for palliation of pain caused by skeletal metastases (61). Our efforts have been mostly concentrated on hypervascular metastases such as those from renal and thyroid carcinoma. Success depends on the ability to occlude the total vascular supply to the tumor while preserving the supply to normal structures.

GENITOURINARY APPLICATIONS

Renal Carcinoma

Embolization of renal carcinoma is now done at MDACC when the patients are not candidates for surgery because of their general medical status or the extent of their metastases. Sequential renal artery embolization that preserves as much renal parenchyma and function as possible has been used in the management of congestive heart failure caused by arteriovenous shunting through the renal carcinoma, and for hypertension, hypercalcemia, polycythemia, and hemorrhage due to renal neoplasm. Selective embolization is especially necessary and effective in patients with an elevated serum creatinine level or a neoplasm in a solitary kidney (76).

Embolization should be done preserving at least 50% of the kidney to maintain adequate function.

At MDACC, in 49 patients with metastases from renal carcinoma, renal artery embolization of the primary neoplasm was used to debulk the tumor in preparation for systemic treatment with 5-FU, mitomycin C, and α-interferon. Embolization proved to be as effective in reducing tumor cell population as nephrectomy. This regimen has a 35% response rate (66). Recently, interleukin-2 has been substituted for mitomycin C in an attempt to decrease myelosuppression, a side effect of mitomycin C.

Adrenal Tumors

Adrenal arterial embolization was performed in nine patients, four with inoperable adrenal cortical carcinomas and five with metastatic adrenal tumors. In eight of these patients, embolization was performed for palliation either to decrease tumor bulk, suppress tumor hormonal function (three patients), or relieve pain (four patients). In four patients in whom it was possible to assess the effect of embolization, a striking reduction in size had occurred in one, the lesions remained stable in size for 12 months in two, and the tumor continued to increase in size in the fourth. A reduction in the production of the cortisol for 12 months was seen in two of three patients with Cushing's syndrome. Adrenal embolization resulted in effective palliation of pain in three of four patients and may have contributed to palliation in the fourth. Apart from a hypertensive episode in one patient, no serious side effects occurred (51).

Carcinoma of the Bladder

Patients with locally advanced bladder carcinoma with or without nodal metastases have been treated with combined IV and intra-arterial CISCA (cisplatin, Cytoxan, and doxorubicin) chemotherapy. Cytoxan (650 mg/m^2) and doxorubicin (50 mg/m^2) were delivered IV on the day the catheters were placed into each internal iliac artery. The next day, after adequate hydration, cisplatin (75–100 mg/m^2) was infused intra-arterially along with mannitol (40 g) IV for diuresis. An overall complete remission rate of 50% and a partial response rate of 18%, for a total response rate of 68%, were achieved (75). This served as the basis for subsequent systemic chemotherapy with CISCA and then with MVAC (methotrexate, vinblastine, Adriamycin, cisplatin).

Carcinoma of the Uterine Cervix

Patients with stages 3 and 4 disease were treated with the intra-arterial (bilateral internal iliac artery) infusion of mitomycin C (10 mg/m^2 over 24 hours every other course), bleomycin (20–40 mg/m^2 over 24 hours), and cisplatin (100 mg/m^2 over 2 hours), while vincristine, a 2-mg bolus, was given IV. After three cycles spaced 3 to 4 weeks apart, the patients were evaluated for further definitive radiation therapy. Forty-four patients had received no prior therapy before intra-arterial chemotherapy was initiated. Thirty-five (76%) of the patients responded to the regimen; 24 (52%) were partial responders and 11 (24%) were complete responders. The 5-year survival rate for the study group was 30%, with a median survival duration of 18 months (57).

Nagata et al. (49) reported the results of infusing both internal iliac arteries in patients with advanced carcinoma of the uterine cervix (stage 3 and higher) with cisplatin (60–70 mg/m^2), doxorubicin (30–40 mg/m^2), 5-FU (500 mg), and mitomycin C (20 mg) or Cytoxan (500 mg) delivered over 30 minutes as a bolus. The approach attempted to downstage the disease prior to surgical resection followed by radiation therapy (50 Gy administered over 5 weeks). There was a decrease in tumor size in 11 of 12 patients; at radical hysterectomy no viable cancer cells were found in the uterus in 6 patients and no extrauterine cancer in 5 additional patients. Sterilization of tumor was therefore possible in advanced stages, suggesting that more patients with cervical carcinoma may become candidates for resection.

GASTROINTESTINAL APPLICATIONS

Hepatocellular Carcinoma

It is our experience that the type of hepatocellular carcinoma (HCC) seen at MDACC, and perhaps in the United States, is different from that treated in Japan (85). Nodular HCC is seen in less than 25% of our patients. This type of tumor can be approached by the direct injection of alcohol or by chemoembolization, but also by surgery, with a 2-year survival rate of approximately 50%. However, there are no randomized studies to compare these different techniques. Advanced, more invasive HCC is more commonly seen at MDACC. Our current regimen consists of cisplatin, 50 to 75 mg/m^2, and doxorubicin, 25 to 40 mg/m^2, infused intra-arterially over 2 hours each, followed by 3 to 4 days of continuous infusion of floxuridine, 50 to 75 mg/m^2, and leucovorin, 15 mg/m^2/d. Treatment with this regimen yielded a response rate of 78% and a median survival period of 11.5 months (56).

Yamada et al. (84), in their series of more than 1,000 patients, including those with large inoperable HCC treated with Gelfoam particles mixed with doxorubicin and mitomycin C, reported survival rates of 51% at 1 year, 28% at 2 years, 13% at 3 years, 8% at 4 years, and 6% at 5 years. Ohishi et al. (50) described their experience in over 500 patients with inoperable HCC. A 4-year survival rate of 20.4% was achieved after treatment with anticancer drugs, gelatin sponge, and iodized oil. From the same group, Uchida et al. (72) reported a 3-year survival rate of 55% in 99 cases of nodular HCC less than 5 cm in diameter that had been treated by subsegmental iodized oil chemoembolization. Subsegmental chemoembolization with iodized oil and anticancer drugs followed by gelatin sponge particles or a mixture of iodized oil and absolute ethanol in 82 patients with nodular HCCs (less than 4 cm in diameter, Childs classes A and B), yielded 1-year and 4-year survival rates of 100% and 67% (44). Ebara et al. (22) reported a 4-year survival rate of 61% in a series of 217 HCCs less than 3 cm in diameter that were treated by percutaneous ethanol injection (PEI). Shiina et al. (67) combined PEI and iodized oil chemoembolization and achieved survival rates of 79% at 1 year and 38% at 5 years.

Metastatic Colorectal Carcinoma

5-FU or 5-FUDR infused through a catheter placed surgically or percutaneously into the hepatic artery yielded response rates ranging from 32 to 88%, depending on the criteria utilized (6). Despite effective control of hepatic disease, extrahepatic metastases were usually the major cause of death. At MDACC, the intra-arterial infusion of floxuridine (100 mg/m^2/d x 5 days) and mitomycin C (10 mg/m^2) yielded a response rate of 61% in previously untreated patients and 45% in patients who had failed to respond to previous IV 5-FU. A response rate of 52% was found with the infusion of floxuridine and cisplatin (100 mg/m^2) (74). The median survival time for the responders was 16 months. Chemoembolization with the combination of Ivalon with floxuridine (800 mg), mitomycin C (10 mg), or cisplatin (150 mg) led to no significant improvement in response rate or survival. Yamashita et al. (86), who treated 68 patients with various hepatic metastases using iodized oil and chemotherapeutic agents, noted a response rate of 22% and a median survival time of 10 months. A similar result was observed by Inoue et al. (33), i.e., a partial response rate of 16% and a median survival period of 11 months. Lang and Brown (41) treated 46 patients with colorectal hepatic metastases using doxorubicin and iodized oil, with 75% selectively administered to different subsegments and 25% into the respective main hepatic artery. In 8 patients the lesions disappeared; 11 patients showed no progression for 12 months; 2 others, for 24 months. Thirteen patients died and 3 were lost to follow-up in the first year. The approach by Kemeny and coworkers is presented in Chapter 115.

Metastatic Ocular Melanoma

Three chemoembolization treatments with Ivalon particles (150 mg) and cisplatin (150 mg) for one lobe of the liver at 1-month intervals have been most effective, resulting in a 46% response rate with a median survival time of 11 months (46). The longest survivor was 5 years from the initial chemoembolization. In the past, these patients lived 2 to 6 months from presentation with hepatic metastases.

Metastatic Leiomyosarcoma

Systemic therapy with ifosfamide and doxorubicin yielded response rates of less than 15%. Fourteen patients with GI leiomyosarcoma metastatic to the liver were treated with hepatic chemoembolization consisting of Ivalon particles suspended in contrast material (150 mg) mixed with cisplatin powder (150 mg) and followed by hepatic artery infusion of vinblastine (10 mg/m^2) once adequate flow was established by a radionuclide study. This usually was possible within 12 to 24 hours after embolization. A tumor response of greater than 50% regression was observed in 70% and lasted 4 to 19 months (median, 9 months) after an average of two procedures, usually performed 4 weeks apart (47).

Metastatic Breast Carcinoma

Several regimens have been used for hepatic artery infusion of chemotherapy in patients with hepatic metastases from carcinoma of the breast, but these are used mostly as second-line treatment after systemic chemotherapy has failed.

Hepatic arterial infusion of cisplatin (120 mg/m^2) over 2 hours at monthly intervals) yielded a 19% response rate among 26 patients, with a median response period of 11 months. When a combination of cisplatin (100 mg/m^2) and vinblastine (1.7 mg/m^2/d for 3.5 days) was used, a partial response rate of 33% was achieved. For the 33 patients who underwent this regimen, a similar median survival period of 11 months was observed (25).

Metastatic Neuroendocrine Tumors

The best results of hepatic artery embolization with Ivalon or Gelfoam segments or powder were observed in patients with metastatic neuroendocrine tumors to the liver. Twenty (87%) of the 23 patients with carcinoid syndrome responded to embolization, with a median response duration of more than 11 months. The symptomatic responses correlated with a decrease in the extent of the hepatic metastases and a decrease in the urine 5-hydroxyindoleacetic acid values to a mean of 41% of pretreatment levels (10).

Of the 20 patients with symptoms from islet cell carcinoma metastatic to the liver, 16 (80%) achieved objective tumor regression after embolization. Sequential and periodic embolization is required for effective palliation (1, 58). Thus far, as many as 21 embolizations have been administered to a patient, and the longest survival in a patient with metastatic neuroendocrine tumor to the liver is now 12 years past presentation.

Chemoembolization of progressive carcinoid hepatic metatases has been successful with doxorubicin, iodized oil, and Gelfoam. Therasse et al. (71) found a complete symptomatic response (average, 29 months) in 70% of 23 patients, and a partial response in 18% of evaluated patients. The biologic response was complete (average, 21 months) in 73% and partial in 18%. The morphologic response was complete in 11% and partial in 24%. The mean survival time was 57 months after the first symptomatic episode of flush, 47 months after the diagnosis of liver metastases, and 24 months after the first treatment.

Microencapsulated cisplatin particles (100 μm in diameter) were prepared by a solvent evaporation technique and contained 46% by weight of cisplatin and poly-(D,L)-lactide. In a 1:1 ratio of chemotherapeutic agent to capsular material, approximately 40% of the cisplatin was released within the first 4 hours after delivery, as determined by in vitro studies. A phase I–II study is under way. There has been dramatic necrosis of hepatic metastases at 50 mg/m^2. In view of the response to the initial dose, 6 patients have been treated with the same dose. Eleven additional patients have been treated, 4 at 75 mg/m^2 and 7 at 100 mg/m^2. Thus far, 11 of 14 have had clinical improvement and 8 of 12 have had a tumor response (Fig. 42.2).

HEAD AND NECK APPLICATIONS

Paranasal Sinuses

Patients with advanced paranasal sinus neoplasms have been treated with combined selective intra-arterial (cisplatin)

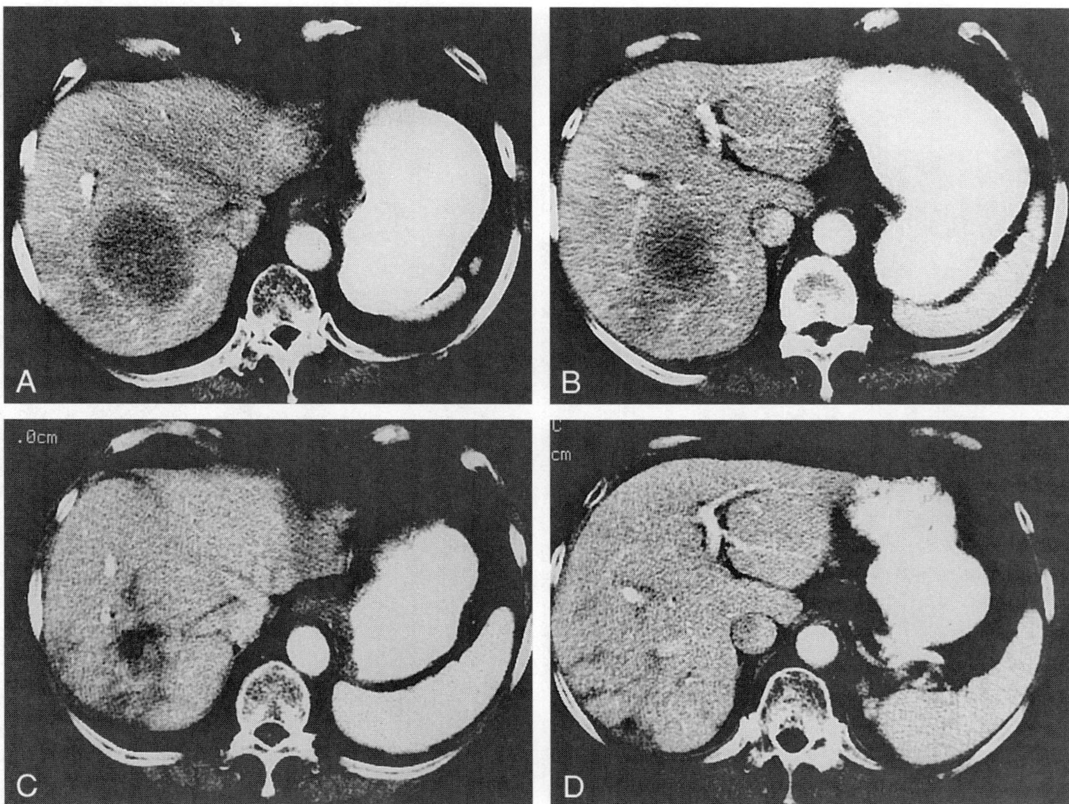

Figure 42.2. Hepatic metastasis from carcinoid tumor of the ileum. **A and B.** Appearance prior to chemoembolization. **C and D.** Appearance after two episodes of chemoembolization with poly-(D,L)-lactide capsules containing cisplatin, 75 mg/m^2. Note the tumor regression, constituting a partial response.

and systemic (5-FU) chemotherapy, which yielded an immediate and satisfactory tumor response rate of 91%. Repetitive uncomplicated catheterization of the pterygoid segment of the internal maxillary artery using a coaxial system with a 2.7-F catheter was essential to success. The effectiveness of intra-arterial chemotherapy seemed to depend on tumor sensitivity and on the ability to encompass the entire tumor within the anatomic territory of the infused artery (43).

Mechanical Devices

VENA CAVA FILTERS

Cancer patients, especially those with hypercoagulability, experience an increased incidence of thrombophlebitis and pulmonary embolism. The percutaneous placement of a vena cava filter is now more frequently the responsibility of the interventional radiologist. It is the optimal therapeutic approach for patients with pulmonary embolism who have a contraindication to anticoagulation or who develop recurrent emboli despite adequate anticoagulation. The filters currently in use are the Greenfield filter (MediTech, Watertown, MA), the bird's nest filter (Cook, Bloomington, IN), the Simon Nitinol filter (Nitinol Medical Technologies, Woburn, MA), the Vena Tech filter (Vena Tech, Evanston, IL) and the Gunther temporary filter (William Cook Europe, Bjaeverskov, Denmark). In in vitro evaluations, Kasmouris et al. demonstrated that the bird's nest filter and the Simon Nitinol filter were most efficient (35), while Hammer et al. concluded that the bird's nest filter had the highest clot-trapping capacity (29).

The stainless steel Greenfield filter, the reference standard since 1972, has been replaced by the titanium Greenfield filter, which is delivered via a 12-F catheter placed through a 14-F sheath; it has not obscured the information at MRI. The success rate of percutaneous placement was 99%; it was placed via the right femoral vein in 70% and via the left femoral or internal jugular vein in the remainder. At 30 days there was a 3% incidence of recurrent pulmonary embolism and 98% caval patency. Incomplete opening was seen in 2% and insertion site hematoma in 1% (20, 63). The bird's nest filter also requires a 12-F insertion system through a 14-F sheath. The clinical incidence of recurrent pulmonary embolism was 2% and the caval patency rate was 97% (20).

METALLIC STENT

The management of patients with stenosis of a tubular structure due to neoplasm or as the result of treatment of a neoplasm led to the development of metallic endoprostheses to reestablish patency. The percutaneous placement of such devices allows the introduction, through catheters, of

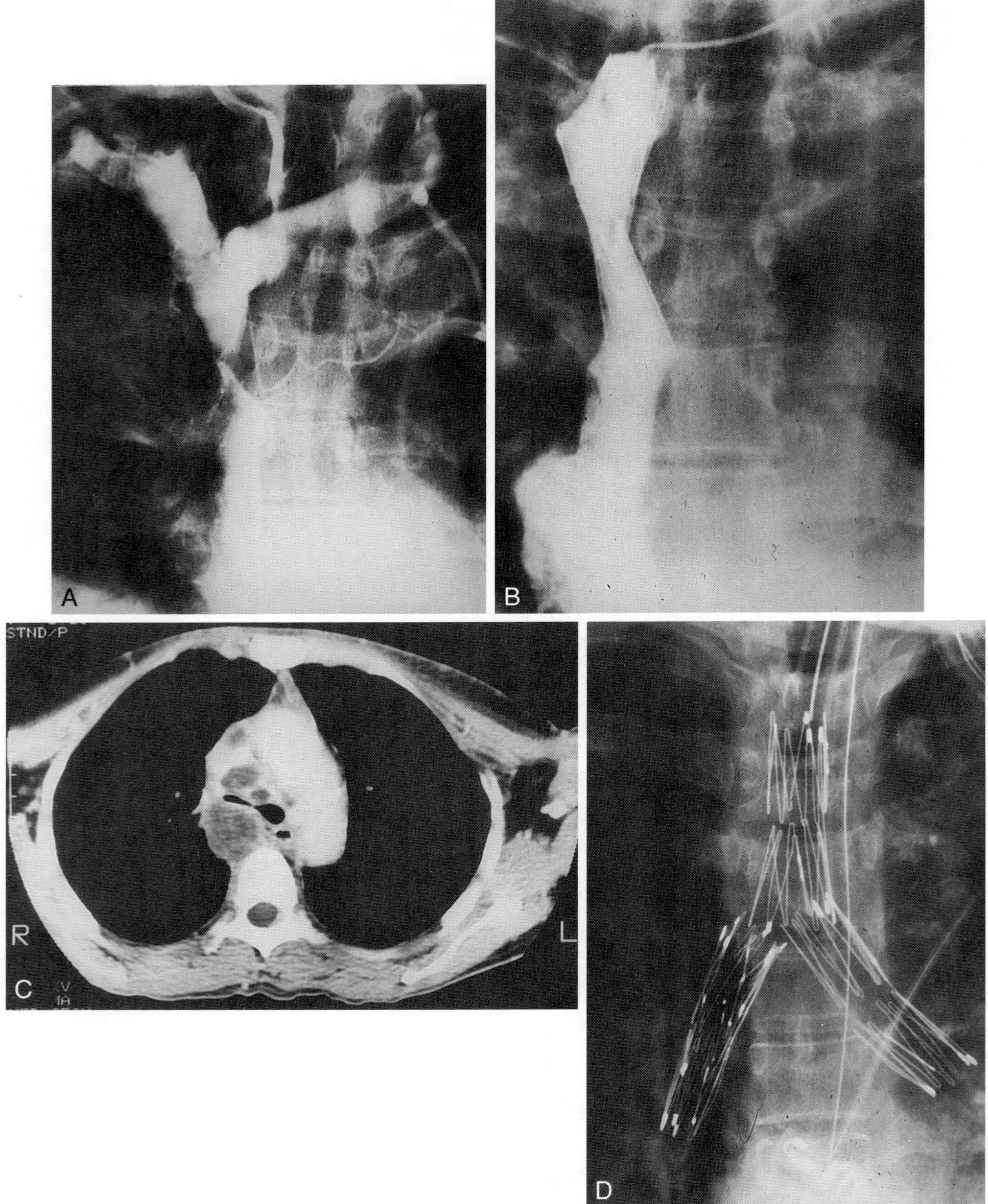

Figure 42.3. Self-expanding Gianturco Z stent. **A.** Carcinoma of the lung encasing and obstructing the superior vena cava. **B.** Patency and flow were reestablished with metallic stents. **C and D.** Carcinoma of the lung. Note marked narrowing of the trachea and main-stem bronchi, which was relieved by placement of self-expanding metallic stents.

relatively small-diameter stents that expand once they are deployed. Metallic stents now available include the self-expandable Gianturco Z stent (Cook, Bloomington, IN), the Wallstent (Medinvent SA, Lausane, Switzerland), and the Nitinol stent (Nitinol Medical Technologies, Woburn, MA), an alloy of nickel and titanium with a thermal memory, a property of an alloy that allows it to be shaped, then annealed so that when it has cooled it can be deformed, but will return to its original shape when heated to a specific temperature (e.g., body temperature); and the balloon-assisted stents, the Palmaz stent (Johnson & Johnson Interventional System, Warren, NJ) and the Strecker stents (Meditech/Boston Scientific, Watertown, MA). In cancer patients, these stents are placed in the vascular system, the biliary ducts, the tracheobronchial tree, and the esophagus. The Gianturco Z stent and the Wallstent are most frequently used.

The Gianturco Z stent is constructed of stainless steel wire (0.046–0.056 cm in caliber) bent in a zig-zag pattern and encircled to form a cylinder. Single stents cannot be deployed precisely, as they tend to spring open into the nonstenotic segment; at least two stents are connected in tandem by monofilament or wire struts and barbs are attached to minimize the risk of migration (19). The Wallstent is constructed of multifilament high-performance medical grade stainless steel alloy woven into a macroporous tube. The filaments (0.008–0.017 cm in diameter) create a flexible and pliable tube that can be elongated and narrowed to fit into a small catheter.

VENOUS STENOSIS

Results of treatment of venous stenosis by using either the Gianturco Z stent (13, 19) or the Wallstent (3) are similar. The stents can effectively palliate symptoms in 68 to 80% of patients with malignant vena cava stenosis (Fig. 42.3, *A* and *B*).

TRACHEOBRONCHIAL STENOSIS

Thirty-six patients with symptomatic tracheobronchial stenosis received Gianturco Z stents (14, 19). Symptoms improved in 28 patients (78%). The overall median survival for patients who showed improvement after receiving stents was 3 months, compared to 1 week for those who did not respond. The complications were minimal. The Z stent may palliate symptoms of tracheobronchial compression in selected cancer patients (Fig. 42.3, *C* and *D*). Because of the greater flexibility, the Wallstent may be the preferred stent in the main-stem bronchi and beyond.

ESOPHAGEAL STENOSIS

Covered expandable Gianturco Z stents were used to treat 119 patients; 132 stent tubes were placed in 116 patients with malignant esophageal neoplasms and 4 stent tubes were placed in 3 patients with benign lesions (28). All patients had aphagia or dysphagia to soft foods. The placement was successful in 100%; 98 (78%) could ingest solid food and 24 (20%) soft food. One hundred four patients died 2 to 80 weeks after stent placement. Complications included obstruction in 13 patients, migration in 12, gastroesophageal reflux in 9, severe pain in 9, and delayed massive bleeding in 4 patients. In 14 patients with esophagorespiratory fistulae the covered stent adequately occluded the communication.

BILIARY DUCT OBSTRUCTION

The advantages of percutaneously placed self-expanding Wallstent (3, 28, 40) and Gianturco Z stents (19) as biliary endoprostheses over internal or external drainage catheters for obstruction due to malignancy include the avoidance of bile leakage, infection, and pain at the skin entry site (62). This approach is indicated even in the presence of cholangitis to accomplish better drainage. The Wallstent is preferred because the tighter mesh is less likely to allow tumor ingrowth. The median survival varies between 3.2 and 7.5 months, with a median stent patency time varying between 3.6 and 6.3 months. Bile encrustation and debris are also responsible for stent obstruction. A stent occlusion rate of 20% for hilar and 5% for common bile duct lesions has been reported (3).

Summary

The percutaneous procedures described represent only a portion of the activities of the interventional radiologist in the diagnosis and management of neoplasms. These techniques, still in their infancy, expand the therapeutic potential of interventional radiology. Tumor debulking is often readily accomplished through this approach. A new drug may be better evaluated by the intra-arterial route to define its effect and toxicity. Targeted microparticles containing chemotherapeutic agents or immunomodifiers to be delivered intraarterially are soon to be available. Interventional radiology assists in the establishment of an accurate diagnosis and therapy with less morbidity and mortality than conventional surgery, and often at a reduced emotional and financial burden for cancer patients.

References

1. Ajani J, Carrasco CH, Charnsangavej C, Samaan NA, Levin B, Wallace S. Islet cell tumors metastatic to the liver: effective palliation by sequential hepatic artery embolization. Ann Surg 1988;108:340.
2. Altemeier WA, Culbertson WR, Fullen WD, Shook CD. Intra-abdominal abscesses. Am J Surg 1973;125:70.
3. Antonucci F, Salomonowitz E, Struckmann G, Siefel M, Largiader J, Zollikofer CL. Placement of venous stents: clinical experience with a self-expanding prosthesis. Radiology 1992;183:493.
4. Aronsen KF, Hellekant C, Holmberg J, Rothman U, Teder H. Controlled blocking of hepatic artery flow with enzymatically degradable microspheres combined with oncolytic drugs. Eur Surg Res 1979;11:99.
5. Ayala AG, Zornoza J. Primary bone tumors: percutaneous needle biopsy. Radiologic-pathologic study of 222 biopsies. Radiology 1983;149:675.
6. Balch CM, Urist MM, Soong S-J, McGregor M. A prospective phase II clinical trial of continuous FUDR regional chemotherapy for colorectal metastases to the liver using a totally implantable drug infusion pump. Ann Surg 1983;198:567.
7. Banner MP, Pollack HM. Hilatation of ureteral stenoses: techniques and experience in 44 patients. AJR 1984;143:789.
8. Barrioz T, Ingrand P, Besson I, de Ledinghen V, Silvain C, Branchart M. Randomised trial of prevention of biliary stent occlusion by ursodeoxycholic acid plus norfloxacin. Lancet 1994;344:581.
9. Benjamin RS, Chawla SP, Carrasco CH, Raymond AK, Murray JA, Armen T, Patel S, Wallace S, Ayala A, Papadopoulos NEJ, Plager C, Romsdahl MM, Martin RG. Preoperative chemotherapy for osteosarcoma with intravenous adriamycin and intra-arterial cisplain. Ann Oncol 1992;3(suppl 2):53.
10. Carrasco CH, Charnsangavej C, Ajani J, Samaan N, Richli W, Wallace S. The carcinoid syndrome: palliation by hepatic artery embolization. AJR 1986;147:149.
11. Carrasco CH, Charnsangavej C, Richli WR, Wallace S. Bone biopsy. In Interventional

Radiology. Edited by RF Dondelinger, P Rossi, JC Kurdziel, S Wallace. Stuttgart: Georg Thieme, 1990, p 58.
12. Carrasco CH, Charnsangavej C, Richli WR, Wallace S. Bone tumors. In Interventional Radiology. Edited by RF Dondelinger, P Rossi, JC Kurdziel, S Wallace. Stuttgart: Georg Thieme, 1990, p 489.
13. Carrasco CH, Charnsangavej C, Wright KC, Wallace S, Gianturco C. Use of the Gianturco self-expanding stent in stenoses of the superior and inferior venae cavae. JVIR 1992;3:409.
14. Carrasco CH, Nesbit JC, Charnsangavej C, Ryan B, Walsh GL, Yasumori K, Lawrence DD, Wallace S. Management of tracheal and bronchial stenoses with the Gianturco stent. Ann Thorac Surg 1994;58:1012.
15. Carrasco CH, Richli WR, Lawrence D, Katz RL, Wallace S. Fine needle aspiration biopsy of lymphoma. Radiol Clin North Am 1990;28:879.
16. Carrasco CH, Zornoza J, Bechtel W. Malignant biliary obstruction: complications of percutaneous biliary drainage. Radiology 1984;152:343.
17. Castellino R, Blank N. Etiologic diagnosis of focal pulmonary infection in immunocompromised patients by fluoroscopically guided percutaneous needle aspiration. Radiology 1979;132:563.
18. Charnsangavej C. Chemoembolization of liver tumors. Semin Intervent Radiol 1993;10:150.
19. Charnsangavej C, Carrasco CH, Wallace S, Gianturco C. Self-expanding endovascular prostheses in the treatment of venous stenoses. In Current Techniques in Interventional Radiology, 2nd ed. Edited by C Cope. Philadelphia: Current Medicine, 1994, p 10.1.
20. Cho KJ, Proctor MC, Greenfield LJ. Efficacy and problems associated with inferior vena cava filters. In Current Techniques in Interventional Radiology, 2nd ed. Edited by C Cope. Philadelphia: Current Medicine, 1994, p 8.1.
21. Dakhil S, Ensminger W, Cho K, Niederhuber J, Doan K, Wheeler R. Improved regional selectivity of hepatic arterial BCNU with degradable microspheres. Cancer 1982;50:631.
22. Ebara M, Kita K, Yoshikawa M, Sugiura N, Ohto M. Percutaneous ethanol injection for patients with small hepatocellular carcinoma. In Primary Liver Cancer in Japan. Edited by T Tobe, H Kameda, M Ohto. Tokyo: Springer, 1992, p 291.
23. Feld R, Eschelman DJ, Sagerman JE, Segal S, Hovsepian DM, Sullivan KL. Treatment of pelvic abscesses and other fluid collections: efficacy of transvaginal sonography guided aspiration and drainage. AJR 1994;163:1141.
24. Fornage B, Faroux MJ, Simatos A. Breast masses: US guided fine-needle aspiration biopsy. Radiology 1987;147:409.
25. Fraschini G, Yap HY, Chuang VP, Hortobagyi GN, Blumenschien GR, Wallace S. Remission consolidation in metastatic breast carcinoma to the liver with hepatic arterial infusion chemotherapy. Proc Am Soc Clin Oncol 1983;2:107.
26. Frei E III, Antman K. Combination chemotherapy, dose and schedule. In Cancer Medicine, 3rd ed. Edited by JF Holland, E Frei III, RC Bast, DW Kufe, DL Morton, RR Weichselbaum. Philadelphia: Lea & Febiger, 1993, p 631.
27. Gerzof SG. Percutaneous drainage technique. In Interventional Radiology. Edited by RF Dondelinger, P Rossi, JC Kurdziel, S Wallace. Stuttgart: Georg Thieme, 1990, p 96.
28. Gordon RL, Ring EJ, LaBerge JM, Doherty MM. Malignant biliary obstruction: treatment with expandable metallic stents. Follow-up of 50 consecutive patients. Radiology 1992;182:697.
29. Hammer FD, Rousseau HP, Joffre FG, Sentenac BP, Tran-Van T, Barthelemy RP. In vitro evaluation of vena cava filters. JVIR 1994;5:869.
30. Hemingway AP, Allison DJ. Complications of embolization: analysis of 410 procedures. Radiology 1988;166:669.
31. Howell SB. Regional chemotherapy. In Cancer Medicine, 3rd ed. Edited by JF Holland, E Frei III, RC Bast, DW Kufe, DL Morton, RR Weichselbaum. Philadelphia: Lea & Febiger, 1993, p 640.
32. Hruby W, Marberger M. Late sequellae of percutaneous nephrostomy. Radiology 1984;152:383.
33. Inoue H, Kobayashi H, Itoh Y, Shinohara S. Treatment of liver metastases by arterial injection of adriamycin/mitomycin C lipiodol suspension. Acta Radiol 1989;30:603.
34. Kaplan WD, D'Orsi CJ, Ensminger WD, Smith EH, Levin DC. Intra-arterial radionuclide infusion: a new technique to assess chemotherapy perfusion patterns. Cancer Treat Rep 1978;62:699.
35. Kasmouris AA, Williams AC, Delichatsios MA, Athanasoulis CA. Inferior vena cava filters: in vitro comparison of clot capture and flow dynamics. Radiology 1988;166:361.
36. Kato T, Nemoto R, Mori H, Takahashi M, Tamakawa Y, Harada M. Arterial chemoembolization with microencapsulated anticancer drug. JAMA 1981;245:1123.
37. Konya A, Szendrői M. Aneurysmal bone cysts treated by superselective embolization. Skeletal Radiol 1992;21:167.
38. Kuligowska E, Keller E, Ferrucci JT. Treatment of pelvic abscesses: value of one-step sonographically guided transrectal needle aspiration and lavage. AJR 1995;164:201.
39. Lamarque JL, Rodiere MJ. Breast biopsy. In Interventional Radiology. Edited by RF Dondelinger, P Rossi, JC Kurdziel, S Wallace. Stuttgart: Georg Thieme, 1990, p 27.
40. Lammer J, Klien GE, Kleinhart R, Hausegger K, Einspieler R. Obstructive jaundice: use of expandable metal endoprostheses for biliary drainage. Radiology 1990;177:789.
41. Lang E, Brown CL. Colorectal metastases to the liver: selective chemoembolization. Radiology 1993;189:417.
42. Laoide RO, Fundell LJ, vanSonnenberg E, D'Agostino H, Oglevie SB, Rosenkrantz H. Treatment of postbiopsy pneumothorax with a self-contained pneumothorax treatment device. Radiology 1994;193:393.
43. Lee Y-Y, Dimery IW, Van Tassel P, De Pena C, Blacklock JB, Goepfert H. Superselective intra-arterial chemotherapy of advanced paranasal sinus tumors. Arch Otolaryngol Head Neck Surg 1989;115:503.
44. Livraghi T, Bolondi L, Lazzaroni G. Percutaneous ethanol injection in the treatment of hepatocellular carcinoma in cirrhosis: a study of 207 patients. Cancer 1992;69:925.
45. Matsui O, Kadoya M, Yoshikawa J, Gabata T, Arai K, Demachi H, Miyayama S, Takashima T, Unoura M, Kogayashi K. Small hepatocellular carcinoma: treatment with subsegmental transcatheter arterial embolization. Radiology 1993;188:79.
46. Mavligit GM, Charnsangavej C, Carrasco CH, Patt YZ, Benjamin RS, Wallace S. Regression of ocular melanoma metastatic to the liver after hepatic artery chemoembolization with cisplatin and polyvinyl sponge. JAMA 1988;260:974.
47. Mavligit GM, Zukiwski AA, Ellis LM, Chuang VP, Wallace S. Effective palliation in patients with gastrointestinal leiomyosarcoma metastatic to the liver by hepatic chemoembolization-infusion with cisplatin and vinblastine. Cancer 1995;75:2083.
48. Mueller PR, van Sonnenberg E, Ferrucci JT. Percutaneous biliary drainage: technical and catheter related problems in 200 procedures. AJR 1982;138:17.
49. Nagata Y, Ishigaki T, Okajima K, Fujiwara K, Kinashi T, Mitumori M, Ooya N, Kitakabu Y, Hiraoka M, Abe M, Takokura K, Konishi I, Takai I, Taii S, Mori T. Transcatheter arterial infusion: therapy combined with radical hysterectomy in the treatment of advanced cervical cancer. Cardiovasc Intervent Radiol 1993;16:14.
50. Ohishi H, Yoshimura H, Uchida H, Sakaguchi H, Yoshioka T, Ohue S, Matsui T, Takaya A, Tsujii T. Transcatheter arterial embolization using iodized oil (lipiodol) mixed with an anticancer drug for the treatment of hepatocellular carcinoma. Cancer Chemother Pharmacol 1989;23(suppl):33.
51. O'Keefe FN, Carrasco CH, Charnsangavej C, Richli WR, Wallace S. Arterial embolization of adrenal tumors: result in nine cases. AJR 1988;151:819.
52. O'Keefe F, Carrasco CH, Charnsangavej C, Richli WR, Wallace S, Freedman RS. Percutaneous drainage and feeding gastrostomies in 100 patients. Radiology 1989;172:341.
53. Oleaga JA, Ring EJ. Interventional biliary radiology. Semin Roentgenol 1981;16:116.
54. Otto RC, Dondelinger RF, Kurdziel JC. Abdominal biopsy. In Interventional Radiology. Edited by RF Dondelinger, P Rossi, JC Kurdziel, S Wallace. Stuttgart: George Thieme, 1990, p 33.
55. Parker SH, Burbank F, Jackman RJ, Aucreman CJ, Cardenas G, Cink MT, Coscia JL Jr, Eklund GW, Evans WP III, Garver PR, Gramm HF, Haas DK, Jacob KM, Kelly KM, Killebrew LK, Lechner MC, Perlman SJ, Smid AP, Tabar L, Taber FE, Wynn RT. Percutaneous large-core breast biopsy: a multi-institutional study. Radiology 1994;193:359.
56. Patt YZ, Charnsangavej C, Boddie A, Cleary K, Carrasco CH, Soski M, Claghorn L, Lambert M, Lamki L, Mavligit G. Treatment of hepatocellular carcinoma with hepatic arterial floxuridine, doxorubicin and mitomycin with or without hepatic artery embolization: factors associated with longer survival. Reg Cancer Treat 1989;2:98.
57. Patton TJ, Kavanagh JJ, Delclos L, Wallace S, Haynie TP, Gershenson DM, Wharton JT, Bass S. Five-year survival in patients given intra-arterial chemotherapy prior to radiotherapy for advanced squamous carcinoma of the cervix and vagina. Gynecol Oncol 1991;42:54.
58. Pentecost MJ, Teitelbaum GP, Katz M, Daniels JR. Chemoembolization in hepatic malignancy. Semin Intervent Radiol 1992;9:28.
59. Ponsky JL, Gauderer MWL, Stellato TA. Percutaneous endoscopic gastrostomy: review of 150 cases. Arch Surg 1983;118:913.
60. Prenshaw RM. A percutaneous method for inserting a feeding gastrostomy tube. Surg Gynecol Obstet 1981;152:659.
61. Reuter M, Heller M, Heise U, Beese M. Transcatheter embolization of tumors of the musculoskeletal system. Fortschr Rontgenstr 1992;156:182.
62. Roddie ME, Adam A. Self-expanding metal stents in the management of bile duct strictures. In Current Techniques in Interventional Radiology. Edited by C Cope. Philadelphia: Current Medicine, 1994, p 5.1.
63. Roehm, JOF, Johnsrude IS, Barth MH, Gianturco C. The bird's nest filter inferior vena cava filter: progress report. Radiology 1988;168:745.
64. Rosenberger A, Adler OB. Mediastinal biopsy. In Interventional Radiology. Edited by RF Dondelinger, P Rossi, JC Kurdziel, S Wallace. Stuttgart: George Thieme, 1990, p 18.
65. Sacks BA, Glotzer DJ. Percutaneous reestablishment of feeding gastrostomies. Surgery 1979;85:575.
66. Sella A, Logothetis CJ, Fitz K, Dexeus FH, Amato R, Kilbourn R, Wallace S. Phase II study of interferon-α and chemotherapy (5-fluorouracil and mitomycin C) in metastatic renal cell cancer. J Urol 1992;147:573.
67. Shiina S, Niwa Y. Percutaneous ethanol injection therapy in the treatment of liver neoplasms. In Current Techniques in Interventional Radiology. Edited by C Cope. Philadelphia: Current Medicine, 1994, p 3.1.
68. Skinner WN. Transthoracic needle biopsy of small peripheral malignant lung lesions. Invest Radiol 1973;8:305.
69. Song HY, Do YS, Han YM, Sung KB, Choi EK, Sohn KH, Kim HR, Kim SH, Min YI. Covered, expandable esophageal metallic stent tubes: experience in 119 patients. Radiology 1994;193:689.
70. Tehranzadeh J, Freiberger RH, Ghelman B. Closed skeletal needle biopsy: review of 120 cases. AJR 1983;140:113.
71. Therasse E, Breittmayer F, Roche A, De Baere T, Indushekar S, Ducreux M, Lasser P, Elias D, Rougier P. Transcatheter chemoembolization of progressive carcinoid liver metastasis. Radiology 1993;187:541.
72. Uchida H, Ohishi H, Matsuo N, et al. Transcatheter hepatic segmental arterial embolization using lipiodol mixed with an anticancer drug and Gelfoam particles for hepatocellular carcinoma. J Cardiovasc Intervent Radiol 1990;13:140.
73. von Sonnenberg E, Mueller PR, Ferrucci JT. Percutaneous drainage of 250 abdominal abscesses and fluid collections. Radiology 1984;151:337.
74. Wallace S, Carrasco CH, Charnsangavej C, Richli WR, Wright K, Ganturco C. Hepatic artery infusion and chemoembolization in the management of liver metastases. J Cardiovasc Intervent Radiol 1990;13:153.
75. Wallace S, Charnsangavej C, Carrasco CH, Logothetis C.Intra-arterial chemotherapy of genitourinary tumors. In Clinical Urography. Edited by HM Pollack. Philadelphia: Saunders, 1990, p 3018.
76. Wallace S, Charnsangavej C, Carrasco CH, Swanson DA. Embolization of malignant renal tumors. In Clinical Urography. Edited by HM Pollack. Philadelphia: Saunders, 1989, p 3003.
77. Wallace S, Medellin H, de Jongh DS, Gianturco C. Systemic heparinization for angiography. AJR 1972;116:204.
78. Wallace S, Yang D, Wallace MJ, Kuang LR, Newman R, Wright K. Microencapsulation. Regional Cancer Treat 1991;4:49.
79. Welch TJ, Sheedy PF, Stephens DH, Johnson CM, Swensen SJ. Percutaneous adrenal biopsy: review of a 10-year experience. Radiology 1994;193:341.
80. Westcott JL. Lung biopsy. In Interventional Radiology. Edited by RF Dondelinger, P Rossi, JC Kurdziel, S Wallace. Stuttgart: Georg Thieme, 1990, p 9.
81. Winkler K, Bielack S, Delling G, Salzer-Kuntschik M, Kotz R, Greenshaw C, Jürgens H, Ritter J, Kusnierz-Glaz C, Erttman R, Gädicke G, Graf N, Ladenstein R, Leyvraz S,

Mertens R, Weinel P. Effect of intra-arterial vs. intravenous cisplatin in addition to systemic adriamycin, high dose methotrexate and ifosfamide on histologic tumor response in osteosarcoma (Study Coss-86). Cancer 1990;66:1703.
82. Woods D, Bechtel W, Charnsangavej C, Haynie TP, Kim EE, Carrasco CH, Wallace S. Gluteal artery occlusion: intra-arterial chemotherapy of pelvic neoplasms. Radiology 1985;155:341.
83. Wright KC, Jahns M, Kasi L, Hashimoto S, Perez-Soler R, Haynie T, Wallace S. Liposome distribution after arterial and venous infusion. Invest Radiol 1987;22:S28.
84. Yamada R, Kishi K, Terada M, Sonomura T, Sato M. Transcatheter arterial chemoembolization for unresectable hepatocellular carcinoma. In Primary Liver Cancer in Japan. Edited by T Tobe, H Kameda, M Ohto. Tokyo: Springer, 1992, p 259.
85. Yamashita Y, Takahashi M, Baba Y, et al. Hepatocellular carcinoma with or without cirrhosis: a comparison of CT and angiographic presentations in the United States and Japan. Abdominal Imaging 1993;18:168.
86. Yamashita Y, Takahashi M, Koga Y, Saito R, Nanakawa S, Hatanaka Y, Sato N, Nakushima K, Urata J, Yoshizumi K, Ito K, Sum S. Prognostic factors in liver metastases after transcatheter arterial embolization or arterial infusion. Acta Radiol 1990;31:269.
87. Yang DJ, Li C, Nikiforow S, Gretzer MB, Kuang L-R, Lopez MS, Vargas K, Wallace S. Diagnostic and therapeutic potential of poly(benzyl-L-glutamate). J Pharm Sci 1994;83:328.
88. Zornoza J, Jonsson K, Wallace S, Lukeman JM. Fine needle aspiration biopsy of retroperitoneal lymph nodes and abdominal masses: an updated report. Radiology 1977;125:87.

SECTION XI

ENDOSCOPY

CHAPTER 43

Gastrointestinal Endoscopy

J. MARK LAWSON AND JOHN BAILLIE

The gastrointestinal (GI) tract is long and tortuous. For the first half of the 20th century, the detection and diagnosis of diseases of the GI tract (and of associated organs, such as the liver and pancreas) relied upon barium contrast radiology, and open surgery. Rigid esophagoscopes and proctoscopes provided only glimpses of the dark tunnels beyond. Semiflexible lens gastroscopes were introduced in the 1930s and used by a few enthusiasts; examinations were incomplete and uncomfortable, and biopsy facilities were inadequate. Subsequently, a miniaturized intragastric camera was used extensively in Japan for detection of early gastric cancer. These techniques have all been superseded in the era of flexible endoscopy, which began in 1958 with the publication by Hirschowicz and colleagues of the first clinical application of a fiberoptic endoscope (50). Commercial versions were introduced in the early 1960s and widely applied for diagnostic purposes in the upper and lower GI tract in the 1970s. This wave of diagnostic application was followed, predominantly in the 1980s, by the development of numerous endoscopically based therapeutic techniques. Within the past 10 years, light-sensitive transistors (charged coupled devices or CCDs) have wrought a new revolution (56). Video endoscopes employ these devices to create high-resolution television images that can be analyzed and manipulated to provide information never before available to endoscopists. These electronic refinements—which include image enhancement (92), reflectance spectrometry (20), and mucosal blood flow mapping (36)—have greatly increased the potential of endoscopy for the diagnosis and treatment of GI cancer.

Diagnostic and therapeutic endoscopy has become a subspecialty of its own. Gastroenterologists and surgeons undertaking such procedures need appropriate supervised training and certification. Because few medical oncologists have had formal endoscopic training, the oncologist and the endoscopist work as a team to investigate and treat GI cancer. Increasingly, GI endoscopy is being performed in the outpatient setting. It is unusual to require more than intravenous sedation; some basic therapeutic procedures (e.g., dilation of esophageal strictures, colonoscopic polypectomy) do not require hospitalization. However, patients undergoing more aggressive endoscopic therapy (e.g., laser ablation of tumors, biliary stent placement) need to be observed in a hospital setting after their procedures.

Diagnostic Endoscopy

The major advances in diagnostic endoscopy have followed refinement of endoscopes and their accessories. Modern endoscopes are much more flexible than their predecessors, allowing them to reach previously inaccessible or poorly visualized areas of the GI tract. However, until recently the small intestine from the distal duodenum to the distal ileum was relatively difficult to view endoscopically; a variety of enteroscopes have recently been developed and are now commercially available (6, 14). Using standard endoscopes, we can directly visualize the esophagus, stomach, duodenum, the last 10 cm of the ileum, and the entire colon. In addition, we can opacify the biliary tree and pancreatic ducts by retrograde injection of contrast agents. Finally, rigid laparoscopy allows us to view the peritoneum and peritoneal surfaces of the liver and small intestine. Technical aspects of these procedures are well described elsewhere (5).

A significant proportion of the work of the GI endoscopist involves a search for, and characterization of, cancers. Sometimes a gut tumor can be diagnosed as malignant with a high degree of confidence solely from the macroscopic appearance at endoscopy. However, other adjuvant techniques such as vital staining and endoscopic ultrasonography can provide additional diagnostic information and material for histologic or cytologic confirmation of the diagnosis. It is almost always necessary to determine the cell type and degree of differentiation to plan the most effective therapy.

BIOPSY AND CYTOLOGY

Samples must be taken from all suspicious lesions. Standard endoscopic biopsies are quite accurate for most mucosal malignancies but yield rates can be increased from the 90–95% range typically obtained with two biopsy specimens to the 95–98% range with more than six specimens (67). Biopsy specimens taken from the rim of a malignant ulcer are often positive, as this area represents the growing edge of the tumor, whereas biopsies of the base show only necrotic material. These specimens are rather small and usually do not penetrate beyond the mucosa. As a result, submucosally spreading and intramural tumors may be missed by the usual biopsy technique. For example, Kaposi's sarcoma (a frequent accompaniment of AIDS) (120), gastric lymphoma, and leiomyoma are rarely diagnosed from specimens taken with standard biopsy forceps (67). When there is evidence that the bowel wall is thickened, larger and deeper specimens than normal can be taken using large-particle (jumbo) forceps, or the submucosa can be accessed by "tunneling": repeated biopsies in the same site allow the endoscopist to tunnel down to the lesion of interest (7). With the use of the "turn and suction" technique described by Levine and Reid, larger endoscopic mucosal biopsy specimens (up to 56% larger) can be obtained; these are particularly helpful in surveillance of flat mucosal areas, as in the case in Barrett's esophagus (67). Endoscopic needle aspiration biopsy is an alternative method of biopsy for mass lesions that has yet to gain widespread acceptance (39). The endoscopist must ensure that the pathologist receives specimens in appropriate fixative. For example, biopsies destined for immunoperoxidase staining (e.g., for lymphoma markers) and electron microscopy require special handling and should not be fixed in standard formalin. It is rarely difficult to target malignant tissue in gross tumors, but more subtle lesions may resist diagnosis.

Brush cytology, alone or in combination with biopsy, can increase the diagnostic yield in malignancy. So-called salvage cytology ensures that no potentially diagnostic material is wasted (40); in one method, washings from the endoscope biopsy channel are centrifuged and the resulting solid pellet is stained for cytologic examination.

TISSUE STAINING

Vital staining with iodine (Lugol's solution), indigo carmine, India ink, or methylene blue highlights the mucosal pattern of the gut (28, 30, 77, 108). Staining with Lugol's solution allows the operator to more accurately predict the extent of esophageal cancer than with the use of endoscopic appearance alone. The combination of methylene blue and the acid-reactive Congo red stain increases the endoscopic detection rate of early gastric cancer from 28% to 89% (30). When used with a magnifying endoscope, dye staining can help identify areas of dysplasia or carcinoma in situ. With the rapid advances being made in electronic imaging analysis, vital staining is likely to regain popularity. Malignant cells have been shown to have an affinity for porphyrins. "Malignant fluorescence" can be detected with the use of intravenously administered hematoporphyrin prior to endoscopy and exposure to blue-violet light (30). Cothren and others have shown that fluorescence of colonic mucosal cells exposed to monochromatic (laser) light may be highly specific for epithelial dysplasia (20, 93). This exciting development, known as "optical biopsy," requires further evaluation but may offer a way to look for dysplasia and carcinoma without the need to take biopsies. The linkage of tissue dyes to monoclonal antibodies offers the hope of improved detection and therapy of neoplasia at an early stage (30). Although tissue staining has broad clinical applications in the detection of early premalignant and malignant lesions, it remains underutilized in Western clinical practice.

ENDOSCOPIC ULTRASOUND

Since the introduction of flexible endoscopic ultrasound (EUS) probes almost 20 years ago, numerous prospective studies have compared its accuracy to that of more traditional imaging methods (11, 48, 57). EUS has the benefits of affording direct access to mucosal lesions, close proximity to submucosal ones, and a superior view of structures within and surrounding the bowel wall. By varying the frequency of the ultrasound signal (e.g., 7.5 MHz, 10 MHz, or 12 MHz), the depth of the image (i.e., millimeters into the bowel wall) can be altered. The resolution of EUS is so good that individual layers of the bowel wall can be identified, which has immediate implications for tumor staging using the TNM system. The marriage of EUS with targeted biopsies is now possible using new phased array endosonoscopes. These tools allow direct histopathologic confirmation of submucosal lesions and local lymph nodes (119). The sensitivity and specificity of EUS in staging local tumor invasion and regional metastases of esophageal and other intra-abdominal malignancies appear to be superior to the sensitivity and specificity of traditional imaging methods, such as computed tomography (CT) or standard ultrasonography (US) (11, 48, 57). The particular strengths of EUS include extremely detailed views of the bowel wall, demonstration of small (<2 cm) lesions of the pancreas (especially islet cell tumors), and demonstration of vascular involvement in pancreatic cancer. Limitations include technical complexity, difficulty in interpretation, inability to accurately differentiate malignancy from inflammatory processes, and difficulty in passing the instrument through strictured areas. At present, the role of EUS in staging esophageal and intra-abdominal malignancies is promising but does not yet warrant dissemination of this complex technology outside specialty referral centers (57).

THERAPEUTIC TECHNIQUES

Gastrointestinal endoscopy during the 1960s focused almost exclusively on diagnosis. However, with the advent of more flexible endoscopes with large instrument channels in the early 1970s, therapy became a possibility. There is now a wide range of therapeutic techniques ranging from snare polypectomy to laser ablation of tumors. The adenoma-carcinoma sequence in the stomach and colon is well established (10, 67, 122); we know that the likelihood of malignant change in polyps increases with size and increasing villous architecture. With electrocautery, polyps can be easily and safely removed and recovered for histologic examination. The search for adenomatous polyps and their removal has become a major focus of colon cancer screening (4, 122). It is now well accepted that removal of these precursor lesions significantly reduces the risk of colon cancer. There is also considerable interest in using therapeutic endoscopy techniques for palliation in patients with malignancies who are unable to undergo definitive surgical management. These techniques include placing plastic or expandable metallic prostheses to bypass obstruction (62, 98, 113), in the esophagus, stomach, bile ducts, and pancreas; debulking luminal tumors using bipolar cautery probes; and laser photocoagulation of obstructing tumors (58, 79). Potentiation of laser energy absorption by administering porphyrins (photodynamic therapy) has not yet proved superior to standard laser therapy for obstructing gut tumors (76, 79). So-called smart lasers that can identify and specifically target abnormal tissue have been developed for laser coronary angioplasty. It is likely that this technology will soon be adapted to allow specific targeting of tumor tissue (76). This has obvious implications for the treatment of small tumors in confined spaces, such as the biliary tree. Smart lasers may eventually offer the potential for cure of small malignant lesions, such as early gastric cancer (107).

Diagnostic and Therapeutic Endoscopy

ESOPHAGUS

Most patients with esophageal neoplasia eventually develop a swallowing disturbance caused by mechanical obstruction, disordered motility, or a combination of the two. The usual complaint is dysphagia (sticking of food or liquid), with or without regurgitation. Painful swallowing (odynophagia) is usually due to mucosal inflammation but can also accompany mechanical obstruction, especially at the gastric cardia. Any patient may have nonspecific signs and symptoms of cancer, such as unexplained weight loss, lassitude, and anemia. There is considerable debate regarding the relative merits of contrast-aided radiology (barium swallow examination) and endoscopy; the choice of initial investigation is often dictated by local availability and expertise. Although endoscopy has the diagnostic edge, as biopsies and cytology specimens can be obtained (see Fig. 112.2, contrast-aided radiology provides valuable complementary information. We prefer that all patients presenting with progressive dysphagia undergo a contrast study prior to endoscopy. The endoscopic literature suggests that endoscopy alone can be used to diagnose cancer in at least 73% of cases, with biopsy and/or cytology increasing the yield to around 95 to 100% (67, 111). False-positive results from cytology occur in between 0.1 and 1% of cases, especially if active inflammation is present (99, 101). Multiple biopsies increase the diagnostic accuracy considerably. If a tight esophageal stricture is present, this usually requires endoscopic dilation for access before biopsy or cytology samples can be taken. Malignant tumors arising in the distal third of esophagus may be either squamous cell carcinoma or adenocarcinoma, the latter arising from ectopic columnar epithelium (Barrett's esophagus). It is vital to identify the cell type, as this determines initial management, squamous tumors being relatively sensitive to irradiation and chemotherapy, compared to adenocarcinoma. Diagnostic laparoscopy is quite sensitive compared to CT in the detection of metastatic esophageal cancer and should be considered preoperatively in patients with comorbid medical illnesses that would increase the risk of surgical therapy (see Chapter 112) (68).

Screening for Esophageal Cancer

Screening strategies for esophageal cancer differ depending on whether the risk factors predispose the patient to squamous or adenocarcinomas. Squamous esophageal cancers are typically seen in patients who smoke, drink heavily, or who have had prior head, neck, or pulmonary neoplasms. Uncommon conditions such as tylosis, celiac disease, the Plummer-Vinson syndrome, lye stricture, and achalasia are predisposing conditions. With the exception of tylosis, no specific screening recommendations exist for conditions predisposing to squamous carcinomas. On the other hand, the presence of metaplastic intestinal epithelium in the esophagus, or Barrett's esophagus, is well recognized to increase the risk of esophageal adenocarcinoma by 20- to 40-fold (46). This risk is similar to a white man's risk of developing lung cancer (31). Over the past three decades the incidence of adenocarcinoma of the esophagus has increased remarkably in white men and is strongly correlated with Barrett's esophagus (3, 31). Screening endoscopy should be considered in any patient with reflux symptoms three or more times per week over a 5-year period, those who have had reflux-related complications, or patients with medically recalcitrant symptoms (31). Once the typical-appearing tongues of reddish mucosa extending above the esophagogastric junction are detected, four-quadrant biopsies are performed every 2 cm to confirm metaplastic intestinal-type mucosa and to evaluate for the presence of dysplasia. Although precise data relating cancer risk to length of Barrett's epithelium are not available, it is now believed that the presence of specialized intestinal epithelium of any length carries an increased cancer risk (15). Specific recommendations for screening strategies have been hampered by numerous complicating factors, including lack of data defining both the true prevalence of Barrett's esophagus in the general population and the incidence of adenocarcinoma in those patients, deficient data on the efficacy of surgery for high-grade dysplasia or cancer, and lack of controlled data demonstrating that a surveillance program improves survival (90). Computer cohort simulations of a population of patients with Barrett's esophagus suggest that if longevity and quality of life are both important considerations, then screening should be performed every 2 to 3 years (90). Other authors have suggested a biennial surveillance program in patients with Barrett's esophagus whose initial biopsies were negative for dysplasia (31). The finding of severe dysplasia on biopsy of Barrett's epithelium probably warrants early rebiopsy and consideration for surgical resection (esophagogastrectomy) (85). Until the natural history of the disease and the effectiveness of surveillance and surgical intervention are better studied, it is difficult to recommend a specific screening program for the patient with Barrett's esophagus.

Palliation of Dysphagia

Beyond initial diagnosis, the role of the GI endoscopist in esophageal cancer is usually to provide palliation for progressive dysphagia. Surgical intervention provides the best palliation by tumor resection and gastric pull-up (49). Unfortunately, few patients are suitable candidates for surgery, but it is important that all undergo appropriate evaluation before the decision is made to pursue a nonsurgical approach. Endoscopic palliation usually involves one of three approaches—dilation, intubation, and debulking procedures.

Dilation is typically accomplished using an endoscopically placed guidewire over which Savary-Gillard plastic dilators are sequentially passed. Although effective, this treatment typically requires frequently repeated procedures because of continued tumor growth. Recent technological advances have led to the development of expandable metal prostheses to stent open the esophageal lumen. These devices appear to avoid many of the complications associated with previously used plastic endoprostheses and offer longer term palliation (62). Drawbacks to the use of these stents have included stent occlusion due to tumor ingrowth and their high initial cost. Trials are currently under way evaluating a new plastic coated expandable metal stent that should prevent tumor ingrowth and provide improved palliation of malignant fistulas connecting to the pulmonary tree. Standard prostheses should be used with caution in patients with significant tracheal compression by a mediastinal tumor, as placing the stent may result in abrupt tracheal obstruction. A lateral chest x-ray should be obtained prior to placement and bronchoscopy should be considered to evaluate tracheal patency. Debulking may involve a number of different techniques, including laser therapy with or without photosensitizing agents, injection of sclerosing agents, and bipolar cautery of the tumor (27, 62, 76, 79, 124).

Endoscopic assessment of postsurgical esophageal strictures requires particular care. When a patient who has undergone esophagogastrectomy for esophageal cancer develops an anastomotic stricture, it can be very difficult to distinguish mediastinal fibrosis from local tumor recurrence, especially on CT. Endoscopic brushings and biopsy may need to be performed repeatedly to yield malignant cells. Endoscopic ultrasound now offers a superior way to image the esophageal wall and adjacent structures, which will undoubtedly improve the accuracy of diagnosis and staging of esophageal malignancy, including recurrence (see Chapter 12) (11, 24, 41, 94).

Benign Tumors

Benign tumors of the esophagus are rare and seldom of clinical significance. However, squamous papillomas associated with human papilloma virus (HPV) infection (111) may grow sufficiently large to become symptomatic. These tumors can be removed by snare cautery. The natural history of this disease, which is increasingly common, is unknown. There is concern that prolonged exposure to HPV may be associated with an increased risk of malignant change, as in the uterine cervix. Long-term follow-up of patients with esophageal papillomas will be needed to determine if this is indeed a risk factor for carcinoma.

An unusual but interesting benign tumor that may cause symptoms is the fibrolamellar polyp (112), which can grow very large indeed. Because fibrolamellar polyps can have a very vascular stalk, large ones are more safely removed by surgery than by endoscopic polypectomy.

STOMACH

Gastric Cancer

Gastric cancers often present insidiously with unexplained weight loss, anorexia, and chronic iron deficiency anemia. They may ulcerate, mimicking benign ulcers. Alternatively, they can be unequivocally malignant-looking exophytic masses or can spread submucosally, causing gross thickening and loss of distensibility of the stomach wall (linitis plastica).

Adenocarcinoma of the stomach is a particular challenge to the GI endoscopist; by the time it causes obvious symptoms such as esophageal or gastric outlet obstruction, bleeding, or marked anorexia and weight loss, the tumor has almost always grown beyond the stage of curative resection. The challenge is to diagnose gastric cancer early. Barium studies have a low detection rate for early gastric cancer of between 1 and 2 per 1,000, and a high false-positive rate (53). Endoscopy in patients over 40 years of age in high-risk areas yields five early gastric cancers per 1,000 patients but reportedly detects only 60% of these lesions at initial examination (106). When early gastric cancer is suspected, the changes may be subtle. As there is a false-negative rate of up to 15%, suspicious lesions must be reexamined and rebiopsied when initial biopsies are negative for malignancy. It is desirable to confirm the benign nature of all gastric ulcers by endoscopy and biopsy, especially as small malignant ulcers may heal transiently. Follow-up endoscopy should be performed 4 to 8 weeks after the initial examination and repeated at regular intervals thereafter until healing is confirmed. As dysplasia is difficult to interpret in gastric mucosa, only the most severe dysplasia should be considered as having malignant potential (67). The natural history of gastric dysplasia is unknown, and there is no consensus regarding the management of early gastric cancer (67, 82).

Gastric adenomas larger than 20 mm in diameter carry a significant risk of malignancy and should be removed endoscopically. For those below 20 mm the risk is small—possibly around 2% (55), but it is good practice to remove these lesions by snare cautery or "hot biopsy" technique. The screening of patients with putative high-risk associations for gastric adenocarcinoma is addressed below.

Gastric lymphoma is frequently difficult to diagnose, although large folds and/or decreased motility seen on barium studies or at endoscopy should raise suspicion of this lesion (67, 102). Superficial mucosal biopsies are inadequate for diagnosis; once thickening of the gastric wall has been confirmed by CT or endoscopic ultrasound, multiple large biopsies should be taken from suspect areas (94). Sufficient biopsies should be taken to allow some material to be sent for immunohistochemical analysis for lymphoma markers. Occasionally, laparotomy is required to obtain full-thickness biopsy specimens of the stomach wall before a diagnosis of lymphoma can be confirmed.

Tumor metastatic to the stomach is unusual, but certain cancers appear to have a predisposition for this site, including adenocarcinoma of breast and malignant melanoma (81). With the increasing prevalence of the acquired immunodeficiency syndrome (AIDS), endoscopists have become familiar with the esophageal, gastric, and colonic lesions of Kaposi's sarcoma (35). The typical histologic appearances are rarely seen in superficial biopsies; suspected Kaposi's sarcoma is another indication for multiple, large-particle biopsies.

Benign Tumors

Excluding congenital abnormalities such as the pancreatic rest, the most common benign tumor of clinical significance seen in the stomach is the leiomyoma (78), which has a characteristic cylindrical shape with an apical depression. Leiomyomas can grow very large; they frequently ulcerate and bleed. Because leiomyomas may undergo malignant degeneration to form leiomyosarcomas, large lesions should be surgically excised. Small neuroendocrine tumors such as carcinoids are an occasional finding in gastric biopsies (42, 67); they are rarely functional. Pathologic gastric acid hypersecretion (the Zollinger-Ellison syndrome) may be caused by a primary gastric gastrinoma. Almost invariably, these lesions are too small to be identified radiologically or by endoscopy. The majority of benign gastric tumors are submucosal—other histologic types include fibroma, lipoma, eosinophilic granuloma, and a variety of cysts—and are therefore difficult to diagnose by mucosal biopsy. Endoscopic ultrasound has proved useful in characterizing these lesions (94).

Endoscopic Treatment

In general, therapeutic endoscopy has not been especially helpful in the management of gastric cancer. Recently, though, several reports have appeared in which mucosal strip biopsy was used to treat early gastric cancer (62). This technique involves elevating flat or slightly raised early gastric malignancies with either the submucosal injection of saline or though the use of a two-channel endoscope to pass forceps to lift the mucosa prior to removal with a snare placed in the second channel. A comparative study of surgery and strip biopsy from Japan found similar 5-year survival rates of 89% and 84%, respectively (62). Careful preoperative staging with endoscopic ultrasound is needed before attempting the strip biopsy technique for early gastric cancer. Unfortunately, experience with this technique remains quite limited in the West. Endoscopically placed prostheses are useful for palliating dysphagia in obstructing tumors of the gastric cardia but have proved less satisfactory for more distal lesions, mainly because of the technical difficulty of inserting them. Expandable metal mesh stents have been used with encouraging results for malignant gastric outlet obstruction (62, 105). Laser therapy can provide palliation in noncircumferential lesions of the gastric cardia (73). However, use of the neodymium:yttrium-aluminum-garnet (Nd-YAG) laser to debulk large, exophytic stomach tumors seldom provides clinical benefit since gastric emptying problems result as much from disordered or absent motility as from mechanical factors. Furthermore, laser therapy in the normally thin-walled stomach carries a significant risk of perforation. Microwave radiation may prove a safer alternative; probes suitable for endoscopic use are being evaluated (61). Laser photocoagulation can occasionally be helpful in management of bleeding from ulcerating tumors.

Screening for Gastric Cancer

Screening of patients at increased risk for gastric cancer is even more contentious than screening for esophageal malignancies. There is no established role for endoscopic surveillance in asymptomatic patients who have undergone gastric surgery, at least within the first 20 years (13, 67). In patients who develop symptoms, any abnormality seen at endoscopy should be biopsied; many invisible early lesions have been detected by routine biopsy close to the gastric stoma. There may be an increased risk of gastric cancer in young patients with pernicious anemia and atrophic gastritis with intestinal metaplasia (4).

Recently, *Helicobacter pylori* infection of the stomach has been associated with the development of mucosa associated lymphoma (MALT) and adenocarcinoma (118). Intestinal metaplasia caused by *H. pylori* is suspected of being a factor in the development of gastric adenocarcinoma (80). Infection with *H. pylori* is easily diagnosed by histopathologic examination of endoscopically obtained gastric biopsy specimens or by using a rapid urease test on gastric tissue. Currently there are no guidelines recommending routine testing for *H. pylori* or treating it when detected in an otherwise asymptomatic patient (80). Controlled studies are needed to assess risk-benefit ratios before any general screening recommendations can be made. Gastric adenomas greater than 2 cm in diameter carry a significant risk of malignancy, which makes endoscopic resection mandatory for large lesions (4). The risk of malignant transformation in multiple gastric adenomatosis of familial polyposis syndromes (e.g., Gardner's syndrome, Peutz-Jeghers syndrome) has yet to be defined.

DUODENUM AND SMALL INTESTINE

Endoscopists tend to consider the duodenum as a separate entity from the remainder of the small intestine, as it is readily accessible with standard endoscopic equipment. Anatomically the duodenum can be divided into four parts, the first part (or bulb) beyond the pylorus leading to the second (D2), third (D3), and fourth (D4) parts. Standard gastroscopes routinely reach D2. As the duodenal papilla is usually located on the medial wall of D2, adequate inspection requires the use of a side-viewing instrument (duodenoscope). A pediatric colonoscope can frequently be advanced to D4 but rarely further (unless this is done at surgery, when the surgeon can feed the endoscope through the loops of small bowel). Until recently, endoscopic evaluation of the jejunum and ileum using peroral endoscopy was difficult, time-consuming, and often unsatisfactory. However, this is changing with the introduction of new "push" enteroscopes, which allow high-quality visualization well down into the jejunum (6, 14, 117). Weighted, Sonde-type enteroscopes are still needed to extend this view into the ileum (6). However, the distal 10 cm or so of ileum remains accessible by colonoscope, if the ileocecal valve can be intubated. Often the best view of the small intestine is obtained by perioperative endoscopy; the surgeon can assist the endoscopist by manually advancing the endoscope through the bowel.

Tumors of the duodenum are uncommon and the majority are benign. It is so rare to find malignancy in duodenal ulcers that they are not biopsied routinely at endoscopy. Occasionally a primary duodenal or pancreatic carcinoma will masquerade as a benign duodenal ulcer; it is usually not long before the true nature of the lesion declares itself. Tumors of the ampulla (duodenal papilla) are discussed in the section on pancreatic and biliary cancers. Metastases to the duodenum from distant cancers are rare.

A variety of benign tumors occur in the duodenum. There have been several case reports of duodenal gastrinoma causing Zollinger-Ellison syndrome (114). Carcinoid tumors are rarely of clinical significance. One common benign tumor is Brunner's gland hyperplasia (84), which has no pathologic significance. Lymphoid nodular hyperplasia (29) is associated with a relative deficiency of intestinal IgA, which encourages small bowel colonization by the protozoan parasite, *Giardia lamblia.* Pathologic dilation of intestinal lymphoid channels, lymphangiectasia (47), results in the formation of submucosal cysts filled with chylous fluid. Again, this is a benign condition. Duodenal adenomas may be solitary, or multiple in familial polyposis syndromes (e.g., Peutz-Jeghers syndrome, Gardner's syndrome) (104). The malignant potential of small bowel adenomas in these syndromes is not zero, as was previously supposed, although it is considerably less than that of the corresponding colon polyps. It has been recommended that patients with multiple duodenal adenomas as part of a familial polyposis syndrome undergo periodic screening endoscopy (97).

Benign and malignant tumors of the small bowel present in the same way, with acute or chronic bleeding or mechanical obstruction, including intussusception. Benign tumors such as leiomyomas bleed because they ulcerate. Intussusception tends to occur when tumors are large enough to cause mechanical irritation but are too small to completely obstruct the lumen of the bowel. Although the small bowel is rarely the target of distant metastases except from melanoma, it may be involved by direct extension of cancer from adjacent organs. Primary lymphoma of the small intestine occurs with increased frequency in patients with gluten-sensitive enteropathy (celiac sprue) (110). Enteroscopy is useful in the diagnosis of certain small bowel tumors, but there is little hope as yet for endoscopic therapy (6, 14). However, percutaneous endoscopic gastrostomy (PEG) tube placement has reportedly been used with good results to palliate small intestinal obstruction in metastatic ovarian cancer. In this situation, the PEG tube is used for decompression and not for feeding. It spares terminally ill patients the added discomfort of a nasogastric tube.

COLON

It is estimated that 4 to 5% of the population in Western society will develop colorectal cancer in their lifetime. This incidence has been increasing worldwide by almost 2% annually (74). Most of these tumors are adenocarcinomas, but other primary neoplasms of the colon (e.g., lymphoma) do occur rarely. The colon can be involved in metastatic tumor by direct extension from adjacent organs, or by hematogenous or lymphatic spread. The discrete nodular lesions of Kaposi's sarcoma may be seen at colonoscopy in patients with AIDS. Since more than 50% of colon cancers present clinically when the tumor is beyond curative resection, considerable effort is being directed toward the identification

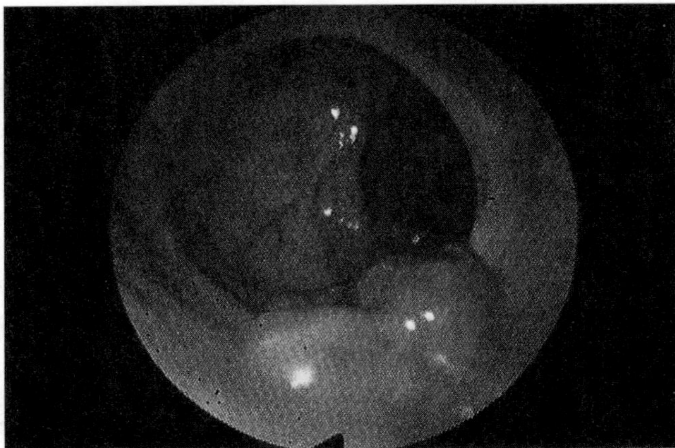

Figure 43.1. Sessile adenocarcinoma of the rectum discovered during colonoscopy in an asymptomatic 50-year-old male. First-degree relatives of patient had had colon cancer.

and screening of patients at increased risk of developing colon cancer (Fig. 43.1). The risk for any individual increases after age 40. Patients with inflammatory bowel disease, a family history of colon cancer (in first-degree relatives), adenomas of the colon, previous colon cancer, and familial polyposis syndromes are at substantially increased risk (18, 52). As the progression of benign adenomatous polyps of the colon to adenocarcinoma is indisputable, the identification and endoscopic removal of polyps is one of the primary objectives of colon cancer screening (10, 122). Mandel and colleagues showed that a definite "stage shift" in Dukes' stage of colon cancer was observed in patients undergoing annual or biennial colonoscopy for adenoma screening (72). The U.S. National Polyp Study of 8,379 patients, published in 1993, added weight to these findings (123). Of 4,121 patients undergoing removal of one or more polyps, 1,422 were randomized to follow-up colonoscopy at 1 and 3 years or at 3 years alone. A low of 11.8 and a high of 37.3 colorectal cancers were expected per 1,000 patients, but in actuality no symptomatic cancers were found, and only 5 asymptomatic cancers were detected, a reduction of 58 to 87%, depending on the reference population. Colon cancer death was reduced 100% in those who underwent colonoscopy. These data support the value of polypectomy in preventing colorectal cancer (122).

Screening Strategies

The studies discussed above provide strong evidence that screening for colorectal cancer with the removal of adenomatous polyps results in improved survival and mortality (72, 74, 122). Now the question is not so much "Does the removal of adenomatous polyps reduce colorectal cancer mortality?" but "How can we can develop an effective, tolerable, and cost-efficient strategy for screening?" (12, 74). A key to developing such a strategy is selecting patients who are most likely to benefit from this screening. Certainly, high-risk subgroups can be identified, such as those with long standing ulcerative colitis, familial polyposis syndromes, a history of colon or other adenocarcinomas in multiple first-degree relatives, prior colon cancer, or adenomatous polyps. Although controversy exists, screening guidelines are available for these high-risk patients (10, 18, 63, 74). Unfortunately, widespread screening of these patients has not significantly lowered the overall colorectal cancer mortality, as almost 75% of patients with the disease have no identifiable predisposing factors. It is in this group of patients that an effective screening strategy is needed if deaths from colorectal cancer are to be reduced or eliminated. Screening of average-risk patients over the age of 50 with yearly fecal occult blood testing and screening sigmoidoscopy every 3 to 5 years is currently recommended by the American Cancer Society and the World Health Organization Collaboration Center for the Prevention of Colorectal Cancer. Clearly, these examinations will identify a proportion of patients with colon polyps and cancer. However, flexible sigmoidoscopy, while three to five times more sensitive than rigid proctoscopy (9), provides access to less than half of the colon. This is of significant concern, as proximal migration of colon cancer is well documented in Western societies (96). These screening recommendations are not widely followed, even by gastroenterologists (1), as only 10% of eligible patients have undergone screening sigmoidoscopy (91). Although most authors agree that double-contrast barium enema examinations can detect most cancers, the ability of this study to demonstrate adenomatous polyps is controversial. In one study, the following were missed on barium enema examinations: 45% of adenomas, 28% of carcinomas in situ, and 26% of invasive carcinomas subsequently detected at colonoscopy (121). Other authors have disputed these findings (33). Colonoscopy and double-contrast barium enema examination with flexible sigmoidoscopy are both acceptable strategies for evaluating the colon for neoplasia. Colonoscopy has the advantage of being more accurate, especially for adenomatous polyps, and can be used to remove premalignant lesions, whereas barium enema examination is slightly safer and less costly. Local expertise and availability often determine which test is chosen. The discovery of polyps on either study mandates colonoscopic removal in most cases. Although advocated by some, routine screening examination of the entire colon by either method in average-risk patients has little support in light of the overwhelming cost of such a program (74). Clearly, an acceptable screening strategy for the general population will have to await advances in molecular biology and cytogenetics that will select out those most likely to benefit. In patients suspected of having colon cancer, flexible sigmoidoscopy followed by double-contrast barium enema examination is probably the minimum acceptable screening. However, colonoscopy is being adopted widely as a more sensitive single-procedure alternative (121).

Epidemiologic studies have led to recent guidelines that patients with multiple adenomatous colon polyps and those with previous colon cancer should be followed up colonoscopically at least every 3 years until no polyps are found, then every 5 years, and that those initially found to have a single small (<1 cm) tubular adenoma may not need further surveillance (9, 123). Carcinoma in patients with long-standing total ulcerative colitis occurs in approximately 8 to 10% of patients at 15 years. It is recommended that surveillance examinations be performed at least every 2 to 3 years after 7 to 10 years of pancolitis, although even these studies may miss the development of a cancer (18, 64, 84). The finding of epithelial dysplasia is significant, particularly when associated with any form of colonic mass (Table 43.1) (8). The risk of GI tract malignancy is slightly increased in patients with Crohn's disease (64), but not sufficiently to justify routine cancer screening. Siblings and offspring of patients with familial polyposis syndromes should be offered colon cancer screening in early adulthood. There is no evidence to justify the routine screening of relatives of patients with sporadic adenomatous polyps.

What will be the effect of aggressive surveillance on the incidence and mortality of colon cancer? To summarize, the previously cited studies suggest that identification and removal of adenomatous polyps have measurable benefit, including a stage shift toward less aggressive cancers and reduced mortality (72, 122, 123). The public has been made aware of the association between cigarette smoking and lung cancer, as well as the benefits of screening for cancers of the breast, uterine cervix, testes, and skin. A major health education effort is needed to encourage those most likely to benefit from colon cancer screening to seek it.

Tumor Ablation

Therapeutic endoscopy can palliate bleeding and/or obstructing colon cancers in selected patients whose comorbid diseases make them unsuitable for conventional surgical management (Fig. 43.2) (74). The surface of acutely or

Table 43.1. Probability of Finding Carcinoma at Surgery in Patients with Chronic Ulcerative Colitis and Dysplasia

Dysplasia grade	Immediate colectomy	Colectomy after some follow-up
High	42% (10/24)	32% (15/47)
Low	19% (3/16)	8% (17/204)

From Bernstein CN, Shanahan F, Weinstein WM. Are we telling patients the truth about surveillance colonoscopy in ulcerative colitis? Lancet 343:71–74, 1994. Reproduced by permission.

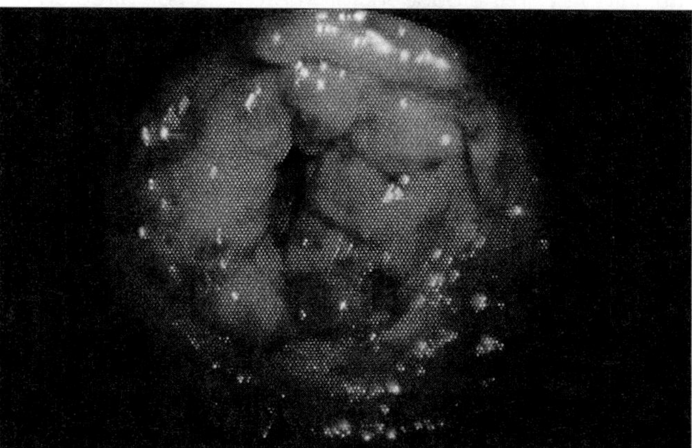

Figure 43.2. Nearly complete rectal obstruction in an elderly male unfit for surgery. Nd-YAG laser photo ablation provided effective palliation by widening the lumen and reducing friability of the tumor.

chronically bleeding tumors can be coagulated using an Nd:YAG laser. This laser can also be used at higher energy levels to vaporize tissue to restore a lumen through obstructing cancers (26). Laser treatment is not without risk; colon perforation is a recognized complication of laser therapy. Photodynamic therapy of colon tumors—using a porphyrin derivative to selectively sensitize tumor cells to laser energy—and technical enhancements such as contact probes remain experimental (74).

BILE DUCTS AND PANCREAS

When managing a patient who presents with symptoms suggestive of pancreatic or biliary cancer, the first goal of the clinician is to define the nature and extent of the problem, as quickly as possible with minimal interference and cost. Twenty years ago most of these cases were diagnosed at laparotomy. Since then, developments in pancreatic and biliary imaging have been spectacular (see Chapter 36), so that diagnosis is often straightforward, allowing more attention to be focused where it is really needed—on treatment.

This section concentrates on the contributions of the GI endoscopist, especially with endoscopic retrograde cholangiopancreatography (ERCP). This method for imaging the biliary tree and pancreas became available before US or CT and was the first modality to provide meaningful radiographs of the pancreas. Developments in scanning techniques have somewhat reduced the relevance of ERCP in pancreatic diagnosis, but its role in bile duct disease has increased markedly because of its therapeutic potential in patients with obstruction due to stones, strictures, and cancer.

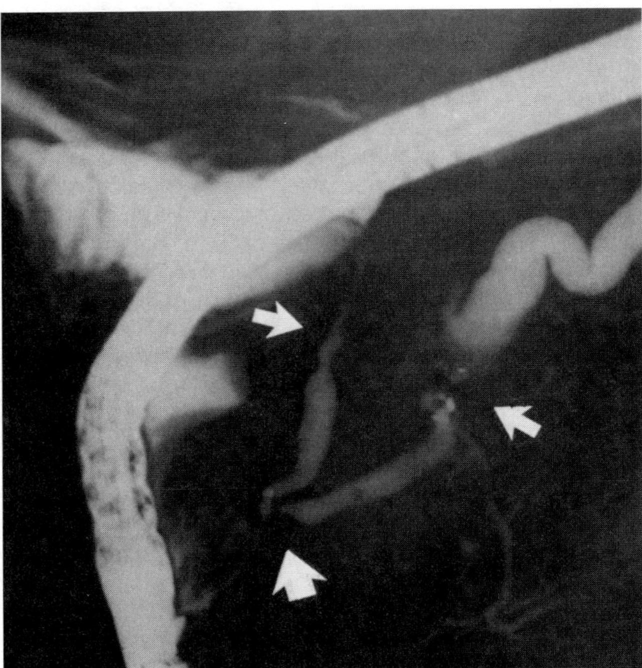

Figure 43.3. Endoscopic retrograde cholangiogram and pancreatogram. The metal tip of the catheter can be seen in the orifice of the papilla. There is a tight stricture of the pancreatic duct in the head, with some upstream dilation. Bile duct is strictured in the same area, a radiographic finding characteristic of pancreatic cancer. *Large arrow*, tip of ERCP cannula. *Smaller arrows*, sites of common bile duct (*left arrow*) and pancreatic duct strictures (*right arrow*).

Technical Aspects of ERCP

ERCP is performed with a lateral-viewing duodenoscope passed under light sedation in a patient lying prone on a standard radiographic table (5). The equipment and all ancillary devices (e.g., catheters, guidewires) are fully disinfected before use. The tip of the endoscope is negotiated into the second part of the duodenum and the papilla of Vater is brought into a direct face-on position. A catheter is advanced through the working channel of the endoscope out into view in the duodenum, where it can be directed into the papilla by combined movements of the endoscope tip and the cannula elevator. Perpendicular insertion into the papilla usually provides a pancreatogram; a more upward path finds the biliary axis. Contrast medium is injected under fluoroscopic guidance, and relevant radiographs are taken in appropriate positions (Fig. 43.3). Fine detail can be obtained by selective deep cannulation of the ducts and their branches. Obstructions (for example, in the bile duct) that appear to be complete radiographically can usually be negotiated with guidewires; these allow subsequent passage of a catheter and demonstration of the ductal systems upstream of the apparent obstruction (Fig. 43.4).

The success rate for cannulating the desired duct or ducts varies with experience. Experts fail in less than 5% of cases, but the success rate may be as low as 70% in the hands of endoscopists who have performed fewer than 100 procedures. Some problems of access to the papilla (e.g., surgical diversions and peripapillary diverticula) make ERCP more difficult, and duct entry may be inhibited by disease such as tumor or stone. The congenital anomaly of pancreas divisum (in which most of the pancreas drains through Santorini's duct and the accessory papilla) occurs in about 7% of the population; in these cases complete pancreatography necessitates cannulation also of the minor papilla, which is technically more demanding.

The main risk involved in diagnostic ERCP (apart from the rare risks of any GI endoscopy procedure) is that of pancreatitis (21). Injection of too much contrast medium under excessive pressure is the commonest cause, but many other factors are involved. The risk of pancreatitis should be less than 3% (depending on one's definition). Injection of contrast medium into an obstructed biliary tree can aggravate infection unless appropriate drainage is provided promptly, preferably by endoscopic techniques. For this reason, training and practice in ERCP should be restricted to those who have ambition or skill to perform all of the therapeutic applications as well as diagnostic indications.

ERCP in Diagnosis

The sensitivity of pancreatography in demonstrating pancreatic cancer is often claimed to be in excess of 90%, by which is meant that an obstructed or strictured duct system is seen, consistent with a mass lesion. Unfortunately, the ra-

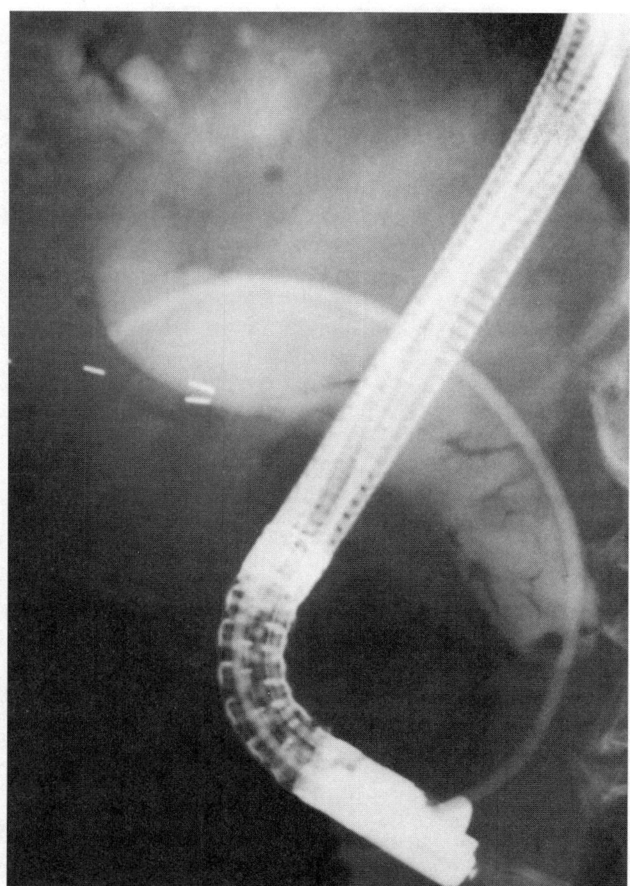

Figure 43.4. After a guidewire has been passed through the malignant bile duct stricture a catheter is slid over it for injection of contrast medium, demonstrating marked upstream dilation.

diographic distinction between chronic pancreatitis and pancreatic cancer (especially when causing complete duct obstruction) is not absolute (88). Thus, pancreatography is more useful in demonstrating pancreatic pathology than in establishing the diagnosis. A good-quality, normal pancreatogram (including first- and second-order branches) makes pancreatic cancer very unlikely, but tumors arising in the uncinate process and islet cell neoplasms are rarely detected (32). ERCP is now most widely used in the investigation and management of patients with biliary obstruction, usually after preliminary US or CT. The double duct sign (contiguous strictures or obstruction of both pancreatic and bile ducts; Fig. 43.1) is almost pathognomonic of pancreatic head cancer (88). Most strictures and obstructions to the bile duct are malignant (apart from those occurring as a result of operative trauma), but there are rare isolated benign strictures that cause diagnostic difficulty. Even more difficult is the detection of cholangiocarcinoma in the presence of multiple strictures in patients with sclerosing cholangitis. Tumors of the gallbladder, hilar nodes, and intrahepatic metastases give fairly characteristic cholangiographic appearances.

Duodenoscopy (with a side-viewing instrument) is the investigation of choice in patients suspected of having tumors in and around the papilla of Vater. Exquisite views are obtained, and the extent of the disease can be judged both from the endoscopic view and from the depth of the strictures on ERCP cholangiography and pancreatography.

Tissue Diagnosis

Tumors of the papilla and deeper lesions invading the duodenum are accessible to standard endoscopic biopsy and cytology techniques. The same probes (or variations) can be passed up the pancreatic and biliary ductal systems (Fig. 43.3). The sensitivity of brushing cytology is 70 to 80% when the lesion can be reached (16). The biopsy yield is lower unless the tumor is exophytic. Attempts are being made to develop new devices such as duct "scrapers" or endoscopic needle aspiration (16, 33). Collection of bile and pancreatic juice for cytology has proved less worthwhile.

Enthusiasm for these ERCP techniques for establishing the diagnosis of cancer has increased recently because more and more patients are being treated without lapa-

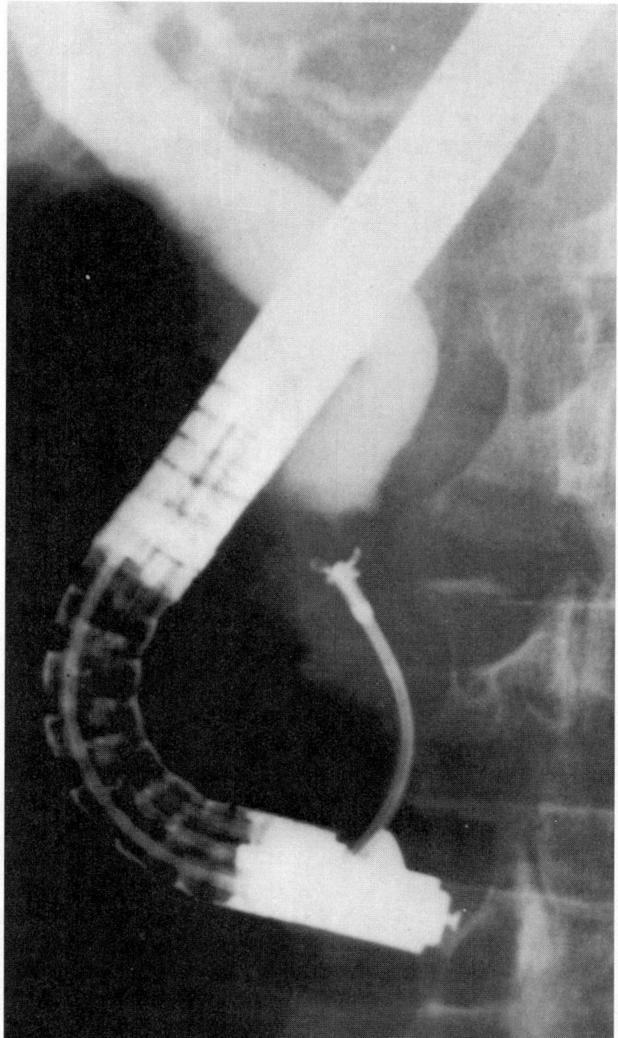

Figure 43.5. Biopsy forceps passed up the bile duct for tissue diagnosis of cholangiocarcinoma.

rotomy, and because alternative tissue techniques (such as percutaneous fine needle aspiration biopsy under CT control) are not always successful (45).

Endoscopic Techniques for Tumor Staging

Staging becomes the most important issue once a tumor has been detected. Unfortunately, most biliary and pancreatic cancers are unresectable at the time of diagnosis (23). Because there are now effective nonoperative methods for palliation, the ability to determine unresectability without laparotomy has become more important. The mere size of a tumor may predict unresectability, but other parameters, such as distant metastases and invasion of major vessels, are more specific. Standard ERCP has little contribution to make in this context, but its fledgling companion—endoscopic ultrasound—may provide a contribution over and above that available from standard US, CT, nuclear magnetic resonance imaging, and angiography (83, 105). Laparoscopy also has an important role to play in the detection of small (<1 cm) peritoneal and liver implants (68).

Endoscopic Treatment

So far the main therapeutic contribution of endoscopy has been in the palliation of malignant obstructive jaundice, using plastic stents (23, 100). Once a guidewire has been passed through a malignant biliary stricture, it is relatively simple to insert a stent across the strictured duct (Figs. 43.6 and 43.7). This technique is now widely used in poor-risk patients with unresectable disease; the success rate for relief of jaundice in patients with low obstruction is 85 to 90%, with minimal complications (115). The main problem with biliary stenting currently is that standard stents (10 or 11.5 Fr) have a tendency to clog after about 4 to 6 months (98, 100). This factor becomes more important as patients with less advanced disease are treated. Approximately 30% of patients with pancreatic cancer treated by endoscopic biliary stenting have needed one or more stent changes (51). Recently, several advances in stent design have been developed that

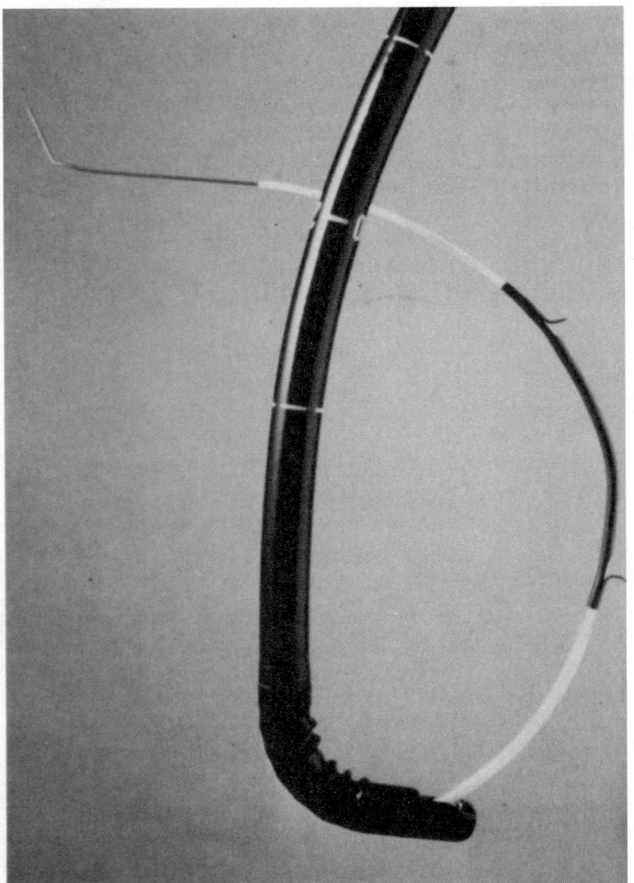

Figure 43.6. Endoscopic equipment for stent insertion: large-channel duodenoscope with a three-layer system comprising a guidewire, catheter, and stent with anchoring flaps.

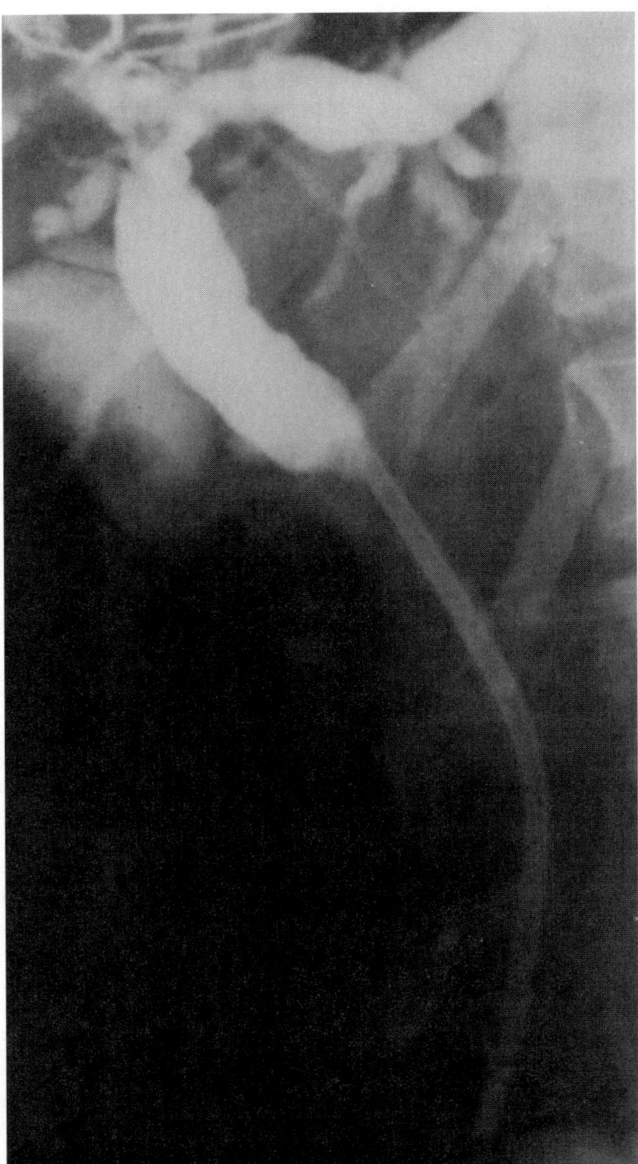

Figure 43.7. Stent placed through a mid-duct cholangiocarcinoma, with good drainage into the duodenum.

appear to prolong the patency rate and enhance the utility of this method for long-term palliation of biliary obstruction. A new Teflon stent lacking side holes, the so-called Tannenbaum or "fir tree" stent, has been reported to have impressive duration of clinical patency (median, 15 months) in patients in whom stents have been placed for malignant biliary obstruction (98). If this patency rate is confirmed in other studies, these stents will most likely replace another innovation in the field of endoscopic palliation of biliary obstruction, the expandable metal stent. These stents also have a prolonged duration of patency (6–9 months) and have resulted in a 28% decrease in procedures for stent replacement (51, 59, 100). They may be deployed from a standard duodenoscope, as they are constrained to less than 3 mm in diameter by the delivery catheter; after release, these stents expand to a diameter of 10 mm. Unfortunately, once fully deployed they are not removable and thus render future surgical biliary bypass technically difficult. Whether the substantial expense of metallic stents when compared with conventional plastic stents is justified is controversial. Randomized controlled trials are under way to further define the roles of these devices in the palliation of malignant biliary obstruction.

Obstructive jaundice can also be relieved by surgical bypass and by percutaneous transhepatic radiologic stenting. The relative roles of these techniques are hotly debated (23). Undoubtedly, results depend considerably on individual expertise, so that each institution tends to develop its own bias. Randomized studies have shown that endoscopic stenting is safer and more effective than the percutaneous transhepatic approach and has substantial short-term advantages over surgical bypass (23). However, these conclusions apply only to the groups of patients in which the studies were performed and should not be extrapolated to other patients—or other centers.

Management of hilar tumors is more troublesome, both technically and conceptually; it is difficult to drain all obstructed segments effectively (89, 115). Endoscopists approach these strictures from below and interventional radiologists from above; increasingly, endoscopists and radiologists work together to insert two or more stents in an attempt to provide comprehensive drainage, thereby reducing the risk of sepsis in undrained segments. Although plastic stents and expandable metal stents are associated with similar success rates initially, the metallic stents require fewer re-interventions (115). Whether drainage of both right and left ductal systems is needed is also hotly debated.

Tumors of the papilla of Vater causing jaundice or pancreatitis can also be managed endoscopically when there are strong contraindications to surgical resection (e.g., advanced age, distant metastases). The tumor can be debulked by snare diathermy or laser, and the obstructed orifices opened by endoscopic diathermy sphincterotomy, with or without stenting. Some patients have been managed successfully for several years, but there is a need for repeated intervention, and some patients have problems with bleeding and eventual duodenal obstruction (100).

Some endoscopists have advocated placing stents in malignant strictures of the pancreatic duct in the hope of relieving pain and improving digestion. The value of this treatment has not been proved except in circumstances when the pain is aggravated by meals (19).

Techniques for tumor destruction have been developed (23). Iridium 192 wires can be placed in the bile duct through endoscopically inserted nasobiliary tubes or stents (brachytherapy). Unfortunately, as with intraoperative or percutaneous iridium treatment, there are no randomized controlled data to prove benefit. Attempts to debulk intraluminal bile duct tumors by laser balloons or other tumor probes are in their infancy. Such techniques may eventually be linked to endoluminal ultrasound probes to demonstrate the depth of tumor invasion and results of treatment.

Peroral Transpapillary Cholangioscopy and Pancreatoscopy

The development of "mother and baby" endoscope systems (Fig. 43.8) now permits direct peroral visualization of the biliary and pancreatic ductal systems. The smallest "miniscopes" can be passed through the intact papilla, but are limited in their functions. Endoscopes large enough (4 mm) to have tip deflection and an operating channel require a sphincterotomy for insertion. Cholangioscopy and pancreatoscopy occasionally permit diagnosis of tumors that have previously escaped detection (especially small mucus-secreting lesions). Tumor destruction and manipulation under

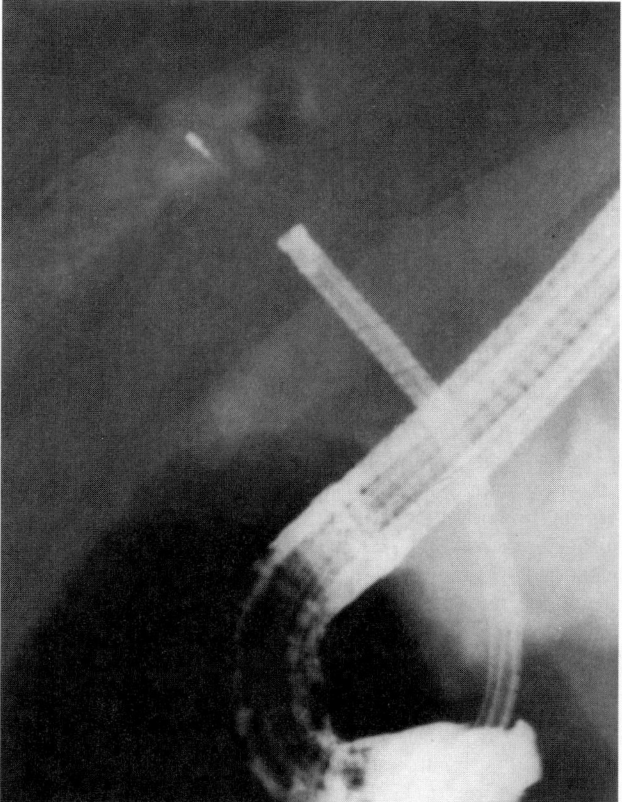

Figure 43.8. "Mother and baby" endoscope system. A small fiberscope is passed through the channel of a larger instrument, allowing direct examination of the bile duct and tissue sampling under direct vision.

direct vision may be possible eventually. Similar instruments and techniques can be applied in the bile duct (and pancreas) in patients who have a suitable stoma formed at surgery or by percutaneous intervention.

Clinical Contexts

Patients with symptoms suggestive of pancreatic cancer (without jaundice) are normally investigated with US, CT and upper GI endoscopy to rule out gastric or duodenal disease. Scans show most pancreatic cancers (because they are large at presentation), and the diagnosis can be confirmed by percutaneous biopsy. Patients in whom pancreatic disease is suspected despite negative or equivocal imaging results should undergo ERCP. Pancreatography will demonstrate tumors of duct origin (and pancreatitis) in some patients with negative imaging results, and a normal examination in this context provides considerable reassurance. In specialty centers, endoscopic ultrasound may provide additional information in difficult cases.

Endoscopic methods make their greatest contribution in the management of jaundice. Percutaneous transhepatic cholangiography is a very effective diagnostic technique, but the endoscopic approach has a greater diagnostic and therapeutic range. Where expertise is available, ERCP will be required in most jaundiced patients, whatever the scans demonstrate, unless there is a clear indication of a hepatocellular cause or need for immediate surgery. Good-quality ERCP is of use in refining the diagnosis (perhaps with tissue confirmation) and starting the treatment process. Stones are managed by sphincterotomy, and strictures by stenting (22, 100). We recommend stenting patients with malignant strictures even if there is a strong possibility of subsequent surgical resection. The risks of stent insertion are probably less than those of leaving instrumented ducts undrained, and it is likely that preoperative drainage may have some beneficial effect on surgical morbidity. Enthusiasm for preoperative external drainage has evaporated after several negative randomized trials (87), but the endoscopic approach is significantly less morbid: bile drains internally, there are none of the risks of transhepatic puncture, and the stent can remain in place for permanent palliation if the decision is eventually made not to attempt resection.

The management of patients with biliary and pancreatic malignancy is a multidisciplinary task. Endoscopists have powerful diagnostic and therapeutic skills, which are most effective if they work closely with colleagues in radiology, surgery, and oncology. It is equally true that more prospective collaborative studies are needed to evaluate and improve our management.

Laparoscopy

Laparoscopy, or direct visualization of the peritoneal cavity using a rigid telescope (laparoscope), is infrequently used by most gastroenterologists, largely because of significant advances in US, CT, and MRI. In addition, ERCP has greatly improved visualization of the biliary tree and pancreas. However, a renaissance may be just around the corner: one spin-off of the current vogue for laparoscopic cholecystectomy is likely to be a renewed appreciation of the diagnostic uses of laparoscopy.

Laparoscopy has been shown to provide a diagnosis in many patients with obscure abdominal pain (38). Indeed, it has been suggested, albeit by supporters of the technique, that no patient should have his or her abdominal pain labeled "psychogenic" unless laparoscopy has been performed. Although innovative Japanese workers have described a sophisticated technique for directly visualizing the pancreas (116), the usual application of the laparoscope in pancreatic disease is to perform peritoneoscopy for staging (68). Patients with adenocarcinoma of the pancreas can be spared major surgery for attempted curative resection if liver and/or peritoneal metastases are seen and biopsied at laparoscopy. The accuracy of laparoscopy for these small tumor implants is frequently superior to that of standard CT (32). Laparoscopic biopsy of tumor nodules can also provide a histologic diagnosis in other cancers such as metastatic esophageal carcinoma, gastric carcinoma, hepatocellular carcinoma, and carcinoma of unknown primary (68). Additionally, it has been used in the staging of Hodgkin's disease for liver involvement (65). This application has not received widespread use as its accuracy is slightly less than that of standard laparotomy.

Perhaps the unique diagnostic value of laparoscopy is in the evaluation of focal, superficial liver lesions. Not only can biopsy of nodules on the liver surface confirm the presence and type of tumor, but it may yield a diagnosis of chronic granulomatous disease such as tuberculosis (2) and brucellosis, or one of the systemic mycoses (95). Peritoneoscopy and biopsy of peritoneal nodules can also provide valuable diagnostic information in ascites, especially if exudative in character (44). To date, there have been few therapeutic applications of laparoscopy in malignancy, but this is certain to change with the rapid development of laparoscopic surgery and the miniaturization of flexible endoscopes and accessories. With increasing endoscopic access to organs and body cavities that previously could be reached only by surgical exploration, the possibilities for laser photoablation, cryosurgery, local irradiation, and surgical procedures performed through the laparoscope seem considerable.

Conclusion

The primary role of GI endoscopy is in the diagnosis of tumors arising in the esophagus, stomach, and large bowel. Refinements in some techniques and concentration on high-risk groups will eventually result in earlier diagnosis and more effective treatment. Table 43.2. The relatively new technology of endoscopic intraluminal ultrasonography provides an intriguing new perspective in staging and enhances the possibility of tumor cure by endoscopic techniques, validated by submucosal scanning. Current crude techniques for palliation of malignant luminal strictures (esophagus and colon) will be refined.

Endoscopic access to the biliary tree and pancreas has equally dramatic diagnostic and therapeutic consequences, which, through lack of training, are not being exploited fully

Table 43.2. Recommendations for Screening for GI Malignancy

Organ	Premalignant condition	Recommendation
Esophagus	Barrett's esophagus	Endoscopy for persistent symptomatic reflux (> 2 yr). If Barrett's epithelium found, enter into screening program (annual EGD* with biopsy).
	Other premalignant conditions (e.g., achalasia, lye stricture)	No established recommendations. EGD for symptoms and/or radiologic abnormalities
Stomach	Atrophic gastritis (pernicious anemia)	No established recommendations.
	Adenomatous polyps	Screening program indicated. Interval not established (every 1–3 yr?).
Duodenum	Familial polyposis (e.g., Gardner's syndrome)	Screening program indicated. Interval not established (annual EGD?).
Colon	Familial polyposis coli	Colectomy indicated. Annual screening colonoscopy if surgery refused.
	Familial hamartomatous polyposis	No established recommendations.
	Nonfamilial (sporadic) adenomatous polyposis	Repeat colonoscopy at 1 yr, then every 3–5 yr, if original polyp > 1 cm or multiple.
	Family history of colon cancer	If two or more 1st-degree relatives affected, screening recommended. No consensus on screening requirements. Baseline colonoscopy at age 50? Start annual rectal examination and fecal blood testing at age 40 instead of 50? One 1st-degree relative affected may not justify early/aggressive screening.
	Ulcerative colitis (UC)	Left-sided colitis only: no screening recommendations. May have increased cancer risk after 20 yr. Pancolitis. Recognized cancer risk. May begin as early as 8 yr after onset of disease. Annual colonoscopy with multiple biopsy sites starting 10–20 yr from onset of UC.

* EGD = Endoscopic gastroduodenoscopy.

at the present time. The spread of these techniques and collaboration with other cancer specialists will provide an increasingly tight focus on specific problems and patients.

References

1. Afridi S, Jafre S, Marshall J. Do gastroenterologists themselves follow the American Cancer Society recommendations for colorectal cancer screening? Am J Gastroenterol 1994;89:2184–2187.
2. Alvarez SZ, Carpio R. Hepatobiliary tuberculosis. Dig Dis Sci 1983;28:193.
3. Armstrong D. Reflux disease and Barrett's oesophagus. Endoscopy 1994;26:9–19.
4. Axon A, Boyle P, Riddell R, Grandjouan S, Hardcastle J, Yoshida S. Summary of a working party on the surveillance of premalignant lesions. Am J Gastroenterol 1994;89:s160–168.
5. Baillie J. Gastrointestinal Endoscopy: Basic Principles and Practice, 1st ed. Oxford: Butterworth-Heinemann, 1992.
6. Berner J, Mauer K, Lewis B. Push and Sonde enteroscopy for the diagnosis of obscure gastrointestinal bleeding. Am J Gastroenterol 1994;89:2139–2142.
7. Bjork JT, Geenen JE, Soergel KH, Parker HW, Leinicke JA, Komorowski RA. Endoscopic evaluation of large gastric folds: a comparison of biopsy techniques. Gastrointest Endosc 1977;24:22.
8. Blackstone M, Riddell RH, Rogers BHG, Levin B. Dysplasia-associated lesions or mass (DALM) detected by colonoscopy in longstanding ulcerative colitis: an indication for colectomy. Gastroenterology 1981;80:366.
9. Bohlman T, Katon R, Lipshultz G, McCool MF, Smith FW, Melnyk CS. Fiberoptic pansigmoidoscopy. An evaluation and comparison with rigid sigmoidoscopy. Gastroenterology 1977;72:644.
10. Bond J. Polyp guideline: diagnosis, treatment, and surveillance for patients with nonfamilial colorectal polyps. Ann Intern Med 1993;119:836–843.
11. Caletti G, Odegaard S, Rosch T, Sivak M, Tio L, Yasuda K. Endoscopic ultrasonography: a summary of the conclusions of the working party for the Tenth World Congress of Gastroenterology, Los Angeles, California, October, 1994. Am J Gastroenterol 1994;89:S138–S143.
12. Carey WD. Colon polyps and cancer in 1994. Am J Gastroenterol 1994;89:823–824. Editorial.
13. Caygill C, Hill M, Kirkham J, Northfield TC. Mortality from gastric cancer following gastric surgery for peptic ulcer. Lancet 1986;1:929.
14. Chong J, Tagle M, Barkin J, Reiner D. Small bowel push-type fiberoptic enteroscopy for patients with occult gastrointestinal bleeding or suspected small bowel pathology. Am J Gastroenterol 1994;89:2143–2146.
15. Clark GW, Smyrk TC, Burdiles P, Hoeft SF, et al. Is Barrett's metaplasia the source of adenocarcinomas of the cardia? Arch Surg 1994;129:609–614.
16. Chung SC. Biliary endoscopy. Curr Opin Gastroenterol. 1992;8:770–778.
17. Colina F, Solis JA, Munoz MT. Squamous papilloma of the esophagus. Am J Gastroenterol 1980;74:410.
18. Connell W, Lennard-Jones J, Williams C. Factors affecting the outcome of endoscopic surveillance for cancer in ulcerative colitis. Gastroenterology 1994;107:934–944.
19. Costamagna G, Gabbrielli A, Mutignani M, Perri V, Crucitti, F. Treatment of obstructive pain by endoscopic drainage in patients with pancreatic head carcinoma. Gastrointest Endosc 1993;39:774–777.
20. Cothren RM, Richards-Kortum R, Sivak MV, et al. Gastrointestinal tissue diagnosis by laser-induced fluorescence spectroscopy at endoscopy. Gastrointest Endosc 1990;36:105.
21. Cotton PB. Complications of ERCP and therapeutic procedures. In Gastrointestinal Emergencies. Edited by MB Taylor. Baltimore: Williams & Wilkins, 1989.
22. Cotton PB. Endoscopy can replace surgery for treatment of many patients with biliary obstruction. NC Med J 1990;5:210.
23. Cotton PB. Management of malignant bile duct obstruction. J Gastroenterol Hepatol 1990;5:63.
24. Dam J. Endosonographic evaluation of the patient with esophageal carcinoma. Chest Clin North Am 1994;4:269–284.
25. Domschke W, Foerster EC, Matek W, Rodl W. Self-expanding mesh stent for esophageal cancer stenosis. Endoscopy 1990;22:134.
26. Eckhauser ML, Imbembo AL, Mansour EG. The role of pre-resectional laser recanalization for obstructing adenocarcinoma of the rectum: comparison of costs and complications. Gastrointest Endosc 1989;21:81.
27. Ell C, Gossner L. Photodynamic therapy: its potential for the treatment of gastrointestinal malignancies and precancerous conditions. Endoscopy 1994;26:262–263.
28. Endo M, Takeshita K, Yoshida, M. How can we diagnose the early stage of esophageal cancer? Endoscopic diagnosis. Endoscopy 1986;18:1.
29. Feller ER, Weiser MM, Schapiro RH. Endoscopic visualization of nodular lymphoid hyperplasia. Gastrointest Endosc 1977;24:37.
30. Fennerty M. Tissue staining. Gastrointest Endosc Clin North Am 1994;4:297–311.
31. Fennerty M, Sampliner R, Garewal H. Barrett's oesophagus-cancer risk, biology and therapeutic management. Aliment Pharmacol Ther 1993;7:339–345.
32. Fockens P, Huibregtse K. Staging of pancreatic and ampullary cancer by endoscopy. Endoscopy 1993;25:52–57.
33. Foutch PG. Diagnosis of cancer by cytologic methods performed during ERCP. Gastrointest Endosc 1994;40:249–252. Editorial.
34. Freedman S. The role of barium enema in detecting colorectal disease: a radiologist's perspective. Postgrad Med 1992;92:245–251.
35. Friedman SL, Wright TL, Altman DF. Gastrointestinal Kaposi's sarcoma in patients with acquired immunodeficiency syndrome. Gastroenterology 1985;89:102.
36. Gana TJ, Soenen GM, Koo J. A controlled study of human resting gastric mucosal blood flow by endoscopic laser-Doppler flowmetry. Gastrointest Endosc 1990;36(3):264.
37. Gasparri G, Caselegno PA, Camandona M, Dei Poli, M, Salizzoni M, Ferrarotti G, Bertero D. Endoscopic insertion of 248 prostheses in inoperable carcinoma of the esophagus and cardia: short-term and long-term results. Gastrointest Endosc 1987;33:354.
38. Goldstein DP. Acute and chronic pelvic pain. Adolesc Gynecol 1989;36:573.
39. Graham DY, Tabibian N, Michaletz PA, et al. Endoscopic needle biopsy: a comparative study of forceps biopsy, two different types of needles, and salvage cytology in gastrointestinal cancer. Gastrointest Endosc 1989;35:207.
40. Graham DY, Spjut HJ. Salvage cytology, a new alternative fiberoptic technique. Gastrointest Endosc 1979;25:137.
41. Grimm H, Binmoeller K, Hamper K, Koch J, Henne-Bruns D, Soehendra N. Endosonography for preoperative locoregional staging of esophageal and gastric cancer. Endoscopy 1993;25:224–230.
42. Gueller R, Haddad JK. Gastric carcinoids simulating benign polyps. Two cases diagnosed by endoscopic biopsy. Gastrointest Endosc 1975;21:153.
43. Guillem JG, Forde KA, Treat MR, Neugut AI, Bodian CA. The impact of colonoscopy on the early detection of colonic neoplasms in patients with rectal bleeding. Ann Surg 1987;206:606.
44. Hall TJ, Donaldson DR, Brennan TG. The value of laparoscopy under local anesthesia in 250 medical and surgical patients. Br J Surg 1980;67:751.
45. Hall-Craggs MA, Lees WR. Fine needle biopsy: cytology, histology or both? Gut 1987;28:233.

46. Haggitt, R. Barrett's esophagus, dysplasia, and adenocarcinoma. Hum Pathol 1994;25:982–993.
47. Hart MH, Vanderhoof JA, Antonson DL. Failure of blind small bowel biopsy in the diagnosis of intestinal lymphangiectasia. J Pediatr Gastroenterol Nutr 1987;6:803.
48. Hawes R. New staging techniques. Endoscopic ultrasound. Cancer 1993;71: 4207–4213.
49. Hennessy TPJ. Choice of treatment in carcinoma of the esophagus. Br J Surg 1988;75:193.
50. Hirschowicz BI, Curtis LE, Peters CW, Pollard HM. Demonstration of a new gastroscope: the "fibrescope." Gastroenterology 1958;35:50.
51. Hoepffner N, Foerster E, Hogemann B, Domschke W. Long term experience in Wallstent therapy for malignant choledochal stenosis. Endoscopy 1994;26:597–602.
52. Hunt RH, Cotton PB, Crespi M, et al. Role of endoscopy in the diagnosis of cancer: a consensus statement prepared by a working party of the International Union Against Cancer. Cancer Res 1989;49:6822.
53. Ichikawa, H. Screening in Cancer. Genova: Union International Contra Cancer, 1978.
54. Imaoka W, Ida K, Katoh T. Is curative endoscopic treatment of early gastric cancer possible? Endoscopy 1986;19:1.
55. Kamiya T, Morishita T, Asa Kura H, Miura S, Munakata, Y, Tsuchiya M. Long term follow up study on gastric adenomas. Cancer 1982;50:2496.
56. Kayrim K, Seidlitz HK, Hagenmuller F, Classen M. Videoendoscopes in comparison with fiberoscopes: quantitative measurements of optical resolution. Endoscopy 1987;19:1567.
57. Kelsey P, Warshaw A. EUS: an added test or a replacement for several? Endoscopy 1993;25:179–181. Editorial.
58. Kiefhaber P. Indications for endoscopic neodymium-YAG laser treatment in the gastrointestinal tract: twelve years' experience. Scand J Gastroenterol 1987;2(suppl 139):53.
59. Knyrim K, Wagner H, Pausch J, Vakil N. A prospective randomized, controlled trial of metal stents for malignant obstruction of the common bile duct. Endoscopy 1993;25: 207–212.
60. Kronborg O, Hage E, Deichgraeber E. The clean colon: a prospective, partly randomized study of the effectiveness of repeated examinations of the colon after polypectomy and radical surgery for cancer. Scand J Gastroenterol 1981;16:879.
61. Kuyama Y, Yamamoto N, Takashimizu Y, et al. Endoscopic microwave treatment. Gastrointest Endosc 1987;33:229.
62. Lambert R. Endoscopic treatment of esophago-gastric tumors. Endoscopy 1994;26: 28–35.
63. Lanspa S, Jenkins J, Cavalieri J, et al. Surveillance in Lynch syndrome: how aggressive? Am J Gastroenterol 1994;89:1978–1980.
64. Lashner B. Cancer in inflamatory bowel disease. Curr Opin Gastroenterol, 1992;8: 683–687.
65. Lefor AT, Flowers JL, Heyman MR. Laproscopic staging of Hodgkin's disease. Surg Oncol 1993;2:217–220.
66. Lewis BS, Waye JD. Total small bowel enteroscopy. Gastrointest Endosc 1987;33: 435.
67. Lightdale CJ. Diagnosis of esophago-gastric tumors. Endoscopy 1994;24:18–23.
68. Lightdale CJ. Laparoscopy for cancer staging. Endoscopy 1992;24:682–686.
69. Lightdale CJ. Endoscopic ultrasonography in the diagnosis, staging, and follow-up of esophageal and gastric cancer. Endoscopy 1992;24:297–303.
70. Lightdale CJ. Clinical applications of laparoscopy in patients with malignant neoplasms. Gastrointest Endosc 1982;28:99.
71. Luk G. Epidemiology, etiology, and diagnosis of colorectal neoplasia. Curr Opin Gastroenterol, 1993;9:19–27.
72. Mandel JS, Bond JH, Church TR, et al. Reducing mortality from colorectal cancer by screening for fecal occult blood. N Engl J Med 1993;328:1365.
73. Maunoury V, Brunetaud JM, Cochelard D, Delette O, Cortot A, Paris JC. Palliative treatment of esophagogastric cancer by laser photoablation. Gastroenterol Clin Biol 1987;11:371.
74. McGahan T, Gilinsky N. Colonic tumors. Endoscopy 1994;26:70–87.
75. Meijssen MA, Tilanus HW, van Blankenstein M, Hop WC, Ong GL. Achalasia complicated by oesophageal squamous cell carcinoma: a prospective study in 195 patients. Gut 1992;33:155.
76. Mion F, Lambert R. Therapeutic endoscopy in the esophagus. Curr Opin Gastroenterol 1992;8:606–612.
77. Mitooka H, Fujimori T, Ohno S, Morimoto S, et al. Chromaoscopy of the colon using indigo carmine dye with electrolyte lavage solution. Gastrointest Endosc 1992;38: 373–374.
78. Morson BC, Dawson IP. Non-epithelial tumours. in Gastrointestinal Pathology. Edited by BC Morson, IP Dawson. Oxford: Blackwell, 1979, p 187–199.
79. Narayan S, Sivak M. Palliation of esophageal carcinoma. Chest Surg Clin North Am 1994;4:347–367.
80. Munoz N. Is *Helicobacter pylori* a cause of gastric cancer? An appraisal of the serological evidence. Cancer Epidemiol Biomarkers Prev 1994;3:445–451.
81. Nelson RS, Lanza F. Malignant melanoma metastatic to the upper gastrointestinal tract. Gastrointest Endosc 1978;24:156.
82. Northfield TC, Swain CP, Kirkham JS, Salmon RR, Bown SG. Controlled trial of Nd-YAG laser photocoagulation in bleeding peptic ulcers. Lancet 1986;1:1113.
83. Pallazzo L, Roseau G, Gayet B, Vilgrain V, et al. Endoscopic ultrasonography in the diagnosis and staging of pancreatic adenocarcinoma. Endoscopy 1993;25: 143–150.
84. Peetze ME, Moseley HS. Brunner's gland hyperplasia. Am Surg 1989;55:474.
85. Peters JH, Clark GW, Ireland AP. Outcome of adenocarcinoma arising in Barrett's esophagus. J Thorac Cardiovasc Surg 1994;108:813–821.
86. Perry J, Baillie J. Failure of colonoscopic surveillance in ulcerative colitis. Gastrointest Endosc 1994;40:655–656.
87. Pitt HA, Gomes AS, Lois JF. Does preoperative percutaneous biliary drainage reduce operative risk or increase hospital cost? Ann Surg 1985;201:545.
88. Plumley TF, Rohrmann TF, Freeny PC, Sivlerstein FE, Ball TJ. Double duct sign: reassessed significance of ERCP. AJR 1982;138:31–35.
89. Polydorou AA, Cairns SR, Dowsett JF, Hatfield AR, Salmon PR, Cotton PB, Russell RC. Palliation of proximal malignant biliary obstruction by endoscopic endoprosthesis insertion. Gut 1991;32:685.
90. Provenzale D, Kemp J, Arora S, Wong J. A guide for surveillance of patients with Barrett's epithelium. Am J Gastroenterol 1994;89:670–680.
91. Ranshoff D. Using colonoscopy to screen for colorectal cancer. Am J Gastroenterol 1994;89:1765–1766. Editorial.
92. Rey JF, Albuisson M, Greff M, Bidart JM, Monget JM. Electronic video endoscopy: preliminary results of image modification. Endoscopy 1988;20:8.
93. Romer TJ, Fitzmaurice M, Cothren RM, et al. Laser induced fluorescence microscopy of normal colon and dysplasia in colonic adenomas: implications for spectroscopic diagnosis. Am J Gastroenterol 1995;90:81–87.
94. Rosch T. Endoscopic ultrasonography. Endoscopy 1992;24:144–153.
95. Saw EC, Shields SJ, Comer TP, Huntington RW. Granulomatous peritonitis due to *Coccidioides immitis*. Arch Surg 1974;108:369.
96. Schottenfeld D, Winawer S. Large intestine. In Cancer Epidemiology and Prevention. Edited by D Schottenfeld, J Fraumeni Jr. Philadelphia: Saunders, 1982, pp 703–727.
97. Schuman BM. Diseases of the duodenum. In Gastroenterologic Endoscopy. Edited by MV Sivak Jr. Philadelphia: Saunders, 1987.
98. Seitz U, Vadeyar H, Soehendra N. Prolonged patency with a new-designed Teflon biliary prothesis. Endoscopy 1994;26:478–482.
99. Shen Q. Diagnostic cytology and early detection. In Carcinoma of the Esophagus and Gastric Cardia. Edited by GJ Huang, WY Kai. Berlin: Springer, 1984, p 156.
100. Sherman S, Gottlieb K, Lehman G. Therapeutic biliary endoscopy. Endoscopy 1994;26:93–112.
101. Shu Y-J. Cytopathology of the esophagus. Acta Cytol 1983;27:7.
102. Shutz WP, Halpern NB. Gastric lymphoma. Surg Gynecol Obstet 1991;172:33–38.
103. Sipponen P, Kekki M, Haapakoski J, Ihamaki T, Siurala M. Gastric cancer risk in chronic atrophic gastritis: statistical calculations of cross-sectional data. Int J Cancer 1985;35:173.
104. Sivak MV Jr, Jagelman DG. Upper gastrointestinal endoscopy in polyposis syndromes: familial polyposis coli and Gardner's syndrome. Gastrointest Endosc 1984;30:102.
105. Snady H. Clinical utility of endoscopic ultrasonography for pancreatic tumors. Endoscopy 1993;25:182–184. Editorial.
106. Stevenson, G. Radiology in the detection of early gastric cancer. In Early Gastric Cancer. Edited by PB Cotton. In Proceedings of the Second BSG SK&F International Workshop, 1981.
107. Suzuki H, Miho O, Watanabe Y, Kohyama M, Nago F. Endoscopic laser therapy in the curative and palliative treatment of upper gastrointestinal cancer. World J Surg 1989;13:158.
108. Tatsuta M, Iishi H, Okuda S. Histological features and recurrence of completely and incompletely healed gastric ulcers classified by the methylene blue dye method. Endoscopy 1987;19:193.
109. Tepperman B, Fitzpatrick P. Second respiratory and upper digestive tract cancer after oral cancer. Lancet 1981;ii:547.
110. Trier JS. Complications of celiac sprue and potentially related diseases with similar intestinal histopathology. Gastroenterology 1978;75:314.
111. Tytgat G. Diagnosis and differential therapy of malignant esophageal stenosis. Internist 1982;23:251.
112. Tytgat GNJ. Benign and malignant tumors of the esophagus. In Gastroenterologic Endoscopy. Edited by MV Sivak Jr. Philadelphia: Saunders, 1987.
113. Vadeyar H, Binmoeller K, Soehendra N. Biliary tract endoscopy. Curr Opin Gastroenterol 1993;9:821–828.
114. Wadas DD, Foutch PG, Manne RK, Sanowski RA. Endoscopic diagnosis of a duodenal gastrinoma. Gastrointest Endosc 1988;34:430.
115. Wagner HJ, Knyrim K, Vakil N, Klose K. Plastic endoprostheses versus metal stents in the palliative treatment of malignant hilar biliary obstruction: a prospective and randomized trial. Endoscopy 1994;25:213–218.
116. Watanabe M, Takatori Y, Ueki K, et al. Pancreatic biopsy under visual control in conjunction with laparoscopy for diagnosis of pancreatic cancer. Endoscopy 1989;21: 105.
117. Waye JD. Small bowel endoscopy. Endoscopy 1992;24:68.
118. Weber DM, Dimoupolos MA, Anandu DP, Pugh WC, Steinbach G. Regression of gastric lymphoma of mucosa-related lymphoid tissue with antibiotic therapy for *Helicobacter pylori*. Gastroenterology 1994;107:1835–1838.
119. Wegener M, Adamek R, Wedmann B, Pfaffenbach B. Endosonographically guided fine-needle aspiration puncture of paraesophagogastric mass lesions: preliminary results. Endoscopy 1994;26:586–591.
120. Weller IVD. AIDS and the gut. Am J Gastroenterol 1986;81:619.
121. Williams CV, Macrae FA, Bartram CI. A prospective study of diagnostic methods in adenoma follow up. Endoscopy 1982;14:74.
122. Winawer SJ, Zauber AG, Ho MN, et al. Prevention of colorectal cancer by colonoscopic polypectomy. N Engl J Med 1977,1993;329.
123. Winawer SJ, Zauber AG, O'Brien MJ, et al. Randomized comparison of surveillance intervals after colonoscopic removal of newly diagnosed adenomatous polyps. N Engl J Med 1993;328:901.
124. Yang GR, Zhao L, Li SS, Qiu SL, Wang Y, Jia J. Endoscopic Nd:YAG laser therapy in patients with early superficial carcinoma of the esophagus and the gastric cardia. Endoscopy 1994;26:681–685.

CHAPTER 44

Bronchoscopy

VICTOR F. TAPSON AND WILLIAM J. FULKERSON, JR.

Introduction

Bronchoscopy permits direct examination of the tracheobronchial tree, and it facilitates the diagnosis and treatment of lung neoplasms and other pulmonary conditions that occur in patients with cancer or immune compromise (3, 14). The advent of flexible fiberoptics has greatly expanded the role and utility of bronchoscopy, allowing outpatient procedures in many patients with only topical anesthesia and minimal sedation. Indications for diagnostic and therapeutic bronchoscopy are listed in Table 44.1.

Tumors

Diagnostic flexible bronchoscopy is perhaps most valuable in evaluating patients with suspected lung cancer, in whom staging for resectability and tissue diagnosis can be obtained with this one procedure. During bronchoscopy, the larynx and vocal cords are carefully examined, and suspicious lesions or vocal cord paralysis can be detected. Left vocal cord paralysis associated with a left-sided lung mass is usually secondary to injury of the left recurrent laryngeal nerve by pathologic adenopathy in the mediastinum. This contraindicates surgical resection.

Next, the proximal and distal trachea as well as the mainstem carina are examined. Involvement of these areas by endobronchial tumor or tumor in the mainstem bronchi within 2 cm of the mainstem carina also prohibit surgical resection. Edema, erythema, extrinsic compression, or splaying of the carina also may indicate submucosal tumor involvement and necessitate biopsy or needle aspiration (10).

The major mediastinal lymph node groups can be sampled transtracheally or transbronchially using a small biopsy needle attached to a flexible catheter (32, 35, 38, 39). The catheter can be passed through the bronchoscope, and the needle can penetrate the bronchial wall under direct vision to obtain cytologic samples of paratracheal or subcarinal lymph nodes (Fig. 44.1). This yields accurate and definitive information for the staging of lung cancer. The sensitivity is comparable to that of computed tomography (CT) with superior specificity. Transbronchial needle aspiration of mediastinal nodes should be performed during diagnostic bronchoscopy for suspected malignancy whenever there is concern for nodal metastasis. The yield with this technique may be highest in the setting of radiographically apparent mediastinal adenopathy, subcarinal adenopathy visualized by CT, and when carinal widening or endobronchial disease is noted bronchoscopically (16). Positive results make surgical staging procedures such as mediastinoscopy unnecessary, and thoracotomies for unresectable disease can be avoided.

After examination of the main bronchi, a detailed inspection of all segmental and proximal subsegmental bronchi in each lung should be performed. If endobronchial abnormalities are detected, the anatomic location and extent of a potential resection can be determined. Synchronous lung cancer may occur in as many as 1 to 2% of patients with bronchogenic carcinoma, and discovery of additional neoplasms almost always drastically changes patient management (31). The discovery of endobronchial metastases by fiberoptic bronchoscopy appears to be more likely in the setting of cough, hemoptysis, or radiographic evidence of atelectasis (2).

The bronchoscopic yield for endobronchially visible carcinoma should exceed 90% (Fig. 44.2) (8, 19). Peripheral mass lesions may be approached by fluoroscopically directed transbronchial biopsy or needle aspiration, but the diagnostic success is less. Positive diagnoses of peripheral mass lesions in 60 to 70% of patients have been reported when combined transbronchial biopsy, cytologic brushings, and cytologic washings are reported (8, 28, 29). Positive results are uncommon, however, for nodules less than 2 cm in diameter. When fiberoptic bronchoscopy is non-diagnostic, a repeat bronchoscopy may occasionally be useful, particularly when endobronchial or extraluminal abnormalities were initially visualized (38). Bronchoscopy is sometimes performed in the setting of an idiopathic pleural effusion; this approach appears to be most useful when there is associated hemoptysis, accompanying lung mass or infiltrate, atelectasis, massive effusion, or cytology-positive effusions without an obvious primary tumor (26).

Transthoracic needle aspiration (TTNA) offers a higher yield than flexible bronchoscopy for diagnosing small, peripheral mass lesions in the chest, but the pneumothorax complication rate is much higher. TTNA obviously supplies no information regarding endobronchial status, and aspiration of central or mediastinal masses is better performed transbronchially than transthoracically. Bronchoscopy is therefore the initial diagnostic procedure of choice for most patients with suspected lung cancer.

Hemoptysis may be a presenting symptom of bronchogenic carcinoma. Approximately 30% of patients with hemoptysis and focal abnormalities on chest radiographs

Table 44.1. Indications for Bronchoscopy

Diagnostic
Persistent atelectasis
Unresolved pneumonia
Radiographic suspicion of neoplasia
Persistent, unexplained cough
Hemoptysis
Abnormal sputum cytology
Diffuse lung disease
Pulmonary infiltrate in an immunocompromised host
Therapeutic
Foreign-body aspiration
Acute lobar collapse
Potential laser therapy
Endobronchial radiotherapy

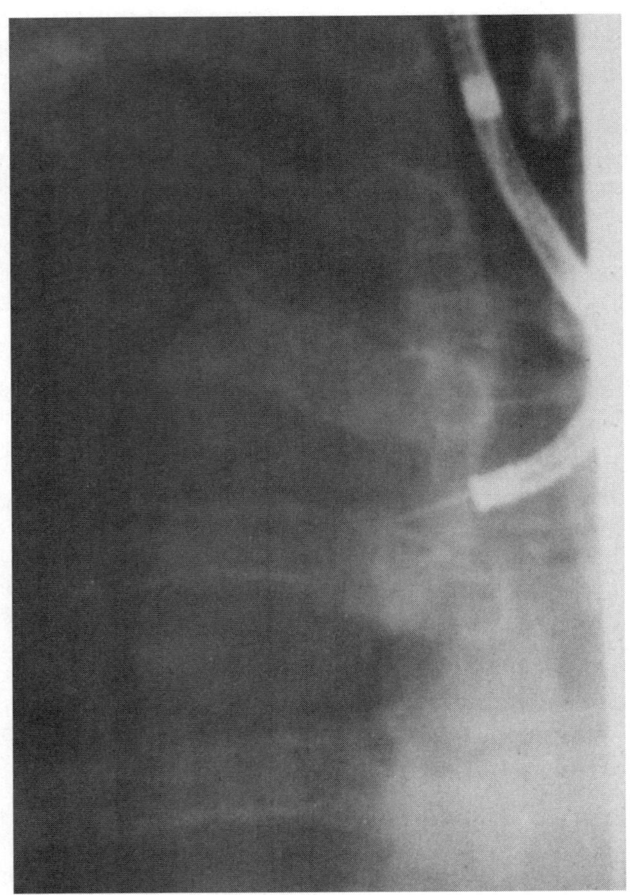

Figure 44.1. Transbronchial needle aspiration of a right paratracheal mass through a flexible bronchoscope.

have cancer at bronchoscopy (24). The utility of bronchoscopy in the evaluation of hemoptysis with a normal or non-localizing chest radiograph is less clear (24, 25); most studies report bronchoscopic diagnoses of cancer in 5% or less of these patients. Age greater than 50 years, history of cigarette use, and duration of hemoptysis longer than 1 week are associated with a cancer diagnosis. CT may be a

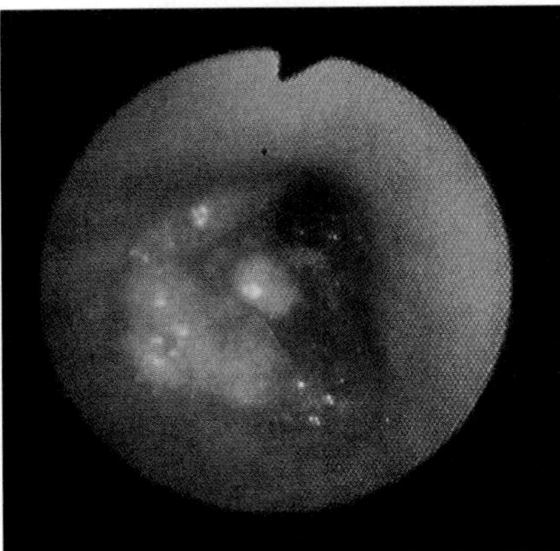

Figure 44.2. Endobronchial squamous cell carcinoma in the bronchus of the left upper lobe.

useful adjunct to fiberoptic bronchoscopy in the setting of hemoptysis (21, 23), but the initial procedure should be bronchoscopy when a high clinical suspicion of carcinoma exists and a radiographic abnormality is present (34).

Pulmonary Infiltrates and Infections

Pulmonary infiltrates and pulmonary infections frequently occur in patients with cancer who are immunocompromised secondary to chemotherapy-induced leukopenia, corticosteroids, or the primary disease process. Physicians must often decide between a course of empiric antibiotic therapy or an invasive diagnostic procedure. When the patient is ill, and particularly when the infiltrates are diffuse and progressive, an invasive approach is often chosen. Bronchoscopy has been widely used to bypass upper airway colonization and obtain diagnostic specimens in immunocompromised patients with pulmonary infiltrates. Several different techniques including the protected specimen brush (PSB), bronchoalveolar lavage, and transbronchial biopsy, can be employed. The concept of the PSB is to avoid contamination during passage of the bronchoscope through the upper airway (41). Using semiquantitative cultures, results from the PSB have been accurate at diagnosing bacterial pneumonia in both animal and clinical studies (12, 13, 27, 40).

In conjunction with quantitative cultures of lavage fluid, bronchoalveolar lavage (BAL) has been used to distinguish pneumonia from bacterial colonization of the upper airways in intubated, mechanically ventilated patients. The bronchoscope is wedged in a segment corresponding to the radiographic abnormality. In a patient with diffuse infiltrates, the right middle lobe or the lingula is often used because their accessibility and anatomic orientation favor the recovery of fluid in supine patients. Physiologic saline solution (100–200 mL) is infused through the bronchoscope into the lung and subsequently suctioned out. Fever and increased pulmonary infiltrates in the area of lavage have been reported, but blood cultures are usually negative. Hemorrhage is unusual and rarely significant. BAL has proven to be effective in diagnosing pneumonia resulting from *Pneumocystis carinii* in patients with hematologic neoplasms and those with the acquired immunodeficiency syndrome; sensitivities range from 85 to 97% (4, 7, 15). The culture of organisms such as *Mycobacterium tuberculosis* and *Legionella pneumophila* is also diagnostic of infection, but quantitative cultures of BAL fluid are necessary to distinguish routine bacterial infections from colonization (37). BAL may be useful for diagnosing fungal pneumonias in immunocompromised patients. Recovery of histoplasma organisms in BAL fluid is considered to be diagnostic of infection, but BAL may be less sensitive than transbronchial biopsy for diagnosing histoplasmosis. *Candida* species frequently colonize the respiratory tract of hospitalized patients, and positive cultures in BAL fluid for candida are not sufficiently diagnostic of true infection. *Aspergillus* species also may colonize the air passages of both normal and immunocompromised hosts without causing infection; thus a firm diagnosis of invasive aspergillus pneumonia requires demonstration of tissue invasion. Kahn and colleagues (19) found that the presence of hyphae in BAL fluid from immunocompromised patients with new pulmonary infiltrates had 53% sensitivity, a 97% specificity, and a 75% predictive value for invasive disease. A positive BAL smear from an immunocompromised host with prolonged neutropenia and focal infiltrate should warrant consideration of antifungal therapy. When possible, however, the patient should have direct biopsy evidence of tissue invasion.

The diagnosis of viral pneumonia may be difficult to make with BAL. Some clinicians accept the diagnosis if BAL fluid cultures reveal virus, but more conclusive information requires the addition of characteristic cytopathologic findings such as the intranuclear inclusions of cytomegalovirus infection. Crawford and colleagues (9) found that viral cultures from the rapidly centrifuged BAL fluid of 33 bone marrow–transplant recipients were positive in 96% of specimens. Confirmatory lung tissue cultures were positive in all cases. Thus, the sensitivity of BAL fluid was 96% and the specificity 100%.

Transbronchial biopsy also has been used to diagnose pulmonary infections. Critically ill patients may be more susceptible to bleeding but, in general, the procedure can be safely performed if coagulation studies are normal and the platelet count is above 100,000/mL. Mechanical ventilation may add a significant risk of pneumothorax to the procedure. Hedemark and colleagues (18) evaluated 39 renal allograft patients with fever and new pulmonary infiltrates using fiberoptic bronchoscopy. Transbronchial biopsy was performed in 17 patients, with specific diagnoses obtained in 9 (53%). In 3 patients (18%), transbronchial biopsy was the only positive bronchoscopic specimen.

Diffuse or focal infiltrates in immunocompromised patients do not always represent infections. Pulmonary hemorrhage, pulmonary edema, lymphangitic carcinomatosis, radiation pneumonitis, and chemotherapy-induced lung disease may complicate the course and treatment of individual patients. Differentiating these diagnoses from infection based on clinical and radiographic findings is often impossible. Bronchoscopy and transbronchial biopsy are usually diagnostic of lymphangitic carcinomatosis, but transbronchial biopsies often are only suggestive or consistent with any of the alternative diagnoses. Open-lung biopsy may be necessary when definitive information is required.

Therapeutic Bronchoscopy

The therapeutic role for flexible and rigid bronchoscopy is expanding. Aspirated foreign bodies in adults are often removable with flexible bronchoscopes using forceps to grasp objects or special basket attachments for retrieval. In small children and some adults, rigid bronchoscopy is preferable. Lobar collapse in hospitalized patients because of retained mucus can often be resolved with bronchoscopic lavage and suctioning.

More appropriate to the cancer physician is the therapeutic role of bronchoscopy in managing endobronchial lesions. Successful treatment of airway obstruction caused by benign and malignant lesions with a Nd-YAG laser has been reported (5, 6, 36). Airway caliber can be improved in 85 to 90% of patients with malignant airway obstruction, and in addition to the vaporization of airway lesions, hemostasis can be achieved in refractory bleeding lesions. The Nd-YAG laser can be used through a flexible bronchoscope; however, most operators agree that a rigid bronchoscope is safer and more effective. Nd-YAG laser treatment of malignant airway lesions is effective but palliative treatment. Major complications include hemorrhage and bronchopleural fistulae, but they are uncommon.

Successful phototherapy of unresectable, endobronchial, malignant neoplasms through the flexible bronchoscope with hematoporphyrin-derivative labelling and argon laser activation has been reported (11, 17). Occasional patients with small lesions, radiographically occult tumors, or carcinoma in situ have shown apparent cure on long-term follow-up (11). This methodology is currently being evaluated in multicenter trials and may be generally available soon.

Endobronchial irradiation brachytherapy, either with implanted ^{198}Au seeds or temporary indwelling catheters containing ^{192}Ir radioactive sources also may offer palliative relief of airway obstruction and control of tumor hemorrhage (20, 22, 30). Objective evidence of airway improvement has been described in approximately 75% of patients. Radiation brachytherapy is easily performed through a flexible bronchoscope under minimal sedation. This treatment may be most appropriate for patients who have failed external beam therapy. Brachytherapy delivers an intensive, short course of radiation to the surrounding area, and it minimizes potential radiation-induced damage to extrapulmonary tissues. The combination of brachytherapy with Nd-YAG laser treatment may offer even greater palliation (1, 33).

Complications of Bronchoscopy

Complications from bronchoscopy are uncommon if patients are carefully selected and screened. Potential complications are listed in Table 44.2, and contraindications to the procedure are listed in Table 44.3. Problems related to med-

Table 44.2. Complications of Bronchoscopy

Laryngospasm
Bronchospasm
Hypoxemia
Cardiac arrhythmias
Fever
Pneumonia
Pneumothorax
Hemorrhage

Table 44.3. Contraindications to Bronchoscopy

Routine
Unstable asthma
Severe hypoxemia
Serious arrhythmia
Unstable angina pectoris
Poor co-operation
Biopsy procedure
Uncorrected bleeding diathesis
Severe pulmonary hypertension
Severe anemia

ications are most often secondary to excessive dosage or an underlying organ-system dysfunction. Patients with significant respiratory or cardiac impairment have an increased risk for subsequent complications, and indications for procedures in these patients should be absolute and the procedure done under the most optimal conditions.

In an average patient, the arterial partial pressure of oxygen falls approximately 20 torr during flexible bronchoscopy. Fever occurs after bronchoscopy in 15 to 20% of patients, and radiographic and clinical evidence of pneumonia occurs in approximately 5%. Patients with near-obstructive endobronchial neoplasms are at increased risk for postprocedural pneumonia. Pneumothorax following transbronchial biopsy has been reported to occur in as many as 5% of patients; however, our experience with routine use of fluoroscopic guidance incurs a frequency of less than 1%. Significant bleeding (i.e., >50 mL) is uncommon after endobronchial or transbronchial biopsy in patients with no evidence of ongoing coagulopathy. Multiple antibiotics may qualitatively alter platelet function, and a preoperative bleeding time is recommended in this patient population. All patients undergoing bronchoscopy should receive supplemental oxygen, and both cardiac rhythm and arterial oxygen saturation should be continuously monitored throughout and immediately following the procedure.

References

1. Allen M, Baldwin J, Fish V, Goffinet D, Cannon W, Mark J. Combined laser therapy and endobronchial radiotherapy for unresectable lung carcinoma with bronchial obstruction. Am J Surg 1985;150:71.
2. Argyros GJ, Torrington KG. Fiberoptic bronchoscopy in the evaluation of carcinoma metastatic to the lung. Chest 1994;105:454.
3. Arroliga AC, Matthay RA. The role of bronchoscopy in lung cancer. Clin Chest Med 1993;14:87.
4. Broaddus C, Dake M, Stulbarg M, Blumfeld W, Hadley W, Golden J, Hopewell P. Bronchoalveolar lavage and transbronchial biopsy for the diagnosis of pulmonary infections in the acquired immunodeficiency syndrome. Ann Intern Med 1985;102:747.
5. Brutinel W, Cortese D, McDougall J, Gillio R, Bergstral H. A two-year experience with the neodymium-YAG laser in endobronchial obstruction. Chest 1987;91:159.
6. Cavaliere S, Foccoli P, Farina P. Nd-YAG laser bronchoscopy. A five-year experience with 1,396 applications in 1,000 patients. Chest 1988;94:15.
7. Clement MJ, Luce JM, Hopewell PC. Diagnosis of pulmonary disease. Clin Chest Med 1988;9:497.
8. Cortese DA, McDougall JC. Biopsy and brushing of peripheral lung cancer with fluoroscopic guidance. Chest 1979;75:141.
9. Crawford S, Bowden R, Hackman R, Gleaves C, Meyers J, Clark J. Rapid detection of cytomegalovirus pulmonary infection by bronchoalveolar lavage and cytocentrifugation culture. Ann Intern Med 1988;108:180.
10. Dreisin R, Albert R, Talley P, Krygen M, Scoggin C, Zwillich C. Flexible fiberoptic bronchoscopy in the teaching hospital: yield and complications. Chest 1978;74:144.
11. Edell E, Cortese D. Bronchoscopic phototherapy with hematoporphyrin derivative for treatment of localized bronchogenic carcinomas: a 5-year experience. Mayo Clin Proc 1987;62:8.
12. Fagon J, Chastre J, Domart Y, Trouillet J, Pierre J, Darne C, Gibert C. Nosocomial pneumonia in patients receiving continuous mechanical ventilation. Am Rev Respir Dis 1989;139:877.
13. Fagon JY, Chastre J, Hance A, Guiget M, Trouillet J, Domart Y, Pierre J, Gibert C. Detection of nosocomial lung infection in ventilated patients: use of a protected specimen brush and quantitative culture techniques in 147 patients. Am Rev Respir Dis 1988;138:110.
14. Fulkerson WJ. Fiberoptic bronchoscopy. N Engl J Med 1984;311:511.
15. Golden J, Holander H, Stulbarg M, Gamsu G. Bronchoalveolar lavage as the exclusive diagnostic modality for pneumocystis pneumonia: a prospective study among patients with acquired immunodeficiency syndrome. Chest 1986;90:18.
16. Harrow E, Halber M, Hardy S, Halteman W. Bronchoscopic and roentgenographic correlates of a positive transbronchial needle aspiration in the staging of lung cancer. Chest 1991;100:1592.
17. Hayata Y, Kato H, Konaka C, Amemiya R, Ono J, Ogawa I, Kinoshita K, Sakai H, Takahashi H. Photoradiation therapy with hematoporphyrin derivative in early and stage 1 lung cancer. Chest 1984;86:169.
18. Hedemark L, Kronenberg R, Rasp F, Simmons R, Peterson P. The value of bronchoscopy in establishing the etiology of pneumonia in renal transplant recipients. Am Rev Respir Dis 1982;126:981.
19. Kahn F, Jones J, Englund D. The role of bronchoalveolar lavage in the diagnosis of invasive pulmonary aspergillosis. Am J Clin Pathol 1986;86:518.
20. Lo T, Beamis J, Weinstein R, Costey G, Andrews C, Webb-Johnson D, Girshovich L, Leibenhaut M. Intraluminal low-dose rate brachytherapy for malignant endobronchial obstruction. Radiother Oncol 1992;23:16.
21. McGuinness G, Beacher JR, Harkin TJ, Garay SM, Rom WN, Naidich DP. Hemoptysis: prospective high-resolution CT/bronchoscopic correlation. Chest 1994;105:1155.
22. Mehta M, Shahab S, Jarjour N, Steinmetz M, Kubsad S. Effect of endobronchial radiation therapy on malignant bronchial obstruction. Chest 1990;97:662.
23. Naidich DP, Funt S, Ettenger NA, Arranda C. Hemoptysis: CT/bronchoscopic correlations in 58 cases. Radiology 1990;177:357.
24. O'Neil K, Lazarus A. Hemoptysis: indications for bronchoscopy. Arch Intern Med 1992;151:171.
25. Poe R, Israel R, Marin M, Ortiz C, Dale R, Wahl G, Kallay M, Greenblatt D. Utility of fiberoptic bronchoscopy in patients with hemoptysis and a non-localizing chest roentgenogram. Chest 1988;93:70.
26. Poe RH, Levy PC, Israel RH, Ortiz CR, Kallay MC. Use of fiberoptic bronchoscopy in the diagnosis of bronchogenic carcinoma. A study in patients with idiopathic pleural effusions. Chest 1994;105:1663.
27. Pollock HM, Hawkins EL, Bonner JR, Sparkman T, Bass JB. Diagnosis of bacterial pulmonary infections with quantitative protective catheter cultures obtained during bronchoscopy. J Clin Microbiol 1983;17:255.
28. Popovich J, Kvale P, Eichenhorn M, Radtke J, Ohorodnik J, Fine G. Diagnostic accuracy of multiple biopsies from flexible fiberoptic bronchoscopy: a comparison of central vs. peripheral carcinoma. Am Rev Respir Dis 1982;125:521.
29. Popp W, Rauscher H, Ritschka L, Redtenbacher S, Zwick H, Dutz W. Diagnostic sensitivity of different techniques in the diagnosis of lung tumors with the flexible fiberoptic bronchoscope. Comparison of brush biopsy, imprint cytology of forceps biopsy, and histology of forceps biopsy. Cancer 1991;67:72.
30. Rabie T, Wilson K, Easley J, Teague R, Bloom K, Lawrence C, Ilaria R. Palliation of bronchogenic carcinoma with 198 Au implantation using the fiberoptic bronchoscope. Chest 1986;90:641.
31. Rohmedder J, Weatherbee L. Multiple primary bronchogenic carcinoma with a review of the literature. Am Rev Respir Dis 1974;109:435.
32. Salathe M, Soler M, Bolliger C, Dalquen P, Perruchoud A. Transbronchial needle aspiration in routine fiberoptic bronchoscopy. Respiration 1992;59:5.
33. Schray M, McDougall J, Martinez A, Cortese D, Brutinel W. Management of malignant airway compromise with laser and low dose rate brachytherapy. The Mayo Clinic experience. Chest 1988;93:264.
34. Set PA, Flower CD, Smith IE, Chan AP, Twentyman OP, Shneerson JM. Hemoptysis: comparative study of the role of CT and fiberoptic bronchoscopy. Radiology 1993;189:677.
35. Shure D, Fedullo P. The role of transcarinal needle aspiration in the staging of bronchogenic carcinoma. Chest 1984;86:693.
36. Stanopoulos I, Beamis J, Martinez F, Vergos K, Shapshay S. Laser bronchoscopy in respiratory failure from malignant airway obstruction. Crit Care Med 1993;21:386.
37. Torres A, Puig de la Bellacasa J, Zaubet A, Gonzalez J, Rodriguez-Roisin R, DeAnta T, Vidal A. Diagnostic value of quantitative cultures of bronchoalveolar lavage and telescoping plugged catheters in mechanically ventilated patients with bacterial pneumonia. Am Rev Respir Dis 1989;140:306.
38. Torrington KG, Poropatich RK. Utility of repeated fiberoptic bronchoscopy for suspected malignancy. Chest 1992;102:1080.
39. Wang K, Brower R, Haponik E, Siegelman S. Flexible transbronchial needle aspiration for staging bronchogenic carcinoma. Chest 1983;84:571.
40. Wimberly N, Bass JB, Boyd BW, Kirkpatrick M, Serio R, Pollock H. Use of a bronchoscopic protective catheter brush for the diagnosis of pulmonary infections. Chest 1982;81:556.
41. Wimberly N, Faling JC, Bartlett JG. A fiberoptic bronchoscopy technique to obtain uncontaminated lower airway secretions for bacterial culture. Am Rev Respir Dis 1979;199:337.

SECTION XII

PRINCIPLES OF SURGICAL ONCOLOGY

CHAPTER 45

Principles of Surgical Oncology

DONALD L. MORTON AND RALPH C. JONES[a]

Introduction

Surgery is the oldest and most frequently used cancer therapy. More patients are cured of cancer by surgery alone than by any other single therapeutic modality. Surgery is the treatment of choice for most localized, solid neoplasms, almost 90% of the 1,252,000 new cancer cases anticipated in 1995.

Over the years, surgical practice has come full circle. Originally, surgeons attempted to treat cancer conservatively by removing only the gross lesion. Unfortunately, this led to unacceptable rates of recurrence and patient mortality. In the late 19th century, surgeons undertook complete en bloc resections and amputations to treat patients with cancerous lesions. These techniques brought improved results, but the procedures were ablative and mutilating. With the advent of complementary treatment modalities—notably radiation therapy in the 1920s and chemotherapy in the 1940s—the attitude toward surgical resection is once again becoming conservative.

The use of chemotherapy and radiation therapy in combination with surgery has considerably reduced the extent of operation needed to manage many types of cancer. Adjuvant chemotherapy alone or in combination with radiation therapy has improved disease-free survival and prolonged life for patients who have been rendered free of gross disease by surgery, but who have a high likelihood of recurrence due to microscopic residual metastatic disease. Randomized clinical trials have demonstrated the benefit of adjuvant chemotherapy in a variety of tumors, including breast cancer, colon cancer, osteogenic sarcoma, testicular cancer, ovarian cancer, and certain lung cancers. Although in some cancers, such as those of the colon, the benefit of adjuvant therapy may be limited, in others, such as testicular and bone cancer, it has doubled or tripled survival rates.

Surgery is most efficacious in the treatment of local disease in the region of the primary tumor and in regional lymphatics. Radical resections and en bloc surgical procedures attempt to encompass gross and microscopic tumor in all adjacent, contiguous anatomic locations. Conventional logic suggests that once a neoplasm has spread from the primary site to a distant organ, surgery should have little role in management of the disease. However, prolonged survival is possible following the surgical resection of metastases in the lung or liver. For example, colon cancer with solitary metastasis in the liver is associated with a 5-year survival rate after surgical resection of up to 40%.

Although surgery is still preferred in a high percentage of cases, it is no longer considered the sole therapy for many neoplasms. Surgery operates by zero-order kinetics, meaning that 100% of cells excised are killed. By contrast, chemotherapy and radiation therapy operate by first-order kinetics: only a fraction of tumor cells are killed with each treatment. The two processes are complementary; surgical resection reduces the tumor burden, thereby reducing the immunosuppressive effects of the tumor and increasing the efficacy of nonsurgical adjuvant therapies intended to eliminate microscopic residual disease and decrease the risk of recurrence.

During the past two decades, major improvements in operative techniques and the use of combined modality therapy have significantly reduced the morbidity and mortality associated with the treatment of solid neoplasms. Breast-preserving surgery has become an alternative to mastectomy in patients with breast carcinoma, limb salvage is often possible in patients with bone and soft tissue sarcomas, and sexual potency/urinary continence can be preserved for patients with prostate cancer. Because surgery is increasingly combined with other treatment modalities, it is essential that most patients with solid neoplasms have their treatment planned by an interdisciplinary team, which includes radiation and medical oncologists, as well as surgical oncologists. The successful surgical oncologist must be able to coordinate and integrate the efforts of the entire oncologic team if he or she is to retain a primary role in the management of the cancer patient.

History of Surgical Oncology

Oncology (from the Greek words *onkos*, meaning mass or tumor, and *logos*, meaning study) is the study of neoplastic diseases. Cancer has plagued humankind, and indeed all multicellular organisms, since antiquity, although not always equally. Early authors suggested that certain families, races, and working classes were predisposed to neoplastic transformations. In 1862, Edwin Smith, an American Egyptologist, discovered the earliest writings on the surgical treatment of cancer (5). Written in Egypt circa 1600 B.C., the treatise was based on teachings possibly dating back to 3000 B.C. The

[a] The views expressed herein are those of the authors and do not necessarily reflect the views of the US Army, US Navy, Department of Defense, or the Uniformed Services University of the Health Sciences.

Egyptian author advised surgeons "to contend" with tumors that might be cured by surgery but "not to treat" those lesions that might be fatal.

Hippocrates (460–375 B.C.) was the first to describe the clinical symptoms associated with cancer. He advised against treating terminal patients, who would enjoy a better quality of life without surgical intervention (19). He also originated the terms "carcinoma" (crab legs tumor) and "sarcoma" (fleshy mass). In the second century A.D., Galen (A.D. 129–199) published his classification of tumors, describing cancer as a systemic disease caused by an excess of black bile (17). Galen cautioned that as a systemic disease, cancer was not amenable to cure by surgical techniques and was, in fact, often followed by patient death. This strong admonition against surgery persisted for more than 1,500 years until pathologists in the 18th century discovered that cancer often grew locally before spreading to other anatomic sites.

During the 18th and 19th centuries, advances in pathologic technique led to an increase in autopsies, which in turn resulted in a better understanding of human physiology. The early work of Morgagni, Le Dran, and Da Salva indicated that there was an initial period of local tumor growth before dissemination. This led to the understanding that not all tumors are systemic and that certain lesions cause death solely by local invasive growth. Percival Pott (1714–1788) was the first to describe a specific etiologic factor associated with cancer development. In 1775, he discovered a high incidence of cancer of the scrotum in chimney sweeps who had reached puberty and recommended a wide local resection to effect its cure. In 1829, Joseph Recamier (1774–1852), a French surgeon, was the first to describe the complicated process of tumor dissemination. The first recorded attempt at elective tumor surgery was performed in 1809 by Ephraim McDowell, an American surgeon. He successfully removed a 22-pound ovarian tumor from a patient, who subsequently survived 30 years. McDowell's work, which included 12 more ovarian resections, encouraged greater interest in elective surgery for cancer patients.

Surgeons were originally hindered in their work by the extreme discomfort of patients during the surgical procedure and by the lack of agents that would reduce the incidence of infection. Crawford Long (1815–1878) was the first to use ether for general anesthesia in 1842, but it was the reported work of John Collins Warren (1778–1856) and William T.G. Morton (1819–1868) that brought the potential of anesthesia to the public's attention. Joseph Lister (1827–1912) was the first to report the use of antisepsis during elective surgery. The work of these doctors opened new frontiers to surgical oncology in the late 1880s by freeing patients from pain and sepsis during and following their operations.

Even with the advent of antisepsis and general anesthesia, surgical oncology in the early 20th century was still associated with a high incidence of patient mortality. Cancer was rarely diagnosed in the early stages, and thus few patients were considered candidates for curative surgery. Those surgeons who did attempt surgical excision of a cancerous lesion were hindered by poor anesthesia, which was associated with high patient mortality. Antibiotics were not yet available, and surgical instruments were crude. Also, the microscope was still rarely used to study frozen tissues or to evaluate surgical margins, because surgeons had greater faith in their own assessment of the tumor. These conditions were not ideal and surgical oncology was associated with a high mortality. Major advances in surgical oncology are summarized in Table 45.1 (17, 19).

Table 45.1 Landmark Advances in Surgical Oncology

Year	Surgery/discovery	Surgeon
1600 B.C.	Edwin Smith papyrus	Unknown
129 A.D.	Cancer as systemic disease	Galen of Pergamum
1543	De humani corporis fabrica	Andreas Vesalius
1775	Etiologic cause of cancer	Percival Pott
1809	Elective oophorectomy	Ephraim McDowell
1829	Metastatic process	Joseph Recamier
1846	Ether as anesthesia	John Collins Warren
1867	Carbolic acid as antisepsis	Joseph Lister
1873	Laryngectomy	Albert Theodore Billroth
1878	Resection of rectal tumor	Richard von Volkman
1880	Esophagectomy	Albert Theodore Billroth
1881	Gastrectomy	Albert Theodore Billroth
1890	Radical mastectomy	William Stewart Halsted
1904	Radical prostatectomy	Hugh H. Young
1908	Abdominoperineal resection	W. Ernest Miles
1909	Thyroid surgery (Nobel Prize)	Theodor Emil Kocher
1910	Craniotomy	Harvey Cushing
1913	Thoracic esophagectomy	Franz Torek
1927	Resection of pulmonary metastases	Georg Divis
1933	Pneumonectomy	Evarts Graham
1935	Pancreaticoduodenectomy	Allen O. Whipple
1945	Adrenalectomy for prostate cancer	Charles B. Huggins

Metastasis

METASTATIC ROUTE OF THE TUMOR

In general, a malignant tumor may spread (*a*) by infiltrating surrounding tissue, (*b*) via the lymphatics, (*c*) by vascular invasion, or (*d*) by implantation in serous cavities (Fig. 45.1). However, many cancers spread by more than one route, and an orderly course of metastasis is not a certainty. For example, patients with breast cancer or melanoma may exhibit distant metastatic disease in the lungs, liver, or skeleton but never develop evidence of lymph node metastases. Metastatic patterns of various human tumors are summarized in Table 45.2.

Direct Extension

Cancer cells may spread by direct extension through tissue spaces. Some neoplasms, such as soft tissue sarcomas and adenocarcinomas of the stomach or esophagus, may extend for considerable distances (10 to 15 cm) along tissue planes beyond the palpable tumor mass. Other neoplasms, such as a basal cell carcinoma of skin, rarely extend for more than a few millimeters beyond the visible margin. Even though some central nervous system (CNS) tumors rarely metastasize, they may permeate nearby brain tissue, and their location can cause death by interfering with vital CNS functions.

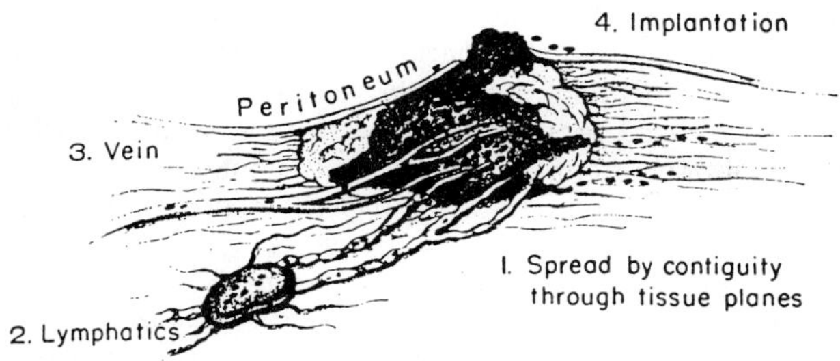

Figure 45.1. The four mechanisms for dissemination of cancer cells from a malignant tumor. (*Source:* Cole et al. (8). Used with permission.)

Table 45.2 Patterns of Neoplastic Spread for Common Human Cancers

Neoplasm	Hematogenous	Lymphatic	Local infiltration (expressed as local recurrence)
Adenocarcinoma			
Breast	4	3	2
Endometrium	1	2	1
Ovary	2	3	4
Stomach	4	4	3
Pancreas	4	4	3
Colon	3	3	1
Kidney	2	2	2
Prostate	3	3	3
Liver	1	1	4
Epidermoid carcinoma			
Lung	4	3	2
Oropharynx	1	3	3
Larynx	1	3	2
Cervix	1	4	3
Transitional cell carcinoma			
Bladder	2	3	4
Cutaneous neoplasm			
Squamous cell carcinoma	1	2	1
Melanoma	3	3	2
Basal cell carcinoma	0	0	1
Sarcoma			
Bone	4	1	1
Soft tissue	4	1	3
Brain neoplasm	0	0	4

0, Does not occur; 1, 1–15%; 2, 15–30%; 3, >30%; 4, >50%.

Lymphatic Spread

Tumor cells can readily enter lymphatics and extend along these channels by permeation or embolism through the regional lymphatics to lymph nodes. Permeation is the growth of a colony of tumor cells along the course of the lymph vessel. This occurs commonly in the skin lymphatics in carcinoma of the breast and in the perineural lymphatics in carcinoma of the prostate.

Spread along the lymphatics by embolism to regional or distant lymph nodes is of great importance. Tumor cells travel by anastomosing lymphatics and generally spread to proximal nodes via collateral lymph channels. Lymph node metastases are first confined to the subcapsular space: at this stage, the node is not enlarged and may appear normal to the naked eye. Gradually, the tumor cells permeate the sinusoids and replace the parenchyma. There is little direct spread from node to node, because the capsule is not penetrated until a late stage. However, when an involved lymph node is more than 3 cm in diameter, tumor has usually extended beyond the capsule into the perinodal fat, indicating an ominous prognosis.

Lymph from the abdominal organs and lower extremities drains into the cisterna chyli and then into the thoracic duct, which finally opens into the left jugular vein. Tumor cells probably pass freely from the lymph to the bloodstream. Originally, oncologists believed that solid neoplasms involved regional lymph nodes and then spread into the bloodstream by drainage through the lymphatics into the thoracic duct and to other parts of the body. An alternative explanation now favored by most oncologists assumes that the presence of cancer cells in regional lymph nodes indicates an unfavorable host–tumor relationship and the likelihood of distant metastases.

Lymphatic involvement is extremely common in epithelial neoplasms of all types, except basal cell carcinoma of the skin, which does not metastasize to regional lymphatics. Sarcomas metastasize to lymph nodes only 2 to 5% of the time.

Vascular Spread

Cancer cells may reach the bloodstream through the thoracic duct or by direct invasion of blood vessels. Capillaries are almost always invaded. Small veins are invaded frequently, but the arteries rarely. This probably is so because the veins form a plexus reaching to subendothelial regions, thus providing a portal of entry through the vein wall. When the vascular endothelium is destroyed, a thrombus forms that is quickly invaded by tumor. This combination of thrombus and tumor may detach to form large tumor emboli. Vascular invasion is common in both carcinomas and sarcomas and is associated with a poor prognosis. Some types of neoplasms have a remarkable tendency to grow as a solid column along the course of veins, for example, renal carcinomas and sarcomas. Renal carcinomas may grow out of the renal vein into the inferior vena cava and up the inferior vena cava to the right atrium, where, amazingly, their removal may still result in long-term survival.

Spread Through Serous Cavities

Tumor cells occasionally gain entrance to serous cavities by growing through the wall of an organ. Many tumor cells can grow in suspension without a supporting matrix and may spread within the peritoneal cavity or attach to serous surfaces. In either case, tumor cells often spread widely when they encounter a space lined with a serous surface. Thus, widespread peritoneal seeding is common with gastrointestinal neoplasms and tumors of ovarian origin. Similarly, malignant gliomas may spread widely within the CNS via cerebral spinal fluid.

HOST RESPONSE TO TUMOR INVASION

Although much is known about the routes of spread, the mechanisms underlying this process remain unclear. Some cancers are metastatic at the time of clinical discovery, whereas others of the same type and in the same organ tissue may remain localized for years. Metastases may dominate the clinical picture while the primary tumor remains latent and asymptomatic. Some patients present with metastatic cancer and no evidence of a primary site. Cerebral metastases from silent cancers in the bronchus or the breast are often mistaken for primary brain tumors.

The generally accepted premise behind cancer surgery is that cancer begins as a local disease and then spreads in an orderly fashion from the primary site to adjacent tissues by direct extension, through the lymphatics to the regional lymph nodes, and via the vascular system to distant sites. The surgical procedure is designed to remove the primary neoplasm and the usual contiguous routes of spread; the aim is to ablate every cancer cell in the body. According to this view of surgical therapy, cure is achieved by the mechanical removal of all cancer cells. However, cancer cells are frequently found in the washings of operative wounds or in postoperative wound drainage in patients undergoing definitive cancer surgery. The observation that many of these patients never develop recurrent cancer suggests the existence of host immune defenses that destroy any tumor cells missed by the surgeon's knife (30, 35). Similarly, apparently viable tumor cells frequently found in the blood or lymphatics of cancer patients seldom lead to metastatic lesions.

Another piece of evidence supporting the existence of host immune defenses is the failure of most attempts to implant primary neoplasms in intracutaneous or subcutaneous areas of the same patient. The incidence of successful tumor growth varies between 10 and 25%, even in patients with advanced malignant disease. The report by Southam's group suggests that this resistance is relative rather than absolute, since challenges of greater than 100 million tumor cells will often result in tumor growth (38).

Prolonged remission is also evidence of an immune defense. Ten to twenty years after successful treatment of the primary tumor, cancer sometimes recurs, with the development of rapidly progressive disease. During the long period of clinical remission, the growth of tumor cells must have been inhibited by host defenses. Host immune mechanisms also may explain the salvage of patients undergoing surgical resection of bloodborne metastases in distant organs, such as the lung or liver. Presumably, these patients also had subclinical metastases, which must have been destroyed by host immune mechanisms.

Finally, there is a significant correlation between cell-mediated immunologic reactivity, measured by the ability to show delayed cutaneous hypersensitivity following sensitization to dinitrochlorobenzene (DNCB), and the postoperative course of cancer patients (21, 29). In one study, more than 95% of control patients with benign neoplasms and those free of disease for at least 5 years following cancer surgery could be sensitized to this chemical (12). However, only 72% of all potential candidates for definitive cancer surgery were able to be sensitized to DNCB; the remaining 28% exhibited cutaneous anergy to the chemical. The anergic patients had a uniformly poor prognosis following surgical therapy: more than 95% either were found to have inoperable disease, because of local or metastatic spread, or developed recurrent disease within 6 months after surgical resection. In contrast, 84% of the DNCB-reactive group had localized tumors that could be resected and were free of disease for at least 6 months following surgery.

This study also reported considerable differences in the pattern of DNCB reactivity according to the histologic type of neoplasm (12). Patients with epidermoid carcinomas of the cervix, mouth, pharynx, or larynx showed a very strong correlation between a positive DNCB response and a good prognosis following cancer surgery. In contrast, most sarcoma patients were immunologically competent whether they were free of disease at 6 months or had early recurrence. These distinct patterns of cutaneous reactivity possibly reflect important differences in the effects of different neoplasms on the immune system.

Immune competence is inversely correlated with tumor burden. Patients who, on sequential testing with DNCB, converted from a reactive to an anergic status usually had progressive cancer, whereas patients who converted from an anergic to a reactive status were observed to establish control of their tumor (12). The immunosuppression caused by cancer appears to be the result of a humoral factor released by the cancer cell or the host's response to the cancer cell. Lymphocytes from cancer patients show depressed functions when compared with those of normal individuals, and the degree of depression is correlated with the extent of the cancer (16, 20). Serum factors from cancer patients inhibit the function of normal lymphocytes in culture. These factors undoubtedly contribute to the immunosuppression observed in cancer patients (7, 15). This defect in systemic immunity can be reversed by successful therapy.

Biopsy Diagnosis of Tumors

The diagnosis of solid tumors depends on locating and performing a biopsy of the lesion. Biopsy evidence will determine the histology of the tumor, which is a prerequisite for planning definitive therapy. Significant therapeutic errors have been made when biopsies were not obtained; for example, radical mastectomies have been performed for fat necrosis. Even when biopsy reports from another hospital are available, the slides of the previous biopsy must be obtained and reviewed prior to the institution of therapy. This is essential, because not infrequently, and particularly in rare neoplasms, an erroneous interpretation may have been made.

Biopsy is easiest when the tumor is near the surface or involves an orifice that can be examined with appropriate visual instruments, such as a bronchoscope, colonoscope, or cystoscope. Carcinomas of the breast, tongue, or rectum can be seen or palpated, and a portion can be excised for definitive diagnosis.

The most difficult cancers to diagnose, and unfortunately the most lethal ones, occur in the internal organs. Space-occupying lesions in the internal organs may grow quite large before causing symptoms. Ultrasonography and computed tomography (CT) scans are the most useful techniques for localizing such lesions. They are important additions to older techniques, such as barium sulfate opacification of the gastrointestinal tract, examination of the bronchial tree by iodinated oil bronchograms, selective arteriography of major vessels supplying internal organs, radioisotopes, and radiopaque dyes that concentrate in various organs such as the liver, gallbladder, kidney, and lymph nodes. Although CT or sonographically directed needle biopsy may be useful in some patients, exploratory surgery is often required to obtain a biopsy and to confirm the exact histologic diagnosis.

Three methods are commonly used for biopsy of suspicious tissue: needle biopsy, incisional biopsy, and excisional or open biopsy. Each has its advantages and disadvantages. Regardless of the method used, the pathologic interpretation of the tumor mass can be valid only if a representative section of tumor is obtained. The oncologist must be aware that a sampling error can occur with needle and incisional biopsies when only a small portion of the total tumor mass is submitted for pathologic examination.

NEEDLE BIOPSY

Needle biopsy is the simplest method and may be used for the biopsy of subcutaneous masses, muscular masses, and some internal organs, such as liver, kidney, and pancreas. Further, this method is inexpensive and causes minimal disturbance of the surrounding tissue. The danger of implanting tumor cells in a needle track during biopsy is extremely small and can be avoided if the location of the needle track is such that it can be excised easily at the time of the definitive surgical procedure. Needle biopsy may be disadvantageous when the specimen is small and not representative of the total tumor, or if the needle misses the space-occupying lesion. Hence, a needle biopsy requires experience to interpret. A negative report for malignant neoplastic disease is always viewed with skepticism and should be followed by incisional or excisional biopsy if there is any doubt. Stereotactic control of needle biopsies of the breast for mammographically demonstrable lesions should essentially eliminate geographic misses.

Needle biopsies can be done with a large-bore needle, such as the Vim Silverman or Tru Cut type. The latter actually obtains a small piece of tissue, which allows the pathologist to study the relation between cancer cells and the surrounding tissue. More common, however, is fine-needle aspiration cytology. In this procedure, a fine needle is inserted into the tumor, and strands of the single cells are obtained for cytologic diagnosis. This procedure is extremely useful for a number of tumors but requires considerable skill to interpret and should be carried out only by an experienced pathologist.

INCISIONAL BIOPSY

Incisional biopsy involves the removal of only a portion of a tumor mass for pathologic examination. It is best performed under circumstances in which, if tumor cells are spilled at the time of biopsy, the incisional wound can be encompassed and totally excised at the time of the definitive surgical procedure. Incisional biopsy includes the removal of portions of the tumor with forceps during endoscopic examination of the bronchus, esophagus, rectum, and bladder, and by suction or curettage from the endometrium. Incisional biopsy is indicated for deeper subcutaneous or muscular tumor masses when needle biopsy fails to establish a diagnosis.

The incisional biopsy is also used when a tumor is so large that total local excision would expose wide tissue planes and prejudice any subsequent adequately wide, locally curative resection. If possible, such a biopsy should take a deep section of tumor, as well as a margin of normal tissue. Incisional biopsies suffer from the same hazard as do needle biopsies: the removed portion may not be representative of all the involved tissue. Hence, a negative biopsy does not preclude the presence of cancer in the remaining mass. Another theoretic objection to the incisional method is the possibility that the surgeon may seed cancer cells into the operative wound or that transected lymphatics and blood vessels may transport the cells to distant sites. Despite these dangers, definitive surgical procedures cannot be planned rationally without knowing the nature of the neoplastic lesion.

EXCISIONAL BIOPSY

Excisional biopsy completely removes the local tumor mass. It is used for small, discrete masses, 2 to 3 cm in diameter, when local removal will not interfere with the wider excision required for permanent local control. Excisional biopsy allows the pathologist to examine the entire lesion. However, this method is contraindicated in large tumor masses because, again, the biopsy procedure often scatters tumor cells throughout a large incision that must be widely and totally encompassed by subsequent definitive surgical procedures. Therefore, excisional biopsy is usually contraindicated for skeletal and soft tissue sarcomas, although it is ideally suited for superficial squamous or basal cell carcinomas and malignant melanomas.

The excisional method is principally used for polypoid lesions of the colon, for thyroid and breast nodules, for small skin lesions, and when the pathologist cannot make a definitive diagnosis from tissue removed by incisional biopsy. An unbiopsied lump is surgically removed when the suspicious character of the lesion, the need for its removal (whatever the diagnosis), and the nonmutilating nature of the operation make such an approach reasonably definitive. Examples of such procedures include hemithyroidectomy for thyroid nodules and a right colectomy for a cecal mass that might be inflammatory or neoplastic. In the latter instance, colonoscopic biopsy is informative only if positive for neoplasm.

Surgeons should always mark the excisional biopsy margins with sutures so that if removal is incomplete and further excision is indicated, they will know where the tumor margin was positive. Biopsy incisions should be closed with meticulous hemostasis because a collecting hematoma can extend tumor cell contamination by widespread infiltration of tissue planes. Contaminated instruments, gloves, gowns, and drapes should be discarded and replaced with noncontaminated substitutes when the definitive procedure immediately follows the biopsy procedure.

Lymph nodes should be carefully selected for biopsy. Cervical lymph nodes should not be biopsied until a careful search for a primary tumor has been made. Nasopharyngoscopy, esophagoscopy, and bronchoscopy are all simple procedures with fiberoptic instruments. A thyroid scan may be required in the workup. Enlargement of the upper cervical nodes by metastases is usually caused by laryngeal, oropharyngeal, and nasopharyngeal primary neoplasms. Supraclavicular nodes more frequently are enlarged from metastases originating in the thoracic or abdominal cavity.

The specimen may be prepared for pathologic examination by either frozen or permanent sections. Frozen sections are made immediately, and pathologic diagnosis can be obtained within 10 to 20 minutes. Frozen sections are used when the diagnosis is required at the time of major surgery and when it is in the patient's best interests to have the definitive resectional surgery carried out at that time.

Occasionally, mediastinoscopy, laparoscopy (peritoneoscopy), thoracoscopy, exploratory thoracotomy, or laparotomy is necessary to obtain adequate representative tissue samples for microscopic examination and confirmation of diagnosis. As a general rule, the neoplastic nature of the disease process must be confirmed by frozen-section examination prior to closure of the wound, regardless of the suspected clinical picture. The surgeon who fails to obtain tissue for frozen-section examination and proceeds immediately to major surgery risks mischaracterizing the neoplastic nature of the pathologic process; the patient will experience the morbidity of operation without enjoying the benefits of an accurate diagnosis.

Staging of Tumors

Accurately staging a cancer is absolutely essential for designing a therapeutic program. It is an important consideration when comparing the results of therapy in different centers, and as therapeutic methods for cancer improve, it is only by comparison of neoplasms at equivalent stages that new forms of therapy can be appropriately evaluated.

The recognized importance of staging has led to a variety of international and national attempts to standardize the staging of the patient with cancer. To date, no single system has been universally accepted. The American Joint Committee on Cancer (AJCC) has recommended a staging system ranging from stage I (carcinoma in situ) to stage IV (distant metastatic spread). Both the AJCC and the Union Cancyum Internationale Contre (UCIC) have adopted a TNM system that defines a cancer in terms of the primary tumor (T), the presence or absence of nodal metastases (N), and the presence or absence of distant metastases (M). Increasing numbers after the T, such as T1, T2, T3, or T4, indicate lesions of increasing size that are associated with a poorer prognosis. The absence of nodal metastasis is designated as N0, the presence of nodal metastasis is N1, and for more extensive nodal involvement, additional numbers may be used. Finally, distant metastases are indicated by adding a subscript 1 following M for metastases, or a subscript 0 for their absence. Thus, a small lesion that has neither spread to regional nodes nor metastasized to distant sites would be designated T1 N0 M0. A larger lesion that involved regional nodes but not distant sites might be identified as T2 N1 M0. A large neoplasm associated with both regional and distant metastases would be designated T3\N1\M1. For some tumor types, such as soft tissue sarcoma, a G for grade of malignancy is added. High-grade tumors are more anaplastic and tend to metastasize sooner.

The TNM system has four chronologic classifications (4). The clinical classification (cTNM or TNM) represents the extent of the disease prior to first definitive treatment, as determined from physical examination, imaging studies, endoscopy, biopsy, surgical exploration, and any other relevant findings. The pathologic classification (pTNM) incorporates the additional information available at the time of surgery and from pathologic examination of a completely resected specimen. It is especially useful in planning adjuvant therapy. The retreatment classification (rTNM) is used to stage a cancer recurring after a disease-free interval; it includes clinical and pathologic evidence. Finally, the autopsy classification (aTNM) is based on postmortem examination.

Unfortunately, one of the great deficiencies of the present staging methods is their inability to indicate subclinical, microscopic metastatic lesions. Many patients who are treated for apparently localized cancers already have disseminated metastases. For example, about half of those patients who have cancer of the breast and who undergo mastectomy have subclinical distant metastasis at the time of the operation.

Selection of Appropriate Therapy

Surgery and radiation are the most successful means of treating cancer localized to the primary site and regional lymph nodes. Since these forms of therapy exert their effect locally, neither is usually considered curative once the disease has metastasized beyond the local region. Both methods are frequently useful as palliative treatments, and occasional long-term survival follows surgical resection of metastases to single organs.

Unlike surgery and radiation therapy, chemotherapy and other forms of systemic therapy, including immunotherapy, hormonal therapy, and cytokines, represent systemic forms of treatment effective against tumor cells already metastatic to distant organ sites.

These systemic therapeutic modalities have a greater chance of curing patients with a minimum number of tumor cells than those with clinically evident disease. Thus, though surgery and radiation therapy cannot be curative unless the tumor is confined locally or regionally, they can decrease the patient's tumor burden so that systemic therapy may become more effective.

During the past several years, enough evidence has accumulated to suggest that multimodal therapy often significantly improves cure rates above those achievable with any single therapeutic modality. Cancer treatment, therefore, should be approached in an interdisciplinary manner. The practice of assigning certain types of neoplasms to surgery, radiation therapy, or medical oncology with a further division into various anatomically oriented specialties should be discontinued.

GOALS OF THERAPY—CURE OR PALLIATION?

The goals of therapy vary with the extent of the cancer. If the cancer is localized without evidence of spread, the goal is to eradicate the cancer and cure the patient. When the cancer has spread beyond local cure, the goal is to control the patient's symptoms and to maintain maximum activity as long as possible. Palliation should be measured in terms of useful life. Diabetes is not cured, but the manifestations of the disease are controlled so that a patient has many years of active and useful life. Goals for the palliation of patients living with cancer are similar.

Patients are generally judged incurable if they have distant metastases or evidence of extensive local infiltration of adjacent organs or structures. However, some patients are potentially curable even if they have distant metastases. For example, patients with solitary pulmonary metastases may be curable by resection, and even those with widespread metastases who have choriocarcinoma may be curable with chemotherapy. Histologic proof of distant metastases should be obtained before the patient is assessed as incurable. Occasionally, an exploratory celiotomy or thoracotomy may be necessary to determine the nature of equivocal lesions in the lungs or liver. In rare situations, the clinical situation may point so overwhelmingly to distant metastases that the patient may be considered incurable without biopsy.

Local extension may be a criterion of incurability. For each anatomic site, there are certain local criteria that place the patient unequivocally in an incurable status, whereas others imply a poor prognosis but are not absolutely indicative of incurability. In equivocal situations after extensive studies have failed to demonstrate metastatic or incurable local extension, the patient deserves the benefit of doubt and should be treated for cure.

PATIENT-RELATED FACTORS

The selection of therapeutic modalities depends not only on the type and extent of cancer, but also on the patient's general condition and the presence of any coexisting disease. Surgery may be contraindicated in a patient who has recently experienced a myocardial infarction. A patient with preexisting diabetes will be much more susceptible to the toxic effects of hormonal therapy with corticosteroids. Renal disease may increase the toxicity of some of the chemotherapeutic drugs, such as methotrexate. In addition, evidence of infection or bleeding may make any form of cancer therapy dangerous, requiring vigorous treatment before the initiation of definitive therapy.

The patient's psychologic makeup and life situation also must be considered. A patient who is unable to accept the realities of a given treatment should be offered an alternative approach when possible. Consultation with a psychiatrist experienced in cancer (a psycho-oncologist) may help the patient deal with the reality of the disease and its treatment (see Chapter 87). This is particularly true for surgical procedures that significantly alter the patient's appearance, such as mastectomy, or that involve a change of organ function, such as colostomy. Experimental forms of therapy should also be avoided in some patients whose noncompliance might jeopardize themselves and the research. Obviously, a patient who is unwilling to tolerate the inconvenience of an intra-arterial catheter and who thus might remove it without medical approval should not undergo such treatment.

Surgical Therapy

Surgical treatment represents the most frequently used and most successful single method of cancer therapy currently available. More patients are cured of cancer by surgery than by any other therapeutic modality. However, only about one-third of cancer patients are cured by surgery alone; with a few notable exceptions, surgical therapy is curative only in those patients whose disease is localized to the primary site and regional nodes.

PREOPERATIVE PREPARATION

Often, the patient's physical condition is relatively poor. Many malignant tumors appear to have a toxic effect on the host disproportionate to the size of the lesion. Patients may have a poor nutritional status because of interference with normal alimentary function, as is true with cancers of the mouth, pharynx, esophagus, intestinal tract, and appended glandular organs. Pain may contribute to anorexia and severe electrolyte disorder. Anemia, vitamin deficiencies, and defects in the coagulation mechanisms must be corrected before an operation can be safely performed.

Every effort should be made to correct nutritional deficiencies, restore depleted blood volume, and correct hypoproteinemia prior to extensive surgical procedures. Total parenteral nutrition (TPN) can be used to prepare the malnourished patient for a major operation, although reconstitution is a slow process, and TPN may chiefly serve to interrupt further deterioration (see Chapter 173). Without correction of critical physiologic and biochemical deficiencies, the operative morbidity and mortality following extensive cancer operations will be excessive.

OPERATIVE CONSIDERATIONS

Once the decision has been made to proceed with surgical therapy, the operative procedure should be planned carefully. It is essential to realize that the best, and often the only, opportunity for cure is at the time of the first operation. If the neoplasm is incompletely excised at that time, tissue planes, lymphatics, and blood vessels are violated and tumor cells are seeded throughout the wound. Any recurrence that follows may be difficult to separate from the inflammatory reaction and scarring that can distort tissue planes to a point where tumor margins are indistinct. Therefore, enucleation or incomplete excision of tumor masses is never indicated as a therapeutic measure.

Prevention of Tumor Cell Implantation

Local recurrence of cancer following surgery may be the result of incomplete removal or spillage of cancer cells into

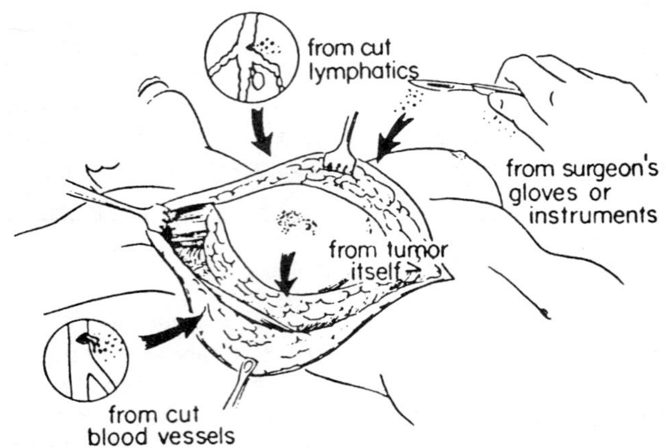

Figure 45.2. The seeding of cancer cells during the operative procedure. (*Source:* Cole et al. (8). Used with permission.)

the operative area. The cancer surgeon must be constantly aware of the danger of possibly transferring cancer cells by inoculation into the surrounding tissues during the course of an operation. As soon as the incision is made, all edges of the wound should be protected with a plastic drape to prevent tumor cell contamination (Fig. 45.2). This precaution is exemplified best when laparotomy or thoracotomy is performed for malignant neoplastic disease within the abdomen or thorax.

Tumor cells may be inadvertently transplanted from the primary site to other sites during the surgical procedure. When a preliminary biopsy has been done, the entire operative field should be reprepared after the biopsy incision is closed. The instruments and gloves used during the biopsy are not used again, because they may have been contaminated. Even the basin of saline solution in which the surgeon's gloved hand is dipped may be contaminated with cancer cells.

If the tumor is entered during an operative procedure with curative intent, the risk of implanting cancer cells into the wound is greatly increased. Should this happen, the operative field must be isolated; the cut surface of the tumor must be cauterized with electrocautery and isolated from the remainder of the wound; and the contaminated knife, instruments, and gloves must be discarded. Then, and only then, can the operation continue through a new plane of dissection that allows a much wider margin around the tumor.

Many different cytotoxic solutions have been used to irrigate the wound following cancer surgery in an effort to sterilize the operative site. None has been effective in decreasing the local recurrence rate, with the exception of 0.5% formaldehyde used to prevent local recurrence from carcinoma of the cervix. Sodium hypochlorite solution, nitrogen mustard, and thiotepa have all been tried, with little success.

The rate of local recurrence in the suture line following resection for carcinoma of the colon is about 10%. There has been some success with various techniques to prevent this local recurrence. Ligation of the bowel with umbilical tape proximal and distal to the tumor, or irrigation of the cut ends of the colon with bichloride of mercury solution and then excision of the edge of each end of the bowel has been used and has decreased the recurrence rate to less than 2%. The use of closed anastomosis and iodized sutures has decreased the anastomotic recurrence rate in the laboratory.

Local recurrence can occur, however, despite every effort to isolate the tumor or avoid spilling cancer cells into the operative field. For example, tumor in local lymphatics may be unrecognized at the time of the initial operation, or bloodborne cells may implant the fresh wound. Usually a local recurrence is associated with systemic disease and is an unfavorable prognostic factor, but this is not always the case, because approximately 20% of the patients whose local recurrences are widely resected survive 5 years.

Prevention of Vascular Dissemination

In the case of most tumors, bloodborne metastases are a major factor in the deaths of patients . Although cancer cells have been identified in the blood of many cancer patients, only a small number of these circulating cancer cells survive owing to host resistance and other factors. Thus, tumor embolism and metastases are not synonymous. In fact, there appears to be little difference in the prognoses of patients with or without tumor cells in their blood preoperatively. Furthermore, manipulation of the tumor at any time in the surgical procedure can greatly increase the number of cancer cells recovered from the blood. There have been reports of a correlation between prognosis and the presence of tumor cells in the blood during the operative procedure, which may be secondary to implantation and growth occurring as a result of the immunosuppression induced by the operation.

Definite measures should be taken to prevent the dissemination of tumor cells during the operation. These can include: avoiding manipulation of the tumor ("no-touch" technique) and early ligation of the vascular pedicle. Since any manipulation of the tumor mass may result in exfoliation of tumor cells into the lymphatics and blood, such manipulation must be kept to a minimum prior to the operative procedure and during preparation of the skin with antiseptic agents, as well as during the operative procedure. Furthermore, it is imperative to use a properly sized incision to minimize unnecessary manipulation of the tumor. One that is too small will not permit the necessary wide excision without excessive handling. Turnbull has reported a significantly higher survival in left colon cancer using the no-touch technique, which combines minimal manipulation, early ligation of the vascular pedicle, and wide excision (40). However, the importance of early ligation of the vascular pedicle has been questioned by other investigators, who reported similar results without the early ligation.

TYPES OF CANCER OPERATIONS

Local Resection

Wide local resection in which an adequate margin of normal tissue is removed with the tumor mass may be adequate treatment for certain low-grade neoplasms that do not metastasize to regional nodes or widely infiltrate adjacent tissues. Basal cell carcinomas and the mixed tumors of the parotid gland are examples of such neoplasms. However, at least some normal tissue surrounding the tumor must be excised to prevent local recurrence.

Neoplasms that spread widely by infiltration into adjacent tissues, such as soft tissue sarcomas and esophageal and gastric carcinomas, must be excised with a wide margin of normal tissue. This wide margin between the line of excision and the tumor mass also acts as a protective barrier against tumor cell spillage into the severed lymphatics and vessels. The greater the width of normal tissue between the plane of dissection and the tumor, the greater is the likelihood of a complete local excision.

If the tumor was previously explored but not removed, or if an incisional biopsy was performed, tumor cells may have been implanted in the incision. It is, therefore, extremely important to remove a wide segment of skin and the underlying muscles, fat, and fascia far beyond the limits of the original incision.

Malignant neoplasms are not well encapsulated. A pseudocapsule composed of a compression zone of neoplastic cells usually covers the tumor. This apparent encapsulation offers a great temptation for simple enucleation, because the tumor may be easily dislodged from its bed. This temptation must be resisted. The surgeon must cut through normal tissue at all times and should never encounter the neoplasm during its removal. Dissection should proceed with meticulous care to avoid tumor cell spillage. Retraction always should be away from, rather than toward, the tumor. The surgeon must make the incision as far as possible from the gross extent of the tumor on all sides, including the deep aspect. Skin, subcutaneous fat, and muscle usually can be sacrificed with impunity and little functional loss. Involvement of major vessels, nerves, joints, or bones may require sacrifice of these structures, and even amputation, in order to obtain a curative result.

When the only therapy is the surgical procedure, the extent of operation should be determined by the concern for adequate margins to achieve cure and not for planning of reconstruction and postoperative function. The problem of reconstruction should be approached as a separate specialized procedure, often requiring the assistance of plastic and reconstructive surgeons and perhaps other special surgical expertise. The definition of adequate margins varies with the type of neoplasm. For example, all deeply situated sarcomas lying between or within muscle groups require the removal of all muscle bundles from their origin to insertion within that particular fascial compartment, all surrounding or adjacent fascia, periosteum, vessels, nerves, and connective tissues, and all skin adjacent to the lesions. This is necessary because sarcomas tend to infiltrate along fascial and muscle planes far beyond the palpable limits of the tumor.

During the operation, visualization of the tumor's extent and/or pathologic evaluation of resected margins may indicate an alteration in the initial operative plan. Decisions regarding the extent of resection are difficult and require experienced judgment. In borderline situations, it is usually better to proceed with a potentially curative resection of the tumor mass unless there is histologic confirmation that the lesion has extended beyond the boundaries of possible surgical resection.

Radical Resection with En Bloc Excision of Lymphatics

Since many neoplasms commonly metastasize by way of the lymphatics, operations have been designed to remove the primary neoplasm and the regional lymph nodes draining that area in continuity with all the intervening tissues. Conditions are best for this type of operation when the collecting nodes of the lymphatic channels draining the neoplasm lie adjacent to the primary site or when there is a single avenue of lymphatic drainage that can be removed without sacrificing vital structures. It is important to avoid cutting across involved lymphatic channels, because such action increases the possibility of local recurrence.

Individually, Meyer and Halsted applied the principle of radical resection with en bloc excision of lymphatics to breast cancer at the turn of the century. This principle has formed the foundation of cancer surgery for many years. At the present time, it is generally agreed that en bloc regional lymph node dissection is indicated for clinical involvement of nodes by metastatic tumor. In many cases, however, the tumor has already spread beyond the regional nodes. Although the cure rates following such procedures may be quite low (20 to 40%), undue pessimism should not prevent such patients from receiving surgical treatment. En bloc removal of the involved nodes offers the only chance for cure and provides significant palliation and local control. Therefore, the surgical oncologist should view regional lymph node involvement not as a contraindication to surgery but as an indication for adjuvant systemic therapy, such as chemotherapy.

Elective Lymph Node Dissection. Due to the high rate of local recurrence following surgical resection when multiple lymph nodes are involved and the high error rate when palpation is used to assess the extent of lymph node involvement, the routine dissection of regional nodes in close proximity to the primary tumor is recommended, even when they are not clinically involved. This recommendation is supported by the microscopic evidence of tumor dissemination in 20 to 40% of carcinomas and melanomas. By resecting the subclinically involved lymph nodes before the disease has progressed to the palpably evident stage, some series suggest improved 5-year survival rates.

This concept of elective or prophylactic lymph node dissection has been challenged because it is not clear whether cure rates are improved if the nodes are removed before they are palpable. Controlled clinical trials directed toward this question in many types of neoplasms are currently underway. Regardless of direct therapeutic benefit, foreknowledge of tumor in regional nodes can affect staging, treatment, and prognosis. For example, patients with breast cancer who have metastases to regional nodes benefit considerably from adjuvant chemotherapy or hormonal therapy. Also, some patients with deep melanomas may become candidates for investigational adjuvant trials only if lymph node metastases are present. Furthermore, a comparison of experimental results from different institutions depends on accurate staging when therapy is initiated.

Extensive Surgical Procedures

Advances in surgical techniques, anesthesia, and supportive care (blood transfusion, antibiotics, and fluid and electrolyte management) have permitted more radical and extensive operative procedures. These procedures sometimes offer a chance for a cure that is not possible by other means and are justified in selected situations when an extensive workup shows no evidence of distant metastases. For example, some slow-growing primary tumors may reach enormous size and may locally infiltrate widely without developing distant metastases. Supraradical operative procedures can be undertaken for these extensive, nearly inoperable tumors, with cure of occasional patients.

Although surgical care, anesthesia, blood replacement, and physiologic monitoring are much improved over the past, these operations should be undertaken only by experienced surgeons who can select those patients most likely to benefit. Procedures such as pelvic exenteration for carcinoma of the cervix recurring after radiation therapy have significantly improved the cure rates for certain neoplasms, but these more radical procedures have often failed significantly to increase cure rates for common solid neoplasms. Moreover, the surgeon must be willing to accept the responsibility for the postoperative emotional rehabilitation of the patient before undertaking such extensive procedures as hemipelvectomy, forequarter amputation, mutilating operations for head and neck carcinomas, and pelvic exenteration.

As an example of radical surgery, pelvic exenteration is a well-conceived operation capable of curing patients with radiation-treated recurrent cancer of the cervix and certain well-differentiated and locally extensive adenocarcinomas of the rectum. This operation removes the pelvic organs (bladder, uterus, and rectum) and all soft tissues within the pelvis. Bowel function is restored with colostomy. Urinary tract drainage is established by anastomosis of ureters into a segment of bowel (ileum or sigmoid colon). The 5-year, relapse-free survival with pelvic exenteration is 25% in this situation.

Surgery of Recurrent Cancer

Surgical resection of localized recurrent neoplasms of low-grade malignancy and slow growth may produce a long period of remission. Surgical procedures are frequently successful in controlling recurrent soft tissue sarcomas, anastomotic recurrences of colon cancer, certain basal and squamous carcinomas of skin, and breast cancer recurrence following lumpectomy. However, surgical resection of the recurrent neoplasm in the patient with metastatic disease is usually unsuccessful and rarely indicated, unless the entire tumor mass can be completely removed.

Routine second-look operations to detect early recurrence of colon cancer were advocated by Gilbertsen and Wangensteen. The results of this second-look procedure were not impressive and do not appear to justify its routine use. However, various tumor markers, such as carcinoembryonic antigen (CEA), have been extremely useful in selecting patients likely to benefit from reoperation. In general, a local recurrence can be treated surgically or with radiation. The surgeon must decide which form of treatment will achieve local control with the lowest morbidity.

Surgery for Metastatic Disease

Although logic would suggest that once a neoplasm has metastasized to a distant site it is no longer curable by surgical resection, experience has shown otherwise. The removal of metastatic lesions in the lung, liver, or brain has occasionally produced a clinical cure. Therefore, in selected patients with slowly growing neoplasms, resections of the metastatic lesions may be indicated, especially if the metastasis is solitary, but even multiple metastases may be successfully resected if their growth rate is slow. Prior to undertaking resection, an extensive laboratory workup should rule out metastatic spread to other body areas.

Some patients with isolated liver metastases may benefit from surgical resection. Resection is recommended for the patient whose primary tumor is controlled and who has no evidence of other metastases. Those patients with a solitary liver metastasis, or metastases located in one lobe, are often successfully treated with resection. Approximately 25% of these patients survive more than 5 years. However, only the minority of patients with colon cancer metastatic to the liver are candidates for this type of treatment. Most of these patients have diffuse disease and are best treated with systemic or intra-arterial chemotherapy.

The results of resection of pulmonary metastatic lesions have been much more satisfactory. In fact, resection of a solitary pulmonary metastasis provides a higher rate of 5-year survival than does resection of primary bronchogenic carcinoma of the lung. Resection of pulmonary metastases may be indicated even when more than one metastatic lesion is present. Many patients die of their pulmonary metastases when resection might have effected a cure.

Tumor Doubling Time. The growth rate of a tumor can be expressed by the time it takes for the tumor to double in volume. The tumor doubling time (TDT) is an accurate and reproducible measure of biologic aggressiveness that can be used to determine the indications for surgical resection of metastatic disease. In essence, TDT represents the balance between the intrinsic proliferative rate of the tumor cell and the patient's immune defense mechanisms.

Collins, in 1956, was the first to describe the method for determining the growth rate of human neoplasms by using serial x-rays (9). In 1971, Joseph, Morton, and Adkins reported the prognostic significance of TDT in evaluating the operability of lung metastases (23). TDT is especially efficacious in treating patients with pulmonary metastases, since these neoplasms tend to be peripherally located and discretely identified on chest radiographs. Thus it is quite easy to obtain accurate serial chest roentgenograms.

Figure 45.3 illustrates the method for calculating the TDT of pulmonary nodules (23). Successive chest roentgenograms are used to measure the changing diameters of the lesion. The greater and lesser diameters are averaged and then plotted against time on semilogarithmic paper. The slope of the line drawn between any two points represents the rate of tumor growth. The horizontal distance between any two doubling points represents the TDT in days.

Although the TDT may vary from 8 to 600 days, most tumors double in 20 to 100 days. In general, patients presenting with a short TDT will have aggressive, fast-growing metastatic lesions. By contrast, patients with long doubling times might have nonaggressive lesions that would be amenable to surgery. Thus, TDT is an important prognostic tool for determining patient selection. Using TDT also makes it possible to monitor the effects of chemotherapeutic agents and to compare different therapeutic regimens.

As discussed in chapter III (Metastatic Tumors in the Thorax), patients with pulmonary metastases can be divided into three survival groups according to TDT (Fig. 45.4) (22, 23, 31). Those patients with TDTs of less than 20 days are not recommended for surgery as it is likely to be ineffective and will not result in long-term survival. Patients with TDTs of 20 to 40 days are not ineligible for surgery, even though their long-term survival rates are not much improved by surgery alone, particularly if a slowing of the TDT is observed following preoperative chemotherapy (22). Patients with TDTs of 40 days or greater will often enjoy long-term survival following resection of the pulmonary lesion.

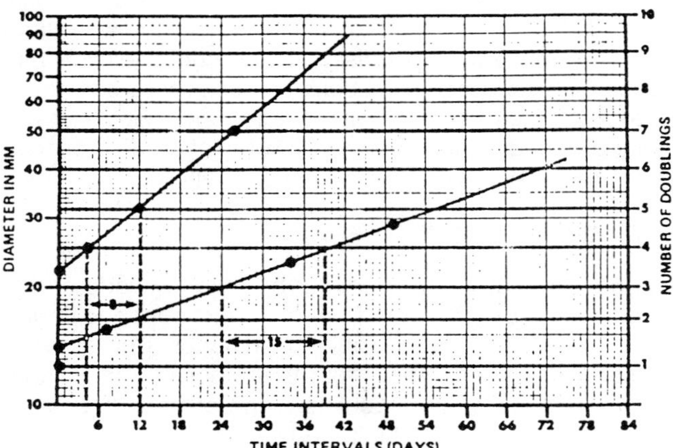

Figure 45.3. Method of calculating tumor doubling time based on direct measurement of the changing diameters of metastatic pulmonary nodules. (*Source:* Joseph (23). Used with permission.)

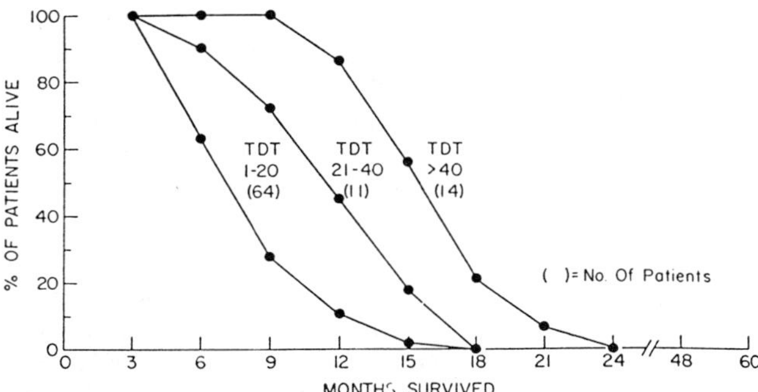

Figure 45.4. Survival curves in 89 untreated patients following the onset of pulmonary metastases, showing three groups defined by tumor doubling time. (*Source:* Joseph (23). Used with permission.)

Palliative Surgery

Surgical procedures are sometimes indicated to relieve symptoms, to reduce the severity of the patient's illness, or to prolong a useful, comfortable life without attempting to cure the patient. A palliative operation is justified to relieve pain, hemorrhage, obstruction, or infection when it can be done without great risk to the patient, and when it improves the quality of life even if it does not prolong it. Surgery that only prolongs a miserable existence certainly does not benefit the patient.

Some examples of palliative surgical procedures are (*a*) colostomy, enteroenterostomy, or gastrojejunostomy to relieve obstruction; (*b*) cordotomy to control pain; (*c*) cystectomy to control infected, bleeding tumors of the bladder; (*d*) amputation for painful tumors of the extremities; (*e*) simple mastectomy for carcinoma of the breast when the tumor is infected, large, ulcerated, and locally resectable, even in the presence of distant metastases; and (*f*) colon resection in the presence of hepatic metastases.

Chemotherapy as an Adjuvant to Cancer Surgery

Even though extensive staging procedures indicate that a tumor localized to the primary site and regional lymph nodes is potentially curable by local therapy (either surgery or radiation), about 60% of malignant tumors ultimately recur. Obviously, patients whose tumors fall into this category have subclinical metastases at the time of diagnosis. The probability of cure may be improved if systemic therapy is coupled to the local treatment. This adjuvant treatment can consist of chemotherapeutic agents, hormones, or, in some instances, immunotherapy using vaccines or nonspecific stimulants.

The rationale for chemotherapy under these circumstances relates to the principles of the log cell-kill hypothesis: a given dose of drug kills a constant fraction of cells, the so-called first-order cell kill. Chemotherapeutic drugs must be given when the number of tumor cells is low enough to permit destruction and at doses that can be tolerated by the patient. The opportunity for cure probably occurs during the early stage of the disease or immediately after surgery when tumor burden is minimal. At the present time, the results of extensive breast cancer trials indicate that adjuvant chemotherapy or hormonal therapy for patients with carcinoma of the breast can improve disease-free and overall survival. Among the neoplasms that respond to adjuvant chemotherapy are breast cancer, osteosarcoma, Ewing's sarcoma, Wilms' tumor, ovarian carcinoma, and colon carcinoma.

Adjuvant chemotherapy has significantly improved surgical results, primarily by its effect on neoplastic cells outside the operative field. Neoadjuvant, induction, or primary chemotherapy—that is, initiated prior to local and regional treatments—affects micrometastatic distant disease and may also significantly kill the primary tumor. The tumor may then be surgically resected or irradiated. When used alone, surgery must encompass the surgical margins of the original tumor.

Combined Modality Therapy

Pediatric oncologists pioneered the use of combined modality therapy—radiation in combination with chemotherapy and surgical therapy—to overcome childhood neoplasms. The cure rate for localized retinoblastoma (see Chapter 98) and other sarcomas in children (see Chapters 139 and 169) has increased dramatically with combined therapy. The cure rate for patients with Wilms' tumor is 75% if surgical therapy is followed by radiation and chemotherapy, an increase of 40% over operation alone (see Chapter 171). Embryonal rhabdomyosarcoma responds best to combinations of radiation, chemotherapy, and operation (see Chapter 169).

Until recently, the effectiveness of multimodality therapy was demonstrated only occasionally for adult neoplasms. A striking example is the approach to skeletal and soft tissue sarcomas (see Chapters 139 and 140). Surgical therapy, the accepted method for management of most skeletal and soft tissue sarcomas of the extremities, has been associated with frequent treatment failure. In the past, even with amputation, approximately 50% of patients with soft tissue sarcomas and 80% of those with bone sarcomas eventually succumbed to distant metastases. In an attempt to improve the results of treatment for sarcomas, a multimodal treatment regimen was developed. Preoperative therapy with intra-arterial doxorubicin followed by radiation caused extensive tumor-cell necrosis in as many as 75% of patients (see Table 140.5 in Chapter 140) (1). The effectiveness of this preoperative therapy permitted local resection of the sarcoma and salvage of a viable functional extremity. Local recurrence rates were as low as with amputation, and long-term results were functionally and psychologically superior. In addition, there was no decrease in survival rate.

Multimodality therapy may also be effective for small, localized breast cancers. In several studies, radiation and minimal surgery were as effective as mastectomy in the control of small breast cancers. Survival and local recurrence rates were the same for both groups, and patients treated with multimodality therapy were spared the physical deformity and psychologic problems of mastectomy (see Chapter 136).

An increasingly important component of a multimodal approach is immunotherapy. The concept of immunostimulation with biologic response modifiers or nonspecific immunomodulators is not new to cancer therapy. Nearly a century ago, William B. Coley developed the basis for nonspecific cancer immunotherapy using mixed bacterial vaccines (Coley's toxins). Since then, whole-cell or cell-fragment tumor vaccines have been introduced for active specific immunotherapy of neoplastic disease; some of these have reached phase III clinical trials. In melanoma, which has been the focus of most cancer vaccine research, immunotherapy is now used as an adjuvant to surgery for local and regional neoplastic disease, and to prolong the survival of patients with distant metastases (see Chapter 79) (28). Cytokines, such as interferon, are being used to modulate the immune response (see Chapter 80) and have proved effective in some diseases, such as myeloid leukemia (see Chapter 143) and hairy cell leukemia (see Chapter 148) (13). Use of colony-stimulating factor is invaluable in accelerating hematopoietic recovery from high-dose chemotherapy or in conjunction with bone marrow transplant protocols (3, 34).

Surgery of the Future

SURGERY AS ADJUVANT THERAPY

Classically, surgery has been first in the order of therapy for solid neoplasms, but increasing evidence suggests that it should be last. Since both chemotherapy and radiation therapy are thought to work by first-order kinetics, resistant clones of neoplastic cells usually remain after these therapies owing to the heterogeneity of the tumor cell population. Heterogeneity is most likely in large tumor masses that have poor perfusion of chemotherapeutic agents and are frequently hypoxic and resistant to radiation therapy. Since surgery works by zero-order kinetics, it efficiently removes the residual cancer cells that are resistant to these other modalities in the local site. Another advantage of this altered sequence of therapy relates to the shrinkage of tumor mass that occurs with preoperative therapy due to the destruction of tumor cells sensitive to chemotherapy or radiation therapy. There have been promising results from preliminary trials using these concepts in bone and soft tissue sarcomas, locally advanced breast cancer, and other neoplasms. A major dividend is the frequent possibility of organ preservation because of a lesser need for radical surgery.

SURGERY AS IMMUNOTHERAPY

A growing neoplasm seems to be able to evade an immune attack by producing specific and nonspecific immunosuppression (30). Specific immunosuppression is caused by antigens shed from the tumor into the blood. These antigens, which circulate alone or as antigen-antibody complexes, can inhibit the lymphocyte-mediated destruction of tumor cells in vitro and may play a similar role in vivo (18). Nonspecific or generalized immunosuppression is attributed to humoral factors produced by or in response to the neoplasm.

Any therapeutic maneuver that lowers tumor burden may reverse specific and nonspecific immunosuppression, thereby altering the immune balance in favor of the patient (Fig. 45.5) (30). In this respect, cancer surgery is immunotherapy because it effectively removes the cancer cell mass that produces the immunodepression and allows the patient's immune responses to recover. Once the tumor mass has been removed, the patient's immune system may deal with clinically silent micrometastases.

This premise suggests that local disease should be considered a manifestation of systemic illness, whether or not the patient has overt metastases. Surgery for apparently localized tumors can favorably affect the host–tumor relationship and may even cure the patient with subclinical distant metastases. By reducing the number of tumor cells, it also increases the curative potential of systemic therapies. Surgery

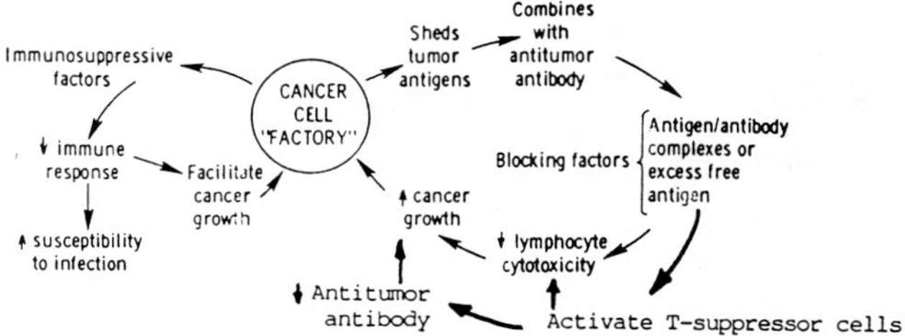

Figure 45.5. Cancer cell "factory" is depicted as a function of immunodepression in the host. Theoretically, cytoreductive cancer therapy interrupts this process, so that the host immune response returns to normal. (*Source:* Morton et al. (30). Used with permission.)

must be considered as part of a multimodal approach to cancer therapy.

SURGERY FOR EARLY DETECTION

In many neoplasms, prognosis depends on the status of the lymph node basin draining the primary tumor. However, the extent and timing of lymph node dissection are still controversial. Sentinel lymphadenectomy is a promising technique for early detection of nodal disease, which is currently under investigation in multicenter trials. Detection of the sentinel node (i.e., the first lymph node draining a primary tumor) was introduced for melanoma (32) and is now being applied to breast carcinoma (14) and other neoplasms (26). Initially, the technique relied on the injection of a vital blue dye at the tumor site and visual tracking of this dye along the lymphatics to the nodal basin. Recently, sentinel node mapping has been facilitated by adding a radiolabeled isotope to the dye and monitoring its path by a handheld gamma probe (25, 41).

Radioimmunoguided surgery (RIGS) using murine monoclonal antibody (MAb) enables surgeons to localize cancer during primary surgery and to evaluate the extent of advanced disease. B72.3, a first-generation IgG anti-TAG (tumor-associated glycoprotein) MAb that was useful in developing RIGS, identified approximately 80% of gastrointestinal and ovarian tumors, as well as 80% of secondary colorectal carcinomas (27). A second-generation murine MAb of the IgG_1 subclass, CC49, reacts with a 200 to 400K glycoprotein complex, TAG-72, which is a human colorectal cancer antigen (2). The antigen affinity of CC49 is eight times that of B72.3, and its efficiency in localizing primary and secondary tumors is reportedly 86% and 97%, respectively (2). A newer MAb, CC83, with even greater antigen affinity is currently under investigation (6).

For RIGS, MAb is conjugated to iodine 125, which has a half-life of about 60 days. Radiolabeled MAb is administered intravenously approximately 2 weeks before surgery. To avoid radioactive uptake by the thyroid gland, a supersaturated solution of potassium iodide is administered 2 days before the monoclonal antibody and continued for 3 weeks. During surgery, the surgeon manipulates the gamma-detecting device, consisting of a detection crystal, a preamplifier, and a signal processor with a digital readout. This device produces audible and numeric displays as it encounters radiolabeled tumor cells. It allows the surgeon to define tumor margins (11), seek out malignant lesions that might have escaped previous detection by CT scan or plain chest x-ray (10), and examine more thoroughly those sites that might contain tumor cells (24, 25).

Radioimmunoguided surgery is efficacious in localizing previously undetected malignant lesions and disseminated disease intraoperatively, and is especially effective in localizing primary and secondary colorectal, gastric, and ovarian carcinomas (6, 24, 39, 42). Although this technique is still in its infancy, it offers great promise for the future.

Surgical Oncology as a Specialty

What is a surgical oncologist (37)? Surgical oncologists are surgeons who devote most of their time to the study and treatment of malignant neoplastic disease. They must possess the necessary knowledge, skills, and clinical experience to perform the standard surgical procedures required by patients with cancer. Surgical oncologists must be able to diagnose all tumors accurately and to differentiate aggressive neoplastic lesions and benign reactive processes. In addition, surgical oncologists should have a firm understanding of radiation oncology, medical oncology, and hematology. They must also be capable of organizing interdisciplinary studies of cancer. Surgical oncologists should be trained in pathology as well, since they will be called on to decide surgical margins and to excise adequate tumor samples for pathologists.

Unfortunately, the Accreditation Council for Graduate Medical Education (ACGME) has not yet granted subspecialty status to surgical oncology. This inaction has retarded growth in the field and, consequently, delayed progress in the treatment of solid neoplasms by surgical therapy. There is a great need for a larger number of trained surgical oncologists who will commit to comprehensive cancer research centers and will work together with other oncologists in multidisciplinary studies of combined modality treatment programs. The full potential of surgical oncology cannot be realized without more trained surgical oncologists and ACGME recognition of subspecialty status.

References

1. Antman KA, Eilber FR, Shiu MH. Soft tissue sarcomas: current trends in diagnosis and management. Curr Prob Cancer 1989;13:339.
2. Arnold MW, Schneebaum S, Berens A, Petty L, Mojzisik C, Hinkle G, Martin EW Jr. Intraoperative detection of colorectal cancer with radioimmunoguided surgery and CC49, a second-generation monoclonal antibody. Ann Surg 1992;216:627.
3. Antman KH. G-CSF and GM-CSF in clinical trials. Yale J Biol Med 1990;63:387.
4. Beahrs OH, Henson DE, Hutter RVP, Kennedy BJ. Manual for Staging of Cancer, 4th ed. Published for the American Joint Committee on Cancer. Philadelphia: Lippincott, 1992.
5. Breasted JH. The Edwin Smith Surgical Papyrus. Chicago: University of Chicago Press, 1930.
6. Burak WE Jr, Schneebaum S, Kim JA, Arnold MW, et al. Pilot study evaluating the intraoperative localization of radiolabeled monoclonal antibody CC83 in patients with metastatic colorectal carcinoma. Surgery 1995;118:103.
7. Chretian PB, Catalona WG, Twomey PL, Sample WF. Correlation of immune reactivity and clinical status in cancer. Ann Clin Lab Sci 1974;4:331.
8. Cole WH, McDonald GO, Roberts SS, Southwick HW. Dissemination of cancer. Prevention and therapy. New York: Appleton-Century-Crofts, 1961.
9. Collins VP, Loeffler RK, Tivey H. Observations on growth rates of human tumors. Am J Roentgenol 1956;76:988.
10. Di Carlo V, Badellino F, Stella M, De Nardi P, et al. Role of B72.3 iodine 125-labeled monoclonal antibody in colorectal cancer detection by radioimmunoguided surgery. Surgery 1994;115:190.
11. De Boeck H, Casteleyn PP, Bossuyt A, Jacobs A. Intraoperative radioactive localization of small bone tumours. Int Orthop 1992;16:172.

12. Eilber FR, Nizze A, Morton DL. Sequential evaluation of general immune competence in cancer patients: correlation with clinical course. Cancer 1975;35:660.
13. Ellis ED, Moormeier JA, Golomb HM. The treatment of hairy cell leukemia: a review. Leuk Lymphoma 1990;1:77.
14. Giuliano AE, Kirgan DM, Guenther JM, Morton DL. Lymphatic mapping and sentinel lymphadenectomy for breast cancer. Ann Surg 1994;220:391.
15. Golub SH. Host Immune Response to Human Tumor Antigens. New York: Plenum, 1976.
16. Gupta RK, Morton DL. Suggestive evidence for in vivo binding of specific antitumor antibodies of human melanomas. Cancer Res 1975;35:58.
17. Hayward OS. The history of oncology. I. Early oncology and the literature of discovery. Surgery 1965;58:460.
18. Hellstrom KE, Hellstrom I. Lymphocyte mediated cytotoxicity to tumor antigens. Adv Immunol 1974;18:209.
19. Hill GJ, 2nd. Historic milestones in cancer surgery. Semin Oncol 1979;6:409.
20. Holmes EC, Golub SH. Immunologic defects in lung cancer patients. J Thorac Cardiovasc Surg 1976;71:161.
21. Holmes EC, Roth JA, Morton DL. Delayed cutaneous hypersensitivity reactions to melanoma antigen. Surgery 1975;78:160.
22. Huth JF, Holmes EC, Vernon SE, Callery CD, Ramming KP, Morton DL. Pulmonary resection for metastatic sarcoma. Am J Surg 1980;140:90.
23. Joseph WJ, Morton DL, Adkins PC. Prognostic significance of tumor doubling time in evaluating operability in pulmonary metastatic disease. J Thorac Cardiovasc Surg 1971;61:23.
24. Kim JA, Triozzi PL, Martin EW, Jr. Radioimmunoguided surgery for colorectal cancer. Oncology 1993;7:55.
25. Krag DN, Meijer SJ, Weaver DL, Loggie BW, Harlow SP, Tanabe KK, Laughlin EH, Alex JC. Minimal-access surgery for staging of malignant melanoma. Arch Surg 1995;130: 654.
26. Levenback C, Burke TW, Gershenson DM, Morris M, et al. Intraoperative lymphatic mapping for vulvar cancer. Obstet Gynecol 1994;84:163.
27. Martin EW Jr, Mojzisik CM, Hinckle GH, Sampsel J, Siddigi MA, Tuttle SE, Sidele-Santanello B, Colchen D, Thurston MO, Bell JG, Ferrara WB, Schlom J. Radioimmunoguided surgery using monoclonal antibody. Am J Surg 1988;156:396.
28. Morton DL, Foshag LJ, Hoon DSB, Nizze JA, Famatiga E, Wanek LA, Chang C, Davtyan DG, Gupta RK, Elashoff R, Irie RF. Prolongation of survival in metastatic melanoma after active specific immunotherapy with a new polyvalent melanoma vaccine. Ann Surg 1992;216:463.
29. Morton DL, Holmes EC, Eilber FR, Wood WC. Immunological aspects of neoplasia: a rational basis for immunotherapy. Ann Intern Med 1971;74:587.
30. Morton DL, Holmes EC, Golub SH. Immunologic aspects of lung cancer. Chest 1977;71:640.
31. Morton DL, Joseph WL, Ketcham AS, Geelhoed GW, Adkins PC. Surgical resection and adjunctive immmunotherapy for selected patients with multiple pulmonary metastases. Ann Surg 1973;178:360.
32. Morton DL, Wen, D-R, Wong JH, Economou JS, Cagle LA, Storm FK, Foshag LJ, Cochran AJ. Technical details of intraoperative lymphatic mapping for early stage melanoma. Arch Surg 1992;127:392.
33. Nieroda CA, Mojzsik C, Sardi A, Ferrara P, Hinckle GR, Thurston MD, Martin EW Jr. The impact of radioimmunoguided surgery (RIGS) on surgical decision making in colorectal cancer. Dis Col Rect 1989;32:927.
34. Peters WP, Kurtzberg J, Atwater S, Borowitz M, Gilbert C, Rao M, Currie M, Shogan J, Jones RB, Shpall EJ, Souza L. Comparative effects of rHuG-CSF and rHuGM-CSF on hematopoietic reconstitution and granulocyte function following high dose chemotherapy and autologous bone marrow transplantation (ABMT). Blood 1988;71:130a.
35. Roberts SS, Hengesh JW, McGrath RG, Valaitis J, McGrew EA, Cole WH. Prognostic significance of cancer cells in circulating blood: a ten-year evaluation. Am J Surg 1967;113:757.
36. Schlom J. Radiolocalization of human mammary tumors in athymic mice by monoclonal antibody. Cancer Res 1983;43:736.
37. Schweitzer RJ, Edwards MH, Lawrence W Jr., Mozden PJ, Scanlon EF, Leffal LD Jr. Training guidelines for surgical oncology. Cancer 1981;48:2336.
38. Southam CM, Brunschwig W, Levin AG, Dixon QS. The effect of leukocytes on transplantability of human cancer. Cancer 1966;19:1743.
39. Surwit EA, Childers JM, Krag DN, Katterhagen, JG, et al. Clinical assessment of ^{111}In-CYT-103 immunoscintigraphy in ovarian cancer. Gynecol Oncol 1993;48:283.
40. Turnbull RB, Jr. The no-touch isolation techniques of resection. JAMA 1975;231:1181.
41. Van der Veen H, Hoekstra OS, Paul MA, Cuesta MA, Meijer S. Gamma probe-guided sentinel node biopsy to select patients with melanoma for lymphadenectomy. Br J Surg 1994;81:1769.
42. Xu G, Zhang M, Liu B, Li Z, Lin B, Xu X, Jin M, Li J, Wu J, Dong Z. Radioimmunoguided surgery in gastric cancer using 131-I labeled monoclonal antibody ^{3}H11. Semin Surg Oncol 1994;10:88.

CHAPTER 46

Vascular Access in Cancer Patients

MICHAIL SHAFIR

Introduction

The management of patients with cancer has evolved rapidly in the second half of this century. Extensive surgical procedures have become safer and easier to undertake mainly due to increase in knowledge and applications of supportive treatment. Central vessels have been cannulated for monitoring of physiologic parameters and delivery of medications, fluids, blood products, and nutrition. The rapid expansion of chemotherapy stimulated research in venous access. The development of total parenteral nutrition also contributed significantly to the search for and development of better and easier access to the central veins. Before 1970, the most commonly used catheters were made of semirigid materials, such as polyvinyl chloride, and were introduced through a cutdown of the cephalic or basilic veins or through subclavian punctures. These catheters were not "tunnelized" and had to be removed after no more than 1 week because of risk of infection and thrombosis. In 1973, Broviac pioneered the use of a barium-impregnated silicone-rubber catheter to be inserted in the right atrium through a subcutaneous tunnel for prolonged parenteral hyperalimentation (1). This technique revolutionized long-term central venous access, as this catheter proved to be less thrombogenic. The segment of catheter in the subcutaneous tunnel between the skin exit site and venous insertion site contains a Dacron cuff that allows fibroblastic ingrowth from the surrounding fat, thus blocking free passage from the skin along the entry path of the catheter to the deeper tissues, decreasing the risk of infection. These two characteristics allow the catheter to remain in the central venous system for prolonged intervals, sometimes years. The first modification to the Broviac catheter was introduced by Hickman, who developed a larger internal diameter catheter, allowing higher infusion flows, for bone marrow transplant patients (2). Shortly thereafter we reported the simultaneous use of two catheters of different length, to allow synchronous access for hyperalimentation through one dedicated line and administration of other fluids and medications through the second line (3) (Fig. 46.1). The next advance occurred with the introduction of double and triple lumen catheters contained in one sheath but with separate external ports. Thus, multiple medications, solutions, and blood products may be administered simultaneously without risking precipitation in the lumina of the catheter.

Subsequently, a totally implantable system was developed in which a catheter similar to the Broviac/Hickman was connected to a reservoir that is positioned in continuity in a subcutaneous pocket. Such devices must be accessed through a noncoring needle; thus, they do not easily permit as high flow infusions as do the external catheters. However, they clearly demonstrate the advantage of a system that has no external component, and, once the incisions are healed, they are aesthetically more appealing. Niederhuber reported the initial series, demonstrating the practicality of this technique in cancer patients (4). More recently, double lumen catheter port systems have been developed with the catheter tips in close vicinity or staggered 3 cm apart in order to allow continuous infusion through both lumina, minimizing contact between solutions.

A larger double-lumen catheter (Permcath), initially intended for hemodialysis, has found its application in oncology. This is a more rigid staggered-tipped double lumen external device that allows high flow as part of a cytapheresis apparatus. It has become very useful for peripheral stem cell collection prior to chemotherapy and for cytapheresis in hematologic malignancies.

Lastly, thinner polyurethane catheters attached to a small port (P.A.S.-PORT) have been utilized. These catheters can be placed through basilic or cephalic veins and tracked with an electromagnetic unit, thus avoiding fluoroscopy during insertion and permitting the placement at the bedside or the office/clinic (5). An external version without a port has been incorporated more recently (PiccCatheter); it represents a new variety of semirigid, less thrombogenic central catheter that can be placed through a peripheral vein and may be

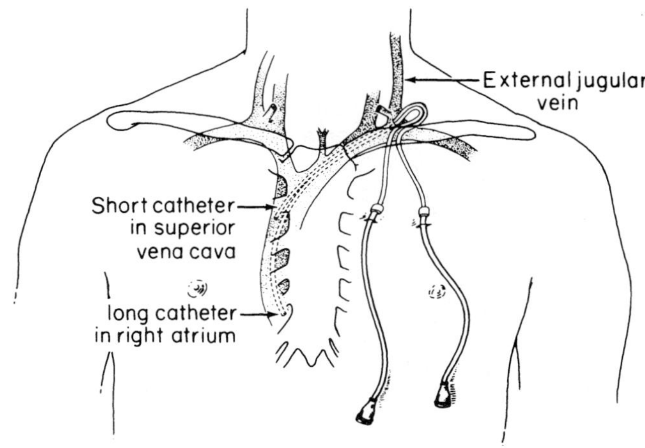

Figure 46.1. Schema of position of catheter tip.

useful for patients who require short- or medium-term central venous access, or for patients in whom a surgical implantation of a port is particularly difficult (e.g., massive chest wall tumor, tracheostomy).

Indications for Central Venous Access in Oncology

Several factors must be considered before the cancer patient receives a central venous access device. If a major surgical procedure is contemplated, a percutaneously placed, short term catheter with one, two or three lumina is indicated. Such a catheter permits rapid fluid resuscitation, blood and blood products transfusion, and multiple medications, as well as the monitoring of central venous pressure during surgery. Postoperatively, all fluids can be administered through this catheter, avoiding the need for multiple peripheral venous punctures.

In the nonsurgical context, the patient's age and type of cancer influences which catheter is preferable. Pediatric patients tend to tolerate an external catheter better than a port. In a child, the aesthetics of an external catheter is not usually an important problem, but the repeated needle puncture of a subcutaneous port might become unbearable. A child may inadvertently pull on an external catheter and accidentally remove it or mechanically disrupt it. Consequently, in a child it is important to make the tunnel sufficiently long and to secure the catheter to the skin at the exit site adequately, to avoid dislodgment or breakage.

In the adult patient, several questions must be asked before determining the type of catheter to be used. (*a*) Does the patient have a severe hematologic malignancy (e.g., acute leukemia)? If so, this patient will require at least a double lumen catheter, preferably of external type, since the treatment will necessitate multiple simultaneous venous access for drugs, fluids, and transfusions of blood and blood products. (*b*) Does the patient require only intermittent central venous access (e.g., for adjuvant chemotherapy of breast or colon cancer)? If so, a totally implanted port catheter system is preferable, since such a device is easier to care for, is aesthetically more appealing, and requires use for short, small volume infusions. (*c*) Does the patient require peripheral cell harvesting and/or bone marrow transplantation and intensive chemotherapy (e.g., for stage IV breast cancer, recurring after prior treatment)? Such a patient will benefit from a larger, double lumen, hemodialysis-type catheter (Permcath) because this catheter allows blood withdrawal at a rapid rate for cytapheresis and rapid infusion of large volumes of fluids if necessary. (*d*) Does the patient require long-term access for opiates for palliation of terminal disease? In this clinical situation, any type of catheter may be used, and the decision is made based on individual circumstances. For instance, if the patient will be cared for at home, an external catheter may be easier, as a relative can be taught to manage the catheter. If the patient is to be cared for in a nursing home or a hospice, any catheter is acceptable, including a thin one placed in the upper extremity vein, with or without a small subcutaneous port (P.A.S.-PORT or Picc).

A particular indication for a long-term access in a patient with adequate peripheral veins, is the anticipated use of doxorubicin because of major damage that can occur in the peripheral veins, or worse, to the surrounding tissues if the drug is extravasated.

In patients with fat arms it is difficult to obtain access to peripheral veins, and such patients should have a central line placed early in the course of treatment.

For patients with "needle phobia," an external catheter may be the ideal access, as no further skin punctures will be necessary. An implanted port can also be a successful alternative when extensive denervation of the skin around the port pocket is performed, thus allowing an almost painless access of the port with a noncoring needle. This technique is advantageous, and patients have minimal discomfort in the hypesthetic area.

When continuous infusion of chemotherapy with a portable pump is indicated, long-term access is ideal, allowing for freedom of the upper extremities that would otherwise be the site of angiocaths.

Techniques for Placement of Central Venous Access Catheters

A variety of approaches are possible, and the decision must be made based on the patient's age, loco-regional pathology at the prospective catheter site, patient's general medical condition [e.g., ability to tolerate transportation to an operating room, to tolerate IV sedation and/or general anesthesia if necessary (particularly in the pediatric patient), patient's preference and surgeon's preference of different techniques].

Some catheters may be placed safely at the bedside or in the office without requiring an operating room. An example is the young patient in excellent general condition and performance status, whose antecubital veins have not been used repeatedly and who requires intermittent small volume chemotherapy administration; a P.A.S.-PORT® or a Picc can be safely placed in such a patient. Also, a hospitalized patient who requires a central line for a short period may have a Picc line placed at the bedside.

All other catheters and ports should be placed in the operating room. The standard approach is by cutdown of an adequately sized vein in relation to the size of the catheter. For single and double lumen catheters, less than 9 French in diameter, the cephalic vein in the deltopectoral groove or the external jugular vein are usually used successfully. If a larger catheter (e.g., Permcat® or double lumen port system) is to be employed, a larger vein, such as the internal jugular may need to be accessed (Fig. 46.2). The surgical cutdown of these veins is possible under local anesthesia and requires only a short incision (6). The catheter exit site or the port pocket location is placed on the anterior chest wall in a position comfortable for the patient (e.g., where the chest wall is flat and where the catheter or the port pocket does not interfere with clothing). For the female patient, it is particularly important to avoid the line of the brassiere straps and to allow the catheter or the port to be covered by the brassiere,

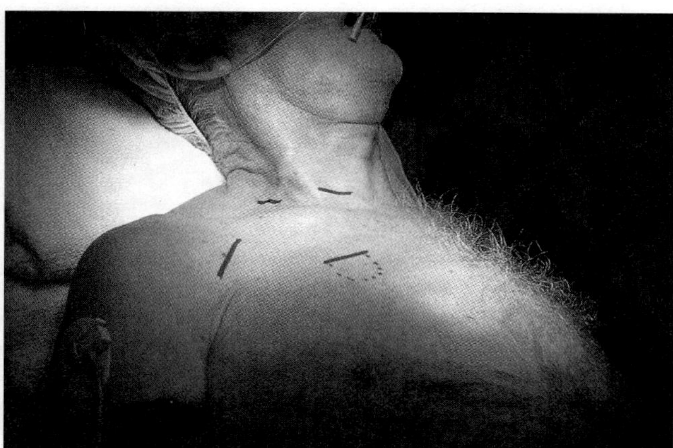

Figure 46.2. Sites of incisions for approach of cephalic, external and internal jugular veins. On anterior chest wall, the site for a port reservoir or exit site and for external catheter is marked.

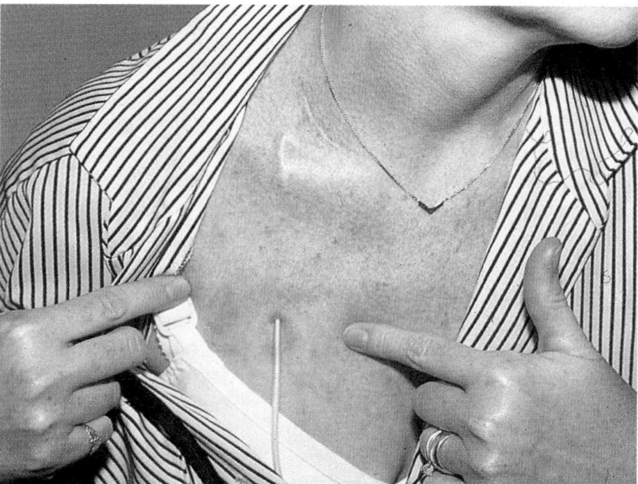

Figure 46.3. Well healed, properly maintained Hickman catheter in right atrium through right external jugular vein.

to permit the use of open collared blouses or dresses (Fig.46.3). This technique is safe and in the experience of this author has never been complicated by hemothorax or pneumothorax.

An alternative technique, much in vogue lately, is to place the catheter in the subclavian vein through a percutaneous puncture, followed by a Seldinger technique, dilating the site over a guide wire and inserting the catheter through a peel-away sheath (7). This technique still requires a second incision for the placement of the port or for the exit site of the catheter; the incidence of hemothorax and/or pneumothorax following this approach is 1–3%. Vascular injury can also occur with the wire, leading to fatal complications (8). Pneumothorax has been reported in 6% of all central venous catheterizations, representing 30% of all catheterization complications (9, 10). Cases of delayed pneumothorax have been reported, emphasizing the need for close monitoring of the patient after a subclavian approach (11). It appears that this technique is indicated primarily when access through the other veins is not possible.

For breast cancer patients who have undergone modified radical mastectomy or partial mastectomy with axillary dissection, it is preferable to access the contralateral side to decrease the risk of edema of the upper extremity if thrombosis should occur.

If a patient has had many prior venous accesses in the upper trunk and neck, or if there are mechanical difficulties secondary to cervical/mediastinal tumors, tracheostomy, massive chest wall tumors, or marked fibrosis secondary to radiation, it may be necessary to approach the inferior vena cava for access. The simplest route is through a saphenous vein cutdown or a femoral vein percutaneous Seldinger technique; the drawback of such an approach is that if thrombosis of the inferior vena cava occurs, significant edema of the lower extremities results. Moreover, the inguinal-femoral area is more difficult to maintain sterile and the incidence of infection is higher (12). Consequently, this anatomic route should be used only when there is no better alternative. Patients who have undergone repeated catheterizations and who may also present with extensive loco-regional tumors that render use of the more common veins impractical may need to be approached through less accessible veins such as the azygos, or intercostals (13).Central approaches directly into the superior vena cava or the right atrium have been described (14). These very invasive techniques have limited applications; they should be considered at the time of thoracotomy for the primary tumor. Other approaches, such as of the inferior epigastric (15), gonadal (16), or lumbar veins (17), have been described, as well as direct catheterization of the inferior vena cava when all other veins are not utilizable (18). All these techniques are clearly more invasive than the more conventional techniques and should be reserved for selected patients in whom the benefit of such a procedure clearly outweighs the risks and complications. For urgent blood and short time infusion needs, in the absence of venous access, a marrow needle may be placed in the iliac or sternal marrow in adults, or the proximal tibia in children.

Complications of Long-term Central Venous Access

Complications related to these foreign bodies implanted for variable periods of time are of a mechanical and/or infectious nature. Because a central venous catheter floats freely in a large vein, thrombosis around the catheter can occur as a result of inflammatory reaction. When thrombosis takes place, secondary infection can easily start. Intraluminal occlusion of the catheter can occur due to thrombosis, IV solution precipitate or inadequate flow. It follows that the nursing care of central venous access devices is of paramount importance; insufficient flow through the catheter, incompatible drug admixture, excessively thick fluid administration (e.g., lipids, undiluted packed cells), or interruption of flow through the catheter may lead to occlusion, which invites a cascade of complications. Major right atrial thrombosis and pulmonary emboli have been reported in patients receiving long-term total parenteral nutrition (19).

Other mechanical complications may occur due to the length and flexibility of the catheter; the tip may become displaced and, secondary to pressure changes in the mediastinum, the catheter tip may "flip" outside of the right atrium or superior vena cava into the contralateral subclavian or internal jugular vein. On occasion, the catheter tip intimately apposes itself to the wall of the superior vena cava, producing withdrawal occlusion, a situation in which infusion is possible but no blood can be withdrawn; this problem can also occur if a fibrin sheath forms around the tip of the catheter, occluding the tip when suction is applied. Withdrawal occlusion is not infrequent and can often be managed by positioning the patient in Trendelenburg and/or attempting blood withdrawal during deep inspiration and other positional changes (elevation of arms, lateral decubitus) to attempt mobilization of the tip of the catheter. Extravasation can occur secondary to thrombosis (Fig 46.4). If the catheter tip lies in the upper half of the superior vena cava, rather than in its distal portion or in the right atrium, the risk of thrombosis is much higher (20). A rare complication of catheter fracture and embolization during strenuous exercise has been reported (21).

Significant bleeding may occur during implantation of a central venous device in thrombocytopenic patients. It is essential to transfuse platelets pre- and intraoperatively in such patients, to maintain adequate local hemostasis. If necessary, vitamin K and fresh-frozen plasma are to be administered perioperatively to normalize coagulation parameters.

Catheter related sepsis is a common occurrence in the cancer patient, in whom immunodepression and bacteremia are often present after therapy. Infections are either (*a*) primary in the catheter or its surgical implantation area, occurring perioperatively or at a later date due to contamination, or (*b*) secondary to infection in other areas of the body with bacteremia and subsequent seeding of the catheter.

Primary infection of the catheter site(s) is usually easy to diagnose; there is new onset of pain and/or erythema, increase of skin temperature, and swelling of the catheter area (these are cardinal signs of any infection: "calor-rubor-dolor-tumor"). There may be serous or purulent discharge around the subcutaneous tunnel exit site or the port (Fig. 46.5). *Staphylococcus epidermidis* is the most frequent organism of these primary infections (22), although more virulent pathogens such as *staphylococcus aureus* can also be responsible (23).

If the external catheter site infection extends to the IV portion of the catheter, or if there is "seeding" of this portion by bacteria originating at a distant focus, a potentially much more serious clinical picture arises. Long-term catheters are often surrounded by a fibrinous, reactive sheath, or by a wide non-occluding thrombus. These structures are a fertile ground for bacterial proliferation (24, 25); if this phenomenon occurs, the clinical picture and management will be different. An infected device can give origin to disseminated foci of infection (26). Internal port systems have been reported to be five times less frequently infected than external catheters (27).

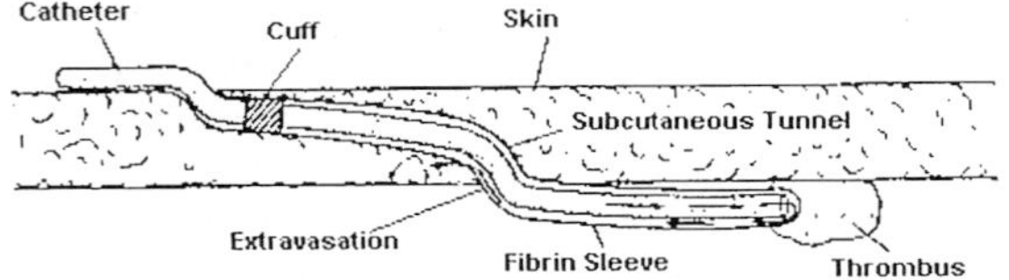

Figure 46.4. Schema of thrombus related extravasation.

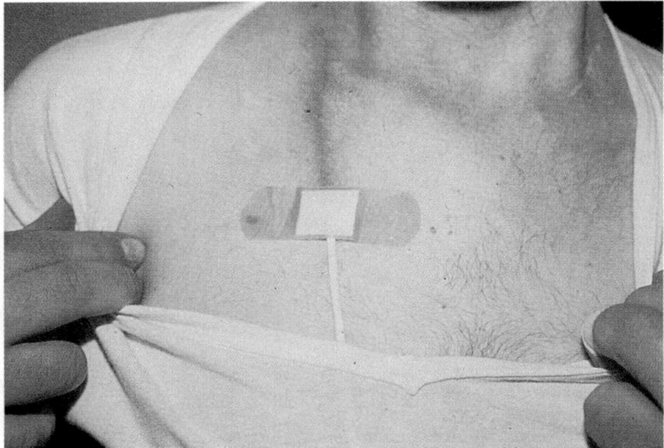
Figure 46.5. Tunnel infection with external catheter.

The differential diagnosis of fever in the patient with a central catheter requires blood cultures through the catheter and from a peripheral vein. If the catheter is the source of infection, there will be a more than 5-fold increase of bacterial colonies from the catheter blood compared to the peripheral one (28). In the absence of these bacteriologic counts, clinical suspicion of catheter-line infection is provided by chills and fever spikes associated with flushing the catheter or infusing medications through it. Catheter sepsis should always be considered when entertaining the diagnosis of drug fever.

Prevention of Complications

Adequate surgical techniques and care of the operative areas and the catheter are of paramount importance in the long-term success of these devices. Placement of central venous catheters must be performed aseptically, whether in the operating room or at the bedside. The patient's hygiene is also important, since it is possible to minimize bacterial contamination. It is difficult to sterilize the operative field in a few seconds; patients should wash with bactericidal soap preoperatively and after implantation of the access device.

Surgical technique must be meticulous and painstaking hemostasis accomplished; if a hematoma should develop, the risk of infection with the foreign body is high. The placement of the catheter in the subcutaneous tunnel must be sufficiently deep in order to avoid skin compression and possible necrosis with catheter extrusion (Fig. 46.6). A deep position of the catheter in the subcutaneous fat also prevents trauma to it and makes it less visible, thus more aesthetically

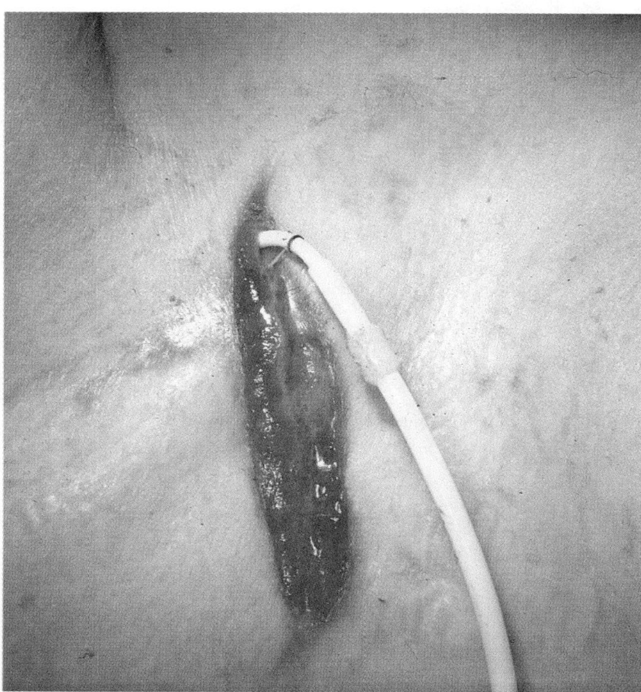

Figure 46.6. Extruded Broviac catheter after pressure necrosis of skin overlying the catheter.

appealing. If a port is placed, the flap of skin overlying it must be of sufficiently homogeneous thickness to permit easy palpation and access. Once the catheter is placed, a chest film or fluoroscopy is essential, to confirm good central positioning. Ideally, the catheter should be in the distal superior vena cava or the right atrium. This position allows for the tip of the catheter to float in a high-flow wide area and minimizes the chances of thrombosis around it. A lower extremity catheter should have its tip in the distal inferior vena cava. Immediately after placement, the catheter should be flushed with 10–20 mL of normal saline to clear it of small amounts of blood. The entire catheter and/or port systems are then filled immediately with heparin. The concentration of heparin varies in different protocols. It seems important to use concentrated heparin (i.e., 1000 or 5000 U/mL) in a volume equal to the capacity of the system in use; this avoids excess heparin in the systemic circulation and allows impregnation or adhesion of heparin to the catheter wall, which reduces the risk of intraluminal thrombosis (29). Every time the catheter is to be used, the heparin must be withdrawn and discarded. When the catheter is utilized for prolonged periods of time, a small dose of heparin can be incorporated in the solution (i.e., in total parenteral nutrition) to reduce thrombosis (30). An alternative method to minimize thrombosis is the daily administration of low dose warfarin (i.e., 1 mg/day), which has been reported to decrease significantly the number of symptomatic thromboses without altering the systemic coagulation parameters (31).

The prevention of infection is critical in the management of these devices. Continuous, reiterative education at all levels is essential. All physicians, nurses, patients, and relatives who may at any time be involved with use of the venous access device must know all aspects of care: strict aseptic technique in dressing, changes of needles, connection of IV solutions, flushing, and changes of caps. Totally occlusive dressings around the exit site of external catheters and around the port when it is accessed are mandatory to decrease external contamination. Transparent sterile dressings have become popular as they allow continuous inspection of the site and create a totally occlusive dressing by self-adhesion in the shape of a mesentery around the catheter or the Huber needle tubing (Fig. 46.7). General medical, nursing, and mechanical common sense is essential. All external tubing, whether permanent or temporary during treatments, must be strongly secured by tape (with redundant loops) to avoid accidental dislodgment, trauma, or traction. It is preferable that the patient does not lie on the side of the accessed vein with the extremity bent since this can impair flow and may increase the incidence of thrombosis. When the catheter is not in use and the patient takes a bath, shower or swims, it is important to change the dressing around the exit site of an external catheter and to maintain the skin overlying a port totally clean.

A common complication is nonthrombotic occlusion of the catheter due to mixtures of incompatible solutions or medications. It is important to avoid concomitant infusions of solutions that are possibly incompatible, even through separate lumina of the catheter, unless their tips are staggered to allow dilution by the flowing blood. If tips are conterminous, precipitation may occur (Fig 46.8).

When a vesicant solution is to be administered, a rapid infusion of normal saline should be given initially to assure that there is no extravasation or resistance to the flow. Then, it is sound practice to administer the drug through a side port ("piggyback"). If a subcutaneous extravasation occurs, severe necrosis can ensue with consequent loss of the device and major morbidity.

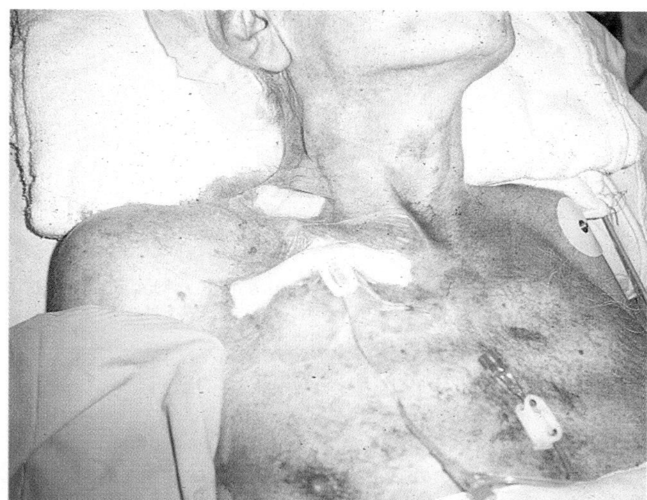

Figure 46.7. Double-lumen Port-A-Cath with transparent dressing, one port accessed with Huber-gripper needle.

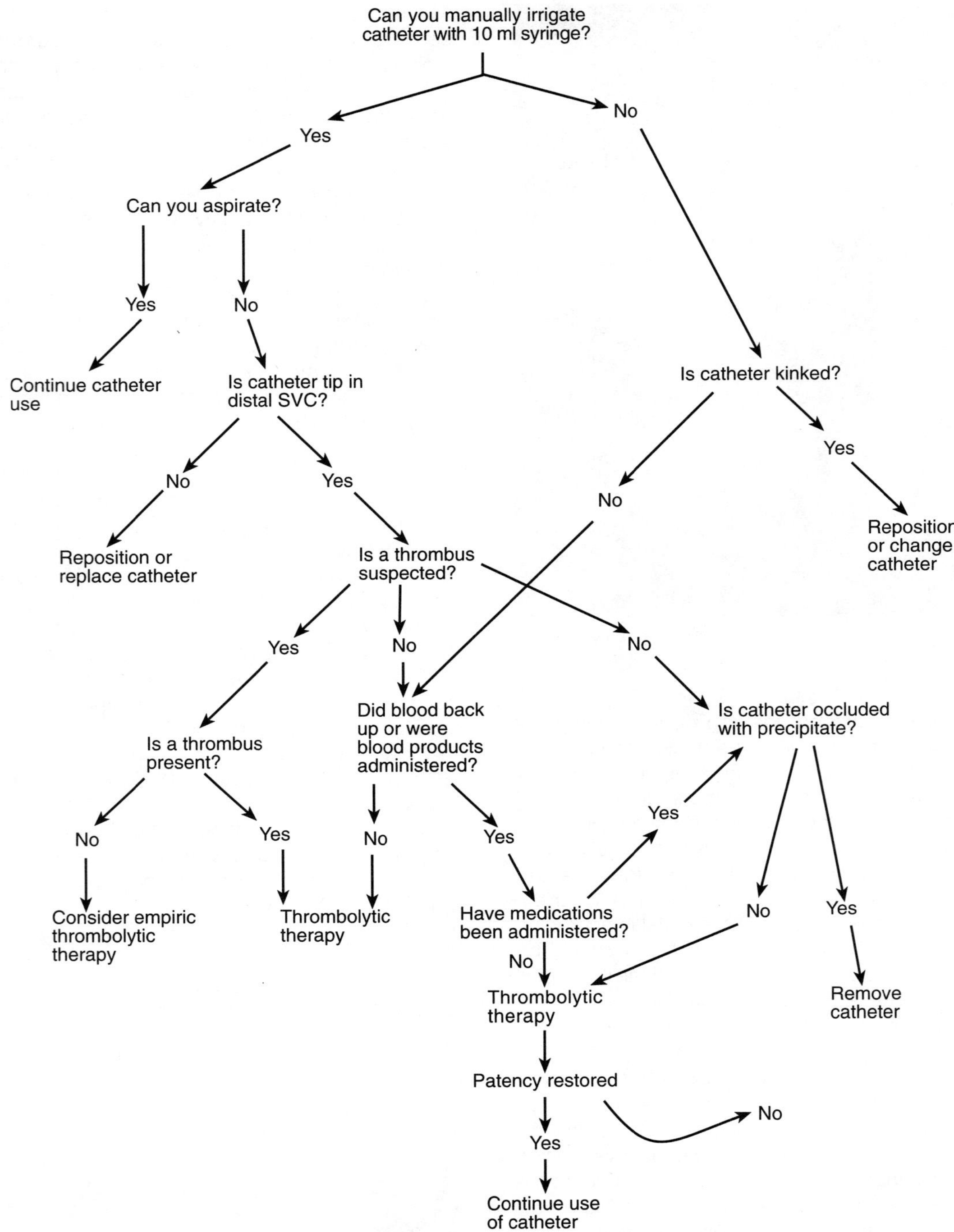

Figure 46.8. Management of malfunctioning central access devices.

Treatment of Complications

The nature of a complication determines the treatment. Thrombosis of the catheter lumen is a common occurrence most frequently due to interruption of infusion for more than 1 min or with a slow infusion of a thick solution. If the diagnosis is made promptly, intermittent withdrawal and injection of normal saline may be successful. If thrombosis is established within the catheter lumen, concentrated heparin may be useful but usually is not. Thrombolytic agents such as urokinase can be successful: 1 or 2 mL of 5,000/U can be gently injected into the port or catheter and left in situ for 20 or 30 min. Frequently, a relatively recent clot will dissolve and catheter patency can be restored. If unsuccessful, a second dose may be given and left for 12 to 24 h before attempting catheter use. The majority of catheters become patent with this treatment (32–34). The algorithm in Figure 46.8 guides the management of an occluded device.

A more serious complication occurs when a major vein

thromboses around the catheter. High percentages of subclavian vein thromboses have been reported (35), but the majority remain asymptomatic unless pulmonary emboli occur. Diagnostic tests are helpful in patients who develop edema of the arm and shoulder, pain along the axillary-subclavian vein, and collateral circulation. The most precise test is a venogram through a distal peripheral vein (not through the catheter, since the thrombosis can spare the distal catheter) (36). Duplex Doppler studies, magnetic resonance imaging, nuclear angiography, and sometimes computed tomographic studies can assist in establishing the extent of thrombosis (37).

Once the diagnosis of major venous thrombosis is established in the symptomatic patient, several therapeutic options exist. The safest standard approach is to remove the catheter, after which the flow may be reestablished through the catheter channel. Anticoagulation will diminish spread of the thrombosis and allow spontaneous lysis at the periphery of the thrombosed segment (38). In an attempt to salvage the catheter, particularly in patients with difficult access, treatment with arm elevation and anticoagulation without removal of the catheter has been reported as successful (39). The successful use of urokinase in a peripheral vein infusion has also been reported (40) but the risk of hemorrhage may not justify its use. Streptokinase and recombinant plasminogen activator are of known value for other intravascular thromboses. Thrombolytic therapy benefits must be evaluated for each patient.

By far the most severe complications are of infectious nature. A frequent occurrence is an exit site infection usually due to *Staphylococcus epidermidis*, for which local care and antibiotics are usually successful, conserving the catheter in situ (41). If the infection is due to *Staphylococcus aureus*, the catheter must be removed because of the virulence of this organism (23).

Tunnel or port-pocket "cellulitis-like" infection without overt purulent contents may be treated with IV antibiotics and local care (Fig. 46.5). If no improvement is seen within 1 or 2 days, however, or if systemic symptoms develop, the catheter must be removed. On occasion, debridement of the area may become necessary. Of all the catheter-related sepsis, the most difficult to manage is of fungal origin, particularly in children (42). It is unusual to manage successfully a patient with a fungus-contaminated catheter without removing it, in addition to using antifungal antibiotics such as Amphotericin B. Prophylactic antifungal treatment is not usually justified, however. When a catheter has been removed as a source of sepsis, it is advisable to treat the patient with antibiotics for several days until blood cultures become negative and all signs and symptoms disappear. Many of these patients, however, have poor venous peripheral access; it is important to maintain only a temporary peripheral or central access until, after sepsis is cured, a new long-term access can be placed.

Results of Long-term Central Venous Catheters in Cancer Patients

The ideal result is represented by a patient who has a correctly placed catheter, properly managed by patient and staff, that stays functional for the entire length of time required, allows blood samples to be drawn, medications and solutions administered through it, without thrombosis or infection occurring. How often does this happen?

Many series report different complications that highlight the difficulties in maintaining ideal central venous access. The first important comparison is between external catheters and ports. A randomized trial of 100 patients with solid tumors found a significantly higher removal rate for external catheters versus ports (20 versus 4%). Infection rates were significantly lower in port patients (12 versus 2.5%) (43). Other retrospective studies tend to confirm the concept that implanted ports are less prone to infection than are external catheters, (44, 45). In children, a prospective study of 144 ports versus 130 external catheters also found superior performance of implanted ports compared to external catheters (46).

This author's initial personal experience with external catheters in 169 patients (182 catheterizations) for hematologic malignancies and solid tumors, in which all catheters were placed by surgical incisions and all were subject to meticulous postoperative care, revealed 10 infections (5.9%) and 6 thromboses (3.5%). Thirteen catheters required replacement secondary to infection and/or catheter occlusion. This emphasizes the safety of external catheters provided there is optimal long-term care (47) (Table 46.1).

In the past $4\frac{1}{2}$ years, 296 central venous access devices have been implanted by the author and surgical residents under his direct supervision (Table 46.2). Wide acceptance

Table 46.1. Initial Experience of One Surgeon with External Long-term Central Venous Catheters

Patients	169
Females	98
Males	71
Age range	12–82
Catheters	
Total	182
Broviac	146
Hickman	36
Diagnoses	
Leukemia	54
Lymphoma	20
Gastrointestinal cancers	24
Gynecologic cancers	14
Head and neck cancers	8
Miscellaneous	19
Site of Venous Access	
External jugular vein	161
Cephalic vein	18
Internal jugular vein	3
Complications	
Infections	10
Thromboses	5
Hematomas at operative site	2
Mechanical disruption of catheter	7
Follow-up (mean, 6 months)	
Functioning	89
Removed	16
Infections	8
End of treatments	8
Died with functioning catheters	77

From Shafir and Hoffman (47).

Table 46.2. Consecutive Central Venous Devices by One Surgeon in 54 Months

Patients	296
Outpatient	119
Inpatient	117
Catheter	
Portacath (single lumen)	187
Portacath (double lumen)	19
Pas-port	6
Broviac/Hickman	16
Double-lumen Hickman	27
Triple-lumen Hickman	11
Permcath	30
Complications requiring removal	26–8.6%
Occlusion	6–2%
Thrombosis	10–3.3%
Infection	10–3.3%

Shafir M., unpublished data.

of the safety and convenience of these devices has led to their increasing use in women undergoing adjuvant treatment for breast cancer, particularly if vasotoxic and histotoxic drugs are to be used.

The quality of life for patients has improved significantly, since these devices allow avoidance of repeated peripheral venous punctures. In one study, the patient's satisfaction was particularly notable with implanted ports (48). Avoidance of occlusion of catheters has been reported by the use of double lumen devices for administration of fluorouracil and leucovorin, a common regimen in gastrointestinal cancer (49).

Nonmetallic ports were evaluated in one study of 78 patients with 369 treatment cycles and a total of 1370 infusion days; there were no infections and 87% of long-term function (50). Successful urokinase and antibiotics, when needed, maintained 94.9% of catheters functional in a prospective study of 177 pediatric oncology patients (51).

The National Cancer Institute's experience with catheter related fungemia in 155 cancer patients has been reported. Of patients treated only with antifungal therapy, 82% had a poor outcome, suggesting that catheters should be removed early in the course of fungal infection (52). The experience of the University of Maryland Cancer Center with 690 external (Hickman) catheters between 1978 and 1987 reported a total of 134,273 catheter days (53). There were 438 noninfectious complications and 603 infections, the majority at the exit site. Infections and bacteremias were treated effectively without removing the catheter.

Conclusion

Long-term central venous catheterization in cancer patients has become an important aspect of the management and treatment. The use of the different devices can be systematized and adapted to the needs of the individual patient. Adequate care of the catheter and patient education are essential factors in successful longevity of the catheter; in patients with small veins, fat arms, or venous thrombosis from prior chemotherapy, the improved quality of life related to the expediency of access to the blood stream cannot be overemphasized.

References

1. Broviac JW, Cole JJ, Schribner BH. A silicone rubber atrial catheter for prolonged parenteral alimentation. Surg Gynecol Obstet 1973;136:602–606.
2. Hickman RO, Buckner CD, Clife RA, Sander JE, Stewart P, Thomas ED. A modified right atrial catheter for access to the venous system in marrow transplant recipients. Surg Gynecol Obstet 1979;148:871–875.
3. Shafir M, Tiefenbrun J. Simultaneous placement of two permanent central venous catheters. Indications and technique. Surg Gynecol Obstet 1983;156,3:369–370.
4. Niederhuber JE, Ensminger W, Gyves JW, Lipeman M, Doan K, Cozzi E. Totally implanted venous and arterial access system to replace external catheters in cancer treatment. Surgery 1982;92:706–712.
5. Finney R, Albrink MH, Hart MB, Rosemurgy AS. A cost-effective peripheral venous port system placed at the bedside. J Surg Res 1992;53:17–19.
6. Raaf JH, Heil D. Open insertion of right atrial catheters through the jugular veins. Surg Gynec Obstet 1993;177:295–298.
7. Jansen RFM, Wigger T, vanGeel BN, van Putten WLJ. Assessment of insertion techniques and complication rates of dual lumen central venous catheters in patients with hematological malignancies. World J Surg 1990;14:101–106.
8. Pessa ME, Howard RJ. Complications of Hickman-Broviac catheters. Surg Gynecol Obstet 1985;161:257–260.
9. Mitchell SE, Clark RA. Complications of central venous catheterization. Am J Roentgenol 1979;133:467–476.
10. Herbst CA Jr. Indications management and complications of percutaneous subclavian catheters. Arch Surg 1978;113:1421–1425.
11. Collin GR, Clarke LE. Delayed pneumothorax: a complication of central venous catheterization. Surg Rounds 1994:589–594.
12. Williard W, Coit D, Lucas A, Groeger JS. Long-term vascular access via the inferior vena cava. J Surg. Oncol 1991;46:162–166.
13. Malt RA, Kempster M. Direct azygos vein and superior vena cava cannulation for parenteral nutrition. J Parenter Enteral Nutr 1983;7:580–581.
14. Oram-Smith JC, Mullen JL, Harken AH, Fitts WT. Direct right atrial catheterization for total parenteral nutrition. Surgery 1978;83:274–276.
15. Maher JW. A technique for the positioning of permanent central venous catheters in patients with thrombosis of the superior vena cava. Surg Gynecol Obstet 1983;156:659–660.
16. Coit DG, Turnbull ADM. Long-term central venous access through the gonadal vein. Surg Gynecol Obstet 1992;175:362–364.
17. Boddie AW Jr. Translumbar catheterization of the inferior vena cava for long-term angio access. Surg Gynecol Obstet 1989;168:55–56
18. Kenney PR, Dorfman GS, Denny DF Jr. Percutaneous inferior vena cava cannulation for long-term parenteral nutrition. Surgery 1985;97:602–604
19. Dollery CM, Sullivan ID, Bauraind O, et al. Thrombosis and embolism in long-term central venous access for parenteral nutrition. Lancet 1994;344:1043–1045.
20. Puel U, Caudry M, Le Metayer P, et al. Superior vena cava thrombosis related to catheter mal position in cancer chemotherapy given through implanted ports. Cancer 1993;72:2248–2252.
21. Roggla G, Linkesch M, Roggla M, et al. A rare complication of a central venous catheter system (Port-a-Cath). A case report of a catheter embolization after catheter fracture during power training. Int J Sports Med 1993;14:345–346.
22. Schuman ES, Winters V, Gross GF, Hayes JF. Management of Hickman catheter sepsis. Am J Surg 1985;149:627–628.
23. Dugdale DC, Ramsey PG. Staphylococcus aureus bacteremia in patients with Hickman catheters. Am J Med 1990;89:137–141.
24. Tenney JH, Moody MR, Newman KA, et al. Adherent microorganisms on luminal surfaces of long-term intravenous catheters. Arch Intern Med 1986;146:1949–1954.
25. Stillman RM, Soliman F, Garcia L, Sawyer PN. Etiology of catheter associated sepsis. Arch Surg 1977;112:1497–1499.
26. Dickinson GM, Bisno AL. Infections associated with indwelling devices: Concepts of pathogenesis of infections associated with intravascular devices. Antimicrob Agents Chemother 1989;33–597–601.
27. Groeger JS, Lucas AB, Thaler HT, et al. Infections morbidity associated with long-term use of venous access devices in patients with cancer. Ann Intern Med 1993;119:1168–1174.
28. Flynn PM, Shenep JL, Stokes DC, Barrett FF. In situ management of confirmed central venous catheter-related bacteremia. Pediatr Infect Dis J 1987;6:729–734.
29. Hoar PF, Wilson RM, Mangano DT, Avery GJ, Szarnicki RJ, Hill JD. Heparin bonding reduces thrombogenicity of pulmonary artery catheters. N Engl J Med 1981;305:993–995.
30. Brismar B, Hardstedt C, Jacobson S, Kager L, Malmborg AS. Reduction of catheter associated thrombosis in parenteral nutrition by intravenous heparin therapy. Arch Surg 1982;117:1196–1199.
31. Bern MM, Lokich JJ, Wallach SR, et al. Very low doses of warfarin can prevent thrombosis in central venous catheters. Ann Intern Med 1990;112:423–428.
32. Wachs T. Urokinase administration in pediatric patients with occluded central venous catheters. J Intraven Nutr 1990;13:100–102.
33. Lawson M, Bottino JC, Hurtubise MR, McCredie KB. The use of urokinase to restore the patency of occluded central venous catheters. Am J Intraven Ther Clin Nutr 1982;5:29–32.
34. Kersen C, DiStefano A, Blumenschein G, et al. Treatment of vascular access catheter occlusion with urokinase infusion. Proc Am Assoc Cancer Res 1988;29:228.
35. Horattas MC, Wright DJ, Fenton AH, et al. Changing concepts of deep vein thrombosis of the upper extremity: report of a series and review of the literature. Surgery 1988;104:561–567.
36. Cassidy FP Jr, Zajko AB, Bron KM, et al. Non-infectious complications of long-term central venous catheters: radiologic evaluation and management. Am J Roentgenol 1987;149:671–675.

37. Wechsler RJ, Spirn PW, Conant EF, et al. Thrombosis and infection caused by thoracic venous catheters: pathogenesis and imaging findings. Am J Roentgenol 1993;160:467–471.
38. Lokich JJ, Becker B. Subclavian vein thrombosis in patients treated with infusion chemotherapy for advanced malignancy. Cancer 1983;52:1586–1589.
39. Moss JF, Wagman LD, Riihimaki DU, Terz JJ. Central venous thrombosis related to the silastic Hickman-Broviac catheters in an oncologic population. J Parenter Enteral Nutri 1989;13:397–400.
40. Fraschini G, Jadeja J, Lawson M, et al. Local infusion of urokinase for the lysis of thrombosis associated with permanent central venous catheters in cancer patients. J Clin Oncol 1987;5:672–678.
41. Raaf JH. Results from use of 826 vascular access devices in cancer patients. Cancer 1985;55:1312–1321.
42. Dato VM, Dajani AS. Candidemia in children with central venous catheters: role of catheter removal and Amphotericin B therapy. Pediatr Infect Dis J 1990;9:309–314.
43. Carde P, Cosset-Delaigue MF, La Planche A, Chareau J. Classical external indwelling central venous catheter versus totally implanted venous access systems for chemotherapy administration: a randomized trial in 100 patients with solid tumors. Eur J Cancer Clin Oncol 1989;25:939–944.
44. Greene FL, Moore W, Strickl G, McFarl J. Comparison of a totally implantable access device for chemotherapy (PortCath) and long-term percutaneous catheterization (Broviac). South Med J 1988;81:580–603.
45. Stanislav GV, Fitzgibbons RJ, Bailey RT, et al. Reliabilty of implantable central venous access devices in patients with cancer. Arch Surg 1991;122:1280–1283.
46. Ingram J, Weitzman S, Greenberg ML, et al. Complications of indwelling venous access lines in the pediatric hematology patient: a prospective comparison of external venous catheters and subcutaneous ports. Am J Pediatr Hematol Oncol 1991;13:130–136.
47. Shafir M, Hoffman KR. Permanent venous access in oncology: a personal experience of 182 consecutive catheterizations. Proc 2nd Congr Eur Soc Surg Oncol 1984.
48. Borst CG, de Kruif AT, van Dam FS, et al. Totally implantable venous access ports: the patient's point of view. A quality control study. Cancer Nurs 1992;15(5):378–381.
49. Flores MR, Berlin N, Austin G, et al. A new complication of permanent indwelling central venous catheters (meeting abstract) Proc Am Soc Clin Oncol 1993;12:1620a.
50. Hoekstra A, Bassot V, Bertoglio S, et al. Clinical evaluation of the cordis vascular access port systems: a multicenter study. Med Oncol Tumor Pharmacother 1993;10(3):131–138.
51. Jones GR, Konsler GK, Dunaway RP, et al. Prospective analysis of urokinase in the treatment of catheter sepsis in pediatric hematology-oncology patients. J Pediatr Surg 1993;28(3):350–357.
52. Lecciones JA, Lee JW, Navarro EE, et al. Vascular catheter associated fungemia in patients with cancer: analysis of 155 episodes. Clin Infect Dis 1992;14:875–883.
53. Newman KA, Reed WP, Schimpff SC, et al. Hickman catheters in association with intensive cancer chemotherapy. Support Care Cancer 1993;1:92–97.

CHAPTER 47

Minimally Invasive Surgery

MICHAEL EDYE, BARRY SALKY, STEVEN M. KELLER,
T. SCOTT JENNINGS, PETER R. DOTTINO, AND NELSON N. STONE

There is an expanding role for minimally invasive surgery (MIS) in the management of neoplastic disease. Practitioners in this growing field come from numerous organ-based subspecialities. The general laparoscopic surgeon is a newcomer but one who practices a broader range of diagnostic and therapeutic procedures. Much of the technology used has been available for some time. Beginning in the late 1980s, the combination of key hardware advances and a new appreciation of the efficacy of less traumatic surgery has led to a paradigm shift in attitudes toward surgical access. Development of safe, effective procedures that do the job, minimize pain, and allow equal access to resection for cure or for maximal enjoyment of a life, perhaps shortened by malignant disease, is the essence of good surgery.

Historical Perspective

Until the beginning of the 1980s, rigid endoscopic techniques to examine the thoracic and peritoneal cavities were largely for diagnostic purposes. Thoracoscopy and peritoneoscopy had been used for most of this century to inspect viscera and obtain samples of tissue and fluid. The development of the Hopkins rod lens system made a crystal clear image possible through a simple, sealed telescope inserted into the body cavity through a cannula. Gynecologists, urologists, and orthopedic surgeons were the first to routinely perform therapeutic endoscopic procedures. Beginning with appendectomy by Semm in 1983 (39) and cholecystectomy, independently by Mühe in 1985 (29) and Mouret in 1987 (28), use of laparoscopic therapeutic techniques has only recently become routine. Early photographs of the laparoscopist at work (20), bent over the eyepiece of a laparoscope, show why. Mouret's first laparoscopic cholecystectomy was performed this way. Holding the laparoscope up to the eye with one hand, the surgeon used the other to manipulate a second instrument. Assistants, unable to see inside, could not help effectively. Complex or prolonged procedures were not undertaken because of lack of assistance and operator comfort. It was impossible to prevent the face of the surgeon from contaminating sterile objects near the eyepiece during any but the shortest of procedures.

The greatest practical stride was the development of small, light, high-resolution video cameras attached to the telescope and connected to a video monitor giving faithful reproduction of the target structures at a distance from the operative field. An image on a screen, physically separate from the eyepiece, allowed two or more operators to stand or sit comfortably, manipulating instruments distant from the screen image. For the surgeon, two handed operative technique was possible for long periods without excessive fatigue.

Now able to see their own movements, assistants could help constructively. Retraction for exposure, countertraction to aid dissection, and concurrent suction to clear the field of blood or smoke increased the sophistication of the surgical technique and, eventually, the complexity of the procedures attempted. Blood vessels could be ligated and divided, anatomic dissection along tissue planes performed, intestine divided, stapled, or sutured, organs freed, and function restored, as in conventional surgery.

The final step leading to the rapid acceptance of minimal access procedures, at least for cholecystectomy, was the realization of the contribution of a lengthy incision to postoperative pain and disability. *Big surgeon, big incision* became an anachronism of surgical dogma, provided a minimal access approach permitted an equally effective operation with no more drawbacks.

One major obstacle was extraction of the operative specimen, which invariably was larger than the small punctures used to gain access to the operative cavity. Morcellation, a technique that reduced the operative specimen to small fragments within a resilient intraperitoneal plastic bag, was devised for instances when the specimen need not be intact. For neoplastic conditions, however, an intact specimen is usually an important goal of the procedure. In these cases, a short incision of sufficient length to allow the removal of the specimen is made in an anatomically or cosmetically ideal site. By using an extraction bag or wound protection device, the specimen does not contaminate the edges of the extraction wound with cells from its surface.

47/A

Minimally Invasive Surgery for Neoplasms of the Abdominal Cavity

MICHAEL EDYE AND BARRY SALKY

Although there may be some place for diagnostic laparoscopy in an endoscopy suite (15), therapeutic procedures require an operating room. Endoscopy access routes may cause less injury, but this is still surgery, with the potential for intraoperative complications requiring adequate staff, equipment, and anesthetic support.

Most procedures are performed under positive-pressure carbon dioxide pneumoperitoneum, which produces a voluminous operating space for ease of operating and eliminates the risk of ignition of inflammable colonic gases by electrosurgical sparks. Nitrous oxide, which supports combustion, is a less irritant substitute for low-pressure laparoscopy under local anesthesia. Elevation of the abdominal wall by mechanical devices, once valveless operating cannulas have been inserted, maintains an air pneumoperitoneum. Constant suction and conventional instrumentation can be used but the operating space is more cramped and postoperative pain due to crushing of tissues may be more marked.

Operating table angle and patient position are varied to suit the target. Rolling the table so that the target organ is uppermost allows gravity to assist in retraction of surrounding mobile structures. With a supine patient in 20° head-down (Trendelenburg) position, the small bowel will slide out of the pelvis, if it is not adherent, exposing the pelvic viscera and rectum. Rolling the patient left side down exposes the root of the small bowel mesentery and terminal ileum enabling vascular pedicle ligation and lymph node clearance for right colon resection. Right side–down tilt exposes the sigmoid colon. Head-up position exposes the stomach and, with left side elevation, the splenic flexure of the colon. Certain approaches to the adrenal or spleen have the patient lying on his or her side, target organ uppermost.

Any instrument inserted into body cavities should be sterile. Its shaft must be smooth and adapted to the shape of the seal through which it passes, so as to prevent gas leaks if positive-pressure pneumoperitoneum is used.

Continuous hemostasis is vital as constant suction is usually not possible (as it produces loss of pneumoperitoneum), and the slightest amount of blood pooling causes image degradation owing to peculiarities of the video circuitry.

A centered image with good color balance, enough light, and no glare is essential to safe operating. Correct orientation of the visual horizon is fundamental to operator comfort and recognition of anatomy. The restrictions of this new operative environment oblige the surgeon to relearn what was once intuitive, without compromising precision of technique.

Limitations of Abdominal MIS

An understanding of the possibilities and limitations of laparoscopic procedures is invaluable, for surgeon and nonsurgeon alike. What may be an inappropriate referral for minimally invasive treatment today may in the near future be a good indication. Similarly, some procedures accomplished laparoscopically will fall into disfavor for lack of clear advantage or obvious inferiority to the conventional counterpart.

Instrumental palpation replaces manual examination of the body cavities afforded by a long incision. This limitation leads to increased reliance on organ imaging techniques in an attempt to exclude synchronous lesions before proceeding with surgery. Operating room use and costs may be higher than with conventional surgery, although laparoscopic equipment prices are certain to drop as more becomes available and competition increases.

Bulky tumors are a major challenge, and a full range of strategies is required to overcome the technical difficulties imposed, including use of angled scopes and table positioning. Dissection in the presence of inflammatory or neoplastic infiltration of vascular pedicles is difficult even in open surgery and may prompt abandonment of a laparoscopic approach.

The presence of dense adhesions following previous surgery, especially recent surgery, may obliterate the peritoneal cavity, necessitating extensive, hazardous adhesiolysis or even conversion to laparotomy if access is not adequate. The temptation to persist with a laparoscopic approach when an open procedure is more expeditious requires application of good surgical judgment.

Most important, there are no long-term data on laparoscopic resection for cure of malignant disease, and comparative studies are essential. Whether this will be accomplished in randomized controlled trials, using procedure registries or historical controls remains to be seen.

Abdominal Operative Strategy

To produce an operative space in the abdomen, gas must be introduced into the peritoneal cavity. In one method, a spring-loaded, blunt-tipped (Veress) needle is inserted just deep to the parietal peritoneum, insufflation is commenced, and the first cannula is inserted blindly. The surgeon may elect to use a technique known as *open laparoscopy*, whereby the peritoneum is exposed through a short incision between the muscle layers and the cannula is inserted under direct vision into the peritoneal cavity. This is advisable if the abdomen is scarred or if it is possible that a viscus is adherent to the back of the abdominal wall.

Cannulas act as a guide to permit instruments to slide in and out of the small punctures. They are inserted with the aid of a central trocar that can be sharp or blunt tipped. They are fitted with a valve to prevent loss of gas during laparoscopy with positive-pressure pneumoperitoneum. Conversely, for thoracoscopy, a valveless sleeve is sufficient, as the operative space is created by letting air in and allowing the lung to collapse.

Subsequent cannulas are inserted under visual control to avoid inadvertent damage to other structures. How many are inserted and of what size, depends on the complexity of the planned procedure. The first cannula used is large enough to accommodate the laparoscope, which is usually 10 mm in diameter. Smaller telescopes (laparoscopes) of 5 and 8 mm diameter that have been in use for many years provide enough illumination for limited diagnostic and therapeutic maneuvers in a small field. More light is necessary for more complex procedures in larger cavities, and the larger telescope is preferred.

A central laparoscope with the operating cannulas positioned at roughly 45° to either side of the optical axis is the most common arrangement. This permits two-handed technique and instrument tips which meet at roughly 90 degrees. A fourth cannula is positioned peripherally for an assistant to retract. Frequently, a fifth cannula is necessary to accommodate a suction apparatus or secondary retraction devices.

Preoperative localization of lesions is essential in the absence of information provided by manual palpation of organs. Although true stereognosis is not feasible, limited palpation is possible using probes and other smooth instruments to stroke the surfaces of structures. Texture, density, and fixity can all be appreciated with practice, but great reliance is placed on the visual appearance of the structures.

While operating, the surgeons should stand in positions that maximize their comfort. The camera, laparoscope, and target structure form an axis. The surgeon stands behind the camera with the video monitor positioned opposite, behind the target.

ANESTHESIA

If the operative site can be exposed with a single retractor, the number of cannulas required is minimized. Assuming the patient is able to cooperate, diagnostic laparoscopy can usually be performed under mild conscious sedation, local anesthesia for the puncture sites, and insufflation with a nonirritant gas such as nitrous oxide (N_2O). At present, such procedures are limited to biopsy of relatively superficial lesions such as peritoneal implants and omental or liver nodules.

Therapeutic laparoscopy usually requires general anesthesia. Full relaxation of the abdominal wall for a lengthy procedure allows maximum utilization of pneumoperitoneum. Multiple punctures through the abdominal wall under local anesthesia and the irritant effect of carbon dioxide (CO_2) on peritoneum may not be tolerated for long periods. Manipulation of retroperitoneal structures and blood vessels with rich autonomic innervation can be very distressing to the conscious patient.

PHYSIOLOGICAL EFFECTS

Cardiac and respiratory function are affected by the degree and duration of alteration in the patient's position and the pressure of insufflated gas. A patient anesthetized supine undergoes vasodilation with venous pooling. When placed in head-up position, venous return falls further, causing a rise in pulse rate and a fall in arterial pressure, which can usually be corrected by blood volume replacement. In the head-down position, venous return increases, often with a slight fall in pulse rate but no change in arterial pressure. If prolonged, pneumoperitoneum and the weight of the abdominal contents restrict diaphragmatic excursions, reducing the functional residual capacity of the lungs, resulting in gas exchange abnormalities and hypoxemia that become more difficult to correct. Pulmonary and cerebral edema are uncommon, but serious, potential complications. In spite of these possibilities, it is rarely necessary to abandon the laparoscopic procedure, as long as blood loss is kept to a minimum, the surgery is progressing expeditiously, and the patient is returned to the supine position when steep tilt is not necessary.

Compared to conventional surgery, evaporative cooling due to exposure of viscera to the air and third-space losses are markedly reduced. Mechanical hyperventilation will correct hypercarbia that may occur with CO_2 insufflation.

Insufflation pressures can vary between 6 and 15 mm Hg. Even patients with impaired left ventricular function can tolerate long periods of low-pressure pneumoperitoneum (6 to 10 mm Hg). Assuming that patients are well-paralyzed, thin, easily distensible abdominal walls require less pressure than a thick, heavy pannus.

CONVERSION TO LAPAROTOMY

As any major laparoscopic procedure may theoretically require conversion, patients should be fit for laparotomy. This is less of an issue in experienced hands, as it is possible to complete the majority of laparoscopic procedures as planned. Conversion should not be considered a mistake, as it demonstrates sound surgical judgment. Possible reasons for conversion from laparoscopy to a conventional procedure include:

Lesions Unsuited to a Laprarascopic Approach

- Technical—invasion of contiguous structures where excision en-bloc is needed and is not laparoscopically practical.
- Size—bulky lesions, difficult to free that, must be kept intact for microscopic examination and need a lengthy extraction incision render irrelevant the advantages of minimal access exposure.
- Anatomy—uncertainty of anatomic relations (e.g., ureteric involvement in inflammatory or neoplastic retroperitoneal infiltration).

Hemmorhage

With good surgical technique, uncontrolled hemorrhage necessitating conversion is rare. If the operative field is constantly obscured by blood, hampering accurate dissection, or if the rate of hemorrhage exceeds the surgeon's ability to control it in a timely fashion, prompt conversion is warranted.

Equipment Failure

Inability to maintain adequate image quality may be due to insufficient light delivery because of defects in the light source, light cable, or video circuitry. Loss of pneumoperitoneum can follow leaks or unexpected exhaustion of the gas supply and leads to a diminishing operative field and smudging of the tip of the scope. The ability to deal promptly with this requires experience, familiarity with the equipment, and mental checklists similar to the formal lists pilots and scuba divers use.

Benefits of MIS

If the surgery proceeds uneventfully, the patient's return to normal activity is usually rapid. Analgesic needs are much reduced (Fig. 47. 1) (10). Earlier return of alimentary function is reported after bowel resection, while improved musculoskeletal activity and respiratory function, as compared with that after open surgery, are well-documented following laparoscopic cholecystectomy. Hospitalization time is shortened.

Wound pain is related to the length, site, and closure method of an incision, and its degree is not directly proportional to the number of incisions. Four or five short incisions seem to be less painful than one incision equal to the sum of their lengths. Once hospitalization is prolonged, the benefits of laparoscopic surgery are less clear and are limited to a reduction of the mid- and long-term complications of dehiscence, incisional hernia, and adhesions.

Laparoscopic Procedures for Neoplastic Disease

As a diagnostic modality, laparoscopy is very effective in the evaluation of ascites of unknown cause, abdominal masses, adenopathy, and liver defects seen on organ imaging. Table 47.1 illustrates the most common malignant diseases identified by laparoscopic biopsy by the authors from 1979 to 1994. Undifferentiated carcinoma was the most common cause of ascites, mass, or liver defects. Ovarian tumor metastases to the liver were not seen in this series. The tendency for lymphoma to present as an abdominal mass, rather than as ascites or a liver deposit, is highlighted. Over this period there has been substantial evolution of diagnostic imaging and biochemical modalities employed to elucidate the nature of neoplastic disorders, and we have observed a decline in the number of diagnostic laparoscopies performed, as have others (4).

Ultrasound and computed tomography (CT)-guided needle biopsy are effective means of providing cellular material for microscopic examination, provided tissue architecture is not central to interpretation. If larger fragments are required, visualization becomes necessary. If percutaneous techniques have failed to provide "diagnostic tissue" (e.g., lymph node, ultrasound, or CT-guided needle aspiration), laparoscopy is the most reliable next step. Sizable fragments of tissue are retrieved under direct vision, allowing better evaluation of cellular architecture with less artifact. Hemostasis is possible; this is not the case with other forms of guided biopsy. Even in the presence of portal hypertension, as in the evaluation of hepatocellular carcinoma with cirrhosis, although the possibility of intra- and post-operative bleeding is never eliminated, careful technique allows avoidance of potentially hazardous varices.

When is laparoscopic biopsy preferable to other modalities? Use of biopsy needles (such as a Trucut) produces satisfactory fragments of tissue from solid organs, usually the liver. If the risk of hemorrhage is too great, or if contiguous structures such as stomach or spleen are too close (as in the left lobe of the liver), percutaneous biopsy is hazardous and a laparoscopic approach more desirable (Fig. 47.2). Large fragments or whole lymph nodes are essential for recognition of tissue architecture in the diagnosis of hematologic malignancy; these can be dissected free and removed in a retrieval bag. Chemotherapy or radiation can start immediately without fear of the wound complications of a laparotomy.

Most areas of the peripheral parts of the liver are accessible. With a patient positioned left side down, after triangular ligament division, the liver falls toward the midline, allowing inspection of the right side of the liver as far as the vena cava. The head of the pancreas can be sampled transduodenally. Pancreatic body and tail can be reached through the lesser sac by division of branches of the gastroepiploic

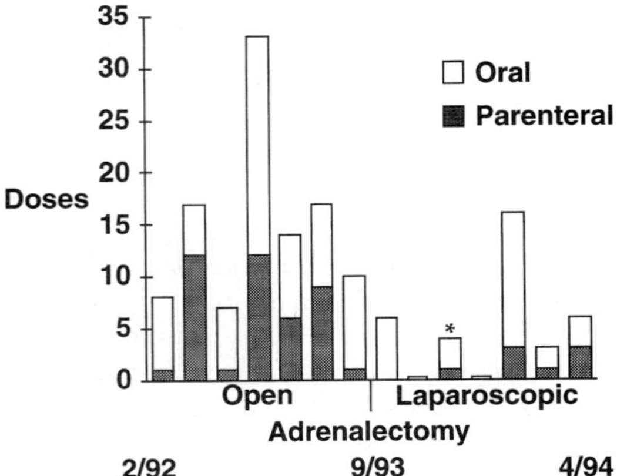

Figure 47.1. Successive adrenalectomies: the columns represent opiate analgesic doses received by each patient in the open and laparoscopic groups. *Asterisk*, conversion to laparotomy. (*Source:* Edye M, Pertsimlidis D. Unpublished data.)

Table 47.1. Indications for Laparoscopic Biopsy (1979–1995) (Salky B, Edye M)

Lesions	Ascites (No. cases) 51	Abdominal mass (No. cases) 61	Liver defects (No. cases) 105
	(%)	(%)	(%)
Carcinoma	45[a]	31	28[b]
Ovarian cancer	23	8	—
Pancreatic cancer	6	8	9
Lymphoma	2	31	3
Hepatocellular cancer	6	—	16
Breast cancer	4	—	7
Mesothelioma	6	—	—
Balance	8	22	37

[a] Carcinomatosis.
[b] Unknown primary lesion.

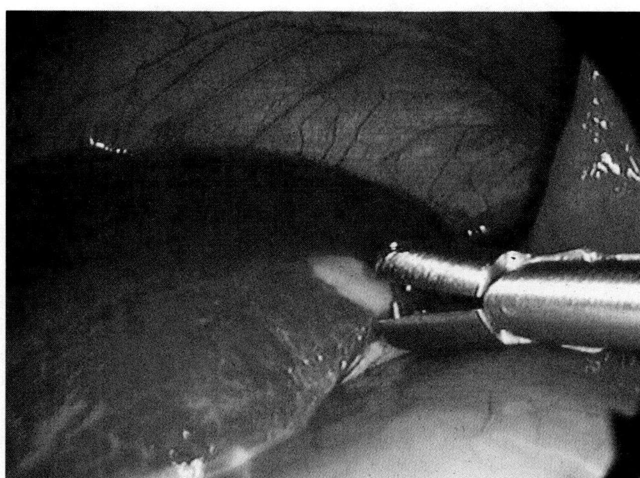

Figure 47.2. Laparoscopic view of biopsy of a 5-mm × 7-mm pancreatic carcinoma metastasis in left lobe of liver, not visible by CT.

arcade along the greater curvature of the stomach. The para-aortic lymph node–bearing regions are accessible with good positioning and careful retraction of the small bowel. In suitable cases, formal excision of a malignant mass that would otherwise require a major incision is possible with little disturbance to the patient and early return to normal activity (Fig. 47.3).

At present, the impact of gastrointestinal MIS is seen principally in the staging of peripancreatic malignancy and resection of colonic tumors. In appropriate hands, laparoscopic adrenalectomy is set to become the method of choice for benign lesions.

PANCREAS

Distal pancreatectomy for benign cystadenoma has been reported (37) and in our experience is a safe, rational procedure in selected cases (36). Before a laparoscopic approach is chosen, preoperative imaging should suggest a nonmalignant process less than 6 to 8 cm in diameter. The relationship of the splenic vessels to the tumor will determine whether concurrent splenectomy will be necessary.

The role for laparoscopic staging in the management of pancreatic malignancy is increasing as the sophistication of laparoscopic approaches to the pancreas develops. The trend is to perform diagnostic laparotomy in fewer patients and to base management on preoperative imaging and laparoscopic findings (31, 35). Laparoscopy can identify the small peritoneal and liver implants, often missed by other organ imaging techniques such as CT but present in 27% of head lesions and 65% of body and tail cancers (see Fig. 47.2) (12).

Sonography can help in the evaluation of suspicious intrahepatic lesions during staging laparoscopy (25). A flexible-tipped 5- to 8-MHz probe laid directly on the liver surface gives ultrasonic images of good resolution. The ability to distinguish a solid lesion from a hemangioma may determine if more biopsies are necessary or whether to proceed to curative resection.

The reported incidence of positive cytology in peritoneal

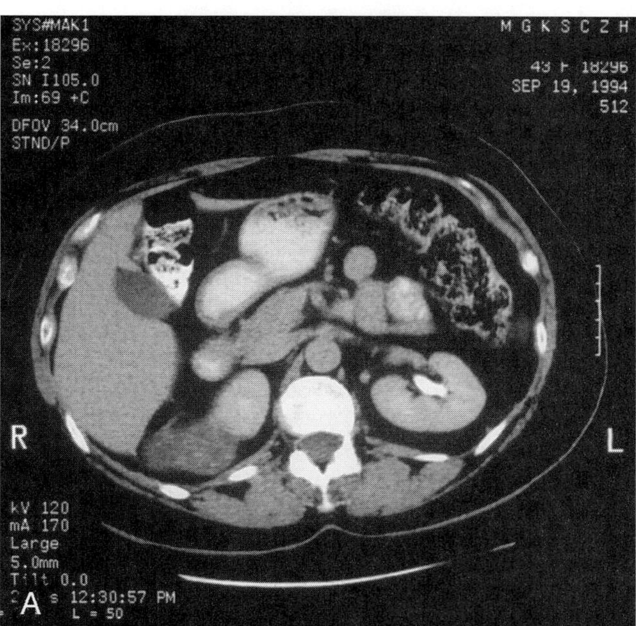

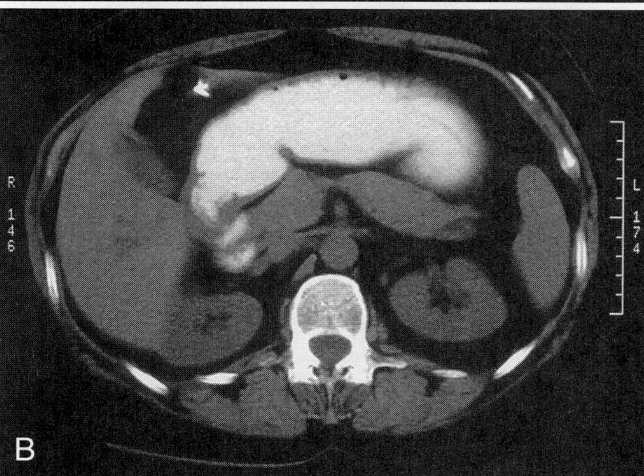

Figure 47.3. **A.** Recurrent granulosa cell tumor of the ovary seen on CT as a subhepatic mass compressing the upper pole of the right kidney and indenting the liver, 9 years after total abdominal hysterectomy and bilateral oophorectomy. The tumor was resected laparoscopically by a flank approach (as for a right adrenalectomy). Patient discharged on second postoperative day. **B.** Appearance after 7 months showing a scarred plane between liver and right kidney and no evidence of recurrent tumor.

washings is as high as 75% in patients who undergo preoperative percutaneous pancreatic biopsy and 19% in those who do not (12). This risk of peritoneal dissemination should be kept in mind in those patients when curative resection is contemplated.

Patients with a short life expectancy are best served by palliation of their most distressing symptoms. Jaundice and itch are usually relieved by an endoscopically placed stent. Vomiting due to gastric outlet obstruction necessitates a drainage procedure—either laparoscopic, conventional, or percutaneous, depending on the lesions and the available expertise. Unresectable jaundiced patients likely to live more than 6 months deserve better palliation than biliary stents that tend to block over time (8), and surgical drainage is preferable.

Van den Bosch and colleagues report patients treated with an endoprosthesis and surviving longer than 6 months had morbidity rates of up to 60% as compared with 5% for those treated with surgical bypass. Advanced age, male sex, liver metastases, and large tumors were found to be unfavorable prognostic factors. Using survival curves calculated from experience with 148 patients, males with liver metastases, regardless of age or tumor size, had little chance of surviving beyond 6 months. Females with similar tumors fared slightly better. Those with small tumors and no liver metastases, especially young women, had a relatively good chance of surviving beyond 6 months. For patients somewhere in between, the outlook was less clear (41).

Conlon and coworkers from the Memorial-Sloan Kettering Cancer Center reported 115 patients with peripancreatic neoplasms and preoperative evaluation suggesting resectability. Of 108 who had complete laparoscopic examination, 67 (62%) had lesions deemed resectable. Of these, 61 (91%) underwent resection (7). That as many as 56% of the whole group were resected probably reflects selection bias introduced by referral of patients with apparently resectable lesions to a cancer center.

Endosurgical options are evolving that may offer safe biliary-enteric and gastroenteric drainage, with many of the advantages of laparoscopic cholecystectomy. The stakes are somewhat higher, since the chief procedure-related morbidity of surgical drainage of the biliary tree is a potentially lethal anastomotic bile leak. Cholecystojejunostomy is a straightforward laparoscopic procedure, but reports have been confined to a few cases (14, 40). Early results are promising; patients report good relief of jaundice and itch. Experimental animal studies are establishing the feasibility of formal laparoscopic palliative bypass of duodenum and bile duct using a Roux-en-Y anastomosis (38), arguably the best form of bilioenteric reconstruction.

Pancreaticoduodenectomy has been described for chronic pancreatitis with pancreas divisum (18). This is a technical tour de force beyond the capacity of the majority of experienced laparoscopic surgeons and is not currently a feasible option for either benign or malignant disease. Similarly, the technical demands of excision of malignant lesions of the gallbladder for cure are such that they should be handled by conventional surgery.

For the group of patients who require palliative care after a diagnosis of incurable foregut cancer or a second group anticipating curative pancreatic resection who require nutritional support during chemoradiation, laparoscopically assisted placement of a feeding jejunostomy tube can be performed as an ambulatory procedure (11). The proponents of this technique assert that creation of a Witzel serosal tunnel reduces the possibility of developing an enterocutaneous fistula. The procedure consists of visual inspection of the peritoneal cavity, peritoneal washings for cytology, and selection of a proximal loop of jejunum, which is exteriorized through a 3- to 4-cm incision prior to fashioning the jejunostomy on the outside. The importance of the laparoscopy to the technique is chiefly the ability to make a broad general assessment of the peritoneal cavity and then facilitate selection of the correct loop of intestine.

Benign head and body lesions, such as insulinoma, that can be identified with intraoperative ultrasound with an accuracy of 90 to 100% (33) may need enucleation or distal pancreatectomy. This is an ideal indication for laparoscopic excision but is still under early evaluation.

COLON

Accepted indications for laparoscopic resection of colonic lesions include endoscopically unresectable, large, benign polyps and potentially obstructing submucosal tumors such as lipomas and premalignant adenomatous polyps. Noncurative resection for carcinoma, when distant metastases are present, is a logical extension of the indications for benign disease, in the hope that the surgical assault on the patient will have less of an impact on recovery while not compromising the safety of the procedure.

The role of laparoscopy in curative resection of colonic malignancy remains controversial. Until long-term results are available, it will not be clear whether laparoscopic surgery offers more than the short-term advantages of reduced hospital stay and rapid return to normal activity. There is uncertainty about the adequacy of resection in low rectal tumors or the possibility of missing intercurrent lesions in an incompletely imaged colon, as may occur with an endoscopically impassable or obstructing malignant stricture.

Endoscopic localization in the sigmoid and transverse colon, and at the flexures, is unreliable (43). An endoscopic photograph showing the lesion near the ileocecal valve is adequate in the right colon, as is a barium contrast study showing the lesion. Small or soft lesions distant from reliable endoscopic landmarks should be tattooed with India ink or methylene blue at the time of diagnosis (23), or at least one day before surgery if resection is indicated. Circumferential injection is essential, as the mesenteric side is impossible to recognize at endoscopy and a tattoo there may be obscured at laparoscopy. If visible, the tattoo is seen on the peritoneal surface as a black or blue stain marking the center of the resection specimen. Apart from signaling what part of the colon to resect, the mark allows the surgeon to avoid handling the lesion and adjacent bowel, so as to prevent shedding of cells into the intestinal lumen or peritoneal cavity.

Early results of laparoscopic colon resection demonstrate acceptable operative morbidity and mortality, shorter hospital stay, and more rapid return to normal activity (2, 16, 24, 42, 45). Resection margins and mesenteric lymph node count, important factors in the determination of adequacy of resection, are no different from those obtained after conventional surgery (Tables 47.2 and 47.3). These reports come from experienced units and their results should not be extrapolated to centers where laparoscopic skills are not finely honed.

The possibility of tumor recurrence in laparoscopic cannula sites is of considerable concern. Recurrence in abdominal wall scar tissue following conventional colonic resection for cure is reported as 0.7% (22). It is not clear from the sporadic reports of similar lesions appearing in cannula sites after laparoscopic resections (5, 44) that this occurs

Table 47.2. Laparoscopic Resections for Colorectal Cancer: Lymph Node Harvest

Investigator	Patients (No.)	Nodes (No. mean)
Monson 1992 (27)	35	10
Peters 1993 (32)	24	7.9
Hoffman 1994 (21)	32	8
Musser 1994 (30)	24	10.6
Puente 1994 (34)	38	11
Salky & Edye (unpublished)	39	9.4

Table 47.3. Mean Lymph Node Retrieval in 39 Colon Resections for Cancer: Historical Open Controls from the Same Institution

Site	Resection	
	Open (No.)	Laparoscopic (No.)
Ileocolic	8	10
Right	13	10
Left	12	10
Sigmoid	6	7
Anterior resection	7	10

Source: Edye M, Salky B. Unpublished data.

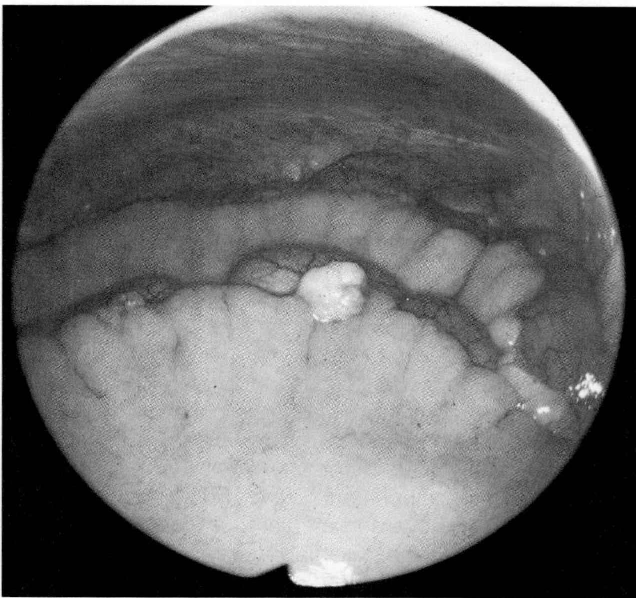

Figure 47.4. Colon cancer metastatic to the small bowel is seen as the large nodule on the mesenteric border of the intestine. Lesions such as these can ulcerate through the intestinal wall, causing perforation or gastrointestinal hemorrhage.

more frequently than could otherwise be expected. Beart reports three such recurrences among 498 resections for cure (0.6%) in the American Society of Colorectal Surgeons registry of laparoscopic colon resections (1). The contribution, if any, of type of access and surgical technique to tumor recurrence in general remains to be determined.

T cell–related immune function, as measured by skin antigen testing in the porcine model, appears better preserved after laparoscopic than after open colectomy (3), although cortisol levels were no different. The abdominal component of the laparoscopic procedure was the same as for the controls. This suggests that the method of access is the chief determinant of the immune response. Correlation in human subjects is still required.

Although the early experience has been very favorable, clinicians should remain circumspect until 5-year follow-up data are available. Whether survival is better, worse, or the same, stage for stage, after laparoscopic than after open surgery will be established only by careful comparative trials. Referrals should be restricted to units that regularly audit their results and have good general laparoscopic and colorectal skills and acceptable morbidity.

STOMACH AND SMALL BOWEL

Local excision of small, benign lesions of the stomach wall (such as leimyomas or stromal tumors) lends itself to a laparoscopic approach and has been reported (6, 26). The operative specimen is small, and resection margins need only be clear of tumor. The chief limitations will be the site and size of the tumor in relation to the esophagus, pylorus, lesser curve, or posterior wall. These factors determine accessibility, the type of gastric closure the surgeon uses, and, thus, the complexity of the procedure.

Gastric resection for malignancy is still in its infancy, with no significant series reported and no long-term follow-up. The operation is technically feasible for benign ulcer disease (19), but it has yet to be demonstrated that an adequate cancer operation is possible laparoscopically, and this approach must be considered experimental at this stage.

Excision of primary small bowel tumors or metastases, if symptomatic from hemorrhage or intestinal obstruction, may be indicated. In addition to localizing the tumor, laparoscopy can identify other peritoneal implants, liver metastases, and synchronous lesions by careful examination of the entire small intestine (Fig. 47.4). An appropriate site is selected for a short incision, delivery of the tumor, resection, and restoration of continuity. There are no large series as yet that establish the benefits of minimizing access in this setting, although, intuitively, reduced postoperative pain and earlier return to normal activity could be expected.

ADRENALECTOMY

The adrenal is an ideal structure for minimally invasive resection. Its retroperitoneal position high on the posterior abdominal wall and, thus, its relative inaccessibility create a problem of surgical access out of proportion to its small size. Benign unilateral functioning adenomas (Cushings and Conn's tumors) and pheochromocytomas are resectable, although the difficulty of laparoscopic dissection increases markedly with lesions greater than 8 cm in diameter. Metastatic neoplasm in or near the adrenal may be resectable (see Fig. 47.3).

Preoperative work-up for functioning adenoma such as lateralizing studies or selective venous sampling is identical to that necessary for open adrenalectomy. Effects of catecholamine excess in patients with pheochromocytoma must be completely blocked (9) and if so do not pose additional intraoperative risk.

Three methods of access have been described. A laparoscopic version of the traditional anterior approach (13) posterolateral to the duodenum on the right or through the transverse mesocolon on the left has the advantage that both sides are accessible without repositioning the patient, although more dissection is required to gain exposure and bleeding may be more troublesome.

In a transperitoneal approach in the lateral decubitus position, described by Gagner (17) (the patient lies on the operating table lesion side up), the viscera are pulled away from the operative field by gravity. On the left, the spleen is reflected from its attachment to the abdominal wall, exposing the adrenal above and medial to the upper pole of the kidney. This carries the potential of injury to the spleen but is the most direct route to the gland. On the right, the liver is mobilized by incising the triangular ligament, exposing the adrenal in the space between vena cava, liver, and right kidney. The colon is rarely even seen, and access to the adrenal vein is straightforward. This approach is also ideal for gaining access to the suprarenal space (see Fig. 47.3*B*) and for visualizing posteroinferior lesions of the liver, by reflecting it medially.

A third approach, also in the lateral decubitus position, involves creation of an operative space posterior to the peritoneal sac by blunt dissection or inflation of a balloon and may be appropriate for small, unilateral lesions.

If patients operated for pheochromocytoma are adequately "blocked," early ligature of the adrenal vein to minimize catecholamine release during handling, contrary to traditional teaching, is not essential. Blood can still escape via the numerous venous collaterals issuing from the gland and parasitic circulation of the tumor.

Using historical controls, postoperative analgesic requirements were reduced to one sixth (see Fig. 47.1) and median postoperative stay was halved in seven consecutive adrenalectomies performed laparoscopically (10). These results have continued: experience now totals 28 unilateral resections.

References

1. Beart R. Proceedings of the American Society of Colorectal Surgeons. Chicago: American Society of Colorectal Surgeons, 1994.
2. Beart RW Jr. Laparoscopic colectomy: status of the art. Dis Colon Rectum 1994;37:S47–S49.
3. Bessler M, Whelan R, Halverson A, Treat M, Nowygrod R. Is immune function better preserved after laparoscopic versus open colon resection? Surg Endosc 1994;8:881–883.
4. Chu CM, Lin SM, Peng SM, Wu CS, Liaw YF. The role of laparoscopy in the evaluation of ascites of unknown origin. Gastrointest Endosc 1994;40:285–289.
5. Cirocco WC, Schwartzman A, Golub RW. Abdominal wall recurrence after laparoscopic colectomy for colon cancer. Surgery 1994;116:842–846.
6. Clancy TV, Moore PM, Ramshaw DG, Kays CR. Laparoscopic excision of a benign gastric tumor. J Laparoendosc Surg 1994;4:277–280.
7. Conlon KC, Dougherty E, Klimstra DS, Brennan MF. Operative laparoscopy in the staging of patients with potentially resectable peripancreatic malignancy. In American College of Surgeons Annual Clinical Congress. Chicago, 1994.
8. Dowsett JF, Russell RCG, Hatfield ARW, et al. Malignant obstructive jaundice: a prospective randomised trial of by-pass surgery versus endoscopic stenting. Gastroenterology 1989;96:A128.
9. Edye MB, Pertsemlidis D. Laparoscopic adrenalectomy. In Color Atlas/Text of Advanced Laparoscopy for Surgeons. Edited by BA Salky. New York: Igaku-Shoin, 1995.
10. Edye MB, Pertsimlidis D. Laparoscopic approaches to adrenalectomy. Proceedings of the Annual Scientific Congress of the Royal Australasian College of Surgeons, Hobart, Australia, 1994.
11. Ellis LM, Evans DB, Martin D, Ota DM. Laparoscopic feeding jejunostomy tube in oncology patients. Surg Oncol 1992;1:245–249.
12. Fernandez del Castillo C, Warshaw AL. Laparoscopy for staging in pancreatic carcinoma. Surg Oncol 1993;2(suppl)1:25–29.
13. Fernndez-Cruz L, Saenz A, Benarroch G, Torres E, Astudillo E. Technical aspects of adrenalectomy via operative laparoscopy. Surg Endosc 1994;8:1348–1351.
14. Fletcher DR, Jones RM. Laparoscopic cholecystjejunostomy as palliation for obstructive jaundice in inoperable carcinoma of pancreas. Surg Endosc 1992;6:147–149.
15. Fockens P, Huibregtse K. Staging of pancreatic and ampullary cancer by endoscopy. Endoscopy 1993;25:52–57.
16. Franklin ME Jr, Ramos R, Rosenthal D, Schuessler W. Laparoscopic colonic procedures. World J Surg 1993;17:51–56.
17. Gagner M, Lacroix A, Bolte E, Pomp A. Laparoscopic adrenalectomy. The importance of a flank approach in the lateral decubitus position. Surg Endosc 1994;8:135–138.
18. Gagner M, Pomp A. Laparoscopic pylorus-preserving pancreatoduodenectomy. Surg Endosc 1994;8:408–410.
19. Goh P, Tekant Y, Kum CK, Isaac J, Shang NS. Totally intra-abdominal laparoscopic Billroth II gastrectomy [letter]. Surg Endosc 1992;6:160.
20. Greene FL, Ponsky JL. Endoscopic surgery. In History of Endoscopic Surgery. Edited by G Berci. Philadelphia: Saunders, 1994, pp 1–5.
21. Hoffman GC, Baker JW, Fitchett CW, Vansant JH. Laparoscopic-assisted colectomy. Initial experience. Ann Surg 1994;219:732–740.
22. Hughes ESR, McDermott FT, Polglase AL, Johnson WR. Tumor recurrence in the abdominal wall scar tissue after large-bowel cancer surgery. Dis Colon Rectum 1983;26:571–572.
23. Hyman N, Waye JD. Endoscopic full quadrant tattoo for the identification of lesions at surgery. Gastrointest Endosc 1991;37:56–58.
24. Jacobs M, Verdeja JC, Goldstein HS. Minimally invasive colon resection (laparoscopic colectomy). Surg Laparosc Endosc 1991;1:144–150.
25. Jakimowicz JJ. Review: Intraoperative ultrasonography during minimal access surgery. J R Coll Surg (Edinb) 1993;38:231–238.
26. Lukaszczyk JJ, Preletz RJ, Jr. Laparoscopic resection of benign stromal tumor of the stomach. J Laparoendosc Surg 1992;2:331–334.
27. Monson JR, Darzi A, Carey PD, Guillou PJ. Prospective evaluation of laparoscopic-assisted colectomy in an unselected group of patients. Lancet 1992;340:831–833.
28. Mouret P. From the first laparoscopic cholecystectomy to the frontiers of laparoscopic surgery. The prospective futures. Dig Surg 1991;8:124–125.
29. Mühe E. Die erste Cholezystektomie durch das Laparoskope. Langenbecks Arch Chir 1986;369:804.
30. Musser DJ, Boorse RC, Madera F, Reed JF. Laparoscopic colectomy: at what cost? Surg Laparosc Endosc 1994;4:1–5.
31. Niederau C, Grendell JH. Diagnosis of pancreatic carcinoma. Imaging techniques and tumor markers. Pancreas 1992;7:66–86.
32. Peters WR, Bartels TL. Minimally invasive colectomy: are the potential benefits realized? Dis Colon Rectum 1993;36:751–756.
33. Pietrabissa A, Shimi SM, Vander Velpen G, Cuschieri A. Localization of insulinoma by laparoscopic infragastric inspection of the pancreas and contact ultrasonography. Surg Oncol 1993;2:83–86.
34. Puente I, Sosa JL, Sleeman D, Desai U, Tranakas N, Hartmann R. Laparoscopic assisted colorectal surgery. J Laparoendosc Surg 1994;4:1–7.
35. Roder JD, Rosch T, Bautz W, Gerhardt P, Siewert JR. Pankreascarcinom praoperative Diagnostik und Indikationsstellung. Chirurg 1994;65:225–231.
36. Salky BA, Edye MB, Gellman L. Laparoscopic distal pancreatectomy and splenectomy for mucinous cystadenoma of the pancreas. In Proceedings of the Annual Scientific Session of the Society of American Gastrointestinal Endoscopic Surgeons. Orlando, 1995, p 63.
37. Sànchez AW, Berry FS, Garcia JC, Weber GR. Laparoscopic treatment of pancreatic serous cystadenoma. Surg Laparosc Endosc 1994;4:304–307.
38. Schöb O, Schlumpf R, Kunz M, Uhlschmid GK, Largiader F. Technique of laparoscopic cholecystojejunostomy with a Roux-en-Y loop. Surg Laparosc Endosc 1993;3:386–390.
39. Semm K. Endoscopic appendicectomy. Endoscopy 1983;15:59–64.
40. Shimi S, Banting S, Cuschieri A. Laparoscopy in the management of pancreatic cancer: endoscopic cholecystojejunostomy for advanced disease. Br J Surg 1992;79:317–319.
41. van den Bosch RP, van der Schelling GP, Klinkenbijl MD, Mulder PG, van Blankenstein M, Jeekel J. Guidelines for the application of surgery and endoprostheses in the palliation of obstructive jaundice in advanced cancer of the pancreas. Ann Surg 1994;219:18–24.
42. Van Ye TM, Cattey RP, Henry LG. Laparoscopically assisted colon resections compare favorably with open technique. Surg Laparosc Endosc 1994;4:25–31.
43. Vignati P. Endoscopic localization of colon cancers. Surg Endosc 1994;8:1085–1087.
44. Walsh DC, Wattchow DA, Wilson TG. Subcutaneous metastases after laparoscopic resection of malignancy. Aust N Z J Surg 1993;63:563–565.
45. Zucker KA, Pitcher DE, Martin DT, Ford RS. Laparoscopic-assisted colon resection. Surg Endosc 1994;8:12–18

47/B
Minimally Invasive Surgery for Thoracic Cancer

STEVEN M. KELLER

Historical Perspective

The introduction of thoracoscopy as a useful and practical procedure is generally attributed to Hans Christian Jacobaeus, who, in 1922, reported insertion of a cystoscope under local anesthesia into the thorax for the diagnosis and treatment of tuberculosis (7). Collapse therapy was accomplished by inducing pneumothorax and lysing adhesions to the parietal pleura with a cautery inserted via a separate incision. Jacobaeus also employed this ersatz thoracoscope to identify nontuberculous disease of the chest. Rigid thoracoscopy became widely accepted; though, with the discovery of antituberculous drugs, interest in the technique waned and the principal use shifted to diagnosis of pleural disease.

The reemergence of thoracoscopy as a valuable and frequently performed procedure can be attributed to three technical advances: single-lung ventilation with a double-lumen endotracheal tube, fiberoptics, and the development of advanced endoscopic instruments. These combine to permit methodical and unhindered visualization of the entire hemithorax and lung surface as well as biopsy or excision of mediastinal, pulmonary, pleural, and esophageal disease. Though video-assisted thoracoscopic surgery (VATS) is currently enjoying the popularity associated with new procedures, novelty must never interfere with delivery of appropriate treatment. Less is not always better.

Technical Aspects

VATS is usually performed following induction of general anesthesia utilizing an endotracheal tube that permits selective, individual ventilation of either lung. The endotracheal tube is constructed with two lumens of different lengths. The distal portion of the tube is positioned in a mainstem bronchus (usually the left), proximal to the lobar orifices. This places the proximal endotracheal lumen above the carina. Occlusive balloons proximal to the endotracheal tube orifices permit selective ventilation of either lung. Correct positioning of the tube is confirmed by auscultation of the chest and direct visualization with a bronchoscope. If the patient is unable to tolerate general anesthesia, VATS may be performed with intravenous sedation and a combination of local and regional (intercostal block) anesthesia; though this technique does not permit such thorough visualization of the chest.

The patient is turned to the lateral decubitus position, and the thoracoscopy port sites are marked. The number of port sites varies with the extent of the procedure. Preparations are made for a thoracotomy in order that conversion to an open procedure, should it become urgently necessary, may be performed expeditiously. Ventilation of the ipsilateral lung is halted, and pneumothorax is induced via a 2-cm incision. Gas insufflation to collapse the lung is unnecessary. Previous obliteration of the pleural space, iatrogenic or pathologic, renders thoracoscopy impossible. The thoracoscope with attached video camera is inserted and the hemithorax inspected. Thoracoscopic operating instruments are inserted through additional small incisions. Including the camera, a pleural biopsy may require only two port sites while pulmonary wedge resection necessitates three ports. More complicated procedures may require as many as five instrument insertion sites. Convenient placement of the port sites locates the instruments and lesion in a "baseball-diamond" pattern, with the camera at home plate and the lesion at second base.

To remove the specimen it is often necessary to enlarge slightly one of the port sites. Tumor implantation at the incision site is more than just a theoretic possibility. More than 20 such cases have already been documented (5, 6, 18). It is, therefore, imperative that any specimen suspected of containing cancer be placed in a protective container before it is removed from the thorax. Upon completion of the procedure, ventilation to the collapsed lung is resumed and a chest tube inserted. The patient is usually extubated in the operating room.

Thoracoscopic instrumentation is sometimes combined with standard techniques to perform true "video-assisted" surgery. The video camera is utilized to monitor an operation performed with regular instruments inserted via an abbreviated thoracotomy incision (8, 12, 14). Access to the chest is gained without spreading the ribs, thus avoiding a maneuver to which many attribute postthoracotomy pain.

Perceived advantages of VATS are decreases in immediate postoperative pain, length of hospitalization, and overall cost. When comparisons are made to historic controls, the former two assumptions appear true; however, differences in total patient charges are less apparent and may vary by procedure. Investigators from the Mayo Clinic reported that the median charge for 64 patients who underwent thoracoscopic wedge resection of a pulmonary nodule was $12,898, while a wedge excision via thoracotomy without prior thoracoscopy in 64 similar patients generated a median cost of $12,502 (1). They attributed the lack of savings (despite shorter median hospital stay) to the cost of thoracoscopic instruments.

Applications

PULMONARY LESIONS

Perhaps the most common indication for VATS is resection of indeterminate pulmonary nodules (1, 10). Nodules greater than 1 cm in diameter and located within 2 cm of the periphery of the lung or the interlobar fissures are easily identified and lend themselves to VATS resection. Techniques similar to those employed to identify nonpalpable breast tumors have been utilized to locate smaller nodules or those located more centrally. Prior to operation such nodules are visualized in the radiology department by CT and their position is marked via injection of methylene blue. Alternatively, the distal end of a percutaneously placed, small-caliber, flexible wire is fixed within the tumor. The surgeon follows either the trail of methylene blue or the wire directly to the nonpalpable nodule.

During the early experience with VATS at the Mayo Clinic, unplanned conversion to open thoracotomy owing to inability to locate the lung nodule thoracoscopically was required in 14% (17/118) of patients (1). Mack and co-workers reported the experience of three surgeons from different institutions who performed 242 thoracoscopies for excision of a pulmonary nodule (10). Only two required conversion to open thoracotomy in order to locate the pulmonary pathology. This reflects the surgeon's ability to determine accurately which nodules can be successfully approached with VATS.

Multiple firings of the GIA stapler (Fig. 47.5) are employed to remove the nodule in continuity with a rim of normal tissue. Morbidity of VATS wedge resection varies from 2 to 6%, median hospitalization ranges from 2 to 3 days (1, 10). Should frozen section analysis of the specimen reveal a primary lung cancer, the appropriate cancer operation is performed (i.e., lobectomy or pneumonectomy). The relatively low frequency of cancer in nodules removed via VATS varies from 34 to 52% (1, 10) and reflects the willingness of physicians to refer patients for VATS resection of x-ray abnormalities that previously they would have observed.

Some surgeons have performed thoracoscopic wedge resections as definitive treatment for T1 non–small cell lung cancers in patients deemed too ill to undergo thoracotomy. Shennib and co-workers documented their experience with 30 poor-risk patients who had one or more of the following: age over 75 years, FEV1 below 1 L or less than 35% predicted, Pao_2 less than 60mm Hg, DCO less than 40% (17). Morbidity was 23% and mortality 3%. Median hospitalization was 6.5 days.

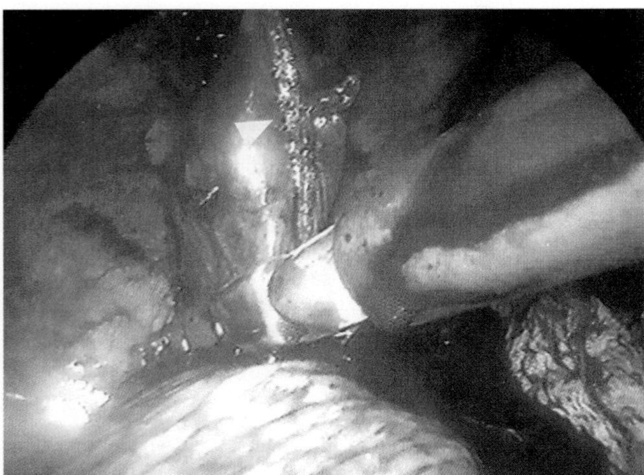

Figure 47.5. Thoracoscopic lung biopsy. Multiple firings of a 12-mm stapler enable a large excisional biopsy of a lung nodule. The jaws of the instrument just to the left of center are clamped around the last attachment of lung. Yellow arrow points to row of staples on specimen.

Video-assisted lobectomy or pneumonectomy has been demonstrated to be technically feasible in the hands of highly skilled and experienced thoracoscopists (8, 12, 14). The morbidity and mortality rates following 75 lobectomies and 4 pneumonectomies were similar to those seen with standard thoracotomy. The postoperative hospitalization may have been slightly reduced, as compared with that usually associated with open procedures. The absence of compelling reasons to perform these video-assisted major surgical procedures has been responsible for their lack of popularity among thoracic surgeons.

The role of VATS in the resection of metastatic pulmonary nodules is uncertain. McCormack and co-workers reviewed the records of 144 patients who underwent resection of lung metastases from colorectal carcinoma and demonstrated that chest radiography and CT underestimate the number of malignant nodules by 54 and 25%, respectively (11). They cautioned that, owing to the inability to palpate the lung during VATS, it is likely that a significant number of metastases will be similarly missed.

PLEURA

Though no reports specifically compare VATS with rigid thoracoscopy, the former has replaced the latter for the diagnosis and treatment of malignant pleural diseases. The magnification of the pleural surface and the flexibility of endoscopic instruments render VATS a superior tool for the diagnosis of pleural lesions. These same features permit obliteration of the pleural space for therapy of malignant pleural effusion via mechanical pleural abrasion, pleurectomy, or chemical pleuradesis. In patients with undiagnosed pleural effusions, VATS inspection of the pleural surface, biopsy, and frozen section followed by immediate pleuradesis may replace the current standard of chest tube insertion, prolonged drainage, and instillation of a sclerosing agent.

ESOPHAGUS

A significant portion of the morbidity and mortality that accompany esophagectomy have been associated with the thoracic portion of the operation. Indeed, the transhiatal esophagectomy popularized by Orringer was specifically designed to avoid the sequela of thoracotomy. The technique of transhiatal esophagectomy has, however, been criticized, since it precludes a "radical cancer operation."

VATS may obviate the objections to esophagectomy without thoracotomy because it permits the performance of an operation that satisfies all oncologic principles. Collard and co-workers reported their experience with 7 patients (2), while Cuschieri documented his experience with an additional 20 (3). The techniques of the two investigators are similar; both describe extensive en bloc resections. The patient is intubated with a double-lumen endotracheal tube and the right lung is allowed to collapse. Utilizing up to five port sites inserted in the right hemithorax, they incise the parietal pleura on either side of the esophagus, staple and transect the azygos vein, ligate the thoracic duct, and perform extensive mediastinal lymph node dissections. Cuschieri advocates concurrent use of the endoscope to identify and elevate the esophagus from the posterior mediastinum. Upon completion of the intrathoracic portion of the procedure, the cervical esophagus is exposed and the stomach is prepared for transfer to the neck. Anastomosis is accomplished in the usual fashion.

Postoperative morbidity and mortality in this group of 27 patients included one death, one anastomotic leak, and five episodes of respiratory failure/pneumonitis. The authors note that these are disappointingly similar to the complications of esophagectomy with thoracotomy. Cuschieri speculates that this may be due to the necessary collapse of the right lung during the VATS portion of the procedure.

The future role of VATS in esophagectomy for cancer is unclear. To replace open thoracotomy, it must be shown safe and cost effective. To supplant transhiatal esophagectomy, perioperative morbidity and long-term survival must be demonstrably superior. Certainly, before attempting VATS resection, a surgeon must be thoroughly familiar with open esophageal surgery.

MEDIASTINUM

Video thoracoscopy has been employed for both biopsy and excision of mediastinal lymph nodes and tumors. Krasna demonstrated the utility of video thoracoscopy in preresection staging of patients with esophageal cancer (9). Thirteen patients underwent prospective VATS staging via the left hemithorax, with biopsy of aortopulmonary window (levels 5 and 6), inferior pulmonary ligament (level 9), and paraesophageal lymph nodes (level 8). Mean hospital stay was 3.3 days. Biopsy results were identical to those obtained during transthoracic esophagectomy and lymph node dissection performed at a later date. The authors concluded that VATS was particularly useful for the stratification of patients with esophageal cancer prior to entry into protocols involving neoadjuvant therapy.

Rendina and co-workers (13) investigated the utility of VATS, mediastinoscopy, and mediastinotomy for the biopsy and diagnosis of 51 patients with mediastinal masses. They concluded that mediastinoscopy was indicated for the biopsy of tumors in the paratracheal region. Anterior mediastinotomy was useful for the biopsy of tumors with extensive invasion of the chest wall, when it could be performed under local anesthesia. In all other instances, they concluded that VATS was the most efficient and least traumatic method by which to establish the diagnosis of mediastinal masses.

VATS excision of 20 mediastinal tumors was reported by Roviaro and co-workers (15). The authors detailed their techniques for removing neurogenic tumors, mediastinal cysts, and thymic tumors. Dissection was accomplished with instruments introduced into the chest via two thoracoscopy ports. The majority of patients required a "utility" submammary thoracotomy, however, to permit removal of the bulky tumor mass from the hemithorax. Two patients (10%) suffered postoperative hemorrhage and both required numerous transfusions and reoperation. The authors speculated that VATS may become the operation of choice to remove noninvasive mediastinal tumors.

OTHER

VATS has been utilized for palliation of a variety of other cancer-related disorders. Cuschieri and co-workers have described their experience with a bilateral splanchnicectomy performed via a posterior approach for the relief of intractable pancreatic cancer pain in three patients (4). Under general endotracheal anesthesia and with the patient prone, the camera and two additional ports were inserted caudad to the inferior angle of the scapula. The sympathetic trunk was visualized and the T5 ganglion identified. The sympathetic trunk was elevated and the medial pleura incised, exposing the main splanchnic roots and greater splanchnic nerve, which were then transected. The process was repeated at the T8 sympathetic ganglion, to expose the lesser roots and the lesser splanchnic nerve. The operation was continued in the contralateral hemithorax during the same anesthesia. The authors report that, in the absence of iatrogenic lung injury, chest tubes were unnecessary. There was no morbidity, and good analgesia was obtained in all three patients.

VATS may be utilized to create a pericardial window in selected patients with cardiac tamponade. Shapira and coworkers described creating a 4-cm × 4-cm pericardial window in three patients with hemodynamically significant pericardial effusions (16). Following general anesthesia, the patient was turned to the right lateral decubitus position and one-lung ventilation was instituted. The camera and two grasping instruments were required. Advantages of this procedure over a subxiphoid approach are direct inspection of both the pleura and pericardial spaces. Disadvantages are the need for general anesthesia and single-lung ventilation, neither of which is tolerated well by these critically ill patients.

Summary

Video thoracoscopy has certainly found a niche in the armamentarium of thoracic surgeons. The extent to which it will be utilized in the treatment of patients with malignant disease, however, will be determined by its effectiveness and cost as when compared with those of established methods. Most important, the potential cure associated with an open cancer resection must not be sacrificed for the length of an incision or a briefer hospitalization period.

References

1. Allen MS, Deschamps C, Lee RE, Trastek VF, Daly RC, Pairolero PC. Video-assisted thoracoscopic stapled wedge excision for indeterminate pulmonary nodules. J Thorac Cardiovasc Surg 1993;106:1048–1052.
2. Collard J-M, Lengele B, Otte J-B, Kestens P-J. En bloc and standard esophagectomies by thoracoscopy. Ann Thorac Surg 1993;56:675–679.
3. Cuschieri A. Endoscopic subtotal oesophagectomy for cancer using the right thoracoscopic approach. Surg Oncol 1993;2:(suppl)1:3–11.
4. Cuschieri A, Shimi SM, Crosthwaite G, Joypaul V. Bilateral endoscopic splanchnicectomy through a posterior thoracoscopic approach. J R Coll Surg (Edinb) 1994;39:44–47.
5. Downey RJ, McCormack PM. Video Assisted Thoracic Surgery Study Group. Proceedings of Society of Thorac Surgery 31st Annual Meeting 1995:abstract 9.
6. Fry WA, Siddiqui A, Pensler JM, Mostafavi H. Thoracoscopic implantation of cancer with a fatal outcome. Ann Thorac Surg 1995;59:42–45.
7. Jacobaeus HC. The practical importance of thoracoscopy in surgery of the chest. Surg Gynecol Obstet 1922;34:289–296.
8. Kirby TJ, Rice TW. Thoracoscopic lobectomy. Ann Thorac Surg 1993;56:784–786
9. Krasna MJ, McLaughlin JS. Thoracoscopic lymph node staging for esophageal cancer. Ann Thorac Surg 1993;56:671–674.

10. Mack MJ, Hazelrigg SR, Landreneu RJ, Acuff TE. Thoracoscopy for the diagnosis of the indeterminate solitary pulmonary nodule. Ann Thorac Surg 1993;56:825–832.
11. McCormack PM, Ginsberg KB, Bains MS, et al. Accuracy of lung imaging in metastases with implications for the role of thoracoscopy. Ann Thorac Surg 1993;56: 863–866.
12. McKenna RJ. Lobectomy by video-assisted thoracic surgery with mediastinal node sampling for lung cancer. J Thorac Cardiovasc Surg 1994;107:879–882.
13. Rendina EA, Venuta F, De Giacomo T, et al. Comparative merits of thoracoscopy, mediastinoscopy, and mediastinotomy for mediastinal biopsy. Ann Thorac Surg 1994;57: 992–995.
14. Roviaro G, Varoli F, Rebuffat C, et al. Major pulmonary resections: pneumonectomies and lobectomies. Ann Thorac Surg 1993;56:779–783.
15. Rovario G, Rebuffat C, Varoli F, Vergani C, Maciocco M, Scalambra SM. Videothoracoscopic excision of mediastinal masses: indications and technique. Ann Thorac Surg 1994;58:1679–1684.
16. Shapira OM, Aldea GS, Fonger JD, Shemin RJ. Video-assisted thoracic surgical techniques in the diagnosis and management of pericardial effusion in patients with advanced lung cancer. Chest 1993;104:1262–1263.
17. Shennib HA, Landreneau R, Mulder DS, Mack M. Video-assisted thoracoscopic wedge resection of T1 lung cancer in high-risk patients. Ann Surg 1993;218:555–560.
18. Walsh GL, Nesbitt JC. Tumor implants after thoracoscopic resection of a metastatic sarcoma. Ann Thorac Surg 1995;59:215–216.

47/C
Minimally Invasive Surgery in Gynecologic Oncology

T. SCOTT JENNINGS AND PETER DOTTINO

The past 20 years have seen the applications of laparoscopy expand from diagnostic and sterilization procedures to include the surgical treatment of most benign gynecologic diseases (28). Recently, investigators have attempted to define the integration of this technology into the management of gynecologic cancer, a realm traditionally dominated by the lower midline incision and long recovery times (14). Gynecologic oncologists, although cognizant of the potential for savings in terms of patient recovery and morbidity that minimally invasive surgery (MIS) may offer, have emphasized the need for caution in the application of this new technology (1, 16, 27). Assessing the benefit of MIS in gynecologic cancer has centered upon two questions: which disease sites are most amenable to improved management by MIS and, even more important, are there data to suggest that MIS may negatively impact the prognosis of these patients?

Historical Note

Investigators at the National Cancer Institute first identified the ability of laparoscopy to safely upstage 36% of patients referred with early ovarian cancer in the 1970s. Serious limitations were found, however, when the "peritoneoscopy" did not demonstrate obvious metastatic disease (18). Similarly, investigators at the Mount Sinai Hospital identified the utility of laparoscopy for surgical end staging in the 1980s, once again with serious limitations on "negative" findings that required laparotomy for more meticulous identification of occult disease (6). The first laparoscopic hysterectomy was reported in 1989 for benign disease (24) and was an important demonstration that relatively major pelvic procedures might be feasible by methods other than laparotomy or vaginal colpotomy. The widespread adoption of laparoscopy for adnexal masses was delayed until more accurate diagnostic imaging techniques such as transvaginal sonography were available. Currently, MIS has become the gold standard by which to manage most benign adnexal disease (3). Accordingly, the same investigators who demonstrated the ability to resect most female reproductive organs were also the first to report the staging of frank ovarian cancer in 1990 (25). In a very short time, nearly all gynecologic oncology procedures other than cytoreduction and exenteration have been demonstrated to be feasible (Table 47.4).

Operative laparoscopy has been, and continues to be, strongly criticized in its application to gynecologic cancer, and this is likely to continue until the benefits of MIS are securely documented. Importantly, however, not only must the procedure be advanced in the hands of a few capable surgeons, but it must be reproducible in surgical suites everywhere. In an attempt to control for both of these needs, some conceptual understanding of MIS in gynecologic cancer is useful. One method of approach is to categorize the reported studies as demonstrated in Table 47.5. In this manner, it may be possible to identify laparoscopic approaches which may truly offer advantages over laparotomy and those which are merely possible but unlikely to benefit the majority of the 50,000 American women who each year are diagnosed with genital tract cancers.

Table 47.4. Laparoscopic Procedures in Gynecologic Oncology Patients for Which Feasibility Studies Have Been Performed

Ovarian carcinoma
Staging of apparent early malignancy
Survey for occult disease prior to second-look laparotomy
Complete surgical end staging after cytotoxic therapy
Cervical carcinoma
Pelvic lymph node sampling
Para-aortic lymph node sampling
Assistance of radical vaginal (Schuata) hysterectomy
Assistance of radical abdominal (Wertheim) hysterectomy
Bilateral oophoropexy prior to definitive irradiation therapy
Endometrial carcinoma
Assistance of vaginal hysterectomy
Pelvic lymph node sampling
Para-aortic lymph node sampling

Table 47.5. Proposed Concept for Integration of Minimally Invasive Surgical Approaches to Cancer

Preclinical models
Computer simulation models (virtual reality)
Animal models
Feasibility studies
Case reports and series, generally by experts in the field
Controlled clinical trials
Attempts to apply rationally new surgical approaches to subgroups of patients, preferably via multi-institutional co-operative groups

Chief Indications

Although many controversial points are raised by the expansion of MIS to gynecologic cancer, and no procedure has yet been validated by controlled clinical trials, a number of procedures appear reproducible and safe in selected subsets of patients who may have much to gain from MIS.

OVARIAN CARCINOMA

In the setting of metastatic ovarian cancer, primary surgical debulking is clearly a cornerstone of therapy that currently leaves little place for minimally invasive approaches. Surgical staging of early ovarian cancer requires intact tumor removal, intraperitoneal inspection, cytologic washings, omental biopsy, pelvic and aortic lymph node biopsy, and biopsy of suspicious peritoneal surfaces, all of which can, technically, be accomplished through the laparoscope. If MIS is to play a role in the staging of these potentially curable early cancers, there must be no question about the adequacy of the specimens or of the procedure. There are now several reports describing laparoscopic staging of early ovarian cancer. The first, in 1990 (25), described a 5-hour staging procedure that was still incomplete by virtue of omitting biopsy of the para-aortic nodes. In 1992, Querleu described two cases of early ovarian cancer in which sampling of the infrarenal para-aortic nodes was successfully completed by laparoscopy (22). These investigators identified important issues regarding the feasibility of laparoscopic aortic lymph node sampling, especially patient selection. Although both of these investigators have demonstrated a possible role for laparoscopy, reports of delay of staging and therapy for patients after laparoscopic management of adnexal masses later found to be malignant are disturbing (16). In addition, cases are now being reported of trocar site metastases after dragging specimens through the unprotected abdominal wall and skin after intraoperative rupture of malignant ovarian masses (8, 13). This will undoubtedly impair the prognosis for these patients, and may seriously retard the application of laparoscopy to patients with early ovarian malignancy. It is imperative that any surgeon who approaches this disease at an early stage with MIS understand the potential for harm to the patient if the procedure is eventually proven inadequate (i.e., the risk of delay in therapy and of potentially preventable death in the setting of early but undetected metastases or poorly understood subtleties of laparoscopy). Further experience in laparoscopic end staging will be needed before a firm recommendation can be made for this indication.

Surgical end staging of patients after chemotherapy for ovarian cancer remains a controversial topic in itself, but it represents the definitive procedure for determination of treatment response in this difficult disease (6). One of the primary critiques of "second-look" laparotomy is the incapacitation of the patient and the potential morbidity of the procedure. MIS is unlikely to improve any survival advantage of surgical end staging that is already possible with open laparotomy, but it may facilitate surgical end staging in two ways. The first is the use of laparoscopy to survey for unsuspected but grossly evident peritoneal disease. Investigators at the Mount Sinai Medical Center have used open laparoscopy prior to formal second-look laparotomy since 1982, sparing a significant percentage of our patients the need for laparotomy in the setting of small-volume (occult) peritoneal metastases (Fig. 47.6) (6). Second, it may be possible to offer complete surgical end staging using operative laparoscopic techniques. In this regard, Canis and co-workers reported that there were no more recurrences in a series of patients deemed free of disease after second-look laparoscopy than those who underwent second-look laparotomy (2). Further studies with long-term follow-up will be necessary to determine if laparoscopic end staging is as sensitive to occult disease as formal second-look laparotomy.

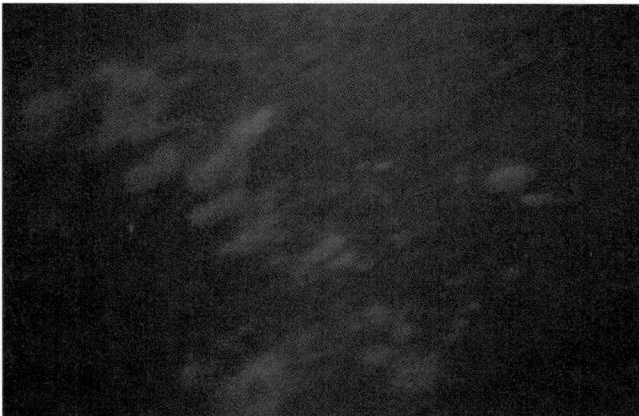

Figure 47.6. Laparoscopic visualization of metastatic nodules less than 1 mm thick on the right hemidiaphragm in a 42-year-old patient after excellent clinical response to intensive chemotherapy for ovarian carcinoma. Biochemical markers and CT were normal immediately preoperatively.

CERVICAL CARCINOMA

Cervical carcinoma is the last gynecologic malignancy still clinically staged by physical examination. Retroperitoneal metastases have been found to be one of the most important prognostic indicators of survival in patients with cervical cancer, yet they are poorly predicted by noninvasive techniques (20, 21). Unlike ovarian, endometrial, and vulvar carcinoma, surgical staging has remained a research tool in the management of cervical cancer owing to the morbidity associated with formal staging laparotomy. Laparoscopic technology now exists to allow sampling of nodal chains in the pelvis, and a number of urologic studies have demonstrated the accuracy of endoscopic pelvic node sampling in prostatic and bladder carcinomas (26). Attention has been turned to the surgical staging of patients with cervical cancer by retroperitoneal endoscopy.

Several investigators have documented encouraging preliminary results with pretreatment laparoscopic lymphadenectomy using both intraperitoneal and extraperitoneal techniques (4, 10, 12, 23). As feasibility studies are completed, it is apparent that laparoscopic pelvic and para-aortic lymph node sampling are viable procedures that are reasonably accurate and remarkably more tolerable for the patient than open lymphadenectomy. In addition to the important prognostic information that laparoscopic node sampling may offer, some patients may see benefits in terms of treatment planning. Some options include offering those patients found to have negative nodes radical surgical resection, with or without neoadjuvant chemotherapy, whereas those with positive nodes may be offered investigational chemoradiation. Few studies have attempted to demonstrate the sensitivity of laparoscopic lymph node sampling in a comparative fashion with open lymphadenectomy. Investigators at the University of Arizona found one microscopic nodal metastasis in the parametria of 5 radical hysterectomy patients that was not detected by laparoscopic lymphadenectomy (4). Investigators at the University of Minnesota, however found no nodal metastases at laparotomy that were not detected by transperitoneal laparoscopic node sampling of 12 patients (12). In a similar series at the Mount Sinai Medical Center, we have found no discordance in pelvic lymph node metastasis among 11 radical surgical specimens following extraperitoneal laparoscopic sampling (15). Dargent extrapolated the false-negative rate of their extraperitoneal sampling procedure to be 3.8% based on the later pelvic sidewall recurrence rate among 105 patients with negative laparoscopic findings (10). Further study of the sensitivity of laparoscopic lymph node sampling procedures for all disease sites will be necessary to fully characterize the utility of these procedures. It appears that laparoscopy may provide the opportunity to sample important regional lymph nodes with minimal surgical trauma; however, neither laparoscopic lymph node sampling nor formal surgical staging is likely to be useful in situations in which lymph nodes have already been proven positive by fine-needle aspiration.

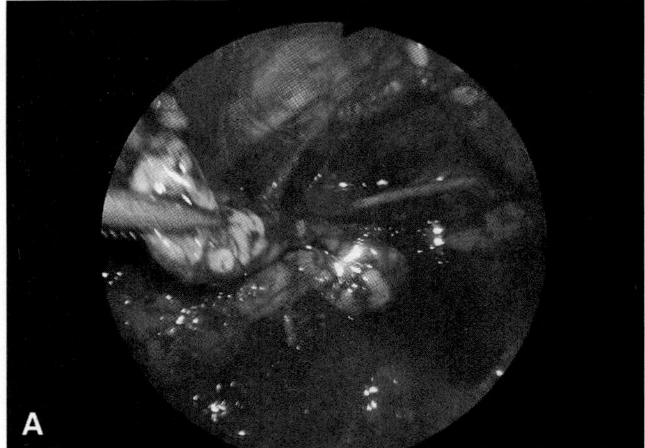

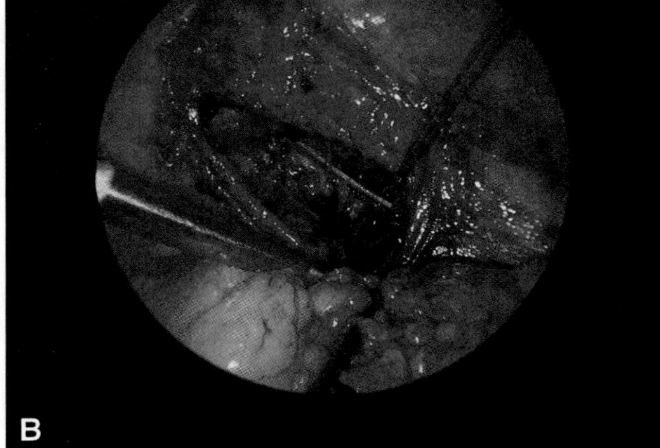

Figure 47.7. **A.** Laparoscopic pelvic lymph node sampling from a 60-year-old patient with clinical stage I endometrial cancer. **B.** Bifurcation of the common iliac artery after the laparoscopic dissection.

ENDOMETRIAL CARCINOMA

Surgical staging, hysterectomy, and bilateral adnexectomy are clearly the mainstays of contemporary management of nearly all patients with endometrial cancer (7). Abdominal laparotomy has been associated with higher surgical morbidity than vaginal surgery (11). The adoption of vaginal hysterectomy for the management of cancer of the uterine corpus has only recently been addressed, since the utility of MIS to sample pelvic and aortic lymph nodes was demonstrated (Fig. 47.7). Authors from both the Universities of Arizona and Tennessee concurrently published the first case reports of surgical staging of endometrial carcinoma with the use of laparoscopic lymphadenectomy and laparoscopically assisted vaginal hysterectomy in 1992 (5, 19). Both teams concluded that the laparoscopic procedures required long operative times (2 to 4 hours) and costly equipment but that these disadvantages might be offset by faster patient recovery and shorter hospital stay. As mentioned earlier, lymph node sampling for malignancies of the pelvis has been aggressively pursued and appears to be sensitive for the detection of lymphatic metastases. If the techniques of laparoscopic hysterectomy, bilateral adnexectomy, and staging can be proven to be both safe and effective, it may be inferred that laparoscopic management of endometrial cancer may offer the patient many of the same benefits that endoscopic treatment offers patients with benign gynecologic diseases. To this end, the multi-institutional co-operative Gynecologic Oncology Group is undertaking a large randomized trial of laparoscopically assisted vaginal hysterectomy and adnexectomy with surgical staging in clinical stage I endometrial cancer, begun in 1995. This is an important study of the first randomized clinical trial using MIS in a specific disease site.

Future of Minimally Invasive Surgery

Even as feasibility studies are completed and clinical trials are commencing in an attempt to study the utility of MIS in gynecologic cancer, new applications are being developed. Laparoscopy has been reported to improve the surgical management of early-stage cervical cancer through the laparoscopic assistance of radical vaginal hysterectomy. Several investigators have advocated a return to the radical vaginal hysterectomy (Schauta's procedure) for women with negative pelvic nodes at laparoscopic assessment, reporting excellent results (9, 17). A small series of laparoscopic abdominal radical hysterectomies in combination with pelvic node sampling was recently reported, although the advantages of this nearly complete abdominal approach over that of radical vaginal surgery are not yet known (28). Other innovative applications of laparoscopy to cervical cancer include laparoscopic pelvic "lid" placement before pelvic irradiation and the laparoscopic suspension of ovaries out of pelvic irradiation fields in an attempt to abrogate radiation toxicity.

Results

Only feasibility studies have been concluded for the application of MIS, and accurate representation of the real complication rates and impact of laparoscopy in each particular disease site or by procedure are remarkably sparse.

Another method to see the results of aggressive application of minimally invasive surgery to patients with gynecologic cancer is to demonstrate the effects of the method in a rather large conglomerate of patients undergoing surgery for known or suspected ovarian, endometrial, or cervical cancer. As these methods were recently learned and taught in our gynecologic oncology service between the years of 1991 and 1993, it is possible to utilize outcome-based methods to demonstrate the effects of incorporating laparoscopy in these patients, both before and after this time period. Comparative analysis of the 12-month academic years of 1990–1991 and 1993–1994 on the academic gynecologic service at Mount Sinai is demonstrated in Table 47.6. The use of laparoscopy was increased dramatically for the 2 years of study concomitantly with a decreased utilization of laparotomy. During this time, a significant decrease ($P < .0001$ by ANOVA) in mean length of stay (LOS) was noted for patients undergoing chemotherapy or palliative care. The improvement in LOS for surgical patients was limited to the four procedures in which laparoscopy was utilized most aggressively, and no improvement was noted for patients managed by laparotomy or vaginal surgical approaches. Despite the shift in surgical approach, no difference was detected in the frequency of surgical complications.

The surgical patients in 1993–1994 were found to have a mean LOS 3.5 days less than the patients in 1990–1991. Owing to this reduction in mean LOS, 1500 fewer hospital days were necessary for the patients on this service. Although not all of this reduction in hospital stay may be attributed to the change in surgical approaches, a large portion of the change does indeed appear to be the result of increased utilization of laparoscopy. The cost to the surgeons for this integration of operative laparoscopy was 24 months of education and refinement of new surgical approaches for a limited number of procedures. The data strongly suggest that aggressive utilization of MIS for patients with gynecologic malignancy may have major medical and economic impact.

Table 47.6. The Impact of Minimally Invasive Surgery on a Gynecologic Oncology Service, 1990–1994

	1990–1991 (12 mo)	1993–1994 (12 mo)	
Total admissions (No.)	776	974	
Surgical admissions (No.)	306	370	
Gynecologic malignancies (No.)	254	263	NSD
Use of postop chemotherapy (%)	22	20	NSD
Length of stay, all (mean days)	6.4	4.8	($P < .0001$)
Length of stay, surgical admits (mean days)	9.9	6.4	($P < .0001$)
Postop complications (%)	7.2	7.6	NSD

NSD = Not significantly different.

Conclusions

The use of MIS in patients with gynecologic cancer is in its infancy but has the potential for improving the recovery of selected patients from the surgical aspects of their therapy, and may lessen the time to initiating adjuvant chemotherapy. Skilled endoscopic surgeons have demonstrated the feasibility of operative laparoscopy for ovarian, cervical, and endometrial cancer, yet the mere feasibility of a surgical procedure does not validate its utility, and controlled clinical trials are necessary to demonstrate where MIS will be of use in this unique patient population. For this reason, it is intuitive that gynecologic oncologists with interest in endoscopic surgery should be encouraged to receive high-quality training that will maximize their current abilities and allow them to lead further development. Controlled trials of laparoscopic surgical staging of endometrial cancer by a co-operative group are now under way in the United States, and more such trials will be needed.

References

1. Barber HRK. Operative laparoscopy: a passing fad? Female Patient 1993;18:10–12.
2. Canis M, Chapron C, Mage G, Pouly JL, et al. Technique et resultats preliminaires du second look per-coelioscopique dans les tumeurs epitheliales malignes de l'ovarie. J Gynecol Obstet Biol Reprod 1992;21:655–663.
3. Canis M, Pouly JL, Mage G, et al. Laparoscopic adnexal surgery: the gold standard. In Women's Health Today. Edited by D Popkin, LJ Peddle. New York: Parthenon, 1994.
4. Childers JM, Hatch K, Surwit EA. The role for laparoscopic lymphadenectomy in the management of cervical carcinoma. Gynecol Oncol 1992;47:38–43.
5. Childers JM, Surwit EA. Combined laparoscopic and vaginal surgery for the management of two cases of stage I endometrial cancer. Gynecol Oncol 1992;45:46.
6. Cohen CJ, Goldberg JD, Holland JF, et al. Improved therapy with cisplatin regimens for patients with ovarian carcinoma as measured by surgical end-staging (second look operation). Am J Obstet Gynecol 1983;145:955–963.
7. Creasman WT, Morrow CP, Bundy L, et al. Surgical pathologic spread patterns of endometrial cancer: a Gynecologic Oncology Group Study. Cancer 1987;60:2035.
8. Crouet H, Heron JF. Dissemination of ovarian cancer during celioscopic surgery. A real danger. Presse-Med 1991;20:1738–1739.
9. Dargent D. A new future for Schuata's operation through presurgical retroperitoneal pelviscopy. Eur J Gynecol Oncol 1987;8:292–296.

10. Dargent D, Arnould P, Roy M. The value and the limits of panoramic retroperitoneal pelviscopy in gynecological cancer. Paper presented at the Annual Meeting of the Society of Gynecologic Oncologists, March 1992.
11. Dicker RC, Greenspan JR, Strouss LT, et al. Complications of abdominal and vaginal hysterectomy among women of reproductive age in the United States. Am J Obstet Gynecol 1982;144:841.
12. Fowler J, Carter, Carlson R, Maslonkowski L, Byers L, Carson L, Twiggs L. Lymph node yield from laparoscopic lymphadenectomy in cervical cancer: a comparative study. Gynecol Oncol 1993;51:187–192.
13. Hsiu JG, Given FT, Kemp GM. Tumor implantation after diagnostic laparoscopic biopsy of serous ovarian tumors of low malignant potential. Obstet Gynecol 1986;68: 90s-93s.
14. Jennings TS, Dottino PR. The application of operative laparoscopy to gynecologic oncology. Curr Opin Obstet Gynecol 1994;6:80–85.
15. Jennings TS, Dottino PR, Beddoe AM. Unpublished data.
16. Maiman M, Seltzer V, Boyce J. Laparoscopic excision of ovarian neoplasms subsequently found to be malignant. Obstet Gynecol 1991;77:563–565.
17. Nezhat C, Burrell M, Nezhat F, et al. Laparoscopic radical hysterectomy with paraaortic and pelvic node dissection. Am J Obstet Gynecol 1992;166:864–865.
18. Ozols RC, Fisher R, Anderson T, et al. Peritoneoscopy in the management of ovarian cancer. Am J Obstet Gynecol 1981;140:611.
19. Photopulos G, Stovall TG, Summitt RL. Laparoscopic-assisted vaginal hysterectomy, bilateral salpingo-oophorectomy, and pelvic lymph node sampling for endometrial cancer. J Gynecol Surg 1992;8:91–94.
20. Pilleron JP, Durand JC, Hamelin JP. Location of lymph node invasion in cancer of the uterine cervix: study of 140 cases treated at the Curie Foundation. Am J Obstet Gynecol 1974;119:453–457.
21. Piver MS, Chung WS. Prognostic significance of cervical lesion size and pelvic node metastases in cervical carcinoma. Obstet Gynecol 1975;46:507–510.
22. Querleu D. Laparoscopic para-aortic node sampling in gynecologic oncology: a preliminary experience. Gynecol Oncol 1993;49:24–29.
23. Querleu D, Leblanc E, Castelain B. Laparoscopic pelvic lymphadenectomy in the staging of early carcinoma of the cervix. Am J Obset Gynecol 1991;164:579–581.
24. Reich H, DeCaprio J, McGlynn F. Laparoscopic hysterectomy. J Gynecol Surg 1989;5: 213.
25. Reich H, McGlynn F, Wilkie W. Laparoscopic management of stage I ovarian cancer: a case report. J Reprod Med 1990;35:601–605.
26. Schuessler WW, Vancaillie TG, Reich H, Griffith DP. Transperitoneal endosurgical lymphadenectomy in patients with localized prostate cancer. J Urol 1991;145:988.
27. Schwartz PE. An oncologic view of when to do endoscopic surgery. Clin Obstet Gynecol 1991;34:467–472.
28. Sedlacek T, Campion MM, Reich H, Sedlacek T. Laparoscopic radical hysterectomy: a feasibility study. Paper presented at the Society of Gynecologic Oncologists, San Fransisco, Feb 21, 1995.
29. Sutton C. Operative laparoscopy. Curr Opin Obstet Gynecol 1992;4:430–438.

47/D

Minimally Invasive Surgery for Urinary Tract Cancer

NELSON N. STONE

The use of minimally invasive surgery (MIS) in urologic oncology is relatively new. The initial application of MIS had been limited to laparoscopic pelvic lymph node dissection (PLND) for prostate cancer staging. Its use has now been applied to nodal assessment of other sites, organ extirpation, and nonsurgical treatment of prostate cancer. Diseases that have either been evaluated or treated by this technology include cancer of the prostate, bladder, kidney, penis, and testis.

Several types of minimally invasive technologies are currently being used in the diagnosis and treatment of urologic cancers. For diagnostic assessment these include ultrasound-guided transrectal needle biopsy of the prostate and of the seminal vesicles, for determining local extent of prostate cancer, and laparoscopic lymph node dissection, for determining nodal status in patients with cancers of the prostate, testis, bladder, and penis. For therapeutic intervention, MIS has been applied to laparoscopic organ removal (nephrectomy) in patients with renal cancer and in the treatment of localized prostate cancer by brachytherapy and cryoablation.

Application

PROSTATE CANCER

Prostate cancer is the most common extrategumental malignancy in men. The American Cancer Society predicts 317,100 new cases in 1996 (4). Of these, 240,000 patients (75%) will be candidates for treatment for apparent localized disease (10, 42). These men are potential candidates for MIS for diagnosis and treatment of this disease.

Staging of localized prostate cancer has always been problematic in that more than 50% will be "upstaged" at the time of surgery. Some 12 to 20% of the clinical T1b to T2c prostate cancers have seminal vesicle involvement (T3c) and 5 to 10% harbor occult pelvic lymph node micrometastases (N+). When Gleason grading criteria are applied, these values can rise as high as 35 and 32%, respectively (1, 6, 11, 23, 26, 30, 31, 37, 49).

Several studies have been done that demonstrate the benefit of analyzing presurgical clinical data using multiple individual and logistic regression analyses. These data have usually been derived from radical prostatectomy series where the significant prognostic variables were determined retrospectively (1, 26, 31, 49). Since final pathologic stage is an important factor in deciding the preferred form of therapy, accurate staging by MIS prior to definitive therapy is critical.

Transrectal ultrasonography of the prostate has been a major benefit to urologists by improving diagnostic yield in patients undergoing prostate biopsy. Grading of tumor histology also significantly affects therapeutic strategy. This technology has also been used to biopsy the seminal vesicles (SVB) to determine if a patient with apparent clinical T1b-T2c disease has T3c disease (45, 49).

SEMINAL VESICLE BIOPSY

The SVB is performed in the office by taking three needle biopsies under ultrasound guidance from each seminal vesicle at the base of the prostate. The tip of the spring-loaded biopsy needle is positioned just outside the posterior wall of the seminal vesicle (on the anterior rectal wall) and fired, sampling both anterior and posterior walls of the seminal vesicles. Patients are prepared as for prostate biopsy with an enema and oral fluoroquinolone prior to the procedure. Anesthesia is not necessary because the rectal wall and prostate are relatively poorly supplied with pain fibers.

Data from radical prostatectomy series where seminal vesicle involvement was determined from the final pathologic specimen can be compared to data obtained from studies where SVB was done prior to treatment (Table 47.7) (1, 26, 29, 30, 31, 49). As can be seen from the data, SVB prior to considering definitive therapy can identify about two-thirds of patients who have involvement of the seminal vesicles (stage T3c) with prostate cancer. If high-risk criteria are used to decide which patients should undergo SVB, the diagnostic yield can be significantly increased. Using multivariate stepwise logistic regression analysis in the author's SVB series, high Gleason score ($P < .0001$), PSA ($P = .007$), and clinical stage ($P = .02$) were all predictors of seminal vesicle involvement. These data (Table 47.8) agree with the

Table 47.7. Frequency of Seminal Vesicle Involvement with Prostate Cancer

Investigator	Patients (No.)	Vesicle involvement (%)
Found by radical prostatectomy		
Zeitman (49)	62	12 (19)
Blackwell (1)	311	50 (16)
Catalona (7)	250	32 (13)
Total	623	94 (15.1)
Detected by transrectal ultrasound-guided biopsy		
Terris (45)	73	8/12 (11/16)[a]
Vallancien (46)	67	11/18 (16/27)[a]
Author's data	157	23 (14.6)
Total	297	42/53 (14/17.8)[a]

[a] First value is amount detected by biopsy; second is seminal vesicle involvement found at subsequent radical prostatectomy.

Table 47.8. Frequency of Seminal Vesicle Involvement Stratified by Gleason Score, PSA, and Clinical Stage

Investigator	Gleason >6 (%)	PSA >10 (%)	Stage >T2b (%)
Author's data	34	20	20
Oesterling (26)	31	13	13[a]
Partin (31)	15	18	Not reported

[a] Represents stage T2c.

data from the radical prostatectomy series when the prognostic variables are similarly stratified (1, 7, 3, 26, 30, 31, 46, 47, 49).

The SVB is well tolerated and results reproducible: all 157 patients in the author's series had confirmed seminal vesicle involvement upon pathologic review. The procedure was associated with transient hematospermia, which was self-limiting. There were no prostatic or seminal vesicle infections and no long-term complications associated with SVB.

These data demonstrate that the SVB can identify patients who are clinical candidates for radical prostatectomy yet harbor microscopic disease in the seminal vesicles. With disease recurrence ranging from 57 to 76% in patients with T3c prostate cancer following radical prostatectomy, other modalities of treatment, such as neoadjuvant hormone therapy, might be worth considering (6, 37, 48). Several investigators found that significant "downstaging" to pathologic T2b could occur with neoadjuvant hormonal therapy (11, 23). In addition, radiation therapy protocols utilizing androgen deprivation or higher-dose radiation therapy via conformal technique might be more appropriate for these patients (48).

The number of patients who might be upstaged by the SVB is not insignificant: with 14.6% of the clinical T1a-T2c prostate cancer patients having seminal vesicle involvement, approximately 27,000 men (0.146 × 183,000 diagnosed with localized disease in 1995) might be correctly identified with T3c disease and offered alternative treatment. Given these results, it seems prudent to recommend SVB for patients who present with localized prostate cancer and have a Gleason score above 4, PSA above 10 ng/ml, or a palpable lesion T2a or greater.

LAPAROSCOPIC PELVIC LYMPH NODE DISSECTION

LPLND is a safe and effective method of removing lymph nodes commonly involved with prostate cancer (28, 29, 35, 39). Rukstalis performed LPLND on patients with clinically localized prostate cancer. In 20 patients, this was followed by an open lymph node dissection with removal of remaining lymph nodes in the dissection area. Using this method he found that the LPLND was able to remove 87 to 95% of the desired lymph nodes (34).

Unlike the open pelvic lymph node dissection, which requires a lower abdominal incision and lengthy hospital stay, the LPLND can be performed through a four-puncture incision. Trocars are passed into the abdominal cavity (either intraperitoneal or extraperitoneal) through which a lens and camera system allows for surgical removal of the obturator nodes. This procedure can usually be accomplished with an overnight hospital stay (40).

Prognostic factors affect the outcome of LPLND in a fashion similar to the manner in which they affect open pelvic lymph node dissections. The overall frequency of positive lymph nodes in the author's series is 10.8%, nearly identical to the rate of 11% reported by Partin in a series of 1,058 men undergoing radical prostatectomy and open staging pelvic lymphadenectomy (31). In our series, multivariate analysis revealed that both SVB and high Gleason score significantly predicted for positive pelvic lymph nodes ($P = .0001$ and $P = .003$, respectively) while PSA and clinical stage were not significant. Positive lymph nodes were found in 32% of patients with Gleason grade 7 or greater as compared with 1.7% for patients with lower-grade lesions, and in 48% of those patients with a positive SVB. These results are similar to Partin's series, in which 25% of patients with Gleason grades of 7 or greater had positive pelvic lymph nodes, as compared with 6% of patients with lesser-grade lesions (31).

A PSA greater than 20 ng/ml was also associated with increased risk (24%) of positive nodes, while those with stages T2b-T2c had a 17% risk of positive nodes. Five patients (3.8%) experienced minor surgical complications from the LPLND. No patient required an exploratory laparotomy for complications. Hospital stay averaged fewer than 2 days.

Patients with pelvic lymph node metastases are considered by many to be destined to develop distant metastases (13, 15, 22, 23, 32, 36, 38). For this reason, controlling the primary disease may not affect the subsequent development of distant metastases in these patients. In an analysis by Leibel, local control of the primary lesion did not decrease the likelihood of developing distant metastases in node-positive patients (24). LPLND can be an important tool for properly selecting node-negative patients for curative therapy, especially those with high-risk criteria who are to undergo radiation therapy, where normally a lymph node analysis is not planned.

These data demonstrate that 10% of patients who present with T1a-T2c prostate cancer have microscopic disease in the pelvic lymph nodes. Using univariate analysis, those patients with positive SVB, combined Gleason grade of 7 or above, or PSA over 20 ng/ml had positive LPLND rates of 48, 32, and 24%, respectively. These patients should undergo staging LPLND prior to instituting curative therapy.

PROSTATE SEED IMPLANTATION

Once patients are properly staged, treatment of localized disease (T1b-T2c) can be initiated. In 1996, the majority (more than 100,000) will have radical prostatectomy. While half as many will be treated by radiation therapy, only a minority will receive brachytherapy (prostate seed implantation).

By the 1980s and early 1990s, technologic advances in ultrasound imaging and three-dimensional (3-D) simulation permitted further refinements in prostate implantation. First, the introduction of the biplanar transrectal ultrasound probe and its incorporation into a treatment device allowed for real time interactive placement of radioactive seeds into the prostate (Fig. 47.8) (17). Second, the development of 3-D simulation software combined with digitalization of postimplant images allowed for accurate, precise determination of dose delivered to both the prostate and contiguous structures (bladder, urethra, and rectum) (Fig. 47.9). These new tools permitted the refinement of interstitial therapy for prostate cancer with a more accurate way of delivering the dose to the prostate gland. This new technique provides an alternative to radical prostatectomy or external-beam therapy for men with localized prostate cancer (2, 3, 5, 9, 14, 19, 20, 21, 33, 41).

The equipment required for interstitial therapy consists of the radioactive isotopes to deliver the radiation to the prostate gland, the instruments to insert these isotopes, and ultrasound hardware to perform the real-time implant. There are two categories of interstitial implants: permanent and temporary implants. Temporary implants require patient isolation and have only limited indications for use, mostly for advanced localized prostate cancer.

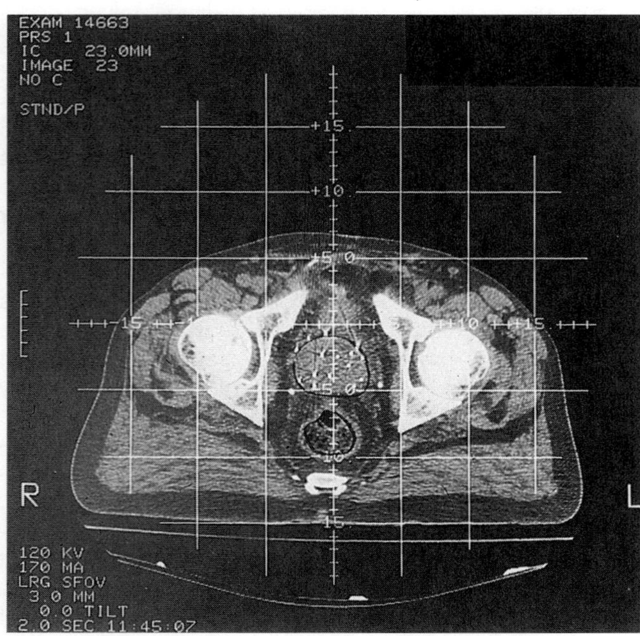

Figure 47.8. CT image through midsection of prostate demonstrating symmetric placement of radioactive seeds.

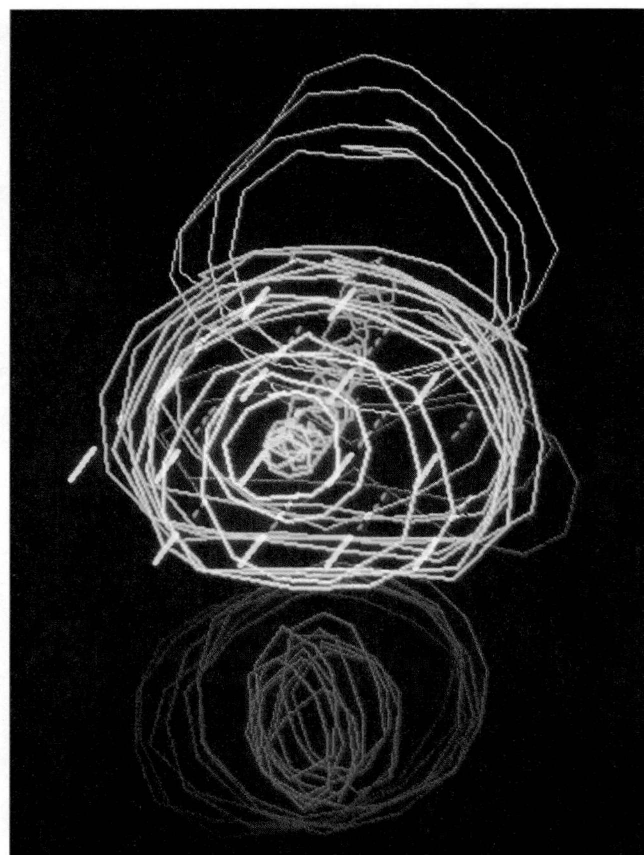

Figure 47.9. Three-dimensional reconstruction of CT images demonstrating accurate distribution of radioactive sources in prostate.

Permanent implants deliver their dose over a long time. Gold (^{198}Au) and iodine (^{125}I) have been used commonly in the past. Palladium (^{103}Pd) is a newer isotope. Because of the difficulty in handling ^{198}Au, owing to its relatively high energy and dose rate, most centers prefer not to implant this isotope. Both ^{125}I and ^{103}Pd have lower energy and longer half lives, 60 and 17 days, respectively.

Generally, ^{125}I is preferred for low-grade tumors, while Pd 103 is chosen for the faster-growing, high-grade lesions. This is based on the dose rate (number of radioactive disintegrations per unit time) for the isotope; however, palladium has less energy (22 keV) than iodine (28 keV) and a shorter depth of delivery of the radiation dose. Thus, palladium is inherently more difficult to implant to ensure adequate dose coverage to the entire gland. For these reasons, ^{125}I is selected for patients who present with a Gleason grade of 3 or under (score below 6) and Pd 103 for patients who have a Gleason grade of 4 (score over 7).

Real-time prostate implantation requires the availability of dedicated ultrasound hardware. Seeds are implanted into the prostate via an applicator (Mick -200 TP, Mick Radio-Nuclear Instruments, Bronx, NY) through which the radioactive sources are passed into a needle or trocar (Mick TP needle) which has been placed in the prostate.

The largest experience using permanent radioisotope implants for localized prostate cancer comes from the Northwest Tumor Institute in Seattle, Washington. Patients with early-stage T1-T2 lesions underwent preplanned ultrasound-guided transperineal implants. ^{125}I was used in 244 patients with Gleason scores of 2 to 6 and ^{103}Pd in 47 patients with Gleason scores of 7 or greater. With a median follow-up of 37 months (range 12 to 78 months) 93% of patients had their PSA fall below 4 ng/ml. Only 5% (14/291) had evidence of local or distant failure (2, 3, 14). Others report similar levels of success for shorter periods (9, 19, 41).

CRYOABLATION OF THE PROSTATE

Cryoablation of the prostate is also a "reborn" minimally invasive surgical technique that owes its renewed appeal to ultrasound imaging. Rather than requiring an open perineal incision or transurethral instillation of liquid nitrogen, transrectal imaging permits percutaneous placement of catheters through which pass liquid nitrogen. The freeze-thaw cycle causes cell death and destruction of the cancer cells. Real-time imaging allows control of the "ice ball" with destruction of prostatic tissue down to capsule and seminal vesicles.

Advantages of cryotherapy include its percutaneous approach and resultant short hospital stay, minimal blood loss, and rapid recovery. Potential candidates include T1b-T3c lesions in patients with newly diagnosed cancers and in those who have failed radiation therapy.

To perform the procedure, general or spinal anesthesia is required and the patient is placed in the dorsal lithotomy position. Five probes are placed under ultrasound guidance through the perineum into the prostate. Liquid nitrogen is circulated through the probes, creating multiple concentric ice balls. The ice balls extend to the anterior rectal wall posteriorly, the seminal vesicles superiorly, and to the prostate apex caudally. Urethral warming (with a special device) is necessary to prevent sloughing and urinary sphincter damage. Suprapubic drainage is required because of the risk of urinary retention associated with the procedure.

Initial experience with this treatment modality has been favorable. Positive biopsy rates at 3 and 12 months following treatment are between 15 and 30%. Significant complications include urethrorectal fistula (0.5 to 3%) and incontinence (3.2 to 10%). Impotence occurs in most patients. Complication rates are higher in association with previous radiation therapy (25, 27).

Summary

MIS has improved quality of life for patients with urologic cancers. Rather than requiring exploratory laparotomy to stage GU cancers, laparoscopy can adequately determine nodal status. In high-risk patients with prostate, bladder, penile and urethral cancer, pelvic lymph node dissection can be performed. Considerably more skill is required to perform LRLND in men with testis cancer. Patients with negative computed tomographic (CT) scans of the retroperitoneum and high-risk T1 or T2 nonseminomatous testicular lesions are candidates for this procedure. The advantages of such an approach are rapid recovery and early institution of chemotherapy in those with a positive result (16, 18, 43, 44).

Organ removal with the laparoscope has generally been limited to the kidney when small renal lesions are present. Laparoscopic removal of a poorly functioning kidney involved with benign disease has become an accepted practice. Laparoscopic nephrectomy for renal cell carcinoma is a controversial procedure, owing to the risks of incomplete removal and the difficulties of organ entrapment, morcellation, and retrieval (8, 12). When problems are solved, more urologists may eventually consider this as an acceptable surgical approach.

It is clear from the preceding discussion that MIS in urologic oncology is an evolving field and more changes are yet to come. Recent advances in technology have enabled the diagnostic and therapeutic modalities to be perfected to their current status. These improvements have improved the quality of life without increasing costs in patients diagnosed with GU cancers. Such improvements have generally been welcomed by treating physicians and patients alike.

References

1. Blackwell KL, Bostwick DG, Meyers RP, Zinke H, Oesterling JE. Combining prostate specific antigen and gland volume to predict more reliable pathological stage: the influence of prostate specific antigen cancer density. J Urol 1994;151:1565.
2. Blasko JC, Ragde H, Grimm PD. Transperineal ultrasound-guided implantation of the prostate: morbidity and complications. Scand J Urol Nephrol 1991;137(suppl): 113–118.
3. Blasko JC, Grimm PD, Radge H. Brachytherapy and organ preservation in the management of carcinoma of the prostate. Semin Radiat Oncol 1993;3:240–249.
4. Boring C, Squires T, Tong T, Montgomery S. Cancer statistics, 1994. CA Cancer J Clin 1994;44:7.
5. Brosman SA, Tokita K. Transrectal ultrasound-guided interstitial radiation therapy for localized prostate cancer. Urology 1991;38:4:372–376.
6. Carter GE, Lieskowsk,G, Skinner D, Petrovich Z. Results of local and/or systemic adjuvant therapy in the management of pathological stage C or D1 prostate cancer following radical prostatectomy. J Urol 1989;142:1266.
7. Catalona WJ, Bigg SW. Nerve-sparing radical prostatectomy: evaluation of results after 250 patients. J Urol 1990;143:538.
8. Clayman RV, Kavoussi LR, Long SR, Dierks SM, Meretyk S, Soper NJ. Laparoscopic nephrectomy: initial report of pelviscopic organ ablation. J Endourol 1990;4:247.
9. Dattoli MJ, Wasserman S, Cash J. Wedding B, Sorace RA, Koval JM. Prostatic brachytherapy using palladium-103 for localized prostate cancer: a report of PSA response and toxicity. Int J Radiat Oncol Biol Phys 1994;30:102A.
10. DeAntoni E, Crawford ED, Stone N, Blum D, Berger E, Eisenberg M, Gambert S, Staggers F. Prostate cancer awareness week: a summary of key findings. Clin Invest Med 1992;16:444.
11. Fair WR, Aprikian A, Sogani P, Reuter V, Whitmore WF. The role of neoadjuvant hormonal manipulation in localized prostate cancer. Cancer 1993;71:1031.
12. Gaur DD. Laparoscopic operative retroperitoneoscopy: use of a new device. J Urol 1992;148:2:1137–1139.
13. Gervasi L, Mata J. Easley J, Wilbanks J, Seale-Hawkins C, Carlton C, Scardino P. Prognostic significance of lymph nodal metastases in prostate cancer. J Urol 1989;134: 332.
14. Grimm PD, Blasko JC, Radge H. Ultrasound guided transperineal implantation of iodine-125 and palladium-103 for the treatment of early stage prostate cancer. Technical concepts in planning, operative technique and evaluation. Urol Clinics NA 1994;2:11.
15. Hanks GE, Krall JM, Pilepilch MV. Comparison of pathologic and clinical evaluation of lymph nodes in prostate cancer. Implications of RTOG data for patient management and trial design and stratification. Int J Radiat Oncol Biol Phys 1992;23:239.
16. Herr HW, Whitmore WF, Sogani PC, Watson RC, Fair WR. Selection of testicular tumor patients for omission of retroperitoneal lymph node dissection. J Urol 1986;135: 500–503.
17. Holm HH, Juul N, Pederson JF, Hansen, Stroyer I. Transperineal iodine-125 seed implantation in prostatic cancer guided by transrectal ultrasonography. J Urol 1983;130: 283–286.
18. Hulbert JC, Fraley EE. Laparoscopic retroperitoneal lymphadenectomy. A new approach to pathologic staging of clinical stage I germ cell tumors of the testis. J Endourol 1992;6:123.
19. Kaye KW, Olson DJ, Payne JT. Detailed preliminary analysis of 125-iodine implantation

for localized prostate cancer using percutaneous approach. J Urol 1995;153: 1020–1025.
20. Kleinberg L, Wallner K, Roy J, Zelefsky M, Arterberry E, Fuks Z, Harrison L. Treatment-related symptoms during the first year following transperineal I-125 prostate implantation. Int J Radiat Oncol Biol Phys 1994;28:985–990.
21. Koprowski CD, Berkenstock KG, Borofski AM, Ziegler JC, Lightfoot MA, Brady LW. External beam irradiation versus 125 iodine implant in the definitive treatment of prostate cancer. Int J Radiat Oncol Biol Phys 1991;21:4:955–966.
22. Kramer S, Cline W, Farnham R, Carson C, Cox E, Hinshaw W, Paulson D. Prognosis of patients with stage D1 prostatic adenocarcinoma. J Urol 1981;125:817.
23. Labrie F, Dupont A, Cusan L, Gomez JL, Diamond P, Koutsieris M, Suburu R, Fadet Y, Lemay M, Tetu B, Emond J, Candas B. Downstaging of localized prostate cancer by neoadjuvant therapy with flutamide and Lupron: the first controlled and randomized trial. Clin Invest Med 1993;16:499.
24. Leibel S, Fuks Z, Zelefsky M, Whitmore W. The effect of local and regional treatment on the metastatic outcome in prostatic carcinoma with pelvic lymph node involvement. Int J Radiat Oncol Biol Phys 1993;28:7.
25. Miller RJ, Cohen JK, Merlotti LA. Percutaneous transperineal cryosurgical ablation of the prostate for the primary treatment of clinical stage C adenocarcinoma of the prostate. Urology 1994;44:170.
26. Oesterling JE, Brendler CB, Epstein JI, Kimball AW, Walsh PC. Correlation of clinical stage, serum prostatic acid phosphatase and preoperative Gleason grade with final pathological stage in 275 patients with clinically localized adenocarcinoma of the prostate. J Urol 1987;138:92.
27. Onik GM, Cohen JK, Reyes GD, Rubinsky B, Chang ZH, Baust J. Transrectal ultrasound guided percutaneous radical cryosurgical ablation of the prostate. Fifth International Prostate Cancer Update. Cancer 1993;72:1291–1299.
28. Parra RO, Andrus C, Boullier J. Staging laparoscopic pelvic lymph node dissection: comparison of results with open pelvic lymphadenectomy. J Urol 1992;147:875.
29. Parra RO, Andrus CH, Boullier JA. Staging laparoscopic pelvic lymph node dissection: experience and indications. Arch Surg 1992;127:1294.
30. Partin AW, Lee BR, Carmichael M, Walsh PC, Epstein JI. Radical prostatectomy for high grade disease: a reevaluation. J Urol 1994;151:1583.
31. Partin AW, Yoo J, Carter HB, Pearson JD, Chan DW, Epstein JI, Walsh PC. The use of prostate specific antigen, clinical and Gleason score to predict pathological stage in men with localized prostate cancer. J Urol 1993;150:110.
32. Paulson DF, Cline W, Koefoot R, Hinshaw W, Stephani S. The Uro-Oncology Research Group Extended field radiation therapy versus delayed hormonal therapy in node positive prostatic adenocarcinoma. J Urol 1982;127:935.
33. Priestly JB, Beyer DC. Guided brachytherapy for treatment of confined prostate cancer. Urology 1992;40:127–132.
34. Rukstalis DB, Gergber GS, Vogelzang NJ, Haraf DJ, Straus FH, Chodak GW. Laparoscopic pelvic lymph node dissection: a review of 103 cases. J Urol 1994;150:640.
35. Schuessler WW, Vancaillie TG, Reich H, Griffith DP. Transperitoneal endosurgical lymphadenectomy in patients with localized prostate cancer. J Urol 1991;145.
36. Smith J, Haynes T, Middleton R. Impact of external irradiation on local symptoms and survival free of disease in patients with pelvic lymph node metastases from adenocarcinoma of the prostate. J Urol 1984;131:705.
37. Stein A, deKernion JB, Smith RB, et al. Prostate-specific antigen levels after radical prostatectomy in patients with organ-confined and locally extensive prostate cancer. J Urol 1992;147:942.
38. Steinberg G, Epstein J, Piantadosi S, Walsh P. Management of stage D1 adenocarcinoma of the prostate: the Johns Hopkins experience 1974 to 1987. J Urol 1990;144: 1425.
39. Stone NN. Principles of laparoscopy. In Management of Urologic Disease. Edited by MJ Droller. St. Louis: Mosby, 1992, p 1260.
40. Stone NN, Stock RG, Unger P. Seminal vesicle biopsy and laparoscopic pelvic lymph node dissection: implications for patient selection in the radiotherapeutic management of prostate cancer. Int J Radiat Oncol Biol Phys 1994;30:1022A.
41. Stone NN, Ramin SA, Wesson MF, Stock R, Unger P, Klein G. Laparoscopic pelvic lymph node dissection combined with real time interactive transrectal ultrasound guided transperineal radioactive seed implantation of the prostate. J Urol 1995;153:1555–1560.
42. Stone NN, DeAntoni EP, Crawford ED. Screening for prostate cancer by digital rectal exam and prostate specific antigen. Urology 1995;44:18–25.
43. Stone NN, Schlussel RN, Waterhouse RL, Unger PU. Laparoscopic retroperitoneal lymph node dissection in stage A nonseminomatous testis cancer. Urology 1993;42: 610–614.
44. Stone NN. Retroperitoneal laparoscopic surgery: ureterolithotomy and retroperitoneal lymph node dissection. In Laparoscopic Urologic Surgery. Edited by LG Gomella, M Kozminski, HN Winfield. New York: Raven, 1994, pp 195–202.
45. Terris MK, McNeal JE, Freiha FA, Stamey TA. Efficacy of transrectal ultrasound guided seminal vesicle biopsies in the detection of seminal vesicle invasion by prostate cancer. J Urol 1993;149:1035.
46. Vallancien G, Bochereau G, Wetzel O, Bretheau D, Prapotnich D, Bougaran J. Influence of preoperative positive seminal vesicle biopsy on the staging of prostatic cancer. J Urol 1994;152:1152–1156.
47. Villers AA, McNeal JE, Redwine EA, Freiha FS, Stamey TA. Pathogenesis and biological significance of seminal vesicle invasion in prostatic adenocarcinoma. J Urol 1990;143:1183.
48. Zeitman AL, Coen JJ, Shipley WW, et al. Adjuvant irradiation after radical prostatectomy for adenocarcinoma of the prostate: analysis of freedom from PSA failure. Urology 1993;42:292–299.
49. Zietman AL, Edelstein RA, Coen JJ, Babayan RK, Krane RK. Radical prostatectomy for adenocarcinoma of the prostate, the influence of preoperative and pathologic findings on biochemical disease-free outcome. Urology 1994;43:828.

SECTION XIII

PRINCIPLES OF RADIATION ONCOLOGY

CHAPTER 48

Biological and Physical Basis of Radiation Oncology

RALPH R. WEICHSELBAUM, GEORGE CHEN, AND DENNIS E. HALLAHAN

Introduction

X-ray production by a cathode-ray tube was first described in 1895 by Roentgen, and the emission of gamma rays by radium was discovered in 1896 by the Curies. The first reports of curative radiotherapy for the treatment of a malignancy appeared at the turn of the century. It was soon recognized that radiation not only led to tumor cures, but also produced adverse effects on normal tissues. Radiobiology had its first clinical application in the 1920s when fractionation was first demonstrated in the successful treatment of laryngeal carcinoma. With the introduction of supervoltage radiotherapy produced by cobalt 60 sources and linear accelerators in the 1950s, increased doses could be delivered to deep tumors without excessive skin injury. In parallel with external beam advances, interstitial and intracavitary techniques of administering radiotherapy have improved over the past 50 years and have resulted in the cure of tumors amenable to brachytherapy. Radiotherapy is likely to have a major impact on the future management of the systemic spread of cancer through treatment with chemotherapy, biologic response modifiers, and wide-field radiotherapy, and in combination with radiolabeled monoclonal antibodies. In addition, technical improvements in radiotherapy will continue to provide an increasing number of uncomplicated local cures.

Ionizing radiation produces its biologic effects by imparting energy to body tissues. Radiations may be subdivided into indirectly and directly ionizing types. In either case, charged particles are ultimately set into motion through the interaction of radiation with matter, and result in the ionization and excitation of tissue atoms and molecules, causing biologic damage.

INDIRECTLY IONIZING RADIATIONS

Photons

X-rays and gamma radiation are part of the electromagnetic spectrum, which includes radiowaves, infrared radiation, and visible and ultraviolet light. Unlike these lower-energy radiations, x-rays and gamma rays ionize the medium through which they travel. The distinction between x-rays and gamma radiation lies in their origin; gamma rays originate from excited or unstable nuclei, while x-rays are produced by electron level transitions in an atom, or through high-kinetic-energy electrons that are rapidly decelerated. Photons exhibit properties of both waves and particles. As such, x-rays are characterized with classic electromagnetic theory variables, such as frequency and wavelength, associated with the oscillating electric and magnetic vectors. In the quantum mechanical description, photons are considered to be packets of energy that are massless but have momentum. The energy of a photon is proportional to its frequency v:

$$E = \mathbf{h}v$$

where **h** is Planck's constant. X-rays have frequencies of approximately 10^{20} Hz. The energy of monochromatic photons is expressed in kiloelectron volts (keV) or million electron volts (MeV). Since therapeutic beams most commonly consist of a distribution or spectra of different energy photons, the highest-energy photons are expressed in kVp (kilovolts peak) or MV (megavolts). In typical spectra, the average photon energy is approximately one third of the maximum. Radiations used in therapy span the energies from 50 kVp (which penetrate superficially) to 25 MV or greater (for deep therapy). In this energy range, the relevant interactions of photons with matter include the photoelectric effect, the Compton effect, and pair production (84, 91). As a result of these interactions, electrons are set into motion, causing additional ionization and excitation of other atoms in the medium.

In the photoelectric effect, an incident photon is completely absorbed by an inner shell electron with the subsequent emission of a photoelectron. The kinetic energy of the ejected electron is equal to the incident photon energy less the electron binding energy. The probability of photoelectric interactions is proportional to Z^3/E, where Z is the atomic number of the material and E the photon energy. At low energies, differential absorption of radiation by high-atomic-number biologic tissues such as bone, can be several times that of adjacent low-Z soft tissues. At megavoltage energies, the probability of interaction through the photoelectric effect is small. A schematic representation of the photoelectric effect is shown in Figure 48.1*A*.

The Compton effect is the dominant interaction in tissue for photons used in modern radiotherapy. In this interaction, the photon behaves like a particle, as it "collides" with an outer loosely bound orbital electron, scattering the incident photon

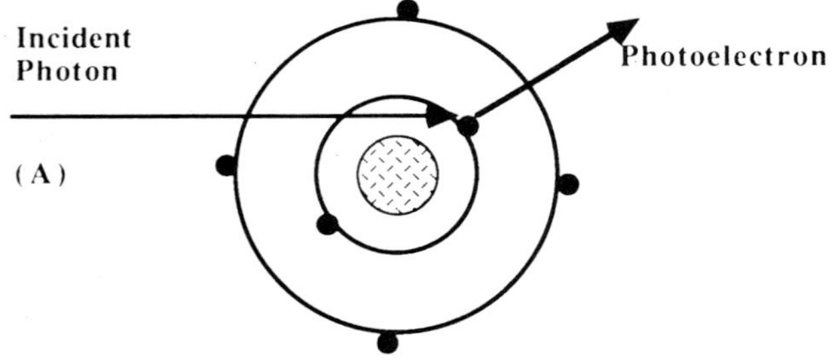

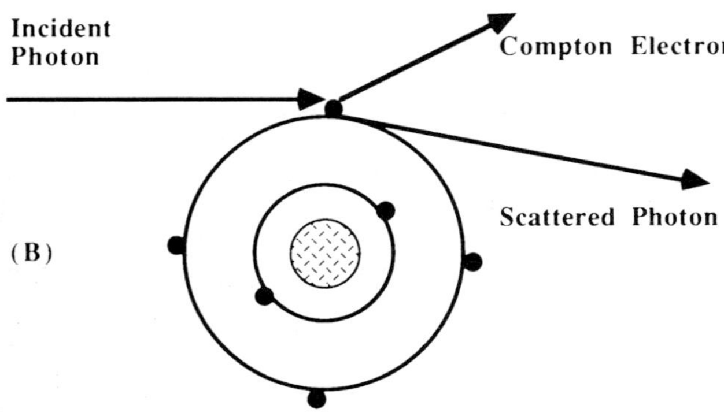

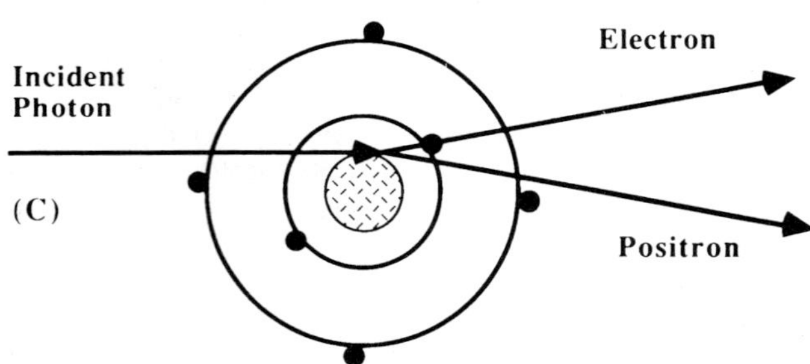

Figure 48.1. Photon interactions with matter. **A.** Photoelectric effect. **B.** Compton effect. **C.** Pair production.

and imparting kinetic energy to the electron. The angle of scatter and the energy of the scattered photon are determined by the kinematics of an elastic collision, where both momentum and energy are conserved. Because the Compton electrons are energetic and are predominantly scattered in the forward direction, megavoltage photon beams exhibit skin sparing. Thus, the first few millimeters of skin absorb less energy, thereby reducing skin erythema. The probability of interaction via the Compton process is independent of the atomic number of the material and decreases approximately as 1/E. The electron density (number of electrons per gram) is the dominant physical parameter in the attenuation of photons by the Compton effect. Since the Z/A ratio (atomic number/atomic weight) ratio of soft tissue and bone are nearly the same, the energy imparted per gram to these tissues is nearly identical. A schematic representation of the Compton effect is shown in Figure 48.1*B*.

At photon energies greater than 1.02 MeV, photons interacting near the strong electric field of the nucleus may lead to the creation of a positron electron pair, with the subsequent disappearance of the incident photon. Pair production increases with increasing energy and atomic number; approximately 15% of the interactions of a 24-MV beam in water are due to pair production. In bone, this percentage rises to approximately 20%. A schematic representation of the pair production process is shown in Figure 48.1*C*. After losing its kinetic energy, the positron is annihilated with an electron, producing two photons traveling in opposite directions.

As a photon beam passes through matter, its intensity diminishes as a result of the interactions described above. A photon beam is attenuated according to an exponential attenuation law:

$$I(x) = I_o e^{-\mu x}$$

where I_o is the initial intensity of the photon beam, I(x) is the intensity after traversing a depth x, and μ is the material's linear attenuation coefficient. High-energy beams are attenuated less than are low-energy beams and thus are the choice for the irradiation of deep tumors. The radiation intensity per unit area from a point source also diminishes as the inverse square of the distance from the source. This dependence is known as the inverse square law.

Free electrons formed by incident photons track through the cell nucleus, producing clusters of ionizations by low-energy secondary electrons. DNA damage is induced by ionizing radiation through direct and indirect interaction with these electrons. Direct damage occurs when the charged particle ionizes DNA without a free radical intermediate, whereas indirect damage occurs when water molecules are ionized, forming hydroxyl radicals, which then ionize DNA. Ionization occurs primarily in cellular water, which subsequently damages DNA.

Radiation Absorbed Dose

The quantification of radiation for therapeutic purposes has evolved over time. Historically, in the early 20th century, units of skin erythema and the roentgen, a measure of ionization produced in air, were used to quantify radiation. Today, dose, the energy absorbed per unit mass, is used to relate a physically measurable quantity with biologic effect. In SI units, the unit of absorbed dose is the gray (Gy), which is defined as the absorption of 1 joule per kilogram (J/kg). One gray is equivalent to 100 centigray (cGy) or 100 rads. Dose is plotted as a function of depth in water, and depth dose curves for different megavoltage energy beams are shown in Figure 48.2.

Sources of Therapeutic Photon Beams

Therapeutic high-energy photon beams (4 to 25 MV) are produced by linear accelerators (Fig. 48.3). In these devices, electrons are accelerated to megavoltage energies by microwave power and the resulting electron beam is focused onto a high atomic number target, producing a forward peaked high-energy photon beam. The photon beam is flattened to provide a large uniform radiation field (approximately 40 cm by 40 cm), which is then collimated by tungsten jaws to the desired rectangular field size. The gantry may be rotated about its axis to direct radiation to the target from the chosen angle. The patient is immobilized in a recumbent position, and is aligned to the radiation beam through optical positioning lasers. High dose rate beams are available, and, typically, a treatment of 200 cGy is delivered to the tumor within a few minutes. Including setup and irradiation, a treatment session of average complexity requires approximately 20 minutes.

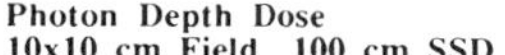

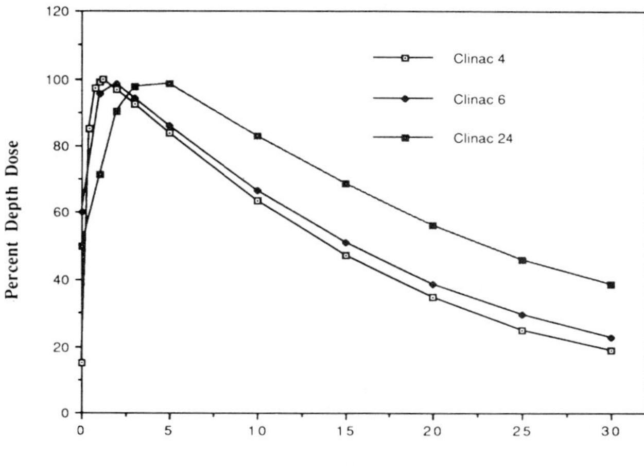

Figure 48.2. Percent depth–dose curves for megavoltage photon radiation, including 4-MV, 6-MV, and 24-MV beams.

Cobalt 60 may also be used to provide megavoltage therapeutic beams (1.25 MeV). Cobalt 60 is artificially produced by irradiating cobalt 59 with neutrons from a nuclear reactor. The treatment head contains pellets of cobalt 60 packed in a stainless steel source housing. A shutter system controlled by a timer is used to control radiation output. Cobalt units provide a dose rate of approximately 100 cGy/min. Since the laws of radioactive decay govern the radiation output of a cobalt treatment unit, such units are considered more stable than are complex linear accelerators. However, the source size is of the order of several centimeters in diameter and the beam penumbra is large in comparison with the sharp penumbra of a linear accelerator beam. The penetration of cobalt 60 beams is slightly less than that of a 4-MV linear accelerator beam.

Neutrons

Several centers throughout the world are investigating the use of neutron beams for radiation therapy (24). Therapeutic neutron beams are usually generated by bombarding a beryllium target with a cyclotron-accelerated proton beam. Like photons, neutrons are indirectly ionizing radiation and are exponentially attenuated. Interactions of neutron beams with tissue include neutron–proton collisions and neutron–nuclei reactions, both of which set heavy charged particles in motion, as shown schematically in Figure 48.4. The density of energy deposition along a charged particle

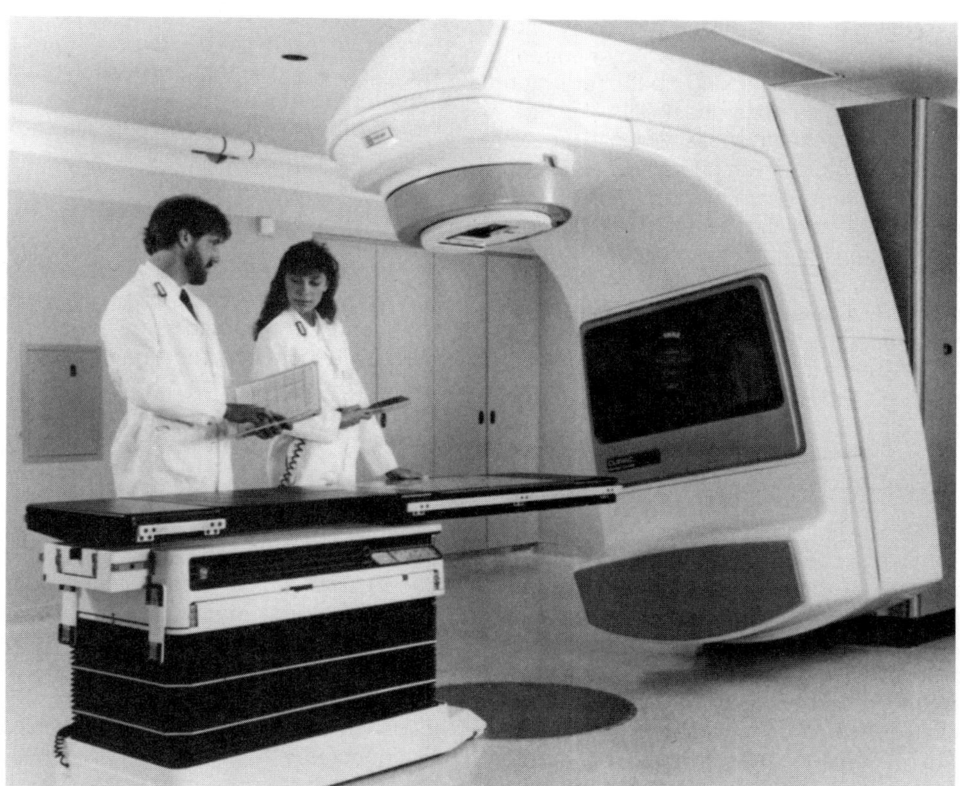

Figure 48.3. A typical modern linear accelerator used in radiation therapy, which produces both photon and electron beams.

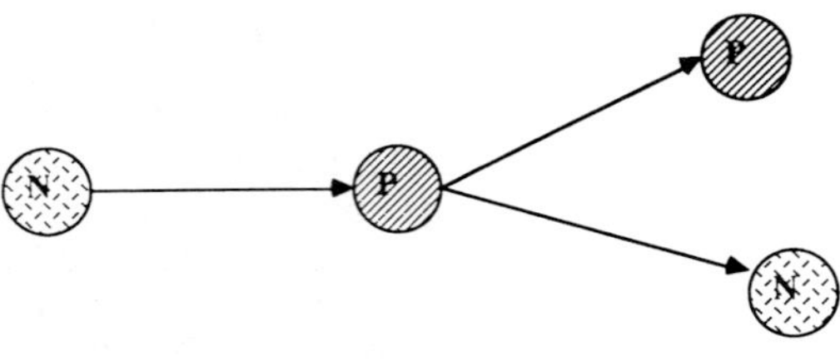

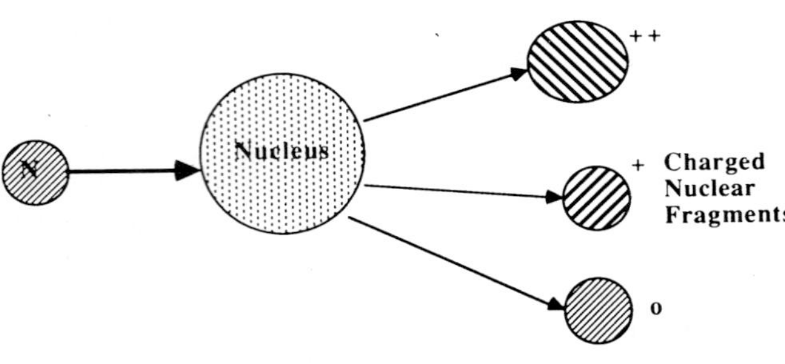

Figure 48.4. Neutron interactions with matter. Heavy charged particles are set into motion, resulting in high LET energy deposition.

track is quantified as its linear energy transfer (LET), and may be expressed in kiloelectron volts per micrometer (KeV/μm). In contrast to the electrons set into motion by photons, heavy charged particles set into motion by neutrons ionize densely along their tracks, making neutrons a high LET radiation. High LET beams cause direct DNA damage, and exhibit a relative biologic effectiveness, which is greater than that of low LET radiations, such as photons or electrons (67). The total dose for neutron beam therapy, therefore, is less than that required for x-irradiation for the same biologic end point. Because neutrons interact primarily with hydrogen nuclei, resulting in proton ejection as opposed to electron ejection, a higher RBE is observed for tissues with a high hydrogen component, such as the central nervous system, and a lower RBE for tissues with few hydrogen nuclei, such as bone. The concept of RBE is discussed in greater detail in the radiobiology section.

Directly Ionizing Radiations

Charged particle beams, or charged particle radiations emitted from radioactive nuclei, may be used for therapeutic applications. Unlike an exponentially attenuated photon beam, the depth of charged particle penetration can be controlled, and tissues beyond this depth are not irradiated, thereby sparing distal normal tissues. The most common directly ionizing therapeutic beam is that of accelerated electrons. Typical depth–dose curves for electron beams are shown in Figure 48.5. As seen, after an initial buildup of dose, peaking at a depth of 2.5 cm, a 12-MeV electron beam

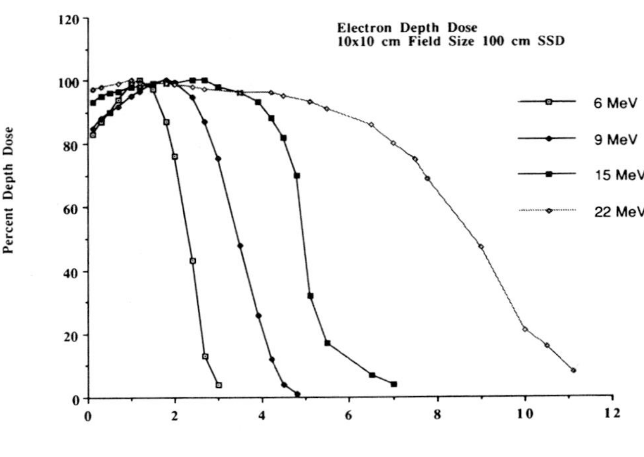

Figure 48.5. Percent depth–dose curves for megavoltage electron beams from a linear accelerator. Energies of electron beams range from 6 MeV to 22 MeV.

dose falls to nearly zero after 6 cm (from 80 to 5% in 2 cm).

Proton and other heavy charged particle beams exhibit a Bragg peak, which is an increased dose deposition near the end of the particle range (Fig. 48.6). If a proton Bragg peak is modified to encompass the tumor dimension in depth, a high dose may be delivered to the target with reduced dose to the proximal tissues, and near zero to distal tissues. Charged particle beam penetration is much more sensitive to the presence of inhomogeneities (e.g., bone or air cavities) than photon beams, resulting in a technically more difficult treatment execution (175). Energies of approximately 250 MeV are needed to generate proton beams of sufficient energy to reach deep tumors (25 cm range). Proton synchrotrons or cyclotrons are used to accelerate protons to these energy levels (162). Currently, there are two proton therapy facilities in the United States, at the Harvard Cyclotron Laboratory (therapy in conjunction with the Department of Radiation Medicine at Massachusetts General Hospital), and a facility at Loma Linda Medical Center. In addition to the dose localization properties associated with a Bragg peak, beams of heavy ions (e.g., carbon or neon) also contain a high LET component. Heavy ion beams for radiation therapy clinical studies were studied at the Lawrence Berkeley Laboratory, and a new accelerator for heavy ion radiotherapy construction has been completed at the National Institute of Radiological Sciences in Chiba, Japan.

BIOLOGIC BASIS OF RADIOTHERAPY

Radiation is randomly deposited within the cell; DNA, however, is the most critical target for cell killing. Radiation-induced DNA damage includes single- or double-strand breaks in the sugar phosphate backbone of the DNA molecule and alterations or loss of nucleotide bases. The formation of cross-links between DNA strands and chromosomal proteins also occurs as a result of radiation exposure. Evidence implicating DNA as the principal target in radiation killing includes (67): (1) Cells are killed by radioactive tritiated thymidine incorporated into DNA. The range of the beta

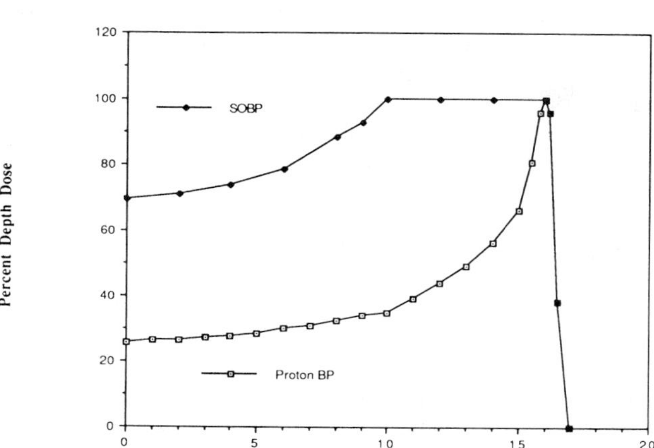

Figure 48.6. Pristine proton Bragg peak (narrow peak) and a spread-out Bragg peak beam (SOBP) used for radiation therapy. Maximum proton energy is 160 MeV. SOBP is generated by interposing variable absorber in the beam as a function of time.

particles is very short and, therefore, is localized in DNA. (2) Halogenated pyrimidines are selectively incorporated into DNA in place of thymine when substituted in cell culture medium. This incorporation greatly increases the radiosensitivity of cells (93). Substituted deoxyuridines are not incorporated into DNA and do not affect radiosensitivity. (3) There is a direct relationship between viral size and radiosensitivity, which correlates with nucleic acid volume. The radiosensitivity of plants has been correlated with mean interphase volume, which is defined as the ratio of nuclear volume to chromosome number (67). The larger the mean chromosome number, the greater is the radiosensitivity. Taken together, these data imply that DNA damage is the primary lethal event from radiotherapy.

The radiobiologic definition of death is the loss of reproductive integrity. Inhibition of the reproductive ability of cells is important to the cancer therapist because the aim of therapeutic radiation is sterilization of malignant tissue. Also, the major long-term effects of radiation on normal tissue result from killing of tissue stem cells and/or vascular endothelial cells. Most cell types do not show morphologic evidence of radiation damage until they attempt to divide. Lethally irradiated cells may undergo several divisions before exhibiting metabolic death and disappearing from the population (171). Exceptions are some populations of unstimulated lymphocytes and spermatogonia, which undergo interphase death at low doses. The concept that cell death may not be expressed for several cell divisions following irradiation has clinical relevance in that very slowly proliferating tumors may persist for months and appear histologically viable. The histologic appearance of malignancy may clear only after tumor cells have had an opportunity to divide. An example of a slowly proliferating tumor that may require up to 24 months after irradiation for accurate histologic prediction of local control is prostate carcinoma (32).

RADIATION SURVIVAL ANALYSIS

Puck and Marcus performed the first clonogenic in vitro radiation survival curves, for HeLa cells, in 1955 (136). Exponentially growing cells are irradiated and immediately trypsinized and a specific cell number is plated onto a dish. After 2 to 3 weeks, colonies are stained, and those with greater than 50 cells are counted as representative of cells that are capable of infinite division (in the case of tumor cells). The surviving fraction is calculated by dividing the number of colonies by the plating efficiency of unirradiated cells. Radiation survival analysis is frequently represented by a graphic representation of the log of surviving fraction versus a linear plot of dose (Fig. 48.7). Resulting radiation survival curves are characterized by an initial shoulder followed by exponential killing at higher doses.

Radiation survival analysis can be studied both in vitro and in vivo. In vivo models examine both the inherent radiosensitivity of tumor cells and environmental influences, such as hypoxia and host immunity. A model commonly used to study radiation effects is the growth delay assay, which measures the time interval required for a tumor exposed to radiation to regrow to a specified volume (Fig. 48.8) (7). An assay that analyzes the dose required to control 50% of tumors is the TCD_{50} assay, which has been widely employed to study tumors in a variety of experimental systems (161). The radiobiologic use of transplantable solid tumor systems in experimental animals has been reviewed by Hall (67). Radiation survival parameters can be assayed for normal tissues

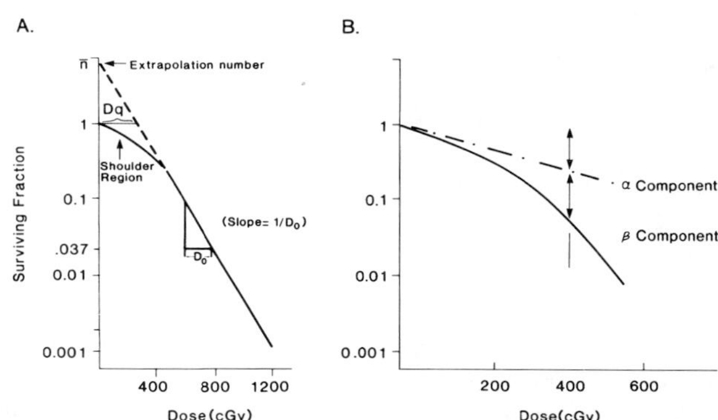

Figure 48.7. Models for survival curve analysis. Experimental data are typically shown as the fraction of cells surviving a dose of radiation plotted on a logarithmic scale while the dosage of radiation is plotted on a linear scale (**A**). When using the multitarget model, the shoulder region is quantified by extrapolation of the exponential portion of the curve to the y-axis intercept. This point is referred to as n (extrapolation number) while a horizontal line drawn from 100% survival to the extrapolation line is referred to as D_q (or quasi-threshold dose). Slope of the terminal portion of the survival curve is quantified by the term D_o, which is the inverse of the slope and designated as the radiosensitivity of the cells or tissue under study. **B.** When using the linear-quadratic models for survival analysis, there are two components for cell killing. The alpha component represents the initial slope, and the beta component represents the terminal slope of the survival curve. The alpha component is proportional to the dose, whereas the beta component is proportional to the square of the dose. The dose at which the alpha and beta components are equal is referred to as the alpha/beta ratio, which, for example, is 400 cGy in **B**.

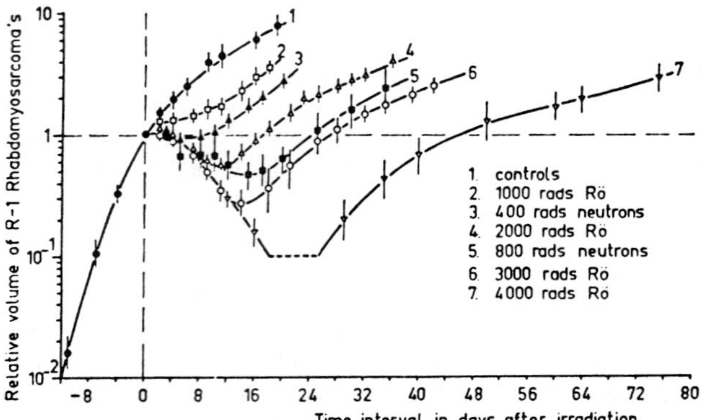

Figure 48.8. Data points represent volume changes observed in tumors in animal models after irradiation. After an initial decrease in the volume size, tumors grow back to the original volume over a time interval referred to as the growth delay. Curve 1 is the growth of an unirradiated control tumor. Curves 2, 4, 6, and 7 represent the growth of tumors irradiated with 1,000, 2,000, 3,000, and 4,000 cGy of photons. Curves 3 and 5 represent the growth of tumors irradiated with 400 and 800 cGy of 152 MeV neutrons. Growth delay is prolonged with increasing dosage and more densely ionizing radiation, such as neutrons. *Source*: Barendsen and Broerse (7).

in vivo as well as for tumors. For acutely responding tissues, in vivo survival is measured by studying clones of normal tissues regrowing in situ (e.g., skin, jejunal crypt cells) or cells transplanted to another site (bone marrow stem cells). To study radiation effects in late-responding tissues, such as the nervous system, functional assays, such as paralysis and death, may be employed.

MODELS OF RADIATION SURVIVAL CURVE ANALYSIS

Radiation survival curves usually graph the dose of radiation on a linear scale and surviving fraction on a logarithmic scale, as shown in Figure 48.7. Two mathematical models are commonly employed to analyze radiation survival data. One analysis of radiation survival data is carried out by a two-component or multitarget model. A two-component survival curve derived from mammalian cells is characterized by an initial shoulder region followed by a terminal exponential region. The reciprocal of the slope is defined by a D_0 value (slope = $1/D_0$). D_0 is referred to as the radiosensitivity of the cell population or tissue under investigation. The fraction of cells surviving the average of one lethal event per cell is defined by Poisson distribution to be one third or 37%. D_0 is the dose required to reduce the surviving fraction to 37% in the exponential portion of the survival curve. The width of the shoulder region is represented by the quantities *n* or D_q. D_q is the quasi-threshold dose, or the point at which killing becomes exponential. The term "radiosensitive" is frequently confused with "radiocurability" and "radioresponsive." Radiocurability is defined as local control in a clinical (or laboratory) setting and implies that the therapeutic ratio is such that curative doses can be applied in a high percentage of cases. Radioresponsiveness refers to how rapidly a tumor disappears after initiation of radiotherapy and is a function of a variety of kinetic parameters, such as the growth fraction, as well as the radiobiologic characteristics of the tumor cells. Small cell carcinoma of the lung is an example of a radioresponsive tumor that requires relatively high doses to be locally controlled. As mentioned previously, prostate carcinoma may regress slowly but is radiocurable in its early stages. Therefore, radioresponsive tumors are not necessarily radiocurable and radiocurable tumors are not necessarily radioresponsive (39, 67, 84).

The linear quadratic model (surviving fraction = $e^{\alpha D - \beta D_2}$) is used to fit radiation survival data to a continuously bending curve where D is dose and α and β are constants. The linear component, a measure of the initial slope, termed alpha, represents single-hit killing kinetics and dominates the radiation response at low doses. The quadratic component of cell killing, termed beta, represents multiple-hit killing kinetics and causes the curve to bend at higher doses. The ratio of alpha to beta is the dose at which the linear and quadratic components of cell killing are equal (Fig. 48.7). The more linear the response to killing of cells at low radiation dose, the higher is the value of alpha and the greater is the radiosensitivity of cells (Fig. 48.7) (67, 195). Neither the linear quadratic nor the two-component model has a firmly established biologic basis. Therefore, they should be viewed only as convenient models for describing a survival curve mathematically. The concept of the mean inactivation dose (D) is an additional measure of intrinsic radiation sensitivity. The calculation of D involves a linear quadratic analysis of survival graphed on linear coordinates. The mean inactivation dose is equal to the area under the curve and is disproportionally influenced by surviving fractions obtained at 100 to 300 cGy (39, 47, 172). Other authors suggest that the surviving fraction at 200 cGy is an important parameter when describing the radiobiologic characteristics of human tumor cells because 200 cGy is a common daily dose used in radiotherapy.

The biologic effectiveness of different types of radiation can be characterized by a parameter known as the relative biologic effectiveness (RBE). RBE is defined as the ratio of a dose of a standard type of radiation to that of a test dose of a different type of radiation that gives the same biologic effect (Fig. 48.9). High LET beams such as neutrons cause direct DNA damage and exhibit a relative biologic effect that is greater

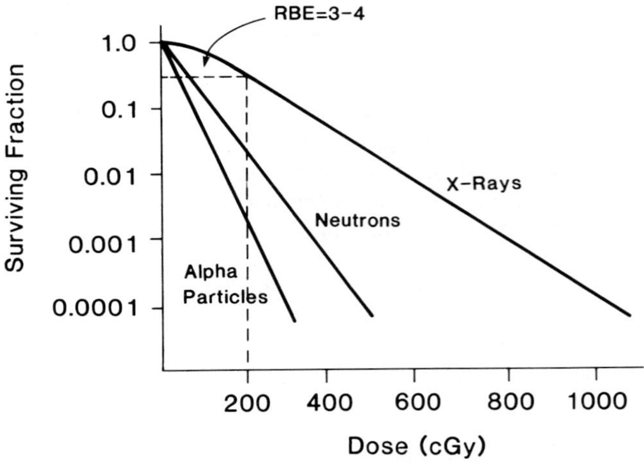

Figure 48.9. Survival curves from mammalian cells exposed to x-rays, neutrons, or alpha particles vary in the shoulder region and terminal slope. The relative biologic effect (RBE) is a ratio of survival at a specific dose for different types of radiation.

than that of low LET radiations, such as photons or electrons. The total dose for neutrons to produce a biologic effect, therefore, is less than that required for x-irradiation (67, 84).

RADIATION SURVIVAL PARAMETERS OF HUMAN TUMOR CELLS

A limitation of the study of in vitro radiobiologic parameters of human tumor cells is that cells that grow in tissue culture might not be representative of the characteristics of the clonogenic cells that make up the host tumor. In addition, in vitro analysis may ignore physiologic conditions within the tumor, such as hypoxia and cell cycle distribution. Nonetheless, the characterization of human tumor cells phenotypically resistant to chemotherapeutic agents in vitro has led to an increase in the understanding of the cellular and molecular biology of chemoresistance. Therefore, an investigation of human tissue cell lines of differing radiosensitivity is useful to understand the basis of the cellular radiation response as one major determinant of clinical radiocurability.

Human tumor cell lines derived from various histologic tumor types have varying degrees of radiosensitivity (56, 90, 119, 187, 190). Cellular radiosensitivity varies between and among tumor types. Most in vitro radiobiologic data have been determined from cell lines passaged many times. To assess the in vitro radiobiologic parameters of early passage human tumor cells derived from patients' tumors prior to radiotherapy, Weichselbaum and colleagues analyzed radiation survival data from 20 early-passage epithelial tumor cell lines established from head and neck carcinoma patients and 13 early-passage mesenchymal tumor lines established from patients with soft tissue sarcomas (185, 186). Both groups of patients were treated with curative-intent radiotherapy and subsequently followed. Tumor cells cultured from head and neck cancer patients exhibited a relatively wide range of radiosensitivities with D_0 values ranging from 100 to 330 cGy. Some patients whose tumors contained radioresistant tumor cells either had a rapid recurrence of their tumors or never had resolution of their disease, with the exception of patients who underwent surgical resection of their tumors. Cell lines derived from patients with soft tissue sarcomas were more radiosensitive, and exhibited less heterogeneity of radiosensitivity than did tumor cell lines derived from patients with head and neck carcinoma. This characterization was true regardless of the method of radiobiologic analysis. More in-field recurrences occurred in head and neck cancer patients as compared with sarcoma patients. A larger number of patients with longer follow-up times is necessary to draw conclusions about the predictive value of individual radiobiologic parameters to local control following radiotherapy. However, the above data suggest that the inherent radiosensitivity/resistance of human tumor cells contributes to radiotherapy success or failure. This concept is supported by the fact that tumor cells cultured from patients' tumors who failed radiotherapy are more radioresistant as a group than are normal fibroblasts (Fig. 48.10) (182, 184, 190). Thus, either radioresistant tumor cells are present at the beginning of therapy and radiosensitive cells are selected against during fractionated treatment, or genes are activated, amplified, or mutated, which renders tumor cells radioresistant during fractionated treatment (Fig. 48.11).

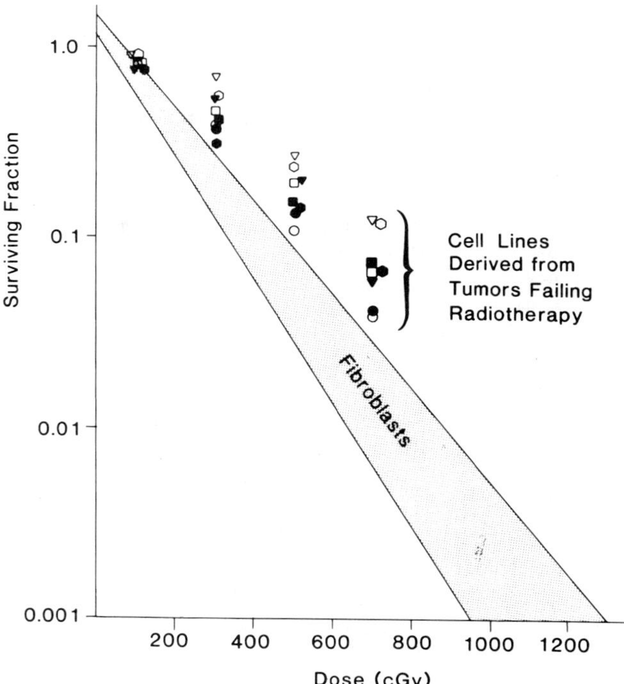

Figure 48.10. The surviving fraction of cell lines derived from tumors that failed radiotherapy are plotted and compared with the range of survival for normal fibroblasts. Each symbol represents a different radioresistant cell line. Data indicate that cells derived from tumors after radiotherapy have survivals that are greater than those for normal fibroblasts. *Source:* Weichselbaum et al. (184).

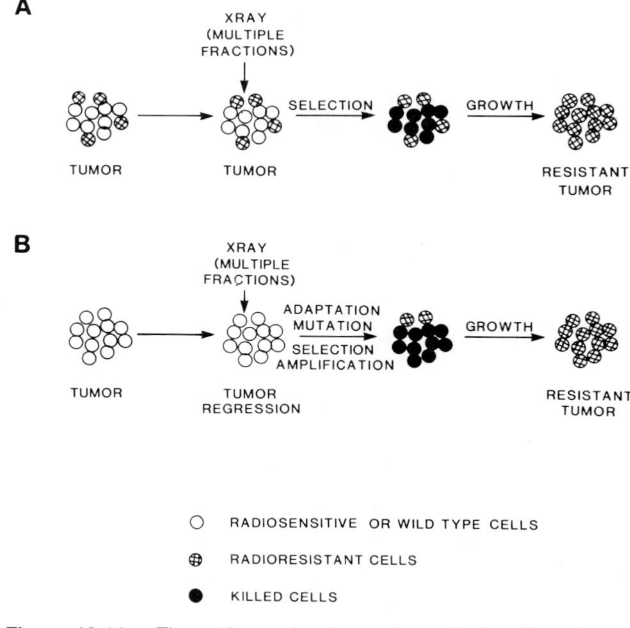

Figure 48.11. Theoretic mechanisms of acquired radioresistance in tumors. **A.** Radioresistant cells are present in a tumor cell population exposed to radiation. After multiple fractions of radiation, radioresistant cells are selected, whereas sensitive cells are killed. After the radioresistant, clonogenic cells regrow, a resistant tumor population is present. **B.** Radioresistant cells are not present before irradiation. Adaptation, mutation, and gene amplification may occur during multiple fractions of irradiation, resulting in radioresistant cells. These cells regrow, resulting in a resistant tumor population.

Repair of Radiation Damage

SUBLETHAL DAMAGE REPAIR

When a population of cells is exposed to ionizing radiation, some cells may not receive damage in a site critical for cell division. Others may have accumulated enough damage in critical sites to be lethal and will die during subsequent mitosis. An initial shoulder on a radiation survival curve suggests that sublethal damage must be accumulated prior to cell death. If additional radiation damage is accumulated before the first sublethal lesion is repaired, the two may interact, resulting in cell death. Sublethal damage repair (SLDR) may be operationally defined as the enhancement in survival when a dose of radiation is separated over a period of time. SLDR may be represented by the extrapolation number (n) of the radiation survival curve when multitarget survival analysis is employed (38-42).

Sublethal damage has been studied in vitro and in vivo. In general, SLDR experiments divide a single dose into two relatively equal doses spaced at variable time intervals. Elkind and colleagues investigated this phenomenon in great detail (38, 43). Figure 48.12 shows results representative of split-dose experiments. An enhancement in survival following two doses separated in time is observed in exponentially growing Chinese hamster cells at 2 hours. This enhancement in survival is due to the rapid repair of SLD and is followed by a subsequent decline in survival at 5 hours and then another increase in survival at 8 hours. This variability in survival is caused by synchronization of the exponentially growing cell populations by the first radiation dose and subsequent treatment with a second dose during the radioresistant S phase (t = 2 hours) or radiosensitive G_2-M phase of the cell cycle (t = 6 hours) (7, 39, 41, 42). The concept of repair of SLD is important during a course of fractionated radiotherapy, because the shoulder region of the survival curve is recapitulated due to SLDR (Fig. 48.12) (35). Fractionation magnifies the surviving fraction after each treatment to an exponent equal to the number of treatments (Table 48.1). Therefore, small differences in survival after each dose may have a great impact on treatment outcome. Most human tumor cell lines studied in vitro have relatively small shoulders (n = 13) (14, 19, 90, 128, 185, 191). However, a large capacity for sublethal repair has been reported for some human tumor cell lines (8, 19).

The ability of tissues to repair sublethal damage has been demonstrated using a variety of normal tissue clonogenic or functional assays (67, 167, 452). The capacity of different

Table 48.1. Calculated Cumulative Survival

Survival fraction	X^{32a} X =	X^{20a} X =
10^{-11}	0.45	0.28
10^{-10}	0.49	0.32
10^{-9}	0.52	0.35
10^{-8}	0.56	0.40
10^{-7}	0.60	0.45
10^{-6}	0.65	0.50
10^{-5}	0.70	0.56

[a] Calculated cumulative survival fraction for either 32 or 20 equal fractions when the fractional survival is varied.
From Hellman (73A) with permission.

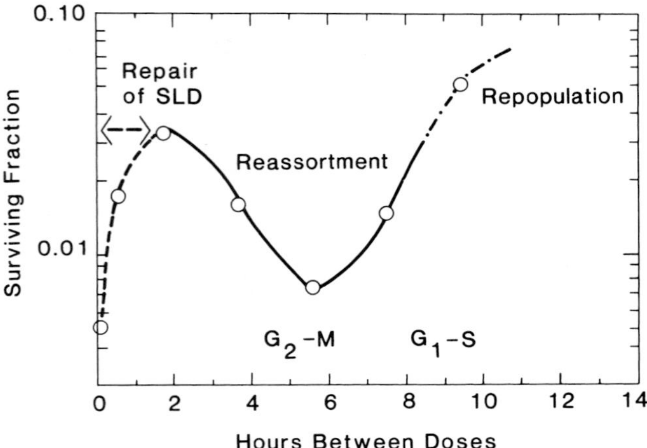

Figure 48.12. The surviving fractions of Chinese hamster cells exposed to two doses of x-rays separated by various time intervals are shown. When the two doses are given together (time between doses = 0 hours), the surviving fraction is equal to that observed after the single larger dose of radiation. As the two doses are separated by time, an enhancement in survival occurs and is interpreted as the repair of sublethal damage (*dashed line*). Subsequent radiation doses result in a reduction in the surviving fraction. This reduction in survival occurs because of more sensitive phases of the cell cycle (G_2 and M). Later time points demonstrate increased surviving fractions due to radiation synchronization of cells and their entry into resistant phases of the cell cycle (G_1 and S). *Source*: Elkind (38, 39).

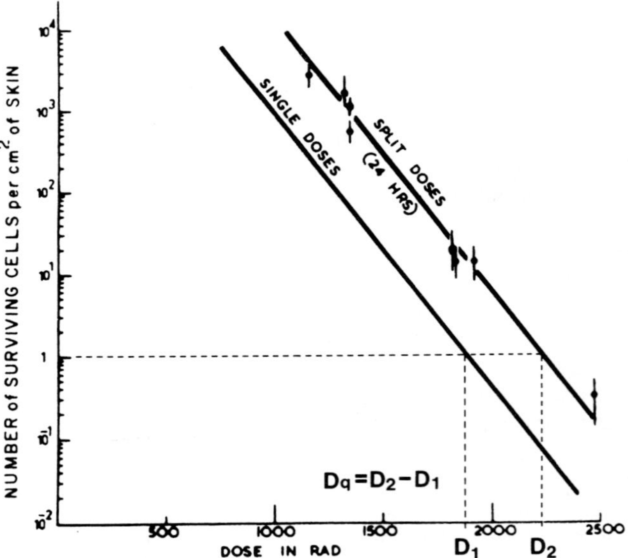

Figure 48.13. Single-dose and two-dose survival curves for epithelial cells. The D_0 is 135 cGy. The ordinate is not the surviving fraction, as in survival curves for cells cultured in vitro, but is the number of surviving cells per square centimeter of skin (plating efficiency is obviously not known in vivo). In the two-dose survival curve, the interval between dose fractions is 24 hours. Although the curves are parallel (similar D_0), their graphic horizontal separation number (n), may then be calculated from D_0 and D_q. *Source*: Withers (194, 195).

cell populations to repair SLD is reflected by the width of the shoulder (or initial slope) of their survival curve. An increase in the total dose required to give the same biologic damage when a single dose (D_1) is split into two doses (total dose D_2) with a time interval between doses to obtain a single biologic end point is the capacity of a normal tissue to repair SLD. The difference in the two doses, $D_2 - D_1$, is a measure of SLDR by the tissue, provided that the two doses are larger than those that generate the shoulder region of the survival curve (67, 194, 195) (Fig. 48.13), $D_2 - D_1 = D_q$. If the D_0 is known, then n can be calculated from the equation $\log_e n = D_q/D_0$.

A clinical example of exploiting the difference in the abilities of various rapidly proliferating normal tissues to repair SLD is demonstrated by the application of fractionated TBI for bone marrow ablation delivered two to three times a day (separated by 4 to 6 hours; total dose 1,200 to 1,320 cGy) in preparation for bone marrow transplantation. The small bowel ($n = 40$) has a large shoulder as compared with the bone marrow, which has a small shoulder ($n = 1$) (52). Thus, the hematopoietic compartment is ablated while the gut is spared due to differences in the repair of SLD. Similar results are obtained at low dose rates.

DOSE RATE EFFECT

Normal tissues tolerate relatively high doses of radiation (3,000 to 6,000 cGy) given over 2 to 7 days during brachytherapy with interstitial or intracavitary ^{137}Cs or ^{226}Ra. The dose rate is usually prescribed 40 to 50 cGy/h at 0.5 cm from the sources. Conversely, ionizing radiation delivered at a higher dose rate (greater than 100 cGy/min), as with external irradiation, must be fractionated over 5 to 7 weeks to be tolerated by normal tissues. Figure 48.14 demonstrates that the D_0 is reduced by more than 2 and the shoulder on the survival curve is also decreased when the dose rate is increased from 0.01 Gy to 1 Gy/min in HeLa cells. This dose rate effect has also been demonstrated in normal tissue cell lines (9, 66).

Photon release from a radioisotope is a random event and is separated by random time intervals. Thus, reduced cell killing by low-dose-rate radiation represents sublethal damage repair and is analogous to irradiation with multiple small fractions. The shoulder region is recapitulated repeatedly with each dose delivered, resulting in magnification of the shoulder region of the survival curve, as demonstrated in Figure 48.15. Constant, low-dose-rate radiation increases the therapeutic ratio during brachytherapy because tumor cells pass through relatively radiosensitive phases of the cell cycle. Also, surrounding tissues receive a lower dose rate than adjacent tumor cells because the dose rate falls off at a rate of the square of the distance from the isotope source. Whole-body, low dose rate radiation has been applied in bone marrow transplantation in a fashion similar to fractioned TBI to take advantage of the differentiated abilities of the gut and bone marrow to repair SLD.

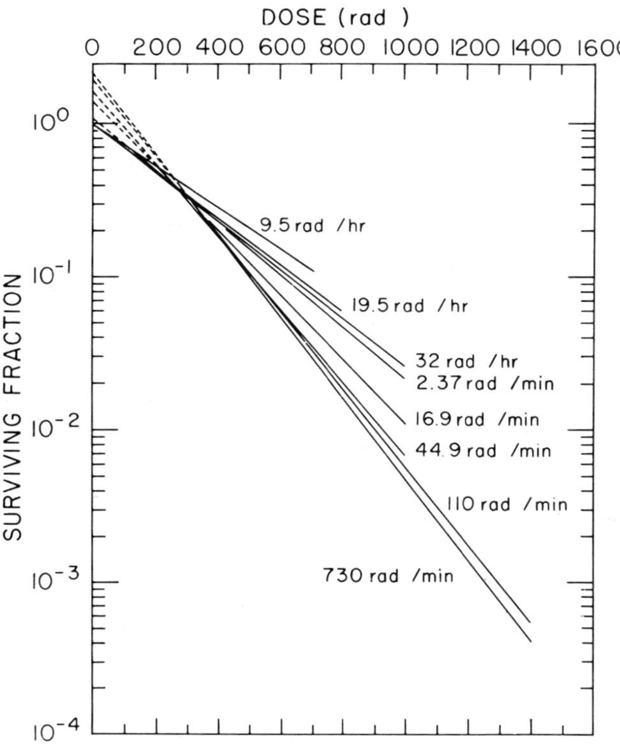

Figure 48.14. Dose rate effect in HeLa cells. Slope of the survival curve steepens as the dose rate increases. The survival curves for HeLa cells exposed to x-rays given at various dose rates are shown. *Source*: Hall (66).

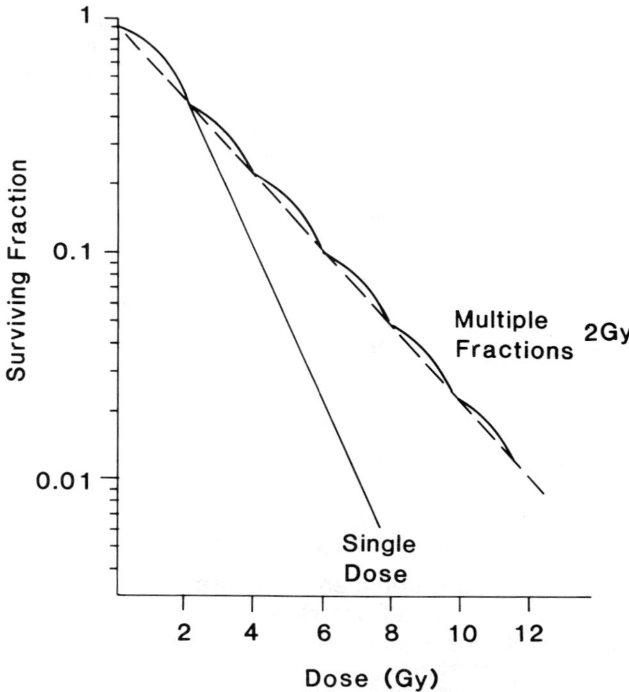

Figure 48.15. Recapitulation of the shoulder on the survival curve during fractionation. When a single-dose survival curve is performed, the terminal exponential region of the survival curve is reached. However, when multiple 2 Gy fractions are given, the shoulder region of the curve is reproduced after each dose due to the repair of sublethal damage. SLDR results in surviving fractions that are greater for a cumulative fractional dose compared with the same dose given in a single fraction.

POTENTIALLY LETHAL DAMAGE REPAIR

Varying environmental conditions can influence cell survival after a dose of x-rays. Thus, damage that is potentially lethal under a given set of conditions may not be lethal if postirradiation conditions are altered (131, 189). The enhancement in survival seen following manipulation of postirradiation conditions is referred to as the repair of potentially lethal damage (PLD). This phenomenon is analogous to the liquid holding recovery observed in bacteria and yeast. Hahn and Little studied PLD repair in density-inhibited stationary phase cultures which they considered more analogous to in vivo tumors than exponentially growing cells (63, 64). Quiescent cells were subcultured at varying time intervals after irradiation. Cells plated immediately after irradiation allow for no PLDR (Fig. 48.16). Delay in subculture allows quiescent cells to repair PLD, resulting in a higher surviving fraction than an immediate subculture. PLDR has also been shown to occur in vivo if the explant of an experimental animal tumor is delayed (64, 105, 141). This effect is reported to be more pronounced in large tumors, presumably because a large proportion of cells are in G_1 or G_0. PLDR has been described to occur principally in the G_1 phase of the cell cycle (17a). Efficient PLDR occurs in a variety of human tumor cell lines in vitro (94, 136, 181, 183, 186, 187). Weichselbaum and colleagues (181, 182, 192) and Guichard and colleagues (62) have suggested that PLDR contributes to radiotherapy failure under certain circumstances.

PLDR and/or SLDR may not be expressed under all conditions in vivo (20). For example, cells must be genetically competent to repair these types of damages, and the tumor environment may affect the proliferative status of tumor cells (183, 189, 192). Also, radiation (or chemotherapy) may induce tumor proliferation, which allows fixation of radiation damage before PLDR or SLDR is complete (181, 189). Therefore, PLDR is likely to be most important in tumor cells of intermediate or high radiosensitivity when cells are quiescent between fractions. The 24-hour PLDR surviving fraction following treatment of human tumor cells in plateau phase culture with a similar dose is referred to as the maximum recovery potential (MRP) (183). Figure 48.16 shows that although two cell lines have different amounts of initial lethal damage induced by a constant radiation dose (a function of D_0 and n), the surviving fraction after a 24-hour delay in subculture (a function of n, D_0, PLDR) may be similar.

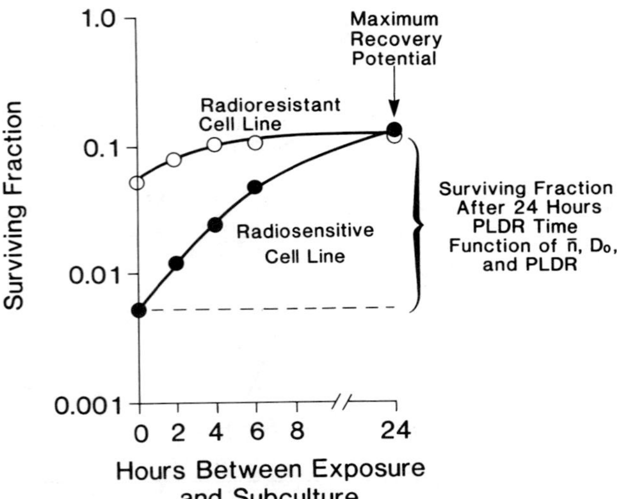

Figure 48.16. Maximum recovery potential (MRP) for radioresistant and radiosensitive cells. Confluent cell lines (noncycling) were irradiated and immediately subcultured, which resulted in an initial surviving fraction (0), which is generally equal or slightly less than the surviving fraction of exponentially growing cells in tissue culture. However, when these irradiated confluent cells are not subcultured for the indicated time intervals, an enhancement in survival, interpreted as STR repair of potentially lethal damage (PLDR), occurs. The surviving fractions of cells after a 24-hour delay in subculture (MRP) of confluent cells is dependent on n, D_0, and PLDR. The initial surviving fraction of cells at 0 hours is dependent on n and D_0 but not on PLDR.

CELL CYCLE AND RADIATION KILLING

Radiation survival analysis of synchronously dividing cells demonstrated that cells irradiated during the G_2 and M phases of the cell cycle are more radiosensitive as compared with cells irradiated during G_1 and S (Fig. 48.17) (148). Thus, irradiation of an asynchronously dividing population of cells results in killing a greater proportion of cells in G_2 and M while surviving G_1 and S cells may progress into more sensitive phases. This phenomenon, referred to as reassortment, results in increased cell killing when subsequent radiation doses are given during sensitive phases of the cell cycle, as illustrated in Figure 48.17 (148). Enhanced cell killing after synchronization and reassortment of irradiated tumor cells suggests a potential benefit from the fractionation of radiotherapy.

One consequence of x-ray exposure is the transient inhibition of cell cycle progression at the G_1/S and G_2/M interfaces of the cell cycle. Such delays likely represent active processes and not simply the deleterious effects of DNA damage. For example, in the yeast *Saccharomyces cerevisiae*, the RAD-9 gene product is responsible for the arrest of cells in G_2 after radiation induced DNA damage (193). It

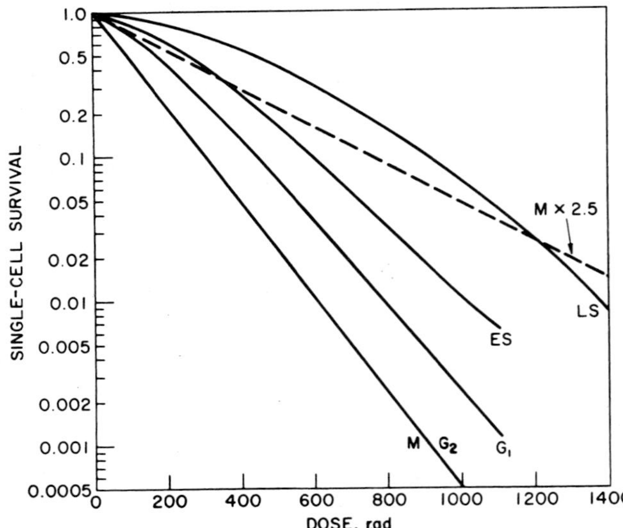

Figure 48.17. Radiation survival curves for Chinese hamster cells irradiated at various stages of the cell cycle. Cells irradiated in G_2 and M are most radiation sensitive, followed by G_1, early S phase (ES), and late S phase (LS). *Dashed line*, survival curve of mitotic cells under hypoxic conditions. *Source*: Sinclair (148).

has been postulated that chromosomal reconstitution, as well as fidelity of DNA replication, requires the cell cycle arrest induced by the RAD-9 gene product. Yeasts that have the RAD-9 gene deleted do not undergo growth arrest and are more sensitive to the killing effect of x-rays than are the wild-type yeast. This suggests that growth arrest is an important function during cellular repair of ionizing radiation damage. X-ray–induced G_1/S cell cycle delays are also seen in mammalian cells, although specific genes associated with this phenotype have not been cloned. However, Fornance and colleagues have cloned several growth-arrest DNA-damage inducible genes, which are expressed following treatments with ultraviolet rays and alkylating agents in mammalian cells, some of which may be analogous in function to RAD-9 in yeast (51). Potentially lethal damage repair (discussed in the previous section) may occur partially as a result of the effects of growth arrest, and repair gene products function to repair x-ray damage.

Molecular Aspects of Radioresistance

Common types of DNA damage induced by ionizing radiation include DNA base damage, as well as DNA single-strand and double-strand breaks. Unrepaired x-ray–induced base damage is frequently mutagenic, whereas unrepaired x-ray induced DNA double-strand breaks are frequently lethal. Studies of x-ray–sensitive rodent cell lines suggest that radiation killing is directly proportional to the rate of rejoining of DNA double-strand breaks (83, 151). Based on these data and data from lower organisms, it is hypothesized that the initial number and/or the rate of rejoining (repair) of some classes of DNA double-strand breaks may be important in cell survival following x-ray exposure. Schwartz and colleagues employed the DNA neutral filter elution assay to study repair of x-ray damage in human tumor cells and reported that radioresistant cell lines rejoined DNA double-strand breaks faster than did more radiosensitive cell lines (145). These data suggest that the neutral elution assay has promise as a rapid assay of human tumor radiosensitivity. Although this assay is relatively simple and rapid, it has been criticized because the doses of radiation employed are nonphysiologic and it is difficult to distinguish various specific classes of DNA double-strand breaks. Only further investigation will clarify the use of neutral elution as an assay predictive of radiotherapy outcome.

Efforts to identify stress response genes have been successful for heat, alkylating agents, and ultraviolet light in mammalian cells, whereas genes that repair gamma-ray–induced double-strand breaks or radiation base damage have not yet been successfully identified in higher eukaryotes. Well-characterized genes that contribute to the repair of gamma-induced radiation damage have been identified in bacteria and lower eukaryotes (12, 26, 178). For example, in *Escherichia coli*, various adverse stimuli can lead to the induction of stress-related genes, such as the ultraviolet- and x-ray–mediated sos response (178). In the sos response, genes coding for DNA repair enzymes are coordinately induced after DNA damage. In this instance, DNA damage leads to the activation of a specific proteinase function of the Rec-A protein that cleaves a repressor protein Lex-A. The Lex-A protein binds to the regulatory region of sos genes, and with its removal by activated Rec-A protein, transcription of these genes occurs. Many sos-genes encode for low abundance transcripts that are rapidly induced by 2- to 10-fold by activated Rec-A protein. The search for a sos-like response in mammalian cells has been limited, since few DNA repair genes have been isolated (95). It is of interest that DNA damage inducible yeast genes RAD-6, -52, and -54 play roles in x-ray damage repair, although RAD-52 is not x-ray inducible (12, 26). In mammalian cells, Herrlich and colleagues reported expression of damage inducible genes following ultraviolet-light exposure (154). Induction of these genes is mediated by various transcription factors, such as c-jun and NF-κB. Recently, Sherman and colleagues observed c-jun and c-fos to be transcriptionally induced by ionizing radiation in a human promyelocytic leukemia cell line (147).

MOLECULAR RADIATION ONCOLOGY

The potential importance of identifying x-ray repair genes to radiotherapy is analogous to the importance of identifying genes that alter cell survival identification following exposure to chemotherapeutic agents (21, 105, 146). Amplification of genes that repair DNA damage or induce growth arrest might be responsible for tumor radioresistance or indirectly influence tumor cell survival following radiation by altering cell cycle distribution. Manipulation of mammalian genes that repair different classes of x-ray–induced DNA damage might increase the therapeutic ratio by increasing tumor cell kill, as well as possibly decreasing normal tissue sequelae following radiotherapy. Identification of gamma DNA repair genes, and the detection of amplification and/or overexpression of these genes, can result in a rapid, accurate prediction of clinical outcome in radiotherapy.

ONCOGENES AND CELLULAR RESPONSE TO RADIATION

Fitzgerald and colleagues reported that leukemia cells transfected with the n-ras oncogene acquired radioresistance, although the radioresistance was dose rate dependent (49). Sklar reported that the intrinsic radiation resistance of NIH-3T3 cells was increased by transfection with *ras* oncogenes activated by missense mutations (149). Chang and colleagues transfected DNA from fibroblasts derived from members of a cancer-prone family displaying the Li-Fraumeni syndrome into NIH 3T3 cells (22). These transfections resulted in transformed colonies when compared with cells transfected with DNA from normal cells. This report was accompanied by the observation of Kasid and colleagues, who reported that when DNA from a radioresistant human laryngeal carcinoma cell line was transfected into NIH 3T3 cells, a human c-raf transcript was identified in the subsequent transformants (88). In the reports from Chang and colleagues and Kasid and colleagues, the human c-raf-1 oncogene appeared to be rearranged in transformed NIH-3T3 cells transfected with human DNA and retained the majority of a presumably unregulated kinase domain of the c-raf gene. Kasid and colleagues followed this work by a report that antisense c-raf RNA partially reversed the radioresistant and tumorigenic phenotypes of raf-sense–transfected human laryngeal carcinoma cells (89). Pirollo and colleagues confirmed this observation and reported that activated c-raf-1 simultaneously conferred both the radioresistant and transformed phenotype on NIH 3T3 cells (133). These investigators also observed that transfection with v-mos oncogene conferred radioresistance on 3T3 cells, whereas transfection of cells with the v-fes and v-abl oncogenes did not. V-mos, like v-raf, is a serine threonine protein kinase, whereas v-fes and v-abl are tyrosine kinases. Pirollo and colleagues hypothesized that activated oncogenes whose protein products are related to serine and threonine phosphorylation effect radioresistance. They suggest that ras confers radioresistance because, in addition to its role as a G-protein and affecting hydrolysis of phosphoinositides, ras transduces signals through a direct regulation of protein kinase C, a serine threonine kinase.

INDUCTION OF CYTOKINES AND RADIATION RESPONSE

Hallahan and colleagues proposed that a cytotoxic protein was induced by x-rays when media decanted following irradiation of tissue cultures of some human sarcoma cell lines were cytotoxic to these as well as to other tumor cell lines (71). ELISA analysis showed that the level of tumor necrosis factor alpha (TNF-α) in the irradiated cultures was elevated over that of nonirradiated cells. This cytotoxicity was reversed by monoclonal antibodies to TNF-α. Increased levels of TNF-α mRNA were detected in TNF-α–producing cell lines. Nuclear run-on studies showed that radiation controlled TNF expression at the level of transcription. Because the media of irradiated cells were cytotoxic to other cell lines, a paracrine effect of TNF induction following x-rays was suggested. The authors proposed that intracellular secretion of TNF following x-ray exposure may also produce autocrine effects on irradiated cells. TNF-α is a polypeptide mediator of the cellular immune response with a wide range of activity. It has a direct effect on human cancer cell lines in vitro, resulting in death and growth inhibition, whereas in some normal cell lines, growth stimulation is observed. The cytotoxic effect of TNF correlates with free radical formation, DNA fragmentation, and microtubial destruction (173, 176). Radiation survival analyses conducted on cell lines that were TNF producing as well as TNF nonproducing were carried out in the presence of varying concentrations of tumor necrosis factor (71). In some cell lines, sublethal concentrations of TNF enhanced killing by radiation, suggesting a radiosensitizing and synergistic effect between TNF and x-rays (70). In other cell lines, additive killing was observed. The interaction between TNF and ionizing radiation may result from saturation of radical scavenging systems within the cell. This fact is supported by reports that cell lines that are resistant to oxidative damage by TNF also have an elevated free radical buffering capacity. Thus, cells that do not exhibit interactive killing between TNF and x-rays may be inherently more resistant to oxidative damage. Production of a cytokine (TNF-α in this instance) within irradiated cells may result in a greater biologic effect after x-ray exposure than is observed from killing produced by the direct effects of ionizing radiation alone. It is also possible that if a cytokine is secreted into adjacent cells or the systemic circulation, its production may have paracrine and endocrine, as well as autocrine, effects. Further analysis will demonstrate whether TNF induction by x-rays is a common occurrence. However, TNF induction and secretion serve as a model for the general concept that radiation-induced cytokines produce killing or protective effects in addition to the effects predicted by the direct effects of radiation on DNA.

The concept of the release of growth factors from endothelial cells following irradiation was advanced by Witte and colleagues (196). In their study, PDGF- and FGF-like growth factors were released following radiation treatment. These authors suggest that, PDGF-like factors secreted from the intima of blood vessels may serve as paracrine factors for the proliferation of smooth muscle cells observed in small arterioles after radiation in vivo. Similarly, FGF secreted after radiation may participate in the abnormal proliferation of endothelial cells that obliterate the lumen of small caliber arterioles in various organs. Secretion of these growth factors may account for some of the long-term effects of radiation secondary to small vessel obliteration. Radiation-mediated endothelial cell killing has been shown to be associated with apoptosis. Apoptosis following irradiation is prevented by the addition of basic fibroblast growth factor or protein kinase C agonists (54, 65).

ACUTE SEQUELAE OF RADIOTHERAPY

The acute sequelae of radiotherapy include common manifestations of radiotherapy, such as dermitis, enteritis, and mucositis. These self-limited processes are typically not of major consequence unless vital organs, such as the brain, pericardium, or lung, are involved. Acute sequelae in these organs may necessitate hospitalization and they are potentially life-threatening. In many instances, acute sequelae resemble an inflammationlike response. The etiology of this inflammationlike response is most likely multifactorial, may include apoptosis of many cell types, and x-ray killing of rapidly proliferating cells, and may be the associated x-ray–mediated induction of inflammatory mediators. Radiation-inducible inflammatory mediators include such cytokines as tumor necrosis factor and interleukin-1 (IL-1) and such cellular adhesion molecules as ICAM-1 (10) and the endothelial leukocyte adhesion molecule, E-selectin (69). E-selectin is crucial for the pathogenesis of tissue injury following the inflammatory response (11, 173). Neutrophils bind to irradiated endothelial cells (25, 36), which is necessary for the extravasation of leukocytes soon after irradiation (117, 150). Normal tissues respond to radiation with increased rolling and adhesion of leukocytes to the endothelium, whereas tumors do not (198). Taken together, these findings indicate that the pathogenesis of acute radiation sequelae is multifactorial, involving cellular depletion and an inflammationlike response.

Woloschak and colleagues described transcriptional induction of IL-1 following x-ray exposure (197). IL-1 is reported to be a radioprotector of hematopoietic cells in vivo (118). The production of various growth factors and cytokines may explain some unusual effects of radiation such as the abscopal effect on hematopoietic cells or the fatigue experienced by patients who undergo localized radiation therapy. Also, secretion of growth factors and cytokines may be an important step in radiation carcinogenesis in normal cells. Inhibition of molecular mediators of deleterious late radiation effects on the normal tissues may increase the therapeutic ratio and presents the possibility of genetic manipulation in clinical radiotherapy.

CELLULAR RADIATION RESPONSE: SIGNAL TRANSDUCTION

Recent data suggest that radiation induction of the early response genes, c-jun, fos, and Egr-1, which act as transcription factors, may initiate a cascade effect with pleiotropic cellular consequences (72, 147). At this time, the initiating events preceding early-response gene induction are unknown, although signaling in prokaryotes includes DNA strand breaks. Posttranslational modification of proteins that activate the early response genes is mediated in part through protein kinase C (72). Also, membrane changes induced by radiation may induce posttranslational changes, such as activation of tyrosine or serine/threonine protein kinases. Thus, biochemical changes within the cell may result in the activation of protein kinase C, the raf-1 protein, or other related kinases that may activate early-response genes and initiate DNA repair processes, cytokine production, cell cycle alteration, and the like (Fig. 48.18). Several previous undescribed proteins induced by ionizing radiation have been described (14). Also, activation of oncogenes by mutation or truncation (through deletion or inversion) may affect radioresistance, especially throughout a fractionated course of radiotherapy. The investigation of the molecular aspects of radiobiology presents exciting possibilities to enhance radiation therapy as a local and systemic modality.

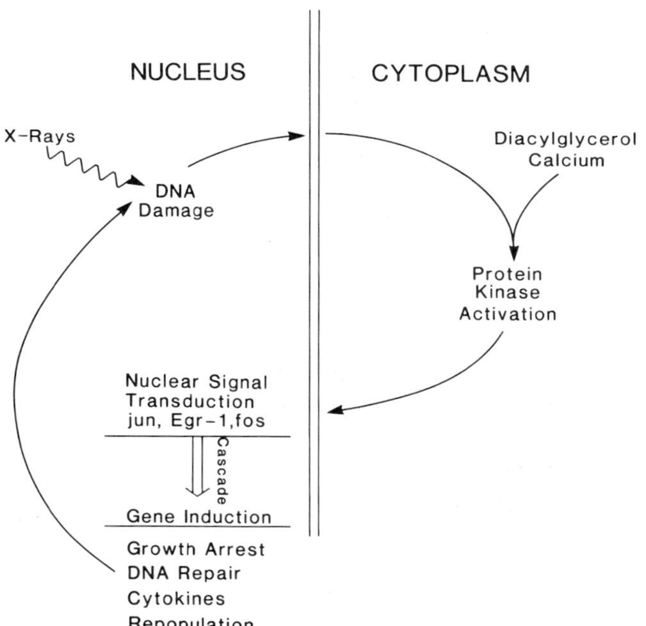

Figure 48.18. Proposed radiation response cycle demonstrating nuclear and cytoplasmic components. Ionizing radiation damage of cellular components results in activation of kinases. Inhibition of these kinases results in attenuation of nuclear signal transduction. The transcription factor genes in jun, Egr-1, and fos may be induced immediately after ionizing radiation damage. These transcription factors induce a cascade of molecular events leading to growth arrest, cytokine production, and repopulation. Kinase activation may also lead to activation of DNA repair enzymes directly. The radiation response cycle is complete when repair enzymes repair DNA damage caused by ionizing radiation.

RADIATION-MEDIATED APOPTOSIS

Apoptosis refers to the process of programmed cell death, which occurs in many physiologic processes, including embryogenesis, the elimination of self-recognizing T cells in the thymus, and the regulation of hematopoiesis (170). In many cells, apoptosis results in activation of a Ca^{++}/Mg^{++} dependent endonuclease, which cleaves DNA into multiples of 180 bp oligonucleosomal fragments. BCl^2 protects against oxidative stress and functions to prevent lipid peroxidation following growth factor withdrawal and may regulate apoptotic signals generated by free radicals, including those produced by ionizing radiation (80). BCl^2 dimerizes with the protein product of a related gene, BAX (120). Recent studies favor a model in which BCl^2 must bind to BAX to exert its antiapoptotic activity. Conditions that disrupt BCl^2/BAX heterodimers result in apoptosis (199). BCl_X, a gene related to BCl^2, has been shown to encode a potent dominant regulator of apoptotic death that suppresses radiation-mediated apoptosis. BCl_{XL}, a large-form splice variant of BCl_X, has been shown to be extremely efficient in suppressing apoptosis (13). BCl_{XS}, a small-form splice variant of BCl_X, has been shown to decrease the antiapoptotic effects of BCl_{XL}. Radiation-mediated apoptosis is associated with down regulation of Bl2 and BCl-X_L, whereas radioresistant cells that do not apoptose demonstrate upregulation of BCl_{XS} after irradiation. Therefore, the regulation of expression of these various proteins may determine susceptibility to apoptosis (156, 157).

Investigation of the effects of radiation apoptosis on radiocurability in murine tumors demonstrated that the induction of radiation-mediated apoptosis in a relatively large percentage of tumor cells correlated with longer growth delays and higher tumor control probabilities as compared with tumors in which radiation induced a small percentage of apoptotic tumor cells (156). These data suggest that increasing the induction of apoptosis in human tumor cells may be desirable in radiotherapy to increase local tumor control (111, 156, 157). Cells from some normal tissues also undergo radiation mediated apoptosis. In addition to thymic, lymphoid, and hematopoietic cells, radiation-induced apoptosis has been reported in stem and undifferentiated progenitor cells of testicular, intestinal, renal, and oligodendrocytic lineage and in the epithelium of the parotid and lacrimal glands (3, 24–26, 74, 158). Endothelial cells undergo apoptosis after exposure to ionizing radiation. A mechanism by which radiation induces apoptosis in endothelial cells has recently been described (65). Ionizing radiation acted directly on membrane preparations devoid of nuclei, stimulating sphingomyelin hydrolysis. These studies provide evidence that apoptotic signaling can be generated by the interaction of ionizing radiation with cellular membranes and suggest an alternative to the hypothesis that direct DNA damage mediates radiation-induced cell kill.

Currently, apoptotic signals from radiation are proposed to originate from damaged DNA. For example, Lowe et al. reported that the p53 gene is required for induction of apoptosis by radiation (and other DNA damaging agents) (106, 107). These investigators suggest that p53 may be critical in sensing DNA damage and may promote apoptosis to rid the organism of damaged cells. Waters et al. reported that BudR incorporation into the DNA of a murine T-cell hybridoma increased both BudR/x-ray–induced DNA strand breaks and apoptosis to a similar degree, lending support to the concept that DNA damage triggers apoptosis (29, 180). Many clinical investigations are directed at employing DNA damaging agents as radiosensitizers (177). One limitation of this approach may be that many tumors lack a functional p53 gene and, therefore, fail to initiate an apoptotic signal following DNA damage. Also, most normal tissues have an intact p53 gene and so may be susceptible to apoptotic signals from damaged DNA.

Growth and Regeneration Kinetics

The percentage of tumor cells detected to be in cycle is called the growth fraction. In human solid tumors, it is usually a small proportion of the total number of cells. If the growth fraction remains constant with time, the growth rate of the tumor is proportional to the growth fraction. If the growth fraction decreases with time, the rate of the tumor growth slows. Solid tumors usually grow at a slower rate as they enlarge and so growth is approximated by the Gompertz formula (79, 186). In circumstances of equilibrium in normal tissues, each mitotic division results in the average of only one new cell. Usually, one daughter is lost by desquamation, or metastasis. By definition, the cell loss factor in a steady state is one. Maximum growth occurs if the cell loss factor is reduced to zero. The only requirement for growth is a reduction from 1.0 in the cell loss factor—that is, an average of fewer than one of two daughter cells of a division is lost. A cell loss factor of less than one is characteristic regeneration of both normal tissue and malignant growth. Tumor growth is usually characterized by cell loss factors that are closer to one than zero.

An index for the potential regeneration of tumors and normal tissue populations is the proliferative activity of the cell population (195). One common measurement of tumor growth is the potential doubling time, which is defined as the time required to double the number of clonogenic cells if the cell loss factor decreases to zero. In this concept, the doubling time is equal to the cell cycle time. Tumors with a high rate of both cell production and loss have the potential for early and rapid regeneration after irradiation or other cytotoxic treatment. Thus, even though a tumor may exhibit slow pretreatment growth, it may regenerate rapidly. Excessive protraction in the time of radiation fractionation or split-course regimens may give inferior local control results if accelerated proliferation occurs during the period when radiation is not given. Clonal proliferation during tumor regression after irradiation was demonstrated by Hermens and Barendsen, who showed an exponential increase in clonogen number in a rat rhabdomyosarcoma during a time of tumor shrinkage (Fig. 48.19) (76). Accelerated repopulation of irradiated tumors and tissues may be associated with the recruitment of quiescent cells into the cell cycle. This effect is associated with radiation-mediated induction of the immediate early genes c-jun and Egr-1 (68).

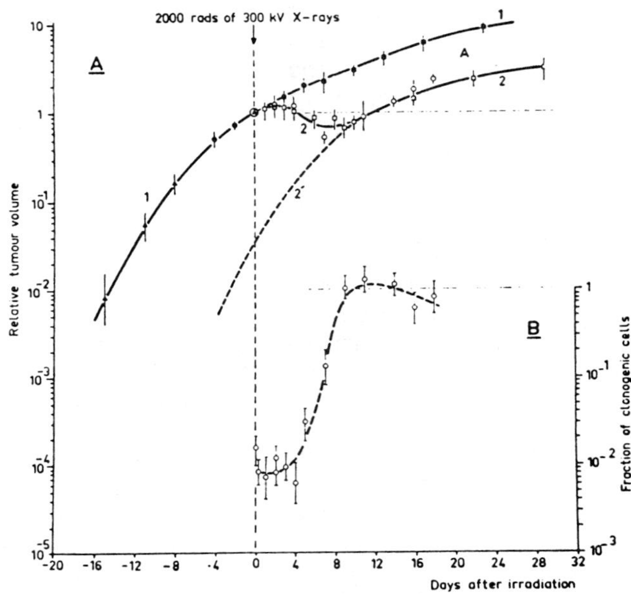

Figure 48.19. Growth curves of rat rhabdosarcoma tumors irradiated in vivo demonstrating accelerated repopulation. **A.** Volume change in the tumor after a single dose of 2,000 cGy. Curve 1 is the growth of an unirradiated tumor. Curve 2 represents regression and regrowth of an irradiated tumor. **B.** Exponential increase in the fractions of clonogenic cells as a function of time after irradiation. Cells were obtained from the tumors irradiated in **A**, and the colony-forming assay was used to determine clonogenic potential. This figure demonstrated that there is an exponential increase in the number of clonogenic cells within 6 to 10 days after irradiating a tumor in vivo and that clonogens can repopulate during tumor regression. *Source*: Hermens and Barendsen (76).

Tumor Hypoxia

As discussed earlier, ionizing radiation interacts with matter to produce short-lived free radicals that result in oxidative damage to the cells. Anoxic cells require two to three times the radiation dose to produce the same amount of cell killing as do well-oxygenated cells (168, 169). As demonstrated in Figure 48.20, the ratio of doses required to produce the same degree of cell killing in anoxic and oxygenated cells is referred to as the oxygen enhancement ratio (OER). The OER is 2.5 to 3 for x-rays but 1.6 for neutrons and 1.0 for alpha particles, since these particulate forms, of radiation directly damage DNA, thus decreasing the need for oxygen fixation of DNA damage.

Thomlinson and Gray observed that tumors "outgrow" their vasculature, resulting in necrotic areas (Chapter 10) and suggested that tumor cells adjacent to the anoxic region may be clonogenic but hypoxic (168, 169). As shown in Figure 48.21, the oxygen tension within the tumor falls with the distance from the capillary, producing a hypoxic region. In

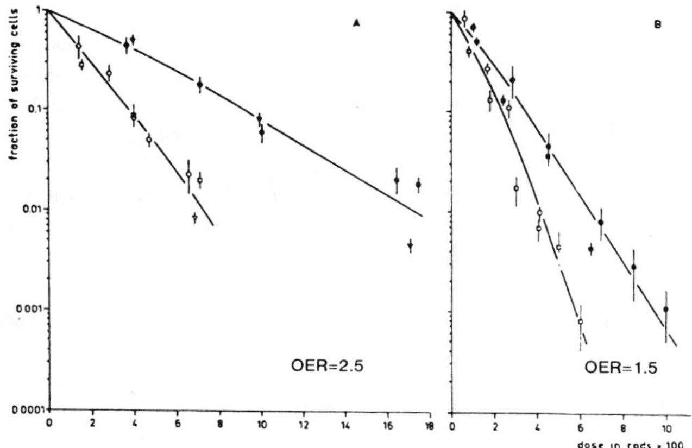

Figure 48.20. Radiation survival curves for cells irradiated under hypoxic and aerated conditions demonstrating the oxygen enhancement ratio (OER). OER is the ratio of the surviving fraction of cells after irradiation under hypoxic conditions. **A.** Oxygen enhancement ratio for cells irradiated with x-rays. **B.** Oxygen enhancement ratio for cells irradiated with neutrons. *Source*: Broerse et al. (15a).

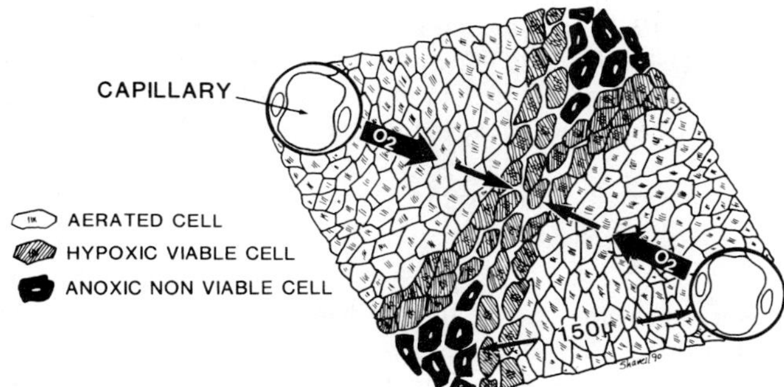

Figure 48.21. Oxygen diffusion through tissue from a capillary resulting in hypoxic cells. Oxygen diffuses an average of 150 Ci from the capillary. Cells beyond this region are anoxic and nonviable. Cells at the periphery of this radius are hypoxic but viable.

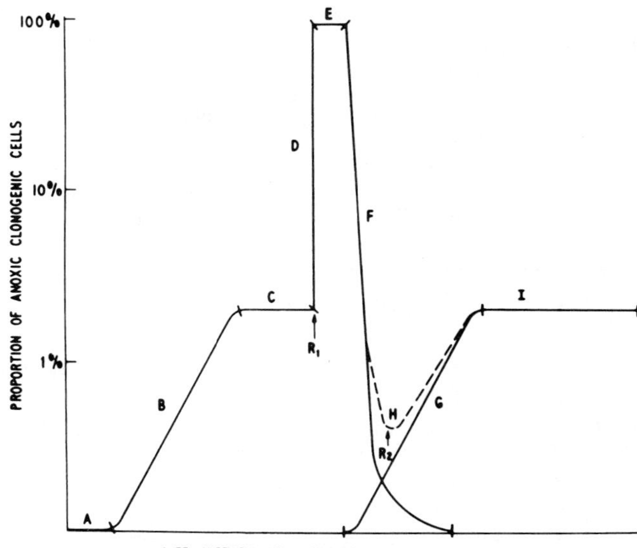

Figure 48.22. A theoretic model demonstrates that the percentage of viable hypoxic cells within a tumor varies as the tumor grows after irradiation. Curve A represents no hypoxic cells in a small tumor, whereas curve B shows the increase in hypoxic cells as the tumor "outgrows" its blood supply. This reaches a plateau region (curve C) that frequently ranges from 10 to 20% in a tumor. R_1 represents the time at which this tumor is exposed to x-rays. This dosage of radiation kills most of the aerated cells while the hypoxic cells survive. Thus, curve D represents the increase in the percentage of hypoxic cells that are clonogenic after irradiation. This increased percentage of hypoxic cells that persists for a short period is represented by curve E. Reoxygenation occurs, and the proportion of hypoxic cells decreases (curve F). Curve G represents regrowth of the tumor after irradiation and shows the increase in proportion of hypoxic cells in the growing tumor. Curve H is an extrapolation of the percentage of hypoxic cells caused by reoxygenation and tumor regrowth. The plateau region is again obtained in curve I. *Source*: Thomlinson (168).

some experimental tumor systems, reoxygenation of hypoxic tumor cells occurs within 24 hours (137). The physiologic mechanism for reoxygenation may involve reduced oxygen utilization by radiation-injured cells or the redistribution of blood flow within the tumor. The potential importance of reoxygenation during multifractionated radiotherapy is demonstrated when considering a theoretic tumor in which 90% of cells are well oxygenated and 10% are hypoxic. If reoxygenation did not occur, the percentage of hypoxic cells eventually would exceed that of aerated cells due to the radioresistance of hypoxic cells. However, if reoxygenation occurs, the percentage of hypoxic cells remains constant (10%) and eventually can be eliminated (86, 137). Thus, reoxygenation provides an advantage to multifractionated radiotherapy by reducing the number of clonogenic hypoxic cells irradiated during each treatment. A theoretical model for tumor reoxygenation was proposed by Thomlinson (Fig. 48.22) (168, 169). In this model, small tumors have no hypoxic component (curve A), but the percentage of hypoxic cells increases as the tumor grows (curve B). A steady state of hypoxia then develops (curve C). Immediately after irradiation, aerated cells are killed, resulting in an increase in the percentage of hypoxic cells (curve D). Following a transient period of hypoxia (curve E), metabolism ceases and more oxygen is available to hypoxic cells (curve F). Tumor regrowth results in a return to the original percentage of hypoxic cells (curves G and I). Curve H represents the optimal time for the second radiation fraction (R_2).

A clinical observation that suggests that hypoxia participates in tumor radioresistance is that severe anemia is associated with worsened local control in a number of tumors. Several studies demonstrated improved survival in intermediate-stage cervical carcinoma patients treated with radiotherapy when hemoglobin concentrations were above 11 grams as compared with patients with lower hemoglobin levels (17, 45, 77). The reduction in survival associated with anemia during radiotherapy is also observed in other tumor types, including endometrial, bladder, and pharyngeal carcinomas (123, 138, 143). Other clinical observations that suggest that hypoxia contributes to radioresistance include hyperbaric oxygen (HBO), which has been used to improve the therapeutic ratio during radiotherapy for hypoxic tumors. HBO was used during the treatment of cervical carcinoma in a Medical Research Council (MRC) trial. The local control was improved by 25% ($p = .0003$) and survival improved by

12% (35). The MRC trial of radiotherapy and HBO (O_2 at 3 A T M) for head and neck cancer also demonstrated a significant improvement in local control and survival (75). Despite the encouraging results, HBO is seldom used because of the technical difficulties associated with irradiating patients while they are in hyperbaric chambers. Also, some hyperbaric oxygen trials have not shown an advantage for HBO as compared with standard treatment.

Hypoxic Tumor Cell Radiosensitizers

Hypoxic tumor cell sensitizers are a class of electron affinic compounds that fix damage induced by ionizing radiation under hypoxic conditions, thereby mimicking oxygen (1). The prototypes of hypoxic cell sensitizers are the nitroimidazole compounds (1, 27–29). The nitroimidazole used in most clinical trials to date is misonidazole. Most studies have demonstrated no benefit from misonidazole despite the fact that it enhances cell killing under hypoxic conditions in vitro (27–29). Possible reasons for the lack of clinical efficacy are that neurotoxicity prevents the obtaining of adequate drug levels, misonidazole may not demonstrate adequate electron affinity (1), and hypoxia is not a cause of radioresistance in human tumors studied in sensitizer trials. Several recently developed nitroimidazole compounds may prove to have greater clinical efficacy because they have less neurotoxicity. One such compound is SR-2508 (etanidazole), which can be given at a dose five times greater than for misonidazole, and has been used in phase I and II trials (28, 29). Further clinical investigation with hypoxic cell sensitizers continues.

The importance of the role of hypoxic tumor cells in radiotherapy is controversial because many of the clinical data comparing HBO and hypoxic cell sensitizers do not compare these modifiers with optimal fractionation schemes, or are negative. Theoretic calculations of potentially hypoxic tumor cells suggest that even a very small proportion of these cells would render most human tumors impossible to control with radiotherapy. It is likely, however, that tumor cell hypoxia plays a role in the failure of radiotherapy to sterilize some human tumors.

Radiation Protectors

A potential means of improving the therapeutic ratio is to develop drugs that protect normal tissues against ionizing radiation while not affecting tumor radiosensitivity (201). One class of drugs under study is sulfhydryl-containing compounds. A prototype compound is the sulfhydryl-containing amino acid cysteine, which demonstrates the property of being a free-radical scavenger. Experimentally, cysteine protects mice from lethal doses of irradiation (126, 127). The proposed mechanisms by which sulfhydryls protect against radiation are at both the chemical level (free-radical scavenging, stabilization of chromatin, and hydrogen ion donation) and at the enzymatic level (enhanced DNA repair, and cell cycle delay) (59). Sulfhydryl compounds have been developed that are less toxic than cystine to humans. They include WR-2721 (S-2[3-aminopropylamino) ethylphosphoric acid, amifostine] which reduces mucositis resulting from radiotherapy when applied topically (97, 200). Infusion of WR-2721 into rodents protected normal tissues while not affecting tumor control (201). One clinical trial demonstrated protection of human bone marrow by WR-2721 in patients receiving hemibody irradiation (30). The radioprotector WR-1065 has demonstrated protection against x-ray–induced double-strand breaks, cytotoxicity, and mutagenicity from cisplatinum (116). Thus, these protectors may be combined with radiotherapy or chemotherapy to reduce the risk of treatment-related carcinogenesis.

Biologic response modifiers that are demonstrated radioprotectors include IL-1 and GM-CSF (118, 121). GM-CSF protects the bone marrow when added after irradiation, acting to enhance the recovery of irradiated bone marrow. These agents are not classic radioprotectors since they do not directly scavenge free radicals, but rather improve bone marrow tolerance by expanding the hematopoietic compartment (IL-1 has been reported to induce free-radical scavengers). Interleukin-1 protects mice from lethal doses of radiation (121) and accelerates the recovery of CFU-E, GM-CFU, BFU-E, and CFU-Meg after irradiation. Interleukin-1 also enhances the survival of lethally irradiated mice treated with allogenic bone marrow cells (121).

Fractionation

Radiation therapy is usually delivered as a series of 180 to 300-cGy fractions in 5 to 6 days for 5 to 8 weeks. The use of fractionation arose from the empiric studies of European radiotherapists and radiobiologists in the early 20th century. Many modifications in fractionation have been attempted since these studies; however, it is generally accepted that fractionation increases the therapeutic ratio (52, 161, 167). The effects of fractionation on tumors and normal tissues depend on the total dose, the fraction size (amount of radiation delivered per dose), the number of treatment sessions, and the overall time of radiation delivery. Repair and regeneration (repopulation) increase the total dose required to achieve a specific level of biologic damage (referred to as an isoeffective dose) when radiation is fractionated (161). Redistribution of cells to radiosensitive phases of the cell cycle and reoxygenation of radioresistant hypoxic cells reduce the dose required for a specific level of biologic damage. In general, the larger the fraction size, the more severe are the late effects of radiotherapy on normal tissues. Acute reactions caused by interruptions in relatively rapid cell renewal systems are not good indicators of late normal tissue effects and are usually not dose limiting in standard fraction schemes. Successful fractionation is a balance between the delivery of a tumoricidal dose without causing acute reactions that are so severe that the duration of radiation therapy is excessively protracted or intolerable long-term normal tissue damage occurs. Various mathematic models have been proposed to equate overall dose, time, fraction size, and achieve an isoeffective dose. The clinical usefulness of these models is controversial.

ALTERATIONS IN FRACTIONATION

Historically, split-course fractionated radiotherapy was one of the first alterations in the fraction schedule attempted. A break of 2 to 3 weeks was established in the middle of the treatment to allow tumor shrinkage and possible reoxygenation. However, clinical results obtained using split-course radiotherapy generally are not superior to, and in some instances are worse than, the results obtained with continuous radiotherapy (124). Accelerated fractionation decreases the overall treatment time to diminish clonogenic proliferation between doses. In accelerated fractionation schedules, treatment is given two to four times a day employing fractions of 150 to 200 cGy per treatment with 4 to 6 hours between fractions (179, 195). Thus, the daily dose is 300 to 600 cGy and the total dose is given in 3 to 4 weeks. Frequently, severe acute normal tissue reactions develop and a break in treatment is required (130, 195). Even when treatment interruption is necessary, the total treatment time is reduced from 6 to 8 weeks to 5 to 6 weeks. Tumors with a relatively short potential doubling time are the most suitable candidates for accelerated fractionation. Clinical gain from an accelerated fractionation schedule has been demonstrated in patients with Burkitt's lymphoma and promising results have been obtained in patients with stages II and III head and neck cancer (116, 195).

Hyperfractionation employs relatively small doses per fraction, usually 100 to 120 cGy administered two or three times a day (116, 195). This approach achieves a small decrease in the overall treatment time. Hyperfractionation delivers an increased number of treatments, 50 to 60 versus 30 to 35. Thus, relatively rapidly dividing cell populations may have a higher proportion of cells in the most sensitive phases of the cell cycle at each treatment. Cells in late-responding normal tissues are slowly proliferating; therefore, after a few fractions, many surviving cells will be concentrated at the most resistant phases of the cell cycle. This concept provides a rationale for a potential differential response in normal tissue versus tumor in hyperfractionated regimens.

Vokes and Weichselbaum (177) and Taylor and colleagues (165) have employed concomitant chemotherapy and radiotherapy on alternative weeks. Preliminary data suggest that increased tumor cell kill achieved by concomitant radiotherapy and chemotherapy overcomes tumor cell proliferation between alternative-week treatments. The goal of these trials will be to shorten the overall treatment time by manipulation of chemotherapy dose and radiotherapy fractionation. Hypofractionation or larger than standard fractions have been employed in melanoma, lung cancer, and head and neck cancer (182). Although tumor regressions frequently are more rapid with large fraction sizes, local control is not necessarily increased and, in fact, may be decreased under some circumstances. For example, Eichhorn employed several fractionation schemes of 400 to 1,000 cGy in lung cancer as compared with 200-cGy fraction sizes (but similar final doses) and found that an increased fraction size actually provided a decrease in tumor sterilization at the time of surgery (37). Byhardt, Greenberg, and Cox compared treatment five times per week with treatment three times per week with slightly larger fraction sizes and found decreased local control in the oral cavity and oropharynx with larger fraction sizes and a smaller number of fractions (18). Increased PLDR at large fraction sizes is one reason suggested for the decrease in local control in these studies (182).

Dose Response and the Therapeutic Ratio

Various levels of radiation yield different tumor-control probabilities, depending on the size and anatomic extent of the lesion. The total number of surviving cells is proportional to the initial number and biologic characteristics of clonogenic cells and the total cell kill achieved with a specified dose of radiation. Dose–response relationships for local control of homogeneous tumor groups have been empirically determined. The higher the doses of radiation delivered, the more likely is tumor control (Table 48.2).

The dose of radiation that can be delivered to a tumor is limited by the probability of serious normal tissue complications. Therefore, the choice of a tumor dose is based on the relative probability of tumor control and normal tissue complications. The potential therapeutic gain can be estimated for an average group of patients based on tumor size, histologic type, and the normal tissues that will be included in the treatment fields. Figure 48.23 shows a theoretic dose–re-

Table 48.2. Relationship of Tumor Diameter and Dose to Percent Local Control

Dose (5×200 cGy/wk)	% Control	
	Squamous cell carcinoma	Adenocarcinoma
5,000	>90% microfoci 50% 2–3-cm nodes	>90% subclinical
6,000	80–90% T1 pharynx and larynx 50% T3–T4 tonsil	
7,000	90% 1–3-cm nodes 80% T3–T4 tonsil	90% axillary

Adapted from Fletcher (49a).

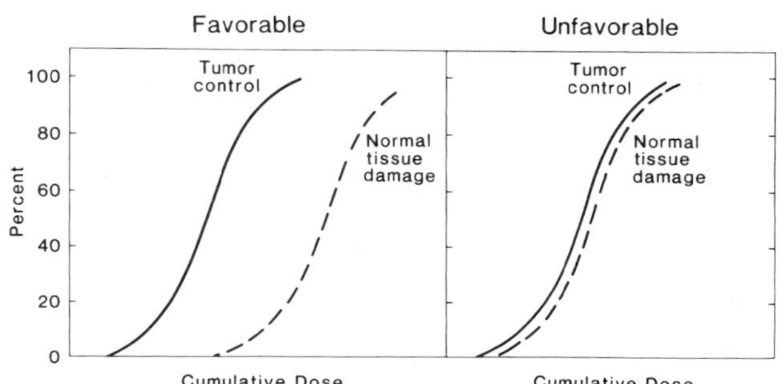

Figure 48.23. Dose control and complication curves in curable and noncurable tumors treated with radiotherapy. The percentages of tumor control and normal tissue damage are sigmoidal. In a radiocurable tumor, such as Hodgkin's disease, the dose required to control a tumor is less than the normal tissue tolerance. This results in a favorable therapeutic ratio. The dosage required to control an unfavorable tumor, such as pancreatic carcinoma, is approximately that of the normal tissue tolerance, resulting in an unfavorable therapeutic ratio. (Courtesy of Varian, Palo Alto, California.)

sponse relationship for tumor control and normal tissue complications. The therapeutic ratio is defined as the percentage of tumor cures obtained at a given level of toxicity for normal tissues. Hill suggests that the therapeutic ratio is better defined in terms of a ratio of radiation doses required to produce a given percentage of tumor control and complications (79). Figure 48.23*A* depicts a favorable therapeutic ratio and Figure 48.23*B* depicts an unfavorable therapeutic ratio. The greater the displacement between the two curves (in the favorable situation), the more radiocurable is the tumor.

CHEMOTHERAPY X-RAY INTERACTION

The use of combined chemotherapy and radiation therapy aims to overcome the lack of tumor radiocurability as a cause of local treatment failure and to eradicate distant micro metastases and gross metastases as a cause of systemic failure. Four theoretic types of interactions between radiation and chemotherapy can occur (54, 152, 153, 177): (1) Spatial cooperation describes the independent activity of each treatment modality—for radiotherapy within the radiation treatment field, against the primary site of disease, and for chemotherapy outside of the radiotherapy field, against presumed metastatic disease. (2) Toxicity independence implies that administration of each treatment modality at a full or nearly full dose without significantly increasing normal tissue damage might result in therapeutic enhancement. No interaction between the two therapy modalities is required, and additive activity would be the expected clinical outcome. (3) The protection of normal tissues from radiation by a systemic agent might increase local control by allowing for the administration of higher doses of radiation. However, increased efficacy will result only if the tumor is exempted from the protective action of the drug. (4) Increased activity in the radiation field may result directly from the interaction of chemotherapy with radiation. In this situation, the drug has been called a sensitizer, enhancer, or potentiator of radiation (34, 152, 153, 177).

Steel proposed terminology to characterize the type and extent of interaction between two agents in the laboratory (152, 153). These concepts are based on the availability of a dose–response curve for each of the single-treatment modality agents and an isobologram analysis of their combined response. Where the drug is inactive by itself, a positive interaction with radiation is referred to as sensitization and a negative interaction as protection. Where the drug has activity by itself and dose–response curves are available for both the drug and the radiation, the interaction can be described as supra-additive (synergistic), additive, or subadditive (34, 152). One common definition of synergy is a reduction in the D_0 when the drug is added to radiation; additivity is defined as a reduction in *n* with no change in D_0 when the drug is added (34). Detailed dose–response curves may be available for only one or none of the two agents. In these instances, a positive interaction is described as enhancement or cooperation and a negative interaction as inhibition or antagonism. Vokes and Weichselbaum suggested the use of the term "enhancement" to describe an increase in the activity of radiation in the presence of chemotherapy, while not attempting to distinguish between additivity and synergy (177).

Table 48.3. Interaction of Radiotherapy and Chemotherapy

Chemotherapy drug and radiation active against different tumor cell subpopulations based on hypoxia, cell cycle specificity, and pH
Decreased tumor cell repopulation following fractionated radiation due to effects of chemotherapy
Increased tumor cell recruitment from G_0 into a therapy-responsive cell cycle phase
Increased tumor cell oxygenation following radiation with improved drug or radiation activity
Improved drug delivery with shrinkage of tumor
Early eradication of tumor cells preventing emergence of drug and/or radiation resistance
Eradication of cells resistant to one treatment modality by the other treatment
Cell cycle synchronization
Inhibition of repair of sublethal radiation damage or inhibition of recovery from potentially lethal radiation damage

From Vokes and Weichselbaum (177).

Possible mechanisms of interaction between chemotherapeutic drugs and radiation have been reviewed in detail and include those listed in Table 48.3 (177). These interactions may be based on differential activity of drug and radiation against specific tumor cell subpopulations, for example, tumor cell hypoxia and cell-cycle phase-sensitivity patterns, or on mechanical factors, such as reduced tumor bulk, leading to improved drug delivery to malignant cells. Other mechanisms require a direct interaction between drug and radiation and include inhibition of repair of radiation damage, cell cycle synchronization, and the elimination of inherently radioresistant cells. A major limitation to the effective combination of chemotherapy and radiotherapy is toxicity, which limits potentially curative doses of either modality. A theoretic limitation of combined therapy is the emergence of drug- and/or x-ray–resistant tumor cells, which may occur as a result of gene alterations induced by drugs, x-rays, or both. It has been suggested that chemotherapy administered concomitantly with radiotherapy may increase rather than decrease the incidence of distant metastases (177).

The halogenated pyrimidines, iododeoxyuridine (IudR) and bromodeoxyuridine (BUdR) are analogues of thymidine that may be incorporated into DNA. The van der Waals forces surrounding the halogen approximate that of the methyl group of thymidine. DNA replaced with BUdR or IUdR is more susceptible to damage by ionizing radiation. Halogenated pyrimidines must be available to cells for several cell divisions prior to irradiation; radiosensitization increases as the percentage replacement of thymidine increases (93, 94). BUdR and IUdR demonstrate equal radiosensitivity, while BUdR produces more sensitization to fluorescent light and, therefore, is used less frequently in clinical trials. Halogenated pyrimidines are under clinical investigation.

Gene Therapy and Radiation

The potential advantage of combining gene therapy with radiotherapy in the treatment of cancer is the accurate delivery of therapeutic agents to tumor cells to induce tumor cell cytotoxicity (4, 33). Gene therapy strategies to enhance the killing of tumor cells by radiation include genes encoding cytokines that interact with radiation. For example, human glioma cells transduced with HSV-tk and exposed to BrdUrd for 24 hours prior to irradiation were more sensitive to radiation than were control cells under the same conditions (92). Cell-based studies examining the efficacy of radiation combined with gene therapy in vivo include the myeloid-derived cells containing TNF regulated by the radiation inducible promoter Egr-1 (188). Conversely, radioprotection of normal tissues can also be achieved by delivering the gene-encoding manganese superoxide dismutase (MnSOD). This gene, placed on the radiation-inducible promoter Egr-1 and delivered to bone marrow stromal cells, results in radioprotection at low doses.

Methods to localize cytotoxic gene therapy for cancer include the use of viral delivery systems that bind tissue specific receptors (87) and of tissue-specific enhancers that limit transcription to certain cell types (109). In spite of these advances, one major obstacle to the efficacy of gene therapy is the lack of spatial and temporal regulation of cytotoxic genes. To achieve spatial and temporal control of gene transcription, localization of ionizing radiation has been used to regulate gene transcription through the promoter/enhancer region of the radiation-inducible gene Egr-1, upstream of TNF cDNA. The Egr-TNF genetic construct was then ligated into the replication-deficient adenovirus type 5 (Ad5) genome, creating the Ad5(Egr-TNF) vector (85, 110). SQ-20B xenografts were inoculated with Ad5(Egr-TNF) twice weekly for 2 weeks in combination with x-rays (5 Gy/d, 4 days a week) to a total dose of 50 Gy (69). Immunohistochemical staining of tumor cryosections demonstrated granular intracytoplasmic staining for TNF and ELISA assay demonstrated in vivo induction of TNF. The combination of Ad5(Egr-TNF) and radiation significantly reduced the mean tumor volume ($p<.05$) as compared with Ad5(Egr-TNF) alone or radiation alone (Fig. 48.24). The interaction between Ad5(Egr-TNF) and radiation results from increasing apoptosis, necrosis, and tumor infiltration by neutrophils.

Localization of TNF by means of genetic radiotherapy avoids potential systemic toxicity while maintaining interactive killing, thereby improving the therapeutic ratio. This regional gene therapy is probably most advantageous for tumors currently treated with radiotherapy, such as gliomas, rectal, and upper aerodigestive tract tumors, because local/regional control leads to cure in a large percentage of these neoplasms with relatively low metastatic potential. Ge-

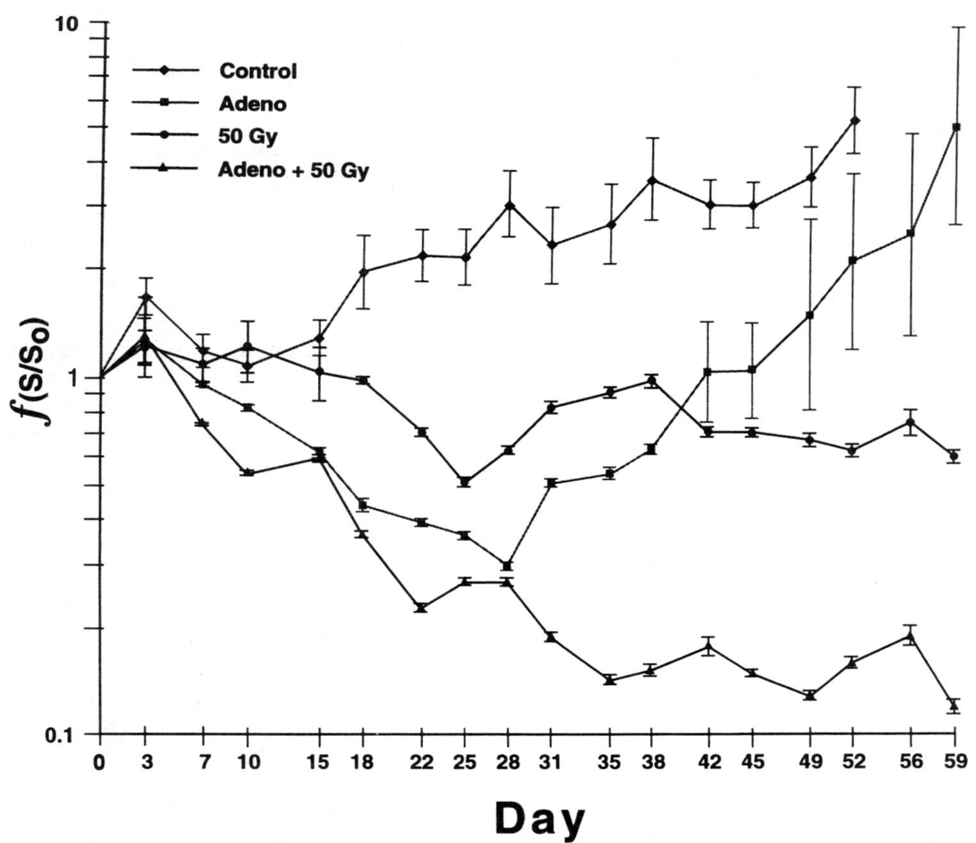

Figure 48.24. In vivo tumor control with Ad5(Egr-TNF) and radiation. Ad5(Egr-TNF) alone produced tumor regression to a mean of 30% of original volume (day 28), whereas radiation alone (50 Gy) reduced mean tumor volume to 51% (day 25). Tumor regrowth to original volume occurred at day 42 and day 58, respectively. Ad5(Egr-TNF) plus 50 Gy reduced mean volume to 16% (day 35), and tumor regrowth did not occur by day 80 ($P < 0.05$).

netic radiotherapy is a new paradigm for the treatment of cancer in that transcription of therapeutic genes can be localized and regulated by ionizing radiation without an apparent increase in local or systemic toxicity. Tumor specificity is achieved through the use of this system, because transcription of Egr-TNF is localized by ionizing radiation, and TNF, in turn, produces tumor-specific cell killing. Egr-TNF is well suited for a radiation-inducible system, because each daily radiation treatment will localize transcription of the therapeutic gene to the tumor volume. Ionizing radiation is effective in inducing gene transcription within a confined volume and time. The concept of activation of genes by x-irradiation, which has a well-defined targeting technology, may lead to broad and essential applications of ionizing radiation with precise spatial and temporal control of gene therapy.

BASIS FOR COMBINING RADIATION AND SURGERY

Radical surgery frequently requires organ removal or amputation, while conservative surgery removes only clinically apparent tumor. Radiation therapy used in combination with conservative surgery eliminates residual microscopic tumor cell extension into normal tissues. The goal of conservative surgery combined with radiotherapy is to avoid the consequences of radical surgery and thus preserve organ function and cosmesis. These goals are achieved not only by reducing the extent of surgery, but also by reducing the radiation dose that would be required to control gross tumor. Examples of cancer in which limited surgery and radiotherapy that have been shown to be effective in organ preservation and cosmesis are localized limb sarcoma and breast cancer (48, 134).

Preoperative radiation therapy is given with the intention of reducing the quantity of viable tumor cells, as well as the anatomic extent of tumor prior to surgery. Preoperative radiotherapy may diminish the risk of wound contamination by malignant cells and theoretically reduce the risk of metastases during tumor manipulation. Tumor regression subsequent to preoperative radiation therapy may increase the resectability of locally advanced disease. Among the limitations of preoperative irradiation are (1) that in general, higher radiation doses can be given postoperatively; and (2) although some patients in a disease category may not require radiotherapy, with current staging methods, it would be used for all patients treated (e.g., Duke's A, B1, and D rectal cancer patients do not require radiotherapy but likely would be included in a preoperative radiotherapy protocol). Examples of the use of preoperative radiation are in the treatment of superior sulcus lung cancer, locally advanced rectal carcinoma, and bladder carcinoma prior to cystectomy or interstitial implantation of radioactive sources (15, 78, 174).

Indications for postoperative radiation therapy include known or suspected residual disease or anatomic sites with a high risk of local recurrence following surgery (112, 176). Anatomic sites in the upper aerodigestive tract with a high incidence of local recurrence after resection are listed in Table 48.4 (49, 112). Table 48.5 demonstrates the influence of surgical margins and postoperative radiotherapy on local recurrence (112). Local recurrence increases significantly if the interval exceeds 7 weeks (112). Thus, the interval should be as short as postoperative wound healing permits, preferably within 2 weeks. The risk of poor wound healing increases with dose (135, 177).

Table 48.4. Number of Patients with Negative Tumor Margins Who Develop Local Recurrences

Site	Total no.	No. recurrences in primary site (%)
Tongue	510	166 (32.5)
Gingiva	134	42 (31.3)
Lip	81	7 (8.6)
Supraglottic larynx	167	42 (25.1)
Palate	137	57 (41.6)
Tonsil	147	61 (41.5)
Pharynx and pyriform sinus	183	68 (37.2)
Buccal mucosa	99	33 (33.3)
Floor of mouth	255	67 (26.3)

From Fletcher (49a).

Table 48.5. Local Control Is Dependent upon Status of Surgical Margins and Preoperative Radiotherapy

Status of margin	Local recurrence without radiotherapy (%)	Recurrence after postoperative radiotherapy (%)
No tumor	39*	2
In situ carcinoma	84.6	—
Close (within 5 mm)	73.7	—
Invasive cancer present	64-73	10.5

* See Table 48.4 for recurrence rate for each site when margins are without tumor.
Adapted from Looser (105a) and Vikram (176).

RADIATION INJURY TO NORMAL TISSUE

The response of normal tissues to radiation may be categorized by the length of time after irradiation that damage appears. Acute radiation injury occurs hours to days after irradiation and is due to interruption of repopulation in rapidly proliferating tissues, such as the oral mucosa or gastrointestinal tract (159). Subacute radiation injury is seen weeks to months after irradiation and is caused by injury to such cells as the type II pneumocytes that exhibit lethality or dysfunction during this time (31).

The pathogenesis of chronic radiation injury is multifactorial: (1) microvascular destruction by radiation results in organ ischemia, fibrosis, and necrosis; (2) stem cells required to replenish cell renewal systems can be reduced in quantity sufficiently to cause organ failure; and (3) the concept of the functional unit theorizes that strategically placed cell death can result in dysfunction of the entire organ. Destruction of a functional unit produces significant morbidity for such systems as the spinal cord and the nephron. Injury to the renal tubule or glomerulus may cause dysfunction of the entire nephron. Myelopathy may result from injury to a microscopic cross section of the spinal cord and does not require injury to the entire organ. These processes act interdependently to cause the pathogenesis of chronic radiation injury. Thus, cell death can result in organ dysfunction if injuries are strategically placed (130, 195). Late tissue injury is usually the dose-limiting event in radiotherapy, although acute and subacute reactions may be dose limiting under certain circumstances, such as radiation pneumonitis, pericarditis, or severe mucositis (31, 159, 160).

The shape of the radiation survival curve varies among normal tissues. Both the initial slopes and the terminal slopes are different for tissues responding to early acute effects and to late long-term effects, as illustrated in Figure 48.25. For doses used during radiotherapy, the shape of the initial slope is extremely important. In general, early-responding tissues have a steeper initial slope as compared with late-responding tissues. This results in a greater surviving fraction in late tissues as compared with early tissues (195). During fractionation of radiotherapy, these differences in surviving fractions are recapitulated daily, resulting in accentuation of the initial slope of the survival curve. Thus, late-responding tissues are spared by fractionation to greater degree than are early tissues.

A tumor's dose curve versus the normal tissue damage paradigm can be confusing. For example, to sterilize a gross tumor a dose sufficient to kill 10^9 to 10^{11} cells must be delivered. A small volume of most normal tissue will tolerate such a dose, depending on the function of the organ. For example, the cervix tolerates much higher doses than does the spinal cord because moderate fibrosis in the cervix usually does not result in severe functional consequences whereas a similar amount of damage in the spinal cord might be catastrophic. Also, fewer cells need to be killed to disrupt the functional unit of the spinal cord than to sterilize most tumors. Therefore, the volume of normal tissue exposed to radiation is critical, and optimal treatment planning is necessary to maintain the most favorable therapeutic ratio possible in a specific clinical situation. The tolerance doses listed in Table 48.6 are adapted and updated from Rubin et al. (141). The $TD_{5/5}$ is known from clinical studies in which 5% of patients developed the listed injury after the entire organ or a significant portion was irradiated using standard fractionation (200 cGy/d for 5 days a week).

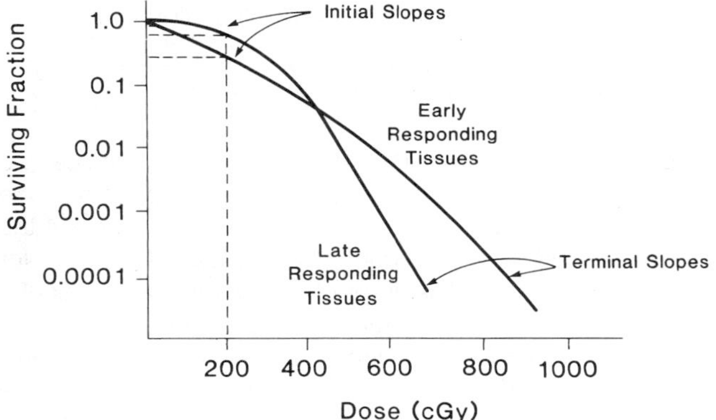

Figure 48.25. Initial slopes and terminal slopes for early- and late-responding normal tissues. Late-responding tissues have a small initial slope followed by a larger terminal slope of the survival curve. In contrast, early-responding tissues have a larger initial slope and smaller terminal slope. Thus, the surviving fraction of late-responding tissues at 200 cGy is greater than that of early-responding tissues. This difference in surviving fraction in the shoulder region of the survival curves of these two tissue types is recapitulated with each fraction of radiotherapy. This results in the risk of radiation injury to late-responding tissues.

Table 48.6. Late Tissue Injury from Radiation

Organs	Injury	$TD_{5/5}$
Bone marrow (TBI)	Aplasia, pancytopenia	250
Liver	Acute and chronic	3000
Stomach	Perforation, ulcer,	4500
	hemorrhage	5000
Brain	Infarction, necrosis	6000
Spinal cord	Infarction, necrosis	4500
Heart	Pericarditis and pancarditis	4500
Lung	Acute and chronic pneumonitis	2000
Kidney	Acute and chronic nephrosclerosis	2000
Esophagus	Ulceration	6000
Rectum	Ulcer, stricture	6000
Salivary glands	Xerostomia	5000
Bladder	Contracture	6000
Ureters	Stricture	7500
Testes	Sterilization	100
Ovary	Sterilization	200-300
Eye		
a) Retina	Blindness	5500
b) Cornea	Ulceration	5000
c) Lens	Cataract	500
Thyroid gland	Hypothyroidism	4500
Peripheral nerves	Neuropathy	6000

Normal tissue tolerance doses in cGy which produce injury in 5% ($TD_{5/5}$) within five years after irradiation. Modified from Rubin (141).

VASCULAR INJURY BY IONIZING RADIATION

Vascular lesions are prominent pathologic findings in normal tissue damage resulting from ionizing radiation. The importance of the vascular component in the pathogenesis of radiation-mediated organ injury was first described at the turn of the century (55, 114). Numerous studies verifying these findings led to the hypothesis by Rubin and Casarett that vascular insufficiency and ischemia are primary components of the pathogenesis of late radiation damage in normal tissues (140). Morphologic and ultrastructural studies have demonstrated that damage to the microvascular endothelium is a predominant lesion in the early phases of radiation injury (46, 81, 99, 139). Depletion of the microvasculature, in turn, leads to vascular insufficiency and ischemia. Organ dysfunction and possibly tissue necrosis are complications of radiotherapy that are life threatening when they appear in vital organs, such as the brain or heart.

Clinical Treatment Planning

The goal of treatment planning is uniformly to irradiate the gross tumor volume and known or suspected routes of disease spread while sparing adjacent radiation-sensitive tissues (125). Treatment planning is a critical link among physics, biology, and clinical radiotherapy. The spatial distribution of radiation delivered depends on the external patient contour, variations in tissue density that affect radiation transport, and the technical details of the planned irradiation, including beam energy and configuration of radiation portals. Because the gross tumor may be irregularly shaped, and a high dose margin around the tumor is needed to treat microscopic disease adequately and account for variations in daily patient setup, an approach based on a three-dimensional image is becoming increasingly important in radiation therapy planning (57, 58, 104, 113). As noted in the previous section, limiting normal tissue volume irradiated is critical to decreasing complications. Both the basic concepts of treatment planning and the more advanced technical considerations related to the planning of three-dimensional treatment are described here.

IMAGING

Imaging plays a central role in radiotherapy, providing geometric information on external patient contour and tumor size, shape, and location relative to adjacent critical structures (57). The process begins with the acquisition of a volumetric computed tomography (CT) scan, where contiguous slices of transaxial image data are acquired with the patient in the treatment position. In a more conventional approach, information on tumor size, shape, and location are transferred from hard-copy films of the CT slices onto AP or lateral radiographs, using bony landmarks visualized on both CT and conventional radiographs. Mapping the target to oblique films is significantly more difficult.

To provide more flexible and precise treatment planning methods, image-based treatment planning approaches that permit the graphic visualization of tumor and anatomy on a computer have been developed. Through interactive manipulation, these displays can provide insights into the optimal approaches for radiation portals. After the CT scan, the image data set are read into the treatment planning computer, on which the radiation therapist identifies and outlines, on each CT image, the target volume to be treated. The external body outline and other critical structures are also defined. These contours are input into a beam's eye view (BEV) program, which permits the display and inspection of the geometry from different viewpoints (58).

The radiotherapist views the target and adjacent critical structures and adjusts the viewpoint to identify beam orientations that fully irradiate the target volume but spare the most critical structure. Figure 48.26 shows a tumor and adjacent normal anatomy from a superior anterior viewpoint. By viewing from obliques, the treatment planner can find an angle that avoids irradiation of the spinal cord while adequately covering the lung target volume with the radiation portal. In addition to determining the optimal beam angle, BEV planning also permits the design of customized shielding blocks to spare uninvolved lung, heart, and cord. Alignment aids (58) may also be generated to assist in the accurate alignment of oblique fields at the time of treatment.

MULTIMODALITY IMAGING

Although CT scanning is the primary imaging modality for radiation treatment planning, magnetic resonance imaging (MRI) provides important complementary information, especially for intracranial and head and neck tumors. Newer modalities, such as PET and SPECT, also provide complementary information (2, 103). Ideally, all imaging data can be cross-correlated to transfer regions of interest from one study to another. For example, mapping the location of the tumor and critical organs from MRI studies to CT scans for treatment planning is desirable for accurate dose calculations and targetry. Other applications of image correlation in radiation oncology (23) include the definition of the preresection tumor volume and its transfer to postoperative scans, in order to adequately treat the tumor bed, and the correlation of the three-dimensional radiation dose distribution with posttherapy imaging studies to evaluate the efficacy of therapy, tumor recurrence, or treatment-related complications.

Image correlation methods for intracranial lesions have been developed by a number of investigators (129, 144). Approaches use either high-precision localization masks, markers, or surfaces (external or internal) to define the trans-

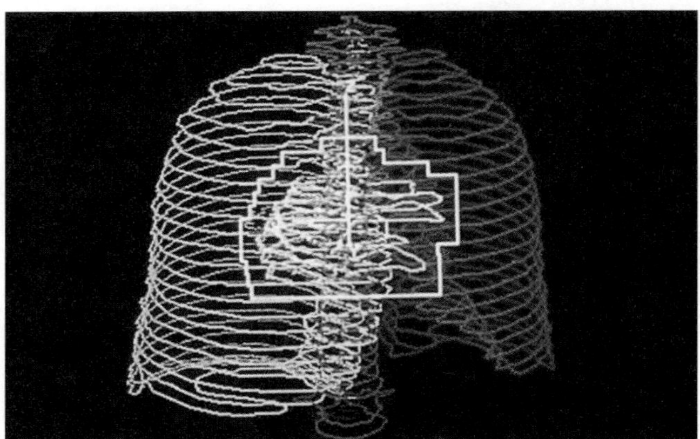

Figure 48.26. A beam's-eye view graphic of a three-dimensional tumor volume contoured on sequential axial CT scans (*white*), depicting its location relative to the right lung (*yellow*), left lung (*blue*), vertebral column (*green*), and spinal cord (*red*). A margin of 1 cm defines a suitable aperture to fully encompass the target volume (*white border*). Rotating the viewing perspectives to oblique angles yields a range of angles that encompasses the target yet avoids the spinal cord.

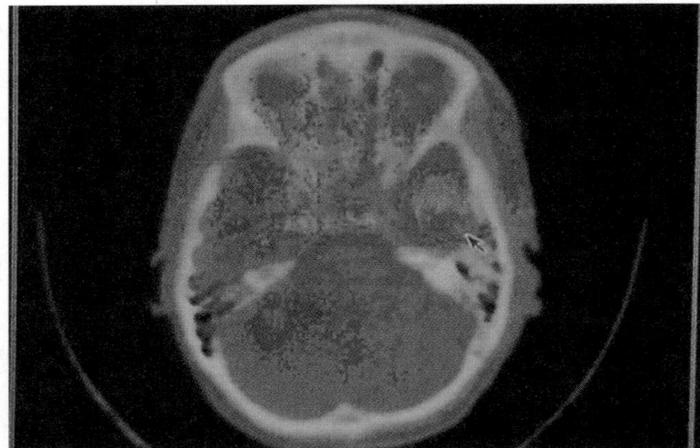

Figure 48.27. Image correlation of two complementary imaging modalities, here magnetic resonance imaging (MRI) of tumor and computed tomography of skull. Positron emission tomography (PET scanning) or single photon emission computed tomography (SPECT) can also be correlated in similar fashion.

formation. Figure 48.27 shows the result of an image correlation technique used in radiation therapy planning, where the high-intensity colored region indicating tumor and edema extracted from an MRI scan has been registered onto the corresponding CT image.

INTERACTIVE TREATMENT PLANNING

Once the tumor and normal anatomy have been defined, the planning process proceeds to choice of radiation type (photons, electrons, or both), radiation energy, and the general arrangement of portals. This is performed interactively on a computer. Variables in the development of a treatment plan include energy and modality of radiation beam, number of portals and their angulation, relative weights of radiation fields, and use of beam-modifying devices (wedges, compensators). These parameters are adjusted interactively to generate an optimized isodose distribution. An optimized isodose distribution uniformly irradiates the target and minimizes dose to normal tissues.

The beam energy is chosen to match the scale of patient anatomy. High-energy photon beams are appropriate for deep-seated tumors in obese patients. Low-megavolt-energy beams are appropriate for lesions of the head and neck. Superficial tumors may be treated with orthovoltage-energy photon beams (100 to 250 kVp) or with electrons. The number of radiation fields to be used in a treatment plan is determined by both physical considerations, such as the acceptability of the resulting dose distribution, and biologic aspects. Figure 48.28 shows the irradiation of a pelvic tumor with one, two, and four fields. In all plans, a dose of 100% is delivered to the center of the tumor. However, in the single-field dose distribution, a maximum of 130% is found within the patient, in tissues proximal to the target, due to the exponential attenuation of radiation and the inverse square effect. The tumor dose ranges from 105 to 97%. When the tumor is treated with a parallel opposed pair of fields, it receives a minimum of 102% and a maximum of 105%, whereas most tissues in the geometric path receive approximately 100% of the dose. Finally, in the four-field box plan, a greater volume of normal tissue is irradiated to a moderate dose level of 60%, whereas the target is enclosed in a rectangular high-dose region. In general, the greater number of radiation fields results in greater sparing of normal tissues to high doses, if each field is treated every day. It was noted previously that an increase in the daily fraction size may dramatically increase tissue complications. In the case of the plans with one field in normal tissue dose, a 3% increase over the tumor dose is delivered. Even if multiple fields are employed and only one field per day is treated (assuming the tumor receives 15% each day), the normal tissue will receive an unnecessarily large fraction size.

The radiation fields exiting from the linear accelerator are rectangular in shape and uniform across the field. The patient's external surface, tissue density differences, and shape and location of the target volume can be highly irregular in three dimensions. In order to achieve a uniformly shaped high-dose region confined to the target, the dose distribution is modified. In the plane perpendicular to the beam direction, high-density, low-melting point blocks are individually shaped for each patient to include the target but exclude adjacent radiation-sensitive tissues. Dose distribution in depth may be adjusted through the use of compensators that account for missing tissue, or through the use of wedges that vary the isodose shape.

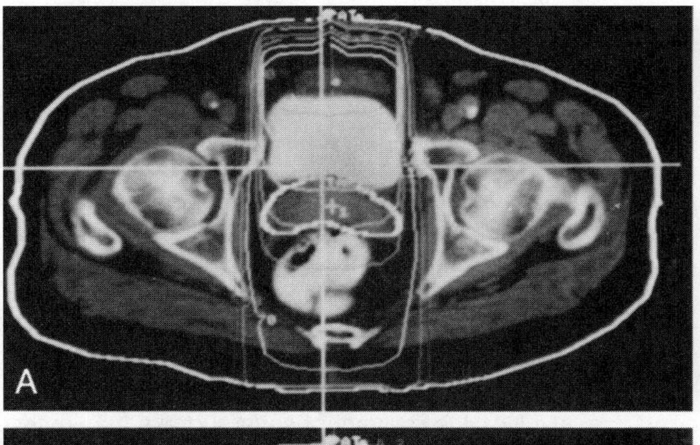

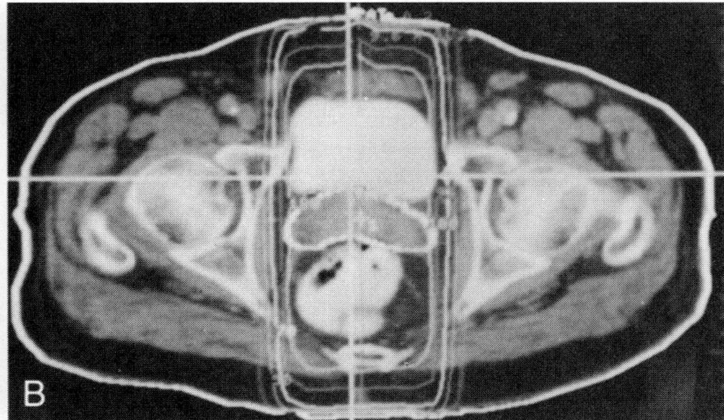

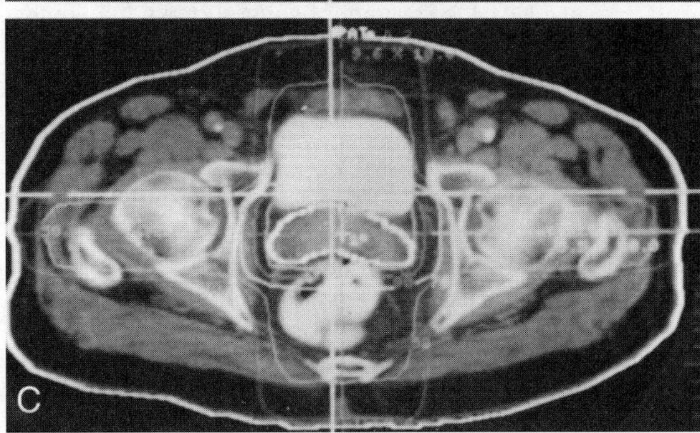

Figure 48.28. Isodose distributions as a function of number of radiation fields. **A.** Single-field irradiation if the target volume (prostate) produces inhomogeneous distribution in the target and a high dose in normal tissues proximal to the target. For this reason, single fields are rarely used for more than very superficial targets. **B.** Two fields, parallel opposed, irradiate bladder and rectum to the same dose as the target. **C.** Four-field irradiation of prostate results in high dose to target and spares normal tissues.

EXAMPLES OF TREATMENT PLANS

Lung

Treatment of nonresectable lung tumors with radiation treatment is common, and Figure 48.29 shows a lung tumor (white outline) in the right lung, near the hilum. A treatment plan is designed to minimize dose to the spinal cord, normal lung, and heart within tolerable dose levels. Isodose lines indicate the relative dose distribution from a four-field treatment plan. Both anterior/posterior opposed fields are used in addition to opposed oblique fields angled to avoid the spinal cord. The dose to the normal lung and spinal cord may be minimized by evaluating various radiation fields that irradiate normal tissues within the tolerance of the organs.

Head and Neck Tumors

Consider the nasopharyngeal carcinoma imaged by CT in Figure 48.30. The gross mass is seen as an asymmetric fullness on the left side. Because of lymphatic drainage in this region, carcinoma of the nasopharynx metastasizes to regional cervical lymph nodes. The treatment volume, therefore, includes both the primary tumor and neck nodes. The initial target volume is treated with opposed lateral photon fields. Critical structures, such as the eyes, portions of the tongue, and brain, are excluded from the port by shielding blocks. The initial dose distribution to the nasopharynx is shown in Figure 48.30*A*. After an initial course of 45 Gy to control subclinical disease, the target is divided into a segment anterior to the cord and treated with opposed lateral photon beams for an additional 25 Gy (Figure 48.30B). The posterior neck nodes are treated with electrons, matched to the photon fields, as shown in Figure 48.30*C*. A composite dose distribution is shown in Figure 48.30*D*.

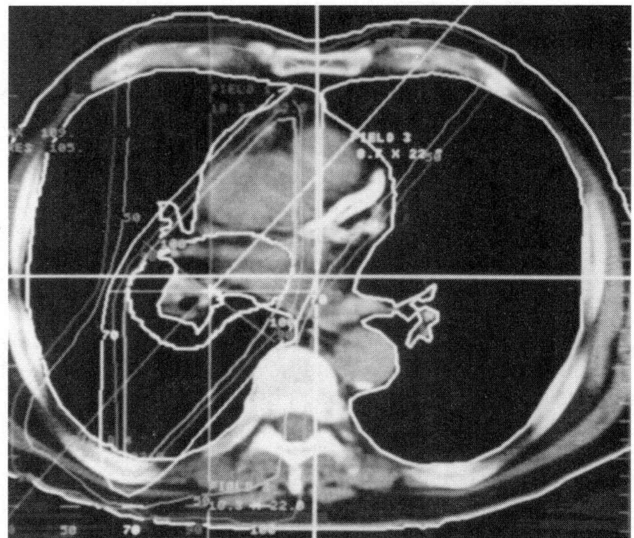

Figure 48.29. Representative lung treatment plan. Field configuration includes AP-PA and parallel opposed oblique portals.

BRACHYTHERAPY

Brachytherapy involves the use of sealed radioactive sources placed in proximity to the tumor (intracavitary technique) or within the tumor volume (interstitial treatment). In Greek, *brachys* means short, and brachytherapy implies a short distance between source and target (82). Because the radioactive sources are placed in direct contact with the tumor, the dose falls off rapidly and dose distribution is more localized than with external beam therapy. Brachytherapy has been used successfully in combination with external beam therapy in the curative treatment of tumors in a variety of primary sites, notably, carcinoma of the cervix, bladder, breast, and head and neck.

Brachytherapy was initially instituted with the use of naturally occurring isotopes, such as radium or radon, but with the availability of artificially produced isotopes in the past few decades, it has been practiced more frequently with cesium 137, iridium 198, and iodine 125. To illustrate one of the more common applications of brachytherapy, consider the irradiation of carcinoma of the cervix with an intracavitary Fletcher-Suit applicator. Intracavitary insertion is the most commonly used brachytherapy technique, and can provide an excellent dose distribution for patients with early-stage disease and normal anatomy (53). The device is shown in Figure 48.31. The tubelike tandem is inserted into the uterus, and the colpostats are positioned against the lateral fornices. In general, the geometric distance of the isodose lines of radioactive material applied in this fashion is similar to the local spread of cervix cancer. The placement of the Fletcher-Suit applicator is performed under anesthesia, with no sources loaded. After verification of proper placement, during which radiographs are taken with dummy sources, the radioactive sources are loaded into the applicator. This technique of "afterloading" minimizes the staff's exposure to radiation during the placement and positioning of the device. Representative dose distributions resulting from a standard loading of the applicator are shown in Figure 48.32. A dose rate of approximately 40 to 50 cGy an hour at specified points is desirable. A boost dose of 25 Gy under this dose-rate condition would require 50 hours of treatment, which is typical. Brachytherapy has also been extensively used in boosting the dose to tumors of the head and neck, breast, prostate, sarcomas, and recently the brain (82). In these instances, plastic catheters are inserted into the target volume, guided by large-gauge needles, followed by the placement of radioactive sources.

High-dose-rate (HDR) remote afterloaded brachytherapy, a new delivery technique that is gaining greater clinical acceptance, involves the delivery of several grays in minutes. Low-dose-rate (LDR) brachytherapy may require several days of hospitalization, whereas HDR can be delivered in a fractionated manner as an outpatient procedure. In HDR remote afterloading, a high-activity source is driven to a predetermined series of positions for specific periods. Furthermore, because of the small source size, smaller-diameter catheters may be used and applied to interstitial and intraluminal sites, such as the bronchus, esophagus, and bile duct, which previously could not be easily treated with LDR techniques. One of the advantages of this computer-operated remote afterloading technique is that the dose distribution can be optimized.

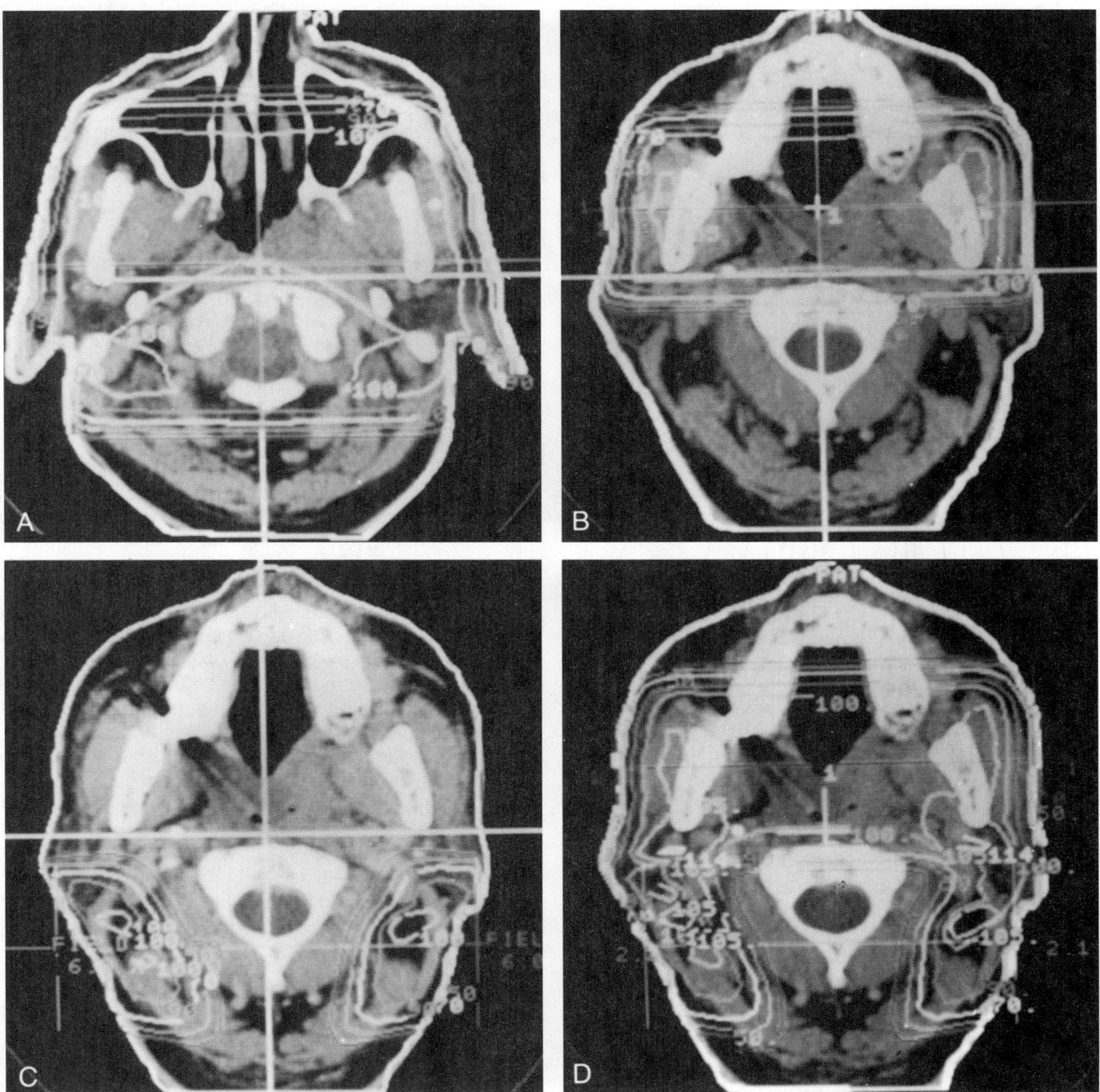

Figure 48.30. Treatment plans for a head and neck case. Target area includes gross lesion and regional nodes and is irradiated with opposed lateral photon fields to approximately 45 Gy (**A**). This is commonly followed by dividing the target volume into two regions, one anterior to the spinal canal and the posterior neck nodes. The anterior target is irradiated with lateral opposed photon fields (**B**), and the neck nodes are irradiated with electron beams (**C**). **D.** Composite distribution.

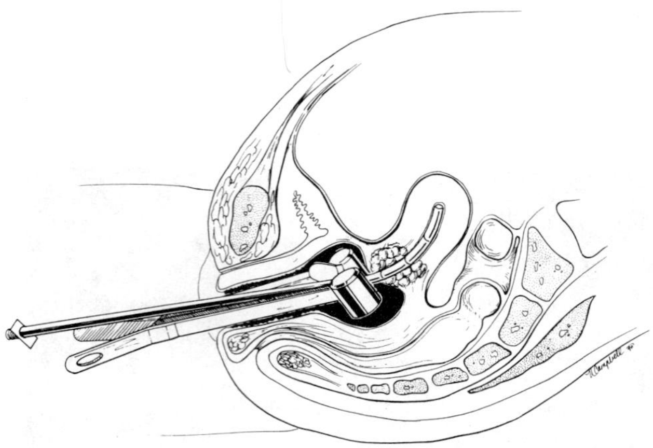

Figure 48.31. Fletcher-Suit applicator. Typically, three sources are placed in the tandem (tube) and one source each into colpostats. (Courtesy of 3M Company.)

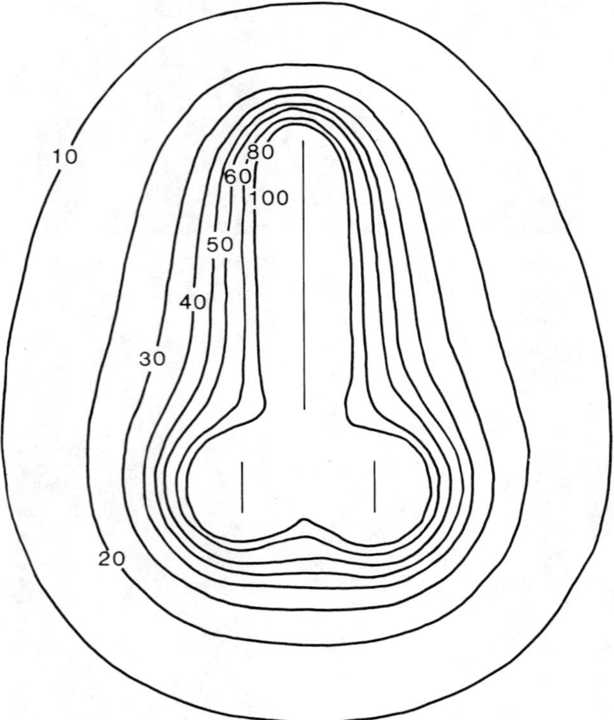

Figure 48.32. Dose distribution from Fletcher-Suit applicator, superimposed on anatomy, frontal view.

Newer Modalities for Radiation Therapy

While primary radiation therapy and therapy in combination with chemotherapy and surgery are curative in a number of sites, some tumors are not well controlled. Investigational approaches to offer more effective radiotherapy include techniques to increase the dose to the tumor without increased morbidity through more effective dose localization, or through biologically more effective radiations, such as high LET beams. These approaches are discussed in the following.

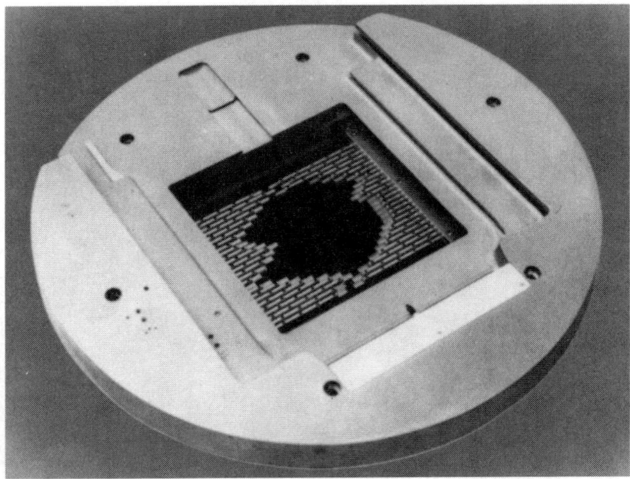

Figure 48.33. Multivane (multileaf) collimator. Individual vanes are controlled by computer and provide field-sharing capabilities similar to that of blocks. (Photograph courtesy of Varian, Palo Alto, California.)

CONFORMAL THERAPY

In the 1960s, Takahashi proposed conformal therapy, a radiation therapy delivery technique in which blocks, the radiation field direction, and the patient might be dynamically controlled during treatment in order to achieve a tightly conforming high-dose region around the target volume (163, 164). More recently, three-dimensional computer simulations of conformal therapy (132, 166) suggest that significant volumes of normal tissue can be spared. Conformal therapy is technically more feasible today with the wide availability of advanced imaging modalities and powerful minicomputers needed to calculate and control the complex movements of linear accelearator systems. The commercial availability of multivane collimators, which make feasible the numerous blocked fields needed to provide good dose localization (Fig. 48.33) and real-time portal field imagers that verify the correct relationship between oblique noncoplanar radiation fields with computer calculations also make dynamic conformal therapy more feasible. Dynamic conformal radiation therapy is under study at a number of institutions, and is likely to be a technologic focus for radiation therapy into the year 2000.

STEREOTACTIC RADIOSURGERY

Stereotactic radiosurgery is a term associated with the irradiation of a CNS lesion in a single fraction. Typically, a stereotactic frame is securely attached to the patient's cranium through the use of pins, and the patient is imaged (CT or MRI). The target is delineated interactively, and single or multiple isocenters are determined. A multiple noncoplanar arc treatment plan is designed to irradiate the lesion (Fig. 48.34). The irradiation is delivered by a standard linear accelerator (73, 108) (with appropriate attachments) or by a gamma knife (102), which is a cobalt 201 source convergent-irradiation device. An advantage of stereotactic technology is the high mechanical precision achievable; the me-

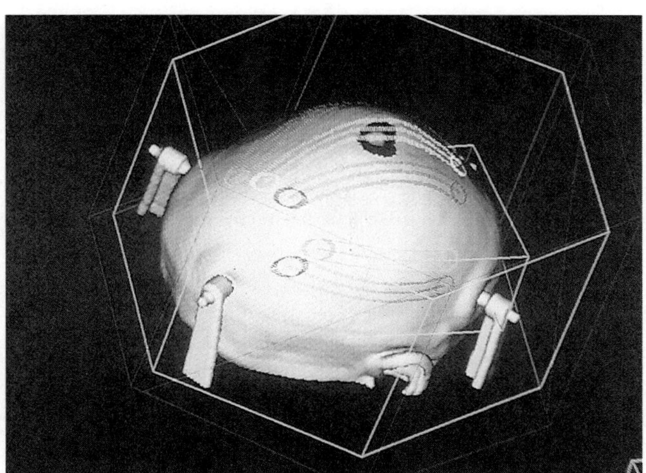

Figure 48.34. Computer treatment planning display of noncoplanar beam arcs that irradiate an arteriovenous malformation using a stereotactic frame and linear accelerator.

chanical accuracy of the alignment of the isocenter with the lesion center is of the order of 1 mm. In single-fraction treatment, several thousand centigrays may be delivered, resulting in necrosis of the lesion. The technique was initially applied for the treatment of arteriovenous malformations and other vascular lesions (155), but more recently, brain tumors or metastases have been treated. Investigational studies using techniques that permit fractionation are under development.

PARTICLE THERAPY

If tumors are large, or are located near tissues damaged by relatively low doses of radiation, it becomes very difficult to deliver tumoricidal doses to the entire tumor volume without compromising the function of adjacent organs (6, 175). In some clinical situations, high-energy proton beams are employed because of the ability to shape the high-dose region in three dimensions (5, 175). Collimation of a proton beam in the plane perpendicular to the beam direction is achieved in the same manner as with photon beams: individually customized shielding blocks are used to shape the radiation portal. Treatment planning simulations suggest that greater doses may be delivered to the tumor with photon beams (16). However, because heavy charged-particle beams have a well-defined range in matter, a proton beam can also be shaped in depth, such that the Bragg peak region is stopped along the distal surface of a three-dimensional target volume, with certain limitations imposed by different tissue densities.

Proton therapy has been shown to be successful in several clinical sites, including choroidal melanoma (115), arteriovenous malformations (AVMs) (96), and juxtaspinal and base-of-skull tumors (5, 6). More than 1,300 patients have been treated for choroidal melanomas at Harvard. In this technique, 70 Gy is delivered in five fractions. Munzenrider reported that the probability of retaining the eye after proton therapy is 89%, and that a large proportion of treated eyes retained useful vision (115).

High LET particle beams (heavy ions and neutrons) induce irreparable and directly lethal changes in chromosome structure almost independently of cellular metabolism or biochemical state. For these reasons, tumors resistant to conventional radiotherapy are relatively more sensitive to high LET radiation. Neutron irradiation may be beneficial for slowly proliferating tumors, hypoxic tumors, and inherently radioresistant tumors.

Trials have shown that neutron therapy is effective in advanced prostate disease (60) and in salivary gland tumors (61). In a randomized trial comparing mixed-beam therapy of neutrons and photons with photons alone in the treatment of stages C and D prostatic cancer, the local control rate found for mixed beam was 77% in comparison with 31% for photons alone. A randomized trial comparing neutron irradiation with photon treatment for inoperable malignant salivary gland tumors has also been conducted. The reported local control was 67% for neutrons and 17% for photons, while survival rates were 62% for neutrons and 25% for photons (142).

MONOCLONAL ANTIBODIES

Radioimmunotherapy utilizes antibodies with specificity against tumor associated antigens to carry radioactive nuclei to tumor. The concept was originally proposed in the late 1940s by Pressman, and interest in it was renewed when Kohler and Millstein devised a technique to produce monoclonal antibodies in the quantities needed for therapy. Many clinical trials using radiolabeled antibodies for both diagnosis and therapy have been conducted (44, 50, 98, 100, 101, 122) and are reviewed in Chapter 83.

Several aspects of radiolabeled monoclonal antibody therapy are appropriate to discuss in the context of radiation oncology. First, an understanding of the radiobiology of tumors and normal tissues is essential in the scientific study of this new modality. Traditionally, this scientific discipline has been an integral part of radiation oncology. Second, a detailed knowledge of the dosimetry of radiolabeled antibodies is essential in both the development and improvement of radioimmunotherapy. Radiation oncologists and therapy physicists historically have been involved in the development of dose calculations for therapeutic applications of radiation.

The dosimetry associated with radioimmunotherapy is unique in that it spans logs of geometric scale. In some therapeutic applications, understanding of the dose on the geometric scale of micrometers to millimeters is required. An example of this is the microdosimetry associated with alpha particle emitting radionuclides conjugated to antibodies. As the antibody/nuclide complex is distributed through the circulatory systems, it may preferentially accumulate in specific organs. Under these conditions, dose variations of the order of centimeters are important, and SPECT-based treatment planning is needed. As the isotope distributes itself throughout the whole body, and irradiates distributed radiation-sensitive tissues, such as bone marrow, whole-body calculations become important. Within the next 5 years, techniques that will accurately calculate dose from radioimmunotherapy appear to be within reach.

References

1. Adams GE. Chemical radiosensitization of hypoxic cells. Br Med Bull 1973;29:48–53.
2. Adler LP. Oncology overview: Selected abstracts on newer radionuclide imaging techniques in oncology: PET and SPECT. In Newer Radionuclide Imaging Techniques in Oncology: PET and SPECT. Bethesda, MD: ICRDB, ICIC, National Cancer Institute.
3. Allan DJ. Radiation-induced apoptosis: its role in a MADCaT (mitosis-apoptosis-differentiation-calcium toxicity) scheme of cytotoxicity mechanisms. Int J Radiat Biol 1992;62:145–152.
4. Anderson WF. Gene therapy for cancer. Hum Gene Ther 1994;5:1–2. Editorial.
5. Austin-Seymour M, Munzenrider J, Goitein M, Verhey L, Urie M, Gentry R, Birnbaum S, Ruotolo D, McManus P, Skates S, et al. Fractionated proton radiation therapy of chordoma and low-grade chondrosarcoma of the base of the skull. J Neurosurg 1989;70:13–17.
6. Austin-Seymour MM. Particle therapy. In Syllabus: Radiation Therapy in the 1990s: Rationale for the Emerging Modalities. Edited by EJ Hall and JD Cox. Oak Brook, IL: Radiological Society of North America, 1989, pp 35–38. RSNA Categorical Course.
7. Barendsen GW, Broerse JJ. Experimental radiotherapy of a rat rhabdomyosarcoma with 15 meV neutrons and 300 kV x-rays. II. Effects of fractionated treatments, applied five times a week for several weeks. Eur J Cancer 1970;6:89–109.
8. Barranco SC, Romsdahl MM, Humphrey RM. The radiation response of human malignant melanoma cells grown in vitro. Cancer Res 1971;31:830–833.
9. Bedford JS, Mitchell JB. Dose-rate effects in synchronous mammalian cells in culture. Radiat Res 1973;54:316–327.
10. Behrends U, Peter RU, Knabe R, Eissner G, Holler E, Bornkamm BW, Caughman SW, Degitz K. Ionizing radiation induces ICAM. J Invest Dermatol 1994;103:726–730.
11. Berg EL, Fromm C, Melrose J, Tsurushita N. Antibodies cross-reactive with E- and P-selectin block both E- and P-selectin functions. Blood 1995;85:31–37.
12. Bohr VA, Evans MK, Fornace AJ Jr. DNA repair and its pathogenetic implications. Lab Invest 1989;61:143–161.
13. Boise LH, Gonzalez-Garcia M, Postema CE, Ding L, Lindsten T, Turka LA, Mao X, Nunez G, Thompson CB. Bcl-x, a Bcl-2-related gene that functions as a dominant regulator of apoptotic cell death. Cell 1993;74:597–608.
14. Boothman DA, Bouvard I, Hughes EN. Identification and characterization of X-ray-induced proteins in human cells. Cancer Res 1989;49:2871–2878.
15. Boulis-Wassif S, Langenhorst BL, Hop WC. The contribution of preoperative radiotherapy in borderline operability rectal cancer. In Adjuvant Therapy Cancer. Edited by SE Jones and SE Salmon. New York: Grune & Stratton, 1979, pp 613–620.

15a. Broerse JJ, Barendsen GW, van Kersen GR. Survival of cultured human cells after irradiation with fast neutrons of different energies in hypoxia and oxygenated conditions. Int J Radiat Biol Relat Stud Phys Chemk Med 1968;13:559.

16. Brown AP, Urie MM, Chisin R, Suit HD. Proton therapy for carcinoma of the nasopharynx: a study in comparative treatment planning. Int J Radiat Oncol Biol Phys 1989;16:1607–1614.
17. Bush RS, Jenkin RD, Allt WE, Beale FA, Bean H, Dembo AJ, Pringle JF. Definitive evidence for hypoxic cells influencing cure in cancer therapy. Br J Cancer Suppl 1978;37:302–306.
18. Byhardt RW, Greenberg M, Cox JD. Local control of squamous carcinoma of oral cavity and oropharynx with 3 vs 5 treatment fractions per week. Int J Radiat Oncol Biol Phys 1977;2:415–420.
19. Carney DN, Mitchell JB, Kinsella TJ. In vitro radiation and chemotherapy sensitivity of established cell lines of human small cell lung cancer and its large cell morphological variants. Cancer Res 1983;43:2806–2811.
20. Castro JR, Chen GT, Blakely EA. Current considerations in heavy charged-particle radiotherapy: a clinical research trial of the University of California Lawrence Berkeley Laboratory, Northern California Oncology Group, and Radiation Therapy Oncology Group. Radiat Res Suppl 1985;8:S263–S271.
21. Chan HS, Thorner PS, Haddad G, Ling V. Immunohistochemical detection of P-glycoprotein: prognostic correlation in soft tissue sarcoma of childhood. J Clin Oncol 1990;8:689–704.
22. Chang EH, Pirollo KF, Zou ZQ, Cheung HY, Lawler EL, Garner R, White E, Bernstein WB, Fraumeni JW Jr, Blattner WA. Oncogenes in radioresistant, noncancerous skin fibroblasts from a cancer-prone family. Science 1987;237:1036–1039.
23. Chen GTY, Pelizzari CA, Levin DN. Image Correlation in Oncology. In Important Advances in Oncology. Edited by VT DeVita and S Hellman. Philadelphia: Lippincott, 1990, pp 131–141.
24. Cohen L, Awschalom M. Fast neutron radiation therapy. Ann Rev Biophys Bioeng 1982;11:359–390.
25. Colden-Stanfield M, Kalinich JF, Gallin EK. Ionizing radiation increases endothelial and epithelial cell production of influenza virus and leukocyte adherence. J Immunol 1994;153:5222–5229.
26. Cole GM, Schild D, Lovett ST, Mortimer RK. Regulation of RAD54- and RAD52-lacZ gene fusions in *Saccharomyces cerevisiae* in response to DNA damage. Mol Cell Biol 1987;7:1078–1084.
27. Coleman CN. Modification of radiotherapy by radiosensitizers and cancer chemotherapy agents. I. Radiosensitizers. Semin Oncol 1989;16:169–175.
28. Coleman CN, Bump EA, Kramer RA. Chemical modifiers of cancer treatment (review). J Clin Oncol 1988;6:709–733.
29. Coleman CN, Wasserman TH, Urtasun RC, Halsey J, Hirst VK, Hancock S, Phillips TL. Phase I trial of the hypoxic cell radiosensitizer SR-2508: the results of the five to six week drug schedule. Int J Radiat Oncol Biol Physi 1986;12:1105–1108.
30. Constine LS, Zagars G, Rubin P, Kligerman M. Protection by WR-2721 of human bone marrow function following irradiation. Int J Radiat Oncol Biol Phys 1986;12: 1505–1508.
31. Cox JD. The Lung and Thymus. In Radiation Oncology, Ratonale, Techniques, Results. Edited by WT Moss and JD Cox. St. Louis: Mosby, 1989, pp 285–311.
32. Cox JD, Kline RW. Do prostatic biopsies 12 months or more after external irradiation for adenocarcinoma, stage III, predict long-term survival? Int J Radiat Oncol Biol Phys 1983;9:299–303.
33. Culver KW, Blaese RM. Gene therapy for cancer (review). Trends Genet 1994;10: 174–178.
34. Dewey WC. In vitro systems: standardization of endpoints. Int J Radiat Oncol Biol Phys 1979;5:1165.
35. Dische S, Anderson PJ, Sealy R, Watson ER. Carcinoma of the cervix—anaemia, radiotherapy and hyperbaric oxygen. Br J Radiol 1983;56:251–255.
36. Dunn MM, Drab EA, Rubin DB. Effects of irradiation on endothelial cell-polymorphonuclear leukocyte interactions. J Appl Physiol 1986;60:1932–1937.
37. Eichhorn HJ. Different fractionation schemes tested by histological examination of autopsy specimens from lung cancer patients. Br J Radiol 1981;54:132–135.
38. Elkind MM. Fractionated dose radiotherapy and its relationship to survival curve shapes. Cancer Treat Rev 1976;3:2–15.
39. Elkind MM. The initial part of the survival curve. Does it predict outcome of fractionated radiotherapy? Radiat Res 1988;114:425–436.
40. Elkind MM, Sutton H. Radiation response of mammalian cells grown in culture. I. Repair of x-ray damage in surviving Chinese hamster cells. Radiat Res 1960;13: 556–593.
41. Elkind MM, Sutton HG. X-ray damage and recovery in mammalian cells in culture. Nature 1959;184:1293–1295.
42. Elkind MM, Sutton-Gilbert H, Moses WB, Alescio T, Swan RB. Radiation response in mammalian cells in culture V: temperature dependence of the repair of x-ray damage in surviving cells (aerobic and hypoxic). Radiat Res 1965;25:359–376.
43. Elkind MM, Witmore GF. Radiobiology of Cultured Mammalian Cells. New York: Gordon & Breach, 1967.
44. Epenetos AA, Britton KE, Mather S, Shepherd J, Granowska M, Taylor-Papadimitriou J, Nimmon CC, Durbin H, Hawkins LR, Malpas JS, Bodmer WF. Targeting of iodine-123-labelled tumour-associated monoclonal antibodies to ovarian, breast, and gastrointestinal tumours. Lancet 1982;2:999–1005.
45. Evans JC, Bergsio P. The influence of anemia on the results of radiotherapy in carcinoma of the cervix. Radiology 1965;84:709–717.
46. Fajardo LF, Berthrong M. Vascular lesions following radiation. Pathol Ann 1988;1: 297–330.
47. Fertil B, Malaise EP. The mean inactivation dose: experimental versus theoretical. Radiat Res 1986;108:222–225.
48. Fisher B, Bauer M, Margolese R, Poisson R, Pilch Y, Redmond C, Fisher E, Wolmark N, Deutsch M, Montague E, Saffer E, Wickerham L, Lerner H, Glass A, Shibata H, Deckers P, Ketcham A, Oishi R, Russell I. Five-year results of a randomized clinical trial comparing total mastectomy and segmental mastectomy with or without radiation in the treatment of breast cancer [scientific misconduct-reanalysis of NSABP protocol B-06 is available via PDQ, CANCERNET, or CANCERFAX]. N Engl J Med 1985;312:665–673.
49. FitzGerald TJ, Daugherty C, Kase K, Rothstein LA, McKenna M, Greenberger JS. Activated human N-ras oncogene enhances x-irradiation repair of mammalian cells in vitro less effectively at low dose rate. Implications for increased therapeutic ratio of low dose rate irradiation. Am J Clin Oncol 1985;8:517–522.

49a. Fletcher GH. Keynote address: The scientific basis of the present and future practice of clinical radiotherapy. Int J Radiat Oncol Biol Phys 1983;9:1073.

50. Foon KA. Monoclonal Antibodies in the Diagnosis and Treatment of Cancer. Seattle, WA: NeoRx.
51. Fornace AJ Jr, Nebert DW, Hollander MC, Luethy JD, Papathanasiou M, Fargnoli J, Holbrook NJ. Mammalian genes coordinately regulated by growth arrest signals and DNA-damaging agents. Mole Cell Biol 1989;9:4196–4203.
52. Fowler JF. Review: Total doses in fractionated radiotherapy—implications of new radiobiologic data (review). Int J Radiat Biol Related Studies Phys Chem Med 1984;46: 103–120.
53. Fu KK, Sneed PK, Leibel SA, Nori D, Peschel RE. Carcinoma of the cervix. In Interstitial Brachytherapy: Physical, Biological and Clinical Considerations. Interstitial Collaborative Working Group. Edited by LL Anderson et al. New York: Raven, 1990.
54. Fuks Z, Persaud RS, Alfieri A, McLoughlin M, Ehleiter D, Schwartz JL, Seddon AP, Cordon-Cardo C, Haimovitz-Friedman A. Basic fibroblast growth factor protects endothelial cells against radiation-induced programmed cell death in vitro and in vivo. Cancer Res 1994;54:2582–2590.
55. Gassmann A. Zur Histologie der Roentgenulcera. Fortschr Rontgenstr 1899;2: 199–207.
56. Gerweck LE, Kornblith PL, Burlett P, Wang J, Sweigert S. Radiation sensitivity of cultured human glioblastoma cells. Radiology 1977;125:231–234.
57. Goitein M, Abrams M. Multi-dimensional treatment planning: I. Delineation of anatomy. Int J Radiat Oncol Biol Phys 1983;9:777–787.
58. Goitein M, Abrams M, Rowell D, Pollari H, Wiles J. Multi-dimensional treatment planning: II. Beam's eye-view, back projection, and projection through CT sections. Int J Radiat Oncol Biol Phys 1983;9:789–97.
59. Grdina DJ, Sigdestad CP. Radiation protectors: the unexpected benefits (review). Drug Metab Rev 1989;20:13–42.
60. Griffin TW. Status of clinical trials with neutron irradiation (review). Imp Adv Oncol 1989;221–34.
61. Griffin TW, Pajak TF, Laramore GE, Duncan W, Richter MP, Hendrickson FR, Maor MH. Neutron vs photon irradiation of inoperable salivary gland tumors: results of an RTOG-MRC Cooperative Randomized Study. Int J Radiat Oncol Biol Phys 1988;15: 1085–1090.
62. Guichard M, Weichselbaum RR, Little JB, Malaise EP. Potentially lethal damage repair as a possible determinant of human tumour radiosensitivity. Radiother Oncol 1984;1:263–269.
63. Hahn GM, Bagshaw MA, Evans RG, Gordon LF. Repair of potentially lethal lesions in x-irradiated density inhibited Chinese hamster cells. Radiat Res 1973;55:280–290.
64. Hahn GM, Little JB. Plateau-phase cultures of mammalian cells: an in vitro model for human cancer. Curr Top Radiat Res Q 1972;8:39–43.
65. Haimovitz-Friedman A, Kan CC, Ehleiter D, Persaud RS, McLoughlin M, Fuks Z, Kolesnick RN. Ionizing radiation acts on cellular membranes to generate ceramide and initiate apoptosis. J Exp Med 1994;180:525–535.
66. Hall EJ. Radiation dose-rate: a factor of importance in radiobiology and radiotherapy (review). Br J Radiol 1972;45:81–97.
67. Hall EJ. Radiobiology for the Radiologist. Philadelphia: Lippincott, 1988, pp 17–160.
68. Hallahan DE. c-jun and Egr-1 participate in DNA synthesis and survival in response to ionizing radiation exposure. J Biol Chem (submitted 1995).
69. Hallahan DE. E-selectin induction by ionizing radiation. Proc Am Assoc Cancer Res (submitted 1995).
70. Hallahan DE, Beckett MA, Kufe D, Weichselbaum RR. The interaction between re-

combinant human tumor necrosis factor and radiation in 13 human tumor cell lines. Int J Radiat Oncol Biol Phys 1990;19:69–74.
71. Hallahan DE, Spriggs DR, Beckett MA, Kufe DW, Weichselbaum RR. Increased tumor necrosis factor alpha mRNA after cellular exposure to ionizing radiation. Proc Natl Acad Sci USA 1989;86:10104–10107.
72. Hallahan DE, Sukhatme VP, Sherman ML, Virudachalam S, Kufe D, Weichselbaum RR. Protein kinase C mediates x-ray inducibility of nuclear signal transducers EGR1 and JUN. Proc Natl Acad Sci USA 1991;88:2156–2160.
73. Hartmann GH, Schlegel W, Sturm V, Kober B, Pastyr O, Lorenz WJ. Cerebral radiation surgery using moving field irradiation at a linear accelerator facility. Int J Radiat Oncol Biol Phys 1985;11:1185–1192.
73a. Hellman S. Cell kinetics, models and cancer treatment: some principles for the radiation oncologist radiology. 1975;114–219.
74. Hendry JH, Potten CS. Intestinal cell radiosensitivity: a comparison for cell death assayed by apoptosis or by a loss of clonogenicity. Int J Radiat Biol Related Studies Phys Chem Med 1982;42:621–628.
75. Henk JM. Does hyperbaric oxygen have a future in radiation therapy? Int J Radiat Oncol Biol Phys 1981;7:1125–1128.
76. Hermens AF, Barendsen GW. Changes of cell proliferation characteristics in a rat rhabdomyosarcoma before and after x-irradiation. Eur J Cancer 1969;5:173–189.
77. Hierlihy P, Jenkin RD, Stryker JA. Anemia as a prognostic factor in cancer of the cervix: a preliminary report. Can Med Assoc J 1969;100:1100–1102.
78. Hilaris BS, Martini N. Multimodality therapy of superior sulcus tumors. Adv Pain Res Ther 1982;4:113.
79. Hill RP. Experimental radiotherapy. In The Basic Science of Oncology. Edited by IF Tannock and RP Hill. Elmsford NY: Pergamon, 1987.
80. Hockenbery DM, Oltvai ZN, Yin XM, Milliman CL, Korsmeyer SJ. Bcl-2 functions in an antioxidant pathway to prevent apoptosis. Cell 1993;75:241–251.
81. Hopewell JW, Calvo W, Jaenke R, Reinhold HS, Robbins ME, Whitehouse EM. Microvasculature and radiation damage (review). Rec Res Cancer Res 1993;130:1–16.
82. Interstitial Collaborative Working Group. Interstitial Brachytherapy: Physical, Biological and Clinical Considerations. Edited by L Lowell et al. New York: Raven, 1990.
83. Jeggo PA, Kemp LM. X-ray-sensitive mutants of Chinese hamster ovary cell line. Isolation and cross-sensitivity to other DNA-damaging agents. Mut Res 1983;112: 313–327.
84. Johns HE, Cunningham J. The Physics of Radiation Therapy. Springfield IL: Charles C. Thomas, 1990.
85. Jones N, Shenk T. Isolation of adenovirus type 5 host range deletion mutants defective for transformation of rat embryo cells. Cell 1979;17:683–689.
86. Kallman RF. Effects of different schedules of dose fractionation on the oxygenation status of a transplantable mouse sarcoma. JNCI 1970;44:369–377.
87. Kasahara N, Dozy AM, Kan YW. Tissue-specific targeting of retroviral vectors through ligand-receptor interactions [see comments]. Science 1994;266:1373–1376.
88. Kasid U, Pfeifer A, Brennan T, Beckett M, Weichselbaum RR, Dritschilo A, Mark GE. Effect of antisense c-raf-1 on tumorigenicity and radiation sensitivity of a human squamous carcinoma. Science 1989;243:1354–1356.
89. Kasid U, Pfeifer A, Weichselbaum RR, Dritschilo A, Mark GE. The raf oncogene is associated with a radiation-resistant human laryngeal cancer. Science 1987;237: 1039–1041.
90. Kelland LR, Bingle L, Edwards S, Steel GG. High intrinsic radiosensitivity of a newly established and characterised human embryonal rhabdomyosarcoma cell line. Br J Cancer 1989;59:160–164.
91. Khan FM. The Physics of Radiation Therapy. Baltimore: Williams & Wilkins, 1984.
92. Kim JH, Kim SH, Brown SL, Freytag SO. Selective enhancement by an antiviral agent of the radiation-induced cell killing of human glioma cells transduced with HSV-tk gene. Cancer Res 1994;54:6053–6056.
93. Kinsella TJ, Mitchell JB, Russo A, Aiken M, Morstyn G, Hsu SM, Rowland J, Glatstein E. Continuous intravenous infusions of bromodeoxyuridine as a clinical radiosensitizer. J Clin Oncol 1984;2:1144–1150.
94. Kinsella TJ, Mitchell JB, Russo A, Morstyn G, Glatstein E. The use of halogenated thymidine analogs as clinical radiosensitizers: rationale, current status, and future prospects: Non-hypoxic cell sensitizers. Int J Radiat Oncol Biol Phys 1984;10: 1399–1406.
95. Kirchgessner CU, Patil CK, Evans JW, Cuomo CA, Fried LM, Carter T, Oettinger MA, Brown JM. DNA-dependent kinase (p350) as a candidate gene for the murine SCID defect. Science 1995;267:1178–1183.
96. Kjellberg RN, Hanamura T, Davis KR, Lyons SL, Adams RD. Bragg-peak proton-beam therapy for arteriovenous malformations of the brain. N Engl J Med 1983;309: 269–274.
97. Kligerman MM, Shaw MT, Slavik M, Yuhas JM. Phase I clinical studies with WR-2721. Cancer Clin Trials 1984;3:217–221.
98. Larson SM, Carrasquillo JA, Krohn KA, Brown JP, McGuffin RW, Ferens JM, Graham MM, Hill LD, Beaumier PL, Hellstrom KE, et al. Localization of 131-labeled p97-specific Fab fragments in human melanoma as a basis for radiotherapy. J Clin Invest 1983;72:2101–2114.
99. Law MP. Radiation-induced vascular injury and its relation to late effects in normal tissue. Adv Radiat Biol 1981;9:37–73.
100. Leibel SA. Targeted radionuclides. In Innovations in Radiation Oncology. Edited by HR Withers and LJ Peters. New York: Springer-Verlag, 1988, pp 2556–2561.
101. Leibel SA, Klein JL, Leichner PK. Radioimmunotherapy: current results and future strategies. In Syllabus: Radiation Therapy in the 1990s: Rationale for the Emerging Modalities. Edited by EJ Hall and JD Cox. 1989, pp 39–44.
102. Leksell L. Stereotactic radiosurgery. J Neurol Neurosurg Psychiat 1983;46:797–803.
103. Levin DN, Hu XP, Tan KK, Galhotra S, Pelizzari CA, Chen GT, Beck RN, Chen CT, Cooper MD, Mullan JF, et al. The brain: integrated three-dimensional display of MR and PET images. Radiology 1989;172:783–789.
104. Lichter A. Clinical practice of modern radiation therapy treatment planning. In Syllabus: A Categorical Course in Radiation Therapy Treatment Planning. Edited by Paliwal and ML Griem. Radiology Society of North America, 1986.
105. Little JB, Hahn GM, Frindel E, Tubiana M. Repair of potentially lethal radiation damage in vitro and in vivo. Radiology 1973;106:689–694.
105a. Looser KG, Shah JP, Strong EW. The significance of possible margins in surgically resected epidermoid carcinoma. Head Neck Surg. 1978;1:107.
106. Lowe SW, Ruley HE, Jacks T, Housman DE. P53-dependent apoptosis modulates the cytotoxicity of anticancer agents. Cell 1993;74:957–967.
107. Lowe SW, Schmitt EM, Smith SW, Osborne BA, Jacks T. p53 is required for radiation-induced apoptosis in mouse thymocytes [see comments]. Nature 1993;362:847–849.
108. Lutz W, Winston KR, Maleki N. A system for stereotactic radiosurgery with a linear accelerator. Int J Radiat Oncol Biol Phys 1988;14:373–381.
109. Manome Y, Abe M, Hagen MF, Fine HA, Kufe DW. Enhancer sequences of the DF3 gene regulate expression of the herpes simplex virus thymidine kinase gene and confer sensitivity of human breast cancer cells to ganciclovir. Cancer Res 1994;54: 5408–5413.
110. McGrory WJ, Bautista DS, Graham FL. A simple technique for the rescue of early region I mutations into infectious human adenovirus type 5. Virology 1988;163:614–617.
111. Meyn RE, Stephens LC, Voehringer DW, Story MD, Mirkovic N, Milas L. Biochemical modulation of radiation-induced apoptosis in murine lymphoma cells (review). Radiat Res 1993;136:327–334.
112. Million RR, Cassissi NJ, Clark JR. Cancer of the head and neck. In Cancer Principles and Practice of Oncology. Edited by VT Devita, S Hellman, and SA Rosenberg. Philadelphia: Lippincott, 1989, pp 488–580.
113. Mohan R, Barest G, Brewster LJ, Chui CS, Kutcher GJ, Laughlin JS, Fuks Z. A comprehensive three-dimensional radiation treatment planning system. Int J Radiat Oncol Biol Phys 1988;15:481–495.
114. Muhsam R. Uber Dermatitis der Hand nach Roentgenbestrahlung (Fingramputation). Arch Klin Chir 1904;74:434–453.
115. Munzenrider JE, Gragoudas ES, McNulty P, Seddon JM. Uveal melanoma: conservative treatment with radiation therapy. In Innovations in Radiation Oncology. Edited by HR Withers and LJ Peters. New York: Springer-Verlag, 1988, pp 41–51.
116. Nagy B, Dale PJ, Grdina DJ. Protection against cis-diamminedichloroplatinum cytotoxicity and mutagenicity in V79 cells by 2-[(aminopropyl)amino]ethanethiol. Cancer Res 1986;46:1132–1135.
117. Narayan K, Cliff WJ. Morphology of irradiated microvasculature: a combined in vivo and electron-microscopic study. Am J Pathol 1982;106:47–62.
118. Neta R, Oppenheim JJ, Douches SD. Interdependence of the radioprotective effects of human recombinant interleukin 1 alpha, tumor necrosis factor alpha, granulocyte colony-stimulating factor, and murine recombinant granulocyte-macrophage colony-stimulating factor. J Immunol 1988;140:108–111.
119. Nilsson S, Carlson J, Larson E, Ponten J. Survival of irradiated glioma cells studied with a new cloning technique. Int J Radiat Biol 1980;37:267.
120. Oltvai ZN, Milliman CL, Korsmeyer SJ. Bcl-2 heterodimerizes in vivo with a conserved homolog, Bax, that accelerates programmed cell death. Cell 1993;74:609–619.
121. Oppenheim JJ, Neta R, Tiberghien P, Gress R, Kenny JJ, Longo DL. Interleukin-1 enhances survival of lethally irradiated mice treated with allogeneic bone marrow cells. Blood 1989;74:2257–2263.
122. Order SE, Stillwagon GB, Klein JL, Leichner PK, Siegelman SS, Fishman EK, Ettinger DS, Haulk T, Kopher K, Finney K, et al. Iodine 131 antiferritin, a new treatment modality in hepatoma: a Radiation Therapy Oncology Group study. J Clin Oncol 1985: 3:1573–1582.
123. Overgaard J, Hansen HS, Jorgensen K, Hjelm-Hansen M. Primary radiotherapy of larynx and pharynx carcinoma–an analysis of some factors influencing local control and survival. Int J Radiat Oncol Biol Phys 1986;12:515–521.
124. Overgaard J, Hjelm-Hansen M, Johansen LV, Andersen AP. Comparison of conventional and split-course radiotherapy as primary treatment in carcinoma of the larynx. Acta Oncol 1988;27:147–152.
125. Paliwal BR, Griem ML. Syllabus: A Categorical Course in Radiation Therapy Treatment Planning. Radiology Society of North America, 1986.
126. Patt HM. Protective mechanisms in ionizing radiation injury. Physiol Rev 1953;33:35.
127. Patt HM, Tyree EB, Straube RL, Smith DE, Scystein E. Protection against x-radiation. Science 1949;110:213.
128. Peckham MJ. In The Biological Basis of Radiotherapy. Edited by GG Steele and GE Adams. New York: Elsevier, 1983, pp 1–15.
129. Pelizzari CA, Chen GT, Spelbring DR, Weichselbaum RR, Chen CT. Accurate three-dimensional registration of CT, PET, and/or MR images of the brain. J Comp Assisted Tomogr 1989;13:20–26.
130. Peters LJ, Brock WA, Travis EL. Radiation Biology at Clinically Relevant Fractions. In Important Advances in Oncology. Philadelphia: Lippincott, 1990, pp 65–83.
131. Phillips RA, Tolmach LJ. Repair of potentially lethal damage in x-irradiated HeLa cells. Radiat Res 1966;29:413–432.
132. Photon Treatment Planning Collaborative Working Group. Evaluation of high energy photon external beam treatment planning: project summary. Int J Radiat Oncol Biol Phys 1991;21.
133. Pirollo KF, Garner R, Yuan SY, Li L, Blattner WA, Chang EH. Raf involvement in the simultaneous genetic transfer of the radioresistant and transforming phenotypes. Int J Radiat Biol 1989;55:783–796.
134. Potter DA, Glenn J, Kinsella T, Glatstein E, Lack EE, Restrepo C, White DE, Seipp CA, Wesley R, Rosenberg S. Patterns of recurrence in patients with high-grade soft-tissue sarcomas. J Clin Oncol 1985;3:353–366.
135. Powers WE, Palmer LA. Biologic basis of preoperative radiation treatment (review). Am J Roentgenol Rad Ther Nuc Med 1968;102:176–192.
136. Puck TT, Marcus PI. Action of x-rays on mammalian cells. J Exp Med 1956;103:653.
137. van Putten LM. Tumour reoxygenation during fractionated radiotherapy; studies with a transplantable mouse osteosarcoma. Eur J Cancer 1968;4:172–182.
138. Quilty PM, Duncan W. The influence of hemoglobin level on the regression and long term local control of transitional cell carcinoma of the bladder following photon irradiation. Int J Radiat Oncol Biol Phys 1986;12:1735–1742.
139. Reinhold HS, Fajardo LF, Hopewell JW. The vascular system. Adv Radiat Biol 1990;14:177–226.
140. Rubin P. Combination therapy—irradiation, surgery, and chemotherapy. JAMA 1966;196:348.
141. Rubin PJ, Cooper R, Phillips TL. Radiation Biology and Radiation Oncology Syllabus (Set RT 1: Radiation Oncology). Chicago: American College of Radiology, 1975.
142. Russell KJ, Laramore GE, Krall JM, Thomas FJ, Maor MH, Hendrickson FR, Krieger JN, Griffin TW. Eight years experience with neutron radiotherapy in the treatment of stages C and D prostate cancer: updated results of the RTOG 7704 randomized clinical trial. Prostate 1987;11:183–193.

143. Rustowski J, Kupsc W. Factors influencing the results of radiotherapy in cases of inoperable endometrial cancer. Gynecol Oncol 1982;14:185–193.
144. Schad LR, Boesecke R, Schlegel W, Hartmann GH, Sturm V, Strauss LG, Lorenz WJ. Three dimensional image correlation of CT, MR, and PET studies in radiotherapy treatment planning of brain tumors. J Comput Assist Tomogr 1987;11:948–954.
145. Schwartz JL, Mustafi R, Beckett MA, Weichselbaum RR. Prediction of the radiation sensitivity of human squamous cell carcinoma cells using DNA filter elution. Radiat Res 1990;123:1–6.
146. Seeger RC, Brodeur GM, Sather H, Dalton A, Siegel SE, Wong KY, Hammond D. Association of multiple copies of the N-myc oncogene with rapid progression of neuroblastomas. N Engl J Med 1985;313:1111–1116.
147. Sherman ML, Datta R, Hallahan DE, Weichselbaum RR, Kufe DW. Ionizing radiation regulates expression of the c-jun protooncogene. Proc Natl Acad Sci USA 1990;87:5663–5666.
148. Sinclair WK. Cyclic x-ray responses in mammalian cells in vitro (review). Radiat Res 1968;33:620–643.
149. Sklar MD. The ras oncogenes increase the intrinsic resistance of NIH 3T3 cells to ionizing radiation. Science 1988;239:645–647.
150. Slauson DO, Hahn FF, Benjamin SA, Chiffelle TL, Jones RK. Inflammatory sequences in acute pulmonary radiation injury. Am J Pathol 1976;82:549–572.
151. Stamato TD, Weinstein R, Giaccia A, Mackenzie L. Isolation of cell cycle-dependent gamma ray-sensitive Chinese hamster ovary cell. Somat Cell Genet 1983;9:165–173.
152. Steel GG. Terminology in the description of drug-radiation interactions. Int J Radiat Oncol Biol Phys 1979;5:1145–1150.
153. Steel GG, Peckham MJ. Exploitable mechanisms in combined radiotherapy-chemotherapy: the concept of additivity. Int J Radiat Oncol Biol Phys 1979;5:85–91.
154. Stein B, Rahmsdorf HJ, Steffen A, Litfin M, Herrlich P. UV-induced DNA damage is an intermediate step in UV-induced expression of human immunodeficiency virus type 1, collagenase, c-fos, and metallothionein. Mol Cell Biol 1989;9:5169–5181.
155. Steiner L. Stereotactic radiosurgery with cobalt-60 gamma unit in the surgical treatment of intracranial tumors and arteriovenous malformations. In Operative Neurological Techniques, vol I. Edited by HH Schmidkek and WH Sweet. Philadelphia: Saunders, 1988, pp 515–528.
156. Stephens LC, Ang KK, Schultheiss TE, Milas L, Meyn RE. Apoptosis in irradiated murine tumors. Rad Res 1991;127:308–316.
157. Stephens LC, Hunter NR, Ang KK, Milas L, Meyn RE. Development of apoptosis in irradiated murine tumors as a function of time and dose. Radiat Res 1993;135:75–80.
158. Stephens LC, Schultheiss TE, Price RE, Ang KK, Peters LJ. Radiation apoptosis of serous acinar cells of salivary and lacrimal glands. Cancer 1991;67:1539–1543.
159. Stevens KR. The stomach and intestines. In Radiation Oncology, Rationale, Techniques. Edited by MWT and JD Cox. St. Louis: Mosby, 1989, pp 362–408.
160. Stewart JR, Fajardo LF. Dose response in human and experimental radiation-induced heart disease. Application of the nominal standard dose (NSD) concept. Radiology 1971;99:403–408.
161. Suit H, Wette R. Radiation dose fractionation and tumor control probability. Radiat Res 1966;29:267–281.
162. Suit HD, Griffin TW, Castro JR, Verhey LJ. Particle radiation therapy research plan. Am J Clin Oncol 1988;11:330–341.
163. Takahashi S. Conformation radiotherapy applied to cancer of uterus. Nippon Acta Radiol 1961;20:2746–2753.
164. Takahashi S. Conformation radiotherapy. Rotation techniques as applied to radiography and radiotherapy of cancer. Acta Radiol Diagn 1965;242.
165. Taylor SG, Murthy AK, Showel J, Caldarelli DD, Hutchinson JC Jr, Holinger LD, Kramer T, Kiel K. Concomitant therapy with infusion of cisplatin and 5-fluorouracil plus radiation in head and neck cancer. NCI Monogr 1988;6:343–345.
166. Ten Haken RK, Perez-Tamayo C, Tesser RJ, McShan DL, Fraass BA, Lichter AS. Boost treatment of the prostate using shaped, fixed fields. Int J Radiat Oncol Biol Phys 1989;16:193–200.
167. Thames HD, Henry JH. Fractionation in Radiotherapy. London: Taylor & Francis, 1987.
168. Thomlinson RH. In Modern Trends in Radiotherapy, vol 1. Edited by TJ Deelay and CAP Wood. London: Butterworth's, 1967, pp 52–72.
169. Thomlinson RH, Gray LH. The histological structure of some human lung cancers and the possible implications for radiotherapy. Br J Cancer 1955;9:539–541.
170. Thompson CB. Apoptosis in the pathogenesis and treatment of disease. Science 1995;267:1456–1462.
171. Thompson LH, Suit HD. Proliferation kinetics of x-irradiated mouse L cells studied with time-lapse photography. I. Experimental methods and data analysis. Int J Radiat Biol Related Studies Phys Chem Med 1967;13:391–397.
172. Tucker SL. Is the mean inactivation dose a good measure of cell radiosensitivity? Radiat Res 1986;105:18–26.
173. Ulich TR, Howard SC, Remick DG, Yi ES, Collins T, Guo K, Yin S, Keene JL, Schmuke JJ, Steininger CN, et al. Intratracheal administration of endotoxin and cytokines: VIII. LPS induces E-selectin expression; anti-E-selectin and soluble E-selectin inhibit acute inflammation. Inflammation 1994;18:389–398.
174. van der Werf-Messing B, Star WM, Menon RS. T(3)N(X)M(O) carcinoma of the urinary bladder treated by the combination of radium implant and external irradiation. A preliminary report. Int J Radiat Oncol Biol Phys 1980;6:1723–1725.
175. Verhey LJ, Munzenrider JE. Proton beam therapy (review). Ann Rev Biophys Bioeng 1982;11:331–357.
176. Vikram B, Strong EW, Shah JP, Spiro R. Failure at the primary site following multimodality treatment in advanced head and neck cancer. Head Neck Surg 1984;6:720–723.
177. Vokes EE, Weichselbaum RR. Concomitant chemoradiotherapy: rationale and clinical experience in patients with solid tumors (published erratum appears in J Clin Oncol 1990 Aug;8(8):1447) (see comments) (review). J Clin Oncol 1990;8:911–934.
178. Walker GC. Mutagenesis and inducible responses to deoxyribonucleic acid damage in *Escherichia coli* (review). Microbiol Rev 1984;48:60–93.
179. Wang CC. Cancer of the head and neck. In Clinical Radiation Oncology. Edited by CC Wang. Littleton, MA: PSG Publishing, 1988, pp 120–179.
180. Warters RL. Radiation-induced apoptosis in a murine T-cell hybridoma. Cancer Res 1992;52:883–890.
181. Weichselbaum R, Little JB, Nove J. Response of human osteosarcoma in vitro to irradiation: evidence for unusual cellular repair activity. Int J Radiat Biol Related Studies Phys Chem Med 1977;31:295–299.
182. Weichselbaum RR. The role of DNA repair processes in the response of human tumors to fractionated radiotherapy (review). Int J Radiat Oncol Biol Phys 1984;10:1127–1134.
183. Weichselbaum RR, Beckett M. The maximum recovery potential of human tumor cells may predict clinical outcome in radiotherapy. Int J Radiat Oncol Biol Phys 1987;13:709–713.
184. Weichselbaum RR, Beckett MA, Schwartz JL, Dritschilo A. Radioresistant tumor cells are present in head and neck carcinomas that recur after radiotherapy. Int J Radiat Oncol Biol Phys 1988;15:575–579.
185. Weichselbaum RR, Beckett MA, Vijayuakumar S, Simon MA, Awan AM, Nachman J, Panje WR, Goldman ME, Tybor AG, Moran WJ, Vokes EE, Ahmed-Swan S, Farhangi E. Radiobiological characterization of head and neck and sarcoma cells derived from patients prior to radiotherapy. Int J Radiat Oncol Biol Phys 1995. In press.
186. Weichselbaum RR, Dahlberg W, Beckett M, Karrison T, Miller D, Clark J, Ervin TJ. Radiation-resistant and repair-proficient human tumor cells may be associated with radiotherapy failure in head- and neck-cancer patients. Proc Natl Acad Sci USA 1986;83:2684–2688.
187. Weichselbaum RR, Dahlberg W, Little JB. Inherently radioresistant cells exist in some human tumors. Proc Natl Acad Sci USA 1985;82:4732–4735.
188. Weichselbaum RR, Hallahan DE, Beckett MA, Masuceri H, Lee Sukhatme V, Kufe D. Radiation targeting of gene therapy preferentially radiosensitizes tumor cells. Cancer Res 1994;54:4266–4269.
189. Weichselbaum RR, Nove J, Little JB. Deficient recovery from potentially lethal radiation damage in ataxia telangiectasia and xeroderma pigmentosum. Nature 1978;271:261–262.
190. Weichselbaum RR, Nove J, Little JB. X-ray sensitivity of fifty-three human diploid fibroblast cell strains from patients with characterized genetic disorders. Cancer Res 1980;40:920–925.
191. Weichselbaum RR, Rotmensch J, Ahmed-Swan S, Beckett MA. Radiobiological characterization of 53 human tumor cell lines. Int J Radiat Biol 1989;56:553–560.
192. Weichselbaum RR, Schmit A, Little JB. Cellular repair factors influencing radiocurability of human malignant tumours. Br J Cancer 1982;45:10–16.
193. Weinert TA, Hartwell LH. The RAD9 gene controls the cell cycle response to DNA damage in *Saccharomyces cerevisiae.* Science 1988;241:317–322.
194. Withers HR. Regeneration of intestinal mucosa after irradiation. Cancer 1971;28:75–81.
195. Withers HR. In Principles and Practice of Radiation Oncology. Edited by CA Perez and LW Brady. Philadelphia: Lippincott, 1987, pp 67–98.
196. Witte L, Fuks Z, Haimovitz-Friedman A, Vlodavsky I, Goodman DS, Eldor A. Effects of irradiation on the release of growth factors from cultured bovine, porcine, and human endothelial cells. Cancer Res 1989;49:5066–5072.
197. Woloschak GE, Chang-Liu CM, Jones PS, Jones C. A modulation of gene expression in Syrian hamster embryo cells following ionizing radiation. Cancer Res 1990;50:339–344.
198. Wu NZ, Ross BA, Gulledge C, Klitzman B, Dodge R, Dewhirst MW. Differences in leucocyte-endothelium interactions between normal and adenocarcinoma bearing tissues in response to radiation. Br J Cancer 1994;69:883–889.
199. Yin XM, Oltval ZN, Korsmeyer SJ. BH1 and BH2 domains of Bcl-2 are required for inhibition of apoptosis and heterodimerization with Bax [see comments]. Nature 1994;369:321–323.
200. Yuhas JM. A more general role for WR-2721 in cancer therapy. Br J Cancer 1980;41:832–834.
201. Yuhas JM, Storer JB. Differential chemoprotection of normal and malignant tissues. JNCI 1969;42:331–335.

CHAPTER 49

Principles of Hyperthermia

DANIEL S. KAPP, GEORGE M. HAHN, AND ROBERT W. CARLSON

Historical Perspective

Hyperthermia as a method of treating cancer has a long history. Many Greek and Roman physicians thought that if they could simply control body temperature they could cure all diseases. Very likely this included cancer, because the pathology of tumor development had been described in the Greek literature. The modern use of this modality is to a large extent based on the well-documented occurrences of spontaneous remission in patients who had febrile episodes and on extensive laboratory data obtained over the last few years. Initial attempts to take advantage of the anticancer activity of hyperthermia involved the use of pyrogens for the induction of high fevers in patients with malignancies. Perhaps the best-known of these studies was that of Coley in 1893, who utilized bacterial toxins to raise the temperature in patients with osteosarcomas and soft tissue sarcomas (12). While he reported quite impressive results, it is not clear whether these involved primarily hyperthermia or, possibly, nonspecific host immune responses. Perhaps more importantly, recent laboratory studies have demonstrated that hyperthermia can inactivate cells, cause tumor regression, cause normal tissue damage, potentiate the effects of radiation therapy, and enhance the action of many anticancer drugs (16, 21, 47).

Biological Rationale

HEAT ALONE

The responses of tumors to hyperthermia involve both cellular and host-related factors. Experimentally, frequently it is not easy to separate these. When cells are exposed to elevated temperatures, they are inactivated in a time- and temperature-dependent fashion. Inactivation starts at 40° to 41°C, at least, for murine cells and tumors. At these low temperatures, cell inactivation continues for only a few hours; beyond that time, the surviving cells appear resistant to further exposure to such temperatures. Studies have shown that this is not a selection of heat-resistant subpopulations but that it results from the induction of a temporary resistance to heat. This transient phenomenon is referred to as *thermotolerance*. However, very prolonged heating at mild temperature (41° to 42°C) overcomes this transient thermotolerance (54).

Above 43°C, for most rodent lines, inactivation is exponential with time and thus resembles cell inactivation by ionizing radiation. Human cells tend to be more resistant, and in some human tumor cell lines this temperature threshold is as high as 44.5°C. Hence, thermotolerance can develop during treatment of human lesions, since tumor temperatures only rarely exceed 44°C. At even higher temperatures, thermotolerance does not develop, but if the cells are returned to 37°C, within a few hours the surviving cells do become resistant. At temperatures between 41° and 42°C, human tumor cell lines may be more sensitive than rodent tumor cells, and a potential therapeutic advantage may be achieved with prolonged heating at these milder temperatures (4).

The development of thermotolerance is accompanied by the preferential synthesis (or de novo synthesis) of a series of proteins referred to as *heat shock proteins*. These molecules are the subject of intense study because of their importance in normal cell function and in various disease states (44). In terms of survival, the effects of thermotolerance can be quite dramatic. For example, exposure for 45 minutes to 45°C kills approximately 99.9% of Chinese hamster cells. If, however, such heating is preceded by a 20-minute exposure at 45°C 4 hours earlier, then the 45-minute 45°C treatment leaves about 50% of the cells as survivors. Clearly, thermotolerance must be taken into account when scheduling fractionated heat treatments of patients. Thermotolerance can also greatly modify the cells' response to some drugs, to heat, and to X irradiation, but it does not seem to have much effect on the cells' response to X irradiation alone (22).

In addition to thermotolerance, there is great variability in genetically determined heat sensitivity of tumor cells. Heat-resistant variants of B16 melanoma cells and of a radiation-induced fibrosarcoma (RIF-1) have been isolated and characterized (1, 23). Very likely, many human neoplasms also contain subpopulations of resistant cells. The frequency of occurrence of such cells appears to be very low; however, there is no evidence of cross-resistance between heat sensitivity and X irradiation or most anticancer drugs. Hence, genetically heat-resistant cells may be of little importance during combination treatments with heat and radiation or chemotherapy.

Interestingly, when malignant cells and normal cells are tested under identical culture conditions, there is little or no difference in their response to heat. The old notion that cancer cells are necessarily more heat sensitive than their normal counterparts does not appear to be correct.

The microenvironment of cells in solid tumors is particularly conducive to heat sensitivity, a finding that may be important in the treatment of such tumors. The combination of low pH, low oxygen tension, and lack of glucose and other nutrients tends to make cells extremely responsive to elevated temperatures (21).

HEAT AND X IRRADIATION

Heat enhances the cytotoxicity of X rays, in both a super additive and a complementary fashion. Super additivity—that is, the increased cytotoxicity observed over that which would be expected on the basis of additivity of the two treatments—is maximum when these are given simultaneously. It decays with time when the treatments are separated by more than 1 or 2 hours, or, in some systems, even less. Complementarity results from the normal findings that cells particularly resistant to radiation tend to be sensitive to heat. Lack of sufficient blood flow causes cells to become hypoxic, and thus, radiation resistant. This lack of blood flow also causes low pH and low nutrient availability, making the hypoxic cells highly susceptible to killing by hyperthermia. An additional feature of complementarity is related to the cells' age response. Cells in the late S phase (i.e., cells that are in the process of completing DNA replication) tend to be quite resistant to X irradiation. The same cells, however, are particularly sensitive to heat. Overall, the results suggest strongly that tumors, provided they can be heated adequately, should be susceptible to the combination of X irradiation and heat (16, 21, 47).

HEAT AND DRUGS

When cells are exposed at elevated temperatures to drugs, their response is frequently very different from that seen at 37°C. Drugs whose rate-limiting reaction is primarily chemical (i.e., not involving enzymes) would, on thermodynamic grounds, be expected to be more efficient at higher temperatures. The rates of alkylation of DNA, or of conversion of a nonreactive species to a reactive one, can be expected to increase as the temperature increases. Tissue culture studies have shown this to be true for the nitrosoureas and cisplatin. For other drugs, there appears to be a threshold at or near 43°C. Below that temperature, drug activity is only mildly enhanced. At higher temperatures, however, cell killing proceeds at a greatly enhanced rate. Two such drugs are bleomycin and doxorubicin. For still other drugs, including most of the antimetabolites, cytotoxicity is not enhanced at elevated temperatures. Indeed, for the topoisomerase inhibitors, drug activity may be reduced at elevated temperatures. In addition, low pH can enhance drug activity. The nitrosoureas and cisplatin are far more effective at low pH ($\approx$6.5) than they are at neutral pH. Tissue culture and animal studies indicate that heat-drug combinations should be quite effective against some tumors. The *in vivo* experiments show that effectiveness of such treatments can be further enhanced by blood flow manipulations to reduce pH (26).

Physics and Physiology of Heating

HEATING METHODS

Whole-Body Heating. Three major methods are now available to achieve reproducible, controlled whole-body hyperthermia: thermal conduction (surface heating), extracorporeal induction, and radiant or electromagnetic induction (42, 53, 55, 65). The tolerance of liver and brain tissue limits the maximum temperature for using whole-body hyperthermia to 41.8° to 42.0°C, but this temperature may be maintained for several hours. All three methods of systemic hyperthermia require general anesthesia or sedation of the patient and careful monitoring for safety, and are all technically demanding.

Methods of whole-body hyperthermia induction by direct thermal conduction have used heated circulating water suits, heating blankets, and hot wax baths. Heating for 2 to 3 1/2 hours is required to achieve a core temperature of 41.8° to 42.0°C. Because the body surface is covered in this technique, access to temperature probes, ECG leads, and intravenous sites is limited. The use of extracorporeal induction requires both a high-flow arteriovenous shunt for vascular access and the availability of an extracorporeal heat exchanger. Extracorporeal heat exchangers, however, allow for rapid induction of hyperthermia in only 30 to 60 minutes, and for accurate temperature control. The patient is readily accessible for monitoring of vital signs and for initiation of supportive interventions.

Techniques are available that use radiant heat, microwave radiation, infrared radiation, or combinations of these to induce whole-body hyperthermia with steady state temperatures of 41° to 42°C. While the power absorption patterns are nonuniform, redistribution of the thermal energy is rapid via the circulatory system.

The toxicities associated with whole-body hyperthermia may be significant, and careful patient selection and supportive care are essential. Sedation or general anesthesia must be used and continuous monitoring of vital signs, core body temperature, ECG, and urine output is necessary. Typically large fluid losses require vigorous replacement. Electrolyte abnormalities, decreases in platelet count, and prolongation of coagulation are common; these changes may be more pronounced with the use of extracorporeal methods of hyperthermia induction. Elevation in liver function tests reflecting mild liver necrosis and increase in serum creatine phosphokinase, reflecting skeletal muscle necrosis, have also been observed. The physiologic response to hyperthermia includes an approximate doubling of cardiac output with an increase in pulse rate but little change in blood pressure. Cardiac arrhythmias, pulmonary edema, and seizures occur occasionally and may be life-threatening. Diarrhea, nausea, and vomiting, posthyperthermia fever, and reactivation of herpes simplex infections are frequently observed.

Equipment Available for Localized (or Regional) Hyperthermia. While many heating modalities are discussed in the literature, almost all local heating is currently delivered by microwave, radiofrequency, or ultrasound equipment. Most microwave equipment works in the 100-MHz to 3-GHz region (*microwaves*, here, is really a misnomer: strictly speaking, most of that range is termed *ultra high frequency*); radiofrequency systems work in the 500-kHz to 15- MHz band, and ultrasound in the 300-kHz to 2-MHz region. The relative merits of each of the techniques are discussed in Table 49.1. Other techniques (radiofrequency inductively coupled, ferromagnetic seeds, lasers) are either little used or in the developmental stage (2, 16, 21, 47).

Table 49.1. Methods of Producing Local-Regional Hyperthermia

Heating Techniques	Advantages	Disadvantages	Applications (as described in the literature)	Commercial availability
Microwaves	Technology very advanced. Heating of large volumes theoretically possible. Multiple applicators, coherent or incoherent, can be utilized. Specialized antennas for heating from body cavities have been developed. Skin cooling feasible. Interstitial use has been demonstrated.	Heating not localized at depth; limited penetration at high frequencies. Possible adverse effects on personnel. Shielding of treatment rooms required, except at medically reserved frequencies (e.g., 915 MHz). Thermometry requires noninteracting probes. Temperature distributions subject to variations in local blood flow. Commercial antennas available are of fixed length. Depth of tissue implant alters specific absorption rate pattern.	Surface or near-surface lesions. Lesions on breast, chest wall, extremities (external applicators). Bladder, prostate, esophagus, cervix, brain, head and neck with specialized or interstitial applicators.	USA—yes Japan—yes Europe—yes
Radiofrequency (direct current or capacitive coupling)	Equipment relatively simple. No special shielding required. Large volumes may be heated. Heating of deep-seated lesions sometimes possible. Interstitial use has been demonstrated. Electrodes not limited in size; insulation easily accomplished.	Fat tissue may heat preferentially. Current flow subject to local electrical tissue characteristics. Temperature distribution additionally subject to blood flow variations. Heating regional with external applicators.	Large-surface tumors; lesions in extremities, lung, pancreas, liver, bladder. Interstitial applications: chest wall, head and neck, prostate, uterine cervical cancer.	USA—no Japan—yes Europe—?
Ultrasound Single transducers	Readily focuses in tissue. Heating possible to 5–10-cm depth with focused transducers. Dynamic systems have been demonstrated. Shielding not required, and no health hazards to personnel. Fat not treatment limiting. In dynamic systems, effects of blood flow can be reduced by minimizing focal volume.	No penetration of tissue–air interfaces. "Shadowing" by bone. Bone tends to heat preferentially. Patients may experience pain during treatment.	Surface lesions; head and neck, and lesions in extremities.	USA—yes Japan—yes Europe—yes
Multiple transducers	Focusing and preferential heating to 20-cm depth has been demonstrated. Dynamic systems can heat larger volumes.	As for single transducers (above).	Brain, prostate, head and neck.	USA—yes Japan—yes Europe—yes

THERMOMETRY

Temperature measurements during heating are subject to two types of errors. First, the measuring device may itself absorb energy, causing the temperature to rise in its immediate vicinity. The sensor may then record (correctly) the temperature but may overestimate tissue values. This problem can occur with both electromagnetic and ultrasound heating devices. In addition, noise in the receiver associated with electromagnetic energy may cause erroneous temperature readings. Optical temperature sensors can minimize or essentially eliminate this problem. Because temperature distributions in tumors and in normal tissue are usually anything but uniform, it is important to obtain many data points during treatment. One way of doing this is to implant one or more hollow catheters into the volume of tissue to be heated and then pass a sensor through the catheter. Catheter material must be chosen carefully, particularly if ultrasound is used to heat the lesion. Automated samplers have been developed that move the sensor at a predetermined rate, so that measurement along a catheter can be made with essentially arbitrary frequency and spatial resolution. In addition, exciting progress has been made in noninvasive monitoring systems, using magnetic resonance techniques in conjunction with microwave (57) or focused ultrasound (11) hyperthermia treatments.

HYPERTHERMIC DOSE

A serious problem in hyperthermia is the definition of *clinically meaningful dose.* Deposition of energy, usually stated in terms of *specific absorption rate,* while useful for quality control and intercomparison of equipment, is not necessarily related to tissue temperature and, therefore, not to cytotoxicity. The effect of nonuniform temperature distributions on cytotoxicity is amplified by the temperature threshold effect discussed earlier, which may vary from tumor to tumor, and from normal tissue to tissue. Attempts to define a unifying biologically based dose concept ("43°C–equivalent minutes") (58), have not been entirely satisfactory, in part because of biologic variations and development of thermotolerance. Although cumbersome, it probably is best to describe treatments in terms of multiple local time-temperature profiles; however, recent thermal dose formulations that have taken into account both the temperature distribution and time at various temperatures have shown good correlations with complete response rates (45) and duration of local tumor control (30). These need to be confirmed in future clinical trials.

Clinical Experience

HEAT ALONE

Local-Regional Heating. In the 1970s, initial studies were undertaken utilizing hyperthermia alone primarily for the treatment of superficial, recurrent, or metastatic tumors. A detailed survey of these trials by Meyer revealed an overall complete response rate of 15%, and the responses were typically of short duration (41); however, several studies (Table 49.2) have suggested that higher complete response rates and longer duration of response were associated with higher intratumor temperatures. For example, Storm and colleagues reported tumor regression in all 12 patients when intratumor temperatures of 46°C or greater were achieved (66). A multi-institutional trial utilizing the annular phased array (BSD Medical, Salt Lake City, UT) reported only one complete and three partial responders among 47 patients treated with hyperthermia alone (52).

Currently, local-regional hyperthermia is rarely employed as the sole treatment for advanced or recurrent malignancies. One possible exception may be symptomatic recurrent chondrosarcoma. Delephin reported excellent tumor responses, with decrease in tumor volumes, noted after 6 months in four patients with pelvic chondrosarcoma treated with local-regional hyperthermia alone (14). The relatively poor blood supply to tumor cells in chondrosarcomas may explain the response of such tumors to hyperthermia. Additional patient accrual and longer-term follow-up will be needed before definitive conclusions can be reached concerning the role of hyperthermia alone in such tumors.

Whole-Body Heating. Early attempts to induce systemic hyperthermia with pyrogens (e.g., Coley's toxin) resulted in occasional tumor responses, but the duration and height of temperature elevations were difficult to predict or control. Since the development of predictable, controlled whole-body hyperthermia techniques, few studies using contemporary criteria of response have been reported. The available studies demonstrate no benefit to controlled whole-body hyperthermia alone in the treatment of cancer (5, 8, 63, 72).

HYPERTHERMIA AS AN ADJUVANT

Radiation Therapy and Local Hyperthermia. The majority of clinical trials comparing hyperthermia as an adjunct to radiation with radiation therapy alone have addressed small superficially located tumors (64). These have the greatest chance of being adequately heated; their temperatures can be readily monitored; and response and normal tissue complications can easily be followed (29). Anderson and Kapp reviewed the clinical studies for superficial tumors treated with radiation therapy alone or in combination with hyperthermia (2). An update of their summary is presented in Table 49.3. In general, an increase in complete response

Table 49.2. Response as a Function of Thermal Parameters for Tumors Treated with Hyperthermia Alone

Authors (yr)	Response criteria	Thermal parameter (°C)	Fields (No.)	Responders (%)	Response duration (median)
Marmour, et al. (1982)	CR plus PR	Ave. at tumor center			
		43–44	23	39	6 WK
		44.1–45	21	48	6 WK
Corry, et al. (1982)	CR plus PR	Maximum at tumor center			
		43–44	15	53	29 D
		45–47	7	42	46 D
		48–50	6	83	250 D
Storm, et al. (1985)	Greater than 25% reduction in tumor size	Highest temperature sustained in			
		tumor 30–60 Min	56	14	NA
		<41.9	29	17	NA
		42–44.9	21	67	NA
		45–50			

Key: CR, complete response; PR, partial response; WK, weeks; D, days; NA, not available.

Table 49.3. Complete Response Rates for Tumors Treated Either with Radiation Therapy Alone or in Combination with Hyperthermia

Authors (yr)	No. Patients (No. fields or lesions)	Type of trial	Radiation dose (Gy)	Complete response rate: Radiation alone (%)	Complete response rate: Radiation plus hyperthermia (%)	P value
A. Local-Regional Metastases from Breast Cancer						
Low-dose radiation						
Hofman, et al. (1984)	23	Nonrandomized	30–50 (median 38)	Not performed	61	——
Steeves, et al. (1986)	(90; 81% breast metastases)	Matched pair	20–56	31	45	<0.05
	20	——	20–56	30	65	<0.05
Lindholm, et al. (1987)	11 (34)	Paired lesions	30	35	66	0.025
van der zee, et al. (1988)	66	Nonrandomized controls (15 fields)	<29	7	24	——
	31	Nonrandomized controls (10 fields)	30–36	20	58	——
Gonzalez, Gonzalez, et al. (1988)	35 (45)	Nonrandomized	18–60 (median 24)	Not performed	60	——
Dragovic, et al. (1989)	30	Nonrandomized	32	Not performed	57	——
Kapp, et al. (1989)	85	Nonrandomized	(median 30.6)	Not performed	68	——
Perez, et al. (1989)[a]	20	Randomized	32	33	55	0.62
Seegenschmiedt, et al. (1989)	49 (95)	Nonrandomized	(mean 36.8)	Not performed	52	——
Full-dose radiation						
Scott, et al. (1984)	17 (34)	Paired lesions	48–66	47[b]	94[b]	——
Perez, et al. (1986)	7	Nonrandomized historical controls (53 patients)	50	51[b]	86[b]	——
Scott, et al. (1988)	54	Nonrandomized	60–70	Not performed	85[b]	——
B. Advanced Neck Node Metastases from Head and Neck Cancers						
Arcangeli, et al. (1985)	38 (81)	Nonrandomized: One lesion in radiation field selected for hyperthermia	40–70	42	79	<0.05
Valdagni, et al. (1986)	27	Historical controls (45 patients: radiation dose ≥60–65 Gy), as	20–70	35	59	0.095
	19	above	≥60	35	68	0.034
Valdagni, et al. (1988)	(36)	Prospectively randomized	64–70	37	82	0.015
Scott, et al. (1988)	41	Nonrandomized	60–70	Not performed	51[b]	——
C. Superficially Located Metastases from Melanoma						
Kim, et al. (1982)	38 (99)	Nonrandomized matched pair and paired lesions	38.5–42.9	46	69	≤0.01
Kim, et al. (1982)	(97)	As for Kim et al., 1982	39.6–40.0	45	66	——
Hofman, et al. (1984)	12	Nonrandomized	30 (6 Gy × 5)	Not performed	73	——

[a] Lesions <3 cm diameter.
[b] Local control at 6 months.

Table 49.3. *(continued)*

Authors (yr)	No. Patients (No. fields or lesions)	Type of trial	Radiation dose (Gy)	Complete response rate: Radiation alone (%)	Complete response rate: Radiation plus hyperthermia (%)	*P* value
Gonzalez Gonzalez, et al. (1986)	(18)	Nonrandomized controls (6 fields)	24 (8 Gy × 3)	50	83	——
Arcangeli, et al. (1987)	17 (38)	Nonrandomized controls	30.0–40.0	53	76	——
Overgaard, Overgaard, et al. (1987)	10 (25)	Matched pair	15–27 (5–9 Gy × 3)	20	73	<0.05
	(67)	Nonrandomized and matched pair	24–27 (8–9 Gy × 3)	59	91	<0.05
Emami, et al. (1988)	18 (49)	Nonrandomized controls (67 lesions)	<20–>60	24	59	0.0003

[a] Lesions <3 cm diameter.
[b] Local control at 6 months.

rates by a factor of 1.5 to 2 has been demonstrated for the combination of radiation therapy plus hyperthermia as compared with radiation therapy alone in local-regional recurrences of breast cancer (see Table 49.3A); advanced neck nodal metastases from head and neck cancers (see Table 49.3B); and for cutaneous, subcutaneous, and peripheral lymph node metastases from melanoma (see Table 49.3C). Although the trials on superficial metastases from breast cancer varied considerably in the hyperthermia treatment regimens employed, complete response rates were remarkably similar when hyperthermia was utilized with similar radiation therapy doses.

Four prospectively randomized trials are of particular interest. A subset analysis from the Radiation Therapy Oncology Group's randomized study of 20 patients with chest wall metastasis from breast cancer and lesions less than 3 cm in diameter showed an improvement in complete response rates for radiation therapy plus hyperthermia as compared with radiation therapy alone (55 vs. 33%, respectively; $P =$ 0.62) (50). Further analysis of all superficial lesions smaller than 3 cm showed, however, a significant improvement in the probability of local control at 12 months. Local control for lesions treated with hyperthermia plus radiation was 80% as compared with 15% for lesions treated with radiation therapy alone ($P = 0.02$) (49). Similarly, the trial reported by Valdagni and colleagues compared full-dose radiation therapy with radiation and either two or six hyperthermia treatments for extensive neck nodal metastases from head and neck cancers and demonstrated a statistically significant difference in complete response rates (37 vs. 82% respectively; $P =$ 0.015) for the combined modality treatment arms (70). Exciting preliminary results have been reported from the collaborative phase III (MRC/ESHO/PMH) trial comparing radiation therapy with or without hyperthermia in the treatment of selected patients (tumors <4 cm diameter and <2.5 cm depth) with primary or recurrent local breast cancers. A joint analysis of 315 patients has revealed a statistically significant increase in complete response rates (60 vs. 40%); a lower relapse rate at 2 years among the complete responders (15 vs. 28%); and no increase in acute or long-term side effects in the patients receiving adjuvant hyperthermia (73). A fourth prospective randomized phase III trial (ESHO 3–85) has been completed, which tested the value of hyperthermia as an adjuvant to radiation therapy in the treatment of superficial metastatic melanomas. Analysis of 128 tumors stratified on size (<4 cm or ≥4 cm) and randomized to radiation alone (second randomization to 8 Gy × 3 or 9 Gy × 3) or radiation plus hyperthermia (43°C for 60 minutes following each radiation treatment) showed a significantly higher 2-year local-regional control rate for the tumors that received adjuvant hyperthermia (46 vs. 28%; $P = 0.008$) (46). Here, too, no significant increase in acute or late reactions was noted in the hyperthermia group.

Similarly, in other trials in which longer-term follow-up (6 months to 5 years) is available, the adjuvant use of hyperthermia resulted in an increase in complete response rates and/or survival, as summarized in Table 49.4. For example, an improvement in 5-year survival rates with the addition of hyperthermia (0 vs. 53%; $P = 0.02$) was recently reported by Valdagni and Amichetti in an update of their study on advanced neck nodal metastases (69). Surprisingly good local control rates have also been obtained for superficial metastases of other selected tumors, including Hodgkin's disease (51), Merkel cell tumors (33), adenoid cystic carcinomas (6), and penile metastases from prostatic cancer. In addition, thermal dose-response relationships for superficial tumors treated with combined radiation-hyperthermia are now better defined (30, 45). This will permit more relevant hyperthermia prescriptions to be used in subsequent trials.

In general, the hyperthermia treatments for superficially located tumors have been well-tolerated, considering the extensive treatment that most of these patients had already undergone and the often advanced nature of their disease (31). Small blisters are often noted following local hyperthermia

Table 49.4. Local Control Rates for Tumors Treated with Radiation Alone or in Combination with Hyperthermia

Authors (yr)	Fields (No.)	Time of follow-up	Local control	
			Radiation alone (%)	Radiation plus hyperthermia (%)
A. Local-Regional Metastases from Breast Cancer				
Low-dose radiation				
Perez, et al. (1986)[a]	70	> 6 mo	31	61
Lindholm, et al. (1987)	34	1 y	30	53
		2 y	30	45
Gonzalez Gonzalez, et al. (1988)	18	>6 mo	33[c]	78[c]
Kapp, et al. (1988)	85	2 y	Not performed	45
Dragovic, et al. (1989)	30	6–32 mo	Not performed	43
Seegenschmiedt, et al. (1989)	95	≥6 mo	Not performed	67
Full-dose radiation				
Scott, et al. (1984)	34	1 y	55	100
Perez, et al. (1986)[b]	95	>6 mo	46	86
B. Advanced Neck Node Metastases from Head and Neck Cancers				
Scott et al. (1984)	10	12 mo	40	100
Arcangeli et al. (1985)	81	24 mo	14	58
Valdagni (1994)	36	60 mo	24	69
			0[d]	53[d]
C. Superficially Located Metastases from Melanoma				
Gonzalez Gonzalez, et al. (1986)	24	≤36 mo	17	83
Arcangeli, et al. (1987)	38	6–24 mo	53	76
Overgaard, Overgaard (1987)	67	18 mo	56	86
Emami, et al. (1988)	116	Not stated	21	57

[a] Dose <40 Gy.
[b] Dose ≥40 Gy.
[c] Maintained (CR plus PR).
[d] Five-year survival rates.

but are mostly self-limited. When the tumors eroded through the skin surface, ulcerations are occasionally noted following regression of the tumors. These ulcerations often require prolonged time for healing, a phenomenon that's possibly related to the extensive radiation therapy, which compromises the vascular supply to the damaged tissue. Rarely is surgical repair of these ulcers required.

Radiation Therapy and Regional Hyperthermia. Several studies on the adjunctive use of hyperthermia with radiation therapy in the treatment of deep-seated malignancies have suggested that improvements in local control or survival can be achieved (Table 49.5). Sugimachi and colleagues compared their results with the adjuvant use of hyperthermia in conjunction with radiation therapy and bleomycin in patients with either unresectable esophageal cancer or patients treated preoperatively for potentially resectable esophageal cancers (67). In the unresectable cases, improvement in 1- and 2-year survival rates were noted as compared with historical controls. For the patients with resectable disease, improvements in 1- to 5-year survival rates were obtained. The 5-year survival rate in the patients treated preoperatively with radiation and bleomycin was 15%, as compared with 43% when hyperthermia was added to the preoperative treatment regimen. Improved survival was noted for patients with early (stage I and II) as well as advanced (stage III and IV) surgically treated cancers.

A prospectively randomized trial reported by Sharma and colleagues demonstrated improved local tumor control in stage II and III squamous cell carcinomas of the uterine cervix with the addition of hyperthermia to standard radiation therapy treatment regimens (60). Similarly, Datta and colleagues demonstrated improved survival at 18 months for stage III and IV squamous cell carcinoma of the head and neck with the addition of hyperthermia to external beam treatment (25%) as compared with external beam treatment alone (8%) (13). In addition, a pilot study on re-treatment of locally recurrent prostatic cancer with external beam radiation therapy and hyperthermia has suggested that long-term local control can be obtained (28).

Two randomized trials have investigated the use of hyperthermia as an adjuvant to preoperative radiation in locally advanced initially unresectable rectal cancers. Berdov and Menteshashvili reported higher complete response rates (16.1 vs. 1.7%), ability to perform radical surgery (55.4 vs. 27.1%), and 5-year survival rates (35.6 vs. 6.6%) in 56 patients randomized to 40 Gy plus hyperthermia, as compared with 59 patients who received preoperative radiation therapy (7). Similarly, in a three-arm randomized trial comparing preoperative radiation plus hyperthermia, preoperative radiation, and surgery alone in locally advanced rectal cancer,

Table 49.5. Survival or Local Control for Deep-Seated Tumors Treated with Either Radiation Therapy or Combination Radiation Therapy and Hyperthermia

Author (yr)	Site: No. Patients	Type of Trial	Radiation dose (Gy)	Follow-up (y)	Survival rate: Radiation (%)	Survival rate: Radiation plus HT (%)	*P* value
Sugimachi, et al. (1988)	Esophageal cancer: unresectable 31 (XRT plus bleomycin plus HT)	Historical controls: 83 (XRT plus bleomycin)	48	1 2	11 1	33 16	<0.05
	Esophageal cancer: preoperative 62 (XRT plus bleomycin plus HT)	Historical controls; 121 (XRT plus bleomycin)	30	1 3 5	45 20 15	66 43 43	<0.05
Sharma, et al. (1989)	Stage II and III SCC of uterine cervix: 50	Prospectively randomized	70 or 45, plus 35 ICR	1.5	50[a]	70[a]	<0.05
Datta, et al. (1990)	Stage III and IV SCC of head and neck	Prospectively randomized	65	1.5	8	25	0.03
Berdov, Menteshashvili (1990)	Locally advanced carcinoma of the rectum: preoperative 56 (XRT plus HT)	Prospectively randomized: 59 (XRT)	40 (80 Gy if lesion remains unresectable)	5	7	36	<0.05
You et al. (1993)	Locally advanced carcinoma of the rectum: preoperative 44 (XRT plus HT)	Prospectively randomized: 38 (XRT); 40 (surgery alone)	30 or 40	5	50 41 (surgery alone)	67	NA
Karasawa et al. (1994)	Locally advanced non-small cell lung cancer: 10 (XRT plus HT); 9 (XRT, plus HT, plus surgery)	Historical controls: 26 (XRT); 4 (XRT plus surgery)	42–80	3	37	7	<0.01

Key: XRT, X-irradiation; HT, hyperthermia; SCC, squamous cell carcinoma; ICR, intracavitary radiation to point A; [a]locally disease free.

You and colleagues reported higher 5-year survival rates with the addition of hyperthermia (67 vs. 50 vs. 41%, for preoperative radiation plus hyperthermia, preoperative radiation, or surgery alone, respectively) (76). Hyperthermia has also been studied in conjunction with preoperative radiation in locally advanced non–small cell lung cancer. Compared to historical controls treated with similar doses of radiation, the hyperthermia-treated patients reportedly had a higher complete response rate (26 vs. 0%; $P<0.005$) and 3-year survival rate (37 vs. 6.7%; $P<0.01$) without an increase in complications (21 vs. 23%) (32).

Multi-institutional studies have also suggested improved local control rates can be obtained when hyperthermia is utilized as an adjunct to radiation therapy for the treatment of deep-seated tumors. Petrovich and colleagues have reported the results of a 14-institution trial conducted in the United States that employed the annular phased array system for regional hyperthermia production in 353 patients with advanced, recurrent, or persistent deep-seated tumors (52). Hyperthermia was used alone or in conjunction with radiation therapy, chemotherapy, chemotherapy and radiation therapy in 4, 12, 13, and 69% of the patients, respectively. Complete responses (10%) and partial responses (17%) were obtained, with the highest complete response rates noted in patients receiving radiation therapy in conjunction with hyperthermia (12 vs. 2%; $P = 0.003$). There was a correlation between complete response rates and increasing radiation dose ($P < 0.001$) but no correlation was noted between thermal dose and response. Of the 195 patients with pain present prior to treatment, 23% had complete pain resolution and 39% had partial pain relief. The treatment was, in general, well-tolerated, but 35% of the patients had some pain during the treatment. Three percent of the patients had elevated heart rates, 2% had anxiety reactions, and 1% noted claustrophobia during treatment. Only 1% of the patients developed infections in the sites of the catheters used for temperature monitoring, and 3% developed blisters within their hyperthermia treatment fields. A second-generation phased array device (Sigma-60, BSD-2000 system) has been developed (BSD Medical, Salt Lake City, UT), which should permit better power localization, and, possibly less patient discomfort. A multi-institutional phase I/II trial is currently ongoing in the United States employing the Sigma-60 system while phase III trials in patients with advanced bladder, rectal, and uterine cervical cancers are being conducted in Holland. Preliminary results of the Dutch trial have demonstrated that a higher percentage of patients treated with full-dose radiation therapy and adjuvant hyperthermia for primary inoperable or recurrent rectal cancer (19 vs. 13%), advanced cervical cancer (78 vs. 56%), or inoperable bladder cancer (79 vs. 41%) were alive at 1 year with local control, as compared with those treated with full-dose radiation alone (71).

Preliminary results of a Japanese seven-institution trial employing the Thermotron RF-8 capacitive heating device (Yamamoto Vinyter, Osaka, Japan) are also noteworthy (27). Treatment given to 177 patients with deep-seated tumors utilized hyperthermia in combination with radiation therapy alone (96 patients) or with radiochemotherapy (81 patients). Maximum intratumor or intracavitary temperatures greater than 42°C were obtained in 77 and 74% of the tumors, respectively. Response rates and symptomatic improvement were felt to be higher than expected for historical controls treated with radiation therapy or chemotherapy alone. No severe side effects were noted. Minor side effects were seen, however, in 37 patients (21%) and consisted mainly of fatty induration, pain, and burns. Preliminary results of a prospectively randomized trial included in this report, which compared preoperative radiation therapy (40 Gy) with and without hyperthermia in primary rectal cancers revealed statistically significant improved total response rates for patients with the addition of hyperthermia. Comparison of these results with historical controls treated with radiation (60 Gy) alone suggested a dose enhancement by hyperthermia of approximately 1.5. Further patient accrual and follow-up in this randomized study is awaited, as is additional patient accrual utilizing this capacitive heating device in the treatment of other deep-seated tumors.

Interstitial Hyperthermia. Excellent results have been obtained utilizing interstitial hyperthermia techniques in conjunction with brachytherapy in the treatment of implantable tumors at a variety of locations. Both radiofrequency local current field techniques and microwave antennas have been employed. Site-specific results of thermobrachytherapy for the more commonly treated sites (head and neck, pelvis, breast and chest wall) are summarized in Table 49.6. In addition, a review of 90 patients with localized tumors treated in a phase I/II trial with interstitial thermoradiotherapy and external-beam radiation therapy revealed a complete response rate at 3 months of 66% and a 1-year local control rate of 64% (59). Multivariate analyses demonstrated that tumor volume and minimum tumor temperature variables including average minimum intratumor temperature and T_{90} (the temperature at or above that of 90% of all measured temperatures) were significantly predictive of complete response. However, it should be borne in mind that high local control rates have also been reported in similar tumors utilizing brachytherapy without the addition of hyperthermia (29). These results, therefore, await confirmation in randomized trials. Recent studies are also exploring the use of continuous "mild" hyperthermia (41°C) throughout the entire low-dose rate brachytherapy treatment. Exciting preliminary results in advanced prostate and gynecologic cancers have been noted (40).

Chemotherapy. The compelling preclinical finding that hyperthermia augments the antitumor activity of many chemotherapeutic agents has been tested in relatively few clinical trials. With rare exceptions, the reported trials have *not* been disease-specific, prospectively randomized clinical trials comparing chemotherapy alone versus chemotherapy plus hyperthermia. The inconvenience, required professional expertise, special equipment, expense, and potential toxicities require clear demonstration of benefit before the addition of hyperthermia should be adopted as standard practice.

At least four types of heat–drug interactions appear to occur in vitro (Table 49.7) (21). In addition, hyperthermia may in some circumstances at least partially overcome selective drug resistance (35, 74, 75). The nature of the heat–drug interaction has important implications for the use of hyperthermia plus chemotherapy in the clinic. Hyperthermia, for instance, may not increase the cytotoxicity of some agents at temperatures that are tolerable using whole-body hyperthermia. In addition, the heat–drug interaction may be influenced by blood flow, time to steady-state temperature, tumor and normal tissue steady-state temperatures, duration of heat-

Table 49.6. Interstitial Thermobrachytherapy: Site-Specific Results

Authors (yr)	HT System (type, freq [MHz])	Site treated: no. CR/total no. tumors (%)			
		Head & neck	Pelvis	Breast & chest wall	Other
Surwit, et al. (1983)	RF, 0.5	——	7/21 (33%)	——	——
Puthawala, et al. (1985)[a]	MW, 915	15/20 (75%)	10/13 (77%)	5/8 (63%)	2/2 (100%)
Vora, et al. (1988)	RF, 0.5	——	10/19 (53%)	——	——
Gautherie, et al. (1989)	MW, 915	24/35 (69%)	23/39 (59%)	11/14 (79%)	3/8 (39%)
Rafla, et al. (1989)	MW, 915	8/15 (53%)	8/14 (57%)	3/6 (50%)	——
Petrovich, et al. (1989)	MW, 915,630	16/23 (70%)	3/4 (75%)	7/9 (78%)	2/8 (25%)
Goffinet, et al. (1990)	RF, 0.5	5/5 (100%)	3/5 (60%)	——	——
Shimm, et al. (1990)	RF, 0.5	8/13 (61%)	14/48 (29%)	——	——
Phromratanapongse, et al. (1990)	MW, 915	22/30 (73%)	7/11 (64%)	0/2 (0%)	2/2 (100%)

Key: HT, hyperthermia; CR, complete response.
[a] Local control rates.

Table 49.7. Types of Heat-Drug Interactions Observed In Vitro

Group		Examples
1	Linear increase in cytotoxicity	Thiotepa, cisplatin, mitomycin C, nitrosoureas
2	Threshold increase in cytotoxicity	Doxorubicin, bleomycin, actinomycin
3	No cytotoxicity at low temperatures; cytotoxicity at high temperatures	Lidocaine, amphotericin B
4	No effect on cytotoxicity	Methotrexate, 5-fluorouracil, vincristine

ing, uniformity of heating, changes in drug pharmacokinetics, and the sequencing of the chemotherapy and hyperthermia.

Whole-Body Hyperthermia. The successful application of hyperthermia in the treatment of systemic neoplasms requires the application of whole-body hyperthermia. Although a number of trials have tested the use of whole-body hyperthermia plus chemotherapy, most trials are small and uncontrolled, include patients with tumors of multiple histologies, and utilize many different chemotherapy regimens.

The available studies document that combined whole-body hyperthermia plus chemotherapy can be safely administered, although some drug toxicities do appear to be increased (9, 15, 37, 39, 48, 53, 72). For instance, in a study of 11 patients with a variety of cancers treated with doxorubicin plus whole-body hyperthermia, two partial responses were achieved and there was a suggestion of enhanced anthracycline cardiac toxicity (9). The same investigator has studied methyl-CCNU (semustine) plus whole-body hyperthermia in 12 patients with melanoma. Three partial responses were observed.

In a series of 132 patients with multiple tumor types treated with a variety of chemotherapeutic agents plus whole-body hyperthermia, no relation between tumor histology or chemotherapeutic agent and response rates was observed (39). The heterogeneous nature of the patient population and treatment, however, made subset analysis difficult.

Preliminary results of a randomized study combining whole-body hyperthermia plus doxorubicin, cyclophosphamide, and vincristine in the treatment of non–small cell lung cancer have been reported by Engelhardt (15). Fifty-five patients were randomized and 44 were "evaluable." The rates of response were 8/22 (36%) with chemotherapy alone and 15/22 (68%) with chemotherapy plus whole-body hyperthermia. Mean duration of response was 105 days with chemotherapy alone and 130 days with the addition of hyperthermia.

Assessment of the impact of whole-body hyperthermia added to chemotherapy in the treatment of cancer remains difficult because of the paucity of nonrandomized and randomized clinical trials. The use of whole-body hyperthermia remains experimental until additional studies are performed.

Regional-Perfusion Chemotherapy Plus Heat. Isolated hyperthermic perfusion chemotherapy has been utilized primarily in the treatment of malignant melanoma of the extremities (19, 36, 56, 61, 62). Melphalan, cisplatin, nitrogen mustard, thiotepa, and actinomycin D have all been administered safely by hyperthermic isolated limb perfusion (36). Most studies have utilized perfusion with melphalan, and all demonstrate benefit from the use of hyperthermic perfusion in association with surgical excision as compared with historical control groups. Limb perfusion requires isolation and cannulation of the arterial supply and venous drainage of the limb, the use of an extracorporeal blood oxygenator, and the use of a heating unit. The complication rates are low when the procedure is performed by an experienced team (36).

With almost 6 years of follow-up, a randomized comparison of surgery, with or without isolated hyperthermic limb perfusion of melphalan, in patients with newly diagnosed intermediate- and high-risk malignant melanoma has documented the advantage of limb perfusion (19). The use of hyperthermic limb perfusion decreased rates of recurrence (48% without perfusion, 11% with perfusion, $P < 0.001$) and decreased the number of melanoma deaths (20% without perfusion, 6% with perfusion; $P < 0.01$). The Swedish Melanoma Study Group randomized trials for recurrent melanoma compared surgery (36 patients) or surgery plus regional hyperthermic melphalan perfusion (33 patients) (20). The study demonstrated decreased subsequent local regional recurrences in the perfusion group (15 patients vs. 24 patients) and significantly improved tumor-free survival for the perfusion group ($P = 0.044$). Median survival time was 57 months in the group perfused as compared with 35 months in the surgery alone control group. Unfortunately, the control arm of these studies did not test normothermic perfusion, so it is unclear how much the hyperthermia contributed to the effect of the melphalan; however, a retrospective analysis of 82 evaluable patients treated with hyperthermic limb perfusion with chemotherapy (mainly melphalan) for advanced melanoma of the limb revealed higher complete response rates in patients treated with higher limb temperatures, supporting the contribution of hyperthermia in limb perfusion treatment (10). The results of an additional and larger, multi-institutional trial of the World Health Organization (WHO), European Organization for Research in Therapy of Cancer (EORTC), and Melanoma Intergroup testing the use of isolated, hyperthermic perfusion with melphalan should be awaited with great interest (68). If this randomized trial also favors the use of perfusion, then an important role for perfusion chemotherapy will be clearly established in the treatment of intermediate-risk melanoma of the extremity. The contribution of hyperthermia to these results needs to be further explored.

Hyperthermic regional perfusion has also been utilized in the treatment of tumors of the liver, brain, and breast and of sarcomas of the extremity. The appropriate role of perfusion therapy in these sites and histologies, however, remains uncertain.

Regional Hyperthermia. The development of clinical systems capable of delivering controlled hyperthermia to local regions by ultrasound, microwaves, or radio frequency energy have allowed the investigation of local-regional hyperthermia plus chemotherapy. A number of studies have been performed over the past decade. Unfortunately, none of those reported with combined chemotherapy plus local-regional hyperthermia is a prospective, randomized trials.

Several series of patients with head and neck cancer treated with chemotherapy plus local hyperthermia have been reported. Fifteen patients with neck node metastasis were treated with either bleomycin or doxorubicin, with or without local hyperthermia (3). All of the lymph node lesions treated with chemotherapy plus hyperthermia responded, while only 25 to 50% of the lymph node lesions treated with doxorubicin or bleomycin alone responded. The rates of complete response also favored the use of hyperthermia. A series of 14 patients with recurrent head and neck cancers were treated with local hyperthermia plus a variety of chemotherapeutic agents (43). Three of the patients experienced complete responses and one a partial response. In another series, 12 patients with pretreated, recurrent squamous cell cancer of the head and neck were treated with bleomycin, cisplatin, and 5-fluorouracil plus local hyperthermia simultaneous with the cisplatin (63). A single patient achieved a complete response.

A series of 69 patients with primary or recurrent cancers of the vulva, vagina, uterine cervix, or ovary received chemotherapy with bleomycin or peplomycin and mitomycin (17). Forty-two of the patients received local hyperthermia concurrent with the chemotherapy. Most patients subsequently received additional surgery or radiation. Although the patients were not randomized to chemotherapy alone or chemotherapy plus radiation, the response rate was higher in those patients receiving hyperthermia (62 vs. 19%), as was survival.

High local regional failure rates, including peritoneal seeding, are noted after surgical treatment of advanced gastric and ovarian cancers. This suggests that intraperitoneal hyperthermic chemotherapeutic perfusions may be of value when used either prophylactically after initial surgical resection or following optimal debulking of recurrent disease. Several studies now support the value of this approach following resection of locally advanced gastric cancers. Koga and colleagues reported two studies, one with a historical control group and one a randomized control study (34). Patients with gastric cancer who had macroscopic serosal invasion and no macroscopic peritoneal metastases were treated either with surgery alone or with continuous hyperthermic peritoneal perfusion with mitomycin C (inflow temperature 44° to 45°C, outflow temperature 40° to 42°C, for 50 to 60 minutes). The 3-year survival rate was significantly higher in the patients treated with hyperthermic perfusion than in the historical controls (73.7 vs. 52.7%; $P < 0.04$). Similarly, in the randomized control study, the survival rate at 30 months was higher in the treated group than in the surgery-only control group (83 vs. 67.3%), but this difference was not statistically significant. The final results of this randomized controlled study revealed 5-year survival rates for the treatment and control groups of 64.2 and 52.5% respectively, with a decrease in peritoneal recurrences in the group receiving the hyperthermic perfusion (24). Fujimura and colleagues have employed continuous hyperthermic peritoneal perfusion with cisplatin and mitomycin in the treatment of 31 patients with gastric cancer with peritoneal dissemination (18). Among the 12 patients in this series who underwent second-look operation following treatment, complete response was noted in four patients, and partial response in one, for an overall response rate of 41%. Phase I studies have also been reported in patients with abdominal recurrence of ovarian cancer, using either intraperitoneal cisplatin or mitomycin C and abdominopelvic hyperthermia accomplished with either the CDHR Helix (25) or the annular phased-array system (38).

Multiple other series of patients treated with chemotherapy plus local-regional hyperthermia are available in the literature. The paucity of studies utilizing consistent chemotherapy in patients with tumors of the same histologic type and site prevent the formulation of even preliminary conclusions regarding the definite value of combination local-regional hyperthermia plus chemotherapy. Randomized clinical trials clearly are needed.

References

1. Anderson RL, Tao TW, Betten DA, and Hahn GM. Heat shock protein levels are not elevated in heat-resistant B16 melanoma cells. Radiat Res 1986;105:240.
2. Anderson RL, Kapp DS. Hyperthermia in cancer therapy: current status. M J Austral 1990;152:310.
3. Arcangeli G, Cividalli, A, Mauro F, Nervi C, Pavin G. Enhanced effectiveness of adriamycin and bleomycin combined with local hyperthermia in neck node metastases from head and neck cancers. Tumori 1979;65:481.
4. Armour EP, McEachern D, Wang Z, Corry P, Martinez A. Sensitivity of human cells to mild hyperthermia. Cancer Res 1993;53:2740.
5. Barlogie B, Corry PM, Yip E, Lippman L, Johnston DA, Khalil K, Tenczynski TF, Reilly E, Lawson R, Dosik G, Rigor B, Hankenson R, Freireich EJ. Total-body hyperthermia with and without chemotherapy for advanced human neoplasms. Cancer Res 1979;39:1481.
6. Barnett TA, Kapp DS, Goffinet DR. Adenoid cystic carcinoma of the salivary gland: management of recurrent, advanced, or persistent disease with hyperthermia and radiation therapy. Cancer 1990;65:2648.
7. Berdov BA, Menteshashvilli GZ. Thermoradiotherapy of patients with locally advanced carcinoma of the rectum. Int J Hyperther 1990;6:881.
8. Bull JM, Lees D, Schuette W, Whang-Peng J, Smith R, Bynum G, Atkinson ER, Gottdiener JS, Gralnick HR, Shawker TH, DeVita VT Jr. Whole-body hyperthermia: a phase-I trial of a potential adjuvant to chemotherapy. Ann of Int Med 1979;90:317.
9. Bull JMC. A review of systemic hyperthermia. Front Radiat Ther Onc 1984;18:171.
10. Cavaliere R, DiFilippo F, Giannarelli D, Caralini S, Anza M, Cavaliere F, Graziano F, Perri P. Hyperthermic antiblastic perfusion in the treatment of local recurrence or "in-transit" metastases of limb melanoma. Semin Surg Oncol 1992;8:374.
11. Cline HE, Hynynen K, Hardy CJ, Watkins RD, Schenck JF, Jolesz FR. MR temperature mapping of focused ultrasound surgery. Magn Reson Med 1994;31:628.
12. Coley WB. The treatment of malignant tumors by repeated inoculations of erysipelas, with a report of ten original cases. Am J Med Sci 1893;105:488.
13. Datta NR, Bose AK, Kapoor HK, Gupta S. Head and neck cancers: results of thermoradiotherapy versus radiotherapy. Int J Hypertherm 1990;6:479.
14. Delepine N, Delepine G, Desbois JC, Sidi J, Jasmin C. Treatment of pelvic chondrosarcoma by an external deep heating device in 12 cases. Abstracts of Papers for the 5th European BSD-Users Conference: Hyperthermia in Clinical Oncology. Rotterdam, The Netherlands, May 19, 1990.
15. Engelhardt R. Summary of recent clinical experience in whole-body hyperthermia combined with chemotherapy. Recent Results Cancer Res 1988;107:200.
16. Field SB, Franconi C (eds.). Physics and Technology of Hyperthermia. Boston: Nijhoff, 1987.
17. Fujiwara K, Kohno I, Sekiba K. Therapeutic effect of hyperthermia combined with chemotherapy on vulvar and vaginal carcinoma. Acta Med Okayama 1987;41:55.
18. Fujimura T, Yonemura Y, Fushida S, Urade M, Takegawa S, Kamata T, Sugiyama K, Hasegawa H, Katayama K, Miwa K, Miyazaki T. Continuous hyperthermic peritoneal perfusion for the treatment of peritoneal dissemination in gastric cancers and subsequent second-look operation. Cancer 1990;65:65.
19. Ghussen F, Kruger I, Smalley RV, Groth W. Hyperthermic perfusion with chemotherapy for melanoma of the extremities. World J Surg 1989;13:598.
20. Hafström L, Rudenstam C-M, Blomquist E, Ingvar C, Jönsson P-E, Lagerlöf B, Lindholm C, Ringborg U, Westman G, Östrup L. Regional hyperthermic perfusion with melphalan after surgery for recurrent malignant melanomas of the extremities. J Clin Oncol 1991;9:2091.
21. Hahn GM. Hyperthermia and Cancer. New York: Plenum, 1982.
22. Hahn GM, Adwankar MK, Basrur VS, Anderson RL. Survival of cells exposed to anticancer drugs after stress. In Stress-Induced Proteins. Edited by ML Pardue, JR Feramisco, S Lindquist. New York: Liss, 1989, pp 223–233.
23. Hahn GM, van Kersen I. Isolation and initial characterization of thermoresistant RIF tumor cell strains. Cancer Res 1988;48:1803.
24. Hamazoe R, Maeta M, Kaibara N. Intraperitoneal thermochemotherapy for prevention of peritoneal recurrence of gastric cancer. Cancer 1994;73:2048.
25. Harari PM, Shimm DS, Gerner EW, Alberts DS. Intraperitoneal chemotherapy plus regional/systemic hyperthermia in the treatment of advanced ovarian cancer. Reg Cancer Treat 1989;2:54.
26. Hiraoka M, Hahn GM. Changes in pH and blood flow induced by glucose and their ef-

fects on hyperthermia with or without BCNU in RIF-1 tumours. Int J Hypertherm 1990;6: 97.

27. Kakehi M, Ueda K, Mukojima T, Hiraoka M, Seto O, Akanuma A, Nakatsugawa S. Multi-institutional clinical studies on hyperthermia combined with radiotherapy or chemotherapy in advanced cancer of deep-seated organs. Int J Hypertherm 1990;6: 719.
28. Kaplan I, Kapp DS, Bagshaw MA. Secondary external-beam radiotherapy and hyperthermia for local recurrence after 125-iodine implantation in adenocarcinoma of the prostate. Int J Radiat Oncol Biol Phys 1990;20(3):551–554.
29. Kapp DS. Site and disease selection for hyperthermia clinical trials. Int J Hypertherm 1986;2:139.
30. Kapp DS, Cox R. Thermal treatment parameters are most predictive of outcome in patients with single tumor nodules per treatment field in recurrent adenocarcinoma of the breast. Int J Radiat Oncol Biol Phys 1995;33:887.
31. Kapp DS, Cox RS, Fessenden P, Meyer JL, Prionas SD, Lee ER, Bagshaw MA. Parameters predictive for complications of treatment with combined hyperthermia and radiation therapy. Int J Radiat Oncol Biol Phys 1992;22:999.
32. Karasawa K, Muta N, Nakagawa K, Hasezawa K, Terahara A, Onogi Y, Sakata K-I, Aoki Y, Sasaki Y, Akanuma A. Thermoradiotherapy in the treatment of locally advanced non-small cell lung cancer. Int J Radiat Oncol Biol Phys 1994;30:1171.
33. Knox SJ, Kapp DS. Hyperthermia and radiation therapy in the treatment of recurrent Merkel cell tumors. Cancer 1988;62:1479.
34. Koga S, Hamazoe R, Maeta M, Shimizu N, Murakami A, Wakatsuki T. Prophylactic therapy for peritoneal recurrence of gastric cancer by continuous hyperthermic peritoneal perfusion with mitomycin C. Cancer 1988;61:232.
35. Konings AWT, Hettinga JVE, Lemstra W, Humphrey GB, Kampinga HH. Sensitizing for *cis*-diamminedichloroplatinum (II) action by hyperthermia in resistant cells. Int J Hypertherm 1993;9:553.
36. Krementz ET, Ryan RF, Carter RD, Sutherland CM, Reed RJ. Hyperthermic regional perfusion for melanoma of the limbs. In Cutaneous Melanoma. Clinical Management and Treatment Results Worldwide. Edited by CM Balch, GW Milton. Philadelphia: Lippincott, 1985, pp 171.
37. Larkin JM. A clinical investigation of total-body hyperthermia as cancer therapy. Cancer Res 1979;39:2252.
38. Leopold KA, Oleson JR, Clarke-Pearson D, Soper J, Berchuck A, Samulski TV, Page RL, Blivin J, Tomberlin JK, Dewhirst MW. Intraperitoneal cisplatin and regional hyperthermia for ovarian carcinoma. Int J Radiat Oncol Biol Phys 1993;27:1245.
39. Maeta M, Koga S, Wada J, Yokoyama M, Kato N, Kawahara H, Sakai T, Hino M, Ono T, Yuasa K. Clinical evaluation of total-body hyperthermia combined with anticancer chemotherapy for far-advanced miscellaneous cancer in Japan. Cancer 1987;59: 1101.
40. Martinez A, Gersten D, Leslie J, Borrego C, Armour E, Corry P. Interstitial thermo-brachytherapy with continuous mild hyperthermia for the treatment of locally advanced or recurring pelvic malignancies. Abstracts of Papers for the Forty-First Annual Meeting of the Radiation Research Society and the Thirteenth Annual Meeting of the North American Hyperthermia Society, Dallas, Texas, March 20–25, 1993, p 122.
41. Meyer JL. The clinical efficacy of localized hyperthermia. Cancer Res 1984;44(suppl):4745S.
42. Millian AJ. Whole-body hyperthermia induction techniques. Cancer Res 1984;44(suppl):4869S.
43. Moffat FL, Rotstein LE, Calhoun K, Langer JC, Makowka L, Ambus U, Palmer JA, Campbell A, Howard V, Mikkelsaar R, Venturi D, Laing D, Falk JA, Falk RE. Palliation of advanced head and neck cancer with radiofrequency hyperthermia and cytotoxic chemotherapy. Can J Surg, 1984;27:38.
44. Morimoto RI, Tissieres A, Georgopoulos C. Stress Proteins in Biology and Medicine. Cold Spring Harbor, 1990.
45. Oleson JR, Samulski TV, Leopold KA, Clegg ST, Dewhirst MW, Dodge RK, George SL. Sensitivity of hyperthermia trial outcomes to temperature and time: implications for thermal goals of treatment. Int J Radiat Oncol Biol Phys 1993;25:289.
46. Overgaard J, Gonzalez Gonzalez D, Hulshof MCCM, Arcangeli G, Dahl O, Molls O, Bentzen S.M. Randomized trial of hyperthermia as adjuvant to radiotherapy for recurrent or metastatic malignant melanoma. Lancet, 1995;345:540.
47. Paliwal BR, Hetzel FW, Dewhirst MW. Biological, Physical and Clinical Aspects of Hyperthermia. New York: American Institute of Physics, 1988.
48. Parks LC, Smith GV. Systemic hyperthermia by extracorporeal induction. In Hyperthermia in Cancer Therapy. Edited by FK Storm. Boston: Hall, 1983.
49. Perez CA, Gillespie B, Pajak T, Hornback NB, Emami B, Rubin P. Quality assurance problems in clinical hyperthermia and impact on therapeutic outcome: a report by RTOG. In Radiation Oncology Center Scientific Report. St. Louis, MO: Mallinckrodt Institute of Radiology, 1987–1988, p 293.
50. Perez CA, Gillespie B, Pajak T, Hornback NB, Emami B, Rubin P. Quality assurance problems in clinical hyperthermia and impact on therapeutic outcome: a report by the Radiation Therapy Oncology Group. Int J Radiat Oncol Biol Phys 1989;16:551.
51. Petersen IA, Kapp DS. Local hyperthermia and radiation therapy in the retreatment of superficially located recurrences in Hodgkin's disease. Int J Radiat Oncol Biol Phys 1990;18:603.
52. Petrovich Z, Langholz B, Gibbs FA, Sapozink MD, Kapp DS, Stewart RJ, Emami B, Oleson J, Senzer N, Slater J, Astrahan M. Regional hyperthermia for advanced tumors: a clinical study of 353 patients. Int J Radiat Oncol Biol Phys 1989;16:601.
53. Pettigrew RT. Cancer therapy by whole-body heating. In Proceedings of the International Symposium on Cancer Therapy by Hyperthermia and Radiation. Edited by M Wizenberg, SF Robinson. Baltimore: American College of Radiology, 1975.
54. Reed RA, Bedford JS. Thermal tolerance. Br J Radiology 1980;53:920.
55. Robins HI, Hugander A, Cohen JD. Whole body hyperthermia in the treatment of neoplastic disease. Radiol Clin North Am 1989;27:603.
56. Rochlin DB, Smart CR. Treatment of malignant melanoma by regional perfusion. Cancer 1965;18:1544.
57. Samulski TV, Clegg ST, Das S, MacFall J, Prescott DM. Application of new technology in clinical hyperthermia. Int J Hypertherm 1994;10:389.
58. Sapareto SA, Dewey WC. Thermal dose determination in cancer therapy. Int J Radiat Oncol Biol Phys 1984;10:787.
59. Seegenschmiedt MH, Martus P, Fietkau R, Iro H, Brady LW, Sauer R. Multivariate analysis of prognostic parameters using interstitial thermoradiotherapy (IHT:IRT): tumor and treatment variables predict outcome. Int J Radiat Oncol Biol Phys 1994;29:1049.
60. Sharma S, Patel FD, Sandhu APS, Gupta BD, Yadav NS. A prospective randomized study of local hyperthermia as a supplement and radiosensitizer in the treatment of carcinoma of the cervix with radiotherapy. Endocuriether/Hyperther Oncol 1989;5:151.
61. Shiu MH, Knapper WH, Fortner JG, Yeh S, Horowitz G, Schnog J, Guerra J, Gould-Rossbach P, Ray C. Regional isolated limb perfusion of melanoma intransit metastases using mechlorethamine (nitrogen mustard). J Clin Oncol 1986;4:1819.
62. Stehlin JS Jr. Hyperthermic perfusion for melanoma of the extremities: experience with 165 patients, 1967 to 1979. Ann NY Acad Sci 1980;335:352.
63. Steindorfer P, Jakse R, Germann R, Schneider G, Berger A, Mischinger HJ, Rehak P. Hyperthermia as an adjuvant to radiation and/or chemotherapy in far advanced recurrences of the head and neck region. Strahlentherapie Onkologie 1987;163:449.
64. Stewart JR. Past clinical studies and future directions. Cancer Res 1984;44(suppl):4902S.
65. Storm FK. Clinical hyperthermia and chemotherapy. Radiol Clin of North Am 1989;27: 621.
66. Storm FK, Baker HW, Scanlon EF, Plenk HP, Meadows PM, Cohen SC, Olson CE, Thomson JW, Khandekar JD, Roe D, Nizze A, Morton DL. Magnetic-induction hyperthermia. Results of a 5-year multi-institutional national cooperative trial in advanced cancer patients. Cancer 1985;55:2677.
67. Sugimachi K, Matsuda H, Ohno S, Fukuda A, Matsuoka H, Mori M, Kuwano H. Long term effects of hyperthermia combined with chemotherapy and irradiation for the treatment of patients with carcinoma of the esophagus. Surg Gynecol Obstet 1988;167: 319.
68. Sutherland CM, Krementz ET, Carter RD, Muchmore JH. Randomized trials of heated perfusion of extremity melanoma. Cancer Treat Res 1988;43:173.
69. Valdagni R, Amichetti M. Report of long-term follow-up in a randomized trial comparing radiation therapy and radiation therapy plus hyperthermia to metastatic lymph-nodes in Stage IV head and neck patients. Int J Radiat Oncol Biol Phys 1994;28:163.
70. Valdagni R, Amichetti M, Pani G. Radical radiation alone versus radical radiation plus microwave hyperthermia for N3 (TNM-UICC) neck nodes: a prospective randomized clinical trial. Int J Radiat Oncol Biol Phys 1988;15:13.
71. van der Zee J, Gonzalez Gonzalez D, van Putten WLJ, Hart AAM, Koper PCM, Treurniet-Donker AD, Wignmaalen AJ, van Dijk JDP, van Rhoon GC. Hyperthermia combined with radiotherapy in deep seated tumors–a Phase III trial. In Abstracts of the Hyperthermia in Clinical Oncology Meeting, Munich, Germany, 1993.
72. van der Zee J, van Rhoon GC, Wike-Hooley JL, Faithfull NS, Reinhold HS. Whole-body hyperthermia in cancer therapy: a report of a phase I-II study. Eur J Cancer Clin Oncol 1983;19:1189.
73. Vernon CC. Hyperthermia as an addition to radiation vs. radiation alone for superficial breast cancer—results of a collaborative Phase III trial. ESHO Newsletter, September 1994, pp 5–7.
74. Wallner KE, Banda M, Li GC. Hyperthermic enhancement of cell kill by mitomycin C in mitomycin C-resistant Chinese hamster ovary cells. Cancer Res 1987;47:1308.
75. Wallner KE, DeGregorio MW, Li GC. Hyperthermic potentiation of *cis*-diamminedichloroplatinum (II) cytotoxicity in Chinese hamster ovary cells resistant to the drug. Cancer Res 1986;46:6242.
76. You Q-S, Wang R-Z, Suen G-Q, Yan F-C, Gao Y-J, Cui S-R, Zhao J-H, Zhao T-Z, Ding, L. Combination preoperative radiation and endocavitary hyperthermia for rectal cancer: long-term results of 44 patients. Int J Hypertherm, 1993;9:19.

CHAPTER 50

Photodynamic Therapy of Cancer

TAYYABA HASAN AND JOHN A. PARRISH

History

Photodynamic therapy (PDT) is largely an experimental modality for the treatment of neoplastic and nonneoplastic diseases. It is based on the light activation of certain dyes that have been previously localized in target tissues. Although PDT has been seriously developed for clinical use only relatively recently, the foundations of the concept were laid as early as the beginning of the 20th century when Raab noted that certain wavelengths of light were lethal to paramecia exposed to acridine and certain other dyes (1). These observations were followed by the work of von Tappeiner on the use of these dyes topically for the treatment of skin lesions (2a, 2b). The most explored group of dyes for PDT, the porphyrins, were investigated by Meyer-Betz as early as 1913 for the accumulation of hematoporphyrin (Hp) and derivatives in rat tumors and PDT effects following systemic administration (3). The diagnostic and tumor margin delineation potential of these molecules was further investigated in the late 1940s and 1950s by Figge et al. (4). PDT in its current form can be viewed as having been initiated by the studies of Lipson and Blades who established that it was an impurity in Hp that was the tumor-localizing agent, and not the parent compound (5). This led to the "synthesis" of hematoporphyrin derivative (Hpd), a mixture of porphyrins produced by the acid treatment of Hp. The exact chemical composition and structure of this mix remain somewhat unclear, although there is general consensus that the active portions consist of porphyrin oligomers with ether and/or ester linkages along with monomeric porphyrins (6, 7). Hpd was further developed for laboratory and clinical investigations through the efforts of Dougherty et al. in the 1970s and 1980s (8–10). Tumors in virtually every anatomic site have been treated with PDT, and most are responsive to the treatment to some extent. Although to date, several thousand patients have been treated with PDT for a variety of neoplasms, randomized clinical trials of this modality were initiated only in 1987 using a purified form of Hpd, Photofrin (PF) (11). These trials, sponsored by Quadra Logic Technologies, Inc. (QLT, Vancouver, Canada) and American Cyanamid Co. (Pearl River, New York), compared the efficacy of PDT with that of other forms of therapy for bladder, esophageal, and lung cancer. Within the past 2 years significant progress has been made worldwide in obtaining regulatory approval for these indications. Currently, PDT with PF is approved in Canada as a second-line treatment for superficial bladder cancer and in the Netherlands for the treatment of early and late esophageal and lung cancer. A fairly broad approval was obtained in Japan for the treatment of early stomach, esophageal, lung, and cervical cancer and cervical dysplasia. In the United States, a panel of the Food and Drug Administration very recently approved for its use in the treatment of advanced esophageal cancer. Requests for approval for treatment of various other indications have been filed in Canada and Europe and are pending.

Overview

Photodynamic therapy is based on the concept (Fig. 50.1) that (*a*) certain photoactivatable compounds, called photosensitizers, can be localized (somewhat preferentially) in neoplastic tissue and (*b*) subsequently, these photosensitizers can be photoactivated with the appropriate wavelength (energy) of light to generate active molecular species such as free radicals and singlet oxygen ($^1O_2$) that are toxic to cells and tissues. A potential advantage of PDT is its inherent dual selectivity. First, selectivity is achieved by an increased concentration of the photosensitizer in target tissue, and second, the irradiation can be limited to a specified volume. Provided that the photosensitizer is nontoxic, only the irradiated areas will be affected, even if the photosensitizer does bind to normal tissues. Selectivity can be further enhanced by binding photosensitizers to molecular delivery systems that have high affinity for target tissue (12). For photoactivation, the wavelength of light is matched to the electronic absorption spectrum of the photosensitizer so that photons are absorbed by the photosensitizer and the desired photochemistry can occur. Except in special situations, where the lesions being treated are very superficial, the range of activating light is typically between 600 and 900 nm. This is because endogenous molecules, in particular hemoglobin, strongly absorb light below 600 nm and would therefore capture most of the incoming photons (13). The net effect would be the impairment of penetration of the activating light through the tissue. The reason for the 900-nm upper limit will become clear in the next section, where the role of ($^1O_2$), the activated state of oxygen, perhaps critical for successful PDT, is discussed.

This chapter provides an overview of the field; excellent reviews and texts on this topic exist (14–16). A brief introduction to the relevant photochemistry is given in the next section so that the mechanisms underlying PDT may be better understood.

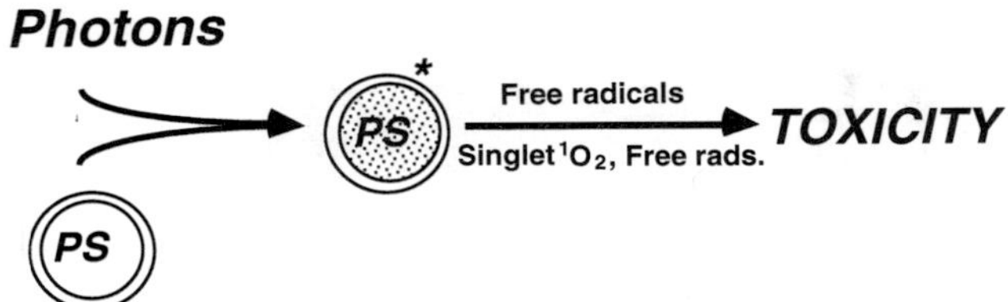

Figure 50.1. A simplified representation of events in photodynamic action. Appropriate energy photons are absorbed by light-activatable molecules, photosensitizers (PS). Activated PS (*) leads to formation of active molecular species that cause cytotoxicity.

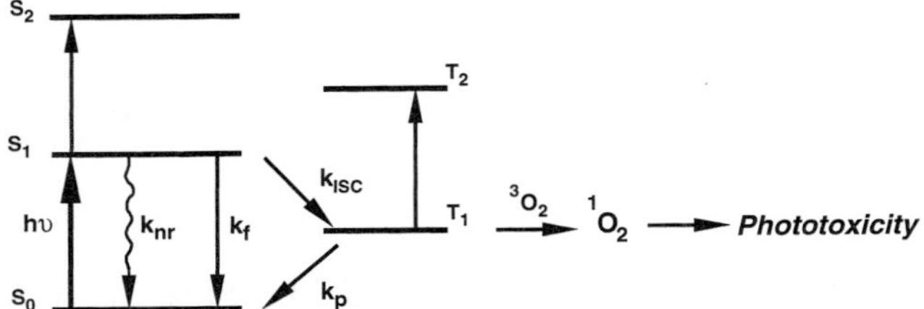

Figure 50.2. A simplified energy level diagram for the photoexcitation of a molecule. S_0, S_1, and S_2 represent singlet electronic states of the molecule. Absorption of a photon (depicted by $h\nu$) results in the excitation of the absorbing molecule from the ground singlet state, S_0, to the first excited singlet state, S_1. Photochemistry may occur from S_1 directly or from the first triplet excited state, T_1, which is generated after intersystem crossing. The molecule can relax back to S_0 from either S_1 or T_1 radiatively or nonradiatively. k_{nr}, k_{isc}, k_f, and k_p represent rate constants for nonradiative decay, intersystem crossing, fluorescence, and phosphorescence, respectively. In general, with conventional light sources only S_1 and T_1 are populated. With high-intensity, pulsed irradiation or with two-wavelength excitation the upper excited states such as S_2 and T_2 may also be populated, giving rise to different photochemistry.

It should be noted that while spatial control of illumination, mentioned above, provides specificity of tissue destruction, it can also be a limitation of PDT. Target sites must be accessible to light delivery systems, and issues of light dosimetry need to be addressed (17). In general, the amenability of lasers to fiber-optic coupling makes the task of light delivery to most anatomic sites manageable, although a precise dosimetry remains elusive. The effective penetration depth, δ_{eff}, of a given wavelength of light is a function of the optical properties such as absorption and scatter of the tissue being interrogated. The fluence (light dose) in a tissue is related to the depth, d, as

$$e^{-d}/\delta_{eff} \quad (18)$$

Typically, the effective penetration depth is about 2 to 3 mm at 630 nm and increases to 5 to 6 mm at longer wavelengths (700–800 nm) (19). These values can be altered by altering the biologic and physical characteristics of the photosensitizer; the relationships are complex. Factors such as self-shielding and photobleaching (self-destruction of the photosensitizer) further complicate precise dosimetry. In general, photosensitizers with longer absorbing wavelengths and higher molar absorption coefficients at these wavelengths are more effective photodynamic agents.

Light Absorption and PDT-Relevant Photochemistry

Light is a form of electromagnetic radiation that covers a wide range of wavelengths, λ, between radio wavelengths in the meter (m) range to gamma rays with wavelengths around 10^{-11} m. Visible light, most relevant to PDT, covers the limited range of 4 to 7×10^{-7} m (400–700 nm). The energy content of light is related to the wavelength of absorption by $E = h\nu = hc/\lambda$ where h is Planck's constant (6.63×10^{-34}J-s), ν is a single frequency, c is the speed of light in vacuum (3.0×10^8 m/s), and λ is a single wavelength.

When light is absorbed, the energy of the absorbed photons causes the absorbing molecule to be electronically excited. (Other processes, such as scatter and reflection, not discussed here, may also occur.) This excitation energy may be converted into heat (kinetic energy) by the collision of the excited molecule with surrounding molecules by radiationless decay. Alternatively, it may be reemitted as fluorescence. The electronic energy levels between which transitions occur by absorption of ultraviolet-visible light (λ = 200–700 nm) may be represented by this simplified energy level diagram presented in Figure 50.2. In the simplified figure, the electronic states are represented by the singlet states S_0 to S_2 and the triplet states T_1 and T_2. (A detailed discussion of the distinction between the singlet and the triplet states is beyond the scope of this chapter. For the purposes of the present discussion, these are two "magnetically" different excited states and arise as a quantum mechanical consequence of electron spin.) With conventional light sources, typical absorption of light by a molecule involves a single photon exciting the molecule to the first excited singlet state, S_1. From this energized state the molecule may initiate photochemistry (depending on the chemical structure) or intersystem cross to an electronically different excited state, the first triplet state, T_1. From S_1 the excited molecule may also relax back to S_0 by radiationless decay or may reemit radiation as fluorescence, which may be used for diagnostic purposes. In general, T_1 is longer lived and chemically more reactive, so that the biologically relevant photochemistry is often mediated by this state. T_1 can initiate photochemical reactions directly, giving rise to reactive free radicals, or transfer its energy to the ground state oxygen molecules ($^3O_2$) to give rise to excited state oxygen molecules, $^1O_2$. This excitation to produce $^1O_2$ requires at least 20 kcal/mole, which places limits on the wavelength of absorption of the photosensitizer. If the energetics are appropriate, photo-oxidative reactions may occur by $^1O_2$ mediation. This photodynamic mechanism of cytotoxicity is the generally accepted one for most photosensitizers currently under investigation, although other competing mechanisms exist. T_1 can also potentially relax to S_0 by radiationless decay or by radiative decay as phosphorescence. Under special circumstances (short pulse, high intensities of irradiation), the upper excited states may be populated and complex photophysical and photochemical processes may originate from these states (21, 22), resulting in increased or decreased phototoxicity which may include oxygen-independent mechanisms (22).

Photosensitizers

By far the majority of clinical experience in PDT has been with PF, and for a long time preclinical studies were dominated by investigations using some form of Hpd. Clinical results with PF have been promising, and this photosensitizer has received regulatory approval in a number of countries. However, it is plagued by prolonged cutaneous phototoxicity, which can last up to 4 to 6 weeks. In addition, it is poorly characterized chemically and has relatively low absorption in the wavelength region of therapeutic interest (600–1,100 nm). These factors, plus an increase in the clinical applications of PDT, have stimulated research in the synthesis and testing of new, non-PF photosensitizers (23) and in improved methods of localizing them (12). Another motivation for the development of new photosensitizing agents has been the possibility of treating larger tumor volumes because of the greater penetration depth of longer wavelengths of light. Therefore, the properties that were aimed for in the development of these sensitizers were improved selectivity, longer wavelengths of light absorption, and increased extinction coefficient (molar absorptivity) at these wavelengths. Although currently there may be over 30 photosensitizers in laboratory investigations, chemically these molecules are similar and are mostly tetrapyrrole compounds. A selected few compounds that are being tested preclinically and clinically are summarized in Table 50.1 and the chemical structures with relevant photophysical properties for some are presented in Figure 50.3.

In general, these newer compounds show somewhat improved selectivity compared to PF and consequently have reduced associated cutaneous phototoxicity. They also have superior photochemical properties in terms of the absorption at longer wavelengths and corresponding extinction coefficients. For example, the chlorins have red-shifted absorption spectra ($\approx$ 650–670 nm, compared with 630 nm for PF) (24) and extinction coefficients in the 3 to 5 $\times$ 10^4 $M^{-1}cm^{-1}$ range compared with the estimated values of 1.5 $\times$ 10^3 $M^{-1}cm^{-1}$ for PF.

Typically, in the application of PDT, presynthesized sensitizers are administered, followed by a delay period that, depending on the photosensitizer, may vary from 60 minutes to 7 days. During this period the photosensitizer is cleared from normal tissues and there is some preferential retention in tumor tissue; light activation then leads to photocytotoxicity, as already discussed. Recently there has been much interest in a different approach where instead of being administered in a presynthesized form, a photosensitizer precursor is administered and the photosensitizer is synthesized in situ in tumors. This is the case with δ-aminolevulinic acid (ALA). ALA is a naturally occurring precursor in the biosynthetic pathway for heme production, shown in Figure 50.4. The last step in the biosynthetic route involves conversion of protoporphyrin IX (PpIX), a photosensitizing species, to heme. Upon exogenous administration of ALA, the feedback control via ALA-synthase (ALAS) is bypassed and ALA can be metabolized to PpIX, which then accumulates in the tissues and can be exploited for PDT (25, 26). Preclinical studies with ALA-induced PpIX (ALA-PpIX) in a variety of systems have been promising in vitro (27) and in the treatment of animal tumor models (28–30). Clinically a variety of cutaneous lesions have been treated after topical application of ALA (31) and patients with oral cancer have been treated following systemic ALA administration (32). Some of the motivation for using ALA-PpIX lies in the brief cutaneous photosensitization ($<$ 24 h) in contrast to PF, and the possibility of oral administration (32–34). Also, ALA is eliminated rapidly from the body (35) and appears to localize primarily in tumor cells (30), in contrast to most other photosensitizers, which localize in the tumor vasculature (see below). Interestingly, when PpIX is administered directly, there is no accumulation in most tumors (14). The reason for the increased tumor accumulation of PpIX synthesized in situ from ALA is not well understood. It has been hypothesized that the activities of some enzymes involved in the heme biosynthetic pathway may differ between tumor and normal tissues. For example, a down-regulated ferrochelatase activity in tumors has been suggested as one mode of concentration of PpIX in tumors. This fact, coupled with the bypassing of ALAS feedback control due to excess exogenous ALA, may then be responsible for the accumulation of PpIX in tumor tissue. Other enzymes may well be involved and may be altered either intrinsically or as a result of some external stimulus. Recent

Table 50.1. Selected Non-PF Photosensitizers and Experimental Clinical Studies

Photosensitizer[a]	Purging (bone marrow, blood)	Cutaneous lesions	Early upper aerodigestive, esoph., bronchus	Gynecology (endometrial, cervical, vulvar)	Ocular tumors neovasculature
ALA-PpIX		X	X	X	
BPD-MA	X	X			X
Porphycenes		X			
MACE		X			
Zn Pc		X	X		X
Tin-etio-purpurin		X	X		X
m-THPC		X	X		
Merocyanine 540	X				

This list is not meant to be exhaustive. Because PDT is rapidly expanding, there are likely to be more applications than listed here.
[a] Abbreviations: ALA-PpIX, δ-aminolevulinic acid-induced protoporphyrin IX; BPD-MA, benzoporphyrin derivative monoacid; MACE, mono-aspartyl chlorin e_6; Zn Pc, zinc phthalocyanine; m-THPC, meso tetra (hydroxyphenyl) chlorin.

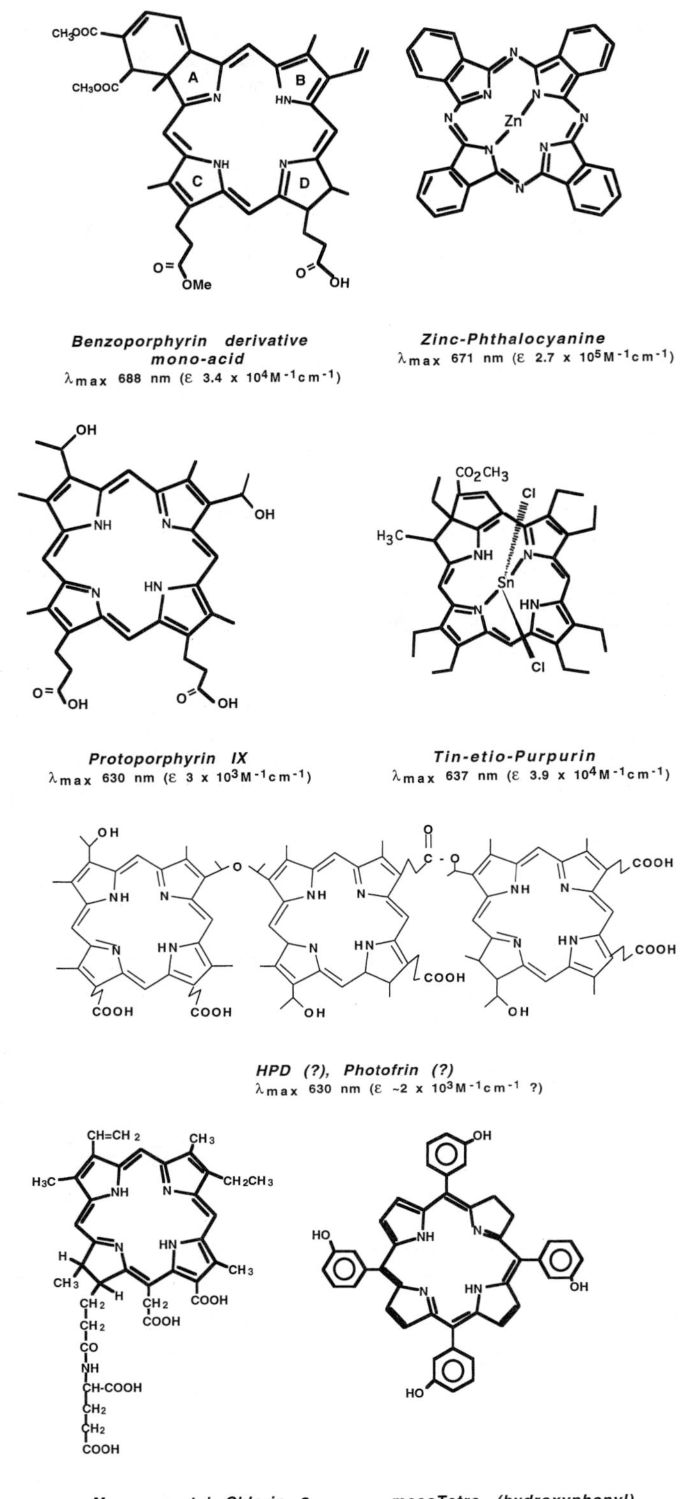

Figure 50.3. Chemical structures of selected photosensitizers. λ_{max}, the PDT-relevant maximum absorption wavelength, and ϵ, the corresponding extinction coefficient, are indicated. Almost all the above molecules have their strongest absorption in the 400-nm region (Soret band). This wavelength is not useful for most clinical situations because of the strong absorption by hemoglobin. In addition, there are other, smaller absorption peaks between 500 nm and 600 nm, some of which are being explored for PDT; however, these are also expected to have strong interference from hemoglobin absorption. (?) indicates the uncertainty of chemical structure for PF.

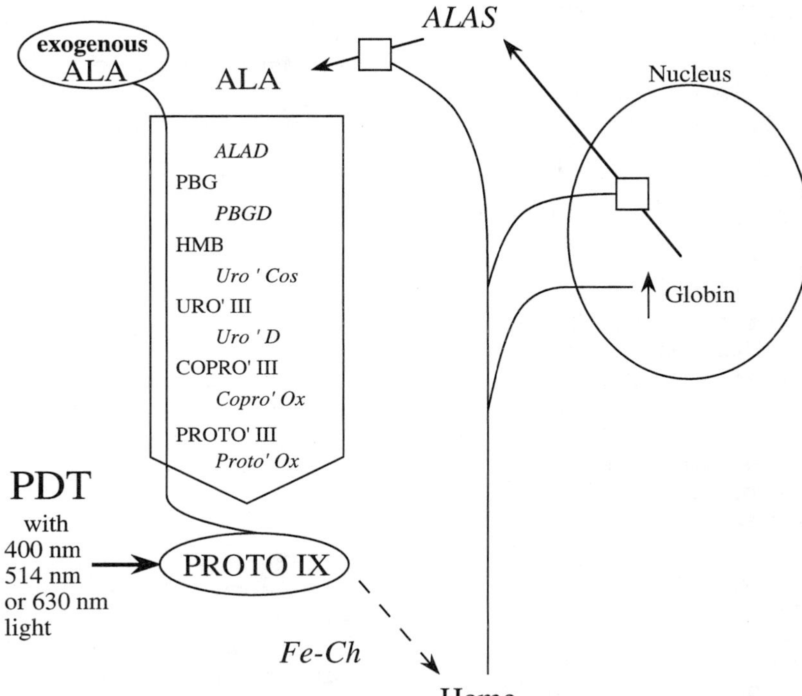

Figure 50.4. A representation of the biosynthetic pathway for the production of heme. Products of biosynthesis at individual steps and relevant enzymes (in *italics*) are indicated. ALA, δ-aminolevulinic acid; *ALAS*, ALA synthase; *ALAD*, ALA dehydratase; PBG, porphobilinogen; *PBGD*, PBG deaminase; HMB, hydroxymethylbilane; *Uro'Cos*, uroporphyrinogen cosynthase; Uro'III, Uroporphyrinogen III; *Uro'D*, uroporphyrinogen decarboxylase; Copro'III, coproporphyrinogen III; *Copro'ox*, coproporphyrinogen oxidase; Proto'III, proporphyrinogen III; *Proto'ox*, protoprophyrinogen oxidase; Proto IX, protoporphyrin IX; *Fe-Ch*, ferrochelatase.

studies show that the mRNA levels of the enzyme coproporphyrinogen oxidase increased 6- to 7-fold in keratinocytes in which differentiation was induced by Ca^{2+} (37). These increased mRNA levels were concomitant with a 100-fold increase in PpIX biosynthesis. The situation is by no means clear. In a recent study, Hua et al. showed that there was no simple relationship between the activities of selected enzymes involved in the heme biosynthesis and PpIX concentrations (38). Finally, in vivo, the accumulation may be related to a combination of these biochemical factors and efflux kinetics. This is an area of active study in ALA PDT that may be clarified in the future.

A different group of photosensitizers that merits brief mention consists of the cationic dyes. In contrast to the porphyrins, which, as will be discussed below, derive their PDT effect in large part via destruction of the tumor vasculature, cationic dyes are believed to be true cellular dyes. The concept here is that the electrical potential across the mitochondrial membrane in tumor cells is much steeper than in normal cells (39). This steep gradient leads to a high accumulation in tumor cells of compounds with a delocalized positive charge. The best developed of the series are the benzophenothiazinium dyes (40, 41). In systematic investigations of these dyes, Cincotta et al. showed high cure rates in two animal models of sarcoma using the cationic photosensitizer 5-ethylamino-9-diethylaminobenzo[*a*]phenothiazinium chloride activated with 652 nm irradiation (41). Minimal damage to surrounding and overlying skin tissue was observed, pointing to the selectivity of this compound. Histologic and fluorescein dye exclusion data indicated minimal damage to the irradiated vasculature within and surrounding the tumor. Cellular uptake of these compounds appears to occur rapidly, within seconds. These preclinical studies are promising, may be useful in various clinical settings, and need to be developed further.

Photosensitizer Transport and Distribution

The accumulation of a photosensitizer in neoplastic tissue relative to normal tissue depends on the photosensitizer, the normal tissue being considered, and, in the laboratory situation, the animal tumor model being investigated. The reason for the preferential accumulation in tumor tissue compared to certain non-RES normal tissue (e.g., skin, muscle) is not clearly understood. It may be due to greater proliferative rates of neoplastic cells, poorer lymphatic drainage, leaky vasculature, or some more specific interaction between the photosensitizer and marker molecules on neoplastic cells. Other factors such as the secretion of vascular endothelial growth factors may be important in photosensitizer accumulation in tumor tissue (42). Immediate tissue effects following photodynamic treatment with most porphyrins suggest that the tumor vasculature is a primary early target (43, 44). Most porphyrin photosensitizers appear to localize in the tumor vasculature (43), and a recent investigation has demonstrated that the neovasculature may play an important role in the preferential accumulation of photosensitizers in neoplastic tissue (45). These observations suggest a possible specific interaction of the photosensitizers with tumor vasculature.

One such suggested specific interaction has been the low-density lipoprotein (LDL) receptor–photosensitizer interaction leading to increased photosensitizer concentrations in neoplastic tissue. It is suggested that LDL receptors on tumor cells and on tumor vascular endothelial cells play a role in the uptake of photosensitizers, a role that may be direct or receptor mediated. This is attributed to increased expression of LDL receptors in malignant cells and neovascular endothelial cells. The increased expression of LDL receptors in malignant cells may be due either to an increased rate of cell proliferation or to an increased rate of membrane turnover without proliferation. The suggestion is that two classes of binding sites exist on lipoproteins for porphyrins (the most frequently used family of photosensitizers), probably located in the apoprotein matrix and the lipid core (46). LDL-associated photosensitizer is then targeted to cellular or vascular components of the tumor. These conclusions are based largely on photosensitizer pharmacokinetics and tissue distribution studies with a number of photosensitizers, primarily PF, the most frequently used photosensitizer clinically.

These pharmacokinetic investigations led to the general agreement that PF initially binds to both albumin and lipoproteins. Initially the binding occurs almost equally to LDL and to high-density lipoproteins (HDL) (46). At longer time periods, the binding occurs almost exclusively to HDL, with a small fraction being associated with LDL. The thought is that association with LDL carries the photosensitizer to tumor tissue. A correlation between LDL receptor level (in neoplastic and reticuloendothelial cells) and PF distribution has been suggested (47). An approximate generalization based on such pharmacokinetic studies with a variety of photosensitizers is that hydrophobic dyes are associated with lipoproteins, while their hydrophilic counterparts bind preferentially to serum proteins such as albumin (48). The significance of this hypothesis was tested in an elegant study by Kongshaug et al. for the distribution of porphyrins with different tumor-localizing ability among human plasma proteins (49). The goal of the study was to ascertain if there was any correlation between the lipophilicity and LDL-binding capability and tumor-localizing ability. The conclusion from this study was that increasing lipophilicity did, in general, increase binding to LDL (Table 50.2). Some exceptions were noted. Protoporphyrin (Pp) and hematoporphyrin (Hp) bind to a similar extent to heavy proteins, even though Hp is significantly more polar than Pp. Similarly, tetraphenylporphine axial disulfonate ($TPPS_{2a}$) binds more extensively to LDL than does the monosulfonated $TPPS_1$, which is significantly less polar. This anomalous behavior was attributed to the asymmetric charge distribution on $TPPS_{2a}$, which may cause a high affinity for a lipid-water interface. The asymmetry of $TPPS_{2a}$ been previously invoked by Kessel et al. as an explanation for their observation the $TPPS_{2a}$ has a higher uptake in cells than does $TPPS_1$ (50). Additionally, the extent of binding to LDL did not always correlate with tumor localization. It was noted that Hp has a higher relative affinity for LDL than does $TPPS_4$ and Pp has an even higher affinity, but Hp and Pp are generally considered inefficient tumor localizers (51). PF has a relative affinity for LDL between that of Hp and that of Pp, but is a good tumor localizer. Similarly, $TPPS_4$, with a very low affinity for LDL and a relatively high affinity for heavy proteins, is an efficient selective tumor localizer (51–53). In studies using both murine models and human plasma, Kessel et al. (54, 55) demonstrated that a relatively hydrophilic compound *N*-aspartyl chlorin e_6 (NPe_6) bound largely to albumin and HDL, and only 1 to 2% bound to LDL. Insofar as successful destruction of mouse tumors has been reported with NPe_6 (56, 57), it is clear that non-LDL modes of photosensitizer localization in tumor tissue are operative and important. In the case of NPe_6, tumor destruction is believed to be dominated by vascular shutdown. Optimal tumor necrosis was not obtained when tumors were irradiated at times of maximal intratumoral photosensitizer concentration. The tumoricidal mechanisms in this study (57) were attributed to vascular shutdown. Factors such as other protein binding, aggregration properties, polarity, pH effects, and the chemical nature of side group photosensitizer and metal ligands are probably equally important determinants of association with lipoproteins. Also, the photosensitizers in serum are probably in a dynamic state as they are transferred between various protein fractions within the same serum.

Table 50.2. Distribution of Porphyrins Among Human Plasma Proteins

Porphyrin	HPLC retention time (min) on RP18[a]	Distribution (%)		
		LDL	HDL	Heavy proteins
Hp	−3	10	55	35
PF	3.6–20	16	70	14
Pp	18	22	41	37
$TPPS_4$	0.05	1–2	18	80
$TPPS_3$	0.35	6	68	26
$TPPS_{20}$	3.95	7	74	19
$TPPS_{2a}$	10.1	36	55	9
$TPPS_1$	20.0	30	60	1

[a] HPLC (high-pressure liquid chromatgraphy) retention time is a measure of hydrophobicity.
Abbreviations: LDL, low-density lipoprotein; HDL, high-density lipoprotein.
Data in table from Kongshaug et al. (49).

The generalization that hydrophobic compounds are transported in vivo via lipoproteins appears to be true for the new photosensitizer family of benzoporphyrin derivatives (Bpd) in experimental clinical use. These compounds absorb strongly around 690 nm and are composed of four structural analogues. The ring A monoacid analogue (Bpd-MA) is the best candidate of the series. Preclinical studies of Bpd-MA biodistribution showed that the majority of the Bpd-MA (55%) was associated with HDL, 15% with LDL, 6% with albumin, and 3% with VLDL (58). Based on preclinical studies, a liposomal preparation of Bpd-MA is currently in phase III clinical trials for cutaneous diseases.

Mechanisms of Tissue Destruction by PDT

For most sensitizers in clinical and preclinical use, three primary mechanisms of PDT-mediated tumor destruction have been proposed: cellular, vascular, and immunologic. The relative contribution of each depends, among other factors, on the nature of the photosensitizer and its localization within the tumor tissue, tumor type (vascularity and macrophage content), and the time after irradiation (which is one determinant of site of localization, e.g., vascular vs. parenchymal). The two best investigated mechanisms are viewed as involving (*a*) direct tumor cell photoinactivation and (*b*) vascular destruction. The PDT response with any photosensitizer is usually a mixture of both effects. For example, using in vivo–in vitro analyses, Henderson and Dougherty (59) have shown that the photosensitizer bacteriochlorophyll *a* has a direct cell kill potential of ≈50% already at the end of the light treatment and exhibits no vascular shutdown until 3 to 4 hours after the end of irradiation. On the other hand, with PF, vascular shutdown begins almost immediately after the initiation of light exposure. Direct cell destruction is expected to dominate when the photosensitizer content is high within the tumor cells at the time of light activation. The actual mechanism of death may then be simple organelle damage, such as membrane lipid peroxidation, disruption of lysosomal membrane, or membrane enzyme inhibition (60). Damage to nuclear components and apoptotic mechanisms of cell death have also been reported (61). Vascular damage is considered the dominant mechanism for most photosensitizers being investigated clinically, and damage is believed to be initiated by release of factors such as eicosanoids, in particular thromboxane (62) histamines, and tumor necrosis factor-α (63). Macroscopically, the vascular PDT response is characterized by acute erythema, edema, blanching, and sometimes necrosis. Microscopically, the tumor tissue is characterized by endothelial cell damage (59, 64), platelet aggregation (64), vasoconstriction, and hemorrhage following PDT. That a clean dissection of the mechanism(s) responsible for PDT-induced tumor destruction is still somewhat murky was pointed out in an elegant recent study by Gomer et al. (65). RIF cells in which PDT resistance had been induced in vitro were implanted in mice and subjected to PF-mediated PDT under typical conditions in which a shutdown of the vasculature is generally believed to be the dominant mode of tumor destruction. As the resistance to PDT was induced within the tumor cells, it was expected that in vivo the tumor response to PDT (via vascular shutdown–induced hypoxia) would be similar for the parent and the resistant cell lines. However, the observation was that the resistance to PDT was maintained in vivo, suggesting that direct cytotoxicity was a major component in the tumor photodestruction. Most of the postulated mechanisms of cell death have been based on in vitro studies. However, the extrapolation from in vitro to in vivo effects is not straightforward. Quite contradictory observations have been made; for example, while PF-mediated PDT in vivo causes platelet aggregation, photosensitization in vitro leads to an inhibition of platelet aggregation (66).

Finally, it has been suggested that the modulation of immune effects may play a role in PDT-induced destruction of tumors (63, 67–73). Nseyo et al. (67) have reported high concentrations of interleukin 1-β, interleukin 2, and TNF-α in the urine of patients treated with PDT for bladder cancer. The reason for the release of these cytokines and the role they may play in PDT are not well understood. In an interesting approach to exploiting immune effects, Steele et al. (68) demonstrated that the selective photodestruction of suppressor T cells using Mab-Hp conjugates resulted in limited increased tumor regression in treated mice as compared to control mice. This enhanced regression was attributed to immune system stimulation after irradiation, leading to increased killing activity of specific cytotoxic T lymphocytes against the target tumor cells. Enhanced natural killer cell activity following PDT was also suggested to be operative by possibly lowering the metastatic potential of surviving tumor cells (69, 70). Increased immunity by colony inhibition assays was also demonstrated in mice treated with benzoporphyrin derivative–mediated PDT (71). Macrophage involvement (TNF-α production) has been reported more recently (63). This is supported by studies that show that tumor-associated macrophages accumulate up to 9 times the PF levels present in tumor cells. This enhanced accumulation is attributed to the association of most porphyrins with LDL (72). In addition to the direct release from macrophages of factors such as TNF-α that may mediate phototoxicity, an indirect mechanism of macrophage-mediated cytotoxicity in PDT has also been suggested (73). According to this hypothesis, initial PDT-induced damage to tumor cells forms exposed lipid fragments. These fragments are then recognized as targets by macrophages. This recognition of possibly reparable cells by macrophages and subsequent phagocytosis is then responsible for tumor cell cytotoxicity. In addition to the above evidence of immune stimulation, immune suppression has also been reported following PDT with both PF and Bpd (74, 75). This observed immune system suppression is being investigated for novel applications such as organ transplantation and the treatment of certain autoimmune diseases.

Photodynamic Therapy and Oxygen

In principle, photodynamic response should occur wherever a photosensitizer and light co-occur. The extent of this response is modulated by the amounts of both the photosensitizer and the light, and in general it varies in a dose-dependent manner for both. There appears to be a threshold component for PDT effects to be lethal (76) below which tissue damage is reparable.

With most photosensitizers under investigation, in addition to amounts of photosensitizer and light, PDT efficacy also appears to be oxygen dependent (77–79). There is general acceptance that in large part this is singlet oxygen mediated. This is based on extrapolation from solution chemistry; the detection of singlet oxygen in vivo has not been possible to date (80). Other species such as hydroxyl radicals and superoxide anion may well be important players (81). The extent of oxygen dependence of PDT effects is somewhat dependent on the nature of the photosensitizer. For example, in sensitization with PF, full effects are obtained when the PO_2 was 5 kPa; this effect is reduced to 50% at 1 kPa Po_2. On the other hand, another photosensitizer, chloroaluminium phthalocyanine (CASPc), shows a much lower dependence on oxygen; the oxygen levels have to be reduced to 0.33 kPa to reduce PDT effects to 50% of the normal values for CASPc.

Under anoxic conditions, the PDT effects are abolished for PF (82). It should be noted that the relationship between tumor blood flow or oxygen concentration and PDT is not a simple one, as demonstrated in the study by Fingar et al. (83), in which the artificial oxygen carrier Fluosel-DA (20%) did not enhance PDT tumor destruction. Similarly, Iinuma et al. (84) demonstrated that in contrast to results from ionizing radiation, pretreatment of animals with nicotinamide, a homogenizer of tumor blood flow and oxygen concentration, did not enhance PDT response.

An interesting consequence of this oxygen dependence is the effect of the fluence rate (the rate of photon delivery) on PDT efficiency. According to the basic laws of photochemistry, within the range of fluence rates for linear photochemistry, there should be no effect of fluence rate on the efficacy of PDT. In a clinical situation, higher subthermal fluence rate has been thought to be favorable because total irradiation time can be shortened. However, as shown in Figure 50.5, reduced efficacy of tumor destruction (78, 79, 84) has been reported when fluence rates, in the range typically applied in clinical studies (≈100–200 mW/cm^2), were used in PDT. This lowered effect was attributed to oxygen depletion during the irradiation due to oxygen consumption in the photochemical reaction.

Depletion of oxygen during photoirradiation has been investigated either by measuring the hypoxic cell fraction in the tumor immediately after PDT (85) or by directly measuring tissue oxygen tension during irradiation using a transcutaneous oxygen electrode (86). This oxygen depletion during PDT has important practical implications and may be an important limitation of PDT. Tumor tissues are not homogeneous and may contain fractions of hypoxic cells, as the induction of neovessels lags tumor growth. In the extreme case, tumor necrosis occurs from lack of nutrients as well as lack of oxygen. It is especially in such hypoxic regions that PDT may be less effective because of the limited availability of oxygen (85). Even for the tumor cells located near blood vessels, oxygen might become depleted when high fluence rates are used, consuming oxygen faster than oxygen is replaced from the circulating blood. This problem can be obviated to some extent by using lower fluence rates or fractionated irradiation, as shown in preclinical studies (77, 78, 84, 87). In studies in an orthotopic rat bladder tumor model, Iinuma et al. showed that at the fluence rate of 100 mW/cm^2 and total cumulative light dose of 30 J/cm^2, PDT mediated by Bpd-MA was enhanced almost 1,000-fold when a light fractionation regimen (690 nm) of 60 seconds on and 60 seconds off was used. At shorter intervals, the enhancement was absent or modest, presumably because oxygen depleted during the initial phase of PDT could not be replenished rapidly enough. Also, for the same fluence (30 J/cm^2) tumor cell cytotoxicity was much enhanced when the fluence rate was 30 mW/cm^2 rather than 100 mW/cm^2. These preclinical studies (Fig. 50.5) appear to suggest that fluence rates lower than those being used currently should produce more efficient clinical PDT response. The problem that has to be addressed, then, is the practicality of treatment times and intervals. Fractionation needs to be accomplished within seconds to minutes and, in contrast to ionizing radiation, is ineffective at longer intervals of hours, possibly because of efficient repair mechanisms following PDT.

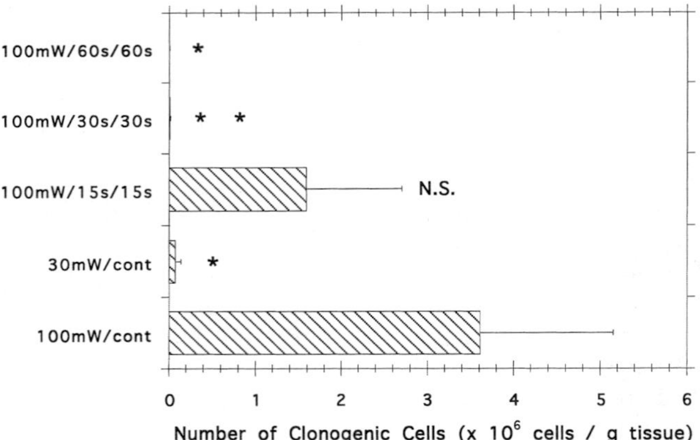

Figure 50.5. The effect of fluence rate and light fractionation on benzoporphyrin derivative monoacid (BPD-MA)–mediated PDT. BPD-MA was administered to rats with NBT II tumors implanted into the bladder wall. One hour later tumors were exposed to a total fluence of 30 J/cm^2 of 690 nm irradiation under the following conditions: 100 mW/cm^2, continuous; 100 mW/cm^2, fractionated 15 s on/15 s off; 100 mW/cm^2, 30 s on/30 s off; 60 s on/60 s off. Tumors were disaggregated 24 hours later and tumor cells were plated for colony formation assay. Colonies (50 cells or more) were counted 9 days later after fixing with methanol and staining with crystal violet. The Wilcoxon rank sum test was used to compare the number of clonogenic cells (with continuous wave PDT at100mW/cm^2. $^*P < .01$, $^{**}P < .05$ (*Source:* Iinuma et al. (84). Reproduced with permission.)

Photodynamic Therapy with Molecular Delivery Systems

An important determinant of successful PDT targeting is the preferential localization of the photosensitizer in neoplastic tissue. In order to optimize photodynamic action, the idea of drug targeting as introduced by Ehrlich (88) has also been applied to PDT. The basic assumption is that these molecular delivery systems have an ability to interact selectively with their targets. In conventional therapy, the drug is subsequently freed to elicit the appropriate biologic response. This is not a prerequisite when macromolecular carrier molecules are used for delivery of photosensitizers in PDT (12).

The rationale for the use of molecular delivery systems for photosensitizers is similar to that for the delivery of chemotherapeutics and toxins. The one important difference is that in PDT, the requirements for specificity of the delivery molecule are less stringent. This is a consequence of the inherent double selectivity mentioned earlier. As long as the delivery agent has preferential (not necessarily exclusive) affinity for the target tissue, improved *selective* photodestruction is expected. Therefore, motivations for carrier-mediated PDT are (*a*) increased concentrations of the photosensitizers at target sites; and (*b*) the possibility of using non-tumor-localizing photosensitizers with efficient photochemistry, thus providing a greater repertoire of usable chemicals. The problems associated with the use of large molecules, such as complicated syntheses, transport barriers, and potential systemic toxicity, are similar for photoconjugates and other conjugates. Although a variety of macromolecular carriers have been used to deliver photosensitizers (12), only two examples, the first using monoclonal antibodies and the second using low-density lipoproteins, will be discussed.

Photoimmunotargeting

Tumor targeting with antibodies is based on (*a*) the assumption that new antigens are present on tumor cells and (*b*) the ability to obtain specific monoclonal antibodies (Mabs) that recognize these antigens. Neoplastic transformation is assumed to generate new and specific antigenic components not present in normal tissue. In practice, this is not always true, and Mabs with uniquely high level of specificity for tumor markers are generally nonexistent (see Chapter 83). Many molecules considered tumor antigens probably represent quantitative differences in glycosylation patterns rather than distinct proteins. Photoimmunoconjugates differ from other immunoconjugates in that in the case of Mab-photosensitizer conjugates, no effector function for the Mab or antibody internalization is required for toxicity because active cytotoxic species can act effectively at the cell membrane level. In cases where drug resistance (e.g., via the enhanced P-glycoprotein pump efflux) may be a problem, Mab-photosensitizer conjugates may be expected to be unaffected as long as binding to the cell surface is not seriously impaired. The potential for cytotoxicity of antigen-negative cells due to the diffusivity of free radicals may also be considered an advantage.

PDT with immunoconjugates has been reviewed recently (12). In contrast to Mab-toxin or Mab-radionuclide conjugates, photoimmunotargeting requires conjugates with high photosensitizer-to-Mab ratios, which makes the syntheses complicated. The goal of any such synthesis should be to retain features essential for both photosensitizer and antibody activities and at the same time allow maximal photosensitizer incorporation. Two basic approaches for the synthesis of antibody-photosensitizer conjugates have been used: (*a*) photosensitizers are linked chemically to Mabs directly, and (*b*) photosensitizers are linked to Mabs via polymers. The development of the latter two-step procedures was motivated by the need for high photosensitizer: Mab ratios without serious impairment of the binding capabilities of the Mab. The photosensitizer is bound to polymeric carriers in the first step, and the carriers are attached to the Mab in a second step. This method allows for a high photosensitizer: Mab ratio with only a small number of attachment sites on the Mab itself and, therefore, in principle, minimal losses in the immunoreactivity of the Mab. A variety of photosensitizer-carrying polymers have been used. These include dextrans (89, 90), polyglutamic acid (PGA) (91–94), polyvinyl alcohols (PVA) (95, 96), and poly[*N*-(2-hydroxypropyl) methacrylamide] (97) and poly-L-lysines (98). Since the antigen-binding capabilities of antibodies largely reside in the Fab portion of the antibodies, conjugation at sites removed from these antigen recognition sites are most desirable, and such site-specific syntheses have recently been developed (89–94).

In the first study of Mab-photosensitizer conjugates (99), the photosensitizer hematoporphyrin (Hp) was coupled directly to a Mab directed against the DBA/2J myosarcoma, M-1. Modestly increased photosensitized inhibition of tumor growth in DBA/2J mice treated with these conjugates and light was demonstrated, compared with controls treated with Hp, Mab, or light alone.

A different approach to photoimmunotargeting was exemplified in a study by Steele et al. (68) in which immune stimulation was demonstrated by targeting T-suppressor cells using a Mab (B16G)-Hp conjugate directed against an epitope on T-suppressor cells in DBA/2J mice. Photosensitized tumor regression, reported in 10 to 40 percent of the mice, was correlated with an increase in the killing activity of specific cytotoxic T lymphocytes against the target tumor cells. Such an exploitation of immune stimulation may be a valuable application of photoimmunotargeting because it circumvents the problems of target accessibility likely to be encountered in solid tumors.

A number of studies report selective and efficient destruction of target cells using photoimmunoconjugates in which large numbers of photosensitizer were linked to Mabs via polymers. T-cell leukemia cells were selectively targeted with a conjugate synthesized from an anti-Leu-1 Mab linked to a chlorin e_6 (Ce_6) derivative, Ce_6-monoethylene diamine monoamide (CMA) via a dextran (89). Photochemical destruction of these same leukemia cells and bladder carcinoma cells using appropriate Mabs bound to CMA via PGA intermediaries instead of dextran has also been reported (91, 92). A different synthetic scheme used PVA as the carrier and a new photosensitizer, Bpd-MA (95). Although this reaction scheme leads to a nonspecific linkage on the Mab, good affinity, specificity, and phototoxicity of the conjugate were reported, probably because of the minimal number of sites on the Mab involved in the linkage. All these investigations suffer from poor conjugate characterization and purification.

More recently, elegant syntheses using PGA and dextran intermediaries have been developed that show clear, site-specific, covalent linkage of the photosensitizer CMA on the heavy chain of the antibody (90, 93). Light- and photosensitizer-dose–dependent killing of target melanoma cells (90) and ovarian cancer cells (from a cell line and from human ovarian cancer patients) (Fig. 50.6) (93) and in a murine mouse model in vivo (94) was shown. A survival advantage in the same murine model was also demonstrated for animals treated with the same immunoconjugate and light dose (Fig. 50.7). In all of the above investigations, the specific site of photosensitizer attachment on the Mab was the carbohydrate moiety.

In addition to Mabs alone, a number of investigators have reported successful targeting in vitro using liposome-Mab conjugates to obtain higher photosensitizer loading (100–102). Because of the size and nature of antibody-lipo-

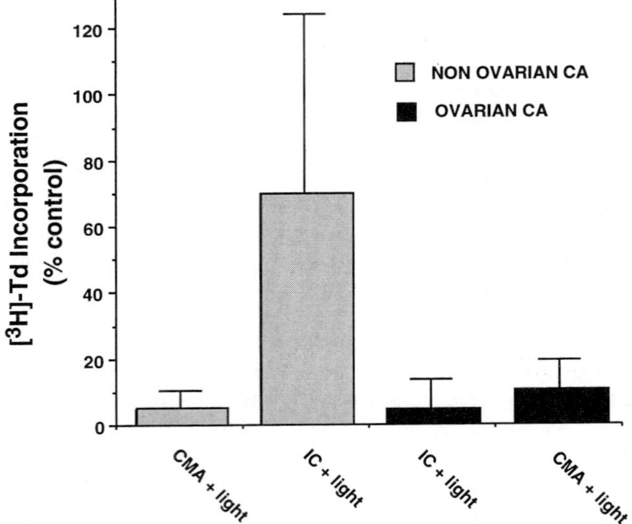

Figure 50.6. Photoimmunotargeting of human ovarian cancer cells ex vivo. Cells from ascites of ovarian and nonovarian cancer patients were treated with immunoconjugate (IC) or the photosensitizer CMA alone for 1 hour, washed with buffer, and irradiated with 25 J/cm^2 of 655 nm light. The IC used the Mab OC125, which recognizes the cell surface antigen CA125 on ovarian cancer cells. OC125 was conjugated to a chlorin derivative CMA via polyglutamic acid. Controls were IC and CMA without irradiation, irradiation alone, or no treatment. The nonovarian cancer cells that showed high cell death were also higher than normal expressors of the relevant antigen CA125. Note that no difference is seen between ovarian and nonovarian cancer cells with CMA and irradiation. (Data from Goff et al. (93); reproduced with permission.)

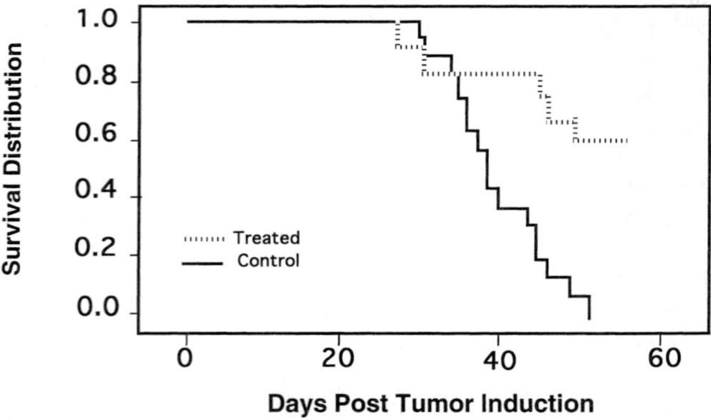

Figure 50.7. Photoimmunotherapy of ovarian cancer in vivo. Ascites (NIH:OVCAR-3 cells)–bearing mice were treated with the same photoimmunoconjugate described in Figure 50.6. Twenty-four hours later, mice in the experimental group were treated with a total of 15 J of 656 nm irradiation interperitoneally with a cylindrically diffusing fiber. The photoimmunotherapy was repeated three times, 1 week apart, and mouse survival of the treated mice was compared with survival of untreated controls. (Unpublished data from Goff and Hasan.)

some conjugates the utility in vivo is likely to be highly limited. In situations such as the treatments of cancers affecting body cavities (e.g., ovarian carcinoma), intravesical application in bladder carcinomas, or extracorporeal treatments, these conjugates may have a role.

In summary, the existing investigations of Mab-photosensitizer conjugates are promising. Better characterized and purified conjugates are needed, along with careful pharmacokinetic information in vivo in appropriate animal models. An aspect that will certainly be explored in the very near future will be the use of Mab-immunoconjugates synthesized with antibody fragments, synthetic Mabs and fragments, single chain and chimeric antibodies. Such experiments will alleviate some of the problems associated with Mab transport and antispecies response.

Targeting with Lipoproteins

Based on the assumption that LDL plays an important role in tumor localization of photosensitizers, one strategy of photochemical targeting of tumor tissue has been to use LDL-complexed photosensitizers. One of the earlier studies along these lines, by Barel et al. (103), used Hp precomplexed to LDL in murine MS-2 fibrosarcoma. An increased delivery of Hp to the mouse tumor was reported with the Hp-LDL complex compared to Hp complexes of HDL, VLDL, or free Hp. Similarly, precomplexing of Bpd-MA with LDL led to a greater accumulation of the photosensitizers in tumors as compared to Bpd administration of an aqueous solution at 3 h. This study (104), which also compared Bpd delivery with complexes of VLDL, HDL, and serum, showed that by 4 hours, the amount of Bpd had decreased for all cases (LDL, VLDL, serum, and free Bpd) except for the HDL complex where an increase was noted. By 24 hours, all three lipoprotein complexes had cleared the tumor. Because skin phototoxicity is a major problem with PF, ratios of tumor to skin (R) are considered important. The R values from this study, summarized in Table 50.3, were optimal at 3 hours.

An alternative way of delivering photosensitizers via the lipoprotein pathway involves the use of liposomes. The concept, although not entirely clear, is that the liposome transfers its photosensitizer content efficiently to the lipoproteins, which then act as the true delivery agents (105). Thus, in a comparison of the administration of aqueous Hp and liposomal Hp, it was demonstrated (106) that the photosensitizer content at 24 hours and 72 hours, was higher for the liposomal delivery than for the aqueous delivery. The tumor to surrounding muscle ratio was also greater for the liposomal preparation. A summary of the photosensitizer content in tu-

Table 50.3. Tumor:Skin Ratios, R, for BPD-MA Delivered in an Aqueous (aq) Formulation and Complexed to Lipoproteins[a]

Formulation	Time		
	3 h	8 h	24 h
BPD-MA(aq)	2.3	4.5	2.8
BPD-MA-LDL	5	2	1.4
BPD-MA-HDL	4	5	1.8
BPD-MA-VLDL	2.5	2.5	3.5

[a] BPD-MA (4 mg/kg) was injected intravenously into tumor-bearing mice and was quantitated by extraction at various time points.
Data from Allison et al. (1990).

Table 50.4. Aqueous and Liposomal Hematoporphyrin Uptake by Tumor and Surrounding Muscle[a]

Tissue	Hp(aq)		HP(lip)	
	24 h	72 h	24 h	72 h
Tumor	1.0	0.6	2.5	2.0
Muscle	0.4	0.3	0.4	0.3
Ratio	2.5	2.0	6.3	6.7

[a] HP (5 mg/kg) was administered to MS-2 fibrosarcoma-bearing mice either in aqueous solution or incorporated into phosphatidylcholine liposomes. Data in table from Jori (106).

mor and surrounding muscle in tissue from this study is given in Table 50.4. Ratios were similar to those reported for Bpd-MA above. Except for PF, the other photosensitizers in experimental clinical use are packaged in liposomes or lipid emulsions. The reason for this is probably as much the lack of solubility of these compounds in the aqueous medium as the desire to deliver them via the LDL pathway.

An expected consequence of photosensitizer delivery with various macromolecular systems is the potentially differing mechanisms of tumor destruction as photosensitizers are delivered to different sites. For example, although albumin and globulins are believed to deliver photosensitizers mainly to the vascular stroma of tumors (105, 107), HDLs apparently deliver photosensitizers to cells via a nonspecific exchange with the plasma membrane. LDLs, as stated earlier, probably deliver a large fraction of the photosensitizer via an active receptor-mediated pathway (105, 108–110). Zhou et al. (111) have suggested that aqueous solutions of Hp lead to predominantly vascular damage, while LDL-mediated PDT leads predominantly to damage of neoplastic cells. An ultrastructure study of PDT with liposome-encapsulated Zn-Pc also claimed predominant tumor cell damage with a delayed and much-reduced vascular damage (112). However, this is not always true. In a recent study of PDT of ocular melanoma in a rabbit model, LDL complexed to Bpd-MA was used. Despite the use of LDL as a carrier, early damage to the vasculature was demonstrated by light and electron microscopy (64). The time that tumors are irradiated following administration of photosensitizer is probably an important determinant of the site of damage.

Perspectives

PDT has been an experimental clinical modality for the past two decades and has typically been used for palliative purposes in advanced cancers where other options have failed. The clinical experience with several thousands of patients who have been treated with PDT is not discussed in any detail in this review because the clinical status has been reviewed comprehensively elsewhere (11). In general, all tumors appear to respond to the treatment; however, cure rates are not easily evaluated for the patient population that was treated with PDT. Limitations of light penetration make this therapy most appropriate for small and/or superficial lesions such as bladder carcinoma in situ, early-stage field cancerization of the oral mucosa, vulvar and early cervical cancers, early lung cancer, Barrett's esophagus, and cancers of the biliary tract. PDT may also have a role to play in the purging of tumor cells from bone marrow (113) or peripheral blood. In certain cases where relatively large solid tumors are in locations with delicate surrounding structures, PDT administered interstitially with multiple fibers may be useful. Examples of such applications are tumors of the brain, prostate, and in specific situations, intraperitoneal carcinomatosis, as in ovarian cancer. Recent regulatory approval of this modality for some indicationshas been encouraging and has stimulated research on new photosensitizers, better methods of localization, and improved sources of light delivery and dosimetry. In the long run, PDT has the potential of being a palliative therapy, a component of combination regimens, or a primary therapy for different indications. The long-term utility will be determined from results of well-designed controlled clinical trials using selectively localized photosensitizers and convenient light sources, such as diode lasers, possibly with built-in light dosimetry components.

Acknowledgments

Partial support of the authors was provided by National Institutes of Health Grant R01 AR40352-03 (T.H.) and Office of Naval Research Contract N00014-94-I-0927 (J.A.P.) during the preparation of this chapter.

References

1. Raab C. Uber die Wirkung Fluroeszierenden Stoffe auf Infusoria. Z Biol 1900;39: 524–526.
2a. von Tappeiner H, Jodlbauer A. Die sensibilisierende Wirkung fluorescierender Substanzen: gesammelte Untersuchungen über die photodynamische Erscheinung. Leipzig: Vogel, 1907.
2b. von Tappeiner HA, Jensionek A. Therapeutische Versuche mit fluorescierenden Stoffen. Münch Med Wochenschr 1903;47:2042–2044.
3. Meyer-Betz F. Untersuchungen über die biologische (photodynamische) Wirkung des Hämatopophyrins und anderer Derivative des Blut- und Gallenfarbstoffs. Dtsch Arch Klin Med 1913;112:476–503.
4. Figge FJ, Wieland GS, Manganielleo LOJ. Cancer detection and therapy: affinity of neoplastic, embryonic, and traumatized tissues for porphyrins and metalloporphyrins. Proc Soc Exp Biol Med 1948;68:640.
5. Lipson RL, Blades EJ. The photodynamic properties of a particular hematoporphyrin derivative. Arch Dermatol 1960;82:508–516.
6. Dougherty TJ, Potter WR, Weishaupt KR. The structure of the active component of hematoprophyrin derivative. In Porphyrin Localization and Treatment of Tumors. Edited by DR Doiron, CJ Gomer. New York: Alan R Liss, 1984.
7. Kessel D, Chou TH. Tumor-localizing components of the porphyrin preparation of hematoporphyrin derivative. Cancer Res 1983;43:1994–1999.
8. Dougherty TJ, Kaufman JE, Goldfarb A, Weishaupt KR, Boyle DG, Mittelman A. Photoradiation therapy for the treatment of malignant tumors. Cancer Res 1978;36: 2628–2635.
9. Dougherty TJ, Lawrence G, Kaufman J, Boyle DG, Weishaupt KR, Goldfarb A. Photoradiation in the treatment of recurrent breast carcinoma. JNCI 1979;62:231–237.
10. Dougherty TJ. Photosensitization of malignant tumors. Semin Surg Oncol 1986;2: 24–37.
11. Marcus SL. Photodynamic therapy of human cancer. Proc IEEE 1992;80:869–886.
12. Hasan T. Photosensitizer delivery mediated by macromolecular carrier systems. In Photodynamic Therapy: Basic Principles and Clinical Applications. Edited by BW Henderson, TJ Dougherty. New York: Marcel Dekker, 1992.
13. Parrish JA, Anderson RR, Urbach F, Pitts D. Optical properties of the skin and eyes. In UV-A: Biological Effects of Ultraviolet Radiation with Emphasis on Human Responses to Longwave Ultraviolet. New York: Plenum, 1978.
14. Dougherty TJ. Photosensitizers Therapy and detection of malignant tumors. J Photochem Photobiol 1987;45:879–889.
15. Henderson BW, Dougherty TJ (editors). Photodynamic Therapy: Basic Principles and Clinical Applications. New York: Marcel Dekker, 1992.
16. Kessel D. Photodynamic Therapy of Neoplastic Disease. Boca Raton, FL: CRC Press, 1990, vols 1 & 2.
17. Wilson BC. Photodynamic therapy: light delivery and dosage for second-generation photosensitizers. In Photosensisitizing Compounds: Their Chemistry, Biology and Clinical Use. Ciba Found Symp 1989;146:60–77.
18. Profio AE, Doiron DR. Transport of light in tisue in photodynamic therapy. Photochem Photobiol 1987;46:591–599.
19. Svaasand LO, Ellingson R. Optical properties of human brain. Photochem Photobiol 1983;38:283–299.

20. Andreoni A, Cubeddu R. De Silvestri S, Laporta P, Svelto O. Two-step laser activation of hematoporphyrin derivative. Chem Phys Lett 1982;88:37–39.
21. Shea CR, Hefetz Y, Gillies R, Wimberly J, Dalickas G, Hasan T. Mechanistic investigation of doxycycline photosensitization by picosecond-pulsed and continuous wave laser irradiation of cells in culture. J Biol Chem 1990;265:5977–5982.
22. Smith G, McGimpsey WG, Lynch MC, Kochevar IE, Redmond RW. Rapid communication: an efficient oxygen independent two-photon photosensitization mechanism. Photochem Photobiol 1994;59:135–139.
23. Gomer CJ. Preclinical examination of first and second generation photosensitizers used in photodynamic therapy. Photochem Photobiol 1991;54:1093–1107.
24. Alian W, Andersson-Engels S, Svanberg K, Svanberg S. Laser-induced fluorscence studies of meso-tetra(hydroxyphenyl)chlorin in malignant and normal tissues in rats. Br J Cancer 1994;70:880–885.
25. Malik Z, Lugaci H. Destruction of erythroleukaemic cells by photoactivation by endogenous porphyrins. Br J Cancer 1987;56:589–595.
26. Divaris DXG, Kennedy JC, Pottier RH. Phototoxic damage to sebaceous glands and hair follicles of mice and after systemic administration of 5-aminolevulinic acid correlates with localized protoporphyrin IX fluorescence. Am J Pathol 1990;136:891–897.
27. Iinuma S, Farshi SS, Ortel B, Hasan T. A mechanistic study of cellular photodestruction with 5-aminolaevulinic acid-induced porphyrin. Br J Cancer 1994;70:21–28.
28. Bedwell J, MacRobert AJ, Phillips D, Bown SG. Fluorescence distribution and photodynamic effect of ALA-induced Pp.IX in the DMH rat colonic tumour model. Br J Cancer 1992;65:818–824.
29. Peng Q, Moan J, Warloe T, Nesland JM, Rimington C. Distribution and photosensitising efficiency of porphyrins induced by application of exogenous 5-aminolaevulinic acid in mice bearing mammary carcinoma. Int J Cancer 1992;52:433–443.
30. Iinuma S, Bachor R, Flotte T, Hasan T. Biodistribution and phototoxicity of 5-aminolevulinic acid-induced Pp.IX in an orthotopic rat bladder tumor model. J Urol 1995;153: 802–806.
31. Kennedy JC, Pottier RH. Endogenous protoporphyrin IX, a clinically useful photosensitizer for photodynamic therapy. J Photochem Photobiol [B] Biol 1992;14:275–292.
32. Grant WE, Hopper C, MacRobert AJ, Speight PM, Bown SG. Photodynamic therapy of oral cancer: photosensitisation with systemic aminolaevulinic acid. Lancet 1993;342:147–148.
33. Mustajoki P, Timonen K, Gorchein A, Seppalainen A, Matikainen E, Tenhunen R. Sustained high plasma 5-aminolaevulinic acid concentration in a volunteer: no porphyric symptoms. Eur J Clin Invest 1992;22:407–411.
34. Loh CS, MacRobert AJ, Bedwell J, Regula J, Krasner N, Bown SG. Oral versus intravenous administration of 5-aminolaevulinic acid for photodynamic therapy. Br J Cancer 1993a;68:41–51.
35. Berlin NI, Neuberger A, Scott JJ. The metabolism of δ-aminolaevulinic acid. 1. Normal pathways, studied with the aid of ^{15}N. Biochem J 1956;64:80–90.
36. Van Hillegersberg R, Hekking-Weijma JM, Wilson JHP, Edixhoven-Bosdijk A, Kort WJ. Adjuvant intraoperative photodynamic therapy diminishes the rate of local recurrence in a rat mammary tumour model. Br J Cancer 1995;71:733–737.
37. Ortel B, Muchnik V, Chen N, Brisette J, Dotto P, Hasan T. Effects of terminal keratinocyte differentiation on ALA-induced endogenous porphyrin production. Presented at the 23rd Annual Meeting of the American Society of Photobiology, Washington, DC, 1995.
38. Hua Z, Gibson SL, Foster TH, Hilf R. Effectiveness of δ-aminolevulinic acid-induced protoporphyrin as a photosensitizer for photodynamic therapy in vivo. Cancer Res 1995;55:1723–1731.
39. Oseroff AR, Ohuoha D, Jasan T, Bommer JC, Yarmush ML. Antibody-targeted photolysis: selective photodestruction of human T-cell leukemia cells using monoclonal antibody-chlorin e6 conjugates. Proc Natl Acad Sci USA 1986;83:8744–8748.
40. Cincotta L, Foley JW, Cincotta AH. Novel red absorbing benzo[a]phenoxazinium and benzo[a]phenothiazinium photosensitizers: in vitro evaluation. Photochem Photobiol 1987;46:751–758.
41. Cincotta L, Foley JW, McEachern T, Lampros E, Cincotta AH. Novel photodynamic effects of a benzophenothiazine on two different murine sarcomas. Cancer Res 1994;54:1249–1258.
42. Roberts, Wg, Hasan T. Tumor-secreted vascular permeability factor/vascular endothelial growth factor influences photosensitizer uptake. Cancer Res 1993;53: 153–157.
43. Nelson JS, Liaw LH, Renstein A, Roberts WG, Berns MW. Mechanism of tumor destruction following photodynamic therapy with hematoporphyrin derivative, chlorin, and phthalocyanine. JNCI 1988;80:1599–1605.
44. Reed MWR, Miller FN, Wieman TJ, Tseng MT, Pietsch CG. A comparison of the effects of photodynamic therapy on normal and tumor blood vessels in the rat microcirculation. Radiat Res 1989;119:542–552.
45. Roberts WG, Hasan T. Role of neovasculature and vascular permeability on the tumor retention of photodynamic agents. Cancer Res 1992;52:924–930.
46. Jori G, Beltramini M, Reddi E, Pagnan A, Tomio L, Tsanov T. Evidence for a major role of plasma lipoproteins as hematoporphyrin carriers in vivo. Cancer Lett 1984;24: 291–297.
47. Kessel D. Porphyrin-lipoprotein association as a factor in porphyrin localization. Cancer Lett 1986;33:183–188.
48. Jori G. In Photodynamic Therapy. Basic Principles and Clinical Aspects. Edited by B Henderson, T Dougherty. New York: Marcel Dekker, 1991.
49. Kongshaug M, Moan J, Brown SB. The distribution of porphyrins with different tumour localising ability among human plasma proteins. Br J Cancer 1989;59:184–188.
50. Kessel D, Thompson P, Saatio K, Nantwi KD. Tumor localization and photosensitization by sulfonated derivatives of tetraphenylporphine. Photochem Photobiol 45: 787–790,1987.
51. Winkelman JW. In Methods in Porphyrin Photosensitization. Edited by D Kessell. New York: Plenum Press, 1985.
52. Evensen JF. In Photodynamic Therapy of Tumors and Other Diseases. Edited by G Jori, C Perria. Padova: Libreria Progetto Editore, 1985.
53. Peng Q, Evensen JF, Rimington C, Moan J. Cancer Lett 1987;36:1.
54. Kessel D. Determinants of photosensitization by mono-L-aspartyl chlorin e6. Photochem Photobiol 1986;49:447–452.
55. Kessel D, Lane-Whitcomb K, Schulz, V Lipoprotein-mediated distribution of N-aspartyl chlorin-E6 in the mouse. Photochem Photobiol 1992;56:51–56.
56. Roberts WG, Shiau, F-Y, Nelson JS, Smith KM, Berns MW. In vitro characterization of monoaspartyl chlorin e6 and diaspartyl chlorin e6 for photodynamic therapy. JNCI 1988;80:330–336.
57. Gomer CJ, Ferrario A. Tissue distribution and photosensitizing properties of mono-L-aspartyl chlorin e6 in a mouse tumor model. Cancer Res 1990;50:3985–3990.
58. Allison BA, Haydn-Pritchard P, Richter AM, Levy JG. The plasma distribution of benzoporphyrin derivative and the effects of plasma lipoproteins on its biodistribution. Photochem Photobiol 1990;52:501–507.
59. Henderson BW, Dougherty TJ. How does photodynamic therapy work? Photochem Photobiol 1992;55:145–157.
60. Dubbelman TMAR. Porphyrin-photosensitized modification of subcellular structures. In Photodynamic therapy of tumors and other diseases. Edited by G Jori, C Perria. Padua: Libreria Progetto Editore, 1985, pp 93–99.
61. Agarwal ML, Larkin HE, Zaidi SIA, Mukhtar H, Oleinick NL. Phospholipase activation triggers apoptosis in photosensitized mouse lymphoma cells. Cancer Res 1993;53: 5897–5902.
62. Fingar VH, Wieman TJ. Studies on the mechanism of photodynamic therapy induced tumor destruction. Proceedings of the SPIC Conference, "Photodynamic Therapy: Mechanisms II", 1990, pp 168–177.
63. Evans S, Matthews W, Perry R, Fraker D, Norton J, Pass HI. Effect of photodynamic therapy on tumor necrosis factor production by murine macrophages. JNCI 1990;82: 34–39.
64. Schmidt-Erfurth U, Bauman W, Gragoudas E, Flotte TJ, Michaud NA, Birngruber R, Hasan T. Photodynamic therapy of experimental choroidal melanoma using lipoprotein-delivered benzoporphyrin. Ophthalmology 1994;101:89–99.
65. Gomer CJ, Ferrario A, Fisher A, Luna M, Rucker N, Wong S. Molecular studies associated with photodynamic therapy mediated oxidative stress. Presented at the 15th Annual Meeting of the American Society for Laser Medicine and Surgery, San Diego, CA, 1995. Abstract 193.
66. Henderson BW, Sweeney J, Gessner T. Endothelial cell production of physiologic mediators in response to PDT in vitro and effects on platelet function. Photochem Photobiol 1991b;53S, 96S.
67. Nseyo UO, Whalen RK, Duncan MR, Berman B, Lundhal SL. Urinary cytokines following photodynamic therapy for bladder cancer: a preliminary report. Urology 1990;36:167–171.
68. Steele JK, Liu D, Stammers AT, et al. Suppressor deletion therapy: selective elimination of T-suppressor cells in vivo using Hp conjugated to a monoclonal antibody permits animals to reject synergeic tumor cells. Cancer Immunol Immunother 1988;26: 125–131.
69. Gover CJ, Ferrario A, Murphree AL. The effect of localized porphyrin photodynamic therapy on the induction of tumour metastasis. Br J Cancer 56:1, 1987:27–32.
70. Gomer CJ, Ferrario N, Hayashi N, Rucker N, Szirth BC, Murphree AL. Molecular, cellular, and tissue responses following photodynamic therapy. Lasers Surg Med 1988;8:450–463.
71. Logan PM, Newton J, Richter A, et al. Immunological effects of photodynamic therapy. SPIE Proc 1990;1203:153–158.
72. Hamblin MR, Newman EL. New trends in photobiology: on the mechanism of the tumour-localising effect in photodynamic therapy. J Photochem Photobiol [B] Biol 1994;23:3–8.
73. Korbelik M, Krosl G. Enhanced macrophage cytotoxicity against tumor cells treated with photodynamic therapy. Photochem Photobiol 1994:60:497–502.
74. Lynch DH, Haddad S, King VJ, et al. Systemic immunosuppression induced by photodynamic therapy is adoptively transferred by macrophages. Photochem Photobiol 1989;49:53–58.
75. Simkin G, Obochi M, Hunt DWC, Chan AH, Levy JG. Effect of photodynamic therapy using benzoporphyrin derivative on the cutaneous immune response. Proc SPIE 1995;2392:23–33.
76. Patterson MS, Wilson BC, Graff R. In vivo tests of the concept of photodynamic threshold dose in normal rat liver photosensitized by aluminum chlorosulphonated phthalocyanine. Photochem Photobiol 1990;51:343–349.
77. Star WM, Marijnissen HPA, van den Berg-block AE, Versteeg JAC, Franken KAP, Reinhold HS. Destruction of rat mammary tumor and normal tissue microcirculation by heamtoporphyrin derivative photoradiation observed in vivo in sandwich observation chambers. Cancer Res 1986;46:2532–2540.
78. Gibson SL, VanDerMeid KR, Murant RS, Raubertas RF, Hilf R. Effect of various photoradiation regimens on the antitumor efficacy of photodynamic therapy for R3230AC mammary carcinomas. Cancer Res 1990;50:7236–7241.
79. Foster TT, Murant RS, Bryant RG, Knox RS, Gibson SL, Hilf R. Oxygen consumption and diffusion effects in photodynamic therapy. Radiat Res 1991;126:296–303.
80. Patterson MS, Madson SJ, Wilson BC. Experimental tests of the feasibility of singlet oxygen luminescence monitoring in vivo during photodynamic therapy. J Photochem Photobiol [B[Biol 1990;5:69–84.
81. Buettner GR, Oberley LW. Apparent production of superoxide and hydroxyl radicals by hematoporphyrin and light as seen by spin-trapping. FEBS Lett 1980;121: 161–164.
82. Henderson BW. Probing the effects of photodynamic therapy through in vivo-in vitro methods. In Photodynamic Therapy of Neoplastic Disease, vol I, pp 169–188. Edited by D. Kessel. Boca Raton, FL: CRC Press, 1990.
83. Fingar VH, Mang TS, Henderson BW. Modification of photodynamic therapy-induced hypoxia by fluosol-DA (20%) and carbon breathing in mice. Cancer Res 1988;48: 3350–3354.
84. Iinuma S, Wagnieres G, Schomacker KT, Bamberg M, Hasan T. The importance of fluence rate in photodynamic therapy with ALA-induced Pp.IX and Bpd-MA in a rat bladder tumor model. Proc SPIE 1995;2392:136–140.
85. Henderson B, Finger VH. Oxygen limitation of direct tumor cell kill during photodynamic treatent of a murine tumor model. Photochem Photobiol 1989;49:299–304.
86. Tromberg BJ, Orenstein A, Kimel S, Barker SJ, Hyatt J, Nelson JS, Berns MW. In vivo tumor oxygenation tension measurements for the evaluation of the efficacy of photodynamic therapy. Photochem Photobiol 1990;52:375–385.
87. Gibson SL, Foster TH, Feins RH, Raubertas RF, Fallon MA, Hilf R. Effects of photodynamic therapy on xenografts of human mesothelioma and rat mammary carcinoma in nude mice. Br J Cancer 1994;69:473–481.
88. Ehrlich P. Collected Studies on Immunity. New York: Wiley, 1906.
89. Oseroff AR, Ohuoha D, Hasan T, et al. Antibody-targeted photolysis: selective photodestruction of human T-cell leukemia cells using monoclonal antibody-chorin e6 conjugates. Proc Natl Acad Sci USA 1986;83:8744–8748.

90. Rakestraw SL, Tompkins RG, Yarmush ML. Antibody-targeted photolysis: in vitro studies with Sn(IV) chlorin e6 covalently bound to monoclonal antibodies using a modified dextran carrier. Proc Natl Acad Sci USA 1990;87:4217–4221.
91. Hasan T, Lin A, Yarmush D, et al. Monoclonal antibody–chromophore conjugates as selective phototoxins. J Controlled Release 1989;10:107–117.
92. Hasan T, Lin CW, Lin A. Laser-induced selective cytotoxicity using monoclonal antibody-chromophore conjugates. Prog Clin Biol Res 1989;288:471–477.
93. Goff B, Bamberg M, Hasan T. Photoimmunotherapy of human ovarian carcinoma cells ex vivo. Cancer Res 1991;51:4762–4767.
94. Goff BA, Hermanto U, Rumbaugh J, Blake J, Bamberg M, Hasan T. Photoimmunotherapy and biodistribution with an OC125-chlorin immunoconjugate in an in vivo murine ovarian cancer model. Br J Cancer 1994;70:474–480.
95. Jiang FN, Jiang S, Liu D, Richter A, Levy JG. Development of technology for linking photosensitizers to a model monoclonal antibody. J Immunol Methods 1990;134: 139–149.
96. Jiang FN, Liu DJ, Neyndorff H, Chester M, Jiang SY, Levy JG. Photodynamic killing of human squamous cell carcinoma cells using a monoclonal antibody-photosensitizer conjugate. JNCI 1991;83:1218–1225.
97. Mew D, Wat CK, Towers GHN, et al. Photoimmunotherapy: treatment of animal tumors with tumor-specific monoclonal antibody-hematoporphyrin conjugates. J Immunol 1983;130:1473–1477.
98. Hamblin MR, Bamberg M, Hasan T. The preparation of site-specific monoclonal antibody hematoporphyrin conjugates via poly-L-lysine linkers. Presented at the 23rd Annual Meeting of the ASP, Washington, DC, 1995.
99. Mew D, Wat CK, Towers GH, Levy JG. Photoimmunotherapy: treatment of animal tumors with tumor-specific monoclonal antibody-hematoporphyrin conjugates. J Immunol 1983;130:1473–1477.
100. Yemul S, Berger C, Estabrook A, Suarez S, Edelson R, Bayley H. Selective killing of T lymphocytes by phototoxic liposomes. Proc Natl Acad Sci USA 1987;84:246–250.
101. Morgan J, Gray AG, Heuhns ER. Specific targeting and toxicity of sulphonated aluminumphthalocyanine photosensitized liposomes directed to cells by monoclonal antibody in vitro. Br J Cancer 1989;59:366–370.
102. Morgan J, MacRobert AJ, Heuhns ER. Phototoxicity of subpopulations of cells in bone marrow by antibody targeted liposomes containing ALSPc (sulphonated aluminum phthalocyanaine). Presented at the Third Biennial Meeting of the International Photodynamic Association, Buffalo, NY, 1990, Abstract.
103. Barel A, Jori G, Perin A, Romandini P, Pagnan A, Biffanti S. Role of high-, low- and very low-density lipoproteins in the transport and tumor-delivery of hematoporphyrin in vivo. Cancer Lett 1992;65:145–150.
104. Allison BA, Pritchard PH, Levy JG. Evidence for low-density lipoprotein receptor-mediated uptake of benzoporphyrin derivative. Br J Cancer 1994;69:833–839.
105. Jori G, Spikes JD. Photothermal sensitizers: possible use in tumor therapy. Int J Biochem 1993;25:1369–1375.
106. Jori G. Factors controlling the selectivity and efficiency of tumour damage in photodynamic therapy. Lasers Med Sci 1990;5:115.
107. Moan J. Porphyrin photosensitization and phototherapy. Photochem Photobiol 1986;43:681–690.
108. Candide C, Reyftmann JP, Santus R, Maziere JC, Morliere P, Goldstein S. Modification of epsiol-amino group of lysines, cholesterol oxidation and oxidized lipid-apoprotein cross-link formation by porphyrin-photosensitized oxidation of human low density proteins. Photochem Photobiol 1988;48:137–146.
109. West CML, West DC, Kumar S, Moore JV. A comparison of the sensitivity to photodynamic treatment of endothelial and tumour cells in different proliferative states. Int J Radiat Biol 1990;58:145–156.
110. Morliere P, Kohen E, Reyftmann JP, Santus R, Kohen C, Maziere JC, Goldstein S, Mengel WF, Dubertret L. Photosensitization by porphyrins delivered to L cell fibroblasts by human serum low density lipoproteins. A microspectrofluorometric study. Photochem Photobiol 1987;46:183–191.
111. Zhou C, Milanesi C, Jori G. An ultrastructural comparative evaluation of tumors photosensitized by porphyrins administered in aqueous solution, bound to liposomes or to lipoproteins. Photochem Photobiol 1988;48:487–492.
112. Milanesi C, Zhou C, Biolo R, Jori G. Zn(II)-phthalocyanine as a photodynamic agent for tumours. II. Studes on the mechanism of photosensitised tumour necrosis. Br J Cancer 1990;61:846–850.
113. Sieber F. Extracorporeal purging of bone marrow grafts by dye-sensitized photoirradiation. In Bone Marrow Processing and Purging. Edited by AP Gee. Boca Raton, FL: CRC Press, 1991, pp 263–280.

SECTION XIV

PRINCIPLES OF MEDICAL ONCOLOGY

CHAPTER 51

Principles of Medical Oncology

JAMES F. HOLLAND, EMIL FREI III, DONALD W. KUFE, AND ROBERT C. BAST, JR.

A medical oncologist is an internist who has undergone additional specialized training. A good medical oncologist is one who applies the thoughtful approach to problem-solving learned as an internist to a body of knowledge that includes patients with cancer. Specific features about individual cancers and their treatments and a reasonable familiarity with the origins, status, and fruits of cancer research at clinical and preclinical levels are requisite (13). More than many internal medicine specialties, a medical oncologist interacts with cognate brother and sister disciplines, particularly surgical and radiation oncology and pathology. The multiple other interfaces include diagnostic radiology, nursing oncology, psycho-oncology, neuro-oncology, gynecologic oncology, rehabilitation medicine, and, for young patients, pediatric oncology. Infectious diseases are common complications of cancers and their treatments, and the parallelism between use of antibiotics and chemotherapeutic agents forges a natural alliance with specialists in infectious disease.

The relationship of medical oncology to hematology is special. Medical oncologists and hematologists both have legitimate interests in neoplastic diseases of the hematopoietic tissues, one because of the commonality with other neoplasms, the other because of the organ system involved. There is a large segment of hematology which is not uniquely related to oncology, however, and the major segment of oncology is not in the province of hematology.

Medical oncology was established as a separate discipline by the American Board of Internal Medicine in 1971. More than 10,000 certified internists have been further certified in the subspecialty of medical oncology. From time to time, since 1971, efforts have been made by others to reamalgamate medical oncology and hematology. The content and orientation of the two subspecialties allow complementarity and coexistence, but the authors are disinclined to the sometimes advocated homogenization. This reticence reflects (*a*) the National Cancer Institute's separate identity from the National Heart, Lung, and Blood Institute; (*b*) research in a far broader field than just hematology; and (*c*) the oncologic practice patient mix, which involves more than 80% of patients with diseases that arise from and affect other body systems. Although many topics and training programs elicit interests in common, the allocation of time to the two disciplines in those institutions that choose to maintain combined training programs should not be equivalent. A separate hematology training track should be available to those whose interests do not focus on neoplasia; a separate medical oncology track should be available to those whose interests are primarily in cancer (13).

The Medical Oncologist's Role

A medical oncologist must understand the pathophysiology of cancers of different sites. All cancers are not identical, and all patients who have cancer are not doomed. Indeed, many patients live with cancer, and, given the present state of our knowledge, many will have to do so until they die. Having cancer is not the same as having a cancer that will kill you, and not a few patients have a neoplastic disease which is relatively less important to their overall health than their cardiovascular disease or some other affliction. Faced with a diagnostic problem, oncologists must try to exclude cancer as the cause, recognizing that some other diseases can mimic cancer. In the endeavor to be certain not to miss the diagnosis of a nonmalignant disease, the medical oncologist must remember that cancer can "do anything." Cancer has replaced syphilis as the great imitator (8). To ascribe a finding to cancer requires histologic proof on at least one occasion. For complex new syndromes appearing in a patient who once had cancer, or presenting de novo, such as pulmonary insufficiency, meningoencephalopathy, or inexplicable pain, it is prudent and usually indispensable to establish that cancer is the proximate cause.

For the patient in whom relatively asymptomatic findings lead to a diagnosis of cancer, it is useful to consider that the day before the discovery, the patient was also living with cancer. It is a source of some encouragement to patients to know that a diagnosis of cancer does not lead immediately nor inevitably to the end of life. The medical oncologist may be able to stress the long-term evolution of a cancer, the several stages which intervene between the carcinogenic stimulus, the mutation at a genetic level, the progressive selection of cells with a survival advantage, and the appearance of an autonomous neoplasm. Since this process usually takes years, and often decades, it is of use to place the neoplastic process in perspective.

The medical oncologist must distinguish between a neoplasm where a chance for cure exists with known information, where a chance for cure is possible in the context of current and ongoing research, or where our present igno-

Table 51.1. Classification of Tumors by Chemotherapeutic Effects[a]

	Curable	Subcurable	Precurable
Curability	>50%	≤50%	Uncommon
Effects on	Metastatic	Micrometastatic	Either
Susceptible tumors	Gigacytomas[b]	Megacytosis[c]	Neither
Role of regional therapy	Helpful	Essential	Insufficient
Drugs	Single or combination	Combination	Mostly untried
Monitoring	Biochemical, anatomic	Usually ineffective	Absent or ineffective

[a] Tumors curable by chemotherapy are defined as at least 50% eradicable by drugs alone. Subcurability indicates the necessity for effective regional therapy in addition to chemotherapy to reach 50% or greater, or in its absence, chemotherapeutic curability of less than 50%. Precurability defines the challenge that lies ahead. Most precurable tumors (except lung and metastatic breast cancer) have been poorly studied with respect to attempts to find more effective chemotherapeutic regimens. Most subcurable tumors, where population data of treated groups demonstrate convincing chemotherapeutic effect, are not susceptible to quantification or monitoring by chemical or present imaging methods.
[b] Tumor masses containing 10^9 cells (or more). Curability is much reduced when tumors reach 10^{12} cells.
[c] Tumor masses containing fewer than 10^9 cells, since clinically detectable metastastic tumors (usually 10^9 or 10^{10} cells) of these types of neoplasms preclude cure.

rance precludes that likelihood. In this context, tumors can be classified therapeutically as curable and precurable (Table 51.1).

There are probably few incurable tumors; the present state of our ignorance just obscures the proper approach to achieving cure (10). It is an axiom that, the day before the first metastatic choriocarcinoma was cured with high-dose methotrexate (7, 12), metastatic cancer in general was considered incurable by most observers. Similar circumstances apply to every neoplastic disease that is now curable (Table 51.2). Other neoplasms are "subcurable" by chemotherapy, insofar as the participation of surgery or radiotherapy is an intrinsic part of the therapeutic process (Table 51.3).

The unexpected benefits of interferon therapy, and then of deoxycoformycin (Pentostatin) and of chlorodeoxyadenosine (cladribin) in hairy-cell leukemia; the unique sensitivity of testicular tumors to cisplatin; the design of combination regimens which lead to high cure rates for childhood cancers and in lymphomas; the initial observations of some responses of renal cell carcinoma and malignant melanoma to interleukin 2; the substantial activity, sometimes striking, of paclitaxel in refractory ovarian cancer are examples of the unpredictability of the next place where dramatic change may become apparent. Old algorithms may fail, but new approaches and new drugs could provide dramatic opportunity for significant advances (Table 51.4).

Table 51.2. Chemotherapeutically Curable Cancers[a]

Choriocarcinoma
Acute lymphocytic leukemia of childhood
Burkitt's tumor
Hodgkin's disease
Acute promyelocytic leukemia
Large follicular center cell (diffuse histiocytic) lymphoma
Embryonal carcinoma of testis
Hairy-cell leukemia (probable)

[a] By definition, at least 50% curable by chemotherapy alone.

Table 51.3. Cancers Subcurable with Chemotherapy[a]

With regional therapy
Wilm's tumor
Osteosarcoma
Ewing's sarcoma
Embryonal rhabdomyosarcoma
Adenocarcinoma of breast[b]
Small-cell carcinoma of lung[b]
Squamous-cell carcinoma of upper aerodigestive tract[b]
Adenocarcinoma of ovary[b]
Without regional therapy
Acute lymphocytic leukemia of adulthood
Acute myeloid leukemia
Lymphomas, some subsets

[a] By definition <50% curable with chemotherapy alone; cure rates obtained with chemotherapy plus regional therapy are significantly superior to those with regional therapy alone (i.e., chemotherapeutic cure of micrometastatic disease only).
[b] Cure rates below 50% in most series.

Clinical Responsibilities

The medical oncologist is often at the junction where final decisions concerning management are made and is frequently the final common pathway through which decisions are implemented. The timing of surgery and radiotherapy, the decision on whether to take curative or palliative approaches, and the decision that watchful waiting is the appropriate approach or that vigorous action is necessary are often entrusted by the patient to the medical oncologist. He or she must have knowledge of the natural history of a disease so as to visualize the likely future and its optimal organization for a specific patient. In addition to a personal library, selected reprints, and access to computer data bases, a medical oncologist is well-advised to construct a data base of patients seen. Not a few of the editors now wish they could recount the details and locate the original charts of yesterday's remembered patients who are relevant to today's problem.

Patients are often influenced by their state of subjective well-being at the moment. It is the responsibility of an oncologist to recognize the often pernicious behavior of the neoplasm in its potential for recurrence and metastasis. In this context the medical oncologist must interact directly with the patient as well as with the chart, films, slides, and other crit-

Table 51.4. Discoveries That Could Lead to Major Advances in Cancer Therapy

1. Liposomes (to carry cytotoxic agents) that have selective affinity for tumor cells and not for organs that exhibit limiting toxicity
2. Monoclonal antibodies with exquisite specificity for tumor-associated antigens, that are not absorbed nonspecifically by other tissues, to carry toxins or radioisotopes, particularly those emitting alpha or beta particles
3. Drugs that suppress oncogene activity
   a. Gene repressors
   b. Antisense RNAs directed to oncogene messenger RNA
   c. Ribozymes that destroy mRNAs of oncogenes
   d. Monoclonal antibodies to gene products
4. Drugs that elicit tumor-suppressor gene activity
   a. Upregulators of suppressor gene function
   b. Gene transfer therapy that can imbue target cells with tumor supressor activity
   c. Polypeptide analogs of tumor suppressor gene products
5. Drugs that inhibit cellular repair mechanisms
   a. Inhibitors of specific and multidrug resistance genes, mRNAs, and derivative proteins
   b. Inhibitors of DNA polymerases, ligases, and topoisomerases involved in DNA repair
   c. Drugs that deplete reductive detoxification processes in cancer cells
   d. Drugs that augment reductive detoxification processes in normal cells
6. Intensification of present therapies to attain greater cytotoxic effects, often using major supportive measures
   a. Increased dose or increased number of drugs
   b. Decreased interval between doses
   c. Design of therapeutic regimens that diminish toxicity by systematic use of cytokines, with or without peripheral progenitor cells
   d. In vitro expansion of peripheral progenitor cells
   e. Cytokines to augment platelet production and mucosal healing
   f. Chemosensitization of neoplasm by gene transfer
7. Drugs that selectively induce programmed cell death (apoptosis) in tumor cells
8. Drugs that block autocrine, paracrine, and endocrine stimulation
   a. Inhibitors of synthesis of, or inactivators of, secretory products that stimulate cancer cell growth
   b. Blockers of receptor sites for hormonal stimulation
   c. Blockers of receptor-stimulated phosphorylation cascades
9. Biochemical or molecular alteration of cancer cells to initiate host immune response against them, and because of similarity to the untreated cancer cell membrane, also initiate lethal immune response against cancer cells not so altered
   a. By gene transfer into tumor cells
   b. By immunization with components of tumor-associated antigens
   c. By alteration of nearby fibroblasts that can thereby attract effective immune defenses to the region of the cancer
10. Drugs that inhibit angiogenesis or that target neoangiogenic vessels
   a. Inhibitors of tumor cell secretion of angiogenic cytokines or neutralizers of such cytokines once secreted
   b. Drugs that selectively localize to neoangiogenic vessels as diagnostic aids, or as therapeutic moieties, alone or as carriers for cytotoxic agents
11. Drugs that inhibit metastasis
   a. Inhibitors of tumor cellular processes that promote metastasis
   b. Restitution of tumor cellular processes that inhibit metastasis
   c. Compounds that interfere with the metastatic cascade, such as inhibitors of (or competitors with) adhesion molecules, and specific protease inhibitors
12. Antiviral treatments for neoplasms when a viral role in pathogenesis may be essential for maintenance of the tumor phenotype
   a. Pharmacologic
   b. Immunologic
   c. Physical
13. Definitive recognition of behavioral, nutritional, environmental, anti-infectious, and chemical measures to prevent cancer: the best therapy for normal individuals
   a. Effective strategies to prevent initiation of tobacco use
   b. Effective measures to discontinue tobacco use
   c. Delineation of dietary constituents including calories, fat, vitamins, and/or supplements that inhibit human cancer of specific types
   d. Recognition and regulation of occupational and environmental exposures that have caused or have a high likelihood of causing human carcinogenesis, sarcomagenesis, lymphomagenesis, or leukemogenesis
   e. Effective antiviral therapy or vaccination to prevent transmission of viral infections associated, probably causatively, with certain cancers (e.g., carcinoma of the cervix, anus, nasopharynx, and probably others)
   f. Search for drugs that, like 13 *cis*-retinoic acid in carcinomas of the upper aerodigestive tract, can prevent cancer in specific populations at high risk for particular tumors
   g. Confirmation of the anti-oncogenic effect of aspirin for colon cancer and expansion of the investigation to other cancers
   h. Search for drugs or dietary constituents that are sufficiently nontoxic and sufficiently broadly active to consider a general population-based trial against cancerogenesis.

ical raw data. Only in such a fashion can advice be tendered with commitment, and with expectation that the patient can be guided to a proper choice. It is unrealistic to expect a patient with a neoplasm to make a choice (informed consent) that is cold and dispassionate, since the very fact of having cancer constitutes a serious emotional burden that may distort ordinary reason. By firsthand intimacy with the diagnosis, the extent of the disease, and the patient's attitudes and infirmities, the medical oncologist can make rational plans and recommendations to the patient and to the other physicians involved.

Many of the other physicians who are involved with a particular patient may concentrate in fields other than surgical or radiation oncology. It is not uncommon—indeed it is often the case—that the patient has a primary family physician or internist who referred the patient to the medical oncologist. In some circumstances cardiologic, pulmonary, neurologic, or other specialists may already have been involved with the patient prior to the recognition of a neoplastic disease. It is incumbent upon the medical oncologist to recognize their interests in, and their continuing role with respect to, the management of patients with multisystem disease. An infectious disease specialist often becomes involved. In the absence of such consultants, however, the medical oncologist must also implement all aspects of internal medicine. Elsewhere, this book contains detailed descriptions of various diseases, the modalities used in their treatment, the pharmacologic, immunologic, neurologic, psychologic, biochemical, epidemiologic, and molecular biologic aspects of cancers, and the complications that cancers cause. Oncologic emergencies, rehabilitation, and the oncologist's relationship to medical informatics and to government are also presented. Familiarity with these topics constitutes a foundation for medical oncology from which the principles derive.

Cancer Prevention

Medical oncologists, because of their knowledge of neoplastic disease and because of their recognition of social, occupational, nutritional and sexual practices that contribute to neoplasia, have a special obligation among physicians to educate the general public, including other professionals with a less intense interest in cancer prevention. Smoking is the principal correctable cancer-inducing activity (see Chapter 27). Medical oncologists should not smoke. Medical oncologists should counsel patients and families about good nutrition (see Chapter 28) and healthy sexual practices (see Chapters 130 and 155). Numerous publications that deal with cancer prevention are available for distribution to patients and families from the National Cancer Institute and the American Cancer Society. The Cancer Information Service (1–800–4–CANCER) will send available publications free of charge.

Familiarity with genetic predispositions to cancer is essential. Many family members immediately fear for their own safety when a relative is diagnosed with a neoplasm. This is entirely appropriate for conditions known to be associated with a genetic predisposition, but not for all types of cancer. It is usually the medical oncologist's responsibility to assess the risk for a particular disease and to conduct the necessary surveillance. Cancer family syndromes and genetic predispositions are set forth in Chapter 12.

Clinical Research

No cancer is so well-treated that an improvement in outcome or therapeutic approach cannot readily be imagined. Thus, research is imperative. Furthermore, therapies that allow preservation of the involved organ are much to be desired, and investigations that have led in many patients to breast preservation, limb salvage, bladder conservation, and avoidance of abdominoperineal resection are major dividends in the treatment of cancers in these organs. Although in these instances it would appear self-evident, measuring the quality of life is now quantitatively valid and has added a major opportunity to reach value judgments (see Chapter 87).

Every established paradigm of medical oncologic management arose from some investigative effort. In many instances, these were one-armed studies that were so successful they became adopted. Examples are methotrexate for choriocarcinoma; vincristine and prednisone induction of acute lymphocytic leukemia; the MOPP regimen for Hodgkin's disease; araC and daunorubicin for acute myeloid leukemia; cisplatin, vinblastine, and bleomycin for testicular cancer; leukovorin and fluorouracil for colon cancer; and many others. After the initial reports of activity, these regimens were often compared with standard programs and demonstrated not only to be highly active, but more active than the prevailing predecessor regimens. Thus, there is a premium on good investigators conducting pioneering observational studies. This is not to say that chemotherapy in the hands of single institutions may not be different from that same regimen when applied by many co-operating physicians in a broad-scale effort. Nonetheless, if a regimen is superior in the hands of many oncologists, it is likely that its utility and validity will be greater in the practice of medical oncology.

To ensure uniformity and reproducibility of procedures, research designs for studies of whatever size should be codified in a written protocol (see Table 51.5). Long after a therapeutic program has been accepted into clinical practice the use of such protocols can be very useful in avoiding omissions, stipulating times for specific procedures, and ensuring that standard doses, thresholds, and end points are used. The possibilities for errors of dosage are sharply diminished when all personnel involved with patient care have access to a written protocol specifying the therapeutic regimen, particularly one that is immediately available on a computer screen. Not only is the oncologist responsible for prescribing the proper drug and dose; pharmacy and nursing intermediacy can serve as additional checks in the system but can also initiate or perpetuate an error for which the oncologist bears contingent responsibility (18) .

Every oncologist's office should be a research station. Every oncologist during his or her training was exposed to, and almost always was a participant in, clinical research. Virtually no regimen or treatment for any tumor is entirely satisfactory, and there is much reason to anticipate that progress would be more rapid if clinical research were accepted as an integral part of the practice of medical oncology so that more would participate than at present. The technology exists in medical informatics (see Chapter 191) for community oncologists to ally themselves with their alma mater or other academic center to participate in diagnostic, preventive, and therapeutic research trials using the expedients of the computer, the electronic mailbox, and facsimile transmission. Those oncologists who claim a work overload so serious that it prevents their devoting the necessary time to participate in clinical research need a partner, for they are depriving themselves and perhaps their patients.

As a part of the commitment to medical oncology, a medical oncologist should reserve a certain number of hours per week for participation in clinical research. This has the virtue of maintaining greater currency with current investigation. Clinical investigation should serve as the bridge to fundamental science and the excitement in the new molecular biologic understanding of the cancer cell. By such association, the medical oncologist in practice may also forestall the burnout syndrome, which is discussed below.

It is not reasonable that an individual in practice devote the same time and energy to clinical research as one who serves full-time on the faculty of a university, research institute, or hospital. A set-aside for research, however, constitutes the same imperative commitment as a set-aside for education and updating. Initiation of one new patient on a protocol every other month should constitute a manageable burden of additional paper work for a practicing oncologist, and, using computer technology, even the paper work can be diminished or eliminated. A patient every other month per medical oncologist would accelerate clinical cancer research by data acquisition on nearly 60,000 more patients per year. Even a fraction of that newly generated information would seem like we'd hit the mother lode. Furthermore, participation in such a study would ordinarily guarantee the patient that he or she was getting a treatment equivalent to (or that is already) the best that is known. Patients with cancer are often apprehensive that they may not receive the best treatment. The medical oncologist can speak with greater authority when a deliberate comparison is being made, since the goal of such studies is toward improvement on the standard, not toward finding treatments that are equally good. Thus, it is not onerous to offer the current best, or, possibly, something better.

Fundamental Science, Clinical Science, and Medical Art

The medical oncologist serves as the principal interface between cancer research in the laboratory and cancer research implementation in the adult patient. Many early chapters in this treatise deal with the structure and aberrant function of the cancer cell, of the cancer process, and of its dissection with molecular and chemical probes. Appreciation of this evolving understanding of science is incumbent on every medical oncologist. A patient with cancer should be viewed in the context of the etiology, pathogenesis, pathology, and biochemistry of the particular neoplastic process.

The effects of the tumor and its products on the structure and function of the patient's normal tissues, including the mind and emotions, define an understanding in depth of the disease process and the patient in whom it takes place. It is not sufficient to order a therapy with the appropriate dose and schedule. A medical oncologist should understand the interaction, so far as it is known, of the administered drug with target molecules, its metabolic pathways, and the chemical or immunologic alteration that one seeks to make. Similarly, it is a given that there be a broad understanding of, and attention to, potential toxicities, which represent the drug's effects on normal tissues. Therapies totally appropriate for someone whose disease might well be cured by judicious application of surgery, radiotherapy, and/or chemotherapy would usually be totally inappropriate if applied to someone with widely metastatic disease for whom no known cure exists. Thus, there is a time ordering of the sequence of therapeutic effort. The nature of therapy with curative intent, which may require a walk through the valley of the shadow of death, is ordinarily of short duration and high intensity. Conservatism means saving a life, not avoiding toxicity. Contrariwise, treatment for palliative purposes would not ordinarily condone similar risks and iatrogenic effects that diminished the quality of life, even temporarily.

Another world of scientific enterprise that materially affects the possibility for curative cancer therapy deals with host support. The availability of powerful antibiotics and the implementation of platelet transfusions were intrinsic to early cures of the acute leukemias. The many new advances in colony-stimulating factors (filgrastim, sargramostim) have already significantly altered the prospect of drug-induced granulocytopenia (see Chapter 82). Continuing search for less cumbersome ways to deal with thrombocytopenia supports the use of single-donor pheresis and study of novel thrombopoietins. Evidence that interleukin 3 shortens drug-induced thrombocytopenia may have heuristic significance. Recombinant thrombopoietin is already in phase I trial. The era of cytokines and their manipulation is just beginning; combinations have not been explored in depth (see Chapters 81 and 82). The impact of cytokines on circulating stem cells ($CD34^+$) is major, making convenient the collection of such marrow repopulating precursors to allow autologous stem cell transfusions as a supplement to, or even as a substitute for, autologous marrow transfusion (see Chapter 85). New antibiotics make granulocytopenia less ominous, and studies of oral prophylaxis with antibiotics and antifungal agents appear to diminish hospital admissions (see Chapter 189). All of these assets allow higher-dose intensity chemotherapy, a characteristic of treatment with curative intent (see Chapters 52 and 54). Some other organ system will next become the limiting toxicity, perhaps the gastrointestinal tract.

The availability of far better antiemetic control makes cancer chemotherapy less dreaded (see Chapter 174). The emergence of psycho-oncology as a widely recognized discipline has also made it possible for patients to strengthen their resolve to undertake approaches aimed at cure or to accept the unlikelihood of cure with greater serenity (see Chapter 87).

Chemotherapy Trials

A number of ethical issues are abrogated by the certainty that a specific patient's disease is or is not potentially curable, given the information presently known. For asymptomatic patients with indolent disease, knowledge of precurability eliminates the need to rush to treatment. Many problems are initially best approached by masterful observation, particularly where age, comorbidity, and equanimity are factors. Where rapid course, portending symptoms, or inquietude prevail, however, therapy is indicated. With metastatic disease for which no cure is known, it is not only ethical but important that systematically designed investigation of new treatments be undertaken early in the course of the patient's disease to determine their activity before toxicity arises from conventional therapies that might limit dosing. Conventional therapies might also elicit resistance of one or another kind, or immune system depression, which might foreclose the opportunity to recognize activity for the candidate compound. A trial of candidate phase II agents prior to conventional chemotherapy for breast cancer has been conducted without significant compromise in response to the established regimen (2). Compounds likely should not be investigated in humans, however, before they have demonstrated greater in vitro activity against human cancer cells than against normal cells, and, ordinarily, activity in vivo against transplanted or spontaneous tumors. The predictive

Table 51.5. Topics To Be Covered in a Clinical Protocol

1. Cover sheet with names and emergency telephone numbers of responsible investigator(s)
2. Schema and synopsis
3. Background history
4. Objectives
5. Patient selection
6. Treatment plan, including changes in dose
7. Registration/randomization, stratification, and data submission
8. Required data at entry, on study, and after
9. Expected toxicity and its treatment
10. Criteria for response, disease progression, and relapse
11. Removal of patients from protocol therapy
12. Drug formulation, availability, and preparation
13. Adverse drug reaction reporting
14. Ancillary therapy
15. Statistical considerations
16. References
17. Model consent form

activity of human tumor xenografts in immunodeficient mice, as contrasted to murine allografts or autochthonous murine tumors, has not been settled (see Chapter 56) (15).

By the same token, for diseases with especially unfavorable outlook and rare therapeutic success, delays in introducing candidate compounds to ensure that they carry little or no risk of toxicity is an unwise investment of resources and time, let alone the patient's short-lived opportunity possibly to benefit. The outcome of unsuccessfully treated cancer is more ominous than the hazards of clinical investigation.

The design of chemotherapy trials is critical to the validity of the data produced. The essentials in the design of a protocol are provided in Table 51.5. Statistical considerations in the design and interpretation of clinical research are detailed in the chapter on clinical trials (see Chapter 26).

The conduct of clinical therapy using intravenous medications which may be toxic to venous wall, and vesicant if extravasated, and, indeed, the care of patients requiring repeated intravenous therapy, commends the use of central venous access. Needle phobia is a perverse part of being under treatment; it can be largely obviated by establishing permanent venous access. Safe administration of the drugs and ready access to blood specimens are the rewards of the operative intervention that establishes central venous access, often with an implanted subcutaneous reservoir. This is particularly necessary when, because of anatomy or obesity, difficult venous access leads to major trauma and time loss in attempting peripheral venous access (see Chapter 46).

Adjuvant and Neoadjuvant Chemotherapy

Most cancer chemotherapy is given to patients with clinically manifest cancer. For a few disease entities, chemotherapy is curative. The advantage of treating patients whose body burden of residual cancer is smaller has proved so persuasive that the profession and patients have accepted the technique of postsurgical chemotherapy, acknowledging that this entails the risk of treating some patients whose body burden is already zero. Thus, adjuvant therapy after surgery has been demonstrated to be curative in several diseases for which surgery alone has low cure rates and chemotherapy alone cannot cure the manifest metastatic condition. Wilms' tumor and osteosarcoma are the prime examples. In many diseases, there is evidence of prolonged disease-free survival and of longer survival, such as stage III breast cancer (1, 4), stage III ovarian cancer (19), and stage III colon cancer (16). Since the adjuvant treatment is aimed at micrometastatic disease remote from the primary tumor, some exploration of applying chemotherapy before surgery has been undertaken in a few types of cancer. In addition to earlier application to the micrometastases, when they may be smaller, this neoadjuvant, induction, or primary chemotherapeutic approach has two additional beneficial characteristics. First, regression of the primary lesion serves as a confirmatory bioassay that the micrometastases will also likely be sensitive (17). Failure of the primary neoplasm to regress affords an opportunity to shift chemotherapeutic treatment while there is still a chance of affecting the micrometastases with a new regimen. Second, regression of the primary tumor may make primary surgery unnecessary, allowing curative radiotherapy, as in some head and neck cancers (see Chapter 105) and a large series of patients with breast cancer in France (12). In other instances, surgery may be technically easier, though not always less radical, since there is no certainty that every cell has been eradicated at the original boundaries. Induction chemotherapy has allowed a major reduction in amputations, however, in favor of limb-sparing surgery (see Chapter 139). Induction chemotherapy may also significantly enhance the effectiveness of radiotherapy.

Surrogate End Points

The medical oncologist must be deeply interested in methods to measure disease progress that anticipate the appearance of symptoms. Recognizing that new therapies will always be forthcoming, it is prudent to anticipate methods to test them that do not depend on such primitive assays as bidimensional measurements of abdominal tumor masses, palpable nodes, and shadows on chest radiographs. These early methods have already been greatly improved by computed tomography, sonography, magnetic resonance imaging, endoscopy, and circulating tumor secretory products that represent marker molecules. Validation of each surrogate marker is desirable, but once established, as for human chorionic gonadotropin, α-fetoprotein, CEA, 5HIAA, calcitonin, PSA, Ca 125, Ca 15–3, Ca 19–9, and other similar compounds that correlate with specific tumor behaviors, the ability to monitor tumor activity is of major value. Recognizing disease progress by marker studies allows identification of inactive therapeutic regimens before clinical failure and provides opportunity for alternative action before the patient has major additional tumor burden, and possibly before symptoms. Marker molecules are not infallible, however, and a tumor cell population may emerge during a cancer relapse from prior therapy that fails to secrete the marker that had been monitored (see Chapter 11).

Palliative therapy no longer requires the patient to have symptoms that require palliation. The more logical construction is to prevent symptoms from appearing, or reappearing, using more discriminant guideposts than palpable or painful tumor. In the future, after the initial treatment, we can confidently anticipate that cancer management will depend upon indirect measures of tumor activity. Thus major therapeutic efforts will be aimed at tumors with a small body burden, and the medical oncologist will be assessing biochemical, molecular biologic, or immunologic surrogates for tumor presence. Some of the reasons for considering patients incurable are that therapeutic efforts have only been made when tumor body burdens exist that would prove too great for cure, even for sensitive tumors. The demonstrated efficacy of adjuvant chemotherapy for breast cancer (see Chapter 136) and of adjuvant chemoimmunotherapy for colon cancer (see Chapter 121) imply that small body burdens of these and other metastatic cancers detected only by markers might be similarly sensitive, even with today's therapies.

Laws of Therapeutics

Certain principles govern the application of therapies no matter what the disease. These were enunciated more than a half century ago by the late Robert F. Loeb, Bard Professor of Medicine at Columbia University's College of Physicians and Surgeons (Table 51.6).

These simple rules have profundity and nearly universal applicability, and they pertain to neoplastic diseases. They must be tempered, however, by an understanding of the neoplastic process. The first law is, If what you're doing is doing good, keep doing it. Vincristine plus prednisone is an excellent induction treatment for acute lymphocytic leukemia of childhood. In 1968, the question was raised, Why not keep administering this highly active induction regimen rather than shifting to antimetabolite management? A cohort of children who were induced into remission by vincristine and prednisone were randomized to continue the induction treatment. They rapidly relapsed, whereas the favorable circumstances for antimetabolite treatment led some of the children randomized to these arms to long-term sustained remissions, and even cures (2). Thus, the first law of therapeutics does not always apply in the context of our knowledge, which is, admittedly, fragmentary, about the effect of successor treatment regimens for cancer. Much of curative oncology relates to the biology of the unseen tumor, about which the current clinical status may not be informative. The first law seems more applicable to clinically recognizable disease.

Table 51.6. Loeb's Rules of Therapeutics

1. If what you are doing is doing good, keep doing it.
2. If what you are doing is not doing good, stop doing it.
3. If you don't know what to do, do nothing.
4. Never make the treatment worse than the disease.

The second law of therapeutics does have considerable universality, however: If what you're doing is not doing good, stop doing it. Most therapeutic regimens have little chance of success if the second monthly cycle of their application has failed to elicit therapeutic benefit. Indeed, most patients show incipient tumor regression after the first cycle, and apprehension rises if that is not observed. It is nonetheless advantageous to undertake a second cycle in most instances, since well-documented early increase in tumor diameter on roentgenographic examinations or increased pain can indeed be followed by tumor regression. If, however, no therapeutic response attends this second cycle, which often represents a total observation time of 6 weeks or longer, it is usually legitimate to infer that a third course will not likely be beneficial. A few therapies are slower, however, and should be considered differently. Before stopping treatment, corroborating information should be sought by direct measurements, by roentgenograms, or by biochemical markers. Increased bony uptake of radionuclides can be a sign of bone healing, even of a previously unsuspected lesion, and is not a suitable end point. The appearance of metastatic disease or its obviously increasing growth despite chemotherapeutic treatment speaks against continuing a treatment, since at least one clone of metastatic cells is clinically resistant to it.

The second law of therapeutics does not extend to toxic effects, however, unless they are life threatening or profoundly disabling. With the medications available today, complete avoidance of toxicity would doom many patients to death from their neoplasm who otherwise can sometimes obtain cure, and oftentimes meaningful remission, by accepting a transient effect of intensive therapy that kills tumor cells and normal cells alike. The patient almost always recovers, but the less resilient tumor may not. Hippocrates' admonition, *Primum non nocere*, is also subject to reassessment in oncology (9). To treat a population of patients at a dose that would avoid toxic harm (i.e., lethal jeopardy) to any patient would surely exact a higher price in depriving others of adequate dose to achieve maximum benefit. Curative and subcurative cancer chemotherapy, as we know it, is always toxic but rarely fatal. Attempts to abrogate toxicity for all by reducing the dose of an established regimen compromises benefit for the majority (5, 6). Dose adjustment for an individual may be prudent, but it must always be considered with respect to other means of mitigating toxicity without dose reduction.

The third law of therapeutics counsels against uninformed action: If you don't know what to do, do nothing. In many circumstances a rush to judgment, or worse, a rush to *do something*, anything, can be disastrous. Aside from oncologic emergencies (see Chapter 190) there is rarely an occasion when observing the evolution of symptoms and findings or seeking consultation with another individual for a fresh viewpoint is contraindicated because of time pressure. In the presence of pain, one should not delay pain relief, but other therapy may be delayed to gain necessary "thinking time." In the presence of a differential diagnosis which includes diseases other than cancer, particularly infections, one must be certain that delay does not risk mortality or morbidity from the other possible disorders. The time invested for observation and consultation should not, thus, be extravagant.

It is an exceptional case, indeed, when a medical oncologist can countenance treatment without a histologic diagnosis. Cytologic diagnoses may provide sufficient information in the presence of unambiguous clinical syndromes, but cytology of the bronchus, stomach, cervix, and body fluids has produced sufficient numbers of false-positive identifications to show that corroborating clinical syndromes are essential. Still, it is extremely useful to have histologic evidence whenever possible.

The fourth law of therapeutics: Never make the treatment worse than the disease. This relates to total life equation and the price the oncologist knows the patient may be obliged to pay in side effects now to attain real effects in the future. Often the patient's vision is foreshortened, since today's disease caused by drug toxicity can be more severe than the original symptoms of the cancer, often excised, for which the treatment is being given. The medical oncologist must ascertain the patient's attitude toward *quality* of life versus *duration* of life. It is a medical oncologist's responsibility to counsel the patient concerning this weighty topic. It is critical to distinguish therapy with curative intent from a palliative orientation. The proper goal is maximal life at maximal quality. It is a modification of the comment that one should die young, as late as possible. For some patients, the toxic effects of treatment outweigh the value of life. This perception is often related directly to age, and treatments imperative for patients in their forties may be inappropriate for patients in their eighties. Pain and disability from cancer may temper the desirability of certain therapies which offer not more than temporary and partial relief. It is not a kindness to defer death only transiently by rescuing a dying patient back to a raft of suffering. Heroic efforts are justified only when a meaningful therapeutic option exists.

It is inappropriate for the medical oncologist to substitute professional judgment for a patient's ardent wishes when the patient desires to terminate efforts—or when the patient passionately strives to accomplish something that is a reasonable therapeutic goal. The medical oncologist must serve as a bastion of reality, however, advising the patient of what is possible and of what is likely. In the course of doing this, the laws of therapeutics and of humanity always include hope.

Truth Telling

Explanations of disease, of anticipated therapies, of protocols in which there is randomization, and of unknowns must be tailored to the intellectual and emotional level of the particular patient. It is never permissible to lie, but it may be prudent not to deposit all the truth, let alone all at once, on a patient who cannot accept the full details and ramifications of diagnosis and management. "Your patient has no more right to all the truth you know than to all the medicine in your saddlebags" was a humane and ethical tenet when advanced by Oliver Wendell Holmes more than a century ago, and it seems still to be (11). It is dishonest to twist facts or to deny specific features such as the existence of metastases. By the same token, it is wrong to deny a patient an opportunity to make final dispositions with respect to self, family, religion, the law, and business by falsely stating that a disease is benign or cured. Families who assert that the patient must not know because he or she could not stand it are usually twice wrong: the patient often knows already, or may be more distraught by being excluded and not knowing; and the patient ordinarily incorporates the information into his or her life equation indistinguishably from other patients. A reading of Tolstoy's *The Death of Ivan Ilyich* should convince any doubting oncologist about the terror of uncertainty and the value of direct and honest, yet humane, interactions with the patient.

When a patient asks, "There is hope, isn't there?," the oncologist can always be enthusiastically positive. Hope is a uniquely human characteristic, which sustains the will to continue, and all oncologists and all patients do hope for a better outcome.

Resuscitation

Several states require that "Do not resuscitate" (DNR) orders be written on patient charts prior to death. In the absence of such orders, when a nurse finds a patient apparently dead she must, by law, initiate emergency calls for resuscitative efforts.

In circumstances where such laws exist, a medical oncologist should be meticulous in writing DNR orders and in explaining them to the family. When death comes from cancer as the expected final event of a gradual deterioration of vital forces, resuscitative efforts do not succeed. When we are unable to keep someone alive, the likelihood of bringing him or her back to meaningful life is infinitesimal. Resuscitative efforts should certainly be applied to patients with cancer who were not anticipated to die, since reversible phenomena such as pulmonary emboli, cardiac arrhythmias, aspiration, and similar events can provoke unexpected death in a patient with a neoplasm just as in any other hospitalized or ambulatory patient. It is, however, in the circumstance of gradual decline and predictable disintegration of body functions that resuscitative efforts place great physical and emotional stress on nursing and ancillary personnel, house staff, attending staff, and the distraught family. Many patients, particularly those apprised of the progress of their disease and elderly ones, can discuss the decision not to resuscitate with equanimity, and, indeed, with a certain personal satisfaction of avoiding the fruitless anguish that such a procedure entails for the surviving family. Many patients are eager to sign living wills or to appoint a health care proxy if these possibilities are presented to them.

Because of the medicolegal implications involved, where particular religious scruples obtain or where families have emotionally uncontrolled members who cannot accept the anticipated death of a loved one, the medical oncologist should spend considerable time planning for the eventual death. Medical oncologists, through their organizations, should also invest effort to alter laws that place significant administrative burdens on them and their colleagues and that infringe on the appropriate professional practice of medicine. DNR forms are a technique of documentation and constitute a further evidence that society has moved medicine to a new plateau of accountability.

The medical oncologist should, however, make known his or her intentions concerning the advisability of resuscitative efforts for each particular patient in advance, to forestall unnecessary trauma to patient, family, and staff, to forestall litigation, and to settle in advance any serious disagreements with patient or family. An impasse might occasion a medical oncologist to find a suitable substitute physician if there is unresolvable conflict concerning the plans surrounding an anticipated death.

DNR orders do not imply that there be diminution of oncologic effort to control or palliate the disease before death. On the other hand, if good medicine indicates that continued efforts are fruitless and only inflict suffering with no prospect of benefit, discontinuation of active therapy should always be accompanied by DNR orders.

Burnout

A sense of frustration can affect anyone who encounters barriers to successful completion of an important task. This is particularly true of intellectual tasks and invisible barriers. When the barrier is a lethal disease about which the oncologist can do little that is effective, the frustration can be all-consuming. Oncologists who encounter several instances of recrudescent or refractory disease in a short time (especially if punctuated by deaths of young or favorite patients uninterrupted by counterbalancing compensatory successes) may well experience frustration, a sense of inadequacy and depression. Frequent repetition of this cyclic phenomenon not uncommonly leads to the syndrome of burnout.

The medical oncologist knows that many of today's cancers are precurable. To the extent that he or she can be involved, actually and conceptually, in the solution to that complex mystery, the frustration is lessened. Cancer research, whether at basic or clinical level, is held in high esteem by our fellow citizens. Group identity—being one of the team—helps to offset the self-deprecation when human tragedies mount despite one's best efforts. The camaraderie of other oncologists who battle the same enemy with the same primitive weapons helps. Another oncologist can understand the trauma and the distress; it is an encounter on familiar terrain.

The appreciation that the horizon is distant and that oncologists are all working intently to proceed there puts present frustration in a more appropriate perspective. Involvement in the systematized academic pursuit, whether in an academic setting, a medical school outreach, an oncology society, or a local collaborative group, provides the security of collegial support, a buddy system, an anchor to windward.

A sound mind in a sound body implies rest, exercise, nutrition, and enjoyment. To ensure the last, the first three are prerequisites. Avocation and vacation are a portion of good mental health, included in the terms *rest* and *exercise*.

Donning the dress uniform of the grand enterprise against cancer, rather than the buckskin of the lone scout, can help imbue the oncologist with the identity and strength of the team. If these stratagems do not help the potentially burnt out oncologist find a new orientation, and a more resilient response to the inevitable future traumas, he or she may well consider an alternative occupation. Many oncologists serve honorably in laboratory, administrative, or pharmaceutical positions, where they are insulated from the vagaries of patients' illnesses. It is better to have a happier oncologist aloof from patient contact than a depressed, and thus impaired, oncologist finally burnt out, still trying to perform at considerable personal discomfort, and perhaps at some patient jeopardy.

Nomenclature: Systeme Internationale (SI) Units

A system of quantitative nomenclature has been adopted in most of the world, except the United States. Soon, it will be impossible to read a medical journal without being thoroughly familiar with SI units. They are presented in Table 51.7 so that readers can have ready access to a source for translation from the old nomenclature, which pervades this treatise.

Summary

The medical oncologist usually serves as the final common pathway for the application of cancer research to patients. A complex corpus of information is available, which expands rapidly, both deeper into the nature of the cancer process and higher into new approaches that provide demonstrated effectiveness in therapy, prevention, or support.

The increasing appreciation that autocrine and paracrine secretions are seemingly ubiquitous and influence the behavior of normal and neoplastic cells provides a variety of new targets for therapy. Many products of oncogenes exert their activity through autocrine or paracrine effects. Tumor suppressor genes and their products offer exceptional promise of elucidating how cellular biochemistry is regulated—or is dysregulated in their absence—and thus may identify valuable targets for therapy. As a starter, the tumor suppressor gene products appear to be among nature's ways of controlling a cell from manifesting cancerous behavior. The tide of fundamental discoveries is already washing away many of the unknowns and the flyspeck observations. It is axiomatic that certain cancers can be cured today without knowing the intimate nature of neoplasia. How better the day, perhaps soon upon us, when we know what we are doing.

Clinical accomplishments have similarly been exceptionally productive in the 40 years since the first cancer was cured with drugs (7, 14). A large assortment of drugs has been provided. A wholly new array of genetically engineered drugs support host function, and others that are cytokines with anticancer activity are still early in their development. Imaging technologies have revolutionized the ability to detect, stage and monitor cancers. Biochemical markers of tu-

Table 51.7. Representative SI (Systeme Internationale) Units for Laboratory Tests of Importance in Oncology

Component	Present reference interval	Present unit	SI conversion factor	SI reference intervals	Unit symbols
Albumin	4.0–6.0	g/dL	10.0	40–60	g/L
α-Fetoprotein, radioimmunoassay	0–20	ng/mL	1.00	0–20	μg/L
Bilirubin					
Total	0.1–1.0	mg/dL	17.10	2–18	μmol/L
Conjugated	0–0.2	mg/dL	17.10	0–4	μmol/L
Calcium	8.8–10.3	mg/dL	0.2495	2.20–2.58	mmol/L
Cholesterol	<200+	mg/dL	0.02586	<5.20	mmol/L
Cortisol	4–19	μg/dL	27.59	110–520	nmol/L
Creatinine	0.6–1.2	mg/dL	88.40	50–110	μmol/L
Fibrinogen	200–400	mg/dL	0.01	2.0–4.0	g/L
Glucose	70–110	mg/dL	0.05551	3.9–6.1	mmol/L
Hemoglobin					
Male	14.0–18.0	g/dL	10.0	140–180	g/L
Female	11.5–15.5	g/dL	10.0	115–155	g/L
Immunoglobulins					
IgG	500–1200	mg/dL	0.01	5.00–12.00	g/L
IgA	50–350	mg/dL	0.01	0.50–3.50	g/L
IgM	30–230	mg/dL	0.01	0.30–2.30	g/L
IgD	<6+	mg/dL	10	<60	mg/L
IgE	20–1000	ng/mL	1.00	20–1000	μg/L
Iron	80–180	μg/dL	0.1791	14–32	μmol/L
Iron-binding capacity	250–460	μg/dL	0.1791	45–82	μmol/L
Lipoproteins					
Low-density (LDL), as cholesterol	50–190	mg/dL	0.02586	1.30–4.90	mmol/L
High-density (HDL), as cholesterol	30–70	mg/dL	0.02586	0.80–1.80	mmol/L
Magnesium	1.8–3.0	mg/dL	0.4114	0.80–1.20	mmol/L
	1.6–2.4	mEq/L	0.500		
Metanephrines (as normetanephrine)	0–2.0	mg/24 hr	5.458	0–11.0	μmol/d
Osmolality	280–300	mOsm/kg	1.00	280–300	nmol/kg
Phosphate (as inorganic P)	2.5–5.0	mg/dL	0.3229	0.80–1.60	mmol/L
Potassium	3.5–5.0	mEq/L	1.00		
		mg/dL	0.2558		
Protein, total	6–8	g/dL	10.0	3.5–5.0	mmol/L
Serotonin	8–21	μg/dL	0.05675	60–80	g/L
Thyroxine, free	0.8–2.8	ng/dL	12.87	0.45–1.20	μmol/L
Tri-iodothyronine (T_3)	75–220	ng/dL	0.01536	10–36	pmol/L
Urate (as uric acid)	2.0–6.0	mg/dL	59.48	1.2–3.4	nmol/L
Urea nitrogen	8–18	mg/dL	0.3570	120–360	μmol/L
Vanillylmandelic acid (VMA)	<6.8	mg/24 hr	5.046	3.0–6.5	mmol/L of urea
				<35	μmol/d

mor behavior are a principal fruit of immunologic study, but immunotherapeutics also holds promise. The partition and disassembly of the patient into a tumor-bearing body that is exposed to highly intensive, even supralethal therapy, regaining viability through reassembly with unexposed marrow or peripheral stem cells extends even farther the ability to deliver a potentially curative lethal injury to the tumor and to salvage the host.

There is probably no cancer in which some progress in diagnosis or therapy has not been achieved in the last decade. Similar achievement has not attended our increased knowledge of cancer prevention. Oncologists must assume greater responsibility for health preservation. Much could be accomplished by applying what is already known about lifestyle, diet, and exercise. Medical facts without political action have been slow to change the tax on health that tobacco levies.

The horizon has never been closer. Although still distant, there are enough promising paths to follow that one of them may prove considerably faster than even reasonable optimism would suppose. The information that serves as our foundation, its rate of accrual, its revelations, and the demonstrated success of translating science to clinical applications augur well for the future of medical oncology, and for cancer patients.

References

1. Bhardwaj S, Holland JF, Norton L. An intensive sequence adjuvant chemotherapy regimen for breast cancer. Cancer Invest 1993;11:6–9, and 1994;12:270–272.
2. Cancer and Leukemia Group B. Unpublished data.
3. Costanza ME, Henderson IC, Berry D, Cirrinciome C, Frei E, Mcintrye OR, Weiss RB. A randomized comparison of single agent induction chemotherapy the standard chemotherapy for stage IV breast cancer: CALGB 8642. Proc Am Soc Clin Oncol 1995;14:104.
4. Early Breast Cancer Trialists' Collaborative Group. Systemic treatment of early breast cancer by hormonal, cytotoxic or immune therapy. Lancet 1992;339:1–15, 1992;339:71–85.

5. Frei E III. Combination cancer therapy: presidential address. Cancer Res 1972;32:2593.
6. Frei E III, Canellos GP. Dose: a critical factor in cancer chemotherapy. Am J Med 1980;69:585.
7. Holland JF. Methotrexate therapy of metastatic choriocarcinoma. Am J Obstet Gynecol 1958;75:195.
8. Holland JF. The diseases that cancer causes. J Chron Dis 1963;16:635.
9. Holland JF. Ethics for a clinical investigator: non primum non nocere. Am J Med 1979;66:554.
10. Holland JF. Karnofsky Memorial Lecture. Breaking the cure barrier. J Clin Oncol 1983;1:75.
11. Holmes OW. Medical Essays "The Young Practitioner."
12. Jacquillat C, Weil M, Baillet F, Borel C, Auclerc G, Maublane MA, Housset M, Forget G, Thill L, Soubrane C, Khayat D. Results of neoadjuvant chemotherapy and radiation therapy in the breast-conserving treatment of 250 patients with all stages of infiltrative breast cancer. Cancer 1990; 66:119.
13. Kennedy BJ, Calabresi P, Carbone PP, Frei E III, Holland JF, Owens AH Jr, Sleisenger MH, Beck JC. Training program in medical oncology. Ann Intern Med 1973;78:127.
14. Li MC, Hertz R, Spencer DB. Effect of methotrexate therapy upon choriocarcinoma and chorioadenoma. Proc Soc Exp Biol Med 1956;93:361.
15. Martin DS, Balis ME, Fisher B, Frei E, Freireich EJ, Heppner GH, Holland JF, Houghton JA, Houghton PJ, Randall KJ, Mittelman A, Youcef R, Sawyer RC, Schmid FA, Stolfi RL, Young CW. Role of murine tumor models in cancer treatment research. Cancer Res 1986;46:2189.
16. Moertel CG, Fleming TR, Macdonald JS. Levamisole and fluorouracil for resected colon carcinoma. N Engl J Med 1990;322:352.
17. Rosen G, Caparos B, Huvos AG, Kosloff C, Nirenberg A, Cacavio A, Marcove RC, Lane JM, Mehta B, Urba C. Preoperative chemotherapy for osteogenic sarcoma: selection of post-operative adjuvant chemotherapy based upon the response of the primary tumor to pre-operative chemotherapy. Cancer 1982;49:1221.
18. Roush W. Dana Farber death sends a warning to research hospitals. Science 1995;269:245–246.
19. McGuire WP, Hoskins WJ, Brady MF, Kucera PR, Partridge EE, Look KY, Clarke-Pearson DL, Davidson M. Cyclophosphamide and cisplatin compared with paclitaxel and cisplatin in patients with stage III and stage IV ovarian cancer. N Engl J Med 1996;334:1.

SECTION XV

PRINCIPLES OF CHEMOTHERAPY

CHAPTER 52

Cytokinetics

ANTONELLA SURBONE, TERESA ANN GILEWSKI, AND LARRY NORTON

Introduction: The Importance of Cytokinetics to the Oncologist

Cytokinetics is the study of the kinetics of growth, a fundamental attribute of all life. Oncology is the study of malignant growth, and is, therefore, fundamentally grounded in cytokinetic facts and principles. All of the cardinal features of a cancer—its proclivity to increase in size, to disseminate, and to destroy the function of normal organs—are dependent on the reproduction of its cells. For this reason, growth kinetic concepts pervade clinical thinking. As evidence we need only refer to the everyday language of clinicians, which is replete with kinetic terms: indolent growth, rapid growth, slow regression ("refractory to therapy"), and brisk regression ("responsive to therapy"). The meanings of these descriptive terms, while somewhat intuitive, are more complex and profound than a superficial familiarity would reveal. Is indolent growth always slow, never to accelerate? Is rapid growth always virulent, never to decelerate? How do the new clinically practical means of quantifying cellular proliferation relate to macroscopic growth patterns? How does growth pattern relate to response to anticancer pharmacotherapy, thought to work by disrupting mitosis? Is there a difference in this regard between the impact of drugs on cancer cells and on such rapidly proliferating host tissues as hematopoietic progenitors and gastrointestinal mucosa?

An exciting development of the past few years has been the asking of these various kinetic questions in experimental treatment protocols. Can prognosis be predicted by pretreatment cytokinetic measurements? Does drug resistance emerge rapidly between diagnosis and the first opportunity to initiate chemotherapy? Is prognosis improved by shrinking a tumor mass as rapidly as possible, even before surgical removal? What is the optimal scheduling of non–cross-resistant chemotherapies? What is the relation between drug dose and the rate of tumor regression? These and similar issues are important to both the cytokineticist in the laboratory and the clinician at the bedside.

The field of cytokinetics actually comprises two related disciplines. The first is the study of cell proliferation, not in the biologic sense of examining how cells divide, but in the numeric sense of studying how fast they divide, how many are dividing, and how biologic measurements, such as DNA content per cell, relate to these kinetic processes. The second aspect of cytokinetics is growth curve analysis, the description of rates of change of cell number over time in both the unperturbed and perturbed (therapeutic) situation. The two disciplines are closely related in that the kinetics of cellular proliferation underlie the kinetics of tumor growth. In addition, both cellular proliferation and tumor growth are now thought to relate to many biologic characteristics of a cancer, including its tendency to invade, to metastasize, and to respond to drug therapy. Hence, this chapter will consider both disciplines—their connections and their clinical implications.

Cell Proliferation

MITOTIC CYCLE: PLM CURVES

Mitosis, or cell division, is the basic biologic process that results in an increase in somatic cell numbers over time. The term "growth" applies to the increasing volume of a cellular population and is measured in units of volume (e.g., cubic centimeters) or weight (e.g., milligrams). Growth is largely the consequence of increasing numbers of cells, but also can be influenced by the increasing size of the individual cells, edema, changes in the context of the extracellular matrix, hemorrhage, and infiltration by host cells, such as leukocytes. The term "proliferation" specifically applies to an increase in the number of cells, which is measured as cell number as a function of time. Cells divide by progressing through a sequence of steps that are collectively called the mitotic cycle. Other names for mitotic cycle are proliferative cycle and cell cycle. Classic autoradiographic techniques were first used to divide the cell cycle into four phases (1, 2). The terms for these phases, described below, are still used today, although the method of assessment is now often biochemical or biophysical, not biologic as in the original usage.

The two key events in mitosis are the synthesis of DNA, which occurs mostly in the S phase or S (for synthesis), and the actual division of the parent cell into two daughters during the M phase or M (for mitosis). The M phase is typified micromorphologically by the metaphase plate. The time gap between cell division and DNA synthesis is gap number 1, or G_1. The time gap between DNA synthesis and cell division is gap number 2, or G_2. Although the term "mitosis" is often used to refer to the M phase, the adjective "mitotic" properly refers to all cells that are engaged in any portion of the whole process of self-replication. This whole process includes the submicroscopic events (G_1, S, G_2) that precede the M phase, as well as the M phase itself. This usage has the advantage of distinguishing cells that provide evidence of their intention to divide, from those cells, called G_0 cells, that do not express that intention.

Cell cycle phases are best understood in the context of their means of quantification. The venerable mitotic index, the counting of metaphase figures in histologic slides, is of real scientific value. However, this is very labor intensive, so it has, unfortunately, decreased in popularity (3). An important variant of the mitotic index, also infrequently applied, is the stathmokinetic technique, in which a mitotic poison is applied prior to counting (4). Of all the older techniques, however, the most important by far is the thymidine labeling index (TLI) (5). Here viable cells are exposed briefly in vitro to a radiolabeled precursor of DNA. The most common thymidine label is tritium ($_3H$), but carbon 14 has also been used. The percentage of tumor cells with autoradiographic grains over their nuclei estimates the fraction of cells that were in S phase during the period of thymidine exposure. Newer variants use monoclonal antibodies directed against proteins expressed during proliferation (see below) to allow mitotic (i.e., cycling) cells to be identified visually (6–8). In all of these techniques, the microanatomy of the specimen is preserved so that the microscopist can actually know that the cell being counted is one of interest.

The highest refinement of the TLI is the percentage of labeled mitoses (PLM) curve. This technique counts, as a function of time after exposure, the number of M phases that contain radioactive label. This measures the cells currently in M phase that had been in S phase during the exposure to radioisotope. The PLM method formerly was used to study human disease, but this application has been curtailed because it requires whole-body exposure to a long-lived radioisotope. In spite of its limitations, the technique has been of fundamental importance in the field of cytokinetics because it directly estimates the durations of phases of the cell cycle. Its theory is illustrated schematically in Figure 52.1. In Figure 52.1*A*, tritiated thymidine is administered as a pulse to label cells in the S phase. As time passes (Fig. 52.1*B*) the labeled cells move beyond S and transverse G_2. At this moment, no M phase cells contain label, so the PLM is zero. Over the next short interval of time (Fig. 52.1*C*) labeled cells enter the M phase. The PLM goes from zero to 100%, as shown in the graph at the bottom of Figure 52.1. The time elapsed from the pulse labeling to the achievement of 100% PLM is equivalent to the sum of the durations of G_2 and M. The time required for the PLM to drop again to zero is the same as the time required for all of the cells labeled during S to pass through their M phases. This is the same as the duration of S phase (Fig. 52.1*D*). If we follow the population through a second generation, the PLM will again rise from zero to 100% (Fig. 52.1*E*). Figures 52.1*C* and 52.1*E* are the same except for a translocation in time, which is equivalent to one full cell cycle.

Actual PLM curves would be as sharp and as precise as is this hypothetic example were cycle lengths homogeneous and invariable, but, unfortunately, they are neither. Another complication is that because of radiopharmacokinetic and other technical considerations, it is rare for label ever to be present in all M phase cells. Thus, sophisticated mathematic methods must be used to estimate phase lengths by model

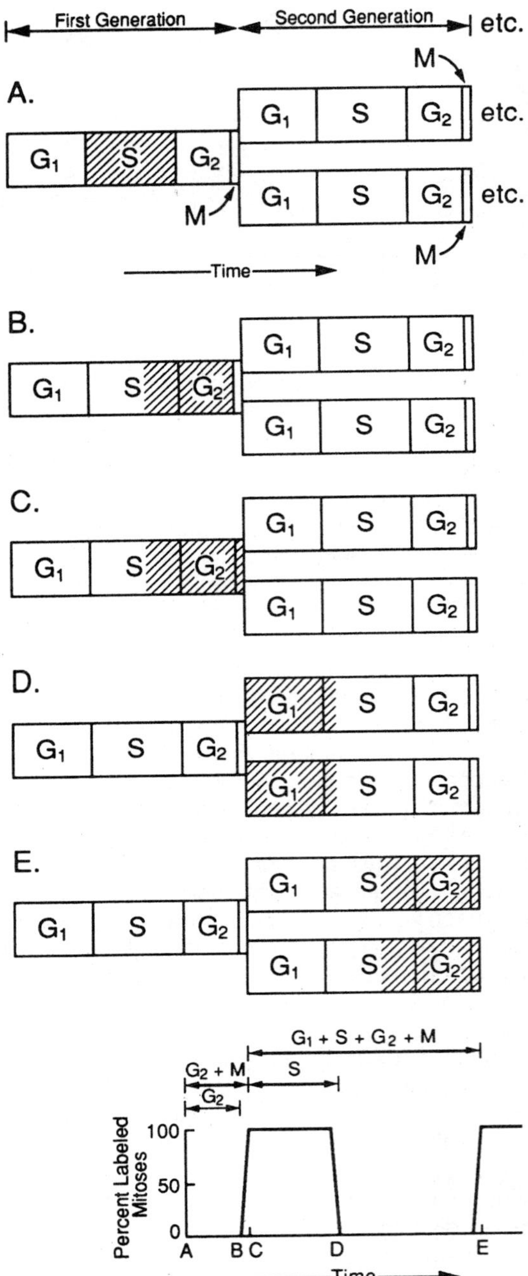

Figure 52.1. The mitotic cycle and percent labeled mitoses curve.

fitting (9). In spite of these limitations, however, almost everything that we now know concerning cycle dynamics has been learned from the PLM method.

CELL CYCLE PHASES AND DNA CONTENT

At its birth, a normal mammalian somatic cell contains a diploid number of chromosomes, and hence diploid (2N) DNA content. Following a successful cell division, the new cell generally experiences a time gap before it begins to engage in measurable DNA synthesis. Some very primitive or embryonic cells enter DNA synthesis immediately, but these are exceptions to the usual pattern. We have termed this gap G_1, but a new cell is properly called G_1 only if it exhibits the biologic intention of entering the S phase. Should the cell never actually progress to the point of starting DNA synthesis, it would properly be classified as G_0. Since both G_0 and G_1 cells are diploid in DNA content, we avoid the presumption of prescience by considering the two phases together. In performing this grouping, we recognize that the lengths of the G_0–G_1 phases are highly variable, fitting a log-normal probability distribution that is skewed markedly to the right, that is, toward longer times. Since the cells on the far right end of the distribution will never divide within the life span of the host, they are the G_0 cells.

This statistical distinction between G_0 and G_1 has biologic correlates. Between their M and S phases, cells prepare to enter S by progressing through defined stages that are dependent on protein synthesis (10). These stages are regulated enzymatically by processes partially sensitive to such extracellular influences as growth factors and the supply of nutrients. Cancer cells may be less dependent on these external signals and conditions than are normal cells, which may account for their ability to grow in suspension cultures without extracellular matrix. This ability may be related to the activity of oncogenes or to the deregulation of suppressor genes, such as p53 or the retinoblastoma gene.

Cells in G_1 have already progressed beyond several preliminary steps to prepare for the S phase, whereas G_0 cells need further time to complete early synthetic events so that they can enter G_1. These differences can be exploited in the laboratory to discriminate G_0 from G_1 cells. G_0 cells tend to be smaller (11), and have lower RNA and protein contents than do G_1 cells, as well as specific, characteristic mRNAs and proteins (12, 13). For example, the Ki67 antigen is present in all mitotic cells (G_1, S, G_2, M), but is not found in G_0 cells (8). Also, G_0 cells do not metabolize the cationic dye rhodamine, which is thought, but has not been proven (14), to reflect the cells' relatively low mitochondrial activity (15). However, G_0 cells, in spite of their distinctive biologic characteristics, can be stimulated by external influences to proceed through the sequence of events that leads them into G_1 and eventually into S. This phenomenon is called recruitment.

After the M phase, but before DNA synthesis begins in earnest, the cell either commits to proliferate by entering the S phase or stops dividing by differentiating into a nonmitotic cell. The ratio $G_1/(G_0 + G_1)$ at any one time defines the proportion of cells entering their next S phase. A particular restriction point at the G_1–S interface, now called Start, may be regulated by the p34cdc2 protein, which may couple with different cyclin proteins (whose levels vary within the cell cycle) to permit, alternatively, a cell's entry into S or its entry into M (16). Normally, the M phase cannot take place unless the S phase has been completed, and the S phase cannot take place unless the M phase has been completed. Abnormalities in this system could result in an unblocking of the normal "block to rereplication," which prevents parts of the genome from being replicated more than once during a single S phase (17). Such abnormalities are one possible etiology for aberrant levels of DNA per neoplastic cell (see below). Once the cell enters the S phase, its progression through the rest of the cycle is largely self-regulated (18). This regulation involves direct controls, in which a step must be completed before the next step commences, as well as indirect feedback loops (19).

The S phase, lasting between 12 and 24 hours in mammalian cells, is generally much less variable than G_0–G_1. Specific regions of chromosomes replicate at specific times, clusters of replication units initiating synchronously, with the whole complex process transpiring in a highly orchestrated manner (20). During S, a cell's DNA content should increase from 2N to 4N. A very small number of S0 cells may actually stop synthesizing DNA before completing S (21). Their ultimate fate is unclear, although it is likely that some can resume S, while others are prevented from proceeding by intrinsic blocks in their self-regulation. Cells completing S enter the second gap, marked by a dramatic diminution in the rate of DNA synthesis. G_2 usually lasts for about 3 hours in mammalian cells, ending when the M phase begins. Rarely, a cell can rest in G_2, and not proceed into actual cell division (22).

The initiation of the M phase may depend on the same molecular trigger as Start, but in a complex interplay with different cyclins and other factors that are actively under investigation (23). The M phase is composed of several parts. In prophase, the cell assumes the shape of a sphere (24). The microtubules and microfilaments of the cell's cytoskeleton rearrange, the Golgi apparatus disperses into small vesicles, protein synthesis drops, and the dispersed chromosomes (duplicated during the S phase) cease metabolic activity and then condense into transportable units (25). During prometaphase, these units orient themselves linearly toward opposite ends of the cell and move to the midplane to form the metaphase plate. In anaphase, spindle fibers attached to kinetochores on each chromosome guide them toward centrosomes in opposite ends of the cell. In telophase, the nuclei reform, the chromosomes decondense, and the cell normally divides into two approximately equal halves, one new nucleus per daughter cell. M is the phase that is least variable in length, lasting about 1 hour in most mammalian cells.

The total duration of the cell cycle, the mitotic cycle time, also called the generation time, varies considerably, but the average in human cancer is between 2 and 4 days. This is in marked contrast with the cell cycle in *Drosophila*, which may take minutes, or with that of mammalian embryos, which may take hours. Some normal cells, such as human neurons, may never divide at all. Cancer is not always a disease of rapid proliferation, but it is always one of persistent proliferation. If a large number of cancer cells are dividing, even if they are dividing with deliberate speed, they will produce many offspring, which, by themselves dividing, will lead to an abnormal accumulation over time. For a given tissue, malignant or benign, the length of the cell cycle in vivo is fairly constant in spite of variations in the number of cycling cells in that population. However, subtle changes in cycle kinetics have been seen in cancers in laboratory animals that are allowed to grow large (26, 27) and phase lengths can shift significantly as cells are cultured in vitro (28).

FLOW CYTOMETRY

The variation in cellular DNA content during the proliferative cycle can be exploited analytically by a collection of automated methods called flow cytometry. Visual procedures, such as mitotic index, TLI, and static Ki-67 staining, are slow, laborious, and subjective. These negative features may change with technological advances in assessing cellularity on slides and in the automated counting of visually distinctive cells (29, 30). At present, however, flow methods are the most rapid and quantitative (31). The major disadvantage of such techniques as flow cytometry, in which the cells being analyzed are not visualized, is that normal stromal cells, normal blood cells, and tumor cells of various types and degrees of oxygenation are all counted together. Another disadvantage is that reliable flow cytometry requires meticulous technique and hence constant attention to quality control. Nevertheless, flow cytometry has become the most widely applied, and the most productive, method of cytokinetic assessment in the modern clinic.

In fluorescence-activated cell sorting, a suspension of individual cells is automatically counted by being allocated into bins by DNA content, RNA content, cell size, antibody label, or combinations of such factors (32, 33). This can be performed on fresh tissue—leukemias, tumor cells in effusions or ascites, enzymatically dispersed solid tumors—or on cells recovered from paraffin-embedded specimens (34). Enzymatic methods of dispersing fresh or fixed solid tumor specimens have been shown to produce high single-cell yields, representative of the tissue as a whole, with low degrees of contamination by cellular debris (35).

Flow cytometry can be used to measure RNA per cell, which, as mentioned above, is helpful in distinguishing G_0 from G_1 cells. Various techniques of tagging cells for the purpose of sorting are being employed. For example, cells can be labeled by the Ki67 antibody (conjugated to a fluorescent dye) (8). Unfixed, viable cells can be exposed to bromodeoxyuridine, which is incorporated during S (36). These cells will then react with an antibromodeoxyuridine antibody tagged with a fluorescent dye, a method that has proved reliable in the study of solid tumors (37). Bromodeoxyuridine can also be administered intravenously (IV) to patients several hours prior to a biopsy. The tissue so recovered can then be examined for an S phase label, or can be exposed to tritiated thymidine to provide a double label, useful for examining phase durations, particularly in leukemia (38).

The primary value of flow cytometry for cytokinetics is in its measurement of DNA content. DNA content is usually assessed by the use of intercalating or base-pair affinity dyes. The standard output of this technique is the DNA flow cytogram, also called a DNA histogram. Standardization of the G_0–G_1 peak for DNA histograms uses diploid cells from the same species as the tissue being studied (39). Human lymphocytes from normal donors are commonly used for many clinical applications. In the assessment of human breast cancer, for instance, lymphocytes are often obtained from normal lymph nodes removed at the time of primary surgery. The completed histogram graphs the relative proportions of cells with 2N DNA (i.e., diploid cells in G_0–G_1), 4N DNA (i.e., tetraploid cells in G_2–M), and DNA content between 2N and 4N, called the S-phase fraction. Another cytometric term in common use is the proliferative index, the fraction of cells that are in either S or G_2 or M.

By measuring DNA content per cell, flow cytometry can also identify cells with abnormal amounts of DNA in the G_0–G_1 peak, termed aneuploid. Categories include near-diploid (2N ± 10%), hypodiploid (less than 2N), simple hyperdiploid (between 2N and 4N), tetraploid (4N), near-tetraploid (4N ± 10%), hypertetraploid (greater than 4N), or combinations, called multiploid. Each aneuploid G_0–G_1 peak is expected to have a corresponding G_2–M peak with twice as much DNA. The DNA index is the ratio between the fluorescence channel of the malignant G_0–G_1 peak and the normal diploid G_0–G_1 peak; less than 0.9 or greater than 1.1 is often considered abnormal. The S-phase fraction may be impossible to measure in the presence of marked aneuploidy, especially if a diploid G_2–M peak overlaps with an aneuploid S. An overview of the literature suggests that ploidy can now be measured in more than 90% of solid tumors, and the S-phase fraction in about 80% of specimens. However, the classification of DNA histograms is not well standardized at present, so interpretations are highly variable, especially when paraffin-embedded rather than fresh source material is used (40).

MITOTIC COMPARTMENTS

When a cell divides, the daughters either must remain in a mitotically quiescent state, enter G_1, or die. There are no other possibilities. Entering G_1 means that the cell has positioned itself to divide again. Such a cell is thereby a member of the proliferative fraction, also called the growth fraction or the growth compartment (41). The second possibility is that the cell enters a prolonged G_0 (or, rarely, S_0 or an arrested G_2), which means that the cell has joined the nonproliferative or quiescent fraction. Classically, the growth fraction is measured by dividing the labeling index by the ratio of the durations of the S phase and the total cycle time (42).

The S-phase fraction as measured by flow cytometry includes S_0 cells in the quiescent fraction. For this and other technical reasons, the S-phase fraction is usually larger than the TLI. It correlates with but is not equivalent to the growth fraction (43). About 2 to 20% of cells in a typical cancer are in S at any point in time. Since the S phase occupies one quarter to one half of the cell cycle, the growth fraction is usually 4 to 80%, with an average of less than 20%. Some normal tissues, such as bone marrow and alimentary mucosa, have larger growth fractions and shorter mitotic cycle times than many cancers, even cancers of those tissues (44, 45).

Nonproliferative cells fall into three categories. Some highly differentiated cells, such as neurons, are permanently nonproliferative but may survive for the whole life of the organism. In distinction, most terminally differentiated cells, such as the polymorphonuclear leukocyte, have a finite life span. The third type of nonproliferative cell is in an unstable G_0, which means that it may be recruited into G_1 with the proper extracellular signal. Stem cells share with neurons the property of living as long as the organism, but, like unstable G_0 cells, they can periodically, or on demand, produce viable progeny (46, 47). Stem cells are also called clonogenic cells because of their capacity for unlimited proliferation. The signal for stem cell recruitment is often from physiologic changes in the environment, such as cell death or cell injury, or extracellular influences such as by drugs or hormones. An operational definition of stem capacity is the ability to form colonies in soft agar (22, 48). Cell culture experiments have found that from 1% to less than 0.1% of the cells in many common tumors have this property, but this may be an underestimate, since in vitro conditions may be more austere than those occurring naturally in vivo. Yet, even though malignant clonogenic cells are a minority population in a cancer, they are the prime target of anticancer therapy since they constantly replenish the whole population. If chemotherapy preferentially kills mitotic cells, termed the "mitotoxicity hypothesis," the ability of tumor stem cells to remain in G_0 for long periods may be one reason for therapeutic failure (49).

The third possible fate for a cell is death. Cells lost from any phase of the cell cycle are collectively called the cell loss fraction (50). Cell loss is important because the growth rate is the difference between cell production and cell loss. Hence, a tumor with high cell loss may appear to be growing slowly, when in fact the rate of mitosis may be high. A well-known clinical example is basal cell epithelioma of the skin, which grows slowly in spite of showing a large number of metaphase figures.

The significance of cell loss may be illustrated by a hypothetic numeric example. Let us imagine a tumor with a growth fraction of 100%, no cell loss, and a mitotic cycle time of 3 days. This tumor will double in size every 3 days. In this case, the generation time is equal to the doubling time, the time it takes the cell number to double in size. If, however, cells are lost from the tumor at one half the rate of cell production, a cell loss fraction of 50%, the tumor will double in 6 days rather than in 3 days. The importance of cell loss goes well beyond the determination of growth rate. Each mitotic cycle carries with it a finite probability of mutation (51). It takes more mitotic cycles for the tumor with a cell loss of 50% to double in size than it does for the tumor with no cell loss. Thus, the rate of cell loss relates directly to the rate of mutations toward biologic properties of clinical importance.

CYTOKINETICS AND BIOLOGIC DIVERSITY

Since 1980 more than 2,000 published studies have assayed the cytokinetics of clinical cancers. There have been major as well as minor applications. A relatively minor use has been in the screening of cytologic specimens for malignant cells. This exercise exploits the observation that with few exceptions (noted below), normal cells are diploid whereas about 70% of clinical cancers are aneuploid. Screening, however, has been of secondary interest in the use of kinetic measurements for correlation with clinical course. The S-phase fraction, thymidine labeling index, and aneuploidy have all been evaluated as prognostic factors. Although the S-phase fraction may be no higher in neoplastic than in some normal tissues, within a given histologic type of cancer, both a high S-phase fraction and aneuploidy are frequently associated with growth that is relatively more rapid, malignant behavior that is relatively more aggressive, and therapeutic response that is relatively poorer.

The reasons for the consistent association of aneuploidy with high S-phase fraction are conjectural. One possibility is that aneuploidy is caused by high S phase activity because it is the consequence of errors in chromosomal construction. The reasoning in this regard is that a high S-phase fraction implies a large number of mitotic cycles per unit of time, which provides more opportunities for erroneous DNA replication. Against this argument is the observation that many normal tissues, such as bone marrow and epithelia, have high S-phase fractions but do not normally become aneuploid. This leaves another possibility, that high S-phase fraction is not the cause of aneuploidy but rather the consequence of the chromosomal abnormalities reflected in the aneuploid state. Such abnormalities may be linked with oncogene activation or suppressor gene inactivation. Some clinically benign tumors are aneuploid, so chromosomal abnormalities do not always mean frank cancerous behavior. Yet aneuploidy is clearly a step in tumor progression: DNA errors lead to growth stimulation, high cell turnover results in more opportunities for error, errors produce increasing genetic aberrancy. The question of how fast mutations accumulate by this process is clinically relevant and will be discussed in the context of growth curve models.

Regardless of the rate of mutations, however, the neoplastic process is so closely related to spontaneous genetic change that tumor progression toward increasing malignancy is regarded as an intrinsic property of cancer (38, 52). The clonal origin of tumors has been well described (53). It has been stated that over 80% of clinical cancers are monoclonal by glucose-6-phosphate dehydrogenase isotype or cytogenetics (54). Yet clonal evolution as the tumors evolve leads to heterogeneity in morphology, metastatic behavior, biochemistry, ploidy, immunogenicity, steroid and growth factor receptors, and drug sensitivity (55). Metastases tend to grow faster than do the primary tumors from which they arise (56, 57). There is ample evidence that cytokinetics either underlies or is a direct covariate of tumor progression. That is, the mechanism relating aneuploidy to S-phase fraction also relates tumor progression to S-phase fraction. This will be illustrated in the discussion of clinical correlates of cytokinetics and further below in the context of the doubling time and the Skipper-Schabel model.

As discussed theoretically above, the third determinant of growth rate, cell loss, is also relevant to the generation of genetic changes. High rates of cell turnover are implicated in carcinogenesis. Elevated levels of thyroid stimulating hormone predispose to thyroid cancer (58). Chronic thermal injury with compensatory hyperplasia (59) and hyperplasia secondary to solar damage (60) lead to skin cancer. Hyperproliferation of the bone marrow in dysmyelopoiesis (61) and in chronic granulocytic leukemia (62) can result in acute leukemia. Hyperproliferation of the epithelium, as of the colon in inflammatory bowel disease and polyps (63), and of the breast in murine models (64) and clinical specimens (65, 66), is also associated with neoplastic transformation. Indeed, chemical carcinogenesis requires a growth promoter (67). It is possible that the hyperproliferation of cancer cells as a compensatory response to chronic antineoplastic drug treatment may predispose to the development of drug resistance in Hodgkin's lymphoma (68) and gastrointestinal cancer (69).

All of the statistical associations among S-phase fraction,

ploidy, cell loss fraction, and clinical behavior are of major scientific interest. It must be cautioned, however, that these associations are not always of practical importance, especially when kinetic parameters are highly correlated with more easily measured prognostic factors, such as tumor size. As is seen with any weak prognostic factor, small studies are often falsely negative. Conversely, false-positive reports may arise via data-driven subset analysis. For example, imagine that a population of patients is divisible into those with some arbitrary factor X and those without X, those with Y and those without Y, those with and without Z, and so on. A small study may show that aneuploidy means poor prognosis in patients with Y but good prognosis in patients without Y, whereas both X and Z seem unrelated to ploidy and prognosis. Here the subset allocation (by Y) is chosen because ploidy seems to be useful within the subset, not because there is a biologic reason to suspect that ploidy and Y should be related. In fact, if ploidy carried no prognostic significance whatsoever, there is a real possibility that some other arbitrary division would distinguish the patients merely by chance. This other arbitrary division could be draped in the illusion of biologic tenability, but it would not prove reproducible in prospective confirmatory studies. Hence, purely statistical phenomena such as these should always be kept in mind when reading conflicting data concerning cytokinetics and clinical behavior.

Breast Cancer

Most invasive adenocarcinomas of the breast are of ductal origin. These have been studied extensively from a cytokinetic viewpoint. Ductal carcinoma in situ is thought to be a true neoplastic lesion that is not yet invasive but has a tendency to progress in that direction. There is some evidence that ploidy and proliferative activity can help identify lesions with greater potential for such progression (70). Regarding frank invasive ductal cancers, the TLIs of primary specimens have been shown to follow a log-normal probability distribution (71). This means that while the majority of TLIs are grouped about a median of 5 to 6%, some very large values are found in a few cases. Nuclear staining with the Ki-67 antigen correlates with thymidine labeling index (72).

As the phenotypic expression of genotypic abnormalities (73), TLI is a fairly stable property of a given breast cancer. That is, TLI values from primary specimens correlate well with values determined from metastatic sites (74). High TLI predicts for the presence of necrosis in the tumor, low estrogen receptor content, anaplastic nuclear and histologic grade, and other predictors of poor clinical outcome. However, a recent analysis of more than 9,000 primary breast cancers failed to find an association between TLI and the most powerful predictors of prognosis: tumor size and lymph nodal involvement (75). Nevertheless, in locally advanced breast cancer, high TLI predicts high metastatic potential, short disease-free interval after intensive treatment, and short survival (76). Similarly, in node-positive breast cancer primarily treated with surgery and subsequently with adjuvant chemotherapy, a low TLI predicted for longer relapse-free and overall survival (77). In node-negative breast cancer patients not receiving adjuvant chemotherapy, a high TLI predicted for recurrence (78). These data are highly controversial since another study with 8-year follow-up failed to show any association between TLI and survival (79). Nevertheless, Italian investigators are currently engaged in a clinical trial in which node-negative patients are assigned to receive adjuvant chemotherapy entirely on the basis of their cancers' TLI measurements (80). The safest statement is that the value of TLI has not been fully established, but that indications are that important biologic information is contained therein, and that further investigation—regarding both the prediction of prognosis and response to chemotherapy—is justified.

As described above, the most commonly measured cytokinetic parameter is now the S-phase fraction by flow cytometry (SPF). TLI and SPF show good correspondence (73, 81). As for TLI, therefore, high SPF in primary disease correlates with low estrogen and progesterone receptor content (81–95), high degree of nodal involvement, increasing nuclear anaplasia (86), and aneuploidy (87-90). The degree of axillary nodal involvement with cancer seems to correlate with high SPF in some studies (91), whereas in others it appears to be independent of axillary nodal status, tumor size, and menopausal status (92). A few studies have reported a higher SPF in patients younger than 50 years of age, notably associated with a poorer prognosis (87, 88, 93). High SPF correlates, albeit weakly, with prognosis following local recurrence in a conserved breast (94).

In node-negative breast cancer, the presence of either high SPF or aneuploidy has been correlated with a higher probability of relapse (95–97). This was only partially confirmed in a prospective series of node-negative breast cancer patients randomized to receive no postoperative adjuvant chemotherapy (91). In that large study, ploidy (measured in 79% of cases) had no prognostic value; SPF (measured in 73% of patients) did, with low SPF predicting longer disease-free survival. However, low SPF correlated so well with small tumor size that its value as an independent predictor remains to be established by further study. That is, both ploidy and SPF may convey prognostic information, but the clinical usefulness of the small magnitude of their impact, especially in light of more powerful covariates, must be considered controversial (98–100). Several studies with median follow-ups of at least 4 years have found that low SPF is an independent predictor of lower relapse rate or longer survival in node-negative disease (87, 90, 93, 101–106). For example, one retrospective analysis of 195 patients with node-negative disease and tumors over 1 centimeter in diameter found that the relapse-free rate was 78% for cases with SPF less than 10%, but 52% for the others (102). Similar data exist for node-positive cases. Yet SPF does not consistently emerge as an independent factor in multivariate analyses (89, 107). In addition, the value of SPF as a prognostic factor sometimes has been limited to subgroups (88, 89, 108–114). It is also of interest to note that for the patients treated by chemotherapy (91), treatment has a positive impact irrespective of the S phase category. Hence, the data are not clear, and great caution regarding the clinical use of SPF must be exercised. In this regard, a consensus review of published data has concluded that SPF is associated with tumor grade, as well as the probability of relapse and survival in node-negative and node-positive disease, but that clinical applications remain indistinct (115).

Ploidy, for all of its theoretic attractiveness, is now known not to be clinically useful. In the subset of stage II patients with estrogen receptor–negative tumors, diploidy has been reported to be a positive prognostic factor (116). Aneuploidy is indeed more common among more poorly differentiated tumors (84, 85, 117–119). For analysis of node-negative and node-positive disease, ploidy has been shown by some to be a prognostic marker (120–124), while others did not confirm it (85, 86, 108, 109, 125, 126). One multisubset analysis was in favor of ploidy, but reported that SPF was a more powerful factor (110). Another subset analysis found prognostic significance of ploidy and estrogen receptor content (127). In node-positive patients, studies with a follow-up of at least 5 years have noted statistically significant differences in relapse-free survival (107) and overall survival (128) in favor of diploid versus aneuploid tumors. Other studies have reported no significant difference in relapse-free or overall survival based on ploidy status (89, 116). Several multivariate analyses found ploidy possibly to be an independent prognostic factor (129, 130, 131), whereas others did not confirm the findings (87, 132). On the contrary, a consensus review of the usefulness of DNA index found that ploidy is a weak prognostic factor, which is not of independent value in multivariate analysis (115).

Several studies have used less common techniques to evaluate the proliferation rate of breast cancers, including in vivo and in vitro labeling with the thymidine analogue 5-bromodeoxyuridine (BrdU) and in vitro staining with anti-Ki-67 antibodies. BrdU labeling seems to correlate well with TLI, large tumor size, poor differentiation, aneuploidy, and high SPF (133, 134), but not estrogen receptor status (134, 135). One study using in vivo BrdU labeling failed to find an association of the values in normal breast tissue and in cancer (136). However, the labeling of the normal cells in premenopausal women was higher than that in older women. Nuclear staining with Ki-67 antigen correlates with TLI (72) and is abundant in cancers with poor estrogen receptor content, aneuploidy, high nuclear grade, and rapid relapse after primary surgery. The relationship between Ki-67 staining and tumor size or histologic grade has not been established (137), although a recent large study found estrogen receptor status, Ki-67 content, tumor size, and nodal status all to be independent prognostic factors (139).

The breast cancer literature is filled with reports of putative prognostic factors that correlate, to various degrees, with proliferative measurements. These include c-erbB2 (HER2/neu), epidermal growth factor receptor (EGFR, HER1), mutant p53, cathepsin D and other proteases, and nm-23 (138, 140) and other mutation suppressors. HER2 is a proto-oncogene, located on chromosome 17q21–22, that is amplified in approximately 30% of primary breast cancers (141). It encodes a 185 kDa glycoprotein with tyrosine kinase activity that is involved in the transduction of signals for growth. Amplification and overexpression of c-erbB2 are observed at all stages of primary breast cancer and in lesions in all metastatic sites. Overexpression of c-erbB2 in node-positive patients correlates with high SPF and aneuploidy (142, 143), but not with TLI (144, 145). Moreover, c-erb-B2 and SPF have been found in some studies to be independent prognostic factors for node-positive breast cancer (146), whereas other studies have not confirmed this observation (147, 148). In ductal carcinoma in situ, c-erbB2 overexpression and high TLI appear to be associated (149). HER1 is thought to be required to maintain normal breast epithelium, but it is overexpressed in 35 to 45% of breast cancers. Some have reported a correlation of HER1 with SPF, ploidy, and Ki-67 staining, but this remains unclear (138, 150). The p53 gene is one of the tumor suppressor genes involved by deletion or inactivation in the development of breast cancer. Wild-type p53 protein arrests cell division at the interface of G_1 and S, binds DNA in a sequence-specific manner, and is a transcriptional activator (151). Mutations of p53 result in the production of an aberrant product with a long half-life and the absence of all of these functions. Investigation of p53 protein (150, 152–154) and proliferative cell nuclear antigen expression in comparison with other measurements of cytokinetics is ongoing (155–157). Cathepsin D is an estrogen-related protein that acts as a peptide growth factor and may facilitate cancer cell migration and invasion (158). Its expression does not correlate with TLI or other proliferative factors (159, 160).

All of these data signify that the growth fraction, as estimated by a large number of currently available techniques, is positively correlated with some aggressive manifestations of breast cancer, but not others, and never strongly or consistently. Hence, factors other than growth fraction alone must be important determinants of the malignant behavior of this disease.

Prostate Carcinoma

Numerous studies have assessed DNA content by flow cytometry in prostate cancer (161–167). The majority of these analyses indicate that ploidy provides prognostic information for localized prostate cancer: Aneuploid tumors recur more frequently than do diploid tumors (162–166). Aneuploidy tends to occur in more advanced stages of disease (168, 169). In a review article, Deitch et al. observed that DNA ploidy may predict tumor volume but does not predict who will profit from radiation therapy for localized disease (169). Aneuploidy and SPF were shown to be significantly related to both large tumor size and a high Gleason score (170, 171). Aneuploidy has also been found in benign tissue in close proximity to high-grade large-volume disease (169). SPF has been assessed by flow cytometry (172), in vivo bromodeoxyuridine labeling (173), and Ki-67 expression (174), but the clinical value of such assessments is uncertain.

Renal Cell Carcinoma

Conflicting data exist regarding the prognostic significance of DNA ploidy in renal cell carcinoma (175–184). Recently, a retrospective univariate analysis of 381 paraffin blocks from 93 primary adenocarcinomas found that DNA ploidy and S-phase fraction were significantly associated with both tumor grade and survival (185). However, when tumor grade was considered, the flow cytometry measurements were not of prognostic significance. The predictive significance of cytokinetics regarding response to therapy can be resolved only by prospective studies.

Bladder Cancer

BrdU labeling has been used to assess the growth fraction in bladder cancer (186), but most studies have used DNA flow cytometry. Walther has reviewed the role of ploidy in predicting and monitoring response to therapy and in screening urine samples for malignancy (187). A number of studies have noted an association between DNA ploidy, tumor grade, and aggressiveness of bladder cancer (187–192). However, it is not clear whether cytokinetics provides any information superior to that afforded by conventional clinical parameters (193, 194). A recent analysis of 448 paraffin specimens of transitional cell bladder cancer found that DNA ploidy was not an independent prognostic factor, although prognosis was predicted by S-phase fraction and mitotic index (194). Recent data on operable muscle-invasive bladder carcinomas do not show ploidy to be a useful prognostic parameter (195). In contrast, one study, DNA image cytometry appeared to be of value in transitional cell carcinomas of the bladder, being particularly useful in predicting the survival of patients with superficial lesions (196).

Testicular Carcinoma

It has been reported that a high DNA index in nonseminomatous germ cell tumors of the testes is associated with advanced disease at presentation (197). Aneuploidy, however, did not correlate with histology or vessel invasion.

Ovarian Cancer

DNA ploidy is not clearly related to the stage of ovarian cancer (198, 199), although, with some exceptions (200), most studies have demonstrated that diploid tumors are associated with a better prognosis (201–206). This association may be less apparent for patients with advanced disease (207). The role of flow cytometry in analyzing ascitic fluid (208) and in monitoring treatment effects is being explored (203). Assessment of S-phase fraction by Ki-67 staining (209), flow cytometry (205, 206, 210, 211), and thymidine labeling has produced variable results (210–215). The role of ploidy in mucinous borderline ovarian tumors has been discussed (216).

Uterine Cancer

In endometrial carcinoma, with few exceptions (217), aneuploidy has been associated with poorly differentiated tumors (218–220) and decreased survival (218, 219, 221, 222). Multiparametric analyses of response to hormonal therapy are ongoing (223). Also of current interest are flow cytometric determinations of levels of expression of epidermal growth factor receptors and c-erbB-2 oncoprotein (222, 224, 225).

Cervical Carcinoma

DNA ploidy and S-phase fraction have an unclear role as prognostic factors in cervical carcinoma (226–231), although some studies have suggested that diploid or tetraploid tumors may have a worse prognosis (232, 233). A recent study has shown a correlation between the Ki-67 index and response to radiation therapy (234).

Colorectal Carcinoma

While Ki-67 immunoreactivity has been used to measure proliferative activity in colorectal carcinoma (235), most studies have used flow cytometry. Both retrospective and prospective data suggest that aneuploid colorectal carcinomas, particularly those in stages A, B, and C, have a worse prognosis (236–244). This is not a universal finding, however (245–247). Several analyses have also noted an increased frequency of aneuploidy in more advanced stages of disease (236, 243, 248–252). Multivariate analyses have indicated that S-phase fraction or stage may be a better prognostic factor than ploidy (253, 254). Abnormal DNA content and high proliferative activity have also been noted in benign colonic mucosa adjacent to the primary tumor by some (255), but not all (256), investigators. Analysis of DNA ploidy as a means of identifying patients with ulcerative colitis at higher risk for developing colorectal cancer is an area of active investigation (257).

Carcinoma of the Pancreas

The cytokinetics of this disease has not been well studied. An analysis of 56 patients indicated that ploidy was an independent prognostic factor with a significant effect on survival (258). In one small study, DNA ploidy did not predict the malignant behavior of insulinomas (259). In another study, ploidy did not differentiate benign serous cystadenomas from mucinous cystic cancers (260).

Hepatoma

The limited information concerning the prognostic importance of DNA flow cytometry for hepatocellular carcinoma is conflicting (261). Some retrospective multivariate analyses found a correlation between ploidy and overall and disease-free survival (262, 263), whereas another showed no association with survival (264). The bromodeoxyuridine labeling index has been correlated with histologic findings from hepatocellular carcinomas and cirrhotic tissues (265, 266).

Gastric and Esophageal Carcinomas

There is a rapidly expanding literature concerning the cytokinetics of esophageal cancer (267–274). The most recent data show cytometric analysis to be of prognostic significance in squamous cell carcinoma of the esophagus (272). Moreover, for patients with gastric carcinoma, the most recent data have found that tumor aneuploidy is associated with decreased survival (275–281). This finding is at variance with older studies that did not find this association (283–285), which may reflect improvements in technique. Also, cytokinetic analysis seems to be associated with histologic differentiation and with symptoms such as weight loss (282). Aneuploidy is present in a greater percentage of tumors of the gastroesophageal junction and cardia than in those of the body and antrum (276, 277). Lymph node involvement is also more common in aneuploid tumors (276, 277, 286). Assessment of proliferative activity by thymidine or bromodeoxyuridine labeling may also be of prognostic significance (278, 279, 287, 288). This is an important body of literature to follow carefully in the coming decade, as more biochemical correlates of prognosis become available and are viewed, together with cytokinetic parameters.

Head and Neck Cancer

There is disagreement in the literature regarding the prognostic significance of DNA ploidy in squamous cell carcinoma of the head and neck (289, 290). Some studies identified a more favorable prognosis for aneuploid tumors (291–293), whereas others found a better outcome for diploid tumors (294). One analysis found no significant association between DNA ploidy and response to chemotherapy (295). Several studies have reported increased radiosensitivity for aneuploid lesions (289). An evaluation of 110 patients with oral cavity lesions noted an increased likelihood of aneuploidy in poorly differentiated and larger tumors (296). Only limited studies with bromodeoxyuridine and thymidine have been performed (297–300). A retrospective examination of 45 patients with adenoid cystic carcinomas of the salivary glands, a tumor type of low malignant potential, found that the majority of tumors were diploid (301).

Lung Carcinoma

Numerous studies of non–small-cell lung carcinoma have found an association between aneuploidy and shorter survival times (302–309). However, other analyses have not confirmed this observation (310, 311). In several studies, ploidy was found to be of prognostic significance for squamous cell carcinomas, but not for non–squamous cell tumors (302, 303). Aneuploidy has also been correlated with phenotypic heterogeneity in non–small-cell lung cancer (312). A recent study demonstrated a role for Ki-67 staining in lung cancers (313). It remains unclear whether TLI is of prognostic significance, although increased p-glycoprotein-170 expression has been noted in tumors with low proliferative activity (314, 315). Limited data are available concerning the prognostic significance of ploidy in small-cell lung cancer (316, 317). The ability of flow cytometry to detect bone marrow micrometastases in patients with small-cell lung cancer is being investigated (318).

Brain Cancer

Determination of high growth fraction by bromodeoxyuridine (BrdU) labeling, Ki-67 staining, and mutant p53 expression (disinhibition of the normal G_1–S blockade) was found to convey prognostic information in several studies of primary brain malignancies (319–323). A prospective study of 174 patients with intracranial gliomas found the BrdU labeling index to be an important predictor of survival for low-grade astrocytomas. This index, in conjunction with the patient's age, was also predictive of survival for glioblastomas and malignant astrocytomas (321). BrdU labeling studies have found that cell proliferation increases after in vitro administration of exogenous growth factors to cultured primary glioma cells (324). Flow cytometry has been used to assess ploidy in meningiomas (325), as well as in stereotactic brain biopsies of several types of lesions (326). In gliomas, aneuploidy has been associated with high histologic grade and poor outcome (320, 327–329). In medulloblastoma, aneuploidy has been associated with poor prognosis (330, 331), but aneuploid medulloblastomas may be more sensitive to treatment (332).

Thyroid Cancer

There is no definite role for DNA ploidy as a prognostic factor in thyroid cancer (333–335). Aneuploidy has been noted in both malignant (336–338) and benign (339, 340) thyroid lesions.

Thymomas

Aneuploidy has been associated with more advanced disease, increased tumor recurrence, and the existence of myasthenia gravis (341).

Sarcomas

There is limited information on the role of DNA analysis for soft tissue and bone sarcomas (342–344). The presence of diploid or near-diploid tumors may be associated with a more favorable prognosis for chondrosarcomas and osteosarcomas (345, 346). Although most malignant tumors are aneuploid (347, 348), benign tumors (including Schwannomas) may be aneuploid as well (349). Aneuploid gastric leiomyosarcomas appear to have a worse prognosis (350). Flow cytometry has also been used to assess ploidy in Kaposi's sarcoma (352) and chromosomal abnormalities in Ewing's sarcoma cell lines (353). Expression of mutant p53 and high proliferative rate appear to be strongly correlated with prognosis in adult soft-tissue sarcomas (354).

Pediatric Tumors

Several studies have noted an unfavorable prognosis for diploid neuroblastomas (355–359). Amplification of the N-*myc* oncogene has also been associated with these diploid tumors (360–363). Recent analysis reveals a correlation between high S phase fraction and near-diploid/near-tetraploid DNA content, N-*myc* amplification, and more advanced disease (364). DNA content of neuroblastomas may also correlate with response to therapy (365). There are few data regarding DNA ploidy and Wilms' tumors (366) or nephroblastomas (367). Most rhabdomyosarcomas are aneuploid. Although DNA content has been correlated with age (368) and clinical stage (369), there is no definite evidence that ploidy is of important prognostic significance. A recent study showed both ploidy and SPF to correlate with poor prognosis in rhabdomyosarcoma (351).

Melanoma

Numerous analyses of patients with primary melanoma indicate a correlation between aneuploidy and higher recurrence rates and/or shorter survival (370–374). For metastatic melanoma, aneuploidy has been associated with both a more favorable prognosis (375, 376) and a worse outcome (372). Evaluation of S-phase fraction by flow cytometry is also of prognostic significance for stage III (374) and metastatic disease (376). For stage II melanoma, slow proliferation as measured by thymidine labeling indicates a significant advantage in relapse-free and overall survival (377). Experimentally, flow cytometry has been used to assess the effect of an autocrine-secreted melanoma-growth-inhibiting activity on the cytokinetics of tumor cells (378).

Hodgkin's Disease

The few studies of Hodgkin's disease that have been reported have noted a low frequency of aneuploidy (379–382). This may be the result of the difficulty encountered in isolating malignant cells from a large population of benign cells of similar composition (383). A recent retrospective analysis of 137 patients with Hodgkin's disease found no correlation between aneuploidy and other prognostic factors, or with survival (383). Although tumors with a high S-phase fraction had a less favorable outcome, this prognostic factor was not independent of others.

Non-Hodgkin's Lymphoma

Non-Hodgkin's lymphoma is such a heterogeneous collection of diseases that it is not surprising that the role of DNA flow cytometry remains ill defined, with many conflicting data (384, 385). Nevertheless, it is clear that aneuploidy is more common in lesions of high grade or of B-cell lineage (382, 386). As a prognostic factor, however, ploidy is neither strong nor independent (387–389). In contrast, most (390–394), but not all (395), studies have shown that S-phase fraction or other measures of proliferative activity are useful prognostically. S-phase fraction has been used to evaluate clinical course (396) and to augment histologic classification (397). In this regard, kinetic labeling with iododeoxyuridine and bromodeoxyuridine (398, 399) and flow cytometric analysis using a monoclonal antibody to an S-phase protein (400) are under investigation. Few data are available regarding the cytokinetics of such uncommon lymphomas as mycosis fungoides (401), nonendemic Burkitt's lymphoma (402), and gastric lymphoma (403).

Multiple Myeloma and Monoclonal Gammopathies

Aneuploidy is frequently found in cases of multiple myeloma, but it has also been found in benign monoclonal gammopathies (404, 405), so it is not an unequivocally distinguishing feature. One recent analysis found aneuploidy in bone marrow cells of 54% of 46 patients with untreated multiple myeloma (406). Only 1 of 15 patients with benign monoclonal gammopathy had aneuploid cells, and this patient had progressed to multiple myeloma 34 months later. In these cases, DNA content did not predict survival. Several studies of malignant disease have noted an association between aneuploidy and decreased survival (407–409), while others have not (410). Thus, a larger number of patients will need to be assessed in this regard. Labeling of bone marrow cells with bromodeoxyuridine and the monoclonal antibody Ki-67 can be used to determine proliferative activity in patients with multiple myeloma and monoclonal gammopathies (411, 412).

Leukemias

Flow cytometric analysis of leukemias has been used primarily for immunophenotypic classification, cytogenetic studies, and the determination of gene rearrangements (413). Regarding the prognostic significance of DNA content, several studies of childhood acute lymphoblastic leukemia (ALL) have noted that the presence of hyperdiploid blasts conveys a more favorable outcome and a better response to therapy (414, 415). Also, lower DNA content in the ALL blasts in children has been associated with a greater frequency of late relapses (416). However, in one trial the TLI of blasts before treatment was of no prognostic significance (417). Flow cytometry could be used to monitor residual disease in certain subgroups of ALL (418). Measurement of S phase activity by bromodeoxyuridine has been employed to assess the sensitivity of ALL cells to cytosine arabinoside and results have been mixed (419).

In ALL in adults, aneuploidy has been associated with a worse outcome (420). Although several studies have used a variety of techniques to assess the cell kinetics of acute myeloid leukemia (AML) and chronic myeloid leukemia, the prognostic value of these measurements remains unclear (421–428). Some have found that aneuploidy predicts a more favorable prognosis, as it does in childhood ALL (420). Bromodeoxyuridine labeling of leukemic promyelocytes revealed a lower labeling index and longer cell cycle than in other types of AML (429). These results were thought to be secondary to the marked expression of transforming growth factor-beta. One recent analysis of AML found that a high proliferative activity, as measured by BrdU labeling and proliferative cell nuclear antigen staining, was a positive prognostic factor for those receiving S-phase–specific drugs prior to being given anthracyclines (430A).

Growth Curve Analysis

The correlations between cytokinetics and clinical behavior support the concept that cell proliferation is intimately associated with the generation of tumor heterogeneity. Cell proliferation is, in addition, the primary mechanism for tumor growth. Anticancer therapy is, of course, intended to reverse growth by killing or removing cancer cells. Both upward and downward changes in the number of cells over time are described by a type of mathematic function called a growth curve. These curves not only summarize clinical course, but relate to the rate of emergence of mutations toward clinically relevant cellular diversity. Through both of these attributes, growth curves are proving useful in explaining human cancer and providing research directions toward improved cancer therapy.

SKIPPER-SCHABEL-WILCOX MODEL

The Skipper-Schabel-Wilcox model, or log-kill model, was the original, and is still the preeminent, model of tumor growth and therapeutic regression (430–431). It is based on the observation that leukemia L1210 in BDF_1 or DBA mice grows exponentially until it reaches a lethal tumor volume of 10^9 cells (1 cubic centimeter) (432). Ninety percent of the leukemia cells divide every 12 to 13 hours. This percentage is the same for both a tiny tumor and a tumor close to the lethal volume. As a result, the doubling time is always constant: if it takes 11 hours for 100 cells to grow into 200 cells, it will take 11 hours for 10^7 cells to grow into 2×10^7 cells. This pattern generalizes for any constant fractional increase: if it takes 40 hours for 10^3 cells to grow into 10^4 cells (an increase by a factor of 10*n*), it will take 40 hours for 10^7 cells to grow into 10^8 cells.

Exponential growth and the concept of the doubling time have concrete clinical implications (433). In the clinically observable range of tumor sizes there is great divergence in their doubling times among histologic types of cancers (434). The most therapeutically responsive human cancers, such as testicular cancer and choriocarcinoma, tend to have doubling times that are less than 1 month long. Less responsive cancers such as squamous cell cancer of the head and neck, seem to double in about 2 months. The relatively unresponsive cancers, such as colon adenocarcinoma, tend to double every 3 months. Clearly, this clinical observation may relate to the higher chemosensitivity of proliferating cells (see below). That is, if a tumor has a high fraction of dividing cells, it will tend to grow faster, and will also tend to be more responsive to drugs that kill dividing cells. Alternatively, tumors with a higher rate of cell loss tend to have a relatively slower growth rate and also a higher rate of mutations toward drug resistance. A combination of many such factors may be relevant. Regardless of the theoretic implications of the basic clinical observation, the unspoken assumption is that the fixed doubling time accurately summarizes the proliferative behavior of a given tumor. This questionable assumption will be examined below.

When a tumor that is growing exponentially and is homogeneous in drug sensitivity is treated with a specific chemotherapy regimen, the fraction of cells killed is always the same regardless of the initial size of the malignant population. This has been demonstrated in experimental animal cancers that do indeed grow exponentially, L1210 being the major example. If a given dose of a given drug reduces 10^6 cells to 10^5, the same therapy applied against 10^4 cells will result in 10^3 survivors. These two cytoreductions are both examples of a one-log kill, which means a 90% decrease in cell number. It was shown quite early that for many drugs the log kill increases with increasing dose (435, 436). Hence, it requires higher drug dosages to eradicate larger inoculum sizes of transplanted tumors. In addition, if two or more drugs are used, the log kills are multiplicative: if a given dose of drug A kills 90% of the cells (a one-log kill) and a given dose of drug B kills 90%, drug A given with drug B should kill 90% of the 10% of cells left after B alone, resulting in a kill of 99% of the cells (a two-log kill). As a numeric example, if treatment A given alone leaves 10^5 cells out of 10^6, and if treatment B given alone does the same, the combination A + B (at full doses of each) should be able to reduce 10^6 cells to 10^4. If treatment C is also a one-log kill therapy, A + B + C against 10^6 cells should leave only 10^3 cells. If A + B + C is used to treat 10^3 cells, only 10^0, or one, cell should remain. Thus, if enough drugs at adequate doses are applied against a tumor of sufficiently small size, the number of cells left after treatment should be smaller than one, which means that the tumor is cured. This concept was of major value in the design of early curative approaches to childhood leukemia (437).

When the concept of fractional kill was applied to the postoperative adjuvant treatment of micrometastases, it engendered enormous optimism (438, 439). After all, micrometastases are very small collections of cancer cells. Indeed, very small solid tumors in the laboratory contain a higher percentage of actively dividing cells than do their larger counterparts (26, 27). It is thought that most chemotherapeutic agents preferentially damage mitotic cells. Hence, the fraction of cells killed in a small tumor should actually be even greater than the fraction of cells killed in a histologically identical tumor of larger size. Therefore, according to the Skipper-Schabel-Wilcox model, if the log-kill estimate is wrong, the error should be in the direction of underestimating the impact of therapy against micrometastases. Small-volume tumors should be cured even more promptly by aggressive combination chemotherapy than would be predicted by the model.

Clinical experience with people, unfortunately, has not entirely confirmed these optimistic predictions. An illustration is the postoperative adjuvant chemotherapy of early-stage breast cancer. By Skipper's model, there would seem to be every reason to believe that aggressive combination chemotherapy should readily cure the micrometastases left after almost curative surgery (440, 441). The adjuvant chemotherapy of breast cancer with active agents at conventional doses does indeed reduce the probability of patients developing stage IV disease, and does result in improved survival. However, in most reports, this effect is relatively modest (442, 443). Is this because the duration of the therapy is not long enough? Assume that a given drug combination causes a one-log kill with each application. Six cycles of that combination should cure tumors of fewer than 10^6 cells. For tumors of exactly 10^6 cells, the six cycles would leave just one cell to regrow. If this were the case, then merely extending the duration of treatment beyond six cycles should kill the remaining cell and thereby increase the cure rate. From a modeling perspective, this same argument generalizes for higher degrees of cell kill and higher tumor cell burdens. Yet durations of exposure to the same chemotherapeutic regimen longer than 4 to 6 months have not improved results in adjuvant chemotherapy (443). Hence, the prediction of the model does not match actual observations.

As a consequence, if we accept the basic tenets of the Skipper-Schabel-Wilcox model, the failure of adjuvant chemotherapy to cure all cases of early breast cancer compels consideration of another possibility for failure to cure. Skipper and colleagues were aware of this divergence between theory and experience and considered that some cells in the tumor are biochemically refractory to the applied dose levels of the agents used. As we explore other models, we will see that it is not always necessary to hypothesize that absolutely refractory cells exist. Nevertheless, the inclusion of the concept of absolutely resistant cells in the Skipper-Schabel-Wilcox model can account for many observations. According to this reasoning, once all sensitive cells are eliminated by a certain length of treatment, continuing the same therapy for a longer duration will not give better results because all the cells left after that course cannot be killed by the drugs. If we assume that such resistance is acquired during a cancer's growth history by tumor progression (see below), the only way to guarantee the absence of resistant cells is to initiate therapy at so small a tumor size that no recalcitrant mutants are as yet present. In L1210, the transplantable mouse leukemia that was used to formulate the Skipper model, drug-resistant cells are rarely found in small aliquots. If this translates into spontaneous human cancer, it means that such cells would have to arise spontaneously at some time between the carcinogenic event and the appearance of larger amounts of tumor (444). If this were true, we would need answer only two questions: When in the course of growth does resistance develop? Can tumors be diagnosed early enough to be able to start treatment when the tumor is still curable (445)?

DELBRUCK-LURIA MODEL

To answer these questions, we must turn to quantitative models of the emergence of drug resistance. Drug resistance by whatever biochemical mechanism was recognized quite early to be important in cancer therapeutics (446), based originally on pioneering experiments in bacteriology. In 1943, Luria and Delbruck found that different bacterial cultures developed resistance to bacteriophage infection at random (and hence different) times in their growth histories, often long before exposure to the viruses (447). Later exposure to the viruses could be used to select the resistant bacteria and thereby measure the percentage of cells that had randomly acquired resistance. They reasoned that those cultures that had experienced a mutation earlier in their histories had more time to develop a high percentage of resistant bacteria. If a bacterium mutates toward property X with probability x at each mitosis, the probability of the cell not developing property X in one mitosis is $1 - x$. In y mitoses, the probability of no mutations occurring is $(1 - x)^y$. If each mitosis produces two viable cells (no cell loss), it takes $N - 1$ mitoses (not $N - 1$ generation times) for one cell to grow into N cells. That is, one mitosis produces two cells, each of these two cells undergoes mitosis (for a cumulative total of three mitoses) to produce four cells, each of these four divides (for a cumulative total of seven mitoses) to produce eight cells, and so on. Hence, the probability of not finding any bacteria with property X in N cells is $\exp[(N - 1) * \ln(1 - x)]$, which is approximately $\exp[-x(N - 1)]$ since x is small. A numeric example of the application of this formula is given below. Within a decade of Delbruck and Luria's original observation regarding bacteria, the same pattern was found by Law to apply to the emergence of methotrexate resistance in L1210 cells (448). Thus, antimetabolite resistance was reasoned to be a trait acquired spontaneously at random times in the pretreatment growth of this cancer.

The more modern view of cancer biology has not diminished enthusiasm for the concept of acquired mutations. Abnormalities of the process regulating the entry of G_1 cells into S could disinhibit replication, producing aberrant levels of DNA per neoplastic cell at each cell division (449–452). By this mechanism, aneuploidy, as well as drug resistance, should be a function of the number of mitoses. Cell loss would actually increase the probability of mutations per given cell number, since more cell divisions would be required to produce that cell number than if no cell loss had occurred.

GOLDIE-COLDMAN MODEL

In a qualitative sense, the kinetic observations of Delbruck, Luria, Law, and others were highly influential in the genesis and development of the concept of combination chemotherapy (453). If tumor cells could acquire resistance to a drug prior to exposure to that drug, then the therapist could be faced with a disease heterogeneous in drug sensitivity even at the time of first diagnosis. Only with combinations of drugs could one hope to eradicate all cells, since it has been deemed unlikely that any one cell could spontaneously become resistant to many different drugs, particularly if they had different biochemical sites of action (454). This concept formed the basis for the development of modern medical oncology. In a quantitative sense, the Delbruck-Luria model was applied again to human cancer in 1979 by Goldie and Coldman (455, 456). They later refined their original model to include multiple sublines with double or higher orders of drug resistance and the presence of cell loss (457). Their analysis contended that there is a high probability that mutations arise over a two-log (100-fold) increase in tumor size. That is, using the expression $\exp[-x(N - 1)]$, which was derived above, at a mutation rate x of 10^{-6} (which is tenable) (458), the probability of no mutants in 10^5 cells is $\exp[-10^{-6}(10^5 - 1)]$, which equals 0.905. Similarly, the probability of no mutants in 10^7 cells is 0.000045.

In this regard, it should be noted that while Goldie and Coldman focused on the property of drug resistance, an even clearer illustration of their concept might be found in the acquisition of metastatic ability. The capacity to metastasize is now established to be a reflection of genetic lability (459). The approximate volume of 10^7 packed cells is 0.01 cubic centimeter. If tumor cells are mixed with benign host tissue (including stromal cells, fibrosis, extracellular secretions, blood and lymphatic vessels, cellular infiltrate, and empty space) at a packing ratio of 1:10, 10^7 cancer cells will occupy a volume of 0.1 cubic centimeter. At a packing ratio of 1:100, which is often more realistic, 10^7 cancer cells would be found in a tumor volume of about 1.0 cubic centimeter. This example of scaling relates directly to clinical data. In primary breast cancer, the best predictor of axillary metastases is tumor size. Only 17% of invasive ductal lesions under 1 centimeter in diameter are metastatic to the axilla, contrasted with 41% of lesions of 2 centimeters in diameter and 68% of tumors of 5 to 10 centimeters (460). For primary breast cancer that does not involve axillary lymph nodes, the probability of eventual metastatic spread increases sharply when the mass in the breast is greater than 1 centimeter in diameter (461). Hence, metastatic ability is conspicuously more common in tumors larger than this critical size. A 1 centimeter spherical tumor contains a volume of slightly over 0.5 cubic centimeter, which is right in the middle of the range of 0.1 to 1.0 cubic centimeter described above. These calculations fit the model with reassuring precision, but they cannot be regarded as proof of the model, since other explanations are possible (see "Mitotoxicity Hypothesis" below).

Regarding drug sensitivity, the Goldie-Coldman model has generated specific, testable predictions. The model predicts that a cancer arising from a single, drug-sensitive malignant cell has a 90% chance of being curable at 10^5 cells. If it has a 90% chance of being curable at that size, it will almost certainly become incurable by the time it grows to 10^7 cells. Thus, tumors larger than 0.1 to 1.0 cubic centimeter should always be incurable with any single agent. This led these authors to the conclusion that the best strategy is to treat as small a tumor as possible as early as possible, that is, perioperatively or even preoperatively. Once treatment is started, as many effective drugs as possible should be applied as soon as possible to prevent cells that are already resistant to one drug from mutating to resistance to others.

These recommendations are intuitive, conforming to established empiric principles of combination chemotherapy (462). They differ from classic principles only in that they concentrate on the emergence of resistance during treatment, as contrasted with the likelihood that resistance is already present at the start of treatment. Most uniquely, they imply that if several drugs cannot be used simultaneously at good therapeutic levels (because of overlapping toxicity or competitive interference), they should be used in a strict alternating sequence. This recommendation is based on several assumptions: that cells sensitive to a given therapy A (and resistant to therapy B) are as sensitive to therapy A as are cells sensitive to therapy B (but resistant to therapy A) are sensitive to therapy B; that the rate of mutation toward biochemical resistance is constant in both sublines (with cells sensitive to A mutating toward resistance to A, and cells sensitive to B mutating to resistance to B); and that the growth pattern and growth rates of the two sublines are equivalent (463). These assumptions fit under the general mathematical term "symmetry." Critical appraisal of the various assumptions and conclusions of the Goldie-Coldman model has raised several interesting points. It would be informative to examine these in some detail to show the relevance of growth curve analysis to clinical problems.

The first assumption that we must question concerns the notion that all chemotherapeutic failure is rooted in absolute drug resistance. Contrary evidence exists: lymphomas and leukemias frequently respond to the same chemotherapy when they relapse after the chemotherapeutic achievement of complete remission. Patients with Hodgkin's disease who achieve complete remission with combination chemotherapy and who relapse 18 or more months later have an excellent chance of attaining complete remission again when the same chemotherapy is reapplied (464). Similarly, after they relapse, breast adenocarcinomas frequently respond to further chemotherapy. The Cancer and Leukemia Group B (CALGB) treated patients with advanced breast cancer with cyclophosphamide, Adriamycin (doxorubicin), and 5-fluorouracil (CAF) with or without tamoxifen (465). Although none of these patients had prior chemotherapy for their advanced disease, some had had prior adjuvant chemotherapy. The response rate, response duration, and overall survival were unaffected by a patient's past history of adjuvant chemotherapy, however. Similarly, patients on trials at the National Cancer Institute in Milan who developed stage IV breast cancer after adjuvant cyclophosphamide, methotrexate, and 5-fluorouracil (CMF) responded as well to CMF for advanced disease as those who previously had been randomized to be treated with radical mastectomy alone (466). From this we may safely conclude that breast cancers that regrow after exposure to adjuvant CMF are not universally resistant to CMF (467). We are now observing that patients experiencing recurrence of stage IV disease after the failure of high-dose chemotherapy (autologous bone marrow transplantation) can benefit in terms of tumor response to the reapplication of conventional doses of chemotherapy drugs. Hence, not all chemotherapeutic failure can be attributable to permanent drug resistance. It is possible that some cancers escape cure because of a temporary absolute drug resistance that reverses over time. It is also possible, however, that cancers can escape cure even though some of their cells are not absolutely resistant. This theme will be developed further as we consider other growth models.

Another prediction from the Goldie-Coldman model that is interesting to examine is that tumors larger than 1.0 cubic centimeter (10^7 cells at a packing ratio of 1:100, 10^9 cells at maximum density packing) cannot be cured with single drugs. Two rapidly growing cancers, gestational choriocarcinoma and Burkitt's lymphoma, both densely packed, have been cured with single drugs (468), even when therapy is initiated at tumor sizes much larger than 1.0 cubic centimeter. Childhood acute lymphoblastic leukemias, other pediatric cancers, adult lymphomas, and germ cell tumors of greater than 10^{10} cells are frequently cured with couplets and triplets of drugs. Hence, the size of 10^7 cells does not always mean incurability.

For the purposes of planning chemotherapy schedules, the Goldie-Coldman model speculates that mutations develop rapidly during the treatable portion of a cancer's growth history. This may seem tenable since in our previous discussion of cell proliferation we established that genetic lability is a key attribute of neoplasia. Yet clinical observations hint at a deeper level of complexity. For example, let us examine metastatic ability as a measure of the rate of mutations. A primary breast cancer left untreated to grow in the breast, as was standard practice in the 19th century, always became metastatic (469). Yet at 30 years of follow-up after radical mastectomy (with no adjuvant chemotherapy), more than 30% of patients are alive and free of disease (470, 471). The mortality rate drops gradually from about 10% per year in the first year to about 2% per year by year 25 (472), but a plateau is reached after 30 years, with a rate of mortality indistinguishable from that of the general population (473, 474). This means that most, if not all, breast cancers have the potential for developing metastases, as was seen in the 19th century before mastectomy was widely used. Indeed, many, but not all, have already done so by the time of initial presentation. Let us consider the case of a primary cancer that is diagnosed in the breast before it has developed metastatic ability. If the cancer cells in the breast are not completely removed or destroyed, will the residual cells mutate rapidly to produce metastatic clones? A protocol of the National Surgical Adjuvant Breast and Bowel Project (NSABP) asked this question (475). Some patients with primary disease were treated by lumpectomy without radiotherapy. The local relapse rate was significant, indicating that residual tumor was left unchecked. Yet such patients did not have a higher metastatic rate (measured by the survival rate) than patients treated adequately de novo by lumpectomy plus immediate radiotherapy or by mastectomy (see Chapter 136). This result is surprising since some metastases from residual cancer should be expected even if that residual disease did not progress in its ability to release metastatic clones. Longer follow-up of this trial might eventually reveal a higher rate of distant metastases. However, the absence at 12 years of a major negative survival impact of local recurrence indicates that tumor can remain in a breast, grow in the breast, and yet not develop metastatic cells at a very high rate. If metastases develop, therefore, the odds are that they have already done so before the time of first clinical presentation.

In a similar vein, the Goldie-Coldman model concludes that for chemotherapy to be effective it must be started as soon as possible after diagnosis. Contradictory evidence exists, however. For example, in an early trial of the treatment of acute leukemia, the response to an antimetabolite was the same if that drug was used first or sequentially after the use of a different antimetabolite (475A). In a randomized trial, the International (Ludwig) Breast Cancer Study Group found that it was equally effective to give node-positive breast cancer patients either 7 months of chemotherapy starting within 36 hours of surgery or 6 months of chemotherapy starting about 4 weeks later (475B). Another trial randomized patients with stage B nonseminomatous testicular cancer after retroperitoneal lymph node dissection either to two cycles of cisplatin combination chemotherapy or to observation (476). At a median follow-up of 4 years, 6% of patients randomized to adjuvant chemotherapy relapsed as compared with 49% of patients randomized to observation. Yet because the response of relapsing cases to subsequent chemotherapy was excellent, there was no significant survival difference between the two approaches. Hence, most testicular carcinomas retained their chemosensitivity in spite of a prolonged period of unperturbed growth. We may conclude, therefore, that for both breast and testicular cancer, cells that are residual after surgery can grow unperturbed and yet not develop drug-resistant mutants at a fast rate.

If, as predicted by the Goldie-Coldman model, adjuvant treatment must be instituted as early as possible after surgery to be effective, all drugs in an adjuvant regimen must be introduced immediately to have a biologic impact. This was questioned in a trial by the CALGB (477, 478). Node-positive patients with primary breast cancer were treated with 8 months of an adjuvant CMF regimen (plus vincristine and prednisone) followed by either more CMFVP or 6 months of vinblastine, Adriamycin, thiotepa, and halotestin (VATH). Patients receiving the crossover therapy had a significantly improved disease-free survival, especially those with four or more involved axillary nodes. Thus, dominant resistance to VATH did not develop in the 8 months of CMFVP treatment in the cells remaining after treatment with CMFVP. It is of note that a trial in Milan found no advantage to adriamycin following CMF for patients with one to three involved nodes (479), which corroborates the CALGB's finding of the relative inactivity of this sequence approach for patients with low degrees of nodal involvement. The implications of the CALGB's results in patients with higher degrees of nodal involvement, including the issues of simultaneous versus sequential therapies, dose scheduling, and optimal duration, are discussed in more detail below.

The assertion most singularly identified with the Goldie-Coldman model is the recommendation for alternating chemotherapy sequences. Has this strategy demonstrated unequivocal advantages? Numerous attempts to improve the prognosis of patients with small-cell lung cancer by alternating chemotherapy sequences have resulted in little or no benefit (480). In the treatment of diffuse aggressive non-Hodgkin's lymphoma, the National Cancer Institute found no advantage to a ProMACE-MOPP hybrid, which delivered eight drugs during each monthly cycle, over a treatment plan delivering a full course of ProMACE (prednisone, methotrexate, Adriamycin, cyclophosphamide, etoposide), which was then followed by MOPP (mechlorethamine, vincristine, procarbazine, prednisone) (481). For advanced Hodgkin's disease, MOPP has been compared with MOPP alternating with Adriamycin, bleomycin, vinblastine, and dacarbazine (ABVD). ABVD is an effective first-line therapy for Hodgkin's disease and is also an effective salvage regimen for patients refractory to MOPP (482, 483). Among chemotherapy-naive patients, MOPP-ABVD was found to be superior to MOPP with regard to complete remission rate, freedom from progression, and survival (484, 485). However, the CALGB found that the complete remission rate and failure-free survival with MOPP-ABVD, although better than with MOPP alone, was not different from that with ABVD alone (486). The superiority of MOPP-ABVD and ABVD over MOPP may have been due to differences in dose received, since only about 40% of MOPP patients received full doses of the cytotoxic agents by the third cycle, whereas these percentages were greater than 70% on ABVD and on MOPP-ABVD. At comparable levels of received dose, there were no clear advantages to the alternation of MOPP and ABVD over ABVD alone. Similarly, the National Cancer Institute found no advantage to MOPP alternating with lomustine, Adriamycin, bleomycin, and streptozocin over MOPP alone (487). An American intergroup trial has found that a hybrid of MOPP-ABVD was superior in complete remission duration, failure-free survival, and overall survival to MOPP followed by ABVD (488). As with MOPP-ABVD in the CALGB trial, however, it is possible that this result may be explained by the observation that patients treated with the hybrid regimen received higher doses because of the necessity to modify for toxicity the doses of MOPP in the regimen that delivered MOPP followed by ABVD. It is also possible that the earlier introduction of Adriamycin in the hybrid might have been advantageous because such an approach could diminish the adverse impact of the emergence of multidrug resistance. These points are discussed in the context of the Norton-Simon model.

As with the lymphomas, in the treatment of breast cancer, alternating cycles that have not resulted in a dosage difference have not proved advantageous. For example, the VATH regimen is active against tumors relapsing from or failing to respond to CMF, and thereby meets the non–cross-resistance requirements of the Goldie-Coldman model (489). In patients with advanced disease, the CALGB found no advantage to CMFVP alternating with VATH over CAF or VATH alone (490). A direct comparison of alternating and sequential chemotherapy in the adjuvant chemotherapy of breast cancer was conducted in Milan. This group had previously generated historically controlled data that suggested a benefit from a sequential approach (491), the rationale for which is discussed below (492). In the more recent study, female patients with stage II breast cancer involving four or more axillary lymph nodes were randomized between two arms (493). Arm I prescribed four 3-week courses of Adriamycin (A) followed by eight 3-week courses of IV CMF (C), symbolized as AAAACCCCCCCC. Arm II stipulated the use of two courses of IV CMF alternated with one course of Adriamycin four times for a total of 12 courses, symbolized as CCACCACCACCA. The total amounts of Adriamycin and CMF in both arms were equal, yet the patients who received arm I had a higher disease-free survival and a higher overall survival than those did on arm II. With total dose controlled, alternating courses of chemotherapy were found to be inferior to a crossover therapy plan. These preliminary results have been confirmed by long-term follow-up analysis (494).

The sequential application of drugs has proved to be a useful strategy in the treatment of leukemias. In adult acute myelogenous leukemia, a high rate of complete remission is obtained with cytarabine plus anthracyclines, but the duration of the responses is short. Postremission maintenance therapy has been shown by the CALGB to be relatively ineffective when given at low doses (495). Moreover, a trial showed that 32 months of postremission therapy were not superior to 8 months of the same therapy (496), similar to the failure of longer courses of adjuvant chemotherapy to improve results achieved by 4 to 6 months of such treatment in breast cancer (443). A randomized trial was recently reported that studied 596 patients out of 1,088 who had achieved complete remission with induction chemotherapy (497). This trial was designed to question the effectiveness of intensive postremission chemotherapy, exploiting the steep dose-response curve for cytarabine (498). The study found that the high-dose regimen was the best of three different dose schedules of cytarabine. Indeed, the best results were comparable to those reported in similar patients undergoing allogeneic bone marrow transplantation during first remission (497, 499). The Children's Cancer Group has reported that intensive induction, followed sequentially by intensive consolidation and later intensification, was superior to other strategies in the treatment of childhood acute lymphoblastic leukemia (500). These observations have major practical and theoretic implications, as they suggest that strategies other than those advocated by the Goldie-Coldman hypothesis may have significant clinical impact.

The foregoing detailed examination of the Goldie-Coldman model illustrates the relevance of growth curve analysis to treatment design. The Goldie-Coldman model is mathematically sensible, and may well be applicable to some aspects of cancer biology. The model is also of major historic importance in that it rekindled interest in the quantitative development of drug resistance. These two points are valid even if several of the model's major predictions have not been sustained by clinical data. One common reason for such a discrepancy between tenable theory and empiric results is the invalidity of underlying assumptions. An assumption of particular consequence in this regard that merits reevaluation concerns the concept of absolute drug resistance.

IMPLICATIONS OF RELATIVE DRUG RESISTANCE

It is now well established that much drug resistance is relative rather than absolute (501). A cell that is absolutely resistant cannot be killed with any pharmacologic dose level of the agent. Relative drug resistance, on the other hand, depends on the dose level employed. In terms of the Skipper-Schabel-Wilcox model, one tumor may experience a log kill of two (99% reduction in cell number) when it is exposed to a certain dose and duration of treatment. Another, more resistant, tumor may experience a log kill of one (90% shrinkage) when it is treated with exactly the same therapy. However, if the dose intensity of chemotherapy against the relatively resistant tumor is increased, the log kill can increase as well (502, 503).

Clinically, even twofold increases in dose level can have profound effects on the curative impact of chemotherapy (501), although this is not always seen with all drugs in all diseases (504). However, in retrospective analyses of the adjuvant chemotherapy of operable breast cancer (505, 506) and the chemotherapy of advanced lymphoma (507), a high dose seems to be a key beneficial variable. The validity of conclusions based on retrospective data has been questioned (508, 509). In randomized trials in childhood acute lymphoblastic leukemia (510), adult germ cell tumors (511), advanced breast cancer (512), and breast cancer in the adjuvant setting (513), the higher-dose regimen has proved superior, however.

From a kinetic viewpoint, the importance of dose is defensible. In many animal experiments, the log kill will be greater for the regimen with a higher dose intensity (514). The concept of dose intensity requires definition. It is not just the total amount of drug received, nor is it just the amount of drug received per unit of time; rather, it is a mathematic combination of both. If regimen I gives X amount of drug over Y days, and if regimen II gives $2X$ amount of drug over Y days, then regimen II is clearly more dose intensive. Regimen III, giving X amount of drug over $Y/2$ days, is also more intensive than regimen I. Although the dose rate of drug delivery of regimen III ($2X/Y$ drug per day) is equivalent to regimen II, regimen II delivers more total drug and thus may be superior to regimen III in clinical efficacy. Hence, dose intensity alone may not account for clinical superiority. Yet sometimes, once a certain minimal total dose is achieved, further increases in total dose are unimportant. For example, a number of trials have shown that durations of adjuvant chemotherapy longer than 4 to 6 months do not improve clinical results in operable breast cancer (515–518). Therefore, once the minimal total dose is determined empirically and adhered to, dose intensity should be an important determinant of cell kill.

The shape of the relationship between cell-killing capacity and dose is not totally clear for any drug, but for some agents, some data suggest a strictly proportional relationship. The randomized trial by the CALGB that treated node-positive patients by one of three plans of CAF adjuvant treatment (cyclophosphamide, doxorubicin, 5-fluorouracil) may be used as an example (513). Let *Z* equal a certain total cumulative dose of chemotherapy: the three regimens gave either 2*Z* over 4 months (plan I), 2*Z* over 6 months (plan II), or *Z* over 4 months (plan III). Plan I was superior to plan III in reducing the rate of recurrence, but no difference between plan I and plan II has as yet been reported. Hence, the total anticancer influence of one of these regimens seems to be strictly proportional to the total dose administered. For plan I it was 2*Z*, the sum of 2*Z* over the first 4 months plus zero for the 2 additional months. Plan II also gave 2*Z* but over the entire 6 months. Plan III delivered half as much total anticancer influence, the sum of *Z* over the first 4 months, then zero for the remaining 2 months. A proportional dose–response relationship would predict that plan III should be inferior to both plan I and plan II. One qualifier in this argument is that if CAF chemotherapy cures some patients, then plan I might eventually prove to be superior to plan II, because the cancer cell killing accomplished at 4 months from 2*Z* given over 4 months should be greater than the cell killing measured at 4 or at 6 months from 2*Z* given over 6 months. For some patients given 2*Z* over 4 months, the log kill might be enough to preclude disease regrowth.

This analysis suggests that clinical treatment failure may be the consequence of insufficient dose intensity (i.e., 2*Z* over 6 months when it could have been given over 4 months). A tumor may relapse because some of its cells, relatively but not absolutely insensitive to the agents applied, are not exposed to enough drug to be eradicated. This is analogous to a bacterial infection relapsing because an insufficient dose intensity of an antibiotic is applied, even though the microorganisms are sensitive in vitro. In both infection and neoplasia, however, prolonged or repeated episodes of low-dose therapy can give rise to absolute resistance by the selection of biochemically resistant cells.

If insufficient dose intensity is a major cause of failure to cure, then it is possible that increased dose intensity itself can improve clinical results (519, 520). This statement is phrased as a possibility rather than as a certainty because it is highly dependent on the host tolerance and on the shape (steepness) of the dose–response curve for each agent for each disease. It also depends on the shape of the curve of tumor volume regression, which is considered in the next section.

GOMPERTZIAN MODEL

The log-kill model was formulated from, and is expressed in terms of, exponential growth. Nodular pulmonary metastases and, much less commonly, measurable lesions in other sites do seem to follow exponential growth during periods of observation that are short in relation to the total life histories of the tumors (521–523). Doubling times, ranging from 1 week to 1 year, with a median of 1 to 3 months, correlate with histologic type, growth fraction, and cell loss fraction. Yet many, if not all, human cancers do not grow exponentially with a constant doubling time (524–526). A nonexponential growth pattern of major importance was first described by Benjamin Gompertz in 1825 (527). In exponential growth, the fixed doubling time means that the growth rate relative to tumor size always remains constant. In Gompertzian growth, however, the doubling time increases steadily as the tumor grows larger. Figure 52.2 illustrates a typical breast cancer (the specifics of this tumor's Gompertzian growth are detailed below). Between 10^2 cells and clinical appreciation at 10^{10} cells, the shape of the growth curve on the semilogarithmic plot deflects downward. An exponential curve would appear as a straight line. The progressive slowing of Gompertzian growth may be more the result of decreased cell production than of increased cell loss in larger tumors (26, 27). A consequence is that if a Gompertzian tumor is erroneously assumed to be exponential, the doubling time during the preclinical phase of growth will be assumed to be too slow (528). The assumption of exponentiality has led to some unrealistic estimates of the time from carcinogenesis to the appearance of clinical disease.

The biologic basis for Gompertzian growth is still unclear. The old concept, that a solid tumor "outgrows" its supply of nutrients and so cannot sustain unimpeded exponential growth, has been challenged by evidence that large tumors, with relatively slow growth rates, often have adequate vascularity. Indeed, neovascularization is an important feature of malignancy (529). A new concept concerns the relation between the cancer cell and its local environment (530). Most cancers are composed of repeating elements—such as branching tree patterns or multiple nodules—that are self-similar over various scales of size. As a fractal geometric pattern, this means that the number of cells is proportional to the tumor volume raised to a power less than or equal to one, that power being a function of the packing ratio. Low packing ratios produce low power constants and, therefore, low ratios of number of cells per volume of tumor. Such tumors, with relatively few cells per microscopic field, tend to be more benign, whereas cancers with densely packed cancer cells and little intervening stroma tend to be more malignant. It has been shown that masses growing in a manner that preserves the power relationship between cell number and volume follow a Gompertzian curve. The rate of deviation from exponentiality is functionally related to the power constant; values close to one give more aggressive growth, and smaller values give Gompertzian curves that plateau at a benign size, as in ductal carcinoma in situ of the breast (530). An interesting aspect of this thesis is that a precancerous mass can suddenly become recognizable as malignant with just a small additional increment in the power constant over a certain threshold. Since the power constant reflects the packing ratio, tumors with widely varying packing ratios can be benign, but once the cellular population is close to a critical degree of tight packing, a further small change toward increased packing could be associated with malignant transformation. The molecular bases of the power constants that define Gompertzian growth is an active topic of study,

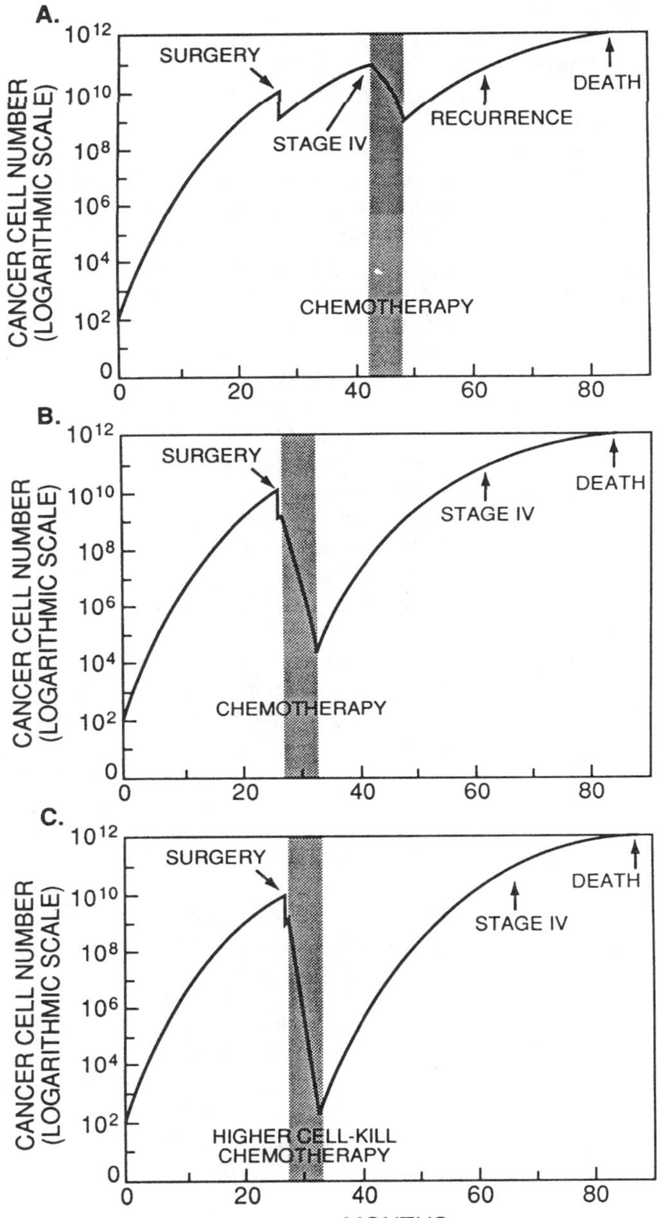

Figure 52.2. Gompertzian model of breast cancer growth.

but current hypotheses concern autocrine and paracrine growth factor loops, which might also determine invasion and metastases (530).

SPEER-RETSKY MODEL

Some of the important characteristics of Gompertzian growth will be illustrated below using a new model of human breast cancer (531). In the 19th century, breast cancer was often followed from diagnosis to death without surgery or any other effective treatment (469). Speer, Retsky, and colleagues used survival histories for such patients, plus the growth histories of mammographic shadows (532), and data for disease-free survival following mastectomy (533), to fit a model in which tumors grow in randomly increasing steps of Gompertzian plateaus (534). This work is interesting because it demonstrates that growth curves that deviate far from exponentiality can fit clinical data. However, the validity of the model has been challenged on several counts. First, it is questionable whether the temporary plateaus that are predicted by the model are ever actually observed (508). Second, the Speer-Retsky model predicts that to maximize the efficacy of postsurgical adjuvant chemotherapy, it should be applied intermittently over a prolonged duration so as to coincide with the presumed growth spurts. This approach, however, proved ineffective in a clinical trial (535). Third, the same clinical data can be fitted more parsimoniously, and with greater accuracy, by a family of simple Gompertzian curves (531). A family of exponential curves could also be fitted to these data, but the model that would result could not account for both disease-free survival and overall survival because the time from relapse to death would be too short. The curve used in Figure 52.2 is the median curve from the family of simple Gompertzian curves mentioned above (531). Note that it takes just $3\frac{1}{2}$ months for the tumor to increase by two logs from 10^2 to 10^4. Yet it takes $5\frac{1}{2}$ months for 10^9 cells to grow just one log to 10^{10}. This is a relevant example of increasing doubling time with increasing tumor volume.

NORTON-SIMON MODEL

The Skipper-Schabel-Wilcox model is so meaningful because it conceptualizes both tumor growth (exponential) and tumor regression (log kill) in response to chemotherapy. We have already discussed the profound implications of the positive association between the rate of tumor regression and the dose intensity of chemotherapy. Experimental and clinical data also indicate that the rate of tumor regression is positively related to the growth rate of the unperturbed tumor just prior to treatment (536, 537). This important observation is corroborated by data showing that the logarithm of the surviving fraction of an experimental neoplasm is negatively correlated with the logarithm of the tumor size at the time of treatment (538).

This concept extends the Skipper-Schabel-Wilcox model. In exponential growth, the growth rate is always proportional to tumor size. If a tumor at size X is growing at rate Y, the same tumor at size $2X$ would grow at rate $2Y$. On a logarithmic scale, these growth rates would appear to be the same since the rate of growth per tumor size (Y/X) is the same in both cases. A rate of regression proportional to growth rate is, therefore, also proportional to tumor size, which results in a constant proportional (or "log") kill. That is, if the tumor at size X shrinks at rate Z to achieve a size $X/2$ in 1 week (a change in size by the proportion of one half), the tumor at size $2X$ treated with the same chemotherapy would shrink at rate $2Z$ to achieve size X in one week (also a change by the proportion of one half). The absolute volume shrinkage would be $X/2$ in the first case and X in the second case, but the proportional change would be one half in both cases (X to $X/2$; $2X$ to X). The distinction between the Skipper-Schabel-Wilcox model and the Norton-Simon model is that in

Gompertzian growth, unlike exponential growth, the growth rate of the unperturbed tumor is always changing. That is, if a tumor at size X grows at rate Y, the same tumor at size $2X$ would not grow at rate $2Y$.

In Figure 52.2 a realistic numeric example illustrates the implications of Gompertzian regression. In Figure 52.2*A* the tumor is observed to grow to clinical diagnosis at 10^{10} cells (about 10 cubic centimeters of packed tumor cells or about 100 cubic centimeters at a packing ratio of 1:10). Let us assume for the purposes of this illustration that 90% of the tumor is in the breast and axillary lymph nodes, and about 10% of the cells are scattered in various micrometastatic sites. The mass in the breast itself would be about 5 centimeters in diameter. If this mass and the axillary contents are removed completely (or destroyed completely with radiotherapy), the total body's burden of tumor is reduced to the 10^9 metastatic cells. Since the 10^9 cancer cells are spread throughout the body, they are invisible to our diagnostic tests. No adjuvant therapy is given. The tumor grows for $13\frac{1}{2}$ months until it reaches about 10^{11} cells in total number, which is large enough for detection as metastases. At this time, chemotherapy is employed, reducing the total cell number to about 10^9 (a two-log kill). A period of remission is experienced but the tumor eventually relapses, leading to death at 10^{12} cells.

Figure 52.2*B* graphs the same tumor, but here the same chemotherapy is applied in the adjuvant setting at a total tumor size of 10^9 cells. The relative rate of growth (the slope of the curve on this semilogarithmic plot) is faster for the tumor at 10^9 cells than it would be for the same tumor at 10^{11} cells. This is clear from inspection of Figure 52.2*A*. According to the Norton-Simon model, the relative rate of regression of the 10^9-cell tumor will be faster as well, even though the dose and schedule of chemotherapy are identical. Figure 52.2*B* shows that the chemotherapy that had caused a two-log kill of 10^{11} cells causes instead a five-log kill of 10^9 cells. The 10^4 cells that result regrow to relapse as stage IV disease at 10^{11} cells and to kill the patient at 10^{12} cells. Comparison of Figures 52.2*A* and 52.2*B* demonstrates a remarkable result. The time from surgery to stage IV is clearly longer when adjuvant chemotherapy is applied. However, the time from surgery to death is identical! The greater fractional kill in the adjuvant setting is counterbalanced by a faster fractional regrowth. This may explain why the adjuvant chemotherapy of breast cancer has less impact on overall survival (a function of eventual tumor body burden) than on disease-free survival. It may also explain why the survival duration of patients with stage IV breast cancer has remained fairly stable in recent decades in spite of more aggressive approaches to management (539–541).

What if another chemotherapy plan, more aggressive but still subcurative, is used in the adjuvant setting against the 10^9 cells? This is illustrated in Figure 52.2*C*. If 10^2 cells are left instead of 10^4, it will take only $3\frac{1}{2}$ months longer for the tumor to reach 10^{12}, since the growth from 10^2 cells to 10^4 cells is very rapid. Hence, adjuvant therapies can differ greatly in log kill, with only a slight impact on eventual clinical results measured years later. This slight impact could easily be lost in the "noise" caused by random fluctuations, especially in clinical data sets of small size. The pessimistic side of this observation is that more aggressive chemotherapy may produce little real clinical benefit. The optimistic side is that, if this model holds, current adjuvant chemotherapies for breast cancer are actually bringing us much closer to total cellular eradication than we might otherwise be led to suspect.

Survival can be improved to a significant degree only when tumor cell populations are actually eradicated or their regrowth is otherwise meaningfully impeded. In our previous discussion of cellular proliferation, we concluded that heterogeneity in drug sensitivity is a characteristic of neoplasia. How can tumor cell eradication be accomplished in a heterogeneous cancer? Gompertzian regression means that slower-growing collections of tumor cells will tend to regress more slowly in response to a given therapy than will the faster-growing tumor cells treated at the same time (542). In a heterogeneous cancer, therefore, the slower-growing clones are also the most kinetically resistant. These slower-growing cells should be in the minority by the time of diagnosis because by then they should have been overgrown by the faster-growing cells. The existence of a population of slow-growing cells may also be the consequence of the hypothetic ability of chemotherapy to differentiate cells that are not killed (543).

The best way to treat a heterogeneous population is to treat the dominant, faster-growing populations as efficiently as possible, and then to treat the numerically inferior, slower-growing populations as efficiently as possible (492). As in the Skipper-Schabel-Wilcox model, the most efficient therapy is the most dose-intensive therapy, giving as much drug as possible over as short a period as possible. This is accomplished much better by crossover therapy than by strict alternation. For example, in the adjuvant breast cancer trial from Milan described above, the alternating plan, CCACCACCACCA, gave eight cycles of CMF over 30 weeks and four cycles of Adriamycin over 33 weeks (494). The crossover plan, AAAACCCCCCCC, gave eight cycles of CMF over 33 weeks and four cycles of Adriamycin over 9 weeks. The dose intensity of the CMF was almost the same, but for Adriamycin it was significantly improved by the crossover. This by itself could account for the superiority of the crossover treatment. A similar result has also been seen in the adjuvant chemotherapy of resected osteosarcoma: Adriamycin alone was superior to Adriamycin alternating with high-dose methotrexate, presumably because the dose intensity of the superior agent (Adriamycin) was impaired by the alternation (544). The results of trials in acute leukemia in adults and children (500) described above are also consistent with the concept of crossover treatment as a means of increasing dose intensity and clinical benefit.

It is important to note that these treatment protocols incorporate two methods of increasing dose intensity. One method is to increase the dose, keeping the time constant. This may be termed "dose escalation." The second, best illustrated by the breast cancer trial (494) and the trial in osteosarcoma (544), is to keep doses constant, but alter the schedule so as to give the doses of the important drugs closer together in time. This may be termed "dose density." AAAACCCCCCCC gives both doxorubicin (A) and cyclophosphamide (C) more densely than CCACCACCACCA. The leukemia trials both escalate doses and use regimens sequentially to increase density, increasing dose intensity by both methods.

In the breast cancer trial from Milan (494), the use of Adriamycin initially might have caused greater cell kill by avoiding the expression of the multidrug-resistance gene, which tends to progress over time, independent of treatment (545, 546). Conversely, the delayed use of Adriamycin might have compromised the efficacy of two other regimens described previously: ABVD following prolonged MOPP for advanced Hodgkin's disease (488) and Adriamycin following 6 months of CMF for primary breast cancer with low degrees of nodal involvement (479). A pilot study in breast cancer used Adriamycin following just 16 weeks of CMFVP in patients with node-positive primary disease (547). The study has established the feasibility of this approach, but the determination of comparative efficacy awaits a randomized trial.

Although the invention and interpretation of clinical trials intended to test cytokinetic principles are fraught with subtleties and complexities, crossover therapy has been successful in the laboratory. The only way to cure 10^8 L1210 cells is by induction with cytosine arabinoside plus 6-thioguanine for two or three courses, followed by one course of high doses of cyclophosphamide and BCNU given simultaneously (548). In the treatment of BDF1 mice bearing the M5076 tumor, the addition of one dose of L-phenylalanine mustard (L-PAM) (a drug that by itself is only weakly active) after four doses of methyl-CCNU doubles the complete remission rate and the median survival (549). The presumed mechanism for this latter effect is that the few cells left after methyl-CCNU induction are L-PAM sensitive, whereas in the untreated situation, most cells are methyl-CCNU sensitive, L-PAM resistant. In general, alkylating agents seem particularly helpful as the crossover therapy.

Goldie and Coldman's prediction of the superiority of alternating chemotherapy assumed stringent conditions of symmetrical tumor cell numbers, growth rates, and mutation rates. Day has performed computer simulations of mutation to drug resistance under asymmetrical conditions (550). He came to a conclusion similar to the Norton-Simon model regarding the expected superiority of a crossover plan (551). By his "worst drug rule," in a coordinated two-regimen plan, the therapy with a lower cell kill per treatment (the worst drug) should be used either first or, if it is used second, for a longer duration. However, the Norton-Simon model qualifies this to specify that the induction therapy must be sufficiently cytoreductive for the residual tumor cell burden to be low. This is another possible reason for the inferiority of ABVD following dose-reduced (and, hence, less cytotoxic) MOPP as compared with a hybrid MOPP/ABV, which could be delivered at fuller dosages (488). The theoretic argument, therefore, would be in favor of an efficient induction followed by one or more aggressive chemotherapeutic crossovers. Indeed, in the treatment of acute lymphocytic leukemia in children, a classic trial demonstrated that induction by vincristine plus prednisone facilitates the anticancer activity of crossover methotrexate (552). The Children's Cancer Study Group trial in childhood leukemia that gave intensive induction, consolidation, and intensification also demonstrated the importance of initial cytoreduction (500).

At present, a number of trials seeking to improve clinical results by increasing dose density and dose escalation are in progress. Many treatment plans are facilitated by the ability of hematopoietic growth factors such as G-CSF and GM-CSF (553)—and other means of hematopoietic reconstitution (554, 555) to permit dose intensification. In the adjuvant chemotherapy of high-risk breast cancer, the Southwest Oncology Group is coordinating an intergroup study of doxorubicin followed by G-CSF–supported high-dose cyclophosphamide versus a more conventional, simultaneous doxorubicin plus cyclophosphamide combination (556). Investigators at Memorial Sloan-Kettering Cancer Center have piloted a regimen giving dose-dense Adriamycin followed by dose-dense paclitaxel followed by dose-dense cyclophosphamide, called ATC (556). Current intergroup plans call for a randomized comparison of this regimen with another form of dose intensification—short-course, high-dose combination chemotherapy with hematopoietic "stem cell" support—in the treatment of women with stage II breast cancer and four to nine involved axillary lymph nodes. An ongoing adjuvant trial in Italy has randomized 718 early-stage breast cancer patients to a combination of cyclophosphamide, epirubicin, and 5-fluorouracil every 21 days or every 14 days with G-CSF support (557). For diffuse large-cell lymphoma, induction Adriamycin, vincristine, prednisone has been followed by sequential high-dose cyclophosphamide, then methotrexate (plus vincristine), then etoposide, then L-PAM (plus total body irradiation), all with GM-CSF support. In a randomized comparison against a standard aggressive combination, the induction-intensification plan proved superior in complete remission rate, failure from relapse, failure from progression, and event-free survival (558).

These cytokinetic considerations may be as applicable to radiation therapy as to chemotherapy. The Gompertzian phenomenon of rapid repopulation of clonogenic cells after cytoreductive treatment is well documented in radiobiology. Moreover, clinical data suggest an acceleration of growth of the remaining viable tumor during the second part of protracted "split-course" radiation therapy (559, 560). In the treatment of head and neck cancer, split-course treatment has been used to allow normal tissues to recuperate from radiation damage. In this treatment plan, it has been observed that an additional radiation dose is needed to overcome tumor regrowth during the rest interval between the split courses. The alternative hypothesis, that the higher radiation dose in split-course treatment could be needed because of increased radioresistance of the tumor following the first part of the split course, is felt to be implausible (561). In fact, the tumor is actually better oxygenated during the second course of treatment, which should render it more radiosensitive (562). Hence, we are left with the likelihood of rapid regrowth between courses, more rapid than could be explained by exponential growth. The mechanism of such rapid regrowth relates to the three parameters that determine Gompertzian growth: mitotic cycle time, growth fraction, and cell loss fraction. Cell-cycle times of 2 to 4 days are commonly measured in head and neck cancers in the unperturbed state and after radiation therapy (563). Nevertheless, the doubling time can decrease from 60 to 4 days because of a persistence of the clonogenic cells (i.e., high growth fraction) resulting from a decrease in their tendency to differentiate or die by apoptosis (i.e., low cell loss fraction). It is important to note that this increase in proliferative parameters is occurring at a time of volume regression induced by the radiotherapy. That is, the observer may see cancer shrinkage while the cells may be experiencing growth acceleration as a means of compensating for the effects of therapy. The same kinetic principles applicable to chemotherapy may be needed to overcome this potential cause of treatment failure. In this regard, a review of studies of head and neck radiotherapy has calculated that the dose of irradiation needed to achieve local control in half of the cases, a standard benchmark, is consistently greater when the treatment is given over a 6-week interval than over a 4-week period (560). This observation is entirely consistent with the principle of dose density described above.

MITOTOXICITY HYPOTHESIS

Both the Skipper-Schabel-Wilcox and Norton-Simon models are based on the observation that the rate of tumor regression is positively related to the rate of unperturbed growth. The most obvious explanation for this observation is the mitotoxicity hypothesis: Tumors regress most rapidly when they are growing most rapidly because more of their cells are then synthesizing DNA and other macromolecules in preparation for mitosis. Such metabolically active cells are thereby at particular risk for cytotoxicity by drugs that interfere with such synthetic processes (564). The intuitive notion is that poisoning the S phase renders cells incapable of progressing successfully through the M phase. This is a dominant idea in cytokinetic thinking, and it undoubtedly has considerable merit. Growth-stimulating substances (i.e., estradiol, epidermal growth factor) increase both cell proliferation and cell kill from Adriamycin in MCF-7 cells in vitro (565). Pharmacologic concentrations of estradiol enhance the cytotoxicity of the chemotherapeutic agent melphalan in hormone-responsive cell lines (566). These observations have been applied clinically, and hormone recruitment schemes have indeed resulted in high local response rates in locally advanced breast cancer (567, 568). However, such treatments have proved only slightly better or no better than chemotherapy alone in metastatic breast cancer, except in data-driven subsets (569, 570). Even when benefits were seen, methodologic issues were raised regarding the analyzability of results (571).

We must be cautious, moreover, in interpreting laboratory data that suggest an enhancement of chemotherapeutic cytotoxicity by manipulations that increase the S-phase fraction. Tamoxifen, which can cause a G_1–S arrest in sensitive cell lines, does antagonize the cytotoxicity of melphalan and 5-fluorouracil, but it does so at dose schedules that do not affect cell proliferation (566). Tamoxifen actually enhances the cytotoxicity of Adriamycin and the alkylating agent 4-hydroxycyclophosphamide in this system. In fact, a broad acceptance of the mitotoxicity hypothesis leaves several cytokinetic enigmas unresolved. For example, only about 5% of the cells in an average breast cancer are in S phase. Thus, even if we use drugs that kill G_1 and G_2 cells, only about 15 to 20% of the tumor mass could possibly be killed by a single exposure to mitotoxic therapy. To get a one-log kill (90% regression) would require more than 10 such exposures (because $[1 - 0.2]^{10.319} = 0.1$). Regressions greater than one log are frequently seen after single treatments with high-dose chemotherapy (555). Even conventional chemotherapy, such as eight exposures to IV CMF, are simulated in Figure 52.2*B* to result in a five-log kill. It may be implausible that such significant cytoreductions are due to mitotoxicity alone. Indeed, cytokinetic analysis of MCF-7 cells exposed to low levels of Adriamycin does not show an immediate S phase reduction (572). There is an accumulation of cells in late S, G_2, and M, but also a block of the G_1 to S transition starting 2 days after treatment.

Another puzzle concerns the effect of chemotherapy on normal host tissues. Chemotherapy is certainly toxic to rapidly dividing bone marrow, alimentary mucosa, and hair follicles. Yet these tissues usually recover from its impact of chemotherapy. Some cancers, however, that are growing no more rapidly than these normal tissues may experience cytoreductions from which they never recover. That is, acute leukemias, malignant lymphomas, choriocarcinomas, and germ cell cancers may be cured by chemotherapy regimens that do not eradicate the patient's normal tissues that have comparable growth kinetics.

There is, at present, no established alternative to the mitotoxicity hypothesis that successfully relates cytokinetics to therapeutic cytotoxicity. One possibility is that chemotherapy could damage G_0 cells that later exhibit their lethal injuries as they are recruited into cycle. Another, perhaps related, possibility is suggested by the thought that the hormonal therapy of responsive cancers works by growth factor perturbation, not by mitotoxicity (573). Could chemotherapy share with hormone therapy this mode of action? Long-term data on the probability of breast-cancer relapse after adjuvant tamoxifen (574) and CMF (515) show similar qualitative changes. Breast cancer is a particularly relevant example because it is modulated by endogenous growth factors secreted by a subset of tumor cells in an individual cancer (575). The concept, however, may be generalizable since growth factors are important in many cancers. In the very genesis of cancer, malignant transformation frequently alters gene expression for growth factors, their receptors, and intracellular signal transduction proteins (576). Leukemogenic drugs, such as alkylating agents, are known to cause cytogenetic abnormalities, frequently at loci coding for products related to growth factors (577). It is even possible that the relation between tumor size and metastatic behavior, described in the context of the Goldie-Coldman model, is a consequence of the dependence of tumor cells on growth factors produced by the supporting stroma (578).

This discussion raises the possibility that chemotherapy, in addition to a gross mitotoxicity, might share with hormonal therapy an influence on growth factor loops (579). When hematopoietic cells are deprived of essential growth factors, they die by "apoptosis," an orderly process of programmed cell death (580, 581). It recently was determined that several chemotherapeutic drugs, as well as other lethal cytotoxins, also cause apoptosis (582). The existence of chemotherapy-induced apoptosis by growth factor disruption could clarify several mysteries. It could explain why the histologic analysis of breast cancers' regressing after chemotherapy does not always reveal a high degree of necrosis (583). It could explain why the TLI of breast cancer appeared not to predict chemosensitivity in locally advanced disease and in the adjuvant setting, an issue that will be further explored in an ongoing adjuvant study in breast cancer utilizing TLI to stratify node-negative patients (584). By implicating host–tumor paracrine interactions, the growth factor hypothesis might explain how tumor resistance to alkylating agents could be operant in vivo but not in vitro (585). The theory would not, moreover, be incompatible with mitotoxicity itself: rapidly growing cells that are dependent on growth factors would be expected to regress most rapidly when their growth-support system is perturbed.

In the laboratory, chemotherapy can influence growth factor pathways. Doxorubicin, for example, may up-regulate epidermal growth factor receptors in HeLa and 3T3 cells (586). Activation of protein kinase C (an intracellular signal of growth factor ligand–receptor interaction) enhances the cytotoxicity of cisplatin without increasing drug uptake (587). In the treatment of human cancer xenografts, antibodies to the epidermal growth factor receptor, which can by themselves inhibit growth (588), synergize with cisplatin (589). Such antibodies also synergize with Adriamycin in the treatment of A431 cells in athymic mice (590). Ongoing clinical trials are exploring the ability of antibodies to HER2 to synergize with doxorubicin plus cyclophosphamide, and of antibodies to HER1 to synergize with paclitaxel.

A consideration of the impact of anticancer therapy on growth factor mechanisms must eventually encompass the diversity of cytokinetic features present in most clinical cancers. For example, clonogenic cells—those cells capable of inexhaustible proliferation—are understood to have cytokinetic parameters that are markedly different from other cancer cells with more limited proliferative capacity. While the clonogenic "stem" cells are overshadowed numerically by the majority of cells in the tumor, these minority cells are the most important to eliminate to prevent tumor recurrence from unstable remission. Malignant clonogenic cells may cycle more quickly than nonclonogenic cells, but this is usually mitigated by a high cell loss fraction. Cell loss from the clonogenic pool is accomplished by differentiation, apoptosis, necrosis, exfoliation, and transportation away from the tumor in blood and lymph. Clearly, these cells differ biologically and cytokinetically from other cancer cells, as determined by genotypic differences that must be exploited to effect a cancer cure. It is, therefore, encouraging that the cytotoxic effects of chemotherapy might extend well beyond crude mitotoxicity. In this regard, cytokinetic analysis may play a key role in unraveling the relationships between cytotoxicity and molecular growth control. It is worthwhile to note that both aspects of cytokinetics, the study of cell proliferation and the analysis of growth curves, are relevant to this field of inquiry.

Conclusion

Cytokinetics is the fundamental physiology of cancer medicine. Its scope is so broad that this chapter merely introduces its basic concepts, laboratory foundations, theoretic underpinnings, clinical relevance, and prospects for future development. This is a rapidly evolving field, both conceptually and technically, that touches all aspects of experimental and practical oncology.

Acknowledgment

The authors are deeply indebted to Stephanie Miranda for her expertise in preparing the manuscript.

References

1. Howard A, Pelc, SR. Nuclear incorporation of 32p as demonstrated by autoradiographs. Exp Cell Res 1951;2:178.
2. Lajtha LG, Oliver R, Ellis F. Incorporation of 32p and adenine 14C into DNA by human bone marrow cells in vitro. Br J Cancer 1954;8:367.
3. Baak JP. A mitosis counting in tumors. Hum Pathol 1990;21:683.
4. Frei E, III, Whang J, Scoggins RB, van Scott EJ, Rall DP, Ben M. The stathmokinetic effect of vincristine. Cancer Res 1964;24:1918.
5. Steel GG. Autoradiographic analysis of the cell cycle: Howard and Pelc to the present day. Int J Rad Biol 1986;49:227.
6. Alama A, Nicolin A, Conte PF, Drewinko B. Evaluation of growth fractions with monoclonal antibodies to human alpha-DNA polymerase. Cancer Res 1987;47:1892.
7. Crocker J. Proliferation indices in malignant lymphomas. Clin Exp Immunol 1989;77:299.
8. Gerdes J, Lemke H, Brisch H, Wacker HH, Schwab U, Stein H. Cell cycle analysis of a cell proliferation-associated human nuclear antigen defined by the monoclonal antibody Ki-67. J Immunol 1984;133:1710.
9. Simon RM, Stroot MT, Weiss GH. Numerical inversion of Laplace transforms with application to percent labeled mitoses experiments. Comput Biomed Res 1972;5:596.
10. Pardee AB. G1 events and regulation of cell proliferation. Science 1989;246:603.
11. Ling MR, Kay JE. Lymphocyte Stimulation. New York: Elsevier, 1965.
12. Baserga R. Growth in size and cell DNA replication. Exp Cell Res 1984;151:1.
13. Darzynkiewicz Z, Traganos F, Melamed MR. New cell cycle compartments identified by multiparameter flow cytometry. Cytometry 1980;1:98.
14. Chaudhary PM, Roninson IB. Expression and acitivity of p-glycoprotein, a multidrug efflux pump, in human hematopoietic stem cells. Cell 1991;66:85.
15. Johnson LV, Walsh ML, Chen LB. Localization of mitochondria in living cells with rhodamine 123. Proc Natl Acad Sci USA 1980;77:990.
16. Broek D, Bartlett R, Crawford K, Nurse P. Involvement of P34cdc2 in establishing the dependency of S phase on mitosis. Nature 1991;349:388.
17. Murray AW. Remembrance of things past. Nature 1991;349:367.
18. Hartwell LH, Weinert TA. Checkpoints: controls that ensure the order of cell cycle events. Science 1989;246:629.
19. Murray AW, Kirschner MW. Dominoes and clocks: the union of two views of the cell cycle. Science 1989;246:614.
20. Laskey RA, Fairman MP, Blow JJ. S phase of the cell cycle. Science 1989;246:609.
21. Darzynkiewicz Z. Age-specific changes in the proliferation of Ehrlich ascites tumor cells grown as solid tumors. Cancer Res 1972;32:628.
22. Gelfant S. Cycling-noncycling cell transitions in tissue aging, immunological surveillance, transformation and tumor growth. Int Rev Cytol 1981;70:1.
23. O'Farrell PH, Edgar BA, Lakich D, Lehner CF. Directing cell division during development. Science 1989;246:635.
24. Folkman J, Moscona A. Role of cell shape in growth control. Nature 1978;273:345.
25. McIntosh JR, Koonce MP. Mitosis. Science 1989;246:622.
26. LaLa PK. Age-specific changes in the proliferation of Ehrlich ascites tumor cells grown as solid tumors. Cancer Res 1972;32:628.
27. Watson JV. The cell proliferation kinetics of the EMT6/M/AC mouse tumor at four volumes during unperturbed growth in vivo. Cell Tissue Kinet 1976;9:147.
28. Baserga R. The Biology of Cell Reproduction. Cambridge MA: Harvard University Press, 1985.
29. Kaman EJ, Smeulders AWN, Verbeek PW, Young IT, Baak JP. Image processing for mitoses in sections of breast cancer: a feasibility study. Cytometry 1984;5:244.
30. Schipper NW, Smeulders AW, Baak JP. Automated estimation of epithelial volume in breast cancer sections. A comparison with the image processing steps applied to gynecological tumors. Pathol Res Pract 1990;186:737.
31. Dressler LG, Bartow S. A DNA flow cytometry in solid tumors: practical aspects and clinical applications. Semin Diagnos Pathol 1989;6:55.
32. Kamensky LA, Melamed MR. Instrumentation for automated examination of cellular specimens. Proc IEEE 1969;57:2007.
33. VanDilla MA, Trujillo TT, Mullaney PF, Coulter JR. Cell microfluorometry. A method for rapid fluorescence measurement. Science 1969;169:1213.
34. Hedley DW, Freidlander ML, Taylor IW, Rigg CA, Musgrove EA. Method for analysis of cellular DNA content of paraffin-embedded pathological material using flow cytometry. J Histochem Cytochem 1983;31:1333.
35. Pallavicini MG. Solid tissue dispersal for cytokinetic analyses. In Techniques for Analysis of Cellular Proliferation. Edited by J. W. Gray, Z. Darzyniewicz. Clifton NJ: Humana, 1986, pp 139–162.
36. Latt SA. Fluorometric detection of DNA synthesis; Possibilities for interfacing bromodeoxyuridine dye techniques with flow fluorometry. J. Histochem. Cytochem 1977;25:913.
37. Meyer JS, Nauert J, Koehm S, Hughes J. Cell kinetics of human tumors by in vitro bromodeoxyuridine labeling. J Histochem Cytochem 1989;37:1449.
38. Raza A, Yasin Z, Grande C. A comparison of the rate of DNA synthesis in myeloblasts from peripheral blood and bone marrows in patients with acute nonlymphocytic leukemia. Exp Cell Res 1988;176:13.
39. Hiddeman WH, Schumann J, Andreeff M, Barlogie B, Herman CJ, Leif RC, Mayall BH, Murphy RF, Sandberg A. A Convention on nomenclature for DNA cytometry. Cytometry 1984;5:445.

40. Joensuu H, Kallioniemi OP. Different opinions on classification of DNA histograms produced from paraffin-embedded tissue. Cytometry 1989;10:711.
41. Mendelsohn ML. The growth fraction: a new concept applied to neoplasia. Science 1960;132:1496.
42. Killman SA. Acute leukemia The kinetics of leukemic blast cells in man. Ser Hematol 1968;1:38.
43. McDivitt RW, Stone KR, Meyer JS. A method for dissociation of viable human breast cancer cells that produces flow cytometric kinetic information similar to that obtained by thymidine labeling. Cancer Res 1984;44:2628.
44. Hoffman J, Post J. In vivo studies of DNA synthesis in human normal and tumor cells. Cancer Res 1967;27:898.
45. Quastler H, Sherman FG. Cell population kinetics in the intestinal epithelium of the mouse. Exp Cell Res 1959;17:420.
46. Bruce WR, Valeriote F. Normal and malignant stem cells and chemotherapy. In The Proliferation and Spread of Neoplastic Cells, Univ. of Texas M. D. Anderson Hospital and Tumor Institute at Houston, 21st Annual Symposium on Fundamental Cancer Research 1967. Baltimore: Williams & Wilkins, 1968, pp 409–422.
47. Till JE, McCulloch GA, Phillips RA, Siminovitch L. Aspects of the regulation of stem cell function. In The Proliferation and Spread of Neoplastic Cells, Univ. of Texas M. D. Anderson Hospital and Tumor Institute at Houston, 21st Annual Symposium on Fundamental Cancer Research 1967. Baltimore: Williams & Wilkins, 1968, pp 235–244.
48. Hamburger A, Salmon SE. Primary bioassay of human myeloma stem cells. J Clin Invest 1977;60:846.
49. Steel GG, Lamerton LF. Cell population kinetics and chemotherapy. In Human Tumor Cell Kinetics. Edited by S Perry. National Cancer Institute Monograph, 1968, p 29.
50. Steel GG. Cell loss as a factor in the growth rate of human tumors. Eur J Cancer 1967;3:381.
51. Novick A, Szilard L. Experiments with the chemostat on spontaneous mutations of bacteria. Proc Natl Acad Sci USA 1950;36:708.
52. Foulds L. The histologic analysis of mammary tumors of mice. II. The histology of responsiveness and progression. The origins of tumors. JNCI 1956;17:713.
53. Iannaccone PM, Weinberg WC, Deamant FD. On the clonal origin of tumors: a review of experimental models. Int J Cancer 1987;39:778.
54. Frei E, III. Models and the clinical dilemma. In Design of Models for Testing Therapeutic Agents. Edited by IJ Fidler, RJ White. New York: Van Nostrand Reinhold, 1982, pp 248–259.
55. Fidler I. Tumor heterogeneity and the biology of cancer invasion and metastases. Cancer Res 1978;38:2651.
56. Charbit A, Malaise EP, Tubiana M. Relation between the pathological nature and the growth rate of human tumors. Eur J Cancer 1971;7:307.
57. Simpson-Herren L, Sanford AH, Holmquist JP. Cell population kinetics of transplanted and metastatic Lewis lung carcinoma. Cell Tissue Kinet 1974;7:349.
58. Wegelin C. Malignant disease of the thyroid gland and its relations to goitre in man and animals. Cancer Rev 1928;3:297.
59. Neve EF. Kangri-burn cancer. Br Med J 1923;2:1255.
60. Groham JH, Helvig EB. In Dermal Pathology. Edited by JH Graham WC Johnson, EB Helvig. New York: Harper & Row, 1972, pp 561–581.
61. Greenberg PL, Mara B. The preleukemic syndrome: correlation of in vitro parameters of granulocytoloiesis with clinical features. Am J Med 1979;66:951.
62. Peterson LC, Bloomfield CD, Brunning RD. Blast crisis as an initial or terminal manifestation of chronic myeloid leukemia. Am J Med 1976;60:209.
63. Parks TG, Bussey HJR, Lockhart-Mummery HE. Familial polyposis coli associated with extracolonic abnormalities. Gut 1970;11:323.
64. De Ome KB, Medina D. A new approach to mammary tumorigenesis in rodents. Cancer 1969;24:1255.
65. Davis HH, Simons M, Davis JB. Cystic disease of the breast: relationship to carcinoma. Cancer 1964;17:957.
66. Sandison AT. An autopsy study of the adult human breast: with special reference to the proliferative epithelial changes of importance in the pathology of the breast. Natl Cancer Inst Monograph 1962;8:1.
67. Ryser HJP. Chemical carcinogenesis. N Engl J Med 1971;285:721.
68. Glicksman AS, Pajak TF, Gottlieb AJ, Nissen N, Stutzman L, Cooper MR. Second malignant neoplasms in patients successfully treated for Hodgkin's disease: a Cancer and Leukemia Group B study. Cancer Treat Rep 1982;66:1035.
69. Boice JD Jr, Greene MH, Killen JY Jr, Ellenberg SS, Keehn RJ, McFadden E, Chen TT, Fraumeni JF Jr. Leukemia and preleukemia after adjuvant treatment of gastrointestinal cancer with semustine (methyl-CCNU). N Engl J Med 1983;309:1079.
70. Mourad WA, Setrakian S, Hales ML, Abdulla M, Trucco G. The argyrophilic nucleolar organizer regions in ductal carcinoma in situ of the breast. The significance of ploidy and proliferative activity analysis using this silver staining techique. Cancer 1994;74: 1739.
71. Meyer JS, Prey MU, Babcock DS, McDivitt RW. Breast carcinoma cell kinetics, morphology, stage, and host characteristics. A thymidine labeling study. Lab Invest 1986;54:41.
72. Kamel OW, Franklin WA, Ringus JC, Meyer JS. Thymidine labeling index and Ki-67 growth fraction in lesions of the breast. Am J Pathol 1989;134:107.
73. Meyer JS, Coplin MD. Thymidine labeling index, flow cytometric S phase measurement, and DNA index in human tumors. Am J Clin Pathol 1988;59:586.
74. Meyer JS, McDivitt RW. Reliability and stability of the thymidine labeling index of breast carcinoma. Lab Invest 1986;54:160.
75. Silvestrini R, Daidone MG, Mastore M, et al. Cell kinetics of 9200 human breast cancer: consistency of basic and clinical results. Proc Am Assoc Cancer Res 1992;33: 238.
76. Silvestrini R, Daidone MG, Valagussa P, Salvadori B, Rovini D, Bonadonna G. Cell kinetics as a prognostic marker in locally advanced breast cancer. Cancer Treat Rep 1987;71:375.
77. Silvestrini R, Daidone MG, Valagussa P, et al. 3H-Thymidine-Labeling Index as a prognostic indicator in node-positive breast cancer. J Clin Oncol 1990;8:1321.
78. Silvestrini R, Daidone MG, Del Bino G, et al. Prognostic significance of proliferative activity and ploidy in node-negative breast cancers. Ann Oncol 1993;4:213.
79. Cooke TG, Stanton PD, Winstanley J, et al. Long-term prognostic significance of thymidine labeling index in primary breast cancer. Eur J Cancer 1992;28:424.
80. Amadori D. Use of cell kinetics to analyze responses in combination therapy studies. New Challenges in Breast Cancer Clinical Trials, November 16, 1994, Philadelphia.
81. McDivitt RW, Stone KR, Craig RB, Palmer JO, Meyer JS, Bauer WC. A proposed classification of breast cancer based on kinetic information derived from a comparison of risk factors in 168 primary operable breast cancers. Cancer 1986;57:269.
82. Dressler LG, Seamer LC, Owens MA, et al. DNA flow cytometry and prognostic factors in 1331 frozen breast cancer specimens. Cancer 1988;61:420.
83. Stal O, Carstensen J, Hatschek T, et al. Significance of S phase fraction and hormone receptor content in the management of young breast cancer patients. Br J Cancer 1992;66:706.
84. Frierson HF. Plidy analysis and S phase fraction determination by flow cytometry of invasive adenocarcinomas of the breast. Am J Surg Pathol 1991;15:358.
85. Frierson HF. Grade and flow cytometric analysis of ploidy for infiltrating ductal carcinomas. Huma Pathol 1993;24:24.
86. Fisher B, Gunduz N, Costantino J, et al. DNA flow cytometric analysis of primary operable breast cancer. Cancer 1991;68:1465.
87. Muss HB, Kute TE, Case LD, Smith R, Boocher C, Long R, Kammire L, Gregory B, Brockschmidt JK. The relation of low cytometry to clinical and biologic characteristics in women with node negative primary breast cancer. Cancer 1989;64:1894.
88. Stal O, Brisfors A, Carstensen J, Ferraud L, Hatschek T, Nordenskjold B, and members of the South-East Sweden Breast Cancer Group Interrelations between cellular DNA content, S phase fraction, hormone receptor status and age in primary breast cancer. Acta Oncol 1992;31:283.
89. Witzig TE, Ingle JN, Schaid DJ, Wold LE, Barlow JF, Gonchoroff NJ, Gerstner JB, Krook JE, Grant CS, Katzmann JA. DNA plidy and percent S phase as prognostic factors in node-positive breast cancer: results from patients enrolled in two prospective randomized trials. J Clin Oncol 1993;11:351.
90. Clark GM, Mathieu M, Owens MA, Dresller LG, Eudey L, Tormey DC, Osborne CK, Gilchrist KW, Mansour EG, Abeloff MD, McGuire WL. Prognostic significance of S phase fraction in good-risk, node-negative breast cancer patients. J Clin Oncol 1992;10:428–432.
91. Dressler LG. DNA flow cytometry measurements have significant prognostic impact in the node negative breast cancer patient: an intergroup study (INT 0076). Treatment of Early Stage Breast Cancer: program and abstracts. NIH Consensus Development Conference, National Cancer Institute and the Office of Medical Applications of Research of the National Institutes of Health, June 18–21, 1990, pp 99–101.
92. Fallenius AG, Franzen SA, Auer GU. Predictive value of nuclear DNA content in breast cancer in relation to clinical and morphologic factors. Cancer 1988;62:521.
93. Dressler LG. Are DNA flow cytometry measurements providing useful information in the management of the node-negative breast cancer patient? Cancer Invest 1992;10: 477–486.
94. Haffty BG, Toth M, Flynn S, Fischer D, Carter D. Prognostic value of DNA flow cytometry in the locally recurrent, conservatively treated breast cancer patient. J Clin Oncol 1992;10:1839.
95. Clark GM, McGuire WL. Steroid receptor and other prognostic factors in primary breast cancer. Semin Oncol 1988;15:20.
96. Meyer JS, Friedman E, McCrate MM, Bauer WC. Prediction of early course of breast carcinoma by thymidine labeling. Cancer 1983;51:1879.
97. Silvestrini R, Daidone MG, Gasparini G. Cell kinetics as a prognostic marker in node-negative breast cancer. Cancer 1985;56:78.
98. Witzig TE, Ingle JN, Cha SS, Schaid DJ, Tabery RL, Wold LE, Grant C, Gonchorff NJ, Katzmann JA. DNA ploidy and the percentage of cells in S phase as prognostic factors for women with lymph node negative breast cancer. Cancer 1994;74:1752–1761.
99. Meyer JD, Province MA. S phase fraction and nuclear size in long term prognosis of patients with breast cancer. Cancer 1994;74:2287–2299.
100. Stal O, Dufmats M, Hatschek T, Carstensen J, Klintenberg C, Rutqvist LE, Skoog L, Sullivan S, Wingren S, Nordenskjold B. S phase fraction is a prognostic factor in stage I breast carcinoma. J Clin Oncol 1993;11:1717–1722.
101. Sigurdsson H, Baldetorp B, Bord A, Dalberg M, Ferno M, Killander D, Olsson H. Indicators of prognosis in node-negative breast cancer. N Engl J Med 1990;322: 1045–1053.
102. O'Reilly SM, Camplejohn RS, Barnes DM, Millis RR, Rubens RD, Richards MA. Node-negative breast cancer: prognostic subgroups defined by tumor size and flow cytometry. J Clin Oncol 1990;8:2040–2046.
103. Dressler LG, Eudey L, Gray R, Tormey DC, McGuire WL, Gilchrist KW, Clark GM, Osborne CK, Mansour EG, Abeloff MD. Prognostic potential of DNA flow cytometry measurements in node-negative breast cancer patients: preliminary analysis of an intergroup study (INT 0076). JNCI Monographs 1992;11:167–172.
104. Merkel DE, Winchester DJ, Goldschmidt RA, August CZ, Wruck DM, Rademaker AW. DNA flow cytometry and pathologic grading as prognostic guides in axillary lymph node-negative breast cancer. Cancer 1993;72:1926–1932.
105. Winchester DJ, Duda RB, August CZ, Goldschmidt RA, Wruck DM, Rademaker AW, Winchester DP, Merkel DE. The importance of DNA flow cytometry in node-negative breast cancer. Arch Surg 1990;125:886–889.
106. Arnerlov C, Emdin SO, Lundgren B, Roos G, Soderstrom J, Bjersing L, Norberg C, Angquist KA. Mammographic growth rate, DNA ploidy and S phase fraction analysis in breast carcinoma. Cancer 1992;70:1935–1942.
107. Hedley DW, Rugg CA, Gelber RD. Association of DNA index and S phase fraction with prognosis of node positive early breast cancer. Cancer Res 1987;47:4729–4735.
108. Ewers S, Attewell R, Baldetorp B, Borg A, Ferno M, Langstrom E, Ryden S, Killander D. Flow cytometry DNA analysis and prediction of loco-regional recurrences after mastectomy in breast cancer. Acta Oncol 1992;31(7):733–740.
109. Stanton PD, Cooke TG, Oakes SJ, Winstanley J, Holt S, George WD, Murray GD. Lack of prognostic significance of DNA ploidy and S phase fraction in breast cancer. Br J Cancer 1992;66:925–929.
110. Ferno M, Baldetorp B, Borg A, Olsson H, Sigurdsson H, Killander D. Flow cytometric DNA index and S phase fraction in breast cancer in relation to other prognostic variables and to clinical outcome. Acta Oncol 1992;31(2):157–165.
111. Ottestad L, Pettersen EO, Nesland JM, Hannisdal E, Fossa SD, Tveit KM. Flow cytometric DNA analysis as prognostic factor in human breast carcinoma. Pathol Res Pract 1993;189:405–410.
112. Hatschek T, Fagerberg G, Stal O, et al. Cytometric characterization and clinical course of breast cancer diagnosed in a population-based screening program. Cancer 1989;64:1074–1081.
113. Ewers S-B, Attewell R, Baldetorp B, Borg A, Langstrom E, Killander D. Prognostic potential of flow cytometric S phase and ploidy prospectively determined in primary breast carcinomas. Breast Cancer Res Treat 1991;20:93–108.

114. Bosari S, Lee AKC, Tahan SR, Figoni MAT, Wiley BD, Heatley GJ, Silverman ML. DNA flow cytometric analysis and prognosis of axillary lymph node-negative breast carcinoma. Cancer 1992;70:1943–1950.
115. Hedley DW, Clark GM, Cornelisse CJ, Killander D, Kute T, Merkel D. Consensus review of the clinical utility of DNA cytometry in carcinoma of the breast. Cytometry 1993;14:482–485.
116. Kute TE, Muss HB, Cooper MR, Case LD, Buss D, Stanley V, Gregory B, Galleshaw J, Booher K. The use of flow cytometry for the prognosis of stage II adjuvantly treated breast cancer patients. Cancer 1990;66:1810.
117. O'Reilly SM, Camplejohn RS, Barnes DM, Millis RR, Allen D, Rubens RD, Richards MA. DNA index, S phase fraction, histological grade and prognosis in breast cancer. Br J Cancer 1990;61:671–674.
118. Feichter GE, Mueller A, Kaufmann M, Haag D, Born IA, Abel U, Klinga K, Kubli F, Goerttler K. Correlation of DNA flow cytometric results and other prognostic factors in primary breast cancer. Int J Cancer 1988;41:823–828.
119. Lawry J, Rogers K, Duncan JL, Potter CW. The identification of informative parameters in the flow cytometric analysis of breast carcinoma. Eur J Cancer 29A:719–723, 1993.
120. Van der Lindeman JC, Baak JPA, Meijer CJLM, Herman CJ. The multivariate prognostic index and nuclear DNA content are independent prognostic factors in primary breast cancer patients. Cytometry 1989;10:56–61.
121. Beerman H, Kluin M, Hermans J, van de Velde CJH, Cornelisse CJ. Prognostic significance of DNA-ploidy in a series of 690 primary breast cancer patients. Int J Cancer 1990;45:34–39.
122. Aaltomaa S, Lipponen P, Papinaho S, Klemi P, Kosma VM, Marin S, Eskelinen M, Alhava E, Syrjanen K. Nuclear morphometry and DNA flow cytometry as prognostic factors in female breast cancer. Eur J Surg 1992;158:135–141.
123. Gnant MFX, Blijham G, Reiner A, Reiner G, Reynders M, Schutte B, van Asche C, Steger G, Jakesz R. DNA ploidy and other results of DNA flow cytometry as prognostic factors in operable breast cancer: 10 year results of a randomised study. Eur J Cancer 1992;28:711–716.
124. Gnant MFX, Blijham GH, Reiner A, Schemper M, Reynders M, Schutte B, van Asche C, Steger G, Jakesz R. Aneuploidy fraction but not DNA index is important for the prognosis of patients with stage I and II breast cancer—10-year results. Ann Oncol 1993;4:643–650.
125. Toikkanen S, Joensuu H, Klemi P. Nuclear DNA content as a prognostic factor in T1–2N0 Breast Cancer. Am J Clin Pathol 1990;93:471–479.
126. Joensuu H, Toikkanen S, Klemi PJ. DNA index and S phase fraction and their combination as prognostic factors in operable ductal breast carcinoma. Cancer 1990;66: 331–340.
127. Ewers SB, Attewell R, Baldetorp B, Borg A, Ferno M, Langstrom E, Killander D. Prognostic significance of flow cytometric DNA analysis and estrogen receptor content in breast carcinomas—a 10 year survival study. Breast Cancer Res Treat 1992;24: 115–126.
128. Kallioniemi O-P, Blanco G, Alavaikko M, Hietanen T, Mattila J, Lauslahti K, Koivula T. Tumour DNA ploidy as an independent prognostic factor in breast cancer. Br J Cancer 1987;56:637–642.
129. Lewis WE. Prognostic significance of flow cytometric DNA analysis in node-negative breast cancer patients. Cancer 1990;65:2315–2320.
130. Clark GM, Dressler LG, Owens MA, Pounds G, Oldaker T, McGuire WL. Prediction of relapse or survival in patients with node-negative breast cancer by DNA flow cytometry. N Engl J Med 1989;320:627–633.
131. Balslev I, Christensen J, Bruun Rasmussen B, Larsen JK, Lykkesfeldt AE, Thorpe SM, Carsten R, Briand P, Mouridsen HT. Flow cytometric DNA ploidy defines patients with poor prognosis in node-negative breast cancer. Int J Cancer 1994;56:16–25.
132. Keyhani-Rofagha S, O'Toole RV, Farrar WB, Sickle-Santanello B, DeCenzo J, Young D. Is DNA ploidy an independent prognostic indicator in infiltrative node-negative breast adenocarcinoma? Cancer 1990;65:1577–1582.
133. Remvikos Y, Vielh P, Padoy E, et al. Breast cancer proliferation measured on cytological samples: a study by flow cytometry of S phase fractions and BrdU incorporation. Br J Cancer 1991;64:501–507.
134. Meyer JS, Koehm S, Hughes JM, et al. Bromodeoxyuridine labeling for S phase measurement in breast carcinoma. Cancer 1993;71:3531–3540.
135. Goodson WH, Waldman F, Ljung B, et al. Bromodeoxyuridine labeling of human breast cancer: preliminary results and inverse association with progesterone receptor content. Proc Am Soc Clin Oncol, vol 9, 1990, p 50.
136. Christov K, Chew KL, Ljung B, et al. Proliferation of normal breast epithelial cells as shown by in vivo labeling with bromodeoxyuridine. Am J Pathol 1991;138:1371–1377.
137. Gasparini G, Reitano M, Bevilacqua P, et al. Relationship of the epidermal growth factor-receptor to the growth fraction (Ki-67 Antibody) and the flow cytometric S phase as cell kinetics parameters, in human mammary carcinomas. Anticancer Res 1991;11:1597–1604.
138. Charpin C, Devictor B, Bonnier P, Andrac L, Lavaut M-N, Allasia C, Piana L. Epidermal growth factor receptor in breast cancer: correlation of quantitative immunocytochemical assays to prognostic factors. Breast Cancer Res Treat 1993;25:203–210.
139. Railo M, Nordling S, von Bougslawsky K, Leivonen M, Kyllonen L, von Smitten K. Prognostic value of Ki-67 immunolabeling in primary operable breast cancer. Br J Cancer 1993;68:579.
140. Steeg PS, De La Rosa A, Flatow U, et al. NM23 and breast cancer metastasis. Breast Cancer Res Treat 1993;25:175.
141. Lupu R, Lippman ME. The role of erbB2 signal transduction pathways in human breast cancer. Breast Cancer Res Treat 1993;27:83.
142. Anbazhagan R, Gelber RD, Bettelheim R, et al. Association of c-erbB-2 expression and S-phase fraction in the prognosis of node positive breast cancer. Ann Oncol 1991;2:47–53.
143. Slamon DJ, Clark GM, Wong SG, Levin WJ, Ullrich A, McGuire WL. Human breast cancer: correlation of relapse and survival with amplification of the Her-2 neu oncogene. Science 1987;235:177–182.
144. Tommasi S, Paradiso A, Mangia A, et al. Biologic correlation between Her-2/neu and proliferative activity in human breast cancer. Anticancer Res 1991;11:1395–1400.
145. French D, Pizzi C, De Marchis L, et al. Proliferative activity and genetic alterations in breast carcinoma. Proc Am Assoc Cancer Res, vol 34, 1993, p 3083.
146. O'Reilly SM, Barnes DM, Camplejohn RS, et al. The relationship between c-erbB-2 expression, S phase fraction and prognosis in breast cancer. Br J Cancer 1991;63: 444–446.
147. Babiak J, Hugh J, Poppema S. Significance of c-erB-2 amplification and DNA aneuploidy: analysis in 78 patients with node-negative breast cancer. Cancer 1992;70: 770–776.
148. Noguchi M, Koyasaki N, Ohta N, et al. Internal mammary nodal status is a more reliable prognostic factor than DNA ploidy and c-erb B-2 expression in patients with breast cancer. Arch Surg 1993;128:242–246.
149. Barnes DM, Meyer JS, Gonzalez JG, et al. Relationship between c-erbB-2 immunoreactivity and thymidine labeling index in breast carcinoma in situ. Breast Cancer Res Treat 1991;18:11–17.
150. Allred DC, Clark GM, Elledge R, Fuqua SAW, Brown RW, Chamness GC, Osborne CK, McGuire WL. Association of p53 protein expression with tumor cell proliferation rate and clinical outcome in node-negative breast cancer. JNCI 1993;85:200–206.
151. Walker RA, Varley JM. The molecular pathology of human breast cancer. Cancer Surv 1993;16:31.
152. Silvestrini R, Benini E, Daidone MG, Veneroni S, Boracchi P, Cappelletti V, Di Fronzo G, Veronesi U. P53 as an independent prognostic marker in lymph node-negative breast cancer patients. JNCI 1993;85:965.
153. Ji H, Lipponen P, Aaltomaa S, Syrjanen S, Syrjanen K. C-erbB-2 oncogene related to p53 expression, cell proliferation and prognosis in breast cancer. Anticancer Res 1993;13:1147–1152.
154. Elledge RM, Fuqua SAW, Clark GM, Pujol P, Allred DC, McGuire WL. Prognostic significance of p53 gene alterations in node-negative breast cancer. Breast Cancer Res Treat 1993;26:225–235.
155. Visscher DW, Wykes S, Kubus J, Crissman JD. Comparison of PCNA/cyclin immunohistochemistry with flow cytometric S phase fraction in breast cancer. Breast Cancer Res Treat 1992;22:111–118.
156. Gillett CD, Barnes DM, Camplejohn RS. Comparison of three cell cycle associated antigens as markers of proliferative activity and prognosis in breast carcinoma. J Clin Pathol 1993;46:1126–1128.
157. Klijn JGM, Berns EMJJ, Bontenbal M, Foekens J. Cell biologic factors associated with the response of breast cancer to systemic treatment. Cancer Treat Rev 1993;19: 45–63.
158. Ravdin PM. Evaluation of cathepsin D as a prognostic factor in breast cancer. Breast Cancer Res Treat 1993;24:219.
159. Paradiso A, Mangia A, Correale M, et al. Cytosol cathepsin-D content and proliferative activity of human breast cancer. Breast Cancer Res Treat 1992;23:63–70.
160. Isola J, Weitz S, Visakorpi T, Holli K, Shea R, Khabbaz N, Kallioniemi O-P. Cathepsin D expression detected by immunohistochemistry has independent prognostic value in axillary node-negative breast cancer. J Clin Oncol 1993;11:36–43.
161. Koss LG, Czerniak B, Herz F, Wersto RP. Flow cytometric measurements of DNA and other cell components in human tumors: a critical appraisal. Hum Pathol 1989;20: 528–548.
162. Blute ML, Nativ O, Zincke H, Farrow GM, Therneau T, Lieber MM. Pattern of failure after radical retropubic prostatectomy for clinically and pathologically localized adenocarcinoma of the prostate: influence of tumor deoxyribonucleic acid ploidy. J Urol 1989;142:1262.
163. Fordham MVP, Burdge AH, Matthews J, Williams G, Cooke T. Prostatic carcinoma cell DNA content measured by flow cytometry and its relation to clinical outcome. Br J Surg 1986;73:400–403.
164. Haugen OA, Mjlnerd O. DNA-ploidy as prognostic factor in prostatic carcinoma. Int J Cancer 1990;45:224.
165. Montgomery BT, Nativ O, Blute ML, Farrow GM, Myers RP, Zincke H, Therneau TM, Lieber MM. Stage B prostate adenocarcinoma: flow cytometric nuclear DNA ploidy analysis. Arch Surg 1990;125:327–331.
166. Nativ O, Winkler HZ, Raz Y, Therneau TM, Farrow GM, Myers RP, Zincke H, Lieber MM. Stage C prostatic adenocarcinoma: flow cytometric nuclear DNA ploidy analysis. Mayo Clin Proc 1989;64:911–919.
167. Ritchie AWS, Dorey F, Layfield LJ, Hannah J, Lovrekovich H, deKernion JB. Relationship of DNA content to conventional prognostic factors in clinically localised carcinoma of the prostate. Br J Urol 1988;62:254–260.
168. Tribukait B. DNA flow cytometry in carcinoma of the prostate for diagnosis, prognosis and study of tumor biology. Acta Oncol 1991;30(2):187–192.
169. Deitch AD, deVere White RW. Flow cytometry as a predictive modality in prostate cancer. Hum Pathol 1992;23:352–359.
170. Vesalainen S, Nordling S, Lipponen P, Talja M, Syrjanen K. Progression and survival in prostatic adenocarcinoma: a comparison of clinical stage, Gleason grade, S phase fraction and DNa ploidy. Br J Cancer 1994;70:309.
171. Fisher HA. Prediction of pathologic stage and postprostatectomy disease recurrence by DNA ploidy analysis of initial needle biopsy specimens of prostate cancer. Cancer 1994;74:2811.
172. Tinari N, Natoli C, Angelucci D, Tenaglia R, Fiorentino B, DiStefano P, Amatetti C, Zezza A, Nicolai M, Iacobelli S. DNA and S phase fraction analysis by flow cytometry in prostate cancer. Cancer 1993;71:1289–1296.
173. Nemoto R, Hattori K, Uchida K, Shimazui T, Nishijima Y, Koiso K, Harada M. S phase fraction of human prostate adenocarcinoma studied with in vivo bromodeoxyuridine labeling. Cancer 1990;66:509–514.
174. Van Weerden WM, Moerings EPCM, van Kreuningen A, de Jong FH, van Steenbrugge GJ, Schroder FH. Ki-67 expression and BrdUrd incorporation as markers of proliferative activity in human prostate tumor models. Cell Prolif 1993;26:67–75.
175. Blute ML, Tsushima K, Farrow GM, Therneau TM, Lieber MM. Transitional cell carcinoma of the renal pelvis: nuclear deoxyribonucleic acid ploidy studied by flow cytometry. J Urol 1988;140:944.
176. Banner BF, Brancazio L, Bahnson RR, Ernstoff MS, Taylor SR. DNA analysis of multiple synchronous renal cell carcinomas. Cancer 1990;66:2180–2185.
177. Tachibana M, Deguchi N, Baba S, Jitsukawa S, Hata M, Tazaki H. Bromodeoxyuridine and deoxyribonucleic acid bivariate analysis in human renal cell carcinoma: does flow cytometric determination predict malignant potential or prognosis of patients with renal cell carcinoma? Am J Clin Pathol 1992;97(suppl 1):S38-S47.
178. Al-Abadi H, Nagel R. Prognostic relevance of ploidy and proliferative activity of renal cell carcinoma. Euro Urol 1988;15:271.
179. Rainwater LM, Hosaka Y, Farrow GM, Lieber MM. Well differentiated clear cell renal carcinoma: significance of nuclear deoxyribonucleic acid patterns studied by flow cytometry. J Urol 1987;137:15–20.

180. Ekfors TO, Lipasti J, Nurmi MJ, et al. Flow cytometric analysis of the DNA profile of renal cell carcinoma. Pathol Res Pract 1987;182:58–62.
181. Currin SM, Lee SE, Walther PJ. Flow cytometric assessment of deoxyribonucleic acid content in renal adenocarcinoma: does ploidy status enhance prognostic stratification over stage alone? J Urol 1990;143:458–463.
182. Ljungberg B, Forsslund G, Stenling R, Zetterberg A. Prognostic significance of the DNA content in renal cell carcinoma. J Urol 1986;135:422–426.
183. Raviv G, Leibovich I, Mor Y, Nass D, Medalia O, Goldwasser B, Nativ O. Localized renal cell carcinoma treated by radical nephrectomy. Influence of pathologic data and the importance of DNA ploidy pattern on disease outcome. Cancer 1993;72:2207.
184. de Riese WT, Crabtree WN, Allhoff EP, Werner M, Liedke S, Lenis G, Atzpodien J, Kirchner H. Prognostic significance of Ki-67 immunostaining in nonmetastatic renal cell carcinoma. J Clin Oncol 1993;11:1804.
185. Masters JRW, Camplejohn RS, Parkinson MC, Woodhouse CRJ, O'Reilly SM. Does DNA flow cytometry give useful prognostic information in renal parenchyma adenocarcinoma? Br J Urol 1992;70:364–369.
186. Nemoto R, Hattori K, Uchida K, Shimazui T, Harada M. Estimation of growth fraction in situ in human bladder cancer with bromodeoxyuridine labeling. Br J Urol 1990;65: 27–31.
187. Walther PJ. The role of flow cytometry in the management of bladder cancer. Hematol/Oncol Clin North Am 1992;6:81–98.
188. Gustafson H, Tribukait B, Esposti PL. DNA pattern, histological grade and multiplicity related to recurrence rate in superficial bladder tumours. Scand J Urol Nephrol 1982;16:135–139.
189. Tribukait B, Gustafson H, Esposti PL. The significance of ploidy and proliferation in the clinical and biologic evaluation of bladder tumours: a study of 100 untreated cases. Br J Urol 1982;54:130–135.
190. Blomjous ECM, Schipper NW, Baak JPA, Vos W, de Voogt HJ, Meijer CJL. The value of morphometry and DNA flow cytometry in addition to classic prognosticators in superficial urinary bladder carcinoma. Am J Clin Pathol 1989;91:243–248.
191. Tribukait B. Flow cytometry in assessing the clinical aggressiveness of genito-urinary neoplasms. World J Urol 1987;5:108–122.
192. Jacobsen AB, Lunde S, Ous S, Melvik JE, Pettersen EO, Kaalhus O, Fossa SD T2/T3 bladder carcinomas treated with definitive radiotherapy with emphasis on flow cytometric DNA ploidy values. Int J Rad Oncol Biol Phys 1989;17:923–929.
193. Lipponen PK, Collan Y, Eskelinen MJ, Pesonen E, Sotarauta M, Nordling S. Comparison of morphometry and DNA flow cytometry with standard prognostic factors in bladder cancer. Br J Urol 1990;65:589–597.
194. Lipponen PK, Nordling S, Eskelinen MJ, Jauhianen K, Terho R, Harju E. Flow cytometry in comparison with mitotic index in predicting disease outcome in transitional-cell bladder cancer. Int J Cancer 1993;53:42–47.
195. Fossa SD, Berner AA, Jacobsen AB, Waehre H, Kvarstein B, Urnes T, Ogreid P, Johanesen TE, Silde J, Nesland JM. Clinical significance of DNA ploidy and S phase fraction and their relation to p53 protein, c-erbB-2 protein and HCG in operable muscle-invasive bladder cancer.
196. Shappers RF, Ploem-Zaaijer JJ, Pauwels RP, Smeets AW, van den Brandt PA, Tanke HJ, Bosman, F.T. Image cytometric DNA analysis in transitional cell carcinoma of the bladder. Cancer 1993;72:182.
197. de Graaff WE, Sleijfer D T, de Jong B, Schraffordt Koops H, Oosterhuis JW. Significance of aneuploid stem lines in nonseminomatous germ cell tumors. Cancer 1993;72:1300–1304.
198. Kuhn W, Kaufmann M, Feichter GE, Rummell HH, Schmid H, Heberling D. DNA flow cytometry, clinical and morphological parameters as prognostic factors for advanced malignant and borderline ovarian tumors. Gynecol Oncol 1989;33:360.
199. Friedlander ML, Taylor IW, Russell P, et al. Ploidy as a prognostic factor in ovarian cancer. Int J Gynecol Pathol 1983;2:55–63.
200. Redman CWE, Finn C, Ward K, Kelly K, Buxton EJ, Varma R, Shortland-Webb W, Luesley DM. Tumour cell activity markers in epithelial ovarian cancer: are biochemical and cytometric indices complementary? Br J Cancer 1990;61:755–758.
201. Rodenburg CJ, Cornelisse CJ, Heintz PA, et al. Tumor ploidy as a major prognostic factor in advanced ovarian cancer. Cancer 1987;59:317–323.
202. Iverson O-E. Prognostic value of the flow cytometric DNA index in human ovarian carcinoma. Cancer 1988;61:971–975.
203. Braly PS, Klevecz RR. Flow cytometric evaluation of ovarian cancer. Cancer 1993;71: 1621–1628.
204. Drescher CW, Flint A, Hopkins MP, Roberts JA. Prognostic significance of DNA content and nuclear morphology in borderline ovarian tumors. Gynecol Oncol 1993;48: 242–246.
205. Kallioniemi O, Punnonen R, Mattila J, Lehtinen M, Koivula T. Prognostic significance of DNA index, multiploidy, and S phase fraction in ovarian cancer. Cancer 1988;61: 334–339.
206. Barnabei VM, Miller DS, Bauer KD, Murad TM, Rademaker AW, Lurain JR. Flow cytometric evaluation of epithelial ovarian cancer. Am J Obstet Gynecol 1990;162: 1584–1592.
207. Friedlander ML, Hedley DW, Swanson C, Russell P. For the Gynecologic Oncology Group of the Clinical Oncology Society of Australia Prediction of long-term survival by flow cytometric analysis of cellular DNA content in patients with advanced ovarian cancer. J Clin Oncol 1988;6:282–290.
208. Rotmensch J, Atcher RW, Schwartz JL, Gardina DJ. Analysis of ascites from patients with ovarian carcinoma by cell flow cytometry. Gynecol Oncol 1992;44:10–12.
209. Huettner PC, Weinberg DS, Lage JM. Assessment of proliferative activity in ovarian neoplasms by flow and static cytometry: correlation with prognostic features. Am J Pathol 1991;141(3):699–706.
210. Kigawa J, Minagawa Y, Ishihara H, Kanamori Y, Terakawa N. Tumor DNA ploidy and prognosis of patients with serous cystadenocarcinoma of the ovary. Cancer 1993;72: 804.
211. Kaern J, Trope CG, Kristensen GB, Pettersen EO. Flow cytometric DNA ploidy and S phase heterogeneity in advanced ovarian carcinoma. Cancer 1994;73:1870.
212. Alama A, Muttini MP, Merlo F, Barbieri F, Conte PF, Nicolo G, Nicolin A. Survival predictors in relapsed ovarian cancer: performance status and cell kinetics. Proc Am Assoc Cancer Res 1990;31:188 (abstract).
213. Silvestrini R, Daidone MG, Bolis G, Fontanelli R, Landoni F, Andreola S, Colombi R. Cell kinetics: a prognostic marker in epithelial ovarian cancer. Gynecol Oncol 1989;35:15–19.
214. Silvestrini R, Daidone MG, Valentinis B, Ferraris E, Di Re E, Raspagliesi F, Landoni F, Scarfone G, Bolis G. Potentials of cell kinetics in the management of patients with ovarian cancers. Eur J Cancer 28(2/3):386–390, 1992.
215. Conte PF, Alama A, Rubagotti A, Chiara S, Nicolin A, Nicolo G, Rosso R, Gaddi M, Ghiringhello B, Tomao S, Foglia G, Ragni N. Cell kinetics in ovarian cancer: relationship to clinicopathologic features, responsiveness to chemotherapy, and survival. Cancer 1989;64:1188–1191.
216. Guerrieri C, Hogberg T, Wingren S, Fristedt S, Simonsen E, Boeryd B. Mucinous borderline and malignant tumors of the ovary. A clinicopathologic and DNA ploidy study of 92 cases. Cancer 1994;74:2329.
217. Geisinger KR, Homesley HD, Morgan TM, et al. Endometrial adenocarcinoma. A multiparameter clinicopathologic analysis including the DNA profile and the sex steroid hormone receptors. Cancer 1986;58:1518–1528.
218. Lindahl B, Alm P, Ferno M, Killander D, Langstrom E, Norgren A, Trope C. Prognostic value of flow cytometrical DNA measurements in stage I-II endometrial carcinoma: correlations with steroid receptor concentration, tumor myometrial invasion, and degree of differentiation. Anticancer Res 1987;7:791–798.
219. Rosenberg P, Wingren S, Simonsen E, Stal O, Risberg B, Nordenskjold B. Flow cytometric measurements of DNA index and S phase on paraffin-embedded early stage endometrial cancer: an important prognostic indicator. Gynecol Oncol 1989;35: 50–54.
220. Mechiorri C, Chieco P, Lisignoli G, Marabini A, Orlandi C. Ploidy disturbances as an early indicator of intrinsic malignancy in endometrial carcinoma. Cancer 1993;72: 165.
221. Iversen OE. Flow cytometric deoxyribonucleic acid index. A prognostic factor in endometrial carcinoma. Am J Obstet Gynecol 1986;155:770–776.
222. Lukes AS, Kohler MF, Pieper CF, Kerns BJ, Bentley R, Rodriguez GC, Soper JT, Clarke-Pearson DL, Bast RC Jr, Berchuck A. Multivariable analysis of DNA ploidy, p53, and HER-2/neu as prognostic factors in endometrial cancer. Cancer 1994;73: 2380.
223. Nguyen HN, Sevin BU, Averette HE, et al: Determination of hormonal response in uterine cancer cell lines by the ATP bioluminescence assay and flow cytometry. Gynecol Oncol 1992;46:55.
224. van Dam PA, Lowe DG, Watson JV, James M, Chard T, Hudson CN, Shepherd JH. Multiparameter flow-cytometric quantitation of epidermal growth factor receptor and c-erbB-2 oncoprotein in normal and neoplastic tissues of the female genital tract. Gynecol Oncol 1991;42:256–264.
225. Prat J, Oliva E, Lerma E, Vaquero M, Matias-Guiu X. Uterine papillary serous adenocarcinoma. A 10-case study of p53 and c-erbB-2 expression and DNA content. Cancer 1994;74:1778.
226. Miller B, Dockter M, El Torky M, Photopulos G. Small cell carcinoma of the cervix: a clinical and flow-cytometric study. Gynecol Oncol 1991;42:27–33.
227. Strang P, Stendahl U, Bergstrom R, Frankendal B, Tribukait B. Prognostic flow cytometric information in cervical squamous cell carcinoma: a multivariate analysis of 307 patients. Gynecol Oncol 1991;43:3–8.
228. Leminen A, Paavonen J, Vesterinen E, Forss M, Wahlstrom T, Kulomaa P, Lehtinen M. Deoxyribonucleic acid flow cytometric analysis of cervical adenocarcinoma: prognostic significance of deoxyribonucleic acid ploidy and S phase fraction. Am J Obstet Gynecol 1990;162:848–853.
229. Jakobsen A. Ploidy level and short-time prognosis of early cervix cancer. Radiother Oncol 1984;1:271–275.
230. Jakobsen A. Prognostic impact of ploidy level in carcinoma of the cervix. Am J Clin Oncol 1984;7:475–480.
231. Dyson JED, Joslin CAF, Rothwell RI, Quirke P, Khoury GG, Bird CC. Flow cytofluorometric evidence for the differential radioresponsiveness of aneuploid and diploid cervix tumours. Radiother Oncol 1987;8:263–272.
232. Rutgers DH, van der Linden PM, van Peperzeel HA. DNA-flow cytometry of squamous cell carcinomas from the human uterine cervix: the identification of prognostically different subgroups. Radiother Oncol 1986;7:249–258.
233. Atkin NB, Richards BM. Clinical significance of ploidy in carcinoma of cervix: its relation to prognosis. Br Med J 1962;2:1445–1446.
234. Nakano T, Oka K. Differential values of Ki-67 index and mitotic index of proliferating cell population. An assessment of cell cycle and prognosis in radiation therapy for cervical cancer. Cancer 1993;72:2401.
235. Shepherd NA, Richman PI, England J. Ki-67 derived proliferative activity in colorectal adenocarcinoma with prognostic correlations. J Pathol 1988;155:213–219.
236. Seckinger D, Sugarbaker E, Frankfurt O. DNA content in human cancer. Arch Pathol Lab Med 1989;113:619–626.
237. Wolley RC, Schreiber K, Koss LG, Karas M, Sherman A. DNA distribution in human colon carcinomas and its relationship to clinical behavior. JNCI 1982;69:15–22.
238. Kokal WA, Gardine RL, Sheibani K, Morris PL, Prager E, Zak IW, Terz JJ. Tumor DNA content in resectable, primary colorectal carcinoma. Ann Surg 1989;209:188–193.
239. Jones DJ, Moore M, Schofield PF. Refining the prognostic significance of DNA ploidy status in colorectal cancer: a prospective flow cytometric study. Int J Cancer 1988;41:206–210.
240. Quirke P, Dixon MF, Claydens AD, Durdey P, Dyson JED, Williams NBS, Bird CC. Prognostic significance of DNA aneuploidy and cell proliferation in rectal adenocarcinomas. J Pathol 1987;151:285–291.
241. Scott NA, Wieand HS, Moertel CG, Cha SC, Beart RW, Lieber MM. Colorectal cancer: duke's stage, tumor site, preoperative plasma CEA level, and patient prognosis related to tumor DNA ploidy pattern. Arch Surg 1987;122:1375–1379.
242. Schute B, Reynders MMJ, Wiggers T, Arends JW, Volovics L, Bosman FT, Blijham GH. Retrospective analysis of the prognostic significance of DNA content and proliferative activity in large bowel carcinoma. Cancer Res 1987;47:5494–5496.
243. Scivetti P, Danova M, Riccardi A, Fiocca R, Dionigi P, Mazzini G. Prognostic significance of DNA content in large bowel carcinoma: a retrospective flow cytometric study. Cancer Lett 1989;46:213–219.
244. Bosari S, Lee AKC, Wiley BD, Heatley GJ, Silverman ML. Flow cytometric and image analyses of colorectal adenocarcinomas: a comparative study with clinical correlations. Am J Clin Pathol 1993;99:187–194.
245. Melamed MR, Enker WE, Banner P, Janov AJ, Kessler G, Darzynkiewicz Z. Flow cytometry of colorectal carcinoma with three-year follow-up. Dis Col Rect 1986;29: 184–186.
246. Fisher ER, Siderits RH, Sass R, Fisher B. Value of assessment of ploidy in rectal cancers. Arch Pathol Lab Med 1989;113:525–528.

247. Offerhaus GJA, De Feyter EP, Cornelisse CJ, Tersmette KWF, Floyd J, Kern SE, Vogelstein B, Hamilton SR. The relationship of DNA aneuploidy to molecular genetic alterations in colorectal carcinoma. Gastroenterology 1992;102:1612–1619.
248. Scott NA, Rainwater LM, Wieand HS, Weiland LH, Pemberton JH, Beart RW, Lieber MM. The relative prognostic value of flow cytometric DNA analysis and conventional clinicopathologic criteria in patients with operable rectal carcinoma. Dis Col Rect 1987;30:513–520.
249. Jass JR, Mukawa K, Gosh HS, Love SB, Capellaro D. Clinical importance of DNA content in rectal cancer measured by flow cytometry. J Clin Pathol 1989;42:254–259.
250. Meling GI, Rognum TO, Clausen OPF, Chen Y, Lunde OC, Schlichting E, Wiig JN, Hognestad J, Bakka A, Havig O, Bergan A. Association between DNA ploidy pattern and cellular atypia in colorectal carcinomas: a new clinical application of DNA flow cytometric study? Cancer 1991;67:1642–1649.
251. Meling GI, Lothe RA, Borresen AL, Graue C, Hauge S, Clausen OP, Rognum TO. The TP53 tumour suppressor gene in colorectal carcinomas. II. Relation to DNA ploidy pattern and clinicopathological variables. Br J Cancer 1993;67:93.
252. Silvestrini R, D'Agnano I, Faranda A, Costa A, Zupi G, Cosimelli M, Quagliuolo V, Giannarelli D, Gennari L, Cavaliere R. Flow cytometric analysis of ploidy in colorectal cancer: a multicentric experience. Br J Cancer 1993;67:1042.
253. Bauer KD, Lincoln ST, Vera-roman, JM, Wallemark CB, Chmiel JS, Madurski ML, Murad T, Scarpelli DG. Prognostic implications of proliferative activity and DNA aneuploidy in colonic adenocarcinomas. Lab Invest 1987;57:329–335.
254. Wiggers T, Arends JW, Schutte B, Volovics L, Bosman FT. A multivariate analysis of pathologic prognostic indicators in large bowel cancer. Cancer 1988;61:386–395.
255. Ngoi SS, Staiano-Coico L, Godwin TA, Wong RJ, DeCosse JJ. Abnormal DNA ploidy and proliferative patterns in superficial colonic epithelium adjacent to colorectal cancer. Cancer 1990;66:953–959.
256. Wersto RP, Greenebaum E, Deitch D, Kersbergen K, Koss LG. Deoxyribonucleic acid ploidy and cell cycle events in benign colonic epithelium peripheral to carcinoma. Lab Invest 1988;58:218–225.
257. Meling GI, Clausen OPF, Bergan A, Schjolberg A, Rognum TO. Flow cytometric DNA ploidy pattern in dysplastic mucosa, and in primary and metastatic carcinomas in patients with longstanding ulcerative colitis. Br J Cancer 1991;64:339–344.
258. Porschen R, Remy U, Bevers G, Schauseil S, Hengels KJ, Borchard F. Prognostic significance of DNA ploidy in adenocarcinoma of the pancreas. Flow cytometric study of paraffin embedded specimens. Cancer 1993;71:3846–3850.
259. Graeme-Cook F, Bell DA, Flotte TJ, Preffer F, Pastel-Levy C, Nardi G, Compton C. Aneuploidy in pancreatic insulinomas does not predict malignancy. Cancer 1990;66: 2365–2368.
260. Unger PD, Danque POV, Fuchs A, Kaneko M. DNA flow cytometric evaluation of serous and mucinous cystic neoplasms of the pancreas. Arch Pathol Lab Med 1991;115:563–565.
261. Fujimoto J, Okamoto E, Yamanaka N, Fujiwara S, Kato T, Mitsunobu M, Toyosaka A. Nuclear DNA analysis of hepatocellular carcinoma. J Jpn Surg Soc 1989;90:1568.
262. Chiu H, Kao HL, Wu LH, Chang HM, Lui WY. Prediction of relapse or survival after resection of human hepatomas by DNA flow cytometry. J Clin Invest 1992;89:539–545.
263. Seckinger D, Sugarbaker E, Frankfurt O. DNA content in human cancer. Arch Pathol Lab Med 1989;113:619–626.
264. Nagasue N, Yamanoi A, Takemoto Y, Kimoto T, Uchids M, Chang YC, Taniura H, Kohno H, Nakamura T. Comparison between diploid and aneuploid hepatocellular carcinomas: a flow cytometric study. Br J Surg 1992;79:667–770.
265. Tarao K, Shimizu A, Harada M, Ohkawa S, Okamoto N, Kini Y, Ito Y, Tamai S, Iimori K, Sugimasa I, Takemiya S, Okamoto T, Inoue T, Kanisawa M. In vitro uptake of bromodeoxyuridine by human hepatocellular carcinoma and its relation to histopathologic findings and biologic behavior. Cancer 1991;68:1789–1794.
266. Tarao K, Shimizu A, Harada M, Kuni Y, Ito Y, Tamai S, Iimori K, Sugimasa Y, Takemiya S, Okamoto T, Motohashi H, Sairenji M, Inoue T, Kanisawa M. Difference in the in vitro uptake of bromodeoxyuridine between liver cirrhosis with and without hepatocellular carcinoma. Cancer 1989;64:104–109.
267. Dorman AM, Walsh TN, Droogan O, Curran B, Hourihane DOB, Hennessy TPJ, Leader M. DNA quantification of squamous cell carcinoma of the oesophagus by flow cytometry and cytophotometric image analysis using formalin fixed paraffin embedded tissue. Cytometry 1992;13:886–892.
268. Edwards JM, Jones DJ, Wilkes SJL, Hillier VF, Hasleton PS. Ploidy as a prognostic indicator in oesophageal squamous carcinoma and its relationship to various histological criteria. J Pathol 1989;159:35–41.
269. Matsuura H, Sugimachi K, Uro H, Kuwano H, Koga Y, Okamura T. Malignant potential of squamous cell carcinoma of the oesophagus predictable by DNA analysis. Cancer 1986;57:1810–1814.
270. Sugimachi K, Hirako I, Takeshi O, Matsuuura H, Endo M, Inokuchi K. Cytophotometric DNA analysis of mucosal and submucosal carcinoma of the oesophagus. Cancer 1984;53:2683–2687.
271. Patil P, Redkar A, Patel SG, Krishnamurthy S, Mistry RC, Deshpande RK, Mittra I, Desai PB. Prognosis of operable squamous cell carcinoma of the esophagus. Relationship with clinicopathologic features and DNA ploidy [published erratum appears in Cancer, 1993;72:2536.). Cancer 1993;72:20.
272. Doki Y, Shiozaki H, Tahara H, Kobayashi K, Miyata M, Oka H, Iihara K, Mori T. DNA flow cytometry of stomach cancer. Prospective correlation with clinicopathologic findings. Cancer 1993;72:1819.
273. Nakamura T, Nekarda H, Hoelscher AH, Bollschweiler E, Harbeck N, Becker K, Siewert JR, Harbec N. Prognostic value of DNA ploidy and c-erbB-2 oncoprotein overexpression in adenocarcinoma of Barrett's esophagus [published erratum appears in Cancer 1994 Oct 15;74(8):2396). Cancer 1994;73:1785.
274. Minu AR, Endo M, Sunagawa M. Role of DNA ploidy patterns in esophageal squamous cell carcinoma. An ultraviolet microspectrophotometric study. Cancer 1994;74: 578.
275. Bronzo R, Heit P, Weissman G, Kahn E, McKilney M. Implications of flow cytometry in malignant conditions of the stomach. Am J Gastroenterol 1989;84:1065–1068.
276. Nanus DM, Kelsen DP, Niedzwiecki D, Chapman D, Brennan M, Cheng E, Melamed M. Flow cytometry as a predictive indicator in patients with operable gastric cancer. J Clin Oncol 1989;7:1105–1112.
277. Johnson H, Belluco C, Masood S, Abou-Azama AM, Kahn L, Wise L. The value of flow cytometric analysis in patients with gastric cancer. Arch Surg 1993;128:314–317.
278. Ohyama S, Yonemura Y, Miyazaki I. Prognostic value of S phase fraction and DNA ploidy studied with in vivo administration of bromodeoxyuridine on human gastric cancers. Cancer 1990;65:116–121.
279. Yonemura Y, Ooyama S, Sugiyama K, Kamata T, De Aretxabala X, Kimura H, Kosaka T, Yamaguchi A, Miwa K, Miyazaki I. Retrospective analysis of the prognostic significance of DNA ploidy patterns and S-phase fraction in gastric carcinoma. Cancer Res 1990;50:509–514.
280. Yoshino H. A study of DNA ploidy patterns of gastric cancers. J Jpn Surg Soc 1988;89:522.
281. Lee KH, Lee JS, Suh C, Ahn MJ, Kim SW, Doh BS, Min YI, Kim BS, Park KC, Lee IC. DNA flow cytometry of stomach cancer. Prospective correlation with clinicopathologic findings. Cancer 1993;72:1819.
282. Rugge M, Sonego F, Panozzo M, Baffa R, Rubio J, Jr., Farinati F, Nitti D, Ninfo V, Ming SC. Pathology and ploidy in the prognosis of gastric cancer with no extranodal metastasis. Cancer 1994;73:1127.
283. Odegaard S, Hostmark J, Skagen DW, et al. Flow cytometric DNA studies in human gastric cancer and polyps. Scand J Gastroenterol 1987;22:1270–1276.
284. Macartney JC, Camplejohn RS, Powell G. DNA flow cytometry of histological material from human gastric cancer. J Pathol 1986;148:273–277.
285. Deinlein E, Schmidt H, Riemann JF, et al. DNA flow cytometric measurements in inflammatory and malignant human gastric lesions. Virch Arch (A) 1983;402:185–193.
286. Korenaga D, Okamura T, Saito A, Baba H, Sugimachi K. DNA ploidy is closely linked to tumor invasion, lymph node metastasis, and prognosis in clinical gastric cancer. Cancer 1988;62:309–313.
287. Kamata T, Yonemura Y, Sugiyama K, Ooyama S, Kosaka T, Yamaguchi A, Miwa K, Miyazaki I. Proliferative activity of early gastric cancer measured by in vitro and in vivo bromodeoxyuridine labeling. Cancer 1989;64:1665–1668.
288. Amadori D, Bonaguri C, Volpi A, Nanni O, Zoli W, Lundi N, Amadori A, Magni E, Saragoni A. Cell kinetics and prognosis in gastric cancer. Cancer 1993;71:1–4.
289. Joensuu H. DNA flow cytometry in the prediction of survival and response to radiotherapy in head and neck cancer. Acta Oncol 1990;29:513–516.
290. Tytor M, Franzen G, Olofsson J. DNA ploidy in oral cavity carcinomas with special reference to prognosis. Head Neck 1989;11:257–263.
291. Lampe HB, Flint A, Wolf GT, et al. Flow cytometry: DNA analysis of squamous cell carcinoma of the upper aerodigestive tract. J Otolaryngol 1987;16:371–376.
292. Goldsmith MM, Cresson DH, Arnold LA, et al. DNA flow cytometry as a prognostic indicator in head and neck cancer. Otolaryngol Head Neck Surg 1987;96:307–316.
293. Goldsmith MM, Cresson DH, Postma DS, et al. Significance of ploidy in laryngeal cancer. Am J Surg 1986;152:396–402.
294. Sickle-Santanello BJ, Farrar WB, Dobson JL, O'Toole RV, Keyhani-Rofaghe S. Flow cytometric analysis of DNA content as a prognostic indicator in squamous cell carcinoma of the tongue. Am J Surg 1986;152:393–395.
295. Campbell BH, Schemmel JC, Hopwood LE, Hoffmann RG. Flow cytometric evaluation of chemosensitive and chemoresistant head and neck tumors. Am J Surg 1990;160: 424–426.
296. Hemmer J, Kreidler J. Flow cytometric DNA ploidy analysis of squamous cell carcinoma of the oral cavity: comparison with clinical staging and histologic grading. Cancer 1990;66:317–320.
297. Browman GP, Daya D, Booker L, Kanclerz A, Goldsmith C. Comparison of bromodeoxyuridine (BRDU), tritiated thymidine (T) and tritiated deoxyuridine (DU) for assessing DNA synthesis labeling index (LI) in tumor fragments of squamous carcinoma of the head and neck (SCHN). Proc Am Assoc Cancer Res 1988;29:26.
298. Forster G, Cooke TG, Cooke LD, Stanton PD, Bowie G, Stell PM. Tumour growth rates in squamous carcinoma of the head and neck measured by in vivo bromodeoxyuridine incorporation and flow cytometry. Br J Cancer 1992;65:698–702.
299. Hirano T, Zitsch R, Gluckman JL. Cell kinetics study of upper aerodigestive tract squamous cell carcinoma using bromodeoxyuridine. Ann Otol Rhinol Laryngol 1993;102:42–46.
300. Cooke LD, Cooke TG, Forster G, Jones AS, Stell PM. Prospective evaluation of cell kinetics in head and neck squamous carcinoma: the relationship to tumour factors and survival. Br J Cancer 1994;69:717.
301. Greiner TC, Robinson RA, Maves MD. Adenoid cystic carcinoma: a clinicopathologic study with flow cytometric analysis. Am J Clin Pathol 1989;92:711–720.
302. Sahin AA, Ro JY, El-Naggar AK, Lee JS, Ayala AG, Teague K, Hong WK. Flow cytometric analysis of the DNA content of non-small cell lung cancer: ploidy as a significant prognostic indicator in squamous cell carcinoma of the lung. Cancer 1990;65: 530–537.
303. Isobe H, Miyamoto H, Shimizu T, Haneda H, Hashimoto M, Inoue K, Mizuno S, Kawakami Y. Prognostic and therapeutic significance of the flow cytometric nuclear DNA content in non-small cell lung cancer. Cancer 1990;65:1391–1395.
304. Zimmerman PV, Bint MN, Hanson GAT, Parsons PG. Ploidy as a prognostic determinant in surgically treated lung cancer. Lancet 1987;2:530–533.
305. Bunn PA, Carney DN, Gazdar AF, et al. Diagnostic and biologic implications of flow cytometric DNA content analysis in lung cancer. Cancer Res 1983;43:5026–5032.
306. Volm M, Drings P, Mattern J, Sonlka J, Vogt-Moykopf I, Wayss K. Prognostic significance of DNA patterns and resistance-predictive tests in non-small cell lung carcinoma. Cancer 1985;56:1396–1403.
307. Volm M, Hahn EW, Mattern J, Muller T, Vogt-Moykopf I, Weber E. Five-year follow-up study of independent clinical and flow cytometric prognostic factors for the survival of patients with non-small cell lung carcinoma. Cancer Res 1988;48:2923–2928.
308. Volm M, Mattern J, Muller T, Drings P. Flow cytometry of epidermoid lung carcinomas: relationship of ploidy and cell cycle phases to survival. A five-year follow up study. Anticancer Res 1988;8:105–112.
309. Tirindelli-Danesi D, Teodori L, Mauro F, Modini C, Botti C, Cicconetti F, Stipa S. Prognostic significance of flow cytometry in lung cancer: a 5 year study. Cancer 1987;60: 844–851.
310. Van Bodegom PC, Baak JPA, Stroet-van Galen S, Schipper NW, Wisse-Brekelmans ECM, Vanderschueren RG, Wagenarr S. The percentage of aneuploid cells is significantly correlated with survival in accurately staged patients with stage I resected squamous cell lung cancer and long-term follow up. Cancer 1989;63:143–147.
311. Ten Velde GPM, Schutte B, Vermeulen A, Volovics A, Reynders MMJ, Bligham GM. Flow cytometric analysis of DNA ploidy level in paraffin embedded tissue of non-small cell lung cancer. Eur J Cancer Clin Oncol 1988;24:455–460.
312. Pujol JL, Simony J, Laurent JC, Richer G, Mary H, Bousquet J, Godard P, Michel FB. Phenotypic heterogeneity studied by immunohistochemistry and aneuploidy in non-small cell lung cancers. Cancer Res 1989;49:2797–2802.

313. Kawai T, Suzuki M, Kono S, Shinomiya N, Rokutanda M, Takagi K, Ogata T, Tamai S. Proliferating cell nuclear antigen and Ki-67 in lung carcinoma. Correlation with DNA flow cytometric analysis. Cancer 1994;74:2468.
314. Alama A, Repetto L, Vaira F, Serrano J, Ardizzoni A, Nicolin A. Analysis of tumor kinetic in non small cell lung cancer (NSCLC): comparison with clinical variables. Proc Am Assoc Cancer Res 1988;29:231.
315. Volm M, Mattern J, Samsel B. Relationship of inherent resistance to doxorubicin, proliferative activity and expression of p-glycoprotein 170, and glutathione s-transferase-in human lung tumors. Cancer 1992;70:764–769.
316. Abe S, Makimura S, Itabashi K, et al. Prognostic significance of nuclear DNA content in small cell carcinoma of the lung. Cancer 1985;56:2025–2030.
317. Oud PS, Pahlplatz MMM, Beck JLM, Wiersma-van Tilburg A, Wagenaar SJ, Vooijs GP. Image and flow DNA cytometry of small cell carcinoma of the lung. Cancer 1989;64:1304–1309.
318. Vredenburgh JJ, Davis B, Ball ED. The detection of low percentages of small cell carcinoma of the lung (SCCL) or breast cancer cells in the bone marrow by two-color flow cytometry. Proc Am Soc Clin Oncol 1990;9;7.
319. Fujimaki T, Matsutani M, Nakamura O, Asai A, Funada N, Koike M, Segawa H, Aritake K, Fukushima T, Houjo S, Tamura A, Sano K. Correlation between bromodeoxyuridine-labeling indices and patient prognosis in cerebral astrocytic tumors of adults. Cancer 1991;67:1629–1634.
320. Nishizaki T, Orita T, Furutani Y, Ikeyama Y, Aoki H, Sasaki K. Flow-cytometric DNA analysis and immunohistochemical measurement of Ki-67 and BUdR labeling indices in human brain tumors. J Neurosurg 1989;70:379–384.
321. Hoshino T, Ahn D, Prados MD, Lamborn K, Wilson CB. Prognostic significance of the proliferative potential of intracranial gliomas measured by bromodeoxyuridine labeling. Int J Cancer 1993;53:550–555.
322. Onda K, Davis RL, Shibuya M, Wilson CB, Hoshino T. Correlation between the bromodeoxyuridine labeling index and the MIB-1 and Ki-67 proliferating cell indices in cerebral gliomas. Cancer 1994;74:1921.
323. van Meyel DJ, Ramsay DA, Casson AG, Keeney M, Chambers AF, Cairncross JG. p53. JNCI 1994;86:1011.
324. Engebraaten O, Bjerkvig R, Pedersen PH, Laerum OD. Effects for EGF, bFGF, NGF and PDGF(bb) on cell proliferative, migratory and invasive capacities of human brain-tumour biopsies in vitro. Int J Cancer 1993;53:209–214.
325. Spaar FW, Ahyai A, Blech M. DNA-fluorescence-cytometry and prognosis (grading) of meningiomas: a study of 104 surgically removed tumors. Neurosurg Rev 1987;10:35.
326. Franzini A, Broggi G, Giorgi C, Caiola L, Allegranza A. Predictive accuracy of cell kinetics data in glial tumors investigated by serial stereotactic biopsy. J Neurosurg Sci 1989;33:43.
327. Spaar FW, Blech M, Ahyai A. DNA-flow fluorescence-cytometry of ependymomas. Report on ten surgically removed tumours. Acta Neuropathol (Berlin) 1986;60:153–160.
328. Darona M, Riccardi A, Mazzini G, et al. Ploidy and proliferative activity of human brain tumors. A flow cytofluorometric study. Oncology 1987;44:102–107.
329. Zaprianov Z, Christov K. Histological grading, DNA content, cell proliferation, and survival of patients with astroglial tumors. Cytometry 1988;9:380–386.
330. Zerbini C, Gelber RD, Weinberg D, Sallan SE, Barnes P, Kupsky W, Scott RM, Tarbell NJ. Prognostic factors in medulloblastoma, including DNA ploidy. J Clin Oncol 1993;11:616.
331. Gajjar AJ, Heideman RL, Douglass EC, Kun LE, Kovnar EH, Sanford RA, Fairclough DL, Ayers D, Look AT. Relation of tumor-cell ploidy to survival in children with medulloblastoma. J Clin Oncol 1993;11:2211.
332. Tomita T, Yasue M, Engelhard HH, et al. Flow cytometric DNA analysis of medulloblastoma. Prognostic implication of aneuploidy. Cancer 1988;61:744–749.
333. Cusick EL, MacIntosh CA, Krukowski ZH, Ewen SWB, Matheson NA. Comparison of flow cytometry with static densitometry in papillary thyroid carcinoma. Br J Surg 1990;77:913–916.
334. Klemi PJ, Joensuu H, Eerola E. DNA aneuploidy in anaplastic carcinoma of the thyroid gland. Am J Clin Pathol 1988;89:154–159.
335. Rainwater LM, Farrow GM, Hay ID, Lieber MM. Oncocytic tumours of the salivary gland, kidney, and thyroid: nuclear DNA patterns studied by flow cytometry. Br J Cancer 1986;53:799–804.
336. Joensuu H, Klemi P, Eerola E, et al. Influence of cellular DNA content on survival in differentiated thyroid cancer. Cancer 1986;58:2462–2467.
337. Tangen KO, Lindmo T, Sorbinho-Simoes M, et al. A flow cytometric DNA analysis of medullary thyroid carcinoma. Am J Clin Pathol 1983;79:172–177.
338. Johannessen JV, Sobrinho-Simoes M, Tangen KO, et al. A flow cytometric deoxyribonucleic acid analysis of papillary thyroid carcinoma. Lab Invest 1981;45:336–341.
339. Greenebaum E, Koss LG, Elequin F, et al. The diagnostic value of flow cytometric DNA measurements in follicular tumors of the thyroid gland. Cancer 1985;56:2011–2018.
340. Cusick EL, Ewen SWB, Krukowski, Matheson NA. DNA aneuploidy in follicular thyroid neoplasia. Br J Surg 1991;78:94–96.
341. Davies SE, Macartney JC, Camplejohn RS, et al. DNA flow cytometry of thymomas. Histopathology 1989;15:77–83.
342. Helio J, Karaharju E, Nordling S. Flow cytometric determination of DNA content in malignant and benign bone tumours. Cytometry 1985;6:165–171.
343. Kreicbergs A, Silvfersward C, Tribukait B. Flow DNA analysis of primary bone tumors. Relationship between cellular DNA content and histopathologic classification. Cancer 1984;53:129–136.
344. Alvegard TA, Berg NO, Baidetorp B, Feno M, Killander D, Ranstam J, Rydholm A, Akerman M. Cellular DNA content and prognosis of high-grade soft tissue sarcoma. The Scandinavian Sarcoma Group experience. J Clin Oncol 1990;8:538.
345. Alho A, Connor JF, Mankin HJ, et al. Assessment of malignancy of cartilage tumors using flow cytometry. A preliminary report. J Bone Joint Surg 1983;65:779–785.
346. Look AT, Douglass EC, Meyer WH. Clinical importance of near-diploid tumor stem lines in patients with osteosarcoma of an extremity. N Engl J Med 1988;318:1567–1572.
347. Bauer HCF, Kreicbergss A, Silfversward C, Triubukait B. DNA analysis in the differential diagnosis of osteosarcoma. Cancer 1988;61:1430–1436.
348. Xiang J, Spanier SS, Benson NA, Brayalan RC. Flow cytometric analysis of DNA in bone and soft tissue tumors using nuclear suspensions. Cancer 1987;59:1951–1958.
349. Agarwal V, Greenebaum E, Wersto R, Koss LG. DNA ploidy of soft tissue tumors and its relationship to histology and clinical outcome. Arch Path Lab Med 1991;115:558–562.
350. Tsushima K, Rainwater LM, Goeilner JR, van Heerden JA, and Lieber MM. Leiomyosarcomas and benign smooth muscle tumors of the stomach: nuclear DNA patterns studied by flow cytometry. Mayo Clinic Proc 1987;62:275.
351. Niggli FK, Powell JE, Parkes SE, Ward K, Raafat F, Mann JR, Stevens MC. DNA ploidy and proliferative activity (S phase) in childhood soft-tissue sarcomas: their value as prognostic indicators. Br J Cancer 1994;69:1106.
352. El-Jabbour J, Wilson G, Henry K, et al. A flow cytometric (FCM) study of 35 Kaposi's sarcomas (KS) from HIV+ patients. Synopses of papers 113a.
353. Boschman GA, Rens W, Manders EMM, et al. Detection of recurrent chromosome abnormalities in Ewing's sarcoma and peripheral neuroectodermal tumor cells using bivariate flow karyotyping. Genes, Chromosomes Cancer 1992;5:375–384.
354. Drobnjak M, Latres E, Pollack D, Karpeh M, Dudas M, Woodruff JM, Brennan MF, Cordon-Cardo C. Prognostic implications of p53 nuclear overexpression and high proliferation index of Ki-67 in adult soft-tissue sarcomas. JNCI 1994;86:549.
355. Gansler T, Chatten J, Varello M, Bunin GR, Atkinson B. Flow cytometric DNA analysis of neuroblastoma. Correlation with histology and clinical outcome. Cancer 1986;58:2453–2458.
356. Taylor SR, Blatt J, Constantino JP, Roadster M, Murphy RF. Flow cytometric DNA anaysis of neuroblastoma and ganglioneuroma: a 10-year retrospective study. Cancer 1988;62:749–754.
357. Oppedal BR, Storm-Mathisen I, Lie SO, Brandtzaeg P. Prognostic factors in neuroblastoma: clinical, histopathologic, and immunohistochemical features and DNA ploidy in relation to prognosis. Cancer 1988;62:772–780.
358. Bourhis J, DeVatharie F, Wilson GD, Hartmann O, Terrier-Lacombe MJ, Boccon-Gibod L, McNally NJ, Lemerle J, Riou G, Benard J. Combined analysis of DNA ploidy index and N-myc genomic content in neuroblastoma. Cancer Res 1991;51:33–36.
359. Brenner DW, Barranco SC, Winslow BH, Shaeffer J. Flow cytometric analysis of DNA content in children with neuroblastoma. J Pediatr Surg 1989;24:204–207.
360. Bourhis J, Dominici C, McDowell H, Raschella G, Wilson G, Castello MA, Plouvier E, Lemerle J, Riou G, Benard J, Hartmann O. M-myc genomic content and DNA ploidy in stage IVS neuroblastoma. J Clin Oncol 1991;9:1371–1375.
361. Dominici C, Negroni A, Romeo A, Castello MA, Clerico A, Scopinaro M, Mauro F, Raschella G. Association of near-diploid DNA content and N-myc amplification in neuroblastomas. Clin Exp Metastasis 1989;7:201–211.
362. Hayashi Y, Kanda N, Inaba T, Hanada R, Nagahara N, Muchi H, Yamamoto K. Cytogenetic findings and prognosis in neuroblastoma with emphasis on marker chromosome. Cancer 1989;63:126–132.
363. Muraji T, Okamoto E, Fujimoto J, Suita S, Nakagawara A. Combined determination of N-myc oncogene amplification and DNA ploidy in neuroblastoma. Complementary prognostic indicators. Cancer 1993;72:2763.
364. Dominici C, Negroni A, Romeo A, et al. Flow cytometric and molecular analysis of proliferative activity and DNA content in neuroblastoma: presence of stationary cells in S phase. Anticancer Res 1992;12:59–64.
365. Look AT, Hayes FA, Nitschke R, McWilliams NB, Green AA. Cellular DNA content as a predictor of response to chemotherapy in infants with unresectable neuroblastoma. N Engl J Med 1984;311:231–235.
366. Rainwater LM, Hosaka Y, Farrow GM, et al. Wilms' tumors. Relationship of nuclear deoxyribonucleic acid ploidy to patient survival. J Urol 1987;138:974–977.
367. Schmidt D, Wiedemann B, Keil W, et al. Flow cytometric analysis of nephroblastomas and related neoplasms. Cancer 1986;58:2494–2500.
368. Dias P, Kumar P, Marsden HB, Gattamaneni HR, Kumar S. Prognostic relevance of DNA ploidy in rhabdomyosarcomas and other sarcomas of childhood. Anticancer Res 1992;12:1173–1178.
369. Kowal-Vern A, Gonzalez-Crussi F, Turner J, Trujillo YP, Chou P, Herman C, Canstelli M, Walloch J. Flow and image cytometric DNA analysis in rhabdomyosarcoma. Cancer Res 1990;50:6023–6027.
370. Von Roenn JM, Kheir SM, Wolter JM, et al. Significance of DNA abnormalities in primary malignant melanomas and nevi, a retrospective flow cytometric study. Cancer Res 1986;46:3192–3195.
371. Kheir SM, Bines SD, Vonroenn JH, Soong SJ, Urist MM, Coon JS. Prognostic significance of DNA aneuploidy in stage I cutaneous melanoma. Ann Surg 1988;207:455–461.
372. Sondergaard K, Larsen JK, Moller U, Christensen L, Hou-Jensen K. DNA ploidy-characteristics of human malignant melanoma analysed by flow cytometry and compared with histology and clinical course. Virch Arch (B) 1983;42:43–52.
373. Bartkowiak D, Schumann J, Otto FJ, Lippold A, Drepper H. DNA flow cytometry in the prognosis of primary malignant melanoma. Oncology 1991;48:39–43.
374. Karlsson M, Boeryd B, Carstensen J, et al. DNA ploidy and S phase in primary malignant melanoma as prognostic factors for stage III disease. Br J Cancer 1992.
375. Muhonen T, Pyrhonen S, Laasonen A, et al. DNA aneuploidy and low S phase fraction as favourable prognostic signs in metastatic melanoma. Br J Cancer 1991;64:749–752.
376. Muhonen T, Pyrhonen S, Laasonen A, Wasenius V, Asko-Seljavaara S, Franssila K, Kangas L. Tumour growth rate and DNA flow cytometry parameters as prognostic factors in metastatic melanoma. Br J Cancer 1992;66:528–532.
377. Costa A, Silverstrini R, Mezzanotte, Vaglini M, Grignolio E, Clemete C, Cascinelli N. Cell kinetics: an independent prognostic variable in stage II melanoma of the skin. Br J Cancer 1990.
378. Weilbach FX, Bogdahn U, Poot M, Apfel R, Behl C, Drenkard D, Martin R, Hoehn H. Melanoma-inhibiting activity inhibits cell proliferation by prolongation of the S phase and arrest of cells in the G2 compartment. Cancer Res 1990;50:6981–6986.
379. Joensuu GH, Klemi PJ, Korkeila E. Prognostic value of DNA ploidy and proliferative activity in Hodgkin's disease. Am J Clin Pathol 1988;90:670–673.
380. Morgan KG, Quirke P, O'Brien CJ, Bird CC. Hodgkin's disease: a flow cytometric study. J Clin Pathol 1988;41:365–369.
381. Anastasi J, Bauer KE, Variakojis D. DNA aneuploidy in Hodgkin's disease: a multiparameter flow-cytometric analysis with cytologic correlation. Am J Patholol 1987;128:573–582.
382. Diamond LW, Nathwani BN, Rappaport H. Flow cytometry in the diagnosis and classification of malignant lymphoma and leukemia. Cancer 1982;50:1122–1135.
383. Erdkamp FL, Breed WP, Schouten HC, Janssen WC, Hoffmann JJ, Wijnen J Th, Bli-

jham GH. DNA aneuploidy and cell proliferation in relation to histology and prognosis in patients with Hodgkin's disease. Ann Oncol 1993;4:75–80.
384. Macartney JC, Camplejohn RS. DNA flow cytometry of non-Hodgkin's lymphomas. Eur J Cancer 1990;26:635–637.
385. Braylan RC. Flow-cytometric DNA analysis in the diagnosis and prognosis of lymphoma. Am J Clin Pathol 1993;99:374–380.
386. Wain SL, Braylan RC, Borowitz MJ. Correlation of monoclonal antibody phenotyping and cellular DNA content in non-Hodgkin's lymphoma; the Southeastern Cancer Study Group experience. Cancer 1987;60:2403–2411.
387. Young GA, Hedley DW, Rugg CA, Iland HJ. The prognostic significance of proliferative activity in poor histology non-Hodgkin's lymphoma: a flow cytometry study using archival material. Eur J Cancer Clin Oncol 1987;23:1497–1504.
388. Cowan RA, Harris M, Jones M, Crowther D. DNA content in high and intermediate grade non-Hodgkin's lymphoma—prognostic significance and clinicopathological correlations. Br J Cancer 60:904, 1989.
389. Lehtinen T, Aine R, Lehtinen M, Kallioniemi OP, Leino T, Hakala T, Leinikki P, Alavaikko M. Flow cytometric DNA analysis of 199 histologically favourable or unfavourable non-Hodgkin's lymphomas. J Pathol 1989;157:27–36.
390. Costa A, Silvestrini R, Giardini R, Messina-Gabrielli G, Boracchi P, Veneroni S. Contribution of 3H-thymidine labeling index and flow cytometric S phase in predicting survival of patients with non-Hodgkin's lymphoma. Br J Cancer 1992;66:680–684.
391. Lindh J, Jonsson H, Lenner P, Roos G. Fraction of S phase cells in blood mononuclear cells in non-Hodgkin's lymphomas—correlation with clinical features and prognosis. Eur J Haematol 1989;42:331–338.
392. Christensson B, Tribukait B, Linder IL, Ullman B, Biberfeld P. Cell proliferation and DNA content in non-Hodgkin's lymphoma. Cancer 1986;58:1295–1304.
393. Christensson B, Lindemalm C, Johansson B, Melistedt H, Tribukait B, Biberfeld P. Flow cytometric DNA analysis: a prognostic tool in non-Hodgkin's lymphoma. Leuk Res 1989;13:307.
394. Silvestrini R, Costa A, Giardini R, Boracchi P, Del Bino G, Marubini E, Rilke F. Prognostic implications of cell kinetics, histopathology and pathologic stage in non-Hodgkin's lymphomas. Hematol Oncol 1989;7:411–422.
395. Cavalli C, Danova M, Gobbi PG, Riccardi A, Magrini U, Mazzini G, Bertoloni D, Rutigliano L, Rossi A, Ascari E. Ploidy and proliferative activity measurement by flow cytometry in non-Hodgkin's lymphomas. Do speculative aspects prevail over clinical ones? Eur J Cancer Clin Oncol 1989;25:1755–1763.
396. Joensuu H, Klemi PJ, Jalkanen S. Biologic progression in non-Hodgkin's lymphomas: a flow cytometric study. Cancer 1990;65:2564–2571.
397. Joensuu H, Klemi PJ, Soderstrom KO, Jalkanen S. Comparison of S phase fraction, working formulation, and Kiel classification in non-Hodgkin's lymphomas. Cancer 1991;68:1564–1571.
398. Yanik G, Yousuf N, Miller M, Swerdlow SH, Lampkin B, Raza A. In vivo determination of cell cycle kinetics of non-Hodgkin's lymphomas using iododeoxyuridine and bromodeoxyuridine. J Histol Cytochem 1992;40:723–728.
399. Witzig TE, Gonchoroff NJ, Greipp PR, Katzmann JA, Stenson MJ, Habermann TM, Colgan JP, Therneau TM, Banks PM. Rapid S phase determination of non-Hodgkin's lymphomas with the use of an immunofluorescence bromodeoxyuridine labeling index procedure. Am J Clin Pathol 1989;91:298–301.
400. Krauss JS, Pantazis CG, Chandler FW. The proliferative fraction in lymph nodes: a comparison of proliferating cell nuclear antigen morphometry to flow cytometry. Ann Clin Lab Sci 1992;22:189–196.
401. Bunn PA Jr, Whang-Peng J, Carney DN, et al. DNA content analysis by flow cytometry and cytogenetic analysis in mycosis fungoides and Sezary's syndrome. J Clin Invest 1980;65:1440–1448.
402. Lehtinen T, Lehtinen M, Aine R, et al. Nuclear DNA content of non-endemic Burkitt's lymphoma. J Clin Pathol 1987;40:1201–1205.
403. Joensuu H, Soderstrom K-O, Klemi PJ, et al. Nuclear DNA content and its prognostic value in lymphoma of the stomach. Cancer 1987;60:3042–3048.
404. Latreille J, Barlogie B, Johnston D, Drewinko B, Alexanian R. Ploidy and proliferative characteristics in monoclonal gammopathies. Blood 1982;59:43–51.
405. Montecucco C, Riccardi A, Merlini G, Mazzini G, Giordano P, Danova M, Ascari E. Plasma cell DNA content in multiple myeloma and related paraproteinemic disorders. Relationship with clinical and cytokinetic features. Eur J Cancer Clin Oncol 1984;20:81–90.
406. Tienhaara A, Pelliniemi TT. Flow cytometric DNA analysis and clinical correlations in multiple myeloma. Am J Clin Pathol 1992;97:322–330.
407. Morgan RJ, Gonchoroff NJ, Katzmann JA, Witzig TE, Kyle RA, Greipp PR. Detection of hypodiploidy using multi-parameter flow cytometric analysis: a prognostic indicator in multiple myeloma. Am J Hematol 1989;30:195–200.
408. Barlogie B, Alexanian R, Gehan EA, et al. Marrow cytometry and prognosis in myeloma. J Clin Invest 1983;72:853–861.
409. Bunn PA, Krasnow S, Makuch RW, Schlam ML, Schechter GP. Flow cytometric analysis of DNA content of bone marrow cells in patients with plasma cell myeloma: clinical implications. Blood 1982;59:528–535.
410. Tafuri A, Meyers J, Lee BJ, Andreeff M. DNA and RNA flow cytometric study in multiple myeloma. Cancer 1991;67:449–454.
411. Girino M, Riccardi A, Luoni R, Ucci G, Cuomo A. Monoclonal antibody Ki-67 as a marker of proliferative activity in monoclonal gammopathies. Acta Haematol 1991;85:26–30.
412. Drach J, Gattringer C, Glassl H, Drach D, Huber H. The biologic and clinical significance of the Ki-67 growth fraction in multiple myeloma. Hematol Oncol 1992;10:125.
413. Geisler CH, Larsen JK, Hansen NE, Hansen MM, Christensen BE, Lund B, Nielsen H, Plesner T, Thorling K, Andersen E, Andersen PK. Prognostic importance of flow cytometric immunophenotyping of 540 consecutive patients with B-cell chronic lymphocytic leukemia. Blood 1991;78(1):1795–1802.
414. Look AT, Roberson PK, Williams DL, Rivera G, Bowman WP, Pui CH, Ochs J, Abromowitch M, Kalwinsky D, Dahl GV, Geroge S, Murphy SB. Prognostic importance of blast cell DNA content in childhood acute lymphoblastic leukemia. Blood 1985;65:1079–1086.
415. Barlogie B, McLaughlin P, Alexanian R. Characterization of hematologic malignancies by flow cytometry. Anal Quant Cytol Histol 1987;9:147–155.
416. Pui CH, Dodge RK, Look AT, George SL, Rivera GK, Abromowitch M, Ochs J, Evans WE, Crist WM, Simone JV. Risk of adverse events in children completing treatment for acute lymphoblastic leukemia: St Jude total therapy studies VIII, IX, and X. J Clin Oncol 1991;9:1341–1347.
417. Murphy SB, Aur RJA, Simone JV, George S, Mauer AM. Pretreatment cytokinetic studies in 94 children with acute leukemia. Relationship to other variables at diagnosis and to outcome of standard treatment. Blood 1977;49:683–691.
418. Tsurusawa M, Kaneko Y, Katano N, Niwa M, Ito M, Fujimoto T. Flow cytometric evidence for minimal residual disease and cytological heterogeneities in acute lymphoblastic leukemia with severe hypodiploidy. Am J Hematol 1989;32:42–49.
419. Katano N, Tsurusawa M, Niwa M, Fujimoto T. Flow cytometric determination with bromodeoxyuridine/DNA assay of sensitivity of S phase cells to cytosine arabinoside in childhood acute lymphoblastic leukemia. Am J Pediatr Hematol/Oncol 1989;11(4):411–416.
420. Barlogie B, Stass S, Dixon D, et al. DNA aneuploidy in adult acute leukemia. Cancer Genet Cytogenet 1987;28:213–228.
421. Raza A, Preisler HD, Day R, Yasin Z, White LM, Lykins J, Barcos M, Bennett J, Browman G, Goldberg J, Grunwald H, Larson R, Vogler R. Direct relationship between remission duration in acute myeloid leukemia and cell cycle kinetics. Blood 1990;76:2;191.
422. Raza A, Preisler H, Lampkin B, Yousuf N, Tucker C, Peters N, White M, Kukla C, Gartside P, Siegrist C, Bismayer J, Barcos M, Bennett J, Browman G, Goldberg J, Grunwald H, Larson R, Vardiman, Vogler R. Biologic significance of cell cycle kinetics in 128 standard risk newly diagnosed patients with acute myelocytic leukaemia. Br J Haematol 1991;79:33–39.
423. Hiddemann W, Buchner T, Andreeff M, Wormann B, Melamed MR, Clarkson BD. Cell kinetics in acute leukemia: a critical reevaluation based on new data. Cancer 1982;50:250–258.
424. Dosik GM, Barlogie B, Smith TL, Gehan EA, Keating MJ, McCredie KB, Freireich EJ. Pretreatment flow cytometry of DNA content in adult acute leukemia. Blood 1980;55:474–482.
425. Riccardi A, Giordano M, Danova M, Girino M, Brugnatelli S, Ucci G, Mazzini G. Cell kinetics with in vivo bromodeoxyuridine and flow cytometry: clinical significance in acute non-lymphoblastic leukaemia. Eur J Cancer 1991;27:882–887.
426. Giordano M, Danova M, Pellicciari, Wilson GD, Mazzini G, Conti AM, Franchini G, Riccardi A, Romanini MGM. Proliferating cell nuclear antigen (PCNA)/cyclin expression during the cell cycle in normal and leukemic cells. Leuk Res 1991;15:965–974.
427. Hart JS, George SL, Frei E, Bodey GP, Nickerson RC, Freireich EJ. Prognostic significance of pretreatment proliferative activity in adult acute leukemia. Cancer 1977;39:1603–1617.
428. Ogawa M, Fried J, Sakai Y, Strife A, Clarkson BD. Studies of cellular proliferation in human leukemia: the proliferative activity generation time, and emergence time of neutrophilic granulocytes in chronic granulocytic leukemia. Cancer 1970;25:1031–1049.
429. Raza A, Yousuf N, Abbas A, Umerani A, Mehdi A, Bokhari SAJ, Sheikh Y, Qadir K, Freeman J, Masterson M, Miller MA, Lampkin B, Browman G, Bennett J, Goldberg J, Grunwald H, Larson R, Vogler R, Preisler H. High expression of transforming growth factor-B long cell cycle times and a unique clustering of S phase cells in patients with acute promyelocytic leukemia. Blood 1992;79(4):1037–1048.
430. Skipper HE, Schabel FM, Jr., Wilcox WS. Experimental evaluation of potential anticancer agents XIII: on the criteria and kinetics associated with "curability" of experimental leukemia. Cancer Chemother Rep 1964;35:1.
430A. Giordano M, Danova M, Mazzini G, et al. Cell kinetics with in vivo bromodeoxyuridine assay, proliferating cell nuclear antigen expression and flow cytometric analysis. Prognostic significance in acute nonlymphoblastic leukemia. Cancer 1993;71:2739.
431. Skipper HE. Laboratory models: the historical perspective. Cancer Treat Rep 1986;70:3.
432. Simpson-Herren L, Lloyd HH. Kinetic parameters and growth curves for experimental tumor systems. Cancer Chemother Rep 1970;54:143.
433. Frei E, III. Models and the clinical dilemma. In Design of Models for Testing Therapeutic Agents. Edited by IJ Fidler, RJ White. New York: Van Nostrand Reinhold, 1982, pp 248–259.
434. Shackney SE, McCormack GW, Guchural GJ, Jr. Growth rate patterns of solid tumors and their relation to responsiveness to therapy: an analytical review. Ann Intern Med 1978;89:107.
435. Goldin A, Venditti JM, Humphreys SR, Mantel N. Influence of the concentration of leukemic innoculum on the effectiveness of treatment. Science 1956;123:840.
436. Roosa R, Weaver CF, DeLamater ED. Importance of transplant size in chemotherapeutic assay with the use of the Gardner lymphosarcoma. Proc Am Assoc Cancer Res 1957;2:243.
437. Holland JF. Clinical studies of unmaintained remissions in acute lymphocytic leukemia. In the Proliferation and Spread of Neoplastic Cells. 21st Annual Symposium on Fundamental Cancer Research 1967, Baltimore, Williams & Wilkens, 1968, pp 453–462.
438. Schabel FM. Concepts for the systemic treatment of micrometastases. Cancer 1975;35:15.
439. Shapiro DM, Fugmann RA. A role for chemotherapy as an adjunct to surgery. Cancer Res 1957;17:1098.
440. Schabel FM. Concepts for the systemic treatment of micrometastases. Cancer 1975;33:15.
441. Shapiro DM, Fugmann RA. A role for chemotherapy as an adjunct to surgery. Cancer Res 1957;17:1098..
442. Early Breast Cancer Trialists' Collaborative Group. Systemic treatment of early breast cancer by hormonal cytotoxic, or immune therapy. Lancet 1992:339:1.
443. Early Breast Cancer Trialists' Collaborative Group. Treatment of Early Breast Cancer: Worldwide Evidence in 1985–1990. A Systematic Overview of All Available Randomized Trials in Early Breast Cancer of Adjuvant Endocrine and Cytotoxic Therapy. New York: Oxford, 1990.
444. Skipper HE. Laboratory models: The historical perspective. Cancer Treat Reports 1986;70:3.
445. DeVita VT. The relationship between tumor mass and resistance to treatment of cancer. Cancer 1983;51:1209.
446. DeVita VT. Principles of chemotherapy. In Cancer: Principles and Practice, 3rd ed. Edited by T DeVita Jr, S Hellman, SA Rosenberg. Philadelphia: Lippincott, 1988, p 279.
447. Luria SE, Delbruck M. Mutations of bacteria from virus sensitivity to virus resistance. Genetics 1943;28:491.
448. Law LW. Origin of resistance of leukaemic cells to folic acid antagonists. Nature 1952;169:628.

449. Broek D, Bartlett R, Crawford K, Nurse D. Involvement of p34[cdc2] in establishing the dependency of S phase on mitosis. Nature 1991;349:388.
450. Hartwell LH, Weinert TA. Checkpoints: Controls that ensure the order of cell cycle events. Science 1989;246:629.
451. Murray AW, Kirschner MW. Dominoes and clocks: the union of two views of the cell cycle. Science 1989;246:614.
452. Murray AW, Remembrance of things past. Nature 1991;349:367.
453. Burchenal JH, Cremer MA, Williams BS, Armstrong RA. Sterilization of leukemic cells in vivo and in vitro. Cancer Res 1951;11:700–705.
454. Frei E, III, Freireich EJ, Gehan E, Pinkel D, Holland JF, Selawry O, Haurani F, Spurr CL, Hayes DM, James GW, Rothberg H, Sodee DB, Rundles RW, Schroeder LR, Hoogstraten B, Wolman IJ, Traggis DG. Studies of sequential and combination antimetabolite therapy in acute leukemia: 6-Mercaptopurine and methotrexate. Blood 1961;18:431.
455. Goldie JH, Coldman AJ. A mathematic model for relating the drug sensitivity of tumors to their spontaneous mutation rate. Cancer Treat Rep 1979;63:1727.
456. Goldie JH, Coldman AJ. Application of theoretical models to chemotherapy protocol design. Cancer Treat Rep 1986;70:127
457. Goldie JH. Scientific basis for adjuvant and primary (neoadjuvant) chemotherapy. Semin Oncol 1987;14:1.
458. Kendal WS, Frost P. Metastatic potential and spontaneous mutation rates: studies with two murine cell lines and their recently induced metastatic variants. Cancer Res 1986;46:6131
459. Poste G, Fidler IJ. The pathogenesis of cancer metastases. Nature (London) 1980;283:139.
460. National Cancer Institute (USA). Surveillance, Epidemiology and End Results (SEER) Program, 1974–1987.
461. Rosen PP, Groshen S. Factors influencing survival and prognosis in early breast carcinoma (T1N0M0-T1N1M0): assessment of 644 patients with median follow-up of 18 years. Surg Clin North Am 1990;70:937.
462. DeVita VT, Young RC, Cannellos GP. Combination vs. single agent chemotherapy: A review of the basis for selection of drug treatment of cancer. Cancer 1975;35:98.
463. Coldman AJ, Goldie JH. A mathematical model of drug resistance in neoplasms. In Drug and Hormone Resistance in Neoplasia. Edited by N Bruchovsky, JH Goldie. Boca Raton, FL: CRC Press, 1982, pp 55–78.
464. Fisher RI, DeVita VT, Hubbard SM, Simon R, Young RC. Prolonged disease-free survival in Hodgkin's disease with MOPP reinduction after first relapse. Ann Intern Med 1979;90:761.
465. Kardinal CG, Perry MC, Korzun AH, Rice MA, Ginsberg S, Wood WC. Responses to chemotherapy or chemohormonal therapy in advanced breast cancer patients treated previously with adjuvant chemotherapy: a subset analysis of CALGB study 8081. Cancer 1988;61:415.
466. Valagussa P, Tancini G, Bonadonna G. Salvage treatment of patients suffering relapse after adjuvant CMF chemotherapy. Cancer 1986;58:1411.
467. Valagussa P, Brambilla C, Zambetti M, Bonadonna G. Salvage treatment after first relapse of breast cancer: a review. Proceedings, Third International Conference on Adjuvant Therapy of Primary Breast Cancer, St. Gallen, Switzerland, 1988, p 9.
468. Iversen OH, Iversen U, Ziegler JL, Bluming AZ. Cell kinetics in Burkitt's lymphoma. Eur J Cancer 1974;10:155.
469. Bloom H, Richardson M, Harris B. Natural history of untreated breast cancer (1804–1933): comparison of treated and untreated cases according to histological grade of malignancy. Br Med J 1962;2:213
470. Adair F, Berg J, Joubert L, Robbins GF. Long-term follow-up of breast cancer patients: the 30-year report. Cancer 1974;33:1145.
471. Ferguson DJ, Meier P, Karrison T, Dawson PJ, Straus FH, Lowenstein FE. Staging of breast cancer and survival rates. An assessment based on 50 years experience with radical mastectomy. JAMA 1982;248:1337.
472. Harris JR, Hellman S. Observations on survival curve analysis with particular reference to breast cancer. Cancer 1986;57:925
473. Brinkley D, Haybittle JL. The curability of breast cancer. Lancet 1975;2:95.
474. Rutqvist LE, Wallgren A, Nilsson B. Is breast cancer a curable disease? A study of 14,731 women with breast cancer from the Cancer Registry of Norway. Cancer 1984;53:1793.
475. Fisher B, Redmond C, Poisson R, et al. Eight-year results of a randomized clinical trial comparing total mastectomy and lumpectomy with or without irradiation in the treatment of breast cancer. N Engl J Med 1989, 320:822.
475A. Frei E III, Freireich EJ, Gehan, E, et al. Studies of sequential and combination antimetabolite therapy in acute leukemia: 6-mercaptopurine and methotrexate. Blood 1961;18:431.
475B. Ludwig Breast Cancer Study Group. Combination adjuvant chemotherapy for node positive breast cancer. N Engl J Med 1988;319:677.
476. Williams S, Stablein D, Einhorn L, Muggia F, Weiss R, Donohue J, Paulson D, Brunner K, Jacobs E, Spaulding J, DeWys W, Crawford E. Immediate adjuvant chemotherapy versus observation with treatment at relapse in pathological stage II testicular cancer. N Engl J Med 1987;317:1433.
477. Korzun A, Norton L, Perloff M, Wood W, Carey R, Rice M, Holland JF, Frei E. Clinical equivalence despite dosage differences of two schedules of cyclophosphamide, methotrexate, 5-fluorouracil, vincristine and prednisone (CMFVP) for adjuvant therapy of node-positive stage II breast cancer. Proc Am Soc Clin Oncol 1988;7:12.
478. Perloff M, Norton L, Korzun A, Wood W, Carey R, Weinberg V, Holland JF. Advantage of an Adriamycin combination plus halotestin after initial CMFVP for adjuvant therapy of node-positive stage II breast cancer. Proc Am Soc Clin Oncol 1986;70:273.
479. Moliterni A, Bonadonna G, Valagussa P, Ferrari L, Zambetti M. Cyclophosphamide, methotrexate, and fluorouracil with or without doxorubicin in the adjuvant treatment of resectable breast cancer with one to three positive axillary nodes. J Clin Oncol 1991;9:1124.
480. Wampler GL, Heim WJ, Ellison NA, Ahlgren JD, Fryer JG. For the Mid-Altantic Oncology Program: comparison of cyclophosphamide, doxorubicin, and vincristine with an alternating regimen of methotrexate, etoposide, and cisplatin/cyclophosphamide, doxorubicin, and vincristine in the treatment of extensive-disease small-cell lung cancer. J Clin Oncol 1991;9:1438.
481. Longo DL, DeVita VT, Jr., Duffey PL, Wesley MN, Ihde DC, Hubbard SM, Gilliom M, Jaffe ES, Cossman J, Fisher RI, Young RC. Superiority of ProMACE-CytaBOM over ProMACE-MOPP in the treatment of advanced diffuse aggressive lymphoma. Results of a prospective randomized trial. J Clin Oncol 1991;9:25.
482. Bonadonna G, Santoro A. ABVD chemotherapy in the treatment of Hodgkin's disease. Cancer Treat Rev 1982;9:21.
483. Santoro A, Bonfante V, Viviani S, Valagussa P, Bonadonna G. Salvage chemotherapy in relapsing Hodgkin's disease. Proc Am Soc Clin Oncol 1984;3:254.
484. Bonadonna G, Valagussa P, Santoro A. Alternating noncross-resistant combination chemotherapy or MOPP in stage IV Hodgkin's disease. Ann Intern Med 1986;104:739
485. Valagussa P, Santoro A, Boracchi P, Viviani S, Bonadonna G. Nine-year results of two randomized studies with MOPP and ABVD in Hodgkin's disease. Multiple regression analysis. Proc Am Soc Clin Oncol 1989;8:976.
486. Canellos GP, Propert K, Cooper R, Nissen N, Andersen J, Antman KH, Santamauro B, Gottlieb AJ. MOPP vs. ABVD vs. MOPP alternating with ABVD in advanced Hodgkin's disease: a prospective randomized CALGB trial. Proc Am Soc Clin Oncol 1988;7:888.
487. Longo DL, Duffey PL, DeVita VT, Jr., Wiernik PH, Hubbard SM, Phares JC, Bastian AW, Jaffe ES, Young RC. Treatment of advanced-stage Hodgkin's disease: alternating noncross-resistant MOPP/CABS is not superior to MOPP. J Clin Oncol 191;9:1409.
488. Glick J, Tsiatis A, Schilsky R, Beck T, Oken M, Peterson B, Fisher R. A randomized phase III trial of MOPP/ABV hybrid vs. sequential MOPP-ABVD in advanced Hodgkin's disease: preliminary results of the Intergroup Trial. Proc Am Soc Clin Oncol 1991;10:941.
489. Hart R, Perloff M, Holland J. One-day VATH (vinblastine, Adriamycin, thiotepa, and halotestin) therapy for advanced breast cancer refractory to chemotherapy. Cancer 1981;48:1522.
490. Aisner J, Korsun A, Perloff M, Chiarieri D, Abrams J, Panasci L, Rice MA, Wood WC. A randomized comparison of CAF, VATH, and VATH alternating with CMFVP for advanced breast cancer, a CALGB study. Proc Am Soc Clin Oncol 1988;7:27.
491. Brambilla C, Rossi A, Valagussa P, Bonadonna G. Adjuvant chemotherapy in postmenopausal women: results of sequential noncross-resistant regimens. World J Surg 1985;9:728.
492. Norton L. Implications of kinetic heterogeneity in clinical oncology. Semin Oncol 1985;12:231.
493. Buzzoni R, Bonadonna G, Valagussa P, Zambetti M. Adjuvant chemotherapy with doxorubicin plus cyclophosphamide, methotrexate, and fluorouracil in the treatment of resectable breast cancer with more than three positive axillary nodes. J Clin Oncol 1991;9:2134.
494. Bonadonna G, Zambetti M, Valagussa P. Sequentialor alternating doxorubicin and CMF regimens in breast cancer with more than three positive nodes. JAMA 1995;273:542–547.
495. Cassileth PA, Lynch E, Hines JD, et al. Varying intensity of postremission therapy in acute myeloid leukemia. Blood 79:1924;1992.
496. Preisler H, Davis RB, Kirshner J, et al. Comparison of three remission induction regimens and two postinduction strategies for the treatment of acute nonlymphocytic leukemia: a Cancer and Leukemia Group B study. Blood 1987;69:1441.
497. Mayer RJ, Davis RB, Schiffer CA, et al. Intensive postremission chemotherapy in adults with acute myeloid leukemia. N Engl J Med 1994;331:896.
498. McCulloch EA, Buick RN, Curtis JE, Messner HA, Senn JS. The heritable nature of clonal characteristics in acute myeloblastic leukemia. Blood 1981;58:105.
499. Bishop JF. Intensified therapy for acute myeloid leukemia. N Engl J Med (editorial) 1994;331:941.
500. Tubergen D, Gilchrist G, Coccia P, Novak L, O'Brien R, Waskerwitz M, Sather H, Bleyer A, Hammond D. The role of intensified chemotherapy in intermediate risk acute lymphoblastic leukemia (ALL) of childhood. Proceedings, Annual Meeting of American Society on Clinical Oncology, vol 9, 1990, p A835.
501. Frei E, Teicher BA, Holden SA, Cathcart KN, Wang YY. Preclinical studies and clinical correlation of the effect of alkylating dose. Cancer Res 1988;48:6417.
502. Bruce WR, Meeker BE, Valeriote FA. Comparison of the sensitivity of normal hematopoietic and transplanted lymphoma colony-forming cells to chemotherapeutic agents administered in vivo. JNCI 1996;37:233.
503. Griswold DP, Jr., Trader MW, Frei E, III, Peters WP, Wolpert MK, Laster WR, Jr. Response of drug-sensitive and -resistant L1210 leukemias to high-dose chemotherapy. Cancer Res 1987;47:2323
504. Tattersall MHN, Parker LM, Pitman SW, Frei E, III. Clinical pharmacology of high-dose methotrexate. Cancer Chemother Rep (Part 3) 1975;6:25.
505. Bonadonna G, Valagussa P. Dose-response effect of adjuvant chemotherapy in breast cancer. N Engl J Med 1981;304:10.
506. Hryniuk WM. The importance of dose intensity in the outcome of chemotherapy. In Important Advances in Oncology 1988. Edited by VT DeVita Jr, S Hellman, SA Rosenberg. Philadelphia: Lippincott, 1988, pp 121–141.
507. DeVita VT, Hubbard SM, Longo DL. The chemotherapy of lymphomas: looking back, moving forward. Richard and Linda Rosenthal Foundation Award Lecture. Cancer Res 1987;47:5810.
508. Henderson IC, Hayes DF, Gelman R. Dose-response in the treatment of breast cancer: a critical review. J Clin Oncol 1988;6:1501.
509. Redmond C, Fisher B, Wieand HS. The methodological dilemma in retrospectively correlating the amount of chemotherapy received in adjuvant therapy protocols with disease-free survival. Cancer Treat Rep 1983;67:519.
510. Pinkel D, Hernandez K, Borella L, Houlton C, Aur R, Samoy G, Pratt C. Drug dosage and remission duration in childhood lymphocytic leukemia. Cancer 1971;27:247.
511. Samson MK, Rivlin SE, Jones SE, Constanzi JJ, LoBuglio AF, Stephens RL, Gehan EA, Cummings GD. Dose-response and dose-survival advantage for high- vs. low-dose cisplatin combined with vinblastine and bleomycin in disseminated testicular cancer. Cancer 1984;53:1029.
512. Tannock IF, Boyd NF, DeBoer G, Erlichman C, Fine S, Larocque G, Mayers C, Perrault D, Sutherland H. A randomized trial of two dose levels of cyclophosphamide, methotrexate, and fluorouracil chemotherapy for patients with metastatic breast cancer. J Clin Oncol 1988;6:1377.
513. Wood WC, Budman DR, Korzun AH, et al. Dose and dose intensity of adjuvant chemotherapy for Stage II, node-positive breast carcinoma. N Engl J Med 1994;330:1253.
514. Bruce WR, Meeker BE, Valeriote FA. Comparison of the sensitivity of normal hematopoietic and transplanted lymphoma colony-forming cells to chemotherapeutic agents administered in vivo. JNCI 1966;37:233.
515. Bonadonna G, Valagussa P, Rossi A, Tancini G, Brambilla C, Zambetti M, Veronesi

U. Ten-year experience with CMF-based adjuvant chemotherapy in resectable breast cancer. Breast Cancer Res Treat 1985;5:95.
516. Henderson IC, Gelman RS, Harris JR, Canellos GP. Duration of therapy in adjuvant chemotherapy trials. Natl Cancer Inst Monograph 1986;1:95.
517. Rivkin SE, Knight WA, McDivitt R, Cruz T, Foulkes M, Osborne CK, Fabian CJ, Costanzi JJ. Adjuvant therapy for breast cancer with positive axillary nodes designed according to estrogen receptor status. World J Surg 1985;9:723.
518. Early Breast Cancer Trialists' Collaborative Group: Systemic treatment of early breast cancer by hormonal, cytotoxic, or immune therapy. Lancet 1992;339:71.
519. DeVita VT Jr. Dose-response is alive and well. J Clin Oncol 1986;4:1157.
520. Frei E, III, Canellos GP. Dose. A critical factor in cancer chemotherapy. Am J Med 1980;69:585.
521. Collins VP, Loeffler K, Tivey H. Observations on growth rates of human tumors. Am J Radiol 1956;76:988.
522. Steel GG. Growth Kinetics of Tumours—Cell Population Kinetics in Relation to the Growth and Treatment of Cancer. Oxford: Clarendon Press, 1977, pp 46–52.
523. Tubiana M. Tumor cell proliferation kinetics and tumor growth rate. Acta Oncol 1989;28:113.
524. Demicheli R. Growth of testicular neoplasm lung metastases: tumor-specific relation between two Gompertzian parameters. Eur J Cancer 1980;16:1603.
525. Spratt JS, Greenberg RA, Heuser LS. Geometry, growth rates and duration of cancer and carcinoma in situ of the breast before detection by screening. Cancer Res 1986;46:970.
526. Sullivan PW, Salmon SE. Kinetics of tumor growth and regression in IgG multiple myeloma. J Clin Invest 1972;51:1697.
527. Laird AK. Dynamics of growth in tumors and normal organisms. Natl Cancer Inst Monograph 1969;30:15.
528. Norton L. Mathematical interpretation of tumor growth kinetics. In Clinical Interpretation and Practice of Cancer Chemotherapy. Edited by EM Greenspan. New York: Raven, 1982, pp 53–70.
529. Folkman J, Shing Y. Angiogenesis. J Biol Chem 1992;267:10931–10934.
530. Gilewski T, Norton L. Cytokinetics of neoplasia. In The Molecular Basis of Cancer. Edited by J Mendelsohn, P Howley, MA Israel, LA Liotta. Philadelphia: Saunders, 1995, pp 143–159
531. Norton LA. Gompertzian model of human breast cancer growth. Cancer Res 1988;48: 7067.
532. Heuser L, Spratt J, Polk H. Growth rates of primary breast cancer. Cancer 1979;43: 1888.
533. Fisher B, Slack N, Katrych D, Wolmark N. Ten-year follow-up results in patients with carcinoma of the breast in a cooperative clinical trial evaluating surgical adjuvant chemotherapy. Surg Gynecol Obstet 1975;140:528.
534. Speer JF, Petrovsky VE, Retsky MW, Wardwell RH. A stochastic numerical model of breast cancer that simulates clinical data. Cancer Res 1984;44:4124.
535. Fisher B, Brown AM, Dimitrov NV, Poisson R, Redmond C, Margolese RG, Bowman D, Wolmark N, Wickerham DL, Kardinal GC, Shibata H, Paterson AHG, Sutherland CM, Robert NJ, Ager PJ, Levy L, Walter J, Wozniak T, Fisher ER, Deutsch M. Two months of doxorubicin-cyclophosphamide with and without interval reinduction therapy compared with 6 months of cyclophosphamide, methotrexate, and fluorouracil in positive-node breast cancer patients with tamoxifen-nonresponsive tumors: results from the National Surgical Adjuvant Breast and Bowel Project B-15. J Clin Oncol 1990;8:1483.
536. Norton L, Simon R. Growth curve of an experimental solid tumor following radiotherapy. JNCI 1977;58:1735.
537. Norton L, Simon R. Tumor size, sensitivity to therapy, and the design of treatment schedules. Cancer Treat Rep 1977;61:1307.
538. Hill RP, Stanley JA. Pulmonary metastases of the Lewis lung tumor—cell kinetics and response to cyclophosphamide at different sizes. Cancer Treat Rep 1977;61:29.
539. Paterson AHG, Lees AW, Hanson J, Szafran O, Cornish F. Impact of chemotherapy on survival in metastatic breast cancer. Lancet 1980;2:312.
540. Powles TJ, Smith IE, Ford HT, Coombes RC, Jones JM, Gazet JC. Failure of chemotherapy to prolong survival in a group of patients with metastatic breast cancer. Lancet 1980;1:580.
541. Tormey D, Carbone P, Band P. Breast cancer survival in single and combination chemotherapy trials since 1968. Proc Am Assoc Cancer Res 1977;18:64.
542. Norton L, Simon R. The Norton-Simon hypothesis revisited. Cancer Treat Rep 1986;70:163.
543. Ross DW, Capizzi RL. Differentiation vs. cytoreduction during remission induction in acute nonlymphoblastic leukemia treated with sequential high-dose ara-c and asparaginase. Cancer 1984;53:1651.
544. Cortes EP, Necheles TF, Holland JF, Carey RW, Blom J, Brunner K, Falkson G, Weinberg V. Adjuvant chemotherapy for primary osteosarcoma: a Cancer and Leukemia Group B experience. In Adjuvant Chemotherapy of Cancer III. Edited by SE Salmon, SE Jones. New York: Grune & Stratton, 1981, pp 201–210.
545. Cordon-Cardo C, O'Brien JP. The multidrug resistance phenotype in human cancer. In Important Advances in Oncology 1991. Edited by VT DeVita Jr, S Hellman, SA Rosenberg. New York: Lippincott, 1991, pp 19–38.
546. Goldstein LJ, Galski H, Fojo A, Willingham M, Lai, S-L, Gazdar A, Pirker R, Green A, Crist W, Brodeur GM, Lieber M, Cossman J, Gottesman MM, Pastan I. Expression of multidrug resistance gene in human tumors. JNCI 1989;81:116.
547. Bhardwaj S, Holland JF, Norton L. Intensive sequenced adjuvant chemotherapy for breast cancer. Proc Am Soc Clin Oncol 1991;10:75.
548. Skipper HE. Analyses of multiarmed trials in which animals bearing different burdens of L1210 leukemia cells were treated with two, three, and four drug combinations delivered in different ways with varying dose intensities of each drug and varying average dose intensities. Southern Res Inst Booklet 7, 1986;42:87
549. Griswold DP, Schabel FM, Jr., Corbett TH, Dykes DJ. Concepts for controlling drug-resistant tumor cells. In Design of Models for Testing Cancer Therapeutic Agents. Edited by IJ Fidler, RJ White. New York: Van Nostrand Reinhold, 1982, pp 215–224.
550. Day RS. Treatment sequencing, asymmetry, and uncertainty: protocol strategies for combination chemotherapy. Cancer Res 1986;46:3876.
551. Norton L, Day R. Potential innovations in scheduling in cancer chemotherapy. In Important Advances in Oncology 1991. Edited by VT DeVita Jr, S Hellman, SA Rosenberg. New York: Lippincott, 1991, pp 57–72.
552. Selawry OS, Hananian J, Wolman IJ, Abir E, Chevalier L, Gourdeam R, Denton R, Gussoff BD, Levy R, Burgert O Jr, Mills SD, Blom J, Jones B, Patterson RB, McIntyre OR, Haurnai FI, Moon JH, Hoogstraten B, Kung FH, Sheehe PR, Frie E III, Holland JF. New treatment schedule with improved survival in childhood leukemia. JAMA 1965;194:187
553. Gabrilove JL. Colony-stimulating factors: clinical status. In Important Advances in Oncology 1991. Edited by VT DeVita Jr, S Hellman, SA Rosenberg. New York: Lippincott, 1991, pp 215–237.
554. Frei E, III, Antman K, Teicher B, Eder P, Schnipper L. Bone marrow autotransplantation for solid tumors—prospects. J Clin Oncol 1989;7:515.
555. Peters WP. High dose chemotherapy and autologous bone marrow support for breast cancer. In, Important Advances in Oncology. Edited by VT DeVita, S Hellman, SA Rosenberg. Philadelphia: Lippincott , 1991, pp 135–150.
556. Hudis C, Lebwohl D, Crown J, Gilewski T, Surbone A, Hakes T, Currie V, Seidman A, Reichman B, Harrison M, Bellettieri R, Hamilton N, Yao TJ, Norton L. Dose-intensive sequential crossover adjuvant chemotherapy for women with high risk node-positive primary breast cancer. In Adjuvant Therapy of Cancer IV. Edited by SE Salmon. Philadelphia: Lippincott, 1993, pp 214–219.
557. Del Mastro L, Garrone O, Sertoli MR, Canavese G, Catturich A, Guenzi M, Rosso R, Venturini M. A pilot study of accelerated cyclophosphamide, epirubicin and 5-fluorouracil plus granulocyte colony stimulating factor as adjuvant therapy in early breast cancer. Eur J Cancer 1994;30A:606
558. Gianni AM, Bregni M, Siena S, Brambilla C, Lombardi F, Gandola L, Tarella C, Stern A, Valagussa P, Bonadonna G. Prospective randomized comparison of MACOP-B vs. rhGM-CSF-supported high-dose sequential myeloablative chemoradiotherapy in diffuse large cell lymphoma. Proc Am Soc Clin Oncol 1991;10:951.
559. Budihna M, Skrk J, Smid L, Furlan L. Tumor cell repopulation in the rest interval of split-course radiation treatment. Strahlentherapie 1980;156:402.
560. Withers HR, Taylor JMG, Maciejewski B. The hazard of accelerated tumor clonogen repopulation during radiotherapy. Acta Oncol 1988;27:131.
561. Andrews RJ. The radiobiology of human cancer radiotherapy. Philadelphia-London-Toronto: Saunders, 1968 p 45.
562. Badib OA, Webster JH. Changes in tumour oxygen tension during radiation therapy. Acta Radiology Ther Phys Biol 1969;8:247.
563. Steel GG. Growth kinetics of tumors. Oxford: Oxford University Press, 1977.
564. Valeriote F, van Putten L. Proliferation-dependent cytotoxicity of anticancer agents: a review. Cancer Res 1975;35:2619
565. Hug V, Johnston D, Finders M, Hortobagyi G. Use of growth-stimulating hormones to improve the in vitro therapeutic index of doxorubicin for human breast cancer. Cancer Res 1986;46:147.
566. Osborne CK, Kitten L, Arteaga CL. Antagonism of chemotherapy-induced cytotoxicity for human breast cancer cells by antiestrogens. J Clin Oncol 1989;7:710.
567. Conte PF, Alama A, Bertelli G, Canavese G, Carnino F, Catturich A, Di Marco E, Gardin G, Jacomuzzi A, Monzeglio C, Mossetti C, Nicolin A, Pronzato P, Rosso R. Chemotherapy with estrogenic recruitment and surgery in locally advanced breast cancer: clinical and cytokinetic results. Int J Cancer 1987;40:490.
568. Swain SM, Sorace RA, Bagley CS, Danforth DN, Jr., Bader J, Wesley MN, Steinberg SM, Lippman ME. Neoadjuvant chemotherapy in the combined modality approach of locally advanced nonmetastatic breast cancer. Cancer Res 1987;47:3889.
569. Conte PF, Pronzato P, Rubagotti A, Alama A, Amadori D, Demicheli R, Gardin G, Gentilini P, Jacomuzzi A, Lionetto R, Monzeglio C, Nicolin A, Rosso R, Sismondi P, Sussio M, Santi L. Conventional vs. cytokinetic polychemotherapy with estrogenic recruitment in metastatic breast cancer: results of a randomized cooperative trial. J Clin Oncol 1987;5:339.
570. Lippman ME. Hormonal stimulation and chemotherapy for breast cancer (editorial). J Clin Oncol 1987;5:331.
571. Lippman ME, Cassidy J, Wesley M, Young RC. A randomized attempt to increase the efficacy of cytotoxic chemotherapy in metastatic breast cancer by hormonal synchronization. J Clin Oncol 1984;2:28.
572. Bontenbal M, Sieuwerts AM, Klijn JGM, Peters HA, Krijnen HLJM, Sonneveld P, Foekens JA. Effect of hormonal manipulation and doxorubicin administration on cell cycle kinetics of human breast cancer cells. Br J Cancer 1989;60:688.
573. Lippman ME, Dickson RB. Growth control of normal and malignant breast epithelium. In Effects of Therapy on Biology and Kinetics of the Residual Tumor, Part A: Pre-Clinical Aspects. Edited by J Ragaz, J Simpson-Herren, ME Lippman, B Fisher. New York: Wiley-Liss, 1990, pp 147–178.
574. Wilson AJ, Baum M, Brinkley DM, Dossett JA, McPherson K, Patterson JS, Rubens RD, Smiddy FG, Stoll BA, Richards D, Ellis SH. Six-year result of a controlled trial of tamoxifen as single adjuvant agent in management of early breast cancer. World J Surg 1985;9:756.
575. Lippman ME, Dickson RB, Bates S, Knabbe C, Huff K, Swain S, McManaway M, Bronzert D, Kasid A, Gelmann EP. Autocrine and paracrine growth regulation of human breast cancer. Breast Cancer Res Treat 1986;7:59.
576. Weinberg RA, Bishop JM, Minna JD, Sharp PA. Gene regulation and oncogenes: AACR special conference in cancer research. Cancer Res 1989;49:2188.
577. Rowley JD, Golomb AM, Vardiman JW. Nonrandom chromosomal abnormalities in acute leukemia and dysmyelopoietic syndromes in patients with previously treated malignant disease. Blood 1981;58:759.
578. Yee D, Rosen N, Favoni RE, Cullen KJ. The insulin-like growth factors, their receptors, and their binding proteins in human breast cancer. Cancer Treat Res 1991;53:93.
579. Norton L. Biology of residual breast cancer after therapy: a kinetic interpretation. In Effects of Therapy on Biology and Kinetics of the Residual Tumor, Part A: Pre-Clinical Aspects. Edited by J Ragaz, L Simpson-Herren, ME Lippman, B Fisher. New York: Wiley-Liss, 1990, pp 109–132.
580. Koury MJ, Bondurant MC. Erythropoietin retards DNA breakdown and prevents programmed death in erythroid progenitor cells. Science 1990;248:378.
581. Williams GT, Smith CA, Spooncer E, Dexter TM, Taylor DR. Haemopoietic colony stimulating factors promote cell survival by suppressing apoptosis. Nature 1990;343:76
582. Barry MA, Behnke CA, Eastman A. Activation of programmed cell death (apoptosis) by cisplatin, other anticancer drugs, toxins and hyperthermia. Biochem Pharmacol 1990;40:2353.
583. Kennedy S, Merino MJ, Swain SM, Lippman ME. The effects of hormonal and chemotherapy on tumoral and nonneoplastic breast tissue. Hum Pathol 1990;21:192.
584. Amadori D. Use of cell kinetics to analyze responses in combination therapy studies. New Changes in Breast Cancer Clinical Trials, November 16, 1994; Warwick Hotel, Philadelphia.
585. Teicher BA, Herman TS, Holden SA, Wang Y, Pfeffer MR, Crawford JW, Frei E III. Tu-

mor resistance to alkylating agents conferred by mechanisms operative only in vivo. Science 1990;247:1457.
586. Zuckiet G, Tritton TR. Adriamycin causes up-regulation of epidermal growth factor receptors in actively growing cells. Exp Cell Res 1983;148:155.
587. Isonishi S, Andrews PA, Howell SB. Increased sensitivity to cis-diamminedichloroplatinum (II) in human ovarian carcinoma cells in response to treatment with 12-0-tetradecanoylphorbol-13-acetate. J Biol Chem 1990;265:3623.
588. Masui H, Kawamoto T, Sato JD, Wolf B, Sato G, Mendelsohn J. Growth inhibition of human tumor cells in athymic mice by antiepidermal growth factor receptor monoclonal antibodies. Cancer Res 1984;44:1002.
589. Aboud-Pirak E, Hurwitz E, Pirak ME, Fellot F, Schlessinger J, Sela M. Efficacy of antibody to epidermal growth factor receptor against KB carcinoma in vitro and in nude mice. JNCI 1988;80:1605.
590. Norton L, Baselga J, Masui H, Hyman J, Kumar R, Mendelsohn J. Growth factor perturbation: a therapeutically exploitable mechanism for chemotherapy action. Proc Am Soc Clin Oncol 1991;10:208.

CHAPTER 53

Drug Resistance and Its Clinical Circumvention

CHARLES S. MORROW AND KENNETH H. COWAN

Introduction

Systemic therapy with cytotoxic drugs is the basis for most effective treatments of disseminated cancers. Additionally, adjuvant chemotherapy can offer a significant survival advantage to selected patients following the treatment of localized disease with surgery or radiotherapy, presumably by eliminating undetected minimal or microscopic residual tumor. However, the responses of tumors to chemotherapeutic regimens vary, and failures are frequent owing to the emergence of drug resistance. Patterns of treatment response and tumor sensitivity are conveniently divided into three groups. First, with modern treatments prompt cytoreduction and cures are common for some intrinsically drug-sensitive tumors such as childhood acute lymphocytic leukemia, Hodgkin's disease, some non-Hodgkin's lymphomas, and testicular cancer. A second group including tumors such as breast carcinomas, small cell lung cancers, and ovarian carcinomas, are also usually highly responsive to initial treatments but more often become refractory to further therapy. Relapses in either group of tumors, particularly during or shortly after the completion of therapy, generally herald the emergence of tumor cells that are resistant to the antineoplastic agents used initially and often to drugs to which the patient was never exposed. Therefore, success with conventional salvage chemotherapies has been limited. Finally, a third common pattern of drug sensitivity is found in tumors that are intrinsically resistant to most chemotherapeutic agents. This group is represented by malignancies such as non-small cell lung cancers, malignant melanoma, and colon cancer. For these tumors, the number of active antineoplastic agents is few, and significant chemotherapeutic responses are effected in a minority of cases.

The phenomenon of clinical drug resistance has prompted studies to clarify mechanisms of drug action and identify mechanisms of antineoplastic resistance. It is expected that through such information drug resistance may be circumvented by rational design of new non-cross-resistant agents, by novel delivery or combinations of known drugs, and by the development of other treatments that may augment the activity of or reverse resistance to known antineoplastics. Multiple mechanisms of antineoplastic failure have been identified using in vitro (tissue culture) and in vivo (animal and xenograft) models of antineoplastic resistance. A list of these general mechanisms of drug resistance is categorized in Table 53.1. Considered are mechanisms involving anatomic, pharmacologic, and host–drug–tumor interactions, which are uniquely pertinent to patients and to in vivo models of drug resistance as well as cellular mechanisms that can be described at the molecular level. These mechanisms are frequently interrelated as, for example, altered gene expression must ultimately underlie most of the cellular and biochemical mechanisms listed in Table 53.1. Furthermore, multiple independent mechanisms of antineoplastic resistance may coexist in a population of tumor cells.

While mechanisms of drug resistance have been largely determined in experimental systems, many have been implicated in at least some examples of clinical chemotherapeutic failure. Evidence that bears upon these mechanisms of resistance as well as strategies to circumvent them are discussed below. First, we discuss the general mechanisms of cellular drug resistance and then some specific examples in the sections that follow. Additionally, the important concepts of resistance to multiple antineoplastic agents, resistance to specific classes of drugs, and resistance mechanisms unique to in vivo situations are discussed.

General Mechanisms of Drug Resistance

Experimental selection of drug resistance by repeated exposure to single antineoplastic agents will generally result in cross-resistance to some related agents of the same drug class. This phenomenon is explained on the basis of shared drug transport carriers, drug-metabolizing pathways, and intracellular cytotoxic targets of these structurally and biochemically similar compounds. Generally, the resistant cells retain sensitivity to drugs of different classes with alternative mechanisms of cytotoxic action (1, 2). Thus, cells selected for resistance to alkylating agents or antifolates will usually remain sensitive to unrelated drugs such as anthracyclines. Exceptions include emergence of cross-resistance to multiple, apparently structurally and functionally unrelated drugs to which the patient or cancer cells were never exposed during the initial drug treatment. Despite apparent differences in the families of drugs associated with multiple drug resistance phenotypes, when the mechanisms underlying these phenotypes are identified, we frequently discover that the involved antineoplastic agents share common metabolic path-

Table 53.1. General Mechanisms of Drug Resistance

Cellular and Biochemical Mechanisms
- Decreased drug accumulation
  - Decreased drug influx
  - Increased drug efflux
  - Altered intracellular trafficking of drug
- Decreased drug activation
- Increased inactivation of drug or toxic intermediate
- Increased repair of drug-induced damage to:
  - DNA
  - Protein
  - Membranes
- Drug targets altered (quantitatively or qualitatively)
- Altered cofactor or metabolite levels
- Altered gene expression
  - DNA mutation, amplification, or deletion
  - Altered transcription, posttranscription processing, or translation
  - Altered stability of macromolecules

Mechanisms Relevant In Vivo
- Pharmacologic and anatomic drug barriers (tumor sanctuaries)
- Host–drug interactions
  - Increased drug inactivation by normal tissues
  - Decreased drug activation by normal tissues
  - Relative increase in normal tissue drug sensitivity (toxicity)
- Host–tumor interactions

ways, efflux transport systems, or sites of cytotoxic action. Conceptually then, the targets of multiple drug resistance mechanisms are similar to the targets of single agent resistance mechanisms.

In this section, we describe broadly defined processes related to drug resistance and a few specific examples. A more comprehensive discussion follows in the sections on resistance to specific classes of drugs.

DECREASED DRUG ACCUMULATION

Decreased intracellular levels of cytotoxic agents is one of the most common mechanisms of drug resistance. This may result from decreased drug influx due to a defective carrier-mediated transport system. Decreased influx via a high affinity folate-transport system (3) as well as via a reduced folate carrier (4) is a well-described cause of methotrexate resistance (5, 6). A deficient membrane transport system has similarly been identified in cells resistant to nitrogen mustard (7). Enhanced drug efflux may also lower intracellular steady state levels of drugs. Cells that are multiply resistant to antineoplastic drugs due to overexpression of the P-glycoprotein drug efflux pump (classical multidrug resistance or MDR) are important examples of this mechanism of resistance (8).

ALTERED DRUG METABOLISM

Modified drug activation, drug inactivation, or cofactors can confer resistance to selected antineoplastic agents. For example, many antimetabolites and some alkylating agents (e.g., cyclophosphamide) are administered as pro-drugs, which must be activated to their cytotoxic forms by the targeted tumor or by other tissues. Resistance to some nucleobase drugs has been associated with decreased conversion of these analogues to their cytotoxic nucleoside and nucleotide derivatives by kinases and phosphoribosyl transferase salvage enzymes (9, 10). Furthermore, enhanced inactivation of pyrimidine and purine analogues by elevated deaminases has been linked to resistance toward these agents (11, 12). Finally, cofactor levels may modify drug toxicity. For example, optimal formation of inhibitory complexes between 5-fluorodeoxyuridine monophosphate (FdUMP) and its target enzyme, thymidylate synthase, require the cofactor 5,10-methylene tetrahydrofolate (13).

INCREASED REPAIR

Cells contain multiple complex systems involved in the repair of membrane and DNA damage. Because such damage may occur as a direct or secondary consequence of cytotoxic drug action, altered intrinsic repair mechanisms can influence drug sensitivity. For example, resistance to cisplatin, a drug whose cytotoxic action is thought to involve intrastrand DNA cross-linkages (see below), has been associated with altered activities presumed to reflect increased DNA repair.

ALTERED DRUG TARGETS

The mechanisms of cell kill of several antineoplastic drugs involve interactions between the drug and an essential intracellular enzyme. These interactions result in alteration or inhibition of normal functions. Quantitative or qualitative changes in these enzyme targets of antineoplastic drugs can compromise drug efficacy. These changes have been demonstrated in several enzymes associated with drug-resistant cells including dihydrofolate reductase (14), thymidylate synthase (15), and topoisomerase II (16).

ALTERED GENE EXPRESSION

The cellular mechanisms of drug resistance outlined above depend upon altered levels or function of key gene products. These alterations may result from changes that occur at any point along the pathways of gene expression and regulation. Indeed, multiple molecular processes have been shown to be involved in examples of drug resistance, including DNA mutation, deletion, or amplification; altered transcriptional or posttranscriptional control of RNA levels; and altered posttranslational modifications of proteins. The prevalence of these changes reflects the phenotypic and genetic instability of cancer cells under the selective, and perhaps mutagenic, pressures of xenobiotic toxin and drug exposure.

Resistance to Multiple Drugs

De novo and acquired cross-resistance to multiple antineoplastic agents can result from several alternative factors and processes. Accordingly, we have grouped the major patterns of cross-resistance into several categories based upon their presumed underlying mechanisms: classical or P-glycoprotein-dependent MDR, multidrug resistance believed to be conferred by the recently described multidrug resistance-associated protein (MRP), multidrug resistance confined to drugs that are topoisomerase II poisons, and multidrug resistance in which the pattern of cross-resistance to particular agents may resemble the other groups but apparently occurs independently of P-glycoprotein, MRP, or topoisomerase II functions. Additionally, more speculative mechanisms of multidrug resistance mediated by nonspecific xenobiotic metabolizing enzymes and cell-to-cell transfer of genetic information are discussed separately.

CLASSICAL (P-GLYCOPROTEIN-DEPENDENT) MDR

An in vitro model of MDR was described by Biedler and Riehm (17) over two decades ago. In these studies cultured cells selected for resistance by exposure to actinomycin D developed cross-resistance to a surprising array of structurally diverse compounds including Vinca alkaloids, puromycin, daunomycin, and mitomycin C. Subsequently, induction of this pattern of cross-resistance has been observed by numerous investigators who have selected cells in the presence of the same and other drugs. Generally, exposure of cells to any of the drugs (many of which are listed in Table 53.2) related to this MDR phenotype can result in cross-resistance to all other members of the phenotype (8). Drug transport studies using parental and MDR cells have demonstrated that the reduced cytotoxicity of these drugs is the result of decreased drug accumulation secondary to enhanced drug efflux (18, 19). Furthermore, the emergence of MDR has been associated with increased levels of a membrane-bound glycoprotein, P-glycoprotein (P-170 or MDR protein).

The consensus view that P-glycoprotein is the energy-dependent drug efflux pump responsible for MDR is supported by pharmacologic, genetic, and biochemical data. First, the expression of P-glycoprotein is associated with concomitant increases in drug efflux and resistance, which are sensitive to metabolic poisons. Furthermore, gene transfer experiments have shown that the expression of P-glycoprotein genes is sufficient to confer drug resistance (20, 21). P-glycoproteins are encoded by members of a multigene family. Analyses of these *mdr* genes have revealed a striking sequence homology between P-glycoproteins and several bacterial transport proteins (22, 23). The deduced amino acid sequences of P-glycoproteins predict the presence of two pairs of six transmembrane domains and two ATP binding sites (Fig. 53.1). Photoaffinity labeling experiments have demonstrated direct binding of drugs to P-glycoprotein (24). Finally, the distribution of P-glycoprotein on the luminal surfaces of normal tissues including renal tubules, colon, small intestine, and bile canuliculi is consistent with its proposed role in excretory transport (25). Thus, P-glycoprotein appears to fulfill the requirements predicted of a membrane-bound energy-dependent drug carrier.

Table 53.2. Cross-resistance Pattern of Classical MDR

Class	Drug
Anthracyclines	Doxorubicin
	Daunorubicin
	Mitoxantrone
Antibiotics	Actinomycin D
	Plicamycin
Antimicrotubule drugs	Vincristine
	Vinblastine
	Colchicine
Epipodophyllotoxins	Etoposide
	Teniposide

P-glycoprotein-associated MDR is subject to significant phenotypic heterogeneity. The relative degree of cross-resistance to the drugs listed in Table 53.2 will vary depending upon the cell line and the selected drug. While the level of drug resistance is roughly correlated with the level of P-glycoprotein expression, protein and RNA levels may be disproportionately higher or lower than expected for the level of resistance observed. Similarly, the magnitude of the drug accumulation defect may appear insufficient to account for the degree of resistance. The phenotypic variability may result from the expression of alternative *mdr* alleles or by differential expression of the different members of the *mdr* gene family. Indeed, the human genome contains two closely related *mdr* genes. However, only one of these genes, *mdr*1 has been shown to confer drug resistance in man (8). Mutations in the coding region of the *mdr*1 gene have been reported to alter the relative resistance patterns of cells (26). Posttranslational modifications of P-glycoprotein may also alter pump function. For example, P-glycoprotein can be phosphorylated by protein kinase C (27, 28) and by a novel membrane-associated protein kinase (29). Specific sites of protein kinase C-mediated phosphorylation are clustered in the linker region between the two halves of P-glycoprotein (28). Transport studies on MDR cells treated with protein kinase C activators and inhibitors as well as with inhibitors of protein phosphatases show that increased phosphorylation of P-glycoprotein is associated with decreased vinblastine accumulation (27, 28, 30). These results indicate that P-glycoprotein phosphorylation status, as determined by the relative levels of opposing protein kinase and protein phosphatase activities, may influence drug efflux pump function, drug resistance, and MDR phenotypic diversity. Other cofactors involved in augmentation of P-glycoprotein function have been proposed but not yet identified (31). Lastly, other mechanisms of drug resistance may coexist with classical MDR.

A thorough understanding of the regulation of P-glycoprotein production and the means to suppress its expression

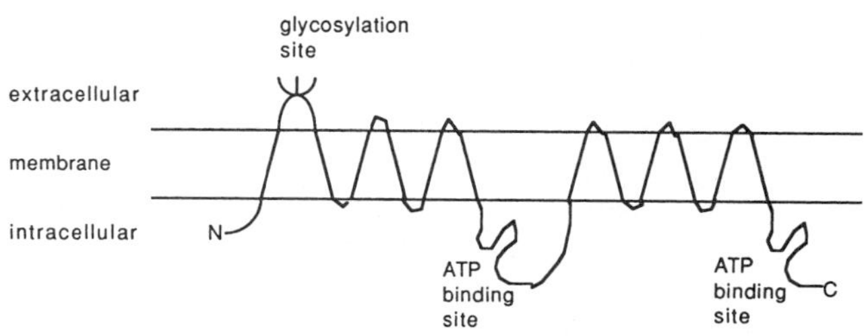

Figure 53.1. Model of P-glycoprotein.

might significantly influence future cancer treatment strategies. Studies addressing this issue have shown that high levels of P-glycoprotein expression in vitro are often associated with *mdr* gene amplification and transcriptional activation (8). Increased expression of P-glycoprotein can also be stimulated by heat shock (32), heavy metals (32), cytotoxic drugs (33–35), regenerating liver (33, 34), differentiating agents (36–38), and repeated exposure to ionizing radiation (39). However, the responses to these treatments appear to vary between species and are cell line specific. Thus, predictable modulation of *mdr* gene expression is not yet possible. Under certain conditions in some cells, *mdr*1 promoter activitiy can be regulated by altered expression of oncogenes (*raf* and *ras*) and the tumor suppressor gene, *p53* (40–44).

Considerable literature has accumulated that concerns the importance of P-glycoprotein in human cancer. P-glycoprotein RNA or protein has been detected in tumor specimens derived from patients with acute and chronic leukemias (45–47), ovarian cancer (48), multiple myeloma (49), breast cancer (50, 51), neuroblastoma (52), soft tissue sarcomas (53), renal cell carcinoma (54), and others (55). Although the numbers of patients with particular tumors in these studies were small, the results have tended to link P-glycoprotein expression with a history of prior therapy (usually with MDR-associated drugs) or toxin exposure, emergence of intrinsic or acquired drug resistance, and treatment outcome. Ma et al. (45) reported that in two patients with ANLL, disease progression with treatment (including an anthracycline) was associated with increasing P-glycoprotein levels in leukemic blasts. In a study of 15 additional patients with ANLL, Sato et al. (46) found that P-glycoprotein was commonly present in leukemic blasts but was more prevalent in blasts derived from patients of poor prognostic groups including those with a history of prior toxin exposure. More recently, three prospective studies have shown that increased P-glycoprotein in patients with AML is associated with decreased complete remission rates and reduced remission duration using conventional chemotherapy (56–58). Although P-glycoprotein was frequently present in tumor specimens from both treated and untreated patients with neuroblastoma, P-glycoprotein RNA tended to be higher in patients treated with regimens that included doxorubicin than in untreated patients (52). Moreover, in patients with advanced neuroblastoma, P-glycoprotein expression has been strongly associated with aggressive biologic behavior, poor treatment response, and poor outcome (59). The impressive correlations between P-glycoprotein expression and aggressive neuroblastoma persisted even when the data were corrected, by multivariant analyses, for other confounding prognostic features. However, the significance of *mdr*1 expression in neuroblastomas is controversial as other data have suggested the opposite—that increased *mdr*1 expression is associated with more favorable clinical variables in patients with neuroblastoma (60). In tumor specimens obtained from patients with childhood ALL (47) and soft tissue sarcomas (53), the presence of P-glycoprotein was associated with anthracycline pretreatment, increased rate of remission induction failure, and increased frequency of relapse. Over 400 tumor specimens were tested for P-glycoprotein RNA levels in a large study (55). Increased levels of P-glycoprotein RNA were more prevalent in tumors that tend to be intrinsically resistant to therapy (colon, renal, adrenal, hepatic, and pancreatic cancers) compared to intrinsically sensitive tumors. Furthermore, P-glycoprotein RNA was often increased in tumors at relapse (acute leukemias, breast cancer, neuroblastoma, pheochromocytoma, and nodular poorly differentiated lymphoma). Additional and prospective studies will be required to confirm the clinical significance of P-glycoprotein in human cancer. However, these preliminary results indicate that P-glycoprotein overexpression is associated with clinical evidence of drug resistance and treatment failure in a significant number of patients. Determinations of P-glycoprotein levels in patients at diagnosis or relapse may have a major role in the design of future treatment protocols.

MULTIDRUG RESISTANCE-ASSOCIATED PROTEIN (MRP)

Similar phenotypes of multiple resistance to antineoplastic agents have been described that are associated with the expression of other membrane proteins. In many of these examples resistance occurs independently of P-glycoprotein expression (61–65). Recently, a gene (MRP) has been isolated from a doxorubicin-selected MDR lung cancer cell line (66). Except for the absence of P-glycoprotein expression, the phenotype of this cell line, which includes the property of reduced drug accumulation, is indistinguishable from classical MDR. The MRP gene encodes a 190-kd transmembrane protein whose structure is strikingly homologous to *mdr*1 and other members of the ATP-binding cassette transmembrane transporter proteins (66, 67). Increased MRP expression is associated with MDR, and decreased MRP expression is associated with reversion to drug sensitivity. Recently, gene transfer experiments have established that MRP can confer MDR (68–70). Transport studies have indicated that MRP is involved in ATP-dependent efflux of native natural product anticancer drugs. Additionally, MRP appears to be (or a component of) an ATP-dependent, glutathione *S*-conjugate transporter (71, 72). Thus, it is suggested that MRP may represent one of the xenobiotic-conjugate efflux pumps and, therefore, may be involved in detoxification of a wide range of cellular poisons including anticancer drugs.

MULTIDRUG RESISTANCE ASSOCIATED WITH TOPOISOMERASE POISONS

Topoisomerases are nuclear enzymes that catalyze the formation of transient single- or double-stranded DNA breaks, facilitate the passage of DNA strands through these breaks, and promote rejoining of the DNA strands (73, 74). As a consequence of these activities, topoisomerases are thought to be critical for DNA replication, transcription, and recombination. The cytotoxicity of drugs that target topoisomerases (topoisomerase poisons) is thought to depend upon the DNA cleavage activities of topoisomerases. There are two classes of mammalian enzymes, topoisomerases I and II. Topoisomerase I catalyzes the formation of single-stranded DNA breaks while topoisomerase II catalyzes both single- and double-stranded breaks. During the cleavage reactions, reversible DNA-topoisomerase complexes (cleavable complexes) can be stabilized by interactions with topoisomerase poisons. The formation of these stabilized DNA-topoisomerase-drug complexes is thought to initiate the production of lethal DNA strand breaks. Of the chemotherapeutic drugs that affect topoisomerase activities, the topoisomerase II poisons have been the most important clinically. A partial list of these agents, which include DNA intercalating and non-intercalating drugs, appears in Table 53.3.

Several laboratories have described a multidrug resistance pattern characterized by resistance of cells to several or all of the drugs listed in Table 53.3 (75, 76). It is readily apparent that many of these topoisomerase II-targeting drugs are also members of the classical MDR phenotype (Table 53.2). However, the pattern of the topoisomerase II-related multidrug resistance differs from the pattern of P-glycoprotein-associated MDR in several important ways. First, resistance to these drugs is not usually associated with a drug transport defect or P-glycoprotein expression. Exceptions to this rule have been described and probably reflect the presence of multiple simultaneous mechanisms of resistance. Additionally, cells that display this topoisomerase II-related resistance phenotype are usually sensitive to antimicrotubule drugs associated with classical MDR including Vinca alkaloids and colchicine unless a concomitant drug transport or microtubule alteration exists. The mechanism of resistance to topoisomerase II poisons is thought to involve altered topoisomerase II activity. Both qualitative and quantitative changes in enzyme activity have been demonstrated in resistant cell lines. Reduced levels of topoisomerase activity have been associated with decreased drug-induced DNA strand breaks as well as reduced drug cytotoxicity (77, 78). Other studies have implicated intrinsic changes in drug-induced catalytic properties or associated cofactors as the basis of drug resistance in some cells (16, 79–81). The nature of the topoisomerase II alterations may influence the cross-resistance patterns observed. For example, cells that develop alterations in topoisomerase II following exposure to m-AMSA (amsacrine) may show cross-resistance to other intercalating topoisomerase II poisons but not to epipodophyllotoxins (80). Collectively, these data indicate that reduced topoisomerase protein levels or selectively altered enzyme activities influencing drug-enzyme interactions may render cells relatively more resistant to drugs by interfering with the formation of stable cleavable complexes and hence cytotoxic DNA strand breaks. Indeed, the normal down-regulation of topoisomerase II in nondividing cells (74) may explain the relative insensitivity to topoisomerase II poisons of some solid tumors containing a large proportion of quiescent cells. Finally, there are two mammalian isozymes of topoisomerase II, a 170-kd form (topoisomerase IIα) and a 180-kd form (topoisomerase IIβ) (82–84). These isozymes differ with respect to their regulation during the cell cycle (85) and their relative sensitivities to topoisomerase II poisons (82, 83). Hence, the relative levels of the specific topoisomerase II isozymes as well as the total topoisomerase II activity may be significant determinants of the sensitivity of tumor cells to topoisomerase II drugs.

Table 53.3. Topoisomerase II Poisons

	Class	Drugs
Intercalators	Epipodophyllotoxins	Etoposide Teniposide
Nonintercalators	Anthracyclines	Doxorubicin Daunorubicin
	Acridine	*m*-AMSA (amsacrine)
	Anthracenedione	Mitoxantrone
	Antibiotic	Actinomycin D
	Ellipticine	9-Hydroxy ellipticine

Sources: Ramani and Dewchand, 1995; Marsh and Center, 1987.

The molecular bases of drug resistance associated with qualitatively altered topoisomerase II have been suggested in several recent reports. Point mutations leading to amino acid substitutions in topoisomerase IIα isolated from cells selected for resistance to topoisomerase II drugs have been described. These mutations are clustered within the conserved ATP binding consensus sequences (86–90) or near the Tyr-804 residue involved in covalent attachment of topoisomerase IIα to DNA (88, 91). Although these topoisomerase IIα mutations are associated with drug resistance in intact cells and, in some cases, with altered enzymatic activities in vitro, the exact mechanism(s) of drug resistance and the relationship of these mutations to a specifically altered enzymatic property are incompletely understood. Moreover, the relevance for clinical drug resistance of these topoisomerase IIα mutations identified in experimentally drug-selected resistant cell lines is unknown. Indeed, one study of topoisomerase IIα derived from leukemic blasts of 15 relapsed patients failed to identify mutations in either of the above two regions implicated in experimental drug resistance (88). Other qualitative alterations in topoisomerase II activity and structure have been described in cell lines selected for resistance to topoisomerase II poisons. These include a selective decrease in nuclear matrix-associated topoisomerase II (92) and a truncated form of topoisomerase IIα (93). Finally, in some resistant cell lines, cytoplasmic or membrane components may be responsible for the altered topoisomerase II activity implicated in the emergence of drug resistance (94).

The cytotoxic agent, camptothecin, has been shown to enhance topoisomerase I-mediated strand breaks. Until recently, host toxicity has prohibited the clinical use of such topoisomerase I poisons. However, the prospect of less toxic analogues of this drug, which maintain a high level of activity against topoisomerase I-rich human cancer cells, has renewed interest in the clinical application of this class of compounds (95). Consequently, the emergence of resistance to these agents may become an increasingly important consideration. There are reports of topoisomerase I mutations derived from cell lines selected for resistance to camptothecin or its derivative, CPT-11 (96–98). In two of these resistant cell lines, the mutant enzyme has altered topoisomerase I activity with a reduced capacity to mediate camptothecin-induced DNA strand breaks (97–99).

MULTIDRUG RESISTANCE ASSOCIATED WITH ALTERED EXPRESSION OF DRUG-METABOLIZING ENZYMES AND DRUG-CONJUGATE EXPORT PUMPS

The emergence of acquired drug resistance may be viewed as an acute or chronic adaptive response of tumor cells to environmental stress, primarily in the form of drug challenge. As discussed above, rapid transient induction of P-glycoprotein may sometimes be mediated by an acute insult such as cytotoxic drug exposure, heavy metal exposure, or heat shock. Alternatively, chronic or repeated exposure to drugs may enhance P-glycoprotein levels by complex, stable genetic changes. In other models and tumor cells, challenges with cytotoxic agents result in alterations in the expression of several genes including those involved in drug metabolism. In the Solt-Farber model of chemical carcinogenesis (100), treatment of rats with various cytotoxins followed by partial hepatectomy results in the appearance of multiple preneoplastic nodules. A number of biochemical changes occur in these nodules, including the overexpression of P-glycoprotein, the induction of several phase II drug-metabolizing (drug conjugating) enzymes, and the down-regulation of some phase I drug-metabolizing (cytochrome P450-dependent mixed function oxidases) enzymes (33, 34). These drug-metabolizing enzymes are generally considered to be involved in the sequential oxidation of xenobiotics to more electrophilic, reactive intermediates followed by the formation of less toxic conjugated compounds, which may be further metabolized or excreted (Fig. 53.2). A similar pattern of P-glycoprotein expression, phase I enzyme suppression, and phase II enzyme induction has been shown in a human breast cancer cell line made multidrug resistant by chronic doxorubicin exposure (101, 102). The emergence of this phenotype appears to represent a programmed cellular stress response, which might offer generalized protection from a variety of exogenous toxins via increased drug efflux secondary to P-glycoprotein expression, decreased drug activation due to reduced phase I enzymes, and increased drug inactivation by phase II enzymes including the glutathione *S*-transferases (GST) and the UDP-glucuronosyl transferases. Of the phase II enzymes, the GSTs have been the most extensively studied.

GSTs (103–105) are comprised of multiple soluble and membrane-associated isozymes that catalyze the conjugation of electrophilic, hydrophobic compounds (R-*X*) with the thiol, glutathione (GSH):

$$\text{R-}X + \text{GSH} \xrightarrow{\text{GST}} \text{R-SG} + \text{H}X$$

Circumstantial evidence has linked the increase in specific GST isozymes or bulk GST activity in cells with resistance to alkylating agents, doxorubicin, and other drugs (104, 105). However, direct evidence that GSTs are responsible for altering drug sensitivities is limited. Another catalytic activity, selenium-independent glutathione peroxidase activity, has been attributed to some isozymes of GST:

$$\text{R-O-OH} + 2\text{GSH} \xrightarrow{\text{GST}} \text{R-OH} + \text{GSSG} + \text{H}_2\text{O}$$

This and other GST-mediated reactions are of interest because of their potential to detoxify oxidative damage to membranes and DNA.

Studies using cell-free preparations of GSTs have identified a limited number of antineoplastic drug substrates of these enzymes. These drugs and other substrates possibly associated with drug-mediated oxidative damage are listed in Table 53.4. Whether GST levels in tumor cells are sufficient to detoxify antineoplastic drugs to a clinically significant extent is a matter of considerable debate. Gene transfer experiments using recombinant GST genes and tissue culture cells have suggested that some GST isozymes may confer a very modest level of resistance to melphalan, chlorambucil, cisplatin (106), and doxorubicin (107). Other gene transfer experiments have failed to confirm any consistent relationship between increased expression of GSTs and resistance

Table 53.4. Some Important Substrates of GSTs Related to Drug Detoxification and Repair of Drug-mediated Damage

Antineoplastic drugs	Products of membrane and DNA oxidation
Nitrogen mustards	Fatty acid hydroperoxides
Chlorambucil	4-Hydroxy alkenals
Melphalan	DNA hydroperoxides
Cyclophosphamide	
Nitrosoureas	
1,3-bis(2-chloroethyl)-1-nitrosourea (BCNU)	
Anthracenedione	
Mitoxantrone	

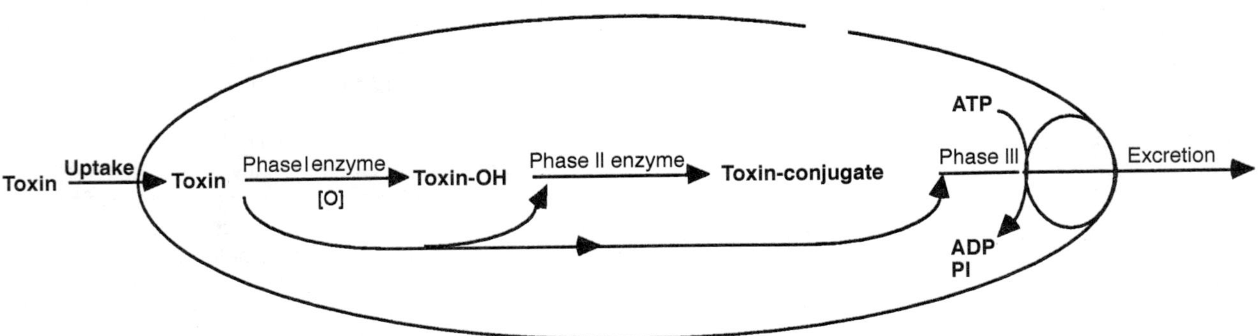

Figure 53.2. Phases I and II drug-metabolizing enzymes.

of breast cancer cells to doxorubicin, cisplatin, melphalan, chlorambucil, or BCNU (31, 108–110).

The importance of drug/xenobiotic-conjugate transporters for cellular export and detoxification of certain compounds has been increasingly appreciated. Conjugation frequently renders the parent drug more hydrophilic and less able to diffuse the plasma membrane, trapping the drug within the cell. While conjugation with glutathionyl or glucuronosyl groups may render some drugs less toxic, these drug conjugates themselves may retain significant toxicity. For example, glutathionyl-cisplatin is itself toxic and an inhibitor of protein synthesis (111). Moreover, drug conjugates may inhibit their conjugating enzyme(s). Thus, the relative resistance of cells expressing drug-metabolizing enzymes may be dependent upon their levels of drug conjugate transporters including the glutathione conjugate transporters (112, 113) and MRP (71, 72).

EMERGENCE OF REFRACTORY TUMORS ASSOCIATED WITH MULTIPLE RESISTANCE MECHANISMS

The backbone of many treatment protocols designed to circumvent the proliferation of resistant tumor cells is the administration of multiple drugs with different structural properties and mechanisms of action. The approach supposes that if enough carefully selected drugs are delivered at optimal doses and intervals, individual clones of cells resistant to one class of drug will be effectively killed by another drug in the regimen. The rapid appearance of refractory tumors despite an initially favorable cytoreductive response suggests that the emergence of multiply resistant tumor cell clones is a common clinical occurrence. We have seen how a single genetic change such as increased P-glycoprotein or altered topoisomerase II can mediate cross-resistance to several but not all useful antineoplastic drugs. Although these mechanisms provide a molecular explanation for broad spectrum resistance, it is clear that many refractory tumor clones must simultaneously develop multiple resistance mechanisms. These mechanisms may arise from multiple independent genetic changes in single cell clones or, as suggested by Cadman (114), from cell-to-cell transfer of genetic information.

RESISTANCE TO ANTICANCER GENOTOXIC TREATMENTS RELATED TO SUPPRESSION OF APOPTOTIC PATHWAYS

The cytotoxicity of several genotoxic anticancer treatments is at least partially due to their abilities to initiate a cascade of events leading to programmed cell death, or apoptosis. As more has been learned of pathways and mechanisms involved in apoptosis, it has become clear that interruption of these pathways can render cells resistant to therapy. In response to certain genotoxic insults, cellular levels of p53 are elevated leading to cell cycle arrest and to apoptosis in some sensitive cells. For example, radiation and etoposide-induced apoptosis were shown to be dependent upon the expression of normal p53 in thymocytes (115, 116). Indeed, thymocytes with deficient normal p53 were relatively resistant to the apoptosis initiated by the treatments that induce DNA strand breaks. In human cells derived from patients with lymphomas, cell lines that have mutant p53 were shown to be relatively resistant to DNA damaging agents when compared to lymphoid cell lines that express wild type p53 (117). These results suggest that abnormal or deficient p53, which are known to be tumorigenic, may also be expected to render tumors more resistant to cytotoxic drug treatment. Consistent with this prediction are the findings that in the hematologic malignancies, AML, MDS, and CLL, p53 mutations are adverse prognostic indicators for response to therapy and survival (118). Additionally, Strasser et al. (119) showed that in proliferating lymphoid cells, DNA-damaging anticancer drugs and radiation induce apoptosis by p53-independent mechanisms. Importantly, expression of Bcl-2 can interrupt apoptosis at a point distal along either the p53-dependent or p53-independent pathways. Indeed the level of Bcl-2 and related proteins as well as the level of late effectors of apoptosis (e.g., the interleukin 1β converting enzymes (ICE) and ICE-like proteases and their putative inhibitors) may govern the level of cellular sensitivity to genotoxic, anticancer drug inducers of programmed cell death (120). Transgenic models of lymphoid tumor cells have shown that high level Bcl-2 expression is associated with prolonged survival and reduced molecular evidence of apoptosis in response to treatment by a variety of anticancer drugs including doxorubicin, methotrexate, ara-C, etoposide, vincristine, cisplatin, and 4-hydroperoxycyclophosphamide (121) and to anticancer drugs that are inhibitors of thymidylate synthase (122). Thus, the expression of *p53, bcl-2*, and other genes potentially associated with apoptosis (e.g., c-*myc and* c-H-*ras* (123, 124)) may contribute significantly to the drug sensitivities of tumor cells. These genes may represent important future targets for the pharmacologic and biologic modulation of drug resistance.

Resistance Factors Unique to Tumor Cells in Vivo: Host-Tumor-Drug Interactions

The failure of chemotherapy to eradicate a tumor in vivo despite exquisite sensitivity to drug in vitro may be due to anatomic or pharmacologic sanctuaries. For example, the failure to deliver adequate amounts of many drugs across blood-brain and -testicular barriers probably accounts for the relatively high frequency of acute lymphoblastic leukemia relapse at these sites (125). In large solid tumors, chemotherapeutic failures are frequently attributed to decreased drug delivery to a tumor that has overgrown its vascular supply. Additionally, development of acidosis and hypoxia in poorly perfused areas of large tumors may interfere with the cytotoxicity of some drugs. Altered pro-drug activation by liver or other normal tissues may profoundly influence the efficacy of drugs such as cyclophosphamide.

A report by Teicher et al. (126) suggests that tumor-host interactions may influence drug pharmacokinetics and tumor resistance in unexpected ways. In this study, tumor cells selected for cyclophosphamide and cisplatin resistance in vivo were normally sensitive to drugs in vitro. When the tumor cells were reimplanted into nude mice in vivo drug resistance was restored. These results suggest that resistant tumors may harbor cellular resistance factors that are operative only in conjunction with host factors and, therefore, mediate resistance by altered drug pharmacokinetics in vivo only. If this novel host-dependent mechanism of tumor resistance proves common, these results would provide one explanation for the failure of conventional in vitro testing to predict clinical responsiveness in all cases.

Approaches to Overcoming Resistance to Specific Groups of Drugs

Approaches to overcome chemotherapeutic failures include efforts to prevent the emergence of drug resistance (Table 53.5). An appreciation of factors that induce resistance mechanisms may lead to the choice of more efficacious treatment regimens. For example, drugs that may have only sporadic activity against a specific tumor yet are likely to select for cross-resistance to more active agents would be avoided. It is hoped that aggressive combination chemotherapy with noncross-reacting drugs will eliminate tumor rapidly enough to prevent the selection of multiply resistant tumor cell clones. Failures of the preventative approach require the incorporation of specific measures aimed at reversing or circumventing drug resistance.

DRUGS ASSOCIATED WITH P-GLYCOPROTEIN-MEDIATED RESISTANCE

Prior to the original descriptions of P-glycoprotein, Tsuruo and co-workers (127) noted that treatment with verapamil of leukemia cells made drug resistant by selection in vincristine or doxorubicin could partially restore antineoplastic drug sensitivity. Furthermore, this verapamil-enhanced antineoplastic cytotoxicity, which was specific for drug-resistant but not sensitive parental cells, was associated with increased accumulation of vincristine and doxorubicin. These results suggested that in the drug-resistant cells vincristine and doxorubicin share a common transport system that is sensitive to modulation by verapamil. This transport system has now been identified as the P-glycoprotein drug efflux pump. Subsequently, numerous agents have been studied that can partially reverse the drug accumulation defects in classically multidrug-resistant cells including several calcium channel blockers, calmodulin inhibitors such as phenothiazines, cyclosporin A, and cyclosporin derivatives, and other drugs (128–135). Although the mechanism(s) by which these agents reverse MDR is incompletely understood, it is believed that direct interactions between these agents and P-glycoprotein interfere with antineoplastic drug efflux activity. Since a considerable clinical experience in the use of MDR-reversing agents has existed for the treatment of other disorders, these agents have been included in several clinical trials designed to enhance the antitumor activity of conventional cancer drugs in refractory human neoplasms.

Several clinical trials have used verapamil as a multidrug resistance-modifying agent. Some efficacy with these regimens has been reported, especially in the treatment of hematologic malignancies. In one study, verapamil in combination with etoposide resulted in 8 of 11 partial responses in pediatric patients with leukemias refractory to MDR drugs (136). However, the levels of P-glycoprotein in these tumors were not assessed. Thus, the relationship between *mdr* gene expression and the efficacy of the reversing agent could not be determined. To address this issue, Dalton and colleagues (137) examined eight patients with myelomas and lymphomas refractory to regimens containing vincristine and doxorubicin. Patient tumors were analyzed for the presence of P-glycoprotein RNA and protein as well as for their responses to treatment regimens consisting of verapamil administered with vincristine, doxorubicin, and dexamethasone. Three patient tumors responded to the verapamil-containing regimens (two transient PRs and one transient CR) and all of these responding tumors were P-glycoprotein positive. A study involving patients with lymphomas demonstrated that P-glycoprotein expression was rare in tumors from newly diagnosed patients but common in refractory tumors from previously treated patients (138). Following treatment with verapamil in combination with doxorubicin- and vincristine-containing regimens, a 72% response rate (28% CR) was observed in refractory patients. Verapamil-containing regimens also showed some efficacy in the treatment with vincristine and doxorubicin of patients with refractory multiple myelomas (5 of 22 patients showed PRs). In this study, a relationship between the administration of verapamil and the reversal of MDR was suggested by the finding that 4 of 10 patient tumors that tested positive for *mdr*1 expression responded, whereas none of 5 patient tumors that tested negative for *mdr*1 expression responded (139). In contrast, the inclusion of verapamil in treatment regimens for colorectal or refractory ovarian cancer has not been effective in enhancing clinical responses to chemotherapy (140, 141). A major factor limiting the usefulness of verapamil as an MDR-reversing agent is dose-limiting cardiac toxicity. It has therefore been difficult to achieve clinical levels of verapamil that are predicted, by in vitro testing, to be necessary for optimal MDR reversal, even when the less cardiotoxic D-isomer of verapamil is used (142).

Several other potential MDR-reversing agents have been used in various pilot studies and include tamoxifen (143,

Table 53.5. Approaches to Overcome or Circumvent Drug Resistance

Prevention	Aggressive multiple agent therapy
	Appreciation of factors that induce resistance mechanisms
Circumvention	Drug screening programs and rational drug design
	Circumvention of drug uptake defects
	Dose escalation
	Drugs that use alternative transport mechanisms
	Agents that reverse increased efflux
	Cofactors that augment drug activation or efficacy
	Inhibition of drug inactivation
	Novel treatment modalities
	Immunotherapy

144), trifluperazine (145), nifedipine (146), quinidine (147), and quinine (148). Recently, cyclosporin and its derivatives have shown considerable promise as MDR-reversing agents in both preclinical and clinical testing (134, 149–152). While toxicities are observed with the use of cyclosporin, these are reversible. Moreover, pharmacologically efficacious levels are achievable and tolerated as reported in several clinical trials. In the treatment of high risk AML patients, good response rates were observed with regimens containing cyclosporin A in combination with high dose ara-C and daunorubicin (151). However, the proportion of responders attributable to the inclusion of cyclosporin versus high dose ara-C and daunorubicin alone could not be assessed. Moreover, no association between MDR phenotype and response was demonstrated. In contrast, a study of a patient with refractory AML showed a relationship between the pharmacological effects of cyclosporin A and the MDR status of the tumor cells. In this report, treatment with cyclosporin A resulted both in enhanced daunorubicin accumulation in P-glycoprotein positive myeloblasts in vitro as well as a transient elimination of P-glycoprotein-positive AML cells in vivo (149). In another anecdotal report, a CR was achieved in a refractory T-cell ALL patient upon treatment with cyclosporin A plus ara-C, methotrexate, and etoposide (153). However, for some tumors such as colorectal carcinomas, the results of attempts to improve therapeutic efficacy with cyclosporin have been disappointing (154).

In addition to their actions on P-glycoprotein-positive tumor cells, cyclosporins can have profound effects on the pharmacokinetics and pharmacodynamics of cytotoxic drugs associated with MDR (135, 155). Indeed, marked increases in area under the curve levels, decreased renal and non-renal clearances, and increased volumes of distribution of etoposide have been observed in patients concomitantly treated with cyclosporin A. The reason for these effects is unknown, but it is suggested they are due to the action of cyclosporins on normal tissues (such as renal, biliary, and endothelial) possibly via cyclosporin interactions with the P-glycoprotein resident within these normal tissues. Toxicities, such as myelosuppression, of MDR-associated drugs may be enhanced when administered with cyclosporins. These toxicities necessitate appropriate reduction in dosage of cytotoxic drugs when they are used in combination with cyclosporins. Because P-glycoprotein is found at high levels in human endothelium and is believed to contribute to the blood-brain barrier (156, 157), cyclosporins may also contribute to some of the neurotoxicities observed when certain MDR-associated drugs are administered with cyclosporins. These pharmacologic issues must be carefully considered in future clinical trials.

Collectively, these trials suggest that the use of MDR-reversing agents may be of some benefit to selected patients with P-glycoprotein-positive refractory tumors. Needed before such reversing drugs can be recommended in standard regimens are additional clinical trials that clearly establish a correlation between improved antitumor response using MDR-reversing agents and the presence of P-glycoprotein in those tumors. Moreover, the pharmacodynamic influence of agents such as cyclosporins on cytotoxic drugs must be carefully defined to achieve appropriate cytotoxic drug dosing. It is necessary to continue the search for reversing agents with improved efficacy and decreased toxicities as well as to determine optimal dosages and schedules. Finally, other preclinical studies indicate that anti-P-glycoprotein antibodies, either covalently linked to cellular toxins (158) or used in conjunction with complement (159), can specifically reduce the burden of P-glycoprotein-positive tumor cells. The clinical utility of these immunologic reagents is a matter for future investigation.

TOPOISOMERASE II POISONS

As discussed above, resistance to topoisomerase II poisons may occur as a consequence of P-glycoprotein overexpression or altered topoisomerase II activities. However, neither of these mechanisms will necessarily result in cross-resistance to all of the topoisomerase II-directed drugs listed in Table 53.3. For example, resistance to epipodophyllotoxins and anthracyclines on the basis of increased P-glycoprotein is not usually associated with resistance to the acridine derivative, amsacrine. Conversely, resistance to amsacrine and other intercalating drugs due to alterations in topoisomerase II protein is not always associated with resistance to the nonintercalating, epipodophyllotoxin class of topoisomerase II poisons (80). Therefore, these data derived from in vitro studies suggest a rationale for administering an alternative class of topoisomerase II poison in selected cases of clinical resistance to another class of topoisomerase II-directed drug.

The cross-resistance patterns of several multidrug-resistant human leukemia cell lines to a series of amsacrine analogues has been reported (160, 161). In these studies resistant cells were selected in the presence of amsacrine or doxorubicin. When compared to their parental cell lines, the resistant cells displayed multiple patterns of cross-resistance to the panel of drugs tested. Most significantly, for some cell lines resistant or cross-resistant to amsacrine, analogues of amsacrine were identified to which resistant cells showed increased sensitivity that approached the level of parental cell sensitivity. Although the precise changes in the resistant cells were not determined, the authors suggested that an altered topoisomerase II with reduced capacity to form stable ternary complexes with drugs and DNA might underlie one resistance pattern. Furthermore, some specific modifications in the putative drug-binding portion of the amsacrine analogues were associated with increased toxicity of the drugs toward amsacrine-resistant cells displaying this pattern. It was suggested that rational design of such analogues might enhance drug interaction with the altered topoisomerase II and thereby augment the clinical efficacy of these drugs in some resistant tumor cells.

RESISTANCE TO FREE RADICAL-MEDIATED DRUG CYTOTOXICITY

Several antineoplastic agents form free radical intermediates that are thought to contribute to drug cytotoxicity. Anthracyclines, such as doxorubicin, are among the most important members of this class of compound. While DNA-intercalating anthracyclines can damage cells by multiple mechanisms including inhibition of nucleic acid synthe-

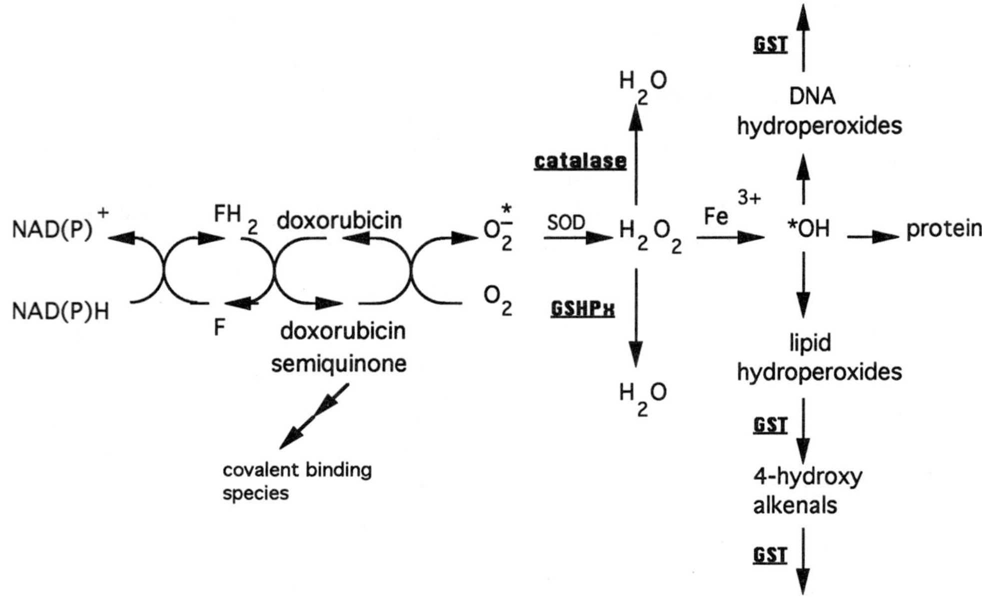

Figure 53.3. Mechanisms of free-radical-dependent doxorubicin toxicity and its reversal. GST, glutathione *S*-transferase; GSHPx, glutathione peroxidase; SOD, superoxide dismutase.

sis, induction of topoisomerase II-mediated DNA strand breaks, and perturbation of cell membranes, these quinone-hydroquinone compounds can also generate toxic-free radical species that may cause cell death. As represented in Figure 53.3, doxorubicin and related drugs can undergo one-electron reductions in reactions catalyzed by a variety of enzymes (162, 163). The semiquinone radical so generated may either form a covalently binding free radical derivative or in the presence of oxygen may be reoxidized to the quinone species in a reaction producing superoxide anion. Decomposition of hydrogen peroxide formed by dismutation of superoxide anion produces the highly reactive hydroxyl radical which may directly damage DNA, lipid, and protein. Thus, cellular factors that limit hydrogen peroxide production or repair peroxidative damage to macromolecules could theoretically confer some resistance to anthracyclines.

The pathways depicted in Figure 53.3 suggest several mechanisms by which tumor cells may become resistant to anthracycline-mediated free radical damage. First, superoxide anion formation is limited in poorly vascularized, relatively hypoxemic tissues such as may exist in the centers of large solid tumors. Second, increased intracellular levels of catalase and glutathione peroxidase (GSHPx) can deplete hydrogen peroxide thus reducing the formation of toxic hydroxyl radicals. Indeed, in comparing parental and MDR-positive MCF-7 cells, Sinha and co-workers (164) have reported an association between increased GSHPx activity and reduced doxorubicin-stimulated hydroxyl radical formation. Furthermore, lowering GSHPx activity by depleting the enzyme's cosubstrate, GSH resulted in enhanced doxorubicin-dependent free radical formation and cytotoxicity (165). Additionally, Kramer et al. (166) found that GSH depletion with buthionine sulfoximine (BSO) could partially restore the doxorubicin sensitivity of MDR-positive MCF-7 cells, presumably by interfering with GSH-dependent reactions including those catalyzed by GSHPx (166). While these results are consistent with the importance of hydrogen peroxide and hydroxyl radical formation in anthracycline cytotoxicity in MCF-7 cells, other investigators have noted that increased catalase, GSH, and GSHPx levels are not always protective of some cells from doxorubicin-mediated damage (167). Finally, increased repair of peroxidative damage to DNA and unsaturated lipids represents another potentially protective mechanism against doxorubicin-dependent hydroxyl radical toxicity. For example, some isozymes of GST exhibit significant lipid hydroperoxidase activity and may also contain limited DNA hydroperoxidase activity (168). Additionally, the highly toxic 4-hydroxy alkenals formed from the decomposition of lipid hydroperoxides are relatively good substrates for some GSTs (169). Thus, overexpression of particular GST isozymes could conceivably contribute to doxorubicin resistance.

The relative importance of free radical generation in tumor cell kill is unknown and the protective mechanisms outlined above are speculative. Nevertheless, the GSH-dependent detoxification pathways are of particular interest as they are subject to pharmacologic manipulation. GSHPx and GST activities can be secondarily reduced by depleting tissue GSH with BSO treatment. Furthermore, the activity of GSTs can be inhibited by the administration of competitive substrates such as ethracrynic acid (170). Such clinical manipulations may enhance tumoricidal activity of doxorubicin but must be viewed cautiously as they may also potentiate drug toxicity toward normal tissues.

ALKYLATING AGENTS AND PLATINUM COMPOUNDS

Resistance to alkylating agents and platinum compounds can be described by at least three broad mechanistic categories including decreased drug accumulation, increased drug inactivation, and enhanced repair of DNA damage. Preclinical studies have indicated that the latter two mechanisms may be circumvented by pharmacologic manipulations. Reactions of electrophilic alkylating agents with thiol-containing compounds represent a relatively general mechanism of antineoplastic inactivation or detoxification. For example, GSH forms conjugate with a variety of alkylating agents in both nonenzymatic and in GST-dependent reactions. Table 53.4 lists some of the compounds whose conjugation with GSH is catalyzed by GSTs in vitro (104). Several laboratories have demonstrated an association between increased bulk GST levels or specific GST isozymes with resistance to drugs such as nitrosoureas (171), chlorambucil, and other nitrogen mustards (106, 172–175). Additionally, increased GSH levels have been correlated with resistance to alkylating agents and cisplatin (176, 177). While the electrophilic cisplatin compound can react directly with GSH, it is unknown whether GSTs can catalyze this reaction. This issue is unresolved by conflicting results that show a correlation between elevated expression of the π isozyme of GST and resistance to cisplatin in some cells (178, 179) but not others (109). Perhaps more relevant to the issue of cisplatin resistance is the finding that glutathionyl-platinum complexes, which are themselves toxic, are exported by an ATP-dependent pump probably identical to one of the glutathione conjugate pumps described previously (111). Thus, these drug exporters should be considered in the design of treatments and formulation of strategies to enhance cisplatin efficacy.

The correlations between GSH or GST levels and drug resistance are variable. Indeed, some investigators have been unable to demonstrate a relationship between the overexpression of multiple isozymes of GST and antineoplastic resistance (31, 108–110). In other studies that have compared paired parental and resistant cell lines, the magnitude of alkylating agent resistance associated with increased GST activity is often modest. While the clinical importance of GST and GSH in alkylating resistance is accordingly debated, existing preclinical data have prompted phase I trials using GST inhibitors or the GSH synthesis inhibitor, BSO, in conjunction with alkylating agents.

Aldehyde dehydrogenase is another drug metabolizing enzyme that has been linked to cyclophosphamide-derivative resistance in murine and human models of drug resistance (180–182). This enzyme converts a metabolite of cyclophosphamide, aldophosphamide, to the inactive compound, carboxyphosphamide, thereby preventing the decomposition of aldophosphamide to its cytotoxic derivative, phosphoramide mustard. Increased expression of aldehyde dehydrogenase has been associated with resistance to cyclophosphamide in vitro. Whether inhibitors of aldehyde dehydrogenase such as disulfiram and diethylaminobenzaldehyde can be used therapeutically to enhance the antitumor effect of cyclophosphamide without undue host toxicity remains to be explored.

Cisplatin toxicity is thought to be mediated primarily by the formation of lethal intrastrand DNA cross-links. Several reports have suggested that increased DNA repair is associated with resistance to this compound. For example, unscheduled DNA synthesis, which is thought to be indicative of DNA repair, is relatively increased in response to cisplatin treatment of cisplatin-resistant ovarian cancer cells when compared to drug-sensitive parental cells (183). In a murine leukemia model, cells selected for cisplatin resistance showed enhanced ability to repair cisplatin-induced intrastrand DNA cross-links (184, 185). Aphidicolin can inhibit an enzyme implicated in DNA repair, DNA polymerase α. Treatment of ovarian carcinoma cells with aphidicolin potentiated the toxicity of cisplatin in resistant but not sensitive cells (183). These results suggest that the coadministration of DNA polymerase α inhibitors with cisplatin may be useful in overcoming cisplatin resistance. The results of ongoing phase I trials using the analogue, aphidicolin glycinate, should help clarify the feasibility of this approach.

ANTIMETABOLITES

The antimetabolites are a clinically important group of cancer drugs used in the treatment of a variety of solid tumors and hematologic malignancies. The cytotoxicities of the antimetabolites stem from their abilities to interfere with key enzymatic steps in nucleic acid metabolism. The discussion that follows concerns three particularly well-studied compounds, the antifolate, methotrexate (MTX) and the pyrimidine analogues, 5-fluorouracil (5FU) and cytosine arabinoside (ara-C, 1-β-D-arabinofuranosylcytosine, cytarabine). Strategies designed to overcome the multiple described mechanisms of cellular resistance to these compounds include dose escalation, pharmacologic manipulation of drug metabolism, and rational design of new antimetabolites.

The clinically important antifolate, MTX, displays significant tumoricidal activity against a variety of human neoplasms such as acute leukemia, osteogenic sarcoma, choriocarcinoma, breast cancer, head and neck cancers, and others (186). Consideration of MTX metabolism and sites of action (Fig. 53.4) serves as the basis for understanding mechanisms of methotrexate resistance. Following uptake by the folate transport systems, MTX can bind avidly to and inhibit its primary enzyme target, dihydrofolate reductase (DHFR). In the presence of adequate thymidylate synthase activity, inhibition of DHFR results in depletion of the reduced folate pools essential for thymidylate and de novo purine synthesis. The cytotoxicity of MTX is significantly influenced by intracellular polyglutamation. MTX polyglutamates are retained preferentially by cells and bind more effectively to DHFR. Additionally, these polyglutamyl derivatives can inhibit other folate-dependent enzymes including thymidylate synthase (187) and 5-aminoimadazole carboxamide ribotide (AICAR) transformylase (188), enzymes involved in thymidylate and de novo purine synthesis, respectively. Therefore, resistance to MTX can result from a number of alternative mechanisms including reduced MTX uptake via a defective folate transport system (6), reduced polyglutamation leading to decreased drug retention as well as reduced inhibition of thymidylate synthase and AICAR transformylase (189), and either elevated levels of DHFR or reduced affinity of DHFR for MTX (190–193). While all of these mechanisms have been described in examples of experimental resistance of cultured cells to MTX, increased DHFR levels secondary to

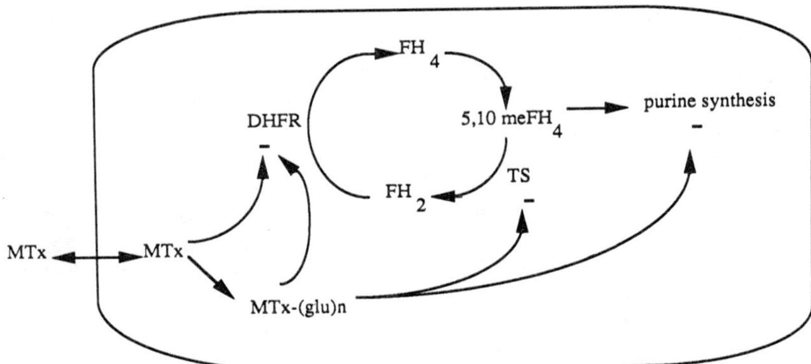

Figure 53.4. Methotrexate metabolism and toxicity. MTx, methotrexate; MTx-(glu)n, plyglutamate methotrexate; DHFR, dehydrofolate reductase; TS, thymidylate synthase; FH_2, dihydrofolate; FH_4, tetrahydrofolate; 5,10 mdFH_4, 5,10-methylene tetrahydrofolate.

gene amplification is the only mechanism identified to date that has been associated with clinical MTX resistance (194–196).

The use of high dose MTX (HDMTX) with subsequent rescue of normal tissues by administration of the reduced folate, leucovorin (*N*5-formyl tetrahydrofolate) has been advocated as an approach that could theoretically circumvent most mechanisms of MTX resistance. At high systemic drug concentrations, cytocidal levels can be achieved by passive diffusion of drug into transport-defective resistant cells. Furthermore, prolonged exposure of cells to high extracellular concentrations of drug can maintain cytotoxic intracellular drug levels in the face of a drug retention defect secondary to decreased polyglutamation. Finally, increased intracellular MTX delivered by HDMTX therapy can saturate DHFR in cells whose resistance is due to amplification of the DHFR gene or due to lowered affinity of DHFR for MTX. Although HDMTX is of proven value in the treatment of ALL and perhaps osteogenic sarcoma, the rationale for the use of this modality in the treatment of other cancers has been recently questioned (197, 198). Indeed, some tumors, as well as normal tissues, are rescued from HDMTX toxicity by leucovorin. In these and other cases, the use of HDMTX with leucovorin rescue offers no therapeutic advantage over regimens that use conventional MTX doses. While early studies suggested that HDMTX improved response rates to chemotherapy of osteogenic sarcoma (199), the contribution of HDMTX therapy to the success of recent multiagent adjuvant protocols is unclear. In contrast, HDMTX is indisputably efficacious in the treatment of ALL. The success of HDMTX in this setting is probably due to the penetration of drug across anatomic and pharmacologic barriers into tumor sanctuaries such as testes and, at very high MTX doses, the central nervous system (125).

In an effort to improve drug efficacy, other inhibitors of DHFR, such as trimetrexate and piritrexim, have been developed (200–202). These lipid-soluble drugs are taken up by cells independently of the folate-carrier system; consequently, their use might obviate transport-mediated antifolate resistance. However, cells that are resistant to MTX on the basis of amplified DHFR will be cross-resistant to trimetrexate. The utility of trimetrexate is further limited by the association of classical MDR with cross-resistance to trimetrexate (203). These results suggest that trimetrexate and drugs of the MDR phenotype share the same P-glycoprotein efflux pump.

Other antifolate compounds capable of inhibiting folate-dependent enzymes besides DHFR have been investigated. One drug, 10-propargyl-5,8-dideazafolate, has shown promise as a thymidylate synthase inhibitor (204). Another drug with potential clinical utility, 5,10-dideazatetrahydrofolate is an effective inhibitor of glycinamide ribonucleoside transformylase, the first folate-dependent enzyme in de novo purine synthesis (205). As these and related antifolates pass through preclinical and clinical testing, they may assume important roles as cytotoxic agents for the treatment of tumors refractory to the conventional antifolate, MTX. Cells resistant to MTX by virtue of increased DHFR expression would be expected to remain sensitive to some but not all of these novel antifolates.

The pyrimidine base, 5-FU, and its deoxynucleoside metabolite, 5-fluoro-2′-deoxyuridine (FdUrd), have been used in the treatment of gastrointestinal tumors, breast cancer, head and neck cancer, and some other malignancies. The metabolism of 5-FU is complex and is partially shown in Figure 53.5 (15). The best characterized mechanism of fluoropyrimidine cytotoxicity involves the inhibition of thymidylate synthase by 5-fluoro-2′-deoxyuridine monophosphate (FdUMP). Additionally, the incorporation of the metabolite, 5-fluorouridine triphosphate (FUTP) into RNA has been correlated with cytotoxicity in some systems. While 5-fluro-2′-deoxyuridine triphosphate (FdUTP) can be incorporated into DNA, the relationship between this process and the cytocidal activity of fluoropyrimidines remains undetermined. Resistance to 5-FU may be conferred by alterations in enzymes involved in fluoropyrimidine metabolism, particularly those

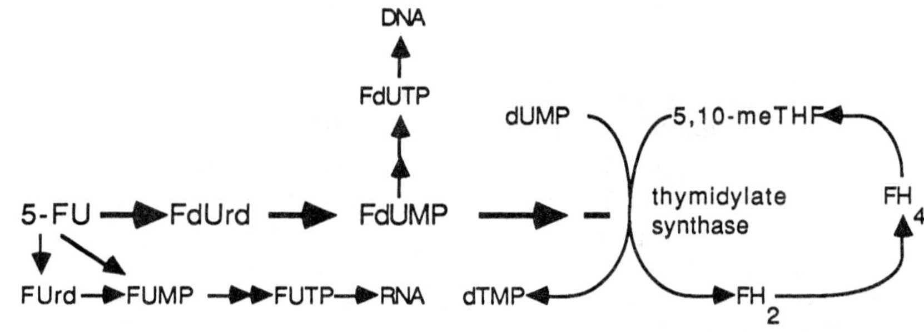

Figure 53.5. 5-Fluorouracil metabolism and toxicity. 5-FU, 5-fluorouracil; FdUrd, 5-fluoro-2′-deoxyuridine; FdUMP and FdUTP, 5-fluoro-2′-deoxyuridine mono- and triphosphate.

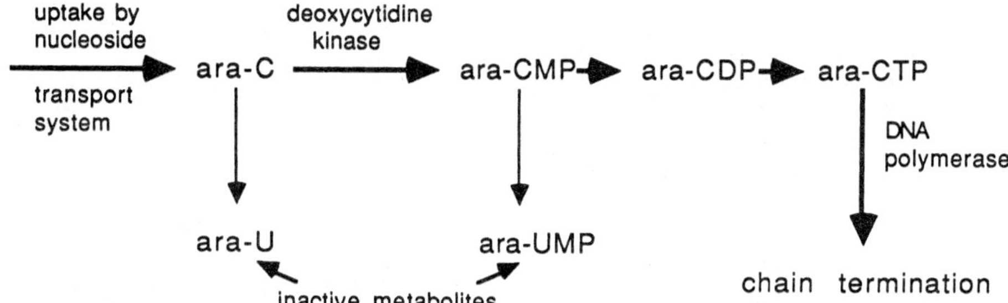

Figure 53.6. Cytosine arabinoside (ara-C) metabolism and toxicity.

enzymes associated with the conversion of 5-FU to the thymidylate synthase inhibitor, FdUMP (15). Furthermore, changes in thymidylate synthase level or its affinity for FdUMP have been associated with 5-FU resistance (206–208).

Several strategies to improve fluoropyrimidine efficacy and overcome resistance have been advanced. It has been suggested that tumor cell killing may be improved by prolonged or continuous exposure to drug (209, 210). Other studies have advocated the coadministration with 5-FU of the reduced folate, leucovorin. The efficacy of this combination stems from leucovorin-dependent increases in intracellular 5,10-methylene tetrahydrofolate (5, 10-meTHF), a cofactor that stabilizes the FdUMP-thymidylate synthase inhibitor complex (211, 212). Synergy between 5-FU and other agents that might be exploited clinically have also been studied. For example, pretreatment of cells with methotrexate enhances the toxicity of 5-FU subsequently administered. Such pretreatment with methotrexate, an inhibitor of de novo purine synthesis (above), has been shown to increase the level of phosphoribosyl pyrophosphate (PRPP). Thus, the expanded pool of PRPP is available for conversion of 5-FU to FUMP and FUTP (Fig. 53.5). It has been suggested that the increased incorporation of FUTP into RNA that results is responsible for the improved cytotoxicity (213, 214). The inhibitor of de novo pyrimidine synthesis, phosphonacetyl-L-aspartate (PALA), has been used with 5-FU in an effort to reduce pyrimidine metabolites that compete for the targets of fluoropyrimidine toxicity (215). Finally, the synergistic interaction between interferon and halogenated pyrimidines has been recently investigated (216).

Ara-C is an important nucleoside antineoplastic agent effective in the treatment of acute leukemias. The metabolism and mechanism of cytotoxicity of ara-C are represented in Fig. 53.6 (217). Following uptake by the nucleoside transport system, ara-C is activated by a series of kinases to ara-CTP, a substrate of DNA polymerase that is incorporated into nascent DNA causing premature chain termination and ultimately cell death. The rate-limiting step in ara-C activation is the S-phase-specific reaction catalyzed by deoxycytidine kinase. The cytotoxic compound, ara-CTP or its precursors (ara-CMP and ara-CDP), can be catabolized by phosphatases or they (ara-C and ara-CMP) can be inactivated by deaminases. Several mechanisms of cancer cell resistance to ara-C have been demonstrated that include, but not confined to the following. Because ara-C activation is cell cycle-dependent, quiescent cells or cells that fail to enter S-phase during the interval of treatment escape the cytotoxicity of ara-C. At suboptimal doses otherwise drug-sensitive tumor cells located in pharmacologic or anatomic sanctuaries may survive ara-C treatment (218). Decreased nucleoside transport has also been implicated in ara-C resistance (219). Additionally, resistance may be conferred by altered drug metabolism such as decreased activation by deoxycytidine kinase (217), increased inactivation by cytidine deaminase (11), or altered DNA polymerase affinity for ara-C (220).

Administration of high dose ara-C represents one approach to overcoming resistance to the drug and has been clinically useful in the treatment of some leukemias refractory to conventional doses of ara-C. Resistance based upon diminished nucleoside transport and pharmacologic/anatomic sanctuaries can be circumvented with high dose drug treatment (218). In resistance secondary to increased drug inactivation by cytidine deaminase, coadministration with ara-C of a cytidine deaminase inhibitor such as tetrahydrouridine may reverse this mode of drug resistance (221). The alternative pyrimidine analogue, ara-AC (arabinofuranosyl-5-azacytosine, fazarabine) has shown activity against a broad range of tumor cells in preclinical testing and has been the subject of two recently completed phase I clinical trials (222, 223). This compound contains a triazine ring, which is resistant to deamination and therefore should theoretically be effective against tumors that are resistant to ara-C due to increased cytidine deaminase activity.

Conclusions and Future Directions

Through the kinds of studies done largely in vitro described in this chapter, many of the mechanisms of antineoplastic drug resistance have been identified. While several of these processes operate in vivo, their relative clinical importance must be better clarified in controlled, prospective examinations of patient tumor specimens and correlations with therapeutic responses to chemotherapy. Nevertheless, these mechanisms have suggested potentially useful approaches to overcoming clinical drug resistance. These approaches include the rational choice of conventional agents or design of novel drugs that are less likely to share resistance mechanisms. Additionally, many of the pathways of antineoplastic drug inactivation or transport are targets for pharmacologic manipulations that may reverse or circumvent the resistance of tumors to some drugs. Despite these efforts, many tumors will remain refractory to conventional chemotherapeutic drugs. Their successful treatment may require novel modalities such as biologic response modifiers. For example, the use of cytokines alone or in combination with adoptive immunotherapy, differentiating agents like retinoic acid, and pharmacologic agents capable of altering the responses of tumors to exogenous and autocrine growth factors may hold promise for the treatment of some cancers. Dose escalation of conventional agents followed by hematologic rescue with cytokines or bone marrow transplantation is assuming a greater role in protocols designed to treat a variety of cancers. Finally, the pathways of signal transduction and programmed cell death have been identified as important determinants of cellular sensitivity to genotoxic drugs. Factors that modulate the pathways of apoptosis may become important targets for future therapeutics aimed at overcoming or circumventing drug resistance.

References

1. Teicher BA, Cucchi CA, Lee JB, et al. Alkylating agents: in vitro studies of cross-resistance patterns in human cell lines. Cancer Res 1986;46:4379.
2. Hill BT, Price LA, Goldie JH. The value of Adriamycin in overcoming resistance to methotrexate in cell culture. Eur J Cancer 1976;12:541.
3. Anthony AC, Kane MA, Portillo RM, Elwood PC, Kolhouse JF. Studies of the role of a particulate folate-binding protein in the uptake of 5-methytetrahydrofolate by cultured human KB cells. J Biol Chem 1985;260:14911.
4. Dixon KH, Lanpher BC, Chiu J, Kelley K, Cowan KH. A novel cDNA restores reduced folate carrier activity and methotrexate sensitivity to transport deficient cells. J Biol Chem 1994;269:17–20.
5. Hill BT, Bailey BD, White JC, Goldman ID. Characteristics of transport of 4-amino antifolates and folate compounds by two cell lines of LY5178Y lymphoblasts, one with impaired transport of methotrexate. Cancer Res 1979;39:2440.
6. Sirotnak FM, Moccio DM, Kelleher LE, Goutsas LJ. Relative frequency and kinetic properties of transport defective phenotypes among methotrexate-resistant L1210 clonal cell lines derived in vivo. Cancer Res 1981;41:4447.
7. Goldenberg GJ, Vanstone CL, Isreals LG, Isle D, Bihler D. Evidence for a transport carrier of nitrogen mustard in nitrogen mustard-sensitive and -resistant L5178Y lymphoblasts. Cancer Res 1970;30:2285.
8. Endicott JA, Ling V. The biochemistry of P-glycoprotein-mediated multidrug resistance. Annu Rev Biochem 1989;58:137.
9. Drahovsky D, Kreis W. Studies on drug resistance. II. Kinase patterns in P815 neoplasms sensitive and resistant to 1-β-D-arabinofuranosyl cytosine. Biochem Pharmacol 1970;19:940.
10. Brockmann RW. Mechanisms of resistance to the anticancer agents. Adv Cancer Res 1963;7:129.
11. Steuart CD, Burke PJ. Cytidine deaminase and the development of resistance to cytosine arabinoside. Nature New Biol 1971;233:109.
12. Hunt SW, Hoffee PA. Amplification of adenosine deaminase gene sequence in deoxycoformycin-resistant rat hepatoma cells. J Biol Chem 1983;258:13185.
13. Houghton JA, Maroda SJ, Phillips JO, Houghton PJ. Biochemical determinants of responsiveness to 5-fluorouracil and its derivatives in xenografts of human colorectal adenocarcinomas in mice. Cancer Res 1981;41:144.
14. Haber DA, Beverly SM, Kiely ML, Schimke RT. Properties of altered dehydrofolate reductase encoded by amplified genes in cultured mouse fibroblasts. J Biol Chem 1981;256:9501.
15. Armstrong RA. Fluoropyrimidine activity and resistance at the cellular level. Boca Raton, FL: CRC Press, 1989.
16. Pommier Y, Kerrigan D, Schwartz RE, Swack JA. Altered DNA topoisomerase II activity in Chinese hamster cells resistant to topoisomerase II inhibitors. Cancer Res 1986;46:3075.
17. Biedler JL, Riehm H. Cellular resistance to actinomycin D in Chinese hamster ovary cells in vitro: cross-resistance, radioautographic, and cytogenetic studies. Cancer Res 1970;30:1174.
18. Juliano RL, Ling V. A surface glycoprotein modulating drug permeability in Chinese hamster ovary cell mutants. Biochim Biophys Acta 1976;455:1252.
19. Riordan JR, Ling V. Genetic and biochemical characterization of multidrug resistance. Pharmacol Ther 1985;28:51.
20. Gros P, Ben Neriah Y, Croop JM, Houseman DE. Isolation and expression of a complimentary DNA that confers multidrug resistance. Nature 1986;323:728.
21. Ueda K, Cardarelli C, Gottesman MM, Pastan I. Expression of a full-length cDNA from the human *mdr1* gene confers resistance to colchicine, doxorubicin, and vinblastine. Proc Natl Acad Sci USA 1987;84:3004.
22. Chen C, Chin JE, Ueda K, et al. Internal depletion and homology with bacterial transport proteins in the *mdr1* gene for multidrug-resistant human cells. Cell 1986;47:381.
23. Gros P, Croop J, Houseman D. Mammalian multidrug resistant gene: complete cDNA sequence indicates strong homology to bacterial transport proteins. Cell 1986;47:371.
24. Safa AR, Glover CJ, Meyers MB, Biedler JL, Felsted RL. Vinblastine photoaffinity labeling of a high molecular weight surface membrane glycoprotein specific for multidrug-resistant cells. J Biol Chem 1986;261:6137.
25. Gottesman MM, Pastan I. Resistance to multiple chemotherapeutic agents in human cancer cells. Trends Pharmacol Sci 1988;9:54.
26. Choi K, Chen C, Kriegler M, Roninson IB. An altered pattern of cross-resistance in multidrug-resistant human cells results from spontaneous mutations in the *mdr1* (P-glycoprotein) gene. Cell 1988;53:519.
27. Chambers TC, McAvoy EM, Jacobs JW, Eilon G. Protein kinase C phosphylates P-glycoprotein in multidrug resistant human KB carcinoma cells. J Biol Chem 1990;265:7679.
28. Chambers TC, Pohl J, Raynor RL, Kuo JF. Identification of specific sites in human P-glycoprotein phosphorylated by protein kinase C. J Biol Chem 1993;268:4592–4595.
29. Staats J, Marquardt D, Center MS. Characteristics of a membrane-associated protein kinase of multidrug-resistant HL60 cells which phosphorylates P-glycoprotein. J Biol Chem 1990;265:4084.
30. Chambers TC, Zheng B, Kuo JF. Regulation by phorbol ester and protein kinase C inhibitors, and by a protein phosphatase inhibitor (okadaic acid), of P-glycoprotein phosphorylation and relationship to drug accumulation in multidrug-resistant human KB cells. Mol Pharmacol 1992;41:1008–1015.
31. Fairchild CR, Moscow JA, O'Brien EE, Cowan KH. Multidrug resistance in cells transfected with human genes encoding a variant P-glycoprotein and glutathione *S*-transferase-pi. Mol Pharmacol 1990;37:801.
32. Chin K, Tanaka S, Darlington G, Pastan I, Gottesman MM. Heat shock and arsenate increase expression of multidrug resistance (*mdr1*) gene in human renal carcinoma cells. J Biol Chem 1990;265:221.
33. Fairchild CR, Ivy SP, Rushmore T, et al. Carcinogen-induced *mdr* overexpression is associated with xenobiotic resistance in rat preneoplastic liver nodules and hepatocellular carcinomas. Proc Natl Acad Sci USA 1987;84:7701.
34. Thorgeirsson SS, Huber BE, Sorrel S, et al. Expression of the multidrug-resistant gene in hepatocarcinogenesis and regeniety liver. Science 1987;236:1120.
35. Chin, KV, Chauhan SS, Pastan I, Gottesman MM. Regulation of mdr RNA levels in response to cytotoxic drugs in rodent cells. Cell Growth Differ 1990;1:361.
36. Morrow CS, Nakagawa M, Goldsmith ME, Madden MJ, Cowan KH. Reversible transcriptional activation of mdr1 by sodium butyrate treatment of human colon cancer cells. J Biol Chem 1994;269:10739–10746.
37. Bates SE, Mickley LA, Chen, YN, et al. Expression of a drug resistant gene in human neuroblastoma cell lines: modulation by retinoic acid-induced differentiation. Mol Cell Biol 1989;9:4337.
38. Mickley LA, Bates SE, Richert, ND, et al. Modulation of the expression of a multidrug resistance gene (*mdr1*/P-glycoprotein) by differentiating agents. J Biol Chem 1989;264:18031.
39. Hill BT, Deuchars K, Hosking LK, Ling V, Whelan RDH. Overexpression of P-glycoprotein in mammalian tumor cell lines after fractionated X irradiation in vitro. JNCI 1990;82:607.
40. Goldsmith ME, Gudas JM, Schneider E, Cowan KH. Wild type p53 stimulates expression from the human multidrug resistance promoter in a p53-negative cell line. J Biol Chem 1995;270:1894–1898.
41. Chen Y, Chen PL, Lee WH. Hot-spot p53 mutants interact specifically with two cellular proteins during progression of the cell cycle. Mol Cell Biol 1994;14:6764–6772.
42. Chin KV, Ueda K, Pastan I, Gottesman MM. Modulation of activity of the promoter of the human MDR1 gene by Ras and p53. Science 1992;255:459–462.

43. Burt RK, Garfield S, Johnson K, Thorgeirsson SS. Transformation of rat liver epithelial cells with v-H-ras or v-raf causes expression of MDR-1, glutathione-*S*-transferase-P and increased resistance to cytotoxic chemicals. Carcinogenesis 1988;9:2329–2332.
44. Zastawany RL, Sakvino R, Chen J, Benchimol S, Ling V. The core promoter region of the P-glycoprotein gene is sufficient to confer differential responsiveness to wild-type and mutant p53. Oncogene 1993;8:1529–1535.
45. Ma DD, Scurr RD, Davey RA, et al. Detection of a multidrug-resistant phenotype in acute non-lymphoblastic leukaemia. Lancet 1987;1(8525):135.
46. Sato H, Gottesman MM, Goldstein LJ, et al. Expression of the multidrug resistance gene in myeloid leukemias. Leuk Res 1990;14:11.
47. Rothenberg ML, Mickley LA, Cole DE, et al. Expression of the *mdr1* gene/P-170 gene in patients with acute lymphoblastic leukemia. Blood 1989;74:1388.
48. Bell DR, Gerlach JH, Kartner N, Buick RN, Ling V. Detection of P-glycoprotein in ovarian cancer. A molecular marker associated with multidrug resistance. J Clin Oncol 1985;3:311.
49. Dalton WS, Grogan TM, Rybski JA, et al. Immunohistochemical detection and quantitation of P-glycoprotein in multiple drug-resistant human myeloma cells: association with level of drug resistance and drug accumulation. Blood 1989;73:747.
50. Keith WN, Stallard S, Brown R. Expression of *mdr1* and GST π in human breast tumors: comparison to in vitro sensitivity. Br J Cancer 1990;61:712.
51. Schneider J, Bak M, Efferth TH, et al. P-glycoprotein expression in treated and untreated breast cancer. Br J Cancer 1989;60:815.
52. Goldstein LJ, Fojo AT, Ueda K, et al. Expression of the multidrug resistant, MDR1, gene in neuroblastoma. J Clin Oncol 1990;8:128.
53. Chan HSL, Thorner PS, Haddad G, Ling V. Immunohistochemical detection of P-glycoprotein: prognostic correlation in soft tissue sarcoma of childhood. J Clin Oncol 1990;8:689.
54. Mickisch G, Bier H, Bergler W, et al. P-170 glycoprotein, glutathione and associated enzymes in relation to chemoresistance of primary human renal cell carcinomas. Urol Int 1990;45:170.
55. Goldstein LJ, Galski H, Fojo A, et al. Expression of a multidrug resistance gene in human cancers. JNCI 1989;81:116.
56. Marie JP, Zittoun R, Sikic BI. Multidrug resistance (mdr1) gene expression in adult acute leukemias. Correlations with treatment and outcome and in vitro drug sensitivity. Blood 1991;78:586.
57. Pirker R, Wallner J, Geissler K, et al. MDR1 gene expression and treatment outcome in acute myeloid leukemia. JNCI 1991;83:708.
58. Campos L, Guyotat D, Archimbaud E, et al. Clinical significance of multidrug resistance P-glycoprotein expression on acute nonlymphoblastic leukemia cells at diagnosis. Blood 1992;79:473.
59. Chan HSL, Haddad G, Thorner PS, et al. P-glycoprotein expression as a predictor of the outcome of therapy for neuroblastoma. N Engl J Med 1991;325:1608.
60. Ramani P, Dewchand H. Expression of *mdr1*/P-glycoprotein and p110 in neuroblastoma. J Pathol 1995;175:13–22.
61. Marsh W, Center M. Adriamycin resistance in HL60 cells and accompanying modification of a surface membrane protein contained in drug-sensitive cells. Cancer Res 1987;47:5080.
62. McGrath T, Latoud C, Arnold ST, et al. Mechanisms of multidrug resistance in HL60 cells. Analysis of resistance-associated membrane proteins and levels of mdr gene expression. Biochem Pharmacol 1989;38:3611.
63. Marquardt D, McCrone S, Center MS. Mechanisms of multidrug resistance in HL60 cells: detection of resistance-associated proteins with antibodies against synthetic peptides that correspond to the deduced sequences of P-glycoprotein. Cancer Res 1990;50:1426.
64. Ohtsu T, Ishida Y, Tobinai K, et al. A novel multidrug resistance in cultured leukemia and lymphoma cells detected by a monoclonal antibody to 85 kDa protein, MRK20. Jpn J Cancer Res 1989;80:1133.
65. Chen, Y.-N., Mickley LA, Schwartz AM, et al. Characterization of Adriamycin resistant human breast cancer cells which display overexpression of a novel resistance-related membrane protein. J Biol Chem 1990;265:10073.
66. Cole SP, Bhardwaj G, Gerlach JH, et al. Overexpression of a transporter gene in a multidrug-resistant human lung cancer cell line. Science 1992;258:1650–1654.
67. Krishnamachary N, Center MS. The MRP gene associated with a non-P-glycoprotein multidrug resistance encodes a 190-kDa membrane-bound glycoprotein. Cancer Res 1993;53:3658–3661.
68. Zaman GJR, Flens MJ, van Leudsden MR, et al. The human multidrug resistance-associated protein MRP is a plasma membrane drug-efflux pump. Proc Natl Acad Sci USA 1994;91:8822–8826.
69. Kruh GD, Chan A, Myers K, et al. Expression complementary DNA library transfer establishes *mrp* as a multidrug reistance gene. Cancer Res 1994;54:1649–1652.
70. Grant CE, Valdimarsson G, Hipfner DR, et al. Overexpresson of multidrug resistance-associated protein (MRP) increases resistance to natural product drugs. Cancer Res 1994;54:357–361.
71. Muller M, Meijer C, Zaman GJR, et al. Overexpression of the gene encoding the multidrug resistance-associated protein results in increased ATP-dependent glutathione *S*-conjugate transport. Proc Natl Acad Sci USA 1994;91:13033–13037.
72. Jedlitschky G, Leier I, Buchholz, Center M, Keppler D. ATP-dependent transport of glutathione *S*-conjugates by the multidrug resistance-associated protein. Cancer Res 1994;54:4833–4836.
73. Zhang H, D'Arpa P, Liu LF. A model for tumor cell killing by topoisomerase poisons. Cancer Cells 1990;2:23.
74. Liu L. DNA topoisomerase poisons as antitumor drugs. Annu Rev Biochem 1989;58:351.
75. Glisson BS. Multidrug resistance mediated through alterations in topoisomerase II. Cancer Bull 1989;41:37.
76. Gupta RS. Genetic, biochemical, and cross-resistance studies with mutants of Chinese hamster ovary cells resistant to anticancer drugs, VM-26 and VP-16–213. Cancer Res 1983;43:1568.
77. Deffie AM, Batra JK, Goldenberg GJ. Direct correlation between DNA topoisomerase II activity and cytotoxicity in Adriamycin-sensitive and resistant P388 leukemia cell lines. Cancer Res 1989;49:58.
78. Per SR, Mattern MR, Mirabelli CK, et al. Characterization of a subline of P388 leukemia resistant to amsacrine: evidence of altered topoisomerase II function. Mol Pharmacol 1987;32:17.
79. Glisson B, Gupta R, Smallwood-Kentro S, Ross W. Characterization of acquired epipodophyllotoxin resistance in a Chinese hamster ovary cell line: loss of drug-stimulated DNA cleavage activity. Cancer Res 1986;46:1934.
80. Zwelling LA, Hinds M, Chan D, et al. Characterization of an amsacrine-resistant line of human leukemia cells. Evidence for a drug-resistant form of topoisomerase II. J Biol Chem 1989;264:16411.
81. Danks MK, Schmidt CA, Cirtain MC, Suttle DP, Beck WT. Altered catalytic activity of and DNA cleavage by DNA topoisomerase II from human leukemia cells selected for resistance to VM-26. Biochemistry 1988;27:8861.
82. Hochhauser D, Harris AL. The role of topoisomerase IIα and β in drug resistance. Cancer Treat Rev 1993;19:181–194.
83. Drake FH, Hofmann GA, Bartus, HF, et al. Biochemical and pharmacological properties of p170 and p180 forms of topoisomerase II. Biochemistry 1989;28:8154–8160.
84. Chung TDY, Drake FH, Tan KB, et al. Characterization and immunological identification of cDNA clones encoding two human DNA topoisomerase II isozymes. Proc Natl Acad Sci USA 1989;86:9431–9435.
85. Woessner RD, Mattern MR, Mirabelli CK, Johnson RK, Drake FH. Proliferation- and cell cycle-dependent differences in expression of the 170-kilodalton and 180-kilodalton forms of topoisomerase II in NIH-3T3 cells. Cell Growth Diff 1991;2:209–214.
86. Bugg BY, Danks MK, Beck WT, Suttle DP. Expression of a mutant DNA topoisomerase II in CCRF-CEM human leukemic cells selected for resistance to teniposide. Proc Natl Acad Sci USA 1991;88:7654–7658.
87. Chan VTW, Ng SW, Eder JP, Schnipper LE. Molecular cloning and identification of a point mutation in the topoisomerase II cDNA from an etoposide-resistant Chinese hamster ovary cell line. J Biol Chem 1993;268:2160–2165.
88. Danks MK, Warmouth MR, Friche E, et al. Single-strand conformational polymorphism analysis of the Mr 170,000 isozyme of DNA topoisomerase II in human tumor cells. Cancer Res 1993;53:1373–1379.
89. Hind M, Deisseroth K, Mayes J, et al. Identification of a point mutation in the topoisomerase II gene from a human leukemia cell line containing an amsacrine-resistant form of topoisomerase II. Cancer Res 1991;51:4729–4731.
90. Lee MS, Wang JC, Beran M. Two independent amsacrine-resistant human myeloid leukemia cell lines share an identical point mutation in the 170-kDa form of human topoisomerase II. J Mol Biol 1992;223:837–843.
91. Patel S, Fisher LM. Novel selection and genetic characterization of an etoposide-resistant human leukaemic CCRF-CEM cell line. Br J Cancer 1993;67:456–463.
92. Fernandez DJ, Danks MJ, Beck WT. Decreased nuclear matrix DNA topoisomerase II in human leukemia cells resistant to VM-26 and m-AMSA. Biochemistry 1990;29:4235–4241.
93. Mirski SEL, Evans CD, Almquist KC, Slovak ML, Cole SP. Altered topoisomerase IIα in a drug-resistant small cell lung cancer cell line selected in VP-16. Cancer Res 1993;53:4866–4873.
94. Campain JA, Padmanabhan R, Hwang J, Gottesman MM, Pastan I. Characterization of an unusual mutant of human melanoma cells resistant to anticancer drugs that inhibit topoisomerase II. J Cell Physiol 1993;155:414–425.
95. Giovanella BC, Stehlin JS, Wall, ME, et al. DNA topoisomerase I-targeted chemotherapy of human colon cancer in xenografts. Science 1989;246:1046.
96. Kubota N, Kanzawa F, Nishio K, et al. Detection of topoisomerase I gene point mutation in CPT-11 resistant lung cancer cell line. Biochem Biophys Res Commun 1992;188:571–577.
97. Tamura HO, Kohchi C, Yamada R, et al. Molecular cloning of a cDNA of a camptothecin-resistant human DNA topoisomerase I and identification of mutation sites. Nucleic Acids Res 1990;19:69–75.
98. Tanizawa A, Pommier Y. Topoisomerase I alteration in a camptothecin-resistant cell line derived from Chinese hamster DC3F cells in culture. Cancer Res 1992;52:1848–1854.
99. Andoh T, Ishii K, Suzuki Y, et al. Characterization of a mammalian mutant with a camptothecin-resistant DNA topoisomerase I. Proc Natl Acad Sci USA 1987;84:5565.
100. Farber E. Cellular biochemistry of the stepwise development of cancer with chemicals. Cancer Res 1984;44:5463.
101. Cowan KH, Batist G, Tulpule A, Sinha BK, Myers CE. Similar biochemical changes associated with multidrug resistance in human breast cancer cells and carcinogen-induced resistance to xenobiotics in rats. Proc Natl Acad Sci USA 1986;83:9328.
102. Fairchild CR, Ivy SP, Kao-Shaw CS, et al. Isolation of amplified and overexpressed DNA sequences from adriamycin-resistant human breast cancer cells. Cancer Res 1987;47:5141.
103. Mannervik B, Danielson UH. Glutathione transferases-structure and catalytic activity. Crit Rev Biochem 1988;23:283.
104. Morrow CS, Cowan KH. Glutathione *S*-transferases and drug resistance. Cancer Cells 1990;2:15.
105. Townsend AJ, Cowan KH. Glutathione *S*-transferases and antineoplastic drug resistance. Can Bull 1989;41:31.
106. Puchalski RB, Fahl WE. Expression of recombinant glutathione *S*-transferase π, Ya or Yb1 confers resistance to alkylating agents. Proc Natl Acad Sci USA 1990;87:2443.
107. Nakagawa K, Saijo N, Tsuchida S, et al. Glutathione *S*-transferase π as a determinant of drug resistance in transfectant cell lines. J Biol Chem 1990;265:4296.
108. Leyland-Jones BR, Townsend AJ, Tu CD, Cowan KH, Goldsmith ME. Antineoplastic drug sensitivity of human MCF-7 breast cancer cells stably transfected with a human alpha class glutathione *S*-transferase gene. Cancer Res 1991;51:587–594.
109. Moscow JA, Townsend AJ. Elevation of the π class glutathione S-transferase activity in human breast cancer cells by transfection of the GSTπ gene and its effect on sensitivity to toxins. Mol Pharmacol 1989;36:22.
110. Townsend AJ, Tu CP, Cowan KH. Expression of human mu or alpha class glutathione *S*-transferases in stably transfected human MCF-7 breast cancer cells: effect on cellular sensitivity to cytotoxic agents. Mol Pharmacol 1992;41:230.
111. Ishikawa T, Ali-Osman F. Glutathione-associated *cis*-diamminedichloroplatinum. II. Metabolism and ATP-dependent efflux from leukemia cells: molecular characterization of glutathione-platinum complex and its biological significance. J Biol Chem 1993;268:20116–20125.
112. Ishikawa T. The ATP-dependent glutathione *S*-conjugate export pump. Trends Biochem Sci 1992;17:463–468.
113. Awasthi S, Singhal SS, Srivastava SK, et al. Adenosine triphosphate-dependent transport of doxorubicin, daunomycin, and vinblastine in human tissues by a mechanism distinct from the P-glycoprotein. J Clin Invest 1994;93:958–965.

114. Cadman EC. The selective transfer of drug-resistant genes in malignant cells. Boca Raton, FL: CRC Press, 1989.
115. Lowe SW, Schmitt EM, Smith SW, Osborne BA, Jacks T. p53 is required for radiation-induced apoptosis in mouse thymocytes. Nature 1993;362:847–849.
116. Clark AR, Purdie CA, Harrison DJ, et al. Thymocyte apoptosis induced by p53-dependent and independent pathways. Nature 1993;362:849–852.
117. Fan S, El-Deiry WS, Bae I, et al. p53 gene mutations are associated with decreased sensitivity of human lymphoma cells to DNA damaging agents. Cancer Res 1994;54: 5824–5830.
118. Wattel E, Preudhomme C, Hecquet B, et al. p53 mutations are associated with resistance to chemotherapy and short survival in hematologic malignancies. Blood 1994;84:3148–3157.
119. Strasser A, Harris AW, Jacks T, Cory S. DNA damage can induce apoptosis in proliferating lymphoid cells via p53-independent mechanisms inhibitable by Bcl-2. Cell 1994;79:329–339.
120. Oltvai ZN, Korsmeyer SJ. Checkpoints of dueling dimers foil death wishes. Cell 1994;79:189–192.
121. Miyashita T, Reed JC. *Bcl*-2 oncoprotein blocks chemotherapy-induced apoptosis in a human leukemia cell line. Blood 1993;81:151–157.
122. Fisher TC, Milner AE, Gregory CD, et al. *Bcl*-2 modulation of apoptosis induced by anticancer drugs: resistance to thymidylate stress is independent of classical resistance pathways. Cancer Res 1993;53:3321–3326.
123. Heiko H, Eick D. Mediation of c-myc-induced apoptosis by p53. Science 1994;265: 2091–2093.
124. Nooter K, Boersman AWM, Oostrum RG, et al. Constitutive expression of c-H-*ras* oncogene inhibits doxorubicin-induced apoptosis and promotes cell survival in a rhabdomyosarcoma cell line. Br J Cancer 1995;71:556–561.
125. Poplack DG, Reaman G. Acute lymphoblastic leukemia in childhood. Pediatr Clin North Am 1988;35:903.
126. Teicher BA, Herman TS, Holden SA, et al. Tumor resistance to alkylating agents conferred by mechanisms operative only in vivo. Science 1990;247:1457.
127. Tsuruo T, Iida H, Yamashiro M, Tsukagoshi S, Sakurai Y. Enhancement of vincristine- and adriamycin-induced cytoxicity by verapamil in P388 leukemia and its sublines resistant to vincristine and Adriamycin. Biochem Pharmacol 1982;31:3138.
128. Akiyama S, Shiraishi N, Kuratomi Y, Nakagawa M, Kuwano M. Circumvention of multidrug resistance in P388 murine leukemia and its circumvention by calcium antagonists. Cancer Res 1985;45:1687.
129. Stewart DJ, Evans WK. Non-chemotherapeutic agents that potentiate chemotherapy efficacy. Cancer Treatment Rev 1989;16:1.
130. Nooter K, Sonneveld P, Oostrum R, et al. Overexpression of the *mdr*1 gene in blast cells from patients with acute myelocytic leukemia is associated with decreased anthracycline accumulation that can be restored by cyclosporin-A. Int J Cancer 1990;45:263.
131. Hu XF, Martin TJ, Bell DR, Luise M, Zalcberg JR. Combined use of cyclosporin A and verapamil in modulating multidrug resistance in human leukemia cell lines. Cancer Res 1990;50:2953.
132. Coley HM, Twentyman PR, Workman P. Improved cellular accumulation is characteristic of anthracyclines which retain high activity in multidrug-resistant cell lines alone or in combination with verapamil or cyclosporin A. Biochem Pharmacol 1989;38: 4467.
133. Boesch D, Gaveriaux C, Jachez B, et al. In vivo circumvention of P-glycoprotein-mediated multidrug resistance of tumor cells with SDZ PSC-833. Cancer Res 1991;51: 4226–4233.
134. Twentyman PR, Bleehen NM. Resistance modification by PSC-833, a novel non-immunosuppressive cyclosporin A. Eur J Cancer 1991;27:1639–1642.
135. Sikic BI. Modulation of multidrug resistance: at the threshold. J Clin Oncol 1993;11: 1629–1635.
136. Cairo MS, Siegel S, Arias N, Sender L. Clinical trial of continuous infusion verapamil, bolus vinblastine and continuous infusion VP-16 in drug-resistant pediatric tumors. Cancer Res 1989;49:1063.
137. Dalton WS, Grogan TM, Meltzer PS, et al. Drug resistance in multiple myeloma and non-Hodgkin's lymphoma: detection of P-glycoprotein and potential circumvention by addition of verapamil to chemotherapy. J Clin Oncol 198;7:415.
138. Miller TP, Grogan TM, Dalton WS, et al. P-glycoprotein expression in malignant lymphoma and reversal of clinical drug-resistance with chemotherapy plus high-dose verapamil. J Clin Oncol 1991;9:17–24.
139. Salmon SE, Dalton WS, Grogan TM, et al. Multidrug-resistant myeloma: laboratory and clinical effects of verapamil as a chemosensitizer. Blood 1991;78:44–50.
140. Dalmark M, Pals H, Johnsen AH. Doxorubicin in combination with verapamil in advanced colorectal cancer. Acta Oncol 1991;30:23–26.
141. Ozols RF, Cunnion RE, Klecker RW, et al. Verapamil and Adriamycin in the treatment of drug-resistant ovarian cancer patients. J Clin Oncol 1987;5:641.
142. Bisset D, Kerr DJ, Cassidy J et al. Phase I and pharmacokinetic study of D-verapamil and doxorubicin. Br J Cancer 1991;64:1168–1171.
143. Stuart NSA, Philip P, Harris AL, et al. High-dose tamoxifen as an enhancer of etoposide cytotoxicity. Clinical effects and in vitro assessment in p-glycoprotein expressing cell lines. Br J Cancer 1992;66:833–839.
144. Trump DL, Smith DC, Ellis PG et al. High-dose oral tamoxifen, a potential multidrug-resistance-reversal agent: phase I trial in combination with vinblastine. JNCI 1992;84: 1811–1816.
145. Miller RL, Bukowski RM, Budd GT, et al. Clinical modulation of doxorubicin resistance by the calmodulin-inhibitor trifluperazine: a phase I/II trial. J Clin Oncol 1988;6: 880.
146. Philip PA, Joel S, Monkman SC, et al. A phase I study on the reversal of multidrug resistance (MDR) in vivo: nifedipine plus etoposide. Br J Cancer 1992;65:267–270.
147. Jones RD, Kerr DJ, Harnett AN, et al. A pilot study of quinidine and epirubicin in the treatment of advanced breast cancer. Br J Cancer 1990;62:133–135.
148. Solary E, Caillot D, Chauffert B, et al. Feasibility of using quinine, a potential multidrug resistance-reversing agent, in combination with mitoxantrone and cytarabine for the treatment of acute leukemia. J Clin Oncol 1992;10:1730–1736.
149. Sonneveld P, Nooter K. Reversal of drug resistance by cyclosporin-A in a patient with acute myelocytic leukaemia. Br J Haematol 1990;75:208–211.
150. Sonneveld P, Durie BGM, Lokhorst HM, et al. Modulation of multidrug-resistant multiple myeloma by cyclosporin. Lancet 1992;340:255–259.
151. List AF, Spier C, Greer J, et al. Phase I/II trial of cyclosporine as a chemotherapy-resistance modifier in acute leukemia. J Clin Oncol 1993;11:1652–1660.
152. Yahanda AM, Adler KM, Fisher GA, et al. Phase I trial of etoposide with cyclosporin as a modulator of multidrug resistance. J Clin Oncol 1992;10:1624–1634.
153. Bertrand Y, Capdeville R, Balduck N, Phillipe N. Cyclosporin A used to reverse drug resistance increases vincristine neurotoxicity. Am J Hematol 1992;40:158–159.
154. Virweij J, Herwijer H, Oosterom R, et al. A phase II study of epidoxorubicin in colorectal cancer and the use of cyclosporin-A in an attempt to reverse multidrug resistance. Br J Cancer 1991;64:361–364.
155. Lum BL, Kaubisch S, Yahanda AM, et al. Alteration of etoposide pharmacokinetics and pharmacodynamics by cyclosporine in a phase I trial to modulate multidrug resistance. J Clin Oncol 1992;10:1635–1642.
156. Thiebaut F, Tsuruo T, Hamada H, et al. Cellular localization of the multidrug-resistance gene product P-glycoprotein in normal human tissues. Proc Natl Acad Sci USA 1987;84:7735–7738.
157. Cordon-Cardo C, O'Brien JP, Casals D, et al. Multidrug-resistance gene (P-glycoprotein) is expressed by endothelial cells at the blood-brain barrier sites. Proc Natl Acad Sci USA 1989;86:695–698.
158. Fitzgerald DJ, Willingham MC, Cardarelli CO, et al. Monoclonal antibody—Pseudomonas toxin congugate that specifically kills multidrug-resistant cells. Proc Natl Acad Sci USA 1987;84:4288.
159. Tong AW, Lee J, Wang RM, Dalton WS, Tsuruo T, Fay JW, Stone MJ. Elimination of chemoresistant multiple myeloma clonogenic colony-forming cells by combined treatment with a plasma cell-reactive monoclonal antibody and a P-glycoprotein-reactive monoclonal antibody. Cancer Res 1989;49:4829.
160. Baguley BC, Holdaway KM, Fray LM. Design of DNA intercalators to overcome topoisomerase II-mediated multidrug resistance. JNCI 1990;82:398.
161. Finlay GJ, Baguley BC, Snow K, Judd W. Multiple patterns of resistance of human leukemia cell sublines to amsacrine analogues. JNCI 1990;82:662.
162. Myers CE, Mimnaugh E, Yeh G, Sinha BK. Biochemical mechanisms of tumor cell kill by the anthracyclines. Amsterdam: Elsevier, 1988.
163. Sinha BK. Free radicals in anticancer drug pharmacology. Chem Biol Interact 1989;69:293.
164. Sinha BK, Katki AG, Batist G, Cowan KH, Myers CE. Differential formation of hydroxy radicals by Adriamycin in sensitive and resistant MCF-7 human breast cancer tumor cells: implications for the mechanism of action. Biochemistry 1987;26:3776.
165. Dusre L, Mimnaugh EG, Myers CE, Sinha BK. Potentiation of doxorubicin cytotoxicity by butathionine sulfoximine in multidrug-resistant human breast cancer cells. Cancer Res 1989;49:511.
166. Kramer RA, Zakher J, Kim G. Role of glutathione redox cycle in acquired and de novo multidrug resistance. Science 1988;241:694.
167. Keizer HG, Rijn J, Pinedo HM, Joenje H. Effect of endogenous glutathione, superoxide dismutase, catalase, and glutathione peroxidase on Adriamycin tolerance of Chinese hamster ovary cells. Cancer Res 1988;48:4493.
168. Ketterer B, Tan KH, Meyers DJ, Coles B. Glutathione transferases: a possible role in the detoxification of DNA and lipid hydroperoxides. London: Taylor and Francis, 1987.
169. Alin P, Danielson UH, Mannervick B. 4-hydroxyalk-2-enals are substrates for glutathione transferases. FEBS Lett 1985;179:267.
170. Tew KD, Bomber AW, Hoffman SJ. Ethracrynic acid and piriprost as enhancers of cytotoxicity in drug-resistant cell lines. Cancer Res 1988;48:3622.
171. Evans CG, Bodell WJ, Tokuda K, Doane-Setzer P, Smith MT. Glutathione and related enzymes in rat brain tumor cell resistance to 1,3-bis(2-chloroethyl)-1-nitrosourea and nitrogen mustard. Cancer Res 1987;47:2525.
172. Robson CN, Lewis AD, Wolf CR, et al. Reduced levels of drug-induced DNA cross-linking in nitrogen mustard-resistant Chinese ovary cells expressing elevated glutathione *S*-transferase activity. Cancer Res 1987;47:6022.
173. Buller AL, Clapper ML, Tew KD. Glutathione *S*-transferases in nitrogen mustard-resistant and -sensitive cell lines. Mol Pharmacol 1987;31:575.
174. Lewis AD, Hickson ID, Robson CN, et al. Amplification and increased expression of alpha class glutathione *S*-transferase-encoding genes associated with resistance to nitrogen mustards. Proc Natl Acad Sci USA 1988;85:8511.
175. Wolf CR, Hayward IP, Lawrie SS, et al. Cellular heterogeneity and drug resistance in two ovarian adenocarcinoma cell lines derived from a single patient. Int J Cancer 1987;39:695.
176. Hamilton TC, Ozols RF, Dabrow MB. Multidrug resistance to alkylating agents and platinum compounds: state of our knowledge. Oncology 1990;4:101.
177. Somfai-Relle S, Suzukake KB, and et al. Reduction in cellular glutathione by buthionine sulfoximine and sensitization of murine tumor cells to L-phenylalanine mustard. Biochem Pharmacol 1984;33:485.
178. Nakagawa K, Yokota J, Wada M, et al. Levels of glutathione *S*-transferase pi mRNA in human lung cancer cell lines correlate with the resistance to cisplatin and carboplatin. Jpn J Cancer Res 1988;79:301.
179. Miyazaki M, Kohno K, Saburi Y, et al. Drug resistance to cis-diammine dichloroplatinum (II) in Chinese hamster ovary cell lines transfected with glutathione *S*-transferase pi gene. Biochem Biophys Res Commun 1990;166:1358.
180. Bunting KD, Lindhahl R, Townsend AJ. Oxazaphosphorine-specific resistance in human MCF-7 breast carcinoma cell lines expressing transfected rat class 3 aldehyde dehydrogenase. J Biol Chem 1994;269:23197–23203.
181. Colvin M, Russo JE, Hilton J, Dulik DM, Fenselau C. Enzymatic mechanisms of resistance to alkylating agents in tumor cells and normal tissues. Adv Enzyme Regul 1988;27:211.
182. Hilton J. Role of aldelyde dehydrogenase in cyclophosphamide-resistant L1210 leukemia. Cancer Res 1984;44:5156.
183. Masuda H, Ozols RF, Gi-Ming L, et al. Increased DNA repair as a mechanism of acquired resistance to cis-diamminedichloroplatinum (II) in human ovarian cancer cell lines. Cancer Res 1988;48:5713.
184. Eastman A, Schulte N. Enhanced DNA repair as a mechanism of resistance to cis-diammine dichloroplatinum (II). Biochemistry 1988;27:4730.
185. Sheibani N, Jennerwein MM, Eastman A. DNA repair in cells sensitive and resistant to cis-diammine dichloroplatinum (II): host cell reactivation of damaged plasmid DNA. Biochemistry 1989;28:3120.
186. Curt GA, Allegra CJ. Methotrexate resistance: mechanisms and implications. Boca Raton, FL: CRC Press, 1989.

187. Allegra CJ, Chabner BA, Drake JC. Enhanced inhibition of thymidylate synthase by methotrexate polyglutamates. J Biol Chem 1985;260:9720.
188. Allegra CJ, Drake JC, Jolivet J, Chabner BA. Inhibition of phosphoribosyl aminoimadazole carboxamide transformylase by methotrexate and dihydrofolic acid polyglutamates. Proc Natl Acad Sci USA 1985;82:4881.
189. Cowan KH, Jolivet J. A methotrexate resistant human breast cancer cell line with multiple defects including diminished formation of methotrexate polyglutamates. J Biol Chem 1984;259:10793.
190. Alt FW, Kellems RE, Bertino JR, Schimke RT. Selective multiplication of dihydrofolate reductase genes in methotrexate resistant variants of cultured murine cells. J Biol Chem 1978;253:1357.
191. Melera PW, Lewis JA, Biedler JL, et al. Antifolate resistant Chinese hamster cells. J Biol Chem 1980;255:7024.
192. Goldie JH, Krystal G, Hartley D, Gudauskas G, Dedhar S. A methotrexate insensitive variant of folate reductase present in two lines of methotrexate resistant L5178Y cells. Eur J Cancer 1980;16:1539.
193. Flintoff WF, Essani K. Methotrexate-resistant Chinese hamster ovary cells contain a dihydrofolate reductase with an altered affinity for methotrexate. Biochemistry 1980;19:4321.
194. Carman MD, Schornagel JH, Rivest RS, et al. Resistance to methotrexate due to gene amplification in a patient with acute leukemia. J Clin Oncol 1984;2:16.
195. Trent JM, Buick RN, Olson S, Horns RC, Schimke RT. Cytologic evidence for gene amplification in methotrexate resistant cells obtained from a patient with ovarian adenocarcinoma. J Clin Oncol 1984;2:8.
196. Curt GA, Carney DN, Cowan KH, et al. Unstable methotrexate resistance in human small cell carcinoma associated with double minute chromosomes. N Engl J Med 1983;308:199.
197. Ackland SP, Schilsky RL. High-dose methotrexate: a critical reappraisal. J Clin Oncol 1987;5:2017.
198. Kamen BA, Winick NJ. High dose methotrexate therapy: insecure rationale? Biochem Pharmacol 1988;37:2713.
199. Jaffe N, Link MP, Cohen D, et al. High dose methotrexate in osteogenic sarcoma. NCI Monogr 1981;56:201.
200. Bertino JR. Folate antagonists: toward improving the therapeutic index and development of new analogues. J Clin Pharmacol 1990;30:291.
201. Lin JT, Bertino JR. Trimetrexate: a second generation folate antagonist in clinical trial. J Clin Oncol 1987;5:2032.
202. Duch DS, Edelstein MP, Bowers SW, Nichol CA. Biochemical and chemotherapeutic studies on 2,4-diamino-6-(2, 5-dimethoxybenzyl)-5-methylpyrido-[2,3-d] pyrimidine (BW 301U), a novel lipid-soluble inhibitor of dihydrofolate reductase. Cancer Res 1982;42:3987.
203. Assaraf YG, Molina A, Schinke RT. Cross-resistance to the lipid soluble antifolate trimetrexate in human carcinoma cells with the multidrug-resistant phenotype. JNCI 1989;81:290.
204. Jackson RC, Jackman AL, Calvert AH. Biochemical effects of a quinazoline inhibitor of thymidylate synthase, CB3717, on human lymphoblastoid cells. Biochem Pharmacol 1983;32:3783.
205. Beardsley GP, Moroson BA, Taylor EC, Moran RG. A new folate antimetabolite, 5,10-dideaza-5,6,7,8-tetrahydrofolate, is a potent inhibitor of de novo purine synthesis. J Biol Chem 1989;264:328.
206. Bapat AR, Zarow C, Danenberg PV. Human leukemic cells resistant to FdUrd contain a thymidylate synthase with lower affinity for nucleotides. J Biol Chem 1983;258:4130.
207. Jenh CH, Geyer PK, Baskin F, Johnson LF. Thymidylate synthase gene amplification in fluorodeoxyuridine resistant mouse cell lines. Mol Pharmacol 1985;28:80.
208. Priest DG, Ledford BE, Day MT. Increased thymidylate synthase in FdUrd resistant cultured hepatoma cells. Biochem Pharmacol 1980;29:1549.
209. Calabro-Jones PM, Byfield JE, Ward JF, Sharp TR. Time-dose relationship for 5-fluorouracil toxicity against human epithelial cancer cells in vivo. Cancer Res 1982;42:4413.
210. Seifert P, Baker LH, Reed ML, Vaitkevicious VK. Comparison of continuously infused FUra with bolus injection in treatment of patients with colorectal carcinoma. Cancer 1975;36:123.
211. Arbuck SG. 5-FU/leucovorin.biochemical modulation that works. Oncology 1987;1:61.
212. Grem JL, Hoth OF, Hamilton JM, King SA, Leyland-Jones B. Overview of current status and future direction of clinical trials with 5-fluorouracil in combination with folinic acid. Cancer Treat Rep 1987;71:1249.
213. Cadman E, Heimer R. Enhanced 5-fluorouracil nucleotide formation after methotrexate. Explanation for drug synergism. Science 1979;205:1135.
214. Cadman E, Heimer R, Davis L. The influence of methotrexate pretreatment on 5-fluorourawcil metabolism in L1210 cells. J Biol Chem 1981;256:1695.
215. Grem JL, King SA, Leyland-Jones B. Biochemistry and clinical activity of *N*-(phosphonacetyl)-L-aspartate: a review. Cancer Res 1988;48:4441.
216. Elias L, Crissman HA. Interferon effects upon the adenocarcinoma MCA 38 and HL-60 cell lines. Antiproliferative responses and synergistic interactions with halogenated pyrimidine antimetabolites. Cancer Res 1988;48:4868.
217. Momparler RL, Onetto-Pothier N. (Ed.). Drug resistance to cytosine arabinoside. Boco Raton, FL: CRC Press, 1989.
218. Capizzi RL, Yang JI, Rathmell JP, et al. Dose-related pharmacologic effects of high-dose ARA-C and its self potentiation. Semin Oncol 1985;12(suppl 3):65.
219. Wiley JS, Jones SP, Sawyer WH, Paterson ARP. Cytosine arabinoside influx and nucleoside transport sites in acute leukemia. J Clin Invest 1981;69:479.
220. Tanaka M, Yoshida S. Altered sensitivity to 1-D-arabinofuranosylcytosine 5′-triphosphate of DNA polymerase from leukemia blasts of acute lymphoblastic leukemia. Cancer Res 1982;42:649.
221. Ho DHW, Carter CJ, Brown NS, et al. Effects of tetrahydrouridine on the uptake and metabolism of 1-D-arabinofuranosylcytosine in human normal and leukemic cells. Cancer Res 1980;40:2441.
222. Heideman RL, Gillespie A, Ford H, et al. Phase I trial and pharmacokinetic evaluation of fazarabine in children. Cancer Res 1989;49:5213.
223. Surbone A, Ford H, JAK, et al. Phase I and pharmacokinetic study of arabinofuranosyl-5-azacytosine (fazarabine, NSC 281272). Cancer Res 1990;50:1220.

CHAPTER 54

Combination Chemotherapy, Dose, and Schedule

EMIL FREI III AND KAREN H. ANTMAN

Introduction

The identification of novel, clinically active agents has been central to progress in cancer chemotherapy. The optimal use of such agents, of which some 40 have been identified over the past 50 years, has been crucial.

Dose is a major determinant of the antitumor activity and toxicology for classical antitumor agents (56). The effect of dose for biotherapeutic agents and hormones is complex and currently under study. In the context of bone marrow transplantation, dose has proven to be curative for some hematologic neoplasms.

The schedule of drug administration may be important to the therapeutic index independent of dose. For example, cytokinetic studies of both experimental and clinical leukemia have led to the improved use of agents such as arabinosyl cytosine (130, 131).

Finally, combination chemotherapy has been critical in the development of curative regimens for the hematologic malignancies, pediatric solid tumors, testicular cancer, and many adjuvant and neoadjuvant regimens (47, 48). Combination chemotherapy trials derive in part from studies of the development of drug resistance (85, 111, 122).

Dose

The fundamental relationship between dose and tumor cell "kill" is a linear log (i.e., exponential) (129). A linear increase in dose of selected chemotherapeutic agents may cause a log reduction of MCF7 human breast cancer cells in culture (Fig. 54.1) (57). Dose is expressed as multiples of the IC_{90} (i.e., the dose or concentration that reduces the number of tumor cells by 90%). This would represent a very good response in terms of tumor regression in the patient. In terms of the "exponential iceberg," it, however, is only the end of the beginning. We still have 10 to 11 logs to go to achieve cure (10, 58).

Dose generally is expressed as dose per unit of time (i.e., dose intensity or rate) (74). Numerous factors influence the dose effect. The major ones are illustrated in Figures 54.1 and 54.2.

FACTORS INFLUENCING THE DOSE EFFECT

Chemotherapeutic Agents

X-irradiation is the best agent in terms of maintaining linearity down through multiple logs of cell "kill" (Fig. 54.1). One reason for decreased resistance to x-irradiation is that it is not subject to the many active membrane transport, enzymatic biotransformation, and other factors that affect many chemotherapeutic agents. Alterations in these functions may serve as a basis for resistance (135). Some degree of curvilinearity in x-irradiation dose-response curves is evident among in vivo studies, mainly because of tumor hypoxia (135, 140).

As a group, alkylating agents are not quite as good as x-irradiation in terms of maintained linearity, but as a generalization, they are considerably superior to the other chemotherapeutic agents (Fig. 54.1). This agrees with observations that induction or selection for resistance occurs rapidly with antimetabolites, whereas in general, extensive selection pressure is required for the alkylating agents (57). Moreover, high levels of resistance are common with the nonalkylating agents, whereas with alkylating agents, it is difficult to achieve resistance of greater than 3- to 15-fold (52, 57).

What is the basis for the curvilinearity of the alkylating agent dose response (Fig. 54.1)? The major factor is heterogeneity with respect to drug resistance. Alkylating agents have some properties resembling those of x-irradiation, which perhaps explains their similarity in terms of dose response. The nonalkylating agents, particularly antimetabolites, may exhibit much greater resistance with increasing doses or concentrations. Part of this is cytokinetic resistance; in other words, cells in certain stages of the mitotic cycle may be resistant to cell-cycle-specific agents, such as arabinosylcytosine (ara-C). Ara-C inhibits DNA synthesis and is not cytotoxic for non-S-phase cells. Thus, the curves presented in Figures 54.1 and 54.2 for ara-C and other cell-

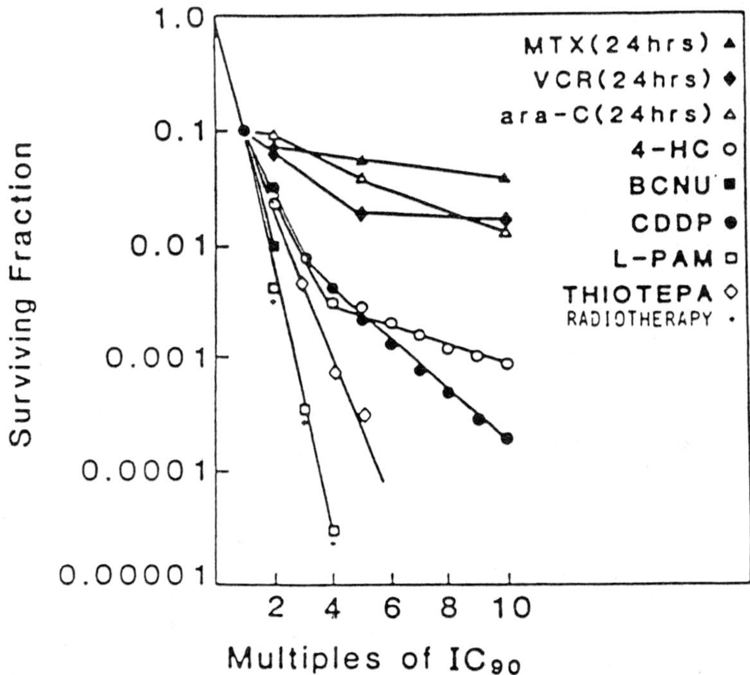

Figure 54.1. Effect of antitumor agent concentration (expressed as multiples of IC_{90}) on surviving fraction of human breast cancer (MCF7) cells in culture (colony assay). *Source*: Frei and colleagues (48).

cycle-specific agents can be straightened slightly by administering such agents over several days, but there remains a substantially greater curvilinearity compared with the alkylating agents (16, 57, 134).

Intrinsic Tumor Cell Sensitivity

Figure 54.2*A* compares the effect of agents on an insensitive tumor compared with a sensitive tumor (53, 56). In general, the more sensitive the tumor is to a given agent, the steeper the dose effect will be. Thus, if unit dose produces a 0.5 log kill, then doubling that dose may produce a 1.0 log tumor cell kill—a limited achievement at best. Clinically, it would represent a partial remission. On the other hand, in a sensitive tumor where unit dose produces a 3 log kill, doubling the dose may produce up to a 6 log kill (128). This is a major achievement in terms of complete response duration and, most importantly, approaching cytoeradication. Clinical trials that demonstrate a major dose effect for sensitive hematologic and embryonic neoplasms but less for common epithelial tumors provide recognition of this intrinsic difference in sensitivity (51, 56).

Tumor Burden

The most consistent adverse prognostic factor regarding response to chemotherapy is tumor burden. The less the tumor burden, the greater the opportunity for response and the steeper the dose-response curve (Fig. 54.2*C*). This has been demonstrated for transplanted tumors in mice. Macroscopic (i.e., palpable) tumors often respond minimally to a given chemotherapy: however, the same tumor at a microscopic tumor burden size may be much more responsive and potentially curable (67).

This assumes that transplanted microscopic disease is similar to autochthonous microscopic metastases in patients. There is substantial experimental and clinical evidence, however, that this is not the case. For example, microscopic tumor may grow and metastasize if tumor angiogenesis has occurred. This occurs rapidly with transplanted tumors that have been selected for growth. For the autochthonous micrometastases that attend the primary tumor, it may take months or years before the mutation(s) occurs that results in angiogenesis factor production and other molecules that are involved in invasion and metastases (see Chapters 9 and 10) (49).

Other postulates for the delay in growth of microscopic metastases include a balanced rate of cell loss (i.e., apoptosis) and cell production. In the resting cell hypothesis, tumor cells remain indolent for long periods of time before replication commences.

The study of microscopic metastases in patients may become increasingly possible with modern molecular techniques addressing the detection and characterization of minimal tumor (67). Some of the kinetics of microscopic disease can be inferred from adjuvant chemotherapy studies. Norton, in particular, has conducted adjuvant studies in patients with breast cancer based on extrapolations and as-

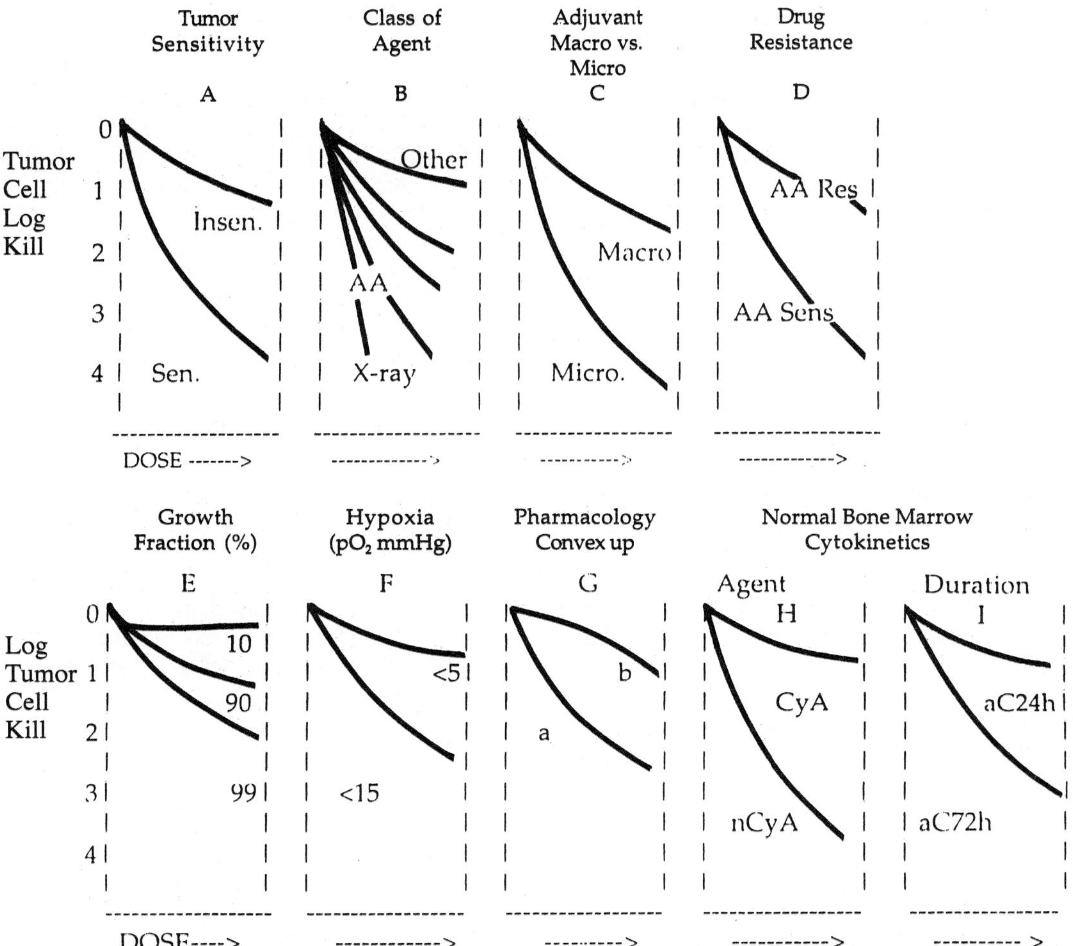

Figure 54.2. Each box represents an important variable affecting the dose response of antitumor agents. Dose or concentration is given in arithmetic form on the *x*-axis. Tumor cell reduction (generally colony assay) is given on the *y*-axis. **A.** Effect of intrinsic chemotherapeutic sensitivity of the tumor. Given a linear log relation between dose and response, "log kill" is profoundly, and most importantly, affected by intrinsic sensitivity. **B.** The effect of different chemotherapeutic agents on dose response (presented in Fig. 54.1). AA, alkylating agent. **C.** Effect of tumor burden on dose and antitumor response (major rationale for adjuvant chemotherapy). Macro, macroscopic (overt) tumor; micro, microscopic (adjuvant) tumor. **D.**, Effect of drug resistance on dose response curve. **E.** Effect of growth fraction on dose-response curves. Growth fraction is a co-variable with vascularity, O_2 tension, and tumor burden. **F.** Tumor hypoxia. Experimental and human solid tumors are commonly found to be hypoxic, and often severely so (O_2 tension, <5 mm Hg). This is known to adversely affect the response to radiotherapy and recently has been found to adversely affect the response to many chemotherapeutic agents. **G.** Pharmacology. The majority of factors that impact on dose-response result in convex curves down, as illustrated in this composite figure. With increasing dose, however, if one saturates an activating mechanism, as can happen with the p450 system with ifosfamide, a convex curve up will result. (See text for other pharmacokinetic factors that affect the dose curve.) **H** and **I.** In the normal marrow, approximately 10% of cells initiate DNA synthesis during a 24-hour period. Largely because of this, cell-cycle-specific agents produce different dose curves compared with non-cell-cycle-specific agents. Also, the duration of cell-cycle-specific agent administration may markedly affect the dose curve. CyA, cell-cycle-active agent; nCyA, non-CyA; aC, araC given by continuous administration for 24 or 72 hours.

sumptions concerning the Gompertzian cytokinetics of microscopic tumor (see Chapter 52).

Drug Resistance

Figure 54.2*D* is a hypothetic plot of the comparative effects of a given agent on sensitive and resistant tumors developed by selection pressure. Resistance usually is expressed as the concentration of drug that is required to produce 50% inhibition in a colony or growth assay (IC_{50}) for the resistant cell line divided by the concentration required (IC_{50}) for the parent sensitive cell line. In Figure 54.2*D*, the IC_{50} for the sensitive cell is approximately one-fifth that of the resistant line (i.e., 5-fold resistance). The situation with drug-induced resistance is comparable to original sensitivity (Fig. 54.2*A*) in that the magnitude of the sensitivity of the cell line correlates directly with the impact of dose. Thus, for cell lines with low levels (3- to 10-fold) of resistance, high-dose therapy that may include a 5- to 10-fold increase in dose may be capable of tumor cytoeradication (i.e., cure).

For a more detailed presentation of drug resistance, see

the combination chemotherapy section later in this chapter and in Chapter 53.

Cytokinetics of the Tumor: The Growth Fraction

Figure 54.2*E* presents the effect of growth fraction on dose curves. Tritiated thymidine autoradiographic studies of experimental tumors have found that the volume doubling time was in excess of the generation time of cycling (i.e., of mitotically active) cells (135, 136). This led to the observation that many cells within tumors are "noncycling," i.e., in G_1, G_0, or commonly, particularly after injury, in G_2. This is referred to as "low" growth fraction (93, 94, 134). Such cells would be substantially less sensitive to cell-cycle-specific agents and variably less sensitive to other chemotherapeutic agents. A solid tumor with a growth fraction of, for example, 10% would be minimally responsive to cell-cycle-specific agents (Fig. 54.2*E*). Repetitive treatments, however, might "recruit" cells into cycle and thus be more effective. Also, prolonged infusion of cell-cycle-specific agents might be effective in low-growth-fraction tumors. The effect of the dose of cell-cycle-specific agents on the log kill of tumor cells is presented in Figure 54.2*E*. On the other hand, a high-growth-fraction tumor such as Burkitt's lymphoma would, with the same treatment, have a multilog response. The molecular biology of the cell cycle is revolutionizing our knowledge in this area and is already impacting on our clinical approaches (discussed later and in Chapter 1 and 52).

Tumor Hypoxia

It has been known since the 1950s that solid tumors commonly are hypoxic. With improved instrumentation, this has been confirmed in both experimental and clinical solid tumors. The hypoxia that is present presumably relates to the suboptimal angiogenesis of solid tumors as well as the high metabolic activity of the tumor cells. Figure 54.2*F* presents the effect of tumor hypoxia on dose.

Radiotherapy has long been known to require molecular oxygen for cytotoxicity. In experimental in vivo systems, "oxic" agents such as perfluorocarbons and hemoglobin solutions may correct the hypoxia and improve the effectiveness of radiotherapy and a variety of chemotherapeutic agents (50, 140).

Pharmacokinetics

Pharmacokinetic factors commonly may affect the dose-response curve. For example, if an inactivating enzyme for the drug becomes saturated, an increase in both the toxicity and antitumor effect with increasing dose could occur (Fig. 54.2*G*). Such an effect has been observed with fluorouracil (23, 50, 119).

Pharmacokinetics may have the opposite effect, as well (i.e., produce a convex down curve if a drug activation system becomes saturated). For example, ifosfamide is activated by the p450, oxygen-dependent, drug-metabolizing enzymes in the liver to the 4-hydroxyl derivative, which is biologically active. The rate of p450 activation is relatively slow for ifosfamide compared with the congener compound cyclophosphamide. With increasing doses of cyclophosphamide, a constant fractional conversion to active 4-OH cyclophosphamide occurs. However, pharmacokinetic studies of ifosfamide indicate that with increasing doses, a decreasing proportion of ifosfamide is converted to the active form, because the p450 enzyme system becomes saturated and an antitumor effect such as that shown in Figure 54.2*G* would result. It is for this reason that ifosfamide is given in three to five fractions per course.

Other factors can produce a convex up curve such as in Figure 54.2*G*. Clinically, for slow-growing tumors, reduction in tumor size with treatment may be delayed and have the appearance of the curve in the figure. On the other hand, where tumor stem-cell assays have been employed, the curve is log linear with dose (109). This presumably results from delay in the clearing of dead tumor and related stromal tissues. With many agents, particularly the alkylators, tumor cells can be rendered nonclonogenic yet undergo several replication cycles before delayed death and resorption occurs.

Curve b in Figure 54.2*G* resembles x-irradiation survival curves, wherein, at low doses, DNA repair produces a "shoulder." Repair of potential lethal damage has been described for a variety of preclinical models (119).

Cytokinetics of Bone Marrow

Because of its cytokinetic activity and relative lack of DNA repair capacity, bone marrow toxicity is dose limiting for many chemotherapeutic agents. The effect of a cell-cycle-specific agent (Fig. 54.2 *H* and *I*), such as ara-C given for 24 hours to mice, produces in the spleen colony assay the curves presented in Figure 54.2*H* (15). With increasing doses, the ara-C effect plateaus at approximately 10%, because that proportion of bone marrow stem cells is out of the mitotic cycle during any given 24-hour period in mice. This applies not only to ara-C but to other cell-cycle-specific agents as well. On the other hand, agents that are non-cycle-dependent, such as the alkylating agents and many antitumor antibiotics, produce a steep dose-response curve that is maintained through multiple logs of normal bone-marrow-stem-cell kill (Fig. 54.2 *H* and *I*) (16).

Important therapeutic principles derive from these studies. Indeed, exploiting the cytokinetic difference between marrow and tumor has been a basis for the construction of clinical trials. For acute myeloid leukemia (AML), a series of clinical trials established the superiority of 5- to 7-day courses of ara-C given at 2- to 3-week intervals as being optimal. The cytokinetic basis for this is that the generation time and growth fraction of AML cells in vivo are such that over 90% of AML cells will have entered DNA synthesis in any 5- to 7-day period (19). The normal marrow recovers rapidly (i.e., within 1 to 2 weeks), and cumulative toxicity does not occur. Treatment of AML with the described dose schedule of ara-C results in rapid disappearance of AML cells from the blood and marrow. For many patients, recovery of the AML cells between courses of ara-C is incomplete compared to normal marrow. This is consistent with in vitro data that AML cells are less susceptible to growth factors such as granulocyte (G) and granulocyte-macrophage colony-stimulating factor (GM-CSF) than the normal marrow. Thus, when marrow CSFs increase in homeostatic response to ara-C-induced myelosuppression, there often is an interval recovery of the normal marrow in contrast to the AML cells, hence the therapeutic advantage (9). Recent studies indicating that mutations in the G-CSF receptor interfere with maturation in congenital neutropenia and AML support this admittedly speculative interpretation (33).

This may explain in part the effectiveness of cell-cycle-active agents such as methotrexate (Mtx) and fluorouracil (FU) in solid tumors. When these agents are employed in metastatic breast cancer, there is a reproducible and major myelosuppression, with rapid recovery. Why should such relatively short courses (e.g., 5 days) be effective in indolent tumors such as breast cancer? The mitotically cycling tumor cells respond to Mtx and FU. These have generation or cell-cycle times of 3 to 5 days; the reason for the slow growth is that only a small proportion are in cycle (i.e., the growth fraction is low, 3 to 10%). As indicated earlier, the marrow is kinetically more active. This explains the fact that for a given course of chemotherapy with FU and/or Mtx, the acute effect is greater on the marrow and gut. These organs, however, recover within a 3- to 4-week interval, whereas the breast in cancer does not. The flux of "resting" tumor cells into cycle over time and lack of interval recovery of the breast cancer cells permits major response to these agents in some patients. As in AML, this difference in recovery could be caused by homeostatic (i.e., growth factor induced) recovery of the normal marrow as compared to breast cancer cells (135, 136).

The basis for the therapeutic index advanced here has not been rigorously proven, and it is in part speculative. Nevertheless, such basic data have influenced the design of clinical trials and are in accord with the therapeutic and toxicologic results of clinical trials involving cell-cycle-specific agents (135).

CLINICAL TRIALS AND DOSE EFFECT

Dose Effect in Sensitive Tumors

Relatively few clinical studies have included dose intensity as an independent, randomized variable. The first was performed in patients with Hodgkin's disease and non-Hodgkin's lymphoma, wherein patients were randomized to a full or half dose of an alkylating agent. The full dose was significantly superior, producing a 60% objective response rate, compared with 10% for the half dose. Toxicity also was increased (15). A similar study was conducted in patients with lymphoma using folic acid antagonists and obtained similar results (51). In acute lymphocytic leukemia, the dose rate of maintenance chemotherapy had a major impact on the duration of response (105). Similarly, in studies of combination chemotherapy in small-cell lung cancer, the dose effect was major (22). Recent comparative studies in patients with metastatic breast cancer affirm the importance of dose and, in one study, provide evidence for improved quality-of-life (137). On the other hand, dose effect is more difficult to achieve in patients with chemotherapy-resistant, epithelial solid tumors for reasons presented in Figure 54.2*A*.

Adjuvant Chemotherapy

Introduction. A number of comparative studies have demonstrated a dose effect in chemosensitive tumors such as acute lymphocytic leukemia, AML, and lymphoma (15, 92, 104, 105). Hryniuk conducted several retrospective studies of dose intensity for a variety of tumors. He found a dose-response effect in essentially all sensitive hematologic neoplasms, but also in the relatively less sensitive tumors such as breast cancer (59, 61, 62). Selected prospective, randomized, comparative studies of dose are nearing completion and provide more rigorous data with respect to the dose effect (121).

It is almost axiomatic for neoplasia that the greater the tumor burden, the worse the prognosis. This is because as a function of increasing size, macroscopic tumor burdens are increasingly adversely affected by growth fraction, hypoxia, diminished blood supply, heterogeneity, and drug resistance (Fig. 54.2) (49, 135, 136). In the adjuvant situation, however, where chemotherapy addresses micrometastatic disease, these factors are eliminated or very much reduced (Fig. 54.2*C*). Accordingly, much more effective killing curves can be achieved in experimental studies in vivo and may be inferred from clinical studies (53, 54).

Cancer and Leukemia Group B Study

Experimental Design and Results. During the past 10 years, several well-designed clinical trials have addressed the issue of dose in the adjuvant situation, particularly in patients with breast cancer. The CALGB study, which began in 1985, included the randomization of patients to three dose levels, the high and low dose of which are included in Figure 54.3 (121). As indicated in the bottom of that figure, the high dose of cyclophosphamide, Adriamycin, and 5-FU (CAF) was exactly twice the low dose. In both arms, four courses of treatment were given, and a retrospective study indicated

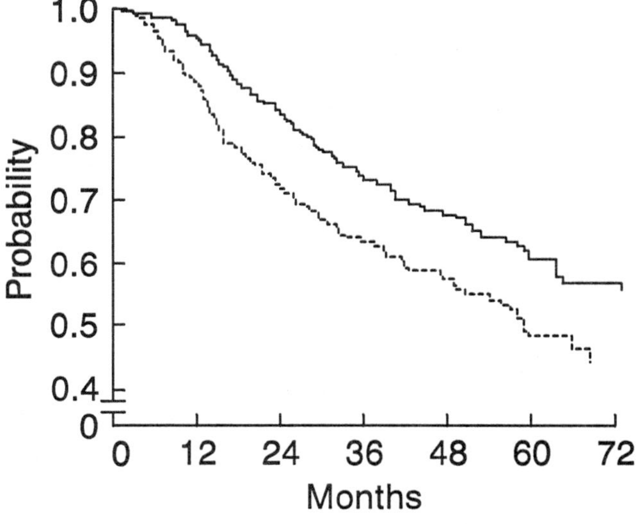

Figure 54.3. CALGB study of two dose levels of cyclophosphamide, Adriamycin, fluorouracil (CAF) in the adjuvant chemotherapy of node-positive breast cancer. HD, high dose; LD, low dose; numbers are dose in mg/m^2.

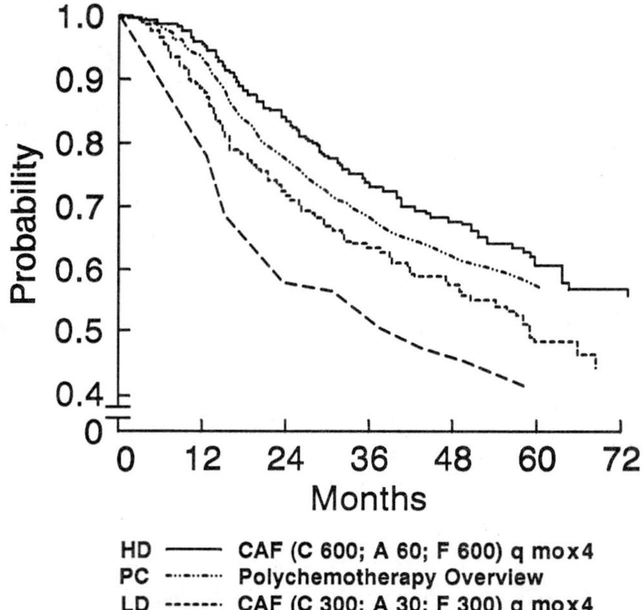

Figure 54.4. Same study as in Figure 54.3 but with the addition of the "no treatment" control arm and the polychemotherapy arm from the overview (see text). CAF—cyclophosphamide, Adriamycin, fluorouracil. HD, high dose; LD, low dose; numbers are dose in mg/m^2.

that 90% of the prescribed dose was actually delivered in both arms. Note that at 5 years, approximately one-half of the patients failed, so the 10% difference between the two curves translates into a 20% difference in reduction for the risk of recurrence.

A control "no chemotherapy" arm is important to interpreting the two CAF dose levels presented in Figure 54.4. We have selected the control arm (the lowest curve in Fig. 54.4) from the overview or meta-analysis (37, 38). It involves all patients with primary node positive breast cancer entered into quantitative, comparative, adjuvant studies and who were randomized to the "no-chemotherapy" arm (37, 38). This control arm represents a historical control and is vulnerable. We believe, however, that its use is appropriate for the following reasons.

1. All trials are interpreted against some "control" or frame of reference, whether randomized, sequenced historical, remote historical, meta-analysis, or even universal experience.
2. Earlier breast cancer adjuvant studies clearly demonstrated the superiority of chemotherapy over no-treatment controls, rendering such controls unethical (11, 45).
3. In the absence of randomization, the best control is the overview or meta-analysis which includes all completed or ongoing comparative studies of adjuvant therapy for primary breast cancer, both published and unpublished (37, 38).
4. The criteria for patient selection, i.e., patients of all ages and menopausal status, with node-positive primary breast cancer, were the same for the overview and the CALGB study.
5. This recurrence-free survival curve from the overview contains 11,000 node-positive control patients.
6. This large number of patients was drawn from the same general pool as the CALGB study, i.e., patients who were entered into prospective clinical trials.
7. The "no-treatment" overview control curve falls in a reasonable position (Fig. 54.4).
8. The polychemotherapy arm of the overview falls between the high- and low-dose curves (Fig. 54.4). "Standard" doses of CAF during the overview time frame were an estimated C 500, A 50, and FU 500 mg/m^2/cycle or the equivalent. CMF, which commonly was used during this period, was considered to be as effective, or slightly less effective, than CAF.

Taken together, these observations make a compelling case for use of the "no-treatment" control in the overview despite the limitations of a nonrandomized control. Derivative analyses may be warranted.

The three recurrence-free survival curves in Figure 54.4 deviate from each other in the first 1 to 2 years, after which the differences are maintained at approximately 10%. Given the 50% who remain recurrence-free, this 10% difference at 5 years translates into a 20% difference in the risk of recurrence. Thus, there is an approximately 20% difference in risk of recurrence between the upper and lower dose curves and a 20% difference between the lower dose and the control (i.e., a 40% spread in risk). While 5 years is a relatively short follow-up for breast cancer, it has been demonstrated, particularly in the overview, that differences in disease-free survival that develop by 5 years are maintained and even augmented at 10 and 15 years for adjuvant breast cancer (37, 38).

Implications of CALGB on Dose Effect in Adjuvant Chemotherapy. These data are further considered in the dose-response context in Figure 54.5*B*. Almost all dose effects follow a sigmoidal distribution curve. With only two points on the curve, position on the sigmoidal curve is uncertain, and a number of possible lines between the two points are possible. With three points, fitting to the sigmoidal curve is more precise. "No treatment" is on the zero-effect line by definition. Because the relative difference between the "no treatment" and low-dose (LD) arm is 20% and between the LD and high-dose (HD) arms an additional 20%, a straight line fit of up to 40% is reasonable (Fig. 54.5*C*). This suggests that a further increase in dose for the same or similar agents of 4- to 5-fold would extrapolate to a greater than 80% reduction in the risk of recurrence. If true, this would have remarkable implications given that substantially higher doses can and are being given to patients with high-risk primary breast cancer (discussed later).

Will it be possible to go from 40 to 80% with similar agents and dose increments, as was possible from 0 to 40%? The curvilinear concentration response effects seen in almost all experimental studies (Fig. 54.1) strongly indicate that every increment of success (i.e., tumor cell kill) makes the next increment more difficult. Indeed, a companion study of the CALGB study demonstrated that the 30% of patients whose tumor cells strongly expressed c-*Erb*-B-2, a growth-factor receptor that is associated with increased proliferative ca-

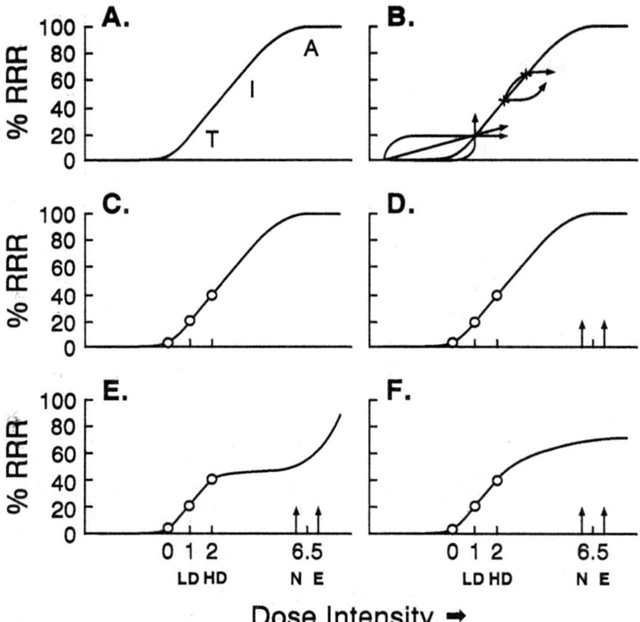

Figure 54.5. Hypothetic sigmoidal dose-response interpretations of CALGB study (see text for running parallel description). RRR, reduction in rate of recurrence; LD, low dose; HD, high dose; N, NSABP; E, ECOG. **A.** Hypothetic sigmoidal dose-response curve. T, threshold; I, intermediate; A, asymptotic. **B.** Multiple possibilities for two points without "anchor." **C.** A more precise fit with three points and an anchor (i.e., "no treatment" point on 0 % RRR line). **D.** Graph in **C** with straight line extrapolation. *Arrows*, current intensification studies. Predicted % RRR greater than 80%. **E.** Bimodal dose-response curve based on *erb*-B2 analysis. **F.** Dose-response curve assuming exponential distribution of risk factors.

pacity, were profoundly affected by dose (5-year recurrence-free survival for LD of 30% and for HD of 80%). For the remaining patients, there was no effect of dose (77). This observation needs to be confirmed. If true, it could readily explain a bimodal curve such as that in Figure 54.5*E*, but heterogeneity with respect to the dose effect is quite certainly multifactorial, which would result in a curve such as that in Figure 54.5*F*.

At this time, the relative contributions of the individual agents to dose effect in the adjuvant chemotherapy of breast cancer remains uncertain. Recent studies, where cyclophosphamide dose was the independent variable, indicate that this dose may not be important (31). For adjuvant cyclophosphamide, methotrexate, fluorouracil (CMF) in breast cancer, c-*Erb*-B-2 does not predict relapse-free or overall survival (58, 66, 76). Thus, the critical correlation between dose and c-*Erb*-B-2 may relate to doxorubicin (82). Supporting this position is the experimental evidence that doxorubicin cytotoxicity increases with increased topoisomerase II expression (70, 82). The genes for topoisomerase II and c-*Erb*-B-2 are in close proximity on the same chromosome. If the two genes were co-amplified and/or co-expressed, it could explain the results of the CAF dose study. Other studies strongly link the dose of doxorubicin to response in metastatic and adjuvant breast cancer (7, 80). The hypotheses implicit in these speculations are the subject of current experiments and include the following (*a*) Is doxorubicin the key player in the dose effect? (*b*) If so, is this effect linked to c-*Erb*-B-2 status? (*c*) Is there linkage between (*a*) and (*b*) and topoisomerase II expression?

In a phase II adjuvant study of high-risk (i.e., 10 or more positive nodes), primary breast cancer, a 72% disease-free survival plateau was observed with intensive trialkylator therapy and stem cell myeloprotection (103). These preliminary results are now the subject of a comparative, multi-institutional study in the CALGB. Mortality in these two HD therapy, high-patient volume studies is 4%.

In patients with 1 to 10 positive nodes, a two-by-two factorial study of the effect of dose of doxorubicin and paclitaxel is underway in the CALGB.

Autologous Bone Marrow Transplantation. This term has become a misnomer. The key element of such research is dose intensity. Moreover, hematopoietic progenitor (i.e., stem) cells are increasingly acquired from the peripheral blood, not the marrow. We prefer the term *HD-SCR* (high-dose stem-cell rescue).

The most compelling evidence regarding dose response relates to HD-SCR studies (54, 143). Alkylating agents and total-body radiotherapy are most commonly employed in this situation, because their dose-limiting toxicity is myelosuppression. Thus, a major (i.e., 5- to 20-fold) increase in dose intensity can be delivered before nonmyelosuppressive toxicity becomes dose limiting.

In this setting, 40 to 60% of patients with metastatic melanoma and colorectal cancer respond to alkylating agents, compared with standard response rates of 10 to 20% (30). In the HD-SCR setting, total-body radiotherapy plus cyclophosphamide produces a 50% cure rate in selected patients who are in first complete remission of AML or early chronic myeloid leukemia. Intensification programs involving, for example, busulphan plus cyclophosphamide are similarly active (117). Allogeneic (see Chapters 85 to 86) or autologous bone marrow transplantation produces significant disease-free survival plateaus (i.e., cures) in patients with previously treated Hodgkin's disease, non-Hodgkin's lymphoma, and acute lymphocytic leukemia (99). This approach currently is being employed in patients with metastatic breast cancer, high-risk primary breast cancer, testicular cancer, ovarian cancer, and small cell lung cancer. In these patients with solid tumor, high response rates, including complete response rates, can be achieved. Documentation of improved survival requires the completion of randomized trials. Toxicity can be major, and this approach should be limited to specialized centers (3, 4, 30, 54, 70, 102).

In terms of the tactical approach to individual patients, dose deserves major emphasis in diseases where curative-intent treatment is possible. Thus, for the leukemias, lymphomas, testicular cancer, childhood solid tumors, and adjuvant treatment of breast cancer, every effort should be made not to compromise dose, even at the risk of significant toxicity. On the other hand, with more resistant tumors, where palliative-intent chemotherapy is indicated, dose should be adjusted primarily based on side effects (i.e., toxicity). With the major dose increases made possible by hematopoietic stem-cell support, significant cure rates can be achieved in some patients who have relapsed after initial therapy.

Schedule of Drug Administration

Until approximately 25 years ago, it generally was thought that chemotherapy should be delivered at maximum safe doses, i.e., to definite (albeit limited) toxicity, and that the schedule of administration made little difference. Laboratory investigations had long established that the therapeutic index of chemotherapeutic agents could be affected by the schedule of drug administration (64).

CYTARABINE

Skipper and Schabel (128–130, performed elegant, quantitative studies in L1210 mouse leukemia of the prototype cell-cycle-phase-specific agent ara-C. They observed that the generation time of the L1210 cells was 12 hours, that the growth fraction approached 100%, and that treatment over a 24-hour period would allow essentially all leukemia cells to enter S (i.e., the ara-C sensitive phase of the cycle). They and others observed that ara-C given over a 24-hour period resulted in a plateau of the dose-toxicity curve (Fig. 54.2*B*), presumably because of "resting" cells in the normal bone marrow, and that by 3 to 4 days, the marrow completely recovered. Twenty-four-hour continuous exposure to ara-C at 4-day intervals did not produce cumulative toxicity (129). Presumably for these cytokinetic reasons, this schedule produced a far greater therapeutic index for ara-C in L1210 leukemia in mice than, for example, longer durations of treatment or other schedules such as daily administration.

Clarkson and colleagues (21) observed that 5 to 7 days of continuous infusion of tritiated thymidine in patients with AML resulted in labeling of over 90% of leukemic cells, thus indicating that this fraction had entered DNA synthesis some time over the 5- to 7-day period. Thus, for AML, continuous infusion for 5- to 7-day courses, with a 2- to 3-week interruption, was extrapolated from the aforementioned preclinical and cytokinetic studies. This treatment with ara-C produced a 30 to 40% complete remission rate in patients with AML, compared with 10% for other schedules such as daily intravenous administration (8, 41). The addition of daunorubicin to ara-C further increased the response rate. Finally, in a comparative study, the CALGB demonstrated a superior complete remission rate for ara-C given by continuous infusion for 7 days along with daunorubicin (41, 106, 148).

METHOTREXATE

Five-day courses of intensive Mtx were developed by Li and colleagues (85) for gestational choriocarcinoma and proved to be curative. Goldin and colleagues (53) demonstrated in L1210 mouse leukemia that intermittent Mtx was superior to continuous (daily) methotrexate. In a randomized, comparative study of patients with acute lymphocytic leukemia (ALL) in complete remission, intermittent Mtx proved to be significantly superior to daily therapy (125). This observation, empiric at the time, is consistent with recent findings by Schimke, indicating that for Mtx, continuous exposure in vitro is the most effective way to produce drug resistance as compared with intermittent Mtx. Moreover, with continuous administration, resistance results from gene amplification compared with a transport defect following intermittent Mtx (109, 120, 121) (for HD Mtx with leucovorin rescue, see the discussion later in this chapter).

FLUOROPYRIMIDINES

In clinical studies, FU classically has been administered by daily pulse doses of 350 to 450 mg/m^2 for 5 days. When treatment is given by continuous infusion over 5 days, twice that dose can be delivered, and both mucositis and diarrhea become dose limiting as compared with bone marrow suppression (124). Fluorodeoxyuridine (FUDR) delivered by continuous infusion is much more toxic; for example, doses in the range of 30 to 50 mg/m^2/d produce toxicity. The biochemical basis for these schedule differences is speculative. There is some evidence that continuous infusion FUDR has a greater effect on DNA synthesis, whereas the other schedules have a relatively greater effect on host tissue RNA and RNA synthesis (55). There are, however, relatively few data regarding the effect of these differences in schedule on the therapeutic index (modulation with leucovorin is discussed later). Longer durations of systemic administration currently are under study (90, 133).

It recently has been reported that mechanisms of action, resistance, and cross-resistance for FU differ depending on whether administration is continuous or pulse (7, 132).

ANTHRACYCLINES

Cardiotoxicity is an important form of delayed toxicity with anthracyclines. Experimental evidence shows that peak concentrations more likely produce cardiotoxicity than the lower concentrations produced by continuous-infusion schedules. The first clinical trial suggesting a dose-schedule effect was the observation by Weiss and Manthel (145) that weekly administration of doxorubicin produced less cardiotoxicity per given total dose than standard, triweekly regimens. Legha and colleagues (86) demonstrated and confirmed in randomized studies that a 4-day, continuous infusion of doxorubicin every 3 weeks is less cardiotoxic than bolus injections. These approaches allow for a 30 to 50% increase in total cumulative dose before cardiotoxicity develops. There also is experimental and preliminary clinical evidence that liposomal doxorubicin may be less cardiotoxic (98).

Two other relevant studies involved the randomization of patients between different schedules of similar regimens. In a SWOG (Southwest Oncology Group) study, continuous infusion DTIC (dimethyl triazene imidazole carboxamide decarbazine) plus doxorubicin was compared with bolus administration. The response rate was identical, but toxicity, including nausea, vomiting, and cardiotoxicity, was substantially less with the continuous-infusion schedule. An adjuvant trial at Memorial Sloan-Kettering corroborated the decreased cardiotoxicity of continuous-infusion doxorubicin, but sarcoma patients receiving the continuous infusion had a higher incidence of relapse (19, 151).

ALKYLATING AGENTS

Most data regarding alkylating agents suggest they are schedule independent. In other words, the antitumor and host effects are dose-related, independent of schedule.

The relative merits (particularly with HD therapy) of bolus versus a 3- to 4-day continuous infusion is debated. In vivo modeling studies indicate that the continuous-infusion approach should be at least as active as bolus (i.e., pulse therapy) (139).

ETOPOSIDE

Etoposide is an inhibitor of topoisomerase II and is selectively active against cells in cycle. It commonly is used in combination chemotherapy, particularly with cisplatin for patients with solid tumors. Its interaction with cisplatin may involve the inhibition of DNA repair. This is consistent with preclinical studies indicating that etoposide must be present both during and immediately following cisplatin to achieve optimal effect.

The optimal dose schedule for etoposide in small cell lung cancer consists of five daily doses every 3 to 4 weeks (131). This is consistent with the earlier discussion of the cytokinetics of bone marrow and tumor and the response to cell-cycle-specific agents (148).

TUBULIN BINDERS

While the vinca alkaloids, vincristine and vinblastine, are cell-cycle-specific, there is little evidence that any one schedule is superior to the standard weekly schedule (6). Based on limited data, the same is true for vinorelbine. The paclitaxel schedule considerations have been dominated by acute histamine-like toxicity, probably related to the vehicle (cremophor), which is relieved by antihistamines and longer durations of infusion. Practical and economic considerations, particularly outpatient use, have emphasized short-term (i.e., 1 to 3 hour) intravenous infusions (7).

NAUSEA, VOMITING, AND SCHEDULE DEPENDENCY

There is evidence that the emetogenic effect of some agents relates to peak concentration. This is particularly true for azacytidine, which at 150 mg/m^2/d for 5 days produces major nausea and vomiting. The same dose rate given as a continuous infusion for 120 hours is less emetogenic and produces the same antileukemic effect. This is also true, though less so, for dacarbazine and cytarabine. There also is evidence that continuous infusion cisplatin may be less emetogenic than the same total dose given by bolus injection.

INTERMITTENT INTENSIVE TREATMENT SCHEDULE AND EFFECT ON THERAPEUTIC INDEX

For most chemotherapeutic agents used alone or in combination, intermittent courses are superior to continuous (i.e., daily) treatment. Definitive studies have not been performed in most instances, but data supporting this position exist for cyclophosphamide and Mtx in Burkitt's lymphoma (48), Mtx and actinomycin D in choriocarcinoma (48), melphalan in myeloma, ara-C in acute myelocytic leukemia, and Mtx in remission maintenance in ALL (48, 125). It also is true for most combination regimens, such as MOPP (mustard, oncovin, procarbazine, and prednisone) treatment for Hodgkin's disease (29), combination chemotherapy for acute myelocytic leukemia (96), and the combination chemotherapy (usually including cyclophosphamide, actinomycin D, and vincristine) for childhood solid tumors (see Chapters 169 and 171).

Experimental and clinical studies both indicate the superiority of intermittent, intensive treatment for rapidly proliferating tumors. Continuous treatment may be superior for the more slow-growing, low-growth-fraction tumors, but more definitive studies are needed (90).

In addition to the foregoing cytokinetic and pharmacologic rationale, immunologic factors may in part explain the superior effect of intermittent treatment. Various facets of immune response are affected by 5-day courses of intensive single-agent or combination chemotherapy given every 3 to 4 weeks (9, 72). Although one study showed the various parameters of immune response were greatly suppressed by 5-day courses of intensive treatment, immunologic recovery was brisk and usually complete by the day 10 following treatment (72). For continuous daily treatment with chemotherapeutic agents, immune suppression initially is less intense, but it tends to be sustained and progressive (9). Consistent with these reports is evidence that intermittent treatment results in fewer infections with organisms of low pathogenicity.

Advances in supportive care have resulted in a novel approach to intermittent intensive chemotherapy. Leukophoresis following marrow recovery from chemotherapy and G-CSF allows the harvest of sufficient stem cells to rescue as many as four courses of moderately intensive chemotherapy with cyclophosphamide and carboplatin for ovarian and lung cancer (141, 142).

Combination Chemotherapy

The most compelling, pragmatic rationale for combination chemotherapy has been its success. Essentially all curative cancer chemotherapy involves a combination of agents. The most compelling, basic-science rationale is tumor cell heterogeneity and its implications for drug resistance. Definitions and quantitation of combination chemotherapy in the clinic are presented here, and preclinical models have been developed.

EXPERIMENTAL MODEL: THE ISOBOLOGRAM

In experimental systems, elaborate mathematic approaches to defining additive effects, synergy, antagonism, and other results have been developed. The isobologram is an in vitro approach to the evaluation of two agents that are employed in combination (Fig. 54.2). Equicytotoxic doses (ED) of drugs 1 and 2 are expressed on co-ordinates. A straight line between the extremes, wherein ED_{50} of drug 1 plus ED_{50} of drug 2 always equals the total of either drug 1 or drug 2, means that the effects are additive. A concave

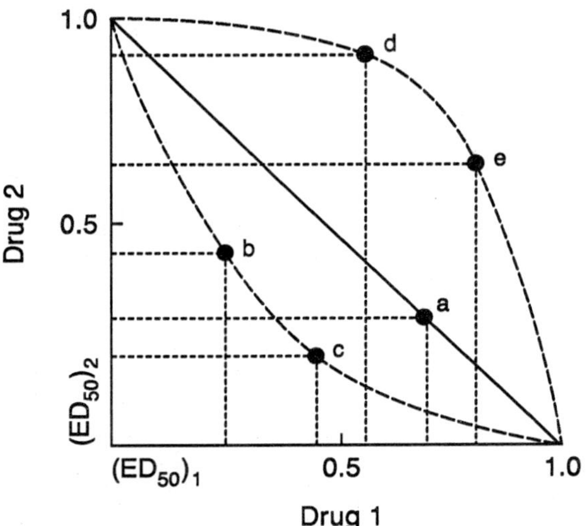

Figure 54.6. Isobologram: the classic way of evaluating the cytotoxic interaction of two agents, with dose effect of drug I and drug II on the *x* and *y* axis, respectively. Various dose or concentration ratios are then evaluated. If a straight line results, the effects are additive; if convex up, antagonistic; if concave down, synergistic.

curve indicates synergy, and a convex curve indicates antagonism. This technique allows the examination of different ratios of combinations (Fig. 54.6).

The isobologram has been modified in several ways, particularly in the direction of simplicity for evaluating in vivo studies. This literature has been superbly reviewed by Rideout and Chou (112).

RELATIONSHIP BETWEEN COMBINATION CHEMOTHERAPY AND DOSE

Before considering the cellular and molecular biologic rationales for combination chemotherapy, it is important to consider the relationship between dose and combination chemotherapy. Most clinical data are consistent with the proposition that effective combinations of chemotherapeutic agents are those that allow an increase in Summation Dose Intensity (SDI) (61).

The two disciplines developed separately, with dose represented by bone-marrow-transplantation-oriented investigators and combination chemotherapy by hematology-oncology-pharmacology researchers. Today, we are witnessing a synthesis of these paradigms, and we propose that dose, or SDI, explains much of what has been achieved in the past with combination chemotherapy. This section also considers the rational interpretation and construction of combination regimens.

Almost without exception, the cure of a given form of clinically evident cancer requires at least three active agents. An active agent is here defined as one that when used alone produces a 40% or greater response rate. Relevant tumors include ALL, AML, Hodgkin's and non-Hodgkin's lymphoma, testicular cancer, choriocarcinoma, Burkitt's lymphoma, Wilm's tumor, and embryonal rhabdomyosarcoma. While very chemosensitive tumors such as choriocarcinoma and localized Burkitt's lymphoma can be cured with one agent, the cure rate generally is higher with combinations of agents, and the more common and generalized forms of these tumors require combinations of three or more agents (17). A valid exception is the rare tumor, hairy-cell leukemia, wherein high cure rates can be achieved with single-agent chemotherapy.

Active agents and their use in appropriate combination and dose are critical to curative therapy (Fig 54.7). The major basic-science rationale for combination chemotherapy is tumor cell heterogeneity (42, 122).

The potential for cure with chemotherapy inversely relates to the tumor burden. Thus, there are many examples where the chemotherapy of clinically evident (i.e., macroscopic) tumor is not curative, whereas the same tumor in microscopic form (i.e., the surgical adjuvant setting) is. These tumors include breast cancer, osteosarcoma, colorectal cancer, ovarian cancer, and Ewing's sarcoma. While single agents can increase long-term tumor-free survival, in selected circumstances (e.g., breast cancer and melphalan), one almost always can do better with combinations, generally of three or more agents (18, 47).

Another exception is bone marrow transplantation. In this case, for the leukemias and lymphomas, two agents or one agent plus total-body irradiation can be curative (discussed later) (143).

Are there tumors that cannot be cured by chemotherapy despite three or more active agents? The only clear example is follicular lymphoma. There are a number of active agents for small cell lung cancer. There is a definite cure rate for small cell lung cancer (limited disease) but it is low (i.e., 5 to 10%).

Supportive care and toxicity have a reciprocal relationship. Lessened morbidity and improved dosing with chemotherapy have been increasingly attained with advances in supportive care. Examples include platelet transfusions, antibiotics, antiemetics, marrow transplantation, and more recently, peripheral-blood stem cells and growth factors (17, 61, 81).

An additional adverse factor is prior chemotherapy. More recent clinical and laboratory observations regarding drug resistance, particularly mechanisms relating to multidrug resistance and apoptosis, bear importantly on this prognostic factor (discussed later) (46, 85, 88).

Given the items discussed, a major objective of research in cancer is the identification of clinically active agents and their integration, where appropriate, into combination and multimodal treatment strategies.

CONCEPT AND APPLICATION OF SDI

Definition and Method of Application

Dose generally means single dose, although it has been used in the past synonymously with *dose rate*. The critical determinants are dose rate and total dose (or duration) of treatment. *Dose rate* and *dose intensity* also are similar, although dose *intensity* has come to mean the dose, schedule, and time relationships as specified by Hyrniuk and colleagues (e.g., dose/m^2/wk) (74, 75). To compare dose rates or intensity within a given study, we employ the time factor in dose rate that is appropriate to the study. When we compare across studies, we keep the time factor constant wherever possible.

In this section, we analyze dose within a given tumor as a function of single agents, combinations, and schedules. Dose intensity (DI) will be expressed and evaluated as follows. It is assumed that active single agents are approximately equiactive within a given tumor. Thus, single active agents given at full dose will have a DI of 1.0. Where there is compelling evidence for major superiority of a component agent in the combination (e.g., cisplatin in testicular cancer), appropriate adjustments are made.

There is compelling evidence that if it is to occur, response does so within the first two or three courses of monthly chemotherapy (discussed later). Similarly, cure, if it is to occur, probably is achieved within the first two or three courses as well. By that time, drug resistance, the major obstacle to cure and discussed later, has developed (79, 128). For these reasons, it is appropriate to select dose rates, whether for single or multiagent chemotherapy, based on the dose prescribed and delivered for a minimum of two to three courses.

We believe that these definitions and approaches are appropriate and meaningful within a given tumor and, to a somewhat more limited extent, across tumors. The operational use of these definitions are presented now and exemplified by Hodgkin's disease.

SDI for Hodgkin's Disease and Non-Hodgkin's Lymphoma

Combination chemotherapy was introduced early and effectively for both Hodgkin's and non-Hodgkin's lymphoma (19, 29). While the initial studies of curative combination chemotherapy were made in ALL, the Hodgkin's protocols are less complex and are used here to introduce the concept of SDI. Response rates for the various treatment programs in this and other discussions are taken from this and another textbook as well as their derivative references (17, 30).

Dose-limiting toxicity is myelosuppression for two of the agents, procarbazine and nitrogen mustard (HN_2), such that toxicity is additive; therefore, the doses of each must be reduced to 0.6y that employed as a single agent (Table 56.1). Prednisone and vincristine, however, have independent dose-limiting toxicity. Therefore, toxicity is not additive, and they can be employed in the MOPP combination at full dose rates (i.e., 1.0).

A total response rate of 40 to 65% can be achieved with each of the individual agents, but complete response rates are low. For the combination of four agents (MOPP), the SDI is 3.2 out of a possible 4.0. This results in a jump from 10 to 70% in the complete response rate and from 0 to 40% in the cure rate. Similar results were obtained for non-Hodgkin's lymphoma and testicular cancer (17).

SDI AND ALL IN CHILDREN

After gestational choriocarcinoma, acute leukemia was the first systemic cancer to be cured. Curative chemotherapy for ALL was introduced in the 1960s, and the cure rate has increased incrementally from 0% in 1960 to from 60 to 80% today (73, 104, 105, 123). Major contributions, including platelet transfusions and central nervous system (CNS) prophylaxis, have been important to this advance; however, systemic treatment with an increasing number of antitumor agents, particularly those that are nonadditive in terms of toxicity, has been critical. Note in Table 54.2 that single agents produce low response rates and no cures. With two dose combinations, a marked increase in complete response rate occurs, but only when nonadditive toxicity allows for increased dose intensity. Cure begins to appear with combinations involving four agents used either concurrently or in close sequence.

Further progress depended on, in addition to CNS prophylaxis, a further increase in the number of agents. With six to nine agents, an SDI of 5 to 7 could be achieved because of nonadditive toxicity. These largely are the nonmyelosuppressive agents, including vincristine, prednisone, asparaginase, Mtx with leucovorin (LCV) rescue, and CNS irradiation. The relationship between the number of agents, SDI, complete response, and cure is presented in a less complex form in Table 54.3 (6, 17, 48, 73, 104, 123).

SDI and Breast Cancer

There are several examples of the negative side of SDI, one of which is metastatic breast cancer. Individual agents with significant activity and their response rates are presented in Table 54.4. Complete responses with single agents are rare (e.g., 5% with doxorubicin). All of these

Table 54.1. Combination Chemotherapy and Summation Dose Intensity in Hodgkin's Disease

Agents(s)	Dose-limiting toxicity	Fraction of Standard Dose	Dose intensity	Total response (%)	Complete response (%)	Cure (%)
M (HN_2)	Marrow	0.6	0.6	60	10	0
O (VCR)	Neuro.	1	1	50	5	0
Proc.	Marrow	0.6	0.6	65	15	0
Pred.	Infection	1	1	40	0	0
MOPP		0.6 + 1 + 0.6 + 1 = 3.2[a]		85	70	40

[a] Summation Dose Intensity.

Table 54.2. Combination Chemotherapy and Summation Dose Intensity in Acute Lymphocytic Leukemia

Agent(s)	Agents (n)	Dose-limiting toxicity		Summation dose intensity[a]	Response: Complete response (%)	Response: Cure (%)
Mtx (M)	1	Marrow	1	1	21	
Mp	1	Marrow	1	1	27	
VCR (V)	1	Neuro.	1	1	47	
P	1	Adr. Cort	1	1	50	
M + Mp	2	—	0.5 + 0.5	1	45	
P + Mp	2	—	1 + 1	2	82	
P + V (VP)	2	—	1 + 1	2	92	
VAMP	4	—	1 + 0.5 + 0.5 + 1	3	95+	15
VP + MpM	4		1 + 1 + 0.5 + 0.5	3	95+	15
VP + MMp + cp	4+		1 + 1 + 0.5 + 0.5 + cp	3+	95+	40
VP + MMp + Asp + Adria + cp	6+		1 + 1 + 0.5 + 0.5 + 1 + 0.8	4.8	95+	75–80
VP + MMp + CPA + Asp + Adria + ML + ara-C + cp	9+		1 + 1 + 0.5 + 0.5 + 0.8 + 1 + 0.8 + 1 + 0.8	7.4	95+	75–80

[a] Dose Intensity. Single agent arbitrarily set at 1. Summation Dose Intensity applies to two or more agents.
Adria—Adriamycin; ara-C—cytosine arabinoside; Asp—asparaginase; cp—central nervous system (CNS) prophylaxis generally with central nervous system irradiation and intrathecal methotrexate; CPA—cyclophosphamide; ML—methotrexate with leucovorin rescue; MMp—methotrexate, 6-mercaptopurine; Mp—6-mercaptopurine; MpM—methotrexate, 6-mercaptopurine; Mtx—methotrexate); P—prednisone; V—vincristine; VAMP—V + Amethopterin (methotrexate) + Mp + P; VCR—vincristine.

Table 54.3. Comparison of Number of Agents and Curative Treatment for Acute Lymphocytic Leukemia in Children

	Chemotherapeutic agents (n)						
	1	2	3	4	5	6	7
Complete response (%)	20–40	40–92	>95	>95	>95	>95	>95
Cure (%)	0	0	Low	15	5–35	75–80	75–80

Table 54.4. Combination Chemotherapy and Summation Dose Intensity in Metastatic Breast Cancer

Agent(s)	Dose-limiting toxicity	Dose rate	Summation dose intensity	Response: PR + CR (%)	Response: CR (%)
CPA	Marrow	1	1	35	0
Methotrexate	Marrow	1	1	25	0
Fluorouracil	Marrow	1	1	25	0
Doxorubicin	Marrow	1	1	50	5
CMF	—	0.5 + 0.33 + 0.33	1.17	50	5
CAF	—	0.5 + 0.7 + 0.33	1.53	75	10

[a] Patients with overt metastases and no prior chemotherapy except in the adjuvant setting.
CAF—cyclophosphamide Adriamycin fluorouracil; CMF—CMF (cytoxan, Mtx, 5-FU); CPA—cyclophosphamide CR—complete response; PR—partial response.

agents have myelosuppression as dose-limiting toxicity; Mtx, FU, and doxorubicin have mucositis as well. Therefore, doses must be reduced proportionately to accommodate the combination. Thus, the SDI for CMF (Cytoxan, Mtx, 5-FU) is only 1.2 (out of a possible 3), and response to CMF is increased only slightly above that for single-agent therapy. CAF has an SDI of 1.5 with an overall response that is somewhat, but not impressively, better than that with the best single agent (i.e., doxorubicin).

SDI, Cisplatin, and Solid Tumors

In the solid epithelial tumors, it is more difficult to evaluate SDIs, because response rates generally are low. The first agent that consistently increased response rates when used in combination was cisplatin. For example, the partial response rate for non-small-cell lung cancer to cisplatin is 20%. For other active agents, such as vindesine, etoposide, FU, and cyclophosphamide, it is in the range of 10 to 20%.

Combinations excluding cisplatin produce a 15 to 20% response rate, whereas several combinations including cisplatin produce response rates of 30 to 40%. Is this because of some biochemical interaction of cisplatin with the other agents, or is it because cisplatin is essentially the only agent with solid tumor activity that is nonmyelosuppressive and therefore can be combined at full dose (17, 24)?

In non-small-cell lung cancer, an opportunity for therapeutic advance is provided by the recent discovery of agents that are active in this disease. In addition to the platinum analogues, these include taxol and taxetere, gemcitibine, CPT111, and vinorelbine. The time-honored principle would be for cisplatin, which is not myelosuppressive, to be used in combination with other agents for which myelosuppression is variably dose limiting. The advent of growth factors that allow for increased dosing of carboplatin and the other agents, however, does not allow for increased dosing of cisplatin. Preliminary studies suggest that taxol, perhaps the best single agent in non-small-cell lung cancer may not produce additive myelosuppression when used with some of the other agents. Clearly, the rationale and construct of combination chemotherapeutic regimens is an ongoing challenge (97).

Alternating (Cycling) Chemotherapy and SDI

Alternating or cycling courses of chemotherapy were proposed many years ago to delay development of drug resistance (59, 85). It was reasoned that resistance takes a finite length of selection pressure before it is stable. Thus, short courses of treatment A might produce resistance that is transient and reverses during treatment B; the same is true for B followed by A. In addition, Goldie and Coldman (62) proposed that cycling therapy might be a way to deliver enhanced dose intensity.

Table 54.5 reviews three studies of cycling therapy. MOPP and ABVD (Adriamycin, bleomycin, vinblastine, dacarbazine) are approximately equally active in the treatment of Hodgkin's disease. The study conducted by the CALGB found that MOPP alternated at monthly intervals with ABVD was slightly less active than ABVD alone and slightly more active than MOPP alone. The alternating regimen does not provide improved dose intensity. This is because both programs are given every other month, which means a dose rate or intensity reduction of 50% (to 0.5) and, therefore, a SDI of only 1.0 (i.e., the same as for the nonalternating programs) (12, 18).

Studies of adjuvant chemotherapy for osteosarcoma illustrate this point. Numerous historical studies indicate that the cure rate for OGS (osteogenic sarcoma) with amputation was only 15 to 20% (90).

It was discovered in the mid-1970s that adjuvant chemotherapy with either HD Mtx with LCV rescue (Mtx/LCV) or doxorubicin resulted in a 40% cure rate. The CALGB then compared doxorubicin and Mtx/LCV alternated at monthly intervals to doxorubicin given monthly. No difference was found, and if SDI is the critical factor, one would not have expected a difference (25, 27, 40, 65, 77, 77a, 91, 114).

Because dose-limiting toxicity was different for doxorubicin and MTX/LCV, it was possible to deliver them in combination without a compromise in dose. This required careful monitoring of the pharmacokinetics of Mtx and renal function. It was predicted that this increase of the SDI to 2.0 would increase the cure rate to 60% ([cure rate for amputation only = 20%] + [increase in cure rate for Mtx/LCV = 20%] + [increase in cure rate for doxorubicin = 20%] = 60%). The actual result was in fact 60%. Subsequent multi-institutional, randomized studies of combined Mtx/LCV and doxorubicin with additional agents resulted in cure rates of 60 to 75%, compared with 15 to 20% for the no-adjuvant-therapy controls (Table 54.5) (25, 40, 65, 77, 77a, 89, 91, 114).

In an older study, patients with ALL were induced into complete remission with vincristine and prednisone and then randomized to receive either concurrent 6-mercaptopurine (6-MP) with Mtx or alternating 6-MP and Mtx at monthly intervals. Concurrent 6-MP with Mtx had to be given at reduced doses because of additive dose-limiting marrow toxicity. Thus, for both programs, SDI of 1.0 was achieved.

Table 54.5. Alternating (Cycling) Chemotherapy and Summation Dose Intensity

	Treatment	Complete response %	DFS %	Toxicity	Dose	Dose rate (SDI)
Hodgkin's Disease stages IIIB & IV	MOPP	70	45	4+	1	1
	ABVD	88	58	2+	1	1
	MOPPalt with ABVD	80	52	3+	0.5 + 0.5[a]	1
Osteosarcoma adjuvant	No chemo.		20	—	—	
	Mtx/LCV		40	1–2+		
	Doxorubicin		40	2–3+	1	1
	Dox alt with Mtx/LCV		40	2–3+	0.5 + 0.5	1
	Dox + Mtx/LCV		60	2–4+	1.0 + 1.0	2
Acute lymphocytic leukemia remission maintenance	Mtx			2+		1
	6MP			2+		1
	Mtx alt. MP			2+		0.5 + 0.5
	Mtx + MP			2+		0.5 + 0.5

ABVD—ABVD (Adriamycin, bleomycin, vinblastine, dacarbazine)

There was no difference in antitumor effect (i.e., in the duration of complete remission) (Table 54.5) (58, 59).

Bonadonna and colleagues (11) compared cycling doxorubicin and CMF with sequential doxorubicin (four courses) followed by CMF (six courses) in the adjuvant chemotherapy of node-positive (i.e., >3) breast cancer. SDI was the same for both programs, but the sequential program was significantly superior to alternating cycles. There is increasingly compelling evidence that nonspecific cross-resistance occurs, probably within 1 to 3 months (discussed later). Thus, in sequential chemotherapy, superior results should occur when the best treatment program (in this case, doxorubicin) is used initially (10, 11).

SDI and HD Chemotherapy with Stem Cell Rescue for Solid Tumors

The evidence that combinations of chemotherapeutic agents are superior to single agents in HD stem-cell growth-factor (HD-SC) programs for solid tumors is substantial, if not quite as rigorously proven as for combination chemotherapy for the hematologic malignancies. The maximum safe dose for total-body irradiation in the marrow transplant situation is approximately 1,200 cGy, depending somewhat on dose rate and shielding technology. Dose-limiting toxicity most commonly is pulmonary. For cyclophosphamide, the maximum safe dose (MSD) that can be delivered is 6.5 to 7.0 g/m^2; dose-limiting toxicity, except myelosuppression, is cardiac. Combining these two programs, total-body irradiation and cyclophosphamide, was possible with minimal compromise in the dose of each modality. Total-body irradiation with cyclophosphamide is the time-honored transplant (also called high-dose, intensification, or conditioning) regimen for the leukemias/lymphomas. More recently, the busulfan/cyclophosphamide combination has been introduced and proven to be as effective as the cyclophosphamide/total-body irradiation program. With this busulfan/cyclophosphamide combination, it also has been possible to employ the nearly full MSD of the individual agents in combination. Finally, combined cyclophosphamide, BCNU, and etoposide in the HD-SC setting has provided significant cure rates for recurrent Hodgkin's and non-Hodgkin's lymphomas (78, 116, 117, 143).

Myelosuppression with chemotherapeutic agents has been the major limitation to their use at full or nearly full doses in combination. What is the SDI potential for combined HD-SC therapy?

We have examined three combination regimens developed at the Dana-Farber Cancer Institute for HD-SC treatment of solid tumors (Table 54.6). The first combination was CBP (cyclophosphamide, BCNU, and cisplatin) (102, 103). The dose-limiting toxicity in the transplant setting for these agents is cardiac for cyclophosphamide, liver and lung for BCNU, and kidney and peripheral nervous system for cisplatin (3). Do these nonoverlapping toxicities allow for improved SDI in the HD-SC setting?

The MSD in the transplant setting for these agents when used alone is presented in Table 54.6 and compared with the MSD when used in the combination. The fraction of the individual doses in combination, as compared with when they are used alone, is presented in the last column. The ratios are high (i.e., 0.93, 0.75, and 1.00). This provides an SDI of 2.7 (out of a maximum of 3). If toxicity were completely additive, the SDI would be 1.0 and if totally independent, 3.0. The selection of the three agents for the CBP combination was based in part on their differing nonmyelosuppressive toxicity in the transplant setting. This strategy in fact worked and allowed for a high SDI, which hopefully will allow for a greater therapeutic effect. Indeed, in a retrospective analysis of single agents versus combinations of agents in the HD marrow protection setting, Antman and Gale (5) observed a consistently higher response rate in patients with solid tumor for the combinations.

The CBP combination had certain problems relating to the

Table 54.6. Dose Intensity of STAMP Regimens (DFCI)

Regimen	Combination	Dose-limiting toxicity	Trans. alone	MSD Transplant when used in triagent	Dose ratio[a]
CBP	CPA	Heart	6,500	6,000	0.93
	BCNU	Liver, lung	800	600	0.75
	Cisplatin	Nerve, kidney	160	160	1.00
		Summation Dose Intensity			**2.7**
CTC	CPA	Heart	6,500	6,000	0.93
	TSPA	Mucositis	800	500	0.63
	Carbo.	Liver	2,000	800	0.40
		Summation Dose Intensity			**2.0**
ICE	IFF	Nerve, kidney	16,000	16,000	1.0
	Carbo.	Liver	2,000	1,800	0.90
	Etoposide	Mucositis	2,500	1,200	0.48
		Summation Dose Intensity			**2.4**

[a] Dose ratio + MSD in combination/MSD when used alone.
MSD—Maximum safe dose; CPA = Cyclophosphamide; IFF = Ifosfamide; Carbo. = Carboplation.

organ toxicity of BCNU and the renal toxicity of cisplatin. To circumvent these limitations and hopefully develop a therapeutically superior program, we conducted a series of phase I studies that culminated in the CTC (cyclophosphamide + thiotepa + carboplatin) program (Table 54.6) (3, 4). The SDI of CTC is 2.0.

The CBP and CTC programs mainly target breast cancer. For a parallel program in lung cancer, we developed the ICE (ifosfamide + carboplatin + etoposide) regimen (Table 54.6). As with the CBP and CTC programs, the SDI in this was high (i.e., 2.4).

Thus, for all three programs, an SDI approaching the maximum of 3.0 could be delivered. Therefore, it appears that for combination chemotherapy in HD setting, high SDIs can be reached because of differing nonmyelosuppressive, dose-limiting toxicity. Therefore, as with standard doses, combination chemotherapy should produce a superior antitumor effect.

It has been suggested that any one of the agents, such as cyclophosphamide, might be as active at maximum high-dose stem cell protection doses as a single agent compared with the combination. The MSD of cyclophosphamide used alone was 6.5 g/m^2. The maximum dose of cyclophosphamide that can be employed in the trialkylator CBP program, however, was 6 g/m^2. Given these figures, it seems most unlikely that cyclophosphamide alone would be as effective as the trialkylator agent combination. This is consistent with the review by Antman and Gale (5) (described earlier).

PRINCIPLES OF COMBINATION CHEMOTHERAPY

The principles of combination chemotherapy may be considered in hypothetical form. If the agents have additive toxicity, the dose must be reduced accordingly: (A+B+C)/3. There are two ways of achieving a higher SDI, in this case full-dose delivery of all three agents (A+B+C). One is by choosing agents with independent nonadditive, nonoverlapping toxicity, and the second involves improved supportive care, such as growth factors and marrow stem cells. Indeed, improved myeloprotection allows for a 4- to 10-fold increase in the dose of selected myelosuppressive agents in the HD-SCR setting (e.g., 4[A+B+C]).

As a generalization, gastrointestinal toxicity is the major dose-limiting toxicity after marrow toxicity. If a gastrointestinal protection approach were to prove successful, the combined use of bone marrow and a gastrointestinal protection approach may affect the therapeutic potential of agents such as doxorubicin and FU, indeed, many chemotherapeutic agents. Pilot studies of gastrointestinal protection agents have been conducted (95).

The next example is the addition of agent D to ABC. If no compromise in dose is necessary, the SDI is increased from 3.0 to 4.0. If, however, there is overlapping toxicity between, for example, C and D, then the dose of each must be reduced to 50% for an SDI of 3.0. If the toxicity of D is additive with A, B, and C, then the dose of each agent must be reduced by 75% to accommodate the combination. What is gained in the number of agents is "neutralized" by the reduction in dose.

An example of the complexities of the dose/number of agents trade-off is the following: Mtx/LCV is active in non-Hodgkin's lymphoma and, properly monitored, can be delivered without significant toxicity (46, 104). In phase II studies, it has been combined with full-dose CHOP (cyclophosphamide, hydroxydaunomycin/doxorubicin, Oncovin, prednisone) without compromise in dose (103). A famous comparative study found that Mtx/LCV plus CHOP was not superior to CHOP and concluded that Mtx/LCV was inactive in that setting (44); however, the doses of two key agents, doxorubicin and cyclophosphamide, were reduced by 33% in the M-CHOP regimen. Thus, an alternative conclusion is that Mtx/LCV is indeed active, because it makes up for a substantial reduction in the dose of these two agents. Thus, there is no conclusion, and the key question (i.e., Does Mtx/LCV added to full-dose CHOP provide a better therapeutic effect?) remains unanswered (75).

The increased number of agents and reduced dose trade-off has been a major consideration in alternating or cycling regimens. Such studies go back almost 40 years and are based on considerations of resistance development (50). Goldie-Coldman placed this approach on a more rational basis in terms of quantitative and theoretic drug resistance considerations (27, 52). Their thesis was that the more active agents, the better, and they suggested that from a practical and toxicologic view, this might be better accomplished by rotating combinations (62).

To our knowledge, no rotating combination has proven to be superior to the appropriate control, because dose rate or intensity is sacrificed to accommodate the increased number of agents (Table 54.5). ABAB is not superior to AAAA, because while the number of agents is doubled, the dose rate for each is halved. This illustrates the principle that an increase in the number of agents with a comparable decrease in dose rate results in no gain in therapeutic effect (51).

The SDI of combination chemotherapy regimens can reach those achieved by HD-SC programs. For example, in Hodgkin's disease, an SDI of 3.2, and in ALL an SDI of 7.4, can be reached because of the large number of active agents, some of which are nonadditive with respect to toxicity (Table 54.1). It is difficult to compare SDIs for HD-SC programs to more standard dose combinations because of the major differences in schedule and duration of treatment; however, the HD-SC setting allows for a 4- to 10-fold increase in dose. Indeed, the 75 and 50% cure rates that can be achieved with combination chemotherapy in ALL and Hodgkin's disease, respectively, compare favorably with HD-SC approaches, but the different settings in which these modalities are employed make comparisons difficult to interpret.

As discussed earlier, there is increasingly compelling evidence that treatment failure, in terms of the potential for cure, occurs relatively early (e.g., after 2 or 3 months) and that while longer treatment may prolong the duration of response by suppressing sensitive tumor cells, it will fail because resistant tumor cells have been induced or selected. This is consistent with adjuvant studies in breast cancer where the duration of chemotherapy was the variable (14). These studies indicate that 12 months of adjuvant chemotherapy is as good as 24 months, that 6 months of CMF is as good as 12, and that 4 months of AC (Adriamycin + cyclophosphamide) is as good as 8 (5). In a study where the total dose of CAF was constant, 4 months was as good as 6 overall and better in the c-*Erb*-2 overexpressing subset of patients (96). On the other hand, one cycle of CMF is not enough. Thus, drug resistance presumably occurs early (i.e., by the second monthly course of therapy but not later than the fourth). These results are in accord with Skipper's cytokinetic analysis of human breast cancer (128). While this may not apply to rotating courses of non-cross-resistant chemotherapy, there is little evidence from clinical trials supporting the rotating, alternating, or cycling approach in general. For breast cancer specifically, there is a marginally positive CALGB study of such rotation and a negative NSABP (National Surgical Adjuvant Breast Program) study.

Shipp and colleagues addressed this issue in patients with non-Hodgkin's lymphoma by studying early changes in gallium scanning (79). They found that if patients did not become gallium negative by the second or third course of chemotherapy, they did not become so subsequently, and relapse was inevitable (16). Preclinical studies indicate that resistance may be induced or selected quickly (i.e., after one or two courses of therapy (20).

Clearly, the information discussed supports short-term intensive therapy. Will rotating, intensive courses of combination chemotherapy (ABC → DEF). So-called double transplant or double HD-SCR therapy, provide for further control of resistant cells? It is an important hypothesis, and appropriate studies addressed to this hypothesis are ongoing. The most mature, relevant (though not HD) study is a NSABP adjuvant trial in node-positive patients with breast cancer. In this study, AC (Adriamycin + cyclophosphamide) for 2 months rotating with CMF for 6 did not prove to be superior to either AC for 2 months or CMF for 6 (71).

Norton has developed a cytokinetic and drug resistance rationale for delayed intensification and the use of agents individually in sequence in HD-SCR studies rather than in concurrent combinations (98) (see Chapter 52).

REAL-TIME PHARMACOKINETICS AND PATIENT SAFETY

Pharmacokinetic studies provide interesting information regarding the dose effect. In general, such studies indicate substantial variation of AUC (area under the plasma curve) per given dose and that the AUC level of drug or active metabolites correlates with toxicity and therapeutic effect. Such results have been found for HD busulfan and BCNU in the transplant setting and for Mtx and 6-MP in acute leukemia (72, 74–76). These results generally support the HD approach and indicate that optimal safety and effectiveness will require pharmacokinetic guidance (42, 43, 66).

INTERPRETATION OF SDI

We do not mean to imply that no important interaction at, for example, a biochemical or cytokinetic level explains the superiority of combination chemotherapy. Rather, we wish to emphasize that such an interaction does not have to be invoked and that clinical data are consistent with the position that the effectiveness of combination chemotherapy results from the dose increase, expressed as SDI.

A significant exception to this is the biochemical interaction that affects response to the sequence of Mtx and FU. This biologic phenomenon results from Mtx inhibition of purine biosynthesis and, hence, an increase in PRPP (phospho-ribosyl pyrophosphate). In turn, this latter effect facilitates the conversion of FU to the nucleotide (i.e., the active metabolic product) (see Chapters 60 and 61).

Clinical trials involving Mtx and FU (plus LCV) indicate higher response rates for the sequence of Mtx to FU and LCV. The LCV plays the dual role of rescuing the Mtx on the one hand and modulating the ternary FU complex on the other. Clinical trials (largely noncomparative) affirm, but do not vigorously establish, the superiority of this sequence.

IMPLICATIONS OF DRUG RESISTANCE FOR SDI

Lack of cross-resistance has been a major rationale for combination chemotherapy from the beginning (77). Almost all resistance, however, is relative to dose. What is the relative impact of tumor cell heterogeneity on dose and combination chemotherapy?

The simplest model for addressing these questions is as follows: take two agents, A and B, that have approximately equal antitumor activity (Fig. 54.8). What are the relative effects of combining A with B as compared with a twofold increase in dose either in terms of tumor cell kill (50)?

The effect of modern concepts of drug sensitivity and drug resistance, as affected by dose and combination chemotherapy have major therapeutic implications. Selected antitumor agents inhibit specific biochemical pathways or damage the product of such pathways. Resistance may occur at the level of an active intermediate. For many years after Law's discovery of Mtx resistance in 1953, resistance was thought to be monofactorial, i.e., it affected primarily the selecting agent and did not cross to the other agents (85). This changed with Ling's discovery of multidrug (largely natural products) resistance in 1983 (69) and, subsequently, with the discovery of other resistance mechanisms to subsets of antitumor agents such as glutathione transferases for the alkylating agents and topoisomerase II enzyme levels and topoisomerase inhibitors (9, 78).

A still more general modern mechanism of drug sensitivity/resistance relates to apoptosis or programmed cell death. The apoptosis concept of drug resistance states that differing cell damage by different chemotherapeutic agents has the common property of triggering the apoptosis or programmed cell death cascade. This is an active process that requires energy, enzymes, and cytostructure for completion and thus is subject to genetic control (83).

The first evidence that apoptosis was important in cancer was the discovery of *bcl*-2 gene, whose product interferes with apoptosis or cell death. There now is definitive evidence that overexpression of the *bcl*-2 gene occurs in the follicular lymphomas, with resultant decrease in tumor cell death. There has long been hematologic evidence that a lack of destruction of tumor cells is the key problem in this tumor (9, 69, 83).

There also now is impressive evidence that the balance of cell proliferation as controlled by cell-cycle-transit molecules and destruction as controlled by apoptosis is fundamental to the proliferative thrust of most tumors (46). Apoptosis can be set in motion by the tumor-suppressor gene, *p53*. The wild-type *p53* gene responds to almost any type of cell damage, such as with differing chemotherapeutic agents (Fig. 54.3), by initiating a cascade that leads to apoptosis. Tumors with wild-type *p53* thus are highly responsive to chemotherapy; these include the leukemias, lymphomas, and testicular cancer. On the other hand, tumors that are minimally or nonresponsive to chemotherapy, such as pancreas, lung, and bowel cancer, have a high incidence of inactivating mutations of *p53*. Thus, the set-point for apoptosis, as determined largely by *p53*, may determine whether a tumor responds to chemotherapy. Whether this would apply to all chemotherapeutic agents is under study (46, 108, 110).

Another recently discovered general mechanism for multidrug resistance is so-called multicellular resistance (1, 84).

Clearly, therapeutic strategies in general, and the relative merits of dose and combination chemotherapy in particular, need to be examined in the context of modern mechanisms of drug sensitivity/resistance.

ADDITIONAL RATIONALE FOR COMBINATION CHEMOTHERAPY

Biochemistry

Metabolic pathways to essential cellular constituents such as nucleic acids can be blocked at sequential or concurrent points in two biochemical pathways. Complementary blockade is defined as inhibition of the metabolic pathway as well as damage to the final product by a second agent. Such considerations provide a major conceptual framework for combination chemotherapy. Unfortunately, and with relatively few exceptions, this approach has not provided greater selectively (i.e., a greater toxic effect to tumor compared with host) (118). For other biochemical approaches, see the discussion of modulation later.

Tumor Cell Heterogeneity and Drug Resistance

The most compelling, basic rationale for combination chemotherapy, or any form of systemic therapy (e.g., endocrine therapy, biotherapy), is tumor cell heterogeneity. While tumors are clonal in origin, the increasing DNA instability that accompanies the onset of neoplasia leads to increased variation of daughter cells, with selection of such cells having greater survival capacity, such as greater metastatic or invasive potential, and of tumor cells with a higher proliferative thrust. Heterogeneity among tumor cells regarding a target site for chemotherapy (e.g., dihydrofolate reductase) will lead to selection of resistant clones. Such heterogeneity also has been demonstrated for hormone receptors and surface antigens. Thus, the selection of resistant cell lines by systemic hormonal manipulation and biotherapeutics, including monoclonal antibody therapy, is likely.

It used to be thought that monodrug resistance occurred (i.e., resistance obtained only for the selecting agent). The recognition of multidrug resistance requires a reexamination of this rationale for combination chemotherapy (88). Thus, p-glycoprotein multidrug resistance relates almost exclusively to natural products, but there is increasing evidence that glutathione transferase and topoisomerase II alterations also may be associated with multidrug resistance. Recent studies of multicellular drug resistance of altered set-point for apoptosis and drug resistance and differences between in vitro and in vivo drug resistance are modifying our approach to and interpretation of combination chemotherapy. In addition, evidence that cell damage may elicit multiple mechanisms of "resistance" (i.e., pleiotropic resistance); that prolonged drug exposure results in stably resistant cell lines; that acute exposure may result in short term, inductive reversible resistance that does not constitute genetic resistance; that tumor cell contact is required for the expression of resistance; and that multiple different mechanisms of cell injury may trigger a final common pathway to cell death (i.e., apoptosis) has necessitated a reexamination of resistance as it affects treatment strategy, particularly combination chemotherapy (46, 84, 88).

Cytokinetics

The discovery that solid tumors contained a large number of potentially clonogenic cells in G_1 or G_0 provided a basis for combination chemotherapy (93, 94, 135, 136) (see the earlier discussion of tumor hypoxia and growth fraction above). Thus, cell-cycle-specific agents were employed for cytotoxicity to mitotically active cells, and agents that were not cell-cycle-specific (i.e., BCNU) were added to damage the noncycling portion of the growth fraction.

Recruitment

Experimentally, one can "recruit" tumor cells in vivo into cycle by reducing tumor size with non-cell-cycle-specific chemotherapy. This probably results from a relative improvement in blood supply and, therefore, an increased growth fraction. This increases susceptibility to cell-cycle-specific agents. While this approach has been widely employed, it has not been proven that such sequential scheduling improves the therapeutic index.

Synchronization

With inhibitors of DNA synthesis or drugs that arrest cells in mitosis, it is possible to synchronize cells in vitro and in vivo, and to exploit this synchronization with a cell-cycle-phase-specific agent. Unfortunately, such approaches also may synchronize host target cells such as the bone marrow, thus providing no improvement in the therapeutic index.

A rationale for recruitment and, perhaps, synchronization is provided by hormone-dependent tumors. Thus, several studies have been conducted in patients with metastatic breast cancer where the cells were arrested cytokinetically with tamoxifen and then pulse stimulated into cycle with an estrogen (115). There is experimental and limited clinical evidence that some degree of tumor-cell synchrony follows this hormonal manipulation. Chemotherapy is ideally delivered at the time of maximum synchronization. The heterogeneity of human tumors regarding the time course of synchronization and recruitment has been a major problem, however, and this approach remains experimental (2).

Pharmacologic Rationale for Combination Chemotherapy

Perhaps the first important clinical example in this area was use of LCV to supply the product of the enzyme dihydrofolate reductase when inhibited by Mtx. There is no question that this approach does rescue the host and allows for the safe delivery of gram quantities of Mtx, provided that the patient is carefully monitored and rescue with LCV is applied appropriately. More commonly, intermediate doses (in the range of 200 to 400 mg/m^2) are employed. There is only one disease, osteogenic sarcoma, wherein Mtx with LCV rescue clearly is superior to standard Mtx. HD Mtx with rescue is not only highly effective against the primary tumor and metastatic disease, it also provides a core component of the highly successful adjuvant combination chemotherapy approach (1, 2) (see Chapter 139).

Non-Hodgkin's lymphoma provides a setting for understanding the Mtx rescue approach; this has been presented earlier (127). In diseases such as breast or head and neck cancer, high- or intermediate-dose Mtx with rescue is effective, and when integrated with combination chemotherapy, it might be more effective. This has not been conclusively demonstrated, however. Indeed, studies in patients with head and neck cancer comparing HD Mtx with intermediate- or even low-dose Mtx have not shown an advantage for the former (141).

Properly applied, LCV rescue after Mtx precludes toxicity. This is true if rescue is delivered by 24 hours. At 36 or 42 hours, such rescue often is incomplete, and toxicity can be major. The biochemical and biologic rationale for HD Mtx with rescue has been the subject of several studies and much discussion, but it remains uncertain (1, 55, 147).

Sanctuary Sites

Sanctuary sites such as the central nervous system may be a basis for combination therapy. Thus, intrathecal Mtx and whole-brain irradiation have been effective in markedly reducing the incidence of meningeal leukemia (83). This also can be accomplished, although perhaps not quite as well, with HD Mtx and LCV rescue, which provides cytotoxic concentrations in the cerebrospinal fluid. In addition, it also can be accomplished with combination intrathecal therapy (104).

Modulation

Of increasing importance has been the modulation approach. Ideally, a modulator is an agent that in itself is nontoxic but, based generally on a biochemical rationale, may improve the therapeutic index of a given chemotherapeutic agent.

A clinically successful example is FU modulated by LCV. The biochemical rationale is that the product of FU, FdUMP, binds to the substrate site of thymidylate synthase, thus inhibiting DNA synthesis and, therefore, cellular replication. The stability and duration of this inhibition directly relate to a third agent, 5,10-methylenetetrahydrofolate, which is a metabolic product of LCV that also binds to thymidylate synthase, producing the so-called ternary complex (FdUMP-TS-5,10-methylenetetrahydrofolate). In preclinical systems both in vitro and in vivo, LCV can favorably modulate the therapeutic index of FU (see Chapters 60 and 61). In clinical trials, four studies comparing FU to FU with LCV indicate an advantage to the latter in patients with metastatic colorectal cancer. In this setting, FU produces a 5 to 15% response rate and FU with LCV a 30 to 50% response rate; two studies also indicate improved survival rates (34). There now is uncontrolled evidence in patients with head and neck cancer and with metastatic breast cancer that FU modulated by LCV is superior to FU alone (35). LCV moderately increases the host effect in the form of mucositis and diarrhea, and this promising approach is now being applied to other tumors. Why there should be an increase in therapeutic effect as compared to toxicity, however, is not known.

Another interesting approach to modulation involves multidrug resistance. Verapamil and several other lipid-soluble heterocycle drugs can inhibit p-glycoprotein and thus decrease the efflux of a number of natural antitumor products (doxorubicin, vincristine, and others) from the cell, thereby increasing cytotoxicity. An increase in p-glycoprotein has been demonstrated in patients with B-cell tumors, AML, sarcoma, and more commonly, in patients who previously received drugs susceptible to multidrug resistance, such as vincristine and doxorubicin. A number of studies addressed to this topic are ongoing (28) (see Chapter 53).

The modulation of alkylating agents and cisplatin also is under study. Glutathione may combine chemically with alkylating agents, thus diminishing their activity. Glutathione production can be decreased by the inhibitor buthionine sulfoxime, which is an approach that preclinically improves the therapeutic index of a number of alkylating agents (79). Similarly, glutathione transferase, which mediates the aforementioned conjugation, can be inhibited by several agents. Hypoxia in solid tumors can be modulated experimentally by perfluorocarbon-oxygen breathing and by oxygen mimics such as the nitroimidazoles (see Chapters 48 and 53). Finally, inhibitors of DNA repair increase the effectiveness of alkylating agents experimentally (32, 39).

BIOTHERAPEUTICS AND COMBINATION CHEMOTHERAPY

The effect of dose schedule and combination therapy for biotherapeutics is currently under study (see Chapters 80 and 81). The mechanisms of the antitumor action of biologic agents, such as tumor necrosis factor (TNF), the interferons, and IL-2, are complex. The effects on immune and inflammatory response may be responsible for their antitumor effects; in addition, the interferons and TNF are directly cytotoxic to tumor cells in culture. While it was hoped that these agents might be employed with limited or no toxicity in the clinical setting, such has not proven to be the case. Indeed, for most of these agents (IL-2, interferons, and TNF), there is a positive correlation between dose and toxicity, and where antitumor effect has been observed, randomization to two dose levels produces significantly greater toxicity at the higher dose but also a significantly greater antitumor effect for Kaposi's sarcoma in HIV-infected patients (see Chapter 155) and for patients with hairy-cell leukemia (see Chapter

148). For TNF, clinical toxicity clearly is dose related. In experimental tumors, there is a steep dose-tumor response curve for TNF (see Chapter 81).

COMBINED CHEMICAL AND BIOLOGICAL THERAPY: THE SOIL AND THE SEED

Combination chemotherapy has depended on the presence of multiple therapeutic targets and chemotherapeutic agents directed at said targets. All other things being equal, the more effective agents that can be delivered without compromise in dose, the better. This point has been emphasized in the SDI concept, where, for example, in ALL some seven to nine chemotherapeutic agents are used in modern regimens, with cure rates approaching 80%. Our developmental research in chemotherapy has focused on the tumor cell per se; however, tumors are composed not only of tumor cells but of intrinsic and critical stromal cells, including vascular structures, supporting matrix molecules, and monocytic chronic inflammatory cells. Paget coined the terms *soil* and *seed*, meaning that the seed (i.e., the tumor cell) had to have the proper soil (i.e., normal tissue) for growth; thus, the soil and seed interaction influenced the distribution of metastases (101). We use these terms in a different context to mean the tumor cells and the supporting stroma of the tumor, i.e., the seed and the soil. Adding the soil to the seed has extended the potential number of therapeutic targets and, hence, the potential for combination chemotherapy.

Folkman has demonstrated the importance of angiogenesis for tumors and the effectiveness of certain antiangiogenic agents in restraining tumor growth (see Chapter 10). The production by tumor cells and adjacent monocytes of matrix metalloproteinases that can destroy supporting structure adjacent to tumors permits tumor invasion through the basement membrane and into the surrounding matrix. Inhibitors of matrix metalloproteinases have been developed that, in experimental systems, have antitumor properties. In a sense, therapy with "oxic" agents such as perfluorocarbons and hemoglobin solutions, which increase oxygen in severely hypoxic tumors, represent a combined soil-seed attack (138, 140).

Teicher and colleagues demonstrated the potential of the combined antisoil-antiseed approach. Several preclinical in vivo model systems demonstrated synergism between combinations of antiangiogenic agents with chemotherapy, combinations of matrix metalloproteinase inhibitors and chemotherapy, and further enhancement by combinations of antiangiogenesis agents, chemotherapy, and oxic agents (36, 138, 140). The mechanism for the antiangiogenesis effect on chemotherapy may relate to the increased entry of small molecules into a tumor.

In summary, the combination of seed and soil approaches extends the purview of combination chemotherapy. Such studies are entering early clinical trials.

ENDOCRINE THERAPY

The dose-response curves for hormonal agents are not as steep as for most chemotherapeutic agents, and these may be complex. For example, low doses of estrogen may stimulate estrogen-receptor-positive breast cancer, whereas higher doses may cause tumor regression.

Moreover, the concept of SDI may not apply to endocrine therapy, or at least to antiestrogen therapy. For example, the combination of tamoxifen and chemotherapy in metastatic breast cancer, and perhaps also in the adjuvant treatment of breast cancer, are subadditive. Dose and schedule considerations for the various hormones are included in the relevant chapters of this text.

References

1. Ackland SP, Schilsky RL. High dose methotrexate: a critical reappraisal. J Clin Oncol 1987;5:2017.
2. Allegra CJ. Antifolates. In Cancer Chemotherapy: Principles and Practice. Edited by BA Chabner, JM Collins. Philadelphia: Lippincott, 1990, p 110.
3. Antman K, Eder JP, Elias A, Ayash L, Shea T, Weisman L, Critchlow J, Schryher SM, Begg C, Teicher BA, Schnipper LE, Frei E III. High dose thiotepa alone and in combination regimens with bone marrow support. Semin Oncol 1990;17:33–37.
4. Antman K, Eder JP, Frei E III. High-dose chemotherapy with bone marrow support for solid tumors. In Important Advances in Oncology. Edited by VT DeVita Jr, S Hellman, SA Rosenberg. Philadelphia: Lippincott, 1987, p, 221.
5. Antman K, Gale RR. Advanced breast cancer: high dose chemotherapy and autotransplants. Ann Intern Med 1988;108:570–574.
6. Beiter A, Schrappe M, Ludlig WD, et al. Chemotherapy of 998 unselected childhood acute lymphocytic leukemia patients. Results and conclusions based on multicenter trials ALL-BFM. Blood 1986;84:3122–3133.
7. Bhardwaj S, Holland JF, Norton L. An intensive sequenced adjuvant chemotherapy regimen for breast cancer. Cancer Invest 1993;11:6–9 (letter 1994;12:270).
8. Bodey GP, Coltman CA. Arabinosyl cytosine (ara-C) vs. combination chemotherapy (COAP) for adult acute leukemia. Proc Am Assoc Res 1972;13:107.
9. Bodey GP, Hersh EM. The problem of infection in patients with malignant disease. In Neoplasia in Childhood. Chicago: Year Book, 1969, p 135.
10. Bonadonna G. Conceptual and practical advances in the management of breast cancer. J Clin Oncol 1989;7:1287–1297.
11. Bonadonna G, Valagussa P, Molitermi A, et al. Adjuvant cyclophosphamide, methotrexate, and fluorouracil in node positive breast cancer: the results of 20 years of follow up. N Engl J Med 1995;332:901–906.
12. Bonadonna G, Valagussa P, Santoro A. Alternating non-cross-resistant combinations of MOPP and ABVD in stage IV Hodgkin's disease: a report of 8 year results. Ann Intern Med 1986;104:739–746.
13. Bonadonna G, Zambetti M, Valagussa P. Sequential or alternating doxorubicin and CMF regimens in breast cancer with more than three positive nodes. Ten year results. JAMA 1995;273:5452–5457.
14. Harris J, Hellman S, Henderson I, Kline C (editors). Breast Diseases. Philadelphia: Lippincott, 1991.
15. Brindley CA, Salvin LG, Lipowska B, Shnider B, Regelson W, Colsky J. Further comparative trial of thiophosphoro-amide and mechlorethamine in patients with melanoma and Hodgkin's disease. J Chron Dis 1964;17:19.
16. Bruce WR, Meeker RE, Valeriote FA. Comparison of the sensitivity of normal hematopoietic and transplanted lymphoma colony-forming cells to chemotherapeutic agents administered in vivo. JNCI 1966;37:233.
17. Cancer: Principles and Practice of Oncology. 3rd ed. Edited by VT DeVita, S Hellman, S Rosenberg. New York: Lippincott, 1989.
18. Canellos GP, Anderson K, Propert K, et al. Chemotherapy of advanced Hodgkin's disease with MOPP, ABVD, or MOPP alternating with ABVD. N Engl J Med 1992;327:1478–1484.
19. Casper ES, Gaynor JJ, Hadju SI, et al. A prospective randomized trial of adjuvant chemotherapy with bolus versus continuous infusion of doxorubicin in patients with high grade extremity soft tissue sarcoma and an analysis of prognostic factors. Cancer 1991;68:1221–1229.
20. Chaudhary PM, Roninson IB. Induction of multidrug resistance in human clones by transient exposure to different chemotherapeutic drugs. JNCI 1993;85:632–639.
21. Clarkson BD, Sakai Y, Kimura T, Ohkita T, Fried J. Studies of cellular proliferation in human leukemia II. Variability in rates of growth and cellular differentiation in acute myelomonoblastic leukemia and effects of treatment. In The Proliferation and Spread of Neoplastic Cells. Baltimore: Williams & Wilkins; 1968, p 295.
22. Cohen MH, Creaven PJ, Fossieck EB Jr, Broder LE, Selawry OS, Johnston AV, Williams CL, Minna JD. Intensive chemotherapy of small cell bronchogenic carcinoma. Cancer Treat Rep 1977;61:349.
23. Collins JM, Dedrick R, King F, Speyer J, Myers C. Nonlinear pharmacokinetic models for 5-fluorouracil in man: intravenous and intraperitoneal routes. Clin Pharmacol Ther 1980;28:235.
24. Colwin M. The alkylating agents and platinum compounds. In Cancer Medicine, 3rd ed. Edited by JF Holland, E Frei III, RC Bast, DW Kufe, DL Morton, RR Weichselbaum. Baltimore: Williams & Wilkins, 1995, pp 773–754.
25. Cortes EP, Holland JF, Wang JJ, et al. Amputation and Adriamycin primary osteosarcoma. N Engl J Med 1974;2912:998–1000.
26. Cortes JE, Pazdur R. Docetaxel. J Clin Oncol 1995;13:2643–2655.
27. Cortes EP, Nechales TF, Holland JF, Carey RW, Blom J, Brunner K, Falkson G, Weinberg V. Adjuvant chemotherapy for primary osteosarcoma: a Cancer Leukemia Group B experience. In Adjuvant Therapy, Cancer III. Edited by SE Salmon, SE Jones. New York: Grune & Stratton, 1981, p 201.
28. Dalton WS, Grogan TM, Meltzer PS, Scheper RJ, Durie BGM, Taylor CW, Miller TP, Salmon SE. Drug resistance and multiple myeloma in non-Hodgkin's lymphoma: detection of p-glycoprotein and potential circumvention by the addition of verapamil to chemotherapy. J Clin Oncol 1989;7:415.

29. DeVita VT Jr, Serpick AA, Carbone PP. Combination chemotherapy in the treatment of advanced Hodgkin's disease. Ann Intern Med 1970;73:881.
30. Dicke KA, Spitzer D, Zander AR. Autologous Bone Marrow Transplantation. Proceedings of the First International Symposium. Houston: The University of Texas M. D. Anderson Hospital and Tumor Institute, 1985.
31. Dimitrou N, Anderson S, Fisher B, el al. Dose intensification and increased total dose of adjuvant chemotherapy for breast cancer. NSABP B-22 study (Abstract). ASCO Proc 1994;13:64.
32. Dong F, Brynes RK, Tidow N, et al. Mutations in the gene for the granulocyte colony stimulating factor receptor in patients with acute myeloid leukemia preceded by severe congenital neutropenia. N Engl J Med 1995;333:487–493.
33. Dolan ME, Moschel RC, Pegg AE. Depletion of mammalian O6-alkylguanine-DNA alkyltransferase activity by O6-benzylguanine provides a means to evaluate the role of this protein in protection against carcinogenic and therapeutic alkylating agents. Proc Natl Acad Sci USA 1990;87:53568–53572.
34. Doroshow JH, Multhauf P, Leong L, Margolin K, Litchfield T, Akman S, Carr B, Bertrand M, Goldberg D, Blayney D, Odujinrin O, DeLap R, Shuster J, Newman E. Prospective randomized comparison of fluorouracil versus fluorouracil and high-dose continuous infusion leucovorin calcium for the treatment of advanced measurable colorectal cancer in patients previously unexposed to chemotherapy. J Clin Oncol 1990;8:491.
35. Dreyfuss AI, Clark JR, Wright JE, Norris CM Jr, Busse PM, Lucarini JW, Fallon BG, Casey D, Andersen JW, Klein R, Rosowsky A, Miller D, Frei E III. Continuous infusion high-dose leucovorin with 5-fluorouracil and cisplatin for untreated stage IV carcinoma of the head and neck. Ann Intern Med 1990;112:167.
36. Connaly JL, Ducamen BS, Schnitt S, Dvorak A, Dvorak H. Principles of cancer pathology. In Cancer Medicine, 3rd ed. Edited by JF Holland, E Frei III, RC Bast, DW Kufe, DL Morton, RR Weichselbaum. Baltimore: Williams & Wilkins, 1993, pp 432–450.
37. Early Breast Clinical Trialists Collaborative Group Systemic treatment of early breast cancer by hormonal, cytotoxic, or immune therapy: 133 randomized studies involving 31,000 recurrences and 24,000 deaths among 75,000 women. Lancet 1992;399: 1–15.
38. Early Breast Clinical Trialists Collaborative Group. Systemic treatment of early breast cancer by hormonal, cytotoxic, or immune therapy. Part II: 133 randomized studies involving 31,000 recurrences and 24,000 deaths among 75,000 women. Lancet 1992;399:71–85.
39. Eder JP, Teicher BA, Holden SA, Cathcart KN, Schnipper LE, Frei E III. Effect of novobiocin on the antitumor activity and tumor cell and bone marrow survivals of three alkylating agents. Cancer Res 1989;49:595.
40. Eilber F, Giuliana A, Eckardt J, Patterson K, Moseley S, Goodnight J. Adjuvant chemotherapy for osteosarcoma: a randomized prospective trial. J Clin Oncol 1987;5:21–26.
41. Ellison RR, Holland JF, Weil M, Jacquillat C, Boiron M, Bernard J, Sawitsky A, Rosner F, Gussoff B, Silver RT, Karanas A, Cuttner J, Spurr CL, Hayes DM, Blom J, Leone LA, Haurani F, Kyle R, Hutchison JL, Forcier J, Moon JH. Arabinosyl cytosine. A useful agent in the treatment of acute leukemia in adults. Blood 1968;32:507–512.
42. Evans WE, Rodman J, Relling MV, et al. Individualized dosages of chemotherapy as a strategy to improve response for acute lymphocytic leukemia. Semin Hematol 1991;28:15.
43. Evans WE, Crom WR. Abromowitch M, Dodge, et al. Clinical pharmacodynamics of high-dose methotrexate in acute lymphocytic leukemia. N Engl J Med 1986;314:471.
44. Fisher R, Gaynor ER, Dahlbeeg S, et al. Comparison of a standard regimen (CHOP) with three intensive chemotherapy regimens for advanced non-Hodgkin's lymphoma. N Engl J Med 1993;328:1002–1006.
45. Fisher B, Redmond CK, Wolmark N. NSABP investigators. Long term results from NSABP trials of adjuvant therapy for breast cancer. In Adjuvant Therapy of Cancer V. Edited by SE Salmon. Orlando: Grune & Stratton, 1987, pp 283–295.
46. Fisher DE. Apoptosis and cancer therapy: crossing the threshold. Cell 1994;778: 539–542.
47. Frei E III. Combination cancer therapy: presidential address. Cancer Res 1972;32: 2593.
48. Frei E III. Curative cancer chemotherapy. Cancer Res 1985;45:6523–6532.
49. Frei E III. Pathobiology of cancer. Sci Am Med 1988;3.12:1–22.
50. Frei E III. Pharmacologic strategies for high dose chemotherapy. In High Dose Cancer Therapy, 2nd ed. Edited by P Armitage, K Antman. Baltimore: Williams & Wilkins, 1995, pp 3–16.
51. Frei E III. Summation dose intensity and combination chemotherapy. Clin Cancer Res 1996 (in press).
52. Frei III E. Therapeutic research in cancer: evolving clinical strategies. In Accomplishments in Oncology, vol 1. Cancer Therapy: Where Do We Go from Here? Philadelphia: Lippincott, 1986, pp 1–6.
53. Frei E III, Antman K, Teicher B. Dose in the adjuvant setting: experimental and clinical considerations. In Adjuvant Chemotherapy of Cancer VI. Edited by SE Salmon. Philadelphia: Saunders, 1990, pp 39–45.
54. Frei III E, Antman K, Teicher B, Eder P, Schnipper L. Bone marrow autotransplantation for solid tumors—prospects. J Clin Oncol 1989;7:515.
55. Frei E III, Blum RH, Pitman SW, Kirkwood JM, Henderson IC, Skarin AT, Mayer RJ, Bast RC, Garnick MB, Parker LM, Canellos GP. High dose methotrexate with leucovorin rescue. Rationale and spectrum of antitumor activity. Am J Med 1980;68:370.
56. Frei E III, Canellos GP. Dose: a critical factor in cancer chemotherapy. Am J Med 1980;69:585–594.
57. Frei E III, Cucchi CA, Rosowsky A, Tantravahi R, Bernal S, Ervin TJ, Ruprecht RM, Haseltine WA. Alkylating agent resistance: in vitro studies with human cell lines. Proc Natl Acad Sci USA 1985;82:2158.
58. Frei E III, Freireich EJ. Progress and perspectives in the chemotherapy of acute leukemia. Adv Chemother 1965;2:269–298.
59. Frei E III, Freireich EJ, Gehan E, et al. Studies of sequential and combined antimetabolite chemotherapy in acute leukemia. 6-mercaptopurine and methotrexate. Blood 1961;18:443–454.
60. Frei E III, Spurr CL, Brindley CO, Selawry O, Holland JF, Rall DP, Wasserman LR, Hoogstraten B, Shnider BI, McIntyre OR, Matthews LB Jr, Miller SP. Clinical studies of dichloromethotrexate (NSC 29630). Clin Pharmacol Ther 1965;6:160.
61. Freireich EJ, Schmidt PJ, Schneiderman MA, Frei E III. A comparative study of the effect of transfusion of fresh and preserved whole blood on bleeding in patients with acute leukemia. N Engl J Med 1959;260:6–11.
62. Goldie JH, Coldman J. Application of theoretical models to chemotherapy protocol design. Cancer Treat Rep 1986;70:127.
63. Goldin A, Venditti J, Humphreys SR, Mantel N. Influence of the concentration of leukemic inoculum on the effectiveness of treatment. Science 1956;123:840.
64. Goldin A, Vendetti JM, Humphreys SB, Mantel N. Modification of treatment schedules in the management of advanced mouse leukemia with amethopterin. JNCI 1956;17: 203.
65. Goorin A, Abelson H, Frei E III. Osteosarcoma: fifteen years later. N Engl J Med 1985;313:1637–1643.
66. Grem JL. Fluorinated pyrimidines. In Cancer Chemotherapy: Principles and Practice. Edited by BA Chabner, JM Collins. Philadelphia: Lippincott; 1990, p 180.
67. Gribben J. Attainment of molecular remission: a worthwhile goal? J Clin Oncol 1994;12:1532–1534.
68. Grochow LB, Jones RJ, Brundett RB, et al. Pharmacokinetics of busulfan: correlation with veno-occlusive disease in patients undergoing bone marrow transplantation. Cancer Chemother Pharmacol 1990;25:55.
69. Harris CC, Holstein M. Clinical implications of p53 tumor suppressor gene. N Engl J Med 1993;329:13–18.
70. Hayes DF. Tumor markers for breast cancer. Ann Oncol 1993;4:407–414.
71. Henderson IC, Hayes DF, Gelman R. Dose-response in the treatment of breast cancer: a critical review. J Clin Oncol 1988;6:1501.
72. Hersh EM, Whitecar JP, McCredie KB, Bodey GP, Freireich EJ. Chemotherapy, immunocompetence, immunosuppression and prognosis in acute leukemia. N Engl J Med 1971;285:1211–1218.
73. Holland JF. Breaking the cure barrier. Karnofsky Award Lecture. J Clin Oncol 1983;1: 75.
74. Deleted in proof.
75. Hryniuk W, Gordon LI, Harrington D, Andersen J, et al. CHOP versus m-BACOD in non-Hodgkin's lymphoma. N Engl J Med 1992;327:1342–1349.
76. Hryniuk WM. The importance of dose intensity in the outcome of chemotherapy. In Important Advances in Oncology 1988. Edited by VT DeVita Jr, S Hellman, SA Rosenberg. Philadelphia: Lippincott, 1988, p 121.
77. Hryniuk W, Bush H. The importance of dose intensity in chemotherapy of metastatic breast cancer. J Clin Oncol 1984;2:1281.
77a. Jaffe N, Frei E III, Traggis D, Bishop Y. Adjuvant methotrexate and citrovorum factor treatment for osteosarcomas. N Engl J Med 1974;291:994–997.
78. Jagannath S, Dicke D, Armitage J, et al. High dose cyclophosphamide, carmustine and etoposide and autologous bone marrow transplantation for relapsed Hodgkin's disease. Ann Intern Med 1986;104:1673–1678.
79. Janicek M, Kaplan W, Neuberg DF, Canellos G, Shipp M. Early restaging gallium scans identify durable responses to induction therapy in high dose patients with aggressive non-Hodgkin's lymphoma (abstract). Blood 1994;84:233A.
80. Jones RB, Holland JH, Bhardwaj S, et al. A phase I-II study of intensive dose Adriamycin for advanced breast cancer. J Clin Oncol 1987;5:172–177.
81. Kessinger A. Reestablishing hematopoiesis after dose intensive therapy with peripheral blood stem cells. In High Dose Cancer Therapy. Edited by P Armitage, K Antman. Baltimore: Williams & Wilkins, 1992, pp 182–195.
82. Keith WN, Douglas F, Wishart GC, McCallum HM, Ceorge WD, Kaye SB, Brown R. Co amplification of *erb*-B2, topoisomerase II alpha and retinoic acid receptor a genes in breast cancer and allelic loss at topoisomerase I on chromosome 20. Eur J Cancer 1993;29A:1469–1475.
83. Kerr JFR, Winterford CM, Harmon BV. Apoptosis—its significance to cancer and cancer therapy. Cancer 1994;73:2013–2026.
84. Kobayashi H, Man S, Graham, Kapitain SJ, Teicher BA, Kerbel RS. Acquired multicellular-mediated resistance to alkylating agents in cancer. Proc Natl Acad Sci USA 1993;90:3294.
85. Law LW. Origin of the resistance of leukemic cells to folic acid antagonists. Nature (Lond) 1956;169:268–275.
86. Legha SS, Benjamin RS, Mackay B, Ewer M, Wallace S, Valdivieso M, Rasmussen SL, Blumenschein GR, Freireich EJ. Reduction doxorubicin and cardiotoxicity by prolonged continuous intravenous infusion. Ann Intern Med 1982;96:133–139.
87. Li MC, Hertz R, Spencer DV. Effect of methotrexate upon choriocarcinoma and chorioadenoma. Proc Soc Exp Biol Med 1956;93:361.
88. Ling V, Kartner N, Sudo T, Siminovitch L, Riordan JR. Multidrug resistance phenotype in Chinese hamster ovary cells. Cancer Treat Rep 1983;67:869.
89. Link MP, Goorin A, Miser AM, Green AA, Pratt CB, Belasco JB, Pritchard J, Malpas JS, Baker A, Kirkpatiricks JA, Ayala A, Shuster J, Abelsonn HT, Simone J, Vietti J. The effect of adjuvant chemotherapy of relapse free survival in patients with osteosarcoma of the extremity. N Engl J Med 1986;314:1600–1608.
90. Lokich J, Anderson N. Infusional cancer chemotherapy: historical evolution and future development at the Cancer Center of Boston. Cancer Invest 1995;13:202–226.
91. Marcove RC, Rosen G. En bloc resection for osteosarcoma. Cancer 1980;45: 3040–3044.
92. Mayer RJ, Davis RB, Schiffer CA, Berg DT, Powell BL, Schulman P, Omura GA, Moore JO, McIntire OR, Frei E III. Intensive postremission chemotherapy for acute myelogenous leukemia. N Engl J Med 1994;331:896.
93. Mendelsohn ML. Autoradiographic analysis of cell proliferation in spontaneous breast cancer of C3H mouse. III. The growth fraction. JNCI 1962;28:1015.
94. Mendelsohn ML. The growth fraction: a new concept applied to tumors. Science 1960;132:1496–1504.
95. Migdalska A, Molineux G, Demuynck H, Evans GS, Ruscetti F, Dexter TM. Growth inhibitory effects of transforming growth factor $\beta 1$ in vivo. Growth Factors 1991;4:239.
96. Muss HB, Thor A, Berry DA, Kute T, Liu ET, Koerner F, Cirrincione CT, Budman DR, Wood WC, Barcos M, Henderson IC. c-*Erb*B-2 expression and response to adjuvant therapy in women with node-positive, early, breast cancer. N Engl J Med 1994;330: 1260–1266.
97. Non-small cell lung cancer. Slide presentation at the American Society of Clinical Oncology, 31st annual meeting, 1995.
98. O'Day SJ, Mazanet R, Salgia R, et al. A phase I study of liposomal encapsulated dox-

orubicin and granulocyte CSF in patients with advanced solid tumors (abstract). Lung Cancer 1994;11(suppl 1):97.

99. O'Reilly R, Esperanza B, Papadopoulis E. Allogeneic bone marrow transplantation. In Cancer Medicine, 3rd ed. Edited by JF Holland, E Frei III, RC Bast, DW Kufe, DL Morton, RR Weichselbaum. Baltimore: Williams & Wilkins, 1995, pp 998–1016.
100. Ozols RF, Hamilton TC, Masuda H, Young RC. Manipulation of cellular thiols to influence drug resistance. In Mechanisms of Drug Resistance in Neoplastic Cells. Bristol-Myers Cancer Symposia, vol 9. Edited by PV Woolley III, KD Tew. San Diego: Academic, 1988, p 289.
101. Puget G. Morton Lecture. Royal College of Surgeons. London. November 1887.
102. Peters WP, Eder JP, Henner WD, Schryber S, Wilmore D, Finberg R, Schoenfeld D, Bast R, Gargone B, Antman K, Anderson J, Anderson K, Kruskall MS, Schnipper L, Frei E III. High-dose combination alkylating agents with autologous bone marrow support: a phase I trial. J Clin Oncol 1986;4:646–651.
103. Peters WP, Ross M, Vredenburgh JJ, Meisenberg B, Marks LB, Winer E, Kurtzberg J, Bast RC, Jones R, Shpall E, Wu K, Rosner G, Gilbert C, Mathius B, Coniglio D, Petros I, Henderson IC, Norton L, Weiss RB, Budman D, Hurd D. High dose chemotherapy and autologous bone marrow support as consolidation after standard-dose adjuvant therapy for high-risk primary breast cancer. J Clin Oncol 1993;11:1132.
104. Pinkel D. The ninth annual David Karnofsky Lecture: treatment of acute lymphocytic leukemia. Cancer 1979;48:1128–1122.
105. Pinkel D, Hernandez K, Borella L, Holton C, Aur R, Samoy G, Pratt C. Drug dosage and remission duration in childhood lymphocytic leukemia. Cancer 1971;27:247.
106. Rai K, Holland JF, Glidewell O, et al. Treatment of acute myelogenous leukemia. A study of the Cancer and Leukemia Group B. Blood 1981;58:1203.
107. Ratain MJ, Plunkett W. Pharmacology. In Cancer Medicine, 3rd ed. Edited by JF Holland, E Frei III, RC Bast, DW Kufe, DL Morton, RR Weichselbaum. Baltimore: Williams & Wilkins, 1995, pp 671–682.
108. Rao L, Debbas M, Sabbitini P, Hockenberry D, Korsmeyer S, White E. The adenovirus E1A proteins induce apoptosis which is inhibited by the E1B, 19K and bcl-2 proteins. Proc Natl Acad Sci USA 1992;89:7742–7746.
109. Rath H, Tolsty T, Schimke RT. Rapid emergence of methotrexate resistance in cultured mouse cells. Cancer Res 1984;44:3303–3307.
110. Reed JC. bcl-2 and the regulation of programmed cell death. J Cell Biol 1994; 124: 1–6.
111. Report to the British Medical Research Council by their Tuberculosis Chemotherapy Trials Committee Various combinations of isoniazid with streptomycin or with PAS in the treatment of pulmonary tuberculosis. Br Med J 1955;435:4911.
112. Rideout DC, Chou TC. Synergism, potentiation, and antagonism in chemotherapy: an overview. In Synergism and Antagonism in Chemotherapy. Edited by TC Chou, DC Rideout. San Diego: Academic, 1991, p 3.
113. Rosen G, Mankin H, Selch M, Forscher C. Bone tumors. In Cancer Medicine, 4th ed. Edited by JF Holland, E Frei III, RC Bast, DW Kufe, DL Morton, RR Weichselbaum. Baltimore: Williams & Wilkins, 1995.
114. Rosen G, Marcove R, Huvos, et al. Primary osteosarcoma: eight year experience with adjuvant chemotherapy. J Cancer Res Clin Oncol 1983;106(suppl):55–67.
115. Ruiz-Cabello J, Derghmans K, Kaplan O, Lippman ME. Hormone dependence of breast cancer cells and the effects of tamoxifen and estrogen. Breast Cancer Res Treat 1995;33:209–17.
116. Santos G. Preparative regimen in bone marrow transplantation. Semin Oncol 1993;20(Suppl 4):4.
117. Santos GW, Tutschka PJ, Brookmeyer R, Saral R, Beschorner WE, Bias WB, Braine HG, Burns WH, Elfenbein GJ, Kaizer H, Mellits D, Sensenbrenner LL, Stuart RK, Yeager AM. Marrow transplantation for acute nonlymphocytic leukemia after treatment with busulfan and cyclophosphamide. N Engl J Med 1983;309:1347–1352.
118. Sartorelli AC, Caresy WA. Combination chemotherapy. In Cancer Medicine, 2nd ed. Edited by JF Holland, E Frei III. Philadelphia: Lea & Febiger, 1982, p 720.
119. Schaaf LJ, Dobbs BR, Edwards TR, Perrier DG. Nonlinear pharmacokinetic characteristics of 5-fluorouracil in colorectal cancer patients. Eur J Clin Pharmacol 1987;32: 411.
120. Schimke RT, Roos DS, Brown PC. Amplification of genes in somatic mammalian cells. Methods Enzymol 1987;151:85.
121. Schimke RT, Sherweed S, Johnston R, Hill A, Rice G, Hoy C, Feder J, Farnham P. On the mechanism of induced gene amplification in mammalian cells. In Mechanisms of Drug Resistance in Neoplastic Cells. Edited by PV Woolley III, KD Tew. San Diego: Academic, 1988, p 29.
122. Schnipper LE. Clinical implications of tumor-cell heterogeneity. N Engl J Med 1986;314:1423–1434.
123. Schorin M, Blattner S, Gelber R, et al. Results of treatment of acute lymphocytic leukemia of childhood. DFCI-Childrens Hospital Consortium Protocol 8501. J Clin Oncol 1994;12:740–747.
124. Seifert P, Baker L, Reed ML, Vaitkevicius VK. Comparison of continuously infused 5-fluorouracil with bolus injection in treatment of patients with colorectal adenocarcinoma. Cancer 1975;36:123–130.
125. Selawry OS, Hananian J, Wolman IJ, Abir E, Chavalier L, Gourdeau R, Denton R, Gussoff BD, Levy R, Burgert O Jr, Mills SD, Blom J, Jones B, Patterson RB, McIntyre OR, Haurani FI, Moon JH, Hoogstraten B, Kung FH, Sheehe PR, Frei E III, Holland JF. (Acute Leukemia Group B). New treatment schedule with improved survival in childhood leukemia. JAMA 1965;194:715–724.
126. Skarin A, Canellos G, Rosenthal D, Case DC, McIntire OR, Pincus G, Moloney W, Frei E III. Improved prognosis of diffuse histiocytic and undifferentiated lymphoma by use of high dose methotrexate alternating with standard agents (M-BACOD). J Clin Oncol 1983;1:9198–9204.
127. Skarin AT, Zuckerman KS, Pitman SW, Rosenthal DS, Moloney W, Frei E III, Canellos GP. High-dose methotrexate with folinic acid in the treatment of advanced non-Hodgkin's lymphoma including CNS involvement. Blood 1977;50:1039–1044.
128. Skipper HE. Cytokinetic analysis of human breast cancer (unpublished data).
129. Skipper HE, Schabel FM Jr, Wilcox WS. Experimental evaluation of potential anticancer agents. XIII. On the criteria and kinetics associated with "curability" of experimental leukemia. Cancer Chemother Rep 1964;35:1.
130. Skipper HE, Schabel FM Jr, Wilcox WS. Experimental evaluation of potential anticancer agents. XXI. Scheduling of arabinosyl cytosine to take advantage of its S-phase specificity against leukemia cells. Cancer Chemother Rep 1967;51:125.
131. Sleviin ML, Clark PI, Joel SP, Malik S, Osborne RJ, Gregory WM, Lowe DG, Rezniak RH, Wrigley PM. A randomized trial to evaluate the effect of schedule of etoposide administration in small cell lung cancer. J Clin Oncol 1989;7:1333.
132. Sobriero AF, Aschele C, Guglielmi AP, Mori AM, Melioli GG, Rosso R, Bertino JR. Synergism and lack of cross resistance between short term and continuous exposure to fluorouracil in human colon adenocarcinoma cells. JNCI 85:1937–1942.
133. Steele G, Tepper J, Motwani BT, Bruchner HW. Adenocarcinoma of the colon and rectum. In Cancer Medicine, 3rd ed. Edited by JF Holland, E Frei III, RC Bast, DW Kufe, DL Morton, RR Weichselbaum. Baltimore: Williams & Wilkins, 1993, pp 1493–1522.
134. Steel GG. Growth Kinetics of Tumors: Cell Population Kinetics in Relation to the Growth in Premedic Cancer. Oxford: Clarendon, 1977.
135. Tannock I. Cancer biology. In The Basic Science of Oncology, 2nd ed. Edited by Tannock and Hill. New York: McGraw-Hill, 1992, pp 139–196.
136. Tannock I. Cell kinetics in chemotherapy: a critical review. Cancer Treat Rep 1978;62: 1117–1127.
137. Tannock IF, Boyd NF, DeBoer G, Erlichman C, Fine S, Larocque G, Mayers C, Perrault D, Sutherland H. A randomized trial of two dose levels of CMF chemotherapy for patients with metastatic breast cancer. J Clin Oncol 1988;6:1377.
138. Teicher BA, Holden SA. A survey of the effect of adding fluosol-DA 20%/O_2 to treatment with various chemotherapeutic agents. Cancer Treat Rep 1987;71:173.
139. Teicher BA, Holden SA, Eder JP, Brann TW, Jones SM, Frei E III. Influence of schedule on alkylating agent cytotoxicity in vivo and in vitro. Cancer Res 1989;49: 5994–5998.
140. Teicher BA, Rose CM. Perfluorochemical emulsions can increase tumor radiosensitivity. Science 1984;223:934.
141. Teppler I, Canistra S, Frei E III, et al. Use of peripheral blood progenitor cells to abrogate the myelosuppression of repeated moderately intensive chemotherapy for ovarian cancer. J Clin Oncol 1993;11:1583–1591.
142. Teppler I, Demetri G, et al. Outpatient treatment with multiple cycles of dose intensive ICE supported by peripheral blood stem cells collected initially during chemotherapy recovery on GCSF (abstract). Blood 1994;84(suppl 1):211A.
143. Thomas ED. Current status of bone marrow transplantation. Transpl Proc 1985;17: 428.
144. Weichselbaum RR, Schmit A, Little JB. Cellular repair factors influencing radiocurability of human malignant tumours. Br J Cancer 1982;44:10.
145. Weiss AJ, Manthel RW. Experience with the use of Adriamycin in combination with other anticancer agents using a weekly schedule, with particular reference to lack of cardiac toxicity. Cancer 1977;40:2046.
146. Wood W, Korzan AH, Cooper R, Younger J, Hart RD, Moore A, Ellerton J, Norton L, Ferree C, Colangelo A, McIntyre OR, Frei E III, Henderson IC. Dose and dose intensity of adjuvant chemotherapy for stage II, node-positive breast carcinoma. N Engl J Med 1994;330:1253–1259.
147. Woods RL, Fox RM, Tattersall MH. Methotrexate treatment of head and neck squamous cell carcinoma—dose response study. Br Med J (Clin Res) 1981;282:600.
148. Wozniak A, Ross W. Epipodophyllatoxins. In Cancer Medicine, 3rd ed. Edited by JF Holland, E Frei III, RC Bast, DW Kufe, DL Morton, RR Weichselbaum. Baltimore: Williams & Wilkins, 1995, pp 774–779.
149. Yates J, Glidewell O, Wiernik P, Cooper MR, Steinberg D, Dosik H, Levy R, Hoagland CI, Henry P, Gottlieb A, Cornell C, Berenberg J, Hutchinson JL, Raich P, Nissen N, Ellison RR, Frelick R, James GW, Falkson G, Silver RT, Haurani F, Green M, Henderson E, Leone L, Holland JF. Cytosine arabinoside with daunorubicin or Adriamycin for therapy of acute myelocytic leukemia. A CALGB study. Blood 1982;60:454–462.
150. Yates JW, Wallare HJ Jr, Ellison RR, Holland JF. Cytosine arabinoside (NSC63878) and daunorubicin (NSC83142) therapy in acute nonlymphocytic leukemia. Cancer Chemother Rep 1973;57:485.
151. Zapulski M, Metch B, Balcerzak S, et al. Phase III comparison of doxorubicin and dacarbazine given by bolus versus infusion in patients with solf tissue sarcomas: a Southwest Group study. JNCI 1991;83:926–932.

CHAPTER 55

Regional Chemotherapy

STEPHEN B. HOWELL

Introduction

Regional chemotherapy refers to the local instillation of drug into a tumor-containing region of the body to increase the ratio of drug exposure for the tumor relative to that for other parts of the body. The amount of tumor cell kill achieved with a dose of drug is a function of how much drug actually reaches critical targets in the tumor cell, and how long cytotoxic concentrations of the drug remain in the environment of the cell. As for cell lines and xenografts, virtually all tumors show increasing cell kill with increasing total drug exposure; for most human tumors the problem is that, in the clinical setting, the total exposures required to produce enough cell kill to be scored as a useful response are often well above what is tolerated by the marrow, gut, and other drug-sensitive normal tissues. The rationale for the use of regional chemotherapy is its potential for increasing the ratio of drug exposure for the tumor relative to that for dose-limiting normal tissues of the body. The clinically useful forms of regional chemotherapy rely on either specific anatomic compartments or localized intra-arterial administration to create a differential drug exposure for tumor and normal tissues.

Pharmacologic Principles of Regional Chemotherapy

PHARMACOLOGIC PRINCIPLES OF INTRACAVITARY THERAPY

The behavior of a drug administered into an extravascular cavity is conveniently described by a two-compartment model (Fig. 55.1) (1). The first compartment represents the tumor-containing cavity, and the second the vascular volume and all the other tissues of the body that are in direct contact with the bloodstream. Total drug exposure is defined as the integral of the area under the concentration times time curve (AUC). The relative advantage of administering a drug by the intracavitary route is determined by the cavity-to-plasma AUC ratio following intracavitary versus intravenous injection, assuming that the drug in the cavity and in the plasma have equal access to the target tumor cell.

Relative Clearances and First-Pass Metabolism

Following rapid intracavitary instillation, the concentration of a drug falls as drug leaks into the plasma, or as it is metabolized in the cavity. Most chemotherapeutic agents undergo little metabolism in the cavity, and for such agents, the rate at which concentration decreases is a function of the volume of the fluid in the cavity, the surface area through which the drug diffuses out of the cavity, the permeability of this surface, and the difference in free drug concentration between the cavity and the plasma. Under steady-state conditions, the cavity-to-plasma concentration ratio is as given by Equation 55.1.

$$\frac{\mathbf{C}_{\text{cavity}}}{\mathbf{C}_{\text{plasma}}} = \frac{(\text{plasma clearance}) + (\text{cavity clearance})}{(\text{cavity clearance})} \qquad (55.1)$$

Since AUC is a function of the product of concentration and time, the clearances also determine the AUC ratio, and anything that either reduces the cavity clearance or increases the plasma clearance will increase the pharmacologic advantage of intracavitary instillation. Thus, the smaller the clearance from the cavity and the greater the clearance from the plasma, the higher will be the AUC ratio. An optimal drug would be one that leaves the cavity very slowly but is promptly removed from the plasma once it reaches the systemic circulation so that it has little time to circulate to the bone marrow and gut, the two most common dose-limiting normal tissues. As a general rule, drugs that have a hard time getting across lipid membranes because they are large, highly ionized, or not very lipid soluble will have low cavity clearances. However, the advantage of intracavitary administration cannot be predicted by these characteristics alone because they also affect plasma clearance, and it is the cavity clearance relative to plasma clearance that determines the pharmacokinetic advantage. Equation 55.1 permits reasonably accurate predictions of the relative advantage of intracavitary instillation.

The AUC ratio is also influenced by the anatomic route of drug absorption from the cavity because this can affect the extent to which the drug is metabolized to an inactive form during transit between the cavity and the systemic compartment. Inactivation of a drug after it has left the tumor-containing cavity but before it reaches the systemic compartment has the same effect on the AUC ratio as does increasing the plasma clearance. The route of absorption is different for each of the major cavities for which regional chemotherapy is used. In the case of the pleural and pericardial cavities, drug is largely absorbed directly into the systemic circulation. In the case of the peritoneal cavity, however, most drugs in the molecular weight range of the

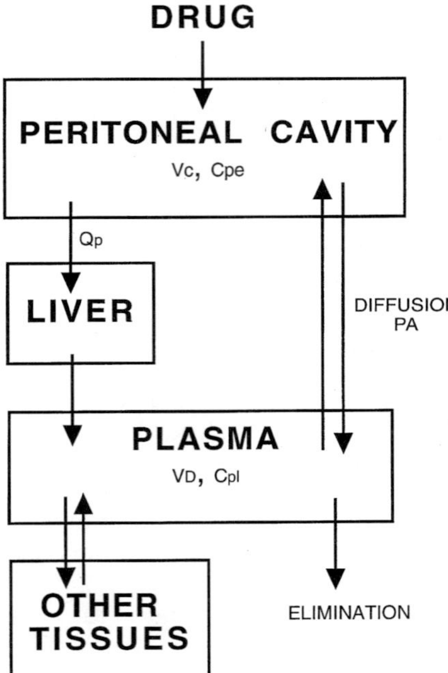

Figure 55.1. Compartmental model of intraperitoneal chemotherapy. V_c is volume of the cavity, C_{pe} is concentration in the peritoneal cavity, Q_p is portal blood flow, *PA* is permeability area product, V_D is apparent plasma volume of distribution, and C_{pl} is concentration in the plasma.

Table 55-1. Ratio of Peritoneal to Plasma Area Under the Curve of Concentration Times Time (AUC) and Major Toxicities

Drug	Mean AUC ratio	Major toxicities
Bleomycin	4	Peritonitis, fever
Carboplatin	6–10	Myelosuppression
Cisplatin	12	Nephrotoxicity
Cytarabine	300–1,000	Myelosuppression
Doxorubicin	400	Peritonitis
Etoposide	65	Myelosuppression
Fluorodeoxyuridine	440–1,300	Myelosuppression
Fluorouracil	400–2,500	Peritonitis and myelosuppression
r-IFN-α2	Unknown	Flulike syndrome
IFN-β	Unknown	Flulike syndrome
r-IFN-γ	Unknown	Flulike syndrome
IL-2	200–1,000	Peritoneal sclerosis
Melphalan	65	Myelosuppression
Methotrexate	92	Myelosuppression
Mitomycin	32	Myelosuppression and peritonitis
Mitoxantrone	1,400	Myelosuppression and peritonitis
Paclitaxel	996	Peritonitis
Teniposide	9.6	Myelosuppression
6-Thioguanine	1,800	Myelosuppression, capillary leak syndrome
ThiotEPA	4.3	Myelosuppression

commonly used antitumor drugs are absorbed primarily via the portal circulation. Most peritoneal perfusion comes from the splanchnic circulation, and the structures that account for the major part of the surface area of the peritoneum, including the visceral peritoneum, the omentum, and the mesentery, drain into the portal circulation. Only the parietal peritoneum drains directly into the systemic circulation, and although a rich network of diaphragmatic lymphatics drains the peritoneal cavity, for drugs with molecular weights less than 1,000 daltons, the flow in the lymphatic channels is so much less than portal flow that quantitatively this probably does not constitute an important route of drug absorption. Drugs that have extensive first-pass metabolism in the liver, such as cytarabine, 5-fluorouracil, 6-thioguanine, and floxuridine, have very much higher AUC ratios following intraperitoneal instillation than drugs with little hepatic metabolism such as cisplatin (Table 55.1).

Tumor Penetration

A chemotherapeutic agent administered by the intracavitary route may have direct access to single cells free in the cavity, but therapeutic efficacy requires that it enter the tumor mass. Figure 55.2 shows a schematic drawing of a tumor nodule growing on a serosal surface. As the drug penetrates from the free surface, it is at risk for being removed or inactivated by (*a*) metabolism in the extracellular fluid, (*b*) uptake and/or metabolism in cells, and (*c*) diffusion into capillaries that enter the nodule from the systemic circulation.

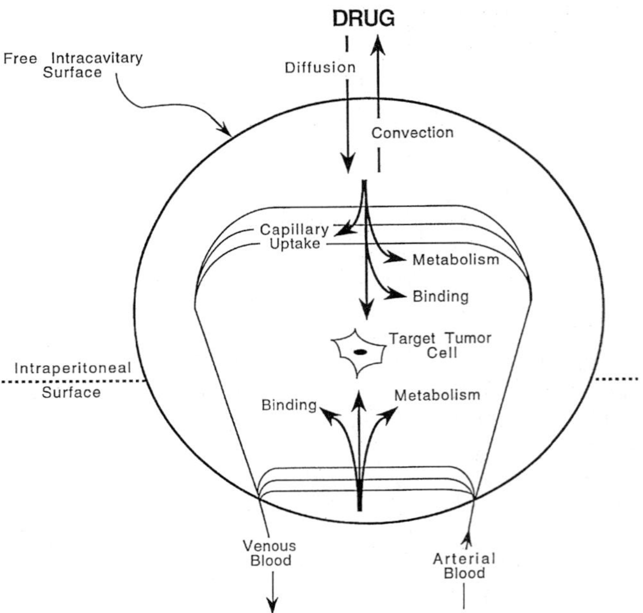

Figure 55.2. Schematic diagram of a tumor nodule growing on a serosal surface, and the processes that control delivery of drug to the target tumor cell by free surface diffusion or systemic capillary blood flow.

Each of these acts as a "sink," reducing the amount of drug available to penetrate deeper into the interstitium. Pharmacokinetic modeling suggests that the capillary area and permeability, blood flow, and the diffusion coefficient of the drug in the tumor are particularly important variables. Tumor capillaries are abnormal and have higher permeability than capillaries in normal tissues, resulting in increased interstitial fluid formation and pressure (2). Since tumor nodules generally have poorly formed or nonfunctional lymphatics, interstitial fluid moves in a radial direction toward the edge of the nodule. Thus, to enter a tumor nodule from the periphery, a drug must move upstream against this convective flow. Since diffusion coefficients for the available chemotherapeutic drugs are low, these considerations lead to the prediction that tumor volume will have a major influence on the success of intracavitary chemotherapy. One can also predict that the profile of drug concentration as a function of distance into the tumor nodule will be more favorable for nonmetabolized drugs entering poorly vascularized nodules, and that the cavity-to-plasma AUC ratio will exceed the tumor-to-plasma AUC ratio.

Clinical experience confirms that tumor volume is a very important determinant of the efficacy of intracavitary chemotherapy. In the case of ovarian carcinoma, intraperitoneal chemotherapy is more effective at increasing survival for patients whose largest tumor nodule is less than 2 cm (3). Direct measurement of cisplatin penetration into millimeter-sized murine colon carcinoma nodules indicates that the advantage of an intraperitoneal over an intravenous injection (IV) is limited to the outermost ≈1.5 mm of the nodule, and that a peritoneal-to-plasma AUC ratio of 12 to 15 is associated with a 1.7-fold increase in drug delivery to such nodules. Even in nodules a few millimeters in diameter, there is marked heterogeneity of actual drug delivery (4).

The significance of the drug "sink" produced by capillary blood flow is given credence by the clinical observation that intraperitoneal chemotherapy produces very little damage to gut even when drug doses are high enough to cause serious bone marrow and other systemic toxicity. Since the crypt cells of the intestinal epithelium are rarely more than 1 mm from the visceral peritoneum, one might expect very high concentrations of drug in the peritoneal cavity to kill these critical stem cells. It is probably the presence of a rich capillary network with relatively high flow rates that protects the gut by siphoning off drug before it can reach the crypt cells.

Intracavitary Drug Distribution

If drugs administered via the intracavitary route are to be effective, they must reach the surface of the tumor. This is often a problem, particularly for intraperitoneal and intrapleural therapy, since tumors in these cavities frequently produce compartmentalizing adhesions. In the peritoneal cavity, adequate drug distribution to even accessible surfaces requires the instillation of large volumes (e.g., 1.4 L/m^2) of drug-containing fluid. The poor results obtained with early attempts at intraperitoneal therapy can be accounted for in part by the use of small volumes of injection. It is currently unclear how best to obtain good drug distribution in the pleural cavity where instillation of large volumes can result in collapse of the lung. Poor distribution probably contributes to the relative lack of success with intrapleural relative to intraperitoneal chemotherapy.

Principles for the Selection of Drugs for Intracavitary Administration

It is unlikely that a single intracavitary instillation of any drug will be curative; clinical programs currently believed to be useful depend on being able to instill drugs repeatedly. In this regard, it is a basic pharmacologic principle of intracavitary therapy that one should use drugs or doses that do not cause extensive chemical injury to the surfaces of the cavity. Such injury is usually associated with fibrosis and adhesion formation, which limits drug access on subsequent administrations.

It is also a basic pharmacologic principle of intracavitary chemotherapy that one should use drugs that have as high a cavity-to-plasma AUC ratio as possible, but whose intracavitary dose is limited by a toxicity that results from the drug's entering the systemic circulation rather than by local compartmental toxicity. This strategy has important advantages. It permits intracavitary dose escalation to the point where the amount of drug leaking into the systemic circulation is equivalent to the systemic AUC that could be produced by an IV injection. If this is done, there is no compromise of drug delivery to those parts of the tumor nodule distant from a free surface, while those portions near the surface receive drug by both capillary flow and free surface diffusion. One would expect this to result in greater total drug delivery and better distribution throughout the nodule. Stated another way, if a drug has a high AUC ratio, for a given amount of systemic toxicity, one can obtain a substantially greater AUC for at least the surface of the tumor without reducing capillary drug delivery by using an intracavitary rather than an IV injection.

Neutralizing Agents

One tactic that can further increase the therapeutic index of intracavitary therapy is to inject a second drug into the systemic compartment that can either neutralize the chemotherapeutic agent before it damages normal cells, or rescue such cells even after the target molecules in the cell have been affected. However, since the neutralizing or rescue agent has the potential of entering the cavity from the systemic compartment, and entering the tumor via capillary flow, the success of this approach depends critically on the concentration of the chemotherapeutic and protective agents actually attained in the tumor, and on the protective agent's being a competitive rather than a noncompetitive antagonist. This approach is facilitated by using an antagonist whose ability to interfere with the cytotoxicity of the agonist is overcome by relatively small increases in the concentration of the agonist. The methotrexate/leucovorin pair is one that is often used (5). Studies with human bone marrow indicated that a concentration of leucovorin that prevents the toxicity of 1 μM methotrexate will not protect against 10 μM methotrexate. Thus, even if the leucovorin equilibrates into the cavity, as long as the intracavitary concentration of methotrexate can be maintained at a level 10-fold higher than that in plasma, the leucovorin should not interfere with the antitumor activity of methotrexate in the cavity.

When sufficient leucovorin is introduced into the systemic circulation to antagonize the effect of methotrexate on bone marrow, it may also be sufficient to antagonize the effect of methotrexate delivered to the tumor nodule by capillary flow. Another tactic is to use a neutralizing agent that is relatively specific for the most sensitive organ in the body. This principle is exemplified by the use of IV thiosulfate in combination with intraperitoneal cisplatin. Thiosulfate is a competitive antagonist that reacts with cisplatin to form a covalently linked product that is neither nephrotoxic nor cytotoxic to the tumor. At the concentrations of both agents usually attained in the plasma, the rate of reaction is much slower than the rate of clearance of free cisplatin through reaction with plasma proteins and renal excretion. In contrast, thiosulfate is extensively concentrated in the kidneys. The result is that when cisplatin is administered in large doses intraperitoneally and thiosulfate by the IV route, there is little neutralization of the cisplatin in the plasma, but excellent protection of the kidneys (6). This tactic reduces, but does not eliminate, the concern that delivery of the neutralizing agent to the tumor by capillary flow may interfere with the effectiveness of the chemotherapeutic agent.

PHARMACOLOGIC PRINCIPLES OF INTRATHECAL CHEMOTHERAPY

Figure 55.3 shows a compartmental model of drug transport between the central nervous system (CNS) and other parts of the body. Since both the volume of the CNS and clearance of drug from the CNS are relatively small, extraordinarily high cerebrospinal fluid (CSF)-to-plasma AUC ratios can be attained by intrathecal (IT) drug administration. Unlike the situation in other cavities, where relatively homogeneous drug distribution is attained by flooding the compartment with drug-containing fluid, drugs can only be administered into the CSF in small volumes (5–18 mL). Drug injected via an Ommaya reservoir into a lateral ventricle must be distributed to the rest of the CSF by bulk flow, and thence by diffusion into the extracellular spaces of the brain. Bulk flow carries drug from the ventricle to the cisterna magnum, and then both down along the spinal cord and up over the cerebrum to the arachnoid granulations, where the CSF is reabsorbed into the venous system. Drug introduced into the lumbar sac is carried by bulk flow to the cisterna magnum; it eventually reaches the ventricles where, in the case of methotrexate, it peaks at 4 to 8 hours.

Abnormalities of CSF flow have been reported in 70% of patients with meningeal neoplasia, and may impair drug distribution (7). Drug can leave the CSF/brain extracellular fluid compartment by (*a*) bulk flow transport along with CSF into the plasma at the arachnoid granulations, (*b*) diffusion into brain and choroid plexus capillaries, or (*c*) metabolism within the CSF/brain compartment. In the case of methotrexate and cytarabine, which are the two agents most commonly used by the IT route, bulk flow accounts for most of the clearance. Neither drug is significantly metabolized in the CSF compartment. The CSF has a volume of approximately 140 mL in subjects more than 3 years old, and the bulk flow absorption of CSF has been reported to be 31.2 mL/h (8). Data from preclinical studies in monkeys indicate that bulk flow dominates the clearance of other water-soluble chemotherapeutic agents, resulting in similar CSF half-lives for many of these drugs (9).

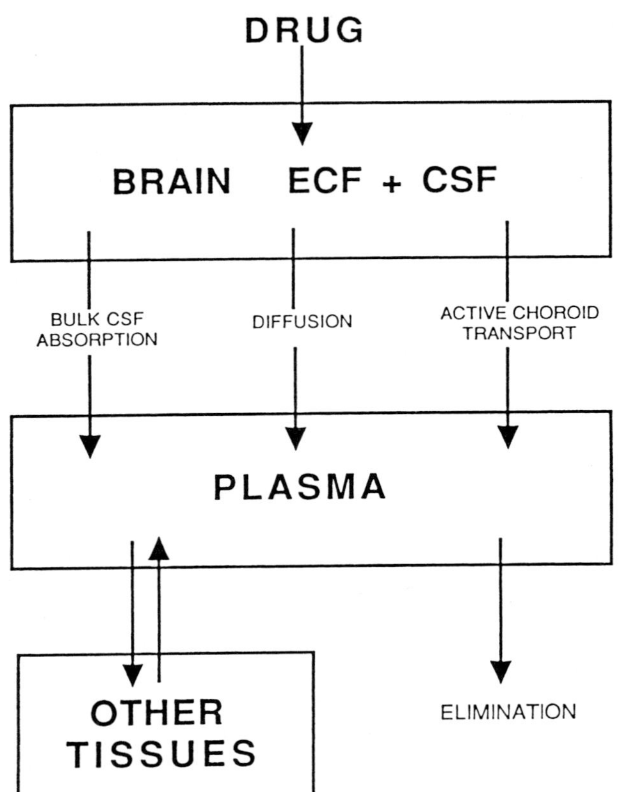

Figure 55.3. Compartmental model of intrathecal chemotherapy and routes by which drug leaves the CSF.

The extent to which anticancer agents in the CSF penetrate into the brain and spinal cord is unknown. Early studies (10–13), suggested that penetration is limited to a few millimeters. More recent studies based on quantitative autoradiography in rabbits (14) have shown deeper penetration, but whether cytotoxic concentrations are attained more than a few millimeters from the surface has not been established. It is clear that penetration is not homogeneous; gray matter regions of both the brain and spinal cord contained higher concentrations than white matter tracts.

The administration of very high doses of drug by the IV route provides a strategy for increasing drug penetration into the CSF to therapeutically effective levels. Although this approach voids the differential drug exposure attainable with IT injection, the presence of meningeal disease often signals the need for systemic therapy as well. This strategy permits more uniform distribution of drug throughout the neuraxis and, since continuous IV infusion is more readily accomplished than frequent IT dosing, longer duration of drug exposure. This approach can be used effectively with both methotrexate and cytarabine.

PHARMACOLOGIC PRINCIPLES OF INTRA-ARTERIAL CHEMOTHERAPY

There is voluminous literature on intra-arterial (IA) therapy. Some aspects of the pharmacokinetic principles underlying IA infusion are counterintuitive, however, accounting in part for the confusion that is prevalent in this field. Many claims for the efficacy of IA therapy are not substantiated by adequate pharmacologic data. The overall relative advantage of an IA as compared with an IV injection of the same drug (R_d) is a composite of the advantage from the point of view of the tumor (R_t) and from the point of view of the systemic circulation (R_s). The reason for considering R_t and R_s separately is that they are controlled by entirely different factors.

Figure 55.4 presents a flow diagram that illustrates the factors that determine the pharmacokinetic advantage of an IA infusion (15). When drug is infused at a constant rate until steady state is reached, then the relative advantage of an IA infusion from the point of view of the tumor located in the infused volume is as given by Equation 55.2.

$$R_t = 1 + Cl_{tb}/Q \quad (55.2)$$

where Cl_{tb} is the total body clearance during an IV infusion and Q is the blood flow to the region. Under the same conditions, the relative advantage from the point of view of the systemic circulation, R_s, is as given by Equation 55.3.

$$R_s = 1 - E \quad (55.3)$$

where E is the extraction ratio, or the fraction of drug entering the perfused organ that is permanently inactivated, bound, or excreted and thus fails to enter the systemic circulation. Equations 55.2 and 55.3 can be combined to yield an expression for the overall relative advantage of an IA infusion (Equation 55.4).

$$R_d = 1 + \frac{Cl_{tb}}{Q(1 - E)} \quad (55.4)$$

Equation 55.4 provides a remarkably simple and powerful tool that allows reasonably accurate prediction of pharmacologic advantage if Cl_{tb}, Q, and E are known or can be measured (16). Equation 55.4 is derived from considerations of the mass of drug moving into and out of the perfused region under steady-state conditions but is equally valid for predicting the advantage of an IA infusion on the basis of total drug exposure (AUC) when clearances are independent of concentration (i.e., when the pharmacokinetics are linear). Table 55.2 lists R_d as a function of flow rate (Q) for some commonly used chemotherapeutic agents.

All of the pharmacokinetic advantage of an IA injection devolves from exposure that occurs during the first pass of the drug through the tumor. Once the drug reaches the venous circulation, then subsequent exposure for the tumor is the same regardless of whether the drug was injected IA or IV. Equation 55.2 indicates that the relative advantage from the point of view of the tumor is controlled solely by total body clearance and the blood flow to the region perfused. This means that R_t values substantially greater than 1 will be obtained only for drugs with relatively high Cl_{tb}, and for tumors in regions receiving relatively low blood flow. This relationship is illustrated in Figure 55.5. The lower the blood flow and the larger the total body clearance, the greater will be the advantage; the relationship is hyperbolic so that while a decrement in blood flow to a well-perfused organ will have little effect on R_t, the same absolute decrement in flow to a poorly perfused organ can strikingly increase R_t. Organ blood flows range from 100 to 1,500 mL/min in humans, leading to the predication that one must select drugs with relatively high total body clearance before R_t can be expected to be very significant.

In contrast to R_t, Equation 55.3 indicates that the only factor influencing the relative advantage from the point of view of the systemic circulation is the extraction ratio. The smaller the fraction of drug injected by the IA route that reaches the

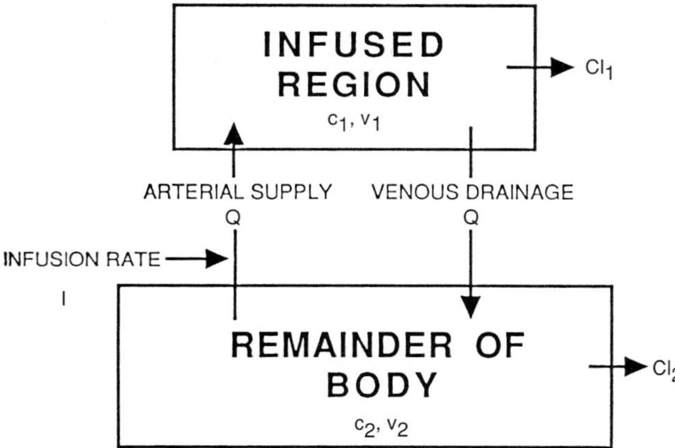

Figure 55.4. Flow diagram illustrating the pharmacokinetics of intra-arterial drug administration. C is the drug concentration in the blood, V is the volume of distribution, Cl is the clearance, Q is the blood flow rate, and i is the infusion rate of the drug. Subscripts 1 and 2 refer to the infused region and the remainder of the body, respectively. Redrawn from Dedrick (15).

Table 55.2. R_d as a Function of Flow Rate for Some Commonly Used Chemotherapeutic Agents

Drug	Cl_{tb}, mL/min	R_d			
		$Q = 1$	$Q = 10$	$Q = 100$	$Q = 1{,}000$
Carmustine	1,000	1,001	101	11	2
Cisplatin	400	401	41	5	1.4
Cytarabine	3,000	3,001	301	31	4
Doxorubicin	900	901	91	10	1.9
Floxuridine	25,000	25,001	2,501	251	26
5-Fluorouracil	4,000	4,001	401	41	5
Methotrexate	200	201	21	3	1.2

Cl_{tb} = total body clearance of drug; R_d = relative advantage compared with IV administration of same drug; Q = blood flow, mL/min, for tumor bed under consideration. From Eckman (100).

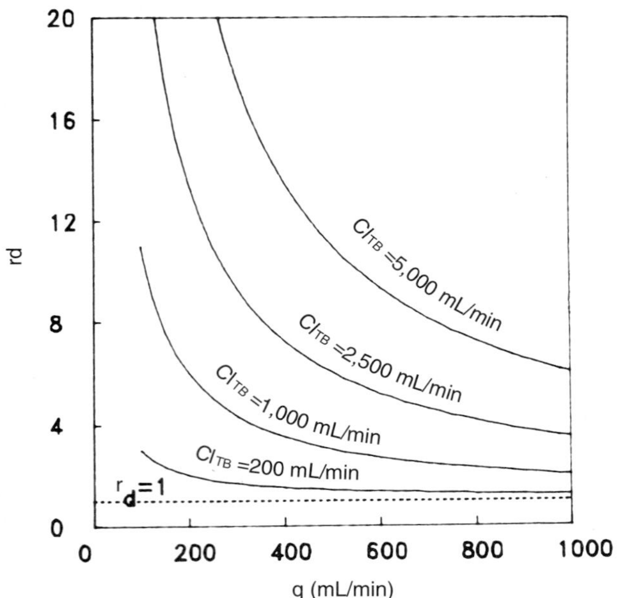

Figure 55.5. Relationship between the pharmacologic advantage of an intra-arterial infusion (R_d), total body clearance (Cl_{tb}), and blood flow (Q) based on Equation 55.4. From Strong (9).

venous circulation, the greater is the advantage. Overall, predicated R_d values are greatest for the IA treatment of tumors in organs with very low blood flows using drugs with high total body clearances and extraction ratios.

Equation 55.4 results in a number of counterintuitive predictions. First, if the extraction ratio is low, as it is for most anticancer drugs injected into organs other than the liver or kidney, then the use of the IA route is of no advantage at all from the point of view of decreasing toxicity to tissues in contact with the systemic circulation. On the other hand, if the target tissue is the only organ that clears the drug from the body, then clearance from the rest of the body is zero and R_d is equal to 1. Under this circumstance, one can anticipate reduced systemic toxicity but no increase in therapeutic response. This has particular relevance for the use of such drugs as floxuridine by hepatic arterial infusion. Another surprising prediction is that R_d is independent of infusion rate and of infusion duration. Although both of these will alter peak regional and plasma drug concentration, R_d varies with regional concentration only to the extent that regional concentration alters the extraction ratio. Thus, the ratio of peak regional to peak plasma concentrations is not an appropriate descriptor of relative advantage.

In using Equation 55.4 to predict the relative advantage of an IA infusion, it is important to recognize that the derivation of the equation is based on the total rate of delivery of biologically active drug to the perfused region. If biologically active drug is carried only in the plasma phase, then the plasma flow and clearance are the relevant parameters; if active drug is partitioned between plasma and blood cells, then total blood flow and blood clearance must be used for prediction. Equation 55.4 is also based on the assumption that the drug is well mixed in the artery at the site of infusion. Recent studies indicate that streaming of drug is common, and that it is critically dependent on catheter position and can result in marked inhomogeneity of tumor exposure following IA injection (15). Finally, the rate at which the concentration changes is a function of the volume of the region and flow rate. Since the volumes of perfused organs are much less than total body volume, concentrations in the perfused organ tend to change more rapidly than plasma concentration.

In addition to permitting predications about the relative advantage of an IA infusion, Equation 55.4 also points to a number of strategies that can be used to increase R_d. Blood flow to an organ can potentially be decreased through the use of balloon catheters or IA-injected particles. Total body clearance can be increased through the use of concurrently administered neutralizing agents or devices that remove drug from the systemic circulation. Finally, isolation of the perfused organ from the systemic circulation has the effect of increasing tumor exposure relative to systemic exposure.

INTRAPERITONEAL CHEMOTHERAPY

Chemotherapeutic agents can be instilled intraperitoneally (IP) via a catheter placed through the skin into the cavity, but it is more common to place a catheter surgically that leads from the cavity up through the fascial planes, and then to a port located in a subcutaneous pocket over the lower anterior rib cage. This type of totally implanted access device permits drug instillation simply by placing a noncoring needle through the skin into the stopper on the top of the port, and is associated with a much lower rate of infection and higher patient acceptance than catheters that protrude through the skin. The average patient with ovarian carcinomatosis absorbs ≈1 liter of fluid from the peritoneal cavity per day, so that there is generally no need to drain the abdomen after drug instillation. This is fortunate because, although access devices permit reliable instillation of drug, fluid drainage is not always feasible.

Table 55.1 presents a list of chemotherapeutic drugs for which information is available on AUC ratio and dose-limiting toxicity following IP instillation. While in principle one would like to select the drug with the highest AUC ratio and greatest activity for a given disease, the pattern of toxicity may restrict the choice. Cisplatin is an example of a drug with a modest AUC ratio that has been extensively used for IP therapy because of its minimal peritoneal toxicity and high level of activity against ovarian carcinoma. In contrast, doxorubicin, despite its much higher AUC ratio, is not useful with IP administration because, at IP doses sufficient to produce cytotoxic plasma concentrations, it causes very severe chemical peritonitis.

OVARIAN CARCINOMA

Intraperitoneal chemotherapy has been used most extensively for the treatment of ovarian carcinoma, a tumor that tends to remain confined to the peritoneal cavity for much of its natural history. A large number of phase I/II studies have demonstrated the technical feasibility of administering quite a variety of different drugs either as single instillations, by repeated exchanges at 6- to 24-hour intervals, or by continuous IP infusion. Based on AUC ratio, toxicity profiles, and activity in ovarian cancer, the following drugs have emerged as prime candidates for IP administration: cisplatin, carboplatin, cytarabine, etoposide, 5-fluorouracil, floxuridine, mitoxantrone, and paclitaxel. Many of these have been tested in phase I/II trials, and it has been possible to define combinations that can be administered safely by the IP route, among which the combination of cisplatin or carboplatin with etoposide has been most extensively tested. Intraperitoneally administered cisplatin, given either as a single agent or in combination with etoposide, can produce pathologically documented complete remissions in ovarian carcinoma patients who have failed IV cisplatin-based regimens (17), suggesting that the IP route can increase drug delivery. This same principle has been demonstrated for several platinum drug-based combinations as well. However, it is now clear that IP treatment with single agents or combinations is much more effective for patients with tumor nodules of less than 2 cm, and ideally of less than 0.5 cm, than it is when larger tumor masses are present. This is consistent with preclinical studies demonstrating limited tumor penetration of drugs (4). Although response rates are lower in patients with bulky disease, IP therapy with cisplatin is usually able to control ascites, probably related to the fact that relatively little kill of tumor obstructing diaphragmatic lymphatics is sufficient to reestablish peritoneal drainage.

The use of IP drug administration as initial therapy for ovarian carcinoma is conceptually attractive, particularly in patients whose tumor has been largely removed by surgery, and a large number of phase II trials have demonstrated promising clinical results. However, only a single randomized trial of IP chemotherapy for ovarian carcinoma has been published to date (18), and no difference in disease-free or total survival was observed when a combination of IP cisplatin/etoposide was compared with IV cisplatin/cyclophosphamide. The significance of this trial is limited by small patient numbers (62) and a heterogeneous patient population. A much more definitive test of the possible benefit of IP chemotherapy is currently under way. The Southwest Oncology Group is conducting a study in patients with resection of all tumor masses of less than 2 cm in which the randomization is to six courses of IV chemotherapy with cisplatin 100 mg/m^2 and cyclophosphamide 600 mg/m^2, or IV cyclophosphamide 600 mg/m^2 in combination with IP cisplatin 100 mg/m^2. The results of this trial are expected in 1996.

Based on the principles outlined, IP chemotherapy is particularly attractive for the treatment of patients with early-stage ovarian carcinoma who remain at high risk of recurrence, and patients who have attained a complete remission with systemic chemotherapy, but whose survival is also limited by a high probability of recurrence. A large randomized study of the latter setting is underway in the European Organization for the Research and Treatment of Cancer (EORTC).

MESOTHELIOMA

Peritoneal mesothelioma is also an attractive target for IP chemotherapy based on the fact that the major management problems in these patients are related to the disease in the peritoneal cavity. Cisplatin-based IP therapy is capable of controlling ascites and producing responses in patients with peritoneal mesothelioma who have failed IV therapy (19, 20), although the response rate and duration of response are less than for ovarian carcinoma. However, the majority of patients relapse in the peritoneal cavity, and there have been no randomized studies documenting prolongation of survival.

COLON AND GASTRIC CARCINOMA

Intraperitoneal chemotherapy has also been used in an attempt to reduce peritoneal and regional lymph node recurrence in patients with resectable colon and gastric carcinomas, the rationale being that microscopic metastases on the peritoneal surface or in draining lymphatics might be susceptible to the high total drug exposures attainable at these sites following IP administration (21). A study of adjuvant IP versus IV 5-fluorouracil performed at the National Institutes of Health (NIH) (22) demonstrated that larger total doses of drug were tolerated when administered by the IP route, and that although there was no increase in time to relapse or total survival, there was a decreased incidence of recurrence on the peritoneal surface. A recent study in which 67 patients with resected stage III or IV gastric carcinoma were randomized to receive 90 mg/m^2 IP cisplatin for four cycles versus no adjuvant therapy failed to show an improvement in survival (23). However, previous work has shown that 50-nm carbon particles are taken up into lymphatics from the peritoneal cavity. Such carbon particles can be used to target mitomycin C to the peritoneal cavity and regional lymphatics. A recent randomized study of 113 gastric carcinoma patients, who had serosal involvement documented at resection, demonstrated a clear improvement in 2- and 3-year survival following a single IP postoperative injection of mitomycin C absorbed to carbon particles (24).

Intrapleural Chemotherapy

Pleural effusions in patients with cancer may be due to direct invasion of the pleural surfaces by tumor, or by elevation of pulmonary or parietal pleural venous or lymphatic pressure due to compression, such as is commonly produced by mediastinal lymphoma. In the latter situation, mediastinal radiation and systemic therapy can relieve compression. The majority of malignant pleural effusions are caused by breast or bronchial carcinomas, however, and systemic therapy is usually ineffective in controlling the effusion. In principle, malignant pleural effusions can be controlled either by completely obliterating the pleural spaces (pleurodesis) or by killing the tumor in the cavity. Operationally, malignant pleural effusions are usually treated by complete drainage followed by instillation of any of a large number of different kinds of compounds. Instillation of highly irritative agents, such as tetracycline, quinacrine, talc, or crude bacterial preparations, is thought to work by causing pleurodesis. Instillation of chemotherapeutic agents, of which bleomycin has been most commonly used, may work either by causing irritation and adhesion or by direct killing of tumor in the cavity. Any strategy directed at pleurodesis requires that the visceral and parietal pleura be effectively brought into contact after instillation of the irritant; thus, nearly complete drainage of the pleural cavity before and for some period after treatment appears to be essential.

Although malignant pleural effusions are common, and a large number of drugs have been used by the intrapleural route, it is difficult to draw any conclusions about relative efficacy because of the problems of documenting the adequacy of drug distribution and making accurate assessments of response (25). In almost all cases, treatment is purely palliative, and survival is determined largely by the course of the underlying disease. The two most commonly used agents are tetracycline and bleomycin (26). Both cause pain on instillation, but few other symptoms, and have the advantage that, since they are nonmyelosuppressive, they can be used concurrently with systemic chemotherapy. Interest has now shifted toward controlling pleural effusions by destroying the intracavity tumor rather than just causing pleurodesis, and recent Lung Cancer Study Group phase II trials have used combinations of cisplatin with cytarabine or mitomycin (27, 28). Pharmacokinetic information is available for only a few drugs, and in a limited number of patients. Reported mean AUC ratios are 47 for free cisplatin, 195 for mitomycin, 10 to 159 for etoposide, and 4 to 28 for teniposide (28, 29). Phase II trials of post-pleurectomy resection in patients with pleural mesothelioma using cisplatin alone or in combination with mitomycin have shown promising results (30).

Intrathecal Chemotherapy

TECHNIQUE

Drugs can be administered into the CSF by injection into the lumbar sac, into a lateral ventricle via an Ommaya reservoir, or by longer-duration infusion via an external or subcutaneously implanted pump linked to an Ommaya reservoir. Administration via an Ommaya reservoir is preferred over injection into the lumbar sac because in up to 24% of even apparently successful lumbar injections, there is leakage of drug from the CSF, whereas delivery into the ventricular CSF via a reservoir is more reliable (31). In addition, with instillation via a reservoir there is a higher probability of good distribution throughout the CSF, response rates are higher and relapse rates are lower (32), and injection of drugs is less painful and more convenient, facilitating frequent dosing. When injected into the lumbar sac, drug distribution to the base of the brain and ventricles is markedly improved by the patient's maintaining a supine position.

METHOTREXATE

Figure 55.6 shows that the relationship between the volume of the CNS and body surface areas is not constant during growth. Children under the age of 3 have a substantially larger CNS volume relative to surface area than do adults, and they need relatively larger doses on a milligram-per-square-meter basis to attain the same total CNS drug exposure (8). Introduction of dosing on the basis of CNS volume rather than body surface area has significantly reduced neurotoxicity and the incidence of meningeal leukemia in children receiving combined IT methotrexate and cranial radiation as prophylaxis (33). Table 55.3 presents a currently recommended dosing regimen. For the treatment of overt meningeal disease, methotrexate is usually injected twice a week until the CSF cytology becomes normal, although a large variety of schedules is used.

When given by the lumbar route, methotrexate distributes into the CSF and brain extracellular fluid and disappears from the lumbar sac with half-lives of 4.5 and 14 hours; CSF ventricular levels reach 1 to 20 μM and greater than 0.1 μM is maintained for 48 hours (8). Shapiro et al. reported that ventricular injection of 6.25 mg/m^2 via an Ommaya reservoir produced peak ventricular levels of 200 μM which declined with a terminal half-life of 8 hours (34). Drug distribution was more reliable, and this route was associated with a lower relapse rate for leukemic meningitis. Methotrexate is cleared more slowly from the lumbar region than from the ventricles, and the lumbar sac concentration may exceed that in the ventricles by four- to fivefold after 4 to 6 hours (11). There is a high variance in the pharmacokinetics of methotrexate in the CSF from patient to patient, and optimal therapy involves the monitoring of CSF methotrexate concentrations (35). In an attempt to avoid high peak methotrexate concentrations and prolong the duration of exposure for this cell cycle phase-specific drug, Bleyer et al. administered methotrexate on a schedule of 1 mg every 12 hours for 3 days via an Ommaya reservoir (36). This schedule maintained the efficacy of IT methotrexate against childhood leukemic meningitis, while significantly reducing the dose required and the neurotoxicity.

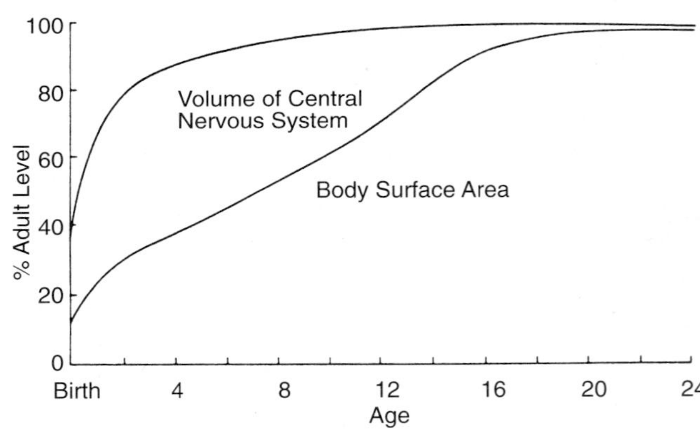

Figure 55.6. Comparison of body surface area and extracellular fluid volume of the CNS during growth. From Bleyer (33).

Table 55.3. Recommended Intrathecal Methotrexate Dose as a Function of Age

Patient age (years)	Dose (mg)
<1	6
1	8
2	10
≥3	12

From Bleyer (33).

Cytotoxic CSF methotrexate concentrations can also be produced by administering high-dose methotrexate IV. During IV infusion of 500 mg/m^2 over 24 hours, the CSF methotrexate concentration averaged 0.6 μM, approximately 33-fold lower than the steady-state plasma concentration (34). Higher CSF concentrations can be attained with larger IV methotrexate doses, particularly when standard doses of the drug are concurrently administered by bolus IT injection. The presence of meningeal leukemia appears to enhance the CSF penetration of methotrexate from the plasma.

Intrathecal injection of methotrexate results in small amounts of drug entering the systemic circulation over a long period, and this can produce systemic toxicity. Oral administration of leucovorin, 7.5 to 9.0 mg every 6 to 12 hours for four to six doses starting concurrently with or 24 hours after IT injection, has been used to limit myelosuppression and mucositis (32, 37), and pharmacokinetic modeling suggests that this should not interfere with the antitumor activity of methotrexate in the CSF.

In 5 to 40% of cases, IT methotrexate causes an acute arachnoiditis that becomes manifest in headache, meningismus, nausea and vomiting, and CSF pleocytosis within a matter of hours to several days after drug injection. In some cases, this may be due to changes in CSF flow dynamics induced by the presence of neoplastic meningitis. Methotrexate can also cause subacute deficits consisting of paresis and paraplegia, cranial nerve palsies, ataxia, visual impairment, altered mentation, and convulsions that evolve over a few days to a week after starting therapy. Necrotizing leukoencephalopathy can develop as a late complication and may vary in severity from mild changes in cognitive functions to dysarthria, dysphagia, spasticity, ataxia, dementia, and coma. Concurrent cranial radiation in children appears to enhance the neurotoxicity of IT methotrexate.

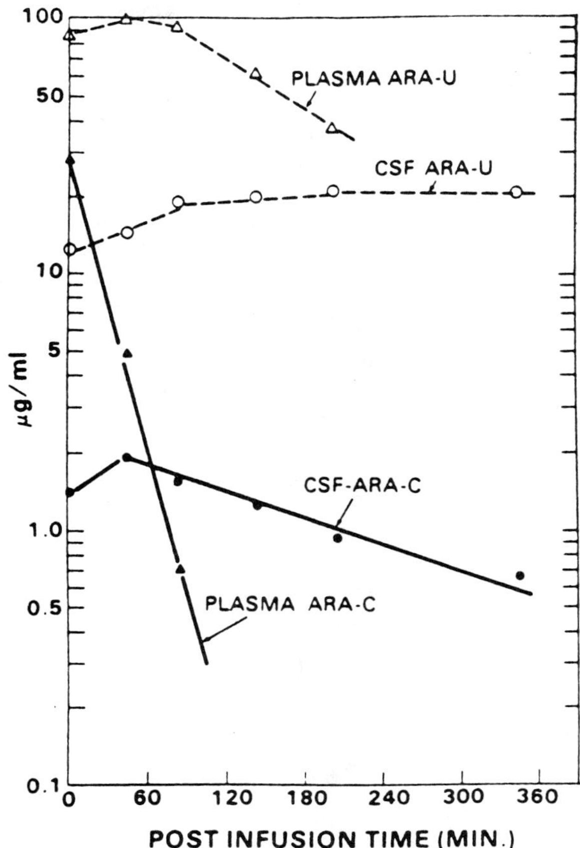

Figure 55.7. Plasma and CSF cytosine arabinoside (ara-C) and uracil arabinoside (ara-U) concentration in plasma and CSF following intravenous administration of cytosine arabinoside (3 g/m^2) over 1 hour. From Lopez (40).

CYTARABINE

Although pharmacokinetic principles indicate that the cytarabine dose, like that for methotrexate, should be based on CNS volume according to age rather than body surface area, the relative lack of cytarabine toxicity permits more latitude. In practice, IT cytarabine is administered in doses of 30 to 100 mg/m^2, generally once or twice weekly. Although pharmacokinetically and cytokinetically sound, multiple-dose or continuous-delivery schedules have not been extensively explored.

When given by injection into a lateral ventricle in a dose of 30 mg, the peak ventricular CSF concentration was in excess of 2 mM and the terminal half-life was 3.4 hours (38). A cytarabine concentration cytotoxic for murine lymphoblasts (0.4 μM) was found to be present in the CSF for more than 24 hours, and no drug was detected in the plasma. Clearance of cytarabine from the CSF is almost entirely by bulk flow; in contrast to plasma, there is very little conversion of cytarabine to uracil arabinoside in the CSF. Following IV injection, cytarabine enters the CSF more readily than does methotrexate, and because of the difference in cytidine deaminase activity, the half-life of cytarabine in the CSF is substantially longer than its half-life in plasma. The CSF cytarabine concentration increases linearly with the IV dose. When cytarabine was given at a dose of 3 g/m^2 over 3 hours, the mean lumbar CSF concentration of 4.4 μM was 12% of simultaneous plasma concentration (39); when given at the same dose over 1 hour, the mean ventricular level was 8.6 μM or 7% of the plasma concentration (40). In the latter case, the CSF half-life was 140 $\pm$ 45 minutes, as compared with a plasma half-life of 17 $\pm$ 2 minutes, suggesting that a therapeutic concentration of cytarabine would be present in the CSF continuously when high-dose IV cytarabine was given every 12 hours. Figure 55.7 shows that, as a result of extensive deamination of cytarabine in the liver, both plasma and CSF levels of the nearly inactive deamination product uracil arabinoside are even higher than the cytarabine concentration. Initial studies of an experimental slow-release formulation indicate that encapsulation of cytarabine in a lipid foam material can result in therapeutic concentrations of CSF cytarabine being maintained for 2 to 3 weeks following a single injection (41).

In general, the toxicity of IT cytarabine is less than that of methotrexate. The common toxicities of IT cytarabine include nausea and vomiting, headache, and fever; paraparesis, paraplegia, and seizures have been reported in patients receiving very high dose rates.

OTHER DRUGS

Hydrocortisone has been added to regimens containing methotrexate and cytarabine in an attempt to reduce the incidence of arachnoiditis. No pharmacokinetic studies of IT administration have been reported, and no information is available on its activity against meningeal neoplasia.

Although thioTEPA has activity when given IT, recent pharmacokinetic studies have called into question the rationale for the use of this route (9). ThioTEPA is quite lipid soluble, and when injected IV, both the native drug and its active metabolite, TEPA, enter the CNS well. TEPA has a substantially longer plasma half-life than thioTEPA, and thus accounts for a significant fraction of the total CNS drug exposure following IV dosing. Monkey studies indicate equivalent AUC in the plasma and both lumbar and ventricular CSF (9). Although ventricular injection of 10 mg of thioTEPA in a patient with meningeal leukemia produced a ventricular exposure that was 273 times higher than plasma exposure, monkey studies suggest that distribution of drug from the ventricles to the lumbar CSF is poor, probably related to the fact that the transcapillary clearance of the drug is greater than CSF bulk flow. In addition, thioTEPA is not converted to TEPA in the CSF, limiting total CNS exposure to active forms of the drug. When thioTEPA is injected IT, its major toxicity is myelosuppression; it can produce mild lower extremity parasthesias shortly following lumbar instillation.

THERAPEUTIC RESULTS

Intrathecal therapy with methotrexate is highly effective in the treatment of leukemic meningitis in children with acute lymphoblastic leukemia, or in the prophylaxis against its development, when used either alone or in combination with cranial radiation (33, 42). In combination with either radiation or other drugs, it can induce remissions in patients with meningeal lymphoma, and provide prophylaxis against the development of this complication (43). Cytarabine is also active against meningeal leukemia when administered IT, even in patients failing IT methotrexate (44). Regimens used for the treatment of neoplastic meningitis associated with childhood leukemia usually combine methotrexate with hydrocortisone and cytarabine (45) and are capable of producing cytologic clearing in 100% of children suffering an isolated CNS relapse of pre–B-cell acute lymphoblastic leukemia (46).

Intrathecal prophylaxis is considered an essential part of the treatment of childhood leukemia, and plays a central role in the management of aggressive forms of childhood and adult lymphoma as well. Recent randomized trials suggest that the use of prolonged triple IT chemotherapy is able to obviate the need for prophylactic cranial radiation in children with acute lymphoblastic leukemia and to improve overall survival (47), but that prophylactic cranial radiation may still be needed for patients who suffer an isolated late bone marrow relapse (48). Several reports have documented the activity of high-dose IV methotrexate or cytarabine against meningeal leukemia and lymphoma (42, 49, 50).

Intrathecal treatment of meningeal carcinomatosis has been much less successful. Response is often difficult to evaluate in these patients since, even with substantial tumor cell kill, fixed neurologic deficits may not improve. In most centers meningeal carcinomatosis is treated with a combination of IT drugs and cranial radiation. Response rates range from 40 to 65%, but relapse is common and median survival is only in the range of 1 to 5 months (32, 37, 51). A randomized study with a relatively small number of patients indicated that cytarabine did not improve the response rate in patients with meningeal carcinomatosis when added to IT methotrexate (32). In a recent randomized trial conducted by the Eastern Cooperative Oncology Group, IT methotrexate was compared with IT thioTEPA in patients with nonleukemic malignancies (52). Only 31% of evaluable patients converted their CSF cytology to negative, and none of 52 patients attained a complete response. There was no significant difference in the toxicity of the two drugs. Intrathecal thioTEPA has produced responses in patients with meningeal neoplasia, but the small numbers of patients studied precludes any useful assessment of its activity relative to that of methotrexate or cytarabine. A phase I study of a lipid-foam–based slow-release formulation of cytarabine suggests activity against solid tumor when drug concentrations are maintained in a therapeutic range for 2 to 3 weeks (41). Assessment of response in patients with meningeal neoplasia is difficult in many studies because concurrent IV therapy was used to treat systemic disease. There is little information from randomized trials on the relative efficacy of single agents or of single agents versus combinations.

Intrapericardial Chemotherapy

Malignant pericardial effusions are commonly treated with one of five modalities of therapy: pericardiocentesis, pericardial sclerosis, systemic chemotherapy, radiation therapy, or surgical creation of a pericardial window. Malignant pericardial effusion often occurs in the setting of widespread carcinomatosis, and one or more of these modalities is usually effective in controlling the effusion for the short subsequent life span. Regional chemotherapy has not been extensively utilized, although intrapericardial administration of cisplatin, carboplatin, methotrexate, 5-fluorouracil, bleomycin, thioTEPA or interleukin-2 appears to be safe and effective in at least some cases. Pharmacologic information is available only for methotrexate where pericardial-to-plasma AUC ratios were found to average 434 (5).

Intra-Arterial Chemotherapy

The most extensive use of IA therapy has been for the treatment of primary and metastatic disease in the liver. Since the liver is the primary site of metabolism of 5-fluorouracil and floxuridine, intrahepatic infusion of these agents represents a special circumstance where there is no increased advantage from the point of view of the tumor, but where extensive first-pass metabolism limits the amount of drug reaching the systemic circulation. This permits perfusions of very long duration, which, in principle, should improve the therapeutic effectiveness of these cell cycle phase-specific drugs. This subject is dealt with in chapter 115. Intrathecal therapy has also been used primarily in the treatment of limb sarcomas and melanomas, carcinomas of the head and neck, and gliomas. With the development of improved catheterization techniques, IA chemotherapy is now also being studied for the treatment of cervical, endometrial, bladder, breast, lung, pancreatic, and prostatic carcinoma.

INTRA-ARTERIAL CHEMOTHERAPY FOR SOFT TISSUE SARCOMA AND OSTEOSARCOMA OF THE EXTREMITIES

Preoperative IA therapy with 3 days of continuous-infusion doxorubicin followed by radiation and surgery for the treatment of limb soft tissue sarcomas has been studied in a series of nonrandomized trials over the past 15 years. This strategy is reported to reduce the need for amputation and the local recurrence rate, but has not changed the rate of failure due to pulmonary metastases when compared with historical controls (53–55). However, doxorubicin must be infused into large arteries in order to avoid vasculitis, and since doxorubicin has little tissue extraction and a relatively long plasma half-life, the rationale for the IA use of this drug is questionable—particularly in light of a complication rate in the range of 7%. Preliminary results of the only randomized trial comparing IA with IV doxorubicin followed by radiation and surgery indicate no superiority for the IA route of administration (41, 56). The value of the use of IV doxorubicin in combination with radiation and surgery has also not been established. With the exception of cisplatin, there is little experience with IA infusion of any other agents for the treatment of soft tissue sarcomas, but a number of studies have been done using isolation/perfusion (see below).

There is substantial controversy about the use of IA cisplatin for the preoperative treatment of osteogenic sarcoma (57, 58). Using catheters positioned in the brachial or femoral arteries, it was found that cisplatin doses of 150 mg/m^2 could be delivered in 3% saline over 2 hours on an every-other-week schedule when very large forced diuresis was employed to protect the kidneys (59). This represents an extraordinarily high dose rate for cisplatin, and this program proved more effective than high-dose methotrexate for induction of initial response (60). The extent of tumor response is greater in patients receiving more than four cycles of treatment, pulmonary metastases have responded in some patients, and the rate of limb salvage in treated patients is high (58, 61–63). The predicted advantage for an IA infusion of cisplatin into a high-flow vessel is not very great, however, and it is unclear whether the IA route is a crucial component of the program. Pharmacokinetic data from a randomized trial comparing IA with IV cisplatin as preoperative treatment for osteogenic sarcoma demonstrated no difference in plasma AUC, renal platinum excretion, or tumor platinum content (12). In addition, in a randomized trial of preoperative treatment that compared two courses of cisplatin, given either IA or IV, in combination with one course of doxorubicin and two doses each of high dose methotrexate and ifosfamide, no difference was found in response (51). The use of IA cisplatin in combination with IV chemotherapy in this setting remains experimental.

INTRA-ARTERIAL CHEMOTHERAPY FOR CARCINOMAS OF THE HEAD AND NECK

Intra-arterial chemotherapy for head and neck carcinomas is attractive because this tumor is often localized, and obtains most of its blood supply from the external carotid artery (64). There is a long history of attempts at IA therapy, but widespread acceptance has been hampered by a high catheter complication rate, progression of tumor outside the infused volume, and the lack of cogent pharmacokinetic data and randomized trials. Comparison of patients receiving 50 mg/m^2 cisplatin by the IA or IV route showed that IA administration was associated with an approximately twofold reduction in peak plasma concentration and AUC, but no difference in tumor platinum content as a function of route of administration (65, 66). Local toxicity rates have also been high. For cisplatin, these include hemialopecia, cranial nerve palsies, visual disturbances, and seizures. Several recent studies have identified tactics for decreasing the rate of catheter complications, and have established that the dose intensity of IA cisplatin can be increased to 150 mg/m^2 IA every 7 days for four doses when used in conjunction with protection of the systemic circulation with the neutralizing agent thiosulfate (67); early results indicate that this can be safely combined with concurrent full-dose-rate radiation therapy (68). This offers the possibility of completing a course of preoperative chemotherapy or definitive treatment with chemoradiotherapy in a period of 1 month as compared with the 3 months required with standard IV administration of cisplatin and 5-fluorouracil. It has also been possible to combine IA cisplatin with 14-day infusions of floxuridine, an agent for which the predicted advantage of regional delivery is very high (69). There have been no randomized studies comparing IA and IV therapy for head and neck carcinoma.

INTRA-ARTERIAL THERAPY FOR PRIMARY CENTRAL NERVOUS SYSTEM TUMORS

The treatment of brain tumors poses a special challenge for IA therapy because a variable portion of the tumor is protected from even high capillary drug concentrations by the blood–brain barrier, and there is marked regional and clonal heterogeneity of drug sensitivity found in glioblastoma multiforme (34). Injection of drug into the carotid artery limits the pharmacologic advantage because of high blood flow; in principle, the use of highly selective supraophthalmic injections can improve the pharmacologic advantage somewhat, and current results support this approach (70). A number of trials using carmustine (BCNU) (71), ACNU (64), PCNU (72), cisplatin (73), carboplatin (74), alone or in combination, have been reported, and it is clear that IA administration results in ipsilateral brain and eye toxicities, including hemiparesis, aphasias, seizures, leukoencephalopathy, brain necrosis, blurring of vision, and blindness. Ocular toxicity may be decreased but not eliminated by administration of the IA injection above the ophthalmic artery (75), and modifications in catheterization techniques to minimize streaming appear to improve distribution (76). Although the occurrence of such regional toxicities strongly suggests increased drug delivery, the actual pharmacologic advantage attained for any of these drugs has not been well documented (77). A randomized phase III study comparing IA with IV BCNU in combination with radiation therapy and with or without IV 5-fluorouracil for the treatment of newly resected gliomas demonstrated unacceptable visual loss and encephalopathy, requiring discontinuation of accrual in the IA arm. In addition, there was no survival advantage for the IA arm (72, 78).

The extent to which the blood–brain barrier is disrupted in brain tumors appears to be quite variable, but drug delivery to most tumors is probably at least partially impeded by tight endothelial junctions that limit drug diffusion. The blood–brain barrier can be transiently opened by the use of hyperosmolar agents, such as mannitol (79) or etoposide (80). In experimental systems, opening the barrier just prior to chemotherapeutic drug administration can increase drug delivery to the brain, but has the potential of increasing delivery to both normal and malignant brain tissue, a situation that yields no increase in selectivity (81). The ability of IA mannitol to open the blood–brain barrier has been documented by the entry of ^{99}Tc, and this strategy has been used in combination with BCNU, ACNU, and cisplatin in phase II trials (79, 82). A single randomized trial comparing IA ACNU and cisplatin with and without prior IA injection of hyperosmolar mannitol demonstrated no survival advantage in patients' malignant gliomas, but a statistically significant improvement in survival of patients with brain metastases from other types of primary tumors (82). There remains substantial controversy about this approach and uncertainty about its therapeutic value.

ISOLATION-PERFUSION CHEMOTHERAPY FOR MELANOMA AND SOFT TISSUE SARCOMA

This strategy for differentially increasing total drug exposure involves cannulating the major artery and vein for all or a portion of a limb, and connecting a pump oxygenator to create a closed circuit into which drug is introduced. Leakage from this closed circuit into the systemic circulation is limited by the application of a constricting bandage at the base of the limb. Although a large number of variations have been employed, by far the greatest experience is with the use of hyperthermic isolation/perfusion with melphalan for the prevention of recurrence of limb melanomas following wide local excision with or without lymph node dissection. A commonly used program involves heating of the blood in the extracorporeal circuit to 39 to 42°C with careful thermistor monitoring of limb temperature. Melphalan is introduced into the circuit as the temperature rises, and perfusion is continued for 1 hour. The extracorporeal circuit is then rinsed with new blood or dextran solution to remove the melphalan, and the vessels are repaired.

Early studies used melphalan dosing regimens that were based on body weight or surface area; a dose of 1 to 1.5 mg/kg was commonly employed. However, neither body weight nor surface area is a good predictor of the blood volume of a limb, and selection of dose based on direct measurement of limb volume (83) or indirect estimation of limb blood volume results in smaller patient-to-patient variance (84). Melphalan has a terminal half-life of 53 minutes in the extracorporeal circuit, and total drug exposure for the circuit ranges from 1,000 to nearly 4,000 μg·min/mL (85). For comparison, IV injection of a maximum tolerated dose of melphalan produces an AUC in the range of 55 μg·min/mL. Although generally 5 to 12% of the volume of the albumin in the extracorporeal circuit leaks into the systemic circulation during a 1-hour perfusion (85, 86), systemic melphalan exposure is insufficient to cause myelosuppression in more than a small fraction of the patients treated.

Although melphalan hyperthermic isolation/perfusion has established activity against advanced limb melanomas and soft tissue sarcomas, its major use has been as an adjuvant to wide local resection of early-stage disease. Despite more than 30 years of experience, only one prospective randomized trial has been completed (86). This study showed a significant decrease in relapse rate (11% versus 48%) and an increase in both disease-free and total survival for patients with operable limb melanomas undergoing melphalan hyperthermic isolation/perfusion. A number of retrospective analyses have shown minimal or no benefit, however, and this form of treatment remains controversial (87, 88). Acute complications of isolation/perfusion include edema, nerve palsy, and skin toxicity, but significant long-term sequelae other than limitation of motion at distal joints are unusual. While a number of other drugs in addition to melphalan have been administered by limb isolation/perfusion, including imidazole carboxamide, doxorubicin, cisplatin (89), etoposide, mechlorethamine, actinomycin D, tumor necrosis factor (TNF), and various interferons, pharmacokinetic information is largely lacking and no comparative studies of efficacy have been conducted. In a recent phase II multicenter study, a regimen of IA recombinant TNF, recombinant interferon-γ and melphalan plus limb hyperthermia was reported to result in a response rate of 100% among 53 patients with in-transit melanoma metastases (complete response rate was 90%) (90).

INTRA-ARTERIAL CHEMOTHERAPY FOR LUNG CANCER

Blood flow in the bronchial arteries constitutes only a small fraction of cardiac output, predicting a relatively big pharmacokinetic advantage for IA infusion via these arteries for the treatment of small-cell and non–small-cell lung cancer. However, the pharmacology is complicated by an unknown but presumably variable effect of pulmonary arterial blood flow and the risk of damage to normal lung tissue; no pharmacokinetic data have been published. A modest but poorly documented clinical experience with bronchial artery infusions, particularly with doxorubicin, mitomycin, and cisplatin has been reported (91). This approach is capable of producing responses, particularly in squamous cell carcinomas, but the existing published information does not permit an assessment of whether such responses increase resectability or alter survival.

INTRA-ARTERIAL CHEMOTHERAPY FOR CARCINOMA OF THE CERVIX, BLADDER, BREAST, AND PROSTATE

Intra-arterial chemotherapy has been used for the local treatment of regional components of a number of other diseases, including carcinoma of the cervix, bladder, breast, and prostate. Only pilot phase I/II studies with small numbers of patients have been reported for any of these diseases. No dose ranging or complete pharmacokinetic studies are available, methodology has not been standardized and, in many cases, the choice of drugs has been based on their activity when given by the IV route rather than the suitability of their pharmacokinetics for administration by the IA route. Nevertheless, reported response rates are high, and clinically important tumor regressions have been observed for each of these diseases. In the case of cervical carcinoma, IA infusion into both internal iliac arteries has been used as neoadjuvant therapy prior to surgery or radiation therapy, or for the management of inoperable or recurrent disease. The greatest experience has been with IA cisplatin, and in combination with either bleomycin, mitomycin, or vincristine, response rates of 71 to 76% with complete responses of 5 to 24% have been reported (92, 93). The goal of IA chemotherapy for bladder cancer is to downstage the disease to permit preservation of the bladder at subsequent surgery in a larger fraction of patients. Intra-arterial infusion via the internal iliac arteries can clearly produce responses (94), but documentation that this permits less extensive resection or has an impact on overall outcome awaits a randomized trial. The possibility of combining IA chemotherapy with local radiotherapy and surgical resection offers a particularly fertile area for investigation (95). Intra-arterial chemotherapy for breast cancer has been directed at improving local control for inflammatory carcinoma and unresectable disease at high risk for regional recurrence. Infusion is accomplished through the internal mammary or subclavian arteries, while the brachial artery is compressed to prevent drug from entering the arm. High response rates have been reported in phase I/II trials (96, 97); one small randomized trial of preoperative IA versus IV epirubicin demonstrated a greater local response rate in the IA arm (98). The role of the IA approach relative to neoadjuvant IV combination chemotherapy remains to be defined.

Cisplatin and doxorubicin have been used on several different schedules for the treatment of inoperable advanced prostatic carcinoma, and one study of 21 patients has reported a complete response rate of 28% with a total response rate of 90% (99). This promising lead needs confirmation.

Overview

Regional therapy is currently part of standard treatment only for the prophylaxis or management of meningeal metastases; the extent to which other forms of regional therapy should be part of standard treatment has not yet been clearly defined. One criticism of regional therapy is that it usually cannot deal with all of the disease in the body. However, tumor burden is an important determinant of treatment outcome for many types of cancer, and under circumstances where regional therapy actually increases drug delivery sufficiently to control the local tumor, there is a reasonable probability that the regional approach will improve the chances for management of the disease by concurrent or subsequent systemic therapy (100). The pharmacologic advantage of regional therapy can be enhanced by a variety of currently available tactics, such as the use of systemic neutralizing agents and modulation of tumor blood flow and regional clearances. Newly evolving technologies for creating slow-release forms of drugs promise additional improvements in the efficacy of regional therapy in the future.

References

1. Dedrick RL, Myers CE, Bungay PM, DeVita VT Jr. Pharmacokinetic rationale for peritoneal drug administration in the treatment of ovarian cancer. Cancer Treat Rep 1978;62:1–11.
2. Jain RK. Barriers to drug delivery in solid tumors. Sci Am 1994;271:58–65.
3. Howell SB, Zimm S, Markman M, Abramson IS, Cleary S, Lucas WE, Weiss RJ. Long term survival of advanced refractory ovarian carcinoma patients with small-volume disease treated with intraperitoneal chemotherapy. J Clin Oncol 1987;5:1607–1612.
4. Los G, Mutsaers PH, van der Vijgh WJ, Baldew GS, de Graaf PW, McVie JG. Direct diffusion of cis-diamminedichloroplatinum (II) in intraperitoneal rat tumors after intraperitoneal chemotherapy: a comparison with systemic chemotherapy. Cancer Res 1989;49:3380–3384.
5. Howell SB, Chu BB, Wung WE, Metha BM, Mendelsohn J. Long-duration intracavitary infusion of methotrexate with systemic leucovorin protection in patients with malignant effusions. J Clin Invest 1981;67:1167–1170.
6. Howell SB, Pfeifle CL, Wung WE, Olshen RA, Lucas WE, Yong JL, Green M. Intraperitoneal cisplatin with systemic thiosulfate protection. Ann Intern Med 1982;97:845–851.
7. Grossman SA, Trump DL, Chen DC, Thompson G, Camargo EE. Cerebrospinal fluid flow abnormalities in patients with neoplastic meningitis. An evaluation using ^{111}indium-DTPA ventriculography. Am J Med 1982;73:641–647.
8. Bleyer WA, Dedrick RL. Clinical pharmacology of intrathecal methotrexate. I. Pharmacokinetics in nontoxic patients after lumbar injection. Cancer Treat Rep 1977;61:703–708.
9. Strong JM, Collins JM, Lester C, Poplack DG. Pharmacokinetics of intraventricular and intravenous N,N',N''-triethylenethiophosphoramide (thiotepa) in rhesus monkeys and humans. Cancer Res 1986;46:6101–6104.
10. Blasberg RG, Patlak C, Fenstermacher JD. Intrathecal chemotherapy: brain tissue profiles after ventriculocisternal perfusion. J Pharmacol Exp Ther 1975;195:73–83.
11. Blasberg RG, Patlak CS, Shapiro WR. Distribution of methotrexate in the cerebrospinal fluid and brain after intraventricular administration. Cancer Treat Rep 1977;61:633–641.
12. Bielack SS, Erttmann R, Looft G, Purfurst C, Delling G, Winkler K, Landbeck G. Platinum disposition after intraarterial and intravenous infusion of cisplatin for osteosarcoma. Cancer Chemother Pharmacol 1989;24:376–380.
13. Patlak CS, Fenstermacher JD. Measurements of dog blood-brain transfer constants by ventriculocisternal perfusion. Am J Physiol 1975;229:877–884.
14. Burch PA, Grossman SA, Reinhard CS. Spinal cord penetration of intrathecally administered cytarabine and methotrexate: a quantitative autoradiographic study. J Natl Cancer Inst 1988;80:1211–1216.
15. Dedrick RL. Arterial drug infusion: pharmacokinetic problems and pitfalls (review). JNCI 1988;80:84–89.
16. Collins JM. Pharmacologic rationale for regional drug delivery. J Clin Oncol 1984;2:498–504.
17. Schneider JG. Intraperitoneal chemotherapy. Obstet Gynecol Clin North Am 1994;21:195–212.
18. Kirmani S, Braly PS, McClay EF, Saltzstein SL, Plaxe SC, Kim S, Cates C, Howell SB. A comparison of intravenous versus intraperitoneal chemotherapy for the initial treatment of ovarian cancer. Gynecol Oncol 1994;54:338–344.
19. Markman M, Cleary S, Pfeifle C, Howell SB. Cisplatin administered by the intracavitary route as treatment for malignant mesothelioma. Cancer 1986;58:18–21.
20. Markman M, Kelsen D. Efficacy of cisplatin-based intraperitoneal chemotherapy as treatment of malignant peritoneal mesothelioma. J Cancer Res Clin Oncol 1992;118:547–550.
21. Lindner P, Heath DD, Shalinsky DR, Howell SB, Naredi P, Hafstrom L. Regional lymphastic drug exposure following intraperitoneal administration of 5-fluorouracil, carboplatin, etoposide. Surg Oncol 1993;2(2):105–112.
22. Sugarbaker PH, Gianola FJ, Speyer JL, Wesley R, Barofsky I, Myers CE. Prospective randomized trial of intravenous v intraperitoneal 5-FU in patients with advanced primary colon or rectal cancer. Semin Oncol 1985;12(3 suppl 4):101–111.
23. Sautner T, Hofbauer F, Depisch D, Schiessel R, Jakesz R. Adjuvant intraperitoneal cisplatin chemotherapy does not improve long-term survival after surgery for advanced gastric cancer. J Clin Oncol 1994;5:970–974.
24. Takahashi T, Hagiwara A, Shimotsuma M. Intraperitoneal chemotherapy with mitomycin C bound to activated carbon particles for patients with advanced gastric cancer. Eur J Surg Oncol 1994;2:183–184.
25. Hausheer FH, Yarbro JW. Diagnosis and treatment of malignant pleural effusion. Semin Oncol 1985;12:54–75.
26. Ostrowski MJ. Intracavitary therapy with bleomycin for the treatment of malignant pleural effusions. J Surg Oncol 1989;(suppl)1:7–13.
27. Rusch VW, Figlin R, Godwin D, Piantadosi S. Intrapleural cisplatin and cytarabine in the management of malignant pleural effusions: a Lung Cancer Study Group trial. J Clin Oncol 1991;9:313–319.

28. Rusch VW, Niedzwiecki D, Tao Y, Manendez-Botet C, Dnistrian A, Kelsen D, Saltz L, Markman M. Intrapleural cisplatin and mitomycin for malignant mesothelioma following pleurectomy: pharmacokinetic studies. J Clin Oncol 1992;10:1001–1006.
29. Montaldo PG, Figoli F, Zanette ML, Sorio R, Zucchetti M, Tirelli U, D'Incalci M. Pharmacokinetics of intrapleural versus intravenous etoposide (VP16) and teniposide (VM26) in patients with malignant pleural effusion. Oncol 1990;47:55–61.
30. Rusch V, Saltz L, Ven Katraman E, Ginsberg R, McCormack P, Burt M, Markman M, Kelsen D. A phase II trial of pleurectomy/decortification followed by intrapleural and systemic chemotherapy for malignant pleural mesothelioma. J Clin Oncol 1994;6: 1156–1163.
31. Kieffer SA, Wolff JM, Prentice WB, Loken MK. Scinticisternography in individuals without known neurological disease. Am J Roentgenol 1971;112:225–236.
32. Hitchins RN, Bell DR, Woods RL, Levi JA. A prospective randomized trial of single-agent versus combination chemotherapy in meningeal carcinomatosis. J Clin Oncol 1987;5:1655–1662.
33. Bleyer WA, Coccia PF, Sather HN, Level C, Lukens J, Niebrugge DJ, Siegel S, Littman PS, Leikin SL, Miller DR, Chard RL, Hammond GD, Childrens' Cancer Study Group. Reduction in central nervous system leukemia with a pharmacokinetically derived intrathecal methotrexate dosage regimen. J Clin Oncol 1983;1:317–325.
34. Shapiro WR, Young DF, Mehta BM. Methotrexate: distribution in cerebrospinal fluid after intravenous, ventricular and lumbar injections. N Engl J Med 1975;293:161–166.
35. Strother DR, Glynn-Barnhart A, Kovnar E, Gregory RE, Murphy SB. Variability in the disposition of intraventricular methotrexate: a proposal for rational dosing. J Clin Oncol 1989;7:1741–1747.
36. Bleyer WA, Poplack DG, Simon RM. "Concentration x Time" methotrexate via a subcutaneous reservoir: a less toxic regimen for intraventricular chemotherapy of central nervous system neoplasms. Blood 1978;51:835–842.
37. Wasserstrom WR, Glass JP, Posner JB. Diagnosis and treatment of leptomeningeal metastases from solid tumors: experience with 90 patients. Cancer 1982;49:759–772.
38. Zimm S, Collins JM, Miser J, Chatterji D, Poplack DG. Cytosine arabinoside cerebrospinal fluid kinetics. Clin Pharmacol Ther 1984;35:826–830.
39. Slevin ML, Piall EM, Aherne GW, Harvey VJ, Johnston A, Lister TA. Effect of dose and schedule on pharmacokinetics of high-dose cytosine arabinoside in plasma and cerebrospinal fluid. J Clin Oncol 1983;1:546–551.
40. Lopez JA, Nassif E, Vannicola P, Krikorian JG, Agarwal RP. Central nervous system pharmacokinetics of high-dose cytosine arabinoside. J Neuro-oncol 1985;3:119–124.
41. Kim S, Chatelut E, Kim JC, Howell SB, Cates C, Kormanik PA, Chamberlain MC. Extended CSF cytarabine exposure following intrathecal administration in Depofoam. J Clin Oncol 1993;11:2186–2193.
42. Abromowitch M, Ochs J, Pui CH, Kalwinsky D, Rivera GK, Fairclough D, Look AT, Hustu HO, Murphy SB, Evans WE, Dahl GV, Bowman WP. High-dose methotrexate improves clinical outcome in children with acute lymphoblastic leukemia: St. Jude total therapy study X. Med Pediatr Oncol 1988;16:297–303.
43. Recht L, Straus DJ, Cirrincione C, Thaler HT, Posner JB. Central nervous system metastases from non-Hodgkin's lymphoma: treatment and prophylaxis. Am J Med 1988;84:425–435.
44. Wang JJ, Pratt CB. Intrathecal arabinosyl cytosine in meningeal leukemia. Cancer 1970;25:531–534.
45. Buchanan GR, Rivera GK, Boyett JM, Chauvenent AR, Crist WM, Vietti TJ. Reinduction therapy in 297 children with acute lymphoblastic leukemia in first bone marrow relapse: a pediatric oncology group study. Blood 1988;72:1286–1292.
46. Winick NJ, Smith SD, Shuster J, Lauer S, Wharam MD, Land V, Buchanan G, Rivera G. Treatment of CNS relapse in children with acute lymphoblastic leukemia: a Pediatric Oncology Group study. J Clin Oncol 1993;11:271–278.
47. Pullen J, Boyett J, Shuster J, Crist W, Land V, Frankel L, Iyer R, Backstrom L, van Eys J, Harris M. Extended triple intrathecal chemotherapy trial for prevention of CNS relapse in good-risk and poor-risk patients with B-progenitor acute lymphoblastic leukemia: a Pediatric Oncology Group study. J Clin Oncol 1993;5:839–849.
48. Buhrer C, Hartmann R, Fengler R, Schober S, Arlt I, Loewke M, Henze G. Importance of effective central nervous system therapy in isolated bone marrow relapse of childhood acute lymphoblastic leukemia. Blood 1994;83(12):3468–3472.
49. Freeman AI, Weinberg V, Brecher ML, Jones B, Glicksman AS, Sinks LF, Weil M, Pleuss H, Hannanian J, Burgert EO, Gilchrist GS, Necheles T, Harris M, Kung F, Patterson RB, Maurer H, Leventhal B, Chevalier L, Forman E, Holland JF. Comparison of intermediate-dose methotrexate with cranial irradiation for the post-induction treatment of acute lymphocytic leukemia in children. N Engl J Med 1983;308:477–484.
50. Morra E, Lazzarino M, Brusamolino E, Pagnucco G, Castagnola C, Bernasconi P, Orlandi E, Corso A, Santagostino A, Bernasconi C. The role of systemic high-dose cytarabine in the treatment of central nervous system leukemia. Cancer 1993;72: 439–445.
51. Winkler K, Bielack S, Delling G, Salzer-Kuntschik M, Kotz R, Greenshaw C, Jurgens H, Ritter J, Kusnierz-Glaz C, Erttmann R. Effect of intraarterial versus intravenous cisplatin in addition to systemic doxorubicin, high-dose methotrexate, and ifosfamide on histologic tumor response in osteosarcoma (study COSS-86). Cancer 1990;66: 1703–1710.
52. Grossman SA, Finkelstein DM, Ruchdeschel JC, Trump DL, Moynihan T, Ettinger DS. Randomized prospective comparison of intraventricular methotrexate and thiotepa in patients with previously untreated neoplastic meningitis. J Clin Oncol 1993;11: 561–569.
53. Eilber FR, Guiliano AE, Huth J, Mirra J, Morton DL. High-grade soft-tissue sarcomas of the extremity: UCLA experience with limb salvage. Prog Clin Biol Res 1985;201: 59–74.
54. Eilber FR, Morton DL, Eckardt J, Grant T, Weisenburger T. Limb salvage for skeletal and soft tissue sarcomas. Cancer 1984;53:2579–2584.
55. Levine EA, Trippon M, Das Gupta TK. Preoperative multimodality treatment for soft tissue sarcomas. Cancer 1993;71:3685–3689.
56. Eilber FR, Guiliano AE, Huth JF, Weisenburger T, Eckardt J. Intravenous IV vs. intraarterial IA adriamycin, 2800r radiation and surgical excision for extremity soft tissue sarcomas: a randomized prospective trial. Proc Am Soc Clin Oncol 1990;9:309.
57. Bielack SS, Bieling P, Erttmann R, Winkler K. Intra-arterial chemotherapy for osteosarcoma: does the result really justify the effort? Cancer Treat Res 1993;62:85–92.
58. Jaffe N. Pediatric osteosarcoma: treatment of the primary tumor with intraarterial cis-diamminedichloroplatinum-II (CDP)—advantages, disadvantages, and controversial issues. Cancer Treat Res 1993;62:75–84.
59. Jaffe N, Knapp J, Chuang VP, Wallace S, Ayala A, Murray J, Cangir A, Wang A, Benjamin RS. Osteosarcoma: intra-arterial treatment of the primary tumor with cis-diammine-dichloroplatinum II (CDP). Cancer 1983;51:402–407.
60. Jaffe N, Robertson R, Ayala A, Wallace S, Chuang V, Anzai T, Cangir A, Wang Y, Chen T. Comparison of intra-arterial cis-diamminedichloroplatinum II with high-dose methotrexate and citrovorum factor rescue in the treatment of primary osteosarcoma. J Clin Oncol 1998;3:1101–1104.
61. Jaffe N, Raymond AK, Ayala A, Carrasco CH, Wallace S, Robertson R, Griffiths M, Wang YM. Effect of cumulative courses of intraarterial cis-diamminedichloroplatin-II on the primary tumor in osteosarcoma. Cancer 1989;63:63–67.
62. Kempf RA, Irwin LE, Menendez L, Chandrasoma P, Groshen S, Melbye W, Moore T, Pentecost M, Quinn M, Sapozink M. Limb salvage surgery for bone and soft tissue sarcoma. A phase II pathologic study of preoperative intraarterial cisplatin. Cancer 1991;68:738–743.
63. Malawer M, Buch R, Reaman G, Priebat D, Potter B, Khurana J, Shmookler B, Patterson K, Schulof R. Impact of two cycles of preoperative chemotherapy with intraarterial cisplatin and intravenous doxorubicin on the choice of surgical procedure for high-grade bone sarcomas of the extremities. Clin Orthopaed Related Res 1991;270: 214–222.
64. Wheeler RH, Ziessman HA, Medvec BR, Juni JE, Thrall JH, Keyes JW, Pitt SR, Baker SR. Tumor blood flow and systemic shunting in patients receiving intraarterial chemotherapy for head and neck cancer. Cancer Res 1986;46:4200–4204.
65. Gouyette A, Apchin A, Foka M, Richards J. Pharmacokinetics of intra-arterial and intravenous cisplatin in head and neck cancer patients. Eur J Cancer Clin Oncol 1986;22:257–263.
66. Sileni VC, Fosser V, Maggian P, Padula E, Beltrame M, Nicolini M, Arslan P. Pharmacokinetics and tumor concentration of intraarterial and intravenous cisplatin in patients with head and neck squamous cancer. Cancer Chemother Pharmacol 1992;30: 221–225.
67. Robbins KT, Storniolo AM, Kerber C, Vicario D, Seagren S, Shea M, Hanchett C, Los G, Howell SB. Phase I study of highly selective supradose cisplatin infusions for advanced head and neck cancer. J Clin Oncol 1994;12:2113–2120.
68. Robbins KT, Vicario D, Seagren S, Weisman R, Pellitteri P, Kerber C, Orloff L, Los G, Howell SB. A targeted supradose cisplatin chemoradiation protocol for advanced head and neck cancer. Am J Surg 1994;168:419–422.
69. Forastiere AA, Baker SR, Wheeler R, Medvec BR. Intra-arterial cisplatin and FUDR in advanced malignancies confined to the head and neck. J Clin Oncol 1993;5: 1601–1606.
70. Nakagawa H, Fugita T, Kubo S, Tsuruzono K, Yamada M, Tokiyoshi K, Miyawaki Y, Kanayama T, Kadota T, Hayakawa T. Selective intra-arterial chemotherapy with a combination of etoposide and cisplatin for malignant gliomas: preliminary report. Surg Neurol 1994;41:19–27.
71. Bashir R, Hochberg FH, Linggood RM, Hottleman K. Pre-irradiation internal cartoid artery BCNU in treatment of glioblastoma multiforme. J Neurosurg 1988;68:917–919.
72. Green SB, Byar DB, Strike TA, Burger PC, Mahaley MS, Mealey J, Pistenmaa DA, Ransohoff J, Robertson JT, Selker RG, Shapiro WR, VanGilder JC. Randomized phase II comparison of PCNU and AZQ for the treatment of primary brain tumors (Study 8120). Proc Am Soc Clin Oncol 1985;4:558.
73. Brambilla Bas M, Boccardo M. Intracarotid cisplatin chemotherapy for high-grade astrocytomas. J Neurosurg Sci 1993;37:83–86.
74. Stewart DJ, Belanger JM, Grahovac Z, Curuvija S, Gionet LR, Autkin SE, Hugenholtz H, Benoit GB, DaSilva VF. Phase I study of intracarotid administration of carboplatin. Neurosurgery 1992;30:512–516.
75. Clayman DA, Wolpert SM, Heros DO. Superselective arterial BCNU infusion in the treatment of patients with malignant gliomas. AJNR 1989;10:767–771.
76. Aoki S, Terada H, Kosuda S, Shitara N, Fujii H, Suzuki K, Kutsukake Y, Tanaka J, Sasaki Y, Okubo T. Supraophthalmic chemotherapy with long tapered catheter: distribution evaluated with intraarterial and intravenous Tc-99m HMPAO. Radiology 1993;188:347–350.
77. Shani J, Bertram J, Russell C, Dahalan R, Chen DCP, Parti R, Ahmadi J, Kempf RA, Kawada TK, Muggia FM, Wolf W. Noninvasive monitoring of drug biodistribution and metabolism: studies with intraarterial Pt-195m-cisplatin in humans. Cancer Res 1989;49:1877–1881.
78. Shapiro WR, Green SB, Burger PC, Selker RG, VanGilder JC, Robertson JT, Mealey J Jr, Ransohff J, Mahaley MS Jr. A randomized comparison of intra-arterial versus intravenous BCNU, with or without intravenous 5-fluorouracil, for newly diagnosed patients with malignant glioma. J Neurosurg 1992;76:772–781.
79. Neuwelt EA, Bigner D, Frenkel EP. The effects of osmotic modification of the blood brain barrier and adrenal steroid administration on methotrexate delivery of gliomas in rats: the blood brain barrier is a factor. Proc Natl Acad Sci USA 1982;79: 4420–4423.
80. Spigelman MK, Zappulla RA, Strauchen JA, Feuer EJ, Johnson J, Goldsmith SJ, Malis LI, Holland JF. 1986 Etoposide induced blood-brain barrier disruption in rats: duration of opening and histological sequelae. Cancer Res 1986;46:1453–1457.
81. Shapiro WR, Shapiro JR. Principles of brain tumor chemotherapy. Semin Oncol 1986;13:56–69.
82. Iwadate Y, Namba H, Saegusa T, Sueyoshi K. Intra-arterial mannitol infusion in the chemotherapy for malignant brain tumors. J Neuro-oncol 1993;15:185–193.
83. Wieberdink J, Benckhuysen C, Braat RP, Van Slooten EA, Olthuis GAA. Dosimetry in isolation perfusion of the limbs by assessment of perfused tissue volume and grading of toxic tissue reactions. Eur J Cancer Clin Oncol 1982;18:905–910.
84. Lejeune FJ, Ghanem GE. A simple and accurate new method for cytostatics dosimetry in isolation perfusion of the limbs based on exchangeable blood volume determination. Cancer Res 1987;47:639–643.
85. Benckhuijsen CF, Varossieau J, Hart AA, Wieberdink J, Noordhoek J. Pharmacokinetics of melphalan in isolated perfusion of the limbs. J Pharmacol Exp Ther 1986;237:583–588.
86. Ghussen F, Kruger I, Smalley RV, Groth W. Hyperthermic perfusion with chemotherapy for melanoma of the extremities. World J Surg 1989;13:598–602.
87. Lejeune FJ, Lienard D, el Douaihy M, Seyedi J, Ewalenko P. Results of 206 isolated limb perfusions for malignant melanoma. Eur J Surg Oncol 1989;15:510–519.
88. Edwards MJ, Soong S, Boddie AW, Balch CM, McBride CM. Isolated limb perfusion for localized melanoma of the extremity. Arch Surg 1990;125:317–321.
89. Fletcher WS, Pommier R, Small K. Results of cisplatin hyperthermic isolation perfu-

sion for stage IIIA and IIIAB extremity melanoma. Melanoma Res 1994;4(suppl 1):17–19.

90. Leinard D, Eggermont AM, Koops H, Schraffordt H, Kroonj BB, Rosenkaimer F, Autier P, Lejeune FJ. Isolated perfusion of the limb with high-dose tumour necrosis factor alpha (TNF-alpha), interferon-gamma (IFN-gamma) and melphalan for melanoma stage III. Results of a multi-centre pilot study. Melanoma Res 1994;4(suppl 1):21–26.
91. Watanabe Y, Shimizu J, Murakami S, Yoshida M, Tsubota M, Iwa T, Kitagawa M, Mizukami Y, Nonomura A, Matsubara F. Reappraisal of bronchial arterial infusion therapy for advanced lung cancer. Jpn J Surgery 1990;20:27–35.
92. Kigawa J, Kanamori Y, Ishihara H, Minagawa Y, Iwamoto K, Terakawa N. Response rate and cell-cycle changes due to intra-arterial infusion chemotherapy with cisplatin and bleomycin for locally recurrent uterine cervical cancer. Am J Clin Oncol 1992;15: 474–479.
93. Patton Jr TJ, Kavanagh JJ, Declos L, Wallace S, Haynie TP, Gershenson DM, Wharton JT, Bass S. Five-year survival in patients given intra-arterial chemotherapy prior to radiotherapy for advanced squamous carcinoma of the cervix and vagina. Gynecol Oncol 1991;42:54–59.
94. Kuriyama M, Takashi Y, Nagatani Y, Shinoda I, Yamamoto N, Nagai T, Ueno K, Takeuchi T, Maeda S, Isogai K. Intra-arterial administration of methotrexate, Adriamycin, and cisplatin as neoadjuvant chemotherapy for bladder cancer. Cancer Chemother Pharmacol 1992;30:S1–S4.
95. Sumiyoshi Y, Yokota K, Akiyama M, Inoue Y, Yoneda F, Tsujimura H, Nakajima M, Yokozeki H, Maebayashi K. Neoadjuvant intra-arterial doxorubicin chemotherapy in combination with low dose radiotherapy for the treatment of locally advanced transitional cell carcinoma of the bladder. J Urol 1994;152(2 pt 1):362–366.
96. Bilbao JI, Rebollo J, Long JM, Mansilla F, Munoz-Galindo L, Vieitz JM. Neoadjuvant intra-arterial chemotherapy in inflammatory carcinoma of the breast. Br J Radiol 1992;65:248–251.
97. Stephens FO. Intraarterial induction chemotherapy in locally advanced stage III breast cancer. Cancer 1990;66:645–650.
98. Takatsuka Y, Yayoi E, Kobayashi T, Aikawa T, Kotsuma Y. Neoadjuvant intra-arterial chemotherapy in locally advanced breast cancer: a prospective randomized study. Osaka Breast Cancer Study Group 1994;1:20–25.
99. Nakamura K, Takashima S, Nakatsuka H, Onoyama Y. Prostate cancer: arterial infusion chemotherapy and alteration of intrapelvic blood flow. Radiology 1992;185: 885–889.
100. Eckman WW, Patlak CS, Fenstermacher JD. A critical evaluation of the principles governing the advantages of intra-arterial infusions. J Pharmacokinet Biopharm 1974;2:257–285.

CHAPTER 56

Animal Models in Drug Development

SAMIR N. KHLEIF AND GREGORY A. CURT

Introduction

The process of cancer drug discovery may begin with either empiric screening or rational drug design. In either case, the necessary steps in drug development that follow the identification of an interesting lead require appropriate animal model systems. Just as screening systems and rational drug design have benefited from recent advances in cell culture technique and molecular biology, so too has the role of animal model systems in drug development. Beyond simply predicting dose-limiting toxicity, drug metabolism or tissue and compartment distribution, animal models are increasingly being used to guide dose escalation in Phase I trials and provide tumor microenvironments that mimic the clinical situation.

The processes of cancer drug discovery and drug development have evolved, and will continue to change, since the first successful use of drugs to treat systemic cancer more than 50 years ago. Basic research in cancer biology has provided new targets for cancer drug development and brought older targets into sharper focus. Of the properties that make a cell malignant (uncontrolled growth, metastasis, dedifferentiation, genetic plasticity, and drug resistance), only uncontrolled growth has been exploited as a target for cancer drug development. Agents that have the potential to interfere with the metastatic cascade, interrupt autocrine and paracrine growth loops, differentiate tumors, or reverse drug resistance are now in preclinical development and early clinical trial. Appropriate and evolving animal model systems will be needed to discover the next generation of cancer drugs and bring them to clinical study. This chapter will discuss the history and future of cancer drug discovery and drug development with special emphasis on the role of animal models in the process.

THE ROLE OF ANIMAL MODELS

In Drug Discovery

Drug Screening. The idea that systemic drugs could treat, and possibly cure, systemic cancer is relatively new in medicine. In the mid 1940s, Gilman's treatment of lymphomas with alkylating agents at Yale and Farber's induction of short remissions in leukemia with antifolates at Harvard led the National Cancer Institute (NCI) to begin a major effort in cancer drug discovery and development. Stated in its simplest terms, the purpose of the initial NCI screen was to select and prioritize drugs for clinical trial (4–6, 17–23, 33, 38, 78, 113, 168, 169).

In 1955, murine leukemia models P388 and L1210 were selected as the initial system in which potential agents would need to demonstrate activity before further development. The reason for this selection was simple. Murine leukemia and lymphoma models were relatively inexpensive and allowed for a relatively high throughput of compounds. Indeed, from the inception of the mouse screen until its first modifications in the mid 1970s, more than 400,000 compounds passed through this screen.

At first, this mouse screening system was empiric. Over time, however, this empiricism became more enlightened with the development of the NCI Drug Information System. This computer-based inventory maintains the structure of each compound screened and its activity in murine model systems. This system has been used to limit the screening of analogues while turning greater attention to novel structures. Importantly, the Drug Information System also maintains discrete databases on compounds provided to NCI on a proprietary basis by pharmaceutical companies, allowing open access of the screen to industry.

From the beginning, however, it was obvious that this system had serious limitations. While most of the active drugs currently used in the treatment of leukemia and lymphoma were initially screened in the L1210 system, screening against rapidly growing leukemic cells could bias selection toward compounds that are preferentially active against rapidly growing tumors with essentially a 100% growth fraction. In fact, it was found that plateau phase cultures were less sensitive to cycle-specific agents than log phase culture, while some classes of clinically useful drugs, such as the alkylators, were active in plateau phase cell lines. The development of drugs active against the solid tumors of adulthood would presumably require a different approach.

The availability of new rodent models enabled the NCI to take further steps toward rational drug screening in 1975 (63). Instead of a single hurdle of activity in murine leukemia, compounds active in this system were subsequently tested against a panel that included transplantable murine tumor models designed to resemble common human solid tumors (including melanoma and lung, colon, and breast cancer) both in histology and cell kinetics. In a step that would presage later changes in the NCI screen, the availability of athymic (nude) mice also allowed the screening of drugs against transplantable human tumors as well (138, 162). Initially, these human tumor xenografts included lung, colon, and breast cancer (52, 97, 121).

Overall, these changes took the NCI screen from a com-

Table 56.1. Origin of DCT Prescreen and Tumor Panel Models

Site tumor	Host of origin	Tumor of origin	Historical description	Site
		Prescreen		
P388 leukemia	DBA/2 mouse	Chemically induced with 3-methyl-cholanthrene	Lymphocytic leukemia	IP
L1210 leukemia	DBA/2 mouse	Chemically induced with 3-methyl-cholanthrene in ethyl ether	Lymphoid leukemia	IP
		Tumor Panel		
Mouse tumors				
B16 melanoma	C57BL/6 mouse	Spontaneous at base of ear	Melanoma	IP
CD8F mammary carcinoma	CD8F female mice	Spontaneous	Mammary adenocarcinoma	SC
Colon 38	C57BL/6 mouse	Induced by 1,2-dimethylhydrazine	Colon carcinoma	SC
Lewis lung carcinoma	C57BL/6 mouse	Spontaneous in the lung	Carcinoma	IV
Human tumor xenografts				
CX-1 colon	Isolated in tissue culture, subsequently maintained in nude mice	Human colon. Untreated primary tumor from 44-year old caucasian female	Adenocarcinoma of the colon	src
LX-1 lung	Isolated and maintained in nude mice	Metastatic lesion from arm of 48-year-old male with oat cell lung carcinoma treated with *Corynebacterium Parvum*, cyclophosphamide (Cytoxan), and radiation.	Carcinoma	src
MX-1 mammary	Isolated and maintained in nude mice	Human breast. Primary tumor from 29-year-old female with no previous chemotherapy. CL-1 line	Carcinoma	src

src, subrenal capsule; IP, intraperitoneal; IV, intravenous; SC, subcutaneous.

pound-oriented toward a more tumor-specific approach. However, the high cost of the transplantable mouse and human xenograft systems (approximately $5,000 per compound) was unsuitable for high capacity screening. Instead, the NCI designed a two-stage system in which the murine leukemia model was maintained as a stage I "prescreen."

Compounds entering the system were first tested against a highly drug-sensitive mouse leukemia. Agents shown active against P388 or L1210 were then tested in a stage II screen against the solid tumor panel. Table 56.1 illustrates the animal tumor panel used in the screen. It includes both the transplantable murine tumor models and the human tumor xenografts. In turn, those agents with the broadest spectrum of activity against solid tumors received priority for phase I clinical trial (Fig. 56.1).

The rationale for this approach was simple. Earlier experience in the NCI murine leukemia-based screen had shown that L1210 and P388 were the most sensitive models for drugs that were subsequently shown to have clinical activity (138). In particular, P388 was more sensitive to compounds of the natural product class than L1210 (64, 148). Thus, most inactive compounds could be screened-out by an inexpensive, high capacity, highly sensitive, less specific prescreen before the presumably more rigorous development in the low capacity, less sensitive, more specific tumor panel. When in full operation, P388 screened some 15,000 compounds each year, of which 500 to 1,000 were advanced into the stage II (solid tumor) phase of testing.

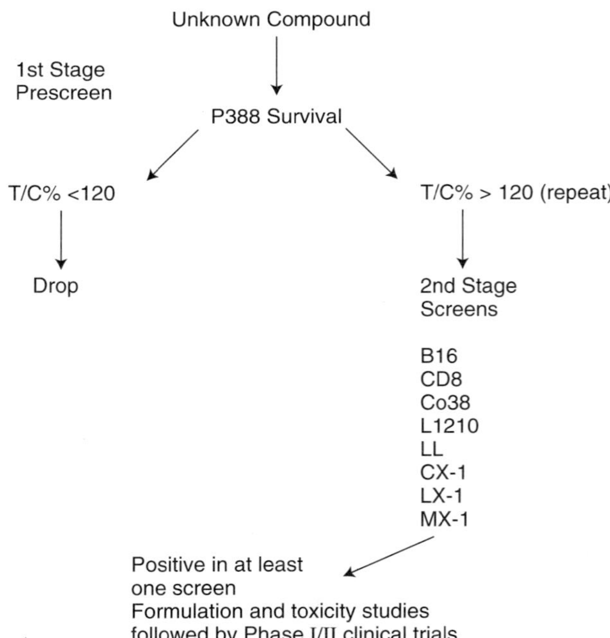

Figure 56.1. National Cancer Institute Drug Screening Strategy 1975–1985.

While the approach appeared a reasonable compromise considering costs and logistics, the limitations remain obvious. The refined screen remained, at its heart, a compound-oriented strategy using a highly sensitive, rapidly dividing leukemia model for initial intake. However, the bias against selection of drugs specifically active in solid tumors remained. For example, fewer than 2% of all agents active against P388 showed significant effects in Lewis lung or colon (38) adenocarcinomas (91, 148).

Most disturbing was the failure of the disease-specific phase II component of the screen to predict for disease-specific clinical activity. Retrospective analysis of solid tumor activity in phase II trials was not predicted by parallel preclinical solid tumor activity. As will be discussed later, if a given drug demonstrated significant preclinical activity in xenograft models of human breast, colon, or lung cancer, this did not predict for clinical activity in patients with these diseases. In addition, the screen identified few active new leads (11, 30, 51, 163). Accepting the limitations of animal models of this type in cancer drug screening and recognizing the need for a preclinical screening system with greater predictive power, the NCI began to focus on a truly disease-oriented approach to drug discovery in the mid 1980s. Ideally, such a screen would be able to detect broadly active or disease-specific drugs.

Because of the high cost and a continued need for a high volume screen, animal models were determined to be impractical. Instead, the development, characterization, and maintenance of an entirely in vitro human tumor cell line screen was initiated (7, 8, 37, 103, 107, 141, 155). In 1985, the NCI screen evolved into its most recent configuration, an in vitro (stage I) screen followed by the more refined in vivo (stage II) screen (Fig. 56.2).

In stage I, agents are tested against a panel of approximately 60 cell lines representing the most common solid tumors of adulthood including lung, breast, colon, renal, and ovarian cancer (21, 23). Drug-resistant tumors are specifically included in the screen. These include the human breast carcinoma selected for multiple drug resistance (mdr) and P388 murine leukemia resistant to natural products, both of which potentially provide additional identification of new agents with particular activity against potentially resistant tumors (31, 71). In stage II, the most sensitive human tumors are tested against the same drug in nude mice. Activity in the nude mouse-human xenograft system in itself is sufficient for further preclinical development including toxicology and formulation, steps that are often the most costly process of drug development.

In summary, the current NCI approach to cancer drug discovery has evolved from a highly empiric compound oriented animal-based screen to a human in vitro panel. An advantage to this approach in addition to its disease orientation and adaptability to high volume screening is its flexibility with respect to natural product extracts. While animal models require relatively large quantities of relatively pure compounds for screening, the in vitro panel can actually be used to purify active compounds from small quantities of natural product extracts.

However, animal models will continue to play a critical role in cancer drug development. Preclinical activity of an antitumor agent in a relevant in vivo system is a sine qua non for clinical testing. As development of anticancer agents turns progressively toward agents that modify biological responses, differentiate tumors, and inhibit metastasis and invasion, animal models will become more important in the future. Immunostimulants and inhibitors of metastasis can only be studied preclinically in the appropriate animal model system.

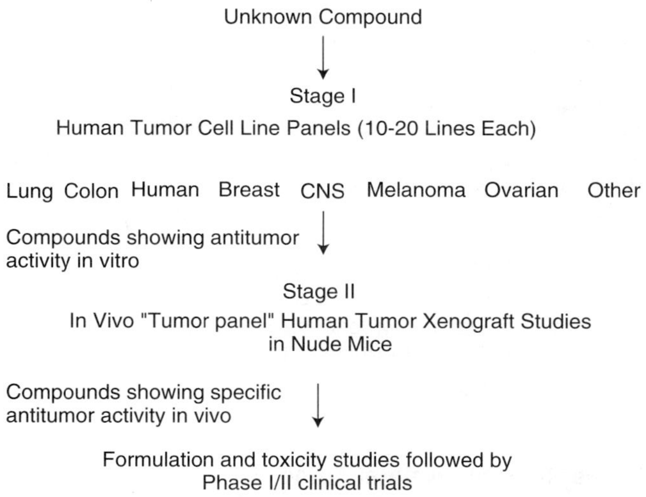

Unknown Compound

↓

Stage I

Human Tumor Cell Line Panels (10-20 Lines Each)

Lung Colon Human Breast CNS Melanoma Ovarian Other

Compounds showing antitumor activity in vitro ↓

Stage II

In Vivo "Tumor panel" Human Tumor Xenograft Studies in Nude Mice

Compounds showing specific antitumor activity in vivo ↓

Formulation and toxicity studies followed by Phase I/II clinical trials

Figure 56.2. National Cancer Institute Drug Screening Strategy 1985–present.

ANIMAL TUMOR MODELS

The selection of the appropriate experimental model is critical to cancer drug discovery and development. The value of the model depends on its validity, selectivity, predictability, and reproducibility (33, 34, 168). In cancer drug development, the animal model is selected to demonstrate the cytotoxic effect of the drug or biological agent on the tumor passage in that model system.

There is no perfect tumor model for any human cancer. Nevertheless, in selecting the best model system, consideration should be given to the genetic stability and heterogeneity of the transplanted cell line, its immunogenicity within the host animal, and the appropriate biologic endpoint (local growth, metastasis, survival). For example, the KHT sarcoma is a tumor with high metastatic potential, making it a very suitable model for the evaluation of a combined modality treatment (164) or inhibitor of metastasis.

In general, animal tumor models can be divided into either spontaneous or artificially transplanted systems. Solid tumors are usually transplanted by the inoculation of cell suspensions by the subcutaneous (SC), intradermal (ID), intramuscular (IM), intraperitoneal (IP), or intravenous (IV) routes. Leukemia models are transplanted only by the SC, IV, or IP routes.

The spontaneous tumor models that are either idiopathic or arise following carcinogenic (28, 29) or viral exposure mimic the clinical situation most closely. Spontaneous tumors are usually measurable only late in their course. Their metastatic pattern is not uniform, and their response to therapy is generally poor. They also resemble human cancers in kinetics and antigenicity.

However, there are significant obstacles to the use of such model systems. For example, a relatively small percentage of animals may develop disease following exposure to carcinogen or virus, and the tumors may have a variable natural course. In addition, the inability to establish accurate staging makes these models quantitatively unsuitable for assessing therapeutic response to an agent given in a uniform fashion. Generally speaking, spontaneous tumor models have their greatest role in studying the biology of carcinogenesis. In the future, they may also be important in the development of chemopreventive or chemosuppressive drugs.

The models with the widest use in experimental therapeutics are the transplanted animal tumor models and the human tumor xenografts. These will be discussed in some detail below.

Transplantable Animal Tumor Models

Early passages of transplanted tumors resemble spontaneous cancer most closely. These early passages show significant heterogeneity in cell kinetics and histology (101, 151). Despite these limitations, such models have been used in drug screening. Because established transplantable tumor models are well characterized and reproducible, they have traditionally been the foundation of cancer drug development (108, 131, 132, 144). How good are they in predicting clinical activity?

Multiple studies have been undertaken to assess the ability of preclinical animal activity to predict antitumor response in man (11, 14, 89). Marsoni and co-workers evaluated the activity of all cytotoxic drugs introduced into phase II clinical trial by the NCI between 1970 and 1985 (99). Of the 75 drugs entered into clinical trial during this period, 24 showed some evidence for clinical activity. One interpretation of these data is that the screen is highly predictive for clinical activity. Approximately 30% of drugs taken to clinical trial showed some evidence of activity. However, 74% of the drugs were active against lymphoma and 35% were active against leukemia. Only minimal activity was observed against solid tumors including those represented in the phase II portion of the screen. Indeed, analysis showed a poor correlation between preclinical in vivo and clinical activity in the same tumors. One must conclude that either animal model systems using transplantable tumors do not predict for clinical activity or that the P388 prescreen effectively selected against compounds specifically active in human solid tumors. The new in vitro human cell line screen will be important in answering these questions, since the initial identification of activity is in a human solid tumor rather than a murine leukemia-lymphoma model system.

A range of methods can be used to evaluate drug effect on tumors in animal models. Tumor size and tumor weight or volume changes are simple and easily reproducible parameters. Morphologic changes and alterations in tumor immunogenicity or invasiveness are other markers of response (62).

In addition, many specific assays have been developed for the measurement of treatment effects on tumors. This section will discuss some assays that can be used to judge tumor response.

Excision Clonogenic Assay. This assay has been used widely as a method to assess what fraction of cells in a tumor population retain proliferative capability after being exposed to a chemotherapeutic agent. This assay is based on the assumption that the proliferative or clonogenic potential of tumor cells reflects the in vivo tumorigenicity of the tumor stem cell (149, 152). Thus, colony number is assumed to be proportionate to the number of viable cells.

The assay itself is straightforward. Tumor-bearing animals are tested with the drug under evaluation. At 24 hours, the tumors are excised from treated and untreated animals. A cell suspension is prepared from every tumor. The proliferative capacity of the cells in each suspension is evaluated by either in vivo inoculation intravenously into test animals of a selected cell suspension dilution (76, 153), or by plating the cells in liquid or agar medium (26, 75, 133). If an animal model is used, colony count is then performed in specific tissues at necroscopy. The lung, liver, and spleen are commonly used for this purpose. If the cells were plated in agar, a colony count is performed in the dish. Colony-forming efficiency (CE) of the inoculated cells is calculated to assess the efficacy of treatment in terms of cell survival.

$$\text{CE} = \frac{\text{number of tumor colonies counted}}{\text{number of tumor cells plated}}$$

The ratio of the CE treated to the CE control is called surviving fraction (SF).

$$\text{SF} = \frac{\text{CE treated}}{\text{CE control}}$$

SF is the best parameter for expressing cell survival results from the excisional biopsy (92, 154).

This assay has the advantage of placing the treated and untreated tumors in identical environments. It is also able to select a resistant population of cells within the tumor at a low drug dose. In addition, excising the tumor 24 hours after exposing the animal to the cytotoxic agent allows giving doses up to the transplant range, which has important implications for the selection of agents for bone marrow transplantation.

TD50 (Endpoint Dilution Assay). TD50 (74, 77, 93) is the tumor cell inoculum that produces tumor growth in 50% of inoculated animals or sites. It is a measurement of the number of cells required to produce tumors from inocula in vivo. The assay is based on the same principles as that of colony formation. A cell suspension is prepared from both treated and untreated animals, with ranges of dilutions for each tumor depending on the expected value of TD50. The suspension is inoculated into groups of test animals subcutaneously, intramuscularly or intradermally for solid tumors, and intraperitoneally or intravenously for leukemias. The percentage of tumor take versus cell number inoculated for each treatment is determined and compared to control animals to determine TD50 (49).

Tumor Growth Delay Assay. Cytotoxic treatment can slow tumor growth and delay disease progression. These effects are measured by the tumor growth delay assay (9, 10, 157). Tumor delay by definition is the time required for the treated tumor to reach a specific size minus the time for the untreated tumor to reach that certain size. This assay involves a very simple technique, little equipment, and can be completed for many types of tumors before animals are lost to metastasis or disease progression. Unlike the survival time assay discussed later, this evaluation does not require death as an endpoint.

The correlation between the growth delay and the amount of cell kill varies with the growth rate of the tumor (10). Thus, when a treatment effect on tumors with different growth rates is assessed, a comparison of absolute growth delay between tumor models is misleading. Therefore, a specific growth delay (growth delay/doubling time of the tumor) reflects more accurately the differences in cell kill. Figure 56.3 illustrates the concept of specific growth delay.

Survival Time Assay. Another parameter that can be used to assess the effect of a drug on tumor in the animal model is the survival time. Survival time is an obvious endpoint, since it combines the sum total of interactions between tumor, drug, and host. Since drug toxicity and tumor growth both have independent effects on survival, a judgment can be made about therapeutic index. However, this approach cannot directly assess cell kill or time-dependent cytotoxicity.

The therapeutic efficacy can be assessed by determining the increase in survival as an effect of the escalating dose of the studied drug. As the dose of an active drug increases, the survival time increases because of increasing logarithmic tumor cell kill. Survival time reaches a maximum point as the toxic effect of the drug outweighs the therapeutic effect and survival times diminish (145). The maximum point of survival is called the optimal point (OP) or the maximum increase in life span (IL). The higher the OP the better the given intervention's therapeutic efficacy. This model also helps in assessing the safety of certain drugs by measuring the therapeutic ratio (TR), that is, the ratio between the optimal dose and that dose that leads to a specific increase in survival time (e.g., IL 20, IL 40, and so on). Therefore, in comparing drugs with the same maximum survival (optimal point), the higher the therapeutic ratio, the safer the drug (145).

A common use of survival to assess drug efficacy or increase in life span is the *T/C* percent ratio. This is defined as the ratio of the survival time of treated animals to the survival time of control, expressed as a percentage. This parameter has been used by the NCI for decision making, setting specific criteria of activity before further development is undertaken. A *T/C* of $>$120 in the solid tumor panel has been used as the benchmark for clinical development (Fig. 56.1) (15, 16, 100, 122).

Animal Tumor Xenografts

Before the availability of athymic or nude mice, human tumors were xenografted in mice immunocompromised by irradiation, thymectomy, or steroids (32, 158, 159). The first nude mice arose spontaneously in a closed, but not inbred, colony of albino mice in a virus laboratory in Ruchill Hospital, Glasgow, Scotland (134) and were described by Isaacson and Cattanach as lacking fur (84). The first xenograft in nude mice was performed by Rygaard and Povlsen in 1969 using a human colon adenocarcinoma (136).

Flanagan initially described the genetic component of immunodeficiency in this important model. He found that the mutant gene (*nu*, for nude) is present on chromosome 11, as

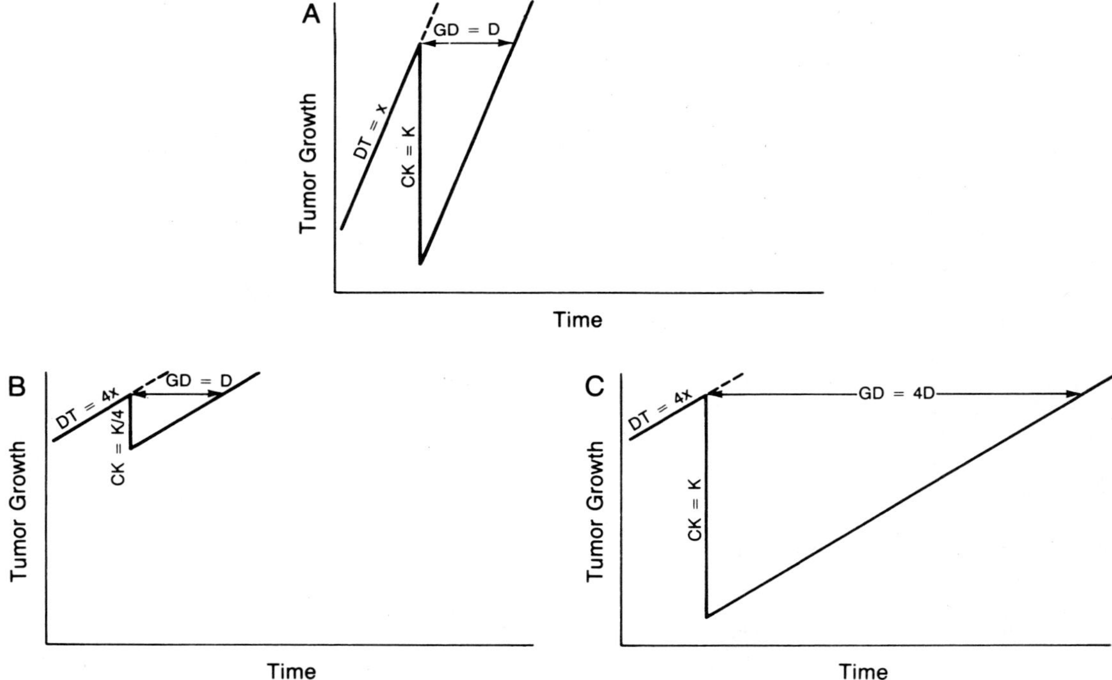

Figure 56.3. Tumor growth in relation to time before and after treatment (**A**). A 4-fold doubling time requires 1/4 of cell kill for the same growth delay (**B**). The same amount of cell kill results in 4-fold increase in growth delay (**C**). DT, doubling time; CK, cell kill; GD, growth delay; K, relative cell kill; D, relative growth delay over time.

an autosomal recessive gene (50). It is responsible for the absence of hair in addition to other abnormalities including retarded growth, low fertility, and short life span (100% mortality within 25 weeks of birth and 45% mortality within 2 weeks of birth) (134). It was not until 1968 that Pantelouris noted that some of the nude mice lacked a thymus gland. These mice were found to have a homozygous mutation *nu/nu*, while both the phenotypically normal +/+ and the heterozygous *nu*/+ had a thymus (124). Immunologically, the *nu/nu* athymic mice have a small number of T cells that are residual after transplacental passage from heterozygous mothers. However, these T cells do not affect the rejection of tissue transplants (or other markers of T cell function) (129). These animals preserve B cell function (147) and exhibit a higher activity of natural killer cells (73, 80). These characteristics led to widespread use of nude mice in tissue transplantation and other areas of biomedical research (50, 53, 82, 118, 135, 137), including their use in human tumor transplantation.

The success of human tumor xenografting into the nude mice and the ability to maintain the histologic and biologic identity of tumors through successive passages in vivo revolutionized many aspects of cancer research, including drug development (83, 114, 128, 140). Transplantation of tumor cell lines into nude mice can be accomplished via multiple routes: subcutaneous, intraperitoneal (59), intravenous, intracranial (58), intrasplenic, renal subcapsular, or through a new orthotopic model by site-specific organ inoculation. Each site has specific advantages and limitations.

Subcutaneous implantation is the predominant site for transplantation of human tumor into the nude mouse because of its simplicity and easy access to tumor. Indeed, it provides the mainstay for in vivo testing of the drug discovery and screening program of the NCI (120).

A tumor cell suspension is usually injected into the flank of the animal. Depending on the clonogenic potential of the tumor, between 106 and 107 cells are required for successful engraftment. Tumors usually require between a few days to a few months to grow depending on the growth rate of the cell line used. Many human tumor xenografts have been established to date, including those from most of the solid tumors affecting adults. Human colon cancer and melanoma have been passaged for the longest time in vivo. Brain tumors have proven the most difficult to maintain (40, 47). Approximately one-half of the brain tumor cell lines have been successfully xenografted into athymic mice (40).

Of interest, subcutaneous xenografts metastasize infrequently and seldom invade adjacent tissues. This may be because of the retention of some host defenses, especially natural killer cell activity (73, 80). Thus, animal survival is not a feasible endpoint for assessing drug efficacy in nude mice, since large tumor burdens prior to death may be associated with discomfort. Instead, the growth delay or the clonogenic assay would be more appropriate in this model. However, it is possible to select primary tumors or perturb the host defense mechanisms to develop models that are locally invasive or metastatic. Metastasis can be enhanced with the depletion of NK cells by pretreating the mice with cyclophosphamide, beta estradiol, or other agents (44, 48, 94).

Human tumor cells undergo kinetic changes after transplantation and passage in the nude mice. Most frequently, the transplanted tumor adapted to growth in animals has a shorter doubling time than the original tumor isolated from a patient (149). Growth rates increase further during subsequent passages (35, 150). The vascularity of the primary and transplanted tumor also differ with transplanted tumors showing better blood supply and less necrosis. This difference could be due to selection of the most rapidly growing cells from a heterogeneous primary animal, secretion of paracrine growth factors, which induce neovascularization, or simply tumor size.

Despite these changes in kinetics of invasive potential, the majority of the xenografted human tumors maintain the morphologic and biochemical characteristics of their original tumors. Therefore, it is expected that chemosensitivity would be similar in both the original and the xenografted human tumor, and that this correlation would predict for both active single agents and active drug combinations. In fact, excellent correlations can be made between average growth delay for human tumors in nude mice treated with the best available drug combinations and complete clinical response rates (46, 61). In increasing order of responsiveness, these correlations have been shown for human xenografts of non-small cell lung cancer (114, 142), colon cancer (119), breast cancer (60), small cell lung cancer (30), and malignant melanoma (51).

Renal Subcapsular Assay (RSC). Unlike the subcutaneous xenograft assay, the renal subcapsular assay has a relatively short and constant period between tumor inoculation and the appearance of a grossly palpable mass. Tumors can usually be assessed in a period of 6 days (3). Therefore, this model is particularly appropriate when a short term in vivo assay is required. Cells are inoculated as a tumor fragment, usually 1 mm in size, under the kidney capsule of the nude mouse, as first described by Bogden and colleagues in 1978 (15). These tumors maintain true morphologic, functional, and growth characteristics of the original tumor from which they were derived (2). For example, they preserve cell-cell contact, maintain the spatial relationship of the tumor, and form a more representative model of human metastasis than the subcutaneous xenograft. Therefore, tumor response can be subsequently assessed by measuring tumor size (growth assay), colony formation by surviving cells (the clonogenic assay), or simply animal survival (1, 14, 39, 42, 156).

While appealing in many ways, the renal subcapsular assay has limitations. The subcapsular area of the kidney is not a totally immunoprivileged site. When sectioned and examined microscopically, variable amounts of tumor mass represent invading lymphocytes (49, 98, 160). Thus, the immunogenicity of a given tumor in a given animal model is an important variable to control, and considerable controversy surrounds the use of this assay (1). However, as will be discussed later, it might be an ideal orthotopic model for renal cell carcinoma (see below) (111).

Intraperitoneal, Microencapsulated Tumor Assay

Because of the limitations of the renal subcapsular assay, and its specific poor adaptability to slow-growing tumors (2,

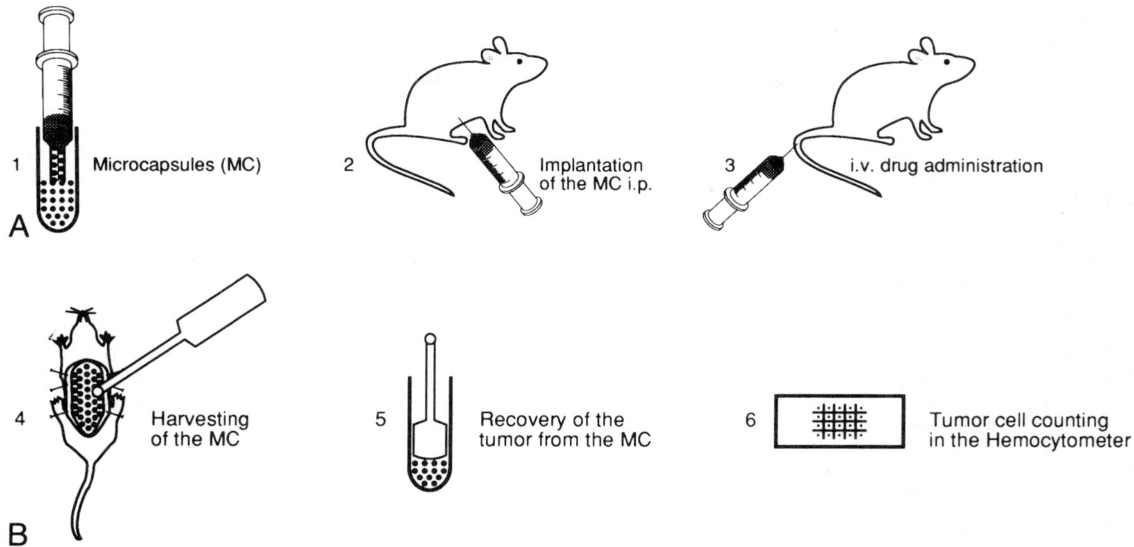

Figure 56.4. Intraperitoneal microencapsulated tumor assay.

Table 56.2. Orthotopic Models for Study of Human Cancers Grown in Athymic Nude Mice

Human cancer organ site of origin	Implantation site in nude mice	Nomenclature
Central nervous system	Percutaneous intracranial implantation into cerebral cortex	Intracranial model
Colon	Wall of cecum	Intracolonic model
Lung	Intrabronchially into right mainstem bronchus	Intrapulmonary model
	Percutaneously into right pleural space	Percutaneous intrathoracic model
Pancreas	Pancreas parenchyma	Intrapancreatic model
Renal	Subrenal capsule	Subrenal capsule model
	Kidney parenchyma	Intrarenal model

12, 43), alternative short-term in vivo assays have been developed. One of the more interesting is the microencapsulated tumor assay which depends on microencapsulation technology. Tumor cells are encapsulated in semipermeable gels that can be formed into microcapsules of (0.05 to 1 mm) (90). These microcapsules can be inoculated into the peritoneal space of experimental animals. Under typical assay conditions using mice, approximately 600 microcapsules are injected into the peritoneum. The semi-permeability of the capsule protects the tumor cells from host cell-mediated immune cytotoxicity, so that athymic (nude) mice need not be used. At the same time, it allows nutrients and systemic cytotoxic agents to diffuse and reach the tumor cells. Anticancer effect is assessed by recovering microcapsules and counting viable tumor cells in treated versus control animals (Fig. 56.4) (67, 68).

The microencapsulation assay is simple, rapid, and relatively inexpensive. For a given analysis, it requires fewer mice when compared to the subcutaneous transplanted tumor assay (68). By definition, tumor cells are evaluated after exposure to drug concentrations that are obtainable in vivo. In addition, the system is adaptable to most solid tumors and, unlike the subcutaneous transplanted tumor assay, uses immunocompetent mice. For these reasons, the microencapsulated tumor assay is being evaluated by the NCI screening program as an in vivo second line screen to follow initial drug leads that pass the in vitro screening system previously described (20).

Orthotopic Xenograft Model. In 1889, after analyzing autopsies from patients with metastatic breast cancer, Paget concluded that metastasis is not a random phenomenon. Rather, he concluded the malignant cells have special affinity for growth in the environment of certain organs, the familiar seed and soil hypothesis (123). Certainly, there exist organ site-specific interactions that are essential for optimal growth and progression of cancer in vivo (77, 106, 117, 126, 127). The orthotopic xenograft model is a system in which tumor cells are implanted at the site of the organ of origin. This organ-specific site presumably provides the tumor cells with an optimal environment for growth and progression. Because of its relevant expense and novelty, this model has as yet not been used widely by the NCI drug screening program. However, it is being used extensively to explore its role as an in vivo evaluation model for cytotoxic agents specific for organ sites such as lung cancer.

Multiple tumor xenografts have already been developed using nude mice, including renal cell carcinoma (44, 45, 112), pancreatic carcinoma (136), certain brain tumors

(139), prostate, colon, and to a larger extent lung cancer (Table 56.2) (102). All of these models are potentially amenable to orthotopic development.

The lung tumor model is the predominant orthotopic model that has been explored by the NCI102 (105), and application of other models is currently underway. In the case of lung cancer, tumor cells in suspension are inoculated through the right main stem bronchus into the right lung in a lightly anesthetized animal (Fig. 56.5). Tumor response can be evaluated by sacrificing the animal and histologically quantifying tumor growth, or as shown in Figure 56.6, non-invasive chest x-ray may be sufficient to provide interim evaluation of tumor response (104).

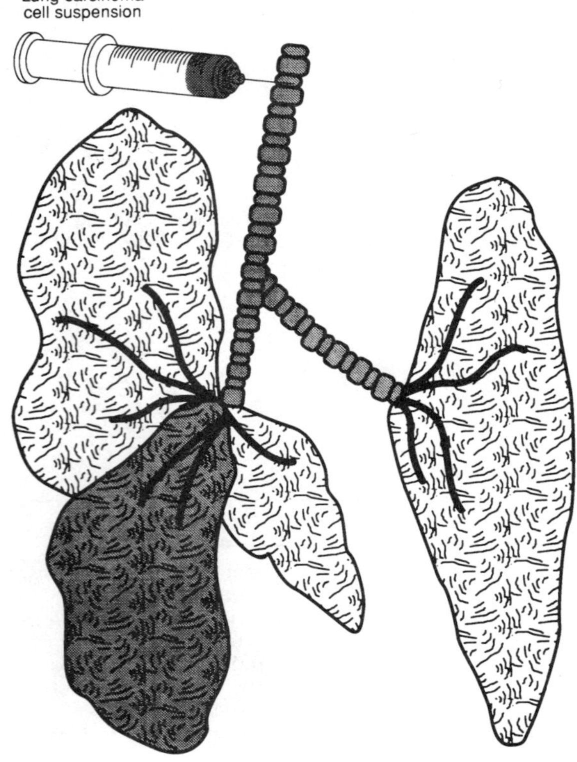

Figure 56.5. Orthotopic in vivo human lung cancer model in athymic nude mice. Intrabronchial tumor cell inoculations. *Shaded area*, tumor.

Another approach toward establishing a lung tumor orthotopic model is through percutaneous intrathoracic implantation (Fig. 56.7) (102). A disadvantage to this model is the finding that as many as 30% of the inoculated tumor grows outside the lung parenchyma, either in the pleural space or the chest wall. Tumor related mortality from the intrabronchial model is higher than that of intrathoracic implantation. Both orthotopic approaches have a much higher tumor mortality than the subcutaneous model of the same tumor cell line (102). The far greater aggressiveness of identical inoculates of lung cancer injected into the bronchus compared with subcutaneous injection is a reflection of Paget's early observation on tumor cell tissue tropism and suggests that orthotopic models may reflect the clinical situation most closely (69, 95, 110, 116).

Hollow Fiber Technology. Recently, the NCI has incorporated semipermeable hollow fiber assays into the in vivo phase of drug development. These hollow fibers allow tumor cells to grow in contact with each other, either in the log or stationary phases of cell growth (Fig. 56.8). The permeability of the fibers can be selected to limit the molecular weight of drug, which can penetrate into the tumor mass. A practical advantage of this system is that more than one tumor type can be implanted into a single animal, allowing more information to be obtained from a single in vivo experiment. In addition, the system may be adaptable to epithelial cells in an attempt to screen for compounds that interfere with angioneogenesis. Because this is an in vivo system, the agent

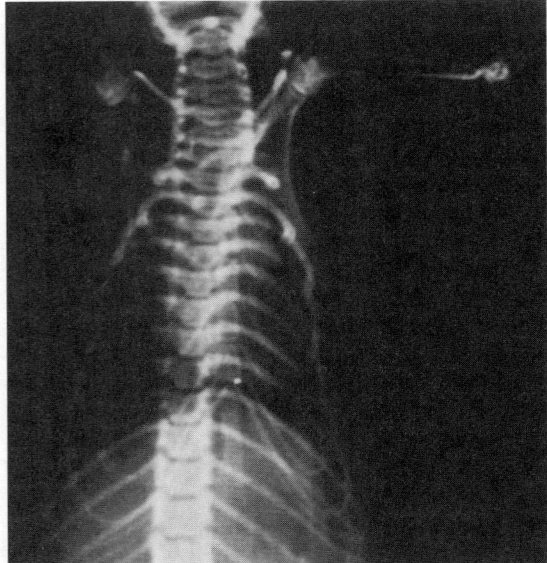

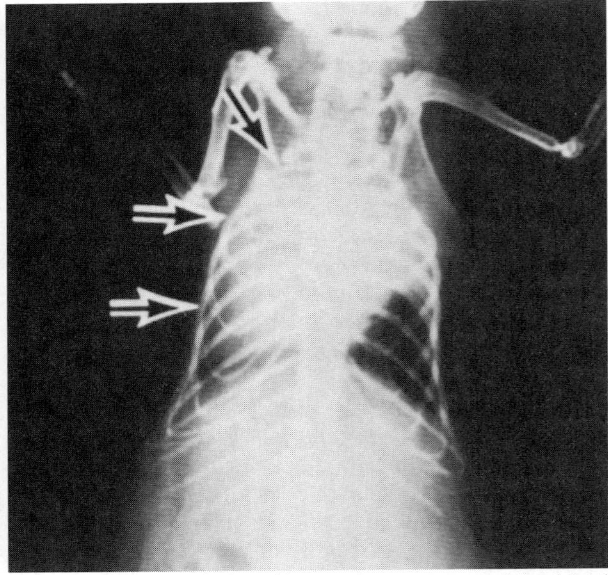

Figure 56.6. X-ray of a lung field of a normal athymic mouse (*left*) and an x-ray showing a right lung carcinoma resulted from intrabronchial inoculation of human lung cancer cell line (*right*). *Arrows*, tumor site.

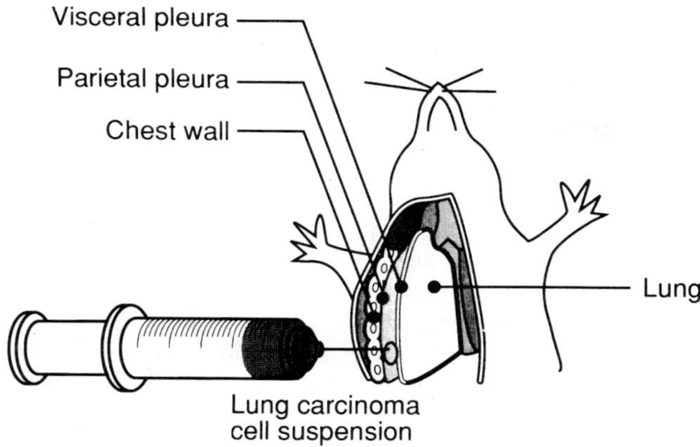

Figure 56.7. Orthotopic in vivo human lung cancer model in athymic nude mice. Percutaneous tumor cell inoculation.

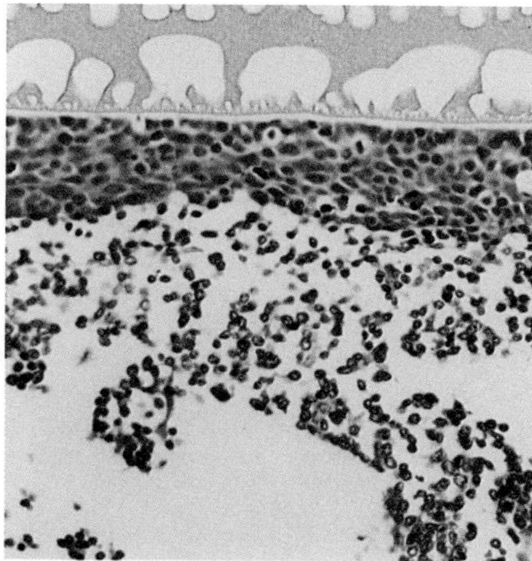

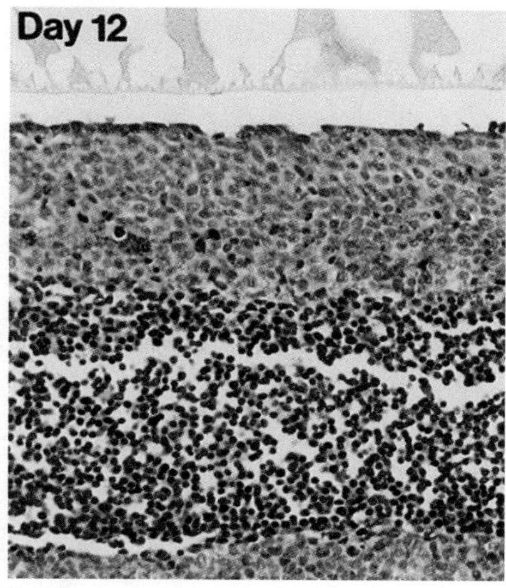

Figure 56.8. Human colon cancer cells grown in vivo in hollow fibers. Day 8 log phase growth. Day 12 stationary growth at confluence. Note central necrotic cells in the confluent tumor.

must be bioavailable to show activity, correcting for the variables of serum protein binding and drug metabolism.

Another potential advantage of hollow fiber technology is that it allows the successful maintenance of allogeneic and xenogeneic cells in immunocompetent hosts, thereby decreasing the costs associated with in vivo drug development considerably.

As currently used in the NCI program, malignant cells derived from patients with breast, kidney, lung, ovary, colon, CNS, hematologic, and melanoma cancers are encapsulated in polyvinylidene fluoride hollow fibers, which exclude molecules with a molecular weight of 500,000 or greater (80A). The fibers are then implanted either subcutaneously or intraperitoneally, with each animal hosting six samples representing three tumor cell lines each, cultured both in the peritoneal and subcutaneous spaces. Already, this technique has shown promise with known active drugs, and hollow fiber technology is increasingly being adapted to the in vivo phase of cancer drug development.

Limitations of Animal Models

IMMUNOGENICITY

The development of immunogenicity to a transplantable tumor model can complicate interpretation of treatment results. The cell kill and animal survival can become exaggerated as a result of this potential for genetic drift over time. Therefore, periodic monitoring is important to quality assurance in maintaining a stable animal model with consistent predictability.

INFECTION

Several viral infections are difficult to control in laboratory animals and require constant vigilance. These infections not only cause a decrease in the reproductive capacity but also can limit the tolerance of the animal to both tumor inoculation and therapeutic interventions. Many effects of viral infection (wasting, cachexia, or growth retardation) can mimic the dose-limiting toxicities of anticancer drugs. The most common viruses that affect laboratory mice are the mouse hepatitis virus (MHV), the Sendai virus, and the pneumonia virus of the mouse (PVM).

MHV is a major cause of death among nude mice (41). Infection can be fatal and usually (55, 56) produces cachexia and necrotizing hepatitis. Infected mice may not tolerate drugs that require hepatic clearance or that are hepatotoxic in themselves.

The Sendai virus is a common murine respiratory virus. It causes a wasting syndrome and death in immunocompromised mice (13, 41, 166). It also causes pulmonary vein thrombosis, suppurative rhinitis, and otitis media. In addition, this virus can lead to squamous metaplasia of the lung that might cause confusion in assessing tumors in these animals (130). Subclinical infection of breeding colonies can occur with no apparent symptoms (56), and continuous monitoring of animals is essential. Like the Sendai virus, PVM can induce squamous cell changes in the bronchus similar to squamous cell cancer (115). Another virus that can affect athymic mice is the mouse leukemia virus that can cause erythroleukemia. Reovirus, polyomavirus, and ectomelia are other pathogens that can affect lab animals.

Because of the high susceptibility of the nude mice for infection, strict isolation and exclusion of infected animals from experiments is essential. In addition, microbiologic monitoring is important to maintain any reproducible experimental animal model system. Microbiologic monitoring includes routine viral isolation and serologic studies on the breeding colonies.

Other Animal Models

TRANSGENIC AND CHIMERIC MICE

The transgenic mouse is the resultant progeny of the pronucleus of a fertilized egg that is injected with a foreign gene. This progeny then carries and expresses this exogenous gene and passes it on in a Mendelian fashion to its descendants (25). Genes can be transferred to the pronucleus by microinjection (24, 66, 79, 85), retroviral infection (86–89, 146), or embryonal stem cell (ESC) transfer (Fig. 56.9) (36, 81, 96). By far, the most efficient of these three strategies is microinjection. ESC provides a means to manipulate and select cells containing the transferred gene in culture prior to insertion into animals. This is accomplished by transferring the gene into ES cells, which are then transplanted into the blastocyst to create a chimeric mouse. If reproductive tissues derived from the embryonal stem cell contribute to the germ line, a transgenic mouse is established from the progeny of the chimeric animals (Fig. 56.10) (65).

The ability to integrate a gene of interest into the genome of an animal, which then expresses it, provides a novel approach for cancer investigation. Tumorigenesis can be studied through a better understanding of interactions between regulation of expressed cellular and viral oncogenes (21). Transgenic mice are excellent models for studying the consequences of oncogene expression in animals, the effect of oncogenes on growth and differentiation, and their potential for cellular transformation. These mice also provide an in vivo preclinical model for gene therapy and gene transfer.

An example of how this technique can be applied to drug development is the recent introduction of drug resistance

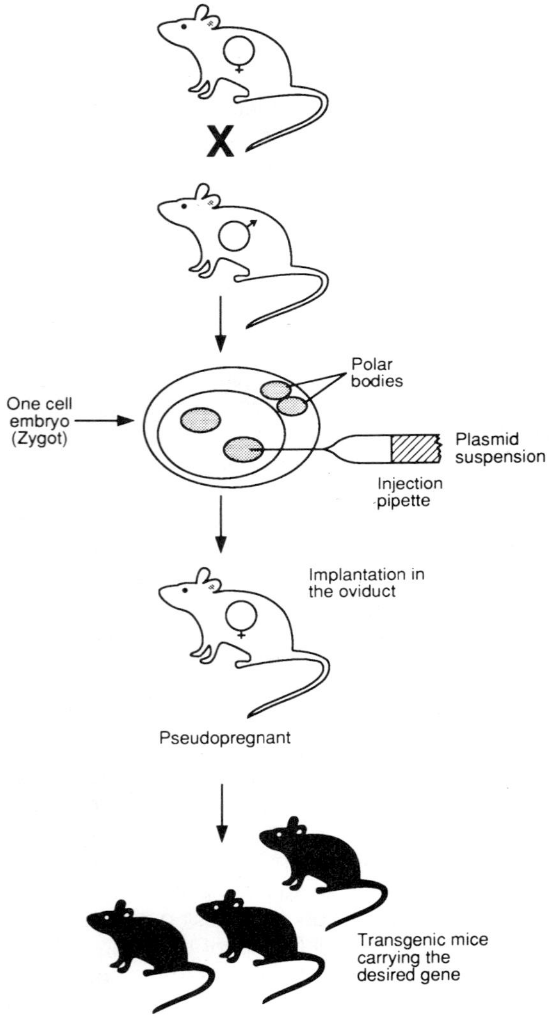

X
Polar bodies
One cell embryo (Zygot)
Plasmid suspension
Injection pipette
Implantation in the oviduct
Pseudopregnant
Transgenic mice carrying the desired gene

Figure 56.9. Transgenic mice production by pronuclear microinjection.

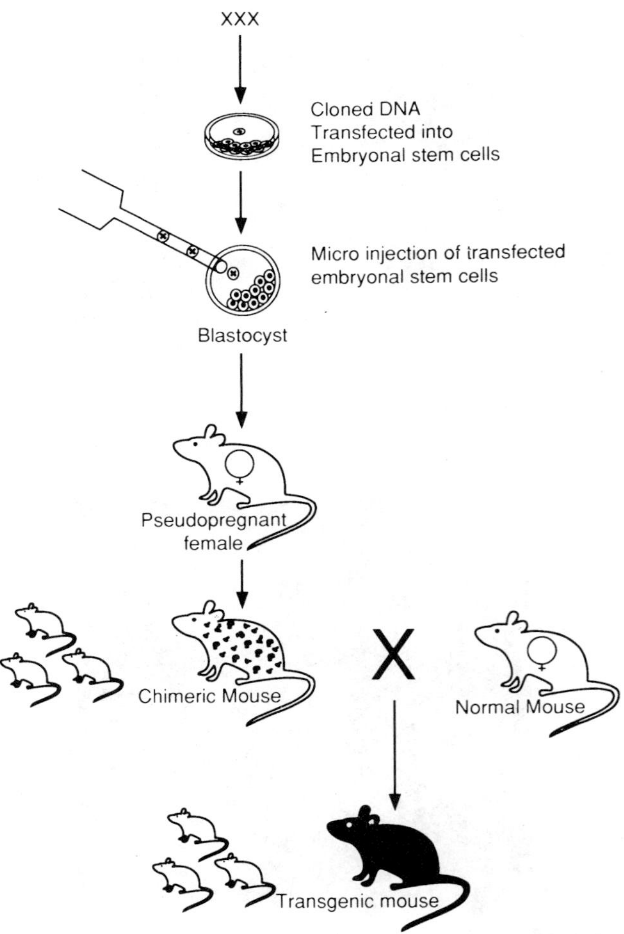

Figure 56.10. Chimeric transgenic mice derived from transfected embryonal stem cell-mediated transfer.

genes into transgenic animals. These genes include the multiple drug resistance (or *mdr* gene), which confirms resistance to a variety of important drugs of the natural product class including VP-16, Adriamycin, and the vinca alkaloids (20).

Because normal cells from transgenic mice transfected with the *mdr* gene express the same surface glycoprotein that confers drug resistance to tumor cells, they are able to tolerate normally lethal doses of anticancer drugs of the natural product class with toxicity. Such animal models may have unique roles in cancer drug development (57, 109). For example, they could be used, in an in vivo system, to screen or further evaluate drugs capable of reversing the resistance phenotype.

ANIMAL MODELS IN CANCER DRUG DEVELOPMENT

The previous section of this chapter has reviewed the role of animal models in cancer drug discovery. Following identification of a compound of interest, animal models continue to be important to the process of cancer drug development, specifically in the area of preclinical toxicology. These studies are done with a 2-fold purpose: 1) to estimate a safe starting dose for phase I clinical trials in man and 2) to predict acute and chronic toxicities in a relevant preclinical animal model. The role of the animal model has evolved in this area as well.

In the 1970s, the NCI used only dogs and monkeys in its preclinical toxicology protocols. Lethal and nonlethal doses were established in both models and chronic toxicity studies undertaken only in dogs. Starting doses for patient studies were calculated as one-third of the lowest toxic dose for the most sensitive animal model, monkey or dog (70).

In 1979, the NCI and the Food and Drug Administration reviewed existing data and agreed that toxicity studies performed largely in mice could safely replace the more costly and time-consuming large animal studies in dog and monkey models.

Currently, the LD10 (the dose of drug lethal to 10% of animals) in mice is tested in a dog model using an MELD10 or mouse equivalent LD10. This dose can be estimated from a conversion equation:

$$\text{dose (in mg/m}^2\text{) in dogs} = \frac{K_m \text{ dog}}{K_m \text{ mouse}} \times \text{dose (in mg/m}^2\text{) in mouse}$$

where K_m is the surface area to weight ratio in each species (54). This is an important equation for dose conversion between species for cancer drug development (Table 56.3). In the absence of severe toxicity in dogs, phase I trials in humans may begin at one-tenth the LD10 in mice. Of course, if severe toxicity is observed in dogs at the mouse LD10, doses are de-escalated to determine the minimally toxic dose in dogs. Clinical studies may then begin at one-third of this dose derived in dogs. Overall, the new NCI toxicology protocol has performed well in predicting safe initial doses for clinical trials, while reducing the reliance on and cost of preclinical large animal toxicology.

A new use of animals in preclinical drug development beyond simple prediction of toxicity has recently gained momentum. This is the use of preclinical pharmacology to guide dose escalation during the conduct of phase I clinical trials. As Collins and co-workers note in a recent excellent review of this concept (27), the rationale for pharmacologically guided dose escalation derives from the simple assumption that similar toxicities will occur at similar drug levels in mice and man. Since both toxicity and efficacy of anticancer drugs is related to total drug exposure, the area under the pharmacokinetic curve (AUC) has been proposed for this purpose.

Table 56.3. Surface Area to Weight Ratios (K_m) of Various Species

Species	Body weight	Surface area	Surface area to weight ratio
	(*kg*)		(K_m)
Mouse	0.02	0.0066	3.0
Rat	0.15	0.025	5.9
Monkey	3	0.24	12
Dog	8	0.40	20
Human			
Child	20	0.80	25
Adult	60	1.6	37

In essence, the AUC is measured in mice following treatment with a given drug at the LD10 dose. This is compared with the AUC in patients entering the first dose of the phase I study, which, as previously discussed, is usually one-tenth the mouse LD10. If the AUC in man is significantly lower than that observed at the LD10 in mice, dose escalation can be accelerated beyond the standard Fibonacci schema. The speed with which dose can be escalated depends upon the therapeutic index of a given agent, but two escalation schemas have been proposed. The first, a geometric mean approach, uses a dose escalation factor equal to the square root of the ratio of the AUC at the mouse LD10 to the AUC in man at the entry dose level. The second schema continues to double doses at each escalation until the AUC in man approaches that seen in the mouse at the LD10. Drug levels would continue to be monitored in all patients on study to be certain that non-linear kinetics would not cause unexpected toxicities.

This hypothesis, of course, assumes that drug metabolism and end organ sensitivity to both parent drug and metabolites are similar in mouse and man. As Collins and others have convincingly demonstrated, these assumptions generally are true so that this approach could potentially save significant time in clinical drug development. In fact, pharmacologically directed dose escalation has been successfully used to accelerate dose escalation in a number of anticancer drugs in phase I clinical trials, including HMBA, merbarone, piraxantrone, and lodoxorubicin.

Conclusions

The use of animals in cancer drug discovery and development has evolved to become both more sophisticated and efficient over the past four decades. Despite contemporary interests and pressure to decrease animal use in research, it is likely that animal models will play an increasingly important role in both cancer drug discovery and development.

To be sure, it is likely that the broad-based in vivo mouse screen using sensitive murine tumor cell lines, and which required several million mice during each year of operation, has been supplanted by more targeted screening systems that no longer require an in vivo model. The current NCI human tumor cell line screen has the theoretic advantage of being able to identify compounds specifically active in a given tumor type (e.g., breast, colon, lung) or histology (e.g. adenocarcinoma or squamous cell cancer). In addition, the assay conditions of the screen will hopefully allow the identification and characterization of new natural products from novel sources.

There are other screening models that require neither animals nor living cells. These screens select biochemical targets that can be purified and then inhibited as part of a screen. Examples include the P170 glycoprotein (screening for compounds that displace active drugs from the binding site, and that could reverse the multiple drug resistance phenotype), inhibitors of DNA topoisomerases or drugs that bind to specific growth factor receptors.

While these new screening systems are now possible because of a better understanding of the biology and growth requirements of cancer cells, they do not supplant animals entirely. Once a screen of any kind has identified an interesting lead, intermediate steps requiring animals will still be required prior to clinical trials in man.

These studies at a minimum include confirming activity against a given tumor in a relevant animal model, growth delay or improved survival in nude mice, inhibition of orthotopic tumor growth, or significant cell kill in the microencapsulation model. The animal model is critical in taking the screen one step closer to the clinic. It confirms that the drug and/or its metabolites reach their target and demonstrate a positive and reproducible therapeutic effect.

While this chapter has focused on cancer drug discovery and development, animal models have a special role in the development of biologic agents. Here the relevant biologic endpoints may not cross species. For example, G-CSF does not affect bone marrow function in mice, while GM-CSF treatment induces a profound leucocytosis in mice. These agents may require animal models closer to man (non-human primates) or other systems, such as the SCID (severe combined immunodeficiency) mouse model, in which the human immune system can be selectively introduced and the effects of biological agents monitored in a controlled, yet essentially human, milieu.

Just as the role of animals in cancer drug discovery has become more refined over time, so too has their role in drug development. The general convertibility of doses between species has decreased the need for larger animals (non-human primates and dogs) during preclinical toxicology. The incorporation of pharmacokinetics into preclinical toxicology has become routine and is appealing for a number of reasons. Such studies provide insights into drug metabolism as it relates to end organ toxicity and can determine whether saturable (non-linear) kinetics contribute to the therapeutic index. Perhaps most interesting is the recent successful application of pharmacologically directed dose escalation to phase I studies in man and the refinement that this approach will give to what has been a largely empiric area of clinical research.

Appropriate use of animal models is essential to the successful, efficient and safe discovery and development of new treatments for patients with cancer. The lessons learned will hopefully have a positive influence on the development of new therapies for other diseases as well.

References

1. Aamdal S, Fostad O, Kaalhus O, Phil A. Chemosensitivity profiles of human cancers assessed by the 6-day SRC assay on serially xenografted tumors. Int J Cancer 1986;37:579.
2. Aamdal S, Fodstad O, Phil A. Human tumor xenografts transplanted under the renal capsule of conventional mice: growth rates and host immune response. Int J Cancer 1984;34:725.
3. Aamdal S, Fodstad O, Phil A. Methodological aspects of the 6-day subrenal capsule assay for measuring response of human tumors to anticancer agents. Anticancer Res 1985;5:329.
4. Ad Hoc review committee proceedings for National Cancer Institute. In Vitro/In Vivo Disease-oriented Screening Project. NCI, National Institutes of Health. Bethesda, MD, September 23–24, 1985.
5. Ad Hoc review committee proceedings for National Cancer Institute. In Vitro/In Vivo Disease-oriented Screening Project. NCI, National Institutes of Health, Bethesda, MD, December 8–9, 1986.
6. Ad Hoc review committee proceedings for National Cancer Institute. In Vitro/In Vivo Disease-oriented Screening Project. NCI, National Institutes of Health, Bethesda, MD, December 8–9, 1989.
7. Alley MC, Hursey ML, Pacula-Cox CM, Stinson SF, McLemore TL, Boyd MR. Suitability of multicellular growth units in soft agar culture for experimental drug evaluations and morphologic examinations. Proc Am Assoc Cancer Res 1989;30:529.
8. Alley MC, Scudiero DA, Monks A, Hursey ML, Czerwinski MJ, Fine DL, Abbott BJ, Mayo JG, Shoemaker RH, Boyd MR. Feasibility of drug screening with panels of human tumor cell lines using a microculture tetrazolium assay. Cancer Res 1988;48:589.
9. Begg AC. Analysis of growth delay data: potential pitfalls. Br J Cancer 1980;41(suppl IV):93.
10. Begg AC. Principles and practices of the tumor growth delay assay. In Rodent Tumor Models in Experimental Cancer Therapy. Edited by RF Kallman. New York: Pergamon, 1987, p 114.
11. Bellet RE, Danna V, Mastrangelo MJ, Berd D. Evaluation of a nude mouse-human tumor panel as a predictive secondary screen for cancer chemotherapeutic agents. JNCI 1979;63:1185.
12. Bennett JA, Pilon VA, MacDowell RT. Evaluation of growth and histology of human tumor xenografts implanted under the renal capsule of immunocompetent and immunodeficient mice. Cancer Res 1985;45:4963.
13. Blandford G, Cureton RJ, Heath RB. Studies of the immune response in Sendai virus infection of mice. J Med Microbiol 1971;4:351.
14. Bogden AE, Griffin W, Reich SD, Constanza ME, Cobb WR. Predictive testing with the subrenal capsule assay. Cancer Treat Rev 1984;11:113.
15. Bogden AE, Haskell PM, LePage DJ, Kelton D, Cobb WR, Esber HJ. Growth of human tumor xenografts implanted under the renal capsule of normal immunocompetent mice. Exp Cell Biol 1979;47:218.
16. Bogden AE, Kelton DE, Cobb WR, Esber HJ. In Proceedings of the Symposium on the Use of Athymic (Nude) Mice in Cancer Res. Edited by DP Houchens and AA Ovejera. New York: Gustav Fisher, 1978, p 231.
17. Boyd MR. National Cancer Institute drug discovery and development. In Accomplishments in Oncology: Cancer Therapy: Where Do We Go From Here? vol 1, no 1. Edited by E Frei and EJ Freireich. Philadelphia: Lippincott, 1986.
18. Boyd MR. NIH new drug program. Proceedings of the IV World Conference on Lung Cancer, Toronto, Canada, August 1985:25–30. Chest 1986;89:355S.
19. Boyd MR. Status of implementation of the NCI human tumor cell line in vitro primary drug screen. Proc Am Assoc Cancer Res 1989;30:652.
20. Boyd MR. Status of the NCI preclinical antitumor drug discovery screen. In Principles and Practice of Oncology Updates. Edited by VT DeVita, S Hellman, and SA Rosenberg. Philadelphia: Lippincott, 1981.
21. Boyd MR, Shoemaker R, Alley M, et al. New NCI disease-oriented drug screening program. In Proceedings of the 5th NCI-EORTC Symposium on New Drugs Cancer Therapy. Amsterdam, 1986.
22. Boyd MR, Shoemaker RH, Cragg GM, Suffness M. New avenues of investigation of marine biologicals in the anticancer drug discovery program of the National Cancer Institute. In Pharmaceuticals and the Sea. Edited by CW Rinehart, KL Rinehart, and LS Shields. Lancaster: Technomic Publishing AG 1988.
23. Boyd MR, Shoemaker RH, McLemore TL, et al. New drug development. In Thoracic Oncology. Edited by J Roth, JC Ruckdescel, and THE Weisenburger. Philadelphia: Saunders, 1989.
24. Brinster RL, Chen HY, Trumbauer ME, Yagle MK, Palmiter RD. Factors affecting the efficiency of introducing foreign DNA into mice by microinjecting eggs. Proc Natl Acad Sci USA 1985;82:4438.
25. Brinster RL, Palmiter RD. Introduction of genes into germ line of animals. Harvey Lect 1985;80:1.
26. Bruce WR, Meeker BE, Valeriote F. A comparison of the sensitivity of normal hematopoietic and transplanted lymphoma colony-forming cells to chemotherapeutic agents administered in vivo. JNCI 1966;37:233.
27. Collins JM, Grieshaber CK, Chabner BA. Pharmacologically guided Phase I clinical trials based on preclinical drug development. JNCI 1990;82:1321.
28. Corbett TH, Griswold DP Jr, Roberts BJ, Peckham JC, Schabel FM Jr. Tumor induc-

tion relationships in development of transplantable cancers of the colon in mice for chemotherapy assays, with a note on carcinogen structure. Cancer Res 1975;35: 2434.
29. Corbett TH, Roberts BJ, Leopold WR, Peckham JC, Wilhoff LJ, Griswold DP Jr, Schabel FM Jr. Induction and chemotherapeutic response of two transplantable ductal adenocarcinomas of the pancreas in C57B2/6 mice. Cancer Res 1984;44:717.
30. Corbett TH, Valeriote FA, Baker LH. Is the P388 murine tumor no longer adequate as a drug discovery model? Invest New Drugs 1987;5:3.
31. Danks MK, Yalowich JC, Bech WT. Atypical multiple drug resistance in a human leukemic cell line selected for resistance to teniposide (VM-26). Cancer Res 1987;47: 1297.
32. Davis AJS, Leuchars E, Wallis V, Koler PC. The mitotic response of thymus-derived cells to antigenic stimulus. Transplantation 1966;4:4348.
33. DeVita VT, Oliverio VT, Muggia FM, et al. The drug development and clinical trials programs of the Division of Cancer Treatment, National Cancer Institute. Cancer Clin Trials 2:195;1979.
34. DeVita VT, Schein PS. The use of drugs in combination for the therapy of cancer. N Engl J Med 1973;288:998.
35. Division of Cancer Treatment Board approves new screening program, natural products concepts. Cancer Lett 1985;11:4.
36. Doetschman TC, Eistetter H, Katz M, Schmidt W, Kemler R. The in vitro development of blastocyst-derived embryonic stem cell lines: formation of visceral yolk sac, blood islands and myocardium. J Embryol Exp Morphol 1985;87:27.
37. Donovick R, Alley AM, Stinson S, McLemore T, Mayo J, Shoemaker R, Fiebig H, Boyd M. Current status and future development of "disease-oriented" panels of human tumor cell lines for use in the NCI anticancer drug screen. Proc Am Assoc Cancer Res 1989;30:611.
38. Driscoll JS. The preclinical new drug research program of the National Cancer Institute. Cancer Treat Rep 1984;68:63.
39. Dumont P, VanderEsch EP, Jabri M, Lejeune F, Atassi G. Chemosensitivity of human melanoma xenografts in immunocompetent mice and its histological evaluation. Int J Cancer 1984;33:447.
40. Dykes DJ, Mayo JG, Abbott BJ, Harrison SD Jr, Laster WR Jr, Simpson-Herren L, Griswold DP Jr, Boyd MR. In vivo growth characteristics of human tumor xenografts from the NCI in vitro "disease-oriented" drug discovery program. Proc Am Assoc Cancer Res 1989;30:614.
41. Eaton GJ, Outzen HC, Custer RP, Johnson FN. Husbandry of the "nude" mouse in conventional and germ-free environments. Lab Anim Sci 1975;25:309.
42. Edelstein MB, Smink T, Ruiter DJ, Visser W, Van Putten LM. Improvements and limitations of the subrenal capsule assay for determining tumour sensitivity to cytostatic drugs. Eur J Cancer Clin Oncol 1984;20:1549.
43. Edelstein MD, Fiebig HH, Smink T, Van Putten LM, Schuchhardt C. Comparison between macroscopic and microscopic evaluation of tumor responsiveness using the subrenal capsule assay. Eur J Cancer Clin Oncol 1983;19:995.
44. Fidler IJ. Rationale and methods for the use of nude mice to study the biology and therapy of human cancer metastasis. Cancer Metastasis Rev 1986;5:29.
45. Fiebig HH, Weigeldt H, Schuchhardt C, Zeschnigk C, Lohr GW. Transplantation of human tumors under the renal capsule of nude, immunocompetent and preirradiated normal mice. In Advances in the Chemotherapy of Gastrointestinal Cancer. Edited by HD Klein and H Kohn. Erlanden: perimed Fachbuch-Verlagsgesellschaft 1984, p 27.
46. Fiebig HH, Schuchhardt C, Henss H, Fiedler L, Lohr GS. Comparison of tumor response in nude mice and in the patients. Behring Inst Mitt 1984;74:343.
47. Fiebig HH, Winterhalter B, Berger D, Wittekind C, Bender K, Selby M, Bittner C, Alley M, Boyd M. Properties of 6 human tumor xenografts in vivo from which cell lines were developed. Proc Am Assoc Cancer Res 1989;30:612.
48. Fine DL, Shoemaker R, Gazdar A, Mayo JG, Fodstad O, Boyd MR, Abbott BJ, Donovan PA. Metastatic models of human tumors in athymic mice: useful models for drug development. Cancer Detect Prev (suppl) 1987;1:291.
49. Finney DJ. Statistical Method in Biological Assay, 2nd ed. London: Charles Griffin, 1964, p 524.
50. Flanagan SP. Nude, a new hairless gene with pleiotropic effects in the mouse. Genet Res 1966;8:295.
51. Fodstad O, Aas N, Phil A. Response to chemotherapy of human, malignant melanoma xenografts in athymic, nude mice. Int J Cancer 1980;25:453.
52. Fogh J, Trempe G. In Human Cells in Vitro New Human Tumor Cell Line. Edited by J Fogh. New York: Plenum, 1975, p 115.
53. Fogh J, Giovanella BC. (eds.) The Nude Mouse in Experimental and Clinical Research. New York: Academic, 1978.
54. Freireich EJ, Gehan EA, Rall DP, Schmidt LH, Skipper HE. Quantitative comparison of toxicity of anticancer agents in mouse, rat, hamster, dog, monkey and man. Cancer Chemother Rep 1966;50:219.
55. Fujiwara K. Spontaneous virus infections of nude mice. In The Nude Mouse in Experimental and Clinical Research. Edited by J Fogh and BC Giovalla, 1982, p 1.
56. Fujiwara K, Takenaka S, Shumiya, S. Carrier state of antibody and viruses in a mouse breeding colony persistently infected with Sendai and mouse hepatitis viruses. Lab Anim Sci 26(suppl 2, part 1):153 1976.
57. Galski H, Sullivan M, Willingham MC, Chin K-V, Gottesman MM, Pastan I, Merlino GT. Expression of a human multidrug resistance cDNA (MDR1) in the bone marrow of transgenic mice: resistance to daunomycin-induced leukopenia. Mol Cell Biol 1989;9: 4357.
58. Gazdar AF, Carney DN, Sims HL, Simmons A. Heterotransplantation of small cell carcinoma of the lung into nude mice: comparison of intracranial and subcutaneous route. Int J Cancer 1981;28:777.
59. Gazdar AF, Shoemaker R, Mayo J, Oie HK, Donovan P, Fine D. Human lung cancer xenografts and metastases in athymic (nude) mice. In Immune-deficient animals in biomedical research, 5th International Workshop. Edited by N Rygaard, N Brunner, N Graem, and M Spang-Thornsen. Basel: Karger, 1987, p 277.
60. Giovanella BC, Stehlin JS, Shepard RC. Experimental chemotherapy of human breast carcinomas heterotransplanted in nude mice. In Proceedings Second International Workshop on Nude Mice. Tokyo: University of Tokyo Press, 1977, p 475.
61. Giovanella BC, Stehlin JS, Shepard RC, Williams LJ. Correlation between response to chemotherapy of human tumors in patients and in nude mice. Cancer 1983;52:1146.
62. Goldin A, Carter SK. Screening and Evaluation of Antitumor Agents. In Cancer Medicine. Edited by JF Holland and E Frei III. Philadelphia: Lea & Febiger, 1982, p 633.
63. Goldin A, Schepartz SA, Venditti JM, et al. Historical development and current strategy of the National Cancer Institute Drug Development Program. In Methods of Cancer Res, vol 16. Edited by VT DeVita, and H Busch. New York: Academic, 1979, p 165.
64. Goldin A, Venditti JM, Macdonald JS, Muggia FM, Henney JE, DeVita VT, Jr. Current results of the screening program at the Division of Cancer Treatment, National Cancer Institute. Eur J Cancer 1981;17:129.
65. Gordon JW. Transgenic animals. Int Rev Cytol 1989;115:171.
66. Gordon JW, Ruddle FH. Gene transfer into mouse embryos: production of transgenic mice by pronuclear injection. Methods Enzymol 1983;101:411.
67. Gorelik E, Alley M, Shoemaker R. A new in vivo short-term assay for evaluation of antitumor chemotherapeutic drugs. Proc Am Assoc Cancer Res 1986;27:389.
68. Gorelik E, Ovejera A, Shoemaker R, Jarvis A, Alley M, Doff R, Mayo J, Herberman R, Boyd M. Microencapsulated tumor assay: new short-term assay for in vivo evaluation of the effects of anticancer drugs on human tumor cell lines. Cancer Res 1987;47: 5739.
69. Goustin AS, Leof EB, Shipley GD, Moses HL. Growth factors and cancer. Cancer Res 1986;46:1015.
70. Grieshaber CK, Marsoni S. Relation of preclinical toxicology to findings in early clinical trials. Cancer Treatment Reports 1986;70:65.
71. Gupta RS. Genetic, biochemical and cross-resistance studies with mutants of Chinese hamster ovary cells resistant to the anticancer drugs, VM-26 and VP16–213. Cancer Res 1983;43:1568.
72. Hart IR. "Seed and soil" revisited: Mechanisms of site-specific metastasis. Cancer Met Rev 1982;1:5.
73. Herberman RB. Natural cell-mediated cytotoxicity in nude mice. In The Nude Mouse in Experimental and Clinical Research. Edited by J Fogh and BC Herbeman. New York: Academic, 1978, p 135.
74. Hill RP. An appraisal in vivo assays of excised tumours. Br J Cancer 1980;41(suppl IV):230.
75. Hill RP. Excision assay. In Rodent Tumor Models in Experimental Cancer Therapy. Edited by RF Kallman. New York: Pergamon, 1987, p 67.
76. Hill RP. The assay of tumour colonies in the lung. In Cell Clones: A Manual of Mammalian Cell Techniques. Edited by C Potten and JH Hendry. London: Churchill Livingstone, 1985, p 208.
77. Hill RP. The TD50 assay for tumour cells. In Cell Clones: A Manual of Mammalian Cell Techniques. Edited by C Potten and JH Hendry. London: Churchill Livingstone, 1985, p 223.
78. Hirschberg E. Patterns of response of animal tumors to anticancer agents. Cancer Res 1963;23:(suppl 5, Part 2):521.
79. Hogan B, Constantini F, Lacy E. Manipulating the mouse embryo: a laboratory manual. Edited by D. Hanahan. Cold Spring Harbor Laboratory Manual. Cold Spring Harbor, NY: Cold Spring Harbor Laboratory Press, 1986.
80. Holden HT, Herberman RB, Santoni A, et al. Natural cell-mediated cytotoxicity in nude mice. In Proceedings of the Symposium on the Use of Athymic Nude Mice in Cancer Res. Edited by DP Houchens and AA Ovejera. New York: Gustav Fischer 1978:p 81.
80a. Hollingshead, MG, Alley MC, CamAlier RF, Abbott BJ, Mayo JG, Malspeis L, Grever MR. In vivo cultivation of tumor cells in hollow fibers. Life Sci 57:131–141, 1995.
81. Hooper M, Hardy K, Handyside A, Hunter S, Monk M. HPRT-deficient (Lesch-Nyhan) mouse embryos derived from germline colonization by cultured cells. Nature 1987;326:292.
82. Houchens DP, Ovejera AA. (eds.). Proceedings of the Symposium on the Use of Athymic Nude Mice in Cancer Res. New York: Gustav Fischer, 1978.
83. Houghton JA, Taylor DM. Growth characteristics of human colorectal tumours during serial passage in immune-deprived mice. Br J Cancer 1978;37:213.
84. Isaacson JH, Cottanach BM. Report. Mouse Newsletter 1962;27:31.
85. Jaenisch R. Infection of mouse blastocysts with SV40 DNA: normal development of the infected embryos and persistence of SV40-specific DNA sequences in the adult animals. Cold Spring Harb Symp Quant Biol 1975;39:375.
86. Jaenisch R. Retroviruses and embryogenesis: microinjection of Moloney leukemia virus into midgestation mouse embryos. Cell 1980;19:181.
87. Jaenisch R, Kahner D, Nobis P, Simon I, Lohler J, Harbers K, Grotkopp D. Chromosomal position and activation of retroviral genomes inserted into the germ line of mice. Cell 1981;24:519.
88. Jaenisch R, Mintz B. Simian virus 40 DNA sequences in DNA of healthy adult mice derived from preimplantation blastocysts infected with viral DNA. Proc Natl Acad Sci USA 1974;71:1250.
89. Jahner D, Jaenisch R. Integration of Moloney leukaemia virus into the germ line of mice: correlation between site of integration and virus activation. Nature 1980;287: 456.
90. Jarvis AP, Grdina TA. Production of biologicals from microencapsulated living cells. BioTechniques 1983;1:22.
91. Johnson RD, Goldin A. The clinical impact of screening and other experimental tumor studies. Cancer Treat Rev 1975;2:1.
92. Jung H, Beck HP, Brammer I, Zywietz F. Depopulation and repopulation of R1H rhabdomyosarcoma of the rat after X-irradiation. Eur J Cancer 1981;17:375.
93. Kallman RF, Silini G, Van Putten LM. Factors influencing the quantitative estimation of the in vivo survival of cells from solid tumors. JNCI 1967;39:539.
94. Kerbel RS, Frost P, Liteplo R, Carlow DA, Elliot BE. Possible epigenetic mechanism of tumor progression: induction of high-frequency heritable but phenotypically unstable changes in the tumorigenic and metastatic properties of tumor cell populations by 5-azacytidine treatment. J Cell Physiol 1984;3:(suppl)87.
95. Korman LY, Carney DN, Citron ML, Moody TW. Secretin/vasoactive intestinal peptide-stimulated secretion of bombesin/gastrin releasing peptide from human small cell carcinoma of the lung. Cancer Res 1986;46:1214.
96. Kuehn MR, Bradley A, Robertson EJ, Evans MJ. A potential animal model for Lesch-Nyhan syndrome through introduction of HPRT mutations into mice. Nature 1987;326: 295.
97. Lee SS, Giovanella BC, Stehlin JS Jr, Brunn JC. Progression of human tumors established in nude mice after continuous infusion of thymidine. Cancer Res 1979;39:2928.
98. Levi FA, Blum JP, Lemaigre G, Bourut C, Reinberg A, Mathe G. A four-day subrenal capsule assay for testing the effectiveness of anticancer drugs against human tumors. Cancer Res 1984;44:2660.

99. Marsoni S, Hoth D, Simon R, Leyland-Jones B, De Rosa M, Wittes RE. Clinical Drug Development: an analysis of phase II Trials 1970–1985. Cancer Treat Rep 1987;71: 71.
100. Martin DS, Fugmann RA, Stolfi RL, Hayworth PE. Solid tumor animal model therapeutically predictive for human breast cancer. Cancer Chemother Rep 1975;5:(part 2)89.
101. McCredie JA, Inch WR, Sutherl RM. Differences in growth and morphology between the spontaneous C3H mammary carcinoma in the mouse and its syngeneic transplants. Cancer 1971;27:635.
102. McLemore TL, Abbott BJ, Mayo JG, Boyd MR. Development and application of new orthotopic in vivo models for use in the U.S. National Cancer Institute's drug screening program. In 6th International Workshop on Immunodeficient Animals in Biomedical Research. Edited by B Wu and JS Zheng. Basel: S. Karger, AG, 1988.
103. McLemore T, Alley M, Liu M, Hubbard W, Adelberg S, Czerwinski M, Yu S, Stinson S, Storeng R, Eggleston J, Boyd M. Histopathologic, biochemical and molecular genetic characterization of four newly established human pulmonary carcinoma cell lines. Proc Am Assoc Cancer Res 1989;30:225.
104. McLemore TL, Eggleston JC, Shoemaker RH, Abbott BJ, Bohlman ME, Liu MC, Fine DL, Mayo JG, Boyd MR. Comparison of intrapulmonary, percutaneous intrathoracic and subcutaneous models for the propagation of human pulmonary and nonpulmonary cancer cell lines in athymic nude mice. Cancer Res 1988;48:2880.
105. McLemore TL, Liu MC, Blacker PC, Gregg M, Alley MC, Abbott BJ, Shoemaker RH, Bohlman ME, Litterst CC, Hubbard WC. Novel intrapulmonary model for orthotopic propagation of human lung cancers in athymic nude mice. Cancer Res 1987;47: 5132.
106. McLemore TL, Liu MC, Blacker PC. Comparison of intrapulmonary, percutaneous intrathoracic and subcutaneous models for the propagation of human pulmonary and non-pulmonary cancer cell lines in athymic nude mice. Cancer Res 1988;48:2880.
107. McLemore T, Storeng R, Adelberg S, Czerwinski M, Yu S, Nhamburo P, Gonzalez F, Hines R, Boyd M. Expression of different cytochrome P450 genes in human lung cancer cell lines. Proc Am Assoc Cancer Res 1989;30:11.
108. McNally NJ, DeRonde J. Radiobiological studies of tumours in situ compared with cell survival. Br J Cancer 1980;41(suppl IV):259.
109. Mickisch GH, Merlino GT, Galski H, Gottesman MM, Pastan I. Transgenic mice that express the human multidrug-resistance gene in bone marrow enable a rapid identification of agents that reverse drug resistance. Proc Natl Acad Sci USA 1991;88:547.
110. Moody TW, Pert CB, Gazdar AF, Carnay DN, Minna JD. High levels of intracellular bombesin characterize human small cell lung carcinoma. Science 1986;214:1246.
111. Naito S, von Eschenhach AC, Fidler IJ. Different growth patterns and biologic behavior of human renal cell carcinoma implanted into different organs of nude mice. JNCI 1987;78:377.
112. Naito S, von Eschenbach AC, Giavazzi R, Fidler IJ. Growth and metastasis of tumor cells isolated from a human renal cell carcinoma implanted into different organs of nude mice. Cancer Res 1986;46:4109.
113. National Cancer Institute planning to switch drug development emphasis from compound to human cancer-oriented strategy. Cancer Lett 1984;10:1.
114. Neeley JE, Ballard ET, Britt AL, Workman L. Characteristics of 85 pediatric tumors heterografted into nude mice. Exp Cell Biol 1983;51:217.
115. Nettesheim P, Schreiber H, Creasia DA, Richter CB. Respiratory infections and the pathogenesis of lung cancer. Recent Results Cancer Res 1974;44:138.
116. Nicolson G. Tumor cell instability, diversification, and progression to metastatic phenotype: from oncogene to oncofetal expression. Cancer Res 1987;47:1473.
117. Nicolson GL. Organ colonization and the cell surface properties of malignant cells. Biochim Biophys Acta 1982;695:113.
118. Nomura T, Oshawa N, Tamaoki N, et al. Proceedings of the Second International Workshop on Nude Mice. Tokyo: University of Tokyo Press, 1977.
119. Nowak K, Peckham MJ, Steel GG. Variation in response of xenografts of colorectal carcinoma to chemotherapy. Br J Cancer 1978;37:576.
120. Ovejera AA. The Use of Human Tumor Xenografts in Large-Scale Drug Screening. In Rodent Tumor Models in Experimental Cancer Therapy. Edited by R F Kallman. 1987, p 218.
121. Ovejera AA, Houchens DP. Human tumor xenografts in athymic nude mice as a preclinical screen for anticancer agents. Semin Oncol 1981;8:386.
122. Ovejera AA, Johnson RK, Goldin A. Growth characteristics and chemotherapeutic response of intravenously implanted Lewis lung carcinoma. Cancer Chemother Rep 1975;5(part 2):111.
123. Paget S. The distribution of secondary growths in cancer of the breast. Lancet 1889;1:571.
124. Pantelouris EM. Absence of a thymus in a mouse mutant. Nature 1968;217:370.
125. Pattengale PK, Stewart TA, Leder A, Sinn E, Muller W, Tepler I, Schmidt E, Leder P. Animal models of human disease. Pathology and molecular biology of spontaneous neoplasms occurring in transgenic mice carrying and expressing activated cellular oncogenes. Am J Pathol 1989;135:39.
126. Poste G. Experimental systems for analysis of the malignant phenotype. Cancer Met Rev 1982;1:141.
127. Poste G, Fidler IJ. The pathogenesis of cancer metastasis. Nature 1980;283:139.
128. Povlsen CO, Rygaard J. Heterotransplantation of human adenocarcinoma of the colon and rectum to the nude mouse: a study of nine consecutive transplantations. Acta Pathol Microbiol Scand 1971;79:159.
129. Raff MC, Wortis HH. Thymus dependence of Theta-bearing cells in the peripheral lymphoid tissue of mice. Immunology 1970;18:1931.
130. Richter CB. In "Morphology of Experimental Respiratory Carcinogenesis." AEC Symposium Series 1971;21:365.
131. Rockwell S. In vivo-in vitro tumor systems: new models for studying the response of tumors to therapy. Lab Anim Sci 1977;27:831.
132. Rockwell S. In vivo-in vitro tumour cell lines: characteristics and limitations as models for human cancer. Br J Cancer 1980;41(suppl IV):118.
133. Rockwell SC, Kallman RF, Fajardo LF. Characteristics of a serially transplanted mouse mammary tumor and its tissue-culture adapted derivative. JNCI 1972;49:735.
134. Rygaard J, Povlsen CO. Athymic (nude) mice. In The Mouse in Biochemical Research, vol. VI. Edited by HL Foster, JD Small, and JG Fox. New York: Academic Press, 1982, p 51.
135. Rygaard J, Povlsen CO. (eds.). Bibliography of the Nude Mouse. Stuttgart/New York: Gustav Fischer Verlag, 1977.
136. Rygaard J, Povlsen CO. Heterotransplantation of a human malignant tumor in nude mice. Acta Pathol Microbiol Scand 1969;77:758.
137. Rygaard J, Povlsen CO. (eds.). Proceedings of the First International Workshop on Nude Mice. Stuttgart: Gustav Fischer Verlag, 1974.
138. Schepartz SA. Memorandum to suppliers of compounds. In Methods of Development of New Anticancer Drugs, National Cancer Institute Monograph 45, DHEW Publication (NIH) 76-1037, 1977, p 155.
139. Shapiro WR, Basler GA, Chernick NL, Posner JB. Human brain tumor transplantation into nude mice. JNCI 1979;62:447.
140. Sharkey FE, Fogh J, Hajdu S, Fitzgerald P, Fogh J. Experience in surgical pathology with human tumor growth in the nude mouse. In The Nude Mouse in Experimental and Clinical Research. Edited by J Fogh and B Giovanella. New York: Academic, 1978, p 188.
141. Shoemaker RH, Monks A, Alley MC, et al. Development of human tumor cell line panels for use in disease-oriented drug screening. In Prediction of Response to Cancer Chemotherapy. Edited by T Hall. New York: Alan Liss, 1988.
142. Shorthouse AJ, Peckham MJ, Smyth JF, Steel GG. The therapeutic response of bronchial carcinoma xenografts: a direct patient-xenograft comparison. Br J Cancer 1980;41(suppl IV):142.
143. Shorthouse AJ, Smyth JF, Steel GG, Ellison M, Mills J, Peckham MJ. The human tumour xenograft—a valid model in experimental chemotherapy? Br J Surg 1980;67: 715.
144. Siemann DW. Satisfactory and unsatisfactory tumor models: factors influencing the selection of a tumor model for experimental evaluation. In Rodent Tumor Models in Experimental Cancer Therapy. Edited by RF Kallman. 1987, p 12.
145. Skipper HE, Schmidt LH. Background: description of criteria, and presentation of quantitative therapeutic data on various classes of drugs obtained in diverse experimental tumor systems. Cancer Chemother Rep 1962;17:1.
146. Soriano P, Jaenisch R. Retroviruses as probes for mammalian developments: allocation of cells to the somatic and germ cell lineages. Cell 1986:46;19.
147. Sprent J, Miller J. Thoracic duct lymphocytes from nude mice: migratory properties and life span. Eur J Immunol 1972;2:384.
148. Staquet MJ, Byar DP, Green SB, Rozencweig M. Clinical predictivity of transplantable tumor systems in the selection of new drugs for solid tumors: rationale for a three-stage strategy. Cancer Treat Rep 1983;67:753.
149. Steel GG. Growth Kinetics of Tumours. Oxford: Oxford University Press, 1977.
150. Steel GG, Courtenay VD, Peckham MJ. The response to chemotherapy of a variety of human tumour xenografts. Br J Cancer 1983;47:1.
151. Steel GG, Adams K, Hodgett J, Janik P. Cell population kinetics of a spontaneous rat tumor during serial transplantation. Br J Cancer 1971;25:802.
152. Steel GG, Stephens TC. Stem cells in tumours. In Stem Cells: Their Identification and Characterization. Edited by CS Pottern. London: Churchill Livingstone, 1983, p 271.
153. Stephens TC. Measurement of tumor cell surviving faction and absolute numbers of clonogens per tumor in excision assays. In Rodent Tumor Models in Experimental Cancer Therapy. Edited by RF Kallman. New York: Pergamon Press, 1987, p 90.
154. Stephens TC, Currie GA, Peacock JH. Repopulation of irradiated Lewis lung carcinoma by malignant cells and host macrophage progenitors. Br J Cancer 1978;38: 573.
155. Stinson SF, Alley MC, Kenney S, Fiebig S, Boyd MR. Morphologic characterization of human carcinoma cell lines. Proc Am Assoc Cancer Res 1989;30:613.
156. Stratton JA, Kucera PR, Micha JP, Rettenmaier MA, Braly PS, Berman ML, Di Saia PJ. The subrenal capsule tumor implant assay as predictor of clinical response to chemotherapy: 3 years of experience. Gynecol Oncol 1984;19:336.
157. Thomlinson RH. An experimental method for comparing treatments of intact malignant tumours in animals and its application to the use of oxygen in radiotherapy. Br J Cancer 1980;14:555.
158. Toolan HW. Successful subcutaneous growth and transplantation for human tumors in X-irradiated laboratory animals. Proc Soc Exp Biol Med 1951;77:572.
159. Toolan HW. Transplantable human neoplasms maintained in cortisone-treated laboratory animals: HS #1, HEP #1, HEP #2, HEP #3, and HENBRH #1. Cancer Res 1954;14:660.
160. Tueni EA, Dumont P, Jacobovitz D, Massi G, Rocmans P, Lejeune F, de Franquer P, Semal P, Klastersky J. Subrenal capsule assay for fresh human tumors in immunocompetent mice; an inappropriate technique for non-small cell lung cancer. Eur J Cancer Clin Oncol 1987;23:1163.
161. Uvarov O. Research with animals: requirements, responsibilities, welfare. Lab Animal 1985;19:51.
162. Venditti JM. Foreword. In Proceedings of the Symposium on the Use of Athymic Nude Mice in Cancer Res. Edited by DP Houchens and AA Ovejera. New York: Gustav Fischer, 1978.
163. Venditti JM. Preclinical drug development: rationale and methods. Semin Oncol 1981;8:349.
164. Venditti JM. The model's dilemma. In Design of Models for Testing Cancer Chemotherapeutic Agents. Edited by IJ Fidler and RJ White. New York: Van Nostrand Reinhold, 1981, p 80.
165. Venditti JM. The National Cancer Institute Drug Discovery Program current and future perspectives. A commentary. Cancer Treat Rep 1983;67:767.
166. Ward JM, Houchens DP, Collins MJ, Young DM, Reagan RL. Naturally-occurring Sendai virus infection of athymic nude mice. Vet Pathol 1976;13:36.
167. Workshop on "Disease-oriented Antitumor Drug Discovery and Development," NIH, Bethesda MD, January 9–10, 1985. Sponsored by Developmental Therapeutics Program, Division of Cancer Treatment, National Cancer Institute.
168. Zubrod CG. Chemical control of cancer. Proc Natl Acad Sci USA 1972;69:1042.
169. Zubrod CG, Schepartz S, Leiter J, et al. The Chemotherapy Program of the National Cancer Institute: History, Analysis and Plans. Cancer Chemother Rep 1966;50:349.

CHAPTER 57

In Vitro and In Vivo Predictive Tests

AXEL-R. HANAUSKE AND DANIEL D. VON HOFF

Introduction

Most patients with cancer require treatment with chemotherapeutic agents in the course of their disease. Current treatment recommendations rest on carefully designed clinical studies of large patient populations that provide the individual patient with a probability of response based on clinically observed response rates. This approach has resulted in major progress in clinical oncology and has helped to identify curative therapeutic regimens for testicular cancer, some leukemias, some malignant lymphomas, and childhood tumors. Successful regimens are now also available for the adjuvant treatment of breast cancer, osteogenic sarcoma, and colorectal cancer. However, there are still many cancers for which therapeutic success rates are only marginal. For this reason, numerous attempts have been made to develop in vitro or in vivo assays that might predict individual therapeutic response or resistance (5, 7, 29, 32, 67, 69, 73).

Predictive assays present a number of problems that are independent of the type of experimental system used. These include the choice of drug concentrations relevant for the clinical situation, intratumor and intertumor heterogeneity in the tumor specimen, determination of how experimental conditions interfered with the physiologic microenvironment of tumor cells that existed in the patient, and selection pressure on tumor cells by the experimental system used. The relationship between inhibition of tumor growth in vitro and a patient's response to chemotherapy (and survival) is obviously quite complex.

Chemosensitivity assays alone would be helpful in patients with curable diseases receiving known effective first-line chemotherapy if they had an excellent predictivity, that is, if they allowed identification of the rare patient with primary resistant disease. However, there is no convincing evidence that any chemosensitivity assay has such a predictive power. In the clinical setting of patients with refractory disease where palliation is the goal, such assays certainly might help patients avoid toxic side effects of agents that are unlikely to be clinically effective. At present, there is no convincing evidence that such assay-guided chemotherapy is superior to a treatment recommendation by an experienced oncologist with regard to patient survival. There is, however, recent evidence that clinical response rates may be superior for in vitro assay–directed chemotherapy than for chemotherapy selected by a clinician (69).

Available Tests

Table 57.1 lists the various in vitro and in vivo tests that have been used to predict patient response or lack of response.

IN VITRO SYSTEMS

Early attempts to establish predictive tests were dependent on the availability of cell culture techniques in the 1950s. The procedures used included evaluation of cell morphology, exclusion of vital dyes, activity of various enzymes, and incorporation of radioactive precursor molecules after incubation of tumor cells with anticancer agents. However, subsequent correlative studies showed that only a minority of tests had predictive value (56, 74). Potential problems that may have confounded the predictive value included a lack of standardization, and an inability to distinguish with accuracy the growth of malignant and nonmalignant cells in explant cultures from primary tumors. In addition, some assays (e.g., tests for oxygen consumption by tumor cells) proved to be too complicated for routine use (45).

Some techniques (Table 57.1) continue to be of interest for the prediction of clinical response.

Dye Techniques

Early attempts to use exclusion of vital dyes, such as trypan blue, eosin, or nigrosin, to predict chemosensitivity were unsuccessful. More recently, Weisenthal and colleagues, and others, have used a combination of fast green dye and hematoxylin-eosin with more promising results, particularly in patients with hematologic malignancies such as chronic lymphocytic leukemia (CLL) (41, 65, 71, 72). No prospective trial of the Weisenthal assay has yet been performed, however, to demonstrate its ability to predict for response or lack of response.

Another assay currently used at the National Cancer Institute to screen for anticancer activity of new chemicals may have some predictive value in screening for hematologic neoplasms (6, 39, 48). It is based on the ability of vital cells to reduce a tetrazolium compound to a blue formazan product which can be measured by photometry in a semiautomated fashion (39). It has been used with monolayer cell cultures and in organ culture systems (6, 39, 48). This assay is relatively simple to use, is rapid, and may be used conve-

Table 57.1. Techniques Used for Predictive Tests

In vitro systems
Dyes
Explant (organoid) cultures
Precursor incorporation
Fluorescence
Cellular adhesive matrix
Intracellular drug concentrations
ATP bioluminescence
Specific molecular markers for resistance
Human tumor cloning assay
In vivo systems
Subrenal capsule
Nude mouse xenograft

niently in screening cell lines in the setting of drug development. However, at present only limited data are available from retrospective studies of primary tumor specimens (28). No final conclusion can be reached regarding the predictive value of this test in the clinical setting.

Explant (Organoid) Cultures

During the early years of development of chemosensitivity assays, short-term organ cultures and explant cultures were used to assess anticancer effects of clinically used drugs (2, 72). Despite some reports on positive clinical correlations, most investigators have subsequently abandoned these techniques because of technical problems and lack of standardization. More recently, staining of tumor cell clusters with fluorescein diacetate has been reported to be predictive for clinical response in a series of 50 patients with a specificity of 84% and a sensitivity of 100% (58). However, those results need to be confirmed in larger prospective studies.

Precursor Incorporation

Incorporation of radiolabeled precursor molecules into cellular macromolecules has long been used to measure cell proliferation and cell death. Specifically, ^{3}H-thymidine incorporation has been used to determine directly the extent of DNA replication (60). This can either be done autoradiographically or by liquid scintillation counting. Autoradiographic determination of the thymidine labeling index is more specific for malignant cells but is too time consuming for general use. However, it will provide information on tumor growth kinetics. DNA histograms might also be used and have the advantage of providing information on the ploidy status. The value of overall determination of ^{3}H-precursor incorporation by liquid scintillation spectrometry after short-term incubation has been heavily debated (21, 42, 47). Encouraging clinical correlations in retrospective trials still need to be confirmed by prospective, randomized correlative studies. Precursor incorporation assays are rapid, relatively inexpensive, and are feasible in the majority of tumor types. However, they do not differentiate between malignant and nonmalignant cells and might lead to false-negative predictions if lethally damaged cells undergo a final division.

Fluorescence

Fluorescent dyes may be used in conjunction with microscopic evaluation methods as an in vitro chemosensitivity assay (58). For this assay, tumor biopsies are not completely disintegrated into single cells. In order to allow for cell-cell interactions to continue, clusters of tumor tissues—termed 'micro-organs'—are prepared using mild mechanical or enzymatic techniques. This method has not yet had a prospective clinical trial, but preliminary results suggest that it may have some predictive value (49). Similarly, other techniques using fluorescent stains on single tumor cell suspensions are still in the area of preclinical investigations (4, 43).

In another approach, cells from primary tumors may be exposed to propidium iodide after drug exposure and the resulting fluorescence determined by flow cytometry (27). This allows for the determination of cell kinetic parameters of individual tumor specimens. Because of technical difficulties in applying flow cytometry to primary tumor specimens, however, data on the predictive value for clinical response are too scarce to permit definitive conclusions

Cellular Adhesive Matrix

The adhesive tumor cell culture system represents a variation of chemosensitivity testing in monolayer cell cultures. Single cells are prepared from biopsies, specimens, or effusions and seeded with medium in multiwell dishes. Adherent cells are exposed to antineoplastic agents for several days. Selectivity for malignant cells is achieved by preparation of the underlying plastic surface with a solution containing fibronectin and fibrinopeptides (3). At the end of the culture period, cells are fixed and stained. The total number of cells is determined and expressed relative to control dishes. In one retrospective series good clinical correlations were obtained with the assay (1). Three-dimensional matrices have also been used when culturing tumor cells for drug testing, but no definitive clinical trial has been published on their predictive value.

Intracellular Drug Concentrations

Only limited information is available on using intracellular drug concentrations to predict patient response. Determination of intracellular drug concentration requires sophisticated methods specific for each compound under investigation. In previously untreated acute nonlymphocytic leukemia, cellular retention of arabinosyl cytidine triphosphate (ara-CTP) has been reported to correlate with longer remission duration in vivo (55). Retention by leukemic cells of less than 20% of ara-CTP 4 hours after removal of arabinosylcytosine from the medium was correlated with a median clinical remission duration of 3 months. For retention of more than 20% of ara-CTP by leukemic blasts, median remission duration was 45 months. Other investigators, however, have not been able to find any correlation between clinical response or remission duration and formation of ara-CTP (54, 57, 59).

There is no definitive evidence for the predictive value of intracellular concentrations of other antineoplastic agents. Determining the predictive value of intracellular drug concentrations is difficult if the compound is clinically used as part of a combination regimen. Effects on tumor response and patient survival might be caused by other components of the combination and does not provide stringent evidence for sensitivity to the drug under investigation.

ATP Bioluminescence

Intracellular ATP is the principal energy source for vital cells and is rapidly consumed in dying cells. A highly sensitive method to determine the amount of intracellular ATP by using the luciferase-luciferin complex has been reported (50). This assay was adapted to determine the viability of established cancer cell lines after cytotoxic treatment and was also found to be suitable for the study of freshly explanted human tumors (40, 61). In principle, tumor tissue is minced, followed by enzymatic disaggregation to give single cells and small clumps, and is plated over an underlayer of agar. This is followed by exposure to various concentrations of cytostatic agents for 6 days. After extraction of the ATP, the luciferase-luciferin complex is used to produce bioluminescence, which is measured and expressed relative to control values. Initial retrospective clinical correlations are promising, with an evaluability rate in excess of 80% and positive as well as negative predictive values comparable to those observed in clonogenic assays (62). Prospective clinical studies have not been completed, and no final conclusion concerning the predictive value of this system in the clinical setting can be made.

Specific Molecular Markers for Resistance

While no molecular markers to predict sensitivity to a specific drug have been identified, great progress has been made to elucidate the molecular mechanisms underlying inherent or acquired resistance to chemotherapeutic agents. Interference with these mechanisms is of potential clinical value because it may offer a specific approach to predict and possibly overcome resistance and may obviate the need for cell culture techniques. Still, this approach would not tell the clinician to which agents a patient's tumor is sensitive and could only be used to exclude drugs from any planned regimen.

Table 57.2 is a summary of important molecular mechanisms of drug resistance. At present, there are no definitive clinical trials available describing how accurately these mechanisms reflect clinical resistance.

Human Tumor Cloning Assay

Clonogenic assays are used to determine the effect of anticancer agents on actively growing tumor cells (35). Contrary to most other assays, inhibition of cellular proliferation is directly used as the experimental endpoint (17, 33). Single-cell suspensions are prepared from tumor biopsy specimens and exposed to anticancer agents. After the cells are washed, they are seeded in a semisolid medium (agar or methylcellulose) to prevent proliferation of nonmalignant cells in the specimen. After 14 to 28 days, some cells will have undergone several divisions and have formed tumor colonies, which can be quantified in a visual or semiautomated fashion.

No other in vitro test system has been investigated as thoroughly as have clonogenic assays. As a result, the potentials and limitations are best known for these types of assays. Retrospective and prospective clinical correlative trials have been performed in more than 2,000 patients. Table 57.3 is a summary of the cumulative results of 2,300 correlations (68). From these data, there is a 69% probability for a patient to have at least a partial response if the tumor specimen is sensitive to the drug in vitro. On the other hand, if a tumor is resistant in vitro, there will be a 91% chance for clinical resistance. These results are comparable to other clinically accepted laboratory tests, e.g., determination of estrogen or

Table 57.2. Molecular Mechanisms of Drug Resistance of Possible Help in the Prediction of Clinical Response

Molecular Alteration	Mechanism	Drug Affected	Reference
Alteration of drug transport			
Expression of P-170 glycoprotein	Increased drug efflux	Miscellaneous ("pleiotropic drug resistance")	Chin et al. (14) Gerlach et al. (29)
Increased enzyme activity			
Glutathione-S-transferase	Drug inactivation	Alkylating agents	Hamilton et al. (33)
Aldehyde dehydrogenase	Drug inactivation	Cyclophosphamide	Hilton (36)
Guanine-O6-alkyl transferase	DNA repair	Nitrosoureas	Ewig et al. (24)
Ribonucleotide reductase	Increase of binding sites	Hydroxyurea	Choy et al. (15)
Decreased enzyme activity			
Deoxycytidine kinase	Drug activation	Arabinosylcytosine (araC) Fludarabine Gemcitabine 2-Chlorodeoxyadenosine	Drahovsky and Kreis (22) Tseng et al. (65) Heinemann et al. (35) Carson et al. (13)
Pyrimidine salvage pathways	Drug activation	5-Fluorouracil	Mulkins and Heidelberger (50)
Topoisomerase II	Decrease of binding sites	Anthracyclines Epipodophyllotoxins	Deffie et al. (21) Hochhauser and Harris (37)
Gene amplification			
Dihydrofolate reductase	Increase of binding sites	Methotrexate	Cowan et al. (18)
Ribonucleotide reductase	Increase of binding sites	Hydroxyurea	Cocking et al. (16)
Thymidylate synthase	Increase of binding sites	5-Fluorouracil	Brown (12)

Table 57.3. Cumulative Results From 2,300 Clinical Correlations Using Clonogenic Assays to Predict Clinical Outcome

Results	No. Patients	%
True positive	512	69
True negative	1,427	91
False positive	226	31
False negative	135	9
Total	2,300	
		Predictive Values
Sensitivity[a]		79
Specificity[b]		86
Positive predictive value[c]		69
Negative predictive value[d]		91

[a] Sensitivity = True positives/True positives + False negatives.
[b] Specificity = True negatives/True negatives + False positives.
[c] Positive predictive value = True positives/True positives + False positives.
[d] Negative predictive value = True negatives/True negatives + False negatives.
Source: Von Hoff (67).

progesterone receptor status in breast cancer patients to predict response to endocrine therapy. Of course, the accuracy of the prediction of clinical resistance depends on the actual response rates in vivo (53, 67). A prospective, randomized trial of assay-guided chemotherapy versus a clinician's choice of drugs in patients with a variety of cancers has shown higher response rates when test results were used in patient management (69). Patients with disseminated malignancies were stratified for performance status, tumor type, and prior chemotherapy. They were then randomized to single agent chemotherapy which was either recommended by a physician or determined by the cloning assay. If progression occurred, patients were crossed over to the other treatment option. A total of 65 patients were randomized to the clinician's choice, while 68 patients were randomized to the assay's choice. However, for a variety of reasons, only 36 and 19 patients, respectively, actually received the treatment they were assigned and were evaluable for response. In the assay-guided arm the largest group of patients inevaluable for response were those with inevaluable in vitro growth. For evaluable patients, one partial response (3%) was noted in the clinician's choice and four in the assay choice (21%). The difference was statistically significant at 0.04. Twenty-six percent of the patients in the assay choice arm had stable disease as compared with 8% in the clinician's choice arm. There was no difference in the survival curves either for the whole group of randomized patients or for the group of actually treated patients who were therefore evaluable for response. This study does provide an encouraging lead for future clinical trials. It pinpoints the need for further improvements in the methodology of cloning assays. Also, it may be of interest to determine the value of assay-guided chemotherapy in less refractory tumors.

Traditional clonogenic systems suffer from a number of significant technical problems, including lack of growth in 40 to 60% of all specimens and a long incubation time (at least 14 days) before results can be made available to the clinician. Furthermore, insufficient data are available on the effect of assay-guided chemotherapy on patient survival. Because most clinically observed responses are partial responses, a significant increase in overall survival is not to be expected.

A combination of ^{3}H-thymidine incorporation and cloning techniques has shown promise by increasing the number of evaluable specimens and decreasing the incubation time (63, 64). With this variation of tumor cloning techniques, the experimental endpoint no longer is direct visualization of clonal proliferation. Instead, the amount of trichloroacetic acid–precipitable radioactivity is determined and taken as representative for cell growth. The relationship between colony counts and tritiated thymidine incorporation is nonlinear, and an algorithm has been developed for conversion (41). However, no prospective clinical trials of that improved system to predict patients' response or lack of response has been performed.

IN VIVO SYSTEMS

The two in vivo systems most commonly used to predict clinical drug activity are the subrenal capsule assay and transplantation of tumor cells into nude mice. Advantages of in vivo techniques include feasibility of testing agents that require metabolic activation and the preservation of three-dimensional tumor structure with cell-cell-interactions. Also, drug effects on cell growth can be determined over several cell cycles and the effects of drug combinations may be studied. Significant disadvantages include the necessity of an animal facility as well as high costs. Extrapolation of assay results to the clinical setting may be hampered by the fact that treatment in animals is usually started at a low tumor burden while patients usually are treated in an advanced stage when the tumor burden is rather high.

Subrenal Capsule Assay

The subrenal capsule assay was developed by Bogden and co-workers for drug testing (9, 10). In principle, small pieces of tumors are implanted under the renal capsule of athymic or of immunocompetent mice. The animals are then treated with chemotherapy, and after 4 to 11 days, size determinations of tumor transplants are performed. Active anticancer agents lead to a decrease in size of tumor transplant relative to untreated controls. Evaluability rates range from 60 to 80%, which is somewhat better than evaluability rates in conventional clonogenic assays (8). However, evaluability depends on the tumor type tested. Some tumors will not grow in this system (19, 23). Retrospective and prospective correlating trials have reported true positives for the assay in the 60 to 83% range and true negatives in the 66 to 95% range (46, 52). In one study, Favre and co-workers compared retrospective and prospective clinical correlations (26). In the retrospective analysis, true correlation with clinical sensitivity was observed in 8 of 11 assays (72%) and true correlation with clinical resistance in 45 of 45 assays (100%). In the prospective series, true prediction for clinical resistance was observed in 26 of 27 assays (96%) and true prediction for clinical sensitivity was found in 19 of 23 tests

(82%). The cumulative analysis gave 98% true resistant correlations and 82% true sensitive correlations.

Nude Mouse Xenograft

Heterotransplantation of human tumors into athymic nude mice has been extensively used in cancer research. Experimental endpoints are a decrease in size of tumor nodules and the prolongation of survival. These endpoints may not correlate with each other. Except for work with cell lines, this assay is too laborious and expensive for routine predictive drug testing. The yield of growing tumors is quite low (15 to 40%) when primary cells are used (6, 11, 47). In contrast to the subrenal capsule assay, tumors implanted in nude mice may require 2 to 3 months to be evaluable for drug testing, a lag time usually not acceptable in the clinical setting. Because of these difficulties there have only been a handful of attempted clinical correlations with the nude mouse xenograft system. None of the studies has been definitive.

Summary

In summary, an ideal predictive chemosensitivity assay should be simple, rapid, reproducible, applicable to all tumor types, and inexpensive. At present, no such system is available. Even the most extensively studied assays more often identify agents that will not work in an individual patient rather than agents that will. Clearly, the lack of active agents in cancer chemotherapy is an important factor in this context, pointing at the dire need to identify new and more active agents. The most important contribution of chemosensitivity assays still lies in the area of research and not in routine clinical use.

References

1. Ajani JA, Baker FL, Spitzer G, Kelly A, Brock W, Tomasovic B, Singletary SE, McMurtrey M, Plager C. Comparison between clinical response and in vitro drug sensitivity of primary human tumors in the Adhesive Tumor Cell Culture System. J Clin Oncol 1987;5:1912.
2. Ambrose EJ, Andrews RD, Easty DM, Field EO, Wylie JA. Drug assays on cultures of human tumour biopsies. Lancet 1962;1:24.
3. Baker FL, Spitzer G, Ajani JA, Brock WA, Lukeman J, Pathak N, Tomasovic B, Thielvoldt D, Williams M, Vines C, Tofilon P. Drug and radiation sensitivity measurements of successful primary monolayer culturing of human tumor cells using cell-adhesive matrix and supplemented medium. Cancer Res 1986;46:1263.
4. Begg AC, Mooren E. Rapid fluorescence-based assay for radiosensitivity and chemosensitivity testing in mammalian cells in vitro. Cancer Res 1989;49:565.
5. Bellamy WT. Prediction of response to drug therapy of cancer. A review of in vitro assays. Drugs 1992;44:690.
6. Bellet RE, Danna V, Mastrangelo MJ, Berd D. Evaluation of a "nude" mouse-human tumor panel as a predictive secondary screen for cancer chemotherapeutic agents. JNCI 1979;63:1185.
7. Black MM, Speer FD. Further observations on the effects of cancer chemotherapeutic agents on the in vitro dehydrogenase activity of cancer tissue. JNCI 1954;14:1147.
8. Bogden AE. The subrenal capsule assay (SRCA) and its predictive value in oncology. Ann Chir Gynaecol 1985;74(suppl 199):12.
9. Bogden AE, Haskell PM, LePage DJ, Kelton DE, Cobb WR, Esber HJ. Growth of human tumor xenografts implanted under the renal capsule of normal immunocompetent mice. Exp Cell Biol 1979;47:281.
10. Bogden AE, Kelton DE, Cobb WR, Esber HJ. A rapid screening method for testing chemotherapeutic agents against human tumor xenografts. In Proceedings of the symposium on the use of athymic (nude) mice in cancer research. Edited by DP Houchens, AA Ovejera. New York: G Fischer, 1978, pp 231–250.
11. Braakhuis BB, Snow GB. Nude mice model as a predictive assay in head and neck cancer. In Head and Neck Cancer, Vol. 1. Edited by PB Chretien, ME Johns, DE Shedd, FW Strong, PH Ward. Philadelphia: Decker, 1985, pp:421–424.
12. Brown R. Gene amplification and drug resistance. J Pathol 1991;163:287.
13. Carson DA, Wasson DB, Beutler E. Antileukemic and immunosuppressive activity of 2-chloro-2′-deoxyadenosine. Proc Natl Acad Sci USA 1984;81:2232.
14. Chin KV, Pastan I, Gottesman MM. Function and regulation of the human multidrug resistance gene. Adv Cancer Res 1993;60:157.
15. Choy BK, Mc Clarty GA, Chan AK, Thelander L, Wright JA. Molecular mechanisms of drug resistance involving ribonucleotide reductase: hydroxyurea resistance in a series of clonally related mouse cell lines selected in the presence of increasing drug concentrations. Cancer Res 1988;48:2029.
16. Cocking JM, Tonin PN, Stokoe NM, Wensing EJ, Lewis WH, Srinivasan PR. Gene for M1 subunit of ribonucleotide reductase is amplified in hydroxyurea-resistant hamster cells. Somatic Cell Mol Genet 1987;13:221.
17. Courtenay VD, Mills J. An in vitro colony assay for human tumours grown in immune-suppressed mice and treated in vivo with cytotoxic agents. Br J Cancer 1978;37:261.
18. Cowan KH, Goldsmith ME, Levine RM, Aitken ST, Douglass E, Clendeninn N, Nienhuis AW, Lippman ME. Dihydrofolate reductase gene amplification and possible rearrangement in estrogen-responsive methotrexate-resistant human breast cancer cells. J Biol Chem 1982;257:15079.
19. Cunningham D, Jack A, McMurdo DF, Soukop H, McArdle CS, Carter DC, Kaye SB. The 6-day subrenal capsule assay is of no value with primary surgical explants from gastric cancer. Br J Cancer 1986;54:519.
20. Daidone MG, Silvestrini R, Sanfilippo O, Zaffaroni N, Varini M, De Lena M. Reliability of an in vitro short-term assay to predict the drug sensitivity of human breast cancer. Cancer 1985;56:450.
21. Deffie AM, Batra JK, Goldenberg GG. Direct correlation between DNA topoisomerase II activity and cytotoxicity in adriamycin-sensitive and -resistant P388 leukemia cell lines. Cancer Res 1989;49:58.
22. Drahovsky D, Kreis W. Studies on drug resistance: II. Kinase patterns in P815 neoplasms sensitive and resistant to 1-beta-D-arabinofuranosylcytosine. Biochem Pharmacol 1970;19:940.
23. Edelstein MB. The subrenal capsule assay: a critical commentary. Eur J Cancer Clin Oncol 1986;22:757.
24. Egawa M, Hisazumi H, Uchibayashi T, Tanaka M, Sasaki T. Comparative study of 3-(4,5-dimethylthiazol-2-yl)-2,5-diphenyltetrazolium bromide and tritiated thymidine in a chemosensitivity test using collagen gel matrix. Urol Res 1993;21:83.
25. Ewig RAG, Kohn KW. DNA damage and repair in mouse leukemia L 1210 cells treated with nitrogen mustard, 1,3-bis (2-chloroethyl)-1-nitrosourea, and other nitrosoureas. Cancer Res 1977;37:2114.
26. Favre R, Mariota L, Drancourt M, Jaquemier J, Delpero JR, Guerinel G, Carcassonne Y. 6-day subrenal capsule assay (SRCA) as a predictor of the response of advanced cancers to chemotherapy. Eur J Cancer 1986;22:1171.
27. Funa K, Dawson N, Jewett PB, Agren H, Ruckdeschel JC, Bunn PA Jr, Gazdar AF. Automated fluorescent analysis for drug-induced cytotoxicity assays. Cancer Treat Rep 1986;70:1147.
28. Furukawa T, Kubota T, Suto A, Takahara T, Yamaguchi H, Takeuchi T, Kase S, Kodaira S, Ishibiki K, Kitajima M. Clinical usefulness of chemosensitivity testing using the MTT assay. J Surg Oncol 1991;48:188.
29. Gellhorn A, Hirschberg E. Investigation of diverse systems for cancer chemotherapy screening. Cancer Res 1955;3(suppl):1.
30. Gerlach JH, Kartner N, Bell DR, Ling V. Multidrug resistance. Cancer Surv 1986;5:25.
31. Glisson B, Gupta R, Hodges P, Ross W. Cross-resistance to intercalating agents in an epipodophyllotoxin-resistant Chinese hamster ovary cell line: evidence for a common intracellular target. Cancer Res 1986;46:1939.
32. Hamburger AW. Use of in vitro tests in predictive cancer chemotherapy. JNCI 1981;66:981.
33. Hamburger AW, Salmon SE. Primary bioassay of human tumor stem cells. Science 1977;197:461.
34. Hamilton TC, Winker MA, Louie KG, Batist G, Behrens BG, Tsuruo T, Grotzinger KR, McKoy WM, Young RC, Ozols RF. Augmentation of adriamycin, melphalan, and cisplatin toxicity in drug resistant and -sensitive human ovarian cancer cell lines by buthionine sulfoximine mediated glutathione depletion. Biochem Pharmacol 1985;34:2583.
35. Hanauske A-R, Hanauske U, Von Hoff DD. The human tumor cloning assay in cancer research and therapy. Curr Probl Cancer 1985;9:1.
36. Heinemann V, Hertel LW, Grindey GB, Plunkett W. Comparison of the cellular pharmacokinetics and toxicity of 2″,2″-difluorodeoxycytidine and 1—D-arabinofuranosylcytosine. Cancer Res 1988;48:4024.
37. Hilton J. Role of aldehyde dehydrogenase in cyclophosphamide-resistant L1210 leukemia. Cancer Res 1984;44:5156.
38. Hochhauser D, Harris AL. The role of topoisomerase II alpha and beta in drug resistance. Cancer Treat Rev 1993;19:181.
39. Hongo T, Fujii Y, Igarashi Y. An in vitro chemosensitivity test for the screening of anti-cancer drugs in childhood leukemia. Cancer 1990;65:1263.
40. Kangas L, Gronroos M, Nieminen AL. Bioluminescence of cellular ATP: A new method for evaluating cytotoxic agents in vitro. Med Biol 1984;62:338.
41. Kern DH, Weisenthal LM. Highly specific prediction of antineoplastic drug resistance with an in vitro assay using suprapharmacologic drug exposures. JNCI 1990;7:582.
42. Khoo SK, Hurst T, Webb MJ, Dickie G, Kearsley J, Parsons PG, Mackay EV. Clinical value of in vitro drug sensitivity testing based on short-term effects of DNA and RNA metabolism in ovarian cancer. J Surg Oncol 1989;41:201.
43. Larsson R, Nygren P, Ekberg M, Slater L. Chemotherapeutic drug sensitivity testing of human leukemia cells in vitro using a semiautomated fluorometric assay. Leukemia 1990;4:567.
44. Laszlo J, Stengle J, Wight K, Burk D. Effects of chemotherapeutic agents on metabolism of human acute leukemia cells in vitro. Proc Soc Exp Biol Med 1958;97:127.
45. Maeenpaeae J, Kangas L, Groenroos M. The subrenal capsule assay for chemosensitivity testing of tumors. A review. Zentralbl Gynaecol 1988;110:989.
46. Mattern J, Volm M. Clinical relevance of predictive tests for cancer chemotherapy. Cancer Treat Rev 1982;9:267.
47. Mosmann T. Rapid colorimetric assay for cellular growth and survival: Application to proliferation and cytotoxicity assays. J Immunol Methods 1983;65:55.
48. Meitner PA. The fluorescent cytoprint assay: a new approach to in vitro chemosensitivity testing. Oncology 1991;5:75.
49. Moyer JD, Henderson JF. Ultrasensitive assay for ribonucleoside triphosphate in 50-1000 cells. Biochem Pharmacol 1983;32:3831.
50. Mulkins MA, Heidelberger C. Isolation of fluoropyrimidine-resistant murine leukemic cell lines by one-step mutation and selection. Cancer Res 1982;42:956.
51. Panje WR, McCormick KJ. Murine subrenal capsule assay: prediction of chemoresponsiveness in head and neck cancer. Laryngoscope 1989;99:41.

52. Parchment RE, Soleimanpour K, Petrose S, Murphy MJ Jr. Pharmacologic validation of human tumor clonogenic assays based on pleiotropic drug resistance: implications for individualized chemotherapy and new drug screening programs. Int J Cell Cloning 1992;10:359.
53. Plunkett W, Iacobini S, Keating MJ. Cellular pharmacology and optimal therapeutic concentrations of 1-beta-D-arabinofuranosylcytosine 5′-triphosphate in leukemic blasts during treatment of refractory leukemia with high-dose 1-beta-D-arabinofuranosylcytosine. Scand J Haematol 1986;34:51.
54. Preisler HD, Rustum Y, Priore RL. Relationship between leukemic cell retention of cytosine arabinoside triphosphate and the duration of remission in patients with acute non-lymphocytic leukemia. Eur J Cancer Clin Oncol 1985;21:23.
55. Roper PR, Drewincko B. Comparison of in vitro methods to determine drug-induced cell lethality. Cancer Res 1976;36:2182.
56. Ross DD, Thompson BW, Joneckis CC, Akman SA, Schiffer CA. Metabolism of ara-C by blast cells from patients with ANLL. Blood 1986;68:76.
57. Rotman B. Fluorescent cytoprinting: A simple nondestructive process for assessing chemosensitivity in micro-organcultures. Proc Am Assoc Cancer Res 1989;30:654.
58. Rustum YM, Riva C, Preisler HD. Pharmacokinetic parameters of 1-beta-D-arabinofuranosylcytosine and their relationship to intracellular metabolism of ara-C, toxicity, and response of patients with acute non-lymphocytic leukemia treated with conventional and high dose ara-C. Semin Oncol 1987;14:141.
59. Sanfilippo O, Silvestrini R, Zaffaroni N, Piva L, Pizzocaro G. Application of an in vitro antimetabolic assay to human germ cell testicular tumors for the preclinical evaluation of drug sensitivity. Cancer 1986;58:1441.
60. Sevin BU, Peng Z, Perras J, Ganjei P, Penalver M, Averette HE. Application of an ATP-bioluminescence assay in human tumor chemosensitivity testing. Gynecol Oncol 1988;31:191.
61. Sevin BU, Perras JP, Averette HE, Donato DM, Penalver M. Chemosensitivity testing in ovarian cancer. Cancer 1993;71:1613.
62. Sugihara K, Collins LA, Homesley HD, Welander CE. An in vitro thymidine incorporation assay for human cancers: Technical details revisited. Int J Cell Cloning 1992;10:344.
63. Tanigawa N, Kern DH, Hikasa Y, Morton DL. Rapid assay for evaluating the chemosensitivity of human tumors in soft agar culture. Cancer Res 1982;42:2159.
64. Tidefelt U, Sundman-Engberg B, Rhedin A-S, Paul C. In vitro drug testing in patients with acute leukemia with incubations mimicking in vivo intracellular drug concentrations. Eur J Haematol 1989;43:374.
65. Tseng W-C, Derse D, Cheng Y-C, et al. In vitro biological activity of 9-β-D-arabinofuranosyl-2-fluoroadenine and the biochemical actions of its triphosphate on DNA polymerases and ribonucleotide reductase from HeLa cells. Mol Pharmacol 1982;21:474.
66. Twentyman PR. Predictive chemosensitivity testing. Br J Cancer 1985;51:295.
67. Von Hoff DD. He's not going to talk about in vitro predictive assays again, is he? JNCI 1990;82:96.
68. Von Hoff DD, Sandbach JF, Clark GM, Turner JN, Forseth BF, Piccart MJ, Colombo N, Muggia FM. Selection of cancer chemotherapy for a patient by an in vitro assay versus a clinician. JNCI 1990;82:110.
69. Von Hoff DD, Weisenthal L. In vitro methods to predict for patient response to chemotherapy. Adv Pharmacol Chemother 1980;17:133.
70. Weisenthal LM, Dill PL, Kurnick NB, Lippman ME. Comparison of dye exclusion assays with a clonogenic assay in the determination of drug-induced cytotoxicity. Cancer Res 1983;43:258.
71. Weisenthal LM, Marsden JA, Dill PL, Macaluso CK. A novel dye exclusion method for testing in vitro chemosensitivity of human tumors. Cancer Res 1983;43:749.
72. Wright JC, Plummer-Cobb J, Gumport S, Golomb FM, Safadi D. Investigation of the relation between clinical and tissue culture response to chemotherapeutic agents on human cancer. N Engl J Med 1957;257:1207.
73. Wright JC, Plummer-Cobb J, Gumport SL, Safadi D, Walker DG, Golomb FM. Further investigation of the relation between the clinical and tissue culture response to chemotherapeutic agents on human cancer. Cancer 1962;15:284.
74. Yarnell M, Ambrose EJ, Shepley K, Tchao R. Drug assays on organ culture of biopsies from human tumours. Br Med J 1964;2:490.

CHAPTER 58

Pharmacology

MARK J. RATAIN AND WILLIAM PLUNKETT

Introduction

For many years the clinical pharmacology of anticancer drugs was poorly understood owing primarily to the lack of sensitive and specific assays for measuring the concentration of these compounds in biologic fluids. The recent development and widespread application of high-performance liquid chromatography and other sophisticated analytic tools now allows measurements of plasma drug (and metabolite) concentrations with a high degree of precision and efficiency. Clinical pharmacokinetic studies of anticancer drugs, particularly new agents, are now performed routinely. Although the pharmacokinetic characteristics of many drugs have been well defined, the application of this information to clinical care still lags far behind other areas in medicine. Plasma concentrations of digoxin, theophylline, aminoglycosides, phenytoin, and many other drugs are monitored routinely to optimize efficacy and reduce toxicity; yet the measurement of doxorubicin or 5-fluorouracil (5-FU) concentrations in plasma is virtually meaningless, since there are no established relationships (of proven therapeutic utility) between pharmacokinetics and clinical effects for these or most other commonly used anticancer drugs. A notable exception is methotrexate: delayed clearance *is* known to be related to an increased risk of severe toxicity.

Pharmacokinetic-pharmacodynamic relationships are difficult to develop, for many reasons. For most antineoplastic agents there is a delay of days to weeks between measurement of drug concentrations and clinical effect. It is therefore necessary to observe patients frequently following chemotherapy administration to accurately assess the drug effect. The maximum observed effect may be significantly less than the true maximum effect, unless patients are seen daily. Although the desired effect of cancer chemotherapy is a reduction in tumor volume, usually optimized by maximizing the dose, the narrow therapeutic index of antineoplastic drugs requires that most dosing strategies focus on minimizing toxicity rather than on optimizing efficacy. Despite these difficulties, significant progress has recently been made in understanding the clinical pharmacodynamics of anticancer drugs, and further studies in this area will no doubt lead to more rational administration of cancer chemotherapy.

This chapter will focus on the principles of clinical pharmacology as they apply to cancer chemotherapy and will attempt to illustrate how an understanding of clinical pharmacokinetics and pharmacodynamics can optimize the therapeutic index of cancer chemotherapy.

General Mechanisms of Drug Action

The initial requirement for drug action is adequate drug delivery to the target site. This depends largely on blood flow in the tumor bed and the diffusion characteristics of the drug in tissue. Delivery may also be influenced, however, by the extent of plasma protein binding and, for orally administered drugs, by absorption and first-pass metabolism in the liver (Fig. 58.1). Blood flow across a capillary bed is directly proportional to the arteriovenous pressure difference and inversely proportional to the geometric and viscous resistances. The geometric resistance to blood flow increases with increasing tumor size, a factor that may limit drug and oxygen delivery to large tumors and thereby diminish the effectiveness of treatment with chemotherapy or radiation (186).

The most common route of drug administration, for both localized and disseminated disease, is intravenous infusion, which, by definition, makes 100% of the drug available in the blood. Drugs may be administered by a number of routes in addition to intravenous infusions, to achieve special pharmacologic and therapeutic goals. Regional administration may be employed to more directly target the drug to the principal tumor site and to achieve a higher drug concentration in the vicinity of the tumor. Intraperitoneal infusion of cisplatin for ovarian cancers, intrapleural administration of interleukin 2 (IL-2) in the treatment of mesothelioma, and intrathecal administration of cytarabine (ara-C) for leukemias are examples of intracavitary drug delivery. Alternatively, intravascular administrations, such as intra-arterial infusion of fluorodeoxyuridine into the hepatic artery for treatment of liver disease has been used to achieve a pharmacologic advantage. Although oral administration is the most convenient and least expensive route, it is associated with problems of inconsistent drug bioavailability, among and within patients. More consistent pharmacokinetics are achieved with subcutaneous or intramuscular drug injection.

Delivery of the drug to the target cell is also dependent upon the rate of removal from the blood. Excretion, either by the kidneys or by the biliary route, constitutes a major clearance mechanism. In addition, many drugs are cleared by metabolism to less effective or inactive metabolites as the blood passes through large organs. Drug binding to plasma

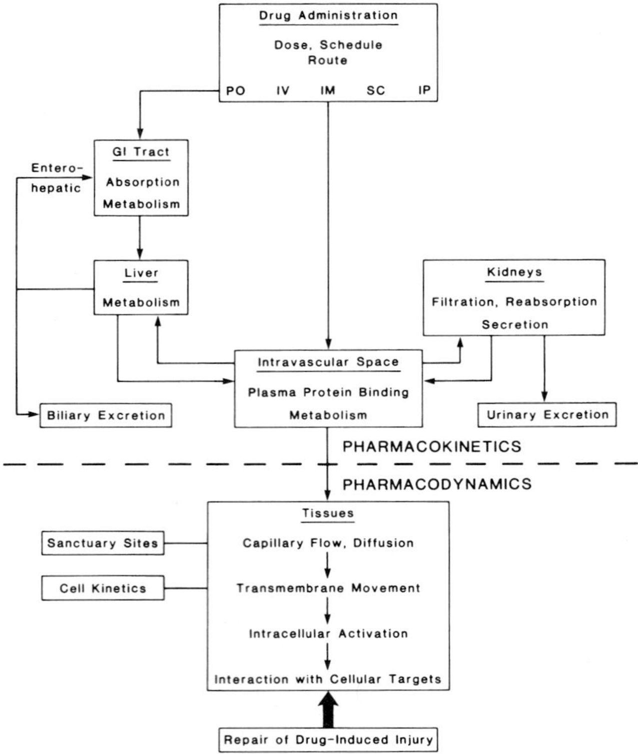

Figure 58.1. Schematic representation of pharmacokinetics and pharmacodynamics. *Pharmacokinetics* represents the distribution, metabolism, and elimination of drugs from the body. *Pharmacodynamics* describes the interaction of drugs with target tissues.

proteins can also effectively lower the concentration of free drug available for entry into target cells to a small fraction of the total concentration in blood.

MEMBRANE TRANSPORT

In order to produce cytotoxicity, most anticancer drugs must be taken up into the cells. A number of mechanisms exist for the passage of drugs across the plasma membrane, including passive diffusion, facilitated diffusion, and active transport systems (78). Passive diffusion of drugs through the lipid bilayer structure of the plasma membrane is a function of the size, lipid solubility and charge of the drug molecule. If the extracellular drug concentration is constant, then drug accumulation by the cell will continue until the rate of drug uptake from the extracellular space is equal to the rate of drug efflux from the cell. At this point, a dynamic equilibrium is reached and intracellular and extracellular drug concentrations are equal. As drug is cleared from the extracellular space, intracellular drug levels will decline if the drug is not bound or metabolized intracellularly. An important feature of the passive diffusion process is that it does not saturate. That is, as the extracellular drug concentration increases, influx into the cell increases proportionally and high intracellular drug levels can be achieved. Passive diffusion, however, is a highly inefficient and nonspecific process that may be a particularly important mechanism of drug uptake when carrier-mediated processes are nonfunctional, as in some cases of methotrexate resistance.

The passage of physiologically important hydrophilic compounds across the plasma membrane is usually mediated by a specific receptor, or carrier, in the plasma membrane that facilitates the translocation of the substance into or out of the cell. Carrier-mediated transport systems are distinguished from passive diffusion by their higher degree of specificity and by the fact that they are saturable at high extracellular drug concentrations, owing to the presence of a finite number of receptor molecules within the membrane. Once all carrier sites become occupied, further increases in extracellular drug concentration will not produce further increments in drug influx unless a component of passive diffusion comes into play. The affinity of the carrier for the substrate can be estimated from the K_m (the drug concentration at which the influx rate is half maximal); the lower the K_m, the higher the carrier affinity. Although carrier-mediated systems enhance the rate of influx into the cell, not all carriers are able to translocate compounds against electrochemical forces and, ultimately, to develop gradients such that the intracellular concentration exceeds the extracellular drug level. To do so requires the expenditure of energy and the coupling of carrier-mediated transport to an energy-requiring reaction, usually hydrolysis of adenosine triphosphate.

Many antineoplastic drugs, particularly those which are structural analogues of natural compounds, gain entry into the cell by carrier-mediated mechanisms. The functional and physiologic characteristics of several nucleoside transporters have been characterized; additional information will be derived as more of these molecules are cloned (96, 134). Naturally occurring nucleosides are transported by both facilitated diffusion and by concentrative mechanisms. Nucleoside analogues, which are important in cancer therapy, also utilize these transporters, but some specificity is emerging (22). For instance, ara-C, floxuridine, and pentostatin appear to utilize equilibrative transporters (40, 99, 100, 217), whereas fludarabine and cladribine appear to be substrates for concentrative transport systems in addition to equilibrative pathways (136). Nucleobase transporters have also been identified, but their roles in the entry of useful antimetabolites such as thiopurines and 5-FU into the cell has not been established (142, 208). Transport of reduced folates and methotrexate is an active energy-dependent process which can be mediated by two distinct mechanisms: (*a*) a membrane-carrier system capable of the rapid transport of reduced folates and of 4-amino analogues of folic acid (187) and (*b*) a group of membrane-bound folate receptors termed the "folate-binding proteins," which are brought into the cell by endocytosis to release ligand before recycling back to the membrane (19, 178). Candidate cDNAs for this function have now been identified (46, 218). Altered methotrexate transport features have recently been described in acute lymphocytic leukemia blasts as a mechanism of acquired resistance (206). Phenylalanine mustard utilizes at least two amino acid transport systems, and its influx can be inhibited by the amino acid substrates specific for these transport carriers (77).

The importance of transmembrane movement of a drug to its pharmacologic effect depends on several factors, including the rate of drug delivery to the tissue, the affinity of the transport process, and the nature of the intracellular biochemical events required for drug action. Though membrane transport can be the rate-limiting step in drug action if it governs the rate at which the drug reaches intracellular targets, this is not always the case. If drug delivery to a cell is slow relative to the influx rate, then the drug effect will be limited primarily by extracellular concentration (i.e., blood flow and diffusion of the drug). Similarly, if, before it can exert a cytotoxic effect, a drug requires intracellular activation, such as phosphorylation of nucleoside analogues or polyglutamylation of methotrexate, then the rate-limiting step in drug action could be activation rather than transport, if the rate of activation is slow relative to the rate of influx into the cell.

Finally, it is important to recognize that membrane transport is frequently bi-directional, so with the final drug concentration in the cell represents the balance between drug influx and drug efflux. These processes may utilize different carrier systems and operate at different rates. Several efflux systems that appear to have importance in cancer chemotherapy are the systems which mediate various forms of multidrug resistance (41, 189).

INTRACELLULAR ACTIVATION

Many anticancer drugs require activation before they are able to exert a cytotoxic effect. The activation process may involve chemical or enzymatic reactions in either normal or tumor tissues (Table 58.1). Cisplatin, for example, undergoes a chemical reaction with water molecules intracellularly that results in the generation of a positively charged aquated species that attacks nucleophilic sites on DNA (114). In contrast, the activation of cyclophosphamide is mediated by hepatic microsomal mixed-function oxidases; in this case, the result is the release of active alkylating species into the systemic circulation (36).

Intracellular activation by tumor cells is a critical determinant of effect for virtually all antimetabolites. Nucleoside antimetabolites such as ara-C (144), fludarabine (145), and cladribine (149) require phosphorylation to active nucleotide triphosphate forms and incorporation into DNA before they are rendered cytotoxic. Nucleobase analogues such as 6-mercaptopurine and 6-thioguanine undergo phosphoribosylation to the nucleoside monophosphate forms, which are active inhibitors of de novo purine nucleotide synthesis. Amination of 6-mercaptopurine to thioguanine monophosphate, followed by phosphorylation, reduction to the deoxynucleotide, and subsequent phosphorylation, results in 2′-deoxythioguanine triphosphate, which is a substrate for incorporation into DNA. Phosphoribosylation also converts 5-FU to the monophosphate, which is then phosphorylated to the diphosphate, reduced to the deoxynucleotide, and dephosphorylated to the active monophosphate (F-dUMP), which inhibits thymidylate synthase. Additionally, the drug may be cytotoxic after incorporation of ribosyl or deoxyribosyl triphosphate, respectively, into RNA or DNA. Although, in its native form, methotrexate is an effective enzyme inhibitor, intracellular conversion of the drug to polyglutamate metabolites significantly increases its potency and facilitates its binding to a number of enzymatic sites (7, 103). Consistent with this is the finding of a more favorable clinical outcome in ALL patients whose blasts accumulate higher levels of methotrexate polyglutamates (201, 216). It is important to note that phosphorylation of nucleic acid analogues and polyglutamylation of methotrexate produces charged molecules that are unlikely to diffuse or to be transported out of cells.

The rate of formation of the activated drug species in cells depends on the rate of transmembrane influx of the drug, the amount and affinity of the activating enzyme(s) in the cell, the extent of competition from naturally occurring substrates of the activating enzymes, and the rate of degradation of the activated drug by catabolic enzymes. For many antimetabolites, membrane transport is rapid, relative to enzymatic activation, and is, therefore, not rate limiting. Once inside the cell, antimetabolites must compete with the natural enzyme substrates for binding and activation. Finally, the activated drug then becomes a substrate for catabolic enzymes in the cell that tend to degrade it to the parent compound or to an inactive metabolite (68). The concentration of active cytotoxic drug in the cell is the result of all these processes.

The pyrimidine nucleoside analogue, ara-C, provides an excellent example of these processes. Ara-C gains entry to the cell by a high-capacity equilibrative nucleoside transport system; transport velocity is nearly proportional to ara-C concentration up to 100 mM (215). This process may limit ara-C activation in cells at plasma ara-C concentrations below 1 μM achieved by standard dose rates (<20 mg/m^2/hr). At higher dose rates, which achieve plasma concentrations greater than 10 μM ara-C (250 mg/m^2/hr), the transport system provides cellular concentrations of ara-C which saturate the rate of ara-C phosphorylation (148). After gaining entry to the cell, ara-C is metabolized in three successive phosphorylation reactions to ara-C triphosphate (ara-CTP), which, after its incorporation by various DNA polymerases into replicating or repairing DNA is inhibitory to cell growth. The initial activating enzyme, deoxycytidine kinase, is found at the lowest specific activity in human leukemic blasts (25) and is believed to be the rate-limiting step in the formation of ara-CTP(29) and thus for incorporation of the drug into DNA. At each phosphorylation step, ara-C and its metabolites

Table 58.1. Activation of Anticancer Drugs

Activation reaction	Drug
Aquation	Cisplatin
Hydrolysis	Irinotecan
Polyglutamylation	Methotrexate
Phosphorylation	Cytarabine Fludarabine Cladribine
Phosphoribosylation	5-Fluorouracil 6-Mercaptopurine 6-Thioguanine
Microsomal oxidation	Cyclophosphamide Ifosfamide Procarbazine
Microsomal reduction	Bleomycin
Demethylation	Dacarbazine Hexamethylmelamine
Acetylation	Amonafide

compete with endogenous deoxycytidine and its nucleotides for enzyme binding. In the case of deoxycytidine kinase, the affinity of the enzyme for ara-C (K_m, 20 μM) is lower than that for deoxycytidine (K_m, 7.8 μM) (25); however, when ATP is the phosphate donor, the enzyme is strongly inhibited by dCTP, but only weakly inhibited by ara-CTP (43). Biochemical modulation strategies which reduce dCTP, and thereby activate dCyd kinase, result in increased ara-CTP formation (72) and improved clinical response (62). Opposing the activation of ara-C are cytidine deaminase and dCMP deaminase, which convert ara-C and ara-CMP, respectively, to inactive uracil derivatives. In addition, the activity of phosphatases such as 5′-nucleotidase, whose activities differ among cell types, may be important determinants of the steady-state ara-CTP concentrations and the rate of elimination of the triphosphate at the end of an ara-C infusion. The response of patients with acute leukemia to the single drug ara-C, either on an intermittent schedule or by continuous infusion, was strongly correlated with the ability of cells to retain ara-CTP (106) or with the steady-state ara-CTP concentrations (61) in blasts during therapy. These findings validate the importance of favorable pharmacokinetic characteristics for response to ara-C in particular and provide a basis for seeking similar pharmacologic modulation strategies with other drugs.

Loss or diminished affinity of an activating enzyme or enhanced activity of a catabolic enzyme may be responsible for drug resistance. In the case of ara-C, cells selected for drug resistance in vitro frequently have lost deoxycytidine kinase activity (14). Although molecular reagents are now available (191) which have permitted the discovery of dCyd kinase deficiencies in selected clinical samples (67), this does not appear to be a major cause of clinical resistance to ara-C, because the blasts of patients with resistant disease accumulate ara-CTP in levels similar to those of responders (147).

DRUG TARGETS

While anticancer drugs have traditionally been classified by mechanisms of action or their origins, they can also be grouped by the target of drug action. There are, essentially, four potential targets: nucleic acids, specific enzymes, microtubules, and hormone and/or growth factor receptors. When nucleic acids are the target, it is generally DNA, rather than RNA, that is presumed to cause cell death. There are several mechanisms by which drugs can bind DNA, the best understood being alkylation of nucleophilic sites within the double helix. Most clinically effective alkylating agents have two moieties capable of developing a charged carbon that binds covalently to negatively charged sites on DNA, such as the O^6 or N^7 positions of guanine. The cross-linking of the two strands of DNA produced by the bifunctional alkylating agents prevents the use of that DNA as a template for further DNA and RNA synthesis leading to inhibition of DNA replication and cell death (20, 107). Although alkylating agents are among the most widely used drugs in clinical oncology, the relationship of pharmacologic parameters to clinical effects for these agents has been ill-defined. In part, this has been due to the lack of sensitive and specific techniques to detect drug–DNA binding in clinical specimens. Studies of chlorambucil-DNA binding in the tumor cells of patients with chronic lymphocytic leukemia have demonstrated considerable heterogeneity in drug–DNA binding among patient samples, but no clear correlation has been shown between amount of drug bound and disease stage or sensitivity to treatment (11), though the drug clearly targets purines (10). In contrast, the formation of cisplatin adducts to DNA has been shown to correlate with cell kill in mammalian tumor cell lines (203). Immunocytochemical methods have been utilized to quantify platinum–DNA adduct formation in either peripheral white blood cells (165) after cisplatin therapy or in buccal cells of patients receiving cisplatin plus carboplatin chemotherapy (15). A subsequent study which used atomic absorption spectroscopy to quantify total cell platinum in lymphocytes indicated a relationship between the adduct levels after the first single-drug dose of either cisplatin or carboplatin and clinical response in 49 patients with 24 different tumor types (164). Although adduct formation in these surrogate cell types was correlated with the response of the tumor to chemotherapy in previously untreated patients, it is difficult to imagine that such determinations will continue to reflect response, as the originally platinum-sensitive tumor becomes resistant to treatment. A second mechanism of drug binding to nucleic acids is intercalation—the insertion of a planar ring structure between two adjacent nucleotide bases of DNA. This mechanism is characteristic of many antitumor antibiotics. The antibiotic molecule is noncovalently (although firmly) bound to DNA and distorts the shape of the double helix, resulting in inhibition of RNA or DNA synthesis (140, 220). Many agents capable of classical intercalation, such as doxorubicin and mitoxantrone, are also inhibitors of topoisomerase II, and may produce DNA strand breaks by inhibition of the reannealing function of this enzyme (170, 204). Indeed, a direct correlation has been noted between DNA topoisomerase II activity and cytotoxicity in doxorubicin-sensitive and -resistant P388 leukemia cells (44). A third mechanism of nucleic acid damage is illustrated by the anticancer drug bleomycin. The amino-terminal tripeptide of the bleomycin molecule appears to intercalate between guanine-cytosine base pairs of DNA. The opposite end of the bleomycin peptide binds Fe (II) and serves as a ferrous oxidase that is able to catalyze the reduction of molecular oxygen to superoxide or hydroxyl radicals that produce DNA strand scission (76, 202). Predictably, the levels in plasma and blood of antioxidant enzymes, such as catalase, peroxidases, and superoxide dismutase, are inversely correlated with chromosomal damage (17).

Enzymes represent the second general category of targets for chemotherapeutic agents. Antimetabolites function as inhibitors of key enzymes in the purine or pyrimidine biosynthetic pathways or as inhibitors of DNA polymerases. The triphosphate of fludarabine, for instance, is known to inhibit both ribonucleotide reductase (135) and DNA ligase I (213), whereas after incorporation into DNA it not only inhibits the function of multiple DNA polymerases (94), DNA primase (24), and DNA ligase I (213), but it is resistant to removal by the proofreading exonuclease activities associated with DNA polymerases (94). Since these enzymes are highly active during DNA replication, antimetabolites tend to be cytotoxic only when present in sufficient concentrations during the vulnerable S phase of the cell cycle. These drugs are, thus, frequently referred to as S-phase–specific. Nevertheless, because these enzymes are also required for repair of damaged DNA, it is likely that antimetabolites which inhibit them will be synergistic with agents which elicit a DNA repair response, regardless of cell cycle stage (180).

The effectiveness of enzyme inhibitors also depends on the amount of the target enzyme, its affinity for the inhibitor, and the extent of competition for enzyme binding from natural substrates. For example, complete saturation of all dihydrofolate reductase–binding sites is required before the enzyme is effectively inhibited. As methotrexate inhibits enzyme activity, dihydrofolate, the natural substrate, accumulates behind the metabolic block and is able to effectively compete with methotrexate for further enzyme binding (214). Thus, much methotrexate, amounts well in excess of the enzyme-binding capacity, is required to effectively inhibit dihydrofolate reductase activity. Similarly, in the case of 5-FU, the dUMP/FdUMP ratio may be an important determinant of optimal inhibition of the target enzyme thymidylate synthase, and high ratios have been associated with lack of tumor response (194). Similarly, the amount of thymidylate synthase expression or activity is an important determinant of 5-FU activity and correlates with therapeutic response (102, 138).

In addition to the enzymes required for purine and pyrimidine biosynthesis, the topoisomerases are important targets of several antineoplastic agents. Topoisomerase I and II catalyze the passage of DNA strands through single- or double-strand breaks in the DNA molecule, respectively, by nicking then reannealing the DNA strands. Topoisomerase inhibitors bind to the enzyme and stabilize the reaction intermediate, the enzyme–DNA cleavable complex. This interference with the DNA breakage-resealing process, which is necessary for both DNA replication and RNA transcription, results in DNA strand breaks that are lethal to the cell. The epipodophyllotoxins etoposide and teniposide are potent inhibitors of topoisomerase II, as are a number of DNA-intercalating agents, including doxorubicin, actinomycin D, and amsacrine (170, 171, 220). Camptothecin, a natural product derived from the Asian tree, *Camptotheca acuminata*, has been shown to be a potent inhibitor of topoisomerase I. Camptothecin itself had an unacceptably low therapeutic index in clinical trials, although several of its semisynthetic derivatives—topotecan, irinotecan (CPT-11), and 9-aminocamptothecin—are now undergoing clinical trials (21).

The microtubule spindle structure provides a third target for chemotherapeutic agents, classically, the vinca alkaloids vincristine and vinblastine, but more recently vinorelbine. The vinca alkaloids exert their cytotoxic effects by binding to specific sites on tubulin, inhibiting assembly of tubulin into microtubules, and ultimately causing dissolution of the mitotic spindle structure (132). The microtubule system of cells performs a variety of other important functions including transport of solutes, cell movement, chromosomal separation, and it provides structural integrity: any of these could potentially be disrupted by tubulin-binding agents (23). The taxanes, a newer class of agents, consist of the natural plant alkaloid paclitaxel and a semisynthetic derivative docetaxel. These novel plant alkaloids inhibit cell division by stimulating tubulin polymerization, thus enhancing the formation and stability of microtubules (172). Paclitaxel-treated cells accumulate large numbers of microtubules, free and in bundles, that disrupt microtubule function and that ultimately cause cell death (92, 116). Although docetaxel appears to be more potent than paclitaxel, the drugs appear to have similar toxicity profiles. Trials are presently being conducted to determine the spectrum of clinical activity of these promising new agents (137, 176, 185).

The search for specific inhibitors of hormone and growth factor receptors has been going on since the demonstration that antiestrogens can be effective treatment for breast cancers that contain the estrogen receptor. Recent studies have also demonstrated an important role for the antiandrogen flutamide in the treatment of prostate cancer (39). As more information becomes available concerning the regulatory properties of growth factors and their cellular receptors, these molecules are likely to become increasingly important targets of novel chemotherapeutic agents (70). One such drug appears to be the polysulfonated naphthylurea, suramin, which has been shown to block the binding to their cellular receptors of a range of tumor growth factors, including platelet-derived growth factor, transforming growth factor–beta, and epidermal growth factor (195). Clinical trials have demonstrated that treatment with suramin can induce antitumor effects in patients with adrenocortical carcinoma, renal cell carcinoma, and prostate cancer.

REPAIR OF DRUG-INDUCED INJURY

Cells that have been damaged by cytotoxic drugs exhibit a variety of repair mechanisms. Indeed, the cytotoxic effects of a drug often represent the balance between injury and repair, and amplified repair mechanisms may account for cellular resistance to certain drugs. The cytotoxicity of alkylating agents reflects the balance between DNA cross-link formation and removal by cellular repair processes. Many cells contain specific enzymes that remove alkyl moieties from DNA and, thus, repair drug damage. A specific example is the protein O^6-alkylguanyltransferase, which repairs DNA injury produced by chloroethylnitrosoureas. Cells containing large amounts of this protein tend to be relatively resistant to these chemotherapeutic agents. Depletion of alkyltransferase activity by exposure of cells to modified purine bases such as O^6-benzylguanine may be effective in circumventing this mechanism of resistance (48, 71). It is now clear that mammalian cells possess a family of such enzymes that are capable of repairing alkylation to specific nucleic acid bases and that the abundance of these in a particular tissue may be responsible for conferring relative sensitivity or resistance to chemotherapeutic alkylating agents (117, 179).

The broader task of protecting the genome from a wide variety of adducts that affect replication and transcription is taken up by the nucleotide excision repair system (32, 88). The increased incidence of cancer associated with inherited diseases such as xeroderma pigmetosum (which is characterized by the lack of effective nucleotide excision repair) attests to the key role of this system in suppressing carcinogenesis due to DNA damage (31). This system has a broad specificity of adducts that it can remove from DNA, ranging from simple methyl groups to bulky adducts, including natural molecules such as psoralen and aminofluorene. Lesions produced by cisplatin and cyclophosphamide are also substrates; an increase in the rate of platinum adduct removal has been associated with drug resistance (221). The mechanism of adduct removal is becoming clear and the various proteins involved are being identified (1, 128). Simply stated, two incisions are made in the adduct-containing DNA strand, about 27 to 29 nucleotides apart. This adduct-containing oligonucleotide is removed as a single piece, and new nucleotides are polymerized in the repair patch by the same DNA polymerases involved in replication. This DNA synthesis phase presents a new opportunity to incorporate nucleoside analogues into DNA of cells not in S phase that otherwise would not be affected. This possibility has given rise to therapeutic strategies which combine agents or modalities that elicit DNA repair with one of the newer nucleoside analogues, such as fludarabine (145) or gemcitabine (146), which inhibit DNA synthesis by various mechanisms and subsequently induce cell death by apoptosis (95).

Cells also contain a variety of free radical–scavenging systems that protect them from the effects of ionizing radiation and drugs that generate oxygen free radicals intracellularly. Catalase, superoxide dismutase, and glutathione peroxidase, key enzymes in the detoxification of reactive oxygen species, may be *deficient* in some tissues (like cardiac muscle), leading to excessive drug toxicity, or *increased* in others, leading to relative drug resistance (51). Some doxorubicin-resistant cells have been shown to have increased activity of superoxide dismutase and sodium-dependent glutathione peroxidase and diminished susceptibility to oxygen radical injury (124). Other studies suggest that expansion of intracellular reduced glutathione pools or increased expression of glutathione transferase may be important mechanisms of alkylating agent resistance in animal and human tumors (5, 80, 127).

Finally, cells may be able to circumvent drug-induced injury by increasing production of target enzymes. In experimental models, exposure of cells to methotrexate or 5-FU can be shown to stimulate production of dihydrofolate reductase or thymidylate synthase, respectively (49, 200). New enzyme production occurs within minutes to hours of drug exposure and is presumed to represent enhanced translation of existing mRNA, rather than transcription of additional message. Amplification of DNA also occurs, and this may be a fundamental mechanism of cellular resistance to antimetabolites and natural products, owing to increased constitutive production of target enzymes or P-glycoprotein (184).

A prerequisite to drug effect at the target tissue is adequate drug delivery. Pharmacokinetics describe the concentration-time history of a drug in the body and can be used to answer fundamental questions about the optimal route and schedule of drug administration. The remainder of this chapter presents the principles of pharmacokinetics and pharmacodynamics and illustrates their importance in cancer chemotherapy.

Principles of Pharmacokinetics

DEFINITIONS

Pharmacokinetics is the study of drug absorption, distribution, metabolism, and excretion. A fundamental concept in pharmacokinetics is drug clearance (i.e., elimination of drugs from the body, a phenomenon analogous to the concept of creatinine clearance). In clinical practice, clearance of a drug is rarely measured directly; rather, it is calculated as either

$$\text{clearance} = \text{dose/AUC} \tag{1}$$

or

$$\text{clearance} = \text{infusion rate}/C_{ss} \tag{2}$$

Area under the concentration-time curve (AUC) represents total drug exposure integrated over time, and it is an important parameter for both pharmacokinetic and pharmacodynamic analyses. As indicated in equation 1, the clearance is simply the ratio of the dose to the AUC, so that the higher the AUC for a given dose, the lower the clearance. If a drug is administered by continuous infusion and steady state is achieved, the clearance can be estimated from a single measurement of the plasma drug concentration (C_{ss}), per equation 2.

Clearance can be considered conceptually to be a function of both distribution and elimination. In the simplest pharmacokinetic model,

$$\text{clearance} = VK \tag{3}$$

where V is volume of distribution and K is elimination constant. V is the volume of fluid in which the dose is initially diluted; thus, the higher the value of V, the lower the initial concentration. K is the elimination constant, which is inversely proportional to the half-life (the interval in which plasma concentration decreases by 50%). When the half-life is short, K is high and plasma concentrations decline rapidly. Thus, both a high V value and a high K result in relatively low plasma concentrations and a high clearance rate.

LINEAR PHARMACOKINETIC MODELS

Although pharmacokinetic analysis can be conducted without specifying any mathematical models (noncompartmental methods), such models are helpful as guides in therapeutic decision making. There are several important properties of drugs that have linear pharmacokinetics (Table 58.2). The key feature of a linear pharmacokinetic model is this:

$$dC/dt = -KC \tag{4}$$

Table 58.2. Characteristics of Drugs with Linear Pharmacokinetics

Half-life is independent of concentration.
Clearance is independent of dose.
Clearance is independent of schedule.

The instantaneous rate of change in drug concentration depends only on the current concentration. The half-life remains constant, no matter how high the concentration.

One implication of this principle is that the drug exposure (AUC) is not affected by changes in drug schedule. For example, the AUC after a 60-mg/m^2 bolus dose of doxorubicin equals the total AUC for three daily (or weekly) bolus doses of 20 mg/m^2, which equals the AUC for the same dose administered as a 96-hour infusion. A second implication is that the AUC is proportional to the dose. Thus, if one measures the AUC for a 60-mg/m^2 dose, one can estimate that the AUC for a 90-mg/m^2 dose in the same patient is 50% higher.

The simplest linear pharmacokinetic model is

$$C(t) = (\text{dose}/V)\, e^{-kt} \quad (5)$$

The relationship is depicted graphically in Figure 58.2. This model assumes that the drug is administered as an instantaneous bolus and that complete distribution of the drug is also instantaneous.

Often, such assumptions are not valid. If the drug is administered as a slow bolus or infusion, the model must be corrected for the infusion duration. During the administration of the drug the concentration is increasing:

$$C(t) = \text{dose}/VKT\,(1 - e^{-kt}) \quad (6)$$

After the infusion is terminated, the drug concentration decay rate is the same as if it had been administered as an instantaneous bolus. Thus, if T represents the infusion time, then the postinfusion drug concentrations can be represented thus:

$$C'(t) = C(T)e^{-k(t-T)} \quad (7)$$

Often, the pharmacokinetic data are more complex than those shown in Figure 58.3, and they may optimally be fitted to a multicompartment model, usually two or three compartments (Fig. 58.3). It must be emphasized that the compartments are theoretical and do not necessarily correlate with any anatomic space or physiologic process.

The widespread availability of nonlinear regression programs makes it relatively easy to analyze pharmacokinetic data (73). Standard pharmacokinetic modeling programs are also available (119). The details of pharmacokinetic modeling are outside the scope of this chapter; though several caveats should be emphasized (118). The validity of pharmacokinetic modeling depends, to a large extent, on the quality of the data entered into the model. Thus, drug infusions must be precisely timed, plasma samples must be obtained on schedule, and analytical methods must be sensitive and specific. The data must be properly weighted to avoid bias due to the increased probability of analytic errors when drug concentrations are near the detection limit of the assay. Results obtained using a specific model should be compared to those using noncompartmental methods. Extrapolation of models outside the known time points must be done with great caution.

NONLINEAR PHARMACOKINETIC MODELS

Nonlinear pharmacokinetic models imply that some aspect of the pharmacokinetic behavior of the drug is sat-

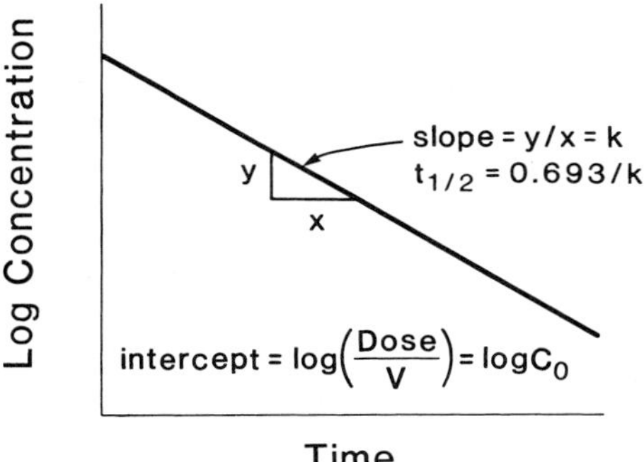

Figure 58.2. Concentration-time plot for one-compartment linear pharmacokinetic mode. C_0 represents the initial concentration, assuming instantaneous administration and distribution. The half-life is $\log_e(2)/k$.

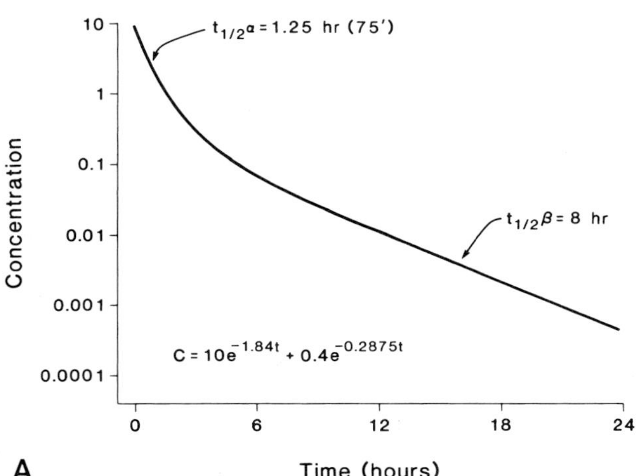

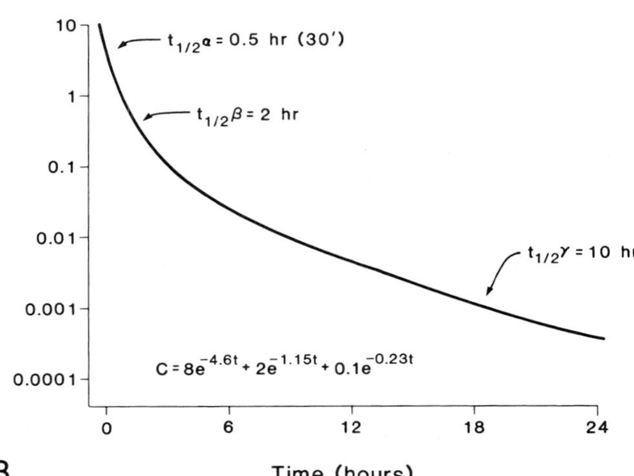

Figure 58.3. Concentration-time plots for representative two-compartment (**A**) and three-compartment (**B**) linear pharmacokinetic models. The two curves are very similar, with $C_0 \approx 10$ for both models. Note that for each "compartment" there is one term and that the corresponding half-life equals $\log_e(2)/k_n$, where k_n is the nth term.

urable. The mathematics of nonlinear models are beyond the scope of this chapter, but the principles are very relevant to several anticancer agents (75, 212). Modifying the schedule of administration of drugs that display nonlinear kinetics may markedly affect the AUC and potentially alter clinical effects, in contrast to the behavior of drugs with linear pharmacokinetics.

Nonlinear pharmacokinetic behavior is due to saturation of a major metabolic pathway. This results in decreased clearance at higher doses, with a disproportionate increase in AUC. The AUC will also increase if the infusion duration is shortened, owing to slower clearance at the higher peak plasma concentrations. This is clearly the case for 5-FU, probably owing to saturation of its conversion to dihydrofluorouracil by the enzyme dihydropyrimidine dehydrogenase (35, 129, 182, 211). Schaaf and colleagues demonstrated that doubling the dose of 5-FU from approximately 7.5 mg/kg to 15 mg/kg (by IV bolus) resulted in a 135% increase in the mean AUC (182). Since 5-FU is used on a variety of schedules, its nonlinear pharmacokinetic behavior may be one factor in its highly schedule-dependent effects. Recently, paclitaxel has also been demonstrated to have nonlinear pharmacokinetics (74, 192). Thus, the AUC is higher, for a fixed dose, when administered by shorter (3-hr vs. 24-hr) infusions, though this does not result in enhanced toxicity (59).

The opposite situation arises when a drug's absorption from the gastrointestinal tract (or renal tubular reabsorption) is saturable. In this case, an increase in dose results in a less than proportional increase in the AUC. Gastrointestinal absorption of drugs that resemble natural compounds is frequently mediated by active transport processes in the gastrointestinal tract that display saturable kinetics. Folate analogues such as methotrexate (MTX) or leucovorin and amino acid analogues such as melphalan are examples of drugs with saturable absorption (6, 28, 199). Cisplatin appears to have nonlinear pharmacokinetics, owing to saturation of its renal tubular reabsorption (69, 162). Forastiere and colleagues demonstrated that free plasma platinum is increased by 42% when the drug is given as a 24-hour continuous infusion, rather than as a 20-minute infusion (69). Prolonged infusion was also associated with a greater than three-fold increase in the free platinum half-life.

Table 58.3. Potential Sources of Interpatient Pharmacokinetic Variability in Cancer Patients

Abnormalities of absorption
Nausea/vomiting
Prior surgery, radiotherapy, or chemotherapy
Concurrent antiemetics affecting gut motility
Patient compliance
Concomitant medications
Abnormalities of distribution
Weight loss
Obesity
Decreased body fat (lipophilic drugs)
Pleural effusions or ascites (methotrexate)
Abnormalities of elimination
Hepatic dysfunction due to tumor replacement or prior (or concurrent) therapy
Renal dysfunction due to malignant involvement or prior (or concurrent) therapy
Concomitant medications
Abnormalities in protein binding
Hypoalbuminemia
Concomitant medications

INTERPATIENT PHARMACOKINETIC VARIABILITY

In describing a drug's pharmacokinetics, it is important to consider the extent of interpatient variability, a value often represented as the coefficient of variation (ratio of standard deviation to mean). Cancer patients may have significant hepatic or renal dysfunction, as well as other abnormalities that lead to alterations in pharmacokinetic parameters (see Table 58.3). Identifying genetic differences in drug metabolism may be particularly relevant to understanding pharmacokinetic variability (16). Such pharmacogenetic variation has been demonstrated to be important in explaining variability observed following administration of 6-mercaptopurine (110, 111), 5-fluorouracil (44, 90), and amonafide (151, 152, 154).

Studies of interpatient pharmacokinetic variability are potentially of great importance for optimizing antineoplastic therapy. Variability in gastrointestinal absorption, is often not considered in the use of orally administered antineoplastic agents, even though drugs such as cyclophosphamide, chlorambucil, melphalan, and etoposide are commonly administered orally for a variety of malignancies. The percentage of a drug absorbed is referred to as its bioavailability (i.e., the ratio of the plasma AUC after oral administration to the plasma AUC after IV administration of a given dose). Bioavailability may be influenced by drug metabolism in the gastrointestinal tract or liver, as well as by absorption. The (6S) isomer of leucovorin, for example, has limited bioavailability, owing primarily to its rapid conversion to 5-methyltetrahydrofolate before it enters the systemic circulation (183). By contrast, the bioavailability of (6R) leucovorin is limited primarily by absorption. Bioavailability is often highly variable and unpredictable (4, 7, 87, 222), and it may be accentuated by concomitant administration of other chemotherapeutic agents, particularly those that produce toxicity to the gastrointestinal mucosa (28).

Variability in drug distribution may be attributed to changes in body size or to the ratio of fat to total body mass (27). In the latter case, there may be altered distribution of lipophilic drugs—among which are included most of the natural product anticancer drugs and their analogues. The best described example of abnormal drug distribution is delayed clearance of methotrexate owing to accumulation and slow release of the drug secondary to ascites or pleural effusions (26). The terminal elimination half-life of doxorubicin, cyclophosphamide, and ifosfamide is prolonged in obese patients (113, 169). In the case of doxorubicin and cyclophosphamide this appears to be due to a reduction in clearance, whereas in the case of ifosfamide, it is related to increased volume of distribution of the drug (113).

Many patients with advanced cancer have abnormalities of liver function or known mass lesions in the liver, often in association with significant malnutrition. Given that many antineoplastic agents are metabolized or excreted by the liver, recognizing altered elimination by the liver becomes important in the optimization of chemotherapy dosing. Unfortunately, altered hepatic elimination or metabolism of drugs is not easily predictable. Clearly, patients with severe hyperbilirubinemia caused by parenchymal replacement or obstruction are likely to have altered elimination (196). However, often, it is not recognized that many patients with normal serum bilirubin levels may have a low drug clearance rate that results in a large AUC and corresponding toxicity. A decrease in serum albumin (in patients with normal serum bilirubin concentrations) has been associated with a decrease in the hepatic elimination of antipyrine—a commonly used marker drug—and of vinblastine (VLB) and trimetrexate (18, 65, 160, 193). Thus, patients whose serum albumin is less than 2.5 g/dl may be at increased risk of toxicity and are potentially candidates for dose reduction of agents requiring hepatic metabolism or excretion. At present, there are few firm guidelines that are useful for accurate dosing of antineoplastic agents in the setting of obvious hepatic disease.

In contrast, alterations in renal function generally correlate with renal clearance of drugs, since renal drug clearance tends to correlate with creatinine clearance. This has been well established for carboplatin: a firm relationship exists between renal function and carboplatin clearance that can be used prospectively to modify the carboplatin dose and avoid excessive toxicity (55, 89, 130).

Abnormalities of protein binding are common, but they rarely affect the clinical outcome. Many anticancer drugs, such as the vinca alkaloids and etoposide, are avidly protein bound (50, 196, 198). Changes in protein binding may affect drug clearance (190). Most important, abnormal protein binding must be considered in the interpretation of measured total plasma drug concentrations, since a decrease in protein binding results in a relative increase in the amount of pharmacologically active free drug (155, 196).

INTRAPATIENT PHARMACOKINETIC VARIABILITY

Although it is well established that *inter*patient pharmacokinetic variability may be significant, the importance of *intra*patient (within a single patient) variability is less clear (126). Oncologists are commonly faced with the clinical situation of increasing myelosuppression after repetitive dosing. This is generally assumed to be due to the cumulative effects of chemotherapy, making the patient more sensitive to subsequent doses. It is also possible that the patient's clearance of the drug(s) may have decreased, however, resulting in increased drug exposure.

Such a situation may arise when either hepatic or renal function changes. Renal function may change owing to progressive disease (ureteral obstruction), complications of therapy (volume depletion), or a direct toxic effect of therapy (e.g., cisplatin). Similarly, renal function may improve over time, reducing the actual level of drug exposure. Changes in hepatic function produce changes in drug clearance, which may result in the appearance of increased toxicity over time, as is the case for vinblastine administered by prolonged continuous infusion (160). Thus, clinicians should carefully review the outcome of prior doses, to minimize the risk of an undesirable outcome owing to intrapatient pharmacokinetic variability.

Another potential source of intrapatient pharmacokinetic variability is circadian rhythm. The best-studied drugs in this regard are 5-FU and 5-fluorodeoxyuridine (93). Petit and colleagues evaluated circadian variability of 5-FU plasma concentrations during a 5-day infusion at a constant dose, and they demonstrated a greater than two-fold difference between maximum and minimum values (139). Similar results were obtained by Harris and colleagues, who demonstrated an inverse correlation between plasma 5-FU concentration and the activity of dihydropyrimidine dehydrogenase, the major catabolic enzyme for 5-FU (90).

DRUG–DRUG INTERACTIONS

Despite the fact that anticancer drugs are almost always given as combination chemotherapy, often in conjunction with antiemetics and/or putative modulators, there have been relatively few studies of this area. One well-studied combination is paclitaxel and cisplatin, an important regimen for ovarian cancer, in which cisplatin reduces paclitaxel clearance if given first (175).

Studies of modulators of drug reactions have also demonstrated that inhibition of clearance may be an unexpected outcome. Such results have been demonstrated for cyclosporine A's effects on clearance of etoposide (115) and clearance of doxorubicin (60, 177) and the effect of IFN-α on 5-FU clearance (42).

Principles of Pharmacodynamics

DEFINITIONS

In a general sense, pharmacodynamics is the study of dose-response relationships (120). Thus, any laboratory or clinical study employing different doses of an agent is addressing a pharmacodynamic question. Examples include exposure of tumor cells in vitro to varying doses of a new agent to evaluate its dose-response relationship and a phase I clinical trial aimed at defining the maximal tolerated dose and dose-limiting toxicities in patients.

In the clinical setting, the results of treatment depend on both pharmacokinetics and pharmacodynamics (Fig. 58.1). A patient may have excessive toxicity at the "standard" dose for either of two reasons. If the patient's "pharmacokinetics" are different from those of the typical patient (e.g., decreased renal clearance of carboplatin), decreased total body clearance may result in a higher than expected drug exposure. The second possibility is that the patient might simply be more sensitive to an average drug exposure—whether owing to prior therapy, poor nutrition, or some other, less well-defined reason(s). It is important to distinguish between these two possibilities. In the first case, lowering the dose will result in an "average" drug exposure, whereas in the second case lowering the dose will result in a lower-than-average drug exposure. Therefore, in the setting of dose reduction, there is a greater possibility of a response in the patient with abnormal pharmacokinetics than in the "sensitive" patient with abnormal pharmacodynamics.

GENERAL PHARMACODYNAMIC PRINCIPLES

In the most general sense, any drug may be considered to have a maximal effect and a median dose (i.e., that required for 50% of the maximal effect). Wagner proposed a generalized sigmoidal model of drug effect (Fig. 58.4), a concept derived from the hypothesis that all drug effects require an initial interaction with a receptor (210).

Most studies that address pharmacodynamic modeling of anticancer agents have addressed phase-specific agents separately (104, 133). It may be adequate to use a simple log-linear model for non–phase-specific agents (105, 188):

$$\text{survival fraction (SF)} = \text{no. of treated cells/no. of control cells} = e^{-KC} \quad (8)$$

This may be referred to as a steep dose-response curve, since the effect continues to increase proportionally as the concentration (C) increases. For any value of K (see equation 8), an increase in C by 2.3/K will result in a 1-log increase in antitumor effect (Fig. 58.5*A*).

The dose-response relationships for phase-specific agents, such as the antimetabolites, are much more complicated. By definition, some cells are out of "phase" and therefore not sensitive (or relatively insensitive) to the effects of the drug during the period of drug exposure. This cannot necessarily be overcome by increasing the dose, but it could be overcome by increasing the duration of drug exposure. The result is the appearance of a plateau in the dose-response curve (Fig. 58.5*B*).

The effects of some antineoplastic agents depend on both the drug concentration and the duration of exposure to that concentration. For some agents, the effect is a function of the product of the concentration and exposure time, analogous to the AUC (58). For antimetabolites and other phase-specific agents, however, the mathematic relationships are much more complex (57, 104, 133). Drug effect tends to be

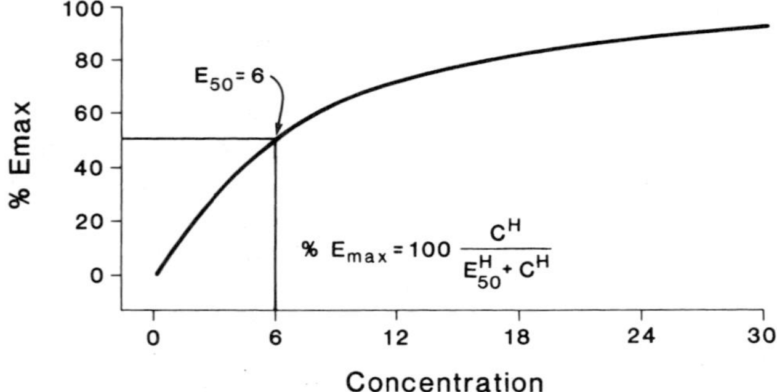

Figure 58.4. Example of E_{max} model as proposed by Wagner (210). The maximum effect is 100%, and a concentration of 6 results in 50% effect. The exponent *H*, also known as the Hill constant, determines the shape of the curve and is usually a value between 1 and 2.

related to duration of exposure *above a threshold concentration.*

Plasma concentrations may be an inadequate predictor of clinical effect for agents that undergo intracellular anabolism to active metabolites, as does ara-C (112). Plasma ara-C concentrations do not appear to correlate with the rate of cellular ara-CTP accumulation or peak ara-CTP concentration in leukemic cells, although the intracellular concentration of ara-CTP is an important determinant of treatment outcome. Thus, knowledge of the plasma pharmacokinetics of ara-C is not likely to be a useful predictor of treatment outcome for individual patients. Pharmacogenetic evaluation may be potentially useful for modeling relationships between 6-mercaptopurine pharmacokinetics and clinical effects, as this drug's conversion to active intracellular 6-thioguanine metabolites by thiopurine methyltransferase is genetically determined (111). Studies in children with acute lymphoblastic leukemia suggest that intracellular levels of 6-thioguanine nucleotides may be an independent predictor of remission duration (110).

PHARMACODYNAMIC MODELING OF CANCER CHEMOTHERAPY

The introduction of pharmacodynamic modeling into clinical oncology has been a slow process. The relationship between toxicity subsequent to high-dose MTX and delayed MTX clearance has led to the routine use of therapeutic drug monitoring of plasma MTX concentrations to guide leucovorin dosing (3). Findings of studies of other drugs have not clearly resulted in a change in clinical practice, though recently, clinical research in this area has increased (156).

Most early pharmacodynamic studies addressed relationships between measurements of drug exposure (AUC, C_{ss}) and toxicity. More recently, investigators have utilized novel pharmacokinetic parameters to model toxicity, such as time above a threshold concentration for etoposide (30) and paclitaxel (74, 97, 192, 219). Other investigators have addressed the importance of active metabolites. This is particularly important for irinotecan, a drug whose metabolism and toxicity patterns are both complex. However, a recent study has suggested that irinotecan-induced diarrhea is secondary to relative deficiency in the glucuronidation of SN-38, its active metabolite (86). Hematologic toxicity has been easier to model than nonhematologic toxicity in Tables 58.4 and 58.5, respectively.

One of the best-characterized drugs is carboplatin, an analogue of cisplatin. Unlike cisplatin, the dose-limiting toxicity of carboplatin is thrombocytopenia, which is a function of drug dose, renal function, pretreatment platelet count, and prior therapy (55). The platelet nadir produced by a dose of carboplatin is related to the carboplatin clearance, which is directly proportional to creatinine clearance. Thus, patients at high risk of severe thrombocytopenia following carboplatin therapy can be identified prospectively and the drug doses can be modified by monitoring glomerular filtration rate.

Etoposide has also been the subject of extensive evaluation. Pharmacodynamic modeling of etoposide is compli-

Table 58.4. Selected Pharmacodynamic Studies of Hematologic Toxicity

Drug	Reference	Pharmacokinetic parameter[a]	Toxicity[b]
Amonafide	Ratain (152, 154)	SP_m	W, P
Carboplatin	Egorin (55)	AUC	P
	Newell (130, 131)	AUC	W, P
Doxorubicin	Ackland (2)	C_{ss}	W
	Piscitelli (141)	AUC	W
	Rushing (177)	AUC	W
Epirubicin	Jakobsen (98)	SP	W
Etoposide	Ratain (155)	C_{ss}	W
	Kunitoh (109)	C_{ss}	N
	Clark (30)	TAT	W, N
	Miller (121, 122, 123)	SP	W, N
	Minami (125)	C_{ss}	W, P
5-Fluorouracil	Au (8)	C_{ss}	W
	Trump (207)	C_{ss}	W
HMBA[c]	Egorin (54)	AUC	P
	Rowinsky (173, 174)	C_{ss}, AUC	P
Menogaril	Egorin (52, 56)	AUC	W, N
	Dodion (47)	AUC, SP	W, N
Paclitaxel	Gianni (74)	TAT	N
	Huizing (97)	TAT	W, N
	Wilson (219)	C_{ss}	N
Topotecan	Grochow (85)	AUC	N
	Stewart (197)	AUC	N, P
	Haas (87)	C_{ss}	N
Trimetrexate	Fanucchi (65)	AUC	P
	Reece (161)	AUC, C_{ss}	P
	Grochow (83, 84)	AUC, SP	P, W
Vinblastine	Ratain (158)	C_{ss}	W

[a] AUC, area under the curve; C_{ss}, "steady-state" concentration during continuous infusion; SP, single point; TAT, time above threshold; SP_m, single point metabolite.
[b] P, thrombocytopenia; W, leukopenia; N, neutropenia.
[c] HMBA, hexamethylene bisacetamide.

cated by the need either to measure free etoposide directly, or to estimate the free etoposide concentration on the basis of measured total plasma etoposide concentration, albumin, and/or bilirubin (155, 198). Many studies have now demonstrated that the extent of leukopenia/neutropenia is correlated with etoposide exposure (13, 109, 121–123, 125, 155). Furthermore, interpatient pharmacodynamic variability may be significant and needs to be considered in future modeling of etoposide and potentially in other drugs (155).

Interest is expanding in trying to optimize cancer chemotherapy by individualizing dosing on the basis of measurements of plasma or tissue drug concentrations. One recent example is the titration of carboplatin dosing discussed above. Other investigators have attempted to optimize the dosing of etoposide (153, 155), teniposide (168), hexamethylene bisacetamide (37, 38), etanidazole (33), melphalan (143), and 5-FU (181) by monitoring plasma drug concentrations during treatment, then using the information obtained to modify the total dose of chemotherapy administered in an attempt to avoid severe toxicity. Although it has not yet been established in a prospective randomized study that this approach will improve the therapeutic index, the studies to date have been very encouraging.

Table 58.5. Selected Pharmacodynamic Studies of Nonhematologic Toxicity

Drug	Reference	Pharmacokinetic parameter[a]	Toxicity[b]
Busulfan	Grochow (82)	AUC	H
Carmustine	Jones (101)	AUC	PU
Cisplatin	Reece (163)	SP, AUC	R
	Ayash (9)	AUC	C
Etanidazole	Coleman (34)	AUC	PN
5-Fluorouracil	Thyss (205)	AUC	NS
	van Groeningen (209)	AUC	NS
	Trump (207)	C_{ss}	MU
Irinotecan	Gupta (86)	RAUC	GI
Paclitaxel	Wilson (219)	C_{ss}	MU

[a] AUC, area under the curve; SP, single point; C_{ss}, "steady-state" concentration during continuous infusion; RAUC, ratio of AUCs of parent drug and metabolites.
[b] H, hepatotoxicity; PU, pulmonary; R, nephrotoxicity; C, cardiac; PN, peripheral neuropathy; NS, not specified; MU, mucositis; GI, gastrointestinal.

FUTURE ROLE OF ANTICANCER PHARMACODYNAMICS

Should the clinical oncologist care about pharmacodynamics? Will therapeutic drug monitoring of antineoplastics be as useful as monitoring of theophylline or aminoglycoside dosing? How will these studies improve the therapeutic index? These are important issues that are currently being addressed.

Our true understanding of dosing of most antineoplastic drugs is primitive. Body surface area is generally the only value used to determine initial dosing, and even that has recently been questioned (81, 166). A history of prior toxicity may be used to adjust dosing for subsequent cycles, although doses are more often reduced than escalated and the magnitude of dose changes is determined empirically, and often arbitrarily.

For drugs with a relatively broad therapeutic index and/or minimal interpatient pharmacokinetic or pharmacodynamic variability, these strategies may not be necessary. As an example, therapeutic drug monitoring of interferon alfa in hairy cell leukemia is unlikely to be useful (79). In contrast, therapeutic drug monitoring of doxorubicin in the adjuvant treatment of breast cancer may potentially help to ensure adequate drug exposure and to minimize the risk of life-threatening toxicity.

An achievable future goal is the individualization of dosing of drugs with polymorphic metabolism. Important examples are 5-FU (45, 66), 6-mercaptopurine (110, 111), amonafide (151, 152), and, possibly, irinotecan (86). To date, most pharmacodynamic studies have focused on toxicity as an end point, primarily owing to the patient populations studied (i.e., patients with refractory tumors enrolled in phase I clinical trials). The potential usefulness of this area is underscored by several studies correlating the clearance of MTX, teniposide, and 6-mercaptopurine with response or survival in acute lymphocytic leukemia (63, 91, 108, 167). Prospective evaluation of plasma (154) or intratumoral (150) concentrations in conjunction with phase II clinical trials may im-

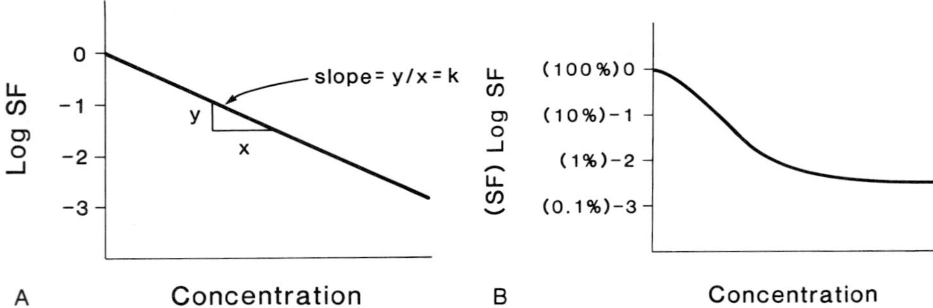

Figure 58.5. Pharmacodynamic plots for drugs with non-saturable (**A**) and saturable (**B**) effects. In the simplest pharmacodynamic model (**A**), there is a linear relationship between dose and log kill. In **B**, there is a maximal effect, resulting in a plateau in the dose-response curve. SF = Survival fraction.

prove our understanding of the relationship between clinical pharmacology and drug efficacy for other tumors as well. Although most studies to date have utilized continuous-infusion chemotherapy, recent strategies have been developed with the aim of optimizing dosing after conventional bolus administration (53, 112, 143, 157, 159, 168). It may eventually become possible to dose routinely toward a target AUC or C_{SS} (or time above a threshold) using principles of therapeutic drug monitoring for guidelines.

The next challenge will be optimizing the use of combination chemotherapy. A prospective randomized study in progress at St. Jude Children's Research Hospital is designed to show that individualized dosing of ara-C, teniposide, and high-dose MTX is superior to conventional dosing for treatment of childhood acute leukemia (64). As studies of the pharmacodynamics of single agents are completed it will become possible to evaluate the pharmacodynamics of drug combinations. As an example, Belani and colleagues recently demonstrated that etoposide does not significantly affect the pharmacodynamics of carboplatin-induced thrombocytopenia (12).

In conclusion, it is hoped that better understanding of the clinical pharmacology of antineoplastics will improve the care of cancer patients. At a minimum, clinicians should understand the basic principles, realizing the limitations of our current approaches.

References

1. Aboussekhra A, Biggerstaff M, Shivji MKK, Vilpo JA, Moncollin V, Podust VN, Protic M, Hubscher U, Egly J-M, Wood RD. Mammalian DNA nucleotide excision repair reconstituted with purified protein components. Cell 1995;80:859.
2. Ackland SP, Ratain MJ, Vogelzang NJ, Choi KE, Ruane M, Sinkule JA. Pharmacokinetics and pharmacodynamics of long-term continuous-infusion doxorubicin. Clin Pharmacol Ther 1989;45:340.
3. Ackland SP, Schilsky RL. High-dose methotrexate: a critical reappraisal. J Clin Oncol 1987;5:2017.
4. Adamson PC, Pitot HC, Balis FM, Rubin J, Murphy RF, Poplack DG. Variability in the oral bioavailability of all-trans-retinoic acid. JNCI 1993;16:993.
5. Ahmad S, Okine L, Le B, Najarian P, Vistica DT. Elevation of glutathione in phenylalanine mustard-resistant murine L1210 leukemia cells. J Biol Chem 1987;262: 15048.
6. Alberts DS, Chang SY, Chen, H-SG, Evans TL, Moon TE. Oral melphalan kinetics. Clin Pharmacol Ther 1979;26:737.
7. Allegra JC, Chabner BA, Drake JC, Lutz R, Rodbard D, Jolivet J. Enhanced inhibition of thymidylate synthase by methotrexate polyglutamates. J Biol Chem 1985;260: 9720.
8. Au, JL-S, Rustum YM, Ledesma EJ, Mittelman A, Creaven PJ. Clinical pharmacological studies of concurrent infusion of 5-fluorouracil and thymidine in the treatment of colorectal carcinoma. Cancer Res 1982;42:2930.
9. Ayash LJ, Wright JE, Tretyakov O, Gonin R, Elias A, Wheeler C, Eder JP, Rosowsky A, Antman K, Frei E. Cyclophosphamide pharmacokinetics: correlation with cardiac toxicity and tumor response. J Clin Oncol 1992;10:995.
10. Bank BB. Studies of chlorambucil-DNA adducts. Biochem Pharmacol 1992;44:571.
11. Bank BB, Kanganis D, Liebes LF, Silber R. Chlorambucil pharmacokinetics and DNA binding in chronic lymphocytic leukemia lymphocytes. Cancer Res 1989;49:554.
12. Belani CP, Egorin MJ, Abrams J, Hiponia D, Eisenberger M, Aisner J, Van Echo DA. A novel pharmacodynamic approach to dose optimization of carboplatin when used in combination with etoposide. J Clin Oncol 1989;7:1896.
13. Bennett CL, Sinkule JA, Schilsky RL, Senekjian E, Choi KE. Phase I clinical and pharmacological study of 72-hour continuous infusion of etoposide in patients with advanced cancer. Cancer Res 1987;47:1952.
14. Bhalla K, Nayak R, Grant S. Isolation and characterization of a deoxycytidine kinase-deficient human promyelocytic leukemic cell line highly resistant to 1-β-D-arabinofuranosylcytosine.
15. Blommaert FA, Michael C, Terheggen PMAB, Muggia FM, Kortes V, Schornagel JH, Hart AAM, den Engelese L. Drug-induced DNA modification in buccal cells of cancer patients receiving carboplatin and cisplatin combination chemotherapy, as determined by an immunocytochemical method: interindividual variation and correlation with disease response. Cancer Res 1993;53:5669.
16. Boddy AV, Idle JR. The role of pharmacogenetics in chemotherapy: modulation of tumor response and host toxicity. Cancer Surv 1993;17:79.
17. Bolzan AD, Bianchi NO, Larramedndy ML, Bianchi MS. Chromosomal sensitivity of human lymphocytes to bleomycin. Influence of antioxidant enzyme activities in whole blood and different blood fractions. Cancer Genet Cytogenet 1992;64:133.
18. Branch RA, Herbert CM, Read AE. Determinants of serum antipyrine half-lives in patients with liver disease. Gut 1973;14:569.
19. Brigle KE, Seither RL, Westin EH, Goldman ID. Increased expression and genomic organization of a folate-binding protein homologous to the human placental isoform in L1210 murine leukemia cell lines with a defective reduced folate carrier. J Biol Chem 1994;269:4267–4272.
20. Brookes P, Lawley PD. The reaction of mono- and bifunctional alkylating agents with nucleic acids. Bio Chem J 1961;80:496.
21. Burris HA, Fields SM. Topoisomerase I inhibitors. An overview of the camptothecin analogues. Hematol Oncol Clin North Am 1994;8:333.
22. Cass C. Nucleoside transport. In Drug Transport in Antimicrobial and Anticancer Chemotherapy. Edited by NH Georgopapadakou. New York: Marcel Dekker, 1994.
23. Cass CE, Beck WT. Vinca alkaloid Pharmacology and Resistance. In Resistance to Antineoplastic Drugs. Edited by D Kessel. Boca Raton, FL: CRC Press, 1989, p 141.
24. Catapano CV, Perrino FW, Fernandes DJ. Primer RNA chain termination induced by 9-β-D-arabinofuranosyl-2-fluoroadenine 5′-triphosphate. A mechanism of DNA synthesis inhibition. J Biol Chem 1993;268:7189.
25. Chabner BA. Cytidine analogues. In Cancer Chemotherapy: Principles and Practice. Edited by BA Chabner, JM Collins. Philadelphia: Lippincott, 1990, p 154.
26. Chabner BA, Stoller RG, Hande K, Jacobs S, Young RC. Methotrexate disposition in humans: case studies in ovarian cancer and following high-dose infusion. Drug Metabol Rev 1978;8:107.
27. Cheymol G. Drug pharmacokinetics in the obese. Fund Clin Pharmacol 1988;2:239.
28. Choi KE, Ratain MJ, Williams SF, Golick JA, Beschorner JC, Fullem LJ, Bitran JD. Plasma pharmacokinetics of high-dose oral melphalan in patients treated with trialkylator chemotherapy and autologous bone marrow reinfusion. Cancer Res 1989;49:1318.
29. Chou T-C, Arlin Z, Clarkson BD, Philips FS. Metabolism of 1-β-D-arabinofuranosylcytosine in human leukemic cells. Cancer Res 1977;37:3561.
30. Clark PI, Slevin ML, Joel SP, Osborne RJ, Talbot DI, Johnson PW, Reznek R, Masud T, Gregory W, Wrigley PF. A randomized trial of two etoposide schedules in small-cell lung cancer: the influence of pharmacokinetics on efficacy and toxicity. J Clin Oncol 1994;12:1427.
31. Cleaver JE. Defective repair replication of DNA in xeroderma pigmentosum. Nature 1968;218:652.
32. Cleaver JE. It was a very good year for DNA repair. Cell 1994;76:1.
33. Coleman CN, Buswell L, Noll L, Riese N, Rose MA. The efficacy of pharmacokinetic monitoring and dose modification of etanidazole on the incidence of neurotoxicity: results from a phase II trial of etanidazole and radiation therapy in locally advanced prostate cancer. Int J Radial Oncol Biol Phys 1992;22:565.
34. Coleman CN, Halsey J, Cox RS, Hirst VK, Blaschke T, Howes AE, Wasserman TH, Urtasun RC, Pajak T, Hancock S, Phillips TL, Noll L. Relationship between the neurotoxicity of the hypoxic cell radiosensitizer SR 2508 and the pharmacokinetic profile. Cancer Res 1987;47:319.
35. Collins J, Dedrick R, King F, Speyer J, Myers C. Nonlinear pharmacokinetic models

for 5-fluorouracil in man: intravenous and intraperitoneal routes. Clin Pharmacol Ther 1980;28:235.
36. Colvin M, Padgett CA, Fenselau C. A biologically active metabolite of cyclophosphamide. Cancer Res 1973;33:915.
37. Conley BA, Egorin MJ, Sinibaldi V, Sewack G, Kloc C, Roberts L, Zuhowski EG, Forrest A, Van Echo DA. Approaches to optimal dosing of hexamethylene bisacetamide. Cancer Chemother Pharmacol 1992;31:37.
38. Conley BA, Forrest A, Egorin MJ, Zuhowski EG, Sinibaldi V, Van Echo DA. Phase I trial using adaptive control dosing of hexamethylene bisacetamide (NSC 95580). Cancer Res 1989;49:3436.
39. Crawford ED, Eisenberger MA, McLeod DG, Spaulding JT, Benson R, Dorr FA, Blumenstein BA, Davis MA, Goodman PI. A controlled trial of leuprolide with and without flutamide in prostate carcinoma. N Engl J Med 1989;321:419.
40. Crawford CR, Ng CYC, Noel LD, Belt JA. Nucleoside transport in L1210 murine leukemia cells. J Biol Chem 1990;265:9732.
41. Dalton WS. Is p-glycoprotein a potential target for reversing clinical drug resistance? Curr Opin Oncol 1994;6:595.
42. Danhauser LL, Freimann JH, Gilchrist TL, Gutterman JU, Hunter CY, Yeomans AC, Markowitz AB. Phase I and plasma pharmacokinetic study of infusional fluorouracil combined with recombinant interferon alfa-2b in patients with advanced cancer. J Clin Oncol 1993;11:751.
43. Datta NS, Shewach DS, Mitchell BS, Fox IH. Kinetic properties and inhibition of human T lymphoblast deoxycytidine kinase. J Biol Chem 1989;264:9359.
44. Deffie AM, Batra JK, Goldenberg GJ. Direct correlation between DNA topoisomerase II activity and cytotoxicity in adriamycin-sensitive and -resistant P388 leukemia cell lines. Cancer Res 1989;49:58.
45. Diasio RB, Beavers TL, Carpenter JT. Familial deficiency of dihydropyrimidine dehydrogenase: biochemical basis for familial pyrimidinemia and severe 5-fluorouracil–induced toxicity. J Clin Invest 1988;81:47.
46. Dixon KH, Lanpher BC, Chiu J, Kelley K, Cowan KH. A novel cDNA restores reduced folate carrier activity and methotrexate sensitivity to transport deficient cells. J Biol Chem 1994;269:17–20.
47. Dodion P, de Valeriola D, Crespeigne N, Peeters B, Wery F, Van Berchem C, Piccart M, Tueni E, Joggi J, Kenis Y. Phase I clinical and pharmacokinetic trial of oral menogaril administered on three consecutive days. Eur J Cancer Clin Oncol 1988;24:1019.
48. Dolan ME, Pegg AE, Moschel RC, Grindey GB. Effects of O^6-benzylguanine analogues on the sensitivity of human colon tumor xenografts to BCNU. Biochem Pharmacol 1993;46:285.
49. Domin BA, Grill SP, Bastow KF, Cheng YC. Effect of methotrexate on dihydrofolate reductase activity in methotrexate resistant human KB cells. Molec Pharmacol 1982;21: 478.
50. Donigian DW, Owellen RT. Interaction of vinblastine, vincristine and colchicine with serum proteins. Biochem Pharmacol 1973;22:2113.
51. Doroshow JH, Locker GY, Myers CE. Enzymatic defenses of the mouse heart against reactive oxygen: alterations produced by doxorubicin. J Clin Invest 1980;65:128.
52. Egorin MJ, Conley BA, Forrest A, Zuhowski EG, Sinibaldi V, Van Echo DA. Phase I study and pharmacokinetics of menogaril (NSC 269148) in patients with hepatic dysfunction. Cancer Res 1987;47:6104.
53. Egorin MJ, Forrest A, Belani CP, Ratain MJ, Abrams JS, Van Echo DA. A limited sampling strategy for cyclophosphamide pharmacokinetics. Cancer Res 1989;49:3129.
54. Egorin MJ, Sigman LM, Van Echo DA, Forrest A, Whitacre MY, Aisner J. Phase I clinical and pharmacokinetic study of hexamethylene bisacetamide (NSC 95580) administered as a five-day continuous infusion. Cancer Res 1987;47:617.
55. Egorin MJ, Van Echo DA, Tipping SJ, Olman EA, Whitacre MY, Thompson BW, Aisner J. Pharmacokinetics and dosage reduction of cis-diammine (1,1-cyclobutanedicarboxylato)-platinum in patients with impaired renal function. Cancer Res 1984;44: 5432.
56. Egorin MJ, Van Echo DA, Whitacre MY, Forrest A, Sigman LM, Engisch KL, Aisner J. Human pharmacokinetics, excretion, and metabolism of the anthracycline menogaril (7-OMEN, NSC 269148) and their correlation with clinical toxicities. Cancer Res 1986;46:1513.
57. Eichholtz H, Trott KR. Effect of methotrexate concentration and exposure time on mammalian cell survival in vitro. Br J Cancer 1980;41:277.
58. Eichholtz-Wirth H. Dependence of the cytostatic effect of adriamycin on drug concentration and exposure time in vitro. Br J Cancer 1980;41:886.
59. Eisenhauer EA, ten Bokkel Huinink WW, Swenerton KD, et al. European-Canadian randomized trial of paclitaxel in relapsed ovarian cancer: high- versus low-dose and long versus short infusion. J Clin Oncol 1994;12:2654.
60. Erlichman C, Moore M, Thiessen JJ, Kerr IG, Walker S, Goodman P, Bjarnason G, DeAngelis C, Bunting P. Phase I pharmacokinetic study of cyclosporin A combined with doxorubicin. Cancer Res 1993;53:4837.
61. Estey EH, Keating MJ, McCredie KB, Freireich EJ, Plunkett W. Cellular ara-CTP pharmacokinetics, response, and karyotype in newly diagnosed acute myelogenous leukemia. Leukemia 1990;4:95.
62. Estey E, Plunkett W, Gandhi V, Rios MB, Kantarjian H, Keating MJ. Fludarabine and arabinosylcytosine therapy of refractory and relapsed acute myelogenous leukemia. Leuk Lymp 1993;9:343.
63. Evans WE, Crom WR, Abromowitch M, Dodge R, Look AT, Bowman WP, George SL, Pui C-H. Clinical pharmacodynamics of high-dose methotrexate in acute lymphocytic leukemia. N Engl J Med 1986;314:471.
64. Evans WE, Rodman J, Relling MV, et al. Individualized dosages of chemotherapy as a strategy to improve response for acute lymphocytic leukemia. Semin Hematol 1991;28:15.
65. Fanucchi MP, Walsh TD, Fleisher M, Lokos G, Williams L, Cassidy C, Vidal P, Chou T-C, Niedzwiecki O, Young CW. Phase I and clinical pharmacology study of trimetrexate administered weekly for three weeks. Cancer Res 1987;47:3303.
66. Fisher TC, Milner AE, Gregory CD, Jackman AL, Aherne GW, Hartley JA, Dive C, Hickman JA. bcl-2 Modulation of apoptosis induced by anticancer drugs: resistance to thymidylate stress is independent of classical resistance pathways. Cancer Res 1993;53:3321.
67. Flasshove M, Tirier C, Heit W, Ayscue L, Mitchell B, Seeber S, Schutte J. Analysis of the deoxycytidine kinase gene in patients with acute myeloid leukemia and resistance to cytosin-arabinoside. Proc Am Assn Cancer Res 1993;34:25.
68. Fleming RA, Milano G, Thyss A, Etienne MC, Renee N, Schneider M, Demard F. Correlation between dihydropyrimidine dehydrogenase activity in peripheral mononuclear cells and systemic clearance of fluorouracil in cancer patients. Cancer Res 1992;52:2899.
69. Forastiere AA, Belliveau JF, Goren MP, Vogel WC, Posner MR, O'Leary GP, Jr. Pharmacokinetics and toxicity evaluation of five-day continuous infusion versus intermittent bolus cis-diamminedichloroplatinum (II) in head and neck cancer patients. Cancer Res 1988;48:3869.
70. Francis GE. Growth and differentiation control. In Cancer Chemotherapy and Biological Reponse Modifiers, Annual 15. Edited by HM Pinedo, DL Longo, BA Chabner. Amsterdam: Elsevier, 1994, p 287.
71. Friedman HS, Dolan ME, Moschel RC, Pegg AE, Felker GM, Rich J, Bigner DD, Schold SC. Enhancement of nitrosurea activity in meduloblastoma and glioblastoma multiforme. JNCI 1992;84:1926.
72. Gandhi V, Estey E, Keating MJ, Plunkett W. Fludarabine potentiates metabolism of cytarabine in patients with acute myelogenous leukemia during therapy. J Clin Oncol 1993;11:11.
73. Garcia-Pena J, Azen SP. A user's experience with a standard non-linear regression program (BMDP 3R). Comput Programs Biomed 1979;10:185.
74. Gianni L, Kearns CM, Giani A, Capri G, Vigano L, Locatelli A, Bonadonna G, Egorin MJ. Nonlinear pharmacokinetics and metabolism of paclitaxel and its pharmacokinetic/pharmacodynamic relationships in humans. J Clin Oncol 1995;13:180.
75. Gibaldi M, Perrier D. Pharmacokinetics, 2nd ed. New York: Marcel Dekker, 1982.
76. Giloni L, Takeshita M, Johnson F, Iden C, Grollman AP. Bleomycin-induced strand scission of DNA: mechanism of deoxyribose cleavage. J Biol Chem 1981;256:8608.
77. Goldenberg GJ, Begleiter A. Membrane transport of alkylating agents. Pharmacol Ther 1980;8:237.
78. Goldman ID. Pharmacokinetics of antineoplastic agents at the cellular level. In Pharmacologic Principles of Cancer Treatment. Edited by BA Chabner. Philadelphia: Saunders, 1982, p 15.
79. Golomb HM, Jacobs A, Fefer A, Ozer H, Thompson J, Portlock C, Ratain M, Golde D, Vardiman J, Burke JS, Brady J, Bonnem E, Spiegel R. Alpha-2 interferon therapy of hairy cell leukemia: a multicenter study of 64 patients. J Clin Oncol 1986;4:900.
80. Green JA, Vistica DT, Young RL, Hamilton TC, Rogan AM, Ozols RF. Potentiation of melphalan cytotoxicity in human ovarian cancer cell lines by glutathione depletion. Cancer Res 1984;44:5427.
81. Grochow LB, Baraldi C, Noe D. Is dose normalization to weight or body surface area useful in adults? JNCI 1990;82:323.
82. Grochow LB, Jones RJ, Brundrett RB, Braine HG, Chen T-L, Saral R, Santos GW, Colvin MO. Pharmacokinetics of busulfan: correlation with veno-occlusive disease in patients undergoing bone marrow transplantation. Cancer Chemother Pharmacol 1990;25:55.
83. Grochow LB, Noe DA, Dole GB, Rowinsky EK, Ettinger DS, Graham ML, McGuire WP, Donehower RC. Phase I trial of trimetrexate glucuronate on a five-day bolus schedule: clinical pharmacology and pharmacodynamics. JNCI 1989;81:124.
84. Grochow LB, Noe DA, Ettinger DS, Doehower RC. A phase I trial of trimetrexate glucuronate (NSC 352122) given every 3 weeks: clinical pharmacology and pharmacodynamics. Cancer Chemother Pharmacol 1989;24:314.
85. Grochow LB, Rowinsky EK, Johnson R, Ludeman S, Kaufmann SH, McCabe FC, Smith BR, Hurowitz L, DeLisa A, Donehower RC, et al. Pharmacokinetics and pharmacodynamics of topotecan in patients with advanced cancer. Drug Metab Dispos Biol Fate Chem 1992;20:706.
86. Gupta E, Lestingi TM, Mick R, Ramirez J, Vokes EE, Ratain MJ. Metabolic fate of irinotecan in humans: correlation of glucuronidation with diarrhea. Cancer Res 1994;54:3723.
87. Haas NB, LaCreta FP, Walczak J, Hudes GR, Brennan JM, Ozols RF, O'Dwyer PJ. Phase I/pharmacokinetic study of topotecan by 24-hour continuous infusion weekly. Cancer Res 1994;54:1220.
88. Hanawalt PC. DNA repair comes of age. Mutation Res 1995;336:101.
89. Harland SJ, Newell DR, Siddik ZH, Chadwick R, Calvert AH, Harrap KR. Pharmacokinetics of cis-diammine-1, 1-cyclobutane dicarboxylate platinum (II) in patients with normal and impaired renal function. Cancer Res 1984;44:1693.
90. Harris BE, Song R, Soong SJ, Diasio RB. Relationship between dihydropyrimidine dehydrogenase activity and plasma 5-fluorouracil levels with evidence for circadian variation of enzyme activity and plasma drug levels in cancer patients receiving 5-fluorouracil by protracted continuous infusion. Cancer Res 1990;50:197.
91. Hayder S, Lafolie P, Bjork O, Peterson C. 6-Mercaptopurine plasma levels in children with acute lymphoblastic leukemia: relation to relapse risk and myelotoxicity. Ther Drug Monitor 1989;11:617.
92. Horwitz SB, Cohen D, Rao S, Ringel I, Shen HJ, Yang CP. Taxol: mechanisms of action and resistance. Monogr Natl Cancer Inst 1993;15:55.
93. Hrushesky WJM, von Roemeling R, Lanning RM, Rabatin JT. Circadium-shaped infusions of floxuridine for progressive metastatic renal cell carcinoma. J Clin Oncol 1990;8:1504.
94. Huang P, Chubb S, Plunkett W. Termination of DNA synthesis by 9-β-D-arabinofuranosyl-2-fluoroadenine: a mechanism for cytotoxicity. J Biol Chem 1990;265:166–176.
95. Huang P, Plunkett W. Fludarabine and gemcitabine-induced apoptosis: incorporation into DNA is a critical event. Cancer Chemother Pharmacol 1995;36:181.
96. Huang Q-Q, Yao SYM, Ritzel MWL, Paterson ARP, Cass CE, Young JD. Cloning and functional expression of a complementary DNA encoding a mammalian nucleoside transport protein. J Biol Chem 1994;269:17757.
97. Huizing MT, Keung AC, Rosing H, vander Kuij V, ten Bokkel Huinink WW, Mandjes IM, Dubbelman AC, Pinedo HM, Beijnen JH. Pharmacokinetics of paclitaxel and metabolites in a randomized comparative study in platinum-pretreated ovarian cancer patients. J Clin Oncol 1993;11:2127.
98. Jakobsen P, Bastholt L, Dalmark M, Pfeiffer P, Petersen D, Gjedde SB, Sandburg E, Rose C, Nielsen OS, Mounidsen HT. A randomized study of epirubicin at four different dose levels in advanced breast cancer. Feasibility of myelotoxicity prediction through single blood-sample measurement. Cancer Chemother Pharmacol 1991;28: 405.
99. Jamieson GP, Snook MB, Bradley TR, Bertoncello I, Wiley JS. Transport and metabolism of 1-β-D-arabinofuranosylcytosine in human ovarian adenocarcinoma cells. Cancer Res 1989;49:309.
100. Jarvis SM, Young JD. Nucleoside transport in rat erythrocytes: two components with

differences in sensitivity to inhibition by nitrobenzylthioinosine and *p*-chloro-mercuriphenyl sulfonate. J Membr Biol 1986;93:1.
101. Jones RB, Matthes S, Shpall EJ, Fisher JH, Stemmer SM, Dufton C, Stephens JK, Bearman SI. Acute lung injury following treatment with high-dose cyclophosphamide, cisplatin, and carmustine: pharmacodynamic evaluation of carmustine. JNCI 1993;21:640.
102. Johnston PG, Fisher ER, Rockette HE, Fisher B, Wolmark N, Drake JC, Chabner BA, Allegra CJ. The role of thymidylate synthase expression in prognosis and outcome of adjuvant chemotherapy in patients with rectal cancer. J Clin Oncol 1994;12:2640.
103. Jolivet J, Schilsky RL, Bailey BD, Drake SC, Chabner BA. Synthesis, retention and biological activity of methotrexate polyglutamates in cultured human breast cancer cells. J Clin Invest 1982;70:351.
104. Jusko WJ. A pharmacodynamic model for cell-cycle-specific chemotherapeutic agents. J Pharmacokinet Biopharm 1973;1:175.
105. Jusko WJ. Pharmacodynamics of chemotherapeutic effect: dose-time-response relationships for phase-nonspecific agents. J Pharm Sci 1987;60:892.
106. Kantarjian H, Estey EH, Plunkett W, Keating MJ, Walters RS, McCredie KB, Freireich EJ. Phase I-II clinical and pharmacologic studies of high-dose cytosine arabinoside in refractory leukemia. Am J Med 1986;81:387.
107. Kohn KW, Spears CL, Doty P. Inter-strand crosslinking of DNA by nitrogen mustard. J Mol Biol 1966;19:266.
108. Koren G, Ferrazini G, Sulh H, Langevin AM, Kapelushnik J, Klein J, Giesbrecht E, Soldin S, Greenberg M. Systemic exposure to mercaptopurine as a prognostic factor in acute lymphocytic leukemia in children. N Engl J Med 1990;323:17.
109. Kunitoh H, Watanabe K. Phase I/II and pharmacologic study of long-term continuous infusion etoposide combined with cisplatin in patients with advanced non-small-cell lung cancer. J Clin Oncol 1994;12:83.
110. Lennard L, Lilleyman JS. Variable mercaptopurine metabolism and treatment outcome in childhood lymphoblastic leukemia. J Clin Oncol 1989;7:1816.
111. Lennard L, Lilleyman JS, Van Loon J, Weinshilboum RM. Genetic variation in response to 6-mercaptopurine for childhood acute lymphoblastic leukaemia. Lancet 1990;336:225.
112. Liliemark JO, Plunkett W, Dixon DO. Relationship of 1-β-D-arabinofuranosylcytosine in plasma to 1-β-D-arabinofuranosylcytosine-5′-triphosphate levels in leukemic cells during treatment with high dose 1-β-D-arabinofuranosylcytosine. Cancer Res 1985;45:5952.
113. Lind MJ, Margison JM, Cerny T, Thatcher N, Wilkinson PM. Prolongation of ifosfamide elimination half-life in obese patients due to altered drug distribution. Cancer Chemother Pharmacol 1989;25:139.
114. Lippard SJ. New chemistry of an old molecule: Cis(Pt (NH3)2 Cl2). Science 1982;218: 1075.
115. Lum BL, Kaubisch S, Yahanda AM, Adler KM, Jew L, Ehsan MN, Brophy NA, Halsey J, Gosland MP, Sikic BI. Alteration of etoposide pharmacokinetics and pharmcodynamics by cyclosporine in a phase I trial to modulate multidrug resistance. J Clin Oncol 1992;10:1635.
116. Manfredi JJ, Horwitz SB. Taxol: an antimitotic agent with a new mechanism of action. Pharmacol Ther 1984;25:83.
117. Matijasevic Z, Boosalis M, Mackay W, Samson L, Ludlum DB. Protection against chloroethylnitrosourea cytotoxicity by eukaryotic 3-methyladenine DNA glycosylase. Proc Nat Acad Sci USA 1993;90:11855.
118. Metzler CM. Estimation of pharmacokinetic parameters: statistical considerations. Pharmacol Ther 1981;13:543.
119. Metzler CM, Elfring GL, McEwen AJ. A User's Manual for NONLIN and Associated Programs. Kalamazoo, MI: The Upjohn Co, 1974.
120. Mick R, Ratain MJ. Statistical approaches to pharmacodynamic modeling: motivations, methods, and misperceptions. Cancer Chemother Pharmacol 1993;33:1.
121. Miller AA, Stewart CF, Tolley EA. Clinical pharmacodynamics of continuous-infusion etoposide. Cancer Chemother Pharmacol 1990;25:361.
122. Miller AA, Tolley EA. Predictive performance of a pharmacodynamic model for oral etoposide. Cancer Res 1994;54:2080.
123. Miller AA, Tolley EA, Niell HB, Griffin JP, Mauer AM. Pharmacodynamics of prolonged oral etoposide in patients with advanced non-small-cell lung cancer. J Clin Oncol 1993;11:1179.
124. Mimnaugh EG, Dusre L, Atwell J, Myers CE. Differential oxygen radical susceptibility of adriamycin-sensitive and -resistant MCF-7 human breast tumor cells. Cancer Res 1989;49:8.
125. Minami H, Shimokata K, Saka H, Saito H, Audo Y, Senda K, Nomura F, Sakai S. Phase I clinical and pharmacokinetic study of a 14-day infusion of etoposide in patients with lung cancer. J Clin Oncol 1993;11:1602.
126. Moore MJ, Erlichman C, Thiessen JJ, Bunting PS, Hardy R, Kerr I, Soldin S. Variability in the pharmacokinetics of cyclophosphamide, methotrexate and 5-fluorouracil in women receiving adjuvant treatment for breast cancer. Cancer Chemother Pharmacol 1994;33:472.
127. Moscow JA, Fairchild CR, Madden MJ, Ransom DT, Wieand HS, O'Brien EE, Poplack DG, Cossman J, Myers CE, Cowan KA. Expression of anionic glutathione-S-transferase and P-glycoprotein genes in human tissues and tumors. Cancer Res 1989;49 1422.
128. Mu D, Park C-H, Matsunaga T, Hsu DS, Reardon JT, Sancar A. Reconstitution of human DNA repair excision nuclease in a highly defined system. J Biol Chem 1995;270 2415.
129. Mukherjee K, Heidelberger C. Studies on fluorinated pyrimidines, IX. The degradation of 5-fluorouracil-6-C14. J Biol Chem 1960;235:433.
130. Newell DR, Pearson AD, Balmanno K, Price L, Wyllie RA, Keir M, Calvert AH, Lewis IJ, Pinkerton CR, Stevens MC. Carboplatin pharmacokinetics in children: the development of a pediatric dosing formula. The United Kingdom Children's Cancer Study Group. J Clin Oncol 1993;11:2314.
131. Newell DR, Siddik ZH, Gumbrell LA, Boxall FE, Gore ME, Smith IE, Calvert AH. Plasma free platinum pharmacokinetics in patients treated with high dose carboplatin. Eur J Cancer Clin Oncol 1987;23:1399.
132. Owellen RJ, Hartke CA, Dickerson RM, Hains FO. Inhibition of tubulin-microtubule polymerization by drugs of the vinca alkaloid class. Cancer Res 1976;36:1449.
133. Ozawa S, Sugiyama Y, Mitsuhashi J, Inaba M. Kinetic analysis of cell killing effect induced by cytosine arabinoside and cisplatin in relation to cell cycle phase specificity in human colon cancer and Chinese hamster cells. Cancer Res 1989;49:3823.
134. Pajor AM, Wright EM. Cloning and functional expression of a mammalian Na^+/nucleoside cotransporter. A member of the SGLT family. J Biol Chem 1992;267:3557.
135. Parker WB, Bapat AR, Shen, J-X, Townsend AJ, Cheng Y-C. Interaction of 2-halogenated dATP analogues (F, Cl, and Br) with human DNA polymerases, DNA primase, and ribonucleotide reductase. Molec Pharmacol 1988;34:485.
136. Paterson ARP, Gati WP, Vijayalakshmi D, Cass CE, Mant MJ, Young JD, Belch AR. Inhibitor-sensitive, Na^+-linked transport of nucleoside analogues in leukemia cells from patients. Proc Am Assoc Cancer Res 1993;34:14.
137. Pazdur R, Kudelka AP, Kavanagh JJ, Cohen PR, Raber MN. The taxoids: paclitaxel (Taxol) and docetaxel (Taxotere). Cancer Treat Rev 1993;19:351–386.
138. Peters GJ, van der Wilt CL, van Groningen CJ, Smid K, Meijer S, Pinedo HM. Thymidylate synthase inhibition after administration of fluorouracil with or without leucovorin in colon cancer patients: implication for treatment with fluorouracil. J Clin Oncol 1994;12:2035.
139. Petit E, Milano G, Levi F, Thyss A, Bailleul F, Schneider M. Circadian rhythm-varying plasma concentration of 5-fluorouracil during a five-day continuous venous infusion at a constant rate in cancer patients. Cancer Res 1988;48:1676.
140. Pigram WJ, Fuller W, Hamilton LD. Stereochemistry of intercalation: interaction of daunomycin with DNA. Nature New Biol 1972;235:17.
141. Piscitelli SC, Rodvold KA, Rushing DA, Tewksbury DA. Pharmacokinetics and pharmacodynamics of doxorubicin in patients with small cell lung cancer. Clin Pharmacol Ther 1993;53:555.
142. Plagemann PGW, Wohlheuter RM, Wolfendin C. Nucleoside and nucleobase transport in animal cells. Biochim Biophys Acta 1988;947:405.
143. Ploin DY, Tranchand B, Guastalla JP, Rebattu P, Chauvin F, Clavel M, Ardiet C. Pharmacokinetically guided dosing for intravenous melphalan: a pilot study in patients with advanced ovarian adenocarcinoma. Eur J Cancer 1992;28A:1311.
144. Plunkett W, Gandhi V. Pharmacokinetics of arabinosylcytosine. J Infus Chemother 1992;2:169.
145. Plunkett W, Gandhi V, Huang P, Robertson LE, Yang L-Y, Gregoire V, Estey E, Keating MJ. Fludarabine: pharmacokinetics, mechanisms of action, and rationales for combination therapies. Semin Oncol 1993;20(suppl 7):2.
146. Plunkett W, Huang P, Xu Y-Z, Heinemann V, Grunewald, Gandhi V. Gemcitabine: metabolism, mechanisms of action, and self-potentiation. Semin Oncol 1995;22 (Supp 4):3
147. Plunkett W, Iacoboni S, Estey E, Danhauser L, Liliemark JO, Keating MJ. Pharmacologically-directed ara-C therapy for refractory acute leukemia. Semin Oncol 1985;12(suppl 3):20.
148. Plunkett W, Liliemark JO, Adams TM, Nowak B, Estey E, Kantarjian H, Keating MJ. Saturation of 1-β-D-arabinofuranosylcytosine triphosphate accumulation in leukemia cells during high-dose 1-β-D-arabinofuranosylcytosine therapy. Cancer Res 1987;47: 3005.
149. Plunkett W, Saunders PP. Metabolism and actions of purine nucleoside analogues. Pharmacol Ther 1991;49:239.
150. Presant CA, Wolf W, Waluch V, Wiseman C, Kennedy P, Blayney D, Brechner RR. Association of intratumoral pharmacokinetics of fluorouracil with clinical response. Lancet 1994;343:1184.
151. Ratain MJ, Mick R, Berezin F, Janisch L, Schilsky RL, Vogelzang NJ, Lane LB. Phase I study of amonafide dosing based on acetylator phenotype. Cancer Res 1993;53: 2304.
152. Ratain MJ, Mick R, Berezin F, Janisch L, Schilsky RL, Williams SF, Smiddy J. Paradoxical relationship between acetylator phenotype and amonafide toxicity. Clin Pharmacol Ther 1991;50:573.
153. Ratain MJ, Mick R, Schilsky RL, Vogelzang NJ, Berezin F. Pharmacologically based dosing of etoposide: a means of safely increasing dose intensity. J Clin Oncol 1991;9: 1480.
154. Ratain MJ, Rosner G, Allen SL, Costanza ME, Van Echo DA, Henderson IC, Schilsky RL. Population pharmacodynamic study of amonafide: a cancer and leukemia group B study. J Clin Oncol 1995;12:741.
155. Ratain MJ, Schilsky RL, Choi KE, Guarnieri C, Grimmer D, Vogelzang NJ, Senekjian E, Liebner MA. Adaptive control of etoposide administration: impact of interpatient pharmacodynamic variability. Clin Pharmacol Ther 1989;45:226.
156. Ratain MJ, Schilsky RL, Conley BA, Egorin MJ. Pharmacodynamics in cancer therapy. J Clin Oncol 1990;8:1739.
157. Ratain MJ, Staubus AE, Schilsky RL, Malspeis L. Limited sampling models for amonafide (NSC 308847) pharmacokinetics. Cancer Res 1988;48:4127.
158. Ratain MJ, Vogelzang NJ. Phase I and pharmacological study of vinblastine by prolonged continuous infusion. Cancer Res 1986;46:4827.
159. Ratain MJ, Vogelzang NJ. A limited sampling model for vinblastine pharmacokinetics. Cancer Treat Rep 1987;71:935.
160. Ratain MJ, Vogelzang NJ, Sinkule JA. Interpatient and intrapatient variability in vinblastine pharmacokinetics. Clin Pharmacol Ther 1987;41:61.
161. Reece PA, Morris RG, Bishop JF. Pharmacokinetics of trimetrexate administered by five-day continuous infusion to patients with advanced cancers. Cancer Res 1987;47: 2996.
162. Reece PA, Stafford I, Russell J, Gill PG. Nonlinear renal clearance of ultrafilterable platinum in patients treated with cis-dichloradiammine platinum (II). Cancer Chemother Pharmacol 1985;15:295.
163. Reece PA, Stafford I, Russell J, Khan M, Gill PG. Creatinine clearance as a predictor of ultrafilterable platinum disposition in cancer patients treated with cisplatin: relationship between peak ultrafilterable platinum plasma levels and nephrotoxicity. J Clin Oncol 1987;5:304.
164. Reed E, Parker RJ, Gill I, Bicher A, Dabholkar M, Vionnet JA, Bostick-Bruton F, Tarone R, Muggia FM. Platinum-DNA adduct in leukocyte DNA of a cohort of 49 patients with 24 different types of malignancies. Cancer Res 1993;53:3694.
165. Reed E, Yuspa SH, Zwelling LA, Ozols RF, Poirier MC. Quantitation of cis-diamminedichloroplatinum 11-DNA-intrastrand adducts in testicular and ovarian cancer patients receiving cisplatin chemotherapy. J Clin Invest 1986;77:545.
166. Reilly JJ, Workman P. Normalization of anti-cancer drug dosage using body weight and surface area: is it worthwhile? A review of theoretical and practical considerations. Cancer Chemother Pharmacol 1993;32:411.

167. Rodman JH, Abromowitch M, Sinkule JA, Rivera GK, Evans WE. Clinical pharmacodynamics of continuous infusion teniposide: systemic exposure as a determinant of response in a phase I trial. J Clin Oncol 1987;5:1007.
168. Rodman JH, Furman WL, Sunderland M, Rivera G, Evans WE. Escalating teniposide systemic exposure to increase dose intensity for pediatric cancer patients. J Clin Oncol 1993;11:287.
169. Rodvold KA, Rushing DA, Tewksbury DA. Doxorubicin clearance in the obese. J Clin Oncol 1988;6:1321.
170. Ross WE, Bradley MO. DNA double-stranded breaks in mammalian cells after exposure to intercalating agents. Biochim Biophys Acta 1981;654:129.
171. Ross W, Rowe T, Glisson B, Yalowich J, Liu L. Role of topoisomerase 11 in mediating epipodophyllotoxin-induced DNA cleavage. Cancer Res 1984;44:5857.
172. Rowinsky EK, Cazenave LA, Donehower RC. Taxol: a novel investigational antimicrotubule agent. JNCI 1990;82:1247.
173. Rowinsky EK, Ettinger DS, Grochow LB, Brundrett RB, Cates AE, Donehower RC. Phase I and pharmacologic study of hexamethylene bisacetamide in patients with advanced cancer. J Clin Oncol 1986;4:1835.
174. Rowinsky EK, Ettinger DS, McGuire WP, Noe DA, Grochow LB, Donehower RC. Prolonged infusion of hexamethylene bisacetamide: a phase I and pharmacological study. Cancer Res 1987;47:5788.
175. Rowinsky EK, Gilbert MR, McGuire WP, Noe DA, Grochow LB, Forastiere AA, Effinger DS, Lubejko BG, Clar B, Sartonius SE, et al. Sequences of taxol and cisplatin: a phase I and pharmacologic study. J Clin Oncol 1991;9:1692.
176. Rowinsky EK, Wright M, Monsarrat B, Sesser GJ, Donehower RC. Taxol: pharmacology, metabolism and clinical implications. Cancer Surv 1993;17:283.
177. Rushing DA, Raber SR, Rodwold KA, Piscitelli SC, Plank GS, Tewskbury DA. The effects of cyclosporine on the pharmacokinetics of doxorubicin in patients with small cell lung cancer. Cancer 1994;74:834.
178. Saikawa Y, Knight CB, Saikawa T, Page ST, Chabner BA, Elwood PC. Decreased expression of the human folate receptor mediates transport-defective methotrexate resistance in KB cells. J Biol Chem 1993;268:5293–5301.
179. Samson LD. The repair of DNA alkylation damage by methyltransferases and glycosylases. Essays Biochem 1992;27:69.
180. Sandoval A, Consoli U, Plunkett W. Differential induction of apoptosis in B and T lymphocytes in response to UV radiation and fludarabine. Proc Am Assn Cancer Res 1995;36:611.
181. Santini J, Milano G, Thyss A, Renee N, Ayela P, Schneider M, Demard F. 5-FU therapeutic monitoring with dose adjustment leads to improved therapeutic index in head and neck cancer. Br J Cancer 1989;59:287.
182. Schaaf LJ, Dobbs BR, Edwards IR, Perrier DG. Nonlinear pharmacokinetic characteristics of 5-fluorouracil (5-FU) in colorectal cancer patients. Eur J Clin Pharmacol 1987;32:411.
183. Schilsky RL, Ratain MJ. Clinical pharmacokinetics of high dose leucovorin calcium after intravenous and oral administration. JNCI 1990;82:1411.
184. Schimke RT. Gene amplification, drug resistance and cancer. Cancer Res 1984;44:1735.
185. Seidman AD. The emerging role of paclitaxel in breast cancer therapy. Clin Cancer Res 1995;1:247.
186. Sevick EM, Jain RK. Geometric resistance to blood flow in solid tumors perfused ex vivo: effects of tumor size and perfusion pressure. Cancer Res 1989;49:3506.
187. Sirotnak FM. Correlates of folate analogue transport, pharmacokinetics and selective antitumor action. Pharmacol Ther 1980;8:71.
188. Skipper HE, Schabel FM, Mellett LB, Montgomery JA, Wilkoff LJ, Lloyd HH, Brockman RW. Implications of biochemical, cytokinetic, pharmacologic, and toxicologic relationships in the design of optimal therapeutic schedules. Cancer Chemother Rep 1970;54:431.
189. Skovsgaard T, Nielsen D, Maare C, Wassermann K. Cellular resistance to cancer chemotherapy. Int Rev Cytol 1994;156:77.
190. Smallwood RH, Mihaly GW, Smallwood RA, Morgan DJ. Effect of a protein-binding change on unbound and total plasma concentrations for drugs of intermediate hepatic extraction. J Pharmacokinet Biopharmacol 1988;16:529.
191. Song JJ, Wlaer S, Chen E, Johnson II, EE, Spychala J, Gribbin T, Mitchell BS. Genomic structure and chromosomal localization of the human deoxycytidine kinase gene. Proc Nat Acad Sci USA 1993;90:431.
192. Sonnichsen DS, Hurwitz CA, Pratt CB, Shuster JJ, Relling MV. Saturable pharmacokinetics and paclitaxel pharmacodynamics in children with solid tumors. J Clin Oncol 1994;12:532.
193. Sotaniemi EA, Pelkonen RO, Mokka RE, Huttunen R, Viljakainen E. Impairment of drug metabolism in patients with liver cancer. Eur J Clin Invest 1977;7:269.
194. Spears CP, Gustavsson BG. Methods for thymidylate synthase pharmacodynamics: serial biopsy, free and total TS, F-dUMP and dUMP, and H4PteGlu and CH2-H4PteGlu assays. Adv Exp Med Biol 1988;244:97.
195. Stein CA, LaRocca RV, Thomas R, McAtee N, Myers CE. Suramin: an anticancer drug with a unique mechanism of action. J Clin Oncol 1989;7:499.
196. Stewart CF, Arbuck SG, Fleming RA, Evans WE. Changes in the clearance of total and unbound etoposide in patients with liver dysfunction. J Clin Oncol 1990;8:1874.
197. Stewart CF, Baker SD, Heideman RL, Jones D, Crom WR, Pratt CB. Clinical pharmacodynamics of continuous infusion topotecan in children: systemic exposure predicts hematologic toxicity. J Clin Oncol 1994;12:1946.
198. Stewart CF, Pieper JA, Arbuck SG, Evans WE. Altered protein binding of etoposide in patients with cancer. Clin Pharmacol Ther 1989;45:49.
199. Straw JA, Szapary D, Wynn WT. Pharmacokinetics of the diastereoisomers of leucovorin after intravenous and oral administration to normal subjects. Cancer Res 1984;44:3114.
200. Swain SM, Lippman ME, Egan EF, Drake JC, Steinberg SM, Allegra CJ. Fluorouracil and high dose leucovorin in previously treated patients with metastatic breast cancer. J Clin Oncol 1989;7:890.
201. Synold TW, Relling MV, Boyett JM, Rivera GK, Sandlund JT, Mahmoud H, Crist WM, Pui C-H, Evans WE. Blast cell methotrexate-polyglutamate accumulation in vivo differs by lineage, ploidy, and methotrexate dose in acute lymphoblastic leukemia. J Clin Invest 1994;94:1996.
202. Takeshita M, Grollman AP, Ohtsubo E, Ohtsubo H. Interaction of bleomycin with DNA. Proc Natl Acad Sci USA 1978;75:5983.
203. Terheggen PMAB, Emondt JY, Floot BGJ, Dijkman R, Schrier PI, den Engelse L. Correlation between cell killing by cis-diamminedichloroplatinum (II) in six mammalian cell lines and binding of a cis-diamminedichloroplatinum (II) DNA antiserum. Cancer Res 1990;50:3556.
204. Tewey KM, Rowe TC, Yang L, Halligan BD, Liu LF. Adriamycin-induced DNA damage mediated by mammalian DNA topoisomerase II. Science 1984;226:466.
205. Thyss A, Milano G, Renee N, Vallicioni J, Schneider M, Demard F. Clinical pharmacokinetic study of 5-FU in continuous 5-day infusions for head and neck cancer. Cancer Chemother Pharmacol 1986;16:64.
206. Trippett T, Schlemmer S, Elisseyeff Y, Goker E, Wachter M, Steinherz P, Tan C, Berman E, Wright JE, Rosowsky A, Schweitzer B, Bertino JR. Defective transport as a mechanism of acquired resistance to methotrexate in patients with acute lymphocytic leukemia. Blood 1992;80:1158.
207. Trump DL, Egorin MJ, Forrest A, Willson JK, Remick S, Tutsch KD. Pharmacokinetic and pharmacodynamic analysis of fluorouracil during 72-hour continuous infusion with and without dipyridamole. J Clin Oncol 1991;9:2027.
208. Ullman B. Mutational analysis of nucleoside and nucleobase transport. In Resistance to Antineoplastic Drugs. Edited by D Kessel. Boca Raton, FL: CRC Press, 1989, p 293.
209. van Groeningen CJ, Pinedo HM, Heddes J, Kok RM, de Jong APJM, Wattel E, Peters GJ, Lankelma J. Pharmacokinetics of 5-fluorouracil assessed with a sensitive mass spectrometric method in patients on a dose escalation schedule. Cancer Res 1988;48:6956.
210. Wagner JG. Kinetics of pharmacologic response: I. Proposed relationships between response and drug concentration in the intact animal and man. J Theoretical Biol 1968;20:173.
211. Wagner JG, Gyves JW, Stetson PL, Walker-Andrews SC, Wollner IS, Cochran MK, Ensminger WD. Steady-state nonlinear pharmacokinetics of 5-fluorouracil during hepatic arterial and intravenous infusions in cancer patients. Cancer Res 1986;46:1499.
212. Wagner JG, Szpunar GJ, Ferry JJ. A nonlinear physiologic pharmacokinetics model: I. Steady-state. J Pharmacokinet Biopharmacol 1985;13:73.
213. Wang S-W, Huang P, Plunkett W, Becker FB, Chan JYH. Dual mode of inhibition of purified DNA ligase I from human cells by 9-β-D-arabinofuranosyl-2-fluoroadenine. J Biol Chem 1992;267:2345.
214. White JC, Goldman ID. Mechanism of action of methotrexate. IV. Free intracellular methotrexate required to suppress dihydrofolate reduction to tetrahydrofolate by Ehrlich ascites tumor cells in vitro. Molec Pharmacol 1976;12:711.
215. White JC, Rathmell JP, Capizzi RL. Membrane transport influences the rate of accumulation of cytosine arabinoside in human leukemia cells. J Clin Invest 1987;79:380.
216. Whitehead VM, Rosenblatt DS, Vuchich MJ, Shuster JJ, Witte A, Beaulieu D. Accumulation of methotrexate and methotrexate polyglutamates in lymphoblasts at diagnosis of childhood acute lymphoblastic leukemia: a pilot prognostic factor analysis. Blood 1990;76:44.
217. Wiley JS, Jones SP, Sawyer WD, Paterson ARP. Cytosine arabinoside influx and nucleoside transport sites in acute leukemia. J Clin Invest 1982;69:479.
218. Williams FMR, Murray RC, Underhill TM, Flintoff WF. Isolation of a hamster cDNA clone coding for a function involved with methotrexate uptake. J Biol Chem 1994;269:5810–5816.
219. Wilson WH, Berg SL, Bryant G, Wittes RE, Bates S, Fojo A, Steinberg SM, Goldspiel BR, Herdt J, O'Shaughnessy J, et al. Paclitaxel in doxorubicin-refractory or mitoxantrone-refractory breast cancer: a phase I/II trial of 96-hour infusion. J Clin Oncol 1994;12:1621.
220. Young RC, Ozols RF, Myers CE. The anthracycline antineoplastic drugs. N Engl J Med 1981;305:139.
221. Zhen W, Link CJ Jr, O'Conner PM, Reed E, Parker R, Howell SB, Bohr VA. Increased gene-specific repair of cisplatin interstrand cross-links in cisplatin-resistant human ovarian cancer cell lines. Molec Cell Biol 1992;12:3689.
222. Zimm S, Collins JM, Riccardi E, O'Neill D, Narang PK, Chabner B, Poplack DG. Variable bioavailability of oral mercaptopurine: is maintenance chemotherapy in acute lymphoblastic leukemia being optimally delivered? N Engl J Med 1983;308:1005.

CHAPTER 59

Toxicology by Organ System

MICHAEL R. GREVER AND CHARLES K. GRIESHABER

Introduction

The treatment of cancer may involve various modalities, including surgery, radiation, and chemotherapy. Newer approaches now under investigation also include anticancer vaccines, agents directed at destroying malignant cells through immunologic mechanisms, and gene therapy. Each form of therapeutic intervention has the potential to produce adverse effects on normal host tissues, and some of these toxicities may be accentuated with combined modality therapy. While other chapters have been devoted to specific classes of agents used in the treatment of cancer, this contribution discusses generalizations regarding the evaluation of toxicity and the organ specificity of the adverse effects from cancer treatment.

The antineoplastic chemotherapeutic drugs have widely diverse chemical structures that are capable of inducing varying degrees of cell destruction by distinct mechanisms of action. They are divided into arbitrary classes based on a combination of their mechanisms of cytotoxicity, chemical structure, and source. Effective clinical use of these antineoplastic agents requires an understanding of toxicology to maximize the adverse effects against tumor cells and minimize the damage to normal host tissue. For example, antimetabolites and other direct cytotoxic agents, which interfere with cell division, have the greatest effect on rapidly dividing cells. Thus, cytotoxic effects are observed both on the tumor cells and those normal host cells with rapid cell-cycle kinetics. The blood-forming hematopoietic cells and gastrointestinal mucosal cells with rapid doubling times are the targets of cytotoxic chemotherapy. Therefore, these antineoplastic agents frequently produce leukopenia, anemia, thrombocytopenia, and mucosal ulceration.

This chapter discusses the basic principles of antineoplastic drug toxicology that have been learned in the rapidly growing fields of experimental oncology and drug development. As such, the purpose is not solely to catalog the myriad of toxic effects associated with use of the commonly employed anticancer chemotherapeutic agents but to describe the principles and procedures through which toxic responses can be anticipated, understood, and possibly surmounted. While the numbers and types of agents under development change both rapidly and constantly, the basic principles involved in toxicology evolve and change more slowly. Therefore, a clear understanding of the latter enables one to maintain pace with the former.

Basic Principles of Preclinical Toxicology

CHEMOTHERAPEUTIC AGENTS

Following the demonstration of encouraging preclinical antitumor activity involving either in vitro or in vivo tumor models, pharmacologic and toxicologic investigations have been targeted at optimizing the proposed clinical trials in humans. The goals of these preclinical toxicologic studies are to establish the safety of new agents in experimental animals and predict primary toxicities as doses escalate.

Preclinical toxicologic testing is the final step in the progression of a chemotherapeutic drug from discovery to initial human studies. While the major goals of preclinical studies are to define a safe starting dose and predict the qualitative toxicities that may be encountered with subsequent dose escalation in patients, toxicologic findings also may result in a decision to forego further investigation of a new anticancer agent. In general, toxicities are expected to occur with the administration of effective agents; however, definition of the therapeutic-to-toxic dose ratio has a major impact on the final decision to pursue new agents into clinical trials.

Chemotherapeutic agents have been dropped from further evaluation based on the results of preclinical toxicologic studies. Several reasons underlie the decisions to discontinue investigation of those anticancer agents, (e.g. data reflecting irreversible or serious degrees of toxicity in a dose range that was dangerously close to the targeted therapeutic levels). Furthermore, appearance of an unacceptable systemic complication (e.g., disseminated intravascular coagulation) also has resulted in discontinuing evaluation for several agents. The appearance of a significant toxic effect in the preclinical setting (e.g., hepatotoxicity or a seizure) does not necessarily preclude entering clinical trials, but it should result in vigorous efforts to further investigate both the cause and potential for circumventing the toxicity (e.g., dose adjustment or schedule variation).

The observation that phase I clinical studies were prolonged was in large part attributable to the empiric dose escalation procedures compounded by safe but ineffective starting doses. This prompted reassessment of the preclinical pharmacologic and toxicologic protocols (25). A commitment was made to expedite the process of preclinical toxicologic assessment with a focus on determining the toxicities likely to be encountered at the proposed clinical doses and with less attention on defining the highly lethal doses. Therefore, the current protocols for developing anticancer drugs determine the maximum tolerable doses and dose-limiting toxicities in rodents and a second animal species. In addition, the pharmacologic parameters (e.g., area under the plasma concentration-time curve) are correlated with the toxicologic data to provide the basis for subsequent pharmacologically guided dose escalation in patients during the phase I trial (24, 25).

The actual protocols for performing preclinical toxicologic studies have changed significantly over the past two decades (51, 81). Numerous schedules of drug administration were examined in a variety of species from 1972 to 1980. The emphasis after 1980, however, focused on initial mouse-lethality studies to define the general toxic dose ranges, followed by further studies in rats and dogs on relatively fixed schedules to refine the various dose levels associated with lethal and nonlethal toxicities. The revised protocols did expedite preclinical evaluation and, with the exception of fludarabine phosphate, generally were successful in providing safe starting doses for phase I studies (51). The predicted acute organ toxicities demonstrated a reasonable correlation between the preclinical and clinical data (25, 40, 51, 80, 81, 111, 115).

Retrospective analyses of preclinical and clinical correlations have confirmed that expressing the dose of a chemotherapeutic agent in mass units per body surface area (e.g., mg/m^2) improves the predictive relationship between dose and toxicity across species (40). Quantitative assessment of toxicity regarding the dose of drug administered is accurately determined using small-animal models (40, 115). Furthermore, the use of small animals may make a significant contribution to providing an early assessment of the therapeutic-to-toxic dose ratio, because the xenograft models for antitumor activity primarily have been established in the murine species (115). The subsequent investigation of qualitative toxicity is better defined by using larger animals which can be carefully assessed for specific organ toxicities by serial blood tests and tissue examinations (80, 111).

While further information occasionally is acquired by completing additional large-animal studies (e.g., monkeys), most agents are adequately characterized by examining preclinical toxicologic data in two animal species (121a). In general, dogs and rats provide better organ-specific toxicity information than mice for predicting human toxicity (51, 80). Myelosuppression most often correlates well between dog and human toxicity profiles. Gastrointestinal toxicity may be more accurately predicted in the rat because the dog is very sensitive to agents inducing this toxicity. Hepatotoxicity and nephrotoxicity are predicted less well by dogs. Pancreatic, cardiac, and pulmonary toxicities are potentially demonstrable but have been underpredicted in acute toxicity studies. The identification of neurologic and cutaneous toxicities probably are the least well predicted from the preclinical models; this reflects the obvious difficulties in assessing the cognitive functions of an animal compared with humans. The sole evidence of neurologic toxicity may manifest at relatively high doses in the animals as gross neurologic dysfunctions (e.g., seizures or hind-limb paralysis). Finally, agents that produce local discomfort or skin irritation may be extremely difficult to evaluate in an animal model.

Preclinical identification of either cardiac or pulmonary toxicity has been attempted by using specific animal models, but these usually require specialized maneuvers (e.g., determining the specific weight of an organ; using physiologic monitoring with blood pressure, pulse, and electrocardiography; measuring a biochemical parameter associated with toxic injury, e.g., hydroxyproline in the lungs following bleomycin) (115). Therefore, use of specialized manipulations or determinations adds significantly to the time and cost that are involved in completing routine toxicologic studies, and these may be better used in comparing various analogues within a chemical class to identify the agent likely to produce the minimum of toxicity in a specific target organ.

There has been substantial interest in the development of in vitro test systems that would predict organ-specific toxicities. The in vitro evaluation of murine and human colony-forming assays is now being attempted to assess the relative myelotoxicity of various experimental agents (34, 35, 50). This type of analysis might have predicted the unanticipated, severe myelosuppression associated with fludarabine monophosphate administration in the early phase I clinical trials. In addition, efforts are underway that use either single-cell suspensions (e.g., cardiac cells) or organ slices (e.g., liver) to develop models for either toxicity or metabolic studies relative to new agents (38, 74). Use of these innovative approaches hopefully will enhance our ability to derive additional predictive information regarding qualitative toxicities (e.g., mechanism of toxicity) but likely will not replace the need for continued use of the whole animal in preclinical toxicologic studies. In fact, comparison of toxicity in the intact animal across species provides extremely valuable information regarding interspecies variation in drug tolerance and metabolism.

BIOLOGIC AGENTS

This diverse category of antineoplastic agents includes anticancer vaccines; monoclonal antibodies, both labeled and unlabeled with radioactive nuclides and conjugated and unconjugated to toxin molecules; cytokines, including the numerous interleukins, interferons, tumor necrosis factor (TNF), and the myriad of growth factors both unconjugated and conjugated to toxin molecules; cytokines in combination with target immunocompetent effector cells (e.g., lymphokine-activated killer and tumor-infiltrating cells); and the numerous potential combinations of these biologic products, either with each other or in combination with cytotoxic chemotherapy or hormonal therapy. The advent of biologic therapy originally promised to usher in relatively well-tolerated and novel modalities for treating malignancy. In fact, however, the observations of significant toxicities in clinical trials are not now surprising and, in many cases, still are being defined.

Development of recommendations for conducting preclinical toxicologic evaluations in this group of novel therapeutic products is quite challenging (44, 120, 127). These products may be highly specific in their targeted interaction and thus can make the choice of an appropriate preclinical animal model difficult. For example, a monoclonal antibody directed against a specific antigen found exclusively in primates could make testing in small animals unproductive. Assessing the effects of a growth factor in a species that is unlikely to have responsive tissue with the appropriate receptor represents an analogous dilemma. Likewise, preclinical models to evaluate the safety of proposed anticancer vaccines are currently under development as promising novel agents move toward early clinical trials (61a, 99a).

The observation that the optimal immunomodulatory dose of a biologic product is not likely to be identical to the maximal tolerated dose adds substantial complexity to the development of an optimal toxicologic protocol (127). Furthermore, development of the optimal therapeutic protocol requires both definition of these important parameters and confirmation that the desired biologic effect has indeed been produced. Adding to the complexity of defining the optimal dose, schedule, and route of administration, the proper sequence of administering the biologic product(s) must be determined (44).

Despite the inherent complexity of determining the preclinical toxicologic and pharmacologic data relevant to these biologic products, acquisition of this information should enhance the likelihood that any subsequent therapeutic trial will be successful (120). In particular, preclinical demonstration of enhanced antitumor activity with combination therapies suggests that an attempted evaluation of enhanced toxicity also is warranted. For example, the in vitro combination of TNF and gamma-interferon produced enhanced tumor-cell cytotoxicity with human colon and pancreatic carcinoma cell lines (110, 113, 114). Because the initial phase I clinical evaluations of each agent administered individually demonstrated tolerable side effects, these two agents were combined in a clinical protocol that had to be discontinued quite early because of unacceptable toxicity of the combination (1). The doses of each agent in the combination were empirically modified to avoid excessive toxicity, but the toxic effects were still observed. Optimal doses and schedules of agents in novel combinations might be determined by using a preclinical in vivo model. While substantial research is needed in this area, the basic approach should provide for preclinical toxicologic testing in appropriate animal models whenever feasible (120).

HORMONAL AGENTS

The number of effective hormonal agents for the treatment of cancer has been somewhat limited. In general, administration of the currently effective agents involves long-term exposure to the drugs. Use of estrogen-blocking agents in the treatment of breast cancer has been extended to involve years of therapy (16). Furthermore, treatment of prostatic carcinoma either with estrogenic agents or androgenic blocking agents also involves prolonged administration. Consequently, the type of toxicologic evaluation that must be considered in dealing with hormonal agents would involve an assessment of both the acute and chronic toxicities that may be attributable to these products. One report suggested a possible increase in the rate of endometrial cancer in patients receiving tamoxifen, but the role of this agent in development of this outcome was not clear (66).

The preclinical toxicologic evaluation of a hormonal agent, which likely will be administered for a protracted period, includes both the short- and long-term administration of the drug to a group of animals. There has been a tendency to administer high doses of these agents in this setting to maximize the likelihood of identifying various toxic events. This approach carries a risk, however, that the exaggerated doses may unmask toxicities that are unlikely to occur at the intended therapeutic doses and thus will miss subtle toxicities resulting from low-dose, prolonged exposure.

The type of toxic event that results from long-term exposure to a hormonal agent may not be evident for an extended period of time (e.g., the development of gynecologic malignancies in the offspring of women treated with stilbestrol appeared decades after their exposure in utero) (56). The cardiovascular effects and enhancement of a risk for thromboembolic events subsequent to estrogenic agents would have been very difficult to assess in a preclinical model (8, 14). Likewise, the effects of endocrine blockade in producing premature menopausal symptoms or decreased libido would not be readily assessed in a preclinical model. Therefore, assessment of the acute and chronic toxic events subsequent to the administration of hormonal agents (e.g., in particular on suspected targeted tissues or the liver) presents a challenge in animal toxicologic protocol design, yet the full toxicity profile ultimately involves completion of the evaluation in a careful, long-term study in humans.

Toxicology: The Bridge Between Preclinical and Clinical Oncology

The clinical relevance of a toxicologic evaluation rests equally with qualitative and quantitative findings. Qualitative findings describe the adverse effects of a drug on organ systems of the host species, whereas quantitative data focus on the determination of doses that produce a specific adverse effect. For example, the dose that produces lethality in 10% of the test animals is identified as the LD_{10}. In addition, the highest nontoxic dose also is quite important. Whereas in the past substantial efforts were directed at determining doses of the drug that produced lethality in specific fractions of the test animals (i.e., LD_{10}, LD_{50}, and LD_{90}), the current emphasis is on defining the maximum tolerable dose and thereby estimating the LD_{10}. In contrast, the highly lethal doses (i.e., LD_{50} and LD_{90}) provide little useful information for further human investigation. More attention now is given to carefully assessing the qualitative toxicities likely to be observed at doses slightly higher than the highest nontoxic dose.

One critical element, which is essential both for safety and efficacy, is selection of the initial human starting dose. The usual determinant of the clinical starting dose is based on the LD_{10} as determined from the murine acute toxicity studies (25, 40, 111). The LD_{10} dose then is converted based on body surface area for interspecies equivalency and termed the $MELD_{10}$ dose (i.e., the murine equivalent LD_{10} dose). In fact, it has been postulated that the $MELD_{10}$ dose in mice and the maximum tolerable dose (MTD) in humans are equitoxic endpoints (25). In retrospective analyses of data at the National Cancer Institute, the risk of exceeding the human

MTD in phase I clinical trials is approximately 1% if the initial starting dose is based on the $MELD_{10}$ data (111). Furthermore, the recent updated analysis of the experience at the National Cancer Institute confirmed that use of two animal species provided a safe starting dose for new agents 97% of the time (121a).

Because there may be substantial variation between species in their tolerance of specific anticancer drugs, a safety factor is used to empirically reduce the probability that the starting dose will be unsafe. The selected starting dose in humans frequently is 10% of the $MELD_{10}$. Before administering the drug to humans, however, the safety of the projected starting dose is confirmed in a second species. If there are no unacceptable toxicities, human trials are scheduled to begin using this dose. On the other hand, if the 1/10 $MELD_{10}$ dose is toxic in the second species, the entry dose in human trials is lowered to a confirmed nontoxic dose, usually by an additional factor of three (i.e., 1/30 $MELD_{10}$).

In recent years, the approach to dose escalation in human phase I clinical trials has been based on pharmacologic data derived during the preclinical study combined with data from the initial patient pharmacokinetic profile obtained in an early phase I trial (24, 25). Therefore, toxicologic studies performed in preparation for human investigation will be complemented by studies designed to provide the area under the plasma-concentration time curve at the $MELD_{10}$ in mice. These data provide a target for dose-escalation maneuvers in patients being treated in the phase I clinical trials.

Most new chemotherapeutic agents customarily have been tested clinically on two relatively fixed schedules: (*a*) single bolus intravenous dosing once every 3 to 4 weeks and (*b*) 5 consecutive days of treatment repeated at 3- to 4-week intervals. Thus, the established, traditional protocols for preclinical toxicology reflect each of these schedules. New, more unique schedules of drug administration are coming into fashion in clinical practice (e.g., continuous intravenous infusion for several hours or days, or prolonged oral administration). There are neither official nor traditional requirements for preclinical toxicity testing using unique administration schedules to possibly uncover unanticipated human toxicities. Good preclinical practice, however, encompasses the testing of drugs for toxic effects on the planned schedules for clinical administration. Thus, close collaboration between the preclinical toxicologist and the clinical investigator is essential.

Evaluation of Toxicity in Humans

GENERALIZATIONS REGARDING TOXICOLOGIC INFORMATION DERIVED FROM ORGANIZED CLINICAL TRIALS

Adverse effects emanating from administration of a therapeutic agent may be either acutely observed or delayed in onset. A correlation may exist between the dose of the drug and the toxic effects. Furthermore, adverse effects may relate to various factors, including the peak plasma concentration, rate of drug delivery, cumulative dose, schedule, or route of drug delivery. Therefore, a complete definition of the toxicity profile of an antineoplastic agent involves observation for both acute and chronic toxicities and correlation of the toxicologic and pharmacologic data.

Various well-defined phases of clinical investigation have been established to provide an organized approach to the drug evaluation process. At each step in the developmental process, the toxicity profile is more accurately defined. In the phase I clinical trial, the ultimate goal is to define the toxicity and pharmacology of a new agent. The dose-limiting toxicity (or toxicities) and the MTD on a particular schedule are established. The dose-limiting toxicity is the adverse effect that limits further escalation of the dose. The MTD has been defined differently in various phase I trials, but in general, it is the dose that results in either serious (i.e., life-threatening) or irreversible toxicity in a predetermined percentage of patients.

The phase II clinical investigation is designed primarily to assess the potential of a new agent to produce a response in a specific type of cancer. There is a strict requirement for evaluable and measurable disease. In general, patients have good performance status and may have had minimal previous treatment for their cancer. These patients more frequently are treated with multiple courses of the new agent at therapeutic levels based on information derived from the phase I trial. Thus, the potential exists for recognizing additional toxicities that are associated with prolonged drug administration (i.e., cumulative toxicity) during this phase of clinical evaluation.

In a phase III clinical investigation, the major objective is to compare both the efficacy and the toxicity of a new therapy with those of standard treatment. In this phase, the new agent may be tested either alone or in a combination with other chemotherapeutic agents. Enrollment in phase III trials is much larger than in other phases of clinical investigation and thus permits a more accurate assessment of the frequency and characterization of treatment-induced toxicities. Furthermore, this large accrual permits recognition of the rare toxic events (e.g., idiosyncratic-type drug-related toxicities or hypersensitivity reactions). Therefore, a relatively complete toxicity profile of a new agent may be constructed following completion of these organized phases of clinical investigation. It is important to add, however, that post-approval (postmarketing) surveillance also is essential to define either unusual or long-term (i.e., late) adverse effects of an agent.

ACTUAL CONDUCT OF PHASE I TRIAL IN HUMANS

During the phase I investigation, acute toxicities are identified and the potential duration and reversibility of the toxicities are defined. While patients with malignancy who have limited therapeutic options may be offered an opportunity to participate in these trials, selection of appropriate patients to accurately evaluate toxicity in a phase I clinical investigation is extremely important. In general, patients should have reasonably good performance status and basically normal organ function. Because the major objective of this phase of clinical investigation is to define organ toxicity, patients with significant pretreatment organ dysfunction will be unevaluable when assessing toxic events. In addition, abnormal organ function may increase the risk of participation in this early phase. After the pharmacologic and toxicologic profiles of a new agent have been characterized, patients with impaired organ function can be entered with appropriate modification of the dose and schedule to further elucidate the appropriate use of the agent under these altered circumstances.

As previously stated, selection of a starting dose in human trials is based on the consideration of several preclinical animal models. Every effort is made to select a safe starting dose, but this conservative approach usually results in an initial dose that is subtherapeutic. Patients entering these trials are confronted with lethal diseases, so it is imperative that every effort be made to arrive as quickly as possible at doses that approximate a biologically effective dose. The procedure for dose escalation of new anticancer agents in the past was simply based on predetermined, fixed increments without a biologic or pharmacologic basis. The current effort stresses the use of pharmacologically guided dose escalation to expedite arrival at an effective yet safe anticancer dose.

Extensive efforts are made to document and characterize the toxicity at each dose level. Cohorts of three to six patients are entered at each dose level on a specific schedule of drug administration. In addition to defining clinical toxicity, most of these patients are concurrently participating in detailed pharmacologic studies. The pharmacokinetic parameters and metabolites of the new agent are identified and important correlations are made between the toxicologic and pharmacologic data.

The procedure for demonstrating the MTD involves careful escalation of doses from an initial starting dose until dose-limiting toxicity is achieved. The phase I investigation is considered to be successfully completed when both the dose-limiting toxicity and the MTD on a specific schedule have been identified. The recommendation of a dose and schedule for further phase II testing should result from data derived from the phase I trial.

ASSESSMENT OF DELAYED TOXICITY

The potential for delayed-onset toxicity must always be appreciated. For example, in the early phase I trials of fludarabine monophosphate, the acute dose-limiting toxicity in patients with solid tumors was reversible myelosuppression (46, 59). The doses subsequently were escalated in patients with refractory forms of leukemia, and a delayed onset of serious neurologic toxicity was observed (22, 46, 138). Approximately 4 to 6 weeks after the administration of high doses of this agent, cortical blindness and coma developed in the patients. Therefore, myelosuppression was the dose-limiting toxicity in the low-dose range, and delayed neurologic toxicity was dose limiting in the high-dose range.

Delayed-onset toxicity is not always easily recognized during phase I clinical investigations. The characteristics of this patient population frequently result in relatively few courses of a drug actually being administered; many of these patients have advanced or refractory disease that is unresponsive to chemotherapy. In the interest of safety, there also is a definite potential for subtherapeutic doses to be delivered during the early portions of the trial. Therefore, many patients who are registered in the phase I clinical investigation receive only one or two courses of the new agent; consequently, either delayed-onset or cumulative toxicities may not be fully appreciated. A recent review of neurotoxicity associated with several purine analogues demonstrated the importance of postmarketing surveillance in recognizing delayed-onset toxicities (21).

The difference in the delayed onset of a toxic event and that emanating from a cumulative total dose also must be distinguished. For example, the neurologic toxicity that resulted from high-dose fludarabine monophosphate was delayed in onset, but it was not simply a function of the total dose. Several patients had received larger total cumulative doses of fludarabine monophosphate administered over a longer time interval, and they did not develop evidence of neurologic toxicity (46). In contrast, cardiac toxicity associated with doxorubicin and pulmonary toxicity produced by bleomycin are examples of toxic events that result from cumulative exposure to the respective drugs (2, 45, 136).

ALTERATION OF THE DOSE-LIMITING TOXICITY

In certain cases, the dose-limiting toxicity may be ameliorated with various interventions. For example, administration of mesna has dramatically reduced bladder toxicity associated with high doses of either cyclophosphamide or ifosfamide (5, 18). Several agents have demonstrated chemoprotection from cisplatin toxicity (12, 41, 43), and use of ICRF-187 may ameliorate cardiotoxicity associated with doxorubicin. Additional maneuvers also may be employed to reduce the potential for cumulative drug-induced cardiotoxicity (123). Finally, use of colony-stimulating factors may markedly reduce the period of myelosuppression associated with high doses of cytotoxic chemotherapy (3, 30, 89). However, postmarketing surveillance for evidence of delayed toxicity that might result from the combined use of these agents is prudent.

When the dose-limiting toxicity has been defined and an intervention subsequently is used to permit additional dose escalation, a new pattern of dose-limiting toxicity may emerge. In the case of either autologous or allogeneic bone marrow transplantation, markedly increased doses of cytotoxic agents are acutely administered, but new limitations are demonstrated with respect to other organ toxicity (i.e., hepatic, pulmonary, or cardiac toxicities) (30, 61a).

Alternating the schedule of drug administration may affect the potential for producing a toxic event. Administration of doxorubicin as a continuous intravenous infusion or a weekly, lower-dose intravenous bolus appears to be effective in reducing the observed cardiac toxicity compared with that from a higher dose as an intravenous bolus on a 3-week schedule (77, 117, 129). Thus, the cardiac toxicity of doxorubicin may result from the higher peak plasma levels achieved with the shorter intravenous bolus administration. While a change in the schedule of administration may lessen toxicity, it is important to ensure that the change also does not alter therapeutic efficacy.

In certain clinical situations, achieving high peak plasma concentrations of a drug may be critically important to produce the desired therapeutic effect. The associated toxicity, however, also may relate to the high plasma concentrations of the drug or its metabolite(s) encountered. For example, administration of high-dose cytosine arabinoside or methotrexate may be beneficial in the treatment of central nervous system leukemia or lymphoma, yet both treatments are associated with the onset of unique types of central nervous system toxicity (9). Under these circumstances, further investigation may provide an optimal dose range that maximizes benefit and minimizes potential for serious toxicity (28).

The Effect of Variation in Drug Metabolism on Toxicity

Variation in drug metabolism among patients may confound the interpretation of clinical data in a study with only a limited number of subjects. Early clinical investigations of amonafide demonstrated discrepancies in the relationship between dose and the onset of myelosuppression in two similar studies (78, 79). These phase I clinical investigations described different MTDs, and consequently, differences in the recommendations for subsequent phase II trials resulted. The pharmacologic data had suggested there was a bimodal population of pharmacokinetic profiles in the patients receiving this agent. Subsequent demonstration of the differences in the acetylation rates of this agent in humans provided a potential metabolic explanation for the variation in doses associated with myelosuppression (49, 101–103).

In the conduct of a phase I clinical trial, the observation of unexpected toxicity frequently is the stimulus for more basic biochemical and pharmacologic investigations. The initial phase I clinical trial of fludarabine monophosphate in patients with solid tumors revealed reversible, but unanticipated, myelosuppression at the initial starting dose (46). In retrospect, there was preclinical evidence suggesting that variability in metabolism existed between species (37, 94). In addition to differences in catabolism, a difference in anabolism existed. Fludarabine monophosphate is rapidly converted to the nucleoside (2-fluoroadenine arabinoside) in vivo (83). In humans, this halogenated derivative of adenine arabinoside is not readily deaminated; in contrast, there is evidence in dogs that the parent nucleoside is deaminated (31). Furthermore, the enzyme responsible for phosphorylation of the 2-fluoroadenine arabinoside (i.e., deoxycytidine kinase) to the triphosphate moiety is approximately tenfold higher in human bone marrow when compared to canine bone marrow. The canine data had been used to select the starting dose in humans. The subsequent biochemical explanation for the enhanced myelosuppressive potential in humans confirms that animal models may indeed be predictive, but original preclinical data must be closely scrutinized for species differences in metabolism.

Complexity of Assessing Treatment-Related Toxicity in Context of Human Disease

The distinction of drug-induced toxicity from the organ dysfunction associated with medical consequences of the underlying malignancy may present a challenge. In the early experiences with high-dose administration of deoxycoformycin (i.e., a potent inhibitor of adenosine deaminase), the onset of neurologic toxicity was difficult to distinguish from the consequences associated with central nervous system involvement with leukemia (48, 100, 122). It became quite clear that the drug was producing central nervous system toxicity when the clinical investigation extended to patients with solid tumors and who lacked evidence of central nervous system malignancy.

In general, careful clinical and laboratory examination of patients entering early clinical trials will provide the basis for assessing toxicities associated with a novel therapeutic agent for the treatment of malignancy. However, extreme caution should be exercised in deciding if a toxic event is treatment induced or a consequence of the underlying disease. Investigators must be aware of the necessity for long-term follow-up to comprehensively characterize the full toxicity profile of a new agent. The long-term consequences of effective chemotherapy also may include diverse problems ranging from endocrine failure to additional catastrophic events (e.g., development of treatment-induced second neoplasms) (4, 15, 23, 55, 62, 65, 67, 99, 104, 106, 118, 139, 140). Certain treatment regimens have been associated with an increased risk of developing a specific type of treatment-induced endocrine failure or cancer. Thus, knowledge of the risk factors is essential to minimize long-term toxic effects of cancer treatment.

Toxicity by Organ System

While each therapeutic agent for the treatment of cancer receives an extensive characterization of its toxicity profile before its approval for marketing, certain generalizations can be made about specific classes of agents (e.g., alkylators, antimetabolites, hormones, antibiotics) with further refinement after extended use. Another approach in understanding cancer drug toxicology focuses on the affected organ systems.

The observation of organ-specific toxicity also has occasionally provided clues for developing a drug to use in a targeted tumor or for therapeutic indications outside the realm of oncology. The production of myelosuppression (in particular, if the toxic profile is restricted to the myeloid elements) has resulted in the selection of agents for therapeutic trials in leukemia. It is noteworthy that the original nitrogen mustards were used empirically in the treatment of leukemia, because they had been found to reduce the leukocyte count in experimental animals (27). The lymphocytotoxicity associated with certain agents (e.g., deoxycoformycin and fludarabine phosphate) clearly led to their subsequent therapeutic development for the lymphoproliferative neoplasms (46, 47, 48,

59, 70). Furthermore, the lymphocytotoxic and other antineoplastic agents have been investigated for their potential use as immunosuppressive agents in the treatment of nonmalignant disorders as well (112).

Agents that have demonstrated toxicity toward normal adrenal gland (e.g., o,p-DDD and Suramin) have been reported to have some antitumor activity in the treatment of adrenal cortical cancer (53, 75). The diabetogenic effects of streptozotocin, which reflected its pancreatic toxicity, were used as a rationale to treat malignant insulinoma (111). In contrast, agents that have been responsible for producing pancreatic toxicities (pibenzimol, L-asparaginase) have not demonstrated any benefit in treating pancreatic carcinoma (71, 98). Therefore, demonstration of organ-specific toxicity does not guarantee efficacy in treating tumors derived from the target organ.

CARDIAC TOXICITY ASSOCIATED WITH CHEMOTHERAPY

Direct injury to the heart may result from either a chemotherapeutic agent or combined modality therapy. These effects may be either acutely encountered or delayed in onset. In general, acute cardiac toxicities are either myocardial tissue injury or electrophysiologic in nature. For example, patients may develop conduction disturbances (e.g., heart block) or rhythm disturbances (e.g., ventricular tachycardia). In contrast, several antineoplastic agents produce a chronic myocardial defect that is associated with congestive heart failure (Table 59.1).

The onset of acute myocardial injury characterized by elevated cardiac enzyme levels and electrocardiographic evidence of ischemic-type injury may be observed during administration of an antineoplastic drug. While clinical evidence of myocardial injury may be silent, the patient also might experience chest discomfort, which is characteristic of an acute ischemic event. The commonly used antimetabolite 5-fluorouracil has produced acute ischemic findings which have been characterized as typical angina, and on occasion, actual evidence of myocardial infarction (20, 39, 88). The frequency of this complication is rare (i.e., 2–5%) with 5-fluorouracil, but other types of agents also have been implicated in producing this type of acute myocardial ischemia (e.g., cisplatin) (32, 33, 126). The mechanism of cardiac ischemia has been postulated to be coronary artery spasm because several patients have had normal coronary artery anatomy demonstrated by angiographic studies following fluorouracil-induced ischemia.

In contrast to the typical clinical picture of acute myocardial ischemia, there have been several independent reports of direct cardiac injury associated with high-dose interleukin-2 therapy (42, 43, 73, 95, 97). In patients receiving this agent, intensive-care precautions have been used, because the patients become acutely ill. Patients have been observed to have either silent or symptomatic acute cardiac toxicity that is associated with chest discomfort and evidence of myocardial injury with elevated cardiac enzyme levels, cardiac dysfunction documented by imaging studies, and electrocardiographic evidence of acute myocardial injury. In addition, patients have had serious ventricular arrhythmias (e.g., ventricular tachycardia) after receiving this biologic product. The proposed mechanism of this cardiac injury has been a myocardial capillary leak syndrome similar to the systemic capillary leakage that results from the administration of interleukin-2.

Conduction disturbances have been reported with the administration of several agents. Amsacrine has been associated with ventricular arrhythmias that possibly were aggravated by electrolyte abnormalities (72, 124). Taxol, which is a novel agent with encouraging antitumor activity in patients with solid tumors, has produced bradycardia (108), and an alert was issued by the National Cancer Institute that in combination with cisplatin, the drug may produce ventricular tachycardia. Clarifying these early reports of potential cardiac toxicity will require further investigation. Taxol is administered with a vehicle (i.e., cremaphor) that also may be responsible for some of the adverse effects.

Both doxorubicin and an experimental agent (i.e., acoda-

Table 59.1. Cardiotoxicity

Drug	Toxic dose range[a]	Comments
Doxorubicin	>550 mg/m^2 (total dose)	Congestive heart failure (cumulative toxic effect), arrhythmias
	<550 mg/m^2 (total dose)	Cardiac toxicity with additional risk factors
Daunorubicin	>550 mg/m^2 (total dose)	Same toxicity as doxorubicin
Mitoxantrone	>100–140 mg/m^2 (total dose)	Congestive heart failure, decreases in LVEF
Cyclophosphamide	>100–120 mg/kg over 2 d	Congestive heart failure, hemorrhagic myocarditis/pericarditis/necrosis
5-Fluorouracil	Conventional dose	Angina/myocardial infarction
Vincristine	Conventional dose	Myocardial infarction
Vinblastine	Conventional dose	Myocardial infarction
Busulfan	Conventional oral daily dose	Endocardial fibrosis
Mitomycin C	Conventional dose	Myocardial damage similar to radiation-induced injury
Cisplatin	Conventional dose	Acute myocardial ischemia
Amsacrine	Conventional dose	Ventricular arrhythmias
Taxol	Conventional dose	Bradycardia
Interferons	Conventional dose	Exacerbates underlying cardiac disease
Interleukin-2	Conventional dose	Acute myocardial injury, ventricular arrhythmias, hypotension

[a] Route of administration is intravenous unless otherwise indicated. Conventional dose is the commonly accepted therapeutic range.
LVEF—Left ventricular ejection fraction.

zole) have prolonged the Q-T interval (11,131). Recognizing the potential for cardiac rhythm disturbances is important to accurately define the need for cardiac monitoring.

Cardiac pump failure may result from both the acute administration of high-dose chemotherapy (e.g., cyclophosphamide in bone marrow transplant dose regimens) and chronically with the administration of the anthracyclines (10, 90). Significant information exists regarding both the mechanism and clinical characteristics of myocardial injury following use of doxorubicin. In general, the incidence of congestive heart failure increases significantly when the total dose of doxorubicin exceeds 550 mg/m^2. Other factors that also increase this risk include a past history of cardiac disease and prior exposure to either chemotherapy or radiation therapy of the mediastinal region (17, 90). In patients with additional risk factors, the total cumulative dose of doxorubicin that can be considered safe is less than 500 mg/m^2. The decision to use an anthracycline in an individual patient involves a comprehensive assessment of the relative importance of that drug in the cancer treatment regimen and the degree of cardiac impairment involved.

The actual mechanism of cardiotoxicity has been considered to result from the generation of reactive oxygen radicals within the cardiac tissue (90). Studies have demonstrated that either administration of ICRF-187 or a change in the drug delivery schedule may reduce the potential for cardiotoxicity associated with anthracycline administration (117, 123, 129). Furthermore, evidence exists that modification of the chemical structure of the anthracycline may reduce the propensity for producing cardiac toxicity. Clinical investigations of other agents (e.g., epirubicin) have demonstrated some potential for a reduction in drug-induced cardiotoxicity (93, 130, 134, 135). These agents were not, however, completely devoid of cardiotoxic effects. The true advantage of these agents over doxorubicin will require further assessment in phase II and III comparative trials.

The contribution of radiation to enhancing the potential for cardiac toxicity may involve several different mechanisms of tissue injury. The combination of thoracic radiation and chemotherapy has been considered to increase the risk of coronary artery disease. Pericardial injury also may be observed in patients with previous exposure to combined modality therapy. Therefore, a careful balance of patients with similar cardiac risk factors must be achieved to eliminate these variables in any comparative assessment of drug-induced cardiotoxicity.

Monitoring the dose of an anthracycline to avoid cardiac toxicity can best be accomplished by considering the individual patient risk factor(s). Serial performance of radionuclide angiocardiography and more invasive cardiac monitoring (e.g., endomyocardial biopsy) may enable the clinician to administer the maximum dose for each individual patient. While no monitoring system can guarantee perfect predictability for the development of cardiotoxicity, aggressive use of these devices may enable additional anthracycline to be administered to those patients who are continuing to derive additional antitumor effect from this drug (13, 133, 143).

The major objective in developing mechanisms to reduce the cardiotoxic potential of antineoplastic therapy will be to enable dose escalation for those agents demonstrating a significant dose-response relationship. Preclinical predictive animal models do exist for evaluating cardiotoxicity, and these should be used to evaluate the effectiveness of new approaches (60).

NEPHROTOXICITY ASSOCIATED WITH CHEMOTHERAPY

In general, renal damage secondary to chemotherapeutic agents predominantly results from injury to the renal tubules (Table 59.2) Substantial information has been developed to explain the pathophysiology of renal injury resulting from chemotherapeutic agents, and clinical approaches have been discovered that may lessen the damage (29).

An important chemotherapeutic agent in the treatment of ovarian, lung, testicular, head and neck, and bladder cancer, cisplatin has been demonstrated to produce dose-related nephrotoxicity (29). This drug-induced nephrotoxicity results from a direct injury involving both the proximal and distal tubules. In addition, there may be an element of vasoconstriction superimposed on the tubular injury. The exact

Table 59.2. Renal Toxicity

Drug	Toxic dose range[a]	Comments
Cisplatin	50–200 mg/m^2	Nephrotoxicity dose limiting, dose-related/cumulative effects on renal tubules, hypomagnesemia/hypocalcemia
Carboplatin	Conventional dose	Renal dysfunction less common than with cisplatin
Carmustine (BCNU)	>1,200 mg/m^2 (total dose)	Renal dysfunction/cumulative dose effect, glomerular sclerosis/tubular atrophy, interstitial fibrosis
Streptozotocin	Conventional dose	Dose-related/cumulative nephrotoxicity, proteinuria early sign nephropathy, interstitial nephritis, tubular atrophy
Cyclophosphamide	>50 mg/kg	Hemorrhagic cystitis (may occur with low-dose daily administration), tubular injury/water retention
Ifosfamide	1.2 gm/m^2/day for 5 days	*See* cyclophosphamide
Methotrexate	Variable	Related to drug and metabolite precipitation, excretion, renal route
Mitomycin C	>30 mg/m^2 (total dose)	Renal insufficiency/hemolytic uremic syndrome

[a] Route of administration is intravenous unless otherwise indicated. Conventional dose is the commonly accepted therapeutic range.

cellular target for toxicity has not been identified, but there is evidence that cellular proteins excreted in the urine of patients experiencing tubular injury include β_2-microglobulin, alanine aminopeptidase, and leucine aminopeptidase, all of which are enzymes specifically located in the proximal tubular cells. Detection of increased excretion of these proteins has been used as a marker of subclinical renal damage related to the drug.

Certain parameters that correlate with degree of nephrotoxicity include drug dose, state of hydration, and concomitant administration of additional nephrotoxic agents (e.g., aminoglycosides). Empirically defined measures for reducing the toxicity of cisplatin include the administration of mannitol, adequate hydration, and use of hypertonic saline. Experimental evidence in animal models has demonstrated that the administration of thiols and thio-ethers may reduce nephrotoxicity without impairing the antitumor response (68).

A structural analogue of cisplatin, carboplatin has been associated with less nephrotoxicity than the parent compound (137). It has been demonstrated, however, that carboplatin may produce renal damage in patients with underlying damage secondary to previous cisplatin (105). Therefore, caution should be exercised in particular when large doses of carboplatin are administered.

While heavy-metal compounds have been associated with renal tubular damage, other agents also are capable of producing intrinsic renal injury (e.g., nitrosoureas, biologic agents including alpha- and gamma-interferon, and interleukin-2) (6, 7, 69, 116, 141).

Use of cisplatin or mitomycin either alone or in combination with other agents has been associated with an infrequent type of renal injury characterized as a microangiopathic-hemolytic process (61, 82). Recognizing this complication is important, because it may be reversible with discontinuation of the responsible agent. Additional benefit also possibly is obtainable if the patient is subjected to plasmapheresis. In general, this type of nephrotoxicity is associated with additional evidence of a hemolytic anemia characterized by mechanical red-cell fragmentation. Similar consequences may also be observed as well with cyclosporine being administered as immunosuppressive therapy following bone marrow transplantation.

Use of high-dose cytotoxic agents such as ifosfamide also has been associated with toxicity to both the kidney and the bladder (5). The discovery of mesna has remarkably reduced the genitourinary toxicity associated with the administration of alkylating agents but, predictably, has unmasked additional dose-limiting toxicities of these agents by permitting larger doses of alkylators to be administered.

HEPATIC TOXICITY ASSOCIATED WITH CHEMOTHERAPY

Despite the predominant role the liver plays in drug detoxification, this organ frequently is the site of drug-induced toxicity (Table 59.3). Hepatotoxicity, however, frequently is reversible with discontinuation of the responsible agent. A myriad of chemotherapeutic agents are capable of producing acute and reversible drug-induced hepatic cell toxicity (125). The histologic pattern of hepatic cell injury associated with most chemotherapeutic agents more often is found in the centrilobular location, and the clinical manifestation of the injury is an elevation of hepatic enzyme levels. Several agents have the potential for producing a specific cholestatic pattern of injury (e.g., anabolic steroids and mercaptopurine) and will have an expected increase in alkaline phosphatase and bilirubin levels.

In addition, a rare but serious hypersensitivity-type hepatocellular injury has been described with dacarbazine that has characteristic histologic features, including eosinophilic infiltration of the hepatic vessels with centrilobular necrosis. The clinical picture is associated with acute onset of upper abdominal pain, ascites, jaundice, and elevated levels of aminotransferases (125). Early recognition and intervention with corticosteroids and discontinuation of dacarbazine are necessary to avoid fatal complications.

Both acute and chronic hepatotoxicity have been clearly documented in association with use of methotrexate, and the chronic toxicity appears to relate to the duration of exposure and the total cumulative dose administered (64, 128). The histologic feature frequently observed with chronic hepatotoxicity is periportal fibrosis leading to cirrhosis (96). Many other agents are capable of producing dose-related acute hepatotoxicity, and the potential for inducing chronic toxicity probably is underappreciated because many of patients with cancer do not receive chronic drug administration. In

Table 59.3. Hepatic Toxicity

Drug	Toxic dose range[a]	Comments
L-Asparaginase	Conventional dose	Elevation of transaminases/alkaline phosphatase levels, diffuse fatty metamorphosis, decreased clotting factors (II, V, VII, IX, and X)
Nitrosoureas	Conventional dose	Elevation of transaminases/alkaline phosphatase levels
6-Mercaptopurine	Conventional dose	Elevation of transaminases/alkaline phosphatase levels, hepatocellular disease
Methotrexate	Conventional dose	Elevation of transaminase levels, portal fibrosis/cirrhosis after total dose >1.5 g
Cytosine arabinoside	Conventional dose	Elevation of transaminases
Hydroxyurea	Conventional dose	Elevation of transaminases/alkaline phosphatase
Mithramycin (Plicamycin)	>30 μg/kg/d or >10 doses	Elevation of transaminases/alkaline phosphatase levels, hemorrhagic diathesis/dose-related decrease in clotting factors (II, V, VII, and X)
Dacarbazine	Conventional dose	Elevation of transaminases, hepatocellular necrosis, hepatic vein thrombosis

[a] Route of administration is intravenous unless otherwise indicated. Conventional dose is the commonly accepted therapeutic range.

contrast, patients with inflammatory joint and skin diseases who receive methotrexate for prolonged periods develop hepatotoxicity (19, 121, 132).

An important clinicopathologic entity called veno-occlusive disease (VOD) of the liver has been associated with high-dose chemotherapy both alone and in association with radiation to the liver (107, 125). The occurrence of VOD has been described in association with bone marrow transplantation, and it is thought to result from the high doses used for the preparative regimen (84, 85). The temporally related onset of VOD is observed within the first 3 to 5 weeks after the preparative regimen. The clinical features of this complication include acute onset of pain in the upper abdomen, ascites, weight gain, and jaundice. The pathologic features may be difficult to demonstrate during the acute setting because of associated thrombocytopenia and coagulation defects. In those patients who die during the first week of the illness, however, the liver demonstrates marked centrilobular necrosis. Furthermore, in those patients who either survive or die later, the characteristic histopathologic lesion is obliteration of the vascular lumen of the central venules (10a).

The frequency of VOD in conjunction with bone marrow transplantation is 20%, with death from complications of this entity occurring in approximately 7 to 50% (107). Preexisting liver disease with abnormalities of liver enzymes result in a 3.4-fold increase in the risk of developing VOD (84). The advent of bone marrow transplantation and hematopoietic growth factors used to enhance the intensity of chemotherapy and administration of combined modality therapy warrant observation for an increased frequency of this complication. It is important to note that a role for monitoring plasma concentrations of busulfan has been recognized as being potentially important in reducing the liver toxicity associated with high doses of this drug (142).

NEUROTOXICITY ASSOCIATED WITH CHEMOTHERAPY

In general, antineoplastic agents have produced either peripheral (i.e., sensory and/or motor) or central neuropathic findings (Table 59.4) The tubulin-binding agents have been known to produce peripheral neuropathy, and taxol, which is the newest active agent from this class, is no exception (108). The tubulin-binding agents demonstrate a dose-dependent relationship to this toxicity and usually result in reversible injury if the drug is discontinued.

Heavy-metal intoxication has been associated with peripheral neuropathy (92). Cisplatin was the first heavy-metal compound to have substantial anticancer activity demonstrated, and its potential for producing neurotoxicity was initially described in 1978 (63). Neurologic toxicity actually is the dose-limiting toxicity that is associated with cisplatin in the treatment of some cancers (43, 54, 87). The patterns of neurotoxicity are both peripheral and central in distribution, with patients developing paresthesia, loss of proprioception or vibration sensation, retrobulbar neuritis, seizures, and ototoxicity. Over the past 10 years, little progress was made in ameliorating the neurologic toxicity associated with this agent.

Central nervous system toxicity associated with chemotherapeutic agents may be transient or devastating in nature. The observation that high-dose cytosine arabinoside produces remarkable results in refractory forms of aggressive leukemia resulted in widespread application of the high-dose regimens. The cerebellar and cerebral toxic events of repeated doses greater than 2 to 3 g/m^2 have been clearly identified as being dose related (36, 58, 76, 91, 109). Recently, the association of age and renal function on the incidence of serious degrees of cytosine (28) arabinoside–induced neurologic toxicity has been better defined (28). Consequently, appropriate dose reductions can be employed for those patients with renal dysfunction or advanced age.

Another promising antimetabolite, fludarabine monophosphate, was demonstrated to have dose-dependent neurotoxic potential. The serious central nervous system toxicity appeared to be associated with a demyelinating process that was clinically delayed in onset (138). The observation of

Table 59.4. Neurotoxicity

Drug	Toxic dose range[a]	Comments
Methotrexate	>12 mg/m^2 IT	Acute meningeal irritation, arachnoiditis/paraplegia, necrotizing leukoencephalopathy
Cytosine arabinoside	>100 mg/m^2 IT	Necrotizing leukoencephalopathy
	$\geqslant 2$–3 g/m^2	Cerebral/cerebellar dysfunction
5-Fluorouracil	Conventional dose	Acute cerebellar syndrome
Vincristine	Conventional dose	Symmetric sensory/motor peripheral neuropathy, cranial nerve motor neuropathy
Cisplatin	Conventional dose	Peripheral neuropathy, ototoxicity
Deoxycoformycin (Pentostatin)	High-dose therapy	Central nervous system toxicity (seizure/coma)
Ifosfamide	High-dose therapy	Central nervous system toxicity (somnolence/confusion/coma)
Fludarabine	Low dose	Peripheral neuropathy/possible central nervous system toxicity
	High dose	Delayed-onset central nervous system toxicity (cortical blindness/coma)
Taxol	Conventional dose	Peripheral neuropathy
Interferons	Conventional dose	Decreased mental status/dizziness and paresthesias
Interleukin-2	Conventional dose	Altered mental status/somnolence

[a] Route of administration is intravenous unless otherwise indicated. Conventional dose is the commonly accepted therapeutic range.
IT—intrathecal.

cortical blindness, coma, and death associated with high-dose administration of this agent almost precluded completing an assessment of the drug's clinical utility. Demonstration of antitumor activity at lower doses fortunately saved this drug from abandonment; however, the potential for low doses of this agent to produce neurologic toxicity has not yet been totally assessed (46, 86). Therefore, caution will need to be exercised with this agent until the total experience with it broadens. Other purine nucleosides appear to have the same propensity for inducing neurologic toxicity (21a).

OTHER TOXICITIES ASSOCIATED WITH CHEMOTHERAPY

The chemotherapeutic agents associated with pulmonary toxicity generally have resulted in the production of interstitial lung injury (Table 59.5) (26). These toxic effects frequently are dose related, but they may be enhanced by prior radiation therapy to the thorax. While idiosyncratic or hypersensitivity reactions may be the cause of pulmonary toxicity in any given patient, it is necessary to review all medications being administered to the patient, because several agents can contribute to the overall toxicity.

The earliest clinical manifestations of pulmonary toxicity may be subtle (e.g., nonspecific cough), and early recognition may prevent irreversible consequences of continued drug administration. Careful monitoring of patients receiving agents that are known to produce pulmonary toxicity also is warranted.

The most frequent toxicities encountered with standard chemotherapeutic agents include the gastrointestinal and hematologic toxicities outlined in Tables 59.6 and 59.7, respectively. The recent application of intensive principles of antiemetic therapy and use of colony-stimulating factors may permit significant dose intensification of these agents (30, 52, 57, 89, 119). Perhaps, the positive contribution of these improved supportive-care measures to lessen toxicity and permit dosing on time will be as important as the actual dose increment achieved.

The toxicologic effects of chemotherapeutic agents on gonadal tissue is critically important in those patients of child-bearing age. The cumulative effects of specific agents on testicular function indicate that certain combination regimens may be more detrimental than others. The teratogenic effects of chemotherapy have been recognized, but long-term follow-up in the children of patients with cancer subsequent to the administration of chemotherapy largely remains unknown. In fact, long-term consequences of chemotherapy regarding the development of secondary neoplasms in patients with cancer is an area requiring intensive study. The problem of defining long-term toxic effects of chemotherapy should be recognized as a product of success deserving careful scrutiny to avoid unnecessary, additional risks without compromising the therapeutic intent.

Table 59.5. Pulmonary Toxicity

Drug	Toxic dose range[a]	Comments
Bleomycin	>400 units (total dose)	Interstitial pneumonitis/fibrosis, dyspnea/cough early symptoms, fine rales early sign/decreased lung volume and vital capacity, toxicity dose and age related
Mitomycin C	Conventional dose	Interstitial pneumonitis
Carmustine (BCNU)	>1 g/m^2 (total dose)	Interstitial pneumonitis, delayed pulmonary fibrosis
Busulfan	Conventional dose	Bronchopulmonary dysplasia/fibrosis onset delayed months to years
Cyclophosphamide	High-dose therapy	Interstitial pneumonitis/fibrosis
Chlorambucil	Conventional dose	Interstitial pneumonitis/fibrosis
Melphalan	High-dose therapy	Interstitial pneumonitis
Cytosine arabinoside	Conventional dose	Pulmonary edema
Methotrexate	Conventional dose	Interstitial pneumonitis
Fludarabine	Conventional dose	Interstitial pneumonitis

[a] Route of administration is intravenous unless otherwise indicated. Conventional dose is the commonly accepted therapeutic range

Table 59.6. Gastrointestinal Toxicity

Drug	Toxic dose range[a]	Comments
Methotrexate	Variable	Nausea and vomiting, mucositis, and ulceration
5-Fluorouracil	Conventional dose	Nausea and vomiting, mucositis, and blood diarrhea
Cisplatin	Conventional dose	Severe nausea and vomiting
Cyclophosphamide	Conventional dose	Nausea and vomiting, diarrhea
Vincristine	Conventional dose	Dose-related constipation/abdominal cramps/adynamic ileus
Doxorubicin	Conventional dose	Nausea and vomiting, mucositis
Hydroxyurea	Conventional dose	Nausea and vomiting, mucositis
Dacarbazine	Conventional dose	Nausea and vomiting
Nitrosoureas	Conventional dose	Nausea and vomiting
Cytosine arabinoside	Conventional dose	Nausea and vomiting, diarrhea, and mucositis

[a] Route of administration is intravenous unless otherwise indicated. Conventional dose is the commonly accepted therapeutic range.

Table 59.7. Hematologic Toxicity

Drug	Level of WBC suppression	Maximum suppression (d)	Time to recovery (d)
Busulfan	Severe	11–30	30–60
Carmustine (BCNU)	Severe	28–42	35–90
Lomustine (CCNU)	Severe	28–42	35–90
Semustine (Methyl-CCNU)	Severe	28–42	35–90
Chlorambucil	Severe	7–14	14–28
Cyclophosphamide	Severe	7–14	21–28
Dacarbazine (DTIC)	Severe	16–25	25–35
Ifosfamide	Severe	10–20	21–35
Mechlorethamine (HN2)	Severe	7–14	14–28
Melphalan (1-PAM)	Severe	7–14	14–28
Carboplatin	Severe	21–28	
Cytosine arabinoside	Severe	12–24	21–30
5-Fluorouracil	Severe	9–14	21–30
Fludarabine	Severe	7–14	14–21
Methotrexate	Severe	7–14	14–21
Daunorubicin	Severe	10–14	21–28
Doxorubicin	Severe	10–14	21–28
Taxol	Severe	8–11	15–21
Hydroxyurea	Moderate	7–10	14–21
Vinblastine	Moderate	5–10	10–21
Mitoxantrone	Moderate	7–14	14–28
Mitomycin C	Moderate	21–42	35–70
Cisplatin	Mild	18–23	21–40

WBC—white blood cell.

Conclusions

This chapter has presented an overview of the basic principles for toxicologic investigation of antineoplastic agents. Appropriate use of animal models will permit reasonable quantitative and qualitative predictions of the toxicities that may be anticipated in humans. Table 59.8 summarizes the basic approach to initiating the necessary preclinical studies for subsequent trials in humans. The process of defining the comprehensive toxicity profile of a new agent will encompass both extensive preclinical and clinical investigations, as previously described in detail.

The study of human toxicology has contributed significantly to the current therapeutic approach of managing patients with cancer. The discovery and development of novel therapeutic agents, combination of biologic products with cytotoxic agents, and use of differentiating agents open new areas for toxicologic investigation. The enormous opportunities on the horizon for truly novel approaches (e.g., gene therapy for cancer, anti-cancer vaccines, ribozymes, and so on) will challenge those investigators responsible for the preclinical toxicologic evaluation of these unique therapeutic products (2a, 74a). The correlation of pharmacologic data with toxicity and efficacy as well as the willingness to implement newer approaches of predicting human toxicity should enhance the contributions yet to be made by this discipline.

Table 59.8. Guide To The Design of Preclinical Toxicology Studies Supporting Early Clinical Investigations on New Anticancer Agents

	Stage 1	Stage 2
Species	Mice	Mice and appropriate second species
Purpose	To establish potential clinical entry dose To determine plasma elimination kinetics and concentration dependency of agent	To determine the safety of the clinical entry dose To forecast the potential toxicities likely to be encountered To establish presence of dose-dependent toxicity To relate plasma pharmacokinetics to predictable biologic effects
Design	Determine MTD (LD_{10}) following bolus dosing and potential clinical schedule Determine plasma elimination kinetics following bolus dosing and continuous administration	Determine toxicity at MTD and $\frac{1}{10}$ MTD on bolus administration and repeated dose scheduling Establish relationship between pharmacokinetics and toxicity observed

MTD—Maximum tolerated dose.

References

1. Abbruzzese JL, Levin B, Ajani JA, Faintrich JS, Pazdur R, Saks S, Edwards C, Gutterman JU. A phase II trial of recombinant human interferon-gamma and recombinant tumor necrosis factor in patients with advanced gastrointestinal malignancies: results of a trial terminated by excessive toxicity. J Biol Resp Modifiers 1990;9:522.
2. Akoun GM, White JP. Treatment-Induced Respiratory Disorders. Edited by MNG Dukes. New York: Elsevier, 1989, p 60.

2a. Anderson WF. Gene therapy for cancer. Hum Gene Ther 1994;5:1–2.

3. Andreeff M, Welte K. Hematopoietic colony-stimulating factors. Semin Oncol 1989;16:211.
4. Andrieu J-M, Ifrah N, Payen C, Fermanian J, Coscas Y, Flandrin G. Increased risk of secondary acute nonlymphocytic leukemia after extended-field radiation therapy combined with MOPP chemotherapy for Hodgkin's disease. J Clin Oncol 1990;8:1148.
5. Antman KH, Elias A, Ryan L. Ifosfamide and mesna: response and toxicity at standard and high-dose schedule. Semin Oncol 1990;17(suppl 4):68.
6. Ault BH, Stapleton FB, Gaber L, Martin A, Roy S, Murphy SB. Acute renal failure during therapy with recombinant human gamma interferon. N Engl J Med 1988;319:1397.
7. Averbuch SD, Austin HA, Sherwin SA, Antonovych T, Bunn PA, Longo DL. Acute interstitial nephritis with the nephrotic syndrome following recombinant leukocyte A interferon for mycosis fungoides. N Engl J Med 1984;310:32.
8. Bailar JC III, Byar DP. Estrogen treatment for cancer of prostate: early results with three doses of diethylstilbesterol and placebo. Cancer 1970;26:257.
9. Balis FM, Poplack DG. Central nervous system pharmacology of antileukemia drugs. Am J Pediatr Hematol Oncol 1989;11:74.
10. Baverman AC, Antin JH, Plappert MT, Cook EF, Lee RT. Cyclophosphamide cardiotoxicity in bone marrow transplantation. J Clin Oncol 1991;9:1215.

10a. Bearman SI. The syndrome of hepatic veno-occlusive disease after marrow transplantion. Blood 1995;85:3005–3020.

11. Bender KS, Shematek JP, Leventhal BG, Kan JS. QT interval prolongation associated with anthracycline cardiotoxicity. J Pediatr 1984;105:442.
12. Berry J, Jacobs C, Sikic B, Halsey J, Borch RF. Modification of cisplatinum toxicity with diethyldithiocarbamate. J Clin Oncol 1990;8:1585.
13. Billingham ME, Bristow MR. Evaluation of anthracycline cardiotoxicity: predictive ability and functional correlation of endomyocardial biopsy. Cancer Treat Symp 1984;3:71.
14. Blackard CE, Byar DP, Jordan WP. Orchiectomy for advanced prostate carcinoma: a re-evaluation. Urology 1973;1:553.
15. Bookman MA, Longo DL, Young RC. Late complications of curative treatment in Hodgkin's disease. JAMA 1988;260:680.
16. Breast Cancer Trials Committee, Scottish Cancer Trials Office (MRC). Adjuvant tamoxifen in the management of operable breast cancer in the Scottish trial. Lancet 1987;ii:171.
17. Bristow MR. Toxic cardiomyopathy due to doxorubicin. Hosp Pract 1982;17:12.

18. Brock N, Pohl J, Stekar J. Detoxification of urotoxic oxazaphosphorines by sulfhydryl compounds. J Cancer Res Clin Oncol 1981;100:311.
19. Chassagne P, Levesque H, Moore N. Methotrexate. Pharmacology applied to the treatment of rheumatoid arthritis. Therapie 1990;45:499.
20. Chaudary S, Song SYT, Jaski BE. Profound, yet reversible, heart failure secondary to 5-fluorouracil. Am J Med 1988;85:454.
21. Cheson BD, Vena DA, Foss FM, Sorensen JM. Neurotoxicity of purine analogs: a review. J Clin Oncol 1994;12:2216–2228.
22. Chun HG, Leyland-Jones BR, Caryk SM, Hoth DF. Central nervous system toxicity of fludarabine phosphate. Cancer Treat Rep 1986;70:1225.
23. Cimino G, Papa G, Tura S, Mazza P, Rossi Ferrini PL, Bosi A, Amadori S, Lo Coco F, D'Arcangelo E, Giannarelli D, Mandelli F. Second primary cancer following Hodgkin's disease: updated results of an Italian multicentric study. J Clin Oncol 1991;9:432.
24. Collins JM, Grieshaber CK, Chabner BA. Pharmacologically guided phase I clinical trials based upon preclinical drug development. JNCI 1990;82:1321.
25. Collins JM, Zaharko DS, Dedrick RL, Chabner BA. Potential roles for preclinical pharmacology in phase I clinical trials. Cancer Treat Rep 1986;70:73.
26. Cooper JAD Jr, Matthay RA. Pneumonitis induced by cytotoxic drugs. In Treatment-Induced Respiratory Disorders, vol 3. Edited by GM Akoun, JP White. New York: Elsevier, 1989, p 51.
27. Dameshek W, Gunz F. Leukemia, 2nd ed. New York: Grune & Stratton, 1964.
28. Damon LE, Mass R, Linher CA. The association between high-dose cytarabine neurotoxicity and renal insufficiency. J Clin Oncol 1989;7:1563.
29. Daugaard G. Cisplatin nephrotoxicity: experimental and clinical studies. Dan Med Bull 1990;37:1.
30. Demetri GD, Griffin JD. Hematopoietic growth factors and high-dose chemotherapy: will grams succeed where milligrams fail? J Clin Oncol 1990;8:761.
31. DeSouza JJV, Grever MR, Neidhart JA, Staubus AE, Malspeis L. Comparative pharmacokinetics and metabolism of fludarabine phosphate (NSC 312887) in man and dog. Proc Am Assoc Cancer Res 1984;25:361.
32. Dixon AC, Nakamura JM, Oishi N, Wachi DH, Fukuyama O. Angina pectoris and therapy with cisplatin, vincristine, and bleomycin. Ann Intern Med 1989;111:342.
33. Doll DC, List AF, Greco FA, Hainsworth JD, Hande KR, Johnson DA. Acute vascular ischemic events after cisplatinum-based combination chemotherapy for germ-cell tumors of the testes. Ann Intern Med 1986;105:48.
34. Du D-L, Volpe DA, Grieshaber CK, Murphy MJ Jr. Comparative toxicity of fostriecin, hepsulfam, and pyrazine diazohydroxide to human and murine hematopoietic progenitor cells in vitro. Invest New Drugs 1991;9:149.
35. Du D-L, Volpe DA, Grieshaber CK, Murphy MJ Jr. Effects of L-phenylalanine mustard and L-buthionine sulfoximine on murine and human hematopoietic progenitor cells in vitro. Cancer Res 1990;50:4038.
36. Early AP, Preisler HD, Slocum H, Rustum YM. A pilot study of high-dose a-β-D-arabinofuranosylcytosine for acute leukemia and refractory lymphoma: clinical response and pharmacology. Cancer Res 1982;42:1587.
37. El Dareer SM, Struck RF, Tillery KF, Rose LM, Brockman RW, Montgomery JA, Hill DL. Disposition of 9-β-D-arabinofuranosyl-2-fluoroadenine in mice, dogs, and monkeys. Drug Metab Dispos 1980;8:60.
38. Frazier JM, Tyson CA, McCarthy C, McCormack JJ, Meyer D, Powis G, Ducat L. Contemporary issues in toxicology: potential use of human tissues for toxicity research and testing. Toxicol Appl Pharmacol 1989;97:387.
39. Freeman N, Costanza M. 5-Fluorouracil associated cardiotoxicity. Cancer 1988;61:36.
40. Freireich EJ, Gehan EA, Rall DP, Schmidt LH, Skipper HE. Quantitative comparison of toxicity of anticancer agents in mouse, rat, hamster, dog, monkey, and man. Cancer Chemother Rep 1966;50:219.
41. Gandara DR, Perez EA, Wiebe U, DeGregorio MW. Cisplatin chemoprotection and rescue: pharmacologic modulation of toxicity. Semin Oncol 1991;18(suppl 3):49.
42. Gaynor ER, Vitek L, Sticklin L, Creekmore SP, Ferraro ME, Thomas JX Jr, Fisher SG, Fisher RI. The hemodynamic effects of treatment with interleukin-2 and lymphokine-activated killer cells. Ann Intern Med 1988;109:953.
43. Kragel AH, Travis WD, Feinberg L, Pittaluga S, Striker LM, Roberts WC, Lotze MT, Yang JJ, Rosenberg SA. Pathologic findings associated with interleukin-2-based immunotherapy for cancer: a postmortem study of 19 patients. Hum Pathol 1990;21:493.
44. Gilewski T, Golomb HM. Design of combination biotherapy studies: future goals and challenges. Semin Oncol 1990;17(suppl 1):3.
45. Ginsberg SJ, Comis RL. The pulmonary toxicity of antineoplastic agents. Semin Oncol 1982;9:34.
46. Grever M, Leiby J, Kraut E, Metz E, Neidhart J, Balcerzak S, Malspeis L. A comprehensive phase I and II clinical investigation of fludarabine phosphate. Semin Oncol 1990;17(suppl 8):39.
47. Grever MR, Leiby JM, Kraut EA, Wilson HE, Neidhart JA, Wall RL, Balcerzak SP. Low-dose deoxycoformycin in lymphoid malignancy. J Clin Oncol 1985;3:1196.
48. Grever MR, Siaw MFE, Jacob WF, Neidhart JA, Miser JS, Coleman MS, Hutton JJ, Balcerzak SP. The biochemical and clinical consequences of 2′-deoxycoformycin in refractory lymphoproliferative malignancy. Blood 1981;57:406.
49. Grever MR, Staubus AE, Malspeis L. Correlation of N-acetylation phenotype with plasma levels of the N-acetylmetabolite of amonafide (NSC 308847). Proc Am Assoc Cancer Res 1990;31:178.
50. Grieshaber CK. Predictions of human toxicity from animal studies. In Mechanisms of Toxicity of Anticancer Drugs: A Study in Human Toxicity. Edited by G Powis, M Hacket. New York: Pergamon, 1991, p 10.
51. Grieshaber CK, Marsoni S. Relation of preclinical toxicology to findings in early clinical trials. Cancer Treat Rep 1986;70:65.
52. Griffin JD. Hemopoietins in oncology: factoring out myelosuppression. J Clin Oncol 1989;7:151.
53. Gutierrez ML, Crooke ST. Mitotane (o,p-DDD). Cancer Treat Rev 1980;7:49.
54. Hansen SW, Helweg-Larsen S, Trojaborg W. Long-term neurotoxicity in patients treated with cisplatin, vinblastine, and bleomycin for metastatic germ cell cancer. J Clin Oncol 1989;7:1457.
55. Hawkins MM. Second primary tumors following radiotherapy for childhood cancer. Int J Radiat Oncol Biol Phys 1990;19:1297.
56. Herbst AL, Ulfelder H, Poskunzes DC. Adenocarcinoma of the vagina: association of maternal stilbestrol therapy with tumor appearance in young women. N Engl J Med 1971;11:284.
57. Herrimann F, Schulz G, Wieser M, Kolbe K, Nicolay U, Noack M, Lindemann A, Mertelsmann R. Effect of granulocyte-macrophage colony-stimulating factor on neutropenia and related morbidity induced by myelotoxic chemotherapy. Am J Med 1990;88:619.
58. Herzig RH, Hines JD, Herzig GP, Wolff SN, Cassileth PA, Lazarus HM, Adelstein DJ, Brown RA, Coccia PF, Strandjord S, Massa JJ, Fay J, Phillips GL. Cerebellar toxicity with high-dose cytosine arabinoside. J Clin Oncol 1987;5:927.
59. Hutton JJ, Von Hoff DD, Kuhn J, Phillips J, Hersh M, Clark G. Phase I clinical investigation of 9-β-D-arabinofuranosyl-2-fluoroadenine 5′-monophosphate (NSC 312887), a new purine antimetabolite. Cancer Res 1984;44:4183.
60. Iatropoulos MJ. Anthracycline cardiomyopathy: predictive value of animal models. Cancer Treat Symp 1984;3:3.
61. Jackson AM, Rose BD, Graff LG, Jacobs JB, Schwartz JH, Strauss GM, Yang JPS, Rudnick MR, Elfenbein IB, Narins RG. Thrombotic microangiopathy and renal failure associated with antineoplastic chemotherapy. Ann Intern Med 1984;101:41.
61a. Jaffee EM, Lazenby A, Pardoll DM. Murine tumor vaccine: models for designing human vaccine trials. Proc AACR 1995;36:495.
62. Jordan VC, Fritz NF, Tormey DC. Endocrine effects of adjuvant chemotherapy and long-term tamoxifen administration on node-positive patients with breast cancer. Cancer Res 1987;47:624.
63. Kedar A, Cohen ME, Freeman AI. Peripheral neuropathy as a complication of cis-dichlorodiammine platinum (II) treatment: a case report. Cancer Treat Rep 1978;62:819.
64. Keim D, Ragsdale C, Heidelberger K, Sullivan D. Hepatic fibrosis with the use of methotrexate for juvenile rheumatoid arthritis. J Rheumatol 1990;17:846.
65. Kellie SJ, Kingston JE. Letter to the editor: ovarian failure after high-dose melphalan in adolescents. Lancet 1987;i:1425.
66. Killackey MA, Hakes TB, Pierce V. Endometrial adenocarcinoma in breast cancer patients receiving antiestrogens. Cancer Treat Rep 1985;69:237.
67. Kirk JA, Raghupathy P, Stevens MM, Cowell CT, Menser MA, Bergin M, Tink A, Vines RH, Silink M. Growth failure and growth-hormone deficiency after treatment for acute lymphoblastic leukemia. Lancet 1987;i:190.
68. Kobayashi H, Hasuda K, Aoki K, Taniguchi S, Baba T. Systemic chemotherapy in tumor-bearing rats using high-dose cis-diamminedichloroplatinum(II) with low nephrotoxicity in combination with angiotensin II and sodium thiosulfate. Int J Cancer 1990;45:940.
69. Kramer R, Boyd MR. Nephrotoxicity of 1-(2-chloroethyl)-3-(trans-4-methylcyclohexyl)-1-nitrosourea (MeCCNU) in the Fischer 344 rat. J Pharmacol Exp Ther 1983;227:409.
70. Kraut EH, Bouroncle BA, Grever MR. Low-dose deoxycoformycin in the treatment of hairy cell leukemia. Blood 1986;68:1119.
71. Kraut EH, Fleming T, Segal M, Neidhart JA. Phase II study of pibenzimol in pancreatic carcinoma. A Southwest Oncology Group study. Invest New Drugs 1991;9:95.
72. Krischer J, Land VJ, Civin CI, Ragub AH, Mahoney DM, Frankel LS. Evaluation of AMSA in children with acute leukemia. Cancer 1984;54:207.
73. Laghi Pasini F, Perri TDI, van der Plas K, Palmer P, Franks CR. Myocardial injury after interleukin-2 therapy. Lancet 1989;i:674.
74. Lampidis TL, Henderson IC, Israel M, Canellos GP. Structural and functional effects of adriamycin on cardiac cells in vitro. Cancer Res 1980;40:3901.
74a. Lange W, Daskalakis M, Finke J, D'Iken. Comparison of different ribozymes for efficient and specific cleavage of BCR/ABL related mRNAs. FEBS Lett 1994;338:174–178.
75. LaRocca RV, Stein CA, Danesi R, Jamis-Dow CA. Suramin in adrenal cancer: modulation of steroid hormone production, cytotoxicity in vitro, and clinical antitumor effect. J Clin Endocrinol Metab 1990;71:497.
76. Lazarus HM, Herzig RH, Herzig GP, Phillips GL, Roessmann U, Fishman DJ. Central nervous system toxicity of high-dose systemic cytosine arabinoside. Cancer 1981;48:2577.
77. Legha SS, Benjamin RS, Mackay B, Ewer M, Wallace S, Valdivieso M, Rasmussen SL, Blumenschein GR, Freireich EJ. Reduction of doxorubicin cardiotoxicity by prolonged continuous intravenous infusion. Ann Intern Med 1982;96:133.
78. Legha SS, Ring S, Raber M, Felder TB, Newman A, Krakoff IH. Phase I clinical investigations of benzisoquinolinedione. Cancer Treat Rep 1987;71:1165.
79. Leiby JM, Malspeis L, Staubus AE, Kraut EH, Grever MR. Amonafide (NSC 308847) A clinical phase I study of two schedules of administration. Proc Am Assoc Cancer Res 1990;29:278.
80. Lowe MC. Large animal toxicological studies of anticancer drugs. In Fundamentals of Cancer Chemotherapy. Edited by K Hellman and S Carter. New York: McGraw-Hill, 1987, p 236.
81. Lowe MC, Davis RD. The current toxicology protocol of the National Cancer Institute. In Fundamentals of Cancer Chemotherapy. Edited by K Hellman, S Carter. New York: McGraw-Hill, 1987, p 228.
82. Lyman NW, Michaelson R, Viscuso RL, Winn R, Mulgaonkar S, Jacobs MG. Mitomycin-induced hemolytic-uremic syndrome. Arch Intern Med 1983;143:1617.
83. Malspeis L, Grever MR, Staubus AE, Young D. Pharmacokinetics of 2-F-ara-A (9-β-D-arabinofuranosyl-2-fluoroadenine) in cancer patients during the phase I clinical investigation of fludarabine phosphate. Semin Oncol 1990;17(suppl 8):18.
84. McDonald GB, Sharma P, Matthews DE, Shulman HM, Thomas ED. Venoocclusive disease of the liver after bone marrow transplantation: diagnosis, incidence, and predisposing factors. Hepatology 1984;4:116.
85. McDonald GB, Shulman HM, Wolford JL, Spencer GD. Liver disease after human marrow transplantation. Semin Liver Dis 1987;7:210.
86. Merkel DE, Griffin NL, Kagan-Hallet K, Von Hoff DD. Central nervous system toxicity with fludarabine. Cancer Treat Rep 1986;70:1449.
87. Mollman JE. Cisplatin neurotoxicity. N Engl J Med 1990;322:126.
88. Monk MR, Sanchez JD, Phelps CD, Miller DM. Myocardial ischemia with fluorouracil and floxuridine therapy. Clin Pharmacy 1987;6:659.
89. Morstyn G, Campbell L, Lieschke G, Layton JE, Maher D, O'Connor M, Green M, Therdan W, Vincent M, Alton K, Souza L, McGrath K, Fox RM. Treatment of chemotherapy-induced neutropenia by subcutaneously administered granulocyte colony-stimulating factor with optimization of dose and duration of therapy. J Clin Oncol 1989;7:1554.

90. Myers CE, McGuire WP, Liss RH, Ifrim I, Grotzinger K, Young RC. Adriamycin: the role of lipid peroxidation in cardiac toxicity and tumor response. Science 1977;197:165.
91. Nand S, Messmore HL Jr, Patel R, Fisher SG, Fisher RI. Neurotoxicity associated with systemic high-dose cytosine arabinoside. J Clin Oncol 1986;4:571.
92. Needleman HL, Schell A, Bellinger D, Leviton A, Allred EN. The long-term effects of exposure to low doses of lead in childhood: an 11-year follow-up report. N Engl J Med 1990;322:83.
93. Nielssen D, Jensen JB, Dombernowsky P, Munck O, Fogh J, Brynjolf I, Havsteen H, Hansen M. Epirubicin cardiotoxicity: a study of 135 patients with advanced breast cancer. J Clin Oncol 1990;8:1806.
94. Noker PE, Duncan GF, El Dareer SM, Hill DL. Disposition of 9—D-arabinofuranosyl-2-fluoroadenine 5′-monophosphate in mice and dogs. Cancer Treat Rep 1983;67: 445.
95. Nora R, Abrams JS, Tait NS, Hiponia DJ, Silverman HJ. Myocardial toxic effects during recombinant interleukin-2 therapy. JNCI 1989;81:59.
96. O'Connor GT, Olmstead EM, Zug K, Baughman RD, Beck JR, Dunn JL, Seal P, Lewandowski JF. Detection of hepatotoxicity associated with methotrexate therapy for psoriasis. Arch Dermatol 1989;125:1209.
97. Osanto S, Cluitmans FHM, Franks CR, Bosker HA, Cleton FJ. Myocardial injury after interleukin-2 therapy. Lancet 1988;ii:48.
98. Patel SR, Kvols LK, Rubin J, O'Connell MJ, Edmonson JH, Ames MM, Kovach JS. Phase I–II study of pibenzimol hydrochloride (NSC 322921) in advanced pancreatic carcinoma. Invest New Drugs 1991;9:53.
99. Pedersen-Bjergaard J, Specht L, Larsen SO, Ersboll J, Struck J, Hansen MM, Hansen HH, Nissen NI. Risk of therapy-related leukemia and preleukaemia after Hodgkin's disease. Lancet 1987;ii:83.
99a. Placke ME, Tosca PJ, Montvic RM, Yarrington JT, Tomaszewski JE. Safety studies of three 13-mer point-mutated ras peptides in rabbits and two recombinant point mutated ras/vaccinia virus constructs in monkeys. Proc AACR 1995;36:492.
100. Poplack DG, Sallan SE, Rivera G, Holcenberg J, Murphy SB, Blatt J, Lipton JM, Venner P, Glaubiger DL, Ungerleider R, Johns D. Phase I study of 2′-deoxycoformycin in acute lymphoblastic leukemia. Cancer Res 1981;41:3343.
101. Ratain MJ, Mick R, Berezin F, Janisch L, Shilsky RL, Williams SF, Smiddy J. Prospective correlation of acetylation phenotype with amonafide toxicity. Proc Am Soc Clin Oncol 1991;10:101.
102. Ratain MJ, Propert K, Costanza M, Allen S, Berezin F, Shilsky RL, Van Echo DA. CALGB-population pharmacodynamic study of amonafide CALGB 8862. Proc Am Assoc Cancer Res 1990;31:181.
103. Ratain MJ, Staubus AE, Shilsky RL, Malspeis L. Limited sampling models for amonafide (NSC 308847) pharmacokinetics. Cancer Res 1988;48:4127.
104. Ravdin PM, Fritz NF, Tormey DC, Jordan VC. Endocrine status of premenopausal node-positive breast cancer patients following adjuvant chemotherapy and long-term tamoxifen. Cancer Res 1988;48:1026.
105. Reed E, Jacob J. Carboplatin and renal dysfunction. Ann Intern Med 1989;110:409.
106. Rivkees SA, Crawford JD. The relationship of gonadal activity and chemotherapy-induced gonadal damage. JAMA 1988;259:2123.
107. Rollins RJ. Hepatic veno-occlusive disease. Am J Med 1986;81:297.
108. Rowinsky EK, Cazenave LA, Donehower RC. Taxol: a novel investigational antimicrotubule agent. JNCI 1990;82:1247.
109. Rudnick SA, Cadman EC, Capizzi RL, Skeel RT, Bertino JR, McIntosh S. High dose cytosine arabinoside (HDARAC) in refractory acute leukemia. Cancer 1979;44:1189.
110. Salmon SE, Young L, Scuderi P, Clark B. Antineoplastic effects of tumor necrosis factor alone and in combination with gamma interferon on tumor biopsies in clonogenic assay. J Clin Oncol 1987;5:1816.
111. Schein P, Anderson T. The efficacy of animal studies on predicting clinical toxicity of cancer chemotherapeutic drugs. Int J Clin Pharmacol 1973;8:228.
112. Schein PS, Winokur S, MacDonald JS, Woolley PV. Long-term complications of cytotoxic and immunosuppressive chemotherapy. In Cancer Medicine, 2nd ed. Edited by JF Holland, E Frei III. Philadelphia: Lea & Febiger, 1982, pp 759–774.
113. Schiller JH, Bittner G, Storer B, Willson JKV. Synergistic antitumor effects of tumor necrosis factor and γ-interferon on human colon carcinoma cell lines. Cancer Res 1987;47:2809.
114. Schmiegel WH, Caesar J, Kalthoff H, Greten H, Schreiber HW, Thiele HG. Antiproliferative effects exerted by recombinant human tumor necrosis factor-α (TNF-α) and interferon-γ (IFN-γ) on human pancreatic tumor cell lines. Pancreas 1988;3:180.
115. Schurig JE, Bradner WT. Small animal toxicology of cancer drugs. In Fundamentals of Cancer Chemotherapy. Edited by K Hellman, S Carter. New York: McGraw-Hill, 1987, p 248.
116. Shalmi CL, Dutcher JP, Feinfeld DA, Chun KJ, Saleemi KR, Freeman LM, Lynn RI, Wiernik PH. Acute renal dysfunction during interleukin-2 treatment: suggestion of an intrinsic renal lesion. J Clin Oncol 1990;8:1839.
117. Shapira J, Gotfried M, Lishner M, Ravid M. Reduced cardiotoxicity of doxorubicin by a 6-hour infusion regimen. Cancer 1990;65:870.
118. Shapiro S, Mealey J Jr. Late anaplastic gliomas in children previously treated for acute lymphoblastic leukemia. Pediatr Neurosci 1989;15:176.
119. Sheridan WP, Wolf M, Lusk J, Layton JE, Souza L, Morstyn G, Dodds A, Maher D, Green MD, Fox RM. Granulocyte colony-stimulating factor and neutrophil recovery after high-dose chemotherapy and autologous bone marrow transplantation. Lancet 1989;ii:891.
120. Sherwin SA, Foon KA, Oldham RK. Animal tumor models for biological response modifier therapy: an approach to the development of monoclonal antibody therapy in humans. In Fundamentals of Cancer Chemotherapy. Edited by K Hellman, S Carter. New York: McGraw-Hill, 1987, p 202.
121. Singh G, Fries JF, Williams CA, Zatarain E, Spitz P, Bloch DA. Toxicity profiles of disease modifying antirheumatic drugs in rheumatoid arthritis. J Rheumatol 1991;18: 188.
121a. Smith AC, Rubinstein L, Koutsoukos A, Christian M, Grieshaber CK, Tomaszewski JE, Grever MR. Evaluation of preclinical toxicity models for phase I clinical trials of anticancer drugs: the NCI experience (1983–1992). Proc AACR 1994;35:2741.
122. Smyth JF, Paine RM, Jackman A, Harrap KR, Chassin MM, Adamson RH, Johns DG. The clinical pharmacology of the adenosine deaminase inhibitor 2′-deoxycoformycin. Cancer Chemother Pharmacol 1980;5:93.
123. Speyer JL, Green MD, Kramer E, Rey M, Sanger J, Ward C, Dubin N, Ferrans V, Stecy P, Zeleniuch-Jacquotte A, Wernz J, Feit F, Slater W, Blum R, Muggia F. Protective effect of the bispiperazinedione ICRF-187 against doxorubicin-induced cardiac toxicity in women with advanced breast cancer. N Engl J Med 1988;319:745.
124. Steuber CP, Holbrook T, Cumitta B, Land VJ, Sexauer C, Krischer J. Toxicity trials of amsacrine (AMSA) and etoposide ± azacitidine (AZ) in childhood acute non-lymphocytic leukemia (ANLL): a pilot study. Invest New Drugs 1991;9:181.
125. Sznol M, Ohnuma T, Holland JF. Hepatic toxicity of drugs used for hematologic neoplasia. Semin Liver Dis 1987;7:237.
126. Talcott J, Herman TS. Acute ischemic vascular events and cisplatin. Ann Intern Med 1987;107:122.
127. Talmadge JE. Therapeutic potential of cytokines: a comparison of preclinical and clinical studies. Prog Exp Tumor Res 1988;32:154.
128. Tolman KG. Hepatotoxicity of antirheumatic drugs. J Rheumatol 1990;22(suppl 1):6.
129. Torti FM, Bristow MR, Howes AE, Aston D, Stockdale FE, Carter SK, Kohler M, Brown BW, Billingham ME. Reduced cardiotoxicity of doxorubicin delivered on a weekly schedule. Ann Intern Med 1983;99:745.
130. Torti FM, Bristow MM, Lum BL, Carter SK, Howes AE, Aston DA, Brown BW, Hannigan JF, Meyers FJ, Mitchell EP, Billingham ME. Cardiotoxicity of epirubicin and doxorubicin: assessment by endomyocardial biopsy. Cancer Res 1986;46:3722.
131. Trump DL, Tutsch KD, Willson JKV, Remick S, Simon K, Alberti D, Grem J, Loeller J, Tormey DC. Phase I clinical trial and pharmacokinetic evaluation of acodazole (NSC 305884), an imidazoquinoline derivative with electrophysiological effects on the heart. Cancer Res 1987;47:3895.
132. Tung JP, Maibach HI. The practical use of methotrexate in psoriasis. Drugs 1990;40: 697.
133. Unverferth DV. Evaluation of anthracycline-induced cardiotoxicity. Cancer Treat Symp 1984;3:67.
134. Villani F, Comazzi R, Genitoni V, Lacaita G, Guindani A, Crippa F, Monti E, Piccinini F, Rozza A, Lanza E, Favalli L. Preliminary evaluation of myocardial toxicity of 4′-deoxydoxorubicin: experimental and clinical results. Drugs Exp Clin Res 1985;11:223.
135. Villani F, Galimberti M, Comazzi R, Crippa F, Bonfante V, Ferrari L, Pacciarini MA. Clinical evaluation of the cardiac toxicity of 4′-deoxy-doxorubicin. Int J Clin Pharmacol Ther Toxicol 1988;26:185.
136. Von Hoff DD, Layard MW, Basa P, Davis HL Jr, Von Hoff AL, Rozencweig M, Muggia FM. Risk factors for doxorubicin-induced congestive heart failure. Ann Intern Med 1979;91:710.
137. Wagstaff AJ, Ward A, Benfield P, Heel RC. Carboplatin: a preliminary review of its pharmacodynamic and pharmacokinetic properties and therapeutic efficacy in the treatment of cancer. Drugs 1989;37:162.
138. Warrell RP Jr, Berman E. Phase I and II study of fludarabine phosphate in leukemia: therapeutic efficacy with delayed central nervous system toxicity. J Clin Oncol 1986;4:74.
139. Watson AR, Rance CP, Bain J. Long term effects of cyclophosphamide on testicular function. Br Med J 1985;29:1457.
140. Waxman J, Terry Y, Rees LH, Lister TA. Gonadal function in men treated for acute leukaemia. Br Med J 1983;287:1093.
141. Weiss RB, Posada JG, Kramer RA, Boyd MR. Nephrotoxicity of semustine. Cancer Treat Rep 1983;67:1105.
142. Yeager AM, Wagner JE Jr, Graham ML, Jones RJ, Santos GW, Grochow LB. Optimization of busulfan dosage in children undergoing bone marrow transplantation: a pharmacokinetic study of dose escalation. Blood 1992;80:2425–2428.
143. Zaret BL, Schwartz PE, Berger HJ, Schwartz RG. Evaluation of doxorubicin cardiotoxicity with radionuclide angiocardiography at rest. Cancer Treat Symp 1984;3: 61.

SECTION XVI

CHEMOTHERAPEUTIC AGENTS

CHAPTER 60

Folate Antagonists

JOSEPH R. BERTINO, BARTON KAMEN, AND ANTONELLA ROMANINI

Introduction

Folate antagonists act as antineoplastic agents by interfering with one or more biosynthetic steps involving folate coenzymes of the tumor cell. Theoretically, a folate antagonist might act in one of several ways; e.g., by competing with folates for uptake into cells, by inhibiting the formation of folate coenzymes, or by inhibiting one or more reactions that are mediated by folate coenzymes. Thus far, however, all the clinically important folate antagonists that have been developed appear to act primarily by inhibiting the enzyme dihydrofolate reductase (DHFR) of the neoplastic cell, thereby inhibiting the formation of the coenzyme tetrahydrofolate. During recent years, several folate antagonists that target either de novo purine synthesis or thymidylate synthase have been developed and are now in clinical trial (see below).

The availability of crystalline pteroylglutamic acid (PGA, folic acid), resulting from a series of research efforts involving several research groups, prompted investigators to test this compound, as well as its diglutamate and triglutamate forms for possible antineoplastic activity. It was soon recognized that administration of these substances not only was ineffective, but possibly even accelerated the course of the disease of patients with chronic myelocytic leukemia and acute leukemia (89, 116). Efforts to treat these leukemias thus turned to creating folate deficiency, and some encouraging results were obtained through use of folate-deficient diets, either alone or in combination with a weak folate antagonist, "x-methyl" folic acid (probably 7-methyl PGA). Soon after, aminopterin (4-amino-4-deoxy PGA) was synthesized and found by Farber and his coinvestigators to be effective in producing remissions in acute leukemia (89). This demonstration was a landmark in cancer chemotherapy: it provided the first demonstration that an antimetabolite could be an effective antineoplastic agent, and provided the stimulus for the development of other antimetabolites as possible antitumor agents.

Since the initial study demonstrating the usefulness of aminopterin in the treatment of acute leukemia of childhood, there has been a sustained interest in, and a continued reevaluation of, this and other folate antagonists. In studies with mice bearing the L1210 leukemia, methotrexate (4-amino-4-deoxy-10-methyl PGA; amethopterin) (MTX) was found to have a more favorable therapeutic index than aminopterin, and thus for the last 40 years, MTX has supplanted aminopterin in the clinic. In recent years, an ever-broadening use for MTX has evolved. The drug has been used not only for the treatment of neoplastic diseases, but also for the treatment of certain nonneoplastic conditions, such as rheumatoid arthritis, asthma, and generalized psoriasis, and as an immunosuppressive agent (6, 245, 276, 302). Although details of therapeutic use are given elsewhere in this text, the broad spectrum of use of this drug deserves emphasis. MTX is the drug of choice in the treatment of choriocarcinoma, where its use provided the first demonstration of drug cure of cancer, and approximately 50% of these patients appear to be cured with the use of MTX alone. MTX is used in curative combination regimens to treat patients with acute lymphocytic leukemia (ALL) and lymphoma, and in combination regimens to treat advanced breast cancer, bladder cancer, and cancer of the head and neck. The drug is also used in high doses with leucovorin (LV) rescue as a component of adjuvant therapies for breast cancer and osteosarcoma. In addition to the clinical usefulness of MTX and other folate antagonists, knowledge of the mechanism of action and the pharmacology of these agents has yielded additional dividends in terms of information on important principles of cancer chemotherapy and mechanisms of drug resistance of general applicability to all types of antineoplastic agents. MTX, the prototype folate antagonist, has probably been studied as intensively as any drug employed in present-day clinical medicine (22).

Chemistry

The two clinically studied 4-aminofolate antagonists, MTX and aminopterin (Fig. 60.1), resemble pteroylglutamate in many of their physical and chemical properties (247, 248). The free acids form yellow or yellowish-orange microcrystals, and are practically insoluble in most organic solvents and sparingly soluble in water. The disodium salts are extremely water soluble, however, and are the most convenient form for parenteral administration. Like PGA, the folic acid antagonists decompose without melting at about 200°C. Both antagonists have characteristic absorption spectra in the ultraviolet and visible regions, which is convenient for identification and for quantitation. The absorption maxima for aminopterin and MTX in dilute alkaline solution (0.1 N sodium hydroxide) are listed in Table 60.1.

Aminopterin, like folic acid, gives a positive Bratton-Marshall reaction after reductive cleavage at the C9—N10 bond; MTX, however, having a methyl substituent on the N10—nitrogen, does not yield a primary aromatic amine on cleav-

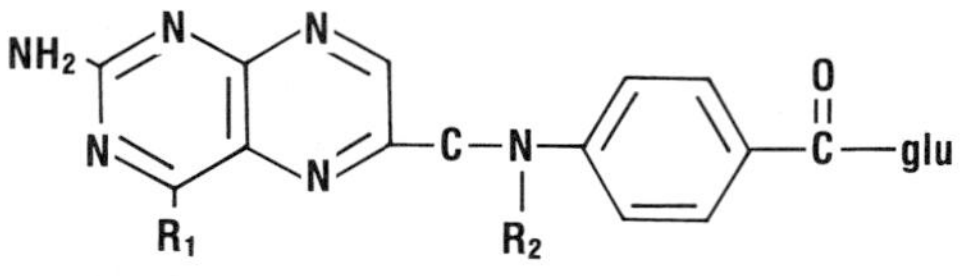

Folic Acid: $R_1 = OH$, $R_2 = H$
Aminopterin: $R_1 = NH_2$, $R_2 = H$
Methotrexate: $R_1 = NH_2$, $R_2 = CH_3$

Figure 60.1. Structure of folic acid (PGA), aminopterin, and MTX.

Table 60.1. Absorption Maxima (nm) and Molar Extinction Coefficients (CE) of Aminopterin and Methotrexate in 0.1 N Sodium Hydroxide Solution

Aminopterin, λ_{max} E × 10^{-3}		MTX, λ_{max} E × 10^{-3}	
nm	CE	nm	CE
260	28.5	257	23.0
284	26.2	302	22.4
370	8.5	370	7.0

age, and thus does not give this color reaction. Alkaline hydrolysis of aminopterin in the absence of oxygen results in deamination at the 4 position, yielding folic acid. Like the parent compound, pteroylglutamate, both compounds are subject to reduction of the pyrazine ring to the dihydro and tetrahydro stages by the use of reducing agents, such as sodium hydrosulfite and sodium borohydride; unlike pteroylglutamate, however, they do not appear to undergo such reduction in vivo. If protected from light, both compounds are stable for several days in aqueous solution as the sodium salts; however, on prolonged storage in solution, they undergo both cleavage and condensation reactions. For most purposes, the purity of commercial preparations is adequate if solutions are freshly prepared. For studies in which a high degree of purity is required, purification treatment by high-performance liquid chromatography or some other means is advisable (215, 240, 287).

Mechanism of Actions

MTX powerfully inhibits a key enzyme in the thymidylate cycle, dihydrofolate reductase (DHFR) (Fig. 60.2) (207, 216). The formation of thymidylate is a key step in the synthesis of DNA, and is the only folate coenzyme–mediated one-carbon transfer reaction in which dihydrofolate, rather than tetrahydrofolate, is the product. Regeneration of tetrahydrofolate is accomplished by DHFR, thus allowing thymidylate and purine biosynthesis to continue. In rapidly dividing cells, the inhibition of thymidylate biosynthesis leads to a decrease in thymidine triphosphate pools, a decrease in DNA synthesis, and eventually cell death (40, 103, 283). Inhibition of tetrahydrofolate formation leading to the inhibition of purine synthesis and rapid cell death has been described as occurring in lymphoblasts treated with high doses of MTX (6, 127).

Methotrexate is required in molar excess to the target en-

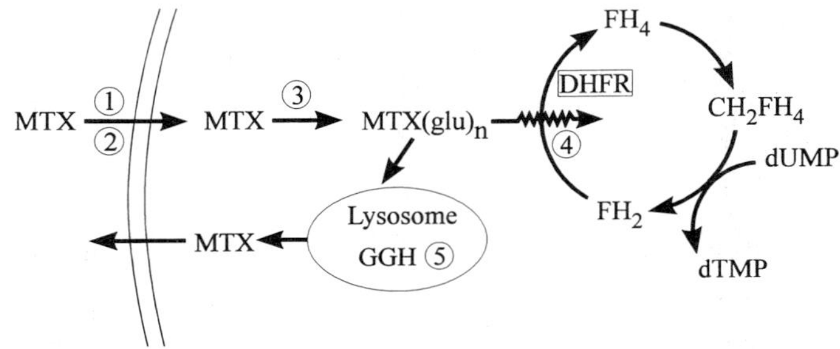

Figure 60.2. Sites of action of MTX and MTX polyglutamates (MTX(glu)N). MTX enters cells by either the reduced-folate carrier (*1*) or the membrane folate binding protein (*2*). MTX is then polyglutamylated by the enzyme folylpolyglutamate synthetase (*3*). MTX $(glu)_n$ is a potent inhibitor of dihydrofolate reductase (DHFR) (*4*). MTX polyglutamates are hydrolyzed to MTX in the lysosome by γ-glutamyl hydrolase (GGH) (*5*). FH_2, dihydrofolate; FH_4, tetrahydrofolate; CH_2FH_4, N5, N10-methylene tetrahydrofolate; dUMP, deoxyuridylate; TMP, thymidine monophosphate; GGH, [γ]-glutamyl hydrolase.

zyme, DHFR, in order to shut off tetrahydrofolate synthesis (258, 299). This concept is important to the present understanding of MTX action. Although the binding of MTX is essentially stoichiometric under ideal conditions (i.e., pH 6.0 and low levels of substrate), in the intact cell, the pH is higher, and blockade of the enzyme results in elevated levels of dihydrofolate and its polyglutamates, thus decreasing the binding of inhibitor to the enzyme (23, 202, 298). Inasmuch as DHFR is in excess in most cells, only a small fraction of the total enzyme need remain catalytically functional to maintain the intracellular reduced folate pool (6, 21).

In recent years, the important role of polyglutamylation as a determinant in MTX sensitivity has been elucidated (Fig. 60.3) (105, 107, 139, 151, 162, 163, 175, 182, 241, 245, 300). A single enzyme, folylpolyglutamate synthetase, appears to be responsible for adding glutamates in γ-carboxyl linkage to both folate coenzyme and MTX and other analogues with a glutamate moiety (45–47, 51, 190, 200, 201). The cDNA for this enzyme was obtained recently (109). This enzyme process, by which up to seven or eight additional glutamate molecules are added to folate coenzymes or MTX, serves to add additional negative charges to these molecules, thus markedly reducing efflux (12). In addition, MTX polyglutamates bind as tightly to DHFR as does MTX, and may dissociate less rapidly from DHFR than MTX (49, 148, 168). Certain human cancer cell lines naturally resistant to MTX, especially to short-term exposures, have been found to have a low capacity to form long-chain MTX polyglutamates (59, 60). In addition, fresh human tumor cells from patients with acute myelocytic leukemia and soft tissue sarcoma, tumors usually refractory to MTX therapy, are unable to form long-chain MTX polyglutamates (172, 173, 176). MTX polyglutamates are also potent inhibitors of other folate-requiring enzymes, including glycinamide ribonucleotide (GAR) and aminoimidazole carboxamide ribonucleotide (AICAR) transformylases and thymidylate synthase (6). Dihydrofolate polyglutamates, and the formylated form of this coenzyme (10-formyl dihydrofolate), which increase after MTX blockage of DHFR, are also potent inhibitors of thymidylate synthase and GAR transformylase (6, 14).

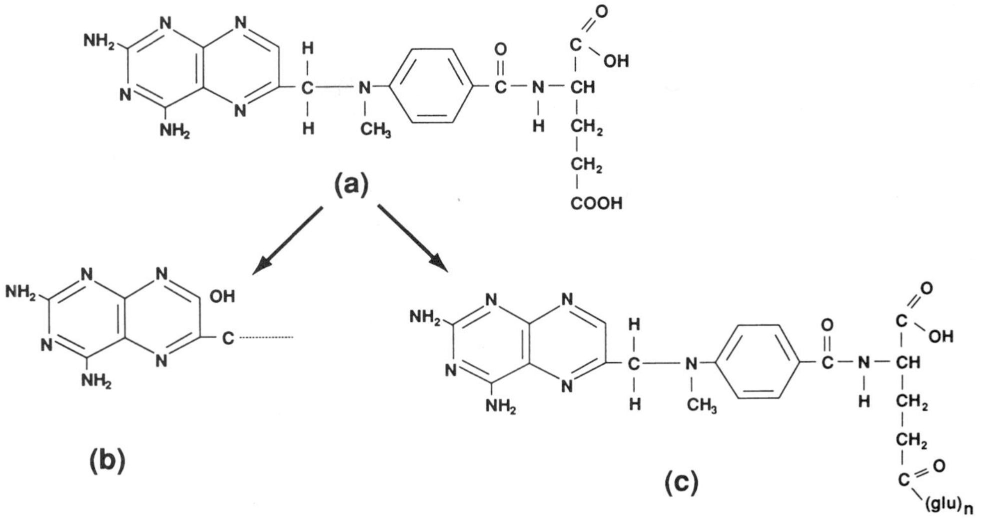

Figure 60.3. Catabolism of MTX. **a.** Methotrexate. **b.** Liver converts MTX to 7-OH MTX. **c.** Bowel bacteria convert MTX to dAMPA (see text).

Biologic Activity

Inhibition of DNA synthesis by MTX and its polyglutamate forms results in "megaloblast" or giant cell formation, followed by cell death with continued inhibition. Mammalian cells require reduced-folate coenzymes for replication; thus, it is not surprising that MTX is capable of preventing DNA synthesis in both normal and neoplastic cells. Folate deficiency can result in apoptosis and/or increased mutagenesis (144).

As a result of the inhibition of DNA synthesis, cell populations are reduced by MTX in proportion to the dose of drug administered and to the duration of exposure to the drug in relation to the growth kinetics of the cell (219). A cell population that has relatively few "resting" or G_0 cells and that accumulates MTX readily as a consequence of polyglutamylation, will be severely affected by a dose of MTX delivered over a period exceeding the generation time of the cell population, assuming the drug gets to the target site in sufficient concentration to inactivate the enzyme (93, 129). A cell population with a large number of G_0 cells would be less affected by the same concentration and time of exposure to MTX if this G_0 fraction were able to enter the proliferating pool when the drug was removed. Thus, MTX, like other inhibitors of DNA synthesis, is most effective when it is employed in the treatment of neoplastic disease characterized by rapidly growing populations with a small percentage of cells in the resting or G_0 phase. Some selectivity, and thus successful use of this drug in certain cancers, has attended the use of high intermittent pulses of the drug, which has little effect on bone marrow and the gastrointestinal tract, organs which, if normal, are characterized by having a substantial number of stem cells "out of cycle" or in the so-called G_0 state. This relative kinetic selectivity may be lost when either the bone marrow or gastrointestinal mucosa is compromised by previous x-ray or drug therapy, or by infiltration with tumor cells or infection.

The effectiveness of MTX against certain tumors (e.g., carcinoma of breast, osteogenic sarcoma) is difficult to explain on the basis of a rapid growth rate. In the latter condition, high-dose therapy appears to be necessary, with LV (folinic acid, citrovorum) rescue. High plasma levels of MTX may lead, by passive diffusion, to a greater intracellular concentration of the drug, resulting in polyglutamate formation. The process results in retention of a high concentration of MTX polyglutamates, thus leading to prolonged inhibition of DHFR. In contrast, normal gut and marrow progenitor cells appear to have a limited capacity to polyglutamylate and thus retain MTX (86, 166).

Other factors that may modify the activity of MTX, in addition to the growth rate of the tumor and retention via polyglutamylation, are the characteristics of MTX transport into cells, its interaction with DHFR, and the rate of turnover of this enzyme (165, 237, 245, 257, 258). In cells with a rapid turnover of enzyme and limited ability to form MTX polyglutamates (e.g., acute granulocytic leukemia blasts), an increase in DHFR may occur, presumably due to decreased degradation of this protein because MTX and MTX polyglutamates are bound to it (24). Recent studies have indicated that this increase may result from the loss of translational regulation of this enzyme; that is, the translation of DHFR protein from its mRNA no longer is inhibited by DHFR when MTX is bound to it (43, 83). These cells may be able to withstand exposure to MTX because this increase in inhibitor-bound DHFR leads to the generation of free enzyme as MTX (Glu_2 or less) rapidly effluxes from cells as the plasma concentration decreases.

Structure–Activity Relationships

The relationships between the structure of folate antagonists and their antitumor activity have been ably summarized, and the relationship between the structure and tightness of binding to the DHFR has also been comprehensively

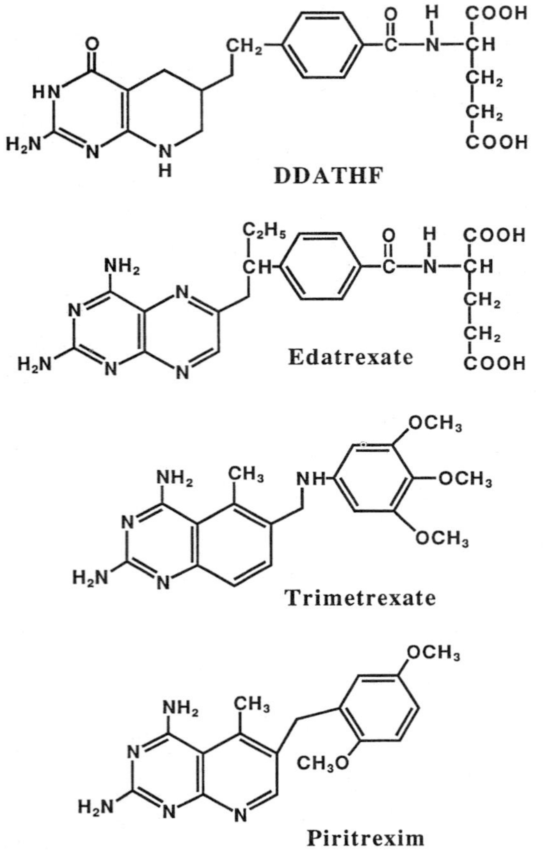

DDATHF

Edatrexate

Trimetrexate

Piritrexim

Figure 60.4. New folate antagonists of current interest.

reviewed and discussed (191–193, 206, 304). Differences between DHFR from mammalian and nonmammalian species, including differing susceptibility to enzyme inhibitors, have been extensively studied, and have led to the development of effective antibacterial and antiprotozoal agents (124, 245, 275).

A great many inhibitors of DHFR have been described, which, unlike aminopterin and MTX, show little or no resemblance to the classic 4-amino-4-deoxypteroylglutamate structure. These include the lipid-soluble antimalarial pyrimethamine (Daraprim), 2,4-diamino-5-(3′,4′-dichlorophenyl)-6-methylpyrimidine (DDMP), "Baker's antifol" (triazinate), and two compounds now in phase II clinical trials, trimetrexate and piritrexim (Fig. 60.4). These "nonclassic" inhibitors bind tightly to this enzyme via hydrophobic interaction, as well as via the 2,4-diaminopyrimidine motif (245). Trimetrexate, together with LV protection, was recently approved for the treatment of *Pneumocystis carinii* pneumonia (PCP) (7).

Resistance to Antifolates

Although the development of effective chemotherapeutic regimens including MTX has significantly improved the therapy of a variety of malignancies (Table 60.2), achieving actual cures is still difficult even in chemotherapy-sensitive diseases. The two problems that represent the major obstacles to the effective treatment of neoplastic disease with MTX, as well as with most other antineoplastic agents, are toxicity and resistance. Resistance to MTX either can be natural or may be acquired after initial response to the drug (172, 264). Resistance to antifolates is also observed in bacteria and protozoa, and often limits the usefulness of these drugs as anti-infectives (245).

Table 60.2. Sensitivity of Neoplastic Diseases to MTX

Sensitive[a]	Moderately sensitive[b]	Not sensitive
Acute lymphocytic leukemia	Head and neck cancer	Renal cell cancer
Acute myelocytic leukemia	Breast cancer	Pancreatic cancer
Burkitt's lymphoma	Bladder cancer	Colon cancer
Choriocarcinoma		
Diffuse large cell lymphoma		

[a] Cures disease or is part of curative regimen.
[b] Greater than 15% response.

Acquired Resistance to MTX

Along with natural resistance, acquired drug resistance remains a major obstacle to effective chemotherapy. For example, 90% of pediatric patients with ALL achieve a complete remission, but 5-year disease-free survival rates are only 70% using MTX-based continuation therapy. Retreatment of these patients with the same agents is less effective because of the development of drug resistance.

Four major mechanisms of resistance to MTX have been described in experimental tumors: an increase in DHFR activity due to amplification of this gene, a decrease in uptake of MTX due to either a decreased influx of MTX or to a decrease of long-chain polyglutamate formation, or a mutation that results in an altered DHFR with decreased binding to MTX (6, 21). Decreased levels of MTX polyglutamates in cells may also result from increased breakdown; indeed, both intrinsic and acquired resistance to MTX in cell lines have been attributed to increased levels of γ-glutamyl hydrolase activity (173, 228).

Amplification of the DHFR gene, resulting in increased levels of the enzyme, has been identified as a common mechanism of acquired MTX resistance. Since the original description of DHFR gene amplification in MTX-resistant mouse tumor cells (8), a number of mouse, hamster, and human MTX-resistant cell lines have been described, with increased DHFR and amplification of the DHFR gene as a mechanism of MTX resistance (53, 94, 229, 269). Unstable or reversible resistance due to gene amplification has usually been associated with the presence of "double minute" or centromereless chromosomes containing the DHFR amplicon, while high-level stable resistance has been associated with an abnormal banding region, often referred to as a homogeneously staining region (HSR) (16, 158–160). It has also been demonstrated that gene amplification as a mechanism of resistance occurs in some patients treated with MTX (36, 58, 111, 125, 289).

Transport resistance as well as DHFR gene amplification is often found as the mechanism of acquired resistance in experimental systems (95, 235, 244). MTX utilizes the reduced-folate carrier system for influx, and uptake is a function of both influx and efflux, as well as polyglutamylation, which leads to retention (42, 66, 105, 119–121, 209, 210). The relationship between the reduced-folate carrier system and a folate-binding protein (folate receptor) present in some epithelial cells and carcinoma is not clear (153). The reduced folate carrier was only recently cloned, and detailed studies of its function, specificity, and regulation are in progress (69, 305).

Although defects in polyglutamylation have been described in several MTX-resistant cell lines, the resistance of these cells has usually been found to be attributable to a combination of mechanisms (54, 236). Recently, cell lines were described that are resistant to MTX solely because of impaired polyglutamylation (223). These cells were obtained by a more clinically relevant selection schedule consisting of short-term, high-dose treatments with MTX, rather than continuous exposure to this drug. Recent studies have indicated that the basis of the defect in these cells is an alteration in the enzyme folylpolyglutamate synthetase (187). Clinical studies have also shown a strong correlation between the amount of MTX polyglutamates formed in blasts and disease-free survival in children with ALL (300, 301).

Although several MTX-resistant cell lines have been found to possess an altered DHFR that has a decreased affinity for MTX, only few altered human DHFRs have been characterized in any detail (64, 65, 71, 98, 113, 114, 138, 195, 196, 269). Point mutations in several cell lines, including human cells, have been detected that cause a change in the binding of MTX to the enzyme, and have usually involved amino acids that bind to the inhibitor by hydrophobic interaction (245). The first mutation of an amino acid in a nonactive site region (trp→gly) associated with MTX resistance in L1210 cells was recently reported (67). Evidence for mutations in the gene for DHFR as a mechanism for resistance in blast cells from patients has not yet been documented, but sensitive methodology (polymerase chain reaction, amplification of DHFR cDNA) to allow sequencing and detection of possible mutations only recently has become available (68, 245). It may be possible to develop antifolates with specificity for altered DHFR enzymes (63, 214, 245). These efforts will be guided by a detailed knowledge of the structure of this enzyme and its interaction with substrates and inhibitors (183–185, 225, 245, 289). It is also possible to convert normal marrow to a state of resistance to MTX by transfection with an altered DHFR in a viral vector (134, 303). These experimental studies open up the possibility of clinical trials with these viral constructs, with the goal of allowing increased doses of MTX to be safely administered to patients with cancer (97).

Pharmacokinetics of MTX

ABSORPTION

In contrast to older studies that demonstrated good absorption at low doses of MTX, recent studies have emphasized the relatively poor and unpredictable nature of absorption of this drug after oral administration (13, 44, 118, 155, 267). The extent of absorption may be less than 50%, even at low doses (<15 mg/m^2). Absorption decreases with increasing oral doses. Following oral administration, peak plasma concentrations may occur 1 to 5 hours after a dose (15 to 30 mg/m^2). Food, nonabsorbable antibiotics, bile salts, and a shortened intestine transit time may decrease the rate and extent of MTX absorption (239, 271). The marked intra- and interpatient variability of MTX absorption may explain the wide variation in oral doses of MTX observed in leukemia patients in remission required to maintain the white blood count between 2,000 and 4,000 μL. Therefore, while oral use of MTX is convenient, unless compliance and/or serum concentrations of drug are measured, some clinicians still favor parenteral administration.

DISTRIBUTION

After intravenous (IV) administration, MTX distributes within an initial volume approximately of 18% (0.18 L/kg of body weight), with a variable steady-state volume of 40 to 80% of body weight (132, 252). The distribution phase (α) $t_{1/2}$ is 30 to 45 min, the renal clearance phase (β) $t_{1/2}$ is 3 to 4 hours, and the $t_{1/2}$ of the third phase, representing reabsorption from the gut and excretion, is 6 to 20 hours (252, 271). MTX binding to plasma proteins, especially to albumin, is approximately 50% (270). The 7-hydroxymetabolite of MTX is 90% bound to plasma proteins, but apparently does not interfere with MTX binding to plasma proteins at concentrations found in patients. The highest tissue-to-plasma concentrations found in humans are in the liver and kidney, followed by the gastrointestinal tract. Higher plasma levels in humans, as compared with mice, are attributed to less rapid excretion in the bile and by the kidney, and a longer residue time in the small intestine (40, 167, 278, 279). Prolonged plasma levels after high-dose MTX infusions in humans have been attributed to decreased transit rate secondary to gastrointestinal obstruction.

Patients with pleural or peritoneal effusions may be at increased risk for developing toxicity to high-dose MTX as a result of "third spacing," or MTX trapping in the infusion, and slow release leading to sustained MTX concentrations in serum (293). This phenomenon is more of a problem when high doses of the drug are administered. In these circumstances, higher doses and prolonged rescue with LV may be necessary, until the serum level of MTX decreases to less than 5×10^{-8} M.

After high doses of MTX (>6 g/m^2), serum concentrations in the range of 10^{-3} to 10^{-4} M are achieved (1, 6, 19, 32, 85, 90, 164). At these concentrations, the active transport of this drug is saturated, limiting further influx of drug to passive diffusion. These high extracellular MTX concentrations inhibit the uptake of reduced folates, including exogenous administered LV, explaining the need for larger doses of LV to reverse MTX action, because of the competitive nature of this interaction at the transport level. Selectivity to high dose MTX regimens likely depends on the intracellular concentration of MTX achieved in the tumor, and subsequent polyglutamylation and retention. Bone marrow and intestinal mucosa have a limited capacity to retain MTX, explaining, in part, the selectivity of this drug for certain tumors. Even with IV administration, there is a wide range in the area under the plasma curve (AUC) produced by a given dose in patients (31, 82, 85, 164).

The passage of MTX from plasma to cerebrospinal fluid (CSF) is poor, and MTX does not achieve cytocidal concentrations in the CSF ($> 5 \times 10^{-8}$ M) after conventional doses (15 to 30 mg/m^2) (81, 84, 251). CSF concentrations after MTX administration are dose related, and cytocidal levels are obtained with doses of 500 mg/m^2 and higher. After high-dose systemic MTX administration, lumbar CSF and ventricular CSF concentrations were similar. When MTX is given by the lumbar route into the CSF, it distributes unreliably into the ventricles, while MTX given by an indwelling ventricular shunt provides reproducible therapeutic drug concentrations ($>10^{-6}$ M) for at least 48 hours (194). An improved dose schedule utilizing the administration of multiple small doses of intrathecal MTX has been suggested (27). Following intrathecal administration, MTX slowly exits into the systemic circulation with a $t_{1/2}$ of 8 to 10 hours (30). The pharmacology of intrathecal MTX and the amount of intraventricular MTX may be altered by overt meningeal leukemia and the position of the patient at the time of lumbar puncture (26).

Among experimental agents, dDMP is highly lipid soluble and crosses the blood–brain barrier readily giving high central nervous system (CNS) levels (123). Other antifolates, including trimetrexate and piritrexim, are only poorly transported into the CNS (135). Although MTX is accumulated poorly into the CSF, even small doses of LV given orally can increase CSF folates significantly. This systemic rescue, especially if given too early after MTX, may rescue cells in the CSF compartment (156, 285).

The clinical observation that irradiation followed by MTX treatment may predispose patients to neurotoxicity (see below) may be a consequence of the effect of radiation therapy on the blood–brain barrier (277).

METABOLISM

The major metabolite of MTX is 7-hydroxy MTX (Fig. 60.3) (79, 170, 265, 273). This hydroxylation process is due to hepatic aldehyde oxidase, and results in a much less active form of MTX, as it is only 1% as potent an inhibitor of DHFR as is MTX (88, 146, 147, 226). The 7-hydroxymetabolite is less water soluble than is MTX, and may contribute to the renal toxicity frequently seen after high doses of the antifolate (140).

A second, less important pathway of metabolism of MTX occurs in the intestine, and the drug is hydrolysed by bacteria to the pteroate (4-amino-4-deoxy-N10-methyl pteroic acid, dAMPA) and glutamic acid (Fig. 60.3) (73, 290). dAMPA, like 7-OH MTX, is also a relatively inactive metabolite with approximately 1/200th the affinity of MTX for DHFR. dAMPA excretion in the urine accounts for only a small percentage of the dose administered (<5%).

As mentioned, the third metabolic product of MTX that occurs via intracellular conversion is MTX polyglutamate. MTX polyglutamates are at least as potent inhibitors of DHFR as is MTX, and have a slower rate of disassociation from DHFR than does MTX (148). MTX polyglutamates are not found in plasma or urine because of the activity of hydrolase(s) (conjugase) in plasma that convert folyl and MTX polyglutamates to monoglutamates. Like MTX, 7-OH MTX is also polyglutamylated intracellularly, and retention of these polyglutamate forms could contribute to MTX cytotoxicity (72, 87, 189, 227).

BILIARY EXCRETION

Following IV administration of doses of 30 to 80 mg/m$_2$, 0.4 to 20% of the administered dose can be recovered in bile. Less than 10% of MTX is recovered in the feces collected over 24 hours (55, 212, 277). The enterohepatic recycling of MTX has been estimated using the D-isomer as a reference marker for nonabsorbable drug (117).

Inadvertent Drug Interactions

Several drugs used in cancer patients, including antibiotics, may increase toxicity when used with MTX, and should be avoided, if possible (135, 136). Obviously, drugs that increase the possibility of bleeding in patients who are at risk of thrombocytopenia, such as aspirin, should be avoided. During recent years, deleterious and even fatal reactions have been reported between MTX and nonsteroidal anti-inflammatory drugs, in particular with naproxen and ketoprofen (11, 62, 256, 286). This increased toxicity may be due to decreased renal elimination, possibly as a result of competition for renal secretion (130). Other commonly used organic drugs may also potentiate MTX toxicity, such as phenylbutazone, salicylate, and probenecid (4, 174). Probenecid increased the efficacy of MTX in tumor-bearing mice, but it has not been used clinically with this goal in mind (260, 261).

Increased toxicity was also reported when trimethoprim, the antibacterial agent, was used together with MTX; presumably this antifolate, with only weak binding affinity to mammalian DHFR, lowers folate stores, especially in patients with subclinical folate deficiency, making marrow cells more susceptible to MTX-induced toxicity (180, 288). Alcohol should also be avoided in patients receiving MTX because of the risk of hepatic fibrosis and cirrhosis.

Clinical Application

CLINICAL DOSAGE SCHEDULES

MTX has been administered on a variety of dosage schedules since its introduction into the clinic over 40 years ago (Table 60.3). Remarkably, there are few carefully controlled studies comparing different dose regimens. In a trial of MTX in patients with head and neck cancer treated with either 50,

Table 60.3. Dosage Schedules Used for MTX

Use	Comment
Oral:	
a. Daily continuous (5–10 mg/d)	Not used anymore
b. Weekly, biweekly (15–25 mg in single or divided doses)	Used mainly to treat psoriasis or rheumatoid arthritis
c. Twice weekly (20–30 mg/m^2)	Used in maintenance treatment of ALL
Parenteral:	
a. Pulse weekly (IV) 30–60 mg/m^2	Used to treat choriocarcinoma, maintenance in ALL
b. "Conventional dose" MTX daily ×5 days 10–20 mg/m^2	
c. Weekly intermediate dose MTX (120–500 mg/m^2), or as part of m BACOD given between cycles (200 mg/m^2), or as a modulating agent (24 hours before 5-FU, 240 mg/m^2). In FAMTX combination, MTX (1000 mg/m^2) is used as modulating agent, followed in 1 hour by 5-FU (1,500 mg/m^2).	Requires LV "rescue," 10–15 mg/m^2 q 6 h for 6 to 8 doses beginning 24–42 hours after MTX
d. High-dose MTX (greater than 500 mg/m^2)	Used in treatment of osteosarcoma (adjuvant) and in ALL (see Table 60.5). *Requires LV "rescue," as above*

Table 60.4. Combination Chemotherapy with MTX

Used With	Result
5-FU	Synergistic if MTX precedes 5-FU by 24 hours (25, 72, 91, 95, 181, 211, 306)
L-Asparaginase	Synergistic if MTX precedes L-asparaginase by 24 hours (null and T-cell leukemia); antagonizes MTX action if used together (35, 131, 149, 178, 309)
Cytosine arabinoside	Additive or synergistic if used together (17, 76). With 6-mercaptopurine, sequencing may be important (MTX increases 6-MP nucleotide levels) (29)
Cyclophosphamide	Additive cytotoxicity if used together (242). With cisplatin, MTX should precede cisplatin because of cisplatin's renal toxicity
Corticosteroids	Synergistic when used together in treatment of ALL
Vinca alkaloids	Additive effects when used together (41, 106, 108, 169, 294)
Bleomycin	Additive effects when used together; mucosal cell toxicity increased (263)
Anthracyclines	Additive effects when used together

500, or 5,000 mg/m^2 with LV "rescue," a trend of dose responsiveness was seen (5 of 24, 5 of 16, 9 of 18, respectively). Some responses were noted with the 5,000 mg/m^2 dose regimen in patients who failed at lower doses (20, 307, 308). The importance of dose scheduling was recently emphasized by an experimental study showing that resistance to high-dose pulse MTX may not extend to continuous low-dose exposure (223). Tumor cells capable of long-chain MTX polyglutamate formation may be more selectively treated with high-dose pulse MTX; e.g., most ALL blasts (287). The marked sensitivity of choriocarcinoma to MTX has also been attributed to the ability of this tumor to form and retain long-chain MTX polyglutamates (6). The relative lack of toxicity of normal renewal tissues to high-dose MTX regimens with LV rescue may reflect the inability of progenitor cells from these tissues to form long-chain polyglutamates of MTX (86, 166).

Determining the optimum dose schedule of MTX is complicated by the use of this drug in combination, thus making it difficult to generalize about a single dose schedule. Sequencing appears to be important when MTX is used with 5-fluorouracil (5-FU) (24-hour pretreatment with MTX appears to be best), with L-asparaginase (again, 24-hour pretreatment is best), and probably with cytosine arabinoside (concurrent treatment may be optimal) and 6-mecaptopurine or 6-thioguanine (pretreatment with MTX may be optimal). Table 60.4 summarizes the use of drug combinations that include MTX.

Current Uses for MTX in the Treatment of Neoplastic Disease

ACUTE LEUKEMIA

Although aminopterin was initially used as a single agent to induce remissions in children with acute leukemia, MTX is now used as part of combination regimens to treat this disease, especially as treatment during remission, and as intrathecal administration for prophylaxis of, as well for treatment of, meningeal leukemia. Early studies by the Acute Leukemia B Group showed that twice-weekly therapy (20 mg/m^2) was superior to continuous daily oral administration for treatment during remission (2). Other dose schedules appear to be even more beneficial, including 5-day courses administered every 3 to 4 weeks, or high-dose regimens with LV rescue (90, 100, 102). Methotrexate and L-asparaginase and MTX/6-mercaptopurine combinations are now commonly employed as part of the treatment of ALL (131, 178, 309). Optimum use of these two combinations requires adequate dosing and correct sequencing (35, 170, 281).

MTX has limited value in the treatment of acute non-lymphocytic leukemia. High-dose regimens with LV rescue have a transient but rapid effect on the peripheral blood count without producing marrow remissions in the large majority of these patients (19, 128). The lack of efficacy of MTX in this disease has been attributed to poor intracellular retention of the drug caused by a lack of polyglutamylation, and an increase of the target enzyme DHFR following treatment with it (24, 172).

LYMPHOMA

Based on phase II studies that indicated that moderate to high doses of MTX with LV rescue could produce transient regressions in patients with large cell lymphoma, MTX (200 mg/m^2 to 3 gm/m^2) with LV rescue has been added to combination regimens for intermediate-grade and high-grade lymphomas (91b, 111, 230). In certain of these regimens (M-BACOD), MTX is used with LV during the leukopenic phase of drug treatment, since the MTX/LV combination has little marrow toxicity (253). Based on experimental studies showing that MTX and cytosine arabinoside produce additive and possibly synergistic effects, this combination has also been utilized in regimens to treat this disease (e.g., COMLA; cyclophosphamide, vincristine, methotrexate, cytosine arabinoside, and LV) (17, 76).

CHORIOCARCINOMA

This neoplasm is unique in that single-drug treatment with either MTX or actinomycin D produces a substantial number of cures (122). The basis for the unusual sensitivity of this tumor to MTX is not entirely clear, but choriocarcinoma cells may accumulate and retain this drug effectively by synthesizing long-chain polyglutamates. Recently, the JAR cell line was shown to have active-receptor coupled uptake (potocytosis) of folates and antifolates (6, 9).

Single-agent curative treatment with intensive 5-day courses of MTX has not resulted in secondary neoplasias in long-term survivors (238). Thus, MTX is not considered carcinogenic. Current data suggest, however, that folate deficiency increases the rate of mutagenesis (144). Current programs for the treatment of this malignancy utilize MTX in combination with other drugs, especially for "poor risk" patients (205) (see Chapter 134).

BREAST CANCER

MTX as a single agent causes regressions of breast cancer in approximately 30% of patients. No single-dose schedule has emerged as the optimum treatment when the drug is used as a single agent, including high-dose treatment with LV rescue. When used with fluorouracil, sequential use of MTX followed by 5-FU has improved response rates to 50%; this sequential combination has improved disease-free survival when used as adjuvant therapy (81) (see Chapter 136). The most frequently used combination regimen is adjuvant therapy and to treat advanced breast cancer is cyclophosphamide, MTX, and 5-FU (CMF).

GASTROINTESTINAL CANCER

MTX as a single agent has limited effectiveness in the treatment of gastrointestinal malignancies (75). Its role in the treatment of these diseases is mainly to modulate, and possibly improve, the effectiveness of 5-FU. In the treatment of gastric cancer, an alternating regimen of doxorubicin with high-dose MTX followed by high-dose 5-FU and LV rescue has resulted in a 35% response rate, with 10% long-time survivors. Data from recent trials using this sequence in colon cancer emphasize the need for a 7- to 24-hour interval between MTX and 5-FU administration, presumably to optimize increases in phosphoribosylpyrophosphate (PRPP) that occur as a consequence of MTX inhibition of purine biosynthesis, to increase 5-FU nucleotide formation (see below) (34, 181, 211, 306). The sequential use of MTX followed by 5-FU 24 hours later has increased the response rate over that of 5-FU alone, with results comparable to those of other regimens that "modulate" 5-FU activity with less or comparable toxicity (181).

GENITOURINARY CANCER

MTX (100 mg/m^2) alone, or MTX in high doses (>0.5 g/m^2) with LV rescue, is clearly active in the treatment of advanced bladder cancer. The response rate reported (approximately 30%) is similar to the response rate of the other most active single drug, cisplatin. Combinations of drugs, including MTX with cisplatin, vinblastine, and doxorubicin (M-VAC), have resulted in a substantial number of long-term clinical remissions (272). This combination is now being further modified and tested as predefinitive (neoadjuvant) treatment in an attempt to improve the cure rates of patients with bladder cancer, and possibly with radiotherapy, to avoid cystectomy.

HEAD AND NECK CANCER

MTX and cisplatin are the two most active single agents for the treatment of patients with advanced carcinoma of the head and neck region. High-dose MTX regimens with LV rescue appear to improve response rates from 30 to 50%, but remission duration and survival are not improved (33). MTX has also been used with 5-FU in this disease, and response rates of 50 to 60% have been reported. The sequence and timing of drug administration have not been shown to affect the response rate, although different patterns of toxicity were observed (33).

LUNG CANCER

MTX as a single agent in conventional doses, or in high doses with LV rescue, has only marginal activity in non–small cell lung cancer (266). This drug does have activity in small cell lung cancer, and has been used in combination regimens to treat that disease (see Chapter 107).

OSTEOGENIC SARCOMA

After studies were reported indicating that high-dose MTX with LV rescue could cause regressions in patients with advanced osteogenic sarcoma, the drug was tested as adjuvant therapy in patients with disease following resection of the tumor, with encouraging results (141, 142). Recent randomized trials of pre- and postdefinitive treatment have demonstrated the beneficial effect of chemotherapy that includes high-dose MTX with LV rescue (77, 177). The single-agent response rate more likely is 20% rather than the 35 to 40% reported in smaller, earlier trials.

Adverse Effects

HEMATOLOGIC TOXICITY

Tissues that are self-renewing—that is, the bone marrow and epithelial cells—are at highest risk for damage by the folate antagonists. Bone marrow progenitor cells of all lineages are affected by MTX, but neutropenia usually predominates. Recovery after a single dose is usually rapid, taking place 14 to 21 days following a nadir that occurs approximately 10 days after drug administration. The effects on marrow are dose related, but there is considerable variability among patients. Subclinical folate deficiency, usually caused by poor nutrition; impaired renal function (pretreatment with cisplatin is a risk factor); a stressed marrow owing to previous x-ray treatment, chemotherapy, or infection; and the use of trimethoprim-sulfa for *P. carinii* prophylaxis may predispose patients to hematologic (and gastrointestinal) toxicity to MTX. Young patients usually tolerate MTX better than do older individuals, a fact presumably related to clearance of the drug by the kidneys. The administration of LV, before 42 hours have elapsed, if in an appropriate dose, may prevent or lessen MTX toxicity, and allow larger doses of the antifolate to be administered (19, 169).

GASTROINTESTINAL TOXICITY

Mucositis is a common side effect of MTX treatment, and usually becomes manifest 3 to 5 days following a dose or course of the drug. This is an early sign of MTX toxicity, and the drug should be discontinued when it occurs. Subsequent doses should not be increased unless the mucositis is grade 1 or less. More severe gastrointestinal toxicity is manifest by diarrhea, which may progress to severe bloody diarrhea. When this occurs in association with neutropenia, patients are at high risk of sepsis and death. Such patients should be hospitalized and managed vigorously with fluids and antibiotics. These severe side effects generally occur in a setting of renal damage, usually a consequence of high doses of MTX, but may also occur in patients treated with conventional doses. MTX blood levels and serum creatinine levels should be followed, and appropriate doses of LV administered, along with the supportive measures instituted (see below). Nausea and vomiting, even with high doses of MTX, are usually mild to moderate, and most patients do not require antinausea medication.

RENAL TOXICITY

Conventional-dose MTX regimens, not requiring LV, were occasionally reported to cause renal toxicity, presumably as a direct effect of MTX on renal tubular epithelium (52). With the introduction of high-dose regimens requiring LV rescue, renal toxicity leading to delayed MTX clearance sometimes resulted in severe marrow and gastrointestinal toxicity, occasionally fatal, especially in adults. This toxicity is believed to be due to precipitation of MTX and its less soluble metabolite, 7-OH MTX, in the tubules, as well as to a possible direct effect of this drug on the renal tubule (140). The use of vigorous hydration, often with osmotic diuresis and alkalinization of urine to increase solubility of MTX and 7-OH MTX, has markedly ameliorated this problem. Occasional patients, even with this regimen (Table 60.5), exhibit renal impairment. Through careful monitoring of MTX and creatinine serum levels, these patients may be identified and larger doses and prolonged duration of LV employed to prevent toxicity.

Table 60.5. Regimen for High-Dose MTX Treatment (>0.5 g/m^2)[a]; Prehydration and Alkalinization of Urine[b]

8 to 12 hours before treatment, patients should receive 1.5 L/m^2 of saline or 5% glucose with 100 mEq HCO_3^- and 20 mEq KCl per liter. Continue until pH of urine is 7.0 or greater at time of MTX administration.

MTX administration

1. 0.5 g to 3.0 g/m^2 as 20- to 30-minute bolus. At 24 hours, begin LV 15 mg/m^2 q 6 h × 6 doses.
2. Jaffe regimen: 1.2 to 6 g/m^2 over 6 hours IV, with continued IV hydration for an additional 18 hours. Begin LV 2 hours after end of MTX infusion, 15 mg/m^2 q 6 h × 7 doses.
3. 36-hour infusion: MTX, 50 mg/m^2, is given as bolus, followed by infusion of MTX over 36 hours at dose of 1.5 g/m^2. LV rescue is started at end of infusion: 200 mg/m^2 over 12 hours as infusion, then 25 mg/m^2 IM q 6 h × 6.

Drug monitoring

MTX levels should be monitored at 24 hours for regimen 1 or 48 hours for regimens 2 and 3. Serum creatinine levels pretreatment and at 24 and 48 hours should also be performed.

For regimen 1, 24-hour levels of MTX of greater than 1×10^{-6} M require additional LV rescue; for regimens 2 and 3, 48-hour blood levels above 5×10^{-7} M should receive additional LV rescue. The dose of LV should be increased to 100 mg/m^2 q 6 h for blood levels of 1×10^{-6} M to 5×10^{-6} M; blood levels above 5×10^{-6} M should receive doses of 200 mg/m^2 or higher. Drug levels should be monitored daily, and LV continued (in decreasing doses as the MTX blood levels fall) until the plasma concentration of MTX is below 1×10^{-8} M.

[a] See references 85, 90, 193, 201, 208, 220, 221, 274.
[b] See references 1, 6, 12.

Extremely high levels of MTX (>1×10^{-5} M) are difficult to rescue, even with high doses of leucovorin (1, 6, 218). Hemodialysis and peritoneal dialysis have proved ineffective in substantially lowering MTX plasma levels (115). Charcoal hemoperfusion columns have been used successfully in a small number of patients (70). Oral charcoal and cholestyramine have also been used to bind MTX in the gut, thus limiting enterohepatic recirculation and toxicity (76, 186). Thymidine (1 to 3 g/m^2/d) is also capable of rescuing patients from MTX toxicity, but this metabolite is not generally available (78, 126, 282). Carboxypeptidase G1, an enzyme capable of cleaving the peptide bond in MTX resulting in glutamate and dAMPA (Fig. 60.3), has also been used experimentally to lower MTX levels, but dAMPA is even less soluble than MTX (188). This enzyme has also been proposed for use as a "rescue" agent, based on studies in experimental tumors (39).

HEPATOTOXICITY

Chronic low-dose continuous treatment with MTX has been associated with portal fibrosis, and in some patients, with frank cirrhosis (310). The basis for this liver damage is not known, but it may result from interference with choline synthesis; acute MTX hepatotoxicity in rats is reversed by choline administration (101). Cirrhosis has been reported in patients with psoriasis, rheumatoid arthritis, and ALL treated with long-term continuous oral MTX (179). Alcohol and other hepatotoxic drugs should be avoided in this patient population. Intermittent schedules with pulse therapy appear to decrease the incidence of fibrosis and cirrhosis (61).

Acute elevations of liver enzymes (SGOT) commonly occur several days after treatment with high-dose MTX, but rapidly return to normal, and do not appear to predict for chronic liver toxicity (295).

CENTRAL NERVOUS SYSTEM TOXICITY

Although intrathecal MTX has been used extensively to treat patients with meningeal leukemia, its use has been associated with neurotoxicity, ranging from mild to severe. In cases of inadvertent overdosing (>100 mg), fatalities have been reported.

The most common side effect of intrathecal MTX administration, made manifest by severe headache, fever, meningismus, vomiting, and CSF pleocytosis, is thought to be caused by a chemical arachnoiditis directly, or perhaps by the release of adenosine, which is a potent autocoid in the CNS. This effect of adenosine has been ameliorated by systemic administration of low doses of methylxanthines, such as aminophyllin and theophylline (18). Dosage adjustment or switching to cytosine arabinoside may be required if these symptoms persist (see Chapter 175).

More serious neurotoxicity has been observed in 5 to 10% of patients receiving 12 to 15 mg/m^2 of MTX intrathecally, consisting of motor paralysis of the extremities, cranial nerve palsies, seizures, and even coma. Inasmuch as these signs are seen mainly in adult patients with active meningeal disease, it is often difficult to distinguish these side effects from meningeal leukemia. This subacute toxicity usually arises during the second or third week of intrathecal treatment, and has been attributed to slow CSF clearance of MTX (27).

A severe chronic demyelinating encephalopathy has also been observed in children treated prophylactically with intrathecal MTX who have also received prophylactic cranial irradiation (>2,000 cGy) (250). These patients develop dementia and limb spasticity, and even coma, months or years after intrathecal MTX treatment. Computed tomography scans show cortical thinning, ventricular enlargement, and diffuse intracerebral calcifications (217). Rarely, encephalopathy has been reported in patients treated only with high-dose IV MTX. Acute transient cerebral dysfunction occurring several days after high-dose systemic MTX treatment has also been reported; in these patients, signs (paresis, aphasia, seizures) usually resolve within 2 to 3 days (104, 143).

In patients who receive a MTX overdose intrathecally (>100 mg), immediate CSF removal with ventricolumbar perfusion is indicated (268). Recently, intrathecal use of carboxypeptidase G2 was shown to decrease mortality markedly in animals given a lethal dose of MTX intrathecally, and may be the preferred treatment for this complication when the enzyme is available (3). Intrathecal or systemic LV is not indicated in these cases, since it is unlikely that this toxicity is attributable to inhibition of DHFR.

PULMONARY TOXICITY

Although uncommon, pulmonary toxicity due to MTX has been described, and has been noted even in patients receiving low-dose oral MTX for rheumatoid arthritis (38, 48, 246, 267). The clinical picture usually consists of cough, dyspnea, fever, and hypoxemia. Chest x-ray films are nonspecific, but show patchy interstitial infiltrates. *Pneumocystis carinii* must be ruled out, especially in patients also receiving steroids. Histologic examinations show diffuse interstitial lymphocytic infiltrates, giant cells, and noncaseating granulomas. In some patients, a peripheral eosinophilia is observed, raising the possibility that this is an allergic pneumonitis. The process may progress to fibrosis, and it is important to discontinue MTX while the pulmonary toxicity is reversible. Some patients have been retreated without recurrence of the problem.

SKIN TOXICITY

Skin toxicity to MTX occurs in 5 to 10% of patients, consisting of an erythematous rash, characteristically noted on the neck and upper trunk. The rash may be pruritic and relatively insignificant, and usually lasts for several days. In other instances, especially when related to other signs of severe MTX toxicity, it may progress to severe bullous formation and desquamation (74). Sun-exposed areas may be more sensitive to MTX (10, 203). A cutaneous vasculitis after intermediate-dose MTX has also been reported (99).

TERATOGENIC AND MUTAGENIC EFFECTS

MTX is known to be a potent abortifacient, especially if administered during the first trimester of pregnancy. However, there is no indication of a higher than normal incidence of fetal abnormalities in women who have been successfully treated with MTX for choriocarcinoma. These women also have not had a higher than normal incidence of secondary malignancies. Thus far, there is no evidence that MTX has any mutagenic or carcinogenic effects (249).

MISCELLANEOUS TOXICITY

Osteoporosis has been reported with chronic low-dose MTX administration (204). Fever seizures, recall of radiation toxicity or phototoxicity, and anaphylactoid reactions have been reported with high-dose administration (112). Pleuritic and left-upper-quadrant pain, presumably attributable to splenic capsule inflammation, has been reported with a moderately high-dose regimen.

New Folate Antagonists Now in Clinical Trial

INHIBITORS OF DHFR

MTX is an extremely potent inhibitor of DHFR, and while it may be possible to develop inhibitors that are more tightly bound or may irreversibly inactivate this enzyme, unless these compounds possess other advantages (i.e., more avid uptake and/or more efficient retention by malignant cells as compared with normal cells) selectivity may not improve. Two types of second-generation folate antagonists are now in clinical trial, "classic" antagonists, whose structures resemble the metabolite folic acid, and "nonclassic" agents, whose structures are markedly different from that of the substrate.

10-Ethyldeazaaminopterin (10-EDAM, Fig. 60.4), developed by Sirotnak and associates, was chosen for clinical trial after detailed structure activity studies demonstrated that hydrophobic substitutions at the N10 position of aminopterin resulted in improved uptake and retention (polyglutamylation) by tumor cells as compared with normal cells (242, 262). The drug is now under active clinical investigation, and encouraging response rates have been noted in patients with non–small cell lung cancer, head and neck cancer, breast cancer, and malignant fibrous histiocytoma (38, 39, 243, 254). One limitation to its use might be that it may be relatively ineffective against MTX-resistant cells, since it utilizes the same carrier mechanism for transport and is polyglutamylated by the same enzyme as is MTX.

In contrast, the nonclassic antifolates, trimetrexate and piritrexim (Fig. 60.4), currently in phase II trials, are also potent inhibitors of DHFR, but enter cells by passive or facilitative diffusion rather than by the reduced-folate transport carrier (135, 154, 213, 255). Consequently, these antifolates are still effective cytotoxic agents against MTX-resistant cells when the mechanism of resistance is impaired transport, decreased polyglutamylation, or even low-level amplification of DHFR (157, 197, 231, 232, 284). Cells resistant to MTX owing to a mutation in the enzyme leading to decreased binding of the inhibitor may or may not be cross-resistant to trimetrexate, depending on the nature of the mutation (245). These drugs also differ from MTX in that they are not substrates for polyglutamate synthetase; therefore, retention depends on other factors. Certain sensitive tumor cells appear to retain trimetrexate in concentrations that are in excess of that required to inhibit DHFR completely, after efflux in drug-free medium. The mechanism of this retention has not been determined. Another intriguing possibility currently under investigation is that some human tumors, either intrinsically or after treatment, may resemble the *Pneumocystis* organism in that they are unable to transport reduced folates and MTX well (5). Similar to the approach currently being taken to treat *Pneumocystis* infections, the coadministration of trimetrexate and LV would be nontoxic to the host, but could be cytotoxic to such tumors (7, 172, 175). Trimetrexate is also under investigation as a modulating agent. Based on experimental studies that showed that trimetrexate followed by 5-FUra and high-dose LV led to synergistic cell kill, when MTX followed by 5-FUra and LV did not, a phase I study of this construction has been completed. Acceptable toxicity and responses were noted even in this phase I investigation (50). Phase II studies are in progress.

INHIBITORS OF OTHER FOLATE ENZYMES

During recent years, other targets for the development of folate antagonists have been identified, including thymidylate synthase, GAR and AICAR transformylase, and methionine synthetase (6). Potent inhibitors of thymidylate synthase and GAR transformylase have been synthesized, and are now under active investigation (Fig. 60.4). The quinazoline inhibitors, IAHQ and CB3717, both showed antitumor activity in experimental systems, and CB3717 also demonstrated activity in phase II clinical trials in breast and ovarian cancer. Renal and hepatic toxicity precluded further testing (92, 137, 152).

Based on a series of structure–activity studies and toxicity studies in animals, another analogue, N-(5-[N-(3,4-dihydro-2-methyl-4-oxoquinazolin-6-ylmethyl)-N-methylamino]-2-thenoyl)-L-glutamic acid (D1694, Tomudex), was chosen for further clinical trials and has shown good clinical activity in colorectal carcinoma (145). Of interest is that these drugs, even more so than MTX, are "pro-drugs," in that polyglutamylation increases cytotoxicity. The potential advantages of folate inhibitors of thymidylate synthase over 5-FU are that these agents are not incorporated into RNA, and that the greater DUMP levels that may result as a consequence of inhibition of this enzyme might increase, rather than decrease, the inhibition of thymidylate synthase (92). Phase I studies have been completed, and phase II studies are in progress. Encouraging antitumor activity has been noted in patients with colon cancer.

5–10–Dideazatetrahydrofolate (dDTHF) (Lometrexol) is also undergoing clinical trials (Fig. 60.4). This compound is also a pro-drug; the addition of glutamates to the molecule markedly increases the inhibition of GAR transformylase (15). dDTHF is extremely potent, and low doses of this agent have produced delayed and prolonged marrow suppression in early clinical trials that was not predicted by rodent toxicity data (57). This may be due to its rapid accumulation by folate receptor positive cells—and to the relatively folate-deficient state of patients in contrast to that of rodent models. Administration of 1 to 5 mg of folic acid before Lometrexol has decreased toxicity (222).

The identification of these and other folate-mediated enzymes as targets for new folate inhibitors, and the demonstration of the antitumor properties of the compounds mentioned, has provided a new impetus for drug development in this field. This work undoubtedly will be guided by computer graphics using crystallographic data from the target enzymes (245).

References

1. Ackland SP, Schilsky RL. High dose methotrexate: a critical reappraisal. J Clin Oncol 1987;5:2017.
2. Acute Leukemia Group B. New treatment schedule with improved survival in childhood leukemia. Intermittent parenteral versus daily oral administration of methotrexate for maintenance of induced remission. JAMA 1965;194:75.
3. Adamson PC, Balis FM, McCully CL, et al. Rescue of experimental intrathecal methotrexate with carboxypeptidase G2. J Clin Oncol 1991;9:670–674.
4. Aherne GN, Prall E, Marks V, Mould G, White WF. Prolongation and enhancement of serum methotrexate concentrations by probenicid. Br Med J 1978;1:1097.
5. Alberto P, Peytremann R, Modenica R, Beretta-Piccoli M. Initial clinical experience with a simultaneous combination of 2-4-diamino 5 (3′,4′-dichlorophenyl)-6-methyl pyrimidine (DDMP) with folinic acid. Cancer Chemother Pharmacol 1978;1:101.
6. Allegra CJ. Antifolates. In Cancer Chemotherapy: Principles and Practice. Edited by BA Chabner, JM Collins. Philadelphia: Lippincott, 1990, p 110.
7. Allegra CJ, Chabner BA, Tuazon CU, Ogata-Araki D, Baird B, Drake JC, Simmons JT, Lack EE, Shelhamer JH, Balis F. Trimetrexate, a novel and effective agent for the treatment of *Pneumocystis carinii* pneumonia in patients with acquired immunodeficiency syndrome. N Engl J Med 1987;317:978.
8. Alt FW, Kellems RE, Bertino JR, Schimke RT. Selective multiplication of dihydrofolate reductase genes in methotrexate-resistant variants of cultured murine cells. J Biol Chem 1978;253:1357.
9. Amadori S, Tribalto M, Pacilli L, De Laurentis C, Papa G, Mandelli F. Sequential combination of methotrexate and L-asparaginase in the treatment of refractory acute leukemia. cancer treat rep 1980;64(8–9):939.
10. Armstrong RB, Poh-Fitzpatrick MB. Methotrexate and ultraviolet radiation. Arch Dermatol 1982;118:177.

11. Badr MZ, Theresa SC. Potentiation of methotrexate induced gastrointestinal toxicity by non-steroidal anti-inflammatory drugs (NSAIDS) and vincristine. Toxicology 1985;29:333.
12. Balinska M, Galivan J, Coward JK. Efflux of methotrexate and its polyglutamate derivatives from hepatic cells in vitro. Cancer Res 1981;41:2751.
13. Balis FM, Savitch JL, Bleyer WA. Pharmacokinetics of oral methotrexate in children. Cancer Res 1983;43:2342.
14. Baram J, Chabner BA, Drake JC, Fitzhugh AL, Sholar PW, Allegra CJ. Identification and biochemical properties of 10-formyl dihydrofolate, a novel folate found in methotrexate-treated cells. J Biol Chem 1988;263:7105.
15. Beardsley GP, Moroson B, Taylor EC, Moran RG. Deaza derivatives of tetrahydrofolic acid: a new class of folate antimetabolite. J Biol Chem 1989;264:328.
16. Beidler JL, Spengler B. A metaphase chromosome anomaly: association with drug resistance and cell-specific products. Science 1976;191:185.
17. Berd D, Cornog J, Deconti RC, Levitt M, Bertino Jr. Long term remission in diffuse histiocytic lymphoma treated with combination sequential chemotherapy. Cancer 1975;35:1050.
18. Bernini JC, Fort DW, Griener JC, Kane BJ, Chappell WB, Kamen BA. The use of aminophylline for methotrexate-induced neurotoxicity: evidence for adenosine receptor blockade. Lancet 1995.
19. Bertino Jr. "Rescue" techniques in cancer chemotherapy: use of leucovorin and other rescue agents after methotrexate treatment. Semin Oncol 1977;2:203.
20. Bertino Jr. Leucovorin rescue revisited (editorial). J Clin Oncol 1990;8:193–195.
21. Bertino Jr. The general pharmacology of methotrexate. In Methotrexate Therapy in rheumatic diseases. Edited by WS Wilke. New York: Dekker, 1989, p 11.
22. Bertino Jr. Karnofsky memorial lecture. "Ode to methotrexate". J Clin Oncol 1993;11:5.
23. Bertino Jr, Boothe BA, Cashmore A, Bieber AL, Sartorelli AC. Studies of the inhibition of dihydrofolate reductase by the folate antagonists. J Biol Chem 1964;239:479.
24. Bertino Jr, Sawicki WL, Cashmore AR, Cadman EC, Skeel RT. Natural resistance to methotrexate in human acute non-lymphocytic leukemia. Cancer Treat Rep 1977;61:667.
25. Bertino Jr, Sawicki WL, Lindquist CA, Gupta VS. Schedule dependent antitumor effects of methotrexate and 5-fluorouracil. Cancer Res 1977;37:327.
26. Blaney SM, Poplack DG, Godwin K, McCully CL, Murphy R, Balis FM. Effect of body position on ventricular csf methotrexate concentration following intralumbar administration. J Clin Oncol 1995;13:177–179.
27. Bleyer WA, Drake JC, Chabner BA. Neurotoxicity and elevated cerebrospinal fluid methotrexate concentration in meningeal leukemia. N Engl J Med 1973;289:770.
28. Bleyer WA, Poplack DG, Simon RM. "Concentration times time" methotrexate via a subcutaneous reservoir: a less toxic regimen for intraventricular chemotherapy of central nervous system neoplasms. Blood 1978;51:835.
29. Bokkerink JPM, Bakker MAH, Hulscher TW, de Abreu RA. Purine de novo synthesis as the basis of synergism of methotrexate and 6-mercaptopurine in human malignant lymphoblasts of different lineages. Biochem Pharmacol 1988;37:2321.
30. Bode U, Magrath IT, Bleyer UA, Poplack DG, Glaubiger DL. Active transport of methotrexate from cerebrospinal fluid in humans. Cancer Res 1980;40:2184.
31. Borsi JD, Moe PJ. Systemic clearance of methotrexate in the prognosis of acute lymphoblastic leukemia in children. Cancer 1987;60:3020.
32. Borsi JD, Sager E, Romelo I, Moe PJ. Rescue after intermediate and high-dose methotrexate. Pediatr Hematol Oncol 1990;7:347.
33. Browman GP, Levine MN, Goodyear MD, Russell R, Archibald SD, Jackson BS, Young Jem, Basrur V, Johanson C. Methotrexate-fluorouracil scheduling influences normal tissue toxicity but not antitumor effects in patients with squamous cell head and neck cancer: results from randomized trial. J Clin Oncol 1988;6:963.
34. Cadman E, Heimer R, Davis L. Enhanced 5-fluorouracil nucleotide formation after methotrexate administration. Explanation for drug synergism. Science 1979;205:1135.
35. Capizzi RL. Schedule-dependent synergism and antagonism between methotrexate and L-asparaginase. Biochem Pharmacol 1974;23:151.
36. Carman MD, Schornagel JH, Rivest RS, Srimatkandata S, Portlock CS, Duffy T, Bertino JR. Resistance to methotrexate due to gene amplification in a patient with acute leukemia. J Clin Oncol 1984;2:16.
37. Carson CW, Cannon GW, Egger JM, Ward JR, Clegg DO. Pulmonary disease during the treatment of rheumatoid arthritis with low-dose pulse methotrexate. Semin Arthritis Rheum 1987;16:186.
38. Casper ES, Christian KL, Schwartz GK, Johnson B, Brennan MF, Bertino JR. Edatrexate in patients with soft tissue sarcoma. Activity in malignant fibrous histiocytoma. Cancer 1993;72:766.
39. Chabner BA, Johns DG, Bertino JR. Enzymatic cleavage of methotrexate provides a method for prevention of drug toxicity. Nature 1972;239:395.
40. Chabner BA, Young RC. Threshold methotrexate concentration for in vivo inhibition of DNA synthesis in normal and tumorous target issues. J Clin Invest 1973;52:1804.
41. Chello PL, Sirotnak FM. Increased schedule dependent synergism of vindisine versus vincristine in combination with methotrexate against L1210 leukemia. Cancer Treat Rep 1981;65:1049.
42. Chello PL, Sirotnak FM, Dorick DM. Alterations in the kinetics of methotrexate transport during growth of L1210 murine leukemia cells in culture. Mol Pharmacol 1980;18:274.
43. Chu E, Takimoto CH, Voeller D, Grem JL, Allegra C. Specific binding of human dihydrofolate reductase protein to dihydrofolate reductase messenger RNA in vitro. Biochemistry 1993;32:4756.
44. Chungi VS, Bourne DWA, Dittert LW. Drug absorption: kinetics of GI absorption of methotrexate. J Pharm Sci 1978;67:560.
45. Cichowicz DJ, Shane B. Mammalian folylpoly-γ-glutamate synthetase: 1. Purification and general properties of the hog liver enzyme. Biochemistry 1987;26:504.
46. Cichowicz DJ, Shane B. Mammalian folyl-γ-glutamate synthetase: 2. Substrate specificity and kinetic properties of the hog liver enzyme. Biochemistry 1987;26:513.
47. Clarke L, Waxman DJ. Human liver folylpolyglutamate synthetase: biochemical characterization and interactions with folates and folate antagonists. Arch Biochem Biophys 1987;256:585.
48. Clarysse AM, Catney WJ, Cartwright GE, Wintrobe MM. Pulmonary disease complicating intermittent therapy with methotrexate. JAMA 1969;209:1861.
49. Clendeninn NJ, Drake JC, Allegra CJ, Welch AD, Chabner BA. Methotrexate (MTX) polyglutamates have a greater affinity and more rapid on-rate for purified human dihydrofolate reductase (DHFR) than MTX. Proc Am Assoc Cancer Res 1985;26:232.
50. Conti JA, Kemeny N, Göker E, Tong W, Colofiore J, Andre M, Ragusa K, Bertino JR. A phase I trial of sequential trimetrexate, fluorouracil and high dose leucovorin in previously treated patients with gastrointestinal carcinoma. J Clin Oncol 1994;12:695.
51. Cook JD, Cichowicz DJ, George S, Lawler A, Shane B. Mammalian folylpoly-γ-glutamate synthetase: 4. In vitro and in vivo metabolism of folates and analogues and regulation of folate homeostasis. Biochemistry 1987;26:530.
52. Condit PT, Chanes RE, Joel W. The renal toxicity of methotrexate. Cancer 1969;23:126.
53. Cowan KH, Goldsmith ME, Levine RM, Aitken SC, Douglass E, Clendenin N, Neinhuis AW, Lippman ME. Dihydrofolate reductase gene amplification and possible rearrangement in estrogen-responsive methotrexate-resistant human breast cancer cells. J Biol Chem 1982;257:15079.
54. Cowan KH, Jolivet J. A methotrexate-resistant human breast cancer cell line with multiple defects, including diminished formation of methotrexate polyglutamates. J Biol Chem 1984;259:10793.
55. Creaven PJ, Hansen HH, Alfred DA, Allen LM. Methotrexate in liver and bile after intravenous dosage in man. Br J Cancer 1973;28:589.
56. Cunningham D, Zalcberg J, Francois E. Tomudex (ZD1694), a new thymidylate synthase inhibitor with good antitumor activity in colorectal cancer. Proc Am Soc Clin Oncol 1994;13:199.
57. Currie VE, Warrell RP, Arlin Z, Tan C, Sirotnak FM, Greene G, Young CW. Phase I trial of 10-deaza-aminopterin in patients with advanced cancer. Cancer Treat Rep 1983;67:149.
58. Curt GA, Carney DN, Cowan KH, Jolivet J, Bailey BD, Drake JC, Chiensong RS, Minna JD, Chabner BA. Unstable methotrexate resistance in human small cell cancer associated with double minute chromosomes. N Engl J Med 1983;308:199.
59. Curt GA, Jolivet J, Bailey BD, Carney DN, Chabner BA. Synthesis and retention of methotrexate polyglutamates by human small cell lung cancer. Biochem Pharmacol 1984;33:1682.
60. Curt GA, Jolivet J, Carney DN, Bailey BD, Drake JC, Clendenin NJ, Chabner BA. Determinants of the sensitivity of human small-cell lung cancer cell lines to methotrexate. J Clin Invest 1985;76:1323.
61. Dahl MGC, Gregory MM, Scheuer PJ. Methotrexate hepatotoxicity in psoriasis—comparison of different dose regimens. Br Med J 1972;1:654.
62. Daly H, Boyle J, Roberts C, Scott G. Interaction between methotrexate and non-steroidal antiinflammatory drugs. Lancet 1986;1:8480.
63. Dedhar S, Freisheim JH, Hynes JB, Goldie JH. Further studies on substituted quinazolines and triazines as inhibitors of a methotrexate-insensitive murine dihydrofolate reductase. Biochem Pharmacol 1986;35:1143.
64. Dedhar S, Goldie JH. Overproduction of two antigenically distinct forms of dihydrofolate reductase in a highly methotrexate-resistant mouse leukemia cell line. Cancer Res 1983;43:4863.
65. Dedhar S, Hartley D, Fitz-Gibbons D, Phillips G, Goldie JH. Heterogeneity in the specific activity and methotrexate sensitivity of dihydrofolate reductase from blast cells of acute myelogenous leukemia patients. J Clin Oncol 1985;3:1545.
66. Dembo M, Sirotnak FM, Moccio DM. Effects of metabolic deprivation on methotrexate transport in L1210 cells: further evidence for separate influx and efflux systems with different energetic requirements. J Membr Biol 1984;78:9.
67. Dicker AP, Waltham MC, Volkenandt M, Schweitzer BI, Otter GM, Schmid FA, Sirotnak FM, Bertino JR. Methotrexate resistance in an in vivo mouse tumor due to a non-active site dihydrofolate reductase mutation. Proc Natl Acad Sci USA 1993;90:11797.
68. Dicker A, Volkenandt M, Adamo A, Barreda C, Bertino JR. Sequence analysis of a human gene responsible for drug resistance: a rapid method for manual and automated direct sequencing of products generated by the polymerase chain reaction. BioTechniques 1989;7:830.
69. Dixon KH, Lanpher BC, Chiu J, Kelley K, Cowan KH. A novel cDNA restores reduced folate carrier activity and methotrexate sensitivity to transport deficient cells. J Biol Chem 1994;269:17–20.
70. Djerassi I. Removal of methotrexate by filtration absorption using charcoal filters or by hemodialysis. Cancer Treat Rep 1977;61:751.
71. Domin BA, Cheng Y, Hakala MT. Properties of dihydrofolate reductase from a methotrexate-resistant subline of human KB cells and comparison with enzyme from KB parent cells and mouse S180 AT/3000 cells. Mol Pharmacol 1982;21:231.
72. Donehower RC, Allegra JC, Lippman ME, Chabner BA. Combined effects of methotrexate and 5-fluoropyrimidine on human breast cancer cells in serum-free cultures. Eur J Cancer 1980;16:655.
73. Donehower RC, Hande KR, Drake JC, Chabner BA. Presence of 2,4-diamino-N10-methyl pteroic acid after high-dose methotrexate. Clin Pharmacol Ther 1979;26:63.
74. Doyle LA, Berg C, Bottino G, Chabner BA. Erythema and desquamation after high-dose methotrexate. Ann Intern Med 1983;98:611.
75. Eastern Cooperative Group in Solid Tumor Chemotherapy. Comparison of antimetabolites in the treatment of breast and colon cancer. JAMA 1967;200:770–778.
76. Edelstein M, Vietti T, Valeriote F. The enhanced cytotoxicity of 1 β-D-arabinosylcytosine and methotrexate. Cancer Res 1975;35:1555.
77. Eilber F, Guliano A, Eckart J, Patterson K, Mosely S, Goodnight J. Adjuvant chemotherapy for osteosarcoma: a randomized prospective trial. J Clin Oncol 1987;5:21.
78. Ensminger WD, Frei E III. The prevention of methotrexate toxicity by thymidine infusions in humans. Cancer Res 1977;37:1857.
79. Erttman R, Bielack S, Landbeck G. Kinetics of 7-hydroxy-methotrexate after high-dose methotrexate therapy. Cancer Chemother Pharmacol 1985;15:101.
80. Erttman R, Landbeck G. Effect of oral cholestyramine on the elimination of high-dose methotrexate. J Cancer Res Clin Oncol 1985;110:48.
81. Ettinger LJ, Chervinsky DS, Freeman A, Creaven PJ. Pharmacokinetics of methotrexate following intravenous and intraventricular administration in acute lymphocytic leukemia and non-Hodgkin's lymphoma. Cancer 1982;50:1676.
82. Evans WE, Crom WR, Abromowitch M, Dodge R, Look AT, Bowman WP, George SL, Pui CH. Clinical pharmacodynamics of high-dose methotrexate in acute lymphocytic leukemia: identification of a relation between concentration and effect. N Engl J Med 1986;314:471.
83. Ercikan E, Banerjee D, Waltham M, Schnieders B, Scotto KW, Bertino JR. Transla-

tional regulation of the synthesis of dihydrofolate reductase. In Chemistry and Biology of Pteridines and Folates. Edited by JE Ayling, MG Nair, CM Baugh. New York: Plenum, 1993, p 537.
84. Evans WE, Hutson PR, Stewart CF, Cairnes DA, Bowman WP, Rivera G, Crom WR. Methotrexate cerebrospinal fluid and serum concentrations after intermediate dose methotrexate infusion. Clin Pharmacol Ther 1983;33:301.
85. Evans WE, Pratt CB, Taylor H, Barker LF, Crom WR. Pharmacokinetic monitoring of high-dose methotrexate. Cancer Chemother Pharmacol 1979;3:161.
86. Fabre I, Fabre G, Goldman ID. Polyglutamylation, an important element in methotrexate cytotoxicity and selectivity in tumor versus murine granulocytic progenitor cells in vitro. Cancer Res 1984;44:3190.
87. Fabre G, Fabre I, Matherly LH, Cano JP, Goldman ID. Synthesis and properties of 7-hydroxymethotrexate polyglutamyl derivatives in Ehrlich ascites tumor cells in vitro. J Biol Chem 1984;259:5066.
88. Fabre G, Seither R, Goldman ID. Hydroxylation of 4-amino-antifolates by partially purified aldehyde oxidase from rabbit liver. Biochem Pharmacol 1986;35:1325.
89. Farber S, Diamond LK, Mercer RD, Sylvester RF Jr, Wolff JA. Temporary remissions in acute leukemia in children produced by folic acid antagonist, 4-aminopteroyl-glutamic acid (aminopterin). N Engl J Med 1948;238:787.
90. Favre R, Monjanel S, Alfonsi M, Pradora JP, Bagarry-Liegey D, Clement S, Imbert AM, Lena N, Colonida d'Istria J, Cano JP, Carcassonne Y. High-dose methotrexate: a clinical and pharmacokinetic evaluation. Chemother Pharmacol 1982;9:156.
91. Fernandes DJ, Bertino JR, Hynes JB. Biochemical and antitumor effects of 5,8-dideazaisopteroylglutamate, a unique quinazoline inhibitor of thymidylate synthetase. Cancer Res 1983;43:1117.
92. Fernandes DJ, Sur P, Kute TE, Capizzi RL. Proliferation-dependent cytotoxicity of methotrexate in murine L5178Y leukemia. Cancer Res 1988;48:5638.
93. Fernandez DJ, Bertino JR. 5-fluorouracil-methotrexate synergy. Enhancement of 5-fluorodeoxyuridylate binding to thymidylate synthase by dihydropteroylpolyglutamates. Proc Natl Acad Sci USA 1980;77:5663.
94. Fischer GA. Increased levels of folic acid reductase as a mechanism of resistance to amethopterin in leukemic cells. Biochem Pharmacol 1961;7:75.
95. Fischer GA. Defective transport of amethopterin (methotrexate) as a mechanism of resistance to the antimetabolite in L5178Y leukemic cells. Biochem Pharmacol 1962;11:1233.
96. Fisher B, Redmond C, Dimitrov NU, Bowman D, Legault-Poisson S, Wickerham DL, Wolmack N, Fisher ER, Margolese R, Sutherland C, Glass A, Foster R, Caplan R. A randomized clinical trial evaluating sequential methotrexate and fluorouracil in the treatment of patients with node negative breast cancer who have estrogen receptor tumors. N Engl J Med 1969;320:473.
97. Flasshove M, Banerjee D Mineishi S, Schlafstein M, Bertino JR, Moore MAS. Retrovirally mediated gene transfer of a mutant dihydrofolate reductase gene into progenitors from human blood. Blood 1993;82:301a.
98. Flintoff WF, Essani K. Methotrexate-resistant Chinese hamster ovary cells contain a dihydrofolate reductase with an altered affinity for methotrexate. Biochemistry 1980;19:4321.
99. Fondevila CG, Milone GA, Pavlovsky S. Cutaneous vasculitis after intermediate dose of methotrexate (IDMTX). Br J Haematol 1989;72:591–592.
100. Frankel LS, Wang YM, Shuster J, Nitschke R, Doering EJ, Pullen J. High dose methotrexate as part of remission maintenance therapy for childhood acute lymphocytic leukemia: a pediatric oncology group pilot study. J Clin Oncol 1983;1:804.
101. Freeman-Narrod M, Narrod SA, Custer RP. Chronic toxicity of methotrexate in rats: partial to complete protection of the liver by choline: brief communication. JNCI 1977;59:1013.
102. Frei E III, Blum RH, Pitman SW, Kirkwood JM, Henderson IC, Skarin AT, Mayer RJ, Bast RC, Garnick MB, Parker LM, Canellos GP. High dose methotrexate with leucovorin rescue. Rationale and spectrum of antitumor activity. Am J Med 1980;68:370.
103. Fridland A. Effect of methotrexate on deoxynucleotide pools and DNA synthesis in human lymphocyte cells. Cancer Res 1974;34:1883.
104. Fritsch G, Urban C. Transient encephalopathy during the late course of treatment with high-dose methotrexate. Cancer 1984;53:1849.
105. Fry DW, Anderson LA, Borst M, Goldman ID. Analysis of the role of membrane transport and polyglutamation of methotrexate in gut and Ehrlich tumor in vivo as factors in drug sensitivity and selectivity. Cancer Res 1983;43:1087.
106. Fry DW, Yalowich JC, Goldman ID. Augmentation of the intracellular levels of polyglutamyl derivatives of methotrexate by vincristine and probenecid in Ehrlich ascites tumor cells. Cancer Res 1982;42:25323.
107. Fry DW, Yalowich JC, Goldman ID. Rapid formation of poly-γ-glutamyl derivatives of methotrexate and their association with dihydrofolate reductase as assessed by high-pressure liquid chromatography in Ehrlich ascites tumor cell in vitro. J Biol Chem 1982;259:257.
108. Fyfe MJ, Goldman ID. Characteristics of the vincristine-induced augmentation of methotrexate uptake in Ehrlich ascites tumor cells. J Biol Chem 1973;248:5067.
109. Garrow TA, Admon A, Shane B. Expression cloning of a human cDNA encoding folylpoly(μ-glutamate) synthetase and determination of its primary structure. Proc Natl Acad Sci USA 1992;89:9151–9155.
110. Ginsberg S, Anderson J, Bloomfield C, Norton L, Barcos M, Gottlieb AJ, Holland J. Therapy of advanced intermediate grade lymphoma with cyclophosphamide, Adriamycin, vincristine and prednisone with or without bleomycin CCAVPB vs CAVP followed by high dose methotrexate or standard dose methotrexate. A randomized trial. Proc Am Soc Clin Oncol 1985;4:202.
111. Göker E, Kheradpour A, Trippett T, Waltham M, Elisseyeff Y, Schnieders B, Bertino JR. Dihydrofolate reductase gene amplification in acute lymphoblastic leukemia is associated with mutations in the p53 gene. Blood 1993;82:38a.
112. Goldberg NH, Romolo JL, Austin EH, Drake J, Rosenberg SA. Anaphylactoid type reactions in two patients receiving high-dose intravenous methotrexate. Cancer 1978;41:52.
113. Goldie JH, Dedhar S, Krystal G. Properties of a methotrexate-insensitive variant of dihydrofolate reductase from methotrexate-resistant L5178Y cells. J Biol Chem 1981;256:11629.
114. Goldie JH, Krystal G, Hartley D, Gudauskas G, Dedhar S. A methotrexate-insensitive variant of folate reductase present in two lines of methotrexate-resistant L5178Y cells. Eur J Cancer 1980;16:1539.
115. Hande KR, Balow DE, Drake JC, Rosenberg SA, Chabner BA. Methotrexate and hemodialysis. Ann Intern Med 1977;87:495.
116. Heinle RW, Welch AD. Experiments with pteroylglutamic acid and pteroylglutamic acid deficiency in human leukemia. J Clin Invest 1948;27:539.
117. Hendel J, Brodthagen H. Entero-hepatic cycling of methotrexate estimated by use of the D-isomer as a reference marker. Eur J Clin Pharmacol 1984;26:103.
118. Henderson ES, Adamson RH, Oliverio VT. The metabolic fate of tritiated methotrexate: 2. Absorption and excretion in man. Cancer Res 1965;25:1018.
119. Henderson GB, Tsuji JM. Methotrexate efflux in L1210 cells: kinetic and specificity properties of the efflux system sensitive to bromosulfophtalein and its possible identity with a system which mediates the efflux of 3′,5′-cyclic AMP. J Biol Chem 1987;262:13571.
120. Henderson GB, Tsuji JM, Kumar HP. Characterization of the individual transport routes that mediate the influx and efflux of methotrexate in CCRF-CEM human lymphoblastic cells. Cancer Res 1986;46:1633.
121. Henderson GB, Tsuji JM, Kumar HP. Transport of folate compounds by leukemic cells: evidence for a single influx carrier for methotrexate, 5-methyltetrahydrofolate, and folate in CCRF-CEM human lymphoblasts. Biochem Pharmacol 1987;36:3007.
122. Hertz R, Lewis J Jr, Lipsett MB. Five years experience with the chemotherapy of metastatic choriocarcinoma and related trophoblastic tumors in women. Am J Obstet Gynecol 1961;82:631.
123. Hill BT, Price LA. dDMP (2,4-diamino-5-(3′,4′-dichlorophenyl)-methylpyrimidine. Cancer Treat Rev 1980;7:95.
124. Hitchings GH, Burchall JJ, Ferone R. The comparative enzymology of dihydrofolate reductase and the design of chemotherapeutic agents. 16th Symposium of the Society of General Microbiology, 1966, p 294.
125. Horns RC Jr, Dower WJ, Schimke RT. Gene amplification in a leukemic patient treated with methotrexate. J Clin Oncol 1984;2:2.
126. Howell SB, Ensminger WD, Krishan A, Frei E III. Thymidine rescue of high-dose methotrexate in humans. Cancer Res 1978;38:325.
127. Hryniuk WM. Purineless death as a link between growth rate and cytotoxicity of methotrexate. Cancer Res 1972;32:1506.
128. Hryniuk WM, Bertino JR. Treatment of leukemia with large doses of methotrexate and folinic acid: clinical-biochemical correlates. J Clin Invest 1969;48:2140.
129. Hryniuk WM, Fischer GA, Bertino JR. S-phase cells of rapidly growing and resting populations. Differences in response to methotrexate. Mol Pharmacol 1969;5:557.
130. Huang KC, Wenczak BA, Liu YK. Renal tubular transport of methotrexate in the rhesus monkey and dog. Cancer Res 1979;39:4843.
131. Hudson MM, Dahl GU, Kalminsky DK, Pui CH. Methotrexate plus asparaginase. An active combination for children with acute non-lymphocytic leukemia. Cancer 1990;65:2615.
132. Huffman DH, Wan SH, Azaranoff DL, Hogstraten B. Pharmacokinetics of methotrexate. Clin Pharmacol Ther 1973;14:572.
133. Isacoff WH, Morrison PF, Aroessty J, Willis KL, Block JB, Lincoln TL. Pharmacokinetics of high-dose methotrexate with citrovorum factor rescue. Cancer Treat Rep 1977;61:1665.
134. Isola LM, Gordon JW. Systemic resistance to methotrexate in transgenic mice carrying a mutant dihydrofolate reductase gene. Proc Natl Acad Sci USA 1986;83:9621.
135. Iven H, Brasch H. Influence of the antibiotics piperacillin deoxycycline and tobramycin on the pharmacokinetics of methotrexate in rabbits. Cancer Chemother Pharmacol 1986;17:218.
136. Iven H, Brasch H. The effects of antibiotics and uricosuric drugs on the renal elimination of methotrexate and 7-hydroxymethotrexate in rabbits. Cancer Chemother Pharmacol 1988;21:337.
137. Jackman AL, Jones TR, Calvert AH. Thymidylate synthetase inhibitors: experimental and clinical aspects. In Experimental and Clinical Progress in Cancer Chemotherapy. Edited by F Muggia. Boston: Martinus Nijhoff, 1985, p 155.
138. Jackson RC, Hart LI, Harrap KR. Intrinsic resistance to methotrexate of cultured mammalian cells in relation to the inhibition kinetics of their dihydrofolate reductase. Cancer Res 1980;36:1991.
139. Jacobs SA, Derr CJ, Johns DG. Accumulation of methotrexate diglutamate in human liver during methotrexate therapy. Biochem Pharmacol 1977;26:2310.
140. Jacobs SA, Stoller RG, Chabner BA, Johns DG. 7-Hydroxymethotrexate as a urinary metabolite in human subjects and rhesus monkeys receiving high dose methotrexate. J Clin Invest 1976;57:534.
141. Jaffe N, Frei E III, Traggis D, Bishop Y. Adjuvant methotrexate and citrovorum-factor treatment of osteogenic sarcoma. N Engl J Med 1974;291:994.
142. Jaffe N, Paed D. Recent advances in the chemotherapy of metastatic osteogenic sarcoma. Cancer 1972;30:1627.
143. Jaffe N, Takaue Y, Anzai T. Transient neurologic disturbances induced by high-dose methotrexate treatment. Cancer 1985;56:1356.
144. James SJ, Basnakian AG, Miller BJ. In vitro folate deficiency induces deoxynucleotide pool imbalance, apoptosis, and mutagenesis in Chinese hamster ovary cells. Cancer Res 1994;54:5075–5080.
145. Jodrell DI, Newell DR, Calvete JA, Stephens TC, Calvert AH. Pharmacokinetic and toxicity studies with the novel quinazoline inhibitor, D 1694. Proc Am Assoc Cancer Res 1990;31:341.
146. Johns DG, Iannotti AT, Sartorelli AC, Booth BA, Bertino JR. The identity of rabbit-liver methotrexate oxidase. Biochim Biophys Acta 1965;105:380.
147. Johns DG, Loo TL. The metabolite of 4-amino-4-deoxy-N10-methylpteroylglutamic acid (methotrexate). J Pharm Sci 1967;56:356.
148. Jolivet J, Chabner BA. Intracellular pharmacokinetics of methotrexate polyglutamates in human breast cancer cells: selective retention and less dissociable binding of 4-NH2-10-CH3-pteroylglutamate 4 and 4-NH2-10-CH3-pteroyl-glutamate 5 to dihydrofolate reductase. J Clin Invest 1983;72:773.
149. Jolivet J, Cole DE, Holcenberg JS, Poplack DG. Prevention of methotrexate cytotoxicity by asparaginase inhibition of methotrexate polyglutamate formation. Cancer Res 1985;45:217.
150. Olivet J, Faucher F, Pinard MF. Influence of intracellular folates on methotrexate metabolism and cytotoxicity. Biochem Pharmacol 1987;36(19):3310–3312.
151. Jolivet J, Schilsky RL, Bailey BD, Drake JC, Chabner BA. Synthesis, retention, and biological activity of methotrexate polyglutamates in cultured human breast cancer cells. J Clin Invest 1982;70:351.

152. Jones TR, Calvert AH, Jackman AL, Brown SJ, Jones M, Harrap KR. A potent antitumor quinazoline inhibitor of thymidylate synthetase: synthesis, biological properties and therapeutic results in mice. Eur J Cancer 1981;17:11.
153. Kamen BA, Capdevila A. Receptor-mediated folate accumulation regulated by the cellular folate content. Proc Natl Acad Sci USA 1986;83:5983.
154. Kamen BA, Eibl B, Cashmore A, Bertino JR. Uptake and efficacy of trimetrexate (TMQ, 2,4-diamino-5-methyl-6-[3,4,5-trimethoxy-anilino-methyl] quinazoline), a nonclassical antifolate in methotrexate-resistant leukemia cells in vitro. Biochem Pharmacol 1984;33:1697.
155. Kamen BA, Whyte-Bauer W, Bertino JR. A mechanism of resistance to methotrexate: NADPH but not NADH stimulation of methotrexate binding to dihydrofolate reductase. Biochem Pharmacol 1983;32:1837.
156. Kamen BA, Vietti T. Letter to the editor. Br J Cancer 1989;60:799.
157. Kano Y, Ohnuma T, Holland JF. Folate requirements of methotrexate-resistant human acute lymphoblastic leukemia cell lines. Blood 1986;68:586.
158. Kaufman RJ, Bertino JR, Schimke RT. Quantitation of dihydrofolate reductase in individual parental and methotrexate-resistant murine cells: use of a fluorescence activated cell sorter. J Biol Chem 1978;253:5852.
159. Kaufman RJ, Brown PC, Schimke RT. Loss and stabilization of amplified dihydrofolate reductase genes in mouse sarcoma S-180 cell lines. Mol Cell Biol 1981;1:1084.
160. Kaufman RJ, Schimke RT. Amplification and loss of dihydrofolate reductase genes in a Chinese hamster ovary cell line. Mol Cell Biol 1981;1:1069.
161. Kearney PJ, Light PA, Preece A, Mott MG. Unpredictable serum levels after oral methotrexate in children with acute lymphoblastic leukemia. Cancer Chemother Pharmacol 1979;3:117.
162. Kennedy DG, Van den Berg HW, Clark R, Murphy RF. The effect of the rate of cell proliferation on the synthesis of methotrexate poly-gamma-glutamates in two human breast cancer cell lines. Biochem Pharmacol 1985;34:3087.
163. Kennedy DG, van den Berg HW, Clarke R, Murphy RF. The effect of leucovorin on the synthesis of methotrexate poly-gamma-glutamates in the MCF-7 human breast cancer cell line. Biochem Pharmacol 1985;34:2897.
164. Kerr IG, Jolivet J, Collins JM, Drake JC, Chabner BA. Test dose for predicting high-dose methotrexate infusions. Clin Pharmacol Ther 1983;33:44.
165. Kessell D, Hall TC, Roberts D, Wodinsky I. Uptake as a determinant of methotrexate response in mouse leukemia. Science 1965;150:752.
166. Koizumi S, Curt GA, Fine RL, Griffin JD, Chabner BA. Formation of methotrexate polyglutamates in purified myeloid precursor cells from normal human bone marrow. J Clin Invest 1985;75:1008.
167. Kristenson L, Weismann K, Hutters L. Renal function and the rate of disappearance of methotrexate from serum. Eur J Clin Pharmacol 1975;8:439.
168. Kumar P, Kisliuk RL, Gaumont Y, Nair MG, Baugh CM, Kaufman BT. Interaction of polyglutamyl derivatives of methotrexate, 10-deazaaminopterin, and dihydrofolate with dihydrofolate reductase. Cancer Res 1986;46:5020.
169. Kyriazis AP, Yagod A, Kyriazis A. A schedule dependency of the combination methotrexate-vinblastine against human urothelial cancer grown in nude mice. Anticancer Res 1989;9:1857.
170. Lankelma J, van der Klein E. The role of 7-hydroxy methotrexate during methotrexate anticancer chemotherapy. Cancer Lett 1980;9:133.
171. Levitt M, Mosher MB, DeConti RC, Farber LR, Skeel RT, Marsh JC, Mitchell MS, Papac RJ, Thomas ED, Bertino JR. Improved therapeutic index of methotrexate with "leucovorin rescue." Cancer Res 1973;33:1729.
172. Li WW, Lin JT, Tong WP, Trippett TM, Brennan MF, Bertino JR. Mechanisms of natural resistance to antifolates in human soft tissue sarcomas. Cancer Res 1992;52:1434.
173. Li WW, Waltham M, Tong W, Schweitzer BI, Bertino JR. Increased activity of γ-glutamyl hydrolase in human sarcoma cell lines: a novel mechanism of intrinsic resistance to methotrexate. In Chemistry and Biology of Pteridines and Folates. Edited by JE Ayling, MG Nair, CM Baugh. New York: Plenum, 1993, p 635.
174. Liegler DG, Henderson ES, Hahn MA, Oliverio VT. The effect of organic acids on renal clearance of methotrexate in man. Clin Pharmacol Ther 1969;10:849.
175. Lin JT, Bertino JR. Update on trimetrexate, a folate antagonist with antineoplastic and antiprotozoal properties. Cancer Invest (in press).
176. Lin JT, Tong WP, Trippett TN, Niedzwieki D, Tao Y, Tan C, Steinherz P, Schweitzer B, Bertino JR. Basis for natural resistance to methotrexate in human acute non-lymphocytic leukemia. Leuk Res 1991;15:1191.
177. Link MP, Goorin AM, Miser AW, Green AA, Pratt CB, Belasco JB, Pritchard J, Malpas JS, Baker AR, Kirkpatrick JA, Ayala AG, Schuster JJ, Abelson HT, Simione JV, Vietti TJ. The effect of adjuvant chemotherapy on relapse-free survival in patients with osteosarcoma of the extremity. N Engl J Med 1986;314:1600.
178. Lobel JS, O'Brien RT, McIntosh S, Aspnes GT, Capizzi RL. Methotrexate and asparaginase combination chemotherapy in refractory acute lymphoblastic leukemia of childhood. Cancer 1979;43:1089.
179. Mackenzie AH. Adverse hepatic effects of methotrexate therapy. In Methotrexate Therapy in Rheumatic Disease. Edited by WS Wilke. New York: Dekker, 1989, p 179.
180. Maricic M, Davis M, Gall EP. Megaloblastic pancytopoenia in a patient receiving concurrent methotrexate and trimethoprim-sulfamethoxazole treatment. Arthritis Rheum 1986;26:133.
181. Marsh JC, Bertino JR, Katz KH, Davis CA, Durivage HJ, Rome LS, Richards F II, Capizzi RL, Farber LR, Pasquale DN, Stuart R, Koletsky AJ, Makuch R, O'Hollaren K. The influence of drug interval on the effect of methotrexate and fluorouracil in the treatment of advanced colorectal cancer. J Clin Oncol 1991;9:371–380.
182. Matherly LH, Barlowe CK, Goldman ID. Antifolate polyglutamylation and competitive drug displacement of dihydrofolate reductase as important elements of leucovorin rescue in L1210 cells. Cancer Res 1986;46:588.
183. Matthews DA, Alden RA, Bolin JT, Freer ST, Hamlin R, Xuong N, Kracut J, Poe M, Williams M, Hoogsteen K. Dihydrofolate reductase X-ray structure of the binary complex with methotrexate. Science 1977;197:452.
184. Matthews DA, Bolin JT, Burridge JM, Filman DJ, Volz KM, Kaufman BT, Beddell CE, Champness JN, Stammers DK, Kraut JK. Refined crystal structures of *E. coli* and chicken liver dihydrofolate reductase containing bound trimethoprim. J Biol Chem 1985;260:381.
185. Matthews DA, Bolin JT, Burridge JM, Filman DJ, Volz KM, Kraut J. Dihydrofolate reductase. The stereochemistry of inhibitor selectivity. J Biol Chem 1985;260:392.
186. McAnena OJ, Ridge JA, Daly JM. Alteration of methotrexate metabolism in rats by administration of an elemental liquid diet: II. Reduced toxicity and improved survival using cholestyramine. Cancer 1987;59:1091.
187. McCloskey DE, McGuire JJ, Russell CA, Ronan BG, Bertino JR, Pizzorno G, Mini E. Decreased folylpolyglutamate synthetase activity as a mechanism of methotrexate resistance in CCRF-CEM human leukemia sublines. J Biol Chem 1991;266:6181.
188. McCullough JL, Chabner BA, Bertino JR. Purification and properties of carboxypeptidase G1. J Biol Chem 1971;246:7203.
189. McGuire JJ, Hsieh P, Bertino JR. Enzymatic synthesis of polyglutamate derivatives of 7-hydroxymethotrexate. Biochem Pharmacol 1984;33:1355.
190. McGuire JJ, Hsieh P, Coward JK, Bertino JR. Enzymatic synthesis of folylpolyglutamates. J Biol Chem 1980;255:5776.
191. Mead JAR. Rational design of folic acid antagonists. In Antineoplastic and Immunosuppressive Agents I. Edited by AC Sartorelli, DG Johns. New York: Springer-Verlag, 1974, p 52.
192. Mead JAR, Wood HB Jr, Goldin A. Relationship of structure to antitumor activity in compounds related to folic acid. Cancer Chemother Rep (Part 2) 1968;1:273.
193. Mead JR, Venditti JM, Schrecker AW, Goldin A, Keresztesy JC. The effect of reduced derivatives of folic acid on toxicity and antileukemic effect of methotrexate in mice. Biochem Pharmacol 1963;12:371.
194. Mehta BM, Glass JP, Shapiro WR. Serum and cerebrospinal fluid distribution of 5-methyltetrahydrofolate after intravenous calcium leucovorin and intra Ommaya methotrexate administration in patients with meningeal carcinomatosis. Cancer Res 1983;43:435.
195. Melera PW, Davide JP, Hession CA, Scotto KW. Phenotypic expression in *E. coli* and nucleotide sequence of two Chinese hamster lung cell cDNAs encoding different dihydrofolate. Mol Cell Biol 1984;4:38.
196. Melera PW, Davide JP, Oen H. Antifolate-resistant Chinese hamster cells: molecular basis for the biochemical and structural heterogeneity among DHFRs produced by drug-sensitive and drug-resistant cell lines. J Biol Chem 1987;262:1978.
197. Mini E, Bertino JR. Biochemical modulation of 5-fluorouracil by metabolites and antimetabolites. In Synergism and Antagonism in Chemotherapy. Edited by TC Chou, D Rideout. San Diego: Academic, 1991, p 449.
198. Mini E, Moroson BA, Franco CT, Bertino JR. Cytotoxic effects of folate antagonists against methotrexate-resistant human leukemic lymphoblast CCRF-CEM cell lines. Cancer Res 1985;45:325.
199. Monjanel S, Rigault JP, Cano JP, Carcassone Y, Favre R. High-dose methotrexate: preliminary evaluation of a pharmacokinetic approach. Cancer Chemother Pharmacol 1979;3:189.
200. Moran RG, Baldwin SW, Taylor EC, Shih C. The 6S- and 6R-diastereomers of 5,10-dideza-5,6,7,8-tetrahydrofolate are equiactive inhibitors of de novo purine synthesis. J Biol Chem 1989;264:21047.
201. Moran RG, Colman PD. Mammalian folylpolyglutamate synthetase. Partial purification and properties of the mouse liver enzyme. Biochemistry 1985;23:4580.
202. Morrison JF. The slow-binding and slow, tight-binding inhibition of enzyme-catalysed reactions. Trends Biochem Sci 1982;7:102.
203. Neiman RA, Fye KH. Methotrexate induced false photosensitivity reaction. J Rheumatol 1985;12.
204. Nesbit M. Acute and chronic effects of methotrexate on hepatic, pulmonary and skeletal systems. Cancer 1976;37:1048.
205. Newland FS. VP-16 in combinations for first-line treatment of malignant germ-cell tumors and gestational choriocarcinoma. Semin Oncol 1985;12:37.
206. Nichol CA, Cavallito JC, Woolley JL, Sigel CW. Lipid-soluble diaminopyrimidine inhibitors of dihydrofolate reductase. Cancer Treat Rep 1976.
207. Nichol CA, Welch AD. Metabolic requirements for formation of citrovorum factor and studies of mechanism of resistance to amethopterin. In Antimetabolites and Cancer. Edited by CP Rhoads. Washington: American Association for the Advancement of Science, 1955, p 63.
208. Nirenberg A, Mosende C, Mehta B, Gisolfi AL, Rosen G. High-dose methotrexate with citrovorum factor rescue: predictive value of serum methotrexate concentrations and corrective measures to avert toxicity. Cancer Treat Rep 1977;61:779.
209. Nixon PF, Bertino JR. Effective absorption and utilization of oral formyltetrahydrofolate in man. N Engl J Med 1972;286:175.
210. Nixon PF, Slutsky G, Nahas A, Bertino JR. The turnover of folate coenzymes in murine lymphoma cells. J Biol Chem 1973;248:5932.
211. Nordic Gastrointestinal Group. Superiority of sequential methotrexate, fluorouracil and leucovorin to fluorouracil alone in advanced symptomatic colorectal carcinoma: a randomized trial. J Clin Oncol 1989;7:1437.
212. Nuernberg B, Koehuke R, Solsky M, Hoffman J, Furst DE. Biliary elimination of low-dose methotrexate in humans. Arthritis Rheum 1990;33:898–902.
213. O'Dwyer PJ, Showmaker DD, Plowman J, Cradock J, Grillo-Lopez A, Leyland-Jones B. Trimetrexate. A new antifol entering clinical trials. Invest New Drugs 1985;3:71.
214. Ohnoshi T, Ohnuma T, Takahashi I, Scanlon K, Kamen BA, Holland JF. Establishment of methotrexate-resistant human acute lymphoblastic leukemia cells in culture and effects of folate antagonists. Cancer Res 1982;42:1655.
215. Oliverio VT. Chromatographic separation and purification of folic acid analogs. Anal Chem 1961;33:263.
216. Osborne MJ, Freeman M, Huennekens FM. Inhibition of dihydrofolic reductase by aminopterin and amethopterin. Proc Soc Exp Biol Med 1958;97:429.
217. Peylan-Ramu N, Poplack DG, Blei CL, Herdt JR, Vermess M, DiChiro G. Computer-assisted tomography in methotrexate encephalopathy. J Comput Assist Tomogr 1977;1:216.
218. Pinedo HM, Zaharko DS, Bull JM, Chabner BA. The reversal of methotrexate cytotoxicity to mouse bone marrow cells by leucovorin and nucleosides. Cancer Res 1976;36:4418–4424.
219. Pinedo HM, Zaharko DS, Bull JM, Chabner BA. The relative contribution of drug concentration and duration of exposure to mouse bone marrow toxicity during continuous methotrexate infusion. Cancer Res 1977;37:445.
220. Pitman S, Landwehr D, Jaffe N, Frei E III. Methotrexate citrovorum (MTX-CF): Effect of alkalinization on nephrotoxicity and of weekly schedule on response. Proc Am Soc Cancer Res 1976;17:129.
221. Pitman SW, Parker LM, Tattersall MHN, Jaffe N, Frei E III. Clinical trial of high-dose methotrexate (NSC-740) with citrovorum factor (NSC-3590)—toxicologic and therapeutic observations. Cancer Chemother Rep 1975;6:43.
222. Pizzorno G, Cashmore AR, Moroson BA, Cross AD, Smith AK, Marling-Cason M,

Kamen BA, Beardsley GP. 5,10-Dideazatetrahydrofolic acid (DDATHF) transport in CCRF-CEM and MA104 cell lines. J Biol Chem 1993;268:1017–1023.
223. Pizzorno G, Mini E, Coronnello M, McGuire JJ, Moroson BA, Cashmore AR, Dreyer RN, Lin JT, Mazzei T, Periti P. Impaired polyglutamylation of methotrexate as a cause of resistance in CCRF-CEM cells after short term, high-dose treatment with this drug. Cancer Res 1988;48:2149.
224. Prasad PD, Mahesh VB, Leibach FH, Ganapathy V. Functional coupling between a bafilomycin A_1-sensitive proton pump and a probenecid-sensitive folate transporter in human placental choriocarcinoma cells. Biochim Biophys Acta 1994;1222: 309–314.
225. Price EM, Smith PL, Klein TE. Photoaffinity analogues of methotrexate as folate antagonist binding probes: 1. Photoaffinity labeling of murine L1210 dihydrofolate reductase and amino acid sequence of the binding region. Biochemistry 1987;26:4751.
226. Redetzki HM, Redetzki JE, Elias AL. Resistance of the rabbit to methotrexate: isolation of a drug metabolite with decreased cytotoxicity. Biochem Pharmacol 1966;15: 425.
227. Rhee MS, Galivan J. Conversion of methotrexate to 7-hydroxymethotrexate polyglutamates in cultured rat hepatic cells. Cancer Res 1986;46:3793.
228. Rhee MS, Wang Y, Nair GM, Galivan J. Acquisition of resistance to antifolates caused by enhanced γ-glutamyl hydrolase activity. Cancer Res 1993;53:2227.
229. Rice GC, Ling V, Schimke RT. Frequencies of independent and simultaneous selection of Chinese hamster cells for methotrexate and doxorubicin (Adriamycin) resistance. Proc Natl Acad Sci USA 1987;84:9261.
230. Rizzoli V, Mangoni L, Caramatti C, Degliantoni G, Costi D. High-dose methotrexate-leucovorin rescue therapy: selected application in non-Hodgkin's lymphoma. Tumori 1985;71:155.
231. Rodenhuis S, McGuire JJ, Narayanan R, Bertino JR. Development of an assay system for the detection and classification of methotrexate resistance in fresh human leukemic cells. Cancer Res 1986;46:6513.
232. Rodenhuis S, McGuire JJ, Sawicki WL, Bertino JR. Effects of methotrexate and of the "nonclassical" folate antagonist trimetrexate on human leukemia cells. Leukemia 1987;1:116.
233. Rosenblatt DS, Whitehead VM, Dupont MM, Vuchich MJ, Vera N. Synthesis of methotrexate polyglutamates in cultured human cells. Mol Pharmacol 1978;14:210.
234. Rosenblatt DS, Whitehead VM, Vuchich MJ, Pottier A, Matiaszuk NV. Inhibition of methotrexate polyglutamate accumulation in cultured human cells. Mol Pharmacol 1981;19:87.
235. Rosowsky A, Wright JE, Cucchi CA, Boeheim K, Frei E III. Transport of a fluorescent antifolate by methotrexate-sensitive and methotrexate resistant human leukemic lymphoblasts. Biochem Pharmacol 1986;35:356.
236. Rosowsky A, Wright JE, Cucchi CA, Lippke JA, Tantrauahi R, Ervin TJ, Frei E III. Phenotypic heterogeneity in cultured human head and neck squamous cell carcinoma lines with low levels of methotrexate resistance. Cancer Res 1985;45:6205.
237. Boss JF, Chaudhuri PK, Ratman M. Differential regulation of folate receptor isoforms in normal and malignant tissues in vivo and in established cell lines. Cancer 1994;73: 2432–2443.
238. Rustin GJS, Rustin F, Dent J, Booth M, Satt S, Bagshane KD. No increase in second tumors after cytotoxic chemotherapy for gestational trophoblastic tumors. N Engl J Med 1983;308:1.
239. Said HM, Hollander D. Inhibitory effect of bile salts on the enterohepatic circulation of methotrexate in the unanesthetized rat: inhibition of methotrexate intestinal absorption. Cancer Chemother Pharmacol 1986;16:121.
240. Salamoun J, Smrz M, Kiss F, Salamounova A. Column liquid chromatography of methotrexate and its metabolites using a post-column photochemical reactor and fluorescence detection. J Chromatogr 1987;419:213.
241. Schilsky RL, Bailey BD, Chabner BA. Methotrexate polyglutamate synthesis by cultured human breast cancer cells. Proc Natl Acad Sci USA 1980;77:2919.
242. Schmid FA, Sirotnak FM, Otter GM, DeGraw JI. Combination chemotherapy with a new folate analog: activity of 10-ethyl-10-deaza-aminopterin compared to methotrexate with 5-fluorouracil and alkylating agents against advanced metastatic disease in murine tumor models. Cancer Treat Rep 1987;71:727–732.
243. Schornagel JH, Cappelaere P, Cognetti F, Verweij J, Clavel M, de Mulder PHM Vermorken, Snow GB. A randomized phase II trial of methotrexate vs 10-ethyl-10-deaza-aminopterin in patients with advanced squamous cell carcinoma of the head and neck. Sixth Symposium on New Drugs 1989:p 462.
244. Schuetz JD, Matherly LH, Westin EH, Goldman ID. Evidence for a functional defect in the translocation of the methotrexate transport carrier in a methotrexate-resistant murine L1210 leukemia cell line. J Biol Chem 1988;263:9840.
245. Schweitzer BI, Dicker AP, Bertino JR. Dihydrofolate reductase as a therapeutic target. FASEB J 1990;4:2441.
246. Searles G, McKendry RJ. Methotrexate pneumonitis in rheumatoid arthritis: potential risk factors. Four case reports and a review of the literature. J Rheumatol 1987;14: 1164.
247. Seeger DR, Cosulich DB, Smith JM Jr, Hultquist ME. Analogs of pteroylglutamic acid. III. 4-Amino derivatives. J Am Chem Soc 1949;71:753.
248. Seeger DR, Smith JM Jr, Hultquist ME. Antagonist for pteroylglutamic acid. J Am Chem Soc 1947;69:2567.
249. Shamberger RC, Rosenberg SA, Seipp CA, Sherins RJ. Effects of high-dose methotrexate and vincristine on ovarian and testicular function in patients undergoing postoperative adjuvant treatment of osteosarcoma. Cancer Treat Rep 1981;65: 739.
250. Shapiro WR, Allen JC, Horten BC. Chronic methotrexate toxicity to the central nervous system. Clin Bull Memorial-Sloan Kettering 1980;10:49.
251. Shapiro WR, Young DF, Mehta BM. Methotrexate distribution in cerebrospinal fluid after intravenous, ventricular and lumbar injections. N Engl J Med 1975;293:161.
252. Shen DD, Azarnoff DL. Clinical pharmacokinetics of methotrexate. Clin Pharmacokinet 1978;3:1.
253. Shipp MA, Harrington DP, Klatt MM, Jochelson MS, Pinkus GS, Marshall JL, Rosenthal DS, Skarin AT, Canellos GP. Identification of major prognostic subgroups of patients with large cell lymphoma treated with mBACOD or M-BACOD. Ann Intern Med 1986;104:757.
254. Shum KY, Kris MG, Gralla RJ, Burke MT, Marks LD, Hellan RT. Phase II study of 10-ethyl-10-deaza-aminopterin in patients with stage III and IV non-small cell lung cancer. J Clin Oncol 1988;6:446.
255. Sigel CW, Macklin AW, Wolley TL, Sigel CW, Macklin AW, Wolley J, Johnson MA, Blum MR, Clendieninn NJ, Everitt BJM, Grebe G, Foss R, Duch DF, Bowers SW, Nichol CA. Preclinical biochemical pharmacology and toxicology of piritrexim, a lipophilic inhibitor of DHFR. Natl Cancer Inst Monogr 1987;5:111.
256. Singh RR, Malaviya AV, Pandey JN, Guleria JS. Fatal interaction between methotrexate and nonsteroidal anti-inflammatory drugs. Lancet 1986;1:8480.
257. Sirotnak FM, Donsbach RC. Differential cell permeability and the basis for selective activity of methotrexate during therapy of the L1210 leukemia. Cancer Res 1973;33: 1290.
258. Sirotnak FM, Donsbach RC. The intracellular concentration dependence of antifolate inhibition of DNA synthesis in L1210 leukemia cells. Cancer Res 1974;34:3332.
259. Sirotnak FM, Donsbach RC. Kinetic correlates of methotrexate transport and therapeutic responsiveness in murine tumors. Cancer Res 1976;36:1151.
260. Sirotnak FM, Moccio DM, Hancock CH, Young CM. Improved methotrexate therapy of murine tumors obtained by probenecid-mediated pharmacological modulation at the level of membrane transport. Cancer Res 1981;41:3944.
261. Sirotnak FM, Moccio DM, Young CW. Increased accumulation of methotrexate by murine tumor cells in vitro in the presence of probenecid by a preferential inhibition of efflux. Cancer Res 1981;41:966.
262. Sirotnak FM, Samuels LL, DeGraw JI. 10-Ethyl-10-deazaaminopterin structural design and biochemical, pharmacologic and antitumor properties. Natl Cancer Inst Monogr 1987;5:127.
263. Skeel RT, Bertino JR. Combination chemotherapy of sarcoma 180 with methotrexate and bleomycin. Cancer Res 1973;33:1028.
264. Sobrero A, Bertino JR. Clinical aspects of drug resistance. Cancer Surv 1986;5:93.
265. Sonneveld P, Schultz FW, Nooter K, Hahlen K. Pharmacokinetics of methotrexate and 7-hydroxymethotrexate in plasma and bone marrow of children receiving low-dose oral methotrexate. Cancer Chemother Pharmacol 1986;18:111.
266. Sorewen JB, Hansen HH. Chemotherapy in adenocarcinoma of the lung. Cancer Surv 1989;8:671.
267. Sostman HD, Matthay RA, Putman C, Smith GJ. Methotrexate induced pneumonitis. Medicine (Baltimore) 1976;55:371.
268. Spiegel RJ, Cooper PR, Blum RH, Speyer JL, McBride D, Mangiardi J. Treatment of massive intrathecal methotrexate overdose by ventriculolumbar perfusion. N Engl J Med 1984;311:386.
269. Srimatkandada S, Medina WD, Cashmore AR, Whyte W, Engel D, Moroson BA, Franco CT, Dube SK, Bertino JR. Amplification and organization of dihydrofolate reductase genes in a human leukemic cell line, K-562, resistant to methotrexate. Biochemistry 1983;22:5574.
270. Steele WH, Stuart JB, Lawrence JR, Calman KC. Methotrexate protein binding. Br J Cancer 1979;40:316.
271. Steinberg SE, Campbell CL, Bleyer WA, Hillman RS. Enterohepatic circulation of methotrexate in rats in vivo. Cancer Res 1982;42:1279.
272. Sternberg CN, Yagoda A, Scherr HI, Watson RC, Ahmed T, Weiselberger LR, Geller N, Hollander PS, Herr HN, Sogani PC. Preliminary results of M-VAC (methotrexate, vinblastine, doxorubicin and cisplatin) for transitional cell carcinoma of the urothelium. J Urol 1985;133:403.
273. Stewart AL, Margison JM, Wilkinson PM, Lucas SB. The pharmacokinetics of 7-hydroxymethotrexate following medium-dose methotrexate therapy. Cancer Chemother Pharmacol 1985;14:165.
274. Stoller RG, Hande KR, Jacobs SA, Rosenberg SA, Chabner BA. Use of plasma pharmacokinetics to predict and prevent methotrexate toxicity. N Engl J Med 1977;297: 630.
275. Stone SR, Morrison JF. Mechanism of inhibition of DHFRs from bacterial and vertebrate sources by various classes of folate analogues. Biochim Biophys Acta 1986;869:275.
276. Storb R, Deeg J, Fisher L, Appelbaum F, Buckner CD, Bensinger W, Clift R, Doney K, Irle C, McGuffin R. Cyclosporine vs methotrexate for graft-vs-host disease prevention in patients given marrow grafts for leukemia: long-term follow-up of three controlled trials. Blood 1988;71:293.
277. Storm AJ, van der Kogel AJ, Nooter K. Effect of X-irradiation on the pharmacokinetics of methotrexate in rats: alteration of the blood-brain barrier. Eur J Cancer Clin Oncol 1985;21:759.
278. Strum WB, Liem HH. Hepatic uptake, intracellular protein binding and biliary excretion of amethopterin. Biochem Pharmacol 1977;26:1235.
279. Strum WB, Liem HH, Muller-Eberhard U. Effect of chemotherapeutic agents on the uptake and excretion of amethopterin by the isolated perfused rat liver. Cancer Res 1978;38:4734.
280. Stuart JFB, Calman KC, Watters J, Paxton J, Whiting B, Lawrence JR, Steele WH, McVie JG. Bioavailability of methotrexate: implications for clinical use. Cancer Chemother Pharmacol 1979;3:239.
281. Tan C, Trippett T, Tong W, Van Syckle K, Göker E, Wollner N, Bertino JR. A pharmacologic guided trial of sequential methotrexate and 6-thioguanine. J Clin Oncol 1994;12:1955.
282. Tattersall MH, Brown B, Frei E III. The reversal of methotrexate toxicity by thymidine with maintenance of antitumor effects. Nature 1975;253:198.
283. Tattersall MH, Jackson RC, Jackson ST, Harrap KR. Factors determining cell sensitivity to methotrexate: studies of folate and deoxyribonucleotide triphosphate pools in five mammalian cell lines. Eur J Cancer 1974;10:819.
284. Taylor IW, Slowiaczek P, Friedlander MI, Tattersall MH. Selective toxicity of a new lipophilic antifolate, BW301U, for methotrexate-resistant cells with reduced drug uptake. Cancer Res 1985;45:978.
285. Thyss A, Milano G, Etienne MC, Paquis P, Roche JL, Grelier P, Schneider M. Evidence for CSF accumulation of 5-methyltetrahydrofolate during repeated courses of methotrexate plus folinic acid rescue. Br J Cancer 1989;59:627–630.
286. Thyss A, Milano G, Kubar J, Namer M, Schneider M. Clinical and pharmacokinetic evidence of a life-threatening interaction between methotrexate and ketoprofen. Lancet 1986;1:256.
287. Tong WP, Rosenberg J, Ludlum DB. Purity of methotrexate. Lancet 1975;2:719.
288. Torosian MH, Mullen JL, Miller EE, Zinnser KR, Buzby GP. Reduction of methotrexate toxicity with improved nutritional status in tumor-bearing animals. Cancer 1988;61: 1731.
289. Trent JM, Buick RN, Olson S, Horns RC Jr, Schimke RT. Cytolic evidence for gene

amplification in methotrexate-resistant cells obtained from a patient with ovarian adenocarcinoma. J Clin Oncol 1984;2:8.
290. Valerino DM, Johns DG, Zaharko DS, Oliverio VT. Studies of the metabolism of methotrexate by intestinal flora. Biochem Pharmacol 1972;21:821.
291. Volger WR, Furtado VP, Huguley CM Jr. Methotrexate for advanced cancer of the breast. Cancer 1968;21:26.
292. Walker RW, Allen JC, Rosen G, Caparros B. Transient cerebral dysfunction secondary to high-dose methotrexate. J Clin Oncol 1986;4:1845.
293. Wan SH, Huffman DH, Azarnoff DL, Stephens R, Hoogstraten B. Effect of route of administration and effusion on methotrexate pharmacokinetics. Cancer Res 1974;34:3487.
294. Warren RD, Nichols AP, Bender RA. The effect of vincristine on methotrexate uptake and inhibition of DNA synthesis by human lymphoblastoid cells. Cancer Res 1977;37:2993.
295. Weber BL, Tanyer G, Poplack DG, Reaman GH, Feusner JH, Miser JS, Bleyer WA. Transient acute hepatotoxicity of high-dose methotrexate therapy during childhood. Natl Cancer Inst Monogr 1987;5:207.
296. Weitman SD, Lark RH, Coney LR, Fort DW, Frasca V, Zurawski VR Jr, Kamen BA. Distribution of the folate receptor GP38 in normal and malignant cell lines and tissues. Cancer Res 1992;52:3396–3401.
297. Weitman SD, Weinberg AG, Coney LR, Zurawski VR Jr, Jennings DS, Kamen BA. Cellular localization of the folate receptor: potential role in drug toxicity and folate homeostasis. Cancer Res 1992;52:6708–6711.
298. Werkheiser WC. The biochemical, cellular, and pharmacological action and effects of the folic acid antagonists. Cancer Res 1963;23:1277.
299. White CJ, Loftfield S, Goldman ID. The mechanism of action of methotrexate: III. Requirement of free intracellular methotrexate for maximal suppression of (14C) formate incorporation into nucleic acids and protein. Mol Pharmacol 1975;11:287.
300. Whitehead VM, Rosenblatt DS, Vuchich MJ, Schuster JJ, Witte A, Beaulieu D. Accumulation of methotrexate and methotrexate polyglutamates in lymphoblasts at diagnosis of childhood acute lymphoblastic leukemia: a pilot prognostic factor analysis. Blood 1990;76:44.
301. Whitehead VM, Vuchich MJ, Lauer SJ, Mahoney D, Carroll AJ, Shuster JJ, Esseltine DW, Payment C, Look AT, Akabutu J, Bowen T, Taylor LD, Camitta B, Pullen DJ. Accumulation of high levels of methotrexate polyglutamates in lymphoblasts from children with hyperdipiod (>50 chromosomes) B-lineage acute lymphoblastic leukemia: a pediatric oncology group study. Blood 1992;80:1316.
302. Wilke NS. Methotrexate Therapy in Rheumatic Disease. New York: Dekker, 1989.
303. Williams DA, Hsieh K, DeSilva A, Mulligan RC. Protection of bone marrow transplant recipients from lethal doses of methotrexate by the generation of methotrexate-resistant bone marrow. J Exp Med 1987;66:210.
304. Williams JW, Duggleby RG, Cutler R, Morrison JF. The inhibition of dihydrofolate reductase by folate analogues: structural requirements for slow- and tight-binding inhibitors. Biochem Pharmacol 1980;29:589.
305. Williams FMR, Murray RC, Underhill TM, Flintoff WF. Isolation of a hamster cDNA clone coding for a function involved in methotrexate uptake. J Biol Chem 1994;269:5810.
306. Wills J, Bleiberg H, Dalesio O, Blijham G, Mulder N, Planting A, Splinter T, Ducz N. An EORTC Gastrointestinal Group evaluation of the combination of sequential methotrexate and 5-fluorouracil combined with Adriamycin in advanced measurable gastric cancer. J Clin Oncol 1986;4:1799.
307. Woods RL, Fox RM, Tattersall MHN. Methotrexate treatment of advanced head and neck cancers. Cancer Treat Rep 1981;65(suppl 1):155–159.
308. Woods RL, Fox RM, Tattersall MHN. Methotrexate treatment of squamous-cell head and neck cancers: dose-response evaluation. Br Med J 1981;282:600.
309. Yap BS, McCredie KB, Benjamin RS, Bodey GP, Freireich EJ. Refractory acute leukemia in adults treated with sequential colaspase and high-dose methotrexate. Br Med J 1978;2:791.
310. Zachariae H, Kragballe K, Sogaard H. Methotrexate-induced cirrhosis. Br J Dermatol 1980;102:407.

CHAPTER 61

Pyrimidine and Purine Antimetabolites

GIUSEPPE PIZZORNO, YUNG CHI CHENG, AND ROBERT E. HANDSCHUMACHER

Introduction

Development of purine and pyrimidine analogues as potential antineoplastic agents evolved from an early presumption that nucleic acids are involved in growth control. Among the first analogues produced and tested for biologic activity were the 5-halogenated pyrimidines, 5-chloro-, 5-bromo-, and 5-iodouracil. Although in original concept these agents were targeted toward the malarial parasite, G. H. Hitchings and his colleague G. B. Elion recognized that these compounds might be valuable in the treatment of cancer, which then was correctly perceived as being a disease of uncontrolled growth (74, 171). These early studies primarily focused on the incorporation of analogue nucleic acid bases into RNA or DNA of bacterial species (117). Concurrent studies on the metabolic activation of these heterocycle analogues, as well as their biochemical targets for growth inhibition and the study of resistance to them afforded many new insights into the intermediary metabolism responsible for the synthesis of DNA and RNA precursors (36). Subsequently, it was recognized that control of these biosynthetic pathways afforded additional targets for therapeutic intervention.

Further development of these analogues was stimulated by the demonstration of quantitative, but not qualitative, differences in the activity of these pathways within normal versus neoplastic tissue. It was also realized that rapid catabolism of these agents to inactive compounds could severely limit anabolic conversion to fraudulent nucleotides. This in itself affords targets for the modulation of cytotoxic activity on a tissue-specific basis.

A virtually complete understanding of enzymes involved in the biosynthesis of purine and pyrimidine nucleotide precursors of RNA and DNA is now at hand (131, 193). This intricate matrix of metabolic reactions operates under a complex web of positive- and negative-feedback controls. Most purine or pyrimidine analogues are active only after metabolic activation to the nucleotide form, so these fraudulent nucleotides not only may be incorporated but also can mimic the natural effector compounds in regulatory pathways. Alternatively, they may deplete critical intermediates, thereby generating enlarged pools of the natural precursors behind a metabolic block and producing effects that can distort the balance of ribonucleoside and deoxyribonucleoside triphosphates. A target of even greater complexity is the incorporation of triphosphates into DNA or RNA and the subsequent modification of these macromolecules. The existence of subtle differences in the specificity and function of the polymerases generates the selectivity of certain purine and pyrimidine nucleotides as anticancer and, more importantly, antiviral agents.

Demonstrating the inhibition of specific enzyme reactions by analogue pyrimidine or purine nucleotides does not ensure that these reactions are rate limiting for tumor growth or responsible for cytotoxicity to either normal or neoplastic tissues. Even though several inhibitory sites have been identified, some having greater apparent sensitivity than others, attribution of a biologic effect to the inhibition of a specific reaction in general is difficult. Similarly, analogues may be incorporated into nucleic acids and either inhibit subsequent replication cycles or result in miscoding; however these mechanisms must be balanced against activity of the DNA editing and repair reactions that can minimize and, in some cases, increase the effects of incorporation.

In addition to purine and pyrimidine analogues, other agents have been developed that inhibit biosynthetic reactions leading to the ultimate nucleic acid precursors. These include PALA, brequinar, acivicin, and hydroxyurea.

Another factor that may affect the action of nucleoside analogues is the rate and nature of the transport systems for both normal and analogue nucleosides in and out of host versus neoplastic tissues. A wide range of neoplastic cell lines have a saturable system that is responsible for the facilitated diffusion of ribonucleosides and deoxyribonucleosides (276). This system essentially equilibrates the cytoplasm with the extracellular milieu. More recently, Na^+-dependent active transport systems for purine and pyrimidine nucleosides have been found in a variety of normal tissues (87, 212, 325). In neoplastic cell lines and some tumors, the Na^+-dependent concentrative mechanisms, if they exist, are nullified by the facilitated diffusion mechanism. These effects are particularly evident with uridine, which is 3- to 10-fold more concentrated in some normal tissues and may be responsible for the selectivity of some antimetabolites.

Pyrimidine Analogues

Pyrimidine analogues include fluorouracil, cytosine arabinoside, 5-azacytidine, and 2′, 2′-difluoro-2′-deoxycytidine.

FLUOROURACIL

Background and Properties

A major motivation for the development of pyrimidine analogues of uracil was the early observation that preneoplastic rat liver and hepatomas incorporated uracil more actively than normal liver (315). Although this may reflect a difference in the relative degradative capacity of these different tissues for uracil, it also provided a focus for the synthetic efforts of Dushinsky and Heidelberger that led to 5-fluorouracil (5-FU) (Fig. 61.1) and a family of related fluorinated pyrimidines (103). This specific site of substitution on the pyrimidine ring was selected because it might inhibit subsequent conversion of a uracil nucleotide to thymine nucleotides. Because insertion of the methyl group occurs on the 5-position, halogen replacement of hydrogen in that position was thought to have a greater chance of inhibiting DNA synthesis and, thus, growth. The selection of fluorine to replace the hydrogen in uracil was based on the similar Van der Waals radii (f = 1.35 A and h = 1.20 A). Unlike earlier syntheses of halogenated pyrimidines that involved simple displacement of the hydrogen with other halogens, chlorine, bromine, or iodine, 5-FU was originally synthesized from an acyclic precursor. This permitted formation of the corresponding 5-fluororotic acid; subsequently, the ribosides and deoxyribosides of FU were prepared (Fig. 61.1). More recently, a direct means of fluorinating FU has been developed that permits positron-emission tomographic (PET) studies with *18*F-FU (369).

As anticipated, the pKa of FU (8.1) is more acidic than that of uracil (9.6); thus, under physiologic conditions, FU partially exists as an anionic species. This is undoubtedly important to the metabolic activation to the nucleotide form via the orotidylate pyrophosphorylase reaction. This uridylate analogue, 5-fluorouridylic acid (FUMP), can then substitute for uridine monophosphate (UMP) in a wide spectrum of intermediary reactions. The product of one of these, fluorodeoxyuridylate (FdUMP), plays a major role by inhibiting displacement of hydrogen from the 5-position of deoxyuridylate and its replacement with a methyl group via a tetrahydrofolate catalyzed reaction (Fig. 61.2) (318). Many of the properties predicted for FU were seen in early studies of bacterial and model tumor systems and remarkably rapid progression to a clinical trial occurred within 2 years of its synthesis (159). These early clinical studies showed enough promise in colon cancer and other solid tumors to sustain 35 subsequent years of further development. A primary focus of this research has been to reduce its very real toxicity for a variety of normal tissues while retaining its antitumor activity. Today, FU remains an important component in the therapy of selected solid tumors, not only as a single agent but also in combination with other compounds that modulate either directly or indirectly the metabolism of pyrimidine nucleotides.

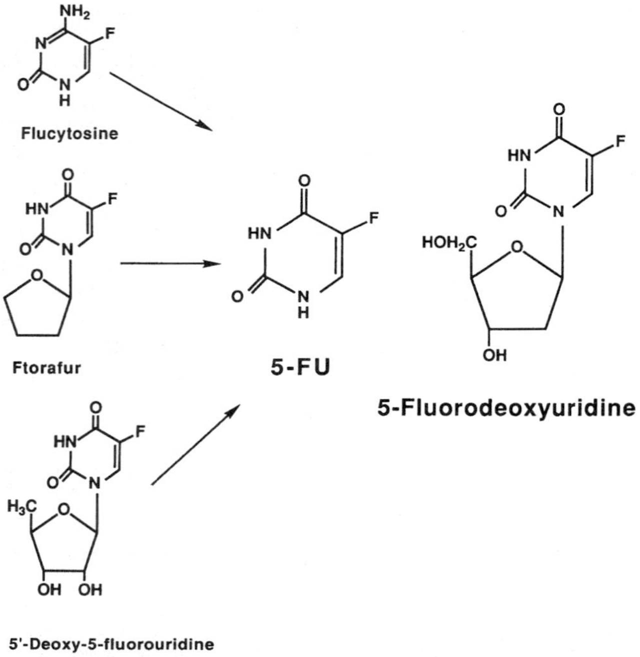

Flucytosine

Ftorafur

5-FU

5-Fluorodeoxyuridine

5'-Deoxy-5-fluorouridine

Figure 61.1. 5-Fluorouracil and analogue structures.

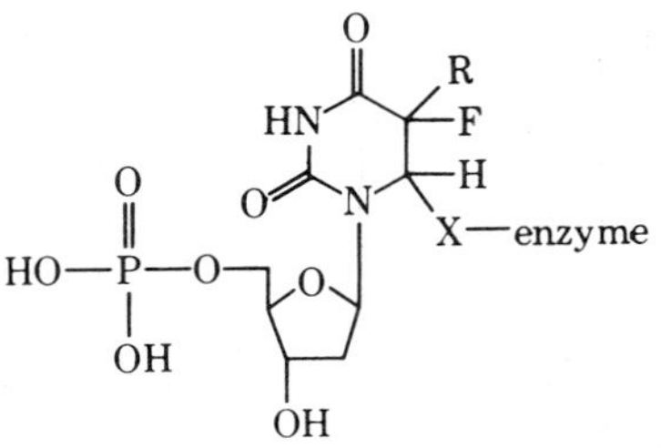

Figure 61.2. Covalent thymidylate synthase–fluorodeoxyuridylate complex; R = H or CH_2FH_4 = methylene tetrahydrofolate.

Cellular Entry and Efflux Mechanisms

Limited evidence suggests that FU enters cells by a carrier-mediated transport mechanism (380). Early reports suggested that a specific mechanism for the transport of uracil existed in the intestine; however, these studies, used methods that made it difficult to distinguish between transport and metabolism. Evidence has been presented for a nonconcentrative transporter in the Novikoff hepatoma that exhibits competitive kinetics between uracil and FU (372). Under conditions in which the FU ring is minimally ionized, enhanced entry of FU occurs if cells are preloaded with uracil, which is consistent with a countertransport mechanism. Using standard analytic techniques, no evidence to date suggests that an alteration of FU entry into cells is responsible for either natural or acquired resistance. However, use of more sophisticated methods has revealed a different picture of 5-FU uptake and retention. Using *19*F-5-FU, a difference in the ability of selected tumors to accumulate free 5-FU was noted to correlate with their response to chemotherapy (301, 319, 373). Extension of these studies to four patients with breast and colon carcinoma indicated a half-life of 0.4 to 2.1 hours for free 5-FU in the tumor compared with a plasma half-life of less than 10 to 15 minutes. Independent studies using gas chromatography–mass spectroscopy (GC-MS) documented free 5-FU concentrations in normal and neoplastic tissue that were at least 10-fold higher than those in plasma. This study also revealed that after an initial, rapid clearance from plasma, it was possible to detect a second, longer half-life of approximately 3.5 hours (280, 365). These new observations on the trapping of 5-FU in tumors lend support to the view that 5-FU is transported into the cells by an active transport mechanism as well (387) as a facilitated diffusion mechanism (98, 372). Free 5-FU also could be concentrated in the cytoplasma (pH, 7.2) from extracellular spaces of tumors rendered acidic by anaerobic glycolysis (pH, 6.2–7.0) by virtue of ionization trapping of this pyrimidine analogue, which has a pKa of 8.1 (251). An alternative source would be a slow liberation of free 5-FU from nucleotides and nucleic acids that sustains an intracellular concentration because of the limited efflux of free 5-FU from the cells. This capacity for trapping free 5-FU may serve as a measure of potential clinical response, and deserves further study.

In contrast to FU, the entry of fluorodeoxyuridine (FdUrd) (Fig. 61.2) into most neoplastic cells involves the saturable but non-concentrative mechanism that is responsible for the facilitated diffusion of a wide spectrum of nucleosides (23). This transporter has been quantified in several cell lines by titration with *p*-nitrobenzylthioinosine (NBMPR). Deletion of this transport mechanism is the basis for resistance to FdUrd (342) or purine nucleoside analogues (55) in at least two cell lines. Such a deletion makes the cells collaterally sensitive to methotrexate and other inhibitors of thymidylate synthase, because they are unable, or limited in their ability, to salvage thymidine, whether naturally available or administered (341). Fluorouridine and FdUrd released from 5-fluorouridylic and 5-fluorodeoxyuridylic by phosphatase action exit the cell via this same facilitated diffusion transporter. Thus, agents that affect this transporter may selectively affect FU cytotoxicity by a differential effect on specific normal or neoplastic cell types. The facilitated diffusion mechanism may play a secondary role in the modulation of FU action in vivo by uridine because this normal nucleoside, but not FUrd or FdUrd, is actively concentrated by a Na^+-dependent system (89). Neoplastic cells appear to be less capable of this transport and are not protected.

Anabolism

Once inside the cell, FU has several possible routes of activation to the nucleotide form (225). In normal tissues, the predominant mechanism appears to be competition with orotate for condensation with pyrophosphorylribose-5-PO_4 (PRPP) via orotidylate pyrophosphorylase to form 5-fluorouridylate (307). In mammalian cells, this protein is a bifunctional enzyme that also catalyzes the decarboxylation of orotidylate to 5′-uridylic acid (307). FU can successfully compete with the very low physiological concentrations of orotate in this reaction because of its acidic pKa (i.e., 8.1), which generates a significant amount of anionic species.

Alternative activation routes of FU follow the salvage pathways for uracil and thymine but these are presumed to be less important in most tissues (80, 174, 288). The first enzyme in the pathway, uridine phosphorylase, condenses ribose-1-P with uracil or FU in a reaction that energetically favors synthesis but normally is catabolic in the cell because further reactions such as PRPP synthesis and phosphatases reduce the concentration of ribose-1-P. The corresponding reaction for thymine uses deoxyribose-1-P, but it is not considered to make a significant contribution to FU activation in current therapeutic regimens. After formation of the nucleoside, phosphorylation by uridine kinase and ATP forms 5-fluorouridine-5-P (FUMP) (Fig. 61.3). Further phosphorylation of FUMP to the diphosphate, FUDP, by nucleotide kinase provides a branch point in FU anabolism (160). Additional phosphorylation of a major portion of FUDP the triphosphate to FUTP provides the substrate for RNA polymerases with consequent incorporation into several forms of RNA (144). Alternatively, FUDP can be reduced to 5-flurodeoxyuridine diphosphate (FdUDP), which is hydrolyzed to the monophosphate FdUMP, which is the covalent inhibitor of thymidylate synthase (318). Some FdUDP is phosphorylated to the triphosphate FdUTP, which is an alternate substrate for thymidine triphosphate dTTP in DNA polymerase reactions; however, high deoxyuridine triphosphate dUTP pyrophosphatase activity converts most of the FdUTP to FdUMP (188). When FU is incorporated into DNA, uracil *N*-glycosylase removes it leaving an apyrimidinic sugar for the process of DNA repair. Errors in this process provide an additional basis for cytotoxicity (188).

Minor amounts of FUDP sugar derivatives have been detected as anabolic products, but their potential to inhibit cell

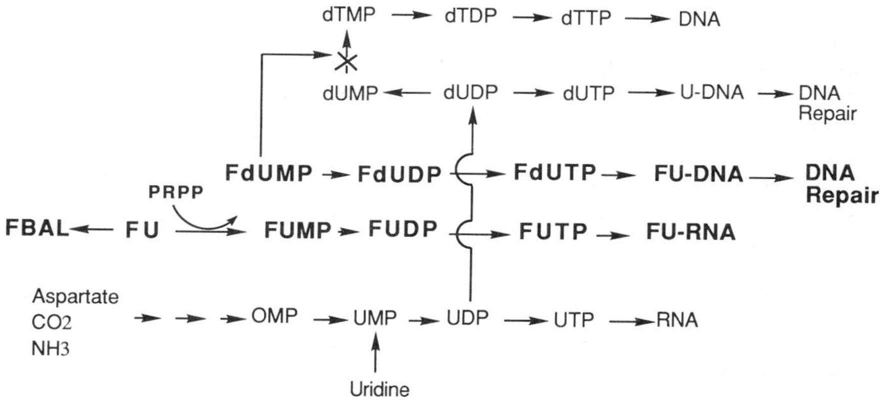

Figure 61.3. Metabolic activation and targets of fluorinated pyrimidines. dT = thymidine (thymine deoxyriboside); MP, DP, TP = mono-, di-, and triphosphate; dTMP also called thymidylate; dU = deoxyuridine; FdU = fluorodeoxyuridine; dUMP and FdUMP also called deoxyuridylate and fluorodeoxyuridylate; FBAL = fluoro-β-alanine; FU = fluorouracil; FUMP also called fluorouridylate; O = orotidine; U = uridine (uracil riboside); OMP also called orotidylate; UMP also called uridylate.

growth or toxicity has not been documented (281, 286). In some of the previously discussed reactions, the analogue FU nucleotides are better substrates than the corresponding uracil derivatives.

Pharmacokinetics

Consideration of FU pharmacokinetics must focus primarily on the balance between anabolism and catabolism. The conversion to nucleotide derivatives is responsible for most, if not all, of its antineoplastic activity, even though it accounts for a very minor portion of the administered drug. Catabolism via the normal degradation pathway for uracil is the immediate fate of more than 80% of an administered dose of FU (96). Therefore, slight alterations in this pathway can greatly affect the very limited amount that is available for conversion to the nucleotide form.

Because of great variability and limited bioavailability via the oral route (10–25%) (71), FU is generally administered intravenously (IV). Dosage depends on the schedule of administration (11). The most common dosage schedules are a monthly course of five daily doses given as an IV bolus of 400 to 600 mg/m^2, or the same dosage given as a single bolus on a weekly basis (122). The limiting toxic effect of these regimens generally is myelosuppression or mucositis. When continuous IV infusion is employed, higher doses are required (1,000–2,000 mg/m^2/d) to sustain steady-state concentrations of FU (1–5 μM) in plasma adequate to achieve therapeutic effects (326). With this route, toxicity is most frequently mucositis, with minimal myelosuppression. Several studies have shown that this regimen is superior to the bolus regimen when FU is given as a single agent (326, 329). Optimal treatment was a 48-hour infusion at weekly intervals, which improved both response and survival. Prolonged infusion of FU for up to 12 weeks at 300 mg/m^2/d also produced a better response than the bolus regimen (220, 221). The most prominent toxicity in this situation was a reversible hand-foot syndrome (221). It was found that during continuous IV infusions, plasma concentrations of FU varied by as much as 10-fold, and subsequent studies have demonstrated that variations in dihydropyrimidine dehydrogenase may be responsible for this effect (156). Because FU is most often used in combination with other agents such as leucovorin and methotrexate, it is important to modify the dosage in each case to limit, but not eliminate, host toxicity. It is generally thought that therapeutic benefit requires a dosage intensity that causes significant host toxicity, a result that has been documented in studies of colorectal cancer (182).

Administered FU has a volume of distribution (Vd) of 0.20 to 0.25 L/kg, which suggests distribution into the extracellular space (129, 224). Good penetration into cerebrospinal fluid, lymph and neoplastic effusions have been documented (75). Since the drug apparently freely permeates cells in culture, it is not clear why the volume of distribution approximates the extracellular space.

The rate of plasma clearance generally is first order with a half-life of 10 to 20 minutes and ranges between 500 and 1,500 mL/min (96). Above a dosage of 800 mg/m^2, clearance may decrease rapidly. Because the primary fate of the drug is catabolism, this decreased clearance undoubtedly reflects saturation of these reactions (236). The circulating concentrations of the initial metabolite, dihydro-5-FU, can be much greater than those of FU, and the fate of this metabolite may affect both pharmacokinetics and response to FU.

Intra-arterial infusion of FU has been used with some success in patients with isolated hepatic metastases. As with systemic therapy, extensive single-pass clearance is achieved (19–51%), but saturation of catabolism occurs when doses are elevated (120). Nevertheless, hepatic FU concentrations considerably in excess of those tolerated systemically can be achieved. The limiting factor in high-dose regimens is cholestatic jaundice and evidence of chemical hepatitis.

The 2′-deoxyriboside of FU, FdUrd, is a very much more potent inhibitor of cell growth than FU in cell culture (361). This presumably reflects the ease with which this compound can be activated by thymidine kinase in a single step to FdUMP, the titrating inhibitor of thymidylate synthase, which after further phosphorylation can also be incorporated into DNA. In both humans and animals, IV bolus injection of FdUrd produces a dose response that is essentially that of FU, because it is cleaved rapidly to an equivalent amount of FU that subsequently experiences the same metabolic fate as directly injected FU. If, however, FdUrd is given by a 14-day continuous infusion, the maximum tolerated dose is approximately 100-fold less (347); however, its therapeutic index is not significantly better than that of FU. Even so, it can be used for isolated hepatic metastases of colon cancer by hepatic artery infusion, because approximately 90% of the drug is cleared in a single pass by the liver, thus reducing systemic effects (120). Using this route, major increases in the hepatic concentrations of intact drug are achieved relative to systemic targets of toxicity.

The only other approved preparation of FU is in a 2 or 5% formulation in ethylene glycol or a water-based cream for topical application to treat epithelial dysplasias, particularly actinic keratoses and early basal cell carcinomas (106). Vulvar and vaginal epithelial neoplasms and genital condylomas also respond to this treatment (206, 336). Insufficient drug is absorbed from these preparations to cause systemic effects, and reports of local drug kinetics have been limited. It is not clear which, if any, of the biochemical mechanisms detailed earlier are responsible for this therapeutic effect, nor has a reason for the rather selective action on lesions been established (except for their presumably more rapid cell kinetics).

Although not directly useful in the treatment of cancer, the 4-amino derivative of FU, 5-fluorocytosine (flucytosine) (Fig. 61.2), is a valuable antifungal agent in systemic infections, which are a common complication of antineoplastic therapy (322). 5-Fluorocytosine is relatively nontoxic in mammalian systems, because it cannot be activated by direct condensation with (PRPP) and, like uracil, is poorly anabolized by uridine-cytidine phosphorylase. However, pathogenic fungi, including *Candida* and *Cryptococcus* species, deaminate 5-fluorocytosine to FU, which is lethal to the organisms by the same mechanisms as in mammalian cells (173). Although resistant strains rapidly emerge, combination therapy with amphotericin B is valuable in systemic fungal infections. Unfortunately, however, some 5-fluorocytosine appears to be converted to FU in the host, presumably by intestinal organisms, and this causes bone marrow depression (i.e., leukopenias and thrombocytopenia) (97). Evidence for its relative stability in humans is the observation that approximately 80% of an oral dose is excreted unchanged in the urine, compared with approximately 5% of a comparable dose of FU.

Several other compounds that serve as prodrugs of FU have also been developed. These include Tegafur (Ftorafur), a 1-(2-tetrahydrofuranyl) derivative of FU that is metabolized to free FU in liver by both cytochrome P_{450} and cytoplasmic activation (17). This agent (Fig. 61.2) appears to produce less myelosuppression, but mucositis and central nervous system toxicity are dose limiting (10). In controlled clinical trials, this agent appears to be equal to or somewhat less effective than FU at a comparable dose (257, 302). However, the favorable bioavailability of the oral formulation has sustained interest in this compound. UTF, a new formulation of Tegafur, is a combination of Ftorafur with uracil in a molar ratio of 1:4. The rationale for this formulation is that uracil inhibits the degradation of 5-FU that is released from Ftorafur (136–138). Response rates in Japanese clinical trials with stomach, colon, and breast cancer have been approximately 20 to 25% with a significantly lower incidence of gastrointestinal symptoms compared with Tegafur alone (272). However, no randomized, controlled study was performed to compare the clinical efficacy of the two drugs. A double-blind, randomized trial of Tegafur and UTF in patients with breast cancer found a 39% response rate for UTF and 21% for Tegafur; adverse effects were similar between the two treatments (353).

Another FU derivative, 5′-deoxy-5-fluorouridine (Fig. 61.1), is cleaved by uridine phosphorylase to liberate FU. Some studies suggest that higher phosphorylase activities are present in neoplastic tissues than their normal counterpart, so selectivity might be expected (13). Clinical trials have revealed activity in breast and colorectal neoplasms but neuro- and cardiotoxicity have limited further studies (8, 161). 5-Fluoro-2-pyrimidinone is another 5-FU pro-drug under investigation. It has been shown to be converted to 5-FU by hepatic aldehyde oxidase (108). This enzymatic conversion did not occur in gastrointestinal tissue or bone marrow, however, suggesting the potential selectivity of 5-fluoro-2-pyrimidinone as an oral pro-drug of 5-FU (152, 214).

Catabolic Reactions

The primary clearance mode of FU is via catabolism along the degradative pathway for uracil (96). Because the products of this pathway do not absorb ultraviolet light, GC-MS, or radioisotopic methods must be employed. The initial reaction is reduction by dihydrouracil dehydrogenase. The liver is a major site of FU metabolism and this is particularly true when the drug is given orally, intraperitoneally, or by intrahepatic arterial infusion. It is now recognized, however, that metabolism in the lung and kidneys may be of equal, or even greater, importance after IV administration (224). These findings have therapeutic relevance, because it was previously felt that hepatic metastases might compromise FU clearance and limit dosage.

Recently, marked circadian variations in the metabolism of FU have been detected and related to 24-hour cyclic variations in dihydrouracil dehydrogenase activity (110, 156). These changes are reflected in the inverse variations of plasma FU concentrations during IV infusions in humans (156, 320). Means to employ these differences in the design of clinical protocols have been outlined (181). Preclinical data in murine models have indicated that less toxicity was encountered during a circadian infusion when the maximal concentration of 5-FU was programmed to occur at 4 AM (40, 299). More recent data indicate that if the maximal concentration is programmed for 9 to 10 PM, even less toxicity is observed than with the previous schedule (240, 284). Several clinical protocols comparing a continuous flat infusion to the circadian schedule have been conducted with 5-FU alone and in combination with leucovorin and/or platinum derivatives (27, 215, 238). A recent study (31) using a 14-day continuous infusion of 5-FU and leucovorin suggests that circadian administration with a maximal infusion rate at 4 AM increases the maximum tolerated dose (MTD) for both agents (5-FU; 250 mg/m^2/d; LV, 20 mg/m^2/d). In patients who experienced grade 2 or higher toxicities with this schedule, the peak of their circadian infusion was moved to 9 to 10 PM. Decreased toxicity was observed (mostly diarrhea and stomatitis), and the MTD for 5-FU increased to 300 mg/m^2/d, a 50% increment over the MTD for a flat continuous infusion (9). In a related finding, familial deficiency of dihydropyrimidine dehydrogenase activity causes severe FU toxicity in patients with this genetic defect (95).

The subsequent metabolic step, catalyzed by dihydropyrimidinase, yields β-fluoroureidopropionic acid. In contrast to the dehydrogenase, this enzyme may be rate-limiting in most normal tissues for the degradation of uracil (and presumably FU) (256). A wide variety of tumors apparently express high levels of this activity because they accumulate the subsequent degradation products β-ureidopropionic acid and β-alanine. A therapeutic advantage has been achieved in model systems by inhibiting this enzyme with 5-ethynyluracil, which is an irreversible inhibitor (90, 314). It will be critical to demonstrate that these enhanced concentrations of 5-FU achieve therapeutic specificity, because earlier clinical studies revealed that thymine formed after thymidine administration inhibited 5-FU catabolism and increased toxicity (discussed later).

α-Fluoro-β-alanine, the counterpart to the final product of uracil catabolism, β-alanine, is the major urinary excretion product of FU (158). In patients with cancer, this has been shown to be conjugated with bile acids and constitutes the primary biliary secretion product of FU (348). It has been suggested that the chenodeoxycholate conjugate may be responsible for the biliary toxicity seen after large-dose, intrahepatic infusion of FU, and cholestasis associated with this conjugate has been demonstrated in isolated, perfused rat livers (348). A summary of FU metabolism is shown in Figure 61.3.

MECHANISMS OF ACTION

Experimental evidence has suggested numerous sites for the biologic action of FU (Fig. 61.3). The relative importance of each varies widely among different normal tissues and neoplasms. Commonly, the effects are divided into DNA or RNA directed toxicity.

RNA

The predominant phosphorylated nucleoside of FU, FUTP, is as good a substrate as uridine triphosphate (UTP) for several RNA polymerase reactions. The degree of FUTP incorporation into RNA bears a direct relationship to its concentration relative to that of the normal substrate, UTP. In cell lines, greater incorporation is associated with reduced clonogenic survival (147, 207). Very substantial amounts of FU replacement of uracil have been reported in each of the RNA species; the highest degree of incorporation generally is seen in the 4S-RNA (144). Some evidence suggests that with a given cell type, the proportion of RNA incorporation in different species depends on the available form of the analogue (FU vs. FUrd), a result that suggests compartmentalization or channeling of the analogue en route to incorporation (330).

What is less clear about incorporation into RNA is its contribution to cytotoxicity. Earlier studies indicated effects on t-RNA acceptor activity, miscoding of protein synthesis, and inhibition of the maturation or processing of ribosomal RNA (228). More recently, attention has focused on the inhibition of processing nuclear RNA to smaller-molecular-weight species (275). Other post-transcriptional effects of FU include inhibiting polyadenylation of mRNA and effects on DNA primase. In some model tumors and tumor lines, there is persuasive evidence that these RNA-directed events can be associated with cytotoxicity, particularly when the effects of extended exposure are monitored (126, 233).

Thymidylate Synthase

The target site that can be defined most clearly is the covalent inactivation of thymidylate synthase by 5-FdUMP (25). This fluorinated deoxyuridylate analogue is formed via the reduction of FUDP by ribonucleotide reductase and dephosphorylation (199). Alternatively, it can be formed directly from 5-FdUrd by thymidine kinase (155) when this FU deoxynucleoside is regionally infused. The earliest studies by Umeda and Heidelberger (361) indicated that in selected cell lines, growth inhibition could be prevented by thymidine but not by uridine. Direct inhibition of the enzyme responsible for the 1-carbon transfer confirmed this site of action (78, 157), and subsequent research identified specific steps in the reaction in which a methylene group from 5–10-methylene-tetrahydrofolate is transferred to the 5-position of 2′-deoxyuridylate (318). These studies elegantly established the formation of a stable ternary covalent complex between the 5′-fluoro-analogue of deoxyuridylate, the reduced folate derivative, and thymidylate synthase (84). The obvious consequence of this inhibition is an induced enzyme deficiency, depletion of dTTP, and the accumulation of dUMP behind the blockade (24, 178, 255). More recently, it has been shown that in some, but not all, tumors or normal tissues, the rate-limiting factor in formation of the abortive ternary complex with FdUMP is availability of the reduced folate derivative (125, 175). When this cofactor is limiting, it is possible to enhance inhibition by the administration of leucovorin (239). The consequence of dTTP depletion generally is considered to be unbalanced growth consequent to reduced DNA synthesis. As might be anticipated, this mode of inhibition would be nullified if thymidine were supplied, because after phosphorylation by thymidine kinase, it would circumvent the site of inhibition. However, thymidine administration in vivo actually can increase the cytotoxic effects of FU in vivo by inhibiting FU catabolism (16).

DNA

Initially, the incorporation of FU into DNA was not detected, and it was assumed to be prevented by the active dUTP phosphatases that also dephosphorylate FdUTP as it formed (188). Subsequently, small quantities of FU could be detected in internucleotide linkages within DNA (208, 250). Like dUTP, FdUTP when it is available, is fully active as a substrate for the several DNA polymerases, but a very active glycosylase is present in most cells that excises any FU or uracil that is incorporated in the place of thymine (174, 188). Mutants have been found that are relatively deficient in this editing function, and it may be that incorporation per se is not the cytotoxic event but that the excision and repair involving a pyrimidine endonuclease generates opportunities for error-prone repair that might again re-incorporate FU or uracil instead of thymine nucleotides (47, 104, 189). Because a considerable accumulation of dUMP occurs behind the blockade of thymidylate synthase, higher concentrations of dUTP are generated, which along with any FdUTP increase the need for an editing function to remove incorporated uracil. Examination of the kinetics of this excision reaction indicates that uracil is removed as much as 30 times more rapidly than FU.

A similar elevation of dUTP concentrations can be achieved by methotrexate therapy via secondary inhibition of thymidylate synthase (145). Under these conditions, uracil incorporation into DNA is also increased, and the potential for error-prone repair is enhanced.

It is not possible to rank the importance of these different potential mechanisms of cytotoxicity (i.e., RNA incorporation, dTTP depletion by thymidylate synthase inhibition, DNA incorporation, or damage to DNA consequent to excision of uracil or FU). In fact, the relative importance of each of these sites may vary, in different cell types. Evidence for high sensitivity to RNA-directed effects is seen in some tumor lines by the inability of thymidine to overcome growth inhibition despite the presence of an active thymidine kinase (220, 352). In these same lines, uridine rescue is more successful than in others where thymidine effectively prevents cytotoxicity, presumably by repleting dTTP.

RESISTANCE

As with most drugs, partial or complete responses of human cancer to FU generally are followed by the eventual regrowth of tumor despite sustained, or even increased, dosages. Understanding some of the factors that contribute to natural or acquired resistance has stimulated several of the approaches to modulating of FU therapy (discussed later). The most prominent mechanism seen in experimental tumors is reduced anabolism of the analogue to nucleotide form (252, 253). This may reflect altered condensation with PRPP or activation via the two-stage salvage pathway involving ribose 1-phosphate or deoxyribose 1-phosphate and the appropriate nucleoside phosphorylase, with subsequent phosphorylation of the resultant nucleoside by uridine or thymidine kinase. Alternatively, lack of sensitivity has been correlated with an increased disappearance rate of FU nucleotides, which were documented in one case to reflect enhanced nucleotide phosphatase activity (127). Other well-documented mechanisms of resistance reflect changes in the thymidylate synthase, with reduced affinity for FdUMP (20), or increases in the rate of synthesis and activity of the enzyme, possibly associated with gene amplification or altered enzyme turnover rates (26). Finally, effective deletion of the facilitated diffusion transport of FdUrd has been shown to confer resistance to this FU derivative but not to FU in a human colon-cancer-cell line (331).

MODULATION OF THERAPY

To improve the limited response rate to therapy with FU (10–25% in the most responsive cancers), various biochemical strategies have been investigated (28). The degree of FU activation by orotidylate pyrophosphorylase is affected by the available concentrations of PRPP. Because alterations of traffic along both the purine and pyrimidine nucleotide biosynthetic pathway affect the available concentrations of PRPP, several drug or metabolite combinations have been shown to modify the activation of FU, presumably by altering the concentration of this ribose-5′-phosphate donor (41, 324, 371). Others have explored depletion of pyrimidine nucleotides by inhibitors of the de novo synthesis of pyrimidines (267). A major focus in this area has been enhancing the efficiency with which the covalent complex of FdUMP with the folate cofactor and thymidylate synthase is formed by supplementation with the reduced folate cofactor (360).

Several current efforts seek to alter the amount of uridine that is available to normal tissues that are the target of FU toxicity, either by administering large doses of uridine or by inhibiting its degradation by uridine phosphorylase (86, 201). These efforts were stimulated by the improved therapeutic index of FU when plasma concentrations of uridine were elevated (232). Some selectivity is achieved, presumably because of uridine's ability to affect selectively the anabolism of FU nucleotides and, thus, its cytotoxic activity. Selectivity may also be consequent to the existence in most normal tissues of a Na^+-dependent, concentrative mechanism for uridine that is either minimal or absent in neoplastic cell lines and, perhaps, in malignant human tumors (87).

PALA

Modulation of the action of FU might be expected if the concentration of normal uracil nucleotides with which it competes in tumors was reduced. Phosphonacetyl-L-aspartic acid (PALA) (Fig. 61.4), has been documented to deplete

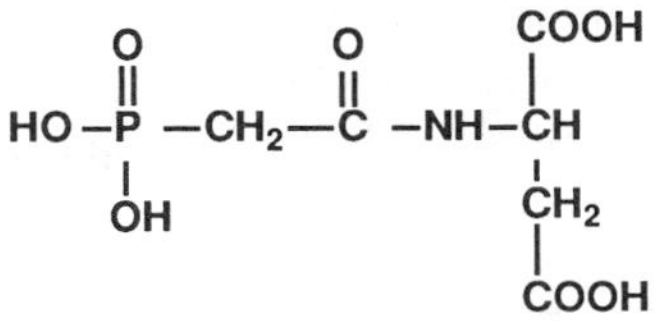

$$HO-P(=O)(OH)-CH_2-C(=O)-NH-CH(COOH)-CH_2-COOH$$

Figure 61.4. PALA [N-(phosphonacetyl)-L-aspartic acid].

the pyrimidine nucleotide pools in most cell types and was a logical candidate to enhance the cytostatic action of FU.

This agent was designed as an analogue of the transitional stage intermediate in the condensation of carbamylphosphate with L-aspartic acid (79). Early studies demonstrated its effectiveness in depleting the cellular pools of pyrimidine nucleotides and as a cytostatic agent for cells in culture (349). Effective reversal of the biochemical and cytotoxic effects could be achieved by supplying uridine to replete pyrimidine nucleotide pools via the salvage pathway (192). Sensitivity to growth inhibition was inversely related to the aspartate transcarbamylase activity of the cell line in question (190, 191), conversely, cell lines selected for resistance often displayed gene-amplified enhancement of enzyme activity (198). In naturally occurring solid tumors, however, such a correlation has not been observed (190). The most consistent correlation appears to be the capacity of the tumor tissue to salvage preformed pyrimidines.

Despite the extreme sensitivity of the target enzyme to PALA, relatively large doses were required both in animals and in human clinical trials to reach dose-limiting toxicity, 1.2–6.0 g/m^2 (6). This undoubtedly reflects poor penetration of this highly charged molecule into cells. It also may reflect the degree of inhibition that is required to make this the rate-limiting reaction in the de novo pathway. Nevertheless, marked reductions of pyrimidine nucleotides were seen in some biopsy specimens of tumors (5) and strong inhibition of the target enzyme also was observed. The drug accumulates in bone but does not cause myelosuppression. This persistence in bone and lack of perceptible metabolism in animals and humans achieves a prolonged biochemical effect on pyrimidine metabolism. The primary limiting toxicity is associated with epithelial tissues (e.g., skin rash, diarrhea, mucositis), but neurotoxicity also has been noted. Despite its potency in animal tumor models, PALA when used as a single agent was found to have minimal antitumor effects on human disease (5).

It was noted, however, that with its profound effect on pyrimidine synthesis de novo, PALA could modulate the action of other agents. Combination therapy with FU was tested as a means to reduce the pools of pyrimidine nucleotides with which FU nucleotides compete. Early studies employed high doses of PALA, and, although biochemically successful (50), serious toxicity and limited therapeutic effects were encountered (123). More recent trials have achieved significantly increased responses in colorectal cancer with much lower doses (250 mg/m^2, 10–20% of the MTD) given on day 1, followed 24 hours later by FU (2600 mg/m^2) as a 24-hour IV infusion and repeated weekly (12, 269). As discussed in Chapter 121, this combination has approximately doubled the response rate in colorectal cancer without serious increase in toxicity. Modulation of FdUrd therapy by PALA also has been documented in a model system (366) and may be applicable to regional infusions of FdUrd with systemic PALA.

Brequinar

A similar approach to modulation employs brequinar (DUP-785), which is an inhibitor of dihydroorotate dehydrogenase. This quinolone carboxylic acid derivative, currently being investigated as an immunosuppressant agent (82, 83, 262, 334), is unique in that it inhibits the only enzyme in the de novo pyrimidine pathway that is found in mitochondria, and it does so in a noncompetitive manner (61, 282). Good activity against a variety of solid tumors was observed in mice (282), and as anticipated by its site of inhibition could be completely overcome by supplementation with uridine. Though minimal clinical activity has been demonstrated when used as a single agent (77, 248), the compound can depress pools of pyrimidine nucleotides in tumors for longer periods than would be the case in normal tissues. This has led to treatment with brequinar before FU (293). In low-dose experimental regimens, this sequential regimen can cure experimental colon neoplasms. Phase I clinical trials of this combination indicate that the desired elevation of plasma uridine concentrations was achieved with no evidence of toxicity (291, 316).

Pyrazofurin and 6-Azauridine

Other inhibitors of de novo pyrimidine synthesis have been examined as single agents and, to a limited degree, in combination with the major antimetabolites FU and araC. After conversion to their respective monophosphates, pyrazofurin (42) and 6-azauridine (340), are potent inhibitors of the final reaction in the de novo pathway, orotidylate decarboxylase. This enzyme is a dual-function protein that also catalyzes the preceding step in the pathway: condensation of orotate with PRPP.

Inhibition by either agent results in the accumulation of orotic acid and orotidine, the dephosphorylation product of orotidylate, in the blood and urine (42). The degree of this accumulation caused by pyrazofurin has been used to quantify the effects of agents that may inhibit earlier steps in the pathway (251, 282). As single agents, both 6-azauridine, administered orally as the triacetyl derivative to facilitate rapid absorption, and pyrazofurin showed limited activity. With both agents, epithelial and erythropoietic toxicity limited their clinical usefulness. The potential use of these compounds in combination with fluorodeoxyuridine (FdUDR) might be considered because thymidine kinase or transport-deficient cells that are resistant to FdUrd would show enhanced sensitivity to inhibitors of de novo synthesis.

5-Ethynyluracil

5-Ethynyluracil is an irreversible inhibitor of dihydropyrimidine dehydrogenase, which is the initial enzyme in the catabolism of 5-FU (300). Because extensive and rapid catabolism through dihydropyrimidine dehydrogenase occurs, 5-ethynyluracil combined with 5-FU was tested in murine and rat models and found to improve the efficacy and therapeutic index of fluoropyrimidines (19, 44). In a rat colorectal-cancer model, 5-ethynyluracil was significantly more effective than either leucovorin or PALA as a modulator of 5-FU (44). The clinical efficacy and toxicity of this new biochemical modulation of 5-FU is now being evaluated.

Allopurinol

Modulation has also been achieved by co-administration of allopurinol and FU (377). After oxidation and conversion to oxypurinol ribonucleotide, allopurinol effectively inhibits orotidylate decarboxylase (22, 140), with accumulation of PRPP and orotate behind the target enzyme, which manifests as orotinuria in patients (22). This accumulation is apparently somewhat tissue-specific and it may selectively enhance the toxicity of FU to neoplastic tissues (324). Initial clinical trials indicated an increased clearance of FU without loss of antitumor activity (132, 180). Allopurinol recently was used in a FU-leucovorin regimen, and the reduced toxicity permitted a dose of FU of 750 mg/m^2 (30, 357). Two studies also have reported that an allopurinol mouthwash used four to six times a day for at least 7 days after FU administration reduced oral toxicity and pain (118, 358).

Acivicin

Another approach to the modulation of pyrimidine nucleotide biosynthesis would be to inhibit the generation of carbamyl phosphate, which is a substrate in the first reaction of the de novo pathway. A glutamine antagonist, acivicin achieves this by blocking the carbamylation of phosphate by covalent alkylation of the enzyme, and it elevates PRPP pools that would favor FU activation. Acivicin also inhibits the conversion of uridine (UTP) to cytidine triphosphate (CTP) and several amide transfer steps in purine biosynthesis because it is a general glutamine analogue (5). No clinical benefits were observed in its use as a single agent, but combination studies with FU or other pyrimidine analogs have been limited thus far.

Methotrexate

Modulation of FU therapy with methotrexate has been widely documented to increase both the cytotoxicity of FU in cell cultures and the inhibition of tumor growth in animal models. Optimal effects have been observed when FU follows the administration of methotrexate (MTX). Two studies indicate improvement in response rate compared with FU alone despite an increased severity of stomatitis and conjunctivitis (230, 261). One study suggested that a 24-hour interval was better than a 1-hour interval between the two drugs (230).

The biochemical basis for this enhanced response is commonly attributed to the expansion of PRPP pools generated by the inhibition of purine synthesis in cells preexposed to MTX (41). This favors greater activation of FU to nucleotide form and subsequent conversion to FdUMP. An augmenting effect is the depletion of thymidylate nucleotides via depletion of tetrahydrofolate derivatives. Reversing the sequence,

FU before MTX, decreases cytotoxicity in tumor cell lines and is less effective in model tumor systems, presumably because the consumption of tetrahydrofolates for thymidylate synthesis is blocked by the FU effect on the synthase (29). Consequently, more reduced folate is available for other reactions. Results from large-scale clinical trials now in progress with MTX followed by FU will determine the ultimate value of this combination and may motivate future efforts to define with greater certainty the responsible biochemical mechanisms.

Leucovorin

Formation of the ternary complex of FdUMP, thymidylate synthase, and folate coenzymes may be limited by the availability of reduced folates in some cell lines and tumors (84, 177). To optimize formation of the covalent complex, large doses of leucovorin (D,L-*N*5-formyl tetrahydrofolate) has been employed to saturate target enzymes with L-5-10-methylene-tetrahydrofolate via conversion of the L-isomer of leucovorin to 5-methyl-tetrahydrofolate (201).

Sound experimental evidence supports the logic of this approach to modulation. Early studies have demonstrated that optimal FU cytotoxicity in cell lines was achieved only when the cells were supplemented with folates to concentrations much greater than those required for optimal growth (125, 360). These effects directly related to the quantity of the ternary complex formed within the cells. The importance of sustaining the folate levels to stabilize the ternary complex could be seen in xenografts of human tumors, in which only transient inhibition of thymidylate synthase with FU would be expected unless supplemental reduced folates were present (179, 360). The importance of polyglutamylation to enhance binding to thymidylate synthase in retaining folates within cells also has been documented using cells that were defective in polyglutamate synthase (309).

If modulation by leucovorin in human disease is to be successful, the enhancement of ternary complex formation must be selective for tumor tissue. In a murine tumor model, leucovorin expanded the reduced folate pools in the tumor but not in bone marrow (379). This result was consistent with the antitumor effect seen without increased host toxicity. In other model systems, however, a consistent improvement in the therapeutic index is not seen. Because of the enhanced inhibition of thymidylate synthase when prior supplementation with leucovorin is employed, the dose of FU must be reduced by approximately 20% (122). Under these conditions, diarrhea and mucositis remain the limiting toxicity.

A wide range of clinical studies have, generally confirmed the increased rate of response to FU therapy in colorectal cancer when supplemented by leucovorin (239, 266). Evidence for increased survival in these trials is limited, however (122). In breast and stomach cancer, the response rate in patients who are not previously treated with FU appears to be increased by the addition of leucovorin; data for other diseases are insufficient to draw conclusions. The generally favorable results obtained in these studies have led to a rather universal addition of leucovorin to FU trials of combination with other drugs. Particularly promising are three studies combining 5-FU-leucovorin with cisplatin in head and neck cancer (239). Despite these positive results, however, carefully controlled studies are needed to assure the validity of this mode of modulation, particularly as other new drugs and modulators are combined with FU-leucovorin regimens.

Thymidine and Uridine

One of the earliest attempts to modulate FU toxicity employed thymidine (267). It might be expected that after conversion to the nucleotide form by thymidine kinase, this nucleoside would be able to rescue tissues from the inhibition of thymidylate synthase and such circumvention of the blockade was documented in some, but not all, cell lines (361). The in vivo extension of these cell culture studies suffered from two limitations. First, thymidine phosphorylase activity in many normal tissues is high. Consequently, the plasma half-life is short at doses below 45 $g/m^2/d$ (267), and large quantities were needed to sustain the plasma concentrations used in the cell culture experiments. A far more serious limitation was the competition for catabolism between FU and the large amounts of thymine generated by phosphorolysis (16). The net effect of thymidine given in large doses was not rescue but rather prolongation of the FU pharmacokinetics without an improved therapeutic effect in most circumstances. It also is interesting to note that myelosuppression replaced mucositis as the dose-limiting toxicity (376).

Modulation of FU therapy with uridine has shown more promise in model systems, but the clinical value of this combination has not been fully tested. In a limited number of cell lines, uridine can prevent the toxicity of FU (283). In vivo studies of uridine modulation not only established the value of uridine rescue but also the importance of a delay in uridine administration for up to 24 hours after FU (232). When given simultaneously in experimental animals, uridine can actually increase the FU toxicity, presumably because it inhibits FU catabolism. Other studies using animal tumor models confirmed that delayed uridine could reduce toxicity without impairing antitumor activity (204, 285). Large doses of uridine were required because of the very short half-life (3–10 minutes).

Based on changes in uridine nucleotide pools, several mechanisms have been postulated for these effects. Thus, one might invoke competition of the enhanced UTP pools with FU nucleotides formed in the period before uridine is administered. Tumor tissues that were less able to augment their uridine nucleotide pool would remain susceptible. Supporting this observation is the documentation of a Na^+-dependent concentrative transport system for uridine in a variety of normal tissues (212, 341). Concentrations of uridine range from 5- to 10-fold greater in liver, spleen, kidney, and, to a lesser degree, in the intestine than they are in plasma (89). Of potential therapeutic importance is the lack of such elevated uridine pools in neoplastic cell lines. Preliminary studies indicate that in general, experimental rodent and human tumors do not have elevated uridine pools. To some degree, these observations may contribute to the tumor specificity of FU (254). Fluorouridine and FdUrd are very poor substrates for this transport system in normal cells (89).

Clinical trials with very large doses of uridine administered

3 to 24 hours after FU by intermittent IV infusion have achieved millimolar concentrations of uridine, and the leukopenia, but not the thrombocytopenia, that is associated with weekly bolus doses of FU was prevented (363). However, these patients require hospitalization and experience fever and phlebitis. Oral uridine (8–12 g/m^2) achieves much lower plasma concentrations (50–80 μM), and the dose-limiting toxicity was diarrhea, not fever (364). Further clinical evaluation of uridine rescue after FU has demonstrated clinical benefit when administration was delayed for at least 24 hours after FU (70).

The practical difficulties that are posed by administering extremely large doses of uridine suggest the value of inhibiting its phosphorolysis. Benzylacyclouridine (BAU), which originally was synthesized as a potential antiviral agent, was found to be a potent inhibitor of uridine phosphorylase (260). Administration of BAU to experimental animals greatly expanded the pool of free uridine in normal tissues, but it had only a minimal effect on pools in murine colon tumor (88). This alteration of uridine homeostasis after FU therapy achieved a better therapeutic effect in this tumor model than the same dose of FU alone, and it actually reduced host toxicity. Clinical trials are planned for this combination, possibly in conjunction with reduced doses of uridine, which has been shown to improve therapy with FU in a murine breast tumor model. A phase I clinical trial demonstrated elevated levels of circulating uridine at non-toxic concentrations of BAU (292). This agent, used either alone or in conjunction with reduced doses of uridine, is now being evaluated in combinations with FU (231).

Other Modulators

Modulation of nucleoside transport has been considered as another approach to improve FU therapy. The facilitated diffusion mechanism for many natural nucleosides as well as analogue derivatives has been shown to be the primary mode of uridine entry and exit in most neoplastic cell lines (276). Very effective inhibition of this process in vitro by nitrobenzylthioinosine nitrobenzyl mercaptopurine riboside (NBMPR) has been extended to in vivo studies by use of the corresponding 5′-phosphate derivative, which improves solubility and is hydrolyzed to NBMPR.

The vasodilatory drug dipyridamole also inhibits this transporter and has been used in combination with FU (147). The rationale is that the access of circulating uridine to the neoplastic cell would be limited and the loss of any fluorouridine formed by phosphatase action on FU nucleotides from the target cell would be restricted. Considerable potentiation of FU action by dipyridamole was seen in culture (146). Limited clinical studies indicate this agent also can affect FU clearance, but it is not established whether an improved therapeutic index of FU can be achieved (147, 304).

Two agents that can modulate host defense mechanisms, levamisole and interferon, have been documented to enhance clinical responses to FU. It is not clear, however, whether the effectiveness of these combinations can be attributed to their activity as immunomodulators. Originally employed as an anthelminic agent, levamisole was an attractive candidate to augment antineoplastic therapy because of its ability to increase the number of functional T cells and activate macrophages in model systems (306). It should be recognized, however, that levamisole has a wide spectrum of activity on both the autonomic and CNS. Although it has limited activity as a single drug, there is convincing evidence from two randomized studies that when combined with FU, the rate of postsurgical disease recurrence in patients with stage C colorectal cancer is reduced and survival increased (209, 242). In general, the toxicity of this combination reflects that of FU, with mucositis and moderate myelosuppression. There is an increased rate of nausea and diarrhea and mild CNS disturbances, but the combination is generally, well tolerated. At present, no clear mechanistic explanation for the basis of the therapeutic effects can be given. Evaluation of this combination with other tumors in which FU has marginal activity is certainly warranted.

The interferons have also been evaluated as a means to recruit host defense mechanisms during FU therapy. The synergistic effects of interferon combined with FU have been observed in human tumor-cell cultures (258) and xenografts in nude mice (250). The enhanced effect of 5-FU, generated by α-interferon, has been attributed to the activation of macrophages in a species specific manner (mouse α-interferon in mice). α- and γ-Interferon have also engendered interest, because they appear to enhance the accumulation of FdUMP in HL-60 and HT-29 cells (111, 323). The increased conversion of 5-FU to FdUMP is reported to relate to an increased activity of pyrimidine nucleoside phosphorylase. Further biochemical studies have documented that 5-FU induces the expression and activity of thymidylate synthase in H630 cells, with no associated changes in thymidylate synthase mRNA levels. γ-Interferon suppresses this 5-FU–mediated elevation in enzyme activity and protein expression (72). A study with α-interferon and leucovorin showed that α-interferon enhances the excision of fluoropyrimidine from DNA following misincorporation, thereby increasing the number of DNA strand breaks (176). Limited clinical studies have been reported with α-interferon in combination with FU. Although initial response rates of 76% were reported in colorectal cancer (370), major increases in the incidence of both mucositis and granulocytopenia required dose reductions of both FU and interferon; subsequent confirmatory studies yielded response rates of only 26 to 35% (279).

CYTOSINE ARABINOSIDE

Background

Cytosine arabinoside (Cytarabin, araC, Cytosar®), is a nucleoside analogue of deoxycytidine that was first synthesized in 1950 and introduced into clinical medicine in 1963 (351). One of the most important drugs in the treatment of acute myeloid leukemia, it also is active against acute lymphocytic leukemia and, to a lesser extent, is useful in chronic myelocytic leukemia and non-Hodgkin's lymphoma (57). It has not proven to be particularly useful in the treatment of nonhematologic neoplasms. Myelosuppression and gastrointestinal epithelial injury are the primary toxic effects of araC. Using high-dose araC regimens, additional toxic effects such as intrahepatic cholestasis and CNS toxicity are frequently observed (43).

Metabolism

Cytosine arabinoside is rapidly deaminated by cytidine deaminase to a much less active compound, arabinosyluracil (Ara U) (58, 65, 67). Ara C enters cells through a carrier-mediated process or simple diffusion (200, 277). At low concentrations of araC ($<2\ \mu M$), the carrier-mediated process predominates. The efficiency of this transport process depends on the binding affinity of araC for the carrier, number of carrier molecules in the membrane, and presence of competing nucleosides sharing the same system. After entering the cells, it is metabolized primarily by the enzymes that normally metabolize deoxycytidine or, in some instances, cytidine (Fig. 61.5).

The enzyme that is responsible for cytarabine monophosphate (AraCMP) synthesis is cytoplasmic deoxycytidine kinase. Mitochondrial deoxypyrimidine nucleoside kinase, which can phosphorylate deoxycytidine and thymidine, does not efficiently phosphorylate araC (64). The activity of the cytoplasmic deoxycytidine kinase is higher in the S phase of the cell cycle. The amount of araCMP formed depends on the relative activity of cytoplasmic deoxycytidine kinase and cytidine deaminase. Tetrahydrouridine is a potent inhibitor of cytidine deaminase, with a K_i value of 10^{-8} M (58, 374). Potentiation of the cytotoxic effect of low araC concentrations by tetrahydrouridine underscores the role of cytidine deaminase in araC metabolism. The enzyme responsible for conversion of araCMP to araCDP is cytidylate-uridylate-deoxycytidylate (CMP-UMP-dCMP) kinase. There are two forms of this enzyme, and both are capable of phosphorylating araCMP. It has been suggested that araCMP could be deaminated to uracil arabinoside monophosphate (araUMP) by dCMP deaminase (227). Whether this pathway is functional in cells is questionable, however, because araCMP is a very poor substrate for dCMP deaminase compared with dCMP. Several mammalian cell lines are partially resistant to araC because of a decreased activity of dCMP deaminase (91, 92). Enzymes responsible for the phosphorylation of araCDP to cytarabine triphosphate (araCTP) are nucleoside diphosphate (NDP) kinases. There are multiple species of NDP kinase activities in human cells (62). Whether a preference exists for one isozyme over another in the phosphorylation of araCDP is unclear, but the formation of araCDP choline in human cells incubated with araC has been reported (45, 210). The enzyme that catalyzes this reversible process is phosphorylcholine cytidyltransferase. Both CDP choline and dCDP choline serve as donors of the phosphorylcholine moiety in phosphatidylcholine synthesis; how araCDP choline participates in or interferes with this reaction is not clear.

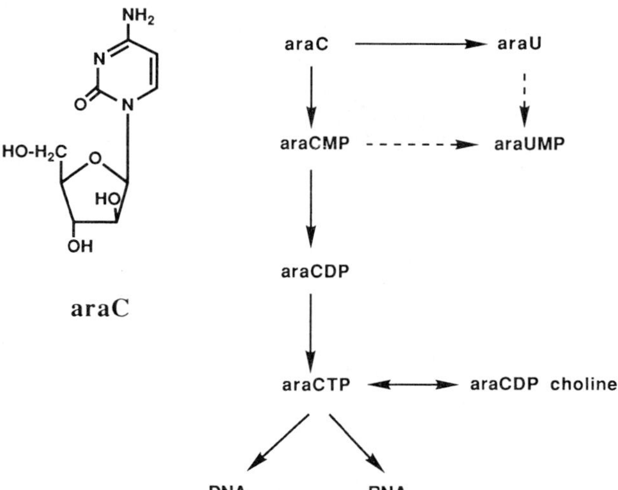

Figure 61.5. Structure and metabolism of arabinosyl cytosine (Ara C).

Major attention also has been focused on the incorporation of AraCTP into DNA in competition with dCTP (139, 244, 362). Elongation of DNA by polymerase α is considerably retarded by the incorporation of araCMP, whereas no significant impact on elongation by DNA polymerase β could be seen after incorporation of a single araC nucleoside residue. However, neither polymerase alone could appreciably elongate the DNA if two consecutive araCMP residues were incorporated. Thus, the behavior of araCTP on DNA polymerase is not only polymerase dependent but also sequence dependent (271, 356).

Mechanism of Action

The primary action of araC is inhibition of nuclear DNA synthesis (15, 243). Mitochondrial DNA synthesis is not affected by araC, even at concentrations 10 times greater than that required to inhibit cell growth by 50%. The possibility remains, however, that the functional nature of mitochondrial DNA may be compromised (61).

Three mechanisms have been suggested to account for the inhibition of nuclear DNA synthesis by araC. The relative importance of each mechanism may depend on the intracellular concentration of araCTP. The first mechanism is inhibition of the initiation of new replication units in chromosomes consequent to the incorporation of araC into the replicon-initiation primer (134). The second mechanism is the retardation of DNA-chain elongation because of the incorporation of araC into DNA (139, 244). This effect is DNA polymerase- and sequence-dependent, as discussed earlier. Reactions catalyzed by DNA polymerase α, and perhaps DNA polymerase δ, are more susceptible than other DNA polymerase activities. The third mechanism, which may become important only when a high dosage araC protocol is used, is the inhibition of DNA primase (274). AraCTP can inhibit the formation of the RNA oligomer required for the initiation of DNA synthesis with K_i values of 25 to 125 μM (depending on the template being used). Although there is no evidence that araCMP can be incorporated into an RNA oligomer in vitro, it has been found that some of the araC that is associated with DNA is alkaline labile (226). This indicates the possibility that araC is incorporated into the RNA primer of DNA, and requires further investigation.

In general, the inhibition of cell growth correlates well with the degree of the incorporation of araC into cellular DNA. The majority of incorporated araCMP is in internucleotide linkage in DNA. The relative ratio of araC in internucleotide compared with chain-terminal positions depends on the concentration of araC; the higher the concentration of araC to which the cells are exposed, the lower the relative amount of internucleotide araC residues. This could result from the higher probability of consecutive araCMPs being incorporated into DNA, which stops further DNA-chain elongation catalyzed by DNA polymerase α as well as DNA polymerase β. The amount of araCMP that is incorporated into DNA also depends on the relative ratio of araCTP to dCTP. Decreases in the intracellular pool of dCTP can increase the amount of araCMP that is incorporated. Exonucleases could remove araC incorporated in terminal positions to limit the cytotoxic effects.

Among other potential targets, araCTP is not a potent inhibitor of ribonucleotide reductase, a key enzyme early in the course of dCTP formation (59). AraCTP can act in lieu of dCTP to activate dCMP deaminase for the deamination of dCMP to dUMP, the substrate for dTMP synthesis. Because araCMP is a poor substrate for dCMP deaminase, the accumulation of araCTP enhances the deamination of dCMP and subsequently decreases the intracellular pool of dCTP (227). This could "self-potentiate" the incorporation of araCTP into DNA. This hypothesis is based on enzyme studies in vitro, but it is substantiated by the observation that cells become resistant to araC because of decreased dCMP deaminase activity (91).

The mechanism of action for araC may be dosage dependent. At noncytotoxic concentrations, araC can cause human promyeloblast HL-60 cell lines to differentiate. It has been suggested that the success of low-dosage araC therapy in patients with myelodysplastic syndrome may result from the differentiation effects of araC (15). When given to patients with leukemia, high doses of araC cause rapid tumor-cell lysis (45). Whether additional mechanisms of araC also play important roles in this protocol is unclear. In patients who receive high doses, the concentration of araU, the deamination product of araC, can exceed 100 μM in plasma (46). The high concentrations of araU may act in concert with araC, and it also may affect cell growth by mechanisms that have not yet been established (381).

Mechanism of Resistance

Cells could become resistant to araC because of decreased activities of the carrier for araC transport, of cytoplasmic deoxycytidine kinase, increased catabolism of araC through the action of cytidine deaminase, increased formation dCTP by ribonucleotide reductase and NDP kinase, or decreased activity of dCMP deaminase which could lead to increased competition by dCTP with araCTP for incorporation into DNA. An increased activity of 3′ to 5′ exonuclease, which could remove the araCMP from the DNA-chain terminus, has also been suggested (211).

5-AZACYTIDINE

Background

5-Azacytidine (5-AC) was first synthesized in 1963, and it was later isolated as a natural product from fungal cultures (154, 343). The clinical utility of this cytidine analogue is primarily in the treatment of acute myelocytic leukemia and myelodysplastic syndrome; occasionally, clinical response has been observed in patients with solid tumors. This compound can promote the expression of genes that are suppressed by hypermethylation (3). This activity suggested use of 5-AC in genetic diseases such as sickle cell anemia and thalassemia, but its usefulness in treating these diseases has been limited by its bone marrow toxicity and concerns over its carcinogenic potential. The major toxicity of 5-AC is leukopenia and, to a lesser degree, thrombocytopenia. Hepatotoxicity has also been reported, particularly in patients with preexisting hepatic dysfunction (57).

Metabolism

The replacement of carbon in position 5 of the heterocyclic ring of cytidine by nitrogen results in a marked chemical instability. The product of the ring opening, *N*-formylamidinoribofuranosyl guanylurea, may recycle to form the parent compound, but it is also susceptible to further decomposition. This tendency to decompose not only may play a role in its mechanism of action but also is troublesome in its clinical use (23). Although 5-AC can be deaminated by cytidine deaminase to 5 azauridine (5-AU), a less toxic compound, the efficiency of this deamination by cytidine deaminase is less than that of cytidine. Nevertheless, inhibition of the deamination by tetrahydrouridine can enhance 5-AC toxicity. 5-AC enters mammalian cells by a facilitated nucleoside transport mechanism that is shared with other nucleosides (294). The initial step in its activation is the conversion to 5 azacytidine monophosphate (5-ACMP) by uridine-cytidine kinase (102). 5-ACMP is further phosphorylated to 5-AC di- and triphosphate by CMP-UMP-dCMP kinases and nucleoside diphosphate kinases, respectively. 5-AC triphosphate, which for several hours is the predominant metabolite in cells treated with 5-AC, can be incorporated into RNA, but its pathway for incorporation into DNA is not well defined. 5-ACDP likely is reduced by ribonucleotide reductase to the corresponding deoxynucleotide diphosphate, which is phosphorylated to 5-AdCTP by nucleoside diphosphate kinases. 5-AdCTP can be efficiently incorporated into DNA by DNA polymerase α and β. The incorporated 5-AdCMP at the 3′ terminus of DNA has less effect on subsequent DNA-chain elongation than the incorporated araCMP at the 3′ terminus of DNA. 5-azadeoxycytidine (5-AdC) also is stabilized against hydrolytic degradation by incorporation into DNA, which could result in part from hydrophobic shielding of the triazine ring from water and other polar nucleophiles within the DNA double helix (355, 356).

A summary of 5-AC metabolism is shown in Fig. 61.6. 5-AC is most cytotoxic to cells in the DNA-synthetic phase of the cell cycle, but the exact mechanism of its cytotoxic action has not been well established. It could inhibit both DNA and RNA synthesis. Incorporation into RNA can inhibit the processing of ribosomal RNA from higher-molecular-weight species, disassembly of polyribosomes, and markedly inhibit protein synthesis. Incorporation into DNA also could inhibit DNA synthesis (73, 217, 218, 368). One important, well-documented effect is the inhibition of DNA methylation because of stoichiometric binding with DNA-methyltransferase after incorporation. The methylation of cytosine

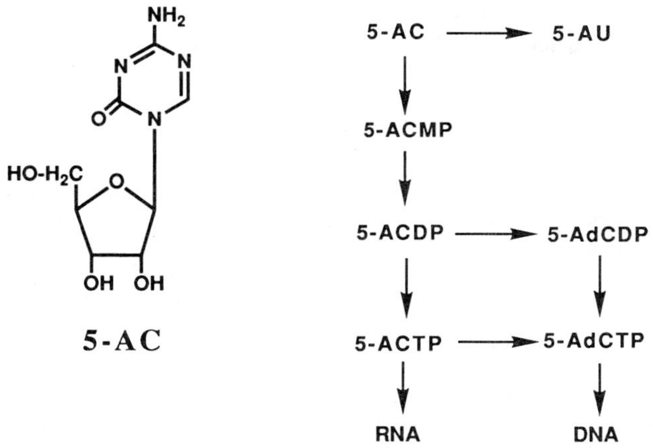

Figure 61.6. Structure and metabolism of 5-azacytidine (5-AC).

residues in DNA is responsible for the inactivation of specific genes; thus, treatment of cells with 5-AC leads to reduced levels of cytosine methylation and enhanced expression of selected genes that are normally suppressed. At minimally cytotoxic concentrations, 5-AC stimulates the differentiation of some tumor cell lines in culture, and it has been suggested for the treatment of genetic diseases that are associated with hypermethylation (see Chapter 141) (3).

Mechanism of Resistance

Cells can become resistant to 5-AC by the reduction or elimination of uridine-cytidine kinase. Decreased nucleoside transport by the facilitated diffusion mechanism also can decrease sensitivity to 5-AC, and cytosine deaminase may play an important role in cell sensitivity as well. In animal models, tumor cells that are resistant to araC because of the deletion of cytoplasmic deoxycytidine kinase activity, a frequent mechanism of cellular resistance to araC, are more susceptible to 5-AC than is the parent tumor line. Sequential treatment with araC and then 5-AC deserves further study, particularly in patients who become refractory to araC.

2′,2′-DIFLUORO-2′-DEOXYCYTIDINE

Background

2′,2′-Difluoro-2′-deoxycytidine (dFdC, Gemcitabine) is a deoxycytidine analogue with two fluorine atoms in the 2′ position of the sugar moiety (Fig. 61.7)(163). First synthesized in 1986, this molecule was initially developed as an antiviral agent because of its potent inhibitory activity against both DNA and RNA viruses (94). Subsequently, its broad spectrum of activity in murine tumors and human tumor xenografts (167) led to evaluating antineoplastic activity in clinical trials.

Phase II clinical trials, using a weekly schedule (30 min infusion) for 3 weeks, repeated every 4 weeks at a dose of 800 to 1250 mg/m^2/wk showed encouraging antitumor activity in ovarian (195, 222), breast (195) and non-small-cell lung cancer (2, 223, 303, 330), with a response rate of approximately 20 to 30%. However, in colorectal (222, 246), gastric (69), pancreatic (48, 53), and renal cancer (222, 237) the activity was less impressive. Encountered toxicities mainly were myelosuppression, nausea, vomiting, skin rash, and a flu-like syndrome.

Metabolism

2′,2′-Difluoro-2′-deoxycytidine requires phosphorylation by deoxycytidine kinase to exert its cytotoxic activity (Fig. 61.7). The major intracellular metabolite is 2′,2′-difluoro-2′-deoxycytidine triphosphate (dFdCTP), lesser amounts of the monophosphate dFdCMP and the diphosphate dFdCDP are

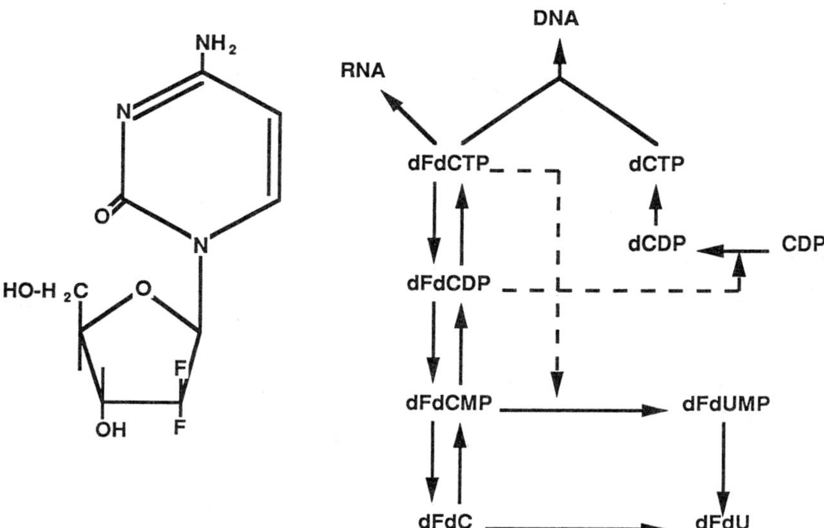

Figure 61.7. Structure, metabolism and actions of 2′, 2′-difluoro-2′-deoxycytidine (dFdC) and its nucleotides. Dashed lines indicate inhibitory actions. Modified from Heinemann et al. (163).

also formed (162). The cellular elimination of dFdCTP was investigated in several human cell lines: CCRF-CEM, K562, and A2780 (295, 311). Elimination of dFdCTP follows a biphasic course, with a short initial half-life followed by a second, slower phase of degradation. The biphasic elimination of dFdCTP differs from the linear monophasic kinetic that is exhibited by the triphosphate of Ara-C (297), arabinosyladenine (333), and arabinosyl-2-fluoro-adenine (85).

Deoxycytidine deaminase inactivates dFdc to 2′,2′-difluoro-2′-deoxyuridine (dFdU), which has no antitumor activity (162). The monophosphate of dFdC also can be deaminated to the uracil derivative dFdUMP by deoxycytidylate deaminase (163).

Pharmacokinetic studies during phase I clinical trials have shown a very rapid half-life (8 min) for dFdc because of deamination over a wide range of dosages (1). The deamination product, dFdU, which is the only metabolite present in the urine, exhibits a biphasic elimination from plasma, with a long terminal phase of 14 hours. The concentration of dFdCTP in mononuclear cells increases in proportion to the dose of dFdc infused up to 250 mg/m^2. Above this dose, the process shows saturation in accumulation of the triphosphate derivative.

Mechanism of Action

2′,2′-Difluoro-2′-deoxycytidine exerts its inhibitory activity on DNA synthesis through several distinct mechanisms. The accumulation of dFdCTP causes a reduction in the deoxyribonucleotide pools in both CCRF-CEM and HT-29 human tumor cells (164, 332). This reflects a direct inhibition of ribonucleotide reductase, caused mainly by dFdCDP; however, dFdCTP was not as inhibitory of the partially purified enzyme (164). Another important mechanism is the incorporation of dFdCTP into DNA; dFdCTP competes with dCTP for incorporation into the C sites of DNA as catalyzed by DNA polymerases α and ϵ. The primer extension pauses one deoxynucleotide after dFdCMP incorporation (185). Moreover, the exonuclease activity of polymerase ϵ was unable to excise nucleotides from DNA containing dFdCMP at either the 3′-end or at an internal position (185). The cytotoxic activity of dFdC strongly correlates with the amount of monophosphate that is incorporated into cellular DNA.

Incorporation of dFdc into RNA has been detected in murine colon 26–10 cells as well as human A2780 and CCRF-CEM cells (313). Although the extent of this incorporation was 2- to 10-fold less than that into DNA, it may play a role in cytotoxicity.

Inhibition of ribonucleotide reductase could have a self-potentiation effect on the inhibitory activity of this drug. The activity of deoxycytidine kinase, which is required for the phosphorylation of dFdc, is regulated by dCTP levels; therefore, a decrease in dCTP pools likely will lead to increased dFdc activation (161). dCTP also is required as an activator of dCMP deaminase, an enzyme that is critical for the catabolism of dFdc nucleotides; thus, a reduction in dCTP could slow the deamination process and prolong the half-life of dFdc nucleotides (163). Finally, dCTP competes with dFdCTP for incorporation into DNA by polymerases α and ϵ, and lower dCTP levels also could enhance dFdc incorporation into DNA as well as increase its inhibitory effect on cell proliferation (185).

To date, only one example of resistance to dFdc has been reported (312). Human ovarian carcinoma A2780 cells that were exposed to increasing concentrations of dFdc became highly resistant to the drug and cross-resistant to Ara-C and 2-chlorodeoxyadenosine and modestly resistant to doxorubicin, vincristine, and *cis*-platinum. Resistant cells did not possess deoxycytidine kinase activity; therefore, they were not able to phosphorylate dFdc as well as the other two nucleoside analogues. Western blot analyses of the cell extract using a polyclonal, anti-deoxycytidine kinase antibody could not detect this protein in the resistant subline.

Purine Analogues

INTRODUCTION

The original syntheses of purine antimetabolites focused on isosteric replacement of oxygen, carbon, or nitrogen in the purine ring, and they were predicated on the same logic as that used for pyrimidines (171). C-N or O-N substitutions gave 8-azaguanine and 2–6-diaminopurine. The first clinically useful agent, however, was 6-mercaptopurine (6-MP) (39), in which the 6-OH of hypoxanthine was replaced with a thiol group (Fig. 61.8). Subsequently, the equivalent analogue of guanine, 6-thioguanine, was prepared (116). Two glutamine analogues, 6-diazo-5-oxo-L-norleucine and azaserine, also made major contributions to our understanding of the purine biosynthetic pathways during that period, but these were not found to be clinically useful (5). Studies of these initial analogues established many of the relevant issues addressed in the subsequent development of purine and pyrimidine analogues (245, 278, 298).

Early studies with 6-MP in model systems quickly demonstrated dependence of the inhibitory activity on metabolic conversion to the corresponding analogue nucleotides by the identification of metabolites and characterization of resistance mechanisms (115). Equally important to the activity

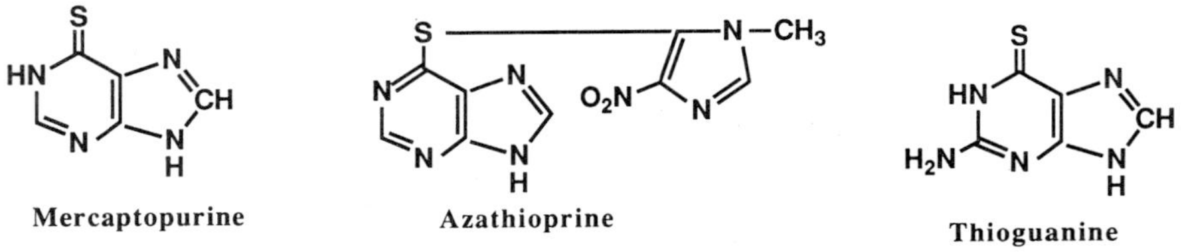

Mercaptopurine

Azathioprine

Thioguanine

Figure 61.8. Purine antimetabolites.

of many purine analogues has been an understanding of the catabolic reactions that limit their availability. Xanthine oxidase, which inactivates 6-MP and thioguanine (278), and adenosine deaminase (4), which is the target for deoxycoformycin and limits the action of arabinosyl adenosine, are of particular relevance.

Two more recently developed purine analogues, acyclovir and ganciclovir, are acyclic nucleoside derivatives and valuable antiviral agents. Along with arabinosyl adenine, these agents are activated by kinase reactions, but they exert their effects on the same spectrum of biochemical reactions as exerted by purine base analogues. Their role in cancer therapy remains to be established.

6-MERCAPTOPURINE

6-Mercaptopurine was among the first purine analogue that demonstrated antineoplastic activity, and it remains useful in the treatment of acute leukemia (354). This derivative of hypoxanthine is a relatively insoluble, amphoteric compound that is stable except in alkaline solutions. Metabolic activation primarily occurs by reaction with 1-pyrophosphoryl-ribose-5-phosphate (PRPP) via hypoxanthine-guanine pyrophosphorylase (HGPRT) to form 6-MP riboside 5′-phosphate, more properly called thioinosine monophosphate (TIMP) (112).

Thioinosine monophosphate (TIMP) is believed to exert its major effect on purine nucleotide metabolism by inhibition of the first step in purine biosynthesis, the formation of 1-NH_2-ribose-5-PO_4, via a pseudo-feedback inhibition in which TIMP mimics the regulatory action of adenine or guanine nucleoside monophosphates (128, 169, 339). An early precursor of purine biosynthesis, 5-amino imidazol-4-carboxamide, which can be converted to the corresponding ribonucleotide, protects cells in culture against the inhibition of growth by 6-MP. This finding is consistent with the view that the primary action is limitation of an early step in de novo synthesis. TIMP also blocks the subsequent metabolism of inosinic acid, which is the initial purine nucleotide, to adenylic acid by inhibiting adenosylsuccinate synthase (112). Similarly, synthesis of guanine nucleotides is reduced by inhibition of the oxidation of inosinic acid to xanthylic acid. TIMP is not incorporated into nucleic acids as such, but minor amounts are converted to thioguanylic acid, which is incorporated into both RNA and DNA. It has not been established, however, that this incorporation is significant to the toxic or antineoplastic actions of 6-MP. A summary of 6-MP metabolism is presented in Figure 61.9.

6-Mercaptopurine is generally administered orally (90 mg/m^2) for several weeks. Absorption is variable, incomplete, and associated with a half-life of 20 to 45 minutes in plasma, where it is minimally bound to serum proteins (387). The rapid turnover largely results from oxidation by xanthine oxidase, which converts it to inactive thiouric acid, the primary urinary excretion product (114). In patients who are receiving allopurinol to control uricemia, the dosage of 6-MP must be reduced by approximately 75% because drug catabolism is sharply reduced with the attendant risks of toxicity (14, 386). No selective advantage in tumor therapy is

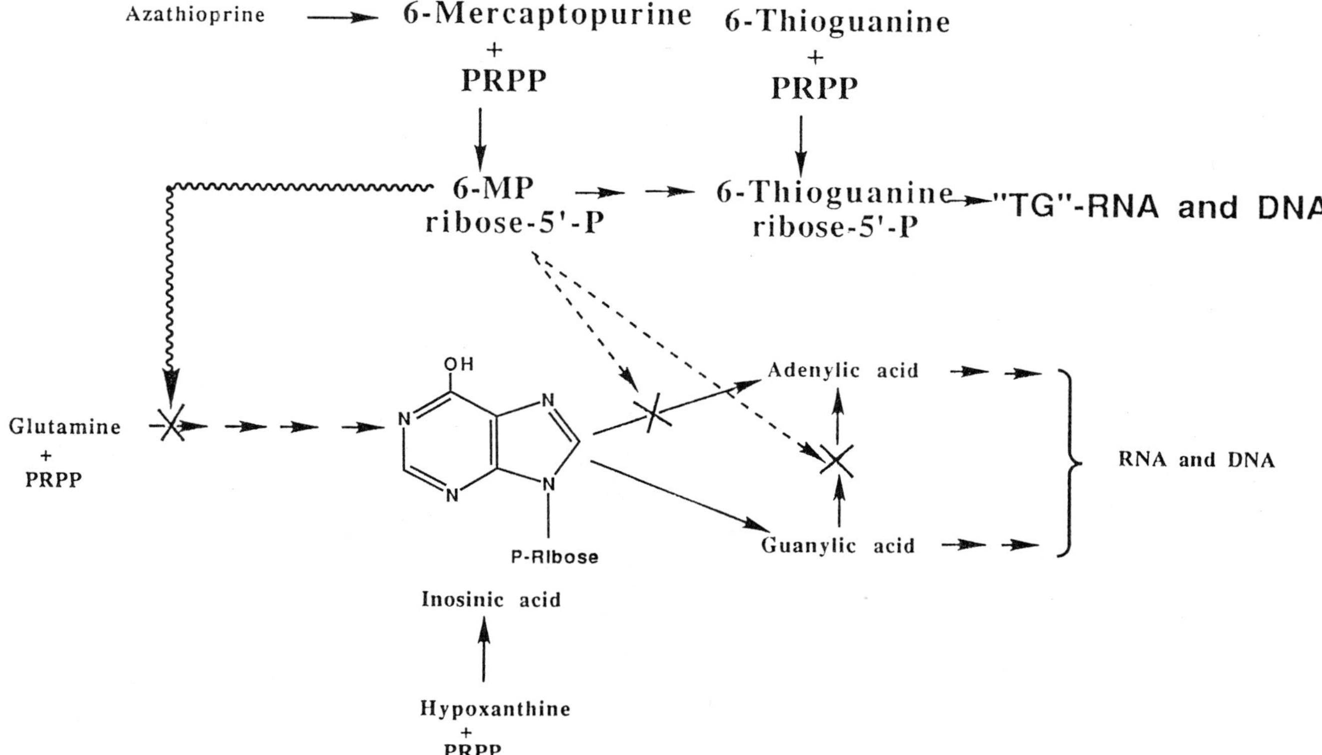

Figure 61.9. Metabolic activation and targets of thiopurines.

achieved by this combination. Another metabolite, the *S*-methyl derivative of 6-MP, is found in cells as methyl mercaptopurine ribonucleotide, where it inhibits purine metabolism; it is excreted in urine as methyl mercaptopurine riboside.

The dose-limiting toxicity of 6-MP is myelosuppression, which is slow in onset (2 to 4 weeks) and rapidly reversed after the dosage is either reduced or discontinued (124, 287). All formed elements (thrombocytes, granulocytes, and erythrocytes) can be affected. Although gastrointestinal mucositis or stomatitis is minimal, approximately 25% of treated patients experience nausea, vomiting, and anorexia, and a small number display hepatotoxicity (109).

Therapeutic action depends on formation of the nucleotide, 6-MP ribonucleoside monophosphate. In experimental tumor systems, resistance commonly is associated with a decreased rate of activation to the nucleotide form, resulting from deletion or modification of HGPRT activity. Limited studies in humans, however, suggest that resistance is caused by increased activity of a 5′-phosphatase that limits the concentration and duration of intracellular 6-MP ribonucleotide (321).

6-Mercaptopurine is effective in combination with prednisone for inducing remission in children with acute lymphoblastic leukemia. Currently, it is a regular component of consolidation and maintenance therapy for this disease (see Chapter 143). It also is of some value in adult acute lymphocytic leukemias (see Chapter 145). It no longer is commonly used in myeloid leukemias of adults, but it does have modest activity in combination therapy (see Chapter 142).

Although many 6-MP derivatives have been synthesized and evaluated in model systems, only one—azathioprine (ImuranR)—, is available at present. This methyl-nitro-imadazole derivative of the thiol group on 6-MP is cleaved in vivo, presumably by thiols, to liberate 6-MP. It generally is not used in cancer therapy, but it remains an important element of immunosuppressant therapy for allograft transplantation and selected autoimmune states (170).

THIOGUANINE

Thioguanine (Fig. 61.8) is the 6-thiol derivative of guanine corresponding to 6-MP, and also depends on activation via HGPRT (354). Unlike 6-MP, however, di- and triphosphates of thioguanine ribonucleotide are formed and incorporated into RNA. After conversion to thioguanine deoxynucleotide triphosphate, it can substitute for deoxyguanosine triphosphate (dGTP) in DNA polymerase reactions (213). This incorporation is thought to be the primary mechanism of cytotoxicity (259). Thioguanylate monophosphate is the predominant acid-soluble nucleotide, but it does not appear to exert the major effects on de novo purine synthesis that have been observed with 6-MP nor deplete pools of normal purine nucleotides.

Like 6-MP, thioguanine, after deamination to thioxanthine by guanase, is readily catabolized to thiouric acid by xanthine oxidase. *S*-Methylation also is observed, yielding *S*-methyl-thioguanine and thioxanthine (305). Dethiolation contributes to metabolism as well, as evidenced by the urinary excretion of $^{35}S\text{-}SO_4$ after administration of ^{35}S-thioguanine. The primary use of thioguanine is in acute myeloid leukemia, where it may be combined with arabinosyl cytosine. Recent studies question its value in this disease, however (105, 234). A summary of thioguanine metabolism is presented in Figure 61.8.

ALLOPURINOL

Allopurinol (4-hydroxypyrazalo-3,4-*d*-pyrimidine) is an important adjuvant to antineoplastic therapy (Fig. 61.10). This agent and its primary metabolite, oxypurinol, are potent inhibitors of xanthine oxidase (113, 344). As such, they limit the formation of uric acid from the degradation of purine nucleotides and nucleic acids. It is interesting to note that oxipurinol is formed by the target enzyme xanthine oxidase and is a potent inhibitor of this enzyme. In addition to this mechanism, allopurinol has been shown to inhibit purine nucleotide biosynthesis by feedback inhibition of the first reaction in the pathway and to deplete pyrophosphoryl ribose-5-PO_4, presumably by formation of the corresponding allopurinol and oxypurinol ribonucleotides (107). These nucleotides are inhibitors of orotidylate decarboxylation as well, and they result in the excretion of urinary orotate and orotidine (197). These actions may relate to the ability of allopurinol to selectively reduce the toxicity of FU to some normal tissues, as described previously.

Although it was originally synthesized as an antineoplastic agent, allopurinol is widely used in the treatment of hyperuricemia that is associated with gout and other metabolic disorders (308). Certain neoplastic states, particularly lympho- and myeloproliferative diseases, also generate hyperuricemia, and allopurinol is an effective means to avoid the associated episodes of gout or uric acid nephropathy (153). This is particularly important in leukemias, lymphomas, and in patients with other bulky disease when chemotherapy produces rapid tumor lysis and its attendant release of purine bases from the nucleic acids.

The elevation of hypoxanthine and xanthine concentrations in plasma by the inhibition of xanthine oxidase is less dangerous than elevated levels of uric acid. This is because these purines are more soluble and less likely to form stones or cause gout. Nevertheless, it generally is recommended that patients who are treated with allopurinol for hyperuricemia also be hydrated and alkalinized when uric acid concentrations rise significantly.

Oral doses of from 300 to 800 mg/d have been recommended and generally are well tolerated. Skin rashes and gastrointestinal disturbances are common and of increased frequency and severity when the allopurinol is given together with ampicillin, but, these effects rarely limit therapy (32). Severe drug-induced fever, vasculitis, and blood dyscrasias of a hypersensitive nature have infrequently occurred (337). Because allopurinol also reduces the rate of metabolic inactivation of oral 6-MP and azathioprine, doses of these purine antimetabolites must be reduced by 50 to 75% to avoid excessive toxicity (387). Oxidation by xanthine oxidase is the primary route of allopurinol metabolism and the relevant site action, but allopurinol also can inhibit the metabolism of drugs such as cyclophosphamide by the mixed function oxidases (367).

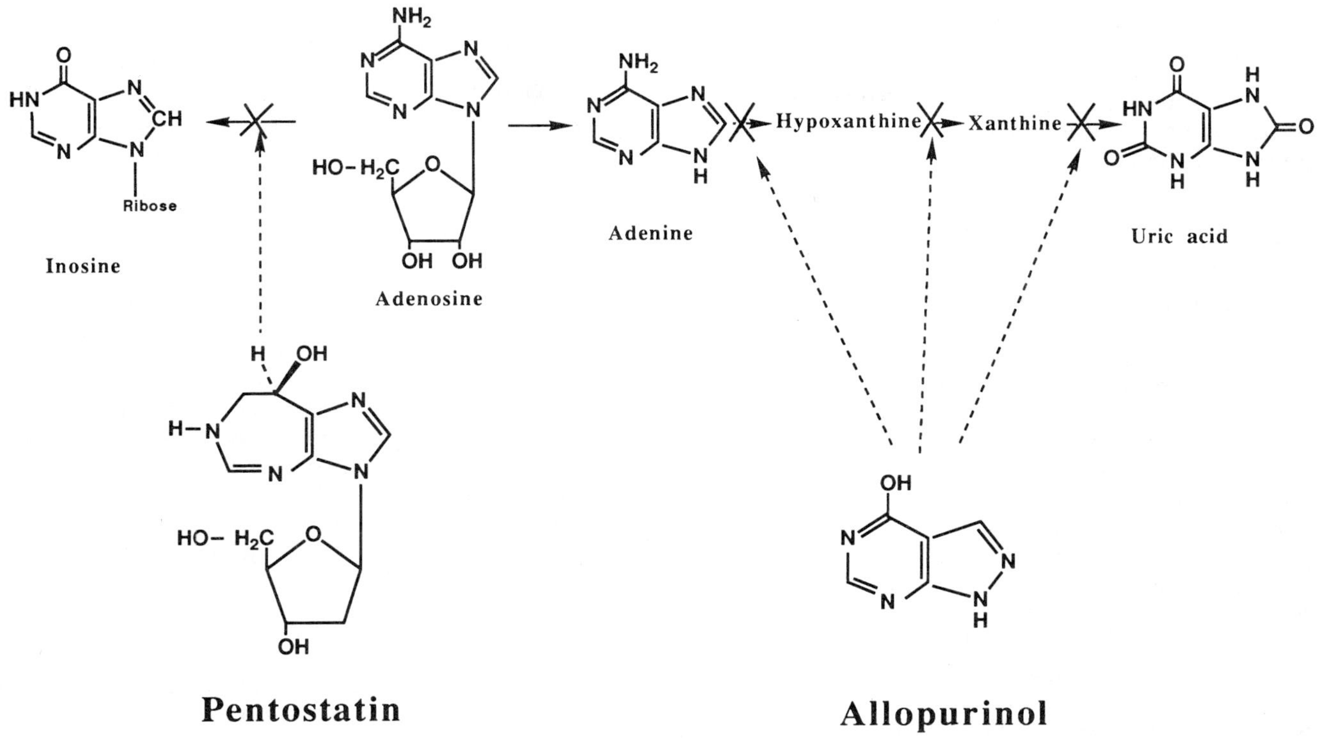

Figure 61.10. Inhibitors of purine nucleoside catabolism.

DEOXYCOFORMYCIN

Background

Deoxycoformycin (pentostatin) is a natural product first isolated in 1974 from the culture of *Streptomyces antibioticus* (Fig. 61.9) (328). Its structure mimics the transitional-state form of adenosine in an adenosine deaminase–catalyzed reaction, and it is one of the most potent inhibitors of adenosine deaminase ($K_i = 10^{-10}$–10^{-12} M depending on the source of the enzyme) (375). Because adenosine deaminase is not essential for cell growth in culture, this compound did not show antitumor activity in preclinical screenings.

The initial clinical development of deoxycoformycin centered on its activity as an adenosine deaminase inhibitor for the potentiation of adenosine arabinoside, which also was deaminated by adenosine deaminase to yield less toxic compounds. During early phase I studies, the profound lymphotoxic effect of deoxycoformycin was noted. Others described a congenital syndrome of severe combined immunodeficiency associated with low or undetectable levels of adenosine deaminase in lymphocytes (135), and these results suggested the importance of adenosine deaminase in lymphocyte function, leading to intensive development of deoxycoformycin as a single agent for the treatment of lymphoproliferative diseases.

The most responsive tumor identified is hairy-cell leukemia, in which durable remissions are achieved in over 90% of patients with a relatively brief course of treatment (see Chapter 148) (205, 345). Other responsive lymphoid diseases include chronic lymphocytic leukemia and prolymphocytic leukemia (see Chapter 147), mycosis fungoides (see Chapter 151), and acute T-cell leukemia/lymphoma (see Chapter 146) (93, 148). Considerable variation exists in the susceptibility of patients to deoxycoformycin toxicity. This includes immunosuppression (268, 270), CNS disturbances, impaired renal function, conjunctivitis, and muscle and joint pain. Impaired renal function and poor performance status place patients at high risk for toxicity even with low dosages of this drug.

Metabolism

Deoxycoformycin enters the cell through the facilitated-diffusion nucleoside carrier. It can be phosphorylated to mono-, di-, and triphosphate nucleotides, and significant incorporation into DNA, but not RNA, has been observed (205). Adenosine kinase and deoxycytidine kinase (335) do not appear to be responsible for the initial phosphorylation, but reversal of the 5′-nucleotidase reaction is a potential basis for nucleotide formation. Definitive statements cannot be made about the enzymology of deoxycoformycin metabolism at this time.

Mechanisms of Action and Resistance

The primary site of action is the inhibition of adenosine deaminase. Because of the inhibition of adenosine deaminase in vivo, deoxyadenosine and adenosine cannot be catabolized efficiently. Consequently, deoxyadenosine phosphorylated metabolites accumulate in many types of cells (241). This imbalance in adenosine derivatives is known to be toxic to cells, and the antitumor activity of deoxycoformycin may result from the combination of direct effects of deoxycoformycin and its metabolites as well as the expanded pools of deoxyadenosine.

The failure of deoxyadenosine to accumulate in cultures treated with deoxycoformycin is why deoxycoformycin was not identified as a potential antitumor compound in cell-culture systems. The degree of deoxyadenosine triphosphate (dATP) accumulation correlated well with cell death caused by deoxycoformycin. Thus, dATP, which is known to be an allosteric inhibitor of ribonucleotide reductase, could result in growth inhibition by generating of an imbalance of deoxynucleotide triphosphate pools. However, additional sites of action for both deoxycoformycin and deoxyadenosine are suggested by the observation that deoxycoformycin and deoxyadenosine are cytotoxic to nondividing cells, which do not require the function of ribonucleotide reductase. One potential site is the depletion of nicotinamide adenine dinucleotide (NAD) in deoxycoformycin- and deoxyadenosine-treated cells. NAD is required for poly-ADP ribosylation, a reaction that is essential to maintain the integrity of DNA and its repair process. Depletion of NAD could reduce the capacity for DNA repair, a constant process in cells, and cause DNA breaks as well as cell death (327, 385).

The second suggested site is inhibition of S-adenosyl homocysteine hydrolase by deoxyadenosine (162, 165). Inhibition of this enzyme decreases the capacity of cells to perform transmethylation, a reaction that is critical for certain macromolecular functions. This mechanism does not require deoxyadenosine to be phosphorylated, and it may play an important role in the toxicity of deoxycoformycin to nonproliferating tissues such as in the liver and CNS.

Deoxycoformycin and deoxyadenosine also decrease ATP levels in some cell systems. In mice, hemolysis after treatment with deoxycoformycin is related to ATP depletion. Deoxycoformycin has also been shown to form phosphorylated metabolites that can be incorporated into DNA; whether these metabolites contribute to deoxycoformycin action, however, is not clear (270).

The mechanism of resistance to deoxycoformycin has not been defined because deoxycoformycin is not cytotoxic in cell culture. The action of deoxycoformycin in vivo results from the combined action of deoxycoformycin and deoxyadenosine, so the mechanism of cellular resistance to deoxyadenosine should be applicable. This could include adenosine kinase deficiency or altered quality or quantity of ribonucleotide reductase.

2-FLUOROADENINE ARABINOSIDE-5′-PHOSPHATE

Background

In the search for more effective compounds than adenine arabinoside (araA, vidarabine), which has limited clinical usefulness because of its rapid deamination by adenosine deaminase, 2-fluoroadenosine arabinoside (fludarabine; 9-β-D-arabinofuranosyl-2-fluoradenine) was synthesized. It has been found to be relatively resistant to adenosine deaminase and has impressive antitumor activities in vivo as well as in cell culture (38). Its limited solubility and consequent difficulties in formulation, led to the synthesis of a pro-drug, the 5′-monophosphate of 2-F-araA (Fludara I.V.).

Fludara I.V. entered clinical trials in 1982, and it is one of the most active agents in the treatment of chronic lymphocytic leukemia (CLL) (149, 196). A high level of activity also has been observed in a variety of indolent lymphoproliferative neoplasms, including low-grade non-Hodgkin's lymphoma, cutaneous T-cell lymphoma, macroglobinemia, and hairy cell leukemia (66, 172, 194). The dose-limiting toxicity during phase I trials is myelosuppression and leukopenia. Delayed onset of severe neurotoxicity also was noted with doses of 96 mg/m^2/d for 5 to 7 days. Other toxicities noted during phase 1 trials included somnolence, mild to moderate nausea and vomiting, and rare but reversible interstitial pneumonitis. Fludara I.V. is converted by phosphatases to 2-F-araA within several minutes of injection; it is not further catabolized in plasma (85).

Metabolism

Transport of F-araA into mouse L1210 cells is mediated by nonconcentrative, high- and low-affinity systems (338). In contrast to these leukemia cells, epithelial crypt cells from mouse intestine possess only a low-affinity system (21), and this difference in transport could be partly responsible for the favorable therapeutic index of 2F-araA against sensitive tumor cells in mice. In future human studies, the potential role of transport systems in determining sensitivity to 2F-araA should be considered. Once 2F araA is taken up by cells, it is phosphorylated to 2 fluoroadenine arabinoside monophosphate (2-F araAMP), not like araA as a substrate of adenosine kinase but by cytoplasmic deoxycytidine kinase (37). Tumor cells lacking cytoplasmic deoxycytidine kinase are resistant to F-araA. Intracellular F-araAMP can be further phosphorylated to the diphosphate F-araADP, but it is not clear which enzyme is responsible for this reaction. AMP kinases likely may be responsible for the further phosphorylation of F-araADP to the triphosphate F-araATP. Nucleoside diphosphate kinases may be the predominant enzyme species responsible for this conversion. F-araATP can be incorporated into DNA in competition with dATP by DNA polymerases. Although DNA polymerases α, β, δ, and γ are all capable of using F-araATP as a substrate, DNA polymerase α has a greater affinity for F-araATP than do other DNA polymerases (296, 359). Once F-araAMP is incorporated into the terminus of the growing DNA chain, the next step of elongation is retarded, regardless of which DNA polymerase is employed (186, 359).

In addition, F-araA also has been shown to be incorporated into RNA (187, 346) but which RNA polymerase is responsible has not been established. The incorporation of F-araA into poly(A+) RNA was 12-fold greater than that into poly (A) RNA. A summary of the metabolism of 2F-araA is shown in Figure 61.11.

Investigations of F-araA as a modulator of ara-C therapy are currently underway. When F-araA is given before ara-C,

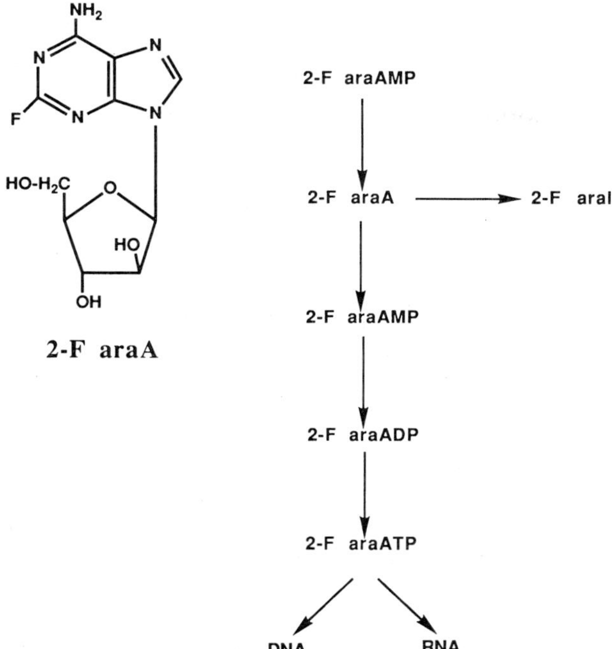

Figure 61.11. Structure and metabolism of 2-fluoro-arabinosyladenine (2-F-Ara A). 2-F-araI represents the dominant inosine derivative.

an increase in the accumulation of ara-CTP occurs in leukemic lymphocytes (142). This modulation of ara-C anabolism probably results from an indirect effect of F-ara-CTP on deoxycytidine kinase that relates to a reduction in the deoxynucleotide pools regulating the enzyme. It also may reflect a direct effect by F-ara-CTP on the activity of deoxycytidine kinase (141, 142). The in vitro accumulation of ara-CTP also has been shown in the lymphocytes of patients with chronic lymphocytic leukemia treated with this sequential combination (143). The results of a clinical study in individuals who are refractory to F-ara-A therapy show partial or minor responses in approximately 35% of patients (143).

Mechanism of Action

The major site of growth inhibition by F-araA is the inhibition of DNA synthesis. Treatment of cells with F-araA is associated with the accumulation of cells at the G1/S phase boundary and in S phase; thus, it is a cell cycle S phase–specific drug. Incorporation of the active metabolite, F-araATP, retards DNA chain elongation. The degree of incorporation of the analog nucleotide depends not only on the type of DNA polymerase but also on the amount of intracellular dATP that competes with F-araATP for incorporation.

Among DNA polymerases in human cells, polymerase α, which is the critical enzyme in nuclear DNA synthesis, is more susceptible to the incorporation of F-araATP. A consequence of this analogue nucleotide incorporation is the retardation of DNA-chain elongation.

F-araATP also is a potent inhibitor of ribonucleotide reductase, the key enzyme responsible for the formation of dATP. This causes a decrease of deoxynucleotides in 2F-araA treated cells, which enhances the incorporation of F-araATP into DNA. This may be considered to be "self-potentiation" of the inhibition of DNA synthesis by F-araATP. In addition, F-araATP was found to be an inhibitor of DNA primase, which is responsible for Okazaki fragment synthesis (274), another important step in DNA synthesis. The inhibition of RNA primer formation for DNA synthesis by F-araATP was recently demonstrated as well (56), but the inhibition of Okazaki fragment formation by F-araATP could conceivably play a role in the inhibition of DNA synthesis by F-araA. In addition, F-araA can inhibit mitochondrial DNA synthesis at concentrations similiar to those that cause cytotoxicity; however, such inhibition does not affect cell growth for several cell generations (56). Thus, the cytotoxicity of F-araA, which usually is estimated by the continuous exposure of cells to drugs for three to four generations, likely does not result from the inhibition of mitochondrial DNA. Also, it has been reported that incubation of normal lymphocytes for 24 hours with 10 μM, but not 1-μM, caused a decrease in both cytoplasmic NAD and ATP concentrations that could be correlated with a decrease in cellular viability (34). The mechanism for the depletion of NAD and ATP by F-araA is not clear, and whether the inhibition of mitochondrial DNA synthesis by F-araA or depletion of NAD and ATP is responsible for the delayed onset of F-araA toxicity observed clinically has not yet been established.

Resistance to F-araA may occur because of decreased uptake, lack of deoxycytidine kinase, increased intracellular concentration of dATP, decreased susceptibility to the activity of ribonucleotide reductase, decreased affinity of DNA polymerase for F-araATP, or increased efficiency of the removal of F-araATP from the 3′ terminus where incorporated into DNA. The potential role of the 3′ and 5′ exonuclease activity of DNA polymerase D and other 3′ and 5′ exonuclease activities in removal of incorporated F-araAMP remains to be defined as a possible mechanism of resistance.

2-CHLORODEOXYADENOSINE

Background

The rationale for the development of 2-chlorodeoxyadenosine, or cladribine (Cl-dAdo, cladribine), was that death of lymphocytes in patients with adenosine deaminase deficiency that was associated with the accumulation of deoxynucleotides. This deoxyadenosine analogue was selected for its resistance to adenosine deaminase. Its specific action on lymphoid cells is attributed to the high level of deoxycytidine kinase and low 5′-nucleotidase activity in these cells (49, 50, 100). This compound is highly cytotoxic to a variety of cell lines in culture, and it has potent antileukemic activity in mice (52, 184). Recently, cladribine was also shown to have potent and lasting effects in the treatment of low-grade B-cell neoplasms such as chronic lymphocytic leukemia, non-Hodgkin's lymphoma, and hairy-cell leukemia (51, 289, 290). In addition, Cl-dAdo has demonstrated clinical activity against acute myeloid leukemia in children, including those with leukemic blast cells in the CNS (317) and in T-cell lymphoproliferative disorders (265). The spectrum of clinical activity is similar to that of Fludara I.V.; however, a few patients who do not respond to F-ara-A are sensitive to

Cl-dAdo (264). The major toxicity encountered is bone marrow suppression that is associated with severe infections. The degree of suppression relates to the rate of administration, cumulative dosage, and tumor burden at the start of therapy (51).

Metabolism

The mechanism of transport for cladribine into a variety of human hematopoietic cell lines was explored using nucleoside transport inhibitors such as dipyridamole and nitrobenzyl thioinosine (NBTI). The transport mechanism appears to be different in different cell lines, an observation based on their differential response to nucleoside transport inhibitors (18). Both NBTI-sensitive and -insensitive nucleoside transporters are involved. Once Cl-dAdo enters cells, it can be phosphorylated by dCyd kinase to 2-Cl-dAMP (150). Subsequently, 2-Cl-dAMP is phosphorylated to 2-Cl-dADP and then to 2-Cl-dATP. The enzymes involved, however, are not established. As 2-Cl-dATP, it can be incorporated into DNA through the action of DNA polymerases by competing with dATP (150). The structure and 2-chlorodeoxyadenosine metabolism of 2-Cl-dAdo are shown in Figure 61.12.

Mechanisms of Action and Resistance

2-Cl-dAdo can inhibit DNA synthesis in growing cells as well as DNA repair in resting cells (183). When growing cells were treated with 2-Cl-dAdo, an accumulation of cells in S-phase was observed, suggesting that inhibition of DNA synthesis could be responsible for the cell-killing effect of the drug. The active metabolite is 2-Cl-dATP which can compete with dATP to be incorporated into the 3′-end of the growing DNA chain. Elongation beyond the incorporated analogue was significantly retarded, and this could partly contribute to its inhibitory activity against DNA synthesis. Furthermore, 2-Cl-dATP is a potent inhibitor of ribonucleotide reductase (273). Levels of intracellular deoxynucleoside triphosphates were found to decrease in cells after exposure to 2-Cl-dAdo (150), which also could contribute to its antitumor activity.

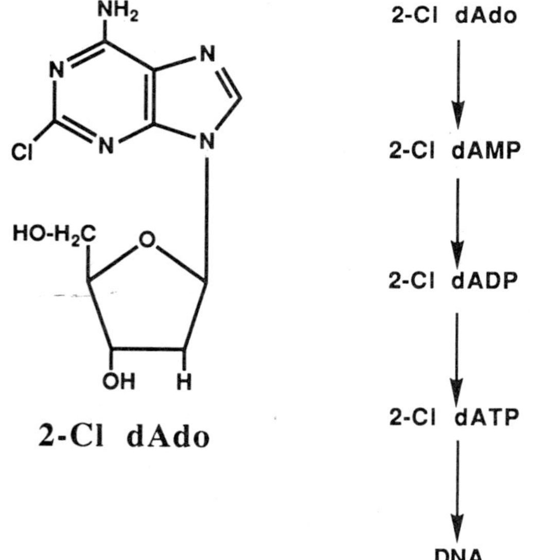

Figure 61.12. Structure and metabolism of 2-chloro-deoxyadenosine (2-C1-dAdo).

The mechanism of resistance is not clear, but it could be similar to that of 2-F-araA. It should be pointed out that although 2-F-araA and 2-Cl-dAdo share many similar features, there are differences in metabolism and mechanisms of action as well.

HYDROXYUREA

Background

Although hydroxyurea was first synthesized in 1869 (102), its biologic activity was not recognized until 60 years later, when it was discovered that hydroxyurea could produce leukopenia, anemia, and megaloblastic changes in the bone marrow of rabbits (310). This simple molecule (Fig. 61.13) has been evaluated in a number of types of cancer, but its principal uses are in myeloproliferative diseases. Currently, it is an initial therapy of choice for chronic myelogenous leukemia; it also is used as therapy for polycythemia vera and hypereosinophilic syndrome. Activity against solid tumors has been demonstrated, but in these cases, it generally is used in combination with other anticancer agents or with radiation (99). A recent report also indicated the ability of hydroxyurea to inhibit human immunodeficiency type I DNA synthesis in activated blood lymphocytes either alone or in combination with zidovudine or dideoxyinosine (ddI), suggesting a possible antiviral application for this compound (133).

Hydroxyurea can be taken orally, and the half-life in plasma is approximately 4 hours (24). It readily crosses the blood-brain barrier. It is excreted predominantly in urine, but the interpatient variability is significant. The full extent and significance of hydroxyurea metabolism in humans has not been well established. It can be degraded by intestinal bacterial urease to form hydroxylamine (NH_2OH), which can interact with acetylcoenzyme A to form acetohydroxamic acid; this metabolite is found in the plasma of patients receiving hydroxyurea therapy (130).

The dose-limiting toxicity of hydroxyurea is myelosuppression. This results from inhibition of DNA synthesis in bone marrow. Toxicity begins within 2 to 5 days, and its duration is short once the drug is discontinued. Gastrointestinal side effects frequently are seen but rarely require discontinuation of therapy at the doses commonly used. Some dermatologic changes such as hyperpigmentation also can occur in patients after extended therapy (99).

Mechanism of Action and Resistance

Hydroxyurea is considered to enter cells by passive diffusion (350). It inhibits cellular DNA synthesis through the inhibition of ribonucleotide reductase, which is the key enzyme

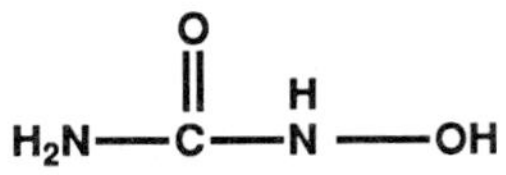

$$H_2N-\overset{O}{\overset{\|}{C}}-\overset{H}{N}-OH$$

Figure 61.13. Hydroxyurea.

responsible for the synthesis of deoxynucleotides (i.e., the building blocks of DNA (81)). The substrates for this reaction are the four ribonucleoside diphosphates; other substrates of the reaction include the diphosphonucleotides of fluoruridine, azacytidine, and thioguanosine (5-FUDP, 5-azaCDP, and 6-ThioGDP). The activity of ribonucleotide reductase is highly regulated by the intracellular concentration of ribonucleoside and deoxyribonucleoside triphosphates. Two models, sequential and intercalating, have been proposed for the interplay of ribonucleotide reductase and deoxynucleoside triphosphates (263). The metabolites of deoxynucleoside analogues such as 2F-araATP and araATP are potent inhibitors of this enzyme as well. The activity of this enzyme plays a key role in controlling the intracellular concentrations of deoxynucleotide triphosphates; thus, it can influence the activation or incorporation of deoxynucleoside antimetabolites such as araC, FUdR, and 2F-araA into DNA.

Inhibition of ribonucleotide reductase by hydroxyurea would not affect the incorporation of these antimetabolites and, therefore, could potentiate their action. Ribonucleotide reductase is composed of two types of protein subunits, M1 and M2. These two proteins are coded by two different chromosomes. M1 protein, which is coded by chromosome 11 and has a molecular weight of 170 KD, does not vary with cell cycle and is responsible for the interaction with nucleotides (35, 229). M2 protein, which is coded by a gene on chromosome 2 in close proximity to the ornithine decarboxylase gene, has a molecular weight of 88 KD and fluctuates throughout the cell cycle, with peak activity in the S phase. The alteration of ribonucleotide reductase activity through the cell cycle primarily is controlled by the amount of M2 protein that binds a stoichiometric amount of iron and a stable organic free radical localized to a tyrosine residue (119, 121, 383). Hydroxyurea inhibits ribonucleotide reductase through inactivation of the tyrosyl free radical on the M2 subunit. This inactivation can be partially prevented by ferrous iron (6). The required concentration of hydroxyurea to inhibit human ribonucleotide reductase by 50% is approximately 0.5 μM.

Because of the inhibition of ribonucleotide reductase by hydroxyurea, pools of deoxynucleotide triphosphates decrease, with concomitant inhibition of DNA synthesis. The cytotoxicity of hydroxyurea is dosage and time dependent. Most cells are accumulated in the S phase and at the G1-S boundary under the influence of hydroxyurea (202, 249).

Cells can become resistant to hydroxyurea because of increased ribonucleotide reductase activity, primarily resulting from increased levels of M2 protein. Levels of M1 protein increase only when high levels of resistance to hydroxyurea are generated. These increases of M1 or M2 proteins generally reflect the overexpression of the proteins because of gene amplification (68, 76, 216, 230, 378). Recently, a human KB cell line that was resistant to hydroxyurea because of gene amplification of the M2 subunit, increased concentrations of M2 mRNA and protein, and increased ribonucleotide reductase activity was found to express collateral sensitivity to 6-thioguanine. The mechanism responsible for this supersensitivity is believed to be an elevated conversion of 6-thioguanine to its triphosphate form (384). As previously hypothesized, alternating use of hydroxyurea with antimetabolites such 6-thioguanine warrants further clinical exploration in the treatment of cancer (63).

References

1. Abbruzzese JL, Grunewald R, Weeks EA, Gravel D, Adams T, Norwak B, Mineishi S, Tarassoff P, Satterlee W, Raber MN, Plunkett W. A phase I clinical, plasma and cellular pharmacology study of Gemcitabine. J Clin Oncol 1991;9:491.
2. Abratt RP, Bezwoda WR, Falkson G, Goedhals L, Hacking D, Rugg TA. Efficacy and safety profile of gemcitabine in non-small cell lung cancer: a phase II study. J Clin Oncol 1994;12:1535.
3. Adams RL, Burdon RH. DNA methylation in eukaryotes. CRC Crit Rev Biochem 1982;13:349.
4. Agarwal RP, Spector T, Parks RE Jr. Tight-binding inhibitors: IV. Inhibition of adenosine deaminase by various inhibitors. Biochem Pharmacol 1977;26:359.
5. Ahluwalia GS, Grem JL, Hao Z, Cooney D. Metabolism and action of amino acid analog anti-cancer agents. Pharmacol Ther 1990;46:243.
6. Akerblom L, Ehrenberg A, Graslsund A, Lankinen H, Reichard P, Thelander L. Overproduction of the free radical of ribonucleotide reductase in hydroxyurea-resistant mousefibroblast 3T6 cells. Proc Natl Acad Sci USA 1981;78:2159.
7. Albert A, Brown DJ. Purine studies. Part I.Stability to acid and alkali. Solubility. Ionization. Comparison with pteridines. J Chem Soc, Part II:2060 1954.
8. Alberto P, Mermillod B, Wever W, Joss R, Cavalli F. A randomized comparison of doxifluridine and fluorouracil in advanced colorectal cancer. Proc Am Soc Clin Oncol 1986;5:94.
9. Anderson N, Lokich J, Bern M, Wallach S, Moore C, Williams D. A phase I clinical trial of combined fluoropyrimidines with leucovorin in a 14-day infusion. Demonstration of biochemical modulation. Cancer 1989;63:233.
10. Ansfield FJ, Kallas GJ, Singson JP. Phase I-II studies of oral segafur (Ftorafur). J Clin Oncol 1983;1:107.
11. Ansfield R, Klotz J, Nealon T, Ramirez G, Minton J, Hill G, Wilson W, Davis H Jr, Cornell G. A phase III study comparing the clinical utility of four regimens of 5-fluorouracil. Cancer 1977;39:34.
12. Ardalan D, Singh G, Silberman H. A randomized Phase I and II study of Short-Term infusion of high-dose fluorouracil with or without n-(phosphonacetyl)-L-aspartic acid in patients with advanced pancreatic colorectal cancers. J Clin Oncol 1988;6:1053.
13. Armstrong RD, Diasio RB. Metabolism and biological activity of 5′-deoxy-5-fluorouridine, a novel fluoropyrimidine. Cancer Res 1980;40:3333.
14. Ascione FJ. Allopurinol with mercaptopurine. Drug Ther 1977;7:69.
15. Au C, Schnider W. The role of low-dosage cytosine arabinoside and aggressive chemotherapy in advanced myelodysplastic syndromes. Cancer 1989;64:1812.
16. Au JL, Rustum YM, Ledesma EJ, Mittelman A, Greaven PJ. Clinical pharmacological studies of concurrent infusion of 5-fluorouracil and thymidine in treatment of colorectal carcinoma. Cancer Res 1982;42:2930.
17. Au JL, Wu AT, Friedman MA, Sadee W. Pharmacokinetics and metabolism of ftorafur in man. Cancer Treat Rep 1979;63:343.
18. Avery TL, Rehg JE, Lumm WC, Harwood FC, Santana VM, Blakley RL. Biochemical pharmacology of 2-chlorodeoxyadenosine in malignant human hematopoietic cell lines and therapeutic effects of 2-bromodeoxyadenosine in drug combinations in mice. Cancer Res 1989;49:4972.
19. Baccanari DP, Davis ST, Knick VC, Spector T. 5-Ethynyluracil (776C85): a potent modulator of the pharmacokinetics and antitumor efficacy of 5-fluorouracil. Proc Natl Acad Sci USA 1993;90:11064.
20. Bapat AR, Zarow C, Danenberg PV. Human leukemic cells resistant to 5-fluoro-2′-deoxyuridine contain a thymidylate synthase with a lower affinity for nucleotides. J Biol Chem 1983;258:4130.
21. Barrueco JR, Jacobsen DM, Chang CH, Brockman RW, Sirotnak FM. Proposed mechanism of therapeutic selectivity of 9-β-D-arabinofuranosyl-2-fluoradenine against murine leukemia based upon lower capacities for transport and phosphorylation in proliferative intestinal epithelium compared to tumor cells. Cancer Res 1987;47:700.
22. Beardmore TD, Kelley WN. Effects of allopurinol and oxipurinol on pyrimidine biosynthesis in man. In Purine Metabolism in Man. Edited by O Sperling, S DeVries, JB Wyngaarden. New York: Plenum, 1974, p 609.
23. Beisler J. Isolation, characterization, and properties of labile hydrolysis product of the antitumor nucleoside 5-azacytidine. J Med Chem 1978;21:204.
24. Belt RJ, Haas CD, Kennedy J, Taylor S. Studies of hydroxyurea administered by continuous infusion: toxicity, pharmacokinetics, and cell synchronization. Cancer 1980;46:455.
25. Berger SH, Hakala MT. Relationship of dUMP and free FdUMP pools to inhibition to thymidylate synthase by 5-fluorouracil. Mol Pharmacol 1984;25:303.
26. Berger SH, Jenh, C-H, Johnson LF, Berger FG. Thymidylate synthase overproduction and gene amplification in fluorodeoxyuridine-resistant human cells. Mol Pharmacol 1985;28:461.
27. Bertheault-Cvitkovic, Levi F, Soussan S, Brienza S, Adam R, Itzakhi M, Misset JL, Bismuth H.Circadian rhythm-modulated chemotherapy with high dose 5-fluorouracil: a pilot study in patients with pancreatic adenocarcinoma. Eur J Cancer 1993;29:1851.
28. Bertino JR, Mini E. Does Modulation of 5-Fluorouracil by Metabolites or Antimetabolites Work in the Clinic? In New Avenues in Developmental Cancer Chemotherapy. Edited by DS Martin. New York: Academic Press, 1987.
29. Bertino JR, Mini E, Fernandes DJ. Sequential methotrexate and 5-fluorouracil: Mechanisms of synergy. Semin Oncol 1983;10:2.
30. Bhalla K, Birkhofer M, Bhalla M, Lutzky J, Hindenburg A, Cole J, Ince C. A phase I study of a combination of allopurinol, 5-fluorouracil and leucovorin followed by hydroxyurea in patients with advanced gastrointestinal and breast cancer. Am. J Clin Oncol 1991;14:509.
31. Bjarnason GA, Kerr IG, Doyle N, Macdonald M, Sone M. Phase I study of 5-fluorouracil and leucovorin by a 14-day circadian infusion in metastatic adenocarcinoma patients. Cancer Chemother Pharm 1993;33:221.
32. Boston Collaborative Drug Surveillance Program Excess of ampicillin rash associated with allopurinol or hyperuricemia. N Engl J Med 1972;286:505.
33. Bowen D, Diasio RB, Goldman ID. Distinguishing between membrane transport and intracellular metabolism of fluorodeoxyuridine in Ehrlich ascites tumor cells by appli-

cation of kinetic and high-performance liquid chromatographic techniques. J Biol Chem 1979;254:5333.

34. Brager PM, Grever MR. 9-β-d-Arabinofuranosyl-2-fluoradenine reduces NAD in normal lymphocytes and neoplastic cells in CLL. Proc Am Assoc Cancer Res 1986;27: 21.
35. Brissenden JR, Caras I, Thelander L, Francke U. The structural gene for the M1 subunit of ribonucleotide reductase maps to chromosome II, band 15 in human and to chromosome 7 in mouse. Exp Cell Res 1988;174:302.
36. Brockman RW. Mechanism of resistance to anticancer agents. Adv. Cancer Res 1963;7:129.
37. Brockman RW, Cheng YC, Schabel FM Jr, Montgomery JA. Metabolism and chemotherapeutic activity of 9-β-D-arabinofuranosyl-2-fluoradenine against murine leukemia L1210 and evidence for its phosphorylation by deoxycytidine kinase. Cancer Res 1980;40:3610.
38. Brockman RW, Schabel FM Jr, Montgomery JA. Biologic activity of 9-β-D-arabinofuranosyl-2-fluoradenine, a metabolically stable analog of 9-β-N-arabinofuranosyl-adenine. Biochem Pharmacol 1977;26:2193.
39. Burchenal JH, Murphy ML, Ellison RR, Sykes MP, Tan TC, Leone LA, Darnofsky DA, Craver LF, Dargeon HW, Rhoads CP. Clinical evaluation of a new antimetabolite, 6-mercaptopurine, in the treatment of leukemia and allied diseases. Blood 1953;8:965.
40. Burns RE, Beland SS. Effect of biological time on the determination of the LD50 of 5-fluorouracil in mice. Pharmacology 1984;28:296.
41. Cadman E, Davis L, Heimer R. Enhanced 5-fluorouracil nucleotide formation following methotrexate: biochemical explanation for drug synergism. Science 1979;205: 1135.
42. Cadman EC, Dix DE, Handschumacher RE. Clinical, biological and biochemical effects of pyrazofurin. Cancer Res 1978;38:682.
43. Calabresi P, Chabner BA. Antineoplastic agents. In The Pharmacological Basis of Therapeutics, 8th ed. Edited by AG Gilman, TW Rall, AS Nies, P Taylor. New York: Pergamon Press, 1990, pp 1231–1232.
44. Cao S, Rustum YM, Spector T. 5-Ethynyluracil (776C85): modulation of 5-fluorouracil efficacy and therapeutic index in rats bearing advanced colorectal carcinoma. Cancer Res 1994;54:1507.
45. Capizzi RL, Cheng YC. Sequential high-dose cytosine arabinoside and asparaginase in refractory acute leukemia. Med Pediatr Oncol 10(S1):221 1982.
46. Capizzi RL, Yang, J-L, Cheng E, Bjornsson T, Sahasrabudhe D, Tan R-S, Cheng YC. Alteration of the pharmacokinetics of high-dose Ara-C by its metabolite, high ara-U in patients with acute leukemia. J Clin Oncol 1983;1:763.
47. Caradonna SJ, Cheng, Y-C. The role of deoxyuridine triphosphate nucleotide hydrolase, uracil-DNA glycosylase, and DNA polymerase in the metabolism of FUdR in human tumor cells. Mol Pharmacol 1980;18:513.
48. Carmichael J, Fink U, Russell RCG, Spittle MF, Harris A, Spiessl G, Blatter J. Phase II study of gemcitabine in patients with advanced pancreatic cancer. Proc Am Soc Clin Oncol 1993;12:227.
49. Carson DA, Kaye J, Matsumoto S, Seegmiller JE, Thompson L. Biochemical basis for the enhanced toxicity of deoxyribonucleosides toward malignant human T cell lines. Proc Natl Acad Sci USA 1979;76:2430.
50. Carson DA, Kaye J, Seegmiller JE. Lymphospecific toxicity in adenosine deaminase deficiency and purine nucleoside phosphorylase deficiency: possible role of nucleoside kinase(s). Proc Natl Acad Sci USA 1977;74:5677.
51. Carson DA, Wasson DB, Beutler E. Antileukemic and immunosuppressive activity of 2-chloro-2′-deoxyadenosine. Proc Natl Acad Sci USA 1984;81:2232.
52. Carson DA, Wasson DB, Kaye J, Ullman B, Martin DW Jr, Robins RK, Montgomery JA. Deoxyadenosine kinase-mediated toxicity of deoxyadenosine analogs toward malignant human lymphoblasts in vitro and toward murine L1210 leukemia in vivo. Proc Natl Acad Sci USA 1980;77:6865.
53. Casper ES, Green MR, Kelaen DP, Heelan RT, Brown TD, Flombaum CD, Trochanowski B, Tarassoff PG. Phase II trial of gemcitabine (2′, 2′-difluorodeoxycytidine) in patients with adenocarcinoma of the pancreas. Invest New Drugs 1994;12: 29.
54. Casper ES, Vale K, Williams LJ, Martin DS, Young CW. Phase I and clinical pharmacological evaluation of biochemical modulation of 5-fluorouracil with n-(phosphonacetyl)-L-aspartic acid. Cancer Res 1983;43:2324.
55. Cass CE, Kolassa N, Uehara Y, Dahlig-Harley E, Harley E, Paterson ARP. Absence of binding sites for the transport inhibitor nitrobenzylthioinosine on nucleoside transport-deficient mouse lymphoma cells. Biochim Biophys Acta 1981;649:769.
56. Catapano CV, Chandler KB, Fernandes DJ. Effects of anticancer agents on primer RNA formation in human leukemia cells (abstract). Proc Am Assoc Cancer Res 1990;31:420.
57. Chabner BA. Cytidine Analogues. In Cancer Chemotherapy: Principles and Practice. Edited by BA Chabner and JM Collins. Philadelphia: Lippincott, 1990, p 154.
58. Chabner BA, Johns DG, Coleman N, Drake JC, Evans WG. Purification and properties of cytidine deaminase from normal and leukemic granulocytes. J Clin Invest 1974;53:922.
59. Chang C-H, Cheng Y-C. Effects of nucleoside triphosphates on human ribonucleotide reductase from molt-4F cells. Cancer Res 1979;39:5087.
60. Chen C-H, Vazquez-Padua M, Cheng Y-C. The effect of anti-HIV nucleoside analogs on mitochondrial DNA and its implication on delayed toxicity. Molec Pharmacol 1991;39:27.
61. Chen S-F, Ruben RL, Dexter DL. Mechanism of action of the novel anticancer agent 6-fluoro-2-(2′-fluoro-1, 1′-biphenyl-4-yl)-3-methyl-4-quinolinecarboxylic acid sodium salt (NSC-368390): inhibition of de novo pyrimidine nucleotide biosynthesis. Cancer Res 1986;46:5014.
62. Cheng YC, Agarwal P, Parks RE. Erythrocytic nucleoside diphosphokinase IV. Evidence for electrophoretic heterogeneity. Biochemistry 1971;10:2139.
63. Cheng YC, Brockman RW. Mechanisms of Drug resistance and collateral sensitivity: bases for development of chemotherapeutic agents. In Development of Target Oriented Anticancer Drugs. Edited by YC Cheng, B Goz, M Minkoff. New York: Raven Press, 1983, pp 107–117.
64. Cheng YC, Domin B, Lee, L-S. Human deoxycytidine kinase. Purification and characterization of the cytoplasmic and mitochondrial isozymes derived from blast cells of acute myelocytic leukemia patients. Biochim Biophys Acta 1977;481:481.
65. Cheng, Y-C, Tan R-S, Ruth JL, Dutschman GE. Cytotoxicity of 2′-fluoro-5-iodo-1-β-d-arabinofuranosylcytosine and its relationship to deoxycytidine deaminase. Biochem Pharmacol 1983;32:726.
66. Cheson BD. Issues for the future development of fludarabine phosphate. Semin Oncol 1990;17:71.
67. Chou TC, Arlin Z, Clarkson BD, Phillips FS. Metabolism of 1-β-d-arabinofuranosylcytosine in human leukemic cells. Cancer Res 1977;37:3561.
68. Choy BK, McClarty GA, Chan AK, Thelander L, Wright JA. Molecular mechanisms of drug resistance involving ribonucleotide reductase: hydroxyurea resistance in a series of clonally related mouse cell lines selected in the presence of increasing drug concentrations. Cancer Res 1988;48:2029.
69. Christman K, Kelsen D, Saltz L. Phase II trial of gemcitabine in patients with advanced gastric cancer. Cancer 1994;73:5.
70. Christman K, Schwartz G, Saltz L, Dougherty J, Casper E, Yao T, Tomasi F, Friedrich C, Martin D, Bertino J, Kelsen D. Uridine (Urd) allows dose-intensification of FAMTX (5-fluorouracil) (FU), adriamycin (A), methotrexate (MTX). (abstract) Proc Am Assoc Clin Oncol 1993;12:200.
71. Christophidis N, Vajda FJE, Lucas I, Drummer O, Moon WJ, Louis WJ. Fluorouracil therapy in patients with carcinoma of the large bowel: a pharmacokinetic comparison of various rates and routes of administration. Clin Pharmacokinet 1978;3:330.
72. Chu E, Koeller DM, Johnston PG, Zinn S, Allegra CJ. Regulation of thymidylate synthase in human colon cancer cells treated with 5-fluorouracil and interferon-γ. Mol Pharmacol 1992;43:527.
73. Cihak A, Vesely J. Prolongation of the lag period preceding the enhancement of thymidine and thymidylate kinase activity in regenerating rat liver by 5-azacytidine. Biochem Pharmacol 1972;21:3257.
74. Clarke DA, Elion GB, Hitchings GH, Stock CC. Structure-activity relationships among purines related to 6-mercaptopurine. Cancer Res 1958;18:445.
75. Clarkson B, O'Connor A, Winston L, Hutchinson D. The physiologic disposition of 5-fluorouracil and 5-fluoro-2′-deoxyuridine in man. Clin Pharmacol Ther 1964;5:581.
76. Cocking JM, Tonin PN, Stokoe NM, Wensing EJ, Lewis WH, Srinivasan PR. Gene for M1 subunit of ribonucleotide reductase is amplified in hydroxyurea-resistant hamster cells. Somat Cell Mol Genet 1987;13:221.
77. Cody R, Stewart D, deForni M, Moore M, Neidhart J, Maurer H, Dallaire B, Grillo-Lopez A. A phase II study of brequinar sodium (DuP 785, NSC 368390) in breast cancer. (abstract) Proc Am Assoc Cancer Oncol 1991;10:61.
78. Cohen SS, Flaks JG, Barner HD, Loeb MR, Lichtenstein J. The mode of action of 5-fluorouracil and its derivatives. Proc Natl Acad Sci (Wash.) 1958;44:1004.
79. Collins KD, Stark GR. Aspartate transcarbamylase interaction with the transition state analog *N*-(phosphonacetyl)-L-aspartate. J Biol Chem 1971;246:6599.
80. Cory J, Breland JB, Carter GL. Effect of 5-fluorouracil on RNA metabolism in Novikoff hepatoma cells. Cancer Res 1979;39:4905.
81. Cory JG. Role of ribonucleotide reductase in cell division. In Inhibitors of Ribonucleoside Diphosphate Reductase Activity. Edited by JG Cory and AH Cory. New York: Pergamon Press, 1989, p 1.
82. Cosenza CA, Cramer DV, Tuso PJ, Chapman FA, Wang HK, Makowka L. Combination therapy with brequinar sodium and cyclosporine synergistically prolongs hamster-to-rat cardia xenograft survival. J Heart Lung Transplant 1994;13:489.
83. Cramer DV, Cahpman FA, Makowka L. The use of brequinar sodium for transplantation. Ann NY Acad Sci 1993;696:216.
84. Danenberg PV, Danenberg KD. Effect of 5, 10-methylenetetrahydrofolate and the dissociation of 5-fluorodeoxyuridylate binding of human thymidylate synthetase: evidence for an ordered mechanism. Biochemistry 1978;17:4018.
85. Danhauser L, Plunkett W, Keating M, Cabanillas F, Greenberg BR, Hutton JJ, Talley R, Von Hoff DD, Balcerzak SP. 9-Fludarabine monophosphate: a potentially useful agent in chronic lymphocytic leukemia. Nouv Rev Fr Hematol, 1988;30:457.
86. Darnowski JW, Handschumacher RE. Enhancement of fluorouracil therapy by the manipulation of tissue uridine pools. Pharmacol Ther 1989;41:381–92.
87. Darnowski JW, Handschumacher RE. Tissue uridine pools. Evidence in vivo of a concentrative mechanism for uridine uptake. Cancer Res 1986;46:3490.
88. Darnowski JW, Handschumacher RE. Tissue-specific enhancement of uridine utilization of 5-fluorouracil therapy in mice by benzylacyclouridine. Cancer Res 1985;45: 5364.
89. Darnowski JW, Holdridge C, Handschumacher RE. Concentrative uridine transport by murine splenocytes: kinetics, substrate specificity, and sodium dependency. Cancer Res 1987;47:2614.
90. Davis S, Knick VC, Baccanari DP, Spector T. 5-Ethynyluracil (5-EU, 776C85) improves the therapeutic index (TI) of 5-fluorouracil (5-FU) against colon 38 and MOPC-315 (abstract). Proc Am Assoc Cancer Res 1993;34:a1684.
91. De Saint Vincent BR, Buttin G. Studies on 1-β-d-arabinofuranosyl-cytosine resistant mutants of Chinese fibroblasts. III. Joint resistance to arabino-furanosylcytosine and to excess thymidine—A semidominant manifestation of deoxyctidine triphosphate pool expansion. Somat Cell Genet 1979;5:67.
92. De Saint Vincent BR, Dechamps M, Butlin G. The modulation of the thymidine triphosphate pool of chinese hamster cells by dCMP deaminase and UDP reductase. J Biol Chem 1980;255:162.
93. Dearden CE, Hoffbrand AV, Ganeshaguru K, Brozovic M, Williams HJ, Traub N, Mills M, Linch DC, Catovsky D. Membrane phenotype and response to deoxycoformycin in mature T-cell malignancies. BMJ 1987;295:873.
94. Delong, D.C. Hertel LW, Tang J. Kroin JS, Wilson JD, Terry J, Lavender, J.F. Antiviral activity of 2′, 2′-difluorodeoxycytidine. Am Soc Miocrobiol, March 24–28, Washington DC, 1986.
95. Diasio RB, Beavers TI, Carpenter JT. Familial deficiency of dihydropyrimidine dehydrogenase. Biochemical basis for familial pyrimidemia and severe 5-fluorouracil-induced toxicity. J Clin Invest 1988;81:447.
96. Diasio RB, Harris BE. Clinical pharmacology of 5-fluorouracil. Clinical Pharmacokinet 1989;16:215.
97. Diasio RB, Lakings DE, Bennett JE. Evidence for conversion of 5-fluorocytosine to 5-fluorouracil in humans: possible factor in 5-fluorocytosine clinical toxicity. Antimicrob Agents Chemother 1978;14:903.
98. Domin BA, Mahony, W.B. 5-Fluorouracil transport into human erythrocytes. (abstract) Proc Am Assoc Cancer Res 199;31:10.l.
99. Donehower RC. Hydroxyurea. In Cancer Chemotherapy: principles and Practice. Edited by BA Chabner, JM Collins. Philadelphia: Lippincott, 1990, pp 154–179.

100. Donofrio J, Coleman MS, Hutton JJ, Daoud A, Lampkin B, Dyminski J. Overproduction of adenine deoxynucleosides and deoxynucleotides in adenosine deaminase deficiency with severe combined immunodeficiency disease. J Clin Invest 1978;62:884.
101. Drake JC, Stoller RG, Chabner BA. Characteristics of the enzyme uridine-cytidine kinase isolated from a cultured human cell line. Biochem Pharmacol 1977;26:64.
102. Dresler WFC, Stein R. Au Uber den Hydroxylharnstoff. Justus Leibigs Ann Chem 1869;150:242.
103. Duschinsky R, Pleven E, Heidelberger C. The synthesis of 5-fluoropyrimidines. J Am Chem Soc 1957;79:4559.
104. Dusenbury CE, Davis MA, Lawrence TS, Maybaum J. Induction of megabase DNA fragments by 5-fluorodeoxyuridine in human colorectal tumor (HT29) cells. Mol Pharmacol 1990;39:285.
105. Dutcher JP, Wiernik PH, Markus S, Weinberg V, Schiffer CA, Harwood KV. Intensive maintenance therapy improves survival in adult acute nonlymphocytic leukemia: an eight-year follow up. Leukemia 1988;2:413.
106. DuVivier A. Topical cytostatic drugs in the treatment of skin cancer. Clin Exp Dermatol 1982;7:89.
107. Edwards NL, Recker D, Airozo D, Fox IH. Enhanced purine salvage during allopurinol therapy: an important pharmacologic property in humans. J Lab Clin Med 1981;98:673.
108. Efange SMN, Alessi EM, Shih HC, Cheng YC, Bardos TJ. Synthesis and biological activities of 2-pyrimidinone nucleosides. 2. 5-halo-2-pyrimidinone 2′deoxyribonucleosides. J Med Chem 1991;28:904.
109. Einhorn M, Davidson I. Hepatotoxicity of 6-mercaptopurine. JAMA 1964;188:802.
110. El Kouni MH, Naguib FNM, Cha S. Circadian rhythm of dihydrouracil dehydrogenase (DHUDase), uridine phosphorylase (UrdPase), and thymidine phosphorylase (dThdPase) in mouse liver. FASEB J., 1989;3:a397.
111. Elias L, Sandoval JM. Interferon effects upon fluorouracil metabolism by HL-60 cells. Biochem Biophys Res Commun 1989;163:867.
112. Elion GB. Biochemistry and pharmacology of purine analogs. Fed Proc 1967;26:898.
113. Elion GB. Enzymatic and metabolic studies with allopurinol. Ann Rheum Dis 1966;25:608.
114. Elion GB, Callahan S, Rundles RW, Hitchings GH. Relationship between metabolic fates and antitumor activities of thiopurines. Cancer Res 1963;23:1207.
115. Elion GB, Hitchings GH. Azathioprine, In handbook of experimental pharmacology. Edited by AC Sartorelli and DG Johns. Berlin: Springer-Verlag, 1975, p 404.
116. Elion GB, Hitchings GH. The synthesis of 6-thioguanine. J Am Chem Soc 1955;77:1676.
117. Elion GB, Hitchings GH, Vander-Werff H. Antagonists of nucleic acid derivatives. VI. Purines. J Biol Chem 1951;192:505.
118. Elzawawy A. Treatment of 5-fluorouracil-induced stomatitis by allopurinol mouthwashes. Oncology 1991;48:282.
119. Engstrom Y, Eriksson S, Jildevik I, Skog S, Thelander L, Tribukait B. Cell cycle-dependent expression of mammalian ribonucleotide reductase. Differential regulation of the two subunits. J Biol Chem 1985;260:9114.
120. Ensminger WD, Rosowsky A, Raso V, Levin DC, Glode,M., Come S, Steel G, Frei E III. A clinical pharmacological evaluation of hepatic arterial infusion of 5-fluoro-2′-deoxyuridine and 5-fluorouracil. Cancer Res 1978;38:3784.
121. Eriksson S, Graslund A, Skog S, Thelander A, Tribukait B. Cell cycle dependent regulation of mammalian ribonucleotide reductase. J Biol Chem, 1984;259:11695.
122. Erlichman C, Fine S, Wong A. A randomized trial of fluorouracil and folinic acid in patients with metastatic colorectal carcinoma. J Clin Oncol 1988;6:469.
123. Erlichman C, Donehower RC, Speyer JL, Klecker R, Chabner BA. Phase I-phase II trial of n-phosphonacetyl-L-aspartic acid given by intravenous infusion and 5-fluorouracil given by bolus injection. JNCI 1982;68:227.
124. Esterhay RJ Jr, Aisner J, Levi JA, Wiernik PH. High-dose 6-mercaptopurine in advanced refractory cancer. Cancer Treat Rep 1978;62:1229.
125. Evans RM, Laskin JD, Hakala MT. Assessment of growth-limiting events caused by 5-fluorouracil in mouse cells and in human cells. Cancer Res 1980;40:4113.
126. Evans RM, Laskin JD, Hakala MT. Effect of excess folates and deoxyinosine on the activity and site of action of 5-fluorouracil. Cancer Res 1981;41:3288.
127. Fernandes DJ, and Carroll CC. Multiple modes of resistance of human CCRF-CEM leukemic cells to 5-fluoro-2′-deoxyuridine. Cancer Res 1983;24:283.
128. Fernandes JF, LePage GA, Lindner A. The influence of azaserine and 6-mercaptopurine on the in vivo metabolism of ascites tumor cells. Cancer Res 1956;16:154.
129. Finch RE, Bending MR, Lant AF. Plasma levels of 5-fluorouracil after oral and intravenous administration in cancer patients. Br J Clin Pharmacol 1979;7:613.
130. Fishbein WN, Carbone PP. Hydroxyurea: mechanisms of action. Science 1963;142:1069.
131. Fox IH. Metabolic basis for disorders of purine nucleotide degradation. Metabolism 1981;30:616.
132. Fox RM, Woods RL, Tattersall MHN, Piper AA, Sampson D. Allopurinol modulation of fluorouracil toxicity. Cancer Chem Pharm 1981;5:151.
133. Franco L, Malykh A, Cara A, Sun D, Winstein JN, Lisziewicz J, Gallo RC. Hydroxyurea as an inhibitor of human immunodeficiency virus-type 1 replication. Science 1994;266:801.
134. Fridland A. Effect of cytosine arabinoside on replicon initiation in human lymphoblasts. Biochem Biophys Res Commun 1977;74:72.
135. Fritsch GL. Adenosine deaminase in disorders of purine metabolism and immune deficiency. Ann NY Acad Sci 1985;451:1.
136. Fujii S, Ikenake K, Fukushima M, Shirasake T. Effect of Uracil and its derivatives on antitumor activity of 5-fluorouracil and 1-(2-tetrahydrofuryl)-5-fluorouracil. Gann 1978;69:763.
137. Fujii S, Kitano S, Ikenaka K, Shirasaka T. Effect of coadministration of clinical doses of 1-(2-tetrahydorfuryl)-5-fluorouracil and level of 5-fluorouracil in rodents. Gann 1979;70:209.
138. Fukui Y, Imabayashi N, Nishi M, Majima K, Yamanura M, Hioki K, Yamamoto M. Clinical study on the enhancement of drug delivery into tumor tissue by using UFT. Jpn J Cancer Chemother 1980;7:2124.
139. Furth JT, Cohen SS. Inhibition of mammalian DNA polymerase by 1-β-D-arabinofuranosylcytosine and the 5′-triphosphate of 9-β-D-arabinofuranosyladenine. Cancer Res 1968;28:2061.
140. Fyfe JA, Miller RL, Krenitsky TA. Kinetic properties and inhibition of orotidine 5′ phosphate decarboxylase. J Biol Chem 1973;248:3801.
141. Gandhi V, Kemena A, Keating MJ, Plunkett W. Fludarabine infusion potentiates arabinosylcytosine metabolism in lymphocytes of patients with chronic lymphocytic leukemia. Cancer Res 1992;52:897.
142. Gandhi V, Plunkett W. Modulation of arabinosyl nucleoside metabolism by arabinosyl nucleotides in human leukemia cells. Cancer Res 1988;48:329.
143. Gandhi V, Robertson LE, Keating MJ, Plunkett W. Combination of fludarabine and arabinosylcytosine for treatment of chronic lymphocytic leukemia: clinical efficacy and modulation of arabinosylcytosine pharmacology. Cancer Chemother Pharm 1994;34:30.
144. Glazer RI, Lloyd LS. Association of cell lethality with incorporation of 5-fluorouracil and 5-fluorouridine into nuclear RNA in human colon carcinoma cells in culture. Mol Pharmacol 1982;21:468.
145. Goulian M, Bleile B, Tseng, B Y. Methotrexate-induced misincorporation of uracil into DNA. Biochemistry 1980;77:1956.
146. Grem JL, Fischer PH. Enhancement of 5–fluorouracil's anticancer activity by dipyridamole. Pharmac Ther 1989;40:349.
147. Grem JL, Fischer PH. Augmentation of 5–fluorouracil cytotoxity in human colon cancer cells by dipyridamole. Cancer Res 1985;45:2967.
148. Grever MR, Chapman RA, Ratanatharathorn V, Slease RB. An investigation of deoxycoformycin in advanced cutaneous T-cell lymphoma. Blood 1986;66(suppl 1):215a.
149. Grever MR, Kopecky KJ, Coltman CA, Files JC, Greenberg BR, Hutton JJ, Talley R. Von Hoff DD, Balcerzak SP. Fludarabine monophosphate: a potentially useful agent in chronic lymphocytic leukemia. Nouv Rev Fr Hematol 1988;30:457.
150. Griffig J, Koob R, Blakley RL. Mechanism of inhibition of DNA synthesis by 2-chlorodeoxyadenosine in human lymphoblastic cells. Cancer Res 1989;49:6923.
151. Guerquin-Kern JL, Leteurtre F., Croisy A, Lloste J.M. pH Dependence of 5-fluorouracil uptake observed by in vivo ^{31}P and ^{19}F nuclear magnetic resonance spectroscopy. Cancer Res 1991;51:5770.
152. Guo X, Chang CN, Chen HX, Zhu JL, Yen Y, Basson MD, Turowski G, Lin TS, Cheng, Y.C. Development of a prodrug of 5-fluorouracil. (abstract) Proc Am Assoc Cancer Res 1993;34:2483.
153. Hande K, Hixon C, Chabner B. Postchemotherapy purine excretion in lymphoma patients receiving allopurinol. Cancer Res 1981;41:2273.
154. Hanka LJ, Evans JS, Mason DJ, Dietz A. Microbiological production of 5-azacytidine: i. Production and biological activity. Antimicrob Agents Chemother 1966;6:619.
155. Harbers E, Chaudhuri NK, Heidelberger C. Studies on fluorinated pyrimidines. VIII. Further biochemical and metabolic investigations. J Biol Chem 1959;234:1255.
156. Harris BE, Ruiling S, Soong S, Diasio RB. Relationship between dihydropyrimidine dehydrogenase activity and plasma 5-fluorouracil levels with evidence for circadian variation of enzyme activity and plasma drug levels in cancer patients receiving 5-fluorouracil by protracted continuous infusion. Cancer Res 50: 197;1990.
157. Hartmann KU, Heidelberger C. Studies on fluorinated pyrimidines. VIII. Inhibition of thymidylate synthetase. J Biol Chem 1961;236:3006.
158. Heggie GD, Sommadossi, J-P., Cross DS, Huster WJ, Diasio RB. Clinical pharmacokinetics of 5-fluorouracil and its metabolites in plasma, urine, and bile. Cancer Res 1987;7:2203.
159. Heidelberger C, Chaudhuri NK, Danneberg P, Mooreh D, Griesbach L, Duschinsky R, Schnitzer RJ, Pleven E. Fluorinated pyrimidines, a new class of tumor-inhibitory compounds. Nature 1957;179:663.
160. Heidelberger C, Danenberg PV, Moran RG. Fluorinated pyrimidines and their nucleosides. Adv Enzymol 1983;54:57.
161. Heier MS, Fossa S. D Wernicke-Korsakoff-like syndrome in patients with colorectal carcinoma treated with high-dose doxifluridine. Acta Neurol Scand 1986;73:449.
162. Heinemann V, Hertel LW, Grindey GB, Plunkett W. Comparison of the cellular pharmacokinetics and toxicity of 2′,2′-difluorodeoxycytidine. Cancer Res 1968;28:1976.
163. Heinemann V, Xu, Y.Z., Chubb S, Sen A, Hertel LW, Grindey GB, Plunkett W. Cellular elimination of 2′, 2′-difluorodeoxycytidine 5′-triphosphate: a mechanism of self-potentiation. Cancer Res 1992;52:533.
164. Heinemann V, Xu, Y.Z., Chubb S, Sen A, Hertel LW, Grindey GB, Plunkett W. Inhibition of ribonucleotide reductase in CCRF-CEM cells by 2′, 2′-difluorodeoxycytidine. Mol Pharmacol 1990;38:567.
165. Helland S, Ueland PM. Effect of 2′-deoxycoformycin infusion on s-adenosylhomocysteine hydrolase and the amount of s-adenosylhomocysteine and related compounds in tissues of mice. Cancer Res 1983;43:4142.
166. Hershfeld MS. Apparent suicide inactivation of human lymphoblast s-adenosylhomocysteine hydrolase by 2′-deoxyadenosineand adenine arabinoside: a basis for direct toxic effects of analogs of adenosine. J Biol Chem 1979;254:22.
167. Hertel LW, Boder GB, Kroin JS, Rinzel SM, Poore GA, Todd GC, Grindey, G.B. Evaluation of the antitumor activity of a (2′-2′-difluoro-2′-deoxycytidine). Cancer Res 1990;50:4417.
168. Hertel LW, Kroin JS, Misner JW, Tustin, J.M. Synthesis of 2-deoxy-2, 2-difluoro-D-ribose and 2-deoxy-2, 2-difluoro-D-ribofuranosyl nucleotides. J Organ Chem 1988;53:2406.
169. Hill DL, Bennett LL Jr. Purification and properties of 5-phosphoribosyl pyrophosphate amidotransferase from adenocarcinoma 758 cells. Biochemistry 1969;8:122.
170. Hillman RS. Hematopoietic agents: growth factors, minerals and vitamins. Edited by LS Goodman and A Gilman. The Pharmacologic Basis of Therapeutics, 8th Edition. Paragamm Press, 1990, p 1277.
171. Hitchings GH, Elion GB. The chemistry and biochemistry of purine analogs. Ann NY Acad Sci 1954;60:195.
172. Hochster H, Cassileth P. Fludarabine phosphate therapy of non-hodgkin's lymphoma. Semin Oncol 1990;17:5.
173. Holt RJ, Newman RL. The antimycotic activity of 5-fluorocytosine. J Clin Pathol 1973;26:167.
174. Houghton JA, Houghton PJ. Elucidation of pathways of 5-fluorouracil metabolism in xenografts of human colorectal adenocarcinoma. Eur J Cancer 1983;19:807.
175. Houghton JA, Maroda SJ Jr, Phillips JO, Houghton PJ. Biochemical determinants of responsiveness to 5-fluorouracil and its derivatives in xenografts of human colorectal adenocarcinomas in mice. Cancer Res 1981;41:144.
176. Houghton JA, Morton CL, Adkins DA, Rahman A. Locus of the interaction among 5-fluorouracil, leucovorin and interferon-α 2a in colon carcinoma cells. Cancer Res 1993;53:4243.
177. Houghton JA, Torrance PM, Radparvar S, Williams LG, Houghton PJ. Binding of 5-flu-

orodeoxyuridylate to thymidylate synthetase in human colon adenocarcinoma xenografts. Eur J Cancer Clin Oncol 1986;22:505.

178. Houghton JA, Weiss KD, Williams LG, Torrance PM, Houghton PJ. Relationship between 5-fluoro-2′-deoxyuridylate, 2′-deoxyuridylate, and thymidylate synthase activity subsequent to 5-fluorouracil administration in xenografts of human colon adenocarcinomas. Biochem Pharmacol 1986;35:1351.
179. Houghton JA, Williams LG, Radparvar A, Houghton PJ. Characterization of the pools of 5, 10-methylenetetrahydrofolates and tetrahydrofolates in xenografts of human colon adenocarcinoma. Cancer Res 1988;48:3062.
180. Howell SB, Wung WE, Taetle R, Hussain F, Romine JS. Modulation of 5-fluorouracil toxicity by allopurinol in man. Cancer 1981;48:1281.
181. Hrushesky W. Circadian timing of cancer chemotherapy. Science 1985;228:73.
182. Hryniuk WM. The importance of dose intensity in the outcome of chemotherapy. Important Adv. Oncol., p 121;1988.
183. Huang M-C, Ashmun RA, Avery TL, Kuehl M, Blakley RL. Effects of cytotoxicity of 2-chloro-2′-deoxyadenosine and 2-bromo-2′-deoxyadenosine on cell growth, clonogenicity, DNA synthesis, and cell kinetics. Cancer Res 1986;46:2362.
184. Huang M-C, Avery TL, Blakley RL, Secrist JA III, Montgomery JA. Improved synthesis and antitumoractivity of 2-bromo-2′-deoxyadenosine. J Med Chem 1984;27:800.
185. Huang P, Chubb S, Hertel LW, Grindey GB, Plunkett W. Action of 2′, 2′-difluorox-eoxycytidine on DNA synthesis. Cancer Res 1991;51:6110.
186. Huang P, Chubb S, Plunkett W. Incorporation of 9-β-D-arabinofuranosyl-2-fluoradenine into DNA and its chain termination effect on DNA synthesis. J Biol Chem., 265: 16617 1990.
187. Huang P, Plunkett W. Preferential incorporation of arabinofuranosyl-2-fluoradenine into poly (A+) RNA and its inhibitory effects on transcription and translation (abstract) Proc Am Assoc Cancer Res 1986;27:21.
188. Ingraham HA, Tseng BY, Goulian M. Mechanism for exclusion of 5-fluorouracil from DNA. Cancer Res 1980;40:998.
189. Ingraham HA, Tseng BY, Goulian M. Nucleotide levels and incorporation of 5-fluorouracil and uracil into DNA of cells treated with 5-fluorodeoxyuridine. Mol Pharmacol 2 1981;1:211.
190. Jayaram HN, Cooney DA, Vistica DT, Kariya S, Johnson RK. Mechanisms of sensitivity of resistance of murine tumors to N-(phosphonacetyl)-L-aspartate (PALA). Cancer Treat Rep 1979;63:1291.
191. Johnson RK, Swyryd EA, Stark GR. Effects of N–(phosphonacetyl)-L-aspartate on murine tumors and normal tissues in vivo and in vitro and the relationship of sensitivity to rate of proliferation and levels of aspartate transcarbamylase. Cancer Res 1978;38:371.
192. Johnson RK, Swyryd EA, Stark GR. Reversal of toxicity and antitumor activity of N-(phosphonacetyl)-L-aspartate by uridine or carbamyl-DL-aspartate in vivo. Biochem Pharmacol 1977;26:81.
193. Jones ME. Pyrimidine nucleotide biosynthesis in animals: genes, enzymes, and regulation of UMP biosynthesis. Ann Rev Biochem 1980;49:253.
194. Kantarjian HM, Redman JR, Keating MJ. Fludarabine phosphate therapy in other lymphoid malignanices. Semin Oncol 1990;17:66–70 .
195. Kaye S, Gemcitabine: current status of phase I and II trials. J Clin Oncol 1994;12: 1527.
196. Keating M. Fludarabine Phosphate in the treatment of chronic lymphocytic leukemia. Semin Oncol 1990;17:49.
197. Kelley W, Beardmore T. Allopurinol: alteration in pyrimidine metabolism in man. Science 1970;169:388.
198. Kempe TD, Swyryd EA, Bruist M, Stark GR. Stable mutant mammalian cells that overproduce the first three enzymes of pyrimidine nucleotide biosynthesis. Cell 1976;9: 541.
199. Kent RJ, Heidelberger C. Fluorinated pyrimidines, ribonucleotide reductase. Mol Pharmacol 1972;8:465.
200. Kessel D, Hall TC, Wodinsky I. Transport and phosphorylation as factors in the antitumor action of cytosine arabinoside. Science 1967;156:1240.
201. Keyomarsi K, Moran R. Folinic acid augmentation of the effects of fluoropyrimidines on murine and human leukemic cells. Cancer Res 1986;46:5229.
202. Kim JH, Gelbard AS, Perez AG. Action of hydroxyurea on the nucleic acid metabolism and viability of HeLa cells. Cancer Res 1967;27:1301.
203. Klubes P, Leyland-Jones B. Enhancement of the antitumor activity of 5-fluorouracil by uridine rescue. Pharmacol Ther 1989;41:289.
204. Klubes PK, Cerna I. Use of uridine rescue to enhance the antitumor selectivity of 5-fluorouracil. Cancer Res 1983;43:3182.
205. Kraut EH, Bouroncle BA, Grever MR. Low-dose deoxycoformycin in the treatment of hairy cell leukemia. Blood 1986;68:1119.
206. Krebs HB. The use of topical 5-fluorouracil in the treatment of genital condylomas. Obstet Gynecol Clin North Am 1987;14:559.
207. Kufe DW, Major PP. 5-Fluorouracil incorporation into human breast carcinoma RNA correlates with cytotoxicity. J Biol Chem 1981;256:9802.
208. Kufe DW, Major PP, Egan EM, Loh E. 5-Fluoro-2′-deoxyuridine incorporation in L1210 DNA. J Biol Chem 1981;256:8885.
209. Laurie JA, Moertel CG, Fleming TR, Wieand HS, Leigh JE, Rubin J, McCormack GW, Gerstner JB, Krook JE, Malliard J, Twito DI, Morton RF, Tschetter LK, Barlow JF. Surgical adjuvant therapy of large-bowel carcinoma: an evaluation of levamisole and the combination of levamisole and fluorouracil. J Clin Oncol 1989;7:1447.
210. Lauzon GJ, Paran JH, Paterson ARP. Formation of l-β-D-arabinofuranosylcytosine diphosphate choline in cultured human leukemic RPMI 6410 cells. Cancer Res 1978;38:1723.
211. Leclerc JM, Cheng, Y-C. Demonstration of activities in leukemic cells capable of removing 1′-β-D-arabinofuranosyl cytosine (araC) from araC incorporated DNA (abstract) Proc Am Assoc Cancer Res 1984;25:19.
212. Lee CW, Cheeseman CI, Jarvis SM. Na^+- and K^+-dependent uridine transport in rat renal brush-border membrane vesicles. Biochim Biophys Acta 1988;942:139.
213. LePage GA. Basic biochemical effects and mechanism of action of 6-thioguanine. Cancer Res 1963;23:1202.
214. Lerner-Tung MD, Chen HX, Guo X, Chang CP, Pizzorno G, Cheng, Y.C. Pharmacokinetic behavior of orally-administered 5-fluoropyrimidinone, a prodrug of 5-fluorouracil (abstract) Proc Am Assoc Cancer Res 1994;35:2575.
215. Levi F, Misset JL, Brienza S, Adam R, Metzger G, Itzakhi M, Caussanel J, Kunstlinger F, Lecouturier S, Descorps-Declere A, Jasmin C, Bismuth H, Reinberg A. A chronopharmacologic phase II clinical trial with 5-fluorouracil, folinic acid, and oxaliplatin using an ambulatory multichannel programmable pump. Cancer 1992;69:893.
216. Lewis WH, Wright JA. Altered ribonucleotide reductase activity in mammalian tissue culture cells resistant to hydroxyurea. Biochem Biophys Res Commun 1974;60:926.
217. Li LH, Olin EJ, Buskirk HH, Reineke LM. Cytotoxicity and mode of action of 5-azacytidine on L1210 leukemia. Cancer Res 1970;30:2760.
218. Li LH, Olin EJ, Fraser TJ, Bhuyan BK. Phase specificity of 5-azacytidine against mammalian cells in tissue culture. Cancer Res 1970;30:2770.
219. Liliemark J, Juliusson G. On the pharmacokinetics of 2-chloro-2′-deoxyadenosine in humans. Cancer Res 1991;51:5570.
220. Lokich J, Ahlgren J, Gullo J, Philips J, Fryer J. A prospective randomized comparison of continuous infusion fluorouracil with a conventional bolus schedule in metastatic colorectal carcinoma: a Mid-Atlantic Oncology Program study. J Clin Oncol 1989;7: 425.
221. Lokich J, Bothe A, Fine N, Perri J. Phase I study of protracted venous infusion of 5-fluorouracil. Cancer 1981;48:2565.
222. Lund B, Kristjansen PEG, Hanson HH. Clinical and preclinical activity of 2′-2′-difluorodeoxycytidine (gemcitabine). Cancer Treat Rev 1993;19:45.
223. Lung B, Anderson H, Walling J, Thatcher N, Hansen, H.D. Phase II study of gemcitabine in non-small cell lung cancer (NSCLC). Lung Cancer 1991;7(suppl):121.
224. MacMillan WE, Wolberg WH, Welling PG. Pharmacokinetics of fluorouracil in humans. Cancer Res 1978;38:3479.
225. Madoc-Jones H, Bruce WR. On the mechanism of the lethal action of 5-fluorouracil on mouse L cells. Cancer Res 28: 1976;1968.
226. Major PP, Egan EM, Beardsley GP, Minden MD, Kufe DW. Lethality of human myeloblasts correlates with the incorporation of arabinofuranosylcytosine into DNA. J Biol Chem 1981;78:3235.
227. Mancini WR, Cheng Y-C. Human deoxycytidylate deaminase. Substrate and regulator specificities and their chemotherapeutic implications. Mol Pharmacol 1983;23: 159.
228. Mandel HG. The incorporation of 5-fluorouracil into RNA and its molecular consequences. Prog Mol Subcell Biol 1969;1:82.
229. Mann GJ, Musgrove EA, Fox RM, Thelander L. Ribonucleotide reductase M1 subunit in cellular proliferation, quiescence, and differentiation. Cancer Res 1988;48:5151.
230. Marsh JC, Bertino JR, Katz KH, Davis CA, Durivage HJ, Rome LS. The influence of drug interval on the effect of methotrexate and fluorouracil in the treatment of advanced colorectal cancer. J Clin Oncol 1991;9:371.
231. Martin DS, Stolfi RL, Sawyer RC. Utility of oral uridine as a substitute for parenteral uridine rescue of 5-fluorouracil therapy, with and without the uridine phosphorylase inhibitor 5-benzylacyclouridine. Cancer Chemother Pharmacol 1989;24:9.
232. Martin DS, Stolfi RL, Sawyer RC, Spiegelman S, Young CW. High-dose 5-fluorouracil with delayed uridine 'rescue' in mice. Cancer Res 1982;42:3964.
233. Maybaum J, Ullman B, Mandel HG, Day JL, Sadee W. Regulation of RNA- and DNA-directed actions of 5-fluoropyrimidines in mouse T-lymphoma (S-49) cells. Cancer Res 1980;40:4209.
234. Mayer RJ. Current chemotherapeutic treatment approaches to the management of previously untreated adults with de novo acute myelogenous leukemia. Semin in Oncol 1987;14:384–396.
235. McClarty GA, Chan AK, Engstrom Y, Wright JA, Thelander L. Elevated expression of M1 and M2 components and drug-induced post transcriptional modulation of ribonucleotide reductase in a hydroxyurea-resistant mouse cell line. Biochemistry 1987;26:8004.
236. McDermott BJ, van der Berg HW, Murphy RF. Nonlinear pharmacokinetics for the elimination of 5-fluorouracil after intravenous administration in cancer patients. Pharmacology 1982;9:173.
237. Mertens WC, Eisenhauer BA, Moore M, Venner P, Stewart D, Muldal A, Wong D. Gemcitabine in advanced renal cell carcinoma. Ann Oncol 1993;4:331.
238. Metzger G, Massari C, Etienne MC, Comisso M, Brienza S, Touitou Y, Milano G, Bastian G, Misset JL, Levi F. Spontaneous or imposed circadian changes in plasma concentrations of 5-fluorouracil coadministered with folinic acid and oxaliplatin: relationship with mucosal toxicity in patients with cancer. Clin Pharm Ther, 1994;56:190.
239. Mini E, Trave F, Rustum YM, Bertino JR. Enhancement of the antitumor effects of 5-fluorouracil by folinic acid. Pharm. Ther 1990;47:1.
240. Minshull M, Gardner MLG. The effect of time of administration of 5-fluorouracil on leukopenia in the rat. Eur J Cancer Clin Onc, 1984;20:857.
241. Mitchell BS, Edwards NL, Koller CA. Deoxyribonucleoside triphosphate accumulation by leukemic cells. Blood 1983;62:419.
242. Moertel CG, Fleming TR, MacDonald JS, Haller DG, Laurie JA, Goodman PJ, Ungerleider JS, Emerson WA, Tormey DC, Glick JH, Veeder MH, Mailliard JA. Levamisole and fluorouracil for adjuvant therapy of resected colon carcinoma. N Engl J Med 1990;322:352.
243. Momparler RL. Effect of cytosine arabinoside 5′-triphosphate on mammalian DNA polymerase. Biochem Biophys Res Commun 1969;34:465.
244. Momparler RL. Kinetic and template studies with 1-β-D-arabinofuranosylcytosine 5′-triphosphate and mammalian deoxyribonucleic acid polymerase. Mol Pharm 1972;8: 362.
245. Montgomery JA. The chemistry and biology of purines and ring analogues. In nucleosides, nucleotides, and their biological applications. Edited by J. Ridout DW Henry, and LM Beacher III. New York: Academic Press, 1984;p 19.
246. Moore DF Jr, Pazdur R, Daugherty K, Tarassoff P, Abbruzzese JL. Phase II study of gemcitabine in advanced colorectal adenocarcinoma. Invest New Drugs 1992;10: 323.
247. Moore EC, Friedman J, Valdivieso M, Plunkett W, Marti JR, Russ J, Loo TL. Aspartatecarbamoyltransferase activity, drug concentrations, and pyrimidine nucleotides in tissue from patients treated with n-(phosphonacetyl)-L-aspartate. Biochem Pharmacol 1982;31:3317.
248. Moore R, Robert F, Cripps M, Ruckdeschel J, Neidhart J, Natale R, Dallaire D, Gyves J. A phase II study of brequinar sodium (DuP 785, NSC 368390) in gastrointestinal (GI) cancers (abstract). Proc Am Soc Clin Onc 1991;10:152.
249. Moran RE, Straus MJ. Cytokinetic analysis of L1210 leukemia after continuous infusion of hydroxyurea in vivo. Cancer Res 1979;39:1616.
250. Morikawa K, Fan D, Denkins YM, Levin B, Gutterman JU, Walker SM, Fidler IJ. Mechanisms of combined effects of γ-interferon and 5-fluorouracil on human colon cancer implanted into nude mice. Cancer Res 1989;49:799.

251. Moyer JD, Handschumacher RE. Selective inhibition of pyrimidine synthesis and depletion of nucleotide pools by n-(phosphonacetyl)-L-aspartate. Cancer Res 1979;39:3089.
252. Mulkins MA, Heidelberger C. Biochemical characterization of fluoropyrimidine-resistant murine leukemic cell lines. Cancer Res 1982;42:965.
253. Mulkins MA, Heidelberger C. Isolation of fluoropyrimidine-resistant murine leukemic cell lines by one-step mutation and selection. Cancer Res 1982;40:1431.
254. Myers CE, Young RC, Chabner BA. Biochemical determinants of 5-fluorouracil response in vivo: the role of deoxyuridylate pool expansion. J Clin Invest 1975;56:1231.
255. Myers CE, Young RC, Johns DG, Chabner BA. Assay of 5-fluorodeoxyuridine 5′-monophosphate anddeoxyuridine 5′-monophosphate pools following 5-fluorouracil. Cancer Res 1974;34:2682.
256. Naguib FNM, el Kouni MH, Cha S. Enzymes of uracil catabolism in normal and neoplastic human tissues. Cancer Res 1985;45:5405.
257. Nakajima T, Takahashi T, Takagi K, Kuno K, andKajitani T. Comparison of 5-fluorouracil with ftorafur in adjuvant chemotherapies with combined inductive and maintenance therapies for gastric cancer. J Clin Oncol 1984;2:1366.
258. Namba M, Miyoshu T, Kanamori T, Nobuhara M, Kimoto T, Ogawa S. Combined effects of 5-fluorouracil and interferon on proliferation of human neoplastic cells in culture. Gann 1982;73:819.
259. Nelson JA, Carpenter JW, Rose LM, Adamson DJ. Mechanisms of action of 6-thioguanine, 6 mercaptopurine and 8-azaguanine. Cancer Res 1975;35:2782.
260. Niedzwicki JG, Chu SH, el Kouni MH, Rowe EC, Cha S. 5-Benzylacyclouridine and 5-benzyloxybenzylacyclouridine, potent inhibitors of uridine phosphorylase. Biochem Pharm 1982;31:1857.
261. Nordic Gastrointestinal Tumor Adjuvant Treatment Group Superiority of sequential methotrexate, fluorouracil and leucovorin to fluorouracil alone in advanced symptomatic colorectal carcinoma: a randomized trial. J Clin Oncol 1989;7:1437.
262. Nozaki S, Ito T, Kamiike W, Uchikoshi F, Yamamoto S, Nakata S, Shirakura R, Miyata M, Matsuda H, Stepkowski, S.M. Effect of brequinar sodium on accelerated cardiac allograft rejection in presensitized recipients. Transplant Proc 1994;26:2333.
263. Nutter LM, Cheng YC. Nature and properties of mammalian ribonucleoside diphosphate reductase. In Inhibitors of Ribonucleoside diphosphate reductase activity. Edited by JG Cory, AH Cory. New York: Pergamon Press, 1989, p 37.
264. O'Brien S, Kantarjian H, Estey E, Koller C, Robertson B, Beran M, Andreeff M., Pierce S, Keating M. Lack of effect of 2-chlorodeoxyadenosine therapy in patients with chronic lymphocytic leukemia refractory to fludarabine therapy. N Engl J Med 1994;330:319.
265. O'Brien S, Kurzrock R, Duvic M, Kantarjian H, Stass S, Robertson, L.E. Estey E, Pierce S, Keating, M.J. 2-Chlorodeoxyadenosine therapy in patients with T-cell lymphoproliferative disorders. Blood 1994;84:733.
266. O'Connell MJ. A phase III trial of 5-fluorouracil and leucovorin in the treatment of advanced colorectal cancer. Cancer 1989;63:1026.
267. O'Dwyer PJ, King SA, Hoth DF, Leyland-Jones B. Role of thymidine in biochemical modulation: a review. Cancer Res 1987;47:3911.
268. O'Dwyer PJ, Marsoni S. Conference on deoxycoformycin: current status and future directions. Cancer Treatment Symposium 1984;2:1.
269. O'Dwyer PJ, Paul AR, Walczak J, Weiner LM, Litwin S, Comic RL. Phase II study of biochemical modulation of fluorouracil by low dose PALA in patients with colorectal cancer. J Clin Oncol 1990;8:1497.
270. O'Dwyer PJ, Wagner B, Leyland-Jones B, Wittes RE, Cheson BD, Hoth DF. 2′-Deoxycoformycin (Pentostatin) for lymphoid malignancies. Ann Intern Med 1988;108:733.
271. Ohno Y, Spriggs D, Matsukage A, Kufe D. Effects of 1-β-D-arabinofuranosylcytosine incorporation on elongation of specific DNA sequences by DNA polymerase β. Cancer Res 1988;48:1494.
272. Ota K, Taguchi T, Kimura K. Report on nationwide pooled data and cohort investigation in UFT phase II study. Cancer Chemother Pharmacol 1988;22:333.
273. Parker WB, Bapat AR, Shen JX, Townsend AJ, Cheng YC. Interaction of 2-halogenated dATP analogs (F, Cl and Br) with human DNA polymerases, DNA primase, and ribonucleotide reductase. Mol Pharmacol 1988;34:485.
274. Parker WB, Cheng YC. Inhibition of DNA primase by nucleoside triphosphates and their arabinofuranosyl analogs. Mol Pharmacol 1987;31:146.
275. Parker WB, Cheng YC. Metabolism and mechanism of action of 5-fluorouracil. Pharmacol Ther 1990;48:381.
276. Paterson ARP, Kolassa N, Cass CE. Transport of nucleoside drugs in animal cells. Pharmacol Ther 1981;12:515.
277. Paterson ARP, Oliver JM. Nucleoside transport. II. Inhibition by *p*-Nitrobenzylthioguanosine and related compounds. Can J Biochem 1971;49:271.
278. Paterson ARP, Tidd DM. 6-Thiopurines. In Handbook of Experimental Pharmacology. Edited by AD Sartorelli and DG Johns. Berlin: Springer-Verlag, 1975, p 384.
279. Pazdur R, Ajani JA, Patt YZ, Winn R, Jackson D, Shepard B, DuBrow R, Campos L, Quaraishi M, Faintuch J, Abbruzzese JL, Gutterman J, Levin B. Phase II study of fluorouracil and recombinant interferon α-2a in previously untreated advanced colorectal carcinoma. J Clin Oncol 1990;8:2027.
280. Peters GJ, Lankelma J, Kok RM, Noordhuis P, van Groeningen CJ, van der Wilt CL, Meyer S, Pinedo, H.M. Prolonged retention of high concentrations of 5-fluorouracil in human and murine tumors as compared with plasma. Cancer Chemother Pharmacol 1993;31:269.
281. Peters GJ, Laurensse E, Lankelma J, Leyva A, Pinedo HM. Separation of several 5-fluorouracil metabolites in various melanoma cell lines: evidence for the synthesis of 5-fluorouracil-nucleotide sugars. Eur J Cancer Clin Oncol 1984;20:1425.
282. Peters GJ, Sharma SL, Laurensse E, Pinedo HM. Inhibition of pyrimidine de novo synthesis by DUP-785 (NSC 368390). Invest New Drugs 1987;5:235.
283. Peters GJ, van Dijk J, Laurensse E, van Groeningen CJ, Lankelma J, Leyva A, Nadal JC, Pinedo HM. In vitro biochemical and in vivo biological studies of the uridine 'rescue' of 5-fluorouracil. Br J Cancer 1988;57:259.
284. Peters GJ, Van Dijk J, Nadal JC, Van Groeningen CJ, Lankelman J, Pineda HM. Diurnal variation in the therapeutic efficacy of 5-fluorouracil against murine colon cancer. In Vivo 1987;1:113.
285. Peters GJ, van Dijk J, van Groeningen CJ, Laurensse EJ, Leyva A, Lankelma J, Pinedo HM. Toxicity and antitumor effect of 5-fluorouracil and its rescue by uridine. Adv Exp Med Biol 195B:121 1986.
286. Peterson MS, Ingraham HA, Goulian M. 2′-Deoxyribosyl analogues of UDP-N-acetylglucosamine in cells treated with methotrexate or 5-fluorodeoxyridine. J Biol Chem 1983;258:10831.
287. Philips FS, Sternberg SS, Hamilton L, Clarke DA. The toxic effects of 6-mercaptopurine and related compounds. Ann NY Acad Sci 1954;60:283.
288. Piper AA, Fox RM. Biochemical basis for the differential sensitivity of human T- and B-lymphocyte lines to 5-fluorouracil. Cancer Res 1982;42:3753.
289. Piro LD, Carrera CJ, Beutler E, Carson DA. 2-Chloro-deoxyadenosine.an effective new agent for the treatment of chronic lymphocytic leukemia. Blood 1988;72:1069.
290. Piro LD, Carrera CJ, Carson DA, Beutler E. Lasting remissions in hairy-cell leukemia induced by a single infusion of 2-chlorodeoxyadenosine. N Engl J Med 1990;322:1117.
291. Pizzorno G, Leffert JJ, Hartigan DJ, Buzaid AC, Marsh JC, Strair RK, Ravikumar TS. Dose-dependent depletion of plasma uridine pools in cancer patients by brequinar treatment. Proc Am Assoc Cancer Res, 33: a2527 1992.
292. Pizzorno G, Marsh JC, Leffert JJ, Handschumacher RE, Calabresi P. Pharmacokinetics of benzylacyclouridine (BAU) in patients with refractory solid tumors (phase I trial). Proc Am Assoc Cancer Res, 1993;34:a127.
293. Pizzorno G, Wiegand RA, Lentz SK, Handschumacher RE. Brequinar potentiates 5-fluorouracil antitumor activity in a murine model colon 38 tumor by tissue specific modulation of uridine nucleotide pools. Cancer Res 1992;52:1660.
294. Plagemann PGW, Behrens M, Abraham D. Metabolism and cytotoxicity of 5-azacytidine in cultured Novikoff rat hepatomaand P388 mouse leukemia cells and their enhancement by preincubation with pyrazofurin. Cancer Res 1978;38:2458.
295. Plunkett W, Gandhi V, Chubb S, Nowak B, Heinemann V, Mineishi S. Sen A, Hertel LW, Grindey, G.B. 2′, 2′-difluorodeoxycytidine metabolism and mechanism of action in human leukemia cells. Nucleosides Nucleotides 1989;8:775.
296. Plunkett W, Huang P, Gandhi V. Metabolism and action of fludarabine phosphate. Semin Oncol, 17(suppl 8):3 1990.
297. Plunkett W, Iacoboni S, Estey E, Danhauser L, Liliemark JO, Keating, M.J. Pharmacologically directed ara-C therapy for refractory leukemia. Semin Oncol 1985;12(suppl 3):20.
298. Plunkett W, Saunders PP. Metabolism and action of purine nucleoside analogs. Pharmacol Ther 1991;49:239.
299. Popovic P, Popovic V, Baughman J. Circadian rhythm and 5-FU toxicity in C3H mice. Biomed Thermol 1982;25:185.
300. Porter DJ, Chestnut WG, Merrill BM, Spector T. Mechanism-based inactivation of dihydropyridine dehydrogenase by 5-ethynyluracil. J Biol Chem 1992;267:5236.
301. Presant CA, Wolf W, Waluch V, Brechner R, Wisemasn C, Blayney D. and Kennedy P. Correlation of clinical tumor response with human tumor 5-fluorouracil pharmacokinetics, measured by 19F magnetic resonance spectroscopy (abstract). Proc Am Soc Clin Oncol 1992;11:301.
302. Queisser W, Schnitzler G, Schaefer J, Arnold, H.,Drings P, Fritze D, Geldmacher J, Hartwich G, Herrmann R, Kempf P, Konig H, Meiser RJ, Nedden R, von Oldershausen HF, Pappas A, Sievers H, Wahrendorf J, Westerhausen M, Witte S. Comparison of ftorafur with 5-fluorouracil in combination chemotherapy of advanced gastrointestinal carcinoma. Recent results. Cancer Res 1981;79:82.
303. Raber RM, Hhong, W.K. Phase I/II study of gemcitabine by 30 minute weekly intravenous infusion x 3 weeks every 4 weeks for non-small cell lung cancer. (abstract) Proc Am Soc Clin Oncol 1993;12:326.
304. Remick SC, Grem JL, Fischer PH, Tutsch KD, Alberti DB, Nieting LM, Tombes MD, Bruggink, J.,Willson JKV, Trump DL. Phase I trial of 5-fluorouracil and dipyridamole administered by seventy-two-hour concurrent continuous infusion. Cancer Res 1990;50:2667.
305. Remy CN. Metabolism of thiopyrimidines and thiopurines: s-Methylation with s-adenosylmethionine transmethylase and catabolism in mammalian tissues. J Biol Chem 1963;238:1078.
306. Renoux G. The general immunopharmacology of levamisole. Drugs 1980;19:89.
307. Reyes P, Guganig ME. Studies on a pyrimidine phosphoribosyltransferase from murine leukemia P1534J. J Biol Chem 1975;250:5097.
308. Rodnan GP, Robin JA, Tolchin SF, Elion GB. Allopurinol and gouty hyperuricemia. JAMA 1975;231:1143.
309. Romanini A, Lin JT, Niedzwiecki D, Bunni M, Priest DG, Bertino JR. Role of folypolyglutamates in biochemical modulation of fluoropyrimidines by leucovorin. Cancer Res 1991;51:789.
310. Rosenthal F, Wislicki L, Koller, L.auUber die Bziehungen von schwertsen Blutgiften zu Abauprodukten desEinweisses: ein Beitrag zum Enstehungmechanismus der pernizosen Anemie. Klin Wochenschr 1928;7:972.
311. Ruiz van Haperen, V.W.T, Veerman G, Boven E, Noordhuis P, Vermorken JD, Peters, G.J. Schedule dependence of sensitivity to 2′, 2′-difluorodeoxycytidine (gemcitabine) in relation to accumulation and retention of its triphosphate in solid tumour cell lines and solid tumours. Biochem Pharmacol 1994;48:1327.
312. Ruiz van Haperen VWT, Veerman G, Eriksson S, Boven E, Stegmann A, Hermsen M, Vermorken JB, Pinedo HM, Peters, G.J. Development and molecular characterization of a 2′, 2′-difluorodeoxycytidine-resistant variant of the human ovarian carcinoma cell line A2780. Cancer Res 1994;54:4138.
313. Ruiz van Haperen VWT, Veerman G, Vermorken JB, Peters, G.J. 2′, 2′-Difluorodeoxycytidine (gemcitabine) incorporation into RNA and DNA of tumour cell lines. Biochem Pharmacol 1993;46:762.
314. Rustum YM, Cao S, Spector T. 5-Ethynyluracil (776C85) is a potent modulator of the therapeutic activity of 5-fluorouracil (abstract) Proc Am Assoc Cancer Res 1993;34:a1686.
315. Rutman RJ, Cantarow A, Paschkis K. Studies in 2-acetylaminofluorene carcinogenesis. III. The utilization of uracil-2-C14 by preneoplastic rat liver and rat hepatoma. Cancer Res 1954;14:119.
316. Sandler AB, Buzaid AC, Pizzorno G, Durivage HJ, Lamb L, Marsh JC, Strair RK, Ravikumar TS. Phase I trial of sequential brequinar and 5-fluorouracil in refractory solid tumors. Proc Am Soc Clin Oncol 1992;11:a366.
317. Santana VM, Hurwitz CA, Blakley RL, Crom WR, Luo X, Roberts, W.M. Complete hematologic remissions induced by 2-chlorodeoxyadenosine in children with newly diagnosed acute myeloid leukemia. Blood 1994;84:1237.
318. Santi DV, McHenry, C.S. and Sommer H. Mechanism of interaction of thymidylate synthetase with 5-fluorodeoxyuridylate. Biochemistry 1974;13:471.
319. Schlemmer HP, Semmler W, Bachert P, Schlag, P.and van Kaick G. Evaluation of early response for in vivo 19F NMR spectroscopy in therapy monitoring of patients with liver metastases of colorectal carcinoma. Radiology 1991;181:210.

320. Schneider M. Circadian rhythm-varying plasma concentration of 5-fluorouracil during a five-day continuous venous infusion at a constant rate in cancer patients. Cancer Res 1988;48:1676.
321. Scholar EM, Calabresi P. Increased activity of alkaline phosphates in leukemic cells from patients resistant to thiopurines. Biochem Pharmacol 1979;28:445.
322. Scholer JJ. Flucytosine. In Antifungal Chemotherapy. Edited by DCE Speller. New York: Wiley, 1980, p:35.
323. Schwartz, E.L, Hoffman M, O'Connor CJ, Wadler S. Stimulation of 5-fluorouracil metabolic activation by interferon-alpha in human colon carcinoma cells, Biochem Biophys Res Commun 1992;182:1232.
324. Schwartz PM, Dunigan JM, Marsh JC, Handschumacher RE. Allopurinol modification of the toxicity and antitumor activity of 5-fluorouracil. Cancer Res 1980;40:1885.
325. Schwenk M, Hegazy E, Lopez Del Pino V. Uridine uptake by isolated intestinal epithelial cells of guinea pig. Biochim Biophys Acta 1984;805:370.
326. Seifert P, Baker L, Reed ML, Vaitkevicius VK. Comparison of continuously infused 5-fluorouracil with bolus injection in treatment of patients with colorectal adenocarcinoma. Cancer 1975;36:123.
327. Seto S, Carrera CJ, Kubota M, Wasson DB, Carson DA. Mechanism of deoxyadenosine and 2-chlorodeoxyadenosine toxicity to non-dividing human lymphocytes. J Clin Invest 1985;75:377.
328. Seto S, Carrera CJ, Wasson DB, Carson DA. Inhibition of DNA repair by deoxyadenosine in resting human lymphocytes. J Immunol 1986;136:2839.
329. Shah A, MacDonald W, Goldie J, Gudauskas G, Brisebois B. 5-Fluorouracil infusion in advanced colorectal cancer: a comparison of three dose schedules. Cancer Treat Rep 1985;69:739.
330. Shani J, Danenberg PV. Evidence that intracellular synthesis of 5-fluorouridine-5′-phosphate from 5-fluorouracil and 5-fluorouridine is compartmentalized. Biochem Biophys Res Commun 1984;122:439.
331. Shepherd CA, Gatzemeier U, Gotfried M. Weynants R, Cottier B. Groen H, Rosso R, Mattson K, Cotes-Funes H, Tonato M, Hatty S, Voi M. An extended phase II study of gemcitabine in non small cell lung cancer. Proc Am Soc Clin Oncol 1993;12:330.
332. Shewach DS, Hahn TM, Chang E, Hertel, L.W. Lawrence, T.S. Metabolism of 2′, 2′-difluoro-2-deoxycytidine and radiation senzitation of human colon carcinoma cells. Cancer Res 1994;54:3218.
333. Shewach DS, Plunkett W. Cellular retention of 9-β-Darabinofuranosyladenine-5′-triphosphate and the pattern of recovery of DNA synthesis in Chinese hamster ovary cells. Cancer Res 1986;46:1581.
334. Shirwan H, Cosenza CA, Wang HK, Wu GD, Makowka L, Cramer DV. Prevention of orthotopic liver allograft rejection in rats with a short-term brequinar sodium therapy. Analysis of intragraft cytokine gene expression. Transplantation 1994;57:1072.
335. Siaw MF, Coleman MS. In vitro metabolism of deoxycoformycin in human T lymphoblastoid cells. Phosphorylation of deoxycoformycin and incorporation into cellular DNA. J Bio Chem 1984;259:9426.
336. Sillman FH, Sedlis A, Boyce JG. A review of lower genital intraepithelial neoplasia and the use of topical 5-fluorouracil. Obstet Gynecol Surv 1985;40: 190.
337. Singer J, Wallace SL. The allopurinol hypersensitivity syndrome: unnecessary morbidity and mortality. Arthritis Rheum 1986;29:82.
338. Sirotnak FM, Chello PL, Dorick DM, Montgomery JA. Specificity of systems mediating transport of adenosine, 9-β-D-arabinofuranosyl-2-fluoradenine, and other purine nucleoside analogues in L1210 cells. Cancer Res 1983;43:104.
339. Skipper HE. On the mechanism of action of 6-mercaptopurine. Ann NY Acad Sci 1954;60:315.
340. Skoda J. Azapyrimidine nucleosides. In Antineoplastic and Immunosuppressive Agents. Edited by AC Sartorelli, DG Johns. Berlin: Springer-Verlag, 1975, p 348.
341. Sobrero AF, Handschumacher RE, Bertino JR. Highly selective drug combinations for human colon cancer cells resistant in vitro to 5-fluoro-2′-deoxyuridine. Cancer Res 1985;45:3161.
342. Sobrero AF, Moir RD, Bertino JR, Handschumacher RE. Defective facilitated diffusion of nucleosides, a primary mechanism of resistance to 5-fluoro-2′-deoxyuridine in the HCT-8 human carcinoma line. Cancer Res 1985;45:3155.
343. Sorm F, Piskala A, Cihak A, Vesely J. 5-Azacytidine, a new highly effective cancerostatic. Experientia 1964;20:202.
344. Spector T, Johns DG. Stoichiometric inhibition of reduced xanthine oxidase by hydroxypyrazolo (3, 4-d) pyrimidines. J Biol Chem 1964;239:2570.
345. Spiers AS, Moore D, Cassileth PA, Harrington DP, Cummings FJ, Neiman RS, Bennett JM, O'Connell MJ. Remissions in hairy-cell leukemia with pentostatin (2′-deoxycoformycin). N Engl J Med 1987;316:825.
346. Spriggs D, Robbins G, Mitchell T, Kufe D. Incorporation of 9-β-D-arabinofuranosyl-2-fluoradenine into HL-60 cellular RNA and DNA. Biochem Pharmacol 1986;35:247.
347. Sugarbaker PH, Klecker RW, Gianola FJ, Speyer JC. Prolonged treatment schedules with intraperitoneal 5-fluorouracil diminish the local-regional nature of drug distribution. Am J Clin Oncol 1986;9:1.
348. Sweeny DJ, Barnes S, Heggie GD, Diasio RB. Metabolism fluorouracil N-choly-2-fluoro-μ-alanine conjugate: previously unrecognized role for bile acids in drug conjugation. Proc Natl Acad Sci USA 1987;84:5439.
349. Swyryd EA, Seaver SS, Stark GR. N-(Phosphonacetyl)-L-aspartate, a potent transition state analog inhibitor as aspartate transcarbamylase, blocks proliferation of mammalian cells in culture. J Biol Chem 1974;49:6945.
350. Tagger AV, Boux J, Wright JA. Hydroxy (14C) urea uptake by normal and transformed human cells:evidence for a mechanism of passive diffusion. Biochem Cell Biol 1987;65:925.
351. Talley RW, Vaitkevicius VK. Megaloblastosis produced by a cytosine antagonist, 1-β-D-arabinofuranosylcytosine. Blood 1963;21:252.
352. Tanaka M, Kimura K, Yoshida S. Increased incorporation of 5-fluorodeoxyuridine into DNA of human T-lymphoblastic cell lines. Gann 1984;75:986.
353. Tashiro H, Nomura Y. Ohsaki A. A double blind comparative study of tegafur (FT) and UFT (a combination of tegafur and uracil) in advanced breast cancer. Jpn J Clin Oncol 1994;24:212.
354. Tidd DM. Antipurines. In Handbook of Experimental Pharmacology. Edited by BW Fox, M. Fox. Berlin: Springer-Verlag, 1984, p 445.
355. Townsend A, Leclerc J-M, Dutschman G, Cooney D, Cheng Y-C. Metabolism of 1-β-D-Arabinofuranosyl-5-Azacytosine and incorporation into DNA of human T-lymphoblastic cells (molt-4). Cancer Res 1985;45:3522.
356. Townsend AJ, Cheng Y-C. Sequence-specific effects of ara-5-aza-CTP and ara-CTP on DNA synthesis by purified human DNA polymerases in vitro: visualization of chain elongation on a defined template. Mol Pharmacol 1987;32:330.
357. Tsavaris N, Bacoyannis C, Milonakis N, Sarafidou M, Zamanis N, Magoulas D, Kosmidis P. Folinic acid plus high-dose 5-fluorouracil with allopurinol protection in the treatment of advanced colorectal carcinoma. Eur J Cancer 1990;26:1054.
358. Tsavaris NB, Komitsopoulou P, Tzannou I, Loucatou P, Tsaroucha-Noutsou A, Kilafis G, Kosmidis P. Decreased oral toxicity with the local use of allopurinol in patients who received high dose 5-fluorouracil. Sel Cancer Ther 1991;7:113.
359. Tseng WC, Derse D, Cheng YC, Brockman RW, Bennett LL Jr. In vitro activity of 9-β-D-arabinofuranosyl-2-fluoradenine and the biochemical actions of its triphosphate on DNA polymerases and ribonucleotide reductase from HeLa cells. Mol Pharmacol 1982;21:474.
360. Ullman B, Lee M, Martin DW Jr, Santi DV. Cytotoxicity of 5-fluoro-2′-deoxyuridine: requirement for reduced folate cofactors and antagonism by methotrexate. Proc Natl Acad Sci USA 1978;75:980.
361. Umeda M, Heidelberger C. Comparative studies of fluorinated pyrimidines with various cell lines. Cancer Res 1968;28:2529.
362. Valeriote F. Cellular aspects of the action of cytosine arabinoside. Med Pediatr Oncol 1982;10(S1):221.
363. Van Groeningen CJ, Peters GJ, Leyva A, Laurensse E, Pinedo HM. Reversal of 5-fluorouracil-induced myelosuppression by prolonged administration of high-dose uridine. J Natl Cancer Inst 1989;81:157.
364. Van Groeningen CJ, Pinedo HM, Heddes J, Kok RM, de Jong APJM, Wattel E, Peters GJ, Lankelma J. Pharmacokinetics of 5-fluorouracil assessed with a sensitive mass spectrometric method in patients on a dose escalation schedule. Cancer Res 1988;48:6956.
365. Van Groeningen CJ, Peters GJ, Nadal JC, Laurensse E, Pinedo HM. Clinical and pharmacologic study of orally administered uridine. J Natl Cancer Inst 1991;83:437.
366. Van Laar JA, Durrani FA, Rustum YM. Antitumor activity of the weekly intravenous push schedule of 5-fluoro-2′-deoxyuridine ± N-phosphonacetyl-L-aspartate in mice bearing advanced colon carcinoma 26. Cancer Res 1993;53:1560.
367. Vesell ES, Passananti GT, Greene F. Impairment of drug metabolism in man by allopurinol and nortriptyline. N Engl J Med 1970;283:1484.
368. Vesely J, Cihak A. 5-Azacytidine: mechanism of action and biological effects in mammalian cells. Pharmacol Ther 1978;2:813.
369. Vine EN, Young D, Vine WH, Wolf W. An improved synthesis of 18F-5-fluorouracil. International Journal of Applied Radiation and Isotopes 1979;30:401.
370. Wadler S, Schwartz EL, Goldman M, Lyver A, Rader M, Zimmerman M, Itri L, Weinberg V, Wiernik PH. Fluorouracil and recombinant α-2a-interferon: an active regimen against advanced colorectal carcinoma. J Clin Oncol 1989;7:1769.
371. Washtien WL. Comparison of 5-fluorouracil metabolism in two human gastrointestinal tumor cell lines. Cancer Res 1984;44:909.
372. Wohlhueter RM, McIvor RS, Plagemann PGW. Facilitated transport of uracil and 5-fluorouracil, and permeation of orotic acid into cultured mammalian cells. J Cell Physiol 1980;104:309.
373. Wolf W, Presant CA, Servic KL, El-Tahtawy A, Albright MJ, Barker PB, Ring R, Atkinson D, Ong RL, King M, Singh M, Ray M, Wiseman C, Blayney D, Shani J. Tumor trapping of 5-FU: in vivo 19F-NMR spectroscopic pharmacokinetics in tumor-bearing humans and rabbits. Proc Natl Acad Sci 1990;87:492.
374. Wolfenden R, Wentworth DF. On the interaction of 3,4,5,6-tetrahydrouridine with human liver cytidine deaminase. Biochemistry 1975;14:5099.
375. Woo PW, Dion HW, Lange SM, Dahl LF, Durham LJ. A Novel adenosine and araA inhibitor,(R)-3-(2-deoxy-βD-erythropento-furanosyl)-3, 6, 7, 8-tetrahydroimidazo (4, 5-d) (1, 3) diazepin-8-o1. J Heterocyclic Chem 1974;11:64.
376. Woodcock TM, Martin DS, Damin LAM, Kemeny NE, Young CW. Combination clinical trials with thymidineand fluorouracil: a Phase I and clinical pharmacologic evaluation. Cancer 1980;45:1135.
377. Woolley PV, Ayoob MJ, Smith FP, Lakey JL, DeGreen P, Marantz A, Schein PS. A controlled trial of the effect of 4-hydroxypyrazolopyrimidine (allopurinol) on the toxicity of a single bolus dose of 5-fluorouracil. J Clin Oncol 1985;3:103.
378. Wright JA, Alam TG, McClarty GA, Tagger AY, Thelander L. Altered expression of M1 and M2 gene amplification in hydroxy-urea resistant hamster, mouse, rat, and human cell line. Somat Cell Mol Genet 1987;13:155.
379. Wright JE, Dreyfuss A, El-Magharbel I, Trites D, Jones SM, Holden SA, Rosowsky A, Frei E III. Selective expansion of 5,10-methylenetetrahydrofolate pools and modulation of 5-fluorouracil antitumor activity by leucovorin in vivo. Cancer Res 1989;49: 2592.
380. Yamamoto S, Kawasaki T. Active transport of 5-fluorouracil and its energy coupling in Ehrlich ascites tumor cells. J Biochem 1981;90:635.
381. Yang JL, Chang EH, Capizzi RL. Effect of uracil arabinoside on metabolism and cytotoxicity of cytosine arabinoside in 25178Y murine leukemia. J Clin Invest 1985;75: 141.
382. Yang, S-W., Huang P, Plunkett W, Becker FF, Chan JYH. Dual Mode of Inhibition of Purified DNA Ligase I from Human Cells by 9-β-D-arabinofuranosyl-2-Fluoroadenosine Triphosphate. J Biol Chem 1992;267:2345.
383. Yang-Feng TL, Barton DE, Thelander L, Lewis WH, Srinivasan PR, Francke U. Ribonucleotide reductase M2 subunit sequences mapped to four different chromosomal sites in humans and mice: functional locus identified by its amplification in hydroxyurea-resistant cell lines. Genomics 1987;1:77.
384. Yen Y, Grill SP, Dutschman GE, Chang CN, Zhou BS, Cheng YC. Characterization of a hydroxyurea-resistant human KB cell line with supersensitivity to 6-thioguanine. Cancer Res 1994;54:3686.
385. Yu J, Matsumoto SS, Yu AL. Inhibition of transcription as a mechanism of lymphocytotoxicity induced by deoxyadenosine and 2′-deoxycoformycin. Cancer Treat Symp 1984;2:75.
386. Zimm S, Collins J, O'Neill D, Chabner BA, Poplack DG. Inhibition of first-pass metabolism in cancer chemotherapy: interaction of 6-mercaptopurine and allopurinol. Clin Pharmacol Ther 1983;34:810.
387. Zimm S, Collins JM, Riccardi R, O'Neill D, Narang PK, Chabner B, Poplack DG. Variable bioavailability of oral mercaptopurine. Is maintenance chemotherapy in acute lymphoblastic leukemia being optimally delivered? N Engl J Med 1983;308: 1005.

CHAPTER 62

Alkylating Agents and Platinum Antitumor Compounds

O. MICHAEL COLVIN

Introduction

The alkylating agents and the platinum antitumor compounds form strong chemical bonds with electron-rich atoms (nucleophiles), such as sulfur in proteins and nitrogen in DNA. While these compounds react with many biological molecules, the primary cytotoxic actions of both classes of agents appear to be the inhibition of DNA replication and cell division produced by their reactions with DNA. However, the chemical differences between these two classes of agents produce significant differences in their antitumor and toxic effects.

Alkylating Agents

The alkylating agents were the first nonhormonal drugs to be used effectively in the treatment of cancer and the story behind the recognition of the antitumor effects of these compounds is a remarkable one. During World War I toxic gases were used as military weapons. The most devastating of these gases was sulfur mustard (Fig. 62.1). The compound was used as a weapon because of its vesicant effects, which produce skin irritation, blindness, and pulmonary damage. However, it was observed that troops and civilians who were exposed to sulfur mustard also developed bone marrow suppression and lymphoid aplasia. Because of these findings, sulfur mustard was evaluated as a topical antitumor agent (3). The closely related, but less toxic, nitrogen mustards of World War II vintage were selected for further study. Trials in patients with lymphoma demonstrated regression of tumors, with relief of symptoms (186, 256, 440). These results encouraged the search for nitrogen mustards that were more effective and less toxic and stimulated efforts to find other chemicals with antitumor activity.

CHEMISTRY OF THE ALKYLATING AGENTS

The alkylating agents are compounds that react with electron-rich atoms in biologic molecules to form covalent bonds. Traditionally, these agents have been divided into two types, those that react directly with biological molecules and those that form a reactive intermediate, which then reacts with the biologic molecules. These types are termed SN1 and SN2, respectively, and are illustrated in Figure 62.2. The terms refer to the kinetics of the reactions; the rate of reaction of an SN1 agent is dependent only on the concentration of the reactive intermediate, while the rate of reaction of an SN2 agent is dependent on the concentration of the alkylating agent and of the molecule with which it is reacting. This distinction has important implications in understanding the cellular and molecular pharmacology of specific alkylating agents. The nitrogen mustards and nitrosoureas are examples of SN1 agents, while busulfan is an SN2 agent.

A large number of chemical compounds are alkylating agents under physiological conditions, and a variety of such compounds have been found to have antitumor activity. While it is not possible to describe all of the compounds that have been used clinically, those compounds that are currently used extensively, look promising in clinical trials, or represent a type of alkylating agent will be discussed.

TYPES OF ALKYLATING AGENTS

Nitrogen Mustards

The most widely used alkylating agents are the nitrogen mustards. While thousands of nitrogen mustards have been synthesized and tested, only five are commonly used in cancer therapy today. These are mechlorethamine (the original "nitrogen mustard"), cyclophosphamide, ifosfamide, melphalan, and chlorambucil, and they are illustrated in Figure 62.3. The characteristic chemical constituent of the nitrogen mustards is the bischloroethyl group and all of the nitrogen mustards react through an aziridinium intermediate as shown in Figure 62.4. The remainder of the molecule is important in determining the physical properties of the molecule and affects the transport, distribution, and reactivity of the specific agents. The importance of the total molecule is demonstrated by cyclophosphamide.

Cyclophosphamide is not a reactive compound, but it undergoes activation in the body. The complex activation scheme (93) is shown in Figure 62.5. The initial activation reaction is carried out by microsomal oxidation in the liver to produce 4-hydroxycyclophosphamide, which is in spontaneous equilibrium with the tautomer, aldophosphamide (151). At physiological pH, this equilibrium is predominantly in the form of 4-hydroxycyclophosphamide (572). This equilibrium mixture diffuses from the hepatocyte into the plasma and is distributed throughout the body. Since 4-hydroxycyclophosphamide is relatively nonpolar, it enters target cells readily by diffusion. Aldophosphamide spontaneously decomposes to produce phosphoramide mustard, which is the first reactive alkylating agent produced in the metabolism of cyclophosphamide. While phosphoramide mustard is also produced extracellularly, this compound is very polar, enters cells poorly, and appears to play relatively little role in the therapeutic and toxic effects of cyclophosphamide. Thus, 4-hydroxycyclophosphamide/aldophosphamide serves as an efficient mechanism to deliver the alkylating phosphoramide mustard into cells. The major reason that cyclophosphamide is the most widely used alkylating agent is that it produces less gastrointestinal and hematopoietic toxicity than other alkylating agents. The basis for this decreased toxicity is the enzyme aldehyde dehydrogenase. This enzyme oxidizes al-

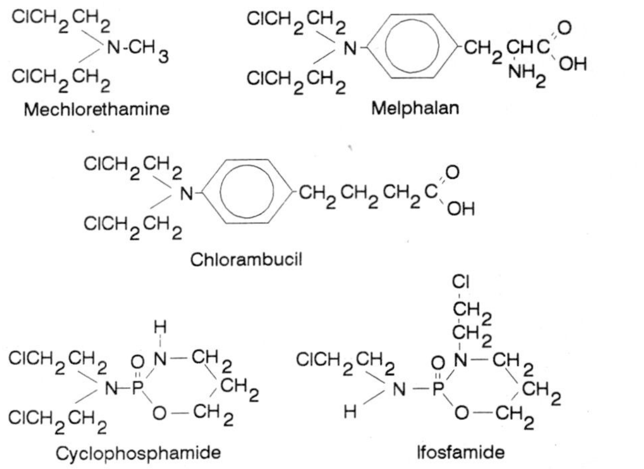

$ClCH_2CH_2{-}S{-}CH_2CH_2Cl$

Figure 62.1. Structure of sulfur mustard (bischloroethylsulfide).

$$RX \longrightarrow R^+ + X^- \xrightarrow{Y^-} RY + X^-$$

S_N1 Reaction

$$RX + Y^- \longrightarrow [\overset{\delta^-}{Y}\cdots R\cdots \overset{\delta^-}{X}] \longrightarrow RY + X^-$$

S_N2 Reaction

Figure 62.2. SN1 and SN2 reactions of alkylating agents.

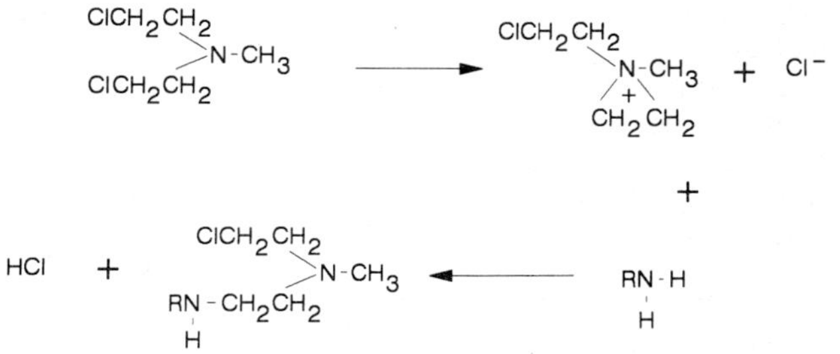

Mechlorethamine

Melphalan

Chlorambucil

Cyclophosphamide

Ifosfamide

Figure 62.3. Structures of nitrogen mustards currently used in therapy.

Figure 62.4. Alkylation mechanism of nitrogen mustards.

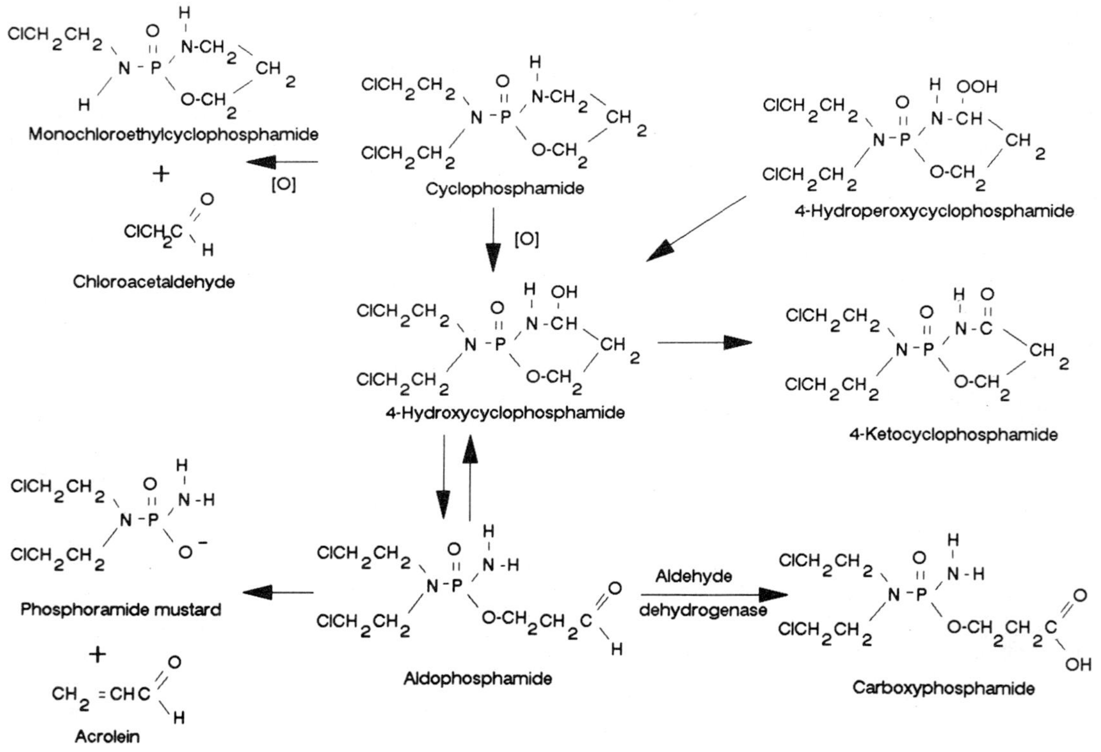

Monochloroethylcyclophosphamide

Chloroacetaldehyde

Cyclophosphamide

4-Hydroperoxycyclophosphamide

4-Hydroxycyclophosphamide

4-Ketocyclophosphamide

Phosphoramide mustard

Acrolein

Aldophosphamide

Aldehyde dehydrogenase

Carboxyphosphamide

Figure 62.5. Metabolism of cyclophosphamide.

dophosphamide to carboxyphosphamide, an inactive product, which is excreted in the urine and accounts for about 80% of an administered dose of cyclophosphamide in any species. This enzyme is found in high concentration in the hepatic cytosol, in primitive hematopoietic cells, and in the stem cells and mucosal absorptive cells in the intestine (459). Administration of an inhibitor of this enzyme to an animal markedly increases the hematopoietic and gastrointestinal toxicity of cyclophosphamide (459).

Ifosfamide is a structural isomer of cyclophosphamide that is being used increasingly in the treatment of testicular tumors and sarcomas (19, 322, 422). This compound undergoes the same metabolic reactions as cyclophosphamide, but the location of the chloroethyl group on the ring nitrogen produces quantitative changes in the metabolism of the drug (53, 91) and subtle changes in the chemical properties of the reactive metabolite, ifosfamide mustard, so that it is less reactive than phosphoramide mustard (52). The primary metabolite, aldoifosfamide, is a substrate for aldehyde dehydrogenase, so that the bone marrow and gastrointestinal tract sparing properties are similar to those of cyclophosphamide. The oxidation of the chloroethyl side chains to produce choroacetaldehyde is a minor metabolic pathway for cyclophosphamide (<10% of dose) but is increased to as much as 50% for ifosfamide. The increased production of chloracetaldehyde has been implicated in the neurotoxicity of ifosfamide (187), and may also contribute to the greater renal and bladder toxicity of ifosfamide. The greater side chain oxidation of ifosfamide and the lesser reactivity of the ifosfamide mustard are consistent with the fact that higher doses of ifosfamide than cyclophosphamide are used clinically.

Melphalan is an alkylating agent that has been used extensively in the treatment of multiple myeloma (31, 97), ovarian cancer (164, 545, 567), and breast cancer (156, 442). Melphalan is an amino acid analogue that has been shown to enter cells and cross the blood-brain barrier through active transport systems. The natural substrates for these systems are amino acids (38, 182, 548), and the entry of melphalan into cells (549) and the central nervous system (195) can be modulated by the presence of certain amino acids in the extracellular fluid (199).

Chlorambucil has been used extensively for the treatment of chronic lymphocytic leukemia (163, 211, 458), ovarian carcinoma (215, 561), and lymphoma (184, 421), but it has been used less often in high-dose combination therapies than the other nitrogen mustards that are described here. This agent is well tolerated by most patients and can be used in patients who have severe nausea and vomiting with cyclophosphamide or melphalan.

Aziridines and Epoxides

Closely related to the nitrogen mustards are the aziridines, which are represented in current therapy by thiotepa, mitomycin C, and AZQ, illustrated in Figure 62.6. These agents presumably alkylate by the same mechanism as the aziridinium intermediates produced by the nitrogen mustards, but the aziridine rings in these compounds are uncharged and not very reactive in vitro.

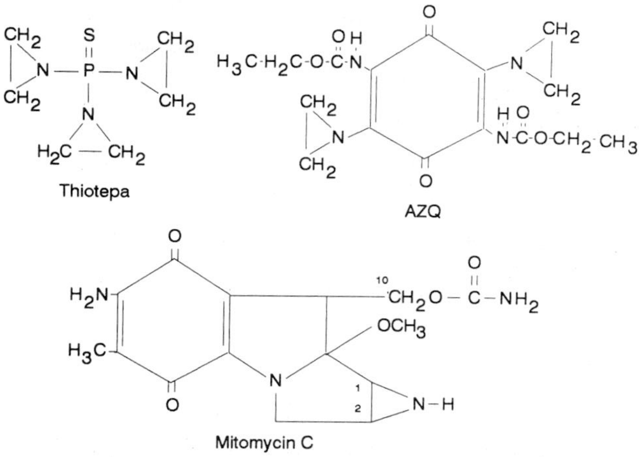

Thiotepa

AZQ

Mitomycin C

Figure 62.6. Structures of aziridine alkylating agents.

Thiotepa (triethylene thiophosphoramide) has been used particularly in the treatment of carcinomas of the breast and ovary and for the intrathecal therapy of meningeal carcinomatosis (194, 203, 406). Thiotepa is oxidatively desulfurated by hepatic microsomes to produce TEPA (370). While TEPA is cytotoxic, it is less so than thiotepa (349). After the clinical administration of thiotepa, both thiotepa and TEPA are found in the blood (208, 224), and the concentration and AUC exposure to TEPA may exceed those of thiotepa (208). The AUC exposure to thiotepa has been shown to correlate with the degree of myelosuppression in patients, while the AUC exposure to TEPA did not (207). Some studies have suggested that a metabolite is produced that is more reactive than the parent compound (133, 516). However, such a metabolite has not been characterized, and the activity of thiotepa may be enhanced by low pH within tumor cells. At the lower pH, the aziridine ring will be protonated and more reactive.

Mitomycin C is a natural product that has been used in the treatment of breast cancer and cancers of the gastrointestinal tract (21, 328, 346, 560). This compound contains an aziridine ring, and appears to exert its cytotoxic effect through the cross-linking of DNA (118, 123, 280). Mitomycin C undergoes reduction in the cell, with enhancement of the affinity of the carbon-1 atom of the aziridine ring for nucleophiles, such as the extracyclic nitrogen atom on guanylic acid in DNA. Following this alkylation, there is displacement of the activated carbamate group on the carbon-≈10 carbon atom of mitomycin C by an extracyclic amino nitrogen of a guanylic acid molecule on the complementary DNA strand to produce an interstrand DNA cross-link (61, 62, 253).

AZQ (diazoquone) was designed to be sufficiently lipophilic to readily cross the blood-brain barrier for the treatment of central nervous system tumors (283). It has demonstrated clinical activity against brain tumors (100, 570), other solid tumors, and leukemia (146). AZQ has been shown to undergo reduction of the quinone ring in cells. This reduction results in protonation of the aziridine rings and enhancement of reactivity of the compound (202, 454).

The epoxides, such as dianhydrogalactitol (80, 204) (Fig. 62.7), are chemically related to the aziridines and alkylate

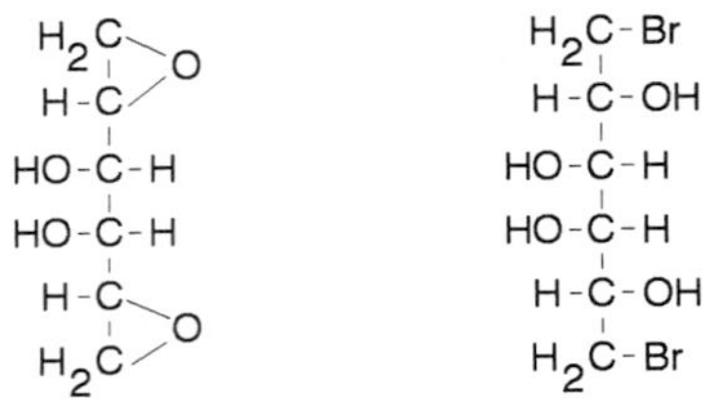

Dianhydrogalactitol Dibromodulcitol

Figure 62.7. Structures of an epoxide alkylating agent (dianhydrogalactitol) and an epoxide prodrug (dibromodulcitol).

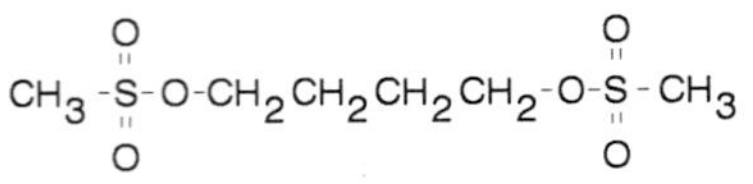

Busulfan

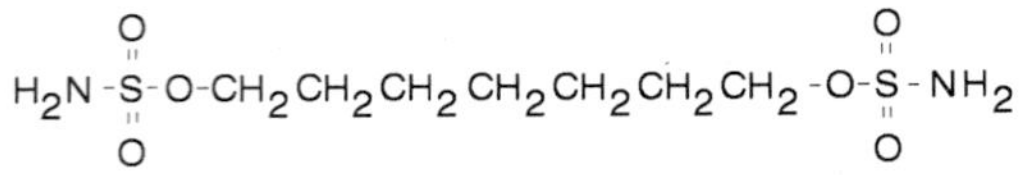

Hepsulfam

Figure 62.8. Structure of alkyl sulfonate (busulfan) and alkyl sulfamate (hepsulfam) agents.

through a similar mechanism of attack of a nucleophile, such as an amino nitrogen, on a carbon of a strained three-member ring. Dibromodulcitol (521) is hydrolyzed to dianhydrogalactitol and thus is a prodrug to an epoxide (476).

Alkyl Sulfonates

The alkyl alkane sulfonate, busulfan (Fig. 62.8), was one of the earliest alkylating agents (205). This compound is one of the few currently used agents that clearly alkylates through an SN2 reaction, as shown in Figure 62.9. Hepsulfam, an alkyl sulfamate analogue of busulfan with a wider range of antitumor activity in preclinical studies (391), is currently in clinical trials. Busulfan has a most interesting, but poorly understood, selective toxicity for early myeloid precursors (139, 165). This selective effect is probably responsible for its activity against chronic myelocytic leukemia (171) and its successful use as a component of bone marrow ablative regimens for bone marrow transplantation of acute myeloid leukemia (464).

Nitrosoureas

The nitrosoureas are a class of alkylating agents that have received considerable attention during the past three decades (111, 251, 469). Several nitrosoureas currently in clinical use or clinical trials are shown in Figure 62.10. These compounds decompose to produce alkylating compounds under physiological conditions. While there are several mechanisms by which this may occur, the predominant mechanism is probably that shown in Figure 62.11, a base catalyzed decomposition to a chloroethyl diazonium moiety (92), which has been shown to react with DNA (291, 327), as

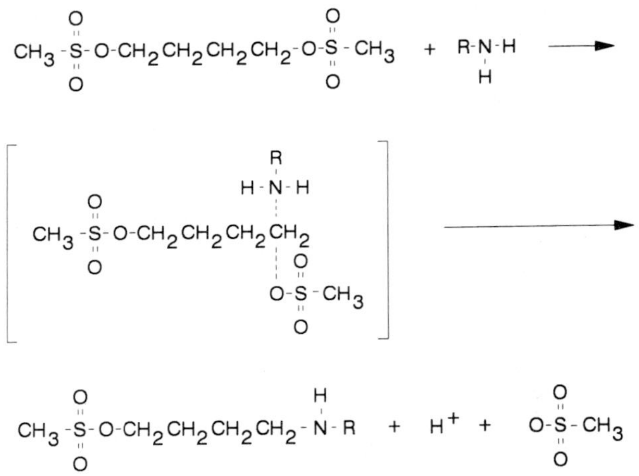

Figure 62.9. Mechanism of alkylation by busulfan.

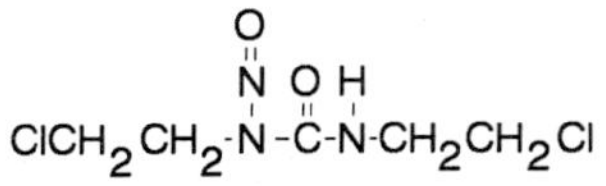

BCNU

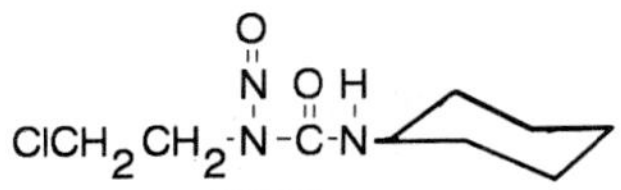

CCNU

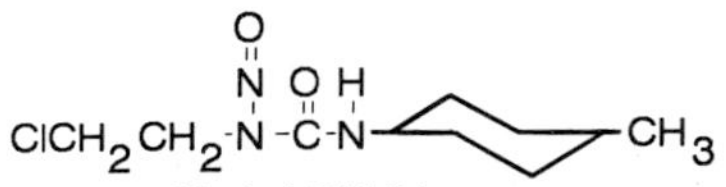

4-Methyl CCNU

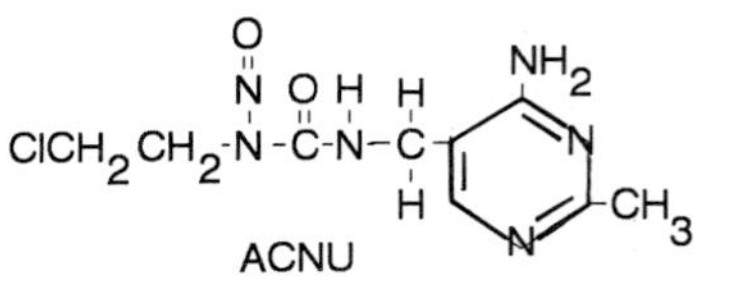

ACNU

Figure 62.10. Structures of nitrosoureas.

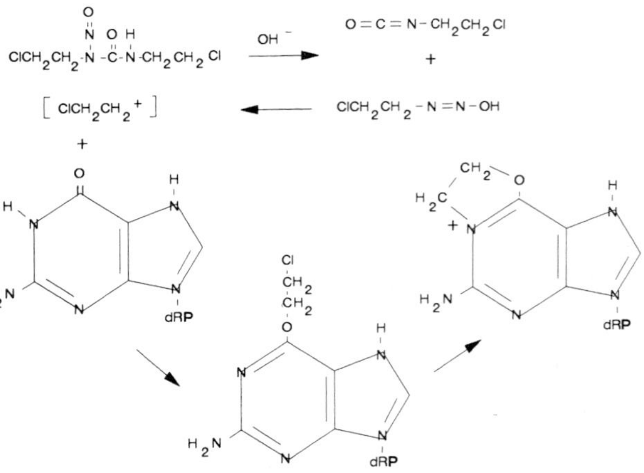

Figure 62.11. Mechanism of nitrosourea activation and alkylation of deoxyguanylic acid.

discussed below. BCNU (carmustine) was the first agent to demonstrate significant activity against a preclinical model of intracerebral tumor (469) and is currently used for the treatment of primary brain tumors (87, 555) and in the treatment of multiple myeloma (122, 539). CCNU (lomustine) and methyl CCNU (semustine) demonstrated greater activity against solid tumors in preclinical studies (468). CCNU is used in the treatment of CNS tumors (299, 306) and lymphomas (254, 308), and methyl CCNU has been used particularly in the treatment of gastrointestinal tumors (2, 86, 175, 537). ACNU, which is more water-soluble than most of the nitrosoureas, has been employed for the intra-arterial and intrathecal treatment of CNS tumors (22, 312, 447) and for solid tumors (261). The clinical use of the nitrosoureas has been limited by marked and prolonged hematopoietic toxicity and by renal toxicity. The development of nitrosoureas with a higher therapeutic index remains a very active area of endeavor (218, 257, 270, 417, 508, 559).

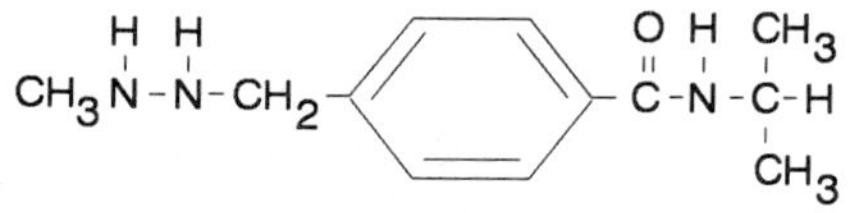

Procarbazine

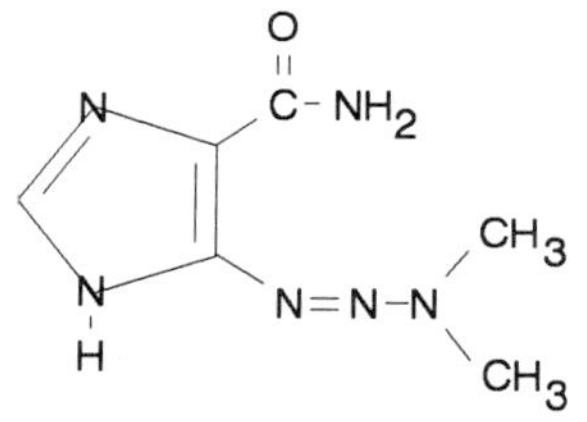

Dacarbazine

Figure 62.12. Structures of monofunctional alkylating agents.

TRIAZENES, HYDRAZINES, AND RELATED COMPOUNDS

These are nitrogen containing compounds that spontaneously decompose or can be metabolized to produce alkyl diazonium intermediates that alkylate biologic molecules. Procarbazine and dacarbazine, which are illustrated in Figure 62.12, are metabolized to reactive intermediates that decompose to produce methyl diazonium, which methylates DNA (24). The metabolism of procarbazine is complex, and there are different pathways through which a reactive methyl group can be produced (24). It is most likely that the pathway responsible for the DNA methylation and cytotoxicity is the generation of methylazoxyprocarbazine (141, 504). The activation of dacarbazine via N-methyl oxidation by a microsomal P_{450} enzyme is illustrated in Figure 62.13 (147, 482, 538). Both procarbazine and dacarbazine are used in the treatment of Hodgkin's Disease (59, 112), procarbazine is a component of combination regimens used for the treatment of primary brain tumors (314), and dacarbazine is used in the treatment of melanoma (see Chapter 138) (158, 285). Procarbazine was originally developed as a monomine oxidase inhibitor, and it can produce central nervous system depression and acute hypertensive reactions after the ingestion of tyramine-rich foods (24). Temozolomide (Fig. 62.13) spontaneously decomposes under physiologic conditions to produce the same active metabolite produced by DTIC (108, 326, 511). This agent can be administered orally and in phase I trials has shown antitumor activity against gliomas and melanomas (368, 382).

Hexamethylmelamine

Hexamethylmelamine (Fig. 62.14) is an active antitumor agent that has been considered to be acting as an alkylating agent because the methyl groups are required for antitumor activity. The methyl groups are hydroxylated with subse-

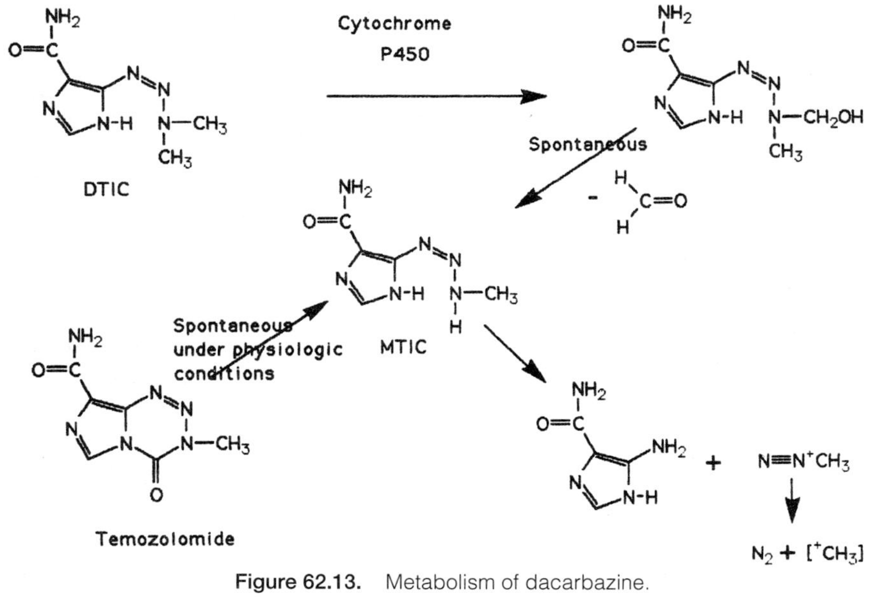

Cytochrome P450

DTIC

Spontaneous

MTIC

Spontaneous under physiologic conditions

Temozolomide

$N_2 + [^+CH_3]$

Figure 62.13. Metabolism of dacarbazine.

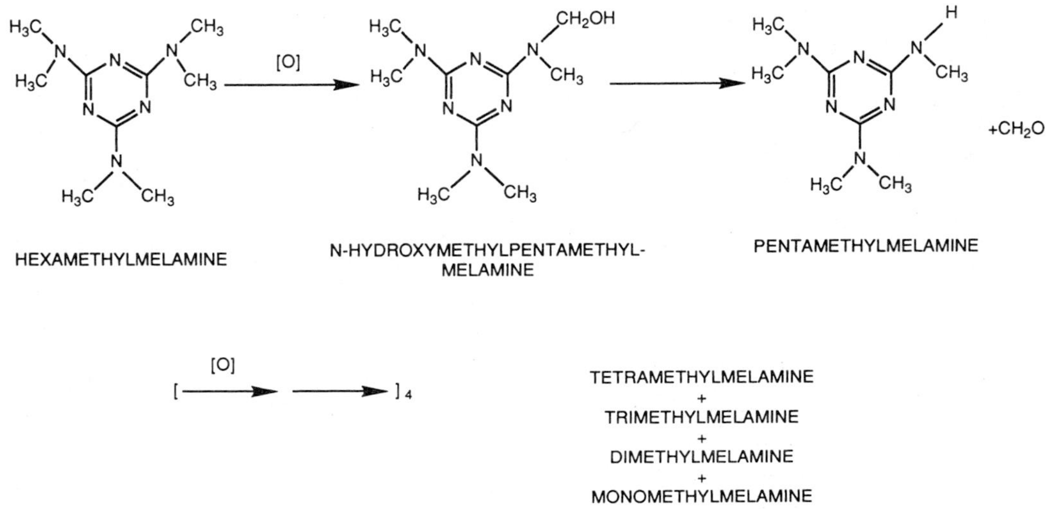

HEXAMETHYLMELAMINE → [O] → N-HYDROXYMETHYLPENTAMETHYLMELAMINE → PENTAMETHYLMELAMINE + CH_2O

[[O] → →]₄ TETRAMETHYLMELAMINE + TRIMETHYLMELAMINE + DIMETHYLMELAMINE + MONOMETHYLMELAMINE

Figure 62.14. Metabolic pathway for hexamethylmelamine resulting in demethylated metabolites.

quent demethylation in vivo (351, 460), a reaction that could generate a reactive methyl group. Analogues in which the methyl groups are hydroxylated are also active (263, 445, 446). Few studies of the cross-resistance of this agent have been carried out, but one study (345) found that O-6-alkyltransferase was not inactivated in vivo by hexamethylmelamine, as would be expected from an O-6 guanyl methylating agent. Therefore, the mechanism of cytotoxic activity of hexamethylmelamine remains in question. The agent does have significant antitumor activity against ovarian cancer (191, 540) and is used primarily in the second line treatment of that tumor.

DECOMPOSITION AND METABOLISM

The alkylating agents react with water and are inactivated by this hydrolysis. The alkylating agents also are inactivated by reaction with thiols, such as glutathione. The reaction of alkylating agents with glutathione can be increased by the enzyme glutathione S-transferase, as will be discussed below in mechanisms of cellular resistance. The alkylating agents also undergo microsomal and other types of xenobiotic metabolism. Such metabolism may activate agents, as described above, inactivate them, or change their physical properties without inactivating them. Nitrosoureas are denitrosated and inactivated by microsomal metabolism (235, 315). Chlorambucil is metabolized to bischoroethylphenylacetic acid, which is an active alkylating agent, and probably contributes to the therapeutic and toxic effects of chlorambucil (5, 144, 344). Mitomycin C must be reductively activated intracellularly to alkylate DNA bases and cross-link the DNA, and glutathione appears to play a role in this process (477).

MECHANISM OF CYTOXICITY

While the alkylating agents react with a number of biologic molecules, including amino acids, thiols, RNA, and DNA, a number of lines of evidence have led to the generally accepted conclusion that the cytotoxic effects of the agents are due to reactions with DNA. Bifunctional agents are much more effective antitumor agents than monofunctional agents, but addition of more than two alkylating groups does not further increase the cytotoxic activity. These observations (325), and the early studies of Brookes and Lawley (67, 68) led to the suggestion that interstrand cross-linking of DNA was responsible for the cytotoxic activity of the bifunctional alkylating agents. A good correlation has been shown between cytotoxicity and the formation of interstrand cross-links by bifunctional alkylating agents. The alkaline elution technique developed by Kohn (145) has been especially important in these studies. More recently, nitrogen mustard interstrand cross-links in oligonucleotides have been chemically characterized (348, 380).

While the alkylating agents can react with virtually all the nitrogens in the DNA bases, there is selectivity, based on the electron density of the nitrogens and the local structure of the DNA. The nitrogen mustards react most readily with the N-7 position of guanylic acid (426). This nitrogen atom has a high electron density, which appears to be enhanced by base stacking in the DNA helical structure (67). Brookes and Lawley suggested that the nitrogen mustard cross-link in DNA was between the N-7 guanine atoms in base-paired G-C sequences in DNA (67). However, two recent studies that examined the cross-linking of oligonucleotides have found the interstrand cross-link of mechlorethamine to occur between the N-7 atoms of guanylic acids in a G-X-C sequence, as illustrated in Figure 62.15 (348, 380). The cross-linking of mitomycin C between two extracyclic guanylic acid amino groups is described above (61). This site of cross-linking may be determined by the orientation of mitomycin C in the minor groove of DNA (62). The reactive species of the nitrosoureas is more reactive than the aziridiniums of the nitrogen mustards and appears to initially alkylate the 0-6 position of guanylic acid (142, 397). According to a mechanism proposed by Ludlum, after a series of rearrangements involving a reactive cyclic five-membered intermediate of the

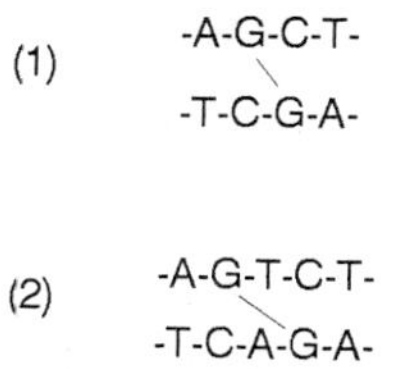

(1) -A-G-C-T-
-T-C-G-A-

(2) -A-G-T-C-T-
-T-C-A-G-A-

Figure 62.15. Interstrand cross-linking of DNA by nitrogen mustards. **A.** Site of cross-linking proposed by Brookes. **B.** Site of cross-linking found by Loechler (331) and Hopkins (307).

N-1, C-6, and O-6 atoms of guanylic acid and two carbons from the chloroethyl group of the nitrosourea (Fig. 62.11), a cross-link is formed between N-1 of guanylic acid and N-3 of a cytidylic acid on the complementary DNA strand (55, 329).

Some alkylating agents, such as procarbazine and dacarbazine, are not bifunctional, but are cytotoxic. The cytotoxic effects of these agents are probably produced by the alkylation of guanylic acid with the subsequent depurination and production of single-strand DNA breaks (542, 543). Bifunctional agents also produce monofunctional alkylations, depurination, and single-strand breaks, but these compounds are cytotoxic at concentrations below those necessary to produce the degree of single-strand breaks associated with cytotoxic levels of monofunctional agents. Kat, Modrich and colleagues (275) have recently provided evidence that active mismatch DNA repair may contribute to the cytotoxicity of monofunctional alkylating agents.

CELLULAR RESISTANCE TO ALKYLATING AGENTS

Cellular resistance to antitumor agents is a critical determinant of the effectiveness of therapy. Resistance mechanisms in normal tissues provide selectivity and an improved therapeutic index. Resistance of tumor cells allows these cells to escape the effects of therapy. Consideration of the pharmacology and chemistry of the alkylating agents predicts three general types of cellular resistance to alkylating agents (Fig. 62.16). These are (*a*) decreased uptake of agents into or increased export out of the cell, (*b*) increased inactivation of agents in the cell, and (*c*) enhanced repair of the DNA damage produced by the alkylating agents. All three of these mechanisms have now been shown to occur. Resistance of tumor cells to mechlorethamine can occur on the basis of decreased transport into the cell (183, 562) and it has also been demonstrated that certain cells resistant to melphalan have decreased active transport of the agent and of amino acids (103, 430). Most alkylating agents enter cells by diffusion, however, and the alkylating agents, with the exception of mitomycin C, are not substrates for the multiple drug resistance (mdr) export system. It seems unlikely, therefore, that decreased cellular uptake or increased export of alkylating agents will prove to be major mechanisms of resistance to most of the alkylating agents.

The second mechanism of cellular resistance to alkylating agents is intracellular inactivation of the agent. As discussed above, the enzyme aldehyde dehydrogenase detoxifies the primary metabolites of cyclophosphamide and ifosfamide, and the presence of this enzyme in bone marrow precursor cells and gastrointestinal epithelial cells protects these organs from toxicity of the agents. Aldehyde dehydrogenase has also been demonstrated to be a mechanism of cyclophosphamide resistance of murine (236), rat (290), and human leukemia cells (94) and human ovarian (398), colon (437), and breast (492) cancer cells.

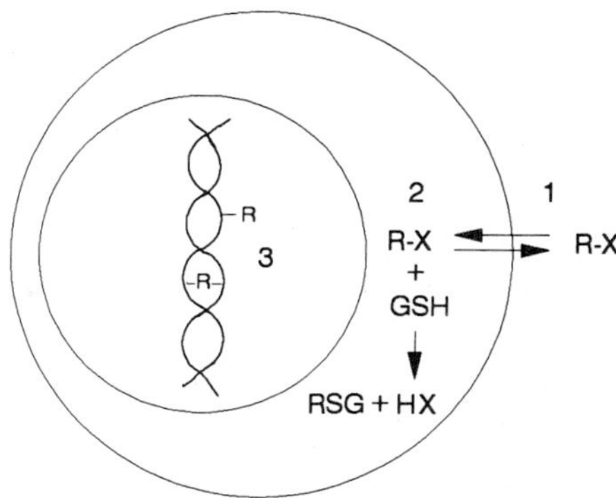

1. Decreased entry into or increased exit of agent from cell
2. Inactivation of agent in cell
3. Enhanced repair of DNA lesions produced by alkylation

Figure 62.16. Mechanisms of resistance to alkylating agents.

An association between cellular resistance to alkylating agents and increased cellular levels of glutathione (74, 167a, 503), and the enzyme glutathione transferase has been described by a number of investigators (72, 364, 377, 427, 444, 517, 556). Glutathione is a thiol-containing tripeptide that is present at millimolar concentrations in many cells, reacts with electrophilic (electron-deficient) molecules, and protects cells from such electrophiles (33, 85, 166). Mulcahy and colleagues (358a) have demonstrated that increased GSH in cells resistant to melphalan is related to increased transcription of gamma-glutamylcysteine synthetase (GCS), the enzyme that catalyzes the rate-limiting step in de novo synthesis of GSH.

While most electrophiles of biologic significance react spontaneously with glutathione, glutathione S-transferase catalyzes the reaction between glutathione and electrophiles. The glutathione conjugates of several alkylating agents have been characterized (120, 121, 569) and their formation shown to be enhanced by glutathione S-transferase.

There are three principal isozymes of glutathione S-transferase, and recent studies indicate that specific isozymes may catalyze the conjugation of different alkylating agents. The alpha isozyme of GST has been found to catalyze the glutathione conjugation of the aziridinium forms of melphalan (58), chlorambucil (85), and phosphosphoramide mustard (116). The GSH conjugation of 4-hydroxycyclophosphamide (394) was found to be enhanced by all three classes of GST, although the alpha isozyme was the most active (116). The mu isozyme has been implicated in the inactivation of BCNU (488). At this time it seems evident that glutathione alone or glutathione plus an appropriate glutathione S-transferase can render cells resistant to alkylating agents and that this mechanism is probably an important mechanism of resistance to electrophilic antitumor drugs, such as the alkylating agents.

Several investigators have demonstrated that buthionine sulfoxime (BSO), an inhibitor of glutathione synthesis, can reduce cellular glutathione levels and sensitize tumors to alkylating agents in vitro and in vivo (167, 297, 389, 566). However, normal cells can also be sensitized by BSO administration (252, 487) to produce significant toxicity. BSO in combination with alkylating agents is now undergoing clinical trials. One recent phase I trial demonstrated that BSO added to a melphalan dose of 15 mg/m^2 increased leukopenia and thrombocytopenia, compared with the same dose of melphalan alone (28). Inhibitors of glutathione S-transferases have been shown to enhance the cytotoxicity of melphalan on cells resistant to alkylating agents (440a) and such inhibitors are being examined in clinical trials. A phase I trial of the GST inhibitor sulfasalazine (201) with melphalan doses of 20 mg/m^2 and greater demonstrated reductions of glutathione and GST levels in the peripheral mononuclear cells of some patients and the main toxicity of the combination was nausea and vomiting. Increased myelosuppression was not seen. An interesting recent observation is that depletion of cellular GSH by BSO changed the mode of cell death produced by alkylating agents from apoptosis to necrosis but did not have this effect with other antitumor agents (152).

An association between increased cellular concentrations of metallothionein and resistance to platinum agents has been established (12, 140), and is probably due to binding of the platinum agents to the multiple thiol groups of this cellular protein. Lazo and colleagues (279) found that transfection-induced increased cellular metallothionein also produced resistance to alkylating agents. Subsequently it has also been shown that increase of metallothionein cellular content by zinc exposure will also increase the resistance of cells to melphalan (465). Fenselau and colleagues (568) have recently demonstrated binding of melphalan to thiol groups in metallothionein. Thus, increased metallothionein content of cells is another mechanism of inactivation of alkylating agents.

Since the cytotoxicity of the alkylating agents appears to be mediated through the alkylation of DNA, the repair of alkylation lesions is an obvious mechanism of resistance to these agents and has been the subject of intense investigation. The best-defined DNA repair resistance to alkylating agents is resistance to the nitrosoureas and other compounds that alkylate the 0-6 position of guanylic acid in DNA. The protein 0-6-alkylguanine-alkyltransferase has been shown to remove alkyl groups from the 0-6 position of guanine and thus prevent the formation of an interstrand cross-link (55, 142, 401). The removed alkyl group is covalently and irreversibly bound to the alkyltransferase, so that the protein can catalyze the removal of only one alkyl molecule and is then rapidly catabolized. A strong association has now been shown between the presence of high levels of this protein in certain normal and tumor cells and the resistance of these cells to nitrosoureas. In particular, it seems clear that elevated 0-6-alkylguanine-DNA-alkyltransferase is a mechanism of resistance to nitrosoureas in human gliomas (9, 55, 150, 473) and other human tumors (65, 101, 331). As described above, the less reactive alkylating agents do not produce DNA cross-links through the 0-6 position of guanylic acid, and elevated alkyltransferase does not confer resistance to these agents.

The fact that the alkyltransferase is irreversibly inactivated by the transfer to it of an alkyl group from the 0-6 position of guanine provides an approach to counteracting this mechanism of resistance. If cells are treated with a monofunctional 0-6 alkylating agent, such as streptozotocin, there follows a period when the 0-6 alkyltransferase activity is decreased. This decrease in activity is due to the removal of alkyl groups from the 0-6 guanine sites on the DNA and a subsequent reduction of the level of active enzyme before enzyme synthesis can restore functional levels of the enzyme. If the cells are treated with a nitrosourea (or other 0-6 guanine alkylating agent) during this period of decreased 0-6 alkyltransferase, the cells are more sensitive to nitrosourea (169). The enzyme will also remove 0-6 alkyl groups from acid-soluble guanine, and compounds such as 0-6 benzylguanine, administered prior to nitrosoureas, will reverse alkyltransferase resistance in cells and animal models (101, 331, 355, 402). Clinical trials have been conducted with the combination of streptozotocin and nitrosourea (392), and clinical trials with 0-6 benzylguanine, which is less toxic than streptozotocin, are now in progress.

Removal of interstrand cross-links from DNA in cells can be shown to occur in studies using alkaline elution and other techniques (99, 292). While excellent progress has been made in understanding the mechanisms of DNA mismatch repair (356), base excision repair (212), and nucleotide excision repair (462), the mechanism by which N7-N7 interstrand alkylating agent cross-links are repaired is not understood. Recently, evidence has been presented that poly(ADP ribose)polymerase is involved in the repair of nitrogen mustard lesions (496). A mammalian tumor cell that is resistant to alkylating agents on the basis of enhanced cross-link repair has not been definitively described. However, there is good evidence that cells that react to alkylation damage by arresting in the G2 phase of the cell cycle can repair DNA during this period and are more resistant to alkylating agents than cells that proceed through mitosis despite alkylation damage. A human tumor cell line has been described that exhibits G_2 arrest in response to alkylating damage and demonstrates increased resistance to nitrogen mustard (376). This cell line was found to have increased accumulation of phosphorylated (and inactivated) cdc2 kinase associated with G_2 arrest after nitrogen mustard treatment. This should allow repair of DNA damage before the cell enters mitosis. This mechanism of resistance to alkylating agents is probably important for some tumor cells but may provide a degree of drug specificity for many other tumors, because normal cells may be more likely to exhibit this protective mechanism. Inhibitors of DNA repair have been shown to enhance the cytotoxicity of alkylating agents (104, 475, 533), and some of these inhibitors are being examined in clinical trials. It seems likely that increased understanding of the DNA repair process will allow more effective utilization of alkylating agents.

In Vivo Resistance

Murine tumors that are resistant to alkylating agents in vivo have been reported. They are not resistant when exposed to the agents in vitro (513). Further studies of these tumors that are resistant to cyclophosphamide, cisplatin, and thiotepa in vivo have demonstrated that the tumors are also resistant to these agents in 3-dimensional in vitro culture, but not in 2-dimensional in vitro culture (288). Such resistance may be acquired rapidly after drug exposure (188a) and may be associated with enhanced metastatic properties (281). The mechanisms responsible for this type of resistance have not yet been established. There may be differences between known cellular resistance factors or between membrane properties in the 3-dimensional milieu, compared with the 2-dimensional configuration. Other potential mechanisms for drug resistance in vivo are poor perfusion of the tumor and changes in the intracellular pH (259). Brain capillaries have been shown to exhibit the mdr resistance protein (225, 362, 509). This fact raises the possibility that capillary endothelial cells, which proliferate under drug exposure along with tumor cells, may be selected for mechanisms of altered transport or inactivation of antitumor agents.

CLINICAL PHARMACOLOGY

Accurate data on the clinical pharmacology of the alkylating agents has become available only in recent years and still remains limited. This is because the newer accurate and definitive methods, such as gas chromatography-mass spectrometry and high performance liquid chromatography, are necessary for many of these measurements.

Cyclophosphamide

After the administration of a systemic dose of 50 mg/kg, plasma levels of the parent compound of up to 400 micromolar may be achieved and decay with a half-life of 3 to 10 hours (132, 262, 268, 500). The rate of metabolism of the parent compound varies considerably among individuals and can be modulated by the administration of compounds that affect the rate of microsomal metabolism, such as phenobarbital (260) or a previous dose of cyclophosphamide (115, 143). However, at conventional doses the clearance rate of the parent compound does not appear to significantly affect the toxicity or therapeutic effect of the agent (484). This independence of effect from the rate of metabolism is probably because the parent compound is not rapidly excreted and continues to be activated, so that the area under the curve (AUC) for systemic exposure to the active metabolites is similar after a given dose.

At the higher doses currently used in bone marrow transplantation regimens, however, the plasma concentrations of cyclophosphamide should be close to the capacity of the microsomal activating enzymes and may go above the renal resorption threshold or be more likely to be metabolized by an alternate and detoxifying metabolic pathway, such as dechlorethylation. Grochow and colleagues (79) have now demonstrated that in patients receiving 4 g/m^2 of cyclophosphamide over 90 minutes and achieving initial plasma concentrations of greater than 500 μM, saturable pharmacokinetics are seen.

These investigators concluded that when the dosing rate equals or exceeds 4 g/m^2 in 90 minutes or the plasma concentration of cyclophosphamide exceeds 150 μM (the lowest Km seen in the patients) nonlinear disposition may occur, with variable exposure to the active metabolites. This study also confirmed previous reports that cyclophosphamide can induce its own metabolism. There has been a recent report (25) that the toxicity and antitumor efficacy of an autologous bone marrow transplant regimen utilizing high doses of cyclophosphamide, thiotepa, and carboplatin were increased when the areas under the plasma concentration curve (AUCs) for cyclophosphamide were lower. This report suggests that patients who metabolize a greater fraction of a large dose of cyclophosphamide may be exposed to a greater quantity of the active metabolites and thus have greater antitumor efficacy and toxicity.

Studies of pharmacokinetics of the critical metabolite 4-hydroxycyclophosphamide have been limited by the difficulty of measuring this molecule (267). Several investigators have measured 4-hydroxycyclophosphamide in patients after cyclophosphamide administration by measuring a fluorescent derivative of acrolein released from 4-hydroxycyclophosphamide on acidification of the sample. These studies have found plasma concentrations of 4-hydroxycyclophosphamide of 1 to 15 micromolar, depending on the dose and time of administration of cyclophosphamide administration, with a half-life of the metabolite of 1 to 6 hours (485, 500, 553, 564). A study has recently been published measuring 4-hydroxycyclophosphamide in patient blood after cyclophosphamide administration, using a very specific gas chromatographic-mass spectrometric technique (10). After a dose of cyclophosphamide of 110 mg/kg over 90 minutes peak concentrations of 9 to 12 micromolar and AUCs of 105 to 110 micromolar hours were measured; a cyclophosphamide dose of 170 mg/kg given as a continuous infusion over 4 days produced plasma concentrations of 1 to 5 micromolar, with a total AUC of about 98 to 110 micromolar hours. These findings are in general agreement with the previous studies using the less specific method.

The majority of a dose of cyclophosphamide ($\approx$70%) is excreted in the urine as the inactive metabolite, carboxyphosphamide (30, 262, 501). Renal function does not significantly affect the toxicity of cyclophosphamide (248), most likely because spontaneous decomposition, and not renal excretion, determines the clearance of the principal active metabolites.

The clinical pharmacology of ifosfamide has been less studied but is similar to that of cyclophosphamide, except that microsomal activation is somewhat slower, and chloroethyl side chain oxidation plays a greater role in its metabolism (63, 366, 375, 552). Thus, for a dose of ifosfamide, lower systemic concentrations of the 4-hydroxy metabolite are achieved than for the same dose of cyclophosphamide (552). Both cyclophosphamide and ifosfamide are well absorbed after oral administration (267, 500). Boddy and coworkers (53) have recently demonstrated that ifosfamide, like cyclophosphamide, can autoinduce its own metabolism.

Melphalan

Alberts and colleagues found that peak plasma levels of 4 to 13 micromolar were present after intravenous administration of a 0.6-mg/kg dose of melphalan, and the half-life ($t_{1/2}\beta$) was 1.8 hours (6). At this dose, the mean AUC for melphalan was 8 micromolar hours. Similar AUC per dose and pharmacokinetics have been demonstrated by other investigators after high intravenous doses of melphalan (282). After conventional oral doses of 0.25 mg/kg, peak plasma levels of up to 0.625 micromolar were found (393). There is variable systemic availability after oral dosing (5, 81, 510), and it has been shown that oral administration of L-leucine or food with melphalan will inhibit absorption of the agent (432, 434). It has been reported that myelosuppression from melphalan is increased in patients with decreased renal function (95). The half-life of melphalan is prolonged in anephric dogs (7), and significant renal clearance of the parent compound in patients has been shown by Reece and colleagues (433).

Chlorambucil

After the oral administration of 0.6 mg/kg of chlorambucil, peak levels of 2 to 6 micromolar parent compound were found at 1 hour by Alberts and colleagues (4, 6). Peak plasma levels of phenylacetic acid mustard of 2 to 4 micromolar occurred at 2 to 4 hours after chlorambucil administration. The plasma half-life ($t_{1/2}\beta$) of chlorambucil was 92 minutes, and that of phenylacetic acid mustard was 145 minutes. At a dose of 0.6 mg/kg of chlorambucil, the plasma AUC of chlorambucil was 3 to 9 micromolar hours (4). Similar values were found by Ehrsson and colleagues (220), who also found a 2- to 4-fold variation in systemic availability of chlorambucil and phenylacetic acid mustard after oral administration of chlorambucil.

Thiotepa

The pharmacokinetics of thiotepa have been studied by Egorin and colleagues (89), after an intravenous injection of 12 mg/m^2. Peak plasma levels of about 5 micromolar were achieved and were found to decay with a $T_{1/2}\alpha$ of 7.7 minutes and a $T_{1/2}\beta$ of 125 minutes. The mean AUC was 9 micromolar hours. Plasma concentrations of TEPA of up to 1 micromolar were found and remained in plasma longer than thiotepa. Henner and colleagues (229) examined the plasma levels of thiotepa after 4-day continuous intravenous infusions of up to 900 mg/m^2. Peak plasma levels of thiotepa of 7 micromolar were initially attained on the first day, and then the levels gradually decreased. Plasma AUC values of up to 600 micromolar hours were achieved. When given intraperitoneally, there is rapid loss of thiotepa from the intraperitoneal cavity and a concomitant increase in plasma levels to those associated with the same dose if given intravenously (551). After intravenous injection, cerebrospinal fluid levels comparable with plasma levels are found (499).

Nitrosoureas

The pharmacokinetics of BCNU have been studied by Levin and colleagues (313). After intravenous infusion of 60 to 170 mg/m^2, peak plasma concentrations of five micromolar were reached and then decayed with an initial half-life of 6 minutes and a second half-life of 68 minutes. Henner and colleagues (228) measured the pharmacokinetics of BCNU after intravenous doses of 600 mg/m^2. The peak plasma level of ultrafilterable BCNU was found to be 4.7 micromolar and the mean AUC was 5.4 micromolar hours. The ultrafilterable BCNU was 23% of the total plasma BCNU. The pharmacokinetics of CCNU after administration of 130 mg/m^2 to patients have also been described (305). The parent compound could not be detected in plasma, but the monohydroxylated metabolites, trans-4-hydroxy CCNU and cis-4-hydroxy CCNU, were found in a ratio of 6 : 4 and at total peak concentrations of about 3 micromolar. The plasma clearance half-lives of the hydroxy-CCNU metabolites varied from 1 to 3 hours between patients.

Busulfan

Because of its insolubility in aqueous solutions, busulfan is available only as an oral preparation. For myeloablative therapy prior to bone marrow transplantation, busulfan is widely used at a dose of 1 mg/kg every 6 hours for 4 days. After a 1 mg/kg dose in adults and older children, there is a considerable variation in bioavailability, with peak plasma levels of 1 to 10 micromolar and elimination half-times between 1 and 7 hours (196, 221, 536). The AUC after a single dose in adults and older children varies between 10 and 80 micromolar hours. However, in young children (age 1–3) the peak plasma concentrations are less (1–5 micromolar), the mean elimination time about 40% faster, and the AUC consistently less at 6 to 17 micromolar hours (197). Grochow and coworkers (196) have demonstrated that AUCs of busulfan greater than one standard deviation from the mean values for all patients are associated with a very high risk of venoocclusive disease of the liver (Fig. 62.17). It has now been demonstrated that pharmacokinetic guided adjustment of the busulfan dose can reduce the incidence and severity of this toxicity (195a, 534).

TOXICITIES

The characteristic toxicities of the alkylating agents are hematopoietic, gastrointestinal, gonadal, and CNS toxicity. However, each of the agents has a characteristic set of toxicities, determined by the reactivity, metabolism, and distribution of the agent, and the clinician should be aware of these idiosyncrasies of the agents.

Hematopoietic Toxicity

In general, the clinical dose-limiting toxicity for alkylating agents is hematopoietic toxicity, particularly suppression of granulocytes and platelets. The nadir of granulocyte depression after alkylating agents is usually 8 to 16 days, and the granulocytes usually return to normal within 20 days after a single dose of the agent (374). Cyclophosphamide and ifosfamide are less hematopoietically toxic than other alkylating agents (360, 374); granulocyte levels return to normal more rapidly, platelets are affected less, and repeated doses of cyclophosphamide and ifosfamide do not produce

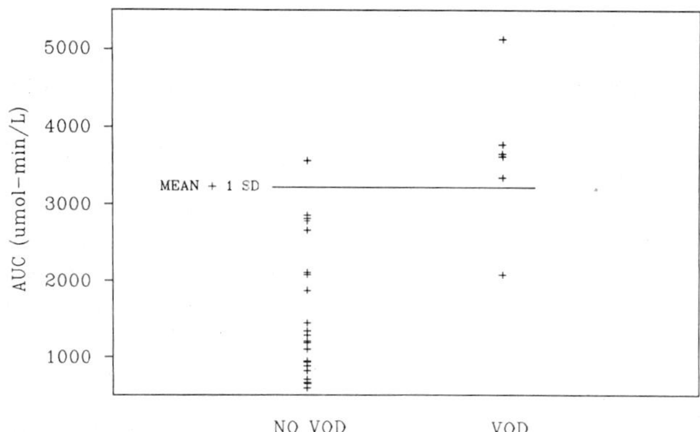

Figure 62.17. Relationship between plasma AUC of busulfan and occurrence of veno-occlusive disease of the liver. *Source:* Grochow et al. (196).

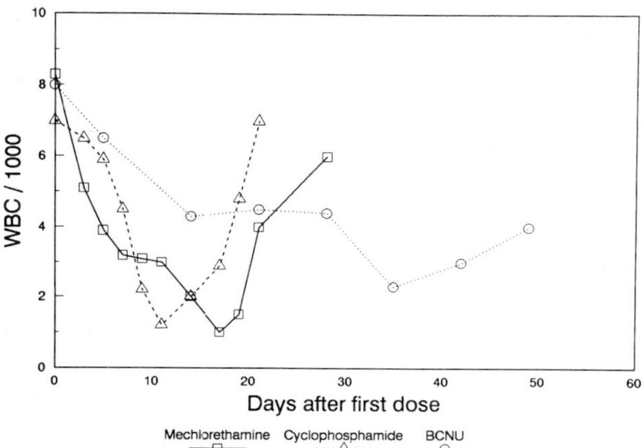

Figure 62.18. Hematopoietic toxicity of alkylating agents.

much cumulative damage and progressive deterioration of the hematopoietic elements. The reduced hematopoietic toxicity of cyclophosphamide and ifosfamide appears to be due to the presence of aldehyde dehydrogenase in the hematopoietic stem cells and the early megakaryocytes, as discussed earlier. In contrast, the nitrosoureas produce severe hematopoietic toxicity, with a delayed onset and nadirs of granulocytes and platelets occurring as late as 45 days (111, 439). Busulfan also produces severe hematopoietic depression, with a selectivity for early myeloid precursors (139, 165). The variations in the cellular patterns and time courses of hematopoietic suppression after the administration of different alkylating agents indicate that the individual agents have selectivity for different hematopoietic precursor cells (Fig. 62.18) (see Chapter 178).

Peptide growth factors, such as granulocyte-macrophage colony-stimulating factor (sargramostim, GM-CSF) and granulocyte colony-stimulating factor (filgrastim, G-CSF), which stimulate the differentiation and proliferation of hematopoietic precursors (507), are now used clinically (see Chapter 82). The degree and duration of granulocyte depression after antitumor drug administration can be reduced by the concomitant use of these growth factors (64, 178, 512). Currently, growth factors that may stimulate the proliferation and restoration of megakaryocytes and platelets are under investigation (289, 324, 428). The use of these factors with the alkylating agents has been particularly attractive because of the steep dose-response curve of the alkylating agents and because, with several alkylating agents, a considerable increase in dose may be administered before another dose-limiting toxicity is reached. For these same reasons combinations of alkylating agents have been used extensively in association with allogeneic and autologous bone marrow transplantation (128, 464). Therefore, current clinical practices are focusing attention on the nonhematopoietic toxicities of the alkylating agents.

Gastrointestinal Toxicity

Damage to the gastrointestinal tract is a toxicity that is being increasingly seen with high-dose regimens (see Chapter 184).

Mucositis, stomatitis, esophagitis, and diarrhea have been seen with high doses of alkylating agents, and in particular after high doses of melphalan and thiotepa or combinations of alkylating agents including melphalan or thiotepa (18, 342, 518). Significant mucositis is unusual even after very high doses of cyclophosphamide or ifosfamide. This lack of gastrointestinal toxicity is probably due to the presence of the enzyme aldehyde dehydrogenase in the epithelial cells of the gastrointestinal tract (459).

Nausea and vomiting are frequent side effects of alkylating agents. While these side effects are not usually life threatening, they are major discomforts to patients and may result in the delay or discontinuation of therapy. The nausea and vomiting are, at least in part, mediated through the central nervous system, and are not due to direct gastrointestinal toxicity (60, 153). These effects are variable between patients, in that some people tolerate high doses of these drugs without nausea and vomiting, while other patients are incapacitated by even low doses of alkylating agents. The frequency of nausea and vomiting does increase as the dose of alkylating agents is increased. Therefore, it is important, especially with the use of increasing doses of alkylating agents, to provide the patient with adequate antiemetic medication. Such medications include phenothiazines, other antiemetics, acute doses of corticosteroids, and more recently, antiserotonin agents (see Chapter 174) (75, 177, 198).

Veno-Occlusive Disease of the Liver

This syndrome is characterized clinically by hepatomegaly, right upper quadrant pain, jaundice, ascites, and a high mortality rate from hepatic failure. Pathologically, the syndrome is associated with subendothelial thickening and narrowing of the hepatic venule lumen (266). This complication has been seen in about 25% of patients receiving high-dose cyclophosphamide and busulfan (Fig. 62.15) or cyclophosphamide and total body irradiation prior to allogeneic or autologous bone marrow transplantation for leukemia or lymphoma (266), and has also been seen after other high-dose alkylating agent therapy (407, 410). Liver transplantation has been used for the treatment of veno-occlusive disease in patients after bone marrow transplantation (see Chapter 183) (373, 441).

Gonadal Damage

A serious toxicity of the alkylating agents is gonadal damage. The characteristic lesion in men, depletion of testicular germ cells with preservation of Sertoli cells, was first described in 1948 in patients treated with mechlorethamine (491). This lesion has subsequently been observed with other alkylating agents (350), and frequently results in aspermia or oligospermia in men treated with drug combinations including alkylating agents (411, 480). However, spermatogenesis and fertility may return after several years (see Chapter 186) (49, 238).

Amenorrhea, associated with disappearance of mature and primordial ovarian follicles, is seen in women treated with alkylating agents (172, 352, 448). The frequency of amenorrhea increases with the age of the woman and is more likely to be irreversible in older women (301).

Pulmonary Damage

Pulmonary damage in the form of interstitial pneumonitis and fibrosis has been associated with almost all of the alkylating antitumor drugs (see Chapter 182). Although the exact mechanism of the pulmonary toxicity is not known, it is presumably due to direct toxicity of the alkylating agents on pulmonary epithelial cells. The typical presentation of this toxicity is the onset of a nonproductive cough and dyspnea, which may progress to tachypnea and cyanosis, and even to severe pulmonary insufficiency and death. This complication was first described in association with busulfan therapy (379), but subsequently it has been described after cyclophosphamide (335, 399, 429), nitrosoureas (27, 240, 319), melphalan (88), chlorambucil (90), and mitomycin C (385). A significant incidence of pulmonary toxicity has been reported in patients receiving high doses of cyclophosphamide, cisplatin, and BCNU (265, 519). Jones and colleagues (265) have reported that the pulmonary toxicity is correlated with the AUC of BCNU and demonstrated in animal studies that coadministration of cyclophosphamide and cisplatin with BCNU increased the AUC of BCNU and the variability of the BCNU AUC, suggesting that the other agents were interfering with the elimination of BCNU.

Hemorrhagic Cystitis

The oxazophosphorines, cyclophosphamide and ifosfamide, produce bladder toxicity, which is not seen with other alkylating agents (see Chapter 180). This toxicity is a hemorrhagic cystitis, which may progress to massive hemorrhage (160, 409). The toxicity has been demonstrated to be due to metabolites of these drugs, which are excreted into the urine. The metabolite principally responsible for this toxicity is acrolein (98), although phosphoramide mustard and chloracetaldehyde may contribute to the effect. Hemorrhagic cystitis is seen more commonly after ifosfamide therapy than cyclophosphamide, partly because higher doses of this agent are used (see above). Renal tubular damage has also been seen after ifosfamide, including a Fanconi's type syndrome, azotemia, elevated serum creatinine, and enzymuria (531).

The systemic administration of thiols can prevent or ameliorate the bladder damage from cyclophosphamide and ifosfamide, because the thiols conjugate the aldehyde functions of acrolein and chloracetaldehyde. The most widely used compound to prevent oxazophosphorine bladder toxicity is the sodium salt of 2-mercaptoethane sulfonate (MESNA) (66). MESNA is usually administered to all patients receiving ifosfamide and to patients who are receiving high-dose cyclophosphamide. Subclinical renal toxicity has been observed in children receiving ifosfamide (422, 424) despite MESNA administration, so that administration of MESNA does not eliminate the need for adequate hydration and careful observation of the patient.

Antidiuresis

An antidiuretic effect is commonly seen in patients receiving doses of cyclophosphamide of 50 mg/kg or greater (54, 107). This syndrome is characterized by a decrease in urine output 6 to 8 hours after drug administration, weight gain, a marked increase in urine osmolality, and a decrease in serum osmolality and sodium concentration. Pericardial and pleural effusions may be seen, and seizures due to hyponatremia have occurred after cyclophosphamide therapy (216), especially if low-sodium replacement fluids have been administered. This antidiuretic syndrome appears to be due to an effect of cyclophosphamide metabolites on the distal renal tubule and is self-limited, with the excess fluid excreted over a period of about 12 hours. Administration of furosemide will promote free water clearance and ameliorate the syndrome (193).

Renal Toxicity

Renal toxicity has proven to be a serious toxicity of the nitrosoureas (217, 470). This effect is dose-related and may produce severe renal failure and death after administration of more than 1,200 mg of BCNU. Elevation of serum creatinine and other clinical evidence of renal toxicity may not be seen until after the completion of therapy. The histology of the kidneys in patients with renal nitrosourea damage is similar to that in radiation nephritis. A case of acute renal failure after melphalan therapy has been reported (273), and increase in creatinine has been described when melphalan was added to high doses of alkylating agents (18).

Alopecia

While the association between an alkylating agent and alopecia was first described with busulfan therapy (47), this toxicity has been predominantly associated with cyclophosphamide and ifosfamide therapy. The alopecia produced by these agents may be quite severe, especially if the agent is given in combination with vincristine or doxorubicin. Regrowth of the hair occurs after cessation of therapy, and may be associated with a change in the texture and color of the hair (173). The structure-function studies of Feil and Lamoureaux (149) suggest that this toxicity is due to the entry of lipophilic metabolites into the hair follicles. This suggestion is consistent with the fact that busulfan, vincristine, and adriamycin are all lipophilic molecules.

Allergic and Hypersensitivity Reactions

Since the alkylating agents react with many biologic molecules, it is not surprising that they would serve as haptenes and produce allergic reactions (96, 302, 455). The most frequent reactions that have been reported have been cutaneous hypersensitivities. Anaphylactic reactions are rare, but they have occurred (271). Patterns of cross-reactivity have not been carefully defined, but cross-reactivity between agents of similar structure, such as the nitrogen mustards, have been described (284, 455).

Cardiotoxicity

The nonhematologic dose-limiting toxicity of cyclophosphamide is cardiac toxicity (70, 486, 495). The fulminant syndrome has been seen most frequently in patients receiving a total dose of cyclophosphamide greater than 200 mg/kg, preparatory to bone marrow transplantation. The clinical course of the syndrome consists of the rapid onset of severe heart failure, which is fatal within 10 to 14 days. The hearts of such patients are dilated, with patchy transmural hemorrhage and pericardial effusion. The microscopic findings consist of interstitial hemorrhage and edema, myocardial necrosis and vacuolar changes, and specific changes in the intramural small coronary vessels (486). Decreased electrocardiographic voltage and a transient increase in heart size is seen in high-dose cyclophosphamide patients without clinical symptoms, and the characteristic pathological findings are present in such patients who die of other causes. Cardiotoxicity and cardiomegaly have been seen in patients receiving lower doses of cyclophosphamide in combination with other alkylating agents (18, 20). Age greater than 50 and previous adriamycin exposure appear to increase the risk of cyclophosphamide cardiotoxicity (495).

Neurotoxicity

In preclinical studies of alkylating agents, convulsions have often been seen (494). At the usual clinical doses of these agents, frank neurotoxicity is not usually seen but drowsiness and alterations of consciousness can be seen (45). With the increasing use of higher doses of alkylating agents and combinations of alkylating agents, more clinical neurotoxicity is being seen (129). At BCNU doses of 1,200 mg/m^2, severe central nervous system toxicity has been seen (505), and the intracarotid administration of BCNU has produced severe eye pain and blindness (565). High-dose busulfan therapy produces seizures, and anticonvulsants are often used prophylactically in these patients (535).

Teratogenecity

Studies carried out in vivo and in embryo cultures have demonstrated that virtually all of the alkylating agents are teratogenic (56, 361). The teratogenic effect is probably due to cytotoxic effects on the embryo by the same mechanisms by which the compounds are toxic to tumor cells (179, 209, 320, 353). The available clinical information indicates that there is a definite risk of a malformed infant if the mother is treated with an alkylating agent during the first trimester of pregnancy (174, 493, 520). In a review of the literature, Nicholson (372) found that of 25 women who had received alkylating agents during the first trimester of pregnancy there were four fetal malformations. However, the administration of alkylation agents during the second and third trimesters is not associated with an increased risk of fetal malformation (309, 372, 384).

Carcinogenesis

Since the initial reports of acute leukemia occurring in patients treated with alkylating agents (239, 300, 451, 452), it has become increasingly obvious that this type of oncogenesis is a significant complication of alkylating agent therapy (see Chapter 188). Several studies have indicated that rate of acute leukemia after alkylating agent therapy may be 10% or higher in certain groups of patients (135, 436, 525). Procarbazine and other methylating agents appear to be the most potent oncogenic agents (117), and melphalan appears to produce a higher rate of acute leukemia than cyclophosphamide (192). The lesser leukemogenic potential of cyclophosphamide may well be related to the hematopoietic stem cell sparing effect of this agent (459). An increased rate of solid tumors is also seen in patients treated with alkylating agents (136, 405, 525). Although sufficient data are not yet available to be certain, it appears that high-dose alkylating agent therapy administered in intermittent pulses over a relatively short period of time is less oncogenic than prolonged alkylating agent therapy.

Immunosuppression

The immunosuppressive effect of alkylating agents was first described by Hektoen and Corper (227) for sulfur mustard. Cyclophosphamide is particularly immunosuppressive (333) and is used for the treatment of autoimmune diseases (32, 304, 522), Cyclophosphamide is also used in preparative regimens for allogeneic transplantation, because of its immunoablative activity (463). Low doses of cyclophosphamide and melphalan can enhance the immune response by selectively inhibiting the immune suppressor cells (43, 119, 386). Because of this effect moderate doses of cyclophosphamide have been used in conjunction with immunotherapy and biologic response modifiers, such as interleukin-2 (42, 354).

The clinical significance of the immunosuppression produced by alkylating agents in their role as antitumor agents is not certain. The two major concerns are susceptibility to infection in the immunosuppressed host and the potential interference with a host immune response to the tumor. The available evidence indicates that most intermittent antitumor regimens do not produce a profound or prolonged immunosuppression (359).

Platinum Antitumor Compounds

The platinum antitumor agents are complexes of platinum with ligands that can be displaced by nucleophilic (electron-

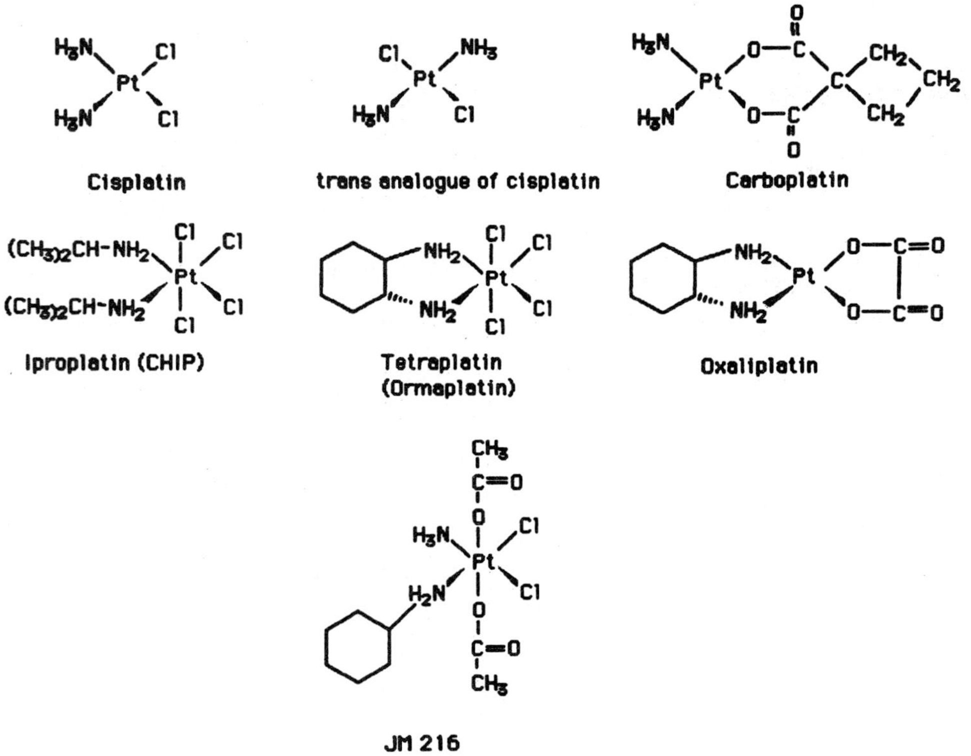

Cisplatin

trans analogue of cisplatin

Carboplatin

Iproplatin (CHIP)

Tetraplatin (Ormaplatin)

Oxaliplatin

JM 216

Figure 62.19. Structures of platinum antitumor agents.

rich) atoms to form strong bonds with covalent characteristics. Thus, like the alkylating agents, the platinum agents form strong chemical bonds with thiol sulfurs and amino nitrogens in proteins and nucleic acids.

The first platinum antitumor compound was discovered by Rosenberg and colleagues (449, 450) while studying the effects of electric current on bacterial growth. The growth inhibition observed was found to be caused by a platinum complex of ammonia and chloride, which was produced in the medium from the platinum electrode. These investigators found several such compounds to have antitumor activity against murine tumors in vivo (450). The most active of these compounds was the one now known as cisplatin (Fig. 62.19).

Cisplatin went into clinical trials in the early 1970s (230, 231, 294, 317, 506), and was found to have significant antitumor activity against testicular cancer, lymphoma, squamous cell carcinoma of the head and neck, ovarian cancer, and bladder cancer. Because of its significant therapeutic effect in these tumors and activity against a number of other solid tumors, it became the most frequently used antitumor agent. Because of the renal and neurotoxicities of cisplatin, there were intensive efforts to devise analogues with less of these toxicities. This work led to the development of carboplatin, which produces primarily hematopoietic toxicity and appears to have an antitumor effect similar to cisplatin (159a, 388, 408, 481, 547), against the tumors against which it has been used. However, many investigators have been reluctant thus far to replace cisplatin with carboplatin in situations where the therapy can be curative, as in the treatment of germ cell tumors. A number of other platinum compounds are currently under investigation and are discussed below.

Chemistry

The platinum compounds that are active antitumor agents can have either four or six ligands (Fig. 62.19), with a square planar or hexahedral configuration, respectively. Those with four ligands have an oxidation state of +2, and those with six ligands an oxidation state of +4. The chloride ligands of cisplatin and the other complexes with the +2 oxidation state can be exchanged for nucleophilic atoms in the biologic milieu, including the nitrogens of the DNA bases. The chloride ligands of the +4 compounds are much less reactive than those of the +2 compounds (200), and it is likely that the +4 compounds are reduced in vivo to produce the reactive +2 complexes (50, 403, 404). The ligand substitution reactions of the square planar complexes occur with retention of the configuration of the platinum complex (219). Since the trans-platinum compounds are essentially inactive as antitumor compounds, the ability of the cis compounds to form certain stereo-specific cross-links probably accounts for their antitumor activity.

In some cis-platinum compounds in clinical use the chloride leaving ligands are replaced with carboxyl ester groups, as in carboplatin and oxaliplatin (Fig. 62.19). These ligands are less readily displaced and, thus, these compounds require higher concentrations for cytotoxicity. The decreased renal and neurologic toxicity of these compounds is also probably due to the fact that they are less chemically reactive than cisplatin. Substitutions on the amino groups alter the lipophilicity and distribution of the agent.

CELLULAR AND MOLECULAR PHARMACOLOGY

While the chloride and carboxyester ligands can probably be directly displaced by biologic atoms, it is likely that, in the biologic milieu, the chloride or carboxy ligands are displaced by water molecules to form the aquo ligand, which is a better leaving group than the chloride or carboxy groups (338). The high chloride content of the extracellular fluid maintains the platinum compounds in the chloride and less reactive form. However, in the lower chloride content of the cell the more reactive aquo species is formed. The loss of a proton produces the hydroxy ligand, which is unreactive (338). The proposed aquation pathway for cisplatin is shown in Figure 62.20. The platinum compounds react with many biologic molecules, but there is considerable evidence that these compounds, like the bifunctional alkylating agents, exert their cytotoxic effect by reacting with DNA and interfering with DNA replication and cell division. Roberts, Pera and colleagues (443) demonstrated that the amount of platinum bound to DNA was directly related to the degree of toxicity of platinum compounds. Zwelling and co-workers (573) demonstrated that the degree of DNA interstrand cross-linking in vitro and in vivo was directly related to the degree of cytotoxicity in rodent tumor cells.

The cis-platinum compounds, like the alkylating agents (125, 126, 154), react with nitrogen atoms of DNA and preferentially react with the N-7 atom of deoxyguanylic acid. Specific adducts of Pt compounds with DNA have now been characterized and studied (443). The consensus of the studies is that the most frequent adducts are dGpdG and dApdG (Fig. 62.21), which result from the cis-platinum complex binding to adjacent deoxyguanylates or an adjacent deoxyadenylate and deoxyguanylate in a strand of DNA, to produce an intrastrand cross-link in both situations. A less common, but perhaps more critical, lesion is the one that results from binding of the platinum atom to the N-7 of a deoxyguanylate in one strand of DNA and to the N-7 atom of a deoxyguanylate in the complementary strand of DNA, thereby producing an interstrand cross-link (Fig. 62.21). Repair of these lesions does occur, and the cytotoxicity to the cell is probably determined by the resultant formation and repair of the lesions (415). As mentioned above, a close correlation between interstrand DNA cross-linking has been demonstrated, but equally precise methods for quantifying intrastrand cross-links in whole cells after drug exposure are not available. Thus, intrastrand DNA cross-links might correlate equally well or better with cytotoxicity. The DNA adducts formed by Pt compounds other than cisplatin have been less well studied but appear to be the same as those formed by cisplatin (287, 416, 502).

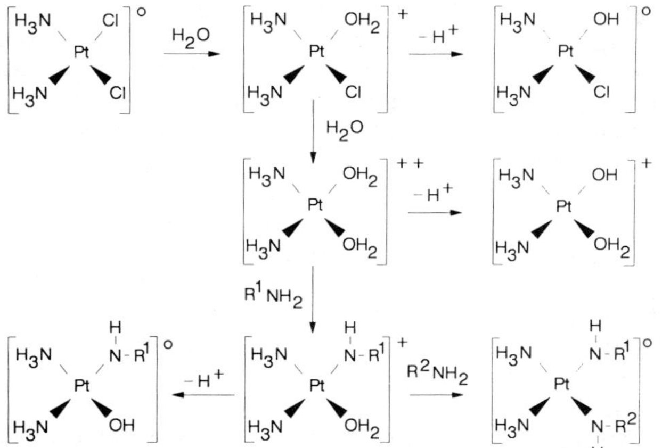

While there is considerable evidence that the formation of DNA adducts is responsible for the cytotoxicity of the platinum antitumor agents, the mechanism through which the cytotoxic effects are mediated is not established. Evidence has been presented that the platinum adducts inhibit replication (414, 546). In a recent paper, Lippard and colleagues (226) have demonstrated that as few as two platinum adducts per genome were sufficient for inhibition of DNA replication by cisplatin. Sorenson and Eastman (489) found that cytotoxicity with cisplatin was correlated with the duration of arrest in the G_2 phase of the cell cycle and postulated that the G_2 arrest was due to the inability of the cells to transcribe the Pt-damaged DNA and produce the mRNA essential for mitosis.

Figure 62.20. Aquation of platinum compounds and reaction with nucleophiles.

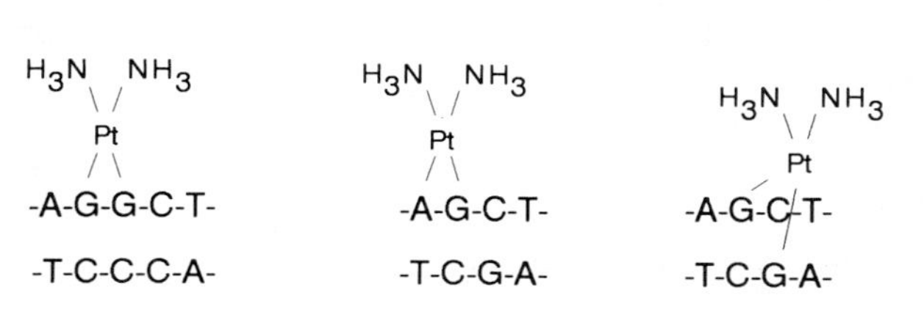

$H_3N\ NH_3$ / Pt	$H_3N\ NH_3$ / Pt	$H_3N\ NH_3$ / Pt
-A-G-G-C-T-	-A-G-C-T-	-A-G-C-T-
-T-C-C-C-A-	-T-C-G-A-	-T-C-G-A-
d(GpG) Adduct	d(ApG) Adduct	Interstrand Crosslink

Figure 62.21. Platinum-DNA adducts.

MECHANISMS OF CELLULAR RESISTANCE TO PLATINUM AGENTS

A number of mechanisms of cellular resistance to platinum compounds have been described. These mechanisms include decreased uptake of the platinum compound into resistant cells, inactivation of the drug by cellular thiol compounds, and enhanced repair of the platinum-related DNA damage.

Decreased cellular uptake of cisplatin by cells resistant to the compound has been described by a number of investigators (15, 246, 323, 347, 472, 515, 557). The uptake of cisplatin into cells is linear for over an hour and does not appear to be an active transport process, although it is partially inhibited by metabolic inhibitors (15). Recently, there has been a report of increased efflux of cisplatin in a resistant cell line (170). Howell and colleagues (334) could not demonstrate changes in the physical properties of the cell membrane of the resistant cells. Thus, while decreased cellular accumulation of the platinum compounds appears to be one type of cellular resistance, the mechanism of this type of resistance remains undefined and may be related to altered binding of the agents to cellular proteins, rather than alteration of passage through the cell membrane (478).

A number of investigators have demonstrated that both rodent and human tumor cells that are selected in vitro or in vivo by exposure to the platinum antitumor compounds frequently demonstrate elevated glutathione levels in association with resistance to these drugs (12, 33, 36, 37, 39, 106, 127, 161, 242, 243, 245, 390, 474). Tumor cell lines derived from patients resistant to therapy with cisplatin have also been found to have elevated glutathione levels (46, 113). In one report the resistant cell line was also found to have elevated activity of gamma-glutamyl transpeptidase, an enzyme in glutathione synthesis (46, 113).

Further evidence that glutathione is involved in resistance to platinum compounds can be inferred from the fact that several investigators have shown that tumor cells can be sensitized to the platinum agents by depletion of cellular glutathione by treatment with buthionine sulfoximine, an inhibitor of glutathione synthesis (11, 14, 210, 245).

The mechanism(s) through which glutathione-associated resistance is mediated have not been definitively elucidated. Andrews and colleagues (11) demonstrated that cisplatin binds to glutathione, and Borch and co-workers (106) have studied the reaction rates of cisplatin with various thiols, including glutathione, and characterized a reaction product in which two glutathiones appeared to be found to each platinum through the cysteine residues of the glutathiones. The thiol platinum ligand is very stable and thus will not react further. Eastman (127) has presented evidence that glutathione may react with monofunctional adducts on DNA to quench the second reactive ligand and prevent cross-link formation. Resistance to cisplatin has also been associated with elevation of glutathione transferase enzyme activity, increased levels of the pi (acidic) isozyme of the protein, and increased levels of the mRNA for the pi isozyme (37, 365, 461, 556). However, the catalysis of the conjugation of glutathione with platinum agents by this enzyme has not been characterized.

Cellular resistance to platinum agents has also been associated with another sulfhydryl-containing protein, metallothionein. Several investigators have found that tumor cells exposed to heavy metals, such as cadmium, develop resistance to cisplatin, which is associated with increased cellular levels of metallothionein (13, 140, 279). In one report, transfection of cells with the metallothionein gene resulted in increased metallothionein levels and resistance of the cells to cisplatin, melphalan, and chlorambucil (279). Imura and colleagues (363) have reported that administration of bismuth subnitrate to mice produced increased levels of metallothionein in the kidneys and resulted in protection of the mice from the renal and gastrointestinal toxicity of cisplatin but did not affect the response of transplanted tumors to cisplatin in the mice. Cisplatin binds to metallothionein in Ehrlich ascites tumor cells (295) and in the liver and kidney of rats (478, 571), and the systemic administration of cisplatin or its hydrolyzed product can induce metallothionein in liver and kidney (148). These findings indicate that metallothionein can protect both tumor and normal cells from cisplatin, although the binding of the drug to this protein has not been characterized.

As with the alkylating agents, there is extensive evidence that enhanced DNA repair can be responsible for resistance to the platinum compounds, and recent work has begun to define specific enzymes involved in this type of resistance (435). Roberts and colleagues (527) first reported that caffeine, a known inhibitor of DNA repair, potentiated cytotoxicity and chromosomal damage in mammalian cells, and shortly thereafter demonstrated that excision repair of cisplatin-damaged DNA does occur in treated cells (162). Many subsequent studies have demonstrated that cells deficient in DNA repair, such as those from patients with xeroderma pigmentosum or Fanconi's anemia, are very sensitive to cisplatin (83, 114, 214, 340, 418, 419).

Agents that are known to inhibit the activity of enzymes involved in the repair of DNA, such as aphidocolin and novobiocin, have been shown to sensitize cells to cisplatin and to reverse the resistance of repair-resistant cell lines (77, 130, 276, 339). The antitumor agents hydroxyurea and cytosine arabinoside, which inhibit DNA repair synthesis, both produce a synergistic cytotoxic effect with cisplatin (157, 524).

There is now considerable evidence that platinum adducts in DNA are repaired by an excision repair mechanism (34, 249) and that the protein product of the human DNA repair gene *ERCC-1* (a homologue of the *E. coli* uvrA gene) is involved (102, 435). Transfection of *ERCC-1* into tumor cells enhances the ability to remove cisplatin from DNA and confers resistance to cisplatin (435). Tumor cells resistant to platinum agents have increased repair capacity (39, 233, 264, 339, 479) and activity of repair enzymes, such as DNA polymerase beta (8, 296) as compared with sensitive lines (232a). It has also been shown that platinum interstrand DNA cross-links are removed more rapidly in cisplatin-resistant cells (232a, 264) and that very sensitive tumor cells may have a decreased ability to remove DNA interstrand cross-links (35). A protein, XPE-BF (xeroderma pigmentosum complementation group E binding factor), which binds to Pt-damaged DNA (82, 84, 250) and may mark it for repair, has been identified. A series of proteins, the Hmg domain proteins, which bind to Pt intrastrand cross-links, produce bending of the DNA, and may inhibit the repair of these lesions has also been described (247, 413). It has also been found that cisplatin-resistant cells can have elevated thymidylate synthase activity and be cross-resistant to 5FU (369) and that c-fos may play a role in the cellular response to Pt agent damage by mediating DNA repair pathways (234, 466, 467).

While it is clear that each of these mechanisms can be associated with the resistance of tumor and normal cells to the platinum agents, the relative roles of these mechanisms in the resistance of tumors to treatment in patients have not been established. Such studies and attempts to overcome resistance with BSO and inhibitors of DNA repair are currently in progress.

CLINICAL PHARMACOLOGY

Analogues in Clinical Use

Both cisplatin and carboplatin are now licensed in the United States and are used extensively. Since the primary toxicity of carboplatin is hematopoietic, it is replacing cisplatin for use in many patients and is being used particularly in situations where nonhematopoietic toxicity should be avoided, such as with bone marrow support (17, 526) or with hematopoietic stimulatory factors. There is no evidence for lack of cross-resistance between these two agents. Iproplatin has been evaluated in phase II trials but was found to be no more effective or less effective than carboplatin, and produced more hematopoietic and gastrointestinal toxicity (167b, 278, 318, 374a, 523, 541, 558). Tetraplatin (ormaplatin) produced severe neurotoxicity in clinical trials (278, 383). Oxaliplatin is similar to tetraplatin in its preclinical toxicity (145a), and because of responses in colon cancer patients during phase II trials (310) is now being evaluated in combination with 5FU and leucovorin in this disease (311). A lipid-soluble platinum compound, JM216 (277, 278) which can be administered orally, is now being evaluated clinically. Some of the new platinum analogues may not be totally cross-resistant with cisplatin due to differences in either cellular uptake (323, 472) or cellular detoxification (396).

Pharmacokinetics

Platinum antitumor compounds have been measured in human plasma and other human tissues as total platinum, as ultrafilterable platinum, and as the specific parent compounds. Total platinum can be measured by using compounds containing the radioactive ^{193}Pt or ^{195}Pt isotopes (110, 303), by trapping the platinum with an ultraviolet absorbing ligand, such as diethyldithiocarbamate (180), or by flameless atomic absorption spectroscopy (105, 180). Ultrafiltration of plasma and other biologic fluids separates the free platinum compounds from those bound to protein. The protein-bound species are biologically inactive and essentially irreversibly bound to the protein (438). Both cisplatin and carboplatin have been measured specifically by separation from other species on HPLC columns and detection by electrochemical detection or by collecting fractions and quantifying the total platinum in each fraction (400, 431). The cisplatinum concentration has been found to be consistently between 60 and 80% of the ultrafilterable platinum and to follow the same kinetics as the ultrafilterable platinum (Fig. 62.22) (237, 400). Carboplatinum represents a higher percentage of the ultrafilterable platinum and follows kinetics similar to the ultrafilterable platinum. Because of the sensitivity, accuracy, and convenience of the method, flameless atomic absorption spectroscopy is the most common technique used to measure the platinum agents. Furthermore, since measuring filterable species appears to measure the reactive compounds, and to approximate closely the measurement of the parent compounds, measurement of ultrafilterable platinum is most commonly used in pharmacokinetic studies.

In pharmacokinetic studies after cisplatin administration, total platinum in the plasma follows a triphasic pattern, with the first phase $t_{1/2}$ about 30 minutes, the second phase $t_{1/2}$ about 60 minutes, and the third phase $t_{1/2}$ greater than 24 hours (40, 105, 237). Measurements of the ultrafilterable platinum indicate that the initial, more rapid clearance phases are due to the renal clearance of filterable platinum,

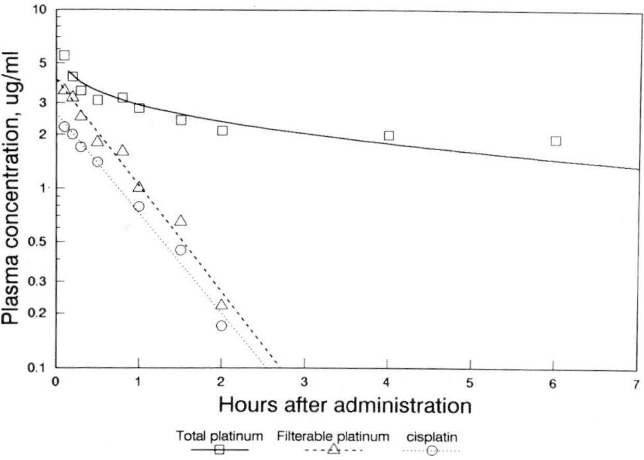

Figure 62.22. Clinical pharmacokinetics of cisplatin after single injection of 100 mg/m^2. (Adapted from Patton et al. (400).)

the majority of which is the parent compound (431). Carboplatin exhibits similar pharmacokinetics, except that the initial half-lives are somewhat longer, less of the total platinum is protein-bound, and a greater percentage of the agent is excreted by the kidneys (378, 431). The pharmacokinetics of total and filterable platinum after iproplatin administration appears to be similar to those of carboplatin (99a). Decreased creatinine clearance results in higher plasma levels of both cisplatin and carboplatin and potentially greater toxicity (134).

After bolus administration of 100 mg/m^2 of cisplatin, initial peak plasma concentrations of 3 to >5 μg/ml are achieved, (400) with this value decreasing to less than 0.2 microgram/ml at 2 hours (Fig. 62.22). After the usual clinical dose of about 300 mg/m^2 of carboplatin, peak plasma levels of about 30 μg/ml are reached, declining to about 5 μg/ml at 2 hours (378, 431).

In typical clinical use, usually in combination with other agents, the platinum antitumor agents are given intravenously, either as a single dose or daily for several days, with repeat courses at 3 to 4 weeks. The agents are given as an infusion over several hours rather than as a bolus dose and, especially with very high doses, may be given as 24-hour or longer infusions. Because of the close relationships between plasma AUC of carboplatin and renal function and between AUC of carboplatin and toxicity, a dosing algorithm based on renal function has been established and is now widely used in the dosing of carboplatin (132a) (see Chapter 58).

Cisplatin and carboplatin have also been administered regionally. There has been considerable experience with the intraperitoneal route, particularly in the treatment of ovarian cancer (343, 411, 490). Very high intraperitoneal concentrations can be obtained, and systemic toxicities can be reduced by the concomitant systemic administration of thiosulfate (244, 336). Cisplatin has also been administered intra-arterially for the treatment of tumors in the extremities (26, 73, 258, 272), brain tumors (159, 307, 497), carcinoma of the head and neck (29, 358), carcinoma of the liver (274), and carcinoma of the bladder (124, 255). Intravesicular instillation of cisplatin has been used for the treatment of superficial cancers of the bladder (51, 241, 316). Cisplatin has also been instilled into the pericardial sac for the treatment of malignant pericardial effusions (155, 337).

TOXICITIES

Renal

The most serious, and usually dose limiting, toxicity of cisplatin is renal (188, 412). This toxicity is manifested clinically by elevated BUN and creatinine, is cumulative with continued cisplatin exposure, and is potentiated by other nephrotoxins (109). Decreases in serum electrolytes have been associated with platinum renal toxicity, including symptomatic hypomagnesemia (471). While the toxicity may remain subclinical, or the renal function return to normal, significant pathological damage appears to persist (185). The pathology of the renal damage is characterized by focal acute tubular necrosis, dilatation of convoluted tubules, thickened tubular basement membranes, formation of casts, and epithelial atypia of the collecting ducts (185, 330). High fluid intake with forced diuresis (78, 223) can reduce the incidence and severity of the renal toxicity. Systemic administration of thiols can reduce renal toxicity of cisplatin in animal models, and in a clinical trial systemic diethyldithiodicarbamate appeared to reduce nephrotoxicity without affecting ototoxicity or myelosuppression (44). The nephrotoxicity of the second generation platinum complexes, such as carboplatin and iproplatin, is markedly less than that of cisplatin.

Ototoxicity

Ototoxicity has been a significant problem with cisplatin. This toxicity is characterized by tinnitus and hearing loss (230, 231, 317, 483). The hearing loss is usually in the high frequency range, 4,000 to 8,000 Hz, but may occur in the lower ranges, which include the speech frequencies (298, 483). Since the higher frequencies are usually involved, the hearing loss may not be symptomatic. Vestibular toxicity does not usually occur but can be seen (48, 563). The ototoxicity of cisplatin is dose-related, and is usually cumulative with subsequent courses of the agent (206, 544). Radiation prior to or simultaneous with the cisplatin administration enhances the toxicity (190, 554), but this additive effect may be less if the cisplatin precedes the radiation (298).

The pathological findings associated with ototoxicity, in both experimental animals and patients, are selective damage to the outer hair cells of the cochlea and lesions in the organ of Corti, the spiral ganglion and cochlear nerve, and the stria vascularis (57, 293, 357, 498). In studies of organ cultures of the cochlear structures the hair cells are very sensitive to very low concentrations of cisplatin (16). Vestibular toxicity is associated with degeneration of the maculae and cristae (563).

Neurotoxicity

The neurotoxicity seen with the administration of cisplatin consists principally of peripheral neuropathy involving both the upper and lower extremities, with paresthesias, weakness, tremors, and loss of taste (550). Seizures and leucoencephalopathy have also been described (69, 76, 168, 420). The neurotoxicity may be persistent (213) and may progress after cessation of cisplatin therapy (200). The quantitative determination of vibratory perception threshold has been reported to correlate with cisplatin neurotoxicity (138).

Particularly severe neurotoxicity has been reported after intra-arterial infusions of cisplatin, with cranial nerve paralysis occurring after intra-arterial infusions for head and neck cancer (168, 420) and severe peripheral neuropathy after lower limb perfusion (71). In experimental animals, severe CNS toxicity was seen when compounds that open the blood brain barrier were administered prior to systemic cisplatin treatment, and intracarotid cisplatin produced damage to the blood-brain barrier and severe neurotoxicity (367). However, severe neurotoxicity was not seen in patients treated with intracarotid cisplatin for primary brain tumors (332). The neurotoxicity of ifosfamide has been reported to be enhanced by prior treatment with cisplatin (423).

Since various pharmacologic maneuvers have been able to control or reduce the nephrotoxicity and severe nausea and vomiting produced by cisplatin, neurotoxicity has become the dose limiting toxicity of cisplatin (387). An interesting observation is that treatment of animals with an ACTH analogue will prevent neurotoxicity from cisplatin and will facilitate the recovery of established neurotoxicity (529, 530), but will not interfere with the antitumor effect of the agent. In a randomized, placebo-controlled clinical trial, this compound appeared to prevent or ameliorate the neurotoxicity of cisplatin (530). Neither carboplatin or iproplatin appear to produce significant neurotoxicity, with the doses used thus far with autologous bone marrow transfusion (371, 395, 532).

Gastrointestinal Toxicity

Severe nausea and vomiting have been a significant problem with cisplatin, occurring in almost all patients receiving the drug (294, 425). The cause of this toxicity is not firmly established. Work in animal models indicates that abdominal visceral innervation and 5-hydroxytryptamine receptors on visceral afferent nerves play a role in mediating this toxicity (222), but there is also evidence that the chemoreceptor trigger zone in the medulla plays a role (232, 341). The use of a dopamine antagonist, metoclopramide, prior to and during cisplatin administration has been effective in controlling this toxicity (189, 269) and the steroids dexamethasone or methylprednisolone alone or in combination with metoclopramide have also been useful (1, 41, 176). More recently antiserotonin analogues such as ondansetron and granisetron have proven highly effective in controlling nausea and vomiting. The gastrointestinal toxicities of carboplatin and iproplatin are much less than those of cisplatin (23, 137, 181).

Immune Effects

In contrast to the alkylating agents, many of which are significantly immunosuppressive, cisplatin appears to have no immunosuppressive effect at the usual clinical doses and may even augment immune function at these doses (435). Monocyte-mediated cytotoxicity was found to be increased in ovarian cancer patients after cisplatin treatment (286), and OKT8+ cytotoxic cells were increased in patients after cisplatin therapy (381).

References

1. Aapro MS, Plezia PM, Alberts DS, Graham V, Jones SE, Surwit EA, Moon TE. Double-blind crossover study of the antiemetic efficacy of high-dose dexamethasone versus high-dose metoclopramide. J Clin Oncol 1984;2:466.
2. Abdi EA, Hanson J, Harbora DE, Young DG, and McPherson TA. Adjuvant chemoimmuno- and immunotherapy in Dukes' stage B2 and C colorectal carcinoma: a 7-year follow-up analysis. J Surg Oncol 1989;40:205.
3. Adair CPJ, Bogg HJ. Experimental and clinical studies on the treatment of cancer by dichloroethylsulfide (mustard gas). Ann Surg 1931;93:190.
4. Alberts DS, Chang SY, Chen H-SG, Larcom BJ, Jones SE. Pharmacokinetics and metabolism of chlorambucil in man: a preliminary report. Cancer Treat Rev 1979;6(suppl):9.
5. Alberts DS, Chang SY, Chen H-SG, Moon TE, Evans TL, Furner RL, Himmelstein K, Gross JF. Kinetics of intravenous melphalan. Clin Pharmacol Ther 1979;26:73.
6. Alberts DS, Chang SY, Chen H-SG, Larcom BJ, Evans TL. Comparative pharmacokinetics of chlorambucil and melphalan in man. Recent Results Cancer Res 1980;74: 124.
7. Alberts DS, Chen H-SG, Benz D, Mason NL. Effect of renal dysfunction in dogs on the disposition and marrow toxicity of melphalan. Br J Cancer 1981;43:330.
8. Ali-Osman F, Berger MS, Rairkar A, Stein DE. Enhanced repair of a cisplatin-damaged reporter chloramphenicol-O-acetyltransferase gene and altered activities of DNA polymerases alpha and beta, and DNA ligase in cells of a human malignant-glioma following in vivo cisplatin therapy. J Cell Biochem 1994;54:11.
9. Ali-Osman F, Srivenugopal K, Berger MS, Stein DE. DNA interstrand cross-linking and strand break repair in human glioma cell lines of varying (1,3-bis(2-chlorethyl)-1-nitrosourea) resistance. Anticancer Res 1990;10:677.
10. Anderson LW, Ludeman SM, Colvin OM, Grochow LB, Strong JM. Quantitation of 4-hydroxycyclophosphamide/aldophosphamide in whole blood. J Chromatogr B: Biomed App 1995;667:247–57.
11. Andrews PA, Murphy MP, Howell SB. Characterization of cisplatin-resistance COLO 316 human ovarian carcinoma cells. Eur J Cancer Clin Oncol 1989;25:619.
12. Andrews PA, Murphy MP, Howell SB. Differential sensitization of human ovarian carcinoma and mouse L1210 cells to cisplatin and melphalan by glutathione depletion. Mol Pharmacol 1986;30:643.
13. Andrews PA, Murphy MP, Howell SB. Metallothionein mediated cisplatin resistance in human ovarian carcinoma cells. Cancer Chemother Pharmacol 1987;19:149.
14. Andrews PA, Schiefer MA, Murphy MP, Howell SB. Enhanced potentiation of cisplatin cytotoxicity in human ovarian carcinoma cells by prolonged glutathione depletion. Chem Biol Interact 1988;65:51.
15. Andrews PA, Velury S, Mann SC, Howell SB. Cis-Diamminendichloroplatinum (II) accumulation in sensitive and resistant human ovarian carcinoma cells. Cancer Res 1988;48:68.
16. Anniko M, Sobin A. Cisplatin: evaluation of its ototoxic potential. Am J Otolaryngol 1986;7:276.
17. Antman K, Eder JP, Elias A, Shea T, Peters WP, Andersen J, Schryber S, Henner WD, Finberg R, Wilmore D. High-dose combination alkylating agent preparative regimen with autologous bone marrow support: the Dana-Farber Cancer Institute/Beth Israel Hospital Experience. Cancer Treat Rep 1987;71:119.
18. Antman K, Eder JP, Elias A, Ayash L, Shea TC, Weissman L, Critchlow J, Schryber SM, Begg C, Teicher BA, Schnipper LE, Frei E III. High-dose thiotepa alone and in combination regimens with bone marrow support. Semin Oncol 1990;17(suppl 3):33.
19. Antman KH, Elias A, Ryan L. Ifosfamide and mesna: response and toxicity at standard- and high-dose schedules. Semin Oncol 1990;17:68.
20. Appelbaum F, Strauchen JA, Graw RG Jr, Savage DD, Kent KM, Ferrans VJ, Herzig GP. Acute lethal carditis caused by high-dose combination chemotherapy: a unique clinical and pathological entity. Lancet 1976;1(7950):58.
21. Arbuck SG, Silk Y, Douglass HO Jr, Nava H, Rustum YM, Milliron S. A phase II trial of 5-fluorouracil, doxorubicin, mitomycin C, and leucovorin in advanced gastric carcinoma. Cancer 1990;65:2442.
22. Arita N, Ushio Y, Hayakawa T, Nagatant M, Huang TY, Izumoto S, Mogami H. Intrathecal ACNU—a new therapeutic approach against malignant leptomengeal tumors. J Neurooncol 1988;6:221.
23. Arseneau J, Blessing JA, Stehman FB, McGehee R. A phase II study of carboplatin in advanced squamous cell carcinoma of the cervix (a Gynecologic Oncology Group Study). Invest New Drugs 1986;4(2):187.
24. Auerbuch SD. Nonclassic alkylating agents. In Cancer Chemotherapy: Principles and Practice. Edited by BA Chabner, JM Collins. Philadelphia: Lippincott, 1990, pp 314–328.
25. Ayash LJ, Wright JE, Tretyakov O, Gonin R, Elias A, Wheeler C, Eder JP, Rosowsky A, Antman K, Frei E III. Cyclophosphamide pharmacokinetics: Correlation with cardiac toxicity and tumor response. J Clin Oncol 1992;10:995.
26. Bacci G, Picci P, Ruggieri P, Mercuri M, Avella M, Capanna R, Brach-Del-Prever A, Mancini A, Gherlinzoni F, Padovani G, Leonossa C, Biagini R, Ferraro A, Ferruzi A, Cazzola A, Manfrini M, Campanacci I. Primary chemotherapy and delayed surgery (neoadjuvant chemotherapy) for osteosarcoma of the extremities. The Instituto Rissoli Experience in 127 patients treated preoperatively with intravenous methotrexate (high versus moderate doses) and intraarterial cisplatin. Cancer 1990;65:2539.
27. Bailey CC, Marsden HB, Jones PH. Fatal pulmonary fibrosis following 1,3-bis(2-chloroethyl)-1-nitrosourea (BCNU) therapy. Cancer 1978;42:74.
28. Bailey HH, Mulcahy RT, Tutsch KD, Arzoomanian RZ, Alberti D, Tombes MB, Wilding G, Pomplun M, Spriggs DR. Phase I clinical trial of intravenous L-buthionine sulfoximine and melphalan: An attempt at modulation of glutathione. J Clin Oncol 1994;12(1):194.
29. Baker SR, Wheeler R. Intraarterial chemotherapy for head and neck cancer. Part 2: clinical experience. Head Neck Surg 1984;6:751.
30. Bakke JE, Feil VJ, Fjelstul CE, Thacker EJ. Metabolism of cyclophosphamide by sheep. J Agric Food Chem 1972;20:384.
31. Barlogie B, Jagannath S, Dixon DO, Cheson B, Smallwood L, Hendrickson A, Purvis JD, Bonnem E, Alexanian R. High-dose melphalan and granulocyte-macrophage colony-stimulating factor for refractory multiple myeloma. Blood 1990;76:677.
32. Barratt TM, Soothill JF. Controlled trial of cyclophosphamide in steroid-sensitive relapsing nephrotic syndrome of childhood. Lancet 1970;2:279.
33. Batist G, Behrens BC, Makuch R, Hamilton TC, Katki AG, Louie KG, Myers CE, Ozols RF. Serial determinations of glutathione levels and glutathione-related enzyme activities in human tumor cells in vitro. Biochem Pharmacol 1986;35:2257.
34. Beck DJ, Popoff S, Sancar A, Rupp WD. Reactions of the UVRABC excision nuclease with DNA damaged by diaminedichloroplatinum (II). Nucleic Acids Res 1985;13: 7395.
35. Bedford P, Fichtinger-Schepman AM, Shellard AA, Walker MC, Masters JR, Hill BT. Differential repair of platinum-DNA adducts in human bladder and testicular tumor continuous cell lines. Cancer Res 1988;48:3019.
36. Bedford P, Shellard SA, Walker MC, Whelan RD, Masters JR, Hill BT. Differential expression of collateral sensitivity or resistance to cisplatin in human bladder carcinoma cell lines pre-exposed in vitro to either x-irradiation or cisplatin. Int J Cancer 1987;40: 681.
37. Bedford P, Walker MC, Sharma HL, Perera A, McAuliffe CA, Masters JR, Hill BT. Factors influencing the sensitivity of two human bladder carcinoma cell lines to cis-diaminedichloroplatinum (II). Chem Biol Interact 1987;61:1.
38. Begleiter A, Lam H-YP, Grover J, Froese E, Goldenberg GJ. Evidence for active transport of melphalan by two amino acid carriers in L5178Y lymphoblasts in vitro. Cancer Res 1979;39:353.
39. Behrens BC, Hamilton TC, Masuda H, Grotzinger KR, Whang-Peng J, Louie KG, Knutsen T, McKoy WM, Young RC. Characterization of a cis-diaminedichloroplatinum (II)-resistant human ovarian cancer cell line and its use in evaluation of platinum analogues. Cancer Res 1987;47:414.
40. Belt RJ, Himmelstein KJ, Patton TF, Bannister SJ, Sternson LA, Repta AJ. Pharmacokinetics of non-protein-bound platinum species following administration of cis-dichlorodiamineplatinum (II). Cancer Treat Rep 1979;63:1515.
41. Benrubi GI, Norvell M, Nuss RC, Robinson H. The use of methylprednisolone and metoclopramide in control of emesis in patients receiving cis-platinum. Gynecol Oncol 1985;21:306.
42. Berd D, Mastrangelo MJ. Effect of low dose cyclophosphamide on the immune system of cancer patients: depletion of CD4+, 2H4+ suppressor-inducer T-cells. Cancer Res 1988;48:1671.
43. Berd D, Mastrangelo MJ. Active immunotherapy of human melanoma exploiting the immunopotentiating effects of cyclophosphamide. Cancer Invest 1988;6:337.
44. Berry JM, Jacobs C, Sikic B, Halsey J, Borch RF. Modification of cisplatin toxicity with diethyldithiocarbamate. J Clin Oncol 1990;8:1585.
45. Bethlenfalvay NC, Bergin JJ. Severe cerebral toxicity after intravenous nitrogen mustard therapy. Cancer 1972;29:366.
46. Bier H, Bergler W, Mende S, Ganzer U. Glutathione content and gamma-glutamyl-transpeptidase activity in squamous cell head and neck cancer xenografts. Arch Otorhinolaryngol 1988;245:166.
47. Bierman HR, Kelly KH, Knudson AG Jr, Maekawa T, Timmis GM. The influence of 1, 4-dimethylsulfonoxy-1, 4-dimethylbutane (CB 2348, di-methyl Myleran) in neoplastic disease. Ann NY Acad Sci 1958;68:1211.
48. Black FO, Myers EN, Schramm VL, Johnson J, Sigler B, Thearle PB, Burns DS. Cisplatin vestibular ototoxicity: preliminary report. Laryngoscope 1982;92:1363.
49. Blake DB, Heller RH, Hsu SH, Schacter BZ. Return of fertility in a patient with cyclophosphamide-induced azoospermia. Johns Hopkins Med J 1976;139:20.
50. Blatter EE, Vollano JE, Krishnan BS, Dabrowiak JC. Interaction of the Antitumor Agents cis,cis,trans-Pt(NH3)C12(OH)2 and cis,cis,trans-Pt IV($(CH_3)_2CHNH_2$) $2Cl_2(OH)_2$ and their reduction products with Pmg DNA. D1. Biochemistry 1984;23: 4817.
51. Blumenreich MS, Needles B, Yagoda A, Sogani P, Grabstald H, Whitmore WF Jr. Intravesical cisplatin for superficial bladder tumors. Cancer 1982;50(5):863.
52. Boal JH, Williamson M, Boyd VL, Ludeman SM, Egan WP. NMR studies of the kinetics of bisalkylation by isophosphoramide mustard: comparisons with phosphoramide mustard. J Med Chem 1989;32:1768.
53. Boddy AV, Cole M, Pearson ADJ, Idle JR. The kinetics of the auto-induction ifosfamide metabolism during continuous infusion. Cancer Chemother Pharmacol 1995;36:53.
54. Bode U, Seif SM, Levine AA. Studies on the antidiuretic effect of cyclophosphamide: vasopressin release and sodium excretion. Med Pediatr Oncol 1980;8:295.
55. Bodell WJ, Tokuda K, Ludlum DB. Differences in DNA alkylation products formed in sensitive and resistant human glioma cells treated with N-(2-chloroethyl)-N-nitrosurea. Cancer Res 1988;48:4489.
56. Bodenstein D, Goldin A. A comparison of the effects of various nitrogen mustard compounds on embryonic cells. J Exp Zool 1948;108:75.
57. Boheim K, Bichler E. Cisplatin-induced ototoxicity: audiometric findings and experimental cochlear pathology. Arch Otorhinolaryngol 1985;242:1.
58. Bolton MG, Colvin OM, Hilton J. Specificity of isozymes of murine hepatic glutathione S-transferase for the conjugation of glutathione with melphalan. Cancer Res (in press).
59. Bonnadonna G, Valgussa P, Santoro A, Viviani S, Bonfante V, Banfi A. Hodgkin's disease: the Milan Cancer Institute experience with MOPP and ABVD. Recent Results Cancer Res 1989;117:169.
60. Borison HL, Brand ED, Orland RK. Emetic action of nitrogen mustard (Mechlorethamine hydrochloride) in dogs and cats. Am J Physiol 1968;192:410.
61. Borowy-Borowski H, Lipman R, Chowdary D, Tomasz M. Duplex oligodeoxyribonucleotides cross-linked by mitomycin C at a single site: synthesis, properties, and cross-link reversibility. Biochemistry 1990;29:2992.
62. Borowy-Borowski H, Lipman R, Tomasz M. Recognition between mitomycin C and specific DNA sequences for cross-link formation. Biochemistry 1990;29:2999.
63. Brade WP, Herdrich K, Varini M. Ifosfamide—pharmacology, safety and therapeutic potential. Cancer Treat Rev 1985;12:1.
64. Brandt SJ, Peters WP, Atwater SK, Kurtzberg J, Borowitz MJ, Jones RB, Shpall EJ,

Bast RC Jr, Gilbert CJ, Oette DH. Effect of recombinant human granulocyte-macrophage colony-stimulating factor on hemotopoietic reconstitution after high-dose chemotherapy and autologous bone marrow transplantation. N Engl J Med 1988;31:869.

65. Brent TP, Houghton PJ, Houghton JA. 06-Alkylguanine-DNA alkyltransferase activity correlates with the therapeutic response of human rhabdomyosarcoma xenografts to 1-(2-chlorethyl)-3-(trans-4-methylcyclohexyl)-1-nitrosourea. Proc Natl Acad Sci USA 1985;82:2985.
66. Brock N. The development of mesna for the inhibition of urotoxic side effects of cyclophosphamide, ifosfamide, and other oxazaphosphorine cytostatics. Recent Results Cancer Res 1980;74:270.
67. Brookes P, Lawley PD. The reaction of mono-and difunctional alkylating agents with nucleic acids. Biochem J 1961;80:486.
68. Brookes P, Lawley PD. The action of alkylating agents on deoxyribonucleic acid in relation to biologic effects of the alkylating agents. Exp Cell Res 1963;9(suppl):512.
69. Bruck W, Heise E, Friede RL. Leukoencephalopathy after cisplatin therapy. Clin Neuropathol 1989;8:263.
70. Buckner CD, Rudolph RH, Fefer A, Clift RA, Epstein RB, Funk DD, Neiman PE, Slichter SJ, Storb R, Thomas ED. High dose cyclophosphamide therapy for malignant disease. Cancer 1972;29:357.
71. Busse O, Aigner K, Wilimzig H. Peripheral nerve damage following isolated extremity perfusion with cis-platinum. Recent Results Cancer Res 1983;86:264.
72. Butler AL, Clapper ML, Tew KD. Glutathione S-transferase in nitrogen mustard-resistant and -sensitive cell lines. Mol Pharmacol 1987;31:575.
73. Calabro A, Singletary SE, Carrasco CH, Legha SS. Intra-arterial infusion chemotherapy in regionally advanced malignant melanoma. J Surg Oncol 1990;43:239.
74. Calcutt G, Conners TA. Tumor sulfhydryl levels and sensitivity to the nitrogen mustard merophan. Biochem Pharmacol 1963;12:839.
75. Carden PA, Mitchell SL, Waters KD, Tiedemann K, Ekert H. Prevention of cyclophosphamide/cytarabine-induced emesis with ondansetron in children with leukemia. J Clin Oncol 1990;8(9):1531.
76. Cattaneo MT, Filipazzi V, Piazza E, Damiani E, Mancarella G. Transient blindness and seizure associated with cisplatin therapy. J Cancer Res Clin Oncol 1988;114:528.
77. Chao CC, Lee YL, Lin-Chao S. Phenotypic reversion of cisplatin resistance in human cells accompanies reduced host cell reactivation of damaged plasmid. Biochem Biophys Res Commun 1990;170:851.
78. Chary KK, Higby DJ, Henderson ES, Swinerton KD. Phase I study of high-dose cis-dichlorodiammineplatinum (II) with forced diuresis. Cancer Treat Rep 1977;61:367.
79. Chen TL, Passos-Coelho JL, Noe DA, Kennedy MJ, Black KC, Colvin OM, Grochow LB. Nonlinear pharmacokinetics of cyclophosphamide in patients with metastatic breast cancer receiving high-dose chemotherapy followed by autologous bone marrow transplantation. Cancer Res 1995;55:810.
80. Chiuten DF, Roseneweig M, Von Hoff DD, Muggia FM. Clinical trials with hexitol derivatives in the U.S. Cancer 1981;47:442.
81. Choi KE, Ratain MJ, Williams SF, Golick JA, Beschorner JC, Fullem LJ, Bitran JD. Plasma pharmacokinetics of high-dose oral melphalan in patients treated with trialkylator chemotherapy and autologous bone marrow. Cancer Res 1989;49:1318.
82. Chu G. Cellular responses to cisplatin. The roles of DNA-binding proteins and DNA repair (review). J Biol Chem 1994;269:787.
83. Chu G, Berg P. DNA cross-linked by cisplatin: a new probe for the DNA repair defect in xeroderma pigmentosum. Mol Biol Med 1987;4:277.
84. Chu G, Chang E. Cisplatin-resistant cells express increased levels of a factor that recognizes damaged DNA. Proc Natl Acad Sci USA 1990;87:3324.
85. Ciaccio PJ, Tew KD, Lacreta FP. The spontaneous and glutathione S-transferase mediated reaction of chlorambucil with glutathione. Cancer Commun 1990;2:279.
86. Clark JL, Barcewicz P, Nava HR, Goodwin PS, Douglass HO Jr. Adjuvant 5-FU and MeCCNU improves survival following curative gastrectomy for adenocarcinoma. Am Surg 1990;56:423.
87. Clayman DA, Wolpert SM, Heros DO. Superselective arterial BCNU infusion in the treatment of patients with malignant gliomas. AJNR 1989;10:767.
88. Codling BW, Chakera TM. Pulmonary fibrosis following therapy with melphalan for multiple myeloma. J Clin Pathol 1972;25:668.
89. Cohen BE, Egorin MJ, Kohlhepp EA, Aisner J, Gutierrez PL. Human plasma pharmacokinetics and urinary excretion of thiotepa and its metabolites. Cancer Treat Rep 1986;70:859.
90. Cole RC, Myers TJ, Klatsky AU. Pulmonary disease with chlorambucil therapy. Cancer 1978;41:455.
91. Colvin M. The comparative pharmacology of cyclophosphamide and ifosfamide. Semin Oncol 1982;9:2.
92. Colvin M, Brundrett RB, Cowens W, Jardine E, Ludlum DB. A chemical basis for the antitumor activity of chloroethylnitrosoureas. Biochem Pharmacol 1976;25:695.
93. Colvin M, Chabner BA. Alkylating Agents in Cancer Chemotherapy: Principles and Practice. Edited by BA Chabner, JM Collins. Philadelphia: Lippincott, 1990, pp 276–313.
94. Colvin M, Russo JE, Hilton J, Dulik DM, Fenselau C. Enzymatic mechanisms of resistance to alkylating agents in tumor cells and normal tissues. Adv Enzyme Regul 1988;27:211–221.
95. Cornwell GG III, Pajak TF, McIntyre OR, Kochna S, Dosik H. Influence of renal failure on myelosuppressive effects of melphalan: cancer and leukemia group B experience. Cancer Treat Rep 1982;66:475.
96. Cornwell GG III, Pajak TF, McIntyre OR. Hypersensitivity reactions to IV melphalan during treatment of multiple myeloma: cancer and leukemia Group B experience. Cancer Treat Rep 1979;63:399.
97. Costa G, Engle RL Jr, Schilling A, Carbone P, Kochua S, Nachman RL, Glidewell O. Melphalan and prednisone: an effective combination for the treatment of multiple myeloma. Am J Med 1973;54:589.
98. Cox PJ. Cyclophosphamide cystitis—identification of acrolein as the causative agent. Biochem Pharmacol 1979;28:2045.
99. Crathorne AR, Roberts JJ. Mechanism of the cytotoxic action of alkylating agents in mammalian cells and evidence for the removal of alkylated groups from deoxynucleic acid. Nature 1966;211:150.
99a. Creaven PJ, Pendylala L, Madajewicz S. Clinical development of iproplatin (CHIP). Drugs Exp Clin Res 1986;12:287.
100. Curt GA, Kelley JA, Kufta CV, Smith BH, Kornblith PL, Young RC, Collins JM. Phase II and pharmacokinetic study of aziridinylbenzoquinone (2,5-diazirindinyl-3, 6-bis(carboethoxyamino)-1, 4-benzoquinone, diaziquone, NSC 182986) in high-grade gliomas. Cancer Res 1983;43:6102.
101. Cussac C, Rapp M, Mounetou E, Madelmont JC, Maurizis JC, Godeneche D, Dupuy JM, Sauzieres J, Baudry JP, Veyre A. Enhancement by O^6-benzyl-N-acetylguanosine derivatives of chloroethylnitrosourea antitumor action in chloroethylnitrosourea-resistant human malignant melanocytes.
102. Dabholkar M, Vionnet J, Bostick-Bruton F, Yu JJ, Reed E. Messenger RNA levels of XPAC and ERCC1 in ovarian cancer tissue correlate with response to platinum-based chemotherapy. JNCI 1994;94:703.
103. Dantzig AH, Fairgrieve M, Slayman CW, Adelberg EA. Isolation and characterization of a CHO amino acid transport mutant resistant to melphalan (L-phenylalanine mustard). Somat Cell Molec Genet 1984;10:113.
104. Das SK, Lau CC, Pardee AB. Comparative analysis of caffeine and 3-aminobenzamide as DNA repair inhibitors in Syrian baby hamster kidney cells. Mutat Res 1984;131:71.
105. DeConti RC, Toftness BAU, Lange RC, Creasey WA. Clinical and pharmacological studies with cis-diamminedichloroplatinum (II). Cancer Res 1973;33:1310.
106. Dedon PC, Borch RF. Characterization of the reactions of platinum antitumor agents with biologic and nonbiologic sulfur-containing nucleophiles. Biochem Pharmacol 1987;36:1955.
107. DeFronzo RA, Braine HG, Colvin M, Davis PJ. Water intoxication in man after cyclophosphamide therapy. Ann Intern Med 1973;78:861.
108. Denny BJ, Wheelhouse RT, Stevens MF, Tsang LL, Slack JA. NMR and molecular modeling investigation of the mechanism of activation of the antitumor drug temozolomide and its interaction with DNA. Biochemistry 1994;33:9045.
109. Dentino M, Luft FC, Yum MN, Williams SD, Einhorn LH. Long term effect of cis-diamminedichloride platinum (CDDP) on renal function and structure in man. Cancer 1978;41:1274.
110. DeSimone PA, Yancey RS, Coupal JJ, Butts JD, Hoeschel JD. Effect of a forced diuresis on the distribution and excretion (via urine and bile) of 195m platinum when given as 195m platinum cis-dichlorodiammineplatinum (II). Cancer Treat Rep 1979;63:951.
111. DeVita VT, Carbone PP, Owens AH Jr, Gold GL, Krant MJ, Edmonson J. Clinical trials with 1,3-bis(2-chloroethyl)-1-nitrosourea, NSC-409962. Cancer Res 1965;25:1876.
112. DeVita VT, Serpick AA, Carbone PP. Combination chemotherapy in the treatment of advanced Hodgkin's disease. Ann Intern Med 1970;73:881.
113. de Vries EG, Jeijer C, Timmer-Bosscha H, Berendsen HH, de Leij L, Scheper RJ, Mulder NH. Resistance mechanisms in three human small cell lung cancer cell lines established from one patient during clinical follow up. Cancer Res 1989;49:4175.
114. Dijt FJ, Fichtinger-Schepman AM, Berends F, Reedijk J. Formation and repair of cisplatin-induced adducts to DNA in cultured normal and repair-deficient human fibroblasts. Cancer Res 1988;48:6058.
115. D'Incalci M, Bolis G, Facchinetti T, Mangioni C, Morasca L, Morazzoni P, Salmona M. Decreased half-life of cyclophosphamide in patients under continual treatment. Eur J Cancer 1979;19:7.
116. Dirven HA, van Ommen B, van Bladeren PJ. Involvement of human glutathione S-transferase isoenzymes in the conjugation of cyclophosphamide metabolites with glutathione. Cancer Res 1994;54:6215.
117. Dorr FA, Coltman CA Jr. Second cancers following antineoplastic therapy. Curr Probl Cancer 1985;9:1.
118. Dorr RT, Bowden GT, Alberts DS, Liddil JD. Interactions of mitomycin C with mammalian DNA detected by alkaline elution. Cancer Res 1985;45:3510.
119. Dray S, Mokyr MB. Cyclophosphamide and melphalan as immunopotentiating agents in cancer therapy. Med Oncol Tumor Pharmacother 1989;6:77.
120. Dulik DM, Colvin OM, Fenselau C. Characterization of glutathione conjugates of chlorambucil by fast atom bombardment and thermospray liquid chromatography/mass spectrometry. Biomed Environ Mass Spectrom 1990;19:248.
121. Dulik DM, Fenselau C, Hilton J. Characterization of melphalan-glutathione adducts whose formation is catalyzed by glutathione S-transferase. Biochem Pharmacol 1986;35:3405.
122. Durie BG, Dixon DO, Carter S, Stephens R, Rivkin S, Bonnet J, Salmon SE, Dabich L, Files JC, Costanzi JJ. Unimproved survival duration with combination chemotherapy induction for multiple myeloma: a Southwest Oncology Group Study. J Clin Oncol 1986;4:1227.
123. Dusre L, Covey JM, Collins C, Sinha BK. DNA damage, cytotoxicity and free radical formation by mitomycin in human cells. Chem Biol Interact 1989;71:63.
124. Eapen L, Stewart D, Danjoux C, Genest P, Futter N, Moors D, Irvine A, Crook J, Aitken S, Gerig L, Peterson R, Rasuli P. Intraarterial cisplatin and concurrent radiation for locally advanced bladder cancer. J Clin Oncol 1989;7:230.
125. Eastman A. Characterization of the adducts produced in DNA by cis-Diaminedichloroplatinum (II) and cis-Dichloro (ethylenediamine) platinum (II). Biochemistry 1983;22:3927.
126. Eastman A. Re-evaluation of interaction of cis-dichloro (ethylenediamine) platinum (II) with DNA. Biochemistry 1986;25:3912.
127. Eastman A. Cross-linking of glutathione to DNA by cancer chemotherapeutic platinum coordination complexes. Chem Biol Interact 1987;61:241.
128. Eder JP, Antman K, Peters W, Henner WD, Elias A, Shea T, Schryber S, Anderson J, Come S, Schnipper L, Frei E III, Antman K. High-dose combination alkylating agent chemotherapy with autologous bone marrow support for metastatic breast cancer. J Clin Oncol 1986;4:1592.
129. Eder JP, Elias A, Shea TC, Schryber SM, Teicher BA, Hunt M, Burke J, Siegel R, Schnipper LE, Frei E III, et al. A phase I-II study of cyclophosphamide, thiotepa, and carboplatin with autologous bone marrow transplantation in solid tumor patients. J Clin Oncol 1990;8:1239.
130. Eder JP, Teicher BA, Holden SA, Cathcart KN, Schnipper LE. Novobiocin enhances alkylating agent cytotoxicity and DNA interstrand cross-links in a murine model. J Clin Invest 1987;79:11524.
131. Eder JP, Wheeler CA, Teicher BA, and Schnippper LE. A phase I clinical trial of novobiocin, a modulator of alkylating agent cytotoxicity. Cancer Res 1991;51:510.
132. Egorin MJ, Forrest A, Belani CP, Ratain MJ, Abrams JS, Van Echo DA. A limited sampling strategy for cyclophosphamide pharmacokinetics. Cancer Res 1989;49:3129.

132a. Egorin MJ, Jodrell DI. Utility of individualized carboplatin dosing alone and in combination regimens. Semin Oncol 1992;19(1 suppl 2):132.
133. Egorin MJ, Snyder SW. Characterization of nonexchangeable radioactivity in L1210 cells incubated with (14C) thiotepa: labeling of phosphatidylethanolamine. Cancer Res 1990;50:4044.
134. Egorin MJ, Van Echo DA, Olman EA, Whitacre MY, Forrest A, Aisner J. Prospective validation of a pharmacologically based dosing scheme for the cis-diamminedichloroplatinum (II) analogue. Cancer Res 1985;45:6502.
135. Einhorn N. Acute leukemia after chemotherapy (melphalan). Cancer 1978;41:444.
136. Einhorn N, Eklund G, Lambert B. Solid tumours and chromosome aberrations as late side effects of melphalan therapy in ovarian carcinoma. Acta Oncol 1988;27:215.
137. Eisenberger M, Hornedo J, Silva H, Donehower R, Spaulding M, Van Echo D. Carboplatin (NSC-241–240): An active platinum analog for the treatment of squamous-cell carcinoma of the head and neck. J Clin Oncol 1986;4:1506.
138. Elderson A, Gerritsen van der Hoop R, Haanstra W, Neijt JP, Gispen WH, Jennekens FG. Vibration perception and thermoperception as quantitative measurements in the monitoring of cisplatin induced neurotoxicity. J Neurol Sci 1989;93(2-3):167.
139. Elson LA. Hematological effects of the alkylating agents. Ann NY Acad Sci 1958;68: 826.
140. Endresen L, Schjerven L, Rugstad HE. Tumours from a cell strain with a high content of metallothionein show enhanced resistance against cis-dichlorodiammineplatinum. Acta Pharmacol Toxicol (Copenh) 1984;55:183.
141. Erikson JM, Tweedie DJ, Ducore JM, Prough RA. Cytotoxicity and DNA damage caused by the azoxy metabolites of procarbazine in L1210 tumor cells. Cancer Res 1989;49:127.
142. Erickson LC, Laurent G, Sharkey NA, Kohn KW. DNA cross-linking and monoadduct repair in nitrosourea-treated human tumour cells. Nature 1980;288:727.
143. Erlichman C, Soldins SJ, Hardy RW, Thiessen JJ, Sturgeon JF, Fine S, Baskerville T. Disposition of cyclophosphamide on two consecutive cycles of treatment in patients with ovarian carcinoma Arzneim-Forsch Drug Res 1988;38:839.
144. Everett JC, Roberts JJ, Ross WCJ. Aryl-2-halogenoalkylamines: part XII. Some carboxylic derivatives of N,N-di-2-chloroethylaniline. J Chem Soc 1953;2386.
145. Ewig RAG, Kohn KW. DNA damage and repair in mouse leukemia L1210 cells treated with nitrogen mustard. 1,3-bis(2-chloroethyl)-1-nitrosourea, and other nitrosoureas. Cancer Res 1977;37:2114.
145a. Extra JM, Espie M, Calvo F, Ferme C, Mignot L, Marty M. Phase I study of oxaliplatin in patients with advanced cancer. Cancer Chemother Pharmacol 1990;25:299.
146. Falletta JM, Cushing B, Lauer S, Bell B, Mahoney DH, Castleberry R, Krance RA. Phase I evaluation of diaziquone in childhood cancer. A Pediatric Oncology Group study. Invest New Drugs 1990;8:167.
147. Farina P, Benfenati BR, Torti L, D'Incalci M, Threadgill MD, Gescher A. Metabolism of the anticancer agent 1-(4-acetylphenyl)-3, 3-dimethyltriazene. Biomed Mass Spectrom 1983;10:485.
148. Farnworth PG, Hillcoat BL, Roos IA. Metallothionein induction in mouse tissues by cis-dichlorodiammineplatinum (II) and its hydrolysis products. Chem Biol Interact 1989;69:319.
149. Feil VS, Lamoureaux CJH. Alopecia activity of cyclophosphamide metabolites and related compounds in sheep. Cancer Res 1974;34:2596.
150. Felker GM, Friedman HS, Dolan ME, Moschel RC, Schold C. Treatment of subcutaneous and intracranial brain tumor xenografts with 0-6-benzylguanine and 1,3-bis(2-chloroethyl)-1-nitrosourea. Cancer Chemother & Pharmacol 1993;32:471.
151. Fenselau C, Kan MN, Rao SS, Myles A, Friedman OM, Colvin M. Identification of aldophosphamide as a metabolite of cyclophosphamide in vitro and in vivo in humans. Cancer Res 1977;37:2538.
152. Fernandes RS, Cotter TG. Apoptosis or necrosis: Intracellular levels of glutathione influence mode of cell death. Biochem Pharm 1994;48:675.
153. Fetting JH, McCarthy LE, Borison HL, Colvin M. Vomiting induced by cyclophosphamide and phosphoramide mustard in cats. Cancer Treat Rep 1982;66:1625.
154. Fichtinger-Schepman AMJ, van der Veer JL, den Hartog JHJ, Lohman PHM, Reedijk J. Adducts of the antitumor drug cis-diamminedichloroplatinum (II) with DNA: formation, identification, and quantitation. Biochemistry 1985;24:707.
155. Fiorentino MV, Daniele O, Morandi P, Aversa SM, Ghiotto C, Paccagnella A, Fornasiero A. Intrapericardial instillation of cis-platin in malignant pericardial effusion. Cancer 1988;62:1904.
156. Fisher B, Sherman B, Rockette H, Redmond C, Margolese R, Fisher ER. L-phenylalanine mustard (L-PAM) in the management of premenopausal patients with primary breast cancer. Cancer 1979;44:847.
157. Fisher RI, Erickson LC. 1-beta-D-arabinofuranosylcytosine and hydroxyurea production of cytotoxic synergy with cis-diamminedichloroplatinum (II) and modification of platinum-induced DNA interstrand cross-linking. Cancer Res 1989;49:1383.
158. Flaherty LE, Redman BG, Chabot GG, Martino S, Gualdoni SM, Heilbrun LK, Valdivieso M, Bradley EC. A phase I-II study of dacarbazine in combination with outpatient interleukin-2 in metastatic malignant melanoma. Cancer 1990;65:2471.
159. Follezou JY, Fauchon F, Chiras J. Intra-arterial infusion of carboplatin in the treatment of malignant gliomas: a phase II study. Neoplasma 1989;36:349.
159a. Forastiere AA. Overview of platinum chemotherapy in head and neck cancer. Semin in Oncol 1994;21(5 suppl 12):20.
160. Forni AM, Koss LG, Geller W. Cytological study of the effect of cyclophosphamide on the epithelium of the urinary bladder in man. Cancer 1964;17:1348.
161. Fram RJ, Woda BA, Wilson JM, Robichaud N. Characterization of acquired resistance to cis-diamminedichloroplatinum (II) in BE human colon carcinoma cells. Cancer Res 1990;50:72.
162. Fravel HN, Roberts JJ. Excision repair of cis-diamminedichloroplatinum (II)-induced damage to DNA of Chinese hamster cells. Cancer Res 1979;39:1793.
163. The French Cooperative Group on Chronic Lymphocytic Leukemia. A randomized clinical trial or chlorambucil versus COP in stage chronic lymphocytic leukemia. Blood 1990;75:1422.
164. Frick JC, Tretter P, Tretter W, Hyman GA. Disseminated carcinoma of the ovary treated by L-phenylalanine mustard. Cancer 1968;21:508.
165. Fried W, Kede A, Barone J. Effects of cyclophosphamide and busulfan on spleen-colony-forming units and on hematopoietic stroma. Cancer Res 1977;37:1205.
166. Friedman HS, Colvin OM, Aisaka K, Popp J, Bossen EH, Reimer KA, Powell JB, Hilton J, Gross SS, Levi R Bigner DD, Griffith OW. Glutathione protects cardiac and skeletal muscle from cyclophosphamide-induced toxicity. Cancer Res 1990;50:2455.
167. Friedman HS, Colvin OM, Griffith OW, Lippitz B, Elion GB, Schold SC Jr, Hilton J, Bigner DD. Increased melphalan activity in intracranial human medulloblastoma and glioma xenografts following buthionine sulfoximine-mediated glutathione depletion. JNCI 1989;81:524.
167a. Friedman HS, Colvin OM, Kaufmann SH, Ludeman SH, Bullock N, Bigner DD, Griffith OW. Cyclophosphamide resistance in medulloblastoma. Cancer Res 1992;52:5373.
167b. Friedman HS, Krischer JP, Burger P, Oakes WJ, Hockenberger B, Weiner MD, Falletta JM, Norris D, Ragab AH, Mahoney DH Jr, et al. Treatment of children with progressive or recurrent brain tumors with carboplatin or iproplatin: a Pediatric Oncology Group randomized phase II study. J Clin Oncol 1992;10:249.
168. Frustaci S, Barzan L, Comoretto R, Tumolo S, Lore G, Monfardini S. Local neurotoxicity after intra-arterial cisplatin in head and neck cancer. Cancer Treat Rep 1987;71: 257.
169. Futscher BW, Micetich KC, Barnes DM, Fisher RI, Erickson LC. Inhibition of specific DNA repair system and nitrosourea cytotoxicity in resistant human cancer cells. Cancer Commun 1989;1:65.
170. Fujii R, Mutoh M, Niwa K, Yamada K, Aikou T, Nakagawa M, Kuwano M, Akiyama S. Active efflux system for cisplatin in cisplatin-resistant human cells. Jpn J Cancer Res 1994;85:426.
171. Galton D. Myleran in chronic myeloid leukaemia. Lancet 1953;1:208.
172. Galton DAG, Till M, Wiltshaw E. Busulfan (1, 4-dimethyl-sulfonoxy-butane, Myleran): summary of clinical results. Ann NY Acad Sci 1958;68:967.
173. Ganci L, Serrou B. Changes in hair pigmentation associated with cancer chemotherapy. Cancer Treat Rep 1980;64:193.
174. Garrett MJ. Teratogenic effects of combination chemotherapy. Ann Intern Med 1974;80:667.
175. Gerard A, Metzger U, Buyse M. Adjuvant therapy in colorectal cancer. Anticancer Res 1989;9:1033.
176. Gez E, Ben Yosef R, Catane R, Brufman G, Biran S. Chlorpromazine and dexamethasone versus high-dose metoclopramide and dexamethasone in patients receiving cancer chemotherapy, particularly cis-platinum: a prospective randomized crossover study. Oncology 1989;46:150.
177. Gez E, Sulkes A, Ochayon L, Gera C, Nathan S, Cass Y, Rubello E, Biran S. Methylprednisolone versus metoclopramide as antiemetic treatment in patients receiving adjuvant cyclophosphamide, methotrexate, 5-fluorouracil (CMF) chemotherapy: A randomized crossover blind study. J Chemother 1989;1:365.
178. Gianni AM, Bregni M, Siena S, Orazi A, Stern AC, Gandola L, Bonadonna G. Recombinant human granulocyte-macrophage colony-stimulating factor reduces hematologic toxicity and widens clinical applicability of high-dose cyclophosphamide treatment in breast cancer and non-Hodgkin's lymphoma. J Clin Oncol 1990;8:768.
179. Gibson JE, Becker BA. Teratogenicity of structural truncates of cyclophosphamide in mice. Teratology 1971;4:141.
180. Goel R, Andrews PA, Pfeifle CE, Abramson IS, Kirmani S, Howell SB. Comparison of the pharmacokinetics of ultrafilterable cisplatin species detectable by derivatization with diethyldithiocarbamate or atomic absorption spectroscopy. Eur J Cancer 1990;26:21.
181. Goldenberg AS, Kelsen D, Dougherty J, Magill G. Phase II study of CHIP chemotherapy in advanced adenocarcinomas of the upper gastrointestinal tract. Invest New Drugs 1990;8:71.
182. Goldenberg GJ, Lee M, Lam H-YP, Begleiter A. Evidence for carrier-mediated transport of melphalan by L5178Y lymphoblasts in vitro. Cancer Res 1977;37:755.
183. Goldenberg GJ, Vanstone CL, Israels LG, Lise D, Bihler I. Evidence for a transport carrier of nitrogen mustard in nitrogen mustard-sensitive and -resistant L51784 lymphoblasts. Cancer Res 1970;30:2285.
184. Galton DAG, Israels LS, Nabarro JDN, Till M. Clinical trials of p-(di-2-chlorethylamino)-phenylbutyric acid (CB 1348) in malignant lymphoma. Br Med J 1955;2:172.
185. Gonzales-Vitale JC, Hayes DM, Cvitkovic E, Sternberg SS. The renal pathology in clinical trials of cis-platinum (II) diamminedichloride. Cancer 1977;39:1362.
186. Goodman LS, Wintrobe MM, Dameshek W, Goodman JJ, Gilman A, McLennan MT. Use of methyl-bis(beta-chlorethyl)amine hydrochloride for Hodgkin's disease, lymphosarcoma, leukemia. JAMA 1946;132:263.
187. Goren MP, Wright RK, Pratt CB, Pell FE. Dechlorethylation of ifosfamide and neurotoxicity. Lancet 1986;II:1219.
188. Gottlieb JA, Drewinko B. Review of the current clinical status of platinum coordination complexes in cancer chemotherapy. Cancer Chemother Rep 1975;59:621.
188a. Graham CH, Kobayashi H, Stankiewicz KS, Man S, Kapitain SJ, Kerbel RS. Rapid acquisition of multicellular drug resistance after a single dose of antitumor alkylating agents. JNCI 1994;86:953.
189. Gralla RJ, Itri LM, Pisko SE, Squillante AE, Kelsen DP, Braun DW Jr, Bordin LA, Braun TJ, Young CW. Antiemetic efficacy of high-dose metoclopramide: Randomized trials with placebo and prochlorperazine in patients with chemotherapy-induced nausea and vomiting. N Engl J Med 1981;305:905.
190. Granowetter L, Rosenstock JG, Packer RJ. Enhanced cis-platinum neurotoxicity in pediatric patients with brain tumors. J Neurooncol 1983;1:293.
191. Greco FA, Johnson DH, Hainsworth JD. A comparison of hexamethylmelamine (altretamine), cyclophosphamide, doxorubicin, and cisplatin (H-CAP) vs. cyclophosphamide, cisplatin (CAP) in advanced ovarian cancer. Cancer Res 1991;18(suppl A):47.
192. Green MH, Harris EL, Gershenson DM, et al. Melphalan may be a more potent leukemogen than cyclophosphamide. Ann Intern Med 1986;105:360.
193. Green TP, Mirkin BL. Prevention of cyclophosphamide-induced antidiuresis by furosemide infusion. Clin Pharmacol Ther 1981;29:634.
194. Greenspan EM. Thio-TEPA and methotrexate chemotherapy of advanced ovarian carcinoma. J Mount Sinai Hosp NY 1968;35:52.
195. Greig NH, Momma S, Sweeney DJ, Smith QR, Rapoport SI. Facilitated transport of melphalan at the rat blood-brain barrier by the large neutral amino acid carrier system. Cancer Res 1987;47:1571.
195a. Grochow LB. Busulfan disposition: the role of therapeutic monitoring in bone marrow transplantation induction regimens. Semin Oncol 1993;20(suppl4):18.
196. Grochow LB, Jones RJ, Brundrett BR, Braine HG, Chen TL, Saral R, Santos GW, Colvin OM. Pharmacokinetics of busulfan: Correlation with veno-occulusive disease in patients undergoing bone marrow transplantation. Cancer Chemother Pharmacol 1989;25:55.

197. Grochow LB, Krivit W, Whitley CB, Blazar B. Busulfan disposition in children. Blood 1990;75:1723.
198. Grunberg SM. Advances in the management of nausea and vomiting induced by non-cisplatin containing chemotherapeutic regimens. Blood Rev 1989;3:216.
199. Groothuis DR, Lippitz BE, Fekete I, Schlageter KE, Molnar P, Colvin OM, Roe CR, Bitner DD, Friedman HS. The effect of an amino acid-lowering diet on the rate of melphalan entry into brain and xenotransplanted glioma. Cancer Res 1992;52:5590.
200. Grunberg SM, Sonka S, Stevenson LL, Muggia FM. Progressive paresthesias after cessation of therapy with very high-dose cisplatin. Cancer Chemother Pharmacol 1989;25:62.
201. Gupta V, Jani JP, Jacobs S, Levitt M, Fields L, Awasthi S, Xu BH, Sreevardhan M, Awasthi YC, Singh SV. Activity of melphalan in combination with glutathione transferase inhibitor sulfasalazine. Cancer Chemother Pharmacol 1995;36:13.
202. Gutierrez PL. Mechanism(s) of bioreductive activation. The example of diaziquone (AZQ). Free Radic Biol Med 1989;6:405.
203. Gutin PH, Levi JA, Wiernik PH, Walker MD. Treatment of malignant meningeal disease with intrathecal thioTEPA: a phase II study. Cancer Treat Rep 1977;61:885.
204. Haas CD, Stephens RC, Hollister M, Hoogstraten B. Phase I evaluation of dianhydrogalactitol (NSC-132313). Cancer Treat Rep 1976;60:611.
205. Haddow A, Timmis GM. Myleran in chronic myeloid leukemia—chemical constitution and biological action. Lancet 1953;1:207.
206. Hadjilaskari P, Fengler R, Hartmann R, Henze G. Ototoxicity of cisplatin in children with malignant diseases. Klin Padiatr 1989;201:316.
207. Hagen B. Pharmacokinetics of thio-TEPA and TEPA in the conventional dose-range and its correlation to myelosuppressive effects. Cancer Chemother Pharmacol 1991;27:373.
208. Hagen B, Neverdal G, Walstad RA, Nilsen OG. Long-term pharmacokinetics of thio-TEPA, TEPA and total alkylating activity following IV bolus administration of thioTEPA in ovarian cancer patients. Cancer Chemother Pharmacol 1990;25:257.
209. Hales BF. Effects of phosphoramide mustard and acroein, cytotoxic metabolites of cyclophosphamide, on mouse limb development in vitro. Teratology 1989;40:11.
210. Hamilton TC, Winker MA, Louie KG, Batist G, Behrens BC, Tsuruo T, Grotzinger KR, McKoy WM, Young RC, Ozols RF. Augmentation of adriamycin, melphalan, and cisplatin cytotoxicity in drug-resistant and sensitive human ovarian carcinoma cell lines by buthionine sulfoximine mediated glutathione depletion. Biochem Pharmacol 1985;34:2583.
211. Han T, Rai KR. Management of chronic lymphocytic leukemia. Hematol Oncol Clin North Am 1990;4:431.
212. Hanawalt PC. Transcription-coupled repair and human disease. Science 1994;266: 1957.
213. Hansen SW, Helweg-Larsen S, Trojaborg W. Long-term neurotoxicity in patients treated with cisplatin, vinblastine, and bleomycin for metastatic germ cell cancer. J Clin Oncol 1989;7:1457.
214. Hansson J, Wood RD. Repair synthesis by human cell extracts in DNA damaged by cis- and trans-diamminedichloroplatinum (II). Nucleic Acids Res 1989;7:8073.
215. Harding M, Kennedy R, Mill L, MacLean A, Duncan I, Kennedy J, Soukop M, Kaye SB. A pilot study of carboplatin (JM8, CBDCA) and chlorambucil in combination for advanced ovarian cancer. Br J Cancer 1988;58:640.
216. Harlow PJ, DeClerck YA, Shore NA, Ortega JA, Carraza A, Heuser E. A fatal case of inappropriate ADH secretion induced by cyclophosphamide therapy. Cancer 1979;44:896.
217. Harmon WE, Cohen HJ, Schneeberger EE, Grupe WE. Chronic renal failure in children treated with methyl CCNU. N Engl J Med 1979;300:1200.
218. Hartley-Asp B, Christensson PI, Gunnarsson K, Gunnarsson PO, Jensen G, Polacek J, Stamvik A. Anti-tumour, toxicological and pharmacokinetic properties of a novel taurine-based nitrosourea (TCNU). Invest New Drugs 1988;6:19.
219. Hartley FR. The Chemistry of Platinum and Palladium, Chapter 11. New York: Wiley, 1973.
220. Hartvig P, Simonsson B, Oberg G, Wallin I, Ehrsson H. Inter- and intraindividual differences in oral chlorambucil pharmacokinetics. Eur J Clin Pharmacol 1988;35:551.
221. Hassan OG, Ehrsson H, et al. Pharmacokinetic and metabolic studies of high-dose busulfan in adults. Eur J Clin Pharmacol 1989;36:525.
222. Hawthorn J, Ostler KJ, Andrews PL. The role of the abdominal visceral innervation and 5-hydroxytryptamine M-receptors in vomiting induced by the cytotoxic drugs cyclophosphamide and cis-platin in the ferret. Q J Exp Physiol 1988;73:7.
223. Hayes DM, Cvitkovic E, Golbey RB, Scheiner E, Helson L, Krakoff IH. High dose cisplatinum diammine dichloride: amelioration of renal toxicity by mannitol diuresis. Cancer 1977;39:1372.
224. Heideman RL, Cole DE, Balis F, Sato J, Reaman GH, Packer RJ, Singher LJ, Ettinger LJ, Gillespie A, Sam J, Poplack DG. Phase I and pharmacokinetic evaluation of thiotepa in the cerebrospinal fluid and plasma of pediatric patients: Evidence for dose-dependent plasma clearance of thiotepa. Cancer Res 1989;49:736.
225. Hegmann EJ, Bauer HC, Kerbel RS. Expression and functional activity of P-glycoprotein in cultured cerebral capillary endothelial cells. Cancer Res 1992;52:6969.
226. Heiger-Bernays WJ, Essigmann JM, Lippard SJ. Effect of the antitumor drug cis-diamminedichloroplatinum (II) and related platinum complexes on eukaryotic DNA replication. Biochemistry 1990;29:8461.
227. Hektoen L, Corper HJ. The effect of mustard gas (dichloroethyl-sulphide) on antibody formation. J Infect Dis 1921;28:279.
228. Henner WD, Peters WP, Eder JP, Antman K, Snipper L, Frei E III. Pharmacokinetics and immediate effects of high-dose carmustine in man. Cancer Treat Rep 1986;70: 877.
229. Henner WD, Shea TC, Furlong EA, Flaherty MD, Eder JP, Elias A, Begg C, Antman K. Pharmacokinetics of continuous-infusion high-dose thiotepa. Cancer Treat Rep 1987;71:1043.
230. Higby DJ, Wallace HJ Jr, Albert DJ, Holland JF. Diaminodichloroplatinum: a phase I study showing responses in testicular and other tumors. Cancer 1974;33:1219.
231. Higby DJ, Wallace HJ Jr, Holland JF. Cis-diamminedichloroplatinum (NSC-119875): a phase I study. Cancer Chemother Rep 1973;57:459.
232. Higgins GA, Kilpatrick GJ, Bunce KT, Jones BJ, Tyers MB. 5-HT3 receptor antagonists injected into the area postrema inhibit cisplatin-induced emesis in the ferret. Br J Pharmacol 1989;97:247.
232a. Hill BT, Scanlon KJ, Hansson J, Harstrick A, Pera M, Fichtinger-Schepman AM, Shellard SA. Deficient repair of cisplatin-DNA adducts identified in human testicular teratoma cell lines established from tumours from untreated patients. Eur J Canc 1994;30A:832.
233. Hill BT, Shellard SA, Fichtinger, Schepman AM, Schmoll HJ, Harstrick A. Differential formation and enhanced removal of specific cisplatin-DNA adducts in two cisplatin-selected resistant human testicular teratomasublines. Anticancer Drugs 1994;5:321.
234. Hill BT, Shellard SA, Hosking LK, Dempke WC, Fichtinger-Schepman AM, Tone T, Scanlon KJ, Whelan RD. Characterization of a cisplatin-resistant human ovarian carcinoma cell line expressing cross-resistance to 5-fluorouracil but collateral sensitivity to methotrexate. Cancer Res 1992;52:3110.
235. Hill DL, Kirk MC, Struck RF. Microsomal metabolism of nitrosoureas. Cancer Res 1975;35:296.
236. Hilton J. Role of aldehyde dehydrogenase in cyclophosphamide-resistant L1210 leukemia. Cancer Res 1984;44:5156.
237. Himmelstein KJ, Patton TF, Belt RJ, Taylor S, Repta AJ, Sternson LA. Clinical kinetics on intact cisplatin and some related species. Clin Pharmacol Ther 1981;29:658.
238. Hinkes E, Plotkin D. Reversible drug-induced sterility in a patient with acute leukemia. JAMA 1973;223:1490.
239. Hochberg MC, Shulman LE. Acute leukemia following cyclophosphamide therapy for Sjogren's syndrome. Johns Hopkins Med J 1978;142:211.
240. Holoye PY, Jenkins DE, Greenberg SD. Pulmonary toxicity in long-term administration of BCNU. Cancer Treat Rep 1976;60:1691.
241. Horn Y, Eidelman A, Walach N, Waron M, Barak F. Intravesical chemotherapy of superficial bladder tumors in a controlled trial with cis-platinum versus cis-platinum plus hyaluronidase. J Surg Oncol 1985;28:304.
242. Hospers GA, Meijer C, de Leij L, Uges DR, Mulder NH, de Vries EG. A study of human small-cell lung carcinoma (hSCLC) cell lines with different sensitivities to detect relevant mechanisms of cisplatin (CDDP) resistance. Int J Cancer 1990;46:138.
243. Hospers GA, Mulder NH, de Jong B, de Ley L, Uges DR, Fichtinger-Schepman AM, Scheper RJ, de Vries EG. Characterization of a human small cell lung carcinoma cell line with acquired resistance to cis-diamminedichloroplatinum (II) in vitro. Cancer Res 1988;48:6803.
244. Howell SB. Intraperitoneal chemotherapy: The use of concurrent systemic neutralizing agents. Semin Oncol 1985;12:17.
245. Hromas RA, Andrews PA, Murphy MP, Burns CP. Glutathione depletion reverses cisplatin resistance in murine L1210 leukemia cells. Cancer Lett 1987;34:9.
246. Hromas RA, North JA, Burns CP. Decreased cisplatin uptake by resistant L1210 leukemia cells. Cancer Lett 1987;36:197.
247. Huang JC, Zamble DB, Reardon JT, Lippard SJ, Sancar A. HMG-domain proteins specifically inhibit the repair of the major DNA adduct of the anticancer drug cisplatin by human excision nuclease. Proc Natl Acad Sci USA 1994;91:10394.
248. Humphrey RL, Kvols LK. The influence of renal insufficiency on cyclophosphamide-induced hematopoietic depression and recovery. Proc Am Assoc Cancer Res 1974;15:84.
249. Husain I, Chaney SG, Sancar A. Repair of cis-platinum-DNA adducts by ABC excinuclease in vivo and in vitro. J Bacteriol 1985;163:817.
250. Hwang BJ, Chu G. Purification and characterization of a human protein that binds to damaged DNA. Biochemistry 1993;32:1657.
251. Hyde KA, Acton E, Skinner WA, Goodman L, Greenberg J, Baker BR. Potential anticancer agents-LX11. The relationship of chemical structure to antileukemia activity with analogues of 1-methyl-3-nitro-1-nitrosoguanidine (NSC-9369). II. J Med Pharm Chem 1962;5:1.
252. Ishikawa M, Sasaki K, Takayanagi Y. Injurious effect of buthionine sulfoximine, an inhibitor of glutathione biosynthesis, on the lethality and urotoxicity of cyclophosphamide in mice. Jpn J Pharmacol 1989;51:146.
253. Iyer VN, Szybalski W. Mitomycin and porfiromycin: chemical mechanisms of activation and cross-linking of DNA. Science 1964;145:55.
254. Jackson DV Jr, Craig JB, Spurr CL, White DR, Muss HB, Cruz JM, Richards F. Powell BL. Vincristine infusion with CHOP-CCNU in diffuse large-cell lymphoma. Cancer Invest 1990;8:7.
255. Jacobs SC, Menashe DS. Intra-arterial chemotherapy for bladder cancer. Prog Clin Biol Res 1990;350:101.
256. Jacobson LP, Spurr CL, Barron ESG, Smith T, Lushbaugh C, Dick GF. Studies on the effect of methyl-bis(beta-chloroethyl)amine hydrochloride on neoplastic diseases and allied disorders of the hematopoietic system. JAMA 1946;132:263.
257. Jacquillat C, Khayat D, Banzet P, Weil M, Avril MF, Fumoleau P, Namer M, Bonneterre J, Kerbrat P, Bonerandi JJ, Bugat R, Monteuquet P, Audhuy B, Cupissol D, Lauvin R, Grosshans E, Vilmer C, Prache C, Bizzari JP. Chemotherapy by fotemustine in cerebral metastases of disseminated malignant melanoma. Cancer Chemother Pharmacol 1990;25:263.
258. Jaffe N, Raymond AK, Ayala A, Carrasco CH, Wallace S, Robertson R, Giffiths M, Wang YM. Effect of cumulative courses of intra-arterial cis-diamminedichloroplatin-II on the primary tumor in osteosarcoma. Cancer 1989;63:63.
259. Jahde E, Glusenkamp KH, Rajewsky MF. Protection of cultured malignant cells from mitoxantrone cytotoxicity by low extrácellular pH: a possible mechanism for chemoresistance in vivo. Eur J Cancer 1990;26:101.
260. Jao JY, Jusko WJ, Cohen JL. Phenobarbital effects on cyclophosphamide pharmacokinetics in man. Cancer Res 1972;32:2761.
261. Japan Radiation–ACNU Study Group. A randomized prospective study of radiation versus radiation versus plus ACNU Study Group. Cancer 1989;63:249.
262. Jardine I, Fenselau C, Appler M, Kan, M-N, Brundrett RB, Colvin M. Quantitation by gas chromatography-chemical ionization mass spectrometry of cyclophosphamide, phosphamide mustard, and nornitrogen mustard in the plasma and urine of patients receiving cyclophosphamide therapy. Cancer Res 1978;38:408.
263. Jarman M, Coley HM, Judson IR, Thornton TJ, Wilman DE, Abel G, Rutty CJ. Synthesis and cytotoxicity of potential tumor-inhibitory analogues of trimelamol (2, 4, 6-tris[(hydroxymethyl)methylamino)-1,3,5-triazine) having electron-withdrawing groups in place of methyl. J Med Chem 1993;36:4;195.
264. Johnson SW, Perez RP, Godwin AK, Yeung AT, Hnadel LM, Ozols RF, Hamilton TC. Role of platinum-DNA adduct formation and removal in cisplatin resistance in human ovarian cancer cell lines. Biochem Pharmacol 1994;47:689.
265. Jones RB, Matthes S, Kemme D, Dufton C, Kernan S. Cyclophosphamide, cisplatin, and carmustine: pharmacokinetics of carmustine following multiple alkylating-agent interactions. Cancer Chemother Pharmacol 1994;35:59.
266. Jones RJ, Lee KS, Beschorner WE, Vogel VG, Grochow LB, Braine HG, Vogelsang

GB, Sensenbrenner LL, Santos GW, Saral R. Venoocclusive disease of the liver following bone marrow transplantation. Transplantation 1987;44:778.

267. Juma FD, Rogers HJ, Trounce JR. The pharmacokinetics of cyclophosphamide, phosphoramide mustard and nor-nitrogen mustard studied by gas chromatography in patients receiving cyclophosphamide therapy. Br J Clin Pharmacol 1980;10:327.
268. Juma FD, Rogers HJ, Trounce JR. Pharmacokinetics of cyclophosphamide and alkylating activity in man after intravenous and oral administration. Br J Clin Pharmacol 1979;8:209.
269. Kahn T, Elias EG, Mason GR. A single dose of metoclopramide in the control of vomiting from cis-dichlorodiammineplatinum (II) in man. Cancer Treat Rep 1978;62:1106.
270. Kaleagasioglu F, Berger MR, Schmahl D, Elsenbrand G. In vitro evaluation of 1-(2-chloroethyl)-1-nitroso-3-(2-hydroxyethyl) urea linked to 4-acetoxy-bisdesmethyltamoxifen, estradiol and dihydrotestosterone. Arzneimittelforschung 1990;40:603.
271. Karchmer RK, Hansen BL. Possible anaphylactic reaction to intravenous cyclophosphamide. JAMA 1977;237:475.
272. Kashdan BJ, Sullivan KL, Lackman RD, Shapiro MJ, Bonn J, Weiss AJ, Gardiner GA Jr. Extremity osteosarcomas: intra-arterial chemotherapy and limb-sparing resection with 2-year follow-up. Radiology 1990;177:95.
273. Kashimura M, Kondo M, Abe T, Shinohara M, Baba S. A case report of acute renal failure induced by melphalan in a patient with ovarian cancer. Gan To Kagaku Ryoho 1986;34:2015.
274. Kasugai H, Kojima J, Tatsuta M, Okuda S, Sasaki Y, Imaoka S, Fujita M, Ishiguro S. Treatment of hepatocellular carcinoma by transcatheter arterial cisplatin and ethiodized oil. Gastroenterology 1989;97:965.
275. Kat A, Thilly WG, Fang WH, Longley MJ, Li GM, Modrich P. An alkylation-tolerant, mutator human cell line is deficient in strand-specific mismatch repair. Proc Natl Acad Sci USA 1993;90:6424.
276. Katz EJ, Andrews PA, Howell SB. The effect of DNA polymerase inhibitors on the cytoxicity of cisplatin in human ovarian carcinoma cells. Cancer Commun 1990;2:159.
277. Kelland LR, Abel G, MeKeage MJ, Jones M, Goddard PM, Valenti M, Murrer BA, Harrup KR. Preclinical antitumor evaluation of bis-acetato-ammine-dichloro-cyclohexylamine platinum (IV): an orally active platinum drug. Cancer Res 1993;53:2581.
278. Kelland LR, McKeage MJ. New platinum agents—a comparison in ovarian cancer. (Review) Drugs Aging 1994;5:85.
279. Kelley SL, Basu A, Teicher BA, Hacker MP, Hamer DH, Lazo JS. Overexpression of metallothionein confers resistance to anticancer drugs. Science 1988;241:1813.
280. Kennedy KA, McGuirl JD, Leondaridis L, Alabaster O. pH Dependence of mitomycin C-induced cross-linking activity in tumor cells. Cancer Res 1985;45:3541.
281. Kerbel RS, Kobayashi H, Graham CH. Intrinsic or acquired drug resistance and metastasis: are they linked phenotypes? J Cell Biochem 1994;56:37.
282. Kergueris MF, Milpied N, Moreau P, Harousseau JL, Larousse C. Pharmacokinetics of high-dose melphalan in adults: influence of renal function. Anticancer Res 1994;14:2379.
283. Khan AS, Driscoll JS. Potential central nervous system antitumor agents. J Med Chem 1976;19:313.
284. Kim HC, Kesarwala HH, Colvin M, Saidi P. Hypersensitivity reaction to a metabolite of cyclophosphamide. J Allergy Clin Immunol 1985;76:591.
285. Kirkwood JM, Ernstoff MS, Giuliano A, Gams R, Robinson WA, Costanzi J, Pouillart P, Speyer J, Grimm M, Spiegel R. Interferon alpha-2a and dacarbazine in melanoma. JNCI 1990;82:1062.
286. Kleinerman ES, Zwelling LA. The effect of cis-diamminedichloroplatinum (II) on immune function in vitro and in vivo.
287. Knox RJ, Friedlos F, Lydall DA, Roberts JJ. Mechanism of cytotoxicity of anticancer platinum drugs: evidence that cis-diamminedichloroplatinum (II) and cis-diammine-(1, 1-cyclobutanedicarboxylato) platinum (II) differ only in the kinetics of their interaction with DNA. Cancer Res 1986;46:1972.
288. Kobayashi H, Man S, Graham CH, Kapitain SJ, Teicher BA, Kerbel RS. Acquired multicellular-mediated resistance to alkylating agents in cancer. Proc Natl Acad Sci USA 1993;90:3294.
289. Kobayashi S, Teramura M, Oshimi K, Mizoguchi H. Interleukin-11. (Review) Leukemia Lymphoma 1994;15:45.
290. Koelling TM, Yeager AM, Hilton J, Haynie DT, Wiley JM. Development and characterization of a cyclophosphamide-resistant subline of acute myeloid leukemia in the Lewis and Brown Norway hybrid rat. Blood 1990;76:1209.
291. Kohn KW. Interstrand cross-linking of DNA by 1,3-bis{2-chloroethyl}-1-nitrosourea and other 1-{2-chloroethyl}-1-nitrosourea and other 1-{2-haloethyl}-1-nitrosoureas. Cancer Res 1977;37:1450.
292. Kohn KW, Steigbigel NH, Spears CL. Cross-linking and repair of DNA in sensitive and resistant strains of E. coli treated with nitrogen mustard. Proc Natl Acad Sci USA 1965;53:1154.
293. Kohn S, Fradis M, Pratt H, Zidan J, Podoshin L, Robinson E, Nir I. Cisplatin ototoxicity in guinea pigs with special reference to toxic effects in the stria vascularis. Laryngoscope 1988;98:665.
294. Kovach JS, Moertel CG, Schutt AJ, Reitemeier RG, Hahn RG. Phase II study of cis-diamminedichloroplatinum (NSC-119875) in advanced carcinoma of the large bowel. Cancer Chemother Rep 1973;57:357.
295. Kraker A, Schmidt J, Krezoski S, Petering DH. Binding of cis-dichlorodiammine platinum(II) to metallothionein in Ehrlich cells. Biochem Biophys Res Commun 1985;130:786.
296. Kraker AJ, Moore CW. Elevated DNA polymerase beta activity in a cis-diamminedichloroplatinum (II) resistant P388 murine leukemia cell line. Cancer Lett 1988;38:307.
297. Kramer RA, Greene K, Ahmad S, Vistica DT. Chemosensitization of L-phenylalaline mustard by the thiol-modulating agent buthionine sulfoximine. Cancer Res 1987;47:1593.
298. Kretschmar CS, Warren MP, Lavally BL, Dyer S, Tarbell NJ. Ototoxicity of preradiation cisplatin for children with central nervous system tumors. J Clin Oncol 1990;8:1:191.
299. Krouwer D, McDermott M, Prados M. Postoperative radiotherapy and radiotherapy combined with CCNU chemotherapy for treatment of brain gliomas. J Neurooncol 1990;8:189.
300. Kyle RA, Pierce RV, Bayrd ED. Multiple myeloma and acute myelomonocytic leukemia. N Engl J Med 1970;283:1121.
301. Kyoma H, Wada T, Nishizawa T, Iwanaga T, Aoki Y. Cyclophosphamide-induced ovarian failure and its therapeutic significance in patients with breast cancer. Cancer 1977;39:1403.
302. Lakin JD, Cahill RA. Generalized urticaria to cyclophosphamide: type I hypersensitivity to an immunosuppressive agent. J Allergy Clin Immunol 1976;58:160.
303. Lange RC, Spencer RP, Harder HC. The antitumor agent cis-P+$(NH_3)_2Cl_2$ distribution studies and dose calculations for 193m Pt. J Nucl Med 1973;14:191.
304. Laros RK Jr, Penner JA. "Refractory" thrombocytopenic purpura treated successfully with cyclophosphamide. JAMA 1971;215:445.
305. Lee FY, Workman P, Roberts JT, Bleehen NM. Clinical pharmacokinetics of oral CCNU (lomustine). Cancer Chemother Pharmacol 1985;14:125.
306. Lefkowitz IB, Packer RJ, Sielgel KR, Sutton LN, Schut L, Evans AE. Results of treatment of children with recurrent medulloblastoma/primitive neuroectodermal tumors with lomustine, cisplatin, and vincristine. Cancer 1990;65:412.
307. Lehane DE, Bryan RN, Horowitz B, DeSantos L, Ehni G, Zubler MA, Moiel R, Rudolph L, Aldama-Leubbert A, Mahoney D, Harper R. Intra-arterial cis-platinum chemotherapy for patients with primary and metastatic brain tumors. Cancer Drug Deliv 1983;1:69.
308. Lennard AL, Carey PJ, Jackson GH, Proctor SJ. An effective oral combination in advanced relapsed Hodgkin's disease prednisolone, etoposide, chlorambucil and CCNU. Cancer Chemother Pharmacol 1990;26:301.
309. Lergier JE, Jiminez E, Maldonado N, et al. Normal pregnancy in multiple myeloma treated with cyclophosphamide. Cancer 1974;34:1018.
310. Levi F, Perpoint B, Garufi C, Focan C, Chollet P, Depres-Brummer P, Zidani R, Brieza S, Itzhaki M, Iacobelli S, et al. Oxaliplatin activity against metastatic colorectal cancer. A Phase II study of 5-day continuous venous infusion at circadian rhythm modulated rate. Eur J Cancer 1993;29A:1280.
311. Levi FA, Zidani R, Vanetzel JM, Perpoint B, Focan C, Faggiuolo R, Chollet P, Garufi C, Itzhaki M, Dogliotti L, et al. Chronomodulated versus foxed-infusion-rate delivery of ambulatory chemotherapy with oxaliplatin, fluorouracil, and folinic acid (leucovorin) in patients with colorectal cancer metastases: a randomized multi-institutional trial. JNCI 1994;86:1608.
312. Levin VA, Chamberlain M, Silver P, Rodriguez L, Prados M. Phase I/II study of intraventricular and intrathecal ACNU for leptomeningeal neoplasia. Cancer Chemother Pharmacol 1989;23:301.
313. Levin VA, Hoffman W, Weinkam RJ. Pharmacokinetics of BCNU in man: a preliminary study of 20 patients. Cancer Treat Rep 1978;62:1305.
314. Levin VA, Silver P, Hannigan J, Wara WM, Gutin PH, David RL, Wilson CB. Superiority of post-radiotherapy adjuvant chemotherapy with CCNU, procarbazine, and vincristine (PCV) over BCNU for anaplastic gliomas. Int J Radiat Oncol Biol Phys 1990;18:321.
315. Levin VA, Stearns J, Byrd A, Finn A, Weinkam RJ. The effect of phenobarbital on the antitumor activity of 1,3-bis(2-chlorethyl)-1-nitrosourea (BCNU), 1-(2-chlorethyl)-3-cyclohexyl-1-nitrosourea (CCNU) and 1-(2-chlorethyl)-3-(2, 6-dioxo)-3-piperidyl-1-nitrosourea (PCNU), and on the plasma pharmacokinetics and biotransformation of BCNU. J Pharmacol Exp Ther 1979;208:1.
316. Liopis B, Gallego J, Mompo JA, Boronat F, Jimenez JF. Thiotepa versus adriamycin versus cis-platinum in the intravesical prophylaxis of superficial bladder tumors. Eur Urol 1985;11:73.
317. Lippman AJ, Helson C, Helson L, Krakoff IH. Clinical trials of cis-diamminedichloroplatinum (NSC-119875). Cancer Chemother Rep 1973;57:191.
318. Lira-Puerto V, Silva A, Morris M, Martinez R, Groshen S, Morales-Canfield F, Tenorio F, Muggia F. Phase II trial of carboplatin or iproplatin in cervical cancer. Cancer Chemother Pharmacol 1991;28:391.
319. Litam JP, Dail DH, Spitzer G, Vellekoop L, Verma DS, Zander AR, Dicke KA. Early pulmonary toxicity after administration of high-dose BCNU. Cancer Treat Rep 1981;65:39.
320. Little SA, Mirkes PE. DNA cross-linking and single-strand breaks induced by teratogenic concentrations of 4-hydroperoxycyclophosphamide and phosphoramide mustard in postimplantation rat embryos. Cancer Res 1987;47:5421.
321. Livingston RB. Current management of unresectable non-small cell lung cancer (Review). Semin Oncol 1994;21:4.
322. Loehrer PJ Sr, Lauer R, Roth BJ, Williams SD, Kalasinski LA, Einhorn LH. Salvage therapy in recurrent germ cell cancer: Ifosfamide and cisplatin plus either vinblastine or etoposide. Ann Intern Med 1988;109:540.
323. Loh SY, Mistry P, Kelland LR, Abel G, Harrap KR. Reduced drug accumulation as a major mechanism of acquired resistance to cisplatin in a human ovarian carcinoma cell line: circumvention studies using novel platinum (II) and (IV) ammine/amine complexes. Br J Cancer 1992;66:1109.
324. Lok S, Foster DC. The structure, biology and potential therapeutic applications of recombinant thrombopoietin. (Review) Stem Cells 1994;12:586.
325. Loveless A, Ross WCJ. Chromosome alteration and tumour inhibition by nitrogen mustards: The hypothesis of cross-linking alkylation. Nature 1950;166:111.
326. Lowe PR, Sansom CE, Schwalbe CH, Stevens MF, Clark AS. Antitumor imidazotetrazines. 25 Crystal structure of 8-carbamoyl-3-methylimidazo (5, 1-d)-1,2,3-tetrazin-4(3H)-one (temozolomide) and structural comparisons with the related drugs (temozolomide) and structural comparisons with the related drugs mitozolomide and DTIC. J Med Chem 1992;35:3377.
327. Ludlum DB, Kramer BS, Wang J, et al. Reaction of 1,3-bis(2-chloroethyl)-1 nitrosourea with synthetic polynucleotides. Biochemistry 1975;14:5480.
328. Lyss AP, Luedke SL, Einhorn L, Luedke DW, Raney M. Vindesine and mitomycin C in metastatic breast cancer. A Southeastern Cancer Study Group Trial. Oncology 1989;46:357.
329. MacFarland JG, Kirk MC, Ludlum DB. Mechanism of action of the nitrosoureas–IV. Synthesis of the 2-haloethylnitrosourea-induced DNA cross-link 1-(3-cytosinyl),2-(1-guanyl)ethane. Biochem Pharmacol 1990;39:33.
330. Madias NE, Harrington JT. Platinum nephrotoxicity. Am J Med 1978;65:307.
331. Magull-Seltenreich A, Zeller WJ. Inhibition of 06-alkylguanine-DNA alkyltransferase in animal and human ovarian tumor cell lines by 06-benzylguanine and sensitization to BCNU. Cancer Chemother Pharmacol 1995;35:262.
332. Mahaley MS Jr, Hipp SW, Dropcho EJ, Bertsch L, Cush S, Tirey T, Gillespie GY. Intracarotid cisplatin chemotherapy for recurrent gliomas. J Neurosurg 1989;70:371.
333. Makinodan T, Snatos GW, Quinn RP. Immunosuppressive drugs. Pharmacol Rev 1970;22:189.
334. Mann SC, Andrews PA, Howell SB. Comparison of lipid content, surface membrane

fluidity, and temperature dependence of cis-diamminedichloroplatinum (II) accumulation in sensitive and resistant human ovarian carcinoma cells. Anticancer Res 1988;8:1211.

335. Mark GJ, Lehimgar-Zadeh A, Ragsdale BD. Cyclophosphamide pneumonitis. Thorax 1978;33:89.
336. Markman M, Cleary S, Howell SB. Nephrotoxicity of high-dose intracavitary cisplatin with intravenous thiosulfate protection. Eur J Cancer Clin Oncol 1985;21:1015.
337. Markman M, Howell SB. Intrapericardial instillation of cisplatin in a patient with a large malignant effusion. Cancer Drug Deliv 1985;2:49.
338. Martin RB. Hydrolytic equilibria and N7 versus N1 binding in purine nucleosides of cis-Diamminedichloroplatinum (II). In Platinum, Gold, and Other Metal Chemotherapeutic Agents. Edited by SJ. Washington, DC: American Chemical Society, 1983, p 231.
339. Masuda H, Ozols RF, Lai GM, Fojo A, Rothenberg M, Hamilton TC. Increased DNA repair as a mechanism of acquired resistance to cis-diamminedichloroplatinum (II) in human ovarian cancer cell lines. Cancer Res 1988;48:5713.
340. Maynard KR, Hosking LK, Hill BT. Use of host cell reactivation of cisplatin-treated adenovirus 5 in human cell lines to detect repair of drug-treated DNA. Chem Biol Interact 1989;71:353.
341. McCarthy LE, Borison HL. Cisplatin-induced vomiting eliminated by ablation of the area postrema in cats. Cancer Treat Rep 1984;68:401.
342. McElwain TJ, Hedley DW, Gordon MY, Jarman M, Millar JL, Pritchard J. High dose melphalan and non-cryopreserved autologous bone marrow treatment of malignant melanoma and neuroblastoma. Exp Hematol 1979;7:50:360.
343. McLay EF, Howell SB. A review: intraperitoneal cisplatin in the management of patients with ovarian cancer. Gynecol Oncol 1990;36:1.
344. McLean A, Woods RC, Catovsky D, Farmer P. Pharmacokinetics and metabolism of chlorambucil in patients with maligant disease. Cancer Treat Rev 1979;6(suppl):33.
345. Meer L, Schold SC, Kleihues P. Inhibition of the hepatic 06-alkylguanine-DNA alkyltransferase in vivo by pretreatment with antineoplastic agents. Biochem Pharmacol 1989;38:929.
346. Menichetti ET, Silva RR, Tummarello D, Miseria S, Torresi U, Cellerino R. Etoposide and mitomycin-C in pretreated metastatic breast cancer. Tumori 1989;75:473.
347. Metcalfe SA, Cain K, Hill BT. Possible mechanism for differences in sensitivity to cisplatinum in human prostate tumor cell lines. Cancer Lett 1986;31:163.
348. Millard JT, Raucher S, Hopkins PB. Mechlorethamine cross links deoxyguanosine residues at 5′ GNC sequences in duplex DNA fragments. J Am Chem Soc 1990;112: 2459.
349. Miller B, Teneholz T, Egorin MJ, Sosnovsky G, Rao NU, Gutierrez PL. Cellular pharmacology of N,N′,N″-triethylene thiophosphoramide. Cancer Lett 1988;41:157.
350. Miller DG. Alkylating agents and human spermatogenesis. JAMA 1971;217:1662.
351. Miller KJ, McGovern RM, Ames MM. Effect of a hepatic activation system on the antiproliferative activity of hexamethylmelamine against human tumor cell lines. Cancer Chemother Pharmacol 1985;15:49.
352. Miller JJ, Williams GF, Leissring JC. Multiple late complications of therapy with cyclophosphamide, including ovarian destruction. Am J Med 1971;50:530.
353. Mirkes PE. Cyclophosphamide teratogenesis: a review. Teratogenesis Carcinog Mutagen 1985;5:75.
354. Mitchell MS, Kempf RA, Harel W, Shau H, Bosell WD, Lind S, Bradley EC. Effectiveness and tolerability of low-dose cyclophosphamide and low-dose intravenous interleukin-2 in disseminated melanoma. J Clin Oncol 1988;6:409.
355. Mitchell RB, Moschel RC, Dolan ME. Effect of 0-6-benzylguanine on the sensitivity of human tumor xenografts to 1,3-bis(2-chloroethyl)-1-nitrosourea and on DNA interstrand cross-link formation. Cancer Res 1992;52:1171.
356. Modrich P. Mismatch repair, genetic stability, and cancer. Science 1994;266:1959.
357. Moroso MJ, Blair RL. A review of cis-platinum ototoxicity. J Otolaryngol 1983;12:365.
358. Mortimer JE, Taylor ME, Schulman S, Cummings C, Weymuller E Jr, Laramore G. Feasibility and efficacy of weekly intra-arterial cisplatin in locally advanced (stage III and IV) head and neck cancers. J Clin Oncol 1988;6:969.
358a. Mulcahy RT, Untawale S, Gipp JJ. Transcriptional unregulation of gamma-glutamylcysteine synthetase gene expression in melphalan-resistant human prostate carcinoma cells. Molecular Pharmacology 1994;46:909.
359. Mullins GM, Anderson PN, Santos GW. High dose cyclophosphamide therapy in solid tumors. Cancer 1975;36:1950.
360. Mullins GM, Colvin M. Intensive cyclophosphamide therapy in solid tumors. Cancer Chemother Rep 1975;59:411.
361. Murphy ML, Del Moro A, Lacon C. The comparative effects of five poly-functional alkylating agents on the rat fetus, with additional notes. Ann NY Acad Sci 1958;68: 762.
362. Nabors MW, Griffin CA, Zehnbauer BA, Hruban RH, Phillips PC, Grossman SA, Brem H, Colvin OM. Multidrug resistance gene (MDR1) expression in human brain tumors. J Neuro Surg 1991;75:941.
363. Naganuma A, Satoh M, Imura N. Prevention of lethal and renal toxicity of cis-diamminedichloroplatinum (II) by induction of metallothionein synthesis without compromising its antitumor activity in mice. Cancer Res 1987;47:983.
364. Nakagawa K, Saijo N, Tsuchida S, Sakal M, Tsunokawa Y, Yokota J, Muramatsu M, Sato K, Terada M, Tew KD. Glutathione-*S*-transferase π as a determinant of drug resistance in transfectant cell lines. J Biol Chem 1990;265:4296.
365. Nakagawa K, Yokota J, Wada M, Sasaki Y, Fujiwara Y, Sakai M, Muramatsu M, Terasaki T, Tsunokawa Y, Terada M, Saijo N. Levels of glutathione S-transferase pi mRNA in human lung cancer cell lines correlate with the resistance to cisplatin and carboplatin. Jpn J Cancer Res 1988;79:301.
366. Nelson RL, Allen LM, Creaven PJ. Pharmacokinetics of divided-dose ifosfamide. Clin Pharmacol Ther 1976;19:365.
367. Neuwelt EA, Glasberg M, Frenkel E, Barnett P. Neurotoxicity of chemotherapeutic agents after blood-brain barrier modification: neuropathological studies. Ann Neurol 1983;14:316.
368. Newlands ES, Blackledge GR, Slack JA, Rustin GJ, Smith DB, Stuart NS, Quarterman CP, Hoffman R, Stevens MF, Brampton MH, et al. Phase I trial of temozolomide (CCRG 81045: m&B 39831: NSC 362856). Br J Canc 1992;65:287.
369. Newman EM, Lu Y, Kashani-Sabet M, Kesavan V, Scanlon KJ. Mechanisms of cross-resistance to methotrexate and 5-fluorouracil in an A2780 human ovarian carcinoma cell subline resistant to cisplatin. Biochem Pharmacol 1988;37:443.
370. Ng SF, Waxman DJ. N,N′,N″-triethylenethiophosphoramide (thio-TEPA) oxygenation by constitutive hepatic P450 enzymes and modulation of drug metabolism and clearance in vivo by P450-inducing agents. Cancer Res 1991;51:2340.
371. Nichols CR, Tricot G, Williams SD, van Besien K, Loehrer PJ, Roth BJ, Akard L, Hoffman R, Goulet R, Wolff SN, et al. Dose-intensive chemotherapy in refractory germ cell cancer—a phase I/II trial of high-dose carboplatin and etoposide with autologous bone marrow transplantation. J Clin Oncol 1989;7:932.
372. Nicholson HO. Cytotoxic drugs in pregnancy. J Obstet Gynaecol Br Commonw 1968;75:307.
373. Nimer SD, Milewicz AL, Champlin RE, Busittil RW. Successful treatment of hepatic venoocclusive disease in a bone marrow transplant patient with orthotopic liver transplantation. Transplantation 1990;49:819.
374. Nissen-Meyer R, Host H. A comparison between the hematological side effects of cyclophosphamide and nitrogen mustard. Cancer Chemother 1960;9:51.
374a. Nitschke R, Pratt C, Harris M, Krischer J, Vietti TJ, Grier H, Kamps W, Toledano S. Evaluation of CHIP (iproplatin) in recurrent pediatric malignant solid tumors. A phase II study. Invest New Drugs 1992;10:93–96.
375. Norpoth K. Studies on the metabolism of isophosphamide (NSC-109724) in man. Cancer Treat Rep 1976;60:437.
376. O'Connor PM, Ferris DK, White GA, Pines J, Hunter T, Longo DL, Kohn KW. Relationships between cdc2 kinase DNA cross-linking, and cell cycle perturbations induced by nitrogen mustards. Cell Growth Diff 1992;3:43.
377. O'Dwyer PJ, LaCreta F, Nash S, Tinsley PW, Schilder R, Clapper ML, Tew KD, Panting L, Litwin S, Comis RL, Ozols RF. Phase I study of thiotepa in combination with the glutathione transferase inhibitor ethacrynic acid. Cancer Res 1991;51:6059.
378. Oguri S, Sakakibara T, Mase H, Shimizu T, Ishikawa K, Kimura K, Smyth RD. Clinical pharmacokinetics of carboplatin. J Clin Pharmacol 1988;28:208.
379. Oliner H, Schwartz R, Rubio F Jr, Dameshek W. Interstitial pulmonary fibrosis following busulfan therapy. Am J Med 1961;31:134.
380. Ojwang JD, Grueneberg DA, Loechler EL. Synthesis of a duplex oligonucleotide containing a nitrogen mustard interstrand DNA-DND cross-link. Cancer Res 1989;49: 6529.
381. Onsrud M, Bosnes V, Graham I. Cis-Platinum as adjunctive to surgery in early stage ovarian carcinoma: effects on lymphoid cell subpopulations. Gynecol Oncol 1986;23: 323.
382. O'Reilly SM, Newlands ES, Glaser MG, Brampton M, Rice-Edwards JM, Illingworth RD, Richards PG, Kennard C, Colquhoun IR, Lewis P, et al. Temozolomide: a new oral cytotoxic chemotherapeutic agent with promising activity against primary brain tumors. Eur J Cancer 1993;29A:940 (erratum Eur J Cancer 29A:15000, 1993).
383. Orourke TJ, Weiss GR, New P, Burris HA, Rodriguez G, Eckhardt J, Hardy J, Kuhn JG, Fields S, Clark GM, Vonhoff DD. Phase I clinical trial of ormaplatin (Tetraplatin, NSC 363812). Anticancer Drugs 1994;5:520.
384. Ortega J. Multiple agent chemotherapy including bleomycin of non-Hodgkin's lymphoma during pregnancy. Cancer 1977;40:2829.
385. Orwoll ES, Kiessling PJ, Patterson JR. Interstitial pneumonia from mitomycin. Ann Intern Med 1978;89:352.
386. Ozer H, Cowens JW, Colvin M, Nussbaum-Blumenson A, Sheedy D. In vitro effects of 4-hydroperoxycyclophosphamide on human immunoregulatory T subset function. 1. Selective effects on lymphocyte function in T-B cell collaboration. J Exp Med 1982;155:276.
387. Ozols RF. Cisplatin dose intensity. Semin Oncol 1989;16:22.
388. Ozols RF. Carboplatin and Taxol (paclitaxel) in advanced ovarian carcinoma. Ann Oncol 1994;6:S39.
389. Ozols RF, Louie KG, Plowman J, Behrens BC, Fine RL, Dykes D, Hamilton TC. Enchanced melphalan cytotoxicity in human ovarian cancer in vitro and in tumor-bearing nude mice by buthionine sulfoximine depletion of glutathione. Biochem Pharmacol 1987;36:147.
390. Ozols RF, Masuda H, Hamilton TC. Mechanisms of cross-resistance between radiation and antineoplastic drugs. NCI Monogr 1988;6:159.
391. Pacheco DY, Stratton NK, Gibson NW. Comparison of the mechanism of action of busulfan with hepsulfam, a new antileukemic agent, in the L1210 cell line. Cancer Res 1989;49:5108.
392. Panella TJ, Smith DC, Schold SC, Rogers MP, Winer EP, Fine RL, Crawford J 2nd, Herndon JE, Trump DL. Modulation of 06-alkylguanine-DNA-alkyltransferase-mediated carmustine resistance using streptozotocin. A phase I trial. Cancer Res 1992;52: 2456.
393. Pallante SL, Fenselau C, Mennel RG, Brundrett RB, Appler M, Rosenshein NB, Colvin M. Quantitation by gas chromatography-chemical ionization-mass spectrometry of phenylalanine mustard in plasma of patients. Cancer Res 1980;40:2268.
394. Pallante SL, Lisek CA, Dulik DM, Fenselau C. Glutathione conjugates Immobilized enzyme synthesis and characterization by fast atom bombardment mass spectrometry. Drug Metab Dispos 1986;14:313.
395. Paolozzi FP, Gaver R, Poiesz BJ, Louie A, Difino S, Comis RL, Newman N, Ginsberg S. Phase I—preliminary Phase II trial of iproplatin, a cisplatin analogue. Invest New Drugs 1988;6:199.
396. Parker RJ, Vionet JA, Bostick-Bruton F, Reed, E Ormaplatin sensitivity/resistance in human ovarian cancer cells made resistant to cisplatin. Cancer Res 1993;53:242.
397. Parker S, Kirk MC, Ludlum DB. Synthesis and characterization of 0-6-(2-chloroethyl)guanine: a putative intermediate in the cytotoxic reaction of chloroethylnitrosoureas with DNA. Biochem Biophys Res Commun 1987;148:1124.
398. Parsons PG, Lean J, Kable EPW, Favier D, Khoo SK, Hurst T, Holmes RS, Bellet AJD. Relationship between resistance to cross-linking agents and glutathione metabolism, aldehyde dehydrogenase isozymes and adenovirus replication in human tumor all lines. Biochem Pharmacol 1990;40:2641.
399. Patel AR, Shah PC, Rhee HL, Sassoon H, Rao KP. Cyclophosphamide therapy and interstitial pulmonary fibrosis. Cancer 1976;38:1542.
400. Patton TF, Repta AJ, Sternson LA. Clinical pharmacology of cisplatin. In Pharmacokinetics of Anticancer Agents in Humans. Edited by MM Ames, G Powis, JS Kovach. New York: Elsevier, 1983.
401. Pegg AE. Mammalian 06—alkylguanine-DNA alkyltransferase: regulation and importance in response to alkylating carcinogenic and therapeutic agents. Cancer Res 1990;50:6119.
402. Pegg AE, Boosalis M, Samson M, Samson L, Moschel RC, Byers TL, Swenn K, Dolan ME. Mechanism of inactivation of human 06-alkylaguanine-DNA alkyltransferase by 06-benzylguanine. Biochemistry 1993;32:1;1998.

403. Pendyala L, Cowens JW, Chheda GB, Dutta SP, Creaven PJ. Identification of cis-dichloro-bis-isopropylamine platinum (II) as a major metabolite of iproplatin in humans. Cancer Res 1988;48:3533.
404. Pendyala L, Walshm JR, Huq MM, Arakali AV, Cowens JW, Creaven PJ. Uptake and metabolism of iproplatin in murine L1210 cells. Cancer Chemother Pharmacol 1989;25:15.
405. Penn I. Second malignant neoplasm associated with immunosuppressive medications. Cancer 1976;37:1024.
406. Perloff M, Hart RD, Holland JF. Vinblastine, adriamycin, thio-TEPA, and Holotestin (VATH). Cancer 1978;42:2534.
407. Peters WP, Eder JP, Henner WD, Schryber S, Wilmore D, Finberg R, Schoenfeld D, Bast R, Gargone B, Antman K, Anderson J, Anderson K, Kruskall MS, Schnipper L, Frei E III. High-dose combination alkylating agents with autologous bone marrow support: a phase I trial. J Clin Oncol 1986;4:646.
408. Pfeiffer P, Bennedbaek O, Bertelsen K. Intraperitoneal carboplatin in the treatment of minimal residual ovarian cancer. Gynecol Oncol 1990;36:306.
409. Philips FS, Sternberg SS, Cronin AP, Vidal PM. Cyclophosphamide and urinary bladder toxicity. Cancer Res 1961;21:1577.
410. Phillips GL, Fay JW, Herzig GP, Herzig RH, Weiner RS, Wolff SN, Lazarus HM, Karanes C, Ross WE, Kramer BS. Intensive 1,3-bis(2-chloroethyl)-1-nitrosourea (BCNU), NSC #4366650 and cryopreserved autologous marrow transplantation for refractory cancer. A Phase I-II study. Cancer 1983;51:1792.
411. Piccart MJ, Abrams J, Dodion PF, Crespeigne N, Schulier JP. Intraperitoneal chemotherapy with cisplatin and melphalan. JNCI 1988;80:1118.
412. Piel IJ, Perlia CP. Phase II study of cis-dichlorodiammineplatinum (II) (NSC-119875) in combination with cyclophosphamide (NSC-26271) in the treatment of human malignancies. Cancer Chemother Rep 1975;59:995.
413. Pil PM, Lippard SJ. Specific binding of chromosomal protein HMG1 to DNA damaged by the anticancer drug cisplatin. Science 1992;256:234.
414. Pinto AL, Lippard SJ. Sequence-dependent termination of in vitro DNA synthesis by cis- and trans-diamminedichloroplatinum (II). Proc Natl Acad Sci USA 1985;82:4616.
415. Plooy AC, van Dijk M, Berends F, Lohman PH. Formation and repair of DNA interstrand cross-links in relation to cytotoxicity and unscheduled DNA synthesis induced in control and mutant human cells treated with cis-diamminedichloroplatinum (II). Cancer Res 1985;45:4178.
416. Poirier MC, Egorin MJ, Fichtinger-Schepman AM, Yushpa SH, Reed E. DNA adducts of cisplatin and carboplatin in tissues of cancer patients. IARC Sci Publ 1988;89:313.
417. Poisson M, Chiras J, Fauchon F, Debussche C, Delattre JY. Treatment of malignant recurrent glioma by intra-arterial infra-ophthalmic infusion of HECNU 1-(2-chloroethyl)-1-nitroso-3-(2-hydroxyethyl) urea. A phase II study. J Neurooncol 1990;8:255.
418. Poll EH, Abrahams PJ, Arwert F, Eriksson AW. Host-cell reactivation of cis-diamminedichloroplatinum (II)-treated SV40 DNA in normal human, Fanconi anaemia and xeroderma pigmentosum fibroblasts. Mutat Res 1984;132:181.
419. Poll EH, Arwert F, Joenje H, Eriksson AW. Cytogenetic toxicity of antitumor platinum compounds in Fanconi's anemia. Hum Genet 1982;61:228.
420. Pomes A, Frustaci S, Cattaino G, DeGrandis D, Bongiovanni LG, Tumolo S, Quadu G. Local neurotoxicity of cisplatin after intra-arterial chemotherapy. Acta Neurol Scand 1986;73:302.
421. Portlock CS, Fischer DS, Cadman E, Lundberg WB, Levy A, Bobrow S, Bertino JR, Farber L. High-dose pulse chlorambucil in advanced, low-grade non-Hodgkin's lymphoma. Cancer Treat Rep 1987;71:1029.
422. Pratt CB, Douglass EC, Etcubanas E, Goren MP, Green AA, Hayes FA, Horowitz ME, Meyer WH, Thompson, EI, Wilimas JA. Clinical studies of ifosfamide/mesna at St. Jude Children's Research Hospital, 1983–1988. Semin Oncol 1989;16(suppl 3):51.
423. Pratt CB, Goren MP, Meyer WH, Singh B, Dodge RK. Ifosfamide neurotoxicity is related to previous cisplatin treatment for pediatric solid tumors. J Clin Oncol 1990;8:1399.
424. Pratt CB, Horowitz ME, Meyer WH, Etcubanas E, Thompson EI, Douglass EC, Wilimas JA, Hayes FA, and Green AA. Phase II trial of ifosfamide in children with malignant solid tumors. Cancer Treat Rep 1987;71:131.
425. Prestayko AW. Cisplatin and analogues: a new class of anticancer drugs. In Cancer and Chemotherapy, vol III, Antineoplastic Agents. Edited by ST Crooke, AW Prestayko. New York: Academic, 1981, p 133.
426. Price CC, Gaucher GM, Koneru P, Shibakawa R, Sowa JR, Yamaguchi M. Relative reactivities for monofunctional nitrogen mustard alkylation of nucleic acid components. Biochim Biophys Acta 1968;166:327.
427. Puchalski RB, Fahl WE. Expression of recombinant glutathione-S-transferase pi, Ya or Yb1 confers resistance to alkylating agents. Proc Natl Acad Sci USA 1990;87:2443.
428. Quesniaux VF. Interleukin 11 (review). Leuk Lymphoma 1994;14:241.
429. Radin AE, Haggard ME, Travis LB. Lung changes and chemotherapeutic agents in childhood. Am J Dis Child 1970;120:337.
430. Redwood WR, Colvin M. Transport of melphalan by sensitive and resistant L1210 cells. Cancer Res 1980;40:1144.
431. Reece PA, Bishop JF, Oliver IN, Stafford I, Hillcoat BL, Morstyn G. Pharmacokinetics of unchanged carboplatin (CBDCA) in patients with small cell lung carcinoma. Cancer Chemother Pharmacol 1987;19:326.
432. Reece PA, Dale BM, Morris RG, Kotasek D, Gee D, Rogerson S, Sage RE. Effect of L-leucine on oral melphalan kinetics in patients. Cancer Chemother Pharmacol 1987;20:256.
433. Reece PA, Hill HS, Green RM, Morris RG, Dale BM, Kotasek D. Renal clearance and protein binding of melphalan in patients with cancer. Cancer Chemother Pharmacol 1988;22:348.
434. Reece PA, Kotasek D, Morris RG, Dale BM, Sage RE. The effect of food on oral melphalan absorption. Cancer Chemother Pharmacol 1986;16:194.
435. Reed E, Kohn KW. Platinum analogues. In Cancer Chemotherapy: Principles and Practice. Edited by BA Chabner, JM Collins. Philadelphia: Lippincott, 1990, p 475.
436. Reimer RR, Hoover R, Fraumeni JF Jr, Young RC. Acute leukemia after alkylating-agent therapy of ovarian cancer. N Engl J Med 1977;297:177.
437. Rekha GK, Sreerama L, Sladek NE. Intrinsic cellular resistance to oxazaphosphorines exhibited by a human colon carcinoma cell line expressing relatively large amounts of a class-3 aldehyde dehydrogenase. Biochem Pharmacol 1994;48:1943.
438. Repta AJ, Long DF. Cisplatin. Current Status and New Developments. Edited by AW Prestayko, ST Crooke, SK Carter. New York: Academic, 1980, p 285.
439. Reyes ES, Talley RW, O'Bryan RM, et al. Clinical evaluation of 1,3-bis-(2-chloroethyl)-1-nitrosourea (BCNU; NSC-409962) with fluoxymesterone (NSC-12165) in the treatment of solid tumors. Cancer Chemother Rep 1973;57:225.
440. Rhoads CP. Nitrogen mustards in treatment of neoplastic disease. JAMA, 1946;131:656.
440a. Rhodes T, Twentyman PR. A study of ethacrynic acid as a potential modifier of melphalan and cisplatin sensitivity in human lung cancer parental and drug-resistant cell lines. Br J Cancer 1992;65:684.
441. Rhodes DF, Lee WM, Wingard JR, Pavy MD, Santos GW, Shaw BW, Wood RP, Sorrell MF, Markin RS. Orthotopic liver transplantation for graft-versus-host disease following bone marrow transplantation. Gastroenterology 1990;99:536.
442. Rivkin SE, Green S, Metch B, Glucksberg H, Gad-el-Mawla N, Constanzi JJ, Hoogstraten B, Athens J, Maloney T, Osborne CK, et al. Adjuvant CMFVP versus melphalan for operable breast cancer with positive axillary nodes: 10-year results of a Southwest Oncology Group Study. J Clin Oncol 1989;7:1229.
443. Roberts JJ, Pera MF. DNA as a target for anticancer coordination compounds. In Platinum, Gold, and the Metal Chemotherapeutic Agents. Edited by JJ Lippard. Washington, DC: American Chemical Society, 1983, p 3.
444. Robson CN, Lewis AD, Wolf CR, Hayes JD, Hall A, Proctor SJ, Harris AL, Hickson ID. Reduced levels of drug-induced DNA cross-linking in nitrogen mustard-resistant Chinese hamster ovary cells expressing elevated glutathione S-transferase activity. Cancer Res 1967;47:6022.
445. Ross D, Langdon SP, Gescher A, Stevens MF. Studies of the mode of action of antitumour triazenes and triazines-V. The correlation of the in vitro cytotoxicity and in vivo antitumor activity of hexamethylmelamine analogues with their metabolism. Biochem Pharmacol 1984;33:1131.
446. Rutty CJ, Judson IR, Abel G, Goddard PM, Newell DR, Harrap KR. Preclinical toxicology, pharmacokinetics and formulation of N2,N4,N6-trihydroxymethyl-N2,N4,N6-trimethylmelamine (trimelamol), a water-soluble cytoxic s-triazine which does not require metabolic activation. Cancer Chemother Pharmacol 1986;17:251.
447. Roosen N, Kiwit JC, Lins E, Schirmer M, Bock WJ. Adjuvant intra-arterial chemotherapy with nimustine in the management of World Health Organization Grade IV gliomas of the brain. Cancer 1984;64:1989.
448. Rose DP, Davis TE. Ovarian function in patients receiving adjuvant chemotherapy for breast cancer. Lancet 1977;1:1174.
449. Rosenberg B, Van Camp L, Krigas T. Nature 1965;98.
450. Rosenberg B, Van Camp L, Trosko JE, Mansour VH. Plantinum compounds: a new class of potent antitumor agents. Nature 1969;222:385.
451. Rosner F, Grunwald H. Multiple myeloma terminating in acute leukemia. Am J Med 1974;57:927.
452. Rosner F, Grunwald H. Hodgkin's disease and acute leukemia. Am J Med 1975;58:339.
453. Rosowsky A, Wright JE, Cucchi CA, Flatow JL, Trites DH, Teicher BA, Frei E III. Collateral methotrexate resistance in cultured human head and neck carcinoma cells selected for resistance to cis-diamminedichloroplatinum (II). Cancer Res 1987;47:5913.
454. Ross D, Siegel D, Gibson NW, Pacheco D, Thomas DJ, Reasor M, Wierda D. Activation and deactivation of quinones catalyzed by DT-diaphorase. Evidence for bioreductive activation of diaziquone (AZQ) in human tumor cells and detoxification of benzene metabolites in bone marrow stroma. Free Radic Res Commun 1990;6:373.
455. Ross WE, Chabner BA. Allergic reaction to cyclophosphamide in a mechlorethamine-sensitive patient. Cancer Treat Rep 1977;61:495.
456. Ross WE, Ewig RA, Kohn KW. Differences between melphalan and nitrogen mustard in the formation and removal of DNA cross-links. Cancer Res 1978;38:1502.
457. Ruckdeschel JC. The future role of carboplatin. (Review) Semin in Oncol 1994;21:114.
458. Rundles RW, Striggle J, Bell W, Corley CC, Frommeyer WB Jr, Greenberg BG, Huguley CM Jr, James GW, Jones R Jr, Larsen WE, Loe BV, Leone LA, Palmer JG, Riser WE Jr, Wilson SJ. Comparison of chlorambucil and Myleran in chronic lymphocytic and granulocytic leukemia. Am J Med 1959;27:424.
459. Russo JE, Hilton J, Colvin OM. The role of aldehyde dehydrogenase isoenzymes in cellular resistance to the alkylating agent cyclophosphamide. In Enzymology and Molecular Biology of Carbonyl Metabolism, vol 2. New York: Liss, 1989, p 65.
460. Rutty CJ, Abel G. In vitro cytotoxicity of the methylmelamines. Chem Biol Interact 1980;29:235.
461. Saburi Y, Nakagawa M, Ono M, Sakai M, Muramatsu M, Kohno K, Kuwano M. Increased expression of glutathione S-transferase gene in cis-diamminedichloroplatinum (II)-resistant variants of a Chinese hamster ovary cell line. Cancer Res 1989;49:7020.
462. Sancar A. Mechanisms of DNA excision repair. Science 1994;266:1954.
463. Santos GW, Sensenbrenner LL, Anderson PN, Burke PJ, Kelin DL, Slavin RE, Schacter B, Borgaonkar DS. HLA-identical marrow transplants in aplastic anemia, acute leukemia, and lymphosarcoma employing cyclophosphamide. Transplant Proc 1976;8:607.
464. Santos GW, Tutschka PJ, Brookmeyer R, Saral R, Beschorner WE, Bias WB, Braine HG, Burns WH, Elfenbein GJ, Kaizer H, et al. Marrow transplantation for acute nonlymphocytic leukemia after treatment with busulfan and cyclophosphamide. N Engl J Med 1983;309:1347.
465. Satoh M, Cherian MG, Imura N, Shimizu H. Modulation of resistance to anticancer drugs by inhibition of metallothionein synthesis. Cancer Res 1994;54:5255.
466. Scanlon KJ, Jiao L, Funato T, Wang W, Tone T, Rossi JJ, Kashani-Sabet M. Ribozyme-mediated cleavage of c-fos mRNA reduces gene expression of DNA synthesis enzymes and metallothionein. Proc Natl Acad Sci USA 1991;88:10591–10595.
467. Scanlon KJ, Kashani-Sabet M, Sowers LC. Overexpression of DNA replication and repair enzymes in cisplatin-resistant human colon carcinoma HCT8 cells and circumvention by azidothymidine. Cancer Commun 1989;1:269.
468. Schabel FM Jr. Nitrosoureas: a review of experimental anti-tumor activity. Cancer Treat Rep 1976;60:665.
469. Schabel FM Jr, Johnston TP, McCaleb GS, et al. Experimental evaluation of potential anticancer agents: VIII. Effects of certain nitrosoureas on cerebral L1210 leukemia. Cancer Res 1963;23:226.
470. Schacht RG, Baldwin DS. Chronic interstitial nephritis and renal failure due to nitrosourea (NU) therapy. Kidney Int 1978;14:661.

471. Schilsky RL, Anderson T. Hypomagnesemia and renal magnesium wasting in patients receiving cisplatin. Ann Intern Med 1979;90:929.
472. Schmidt W, Chaney SG. Role of carrier ligand in platinum resistance of human carcinoma cell lines. Cancer Res 1993;53:799.
473. Schold SC Jr, Brent TP, von Hofe E, Friedman HS, Mitra S, Bigner DD, Swenberg JA, Kleihues P. 06-alkylguanine-DNA alkyltransferase and sensitivity to procarbazine in human brain-tumor xenografts. J Neurosurg 1989;70:573.
474. Sekiya S, Oosaki T, Andoh S, Susuki N, Akaboshi M, Takamizawa H. Mechanisms of resistance to cis-diamminedichloroplatinum (II) in vitro. Cancer Res 1988;48:6803.
475. Selby CP, Sancar A. Molecular mechanisms of DNA repair inhibition by caffeine. Proc Natl Acad Sci USA 1990;87:3522.
476. Sellei C, Ecklardt S, Horvath IP, Kralovanszky J, Institoris L. Clinical and pharmacologic experience with dibromodulcitol (NSC-104800), a new antitumor agent. Cancer Chemother Rep 1969;53:377.
477. Sharma M, He QY, Tomasz M. Effects of glutathione on alkylation and cross-linking of DNA by mitomycin C. Isolation of a ternary glutathione-mitomycin-DNA adduct. Chem Res Toxicol 1994;7:401.
478. Sharma RP, Edwards IR. Cis-Platinum: subcellular distribution and binding to cytosolic proteins. Biochem Pharmacol 1983;32:2665.
479. Sheibani N, Jennerwein MM, Eastman A. DNA repair in cells sensitive and resistant to cis-diamminedichloroplatinum (II): host cell reactivation of damaged plasmid DNA. Biochemistry 1989;28:3120.
480. Sherins RJ, DeVita VT. Effect of drug treatment for lymphoma on male reproductive capacity. Ann Intern Med 1973;79:216.
481. Skarlos, D.v, Samantas E, Kosmidis P, Fountzilas G, Angelidou M, Palamidas P, Mylonakis N, Provata A, Papdakis E, Klouvas G, et al. Randomized comparison of etoposide-cisplatin vs. etoposide-carboplatin and irradiation in small-cell lung cancer. A Hellenic Cooperative Oncology Group Study. Ann Oncol 1994;5:601.
482. Skibba JL, Beal DD, Ramirez G, Bryan T. N-Demethylation of the antineoplastic agent 4(5)-(3,3-dimethyl-1-triazeno)imidazole-5(4)-carboxamide by rats and man. Cancer Res 1970;30:147.
483. Skinner R, Pearson AD, Amineddine HA, Mathias DB, Craft AW. Ototoxicity of cisplatinum in children and adolescents. Br J Cancer 1990;61:927.
484. Sladek N. Therapeutic efficacy of cyclophosphamide as a function of its metabolism. Cancer Res 1972;32:535.
485. Sladek NE, Doeden D, Powers JF, Krivit W. Plasma concentrations of 4-hydroxycylophosphamide and phosphoramide mustard in patients repeatedly given high doses of cyclophosphamide in preparation for bone marrow transplantation. Cancer Treat Rep 1984;68:1247.
486. Slavin RE, Millan JC, Mullins GM. Pathology of high dose intermittent cyclophosphamide therapy. Hum Pathol 1975;6:693.
487. Smith AC, Liao JT, Page JG, Wientjes MG, Grieshaber CK. Pharmacokinetics of buthionine sulfoximine (NSC 326231) and its effect on melphalan-induced toxicity in mice. Cancer Res 1989;49:5385.
488. Smith MT, Evans CG, Doane-Setzer P, Castro VM, Tahir MK, Mannervik B. Denitrosation of 1,3-bis(2-chlorethyl)-1-nitrosourea by class mu glutathione transferases and its role in cellular resistance in rat brain tumor cells. Cancer Res 1989;49:2621.
489. Sorenson CM, Eastman A. Influence of cis-diamminedichloroplatinum (II) on DNA synthesis and cell cycle progression in excision repair proficient and deficient Chinese hamster ovary cells. Cancer Res 1988;48:6703.
490. Speyer JL, Beller U, Colombo N, Sorich J, Wernz JC, Hochster H, Green M, Porges R, Muggia FM, Canetta R, Beckman EM. Intraperitoneal carboplatin: favorable results in women with minimal residual ovarian cancer after cisplatin therapy. J Clin Oncol 1990;8:1335.
491. Spitz S. The histological effects of nitrogen mustards on human tumors and tissues. Cancer 1948;1:383.
492. Sreerama L, Sladek NE. Identification of a methylcholanthrene-induced aldehyde dehydrogenase in a human breast adenocarcinoma cell line exhibiting oxazaphosphorine-specific acquired resistance. Cancer Res 1994;54:2176.
493. Steege JF, Caldwell DS. Renal agenesis after first trimester exposure to chlorambucil. South Med J 1980;73:1414.
494. Steinberg SS, Philips FS, Scholler J. Pharmacological and pathological effects of alkylating agents. Ann NY Acad Sci 1958;68:811.
495. Steinherz LJ, Steinherz PG. Cyclophosphamide cardiotoxicity. Cancer Bull 1985;37: 231.
496. Stevnsner T, Ding R, Smulson M, Bohr VA. Inhibition of gene-specific repair of alkylation damage in cells depleted of poly(ADP-ribose) polymerase. Nucleic Acids Res 1994;22:4620.
497. Stewart DJ, Grahovac Z, Hugenholtz H, Russell N, Richard M, Benoit B. Combined intra-arterial and systemic chemotherapy for intracerebral tumors. Neurosurgery 1987;21:207.
498. Strauss M, Towfight J, Lord S, Lipton A, Harvey HA, Brown B. Cis-platinum ototoxicity: clinical experience and temporal bone histopathology.
499. Strong JM, Collins JM, Lester C, Poplack DG. Pharmacokinetics of intraventricular and intravenous N,N',N''-triethylenethiophosphoramide (thiotepa) in rhesus monkeys and humans. Cancer Res 1986;46(12 Pt 1):6101.
500. Struck RF, Alberts DS, Horne K, Phillips JG, Peng YM, Roe DJ. Plasma pharmacokinetics of cyclophosphamide and its cytotoxic metabolites after intravenous versus oral administration in a randomized, crossover trial. Cancer Res 1987;47:2723.
501. Struck RF, Kirk MC, Mellett LB, El-Dareer S, Hill DL. Urinary metabolites of the antitumor agent cyclophosphamide. Molec Pharmacol 1971;7:519.
502. Sundquist WI, Lippard SJ, Stollar BD. Monoclonal antibodies to DNA modified with cis- or trans-diamminedichloroplatinum (II). Proc Natl Acad Sci USA 1987;84:8225.
503. Suzukaka D, Petro BJ, Vistica DT. Reduction in glutathione content of L-PAM resistant L1210 cell confers drug sensitivity. Biochem Pharmacol 1982;31:121–124.
504. Swaffar DS, Horstman MG, Jaw JY, Thrall BD, Meadows GS, Harker WG, Yost GS. Methoxyprocarbazine, the active metabolite responsible for the anticancer activity of procarbazine against L1210 leukemia. Cancer Res 1989;49:2442.
505. Takvorian T, Parker LM, Hochberg FH, Zervas NP, Frei E III, Canellos GP. Single high-dose of BCNU with autologous bone marrow (ABM). Proc AACR and Am Soc Clin Oncol 1980;21:341.
506. Talley RW, O'Bryan RM, Gutterman JU, Brownlee RW, McCredie KB. Clinical evaluation of toxic effects of cis-diamminedichloroplatinum (NSC-119875)—phase I clinical study. Cancer Chemother Rep 1973;57:465.
507. Talmadge JE, Tribble H, Pennington R, Bowersox O, Schneider MA, Castelli P, Black PL, Abe F. Protective, restorative, and therapeutic properties of recombinant colony-stimulating factors. Blood 1989;73:2093.
508. Tapiero H, Yin MB, Catalin J, Paraire M, Deloffre P, Rustum Y, Bizzari JP, Tew KD. Cytotoxicity and DNA damaging effects of a new nitrosourea, fotemustine, diethyl-1-(3-{2-chloroethyl}-3-nitrosoureido) ethylphosphonate-S10036. Anticancer Res 1989;9: 1617.
509. Tatsuta T, Naito M, O'Hara T, Sugawara I, Tsuruo T. Functional involvement of P-glycoprotein in blood-brain barrier. J Biol Chem 1992;267:29383.
510. Tattersall MHN, Weinberg A. Pharmacokinetics of melphalan following oral or intravenous administration in patients with malignant disease. Eur J Cancer 1978;14:507.
511. Taverna P, Catapano CV, Citti L, Bonfanti M, D'Incalci M. Influence of 06-methylguanine on DNA damage and cytotoxicity of temozolomide in L1210 mouse leukemia sensitive and resistant to chloroethylnitrosoureas. Anticancer Drugs 1992;3:401.
512. Taylor KM, Jagannath S, Spitzer G, Spinolo JA, Tucker SL, Fogel B, Cabanillas FF, Hagemeister FB, Souza LM. Recombinant human granulocyte colony-stimulating factor hastens granulocyte recovery after high-dose chemotherapy and autologous bone marrow transplantation in Hodgkin's disease. J Clin Oncol 1989;7:1791.
513. Teicher BA, Herman TS, Holden SA, Wang YY, Pfeffer MR, Crawford JW, Frei E III. Tumor resistance to alkylating agents conferred by mechanisms operative only in vivo. Science 1990;24:1457.
514. Teicher BA, Holden SA, Eder JP, Herman TS, Antman KH, Frei E. Preclinical studies relating to the use of thiotepa in the high-dose setting alone and in combination. Semin Oncol 1990;Feb 17(1 suppl 3):18.
515. Teicher BA, Holden SA, Kelley MJ, Shea TC, Cucchi CA, Rosowsky A, Henner WD, Frei E III. Characterization of a human squamous carcinoma cell line resistant to cis-diamminedichloroplatinum (II). Cancer Res 1987;47:388.
516. Teicher BA, Waxman DJ, Holden SA, Wang YY, Clarke L, Alvarez-Sotomayor E, Jones SM, Frei E 3rd. Evidence for enzymatic activation and oxygen involvement in cytotoxicity and antitumor activity of N,N,N triethylenethiophosphoramide. Cancer Res 1989;49:4996.
517. Tew KD, Bomber AM, Hoffman SJ. Ethacrynic acid and piriprost as enhancers of cytotoxicity in drug resistant and sensitive cell lines. Cancer Res 1988;48:3622.
518. Thatcher D, Lind M, Morgenstern G, Carr T, Chadwick G, Jones R, Craig P. High-dose, double alkylating agent chemotherapy with DTIC, melphalan, or ifosfamide and marrow rescue for metastatic malignant melanoma. Cancer 1989;63:1296.
519. Todd NW, Peters WP, Ost AH, Roggli VL, Piantadosi CA. Pulmonary drug toxicity in patients with primary breast cancer treated with high-dose combination chemotherapy and autologous bone marrow transplantation. Am Rev Resp Dis 1993;147:1264.
520. Toledo TM, Harper RC, Moser RH. Fetal effects during cyclophosphamide and irradiation therapy. Ann Intern Med 1971;74:87.
521. Tormey DC, Falkson G, Simon RM. A randomized comparison of two sequentially administered regimens to a single regimen in metastatic breast cancer. Cancer Clin Trials 1979;2:247.
522. Townes AS, Sowa JM, Schuman LE. Controlled trial of cyclophosphamide in rheumatoid arthritis (RA): an 11-month double-blind crossover study. Arthritis Rheum 1972;15:129.
523. Trask C, Silverstone A, Ash CM, Earl H, Irwin C, Bakker A, Tobias JS. A randomized trial of carboplatin versus iproplatin in untreated advanced ovarian cancer. J Clin Oncol 1991;9:1131.
524. Trujillo JM, Yang LY. Synergism of 1-beta-D-arabinofuranosylcytosine and cis-diamminedichloroplatinum in their lethal efficacies against seven established cancer cell lines of gastrointestinal origin. Anticancer Res 1989;9:197.
525. Tucker MA, Coleman CN, Cox RS, Varghese A, Rosenberg SA. Risk of second cancers after treatment for Hodgkin's disease. N Engl J Med 1988;318:76.
526. van Besien K, Nichols CR, Tricot G, Langefeld C, Miller ME, Akard L, English DK, Graves VL, Cheerva A, McCarthy LJ, et al. Characteristics of engraftment after repeated autologous bone marrow transplantation. Exp Hematol 1990;18:785.
527. Van Den Berg HW, Roberts JJ. Post-replication repair of DNA in Chinese hamster cells treated with cis platinum (II) diamine dichloride. Enhancement of toxicity and chromosome damage by caffeine. Mutat Res 1975;33:279.
528. van der Hoop R, deKoning P, Boven E, Neijt JP, Jennekens FG, Gispen WH. Efficacy of the neuropeptide ORG 2766 in the prevention and treatment of cisplatin-induced neurotoxicity in rats. Eur J Cancer Clin Oncol 1988;24:637.
529. van der Hoop RG, Hamers FP, Neijt JP, Veldman H, Gispen WH. Protection against cisplatin induced neurotoxicity by ORG 2766: histological and electrophysiological evidence. J Neurol Sci 1994;126:109.
530. van der Hoop RG, Vecht CJ, van der Burg ME, Elderson A, Boogerd W, Heimans JJ, Vries EP, van Houwelingen JC. Prevention of cisplatin neurotoxicity with an ACTH(4-9) analogue in patients with ovarian cancer. N Engl J Med 1990;322:89.
531. Van Dyk JJ, Falkson HC, Van der Merwe AM, Falkson G. Unexpected toxicity in patients treated with iphosphamide. Cancer Res 1972;32:921.
532. van Zandwijk N, Ten Bokkel Huinink WW, Wanders J, Simonetti G, Dubbelman R, Franklin H, van Tinteren H, McVie JG. Dose-finding studies with carboplatin, ifosfamide, etoposide, and mesna in non-small cell lung cancer. Semin Oncol 1990;17: 16.
533. van Zeeland AA, Bussmann CJ, Degrassi F, Filon AR, van Kasteren van Leeuwen AC, Palitti F, Natarajan AT. Effects of aphidicolin on repair replication and induced chromosomal aberrations in mammalian cells. Mutat Res 1982;92(1-2):379.
534. Vassal G. Pharmacologically-guided dose adjustment of busulfan in high-dose chemotherapy regimens—rationale and pitfalls. Anticancer Res 1994;14:2363.
535. Vassal G, Deroussent A, Hartmann O, Challine D, Benhamou E, Valiteau-Couanet D, Brugleres L, Kalifa C, Gouyette A, Lemerle J. Dose-dependent neurotoxicity of high-dose-busulfan in children: a clinical and pharmacological study. Cancer Res 1990;50:6203.
536. Vassal G, Gouyette A, Hartmann O, et al. Pharmacokinetics of high-dose busulfan in children. Cancer Chemother Pharmacol 1989;24:386.
537. Vaughan C, Chapman J, Chinn B, Ward D, Groshko G, Maniscalco B, Reznik S, Piper D. Activity of 5-fluorouracil, mitomycin C, and methyl CCNU in inoperable adenocarcinoma of pancreas. Am J Clin Oncol 1989;12:49.
538. Vaughan K, Tang Y, Lianos G, Horton JK, Simmonds RJ, Hickman JA, Stevens MFG. Studies of the mode of action of antitumor triazenes and trizines. 6. 1-Aryl-3(hydroxymethyl-3-methyltriazenes: synthesis, chemistry, and antitumor properties. J Med Chem 1984;27:357.

539. Ventura GJ, Barlogie B, Hester JP, Yau JC, LeMaistre CF, Wallerstein RO, Spinolo JA, Dicke KA, Horwitz LH, Alexantan R. High dose cyclophosphamide, BCNU and VP-16 with autologous blood stem cell support for refractory multiple myeloma. Bone Marrow Transplant 1990;5:265.
540. Vergote I, Himmelmann A, Frankendal B, Scheistroen M, Valachos K, Trope C. Hexamethylmemamine as second-line therapy in cisplatin-resistant ovarian cancer (see comments). Gynecol Oncol 1992;47:279,282.
541. Vermorken JB, Gundersen S, Clavel M, Smyth JF, Dodison P, Renard J, Kaye SB. Randomized phase II trial of iproplatin and carboplatin in advanced breast cancer. Ann Oncol 1993;4:303.
542. Verly WG. Monofunctional alkylating agents and apurinic sites in DNA. Biochem Pharmacol 1974;23:3.
543. Verly WG, Paquette Y. An endonuclease for depurinated DNA in *Escherichia coli* B. Can J Biochem 1972;50:217–224.
544. Vermorken JB, Kapteijn TS, Hart AA, Pinedo HM. Ototoxicity of cis-diamminedichloroplatinum (II): influence of dose, schedule and mode of administration. Eur J Cancer Clin Oncol 1983;19:53.
545. Viens P, Maraninchi D, Legros M, Oberling F, Philip T, Herve P, Plagne R, Dufour P, Bergerat JP, Guastalla JP, Rozenbaum A, Carcassonne Y. High dose melphalan and autologous marrow rescue in advanced epithelial ovarian carcinomas: a retrospective analysis of 35 patients treated in France. Bone Marrow Transplant 1990;5: 227.
546. Villani G, Hubscer U, Butour JL. Sites of termination of in vitro DNA synthesis on cis-diamminedichloroplatinum treated single stranded DNA: a comparison between *Escherichia coli* DNA polymerase I and eucaryotic DNA polymerases alpha. Nucleic Acids Res 1988;16:4407.
547. Viren M, Liippo K, Ojala A, Helle L, Hinkka S, Huovinen R, Jakobsson M, Jarvinen M, Paloheimo S, Salmi R, et al. Carboplatin and etoposide in extensive small cell lung cancer. Acta Oncol 1994;33:921.
548. Vistica DT, Rabon A, Rabinowitz M. Effects of L-alpha-amino-gamma-guanidinobutyric acid on melphalan therapy of the L1210 murine leukemia. Cancer Lett 1979;6: 345.
549. Vistica DT, Toal JN, Rabinowitz M. Amino acid conferred protection against melphalan: characterization of melphalan transport and correlation of uptake with cytotoxicity in cultured L1210 murine leukemia cells. Biochem Pharmacol 1978;27:2865.
550. Von Hoff DD, Schilsky R, Reichert CM, Reddick RL, Rozencweig M, Young RC, Muggia FM. Toxic effects of cis-dichlorodiammineplatinum (II) in man. Cancer Treat Rep 1979;63(9-10):1527.
551. Wadler S, Egorin MJ, Zuhowski EG, Tororello L, Salva K, Runowicz CD, Wiernik PH. Phase I clinical and pharmacokinetic study of thiotepa administered intraperitoneally in patients with advanced malignancies. J Clin Oncol 1989;7:132.
552. Wadler T, Heydrich D, Jork T, Voelker G, Hohorst HJ. Comparative study on human pharmacokinetics of activated ifosfamide and cyclophosphamide by a modified fluorometric test. Cancer Res Clin Oncol 1981;100:95.
553. Wagner T, Heydrich D, Voelcker G, Hohorst HJ. Characterization and quantitative estimation of activated cyclophosphamide in blood and urine. Cancer Res Clin Oncol 1980;96:79.
554. Walker DA, Pillow J, Waters KD, Keir E. Enhanced cis-platinum ototoxicity in children with brain tumours who have received simultaneous or prior cranial irradiation. Med Pediatr Oncol 1989;17:48.
555. Walker MD, Alexander E Jr, Hunt WE, MacCarty CS, Mahaley MS Jr, Mealey J Jr, Norrell HA, Owens G, Ransohoff J, Wilson CB, Gehan EA, Strike TA. Evaluation of BCNU and/or radiotherapy in the treatment of anaplastic gliomas. A cooperative clinical trial. J Neurosurg 1978;49:333.
556. Wang YY, Teicher BA, Shea TC, Holden SA, Rosbe KW, Al-Achi A, Henner WD. Cross-resistance and glutathione-S-transferase-pi levels among four human melonoma cell lines selected for alkylating agent resistance. Cancer Res 1989;49:6185.
557. Waud WR. Differential uptake of cis-diamminedichloroplatinum (II) by sensitive and resistant murine L1210 leukemia cells. Cancer Res 1987;47:6549.
558. Weiss G, Green S, Alberts DS, Thigpen JT, Hines HE, Hanson K, Pierce HI, Baker LH. Second-line treatment of advanced measurable ovarian cancer with iproplatin: a Southwest Oncology Group Study. Eur J Cancer 1991;27:135.
559. Whittle IR, MacPherson JS, Miller JD, Smyth JF. The disposition of TCNU (tauromustine) in human malignant glioma. J Neurosurg 1990;72:721.
560. Wils J, Bleiberg H. Current status of chemotherapy for gastric cancer. Eur J Cancer Clin Oncol 1989;25:3.
561. Wiltshaw E. Chlorambucil in the treatment of primary adenocarcinoma of the ovary. J Obstet Gynecol Br Commonw 1964;72:586.
562. Wolpert MK, Ruddon RW. A study on the mechanisms of resistance to nitrogen mustard (HN2) in Ehrlich ascites tumor cells: comparison of uptake of HN2-^{14}C. Cancer Res 1969;29:873.
563. Wright CG, Schaefer SD. Inner ear histopathology in patients treated with cis-platinum. Laryngoscope 1982;92:1408.
564. Wright JE, Tretyakov O, Ayash LJ, Elias A, Rosowsky A, Frei E. Analysis of 4-hydroxycyclophosphamide in human blood. Anal Biochem 1995;224.
565. Yamada K, Bremer AM, West CR, Ghoorah J, Park HC, Takita H. Intra-arterial BCNU therapy in the treatment of metastatic brain tumor from lung carcinoma. Cancer 1979;44:2000.
566. Yao K, Godwin AK, Ozols RF, Hamilton TC, O'Dwyer PJ. Variable baseline gamma-glutamylcysteine synthetase messenger RNA expression in peripheral mononuclear cells of cancer patients, and its induction by buthionine sulfoximine treatment. Cancer Res 1993;53:3662.
567. Young RC, Walton LA, Ellenberg SS, Homesley HD, Wilbanks GD, Decker DG, Miller A, Park R, Major F Jr. Adjuvant therapy in stage I and stage II epithelial ovarian cancer. N Engl J Med 1990;322:1021.
568. Yu X, Wu Z, Fenselau C. Covalent sequestration of melphalan by metallothionein alkylation of cysteines. Biochemistry 1995;34:3377.
569. Yuan ZM, Fenselau C, Dulik DM, Martin W, Emary WB, Brundrett RB, Colvin OM, Cotter RJ. Laser desorption electron impact: application to a study of the mechanism of conjugation of glutathione and cyclophosphamide. Anal Chem 1990;62:868.
570. Yung WK, Harris MI, Bruner JM, Feun LG. Intravenous BCNU and AZQ in patients with recurrent malignant gliomas. N Neurooncol 1989;7:237.
571. Zelazowski AJ, Garvey JS, Hoeschele JD. In vivo and in vitro binding of platinum to metallothionein. Arch Biochem Biophys 1984;229:246.
572. Zon G, Ludeman SM, Brandt JA, Boyd VL, Ozkan G, Egan W, Shao KL. NMR spectroscopic studies of intermediary metabolites of cyclophosphamide. A comprehensive kinetic analysis of the interconversion of cis- and trans-4-hydroxycyclophosphamide with aldophosphamide and the concomitant partitioning of aldophosphamide between irreversible fragmentation and reversible conjugation pathways. J Med Chem 1984;27:466.
573. Zwelling LA, Anderson T, Kohn KW. DNA-protein and DNA interstrand cross-linking by cis- and trans-platinum (II) diamminedichloride in L1210 mouse leukemia cells and relation to cytotoxicity. Cancer Res 1979;39:365.

CHAPTER 63

Anthracyclines and DNA Intercalators

CHARLES MYERS

Historical Background

DNA intercalators represent one of the most important classes of anticancer drugs, second only to the alkylating agents in their overall utility in clinical oncology (Table 63.1). The term *DNA intercalation* is used to describe the process by which drugs with a planar aromatic ring structure insert themselves in the space between the successive DNA base pairs. This binding is reversible and is stabilized by the hydrophobic interaction between the opposed aromatic rings of the drug and those of the adjacent DNA bases. In addition, the binding may be enhanced by ionic binding between the drug and charge centers on the DNA double helix. The first intercalator to reach wide usage in oncology was actinomycin D, followed by daunorubicin (5, 32). However, interest in this drug class really may be dated from the discovery of doxorubicin (Adriamycin). While actinomycin D and daunorubicin were antitumor agents with utility in a narrow spectrum of tumors, doxorubicin soon proved its value in a wide range of cancers, including such common neoplasms as carcinoma of the breast, ovary, and lung, as well as both lymphomas and sarcomas. This discovery was followed by much theoretic work on structural requirements for DNA intercalation and the development of ground rules for the rational synthesis of DNA intercalating agents (5, 32). It is ironic that while this rational approach has led to the development of agents such as amsacrine and mitoxantrone, none of these agents has matched the broad antitumor spectrum of doxorubicin (5, 32).

Mechanism of Action

Efforts to understand the basis for the antitumor activity of anthracyclines naturally included a focus on the impact of drug intercalation on DNA double helix structure (Table 63.2). Normally, the spacing between base pair planes in the DNA double helix is approximately 2.5Å. The planar aromatic chromophore of doxorubicin itself is approximately 2.5Å. Thus, intercalation of doxorubicin between base pair planes results in at least a doubling of the usual spacing between them. As a direct consequence of this spreading of base pair planes, the DNA helix undergoes unwinding. If the DNA exists in a supercoiled state, the supercoiling will also undergo a degree of unwinding. Thus, one invariant consequence of intercalation is an alteration of DNA topology. DNA intercalators may be characterized by a range of physical properties, including unwinding angle, binding affinity and the kinetics of DNA association and dissociation. Within a family of drugs, such as the anthracyclines, loss of activity may be observed when the ability to intercalate is lost. However, in general, the correlation between any of these physical constants and clinical utility of intercalators has been disappointing. Thus, DNA intercalators have been synthesized with much greater affinity for DNA than the intercalators in current clinical use, but these high-affinity binders almost always have been potent cytotoxins without a useful therapeutic index. For example, cyanomorpholino-doxorubicin binds covalently to the minor groove of DNA, and this results in a marked increase in cytotoxicity to tumor cells in tissue culture compared with doxorubicin, but the overall efficacy is not improved because toxicity also increases (26, 99).

For these reasons, much of the work in intercalator development has focused on the impact of intercalators on DNA function rather than its structure (32). These drugs were quickly shown to alter the function of DNA and RNA polymerases in a range of experimental models. The drug concentrations required to elicit these effects, however, were uniformly outside the clinically useful range. The only exception to this appears to be actinomycin D, where inhibition of RNA synthesis and, secondarily, protein synthesis appears to be the major mechanism of tumor cell kill, although this drug does trigger topoisomerase II–associated DNA breaks. A series of studies that documented effects of these drugs on nucleolar structure and in chromosomal organization followed. Again, however, a convincing relationship was never established between these effects and clinical utility of a given intercalator.

The degree of DNA supercoiling has been shown to play an important role in chromosomal structure and gene activity. As might be expected, the degree of DNA supercoiling therefore is under the control of enzymes. Because one major effect of all intercalators is to alter DNA supercoiling, it should not be surprising that this effect should trigger activity of the enzymes responsible for regulating DNA topology. One enzyme so affected is topoisomerase II (Fig. 63.1). This enzyme helps control the topology of DNA by allowing one strand to pass through the other (5, 101). This strand passing also is important in the decatenation of chromosomes after DNA replication but before mitosis. The steps in this process include first the establishment of a protein–DNA covalent bond between a tyrosine in the enzyme and phosphates in the backbone of the DNA helix (Fig. 63.1). This is followed by a double-stranded cut, with the cut strands held together by the protein–DNA covalent bond until strand passing has completed. This is followed by rejoining of the cut DNA strands and dissociation of the enzyme. In mammalian cells, one major function of topoisomerase II is the decatenation of daughter strands after DNA replication in preparation for mitosis. Amsacrine, the anthracyclines, and other intercalators have been shown to arrest this process after formation of the protein-associated double-strand cut (5, 101). The net effect is the formation of stable protein-associated double-stranded cuts. In addition to these intercalators, nonintercalating drugs such as etoposide and teniposide also cause similar topoisomerase II–associated

Table 63.1. DNA Intercalators in Clinical Use

Daunorubicin
Doxorubicin
Epirubicin
Idarubicin
Dactinomycin
Mitoxantrone
Amsacrine

Table 63.2. Characteristics Shared by Most Clinically Used DNA Intercalators

Possess at least three planar aromatic rings
Trigger topoisomerase II–associated DNA breaks
Exhibit redox metabolism
Cross-resistance based on *mdr* gene expression or altered topoisomerase II
High tissue-to-plasma ratios
Most intracellular drug is nuclear in location
Terminal half-life of 25 to 50 hours
Radiation sensitization

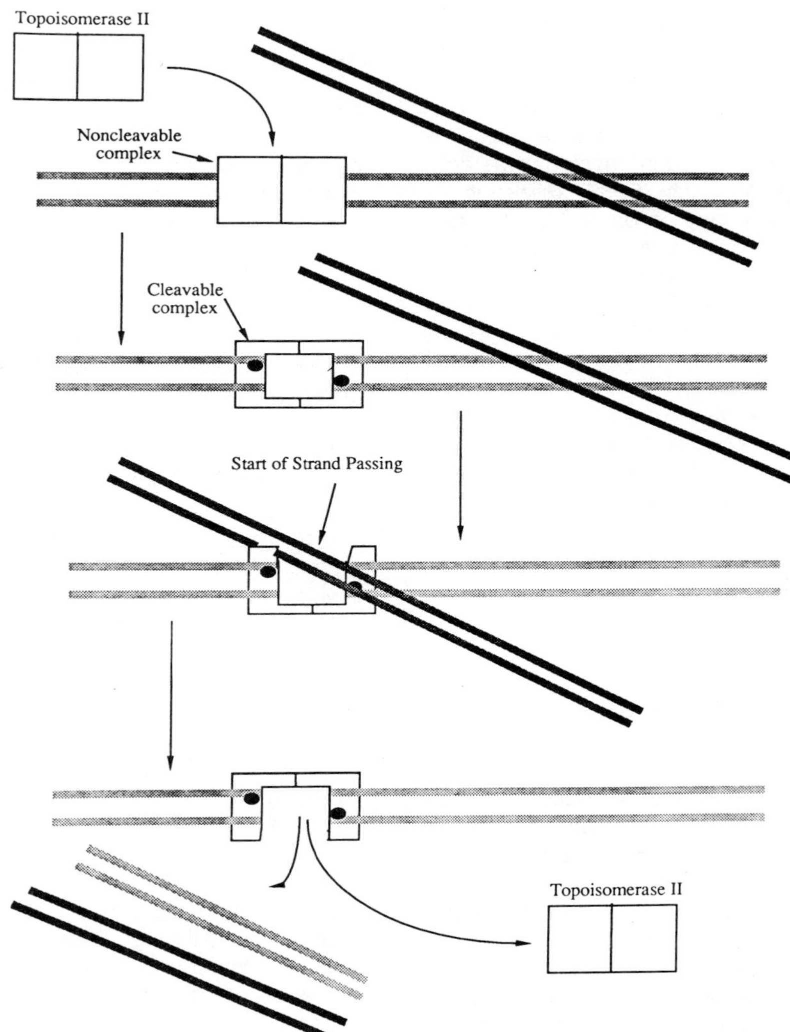

Figure 63.1. Action of topoisomerase II. The enzyme forms a covalent bond with DNA, first creating a noncleavable, then a cleavable, complex. DNA intercalators arrest the enzyme at this stage, creating protein-associated DNA breaks. Under normal conditions, topoisomerase II will then allow one strand to pass through the other and then reseal the break (see Figs. 64.1 and 64.2.).

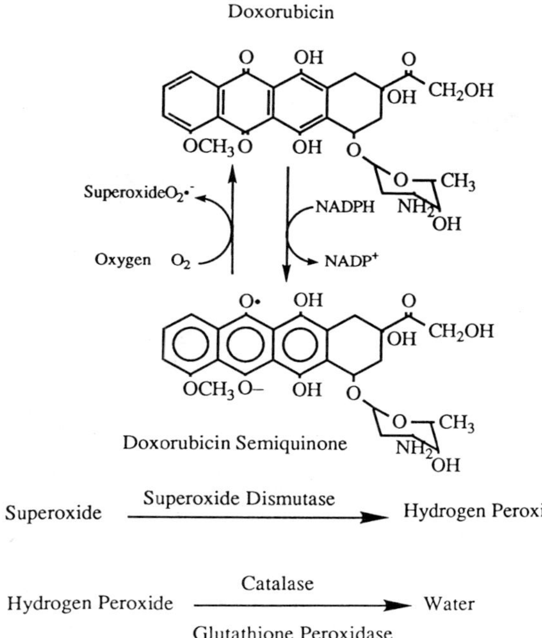

Figure 63.2. Doxorubicin redox cycle and detoxification pathway. The upper portion shows the one electron reduction of doxorubicin to its corresponding semiquinone. This drug-free radical then donates this extra electron to molecular-oxygen-generating superoxide. The lower portion shows the enzymatic pathways for detoxification of superoxide and hydrogen peroxide to water.

double-strand breaks (see Chapter 64). There now is strong evidence that topoisomerase-mediated DNA damage is one of the major mechanisms by which DNA intercalators kill cells. First, topoisomerase-mediated DNA damage is triggered by drug concentrations that are clinically relevant. Second, there is a good correlation between cytotoxicity and DNA damage. Third, cell lines that have altered topoisomerase II activity are resistant to a wide range of intercalating agents.

Most of the clinically useful intercalators also possess the capacity to undergo metabolism, which leads to the generation of free radicals; one of the most difficult issues in this field has been to determine the relative contribution of drug-induced free radical formation and DNA intercalation to both antitumor activity and host toxicity (Table 63.1) (32). There are several reasons for the free radical generating properties of these agents (71). Some, such as the anthracyclines, are quinones, which in general are easily reduced to the corresponding semiquinone free radicals. This chemistry has been best worked out for anthracyclines, where it leads to a rich range of products, including potential DNA alkylating structures and a range of reactive oxygen products including superoxide, hydrogen peroxide, and the hydroxyl radical (Fig. 63.2). These compounds are able to cause severe cell injury by damaging membranes. Oxygen radical damage to membranes can occur in at least two sites. First, oxygen radicals attack and destroy the double bonds in unsaturated fatty acids. Within the phospholipids of the cell membrane, the fatty acids at the 2 position are predominantly unsaturated and are the major site of free radical attack. This process is termed *lipid peroxidation*, in that one of the intermediate products is a lipid peroxide. There is a wide range of proteins that are critical to membrane structure. Some of these contain thiol groups very sensitive to oxidation, and these have been shown to also be destroyed by free radical attack. In addition, some of these agents form complexes with transition metal ions such as iron and copper, and the resulting metal complexes can act as redox catalysts. This has been demonstrated for the anthracyclines (Fig. 63.3). Finally, aromatic hydrocarbons frequently are disposed of by the microsomal mixed function oxidases (71). This process can result in the formation of quinones, diols, and epoxides, all of which can be chemically quite reactive with DNA and other cellular constituents and which thus can cause cell kill or sublethal injury leading to carcinogenesis. The latter has been demonstrated for 9-methoxyellipticine, one of the early intercalators introduced into clinical trial. There is general agreement that free radical formation forms the basis for anthracycline cardiac toxicity; this is reviewed in more detail later. For doxorubicin, there is strong evidence that free radical formation is involved in the ability of the drug to kill breast cancer cell lines in vitro (85). Two of the clinically useful DNA intercalators, amsacrine (75, 80) and mitoxantrone (60, 61, 74), are much less active in redox reactions, and this has been proposed as one of the reasons for the lower frequency of cardiomyopathy in patients treated with these agents.

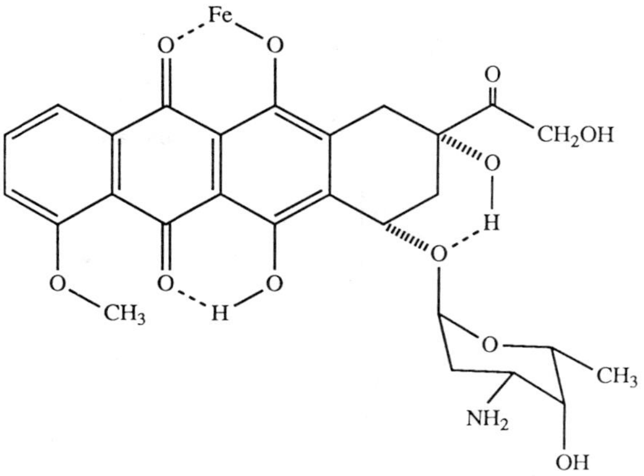

Figure 63.3. The structure of the doxorubicin–iron complex. Iron is bound to the oxygens attached to C-10 and C-11 of doxorubicin.

Cross-resistance between intercalators is a common event. Resistance to anthracyclines, mitoxantrone, amsacrine, and actinomycin D has been associated with expression of the *mdr* gene product (9, 57, 58). This membrane protein mediates drug efflux and is a common basis for cross-resistance (see Chapter 53). As might be expected from the importance of topoisomerase II in tumor cell kill, altered topoisomerase II also has been reported to be the basis for broad resistance to agents including intercalators (9).

Anthracyclines

The anthracyclines are second only to the alkylating agents in the breadth of their antitumor spectrum. Their dis-

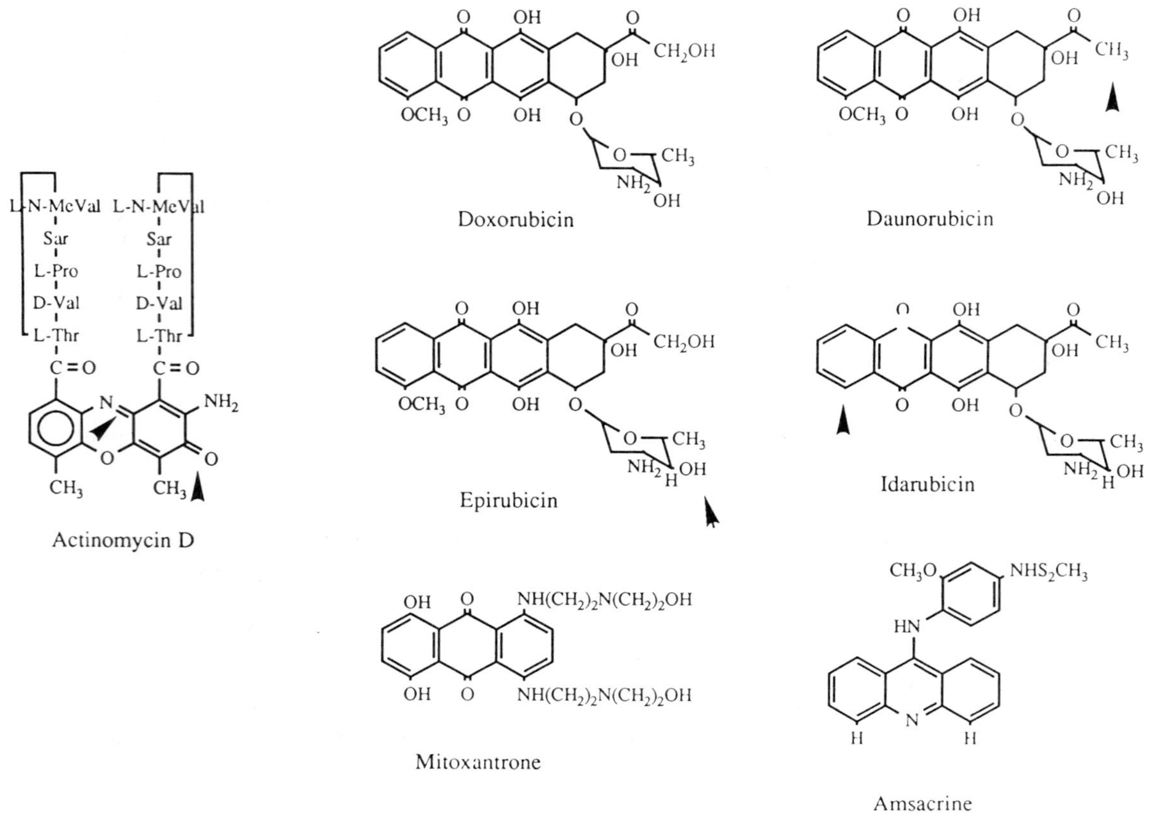

Figure 63.4. DNA intercalators in clinical use. *Arrows* on actinomycin D show sites of potential redox cycling. *Arrows* on the anthracyclines show step by step the changes in structure compared with doxorubicin.

covery and the initial description of their biology was made by Di Marco and colleagues (33) and Arcamore and colleagues (1). The initial clinical investigations were conducted by Bonadonna and colleagues (15a). Both are antibiotics produced by *Streptomyces* species. Daunorubicin was named for the Daunos tribe, native to the region where the original soil sample was obtained. The commercial name for doxorubicin, Adriamycin, derives from the soil sample that came from the Adriatic shore. The structures of the clinically used anthracyclines are shown in Figure 63.4. These drugs are composed of a four-ring chromophore attached to the amino sugar, daunosamine. The chromophore is composed of three planar rings, which are responsible for the ability of the drug to intercalate. In addition, the chromophore contains hydroxyquinone functionality on the middle two rings. It is this hydroxyquinone functionality that is responsible for the intense color of these compounds, their intense fluorescence, their free radical properties, and their ability to chelate transition metal ions (Fig. 63.3; see also Chapter 190) (48).

ROUTES OF ADMINISTRATION, SCHEDULE, AND PHARMACOKINETICS

The clinically used anthracyclines have poor or erratic oral bioavailability and thus traditionally are given parenterally. The only exception to this is idarubicin, which appears to have good bioavailability and be well tolerated orally (42, 89). When extravasated, the anthracyclines cause extensive local injury, which renders them appropriate only for intravenous use. Within 3 hours of administration, tissue levels exceed that of plasma, reaching tissue-to-plasma ratios as high as 100 (39, 87, 95). Within cells, greater than 80% of the drug is found within the nucleus (22). The anthracyclines are highly fluorescent, and cells exposed to anthracyclines typically show an intense nuclear fluorescence.

Thus, within a short time of administration, the bulk of the administered dose of drug in the body is bound to DNA, from which it is only slowly released. All anthracyclines undergo, to a variable degree, reduction of the side chain to the corresponding alcohol, daunorubicinol or doxorubicinol, within the liver (47, 98). In the case of daunorubicinol, the formation of this metabolite is rapid enough that plasma daunorubicinol concentrations usually exceed those of the parent daunorubicin. These events dominate the plasma pharmacokinetics of the anthracyclines. The plasma disappearance curve for the anthracyclines typically is sharply biphasic, with a rapid early distributive phase. This is followed by a terminal phase with half-lives on the order of 24 to 48 hours that is dominated by the slow release of drug bound to DNA (17, 19). During this time period, plasma levels usually are much lower than simultaneously measured tissue levels (87, 95).

Renal elimination, although enough to color the urine reddish, is not quantitatively significant for the anthracyclines. The liver is known to be a major site of metabolism, with the major metabolites being the reduction of the side-chain ketone to an alcohol. For epirubicin, hepatic glucuronidation also appears to be important (79). Despite the major role played by the liver in drug clearance, it is not clear that drug dosages need to be reduced in the face of abnormal liver functions.

Anthracyclines have been given by a range of schedules, including bolus administration every 28 days, once a week, daily for 3 to 4 days and by continuous infusion for various times (55, 90). The tolerated drug dose appears to be relatively independent of schedule. For example, 60 mg/m^2 of doxorubicin results in similar overall toxicity whether given by bolus or by 96-hour infusion (55). The specific dose-limiting toxicity does shift, however. With bolus administration of doxorubicin, dose-limiting toxicity generally is myelosuppression, while with a 96-hour infusion, mucositis becomes more of a problem. There is evidence from clinical trials to suggest that prolonged infusions may be less cardiotoxic than large, monthly, bolus-dose administration (55, 90, 95). The effect of schedule on antitumor activity is less clear. Available evidence does not suggest a difference of response rate in breast cancer if the drug is given by either monthly or weekly bolus or 96-hour infusion.

While dose intensification has been extensively applied to the use of alkylating agents, anthracyclines have been subjected to only limited study (56a). One trial suggested that with co-administration of G-CSF, it may be possible to administer much larger doses of doxorubicin: patients with breast cancer tolerated as much as 180 mg/m^2 of doxorubicin every 2 weeks as a single agent with a response rate of 80% (18, 19).

PATTERNS OF TOXICITY

The major toxicities of the anthracyclines include myelosuppression, mucositis, hair loss, cardiac toxicity, and severe local injury on extravasation.

Cardiac Toxicity

Of the possible toxicities, cardiac toxicity has been the most studied. As a result, the mechanism of this side effect is known, and means are available for its prevention.

The cardiac toxicity of the anthracyclines can manifest in two distinct clinical syndromes. The drugs can precipitate an acute myocarditis-pericarditis syndrome in which the patient develops rapidly progressive heart failure and arrhythmias that can be associated with fever and pericarditis. This syndrome can appear after only 1 to 3 doses of doxorubin and can result in sudden death within 7 to 14 days after a dose of an anthracycline. The second manifestation of cardiac toxicity is a gradual loss of myocardial function with cumulative dosage of anthracycline. Endocardial biopsies performed after various total dosages of doxorubicin suggest a linear relationship between total dose administered and the amount of cardiac tissue lost (14); however, the incidence of clinically evident congestive heart failure increases exponentially with total dose of anthracycline administered (96, 97). This may result from the fact that the heart has physiologic reserves that must be exceeded before clinically evident congestive heart failure is manifest. Each anthracycline appears to have its own unique quantitative relationship between total dose and degree of myocardial damage so that 550 mg/m^2 of doxorubicin is equivalent to 900 mg/m^2 of daunorubicin, both giving an approximate risk for congestive heart failure of 5% (96, 97). Each anthracycline also differs in its potency as an anticancer agent and when this is taken into consideration, the clinically used anthracyclines appear to be equally cardiotoxic when given at doses of equivalent therapeutic effectiveness.

In the face of this information, it has been customary to limit the total dose of anthracycline administered. These limits usually have been set at a risk of 5% or the equivalent of 550 mg/m^2 of doxorubicin. This practice has been useful in limiting the risk of cardiac toxicity. However, there is considerable individual variation in susceptibility to anthracycline cardiac toxicity, with some individuals developing toxicity at total doxorubicin doses below 300 mg/m^2 while others are without symptoms at doxorubicin doses above 800 mg/m^2 (14, 88). It is clear that optimum practice requires monitoring each patient for cardiac toxicity and individualizing the use of the drug. Two techniques have been accepted for this purpose. Endocardial biopsies may be made and used to quantify the degree of cardiac damage pathologically: a useful alternate to this is to measure the ejection fraction with an ECG-gated blood pool scan (14, 88) (see Chapter 181).

The role of this redox chemistry in anthracycline cardiac toxicity is well worked out and illustrative of how drug-induced free radical damage can occur. The flavin-centered reductases are the enzyme family most commonly associated with reduction of the anthracyclines to their corresponding semiquinone free radicals (4). These enzymes include cytochrome P450 reductase, xanthine oxidase, and mitochondrial NADH oxidase. Cardiac tissue is a rich source of these enzymes with doxorubicin free radical formation being demonstrated in both cardiac cytosol and mitochondrial fractions (34–36). However, these enzymes are so widely distributed in normal tissue that their presence or absence is not sufficient to explain the unusual sensitivity of cardiac tissue. Superoxide and hydrogen peroxide are generated at many points in normal intermediary aerobic metabolism. As a result, all aerobic organisms possess enzymatic machinery to detoxify these reactive oxygen species. The detoxification pathway involves the sequential conversion of each reactive species to water (Fig. 63.2). The first step in this process is the conversion of superoxide to hydrogen peroxide by the enzyme superoxide dismutase. The second step is the conversion of hydrogen peroxide to water. This step can be accomplished by either catalase or the enzyme glutathione peroxidase. The latter uses the thiol-containing tripeptide, glutathione, to reduce hydrogen peroxide to water. Cardiac tissue is relatively unusual in that it contains very little catalase and seems to depend solely on glutathione peroxidase for the reduction of hydrogen peroxide to water (37). However, following the administration of doxorubicin, there is a rapid reduction in glutathione peroxidase activity (37). Thus, at the same time that doxorubicin initiates the formation of both superoxide and hydrogen peroxide, it abrogates the major means available for cardiac tissue to dispose of these reactive oxygen species.

The first indication that this picture was not the complete explanation for anthracycline cardiac toxicity came from the observation that agents which are active free radical scavengers, such as *N*-acetylcysteine, were not able to block chronic cardiac toxicity in humans (70). The missing factor proved to be the interaction of doxorubicin and other anthracyclines with iron (70). These drugs are powerful chelators of iron, with measured affinity constants of 10^{33}. In addition, the resulting iron complexes are able to bind to cell membranes and DNA and cause extensive local free radical damage through hydroxyl radical formation (43, 49–51, 68, 69, 72, 73). Because hydroxyl radical formation occurs in the immediate vicinity of the biologic target, general free radical scavengers such as *N*-acetylcysteine and vitamin E are destined to be inefficient. Instead, the only successful approach appears to make the iron unavailable to the anthracycline (28–31, 50, 94). ICRF-187, ADR 529, or Zinocord is an EDTA derivative in which the metal chelating structures of EDTA have been fused into amide rings, creating a nonchelating nonpolar drug that readily diffuses throughout the body (Fig. 63.5). In the presence of the doxorubicin–iron complex, dexrazoxane undergoes prompt hydrolysis to the corresponding carboxylamine, which accepts the iron from the anthracycline–iron complex with the regeneration of free doxorubicin (52, 53). As a result, dexrazoxane is effective in preventing iron-mediated free radical damage initiated by doxorubicin (88).

The pathology and physiology of anthracycline cardiac toxicity is distinctive. In the normal cardiac contractile cycle, the wave of electrical depolarization passes down the sarcoplasmic reticulum. This results in release of calcium bound to the sarcoplasmic reticulum, which then diffuses to the contractile elements and triggers mechanical contraction by activating a calcium-dependent ATPase. The subsequent relaxation involves rebinding of the calcium by the sarcoplasmic reticulum. The sarcoplasmic reticulum has been shown to be a site of avid anthracycline free radical formation (34–36). This free radical formation results in oxidative damage to the sarcoplasmic reticulum membrane and thus defective calcium binding (84). The result is defective relaxation following contraction and an elevated level of free calcium (84). As with skeletal muscles, heart muscle contains proteases activated by elevated calcium. This sequence of events results in the loss of muscle fibers and, consequently, myocardial contractility seen following anthracycline administration. In addition, it explains the pathologic hallmarks of this toxicity which includes dilation of the sarcoplasmic reticulum and fragmentation and loss of myofibrils (14).

At present, there are two approaches that appear to successfully limit the severity of anthracycline cardiac toxicity. First, the cardiac toxicity of these drugs appears to relate to peak drug level; thus, bolus administration every 4 weeks results in a greater risk of cardiac toxicity than weekly bolus administration or 96-hour infusions (55, 90). The second approach depends on co-administration of dexrazoxane. This analogue of EDTA is an effective chelator of transition metal

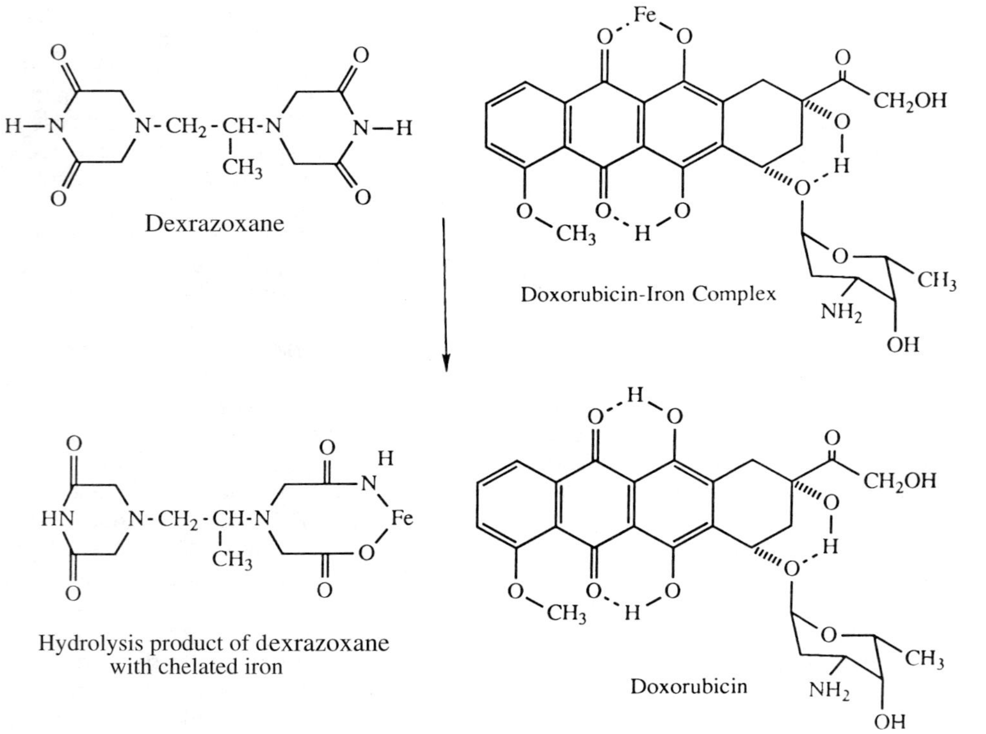

Figure 63.5. The reaction by which dexrazoxane (formerly ADR 529 or ICRF-187) removes iron chelated to doxorubicin.

ions such as iron and copper because these transition metal ions are critical catalysts of oxygen free radical reactions. It has been proposed that dexrazoxane lessens the cardiac toxicity of the anthracyclines by limiting free radical damage to the heart. At present, it is not clear which approach is more effective.

Myelosuppression

In clinical practice, the most common dose-limiting toxicity of the anthracyclines is granulocytopenia. Although lymphopenia, thrombocytopenia, and anemia also occur, they are less severe and rarely dose limiting. While the precise mechanism of this hematopoietic toxicity has not been determined, dexrazoxane did not alter the lymphocytopenia and granulocytopenia; thus, this mechanism has been assumed not to be a result of free radical formation by the drug but rather a consequence of DNA intercalation (88). Clinical trial has demonstated that G-CSF may be highly effective in diminishing the duration of granulocytopenia, thereby allowing a doubling in the maximum tolerated dose intensity of doxorubicin (see Chapter 82), but not the total dose, which is determined by cardiotoxicity (18, 19).

Mucositis

Drugs of this family can cause inflammation and ulceration of oropharynx, esophagitis, colitis, and occasionally, vulvitis. When doxorubicin is given by 96-hour infusion rather than bolus administration, mucositis rather than hematopoietic toxicity may become dose limiting (55, 90).

Extravasation Injury

Leakage of currently used anthracyclines into the subcutaneous tissues results in the development of local tissue necrosis, which heals only with difficulty (Fig. 63.6) (39). In severe cases, the resulting ulcer can continue to extend over many months, resulting in severe disability and even loss of a limb. This process appears to depend on the fact that the drug binds tightly to the subcutaneous tissues, causing local injury. Following cell death, the drug is released and binds to the next tissue layer, and the process thus repeats itself. A wide range of therapeutic approaches have been advocated, ranging from cold compresses to wide surgical excision of involved tissue followed by skin grafting. However, none of these proposals has been subjected to rigorous clinical trial. The best approach appears to be prevention by ensuring that the drug is administered through a freely flowing, newly placed, intravenous line or an indwelling central venous catheter.

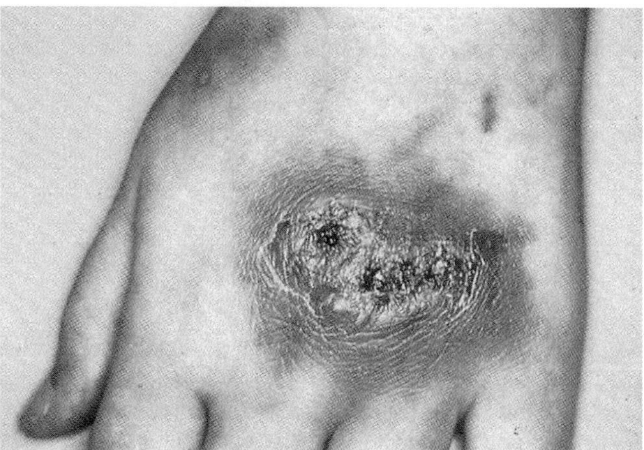

Figure 63.6. Necrosis and inflammation from extravasation of doxorubicin.

Hair Loss

The mechanism by which anthracyclines cause hair loss, a nearly universal toxicity, is unknown. Local scalp hypothermia has been advocated but has not seen wide use.

ANTITUMOR SPECTRUM

The most important activities for doxorubicin are in breast cancer, sarcoma, Hodgkin's and non-Hodgkin's lymphoma, pediatric solid tumors, myeloma, and acute lymphocytic and myeloid leukemias. It has definite, albeit less compelling, activity in stomach, small cell, ovary, endometrial, transitional cell, and thyroid carcinomas, as well as carcinoid and malignant thymoma. In addition, liposome-encapsulated doxorubicin has shown promising activity in AIDS-related Kaposi's sarcoma (51b). Doxorubicin is uncommonly used alone, but it is a component of many combination chemotherapy regimens, particularly with cyclophosphamide, cisplatin, the vinca alkaloids, fluorouracil, or methotrexate.

Daunorubicin currently is used in combination with cytosine arabinoside in the treatment of acute myeloid leukemia and with vincristine and prednisone in acute lymphocytic leukemia.

Idarubicin has been approved for the same indications as daunorubicin because of a series of randomized clinical trials indicating superior results with idarubicin compared with daunorubicin in the treatment of leukemia (3, 11, 12, 23, 24). In addition, idarubicin has shown activity in non-Hodgkin's lymphomas. Orally administered idarubicin has proven active in breast cancer (7, 8, 42). Its value for this indication as compared to epirubicin or doxorubicin is not clear, except for the availability of an oral route of administration. Activity also has been seen in non-small-cell carcinoma of the lung (1).

Epirubicin, which is widely used in Europe, has antitumor activity similar to doxorubicin in breast cancer (77). Its activity against other tumors is less clearly defined, but responses have been seen in acute leukemias, sarcomas, and carcinomas of the lung and ovary (6, 15, 25, 66, 67). It has been claimed to possess reduced cardiac toxicity compared with doxorubicin, and this assertion has been contested (66, 67). Until this issue is settled, epirubicin seems to offer no significant advantage over doxorubicin.

Methoxymorpholinodoxorubicin, a new analogue that is significantly more potent than doxorubicin, is undergoing phase II trials in 1995.

INTERACTIONS

Anthracyclines can sensitize normal tissues to radiation damage (32). This effect appears to be fairly general but is a particular problem in certain treatment situations. First, doxorubicin has been shown to increase the severity of radiation pneumonitis. Second, exposure of the heart to greater than 2,000 cGy effectively doubles the cardiac toxicity of a given cumulative dose of doxorubicin (13). Third, doxorubicin has been shown to worsen the severity of radiation damage to oral and esophageal mucosa. Fourth, anthracyclines can trigger radiation recall in the skin with resultant erythema and folliculitis.

The anthracyclines may be readily co-administered with most other anticancer drugs without significant problem—a factor that has played a role in their wide use in combination chemotherapy. In experimental animals and tissue culture, exposure to doxorubicin and drugs such as BCNU or acetaminophen, which deplete tissue thiols, has been reported to cause acute death of liver cells. To date, this interaction has not been noted clinically.

Dactinomycin (Actinomycin D)

Dactinomycin consists of two symmetric polypeptide chains attached to a phenoxazone, a planar three ring system (Fig. 63.4). As might be expected, it is the planar aromatic phenoxazone ring system that is responsible for the ability of this compound to intercalate DNA. Dactinomycin exhibits considerable DNA sequence specificity, with the most stable DNA complexes forming with the sequence dATGCAT (21, 64, 81, 91). This binding appears to be highly effective at blocking RNA synthesis, with elongation of RNA strands more affected than chain initiation or release. As with the anthracyclines, dactinomycin also exhibits redox chemistry (46, 81, 82). In this case, the drug possesses a quinoneimine functionality that can be reduced to the corresponding semiquinone. Little is known about the consequences of this reduction, but antitumor activity in a series of dactinomycin analogues correlated with redox potential rather than DNA binding affinity.

ROUTES OF ADMINISTRATION, SCHEDULE, AND PHARMACOKINETICS

Dactinomycin may only be administered intravenously. The drug crosses cell membranes by free diffusion, although in the presence of the *mdr* gene product, the drug is susceptible to active efflux (16). Within cells, most of the drug is tightly bound to DNA. As with the anthracyclines, DNA binding dominates the pharmacokinetics of actinomycin D. The initial phase of actinomycin D plasma clearance involves rapid distribution of the drug to tissues (10, 93). The second phase has a half-life of 36 hours and is determined by the slow dissociation of the DNA-bound drug. While no metabolites have been detected, urinary and biliary clearance of parent drug accounts for less than half the administered dose. From this, our knowledge of the pharmacokinetics of actinomycin D clearly is far from complete. The usual clinical dose is 10 to 15 μg/kg/d for 5 days.

PATTERNS OF TOXICITY

Dactinomycin causes nausea, vomiting, diarrhea, mucositis, and alopecia. The most common dose-limiting toxicity is granulocytopenia and thrombocytopenia, with a nadir 10 to 14 days following drug administration. As with the anthracyclines, extravasation of actinomycin D is associated with severe local injury.

ANTITUMOR SPECTRUM

At present, the use of actinomycin D is limited to pediatric cancers. Useful activity is seen in Wilms' tumor, rhabdomyosarcoma, Ewing's sarcoma, and neuroblastoma and has been described in gestational choriocarcinoma and embryonal carcinoma (44, 63, 92, 100).

INTERACTIONS

Dactinomycin causes radiation sensitization (27, 64). In addition, it can trigger a recall phenomenon at sites of previous radiation therapy. This can result in severe skin reactions or compromise of organ function. Corticosteroids have been used to treat these complications.

Mitoxantrone

Mitoxantrone (Fig. 63.4) is a member of the anthracenedione family of DNA intercalators. This drug class is completely synthetic in origin and was developed as part of the search for anthracycline analogues. As with the anthracyclines, mitoxantrone has a chromophore composed of three planar aromatic rings. Also, as with the anthracyclines, the chromophore is a hydroxyquinone. In place of the daunosamine sugar characteristic of the anthracyclines, mitoxantrone has two identical aminoalkyl side chains. As a result, mitoxantrone possesses the ability to intercalate into DNA and to trigger topoisomerase II–dependent DNA cleavage, and this probably is the mechanism of tumor cell kill (41). While it can undergo reduction to the corresponding semiquinone, the redox potential for this reaction is such that it is not favored (60, 61, 74). In addition, while mitoxantrone is able to bind copper and iron as can the anthracyclines, the resultant complexes appear to be unable to catalyze free radical damage to cell membranes. As a result, mitoxantrone does not cause lipid peroxidation in cardiac tissue and is less cardiotoxic than doxorubicin (54).

ROUTES OF ADMINISTRATION, SCHEDULE, AND PHARMACOKINETICS

Mitoxantrone appears to enter cells by free diffusion. Inside cells, most of the drug exists bound to DNA. As with the anthracyclines, DNA binding dominates the pharmacokinetics of mitoxantrone. The initial distribution of the drug occurs with a half-life of 1 to 2 hours followed by a terminal half-life of 23 to 42 hours, limited by the slow dissociation of the drug from DNA40. Parent drug eliminated in urine and stool accounts for less than 30% of the drug administered. While the metabolism of this drug is incompletely described, side-chain oxidation to inactive mono- and dicarboxylic acid metabolites has been described. Common schedules of administration appear to be patterned after those used for the anthracyclines. For acute myeloid leukemia, a dose of 12 mg/m^2/d for 3 days has been used in combination with cytosine arabinoside. For carcinoma of the breast, the typical schedule is 12 to 14 mg/m^2 once every 3 weeks. In lymphocytic neoplasms, 10 to 15 mg/m^2/d for 3 days in association with vincristine and prednisone have been used.

PATTERNS OF TOXICITY

Dose-limiting toxicity is granulocytopenia, with recovery typically complete by day 14 after usual doses. The drug also can cause thrombocytopenia, nausea, and vomiting. Because of its intense blue color, the drug can cause bluish discoloration of the sclera, fingernails, and urine. In contrast to the anthracyclines, extravasation injury is uncommon. While cardiac toxicity has been seen in patients receiving mitoxantrone, this has been most common in patients who were previously treated with doxorubicin or daunorubicin (54). Previous chest-wall irradiation and underlying cardiac disease are other risk factors associated with cardiac toxicity of mitoxantrone. Liver injury also can occur, and this has been associated with lipid peroxidation and other in vitro evidence of free radical injury (40, 65). The enzymatic basis for such free radical formation is not clear. Mucositis is similar to the anthracyclines, but alopecia, nausea, and vomiting are less.

ANTITUMOR SPECTRUM

Antitumor activity of mitoxantrone appears to be limited to breast cancer, leukemias, and lymphomas.

INTERACTIONS

Synergy between cytosine arabinoside and mitoxantrone has been reported in acute myeloid leukemia.

Amsacrine

Amsacrine (m-AMSA) is a derivative of acridine and thus, as with mitoxantrone, is a totally synthetic drug. Again, as with other drugs in this family, the ability of this drug to intercalate into DNA depends on the presence of a three-ring planar aromatic chromophore (Fig. 63.4). This drug is effective at triggering topoisomerase II–dependent protein-associated DNA breaks; available evidence strongly suggests that this is the mechanism of tumor cell kill (59). While this drug can cause cardiac toxicity, this side effect likely is not the result of drug-induced free radical production, because amsacrine is a poor substrate for one electron reduction (2, 45, 83). Hypokalemia potentiates the cardiac arrhythmias. Evidence exists that drug metabolism may play a part in maximizing DNA breakage, but a responsible metabolite has yet to be identified (102).

ROUTES OF ADMINISTRATION, SCHEDULE, AND PHARMACOKINETICS

As with the other DNA intercalators, m-AMSA rapidly enters cells, where the bulk of the drug may be found bound to DNA. As a result, tissue concentrations are typically 3 to 10 times higher than those of plasma. The pharmacokinetics of m-AMSA are very different from the other drugs in this class (20, 56, 75, 76). The terminal half-life is on the order of 4 to 8 hours rather than the 25- to 50-hour half-lives found for the anthracyclines dactinomycin and mitoxantrone. In addition, there is strong evidence that glutathione conjugation by glutathione transferase plays an important role in drug inactivation (75, 80). First, drugs that inhibit the steps in glutathione conjugation significantly alter drug clearance. Second, in rodents, 70 to 80% of the administered dose appears in the bile, and 70–80% of the drug in the bile appears as a glutathione conjugate. In addition, drug administration results in sufficient glutathione consumption to cause depletion of hepatic glutathione. Finally, an m-AMSA resistant breast cancer cell line exhibited a nearly 10-fold increase in the expression of glutathione transferase π in the absence of expression of the *mdr* gene product. Because of the importance of hepatic metabolism, the dose of this drug should be adjusted in the presence of liver function abnormalities (75, 80). The usual dose is 120 mg/m^2 IV daily for 5 days. In addition, 75 to 150 mg/m^2 have been administered as a continuous infusion over 72 hours without any significant alteration in the pattern of toxicity or loss in antitumor efficacy.

PATTERNS OF TOXICITY

The most common dose-limiting toxicities of m-AMSA are mucositis and myelosupression with relative platelet sparing. Alopecia, as well as mild to moderate nausea and vomiting also are common. Hepatic toxicity has been noted but usually is limited to asymptomatic transaminitis. This may be the consequence of the extensive hepatic metabolism of m-AMSA (75, 80). Amsacrine also can cause cardiac toxicity (2, 45, 78, 83). This can manifest as two distinct syndromes. First, patients who have had previous exposure to anthracyclines can have a cardiomyopathy precipitated by m-AMSA administration. Second, the drug can result in a wide range of arrhythmias. The risk of the latter appears to markedly diminish if normal serum potassium levels are maintained.

ANTITUMOR SPECTRUM

This drug has its major use in the treatment of the myeloid leukemias. Activity also has been noted in a range of lymphomas, but it has not seen wide use in their treatment.

INTERACTIONS

The drug–drug interactions with m-AMSA have not been clearly defined in humans. However, in view of the clear documentation of the role of hepatic metabolism in drug clearance, caution should be exercised with co-administration of this drug with certain other agents. In animal models, cimetidine and phenobarbital, two drugs that alter microsomal mixed function oxidases, clearly alter m-AMSA clearance

(75,80). Buthionine sulfoximine, an agent that blocks glutathione synthesis, also alters m-AMSA clearance. Co-administration of m-AMSA with drugs that alter hepatic glutathione should be approached with caution. The nitrosoureas block glutathione reduction and thus are potentially a problem. In addition, acetaminophen is well known to deplete hepatic glutathione and should be used with caution.

References

1. Arcamone F, Cassinelli G, Fantini G, Grein A, Orezzi P, Pol C, Spalla C. Adriamycin, 14-hydroxy daunomycin, a new antitumor antibiotic from *S. peucetius* var. *Caesius*. Biotechnol Bioeng 1969;11:1101.

1a. Ardizzoni A, Pennucci C, Fusco V, Gulisano M, Bonavia M, Pronzato P, De Palma M, Serrano J, Rosso R. Oral chemotherapy for poor risk small-cell lung cancer patients with combined idarubicin and etoposide. Anticancer Res 1989;9:937.

2. Arlin Z, Mehta R, Feldman E, Sullivan P, Pucillo A. Amsacrine treatment of patients with supraventricular arrhythmias and acute leukemia. Cancer Chemother Pharmacol 1987;19:163.

3. Arlin ZA. Idarubicin in acute leukemia: an effective new therapy for the future. Semin Oncol 1989;16:35.

4. Bachur NR, Gordon SL, Gee MV. Anthracycline antibiotic augmentation of microsomal electron transport and free radical formation. Mol Pharmacol 1977;13:901.

5. Baguley BC. DNA intercalating anti-tumour agents. Anticancer Drug Des 1991;6:1.

6. Banham SW, Henderson AF, Bicknell S, Hughes J, Milroy R, Monie RD. High dose epirubicin chemotherapy in untreated poorer prognosis small cell lung cancer. Respir Med 1990;84:241.

7. Bastholt L, Dalmark M, Jakobsen A, Gadeberg CC, Sandberg E, Mouridsen HT. Oral idarubicin in the treatment of advanced breast cancer. Acta Oncol 1989;28:893.

8. Bastholt L, Dalmark M, Jakobsen A, Gadeberg CC, Sandberg E, Mouridsen H. Weekly oral idarubicin in postmenopausal women with advanced breast cancer. A phase II study. Acta Oncol 1990;29:143.

9. Beck WT. Mechanisms of multidrug resistance in human tumor cells. The role of P-glycoprotein, DNA topoisomerase II, and other factors. Cancer Treat Rev 1990;17(suppl a):11.

10. Benjamin RS, Burgass MA. A pharmacokinetically based phase 1–2 study of single dose actinomycin D (NSC-3053). Cancer Treat Rep 1976;60:289.

11. Berman E, Heller G, Santorsa J, McKenzie S, Gee T, Kempin S, Gulati S, Andreeff M, Kolitz J, Gabrilove J, et al. Results of a randomized trial comparing idarubicin and cytosine arabinoside with daunorubicin and cytosine arabinoside in adult patients with newly diagnosed acute myelogenous leukemia. Blood 1991;77:1666.

12. Berman E, Raymond V, Daghestani A, Arlin ZA, Gee TS, Kempin S, Hancock C, Williams L, Stevens YW, Clarkson BD, Young C. 4-demethoxydaunorubicin (idarubicin) in combination with 1-beta-D-arabinofuranosylcytosine in the treatment of relapsed or refractory acute leukemia. Cancer Res 1989;49:477.

13. Billingham ME, Bristow MR, Glatstein E, Mason JW, Masek MA, Daniels JR. Adriamycin cardiotoxicity: endomyocardial biopsy evidence of enhancement by irradiation. Am J Surg Pathol 1977;1:17.

14. Billingham ME, Mason JW, Bristow MR, Daniels JR. Anthracycline cardiomyopathy monitored by morphologic changes. Cancer Treat Rep 1978;62:865.

15. Blackstein M, Eisenhaver EA, Wierzbick R, Yoshida S. Epirubicin in extensive small-cell lung cancer: a phase II study in previously untreated patients: a National Cancer Institute of Canada Clinical Trials Group Study (see comments). J Clin Oncol 1990;8:385.

15a. Bonadonna G, Monfardini S. De Lena M, Fossati-Bellani F. Clinical evaluation of Adriamycin, a new antitumor antibiotic. Br Med J 1969;3:503.

16. Bowen D, Goldman ID. The relationship among transport, intracellular binding, and inhibition of RNA synthesis by actinomycin D in Ehrlich ascites tumor cells in vitro. Cancer Res 1975;35:3054.

17. Brenner DE, Wiernik PH, Wesley M, Bachur NR. Acute doxorubicin toxicity. Relationship to pretreatment liver function, response, and pharmacokinetics in patients with acute nonlymphocytic leukemia. Cancer 1984;53:1042.

18. Bronchud MH, Howell A, Crowther D, Hopwood P, Souzal L, Dexter TM. The use of granulocyte colony-stimulating factor to increase the intensity of treatment with doxorubicin in patients with advanced breast and ovarian cancer. Br J Cancer 1989;60:121.

19. Bronchud MH, Margison JM, Howell A, Lind M, Lucas SD, Wilkinson PM. Comparative pharmacokinetics of escalating doses of doxorubicin in patients with metastatic breast cancer. Cancer Chemother Pharmacol 1990;25:435.

20. Brons PP, Wessels JM, Linssen PC, Haanen C, Speth PA. Determination of amsacrine in human nucleated hematopoietic cells. J Chromatogr 1987;422:175.

21. Brown S, Mullis K, Levenson C, Shafer RH. Aqueous solution structure of an intercalated actinomycin D-dATGCAT complex by two dimensional and one dimensional proton NMR. Biochemistry 1984;23:403.

22. Calendi E, DiMarco A, Reggiani M, Scarpinato B, Valentini L. On physico-chemical interactions between daunomycin and nucleic acids. Biochim Biophys Acta 1965;103:25.

23. Carella AM, Berman E, Maraone MP, Ganzina F. Idarubicin in the treatment of acute leukemias. An overview of preclinical and clinical studies. Haematologica 1990;75:159.

24. Carella AM, Pungolino E, Piatti G, Gaozza E, Nati S, Spriano M, Giordano D, D'Amico T, Damasio E. Idarubicin in combination with intermediate-dose cytarabine in the treatment of refractory or relapsed acute leukemias. Eur J Haematol 1989;43:309.

25. Casadio M, Lelli G, Giordani S, Beltri B, Blotta A, Busutti L, Ramini R, Falcone F, Pannuti F. Small cell bronchogenic carcinoma: a cyclical alternating combination of epirubicin plus cisplatin and cyclophosphamide plus etoposide. J Chemother 1990;2:199.

26. Cramer SC, Rhodes RH, Acton EM, Tokes ZA. Neurotoxicity and dermatotoxicity of cyanomorpholinyl Adriamycin. Cancer Chemother Pharmacol 1989;23:71.

27. D'Angio GJ, Farber S, Maddock CL. Potentiation of x-ray effects by actinomycin D. Radiology 1973;73:175.

28. Demant EJF. Binding of adriamycin-FE^{3+} complex to membrane phospholipids. Eur J Biochem 1984;142:571.

29. Demant EJF. Mobilization of ferritin-iron by Adriamycin. FEBS Lett 1984;176:97.

30. Demant EJF. Transfer of ferritin-bound iron to Adriamycin. FEBS Lett 1984;176:97.

31. Demant EJF, Nørskov-Lauritsen N. Binding of transferrin-iron by Adriamycin at acidic pH. FEBS Lett 1986;196:321.

32. Denny WA. DNA-intercalating ligands as anti-cancer drugs: prospects for future design. Anticancer Drug Des 1989;4:241.

33. DiMarco A, Gaetani M, Orezzi P, Scarpinato B, Silvestrini R, Soldati M, Dasdia T, Valentini L. Daunomycin, a new antibiotic of the rhodomycin group. Nature 1964;201:706.

34. Doroshow JH. Anthracycline antibiotic-stimulated superoxide, hydrogen peroxide, and hydroxyl radical production by NADH dehydrogenase. Cancer Res 1983;43:4543.

35. Doroshow JH. Effect of anthracycline antibiotics on oxygen radical formation in rat heart. Cancer Res 1983;43:460.

36. Doroshow JH, Davies KJ. Comparative cardiac oxygen radical metabolism by anthracycline antibiotics, mitoxantrone, bisantrene, 4′-(9-acridinylamino)-methanesulfon-m-anisidide, and neocarzinostatin. Biochem Pharmacol 1983;32:2935.

37. Doroshow JH, Locker GY, Myers CE. The enzymatic defenses of the mouse heart against reactive metabolites. J Clin Invest 1980;65:128.

38. Dorr RT. Antidotes to vesicant endomyocardial extravasations. Blood Rev 1990;4:41.

39. Dorr RT, Dordal MS, Koenig LM, Taylor CW, McCloskey TM. High levels of doxorubicin in the tissues of a patient experiencing extravasation during a 4-day infusion. Cancer 1989;64:2462.

40. Duthie SJ, Grant MH. The toxicity of menadione and mitoxantrone in human liver-derived Hep G2 hepatoma cells. Biochem Pharmacol 1989;38:1247.

41. Ehninger G, Schuler U, Proksch B, Zeller KP, Blanz J. Pharmacokinetics and metabolism of mitoxantrone. A review. Clin Pharmacokinet 1990;18:365.

42. Elbaek K, Ebbehoj E, Jakobsen A, Juul P, Rasmussen SN, Bastholt L, Dalmark M, Steiness E. Pharmacokinetics of oral idarubicin in breast cancer patients with reference to antitumor activity and side effects. Clin Pharmacol Ther 1989;45:627.

43. Eliot H, Gianni L, Myers C. Oxidative destruction of DNA by Adriamycin-iron complex. Biochemistry 1984;23:928.

44. Farber S. Chemotherapy in the treatment of leukemia and Wilm's tumor. JAMA 1966;198:826.

45. Feldman EJ, Arlin ZA, Sullivan P, Engelking C. Preventing amsacrine-induced cardiac arrhythmias. (Letter) J Clin Oncol 1987;5:2041.

46. Flitter WD, Mason RP. The enzymatic reduction of actinomycin D to a free radical species. Arch Biochem Biophys 1988;267:632.

47. Forrest GL, Akman S, Krutzik S, Paxton RJ, Sparkes RS, Doroshow J, Felsted RL, Glover CJ, Mohandas T, Bachur NR. Induction of a human carbonyl reductase gene located on chromosome 21. Biochim Biophys Acta 1990;048:149.

48. Gianni L, et al. The biochemical basis of anthracycline toxicity and antitumor activity. In Reviews in Biochemical Toxicology. Edited by E Hodgson, JR Bend, RM Philport. Amsterdam: Elsevier, 1983, p 1.

49. Gianni L, Vigano L, Lanzi C, Niggeler M, Malatesta V. Role of daunosamine and hydroacetyl side chain in reaction with iron and lipid peroxidation by anthracyclines. JNCI 1988;80:1104.

50. Gianni L, Vigano L, Niggeler M, Levi S, Arosio P. Human ferritin (HLF) as iron source for lipid peroxidation by Adriamycin (Adr). San Francisco, Proc AACR 1988.

51. Gianni L, Zweier JL, Levy A, Myers CE. Characterization of iron-mediated electron transfer from Adriamycin to molecular oxygen. Biol Chem 1985;260:6820.

51a. Groen HJM, Proz JP, Hauauske AR, Verwey J, van Oosterom AT, Di Palms M, Marby M, Sorio R, Pacciarini MA, Lassus M, de Vries EGE. A feasibility study with FCE 23762 every 4 weeks in adults with solid tumors. Proc Am Soc Clin Oncol 1995;14:1515.

51b. Harrison M, Tomlinson D, Stewart S. Liposomal-entrapped doxorubicin: an active agent in AIDS-related Kaposi's sarcoma. J Clin Oncol 1995;13:914.

52. Hasinoff BB. The interaction of the cardioprotective agent ICRF-187 ((+)-1, 2-bis(3, 5,-dioxopiperazinyl-1-yL)propane); its hydrolysis product (ICRF-198); and other chelating agents with the Fe(III) and Cu(II) complexes of Adriamycin. Agents Actions 1989;26:378.

53. Hasinoff BB, Davey JP. The iron(III)-Adriamycin complex inhibits cytochrome c oxidase before its inactivation. Biochem J 1988;250:827.

54. Henderson IC, Allegra JC, Woodcock T, Wolff S, Bryan S, Cartwright K, Dukart G, Henry D. Randomized clinical trial comparing mitoxantrone with doxorubicin in previously treated patients with metastatic breast cancer. J Clin Oncol 1989;7:560.

55. Hortobagyi GN, Frye D, Buzdar AV, Ewer MS, Fraschini G, Hug V, Ames F, Montague E, Carrasco CH, MacKay B, Benjamin RS. Decreased cardiac toxicity of doxorubicin administered by continuous intravenous infusion in combination chemotherapy for metastatic breast carcinoma. Cancer 1989;63:37.

56. Jehn U, Heinemann V. Intermediate-dose Ara-C/m-AMSA for remission induction and high-dose Ara-C/m-AMSA for intensive consolidation in relapsed and refractory adult acute myelogeneous leukemia. Hamatol Bluttransfus 1990;33:333.

56a. Jones RB, Holland JF, Bhordwaj S, Norton L, Wilfinger C, Strashun A. A phase I-II study of intensive-dose Adriamycin for advanced breast cancer. J Clin Oncol 1987;5:172.

57. Juranka PF, Zastawny RL, Ling V. P-glycoprotein: multidrug-resistance and a super-family of membrane-associated transport proteins. Faseb J 1989;3:2583.

58. Kane SE, Pastan I, Gottesman MM. Genetic basis of multidrug resistance of tumor cells. J Bioenerg Biomembr 1990;22:593.

59. Kawamata J, Imanishi M. Interaction of actinomycin with DNA. Nature 1960;187:1112.

60. Kharasch ED, Novak RF. Bis(alkylamino)anthracenedione antineoplastic agent metabolic activation by NADPH-cytochrome P-450 reductase and NADH dehydrogenase: diminished activity relative to anthracyclines. Arch Biochem Biophys 1983;224:682.

61. Kharasch ED, Novak RF. Mitoxantrone and ametantrone inhibit hydroperoxide-dependent initiation and propagation reactions in fatty acid peroxidation. J Biol Chem 1985;260:10645.

62. Lefevre D, Riou JF, Ahomadegbe JC, Zhou DY, Bernard J, Riou G. Study of molecu-

lar markers of resistance to m-AMSA in a human breast cancer cell line. Decrease of topoisomerase II and increase of both topoisomerase I and acidic glutathione S transferase. Biochem Pharmacol 1991;41:1967.
63. Lewis J. Chemotherapy of gestational choriocarcinoma. Cancer 1972;30:1517.
64. Littman P, Rosenstock JG, Bailey C. Radiation myelitis following craniospinal irradiation with concurrent actinomycin D therapy. Oncology 1978;5:145.
65. Llesuy SF, Arnaiz SL. Hepatotoxicity of mitoxantrone and doxorubicin. Toxicology 1990;63:187.
66. Macchiarini P, Chella A, Riva A, Mengozzi G, Silvano G, Solfanelli S, Angeletti CA. Phase II feasibility study of high dose epirubicin-based regimens for untreated patients with small-cell lung cancer. Am J Clin Oncol 1990;13:495.
67. Macchiarini P, Danesi R Mariotti R, Marchetti A, Fazzi P, Bevilacqua G, Mariani M, Giuntini C, Del Tacca M, Angeletti CA. Phase II study of high-dose epirubicin in untreated patients with small-cell lung cancer. Am J Clin Oncol 1990;13:302.
68. Muindi J, Sinha BK, Gianni L, Myers C. Thiol dependent DNA damage produced by anthracycline-iron complexes The structure activity relationships and molecular mechanisms. Mol Pharm 1985;27:356.
69. Muindi JRF, Sinha BK, Gianni L, Myers CE. Hydroxyl radical production and DNA damage induced by anthracycline iron complex. FEBS Lett 1984;172:226.
70. Myers CE, Borow R, Palmeri S, Jenkins J, Gorden B, Locker G, Doroshow J, Epstein S. A randomized controlled trial assessing the prevention of doxorubicin cardiomyopathy by N-acetylcysteine. Semin Oncol 1983;10:53.
71. Myers CE, Cowan K, Sinha B, Chabner B. The phenomenon of pleiotropic drug resistance. In Important Advances in Oncology. Edited by VT DeVita, S Rosenberg, S Hellman. Philadelphia: Lippincott, 1987, p 27.
72. Myers CE, Gianni L, Simone CB, Klecker R, Greene R. Oxidative destruction of erythrocyte ghost membranes catalyzed by the doxorubicin-iron complex. Biochemistry 1982;21:1707.
73. Myers CE, Gianni L, Zweier J, Muindi J, Sinha BK, Eliot H. The role of iron in Adriamycin biochemistry. Fed Proc 1986;45:2792.
74. Novak RF, Kharasch ED. Mitoxantrone propensity for free radical formation and lipid peroxidation–implications for cardiotoxicity. Invest New Drugs 1985;3:95.
75. Paxton JW, Evans PC, Hardy JR. The effect of cimetidine, phenobarbitone and buthionine sulphoximine on the disposition of N-5-dimethyl-9-[(2-methoxy-4-methylsulphonylamino)phenylamino)-4-acridinecarboxamide] (CI-921) in the rabbit. Cancer Chemother Pharmacol 1989;23:291.
76. Petros WP, Rodman JH, Mirro J Jr, Evans WE. Pharmacokinetics of continuous-infusion amsacrine and teniposide for the treatment of relapsed childhood acute nonlymphocytic leukemia. Cancer Chemother Pharmacol 1991;27:397.
77. Porzsolt F, Kreuser ED, Meuret G, Mende S, Buchelt L, Redenbacher M, Heissmeyer HH, Strigl P, Hiemeyer V, Krause HH, Fleischer K, Saumweber G, Leichtle R, Matischok B, Gaus W, Heimpel H. High-intensity therapy versus low-intensity therapy in advanced breast cancer patients. Cancer Treat Rev 1990;17:287.
78. Puccio CA. Amsacrine is safe in patients with ventricular ectopy. Am J Hematol 1988;28:197.
79. Robert J, David M, Granger C. Metabolism of epirubicin to glucuronides: relationship to the pharmacodynamics of the drug. Cancer Chemother Pharmacol 1990;27:147.
80. Robertson IG, Kestell P, Dormer RA, Paxton JW. Involvement of glutathione in the metabolism of the anilinoacridine antitumour agents CI-921 and amsacrine. Drug Metabol Drug Interact 1988;6:371.
81. Sehgal RK, Sengupta SK, Waxman DJ, Tauber AI. Enzymic and chemical reduction of 2-deaminoactinomycins to free radicals. Anticancer Drug Des 1985;1:13.
82. Sengupta SK, Kelly C, Sehgal RK. Reverse and symmetrical analogues of actinomycin D: metabolic activation and in vitro and in vivo tumor growth inhibitory activities. J Med Chem 1985;28:620.
83. Shinar E, Hasin Y. Acute electrocardiographic changes induced by amsacrine. Cancer Treat Rep 1984;68:1169.
84. Singal PK, Pierce GN. Adriamycin stimulates low affinity CA^{2+} binding and lipid peroxidation but depresses myocardial function. Am J Physiol 1986;250:H419.
85. Sinha BK, Katki AG, Batist G, Cowan KH, Myers CE. Adriamycin-simulated hydroxyl radical formation in human breast tumor cells. Biochem Pharm 1987;36:793.
86. Sobell HM, Jain SC. Stereochemistry of actinomycin D binding to DNA: II. Detailed molecular model of actinomycin-DNA complex and its implications. J Mol Biol 1972;68:21.
87. Speth P, Linssen PCM, Holdrinet RSG, Haanen C. Plasma and cellular Adriamycin concentrations in patients with myeloma treated with 96 hour continuous infusion. Clin Pharmacol Ther 1987;41:661.
88. Speyer JL, Green MD, Kramer E, Rey M, Sanger J, Ward C, Dubin N, Ferrans V, Stecy P, Zeleniuch-Jacquotte A, Wernz J, Feit F, Slater W, Blum R, Muggia F. Protective effect of the bispiperazinedione, ICRF-187, against doxorubicin-induced cardiac toxicity in women with advanced breast cancer. N Engl J Med 1988;319:745.
89. Stewart DJ, Grewaal D, Green RM, Verma S, Maroun JA, Redmond D, Robillard L, Gupta S. Bioavailability and pharmacology of oral idarubicin. Cancer Chemother Pharmacol 1991;27:308.
90. Sweatman TW, Lokich JJ, Israel M. Clinical pharmacology of continuous infusion doxorubicin. Ther Drug Monit 1989;11:3.
91. Takusagawa F, Goldstein BM, Youngster S, Jones RA, Berman HM. Crystallization and preliminary x-ray study of a complex between dATGCAT and actinomycin D. J Biol Chem 1984;259:4714.
92. Tan CT, Dargen HW, Burchenal JH. The effect of actinomycin D on cancer in childhood. Pediatrics 1959;24:544.
93. Tattersall MH, Sodergren JE, Sengupta SK, Trites DH, Modest EJ, Frei E III. Pharmacokinetics of actinomycin D in patients with malignant melanoma. Clin Pharmacol Ther 1975;17:701.
94. Thomas CE, Aust SD. Release of iron from ferritin by cardiotoxic anthracycline antibiotics. Arch Biochem Biophys 1986;248:684.
95. Timour Q, et al. Doxorubicin concentrations in plasma and myocardium and their respective roles in cardiotoxicity. Cardiovasc Drugs Ther 1988;1:559.
96. Von Hoff DD, Layard MW, Basa P, Davis HL Jr, Von Hoff AL, Rozencweig M, Muggia FM. Risk Factors for doxorubicin-induced congestive heart failure. Ann Intern Med 1979;91:710.
97. Von Hoff DD, Rozencweig M, Layard M, Slavik M, Muggia FM. Daunomycin-induced cardiotoxicity in children and adults. Am J Med 1977;62:200.
98. Wermuth B. Aldo-keto reductases. Prog Clin Biol Res 1985;174:209.
99. Westendorf J, Aydin M, Groth G, Weller O, Marquardt H. Mechanistic aspects of DNA damage by morpholinyl and cyanomorpholinyl anthracyclines. Cancer Res 1989;49:5262.
100. Wolf JA, D'Angio G, Hartman J, Krivit W, Newton WA Jr. Long-term evaluation of single vs multiple courses of actinomycin D therapy of Wilms' tumor. N Engl J Med 1974;290:84.
101. Zhang H, D'Arpa P, Lui LF. A model for tumor cell killing by topoisomerase poisons. Cancer Cells 1990;2:23.
102. Zwelling LA, Slovak ML, Doroshow JH, Hinds M, Chan D, Parker E, Mayes J, Sic KL, Meltzer PS, Trent JM. HT1080/DR4: a P-glycoprotein-negative human fibrosarcoma cell line exhibiting resistance to topoisomerase II-reactive drugs despite the presence of a drug-sensitive topoisomerase II. JNCI 1990;82:1553.

CHAPTER 64

Epipodophyllotoxins

ANTOINETTE J. WOZNIAK AND WARREN E. ROSS

Introduction

The epipodophyllotoxins etoposide (VP-16) and teniposide (VM-26) are semisynthetic derivatives of podophyllotoxin. Both of these compounds exhibit a wide spectrum of antitumor activity, and the former, in particular, is now widely used in the treatment of both hematologic and solid neoplasms. In the past decade a great deal has been learned of the mechanism of action, disposition, and clinical role of the epipodophyllotoxins. This chapter focuses mainly on etoposide, since that was the compound initially commercially available in the United States and the one that has received the most extensive clinical testing.

History of Development

The history of the discovery of the epipodophyllotoxins is of considerable interest and was recently reviewed (40). The parent compound, podophyllotoxin, is derived from the American mandrake, *Podophyllum peltatum.* Extracts from the root of this plant were used in Europe and the United States in the early 19th century and were valued for their activity as cathartics and anthelminthics. The principal active species of these extracts, podophyllotoxin, was structurally characterized in 1951. By this time its medicinal use was limited to the treatment of condylomata acuminata. Chemists at Sandoz Laboratory hypothesized that glucoside derivatives of podophyllotoxin might be less toxic and more active than the parent compound, and in 1954 they succeeded in identifying such glucosides in the *Podophyllum* plants. Some of these glucosides fulfilled the expectations regarding activity and toxicity, and further synthetic efforts led to the compound demethylepipodophyllotoxin-benzylidene-glucoside (DETBG). This compound was significant not only for its excellent activity in animal leukemia models, but also because its mechanism of action differed from that of podophyllotoxin. As early as 1946, the action of podophyllum, the extract containing podophyllotoxin, was identified as the arrest of cells in metaphase of mitosis. This results from the binding of podophyllotoxin to tubulin, causing the inhibition of micro tubule assembly. In contrast, DETBG, and the epipodophyllotoxins that followed, inhibit the entry of cells into mitosis. Further synthetic efforts by the Sandoz group led to the synthesis of teniposide, in 1955, and 2 years later etoposide. Although the former was marketed in Europe in the mid-1970s, its place in antitumor therapy has been eclipsed by that of etoposide, whose development was facilitated by Sandoz licensing the compound to Bristol Myers in 1978. It was not until 1983, however, 16 years after its synthesis, that etoposide was approved by the Food and Drug Administration (FDA) for treatment of testicular cancer.

Mechanism of Action

The mechanism of the epipodophyllotoxins' antineoplastic effect is based principally on a unique interaction with the nuclear enzyme DNA topoisomerase II, which leads to DNA damage (33, 34). This enzyme catalyzes the double stranded breaking and resealing of DNA, thereby allowing the passage of one double helical segment of DNA through another (Fig. 64.1). The enzyme's actions are adenosine triphosphate (ATP) dependent and result in changes in DNA topology, such as unknotting, relaxation, and decatenation. The principal cellular function of this enzyme is to catalyze the separation of daughter DNA strands just prior to mitosis. Like the DNA intercalating agents, the epipodophyllotoxins interact with DNA topoisomerase II and/or DNA in such a way as to prevent the DNA resealing action, thereby creating a DNA–protein cross-link for as long as drug is present. This cross-link has been designated a "cleavable complex" because when exposed to denaturing agents, a frank DNA double stranded break is revealed (Fig. 64.2). The precise mechanism by which the epipodophyllotoxins inhibit the resealing action is unknown.

As a drug target, DNA topoisomerase II occupies a unique niche in antineoplastic therapy. Cytotoxicity results not from inhibition of enzyme activity, but rather from the creation of a form of DNA damage by virtue of the drug's perturbation of enzyme function. One consequence of this, addressed below, is that drug potency increases in parallel with intracellular enzyme content.

The cellular consequences of cleavable complex formation include chromosomal aberrations, arrest of cell cycle progression in G2 phase, and finally cell death. Cell death may occur via apoptosis or programmed cell death (46). Maximal cytotoxicity is observed when cells are treated in S phase (13). Quiescent cells are usually less sensitive than proliferating ones owing principally to reduction in intracellular topoisomerase II content accompanying quiescence (43).

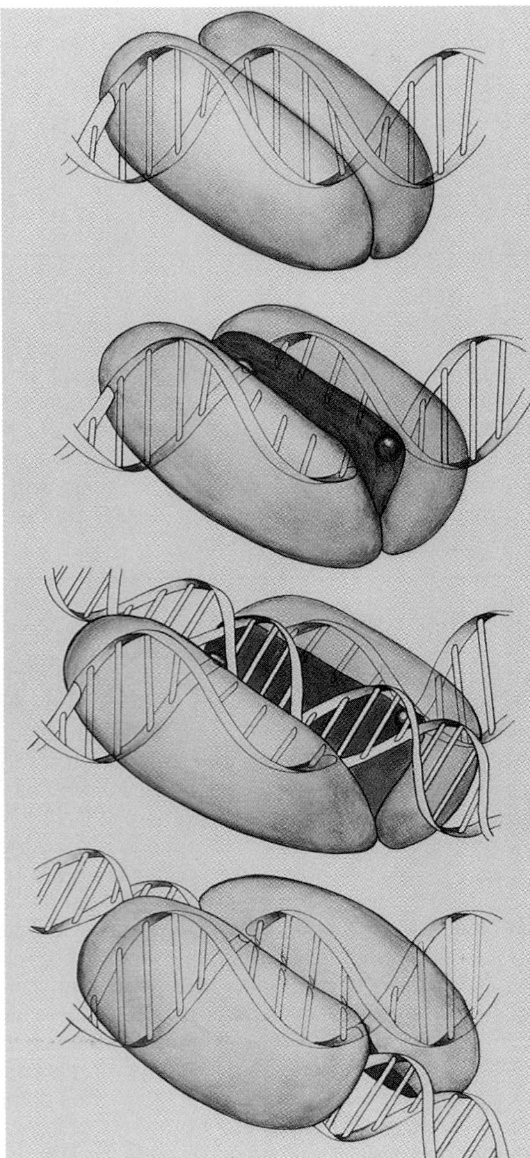

Figure 64.1. A schematic representation of steps leading to DNA strand passage by topoisomerase II. (For simplicity, only the presumed catalytic area of the enzyme is shown.) Following noncovalent attachment, the enzyme cleaves the sugar phosphate backbone and becomes covalently attached at the 5′ (represented by small spheres) of the break site. The dimeric structure of the enzyme appears well-suited for allowing passage of a second DNA duplex through the break site.

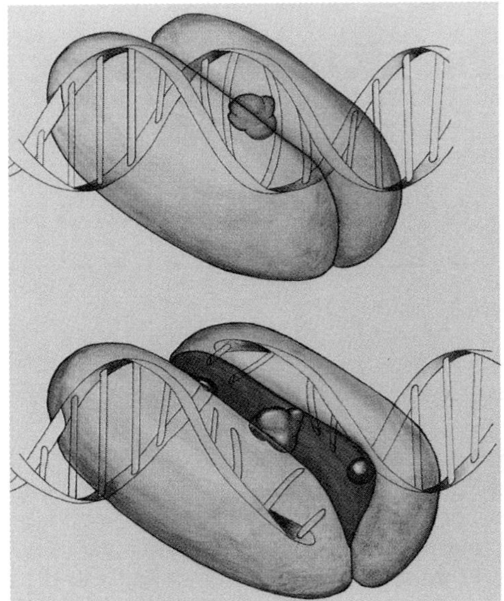

Figure 64.2. A proposed model of how the presence of drug may independently affect topoisomerase II–mediated DNA cleavage and strand passage. Drug binding to DNA is presumed. Cleavable complex formation could result from an altered relationship between the cleaved DNA strands and the catalytic center for the enzyme.

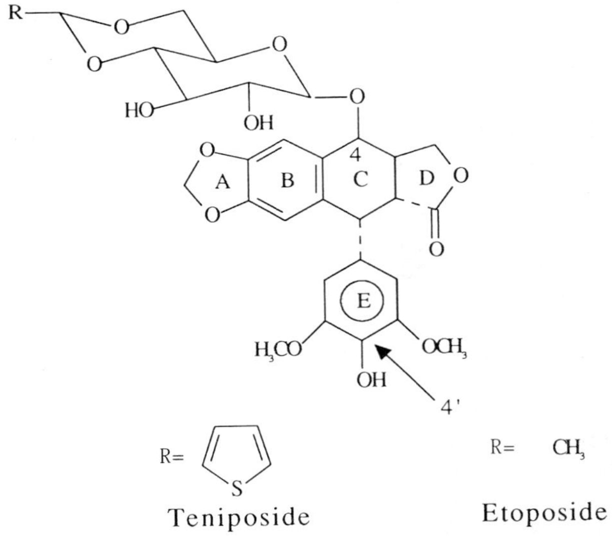

Teniposide

Etoposide

Figure 64.3. Chemical structure of podophyllotoxin derivatives.

Structure–activity relationships of the epipodophyllotoxins are of particular interest when compared to the parent podophyllotoxin since they have quite different mechanisms of action (Fig. 64.3). The three structural differences between podophyllotoxin and its semisynthetic derivatives that are responsible for the change in drug target from tubulin to DNA topoisomerase II are: demethylation at position 4′, epimerization in position C-4, and the presence of a glucopyranose at C-4. It is of note that these two mechanisms of action on tubulin and DNA topoisomerase II form the poles of a continuum, and a number of structural congeners share both mechanisms. Neither etoposide nor teniposide exhibits significant tubulin binding. Computer-assisted comparisons of the structures of the epipodophyllotoxins with those of intercalating agents suggest considerable similarity, and also suggest that the relationship of the glucopyranose ring and the pendant E ring to the polycyclic array represented by rings A through D are of importance in the interaction of the drug with topoisomerase II and DNA (25).

Cellular resistance to epipodophyllotoxins can occur for a

variety of reasons. The drugs are one of the known substrates for the mdr protein, which actively pumps drugs out of cells. This phenomenon, described elsewhere in this book, can occur as a result of cellular exposure to epipodophyllotoxins or a variety of other known substrates for the transport protein. Resistance can also result from a decrease in intracellular topoisomerase II content, either as a natural consequence of cellular quiescence or from loss of one of the two alleles encoding the enzyme. Alterations in the topoisomerase molecule conferring drug resistance, presumably resulting from genetic mutation, can also give rise to cellular resistance (42). Each of the above mechanisms has been studied in experimental cell culture systems. Studies of human tumor cells of hematopoietic origin indicate that intracellular topoisomerase II content is highly variable, and that this heterogeneity could account in part for differences in tumor response (4, 30).

Pharmacokinetics

The majority of pharmacokinetic studies done with etoposide show a biexponential decay following bolus intravenous (IV) administration (12). The terminal elimination half-life is 4 to 8 hours and is independent of the dose. The volume of distribution of etoposide is 7 to 17 L/m^2 in adults (10). Inter- and intrapatient variability exists with regard to these pharmacokinetic parameters. Both the area under the concentration versus time curve (AUC) and the peak plasma concentration of etoposide are dose dependent. There is no drug accumulation with consecutive daily dosing of the drug. Whether the drug is given as a bolus or by continuous infusion, there is essentially no change in the pharmacokinetics.

Etoposide is also available in oral form. There have been different formulations, including a drink ampule, a lipophilic capsule, and a hydrophilic soft gelatin capsule. The peak drug concentration occurs approximately 1 hour after administration. The bioavailability of the drug is about 50%, but wide variability exists, requiring individual dose optimization per patient. There are no statistically significant differences in any pharmacokinetic parameters when the IV and oral routes of administration are compared (39). It is suggested that when doses of etoposide above 200 mg are administered orally, they should be divided to allow for maximum absorption (22). Food does not interfere with etoposide absorption (21).

Etoposide phosphate is a newly developed water-soluble derivative of etoposide. The modification consists of the addition of a phosphate at the 4 position in the E ring (35). The compound is rapidly and completely converted to etoposide following parenteral administration and is biologically and pharmacokinetically equivalent to etoposide. Its advantage is that it can be administered as a bolus, at high concentrations, or as a continuous infusion more easily than the standard formulation.

Approximately 30 to 50% of etoposide is recovered in the urine as unchanged drug. Fecal elimination may account for 16% of the administered dose but biliary excretion is minimal (12). Etoposide is highly protein bound and is metabolized by the liver. A number of metabolites, none of therapeutic importance, have been discovered, including the hydroxy-acid derivatives, cis(picro)-lactone, and the glucuronide and sulfate conjugates of the parent compound (10). One cannot account for the majority of the etoposide dose in some patients. Etoposide has very poor penetration into the cerebrospinal fluid.

There are no specific dose reductions that are recommended for etoposide in patients with hepatic dysfunction, although patients with elevated liver enzymes do tend to exhibit increased neutropenia. Impaired renal function results in decreased drug clearance and increased myelotoxicity (3, 41). It has been suggested that the etoposide dose be decreased by 30% in patients with serum creatinine levels greater than 1.4 mg/dL (41). Low serum albumin levels, prior therapy with cisplatin, and advanced age have also been associated with decreased drug clearance and increased drug AUC.

Teniposide is available only in the IV form. Depending on the study, teniposide was found to follow either a two- or a three-compartment model. The elimination half-life varies according to the compartment model (6–10 hours vs 20–48+ hours) (10). The volume of distribution of teniposide is 8 to 30 L/m^2. The drug is highly protein bound. Both the plasma clearance and the renal clearance are greater for etoposide than for teniposide. The majority of the initial dose of etoposide (30–70%) is accounted for by excretion, but only 5 to 20% of teniposide is accounted for as unchanged drug. Biliary excretion is minimal. The differences between the two drugs have been explained by the reduced renal clearance of teniposide as compared to etoposide, and the higher protein binding of teniposide (2). Very little is known about the metabolism of the drug. Various metabolites have been described, including the hydroxy acid, the cis-isomer, and the aglycone glucuronide. Teniposide penetrates very poorly into the cerebrospinal fluid.

Schedule Dependence

Several studies have addressed the dose scheduling of etoposide. Table 64.1 summarizes the Phase I etoposide studies. Based on these and subsequent studies, it appears more efficacious to give etoposide daily for 3 to 5 days rather than once or twice a week. In a study by Cavalli et al. the response rate increased (by 20–65%) when etoposide was given for 3 days as opposed to a single weekly dose (8). Slevin et al. conducted a randomized trial to evaluate the effect of schedule on the activity of etoposide in small cell lung cancer (37). Patients received either etoposide, 500 mg/m^2 as a continuous infusion over 24 hours, or 100 mg/m^2 as a 2 hour infusion daily for 5 days. There was a marked difference in response rate, 10% versus 89%: The pharmacokinetics were similar in both arms, indicating the superiority of the 5-day schedule.

Interest in etoposide schedule dependence has led to trials of long-term daily oral administration. The maximally tolerated dose is 50 mg/m^2/for 21 days (19). Protracted oral administration of etoposide has resulted in less hematologic

Table 64.1. Summary of Phase 1 Studies with Etoposide

Schedule	Reference
Intravenous	
290 mg/m^2 IV weekly	Creaven and Allen (12)
200–250 mg/m^2 IV weekly	Cavalli et al. (8)
69–86 mg/m^2 IV twice weekly for 3 wk	Nissen et al. (27)
125–140 mg/m^2 IV q2d × 3	Eagan et al. (14)
45 mg/m^2 IV daily for 7 d	Nissen et al. (27)
60 mg/m^2 IV daily for 5 d	Tucker et al. (45)
Infusion	
125 mg/m^2 daily as continuous infusion for 5 d	Aisner et al. (1)
Oral	
300–400 mg/m^2 PO (capsule) over 5 d	Falkson et al. (16)
120 mg/m^2 PO (drinking ampule) daily for 5 d	Nissen et al. (26)
100–130 mg/m^2 PO (capsule) daily for 5 d	Lau et al. (24)

toxicity without sacrificing antineoplastic effect. Evidence indicates that this schedule can evoke responses in patients with malignant neoplasms (i.e., small cell lung cancer, germ cell tumors, lymphoma) in whom traditional dosing schemes of etoposide have failed (18). Prolonged infusion of low-dose etoposide is also being evaluated to avoid the high peak serum levels that may result in more hematologic toxicity (44). The optimal schedule for delivering etoposide has not been determined.

The scheduling of teniposide in humans has not been studied extensively. There is some suggestion in animal studies that the dosing of teniposide is schedule dependent. Based on a Phase I trial, the suggested dose is 67 mg/m^2 given IV once a week. Teniposide has also been given on a daily schedule and by continuous infusion.

Toxic Effects

The primary dose-limiting toxic effect of etoposide is hematologic. Neutropenia occurs in 7 to 10 days, with complete recovery usually occurring by day 20. Thrombocytopenia also occurs but is less frequent. There is no cumulative bone marrow toxicity.

Gastrointestinal toxic effects occur in about 20% of patients and may include nausea, vomiting, diarrhea, and anorexia. The nausea and vomiting are usually mild and can be controlled with antiemetics. There is more gastrointestinal toxicity associated with the oral formulation of the drug. Mucositis is unusual at conventional doses; however, when etoposide is used in high doses (> 1 g/m^2), oropharyngeal mucositis is the dose-limiting toxicity (29). Transient elevations in bilirubin, alkaline phosphatase, and aminotransferase levels can occur with the administration of etoposide in high doses.

Alopecia is frequent and reversible. Occasionally acute side effects including fever, chills, hypotension, bronchospasm, anaphylaxis, and vasomotor response have been attributed to etoposide. The hypotension can be associated with the rate of administration of the drug.

Peripheral neuropathy is uncommon but may increase in frequency when etoposide is administered with a vinca alkaloid. There have been case reports of phlebitis, acute dystonia, and radiation recall (17).

Cardiac toxicity has been reported; however, the patients involved had previous histories of cardiac disease and mediastinal irradiation, so the importance of the cardiac toxic effects of etoposide is unknown (1, 36).

The major toxic effects of teniposide parallel those of etoposide and include leukopenia, thrombocytopenia, alopecia, gastrointestinal and neurologic toxic effects and acute hypersensitivity reactions. There has been a report of hyaline membrane disease (11).

Secondary leukemia has been described in patients treated with etoposide or teniposide. The overall cumulative risk for developing leukemia has been reported to be 3.8% at 6 years. This leukemia is predominantly monocytic or myelomonocytic (FAB M4/M5) and is usually characterized by the absence of a preleukemic syndrome, a shorter latency period, and frequent cytogenetic abnormalities involving 11q23 (47). There are data that indicate that the most important risk factor for developing leukemia is not the total dose of drug but rather the schedule of administration (31).

Clinical Spectrum of Activity

ETOPOSIDE

Etoposide has a wide range of activity. Composite single-agent response rates of greater than 20% for etoposide have been reported in small cell lung cancer, testicular cancer, gestational choriocarcinoma, Hodgkin's and non-Hodgkin's lymphomas, acute myelogenous leukemia, acute myelomonocytic leukemia, Kaposi's sarcoma, neuroblastoma, Ewing's sarcoma, Wilms' tumor, and rhabdomyosarcoma (23). In combination with other agents, etoposide is used as first-line therapy in the treatment of a number of cancers.

Small Cell Lung Cancer

Etoposide is the single most active agent in the treatment of small cell lung cancer and is generally used in combination with other drugs. Some of the more common treatment regimens are listed in Table 64.2. The combination of etoposide and cisplatin yields response rates (86–95%) equivalent to or better than those achieved with non-etoposide-containing regimens. This drug combination has also produced encouraging responses (55% response rate, median duration of 22 weeks) in previously treated patients (15). Oral etoposide has been used in the treatment of small cell lung cancer in elderly patients, with good response rates (>70%) and acceptable toxicity (38). Despite initial regressions, relapse usually occurs (see Chapter 107).

Testicular Cancer

Etoposide has proved very useful in the treatment of testicular cancer. Interest in using it as a first-line agent grew when it was reported to produce responses in tumors that

Table 64.2. Common Etoposide-Containing Regimens for Small Cell Lung Cancer

CAE	
Cyclophosphamide	1,000 mg/m² IV on day 1
Doxorubicin (Adriamycin)	45 mg/m² IV on day 1
Etoposide (VP-16)	50 mg/m² IV on days 1–5
Repeat cycle every 3 wk	
CEV	
Cyclophosphamide	1,000 mg/m² IV on day 1
Etoposide	50 mg/m² IV on day 1; 100 mg/m² PO on day 2–5
Vincristine	1.4 mg/m² IV on day 1
Repeat cycle every 3 wk	
VAM	
Etoposide	200 mg/m² IV on day 1
Doxorubicin	50 mg/m² IV on day 1
Methotrexate	30 mg/m² IV on day 1
CAVE	
Cyclophosphamide	1,000 mg/m² IV on day 1
Doxorubicin	50 mg/m² IV on day 1
Vincristine	1.5 mg/m² IV on day 1
Etoposide	60 mg/m² IV on days 1–5
Repeat cycle every 3 wk	
EP	
Etoposide	100 mg/m² IV on days 1–3, *or* 50–100 mg/m² IV on day 1–5
Cisplatin	25 mg/m² IV on days 1–3, *or* 20 mg/m² IV on days 1–5, *or* 75–100 mg/m² on day 1
Repeat cycle every 3 wk	
CAV/EP	
Cycle of CAV (cyclophosphamide, doxorubicin, vincristine) alternating every 3 wk with a cycle of EP (etoposide, cisplatin)	
E/Carboplatin	
Etoposide	100 mg/m² IV on days 1–3
Carboplatin	300 mg/m² IV on day 1
Repeat cycle every 4 wk	
ICE	
Ifosfamide plus Mesna	5,000 mg/m² IV over 24 h on day 1
Carboplatin	300 mg/m² IV on day 1
Etoposide	120 mg/m² IV on days 1, 2; 240 mg/m² PO on day 3
Repeat cycle every 4 wk	

were resistant to standard PVB (cisplatin, vinblastine, bleomycin) chemotherapy. The etoposide-containing regimen, BEP (Table 64.3), has produced better responses and improved survival, particularly among patients with advanced disease (63% vs. 38% disease free, BEP and PVB, respectively) (48). The two-drug combination of etoposide and cisplatin is being evaluated as first-line therapy for patients with low-volume metastatic disease. VIP (VP-16, ifosfamide, cisplatin) is an important salvage regimen in the treatment of refractory testicular cancer.

Hematologic Malignancies

Etoposide has been used in combination with other drugs to treat acute nonlymphocytic leukemia (ANLL) in children and adults. There have been promising results in the treatment of both refractory and relapsed ANLL (28–51% complete remission rate). Many of the multidrug regimens that are being used to treat non-Hodgkin's lymphoma also contain etoposide. Etoposide is clearly active, but exactly what it adds to the treatment of this disease remains to be resolved. Etoposide-containing regimens have also been used in salvage therapy for Hodgkin's lymphoma, with variable results (13–67% complete response rate). Table 64.3 lists some of the common drug combinations used in hematologic malignancies.

Table 64.3. Common Etoposide-Containing Regimens for a Variety of Cancers

Testicular Carcinoma	
BEP	
Bleomycin	30 units IV on days 1, 8, 15
Etoposide	100 mg/m² IV on days 1–5
Cisplatin	20 mg/m² IV on days 1–5
Repeat cycle every 3 wk for 4 cycles	
VIP	
Etoposide	75 mg/m² IV on days 1–5
Ifosfamide plus Mesna	1,200 mg/m² IV on days 1–5
Cisplatin	20 mg/m² IV on days 1–5
Repeat cycle every 3 wk	
Acute Myeloid Leukemia	
Etoposide	100–150 mg/m² IV on days 1–5
Mitoxantrone	10 mg/m² IV on days 1–5
Etoposide	100 mg/m² IV on days 1–5
Amsacrine	100 mg/m² IV on days 1–5
Non-Hodgkin's Lymphoma	
ProMACE-CytaBOM	
Cyclophosphamide	650 mg/m² IV on day 1
Doxorubicin	25 mg/m² on day 1
Etoposide	120 mg/m² on day 1
Cytarabine	300 mg/m² on day 8
Bleomycin	5 mg/m² on day 8
Vincristine	1.4 mg/m² on day 8
Methotrexate with leucovorin	120 mg/m² on day 8
Prednisone	60 mg/m² PO daily for 2 wk
Cotrimoxazole	2 tablets PO twice daily during therapy
Repeat cycle every 3 wk	
EPOCH	
Etoposide	50 mg/m²/d continuous infusion for 96 h
Doxorubicin	10 mg/m²/d continuous infusion for 96 h
Vincristine	0.4 mg/m²/d continuous infusion for 96 h
Cyclophosphamide	750 mg/m² IV on day 6
Prednisone	60 mg/m² PO daily for 2 wk
Repeat cycle every 4 wk	
Hodgkin's Lymphoma	
CHOPE	
Cyclophosphamide	750 mg/m² IV on day 1
Doxorubicin	50 mg/m² IV on day 1
Vincristine	1.4 mg/m² IV on days 1 and 8
Prednisone	100 mg/day PO on days 1–5
Etoposide	80 mg/m² IV on days 1–3
Repeat cycle every 3 wk	

Other Malignancies

There is high single-agent activity for etoposide in epidemic Kaposi's sarcoma. The drug is being evaluated in the treatment of breast cancer, hepatocellular carcinoma, head and neck cancer, gliomas, gestational choriocarcinoma, ovarian cancer, prostate cancer, gastric cancer, and histiocytosis X.

Bone Marrow Transplantation

Etoposide is an ideal candidate for use in bone marrow transplantation since it has little extramedullary toxicity and it has activity in a number of hematologic malignancies. In a Phase I study of autologous bone marrow transplantation (BMT) in advanced refractory neoplasms 2,400 mg/m^2 was the maximally tolerated dose, and recovery from myelosuppression occurred within 16 days of bone marrow infusion (49). High-dose etoposide with autologous BMT has been most successfully used in the treatment of Hodgkin's disease. Etoposide (60 mg/kg) and total body irradiation have been used with good preliminary results in allogenic bone marrow transplantation of patients with hematologic malignancies (6). It has also been combined with other chemotherapeutic agents and used for allogenic and autologous BMT (5). Additional studies need to be done regarding the use of etoposide and its ultimate role in BMT. Etoposide has also been used as an in vitro purging agent for the treatment of acute leukemia with autologous BMT (9).

TENIPOSIDE

Teniposide has been used primarily in the pediatric population, probably as a result of its course of development rather than of its activity as an antineoplastic agent. Teniposide has received its most extensive evaluation in childhood leukemia, particularly acute lymphocytic leukemia (ALL). It has very modest activity as a single agent. Teniposide has primarily been used in combination with cytosine arabinoside because some preclinical data suggest there is synergistic activity when the two drugs are administered together (32). There have clearly been responses in patients with ALL in whom previous therapy failed. Teniposide is being used as a first-line agent in many multidrug protocols for the treatment of both childhood and adult leukemia. The drug's impact on this disease, however, is still to be determined (20). Teniposide has also been incorporated into ablation regimens administered prior to BMT. It is an active agent in other hematologic malignancies, such as Hodgkin's and non-Hodgkin's lymphoma.

Teniposide has been shown to be very active in small cell lung cancer when used in untreated patients. In one study teniposide, 60 mg/m^2 given IV daily for 5 days, resulted in a 90% overall response rate (30% complete response rate) (7). It is unclear as to whether it offers any advantage over other drugs in the treatment of this disease.

Although teniposide penetrates poorly into the cerebrospinal fluid, it can accumulate in brain tumor tissue, and responses have been observed in brain tumors. It has been used in combination with cisplatin in the treatment of neuroblastoma (28). Teniposide has also demonstrated activity in bladder cancer, epidemic Kaposi's sarcoma, and gynecologic malignancies. Teniposide requires further evaluation with regard to optimal dose and scheduling to determine its activity in other malignancies.

The Future of Epipodophyllotoxins

There is good reason to believe that the clinical role of epipodophyllotoxins will expand considerably in the next few years. The availability of an oral preparation and possibly the water-soluble etoposide phosphate, concomitant with a better appreciation of the drug's schedule dependency, could increase the drug's spectrum of activity. Further understanding of its mechanisms of cytotoxicity and drug resistance may also yield methods of modulating activity to advantage. For example, topoisomerase I inhibitors can be combined sequentially with etoposide for a potentially efficacious drug combination. Finally, it is worth noting that the structure–activity relationships of epipodophyllotoxin congeners, especially with respect to topoisomerase inhibition, are only beginning to be explored. Similarities in structure with intercalating agents, a class of drugs sharing the epipodophyllotoxins' mechanism of action, hint at potentially useful synthetic pathways. Undoubtedly other opportunities will become apparent as more effort is invested.

References

1. Aisner J, Van Echo DA, Whitacre M, Wiernik PH. A phase I trial of continuous infusion VP16-213 (etoposide). Cancer Chemother Pharmacol 1982;7:157.
2. Allen LM, Creaven PJ. Comparison of the human pharmacokinetics of VM-26 and VP-16, two antineoplastic epipodophyllotoxin glucopyranoside derivatives. Eur J Cancer 1975;11:697.
3. Arbuck SG, Douglass HO, Crom WR, Goodwin P, Silk Y, Cooper C, Evans WE. Etoposide pharmacokinetics in patients with normal and abnormal organ function. J Clin Oncol 1986;4:1690.
4. Bakic M, Beran M, Andersson BS, Silberman L, Estey E, Zwelling LA. The production of topoisomerase II–mediated DNA cleavage in human leukemia cells predicts their susceptibility to 4′-(9-acridinylamino)methanesulfon-m-anisidide (m-AMSA). Biochem Biophys Res Commun 1986;134:638.
5. Blume KG, Forman SJ. High-dose etoposide (VP-16)–containing preparatory regimens in allogeneic and autologous bone marrow transplantation for hematologic malignancies. Semin Oncol 1992;19(suppl 13):63–66.
6. Blume KG, Forman SJ, O'Donnell MR, Doroshow JH, Krance RA, Nademanee AP, Snyder DS, Schmidt GM, Fahey JL, Metter GE, Hill LR, Findley DO, Sniecinski IJ. Total body irradiation and high-dose etoposide: a new preparatory regimen for bone marrow transplantation in patients with advanced hematologic malignancies. Blood 1987;69:1015.
7. Bork E, Hansen M, Dombernowsky P, Hansen SW, Pedersen AG, Hansen HH. Teniposide (VM26) an overlooked highly active agent in small-cell lung cancer: results of a phase II trial in untreated patients. J Clin Oncol 1986;4:524.
8. Cavalli F, Sonntag RW, Jungi F, Senn HJ, Brunner KW. VP-16-213 monotherapy for remission induction of small cell lung cancer: a randomized trial using three dosage schedules. Cancer Treat Rep 1978;62:473.
9. Ciobanu N, Paietta E, Andreef M, Papenhausen P, Wiernik PH. Etoposide as an in vitro purging agent for the treatment of acute leukemias and lymphomas in conjunction with autologous bone marrow transplantation. Exp Hematol 1986;14:626.
10. Clark PI, Slevin ML. The clinical pharmacology of etoposide and teniposide. Clin Pharmacokinet 1987;12:223.
11. Commers JR, Foley JF. Pulmonary hyaline membrane disease occurring in the course of VM-26 therapy. Cancer Treat Rep 1979;63:2093.
12. Creavean PJ, Allen LM. EPEG: a new antineoplastic epipodophyllotoxin. Clin Pharmacol Ther 1975;18:221.
13. Drewinko B, Barlogie B. Survival and cycle-progression delay of human lymphoma cells in vitro exposed to VP-16-213. Cancer Treat Rep 1976;60:1295.
14. Eagan RT, Ahmann DL, Hahn RG, O'Connell MJ. Pilot study to determine an intermittent dose schedule for VP-16-213. Proc Am Cancer Res 1975;16:55.
15. Evans WK, Osoba D, Feld R, Shepard FA, Bazos MJ, Deboer G. Etoposide (VP-16) and cisplatin: an effective treatment for relapse of small cell lung cancer. J Clin Oncol 1985;3:65.
16. Falkson G, Van Dyk JJ, Van Eden EB, Van Der Merwe AM, Van Den Bergh JA, Falkson HC. A clinical trial of the oral form of 4′-demethylepipodophyllotoxin-β-D-ethydine glucoside (NSC 141540) V.P.16-213. Cancer 1975;35:1141.
17. Fleming RA, Miller AA, Stewart CF. Etoposide: an update. Clin Pharm 1989;8:274.

18. Greco FA. Etoposide: seeking the best dose and schedule. Semin Oncol 1992;19(suppl 14):59.
19. Greco FA, Johnson DH, Hainsworth JD. Chronic daily administration of oral etoposide. Semin Oncol 1990;17(suppl 2):71.
20. Grem JL, Hoth DF, Leyland-Jones B, King SA, Ungerleider RS, Wittes RE. Teniposide in the treatment of leukemia: a case study of conflicting priorities in the development of drugs for fatal diseases. J Clin Oncol 1988;6:351.
21. Harvey VJ, Slevin ML, Joel SP, Johnston A, Wrigley PFM. The effect of food and concurrent chemotherapy on the bioavailability of oral etoposide. Br J Cancer 1985;52: 363.
22. Harvey VJ, Slevin ML, Joel SP, Johnston A, Wrigley PFM. The effect of dose on the bioavailability of oral etoposide. Cancer Chemother Pharmacol 1986;16:178.
23. Issell BF, Rudolph AR, Louie AC. An overview. In Etoposide (VP-16) Current Status and New Developments. Edited by BF Issell. London: Academic Press, 1984.
24. Lau ME, Hansen HH, Nissen NI, Pederson H. Phase I trial of a new form of an oral administration of VP 16-213. Cancer Treat Rep 1979;63:485.
25. Macdonald TL, Lehnert EK, Loper JT, Chow K-C, Ross WE. On the mechanism of interaction of DNA topoisomerase II with Chemotherapeutic Agents. In DNA Topoisomerases in Cancer Chemotherapy. Edited by M Potmesil. London: Oxford University Press, 1989.
26. Nissen NI, Dombernowsky P, Hansen HH, Larsen V. Phase I clinical trial of an oral solution of V.P.16-213. Cancer Treat Rep 1976;60:943.
27. Nissen NI, Larsen V, Pedersen H, Thomsen K. Phase I clinical trial of a new antitumor agent, 4′-demethylepipodophyllotoxin 9-(4,6-0-ethylidene-β-D-glucopyranoside) (NSC 141540; VP-16-213) Cancer Chemother Rep 1972;56:769.
28. O'Dwyer PJ, Alonso MT, Leyland-Jones B, Marsoni S. Teniposide: a review of 12 years experience. Cancer Treat Rep 1984;68:1455.
29. Postmus PE, Mulder NH, Sleijfer DT, Meinesz AF, Vriesendorp R, de Vries EG. High-dose etoposide for refractory malignancies: a phase I study. Cancer Treat Rep 1984;68:1471.
30. Potmesil M, Hsiang YH, Liu LF, Bank B, Grossberg H, Kirschenbaum S, Forlenza TJ, Penziner A, Kanganis D, Knowles D, Traganos F, Silber R. Resistance of human leukemic and normal lymphocytes to drug-induced DNA cleavage and low levels of DNA topoisomerase II. Cancer Res 1988;48:4716.
31. Pui C-H, Ribeiro RC, Hancock ML, Rivera GK, Evans WE, Raimondi SC, Head DR, Behm FG, Mahmoud MH, Sandlund JT, Crist WM. Acute myeloid leukemia in children treated with epipodophyllotoxins for acute lymphoblastic leukemia. N Engl J Med 1991;325:1682–1687.
32. Rivera G, Avery T, Roberts D. Response of L1210 to combinations of cytosine arabinoside and VM-26 or VP-16-213. Eur J Cancer 1975;11:639.
33. Ross WE, Rowe T, Yalowich J, Glisson B, Liu L. Role of topoisomerase II in mediating epipodophyllotoxin-induced DNA cleavage. Cancer Res 1984;44:5857.
34. Ross WE, Sullivan DM, Chow K-C. Altered function of DNA topoisomerases as a basis for antineoplastic drug action. In Important Advances in Oncology. Edited by V DeVitae. Phildadelphia: Lippincott, 1988.
35. Schacter LP, Igwemezie LN, Seyedsadr M, Morgenthien E, Randolph J, Albert E, Santabarbara P. Clinical and pharmacokinetic overview of parenteral etoposide phosphate. Cancer Chemother Pharmacol 1994;34(suppl):58–63.
36. Schechter JP, Jones SE, Jackson RA. Myocardial infarction in a 27-year old woman: possible complication of treatment with VP-16-213 (NSC-141540), mediastinal irradiation or both. Cancer Chemother Rep 1975;59:887.
37. Slevin ML, Clark PI, Joel SP, Malik S, Osborne RJ, Gregory WM, Lowe DG, Reznek RH, Wrigley PF. A randomized trial to evaluate the effect of schedule on the activity of etoposide in small-cell lung cancer. J Clin Oncol 1989;7:1333.
38. Smit EF, Carney DN, Harford P, Sleijfer DT, Postmus PE. A phase II study of oral etoposide in elderly patients with small cell lung cancer. Thorax 1989;44:631.
39. Smyth RD, Pfeffer M, Scalzo A, Comis RL. Bioavailability and pharmacokinetics of etoposide (VP-16). Semin Oncol 1985;12(suppl 2):48.
40. Stahelin H, von Wartburg A. From podophyllotoxin glucoside to etoposide. Prog Drug Res 1989;33:169.
41. Stewart CF. Use of etoposide in patients with organ dysfunction: pharmacokinetic and pharmacodynamic considerations. Cancer Chemother Pharmcol 1994;34(suppl.): 76–83.
42. Sullivan DM, Latham MD, Ross WE. Proliferation dependent topoisomerase II content as a determinant of anti-neoplastic drug action. Cancer Res 1987;47:3973.
43. Sullivan DM, Latham MD, Rowe TC, Ross WE. Purification and characterization of an altered topoisomerase II from a drug resistant Chinese hamster ovary cell line. Biochem 1989;28:5680.
44. Thompson DS, Hainsworth JD, Hande KR, Halzmer MC, Greco FA. Prolonged administration of low-dose, infusional etoposide in patients with etoposide-sensitive neoplasms: a Phase I/II study. J Clin Oncol 1993;11:1322.
45. Tucker RD, Ferguson A, Van Wyk C, Sealy R, Hewitson R, Levin W. Chemotherapy of small cell carcinoma of the lung with V.P.-16-213. Cancer 1978;41:1710.
46. Walker PR, Smith C, Youdale T, LeBalanc J, Whitfield JF, Sikorska M. Topoisomerase II-reactive chemotherapeutic drugs induce apoptosis in thymocytes. Cancer Res 1991;51:1078.
47. Whitlock JA, Greer JP, Lukens JN. Epipodophyllotoxin-related leukemia: identification of a new subset of secondary leukemia. Cancer 1991;68:600.
48. Williams SD, Birch R, Einhorn LH, Irwin L, Greco FA, Loehrer PJ. Treatment of disseminated germ-cell tumors with cisplatin, bleomycin and either vinblastine or etoposide. N Engl J Med 1987;316:1435.
49. Wolff SN, Mckay CM, Fer MF, Hande KR, Hainsworth JD, Greco FA. High dose VP-16-213 and autologous bone marrow transplantation for refractory malignancies: a phase I study. J Clin Oncol 1983;1:701.

CHAPTER 65

DNA Topoisomerase I Inhibitors

ROBERT SILBER

Introduction

The DNA topoisomerases are a group of enzymes present in eukaryotes and prokaryotes that alter DNA topology by causing and resealing DNA strand breaks. They relax superhelical turns, interconvert knotted rings, and intertwist complementary viral sequences into DNA. Since their discovery by Wang in 1971 (1), DNA topoisomerases have been shown to be essential for such events as replication, transcription, and mitosis. These enzymes are also needed for recombination, DNA insertions, and viral replication. While multiple DNA topoisomerases (numbered I–V) have been described, topoisomerases I and II have been the most extensively characterized, largely because they are the targets of chemotherapeutic agents (2). Inhibitors of DNA topoisomerase I are a promising new class of antineoplastic drugs that are presently undergoing intensive clinical investigation (3–9). DNA topoisomerase II-directed antitumor drugs are discussed in Chapter 63.

DNA Topoisomerase I

Topoisomerase I is a 100-kd protein (10) whose gene has been mapped to chromosome 20q12–13.2 (11). The cDNA encodes for a 765-amino acid polypeptide (12). The localization of topoisomerase I is in keeping with the enzyme's function of relaxing supercoiled DNA (13, 14) for a variety of crucial cellular processes. Its presence in the nucleolus (15, 16) is appropriate for its activity with ribosomal RNA.

A role in transcription is supported by several lines of evidence. These include the following: (*a*) preferential interaction with transcriptionally active DNA which contains topoisomerase I cleavage sites (16); (*b*) impaired transcription in yeast with mutations in the topoisomerase I gene (17, 18); (*c*) possible association with RNA polymerase in a functional complex (19); and (*d*) evidence that the topoisomerase I inhibitor camptothecin also inhibits RNA synthesis (20, 21).

Additional functions for topoisomerase I involving DNA have been established. The enzyme may serve as a swivellase for DNA replication by removing torsional stress (22, 23). It is able to function as a swivel during the elongation phase of DNA replication (24). A role in DNA recombination and repair has been suggested by the demonstration that in vitro it can ligate exogenous DNA fragments with a 5′-OH end (25, 26). Topoisomerase I may play a role in maintaining genomic stability in the cell (27).

A function for topoisomerase I in virus–cell interactions is suggested by several findings. The enzyme is required for vaccinia virus replication (28). It has also been isolated from HIV virus and equine infectious anemia particles (29). Hot spots for topoisomerase I cleavage, at the sites of SV40 virus insertion, have led to the suggestion that it acts to release the virus from host DNA (30). The enzyme also mediates the integration of hepadnavirus DNA in vitro (31).

Topoisomerase I relaxes supercoiled DNA (13, 14) by making single strand breaks in DNA (32), usually adjacent to a thymine. In the first step of the reaction, the enzyme attaches to double-stranded DNA by stacking in DNA grooves rather than by intercalating (2). The enzyme causes *transient* breaks in one strand of the DNA; it remains covalently bound to the nicked DNA's 3-phosphoryl terminus by its tyrosine 723. The intact DNA strand rotates around the cleavage site. In the absence of an inhibitor, the nicks are then sealed in the final, *religating* phase of the reaction (33, 34). During the relaxation reaction the topoisomerase I–DNA complex, referred to as the *noncleavable complex* (Fig. 65.1), is in reversible equilibrium with the covalent adduct topoisomerase I–DNA. This *cleavable complex* is the primary target for the topoisomerase I inhibitors used in cancer chemotherapy (2).

Topoisomerase I–Targeted Drugs

CAMPTOTHECINS

Camptothecin was isolated from the stem wood of the Chinese tree *Camptotheca acuminata* by Wall and co-workers in 1966 (35). In 1970 camptothecin was shown to inhibit macromolecular synthesis. The inhibition of RNA synthesis is reversible, while DNA synthesis inhibition is concentration dependent and reversible only at high concentrations of the drug (20, 21). Topoisomerase I was shown to be the drug's molecular target in 1985 (36). The elevated levels of this enzyme in some human tumor tissues as compared to their normal counterparts make topoisomerase I an attractive target for chemotherapy (37–39). In addition, the enzyme is expressed continuously during the cell cycle (40), providing some rationale for the use of its inhibitors for slow-growing tumors. The mechanism by which camptothecin, a cell–cycle specific inhibitor that is 1,000-fold more cytotoxic to cells

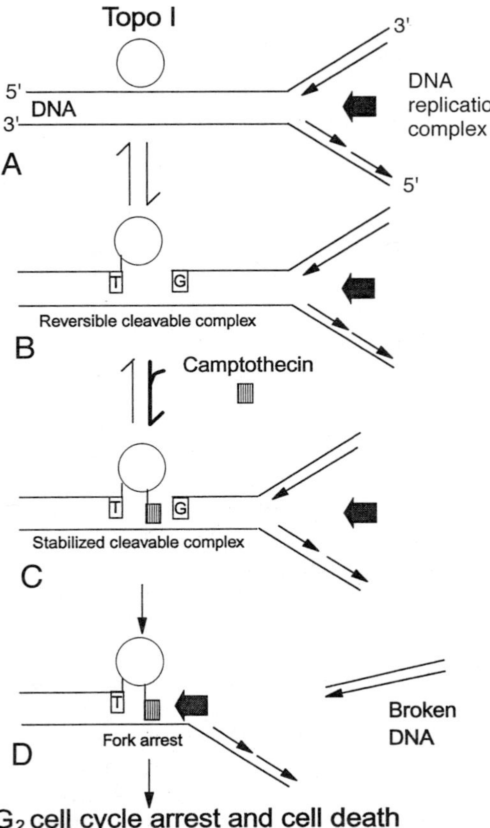

Figure 65.1. A model for the mechanism of topoisomerase I inhibition by camptothecin (**A**) Topoisomerase I (Topo I) is shown in contact with DNA upstream of the cleavage site and of the DNA polymerase replication complex. During a relaxation reaction the Topo I–DNA noncovalent complex is in equilibrium with the reversible cleavable complex (**B**). Topo I, after generating transient breaks in a transesterification reaction, is covalently linked to DNA (B). Under physiologic conditions the breaks are resealed and DNA synthesis continues. An inhibitor, such as camptothecin, shifts the equilibrium to the now stabilized reversible cleavable complex (**C**), and resealing cannot take place. This fork-collision model depicts the dependence of drug cytotoxicity on DNA synthesis (**D**). The Topo I–camptothecin–DNA reversible complex is oriented so that the transiently cleaved strand is complementary to the leading strand of newly synthesized DNA. Upon collision of the inhibitor-stabilized complex with the DNA replication complex, DNA breakage becomes irreversible and fork replication is arrested. This series of events triggers cell cycle arrest at G_2 and cell death. Source: Modified with permission from Chen and Liu (2) and Pommier et al. (118).

in S phase than to cells in the G_1 or G_2 phase of the cell cycle (41), would affect quiescent cells is unknown.

Natural camptothecin, that is, the 20(S) form, inhibits the religating step of the topoisomerase I reaction (Fig. 65.1) (36, 42). It traps the covalent Topo I–DNA complex at sites that have a guanine at their 5′ terminus (43–46). The stable topoisomerase I–camptothecin–DNA ternary *cleavable complex* is thought to be ultimately responsible for the drug's cytotoxicity (2). The current explanation of this effect is based on the stabilization of the cleavable complex by the drug and the requirement for ongoing DNA synthesis for cell killing by camptothecin (47, 48). This "fork-collision" model (Fig. 65.1) postulates that camptothecin increases the concentration of cleavable complex, which is oriented so that the transiently broken DNA strand becomes complementary to the leading strand of DNA synthesis (2, 49, 50). This in turn leads to irreversible replication, fork arrest, and fork breakage. The cell is arrested in the G_2 phase of the replication cycle and subsequently dies (51). The model may explain the protection against camptothecin toxicity by topoisomerase II inhibitors. The precise sequence of the events leading to the final apoptotic event remains unknown. The fork-collision model does not explain all the cellular effects of camptothecin, such as its causing increases in c-*fos* and c-*jun* mRNA, which are independent of DNA synthesis (52, 53).

The structure of camptothecin (NSC 94600) and that of four derivatives in clinical trials is shown in Figure 65.2. The many camptothecin analogues synthesized by Wall, Wani, and co-workers (54–56) have allowed structure–activity correlations to be determined (56–58). Substitutions in the 12 position of the A ring decrease cytotoxicity, while an amino group in the 9 position, or an ethylenedioxy substitution in the 10–11 positions, increases it. The presence of a hydrophilic hydroxyl or nitro group at the 9, 10, or 11 position enhances aqueous solubility. The chiral group in the 20 position imparts stereospecificity to the interaction with topoisomerase I. 20-(R)-camptothecin neither inhibits the enzyme nor manifests cytotoxicity. Derivatives modified in the E ring show that activity is lost when the 21-lactone is changed to a 21-lactim. The E ring lactone and the α-hydroxyl group at position 20 are required for effective stabilization of the cleavable DNA–enzyme–drug complex needed for cytotoxicity. Opening of the 20-hydroxy-21-lactone structure by increasing the pH yields the hydroxy acid form (59) and abolishes the drug's cytotoxicity. As discussed below, this finding has considerable clinical significance.

The synthesis of 9-aminocamptothecin (NSC 603071) yielded a compound that causes a significantly higher number of breaks in DNA (57, 58) and also has greater cytotoxicity than the parent drug. Both drugs are essentially insoluble in water.

The insolubility of camptothecin led to the synthesis of derivatives containing water-solubilizing groups, three of which are now in clinical trials. Irinotecan (NSC 616348, CPT-11, 7-ethyl-10-{4-(1-piperidino)-1-piperidino)carbonyloxycamptothecin}, the first semisynthetic derivative, was developed in Japan (60). This is a water-soluble prodrug, converted in vivo to its active metabolite (SN-38) (7-ethyl-10-hydroxycamptothecin) (61, 62). The introduction of a stable side-chain at the 9 position of the A ring of 10-hydroxycamptothecin yielded another water-soluble drug, topotecan (NSC 609699, SKF 104864, 9-dimethylaminomethyl-10-hydroxycamptothecin) (63).

The latest, totally synthetic water-soluble camptothecin analogue, GG211 (GI147211, 7-(methylpiperazinomethylene)-10, 11-ethylenedioxy-20(S)-camptothecin dihydrochloride), also has significant antitumor activity in xenograft models (64).

There are a few drugs not belonging to the camptothecin family that inhibit topoisomerase I (and in some cases also DNA topoisomerase II). They have a different DNA se-

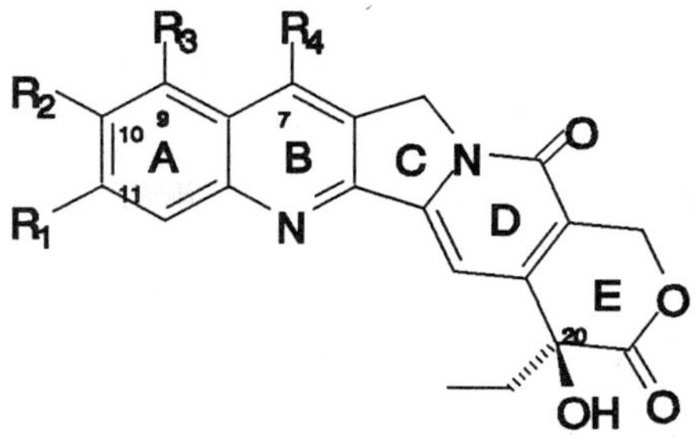

Substitution/ position	R_1/ 11	R_2/ 10	R_3/ 9	R_4/ 7
Camptothecin	H	H	H	H
9-amino-20(S)-camptothecin	H	H	NH_2	H
Irinotecan	H	{4-(1-piperidino)-1-piperidino}carbonyloxy	H	C_2H_5
SN-38	H	OH	H	C_2H_5
Topotecan	H	OH	$(CH_3)_2NCH_2$-	H
GG211	O-CH_2-CH_2-O		H	methylpiperazino methylene

Figure 65.2. Structure of camptothecin, 9-amino-20(5)-camptothecin, irinotecan, SN-38, topotecan, and GG211.

quence selectivity from the camptothecins; some of them are minor groove binders (2). None of these has reached a comparable stage of clinical development.

Preclinical Studies

Some of the antileukemia and antitumor properties of camptothecin were reported at the time of the compound's purification from its natural source (35). It had activity against murine L1210, L5178, and K1964 leukemias, and the Walker 256 carcinosarcoma in the rat (65). Camptothecin showed no cross-resistance with other antitumor drugs (doxorubicin, BCNU, 6-mercaptopurine, cytosine arabinoside, and L-asparaginase, among others) available at the time (66). These features led to the early clinical studies discussed below. Recent reports also show complete growth inhibition by camptothecin in 11 of 14 human cancer xenograft lines in nude mice (67, 68), as well as activity against melanoma and lung adenocarcinoma xenograft lines in a central nervous system model of metastasis (68).

Studies with human xenografts have shown an unprecedented efficacy for 9-aminocamptothecin. Complete remissions were found in colon (37), breast, and non-small cell lung carcinoma, as well as in melanoma cell lines (67). The drug was effective in both small and bulky tumors, with remission lasting the animal's life span in many instances.

Irinotecan caused partial regressions of human gastric, colon, and lung squamous cell carcinomas and complete regressions of a breast carcinoma cell line in nude mice (69); it was also active against rhabdomyosarcoma xenografts and many murine neoplasms. These include pancreatic adenocarcinoma 03, NH134 hepatoma, Lewis lung carcinoma, and Meth A fibrosarcoma (70, 71).

Topotecan has shown activity against a variety of murine tumors (4–6, 63) as well as against xenografts of colon cancer, osteogenic sarcoma and rhabdomyosarcoma (72). The in vivo efficacy of GG221 (GI147211) was established using xenografts of HT 29 colon carcinoma lines as well as ovarian, lung, and epidermoid tumors (64, 73). Based on these results, pharmacokinetic studies were undertaken in patients (74).

Clinical Trials and Pharmacokinetics

CAMPTOTHECIN AND 9-AMINOCAMPTOTHECIN

The early clinical studies (75–78), performed from 1970 to 1972, used the soluble camptothecin sodium salt (NSC 100880) in either single intermittent doses, weekly doses, or daily (×5 days) schedules. Phase I trials showed promise, with responses in five of 16 patients with far advanced colon, stomach, and non-small cell lung cancer or melanoma. Toxic effects included myelosuppression, nausea, vomiting, and diarrhea, as well as hemorrhagic cystitis. Subsequent Phase II trials showed very low response rates and severe toxic effects, including severe hemorrhagic cystitis, with single dosing and daily ×5 schedules (78). No other clinical studies were reported over the next 15 years. Explanations are now available for these early results that almost scuttled further studies with camptothecin. The hemorrhagic cystitis may have stemmed from the effect of pH on the equilibrium between the lactone (closed) form and the hydroxy acid (open) form of the drug. Below pH 5 the lactone predominates; at a higher pH it changes to the far less active hydroxy acid (59). Interconversion of the open form of camptothecin to the active lactone at the acidic pH of urine may have caused the cystitis. The relative ineffectiveness of the drug in the early trials is consistent with the later awareness that the sodium salt of camptothecin has only 1/1,000th the potency of the parent drug.

The encouraging responses observed recently with camptothecin in the xenograft models discussed above prompted a Phase I clinical trial of purified 20(S)-camptothecin (NSC 94600) administered orally. In 52 patients with a variety of tumors, there was one complete remission, in a heavily pretreated patient with lymphoma. Objective responses were seen among five patients with non-small cell lung and ovarian cancer; no responses were seen in patients with colon carcinoma (79).

The relatively water-insoluble analogue 9-aminocamptothecin was also taken to clinical trial because of its efficacy in human colon cancer xenografts (69) and the earlier remissions and lesser degree of drug resistance observed with 9-aminocamptothecin than with camptothecin (67). This drug is more cytotoxic and breaks more DNA strands than irinotecan or topotecan in human colon cancer HT-29 cell lines (80).

IRINOTECAN

Irinotecan is the most advanced of the camptothecins in clinical investigation. Phase I studies in Japan, France, and the United States have established the dose-limiting toxic effects and partially defined the maximally tolerated dose (4, 6, 7). Diarrhea and myelosuppression were the most serious toxic side effects. Intermittent doses caused severe diarrhea, while repeated daily doses were associated with neutropenia, thrombocytopenia, and anemia. Pulmonary toxicity, possibly drug related, was also found infrequently. Encouraging antitumor effects were observed in the Phase I trials. Partial remissions were seen in patients with colon, cervical, esophageal, renal cell, breast, and ovarian cancer. There were also responses in non-small cell lung cancer and in head and neck cancer. The use of loperamide to control the diarrhea, which may be a parasympathetic reaction, has allowed high dose escalation of irinotecan therapy (81). Because of this wide range of activity, many phase II trials were undertaken. Some of the preliminary results of these studies conducted in Japan are summarized in Table 65.1 (82–92). Partial remissions were observed in colorectal and gastric cancer (86–88). Recently, the drug's effectiveness in untreated, treated, and metastatic colorectal cancer has been confirmed in studies conducted in France and in the United States. Phase II studies show occasional complete remissions in ovarian and cervical cancer and in pretreated patients with non-Hodgkin's lymphoma. Partial remissions were seen more commonly in these and other neoplasms.

With the use of recombinant granulocyte colony-stimulating factor (G-CSF), the dose of irinotecan could be increased by 33% in patients with non-small cell lung cancer (93). Combinations with other active agents are being explored. Five of 15 patients with metastatic colorectal cancer had experienced disease regression after treatment with a combination of irinotecan and 5-fluorouracil (94). Irinotecan has also been given with cisplatin (93, 95) and etoposide (96).

Irinotecan, the prodrug, is converted to the active metabolite SN-38 by carboxylesterases in plasma, intestinal mucosa, and liver (62). It is possible that these activities may be important in both drug activation and in causing side effects. Irinotecan and SN-38, like camptothecin, exist in either the

Table 65.1. Phase II Studies of Irinotecan

Tumor type	Dose/schedule	Prior treatment	No. of patients	Response (No.)		Reference
				Complete	Partial	
Lung cancer						
NSCLC	100 mg/m^2 weekly	No	72	0	23	82, 83
SCLC	100 mg/m^2 weekly	Yes	15	2	7	84
SCLC	100 mg/m^2 weekly	Yes/No	27	0	7/4	85
Colorectal	100 mg/m^2 weekly or every 2 wk	NR	36	0	12	86
Colorectal	100 mg/m^2 weekly, or 150 mg/m^2 every 2 wk	Yes/No	63	0	17	87
Gastric cancer	100 mg/m^2 weekly or 150 mg/m^2 every 2 wk	Yes/No	60	0	14	88
Ovarian cancer	100 mg/m^2 weekly, or 150 mg/m^2 every 2 wk, or 250 mg/m^2 every 3–4 wk	Yes	14	1	2	89
Cervical cancer	100 mg/m^2 weekly, or 150 mg/m^2 every 2 wk	Yes, with XRT	55	5	9	90
Non-Hodgkin's lymphoma	40 mg/m^2 for 3 days weekly	Yes	51	8	15	91
Non-Hodgkin's lymphoma	200 mg/m^2 every 3–4 wk 40 mg/m^2 × 5 d q 3–4 wk 40 mg/m^2 × 3 d/wk 20 mg/m^2 bid × 7 d q 3–4 wk	Yes	29	4	3	92

Abbreviations: SCLC, small cell lung cancer; NSCLC, non-small cell lung cancer.

open or closed lactone (active) forms. The half-life of the total and lactone forms of irinotecan is somewhat shorter than that of SN-38 (7.9 vs. 13 hours for the total form and 6.3 vs. 11.5 hours for the lactone, respectively [97]). Irinotecan and SN-38 are eliminated mainly by the biliary route, with extensive enterohepatic recirculation of irinotecan, resulting in a second peak of SN-38 in the plasma. Renal elimination accounts for about 37% of administered drug (98).

TOPOTECAN

Numerous Phase I trials with topotecan, using several dosing schedules, showed that myelosuppression was generally the dose-limiting toxic effect. Neutropenia and thrombocytopenia occurred, the latter more commonly with prolonged infusion schedules (4–7, 99–100). Alopecia occurred in more than 80% of cases, low-grade fever in 15%, and rash in 14%. Fatigue was noted in 10%, anorexia in 10%, and liver function abnormalities and mucositis in less than 5%. These studies showed some complete responses in patients with non-small cell lung cancer, acute myeloblastic leukemia, and chronic myelocytic leukemia in the blastic phase (100). Minor responses were noted in many other cancers, among them small cell lung cancer, ovarian cancer, esophageal cancer, renal cancer, squamous cell skin cancer, prostate cancer, and some cases of acute myeloid leukemia. The addition of G-CSF after the topotecan infusions were completed lessened the severity of the neutropenia and allowed dose escalation in Phase II trials.

Several pharmacologic studies have been performed with topotecan (3–7, 99–102). These show that like the other camptothecins, this drug is active in the lactone form. In the circulation, the drug is rapidly hydrolyzed to the open carboxylate form. Both forms of the drug have biexponential elimination curves with a half-life of about 3.4 hours (4–6), with 40% of the drug eliminated in the urine.

Phase II trials with topotecan given at the maximum tolerated dose (MTD) of 1.5 mg/m^2 × 5 days every 3 to 4 weeks (103–106) have shown only partial responses in colorectal, ovarian, renal cell, and prostate cancer (Table 65.2). Responses have also been observed in leiomyosarcoma and in extensive stage small cell lung cancer (107, 108). It is possible that the long-term infusion approach (99) may offer a better response rate in tumors.

Trials have also been initiated testing topotecan in combination with etoposide (109) and with (110) cisplatin. While synergism between topotecan and these drugs was observed in preclinical studies, there may also be additive hematologic toxicity when these combinations are used clinically.

GG211

The results of the only Phase I study of GG221 reported to date indicate that hematologic toxicity is also dose-limiting for this water-soluble camptothecin analogue. No cumulative hematologic toxicity was observed in up to seven cycles of therapy. Pharmacokinetics revealed a plasma half-life of 4.72 hours (111).

Mechanisms of Resistance to the Camptothecins

Resistance to the camptothecins in tissue culture lines may occur by a variety of mechanisms: (*a*) An altered expression of topoisomersase I causes a decrease in enzyme level or a mutated enzyme with an altered affinity for DNA (112). In the well-characterized human acute lymphoblastic leukemia cell line CPT K-5, two mutations have been discovered in the cDNA of the DNA topoisomerase I gene, both resulting in aspartic acid to glycine substitutions (113). (*b*) Overexpression of the MDR1 gene decreases the cellular content of many drugs via the p170 membrane pump. Topotecan is a substrate for this MDR1 gene product, while camptothecin and 9-aminocamptothecin, irinotecan, and possibly GG211 (64) overcome MDR1-mediated resistance in tissue culture lines (114–116). (*c*) A failure to convert the prodrug irinotecan to the active agent SN-38 (117) is perhaps an additional cause for resistance. (*d*) Selection of cells with a lengthened cell cycle time may also lead to resistance to this highly cycle-specific drug.

Future Prospects

The camptothecins emerge as a class of compounds with considerable promise for the treatment of cancer. The encouraging results of Phase I and Phase II trials, which show a broad spectrum of antitumor activity in patients with usually chemoresistant tumors such as colon and non-small cell lung cancer, must be further evaluated. Future studies will optimize treatment schedules and routes of administration. The extent of benefit derived from growth factor support will be established further. The potential of combinations with other drugs and radiation therapy will be determined. Randomized trials may then be required to establish relative value. Tools are now available to investigate the determinants of resistance in a clinical setting. A better understand-

Table 65.2. Phase II Studies of Topotecan

Tumor type	Dose/schedule	Prior treatment	No. of patients	Response	Reference
Colorectal cancer	1.5 mg/m^2/d × 5 d every 3 wk	No	16	1 PR	103
Ovarian cancer	1.5 mg/m^2/d × 5 d every 3 wk	Yes	28	4 PR	104
Renal cell cancer	1.5 mg/m^2/d × 5 d every 4 wk	No	15	2 MR, 7 SD	105
Prostate cancer	1.5 mg/m^2/d × 5 d every 3 wk	Yes	28	2 PR, 8 SD	106

Abbreviations: PR, partial response; MR, minor response; SD, stable disease.

ing of how the inhibitors work will emerge from the available crystalline forms of the enzyme, which may allow future rational drug design.

References

1. Wang JC. Interaction between DNA and an *Escherichia coli* protein omega. J Mol Biol 1971;55:523–533.
2. Chen AY and Liu LF. DNA topoisomerases: essential enzymes and lethal targets. Annu Rev Pharmacol Toxicol 1994;34:191–218.
3. Pommier Y. DNA topoisomerase I and II in cancer chemotherapy: update and perspectives. Cancer Chemother Pharmacol 1993;32:103–108.
4. Creemers CG, Lund B, Verweij J. Topoisomerase I inhibitors: topotecan and irenotecan. Cancer Treat Rev 1994;20:73–96.
5. Slichenmyer WJ, Rowinsky EK, Donehower RC, Kaufmann SH. The current status of camptothecin analogues as antitumor agents. JNCI 1993;85:271–291.
6. Burris HA 3rd, Fields SM. Topoisomerase I inhibitors: an overview of the camptothecin analogs. Hematol Oncol Clin North Am 1994;8:333–355.
7. Von Hoff DD, Burris HA 3rd, Eckerdt J, Rothenberg M, Fields SM, Chen SF, Kuhn JG. Preclinical and phase I trials of topoisomerase I inhibitors. Cancer Chemother Pharmacol 1994;34(suppl):S41–S45.
8. Potmesil M. Camptothecins: from bench research to hospital wards. Cancer Res 1994;54:1431–1439.
9. Costin D, Potmesil M. Preclinical and clinical development of camptothecins. Adv Pharmacol 1994;29B.
10. Miller KG, Miller KG, Liu LF, Englund PT. A homogeneous type II DNA topoisomerase from HeLa cell nuclei. J Biol Chem 1981;256:9334–9339.
11. Juan CC, Hwang JL, Liu AA, Whang-Peng J, Knutsen T, Huebner K, Croce CM, Zhang H, Wang JC, Liu LF. Human DNA topoisomerase I is encoded by a single-copy gene that maps to chromosome region 20q12–13.2. Proc Natl Acad Sci USA 1988;85:8910–8913.
12. D'Arpa P, Machlin PS, Ratrie H III, Rothfield NF, Cleveland DW, Earnshaw WC. cDNA cloning of human DNA topoisomerase I: catalytic activity of a 67.7-kDa carboxyl-terminal fragment. Proc Natl Acad Sci USA 1988;85:2543–2547.
13. Wang JC. DNA topoisomerase: why so many? J Biol Chem 1991;266:6659–6662.
14. Champoux JJ. Mechanistic aspects of type-I topoisomerases. In Topology and its Biological Effects. Edited by JC Wang , NR Cozzarelli, Cold Spring Harbor, NY: Cold Spring Harbor Laboratory Press, 1990, pp 217–242.
15. Muller MT, Pfund WB, Mehta VB, Trask DK. Eukaryotic type I topoisomerase is enriched in the nucleolus and catalytically active on ribosomal DNA. EMBO J 1985;4: 1237–1243.
16. Fleischmann G, Pflugfelder G, Steiner EK, Javaherian K, Howard GC, Wang JC, Elgin SC. Drosophila DNA topoisomerase I is associated with transcriptionally active regions of the genome. Proc Natl Acad Sci USA 1984;81:6958–6962.
17. Brill SJ, Sternglanz R. Transcription-dependent DNA supercoiling in yeast DNA topoisomerase mutants. Cell 1988;54:403.
18. Trash C, Voelkel K, DiNardo S, Sternglanz R. Identification of *Saccharomyces cerevisiae* mutants deficient in DNA topoisomerase I activity. J Biol Chem 1984;259: 1357–1377.
19. Rose KM, Szopa J, Han FS, Cheng YC, Richter A, Scheer U. Association of DNA topoisomerase I and RNA polymerase I: a possible role for topoisomerase I in ribosomal gene transcription. Chromosoma 1988;96:411.
20. Kessel D. Effects of camptothecin on RNA synthesis in leukemia L1210 cells. Biochim Biophys Acta 1971;246:225–232.
21. Horwitz SB, Chang C-K, Grollman AP. Studies on camptothecin: effects on nucleic acid and protein synthesis. Mol Pharmacol 1971;7:632–644.
22. Wu H-Y, Shyy SH, Wang JC, Liu LF. Transcription generates positively and negatively supercoiled domains in the template. Cell 1988;53:433–440.
23. Tsao Y-P, Wu H-Y, Liu LF. Transcription-driven supercoiling of DNA: direct biochemical evidence from in vitro studies. Cell 1989;56:111–118.
24. Yang L, Wold MS, Li JJ, Kelly TJ, Liu LF. Roles of DNA topoisomerases in SV40 DNA replication in vitro. Proc Natl Acad Sci USA 1987;84:950–954.
25. Been MD, Champoux JJ. DNA breakage and closure by rat liver type I topoisomerase: separation of the half-reactions by using a single-stranded DNA substrate. Proc Natl Acad Sci USA 1981;78:2883–2887.
26. Champoux JJ. DNA Topology and its biological effects. Cold Spring Harbor, NY: Cold Spring Harbor Laboratory Press, 1990:217–242.
27. Wang JC, Caron PR, Kim RA. The role of DNA topoisomerases in recombination and genome stability: a double-edged sword? Cell 1990;62:403.
28. Shuman S, Moss B. Identification of a vaccinia virus gene encoding a type I DNA topoisomerase. Proc Natl Acad Sci USA 1987;84:7478.
29. Priel E, Showalter SD, Roberts M, Oroszlaan S, Segal S, Aboud M, Blair DG. Topoisomerase I activity associated with human immunodeficiency virus (HIV) particles and equine infectious anemia virus core. EMBO J 1990;9:4167–4172.
30. Bullock P, Champoux JJ, Botchan M. Association of crossover points with topoisomerase I cleavage sites: a model for nonhomologous recombination. Science 1985;230:954–958.
31. Wang H-P, Rogler CE. Topoisomerase I-mediated integration of hepadnavirus DNA in vitro. J Virol 1991;65:2381–2392.
32. Champoux JJ. Strand breakage by the DNA untwisting enzyme results in covalent attachment of the enzyme to DNA. Proc Natl Acad Sci USA 1977;74:3800–3804.
33. Champoux JJ. Mechanism of the reaction catalyzed by the DNA untwisting enzyme attachment of the enzyme to 3′-terminus of the nicked DNA. J Mol Biol 1978;118: 441–446.
34. Champoux JJ. Mechanism of catalysis by eukaryotic DNA topoisomerase I. Adv Pharmaco 1994;29A:71–82.
35. Wall ME, Wani MC Cook CE, Palmer KH, McPhail AT, Sim GA. Plant antitumor agents, I: the isolation and structure of camptothecin, a novel alkaloidal leukemia and tumor inhibitor from *Camptotheca acuminata*. J Am Chem Soc 1966;88:3888–90.
36. Hsiang YH, Hertzberg R, Hecht S, Liu LF. Camptothecin induces protein-linked DNA breaks via mammalian DNA topoisomerase I. J Biol Chem 1985;260:14873–14878.
37. Giovanella BC, Stehlin JS, Wall ME, Wani MC, Nicholas AW, Liu LF, Silber R, Potmesil M. DNA topoisomerase I-targeted chemotherapy of human colon cancer in xenografts. Science 1989;246:1046–1048.
38. Hirabayashi N, Kim R, Nishiyama M, Aogi K, Saeki S, Toge T, Okada K. Tissue expression of topoisomerase I and II in digestive tract cancers and adjacent normal tissues. Proc Am Assoc Cancer Res 1992;33:436. (Abstract)
39. Husain I, Mohler JL, Seigler HF, Besterman JM. Elevation of topoisomerase I messenger RNA, protein, and catalytic activity in human tumors: demonstration of tumor-type specificity and implications for cancer chemotherapy. Cancer Res 1994;54: 539–546.
40. Heck MM, Hittelman WN, Earnshaw WC. Differential expression of DNA topoisomerase I and II during the eukaryotic cell cycle. Proc Natl Acad Sci USA 1988;85: 1086–1090.
41. Liu LF. Topoisomerase I-targeting drugs.mechanism of inhibition and cytotoxicity. In Vth World Conference on Clinical Pharmacology and Therapeutics. Highlights of a Satellite Symposium: approaches to Cancer Treatment by Topoisomerase I Inhibitors. Edited by T Taguchi, JC Wang. Tokyo: BIOMEDIS, 1992, pp 6–9.
42. Hsiang Y-H, Liu LF. Identification of mammalian DNA topoisomerase I as an intracellular target of the anticancer drug camptothecin. Cancer Res 1988;48:1722–1726.
43. Hsiang Y-H, Lihou MG, Liu LF. Arrest of replication forks by drug-stabilized topoisomerase I-DNA cleavable complexes as a mechanism of cell killing by camptothecin. Cancer Res 1989;49:5077–5082.
44. D'Arpa P, Beardmore C, Liu LF. Involvement of nucleic acid synthesis in cell killing mechanisms of topoisomerase poisons. Cancer Res 1990;50:6919–6924.
45. Jaxel C, Kohn KW, Pommier Y. Topoisomerase I interaction with SV40 DNA in the presence and absence of camptothecin. Nucleic Acids Res 1988;16:11157–11170.
46. Jaxel C, Capranico G, Kerrigan D, Kohn KW, Pommier Y. Effect of local DNA sequence on topoisomerase I cleavage in the presence or absence of camptothecin. J Biol Chem 1991;266:20418–20423.
47. Jaxel C, Capranico G, Waserman K, Kerrigan D, Kohn KW, Pommier Y. DNA sequence at sites of topoisomerase I cleavage induced by camptothecin in SV40 DNA. In DNA topoisomerases in cancer. Edited by M Potmesil, KW Kohn. New York: Oxford, 1991, pp 182–195.
48. Porter SE, Champoux JJ. The basis for camptothecin enhancement of DNA breakage by eukaryotic topoisomerase I. Nucleic Acids Res 1989;17:8521–8532.
49. Zhang H, D'Arpa P, Liu LF. A model for tumor cell killing by topoisomerase poisons. Cancer Cells 1990;2:23–27.
50. Tsao Y-P, Russo A, Nyamuswa G, Silber R, Liu LF. Interaction between replication forks and topoisomerase I-DNA cleavable complexes: studies in a cell-free SV40 DNA replication system. Cancer Res 1993;53:1–8.
51. Tsao Y-P, D'Arpa P, Liu LF. The involvement of active DNA synthesis in camptothecin-induced G2 arrest: altered regulation of p34cdc2/-cyclin B. Cancer Res 1992;52: 1823–1829.
52. Stewart AF, Herrera RE, Nordheim A. Rapid induction of C-fos transcription reveals quantitative linkage of RNA polymerase-II and DNA topoisomerase-I enzyme activities. Cell 1990;60:141–149.
53. Kharbanda S, Rubin E, Gunji H, Hinz H, Giovanella B, Pantazis P, Kufe D. Camptothecin and its derivatives induce expression of the c-*jun* protooncogene in human myeloid leukemia cells. Cancer Res 1991;51:6636–6642.
54. Wani MC, Ronman PE, Lindley JT, Wall ME. Plant antitumor agents. 18. Synthesis and biological activity of camptothecin analogues. J Med Chem 1980;23:554–560.
55. Wall ME, Wani MC, Nicholas AW, Manikumar G, Tele C, Moore L, Truesdale A, Leitner P, Besterman JM. Plant antitumor agents. 30. Synthesis and structure activity of novel camptothecin analogs. J Med Chem 1993;36:2689–2701.
56. Wall ME, Wani MC. Topoisomerase I inhibitors camptothecin and analogs. In Cancer Chemotherapeutic Agents. Edited by WO Foye. Washington DC: ACS Books, 1993.
57. Jaxel C, Kohn KW, Wani MC, Wall ME, Pommier Y. Structure-activity study of the actions of camptothecin derivatives on mammalian topoisomerase I: evidence for a specific receptor site and for a relation to antitumor activity. Cancer Res 1989;49: 1465–1469.
58. Hsiang Y-H, Liu LF, Wall ME, Wani MC, Nicholas AW, Manikumar G, Kirschenbaum S, Silber R, Potmesil M. DNA topoisomerase I-mediated DNA cleavage and cytotoxicity of camptothecin analogs. Cancer Res 1989;49:4385–4389.
59. Hertzberg RP, Caranfa MJ, Holden KG, Jakas DR, Gallagher G, Mattern MR, Mong SM, Bartus JO, Johnson RK, Kingsbury WD. Modification of the hydroxy lactone ring of camptothecin: inhibition of mammalian topoisomerase I and biological activity. J Med Chem 1989;32:715–720.
60. Kawato Y, Aonuma M, Hirota Y, Kuga H, Sato K. Intracellular roles of SN-38, a metabolite of the camptothecin derivative CPT-11, in the antitumor effect of CPT-11. Cancer Res 1991;51:4187–4191.
61. Kunimoto T, Nitta K, Tanaka T, Uehara N, Baba H, Takeuchi M, Yokokura T, Sawada S, Miyasaka T, Mutai M. Antitumor activity of 7-ethyl-10-{4-(1-piperidino)-1-piperidino}-carbonyloxy-camptothecin, a novel water-soluble derivative of camptothecin, against murine tumors. Cancer Res 1987;47:5944–5947.
62. Kaneda N, Nagata H, Furuta I, Yokokura Y. Metabolism and pharmacokinetics of the camptothecin analogue CPT-11 in the mouse. Cancer Res 1990;50:1715–1720.
63. Kingsbury WD, Boehm JC, Jakas DR, Holden KG, Hecht SM, Gallagher G, Caranfa MJ, McCabe FL, Faucette LF, Johnson RK, Hertzberg RP. Synthesis of water-soluble (aminoalkyl) camptothecin analogues: inhibition of topoisomerase I and antitumor activity. J Med Chem 1991;34:98–107.
64. Emerson DL, McIntyre G, Jones AC, LeRay JD, Onori J, Andrews JL. The antitumor activity of 7-(4-methylpiperazinomethylene)-10, 11-ethylenedioxy-20(S)-camptothecindihydrochloride, (GI 147721 1C). Proc Am Assoc Cancer Res 1994;35:47. (Abstract)
65. DeWys WD, Humphreys SR, Goldin A. Studies on therapeutic effectiveness of drugs with tumor weight and survival time indices of Walker 256 carcinosarcoma. Cancer Chemother Rep 1968;52:229–242.
66. Venditti JM, Abbott BJ. Studies of oncolytic agents from natural sources: correlation of activity against animal tumors and clinical effectiveness. Lloydia 1967;30:332–338.
67. Giovanella BC, Hinz HR, Kozielski AJ, Stehlin JS Jr, Silber R, Potmesil M. Complete growth inhibition of human cancer xenografts in nude mice by treatment with 20-(S)-camptothecin. Cancer Res 1991;51:3052–3055.
68. Potmesil M, Giovanella BC, Wall ME, Liu LF, Silber R, Stehlin JS, Wani MC, Hochster H. Preclinical and clinical development of DNA topoisomerase I inhibitors in the United States. In Molecular biology of DNA topoisomerases and its application to

chemotherapy. Edited by T Andoh, H Ikeda, M Oguro. Nagoya, Japan: CRC Press, 1993, pp 301–311.

69. Houghton PJ, Cheshire PJ, Hallman JC, Bissery MC, Mathieu-Boue A, Houghton JA. Therapeutic efficacy of the topoisomerase I inhibitor 7-ethyl-10-(4-[1-piperidino]-1-piperidino)-carbonyloxy-camptothecin against human tumor xenografts: lack of cross-resistance in vivo in tumors with acquired resistance to the topoisomerase I inhibitor 9-dimethylaminomethyl-10-hydroxycamptothecin. Cancer Res 1993;53(12): 2823–2829.
70. Tsuruo T, Matsuzaki M, Saito H, Yokokura T. Antitumor effect of CPT-11, a new derivative of camptothecin, against pleiotropic drug-resistant tumors in vitro and in vivo. Cancer Chemother Pharmacol 1988;21:71–74.
71. Kawato Y, Furuta T, Aonuma M, Yasuoka M, Yokoura T, Matsumoto K. Antitumor activity of a camptothecin derivative, CPT-11, against human tumor xenografts in nude mice. Cancer Chemother Pharmacol 1991;28:192–198.
72. Houghton PJ, Cheshire PJ, Myers L, Houghton JA. Evaluation on 9-dimethylaminomethyl-10-hydroxycamptothecin (topotecan) against xenografts derived from adult and childhood tumors. Cancer Chemother Pharmacol 1992;31:229–239.
73. Peel MR, Besterman J, Croom DK, Emerson DL, Leitner P, Luzzio MJ, McIntyre G, Milstead MW, Morton BS, Nanthakumar SS, Sisco JM, Sternbach DD, Tong WQ, Uehling DE, Vuong A. 7-Thiomethylcamptothecins as water soluble topoisomerase I inhibitors. Proc Am Assoc Cancer Res 1994;35:453. (Abstract)
74. Kunka RL, Eckardt JR, Verweij J, DePee SP, Littlefield D, Selinger KA, Wissel PS. Use of pharmacokinetics as a tool in predicting toxicity of GG211, a new topoisomerase I inhibitor. Proc Am Soc Clin Pharm Therap 1995 (in press).
75. Gottlieb JA, Guarino AM Call JB, Oliverio VT, Block JB. Preliminary pharmacologic and clinical evaluation of camptothecin sodium (NSC-100880). Cancer Chemother Rep 1970;54:461–470.
76. Gottlieb JA, Luce JK. Treatment of malignant melanoma with camptothecin (NSC-100880). Cancer Chemother Rep 1972;56:103–105.
77. Muggia FM, Creavan PJ, Hansen HH, Cohen MH, Sealwry OS. Phase I clinical trial of weekly and daily treatment with camptothecin (NSC-10080): correlation with preclinical studies. Cancer Chemother Rep 1972;56:515–521.
78. Moertel CG, Schutt AJ, Reitemeier RJ, Hahn RG. Phase II study of camptothecin (NSC-100880) in the treatment of advanced gastrointestinal cancer. Cancer Chemother Rep 1972;56:95–101.
79. Stehlin JS, Natelson EA, Hinz HR, Giovanella BC, de Ipolyi PD, Fehir KM, Trezona TP, Vardeman DM, Harris NJ, Marcee AK, Kozeilski AJ, Ruiz-Razura A. Phase I clinical trial and pharmacokinetics results with oral administration of 20(S)-Camptothecin. In Camptothecins: new anticancer agents. Edited by M Potmesil, H Pinedo. Boca Raton FL: CRC Press. 1995, pp 59–66.
80. Tanizawa A, Fujimori A, Fujimori Y, Pommier Y. Comparison of topoisomerase I inhibition, DNA damage, and cytotoxicity of camptothecin derivatives presently in clinical trials. JNCI 1994;86:836–843.
81. Abigerges D, Armand JP, Chabot GG, Da Costa L, Fadel E, Cote C, Herait P, Gandia D. Irinotecan (CPT-11) high-dose escalation using intensive high-dose loperamide to control diarrhea. JNCI 1994;86:446–449.
82. Fukuoka M, Niitani H, Suzuki A, Motomiya M, Hasegawa K, Nishiwaki Y, Kuriyama T, Ariyoshi Y, Negoro S, Masuda N, Nakajima S, Taguchi T. A phase II study of CPT-11, a new derivative of camptothecin, for previously untreated non-small-cell lung cancer. J Clin Oncol 1992;10:16–20.
83. Fukuoka M, Masuda N, Takada M, Kodama N, Kawahara M, Furuse K. Dose-intensive chemotherapy in extensive-stage small cell lung cancer. Semin Oncol 1994;21: 43–47.
84. Masuda N, Fukuoka M, Kusunoki Y, Matsui K, Takifuji N, Kudoh S, Negoro S, Nishioka M, Nakagawa K, Takada M. CPT-11: a new derivative of camptothecin for the treatment of refractory or relapsed small-cell lung cancer. J Clin Oncol 1992;10: 1225–1229.
85. Negoro S, Fukuoka M, Niitani H, Taguchi T. Phase II study of CPT-11, a new camptothecin derivative, in small cell lung cancer (SCLC). Proc Am Soc Clin Oncol 1991;10:241. (Abstract)
86. Ogawa M, Taguchi T. Clinical studies with CPT-11: the Japanese experience. Ann Oncol 1992;3(suppl 1):118. (Abstract)
87. Shimada Y, Yoshino M, Wakui A, Nakao I, Futatsuki K, Sakata Y, Kambe M, Taguchi T, Ogawa N. Phase II study of CPT-11, a new camptothecin derivative, in metastatic colorectal cancer. CPT-11 Gastrointestinal Cancer Study Group. J Clin Oncol 1993;11:909–913.
88. Kambe M, Wakui A, Nakao I, Futatsuki K, Sakata Y, Yoshino M, Shimada Y, Taguchi T and CPT-11 Gastrointestinal Cancer Study Group, Japan. A late phase II study of irinotecan (CPT-11) in patients with advanced gastric cancer. Proc Am Soc Clin Oncol 1993;12:198. (Abstract)
89. Takeuchi S, Noda K, Yakushiji M, and CPT-11 Study Group on Gynecologic Malignancy, Japan. Late phase II study of CPT-11, topoisomerase I inhibitor, in advanced cervical carcinoma (CC). Proc Am Soc Clin Oncol 1992;11:224. (Abstract)
90. Takeuchi S, Takamizawa H, Takeda Y, Okawa T, Tamaya T, Noda K, Sugawa T, Sekiba K, Yakushiji M, Taguchi T. Clinical study of CPT-11, camptothecin derivative, on gynecological malignancy. Proc Am Soc Clin Oncol 1991;10:189. (Abstract)
91. Tsuda H, Takatsuki K, Ohno R, Masaoka T, Okada K, Shirakawa S, Ohashi Y, Ohta K, Taguchi T and the CPT-11 Study Group on Hematological Malignancy, Japan. A late phase II trial of a potent topoisomerase I inhibitor, CPT-11, in malignant lymphoma. Proc Am Soc Clin Oncol 1992;11:316. (Abstract)
92. Ohno R, Okada K, Masaoka T, Kuramoto A, Arima T, Yoshida Y, Ariyoshi H, Ichimaru M, Sakai Y, Oguro M. An early phase II study of CPT-11: a new derivative of camptothecin, for the treatment of leukemia and lymphoma. J Clin Oncol 1990;8: 1907–1912.
93. Masuda N, Fukuoka M, Kudoh S, Kusunoki Y, Matsui K, Nakagawa K, Hirashima T, Tamanoi M, Nitta T, Yana T, Negoro S. Phase I study of irinotecan and cisplatin with granulocyte colony-stimulating factor support for advanced non-small-cell lung cancer. J Clin Oncol 1994;12:90–96.
94. Shimada Y, Sasaki Y, Sugano K, Shirao K, Kondo H, Yokota T, Saito D, Tamura T, Ohe Y, Shinkai T, Eguchi K, Saijo N, Shintani S. Combination phase I study of CPT-11 (irinotecan) combined with continuous infusion of 5-fluorouracil (5FU) in metastatic colorectal cancer. Proc Am Soc Clin Oncol 1993;12:196. (Abstract)
95. Fukuoka M, Masuda N. Clinical studies of irinotecan alone and in combination with cisplatin. Cancer Chemother Pharmacol 1994;34(suppl):S105–S111.
96. Masuda N, Fukuoka M, Kudoh S, Matsui K, Kusunoki Y, Takada M, Nakagawa K, Hirashima T, Tsukada H, Yana T, Yoshikawa A, Kubo A, Matsuura E, Nitta T, Takifuji N, Terakawa K, Negoro S. Phase I and pharmacologic study of irinotecan and etoposide with recombinant human granulocyte colony-stimulating factor support for advanced lung cancer. J Clin Oncol 1994;12:1833–1841.
97. Rothenberg ML, Kuhn JG, Burris HA, Morales MT, Nelson J, Eckardt JR, Rock MK, Terada K, Von Hoff DD. A phase I and pharmacokinetic trial of CPT-11 in patients with refractory solid tumors. Proc Am Soc Clin Oncol 1992;11:113. (Abstract)
98. Rowinski EK, Grochow LB, Ettinger DS, Sartorius SE, Lubejko BG, Chen TL, Rock MK, Donehower RC. Phase I and pharmacological study of the novel topoisomerase I inhibitor 7-ethyl-10-{4-(1-piperidino)-1-piperidino} carbonyloxycamptothecin (CPT-11) administered as a ninety-minute infusion every 3 weeks. Cancer Res 1994;54: 427–436.
99. Hochster H, Liebes L, Speyer J, Sorich J, Taubes B, Oratz R, Wernz J, Chachoua A, Raphael B, Vinci RZ, Blum RH. Phase I trial of low-dose continuous topotecan infusion in patient with cancer: an active and well-tolerated regimen. J Clin Oncol 1994;12:553–559.
100. Kantarjian HM, Beran M, Ellis A, Zwelling L, O'Brien S, Cazanave L, Koller C, Rios MB, Plunkett W, Keating MJ, Estey E. Phase I study of topotecan, a new topoisomerase I inhibitor, in patients with refractory or relapsed acute leukemia. Blood 1993;81: 1146–1151.
101. Verweij J. Lund B, Beijnen J, Planting A, de Boer-Dennert M, Koier I, Rosing H, Hansen H. Phase I and pharmacokinetics study of topotecan, a new topoisomerase I inhibitor. Ann Oncol 1993;4:673–678.
102. Rowinski EK, Grochow LB, Hendricks CB, Ettinger DS, Forastiere AA, Hurowitz LA, McGuire WP, Sartorius SE, Lubejko BG, Kaufmann SH, Donehower RC. Phase I and pharmacologic study of topotecan: a novel topoisomerase I inhibitor. J Clin Oncol 1992;10:647–656.
103. Verweij J, Wanders J, Calabresi F, Franklin H, Kaye SB. Phase II study with topotecan in colorectal cancer. In Proceedings of the EORTC Early Drug Development Meeting. Bruxelles: European Organization for Research and Treatment of Cancer, 1993, p 31.
104. Kudelka A, Edwards C, Freedman H, Wallin B, Hord M, Howell E, Harper K, Raber M, Kavanagh J. An open phase II study to evaluate the efficacy and toxicity of topotecan administered intravenously as 5 daily infusions over 21 days to women with advanced epithelial ovarian carcinoma. Proc Am Soc Clin Oncol 1993;12:259.
105. Lison D, Motzer RJ, O'Moore P, Nanus D, Bosi GJ. A phase II study of topotecan in advanced renal cell carcinoma. Proc Am Soc Clin Oncol 1993;12:248.
106. Giantonio BJ, Koslerowsky R, Ramsey HE, Fox SC, McAleer CA, Roethke S, Ozols RF, Hudes GR. Phase II study of topotecan (TT) for hormone refractory prostate cancer (HRPC). Proc Am Soc Clin Oncol 1993;12:247.
107. Eisenhauer EA, Wainman N, Boos G, McDonald D, Bramwell V. Phase II trials of topotecan in patients (pts) with malignant glioma and soft tissue sarcoma. Proc Am Soc Clin Oncol 1994;13:175.
108. Schiller JH, Kim K, Johnson D. Phase II study of topotecan in extensive stage small cell lung cancer. Proc Am Soc Clin Oncol 1994;13:330.
109. Anzai H, Frost P, Abbruzzese JL. Synergistic cytotoxicity with combined inhibition of topoisomerase (Topo) I and II. Proc Am Assoc Cancer Res 1992;33:431. (Abstract)
110. Miller AA, Hargis JB, Fields S, Lilenbaum RC, Rosner GL, Schilsky RL. Phase I study of topotecan and cisplatin in patients with advanced cancer (CALGB) 9261. Proc Am Soc Clin Oncol 1993;12:399. (Abstract)
111. Eckardt JR, Rodriguez GI, Burris PS, Wissel PS, Fields SM, Rothenberg ML, Smith I, Thurman A, Kunka RJ, DePee SP, Littlefield D, White LJ, Von Hoff DD. A phase I and pharmamcokinetic study of the topoisomerase I inhibitor GG211. Proc Am Soc Clin Oncol 1995;14:476(#1544). (Abstract)
112. Andoh T, Okada K. Drug resistance mechanisms of topoisomerase I drugs. Adv Pharmacol 1994;29A:93–103.
113. Tamura H, Kohcht C, Yamada R, Ikeda T, Koiwai O, Patterson E, Keene JD, Okada K, Kjeldsen E, Nishikawa K, Andoh T. Molecular cloning of a cDNA of a camptothecin-resistant human DNA topoisomerase-I and identification of mutation sites. Nucleic Acids Res 1991;19:69–75.
114. Potmesil M, Giovanella BC, Liu LF, Wall ME, Silber R, Stehlin J, Hsiang Y-H, Wani M. Preclinical studies of DNA topoisomerase I–targeted 9-amino and 10, 11-methylenedioxy camptothecins. In DNA topoisomerases in cancer. Edited by M Potmesil, KW Kohn. New York: Oxford University Press. 1991, p 299.
115. Chen A, Yu C, Potmesil M, Wall ME, Wani MC, Liu LF. Camptothecin overcomes MDRI-mediated resistance in human KB carcinoma cells. Cancer Res 1991;51: 6039–6044.
116. Hendricks CB, Rowinski EK, Grochow LB, Donehower RC, Kaufmann SH. Effect of P-glycoprotein expression on the accumulation and cytotoxicity of topotecan (SK&F 104864), a new camptothecin analogue. Cancer Res 1992;52:2268–2278.
117. Saijo N, Nishio K, Kubota N, Kanzawa F, Shinkai T, Karato A, Sasaki Y, Eguchi K, Tamura T, Ohe Y, Oshita F, Nishio M. 7-Ethyl-10-{4-(1-piperidino)-1-piperidino}carbonyloxycamptothecin: mechanism of resistance and clinical trials. Cancer Chemother Pharmacol 1994;34(suppl):S112–S117.
118. Pommier Y, Tanizawa A, Kohn KW. Mechanisms of topoisomerase I inhibition by anticancer drugs. Adv Pharmacol 1994;29B:73–92.

CHAPTER 66

Anticancer Drugs from Plants: *Vinca* Alkaloids and Taxanes

WILLIAM T. BECK, CAROL E. CASS, AND PETER J. HOUGHTON

The treatments of many diseases owe much to the important medicines that have been derived from plants, and the treatment of cancer is no exception. Unique classes of natural product anticancer drugs have been derived from plants. As distinct from those agents derived from bacterial and fungal sources, the plant products, represented by the *Vinca* and *Colchicum* alkaloids, as well as other plant-derived products such as paclitaxel (Taxol) and podophyllotoxin, do not target DNA. Rather, they either interact with intact microtubules, integral components of the cytoskeleton of the cell, or with their subunit molecules, the tubulins. In this chapter we will focus attention on the clinically useful plant products: the *Vinca* alkaloids, primarily vinblastine (VLB), vincristine (VCR), and vinorelbine (Navelbine), as well as the two taxanes recently introduced, paclitaxel (Taxol) and docetaxel (Taxotere).

It has been customary in chapters on plant alkaloids to include the epipodophyllotoxins teniposide (VM-26) and etoposide (VP-16–213), as they are semisynthetic derivatives of podophyllotoxin, another plant-derived antimitotic agent. However, while podophyllotoxin has essentially the same mechanism of action as colchicine, it is not an alkaloid (it has no nitrogen). Further, the antitumor mechanism of the epipodophyllotoxins is distinct from that of the parent compound: Whereas podophyllotoxin inhibits microtubule polymerization, its glucoside derivatives teniposide and etoposide target DNA and in fact inhibit the essential nuclear enzyme, DNA topoisomerase II (142, 265). Because of these facts and because of their clinical importance, the epipodophyllotoxins are considered elsewhere (see Chapter 64).

The major areas of *Vinca* alkaloid pharmacology that require updating from the previous edition of this book are those concerning the mechanisms by which tumor cells express resistance to these agents, their clinical pharmacology, and their usage. Clinical studies with newer *Vinca* alkaloids, especially Navelbine, will also be discussed, and we will identify the important place of the *Vinca* alkaloids in clinical oncology. We will also provide an overview of the pharmacology, pharmacokinetics, toxicity, and usefulness of the taxanes and update current knowledge of their actions, clinical uses, and tumor cell resistance to them. Major clinical effort since the last edition has focused on phase I, II, and III studies of vinorelbine and the taxanes paclitaxel and docetaxel, and these studies will be detailed in this chapter.

Vinca Alkaloids

HISTORY AND CHEMISTRY

The history of the *Vinca* alkaloids and the story of their discovery is well known (118, 119). Because of a folklore that had developed about the oral hypoglycemic properties of extracts of the periwinkle plant, they were studied independently by two different laboratories. The plants had no antidiabetic actions but were shown to cause granulocytopenia and bone marrow depression in rats, and were subsequently found to prolong the life of mice bearing a transplantable lymphocytic leukemia. The investigators quickly saw the possibilities and began vigorous development of these agents, and in a relatively short time VCR and VLB were isolated and put into clinical trial.

The chemistry of the *Vinca* alkaloids has been reviewed extensively (51, 154, 189).These agents are derived from the periwinkle plant, *Catharanthus roseus* G. Don (frequently known as *Vinca rosea* Linn). The *Vinca* alkaloids are dimeric compounds in which indole and dihydroindole nuclei are joined together with other complex ring systems. Modifications have been made on both the velbanamine (catharanthine) and vindoline moieties (189). The basic structures of the major (in terms of clinical utility) *Vinca* alkaloids, VCR, VLB, and the semisynthetic derivatives vindesine (VDS), vinzolidine, and vinorelbine (VRLB), are shown in Figure 66.1. Note that VCR and VLB differ only in the presence of a formyl or methyl group, respectively, in the vindoline moiety. As will be seen later, this apparently modest difference in structure, which does not alter in any fundamental way the mechanism of action of and binding to tubulin, is of considerable significance with regard to the clinical spectrum of antitumor efficacy and clinical toxicity of these drugs. The molecular alterations in vinorelbine differ from those of other *Vinca* alkaloids: Although the vindoline moiety of vinorelbine is the same as that of VLB, the catharanthine moiety has been changed, with an 8-membered ring replacing the hydroxyl and 9-membered ring; as a consequence, the overall lipophilicity of this compound is significantly increased compared to the other *Vinca* alkaloids.

MECHANISM OF ACTION

Among the many biochemical effects seen after exposure of cells and tissues to the *Vinca* alkaloids are disruption of

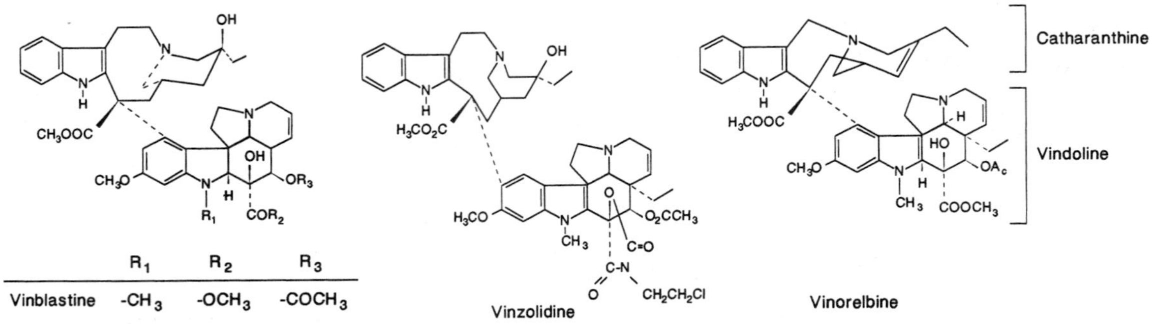

	R_1	R_2	R_3
Vinblastine	$-CH_3$	$-OCH_3$	$-COCH_3$
Vincristine	-CHO	$-OCH_3$	$-COCH_3$
Vindesine	$-CH_3$	$-NH_2$	-H

Vinzolidine

Vinorelbine

Catharanthine

Vindoline

Figure 66.1. Chemical structures of *Vinca* alkaloids.

microtubules, inhibition of synthesis of proteins and nucleic acids, elevation of oxidized glutathione, alteration of lipid metabolism and the lipid content of membranes, elevation of cyclic adenosine monophosphate (cAMP), and inhibition of calcium-calmodulin–regulated cAMP phosphodiesterase (6, 45, 54, 55, 125, 126, 150, 157, 190, 204, 213, 222, 256, 261, 262). The *Vinca* alkaloids are relatively hydrophobic molecules that partition into lipid bilayers in the uncharged state, altering the structure and function of membranes (129, 180, 239, 240). Of their diverse effects, their only well-documented direct action is disruption of microtubules, which results from their reversible binding to tubulin, the subunit protein of microtubules. At pharmacologically active concentrations, most of the biochemical effects associated with exposure to the *Vinca* alkaloids are probably secondary to disruption of microtubules, although it is possible that drug-induced changes in lipid bilayers may alter some membrane-dependent processes. At high intracellular concentrations, these compounds induce formation of large crystalline aggregates that are composed of tubulin and drug (20, 21, 31). Despite their many biochemical actions, the antineoplastic activity of the *Vinca* alkaloids is usually attributed to their ability to disrupt microtubules, causing dissolution of mitotic spindles and metaphase arrest in dividing cells (Fig. 66.2) (30, 83, 110, 131, 139, 150, 186, 248). However, disruption of microtubules also leads to toxicity in nonmitotic neoplastic cells, and although the *Vinca* alkaloids are classified as mitotic inhibitors, their antineoplastic activity in the clinical treatment of cancer probably arises from perturbation of a variety of microtubule-dependent processes (132, 148, 149, 220, 221), as well as from disruption of the cell cycle and induction of programmed cell death (see below) (344–395).

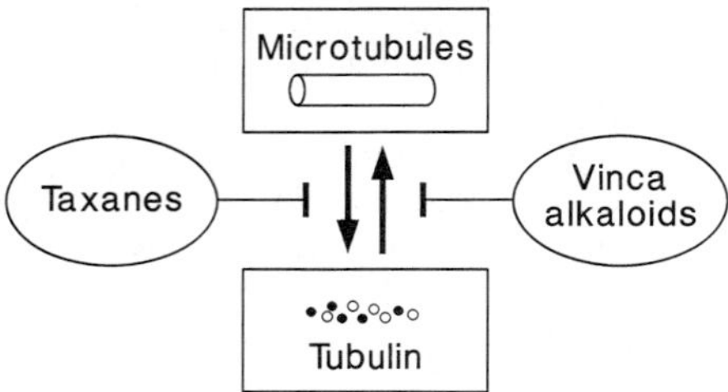

Figure 66.2. Schematic representation of the different actions of *Vinca* alkaloids and taxanes on tubulin/microtubule dynamics. *Vinca* alkaloids block polymerization of tubulins and promote depolymerization, whereas taxanes block microtubule depolymerization.

Microtubules are involved in many cellular processes besides mitosis, and exposure to *Vinca* alkaloids gives rise to diverse biologic effects, many of which could impair essential functions, both in dividing and in nondividing cells (67). Morphologic changes and cell death after treatment with VCR or VLB have been seen in nondividing normal and leukemic lymphocytes, in cultured leukemic cells during interphase, and in G_1- and S-phase cells (132, 148, 149, 220, 221). Chemotaxis in human monocytes and directional migration of cultured tumor cells are inhibited by *Vinca* alkaloids (155, 270). Microtubules are required for the transport of various metabolites and the movement of organelles, including mitochondria and secretory granules, along neuronal processes (210). Exposure of nervous tissue to *Vinca* alkaloids inhibits axonal transport, causing neurotoxicity (42, 92). The *Vinca* alkaloids also inhibit secretory processes, apparently as a result of perturbations in membrane trafficking with disruption of the cytoskeleton (232). Platelets, which depend on the integrity of the peripheral ring of microtubules for their discoidal shape, become spherical after treatment with *Vinca* alkaloids (16, 259). These few examples illustrate that the *Vinca* alkaloids exert a variety of potentially cytotoxic effects that are unrelated to mitotic inhibition.

Although the effects of the *Vinca* alkaloids on the organization and function of microtubules have been extensively characterized, establishing the nature and number of *Vinca* alkaloid binding sites on tubulin has been difficult because of methodological problems (67, 261, 262). However, it appears that each heterodimer of α-β-tubulin possesses a single "*Vinca*-specific" site of high intrinsic affinity and an unknown number of nonspecific sites of low affinity (171, 228). Attempts to compare the tubulin-binding capabilities of different *Vinca* alkaloids are also complicated by differences in assay conditions and methods of analysis of ligand-binding data (96, 171, 172, 228). Nevertheless, some generalizations can be made. For example, the relative strength of drug binding to *Vinca*-specific sites on the α- and β-heterodimers of tubulins is VCR > vindesine > VLB (136, 180, 183). Also, VCR and VLB are more potent inhibitors of in vitro assembly than VRLB (72). It should also be noted that both the velbanamine and vindoline moieties are required for site-specific binding of the *Vinca* alkaloids to tubulin (180).

From the several effects of VLB on assembly of microtubules in vitro, it is generally assumed that the *Vinca* alkaloids disrupt microtubules by more than one mechanism (121, 263). At low concentrations, VLB inhibits microtubule formation in a "substoichiometric" fashion in that assembly is blocked by binding of only a few molecules to high-affinity sites on tubulin heterodimers located at the ends of microtubules (263). It has been estimated that binding of *Vinca* alkaloids by this mechanism to only 1 to 2% of total tubulin could reduce microtubules by 50% (261). At higher concentrations, disassembly results from binding of VLB to tubulin heterodimers located along the microtubule surface, through stoichiometric interaction with *Vinca*-specific sites of reduced affinity and/or nonspecific ionic interaction (229, 263). According to current theories of microtubule assembly, microtubules are dynamic, inherently polar structures that rapidly assemble and disassemble, depending on conditions at the ends (101, 163–165). In cells, one end is usually anchored to an organizing center and the other end may be either slowly growing by addition of tubulin heterodimers or rapidly shrinking (209). Conversion between the two states, which is thought to be controlled by specialized proteins, occurs infrequently. At any given time, cells contain mixed populations of microtubules of different stability, and in at least one experimental system, there are differences among these populations in intrinsic sensitivity to *Vinca* alkaloids (24, 162, 223).

Although there is no question that the *Vinca* alkaloids disrupt microtubules, the biologic mechanisms underlying the antineoplastic activity of these drugs are less certain. In actively proliferating cells, the mechanism of cytotoxicity of the *Vinca* alkaloids is usually considered to be disruption of the mitotic spindle, resulting in metaphase arrest and, ultimately, cell death (30, 83, 131, 150, 186). In support of this mechanism, correlations have been shown in studies with cultured cells between dissolution of mitotic spindles and cytotoxicity, and between the accumulation of mitotic figures and the concentration and duration of drug exposure (30, 110, 139, 248). Among anticancer drugs, the *Vinca* alkaloids are classified as mitotic inhibitors, with their primary site of action being M phase of the cell cycle, although it is by no means certain that mitotic inhibition is the predominant cytotoxic mechanism in vivo. New studies suggest that disruption of the cell cycle may lead to cell death through initiation of programmed cell death pathways, known as *apoptosis* (344–348, 394). Indeed, it is now generally accepted that cell death in response to treatment with certain anticancer drugs, cytokines, and ionizing radiation represents the culmination of a complex set of biochemical and molecular events that in many instances is due to activation of a programmed cell death pathway that involves p53 and other proteins (349), and there is some evidence to suggest that these pathways are activated in tumor cells following treatments with *Vinca* alkaloids (344, 395).

The many biologic actions of the clinically active *Vinca* alkaloids are seen over a wide range of drug concentrations, and there are selective effects in various normal and neoplastic tissues. Since VCR, vindesine, and VLB exhibit similar potencies against preparations of tubulin isolated from the same tissue, in vivo differences in biologic activity must be due either to heterogeneity of expression of various tubulin isoforms in different tissues or to differences in processes that influence interaction with tubulin by affecting drug binding (e.g., microtubule-associated proteins, cytoplasmic cofactors) or by limiting the availability of drug (e.g., permeation) (28, 66, 73, 100, 105, 120, 181). A key determinant of the pharmacologic activity of the *Vinca* alkaloids in different tissue types appears to be cellular retention of drug. For example, greater retention of VCR through stronger binding to tubulin of neoplastic tissues (relative to normal tissues) is responsible for the selective action of VCR against xenografts of human rhabdomyosarcoma (106–108). The greater potency of VCR relative to VLB can be explained by differences in cellular retention of the two drugs, particularly during drug exposures of limited duration (73, 74, 91, 138). VCR and VLB are equitoxic against cultured leukemic cells during continuous exposures, whereas VCR is more potent during exposures of short duration, because cellular retention of VCR is greater than that of VLB (73, 90). The same can be said for VRLB: The chemical change on the catharanthine ring, described above, makes the molecule more lipophilic with greater tissue retention and greater affinity for mitotic rather than axonal microtubules (350). Because the antitumor effect of VRLB is similar to that of VLB and VCR, this decreased effectiveness of VRLB on axonal microtubules may be a factor in the drug's decreased neurotoxicity (discussed below).

VINCA ALKALOID RESISTANCE

Resistance of tumor cells to the cytotoxic actions of the *Vinca* alkaloids has been well-described experimentally and appears to have clinical correlates (7–9, 38, 58, 87). In nearly all instances, *Vinca* alkaloid resistance derived in cells in culture is associated with cross-resistance to a variety of natural product antitumor drugs of different structure and mechanisms of action (but see below). For example, as seen in Table 66.1, human leukemic lymphoblasts selected for resistance to VLB are cross-resistant to other *Vinca* alkaloids and colchicine but not to another tubulin-binding drug, podophyllotoxin. Of interest, however, is the fact that the cells are cross-resistant to the podophyllotoxin derivatives teniposide and etoposide. They are also cross-resistant to the DNA intercalators doxorubicin, daunorubicin, dactinomycin, and mitoxantrone, but no cross-resistance is seen to other agents that damage DNA either directly (BCNU, bleomycin) or indirectly (methotrexate, 6-mercaptopurine). This profile of cross-resistance properties typifies the "classic" multidrug resistance (MDR) phenotype (14, 59). MDR associated with overexpression of P-glycoprotein (Pgp-MDR) is the subject of several recent reviews (69, 167, 251, 281, 396–401). Recent studies of vinorelbine-resistant bladder carcinoma cells revealed a different phenotype than that described above: Those cells expressed cross-resistance to other *Vinca* alkaloids, colchicine, and paclitaxel, but not to other natural product drugs such as doxorubicin, daunorubicin, or etoposide (315). By contrast, a K562 leukemia cell

Table 66.1. Cross-resistance of CEM/VLB$_{100}$ Human Leukemic Lymphoblasts Selected for Resistance to Vinblastine

Drug	Degree of resistance[a]
Vinblastine	186
Vincristine	2,023
Vindesine	1,186
Colchicine	20
Podophyllotoxin	0.8
Etoposide	44
Teniposide	32
Doxorubicin	152
Daunorubicin	44
Mitoxantrone	21
Dactinomycin	49
Bleomycin	3.2
Bischloroethylnitrosourea	0.5
Methotrexate	2.1
6-Mercaptopurine	1.0

[a] Drug-sensitive CEM and MDR CEM/VLB$_{100}$ cells were tested for their sensitivity to the drugs shown in a 48-hour growth inhibition assay, and the 50% inhibitory concentrations (IC_{50}) were determined. The degree of resistance is the ratio of the IC_{50} for the resistant cells over that of the sensitive cells. Data compiled from Danks et al. (59) and Beck et al. (15), with permission.

line also selected for vinorelbine resistance in the same study apparently displayed the classic, P-glycoprotein-expressing MDR phenotype (315). In another recent study, P388 mouse leukemia cells were selected for resistance to VRLB (321). These Navelbine-resistant cells (P388/NVB), which were about 30-fold resistant to VRLB in vitro, were cross-resistant to other MDR-type drugs, but not to alkylating agents or antimetabolites, and overexpressed Pgp.

Although the *Vinca* alkaloids bind to tubulin and disrupt microtubules, most tumor cells express resistance to these agents through a mechanism that does not appear to involve alterations in tubulin binding. When studied in tumor cells in vitro, resistance to the *Vinca* alkaloids appears to be due primarily to their decreased accumulation and retention (8). The altered cellular pharmacology is mediated by the action of a protein, termed P-glycoprotein (Pgp or P170), that is expressed in the plasma membranes of the drug-resistant tumor cells (7, 9, 38). This protein (Fig. 66.2), encoded by the *MDR1* gene, spans the membrane 12 times and most likely forms a pore or channel in the membrane through which drugs are transported (43, 76, 85, 93). P-glycoprotein appears to bind the *Vinca* alkaloids and extrudes them from the tumor cell through a process that requires energy (8, 13, 48, 49, 206, 230). This is the most likely mechanism behind the cross-resistance to the other natural product drugs listed in Table 66.1, although alternative mechanisms have been proposed (9). It is now known that many of the drugs that can circumvent *Vinca* alkaloid resistance or MDR (see below) also bind to P-glycoprotein and compete with the anticancer drug for binding to this protein (191, 192, 205, 269). The putative binding sites on P-glycoprotein for *Vinca* alkaloids, other anticancer drugs, and modulators of MDR are not known, although recent evidence suggests that these sites reside in or around the 11th and 12th transmembrane domains of the protein (369, 406), or possibly a binding site is made by bringing both halves of the protein together (367). Other evidence suggests that the process of drug export from the P-glycoprotein-expressing tumor cell requires energy derived from ATP, which also binds to this protein (8, 50, 60, 104). Indeed, Pgp has been shown to be an ATPase (404, 405). Hydrolysis of ATP or phosphorylation of P-glycoprotein may cause a conformational change in the protein which, in turn, could affect drug binding or even provide energy to actively extrude the *Vinca* alkaloid from the cell.

Much has been learned recently about the regulation of expression of the *MDR1* gene. Mechanisms and factors involved in transcriptional regulation of *MDR1* expression have been reported (352–354), as have studies on posttranscriptional regulation of Pgp function (355, 356). Drugs and modulators that are P-glycoprotein substrates or inhibitors (357–360), as well as DNA-damaging agents (359, 361, 362) can induce expression of *MDR1*/Pgp. These findings indicate that expression and activity of P-glycoprotein can be up-regulated by agents that are or have been used to affect clinical MDR. Other work has revealed that the cell cycle checkpoint protein p53 (349), may also play a role in *MDR1* expression (363–365), and therefore in regulating aspects of MDR. Mutations in the promoter of the *MDR1* gene have been shown to be associated with up-regulation of *MDR1* in osteosarcoma (366). Finally, other recent studies have contributed to our better understanding of Pgp topology (367), domains (365), and drug-binding sites (369). The importance of all of these studies lies in the fact that expression of the *MDR1* gene is regulable. That anticancer drugs and ionizing radiation can, under certain circumstances, up-regulate expression of *MDR1* suggests a potential mechanism behind its overexpression in some tumors in patients treated with these agents. Additionally, the up-regulation mediated by MDR modulators also suggests that their continued usage may be self-limiting.

As will be discussed below, MDR due to overexpression of the *MDR1* gene may have clinical correlates, as P-glycoprotein is expressed in many different tumors (41, 87, 370). Also, certain classes of clinically available membrane-active drugs have been shown to be able to "reverse" or overcome this form of drug resistance in vitro, and efforts have been made to determine whether such reversal can be achieved clinically (10, 11, 58, 371–375).

Further, in contrast to *Vinca* alkaloid-resistant murine tumors developed experimentally, a human rhabdomyosarcoma xenograft selected for VCR resistance in vivo did not express P-glycoprotein (104). Rather, this tumor was shown to express an altered β-tubulin, which most likely accounted for the decreased VCR binding (104). An alteration in tubulin isoforms has only been shown in vitro in rodent cells selected for resistance to Taxol and colchicine and griseofulvin, but no evidence was presented that those cells expressed P-glycoprotein (33, 34, 124). As will be detailed in the section on Taxol, the mechanism behind selection of one form of resistance versus another is not immediately apparent. It is worth noting, however, that vinorelbine-resistant bladder carcinoma cells did not express *MDR1* or P-glycoprotein; rather, the tubulins in these cells appeared to be altered so that the depolymerization kinetics of the resistant cells differed from those of the sensitive cells (315).

Novel drug resistance-associated proteins have been identified that may have an impact on the cellular and clini-

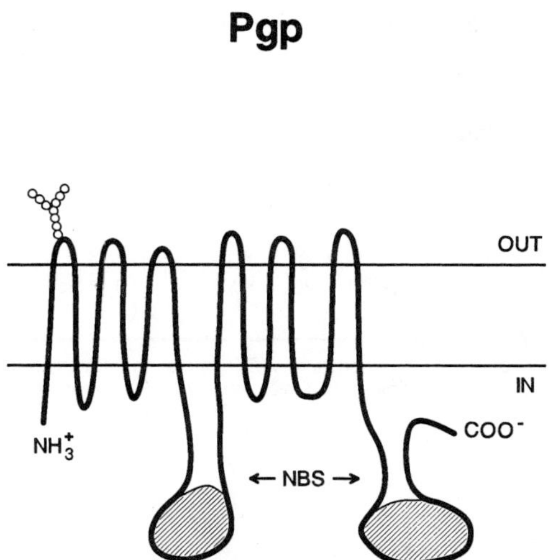

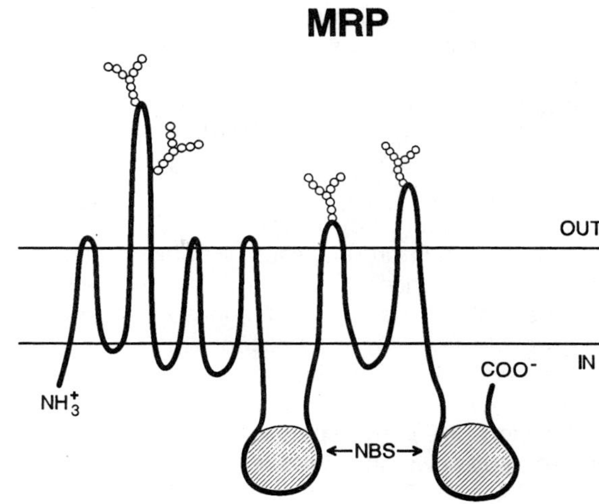

Figure 66.3. Proposed models of P-glycoprotein (Pgp) and the multidrug resistance-associated protein (MRP) in the cell membrane. Both proteins span the membrane 12 times, have major glycosylation sites (*open circles*), and two potential ATP (nucleotide)-binding sites (NBS). The model of Pgp is adapted from Chen et al. (43) and Gros et al. (93), and the model for MRP is adapted from Flens et al. (343), with permission.

cal resistance to the *Vinca* alkaloids. One, termed MRP, for *m*ultidrug *r*esistance-associated *p*rotein, has been cloned and characterized by several laboratories since 1992 (376–379). The protein encoded by the MRP cDNA is a 190-kd membrane protein that, when the full-length cDNA is expressed in cells, confers multidrug resistance to doxorubicin, VCR, etoposide, and colchicine (376–379). In this regard, MRP expression has been shown to be increased in relapsed or chemotherapy-refractory leukemias (383–388).

Compared to Pgp, MRP has similar and dissimilar features. For example, MRP, like Pgp, is a member of the ABC casette transporter family, but it is more closely related to the *Leishmania* homologue than to human Pgp (376). While MRP, like Pgp, also spans the plasma membrane 12 times, it apparently is not comprised of two homologous halves, as is the case for Pgp; rather, in terms of membrane spanning, each "half" of MRP is asymmetric with a distribution of 8 plus 4 transmembrane segments (Fig. 66.3) (376, 382). The gene for MRP has been shown to be located on chromosome 16p13.1 (376), whereas *MDR1* is located on chromosome 7q21.1 (380). MRP appears to be a transporter for leukotriene C_4 and glutathione (381). This functional and physiologic role for MRP may be related to its unusual transmembrane distribution of "8 plus 4," discussed above.

More recently, another protein associated with MDR, called LRP, for *l*ung cancer *r*esistance-associated *p*rotein, of 110 kd, has been identified and cloned (411, 412). LRP, named because it was first identified in drug-resistant lung tumor cells, appears to be one of four major "vault" proteins whose function is unknown (413), but its relation to MDR is presently unclear. The chromosomal localization of the LRP gene has been shown to be near that of MRP, on chromosome 16p13.1–16p11.2 (412). The chromosomal proximity of these genes suggests a common function and also provides a conceptual framework to explain their overexpression under similar circumstances. The roles of both MRP and LRP in clinical drug resistance will be defined over the next few years.

MODULATION OF *VINCA* ALKALOID RESISTANCE

This subject has been reviewed in substantial detail over the past several years and will only be summarized here (10–12, 79, 372, 374, 389). One of the first compounds shown to reverse what we now know to be Pgp-MDR was a detergent, Tween 80 (189). However, interest in modulation of MDR grew after the important observation by Tsuruo and colleagues that verapamil, a membrane-active drug used in cardiology, could sensitize VCR-resistant cells to the cytotoxic actions of VCR and VLB, both in vitro and in mice bearing VCR-resistant Ehrlich ascites tumors (247). Because verapamil blocks the voltage-gated Ca^{2+} current (the slow calcium channels) in excitable tissues, other calcium channel blockers and calmodulin antagonists were quickly studied for their ability to circumvent Pgp-MDR. Many, if not most, of these agents were found to have varying degrees of activity in experimental systems.

Drugs belonging to the classes of calcium channel blockers and calmodulin inhibitors do not appear to reverse *Vinca* alkaloid resistance or Pgp-MDR through direct inhibition of either voltage-gated calcium channels or calmodulin activity (137, 173, 264). Where it has been examined, these and other classes of compounds shown to reverse Pgp-MDR all appear to work by competing with the anticancer drug for binding to P-glycoprotein (10, 12, 48). Indeed, verapamil and progesterone, another modulator of Pgp-MDR, both bind directly to P-glycoprotein (112, 191, 192, 205, 269). As a consequence of this competition, the efflux of the anticancer drug, e.g., VCR, from the resistant tumor cell is blocked, and its levels in the cell rise to levels that are apparently cytotoxic (15, 247). Although these data appear to strongly support the proposition that interaction with Pgp is the major mechanism by which these agents block Pgp function, recent results of Wadkins and Houghton suggest that indirect effects of modulators on the lipid structure of the plasma membrane are also potentially important contributors to modulator action (333).

There are many clinically available compounds that modulate or circumvent experimental Pgp-MDR, and therefore *Vinca* alkaloid resistance, and they reflect a variety of chemical structures and different drug classes, including detergents, progestational and antiestrogenic agents, antibiotics, antihypertensives, antimalarials, and immunosuppressive agents such as cyclosporin A. More recent studies have shown that nonimmunosuppressive analogues of cyclosporin A (e.g., SDZ PSC833) can also effectively inhibit P-glycoprotein function (407). The specific compounds are discussed in recent reviews and will not be detailed here (10–12, 79, 372, 374, 389). Several clinical trials of modulators of MDR have been conducted and are discussed below. Although this is an important and active field of research, there are some serious concerns that may limit its full development (11, 390–393). P-glycoprotein, which is central to *Vinca* alkaloid resistance and MDR, is also expressed in such normal tissues as liver, kidney, small intestine, and colon (47, 241). Drugs that bind to and inhibit tumor cell P-glycoprotein will also do the same to the P-glycoprotein of these normal tissues, consequently increasing their levels of the anticancer drug and causing unacceptable tissue toxic effects. Indeed, using VCR-treated mice bearing human tumor xenografts, Horton and colleagues showed that administration of verapamil at levels necessary to reverse MDR in vitro caused substantial increases in VCR levels in kidney, small intestine, and liver and increased the overall toxicity of VCR to the mice (102). This important observation, which was replicated in subsequent clinical trials by List et al. (371) and Lum et al. (373), draws attention to the potential problems associated with circumvention of *Vinca* alkaloid resistance, and challenges investigators not only to design creative therapeutic protocols to obtund the potential toxic effects associated with the use of modulators, but also to devise new strategies to circumvent Pgp-MDR (11). Too little is known at present about reversal of MRP- and LRP-associated forms of MDR to warrant comment. Efforts to reverse clinical multidrug resistance with modulators all focus on Pgp-associated MDR and are discussed below in the section Clinical Resistance to the *Vinca* Alkaloids.

PHARMACOLOGY AND PHARMACODYNAMICS

The pharmacokinetics of the *Vinca* alkaloids in humans have been determined by detection in body fluids of ^{3}H-labeled drugs and their derivatives, and by immunoassay using antiserum raised against *Vinca* alkaloids (18, 26, 29, 113, 128, 145, 174, 176, 182, 218, 225, 226), as well as by high-performance liquid chromatography (HPLC) (303). These approaches differ in their resolution and reliability. The interpretation of results obtained with ^{3}H-labeled *Vinca* alkaloids is compromised by chemical instability of these compounds. For example, both VLB and VCR undergo spontaneous degradation under relatively mild conditions, forming a variety of structurally related products that can be separated using HPLC (227, 243). The extent to which the formation of degradation products, some of which have biologic activity (e.g., 4-deacetylvinblastine), occurs in vivo is unknown. The detection of *Vinca* alkaloids by radioimmunoassay, which has been used most frequently in pharmacokinetic studies, has the advantage of greater sensitivity, allowing detection of material in body fluids at nanomolar concentrations (177, 179, 193, 224). However, because the polyclonal antisera raised against the *Vinca* alkaloids, usually VLB, cannot distinguish between parent drug and its structurally related derivatives, the various radioimmunoassays currently in use for pharmacokinetic studies cannot provide information on the formation of degradative products or metabolites.

Table 66.2. Pharmacokinetic Values for Parenteral Administration of *Vinca* Alkaloids in Humans

Parameter	VCR	VLB	VDS	VRB	VZL
$t_{1/2}\alpha$ (min)	2–6	2–6	1–3	1–3	0.39
$t_{1/2}\beta$ (h)	2.27	1.64	0.91	1.9	1.8
$t_{1/2}\gamma$ (h)	85	24.8	24.2	27.7–44.7	159
Vd_{ss} (L/kg)	8.42	27.3	8.84	75.6	11.4
Clearance (L/kg/h)	0.106	0.252	0.74	1.28	0.06
Urinary elimination (%)	10–20	<10	<10	<8	13.6

Abbreviations: VCR, vincristine; VLB, vinblastine; VDS, vindesine; VRB, vinorelbine; VZL, vinzolidine; Vd_{ss}, volume of distribution at steady state.
Data in table from Armand and Marty (2), Kreis et al. (127), Nelson et al. (176), and Marquet et al. (402).

When administered by intravenous bolus injection, the normal route of administration, the *Vinca* alkaloids exhibit triphasic serum decay patterns in humans (26, 174–176). The pharmacokinetic parameters for the various *Vinca* alkaloids are summarized in Table 66.2. In adult cancer patients, the mean half-lives of the first two phases are about the same for VCR, VLB, vindesine, and VRLB (1–5 minutes and 1–2 hours), whereas that of the terminal phase differs by approximately 4-fold for VCR (about 85 hours), VRLB (about 27–44 hours), VLB (about 25 hours), and vindesine (about 24 hours). Following IV administration, the initial rapid clearance of the *Vinca* alkaloids from plasma is due to uptake of drug by various tissues, particularly blood elements such as platelets (18, 26, 182). The terminal phase of clearance from plasma represents the slow release of drug from various tissues where it has been sequestered, presumably through binding to tubulin. The range of values obtained for the terminal clearance phase, particularly with VCR, is large (174, 176). The greater potency of VCR has been attributed to prolonged exposures of sensitive tissues resulting from its slow clearance, relative to that of the other *Vinca* alkaloids (29, 174, 176). At the doses currently used in therapy for adults, the plasma peak concentrations, which persist for only a few minutes, are between 100 and 500 nM, and the steady-state concentrations are 1 to 2 nM (26, 174). The values found for the volumes of the central compartment differ significantly: vindesine is equivalent to the plasma volume (5.4% of body weight), whereas VCR and VLB greatly exceed the plasma volume (32.8 and 70% of body weight, respectively) (174, 176).

The *Vinca* alkaloids are excreted primarily by the hepatobiliary route (113, 130, 184). Cancer patients with impaired liver function exhibit reduced clearance of VCR, resulting in higher steady-state concentrations of drug and prolongation of the terminal elimination phase (63, 250). In such patients a reduction in drug dosage is recommended to reduce VCR-related neurotoxicity (63).

The *Vinca* alkaloids are sometimes given by continuous intravenous infusion in an effort to maintain pharmacologically effective serum drug levels for a longer period. Although a variety of different schedules have been used, the administration of VCR, VLB, or vindesine by infusion generally results in steady-state concentrations of drug that are higher than those achieved after intravenous bolus injection (115, 116, 145, 177, 195, 268).

The pharmacokinetics of vinzolidine have been studied after either oral administration or intravenous bolus injection of tritium-labeled drug (128, 218). After oral administration, vinzolidine is rapidly absorbed, with an absorption half-life of 1 hour and a peak at 4 hours. The serum decay curve is biphasic, with half-lives of 10.5 and 172 hours. After intravenous administration, the pharmacokinetics of vinzolidine resemble those of VLB, except that the volume of distribution is much larger (about 15–20 times the blood volume). The terminal half-life for elimination of vinzolidine from plasma is about 23 hours.

Finally, the pharmacokinetics of vinorelbine have been studied extensively. Following IV administration the compound exhibits a triphasic plasma disappearance (277), as is common for *Vinca* alkaloids, and the basic parameters are listed in Table 66.2. VRLB is metabolized in the liver and its metabolites are excreted in the bile; indeed, the clearance of VRLB is similar to that of hepatic blood flow (277), indicating that the drug is extracted by the liver. Of importance, VRLB is the first *Vinca* alkaloid that has demonstrated oral effectiveness (277): Absorption after oral administration is rapid, reaching peak plasma levels in the first 1 to 2 hours, with concentrations of approximately 70 to greater than 800 ng/mL (about 0.09 to more than 1.03 μM) (277); these concentrations also reflect the large intra- and interindividual variability of VRLB pharmacokinetics. The doses show in general both dose and time dependence (277), and the plasma disappearance is biphasic. The pharmacokinetics of oral VRLB are similar to those of an IV bolus dose: high clearance rate, a large volume of distribution, and a long terminal half-life (277).

TOXIC EFFECTS AND DOSES

The toxic effects of the *Vinca* alkaloids in humans are well documented and are related to the drug, route of administration, and dose (29, 52, 53, 123, 158). The toxic effects of the *Vinca* alkaloids differ significantly, despite similarities in biochemical activities. The dose-limiting toxic effect of VCR is neurologic, with extensive peripheral neuropathy occurring at higher doses (199, 211). Similar neurotoxicity is also seen with VLB, but, at the dosages used clinically, to a much lesser extent since its dose-limiting toxic effect is myelosuppression. Early symptoms of neurotoxicity are numbness and painful paresthesias in the fingers and toes and depression of the Achilles tendon reflex, followed, if treatment continues, by severe muscle weakness and uncoordinated movements. The dose-limiting toxicity of VLB is myelosuppression, with the nadir of leukopenia 5 to 9 days after administration and recovery occurring within 14 to 21 days. Myelosuppression is rare with VCR, probably because dosages are limited by neurotoxicity. Vindesine is both myelosuppressive and neurotoxic, and the neurotoxicity is less severe than that seen with VCR (29, 39). Vinorelbine is myelosuppressive with mild, reversible neurotoxicity (23). Nausea and vomiting are frequently seen in patients receiving VLB or vindesine, and constipation, resulting from neurotoxicity, can occur in patients receiving VCR. In elderly patients, particularly those with a tendency toward constipation, prophylactic cathartics are indicated. Alopecia and irritation at sites of IV administration are also common. For all of the *Vinca* alkaloids, dose reduction should be considered in patients with impaired liver function since the primary excretory route is hepatobiliary (113, 130, 184). Toxic effects, particularly neurotoxicity and myelosuppression, are increased when the *Vinca* alkaloids are administered by continuous IV infusion. Severe neurologic and hematologic toxic effects are seen with infusion of high doses of VCR, although lower doses are reasonably well tolerated (114, 116, 255). Neurotoxicity is seen during infusion of VLB and vindesine, and the major toxic effect during infusion of VLB is myelosuppression (177, 195, 268). Specific toxic effects are discussed below in relation to drug and dose.

VCR and VLB are most frequently administered by direct IV injection or through tubing of a running IV infusion. Administration is complete within 1 minute. Extravasation may cause irritation, and the local application of hyaluronidase and moderate heat to the area of leakage helps dispersion of drug and may minimize discomfort and the possibility of cellulitis. Both agents are given at intervals of 7 days until moderate or limiting toxic effects occur. In preclinical models the scheduling of VCR has been shown to affect antitumor activity markedly (105). The usual dose of VCR in adults is 1.4 mg/m^2; it is 2 mg/m^2 in children (>10 kg). Many protocols stipulate a maximum single dose of 2 mg. For smaller children a dose of 0.05 mg/kg every 7 days is used. The plasma concentrations of VCR are related to serum alkaline phosphatase levels, which may influence the neurotoxicity of VCR (63). For VLB the usual doses are 4 to 5 mg/m^2 every week, although, because of variable leukopenia, an escalating schedule has been suggested. Alternative routes of administration of both VLB and VCR have been reported. Oral administration of VLB was unpredictable, not very effective, and potentially severely toxic (70). VLB, 1.4 to 2.0 mg/m^2/d administered as a 5-day continuous IV infusion, resulted in unacceptable myelosuppression at dosages above 1.8 mg/m^2/d in patients with refractory breast cancer (268). A similar study in patients with testicular cancer (3 mg/m^2/d) resulted in frequent nonhematologic toxic effects, including inappropriate secretion of antidiuretic hormone, paralytic ileus, mucositis, neuropathy, and Raynaud's syndrome (44). Nonhematologic toxic effects correlated directly with steady-state plasma levels. Toxic effects were more severe in patients with plasma levels of 8.5 ng/mL than in a group with a mean steady-state level of 5.8 ng/mL. VCR given as continuous infusion for up to 5 days has caused primarily neuropathy, hyponatremia, and leukopenia, with dose-limiting toxic effects occurring at 0.5 mg/m^2/d (117). Although responses have been reported in a number of hematologic and solid tumors, the value of prolonged infusion of VLB and VCR relative to bolus administration remains to be demonstrated conclusively at both the preclinical and clinical levels.

Most studies with vindesine have used this agent at weekly intervals at a dose level between 2 and 5 mg/m^2. Exceptions have been in acute lymphoblastic leukemia (ALL), where in one study 2 mg/m^2 was administered daily for 5 days, and in another study 0.5 mg/m^2 was given every 12 hours for 5 days (151, 236). There is some suggestion that continuous infusion of vindesine may be superior to bolus administration in terms of therapeutic efficacy. A 5-day continuous infusion of vindesine (1.0–1.4 mg/m^2/d) was associated with an objective response rate of 25% in patients with refractory breast cancer, whereas bolus administration (3–4 mg/m^2) yielded a 7% response rate. Further, 4 of 11 patients whose disease progressed while they were taking vindesine by bolus achieved partial remission when treated with continuous infusion (266). A similar observation has been made in patients with ALL (160).

The toxicity of VRLB has been summarized recently (417, 419). Compared to the other *Vinca* alkaloids, VRLB is well tolerated and safe in the outpatient setting. The primary toxic effects of VRLB are hematologic, granulocytopenia being dose-limiting, with 64% of patients experiencing grade 3 or 4 granulocytopenia. Grade 3 or 4 leukopenia was also reported in 50% of the patients. Despite these toxic effects, complications such as fever and infection were relatively uncommon in three trials comprising more than 300 patients. Of importance, this hematologic toxic effect from VRLB appears to be noncumulative, and patients recover rapidly. Hematologic nadirs are usually seen on day 14 when the drug is given on a once-per-week schedule. In addition to the hematologic effects, nonhematologic toxic effects due to VRLB have been observed and consist of asymptomatic and transient elevations of liver enzyme serum levels, grade 3 or 4 elevation of bilirubin levels in 6% of patients, and elevated alkaline phosphatase levels in essentially all patients (99%). Although these latter changes were primarily grade 1 or 2, grade 3 or 4 alkaline phosphatase levels were seen in about a fourth of the patients. Of clinical importance, VRLB administration produces a generally low frequency of severe toxicity. Phase II studies of IV vinorelbine were initiated at 30 mg/m^2 weekly until either disease progression or severe toxic effects occurred. Leukopenia and neutropenia have been the most significant side effects, the latter being observed in 42% of cycles. However, the neutropenia was not cumulative and was of short duration (156). Preclinical studies indicated that vinorelbine retained both toxicity and antitumor activity when given orally. The maximum tolerated dose of oral vinorelbine in a phase I trial was determined to be approximately 80 to 100 mg/m^2 (71, 249). Again, noncumulative leukopenia was limiting, with no unpredictable toxic effects. Nausea, vomiting, and neurotoxicity were mild and did not alter drug administration or absorption (2).

The pharmacokinetics of parenterally administered *Vinca* alkaloids have been determined using either a sensitive radioimmunoassay or radiolabeled material. Bolus administration is characterized by a rapid initial elimination from serum, tight tissue binding, and a relatively long terminal half-life. Pharmacokinetic parameters are summarized in Table 66.2 (127, 156, 176).

CLINICAL USES: VCR, VLB, VRLB, AND OTHER NEWER *VINCA* ALKALOIDS

Vinca alkaloids have been incorporated into combination chemotherapy protocols, based not only on their lack of cross-resistance with drugs that alkylate DNA, but also on their different mechanism of action. VCR has the added advantage that its limiting toxic effect is peripheral neuropathy, whereas VLB may cause additive myelosuppression with other myelosuppressive agents. The use of VCR and VLB in combination therapy extends beyond the spectrum of cancers for which definitive activity has been demonstrated. VCR is approved as a component of combination therapy for use in Hodgkin's lymphoma, non-Hodgkin's lymphomas (including lymphocytic, mixed cell, histiocytic, undifferentiated, nodular, and diffuse), rhabdomyosarcoma of childhood, neuroblastoma, and Wilms' tumor (nephroblastoma) (3, 65, 144, 146, 233, 233a, 253). VLB has a similar spectrum of activity for Hodgkin's and non-Hodgkin's lymphomas and has been used in advanced mycosis fungoides, advanced testicular carcinoma, Kaposi's sarcoma, and histiocytosis X (36, 37, 169, 254).

Four other *Vinca* alkaloids have been introduced into the clinical treatment of cancer: vindesine, vinzolidine, vinepedine, and vinorelbine. While these agents were undergoing clinical trial, most clinical activity focused on vinorelbine, and those studies will be detailed below. Vindesine (4-desacetylvinblastine carboxy amide; Figure 66.1), an extensively studied analogue, was selected for clinical evaluation based on its VCR-like spectrum of activity against murine tumors, and its greater activity against the murine B16 melanoma (86). Preclinical data also suggested that cross-resistance between VCR and vindesine was not absolute. It has been shown clinically that vindesine has activity against hematologic malignancies, causing responses in VCR-resistant disease. Mathé and colleagues initially reported six complete responses in 15 patients with VCR-resistant acute lymphocytic leukemia (160). Of interest was that two complete responses were obtained by administration of vindesine as a 48-hour infusion in patients not responsive to bolus administration of this agent. Several other studies have confirmed the lack of complete cross-resistance with VCR in hematologic malignancies, although this is less apparent in the treatment of solid tumors (133, 151, 231, 252). Vindesine has also shown activity against resistant hematologic malignancies, breast carcinoma, malignant melanoma, and adenocarcinoma of the lung (75, 81, 109, 133, 151, 178, 196, 231, 252).

Vinzolidine (3′(2-chloroethyl)-3-de(methoxycarbonyl)-3-deoxy-2′, 4′-dioxospiro[oxazolidine-5′′, 3-*Vinca*leukoblastine]) was developed for clinical trial because it had greater therapeutic activity in murine tumors than either VCR or VLB. In rhesus monkeys, bioavailability was 2.5-fold that of VLB after oral administration (32). Vinzolidine has a substituted oxazolidine dione ring at the 4′ position of the vindoline moiety. The β-chloroethyl side chain is nonfunctional with respect to alkylation but increases the lipophilicity of the molecule. In vitro studies of vinzolidine activity suggested a lack of cross-resistance with VLB and potential activity in gastrointestinal, breast, and lung carcinoma and in melanoma (135, 235). Phase I studies have revealed primarily hematologic, gastrointestinal, and neurologic toxic effects (32, 204). Hematologic toxic effects have been dose-limiting, and marked variation in tolerance between patients was observed. Unpredictable and severe toxicity of oral dosing schedules has led to early closure of several studies. Variable toxicity appears to relate to marked differences either in the terminal half life of vinzolidine in patients (35–100 hours), or in erratic absorption. In early trials, oral administration demonstrated some activity against both Hodgkin's and non-Hodgkin's lymphoma, Kaposi's sarcoma, adenocarcinoma of pancreas, breast, and both squamous cell and adenocarcinoma of the lung (32, 204, 212). Parenteral trials have shown more predictable toxicity, which has been predominantly hematologic, with responses reported in melanoma, renal, and breast carcinoma (237).

Vinca alkaloids with modifications of the velbanamine (catharanthine) moiety have generally been associated with reduced potency. For example, the natural alkaloids 4′-deoxyvinblastine and 4′-deoxyleurosidine were less active mitotic inhibitors in vitro and less potent against rodent tumors in vivo. Leurosidine (epimeric at C-4′) was also less potent than VLB against P1534 leukemia in mice. However, leurosidine and 4′-deoxyleurosidine demonstrated high therapeutic index against P1534 leukemia and B16 melanoma, with activity equal or superior to that of VLB (119). Vinepidine, 4′-deoxyepivincristine, epimeric at C-4′, differs from deoxyleurosidine in the substitution of a formyl group at the N-atom of the vindoline moiety. These modifications to the velbanamine moiety imparted some new activities to a *Vinca* alkaloid. In mice, vinepidine was more potent than VCR, and in vitro vinepidine demonstrated 50- to 100-fold less potency in the rat midbrain cell culture assay, which has an excellent correlation with *Vinca* alkaloid-induced neuropathy in man (25, 244). Vinepidine was therefore selected for clinical evaluation based on a VCR-like preclinical spectrum of activity in vivo and lack of potential neurotoxicity as determined from an in vitro assay. However, in clinical studies using a weekly administration schedule, neurotoxicity was observed, and this drug was not evaluated further (170). Whether neurotoxicity was due to cumulative effects caused by slower elimination or metabolism using this schedule is not known. Preclinical data indicated that the drug accumulated in tumor tissue even at very low plasma concentrations, raising the possibility that continuous infusion may achieve adequate levels in tumor while reducing the toxicity to the host (170).

Vinorelbine (Navelbine; 3′,4′-didehydro-4-deoxy-C′-nor-Vincaleucoblastine; 5′-nor-anhydrovinblastine) demonstrated a profile of activity against murine tumors similar to that of other *Vinca* alkaloids, and also showed activity against five human tumor xenografts in nude mice. Further, no neurotoxicity, demyelination, or muscle degeneration was observed in monkeys (156). In a phase I evaluation the dose-limiting toxic effect was leukopenia, and 2 of 16 patients with refractory lymphomas experienced partial responses (159). Vinorelbine has shown considerable activity in non-small cell lung cancer when administered weekly at 30 mg/m^2. The overall objective response rate was 33% (62). Significant activity of IV vinorelbine was demonstrated against predominantly untreated advanced breast carcinoma (52% objective responses), with 4 of 24 patients having a complete response (35). The response rate in heavily pretreated patients was 38% (157).The current status of VRLB in breast cancer was recently summarized in symposium proceedings (297). The response rate of advanced (stages III and IV), previously untreated Hodgkin's lymphoma was 90%, and 5 of 25 evaluable patients with previously treated ovarian cancer had objective responses (82, 156). Because of its distribution to the lung and relatively low incidence of severe neurotoxicity, VRLB has been shown to have significant activity in non-small-cell lung cancer, and its use in the adjuvant and neoadjuvant setting in the treatment of this disease was summarized recently. Preclinical and clinical studies have shown that vinorelbine is well absorbed orally and has not been associated with erratic or unpredictable toxic effects, as was found with vinzolidine (71).

CLINICAL RESISTANCE TO THE *VINCA* ALKALOIDS

In cell culture systems, cross-resistance between *Vinca* alkaloids is common, although not absolute; the degree of resistance may depend on the specific agent. In patients, drug effectiveness may also be a function of dose, route of administration, and pharmacokinetic factors, all of which compound the difficulties in interpreting whether cross-resistance between *Vinca* alkaloids occurs in clinical cancer. VCR-resistant acute lymphoblastic leukemia was shown to be responsive to vindesine, and several other studies support this (160). Vindesine infusion was also active in some patients who did not respond to bolus administration, and similar observations have been made with VCR and VLB. This suggests that, as in vitro, the degree of resistance between *Vinca* alkaloids may differ, and that dose and intensity of therapy may determine the response rate in *Vinca*-resistant disease.

Several mechanisms of resistance to *Vinca* alkaloids were discussed above. The best characterized is that mediated by P-glycoprotein, thought to act as an energy-dependent drug efflux pump. There are now many reports documenting the presence of P-glycoprotein in patients' tumors by analysis of RNA transcripts or using immunologic methods (4, 17, 27, 40, 41, 58, 77, 78, 84, 87, 88, 122, 147, 168, 208, 219). The presence of P-glycoprotein has been correlated with poor outcome in childhood rhabdomyosarcoma and neuroblastoma in some studies (40, 41) but not in others (403), and definitive relationships have not been established for other tumor types. The incidence of P-glycoprotein-positive human cancers is summarized in Table 66.3. The apparent differences in detection of P-glycoprotein may reflect the sensitivity of RNA analysis compared to immunologic techniques, and even immunologic methods have proved to have a fairly high degree of interlaboratory variability, especially for detection of low levels of P-glycoprotein (408). At

Table 66.3. Incidence of Detection of Biochemical Markers of P-Glycoprotein-Mediated Multidrug Resistance in Human Cancer

Tumor	Treatment status (positive total)			Method[a]
	Untreated	Treated	Not defined	
Breast Ca.	2/12	8/11	5/16	1
	9/57	2/2	0/5	R
Colon Ca.			6/54	1/W
	35/41		10/20	R
Ovarian Ca.		2/5	6/66	I/W
	0/56	3/10	0/16	R
Renal cell Ca.	0/4		3/13	I
	72/88		7/8	R
Lung Ca.	0/19			R
(NSCLC)	7/19			R
Neuroblastoma	35/78	32/52		R
Myeloma	4/7	7/13		I
Sarcoma	0/11	4/4		R
			9/30	I
Pheochromocytoma	25/34			R

[a] I, detection by immunocytochemistry; W, Western blot; R, RNA slot blot. Data compiled from references 4, 17, 40, 58, 77, 78, 84, 87, 88, 122, 147, 168, 208, and 219.

this time there is limited information regarding the significance of these data. However, several clinical trials have been initiated using agents that have reversed P-glycoprotein-mediated MDR in cultured cells, as recently summarized by several authors (12, 370–373, 389–391). Initial studies with verapamil showed that concentrations of modulator required in vitro (5–10 μM) could not be sustained in patients (22, 185). Its use was limited by its intrinsic pharmacologic activity, causing heart block. Transient responses were observed in pediatric patients treated with a 6-day continuous infusion of verapamil (0.005 mg/kg/min) with bolus VLB (2 mg/m^2) and a 5-day continuous infusion of VP-16 (200 mg/m^2/d). However, the study design prevented any conclusions from being drawn regarding the role of verapamil. In P-glycoprotein-positive, drug-resistant myeloma, there is some indication that simultaneous infusion of verapamil with VCR and doxorubicin may elicit transient responses in some patients (57). Other modulators of P-glycoprotein-mediated MDR that have been tried clinically include Bepridil, R-verapamil, trifluoperazine, cyclosporin A, acrivastine, and amiodarone (12, 389–391, 397, 401). Clearly, this concept of modulation should be thoroughly evaluated in controlled, randomized trials. However, there are few preclinical data to support therapeutic selectivity, and P-glycoprotein may play an important role in protecting certain normal tissues in man and rodents (56, 89, 102).

Reversal of clinical MDR has been reviewed (12, 370–372, 389–393). Major concerns of clinical MDR modulator studies relate to tumor type, accessibility of Pgp, ability to measure Pgp reliably in patients' tumors, and the presence in clinical specimens of other proteins that can confer MDR on a tumor cell. Several important clinical trials of Pgp modulators have been performed (7, 8, 371, 373), and these have used either cyclosporin A or its nonimmunosuppressive analogue, PSC 833, in two-arm studies: doxorubicin or etoposide with or without a modulator. The key finding is that the modulator increases the plasma levels and half-lives of the anticancer agents, possibly through inhibition of hepatic Pgp. This will also be discussed below in studies of paclitaxel and r-verapamil (332).

Since 1989, many studies of *MDR1*/Pgp in tumors from patients have demonstrated an increased expression of either *MDR1* or Pgp either de novo in tumors derived from tissues that normally express this gene, or, importantly, after therapy (reviewed in references 11, 12, 59–61). Chan et al. showed a strong association of Pgp positivity (by immunostaining) and disease outcome in rhabdomyosarcoma and neuroblastoma (62, 63), suggesting that Pgp expression is highly associated with disease progression. However, it is now clear that *MDR1*/Pgp is not expressed in many tumors in which clinical drug resistance has been documented (reviewed in (2, 9–12, 59)), suggesting either that there are other mechanisms of clinical MDR (e.g., MRP [383, 385–388] or LRP [409, 410]), or that there is interassay (or interlaboratory) variability in measuring MDR-associated markers, a focus of a Pgp/*MDR1* methods standardization workshop (408).

Critical factors in clinical MDR modulator studies have been discussed by Sikic (389), and include end point (e.g., clinical improvement, drug toxicity, altered drug pharmacokinetics) and Pgp status (i.e., mechanism of resistance) of the tumor. Many clinical trials of modulators of MDR (9–12) have not been successful because these and other factors have not been considered. However, key studies from the laboratories of Dalton (58) and of Sikic (389, 408) showed clearly that the addition of a modulator of MDR increases the plasma half-life of the anticancer drug, possibly through inhibition of the biliary excretion of the oncolytic agent, showing for the first time that modulators of Pgp have significant pharmacokinetic actions that necessitate decreasing the dose of the anticancer drug administered. Together, these observations raise a cautionary flag and provide several explanations for the lack of concordance between Pgp expression and clinical MDR in some instances.

Taxanes: Paclitaxel (Taxol) and Docetaxel (Taxotere)

Much effort has recently gone into the chemistry and clinical trials of the taxanes. These agents, typified by paclitaxel and the semisynthetic analogue, Taxotere, have been the subject of intense clinical scrutiny, and their chemistry, biochemical actions, pharmacology, and clinical activities are the subject of several recent excellent reviews and monographs (271–274, 294–296).

HISTORY AND CHEMISTRY

Taxol (paclitaxel) was isolated in 1971 from the bark of the Western yew, *Taxus brevifolia* Nut (Taxaceae), and was found to have antitumor and antileukemic activity (103). It has subsequently been found in the roots, leaves, and stems of this tree and related members of the yew family (103). As seen in Figure 66.4, Taxol is a complex ester with an unusual

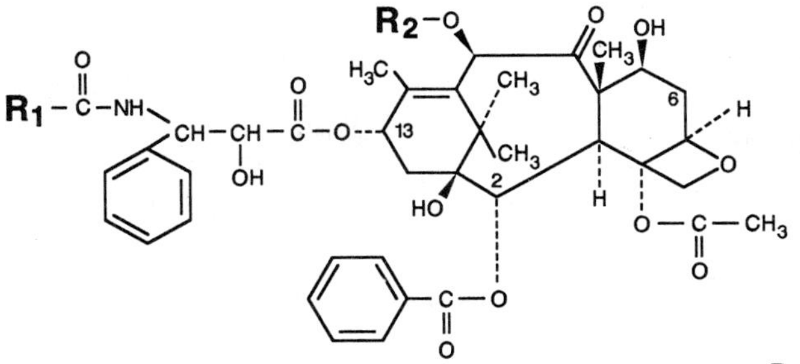

	R_1	R_2
Taxol (Paclitaxel)	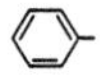 (phenyl)	$CH_3\text{-}C(=O)\text{-}O\text{-}$
Taxotere (Docetaxel)	$(CH_3)_3\text{-}O\text{-}$	H-

Figure 66.4. Chemical structures of the taxanes paclitaxel and docetaxel.

structure consisting of an oxetan ring attached to a derivative of taxane. Because of its unusual mechanism of action, it has become an important tool for investigating microtubule function. Its unique action and spectrum of antitumor activity have earned it a place in experimental therapeutics, and it is presently undergoing clinical trials. The major barrier to Taxol's earlier clinical development was its low abundance in the yew trees, since chemical synthesis had not been possible; there simply was not enough Taxol to do the appropriate trials. This situation has changed because of the development of novel synthetic methods and the identification of new sources of the taxanes. For example, docetaxel (Taxotere) is extracted from the leaves of the European yew tree (271, 272), leaves being a renewable resource. Thus, much progress has been made in basic and clinical studies of the taxanes (271, 272, 294–296).

MECHANISM OF ACTION

Among antineoplastic drugs that interfere with microtubules, paclitaxel exhibits a unique mechanism of action and for this reason has been studied extensively (19, 103, 152, 200). Taxol promotes assembly of microtubules by shifting the equilibrium between soluble tubulin and microtubules toward assembly, reducing the critical concentration of tubulin required for assembly (Fig. 66.2) (215, 216). The result is stabilization of microtubules, even in the presence of conditions (e.g., low temperature, high calcium) that normally promote disassembly of microtubules (134, 207, 215, 216, 245). The remarkable stability of microtubules induced by Taxol is damaging to cells because of the perturbation in the dynamics of various microtubule-dependent cytoplasmic structures that are required for such functions as mitosis, maintenance of cellular morphology, shape changes, neurite formation, locomotion, and secretion (5, 61, 80, 99, 111, 124, 140, 141, 158, 166, 194, 198, 201, 203, 216, 246). Microtubules are the only known biochemical targets of Taxol, and the many biologic effects observed in Taxol-treated cells are thought to arise from perturbations of microtubule dynamics.

Interaction of paclitaxel with microtubules occurs by reversible, high-affinity binding of the drug to polymerized microtubules (46, 134, 153, 187, 188). The stoichiometry of binding is approximately 1 mole of Taxol per mole of polymerized tubulin, and the binding site for Taxol is distinct from the binding sites for the *Vinca* alkaloids, colchicine, or podophyllotoxin (134, 188, 217). Cells treated with pharmacologic levels of Taxol (0.1–10 μM) are arrested in the G_2 and M phases of the cell cycle and contain disorganized arrays of microtubules, often aligned in parallel bundles (80, 98, 99, 201, 216). Treatment of mitotic cells with Taxol results in the formation of abnormal spindle asters (61, 166, 201). Studies of the effects of low concentrations (0.25 μM) of Taxol on cultured cells, under conditions of minimal inhibition of DNA, RNA, and protein synthesis, demonstrated that Taxol specifically blocks progression of cells through the cell cycle in M phase, indicating that mitosis exhibits high sensitivity to Taxol (215). Higher concentrations of Taxol result in damage to interphase cells, with formation of microtubule bundles and loss of a variety of cell functions known to be dependent on microtubules. Recent studies with different photoaffinity analogues of Taxol have revealed that the analogues specifically bind to β-tubulin at amino acid residues 1–31 (404) and 217–231 (403). These results suggest that Taxol has at least two tubulin contact domains that eventually may provide insights into the actions of the drug and spur development of more specific inhibitors.

RESISTANCE TO TAXOL

Resistance to paclitaxel has been described in cells in culture, and it appears to take two forms. In one, resistance is associated with alterations or mutations in α- and β-tubulins (311, 312), whereas in another, Taxol resistance is associated with overexpression of P-glycoprotein and the MDR phenotype (33, 94, 95, 202, 218). Recent studies indicate that these distinct lesions can coexist in the same resistant cell lines (312). The Taxol-resistant cells that express altered tubulins were selected after mutagenesis of the cells by ultraviolet irradiation, whereas the Taxol resistant cells that overproduced P-glycoprotein were selected for resistance by long-term growth in sublethal concentrations of the drug (33, 94, 95, 202, 218). However, it is unlikely that the selection conditions played a major role in the type of resistance obtained, since other cell lines that expressed a "classic" Pgp-MDR phenotype were selected for resistance after mutagenesis by exposure to ethylmethanesulfonate (1). More recent studies also revealed that selection for Taxol resistance led to expression of *MDR1* and Pgp as well as decreased β-tubulin (311, 312). That β-tubulin expression is decreased is consistent with the finding that this subunit is the target for Taxol (403, 404).

DOSE AND PHARMACOKINETICS

Taxol is formulated in dehydrated alcohol, cremophor EL (1:1), at a concentration of 6 mg/mL. The drug is diluted to a final concentration of 0.03 ro 0.6 mg/mL in 0.9% sodium chloride or 5% dextrose solution. In the concentration range 0.3 to 1.2 mg/mL, Taxol is stable for at least 12 hours. The frequency of hypersensitivity reactions appears to relate to the rate of administration during infusion. Schedules, recommended doses and limiting toxicities of Taxol derived from phase I studies are given in Table 66.4. Based on this information, the National Cancer Institute recommended that phase II trials utilize 24-hour infusion, with prophylactic premedication with dexamethasone (20 mg) given 14 and 7 hours prior to Taxol, and with diphenhydramine (50 mg IV) and cimetidine or ranitidine (300 or 50 mg IV) given 30 minutes before Taxol. For treatment of renal cell carcinoma the dose was 250 mg/m^2 every 3 weeks (242). In patients with refractory ovarian carcinoma, whose hematopoietic tolerance is reduced, dose escalation has started at 110 mg/m^2. Of significance is that responses have occurred at this relatively low dose, whereas dose levels of 200 to 250 mg/m^2 appear to be safe in previously untreated patients.

Pharmacokinetic parameters for paclitaxel and docetaxel have been obtained in multiple clinical trials and have been summarized. Results from some of these studies are outlined in Tables 66.5 and 66.6. Paclitaxel is highly bound to plasma albumin, ranging from 88 to 98% bound. The elimination of paclitaxel in urine is low, with only 2 to 10% recovered unchanged in urine. Approximately 70% of drug was recovered fecally, with 6α-hydroxypaclitaxel constituting the major component. The elimination of paclitaxel in humans is saturable when administered as short infusions (<6 hours) or when high dosage levels (>300 mg/m^2) are administered over 24 hours. Table 66.5 summarizes pharmacokinetic parameter estimates for paclitaxel from studies where compartmental analyses were undertaken. Paclitaxel clearance has been shown to be variable (5- to 7-fold) between patients given the same dose. The primary route of elimination in both rodents and humans appears to involve hepatic metabolism and subsequent biliary elimination. 6α-hydroxypaclitaxel appears to be the predominant metabolite, formed by hepatic CYP2C8 enzyme, whereas the enzyme responsible for catalyzing hydroxylation of the C-13 side chain benzyl moiety is hepatic CYP3A4. In general, metabolites are less potent cytotoxic agents than the parent drug.

The semisynthetic taxane docetaxel appears to be less protein bound than paclitaxel. As for paclitaxel, the predominant route of elimination is by hepatic metabolism and biliary excretion. Less than 10% of docetaxel is excreted unchanged in urine. Although complete characterization of its metabolism is unavailable, inhibition studies suggest that the CYP3A family of hepatic enzymes is involved in docetaxel metabolism in humans. Pharmacokinetic parameter analyses (Table 66.6) indicate that estimates of plasma clearance

Table 66.4. Phase I Studies of Paclitaxel (Taxol)

Schedule	Maximum tolerated dose (mg/m^2)	Recommended phase II dose (mg/m^2)	Dose-limiting toxic effect	Other principal effects
1–6-h infusion every 21 d	265	210	Neutropenia	Neuropathy, mucositis, arthralgias/myalgias, hypersensitivity reactions
1–6-h infusion every 21 d	275	250	Neutropenia, neuropathy	Hypersensitivity reactions, alopecia, mucositis
24-h infusion every 21 d	275	250	Neutropenia, neuropathy	Hypersensitivity reactions
3-h infusion every 21 d	190		Hypersensitivity reactions	Leukopenia, nausea, alopecia
6-h infusion every 21 d	275	225	Neutropenia	Arthralgias/myalgias, mucositis, alopecia, neuropathy, hypersensitivity reactions
24-h infusion every 21 d	200		Neutropenia	Alopecia, nausea, vomiting
1-h infusion × 5 d every 21 d	40	20	Neutropenia	Alopecia, diarrhea
1–6-h infusion × 5 d every 21 d	40	30	Neutropenia	Hypersensitivity reactions, nausea, vomiting, alopecia, mucositis, thrombocytopenia
24-h infusion every 14–21 d	390	310	Mucositis	Neutropenia, hypersensitivity reactions, neuropathy
24-h infusion + cisplatin every 21 d	135–170 + 75 (cisplatin)	135–170 + 75 (cisplatin)	Neutropenia	Arthralgias/myalgias, alopecia, cardiac, hypersensitivity reactions, neuropathy

From Rowinsky et al. (200). Used with permission.

Table 66.5. Pharmacokinetic Parameters of Paclitaxel (Taxol)

Dose (mg/m^2)	T^a (h)	$t\frac{1}{2}\alpha^b$ (min)	$t\frac{1}{2}\beta^b$ (h)	$t\frac{1}{2}\gamma^b$ (h)	CL^b ($mL/min/m^2$)	$Vd_{ss}{}^b$ (L/m^2)	Vc^b (L/m^2)	Dose (mg/m^2)	$C_{peak}{}^b$ (μM)	AUC^b ($\mu M{\cdot}h$)
15–265	1 or 6	16 ± 9	6.4 ± 3.9		253 ± 274	67 ± 55	8.6 ± 6.6	170[c]	2.2–5.9	18.1–48.5
								212	2.6–3.5	19.7–22.9
								265	3.9–13	27.3–97.2
175–275	6	23 ± 9	8.4 ± 1.9		134 ± 36.9	60 ± 13		175	2.0–4.4	18.8–29.9
								200	5.2–5.4	25.5–29.3
								230	2.3–5.1	21.1–36.2
								275	5.5–10.1	41.3–75.4
175–275	6	29 ± 18	4.3 ± 2.5		232 ± 102	49 ± 18	19.2 ± 5.8	175	1.5–1.9	9.4–10.3
								225	2.4–4.8	13.5–32.7
								250	1.4–3.5	10.6–22.4
								275	4.1–7.3	33.7–47.4
200–275	24	20 ± 10	3.3 ± 0.7		359 ± 78	119 ± 67		200	0.51–0.64	9.4–13.9
								250	0.77–0.97	11.6–17.6
								275	0.67–1.27	11.7–20.1
135 or 175	3	14 ± 7	1.8 ± 0.7	16.3 ± 8.9	260 ± 69	98 ± 49		135	1.9–3.5	6.9–13.0
								175	2.8–5.9	12.5–21.1
	24	7 ± 6	2.1 ± 0.5	29.7 ± 19.2	380 ± 98	398 ± 268		135	0.20–0.25	7.2–7.4
								175	0.31–0.61	6.0–12.2
135–225	3			6.5–9.2[d]	190–274[d]		3.8 ± 0.3[e]	135	3.3 ± 0.4	10.9 ± 1.1
								175	5.9 ± 0.9	18.5 ± 3.0
								225	7.6 ± 1.9	24.3 ± 6.8
	24			14.6–16.2[d]	232–232[d]			135	0.3 ± 0.1	12.4 ± 2.2
								175	0.5 ± 0.1	16.0 ± 4.4
210–300	3	11–16[d]	1.5–1.8[d]	9.8–12.9[d]	126–198[d]	33–68[d]		210	6.0 ± 2.0	22.4 ± 6.7
								250	9.2 ± 2.0	31.2 ± 5.6
								300	14.2 ± 3.4	48.7 ± 11
200–420	24				202 ± 130	72 ± 60	8.8 ± 32	200	1.06–1.26	29.2–29.6
								250	0.31–1.56	9.4–37.3
								290	0.63–2.31	14.6–46.9
								350	0.54–2.61	13.2–71.3
								420	1.18–6.77	28.9–115

Abbreviations:T, time; t½, half-time; CL, clearance; Vd_{ss}, volume distribution at steady state; Vc, central volume; C, plasma concentration; AUC, area under the curve.
[a] Duration of continuous infusion.
[b] Mean ± standard deviation or range (unless otherwise indicated).
[c] Only 6-hour infusion data are presented.
[d] Range of harmonic means of the two or three different dosages.
[e] A three-compartment model incorporating saturable distribution and saturable elimination was fitted to plasma paclitaxel and 6α-hydroxypaclitaxel concentrations simultaneously in 15 patients. Parameters describing metabolite disposition were fixed for the remaining 15 patients without metabolite data.
[f] A two-compartment model incorporating saturable distribution and saturable elimination was used to fit the plasma concentration versus time data.
Median [range] results for the primary pharmacokinetic parameters were: Vm_{I-60} ($\mu mol{\cdot}h^{-1}$) 31.9 [2.9–47.4]; Km_{1-0} (μM) 2.16 [0.64–4.81]; Vm_{3-2} ($\mu mol{\cdot}h^{-1}$) 26.9 [6.0–142.7]; Km_{1-2} (μM) 0.454 [0.103–1.08]; K_{2-1} (hr^{-1}) 0.254 [0.052–1.04]; V_e (L/m^2) 8.3 [2.9–20.0]
Adapted from Sonnischen and Relling (273), with permission.

(267–369 $mL/min/m^2$) and Vd_{ss} of docetaxel are comparable to estimates for paclitaxel. Pharmacokinetic data for docetaxel suggest that the elimination and distribution of this drug are both linear processes, with linear increases in AUC or steady-state concentrations of docetaxel over the range of clinically used dosages.

TOXIC EFFECTS OF PACLITAXEL AND DOCETAXEL USED CLINICALLY

Dose-limiting and other toxic effects of Taxol are listed in Table 66.4. The onset of neutropenia, which is not schedule dependent, usually begins by day 8; the nadir of neutrophil counts occurs around days 8 to 11, with rapid recovery by day 21. Fever and sepsis have been infrequent. Although neutropenia does not appear to be cumulative, severe neutropenia has been reported consistently in heavily pretreated patients with ovarian cancer (161). Significant anemia and thrombocytopenia appear to occur infrequently. Type 1 hypersensitivity reactions occurred in early phase I trials, the predominant manifestations being hypotension, dyspnea with bronchospasm, and urticaria. Other adverse effects included abdominal and extremity pain, angioedema, diaphoresis, generalized erythema, and pruritus. It is possible that the hypersensitivity reactions are caused by formulation of Taxol with cremophor, as other agents with similar formulation (teniposide, cyclosporin) have also been associated with reactions attributed to the release of histamine (143).

For docetaxel, the most common toxic effect seen in several trials in women with breast carcinoma was neutropenia, with grade 4 neutropenia occurring in the majority of patients. For most patients neutropenia was of short duration, allowing retreatment on schedule. Other toxic effects in-

Table 66.6 Pharmacokinetic Parameters of Docetaxel (Toxotere)

Dose (mg/m^2)	T[a] (h)		$t_{1/2}\alpha$[b] (min)	$t_{1/2}\beta$[b] (h)	$t_{1/2}\gamma$[b] (h)	CL[b] (mL/min/m^2)	Vd_{ss}[b] (L/m^2)	Dose (mg/m^2)	C_{peak}[b] (μM)	AUC[b] (μM·h)
12–16/d ×5	1		7 ± 2		4.8 ± 4.9[c]	675 ± 488	126 ± 140	12	0.07–0.35	0.70 ± 0.41
								14	0.27–0.64	0.48 ± 0.15
								16	0.32–0.98	0.59 ± 0.39
								16	0.26–0.85	0.72 ± 0.30
20–90	24			0.2–2.3[d]		625–1,313[e] (mL/min)	9.1–168	20	0.11	1.14
								40	0.14–0.21	2.65–2.77
								55	0.07–0.28	1.47–4.06
								70	0.19–0.41	3.59–5.58
								90	0.33–0.71	7.36–12.15
20–115	1–2[f]				13.5 ± 7.5	351 ± 88	72 ± 40	20	1.01	1.19
								30	0.79 ± 0.56	1.56 ± 0.42
								40	0.52	0.83
								55	1.01 ± 0.47	1.76
								70	2.36 ± 0.40	3.45 ± 1.05
								85	3.00 ± 1.14	5.07 ± 1.14
								100	2.98 ± 0.43	7.34 ± 0.66
								115	3.32 ± 1.15	6.42 ± 0.20
100	2		3 ± 2	1.1 ± 0.5	12.4 ± 10.0	267 ± 80	99 ± 88	100	2.57 ± 0.89[g]	6.44 ± 1.48
	6		4 ± 4	0.9 ± 0.3	11.4 ± 6.0	333 ± 90	82 ± 48	100	0.99 ± 0.28[g]	8.42 ± 2.85
70–115	1–2	NONMEN[h]	4.5	0.64	12.2	353	124[e]			
		NMPL	2.2	0.34	7.9	369	83.2[e]			

Abbreviations: T, time; $t_{1/2}$, half-time; CL, clearance; Vd_{ss}, volume of distribution at steady state; C, plasma concentration; AUC, area under the curve.
[a] Duration of continuous infusion.
[b] Mean ± standard deviation or range (unless otherwise indicated).
[c] Model parameterization limited to assay sensitivity.
[d] Monoexponential model used to describe data.
[e] Estimates not adjusted to body surface area.
[f] Infusion duration and product formulation varied to minimize exposure of diluent (polysorbate 80).
[g] Average concentration during infusion.
[h] Population-based analysis using either nonlinear mixed effects modeling (NONMEM) or nonparametric maximum likelihood estimation (NMPL).
Adapted from Sonnischen and Relling (273), with permission.

cluded alopecia, nausea, stomatitis, diarrhea, skin rash, and asthenia. Acute hypersensitivity reactions, characterized by mild transient rash or flushing, occurred in the majority of patients, although more serious manifestations were rare (295). As with paclitaxel, antihistamines and/or glucocorticoids have been used as premedication. Docetaxel appears to have one toxic effect that is not shared with paclitaxel. Patients receiving more than four cycles of docetaxel had fluid retention, manifested by development of peripheral edema, pleural effusion, or both. Further studies showed that peripheral edema was reversible, progressed only slowly if therapy was continued, and could be largely controlled through the use of diuretics. Other data indicated that edema may occur at a higher cumulative dose and was less frequent in patients premedicated with glucocorticoids. Similar approaches appear to control pleural effusions, hence in later studies the fluid retention syndrome rarely resulted in discontinuation of treatment (295).

CLINICAL USES AND CLINICAL RESISTANCE

Paclitaxel entered clinical phase I trials in 1983. A high prevalence of acute hypersensitivity reactions necessitated discontinuation of many trials. However, concomitant administration of steroids, histamine H_1 and H_2 receptor antagonists, and prolonged infusion (6–24 hours) have been used successfully. In early phase I trials, significant activity was demonstrated in refractory ovarian carcinoma, breast carcinoma, melanoma, non-small-cell lung carcinoma, and adenocarcinoma of unknown origin. Minor responses were observed in gastric, colon, and head and neck carcinomas as well as in lymphoblastic and myeloblastic leukemias (reviewed by Rowinsky and colleagues [200]). Phase II trials are ongoing in refractory ovarian carcinoma, where an objective response rate of 30% has been reported (161). Confirmatory studies have reported a 37% response rate, and 33% of patients with documented platinum resistance have responded. Paclitaxel has limited value in renal cell carcinoma, where no responses were observed in 18 patients receiving high doses of this drug (68).

Phase II studies have demonstrated that paclitaxel has broad activity against many types of cancer. In chemotherapy-naive patients with urothelial cancer, paclitaxel induced an objective response rate of 42%, with 7 complete responses in 26 patients (296). Phase II studies have most commonly used paclitaxel at a dose of 250 mg/m^2 delivered over 24 hours with G-CSF support. When used in the treatment of squamous carcinoma of head and neck, paclitaxel produced a response rate of 40%, and when used to treat previously treated germ cell tumors, a 26% response rate was obtained. Paclitaxel has also demonstrated significant activity against carcinoma of the esophagus, with a 36% objective response rate in adenocarcinoma and a 22% objective response rate in squamous cell histologies, respectively. Activity has also been demonstrated against both small cell (SCLC) and non-small-cell lung cancer (NSCLC). Response rates for NSCLC range from 21 to 24%, with 34% of SCLCs demonstrating objective responses. Phase II trials of paclitaxel have shown significant activity in breast cancer patients who had received one prior therapy. The overall response rate was 56%, with 12% of patients having a complete response. From these studies it is clear that paclitaxel will play a significant role in the primary treatment of several types of cancer, although at present it is not clear whether the schedule of administration can alter efficacy. Paclitaxel has been administered over 1, 3, 24 and 96 hours. Preliminary results suggest that a 96-hour infusion can induce a partial response in breast cancer that was refractory to paclitaxel administered by 3-hour infusion (296). The predominant focus is now the evaluation of paclitaxel in combination with other agents. In the treatment of breast cancer, paclitaxel is being administered with cisplatin, cyclophosphamide, or doxorubicin as two-drug combinations. Although data are preliminary and based on relatively few evaluable patients, the combination of paclitaxel and cisplatin appears to induce a high rate of objective responses (296). Of note is the potential for paclitaxel to decrease the clearance of doxorubicin, causing greater than anticipated toxic effects. For ovarian cancer paclitaxel is being combined with cisplatin or carboplatin, and ifosfamide.

Less clinical information is available for docetaxel. In ovarian cancer response rates vary from 13 to 37% according to the pretreatment status of patients. In breast carcinoma, paclitaxel has demonstrated significant and consistent activity. In five trials (four multicenter) the overall response rate was 59% when docetaxel was administered at 100 mg/m^2 over 1 hour every 3 weeks (296). In patients whose disease relapsed while they were taking other therapies, the response rate was 49%. Of note was that in patients whose disease progressed while they were taking doxorubicin or an anthacenedione, the response rate was 43% in 83 patients. In chemotherapy-naive patients with NSCLC the overall response rate was 30% and in patients with platinum-refractory disease it was 20%. As for paclitaxel, the response rates for docetaxel in treatment of melanoma are relatively low (12–14%), and no significant activity has been demonstrated in colon cancer (296).

Relatively little information is available to determine cross-resistance patterns to Taxol in human tumors. However, as preclinical studies have demonstrated that Taxol resistance is associated with the multidrug resistance phenotype, one would anticipate cross-resistance with *Vinca* alkaloids and possibly epipodophyllotoxins and certain other natural products (94, 95, 202). A relatively high response rate in ovarian carcinoma refractory to cisplatin suggests little or no cross resistance between this agent and Taxol.

Summary

The *Vinca* alkaloids are important oncolytic agents that have a significant important place in the chemotherapy of many neoplastic diseases. In this chapter we have updated current knowledge about *Vinca* alkaloid action and reviewed the current status of clinical trials with newer *Vinca* alkaloids. With VCR and VLB used as a paradigm, it is evident that small modifications of the chemical structure of these agents have substantial effects on their clinical efficacy and toxicity without altering in any fundamental way their mechanism of action, which entails binding to tubulin and causing microtubule depolymerization. The toxicity of the *Vinca* alkaloids is also related to dose and route of administration. *Vinca* alkaloid resistance is associated with a broad cross-resistance to many natural product compounds, a phenomenon known as multidrug resistance. Resistance to *Vinca* alkaloids in vitro can be due not only to overexpression of the *MDR1* gene and its product, P-glycoprotein, but also to other resistance-associated proteins such as MRP; moreover, a recent study indicated that resistance to Navelbine can be due either to *MDR1* expression or to altered tubulin dynamics. Expression of P-glycoprotein is seen in a number of different types of tumors from patients, and frequently increases after therapy that includes *Vinca* alkaloids; the extent of clinical MRP expression is just beginning to be documented, as reagents to measure it have only recently become available. Efforts over the next few years will focus not only on the development of newer, non-cross-resistant *Vinca* alkaloids, but also on the development of agents that may be effective in circumventing clinical multidrug resistance.

Paclitaxel has a unique mechanism of action, stabilization of microtubules. Supply problems have been largely resolved, permitting substantial basic and clinical research efforts with paclitaxel and docetaxel. It is clear that the former is a substrate for *MDR1*; as a consequence, several clinical trials have been initiated to evaluate the effectiveness of PSC833, the nonimmunosuppressive cyclosporin A analogue, in reversing clinical MDR. The taxanes have shown activity in a number of tumors, and paclitaxel appears to be especially effective in ovarian and breast carcinomas. Clinical trials with these agents continue.

References

1. Akiyama SI, Fojo A, Hanover JA, Pastan I, Gottesman MM. Isolation and genetic characterization of human KB cell lines resistant to multiple drugs. Somat Cell Genet 1985;11:117.
2. Armand JP, Marty M. Navelbine: a new step in cancer chemotherapy? Semin Oncol 1989;2:41.
3. Bagley CM Jr, DeVita VT Jr, Berard CW, Canellos GP. Advanced lymphosarcoma intensive cyclical chemotherapy with cyclophosphamide, vincristine, and prednisone. Ann Intern Med 1972;76:227.
4. Baker RM, Fredericks WJ, Chen Y, Murawski MJ, Meegan RL, Rustum YM, Karakousis C, Piver MS. Detection of P-glycoprotein in human tumors by immunoblot analysis. In Drug Resistance Mechanisms and Reversal. Edited by E Mihich. New York: Wiley, 1990, p 167.
5. Baum SG, Wittner M, Nadler JP, Horwitz SB, Dennis JE, Schiff PB, Tanowitz HB. Taxol, a microtubule stabilizing agent, blocks the replication of *Trypanosoma cruzi.* Proc Natl Acad Sci USA 1981;78:4571.
6. Beck WT. Increase by vinblastine of oxidized glutathione in cultured mammalian cells. Biochem Pharmacol 1980;29:2333.
7. Beck WT. *Vinca* alkaloid-resistant phenotype in cultured human leukemic lymphoblasts. Cancer Treat Rep 1983;67:875.
8. Beck WT. Cellular pharmacology of *Vinca* alkaloid resistance and its circumvention. Adv Enzyme Regul 1984;22:207.
9. Beck WT. The cell biology of multiple drug resistance. Biochem Pharmacol 1987;36: 2879.
10. Beck WT. Multidrug resistance and its circumvention. Eur J Cancer 1990;26:513.
11. Beck WT. Strategies to circumvent multidrug resistance due to P-glycoprotein or to altered DNA topoisomerase II. Bull Cancer 1990;77:1131.
12. Beck WT. Modulators of P-glycoprotein-associated multidrug resistance. In Molecular and Clinical Advances in Anticancer Drug Resistance. Edited by RF Ozols. Norwell, MA: Kluwer Academic, 1991, p 151.
13. Beck WT, Cirtain MC, Lefko JL. Energy-dependent reduced drug binding as a mech-

anism of *Vinca* alkaloid resistance in human leukemic lymphoblasts. Mol Pharmacol 1983;24:485.
14. Beck WT, Cirtain MC, Danks MK, Felsted RL, Safa AR, Wolverton JS, Suttle DP, Trent JM. Pharmacological, molecular, and cytogenetic analysis of "atypical" multidrug-resistant human leukemic cells. Cancer Res 1987;47:5455.
15. Beck WT, Cirtain MC, Look AT, Ashmun RA. Reversal of *Vinca* alkaloid resistance but not multiple drug resistance in human leukemic cells by verapamil. Cancer Res 1986;46:778.
16. Behnke O. An electron microscope study of the rat megacaryocyte: II. Some aspects of platelet release and microtubules. J Ultrastruct Res 1969;26:111.
17. Bell DR, Gerlach JH, Kartner N, Buick RN, Ling V. Detection of P-glycoprotein in ovarian cancer: a molecular marker associated with multidrug resistance. J Clin Oncol 1985;3:311.
18. Bender RA, Castle MC, Margileth DA, Oliverio VT. The pharmacokinetics of (^{3}H]-vincristine in man. Clin Pharmacol Ther 1977;22:430.
19. Bender RA, Hamel E, Hande KR. Plant alkaloids. In Cancer Chemotherapy: Principals and Practice. Edited by BA Chabner, JM Collins. Philadelphia: Lippincott, 1990, p 253.
20. Bensch KG, Malawista SE. Microtubule crystals: a new biophysical phenomenon induced by *Vinca* alkaloids. Nature 1968;218:1176.
21. Bensch KG, Malawista SE. Microtubular crystals in mammalian cells. J Cell Biol 1969;40:95.
22. Benson AB, Trump DL, Koeller JM, Egorin MI, Olman EA, Witte RS, Davis TE, Tormey DC. Phase I study of vinblastine and verapamil given by concurrent iv infusion. Cancer Treat Rep 1985;69:795.
23. Besenval M, Delgado M, Demarez JP, Krikorian A. Safety and tolerance of Navelbine in phase I–II clinical studies. Semin Oncol 1989;16:37.
24. Binet S, Fellous A, Lataste H, Krikorian A, Couzinier JP, Meininger V. In situ analysis of the action of Navelbine on various types of microtubules using immunofluorescence. Semin Oncol 1989;16:5.
25. Boder GB, Bromer WW, Poore GA, Thompson GL, Williams DC. Comparative cellular responses to semisynthetic and natural *Vinca* alkaloids. Proc Am Assoc Cancer Res 1982;23:201.
26. Bore P, Rahmani R, van Cantfort J, Focan C, Cano JP. Pharmacokinetics of a new anticancer drug, Navelbine, in patients. Cancer Chemother Pharmacol 1989;23:247.
27. Bouris J, Benard J, Hartman O, Boccon-Gibod L, Lemerle J, Riou G. Correlation of MDR1 gene expression with chemotherapy in neuroblastoma. JNCI 1989;81:1401.
28. Bowman LC, Houghton JA, Houghton PJ. GTP influences the binding of vincristine in human tumor cytosols. Biochem Biophys Res Commun 1986;135:695.
29. Brade W. Critical review of pharmacology, toxicology, pharmacokinetics of vincristine, vindesine, vinblastine. In Proceedings of the International *Vinca* Alkaloid Symposium: Vindesine. Edited by W Brade, GA Nagel, S Seeber. Basel: Karger, 1980, p 95.
30. Bruchovsky N, Owen AA, Becker AJ, Till JE. Effects of vinblastine on the proliferative capacity of L cells and their progress through the division cycle. Cancer Res 1965;25:1232.
31. Bryan J. Vinblastine and microtubules: II. Characterization of two protein subunits from the isolated crystals. J Mol Biol 1972;66:157.
32. Budman DR, Schulman P, Marks M, Vinciguerra V, Weiselberg L, Kreis W, Degnan TJ. Phase I trial of vinzolidine. Cancer Treat Rep 1984;68:979.
33. Cabral F, Abraham I, Gottesman MM. Isolation of a Taxol-resistant Chinese hamster ovary cell mutant that has an alteration in α-tubulin. Proc Natl Acad Sci USA 1981;78:4388.
34. Cabral F, Sobel ME, Gottesman MM. CHO mutants resistant to colchicine, colcemid or griseofulvin have an altered α-tubulin. Cell 1980;20:29.
35. Cannobio L, Pastorino G, Gasparini G, Brema F, Fosser V, Boccardo F. Phase II study of Navelbine in advanced breast cancer patients. In Second International Congress of Neo-Adjuvant Chemotherapy (Paris), 1988, p 15.
36. Carbone PP, Kaplan HS, Musshoff K, Smither DW, Tubiana M. Report of the committee on Hodgkin's disease staging classification. Cancer Res 1971;31:1860.
37. Carter SK, Livingston RB. Single-agent therapy for Hodgkin's disease. Arch Intern Med 1973;131:377.
38. Cass CE, Beck WT. *Vinca* alkaloid pharmacology and resistance. In Resistance to Antineoplastic Drugs. Edited by D Kessel. Boca Raton: CRC, 1989, p 141.
39. Cersosimo RJ, Bromer R, Licciardello JTW, Hong WK. Pharmacology, clinical efficacy and adverse effects of vindesine sulfate, a new *Vinca* alkaloid. Pharmacotherapy 1983;3:259.
40. Chan HSL, Thorner PS, Haddad G, DeBoer G, Lin S, Yeger H, Ondrusek N, Ling V. Increased P-glycoprotein expression in advanced neuroblastoma correlates with adverse outcome of therapy. Proc Am Assoc Cancer Res 1990;31:372.
41. Chan HSL, Thorner PS, Haddad G, Ling V. Immunohistochemical detection of P-glycoprotein: prognostic correlation in soft tissue sarcoma of childhood. J Clin Oncol 1990;8:689.
42. Chan SY, Worth R, Ochs S. Block of axoplasmic transport in vitro by *Vinca* alkaloids. J Neurobiol 1980;11:251.
43. Chen C-J, Chin JE, Ueda K, Clark DP, Pastan I, Gottesman MM, Roninson IB. Internal duplication and homology with bacterial transport proteins in the mdr1 (P-glycoprotein) gene from multidrug-resistant human cells. Cell 1986;47:381.
44. Chong DCK, Logothetis CJ, Savaraj N, Fritsche HA, Gietner AM, Samuels ML. The correlation of vinblastine pharmacokinetics to toxicity in testicular cancer patients. J Clin Pharmacol 1988;28:714.
45. Cline MJ. Effect of vincristine on synthesis of ribonucleic acid and protein in leukaemic leucocytes. Br J Haematol 1968;14:21.
46. Collins CA, Vallee RB. Temperature-dependent reversible assembly of Taxol-treated microtubules. J Cell Biol 1987;105:2847.
47. Cordon-Cardo C, O'Brien JP, Casals D, Rittman-Grauer L, Biedler JL, Melamed MR, Bertino JR. Multidrug resistance gene (P-glycoprotein) is expressed by endothelial cells at blood-brain barrier sites. Proc Natl Acad Sci USA 1989;86:695.
48. Cornwell MM, Pastan I, Gottesman MM. Certain calcium channel blockers bind specifically to multidrug-resistant human KB carcinoma membrane vesicles and inhibit drug binding to P-glycoprotein. J Biol Chem 1987;262:2166.
49. Cornwell MM, Safa AR, Felsted RL, Gottesman MM, Pastan I. Membrane vesicles from multidrug-resistant human cancer cells contain a specific 150- to 170-kDa protein detected by photoaffinity labeling. Proc Natl Acad Sci USA 1986;83:3847.
50. Cornwell MM, Tsuruo T, Gottesman MM, Pastan I. ATP-binding properties of P-glycoprotein from multidrug-resistant KB cells. FASEB J 1987;1:51.
51. Creasey WA. *Vinca* alkaloids and colchicine. In Antineoplastic and Immunosuppressive Agents, II. Edited by AC Sartorelli, DG Johns. New York: Springer-Verlag, 1975, p 670.
52. Creasey WA. The *Vinca* alkaloids. In Antibiotics, V-2. Edited by FE Hahn. Berlin: Springer-Verlag, 1979, p 414.
53. Creasey WA. The *Vinca* alkaloids and similar compounds. In Cancer and Chemotherapy 3. Edited by ST Crooke, AW Prestayko. New York: Academic, 1981, p 79.
54. Creasey WA, Markiw ME. Biochemical effects of the *Vinca* alkaloids: II. A comparison of the effects of colchicine, vinblastine and vincristine on the synthesis of ribonucleic acids in Ehrlich ascites carcinoma cells. Biochim Biophys Acta 1964;87:601.
55. Creasey WA, Markiw ME. Biochemical effects of the *Vinca* alkaloids: III. The synthesis of ribonucleic acid and the incorporation of amino acids in Ehrlich ascites cells in vitro. Biochim Biophys Acta 1965;103:635.
56. Croop JM, Raymond M, Haber D, DeVault A, Arceci RJ, Gros P, Housman DE. The three mouse multidrug resistance (mdr) genes are expressed in a tissue-specific manner in mouse normal tissues. Mol Cell Biol 1989;9:1346.
57. Dalton WS, Grogan TM, Meltzer PS, Scheper RJ, Salmon SE. Drug-resistance in multiple myeloma and non-Hodgkin's lymphoma: detection of P-glycoprotein and potential circumvention by addition of verapamil to chemotherapy. J Clin Oncol 1989;7:415.
58. Dalton WS, Grogan TM, Rybski JA, Scheper J, Richter L, Kailey J, Broxterman HJ, Pinedo HM, Salmon SE. Immunohistochemical detection and quantitation of P-glycoprotein in multiple drug-resistant human myeloma cells: association with level of drug resistance and drug accumulation. Blood 1989;73:747.
59. Danks MK, Yalowich JC, Beck WT. Atypical multiple drug resistance in a human leukemic cell line selected for resistance to teniposide (VM-26). Cancer Res 1987;47:1297.
60. Danto K. Active outward transport of daunomycin in resistant Ehrlich ascites tumor cells. Biochim Biophys Acta 1973;323:466.
61. De Brabander M, Geuens G, Nuydens R, Willebrords R, De Mey J. Taxol induces the assembly of free microtubules in living cells and blocks the organizing capacity of the centrosomes and kinetochore. Proc Natl Acad Sci USA 1981;78:5608.
62. Depierre A, Lemarie E, Dabouis G, Samak R, Krikorian A, Besenval M. Phase II study of Navelbine (NVB) in non small cell lung cancer (NSCLC). Proc Am Soc Clin Oncol 1988;7:201.
63. Desai ZR, Van den Berg HW, Bridges JM, Shanks RG. Can severe vincristine neurotoxicity be prevented? Cancer Chemother Pharmacol 1981;8:211.
64. DeVita VT Jr, Hellman S, Rosenberg SA, eds. Cancer: Principles and Practice of Oncology, 2nd ed. Philadelphia: Lippincott, 1985.
65. DeVita VT Jr, Serpick AA, Carbone PP. Combination chemotherapy in the treatment of advanced Hodgkin's disease. Ann Intern Med 1970;73:881.
66. Donoso JA, Haskins KM, Himes RH. Effect of microtubule-associated proteins on the interaction of vincristine with microtubules and tubulin. Cancer Res 1979;39:1604.
67. Dustin P. Microtubules, 2nd ed. Berlin: Springer-Verlag, 1984.
68. Einzig AI, Gorowski E, Sasloff J, Wiernik PH. Phase II trial of Taxol in patients with renal carcinoma. Proc Am Assoc Cancer Res 1988;29:884.
69. Endicott JA, Ling V. The biochemistry of P-glycoprotein-mediated multidrug resistance. Annu Rev Biochem 1989;58:137.
70. Falkson G, Van Dyk JJ, Falkson FC. Oral vinblastine sulfate (NSC49842) in malignant disease. S Afr Cancer Bull 1968;12:78.
71. Favre R, Delgado M, Besenval M, Saraga J, Danet S, Krikorian A. Phase I trial of escalating doses of orally administered Navelbine (NVB): Part II. Clinical results. Proc Am Soc Clin Oncol 1989;8:A246.
72. Fellous A, Ohayon R, Vacassin T, Lataste H, Krikorian H, Couzinier JP, Meininger V. Biochemical effects of Navelbine on tubulin and associated proteins. Semin Oncol 1989;2(suppl 4):9.
73. Ferguson PJ, Cass CE. Differential cellular retention of vincristine and vinblastine by cultured human promyelocytic leukemia HL-60/C1 cells: the basis of differential toxicity. Cancer Res 1985;45:5480.
74. Ferguson PJ, Phillips JR, Selner M, Cass CE. Differential activity of vincristine and vinblastine against cultured cells. Cancer Res 1984;44:3307.
75. Ferrazzi E, Zagonel V, Vinante O, Galligioni E, Pappagallo GL, Cartei G. Vindesine in the treatment of squamous cell carcinoma (WHO I), adenocarcinoma (WHO III), and large cell carcinoma (WHO IV) of the lung. Tumori 1982;68:531.
76. Ferro-Luzzi Ames G. The basis of multidrug resistance in mammalian cells: homology with bacterial transport. Cell 1986;47:323.
77. Fojo AT, Shen D-W, Mickley LA, Pastan I, Gottesman MM. Intrinsic drug resistance in human kidney cancer is associated with expression of a human multidrug-resistance gene. J Clin Oncol 1987;5:1922.
78. Fojo AT, Ueda K, Slamon DJ, Poplack DG, Gottesman MM, Pastan I. Expression of a multidrug-resistance gene in human tumors. Proc Natl Acad Sci USA 1987;84:265.
79. Friche E, Skovsgaard T, Dano K. Multidrug resistance: drug extrusion and its counteraction by chemosensitizers. Eur J Haematol 1989;42:59.
80. Fuchs DA, Johnson RK. Cytologic evidence that Taxol, an antineoplastic agent from *Taxus brevifolia*, acts as a mitotic spindle poison. Cancer Treat Rep 1978;62:1219.
81. Garewal HS, Brooks RJ, Jones SE, Miller TP. Treatment of advanced breast cancer with mitomycin C combined with vinblastine or vindesine. J Clin Oncol 1983;1:772.
82. George M, Heron JF, Kerbrat P, Chauvergne J, Lebrun D, Guastalla JP. Phase II study of Navelbine (NVB) in advanced ovarian cancer (ADOVA). Proc Am Soc Clin Oncol 1988;7:a553.
83. George P, Journey LJ, Goldstein MN. Effect of vincristine on the fine structure of HeLa cells during mitosis. JNCI 1965;35:355.
84. Gerlach JH, Bell DR, Karakousis C, Slocum HK, Kartner N, Rustum YM, Ling V, Baker RM. P-glycoprotein in human sarcoma: evidence for multidrug resistance. J Clin Oncol 1987;5:1452.
85. Gerlach JH, Endicott JA, Juranka PF, Henderson G, Sarangi F, Deuchars KL, Ling V. Homology between P-glycoprotein and a bacterial haemolysin transport protein suggests a model for multidrug resistance. Nature 1986;324:485.
86. Gerzon K. Dimeric catharanthus alkaloids. In Anticancer Agents Based on Natural Product Models. Edited by JM Cassidy, JD Douros. New York: Academic, 1980, p 271.
87. Goldstein LJ, Fojo AT, Ueda K, Crist W, Green A, Brodeur G, Pastan I, Gottesman

MM. Expression of the multidrug resistance, MDR1, gene in neuroblastomas. J Clin Oncol 1990;8:128.

88. Goldstein LJ, Galski H, Fojo A, Willingham M, Lai S-L, Gazdar A, Pirker R, Green A, Crist W, Brodeur GM, Lieber M, Cossman J, Gottesman MM, Pastan I. Expression of a multidrug resistance gene in human cancers. JNCI 1989;81:116.
89. Gottesman MM, Pastan I. The multidrug transporter, a double-edged sword. J Biol Chem 1988;263:12163.
90. Gout PW, Noble RL, Bruchovsky N, Beer CT. Vinblastine and vincristine-growth-inhibitory effects correlate with their retention by cultured Nb2 node lymphoma cells. Int J Cancer 1984;34:245.
91. Gout PW, Wijcik LL, Beer CT. Differences between vinblastine and vincristine in distribution in the blood of rats and binding by platelets and malignant cells. Eur J Cancer 1978;14:1167.
92. Green LS, Donoso JA, Heller-Bettinger IE, Samson FE. Axonal transport disturbances in vincristine-induced peripheral neuropathy. Ann Neurol 1977;1:255.
93. Gros P, Croop J, Housman D. Mammalian multidrug resistance gene: complete cDNA sequence indicates strong homology to bacterial transport proteins. Cell 1986;47:371.
94. Gupta RS. Taxol resistant mutants of Chinese hamster ovary cells: genetic biochemical, and cross-resistance studies. J Cell Physiol 1983;114:137.
95. Gupta RS. Cross-resistance of vinblastine- and Taxol-resistant mutants of Chinese hamster ovary cells to other anticancer drugs. Cancer Treat Rep 1985;69:515.
96. Hains FO, Dickerson RM, Wilson L, Owellen RJ. Differences in the binding properties of *Vinca* alkaloids and colchicine to tubulin by varying protein sources and methodology. Biochem Pharmacol 1978;27:71.
97. Hande K, Gay J, Gober J, Greco FA. Toxicity and pharmacology of bolus vindesine injection and prolonged vindesine infusion. Cancer Treat Rev 1980;7:25.
98. Hausmann K, Linnenbach M, Patterson DJ. The effects of Taxol on microtubular arrays: in vivo effects on heliozoan axonemes. J Ultrastruct Res 1983;82:212.
99. Herman B, Langevin MA, Albertini DF. The effects of Taxol on the organization of the cytoskeleton in cultured ovarian granulosa cells. Eur J Cell Biol 1983;31:34.
100. Himes RH, Kersey RN, Heller-Bettinger I, Samson FE. Action of the *Vinca* alkaloids vincristine, vinblastine, and desacetyl vinblastine amide on microtubules in vitro. Cancer Res 1976;36:3798.
101. Horio T, Hotani H. Visualization of the dynamic instability of individual microtubules by dark-field microscopy. Nature 1986;321:605.
102. Horton JK, Thimmaiah KN, Houghton JA, Horowitz ME, Houghton PJ. Modulation by verapamil of vincristine pharmacokinetics and toxicity in mice bearing human tumor xenografts. Biochem Pharmacol 1989;38:1727.
103. Horwitz SB, Liao L-L, Greenberger L, Lothstein L. Mode of action of Taxol and characterization of a multidrug-resistant cell line selected with Taxol. In Resistance to Antineoplastic Drugs. Edited by D Kessel. Boca Raton, FL: CRC, 1989, p 109.
104. Houghton JA, Houghton PJ, Hazelton BJ, Douglass EC. In situ selection of a human rhabdomyosarcoma resistant to vincristine with altered α-tubulins. Cancer Res 1985;45:2706.
105. Houghton JA, Meyer WH, Houghton PJ. Scheduling of vincristine: drug accumulation and response of xenografts of childhood rhabdomyosarcoma determined by frequency of administration. Cancer Treat Rep 1987;71:717.
106. Houghton JA, Williams LG, Dodge RK, George SL, Hazelton BJ, Houghton PJ. Relationship between binding affinity, retention and sensitivity of human rhabdomyosarcoma xenografts to *Vinca* alkaloids. Biochem Pharmacol 1987;36:81.
107. Houghton JA, Williams LG, Houghton PJ. Stability of vincristine complexes in cytosols derived from xenografts of human rhabdomyosarcoma and normal tissues of the mouse. Cancer Res 1985;45:3761.
108. Houghton JA, Williams LG, Torrance PM, Houghton PJ. Determinants of intrinsic sensitivity to Vinca alkaloids in xenografts of pediatric rhabdomyosarcomas. Cancer Res 1984;44:582.
109. Houwen B, Ockhuizen TH, Marrink J, Nieweg HO. Vindesine therapy in melphalan-resistant multiple myeloma. Eur J Cancer Clin Oncol 1981;17:227.
110. Howard SMH, Theologides A, Sheppard JR. Comparative effects of vindesine, vinblastine, and vincristine on mitotic arrest and hormonal response of L1210 leukemia cells. Cancer Res 1980;40:2695.
111. Howell SL, Hii CS, Shaikh S, Tyhurst M. Effects of Taxol and nocodazole on insulin secretion from isolated rat islets of Langerhans. Biosci Rep 1982;2:795.
112. Huang Yang C-P, DePinho SG, Greenberger LM, Arceci RJ, Horwitz SB. Progesterone interacts with P-glycoprotein in multidrug-resistant cells and in the endometrium of gravid uterus. J Biol Chem 1989;264:782.
113. Jackson DV Jr, Castle MC, Bender RA. Biliary excretion of vincristine. Clin Pharmacol Ther 1978;24:101.
114. Jackson DV Jr, Chauvenet AR, Callahan RD, Atkins JN, Trahey TF, Spurr CL. Phase II trial of vincristine infusion in acute leukemia. Cancer Chemother Pharmacol 1985;14:26.
115. Jackson DV Jr, Sethi VS, Long TR, Muss HB, Spurr CL. Pharmacokinetics of vindesine bolus and infusion. Cancer Chemother Pharmacol 1984;13:114.
116. Jackson DV Jr, Sethi VS, Spurr CL, White DR, Richards F 2nd, Stuart JJ, Muss HB, Cooper MR, Castle MC. Pharmacokinetics of vincristine infusion. Cancer Treat Rep 1981;65:1043.
117. Jackson DV Jr, Sethi VS, Spurr CL, Willard V, White DR, Richards F 2nd, Stuart JJ, Muss HB, Cooper MR, Homesley HD, Jobson VW, Castle MC. Intravenous vincristine infusion: phase I trial. Cancer 1981;48:2559.
118. Johnson IS. Historical background of *Vinca* alkaloid research and areas of future interest. Cancer Chemother Rep 1968;52:455.
119. Johnson IS, Armstrong JG, Gorman M, Burnett JP Jr. The *Vinca* alkaloids: a new class of oncolytic agents. Cancer Res 1963;23:1390.
120. Jordan MA, Himes RH, Wilson L. Comparison of the effects of vinblastine, vincristine, vindesine, and vinepidine on microtubule dynamics and cell proliferation in vitro. Cancer Res 1985;45:2741.
121. Jordon MA, Margolis RL, Himes RH, Wilson L. Identification of a distinct class of vinblastine binding sites. Cancer Chemother Pharmacol 1982;8:215.
122. Kanamaru H, Kalehi Y, Yoshida O, Nakanishi S, Pastan I, Gottesman MM. MDR1 RNA levels in human renal cell carcinomas. Correlation with grade and prediction of reversal of doxorubicin resistance by quinidine in tumor explants. JNCI 1989;81:844.
123. Kaplan RS, Wiernik PH. Neurotoxicity of antineoplastic drugs. Semin Oncol 1982;9:103.
124. Keller HU, Zimmermann A. Shape changes and chemokinesis of Walker 256 carcinosarcoma cells in response to colchicine, vinblastine, nocodazole and Taxol. Invasion Metastasis 1986;6:33.
125. Kennedy MS, Insel PA. Inhibitors of microtubule assembly enhance beta-adrenergic and prostaglandin E1-stimulated cyclic AMP accumulation in S49 lymphoma cells. Mol Pharmacol 1979;16:215.
126. Kotani M, Koizumi Y, Yamada T, Kawasaki A, Akabane T. Increase of cyclic adenosine 3′,5′-monophosphate concentration in transplantable lymphoma cells by *Vinca* alkaloids. Cancer Res 1978;38:3094.
127. Kreis W, Budman DR, Freeman J, Milazzo J, Bergstrom RF, Nelson R. Clinical pharmacology studies with iv administered ^{3}H-vinzolidine. Proc Am Assoc Cancer Res 1988;29:216.
128. Kreis W, Budman DR, Schulman P, Freeman J, Greist A, Nelson RL, Marks M, Kevill L. Clinical pharmacology of vinzolidine. Cancer Chemother Pharmacol 1986;16:70.
129. Kremmer T, Holczinger L. Investigation of *Vinca* alkaloid-plasma membrane interactions by detergent gel chromatography. J Chromatogr 1980;191:287.
130. Krikorian A, Rahmani R, Bromet M, Bore P, Cano JP. Pharmacokinetics and metabolism of Navelbine. Semin Oncol 1989;16:21.
131. Krishan A. Time-lapse and ultrastructure studies on the reversal of mitotic arrest induced by vinblastine sulfate in Earle's L-cells. JNCI 1968;41:581.
132. Krishan A, Frei E III. Morphological basis for the cytolytic effect of vinblastine and vincristine on cultured human leukemic lymphoblasts. Cancer Res 1975;35:497.
133. Krivit W, Chilcote R, Pyesmany A, Anderson J, Hammond D. An initial report of a phase III trial comparing vindesine and vincristine for acute lymphocytic leukemia of childhood. Cancer Chemother Pharmacol 1979;2:267.
134. Kumar N. Taxol-induced polymerization of purified tubulin. J Biol Chem 1981;256:10435.
135. Lathan B, Von Hoff DD, Melink TJ, Kisner DL. Screening phase I drugs in the human tumor cloning system (HTCS) to pinpoint areas of emphasis in phase II studies. In Human Tumor Cloning. Edited by SE Salmon, JM Trent. New York: Grune & Stratton, 1984, p 669.
136. Lee JC, Harrison D, Timasheff SN. Interaction of vinblastine with calf brain microtubule protein. J Biol Chem 1975;250:9276.
137. Lee SC, Deutsch C, Beck WT. Comparison of ion channels in multidrug-resistant and -sensitive human leukemic cells. Proc Natl Acad Sci USA 1988;85:2019.
138. Lengsfeld AM, Dietrich J, Schultze-Maurer B. Accumulation and release of vinblastine and vincristine by HeLa cells: light microscopic, cinematographic, and biochemical study. Cancer Res 1982;42:3798.
139. Lengsfeld AM, Schultze B, Maurer W. Time-lapse studies on the effect of vincristine on HeLa cells. Eur J Cancer 1980;17:307.
140. Letourneau PC, Ressler AH. Inhibition of neurite initiation and growth by Taxol. J Cell Biol 1984;98:1355.
141. Letourneau PC, Shattuck TA, Ressler AH. Branching of sensory and sympathetic neurites in vitro is inhibited by treatment with Taxol. J Neurosci 1986;7:1912.
142. Loike JD, Horwitz SB. Effects of VP-16–213 on the intracellular degradation of DNA in HeLa cells. Biochemistry 1976;15:5443.
143. Lorenz W, Reiman HJ, Schmal A, Dormann P, Neugebauer E, Doenicke A. Histamine release in dogs by cremophor EL and its derivatives: oxyethylated oleic acid is the most effective constituent. Agents Actions 1977;7:63.
144. Lowenbraun S, DeVita VT Jr, Serpick AA. Combination chemotherapy with nitrogen mustard, vincristine, procarbazine, and prednisone in lymphosarcoma, and reticulum cell sarcoma. Cancer 1970;25:1018.
145. Lu K, Yap H-Y, Loo TL. Clinical pharmacokinetics of vinblastine by continuous intravenous infusion. Cancer Res 1983;43:1405.
146. Luce JK, Gamble JF, Wilson HE, Monto RW, Isaacs BL, Palmer RL, Cottman CA Jr, Hewlett JS, Gehan EA, Frei E III. Combined cyclophosphamide, vincristine and prednisone therapy of malignant lymphoma. Cancer 1971;28:306.
147. Ma DD, Davey RA, Harman DH, Isbister JP, Scurr RD, Mackertich SM, Dowden G, Bell DR. Detection of a multidrug resistant phenotype in acute nonlymphoblastic leukaemia. Lancet 1987;1:135.
148. Madoc-Jones H, Mauro F. Interphase action of vinblastine and vincristine: differences in their lethal action through the mitotic cycle of cultured mammalian cells. J Cell Physiol 1968;72:185.
149. Madoc-Jones H, Mauro F. Site of action of cytotoxic agents in the cell life cycle. In Antineoplastic and Immunosuppressive Agents. Part 1. Handbook of Experimental Pharmacology XXXVIII/1. Edited by AC Sartorelli, DG Johns. Berlin: Springer-Verlag, 1974, p 205.
150. Malawista SE, Bensch KG, Sato H. Vinblastine and griseofulvin reversibly disrupt the living mitotic spindle. Science 1968;160:770.
151. Mandelli F, Amadori S, Giona F, Antonietta M, Spiriti A, Pastore S, Meloni G, Paolucci G. Vindesine in the treatment of refractory hematologic malignancies: a phase II study. Leuk Res 1982;6:649.
152. Manfredi JJ, Horwitz SB. Taxol: an antimitotic agent with a new mechanism of action. Pharmacol Ther 1984;25:83.
153. Manfredi JJ, Parness J, Horwitz SB. Taxol binds to cellular microtubules. J Cell Biol 1982;94:688.
154. Marantz R, Ventilla M, Shelanski M. Vinblastine-induced precipitation of microtubule protein. Science 1969;165:498.
155. Mareel MM, Storme GA, De Bruyne GK, Van Cauwenberge RM. Vinblastine, vincristine and vindesine: anti-invasive effect on MO4 mouse fibrosarcoma cells in vitro. Eur J Cancer Clin Oncol 1982;18:199.
156. Marty M, Extra JM, Leandri S, Besenval M, Krikorian A. Advances in *Vinca*-alkaloids: navelbine. Nouv Rev Fr Hematol 1989;31:77.
157. Marty M, Leandri S, Extra JM, Espie M, Besenval M. A phase II study of vinorelbine (NVB) in patients (PTS) with advanced breast cancer (BC). Proc Am Assoc Cancer Res 1989;30:256.
158. Masurovsky EB, Peterson ER, Crain SM, Horwitz SB. Morphological alterations in dorsal root ganglion neurons and supporting cells of organotypic mouse spinal cord-ganglion cultures exposed to Taxol. Neuroscience 1983;10:491.
159. Mathé G, Delgado M, Ribaud P, Gouveia J. Discovery of a new *Vinca* alkaloid: navelbine (NVB). J Chemother. Infect Dis Malignancies 1989;1:a478.
160. Mathé G, Misset JL, De Vassal F, Gouveia J, Hayat M, Machover D, Belpomme D, Pico JL, Schwarzenberg L, Ribaud P, Musset M, Jasmin C, De Luca L. Phase II clinical trial with vindesine for remission induction in acute leukemia, blastic crisis of

chronic myeloid leukemia, lymphosarcoma, and Hodgkin's disease: absence of cross resistance with vincristine. Cancer Treat Rep 1978;62:805.
161. McGuire WP, Rowinsky EK, Rosenshein NB, Grundine FC, Ettinger DS, Armstrong DK, Donehower RC. Taxol: a unique antineoplastic agent with significant activity in advanced ovarian epithelial neoplasms. Ann Intern Med 1989;111:273.
162. Meininger V, Binet S, Chaineau E, Fellous A. In situ response to *Vinca* alkaloids by microtubules in cultured post-implanted mouse embryos. Biol Cell 1990;68:21.
163. Mitchison T, Kirschner M. Dynamic instability of microtubule growth. Nature 1984;312:237.
164. Mitchison T, Kirschner M. Microtubule assembly nucleated by isolated centrosomes. Nature 1984;312:232.
165. Mitchison TJ. Microtubule dynamics and kinetochore function in mitosis. Annu Rev Cell Biol 1988;4:527.
166. Mole-Bajer J, Bajer AS. Action of Taxol on mitosis: modification of microtubule arrangements and function of the mitotic spindle in Haemanthus endosperm. J Cell Biol 1983;96:527.
167. Moscow JA, Cowan KH. Multidrug resistance. JNCI 1988;80:14.
168. Moscow JA, Fairchild CR, Madden MJ, Ransom DT, Wieand HS, O'Brien EE, Poplack DG, Cossman J, Myers CE, Cowan KH. Expression of anionic glutathione-S-transferase and P-glycoprotein genes in human tissues and tumors. Cancer Res 1989;49: 1422.
169. Muggia FM. New drugs in the treatment of testicular cancer. In Therapeutic Progress in Ovarian Cancer, Testicular Cancer and the Sarcomas. Edited by AT Van Oosterom, FM Muggia. Boston: Martinus Nijhoff, 1979, p 507.
170. Mullin K, Houghton PJ, Houghton JA, Horowitz ME. Studies with 4'-deoxyepivincristine (vinepidine), a semi synthetic *Vinca* alkaloid. Biochem Pharmacol 1985;34: 1975.
171. Na GC, Timasheff SN. Interaction of vinblastine with calf brain tubulin: multiple equilibria. Biochemistry 1986;25:6214.
172. Na GC, Timasheff SN. Interaction of vinblastine with calf brain tubulin: effects of magnesium ions. Biochemistry 1986;25:6222.
173. Nair S, Samy TS, Krishan A. Calcium, calmodulin, and protein content of adriamycin-resistant and -sensitive murine leukemic cells. Cancer Res 1986;46:229.
174. Nelson RL. The comparative clinical pharmacology and pharmacokinetics of vindesine, vincristine, and vinblastine in human patients with cancer. Med Pediatr Oncol 1982;10:115.
175. Nelson RL, Dyke RW, Root MA. Clinical pharmacokinetics of vindesine. Cancer Chemother Pharmacol 1979;2:243.
176. Nelson RL, Dyke RW, Root MA. Comparative pharmacokinetics of vindesine, vincristine and vinblastine in patients with cancer. Cancer Treat Rev 1980;7:17.
177. Ohnuma T, Norton L, Andrejczuk A, Holland JF. Pharmacokinetics of vindesine given as an intravenous bolus and 24-hour infusion in humans. Cancer Res 1985;45:464.
178. Osterlind K, Horbov S, Dombernowsky P, Rorth M, Hansen HH. Vindesine in the treatment of squamous cell carcinoma, adenocarcinoma, and large cell carcinoma of the lung. Cancer Treat Rep 1982;66:305.
179. Owellen RJ, Blair M, Van Tosh A, Hains FC. Determination of tissue concentrations of *Vinca* alkaloids by radioimmunoassay. Cancer Treat Rep 1981;65:469.
180. Owellen RJ, Donigian DW, Hartke CA, Hains FO. Correlation of biologic data with physico-chemical properties among the *Vinca* alkaloids and their congeners. Biochem Pharmacol 1977;26:1213.
181. Owellen RJ, Hartke CA, Dickerson RM, Hains FO. Inhibition of tubulin-microtubule polymerization by drugs of the *Vinca* alkaloid class. Cancer Res 1976;36:1499.
182. Owellen RJ, Hartke CA, Hains FO. Pharmacokinetics and metabolism of vinblastine in humans. Cancer Res 1977;37:2597.
183. Owellen RJ, Owens AH Jr, Donigian DW. The binding of vincristine, vinblastine and colchicine to tubulin. Biochem Biophys Commun 1972;47:685.
184. Owellen RJ, Root MA, Hains RO. Pharmacokinetics of vindesine and vincristine in humans. Cancer Res 1977;37:2603.
185. Ozols RF, Cunnion RE, Klecker RW Jr, Hamilton TC, Ostchega Y, Parillo JE, Young RC. Verapamil and adriamycin in the treatment of drug-resistant ovarian cancer patients. J Clin Oncol 1987;5:641.
186. Palmer CG, Livengood D, Warren AK, Simpson PJ, Johnson IS. The action of Vincaleukoblastine on mitosis in vitro. Exp Cell Res 1960;20:198.
187. Parness J, Asnes CF, Horwitz SB. Taxol binds differentially to flagellar outer doublets and their reassembled microtubules. Cell Motility 1983;3:123.
188. Parness J, Horwitz SB. Taxol binds to polymerized tubulin in vitro. J Cell Biol 1981;91: 479.
189. Pearce HL. Medicinal chemistry of bisindole alkaloids from *Catharanthus*. In The Alkaloids, vol. 37. Edited by A. Brossi. Orlando: Academic, 1990, p 145.
190. Pike MC, Kredich NM, Snyderman R. Influence of cytoskeletal assembly on phosphatidylcholine synthesis in intact phagocytic cells. Cell 1980;20:373.
191. Qian X-D, Beck WT. Binding of an optically pure photoaffinity analogue of verapamil, LU-49888, to P-glycoprotein from multidrug-resistant human leukemic cell lines. Cancer Res 1990;50:1132.
192. Qian X-D, Beck WT. Progesterone photoaffinity labels P-glycoprotein in multidrug resistant human leukemic lymphoblasts. J Biol Chem 1990;265:18753.
193. Rahmani R, Martin M, Barket J, Cano JP. Radioimmunoassay and preliminary pharmacokinetic studies in rats of 5'-noranhydrovinblastine (Navelbine). Cancer Res 1984;44:5609.
194. Rainey WE, Kramer RE, Jason JI, Shay JW. The effects of taxol, a microtubule-stabilizing drug, on steroidogenic cells. J Cell Physiol 1985;123:17.
195. Ratain MJ, Vogelzang NJ. Phase I and pharmacological study of vinblastine by prolonged continuous infusion. Cancer Res 1986;46:4827.
196. Retsas S, Newton KA, Westbury G. Vindesine as a single agent in the treatment of advanced malignant melanoma. Cancer Chemother Pharmacol 1979;2:257.
197. Riehm H, Biedler JL. Potentiation of drug effect by Tween 80 in Chinese hamster cells resistant to actinomycin D and daunomycin. Cancer Res 1972;32:1. 195.
198. Roberts RL, Nath J, Friedman MM, Gallin JI. Effects of Taxol on human neutrophils. J Immunol 1982;129:2134.
199. Rosenthal S, Kaufman S. Vincristine neurotoxicity. Ann Intern Med 1974;80:733.
200. Rowinsky EK, Cazenave LA, Donehower RC. Taxol: a novel investigational antimicrotubule agent. JNCI 1990;82:1247.
201. Rowinsky EK, Donehower RC, Jones RJ, Tucker RW. Microtubule changes and cytotoxicity in leukemic cell lines treated with Taxol. Cancer Res 1988;48:4093.
202. Roy SN, Horwitz SB. A phosphoglycoprotein associated with Taxol resistance in J774.2 cells. Cancer Res 1985;45:3856.
203. Roytta M, Laine K-M, Harkonen P. Morphological studies on the effect of Taxol on cultured human prostatic cancer cells. Prostate 1987;11:95.
204. Rudolph S, Greengard P, Malawista SE. Effect of colchicine on cyclic AMP levels in human leukocytes. Proc Natl Acad Sci USA 1977;74:3404.
205. Safa AR. Photoaffinity labeling of the multidrug-resistance-related P-glycoprotein with photoactive analogs of verapamil. Proc Natl Acad Sci USA 1988;85:7178.
206. Safa AR, Glover CJ, Meyers MB, Biedler JL, Felsted RL. Vinblastine photoaffinity labeling of a high molecular weight surface membrane glycoprotein specific for multidrug-resistant cells. J Biol Chem 1986;261:6137.
207. Salmon ED, Wolniak SM. Taxol stabilization of mitotic spindle microtubules: analysis using calcium-induced depolymerization. Cell Motil 1984;4:155.
208. Salmon SE, Grogan TM, Miller T, Scheper R, Dalton WS. Prediction of doxorubicin resistance in vitro in myeloma, lymphoma, and breast cancer by P-glycoprotein staining. JNCI 1989;81:696.
209. Sammak PJ, Borisy GG. Direct observation of microtubule dynamics in living cells. Nature 1988;332:724.
210. Samson FE Jr. Mechanism of axoplasmic transport. J Neurobiol 1971;2:347.
211. Sandler SG, Tobin W, Henderson ES. Vincristine-induced neuropathy: a clinical study of fifty leukemic patients. Neurology 1969;19:367.
212. Sarna G, Mitsuyasu R, Figlin R, Ambersely J, Groopman J. Oral vinzolidine as therapy for Kaposi's sarcoma and carcinomas of lung, breast, and colon/rectum. Cancer Chemother Pharmacol 1985;14:12.
213. Schellenberg RR, Gillespie E. Effects of colchicine, vinblastine, griseofulvin and deuterium oxide upon phospholipid metabolism in concanavalin A-stimulated lymphocytes. Biochim Biophys Acta 1980;619:522.
214. Schibler MJ, Cabral F. Taxol-dependent mutants of Chinese hamster ovary cells with alterations in α- and β-tubulin. J Cell Biol 1986;102:1522.
215. Schiff PB, Fant J, Horwitz SB. Promotion of microtubule assembly in vitro by Taxol. Nature 1979;277:665.
216. Schiff PB, Horwitz SB. Taxol stabilizes microtubules in mouse fibroblast cells. Proc Natl Acad Sci USA 1980;77:1561.
217. Schiff PB, Horwitz SB. Taxol assembles tubulin in the absence of exogenous guanosine 5'-triphosphate or microtubule-associated proteins. Biochemistry 1981;10:3247.
218. Schilber MJ, Cabral F. Taxol-dependent mutants of Chinese hamster ovary cells with alterations in α- and β-tubulin. J Cell Biol 1986;102:1522.
219. Schneider J, Bak M, Efferth TH, Kaufmann M, Mattern J, Volm M. P-glycoprotein expression in treated and untreated human breast cancer. Br J Cancer 1989;60:815.
220. Schrek R. Cytotoxicity of vincristine to normal and leukemic cells. Am J Clin Pathol 1974;62:1.
221. Schrek R, Stefani SS. Toxicity of microtubular drugs to leukemic lymphocytes. Exp Mol Pathol 1981;34:369.
222. Schroeder F, Fontaine RN, Feller DJ, Weston KG. Drug-induced surface membrane phospholipid composition in murine fibroblasts. Biochim Biophys Acta 1981;643:76.
223. Schulze E, Kirschner M. New features of microtubule behaviour observed in vivo. Nature 1988;324:356.
224. Sethi VS, Burton SS, Jackson DV. A sensitive radioimmunoassay for vincristine and vinblastine. Cancer Chemother Pharmacol 1980;4:183.
225. Sethi VS, Jackson DV Jr, White DR, Richards F II, Stuart JJ, Muss HB, Cooper MR, Spurr CL. Pharmacokinetics of vincristine sulfate in adult cancer patients. Cancer Res 1981;41:3551.
226. Sethi VS, Kimball JC. Pharmacokinetics of vincristine sulfate in children. Cancer Chemother Pharmacol 1981;6:111.
227. Sethi VS, Thimmaiah KN. Structural studies on the degradation products of vincristine dihydrogen sulfate. Cancer Res 1985;45:5386.
228. Singer WD, Hersh RT, Himes RH. Effect of solution variables on the binding of vinblastine to tubulin. Biochem Pharmacol 1988;37:2691.
229. Singer WD, Jordan MA, Wilson LA, Himes RH. Binding of vinblastine to stabilized microtubules. Mol Pharmacol 1989;36:366.
230. Skovsgaard T. Mechanism of cross-resistance between vincristine and daunorubicin in Ehrlich ascites tumor cells. Cancer Res 1978;38:4722.
231. Smith IE, Hedley DW, Powles TJ, McElwain TJ. Vindesine: a phase II study in breast carcinoma, malignant melanoma, and other tumors. Cancer Treat Rep 1978;62:1427.
232. Sterle M, Pipan N. Influence of antimicrotubular drugs on the Golgi apparatus of stomach secretory mucoid cells and small intestine absorptive cells. Virchows Arch [Cell Pathol] 1990;58:317.
233. Sullivan MP, Nora AH, Kulapongs P, Lane DM, Windmiller J, Thurman WG. Evaluation of vincristine sulfate and cyclophosphamide chemotherapy for metastatic neuroblastoma. Pediatrics 1969;44:685.
233a. Sutow WW, Sullivan MP. Successful chemotherapy for childhood rhabdomyosarcoma. Tex Med 1970;66:78.
234. Takasugi BJ, Jones SE, Robertone AB. Phase II trial of vinzolidine, an oral *Vinca* alkaloid, in Hodgkin's disease and non-Hodgkin's lymphoma. Cancer Treat Rep 1984;68:1399.
235. Takasugi BJ, Salmon SE, Nelson RL, Young L, Liu RM. Antitumor activity of vinzolidine in the human tumor clonogenic assay and comparison with vinblastine. Invest New Drugs 1984;2:49.
236. Tan C. Clinical and pharmacokinetic studies of vindesine in 50 children with malignant disease. In Current Chemotherapy: Proceedings of the 10th International Congress of Chemotherapy, vol 2. Edited by W Siegenthaler, R Luthy. Washington DC: American Society of Microbiology, p 1326.
237. Taylor CW, Salmon SE, Satterlee WG, Alberts DS, Robertone AB, Peng YM. Intravenous vinzolidine (IV VZL). A phase I and pharmacokinetic study. Proc Am Assoc Cancer Res 1988;29:325.
238. Taylor CW, Salmon SE, Satterlee WG, Robertone AB, McCloskey TM, Holdsworth MT, Plezia PM, Alberts DS. A phase I and pharmacokinetic study of intravenous vinzolidine. Invest New Drugs 1990;8:S51.
239. Ter-Minassian-Saraga L, Madelmont G. Enhanced hydration of ipalmitoylphosphatidylcholine multibilayer by vinblastine sulphate. Biochim Biophys Acta 1983;728: 394.
240. Ter-Minassian-Saraga L, Madelmont G, Hort-Legrand C, Metral S. Vinblastine and vincristine action on gel-fluid transition of hydrated DPPC. Biochem Pharmacol 1981;30:411.

241. Thiebaut F, Tsuruo T, Hamada H, Gottesman MM, Pastan I, Willingham MC. Immunohistochemical localization in normal tissues of different epitopes in the multidrug transport protein P170: evidence for localization in brain capillaries and cross reactivity of one antibody with a muscle protein. J Histochem Cytochem 1989;37:159.
242. Thigpen JT, Blessing J, Ball H, Hummel S, Barret R. Phase II trial of Taxol as second-line therapy for ovarian carcinoma. A Gynecologic Oncology Group study. Proc Am Soc Clin Oncol 1990;9:604.
243. Thimmaiah KN, Sethi VS. Chemical characterization of the degradation products of vinblastine dihydrogen sulfate. Cancer Res 1985;45:5382.
244. Thompson GL, Boder GB, Bromer WW, Grindey GB, Poore GA. A novel potent *Vinca* analog with unique biological properties. Proc Am Assoc Cancer Res 1982;23:201.
245. Thompson WC, Wilson L, Purich DL. Taxol induces microtubule assembly at low temperature. Cell Motil 1981;1:445.
246. Thuret-Carnahan J, Bossu J-L, Feltz A, Langley K, Aunis D. Effect of Taxol on secretory cells: functional, morphological, and electrophysiological correlates. J Cell Biol 1985;100:1863.
247. Tsuruo T, Iida H, Tsukagoshi S, Sakurai Y. Overcoming of vincristine resistance in P388 leukemia in vivo and in vitro through enhanced cytotoxicity of vincristine and vinblastine by verapamil. Cancer Res 1981;41:1967.
248. Tucker RW, Owellen RJ, Harris SB. Correlation of cytotoxicity and mitotic spindle dissolution by vinblastine in mammalian cells. Cancer Res 1977;37:4346.
249. Tueni E, Dodion P, Piccart M, Wery F, Kerger J, Delgado M. A new oral phase I trial with Navelbine (NVB) administered on a weekly schedule. Proc Am Assoc Cancer Res 1990;31:207.
250. Van den Berg HW, Desai ZR, Wilson R, Kennedy G, Bridges JM, Shanks RG. The pharmacokinetics of vincristine in man: reduced drug clearance associated with raised serum alkaline phosphatase and dose-limited elimination. Cancer Chemother Pharmacol 1982;8:215.
251. van der Bliek AM, Borst P. Multidrug resistance. Adv Cancer Res 1989;52:165.
252. Vats TS, Mehta P, Trueworthy RC, Smith SD, Klopovich P. Vindesine and prednisone for remission induction in children with acute lymphocytic leukemia. Cancer 1981;47:2789.
253. Vietti TJ, Sullivan MP, Haggard ME, Holcomb TM, Berry DH. Vincristine sulfate and radiation therapy in metastatic Wilms' tumor. Cancer 1970;25:12.
254. Volberding PA, Abrams D, Conant M, Kaslow K, Vranizan K, Ziegler J. Vinblastine therapy for Kaposi's sarcoma in the acquired immunodeficiency syndrome. Ann Intern Med 1985;103:335.
255. Watanabe K, West WL. Calmodulin, activated cyclic nucleotidephosphodiesterase, microtubules, and *Vinca* alkaloids. Fed Proc 1982;41:2292.
256. Watanabe K, Williams EF, Law JS, West WL. Effects of *Vinca* alkaloids on calcium-calmodulin regulated cyclic adenosine 3′,5′-monophosphate phosphodiesterase activity from brain. Biochem Pharmacol 1981;30:335.
257. Weber W, Nagel GA, Nagel-Studer E, Albrecht R. Vincristine infusion: a phase I study. Cancer Chemother Pharmacol 1979;3:49.
258. Weiss HD, Walker MD, Wiernik PH. Neurotoxicity of commonly used antineoplastic agents. N Engl J Med 1974;291:127.
259. White JG. Effects of colchicine and *Vinca* alkaloids on human platelets: I. Influence on platelet microtubules and contractile function. Am J Pathol 1968;53:281.
260. Deleted in proof.
261. Wilson L. Microtubules as drug receptors: pharmacological properties of microtubule protein. Ann NY Acad Sci 1975;253:213.
262. Wilson L, Bamburg JR, Mizel SB, Grisham LM, Creswell KM. Interaction of drugs with microtubule proteins. Fed Proc 1974;33:158.
263. Wilson L, Jordan MA, Morse A, Margolis RL. Interaction of vinblastine with steady-state microtubules in vitro. J Mol Biol 1982;159:125.
264. Yamashita N, Hamada H, Tsuruo T, Ogata E. Enhancement of voltage-gated Na^+ channel current associated with multidrug resistance in human leukemia cells. Cancer Res 1987;47:3736.
265. Yang L, Rowe TC, Liu LF. Identification of DNA topoisomerase II as an intracellular target of antitumor epipodophyllotoxins in Simian virus 40-infected monkey cells. Cancer Res 1985;45:5872.
266. Yap HY, Blumenschein GR, Bodey GP, Hortobagyi GN, Buzdar AU, DiStefano A. Vindesine in the treatment of refractory breast cancer: improvement in therapeutic index with continuous 5-day infusion. Cancer Treat Rep 1981;65:775.
267. Yap HY, Blumenschein GR, Keating MJ, Hortobagyi GN, Tashima CK, Loo TL. Vinblastine given as a continuous 5-day infusion. Cancer Treat Rep 1980;64:279.
268. Young JA, Howell SB, Green MR. Pharmacokinetics and toxicity of 5-day continuous infusion of vinblastine. Cancer Chemother Pharmacol 1984;12:43.
269. Yusa K, Tsuruo T. Reversal mechanism of multidrug resistance by verapamil: direct binding of verapamil to P-glycoprotein on specific sites and transport of verapamil outward across the plasma membrane of K562/ADM cells. Cancer Res 1989;49:5002.
270. Zakhireh B, Malech HL. The effect of colchicine and vinblastine on the chemotactic response of human monocytes. J Immunol 1980;125:2143.
271. Verweij J, Clavel M, Chevalier B. Paclitaxel (Taxol) and docetaxel (Taxotere): not simply two of a kind. Ann Oncol 1994;5:495.
272. Gelmon K. The taxoids: paclitaxel and docetaxel. Lancet 1994;344:1267.
273. Sonnichsen DS, Relling MV. Clinical pharmacokinetics of paclitaxel. Clin Pharmacokinet 1994;27:256.
274. Arbuck SG, Dorr A, Friedman MA. Paclitaxel (Taxol) in breast cancer. Hematol Oncol Clin North Am 1994;8:121.
275. Donehower RC, Rowinsky EK. An overview of experience with Taxol (paclitaxel) in the USA. Cancer Treat Rev 1993;19:63.
276. Otter GM, Sirotnak FM. Effective combination therapy of metastatic murine solid tumors with edatrexate and the Vinca alkaloids, vinblastine, navelbine and vindesine. Cancer Chemother Pharmacol 1994;33:286.
277. Zhou XJ, Bore P, Monjanel S, Sahnoun Z, Favre R, Durand A, Rahmani R. Pharmacokinetics of navelbine after oral administration in cancer patients. Cancer Chemother Pharmacol 1991;29:66.
278. Perez RP, Hamilton TC, Ozols RF, Young RC. Mechanisms and modulation of resistance to chemotherapy in ovarian cancer. Cancer Suppl 1993;71:1571.
279. Hahn SM, Liebmann JE, Cook J, Fisher Y, Goldspiel B, Venzou D, Mitchell JB, Kaufman D. Taxol in combination with doxorubicin or etoposide. Cancer 1993;72:2705.
280. Abrams JS, Moore TD, Friedman M. New chemotherapeutic agents for breast cancer. Cancer Suppl 1994;74:1164.
281. Vokes EE, Drinkard LC, Samuels BL, Hoffman PC, Watson W, Bitan JD, Haraf DJ, Ferguson MF, Golomb HM. A phase II study of cisplatin, 5-fluorouracil, and leucovorin augmented by vinorelbine (Navelbine) for advanced non-small cell lung cancer: rationale and study design. Semin Oncol 1994;5:79.
282. Crawford J. Vinorelbine (Navelbine) in non-small cell lung cancer: future directions. Semin Oncol 1994;5:85.
283. Garbo C, Kreuser ED, Zouboulis CC, Stadler R, Orfanos CE. Combined treatment of metastatic melanoma with interferons and cytotoxic drugs. Semin Oncol 1992;19:63.
284. Alexanian R, Dimopoulos M. The treatment of multiple myeloma. N Engl J Med 1994;330:484.
285. Arbuck SG, Canetta R, Onetto N, Christian MC. Current dosage and schedule issues in the development of paclitaxel (Taxol). Semin Oncol 1993;20:31.
286. Rowinsky EK, Eisenhauer EA, Chaudhry V, Arbuck SG, Donehower RC. Clinical toxicities encountered with paclitaxel (Taxol). Semin Oncol 1993;20:1.
287. Rowinsky EK, Donehower RC. The clinical pharmacology of paclitaxel (Taxol). Semin Oncol 1993;20:16.
288. Beijinen JH, Hulzing MT, ten Bokkel Huinink WW, Veenhof CHN, Vermorken JB, Glaccone G, Pinedo HM. Bioanalysis pharmacokinetics, and pharmacodynamics of the novel anticancer drug paclitaxel (Taxol). Semin Oncol 1994;5:53.
289. Forasteire AA. Paclitaxel (Taxol) for the treatment of head and neck cancer. Semin Oncol 1994;21:49.
290. O'Shaughnessy JA, Fisherman JS, Cowan KH. Combination paclitaxel (Taxol) and doxorubicin therapy for metastatic breast cancer. Semin Oncol 1994;21:19.
291. Ozols RF. Treatment of ovarian cancer: current status. Semin Oncol 1994;21:1.
292. Caldas C, McGuire WP III. Paclitaxel (Taxol) therapy in ovarian carcinoma. Semin Oncol 1993;20:50.
293. Effinger DS. Overview of paclitaxel (Taxol) in advanced lung cancer. Semin Oncol 1993;20:46.
294. Fisherman JS, McCabe M, Noone M, Ognibene F, Goldspiel B, Venzon DJ, Cowan KH, O'Shaughnessy JA. Phase I study of Taxol, doxorubicin, plus granulocyte-colony stimulating factor in patients with metastatic breast cancer. JNCI 1993;15:189.
295. Aapro MS. Docetaxel (Taxotere): a highly active taxoid with manageable toxicity. Semin Oncol 1995;22:1.
296. Ozols RF. The emerging role of paclitaxel in cancer chemotherapy. Semin Oncol 1995;22:1.
297. Abeloff MD. Vinorelbine (navelbine) in the treatment of breast cancer: a summary. Semin Oncol 1995;22:1.
298. Crawford J, O'Rourke MA. Vinorelbine (navelbine)/carboplatin combination therapy: dose intensification with granulocyte colon-stimulating factor. Semin Oncol 1994;21:73.
299. Roth BJ, Yeap BY, Wilding G, Kasimis B, McLeod D, Loehrer PJ. Taxol in advanced, hormone-refractory carcinoma of the prostate. Cancer 1993;72:2457.
300. Wall ME, Wani MC. Camptothecin and Taxol: discovery to clinic. Thirteenth Bruce F Cain Memorial Award Lecture. Cancer Res 1995;55:753.
301. Pisters KMW, Kris MG, Gralla RJ, Hilaris B, McCormack PM, Bains MS, Martini N. Randomized trial comparing postoperative chemotherapy with vindesine and cisplatin plus thoracic irradiation with irradiation alone in stage III (N2) non-small cell lung cancer. J Surg Oncol 1994;56:236.
302. Sørensen JB, Hansen HH. Is there a role for vindesine in the treatment of non-small cell lung cancer. Invest New Drugs 1993;11:103.
303. Debal V, Morjani H, Millot J-M, Angiboust J-F. Determination of vinorelbine (navelbine) in tumour cells by high-performance liquid chromatography. J Chromatog 1992;581:93.
304. Kuebler JP, Whitehead RP, Ward DL, Hemstreet GP III, Bradley EC. Treatment of metastatic renal cell carcinoma with recombinant interleukin-2 in combination with vinblastine or lymphokine-activated killer cells. J Urol 1993;150:814.
305. Kantoff PW, Scher HI. Chemotherapy for metastatic bladder cancer. Hematol Oncol Clin North Am 1992;6:195.
306. Caplow M, Shanks J, Ruhlen R. How Taxol modulates microtubule disassembly. J Biol Chem 1994;269:23399.
307. Thigpen JT, Vance RB, Khansur T. Second-line chemotherapy for recurrent carcinoma of the ovary. Cancer Suppl 1993;71:1559.
308. Glantz MJ, Choy H, Kearns CM, Mills PC, Wahlberg LU, Zuhowski EG, Calabresi P, Egorin MJ. Paclitaxel disposition in plasma and central nervous systems of humans and rats with brain tumors. JNCI 1995;87:1077.
309. Knick VC, Eberwein DJ, Miller CG. Vinorelbine tartrate and paclitaxel combinations: enhanced activity against in vivo P388 murine leukemia cells. JNCI 1995;87:1072.
310. Danesi R, Figg WD, Reed E, Myers CE. Paclitaxel (Taxol) inhibits protein isoprenylation and induces apoptosis in PC-3 human prostate cancer cells. Mol Pharmacol 1995;47:1106.
311. Bhalla K, Huang Y, Tang C, Self S, Ray S, Mahoney ME, Ponnathpur V, Tourkina E, Ibrado AM, Bullock G, Willingham MC. Characterization of a human myeloid leukemia cell like highly resistant to taxol. Leukemia 1994;8:465.
312. Riou J-F, Petitgenet O, Aynié I, Lavelle F. Establishment and characterization of docetaxel (Taxotere) resistant human breast carcinoma (Calc 18/TXT) and murine leukemic (P388/TXT) cell lines. Proc Am Assoc Cancer Res 1994;35:339.
313. Walle T, Walle UK, Kumar GN, Bhalla KN. Taxol metabolism and disposition in cancer patients. Drug Metab Dispos 1995;23:506.
314. Hennequin C, Giocanti N, Favaudon V. S-phase specificity of cell killing by docetaxel (Taxotere) in synchronised HeLa cells. Br J Cancer 1995;71:1194.
315. Debal V, Allam N, Morjani H, Millot JM, Braguer D, Breillout F, Manfait M. Characterisation of a navelbine-resistant bladder carcinoma cell line cross-resistant to taxoids. Br J Cancer 1994;70:1118.
316. Degardin M, Bonneterre J, Hecquet B, Pion J-M, Adenis A, Horner D, Demaille A. Vinorelbine (Navelbine) as a salvage treatment for advanced breast cancer. Ann Oncol 1994;5:423.
317. Depierre A, Lemarie E, Dabouis G, Garnier G, Jacoulet P, Dalphin JC. A phase II study of navelbine (vinorelbine) in the treatment of non-small-cell lung cancer. Am J Clin Oncol 1991;14:115.
318. Coltman CA Jr. Vinorelbine (Navelbine): a new agent for the treatment of non-small-cell lung cancer: a summary. Semin Oncol 1994;21:1.
319. Vokes EE, Rosenberg R, Jahanzeb M, Craig J, Gralla R, Belani C, Jones S, Bigley J, Hohneker J. Oral vinorelbine (Navelbine) in the treatment of advanced non-small cell lung cancer: a preliminary report. Semin Oncol 1994;21:35.

320. Le Chevalier T, Pujol J-L, Douillard J-Y, Alberola V, Monnier A, Riviere A, Lianes P, Chomy P, Cigloari S, Besson F, Berthaud P, Brisgand D. A three-arm trial of vinorelbine (Navelbine) plus cisplatin, vindesine plus cisplatin, and single-agent vinorelbine in the treatment of non-small cell lung cancer: an expanded analysis. Semin Oncol 1994;21:28.
321. Adams DJ, Knick VC. MDR and non-MDR forms of cellular resistance to 5′-nor-anhydrovinblastine (Navelbine). Proc Am Assoc Cancer Res 1992;33:462.
322. Lavelle F, Bissery MC, Combeau C, Riou JF, Vrignaud P, Andre S. Preclinical evaluation of docetaxel (Taxotere). Semin Oncol 1995;22:3.
323. Budman DR. New Vinca alkaloids and related compounds. Semin Oncol 1992;19: 639.
324. Hei TK, Piao CQ, Geard CR, Hall EJ. Taxol and ionizing radiation: interaction and mechanisms. Int J Radiat Oncol Biol Phys 1994;29:267.
325. Kelland LR, Abel G. Comparative in vitro cytotoxicity of Taxol and Taxotere against cisplatin-sensitive and -resistant human ovarian carcinoma cell lines. Cancer Chemother Pharmacol 1992;30:444.
326. Waud WR, Gilbert KS, Harrison SD, Griswold DP. Cross-resistance of drug-resistant murine P388 leukemias to Taxol in vivo. Cancer Chemother Pharmacol 1992;31:255.
327. Nicolett, MI, Lucchini V, D'Incalci M, Giavazzi R. Comparison of paclitaxel and docetaxel activity on human ovarian carcinoma xenografts. Eur J Cancer 1994;30A:691.
328. Hill BT, Whelan RDH, Shellard SA, McClean S, Hosking LK. Differential cytotoxic effects of docetaxel in a range of mammalian tumor cell lines and certain drug resistant sublines *in vitro*. Invest New Drugs 1994;12:169.
329. Bissery M-C, Guénard D, Guéritte-Voegelein F, Lavelle F. Experimental antitumor activity of taxotere (RP 56976, NSC 628503), a taxol analogue. Cancer Res 1991;51: 4845.
330. Fjällskog M-L, Frii L, Bergh J. Paclitaxel-induced cytotoxicity: the effects of cremophor EL (castor oil) on two human breast cancer cell lines with acquired multidrug resistant phenotype and induced expression of the permeability glycoprotein. Eur J Cancer 1994;30A:687.
331. Steren A, Sevin BU, Perras J, Ramos R, Angioli R, Nguyen H, Koechli O, Averette HE. Taxol as a radiation sensitizer: a flow cytometric study. Gynecol Oncol 1993;50:89.
332. Berg SL, Tolcher A, O'Shaughnessy JA, Denicoff AM, Noone M, Ognibene FP, Cowan KH, Balis FM. Effect of R-verapamil on the pharmacokinetics of paclitaxel in women with breast cancer. J Clin Oncol 1995;13:2039.
333. Wadkins RM, Houghton PJ. The role of drug-lipid interactions in the biological activity of modulators of multi-drug resistance. Biochim Biophys Acta 1993;1153:225.
334. Nicolaou KC, Yang Z, Liu JJ, Ueno H, Nantermet PG, Guy RK, Claiborne CF, Renaud J, Couladouros EA, Paulvannan K, et al. Total synthesis of Taxol. Nature 1994;367: 630.
335. Geard CR, Jones JM. Radiation and Taxol effects on synchronized human cervical carcinoma cells. Int J Radiat Oncol Biol Phys 1994;29:565.
336. Tishler RB, Schiff PB, Geard CR, Hall EJ, Phil D. Taxol: a novel radiation sensitizer. Int J Radiat Oncol Biol Phys 1992;22:613.
337. Choy H, Rodriguez RF, Koester S, Hilsenbeck S, von Hoff DD. Investigation of Taxol as a potential radiation sensitizer. Cancer 1993;71:3774.
338. Hei TK, Piao CQ, Geard CR, Hall EJ. Taxol and ionizing radiation: interaction and mechanisms. Int J Radiat Oncol Biol Phys 1994;29:267.
339. Liebmann J, Cook JA, Fisher J, Hague D, Mitchell JB. In vitro studies of Taxol by a radiation sensitizer in human tumor cells. JNCI 1994;86:441.
340. Milas L, Hunter NR, Mason KA, Kurdoglu B, Peters LJ. Enhancement of tumor radio response of a murine mammary carcinoma by paclitaxel. Cancer Res 1994;54: 3506.
341. Mason KA, Milas L, Peters LJ. Effect of paclitaxel (Taxol) alone and in combination with radiation on the gastrointestinal mucosa. Int J Radiat Oncol Biol Phys 1995;32: 1381.
342. Steren A, Sevin BU, Perras J, Angioli R, Nguyen H, Guerra L, Koechli O, Averette HE. Taxol sensitizers human ovarian cancer cells to radiation. Gynecol Oncol 1993;48: 252.
343. Flens MJ, Izquierdo MA, Scheffer GL, Fritz JM, Meijer CJLM, Scheper RJ, Zaman GJR. Immunochemical detection of the multidrug resistance-associated protein MRP in human multidrug-resistant tumor cells by monoclonal antibodies. Cancer Res 1994;54:4557.
344. Tsukidate K, Yamamoto K, Snyder JW, Farber JL. Microtubule antagonists activate programmed cell death (apoptosis) in cultured rat hepatocytes. Am J Pathol 1993;143:918.
345. Stewart BW. Mechanisms of apoptosis: integration of genetic, biochemical, and cellular indicators. JNCI 1994;86:1286.
346. Green DR, Bissonnette RP, Cotter TG. Apoptosis and cancer. Import Adv Oncol 1994;1994:37.
347. Kerr JF, Winterford CM, Harmon BV. Apoptosis: its significance in cancer and cancer therapy. Cancer 1994;23:2013 (published erratum Cancer 1994;73:3108).
348. Fisher DE. Apoptosis in cancer therapy: crossing the threshold. Cell 1994;78:539.
349. Hartwell LH, Kastan MB. Cell cycle control and cancer. Science 1994;266:1821.
350. Binet S, Chaineau E, Fellous A, Lataste H, Krikorian A, Couzinier JP, Meininger V. Immunofluorescence study of the action of navelbine, vincristine and vinblastine on mitotic and axonal microtubules. Int J Cancer 1990;46:262.
351. Roninson IB, ed. Molecular and Cellular Biology of Multidrug Resistance in Tumor Cells. New York: Plenum, 1991.
352. Cornwell MM, Smith DE. SP1 activates the MDR1 promoter through one of two distinct G-rich regions that modulate promoter activity. J Biol Chem 1993;268:19505.
353. Madden MJ, Morrow CS, Nakagawa M, Goldsmith ME, Fairchild CR, Cowan KH. Identification of 5′ and 3′ sequences involved in the regulation of transcription of the human mdr1 gene in vivo. J Biol Chem 1993;268:8290.
354. Yu L, Cohen D, Piekarz RL, Horwitz SB. Three distinct nuclear protein binding sites in the promoter of the murine multidrug resistance mdr1b gene. J Biol Chem 1993;268: 7520.
355. Chambers TC, Phol J, Raynor RL, Kuo JF. Identification of specific sites in human P-glycoprotein phosphorylated by protein kinase C. J Biol Chem 1993;268:4592.
356. Orr GA, Han EK, Browne PC, Nieves E, O'Connor BM, Yang CP, Horwitz SB. Identification of the major phosphorylation domain of murine mdr1b P-glycoprotein: analysis of the protein kinase A and protein kinase C phosphorylation sites. J Biol Chem 1993;268:25054.
357. Mickley LA, Bates SE, Richert ND, Currier S, Tanaka S, Foss F, Rosen N, Fojo AT. Modulation of the expression of a multidrug resistance gene (mdr-1/P-glycoprotein) by differentiating agents. J Biol Chem 19089;264:18031.
358. Kohno K, Sato S, Takano H, Matsuo K, Kuwano M. The direct activation of human multidrug resistance gene (MDR1) by anticancer agents. Biochem Biophys Res Commun 1989;163:1415.
359. McClean S, Hill BT. Evidence of post-translational regulation of P-glycoprotein associated with the expression of a distinctive multiple drug-resistant phenotype in Chinese hamster ovary cells. Eur J Cancer 1993;29A:2243.
360. Bhat UG, Winter MA, Pearce HL, Beck WT. A structure-function relationship among reserpine/yohimbine analogs in their ability to increase expression of MDR1 and P-glycoprotein in a human colon carcinoma cell line. Mol Pharmacol 1995;48:682.
361. Chaudhary PM, Roninson IB. Induction of multidrug resistance in human cells by transient exposure to different chemotherapeutic drugs. JNCI 1993;85:632.
362. Lu T, Beck WT. Rapid induction of *mdr1* expression following ionizing radiation in the human colon carcinoma cell line DLD-1. Proc Am Assoc Cancer Res 1995;36:606.
363. Chin KV, Ueda K, Pastan I, Gottesman MM. Modulation of activity of the promoter of the human MDR1 gene by Ras and p53. Science 1992;255:459.
364. Zastawny RL, Salvino R, Chen J, Benchimol S, Ling V. The core promoter region of the P-glycoprotein gene is sufficient to confer differential responsiveness to wild-type and mutant p53. Oncogene 1993;8:1529.
365. Nguyen KT, Liu B, Ueda K, Gottesman MM, Pastan I, Chin K-V. Transactivation of the human multidrug resistance (MDR1) gene promoter by p53 mutants. Oncol Res 1994;6:71.
366. Stein U, Walther W, Wunderlich V. Point mutations in the mdr1 promoter of human osteosarcomas are associated with *in vivo* responsiveness to multidrug resistance relevant drugs. Eur J Cancer 1994;30:1541.
367. Zhang J-T, Ling V. Membrane orientation of transmembrane segments 11 and 12 of MDR- and non-MDR-associated P-glycoproteins. Biochim Biophys Acta 1993;1153: 191.
368. Buschman E, Gros P. Functional analysis of chimeric genes obtained by exchanging homologous domains of the mouse mdr1 and mdr2 genes. Mol Cell Biol 1991;11:595.
369. Greenberger LM. Major photoaffinity drug labeling sites for iodoaryl azidoprazosin in P-glycoprotein are within, or immediately C-terminal to, transmembrane domains 6 and 12. J Biol Chem 1993;268:11417.
370. Arceci RJ. Clinical significance of P-glycoprotein in multidrug resistance malignancies. Blood 1993;81:2215.
371. List AF, Spier C, Greer J, Wolff S, Hutter J, Dorr R, Salmon S, Futscher B, Baier M, Dalton W. Phase I/II trial of cyclosporine as a chemotherapy-resistance modifier in acute leukemia. J Clin Oncol 1993;11:1652.
372. Raderer M, Scheithauer W. Clinical trials of agents that reverse multidrug resistance. Cancer 1993;72:3553.
373. Lum BL, Fisher GA, Brophy NA, Yahanda AM, Adler KM, Kaubisch S, Halsey J, Sikic BI. Clinical trials of modulation of multidrug resistance. Cancer 1993;72:3502.
374. Ford JM, Hait WN. Pharmacology of drugs that alter multidrug resistance in cancer. Pharmacol Rev 1990;42:155.
375. Tew KD, Houghton PJ, Houghton JA. Modulation of P-glycoprotein-mediated multidrug resistance. In Preclinical and Clinical Modulation of Anticancer Drugs. Edited by KD Tew, PJ Houghton, JH Houghton. Boca Raton FL: CRC, 1993:125.
376. Cole SPC, Bhardwaj G, Gerlach JH, Mackie JE, Grant CE, Almquist KC, Stewart AJ, Kurz EU, Duncan AMV, Deeley RG. Overexpression of a transporter gene in a multidrug-resistant human lung cancer cell line. Science 1992;258:1650.
377. Kruh GD, Chan A, Myers K, Gaughan K, Miki T, Aaronson SA. Expression of complementary DNA library transfer establishes *mrp* as a multidrug resistance gene. Cancer Res 1994;54:1649.
378. Zaman GJR, Flens MJ, van Leusden MR, de Haas M, Mülder HS, Lankelma J, Pinedo HM, Scheper RJ, Baas F, Broxterman HJ, Borst P. The human multidrug resistance-associated protein MRP is a plasma membrane drug-efflux pump. Proc Natl Acad Sci USA 1994;91:8822.
379. Grant CE, Valdimarsson G, Hipfner D, Almquist KC, Cole SPC, Deeley RG. Overexpression of multidrug resistance-associated protein (MRP) increases resistance to natural product drugs. Cancer Res 1994;54:357.
380. Callen DF, Baker E, Simmers RN, Seshadri R, Roninson IB. Localization of the human multiple drug resistance gene, MDR1, to 7q21.1. Hum Genet 1987;77:122.
381. Müller M, Meijer C, Zaman GJR, Borst P, Scheper RJ, Mulder NH, de Vries EGE, Jansen PLM. Overexpression of the gene encoding the multidrug resistance-associated protein results in increased ATP-dependent glutathione S-conjugate transport. Proc Natl Acad Sci USA 1994;91:13033.
382. Flens MJ, Izquierdo MA, Scheffer GL, Fritz JM, Meijer CJLM, Scheper RJ, Zaman G Jr. Immunochemical detection of the multidrug resistance-associated protein MRP in human multidrug-resistant tumor cells by monoclonal antibodies. Cancer Res 1994;54:4557.
383. Schneider E, Cowan KH, Bader H, Toomey S, Schwartz GN, Karp JE, Burke PJ, Kaufmann SH. Increased expression of the multidrug resistance-associated protein gene in relapsed acute leukemia. Blood 1995;85:186.
384. Friche E, Nissen NI, Beck WT. MRP gene expression in heavily chemotherapy treated AML patients. Proc Am Assoc Cancer Res 1995;36:217.
385. Schuurhuis GJ, Broxterman HJ, Ossenkoppele GJ, Baak JPA, Eekman CA, Kuiper CM, Feller N, Heijningen TH Mv, Klumper E, Oieters R, Lankelma J, Pinedo HM. Functional multidrug resistance phenotype associated with combined overexpression of Pgp/MDR1 and MRP together with 1-β-D-arabinofuranosylcytosine sensitivity. clin cancer res 1995;1:81.
386. Beck J, Niethammer D, Gekeler V. High mdr-1- and mrp-, but low topoisomerase ii-gene expression in B-cell chronic lymphocytic leukaemias. Cancer Lett 1994;86:135.
387. Burger H, Nooter K, Zaman GJR, Sonneveld P, Wingerden KE, Oostrum RG, Stoter G. Expression of the multidrug resistance-associated protein (mrp) in acute and chronic leukemias. Leukemia 1994;8:990.
388. Hart SM, Ganeshaguru K, Hoffbrand AV, Prentice HG, Mehta AB. Expression of the multidrug resistance-associated protein (mrp) in acute leukaemia. Leukemia 1994;8: 2162.
389. Sikic BI. Modulation of multidrug resistance: at the threshold. J Clin Oncol 1993;11: 1629.
390. Kaye SB. P-glycoprotein (p-gp) and drug resistance: time for reappraisal? Br J Cancer 1993;67:641.
391. Murren JR, Hait WN. Why haven't we cured multidrug resistant tumors? Oncol Res 1992;4:1.

392. Beck, WT. Do anti-p-glycoprotein antibodies have a future in the circumvention of multidrug resistance? JNCI 1991;83:1364.
393. Beck WT. Circumvention of multidrug resistance with anti-p glycoprotein antibodies: clinical potential or experimental artifact? JNCI 1995;87:73.
394. O'Connor PM, Kohn KW. A fundamental role for cell cycle regulation in the chemosensitivity of cancer cells? Semin Cancer Biol 1992;3:409.
395. Harmon BV, Takano YS, Winterford CM, Potten CS. Cell death induced by vincristine in the intestinal crypts of mice and in a human burkitt's lymphoma cell line. Cell Prolif 1992;25:523.
396. Pastan I, Gottesman MM. Function and regulation of the human multidrug resistance gene. Adv Cancer Res 1993;60:157.
397. Licht T, Pastan I, Gottesman M, Hermann F. P-glycoprotein-mediated multidrug resistance in normal and neoplastic hematopoietic cells. Ann Hematol 1994;69:159.
398. Gottesman MM, Pastan I. Biochemistry of multidrug resistance mediated by the multidrug transporter. Annu Rev Biochem 1993;62:385.
399. Patel NH, Rothenberg ML. Multidrug resistance in cancer chemotherapy. invest. New Drugs 1994;12:1.
400. Nooter K, Sonneveld P. Clinical relevance of p-glycoprotein expression in haematological malignancies. Leuk Res 1994;18:233.
401. Bellamy WT, Dalton WS. Multidrug resistance in the laboratory and clinic. Adv Clin Chem 1994;31:1.
402. Marquet P, Lachatre G, Debord J, Eichler B, Bonnaud R, Nicot G. Pharmacokinetics of vinorelbine in man. Eur J Clin Pharmacol 1992;42:545.
403. Kuttesch JF JR, Parham DM, Luo X, Meyer WH, Bowman L, Shapiro DN, Pappo AS, Crist WM, Beck WT, Houghton PJ. P-glycoprotein expression at diagnosis does not correlate with response or outcome in childhood rhabdomyosarcoma. J Clin Oncol 1996;14:886.
404. Sharom FJ, Yu X, Chu JW, Doige CA. Characterization of the atpase activity of p-glycoprotein from multidrug-resistant chinese hamster ovary cells. Biochem J 1995;308:381.
405. Urbatsch IL, Al-Shawi MK. Senior AE. Characterization of the atpase activity of purified chinese hamster p-glycoprotein. Biochemistry 1994;33:7069.
406. Zhang X, Collins KI, Greenberger LM. Functional evidence that transmembrane 12 and the loop between transmembrane 11 and 12 form part of the drug-binding domain in p-glycoprotein encoded by mdr1. J Biol Chem 1995;270:5441.
407. Friche E, Jensen PB, Nissen NI. Comparison of cyclosporin a and sdz psc833 as multidrug-resistance modulators in a daunorubicin-resistant ehrlich ascites tumor. Cancer Chemother Pharmacol 1992;30:235.
408. Beck WT, Grogan TM, Willman CL, Cordon-Cardo C, Parham DM, Kuttesch JF, Andreeff M, Bates S, Boyett JM, Brophy N, Broxterman HJ, Chan HSL, Dalton WS, Dietel M, Fojo AT, Gascoyne RD, Head D, Houghton PJ, Srivastava DK, Lehnert M, Leith C, Paietta E, Pavelic ZP, Rimzsa L, Roninson IB, Sikic BI, Twentyman PR, Warnke R, Weinstein R. Methods to detect p-glycoprotein-associated multidrug resistance in Patients' Tumors: consensus recommendations. Cancer Res (in press).
409. Izquierdo MA, VD Zee AGJ, Vermorken LB, VD Valk P, Belien JAM, Giaccone G, Scheffer GL, Flens MJ, Pinedo HM, Kenemans P, Meijer CJLM, De Vries EGE, Scheper RJ. Identification of a new drug resistance-associated marker of poor response to chemotherapy and shorter survival in ovarian carcinoma. JNCI 1995;87:1230.
410. List AF, Spier CS, Grogan TM, Johnson C, Roe D, Greer JP, Wolff SN, Broxterman HJ, Scheffer GL, Scheper RJ, Dalton WS. Overexpression of the major vault transporter protein lrp predicts treatment outcome in AML. Clin Cancer Res (in press).
411. Vasu SK, Kedersha NL, Rome LH. CDNA cloning and disruption of the major vault protein alpha gene (MVPA) in *Dictyostelium discoideum*. J Biol Chem 1993;268:15356.
412. Scheffer GL, Wijngaard PLJ, Fiens MJ, Izquierdo MA, Slovak ML, Pinedo HM, Meijer CJLM, Clevers HC, Scheper RJ. The drug resistance related protein LRP is the human major vault protein. Nature Med 1995;1:578.
413. Rome L, Kedersha N, Chugani D. Unlocking vaults: organelles in search of a function. Trends Cell Biol 1991;1:47.
414. Sonnischen DS, Relling MV. Paclitaxel and Docetaxel. Pharmacokinetics and Pharmacodynamics of Anticancer Agents. Edited by LB Grochow, NM Ames. Baltimore: Williams & Wilkins (in press).
415. Jones AL, Smith IE. Navelbine and the anthrapyrazoles. Breast Cancer 1994;8:141.
416. Shepherd DF. Vinorelbine (Navelbine) in the adjuvant and neoadjuvant treatment of non-small cell lung cancer. Semin Oncol 1994;21:64
417. Hohneker JA. A summary of vinorelbine (Navelbine) safety data from North American clinical trials. Semin Oncol 1994;21:42.
418. Wargin WA, Lucas VS. The clinical pharmacokinetics of vinorelbine (Navelbine). Semin Oncol 1994;21:21.
419. Borris HA III, Fields S. Summary of data from in vitro and phase I vinorelbine (Navelbine) studies. Semin Oncol 1994;21:14.

CHAPTER 67

Asparaginase

JOANNE KURTZBERG

Introduction

"Enzymes far exceed man-made catalysts in their reaction specificity, their catalytic efficiency, and their capacity to operate under mild conditions of temperature and hydrogen-ion concentration" (66). As drugs, enzymes also have unique disadvantages. They must be extensively purified to eliminate contaminating toxic materials, such as endotoxins; they are often rapidly degraded in the body; they have limited distribution because of their size; and they are often immunogenic. Despite these problems, L-asparaginase (L-Asp has become an important chemotherapeutic agent in the treatment of acute lymphoblastic leukemia (ALL) and other lymphoid malignancies (21). It has demonstrated effectiveness in induction, as well as in subsequent phases of various multiagent chemotherapeutic regimens. Because L-Asp is generally not myelosuppressive and is not cross-resistant with other antineoplastic agents, it is easily added to combination chemotherapy protocols. Extensive use of L-Asp in children does not appear to be associated with the development of late adverse effects. The major limitation to the use of L-Asp is dose-limiting clinical hypersensitivity, which develops in 3 to 78% of patients treated with native forms of the enzyme (28, 34, 64, 72). Recent technologic advances have enabled pharmacologic studies of L-Asp, which should improve our understanding of treatment failures and allow for the development of more rational dosing schedules in individual patients.

The potential for asparaginase treatment stemmed from the observation of Kidd in 1953, who described an activity in guinea pig sera that caused regression of transplanted lymphomas in mice and rats (49, 50). This cytolytic activity was not present in horse or rabbit serum. Other unrelated developments during this period contributed to the discovery by Broome, in 1961, that the antilymphoma activity in guinea pig sera was due to L-Asp (14). These included the observations that certain experimental neoplasms, Walker carcinosarcoma 256 and L5178 leukemia, were found to require asparagine, an amino acid previously considered nonessential, to support growth in tissue culture (18, 29). Three years later, Mashburn and Wriston showed that L-Asp isolated from *Escherichia coli* (*E. coli*) exhibited antitumor activity similar to that found in guinea pig sera (16, 70). This finding provided a practical source for the production of large quantities of the enzyme for preclinical and clinical investigations (17, 44, 85, 99).

Today, L-Asp utilized in the clinic is available in three preparations, two unmodified or native forms, both purified from bacterial sources, and one form modified from one of the native preparations. The native preparations are derived from *E. coli* (marketed commercially by Merck & Co. as Elspar), or *Erwinia chrysanthemi*. (*Erwinia*), (available as *Erwinia* L-asparaginase from Ogden BioServices Pharmaceutical Repository in the United States) for patients allergic to the *E. coli* product. The *Erwinia* product is commercially available in Canada and Europe as Erwinase marketed by Porton. Both native preparations are approved for use in the therapy of patients in the front line and at relapse. A third preparation, PEG–L-asparaginase (nonproprietary name pegasparaginase), is a chemically modified form of the enzyme in which native *E. coli* L-Asp has been covalently conjugated to monomethoxypolyethylene glycol (PEG). Pegasparaginase (available commercially from Rhone-Poulenc Rorer as Oncaspar) is approved by the Food and Drug Administration (FDA) for use in combination chemotherapy for the treatment of patients with ALL who are hypersensitive to native (unmodified) forms of *E. coli* L-Asp.

Mechanism of Action, Chemistry, and In Vitro Activity

L-Asp catalyzes the hydrolysis of L-asparagine to L-aspartic acid and ammonia, resulting in the depletion of serum L-asparagine. Plasma asparagine is essentially undetectable throughout the entire period in which asparaginase is present. Leukemic lymphoblasts and certain other tumor cells, which lack or have very low levels of L-asparagine synthetase, do not synthesize L-asparagine de novo and rely on L-asparagine supplied in the serum for survival. Early in the development of L-Asp, it was speculated that the enzyme might selectively kill leukemic cells without affecting normal cells that have the ability to synthesize L-asparagine de novo via induction of the enzyme asparagine synthetase. This turned out to be a simplistic paradigm as resistance to the drug emerged, primarily via derepression of the L-asparagine synthetase gene in tumor cells (45, 103). Preclinical and clinical synergies between asparaginase and cytosine arabinoside have been attributed to lowered activity of asparagine synthetase secondary to increased methylation of cytosine residues in the gene encoding this enzyme (74, 90, 106).

L-Asp has been isolated and characterized from various microorganisms, including many gram-negative bacteria,

Table 67.1. Properties of Therapeutic Asparaginases

	E. coli		Erwinia
	Native	PEG	
Activity[a] (IU/mg protein)	280–400	280–400	650–700
K_m (μM)—L-asparaginase	12	12	15
K_m (μM)—L-glutamine	3,000	3,000	1,400
Ratio maximal activity L-Gln/L-Asp	0.03	0.03	0.10
Molecular weight	141,000		138,000
pI	5.0	5.0	8.7
Half-life (days)	0.6–1.0	6.0–7.0	0.5
Duration of asparagine depletion[b]			
In naive patients	7–10 days	14–35 days	5–7 days
In exposed patients[c]	2–3 days	5–14 days	1–2 days
In hypersensitive patients	0 days	1–3 days	0 days

L-Asp, L-Gln, and pI refer to L-asparaginase, L-glutaminase, and isoelectric point respectively.
[a] One international unit hydrolyzes 1 micromole of asparagine per minute.
[b] After a single dose of 25,000 IU/m^2 of native *E. coli* or *Erwinia* or 2,500 U/m^2 of PEG in front-line–naive, asparaginase-exposed, or clinically hypersensitive patients.
[c] Prior therapy with native *E. coli* asparaginase without a history of clinical hypersensitivity.

mycobacteria, yeasts, and molds, as well as from plants and from the plasma of certain vertebrates (104, 105, 107). Not all enzymes have been found to have useful antitumor activity. *E. coli* produces two L-asparaginases, EC-1 and EC-2; however, only the EC-2 enzyme has substantial antitumor activity (16). *Serratia marcescens* and *Vibrio succinogenes* produce L-Asp with activity against lymphomas (32, 98), but resources have never been directed toward the large-scale production of these enzymes to conduct studies in the clinic. Most L-asparaginases (except for the enzyme found in guinea pig serum) can hydrolyze L-glutamine as well as L-asparagine, although the *Km* for L-glutamine is 3 to 9% of that for L-asparagine (71). The toxicity and spectrum of activity differences observed with different preparations of the enzyme may be due, in part, to differences in L-glutaminase activity also contained in these preparations, as L-glutamine depletion can potentially enhance the antitumor activity of the enzyme, while the hydrolysis of L-glutamine, which produces glutamic acid (monosodium glutamate), may contribute to clinical toxicity, especially neurotoxicity.

The purified *E. coli* L-Asp molecule has a molecular weight of 138,000 to 141,000 daltons, and is composed of four identical subunits with an active site on each subunit, while the purified *Erwinia* enzyme has a molecular weight of 138,000 daltons. Both enzymes have high activity and stability and are readily freed from endotoxin. The enzymes from both *E. coli* and *Erwinia* have a low *Km* for L-asparagine and are not inhibited by high concentrations of aspartic acid and ammonia. They differ in isoelectric point and they lack antigenic cross-reactivity. The L-glutaminase activity of *E. coli* and *Erwinia* L-asp is minor compared with L-asparaginase activity with maximal rates of hydrolysis of L-glutamine ranging between 3 and 9% of the activity for L-asparagine. The *Km* for glutamine is 100 times greater than that for asparagine, but high doses of asparaginase will deplete circulating glutamine in animals and patients (71). Guinea pig asparaginase has no glutaminase activity but has never been available in sufficient quantitites for clinical trials. The purification (104) and properties of the *E. coli* and *Erwinia* enzymes have been extensively reviewed and are summarized in Table 67.1 (18, 19, 29, 99, 104).

Preclinical studies in the late 1950s and early 1960s showed that L-Asp was effective against more than 50 murine tumors, including rat and canine lymphosarcomas, rat fibrosarcoma, Walker's carcinosarcoma, and Jensen's sarcoma (19, 101). The majority of susceptible tumors were of lymphoid origin. Laboratory studies have demonstrated that lymphoid tumors of the T-cell lineage are more sensitive to asparaginase-induced cytotoxicity than are those of the B-cell lineage; however this observation has not been formally investigated in clinical trials (29, 52).

CLINICAL HISTORY

L-Asp was first used clinically in 1966 when an 8-year-old boy with multiply relapsed ALL achieved a short, but definite, clinical response following the administration of partially purified guinea pig L-Asp (33). Subsequently, the *E. coli*–derived drug was taken into phase I and II trials in children and adults (18, 27, 30, 39, 42, 46, 73, 75, 78, 92–94, 100). Response rates of 30 to 65% were achieved in patients with relapsed ALL who were treated with L-Asp as a single agent; however, the duration of remission was very short, averaging about 60 days (73). Response rates were generally higher in children than in adults.

L-asp has also been shown to improve event-free survival when used during the intensification/consolidation phases of ALL treatment protocols (28, 31, 72). It has some efficacy in patients with other hematologic malignancies, such as acute myeloid leukemia and non-Hodgkin's lymphoma (27, 65, 67, 95), but indications other than ALL have not been formally investigated. No responses to L-Asp have been reported for patients with nonlymphoid solid tumors. Adults with ALL do not tolerate L-Asp as well as do children, thus limiting enthusiasm for clinical trials in older patients (23, 37, 51, 67, 91, 102).

Because of its low myelosuppressive activity and non–cross-resistance with other antitumor agents, L-Asp was incorporated into combination chemotherapy protocols for the treatment of relapsed patients with ALL in the late 1960s and early 1970s (25, 40, 53, 67, 82, 92, 95). The reinduction rate for children with relapsed ALL ranges from 30 to 75% with the three-drug combination regimen of vincristine, prednisone, and L-Asp but is dependent on the intensity of front-line therapy (25, 53, 92). The addition of an anthracycline (daunomycin, doxorubicin) to vincristine, prednisone, and L-Asp improves the reinduction rate to 80 to 95% for these patients (1, 15, 83). The highest reinduction rates were achieved when PEG–L-asp was the therapeutic asparaginase utilized in the treatment protocol (1).

Shortly after studies in patients with relapsed ALL demonstrated its safety and efficacy for these patients, L-asp, in combination with vincristine, prednisone, with or without an anthracycline, was added to the front-line therapy of patients with ALL in induction. Beginning in the late 1970s, asparaginase intensification was also added to front-line therapy (87). It is now common practice to incorporate L-asp into ALL induction therapy using a variety of doses and dosing schedules, but formal dose-response studies have not been conducted and the optimum dose delivery and schedule have not been defined. This is attributable in large part to the fact that over 90% of children with newly diagnosed ALL achieve remission following combination chemotherapy with vincristine and prednisone, and because of the overall rarity of the disease, it is inherently difficult to conduct a statistically valid study of the efficacy of additional agents in first-remission induction of ALL.

A single dose-response study performed by the Children's Cancer Study Group (CCSG) in 1976 showed that children treated with total cumulative doses of more than 6,000 U/m^2 in induction had a greater probability of achieving a second remission than did children treated with less than 3,000 U/m^2 (34, 87). In humans, native L-Asp preparations are cleared from the plasma with a half-life ($t_{1/2}$) of 18 to 24 hours, making it necessary to administer the enzyme every 2 to 5 days to replenish continuous asparagine depletion. In 1979, Nesbit et al. showed that L-Asp administered intramuscularly (IM) was as effective as the intravenous (IV) route of administration, with reduced anaphylaxis (72). Currently, the preferred route of administration for L-Asp in children with ALL is intramuscular.

In the past 10 years, two randomized trials designed to evaluate the efficacy of intensified L-Asp therapy in the front-line therapy of childhood ALL have been reported. In 1983, Sallan et al. reported the results of a randomized trial in patients newly diagnosed with B-precursor ALL (DFCI 77–01), which demonstrated that patients treated with L-Asp intensification (25,000 IU/m^2 per week for 20 to 30 weeks) in combination with other chemotherapeutic agents significantly improved disease-free and event-free survival as compared with patients treated without L-Asp (87). The results were similar in both high- and low-risk patients with B-precursor disease. The inability to complete the prescribed asparaginase therapy by patients randomized to receive the drug was associated with a higher probability of leukemic relapse. Event-free survival at a median follow-up of 9.3 years was 71 ± 9% for the patients treated with asparaginase compared with 31 ± 11% for those not receiving asparaginase (86). Subsequent nonrandomized trials designed to improve event-free survival in high-risk T and B-lineage patients confirmed the efficacy of multiagent combination chemotherapy protocols that included intensification with L-Asp (28, 88). In 1987, the Pediatric Oncology Group (POG) conducted a randomized trial (POG 8704) designed to evaluate the efficacy of high-dose L-Asp consolidation (25,000 IU a week for 20 weeks) as part of a multiagent chemotherapy regimen in patients newly diagnosed with T-lineage ALL or advanced-stage lymphoblastic lymphoma. In this study as well, patients treated with the L-Asp–containing regimens achieved improved disease-free survival as compared with patients treated without L-Asp (7). Further incorporation of asparaginase intensification into front- and second-line therapy is likely to occur in the near future.

Asparaginase has also been shown to be effective against meningeal leukemia (18, 41). The enzyme can be given intrathecally, but this is usually not needed since asparagine is depleted from the cerebro spinal fluid (CSF) by diffusion into the circulation as a result of the concentration gradient between the plasma and CSF (12, 84).

TOXICITY

L-Asp has a distinct toxicity profile, characterized primarily by immune mediated hypersensitivity reactions and adverse events related to the inhibition of protein synthesis. Toxicities occur with similar frequencies with all commercially available asparaginases, with the exception of decreased allergic reactions with PEG–L-Asp. Unlike many chemotherapeutic agents, L-Asp causes little bone marrow depression, and usually does not affect the gastrointestinal or oral mucosa or hair follicles.

Normal tissues with high rates of protein synthesis (e.g., liver, pancreas, and coagulation system) are most frequently affected by L-Asp therapy. The majority of patients experience some evidence of chemical hepatotoxicity, made manifest by decreases in serum albumin, fibrinogen, and serum lipoprotein levels, and increases in serum liver enzyme levels and bilirubin. Hepatic function usually returns to normal when the drug is cleared or discontinued. Clinical hepatotoxicity is rarely dose limiting. Effects on the coagulation system (hypofibrinogenemia, decreased antithrombin 3, coagulopathy, thromboses) evidenced by imbalances in the formation of clotting factors are common side effects of L-Asp therapy. Despite the high frequency of chemical abnormalities, bleeding episodes or thromboses are infrequently reported and rarely require discontinuation of therapy. L-Asp can adversely affect both the endocrine (insulin-secreting) and exocrine (digestive enzyme–secreting) cells of the pancreas. Some patients develop signs and symptoms of diabetes due to decreased synthesis of insulin. Hyperglycemia may be more severe when L-Asp is administered in combination with prednisone, but the risk can be reduced if L-Asp is administered after the prednisone (79, 93). Up to 15% of L-Asp treated patients experience acute pancreatitis that becomes manifest as anorexia, nausea and vomiting, and abdominal pain (24). Approximately 2 to 5% of children experience life-threatening clinical pancreatitis, which prohibits further exposure to the drug. Ten percent develop transient hyperamylasemia with mild abdominal discomfort that spontaneously resolves over a few days, which is not a dose-limiting complication. Nonspecific gastrointestinal toxicity (nausea, vomiting, and anorexia) is common in older children and adults treated with intensified asparaginase therapy. Neurotoxicity (depression, lethargy, fatigue, somnolence, confusion, irritability, agitation, dizziness) occurs in up to 25% of adult patients treated with L-Asp, (81), but is less common in children. L-Glutamic acid (monosodium glutamate), a product of the L-Asp reaction, has well-established neurotoxicity. Neurotoxicity may also result from a lack of L-asparagine or L-glutamine in the brain. Blood ammonia levels can be quite high during treatment with L-Asp (ammonia is a product of the L-Asp reaction). A relationship between high blood ammonia levels and either liver toxicity or cerebral dysfunction (e.g., encephalopathy) has not been established. Azotemia occurs frequently in patients receiving L-Asp; however, they rarely experience renal failure.

HYPERSENSITIVITY

Very early in the development of L-Asp it became apparent that the dose-limiting toxicity of the enzyme was clinical hypersensitivity. The most common clinical manifestation of hypersensitivity is urticaria; however, the spectrum of allergic reactions ranges from localized erythema at the injection site to systemic anaphylaxis with subsequent death. Risk factors for L-Asp hypersensitivity include doses above 6,000 IU/m^2 a day (46), IV rather than IM administration (72), repeated courses of treatment (96), and single-agent rather than combination chemotherapy (76). The last observation is probably related to the fact that combination therapy produces immunosuppression, which blunts or obliterates an immune response to asparaginase. Grading of clinical hypersensitivity reactions is not necessarily consistent among treating physicians. A suggested classification system is shown in Table 67.2. Reexposure to asparaginase is generally possible after a grade I or II reaction after premedication with antihistamines, however, the clearance of the drug is significantly shortened. An alternative asparaginase preparation should be used in patients experiencing grade III or IV reactions.

Because the onset of a hypersensitivity reaction often requires discontinuation of treatment, alternative forms of L-Asp that are non-cross-reactive with the *E. coli* preparation were investigated in the clinic early in the development of this therapy. Wade et al. were the first to show that L-Asp isolated from *Erwinia chrysanthemi* exhibited antitumor activity equivalent to that produced by *E. coli* (98). *Erwinia* L-Asp was first used in 1970 as an alternative for the *E. coli*–derived enzyme in patients who had developed hypersensitivity during treatment (11), and for many years thereafter *Erwinia* L-Asp was the only alternative L-Asp product available for continuing L-Asp treatment in these patients. However, *Erwinia* L-Asp itself also causes hypersensitivity. The incidence of severe allergic reaction to *Erwinia* L-Asp is about 2% in children who have never been exposed to L-Asp, and increases to about 18 to 23% in children with prior allergy to *E. coli* L-Asp during initial induction therapy (13, 28, 68). With intensification of asparaginase therapy, rates of allergic reactions to *Erwinia* parallel those seen with *E. coli* and increase to as high as 75%. Attempts to intensify asparaginase therapy with repetitive doses of either *E. Coli* or *Erwinia*-derived asparaginases led to clinical hypersensitivity reactions in 25 to 80% of patients. In POG study 8602 (ALinC 14), investigators

Table 67.2. Grading of Asparaginase Hypersensitivity Reactions

Grade 0	No reaction
Grade 1	Mild local reaction (<10 cm, <24 hours)
Grade 2	Urticaria
Grade 3	Bronchospasm, serum sickness, severe local reaction (>10 cm, >24 hours)
Grade 4	Hypotension, anaphylaxis

attempted to test an L-Asp intensification regimen in children with newly diagnosed ALL (64). L-Asp was given during the first 2 weeks of induction therapy and, after a 3-week break, weekly at a dose of 10,000 IU/m^2 for 20 weeks during consolidation. Two percent of patients in induction and 78% of patients during consolidation experienced clinical allergic reactions to *E. coli* L-Asp. The majority of these patients were switched to *Erwinia* L-Asp, but subsequently (after two or more doses) also became allergic to the *Erwinia*-derived preparation. Only 11% of the children entered into the study completed 20 of 24 prescribed asparaginase doses. In contrast, regimens using intensified asparaginase without a break in therapy between induction and consolidation have demonstrated clinical hypersensitivity rates of 20 to 35% (7, 28, 87, 88).

In the mid-1970s, several groups began chemically modifying L-Asp in various ways in an attempt to identify a form of the enzyme that was less immunogenic while retaining good antitumor activity (6, 97). Abuchowski and colleagues had developed a technique for altering the immunogenicity and pharmacokinetics of various proteins by covalently attaching polyethylene glycol (PEG) (2, 4, 5). In 1979, they showed that a PEG conjugate of *E. coli*-derived L-Asp caused tumor regression in transplanted mice with less immunogenicity than the unmodified, native *E. coli* product despite an increased serum *t*1/2 (3, 6). Pegasparaginase was entered into clinical trials in 1984 and has since been administered to more than 1,000 patients with ALL (10, 36, 38, 43, 48, 54–63). The PEG-conjugated enzyme is less immunogenic than either of the available native products and can be administered safely to most patients with allergic reactions to *E. coli* or *Erwinia* L-Asp (35, 62, 80). Furthermore, the longer serum $t_{1/2}$ of pegasparaginase allows for a longer interval between doses (62).

During a phase I dose-escalation study, 31 adult patients with advanced-stage hematologic malignancies received pegasparaginase by IV infusion over 60 minutes (doses ranging from 500 IU/m^2 to 8,000 IU/m^2 every 2 weeks (43, 48). Major toxicities were hypoalbuminemia and hepatic dysfunction. Three patients developed anaphylactic reactions; two of these had a prior history of hypersensitivity to native L-Asp preparations. There was no clear relationship between the dose of pegasparaginase and toxicity; however, the maximum tolerated dose was not reached in this study. Responses were seen in patients with lymphoma and ALL.

In an early multicenter phase II trial, children or young adults with ALL or acute undifferentiated leukemia in bone marrow relapse received a single dose of pegasparaginase in a 14-day up-front therapeutic window prior to standard multiagent induction chemotherapy (36). The 28-day induction regimen included pegasparaginase 2000 IU/m^2 injected IM once every 2 weeks plus IV vincristine and prednisone beginning on day 14 with or without doxorubicin and intrathecal chemotherapy on day 14. All patients had been heavily pretreated with native L-Asp preparations during previous induction therapies, including nine patients who had developed hypersensitivity reactions. The response rate (CR + PR) was 30% on day 14 when pegasparaginase was used as a single agent and 61% on day 35 following the multiagent induction regimen. Mild (grade 2 or lower by NCI Common Toxicity Criteria [CTC]) asp-associated hypersensitivity reactions occurred in one of nine (11%) hypersensitive patients and 5 of 33 (15%) nonhypersensitive patients. The most common nonallergic toxicities were elevated transaminases and coagulation abnormalities. There were no new or unusual L-Asp–related toxicities reported. The results of this study showed that pegasparaginase could be safely administered to patients with and without known hypersensitivity to native L-Asp preparations, and that pegasparaginase was effective when administered every 2 weeks (compared with three times per week for native preparations) during reinduction therapy. PEG-asparaginase also showed activity against cutaneous T-cell malignancies and chronic lymphoblastic leukemia (CLL) in anecdotal patients treated on a concurrent compassionate-use protocol. In the course of clinical development, 33 patients received prolonged therapy with pegasparaginase under maintenance protocols. In the majority of cases, L-Asp was administered intermittently as a single agent at a dose of 2,500 IU/m^2 for up to 2 years. No new or unexpected toxicities were observed after prolonged use of the enzyme.

A randomized trial designed to compare the safety, efficacy, and feasibility of administering pegasparaginase versus native *E. coli* L-Asp as part of a standard induction regimen in children with ALL in second relapse was conducted by the Pediatric Oncology Group (POG 8866) from 1988 to 1992 (54). All 76 patients enrolled in this study had been previously treated with native L-Asp as part of their front-line therapy. Of the 74 evaluable patients, 35 without prior hypersensitivity to L-Asp were randomized to treatment with either pegasparaginase (2,500 IU/m^2 IM every 2 weeks) or native *E. coli* (10,000 IU/m^2 IM three times per week) in combination with a standard 28-day induction regimen of weekly vincristine and daily prednisone. Thirty-nine patients with a history of hypersensitivity were not eligible for randomization and were directly assigned to treatment with pegasparaginase in combination with vincristine and prednisone. The overall CR rate was 40% with no significant differences among the three treatment groups. Two patients, not previously hypersensitive to native asparaginase and randomized to the native *E. coli* arm, experienced severe (CTC grade 3 or higher) hypersensitivity reactions to native L-Asp, were crossed over to pegasparaginase, and subsequently achieved a complete remission. Interestingly, pharmacokinetic studies of one of these patients demonstrated the phenomenon of "silent hypersensitivity" with subtherapeutic serum asparaginase levels during continued dosing with the native drug during the week prior to his clinical allergic reaction (Fig. 67.1). No unexpected serious adverse reactions were seen in the patients treated with pegasparaginase, and, in general, nonallergic L-asp related toxicities were similar among all three treatment groups.

The lack of new or unusual toxicity in the POG 8866 study and other trials in patients with relapsed ALL led to the evaluation of the biweekly dosing schedule of pegasparaginase in patients newly diagnosed with ALL in front-line pilot studies conducted by the Pediatric Oncology Group, Dana Farber Cancer Institute, and the Children's Cancer Group between 1992 and 1994. Increased toxicity, specifically related

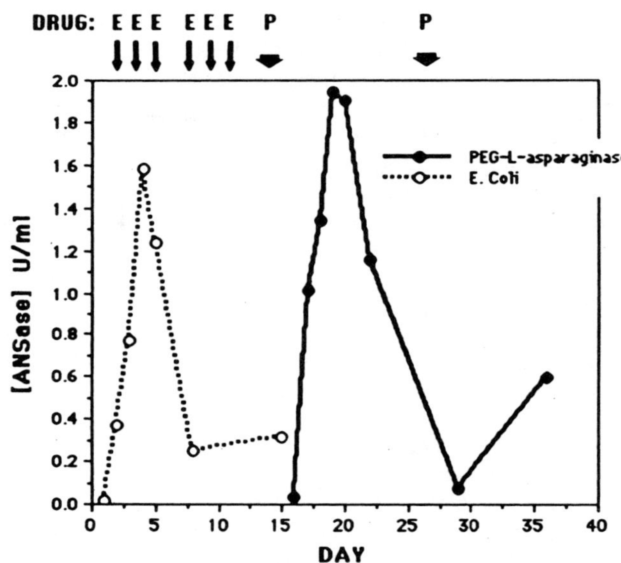

Figure 67.1. Asparaginase pharmacokinetics in ASP-304 patient 1003. Crossover from *E. coli* to PEG–L-asparaginase. Silent hypersensitivity (period during which serum asparaginase levels fell despite continued dosing, indicated by three large arrows) occurred in this relapsed, previously exposed, but non-allergic patient during the second week of dosing with Elspar. The asparaginase was cleared by anti-asparaginase antibodies measurable in the patient's serum after 7 days of therapy. Subsequently (on day 12), the patient experienced a grade III clinical hypersensitivity reaction to Elspar and was switched to pegasparaginase. After PEG dosing, serum asparaginase levels rose appropriately and the patient achieved a complete remission.

to L-asparagine depletion (e.g., pancreatitis, hypoproteinemic syndromes), was observed in this group of L-Asp–naive patients treated with the biweekly dosing schedule. Particularly affected was a subset of patients with high-risk disease on prolonged pegasparaginase therapy in combination with intermediate dose methotrexate, IV 6-mercaptopurine, and IV cytosine arabinoside (56). Despite the increased nonallergic toxicity, fewer hypersensitivity reactions were observed as compared with historic controls who had received native L-Asp preparations as front-line therapy.

As part of a clinical study conducted at Dana Farber Cancer Institute (Study 8701), Asselin et al. prospectively evaluated the in vitro and in vivo efficacy of the three most widely used L-Asp preparations to determine if evidence of an early biologic response could predict long-term outcome (8, 9). Children newly diagnosed with ALL were randomized to receive a single dose of *E. coli* L-Asp, *Erwinia* L-Asp or pegasparaginase on day 0 of a 5-day investigational window prior to the initiation of standard induction chemotherapy. The induction remission regimen included two sequential doses of IV doxorubicin, weekly IV vincristine, a single IV dose of methotrexate (randomized to high dose or standard dose), daily IV prednisone, and two doses of intrathecal cytosine arabinoside. All three types of L-Asp produced equivalent leukemic cell kill in both the in vitro and in vivo assays. These are the first data available demonstrating equivalent efficacy among the three preparations (9). The data also suggested a correlation between in vitro response and the absence of future leukemic relapse. Among the patients classified as nonresponders, 36% had a clinical relapse whereas none of the patients classified as in vitro responders relapsed. Although the sample sizes were too small to demonstrate a statistically significant relationship, the trend suggested that a lack of early response in vitro to L-Asp as a single agent was predictive of a higher risk of relapse. The incidence of acute toxicity due to L-Asp was low in this study and equivalent among the three preparations.

ASPARAGINASE-PHARMACOLOGY

Extensive pharmacologic testing has been conducted as part of the clinical evaluation of pegasparaginase. Because the technology for studying the pharmacology of L-asparaginases was not available when the drug was being developed, this provided an incentive to study the pharmacology of native forms of the enzyme as well.

A pharmacologic assessment of L-Asp was conducted in 27 evaluable patients as part of the phase I study conducted at M.D. Anderson Cancer Center (43, 48). The patients in this study were dosed intravenously. The mean serum $t_{1/2}$ of pegasparaginase was shown to be approximately 15 days. This compared with a mean $t_{1/2}$ of about 24 hours for the unmodified *E. coli* preparation and 10 hours for *Erwinia* L-Asp (48). The rate of total clearance of pegasparaginase was 17-fold lower than that of the unmodified enzyme, while the volume of distribution was similar for the two preparations. Preliminary studies showed that L-asparagine levels were undetectable immediately following the 1-hour infusion of pegasparaginase and remained low during the 14-day interval between doses (43).

Asselin et al. described comparative pharmacokinetics of the three L-Asp preparations (10). Single IM doses of 25,000 IU/m^2 or *E. coli* and *Erwinia* L-Asp were compared with 2,500 IU/m^2 of pegasparaginase in children newly diagnosed with ALL treated using an up front 5-day investigational window of L-Asp therapy. Serum L-Asp levels were monitored for 28 days. The serum half-lives of the three preparations, as well as the duration of L-asparagine depletion following administration of the enzyme, are shown in Table 67.3. The data show that the $t_{1/2}$ of L-Asp is dependent on the enzyme preparation used. The $t_{1/2}$ of *Erwinia* L-Asp was significantly shorter ($p<.001$) while the $t_{1/2}$ of pegasparaginase was significantly longer ($p<.001$) than that of the standard *E. coli* L-Asp preparation. The duration of L-asparagine depletion following administration of the different L-Asp preparations correlated with the serum $t_{1/2}$ of the enzyme (i.e., shortest for the *Erwinia* preparation and longest for pegasparaginase). The L-Asp preparation-dependent pharmacokinetics observed in this study provide important information for establishing an appropriate dosing schedule for L-Asp. The longer $t_{1/2}$ following administration of pegasparaginase affirms the less frequent dosing schedule for this preparation; however, the shortened $t_{1/2}$ of the $t_{1/2}$ of the *Erwinia* preparation as compared with the *E. coli* preparation suggests that the accepted dosing schedule for *Erwinia* L-Asp, which is identical to that for *E. coli* L-Asp, might not be optimal.

Several investigators have shown that patients who develop a hypersensitivity reaction to native L-Asp preparations

Table 67.3. Serum Half-Life ($t_{1/2}$) of Three L-Asparaginase Preparations in Children Newly Diagnosed with ALL

L-Asparaginase preparation	Dose (IU/m^2)	$t_{1/2}$ (days)	L-Asparagine depletion (days)
E coli	25,000	1.28 ± 0.35	7–10
Erwinia	25,000	0.65 ± 0.13	5–7
Pegasparaginase	2,500	5.73 ± 3.24	>28

From Asselin (10 and unpublished data).

Table 67.4. Relationship Between Anti-L-Asparaginase Antibody Level and Clearance of Pegasparaginase

Patient population	Parameter	Antibody titer		*p* value
		Low	High	
Hypersensitive	$t_{1/2}$	4.99	1.43	.002
	AUC	10.52	5.12	.004
Nonhypersensitive	$t_{1/2}$	7.33	3.15	.003
	AUC	11.61	4.14	.002
Total	$t_{1/2}$	7.04	2.38	.001
	AUC	11.26	4.80	.001

AUC, area under the curve.
Modified from Kurtzberg (59).

have a decreased $t_{1/2}$ for the enzyme (18, 60, 67, 77, 89). Asselin et al. showed in their study that patients who had a hypersensitivity reaction to L-Asp also demonstrated a decreased $t_{1/2}$ for pegasparaginase as compared with naive patients (1.82 ± 0.26 days versus 5.73 ± 3.24 days respectively) (60). However, native L-Asp was cleared much faster ($t_{1/2}$ could not be calculated) than pegasparaginase in hypersensitive patients who were dosed with native asparaginase preparations after premedication with antihistamines to ameliorate clinical allergy, suggesting a potential benefit for the polyethyleneglycolated (pegalated) asparaginase.

As part of the POG 8866 study described above, plasma L-Asp levels and anti–L-Asp antibody titers were evaluated in children with ALL in relapse treated with L-Asp (54). The data showed that there was a clear correlation between anti–L-Asp antibody titer and clearance of L-Asp (Table 67.4A and B) (10). More than 50% of the nonallergic patients developed anti–L-Asp antibodies during induction, which resulted in increased clearance of both native and pegasparaginase preparations. In this regard, clearance of native asparaginase was so rapid that levels could not be detected in serum 20 minutes after a dose and produced no asparagine depletion, whereas clearance of PEG-modified asparaginase decreased the $t_{1/2}$ from approximately 6 to 1 to 3 days, still depleting asparagine for 5 to 14 days. Baseline antiasparaginase antibody titers were not predictive of asparaginase clearance, but maximal titer over a 4-week treatment period was predictive. This phenomenon of increased anti–L-Asp antibody formation without clinical evidence of hypersensitivity is called silent hypersensitivity.

An association between high anti–L-Asp levels and decreased rates of remission induction in leukemic patients has been demonstrated in recent studies (26, 60). The data suggest that elevated anti–L-Asp antibody titer in both clinically hypersensitive and nonhypersensitive patients can (by neutralizing L-Asp activity and/or increasing clearance) cause suboptimal L-asparagine depletion and diminished efficacy. In open-label, multicenter, clinical and pharmacokinetic trials (Enzon 305/307), pegasparaginase was incorporated into multiagent remission induction regimens for children with ALL (35). Patients in relapse or remission and those newly diagnosed were included in the study. The initial cohort of hypersensitive patients and all nonhypersensitive patients treated on the study were dosed with pegasparaginase 2,500 IU/m^2 every other week. Pharmacologic parameters (L-Asp and L-asparagine levels and anti–L-Asp antibody titers) were obtained prestudy and on specified days during the treatment period. After analysis of the data from the initial cohort of hypersensitive patients, subsequent hypersensitive patients were treated with weekly doses of pegasparaginase. Hypersensitive patients developed higher levels of anti–L-Asp than either of the other patient groups, and the presence of these antibodies was associated with increased clearance of pegasparaginase.

As shown in Table 67.6, serum L-Asp levels correlated with the duration of L-asparagine depletion in these patient subgroups. In naive patients, 100% (six of six) had continuous L-asparagine depletion for the entire 14-day interval between dosing. This compares with 85% (28 of 33) of previously exposed nonhypersensitive patients. In contrast, only 59% of the hypersensitive patients had L-asparagine depletion for 14 days. For previously exposed, nonhypersensitive and hypersensitive subgroups, respectively, 94% (31 of 33) and 88% (22 of 25) of patients were continuously depleted of L-asparagine for 7 days. Twelve of 13 hypersensitive patients dosed weekly maintained asparagine depletion for 7 days or longer (Table 67.6).

Table 67.5. Relationship Between Anti-L-Asparaginase Antibody Level and L-Asparaginase Level

Pharmacologic parameter	Patient group		
	L-Asp naive	Previously exposed nonhypersensitive	Hypersensitive
L-Asp AUC	11.86 ± 3.4	14.93 ± 1.3	8.13 ± 1.2
Baseline anti–L-Asp level	0.2 ± 0.2	0.4 ± 0.2	1.5 ± 0.2
Highest anti–L-Asp level	0.5 ±	0.68 ± 0.2	1.0 ± 0.3

AUC, area under the curve.

The most common toxicities associated with the use of pegasparaginase in these multiagent chemotherapy regimens were hepatotoxicity and coagulation abnormalities. Hemorrhagic and thrombotic events were not seen. Hypersensitive patients were less likely to experience serious L-Asp–related toxicities than nonhypersensitive or naive patients, probably due to a shorter $t_{1/2}$ for L-Asp and a shorter period of L-asparagine depletion. Hypersensitivity reactions were seen in both hypersensitive and nonhypersensitive patients. The majority of patients hypersensitive to the native drug were successfully treated with pegasparaginase without developing a clinical hypersensitivity reaction.

As part of POG study 9310, the safety, efficacy, and pharmacology of L-Asp were compared in patients randomized to pegasparaginase (2500 IU/m^2) administered weekly versus every 2 weeks in combination with a standard induction regimen in children with relapsed ALL (1). The induction scheme included prednisone, vincristine, doxorubicin, and L-Asp with triple intrathecal therapy (cytosine arabinoside, methotrexate, hydrocortisone). Response data were available for 128 patients. Of these, the overall CR rate was 87% in patients who received pegasparaginase weekly and 82% in patients who received pegasparaginase once every 2 weeks ($P = .02$). Response significantly correlated with mean plasma L-Asp levels ($P = .01$). Hypoalbuminemia (56%) and hypofibrinogenemia (50%) were common nonallergic toxicities. Hypersensitivity (mostly grade 1) occurred in 5% of the patients. The results of this study suggest that pegasparaginase administered weekly may be superior to the enzyme administered once every 2 weeks in relapsed patients, and that plasma L-Asp and anti–L-Asp levels correlate with response rate.

DRUG INTERACTIONS

A series of laboratory and clinical investigations with asparaginase in combination with methotrexate (MTX) and cytosine arabinoside (ara-C) illustrate interactions between these drugs (21). When administered together, inhibition of protein synthesis produced by L-Asp appears to diminish the cytotoxic effect of these antimetabolites. Conversely, the de-

Table 67.6. Number of Patients Demonstrating Continuous L-Asparagine Depletion Following Pegasparaginase Therapy

Dosing schedule	Patient group					
	L-Asp naive		Previously exposed nonhypersensitive		Hypersensitive	
	7 days	14 days	7 days	14 days	7 days	14 days
Every other week (every 14 days)	6/6 (100%)	6/6 (100%)	31/33 (94%)	28/33 (85%)	22/25 (88%)	9/17 (57%)
Weekly (every 7 days)	NA	NA	NA	NA	12/13 (92%)	NA

NA = not applicable
From Kurtzberg J, Asselin B. Unpublished data.

layed administration of asparaginase following the administration of either of these drugs results in pharmacologic synergy. These schedule and time-dependent effects between a preceding dose of asparaginase and a subsequent dose of MTX appear to be related to an asparaginase effect on MTX polyglutamylation (48), a biochemical effect linked to the cellular retention of MTX and its ultimate cytotoxic effect. Clinical studies have shown that administering L-Asp 9 to 10 days before methotrexate enhanced the antitumor activity of methotrexate with reduced gastrointestinal and hematologic toxicity (22, 69, 106). Schedule-dependent synergy associated with high-dose cytosine arabinoside and L-Asp has also been observed, suggesting the capacity of asparaginase to improve the therapeutic index for high dose ara-C in patients with acute myeloid leukemia (20).

Conclusions

In summary, L-asparaginase is an important drug in the treatment of patients with lymphoid malignancies. It does not appear to cause late effects and is not myelosuppressive, rendering it an ideal agent for combination chemotherapy regimens for children with leukemia. Recent technologic advances have enabled detailed pharmacokinetic and pharmacodynamic studies of various asparaginase preparations. Taken together, these data indicate that pharmacokinetic and pharmacodynamic factors have a considerable impact on the efficacy of L-Asp therapy, and that defining the optimum dose and dosing schedule of the different asparaginase preparations that are used in the clinic will require an evaluation of pharmacologic end points, at least in patients who were previously treated with L-Asp. The message from these studies suggests that a pharmacologically guided, individualized approach to L-Asp therapy might achieve the best therapeutic outcome. These types of studies, it is hoped, will become the focus of future asparaginase-based treatment protocols.

References

1. Abshire T, Pollock B, Billett A, Bradley P, Buchanan G. Weekly polyethylene glycol conjugated (PEG) L-asparaginase (ASP) produces superior induction remission rates in childhood relapsed acute lymphoblastic leukemia (rALL): a Pediatric Oncology Group (POG) study 9310. Proc Am Soc Clin Oncol 1995;14:344.
2. Abuchowski A, Davis F, Davis S. Immunosuppressive properties and circulating life of Achromobacter glutaminase-asparaginase covalently attached to polyethylene glycol in man. Cancer Treat Rep 1981;65:1077–1091.
3. Abuchowski A, Kazo G, Verhoest C, et al. Cancer therapy with chemical modified enzymes. I. Antitumor properties of polyethylene glycol-asparaginase conjugates. Cancer Biochem Biophys 1984;7:175–186.
4. Abuchowski A, McCoy J, Palczuk N, van Es T, Davis F. Effect of covalent attachment of polyethylene glycol on immunogenicity and circulation life of bovine liver catalase. J Biol Chem 1977;252:3582–3586.
5. Abuchowski A, van Es T, Palczuk N, Davis F. Alteration of immunological properties of bovine serum albumin by covalent attachment of polyethylene glycol. J Biol Chem 1977;252:3578–3581.
6. Abuchowski A, van Es T, Palczuk N, McCoy J, Davis F. Treatment of L5178Y tumor-bearing BDF_1 mice with a nonimmunogenic L-glutaminase–L-asparaginase. Cancer Treat Rep 1979;67:1127–1132.
7. Amylon M, Caroll A, Link M, Katz J, JJS. Second malignancies in children treated with teniposide (VM-26) for T-cell lymphoid malignancy: a role for asparaginase? (a Pediatric Oncology Group (POG) study). Blood 1992;80:206a.
8. Asselin B, Kreissman S, Coppola D, et al. Efficacy, toxicity and implications of a single dose of asparaginase administered to naive patients prior to multiagent chemotherapy for remission induction of childhood acute lymphoblastic leukemia. In preparation.
9. Asselin B, Ryan D, Frantz C, et al. In vitro and in vivo killing of acute lymphoblastic leukemia cells by L-asparaginase. Cancer Res 1989;49:4363–4368.
10. Asselin B, Whitin J, Coppola D, Rupp I, Sallan S, Cohen H. Comparative pharmacokinetic studies of three asparaginase preparations. J Clin Oncol 1993;11: 1780–1786.
11. Beard M, Crowther D, Galton D, et al. L-Asparaginase in treatment of acute leukemia and lymphosarcoma. Br Med J 1970;1:191–195.
12. Berg S, Balis F, McCully C, Godwin K, Poplack D. Pharmacokinetics of PEG-L-asparaginase and plasma and cerebrospinal fluid L-asparagine concentrations in the rhesus monkey. Cancer Chemother Pharmacol 1993;32:310–314.
13. Billett A, Carls A, Gelber R, Sallan S. Allergic reactions to *Erwinia* asparaginase in children with acute lymphoblastic leukemia who had previous allergic reactions to *Escherichia coli* asparaginase. Cancer 1992;70:201–206.
14. Broome J. Evidence that the L-asparaginase activity of guinea pig serum is responsible for its antilymphoma effects. Nature 1961;191:1114–1115.
15. Buchanan G, Boyett J, Rivera G. Reinduction therapy in 273 children with acute lymphoblastic leukemia (ALL) in first bone marrow (BM) relapse: a Pediatric Oncology Group Study. Proc Am Soc Clin Oncol 1987;6:146.
16. Campbell H, Mashburn L. L-Asparaginase EC-2 from *Escherichia coli.* Some substrate specificity characteristics. Biochemistry 1969;9:3768–3775.
17. Campbell H, Mashburn L, Boyse E, Old L. Two L-asparaginases from E. coli B, their separation, purification and antitumor activity. Biochem Genet 1967;6:721–730.
18. Capizzi R, Bertino J, Skeel R, et al. L-Asparaginase: clinical, biochemical, pharmacological and immunological studies. Ann Intern Med 1971;74:893–901.
19. Capizzi R, Cheng Y-C. Therapy of neoplasia with asparaginase. In Enzymes as Drugs. Edited by J Holcenberg, J Roberts. New York: Wiley, 1981, pp 1–24.
20. Capizzi R, Davis R, Powell B, et al. Synergy between high-dose cytarabine and asparaginase in the treatment of adults with refractory and relapsed acute myelogenous leukemia—a Cancer and Leukemia Group B study. J Clin Oncol 1988;6: 499–507.
21. Capizzi R, JSH. Asparaginase. In Cancer Medicine. Edited by J Holland, E Fries. Philadelphia: Lea & Febiger, 1993, pp 796–805.
22. Capizzi R, Keiser L, Sartorelli A. Combination chemotherapy—Theory and practice. Semin Oncol 1977;4:227–253.
23. Capizzi R, Poole M, Cooper M. Treatment of poor risk acute leukemia with sequential high-dose ara-C and asparaginase. Blood 1984;63:694–700.
24. Chabner B. Enzyme therapy. L-asparaginase. In Cancer Chemotherapy: Principles and Practice. Edited by B Chabner, J Collins. Philadelphia: Lippincott, 1990, pp 397–407.
25. Chesselis J, Cornbleet M. Combination chemotherapy for bone marrow relapse in childhood lymphoblastic leukemia. Med Pediatr Oncol 1979;6:359–365.
26. Cheung N, Chau I, Coccia P. Antibody response to *Escherichia coli.* L-asparaginase. Prognostic significance and clinical utility of antibody measurement. Am J Pediatr Hematol Oncol 1986;8:99–104.
27. Clarkson B, Krakoff I, Burchenal J, et al. Clinical results of treatment with *E. coli.* L-asparaginase in adults with leukemia, lymphoma, and solid tumors. Cancer 1970;25: 279–305.
28. Clavell L, Gelber R, Cohen H, et al. Four agent induction and intensive asparaginase therapy for treatment of childhood acute lymphoblastic leukemia. N Engl J Med 1986;315:657–663.
29. Cooney D, Handschumacher R. L-asparaginase and L-asparagine metabolism. Ann Rev Pharmacol 1970;10:421–440.
30. Crowther D. L-asparaginase and human malignant disease. Nature 1971;229:168.
31. Desai S, Barr R, Andrew M, deVeber L, Pai M. Management of Ontario children with acute lymphoblastic leukemia by the Dana-Farber Cancer Institute protocols. Can Med Assoc J 1989;141:693–697.
32. Distasio J, Niedeman R, Kafkewitz D, Goodman D. Purification and characterization of L-asparaginase with anti-lymphoma activity from Vibrio succinogenes. J Biol Chem 1976;251:6929–6932.
33. Dolowy W, Henson D, Cornet J, Sellin H. Toxic and antineoplastic effects of L-asparaginase. Cancer 1966;19:1813–1819.
34. Ertel I, Nesbit M, Hammond D, Weiner J, Sather H. Effective dose of L-asparaginase for induction of remission in previously treated children with acute lymphocytic leukemia: a report from Childrens Cancer Study Group. Cancer Res 1979;39: 3893–3896.
35. Ettinger L, Asselin B, Poplack D, Kurtzberg J. Toxicity profile of PEG–L-asparaginase in native L-asparaginase-hypersensitive and non-hypersensitive patients (pts) with acute lymphoblastic leukemia (ALL). International Society of Pediatric Oncology (SIOP) 25th Meeting, 1993.
36. Ettinger L, Kurtzberg J, Voute P, Jurgens H, Halpern S. Open-label, multicenter study of PEG–L-asparaginase for the treatment of acute lymphoblastic leukemia. Cancer 1995 (in press).
37. Gahrton G, Engstedt L, Franzen S, et al. Induction of remission with L-asparaginase, cyclophosphamide, cytosine arabinoside, and prednisolone in adult patients with acute leukemia. Cancer 1974;34:472–479.
38. Graham M, Chaffee S, Stewart A. Feasibility of consolidation therapy with PEG–L-asparaginase after bone marrow transplant for acute lymphoblastic leukemia in second or subsequent remission. Proc Am Soc Clin Oncol 1993;12:324.
39. Haskell C, Canellos G, Leventhal B, Carbone P, Block J. L-Asparaginase therapeutic and toxic effects in patients with neoplastic disease. N Engl J Med 1969;2810:2578.
40. Herson J, Starling K, Dyment P, Humphrey G, Pullen J, Vats T. Vincristine and prednisone vs vincristine, L-asparaginase, and prednisone for second remission induction of acute lymphocytic leukemia in children. Med Pediatr Oncol 1979;6:317–323.
41. Hill J, Loeb E, MacLellan A, et al. Responses to highly purified L-asparaginase during therapy of acute leukemia. Cancer Res 1969;29:1573.
42. Hill J, Roberts J, Loeb E, Khan A, MacLellan A, Hill R. L-Asparaginase therapy for leukemia and other malignant neoplasms. JAMA 1967;202:882–888.
43. Ho D, Brown N, Yen A. Clinical pharmacology of polyethylene glycol–L-asparaginase. Drug Metab Dispos 1986;14:349–352.
44. Ho D, Thetford B, Carter C, Frei E. Clinical pharmacologic studies of L-asparaginase. Clin Pharmacol Therapeut 1970;11:408–417.
45. Ho D, Whitecar J, Luce J, Frei E. L-Asparagine requirement and the effect of L-asparaginase on the normal and leukemic human bone marrow. Cancer Res 1970;30: 466–472.
46. Jaffe N, Traggis D, Das L, et al. Favorable remission induction rate with twice week doses of L-asparaginase. Cancer Res 1971;33:1–4.
47. Jolivet J, Cole D, Holcenberg J, Poplack D. Prevention of methotrexate cytotoxicity by asparaginase inhibition of methotrexate polyglutamate formation. Cancer Res 1985;45:217.

48. Keating M, Holmes R, Lerner S, Ho D. L-asparaginase and PEG asparaginase—past, present, and future. Leukemia Lymphoma 1993;10:153–157.
49. Kidd J. Regression of transplanted lymphomas induced in vivo by means of normal guinea pig serum. I. Course of transplanted cancers of various kinds in mice and rats given guinea pig serum, horse serum, or rabbit serum. J Exp Med 1953;98:565–582.
50. Kidd J. Regression of transplanted lymphomas induced in vivo by means of normal guinea pig serum. II. Studies on the nature of the active serum constituent; histological mechanism of the regression; tests for effects of guinea pig serum on lymphoma cells, in vitro discussion. J Exp Med 1953;98:583–606.
51. Killander D, Dohlwitz A, Engstedt L. Hypersensitive reactions and antibody formation during L-asparaginase treatment of children and adults with acute leukemia. Cancer 1976;37:220–228.
52. Koishi T, Minowada J, Henderson E, Ohnuma T. Distinctive sensitivity of some T-leukemia cell lines to L-asparaginase. Gann 1984;75:275–283.
53. Kung F, Nyhan W, Cuttner J, et al. Vincristine, prednisone and L-asparaginase in the induction of remission in children with acute lymphoblastic leukemia following relapse. Cancer 1978;41:428–434.
54. Kurtzberg J. International multicenter study of PEG–L-asparaginase for reinduction therapy for children with acute lymphoblastic leukemia. Blood 1992;80:206a.
55. Kurtzberg J. A new look at PEG–L-asparaginase and other asparaginases in hematological malignancies. Chemotherapy Foundation Symposium XI Innovative Cancer Chemotherapy for Tomorrow. Cancer Invest 1993;12:59–60.
56. Kurtzberg J. Pediatric Oncology Group Protocol 9406, unpublished.
57. Kurtzberg J, Asselin B, Berg S, Graham M, Balis F, Poplack D. Pharmacokinetics of PEG–L-asparaginase in pediatric patients with known hypersensitivity to native L-asparaginase. Proc Am Assoc Cancer Res 1992;33:210.
58. Kurtzberg J, Asselin B, Graham M, Fisherman J, Sallan S, Poplack D. L-Asparaginase therapy in the 90's: new insights into pharmacology should guide future applications. Proc Am Soc Pediatr Hematol Oncol 1993;2:18–19.
59. Kurtzberg J, Asselin B, Pollack B, Bernstein M, Buchanan G. PEG–L-asparaginase vs. native *E. coli*. Asparaginase for reinduction of relapsed acute lymphoblastic leukemia (ALL): POG #8866 phase II trial. Proc Am Soc Clin Oncol 1993;12:325.
60. Kurtzberg J, Asselin B, Poplack D, et al. PEG–L-asparaginase (PEG-ASP) pharmacology in pediatric patients with acute lymphoblastic leukemia (ALL). Proc Am Soc Clin Oncol 1994;13:114.
61. Kurtzberg J, Asselin B, Poplack D, et al. Antibodies to asparaginase alter pharmacokinetics and decrease anzyme activity in patients on asparaginase therapy. Proc Am Assoc Cancer Res 1993;34:304.
62. Kurtzberg J, Friedman H, Asselin B, et al. The use of polyethylene glycol-conjugated L-asparaginase (PEG-Asp) in pediatric patients with prior hypersensitivity to native L-asparaginase. Proc Am Soc Clin Oncol 1990;9:219.
63. Kurtzberg J, Moore J, Scudiery D, Franklin A. A phase II study of polyethylene glycol (PEG) conjugated L-asparaginase in patients with refractory acute leukemias. Proc Am Assoc Cancer Res 1988;29:213.
64. Land V, Schuster J, Pullen J, et al. Proc Am Soc Clin Oncol 1989;8:215.
65. Land V, Sutow W, Dyment P. Remission induction with L-asparaginase, vincristine, and prednisone in children with acute nonlymphoblastic leukemia. Med Pediatr Oncol 1976;2:191–198.
66. Lehinger A. The molecular logic of living organisms. Biochemistry 1970;8–13.
67. Leventhal B, Henderson E. Therapy of acute leukemia with drug combinations which include asparaginase Cancer 1971;28:825–829.
68. Liu Y-P, Chabner B. Enzyme therapy: L-asparaginase. In Pharmacologic Principles of Cancer Treatment. Edited by B Chabner. Philadelphia: Saunders, 1982, p 435.
69. Lobel J, O'Brien R, McIntosh S, Aspnes G, Capizzi R. Methotrexate and asparaginase combination chemotherapy in refractory acute lymphoblastic leukemia of childhood. Cancer 1979;43:1089–1094.
70. Mashburn L, Wriston J. Tumor inhibitory effect of L-asparaginase from Escherichia coli. Arch Biochem Biophys 1964;105:451.
71. Miller H, Slaser J, Balis M. Amino acid levels following L-asparaginase amidohydrolase (EC.3.5.1.1.) therapy. Cancer Res 1969;29:183–187.
72. Nesbit M, Chard R, Evans A, Karon M, Hammond G. Evaluation of intramuscular versus intravenous administration of L-asparaginase in childhood leukemia. Am J Pediatr Hematol Oncol 1979;1:9–13.
73. Nesbit M, Ertel I, Hammond G. L-asparaginase as a single agent in acute lymphocytic leukemia: survey of studies from Childrens Cancer Study Group. Cancer Treatment Reports 1981;65(suppl 4):101–107.
74. Nyce J. Drug-induced DNA hypermethylation and drug resistance in human tumors. Cancer Res 1989;49:5829.
75. Oettgen H, Old L, Boyse E, et al. Inhibition of leukemia in man by L-asparaginase. Cancer Res 1967;27:2619–2631.
76. Oettgen H, Stephenson P, Schwartz M, et al. Toxicity of *E. coli* L-asparaginase in man. Cancer 1979;25:253–278.
77. Ohnuma T, Holland J, Freeman A, Sinks L. Biochemical and pharmacological studies with asparaginase in man. Cancer Res 1970;30:2297–2304.
78. Ohnuma T, Rosner F, Levy R, et al. Treatment of adult leukemia with L-asparaginase (NSC-109229). Cancer Chemother Rep 1971;55:269.
79. Ortega J, Nesbit M, MH D, et al. L-Asparaginase vincristine and prednisone for induction of first remission in acute lymphocytic leukemia. Cancer Res 1977;37:535–540.
80. Park Y, Abuchowski A, Davis S. Pharmacology of *Escherichia coli*–L-asparaginase polyethylene glycol adduct. Anticancer Res 1981;1:373–375.
81. Pochedly C. Neurotoxicity due to CNS therapy for leukemia. Med Pediatr Oncol 1972;3:101–115.
82. Rausen A, Glidewell O, Holland J, et al. Superiority of L-asparaginase combination chemotherapy in advanced acute lymphocytic leukemia of childhood. Cancer Clin Trials 1979;1:137–144.
83. Reaman G, Ladisch S, Echelberger, Poplack D. Improved treatment results in the management of single and multiple relapses of acute lymphoblastic leukemia. Cancer 1980;45:3090–3094.
84. Riccardi R, Holcenberg J, Glaubiger D, Wood J, Poplack D. L-Asparaginase pharmacokinetics and asparagine levels in cerebrospinal fluid of Rhesus monkeys and humans. Cancer Res 1981;41:4554.
85. Roberts J, Prager M, Bachynsky N. The antitumor activity of *Escherichia coli* L-asparaginase. Cancer Res 1966;26:2213–2217.
86. Sallan S, Gelber R, Kimball V, Donnelly M, Cohen H. More is better! Update of Dana-Farber Cancer Institute/Children's Hospital childhood acute lymphoblastic leukemia trials. Haematol Blood Transfusion 1990;33:459–466.
87. Sallan S, Hitchcock-Bryan S, Gelber R, Cassady J, Frei E, Nathan D. Influence of intensive asparaginase in the treatment of childhood non–T-cell acute lymphoblastic leukemia. Cancer Res 1983;43:5601–5607.
88. Schorin M, Blattner S, Gelber R, et al. Treatment of childhood acute lymphoblastic leukemia: results of Dana-Farber Institute children's hospital acute lymphoblastic leukemia consortium protocol. J Clin Oncol 1994;12:740–747.
89. Schwartz M, Lash E, Oettgen H, Tomao F. L-Asparaginase activity in plasma and other biological fluids. Cancer 1970;25:244–252.
90. Schwartz S, Morgenstern B, Capizzi R. Schedule dependent synergy and antagonism between high-dose 1—D-arabinofuranosylcytosine and asparaginase in the L5178Y murine leukemia. Cancer Res 1982;42:2191.
91. Shetty P, Kurkure P, Dasgupta A. Intermediate dose methotrexate and sequential L-asparaginase for treatment of refractory acute lymphocytic leukemia. Indian J Cancer 1984;21:46–49.
92. Sutow W, Garcia F, Starling K, Williams T, Lane D, Gehan E. L-Asparaginase therapy in children with advanced leukemia. Cancer 1971;28:819–824.
93. Sutow W, George S, Lowman J, et al. Evaluation of dose and schedule of L-asparaginase in multidrug therapy of childhood leukemia. Med Pediatr Oncol 1976;2:387–395.
94. Tallal L, Tan C, Oettgen H, et al. *E. coli* L-asparaginase in the treatment of leukemia and solid tumors in 131 children. Cancer 1970;25:306–320.
95. Tan C, Haghbin M, Gee T, Clarkson B, Murphy M. Combination therapy involving L-asparaginase in acute leukemia. Bibl Haematol 1973;39:1074–1084.
96. Trueworthy R, Sutow W, Pullen J. Repeated use of L-asparaginase in multidrug therapy of childhood leukemia. Med Pediatr Oncol 1978;4:91–97.
97. Uren J, Ragin R. Improvement in the therapeutic, immunological, and clearance properties of *Escherichia coli* and *Erwinia carotovora*. L-asparaginases by attachment of poly-DL-alanyl peptides. Cancer Res 1979;39:1927–1933.
98. Wade H, Elsworth R, Herbert D, Keppie J, Sargeant K. A new L-asparaginase with antitumor activity. Lancet 1968;2:776–777.
99. Whelan H, Wriston H. Purification and properties of asparaginase from *Escherichia coli* B. Biochemistry 1969;8:2386–2393.
100. Whitecar JJ, Bodey G, Harris J, Freireich E. Current concepts: L-asparaginase. N Engl J Med 1969;282:732.
101. Winston JJ, Yellin T. L-asparaginase: a review. Adv Enzymol 1973;39:185–248.
102. Woodruff R, Lister T, Paxton A. Combination chemotherapy for haematological relapse in adult acute lymphoblastic leukemia (ALL). Am J Hematol 1978;4:173–177.
103. Worton K, Kerbel R, Andrulis I. Hypomethylation and reactivation of the asparagine synthetase gene induced by L-asparaginase and ethyl methanesulfonate. Cancer Res 1991;51:985–989.
104. Wriston JJ. Asparaginase. Methods Enzymol 1985;113:608–618.
105. Wriston JJ, Yellin T. L-asparaginase: a review. Adv Enzymol 1973;39:185–200.
106. Yap B, McCredie K, Benjamin R, Bodey G, Freireich E. Refractory acute leukemia in adults treated with sequential collaspase and high-dose methotrexate. Br Med J 1978;2:791–793.
107. Yurel E, Peru D, Wriston JJ. On the distribution of plasma L-asparaginase. Experientia 1983;39:383–385.

CHAPTER 68

Antitumor Activity of Polyanions

CHARLES MYERS

Introduction

Interest in polyanions as possible antineoplastic agents has recently been stimulated by studies which indicate that suramin has antitumor activity both in vitro and in vivo. These are not new drugs, however, and their history is tied to the development of modern pharmacology and modern concepts of drug development. In the first decade of this century, Paul Ehrlich conducted a series of investigations which led to the idea that a drug's specificity is the result of a match between its three-dimensional structure and that of its cellular receptor (20). During that same time period, he also played a major role in the development of the concepts of drug screening and preclinical drug development. These twin developments paved the way for the modern concept of drug efficacy, which involves minimizing toxicity while maximizing therapeutic activity. When Ehrlich initiated his program to test dyes for therapeutic activity, one of the targets he selected was trypanosomiasis. By 1904, he had identified the sulfonated cotton dye, trypan red, as an agent with considerable activity. The major disadvantage of trypan red was that it stained the mice an intense red. This observation triggered an extensive search for a better compound, and by 1908, trypan blue had emerged as a second agent with worthwhile activity. However, this agent stained mice blue. The focus then shifted to finding related structures that were colorless but that preserved the antitrypanosomal activity of these two dyes.

Bayer & Co. screened in excess of 1,000 structures for antitrypanosomal activity before coming upon suramin in 1917, some two years after Dr. Ehrlich's death (19). The sequence of structures leading to the synthesis of suramin is shown in Figure 68.1. Since that time, it has been estimated that more than 2,500 additional structural variations have been synthesized without the emergence of an analog superior to suramin in the treatment of trypanosomiasis.

The activity of suramin in trypanosomiasis immediately triggered a wide range of interest in other potential therapeutic uses of sulfonated dyes and other polyanions that has been ably reviewed by Regelson (77, 78). Between 1908 and 1924, both sulfonated dyes and naturally occurring polysulfated polymers such as the glycosaminoglycan chondroitin sulfate, were tested for antitumor activity. Unfortunately, the results were inconsistent; and there followed a waning of interest in the antitumor activity of these compounds. However, there continued to be scattered observations of antitumor potential of polyanionic compounds, such as the demonstration in 1937 by Peters that suramin had activity in murine lymphosarcoma (77, 78). In the late 1960's, interest in polyanions was renewed and advances in animal tumor models allowed for more comprehensive preclinical evaluation (77, 78). Several compounds elicited interest, including dextran sulfate, heparinoids of various types, and pyran copolymer among others. While none of these survived to become clinically useful anticancer drugs, perhaps some reevaluation of their activity may be in order given the advances in supportive care and clinical pharmacology which have made suramin administration possible.

Mechanism of Action

NATURALLY OCCURRING POLYANIONS REGULATING CELL GROWTH AND DIFFERENTIATION

The antitumor activity of suramin and other polyanionic drugs is best understood by considering first the naturally occurring polyanions that control cell growth and differentiation. The most prominent of these are the heparan sulfate proteoglycans, a diverse family of anionic macromolecules involved in the regulation of cell growth and differentiation (15, 31, 45, 51, 55, 56, 80, 92, 93).

Proteoglycans consist of a core protein to which glycosaminoglycan chains are covalently linked. In broad terms, the core proteins have importance for intracellular trafficking and the localization of the mature proteoglycan, while the glycosaminoglycan chains, being anionic and hydrophilic, are frequently involved in interactions with a variety of proteins, including enzymes, growth factors, and components of the extracellular matrix.

The sulfated polysaccharide chains of heparan sulfate consist almost entirely of alternating *N*-acetylglucosamine and uronic acid moieties (glucuronic and iduronic acid). During biosynthesis, a number of chemical and configurational modifications are imposed on these units, leading to a wide range of potential structures. Importantly, rather than being modified at random, the mature glycosaminoglycan chains have been shown to exist as ordered polymeric structures with regions of high and low sulfation along the chain. A schematic representation of the formation of these domains is shown in Figure 68.2.

The regions of most extensive modification have been identified as being involved in many of the biologic activities of heparan sulfates. It is clear that remarkable specificity in structure-activity relationships can occur. An example of

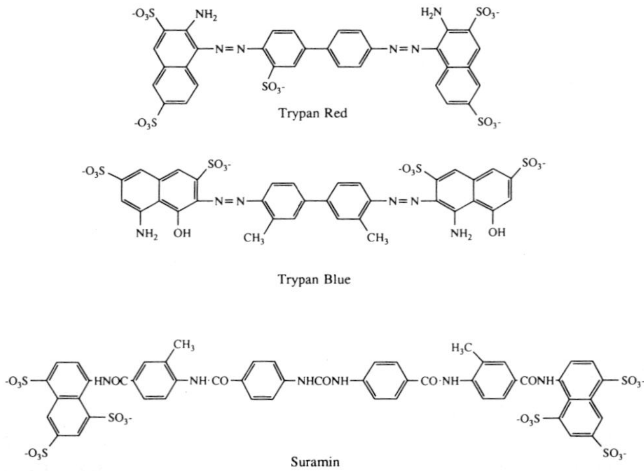

Trypan Red

Trypan Blue

Suramin

Figure 68.1. The development of suramin. Trypan red was the first in a series of dyes active against trypanosomiasis. This was followed by the development of trypan blue and, finally, suramin. A major theme common to all three compounds is the presence of sulfonic acid groups.

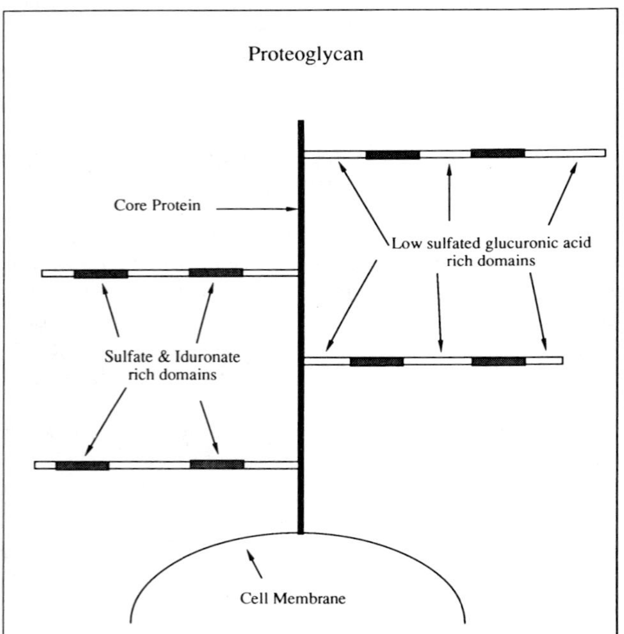

Figure 68.2. Structure of heparan sulfate-containing proteoglycans. The core protein is anchored to the cell membrane. The heparan sulfate chains are attached to the core protein at various points along the protein chain. Within the heparan sulfate chains, there are regions rich in both sulfate and iduronate separated by regions low in sulfate and rich in glucuronic acid. Most of the biologic activity of the heparan sulfates appears to arise from the highly sulfated regions.

ANTIANGIOGENIC PENTASACCHARIDE

ANTITHROMBIN III BINDING PENTASACCHARIDE

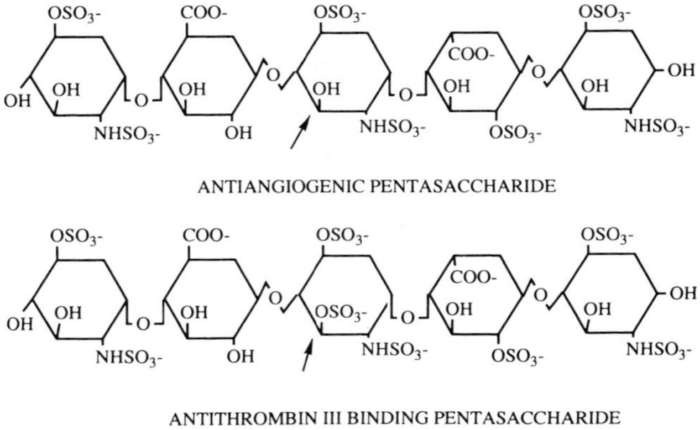

Figure 68.3. Heparan sulfate structure determines biologic activity. The pentasaccharide sequence shown at the top has been reported to inhibit angiogenesis but does not alter coagulation. The lower pentasaccharide shows high affinity for antithrombin III. The *arrows* show the only site where these two pentasaccharides differ.

such specificity may be seen by comparing a pentasaccharide sequence which has little anticoagulant action but exhibits antiangiogenic activity to a similar pentasaccharide sequence that has anticoagulant activity by its ability to interact with antithrombin III (Fig. 68.3) (3, 5, 11, 12, 25, 33, 67, 72, 73, 82, 100).

Heparan sulfate and heparin contain the same disaccharide repeat structure of *N*-acetylglucosamine and uronic acid but differ in the extent of *N*-sulfation, with heparan sulfates typically exhibiting 45 to 55% *N*-sulfation compared with over 80% for heparin. Both polymers may contain similar functional domains such as illustrated in Figure 68.3 and have similar biologic effects (Table 68.1). For example, the antithrombin III–binding sequence shown in Figure 68.3 represents approximately 10% of heparin but can also be found in many heparan sulfate preparations. Thus, while the two families of polymers may be distinguished based on degree of sulfation, they can have similar effects when added to biologic systems and are often used interchangeably.

The binding of anionic polysaccharide chains to proteins typically involves the interaction between negatively charged groups on the carbohydrate and positively charged amino acids in the protein ligand. Sequences of amino acids that have affinity for heterogeneous populations of heparan sulfate or heparin have been identified for a number of proteins. Figure 68.4 shows one such amino acid sequence identified in basic fibroblast growth factor, an important mitogen for endothelial cells (4, 24). However, the structural features of the binding of glycosaminoglycan oligosaccharides have yet to be characterized in many instances because of the lack of any simple, widely available means for the sequence determination of sulfated oligosaccharides.

A detailed consideration of the biology of heparan sulfates (Table 68.1) is beyond the scope of this chapter, and the reader is referred to several recent comprehensive reviews on the subject (15, 31, 45, 51, 55, 56, 80, 92, 93). We confine ourselves here to some of the growth regulatory effects of these molecules that have particular bearing on the observed antiproliferative activity of suramin in patients with cancer.

Direct nuclear actions of heparan sulfates have been proposed in hepatocytes, where an accumulation of oligosaccharides enriched in an unusual glucuronic acid 2–sulfate residue were preferentially translocated to the nucleus following endocytosis of the proteoglycan (22, 23, 41, 81). Increased levels of this nuclear-targeted heparan sulfate were

Table 68.1. Biologic Actions of Heparan Sulfate

1. Extracellular matrix organization
2. Basement membrane organization and regulation of permeability
3. Cell attachment, spreading, and migration
4. Growth and differentiation
5. Membrane localization of enzymes (e.g., acetylcholine esterase, lipoprotein lipase)
6. Localization of cytokines in pericellular domain (IL-3, GM-CSF, bFGF, TGF-β)
7. Anticoagulation
8. Modulation of angiogenesis

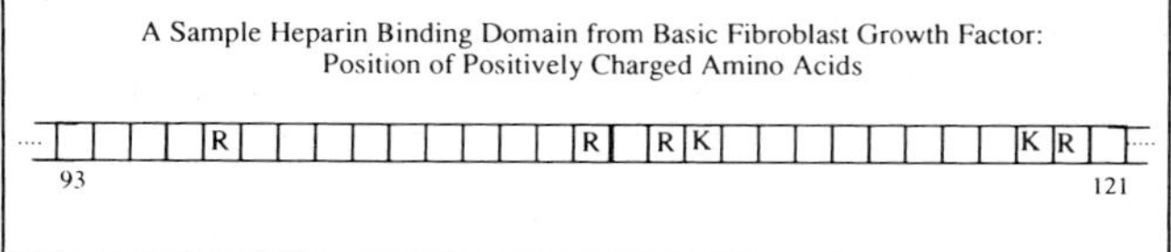

Figure 68.4. Heparan sulfate binding region of basic fibroblast growth factor. The postively charged amino acids are arginine(R) and lysine(K). Because heparan sulfate binding to a protein is likely to involve interactions between the negatively charged sulfates in heparan and positively charged amino acids, we have shown the positions of lysine and arginine; it is likely that one or more of these positively charged amino acids are also involved in the binding to suramin through the drug's sulfonic acid groups.

accompanied by an arrest in cell cycle at the G1 to S transition. An extensive and growing list of growth factors has been found to display an affinity for either heparan sulfate or heparin (Table 68.2). In some instances, the interaction between cytokine and polysaccharide has functional importance. For example, bone marrow stromal heparan sulfate is capable of binding and presenting the growth factors IL-3 and GM-CSF in active form to hemopoietic progenitor cells (79). It has been proposed that heparan sulfates in the bone marrow act to localize and present these cytokines in a paracrine fashion.

The sequestration and localization of basic fibroblast growth factor, an important mitogen for endothelial cells, in basement membranes and extracellular matrix has also been documented, and this interaction restricts the bioavailability of the cytokine while simultaneously protecting it from enzymatic degradation (4, 24, 45, 92, 93). Recently, it has been shown that both the interaction of basic fibroblast growth factor with its high-affinity receptor and its mitogenic activity in vitro require the association of the cytokine with a heparin-like molecule (101).

A further novel mechanism for modulation of growth factor activity by heparan sulfate has been suggested by studies involving transforming growth factor-β (TGF-β) (61). A variable proportion of serum TGF-β is bound in an inert complex with α-*S*-macroglobulin. Heparinoids lead to the dissociation of active TGF-β from the complex, making the cytokine available for interaction with cell surface receptors.

As these examples illustrate, heparan sulfates are important constituents of the cell membrane and the pericellular matrix. They are thus ideally placed to regulate the availability of a range of polypeptides to cell surface receptors.

Table 68.2. Cytokines that Bind to Heparan Sulfate

Growth factor	Study
Fibroblast growth factor (FGF) family	
Acidic FGF	46
Basic FGF	4
Int-2	9
Hst/K-FGF	18
FGF-5	104
FGF-6	60
KGF (Keratinocyte GF)	27
Epidermal growth factor (EGF) family	
Amphiregulin	83
Heparin-binding EGF-like GF	37
Platelet-derived growth factor (PDGF)	59
Macrophage inflammatory peptide-2 family	99
Neuronal growth factors	
Schwann cell mitogen	74
Glial maturation factor-β	54
Hemopoietic growth factors	
IL-3	79
GM-CSF	79
Leukemia-derived transforming GF	103
Insulin-like growth factor 2	65
Hepatocyte growth factor	34
Midkine factor family	
Heparin-binding growth-associated molecule	62
Pleiotropin	52
Heparin-binding neurotropic factor	48
OSF-1	89
Retinoic acid induced heparin-binding protein	91
Heparin-binding growth factor-8	64

AUTOCRINE GROWTH STIMULATION AND MALIGNANT TRANSFORMATION

One of the most important advances in cancer research over the past 15 years has been the identification of the genetic basis of malignant transformation (i.e., the identification of oncogenes). This has been followed by a description of some of the mechanisms by which the oncogenes accomplish malignant transformation. An important step in this process was the proposal in 1980 of autocrine growth as a mechanism of malignant transformation (87). In autocrine growth, a cell normally dependent on growth signals from other cells becomes independent of such control by producing the cytokines needed to stimulate its own growth (Fig. 68.5). An example of this mechanism is the transformation of fibroblasts by the simian sarcoma virus. Fibroblasts have receptors for platelet-derived growth factor (PDGF), and this cytokine will stimulate fibroblast growth. The simian sarcoma virus possesses the *sis* oncogene, and expression of this oncogene results in the production of the *sis* gene product, a protein similar in structure to the β chain of PDGF (32, 98). This protein then binds to the PDGF receptor and stimulates growth and transformation, both of which are reversed by addition of anti-PDGF antibody. Of the cytokines listed in Table 68.2, several fibroblast growth factor family members, epidermal growth factor family, IL-3, GM-CSF, and insulin-like growth factor 2, as well as PDGF have been shown to mediate transformation by autocrine mechanisms. A significant majority of those cytokines documented to be involved in autocrine growth are heparin-binding growth factors.

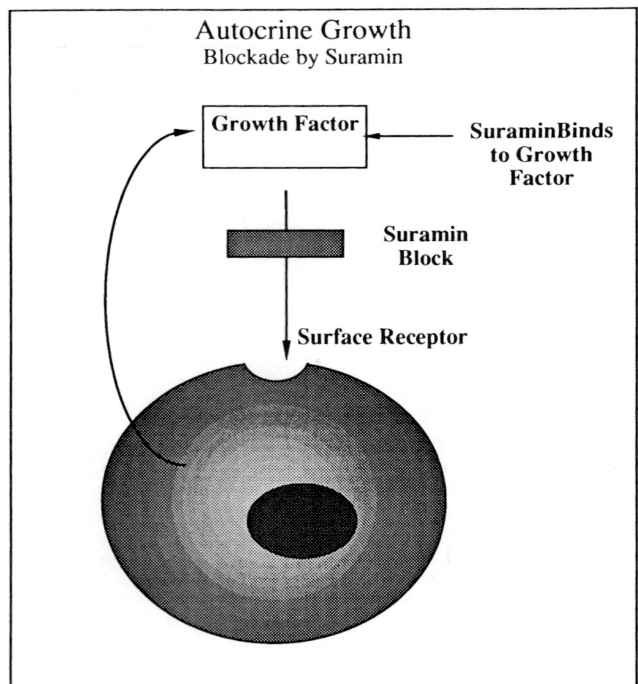

Figure 68.5. The mechanism by which autocrine growth occurs. The cell in question elaborates and secretes into the surrounding medium a peptide growth factor for which it possesses a functional receptor. The consequence is self-stimulation of cellular proliferation. For a majority of the peptide growth factors where such a process has been invoked, suramin binds to the growth factor in question and prevents its association with its cell surface receptor.

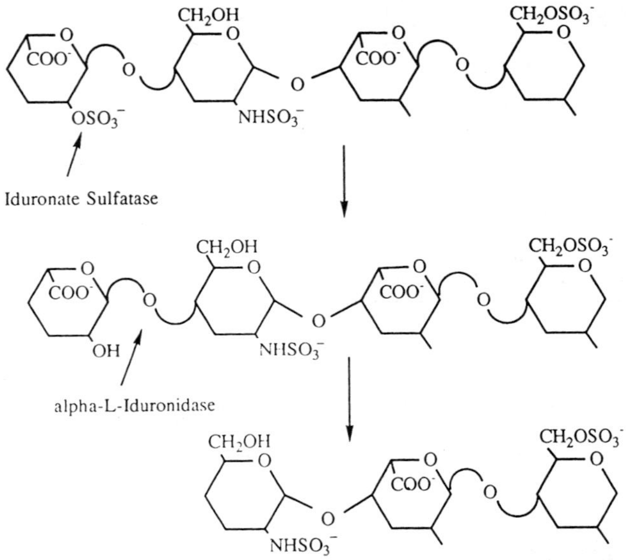

Figure 68.6. Inhibition of heparan sulfate and dermatan sulfate degradation by suramin. The first step in the degradation of the iduronate-containing regions is an O-desulfation reaction involving the enzyme iduronate sulfatase. The next step involves cleavage of the carbohydrate chain by α-L-iduronidase. Suramin arrests this process by inhibiting iduronate sulfatase. The result is a relative sparing of the highly sulfated regions. Hunter's syndrome is an inborn error in glycosaminoglycan degradation characterized by a lack of this same enzyme. Both Hunter's syndrome and suramin administration result in accumulation of the two glycosaminoglycans possessing sulfated iduronic acid residues: heparan sulfate and dermatan sulfate.

RELATIONSHIP OF HEPARAN SULFATE BIOLOGY TO SURAMIN ACTION

The ability of the *sis* oncogene to transform fibroblasts by an autocrine mechanism was first reported in 1984. Within that same year, it was shown that suramin could promptly reverse the transformation of fibroblasts by this oncogene. Suramin has been shown to bind to PDGF and to the *sis* oncogene and thus to prevent these peptides from binding to the cell surface receptor (7, 28, 32, 40, 43, 44, 97, 98). Suramin has subsequently been shown to reverse malignant transformation by hst/K-fgf as well as the v-*sis* gene product (66). This observation has led to the suggestion that suramin acts as an analogue of heparan sulfate. Indeed, a comparison of the known effects of suramin suggest that it acts as an agonist or antagonist of heparan sulfate for most of the functions listed in Table 68.1. In this hypothesis, the sulfonic acid groups of suramin must substitute for the sulfate groups on heparan sulfate.

The ability of suramin to bind to heparin-binding sites within proteins may account for suramin's ability to inhibit a number of glycosaminoglycan degradative enzymes. A step in the degradation of functionally important iduronate and sulfate-rich regions of heparan sulfate is desulfation by iduronate sulfatase. This is then followed by enzymatic cleavage of the carbohydrate chain (Fig. 68.6). In vitro, suramin has been shown to be a powerful inhibitor of iduronate sulfatase. A genetic defect in this enzyme results in Hunter's syndrome, a mucopolysaccharidosis that is associated with the accumulation of heparan and dermatan sulfate. This has enabled an animal model for mucopolysaccharidosis to be created by administering suramin to rats (16, 75, 76). We have noted that suramin administration to patients also results in elevated heparan and dermatan sulfate levels in blood and urine (39). Under certain conditions, this can become severe enough to result in anticoagulation, although in most cases, the anticoagulation seen with suramin results from a direct action of the drug. Also, because iduronate sulfatase is a lysosomal enzyme and heparan degradation normally occurs within the lysosome, suramin administration results in accumulation of both heparan and dermatan sulfate within the lysosomes throughout the body (38, 39, 75, 76).

Because heparan sulfate may either inhibit or stimulate cell growth, the accumulation of heparan sulfate seen in patients receiving suramin might either enhance or antagonize the antitumor activity of suramin. For this reason, we have isolated heparan sulfate from patients undergoing treatment with suramin. This material has considerable activity against a range of human tumor cells.

IN VITRO ANTITUMOR ACTIVITY OF SURAMIN

The antitumor activity of suramin has been reported in a wide range of tumor types in vitro, with the most impressive activity being reported in carcinomas of the prostate, stomach, endometrium, ovary and lung (nonsmall cell), glioma, melanoma, rhabdomyosarcoma, osteogenic sarcoma, and non-Hodgkin's lymphomas (2, 13, 17, 21, 29, 47, 49, 68–70, 86, 94, 96, 102). In cell cultures, one striking property is that maximal antitumor activity requires prolonged contact. For prostate cancer, which we have recently studied in some depth, drug effects are reversible after 3 days of exposure. After 6 days, however, cells proceed to die even days after drug removal. Combination with other active agents may be synergistic or antagonistic (59). Suramin used before radiotherapy of two prostate cancer cell lines inhibited radiation-induced cell death, whereas after radiation exposure, it enhanced cytotoxicity (85).

In general, caution must be applied when considering the relevance of in vitro antitumor activity to clinical cancer treatment. This is especially so for suramin. The activity of this drug may result from its action on cytokines, and little is known about how well the cytokine levels in vitro match those in patients. It is particularly likely that tissue culture media are lacking growth factors present in patients that might plausibly alter the effectiveness of suramin. The only solution presently available is to perform phase II trials in each of the tumors listed earlier.

Routes of Administration, Distribution, Pharmacokinetics, and Implications for Scheduling

Suramin drug is not absorbed after oral administration and so must be given parenterally. This drug is chemically stable in all commonly used intravenous infusion media (6). In all current trials of suramin as an anticancer agent, therapy has been administered intravenously. The administered drug binds tightly to plasma proteins and is greater than 99.7% protein bound at blood levels below 200 μg/mL (8). As blood levels increase above 200 μg/mL, free drug levels increase rapidly, as does toxicity of the drug. In addition to extensive binding to plasma proteins, animal studies of suramin administration have shown that the drug accumulates in tissues, particularly the kidney and adrenal gland. The levels of suramin in most other tissues reflect circulating plasma levels.

The plasma pharmacokinetics of suramin may be accounted for by a three-compartment model. In 71 patients studied at the NCI, total body clearance was 0.331 ± 0.138 mL/h/kg with a volume of distribution at steady state of 32.2 ± 11.8 L. The alpha, beta, and gamma half-lives were 2.2 ± 0.48 hours, 1.3 ± 0.47 days, and 42 ± 23 days, respectively. For each of these values, there is significant variation, and this leads to considerable patient-to-patient variability in blood levels attained following any given drug dose. As a result, current treatment protocols require drug level monitoring to ensure safe drug administration. Figure 68.7 illustrates how suramin levels typically decline after a bolus dose, with a rapid early decline reflecting the two early compartments followed by a very gradual decline that can be followed for months. It is conventional wisdom that with a drug, having a terminal half-life of this length, it should be relatively easy to maintain consistent blood levels with an intermittent bolus schedule. Figure 68.7 illustrates nicely how the rapid early decline in blood levels from the three-compartment behavior makes this more complicated than the long terminal half-life might indicate. At present, there is no known drug metabolism, and renal elimination of the parent drug is the only documented pathway of drug clearance.

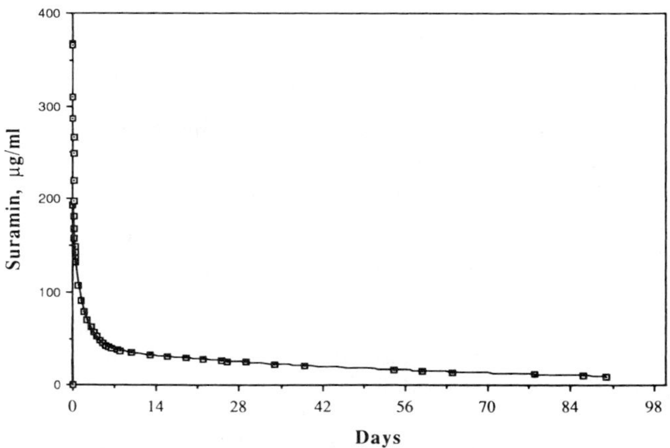

Figure 68.7. An example of the three-compartment behavior of suramin. This is a computer simulation of the blood levels to be expected after a single bolus dose of 1500 mg of suramin to a patient who weighs 70 kg and has the pharmacokinetic parameters of an average patient.

In early trials with suramin, the drug was administered as a weekly bolus at a fixed dose rate. These trials revealed an unacceptable frequency of neurotoxicity associated with blood levels above 350 μg/mL. After the patient-to-patient variability in drug disposition became apparent, it became customary to measure blood levels after initial drug administration and adjust subsequent dosing to keep blood levels below 300 μg/mL. Initially, drug dose was adjusted based on a simple nomogram constructed from a one-compartment model. The pharmacokinetic data arising from these early trials allowed documentation of the three-compartment behavior of suramin's pharmacokinetics and a determination of the variability of each pharmacokinetic parameter (14, 88). This information has allowed a more sophisticated approach to dose adjustment. Currently, best control of suramin blood levels has been obtained by two groups using Bayesian techniques (42, 53). A full discussion of the Bayesian approach is beyond the scope of this chapter and the reader is referred to several recent reviews (71).

The clinical protocols yielding the highest response rate appear to be those that give prolonged exposure to drug levels in excess of 100 μg/ml. This has been accomplished by either bolus or continuous infusion protocols in which the drug is administered for as long as 8 weeks.

Patterns of Toxicity

Most anticancer agents are limited by toxicity that is evident in a few organs consistently involved when full doses of the drug is administered. In contrast, suramin can cause a wide range of toxicities, but it is uncommon for a patient to manifest all or even most of the possible side effects. In addition, the toxicity of the drug appears to depend on blood drug level and to escalate rapidly at blood levels in excess of 200 to 225 μg/mL. In an elderly male population with prostate cancer, drug levels below 200 μg/ml are associated with a frequency of serious or life-threatening side effects of less than 20%, while at blood levels between 275 to 300 μg/mL the frequency may reach as high as 70 to 80%.

ADRENAL CORTICAL FAILURE

Suramin can cause destruction of the normal adrenal cortex in both humans and in a wide range of experimental animals (26). Adrenal medullary function is preserved. Suramin accumulates within the adrenal gland, and this probably plays some role in the development of this toxicity. The natural history of this toxicity has not been documented, but individual patients have had recovery of apparently normal adrenal function six or more months after suramin administration was discontinued.

NEUROTOXICITY

This drug causes three distinct patterns of neurotoxicity. The first to be noted was an acute, demyelinating peripheral neuropathy resembling acute Guillain-Barré syndrome seen only in patients with prolonged blood levels in excess of 350 μg/mL (88). Second, blood levels between 200 to 300 μg/mL are associated with stocking-glove paresthesias very similar to those caused by the vinca alkaloids. Regardless of severity, this neuropathic syndrome improves, usually dramatically, over 6 to 12 months following discontinuation of suramin.

A third neuropathic syndrome has been seen only in protocols where drug administration has continued beyond one month. This syndrome presents as proximal muscle weakness suggestive of a myopathy, but markers of muscle injury are absent and nerve conduction changes observed. This neuropathic syndrome typically continues to progress after drug administration has been discontinued, sometimes for more than a month. Recovery is very gradual over 4 to 9 months.

RENAL INJURY

Suramin causes a 25 to 50% decline in creatinine clearance in most patients. There is usually complete or nearly complete recovery in patients who have normal renal function to start with. More severe renal functional abnormalities have been noted in patients who become septic during suramin administration. However, in such cases, the patients have usually been hypotensive and have received aminoglycoside antibiotics. From such cases, it is difficult to determine the relative contribution of suramin. In addition, suramin may cause proteinuria. This rarely exceeds 1 g per 24 hours and does not result in a nephrotic syndrome.

As mentioned, suramin accumulates in the kidneys to a considerable degree. While the mechanism of this accumulation is not known, it undoubtedly plays a role in the nephrotoxicity observed. The drug has been shown to accumulate within the renal tubular lysosomes, and this is followed by the degeneration of the renal tubular cells.

ANTICOAGULATION

Suramin inhibits factors V, VIII, IX, X, XI, and XII, while thrombin, prothrombin, and factor VII are unaffected. The inhibition of factor V is irreversible, while the effect of suramin on the other coagulation factors is readily reversible on dilution.

As a result of these changes, patients receiving suramin often experience prolongation of prothrombin time, activated partial thromboplastin time, and thrombin clotting times. An unusual aspect is that the thrombin-clotting-time abnormalities caused by suramin do not correct with toluidine blue or while those caused by heparin do.

In practice, we have found that the risk of hemorrhage is markedly reduced if administration of suramin is discontinued when the prothrombin time exceeds 17 seconds. Tumor-induced diffuse intravascular coagulation can be a problem with prostate carcinoma. At present, guidelines have not been developed for safe use of suramin in this situation.

BACTERIAL INFECTIONS

While suramin may induce neutropenia, it is uncommon for the absolute neutrophile count to drop below 1,000 cells/mL. Nevertheless, it is apparent that prolonged exposure to suramin levels of 270 to 300 μg/mL is associated with an increased risk of bacterial infections. In our prostate cancer population, these have typically arisen from either the urinary tract or the catheter used for intravenous drug administration. Catheter-related infections appear to be less frequent when suramin is given by intermittent IV bolus administration compared to continuous intravenous infusion. Suramin has been demonstrated to impair both the rate of phagocytosis and the killing of bacteria by neutrophils, and this may be the mechanism underlying the increase in bacterial infections (35, 36, 84, 90, 95).

LYMPHOCYTOPENIA

Lymphocytopenia occurs in up to 80% of patients exposed to blood levels of 275 to 300 μg/mL and seems to be selective for T cells. Nevertheless, opportunistic infections have been relatively uncommon in patients treated with suramin. Suramin binds IL-2 and prevents its association with the T-cell receptor. Because T cells undergo programmed cell death in vitro when IL-2 is removed, this provides a possible explanation and mechanism for blocking the toxicity of suramin for T cells. In fact, addition of excess IL-2 dramatically lessens the toxicity of suramin for T cells (63).

THROMBOCYTOPENIA

Suramin may induce thrombocytopenia; platelet counts below 50,000 are relatively uncommon, however. In addition, thrombocytopenia is usually self-limiting and resolves despite persistent blood levels of suramin. Bone marrow biopsies in patients with suramin-induced thrombocytopenia reveal normal megakaryocytes with normal budding, suggesting that the thrombocytopenia results from an accelerated peripheral clearance of platelets. Suramin-induced thrombocytopenia is usually a dose-limiting toxicity only in patients with preexisting thrombocytopenia because of marrow replacement, previous radiation or chemotherapy, or tumor-induced diffuse intravascular coagulation.

VORTEX KERATOPATHY

Suramin-induced lysosomal accumulation of heparan and dermatan sulfate occurs in the corneal epithelium (38). As a result, every patient receiving suramin has a vortex keratopathy that can be detected by slit-lamp examination. In most cases, the only symptom associated with this is the appearance of a ring around bright lights. In an occasional patient, pitting of the corneal epithelium occurs, resulting in a gritty sensation, photophobia, and excess tearing. This complication has resolved completely in every case without residual eye damage. Until the corneal epithelium has healed, symptomatic relief may be given with dark glasses, methylcellulose eye drops, and soft contact lenses.

SKIN RASH

Suramin induces a skin rash in the majority of patients who receive the drug. This rash is a mildly pruritic, erythematous, macular eruption that typically starts on the chest and back and can spread to involve the extremities. The rash usually presents during the first two weeks following initiation of suramin treatment. This toxicity is nearly always self-limiting and resolves in the face of continued suramin administration. In the occasional severe case, the rash can be severe enough to lead to desquamation. In such severe cases, the rash is associated with fever and thrombocytopenia.

EDEMA

Ankle edema has developed in individual patients with intact lymphatic and venous drainage to the lower extremities and with a serum albumin level within the normal range. Edema can become a significant problem if the patient also has any of these other problems. The physiologic basis for this complication is unknown.

LIVER INJURY

Suramin may cause mild elevation of the hepatic enzymes and bilirubin, but it rarely causes severe injury in the absence of other sources of liver injury. Patients with ongoing liver injury from other causes can exhibit a marked decline in liver function with suramin administration, however.

Antitumor Spectrum

The efficacy of suramin in prostate cancer has received the greatest attention. In patients with measurable soft-tissue disease, the combined PR and CR rate has ranged between ~15 to greater than 50%. However, soft-tissue involvement is seen in only 15% of patients with prostate cancer. In the more common presentation of bone involvement alone, the major evidence of suramin's antitumor activity has been the decline seen in prostate specific antigen (PSA). In the initial trial of suramin in prostate cancer at the NCI, approximately one third of the patients experienced a decline of their pretreatment PSA of 75% or greater by 8 weeks after therapy was initiated. Declines of PSA of this magnitude were associated with a dramatic shift in survival, with greater than 80% of the patients alive at one year and greater than 60% at two years for the responders compared to a median survival of less than 40 weeks for nonresponders. In this trial, the drug was infused over a two week period. Subsequent trials have reported response rates between 40 and 60% (1, 20). These phase II results are sufficiently promising that suramin should receive additional evaluation in the treatment of metastatic prostate carcinoma.

Because suramin induces depletion of splenic lymphocytes and thymic atrophy in mice, it is perhaps not surprising that suramin has shown clear activity against a range of lymphomas. The first response was noted in the trial of suramin as an agent to treat AIDS (10). In that trial, a patient with non-Hodgkin's lymphoma went into complete remission, which has continued for more than four years. We have treated 10 patients with nodular lymphomas who had been heavily pretreated and have seen five partial responses. In addition, we have treated two patients with thymoma who had failed radiation therapy and conventional chemotherapy programs, both of whom experienced PRs on suramin. Finally, one out of five patients with HTLV-1-associated T-cell leukemia experienced a PR from suramin as a single agent that lasted nearly five months (50).

Early in our work with suramin, we evaluated the drug in adrenal carcinoma and observed a response rate below 20%. It is now possible to administer suramin in a much more dose-intense fashion, however, and its activity in this disease should probably be reevaluated. Suramin has not been subjected to phase II trial in most of the tumor types against which it exhibits activity in vitro.

INTERACTIONS

Suramin has been shown to interact synergistically with alkylating agents with regard to antitumor activity murine models, without evidence of additive toxicity (70). There is more extensive information about the interaction of suramin with doxorubicin (21, 30, 70). Here again, there does not appear to be additive toxicity, but antitumor activity of the two compounds ranges from additive to synergistic over a range of tumor types, including human breast cancer and prostate cancer cell lines. Synergy has also been seen with tumor necrosis factor, but not with γ-interferon (30, 57).

SUMMARY

A nearly infinite number of anionic polyelectrolytes can be synthesized. The understanding of suramin's mechanism of action by electrostatic association with highly charged basic proteins offers the possibility that designer molecules could be synthesized (or may already exist in nature or polymer inventories) with more selective antineoplastic action.

References

1. Ahmann FR, Schwartz J, Dorr R, Slamon S. Suramin in hormone resistant metastatic prostate cancer: significant anticancer activity but unanticipated toxicity. Proc Am Soc Clin Oncol 1991;10:574. Abstract.
2. Alberts D, Miranda E, Dorr R, Nichols N, Ketcham M, MacNeal W, Hatch K, Surwit E, Childers J, Taylor C, Ahmann R, Salmon S. Phase II, pharmacokinetic and human tumor cloning assay study of suramin in advanced ovarian cancer. Proc Am Soc Clin Oncol 1991;10:609. Abstract.
3. Barzu T, Lormeau JC, Petitou M, Michelson S, Choay J. Heparin-derived oligosaccharides: affinity for acidic fibroblast growth factor and effect on its growth-promoting activity for human endothelial cells. J Cell Physiol 1989;140:538.
4. Baird A, Schubert D, Ling N, Guillemin R. Receptor-and heparin-binding domains of basic fibroblast growth factor. Proc Natl Acad Sci USA 1988;85:2324.
5. Beguin S, Choay J, Hemker HC. The action of a synthetic pentasaccharide on thrombin generation in whole plasma. Thromb Haemost 1989;61:397.
6. Beijnen JH, Van Gijn R, Horenblas S, Underberg WJ. Chemical stability of suramin in commonly used infusion fluids. DICP 1990;24:1056.
7. Betsholtz C, Johnsson A, Heldin CH, Westermark B. Efficient reversion of simian sarcoma virus transformation and inhibition of growth factor-induced mitogenesis by suramin. Proc Natl Acad Sci USA 1986;83:6440.
8. Bos OJ, Vansterkenburg EL, Boon JP, Fischer MJ, Wilting J, Janssen LH. Location and characterization of the suramin binding sites of human serum albumin. Biochem Pharmacol 1990;40:1595.
9. Burgess WH, Maciag T. The heparin binding (fibroblast) growth factor family of proteins. Annu Rev Biochem 1989;58:575.
10. Cheson BD, Levin AM, Mildvan D, Kaplan LD, et al. Suramin therapy in AIDS and related disorders. Report of the US Suramin Working Group. JAMA 1987;258:1347.
11. Choay J. Chemically synthesized heparin-derived oligosaccharides. Ann NY Acad Sci 1989;556:61.
12. Choay J. Structure and activity of heparin and its fragments: an overview. Semin Thromb Hemost 1989;15:359.
13. Coffey RJ, Goustin AS, Soderquist AM, Shipley GD, et al. Transforming growth factor alpha and beta expression in human colon cancer lines: implications for an autocrine model. Cancer Res 1987;47:4590.
14. Collins JM, Klecker RJ, Yarchoan R, Lane HC, et al. Clinical pharmacokinetics of suramin in patients with HTLV-III/LAV infection. J Clin Pharmacol 1986;26:22.
15. Conrad HE. Structure of heparan sulfate and dermatan sulfate. Ann NY Acad Sci 1989;556:8.
16. Constantopoulos G, Rees S, Cragg BG, Barranger JA, et al. Suramin-induced storage disease. Mucopolysaccharidosis. Am J Pathol 1983;113:266.
17. Culouscou JM. Garrouste F, Remacle Bonnet M, Mettetini D, Marvaldi J, Pommier G. Autocrine secretion of a colorectum-derived growth factor by HT-29 human colon carcinoma cell line. Int J Cancer 1988;42:895.
18. Dell-Bovi P, Basilico C. Isolation of a rearranged human transforming gene following transfection of Kaposi sarcoma DNA. Proc Natl Acad Sci USA 1987;84:5660.
19. Dressel J, Oesper RE. The discovery of germanin by Oskar Dressel and Richard Kothe. J Chem Educ 1961;38:620.
20. Eisenberger M, Reyno LM, Jodrell D, Sinibaldi V, Tkaczuk KH, Sridhara R, Zubowski EG, Lowitt MH, Jacobs SC, Egorin MJ. Suramin, an active drug for prostate cancer: interim observations in a phase I trial. JNCI 1993;85:611. (Erratum: JNCI 1994;86: 639.)
21. Favoni RE, Russo R, Pirani P, repetto L, Nicolin A, Miglietta L. Synergistic activity of suramin and doxorubicin on human breast cancer cell lines. Proc Am Cancer Res 1991;32:2282.
22. Fedarko NS, Conrad HE. A unique heparan sulfate in the nuclei of hepatocytes: structural changes with the growth state of the cells. J Cell Biol 1986;102:587.
23. Fedarko NS, Ishihara M, Conrad HE. Control of cell division in hepatoma cells by exogenous haparan sulfate proteoglycan. J Cell Physiol 1989;139:287.
24. Feige JJ, Bradley JD, Fryburg K, Farris J, Cousens LC, Barr PJ, Baird A. Differential efforts of heparin, fibronectin, and laminin on the phosphorylation of basic fibroblast growth factor by protein kinase C and the catalytic subunit of protein kinase A. J Cell Biol 1989;109:3105.
25. Ferro DR, Provasoli A, Ragazzi M, Casu B, Torri G, Bossennec V, Perly B, Sinay P, Petitou M, Choay J. Conformer populations of L-iduronic acid residues in glycosaminoglycan sequences. Carbohydr Res 1990;195:157.
26. Feuillan P, Raffeld M, Stein CA, Lipford N, et al. Effects of suramin on the function and structure of the adrenal cortex in the cynomoigus monkey. J Clin Endocrinol Metab 1987;65:153.
27. Finch P, Rubin J, Miki T. Human KGF in FGF-related with properties of a paracrine effector of epithelial cell-growth. Science 1988;245:752.
28. Fleming TP, Matsui T, Molloy CJ, Robbins KC, Aaronson SA. Autocrine mechanism for v-*sis* transformation requires cell surface localization of internally activated growth factor receptors. Proc Natl Acad Sci USA 1989;86:8063.
29. Forgue-Lafitte ME, Coudray AM, Breant B, Mester J. Proliferation of the human colon carcinoma cell line HT29: autocrine growth and deregulated expression of the c-myc oncogene. Cancer Res 1989;49:6566.
30. Fruehauf JP, Myers CE, Sinha BK. Synergistic activity of suramin with tumor necrosis factor alpha and doxorubicin on human prostate cancer cell lines. JNCI 1990;82: 1206.
31. Gallagher JT, Turnbull JE, Lyon M. Heparan sulphate proteoglycans. Biochem Soc Trans 1990;18:207.
32. Garrett JS, Coughlin SR, Niman HL, Tremble PM, et al. Blockade of autocrine stimulation in simian sarcoma virus-transformed cells reverses down-regulation of platelet-derived growth factor receptors. Proc Natl Acad Sci USA 1984;81:7466.
33. Gettins P, Choay J. Examination, by 1H-nmr spectroscopy, of the binding of a synthetic high-affinity heparin pentasaccharide to human antithrombin III. Carbohydr Res 1989;185:69.
34. Gohda E, Tsubouchi H, Nakayama H, et al. Purification and partial characterization of hepatocyte growth factor from plasma of a patient with fulminant hepatic failure. J Clin Invest 1988;81:414.
35. Hart PD, Young MR, Jordan MM, Perkins WJ, et al. Chemical inhibitors of phagosome-lysosome fusion in cultured macrophages also inhibit saltatory lysosomal movements. A combined microscopic and computer study. J Exp Med 1983;158:477.
36. Heyneman RA. Inhibition by suramin of the NADPH oxidase from horse polymorphonuclear leukocytes. Vet Res Commun 1987;11:149.
37. Higashiyama S, Abraham JA, Miller J, Fiddes JC, Klagsbrun M. A heparin-binding growth factor secreted by macrophage cells that is related to EGF. Science 1991;251:936.
38. Holland EJ, Stein CA, Palestine AG, LaRocca RV, Chan CC, Kuwabara T, Myers CE, Thomas R, McAtee N, Nussenblatt RN. Suramin keratopathy. Am J Ophthalmol 1988;106:216.
39. Horne MK III, Stein CA, LaRocca RV, Myers CE. Circulating glycosaminoglycan anticoagulants associated with suramin treatment. Blood 1988;72:273.
40. Huang SS, Huang JS. Rapid turnover of the platelet-derived growth factor receptor in *sis*-transformed cells and reversal by suramin. Implications for the mechanism of autocrine transformation. J Biol Chem 1988;263:2608.
41. Ishihara M, Fedarko NS, Conrad HE. Transport of heparan sulfate into the nuclei of hepatocytes. J Biol Chem 1986;261:3575.
42. Jodrell JI, Reyno LM, Sridhara R, Eisenberger MA, Tkaczuk KH, Zubowski EG, Sinibaldi VJ, Novak MJ, Egarin MJ. Suramin: development of a population pharmacokinetic model and its use with intermittent short infusions to control plasma drug concentration in patients with prostate cancer. J Clin Oncol 1994;12:166.
43. Johnsson A, Betsholtz C, Heldin CH, Westermark B. The phenotypic characteristics of simian sarcoma virus-transformed human fibroblasts suggest that the v-*sis* gene product acts solely as a PDGF receptor agonist in cell transformation. EMBO J 1986;5:1535.
44. Keating MT, Escobedo JA, Fantl WJ, Williams LT. Lingand activation causes a phosphorylation-dependent change in platelet-derived growth factor receptor conformation. Trans Assoc Am Physicians 1988;101:24.
45. Klagsbrun MT. The affinity of fibroblast growth factors (FGFs) for heparin, FGF-heparan sulfate interactions in cells and extracellular matrix. Curr Opin Cell Biol 1990;2: 857.
46. Klagsbrun M, Shing Y. Heparin affinity of anionic and cationic capillary endothelial cell growth factors: analysis of hypothalamus-derived growth factors and fibroblast growth factors. Proc Natl Acad Sci USA 1985;82:805.
47. Kopp R, Pfeiffer A. Suramin alters phosphoinositide synthesis and inhibits growth factor receptor binding in HT-29 cells. Cancer Res 1990,50:6490.
48. Kovesdi I, Fairhurst JL, Kretschmer PJ, Bohlem P. Heparin-binding neurotrophic factor and MK. Members of a new family homologous, developmentally regulated proteins. Biochem Biophys Res Commun 1990;172:850.
49. LaRocca RV, Cooper MR, Uhrich M, Danesi R, et al. Use of suramin in treatment of prostate carcinoma refractory to conventional hormonal manipulation. Urol Clin North Am 1991;8:123.
50. LaRocca RV, Myers CE, Stein CA, Cooper MR, Uhrich M. Effect of suramin in patients with refractory nodular lymphomas requiring systemic therapy. Proc Am Soc Clin Oncol 1990;9:1041. Abstract.
51. Leblond CP, Inoue S. Structure, composition, and assembly of basement membrane. Am J Anat 1989;185:367.
52. Li YS, Milner PG, Chauham AK, Watson MA, Hoffman RM, Kodner CM, Milbrandt J, Deuel TF. Cloning and expression of a developmentally regulated protein that induces mitogenic and neurite outgrowth activity. Science 1990;250:1690.
53. Lieberman R, Katzper M, Cooper M. Population pharmacokinetic analysis and Bayesian forecasting during suramin therapy in prostate cancer: one-versus two-compartment PK models. Proc Am Soc Clin Oncol 1990;9:262.
54. Lim R, Miller JF, Zaheer A. Purification and characterization of glia maturation factor beta: a growth regulator for neurons and glia. Proc Natl Acad Sci USA 1989;86:3901.
55. Lindahl U. Approaches to the synthesis of heparin. Haemostatis 1990;1:146.
56. Lindahl U, Kusche M, Lidholt K, Oscarsson LG. Biosynthesis of heparin and heparan sulfate. Ann NY Acad Sci 1989;556:36.
57. Liu S, Ewing MW, Anglard P, Trahan E, LaRocca RV, Meyers CE, Linehan WM. The effect of suramin, tumor necrosis factor and interferon gamma on human prostate carcinoma. J Urol 1991;145:389.
58. Lopez-Lopez R, van Risswijk RE, Wagstaff J, Pinedo HM, Peteys GJ. The synergistic and anatogonistic effects of cytotoxic and biological agents on the in vitro antitumour effects of suramin. Eur J Cancer 1994;30A:1545.
59. Marez A, NuGuyen T, Chevallier B, et al. Platelet derived growth factor is present in human placenta: purification from an industrially processed fraction. Biochemie 1987;69:125.
60. Maris I, Adelaide J, Raybaud F, Mattei MG, Coulier F, Planche J, de Lapeyriere O, Birnbaum D. Characterization of the HST-related FGF-6 gene, a member of the fibroblast growth factor family. Oncogene 1989;4:335.
61. McCaffrey TA, Falcone DJ, Brayton CF, Agarwal LA, Welt F, Weksler BB. TGF-β activity is potentiated by heparin via dissociation of TGF—alpha 2 macroglobulin inactive complex. J Cell Biol 1988;109:441.
62. Merenmies J, Rauvala H. Molecular cloning of the 18 kDa growth associated protein of developing brain. J Biol Chem 1990;265:16721.
63. Mills GB, Zhang N, May C, Hill M, Chung A. Suramin prevents binding of interleukin 2 to its cell surface receptor: a possible mechanism for immunosuppression. Cancer Res 1990;50:3036.
64. Milner PG, Li YS, Hoffman RM, Kodner CM, SSiegel NR, Deuel TF. A novel 17 kD heparin-binding growth factor (HBGF-8) in bovine uterus: purification and *N*-terminal amino acid sequence. Biochem Biophys Res Commun 1989;165:1096.
65. Mohan S, Jennings JC, Linkhart TA, Baylink DJ. Primary structure of human skeletal growth factor: homology with IGF-II. Biochem Biophys Acta 1988;966:44.
66. Moscatelli D, Quarto N. Transformation of NIH 3T3 cells with basic fibroblast growth factor of the hst/K-fgf oncogene causes down regulation of the fibroblast growth factor receptor: reversal of morphological changes and restoration of receptor number by suramin. J Cell Biol 1989;109:2519.
67. Mourey L, Samama JP, Delarue M, Choay J, Lormeau JC, Petitou M, Moras D. Antithrombin III: structural and functional aspects. Biochimie 1990:72–599.
68. Nakaiima M, deChavigny A, Johnson CE, Hamada J, Stein CA, Nicolson GL. Suramin. A potent inhibitor of melanoma heparanase and invasion. J Biol Chem 1991;266: 9661.
69. Olivier S, Formento P, Fischel JL, Etienne MC, Milano G. Epidermal growth factor receptor expression and suramin cytotoxicity in vitro. Eur J Cancer 1990;26:867.
70. Osswald H, Youssef M. Suramin enhancement of the chemotherapeutic actions of cy-

clophosphamide or adriamycin of intramuscularly-implanted Ehrlich carcinoma. Cancer Lett 1979;6:337.
71. Peck CC, Rodman JH. Analysis of pharmacokinetic data for individualizing patient dosage regimens. In: Evans WE, Schentag JJ, Jusko WJ. Applied Pharmacokinetics: The Principles of Therapeutic Drug Monitoring. Vancouver, WA: Applied Therapeutics, 1986:55.
72. Petitou M, Lormeau JC, Choay J. Chemical synthesis of glycosaminoglycans: new approaches to antithrombotic drugs. Nature 1991;350:30.
73. Ragazzi M, ferro DR, Perly B, Sinay P, Petitou M, Choay J. Conformation of the pentasaccharide corresponding to the binding site of heparin for antithrombin III. Carbohydr Res 1990;195:169.
74. Ratner N, Hong DM, Lieberman MA, Bunge RP, Glaser L. The neuronal cell-surface molecule mitogenic for Schwann cells is a heparin-binding protein. Proc Natl Acad Sci USA 1988;895:6992.
75. Rees S, Constantopoulos G, Brady R. The suramin-treated rat as a model of mucopolysaccharidosis: reversibility of biochemical and morphological changes in the liver. Virchows Arch [b] 1986;51:235.
76. Rees S, Constantopoulos G, Brady RO. The suramin-treated rat as a model of mucopolysaccharidosis. Variation in the reversibility of biochemical and morphological changes among different organs. Virchows Arch [b] 1986;52:259.
77. Regelson W. The antimitotic activity of polyanions. Adv Chemother 1968;3:303.
78. Regelson W. The biologic activity of polyanions: past history and new prospectives. J Polymer Sci 1979;1979:483.
79. Roberts R, Gallagher J, Spooncer E, Allen TD, Bloomfield F, Dexter TM. Heparan sulfate bound growth factors: a mechanism for stromal cell mediated hematopoiesis. Nature 1988;332:376.
80. Rosenberg RD. Biochemistry of heparin antithrombin interactions, and the physiologic role of this natural anticoagulant mechanism. Am J Med 1989;87:25.
81. Shaklee PN, Glass JH, Conrad HE. A sulfatase specific for glucuronic acid 2-sulfate residues in glycosaminoglycans. J Biol Chem 1985;260:9146.
82. Shore JD, Olson ST, Craig PA, Choay J, Bjork I. Kinetics of heparin action. Ann NY Acad Sci 1989k;556:75.
83. Shoyab M, Plowman GD, McDonald VL, Bradley JG, Todaro GJ. Structure and function of human amphiregulin. A member of the EGF family. Science 1989;243:1074.
84. Sipka S, Danko K, Nagy P, Taskov V, Denes L, Czirjak L, Szegedi G. Effects of suramin on phagocytes in vitro. Ann Hematol 1991;63:45.
85. Sklar GN, Eddy HA, Jacobs SC, Kyprianov N. Combined antitumor effect of suramin plus irradiation in human prostate cancer cells: the role of apoptosis. J Urol 1993;150: 1526.
86. Spigelman Z, Dowers A, Kennedy S, DiSorbo D, et al. Antiproliferative effects of suramin on lymphoid cells. Cancer Res 1987;47:4694.
87. Sporn MB, Todaro GJ. Autocrine secretion and malignant transformation of cells. N Engl J Med 1908;303:878.
88. Stein CA, LaRocca RV, Thomas R, McAtee N, Myers CE. Suramin: an anticancer drug with a unique mechanism of action. J Clin Oncol 1989;7:499.
89. Tezuka K, takeshita S, Hakeda Y, Kumegawa M, Kikuno R, Hashimoto-Gotoh T. Isolation of mouse and human cDNA clones encoding a protein expressed specifically in osteoblasts and brain tissue. Biochem Biophys Res Commun 1990;173:246.
90. Toshkov A, Neychev H, Dimov V. Suramin increases the nonspecific antibacterial resistance through macrophage activation. Acta Microbiol Bulg 1986;19:13.
91. Tsutsui J, Uehara K, Kadomatsu K. A new family of heparin-binding factors: strong conversation of midkine (MK) sequences between the human and the mouse. Biochem Biophys Res Commun 1990;176:792.
92. Vlodavsky I, Fuks Z, Ishai-Michaeli R, Bashkin P, Levin E, Korner G, bar-Shavit R, Klagsbrun M. Extracellular matrix-resident basic fibroblast growth factor: implication for the control of angiogenesis. J Cell Biochem 1991;45:167.
93. Vlodavsky I, Korner G, Ishai MR, Bashkin P. Extracellular matrix-resident growth factors and enzymes: possible involvement in tumor metastasis and angiogenesis. Cancer Metastasis Rev 1990;9:203.
94. Walz TM, Abdiu A, Wingrem S, Smeds S, Larsson SE, Wasteson A. Suramin inhibits growth of human osteosarcoma xenografts in nude mice. Cancer Res 1991;51:585.
95. Warr GA, Jakab GJ. Lung macrophage defense responses during suramin-induced lysosomal dysfunction. Exp Mol Pathol 1983;38:193.
96. Wellstein A, Zugmaier G, Califano JA III, Kern F, Palk S, Lippman ME. Tumor growth dependent on Kaposi's sarcoma-derived fibroblast growth factor inhibited by pentosan polysulfate. JNCI 1991;83:716.
97. Westermark B, Heldin CH. Platelet-derived growth factor as a mediator of normal and neoplastic cell proliferation. Med Oncol Tumor Pharmacother 1986;3:177.
98. Williams LT, Tremble PM, Lavin MF, Sunday ME. Platelet-derived growth factor receptors from a high affinity state in membrane preparations. Kinetics and affinity cross-linking studies. J Biol Chem 1984;259:5287.
99. Wolpe SD, Cerami A. Macrophage inflammatory proteins 1 and 2: members of a novel superfamily of cytokines. FASEB J 1989;3:2565.
100. Wright TC Jr, Castellot JJ Jr, Petitou M, Lormeau JC, Karnovsky MJ. Strucutral determinants of heparin's growth inhibitory activity. Interdependence of oligosaccharide size and charge. J Biol Chem 1989;264:534.
101. Yayon A, Klagsbrun M, Esco JD, Leder P, Ornitz DM. Cell surface heparin-like molecules are required for binding of basic fibroblast growth factor to its high affinity receptor. Cell 1991;64:841.
102. Zabrenetzky VS, Kohn EC, Roberts DD. Suramin inhibits laminin-and thrombospondin-mediated melanoma cell adhesion and migration and binding of these adhesive proteins to sulfatide. Cancer Res 1990;50:5937.
103. Zack J, Smith RG, Ozanne B. Characterization of a leukemia-derived transforming growth factor. Leukemia 1987;1:737-745.
104. Zhan X, Bates B, Hu XG, Goldfar M. The human FGF-5 oncogene encodes a novel protein related to fibroblast growth factor. Mol Cell Biol 1988;88:3487.

SECTION XVII

PRINCIPLES OF ENDOCRINE THERAPY

CHAPTER 69

Steroid Hormone Binding and Hormone Receptors

ELWOOD V. JENSEN AND EUGENE R. DESOMBRE

Introduction

It has long been recognized that some human cancers are hormone-dependent in that their growth is influenced by variations in levels of steroid sex hormones, and they undergo regression after removal of glands producing these supporting agents. In the case of breast cancer, as early as 1836 Cooper (22) observed a correlation between tumor growth and the menstrual cycle, and in 1896 Beatson (9) reported the regression of metastatic lesions after oophorectomy in some premenopausal patients. For postmenopausal women, where breast cancer occurs most frequently, Huggins and Bergenstal (58) demonstrated in 1952 that excision of the adrenal glands can provide significant remission of metastatic disease, and Luft and Olivecrona (86) obtained similar regression after hypophysectomy. For prostatic cancer, Huggins and Hodges (59) reported in 1941 that most patients with advanced disease show striking remissions after orchiectomy or the administration of estrogenic hormones.

Hormone deprivation, by surgical ablation of steroidogenic glands, or alteration of the endocrine milieu, by administration of hormone antagonists or inhibitors of hormone biosynthesis, provides effective palliative treatment for patients whose metastatic tumors are of the hormone-dependent type. In contrast to prostatic cancer, in which the majority of tumors respond to endocrine therapy, less than one third of the patients with advanced breast cancer show objective remission to hormonal manipulation. Thus, there has been a need for some means to predict which breast tumors are hormone-dependent, so that endocrine therapy can be restricted to those persons it can help, and patients with nondependent tumors can be placed directly on other kinds of treatments.

Recognition that steroid sex hormones exert their actions in so-called target tissues in combination with intracellular receptor proteins, and that nontarget tissues generally contain only small amounts of such receptors, suggested an approach to predicting hormone dependency in breast cancers (63). In the early 1970s, it was reported (32, 61, 82, 87) that determination of the estrogen receptor content of an excised specimen of a primary or metastatic tumor indicates the likelihood of response to endocrine therapy for the majority of breast cancer patients with advanced disease. Tumors containing estrogen receptors were then shown to have a better chance of response if they also had progestin receptors (56). It was also found that the receptor content of the primary tumor is an indicator of the risk of cancer recurrence in mastectomy patients with no evident metastases (75, 139). Thus, determination of estrogen and progestin receptors in primary and metastatic breast cancers, as a guide to prognosis and therapy selection, has become standard medical practice (28). There is also a relation between the presence of estrogen receptors in the primary tumor and the site where the first metastases are most likely to appear (128, 139).

Receptor Proteins in Steroid Hormone Action

During the 3 decades since the discovery of steroid hormone receptors, much progress has been made toward an understanding of the nature of receptor proteins and of their role in the action of hormones in target cells (8, 13, 60, 144). Receptor proteins were first demonstrated for the estrogens by the ability of target tissues, especially the rodent uterus, to take up and bind labeled estradiol without chemical alteration of the steroid itself (65). Similar binding studies, both in vivo and in vitro, soon established the existence of specific receptors for all classes of steroid hormones (44, 60, 83). Unlike receptors for peptide hormones, which are located in the cell membrane and require a second messenger to transmit the regulatory signal to the eventual site of action, receptors for steroid hormones reside within the target cell. Here they are loosely held until association with the hormone converts them to an activated form that can bind tightly in the genome to stimulate RNA synthesis (62).

During recent years, techniques of molecular biology and immunology have provided detailed knowledge about receptor structure and function (34, 78). Cloning of the cDNAs for various steroid hormone receptors has led to elucidation of their primary structures.

With the aid of deletion mutants, different domains in the molecule have been identified and correlated with specific aspects of receptor function. Steroid receptors belong to a general family of intracellular proteins that mediate the actions of many important cell regulators, including the gonadal and adrenal hormones (Fig. 69.1), vitamin D, ecdysone, thyroid hormone, and retinoic acid (107). Al-

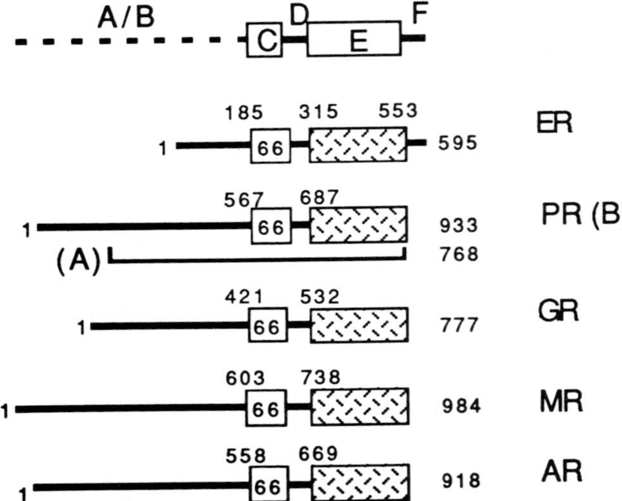

Figure 69.1. Structures of human receptor proteins for gonadal and adrenal hormones. Top diagram shows the six functional domains: A/B, F, modulating regions; C, DNA-binding region; D, "hinge" region; E, hormone-binding region. *Boxes*, highly conserved domains; *thin black lines*, regions of low homology. Position of each domain boundary is given as the number of amino acids from the amino terminus (left). For these receptors, the C domain contains 66 amino acids. Receptors are estrogen (ER), progestin (A and B forms) (PR), glucocorticoid (GR), mineralocorticoid (MR), and androgen (AR).

though these receptor proteins vary in size from 427 amino acids for vitamin D to 984 for mineralocorticoid, corresponding to molecular weights of 47.5 to 107 kD, they are composed of comparable units. Each contains a DNA-binding domain of 66 to 68 amino acids (C), showing a high degree of homology throughout the family; a ligand-binding domain (E) with some homology; a small hinge region (D) joining these two domains; and variable regions (A/B, F) showing little homology. Avian and human progestin receptors are unique in that they come in two sizes; the B form consists of the A protein plus an additional unit at the N terminus. Through a pair of zinc fingers in the C region, the activated steroid-receptor complex, in dimeric form, binds to a hormone response element (HRE) in the target gene, located upstream from the transcription site, to enhance RNA synthesis, apparently acting in concert with other transcription factors.

The conversion of the native receptor protein to a functional transcription factor has been the subject of much investigation (49), as the concept of hormone-induced receptor transformation identified, for the first time, a biochemical role for the steroid (62). It is now established that the activation process involves the removal of a dimeric heat shock protein (15, 122), which obscures the DNA-binding region in the native receptor, as well as of other macromolecular and micromolecular factors that make up the native receptor conglomerate (114, 132). Just how interaction with the steroid can effect this disaggregation under physiologic conditions, the role of phosphorylation in the activation phenomenon, and the precise mechanism by which transformed receptor enhances transcription in target genes remains unclear.

Measurement of Estrogen and Progestin Receptors

STEROID BINDING METHODS

The first correlations of hormone receptors with breast cancer response to endocrine therapy involved uptake of radioactive hormone by tumor tissue after administration of tritiated hexestrol to patients (37), or on incubation of excised tumor slices with tritiated estradiol at 37°C, in the presence and absence of either excess unlabeled hormone or an antiestrogen to distinguish between specific and nonspecific binding (61, 68). When it was found that, before exposure to hormone, the receptor in target cells is not tightly held and appears in the supernatant fraction of tissue homogenates, this protein could be detected conveniently by adding excess tritiated estradiol to tumor cytosol and counting the protein-bound radioactivity. Several procedures have been developed for distinguishing between bound steroid and the excess unbound hormone. These include identification of the steroid-receptor complex by sedimentation in sucrose gradients (61, 67), or by electrophoresis (137) or isoelectric focusing (143) on gels; precipitation of the complex with protamine sulfate (16) or adsorption on hydroxylapatite (43, 54); and the removal of unbound hormone by adsorption on dextran-coated charcoal (DCC) (77) or immobilized antibody to the steroid (14, 36). Each of these techniques has advantages and drawbacks.

Many of the earlier measurements of receptors in breast cancers were done with the sedimentation technique. This procedure, while most informative, is too costly and time consuming to be employed for routine assays. Moreover, the values as originally obtained, although self-consistent, did not indicate directly the total binding capacity of the cytosol; however, they can be readily corrected to provide this value (67). As receptor assays were undertaken on a larger scale, most laboratories adopted the dextran-coated charcoal procedure. Because DCC causes some dissociation of steroid from the receptor, the preferred technique involves incubating cytosol aliquots with several hormone concentrations, in each case plotting the ratio of bound to free steroid against the amount bound, according to Scatchard's method (124), and extrapolating the best linear plot (Fig. 69.2) (142). The intercept with the abscissa gives the total binding capacity, and the reciprocal of the slope indicates the dissociation constant of the complex, thus distinguishing high-affinity binding to receptor from weaker, nonspecific interactions. A disadvantage of such titration procedures is that they require a larger tumor specimen than often is available, especially with metastatic cancers. For such cases, a single high concentration of hormone can be employed, although a single point saturation assay is less accurate and informative than is a multipoint determination. A further problem with the DCC procedure is that the free steroid concentration, calculated as the difference between the total (original) and bound concentrations, is often overestimated, and thus the bound/free ratio underestimated, when there is nonspecific

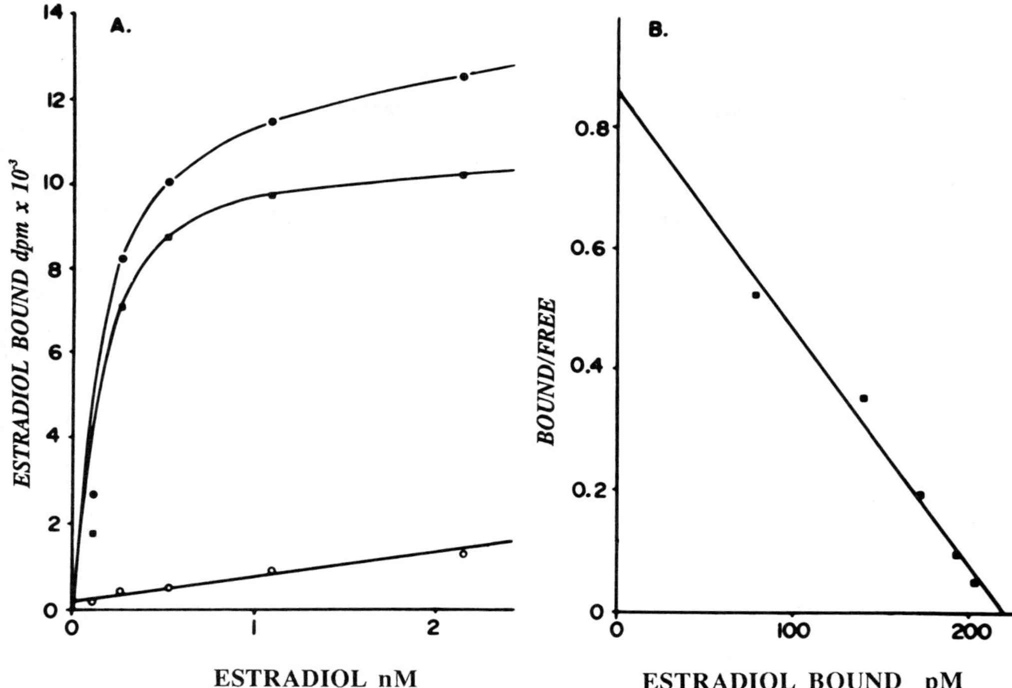

Figure 69.2. Titration analysis of estrogen receptors in human breast carcinoma. **A.** Aliquots (100 μl) of cytosol prepared from a frozen powder of human breast cancer were incubated with 100 μl of buffer containing increasing amounts of [^{3}H]estradiol, in the presence (*open circle*) or absence (*closed circle*) of a 200-fold excess of diethylstilbestrol. After adsorption of unbound steroid on dextran-coated charcoal, the specific binding (*closed box*) was obtained by the difference in soluble radioactivity in the presence and absence of competitor. **B.** The titration data from A were plotted according to the method of Scatchard (124), the free steroid concentration being calculated by the difference between the bound radioactivity and that originally present. The binding capacity is calculated from the intercept on the abcissa, and the dissociation constant (0.21 nM) from the slope of the line. *Source:* Wittliff et al. (142).

association with substances other than the receptor (127).

The foregoing assay procedures were mostly developed for estrogen receptor (ER), but many of them have been applied for the determination of progestin receptor (PR) as well. Most progestin receptor assays have employed the DCC technique.

All steroid-binding procedures suffer from two inherent disadvantages: (*a*) steroid hormone receptors are labile proteins that easily lose binding capacity during storage and processing of the tumor specimen, and (*b*) unless some kind of ligand-exchange procedure is carried out, they do not detect receptor that is already occupied by endogenous hormone or by endocrine agents used in therapy. Binding loss can be minimized by rapidly cooling the specimen after excision, storing it at −80°C or below, pulverizing it in liquid nitrogen, and homogenizing briefly with cooling with a Polytron apparatus in a medium containing traces of a sulfhydryl compound to protect against heavy metals, which inactivate the receptor. Techniques for exchanging endogenous ligand have been developed (6, 16, 145), but these often cause some loss of binding, and they introduce an additional step into the assay procedure.

IMMUNOCHEMICAL METHODS

With the availability of monoclonal antibodies to human estrogen (47, 48) and progestin (33, 46) receptors, it became possible to utilize techniques of immunochemistry and immunocytochemistry for measuring these proteins in breast cancers. Because these antibodies recognize occupied as well as unoccupied receptor, and, in some cases, receptor that has lost steroid-binding ability, immunochemical methods can overcome many of the difficulties inherent in binding techniques. Moreover, they eliminate the need for radioactivity. Two immunochemical procedures for receptor analysis have been developed (64): a sandwich-type enzyme immunoassay (EIA) (105), for measuring receptor in tumor cytosols, and an immunocytochemical assay (ICA) (73) that detects receptor in individual cells of a tumor section or fine-needle aspirate. Kits for either type of assay for estrogen and progestin receptors are now available from Abbott Laboratories and are widely used throughout the world. Early experience with immunoassay for estrogen receptors is summarized in a supplemental issue of *Cancer Research* (115), whereas the immunocytochemical assay for estrogen and progestin receptors is discussed in detail in a recent monograph (109). A direct comparison of the EIA procedure with the usual steroid-binding technique attests to the superiority of the immunochemical assay (55).

In the enzyme immunoassay for estrogen and progestin receptors in tumor cytosol, one monoclonal antibody,[a]

[a] In the original Abbott EIA for estrogen receptor (105), antibody D547 was used to adsorb the receptor and D75 served as the enzyme-labeled reagent; more recently, D75 has been replaced by H222 as the labeled antibody (64). In the EIA for progestin receptor (46), KD68 and JZB39 are used as the anchor and label, respectively.

bound to a polystyrene bead, adsorbs the receptor from the diluted cytosol (Fig. 69.3). The immobilized receptor is then treated with a second monoclonal antibody, which binds to a different region of the receptor molecule and is linked to an enzyme (horseradish peroxidase) that gives rise to a yellow color when exposed to substrate (hydrogen peroxide plus *o*-phenylenediamine). The color intensity is read in a colorimeter, and the receptor content of the cytosol calculated from a standard curve obtained with lyophilized cytosol from MCF-7 breast tumor cells for estrogen receptor and from T47D cells for progestin receptor. The steroid-binding capacity of each reference standard is originally determined by DCC assay. Because the cytosol can be diluted extensively, analyses can be done with very small tumor samples, even with fine-needle aspiration biopsies (90). Immunoassay can be carried out on specimens from patients receiving tamoxifen therapy, where steroid-binding techniques fail to detect receptor. However, tumor specimens from tamoxifen-treated patients show abnormally high values on immunoassay (90) because the antiestrogen exposes an additional epitope in the receptor for the antibody (H222) that is used as the marker in the EIA (92).

The immunocytochemical assays employ the peroxidase-antiperoxidase method of Sternberger (134), in which frozen tumor sections, after gentle fixation, are treated, first with an antireceptor antibody, then with a bridging antibody (goat antirat immunoglobulin), and finally with peroxidase-antiperoxidase (PAP) reagent. Subsequent treatment with hydro-

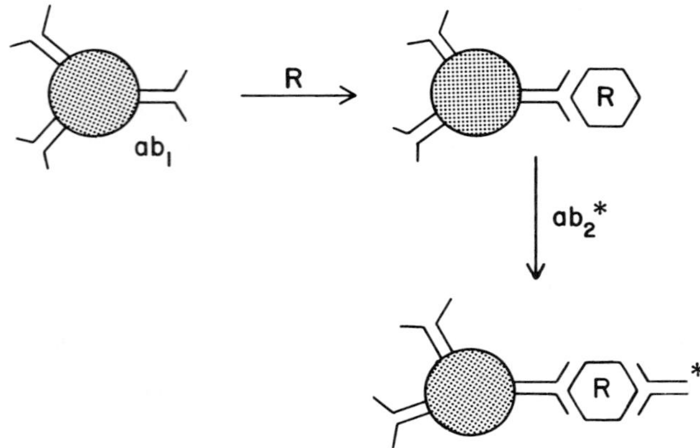

Figure 69.3. System for the immunochemical determination of receptors. A polystyrene bead, coated with one monoclonal antibody preparation, adsorbs the receptor (R, occupied or unoccupied) from the diluted cytosol. The receptor thus bound then reacts at a different site with a second antibody that has been labeled with an enzyme (*) that serves as the basis for a colorimetric assay. *Source:* Greene et al. (48).

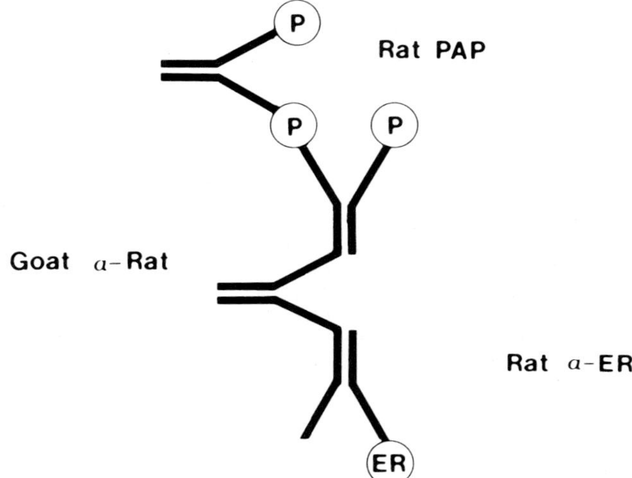

Figure 69.4. Schematic representation of the immunocytochemical assay (ERICA) for estrogen receptor in a tissue section, using goat antirat immunoglobulin as a bridge between the peroxidase/antiperoxidase reagent (P) and the monoclonal antibody bound to receptor in the tissue.

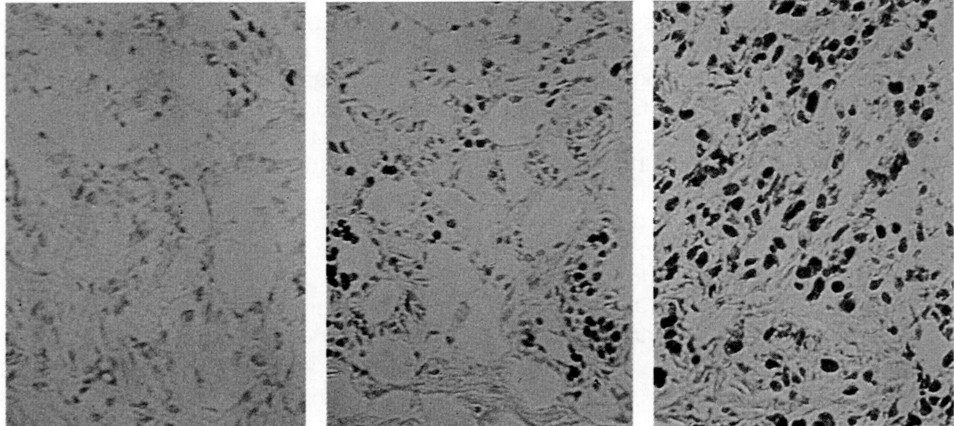

Figure 69.5. Immunocytochemical identification of estrogen receptors in 8 μm frozen sections of human breast cancers using monoclonal antibody H222 and the method of King et al. (73), except that fixation was in picric acid-paraformaldehyde rather than ethanol. Cancers show low (left), moderate (center), or high (right) proportions of receptor-containing cells. ×100. *Source:* DeSombre et al. (31).

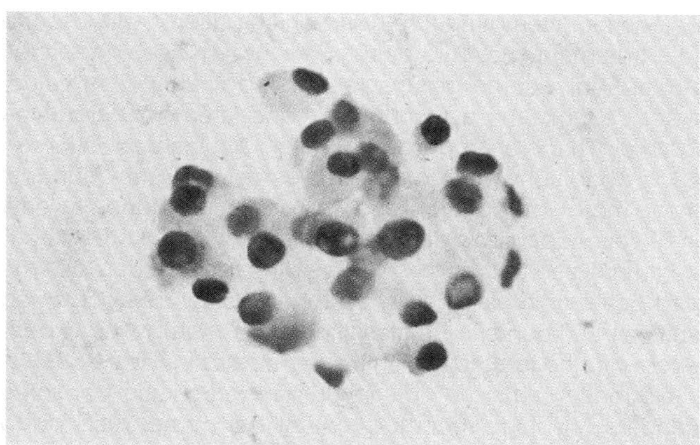

Figure 69.6. Similar to 69.5 with a fine needle aspiration biopsy of an ER-rich human breast cancer. ×250.

gen peroxide and *p*-diaminobenzidine produces a brown stain in the cells where the receptor has retained the antibody and, thereby, the PAP reagent (Fig. 69.4). Abbott immunocytochemical assays for estrogen (ERICA) and progestin (PRICA) receptors use antibodies H222 and KD68, respectively. Counter-staining is with hematoxylin to delineate cell nuclei (Fig. 69.5).

Because immunocytochemical procedures detect receptors in individual cells, they can be used with very small tumor sections or fine-needle aspiration biopsies of either bone marrow (10) or tumor (12, 50, 95, 141) (Fig. 69.6). For estrogen receptor, the ERICA technique is most dependable and sensitive with frozen sections of tumors, although it has been used successfully with paraffin-embedded specimens if the tissue was fixed in a special way with cold buffered formalin (125) or Bouin's solution (27, 113). Specimens fixed in formalin in the usual way can yield erratic results, so negative staining patterns are of questionable significance. However, subjecting the section to enzymatic digestion with trypsin (4, 53), pronase (18), or DNase (126) permits the use of conventionally fixed tissues and thus the assay of archival samples of breast cancers. It has since been found (101) that, after brief ficin predigestion, routinely processed, paraffin-embedded tumor sections give excellent results if antibody D73 rather than H222 is used in the ERICA procedure. In contrast to estrogen receptor, ICA analysis of progestin receptor is reported to work well with embedded specimens without the need for special fixation (104).

In attempts to quantify the results of immunocytochemistry, staining descriptions have been proposed that consider both the proportion of receptor-containing cells and the degree of staining. These include the H Score (93) and the staining intensity index (SII) (94), in which individual cells are assigned to different staining categories and the percentage of cells in each group, multiplied by an intensity factor, is totaled. Such characterization of tumors has proved quite successful in predicting prognosis for recurrence and response to therapy. More recent developments, involving use of automated optical instrumentation, are the SAMBA computed image analysis (17, 21) and the receptogram (109, 129), each of which yields characteristic patterns derived from a combination of receptor concentration (measured optical density, MOD) and receptor content (integrated optical density, IOD) of individual tumor cells.

Receptors and Response to Endocrine Therapy

ESTROGEN RECEPTORS

The rationale of estrogen receptor (ER) determination to identify hormone-dependent breast cancers originated in the observations of the uptake and binding of tritiated estrogens by female reproductive tissues of experimental animals, and the subsequent realization that steroid hormones require receptor proteins to exert their biologic actions. Early studies demonstrated that, when injected with tritiated hexestrol, patients who subsequently responded favorably to adrenalectomy incorporated more radioactivity into their tumors than did those who did not respond (37). With the advent of techniques for determining estrogen binding by tissues in vitro, and then by receptor in the cytosol fraction of tissue homogenates, it became possible to examine excised specimens of breast cancers for the correlation of receptor levels with clinical response. Four early reports (32, 61, 82, 87) established that patients whose tumors lacked detectable ER rarely responded to either endocrine ablation or hormone manipulation (3 of 71 = 4%), whereas most patients with ER-containing cancers (42 of 49 = 86%) received benefit from such treatment. In 1974, investigators from 14 groups in various countries reported similar findings at a workshop sponsored by the Breast Cancer Task Force of the U.S. National Cancer Institute (97). Despite the different procedures used for determining estrogen binding, the conclusions were in substantial agreement: about 60% of patients with ER-positive cancers showed objective remission to some type of endocrine therapy, as compared with less than 10% of those with ER-negative tumors.

As methods for the measurement of receptor proteins became more sensitive, it was found that most breast cancers contain small amounts of estrogen receptor. However, tumors with lower receptor content rarely respond to endocrine therapy, so that quantitative ER levels are important (30, 66, 67, 80, 106, 108). For example, of 160 treated patients studied from 1966 to 1976 at the University of Chicago (29), very few objective remissions were observed in patients whose tumors contained less than a certain amount of receptor (Fig. 69.7). This critical level appears to be lower in premenopausal women, either because more of the receptor is occupied by endogenous hormone and is not detected by binding assay or because the actual production of receptor may be reduced in the presence of higher serum levels of hormone (51). Because tumors with definite but low receptor content rarely respond to endocrine manipulation, it is more realistic to classify patients as receptor-rich or receptor-poor, rather than as positive or negative. If the low receptor cancers are considered receptor-poor rather than positive, the remaining ER-rich cancers show a response rate to endocrine ablation of 71% as compared with 3% in the ER-poor group (29).

When the determination of estrogen receptors in breast

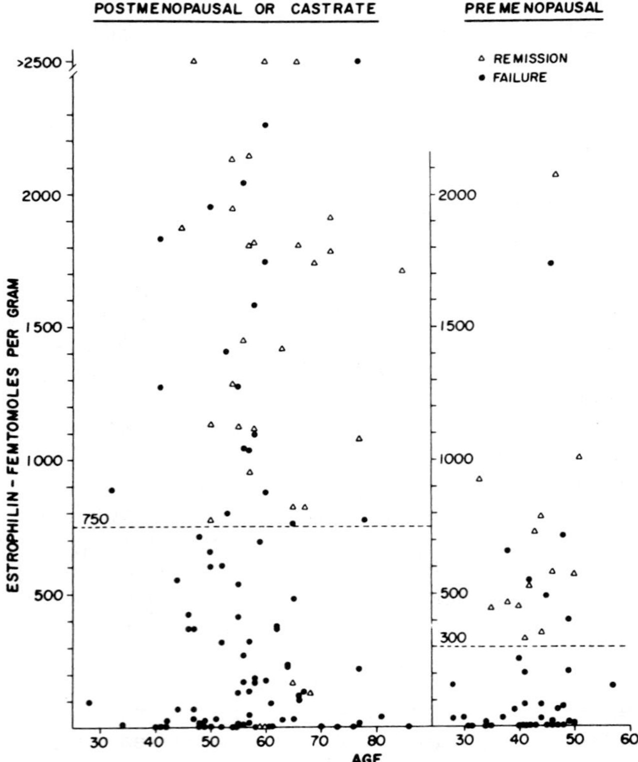

Figure 69.7. Correlation of cytosol ER content with objective remissions to endocrine therapy for 160 patients with metastatic breast cancer. Assays were carried out by sucrose gradient ultracentrifugation using nonsaturating concentrations of tritiated estradiol. When receptor values are corrected to saturation (67), the division between receptor-rich and receptor-poor tumors occurs at about 2.5 pmol per gram of tumor for postmenopausal patients and 1.0 pmol/g for premenopausal patients. With the amount of protein usually found in breast tumor cytosols, these results suggest that the optimal dividing level for postmenopausal patients is about 50 fmol ER per milligram of cytosol protein. *Source:* DeSombre et al. (29).

cancers became a routine clinical procedure, the correlations with patient response generally were not as favorable as those just described or those in the original reports. A somewhat higher proportion of patients with ER-negative tumors were found to respond to endocrine therapy, probably because assays carried out in central laboratories on specimens sent in from different sources provide more chance for the labile receptor protein to lose its binding capacity during tissue collection, storage, and processing. The lower response rate among the so-called positive tumors (often quoted as 50% or less) is attributable, at least in part, to the way positivity has been defined. For reasons more of convenience than of scientific merit, receptor content is expressed in relation to total cytosol protein, a parameter that varies with the serum content of the tumor. Despite evidence that breast cancers with low receptor levels rarely respond to endocrine therapy, tumors originally were considered to be ER-positive if they contained 3 fmol of receptor per milligram of cytosol protein, about the level of detectability. With this definition, many investigators found that 70 to 80% of breast cancers were called ER positive, which is not a very useful criterion in attempting to predict which patients will respond to a treatment known to benefit fewer than 35% of the total. Accordingly, some groups readjusted the dividing value, first to 10 fmol/mg cytosol protein and later to 20 and even 30 fmol. This is an improvement, although the data in Figure 69.7, when converted to femtomoles per milligram, suggest that a more appropriate value would be even higher, at least in postmenopausal patients. Of more than 1,300 breast cancers analyzed at the University of Chicago, about two thirds had detectable estrogen receptor, but only 35% contained sufficient amounts to be classified as ER-rich by the experience with the treated patients summarized in Figure 69.7.

No matter what the optimal cutoff level should be, some cancers with high receptor content still do not respond to hormonal manipulation (29, 88). Explanations include the possibility that the receptor protein in these tumors binds hormone but is otherwise nonfunctional, that tumor cells have escaped from hormone dependency without shutting down receptor synthesis (this appears to be the case in some autonomous rat mammary tumors [7]), or that the cancer is a mixture of hormone-dependent and autonomous cells, with the former responsible for a positive receptor assay but the latter precluding a significant response to endocrine therapy. Both by multiple sampling (25, 136) and by immunocytochemistry (31, 64, 73) (compare Fig. 69.5), many, if not most, breast cancers are seen to be heterogeneous, showing both ER-containing and noncontaining cells. A good response may be observed only with tumors in which the proportion of ER-containing cells is so great that their regression following endocrine treatment results in a significant overall remission of the cancer.

The immunocytochemical procedure for determining steroid receptors in tumor specimens not only has the advantage of being applicable to small tissue samples, but, by identifying receptor in individual cells, it also gives a valuable indication of the relative numbers of ER-positive and ER-negative cells in the tumor. A high proportion of negative cells is associated with poor prognosis (138). When semiquantitative criteria for distinguishing between positive and negative tumors are employed, ICA appears to to be somewhat superior to biochemical methods; in two studies (94, 110), the response rates in the ER-positive group were 72 and 80%, respectively, as compared with 4 and 8% in those with low staining indices. In 336 patients studied in nine different laboratories, the overall response rate in the ER-positive group was 74% by ERICA, as compared with 65% by DCC assay (3). Included in this summary are results obtained with fine-needle aspiration biopsy (10, 12).

Although a subpopulation of autonomous cells may be the reason why some tumors with intermediate ER levels are unresponsive to hormone manipulation, this explanation seems less likely for nonresponding cancers with high ER content in which few receptor-free cells would be expected. As discussed in the next section, analysis of the progestin receptor content of a tumor has been utilized with some success as a measure of functional estrogen receptor (56), but many PR-containing cancers still do not respond. There is growing evidence that the estrogen receptor protein may be aberrant in many breast tumors (42, 98). Early studies of the association of ER complexes with nuclei in vivo (79), in whole cells

(133), or in nuclear suspensions (89), as well as immunohistochemical detection of estradiol-induced translocation of receptor from cytoplasm to nucleus in tumor sections (116), have demonstrated impaired interaction with the nucleus in some ER-containing breast cancers. In cases where clinical correlations could be made, deficient nuclear binding was associated with poor response to endocrine therapy. It has been shown that some human tumors contain either truncated (131) or apparently normal (38, 102) estrogen receptors that bind hormone and react with antibody but cannot bind to an estrogen response element or induce a growth response.

With techniques of molecular biology, abnormalities have been demonstrated in the receptor mRNAs of various breast cancers and, in some cases, in the proteins expressed from them. Many of these involve truncations or exon deletions in regions coding for the steroid-binding domain (E, Fig. 69.1) (39, 40, 103), although a point mutation in the B region has also been reported (81). In T47D cells, postulated to be a model for the transition from an estrogen-responsive to an estrogen-resistant state, deletions involving the DNA-binding domain (C) have been detected (45, 140). A receptor lacking exon 7 has been identified in ER+/PR− breast cancers, which cannot induce transcription in a responsive gene construct but which can inhibit the ability of the wild-type receptor to do so (40). As discussed below, a variant receptor, lacking the 5 exon and showing transcriptional activity without the need for ligand, has been demonstrated in some ER−/PR+ breast cancers (39).

The significance of variant receptors in the clinical management of breast cancer patients remains to be elucidated, but these findings offer promise for achieving better correlation of receptor assays with response to therapy and a clearer understanding of the progression from hormone-dependent to hormone-resistant disease (41, 70, 130). Mutant receptors may also shed light on the phenomenon of acquired tamoxifen resistance, which limits the use of this agent for the long term treatment of some patients. Although neither the constitutively active $\Delta 5$ deletion mutant from ER−/PR+ tumors (24) nor a number of other ER variants studied (111) appears to be responsible for tamoxifen resistance in human breast tumors, the identification of mutant receptors, with which the antiestrogen acts as an agonist rather than an antagonist (71, 91), may provide a clue to how formerly responsive cancers escape from control.

Because many patients with advanced breast cancer do not have readily accessible metastatic lesions for analysis, it was of interest to determine whether receptor analysis of the primary tumor at the time of mastectomy can predict response to endocrine therapy if the cancer recurs in disseminated form. Early studies indicated that metastases generally, but not always (79), resemble the primary cancer in their receptor content, and that the mastectomy specimen can be used for prediction of response to therapy at a later time (11, 30, 106). This conclusion has been confirmed in many studies, and analysis of primary tumors at the time of mastectomy is done routinely.

Early studies on patients being treated with cytotoxic chemotherapy suggested that those with ER-negative breast cancers may respond more favorably to chemotherapy than will those with ER-positive cancers (84, 85). Although some laboratories reported similar findings, which are consistent with the impression that ER-negative tumors are more aggressive, are less differentiated, and grow more rapidly, most workers could not confirm these observations. Not only did several investigators find no correlation of receptor status with response to chemotherapy (52, 69, 118, 119), but others actually observed a higher response rate among the ER-positive group (23, 72, 121). The significance of some of these studies is limited by their use of either 3 or 5 fmol/mg protein as the definition of an ER-positive tumor, but others employed more reasonable criteria, so one must conclude that an inverse relation between ER positivity and response to cytotoxic chemotherapy has not been established.

PROGESTIN RECEPTORS

Since the failure of some ER-containing breast cancers to respond to endocrine treatment might result from the receptor's being nonfunctional, it was proposed that progestin receptor (PR), known to be produced by estrogen action in female reproductive tissues (117), might serve as a measure of functional estrogen receptor (56). It was found that breast cancers containing both estrogen and progestin receptors show a higher response rate (81%) than those having ER alone (41%) (96, 100, 106). In these studies, the ER-positive category has included receptor-poor cancers, which do not respond, so part of the effect may result from the fact that PR-positive tumors in general are those that also have a higher ER content. Nonetheless, the determination of PR in addition to ER appears to be of value, and analysis of both receptors is generally recommended (28).

A small number of breast cancers are found to be ER negative, PR positive; some of these respond to endocrine therapy (106). This observation is difficult to reconcile with the accepted view that PR synthesis depends on estrogen action. However, it has been reported that many such tumors, especially in premenopausal patients, actually do contain estrogen receptors that are not detected by steroid-binding assay unless the cytosol is first treated with charcoal (123). In some instances, ER-positive, PR-negative tumors have been found to contain an aberrant RNA for estrogen receptor that lacks exon 5 in the steroid-binding domain; expression of this gives a truncated protein showing ligand-independent transcriptional activity (39). Such a constitutively active receptor would preclude the need for estrogenic stimulation for the synthesis of progestin receptor.

Receptors and Prognosis for Cancer Recurrence

The observation (75,139) that mastectomy patients with ER-positive primary tumors show a lower incidence of recurrence of advanced disease, and a longer disease-free interval if they do recur, opened a new dimension in the application of receptor analysis to the clinical management of breast cancer (Fig. 69.8). This prognostic criterion appears to be independent of tumor size or nodal status and permits the classification of patients into three groups as to the risk of recurrence: low (ER positive, node negative); intermediate (ER negative, node negative, and ER positive, node positive), and high (ER negative, node positive) (19, 31). This information is of value in the choice of adjuvant or prophylactic therapy after mastectomy. Patients in the high-risk group can justifiably be treated aggressively with cytotoxic chemotherapy, whereas those in the low-risk group can be spared this discomfort and receive either no treatment or a nontraumatic endocrine therapy, such as tamoxifen. The presence of progesterone receptors also was found to predict disease-free survival and may be superior to estrogen receptor (112), especially with stage II primary cancers (20, 100).

Although a relation between the presence of ER and/or PR and the duration of the disease-free interval has been observed in many laboratories, some investigators failed to confirm these findings (2, 26, 35, 57, 120), while others concluded that only ER is of prognostic value (135). It was also found that differences in disease-free survival, observed during the first few years after mastectomy, disappear after a longer time (1). Thus, there has been some controversy over the value of receptor assays in the prognostication for cancer recurrence. It has been suggested that, for the best prediction, one should consider a combination of receptor content with other parameters, such as nuclear grade, tumor size, and ploidy (99).

As in the case of response to therapy, the usefulness of biochemical receptor assays for prognostic information has been hampered by arbitrary definitions of positive and negative tumors and by the fact that most cancers are mixtures of receptor-containing and noncontaining cells. With immunocytochemical procedures, which consider both the staining intensity and the number of cells stained, the prognostic value of receptor determinations appears to be greatly enhanced. The ERICA procedure was found to be equivalent (5, 31) or superior (3, 74) to biochemical ER determination, and, after a 5-year observation period, the ICA, but not the DCC assay, was still able to distinguish between higher- and lower-risk groups (74). In these studies, ER rather than PR had the highest prognostic significance.

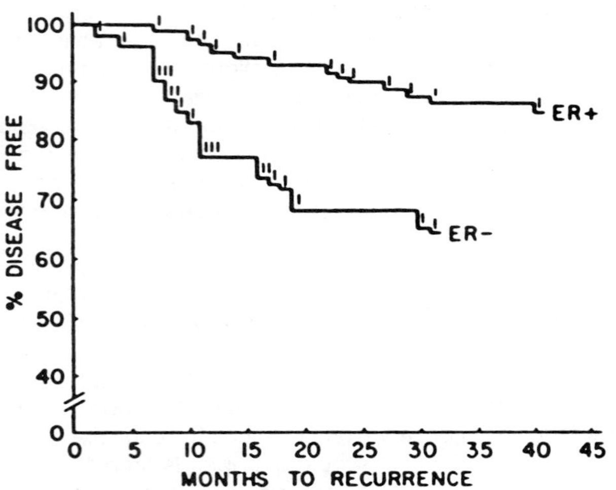

Chart 1. ER and recurrence in all patients.

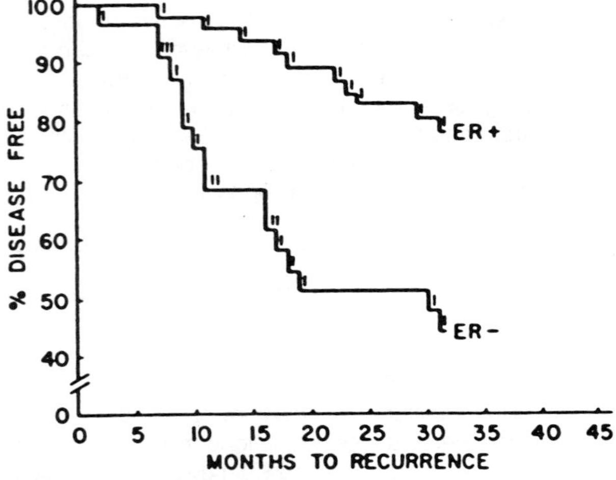

Figure 69.8. Relation of ER status of the primary tumor to the time of appearance of first metastases after mastectomy. Chart 1: 145 patients irrespective of nodal involvement. Chart 2: 74 patients with one or more positive axillary nodes. ER negative = <10 fmol/mg cytosol protein by DCC assay. *Source:* Knight et al. (75).

Receptors and Site of First Metastases

Not only do estrogen and progestin receptor assays on primary breast cancers furnish useful information about the

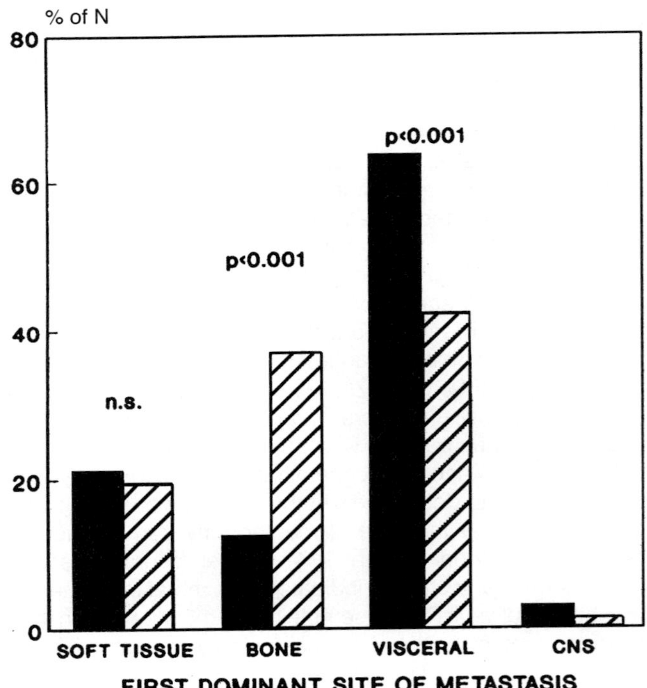

Figure 69.9. The location of first metastases in relation to the estrogen receptor status of the primary breast cancer. ER negative = <10 fmol/mg cytosol protein by DCC assay. *Source:* Koenders et al. (76).

prognosis for recurrence and the response of metastases to endocrine therapy, but they also provide a clue as to the most probable location where the first metastases will appear. The early observations (128, 139) that ER-positive primary tumors show a greater tendency to spread to bone, and ER-negative cancers to lung and liver, have been widely confirmed (76) (Fig. 69.9). Both estrogen and progestin receptors show similar patterns, but ER appears to be the only independent prognostic factor for this phenomenon (76).

Summary

Determination of estrogen and progestin receptors in excised breast cancer tissue provides information concerning the response of the patient to endocrine therapy, the risk of recurrence of advanced disease, and the probable site of first metastases. Such assays have been of considerable value, but their usefulness has been limited by the lability of the steroid-binding capacity of the receptor, the heterogeneity of many tumor specimens, and the use of less than an optimal definition of receptor positivity. The recent development of immunochemical assays, and especially of immunocytochemical techniques that identify receptor with individual cancer cells, promises to overcome many of these deficiencies and to enhance the utility of receptor measurements in the clinical management of breast cancer patients. In some cases, mutant forms of the receptor may be responsible for poor correlation; a simple procedure for the routine identification of such receptor variants would be a valuable asset.

Acknowledgments

Preparation of this chapter was supported by a grant (RDP-53B) from the American Cancer Society.

References

1. Aamdal S, Børmer O, Jørgensen O, Høst H, Eliassen G, Kaalhus O, Pihl A. Estrogen receptors and long-term prognosis in breast cancer. Cancer 1984;53:2525–2529.
2. Alanko A, Heinonen E, Scheinin T, Tolppanen EM, Vihko R. Significance of estrogen and progesterone receptors, disease-free interval, and site of first metastasis on survival of breast cancer patients. Cancer 1985;56:1696–1700.
3. Allred DC, Bustamante MA, Daniel CO, Gaskill HV, Cruz AB Jr. Immunocytochemical analysis of estrogen receptors in human breast carcinomas. Arch Surg 1990;125: 107–113.
4. Andersen J, Ørntoft TF, Poulsen HS. Immunohistochemical demonstration of estrogen receptors (ER) in formalin-fixed, paraffin-embedded human breast cancer tissue by use of a monoclonal antibody to ER. J Histochem Cytochem 1988;36:1553–1560.
5. Andersen J, Thorpe SM, King WJ, Rose C, Christensen I, Rasmussen BB, Poulsen HS. The prognostic value of immunohistochemical estrogen receptor analysis in paraffin-embedded and frozen sections versus that of steroid-binding assays. Eur J Cancer 1990;26:442–449.
6. Anderson JN, Clark JH, Peck EJ Jr. Oestrogen and nuclear binding sites. Determination of specific sites by [^{3}H]oestradiol exchange. Biochem J 1972;126:561–567.
7. Arbogast LY, DeSombre ER. Estrogen-dependent in vitro stimulation of RNA synthesis in hormone-dependent mammary tumors of the rat. JNCI 1975;54:483–485.
8. Beato M. Gene regulation by steroid hormones. Cell 1989;56:335–344.
9. Beatson GT. On the treatment of inoperable cases of carcinoma of the mamma: suggestions for a new method of treatment with illustrative cases. Lancet 1896;2: 104–107.
10. Berger U, Mansi JL, Wilson P, Coombes RC. Detection of estrogen receptor in bone marrow from patients with metastatic breast cancer. J Clin Oncol 1987;5:1779–1782.
11. Block GE, Ellis RS, DeSombre E, Jensen E. Correlation of estrophilin content of primary mammary cancer to eventual endocrine treatment. Ann Surg 1978;188: 372–375.
12. Burton GV, Flowers JL, Cox EB, et al. Estrogen receptor determination by monoclonal antibody in fine needle aspiration breast cancer cytologies: a marker of hormone response. Breast Cancer Res Treat 1987;10:287–291.
13. Carson-Jurica MA, Schrader WT, O'Malley BW. Steroid-receptor family: structure and functions. Endocrine Rev 1990;11:201–220.
14. Casteñeda E, Liao S. The use of anti-steroid antibodies in the characterization of steroid receptors. J Biol Chem 1975;250:883–888.
15. Catelli MG, Binart N, Jung-Testas I, Renoir JM, Baulieu E-E, Feramisco JR, Welch WJ. The common 90-kD protein component of nontransformed "8S" steroid receptors is a heat shock protein. EMBO J 1985;4:3131–3135.
16. Chamness GC, Huff K, McGuire WL. Protamine-precipitated estrogen receptor: a solid-phase ligand exchange assay. Steroids 1975;25:627–635.
17. Charpin C, Martin P-M, Jacquemier J, Lavaut MN, Pourreau-Schneider N, Toga M. Estrogen receptor immunocytochemical assay (ER-ICA): computerized image analysis system, immunoelectron microscopy, and comparisons with estradiol binding assays in 115 breast carcinomas. Cancer Res 1986;46:4271s–4277s.
18. Cheng L, Binder SW, Fu YS, Lewin KJ. Demonstration of estrogen receptors by monoclonal antibody in formalin-fixed breast tumors. Lab Invest 1988;58:346–353.
19. Clark GM, McGuire WL. Steroid receptors and other prognostic factors in primary breast cancer. Semin Oncol 1988;15:20–25.
20. Clark GM, McGuire WL, Hubay CA, Pearson OH, Marshall JS. Progesterone receptors as a prognostic factor in stage II breast cancer. N Engl J Med 1983;309: 1343–1347.
21. Cohen O, Brugal G, Seigneurin D, Demongeot J. Image cytometry of estrogen receptors in breast carcinomas. Cytometry 1988;9:579–587.
22. Cooper AP. The Principles and Practice of Surgery. London: Cox, 1836, pp 333–335.
23. Corle DK, Sears ME, Olson KB. Relationship of quantitative estrogen-receptor level and clinical response to cytotoxic chemotherapy in advanced breast cancer. Cancer 1984;54:1554–1561.
24. Daffada AAI, Johnston SRD, Smith IE, Detre S, King N, Dowsett M. Exon 5 deletion variant estrogen receptor messenger RNA expression in relation to tamoxifen resistance and progesterone receptor/pS2 status in human breast cancer. Cancer Res 1995;55: 288–293.
25. Davis BW, Zava DT, Locher GW, Goldhirsch A, Hartmann WH. Receptor heterogeneity of human breast cancer as measured by multiple intratumoral assays of estrogen and progesterone receptor. Eur J Cancer Clin Oncol 1984;20:375–382.
26. Daxenbichler G, Forsthuber E-P, Marth C, et al. Steroid hormone receptors and prognosis in breast cancer. Breast Cancer Res Treat 1988;12:267–273.
27. De Rosa CM, Ozzello L, Greene GL, Habif DV. Immunostaining of estrogen receptor in paraffin sections of breast carcinomas using monoclonal antibody D75P3γ: effects of fixation. Am J Surg Pathol 1987;11:943–950.
28. DeSombre ER, Carbone PP, Jensen EV, McGuire WL, Wells SA Jr, Wittliff JL, Lipsett MB. Steroid receptors in breast cancer. N Engl J Med 1979;301:1011–1012.
29. DeSombre ER, Greene GL, Jensen EV. Estrophilin and endocrine responsiveness of breast cancer. In Progress in Cancer Research and Therapy. Vol 10: Hormones, Receptors and Breast Cancer. Edited by WL McGuire. New York: Raven, 1978, pp 1–14.
30. DeSombre ER, Jensen EV. Estrophilin assays in breast cancer: quantitative features and application to the mastectomy specimen. Cancer 1980;46:2783–2788.
31. DeSombre ER, Thorpe SM, Rose C, Blough RR, Andersen KW, Rasmussen BB, King WJ. Prognostic usefulness of estrogen receptor immunocytochemical assays for human breast cancer. Cancer Res 1986;46:4256s–4264s.
32. Englesman E, Persijn JP, Korsten CB, Cleton FJ. Oestrogen receptors in human breast cancer tissue and response to endocrine therapy. Br Med J 1973;2:750–752.
33. Estes, PA, Suba EJ, Lawler-Heavner, et al. Immunologic analysis of human breast cancer progesterone receptors. 1. Immunoaffinity purification of transformed receptors and production of monoclonal antibodies. Biochemistry 1987;26:6250–6262.
34. Evans RM. The steroid and thyroid hormone receptor superfamily. Science 1988;240: 889–895.
35. Fisher B, Redmond C, Fisher ER, Caplan R. Relative worth of estrogen or progesterone receptor and pathologic characteristics of differentiation as indicators of prognosis in node negative breast cancer patients: findings from National Surgical Adjuvant Breast and Bowel Project protocol B-06. J Clin Oncol 1988;6:1076–1087.
36. Fishman J, Fishman JH, Nisselbaum JS, Menendez-Botet C, Schwartz MK, Martucci C, Hellman L. Measurement of the estradiol receptor in human breast tissue by the immobilized antibody method. J Clin Endocrinol Metab 1975;40:724–727.
37. Folca PJ, Glascock RF, Irvine WT. Studies with tritium-labelled hexoestrol in advanced breast cancer. Comparison of tissue accumulation of hexoestrol with response to bilateral adrenalectomy and oophorectomy. Lancet 1961;2:796–798.
38. Foster BD, Cavener DR, Parl FF. Binding analysis of the estrogen receptor to its specific DNA target site in human breast cancer. Cancer Res 1991;51:3405–3410.
39. Fuqua SAW, Fitzgerald SD, Chamness GC, et al. Variant human breast tumor estrogen receptor with constitutive transcriptional activity. Cancer Res 1991;51:105–109.
40. Fuqua SAW, Fitzgerald SD, Allred DC, et al. Inhibition of estrogen receptor action by a naturally occurring variant in human breast tumors. Cancer Res 1992;52:483–486.
41. Fuqua SAW, Wiltschke C, Castles C, Wolf D, Allred DC. A role for estrogen-receptor variants in endocrine resistance. Endocrine-Related Cancer 1995;2:19–25.
42. Fuqua SAW, Wolf DM. Molecular aspects of estrogen receptor variants in breast cancer. Breast Cancer Res Treat 1995;35:233–241.
43. Garola RE, McGuire WL. A hydroxylapatite micromethod for measuring estrogen receptor in human breast cancer. Cancer Res 1978;38:2216–2220.
44. Gorski J, Gannon F. Current models of steroid hormone action: a critique. Annu Rev Physiol 1976;38:425–450.
45. Graham ML II, Krett NL, Miller LA, et al. T47D_{CO} cells, genetically unstable and containing estrogen receptor mutations, are a model for the progression of breast cancers to hormone resistance. Cancer Res 1990;50:6208–6217.
46. Greene GL, Harris K, Bova R, Kinders R, Moore B, Nolan C. Purification of T47D human progesterone receptor and immunochemical characterization with monoclonal antibodies. Mol Endocrinol 1988;2:714–726.
47. Greene GL, Nolan C, Engler JP, Jensen EV. Monoclonal antibodies to human estrogen receptor. Proc Natl Acad Sci USA 1980;77:5115–5119.
48. Greene GL, Sobel NB, King WJ, Jensen EV. Immunochemical studies of estrogen receptors. J Steroid Biochem 1984;20:51–56.
49. Grody WW, Schrader WT, O'Malley BW. Activation, transformation, and subunit structure of steroid hormone receptors. Endocrine Rev 1982;3:141–163.
50. Hawkins RA, Sangster K, Tesdale A, Levack PA, Anderson EDC, Chetty U, Forrest APM. The cytochemical detection of oestrogen receptors in fine needle aspirates of breast cancer; correlation with biochemical assay and prediction of response to endocrine therapy. Br J Cancer 1988;58:77–80.
51. Helin HJ, Isola JJ, Helle MJ, Adlercreutz H. Influence of endocrine status on bio-

chemical and immunocytochemical estrogen and progesterone receptor assays in breast cancer patients. Breast Cancer Res Treat 1988;12:67–73.
52. Hilf R, Feldstein ML, Savlov ED, Gibson SL, Seneca B. The lack of relationship between estrogen receptor status and response to chemotherapy. Cancer 1980;46: 2797–2800.
53. Hiort O, Kwan PWL, DeLellis RA. Immunohistochemistry of estrogen receptor protein in paraffin sections. Am J Clin Pathol 1988;90:559–563.
54. Hoffman PG, Jones LA, Kuhn RW, Siiteri PK. Progesterone receptors: saturation analysis by a solid phase hydroxylapatite adsorption technique. Cancer 1980;46: 2801–2804.
55. Holmes FA, Fritsche HA, Loewy JW, Geitner AM, Sutton RC, Buzdar AU, Hortobagyi GN. Measurement of estrogen and progesterone receptors in human breast tumors: enzyme immunoassay versus binding assay. J Clin Oncol 1990;8:1025–1035.
56. Horwitz KB, McGuire WL, Pearson OH, Segaloff A. Predicting response to endocrine therapy in human breast cancer: a hypothesis. Science 1975;189:726–727.
57. Howat JMT, Harris M, Swindell R, Barnes DM. The effect of oestrogen and progesterone receptors on recurrence and survival in patients with carcinoma of the breast. Br J Cancer 1985;51:263–270.
58. Huggins C, Bergenstal DM. Inhibition of human mammary and prostatic cancers by adrenalectomy. Cancer Res 1952;12:134–141.
59. Huggins C, Hodges CV. Studies on prostatic cancer. 1. The effect of castration, of estrogen and of androgen injection on serum phosphatases in metastatic carcinoma of the prostate. Cancer Res 1941;1:293–297.
60. Jensen EV. Steroid hormone receptors. Curr Topics Pathol 1991;83:365–431.
61. Jensen EV, Block GE, Smith S, Kyser K, DeSombre ER. Estrogen receptors and breast cancer response to adrenalectomy. Natl Cancer Inst Monogr 1971;34:55–70.
62. Jensen EV, DeSombre ER. Estrogen-receptor interaction. Science 1973;182: 126–134.
63. Jensen EV, DeSombre ER, Jungblut PW. Estrogen receptors in hormone-responsive tissues and tumors. In Endogenous Factors Influencing Host-Tumor Balance. Edited by R Wissler, TL Dao, S Wood Jr. Chicago: University of Chicago Press, 1967, pp 15–30, 68.
64. Jensen EV, Greene GL, DeSombre ER. The estrogen-receptor immunoassay in the prognosis and treatment of breast cancer. Lab Manag 1986;24:25–42.
65. Jensen EV, Jacobson HI. Basic guides to the mechanism of estrogen action. Rec Prog Hormone Res 1962;18:387–414.
66. Jensen EV, Polley TZ, Smith S, Block GE, Ferguson DJ, DeSombre ER. Prediction of hormone dependency in human breast cancer. In Estrogen Receptors in Human Breast Cancer. Edited by WL McGuire, PP Carbone, EP Vollmer. New York: Raven, 1975, pp 37–55.
67. Jensen EV, Smith S, DeSombre ER. Hormone dependency in breast cancer. J Steroid Biochem 1976;7:911–917.
68. Johansson H, Terenius L, Thorén L. The binding of estradiol-17β to human breast cancers and other tissues in vitro. Cancer Res 1970;30:692–698.
69. Jonat W, Maass H, Stolzenbach G, Trams G. Estrogen receptor status and response to polychemotherapy in advanced breast cancer. Cancer 1980;46:2809–2813.
70. Jordan VC, Catherino WH, Wolf DM. Drug resistance to tamoxifen: mutant estrogen receptors as a potential mechanism of tamoxifen-stimulated tumor growth. Endocrine-Related Cancer 1995;2:45–51.
71. Jordan VC, Catherino WH, Wolf DM. A mutant receptor as a mechanism of drug resistance to tamoxifen treatment. Ann NY Acad Sci 1995;761:138–147.
72. Kiang DT, Frenning DH, Goldman AI, Ascensao VF, Kennedy BJ. Estrogen receptors and responses to chemotherapy and hormonal therapy in advanced breast cancer. N Engl J Med 1978;299:1330–1334.
73. King WJ, DeSombre ER, Jensen EV, Greene GL. Comparison of immunocytochemical and steroid-binding assays for estrogen receptor in human breast tumors. Cancer Res 1985;45:293–304.
74. Kinsel LB, Szabo E, Greene GL, Konrath J, Leight GS, McCarty KS Jr. Immunocytochemical analysis of estrogen receptors as a predictor of prognosis in breast cancer patients: comparison with quantitative biochemical methods. Cancer Res 1989;49: 1052–1056.
75. Knight WA III, Livingston RB, Gregory EJ, McGuire WL. Estrogen receptor as an independent prognostic factor for early recurrence in breast cancer. Cancer Res 1977;37:4669–4671.
76. Koenders PG, Beex LVAM, Langens R, Kloppenborg PWC, Smals AGH, Benraad TJ. Steroid hormone receptor activity of primary human breast cancer and pattern of the first metastasis. Breast Cancer Res Treat 1991;18:27–32.
77. Korenman SG, Dukes BA. Specific estrogen binding by the cytoplasm of human breast carcinoma. J Clin Endocrinol Metab 1970;30:639–645.
78. Kumar V, Green S, Stack G, Berry M, Jin J-R, Chambon P. Functional domains of the human estrogen receptor. Cell 1987;51:941–951.
79. Leake RE, Laing L, Calman KC, MacBeth FR, Crawford D, Smith DC. Oestrogen-receptor status and endocrine therapy of breast cancer: response rates and status stability. Br J Cancer 1981;43:59–66.
80. Leclercq G, Heuson JC, Deboel MC, Mattheiem WH. Oestrogen receptors in breast cancer: a changing concept. Br Med J 1975;1:185–189.
81. Lehrer S, Sanchez M, Song HK, et al. Oestrogen receptor B-region polymorphism and spontaneous abortion in women with breast cancer. Lancet 1990;335:622–624.
82. Leung BS, Fletcher WS, Lindell TD, Wood DC, Krippaehne WW. Predictability of response to endocrine ablation in advanced breast carcinoma. Arch Surg 1973;106: 515–519.
83. Liao S. Cellular receptors and mechanisms of action of steroid hormones. Int Rev Cytol 1975;41:87–172.
84. Lippman ME, Allegra JC. Quantitative estrogen receptor analyses: the response to endocrine and cytotoxic chemotherapy in human breast cancer and the disease-free interval. Cancer 1980;46:2829–2834.
85. Lippman ME, Allegra JC, Thompson EB, et al. The relation between estrogen receptors and response rate to cytotoxic chemotherapy in metastatic breast cancer. N Engl J Med 1978;298:1223–1228.
86. Luft R, Olivecrona H. Experiences with hypophysectomy in man. J Neurosurg 1953;10:301–316.
87. Maass H, Engel B, Hohmeister L, Lehmann F, Trams G. Estrogen receptors in human breast cancer tissue. Am J Obstet Gynecol 1972;113:377–382.
88. Maass H, Jonat W, Stolzenbach G, Trams G. The problem of nonresponding estrogen receptor-positive patients with advanced breast cancer. Cancer 1980;46: 2835–2837.
89. MacFarlane JK, Fleiszer D, Fazekas AG. Studies on estrogen receptors and regression in human breast cancer. Cancer 1980;45:2998–3003.
90. Magdelenat H, Merle S, Zajdela A. Enzyme immunoassay of estrogen receptors in fine needle aspirates of breast tumors. Cancer Res 1986;46:4265s–4267s.
91. Mahfoudi A, Roulet E, Dauvois S, Parker MG, Wahli W. Specific mutations in the estrogen receptor change the properties of antiestrogens to full agonists. Proc Natl Acad Sci USA 1995;92:4206–4210.
92. Martin PM, Berthois Y, Jensen EV. Binding of antiestrogens exposes an occult antigenic determinant in the human estrogen receptor. Proc Natl Acad Sci USA 1988;85: 2533–2537.
93. McCarty KS Jr, Szabo E, Flowers JL, et al. Use of a monoclonal anti-estrogen receptor antibody in the immunohistochemical evaluation of human tumors. Cancer Res 1986;46:4244s–4248s.
94. McClelland RA, Berger U, Miller LS, Powles TJ, Coombes RC. Immunocytochemical assay for estrogen receptor in patients with breast cancer: relationship to a biochemical assay and to outcome of therapy. J Clin Oncol 1986;4:1171–1176.
95. McClelland RA, Berger U, Wilson P, et al. Presurgical determination of estrogen receptor status using immunocytochemically stained fine needle aspirate smears in patients with breast cancer. Cancer Res 1987;47:6118–6122.
96. McGuire WL. Hormone receptors: their role in predicting prognosis and response to endocrine therapy. Semin Oncol 1978;5:428–433.
97. McGuire WL, Carbone PP, Vollmer EP (eds). Estrogen Receptors in Breast Cancer. New York: Raven, 1975.
98. McGuire WL, Chamness GC, Fuqua SAW. Abnormal estrogen receptor in clinical breast cancer. J Steroid Biochem Mol Biol 1992;43:243–247.
99. McGuire WL, Clark GM. Prognostic factors for recurrence and survival in axillary node-negative breast cancer. J Steroid Biochem 1989;34:145–148.
100. McGuire WL, Clark GM, Dressler LG, Owens MA. Role of steroid hormone receptors as prognostic factors in primary breast cancer. NCI Monogr1986;1:19–23.
101. Miller RT, Hapke MR, Greene GL. Immunocytochemical assay for estrogen receptor with monoclonal antibody D753Pγ in routinely processed formaldehyde-fixed breast tissue. Cancer 1993;71:3541–3546.
102. Montgomery PA, Scott GK, Luce MC, Kaufmann M, Benz CC. Human breast tumors containing non-DNA-binding immunoreactive (67 kDa) estrogen receptor. Breast Cancer Res Treat 1993;26:181–189.
103. Murphy LC, Dotzlaw H, Hamerton J, Schwarz J. Investigation of the origin of variant, truncated estrogen receptor-like mRNAs identified in some human breast cancer biopsy samples. Breast Cancer Res Treat 1993;26:149–161.
104. Müller-Holzner E, Zeimet A, Müller LC, Daxenbichler G, Dapunt O. Monoclonal technique to aid decision on endocrine therapy in breast cancer. Lancet 1989;1: 1147–1148.
105. Nolan C, Przywara LW, Miller LS, Suduikis V, Tomita JT. A sensitive solid-phase enzyme immunoassay for human estrogen receptor. In Current Controversies in Breast Cancer. Edited by FC Ames, GR Blumenschein, ED Montague. Austin: University of Texas Press, 1984, pp 433–441.
106. Osborne CK, Yochmowitz MG, Knight WA III, McGuire WL. The value of estrogen and progesterone receptors in the treatment of breast cancer. Cancer 1980;46: 2884–2888.
107. Parker MG (ed). Nuclear Hormone Receptors. London: Academic, 1991.
108. Paridaens R, Sylvester RJ, Ferrazzi E, Legros N, Leclercq G, Heuson JC. Clinical significance of the quantitative assessment of estrogen receptors in advanced breast cancer. Cancer 1980;46:2889–2895.
109. Pertschuk LP. Immunocytochemistry for Steroid Receptors. Boca Raton, FL: CRC, 1990.
110. Pertschuk LP, Eisenberg KB, Carter AC, Feldman JG. Immunohistologic localization of estrogen receptors in breast cancer with monoclonal antibodies. Correlation with biochemistry and clinical endocrine response. Cancer 1985;55:1513–1518.
111. Pfeffer U, Fecarotta E, Vidali G. Coexpression of multiple estrogen receptor variant messenger RNAs in normal and neoplastic breast tissues and in MCF-7 cells. Cancer Res 1995;55:2158–2165.
112. Pichon M-F, Pallud C, Brunet M, Milgrom E. Relationship of presence of progesterone receptors to prognosis in early breast cancer. Cancer Res 1980;40:3357–3360.
113. Poulsen HS, Ozzello L, King WJ, Greene GL. The use of monoclonal antibodies to estrogen receptors (ER) for immunoperoxidase detection of ER in paraffin sections of human breast cancer tissue. J Histochem Cytochem 1985;33:87–92.
114. Pratt WB. Interaction of hsp90 with steroid receptors: organizing some diverse observations and presenting the newest concepts. Mol Cell Endocrinol 1990;74: C69–C76.
115. Pusztay HM, McDonald EM (eds). Symposium on estrogen receptor determination with monoclonal antibodies. Cancer Res 1986;46:4233s–4312s.
116. Raam S, Robert N, Pappas CA, Tamura H. Defective estrogen receptors in human mammary cancers: their significance in defining hormone dependence. JNCI 1988;80:756–761.
117. Rao BR, Wiest WG, Allen WM. Progesterone receptor in rabbit uterus. Characterization and 17β-estradiol augmentation. Endocrinology 1973;92:1229–1240.
118. Rosenbaum C, Marsland TA, Stolbach LL, Raam S, Cohen JL. Estrogen receptor status and response to chemotherapy in advanced breast cancer. Cancer 1980;46: 2919–2921.
119. Rubens RD, Hayward JL. Estrogen receptors and response to endocrine therapy and cytotoxic chemotherapy in advanced breast cancer. Cancer 1980;46:2922–2924.
120. Rydén S, Fernö M, Borg Å, Hafström L, Möller T, Norgren A. Prognostic significance of estrogen and progesterone receptors in stage II breast cancer. J Surg Oncol 1988;37:221–226.
121. Samal BA, Brooks SC, Cummings G, et al. Estrogen receptors and responsiveness of advanced breast cancer to chemotherapy. Cancer 1980;46:2925–2927.
122. Sanchez ER, Toft DO, Schlesinger MJ, Pratt WB. Evidence that the 90-kDa phosphoprotein associated with the untransformed L-cell glucocorticoid receptor is a murine heat shock protein. J Biol Chem 1985;260:12398–12401.
123. Sarrif AM, Durant JR. Evidence that estrogen-receptor-negative, progesterone-receptor-positive breast and ovarian carcinomas contain estrogen receptor. Cancer 1981;48:1215–1220.
124. Scatchard G. The attraction of proteins for small molecules and ions. Ann NY Acad Sci 1949;51:660–672.

125. Shimada A, Kimura S, Abe K, et al. Immunocytochemical staining of estrogen receptor in paraffin sections of human breast cancer by use of monoclonal antibody: comparison with that in frozen sections. Proc Natl Acad Sci USA 1985;82:4803–4807.
126. Shintaku IP, Said JW. Detection of estrogen receptors with monoclonal antibodies in routinely processed formalin-fixed paraffin sections of breast carcinoma. Am J Clin Pathol 1987;87:161–167.
127. Siiteri PK. Receptor binding studies. Science 1984;223:191–193.
128. Singhakowinta A, Potter HG, Buroker TR, Samal B, Brooks SC, Vaitkevicius VK. Estrogen receptor and natural course of breast cancer. Ann Surg 1976;183:84–88.
129. Sklarew RJ, Bodmer SC, Pertschuk LP. Quantitative imaging of immunocytochemical (PAP) estrogen receptor staining patterns in breast cancer sections. Cytometry 1990;11:359–378.
130. Sluyser M. Role of estrogen receptor variants in the development of hormone resistance in breast cancer. Clin Biochem 1992;25:407–414.
131. Sluyser M, Wittliff JL. Influence of estrogen receptor variants in mammary carcinomas on the prognostic reliability of the receptor assay. Mol Cell Endocrinol 1992;85:83–88.
132. Smith DF, Toft DO. Steroid receptors and their associated proteins. Mol Endocrinol 1993;7:4–11.
133. Spelsberg TC, Graham ML II, Berg NJ, Umehara T, Riehl E, Coulam CB, Ingle JN. A nuclear binding assay to assess the biological activity of steroid receptors in isolated animal and human tissues. Endocrinology 1987;121:631–644.
134. Sternberger LA. Immunocytochemistry. New York: Prentice-Hall, 1974.
135. Sutton R, Campbell M, Cooke T, Nicholson R, Griffiths K, Taylor I. Predictive power of progesterone receptor status in early breast carcinoma. Br J Surg 1987;74:223–226.
136. Van Netten JP, Algard FT, Coy P, et al. Heterogeneous receptor levels detected via multiple microsamples from individual breast cancers. Cancer 1985;56:2019–2024.
137. Wagner RK. Characterization and assay of steroid hormone receptors and steroid-binding serum proteins by agar gel electrophoresis at low temperature. Hoppe-Seyler's Z Physiol Chem 1972;353:1235–1245.
138. Walker KJ, Bouzubar N, Robertson J, et al. Immunocytochemical localization of estrogen receptor in human breast tissue. Cancer Res 1988;48:6517–6522.
139. Walt AJ, Singhakowinta A, Brooks SC, Cortez A. The surgical implications of estrophile protein estimations in carcinoma of the breast. Surgery 1976;80:506–512.
140. Wang Y, Miksicek RJ. Identification of a dominant negative form of the human estrogen receptor. Mol Endocrinol 1991;5:1707–1715.
141. Weintraub J, Weintraub D, Redard M, Vassilakos P. Evaluation of estrogen receptors by immunocytochemistry on fine-needle aspiration biopsy specimens from breast tumors. Cancer 1987;60:1163–1172.
142. Wittliff JL, Fisher B, Durant JR. Establishment of uniformity in steroid receptor analyses used in cooperative clinical trials of breast cancer treatment. Recent Results Cancer Res 1980;71:198–206.
143. Wrange Ö, Nordenskjöld B, Gustafsson J-Å. Cytosol estradiol receptor in human mammary carcinoma: an assay based on isoelectric focusing in polyacrylamide gel. Anal Biochem 1978;85:461–475.
144. Yamamoto KR. Steroid receptor regulated transcription of specific genes and gene networks. Annu Rev Genet 1985;19:209–252.
145. Zava DT, Harrington NY, McGuire WL. Nuclear estradiol receptor in the adult rat uterus: a new exchange assay. Biochemistry 1976;15:4292–4297.

CHAPTER 70

Hormone Physiology and Endocrine Ablation

B. J. KENNEDY

Introduction

The removal of endogenous hormones can significantly alter the course of some cancers. Ablation of an endocrine gland may result in the decrease or disappearance of one or more hormonal factors essential for the continuing growth of the neoplasm. Because of the biologic differences of tumors within a specific type, not all patients respond favorably to hormonal manipulation. Measurement of biologic factors, such as receptors in breast cancer, and assessment of the response to prior hormonal therapies allow judicious selection of patients for appropriate ablative procedures and their subsequent alternatives.

Female Breast Cancer

The various modalities of endocrine therapy utilized in the treatment of breast cancer can be classified as ablative, additive, competitive, and inhibitive. The estrogenic hormone is a major factor in the stimulation and growth of some breast cancers. When estrogens are first employed in the treatment of menopausal symptoms, careful examination of the breasts during the first few months is recommended, since an existing small cancer could be stimulated by such hormonal therapy. The administration of androgenic hormone can also stimulate the growth of breast cancer, since that hormone is converted to small amounts of estrogen. This accounts for the induction of hypercalcemia in the initial hormonal treatment of patients with advanced osseous metastases. Administration of small physiologic doses of estrogenic hormone in premenopausal women may also stimulate breast cancer growth, as may the use of contraceptive estrogen. Hence, before such therapy is begun and a few months later, a breast examination may detect an early breast cancer.

The administration of massive doses of estrogen (additive therapy) may cause regression of advanced breast cancer at all ages, but in the postmenopausal patient estrogenic hormone in a large dose (e.g., >3 mg/day of diethylstilbesterol [DES]) in the past played a major role in the treatment of advanced disease. Competitive therapy with the estrogen antagonist tamoxifen replaced the role of DES in breast cancer management both as an adjuvant therapy and as treatment for disseminated disease. Although tamoxifen has replaced the use of estrogenic hormones, the latter may still have a role, since the mechanisms of action are different. Progestogens also suppress breast cancer growth and as additive therapy are used in managing advanced disease. The utilization of additive, inhibitive, and competitive hormones is an essential part of the selective sequential use of hormonal therapies.

Since the biologic behavior of carcinoma of the breast in some females is dependent on hormonal factors, alteration of those hormonal factors can stimulate or inhibit growth of the cancer. By measuring estrogen receptors (ER) of primary breast cancer and its metastases, the response to hormone manipulation can be predicted with reasonable accuracy. Those with ER-positive tumors or metastases are candidates for hormonal therapies. Tumors that lack receptors or have low ER levels have less than a 3% chance of responding to ablative therapy (14).

The removal of hormonal factors involved in the stimulation or maintenance of tumor growth may result in tumor regression. This can be accomplished by ablating hormone production directly or indirectly. Three ablative procedures have been employed—ovariectomy, adrenalectomy, and hypophysectomy.

OVARIECTOMY

In approximately one third of all premenopausal women with breast cancer, estrogenic hormones in physiologic amounts produced by the patient are a significant factor in the maintenance of tumor growth. Removal of these hormones by bilateral ovariectomy may produce objective improvement in breast cancer.

Castration was first employed in 1896, but only recently has the role of this procedure been clarified in the sequential selection of therapies for breast cancer. That castration should be carried out at the time of recurrence of breast cancer (therapeutic castration) rather than at the time of the initial mastectomy ("prophylactic" or adjuvant castration) has been established (13). A comparison study of patients who underwent castration at the time of mastectomy and those who underwent therapeutic castration when the disease recurred found that survival from mastectomy to death was not different between the two groups. Although castration at the time of mastectomy did delay the onset of metastases, it did not prevent the recurrence of the cancer. In this sense it was a form of adjuvant therapy. Furthermore, when the disease recurred in these patients, the interval from recurrence to death was much shorter than in patients who underwent a therapeutic castration. Hence, castration at the time of mastectomy has not increased the curability of breast cancer by conventional surgical or radiologic methods. Castration is of benefit, however, in that castrated patients have had a longer survival time than of noncastrated patients.

When prophylactic (adjuvant) castration was carried out and the cancer later recurred, there was no information available regarding the hormonal characteristics of the tumor. This index of the biologic nature of the cancer was lost. Without this information, an appropriate selection of future therapies was formerly impossible. The introduction of testing for the estrogen and progesterone receptors provided important biologic information for selection of therapies. A high response rate (about two thirds of patients) to castration, hypophysectomy, adrenalectomy, or antiestrogen therapy was assured for metastatic disease. Castration at the time of mastectomy is no longer routinely employed.

Castration is primarily of value in premenopausal women with advanced primary, recurrent, or distant metastatic cancer of the breast. The nature of the tumor response to therapeutic castration consists of a decrease in size of skin, liver, or lung metastases, recalcification of osseous lesions, and a decrease in size of a primary tumor. Central nervous system metastases are less likely to respond. The reported rates of regression of metastatic disease in premenopausal women vary from 24.5 to 50%. The culling of results of 12 different studies revealed an average regression rate of 40%. By limiting ovariectomy to those patients whose cancers expressed high ER levels, the objective response rate can be increased to approximately 64%. The median duration of such improvement is 9 months (range from 4 months to 6 years). Patients who respond to therapeutic castration live longer than do nonresponders. Although some investigators have reported regression of tumor following castration in postmenopausal women, in most such patients it was less than 2 years since the last menstrual period. Castration is of no value in truly postmenopausal women.

The presence of ER and the type of tumor response to therapeutic castration are significant indices of the nature of the breast cancer and provide a guide to the selection of other hormonal therapies. In nonresponders to castration, the formidable methods of secondary hormonal ablative therapy are avoided. Patients who do not respond to therapeutic castration become candidates for chemotherapy and other supportive measures. Patients who demonstrate an unequivocal objective response following a therapeutic castration may, on reactivation of the disease, be candidates for hypophysectomy, bilateral adrenalectomy, aminoglutethimide therapy, adrenal cortical hormone administration, or estrogen antagonists.

The procedure of bilateral ovariectomy is relatively simple. A hysterectomy need not be performed concomitantly. Although castration can be performed by radiotherapy, surgical ovariectomy is complete and removes any doubt that the ovaries might have a residual function. Furthermore, for complications such as hypercalcemia or severe bone pain, which require an immediate antitumor effect, surgical castration is preferable.

Castration in premenopausal women induces an artificial menopause. This is frequently more intense than a spontaneous menopause, but of shorter duration. In patients who respond to castration, no replacement therapy with estrogenic or androgenic hormones should be undertaken. Even women who had ER-negative tumors and who were castrated should not be given estrogenic hormones, since such tumors may have contained a small percentage of ER-positive cells.

In a patient who undergoes ovariectomy but whose cancer fails to improve, it could be inferred that the estrogenic hormone plays no role in the growth pattern of that disease. Once this has been established, replacement therapy with estrogenic hormone might seem appropriate to relieve the patient of severe menopausal symptoms. Such therapy could be detrimental to the course of the patient's disease, however.

Most breast cancers are a mixture of ER-positive and ER-negative cells. This has been clearly demonstrated with the monoclonal assay method for measuring ER immunocytochemically (18). Hence, the administration of estrogens for menopausal symptoms could result in stimulating those few receptor-positive cells that exist in an apparently ER-negative tumor. If the menopausal symptoms are sufficiently severe as to require hormonal therapy, the use of a progestogen is effective.

The role of tamoxifen in lieu of oophorectomy has been considered in receptor-positive patients. Oophorectomy would be preferable, especially in younger women, whereas tamoxifen can still be employed for later relapses.

ADRENALECTOMY

Bilateral adrenalectomy was performed for the management of advanced breast cancer in the female. Although a procedure of the past, its review provides further understanding of the endocrine aspects of breast cancer. Removal of estrogenic hormone produced by the adrenals resulted in an antitumor effect, especially in premenopausal patients who had previously demonstrated a response to castration or who had receptor-positive tumors.

Bilateral adrenalectomy was first introduced in 1951, and hypophysectomy as an alternative to adrenalectomy was introduced in 1954. Both procedures were employed in similar circumstances. The degree of morbidity and the tumor sites were factors in determining which ablative procedure was preferred. For example, a patient with extensive skull metastases was a better candidate for adrenalectomy. A patient with abdominal metastases withstood hypophysectomy more easily. The mortality rate for both procedures was low.

The results of adrenalectomy for female breast cancer reported by several investigators were comparable. A collaborative study comparing bilateral adrenalectomy and hypophysectomy revealed a regression rate of 28.4% and 32.6%, respectively (16). The difference was not significant. Fracchia and colleagues had a regression rate of 32.4% following adrenalectomy (6). These figures reflect the overall regression rate in breast cancer without specific selection of the patient as a candidate for the procedure on the basis of prior response to other hormone therapy or receptor status.

Knowledge of ER content of the tumor plus observations of the response to prior endocrine therapy could predict which patient would benefit from adrenalectomy. The premenopausal patient with a long cancer-free interval following mastectomy, who had mainly osseous or soft tissue disease and who responded favorably to therapeutic castration, would most likely benefit from adrenalectomy. Postmenopausal women who developed primary breast cancer before menopause and women who responded to hormone therapy also had a high rate of regression following adrenalectomy. Utilization of adrenalectomy in advanced cancer was recommended primarily for those female patients whose disease had reactivated following objective improvement as the result of castration or estrogen therapy and in whom the ER status was positive. In view of the low response rate (≤16%) in patients who failed to respond to castration and the lack of response in ER-negative tumors, the employment of this formidable procedure was of little value.

Aminoglutethimide inhibits the biosynthesis of adrenocortical steroids (see Chapter 74). More important, it is an inhibitor of the enzyme aromatase, which converts adrenal androgens to estrogen. The net result is a decrease in estrogens, androgens, and other adrenal steroids (19). Hydrocortisone replacement is required. The response rate (30–53%) and duration (10–17 months) are similar to results of adrenalectomy. The employment of this "medical adrenalectomy" made adrenalectomy a procedure of the past (20).

HYPOPHYSECTOMY

Hypophysectomy had a specific role in the management of advanced female breast cancer (12). The effective utilization of hypophysectomy was dependent on specific selection of patients. Hypophysectomy was carried out at the time of reactivation of the disease in premenopausal women who had responded favorably to surgical castration or in postmenopausal patients who had responded to estrogen therapy. The presence of ER-positive metastases plus a response to prior endocrine therapy almost assured a response to hypophysectomy.

Hypophysectomy removes adrenocorticotropic and gonadotropic hormones and secondarily eliminates adrenal function. Therefore, the expected antitumor results of hypophysectomy and adrenalectomy were similar. Approximately 20% of patients who had undergone oophorectomy followed by adrenalectomy had a subsequent remission after hypophysectomy, which suggested that prolactin may be a factor in tumor growth.

The previous response to hormone therapy was a factor in the subsequent response to hypophysectomy. More than 55% of patients responding to therapeutic castration improved after hypophysectomy (12). In postmenopausal women who experienced a response to estrogenic or androgenic therapy, more than 70% improved. More specific selection of patients was improved by the added information of ER content of the tumor.

As with adrenalectomy, the use of aminoglutethimide and hydrocortisone replaced hypophysectomy. The use of these two major ablative procedures represents an historical era in the evolution of hormonal therapies for breast cancer. The sequential use of endocrine therapies plays a significant role in the overall management of breast cancer (18).

NEW AGENTS

Alternative endocrine methods to treat breast cancer continue to be exploited (8). Inhibitors of the aromatase enzyme system do not require cortisol replacement. Antiestrogens, such as toremifene, resemble the effect of tamoxifen. The antiprogestins mifepristone (RU 486) and onapristone have an antitumor effect mediated through progesterone receptors. Various luteinizing hormone–releasing hormone (LHRH) analogues have been developed for the treatment of metastatic breast and prostate cancers. Their end result is to decrease blood estrogen or testosterone levels, equivalent to medical castration. Among these are buserelin, goserelin, and leuprolide.

Male Breast Cancer

Carcinoma of the male breast is effectively controlled by hormonal measures. The low incidence of this disease does not allow the accurate determination of incidence of regression. Since growth of male breast cancer is in part dependent on androgenic hormones, the antitumor endocrine measures of advanced disease are directed toward removal of androgenic hormones or toward blocking their actions.

Orchiectomy is reserved for recurrent or advanced breast cancer in men of any age. With removal of the androgenic hormones, primary tumor masses and lymph node, lung and skin metastases decrease in size or disappear. Osseous lesions recalcify. Central nervous system lesions are less apt to respond. The regression rate of male breast cancer after castration is 68% (21).

Adrenalectomy and hypophysectomy offered a further method of control of male breast cancer. Although the results of these ablative procedures were derived from a small number of patients, hypophysectomy or adrenalectomy were associated with a response rate of 50% and 53%, respectively (15).

Male breast cancers are often hormone dependent. ER positivity has been demonstrated in more than 85% of men with breast carcinoma (4). This higher rate compared to that in women may be due partly to a lower level of serum estrogen, which makes the receptor sites available for binding (11).

An objective tumor response after bilateral orchiectomy was first observed in 1942. The subsequent overall response rate of 55% was not age related, as is the response to oophorectomy in women (11). Orchiectomy is not only the oldest but also one of the most effective means of palliative therapy. It is safe, lacks significant side effects, and overall is less expensive. A response to orchiectomy increases the likelihood of response to secondary hormonal ablation or therapies. Adrenalectomy or hypophysectomy were replaced by aminoglutethimide and hydrocortisone. Additive hormonal therapies including DES, megestrol and medroxyprogesterone, or corticosteroids provided alternatives or secondary options.

The estrogen antagonist tamoxifen has been found to produce objective response rates about equal to that of orchiectomy (1, 11). It is more acceptable psychologically. Other effective therapies include LHRH analogues, with or without antiandrogen agents.

In males with carcinoma of the breast, androgenic hormones are not employed in treatment since stimulation of the cancer may occur.

Cancer of the Prostate

The growth of carcinoma of the prostate is largely dependent on androgenic hormones. The removal of androgens results in tumor regression; administration of androgens stimulates the growth of the cancer. Hence, hormonal therapy is essential in the management of this tumor.

There appears to be little advantage in beginning hormonal therapy in prostate cancer prior to the onset of symptoms or before active progression of the disease becomes manifest (22). Castration or estrogen therapy at the time of prostatectomy for early lesions is not indicated. With advanced disease, a typical remission following hormonal therapy consists of relief of bone pain, reduction of urinary tract symptoms, regression in the size of the prostate gland, and return of elevated serum acid phosphatase or prostate-specific antigen (PSA) levels to normal. Osseous metastases may disappear entirely and be replaced by new bone. Soft tissue metastases decrease in size or disappear.

Bilateral scrotal orchiectomy is the most direct means of removing the major portion, 90 to 95%, of testosterone in the human male (10). It remains the standard with which all other modalities of hormonal manipulation must be compared. It is the simplest, fastest, least costly, and for some clinicians the method of choice for recurrent prostate cancer (9).

The duration of remission induced by orchiectomy varies widely among patients. Because of the view of the dramatic general improvement exhibited in the majority of patients, most observers assume that treated patients live longer. Ordinarily, reactivation of the tumor occurs within 2 or 3 years. Orchiectomy has the advantage of ensuring complete removal of the testicular stimulus to continued prostatic growth and requires no further patient compliance in taking regular medication. Radiation therapy is ineffective in suppressing androgen production by the testes.

DES is an inexpensive but effective synthetic estrogen that is able to decrease plasma testosterone levels to those of a postorchiectomy patient by suppressing the pituitary secretion of LH. The antitumor effects are similar to those of orchiectomy. The feminizing effects and vascular complications from estrogen hormones have been regarded as disadvantages. The combination of estrogen therapy and castration has no real advantage over the separate use of these agents.

Castration in the male may carry a greater emotional impact than the same procedure in the female. Nevertheless, the antitumor effect usually outweighs the aesthetic disadvantage of orchiectomy, which can be partially assuaged by testicular prostheses. Sexual activity may have terminated by the time orchiectomy is considered. The psychological impact of castration is variable and may be profoundly disturbing to some. This disappointment is usually short-lived. If benefit from castration results, the change in disease status compensates for and displaces the depression concerning castration. If benefit does not occur, the disease prognosis and concern with continuing pain and disability ordinarily eliminate energies for sexual activity.

Bilateral adrenalectomy removed steroidal sex hormones of adrenal origin and produced regression of advanced carcinoma of the prostate in patients responding to orchiectomy. Since the duration of such improvements was short, this procedure has been abandoned. In lieu of adrenalectomy, massive doses of corticosteroids have been employed, resulting in subjective improvement but relatively poor objective improvement. Hypophysectomy, the effect of which is similar to that of adrenalectomy, was used infrequently.

Several innovative hormonal therapies have been studied. Ketoconazole, an antimycotic imidazole derivative, inhibits the cytochrome P450–related steroid hormone biosynthetic enzymes. Castration levels of testosterone are achieved, but adrenal insufficiency is promoted. Various progestational steroids also have been used for primary endocrine therapy and are regarded as antiandrogens. They inhibit the release of LH, but also block androgen receptors (2).

The most dramatic recent advances in the hormonal treatment of advanced prostate cancer have been the introduction of the luteinizing hormone-releasing hormone agonists and androgen blockers, such as flutamide, with results comparable to those of orchiectomy (2, 3, 7, 17, 23). The LHRH analogues offer a complete medical castration. Nonsteroidal antiandrogens block the binding of testosterone and dihydrotestosterone to their intracellular receptors. Both agents are expensive. There is some controversy as to whether total androgen blockade achieved by combining those agents is more effective than their single use. The combination of LHRH analogue leuprolide plus the antiandrogen flutamide was associated with significant improvements in progression-free survival and survival, compared to the use of leuprolide alone (5).

Replacement Therapy

The use of ablative procedures in cancer therapy removes a variety of endocrine substances. The resulting impact on endocrine physiology is formidable and requires careful consideration of the replacement requirements.

OVARIECTOMY

Following bilateral ovariectomy in the young menstruating woman, the patient undergoes an abrupt and highly symptomatic menopause, but fortunately it is of shorter duration than physiologic menopause. It is mandatory that estrogenic or androgenic hormones not be employed as replacement therapy in women with breast cancer, since oophorectomy was introduced primarily to remove the estrogenic hormones. Since the cancer is dependent in part on estrogens for its growth, the administration of estrogens or androgens could result in stimulation of tumor growth and exacerbation of the cancer. Even in patients with ER-negative tumors, the use of estrogenic hormones for the treatment of menopausal symptoms (spontaneous or induced menopause) is not recommended. In the patient who experiences an objective improvement of advanced breast cancer, the menopausal symptoms are managed with sedatives, tranquilizers, or progestogens.

ORCHIECTOMY

Orchiectomy results in less physiologic alteration in the male than does castration in the female. However, the variable degree of impotency induced, gynecomastia, and the loss of the testes do represent emotional stresses that require support. Under no condition should a patient who underwent orchiectomy with objective tumor response be given androgenic hormone as replacement therapy.

ADRENALECTOMY OR HYPOPHYSECTOMY

These major endocrine ablative procedures are no longer employed in management of advanced cancers. If performed, reference to an appropriate endocrine text is recommended.

AMINOGLUTETHIMIDE

The standard medical adrenalectomy regimen includes aminoglutethimide, 250 mg q.i.d., plus hydrocortisone, 40 mg/d in divided doses. Hydrocortisone replacement is required to prevent the reflex rise in adrenocorticotropic hormone (ACTH) which can overcome the blockade in steroidogenesis (18).

Conclusion

Ablative endocrine procedures in advanced breast and prostate cancers can play a significant role in the management of these cancers. Their employment should be considered along with the many hormonal therapies now available that can induce medical castration and block the effect of hormones.

References

1. Bezwoda WR, Hesdorffer C, Dansey R, deMoor N, Derman DP, Browde S, Lange M. Breast cancer in men. Cancer 1987;60:1337–1340.
2. Catalona WJ. Management of cancer of the prostate. N Engl J Med 1994;331:996–1004.
3. Denis L. Prostate cancer: primary hormonal treatment. Cancer 1993;71:1050–1058.
4. Donnegan WL. Cancer of the breast in men. CA 1991;41:339–353.
5. Eisenberger MA, Crawford ED, Wolf M, Blumenstein B, McLeod DG, Benson R, Dorr FA, Benson M, Spaulding JT, investigators of the National Cancer Institute Intergroup Study #0036 Prognostic factors in stage D2 prostate cancer: important implications for future trials: results of a cooperative intergroup study (INT.0036). Semin Oncol 1994;21:613–619.
6. Fracchia AA, Randalla HT, Farrow JN. The results of adrenalectomy in advanced breast cancer in 500 consecutive patients. Surg Gynecol Obstet 1967;125:747–756.
7. Geller J, Albert J, Vik A. Advantages of total androgen blockade in the treatment of advanced prostate cancer. Semin Oncol 1988;15:53–61.
8. Glauber JG, Kiang DT. The changing role of hormonal therapy in advanced breast cancer. Semin Oncol 1992;19:308–316.
9. Greenberg RE, Charles RS, Samaha AM, Chelsky M, Rosen S. Surgical management of recurrent genitourinary malignancies. Semin Oncol 1993;20:474–492.
10. Griffiths K, Eaton CL, Harper ME, Turkes A, Peeling WB. Hormonal treatment of advanced disease: some newer aspects. Semin Oncol 1994;21:672–687.
11. Jaiyesimi IA, Buzdar AU, Sahin AA, Ross MA. Carcinoma of the male breast. Ann Intern Med 1992;117:771–777.
12. Kennedy BJ, French L. Hypophysectomy in advanced breast cancer. Am J Surg 1965;110:411–415.
13. Kennedy BJ, Mielke PW Jr, Fortuny IE. Therapeutic castration versus prophylactic castration in breast cancer. Surg Gynecol Obstet 1964;118:524–540.
14. Kiang DT, Kennedy BJ. Factors affecting estrogen receptors in breast cancer. Cancer 1977;40:1571–1576.
15. Liechty RD, David J, Glysteen J. Cancer of the male breast: forty cases. Cancer 1967;20:1617–1625
16. MacDonald I. Endocrine ablation in disseminated mammary carcinoma. Surg Gynecol Obstet 1962;115:215–222.
17. McLeod DG. Antiandrogenic drugs. Cancer 1993;71:1046–1049.
18. Rausch DJ, Kiang DT, Kennedy BJ. Guidelines for the management of breast cancer: a treatment summary. In Breast Cancer. Edited by BJ Kennedy. New York: Liss, 1989, pp 225–239.
19. Santen RJ, Worgul TJ, Lipton A, Harvey H, Boucher A, Samojlik E, Wells SA. Aminoglutethimide as treatment of postmenopausal women with advanced breast carcinoma. Ann Intern Med 1982;96:94–101.
20. Santen RJ, Worgul TJ, Samojlik E, Interrante A, Boucher AE, Lipton A, Harvey HA, White DS, Smart E, Cox C, Wells SA. A randomized trial comparing surgical adrenalectomy with aminoglutethimide plus hydrocortisone in women with advanced breast cancer. N Engl J Med 1981;305:545–551.
21. Treves N. The treatment of cancer, especially inoperable cancer of the male breast by ablative surgery and hormone therapy. Cancer 1959;12:820–832.
22. Veterans Administration Cooperative Urological Group. Treatment and survival of patients with cancer of the prostate. Surg Gynecol Obstet 1967;124:1011–1017.
23. Waxman J. Gonadotrophin releasing hormone analogues for prostatic cancer: an overview. Semin Oncol 1988;15:366–370.

CHAPTER 71

Hypothalamic and Other Peptide Hormones

ANDREW V. SCHALLY AND ANA MARIA COMARU-SCHALLY

Analogues of Peptide Hormones

INTRODUCTION: HYPOTHALAMO–HYPOPHYSIAL RELATIONSHIP, HYPOTHALAMIC HORMONES, AND OTHER PEPTIDES

It has been known since the 1930s that the anterior pituitary gland secretes several hormones that stimulate the thyroid, the gonads, and the adrenal cortex, and regulate various bodily processes. However, the mechanisms of the control of pituitary function were still not completely understood even in the 1950s and several theories existed concerning this control. Harris (42) assembled anatomic and physiologic evidence that the hypothalamic portion of the brain secreted neurohormones that traversed the portal vessels to regulate the secretion of pituitary hormones. This theory seemed to explain most experimental facts. In the mid 1950s, one of us (A.V.S.) became interested in the hypothalamus, and inspired by Harris's neurohormonal theory, set about to prove it. This work extended over 23 years.

It is well established now that the hypothalamic hormones stimulate or inhibit the release of various anterior pituitary hormones (112, 114). The discovery of several of these hypothalamic hormones and their isolation, structural identification, and synthesis furnished the evidence for the theory of neurohumoral control of the pituitary gland put forward by Harris (42). Hypothalamic hormones are known to influence growth, reproduction, lactation, metabolism, gastrointestinal function, and the response to stress. Basal release of some hypothalamic hormones, including luteinizing hormone-releasing hormone (LH-RH), into hypophysial portal blood is pulsatile and surges occur before such events as ovulation (55). LH-RH pulses are activated at the time of puberty. Some hypothalamic peptide hormones are also produced in the extra-hypothalamic brain areas (where they may serve as neurotransmitters) and in endocrine-like cells of non-neural tissues. Thus, somatostatin is present in discrete cells of the pancreas, gastric mucosa, duodenum, and other tissues, and may, through paracrine control, play an important role in the regulation of the endocrine pancreas and gastrointestinal tract. Mammalian bombesin-like peptides, such as gastrin-releasing peptide (GRP) and neuromedin B, are found in the gastrointestinal tract, the brain (including the hypothalamus), and various tumors and appear to produce mitogenic effects (114, 119, 127, 130). The understanding of functions of these peptide hormones, combined with the development of synthetic analogues, should enable the clinician to diagnose and treat a variety of cancers much more successfully than in the past.

Agonists of Luteinizing Hormone-Releasing Hormone (LH-RH)

EARLY STUDIES AND THE BASIS OF ONCOLOGIC APPLICATIONS

Twenty-four years have passed since our laboratory accomplished the isolation, determination of structure, and synthesis of the hypothalamic hormone controlling the secretion of both LH and follicle-stimulating hormone (FSH) from the anterior pituitary gland (115). The discovery of LH-RH, also called gonadotropin-releasing hormone (GnRH), has led to many practical clinical uses (114, 117, 119). Since 1972, systematic work has been proceeding to synthesize agonistic and antagonistic analogues of LH-RH. A strong interest in medical applications of LH-RH derivatives stimulated this undertaking. However, at that time we could not imagine the impact and the variety of applications, including major uses in oncology, that LH-RH analogues would eventually have. The investigation of the effects of LH-RH analogues on various cancers began in the late 1970s. In the past 23 years, more than 3,000 analogues of LH-RH have been synthesized (117). Many agonistic analogs more potent than the parent hormone have been made (49, 114, 117).

A number of LH-RH analogues substituted in positions 6, 10, or both are much more active than LH-RH (114, 117). Among the agonists being used clinically are [D-Trp^6]LH-RH (Decapeptyl, Triptorelin), [D-Leu^6, Pro^9-NHEt]LH-RH (Leuprolide, Lupron), [D-Ser(Bu^t)^6, Pro^9-NHEt]-LH-RH (Buserelin, Suprefact), [D-Ser(Bu^t)^6, Aza-Gly^{10}]LH-RH (Goserelin, Zoladex), and [D-Nal (2)^6]LH-RH (Nafarelin, Synarel) (Table 71.1), These agonists are 50 to 100 times more potent than LH-RH and also possess prolonged activity (117, 119).

Although an acute injection of superactive agonists of LH-RH induces a marked and sustained release of LH and FSH, chronic administration produces inhibitory effects through a process of "down-regulation" of pituitary receptors for LH-

Table 71-1. LH-RH Agonists in Clinical Use

LH-RH	Structure									
	1	2	3	4	5	6	7	8	9	10
	pyro-Glu	His	Trp	Ser	Tyr	Gly	Leu	Arg	Pro	Gly-NH_2
Buserelin (Hoechst)	----------	----------	----------	----------	----------	D-Ser(Bu^t)	----------	----------	----------	Ethylamide
Nafarelin (Syntex)	----------	----------	----------	----------	----------	D-(2-Nal)	----------	----------	----------	----------
Leuprolide (Abbott-Takeda)	----------	----------	----------	----------	----------	D-Leu	----------	----------	----------	Ethylamide
Zoladex; Goserelin (ICI)	----------	----------	----------	----------	----------	D-Ser(Bu^t)	----------	----------	----------	Az-Gly-NH_2
Decapeptyl, Triptorelin (Debiopharm; Ipsen-Beaufour; Ferring; Aché)	----------	----------	----------	----------	----------	D-Trp	----------	----------	----------	----------

The abbreviations of the amino acids are in accord with the recommendations of the IUPAC-IUB JCBN. In addition: LH-RH = luteinizing hormone-releasing hormone; Az-Gly = AZA-Glycine; Nal(2) = 3-(2-naphthyl)alanine; Bu^t = *o*-tert butyl; Ethylamide, —NH—CH_2—CH_3 (NHEt in text).

RH, desensitization of the pituitary gonadotrophs, and reduction in gonadal receptors for LH and FSH (6, 114, 117, 119, 126). The continuous administration of high doses of LH-RH agonists causes a suppression of circulating levels of LH (bioactive but not always radioimmunoactive) and of sex steroid levels (76). Thus, the inhibition of pituitary and gonadal function that occurs after chronic administration of agonists of LH-RH, and which creates a state of sex steroid deprivation by eliminating the stimulatory effects of estrogen or testosterone, is the main basis for the oncologic application of LH-RH analogues (116, 117, 119).

DEVELOPMENT OF SUSTAINED-DELIVERY SYSTEMS

Initially, super-agonists of LH-RH were given daily by the subcutaneous (SC) or intranasal route (76, 117, 119). However, intranasal absorption is only about 2% and daily injections are inconvenient. Subsequently, long-acting delivery systems for [D-Trp^6]LH-RH and other agonists in microcapsules of poly(DL-lactide-co-glycolide) (PLG) or different polymers designed to release a controlled dose of the peptide (usually 100 μg) over a 30-day period were developed (83, 116, 117, 119, 124, 139). These microcapsules contain 2 to 6% analogue and 94 to 98% of biodegradable, biocompatible polymer(DL-lactide-co-glycolide). Spherical microcapsules are prepared by a phase separation process.

Another form of sustained delivery system consists of microparticles (microgranules) containing the peptide analogues (119). The microparticles were obtained by the cryogenic grinding of extruded polymer containing the homogeneously dispersed peptide and the sieving of the particles. This process results in particles of amorphous shape in a large variety of sizes, but it does not involve the use of solvents such as Freon, which may be banned in the future on environmental grounds. For administration, the microcapsules or microgranules are suspended in an injection vehicle containing 2% carboxymethylcellulose or D-mannitol and 1% Tween 20 or 80 in water and injected intramuscularly (IM) once a month through an 18-gauge (or smaller) needle (119). Depot preparations of Lupron containing 3.75 to 7.5 mg leuprolide microspheres (124) injectable IM or of Zoladex (goserelin, 3.6 mg) in cylindrical rods of the polymer PLG (111, 139) injectable SC through a 14- or 16-gauge needle, and polyhydroxybutyrate tablets containing 3.6 to 5 mg of Buserelin which are implantable SC are also available (119).

The mechanism of peptide release from sustained delivery systems (microcapsules and microgranules) after IM injection, was studied by histologic and immunohistochemical approaches (119). It was determined that the diffusion of the peptides from the aqueous channels in PLG was negligible and that the peptide release from the PLG microcapsules and microparticles was controlled mostly by the speed of the biodegradation of the polymer matrix (119). Sustained delivery formulations are capable of maintaining therapeutic levels of peptides for 4 weeks, and improved depot preparations, which can release the analogues for 60 days, are being prepared. Delayed delivery systems developed for monthly administration are efficacious, reliable, and convenient and also increase the patient's compliance.

CURRENT USES OF LH-RH AGONISTS

Chronic administration of LH-RH agonists is being utilized to induce the regression of endocrine-dependent malignant neoplasms, especially prostate and breast cancer (19, 50–53, 74, 80, 110, 117–119, 124, 139). LH-RH agonists are under study for the treatment of endometrial cancer (24). Reduction of sex steroid levels by LH-RH agonists can be also used for the treatment of idiopathic precocious puberty (117, 119). The inhibition of LH and ovarian steroidogenesis provides the basis for the therapeutic use of LH-RH agonists in diseases and conditions that result from inappropriate hormone levels or that can be treated by the suppression of estrogens. These applications include endometriosis, uterine fibroids (leiomyomas), polycystic ovarian disease (PCOD), dysfunctional uterine bleeding, and hirsutism (24, 117, 119). LH-RH agonists are also used in assisted reproductive technology for in vitro fertilization and embryo transfer (IVF-ET) (82) or gamete intrafallopian transfer (GIFT), and for the development of new contraceptive methods (117, 119).

PHARMACOKINETICS AND METABOLISM

LH-RH agonists are degraded and eliminated from plasma several times more slowly than is natural LH-RH, the half-life of which in humans is 8 minutes (3, 117). The binding affinity of some LH-RH agonists to LH-RH receptors is about 10 times higher than that of LH-RH (49, 117, 119). In normal volunteers, the plasma half-life of D-Trp-6-LH-RH was 7.6 hours. The plasma clearance of D-Trp-6-LH-RH was reported to be 161 to 508 mL/min (3). A single IM injection of the 3.75 mg of depot preparation of microcapsules of D-Trp-6-LH-RH liberating 100 μg/d results, after an initial peak, in D-Trp-6-LH-RH concentrations of 200 to 500 pg/mL lasting for about 4 to 5 weeks (119). Labeled LH-RH analogues accumulate primarily in the liver and kidneys (the main degrading organs) and the pituitary, the biologic target (117, 119).

SIDE EFFECTS AND TOXICOLOGY

The main side effects caused by chronic administration of LH-RH agonists are those that can be attributed to sex-hormone deficiency (117, 119). These consist of impotence and loss of libido in men and "hot flashes" or climacteric-like vasomotor phenomena in both sexes. Episodes of temporary "flare-up" in disease that are manifest by an increase in bone pain during the first week of administration have been reported in 2 to 20% of patients with prostate cancer. None of the patients with prostate cancer develops gynecomastia or thromboembolic episodes, in contrast to treatment with diethylstilbestrol. The acute toxicity of LH-RH agonists is extremely low.

LH-RH Antagonists

THEORETICAL CONSIDERATIONS AND EARLY STUDIES

LH-RH antagonists represent another class of peptide analogues that may be useful for the treatment of hormone-dependent cancers (116–119). These antagonists act on the same receptor sites as LH-RH and cause an immediate inhibition of the release of gonadotropins and sex steroids (24, 116–119). While repeated administration of LH-RH agonists is necessary for the inhibition of LH and sex steroids, this effect can be induced with a single injection of a potent LH-RH antagonist (116–119). During agonist administration, a transient LH and sex steroid release that precedes the secretion blockade may result in a flare-up of disease, whereas the antagonists induce an immediate suppression. The use of antagonists prevents flare-up phenomena, which can occur in some cancer patients (116–119). Antagonistic analogues of LH-RH were developed for contraception (49, 116–119). Since 1972, hundreds of LH-RH antagonists have been synthesized and assayed in animals. Some of the more potent early antagonists were also tested in humans (116–119). [D-Phe2, D-Trp3, D-Phe6]-LH-RH was the first inhibitory analogue found to be active in humans (116–119). Insertion of D-arginine, into position 6 of LH-RH antagonists increased the inhibitory activity, [Ac-D-(4Cl)-Phe^{1,2}, D-Trp^3, D-Arg^6, D-Ala^{10}]LH-RH being active at doses of 1 to 3 μg in rats (49, 116–119). However, antagonists with D-Arg or related basic residues in position 6 induce histamine liberation, resulting in transient edema and other anaphylactoid reactions (49, 116–119). These side effects delayed clinical use of earlier LH-RH antagonists in humans.

Table 71-2. Modern LH-RH Antagonists

Trivial or INN Name	
SB-75 (Cetrorelix)	[Ac-D-Nal(2)^1, D-Phe(4Cl)^2, D-Pal(3)^3, D-Cit^6, D-Ala^{10}]LH-RH
Antide	[N-Ac-D-Nal(2)^1, D-Phe(4Cl)^2, D-Pal(3)^3, Lys(Nic)^5, D-Lys(Nic)^6, Lys-(iPr)^8, D-Ala^{10}] LH-RH
Nal-Glu Antagonist	[Ac-D-Nal(2)^1, D-Phe(4Cl)^2, D-Pal(3)^3, Arg^5, D-Glu^6(AA), D-Ala^{10}]LH-RH
Azaline B	[Ac-D-Nal^1, D-Phe(4Cl)^2, D-Pal^3, Aph^5(Atz), Aph^6(Atz), Ilys^8, D-Ala^{10}]GnRH
Detirelix	[N-Ac-D-Nal(2)^1, D-Phe(4Cl)^2, D-Trp^3, D-hArg(Et$_2$)^6, D-Ala^{10}]GnRH

Abbreviations: The abbreviations of the amino acids are in accordance with the recommendations of the IUPAC-IUB JCBN. In addition: LH-RH = luteinizing hormone-releasing hormone; D-Glu^6(AA), 4-(p-methoxy-benzoyl)-D-2-aminobutyric acid; Cit = citrulline (2-amino-5-ureidopentanoic acid); Nal(2), 3-(2-naphthyl)alanine; Pal(3) = 3-(3-pyridyl)alanine; Phe(4Cl) = 4-chlorophenylalanine; Ac = acetyl; Lys(Nic) = N$^\epsilon$-nicotinoyllysine; Lys-(iPr) = N$^\epsilon$-isopropyllysine.
For comparison with the amino acids sequence of LH-RH, see Table 71-1.

MODERN LH-RH ANTAGONISTS

Modern antagonists possess modifications in positions 1, 2, 3, 6, 10, and others (2, 13, 49, 68, 107). To eliminate the undesirable edematogenic effect of the LH-RH antagonists containing basic D-amino acids at position 6, new analogues with D-ureidoalkyl amino acids, such as D-Cit, D-Hci, at position 6 were synthesized in our laboratory and tested in several in vitro and in vivo systems (2, 117, 119). Among these antagonists [Ac-D-Nal (2)^1 D-Phe (4Cl)^2, D-Pal (3)^3, D-Cit^6, D-Ala^{10}]-LH-RH (SB-75) (Cetrorelix) (Table 71.2) appeared to be the most active in vivo in rats and did not exert any edematogenic effects, even at a dose of 1.5 mg/kg (2, 117, 119).

Other groups have also reported different structural modifications that diminish anaphylactoid toxicity. Antagonists such as antide [N-Ac-D-Nal (2)^1, D-Phe (4Cl)^2, D-Pal (3)^3, Lys (Nic)^5, D-Lys (Nic)^6, Lys (iPr)^8, D-Ala^{10}]-LH-RH) (68) and Nal-Glu antagonist ([Ac-D-Nal (2)^1, D-Phe (4Cl)^2, D-Pal (3)^3, Arg^5, D-Glu^6(AA), D-Ala^{10}]LH-RH) (107) (Table 71.2) were potent, although subsequently the former analogue was shown to have solubility problems and the latter caused some side effects in clinical trials. Among other antagonists considered for development are Azaline B ([Ac-D-Nal^1, D-Phe (4Cl)^2, D-Pal^3, Aph^5 (Atz), Aph^6(Atz), Ilys^8, D-Ala^{10}]-GnRH) (13) and Detirelix ([N-Ac-D-Nal (2)^1, D-Phe (4Cl)^2, D-Trp^3, D-hArg (Et$_2$)^6, D-Ala^{10}]) Gn-RH (1).

CURRENT CLINICAL STATUS OF LH-RH ANTAGONISTS

Phase I clinical studies indicated that Cetrorelix given intravenously (IV), SC, or IM in doses of 300 to 1,200 μg inhibited LH and FSH release in postmenopausal women and cause no allergic reactions or side effects (33). Maximal inhibition was observed 6 to 12 hours after administration. After SC injection of 300 μg of Cetrorelix every 12 hours for 3 days, a marked decrease in the levels of both gonadotropins was observed. A fall in LH and FSH also was produced in patients with gonadal dysgenesis who were given 300 μg of this antagonist (33). Normal men showed a major fall in serum LH, FSH, and total and free serum testosterone levels for 12 to 24 hours after SC administration of 300 μg Cetrorelix (33). These findings are in agreement with the results of Behre et al. (5) and Klingmuller et al. (54), who also studied the effects of Cetrorelix in normal men. Cetrorelix seemed to have the higher suppressive rate than other antagonists, such as Nal-Glu or Detirelix, and even in large doses of up to 5 mg only occasionally caused minimal erythema, in contrast to Nal-Glu antagonist, which produced local side effects (5, 33, 54). In patients with benign prostate hyperplasia (BPH) or advanced prostate carcinoma (D2), treatment with 500 mg Cetrorelix b.i.d. produced a persistent inhibition of serum LH and FSH levels and a fall in serum testosterone levels (32, 34). (See section on prostate cancer.) Cetrorelix has also been used in an in vitro fertilization-embryo transfer program (IVF-ET) and it prevented premature LH surge in all of the 17 patients studied (82).

Several prototypes of sustained delivery systems (microcapsules and microgranules) of Cetrorelix in PLG have been produced and tried in experimental animals (114, 118, 119, 128). Other sustained release formulations of Cetrorelix (depot) have also been developed by Asta Medica and shown to be effective in normal volunteers. Clinical studies in patients with prostate cancer are in progress.

The efficacy of Cetrorelix in patients with breast cancer and ovarian cancer still remains to be demonstrated and will be the subject of intensive investigations (24). Our recent work with Cetrorelix in patients with advanced prostate cancer and paraplegia due to metastatic invasion of spinal cord (35) suggests that LH-RH antagonists could be indicated for patients with extensive metastases in whom the LH-RH agonists cannot be used as single agents, because of the possibility of flare-up. LH-RH antagonists might also be useful for other clinical indications in which inhibition of sex steroids is desirable.

LH-RH ANALOGUES CARRYING CYTOTOXIC RADICALS

Additional new classes of antitumor drugs are being developed based on LH-RH analogues bearing various cytotoxic radicals, such as melphalan (Mel), metal complexes related to cisplatin, anthraquinone derivatives, doxorubicin, methotrexate, and other chemotherapeutic agents (48, 114, 118–120). LH-RH agonists and antagonists carrying various cytotoxic radicals are designed as targeted chemotherapeutic agents intended for the treatment of cancers that contain receptors for LH-RH. Early compounds of this class were or have been already reported by us (48, 103, 114, 118–120). Such analogues exert the effect of LH-RH agonists or antagonists and, at the same time, might act as chemotherapeutic agents targeted to the tumor cells by their peptide portions for which binding sites are present on the tumor cell membranes. It is assumed that a peptide containing a cytotoxic radical can be bound to the membrane receptors and internalized. Thus, cytotoxic analogue T-98 containing an anthraquinone derivative coupled to [D-Lys^6]LH-RH is internalized by rat pituitary cells (103). A similar internalization could occur in prostate or breast cancers, which contain receptors for LH-RH. After endocytosis, such a compound could interfere with intracellular events in cancer cells. These analogues may also kill cancer cells by membrane action on the cell surface, without entering the cell (48, 103, 120). An advantage of using doxorubicin as a radical for linking to peptide analogues is that anthracycline antibiotics may be cytotoxic without entering the cells (103, 120).

The damage inflicted by cytotoxic analogues to pituitary LH- and FSH-secreting cells would not be deleterious to the cancer patient, since hypophysectomy has been used for treatment of some cancers. Our work indicates that in the pituitary cell superfusion system, cytotoxic LH-RH analogues selectively affect LH cells but not GH and PRL cells (103). A possible damage to other cells (e.g., corticotrophs, thyrotrophs) could be also alleviated by replacement therapy (103). The agonistic and antagonistic analogues containing cytotoxic radicals show high biologic activity in vitro and in vivo (48, 120). Some agonists and antagonists containing cytotoxic radicals were found to bind with high affinity to the LH-RH receptors in human breast cancers and prostate cancers. In cytotoxicity tests in cultures of human breast cancer and prostate cancer cell lines, some analogues containing cytotoxic groups powerfully inhibited the ^{3}H-thymidine incorporation into DNA (48, 120). Various cytotoxic LH-RH analogues were tested in vivo and shown to inhibit the growth of estrogen-independent MTX mouse mammary carcinoma (135) and Dunning rat prostate cancers (86). Because the antitumor action may be exerted to a greater degree locally, or at least at more selective sites that have the cell membrane receptors, the peripheral toxicity on normal cells that do not bind cytotoxic analogues would be reduced. In addition to prostate and breast cancers such compounds could be tried for the treatment of ovarian and endometrial cancer (24). The availability of cytotoxic compounds linked to hormonal peptides such as LH-RH that can be targeted to certain cancers possessing receptors for those peptides and, therefore, are more selective for killing cancer cells, could be of significant practical therapeutic importance. This approach might extend the utility of analogues of LH-RH from the current palliation toward an eventual cure.

Mode of Action of LH-RH Analogues

PITUITARY-GONADAL AXIS

LH-RH analogues are widely used in oncology, and their mode of action is almost completely understood. The mechanism of action of these analogues is mainly based on the inhibition of pituitary and gonadal function, but direct effects on various tumors may also play a role (24, 117–119).

Acute administration of LH-RH or LH-RH agonists produces an intense stimulation of pituitary LH and FSH release, but continuous treatment with LH-RH agonists causes a down-regulation (a decrease in the number) of LH-RH receptors and an uncoupling of the LH-RH signal transduction mechanism (6, 24, 44, 116–120). This results in a desensitization of gonadotrophs and a marked reduction in the secretion of bioactive LH and FSH. This state is reversible and is called "selective medical hypophysectomy" (24). The decrease in circulating LH and FSH, together with down-regulation of gonadal receptors for LH and FSH, produces a complete inhibition of testicular or ovarian function. This state is called "chemical or medical castration" (24, 101, 116–119). The key advantage of the medical castration achieved by LH-RH agonists is its reversibility and the possible avoidance of surgery, radiation therapy, or chemotherapy (24, 119). In addition, various extrapituitary tissues, including the prostate and ovaries, as well as many tumors, contain specific receptors for LH-RH, which might permit direct inhibitory actions of LH-RH super-agonists (24-26, 116–119).

The principal mechanism of action of LH-RH antagonists, which inhibit gonadotrophin secretion from the start of the administration, is the competitive blockade of LH-RH receptors, but recent experimental evidence documents that treatment with the LH-RH antagonist Cetrorelix down-regulates pituitary receptors in rats (24, 119, 128). This phenomenon may also occur clinically. The down-regulation of pituitary LH-RH receptors is also reversible, and a complete recovery occurs 3 to 7 months after cessation of treatment with antagonists (24).

The effects of LH-RH agonists were evaluated in a variety of studies carried out since 1976. In the female rat, chronic administration of LH-RH agonists decreased the ovarian and uterine weights, reduced the concentration of plasma estradiol and progesterone, and produced various antifertility effects (24, 116–119). Inhibition of the growth of DMBA-induced mammary tumors (80) was also demonstrated. The effects of chronic administration of LH-RH agonists were similar to those of ovariectomy and suggested a nonsurgical type of endocrine treatment of breast cancer (24). The administration of LH-RH agonists to premenopausal women initially increases plasma levels of gonadotropin, estradiol, and progesterone. However, after several weeks of administration of LH-RH agonists, sex-steroid levels are reduced to the postmenopausal range, but plasma estrone, androstanedione, and testosterone, while decreased, are somewhat above the levels in ovariectomized or postmenopausal women (24, 80, 117, 119). The effects of Decapeptyl, Zoladex, Buserelin, and leuprolide are similar (80), although the response to analogues may vary as a function of potency, Decapeptyl being apparently the most potent (119). The use of sustained-release preparations greatly increases biologic response (117–119).

The chronic administration of LH-RH agonists to male rats was shown to result in decreased plasma gonadotropin and testosterone levels, as well as in atrophy of testes, seminal vesicles, and prostatic tissue (6, 116, 117). This suggested that chronic administration of LH-RH agonists might mimic the effects of orchidectomy in prostatic cancer. Administration of LH-RH agonists to the human male initially results in a rise of FSH, LH, and testosterone, but after 4 to 6 weeks of treatment, plasma testosterone levels are reduced to castration levels (6, 117). In addition to the fall in immunoassayable LH, treatment with LH-RH agonists causes secretion of an LH with decreased biologic potency (6).

The mechanism of pituitary LH release in response to LH-RH is not completely understood. The first step in the action of LH-RH involves its binding to a plasma membrane receptor, which causes a microaggregation of receptors and complex formation (44). The complex formation formed is then internalized and degraded, although this internalization is not necessary for the liberation of the gonadotropins. Calcium and the products of phosphoinositide metabolism have been implicated as second messengers (44). The LH-RH receptor is coupled to a GTP-binding protein ("G protein") that can activate phospholipase C, which leads to the production of diacylglycerol and the activation of protein kinase C (44). Recent studies show that multiple G proteins are involved in the action of LH-RH on the gonadotrope. Activation of G protein stimulates LH release and inositol phosphate production (44).The complete mechanisms still remain to be elucidated.

DIRECT EFFECTS

Clinical evidence indicates that in patients with advanced breast or prostate cancer, medical castration produced by the chronic administration of LH-RH analogues accounts for most benefits derived from the treatment (24, 116–118). However, there is also evidence that LH-RH agonists and antagonists can exert direct effects on tumor cells (24). An exploitation of these effects may improve the results of therapy. The concept of the direct action of LH-RH analogues on cancers is based on evidence provided by clinical results, the detection of high-affinity binding sites for LH-RH in various cancers, and the effects on tumor cell lines in cultures.

Medical castration should not benefit postmenopausal women with breast cancer. However, Harris and colleagues (41) reported that 7 of 28 postmenopausal women with advanced breast cancer showed partial responses or stabilization of disease after Zoladex treatment, although the authors suggest that the reduction in peripheral estradiol, and not direct action on the tumors, may have been responsible for these effects. Schwartz and colleagues (123) and Plowman and colleagues (90) also reported responses in postmenopausal women treated with LH-RH agonists. Recently, Saphner and colleagues obtained an 11% response rate in postmenopausal women treated with Zoladex (111). Similarly, medical castration should not benefit patients with estrogen receptor (ER)-negative tumors. However, therapy with Zoladex depot of 118 premenopausal women with advanced breast cancer showed a response in 33% of ER-negative tumors (50). Manni and colleagues also noted responses in ER-negative premenopausal patients treated with leuprolide (74).

RECEPTORS FOR LH-RH IN VARIOUS TUMORS

Direct effects of LH-RH analogues could be mediated by receptors found on tumor cells. Specific membrane receptors for LH-RH have been found in various animal and human cancers. Both Dunning rat prostate cancers and specimens of human prostate cancers exhibited two types of receptors for D-Trp-6-LH-RH, one with high affinity and low capacity and one with low affinity and high capacity (25, 116, 118). Binding sites for LH-RH were also detected in LNCaP and DU-145 human prostate cancer lines (65, 95). Various investigators found LH-RH receptors in several human mammary carcinoma cell lines (10, 23, 77, 140). In 260 of 500 samples of human breast cancer (52%), two classes of D-Trp-6-LH-RH membrane receptor sites were also detected, one class showing high affinity and low capacity, and the other class showing low affinity and high capacity (26). MTX rat mammary cancers show low-affinity and high-capacity receptors for D-Trp-^{6}LH-RH (131). Both high-affinity and low-affinity LH-RH receptors were found in human ovarian epithelial cancers and in EFO-21 and EFO-27 human ovarian cancer lines (24). In human endometrial carcinomas and in HEC-1A and Ishikawa endometrial cancer lines, the presence of high-affinity membrane receptors for D-Trp-6-LH-RH was established (24). LH-RH receptors were similarly found in human pancreatic cancers (121). The expression of LH-RH receptor gene in human breast, ovarian, and prostate cancer cell lines was also demonstrated (24, 43, 46, 66). These findings provide a rationale for the use of therapeutic approaches based on LH-RH analogues in malignancies in which specific receptors for LH-RH are found.

INHIBITION OF GROWTH OF TUMOR CELL LINES

Observations on growth inhibition of cultured tumor cells by LH-RH analogues strongly support the concept of their direct effects. Original reports that LH-RH agonists inhibit human breast cancer cell growth (77) and suppress the proliferation of a human prostate cancer cell line (69) have been confirmed and extended. Significant inhibition of human breast and prostatic cancer cells by LH-RH agonists is now well documented (43, 53, 65, 69, 77, 95, 125). These results suggest a regulatory role of LH-RH-like peptides in tumor growth. Since LH-RH is not present in the general circulation in significant concentrations, the effects had to be attributed to some local forms of LH-RH. Thus, immunoreactive LH-RH-like peptides were found in cultured breast cancer cells (10). The presence of LH-RH immunoreactivity and mRNA for LH-RH in human mammary cancer cells also implied that LH-RH may play a role in the growth of mammary tumors (43). Subsequently, the evidence for production of an LH-RH-like peptide and/or expression of mRNA for LH-RH was obtained in human prostate cancer and human ovarian cancer lines (46, 66). If these LH-RH-like peptides function as local regulators of tumor growth, exploiting them may lead to improved therapy. LH-RH agonists and antagonists might inhibit the growth of tumor cells by nullifying the action of endogenous LH-RH-like peptides. New LH-RH antagonists such as Cetrorelix cause a marked inhibition of proliferation of mammary, ovarian, and endometrial cancer cell lines (24, 125, 142). Various observations suggest that direct inhibitory effects of LH-RH antagonists on tumor cells could be greater than those of agonists, and this might also occur in a clinical setting.

Somatostatin Analogues

Tetradecapeptide somatostatin (Fig. 71.1) has many biologic actions, inhibits a large variety of cells, and appears to be an endogenous antiproliferative agent (61, 113, 114). The clinical potential of somatostatin has been appreciated for more than 20 years. Various studies demonstrated the inhibitory effects of somatostatin in patients with acromegaly; endocrine pancreatic tumors, such as insulinomas and glucagonomas; ectopic tumors, such as gastrinomas; and vasoactive intestinal peptide (VIP)-producing tumors (113). However, the half-life of somatostatin is very short, so that its therapeutic use is impractical (113).

Several groups synthesized somatostatin analogues with more selective and prolonged activities (4, 11, 137). Veber et al. carried out conformational analysis, and designed several analogues by replacing 9 of the 14 amino acids of somatostatin with a single proline residue (Fig. 71.1) (137). Some of the resulting hexapeptide analogues, including cyclo(-Pro-Phe-D-Trp-Lys-Thr-Phe), were much more potent than somatostatin in inhibiting GH, insulin, and glucagon release (113, 137). However, some of these analogues did not reveal antitumor activities in various tumor models (113). Bauer and colleagues synthesized another series of highly potent octapeptide analogues of somatostatin (4). They incorporated the sequence 7 to 10 of somatostatin, Phe-D-Trp-Lys-Thr, proposed as essential by Veber and colleagues

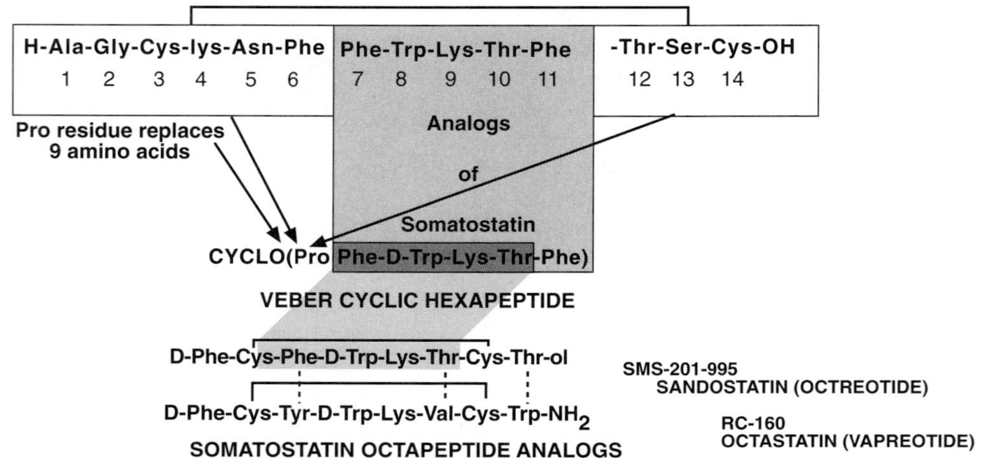

Figure 71.1 Structural relationship of somatostatin, Veber Hexapeptide, and octapeptide analogues Sandostatin and Octastatin.

(137) into a series of cystine-bridged analogues of which D-Phe-Cys-Phe-D-Trp-Lys-Thr-Cys-Thr-OL, containing a C-terminal amino alcohol was the most active (Fig. 71.1) (4). This analogue, designated SMS-201–995 (Sandostatin, octreotide) was 45 to 70 times more potent than somatostatin in tests on inhibition of GH secretion, and more selective.

Nearly 300 analogues of somatostatin, designed specifically for antitumor activity, were synthesized by our group (11, 113). The activity of some somatostatin analogues was enhanced by the incorporation of Tyr and Val in positions corresponding to residues 7 and 10 respectively, of somatostatin 14 (SS 14). Thus, the analogues D-Phe-Cys-Tyr-D-Trp-Lys-Val-Cys-Thr-NH_2 (RC-121) and D-Phe-Cys-Tyr-D-Trp-Lys-Val-Cys-Trp-NH_2 (RC-160) (Fig.71.1) were about 100 times more potent than SS 14 in tests for inhibition of GH release in vivo in rats and possessed a prolonged duration of action. RC-160 has been shown to be a powerful tumor growth suppressor in various experimental models of pancreatic, prostatic, colorectal, gastric, and mammary cancers (87, 88, 99, 100, 113, 114, 132, 133). Somatostatin analogue RC-160 also inhibited the growth of human glioblastomas and human small cell and non-small cell lung carcinomas in nude mice (88, 114). Sandostatin is known to selectively inhibit the growth of various endocrine tumors and is the analogue of somatostatin most extensively investigated in clinical trials (61). Sandostatin and other somatostatin analogues have been used for the treatment of acromegaly; endocrine tumors of the gastroenteropancreatic system, including carcinoid tumors; insulinomas; glucagonomas; gastrinomas; and VIPomas (59, 61, 62, 113). RC-160 and BIM-23014 (Somatulin; 3(2-naphthyl)-D-Ala-Cys-Tyr-D-Trp-Lys-Val-Cys-Thr-NH_2) are also being evaluated clinically for their antitumor activities. Hofland et al. reported that RC-160 was much more potent than Sandostatin or BIM 23014 in tests on inhibition of the release of GH from human pituitary adenoma cells and gastrin from human gastrinoma cells in vitro (45). The difference in potencies may be due to the higher affinity of RC-160 for somatostatin receptors as compared with Sandostatin. Attempts are being made to use modern somatostatin analogues for the therapy of human breast cancer, prostate cancer and carcinoma of exocrine pancreas, colorectal cancer, and gastric cancer, as well as brain tumors and lung cancer (61, 72, 75, 81, 87, 88, 93, 94, 99, 100, 109, 113, 114, 129, 132, 133, 138). (See the sections on specific neoplasms.)

SIDE EFFECTS

The side effects of somatostatin analogues consist mainly of steatorrhea, which can be controlled; malabsorption; gastrointestinal cramps; and occasional nausea. Somatostatin inhibits gallbladder contractions. and some patients treated with Sandostatin were reported to develop gallstones, but the incidence has not been clearly established. Somatostatin analogues are much less toxic than adjuvant chemotherapy (119).

MECHANISMS OF ANTITUMORAL ACTION OF SOMATOSTATIN ANALOGUES

It is likely that somatostatin analogues, by virtue of having a wide spectrum of activities (which include the suppression of the secretions of the pituitary, pancreas, stomach, and gut; interference with growth factors; and direct antiproliferative effects on some tissues), inhibit various tumors through multiple mechanisms (113). The fall in GH levels induced by somatostatin analogues causes a reduction in the production of insulin-like growth factor (IGF-I), which could be of major importance for the inhibition of growth of various tumors. IGF-I and -II and other growth factors, including epidermal growth factor (EGF) and transforming growth factor-α (TGF-α), appear to be involved in the proliferation of both normal and neoplastic cells (27, 28, 30, 36, 67, 71, 91, 92, 104, 113). The administration of RC-160 also causes the down-regulation of the receptors for EGF on various experimental tumors (87, 88, 114). In the Mia PaCa-2 human pancreatic cancer cell line, somatostatin reverses the stimulatory effect of EGF on the phosphorylation of the tyrosine kinase portion of the EGF receptor and on cell growth (64). Analogues RC-160 and RC-121, but not Sandostatin, cause dephosphorylation of EGF receptor and inhibit the EGF-induced growth of cultured MIA PaCa-2 cells more powerfully than does somatostatin (64, 113). These observations indicate that some somatostatin analogues act as growth inhibitors in cancer cells through the activation of tyrosine phosphatase (8, 9, 64, 113) (see also below). Thus, somatostatin analogues appear to exert some of their effects by mechanisms involving interference with the transmission of intracellular signals that regulate cell growth (64, 113). In conclusion, oncological applications of somatostatin analogues are based on multiple effects, and several mechanisms of action are likely.

RECEPTORS FOR SOMATOSTATIN

Somatostatin induces its biologic effects by interacting with specific receptors that are coupled to a variety of signal transduction pathways including adenylate cyclase, Ca^{2+} channels, and protein dephosphorylation (8, 9, 64, 115, 129). High- or low-affinity SS 14 receptors were identified in various normal human tissues; animal and human neoplasms, including such brain tumors as meningiomas and differentiated glia-derived tumors (astrocytomas and oligodendrogliomas); pituitary tumors; hormone-producing gastrointestinal tumors; breast cancers; small cell lung carcinoma cell lines; pancreatic cancer and colorectal cancer; human prostate cancers; and human ovarian cancers (28, 56, 57, 61, 62, 104, 105, 129).

Recently, five subtypes of somatostatin receptor, SSTR-1 to SSTR-5, were cloned and functionally characterized (8, 9, 81). They belong to the guanine nucleotide-binding regulatory protein (G-protein)-linked receptor family. They all bind somatostatin-14 and somatostatin-28 with similar affinity, but show major differences in their affinities for various somatostatin analogues (8, 9, 81). Sandostatin (octreotide) and RC-160 have a high binding affinity for somatostatin receptor subtype SSTR-2 and can induce a stimulation of tyrosine phosphatase activity and an inhibition of the proliferation of the cells expressing SSTR-2 gene (8). This implicates tyrosine phosphatase as a transducer of the growth inhibition signal. Since mRNAs of receptor subtypes are variably expressed in different pancreatic and colon cancer cell lines, this indicates the necessity for a precise determination of receptor subtypes in tumor tissue before therapy with analogues. RC-160 also exhibited moderate to high affinities for SSTR-3 and -5 and low affinity for SSTR-1 and -4 (9). In SSTR-5-expressing cells, the phosphatase pathway was not involved in the inhibitory action of RC-160 on cell growth and the phosphoinositide/calcium pathway could be implicated in this effect. Thus, both SSTR-2 and SSTR-5 receptor subtypes bind RC-160 with high affinity, but mediate the inhibition of cell growth induced by this analogue by distinct mechanisms (9).

LOCALIZATION OF TUMORS AND METASTASES BY SCINTIGRAPHY WITH RADIOLABELED SOMATOSTATIN ANALOGUES

Radioiodinated analogues of somatostatin, such as [^{111}In-DTPA-D-Phe^{1}]-octreotide (OctreoScan) and [^{123}I-Tyr^{3}]-octreotide have been used clinically for the localization of tumors containing receptors for somatostatin (56, 57, 62, 81). Tc-99m labeled RC-160 or ^{111}In-DTPA-RC-160 also could be used. Thus, the presence of somatostatin receptors may permit the localization of some tumors and metastases using scanning techniques (56, 57, 62). Information about membrane receptor levels may make feasible the planning of therapy with analogues. Lamberts et al. used ^{123}I-Tyr^{3}-octreotide for the scanning of five patients with endocrine pancreatic tumors, and found that this procedure was valuable in the localization of primary tumors, as well as their often clinically unrecognized metastases (62). Recently, Krenning et al. (57) reported the Rotterdam experience with somatostatin receptor scintigraphy in more than 1,000 patients. It was stated that various primary tumors, both neuroendocrine or non-neuroendocrine, containing high numbers of somatostatin receptors, can be localized in vivo.

In addition, metastases can be also visualized by scintigraphy with radiolabeled somatostatin analogue octreotide (57). Neuroendocrine tumors that could be readily localized with OctreoScan included GH- and TSH-producing pituitary tumor, gastrinomas, insulinomas, glucagonomas, unclassified apudomas, medullary thyroid carcinoma, neuroblastomas, pheochromocytomas, carcinoids, and small cell lung cancer (57). Non-neuroendocrine tumors that contained somatostatin receptors and that could be localized by in vivo scintigraphy included non-small cell lung cancer, meningiomas, breast cancer, and astrocytomas, but not exocrine pancreatic tumors (57). The value of scintigraphy as a conventional diagnostic technique for tumors such as breast cancer still has to be established (57). Other radiolabeled somatostatin analogues such as RC-160 have yet to be evaluated clinically. Scintigraphy should help to determine in therapeutic trials with somatostatin analogues which patients are likely to benefit from the treatment. In many cases, a positive scintigram predicted a good response to treatment with octreotide (57). A somatostatin analogue labeled with an appropriate radionuclide, such as rhenium^{186}, might be also used in cancer therapy. The presence of binding sites for somatostatin in certain cancers could also be utilized for targeting various chemotherapeutic agents linked to suitable somatostatin analogues, acting as carriers for these cytotoxic radicals (120).

Antagonists of Bombesin and Gastrin-Releasing Peptide

The bombesin-like peptides make up a large family of peptides found in amphibians and humans. The tetradecapeptide bombesin (Table 71.3), isolated from the skin of the frog *bombina* in 1970 (127, 130), was the first family member to be characterized. Subsequently, two mammalian bombesin-like peptides have been characterized, gastrin-releasing peptide (GRP), which is related to bombesin, and neuromedin B, which is related to amphibian ranatensin (127). Recent evidence suggests that bombesin-like peptides can function as growth factors and, through autocrine or paracrine mechanisms, may modulate the growth of some benign and neoplastic tissues. Bombesin can release gastrin and exert other pharmacologic effects on the gastrointestinal tract in mammals (119, 130). Bombesin-like immunoreactivity is widely distributed in mammalian brain, including the hypothalamus, lung, and GI tract (130). GRP is a 27-amino acid peptide isolated from porcine stomach (127, 130). The carboxyl-terminal decapeptide of GRP is identical to that of bombesin, except that residue number 20 in GRP is histidine instead of glutamine, found in position 7 of bombesin (Table 71.3). GRP and GRP (14-27) possess all the biologic and immunologic activities of bombesin (130). GRP is widely distributed in human fetal lung and GI tract and in rat brain, especially the hypothalamus (130). Neuromedin B, isolated from the porcine spinal cord, exists both in the short form (10 amino acids) and long form (32 amino acids) and has phenylalanine in the penultimate position from the C terminus, instead of leucine found in bombesin

Table 71-3.

Bombesin														
pGlu -	Gln -	Arg -	Leu -	Gly -	Asn -	Gln -	Trp -	Ala -	Val -	Gly -	His -	Leu -	Met -	NH_2
1	2	3	4	5	6	7	8	9	10	11	12	13	14	
Gastrin-releasing peptide (human)														
Val -	Pro -	Leu -	Pro -	Ala -	Gly -	Gly -	Gly -	Thr -	Val -	Leu -	Thr -	Lys -		
Met -	Tyr -	Pro -	Arg -	Gly -	Asn -	His -	Trp -	Ala -	Val -	Gly -	His -	Leu -	Met -	NH_2
14	15	16	17	18	19	20	21	22	23	24	25	26	27	

In analogues, ψ (psi) indicates a reduced (pseudo) peptide bond (—CH_2—NH—).

and GRP. Neuromedin B is distributed in various areas of the brain and in the GI tract (127).

From an oncologic point of view, the most interesting action of bombesin/GRP and neuromedin B is their ability to act as growth factors in normal and tumoral tissues. The link between bombesin/GRP and SCLC was discovered by Cuttitta, Moody, Minna, and colleagues, who found that SCLC cells both secrete and respond to bombesin-like peptides (19, 78, 79). Many SCLC lines express neuromedin B and its receptors (127). Since bombesin-like peptides are produced also in other cancers, such as breast, prostatic, and pancreatic cancer, and could act as autocrine growth factors, the development of hormonal therapy based on bombesin antagonists should be considered (87, 88, 96, 98, 100, 114, 119, 121, 127).

RECEPTORS FOR BOMBESIN/GRP

Three receptor subtypes associated with the bombesin-like peptides have been described and cloned (40, 127). They are classified as the GRP-preferring subtype found in the gut and in the central nervous system (CNS) the neuromedin B-preferring subtype, present in the GI tract and in some SCLCs; and the bombesin receptor subtype 3, present in lung cancer cell lines, the natural ligand of which is not yet known (127). GRP receptor subtypes bind GRP and bombesin with high affinity and neuromedin B with lower affinity. In contrast, the neuromedin B receptor subtype has a higher affinity for neuromedin B than for GRP or bombesin. All three subtypes are coupled through G proteins to effectors, including phospholipase C (127). Specific receptors for bombesin/GRP have been also demonstrated in human breast cancer biopsies (40), and in various human breast cancer and pancreatic cancer cell lines (96, 134, 141, 143). In some SCLCs, the mitogenic effects of bombesin-like peptides may be mediated by neuromedin B rather than GRP (127).

The activation of protein kinase C is involved in the transduction of the mitogenic signal of bombesin/GRP. Binding of bombesin/GRP to the receptors causes a rapid mobilization of Ca^{2+} from intracellular stores and an increase in the concentration of cytosolic Ca^{2+} (119, 127, 130).

ANTAGONISTS OF BOMBESIN/GRP

The discovery that bombesin/GRP function as autocrine growth factors for SCLC and other tumors stimulated the development of antagonists for the hormonal treatment of these malignancies. Several laboratories synthesized antagonists based on the tetradecapeptide sequence of bombesin, the COOH-terminal amino acid sequence of mammalian GRP, or broad-spectrum antagonists (12, 16, 17, 63, 98, 100). In addition to SCLC, bombesin/GRP antagonists might also find application in the treatment of colorectal, gastric, pancreatic, mammary, prostatic, and other cancers (87, 88, 100, 114, 118, 119, 121).

Early bombesin antagonists were analogues of substance P, such as [D-Arg^{1}, D-Phe^{5}, D-Trp^{7,9}, Leu^{11}] substance P, which had relatively low potency (63, 119). A second class of bombesin antagonists consisted of [D-Phe^{12}]-substituted bombesin analogues (119), but they were active only in large doses. The first competitive and specific bombesin/GRP receptor antagonists were based on the replacement of Met-14 residue by Leu and the introduction of a reduced peptide bond between positions 13 and 14 (16, 17). [Leu^{13} ψ(CH$_2$NH)Leu^{14}]-bombesin was active in a nanomolar range. Shorter-chain nonapeptide analogues of bombesin (6-14) with reduced ψ13–14 peptide bond, such as D-Phe^{6}, Leu$^{13}\psi$(CH$_2$NH)Leu^{14}-bombesin (6-14), were even more potent (17).

More than 100 pseudo (ψ13–14) bombesin (6–14) antagonists with different modifications at positions 6, 7, and 14 have been synthesized in our laboratory and evaluated for antitumor activity. D-Tetrahydrocarbolinecarboxylic (D-Tpi) acid residue, a constrained structural analogue of Trp, was introduced in position 6 of Leu^{14} or Phe^{14} bombesin (6–14), producing such analogues as D-Tpi^{6}, Leu^{13}, ψ(CH$_2$NH)-Leu^{14}-bombesin (6-14) (RC-3095) (98). Bombesin/GRP antagonist RC-3095 and related analogues blocked the binding of bombesin to the receptors on Swiss 3T3 cells and on human tumors including SCLC, gastric, pancreatic, and prostatic cancers, and effectively suppressed the growth of MTX breast cancers in mice, nitrosamine-induced pancreatic cancers in hamsters, and various human cancer lines, such as HT-29 colon cancer; PC-82, PC-3, and DU-145 prostate cancer; MKN-45 gastric carcinoma; CFPAC-1 pancreatic cancer; H69 SCLC; and MCF-7 MIII breast cancer xenografted into nude mice (87, 88, 96, 98, 114, 133, 134, 141, 143). The antitumor effects of RC-3095 could be linked to a significant decrease in the binding capacity of EGF receptors in these tumors (87, 88, 100, 114). RC-3095 also could inhibit proliferation of CFPAC-1 pancreatic cancer, Hs746T and MKN45 gastric cancer and MCF7 MIII breast cancer cell lines in vitro (87, 96, 141).

In order to develop still more powerful antagonists, several bombesin pseudononapeptides with a structure similar to that of RC-3095, but with modified C and N termini, have been also synthesized in our laboratory (12). Among them, Hca^{6}, Leu^{13}, ψ(CH$_2$N)Tac^{14}-BN (6-14) (RC-3940-II) and (D-Phe^{6}-Leu^{13}, ψ(CH$_2$N)Tac^{14}-BN (6-14)(RC-3950-II) showed a higher binding affinity to the receptors on tumor cells and greater antitumor activity than RC-3095. Since antagonists of this class inhibit the growth of various tumors in animal cancer models, some of them may have clinical applications. Ongoing clinical studies will determine the possible application of bombesin/GRP antagonists in the treatment of various cancers.

Antagonists of Growth Hormone-Releasing Hormone (GH-RH)

Growth hormone-releasing hormone (GH-RH) was first isolated from human pancreatic tumors that caused acromegaly (38, 106), and later from animal and human hypothalami (39). Two major forms were characterized: GH-RH (1–44)NH$_2$ and GH-RH (1–40) (39). Virtually full intrinsic biologic activity is present in the 29 *N*-terminal amino acid residues (GH-RH (1–29)NH$_2$). Various potent agonistic analogues of GH-RH (1–29)NH_2 intended for potential clinical and veterinary applications have been synthesized (144). Specific antagonists of human GH-RH are also needed clinically for the treatment of disorders caused by the excessive secretion of growth hormone, for example, acromegaly. However, the main applications of GH-RH antagonists might be in the field of cancer. Thus, GH-RH antagonists are designed to block the binding and action of GH-RH, which stimulates the secretion of GH. In turn, GH activates the production of insulin-like growth factor I (IGF-I) by the liver and other tissues. By suppressing GH secretion, antagonists of GH-RH should decrease the synthesis of hepatic IGF-I. GH-RH antagonists might also lower the autocrine or paracrine production of IGF-I by various tumors, which could lead to the inhibition of cancer proliferation (89, 144).

IGF-I can act as endocrine, paracrine, or autocrine growth factor for various human cancers (113). The involvement of IGF-I in breast cancer, colon cancer, bone tumors, and other malignancies is well established (30, 36, 67, 91, 113, 114, 118, 119). The receptors for IGF-I are present in various human tumors, including breast cancers (27, 28, 67, 91, 115); lung cancers, both SCLC and non-SCLC (71, 72); colon cancers (91, 100); osteogenic sarcomas (89, 92); pancreatic cancers (93, 94); and prostate cancers (118). The presence of IGF-I receptors in these tumors appears to be related to the malignant transformation and proliferation of these cancers (27, 28, 30, 67, 71, 72, 91, 99). GH-RH antagonists could be given alone or in combination with somatostatin analogues (92). The use of a combination of both analogues could achieve a more complete suppression of IGF-I levels (92). GH-RH antagonists could be also used for the suppression of the growth of tumors that do not express somatostatin receptors, such as osteosarcomas (92).

In the course of the synthesis of various analogues of hGH-RH (1–29)NH_2, it was found that the replacement of Ala_2 by D-Arg_2 produced antagonists (108). An early GH-RH antagonist, [Ac-Tyr^1, D-Arg^2]hGHRH (1–29)NH_2, was able to inhibit the GH-RH-stimulated adenylate cyclase activity in rat pituitary cells (108). This antagonist was also reported to block GH-RH-stimulated GH secretion after injection into rats (70).

We have synthesized and tested biologically antagonists of human growth hormone-releasing hormone (hGH-RH)1–29, which contained D-Arg^2, Phe $(4Cl)^6$, Abu^{15}, Nle^{27}, and Agm^{29} substituents (144). In the superfused rat pituitary cell system, all the analogues inhibited more powerfully the GH-RH-induced growth hormone (GH) release than did the standard GH-RH antagonist. Thus new antagonist [Ibu^0, D-Arg^2, Phe $(4Cl)^6$, Abu^{15}, Nle^{27}]hGHRH (1-28)Agm (MZ-4–71), inhibited GH release at 3×10^{-9} M concentrations (144). This analogue was also found to bind with high affinity to rat pituitary GH-RH receptors. In vivo, our GH-RH antagonists induced a significantly greater inhibition of GH release than did the standard antagonist (144). We have also shown that antagonists such as MZ-4-71 inhibit the growth of human osteosarcomas in nude mice and MTX breast tumors in mice (89). Since the IGF-I concentrations in such tumors as osteosarcomas were decreased by therapy with GH-RH antagonists, this class of analogues may inhibit tumor growth not only by suppressing the GH-stimulated IGF-I levels, but also directly by interfering with the autocrine secretion of IGF-I by tumor cells. In view of their high antagonistic activity and prolonged duration of action, new antagonists of GH-RH may find clinical applications, including the treatment of IGF-I-dependent tumors.

Treatment of Various Tumors with Peptide Analogues

CLINICALLY LOCALIZED PROSTATE CANCER

For the past 14 years, LH-RH agonists have been mostly used for the palliative treatment of patients with advanced (stages C and D) prostate cancer (18, 19, 21, 51, 83, 85, 118, 119, 124, 126). The treatment options for patients with clinically localized prostate cancer include radical prostatectomy, radiation therapy, watchful waiting, and hormonal therapy (14). Potentially curative treatments, such as radical prostatectomy or radiation therapy, are recommended for those men with clinically localized prostate cancer who have a life expectancy of more than 10 years (14). Watchful waiting is considered a reasonable choice for patients with a life expectancy of less than 10 years who present with low-grade, early-stage prostate cancer (14). However, the optimal primary therapy for patients with clinically localized prostate cancer still remains to be determined (14) and LH-RH analogues could be considered for patients who are unsuitable candidates for more aggressive treatment.

LOCALLY ADVANCED PROSTATE CANCER

Some controversy also exists with respect to the best treatment strategy for patients with locally advanced prostate cancer. Cancer that has spread beyond the capsule of the prostate has a much lower chance of cure with radical prostatectomy or radiation therapy. Several studies have shown a promising effect of treatment with LH-RH agonist in combination with an antiandrogen (flutamide), prior to radical prostatectomy in patients with clinical stage C prostate cancer (122). The aim of endocrine therapy is to achieve downstaging and diminish morbidity following the operation and to improve the overall survival (122). Although in one such study, the downstaging was confirmed pathologically in only 13% of patients, this may still have implications for survival (122). Results of a phase III trial on the combined use of Zoladex and flutamide before and during radiation therapy for locally advanced prostatic cancer indicated after 3 years' follow-up, a significant local control of the disease and no clinical progression, no positive rebiopsy, and prostate-specific antigen (PSA) levels below 4 ng/ml (97).

ADVANCED PROSTATE CANCER

Carcinoma of the prostate is androgen dependent in about 70% of all cases (21, 116, 119, 124, 126). A large percentage of patients with prostate cancer already have metastatic disease when first diagnosed. The management of advanced (stages C and D) prostate cancer is palliative and is based on therapies that produce androgen deprivation (85, 119, 126). The aim of endocrine therapy is to improve the quality of life and prolong survival.

Primary endocrine treatment modalities for advanced adenocarcinoma of the prostate include orchiectomy, and administration of estrogens (diethylstilbestrol; DES), antiandrogens, such as cyproterone acetate, or flutamide and LH-RH agonists (85). Combinations of progestational steroids (e.g., megestrol acetate with DES) are occasionally used (118, 119). Currently, bilateral orchiectomy or the administration of LH-RH agonists has become a standard therapy for advanced prostate cancer (21). The elimination or inhibition of testicular androgen secretion can induce a high degree of initial response. Nevertheless, surgical castration is associated with a psychologic impact, and estrogens, such as DES, have serious cardiovascular, hepatic, and mammotropic side effects (119). Treatment with LH-RH agonists is as effective as orchiectomy and offers the advantage of avoiding castration (14, 18, 119).

USE OF LH-RH AGONISTS ALONE AND IN COMBINATION WITH ANTIANDROGENS

Based on the finding of Redding and Schally in 1981 that D-Trp-6-LH-RH inhibited the growth of transplantable rat prostatic tumors (101), the first demonstration of successful palliation with LH-RH analogues in patients with advanced prostate cancer was done in a collaborative trial at the Royal Victoria Hospital in Montreal by Tolis and collaborators (136). This demonstration that LH-RH analogues were safe and effective alternatives to orchiectomy was followed by many confirmations, which have been reviewed (118, 119, 124). However, early daily injections were inconvenient and occasionally produced compliance problems. The development of long-acting sustained-release formulations permitted excellent results with injections on a monthly basis (18, 83, 85, 117–119, 124, 126).

It is now well established that chronic administration of the potent long-acting agonistic analogue of LH-RH, such as leuprolide, Decapeptyl, Zoladex, or Buserelin, provides effective palliative therapy in patients with advanced prostate cancer (18, 119, 124, 126). Acceptance of LH-RH analogues is excellent, and in a recent survey of patients with prostatic cancer who were offered a choice between orchidectomy and LH-RH agonists, the analogues were selected by more than 70% of the patients as primary treatment (18). Nevertheless, since superactive agonists of LH-RH initially induce a marked release of LH, FSH, and sex steroids, some episodes of occasional temporary flare-up of the disease during the first week of administration have been reported (19, 35, 60, 119). Thus, an elevation in prostate acid phosphatase and an increase in bone pain may occur (19, 35, 58, 119). The worsening of clinical symptoms occurs in about 10% of patients, and the expanding tumor may cause spinal cord or cauda equina damage, with possible paraplegia (35, 119). Administration of DES or flutamide for 7 days before and during the first 14 days of therapy with LH-RH agonists will prevent disease flare-ups (35, 60, 119). Cyproterone acetate or the nonsteroidal antiandrogen nilutamide (Anandron) can also prevent disease flare-ups in prostate cancer patients treated with LH-RH agonists (58, 118).

The combination of orchiectomy with surgical adrenalectomy to eliminate adrenal androgens was proposed by Huggins and Scott more than 50 years ago (21). The concept was that adrenal androgen may stimulate the growth of prostate tumors. Antiandrogens, which neutralize the effect of endogenous androgens, have been used for many years in the management of prostate cancer in men; for reviews, see Sogani and Fair (126). Labrie et al. (60) reintroduced the concept of total androgen blockade and proposed the use of the combination of an LH-RH agonist and antiandrogen for the treatment of advanced prostate cancer. In a trial conducted in 603 men with disseminated D2 prostate cancer, the combination of leuprolide with flutamide produced a small increase in progression-free survival and median length of survival as compared to therapy with leuprolide alone (19).

A phase III, European Organization for Research and Treatment of Cancer (EORTC) study (30853) compared a total of 327 patients with metastatic prostatic cancer subjected to bilateral orchiectomy or treated with Zoladex depot combined with flutamide. There was a significant increase in time to progression after the combination treatment, but no differences in survival time were found (51). Meta-analysis of 23 trials showed an advantage of the LH-RH agonist therapy in combination with an antiandrogen over orchiectomy, particularly in time to progression (21). These trials also showed a small but distinct improvement in survival with the combination treatment (21).

LH-RH ANTAGONISTS

Various studies on Dunning R-3327 experimental prostate cancer models in rats showed that the LH-RH antagonist Cetrorelix caused a greater inhibition of tumor growth than did agonist D-Trp-6-LH-RH (118, 119, 128). In nude mice bearing xenografts of PC-82 human prostate adenocarcinoma, Cetrorelix caused a greater decrease in tumor growth, serum testosterone, and prostate-specific antigen (PSA) levels than did the agonist (118, 119). Cetrorelix was also markedly more effective and more rapid in suppressing the proliferation of androgen-independent Dunning R-3327-AT-1 tumor cells in vitro than the agonist (118). LH-RH antagonists may prove to be superior to the agonists for prostate cancer treatment (114).

Since 1988, we have been carrying out various clinical studies with the antagonist Cetrorelix in patients with benign prostatic hyperplasia and advanced prostate cancer (32, 34, 35, 114, 117, 119). Clinical trials indicate that a persistent inhibition of testosterone levels can be maintained in patients with advanced prostatic cancer (stages C and D_2) treated with 500 μg Cetrorelix b.i.d. for several months. After the first week of therapy, a significant decrease in bone pain, relief in urinary outflow obstruction, and reversal of the signs of prostatism were observed (34). Subjective improvement continued during the following weeks of treatment so that the patients no longer required analgesic (34). The serum levels of PSA, acid, and alkaline phosphatase gradually fell, achieving nearly normal values at 6 weeks. In patients with stage C disease, there was a large decrease in prostate size as measured by ultrasonography (34). An improvement in obstructive symptoms of prostatism and prolonged inhibition of serum testosterone to castration levels were also induced in patients with benign prostate hyperplasia (BPH) after SC administration of 500 μg of Cetrorelix b.i.d (34). Clinical improvement of patients with advanced prostate cancer and the absence of side effects indicate that Cetrorelix should be further evaluated for the therapy of prostate carcinoma. In addition, the rapid shrinkage of the prostate and concomitant improvement in obstructive symptoms of prostatism obtained with Cetrorelix in patients with BPH may decrease the morbidity of prostatic surgery and offer a therapeutic alternative for men who are considered poor surgical risks (34).

In view of favorable clinical results, we evaluated the response to Cetrorelix in five patients with advanced carcinoma of the prostate and paraplegia due to metastatic compression of spinal cord or cauda equina, who could not be treated with LH-RH agonists because of the risk of flare-up (35). Cetrorelix was given at two different dose regimens. Three patients were given 500 μg b.i.d. and two received 5 mg b.i.d. for 2 days and then 800 μg b.i.d. In all patients, the neurologic symptoms regressed. The neurologic improvement continued during the treatment and at 3 months all the patients were able to walk with the aid of a cane. In one patient, myelography showed that the spinal cord compression had disappeared and prostatic volume assessed by ultrasonography showed a significant decrease. Bladder function greatly improved in all five patients during treatment with Cetrorelix. Baseline levels of LH, FSH, and testosterone fell after the first day of therapy with Cetrorelix, and persistent inhibition of gonadotropins and testosterone was maintained during the subsequent 3 months of therapy (35). The high levels of PSA gradually decreased by 42 to 96%. Although one patient continued to show clinical improvement during 13 months of therapy with Cetrorelix, he withdrew from the study for nonmedical reasons. After discontinuing the medication, he relapsed and died 6 months later. Our results show that Cetrorelix and related LH-RH antagonists might be particularly useful for patients with prostate cancer and metastases in the brain, spine, liver, and bone marrow, in whom the LH-RH agonists cannot be used as single drugs because of the possibility of flare-up (35).

RELAPSE FROM ANDROGEN CONTROL

It has been documented in thousands of patients with advanced prostate carcinomas that LH-RH agonists provide effective palliative therapy resulting in objective stable disease or partial remission (18, 114, 118, 119). However, all hormonal therapies aimed at androgen deprivation, including orchiectomy, antiandrogens, LH-RH analogues and their combination, provide remissions of only limited duration. Most patients with advanced prostatic carcinoma relapse in 18 to 36 months (18, 119, 124, 126). These patients finally die, apparently of androgen-independent prostatic cancer. The mechanism responsible for the relapse of prostate cancer may involve selective proliferation of clones of androgen-independent cancer cells that were present within a predominantly androgen-sensitive but heterogeneous tumor (47). Although hormone-dependent tumor cells stop growing after androgen elimination, the testosterone-insensitive cells are capable of proliferation, and eventually become predominant (47). Therapeutic options are limited for patients who relapse from androgen control (14, 126). Chemotherapy shows poor response rates and significant toxicity (see Chapter 126). Suramin is being tried (14, 18, 126) (see Chapter 68).

Growth factors including EGF, TGF-α, and IGF-I may play a role in the growth and progression of prostate cancer (14, 114, 118, 119). Several human prostate cancer cell lines were shown to secrete and respond to EGF and TGF-α (114, 118). A stimulatory effect of IGF-I has been also demonstrated in the androgen-independent prostate cancer cell line PC-3. Receptors for EGF, IGF-I, and bombesin/GRP have been demonstrated on prostate cancer cells (113). Interference with the action, secretion, signal transmission, or receptors of endogenous growth factors, such as IGF-I or EGF, by somatostatin analogues or bombesin/GRP antagonists could inhibit the growth of androgen-independent prostate cancers and delay the relapse (113, 118).

In nude mice with transplanted hormone-dependent human prostate cancer PC-82, bombesin antagonist RC-3095 and the combination of D-Trp-6-LH-RH and RC-160 caused a greater inhibition of tumor growth than did D-Trp-6-LH-RH alone (113). Similarly, in nude mice bearing xenografts of the androgen-independent human prostate cancer cell line PC-3 or DU-145, tumor growth was significantly reduced by somatostatin analogue RC-160 and bombesin antagonist RC-3095 (113). In all three prostate cancer models, administration of RC-160 and RC-3095 produced a significant down-regulation of EGF receptors (113). Our results suggest that somatostatin analogue RC-160 and bombesin/GRP antagonist RC-3095 can inhibit the growth of androgen-independent prostate cancer when the therapy is started early (113).

Bombesin antagonists still have to be evaluated clinically in patients with prostate cancer. However, seven patients with prostate cancer (stage D-2), who relapsed after 2 to 7 years of therapy with D-Trp-6-LH-RH alone, were treated using a combination of the somatostatin analogue RC-160 (1 mg t.i.d.) and D-Trp-6-LH-RH and three showed stabilization of disease (32, 118). The elevated serum PSA and prostatic acid phosphatase levels declined in some patients during this treatment. In one patient, this remission has been maintained so far for 18 months (32, 118). Other patients had remissions for a few months, but then showed progressive deterioration and died. These preliminary results suggest the need for a further evaluation of this approach aimed at delaying relapse time and prolonging survival in patients with prostate cancer who no longer respond to androgen deprivation therapy.

PERSPECTIVES FOR IMPROVEMENT OF THERAPY WITH PEPTIDE ANALOGUES

Two classes of analogues consisting of LH-RH agonists and antagonists that safely produce medical castration are now available. New LH-RH antagonists may offer advantages in therapy because of speedy action and avoidance of flare-ups (2, 32–35, 114, 118, 128). In addition, the antagonists may exert greater direct inhibitory effects on prostate cancer than the agonists, but this still has to be shown clinically. Future clinical studies using combinations of LH-RH analogues with somatostatin analogues or bombesin/GRP antagonists might reveal effective combinations of peptides that could delay the relapse and prolong survival. In addition, the ongoing development of LH-RH analogues as carriers for targeted cytotoxic radicals, such as doxorubicin derivatives, could result in therapeutic agents endowed with both a hormonal action and a local tumoricidal effect (48, 114). This approach, which remains to be tested clinically, may open up a new area of therapy and convert the current palliation into an eventual cure.

Breast Cancer

Breast cancer is the most common malignancy among American women and is responsible for about 46,000 deaths annually (7). Approximately 30% of unselected premenopausal patients with breast cancers have estrogen-dependent tumors and can be treated by hormonal manipulations, which include surgical oophorectomy (24). The antiestrogen tamoxifen may constitute a useful therapy in premenopausal women with advanced breast cancer, particularly those with ER-positive tumors (110). Tamoxifen has shown clear benefits in postmenopausal women with breast cancer (110), probably because of direct inhibition of the action of residual estrogens on tumors (110). However, tamoxifen does not completely antagonize the effect of ovarian estrogens (110) and may contribute to an increase in endometrial carcinomas. Surgical oophorectomy is invasive and irreversible (24). Consequently, new approaches to produce rapid estrogen deprivation are being explored. Several experimental studies in rat and mouse models of mammary tumors showed that analogues of LH-RH, by creating a state of sex-steroid deficiency, might be useful for the treatment of estrogen-dependent breast cancer (80, 116). Various clinical trials conducted since 1982 with Decapeptyl, Buserelin, Zoladex, or leuprolide in women with metastatic breast cancer revealed frequent objective responses in premenopausal patients with ER-positive tumors (24, 52, 53, 74, 80, 117, 139). Responses to LH-RH analogues in a small percentage of postmenopausal women, amounting to an overall response rate of about 8 to 11% (24, 41, 74, 90, 111, 117, 123), are incompletely understood, but can be tentatively explained by a hypothesis of direct effects of LH-RH agonists on tumors (24). This issue is still controversial, although LH-RH agonists have been shown to have direct inhibitory effects on some human breast cancer cell lines in vitro, and receptors for LH-RH have been demonstrated in cell lines and in primary breast tumors (23, 24, 43, 77). The responses of postmenopausal women (41, 74, 90, 123) and ER-negative patients (50, 74) to LH-RH agonists are discussed in the section on the mode of action.

At present, LH-RH agonists are mainly targeted at premenopausal women with breast cancer in whom a clear suppression of ovarian estrogen can be obtained (80). This indication is supported by recent studies. Tumor remissions after Zoladex therapy occurred primarily in about 50% of women with well-differentiated, slow-growing, and ER-positive disease (80, 139). A large recent trial by Kaufmann and colleagues in premenopausal women with breast cancer, utilizing depot implants of Zoladex, demonstrated 53% objective tumor responses (50). Santen and colleagues summarized these various studies and calculated a 41% objective response rate in unselected premenopausal patients and 51% in women with ER-positive tumors (110). Overall results suggest that "medical oophorectomy" with LH-RH agonists is effective in women with estrogen-dependent breast cancers. There was a remarkable lack of significant clinical toxicity with LH-RH agonists. The phenomenon of tumor flare has not been clearly documented in women with breast cancer during therapy with LH-RH agonists (110).

COMBINATION THERAPY

The combination of an LH-RH analogue with an antiestrogen in the treatment of breast cancer might provide complete "estrogen blockade." Walker et al. (139) have reported that a combination of Zoladex, in long-acting depot preparations, and tamoxifen can be safely used in premenopausal women with breast cancer. Significantly greater lowering of serum estradiol and FSH was obtained with the combination (139). The use of aromatase inhibitors in combination with LH-RH agonists has also been suggested in patients who relapse on treatment with LH-RH agonists alone (24).

FUTURE DIRECTIONS: SOMATOSTATIN ANALOGUES, BOMBESIN/GRP ANTAGONISTS, AND LH-RH ANTAGONISTS

Growth factors such as EGF and IGF-I, bombesin-like peptides, growth hormone (GH), and prolactin (PRL) may be involved in breast cancer growth (27, 28, 36, 67, 113, 114, 116). Receptors for somatostatin are found in about 30% of human breast cancer specimens (26). The presence of receptors for somatostatin (SS-R) in human breast cancer is associated with a good prognosis (28, 104). The relapse-free survival for patients with tumors containing SS-R was significantly longer than for patients with SS-R-negative tumors; after 5 years, 82 versus 46% were disease-free (28). Manni and colleagues evaluated the effects of combined somatostatin analogue Sandostatin and bromocriptine therapy in postmenopausal women with advanced breast cancer (75). They concluded that combined Sandostatin and bromocriptine therapy can suppress GH, IGF-I, and PRL secretion in most patients (75), but only one patient experienced disease stabilization. Vennin and colleagues also used Sandostatin to treat 16 postmenopausal patients with advanced breast cancer and obtained tumor stabilization in three (138). Combinations of Sandostatin and tamoxifen are also being tried. Other somatostatin analogues have not been tested clinically, but results in animal models of breast cancer demonstrate that treatment with agonist D-Trp-6-LH-RH or LH-RH antagonist Cetrorelix in combination with somatostatin analogue RC-160 strongly inhibits tumor growth (113, 114, 131). These findings suggest the merit of further therapeutic trials in patients with combinations of LH-RH and somatostatin analogues.

Various studies demonstrate that bombesin/GRP may be involved in the function and growth of human breast cancer (40, 134, 141, 143). Bombesin stimulates proliferation of MCF-7 MIII and MDA-MB-231 human breast cancer lines (141), and this effect can be inhibited by bombesin/GRP antagonists. Specific receptors for bombesin/GRP have been demonstrated in 33 of 100 human breast specimens and in various human breast cancer cell lines (40, 134, 141, 143). It has been also shown that bombesin/GRP antagonist RC-3095 inhibits the growth of estrogen-dependent and estrogen-independent MTX mammary cancer in mice, and of MCF-7 MIII human breast cancer in nude mice (134, 143). The inhibitory effect of the bombesin antagonist on the growth of these breast cancers was linked with a major decrease in EGF receptor levels in tumors (134, 143). Bombesin receptor antagonists, such as RC-3095, might be useful for therapy of ER-negative breast cancers, alone or in combination with other agents.

New antagonistic analogues of LH-RH, such as Cetrorelix, cause an immediate inhibition of the pituitary-gonadal axis and await therapeutic trials in women with breast cancer to establish their clinical efficacy. In vitro studies on breast cancer cell lines suggest that antagonists, such as Cetrorelix, may directly inhibit cell proliferation under conditions in which the agonists have no effect (23, 114, 125). It has been demonstrated that Cetrorelix inhibits the growth of DMBA-induced mammary tumors in rats and transplanted estrogen-dependent and -independent MTX mammary tumors in mice, as well as MCF-7-MIII human breast cancers in nude mice (114, 131, 140). In many tests, Cetrorelix proved to be more efficacious and to act more rapidly than the agonist D-Trp-6-LH-RH (114). Thus, the LH-RH antagonist Cetrorelix could be of potential clinical value in the treatment of breast cancer. Future therapies of breast cancer could also be based on the use of cytotoxic LH-RH analogues or antagonists of GH-RH (114, 135, 144).

Epithelial Ovarian Cancer

Epithelial ovarian cancer is the most common cause of death from gynecologic cancer in the United States (7). Treatment based on surgery, chemotherapy, and steroids is not very effective, and new approaches must be explored (24, 84). Ovarian cancer may be dependent on LH and FSH (24, 114, 116, 142). Experimental and clinical findings indicate that suppression of the secretion of gonadotropins produced by LH-RH agonists may inhibit the growth of ovarian epithelial cancers (24, 84, 114, 116). Some of the inhibitory effects of LH-RH agonists could be direct since specific binding sites for LH-RH and its analogues have been found in 80% of surgically removed human ovarian carcinoma specimens, as well as in EFO-21 and EFO-27 human ovarian cancer cell lines (24). The agonist [D-Trp-6]-LH-RH at 10^{-9} M concentrations significantly reduced proliferation of EFO cell lines in culture (24). The expression of mRNA for LH-RH and LH-RH receptors in these cell lines (46) supports the view that local LH-RH-like substances may be involved in the proliferation of ovarian cancer.

Parmar and colleagues were the first to report that chronic treatment with [D-Trp-6]LH-RH microcapsules can induce the regression of advanced ovarian cancer (84). When 41 unselected patients with advanced epithelial ovarian cancer (FIGO stage III or IV) were treated with D-Trp-6-LH-RH, there was a marked suppression of LH and FSH, and about 26% of patients showed partial remission or stabilization of disease (84). This treatment offers a nontoxic alternative to patients who do not tolerate chemotherapy or who have progressive disease following chemotherapy (84). These findings were confirmed by other phase II studies (24). A large controlled multicenter trial with D-Trp-6-LH-RH in about 200 patients with advanced ovarian cancer is now in progress in Europe, but it is still too early to evaluate the effects on survival time (24). However, recent experimental results indicate that the LH-RH antagonist Cetrorelix inhibits the growth of human epithelial ovarian cancers better than agonist D-Trp-6-LH-RH (114, 142) and, therefore, may be more efficacious clinically. Administration of Cetrorelix inhibited the growth of xenografted OV-1063 and UCI-107 human epithelial ovarian cancer lines in nude mice (73, 142). Studies in vitro indicated that Cetrorelix binds to LH-RH receptors on OV-1063 and EFO-21 cells and can inhibit their proliferation (24, 142). It is possible that inhibitory effects of Cetrorelix on ovarian cancers are exerted not only through the suppression of the pituitary-gonadal axis, but also directly (24). In view of a strong inhibitory effect on the growth of ovarian cancers, LH-RH antagonists, such as Cetrorelix, might be considered for hormonal therapy of advanced ovarian carcinoma.

Endometrial Carcinoma

Endometrial carcinoma is the fourth most common cancer in American women (7, 24, 114). Surgery or radiotherapy is successful in 75% of patients, but new methods are needed for advanced (FIGO stage III or IV) or relapsed cases (24). The involvement of estrogens in the pathogenesis of endometrial adenocarcinoma is well recognized (24, 114, 116). LH-RH analogues could influence endometrial cancer mainly by estrogen deprivation through medical castration, although the incidence of this neoplasm is much higher in postmenopausal women. However, the direct effect of LH-RH analogues on tumors must be also considered since about 80% of human endometrial carcinomas show specific high-affinity membrane receptors for LH-RH (24). High-affinity binding sites for LH-RH are also present in HEC-1A and Ishikawa human endometrial cancer cell lines (24). [D-Trp-6]LH-RH and antagonist Cetrorelix can significantly inhibit the proliferation of both cell lines (24). The growth inhibition produced by Cetrorelix is associated with an induction of apoptosis. These findings provide an additional rationale for the use of therapeutic approaches based on LH-RH analogues in this cancer (24, 114). In a phase II trial in patients with recurrent endometrial cancer, administration of depot leuprolide or goserelin led to a partial or complete remission in six patients (35%) (29). Phase II trials with [D-Trp-6]LH-RH also look encouraging (24). Cytotoxic analogues of LH-RH might also provide a targeted chemotherapy with higher efficacy and/or less systemic toxicity than conventional regimens (24, 114).

Exocrine Pancreatic Cancer

Carcinoma of the pancreas has a very poor prognosis and the 5-year survival rate is about 2% (15, 31, 93, 94, 109, 113, 114, 116, 121). Only 15 to 20% of tumors are resectable and radiation and chemotherapy are of limited effectiveness (15, 94, 109). Therefore, it is essential to develop more effective therapy (15). Various experimental and clinical findings indicate that the growth of exocrine pancreatic cancer may be influenced by GI, hormones, growth factors, and sex steroids. These studies have been reviewed extensively (94, 114, 116, 120, 121). That the growth of experimental pancreatic tumors can be inhibited by hormonal manipulations, such as the administration of analogues of LH-RH and somatostatin, was first reported by Redding and Schally in 1984 (102). Attempts are being made to develop a hormonal therapy for exocrine cancer of the pancreas based on somatostatin analogues, bombesin/GRP antagonists, and LH-RH agonists or antagonists, singly or in combination (15, 93, 96, 99, 109, 114, 116, 132, 133). Somatostatin analogues suppress the secretion and/or action of GI hormones (gastrin, secretin, and cholecystokinin), which might influence the growth of the malignant cells of the pancreas (113, 116, 129). Somatostatin analogues also inhibit the action or secretion of growth factors, such as EGF, TGF-α, and IGF-I, which appear to be involved in neoplastic processes (113, 114). Direct antiproliferative actions of somatostatin analogues may be mediated by specific high-affinity receptors located on pancreatic tumor cells (64, 129). Analogue RC-160 inhibits the growth of the Mia PaCa-2 cell line in cultures and stimulates the dephosphorylation of the EGF receptor (64). The existence of five different subtypes of somatostatin receptors makes imperative the identification of the subtype variably expressed in pancreatic cancers before selecting the somatostatin analogue for therapy (8). Thus, RC-160 has a high affinity for SSTR-2, and can induce a stimulation of tyrosine phosphatase activity and inhibition of proliferation of cells expressing this subtype of receptor (8, 9). Various reports indicate that bombesin and GRP can influence the release of GI hormones, promote pancreatic secretion and growth, and stimulate pancreatic carcinogenesis (96, 121, 133). Thus, bombesin stimulates the growth of CFPAC-1 and other human pancreatic cancer cells in vitro, probably through high-affinity binding sites for bombesin found on these cells (96). Receptors for bombesin are found in BOP-induced pancreatic cancers as well (121, 133). Sex steroids may also play a role in the growth of the cancerous pancreas (31, 121) and LH-RH agonists could create a state of sex steroid deprivation (117) or exert a direct effect on LH-RH receptors present in pancreatic cancer (121).

Numerous studies showed that a marked inhibition of tumor growth with apoptosis occurs in hamsters with BOP-induced pancreatic cancer after treatment with microcapsules of somatostatin analogue RC-160 or D-Trp-6-LH-RH (121, 132, 133). The increase in the dosage of RC-160 led to greater regression of tumors. The combination of both peptides produced the best therapeutic results (132). Treatment with RC-160 plus 5-FU also produced greater tumor inhibition than 5-fluorouracil (5-FU) or the analogue alone (114, 121). LH-RH antagonist Cetrorelix likewise causes a powerful inhibition of pancreatic tumor growth (132). In nude mice bearing xenografts of MIA PaCa-2 human cancer cell line, a combination of RC-160 and D-Trp-6-LH-RH inhibited tumor growth better than RC-160 alone, and Cetrorelix also decreased tumor weight and volume (99). Our findings suggest that the combination of RC-160 and LH-RH analogues might increase the therapeutic response.

The inhibitory effect of bombesin antagonist RC-3095 on hamster ductal pancreatic cancers was demonstrated in several experiments (114, 121, 133) and was invariably linked to a major down-regulation of EGF receptors. Chronic administration of bombesin/GRP antagonist RC-3095 inhibits the growth of CFPAC-1 and other human pancreatic cancer cells transplanted to nude mice (96, 121). Bombesin antagonist RC-3095 also powerfully inhibited the bombesin-stimulated growth of various pancreatic cancer cells in vitro (96). Other bombesin/GRP antagonists such as RC-3940-II, with high binding affinity to pancreatic cancers were even more potent than RC-3095 in inhibiting the growth of human pancreatic adenocarcinoma cells in vivo and in vitro (12). These findings suggest the merit of continued evaluation of bombesin/GRP antagonists for the possible development of new approaches to treatment of pancreatic cancer.

On the basis of experimental observations that administration of D-Trp-6-LH-RH inhibits the growth of pancreatic cancers, this analogue was tried clinically in patients with inoperable pancreatic cancer. In some it produced clinical improvement, but the increase in survival time was small (31, 121). In phase I and II clinical trials, RC-160 was used as a single drug in patients with inoperable pancreatic cancer (93, 121). In the first study, RC-160 was given SC three times a day at a dose of 500 μg. In the second trial, an escalating regimen up to 6 mg/d by continuous infusion was used. In both studies, which included over 40 patients, nearly 30% of patients showed radiologic evidence of tumor stabilization for up to 6 months, with improvement in quality of life, particularly analgesic requirements. None of the 9 patients developed gallstones (93, 121). However, RC-160 alone, even in large doses, does not appear to be adequate for inducing an effective palliation in most patients (121). Our present view is that for therapy of pancreatic cancer, RC-160 must be used in combination with other peptides or drugs, such as 5-FU, as shown experimentally (113, 121). Rosenberg et al. (109) reported that a combination of Sandostatin with tamoxifen prolonged the survival of patients with pancreatic cancer. Bombesin antagonists should be also tried, and clinical trials with RC-3095 and other antagonists are planned.

Improved cytotoxic compounds containing doxorubicin linked to somatostatin analogues or bombesin/GRP antagonists that can be targeted to pancreatic cancers are being developed (120). Such cytotoxic analogues could be considered for the treatment of patients with advanced pancreatic cancer who do not respond to other therapies.

Colorectal Cancer

Colorectal cancer is the second most common malignant tumor in the United States (7). Advanced disseminated colon cancer is difficult to treat, and every year about 56,000 patients die of this disease in the United States (7, 114). New treatment modalities are needed for the treatment of advanced disseminated colorectal cancer (100). Gastrointestinal hormones, especially gastrin; growth factors, such as EGF, IGF-I, and TGF-α; and sex steroids may be involved in tumorigenesis of the colon (91, 100, 113, 114). The incidence of colon cancer is increased in acromegalics, suggesting that excessive secretion of GH or IGF-I may be a factor (113). IGF-I receptors were found in human colon carcinomas (91, 113). Consequently, an approach similar to that for pancreatic cancer could also be tried in colorectal cancer based on hormonal manipulations, such as the use of analogues of somatostatin and LH-RH or antagonists of bombesin/GRP and aimed at inhibiting GI hormones, growth factors, and sex steroids (113, 114). Somatostatin analogue RC-160 inhibits the growth of experimental murine and human colon cancers in vivo and hepatic metastases of these cancers (100). Binding sites for bombesin/GRP are found in human and murine colon cancer cell lines (100). Bombesin antagonists RC-3095 and RC-3440 strongly inhibit the growth of HT-29 human colon cancers in nude mice and down-regulate EGF receptors (100). The modest reduction in growth of this tumor induced by agonists [D-Trp-6]LH-RH may be due to sex steroid deprivation (100, 114). Bombesin/GRP antagonists and somatostatin analogues could be considered for the development of hormonal therapies of colon cancer. Clinical trials with somatostatin analogues Sandostatin and RC-160 or bombesin antagonist RC-3095 have been started or planned, but no data are available at present.

Gastric Cancer

Patients with unresectable stomach cancer have a poor prognosis and new therapeutic approaches are needed (114). Gastrointestinal hormones, especially gastrin and growth factors, such as EGF, TGF-α and IGF-I, appear to be implicated in the growth of human gastric adenocarcinoma (87). Our results and those of others indicate that somatostatin analogues such as RC-160 and Sandostatin inhibit the growth of MKN-45 human gastric cancer xenografts in nude mice (87, 114). Bombesin receptors have been found in human gastric cancer, as well as in MKN-45 and Hs746T gastric cancer cell lines, and bombesin stimulated the growth of Hs746T cells in vitro (87, 114). Bombesin/GRP antagonists inhibited the growth of MKN-45 and HS746T human gastric cancer cells implanted in nude mice or cultured in vitro (87, 114). Binding sites for EGF were down-regulated in tumor cells after treatment with RC-3095 or RC-160. On the basis of these findings, Sandostatin and other somatostatin analogues are being tried in patients with advanced gastric cancer. Trials with bombesin antagonists are still in the planning stage.

Brain Tumors

Brain tumors are responsible for about 12,000 deaths annually in the United States (9, 114). Benign tumors, such as meningiomas, can be treated by surgery, but therapeutic modalities for primary brain tumors, such as malignant astrocytomas (glioblastomas), need to be improved. That meningiomas and other brain tumors are hormone sensitive is supported by much evidence (88, 113, 114). On the basis of the frequent detection of receptors for progesterone in meningiomas, the antiprogestin mifepristone (RU486) is being used in clinical trials for the treatment of this tumor and may be a therapeutic option in the case of unresectable meningiomas (37).

The presence of receptors for EGF and IGF-I and -II in human brain tumors is also well established (30, 113, 114). Thus, growth factors may be involved in the proliferation of brain tumors. Various brain tumors, including astrocytomas and meningiomas, also contain significant levels of high-affinity receptors for somatostatin (56, 57, 61, 105, 129) and bombesin/GRP (88). Radioiodinated somatostatin analogues can label somatostatin receptors in various tumors, including meningiomas and astrocytomas, in vivo and, therefore, can be used for tumor localization (56, 57). These findings prompted investigations to determine whether somatostatin analogues or a bombesin antagonist could inhibit the growth of brain tumors (88, 114). We demonstrated that somatostatin analogue RC-160 and bombesin/GRP antagonist RC-3095 inhibited the proliferation of various human glioblastomas transplanted into nude mice or cultured in vitro (88). The survival time of animals inoculated with tumor cells orthotopically into the brain was significantly prolonged by treatment with RC-3095 (88). Somatostatin analogues, such as RC-160, and apparently also bombesin antagonists, can penetrate the blood-brain tumor barrier (88,114). Somatostatin analogues and bombesin/GRP antagonists could be considered for the development of new approaches to the treatment of some brain tumors by hormonal manipulations.

Lung Cancer

Lung cancer is the leading cause of cancer-related deaths in the United States and in the western world (9, 114). Small cell lung carcinoma (SCLC) accounts for 20 to 25% of all cases of lung cancer (78). Most cases of SCLC are already metastatic at the time of diagnosis, and although chemotherapy can be used, long-term survival is infrequent (78). The outlook for patients with non-SCLC (which includes the three remaining major histologic subtypes of lung cancer, squamous, adenocarcinoma, and large cell carcinoma) is likewise poor (81). Therefore, new therapeutic modalities are needed for both SCLC and non-SCLC.

The development of hormonal therapy based on bombesin/GRP antagonists or somatostatin analogues could be considered for SCLC (114). SCLC can secrete bombesin-like peptides, including GRP and neuromedin B, which function like autocrine growth factors and stimulate the growth of this tumor (20, 78, 79). High-affinity receptors for bombesin-like peptides have been identified in several SCLC lines (79, 114, 127). Potent bombesin/GRP antagonists active in vitro and in vivo have been synthesized (12, 16, 17, 63, 98, 114, 119). These bombesin/GRP antagonists block the signals mediated by bombesin-like peptides and inhibit the growth of SCLC in vivo and in vitro (12, 16, 17, 63, 98, 114).

In addition, growth factors, such as EGF, TGF-α and IGF-I, appear to play a role in the proliferation and progression of lung cancer (71, 114). It has been demonstrated that several human SCLC and non-SCLC cell lines secrete and respond to IGF-I, EGF, and TGF-α through specific receptors (71, 114). Somatostatin receptors are also expressed in SCLC (81). Scintigraphy with ^{111}In-pentetreotide can localize primary tumors in patients with non-SCLC (57, 81). Bombesin/GRP antagonists suppress the growth of SCLC, but not of non-SCLC xenografts in nude mice, whereas somatostatin analogue RC-160 can inhibit both tumor types by decreasing the levels of IGF-I and EGF or their receptors (114). This raises the possibility that these peptide analogues could be used selectively in the treatment of various subclasses of lung cancer. Such peptides as RC-160 or RC-3095 should have markedly reduced side effects as compared with combination chemotherapeutic agents. Future studies will determine their possible application in the treatment of SCLC (81). It has been demonstrated that octreotide reduced IGF-I levels in patients with SCLC (72). Clinical trials with various bombesin antagonists and somatostatin analogues are planned for the near future.

Bone Cancers

The most common primary tumors of bone and cartilage are typified by osteogenic sarcomas and chondrosarcomas (22). The treatment for these sarcomas includes chemotherapy, radiotherapy, and radical surgery, but there is much room for therapeutic improvement. The growth of osteosarcomas and chondrosarcomas appears to be dependent on IGF-I or GH (89, 92). In rats bearing transplanted Swarm chondrosarcomas, analogues of somatostatin significantly reduced tumor growth (113). It was also shown that the proliferation of osteosarcomas in cell cultures is enhanced by IGF-I and that hypophysectomy inhibits the metastatic behavior of a murine osteosarcoma (92). The receptors for IGF-I are present on osteosarcomas (89, 92). An approach to lower IGF-I secretion based on somatostatin analogues (113) or antagonists of GH-RH (144) might be beneficial for the treatment of osteosarcomas. However, somatostatin analogues do not adequately suppress IGF-I levels (92), and somatostatin receptors are absent in some osteosarcomas (92). Our recent results indicate that GH-RH antagonists inhibit the growth of human osteosarcomas transplanted into nude mice or cultured in vitro, possibly by interfering with the secretion of IGF-I (89). The findings suggest that GH-RH antagonists should be considered for the therapy of osteosarcomas.

References

1. Andreyko JL, Monroe SE, Marshall LA, Fluker MR, Nerenberg CA, Jaffe RB. Concordant suppression of serum immunoreactive luteinizing hormone (LH), follicle-stimulating hormone, α subunit, bioactive LH, and testosterone in postmenopausal women by a potent gonadotropin releasing hormone antagonist (Detirelix). J Clin Endocrinol 1992;74:399–405.
2. Bajusz S, Csernus VJ, Janaky T, Bokser L, Fekete M, Schally AV. New antagonists of LHRH: II. Inhibition and potentiation of LHRH by closely related analogues. Int J Peptide Prot Res 1988;32:425–435.
3. Barron JL, Millar RP, Searle DI. Metabolic clearance and plasma half-disappearance time of D-Trp6 and exogenous luteinizing hormone-releasing hormone. J Clin Endocrinol Metab 1982;54:1169–1173.
4. Bauer W, Briner U, Doepfner W, Haller R, Huguenin R, Marbach P, Petcher TJ, Pless J. SMS-201-995. A very potent and selective octapeptide analogue of somatostatin with prolonged action. Life Sci 1982;31:1133–1140.
5. Behre HM, Klein B, Steinmeyer E, McGregor GP, Voigt K, Nieschlag E. Effective suppression of luteinizing hormone and testosterone by single doses of the new gonadotropin-releasing hormone antagonist Cetrorelix (SB-75) in normal men. J Clin Endocrinol Metab 1992;75:393–398.
6. Bhasin S, Swerdloff RS. Mechanisms of gonadotropin-releasing hormone agonist action in the human male. Endocr Rev 1986;7:106–114.
7. Boring C, Squires TS, Tong T, Montgomery S. Cancer statistics 1994. Ca—A Cancer J Clin 1994;44:7–26.
8. Buscail L, Delesque N, Estève JP, Saint-Laurent N, Prats H, Clerc P, Robberecht P, Bell GI, Liebow C, Schally AV, Vaysse N, Susini C. Stimulation of tyrosine phosphatase and inhibition of cell proliferation by somatostatin analogues: mediation by human somatostatin receptor subtypes SSTR1 and SSTR2. Proc Natl Acad Sci USA 1994;91:2315–2319.
9. Buscail L, Estève J-P, Saint-Laurent N, Bertrand V, Reisine T, O'Carroll A-M, Bell GI, Schally AV, Vaysse N, Susini C. Inhibition of cell proliferation by the somatostatin analogue RC-160 is mediated by SSTR2 and SSTR5 somatostatin receptor subtypes through different mechanisms. Proc Natl Acad Sci USA 1995;92:1580–1584.
10. Butzow R, Huktaniemi I, Clayton R, Wahlstrom T, Andersson LC, Seppala M. Cultured mammary carcinoma cells contain gonadotropin-releasing hormone-like immunoreactivity, GNRH binding sites and chorionic gonadotropin. Int J Cancer 1987;39: 498–501.
11. Cai RZ, Szoke B, Lu R, Fu D, Redding TW, Schally AV. Synthesis and biological activity of highly potent octapeptide analogues of somatostatin. Proc Natl Acad Sci USA 1986;83:1896–1900.
12. Cai, R-Z, Reile H, Armatis P, Schally AV. Potent bombesin antagonists with C-terminal Leu $\psi(CH_2N)$-Tac-NH_2 or its derivatives. Proc Natl Acad Sci USA 1994;91: 12664–12668.
13. Campen CA, Lai MT, Kraft P, Kirchner T, Phillips A, Hahn DW, Rivier J. Characterization of a new, selective GnRH antagonist with potent antiovulatory activity and extremely low anaphylactoid activity (Abstract 869). 74th Meeting Endocrine Society, San Antonio, June 1992, p 269.
14. Catalona WJ. Management of cancer of the prostate. N Engl J Med 1994;331: 996–1004.
15. Comaru-Schally AM. Intervention-high-priority research approaches for prevention and for intervening in early pancreatic cancer. Int J Pancreatol 1994;16:307–309.
16. Coy DH, Heinz-Erian P, Jiang J, Sasaki Y, Taylor J, Moreau JP, Wolfrey WT, Gardner JD, Jensen RT. Probing peptide backbone function in bombesin. A reduced peptide bond analogue with potent and specific receptor antagonist activity. J Biol Chem 1988;263:5056–5060.
17. Coy DH, Taylor JE, Jiang N-Y, Kim SH, Wang L-H, Huang S, Moreau JP, Gardner JD, Jensen RT. Short-chain pseudopeptide bombesin receptor antagonists with enhanced binding affinities for pancreatic acinar and Swiss 3T3 cells display strong antimitotic activity. J Biol Chem 1989;264:14691–14697.
18. Crawford DE. Hormonal therapy of prostatic carcinoma. Defining the challenge. Oncology 1990;66:1035–1038.
19. Crawford ED, Eisenberger MA, McLeod DG, Spaulding JT, Benson R, Dorr FA, Blumenstein BA, Davis MA, Goodman PJ. A controlled trial of leuprolide with and without flutamide in prostatic carcinoma. N Engl J Med 1989;321:419–424.
20. Cuttitta F, Carney DN, Mulshine JW, Moody TW, Fedorko J, Fischler A, Minna JD. Bombesin-like peptides can function as autocrine growth factors in human small cell lung cancer. Nature (Lond) 1985;316:823–826.
21. Denis L. Role of maximal androgen blockade in advanced prostate cancer. Prostate 1994;5(suppl):17–22.
22. Dorfman HD, Czerniak B. Bone cancers. Cancer 1995;75:203–210.
23. Eidne KA, Fanagan CA, Harris NS, Millar RP. Gonadotropin-releasing hormone (GnRH)-binding sites in human breast cancer cell lines and inhibitory effects of GnRH antagonists. J Clin Endocrinol Metab 1987;64:425–432.
24. Emons G, Schally AV. The use of luteinizing hormone releasing hormone agonists and antagonists in gynecological cancers. Hum Reprod 1994;9:1364–1379.
25. Fekete M, Redding TW, Comaru-Schally AM, Pontes AE, Connelly RW, Srkalovic G, Schally AV. Receptors for luteinizing hormone-releasing hormone, somatostatin, prolactin and epidermal growth factor in rat and human prostate cancers and in benign prostatic hyperplasia. Prostate 1989;14:191–208.
26. Fekete M, Wittliff JL, Schally AV. Characteristics and distribution of receptors for [D-Trp6]-luteinizing hormone-releasing hormone, somatostatin, epidermal growth factor, and sex steroids in 500 biopsy samples of human breast cancer. J Clin Lab Anal 1989;3:137–147.
27. Foekens JA, Portengen H, Janssen M, Klijn JGM. Insulin-like growth factor-1 receptors and insulin-like growth factor-1-like activity in human primary breast cancer. Cancer 1989;63:2139–2147.
28. Foekens JA, Portengen H, van Putten WLJ, Trapman AMAC, Reubi JC, Alexieva-Figusch J, Klijn JGM. Prognostic value of receptors for insulin-like growth factor 1, somatostatin, and epidermal growth factor in human breast cancer. Cancer Res 1989;49:7002–7009.
29. Gallagher CJ, Oliver RTD, Oram DH, Fowler CG, Blake PR, Mantell BS, Slevin, ML and Hope-Stone HF. A new treatment for endometrial cancer with gonadotrophin-releasing hormone analogue. Br J Obstet Gynaecol 1991;98:1037–1041.

30. Gammeltoft A, Ballotti R, Kowalski A, Westermark B, van Obberghen E. Expression of two types of receptors for insulin-like growth factors in human malignant glioma. Cancer Res 1988;48:1233–1237.
31. Gonzalez-Barcena D, Ibarra-Olmos MA, Garcia-Carrasco F, Gutierrez-Samperio C, Comaru-Schally AM, Schally AV. Influence of D-Trp-6-LH-RH on the survival time in patients with advanced pancreatic cancer. Biomed Pharmacother 1989;43:313–317.
32. Gonzalez-Barcena D, Vadillo-Buenfil M, Gomez-Orta F, Martinez ME, Fuentes Garcia M, Cardenas Cornejo I, Comaru-Schally AM, Schally AV. Treatment of patients with advanced prostatic cancer with LH-RH antagonist SB-75 and of the relapse by the combination of agonist D-Trp-6-LH-RH and somatostatin analogue RC-160 (Abstract 135). Program of the Annual Meeting Endocrine Society, Las Vegas, 1993;135, p 389.
33. Gonzalez-Barcena D, Vadillo Buenfil M, Garcia Procel E, Guerra-Arguero L, Cardenas Cornejo I, Comaru-Schally AM, Schally AV. Inhibition of luteinizing hormone, follicle-stimulating hormone and sex steroid levels in men and women with a potent antagonist analogue of luteinizing hormone-releasing hormone, Cetrorelix (SB-75). Eur J Endocrinol 1994;131:286–292.
34. Gonzalez-Barcena D, Vadillo-Buenfil M, Gomez Orta F, Fuentes Garcia M, Cardenas-Cornejo I, Graef-Sanchez A, Comaru-Schally AM, Schally AV. Responses to the antagonistic analogue of LH-RH (SB-75) (Cetrorelix) in patients with benign prostatic hyperplasia and prostatic cancer. Prostate 1994;24:84–92.
35. Gonzalez-Barcena B, Vadillo-Buenfil M, Cortez-Morales A, Fuentas-Garcia M, Cardenas-Cornejo I, Comaru-Schally AM, Schally AV. LH-RH antagonist SB-75 (Cetrorelix) as primary single therapy in patients with advanced prostatic cancer and paraplegia due to metastatic invasion of spinal cord. Urology 1995;45:275–281.
36. Goustin AS, Loef EB, Shipley GS, Moses HL. Growth factors and cancer. Cancer Res 1986;46:1015–1029.
37. Grunberg SM, Weiss MH, Spitz IM, Ahmadi J, Sadun A, Russell CA, Lucci L, Stevenson LL. Treatment of unresectable meningiomas with the antiprogesterone agent mifepristone. J Neurosurg 1991;74:861–866.
38. Guillemin R, Brazeau P, Böhlen P, Esch F, Ling N, Wehrenberg W. Growth hormone-releasing factor from a human pancreatic tumor that caused acromegaly. Science 1982;218:585–587.
39. Guillemin R, Zeytin F, Ling N, Böhlen P, Esch F, Brazeau P, Bloch B, Wehrenberg WB. Growth hormone-releasing factor: chemistry and physiology. Proc Soc Exp Biol Med 1984;175:407–413.
40. Halmos G, Wittliff JL, Schally AV. Characterization of bombesin/GRP receptors in human breast cancer and their relationship to steroid receptor expression. Cancer Res 1995;53:280–287.
41. Harris AL, Carmichael J, Cantwell BMJ, Dowsett M. Zoladex Endocrine and therapeutic effects in post-menopausal breast cancer. Br J Cancer 1989;59:97–99.
42. Harris GW. Neural Control of the Pituitary Gland. London: Arnold, 1955.
43. Harris NS, Dutlow C, Eidne K, Dong, K-W, Roberts J, Millar RP. Gonadotropin-releasing hormone gene expression in MDA-MB-231 and ZR-75-1 breast carcinoma cell lines. Cancer Res 1991;51:2577–2581.
44. Hawes BE, Conn PM. Assessment of the role of G proteins and inositol phosphate production in the action of gonadotropin-releasing hormone. Clin Chem 1993;39: 325–332.
45. Hofland LJ, Van Koetsveld PM, Waaijers M, Zuyderwijk J, Lamberts SWJ. Relative potencies of the somatostatin analogues octreotide, BIM-23014, and RC-160 on the inhibition of hormone release by cultured human endocrine tumor cells and normal rat anterior pituitary cells. Endocrinology 1994;134:301–306.
46. Irmer G, Bürger C, Müller R, Ortmann O, Peter U, Kakar SS, Neill JD, Schulz, K-D, Emons G. Expression of the messenger ribonucleic acids for luteinizing hormone-releasing hormone and its receptor in human ovarian epithelial carcinoma. Cancer Res 1995;55:817–822.
47. Isaacs JT. The timing of androgen ablation therapy and/or chemotherapy in the treatment of prostatic cancer. Prostate 1984;5:1–17.
48. Janàky T, Juhèsz A, Bajusz S, Csernus V, Srkalovic G, Bokser L, Milovanovic SR, Redding TW, Rékasi A, Nagy N, Schally AV. Analogues of luteinizing hormone-releasing hormone containing cytotoxic groups. Proc Natl Acad Sci USA 1992;89:972–976.
49. Karten MJ, Rivier JE. Gonadotropin-releasing hormone analogue design. Structure-function studies toward the development of agonists and antagonists: rationale and perspective. Endocr Rev 1986;7:44–66.
50. Kaufmann M, Jonat W, Kleeburg U, Eirmann W, Janicke F, Hilfrich J, Kreienberg R, Albrecht M, Weitzel HK, Schmid H, Strunz P, Schachner-Wunschmann E, Bastert G, Maass H. The German Zoladex trial group: goserelin, a depot gonadotropin releasing hormone agonist in the treatment of premenopausal patients with metastatic breast cancer. J Clin Oncol 1989;7:1113–1119.
51. Keuppens F, Denis L, Smith P, Pinto Carvalho A, Newling D, Bond A, Sylvester R, De Pauw M, Vermeylen K, Ongena P, the EORTC GU Group. Zoladex and Flutamide Versus Bilateral Orchiectomy. Cancer 1990;66:1045–1057.
52. Klijn JGM, de Jong FH. Treatment with a luteinizing hormone-releasing hormone analogue (Buserelin) in premenopausal patients with metastatic breast cancer. Lancet 1982;1:1213–1216.
53. Klijn JGM, de Jong FH, Lamberts FW, Blankenstein MA. LHRH agonist treatment in clinical and experimental human breast cancer. J Steroid Biochem 1985;23:867–873.
54. Klingmuller D, Schepke M, Enzweiler C, Bidlingmaier F. Hormonal responses to the new potent GnRH antagonist Cetrorelix. Acta Endocrinol 1993;128:15–18.
55. Knobil E. The neuroendocrine control of the menstrual cycle. Recent Prog Horm Res 1980;36:53–88.
56. Krenning EP, Breeman WAP, Kooij PPM, Lameris JS, Bakker WH, Koper JW, Ausema L, Reubi JC, Lamberts SWJ. Localisation of endocrine-related tumors with radioiodinated analogue of somatostatin. The Lancet 1989;1:242–244.
57. Krenning EP, Kwekkeboom DJ, Bakker WH, Breeman WAP, Kooij PPM, Oei HY, van Hagen M, Postema PTE, de Jong M, Reubi JC, Visser TJ, Reijs AEM, Hofland LJ, Koper JW, Lamberts SWJ. Somatostatin receptor scintigraphy with [^{111}In-DTPA-D-Phe^{1}]- and [^{123}I-Tyr^{3}]-octreotide: the Rotterdam experience with more than 1000 patients. Eur J Nucl Med 1993;20:716–731.
58. Kuhn JM, Billebaud T, Navratil H, Moulonguet A, Fiet J, Grise P, Louis JF, Costa P, Husson JM, Dahan R, Bertagna C, Edelstein R. Prevention of the transient adverse effects of a gonadotropin-releasing hormone analogue (Buserelin) in metastatic prostatic carcinoma by administration of an antiandrogen (Nilutamide). N Engl J Med 1984;321:413–418.
59. Kvols LD, Moertel CG, O'Connell MJ, Schutt AJ, Rudin J, Hahn RG. Treatment of the malignant carcinoid syndrome. N Engl J Med 1986;315:663–666.
60. Labrie F, Dupont A, Belanger A, Lachance R. Flutamide eliminates the risk of disease flare in prostatic cancer patients treated with a luteinizing hormone-releasing hormone agonist. J Urol 1987;138:804–806.
61. Lamberts SWJ. The role of somatostatin and its analogues in the diagnosis and treatment of tumors. Endocr Rev 1991;12:450–482.
62. Lamberts SWJ, Hofland LJ, van Koetsveld PM, Reubi J-C, Bruining HA, Bakker WH, Krenning EP. Parallel in vivo and in vitro detection of functional somatostatin receptors in human endocrine pancreatic tumors: consequences with regard to diagnosis, localization and therapy. J Clin Endocrinol Metab 1990;71:566–574.
63. Langdon S, Seithi T, Ritchie A, Muir M, Smythe J, Rozengurt E. Broad spectrum neuropeptide antagonists inhibit the growth of small cell lung cancer in vivo. Cancer Res 1992;52:4554–4557.
64. Liebow C, Reilly C, Serrano M, Schally AV. Somatostatin analogues inhibit growth of pancreatic cancer by stimulating tyrosine phosphatase. Proc Natl Acad Sci USA 1989;86:2003–2007.
65. Limonta P, Dondi D, Moretti RM, Maggi R, Motta M. Antiproliferative effects of luteinizing hormone-releasing hormone agonists on the human prostatic cancer cell line LNCaP. J Clin Endocrinol Metab 1992;75:207–212.
66. Limonta P, Dondi D, Moretti RM, Fermo D, Garattini E, Motta M. Expression of luteinizing hormone-releasing hormone mRNA in the human prostatic cancer cell line LNCaP. J Clin Endocrinol Metab 1993;76:797–800.
67. Lippman ME, Dickson RB, Gelmann EP, Rosen N, Knabbe C, Bates S, Bronzert D, Huff K, Kasid A. Growth regulatory peptide production by human breast carcinoma cells. J Steroid Biochem 1988;29:79–88.
68. Ljungqvist A, Feng DM, Hook W, Shen ZX, Bowers C, Folkers K. Antide and related antagonists of luteinizing hormone release with long action and oral activity. Proc Natl Acad Sci USA 1988;85:8236–8240.
69. Loop SM, Gorder CA, Lewis SM, Drivdahl RH, Ostenson RC. Growth inhibition of human prostate tumor cells by an agonist of gonadotrophin-releasing hormone. Prostate 1995;26:179–188.
70. Lumpkin MD, McDonald JK. Blockade of growth hormone-releasing factor (GRF) activity in the pituitary and hypothalamus of the conscious rat with a peptidic GRF agonist. Endocrinology 1989;124:1522–1531.
71. Macaulay VM, Everard MJ, Teale D, Troutt PA, van Wyk JJ, Smith IE, Millar JL. Autocrine function of insulin-like growth factor I in human small cell lung cancer cell lines and fresh tumor cells. Cancer Res 1990;50:2511–2517.
72. Macaulay VM, Smith LE, Everard MJ, Teale JD, Reubi J-C, Millar JL. Experimental and clinical studies with somatostatin analogue octreotide in small cell lung cancer. Br J Cancer 1991;64:451–456.
73. Manetta A, Gamboa-Vujicic G, Paredes P, Emma D, Liao S, Leong L, Asch B, Schally A.V. Inhibition of growth of human ovarian cancer in nude mice by luteinizing hormone-releasing hormone antagonist (SB-75). Fertil Steril 1995;63:282–287.
74. Manni A, Santen R, Harvey H, Lipton A, Max D. Treatment of breast cancer with gonadotropin-releasing hormone. Endocrine Rev 1986;7:89–94.
75. Manni A, Boucher AE, Demers LM, Harvey HA, Lipton A, Simmonds MA, Bartholomew M. Endocrine effects of combined somatostatin analogue and bromocriptine therapy in women with advanced breast cancer. Breast Cancer Res Treat 1989;14:289–298.
76. Meldrum DR, Tasao Z, Monroe SE, Braustein GD, Sladek J, Lu JKH, Vale W, Rivier J, Judd HL, Chang RJ. Stimulation of LH fragments with reduced bioactivity following GnRH agonist administration in women. J Clin Endocrinol Metab 1984;58:755–757.
77. Miller WR, Scott WN, Morris R, Fraser HM, Sharpe RM. Growth of human breast cancer cells inhibited by a luteinizing hormone-releasing hormone agonist. Nature 1985;313:231–233.
78. Minna JD. Neoplasms of the lung. In Harrison's Principles of Internal Medicine. 11th ed. Edited by E Braunwald, KJ Isselbacher, RG Petersdorf, JD Wilson, JB Martin, AS Fauci. New York: McGraw Hill, 1987, pp 1115–1123.
79. Moody TW, Carney DN, Cuttitta F, Quattrocchi K, Minna JD. High affinity receptors for bombesin/GRP-like peptides on human small cell lung cancer. Life Sci 1985;37: 105–113.
80. Nicholson RI, Walker KJ, Walker RF, Read GF, Turkes A, Robertson JFR, Blamey RW. Review of the endocrine actions of LHRH analogues in premenopausal women in breast cancer. Horm Res 1989;32:198–224.
81. O'Byrne KJ, Halmos G, Pinski J, Groot K, Szepeshazi K, Schally AV, Carney DN. Somatostatin receptor expression in lung cancer. Eur J Cancer 1994;30A:1682–1687.
82. Olivennes F, Fanchin R, Bouchard P, de Ziegler D, Taieb J, Selva J, Frydman R. The single or dual administration of the gonadotropin-releasing hormone antagonist Cetrorelix in an in vitro fertilization-embryo transfer program. Fertil Steril 1994;62: 468–476.
83. Parmar H, Lightman SL, Allen L, Phillips RH, Edwards L, Schally AV. Randomised controlled study of orchidectomy vs. long-acting D-Trp-6-LH-RH microcapsules in advanced prostatic carcinoma. Lancet 1985;2:1202–1205.
84. Parmar H, Phillips RH, Rustin G, Lightman SL, Schally AV. Therapy of advanced ovarian cancer with D-Trp6-LH-RH (Decapeptyl) microcapsules. Biomed Pharmacother 1988;42:531–538.
85. Peeling WB. Phase III studies to compare goserelin (Zoladex) with orchiectomy and with diethylstilbestrol in treatment of prostatic carcinoma. Urology 1989;33:45–52.
86. Pinski J, Schally AV, Yano T, Szepeshazi K, Halmos G, Groot K, Comaru-Schally AM, Radulovic S, Nagy A. Inhibition of growth of experimental prostate cancer in rats by LH-RH analogues linked to cytotoxic radicals. Prostate 1993;23:165–178.
87. Pinski J, Halmos G, Yano T, Szepeshazi K, Qin Y, Ertl T, Schally AV. Inhibition of growth of MKN45 human gastric-carcinoma xenografts in nude mice by treatment with bombesin/gastrin-releasing-peptide antagonist (RC-3095) and somatostatin analogue RC-160. Int J Cancer 1994;57:574–580.
88. Pinski J, Schally AV, Halmos G, Szepeshazi K, Groot K. Somatostatin analogues and bombesin/gastrin-releasing peptide antagonist RC-3095 inhibit the growth of human glioblastomas in vitro and in vivo. Cancer Res 1994;54:5895–5901.
89. Pinski J, Schally AV, Groot K, Halmos G, Szepeshazi K, Zarandi M, Armatis K. Inhibition of growth of human osteosarcomas by antagonists of growth hormone-releasing hormone. JNCI 1995;87:1787–1794
90. Plowman PN, Nicholson RI, Walker KJ. Remission of postmenopausal breast cancer

during treatment with the luteinizing hormone releasing hormone agonist ICI 118630. Br J Cancer 1986;54:903–909.
91. Pollak M, Baer K, Richard M. Presence of somatomedin receptors on primary human breast and colon cancer. Cancer Lett 1987;38:223–230.
92. Pollak M, Polychronakos C, Richard M. IGF-I is a potent mitogen for human osteogenic sarcoma. JNCI 1990;82:301–305.
93. Poston GJ, Schally AV. Somatostatin analogues and pancreatic cancer. Int J Pancreatology 1993;14:64–66.
94. Poston GJ, Gillespie J, Guillou PJ. The biology of pancreatic cancer. Gut 1991;32: 800–812.
95. Qayum A, Gullick W, Clayton RC, Sikora K, Waxman J. The effects of gonadotrophin releasing hormone analogues in prostate cancer are mediated through specific tumor receptors. Br J Cancer 1990;62:96–99.
96. Qin Y, Ertl T, Cai R-Z, Halmos G, Schally AV. Inhibitory effect of bombesin receptor antagonist RC-3095 on the growth of human pancreatic cancer cells in vivo and in vitro. Cancer Res 1994;54:1035–1041.
97. Radiation Therapy Oncology Group. Phase III trial of androgen suppression before and during radiation therapy for locally advanced prostatic cancer (Abstract Report of RTOG 8610). Prostate Suppl 1994;5:2–3.
98. Radulovic S, Cai R-Z, Serfozo P, Groot K, Redding TW, Pinski J, Schally AV. Biological effects and receptor binding affinities of new pseudononapeptide bombesin/GRP receptor antagonists with N-terminal D-Trp or D-Tpi. Int J Peptide Protein Res 1991;38:593–600.
99. Radulovic S, Comaru-Schally AM, Milovanovic S, Schally AV. Somatostatin analogue RC-160 and LH-RH antagonist SB-75 inhibit growth of MIA PaCa-2 human pancreatic cancer xenografts in nude mice. Pancreas 1993;8:88–97.
100. Radulovic S, Schally AV, Reile H, Halmos G, Szepeshazi K, Groot K, Milovanovic S, Miller G, Yano T. Inhibitory effects of antagonists of bombesin/gastrin-releasing peptide (GRP) and somatostatin analogue (RC-160) on growth of HT-29 human colon cancers in nude mice. Acta Oncol 1994;33:693–701.
101. Redding TW, Schally AV. Inhibition of prostate tumor growth in two rat models by chronic administration of D-Trp-6-LH-RH. Proc Natl Acad Sci USA 1981;78: 6509–6512.
102. Redding TW, Schally AV. Inhibition of growth of pancreatic carcinomas in animal models by analogues of hypothalamic hormones. Proc Natl Acad Sci USA 1984;81: 248–252.
103. Rékàsi Z, Szöke B, Nagy A, Groot K, Rékàsi ES, Schally AV. Effect of luteinizing hormone-releasing hormone analogues containing cytotoxic radicals on the function of rat pituitary cells: tests in a long term superfusion system. Endocrinology 1993;132: 1991–2000.
104. Reubi JC, Torhorst J. The relationship between somatostatin, epidermal growth factor, and steroid hormone receptors in breast cancer. Cancer 1989;64: 1254–1260.
105. Reubi JC, Maurer R, Klijn JGM, Stefanko SZ, Foekens JA, Blaauw G, Blankenstein MS, Lamberts SWJ. High incidence of somatostatin receptors in human meningiomas: biochemical characterization. J Clin Endocrinol Metab 1986;63:433–438.
106. Rivier J, Spiess J, Thorner M, Vale W. Characterization of a growth hormone-releasing factor from a human pancreatic islet tumour. Nature (Lond.) 1982;300:276–278.
107. Rivier JE, Porter J, Rivier CL, Perrin M, Corrigan A, Hook WA, Siraganian RP, Vale WW. New effective gonadotropin releasing hormone antagonists with minimal potency for histamine release in vitro. J Med Chem 1986;29:1846–1851.
108. Robberecht P, Coy DH, Waelbroeck M, Heiman ML, de Neef P, Camus J-C, Christophe J. Structural requirements for the activation of rat anterior pituitary adenylate cyclase by growth hormone-releasing factor (GRF): discovery of (N-Ac-Tyr[1], D-Arg[2])-GRF (1-29)-NH_2 as a GRF antagonist on membranes. Endocrinology 1985;117: 1759–1764.
109. Rosenberg L, Barkun AN, Denis MH, Pollak M. Low dose octreotide and tamoxifen in the treatment of adenocarcinoma of the pancreas. Cancer 1995;75:23–28.
110. Santen RJ, Manni A, Harvey H, Redmond C. Endocrine treatment of breast cancer in women. Endoc Rev 1990;11:221–265.
111. Saphner T, Troxel AB, Tormey DC, Neuberg D, Robert NJ, Pandya KJ, Edmonson JH, Rosenbluth RJ, Abeloff MD. Phase II study of goserelin for patients with postmenopausal metastatic breast cancer. J Clin Oncol 1993;11:1529–1535.
112. Schally AV. Aspects of hypothalamic regulation of the pituitary gland. Science 1978;202:18–28.
113. Schally AV. Oncological application of somatostatin analogues. Cancer Res 1988;48: 6977–6985.
114. Schally AV. Hypothalamic hormones: from neuroendocrinology to cancer therapy. Anti-Cancer Drugs 1994;5:115–130.
115. Schally AV, Kastin AJ, Arimura A. Hypothalamic FSH and LH-regulating hormone. Structure, physiology and clinical studies. Fertil Steril 1971;22:703–721.
116. Schally AV, Comaru-Schally AM, Redding T. Antitumor effects of analogues of hypothalamic hormones in endocrine-dependent cancers. Proc Soc Exp Biol Med 1984;175:259–281.
117. Schally AV, Bajusz S, Redding TW, Zalatnai A, Comaru-Schally AM. Analogues of LHRH. The present and the future. In GnRH Analogues in Cancer and in Human Reproduction, Basic Aspects, vol 1. Edited by BH Vickery, V Lunenfeld. Boston: Kluwer, 1989, pp 5–31.
118. Schally AV, Comaru-Schally AM, Gonzalez-Barcena D. Present status of agonistic and antagonistic analogues of LH-RH in the treatment of advanced prostate cancer. Biomed Pharmacother 1992;46:465–471.
119. Schally AV, Radulovic S, Comaru-Schally AM. Experimental and clinical studies in hormone dependent cancers. In Endocrine Tumors. Edited by E Mazzaferri, N Samaan. Boston: Blackwell, 1993, pp 49–73.
120. Schally AV, Nagy A, Cai R-Z, Reile H, Radulovic S, Qin Y, Szepeshazi K, Halmos G, Comaru-Schally AV. Combined hormonal therapy and chemotherapy for pancreatic cancer. Use of cytotoxic peptide analogues for targeted chemotherapy. Int J Pancreatol 1994;16:277–280.
121. Schally AV, Szepeshazi K, Qin Y, Halmos G, Ertl T, Groot K, Cai R-Z, Liebow C, Poston GJ. Antitumor effects of analogues of somatostatin and antagonists of bombesin/GRP in experimental models of pancreatic cancer. Int J Pancreatol 1994;16:60–64.
122. Schulman CC. Neoadjuvant androgen blockade prior to prostatectomy: a retrospective study and critical review. Prostate Suppl 1994;5:9–14.
123. Schwartz L, Guiochet N, Keiling R. Two partial remissions induced by LHRH analogue in two postmenopausal women with metastatic breast cancer. Cancer 1988;62: 2498–2500.
124. Sharifi R, Soloway M. Leuprolide Study Group: clinical study of leuprolide depot formulation in the treatment of advanced prostate cancer. J Urol 1990;143:68–72.
125. Sharoni Y, Bosin E, Miinster A, Levy J, Schally AV. Inhibition of growth of human mammary tumor cells by potent antagonists of luteinizing hormone-releasing hormone. Proc Natl Acad Sci USA 1989;86:1648–1651.
126. Sogani PC, Fair WR. Treatment of advanced prostatic cancer. Urol Clin North Am 1987;14:253–271.
127. Spindel ER, Giladi E, Segerson TP, Nagalla S. Bombesin-like peptides: of ligands and receptors. Rec Progr Horm Res 1993;48:365–391.
128. Srkalovic G, Bokser L, Radulovic S, Korkut E, Schally AV. Receptors for luteinizing hormone-releasing hormone (LH-RH) in Dunning R3327 prostate cancers and rat anterior pituitaries after treatment with a sustained delivery system of LH-RH antagonist SB-75. Endocrinology 1990;127:3052–3060.
129. Srkalovic G, Cai RZ, Schally AV. Evaluation of receptors for somatostatin in various tumors using different analogues. J Clin Endocrin Metab 1990;70:661–669.
130. Sunday ME, Kaplan LM, Motoyama E, Chin WW, Spindel ER. Biology of disease, gastrin-releasing peptide (mammalian bombesin) gene expression in health and disease. Lab Invest 1988;59:5–24.
131. Szende B, Srkalovic G, Groot K, Lapis K, Schally AV. Growth inhibition of mouse MXT mammary tumor by the luteinizing hormone-releasing hormone antagonist SB-75. JNCI 1990;82:513–517.
132. Szende B, Srkalovic G, Schally AV, Lapis K, Groot K. Inhibitory effects of analogues of luteinizing hormone-releasing hormone (LH-RH) and somatostatin on pancreatic cancers in hamsters: events which accompany tumor regression. Cancer 1990;65: 2279–2290.
133. Szepeshazi K, Schally AV, Cai R-Z, Radulovic S, Milovanovic S, Szoke B. Inhibitory effect of bombesin/gastrin-releasing peptide antagonist RC-3095 and high dose of somatostatin analogue RC-160 on nitrosamine induced pancreatic cancers in hamsters. Cancer Res 1991;51:5980–5986.
134. Szepeshazi K, Schally AV, Halmos G, Groot K, Radulovic S. Antagonist of bombesin/GRP releasing peptide inhibits growth of estrogen dependent and independent MXT mammary cancer in mice. JNCI 1992;84:1915–1922.
135. Szepeshazi K, Schally AV, Juhasz A, Nagy A, Janaky T. Effect of LH-RH analogues containing cytotoxic radicals on growth of estrogen independent MXT mouse mammary carcinoma in vivo. Anti-Cancer Drugs 1992;3:109–116.
136. Tolis G, Ackman D, Stellos A, Mehta A, Labrie F, Fazekas A, Comaru-Schally AM, Schally AV. Tumor growth inhibition in patients with prostatic carcinoma treated with luteinizing hormone-releasing agonists. Proc Natl Acad Sci USA 1982;79:1658–1662.
137. Veber DF, Freidinger RM, Schwenk-Perlow D, Paleveda WJ Jr, Holly RW, Strachan RG, Nutt RF, Arison BH, Homnick C, Randall WC, Glitzer MS, Saperstein R, Hirschmann R. A potent cyclic hexapeptide analogue of somatostatin. Nature (Lond) 1981;292:55–58.
138. Vennin PH, Peyrat JP, Bonneterre J, Louchez MM, Harris AG, Demaille A. Effect of the long-acting somatostatin analogue SMS 201-995 (Sandostatin) in advanced breast cancer. Anticancer Res 1989;9:153–156.
139. Walker KJ, Walker RF, Turkes A, Robertson JRF, Blamey RW, Griffiths K, Nicholson RI. Endocrine effects of combination antioestrogen and LH-RH agonist therapy in premenopausal patients with advanced breast cancer. Eur J Cancer Clin Oncol 1989;25:651–654.
140. Yano T, Korkut E, Pinski J, Szepeshazi K, Milovanovic S, Groot K, Clarke R, Comaru-Schally AM, Schally AV. Inhibition of growth of MCF-7 MIII human breast carcinoma in nude mice by treatment with agonists or antagonists of LH-RH. Breast Cancer Res Treat 1992;21:35–45.
141. Yano T, Pinski T, Groot K, Schally AV. Stimulation by bombesin and inhibition by bombesin/gastrin-releasing peptide antagonist RC-3095 of growth of human breast cancer cell lines. Cancer Res 1992;52:4545–4547.
142. Yano T, Pinski J, Halmos G, Szepeshazi K, Groot K, Schally AV. Inhibition of growth of OV-1063 human epithelial ovarian cancer xenografts in nude mice by treatment with luteinizing hormone-releasing hormone antagonist SB-75. Proc Natl Acad Sci USA 1994;91:7090–7094.
143. Yano T, Pinski J, Szepeshazi K, Halmos G, Radulovic S, Groot K, Schally AV. Inhibitory effect of bombesin/gastrin releasing peptide antagonist RC-3095 and luteinizing hormone-releasing hormone antagonist SB-75 on the growth of MCF-7 MIII human breast cancer xenografts in athymic nude mice. Cancer 1994;73:1229–1238.
144. Zarandi M, Horvath JE, Halmos G, Pinski J, Nagy A, Groot K, Schally AV. Synthesis and biological activities of highly potent antagonist of growth hormone-releasing hormone. Proc Natl Acad Sci 1994;91:12298–12303.

CHAPTER 72

Corticosteroids

ROBERT A. SCHWARTZMAN AND JOHN A. CIDLOWSKI

Hormones of the Adrenal Cortex

For nearly 40 years cortisol and its synthetic analogues have been in widespread clinical use. A great deal of knowledge has been gained on the physiology, biochemistry, and pharmacology of steroids over this period, and numerous publications discuss the therapeutic uses and toxicologic hazards of corticosteroids. This chapter will review the physiologic and pharmacologic actions of corticosteroids and then discuss the use of these agents in the treatment of various neoplasms. Finally, the mechanism of action of these hormones will be considered in the context of their therapeutic efficacy.

The necessity of functional adrenal glands for survival was discovered in the 1850s based on observations by Addison (1) of patients with destructive diseases of the adrenal gland and experiments done by Brown-Séquard (2) on adrenalectomized animals. By the 1930s it was noted that the effects of adrenal insufficiency could be divided into two categories: those due to electrolyte imbalances and those resulting from altered carbohydrate metabolism (3, 4). In 1932 Cushing (5) described the syndrome of hypercorticism. In the 1940s and 1950s the discovery of adrenocorticotropic hormone (ACTH) in the anterior pituitary and its role in the stimulation of the adrenal cortex was made (6, 7). The regulation of ACTH release was found to depend on a precise balance between the negative feedback of adrenal corticosteroids and positive stimulation from the nervous system; both effects are mediated at the level of the hypothalamus (8). During these same years several bioactive steroids were isolated from the adrenal cortex and their structures were elucidated, including the principal active corticosteroids in humans, cortisol and aldosterone (9, 10).

In 1949, Hench (11) announced the dramatic effects of cortisol and ACTH in the treatment of rheumatoid arthritis. This observation evoked wide interest, and therapeutic applications of these hormones were subsequently extended to a wide variety of diseases. This surge in clinical investigation prompted an equally large amount of study on the basic sciences of these compounds. During the 1950s most of the biochemistry involved in the synthesis and metabolism of adrenocortical steroids was elucidated, and most of the synthetic analogues available today were developed. Along with these advances, practical methods for plasma cortisol determinations were developed, allowing rapid advances in the field of corticosteroid therapy.

Synthetic analogues of the adrenocortical steroids were eventually developed that separated the anti-inflammatory potency of these compounds from their effects on electrolyte metabolism. However, chemists have not been able to separate desirable clinical effectiveness from toxicity. Consequently, these drugs are very powerful but have slow cumulative toxic side effects on many tissues, which may not be apparent until made manifest in a catastrophic manner.

ADRENAL ANATOMY

The adrenal cortex is composed of three zones, the divisions of which are not clear-cut in humans. The outer zone is the zona glomerulosa, which is responsible for aldosterone synthesis and which is controlled both morphologically and biochemically by sodium, potassium, and angiotensin levels. Cortisol is produced in the inner zones, the zona fasciculata and the zona reticularis, which, along with the zona glomerulosa to a lesser extent, are regulated primarily by ACTH from the pituitary.

SECRETED STEROIDS

All five classes of steroid hormones are produced in the adrenal cortex in varying amounts: the glucocorticoids, mineralocorticoids, and progestins, which contain 21 carbons; the androgens, which contain 19 carbons; and the estrogens, which contain 18 carbons. The amounts of progestins, androgens, and estrogens produced in the adrenal cortex represent only a minor percentage of the total amount of each steroid synthesized in the body; thus, they will not be discussed further in this chapter. The glucocorticoids and the mineralocorticoids are made almost exclusively in the adrenal cortex and therefore represent its major biologic product. The physiologic role of glucocorticoids includes the control of glucose metabolism, gluconeogenesis, and modulation of the immune system. The major human form is cortisol and to a lesser extent corticosterone. The mineralocorticoids are crucial in mineral and water metabolism; the major bioactive forms in humans are aldosterone and deoxycorticosterone.

BIOSYNTHETIC PATHWAYS

The steps in the biosynthesis of corticosteroids have been elucidated and are presented in simplified form in Figure 72.1. The synthesis of all steroids begins with cholesterol (12), which is converted to various steroid molecules in a series of reactions that are mediated by several cytochrome P-450 enzymes (13). The adrenal cortex can synthesize cholesterol to some extent; however 60 to 80% of the choles-

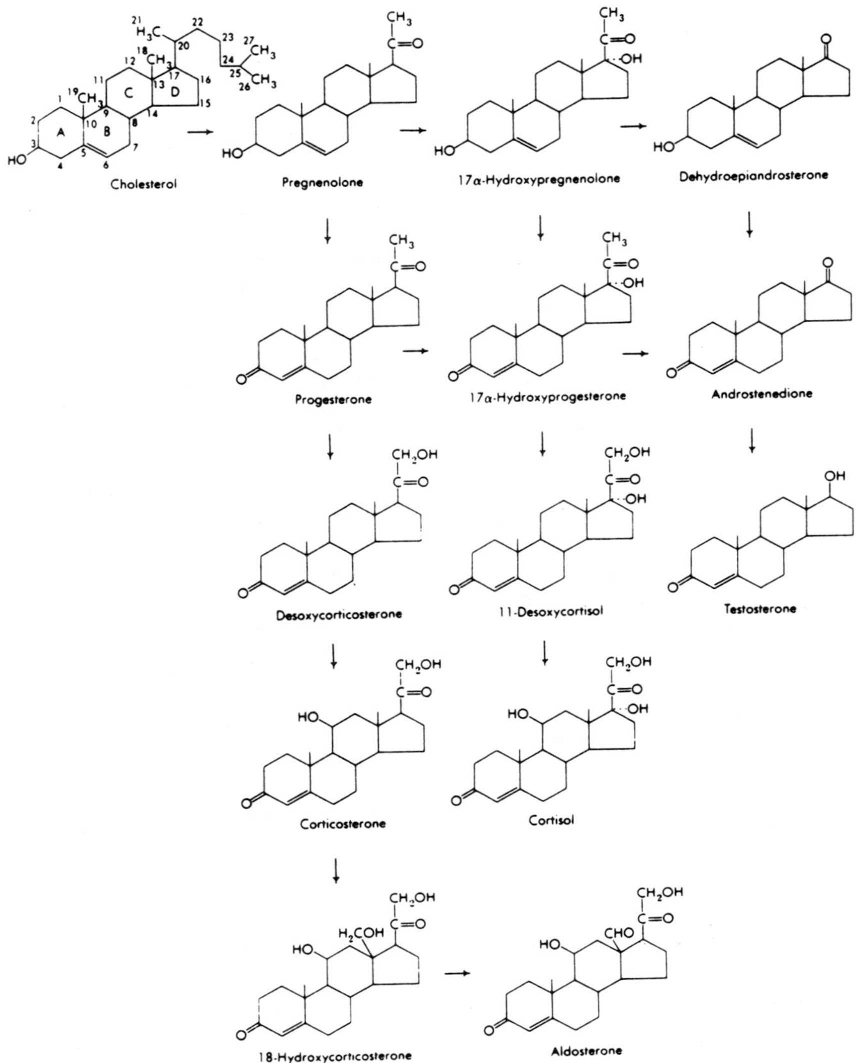

Figure 72.1. Principal pathways for biosynthesis of adrenocorticosteroids. From Haynes and Murad (229).

terol used in steroid synthesis originates from sources outside the adrenal cortex (14). This cholesterol is derived primarily from the cholesterol that is circulating in plasma bound to low-density lipoproteins, for which the adrenal cortex has a large number of receptors. Once synthesized, the corticosteroids are not stored within the adrenal cortex but are rapidly secreted. The adrenal cortex contains only enough steroid to maintain normal serum corticosteroid levels for a few minutes once synthesis is halted. Therefore, the rate of corticosteroid synthesis is essentially equal to the rate of secretion from the adrenal gland.

Control of Corticosteroid Secretion

GLUCOCORTICOIDS

The rate of synthesis of corticosteroids is controlled by the peptide hormone ACTH (15). This hormone, synthesized and secreted from the corticotrophs (basophilic cells) of the anterior pituitary gland, affects all three zones of the adrenal cortex. High levels of ACTH can lead to hyperplasia and hypertrophy of the adrenal cortex and a continuous high output of cortisol and corticosterone. A lack of ACTH results in atrophy of the cortex and decreased secretion of both cortisol and corticosterone. In contrast, aldosterone levels are not significantly affected by changes in ACTH because the zona glomerulosa is least affected by ACTH. ACTH acts through the classical mechanism of action of peptide hormones [i.e., ACTH binds to specific receptors that are located in the adrenal cell membrane and subsequently exerts its effects through an increase in intracellular cyclic adenosine monophosphate (cAMP) and other second messengers (16)]. ACTH acts on the adrenal cortex to increase steroid synthesis and secretion, in part by increasing the number of low-density lipoprotein (LDL) receptors (17). The principal site of action of ACTH is on the side chain cleavage reaction that converts cholesterol to pregnenolone. ACTH stimulates the rate of this reaction by increasing the availability of cholesterol as a substrate for this enzymatic reaction, as well as by increasing the synthesis of the cytochrome P-450 side chain cleavage enzyme (18, 19).

ACTH secretion from the anterior pituitary gland is positively regulated by corticotropin releasing factor (CRF), which is secreted from the median eminence of the hypothalamus (20). Neural signals converge on the hypothalamus to cause the release of CRF, which travels via a vascular connection to the pituitary gland where it stimulates the synthesis and release of the polyprotein precursor to ACTH, pro-opiomelanocortin (POMC). The POMC protein is cleaved into several bioactive peptides that are secreted from the corticotrophs along with ACTH, including β-lipotropin and β-endorphin. Negative feedback control is exerted on ACTH levels by glucocorticoids, which act at the level of both the pituitary gland and the hypothalamus (21). Glucocorticoids suppress POMC synthesis and decrease ACTH stores in secretory granules. High levels of glucocorticoids cause corticotropic cell degeneration. Following adrenalectomy or in patients with Addison's disease, when glucocorticoid levels are low, the concentration of ACTH in the plasma remains high. ACTH levels can, however, still be stimulated by CRF, indicating that ACTH remains under nervous control in the absence of negative feedback. In addition to the described endocrine feedback loops, the ACTH/glucocorticoid pathway can be stimulated by cytokines such as interleukin 1β, which appears to exert its effect at the level of the hypothalamus to increase CRF secretion (22).

Frequent measurement of plasma cortisol levels has revealed that the level of this steroid fluctuates irregularly (23). These spontaneous changes are the result of rapid increases in the cortisol secretion rate that occur 7 to 13 times a day. These increases, although irregular, occur in a reproducible pattern for any given person. The slope of the rise in secretion rate is constant for any individual and averages around 50 μg/min. The decline of these peaks of cortisol levels occurs in a semilog fashion, indicating that this spontaneous secretion occurs in an "on/off" manner. Thus, the total amount of cortisol secreted throughout the day reflects the number of episodes of high secretion that occur rather than changes in the secretion rate. This spontaneous rhythm of cortisol secretion results in minimal plasma cortisol levels 1 to 2 hours after the onset of sleep, with a rise occurring during sleep to maximum levels at the time of awakening and a fall in plasma levels during the day. This secretion pattern is due to an intrinsic function of the hypothalamus and is not subject to glucocorticoid-induced negative feedback. Although the specific mechanism responsible for this intrinsic rhythm is unknown, the major factors that affect the pattern appear to be timing of sleep, feeding, and exposure to light.

Stress also stimulates ACTH production and subsequent adrenal steroid secretion (24). These stimuli can be psychologic (e.g., anticipation, fear, depression) or physical (e.g., exercise, hypoglycemia, surgery, burns, cold, hypotension). If the sensory connections that mediate these stimuli are blocked, no adrenal stimulation occurs (25). There is a quantitative relationship between the intensity of the stressful stimulus and the adrenal response (26); however, pretreatment with glucocorticoid can inhibit this effect through negative feedback mechanisms (27).

MINERALOCORTICOIDS

The major physiologic regulator of aldosterone levels is the renin-angiotensin system (28). Renin, a protein made in the kidney, converts angiotensinogen to angiotensin I, a tetradecapeptide that is subsequently converted by other factors to the active peptides angiotensin II and III. Angiotensin II and III stimulate aldosterone biosynthesis through interaction with cell surface receptors in the zona glomerulosa. This effect is mediated by changes in intracellular calcium but not by changes in cAMP levels (29). Another effect of angiotensin is to increase peripheral arterial resistance, which in turn increases blood pressure (30). Changes in blood pressure then feed back on renin secretion, the control mechanism of which has not been established but which appears to involve kidney baroreceptors as well as sympathetic innervation and serum sodium and potassium levels.

A second control of mineralocorticoid synthesis is serum sodium and potassium levels. Increases in serum potassium increase aldosterone secretion. Potassium acts directly on the adrenal gland to stimulate some of the early steps in steroid biosynthesis and may also affect renin release (31). Low serum sodium also increases aldosterone secretion, but its action does not appear to be a major regulator of mineralocorticoid secretion because serum sodium concentration changes little with changes in total volume.

Pharmacokinetics of Corticosteroids

RATE OF SECRETION

Cortisol, the major glucocorticoid in humans, is secreted at a rate of 15 to 20 mg/day in men and at an approximately 10% lower rate in women (32). The less abundant glucocorticoid corticosterone is secreted at a rate of 4 mg/day, although it can rise to as high as 40 mg/day with ACTH stimulation. The two main mineralocorticoids, aldosterone and deoxycorticosterone, are secreted at the rates of 50 to 200 and 16 to 40 μg/day, respectively.

METABOLISM

The corticosteroids are metabolized through a variety of chemical transformations that destroy physical activity and result in increased water solubility to enhance their urinary excretion (33). The majority of serum cortisol is reduced to dihydrocortisol and then to tetrahydrocortisol, which is then conjugated to glucuronic acid. About 10% of cortisol is converted to the 17-ketosteroid, which is then conjugated to sulfate. Most of the circulating aldosterone is converted to the tetrahydroglucuronide derivative. About 70% of corticosteroid metabolism occurs in the liver, and certain diseases of the liver can allow increased levels of free hormone to occur due to the decrease in metabolism, as well as to the decrease in serum steroid-binding proteins that often occurs during liver disease.

PLASMA CLEARANCE

The plasma clearance of cortisol is rapid, with a half-life of 66 minutes at normal hormone levels (23). With large steroid loads, however, the half-life increases to 120 minutes. The volume of distribution (VD) changes in a similar fashion, with a VD of 10 L under normal conditions and a VD that can be greater than total body water with large steroid loads. Corticosterone turns over even more rapidly than cortisol, and the clearance rates of both steroids are unaffected by acute stress or adrenal insufficiency. The plasma half-life of aldosterone is less than 20 minutes.

EXCRETION

Cortisol excretion in urine is relatively low, <100 μg/day, primarily because 80 to 90% of filtered cortisol is reabsorbed, mostly from the distal tubule (34). In contrast, conjugated metabolites are filtered and excreted with no reabsorption. Over 90% of secreted glucocorticoid is ultimately excreted in urine. Less than 10% of the secreted aldosterone appears in the urine in the free form. The majority is excreted as glucuronide derivatives.

TRANSPORT IN BLOOD

Cortisol is found in the plasma predominantly in three forms: free; bound to corticosteroid-binding globulin (CBG), a glycoprotein with a molecular weight of 51,700; or bound to albumin. CBG is found in the plasma at a level of 40 mg/L (0.8 μM) and binds about 70% of plasma cortisol (14 μg/dL). Cortisol binds to CBG with high affinity (kd = 2.4×10^{-7} M; half-life of steroid binding = 5 days). CBG can bind other steroids, including progesterone, prednisolone, and aldosterone. These steroids compete for binding sites on CBG, and high levels of one steroid will displace the others. For example, therapeutic levels of prednisone displace 35% of CBG-bound cortisol. In contrast, many of the synthetic glucocorticoids, including dexamethasone, fail to bind CBG. Albumin, a protein of molecular weight 69,000, exists in plasma at a concentration of 40 g/L (0.5–0.6 mM). It has a low affinity for cortisol (kd = 10^{-5} M) and binds only 20% of plasma cortisol. Thus, at low serum cortisol levels most of the cortisol is bound to CBG. However, CBG-binding capacity is saturated at a cortisol concentration of 28 μg/dL, a level that is frequently exceeded in stressed patients. At these higher levels there is an increase in albumin-bound and free cortisol levels, whereas CBG-bound cortisol remains the same. The free fraction of cortisol is 1 μg/dL at a normal total plasma cortisol of 20 μg/dL, although this value can rise to as high as 15–50 μg/dL after ACTH stimulation. The active form of cortisol is considered to be the free form because protein-bound cortisol cannot easily pass through cell membranes. There is rapid equilibration between the bound and free fractions of cortisol so the bound fraction acts as a reservoir. The fact that total plasma cortisol falls below 5 μg/dL at night exemplifies how rapidly cortisol can leave the plasma. Aldosterone does not have a specific binding protein but does bind weakly to albumin, producing a normal plasma aldosterone level of 0.006 μg/dL (0.17 nM). Other steroids with mineralocorticoid activity, such as corticosterone and 11-deoxycorticosterone, do bind CBG. CBG-bound corticosteroids are not susceptible to metabolism.

Steroid Synthesis Inhibitors

There are several inhibitors of steroid biosynthesis that are used clinically to treat corticosteroid hypersecretion or to eliminate the synthesis of a specific class of steroids (35). Metyrapone blocks the 11β-hydroxylation of steroids (36). Synthesis therefore terminates after the formation of 11-deoxycortisol, the immediate precursor to cortisol. This compound does not negatively feed back on ACTH secretion so serum ACTH and 11-deoxycortisol levels remain high. Metyrapone also inhibits synthesis of aldosterone, but no sodium balance problems accrue because synthesis of 11-deoxycortisone, which has mineralocorticoid activity, remains intact. Aminoglutethimide inhibits the conversion of cholesterol to 20α-hydroxycholesterol and blocks the synthesis of both cortisol and aldosterone, as well as other classes of steroid hormones (37). Mitotane is an adrenocorticolytic drug, the mechanism of action of which has not been elucidated (38). Mitotane selectively attacks adrenocortical cells and causes a rapid decrease in plasma corticosteroid levels. Several new compounds, the aromatase inhibitors, have recently come into use as steroid synthesis inhibitors, exhibiting increased potency and selectivity. These compounds, which include pyridoglutethimide, 4-hydroxyandrostenedione, and fadrazole, can effectively lower estrogen levels while abrogating the need for corticosteroid replacement (39) (see Chapter 74).

Pharmaceutical Derivatives

The molecular shape of steroid hormones is a critical determinant of physiologic activity. Organic chemists have studied the structure-activity relationships of these molecules and have synthesized a myriad of cortisol analogues with varying potencies that effectively separate the glucocorticoid and mineralocorticoid activities of the natural corticosteroids. This has made the synthetic glucocorticoids clinically useful, even though it has not been possible to separate glucocorticoid activity from the toxic side effects of these molecules. Table 72.1 lists some of the available natural and synthetic corticosteroids with their relative ratio of specificity and equivalent doses. All corticosteroids are absorbed readily from the gastrointestinal tract. Water-soluble esters are given intravenously (IV) to achieve absorption rapidly, whereas high plasma concentrations while intramuscular injection provides more prolonged effects. Corticosteroids are also well absorbed from several sites of topical application, and large doses can lead to systemic absorption.

Changes in steroid activity also result in changes in absorption, plasma protein binding, and clearance rates. There is wide variability in the free fraction of synthetic steroids from patient to patient at comparable total plasma concentrations. There is also variability in patient sensitivity to generation of Cushing-like symptoms. These differing sensitivi-

Table 72.1. Relative Potencies and Equivalent Doses of Corticosteroids

Compound	Relative anti-inflammatory potency	Relative sodium-retaining potency	Duration of action[a]	Approximate equivalent dose[b] (mg)
Cortisol	1	1	S	20
Cortisone	0.8	0.8	S	25
Corticosterone	0.4	15	S	—
Fludrocortisone	10	125	S	—
Prednisone	4	0.8	I	5
Prednisolone	4	0.8	I	5
6α-methylprednisolone	5	0.5	I	4
Triamcinolone	5	0	I	4
Paramethasone	10	0	L	2
Betamethasone	25	0	L	0.75
Dexamethasone	25	0	L	0.75
Deoxycorticosterone	0.2	100	—	—
Aldosterone	0.3	3000	—	—

[a] S, short or 8- to 12-h biologic half-life; I, intermediate or 12- to 36-h biologic half-life; L, long or 36- to 72-h biologic half-life [see Rose and Saccar (230)].
[b] These dose relationships apply only to oral or intravenous administration; relative potencies may differ greatly when injected intramuscularly or into joint spaces.
From Haynes and Murad (229).

ties are reflected in different plasma corticosteroid concentrations, suggestive of pituitary resistance to corticosteroid feedback. Additionally, differences in the pharmacokinetics of glucocorticoids between men, women, and children should be kept in mind in terms of therapy (40, 41).

Physiologic and Pharmacologic Effects of Corticosteroids

The primary role of the corticosteroids is to maintain homeostasis within the body and to provide the body with the capacity to resist environmental changes and invasion of foreign substances. The effects of corticosteroids on the human body are widespread and include profound alterations in carbohydrate, protein, and lipid metabolism, as well as effects on electrolyte and water balance. Corticosteroids also exert effects on all of the major systems of the body, including the cardiovascular, musculoskeletal, nervous, and immune systems, and other tissues and organs. Because so many systems are sensitive to corticosteroid levels, tight regulatory control is exerted on the system. The direct effects of corticosteroids are sometimes difficult to separate from their complex relationship with other hormones, in part due to the permissive action of low levels of corticosteroid on the effectiveness of certain hormones, including catecholamines and glucagon. Nevertheless, the effects of corticosteroids can be classified into two general categories: the effects of glucocorticoids (intermediary metabolism, inflammation, immunity, wound healing, myocardial and muscle integrity) and the effects of mineralocorticoids (salt, water, and mineral metabolism). Although the following section will discuss the separate effects of glucocorticoids and mineralocorticoids, it must be emphasized that the natural steroids possess both glucocorticoid and mineralocorticoid activity to some extent. The ratio between the two activities ranges from all glucocorticoid and almost no mineralocorticoid activity (cortisol) to all mineralocorticoid and almost no glucocorticoid activity (aldosterone).

INTERMEDIARY METABOLISM

Glucocorticoids stimulate the conversion of protein to carbohydrate through gluconeogenesis and promote the storage of carbohydrate as glycogen. The increase in urinary nitrogen after an increase in glucocorticoids is the result of amino acid breakdown as a source of carbon for gluconeogenesis. Adrenalectomized animals are able to function normally as long as food (i.e., free amino acids) is available. Upon starvation, however, these animals cannot mobilize amino acids from muscle or serum protein, indicating that cortisol plays a role in mobilizing amino acids from proteins in plasma and muscle (42). Glucocorticoids cause an elevation in plasma glucose as a result of the increase in liver gluconeogenesis (43), which in turn promotes the formation of glycogen in the liver (44). Prolonged doses of glucocorticoids lead to a diabetic-like state due to the increase in plasma glucose, whereas low glucocorticoid concentrations lead to hypoglycemia, decreased glycogen stores in muscle and liver, and hypersensitivity to insulin. Glucocorticoids also decrease facilitated uptake of glucose in peripheral tissues to provide more glucose for glycogen formation in the liver. This effect is particularly prevalent in leukocytes and may be a major contributing factor to the rapid elevation in blood glucose after steroid administration. The complex mechanisms for the peripheral effects of glucocorticoids are unknown, but chronic administration can result in the atrophy of lymphatic tissue and muscle, osteoporosis, and thinning of the skin. Amino acids are funneled to the liver for glucose and glycogen formation. Glucocorticoids also have a direct effect on gene expression in the liver to increase the synthesis of a number of enzymes required for the biosynthesis of glucose and glycogen.

There are two established effects of glucocorticoids on lipid metabolism. One is the redistribution of body fat in hypercorticism; the other is facilitation of effects of lipolytic agents. Large doses of glucocorticoids lead to formation of fat depots on the back of the neck, the supraclavicular area, and the face, with a concomitant loss of fat in the extremities (45). The mechanism for this effect is not understood, although these apparently paradoxical responses may result from differences in the number of glucocorticoid receptors in these different types of fat cells (46). By this hypothesis, cells with fewer receptors would be spared the effects of glucocorticoids on glucose transport, and, therefore, glucose and triglyceride accumulation would occur in response to the rise in insulin levels. In contrast, fat cells containing higher levels of receptor (perhaps in the periphery) would respond to the high glucocorticoid level by decreasing glucose uptake and would not accumulate triglycerides. Alternatively, cells in the extremities may be less sensitive to insulin (47). The mobilization of fat from peripheral depots by epinephrine and other lipolytics is severely blunted in the absence of glucocorticoids (48). Cortisol facilitates the response of adipocytes to the rise in cyclic AMP (cAMP) induced by these agents rather than creating a larger increase in the amount of cAMP.

ELECTROLYTE AND WATER BALANCE

The major effect of mineralocorticoids is the regulation of electrolyte excretion in the kidney (49). Aldosterone treatment results in increased sodium reabsorption from tubular fluid and an increase in excretion of potassium and hydrogen. Similar effects on cation transport in most other tissues account for all the systemic activity of mineralocorticoids. The primary features of excess mineralocorticoids are positive sodium balance, increased extracellular fluid volume, normal or slightly high plasma sodium, hypokalemia, and alkalosis. Under conditions of hypocorticism there is renal loss of sodium, hyponatremia, hyperkalemia, and a decrease in extracellular fluid volume and cellular hydration. The 1% decrease in sodium reabsorption that occurs in hypocorticism is enough to cause profound cardiovascular changes, resulting in circulatory collapse, renal failure, and ultimately in death. Aldosterone modulates sodium levels by acting through mineralocorticoid receptors, located in the distal tubules of the kidney, to increase the permeability of the apical membrane of the cells lining the cortical collecting tube. Aldosterone also increases activity of the sodium/potassium-ATPase in the serosal membrane (50). These changes allow more sodium to be reabsorbed and generate a higher negative potential in the lumen, which is the driving force for increased potassium and hydrogen excretion. Mineralocorticoids also increase calcium and magnesium excretion, probably due to volume expansion. Prolonged aldosterone treatment results in sodium "escaping," a cessation of sodium changes, while potassium and hydrogen loss continues to occur. The mechanism for this effect is unknown but may involve mineralocorticoid receptor down-regulation and subsequent cessation of hormonal responsiveness.

Glucocorticoids have effects on the kidney that differ from the effects of mineralocorticoids. Glucocorticoids increase water diuresis, glomerular filtration rate, and renal plasma flow. Although increases in sodium retention and potassium excretion occur with cortisol, there seems to be no increase in hydrogen excretion. The major renal complications of glucocorticoid therapy are nephrocalcinosis, nephrolithiasis, and increased stone formation from the increase in urinary concentrations of calcium and uric acid (51).

Electrolyte changes also occur in tissues other than the kidney in response to mineralocorticoid treatment. These affected tissues include gastrointestinal mucosa (52), salivary and sweat glands (53), and exocrine pancreas. In these tissues, a longer onset period is required to detect significant responses to aldosterone, and no sodium "escape" occurs after prolonged hormone administration. Aldosterone apparently does not cause changes in intestinal electrolyte absorption (54), but glucocorticoids increase sodium and water absorption and potassium secretion. Both glucocorticoid and mineralocorticoid receptors are present in the mucosa, but dexamethasone can bind to both receptor types whereas aldosterone can only bind to its own receptor. Cortisol also increases gastric acid secretion and blood flow to the gastric mucosa, while decreasing the rate of gastric cell proliferation. High doses of glucocorticoids may cause peptic ulceration or aggravate preexisting ulcers (55).

ENDOCRINE SYSTEM

In addition to the effects on ACTH secretion previously described, corticosteroids influence the action of several other hormones. Cortisol increases growth hormone secretion in patients with acromegaly (56). In contrast, the spontaneous secretion of growth hormone is inhibited in hypercorticism (57). Growth failure is observed with prolonged glucocorticoid treatment in children. This response is apparently due to decreased maturation of the epiphyseal plates and a decrease in long bone growth (58). Corticosteroids depress the secretion of thyroid-stimulating hormone in patients with myxedema (59), and reduce the physiologic effectiveness of thyroxine (60). High doses of steroid decrease leutinizing hormone release in response to leutinizing hormone-releasing hormone (61). Corticosteroids also have been shown to potentiate the β-adrenergic effects of catecholamines and stimulate the synthesis of epinephrine from norepinephrine (62). Other systemic effects of high doses of glucocorticoids include adrenocortical insufficiency upon glucocorticoid removal (63), steroid-induced diabetes (64), hyperlipidemia (65), high glucagon levels (66), and hypocalcemia (67).

CARDIOVASCULAR SYSTEM

The major effects of corticosteroids on the cardiovascular system are due to their influence on plasma volume, electrolyte retention, epinephrine synthesis, and angiotensin levels, which together result in the maintenance of normal blood pressure and cardiac output. However, the hypotension that occurs from corticosteroid deficiency cannot be totally explained by these factors. Corticosteroids have effects on myocardial responsiveness, arteriolar tone, and capillary permeability. Hypocorticism leads to increased capillary permeability, inadequate vasomotor response, and decrease in cardiac output and cardiac size. Hypercorticism leads to chronic arterial hypertension (68). The mechanism responsible for this effect is unclear, but it is specific for mineralocorticoid activity and may be due to prolonged, excessive sodium retention. Hypertension can also be induced by glucocorticoids. The mechanism for this response is also unknown, but glucocorticoids influence many factors, including increased filtration fraction and glomerular hypertension, increased angiotensinogen synthesis, decreased prostaglandin synthesis that leads to decreased vasodilation, increased responsiveness to vasopressors, and increased synthesis of atrial natriuretic peptide. There is a fair amount of evidence that glucocorticoids potentiate atherosclerosis and thromboembolic complications (69, 70).

MUSCULOSKELETAL SYSTEM

Normal corticosteroid levels are required for muscle maintenance; however, either excess glucocorticoid or mineralocorticoid can lead to muscle abnormalities (71, 72). High aldosterone levels cause muscle weakness due to hypokalemia. High glucocorticoid levels cause muscle wasting due to catabolic effects on protein metabolism as described previously. Corticosteroid insufficiency results in decreased work capacity of striated muscle, weakness, and fatigue. This response reflects an inadequacy of the circulatory system rather than electrolyte and carbohydrate imbalances.

The most debilitating effect of glucocorticoids on bone is induction of osteoporosis (73, 74). This response results from a decrease in osteoblast activity, as well as from a decrease in gastrointestinal absorption of calcium. The decrease in serum calcium causes increased secretion of parathyroid hormone, which in turn stimulates osteoclast activity. Therefore, glucocorticoids act to decrease bone formation, as well as to increase bone resorption. Other effects of high doses of glucocorticoids on the musculoskeletal system include aseptic or avascular necrosis of bone and spontaneous tendon rupture presumably through an effect on collagen metabolism (69, 75, 76).

CENTRAL NERVOUS SYSTEM

Corticosteroids affect the nervous system indirectly in a number of ways by maintaining normal plasma glucose levels, adequate circulation, and normal electrolyte levels. Direct effects of corticosteroids on the central nervous system are not well defined; however, changes in corticosteroid levels do influence mood, behavior, electroencephalograph patterns, and brain excitability. Chronic glucocorticoid treatment has been shown to cause cell death in hippocampal neurons in rats, but it is unknown whether such a response occurs in humans (77). Patients with Addison's disease are subject to apathy, depression, irritability, and psychosis (78). These symptoms are alleviated by glucocorticoid treatment but not by mineralocorticoids. Individuals with Cushing's disease are known to develop neuroses and psychoses that are reversible with the removal of excess hormone (79). Increases in brain excitability in hypercorticism and after mineralocorticoid treatment are due to electrolyte imbalances. However, the increase in brain excitability induced by cortisol is not due to changes in sodium concentration. Chronic glucocorticoid treatment can also result in pseudotumor cerebri, primarily in children (80).

HEMATOLOGIC EFFECTS

Corticosteroids increase hemoglobin and red cell content of blood as demonstrated by the occurrence of polycythemia in Cushing's disease and mild normochromic anemia in Addison's disease. These steroids may retard erythrophagocytosis. Corticosteroids also affect circulating white cells (81). Glucocorticoid treatment results in increased polymorphonuclear leukocytes in blood as a result of increased rate of entrance from marrow and a decreased rate of removal from the vascular compartment. In contrast, the lymphocytes, eosinophils, monocytes, and basophils decrease in number after administration of glucocorticoids. A single dose of cortisol results in a 70% decrease in lymphocytes and a 90% decrease in monocytes, which occurs 4 to 6 hours after treatment and persists for about 24 hours. Cell numbers then rise 24 to 72 hours after treatment (82). The decrease in lymphocytes, monocytes, and eosinophils is thought to be due to redistribution of these cells rather than to their destruction, although recent data suggest that certain lymphocyte subpopulations undergo apoptosis in response to glucocorticoids (83). The T lymphocytes are more sensitive to glucocorticoids than are B lymphocytes, and certain T cell subpopulations are more sensitive to glucocorticoids than others. Decrease in basophils occurs by an unknown mechanism.

ANTI-INFLAMMATORY EFFECTS

Glucocorticoids prevent or suppress the full inflammatory reaction to infectious, physical, or immunologic agents (84). The local heat, redness, swelling, and tenderness typically associated with an inflammatory response do not develop. Glucocorticoids inhibit the early events in the process, including edema, cellular exudation, fibrin deposition, capillary dilatation, migration of leukocytes into the area, and phagocytic activity. Later events are also inhibited, including capillary and fibroblast proliferation, deposition of collagen, and cicatrization. The mechanism is not clearly understood, but it is of great therapeutic relevance.

A major effect of glucocorticoids on the inflammatory process is inhibition of recruitment of neutrophils and monocytes (85). The tendency of neutrophils to adhere to capillary endothelial cells, which is mediated by prostaglandins, is also decreased. This is due to inhibition of the normal increase in expression of endothelial adhesion molecules (i.e., ELAM-1, ICAM-1) (86). Glucocorticoids decrease the synthesis and release of prostaglandins by inducing a protein (lipocortin) that inhibits phospholipase A2, which is an enzyme involved in the synthesis of prostaglandins. Glucocorticoids also inhibit synthesis of plasminogen activator and migration inhibitory factor (87, 88), stabilize lysosomes [thereby decreasing the release of irritating hydrolytic enzymes and histamine (89, 90)], and also decrease binding of chemokines that attract white blood cells (91). Glucocorticoids slow wound healing by blocking the normal inflammatory reaction of breaking down and disorganizing collagen.

IMMUNE SYSTEM

It has been known for a long time that hypocorticism results in hypertrophy of lymphoid tissue (i.e., thymus, spleen, lymph nodes) and that hypercorticism leads to decreases or total loss of these tissues (92). Glucocorticoids induce rapid lysis of lymphatic tissue in rats and mice, but these effects occur only at suprapharmacologic doses in man. The effects that are seen in humans, therefore, may be due to changes in the rate of formation or destruction of lymphoid cells, which only become manifest over a longer period of time. More acute effects of glucocorticoid on lymphoid cells in man are probably due to sequestration of the cells rather than to cell lysis, although recent reports suggest that certain types of activated T lymphocytes are susceptible to glucocorticoid-induced apoptosis (83). In contrast to normal human lymphocytes, acute lymphocytic leukemias and other malignancies respond to glucocorticoid treatment with lymphocytolysis as is seen in rodents. Glucocorticoids decrease the secretion of interleukin 1 and other mediators of immune response, inhibit lymphocyte participation in delayed hypersensitivity reactions, and interfere with the rejection of immunologically incompatible graft tissue (93). This is probably due to decreases in leukocyte recruitment. High doses of glucocorticoids inhibit immunoglobulin synthesis, kill B cells (94), and decrease production of certain components of the complement system (95).

OTHER EFFECTS

Other effects of prolonged glucocorticoid therapy include ophthalmologic [posterior subcapsular cataracts (96), increased intraocular pressure (97)] and dermatologic [redistribution of subcutaneous fat, hirsutism, alopecia, impaired wound healing, purpura, purple striae, and acneiform eruptions (98)] problems. Long-term glucocorticoid treatment, with the concomitant immunosuppression, also leaves patients susceptible to invasive diseases such as Kaposi's sarcoma (99) and fungal infections (100).

Corticosteroids in the Treatment of Neoplasms

Once corticosteroids became available, many experiments were done to test the effect of these compounds on experimental neoplasms. It was first discovered that cortisone caused tumor regression in a transplantable mouse lymphosarcoma (101), and this finding was soon extended to a wide variety of mouse lymphatic tumors. The effects of corticosteroids were also evaluated on many nonendocrine and nonlymphoid transplantable rodent tumors. Pharmacologic doses of steroid inhibited growth of various tumor systems (102). Tissue culture studies subsequently confirmed that lymphoid cells were the most sensitive to glucocorticoids and responded to treatment with decreases in DNA, RNA, and protein synthesis (103). Studies of proliferating human leukemic lymphoblasts supported the hypothesis that glucocorticoids have preferential lymphocytolytic effects (104). The mechanism of action was initially thought to be due to a decrease in glucose transport and/or phosphorylation, which would lead to decreased energy utilization from the lack of glucose (105). However, it has recently been discovered that glucocorticoids induce apoptosis in certain lymphoid cell populations (106). Despite an incomplete understanding of the mechanism of action of glucocorticoids, it is clear that these steroids have great clinical value in the treatment of neoplasms of lymphoid origin and, to a much lesser extent, other endocrine-responsive cancers. Glucocorticoids also serve a function in the treatment of several frequently occurring side effects of malignancies, as well as for general palliative therapy.

NEOPLASMS TREATED WITH CORTICOSTEROIDS

Acute Lymphoblastic Leukemia

Early studies of acute lymphoblastic leukemia treated with prednisone alone showed that 50% of the affected children responded with prompt clinical improvement and remission (107). However, the duration of remission was short (<1 year), and relapse was inevitable, often coinciding with the appearance of steroid resistance. For these reasons, multiple drug therapy was initiated which involves combining prednisone with other cytotoxic agents. Today more than 90% of children (108, 109) and 60 to 80% of adults (110–113) achieve remission with regimens that contain vincristine and prednisone or prednisolone. The inclusion of other agents, such as daunorubicin, L-asparaginase, cytosine arabinoside, doxorubicin, and cyclophosphamide, may or may not increase this rate of remission but does appear to prolong remission.

Once remission is achieved, a 2- to 3-year program of maintenance therapy follows that involves regular intensive chemotherapy sessions that include glucocorticoids (109, 111, 114). Prophylactic treatment to prevent relapse in the central nervous system is often administered, consisting of cranial radiotherapy and intrathecal treatment with prednisone, methotrexate, and cytosine arabinoside (115, 116). With this approach, more than 50% of children appear to be cured (no relapse within 5 years) (see Chapter 164). The success rate is considerably lower in adults; only 15 to 30% of adults appear to be cured (see Chapter 145).

In refractory cases, or in cases of relapse, which occurs in approximately 20% of children with acute lymphoblastic leukemia, reinduction involves more aggressive combination chemotherapy, again including a glucocorticoid (115, 117, 118). Treatment with high doses of methylprednisolone alone (1 g/m^2 for 5–8 days) has also been shown to be effective with little toxicity (119). However, overall survival rates after relapse are much lower, averaging 35 to 65% in children (115, 116, 118) and less in adults (117).

Acute Myeloid Leukemia

Glucocorticoids appear to have little if any value in the treatment of acute myeloid leukemia. Use of glucocorticoids as a single agent results in <10% complete remission (120). Glucocorticoids have been included in some combination chemotherapies, with accompanying complete remission rates of 64 to 82% (117, 121, 122). However, the importance of glucocorticoids in combinations such as these requires further study.

Chronic Lymphocytic Leukemia

Typical B-cell chronic lymphocytic leukemia in the early stage of progression responds well to combination chemotherapy including an alkylating agent (usually chlorambucil) plus or minus prednisolone (123, 124) (see Chapter 147). Advanced stages of the disease sometimes require the addition of an anthracycline and a vinca alkaloid for successful therapy. One commonly used combination is cyclophosphamide, doxorubicin, vincristine, and prednisolone (CHOP) (125). Fludarabine appears to be effective in both untreated and refractory cases of chronic lymphocytic leukemia (126–128). Corticosteroids are particularly useful if the neoplasm is associated with autoimmune hemolytic anemia, neutropenia, and thrombocytopenia with hemorrhagic complications (129). Glucocorticoids alleviate the lymphadenopathy and hepatosplenomegaly that are often associated with this condition.

Chronic Myeloid Leukemia

Chronic myeloid leukemia in the chronic phase presents no indication for corticosteroids. Blast transformation is characterized by increased splenomegaly, bone pain, and deposits of leukemia outside the lymphohematopoietic system. Approximately 20 to 30% of cases show blast cells that resemble those of acute lymphoblastic leukemia. The remainder of cases are myeloblastic, although a proportion have phenotypic features of both types (see Chapter 143).

Transformed lymphoblastic cells generally respond to the same treatments that are used in acute lymphoblastic leukemia. Some patients enter complete remission but most return to the chronic phase. This chronic phase is brief; blastic transformation reappears and becomes increasingly difficult to treat due to the development of resistant cell types.

Hodgkin's Lymphoma

Hodgkin's lymphoma is a solid tumor found to be curable by chemotherapy. Corticosteroids alone were found to achieve worthwhile objective results in 66% of Hodgkin's lymphoma patients resistant to alkylating agents (130). Combination chemotherapy, with mustine, vincristine, procarbazine, prednisone (MOPP), was the first treatment to effectively cause complete remission, and probably cures, in a majority of patients (131). Since then other regimens, most of which contain a glucocorticoid component, have been found to be as effective as MOPP (132). One combination that does not contain a glucocorticoid, doxorubicin, bleomycin, vinblastine, and dacarbazine (ABVD), is at least as effective as MOPP and has a lower incidence of certain side effects (133) (see Chapter 149).

Recent studies have shown that treatment of early stage Hodgkin's lymphoma with radiotherapy is more effective than chemotherapy (134, 135). Advanced stage disease treated with MOPP, ABVD, or other similar combinations exhibits a complete response rate of 55 to 75% (136–138). Aggressive salvage therapies for relapsed or refractory Hodgkin's disease that contain a glucocorticoid have a complete response rate around 30 to 50% (139–141).

Non-Hodgkin's Lymphoma

Corticosteroids used as single agent therapy produce temporary responses in patients with non-Hodgkin's lymphoma; they are therefore included in virtually every complex regimen used for the treatment of non-Hodgkin's lymphoma (142). These regimens differ according to lymphoma histologic subtype and stage (see Chapter 150). Patients with disseminated lymphomas treated with recent generations of drug combinations have 3- to 4-year survival rates of 30 to 70% (143). One recent study indicates that the use of interferon α-2b in combination with a typical glucocorticoid-containing drug regimen produces good results (85% overall response rate and 86% 3-year survival rate) (144). If the tumor is located within the central nervous system, dexamethasone is preferred instead of prednisone to decrease tumor swelling (142).

Multiple Myeloma

The standard therapy for multiple myeloma is melphalan and prednisone, which results in a 50% response rate (145) (see Chapter 152). Complete remission is rare, however, and the median survival is only 24 to 30 months. Combination chemotherapies have also been used (146, 147). These treatments have a higher complete response rate, but the median survival time is not significantly different from treatment with melphalan and prednisone. A combination of vincristine, Adriamycin, and dexamethasone (VAD) appears to be effective, especially in refractory cases (148, 149). A recent study indicates that treatment of multiple myeloma with intermittent dexamethasone administration leads to an overall response rate of 43% (150). Although this is about 15% less than the results of VAD therapy, there is a much lower incidence of serious complications, suggesting that dexamethasone alone may be a simple, effective, and safe therapy for multiple myeloma. Very high doses of glucocorticoids alone may be temporarily useful, albeit toxic, in cases of progressive or resistant disease, or if bone marrow reserve is limited. These doses can be as high as 1 g/m^2/day for prednisone and 40 mg/m^2/day for dexamethasone. High dose melphalan plus methylprednisolone with autologous bone marrow transplantation as consolidation after conventional chemotherapy has resulted in a 75% complete remission rate and an estimated 54 month survival rate of 63% (151). Interferon-α has been used as a single agent and in combination with other treatments with some apparent success (145, 152). The use of interferon-μ along with a glucocorticoid for maintenance therapy, appears to prolong remission duration (153).

Breast Cancer

Glucocorticoids are never used as the sole treatment for breast cancer because of the low response rate (<25%) and the deleterious side effects that result from the high doses needed (154) (see Chapter 136). Nevertheless, glucocorticoids are included in various regimens of combination chemotherapy. The cyclophosphamide, methotrexate, and 5-fluorouracil (CMF)-type regimens, with and without other drugs such as prednisone, result in tumor regression in 50 to 80% of patients and complete response in 15 to 20% (155). Although palliation of symptoms occurs in a majority of patients, only a small percentage benefit by prolonged survival. The impact on median survival is no more than 2 to 3 months.

The role of prednisone in the effectiveness of the cyclophosphamide, methotrexate, 5-fluorouracil, and prednisone (CMFP) regimen is unclear. Some trials comparing CMF and CMFP found that the response to CMFP in premenopausal, node-positive women was not different from the response to CMF (156, 157). Another comparison trial of CMF versus CMFP found that the inclusion of prednisone resulted in a longer time to treatment failure and a longer survival time (158). However, this may be due to the higher average dose of CMF in the CMFP patients. A trial of radiation treatment plus or minus prednisone found that radiation and prednisone together had a significant increase over radiation alone in disease-free and overall survival in premenopausal women over 45 (159). A trial of high-dose chemotherapy involving an 11 drug combination including prednisone resulted in a very high response rate (overall response, 92%; complete response, 73%), but median survival time was not markedly increased from other studies (160). An intensive 8-drug combination with autologous bone marrow transplantation and locoregional radiotherapy tested on patients with at least 5 involved lymph nodes resulted in a 5-year disease-free survival rate of 84% (161). The efficacy of the glucocorticoids in such regimens may be due, at least in part, to the improved tolerance of cytotoxic drugs. As a milder treatment for metastatic breast cancer patients who do not consent to aggressive cytotoxic chemotherapy, the combination of mitoxantrone, leukovorin, 5-fluorouracil, and prednisone induced tumor regression in 67% of patients with a complete response in 25% (162).

Other Uses

Hydrocortisone replacement (approximately 40 mg/day) is indicated after either surgical adrenalectomy or medical adrenalectomy via steroid synthesis inhibitors is performed to eliminate circulating steroids in cases of breast cancer, prostate cancer, and ectopic ACTH excess (154, 163, 164). Hemangiomas in infants are often treated with injections of glucocorticoids (165, 166). Thymomas are often treated with glucocorticoids either alone or in combination with cytotoxic drugs (167, 168) (see Chapter 109). Other tumors that have been treated with combination chemotherapy involving a glucocorticoid include medulloblastoma, primitive neuroectodermal tumors, and ependymomas (169, 170).

SYMPTOMATIC USES OF CORTICOSTEROIDS

Palliative Care

Glucocorticoid treatment produces rapid symptomatic improvements in critically ill patients, including temporary relief of fever, sweats, lethargy, weakness, and other nonspecific effects of cancer. Glucocorticoids also cause mild euphoria, a general feeling of well being, and a stimulation of appetite (171, 172). These effects are transient, and only short-term treatment is possible due to side effects of the high doses. Also, when glucocorticoids are withdrawn, adrenocortical insufficiency and patient discomfort can occur. For these reasons corticosteroid treatment is normally reserved for patients whose life expectancy is brief (a few weeks or less). Doses of 25 mg/day prednisolone are used initially with a decrease to 7.5 to 15 mg/day for maintenance of effects.

Hypercalcemia

Hypercalcemia is a common complication of many malignancies (173). It is caused in many cases by increased bone resorption and renal calcium reabsorption and is thought to be due to many factors that may be secreted by various tumors (see Chapters 77 and 102), especially those of lymphoid origin. Although glucocorticoids do not lower normal calcium levels, glucocorticoids in large doses have been used for treatment of hypercalcemia (100 mg/day prednisolone, 400 mg/day hydrocortisone). The mechanisms by which glucocorticoids reduce serum calcium are thought to be cytolytic action on lymphoid cells, decrease in lymphokine secretion, and inhibition of vitamin D action on calcium metabolism. Glucocorticoids are most effective on hypercalcemia that is secondary to high vitamin D levels. They are less effective in patients with solid tumors. The results in treatment of patients with multiple myeloma have been inconsistent. Glucocorticoids are therefore a poor choice except in cases of vitamin D-mediated hypercalcemia.

Central Nervous System Tumors

Neurologic symptoms from primary and metastatic brain and spinal cord tumors are partially due to peritumoral edema (174). Glucocorticoids can ameliorate these symptoms in about 70 to 80% of cases after several days of treatment (175–177). There is evidence that glucocorticoids cause both a decrease in edema production and an increase in edema reabsorption. Dexamethasone is the recommended steroid for this treatment because it contains no mineralocorticoid activity and is highly potent (see Chapter 175). A dose of 16 mg/day is used with an increase to 100 mg/day if no response occurs. This dose is continued until the maximum response is obtained. Doses are then decreased gradually and are maintained at the smallest effective dose. In a cautionary note, recent findings suggest that currently used doses are greatly in excess of the therapeutic level since 2 to 4 mg of dexamethasone/day was found to be sufficient for controlling edema during radiotherapy for brain metastases (178, 179). Glucocorticoid effects on the brain and spinal cord are short lived and only increase survival time slightly unless other measures, such as radiotherapy and surgery, are taken. Glucocorticoids are often administered during these therapies to alleviate the edema that is normally induced by these treatments. Preliminary evidence suggests that glucocorticoids might decrease the amount of cytotoxic drug that gets to the tumor by decreasing capillary permeability. Because of the extensive use of glucocorticoids in treating central nervous system tumors, this issue must be studied further (180).

Antiemetic Action

Glucocorticoids have been shown to decrease the severity of chemotherapy-induced emesis (181, 182). Both dexamethasone (8–20 mg) and methylprednisolone (125–250 mg) have been used successfully, with vomiting episodes reduced by as much as 74%.

Glucocorticoids are most effective when used at low doses to enhance the antiemetic efficacy of other drugs (183, 184). Recent findings suggest that the combination of glucocorticoids with serotonin receptor antagonists (e.g., ondansetron, granisetron, tropisetron) is extremely effective (185–187). The mechanism by which antiemesis occurs is unknown, but it may be associated with decreases in prostaglandin synthesis. Alternatively, glucocorticoids may act directly on the chemoreceptor trigger zone by modifying capillary permeability or stabilizing lysosomal membranes.

Dyspnea Caused by Lymphangitic Carcinomatosis

The dyspnea caused by lymphangitic carcinomatosis may be a result of tumor edema and is effectively relieved in most cases by glucocorticoid treatment (188). If the primary tumor is chemosensitive, then cytotoxic agents are also given. Prednisone is initially given at a dose of 60–100 mg/day and is then reduced rapidly to the minimum level that maintains the response. The benefits of this treatment may be short lived, and high doses may be indicated with the attendant danger of long-term complications.

Other Uses of Glucocorticoids

Acute upper airway obstruction can result from direct tumor growth or by compression from thyroid, lung, and esophageal cancers. This obstruction can be reduced by glucocorticoid treatment either alone or in combination with radiotherapy (189, 190). Other cancer-related obstructions and mass effects can be partially controlled by glucocorticoids. These include superior vena cava syndrome; lymphedema; liver metastases; masses in the pelvis, mediastinum, or retroperitoneum; and blockages of the large bowel or ureter (191). Therapeutic effects are due to reduction in peritumoral inflammation and edema. The pain that can accompany bone metastases or metastatic arthralgia from a variety of solid tumors often responds to glucocorticoid treatment (192). Several chemotherapeutic agents (mitomycin, bleomycin, busulfan, carmustine), as well as radiotherapy, are associated with pulmonary toxicity. This lung injury can be decreased at least partially by preventive glucocorticoid administration during chemotherapy. This treatment is most effective during mitomycin therapy. Dexamethasone (10–12 mg at each treatment) during mitomycin chemotherapy for non-small cell lung cancer was found to effectively prevent lung injury (193). A decrease in the antineoplastic effect of mitomycin was observed, suggesting that further study on this type of treatment is necessary. Loss of vision associated with pseudotumor cerebri can be treated with glucocorticoids (194, 195).

Mechanism of Glucocorticoid Action

The biologic effects of all of the steroid hormones are mediated by intracellular receptor proteins that are specific for each steroid (196). The glucocorticoid receptor, a cytoplasmic protein with approximate molecular weight of 98,000, is present in all tissues that are targets of glucocorticoid action (197). The concentration of glucocorticoid receptors in a given cell depends on many factors, including cell type, state of differentiation, phase of the cell cycle, endocrine status, and age. Glucocorticoid receptors are required for glucocorticoid-induced changes to occur, but hormonal sensitivity is not guaranteed by the presence of receptors. There is, in general, a good correlation between the concentration of glucocorticoid receptors in a cell and the cellular sensitivity to glucocorticoids. However, other factors may modulate glucocorticoid sensitivity, including the presence of nonfunctional or modified receptors and other cellular factors that modify receptor function.

The current model for glucocorticoid action (Fig. 72.2) starts with the passive diffusion of glucocorticoids into the cell. The steroid then binds noncovalently and with high affinity to the glucocorticoid receptor in the cytoplasm. Ligand binding causes the receptor to undergo a process called activation or transformation in which a conformational change in the receptor is thought to occur (see Chapter 69). The receptor dissociates from the nonsteroid-binding subunits with which it is normally associated, unmasking the DNA-binding domain of the receptor protein. The steroid-receptor complex then translocates to the nucleus where it binds to specific DNA sequences called glucocorticoid-regulatory elements (GREs). After binding to a GRE, the steroid-receptor complex alters the transcription rate of specific genes near to or in which the GRE is located. A typical glucocorticoid-responsive gene is shown in Figure 72.3. The GRE, shown with the consensus DNA sequence, is located in the 5′-regulatory region of the gene where a glucocorticoid receptor bound to the GRE can interact with transcription factors that bind to other regulatory elements, such as the TATA and CAAT boxes, which are also present in this re-

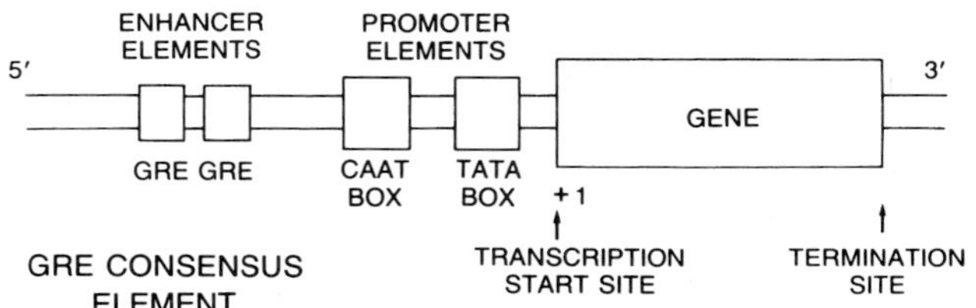

Figure 72.2. Mechanism of action of steroid hormones. S, steroid; R, receptor.

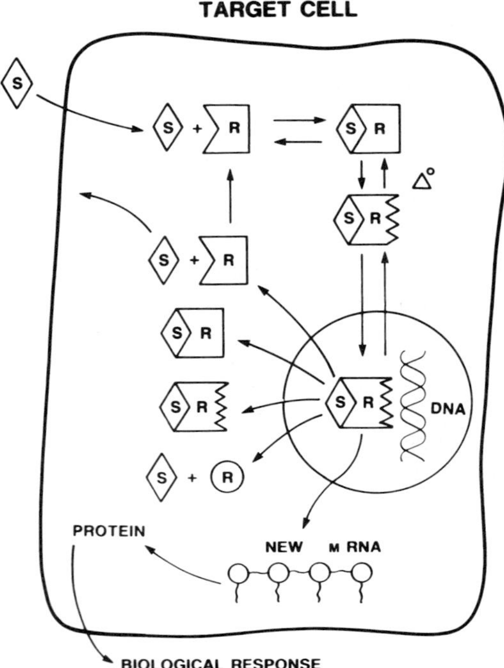

Figure 72.3. Structural requirements for glucocorticoid regulation of gene transcription. GRE, glucocorticoid responsive element; N, nucleoside, unspecified.

gion. In this fashion glucocorticoids can increase the transcription rate of a positive GRE-containing gene or decrease the transcription rate of a negative GRE-containing gene. These alterations in the transcription rate lead to changes in the amount of messenger RNA and ultimately the level of protein that is synthesized from these genes, and thus alter cellular functions. Recent data in experimental systems suggest that glucocorticoid receptors can interfere with AD1 and NF KB signaling pathways, although there is no direct evidence for these pathways in humans.

One important aspect of receptor regulation that is especially relevant to glucocorticoid therapy is glucocorticoid-induced down-regulation (tachyphylaxis) of the glucocorticoid receptor. The ability of glucocorticoid to down-regulate its own receptor is mediated by the receptor itself (198). The maximum effect is a 50 to 75% decrease in receptor protein, which is reflected by a decrease in receptor messenger RNA that occurs within 24 hours of treatment. Long-term administration of glucocorticoids is not only associated with down-regulation of the glucocorticoid receptor but also with decreased function of other genes that are glucocorticoid sensitive (199). This phenomenon implies that continuous glucocorticoid treatment can have widespread deleterious effects on cell function and may explain why alternate day glucocorticoid therapy is associated with a lesser risk of unwanted side effects (200, 201). These results indicate that it may be important, in terms of efficacy and safety, to administer therapeutic doses of glucocorticoids in a manner that simulates the natural diurnal rhythm of glucocorticoid secretion.

ANTICORTICOSTEROIDS

Steroid receptor antagonists have been synthesized that inhibit the action of receptor ligands. Most of these antagonists are modified steroids that are competitive inhibitors of the receptor. The antagonist forms a complex with the receptor and then interferes with one or more of the normal functions of a ligand-bound receptor by not translocating to the nucleus, not binding to the appropriate DNA sequences with high affinity, or not affecting transcription rates. The best characterized antiglucocorticoids are the steroid metabolite cortexolone (11-deoxycortisol) and the antiprogestin RU-486 (202). The antiprogestin effects of mefipristone (RU-486) are used clinically for the induction of abortions. The antiglucocorticoid effects of RU-486 are under investigation as a treatment for hypercorticism and as an antineoplastic agent for meningioma, breast cancer, prostate cancer, and hepatoma. Spironolactone is a commonly used antimineralocorticoid. Recent reports suggest that antimineralocorticoids may be useful in the treatment of diseases involving blood pressure and body fluid regulation (203).

CORTICOSTEROID RESISTANCE

Since it was discovered that glucocorticoids have a specific cytolytic effect on human leukemic and lymphomatous tissue, the medical significance of glucocorticoid receptors in these tissues has been studied. The fact that not all leukemia patients respond to glucocorticoid treatment, combined with the observation that some patients cease to respond during therapy, has prompted investigators to try to identify a relationship between glucocorticoid receptor concentration and clinical responsiveness (204, 205). Various human and mouse lymphoid cell lines, including CEM-C7 (206), P1798 (207), and S49.1 (208), have been extensively studied to determine how these cells become resistant to glucocorticoids. In almost every single case of resistance in mouse cells, the cause is a defective glucocorticoid receptor or a large decrease in receptor number (209). Until recently, however, resistant human leukemia cell lines have not been found to contain major defects in the glucocorticoid receptor, such as those described in mouse lymphoma cell lines. With the advent of molecular analysis of the glucocorticoid receptor gene, it has become possible to determine that resistant variants of the human T cell-derived CEM cell line, which is by far the most extensively studied human leukemia cell line, do contain mutations in the glucocorticoid receptor (210). Additional findings of glucocorticoid receptor mutations have been reported for multiple myeloma cell lines (211, 212). These mutations are often subtle, in some cases involving a single nucleotide base pair change (213). No consistent relationship has been found between glucocorticoid receptor number and sensitivity to lymphocytolysis (214). The correlation is strongest for acute lymphocytic leukemia and non-Hodgkin's lymphoma (215). Other diseases, notably acute myeloid leukemia (121, 216), have no correlation. For chronic lymphocytic leukemia, the results are inconsistent (217, 218). The lack of a consistent relationship between receptor number and sensitivity to glucocorticoid therapy suggests that some factor(s) other than the presence of glucocorticoid receptors may mediate the susceptibility of lymphoid cells to glucocorticoid-induced lymphocytolysis.

GLUCOCORTICOID-INDUCED LYMPHOCYTOLYSIS

For many years it has been known that glucocorticoids induce massive lymphocytolysis in rats and mice, resulting in significant reductions in the size of lymphoid tissues, including thymus, spleen, and lymph nodes. This phenomenon has been widely studied, especially in rodent thymus, where immature thymocytes are available in high numbers and die rapidly after glucocorticoid treatment. This form of cell death has been found to be identical both morphologically and biochemically with a specific form of cell death known as apoptosis, or programmed cell death (219). Apoptosis is associated with many physiologic processes, including embryogenesis, morphogenesis, normal tissue turnover, and cell-mediated immunity, and is induced by many different signals in these various systems (220). Morphologic characteristics of apoptosis include cellular condensation and internucleosomal chromatin degradation, followed by fragmentation into apoptotic bodies that are phagocytosed by neighboring cells or circulating macrophages.

Recent studies have shown that glucocorticoid-induced apoptosis occurs only in lymphocytes and is mediated by the glucocorticoid receptor (221–223). However, not all lymphocytes are sensitive. Immature T cells and some B cells are very sensitive to apoptosis, whereas mature T cells are not. Those cells that are responsive start to die within 8 hours of glucocorticoid treatment in vivo. Nearly all immature thymocytes are dead within 48 hours of treatment.

In contrast, the sensitivity of human lymphocytes to glucocorticoid-induced apoptosis appears to be quite different. Although these cells do respond to glucocorticoids, they do not die with the same kinetics as rodent lymphocytes. The marked lymphocytopenia observed after glucocorticoid treatment is mostly due to redistribution of lymphocytes into other tissues and is returned to normal within 24 hours. This difference in species sensitivity to lymphocytolysis is not well understood.

Although human lymphocytes are generally more resistant to lymphocytolysis, certain subpopulations do lyse in response to glucocorticoids. These include cortical and medullary thymocytes, mature Th cells, natural killer cells and cytotoxic T lymphocytes, and immature B cells (81). More important, several malignant hematopoietic cells are sensitive to glucocorticoid-induced apoptosis. These include multiple myeloma (224), acute lymphoblastic leukemia (225), chronic lymphocytic leukemia (226, 227), and acute myeloid leukemia (228). Several investigators have demonstrated that some human leukemic cells, notably acute and chronic lymphocytic leukemia and acute myeloid leukemia, show morphologic and biochemical signs of apoptosis upon death (226, 228). The difference between normal and malignant human lymphocytes that causes the increased susceptibility of malignant cells to apoptosis is unknown. Targeted apoptosis is developing into an important tool in the repertoire of cancer therapy techniques. Much study remains to be done on the phenomenon of apoptosis to determine the mechanism and specificity of this therapeutically useful process.

References

1. Addison T. On the constitutional and local effects of disease of the suprarenal capsules. London: Samual Highly, 1855.
2. Brown-Séquard CE. Recherches experimentales sur la physiologie et la pathologie des capsules surrénales. C R Acad Sci D (Paris) 1856;43:422.
3. Britton SW, Silvette H. Some effects of corticoadrenal extract and other substances on adrenalectomized animals. Am J Physiol 1931;99:15–32.
4. Harrop GA, Soffer LJ, Ellsworth R, Trescher JH. Studies on the suprarenal cortex. III. Plasma electrolytes and electrolyte excretion during suprarenal insufficiency in the dog. J Exp Med 1933;58:17–38.
5. Cushing H. The basophil adenomas of the pituitary body and their clinical manifestations. Bull Johns Hopkins Hosp 1932;50:137–195.
6. Bell PH, Howard KS, Shepherd RG, Finn BM, Misenhelder JH. Studies with corticotropin. II. Pepsin degradation of β-corticotropin. J Am Chem Soc 1956;78: 5059–5066.
7. Li CH, Evans HM, Simpson ME. Adrenocorticotropic hormone. J Biol Chem 1943;149: 413–424.
8. Ingle DJ, Higgins GM, Kendall EC. Atrophy of the adrenal cortex in the rat produced by administration of large amounts of cortin. Anat Rec 1938;71:363–372.
9. Reichstein T, Shoppee CW. The hormones of the adrenal cortex. Vitam Horm 1943;1: 346–413.
10. Simpson SA, Tait JF, Wettsteon A, et al. Konstitution de aldosterons des neuen mineralocorticoids. Experientia 1954;10:132–133.
11. Hench PS, Kendall EC, Slocumb CH, Polley HF. The effect of a hormone of the adrenal cortex (17-hydroxy-11-dehydrocorticosterone; compound E) and of pituitary adrenocorticotropic hormone on rheumatoid arthritis. Proc Staff Meet Mayo Clin 1949;24:181–197.
12. Caspi E, Dorfman RI, Khan BT, Rosenfeld G, Schmid W. Degradation of corticosteroids. VI. Origin of the carbon atoms of steroid hormones biosynthesized in vitro in the bovine adrenal from acetate-1-C14. J Biol Chem 1962;237:2085–2088.
13. Kimura T, Suzuki K. Components of the electron transport system in adrenal steroid-hydroxylase. Isolation and properties of non-heme iron protein (adrenodoxin). J Biol Chem 1967;242:485–491.
14. Gwynne JT, Strauss III JF. The role of lipoprotein in steroidogenesis and cholesterol metabolism in steroidogenic glands. Endocr Rev 1982;3:299–329.
15. Kimura T. ACTH stimulation of cholesterol side chain cleavage activity of adrenocortical mitochondria. Mol Cell Biochem 1981;36:105–122.
16. Haynes RC Jr. The activation of adrenal phosphorylase by the adrenocorticotropic hormone. J Biol Chem 1958;233:1220–1222.
17. Brown MS, Kovanen PT, Goldstein JL. Receptor-mediated uptake of lipoprotein-cholesterol and its utilization for steroid synthesis in the adrenal cortex. Recent Prog Horm Res 1979;35:215–257.
18. Gwynne JT, Mahaffee D, Brewer HB, Ney RL. Adrenal cholesterol uptake from plasma lipoproteins; regulation by corticotropin. Proc Natl Acad Sci USA 1976;73: 4329–4333.
19. Simpson ER, Mason JI, John ME, Zuber MX, Rodgers RJ, Waterman MR. Regulation of the biosynthesis of steroidogenic enzymes. J Steroid Biochem 1987;27:801–805.
20. Grossman A, Perry L, Schally AV, et al. New hypothalamic hormone, corticotropin-releasing factor, specifically stimulates the release of adrenocorticotropic hormone and cortisol in man. Lancet 1982;1:921–922.
21. Gann DS, Dallman MF, Engleland WC. Reflex control and modulation of ACTH and corticosteroids. Int Rev Physiol 1981;24:157–199.
22. Ericsson A, Kovacs KJ, Sawchenko PE. A functional anatomical analysis of central pathways subserving the effects of interleukin-1 on stress-related neuroendocrine neurons. J Neurosci 1994;14:897–913.
23. Weitzman ED, Fukushima D, Nogeire C, Roffwarg H, Gallagher TF, Hellman L. Twenty-four hour pattern of the episodic secretion of cortisol in normal subjects. J Clin Endocrinol Metab 1971;33:14–22.
24. Czeisler CA, Ede MCM, Regenstein QR, Kisch ES, Fang VS, Ehrlich EN. Episodic 24-hour cortisol secretory patterns in patients awaiting elective cardiac surgery. J Clin Endocrinol Metab 1976;42:273–283.
25. George JM, Reier CE, Lanese RR, Rower JM. Morphine anesthesia blocks cortisol and growth hormone response to surgical stress in humans. J Clin Endocrinol Metab 1974;38:736–741.
26. Vaughan GM, Becker RA, Allen JP, Goodwin CW Jr, Pruitt BA Jr, Mason AD Jr. Cortisol and corticotrophin in burned patients. J Trauma 1982;22:263–273.
27. Copinschi G, L'Hermite M, LeClerq R, et al. Effects of glucocorticoids on pituitary hormone responses to hypoglycemia. Inhibition of prolactin release. J Clin Endocrinol Metab 1975;40:442–449.
28. Davis JD. Regulation of aldosterone secretion. In The Adrenal Cortex. Edited by AB Eisenstein. Boston: Little, Brown, 1967.
29. Elliott ME, Alexander RC, Goodfriend TL. Aspects on angiotensin action in the adrenal. Key roles for calcium and phosphatidylinositol. Hypertension 1982;4:52–58.
30. Blair-West JR, Coghlan JP, Denton DA, et al. A dose-response comparison of the actions of angiotensin II and angiotensin III in sheep. J Endocrinol 1980;87:409–417.
31. Cannon PJ, Ames RP, Laragh JH. Relation between potassium balance and aldosterone secretion in normal subjects and in patients with hypertensive or renal tubular disease. J Clin Invest 1966;45:865–879.
32. New MI, Seaman MP, Peterson RE. A method for the simultaneous determination of the secretion rates of cortisol, 11-desoxycortisol, corticosterone, 11-desoxycorticosterone and aldosterone. J Clin Endocrinol Metab 1969;29:514–522.
33. Bondy PK. The adrenal cortex. In Metabolic Control and Disease, 8th ed. Edited by PK Bondy and LE Rosenberg. Philadelphia: Saunders, 1980, pp 1427–1499.
34. Scurry MT, Sheart L. Stop-flow analysis of the reabsorption of cortisol. Endocrinology 1969;84:681–682.
35. Manni A. Clinical use of aromatase inhibitors in the treatment of breast cancers. J Cell Biochem Suppl 1993;17G:242–246.
36. Cheng SC, Harding BW, Carballeira A. Effects of metyrapone on pregnenolone

biosynthesis and on cholesterol-cytochrome P-450 interaction in the adrenal. Endocrinology 1974;94:1451–1458.
37. Touitou Y, Bogdan A, Legrand JC, Desgrez P. Aminoglutethimide and glutethimide's effects on 18-hydroxycorticosterone biosynthesis by human and sheep adrenals in vitro. Acta Endocrinol 1975;80:517.
38. Hogan TF, Citrin DL, Johnson BM, Nakamura S, Davis TE, Borden EC. *o,p'*-DDD (mitotane) therapy of adrenal corticol carcinoma. Cancer 1978;42:2177–2181
39. Perez N, Borja J. Aromatase inhibitors: clinical pharmacology and therapeutic implications in breast cancer. J Int Med Res 1992;20:303–312.
40. Ito S, Kusunoki Y, Oka T, Ito Y, Okuno A, Yoshioka H. Pharmacokinetics of high-dose methylprednisolone in children. Dev Pharmacol Ther 1992;19:99–105.
41. Lew KH, Ludwig EA, Milad MA, et al Gender-based effects on methylprednisolone pharmacokinetics and pharmacodynamics. Clin Pharmacol Ther 1993;54:402–414.
42. Kaplan SA, Nagareda Shimizu CS. Effects of cortisol on amino acids in skeletal muscle and plasma. Endocrinology 1963;72:267–272.
43. Rizza RA, Mandarino LJ, Gerich JE. Cortisol-induced insulin resistance in man: impaired suppression of glucose production and stimulation of glucose utilization due to a post receptor defect of insulin action. J Clin Endocrinol Metab 1982;54:132–138.
44. Lecocq FR, Mebane D, Madison LL. The acute effect of hydrocortisone on hepatic glucose output and peripheral glucose utilization. J Clin Invest 1964;43:237–246.
45. Rimsza ME. Complications of corticosteroid therapy. Am J Dis Child 1978;132: 806–810.
46. Miller LK, Kral JG, Strain GW, Zumoff B. Differential binding of dexamethasone to ammonium sulfate precipitates of human adipose tissue cytosols. Steroids 1987;49: 507–522.
47. Fain JN, Czech MP. Glucocorticoid effects on lipid mobilization and adipose tissue metabolism. In Adrenal Gland, vol 6, sect 7, Endocrinology. Handbook of Physiology. Edited by H Blashko. Washington, DC: American Physiological Society, 1975, p 169.
48. Shafrir E, Steinberg D. The essential role of the adrenal cortex in the response of plasma free fatty acids, cholesterol and phospholipids to epinephrine injection. J Clin Invest 1960;39:310–319.
49. Mulrow PJ, Forman BH. The tissue effects of mineralocorticoids. Am J Med 1972;53: 561–572.
50. Marver D. Aldosterone action in target epithelia. Vitam Horm 1980;38:55–117.
51. Kobayashi O, Wada H, Utsumi J. Urinary lithiasis in children treated with adrenocorticosteroid hormone. Acta Med Biol 1967;15:91–105.
52. Foster ES, Zimmerman TW, Hayslett JP, Binder HJ. Corticosteroid alteration of active electrolyte transport in rat distal colon. Am J Physiol 1983;245: G668–G675.
53. Blair-West JR, Coghlan JP, Denton DA, Goding JR, Wright RD. The effect of adrenal corticoid steroids on parotid salivary secretion. In Salivary Glands and their Secretions. Proceedings of International Conference, Washington, DC, Aug 1962. New York: Pergamon, 1964, p 253.
54. Charney AN, Kinsey MD, Myers L, Giannella RA, Gots RE. Na+-K+-activated adenosine triphosphatase and intestinal electrolyte transport. J Clin Invest 1975;56: 653–660,
55. Messer J, Reitman D, Sacks H, Smith H, Chalmers T. Association of adrenocorticosteroid therapy and peptic ulcer disease. N Engl J Med 1983;309:21–25.
56. Bridson WE, Kohler PO. Cortisol stimulation of growth hormone production by human pituitary tissue in culture. J Clin Endocrinol Metab 1970;30:538–540.
57. Stiel JN, Island DP, Liddle GW. Effect of glucocorticoids on plasma growth hormone in man. Metabolism 1970;19:158–164.
58. Lucky AW. Principles of the use of glucocorticoids in the growing child. Pediatr Dermatol 1984;1:226–235.
59. Wilber JF, Utiger RD. The effect of glucocorticoids on thyrotropin secretion. J Clin Invest 1969;48:2096–2103.
60. Burr WA, Ramsden DB, Griffiths RS, et al. Effect of a single dose of dexamethasone on serum concentrations of thyroid hormones. Lancet 1976;2:58–61.
61. Sakakura M, Takebe K, Nakagawa S. Inhibition of leutinizing hormone secretion by synthetic LHRH by long-term treatment with glucocorticoids in human subjects. J Clin Endocrinol Metab 1975;40:774–779.
62. Ellul-Micallef R, Fenech FF. Effect of intravenous prednisolone in asthmatics with diminished adrenergic responsiveness. Lancet 1975;2:1269–1271.
63. Cope CL. The adrenal cortex in internal medicine. Br Med J 1966;2:847–853.
64. Alavi IA, Sharma BK, Pillay VKG. Steroid-induced diabetic ketoacidosis. Am J Med Sci 1971;262:15–23.
65. Pennisi AJ, Fiedler J, Lipsey A, Mickey R, Melekzadeh MH, Fine RN. Hyperlipidemia in pediatric renal allograft patients. J Pediatr 1975;87:249–251.
66. Melby JC. Clinical pharmacology of systemic corticosteroids. Annu Rev Pharmacol Toxicol 1977;17:511–527.
67. Eberlein WR, Bongiovanni AM, Rodriguez CS. Diagnosis and treatment: the complications of steroid treatment. Pediatrics 1967;40:279–282.
68. Krakoff LR. Glucocorticoid excess syndromes causing hypertension. Cardiol Clin 1988;6:537–545.
69. David DS, Grieco MH, Cushman P Jr. Adrenal glucocorticoids after twenty years–a review of their clinically relevant consequences. J Chronic Dis 1970;22:637–711.
70. Kalbak K. Incidence of arteriosclerosis in patients with rheumatoid arthritis receiving long-term corticosteroid therapy. Ann Rheum Dis 1972;31:196–200.
71. Askari A, Vignos PJ, Moskowitz RW. Steroid myopathy in connective tissue disease. Am J Med 1976;61:485–492.
72. Mandel S. Steroid myopathy. Insidious cause of muscle weakness. Postgrad Med 1982;72:207–210, 213–215.
73. Ringe JD. Glucocorticoid-induced osteoporosis. Clin Rheumatol 1989;2(suppl 8):109–115.
74. Libanati CR, Baylink DJ. Prevention and treatment of glucocorticoid-induced osteoporosis. A pathogenetic perspective. Chest 1992;102:1426–1435.
75. Richards JM, Santiago SM, Klanstermeyer WB. Aseptic necrosis of the femoral head in corticosteroid-treated pulmonary disease. Arch Intern Med 1980;140:1473–1475.
76. Chan-Lam D, Prentice AG, Copplestone JA, Weston M, Williams M, Hutton CW. Avascular necrosis of bone following intensified steroid therapy for acute lymphoblastic leukaemia and high-grade malignant lymphoma. Br J Haematol 1994;86:227–230.
77. Masters JN, Finch CE, Sapolsky RM. Glucocorticoid endangerment of hippocampal neurons does not involve deoxyribonucleic acid cleavage. Endocrinology 1989;124: 3083–3088.
78. Carpenter WT Jr, Gruen PH. Cortisol's effects on human mental functioning. J Clin Psychopharmacol 1982;2:91–101.
79. Hall RCW, Popkin MK, Stickney SK, Gardner ER. Presentation of the steroid psychoses. J Nerv Ment Dis 1979;167:229–236.
80. Weisberg LA, Chatorian AM. Pseudotumor cerebri of childhood. Am J Dis Child 1977;131:1243–1248.
81. Cupps TR, Fauci AS. Corticosteroid-mediated immunoregulation in man. Immunol Rev 1982;65:133–155.
82. Pountain GD, Keogan MT, Hazleman BL, Brown DL. Effect of single dose compared with three days' prednisolone treatment of healthy volunteers: contrasting effects on circulating lymphocyte subsets. J Clin Pathol 1993;46:1089–1092.
83. Schwartzman RA, Cidlowski JA. Glucocorticoid-induced apoptosis of lymphoid cells. Int Arch Allergy Immunol 1994;105:347–354.
84. Schleimer RP. An overview of glucocorticoid anti-inflammatory actions. Eur J Clin Pharmacol 1993;45(suppl 1):S3–S7.
85. Parrillo JE, Fauci AS. Mechanisms of glucocorticoid action on immune processes. Annu Rev Pharmacol Toxicol 1979;19:179–201.
86. Cronstein BN. The pharmacology of antiinflammatory agents: a new paradigm. Mt Sinai J Med 1993;60:209–217.
87. Balow JE, Rosenthal AS. Glucocorticoid suppression of macrophage migration inhibitory factor. J Exp Med 1973;137:1031–1041.
88. Granelli-Piperno A, Vassali JD, Reich E. Secretion of plasminogen activator by human polymorphonuclear leukocytes. Modulation by glucocorticoids and other effectors. J Exp Med 1977;146:1693–1706.
89. Saavedra-Delgado AM, Mathews KP, Pan PM, Kay DR, Muilenberg ML. Dose-response studies of the suppression of whole blood histamine and basophil counts by prednisone. J Allergy Clin Immunol 1980;66:464–471.
90. Spath JA, Lefer AM. Effects of dexamethasone on myocardial cells in the early phase of acute myocardial infarction. Am Heart J 1975;90:50–55.
91. Skubitz KM, Craddock PR, Hammerschmidt DE, August JT. Corticosteroids block binding of chemotactic peptide to its receptor on granulocytes and cause disaggregation of granulocyte aggregates in vitro. J Clin Invest 1981;68:13–20.
92. Fauci AS, Dale DC, Balow JE. Glucocorticosteroid therapy: mechanisms of action and clinical considerations. Ann Intern Med 1976;84:304–315.
93. Gillis S, Crabtree GR, Smith KA. Glucocorticoid-induced inhibition of T cell growth factor. J Immunol 1979;123:1632–1638.
94. Grayson J, Dooley NJ, Koski IP, Blaese RM. Immunoglobulin production induced in vitro by glucocorticoid hormones. T cell-dependent stimulation of immunoglobulin production without B cell proliferation in cultures of human peripheral lymphocytes. Clin Invest 1981;68:1539–1547.
95. Caren LD, Rosenberg LT. Steroids and serum complement in mice: influence of hydrocortisone, diethylstilbestrol, and testosterone. Science 1966;152:782–783.
96. Lubkin VL. Steroid cataract–a review and a conclusion. J Asthma Res 1977;14:55–59.
97. Giles CL. The ocular complications of steroid therapy. Mich Med 1967;66:298–301.
98. Truhan AP, Ahmed AR. Corticosteroids: a review with emphasis on complications of prolonged systemic therapy. Ann Allergy 1989;62:375–391.
99. Trattner A, Hodak E, David M, Sandbank M. The appearance of Kaposi sarcoma during corticosteroid therapy. Cancer 1993;72:1779–1783.
100. Walsh TJ, Lee JW, Roilides E, Pizzo PA. Recent progress and current problems in management of invasive fungal infections in patients with neoplastic diseases. Curr Opin Oncon 1992;4:647–655.
101. Heilman FR, Kendall EC. The influence of 11-dehydro-17-hydroxycorticosterone (compound E) on the growth of malignant tumor in the mouse. Endocrinology 1944;34:416–426.
102. Vollmer EP. A viewpoint on animal tumors as test systems for steroids. In: Hormonal steroids, biochemistry, pharmacology, and therapeutics. Proc First Int Cong Horm Steroids 1965;2:351.
103. Baxter GD, Collins RJ, Harmon BV, et al. Cell death by apoptosis in acute leukemia. J Pathol 1989;158:123–129.
104. Ernst P, Killman S. Perturbation of generation of human leukemic blast cells by cytostatic therapy in vivo: effect of corticosteroids. Blood 1970;36:689–705.
105. Rosen JM, Fina JJ, Millholland RJ, Rosen F. Inhibition of glucose uptake in lymphosarcoma 1798 by cortisol and its relationship to the biosynthesis of deoxyribonucleic acid. J Biol Chem 1970;245:2074–2080.
106. Cohen JJ. Lymphocyte death induced by glucocorticoids. In: Schleimer RP, Claman HN, Oronsky AL, eds. Anti-inflammatory steroid action: basic and clinical aspects. San Diego: Academic, 1989, p 110.
107. Vietti TJ, Sullivan MP, Berry DH, Haddy TB, Haggard ME, Blattner RJ. The response of acute childhood leukemia to an initial and a second course of prednisone. J Pediatr 1965;66:18–26.
108. Koizumi S, Fujimoto T. Improvement in treatment of childhood acute lymphoblastic leukemia: a 10-year study by the Children's Cancer and Leukemia Study Group. Int J Hematol 1994;59:99–112.
109. Yang CP, Lin ST, Liang DC, et al. Treatment of childhood acute lymphoblastic leukemia with protocol TCL-842 in Taiwan: the Taiwan Children's Cancer Study Group. J Formos Med Assoc 1993;92:431–439.
110. Bassan R, Battista R, Montaldi A, et al. Reinforced HEAV'D therapy for adult acute lymphoblastic leukemia: improved results and revised prognostic criteria. Hematol Oncol 1993;11:169–177.
111. Todeschini G, Meneghini V, Pizzolo G, et al. Relationship between daunorubicin dosage delivered during induction therapy and outcome in adult acute lymphoblastic leukemia. Leukemia 1994;8:376–381.
112. Nagura E, Kimura K, Yamada K, et al. Nation-wide randomized comparative study of doxorubicin, vincristine and prednisolone combination therapy with and without L-asparaginase for adult acute lymphoblastic leukemia. Cancer Chemother Pharmacol 1994;33:359–365.
113. Bassan R, Battista R, Viero P, et al. Intensive therapy for adult acute lymphoblastic leukemia: preliminary results of the idarubicin/vincristine/L-asparaginase/prednisolone regimen. Semin Oncol 1993;20(suppl 8):39–46.
114. Sabbath KD, Weitberg AB, Calabresi P. Potentially curable neoplasms. Dis Mon 1986;32:593–652.
115. Winick NJ, Smith SD, Shuster J, et al. Treatment of CNS relapse in children with acute lymphoblastic leukemia: a Pediatric Oncology Group study. J Clin Oncol 1993;11: 271–278.

116. Buhrer C, Hartmann R, Fengler R, et al. Importance of effective central nervous system therapy in isolated bone marrow relapse of childhood acute lymphoblastic leukemia. BFM (Berlin-Frankfurt-Munster) Relapse Study Group. Blood 1994;83: 3468–3472.
117. Martino R, Brunet S, Sureda A, Mateu R, Altes A, Domingo-Albos A. Treatment of refractory and relapsed adult acute leukemia using a uniform chemotherapy protocol. Leuk Lymphoma 1993;11:393–398.
118. Sadowitz PD, Smith SD, Shuster J, Wharam MD, Buchanan GR, Rivera GK. Treatment of late bone marrow relapse in children with acute lymphoblastic leukemia: a Pediatric Oncology Group study. Blood 1993;81:602–609.
119. Ryalls MR, Pinkerton CR, Meller ST, Talbot D, McElwain TJ. High-dose methylprednisolone sodium succinate as a single agent in relapsed childhood acute lymphoblastic leukaemia. Med Pediatr Oncol 1992;20:119–123.
120. Lowenthal RM, Jestrimski KW. Corticosteroid drugs: their role in oncological practice. Med J Austr 1986;144:81–85.
121. Steuber CP, Civin C, Krischer J, et al. A comparison of induction and maintenance therapy for acute nonlymphocytic leukemia in childhood: results of a Pediatric Oncology Group study. J Clin Oncol 1991;9:247–258.
122. Nagura E, Kimura K, Yamada K, et al. Nationwide randomized comparative study of daunorubicin and aclarubicin in combination with behenoyl cytosine arabinoside, 6-mercaptopurine, and prednisolone for previously untreated acute myeloid leukemia. Cancer Chemother Pharmacol 1994;34:23–29.
123. French Cooperative Group on Chronic Lymphocytic Leukemia Therapy of chronic lymphocytic leukemia patients. Results from the French cooperative trials. Nouv Rev Fr Hematol 1988;30:443–448.
124. Binet JL. Treatment of chronic lymphocytic leukemia. French Co-operative Group on CLL. Bailleres Clin Haematol 1993;6:867–878.
125. Anonymous. Is the CHOP regimen a good treatment for advanced CLL? Results from two randomized clinical trials. French Cooperative Group on Chronic Lymphocytic Leukemia. Leuk Lymphoma 1994;13:449–456.
126. O'Brien S, Kantarjian H, Beran M, et al. Results of fludarabine and prednisone therapy in 264 patients with chronic lymphocytic leukemia with multivariate analysis-derived prognostic model for response to treatment. Blood 1993;82:1695–1700.
127. Keating MJ, O'Brien S, Robertson L, Huh Y, Kantarjian H, Plunkett W. Chronic lymphocytic leukemia–correlation of response and survival. Leuk Lymphoma 1993;11(suppl 2):167–175.
128. Anonymous Comparison of fludarabine, cyclophosphamide/doxorubicin/prednisone, and cyclophosphamide/doxorubicin/vincristine/prednisone in advanced forms of chronic lymphocytic leukemia: preliminary results of a controlled clinical trial. The French Cooperative Group on Chronic Lymphocytic Leukemia. Tumori 1993;79: 195–197.
129. Johnson LE. Chronic lymphocytic leukemia. Am Fam Physician 1988;38:167–176.
130. Hall TC, Choi OS, Abadi A, Krant MJ. High-dose corticoid therapy in Hodgkin's disease and other lymphomas. Ann Intern Med 1967;66:1144–1153.
131. DeVita VT, Serpick AA, Carbone PP. Combination chemotherapy in the treatment of advanced Hodgkin's disease. Ann Intern Med 1970;73:881–895.
132. Hoppe RT. The contemporary management of Hodgkin disease. Radiology 1988;169:297–304.
133. Bonadonna G, Santoro A, Bonfante V, Valagussa P. Cyclic delivery of MOPP and ABVD in stage IV Hodgkin's disease: rationale, background studies, and recent results. Cancer Treat Rep 1982;66:881–887.
134. Noordijk EM, Carde P, Mandard AM, et al. Preliminary results of the EORTC-GPMC controlled clinical trial H7 in early-stage Hodgkin's disease. EORTC Lymphoma Cooperative Group. Groupe Pierre-et-Marie-Curie. Ann Oncol 1994;2(suppl 5):107–112.
135. Climino G, Biti GP, Cartoni C, Magrini SM. Chemotherapy versus radiotherapy in early-stage Hodgkin's disease: evidence of a more difficult rescue for patients relapsed after chemotherapy. Eur J Cancer 1992;28A:1853–1855.
136. Canellos GP, Anderson JR, Propert KJ, et al. Chemotherapy of advanced Hodgkin's disease with MOPP, ABVD, or MOPP alternating with ABVD. N Engl J Med 1992;327: 1478–1484.
137. Cullen MH, Stuart NS, Woodroffe C, et al. ChIVPP/PABIOE and radiotherapy in advanced Hodgkin's disease. The Central Lymphoma Group. J Clin Oncol 1994;12: 779–787.
138. Somers R, Carde P, Henry-Amar M, et al. A randomized study in stage IIIB and IV Hodgkin's disease comparing eight courses of MOPP versus an alteration of MOPP with ABVD: a European Organization for Research and Treatment of Cancer Lymphoma Cooperative Group and Groupe Pierre-et-Marie-Curie controlled clinical trial. J Clin Oncol 1994;12:279–287.
139. Pfreundschuh MG, Rueffer U, Lathan B, et al Dexa-BEAM in patients with Hodgkin's disease refractory to multidrug chemotherapy regimens: a trial of the German Hodgkin's Disease Study Group. J Clin Oncol 1994;12:580–586.
140. Fairey AF, Mead GM, Jones HW, Sweetenham JW, Whitehouse JM. CAPE/PALE salvage chemotherapy for Hodgkin's disease patients relapsing within 1 year of ChIVPP chemotherapy. Ann Oncol 1993:857–860.
141. Smith MR, Khanuja PS, al-Katib A, et al. Continuous infusion ABDIC therapy for relapsed or refractory Hodgkin's disease. Cancer 1994;73:1264–1269.
142. Longo DL, Hathorn J. Current therapy for diffuse large-cell lymphoma. Prog Hematol 1987;15:115–136.
143. Juliusson G, Abrahamsen AF, Cavallin-Stahl E, et al. Management of non-Hodgkin lymphoma in adults in Scandinavia, United Kingdom, and the Netherlands. Acta Oncol 1989;28:135–140.
144. Solal-Celigny P, Lepage E, Brousse N, et al. Recombinant interferon alfa-2b combined with a regimen containing doxorubicin in patients with advanced follicular lymphoma. Groupe d'Etude des Lymphomes de l'Adulte. N Engl J Med 1993;329: 1608–1614.
145. Oken MM. Standard treatment of multiple myeloma. Mayo Clin Proc 1994;69:781–786.
146. Niesvizky R, Siegel D, Michaeli J. Biology and treatment of multiple myeloma. Blood Rev 1993;7:24–33.
147. MacLennan ICM, Drayson M, Dunn J. Multiple myeloma. BMJ 1994;308:1033–1036.
148. Barlogie B, Smith L, Alexanian R. Effective treatment of advanced multiple myeloma refractory to alkylating agents. N Engl J Med 1984;310:1353–1356.
149. Barlogie B, Vesole DH, Jagannath S. Salvage therapy for multiple myeloma: the University of Arkansas experience. Mayo Clin Proc 1994;69:787–795.
150. Alexanian R, Dimopoulos MA, Delasalle K, Barlogie B. Primary dexamethasone treatment of multiple myeloma. Blood 1992;80:887–890.
151. Cunningham D, Paz-Ares L, Milan S, et al. High-dose melphalan and autologous bone marrow transplantation as consolidation in previously untreated myeloma. J Clin Oncol 1994;12:759–763.
152. Ganjoo RK, Johnson PW, Evans ML, et al. Recombinant interferon-alpha 2b and high dose methyl prednisolone in relapsed and resistant multiple myeloma. Hematol Oncol 1993;11:179–186.
153. Palumbo A, Boccadoro M, Garino LA, Gallone G, Frieri R, Pileri A. Interferon plus glucocorticoids as intensified maintenance therapy prolongs tumor control in relapsed myeloma. Acta Haematol 1993;90:71–76.
154. Manni A. Endocrine therapy of breast and prostate cancer. Endocrinol Metab Clin North Am 1989;18:569–592.
155. Henderson IC, Hayes DF, Come S, Harris JR, Canellos G. New agents and medical treatments for advanced breast cancer. Semin Oncol 1987;14:34–64.
156. Tormey DC, Gelman R, Band PR, et al. Comparison of induction chemotherapies for metastatic breast cancer. An Eastern Cooperative Oncology Group Trial. Cancer 1982;50:1235–1244.
157. Ludwig Breast Cancer Study Group. A randomized trial of adjuvant combination chemotherapy with or without prednisone in premenopausal breast cancer patients with metastases in one to three axillary lymph nodes. Cancer Res 1985;45: 4454–4459.
158. Eastern Cooperative Oncology Group Adjuvant systemic therapy in premenopausal (CMF, CMFP, CMFPT) and postmenopausal (observation, CMFP and CMFPT) women with node positive breast cancer. In Adjuvant Therapy of Cancer, IV. Edited by SE Jones, SE Salmon. Orlando: Grune & Stratton, 1984:359–368.
159. Meakin JW, Allt WEC, Beale FA. Ovarian irradiation and prednisone following surgery and radiotherapy for carcinoma of the breast. Breast Cancer Res Treat 1983;3(suppl): S45–S48.
160. Tormey DC, Kline JC, Palta M. Short term high density systemic therapy for metastatic breast cancer. Breast Cancer Res Treat 1985;5:177–188.
161. De Graaf H, Willemse PH, de Vries EG, et al. Intensive chemotherapy with autologous bone marrow transfusion as primary treatment in women with breast cancer and more than five involved axillary lymph nodes. Eur J Cancer 1994;30A:150–153.
162. Carmo-Pereira J, Costa FO, Henriques E. Mitoxantrone, folinic acid, 5-fluorouracil and prednisone as first-line chemotherapy for advanced breast carcinoma. A phase II study. Eur J Cancer 1993;29A:1814–1816.
163. Grayhack JT, Keeler TC, Kozlowski JM. Carcinoma of the prostate: hormonal therapy. Cancer 1987;60:589–601.
164. Santen RJ, Misbin RI. Aminoglutethimide: review of pharmacology and clinical use. Pharmacotherapy 1981;1:95–120.
165. Bilyk JR, Adamis AP, Mulliken JB. Treatment options for periorbital hemangioma of infancy. Int Ophthalmol Clin 1992;32:95–109.
166. Iwanaka T, Tsuchida Y, Hashizume K, Kawarasaki H, Utsuki T, Komuro H. Intralesional corticosteroid injection with short-term oral prednisolone for infantile hemangiomas of the eyelid and orbit. J Pediatric Surg 1994;29:482–486.
167. Papatestas AE, Pozner J, Genkins G, Kornfeld P, Matta RJ. Prognosis in occult thymomas in myasthenia gravis following transcervical thymectomy. Arch Surg 1987;122:1352–1356.
168. Park HS, Shin DM, Lee JS, et al. Thymoma. A retrospective study of 87 cases. Cancer 1994;73:2491–2498.
169. Wang KC, Lee JI, Cho BK, et al. Treatment outcome and prognostic factors of medulloblastoma. J Korean Med Sci 1994;9:64–73.
170. Geyer JR, Zeltzer PM, Boyett JM, et al. Survival of infants with primitive neuroectodermal tumors or malignant ependymomas of the CNS treated with eight drugs in one day: a report from the Childrens Cancer Group. J Clin Oncol 1994;12:1607–1615.
171. Tchekmedyian NS. Clinical approaches to nutritional support in cancer. Curr Opin Oncol 1993;5:633–638.
172. Lai YL, Fang FM, Yeh CY. Management of anorexic patients in radiotherapy: a prospective randomized comparison of megestrol and prednisolone. J Pain Symptom Manage 1994;9:265–268.
173. Attie MF. Treatment of hypercalcemia. Endocrinol Metab Clin North Am 1987;18: 807–828.
174. Edwards MSB, Prados M. Current management of brain stem gliomas. Pediatr Neurosci 1987;13:309–315.
175. Weissman DE. Glucocorticoid treatment for brain metastases and epidural spinal cord compression: A review. J Clin Oncol 1988;6:543–551.
176. Andersen C, Astrup J, Gyldensted C. Quantitative MR analysis of glucocorticoid effects on peritumoral edema associated with intracranial meningiomas and metastases. J Comput Assist Tomagr 1994;18:509–518.
177. Sorensen S, Helweg-Larsen S, Mouridsen H, Hansen HH. Effect of high-dose dexamethasone in carcinomatous metastatic spinal cord compression treated with radiotherapy: a randomised trial. Eur J Cancer 1994;30A:22–27.
178. Hildebrand J, Gangji D. Supportive care of neurologic complications. Curr Opin Oncol 1992;4:632–641.
179. Vech CJ, Hovestadt A, Verbiest HB, van Vliet JJ, van Putten WJ. Dose-effect relationship of dexamethasone on Karnofsky performance in metastatic brain tumors: a randomized study of doses of 4, 8, and 16 mg per day. Neurology 1994;44:675–680.
180. Wolfson AH, Snodgrass SM, Schwade JG, et al. The role of steroids in the management of metastatic carcinoma to the brain. A pilot prospective trial. Am J Clin Oncol 1994;17:234–238.
181. Aapro MS. Corticosteroids as antiemetics. Recent Results Cancer Res 1988;108: 102–111.
182. Tonato M, Roila F, Del Favero A, Ballatori E. Antiemetics in cancer chemotherapy: historical perspective and current state of the art. Support Care Cancer 1994;2:150–160.
183. Buzdar AU, Esparza L, Natale R, et al. Lorazepam-enhancement of the antiemetic efficacy of dexamethasone and promethazine. A placebo-controlled study. Am J Clin Oncol 1994;17:417–421.
184. Misra R, Agarwal N. Effective control of cisplatin induced emesis by combination regimen. Indian J Cancer 1994;31:19–22.
185. Aapro MS. Controlling emesis related to cancer therapy. Eur J Cancer 1991;27: 356–361.
186. Tsavaris N, Mylonakis N, Bacoyiannis C, Katsikas M, Lioni A, Kosmidis P. Comparison of ondansentron versus ondansentron plus methylprednisolone as antiemetic

prophylaxis during cisplatin-containing chemotherapy. J Pain Symptom Manage 1994;9:254–258.
187. Sorbe B, Hogberg T, Himmelmann A, et al. Efficacy and tolerability of tropisetron in comparison with a combination of tropisetron and dexamethasone in the control of nausea and vomiting induced by cisplatin-containing chemotherapy. Eur J Cancer 1994;30A:629–634.
188. Geimer NF, Donegan WL. Role and mechanism of corticosteroid therapy in breast cancer. Rev Endocrine-Related Cancer 1980;6:5.
189. Canellos GP, Cohen G, Posner M. Pulmonary emergencies in neoplastic disease. In: Yarbro J, ed. Oncologic emergencies. New York: Grune and Stratton, 1981, pp 301–322.
190. Walsh TD, West TS. Controlling symptoms in advanced cancer. Br Med J 1988;296: 477–481.
191. Breutman D, Harris J. Oncologic emergencies Part I: SVC syndrome, spinal cord compression. J Crit Illness 1988;3:31.
192. Zimmermann M, Drings P. Guidelines for therapy of pain in cancer patients. Rec Results Cancer Res 1984;89:1–12.
193. Spain RC. The case for mitomycin in non-small cell lung cancer. Oncology 1993;50(suppl 1):35–50.
194. Liu GT, Glaser JS, Schatz NJ. High-dose methylprednisolone and acetazolamide for visual loss in pseudotumor cerebri. Am J Ophthalmol 1994;118:88–96.
195. Char DH, Miller T. Orbital pseudotumor. Fine-needle aspiration biopsy and response to therapy. Ophthalmology 1993;100:1702–1710.
196. Carson-Jurica MA, Schrader WT, O'Malley BW. Steroid receptor family: structure and functions. Endocr Rev 1990;11:201–220.
197. Burnstein KL, Cidlowski JA. Regulation of gene expression by glucocorticoids. Annu Rev Physiol 1989;51:683–699.
198. Burnstein KL, Jewell CM, Cidlowski JA. Human glucocorticoid receptor cDNA contains sequences sufficient for receptor down-regulation. J Biol Chem 1990;265: 7284–7291.
199. Berkovitz GD, Carter KM, Migeon CJ, Brown TR. Down-regulation of the glucocorticoid receptor in cultured human skin fibroblasts: implications for the regulation of aromatase activity. J Clin Endocrinol Metab 1988;66:1029–1036.
200. Walton J, Watson BS, Ney RL. Alternate-day versus shorter-interval steroid administration. Arch Intern Med 1970;126:601–607.
201. Talar-Williams C, Sneller MC. Complications of corticosteroid therapy. Eur Arch Otorhinolaryngol 1994;251:131–136.
202. Weiss BD. RU486 The progesterone antagonist. Arch Fam Med 1993;2:63–69.
203. Waeber B, Nussberger J, Brunner HR. Clinical applications of antimineralocorticoids. J Steroid Biochem 1988;31:739–744.
204. McCaffrey R, Lillquist A, Bell R. Abnormal glucocorticoid receptors in acute leukemia cells. Blood 1982;59:393–400.
205. Pui CH, Dahl GV, Rivera G, Murphy S-B, Costlow ME. The relationship of blast cell glucocorticoid receptor levels to response to single-agent steroid trial and remission response in children with ALL. Leuk Res 1984;8:579–585.
206. Harmon JM, Thompson EB, Baione UA. Analysis of glucocorticoid-resistant human leukemic cells by somatic cell hybridization. Cancer Res 1985;45:1587–1593.
207. Stevens J, Stevens Y-N, Haubenstock H. Molecular basis of glucocorticoid resistance in experimental and human leukemia. In: Litwack G, ed. Biochemical actions of hormones. New York: Academic Press, 1983, pp 383–446.
208. Sibley CH, Tomkins GM. Mechanisms of steroid resistance. Cell 1974;2:221–227.
209. Sibley CH, Yamamoto KR. Mouse lymphoma cells: mechanism of resistance to glucocorticoids. In Glucocorticoid Hormone Action. Edited by JJ Baxter and GG Rousseau. Heidelberg: Springer-Verlag, 1979, pp 357–376.
210. Powers JH, Hillman AG, Tang DC, Harmon JM. Cloning and expression of mutant glucocorticoid receptors from glucocorticoid-sensitive and -resistant human leukemic cells. Cancer Res 1993;53:4059–4065.
211. Moalli PA, Pillay S, Weiner D, Leikin R, Rosen ST. A mechanism of resistance to glucocorticoids in multiple myeloma: transient expression of a truncated glucocorticoid receptor mRNA. Blood 1992;79:213–222.
212. Moalli PA, Pillay S, Krett NL, Rosen ST. Alternatively spliced glucocorticoid receptor messenger RNAs in glucocorticoid-resistant human multiple myeloma cells. Cancer Res 1993;53:3877–3879.
213. Homo-Delarche F. Glucocorticoid receptors and steroid sensitivity in normal and neoplastic human lymphoid tissues: a review. Cancer Res 1984;44:431–437.
214. Junker K. Glucocorticoid receptors of lymphoid cells. Cell biological and clinical aspects. Dan Med Bull 1986;1:12–23.
215. Quddus FF, Levanthal BG, Boyet JM, Pullen DJ, Crist NM, Borowitz MJ. Glucocorticoid receptors in immunological subtypes of childhood acute lymphocytic leukemia cells: a Pediatric Oncology Group study. Cancer Res 1985;45:6482–6486.
216. Koeffler HP, Golde DW, Lippman ME. Glucocorticoid sensitivity and receptors in cells of human myelogenous leukemia lines. Cancer Res 1980;40:563–566.
217. Homo F, Durant S, Duval D, Marie JP, Zittoun R, Harrouseau, JL. Glucocorticoid receptors and hormonal responsiveness of human blood and bone-marrow cells in non-lymphocytic leukemia. J Steroid Biochem 1981;15:479–485.
218. Weiss C, Ho AD, Hiller E, et al. Prognostic significance of glucocorticoid receptor determination in patients with chronic lymphocytic leukemia and immunocytoma–lack of a positive correlation between receptor levels and clinical responsiveness. Leuk Res 1990;14:327–332.
219. Schwartzman RA, Cidlowski JA. Apoptosis: the biochemistry and molecular biology of programmed cell death. Endocr Rev 1993;14:133–151.
220. Walker NI, Harmon BV, Gobe GC, Kerr JFR. Patterns of cell death. Methods Achiev Exp Pathol 1988;13:18–54.
221. Compton MM, Cidlowski JA. Rapid in vivo effects of glucocorticoids on the integrity of rat lymphocyte genomic deoxyribonucleic acid. Endocrinology 1986;118:38–45.
222. Schwartzman RA, Cidlowski JA. Internucleosomal DNA cleavage activity in apoptotic thymocytes: detection and endocrine regulation. Endocrinology 1991;128: 1190–1197.
223. Schwartzman RA, Cidlowski JA. Mechanism of tissue-specific induction of internucleosomal deoxyribonucleic acid cleavage activity and apoptosis by glucocorticoids. Endocrinology 1993;133:591–599.
224. Barlogie B. Pathophysiology of human multiple myeloma–recent advances and future directions. Curr Top Microbiol Immunol 1992;182:245–250.
225. Alnemri ES, Fernandes TF, Haldar S, Croce CM, Litwack G. Involvement of Bcl-2 in glucocorticoid-induced apoptosis of human pre-B-leukemias. Cancer Res 1992;52: 491–495.
226. Galili U, Leizerowitz R, Moreb J, Gamliel H, Gurfel D, Polliack A. Metabolic and ultrastructural aspects of the in vitro lysis of chronic lymphocytic leukemia cells by glucocorticoids. Cancer Res 1982;42:1433–1440.
227. McConkey DJ, Aguilar-Santelises M, Hartzell P, et al. Induction of DNA fragmentation in chronic B-lymphocytic leukemia cells. J Immunol 1991;146:1072–1076.
228. Baxter GD, Harris AW, Tomkins GM, Cohn M. Glucocorticoid receptors in lymphoma cells in culture: relationship to glucocorticoid killing activity. Science 1971;171:189.
229. Haynes RC Jr, Murad F. Adrenocorticotropic hormone; adrenocortical steroids and their synthetic analogs; inhibitors of adrenocortical steroid biosynthesis. In The Pharmacological Basis of Therapeutics, 7th ed. Edited by AG Gilman, LS Goodman, TW Rall, and F Murad. New York: Macmillan, 1985, pp 1459–1489.
230. Rose LI, Saccar C. Choosing corticosteroid preparations. Am Fam Physician 1978;17:198–204.

CHAPTER 73

Estrogens and Antiestrogens

V. CRAIG JORDAN

Introduction

It has been known since the turn of the century (11) that approximately one-third of premenopausal women with advanced breast cancer will respond to oophorectomy. Advances in the understanding of reproductive endocrinology and steroid biochemistry during the early decades of the 20th century permitted the development of specific strategies to restrict the availability of estrogen, the hormone widely believed to be responsible for the development of breast carcinoma (49). Breast cancer in postmenopausal women responds to hypophysectomy (109) and adrenalectomy (52), but paradoxically high-dose therapy with synthetic estrogens like diethylstilbestrol (DES) (25) and trianisylchorethylene (TACE) (130) causes breast tumor regression (44, 138) (Fig. 73.1). However it was unclear which patient would respond until the discovery of the estrogen receptor (ER) (56, 131) and the development of models (40, 57) to describe the subcellular actions of estrogen in its target tissues—uterus, vagina, pituitary gland, breasts, and in some breast cancers (99).

Studies of the structure-activity relationships of estrogens have provided the medical community with cheap, simple molecules that have proved to have powerful biologic effects in a woman's target tissues. The wide application of estrogens in the gynecologic community has resulted in the realization that estrogens might cause a number of cancers in target tissues (49).

As early as 1936, Lacassagne predicted that a therapeutic agent might be found that could block the stimulatory effects of estrogen in breast tissue (80). The nonsteroidal antiestrogen MER 25 (Fig. 73.2) was first described by Lerner and coworkers in 1958 (83). This discovery provoked clinical testing for a variety of applications, but trials were stopped because of toxic side effects (82). Nevertheless, in response to the encouraging clinical findings the pharmaceutical industry synthesized a wide range of compounds in the 1960s but there were few clinical successes. One notable exception was clomiphene (Clomid[reg]) (Fig. 73.2), a mixture of cis and trans geometric isomers of a substituted triphenylethylene (note the similarity to the structure of TACE). Although clomiphene is an antifertility agent in rodents (51) the compound was shown to induce ovulation in women (43). Clomiphene is routinely used as a profertility agent in subfertile women with a functioning hypothalamo-pituitary-ovarian axis (53).

Several antiestrogens (81) were tested as therapeutic agents to control the growth of advanced breast cancer in postmenopausal women, but only tamoxifen (ICI 46474, Nolvadex) (17, 139) was developed further because of demonstrated efficacy and a low incidence of side effects.

Tamoxifen

GENERAL PHARMACOLOGY IN THE LABORATORY

Tamoxifen is the trans geometric isomer of a substituted triphenylethylene with well-characterized antifertility (47) and antitumor (68) activity in the rat. As a group, the triphenylethylene-type antiestrogens have an extremely interesting species-specific pharmacology (39). In short-term tests in the mouse, tamoxifen can cause increases in uterine wet weight and vaginal cornification. In contrast, tamoxifen is classified as a pure antiestrogen in the chick. Tamoxifen exhibits the properties of a partial estrogen agonist/antagonist in rats and women. It is this balance of biologic properties that is key to the current strategies for the use of tamoxifen.

MODE OF ACTION IN BREAST CANCER

Tamoxifen is a competitive inhibitor of estradiol binding to the ER (59). Estradiol causes the proliferation of ER-positive breast cancer cells in culture, and tamoxifen can reversibly prevent estrogen-stimulated growth (87). Similarly, tamoxifen will prevent estrogen-stimulated growth of ER-positive breast cancer cells transplanted into immune deficient (athymic) mice (106).

Estrogens are believed to modulate cell growth by causing an increase in stimulatory growth factors (e.g., transforming growth factor alpha [TGF-α]) and a decrease in inhibitory growth factors (e.g., the family of transforming growth factors beta [TGF-β]) (24). These growth factors are thought to initiate, or prevent, progress through the cell cycle by interaction with their respective membrane receptors. The regulatory mechanism functions as an autocrine loop. There are also paracrine (cell–cell) influences of growth factors (e.g., insulinlike growth factor 1 [IGF-1]) that can play a role in modulating the replication of epithelial cells.

Antiestrogens negate the stimulatory effects of estrogen by blocking the ER, causing the cell to be held at the G1 phase of the replicative cycle (Fig. 73.3) (105). Tamoxifen also causes a decrease in the circulating levels of IGF-1 (18).

A variety of alternate, non-ER-mediated biochemical inter-

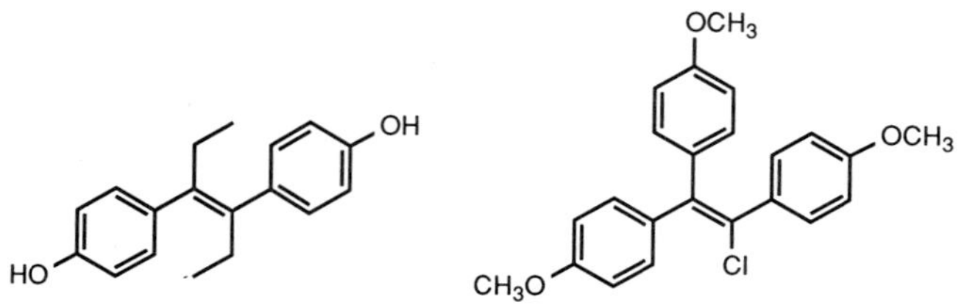

Diethylstilbestrol (DES) TACE

Figure 73.1. The structure of synthetic estrogens.

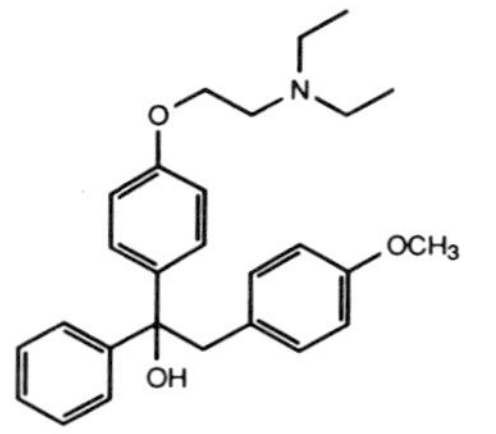

Ethamoxytriphetol (MER 25)

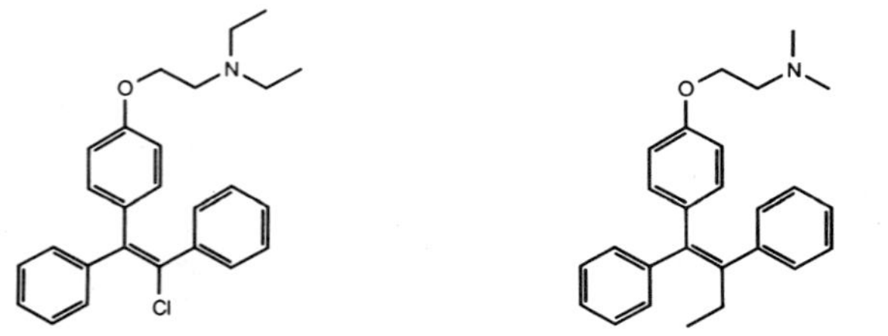

Clomiphene (cis and trans isomers) Tamoxifen (trans isomer)

Figure 73.2. The structure of nonsteroidal antiestrogens.

actions have been described for antiestrogens that might also contribute to the antitumor activity of tamoxifen. This topic has recently been reviewed (73).

CLINICAL PHARMACOLOGY

Tamoxifen (Nolvadex[reg]) is available in 10 mg tablets as the citrate salt. Treatment schedules vary depending on the country and their initial clinical trials evaluating the drug. Schedules of 10 mg b.i.d. are recommended in the United States, although 10 mg t.i.d. and 20 mg b.i.d. are routinely used in other countries. Doses above 100 mg b.i.d. have been used to treat breast cancer, but retinal degeneration has been reported (75). In general, the high therapeutic index has permitted such wide variations in dosage. There is a low incidence of side effects, the most frequent of which is hot flashes (39).

Tamoxifen is rapidly absorbed and attains steady-state serum levels within 4 to 6 weeks (64). The drug is extensively metabolized (Fig. 73.4) to N-desmethyltamoxifen (major metabolite) and 4-hydroxytamoxifen (minor metabolite). Both metabolites have the potential (118) to be converted to 4-hydroxy-N-desmethyltamoxifen, which is also a minor metabolite (85, 86). Nevertheless, 4-hydroxylated triphenylethylenes have high affinity for the ER (67) and may play a significant role in the antitumor actions of tamoxifen (29).

Tamoxifen has a long serum half-life (7 days) and N-desmethyltamoxifen has a serum half-life of 14 days (107). This long serum half-life is probably why a clinical response has not been routinely documented when tamoxifen therapy is discontinued.

Tamoxifen exhibits weak estrogen-like properties in postmenopausal women (39, 71). There is a partial decrease in luteinizing hormone (LH) and follicle-stimulating hormone (FSH) levels, increases in sex hormone-binding globulin (SHBG) levels, decreases in antithrombin III, some changes in vaginal cytology, and hyperplasia of the endometrium (although the last is not consistently reported). Tamoxifen causes ovarian stimulation in premenopausal women with ovulatory cycles and increases in steroidogenesis (97, 114, 125, 126). Women are at risk for pregnancy during tamoxifen therapy. Tamoxifen is not recommended if a woman is pregnant, and patients should be counseled about the need for barrier contraception. Clinical cases of teratogenesis have not been reported with tamoxifen.

USE IN ADVANCED BREAST CANCER

Tamoxifen is the endocrine treatment of choice for metastatic disease in postmenopausal patients (39). Approximately one third of patients respond, and the response rate is similar to that seen with DES therapy (54). However, side effects are reported to be lower with tamoxifen than with DES. The most prevalent side effects noted with DES are nausea (51%), edema (53%), vaginal bleeding (15%), and incontinence (10%). In contrast, hot flashes (29%) are the side effect most commonly reported during tamoxifen therapy. Patients with ER-positive disease are more likely to benefit from tamoxifen therapy (39). Correlation of clinical response and ER status indicates that 48% (159/333) of patients with ER-positive disease had partial or complete responses, whereas only 13% (17/129) of ER-negative patients had responses. A variety of combinations of other hormonal agents and combination chemotherapy have been examined (39), but tamoxifen is usually administered as monotherapy. Prospective randomized clinical trials of tamoxifen versus either megestrol acetate, 40 mg four times daily (101), or medroxyprogesterone acetate, 300 mg three times daily (136), indicate similar response rates, but the author recommends tamoxifen as first-line endocrine therapy based on side effects and time to progression. Aminoglutethimide (plus hydrocortisone) produces response rates similar to those seen with tamoxifen (2), and a combination is not superior to either agent alone. However, the toxic effects are significantly greater in patients taking aminoglutethimide. Aminoglutethimide can be an effective second-line agent following tamoxifen (128).

Tamoxifen is effective in the treatment of advanced disease in premenopausal women (97, 125). Small randomized trials have demonstrated that tamoxifen produces a response rate and overall survival similar to what is seen after oophorectomy (14, 55). Regrettably, the patient population is too small to demonstrate whether any benefit would preferentially accrue from one treatment approach in comparison to the other. However, tamoxifen does cause increases in circulating estradiol levels (97, 114, 125, 126) that could

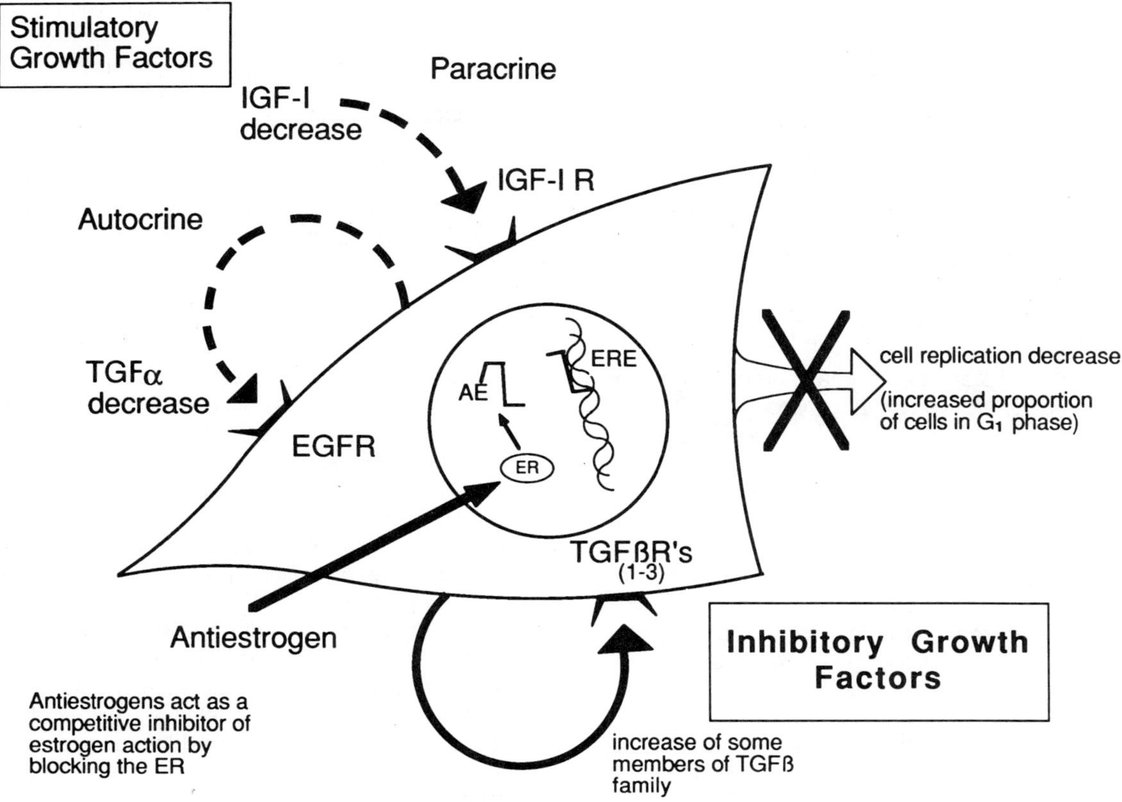

Figure 73.3. The mode of action of antiestrogens in inhibiting replication in a breast cancer cell. Antiestrogens (AE) can bind to the estrogen receptor (ER). This produces an incomplete change in the tertiary structure of the ER (60) so that there is an altered interaction with the estrogen response elements (ERE) on the DNA. As a response to the binding of AE to ER there is a decrease in the production of transforming growth factor alpha (TGF-α) but an increase in the production of some members of the transforming growth factor beta (TGF-β) family. Studies in breast cancer patients demonstrate that tamoxifen can down-regulate TGF-α (104), but there is an induction of TGF-β (15) in the tumor. Antiestrogens also cause a decrease in insulin-like growth factor 1 (IGF-1) (18) that may stimulate cell replication from adjacent cells (paracrine) or organs (endocrine). Cell culture studies have demonstrated that antiestrogens cause an arrest in the G1 phase of the cell cycle (106).

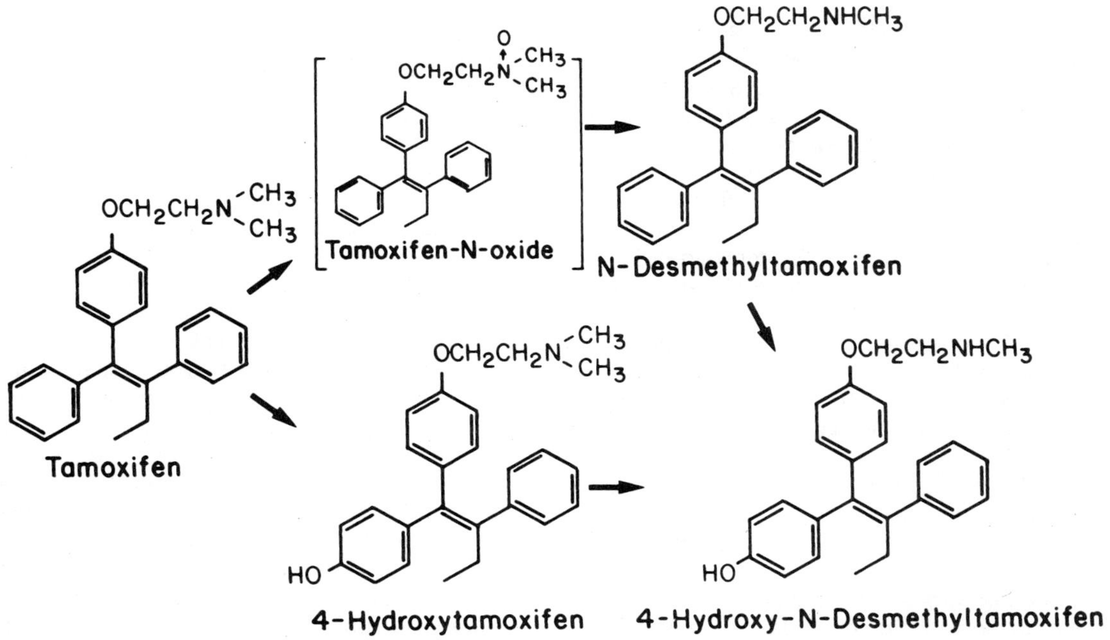

$OCH_2CH_2N(CH_3)_2$ — **Tamoxifen**

$OCH_2CH_2N^{+}(O^{-})(CH_3)_2$ — [**Tamoxifen-N-oxide**]

$OCH_2CH_2NHCH_3$ — **N-Desmethyltamoxifen**

$OCH_2CH_2N(CH_3)_2$, HO — **4-Hydroxytamoxifen**

$OCH_2CH_2NHCH_3$, HO — **4-Hydroxy-N-Desmethyltamoxifen**

Figure 73.4. The metabolites of tamoxifen.

potentially reduce the efficacy of the antiestrogen. Recent laboratory studies (63) have, however, demonstrated that much higher levels of estradiol than are noted clinically are required to reverse the actions of tamoxifen. Nevertheless, combinations of tamoxifen and luteinizing hormone-releasing hormone (LHRH) agonists (to reduce ovarian steroidogenesis by preventing LH release from the pituitary gland) are being evaluated (117). Tamoxifen is currently available in the United States to treat ER-positive disease in premenopausal women.

USE AS ADJUVANT THERAPY

The low incidence of side effects was an important factor when the Eastern Cooperative Oncology Group (ECOG) established their adjuvant trial of tamoxifen in elderly patients who would be unable to cope with the rigors of chemotherapy (20). Similar adjuvant trials with tamoxifen were conducted in the United Kingdom (1, 6–8, 115, 116), Canada (112), and some countries in Europe (96, 120, 122).

In the main, a conservative course of 1 or 2 years of adjuvant tamoxifen was selected. However, this decision was based on a number of reasonable concerns. Patients with advanced disease usually respond to tamoxifen for perhaps 1 or 2 years so that it was expected that ER-negative disease would be encouraged to grow prematurely during adjuvant therapy. If this occurred, then the physician would have already used a valuable palliative drug and would only have combination chemotherapy to slow the relentless growth of recurrent disease. A related argument involved the changing strategy for the application of combination chemotherapy. Recurrent treatment cycles (2 years) were found to be of no long-term benefit for the patient. The strategy was formulated that an aggressive course of short-term treatment (6 months), with the most active cytotoxic drugs, could have the best chance to kill tumor cells before the premature development of drug resistance. Using the same argument, there was an intuitive reluctance to use long-term tamoxifen therapy because this would lead to premature drug resistance. Longer might not be better. Finally, there was a sincere concern about the side effects of adjuvant therapy and the ethical issue of treating patients in whom disease "might" not recur. Although this argument primarily focused on chemotherapy and node-negative patients, it is fair to say that very few patients in the mid-1970s had received extended therapy with tamoxifen, so that long-term side effects were in the main unknown. The majority of tamoxifen-treated patients, up to that point, had received only about 2 years of treatment for advanced disease before drug resistance occurred. Potential side effects—thrombosis, osteoporosis, or other phenomena—were only of secondary importance. The use of tamoxifen in the disease-free patient would change that perspective.

The overall success of 1 or 2 years of adjuvant tamoxifen therapy has recently been evaluated in a meta-analysis of randomized clinical trials (27). Two conclusions can be drawn. Tamoxifen confers a survival advantage to postmenopausal women, whereas combination chemotherapy confers a survival advantage to premenopausal women. Unfortunately, it is not possible to draw a definite conclusion about whether 1 year or 2 years of tamoxifen therapy is of value.

Based on laboratory studies demonstrating the value of long-term or indefinite tamoxifen therapy (62), clinical trials organizations are in the process of evaluating this treatment strategy.

Clinical experience with long-term tamoxifen therapy has been garnered from nationwide clinical trials with and without chemotherapy in pre- and postmenopausal patients with node-positive and node-negative disease.

CHEMOTHERAPY PLUS TAMOXIFEN

ECOG has evaluated the duration of tamoxifen therapy in postmenopausal patients, all of whom received combination chemotherapy (cyclophosphamide plus methotrexate plus fluorouracil, CMF). An early analysis (30) has demonstrated an increase in disease-free survival with 5 years versus 1 year of tamoxifen. The 5-year arm has now gone through a second randomization to evaluate the value of indefinite tamoxifen therapy. A similar study in premenopausal women has been reported (132).

The National Surgical Adjuvant Breast and Bowel Project (NSABP) clinical trials organization has conducted a registration study of 2 years of combination chemotherapy with L-phenylalanine mustard (melphelan, L-PAM) and fluorouracil (5-FU) and tamoxifen plus an additional year of tamoxifen alone (36) to build on the successes of their earlier trials, which demonstrated the efficacy of tamoxifen in receptor-positive postmenopausal patients. Overall, these investigators concluded that 3 years of tamoxifen conferred a significant advantage over 2 years of tamoxifen.

A report from Italy has demonstrated that the addition of combination chemotherapy of CMF (six cycles followed by 4 courses of epirubicin) to long-term tamoxifen (5 years) for the treatment of ER-positive, node-positive disease does not seem to improve significantly the clear-cut effectiveness of tamoxifen alone in preventing recurrence (10). In contrast, NSABP protocol B16 shows benefit for tamoxifen-treated postmenopausal patients with the addition of an adriamycin-containing chemotherapy regimen (37).

TAMOXIFEN ALONE

Although the 2-year adjuvant tamoxifen study conducted by the Nolvadex Adjuvant Trial Organization (NATO) demonstrates a survival advantage for women (7, 8), current clinical trials are evaluating a longer duration of tamoxifen therapy. A small randomized clinical trial comparing 3 years of tamoxifen to no treatment has demonstrated a survival advantage for ER-positive patients receiving tamoxifen (23). Similarly, a Scottish trial that has compared 5 years of tamoxifen to no treatment has demonstrated a survival advantage for patients taking tamoxifen (12). The Scottish trial is particularly interesting because it addresses the question of whether to administer tamoxifen early or to save the drug until recurrence. Most patients in the control arm received tamoxifen at recurrence. Since an overall survival advantage is observed for patients receiving adjuvant tamoxifen, this demonstrates that early resistance to tamoxifen does not occur. The Scottish study included a mixture of node-positive and node-negative patients, but the greatest effect was observed in the node-positive cohort. The problem with being able to demonstrate a significant advantage for the node-negative group is the statistical power necessary to show an effect, because of the low frequency of recurrence.

The NSABP has focused attention on the use of adjuvant tamoxifen to delay the recurrence of ER-positive node-negative disease (35). Tamoxifen increases the disease free survival, and the antiestrogen is active in premenopausal women. The NSABP protocol B14 used an initial treatment period of 5 years of tamoxifen, but the patients will now continue tamoxifen for another 5 years. At present no overall survival advantage has been noted, but the preliminary analysis at 4 years is probably premature.

In summary, multiple clinical trials have demonstrated the effectiveness and safety of long-term tamoxifen therapy for treating breast cancer. The trials that are currently underway will provide additional reassurance to both patients and physicians about the safety of tamoxifen in node-negative disease where only a minority of patients will have a recurrence (63).

TOXICOLOGICAL CONSIDERATIONS IN POSTMENOPAUSAL WOMEN

Several concerns have been expressed about the biologic consequences of long-term tamoxifen treatment for women with breast cancer. One concern about adjuvant tamoxifen in premenopausal women is the rise in circulating estrogen levels (69). This does not appear to affect the efficacy of the drug as an antitumor agent. However, premenopausal women must be counseled about the need to use barrier contraception, as they are at risk for pregnancy. In the main, the toxicologic concerns (Table 73.1) are minor compared with the ability of tamoxifen to control the recurrence of a fatal disease (60).

OPHTHALMIC EFFECTS

Triphenylethylenes are known to cause cataracts in rats during long-term therapy. Clomiphene is particularly active, and ocular effects have been noted with tamoxifen (39).

A recent evaluation (89) of patients receiving tamoxifen, 10 mg/d, for up to 2 years noted no ocular changes. Nevertheless, high-dose tamoxifen therapy has been associated with retinal changes (keratopathy and multiple paramacular refractile lesions in the nerve fiber and inner plexiform layers) (75), and it may be possible that accumulated toxicity will occur with decades of tamoxifen therapy. At present there appears to be little evidence that severe ocular changes occur. Regular eye examinations are not recommended, although patients should be questioned about changes in visual acuity. Patients with preexisting macular degeneration should be carefully evaluated when starting tamoxifen therapy (108).

Table 73.1. Potential Concerns About the Use of Long-term Tamoxifen Therapy in Postmenopausal Patients

Ophthalmic
Antiestrogenic effects
Osteoporosis
Atherosclerosis
Estrogenic effects
Thromboembolic disorders
Uterine stimulation
Liver carcinogenesis

ANTIESTROGENIC EFFECTS

Osteoporosis

Estrogen is important to maintain bone in premenopausal women. After menopause, hormone replacement therapy is often recommended to prevent the development of osteoporosis. Clearly, the long-term administration of an antiestrogen has the potential to precipitate premature osteoporosis.

Some but not all animal studies show that tamoxifen has estrogenic effects in bone (31, 74, 134). Clinical studies show that 2 years of adjuvant tamoxifen therapy does not decrease bone density (32, 92, 110, 133), and there is evidence to suggest that tamoxifen is beneficial and maintains bone in the lumbar spine and the neck of the femur (79, 91, 140).

Atherosclerosis

Estrogen lowers low density lipoprotein (LDL) cholesterol levels and raises high-density lipoprotein (HDL) cholesterol levels. It is possible that this change in blood lipids is responsible for the decrease in myocardial infarction observed in premenopausal women when compared to men. Following menopause, women are at the same risk for coronary heart disease as men. It can be argued that the long-term administration of an antiestrogen could produce a population at risk for premature coronary heart disease. However, the estrogen-like effects of tamoxifen (39) lower the circulating levels of cholesterol in female patients (4, 9, 13, 16, 93–95, 121).

A recent analysis of the Scottish clinical trial of 5 years of adjuvant tamoxifen showed a significant decrease in fatal myocardial infarction (98).

ESTROGENIC EFFECTS

The fact that tamoxifen has an appropriate level of estrogenic activity may be a two-edged sword. The administration of estrogen to women is known to increase the risk for thrombosis and endometrial carcinoma. Clearly, information is required to evaluate the safety of long-term tamoxifen therapy.

Thromboembolic Disorders

There are several anecdotal reports associating the administration of tamoxifen for advanced breast cancer with subsequent thromboembolic episodes (50, 88, 102). Similarly, an association between adjuvant tamoxifen therapy given with chemotherapy and thrombosis has been reported (30). A recent study reported from Sweden showed no significant increases in thromboembolic disorders during long-term tamoxifen monotherapy (123). Nevertheless, decreases in antithrombin III levels have been noted in postmenopausal patients treated with tamoxifen for advanced (28) or node-positive breast cancer (70), although most patients have values well within the normal range. Decreases in antithrombin III levels rarely reach the level of clinical concern (>30% decrease). However, patients with a known history of thromboembolic disorders should be carefully evaluated before a decision is made to use long-term tamoxifen therapy (16).

Uterine Stimulation

Tamoxifen is known to produce some estrogen-like effects in postmenopausal women (39), but very little is known about the long-term stimulatory effects of tamoxifen on the human uterus (19, 103). Recent research demonstrated increases in endometrial thickness, hyperplasia, and fibroids during several years of tamoxifen therapy (73, 77).

One particular focus of current research is the effect of tamoxifen on endometrial carcinoma. Tamoxifen does have some efficacy in the treatment of endometrial carcinoma (129). Nevertheless, the findings that ER- and PgR-positive human endometrial carcinoma can have enhanced growth in athymic mice with tamoxifen (124) and other antiestrogens has raised justifiable concerns about the safety of long-term tamoxifen therapy. Indeed animals bitransplanted with an MCF-7 breast tumor and endometrial carcinoma had target–site specific effects with tamoxifen. Estradiol-stimulated growth of the breast tumor is controlled by tamoxifen, whereas the endometrial tumor grows more rapidly (41).

The clinical situation is more complex. Only about one-third of endometrial tumors are hormone responsive, although it is widely believed that estrogen stimulation is responsible for the promotion of all early disease (49). Endometrial carcinoma has been reported to occur in patients receiving adjuvant tamoxifen therapy (78), but this is unremarkable, as breast and endometrial carcinoma are known to be associated. The Stockholm (38) and NSABP (34) adjuvant trials of tamoxifen noted an increase in endometrial carcinoma compared to rates in a control arm. However, a review of the literature uncovered over 200 cases of endometrial carcinoma worldwide that were associated with tamoxifen therapy in the past decade (3). Most cases are stage 1 (82%), grade I or II disease (80%), which is consistent with the Surveillance, Epidemiology, and End Results (SEER) report of 74% and 79% for stage I and grade I or II endometrial carcinoma. There is a modest increase in endometrial carcinoma associated with tamoxifen that is estimated to be less than 3/1,000 woman-years. There is no strong association with duration of therapy, and tamoxifen is not associated with high-grade, poor prognosis disease (3, 5). All cases of persistent vaginal bleeding should be followed up with a gynecologic examination and an endometrial biopsy. It is clear, though, that patients should not be denied the advantages of tamoxifen to control the recurrence of breast cancer because of the potential complication of endometrial carcinoma, which has a good prognosis.

Liver Carcinogenesis

Tamoxifen produces DNA adducts in the rat liver (45), and lifetime treatment with greater than 3 g/kg causes carcinogenesis in the liver (42, 141). The relevance of these laboratory findings for the treatment of human disease has been discussed (72); however, an increase in human hepatocellular carcinoma has not been noted since tamoxifen was introduced into the market in 1978 (100).

TAMOXIFEN IN THE PREVENTION OF BREAST CANCER

Tamoxifen will prevent carcinogenesis in rodent models of mammary cancer (61, 71). These laboratory data, in conjunction with the efficacy of tamoxifen in producing a significant survival advantage in postmenopausal women (27) and in preventing (13, 35, 38) the appearance of second primary breast cancers, have increased enthusiasm for the use of tamoxifen as a preventive in women at risk for breast cancer (21, 33, 90). The carcinogenic insult that initiates breast cancer probably occurs during the reproductive years. Tamoxifen could not be used as a true preventive because the timing of the event is unknown and the unrestricted use of tamoxifen in young women of reproductive age (20–40 years) would be unwise. Clinical trials that are each recruiting 16,000 to 20,000 women volunteers are now proceeding in the United States, United Kingdom, and Italy (60, 65). A pilot study in healthy, high-risk women has proved successful (111), although compliance is seen as the major obstacle to conducting a successful nationwide clinical trial on tens of thousands of women.

New Agents

The success of tamoxifen in the treatment of all stages of breast cancer has focused attention on the possibility of developing additional drugs with different pharmacologic properties. Several novel compounds are being evaluated in the laboratory and the clinic (73), but only three compounds, toremifene, droloxifene, and ICI 182780 (Fig. 73.5), merit comment at present.

TOREMIFENE

Toremifene is a structural derivative of tamoxifen with similar antiestrogenic and estrogenic properties in laboratory animals. The drug is active against carcinogen-induced rat mammary tumors and exhibits the properties of a tumoristatic agent (76, 119). Interestingly, toremifene has been reported to have activity against a hormone-independent mouse uterine sarcoma. However, no antitumor action can be demonstrated in hormone-independent breast tumors.

The metabolism of toremifene has been described in both animals and patients. In general, toremifene is highly protein bound, which could explain the long serum half-life. The principal metabolite of toremifene is N-desmethyltoremifene. 4-Hydroxytoremifene is a minor metabolite but has a high affinity for the ER (127). Toremifene is less potent than tamoxifen, and consequently clinical studies are using a higher dose than during tamoxifen therapy. Phase II studies indicate that 60 mg of toremifene given as a single daily dose is effective for the treatment of ER-positive advanced

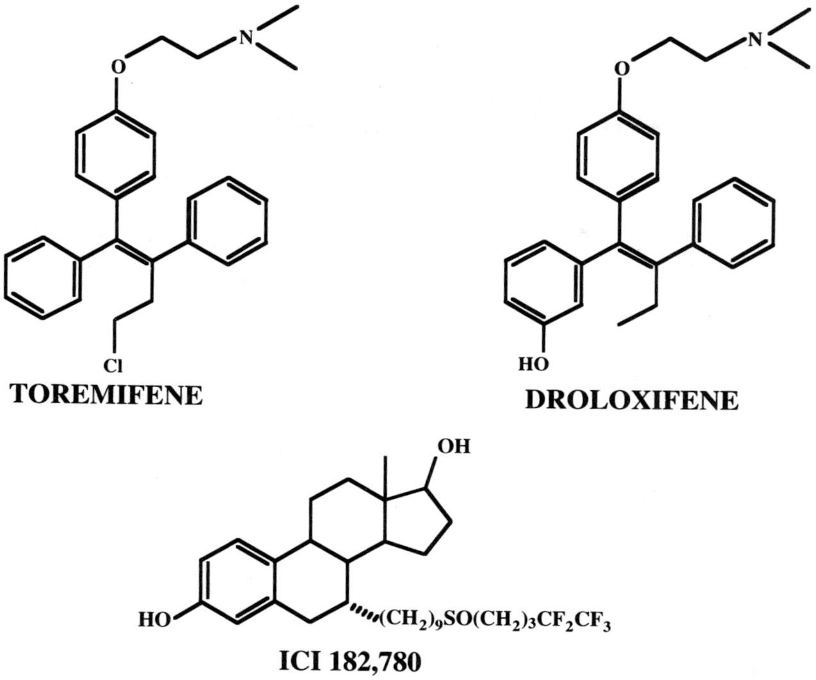

TOREMIFENE

DROLOXIFENE

HO ... $(CH_2)_9SO(CH_2)_3CF_2CF_3$

ICI 182,780

Figure 73.5. Antiestrogens being evaluated as potential breast cancer therapeutic agents.

breast cancer (135). Currently clinical trials are evaluating high-dose (100–240 mg/d) toremifene therapy. Interestingly, no liver cancer has been described during laboratory tests (46). This property may ultimately make toremifene the agent of choice should the studies to prevent breast cancer with tamoxifen prove to be successful but are terminated if an unacceptably high incidence of hepatocellular carcinoma (or some other side effect) is detected at a later date.

DROLOXIFENE

Droloxifene has been extensively studied in the laboratory (48) and has proved to be an effective antiestrogen with high affinity for the ER and antitumor properties both in vivo and in vitro. There is no evidence that droloxifene causes hepatic tumors in rats (48). Droloxifene is effective in the treatment of advanced breast cancer in postmenopausal women in the dose range of 20 to 100 mg/d (113).

PURE ANTIESTROGENS

The compound ICI 182780 exhibits no estrogen-like effects in laboratory tests, but it is effective in controlling estrogen-stimulated growth (137). Preliminary clinical studies demonstrate that daily injections of 5 mg of ICI 182780 can reduce the Ki 67 labeling index of breast cancer in situ and reduce PgR levels (22). Studies in primates have demonstrated almost complete antiuterotrophic actions (26).

The pure antiestrogens may offer clinical advantages over tamoxifen by decreasing tumor cell invasion, tumor flare (which is especially problematic in patients with bone metastases), and the stimulation of occult endometrial carcinoma. Overall, this class of drugs could have a role as second-line therapy in patients in whom primary tamoxifen treatment fails. Long-term application as adjuvant therapy in node-negative disease appears unlikely because of the high probability of developing early atherosclerosis and osteoporosis.

Conclusion

The past 20 years have seen the development of antiestrogens as an important new class of drugs (84). Tamoxifen has found ubiquitous applications as the front-line endocrine therapy in the treatment of all stages of breast cancer. Current clinical and laboratory research is focused on the evaluation of long term adjuvant therapy (60, 66). Several novel antiestrogens with different pharmacologic properties are being evaluated in the clinic, not only as breast cancer therapies, but also for the treatment of osteoporosis (58).

References

1. Abram WP, Baum M, Berstock DA, CRC Adjuvant Trial Working Party. Cyclophosphamide and tamoxifen as adjuvant therapies in the management of breast cancer. Br J Cancer 1988;57:604–607.
2. Alonso-Munoz MC, Ojeda-Gonzalez MB, Beltron-Fabregat M, Dorca-Ribugent J, Lopez-Lopez L, Borras-Balada J, Cardenal-Alemany F, Gomez-Batiste X, Fabregat-Mayol J, Viladiu-Quemada P. Randomized trial of tamoxifen versus aminoglutethimide and versus combined tamoxifen and aminoglutethimide in advanced postmenopausal breast cancer. Oncology 1988;45:350–353.
3. Assikis VJ, Jordan VC. Gynecological effects of tamoxifen and the association with endometrial cancer. Int J Gynecol Obstet 1995;49:241–257.
4. Bagdade JD, Wolter J, Subbaiah PV, Ryan W. Effect of tamoxifen treatment on plasma lipids and lipoproteins lipid composition. J Clin Endocrinol Metab 1990;70:1132–1135.
5. Barakat RR, Wong G, Curtin JP, Vlamio V, Hoskins WJ. Tamoxifen use in breast cancer patients who subsequently develop corpus cancer is not associated with high incidence of adverse histological features. Gynecol Oncol 1994;55:164–168.
6. Baum M, Nolvadex Adjuvant Trial Organization. Controlled trial of tamoxifen as single adjuvant agent in management of early breast cancer. Lancet 1983;1:257–261.
7. Baum M, Nolvadex Adjuvant Trial Organization. Controlled trial of tamoxifen as single adjuvant agent in management of early breast cancer. Lancet 1985;1:836–839.
8. Baum M, Nolvadex Adjuvant Trial Organization. Controlled trial of tamoxifen as a single adjuvant agent in management of early breast cancer. Br J Cancer 1988;57:608–611.

9. Bertelli G, Pronzato P, Amoroso D, Cusimano MP, Conte PF, Montagma G, Bertolini S, Rosso R. Adjuvant tamoxifen in primary breast cancer: influence on plasma lipids and antithrombin III levels. Breast Cancer Res Treat 1988;12:307–310.
10. Boccardo F, Rubagotti A, Bruzzi P, Cappellini M, Isola G, Nenci I, Piffanelli A, Breast Cancer Adjuvant Chemo-Hormone Therapy Cooperative Group. Chemotherapy versus tamoxifen versus chemotherapy plus tamoxifen in node-positive, estrogen receptor–positive breast cancer patients: results of a multicentric Italian study. J Clin Oncol 1990;8:1310–1320.
11. Boyd S. On oophorectomy in cancer of the breast. Br Med J 1990;2:1161–1167.
12. Breast Cancer Trials Committee, Scottish Cancer Trials Office (MRC) Adjuvant tamoxifen in the management of operable breast cancer: the Scottish trial. Lancet 1987;2:171–175.
13. Bruning PF, Boufrer JMG, Hart AAM, de Jorg-Bakker M, Linders D, Van Loor J, Nooyen WJ. Tamoxifen, serum lipoproteins and cardiovascular risk. Br J Cancer 1988;58:497–499.
14. Buchanan RB, Blamey RW, Durrent KR, Howell A, Paterson AG, Preece PE, Smith DC, Williams CJ, Wilson RG. A randomized comparison of tamoxifen with surgical oophorectomy in premenopausal patients with advanced breast cancer. J Clin Oncol 1986;4:1326–1330.
15. Butta A, MacLennan K, Flander KC, Sacks NPM, Smith I, McKinna A, Dowsett M, Wakefield LM, Sporn MB, Baum M, Colletta AA. Induction of transforming growth factor in human breast cancer in vivo following tamoxifen treatment. Cancer Res 1992;52:4261–4264.
16. Caleffi M, Fentiman IS, Clark GM, Wang DY, Needham J, Clark K, LaVille A, Lewis B. Effect of tamoxifen on estrogen binding, lipid and lipoprotein concentrations and blood clotting parameters in premenopausal women with breast pain. J Endocrinol 1988;119:335–339.
17. Cole MP, Jones CTA, Todd IDH. A new antioestrogenic agent in late breast cancer: an early clinical appraisal of ICI 46474. Br J Cancer 1971;25:270–275.
18. Colletti RB, Roberts JD, Devlin JT, Copeland KC. Effect of tamoxifen on insulin-like growth factor 1 in patients with breast cancer. Cancer Res 1989;49:1882–1884.
19. Cross SS, Ismail SM. Endometrial hyperplasia in an oophorectomized woman receiving tamoxifen therapy: case report. Br J Obst Gynaecol 1990;97:190–192.
20. Cummings FJ, Gray R, Davis TE, Tormey DC, Harris JE, Falkson G, Arsenau R. Adjuvant tamoxifen treatment of elderly women with stage II breast cancer. Ann Intern Med 1985;103:324–329.
21. Cuzick J, Wang DY, Bulbrook RD. The prevention of breast cancer. Lancet 1986;1: 83–86.
22. DeFriend DJ, Howell A, Nicholson RI, Anderson E, Dowsett M, Mansel RE, Blamey RW, Bundred NJ, Robertson JF, Saunders C, Baum G, Walton P, Sutcliff F, Wakeling AE. Investigation of a new pure antiestrogen (ICI 182780) in women with primary breast cancer. Cancer Res 1994;54:408–414.
23. Delozier T, Julien JP, Juret P, Veyret C, Covette JE, Grai Y, Olliver JM, deRanieri E. Adjuvant tamoxifen in postmenopausal breast cancer: preliminary results of a randomized trial. Breast Cancer Res Treat 1986;7:105–109.
24. Dickson RB, Lippman ME. Estrogenic regulation of growth and polypeptide growth factor secretion in human breast carcinoma. Endocr Rev 1987;8:29–43.
25. Dodds EC, Lawson W, Noble RL. Biological effects of the synthetic oestrogenic substance 4:4′-dihydroxy-α: β diethylstilbene. Lancet 1938;1:1389–1391.
26. Dukes M, Waterton JC, Wakeling AE. Antiuterotrophic effects of the pure antiestrogen ICI 182780 in adult female monkeys (Macaca nemistria): quantitative magnetic resonance imaging. J Endocrinol 1993;138:203–210.
27. Early Breast Cancer Trialists' Collaborative Group. Effect of adjuvant tamoxifen and of cytotoxic therapy on mortality in early breast cancer. Lancet 1992;339:1–15.
28. Enck RE, Rios CN. Tamoxifen treatment of metastatic breast cancer and antithrombin III levels. Cancer 1984;53:2607–2609.
29. Etienne MC, Milano G, Fischel JL, Frenay M, Francois E, Formento JL, Gioanni J, Namer M. Tamoxifen metabolism: pharmacokinetics and in vitro study. Br J Cancer 1989;60:30–35.
30. Falkson HC, Gray R, Wolberg WH, Gilchrist KW, Harris JE, Tormey DC, Falkson G. Adjuvant trial of 12 cycles of CMFPT followed by observation or continuous tamoxifen versus four cycles of CMFPT in postmenopausal women with breast cancer: an ECOG Phase III study. J Clin Oncol 1990;8:599–607.
31. Feldman S, Minne HW, Parvizi S, Pfeifer M, Lempert UG, Bauss F, Ziegler R. Antiestrogen and antiandrogen administration reduce bone mass in the rat. Bone Mineral 1989;7:245–254.
32. Fentiman IS, Caleffi M, Rodin A. Bone mineral content of women receiving tamoxifen for mastalgia. Br J Cancer 1989;60:262–264.
33. Fentiman IS, Powles TJ. Tamoxifen and benign breast problems. Lancet 1987;2: 1070–1072.
34. Fisher B, Costantino JP, Redmond CK, Fisher ER, Wickerham DL, Cronin WM, other NSABP contributors. Endometrial cancer in tamoxifen treated breast cancer patients: findings from the National Surgical Adjuvant Breast and Bowel Project (NASPB) B-14. JNCI 1994;80:527–534.
35. Fisher B, Costantino J, Redmond C, other members of the NSABP. A randomized clinical trial evaluating tamoxifen in the treatment of patients with node-negative breast cancer who have estrogen receptor positive tumors. N Engl J Med 1989;32:479–484.
36. Fisher B, other NSABP investigators. Prolonging tamoxifen for primary breast cancer: findings from the National Surgical Adjuvant Breast and Bowel Project clinical trial. Ann Intern Med 1987;106:649–654.
37. Fisher B, Redmond C, Legault-Poisson S, Dimitrov NV, Brown A, Wickerham DL, Wolmark N, Margolese RG, Bowman D, Glass AG, Kardinal CG, Robindaux A, Jochimsen P, Cronin W, Duetsch M, Fisher ER, Myers DB, Hoehn JL. Postoperative chemotherapy and tamoxifen compared with tamoxifen alone in the treatment of positive-node breast cancer patients aged 50 years and older with tumors responsive to tamoxifen: results from the National Surgical Adjuvant Breast and Bowel Project B-16. J Clin Oncol 1990;8:1005–1018.
38. Fornander T, Rutqvist LE, Cedermark BV, Glas U, Mattson A, Silversward JD, Skoog L, Somell A, Theve T, Wilking N, Askergren J, Hjolmar ML. Adjuvant tamoxifen in early breast cancer: occurrence of new primary cancers. Lancet 1989;1:117–120.
39. Furr BJA, Jordan VC. The pharmacology and clinical uses of tamoxifen. Pharmacol Ther 1984;25:127–205.
40. Gorski J, Welshons W, Sakai D. Remodeling the estrogen receptor model. Mol Cell Endocrinol 1984;36:11–15.
41. Gottardis MM, Robinson SP, Satyaswaroop PG, Jordan VC. Contrasting actions of tamoxifen on endometrial and breast tumor growth in the athymic mouse. Cancer Res 1988;48:812–815.
42. Greaves P, Goonetilleke R, Nunn G, Topham J, Orton T. Two year carcinogenicity study of tamoxifen in Alderley Park Wistar-derived rats. Cancer Res 1993;53: 3919–3924.
43. Greenblatt RB, Barfield WE, Jungck EC, Ray AW. Induction of ovulation with MRL-41: preliminary report. JAMA 1961;178:101–104.
44. Haddow A, Watkinson JM, Paterson E. Influence of synthetic oestrogens upon advanced malignant disease. Br Med J 1944;ii:393–398.
45. Han X, Liehr JG. Induction of covalent DNA adducts in rodents by tamoxifen. Cancer Res 1992;52:1360–1363.
46. Hard GC, Iatropoulos MJ, Jordan K, Radi L, Katenberg OP, Imondi AR, Williams GM. Major differences in the hepatocarcinogenicity and DNA adduct forming ability between toremifene and tamoxifen in female Crl: CD (BR) rats. Cancer Res 1993;53: 4534–4541.
47. Harper MJK, Walpole AL. A new derivative of triphenylethylene: effect on implantation and mode of action in rats. J Reprod Fertil 1967;13:101–119.
48. Hasmann M, Rattel B, Loser R. Preclinical data for droloxifene. Cancer Letts 1994;84: 101–106.
49. Henderson BE, Ross R, Bernstein L. Estrogens as a cause of human cancer: the Richard, Hilda Rosenthal Foundation Award Lecture. Cancer Res 1988;48:246–253.
50. Hendrick A, Subraminian V. Tamoxifen and thromboembolism. JAMA 1980;243: 514–515.
51. Holtkamp DE, Greslin JG, Root CA, Lerner LJ. Gonadotrophin inhibiting and antifecundity effects of chloramiphene. Proc Soc Exp Biol Med 1960;105:197–201.
52. Huggins C, Bergenstad DM. Inhibition of human mammary and prostatic cancers by adrenalectomy. Cancer Res 1952;12:134–141.
53. Huppert LC. Induction of ovulation with clomiphene citrate. Fertil Steril 1979;31:1–8.
54. Ingle JN, Ahmann DL, Green SJ, Edmonson JH, Bisel HF, Kvols LK, Nichols WC, Creagon ET, Hahn RG, Rubin J, Frytack S. Randomized clinical trial of diethylstilbestrol versus tamoxifen in postmenopausal women with advanced breast cancer. N Engl J Med 1981;304:16–21.
55. Ingle JN, Krook JE, Green SJ, Kukista TP, Everson LK, Ahman DL, Chang MN, Bisel HF, Windschitl HE, Twito DI, Pfeiffe MM. Randomized trial of bilateral oophorectomy versus tamoxifen in premenopausal women with metastatic breast cancer. J Clin Oncol 1986;4:178–185.
56. Jensen EV, Jacobson HI. Basic guides to the mechanism of estrogen action. Recent Prog Horm Res 1962;18:387–414.
57. Jensen EV, Suzuki T, Kawashima T, Stumpf WE, Jungblut PW, DeSombre ER. A two step mechanism for the interaction of estradiol with rat uterus. Proc Natl Acad Sci USA 1968;59:632–638.
58. Jordan VC. Alternate antiestrogens and approaches to the prevention of breast cancer. J Cell Biochem 1995;22:51–57.
59. Jordan VC. Biochemical pharmacology of antiestrogen action. Pharm Rev 1984;36: 245–276.
60. Jordan VC. A current view of tamoxifen for the treatment and prevention of breast cancer. Br J Pharmacol 1993;110:507–517.
61. Jordan VC. Effect of tamoxifen (ICI 46, 474) on initiation and growth of DMBA-induced rat mammary carcinomata. Eur J Cancer 1976;12:419–424.
62. Jordan VC. Laboratory studies to develop general principles for the adjuvant treatment of breast cancer with antiestrogens: problems and potential for future clinical applications. Breast Cancer Res Treat 1983;3(suppl 1):73–86.
63. Jordan VC. Long-term adjuvant tamoxifen therapy for breast cancer. Breast Cancer Res Treat 1990;15:125–1136.
64. Jordan VC. Metabolites of tamoxifen in animals and man: identification, pharmacology and significance. Breast Cancer Res Treat 1982;2:123–128.
65. Jordan VC. Tamoxifen: Toxicities and drug resistance during the treatment and prevention of breast cancer. Annu Rev Pharmacol Toxicol 1995;35:195–211.
66. Jordan VC. (ed) Long-Term Tamxoifen Treatment for Breast Cancer. Madison: University of Wisconsin Press, 1994.
67. Jordan VC, Collins MM, Rowsby L, Prestwich G. A monohydroxylated metabolite of tamoxifen with potent antioestrogenic activity. J Endocrinol 1977;75:305–316.
68. Jordan VC, Dowse LJ. Tamoxifen as an antitumour agent: effect on oestrogen binding. J Endocrinol 1976;68:297–303.
69. Jordan VC, Fritz NF, Langan-Fahey SM, Thompson M, Tormey DC. Alteration of endocrine parameters in premenopausal women with breast cancer during long term adjuvant therapy with tamoxifen as a single agent. JNCI 1991;8l3:1488–1491.
70. Jordan VC, Fritz NF, Tormey DC. Long-term adjuvant therapy with tamoxifen: effects on sex hormone binding globulin and antithrombin III. Cancer Res 1987;47: 4517–4519.
71. Jordan VC, Lababidi MK, Mirecki DM. The antiestrogenic and antitumor properties of prolonged tamoxifen therapy in C3H/OUJ mice. Eur J Cancer 1990;26:718–721.
72. Jordan VC, Morrow M. Should clinicians be concerned about the carcinogenic potential of tamoxifen. Eur J Cancer 1994;30A:1714–1721.
73. Jordan VC, Murphy CS. Endocrine pharmacology of antiestrogens as antitumor agents. Endocr Rev 1990;11:578–610.
74. Jordan VC, Phelps E, Lindgren JU. Effect of antiestrogens on bone in castrated and intact female rats. Breast Cancer Res Treat 1987;10:31–35.
75. Kaiser-Kupfer MI, Lippman ME. Tamoxifen retinopathy. Cancer Treat Rep 1978;62: 315–320.
76. Kangas L, Nieminen AL, Blanco G, Grontroos M, Kallico S, Karjalianen M, Perila M, Sondervall M, Toivola T. A new triphenylethylene compound Fc-1157a II. Antitumor effects. Cancer Chemother Pharmacol 1986;17:109–113.
77. Kedar RP, Bourne TH, Powles TJ, Collins WP, Ashley SE, Cosgrove DO, Campbell S. Effects of tamoxifen on uterus and ovaries of postmenopausal women in a randomized breast cancer prevention trial. Lancet 1994;343:1318–1321.
78. Killackey MA, Hakes TB, Pierce VK. Endometrial adenocarcinoma in breast cancer patients receiving tamoxifen. Cancer Treat Rep 1985;69:237–238.
79. Kristensen B, Ejlertsen B, Dalgaard P, Larsen L, Holmegaard SN, Transbol, I, Mouridsen, HT. Tamoxifen and bone metabolism in postmenopausal low risk breast cancer patients: a randomized study. J Clin Oncol 1994;12:992–997.
80. Lacassagne A. Hormonal pathogenesis of adenocarcinoma of the breast. Am J Cancer 1936;27:217–225.

81. Legha SS, Carter SK. Antiestrogens in the treatment of breast cancer. Cancer Treat Rev 1976;3:205–216.
82. Lerner LJ. The First Non-Steroidal Antioestrogen-MER-25. In: Sutherland RL, Jordan VC: Non-Steroidal Antioestrogens: molecular Pharmacology and Antitumour Activity. Sydney, Australia: Academic Press, 1981, p.1.
83. Lerner LJ, Holthaus FJ Jr, Thompson CR. A non-steroidal estrogen antagonist 1-(*p*-2-diethylaminoethoxyphenyl)-1-phenyl-2-*p*-methoxyphenylethanol. Endocrinology 1958;63:295–318.
84. Lerner LJ, Jordan VC. Development of antiestrogens and their use in breast cancer: eighth Cain Memorial Award Lecture. Cancer Res 1990;50:4177–4189.
85. Lien EA, Solheim E, Kvinnsland S, Veland PM. Identification of 4-hydroxy N-desmethyltamoxifen as a metabolite in human bile. Cancer Res 1988;48:2304–2308.
86. Lien EA, Solheim E, Lea OA, Lundgren S, Kvinnsland S, Ueland PM. Distribution of 4-hydroxy-N-desmethyl tamoxifen and other tamoxifen metabolites in human biological fluids during tamoxifen treatment. Cancer Res 1989;49:2175–2183.
87. Lippman ME, Bolan G. Oestrogen-responsive human breast cancer in long term tissue culture. Nature 1975;256:592–593.
88. Lipton A, Harvey HA, Hamilton RW. Venous thrombosis as a side effect of tamoxifen treatment. Cancer Treat Rep 1984;68:887–889.
89. Longstaff S, Sigurdson H, O'Keefe M, Ogston S, Preece P. A controlled study of the ocular effects of tamoxifen in conventional dosage in the treatment of breast carcinoma. Eur J Cancer Clin Oncol 1989;25:1805–1808.
90. Love RR. Prospect for antiestrogen chemoprevention of breast cancer. JNCI 1990;90:18–21.
91. Love RR, Mazess RB, Barder HS, Epstein S, Newcomb PA, Jordan VC, Carbone PP, Demets DL. Effects of tamoxifen on bone mineral density in postmenopausal women with breast cancer. N Engl J Med 1992;326:852–856.
92. Love RR, Mazess RB, Tormey DC, Barden HS, Newcomb PA, Jordan VC. Bone mineral density in women with breast cancer treated for at least two years with tamoxifen. Breast Cancer Res Treat 1988;12:297–302.
93. Love RR, Newcomb PA, Wiebe DA, Surawicz TS, Jordan VC, Carbone PP, DeMets DL. Lipid and lipoprotein effects of tamoxifen therapy in postmenopausal patients with node negative breast cancer. JNCI 1990;82:1327–1339.
94. Love RR, Wiebe DA, Feyzi JM, Newcomb PA, Chappell RJ. Effects of tamoxifen on cardiovascular risk factors in postmenopausal women after 5 years of treatment. JNCI 1994;86:1534–1539.
95. Love RR, Wieibe DA, Newcomb PA, Cameron H, Leventhal H, Jordan VC, Feyzi J, DeMets DL. Effects of tamoxifen on cardiovascular risk factors in postmenopausal women. Ann Intern Med 1991;115:860–864.
96. Ludwig Breast Cancer Group. Randomized trial of chemoendocrine therapy, endocrine therapy and mastectomy alone in postmenopausal patients with operable breast cancer and axillary node metastases. Lancet 1984;1:1256–1260.
97. Manni A, Pearson OH. Antiestrogen-induced remission in premenopausal women with stage IV breast cancer: effects on ovarian function. Cancer Treat Rep 1980;64: 779–785.
98. McDonald CC, Stewart HJ. Fatal myocardial infarction in the Scottish adjuvant tamoxifen trial. Br Med J 1991;303:435–437.
99. McGuire WL, Carbone PP, Vollmer EP. Estrogen Receptors in Human Breast Cancer. New York: Raven, 1975.
100. Muhleman K, Cook LS and Weiss, N. The incidence of hepatocellular carcinoma in US white women with breast cancer after the introduction of tamoxifen in 1977. Breast Cancer Res Treat 1994;30:201–204.
101. Muss HB, Wells HB, Paschold EH, Black WR, Cooper MR, Capizzi RL, Christian R, Cruz JM, Jackson DV, Powell BL, Richards R, White DR, Zekan PJ, Spurr CL, Pope E, Case D, Morgan TM. Megestrol acetate versus tamoxifen in advanced breast cancer 5-year analysis: a phase III trial of the Piedmont Oncology Association. J Clin Oncol 1988;6:1098–1106.
102. Nevasaari K, Heikkinen M, Taskinen P. Tamoxifen and thrombosis. Lancet 1978;2: 946–947.
103. Neven P, DeMuylder X, Von Belle Y, Vanderick G, De Muylder E. Hysteroscopic follow-up during tamoxifen treatment. Eur J Obstet Gynecol Reprod Biol 1990;35: 235–238.
104. Noguchi S, Motomura K, Inaji H, Imaoka S, Koyama H. Down regulation of transforming growth factor alpha by tamoxifen in human breast cancer. Cancer 1993;72: 131–136.
105. Osborne CK, Boldt DH, Clark GM, Trent JM. Effects of tamoxifen on human breast cancer cell kinetics: accumulation of cells in early G1 phase. Cancer Res 1983;43: 3583–3585.
106. Osborne CK, Hobbs K, Clark GM. Effect of estrogens and antiestrogens on growth of human breast cancer cells in athymic mice. Cancer Res 1985;45:584–590.
107. Patterson JS, Settatree RS, Adam AK, Kemp JV. Serum concentrations of tamoxifen and major metabolites during long-term Nolvadex therapy, correlated with clinical response. In: Mouridsen HT, Palshoff T: Breast Cancer: Experimental and Clinical Aspects. Oxford, England: Pergamon Press, 1980, p. 89.
108. Pavlidis NA, Petris C, Brassoulis E, Klouvas G, Psilos C, Rempopis J, Petrositsos G. Clear evidence that long term, low dose tamoxifen treatment induces occular toxicity. Cancer 1992;69:2961–2964.
109. Pearson OH, Ray BS, Harold CC. Hypophysectomy in the treatment of advanced cancer. JAMA 1956;161:17–21.
110. Powles TJ, Hardy JR, Ashley SE, Farrington GM, Cosgrove D, Davey JB, Dowsett M, McKinna JA, Nash AG, Sinnett HD, Tillyer CR, Treleven JG. A pilot trial to evaluate the acute toxicity and feasibility of tamoxifen for prevention of breast cancer. Br J Cancer 1989;60:126–131.
111. Powles TJ, Jones AL, Ashley SE, O'Brien MER, Tidy VA, Treleaven J, Cosgrove D, Nash AG, Sacks N, Baum M, McKinna JA, Davey JB. The Royal Marsden Hospital pilot tamoxifen chemoprevention trial. Breast Cancer Res Treat 1994;31:73–82.
112. Pritchard KI, Meakin JW, Boyd NF, Ambus K, DeBoer G, Dembo AJ, Paterson AHG, Sutherland DJA, Wilkinson RH, Bassett AA, Evans WK, Beale FA, Clark RM, Keane TJ. A randomized trial of adjuvant tamoxifen in postmenopausal women with axillary node positive breast cancer. In: Jones SE, Salmon SE: Adjuvant Therapy of Breast Cancer, 4th edition. New York: Grune & Stratton, 1984, p. 339.
113. Rausching W, Pritchard KI. Droloxifene, a new antiestrogen: its role in metastatic breast cancer. Breast Cancer Res Treat 1994;31:83–94.
114. Ravdin PM, Fritz NF, Tormey DC, Jordan VC. Endocrine status of premenopausal node positive breast cancer patients following adjuvant chemotherapy and long-term tamoxifen. Cancer Res 1988;48:1026–1029.
115. Ribeiro G, Palmer MK. Adjuvant tamoxifen for operable carcinoma of the breast: report of a clinical trial by the Christie Hospital and Holt Radium Institute. Br Med J 1983;286:827–830.
116. Ribeiro G, Swindell R. The Christie Hospital tamoxifen (Nolvadex) adjuvant trial for operable breast carcinoma: seven year results. Eur J Cancer Clin Oncol 1995;21: 897–900.
117. Robertson JFR, Walker KJ, Nicholson RI, Blamey RW. Combined endocrine effects of LH-RH agonist (Zoladex[reg]) and tamoxifen (Nolvadex[reg]) therapy in premenopausal women with breast cancer. Br J Surg 1989;76:1262–1265.
118. Robinson SP, Langan-Fahey SM, Jordan VC. Implications of tamoxifen metabolism in the athymic mouse for the study of antitumor effects upon human breast cancer xenografts. Eur J Cancer Clin Oncol 1989;25:1769–1776.
119. Robinson SP, Mauel DA, Jordan VC. Antitumor actions of toremifene in the 7, 12 dimethylbenzanthracene (DMBA)-induced rat mammary tumor model. Eur J Cancer Clin Oncol 1988;24:1817–1821.
120. Rose C, Thorpe SM, Andersen KW, Pederson BV, Mouridsen HT, Blicher-Toft M, Rasmussen BB. Beneficial effect of adjuvant tamoxifen therapy in primary breast cancer patients with high oestrogen receptor values. Lancet 1985;1:16–19.
121. Rossner S, Wallgren A. Serum lipoproteins after breast cancer surgery and effects of tamoxifen. Atherosclerosis 1984;53:339–346.
122. Rutqvist LE, Cedermark B, Glas U, Johansson H, Nordenskjold B, Skoog L, Sommell A, Theve T, Friberg S, Askergren J. The Stockholm trial on adjuvant tamoxifen in early breast cancer. Breast Cancer Res Treat 1987;10:255–266.
123. Rutqvist LE, Mattsson A. Cardiac and thromboembolic morbidity among postmenopausal women with early stage breast cancer in a randomized trial of adjuvant tamoxifen. JNCI 1993;85:1398–1406.
124. Satyaswaroop PG, Zaino RJ, Mortel R. Estrogen-like effects of tamoxifen on human endometrial carcinoma transplanted into nude mice. Cancer Res 1984;44: 4006–4010.
125. Sawka CA, Pritchard KI, Paterson DJA, Thomsen DB, Shelley WE, Myers RE, Mobbs BG, Malkin A, Meakin JW. Role and mechanism of action of tamoxifen in premenopausal women with metastatic breast cancer. Cancer Res 1986;46:3152–3156.
126. Sherman BM, Chapler JK, Crickard K, Wycoff D. Endocrine consequences of continuous antiestrogen therapy with tamoxifen in premenopausal women. J Clin Invest 1979;64:398–404.
127. Sipila H, Kangas L, Vuorilehto L, Kalapudas A, Eloranta M, Sondervall M, Toivola R, Antila M. Metabolism of toremifene in the rat. J Steroid Biochem 1990;36:211–215.
128. Smith IE, Harris AL, Morgan M, Ford HT, Gazet J-C, Harmer CL, White H, Parsons CA, Villardo A, Walsh G, McKinna JA. Tamoxifen versus aminoglutethimide in advanced breast carcinoma: a randomized crossover trial. Br Med J 1981;283:1432–1434.
129. Swenerton KD. Treatment of advanced endometrial adenocarcinoma with tamoxifen. Cancer Treat Rep 1980;64:805–811.
130. Thompson CR, Werner HW. Studies of estrogen tri-p-anisylchlorethylene. Proc Soc Exp Biol Med 1951;77:494–497.
131. Toft D, Gorski J. A receptor molecule for estrogens: isolation from the rat uterus and preliminary characterization. Proc Natl Acad Sci USA 1966;55:1574–1581.
132. Tormey DC, Gray R, Abeloff MD, Roseman DL, Gilchrist KW, Barylak EJ, Stott P, Falkson G. Adjuvant therapy with a doxorubicin regimen and long-term tamoxifen in premenopausal breast cancer patients: an Eastern Cooperative Oncology Group Trial. J Clin Oncol 1992;10:1848–1856.
133. Turken S, Siris E, Seldin E, Seldin D, Flaster E, Hyman G, Lindsay R. Effects of tamoxifen on spinal bone density in women with breast cancer. JNCI 1989;81: 1086–1088.
134. Turner RT, Wakley GK, Hannon KS, Bell NA. Tamoxifen prevents the skeletal effects of ovarian hormone deficiency in rats. J Bone Mineral Res 1987;2:449–456.
135. Valavaara R, Pyrhonen S, Heikkinen M, Rissanen P, Blanco G, Tholix E, Nordman E, Taskinen P, Holsi L, Hajba A. Toremifene a new antiestrogenic compound for the treatment of advanced breast cancer: Phase II study. Eur J Cancer Clin Oncol 1988;24:785–790.
136. van Veelen H, Willemse PH, Tjabbes T, Sweitzer MJH, Sleijfer DT. Oral high-dose medroxyprogesterone acetate versus tamoxifen. Cancer 1986;58:7–13.
137. Wakeling AE, Dukes M, Bowler J. A potent specific pure antiestrogen with clinical potential. Cancer Res 1991;51:3867–3873.
138. Walpole AL, Paterson E. Synthetic oestrogens in mammary cancer. Lancet 1949;2: 783–786.
139. Ward HWC. Antioestrogen therapy for breast cancer: a trial of tamoxifen at two dose levels. Br Med J 1973;i:13–14.
140. Ward RL, Morgan G, Dalley D, Kelly PJ. Tamoxifen reduces bone turnover and prevents lumbar spine and proximal femoral bone loss in early postmenopausal women. Bone Min 1993;22:87–94.
141. Williams GM, Iatropoulos MJ, Djordjevic MV, Kaltenberg OP. The triphenylethylene drug tamoxifen is a strong liver carcinogen in the rat. Carcinogenesis 1993;14: 315–317.

CHAPTER 74

Clinical Use of Aromatase Inhibitors in Breast Carcinoma

HAROLD A. HARVEY AND ANDREA MANNI

Antiestrogens are the mainstay of palliative endocrine therapy in women with metastatic hormone-dependent breast cancer. Patients who respond but whose disease later progresses on this form of therapy frequently respond to second-line endocrine treatment. It is thus important to develop effective second-line therapies that interfere with hormonal action through mechanisms other than blockade of the estrogen receptor. A new class of compounds, the aromatase inhibitors, may provide just such an approach to the endocrine treatment of breast cancer. Increasing use of these agents has essentially eliminated the need for major endocrine ablative procedures such as adrenalectomy or hypophysectomy as palliative therapy for metastatic breast cancer.

In postmenopausal or castrated women, the major source of estrogen derives not from the ovaries but from the conversion of the adrenal hormone androstenedione to estrone. This enzymatic conversion occurs at extra-adrenal or peripheral sites such as fat, liver, and muscle and is catalyzed by the aromatase enzyme complex. Some breast cancer tissues also contain aromatase.

The clinical availability of potent aromatase inhibitors which further lower the levels of circulating and intratumoral estrogens are emerging as potentially useful agents in the treatment of postmenopausal women with hormone-sensitive breast cancer. In this chapter we will discuss recent advances in our knowledge of the molecular biology, cellular expression, and physiologic importance of the enzyme aromatase. We will also discuss the preclinical studies and results of clinical trials of those aromatase inhibitors that are farthest along in development.

Biology of Aromatase

GENE STRUCTURE AND REGULATION

Aromatase consists of a complex containing a cytochrome P_{450} protein as well as the flavoprotein NADPH cytochrome P_{450} reductase (59). The gene coding for the cytochrome P_{450} protein (P_{450}AROM) exceeds 70 kilobases (kb) and is the largest of the cytochrome P_{450} family of steroidogenic genes, comprising 10 exons and intervening introns of varying lengths (60). The cDNA of the aromatase gene contains 3.4 kb and encodes a polypeptide of 503 amino acids with a molecular weight of 55 kds. Approximately 30% homology exists with other cytochrome P_{450} proteins. Because its overall homology to other members of the P_{450} superfamily is low: aromatase belongs to a separate gene family designated CYP19. Aromatase expression occurs in many organs including ovary, placenta, hypothalamus, liver, muscle, adipose tissue, and the cancerous breast tissue itself (1, 59). Aromatase expression is controlled by multiple agents, which include cytokines, cyclic nucleotides, gonadotropins, phorbol esthers, glucocorticoids, and growth factors (7). Such regulation is associated with comparable changes in the levels of P_{450} AROM mRNA (20, 59). By contrast, the NADPH–cytochrome P_{450} reductase component is much less markedly affected. At least four major promoter sites have been identified which account for the tissue-specific regulation of the human P_{450} AROM gene (7). Of particular relevance to breast cancer, a unique promoter, 1.4, has been identified in breast adipose tissue (40). This observation raises the possibility that, by blocking promoter 1.4 directed gene transcription, it may be possible to achieve tissue-selective estrogen withdrawal without subjecting the patient to whole-body chemical castration.

Aromatase catalyzes three separate steroid hydroxylations involved in the conversion of androstenedione to estrone. The first two give rise to 19-hydroxy and 19-aldehyde structures, and the third, although still controversial, probably also involves the C-19 methyl group with release of formic acid (23).

SITES OF ESTROGEN BIOSYNTHESIS

Ovary

In premenopausal women the ovary is the most important site of aromatase and estrogen production. Luteinizing hormone (LH) controls the producton of androstenedione by the theca cell compartment, while follicle-stimulating hormone (FSH) up-regulates aromatase expression in granulosa cells. Acting in concert, LH stimulates production of the substrate for aromatase while FSH increases the amount of the enzyme so that estradiol production can increase by eight- to ten-fold at the time of ovulation. Attempts to interrupt ovarian estrogen biosynthesis with first-generation aromatase inhibitors have failed because of the reflex increases in FSH and LH secretion which counteract the inhibitory action of

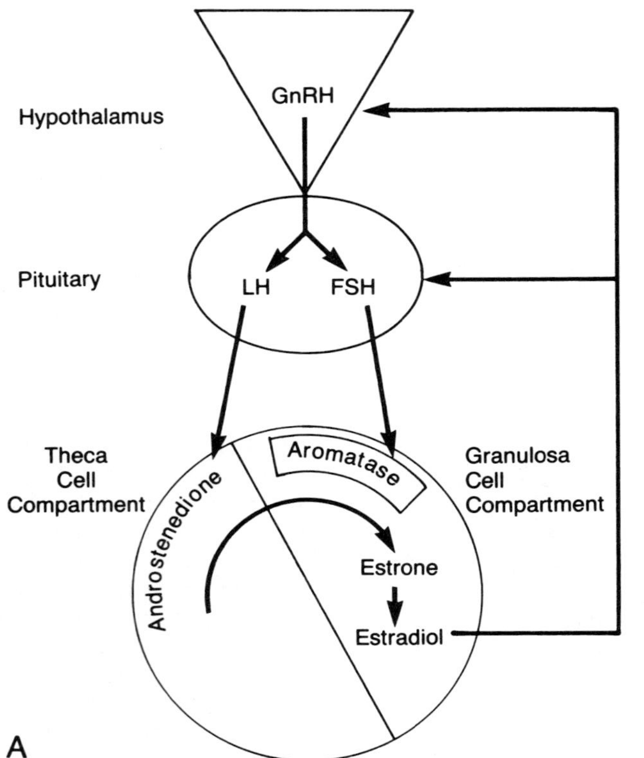

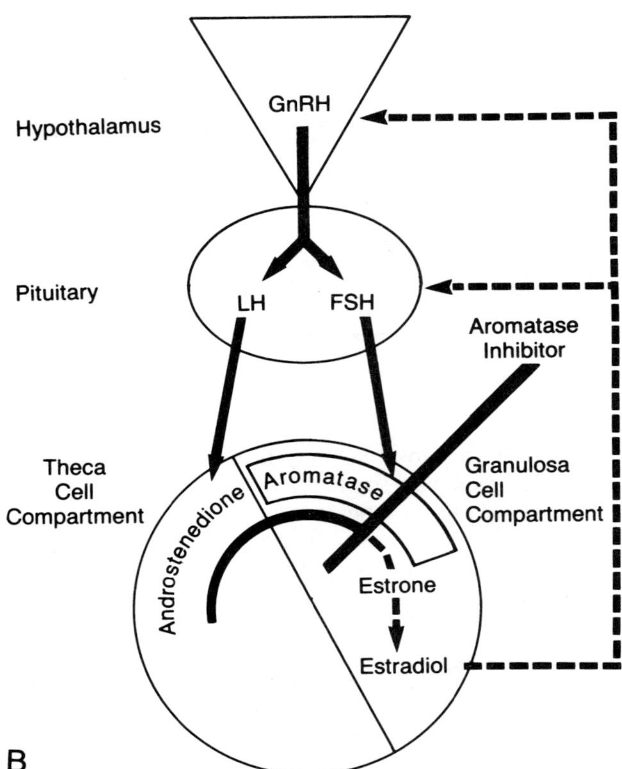

Figure 74.1. **A.** Diagrammatic representation of the hypothalamic-pituitary-ovarian axis. The triangle represents the hypothalamus; the ovoid, the pituitary; and the circle, the ovary. (Key: GnRH, gonadotropin-releasing hormone; LH, luteinizing hormone; FSH, follicle stimulating hormone). As indicated, the ovary is divided into the theca-cell compartment, where androstenedione is synthesized, and the granulosa-cell compartment which contains the majority of the aromatase enzyme. **B.** Blockade of aromatase interrupts the negative feedback inhibition by estradiol of GnRH, LH, and FSH. Consequently, LH increases and stimulates greater production of androstenedione. FSH stimulates increased production of the aromatase enzyme. These two actions are generally sufficient to overcome the inhibitory effects of most aromatase inhibitors.

the drug (Fig. 74.1) (50). It is conceivable that, with the introduction of more potent aromatase inhibitors, it may be possible to block ovarian steroidogenesis.

Extraglandular Aromatase

In postmenopausal women, estrogen synthesis takes place nearly exclusively in extraglandular tissues. Androstenedione, produced primarily by the adrenal—and to a negligible extent by the ovary (35)—is converted to estrone by aromatase in the periphery, such as in adipose tissue. The enzyme 17β—hydroxysteroid dehydrogenase then converts estrone to estradiol. Estrone can also be conjugated into estrone sulfate to form a slowly turning over storage pool with a potential for back-conversion to estrone. Through the androstenedione-to-estrone pathway, postmenopausal women produce approximately 100 μg of estrone per day, and more, if they are obese (36). A substantial fraction of estrone is converted to estradiol to produce circulating concentrations of 10 to 20 pg/ml (Fig. 74.2).

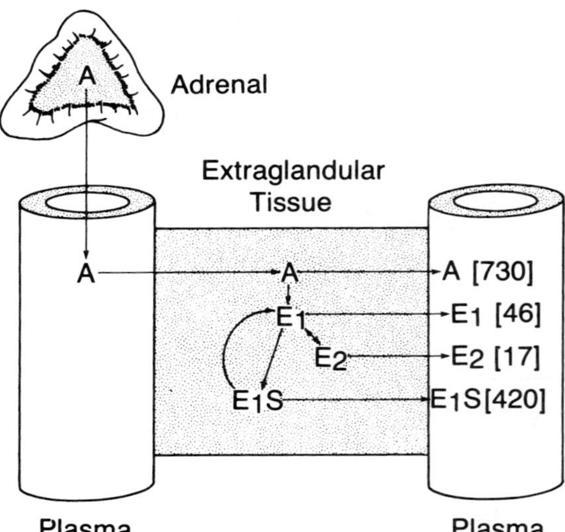

Figure 74.2. Sources of estrogen in postmenopausal women. Adrenal gland secretes androstenedione (A), which enters plasma and then tissue. Extraglandular tissues contain the enzymes necessary to convert A to estrone (E_1) and to estradiol (E_2) or to estrone sulfate (E_1S). These steroids then reenter plasma to circulate at levels indicated within the brackets and expressed as picograms per milliliter.

Local Estrogen Synthesis in Breast Tumors

The levels of estradiol in human breast tumor tissues are an order of magnitude higher than those in plasma (18, 22).

The mechanisms responsible for maintenance of high tissue estradiol concentrations are not completely defined but are likely to involve local production of estradiol by the tumor itself (53). Several investigators have identified aromatase activity in human breast tumors (38, 42). On the other hand, it has been argued that this degree of activity is so low that a meaningful level of estradiol cannot be synthesized locally (3). As we will discuss below, however, aromatase expression is heterogeneous: high activity is present in focal clusters of specific cell types. Therefore, the biochemical measurement in tissue homogenates is likely to underestimate the importance of this enzyme because of dilution by cells and extracellular tissues that have negligible activity. An additional pathway of local estrogen production by the tumor could involve the enzyme sulfatase, which catalyzes the conversion of estrone sulfate to estrone. Levels of this enzyme are actually higher in human breast tumors than those of aromatase; however, the affinity of sulfatase for the substrate is much lower than that of aromatase (53). Therefore, the relative importance of sulfatase versus aromatase for estradiol biosynthesis in situ in human breast cancer tissue remains to be defined (Fig. 74.3).

Heterogeneous Cellular Expression of Aromatase by Normal and Malignant Breast Tissue

Using competitive RT-PCR, Bulun and Simpson quantified P_{450} AROM transcripts in breast adipose tissue from mastectomy specimens. They observed that the highest transcript levels were localized to tumor-bearing quadrants. In addition, using quantitative morphometry, they found the highest proportions of adipose stromal cells (versus adipocytes) in these quadrants (7). Their data suggest that regional differences in relative proportions of histologic components of the breast tissue (i.e., adipocytes versus stromal cells) are the primary cause of estrogenic concentration gradients, since regions containing a higher number of stromal cells are the sites of elevated P_{450} AROM transcript levels. The authors postulate that, once neoplastic transformation has occurred, tumor growth is promoted by locally increased estrogen levels. Secretory products of the tumor stimulated by estrogens may, in turn, further increase aromatase gene expression in the surrounding adipose tissue. Thus, a positive-feedback loop may be created whereby locally produced estrogens and tumor-derived factors act in a paracrine-autocrine fashion to sustain growth and development of the tumor. A similar physiologic construct is also suggested by Santen and co-workers who analyzed aromatase expression by human breast tumors using immunohistochemistry (56). They observed that the highest degree of aromatase expression occurred in stromal spindle cells, whereas tumor epithelial, stromal, inflammatory, and normal breast elements contained lesser amounts (Fig. 74.4). Furthermore, a statistically significant correlation was found between biochemical measurements of aromatase and the stromal spindle cell histologic score (56). Heterogeneity in aromatase expression by human breast cancers has also been reported by other investigators, at both the message and the protein level (19, 37). In the aggregate, these observations provide further support for the possibility that human breast tumors contain biologically relevant amounts of aromatase, exerting autocrine or paracrine effects.

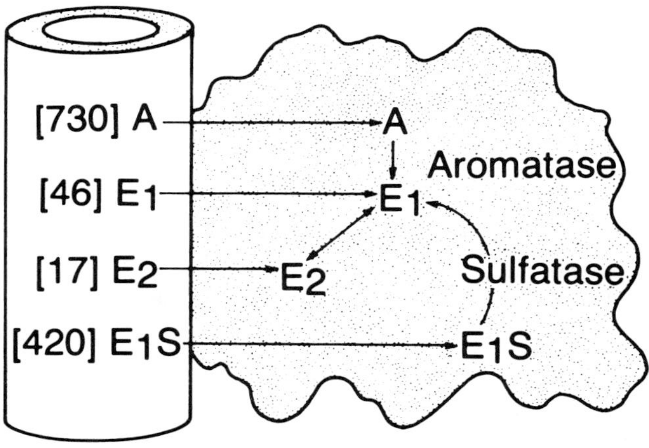

Figure 74.3. Diagrammatic representation of the biosynthetic pathways for estrogen production locally in breast tumors. The shaded area indicates breast tumor tissue. Symbols are the same as for Figure 74.2.

Historical Development of Aromatase Inhibitors

Inasmuch as aminoglutethimide is the prototype of later aromatase inhibitors, it is useful first to review the information gleaned from the early experimental and clinical experience with this agent.

Aminoglutethimide, a derivative of the sedative agent glutethimide, was initially introduced into clinical medicine as an anticonvulsant and was later recognized to be an inhibitor of cytochrome P_{450} *N* mediated steroid hydroxylations, particularly those involving the cholesterol side-chain cleavage enzyme (8). The first clinical use of aminoglutethimide as therapy for breast cancer attempted to produce a "medical adrenalectomy" by blocking cholesterol side-chain cleavage (47). Replacement glucocorticoid was added to compensate for the inhibition of cortisol biosynthesis. Only later it was recognized that the estrogen-lowering effect induced by the aminoglutethimide and glucocorticoid regimen was due primarily to inhibition of the aromatase enzyme (9, 63). This conclusion was inferred from the unexpected observation that androstenedione levels were unchanged, since blockade of cholesterol side-chain cleavage activity should have resulted in suppressed adrenal androgen secretion (52). Indeed, direct isotopic kinetic studies in patients confirmed the activity of aminoglutethimide as an aromatase inhibitor in vivo (49). The effects of this compound, however, are rather nonspecific, since the drug affects a number of hydroxylation steps in the metabolic conversion of cholesterol to active steroid products (Fig. 74.5).

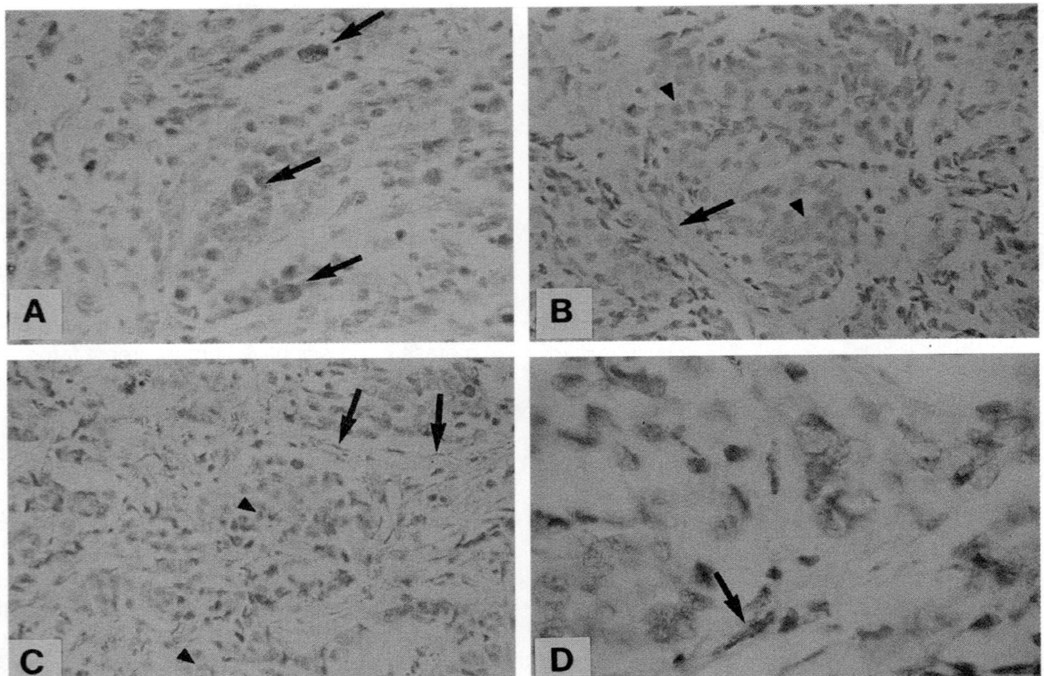

Figure 74.4. Aromatase immunohistochemistry color photomicrographs (modified from Santen et al. (56) with permission). **A.** A section of human breast tumor stained with antiaromatase antibody. Several isolated tumor epithelial cells are present with densely stained cytoplasm (*arrows*; objective magnification ×40). **B.** Control section of human breast tumor stained with an irrelevant antibody, antineuropeptide-Y. Neither tumor cells (*arrowheads*) nor stromal spindle cells (*arrow*) are stained (objective magnification ×40). **C.** A section of human breast tumor stained with antiaromatase antibody. In this area, the stromal spindle cells surrounding groups of tumor epithelial cells exhibit positive staining (*arrows*). Tumor cells are unstained (*arrowheads*; objective magnification ×40). **D.** A photomicrograph of greater magnification from the periphery of a group of tumor epithelial cells that did not exhibit staining for aromatase. At their periphery, however, is a stromal spindle cell with densely stained cytoplasm (*arrow*).

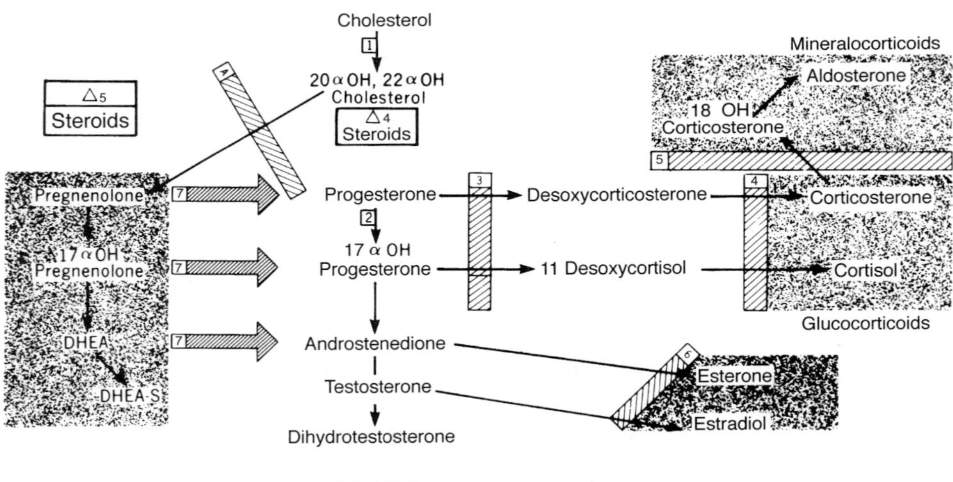

Figure 74.5. Effects of aminoglutethimide on various steroidogenic steps. The numbers in boxes identify several enzymes: (*a*) 20- and 22-hydroxylase; (*b*) 17α-hydroxylase; (*c*) 21-hydroxylase; (*d*) 11-hydroxylase; (*e*) 18-hydroxylase; (*f*) aromatase; (*g*) 3β-ol-dehydrogenase/δ-4,δ-5-isomerase. Aminoglutethimide blocks several of these steps, which can lower the levels of the steroids shown in the shaded boxes. The primary effect of aminoglutethimide is to block step 6—the aromatase enzyme—which converts androgens to estrogens.

CLINICAL EFFICACY

An overall compilation of clinical responses to aminoglutethimide plus glucocorticoid in women with breast cancer reveals results similar to those expected from other forms of endocrine therapy. That is, approximately a third of all patients experience either complete or partial tumor regression, while for patients with estrogen receptor–positive tumors the response rate is 54%. The mean duration of reponse is 13 months and mean survival 20 months. Soft tissues respond most frequently, followed by lymph nodes, bone, lung/pleura, viscera, and liver (47).

Randomized comparative trials of aminoglutethimide plus hydrocortisone versus other endocrine therapies provide a more precise assessment of efficacy. The aminoglutethimide regimen was equally effective when compared to surgical adrenalectomy (51) or transsphenoidal hypophysectomy in small controlled trials (30). Similarly, when compared to tamoxifen, aminoglutethimide plus hydrocortisone produces responses as frequently, and for a comparable duration (43). A trend toward greater healing of osteolytic lesions was observed with aminoglutethimide plus hydrocortisone than with tamoxifen.

Although the efficacy of aminoglutethimide plus hydrocortisone is similar to that of other agents, cross-resistance between aminoglutethimide plus hydrocortisone and tamoxifen or progesterone therapy is not complete. Overall, 31% of patients treated initially with tamoxifen later respond objectively to aminoglutethimide plus hydrocortisone. Patients can be subdivided into those that initially respond to tamoxifen and later relapse, and those whose disease initially progresses. Fifty percent of patients who initially respond objectively to tamoxifen and later relapse experience an objective response to aminoglutethimide plus hydrocortisone. On the other hand, only 25% of tamoxifen nonresponders were objectively benefitted by aminoglutethimide plus hydrocortisone. Although somewhat controversial, responders to progestin therapy also may benefit from aminoglutethimide plus hydrocortisone upon relapse (43).

SIDE EFFECTS

Patients receiving the standard dose of aminoglutethimide 1000 milligram a day experience a wide range of side effects during the induction of therapy (Fig. 74.6). The major problems include drug rash, fever, and lethargy. Skin rash is a particularly important side effect but it resolves spontaneously, even without discontinuation of therapy in the majority of patients. Approximately a third of women require mineralocorticoid replacement with 9α-fluorohydrocortisone (Florinef), because of the inhibition of aldosterone production (51). Another 5% of patients require thyroxine supplementation because of the inhibitory effects of aminoglutethimide on thyroid hormone synthesis, a cytochrome P_{450} *N* dependent process (48). In the remainder, thyroid-stimulating hormone (TSH) levels increase sufficiently to completely overcome the blockade of thyroxine biosynthesis.

The various side effects preclude continuing treatment in 8 to 15% of patients, particularly elderly women; however, many of these symptoms resolve completely or diminish in severity with treatment for longer than 6 weeks (Fig. 74.6). One possible basis for the reduction in side effects over time is the fact that aminoglutethimide accelerates its own metabolism from 12 hours to approximately 7 hours, presumably through hepatic enzyme induction (41).

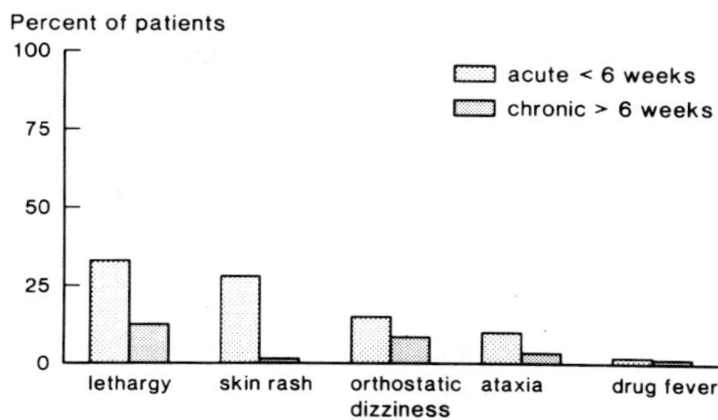

Figure 74.6. Side effects observed in 129 patients receiving 1,000 mg of aminogluthethimide and 40 mg of hydrocortisone daily. Signs or symptoms scored in patients receiving the drug for less than 6 weeks and more than 6 weeks.

The frequency and severity of side effects from aminoglutethimide, particularly when compared to tamoxifen, has led to attempts either to reduce the dose of aminoglutethimide (62) or else to develop less toxic compounds.

Development of Improved Aromatase Inhibitors

The successful use of aminoglutethimide provided an impetus to investigate further the concept of inhibiting estrogen biosynthesis as a means of treating breast cancer. The problem of the multiple actions of aminoglutethimide, its associated side effects, and the need for exogenous glucocorticoid spurred interest in the development of second- and third-generation aromatase inhibitors. Progressively, these newer compounds are demonstrating increasing potency, greater specificity, and reduced toxicity compared with aminoglutethimide. For example, compounds such as 4-hydroxyandrostenedione originally studied by Brodie and colleagues were designed as selective inhibitors of aromatase (6). A wide variety of such compounds are now under study, and the most clinically promising ones will be reviewed.

Classification

A convenient classification divides inhibitors into the mechanism-based, or "suicide," inhibitors and those of the competitive type. Suicide inhibitors initially compete with the natural substrate (i.e., androstenedione and testosterone) for binding to the active site of the enzyme. The enzyme, then, specifically acts upon the inhibitor to yield reactive alkylating species, which form covalent bonds at or near the active site of the enzyme. Through this mechanism, the enzyme is irreversibly inactivated. Competitive inhibitors, on the other hand, bind reversibly to the active site of the enzyme and prevent product formation only as long as the inhibitor occupies the catalytic site. Whereas mechanism-based inhibitors are exclusively steroidal in type, competitive inhibitors consist both of steroidal and nonsteroidal compounds.

Mechanism-based or suicide inhibitors should be preferable to competitive inhibitors because of their irreversible nature. Theoretically, their duration of action in vivo should be prolonged and related primarily to the rate at which new enzyme can be synthesized.

In seeking effective aromatase inhibitors, two considerations are paramount: intrinsic biologic activity and specificity of inhibition. Generally speaking, nonsteroidal inhibitors are more likely than steroidal compounds to lack specificity since they have a potential for blocking several cytochrome P_{450}-mediated steroid hydroxylations. On the other hand, steroidal inhibitors or their metabolites have greater potential for producing estrogen, androgen, glucocorticoid or progestin agonist or antagonistic effects through the inherent properties of their structures. The most promising aromatase inhibitors presently in clinical trials are shown in Figure 74.7.

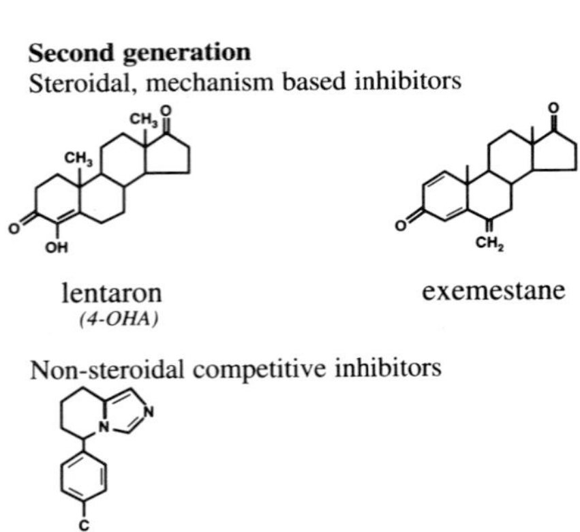

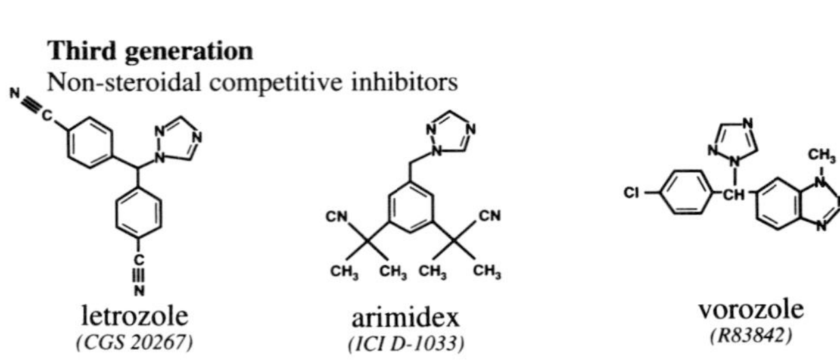

Figure 74.7. Structure and classification of representative aromatase inhibitors. Compounds are shown in approximate order of increasing specificity and potency of aromatase inhibition.

MECHANISM-BASED (SUICIDE) INHIBITORS

4-Hydroxyandrostenedione

Lentaron (Formestane; 4-OHA; 4-hydroxyandrost-4-ene-3,17-dione) is a structural analog of androstenedione. It was the first steroidal suicide-type aromatase inhibitor to enter clinical trials. Using the placental aromatase assay system in vitro 4-OHA was shown to be 60-fold more potent than aminoglutethimide (Ki = $4.1 \times 10^{-3}S^{-1}$). Extensive studies revealed no estrogenic, antiestrogenic, or antiandrogenic properties (4); however, transformation to 4-hydroxytestosterone occurs, and androgenic effects can be demonstrated under certain circumstances (5).

4-Hydroxyandrostenedione (Lentaron) has been studied extensively in postmenopausal women with breast cancer. In a phase I study, postmenopausal women received 500 to 1,000 mg of 4-OHA by weekly intramuscular injection (10). Although the drug has a short plasma half-life, concentrations of drug during chronic therapy and 1 week after the last injection ranged from 0.7 to 23.2 ng/ml (mean, 7.8 $\pm$ 1.1) ng/ml. During therapy, plasma estradiol levels fell from 7.2 $\pm$ 0.8 (SEM) pg/ml to 2.6 to 2.8 pg/ml from 1 to 4+ months after initiating treatment.

Data from four phase II clinical trials of 4-OHA demonstrated a 33% objective regression rate of breast cancer in postmenopausal patients previously treated with multiple endocrine therapies. Toxicity included six patients with sterile abscesses due to intramuscular injections, two of sufficient severity to warrant discontinuation of therapy. No androgenic effects were observed (26).

Höffken and colleagues conducted a large trial of 4-OHA in postmenopausal women (33). Patients initially received 500 mg intramuscularly every 2 weeks for 6 weeks and then 250 mg every 2 weeks thereafter. Plasma estradiol levels fell from baseline values of 10 to 11 pg/ml to levels of approximately 4 pg/ml for up to 7 months of therapy. The drug appeared specific, since no reduction of cortisol or symptoms of cortisol deficiency were observed. Of 86 evaluable patients, there were two complete and 19 partial remissions (24%), and 26 experienced disease stabilization (30%). Side effects included minor systemic symptoms in 11% (hot flashes, constipation, alopecia, pruritus) and local symptoms in 8% (pruritus, local pain, erythema). These side effects resulted in discontinuation of therapy in only 2% of patients. Phase III trials are now ongoing to compare this inhibitor with standard endocrine therapies. In general, 4-OHA is better tolerated than aminoglutethimide.

4-Hydroxyandrostenedione has also been given orally. Even though there is a marked first-pass effect with conversion in the liver to a glucuronidated derivative, oral doses of 250 mg reduce plasma estradiol by 53% and doses up to 1000 mg produce no further suppression. The response rate after 3 months' therapy was 33%, and the only serious side effect from the oral dosage was leukopenia in a single patient (Table 74.1) (15).

Exemestane (6-methyleneandrosta-1,4-diene-3,17-dione) is also a mechanism-based inhibitor and has been studied in patients. Single-dose administration reveals a major reduction of plasma estrogens with this compound (21).

Table 74.1. Nonrandomized Studies of 4-Hydroxyandrostenedione in Postmenopausal Women with Breast Carcinoma

Dose	Number of patients	Overall objective responses	Median duration response	Mean duration survival	Comments	Ref
250 mg I.M. every other week	55	33%	12 mo	—		20
500 mg I.M. weekly	52	33%	10 mo		Dose escalated to 1000 mg weekly in 11 non-responders; sterile abscesses in 6 patients	20
500 mg I.M. every other week	86	24%	13+	—	Dose reduced to 250 I.M. every other week after 6 weeks	38
500 mg p.o. daily	24	33%	—	—	No significant toxicity and side effects minimal	20

Table 74.2. New Aromatase Inhibitors Reaching Clinical Trials

Compound	Potency for aromatase			Clinical studies			Clinical status
	Inhibitor type	Ki[a]	K inact[c]	Selectivity	Dose	Toxicity	
Lentaron	Mechanism-based		$4.1 \times 10^{-3}S^{-1}$	+ +	500/250 mg IM q 2 wk	+ +	Commercially available
Exemestane	Mechanism-based	26 nM	$1.8 \times 10^{-4}S^{-1}$	+ +			Phase I
Pyrido-glutethimide	Competitive	1100 nM		+	200–400 mg bid	+ +	Phase II
Fadrozole	Competitive	0.19 nM		+ +	1 mg bid	+	Phase III
Letrozole	Competitive	—		+ + +	0.5, 2.5 mg q d	+	Phase III completed
Vorozole	Competitive	0.70 nM		+ + +	2.5 mg PO q d	+	Phase III
Arimidex	Competitive	15 nm		+ + +	1, 10 mg q d	+	Commercially available

[a] Inhibitory constant.
[b] Rate constant for inactivation of the enzyme (S = seconds).
[c] IC50.

COMPETITIVE INHIBITORS

Pyridoglutethimide (Rogletimide)

Pyridoglutethimide (rogletimide; 3-ethyl-3-(4-pyridyl) piperidine-2,6-dione) is a nonsteroidal compound resulting from modifications of the structure of aminoglutethimide intended to enhance specificity and to reduce side effects (Fig. 74.7) (24). This agent has a Ki for aromatase (1,100 nM), somewhat higher than that of aminoglutethimide (600 nM), but does not inhibit cholesterol side-chain cleavage at concentrations of up to 50 μg/ml. Tests of central nervous system (CNS) activity in animals suggest that sedative properties, so prominent with aminoglutethimide, are lacking. This agent also reduces the growth of NMU-induced mammary tumors in rats. Further studies with this compound are ongoing, and new, more potent, congeners are being developed.

Phase I trials of oral pyridoglutethimide at twice daily doses ranging from 200 to 500 mg showed significant suppression of serum and urine estrogen levels without significant changes in serum aldosterone and cortisol levels (16). Reported side effects included nausea, fatigue, and hot flashes. Preliminary data from two randomized phase II trials, comparing 200 and 300 mg versus 400 mg twice daily suggest that pyridoglutethimide is tolerated better than aminoglutethimide (25, 29).

Second- and Third-Generation Nonsteroidal Competitive Inhibitors.

A variety of other nonsteroidal competitive inhibitors of aromatase are currently being investigated. The imidazole compounds have potent effects on a number of cytochrome P_{450}-mediated steroid hydroxylation steps. Ketoconazole, for example, blocks C_{17-20} hydroxylase at low concentrations and aromatase at high concentrations (65). This observation suggested that, theoretically, compounds could be found which would exert relatively specific effects on certain P_{450}-mediated steroid hydroxylations with little activity on others. In fact, the several new compounds discussed below are indeed potent competitive inhibitors of aromatase but lack significant cholesterol side-chain cleavage activity. Specificity is not absolute, since high concentrations of drug may block other P_{450}-mediated steps as well (Table 74.2).

Fadrozole. Fadrozole (CGS 16949A; 4-(5,6,7,8-tetrahydroimidazo[1,5a]-pyridin-5yl)benzonitrile monohydro-chloride) (Fig. 74.7) is a highly potent inhibitor of aromatase with a Ki of 0.19 nM (versus 600 nM for aminoglutethimide) (55, 61). Cholesterol side-chain cleavage activity is minimal but C_{11}-hydroxylase inhibitory effects are observed in vitro at high drug concentrations (i.e., 10^{-6} M). Negligible toxicity was observed in animal studies (57).

Initial dose-seeking studies conducted in patients demonstrated effective aromatase inhibition at doses of 1.8 to 4.0 mg daily (54). A phase II study then compared doses of 0.6 mg three times daily, 1 mg twice daily, and 2 mg twice daily. Maximal suppression of plasma and urinary estrogens occurred at a dose of 1.0 mg twice daily, and minimal effects on cortisol secretion were observed. Basal cortisol and adrenocorticotropin (ACTH) levels were unaffected, and cortisol levels increased to more than 20 μg/dl after exogenous synthetic C_{1-24} ACTH (Cortrosyn) administration in all patients. Basal levels of aldosterone also remained stable following administration of all three drug doses. There were no changes in urinary or plasma sodium or potassium, nor in standing blood pressure to suggest a clinical state of aldosterone deficiency; however, Cortrosyn-stimulated aldosterone levels were significantly blunted at all three doses (55).

Clinical data from several phase II trials of fadrozole are now available. The overall objective response rate in postmenopausal patients with advanced breast cancer ranges from 3 to 23%. In one trial, objective regressions were recorded in 11 of 54 patients (20%) (31). Twenty-eight percent of 18 patients treated by Possinger and colleagues experienced an objective response (45). Falkson's group reported a response rate of 23% (10% complete responses, 13% partial responses) among 78 patients (46). All studies report a higher rate of disease stabilization and the median time to treatment failure ranges from 4 to 16 months. It should be noted that most patients enrolled in these early trials had received several prior endocrine and other therapies. Toxicity attributed to this agent is mild and consists mainly of nausea, anorexia, fatigue, and hot flashes. The potency of the compound, its relatively specific effects on aromatase, and its lack of toxicity suggest that it may represent a major improvement over aminoglutethimide for treatment of patients with breast cancer.

Two large multicenter phase III trials in the United States comparing fadrozole hydrochloride to megesterol acetate in patients who have received only tamoxifen as prior hormone therapy have been completed that have now accrued a total of approximately 600 patients. Final clinical results have not yet been published, but it is anticipated that fadrozole will prove to be of equal or greater efficacy with significantly reduced toxicities such as fluid retention, weight gain, hypertension, and thromboembolic phenomena.

Vorozole. Vorozole (R83842; R76713; vorozole(s)-(6-[4-chlorophenyl)(1H-1,2,4-triazol-1-yl)methyl]-1-methyl-1H-benzotriazole)] (Fig. 74.7) represents another highly potent and specific aromatase inhibitor with little toxicity in animal studies (66). The Ki for placental aromatase is 0.8 nM, and this agent is approximately 500-fold more potent than aminoglutethimide. From animal data, vorozole appears to be highly specific for aromatase without having major effects on other cytochrome P_{450}-mediated steroid hydroxylations. Phase I clinical studies revealed an acute reduction of plasma estradiol to undetectable levels in normal men receiving one 10-mg dose and a 64% reduction in premenopausal women (12). Goss and co-workers reported a phase II study of vorozole in an oral dose of 2.5 mg daily given to postmenopausal women with metastatic breast cancer. Treatment-related side effects were mild and included malaise, anorexia and nausea, hot flashes, fluid retention, vaginal infection, alopecia, lightheadedness, and one allergic reaction causing lip swelling. There was profound suppression of serum estradiol and estrone from pretreatment levels. Of 27 evaluable patients, 3 (11%) had partial remission of their disease for 14, 15, and 16 months, respectively, and 14 achieved disease stabilization for a median duration of 12 months (28).

Letrozole. Letrozole (CGS 20267; [4,4′-(1H-1,2,4-triazol-1-yl-methylene)-bis-benzonitrile]) (Fig. 74.7), another nonsteroidal competitive aromatase inhibitor, is more potent than fadrozole and more selective in its inhibition of aromatase. Significantly, aldosterone production in vitro is inhibited only at concentrations 10,000 times higher than those required for inhibition of estrogen production. In vivo, letrozole is 10 to 30 times more potent than fadrozole in an assay that measures inhibition of androstenedione-induced uterine hypertrophy. When administered orally to adult female rats at a dose of 1 mg/kg per day for 14 days, letrozole decreases uterine weight to that observed after a surgical ovariectomy. At doses 1,000 times more than the concentration required to cause a 50% inhibition of the aromatase enzyme, letrozole does not significantly suppress either aldosterone or corticosterone in rats (2). Letrozole also causes significant regression of DMBA-induced rat mammary tumors (58).

In a study of healthy male volunteers letrozole in doses as small as 0.002 mg was effective in suppressing estrogen. Maximal suppression was achieved with doses of 0.25 mg. The agent is specific for aromatase, since there were no changes in aldosterone or cortisol at any of the time points studied (64). Two dose-seeking phase-I trials of letrozole in postmenopausal women with advanced breast cancer have been reported. In one trial, single daily doses of 0.1, 0.5, and 2.5 mg were administered to 21 patients. Treatment was well tolerated, and no clinically significant toxicities were observed. Hormonal studies revealed no significant changes in FSH, LH, TSH, cortisol, 17-γ-hydroxyprogesterone, androstenedione, or aldosterone levels. Seven patients (33%) achieved an objective response (1 complete, 6 partial). Five patients (24%) had stabilization of their disease (34). Lipton and co-workers also performed a phase I study in 23 heavily pretreated postmenopausal patients who were given letrozole in doses ranging from 0.1 to 5.0 mg once daily. Again, no clinically significant toxicities were observed. Letrozole at all doses tested produced remarkably prompt and profound suppression of plasma estrone, estradiol, estrone sulfate, and urine estrone and estradiol (14). Suppression became evident within 24 hours of the initial dose, and there was greater than 90% suppression of both plasma and urinary estrogens within 2 weeks (Fig. 74.8). Letrozole did not compromise glucocorticoid or mineralocorticoid production or thyroid function. Of 21 evaluable patients, there were two partial responses and 7 patients with stable disease. Thus, preliminary clinical experience with letrozole suggests that this drug is a well-tolerated, potent, and specific inhibitor of estrogen biosynthesis in postmenopausal patients with metastatic breast cancer (39). These encouraging results

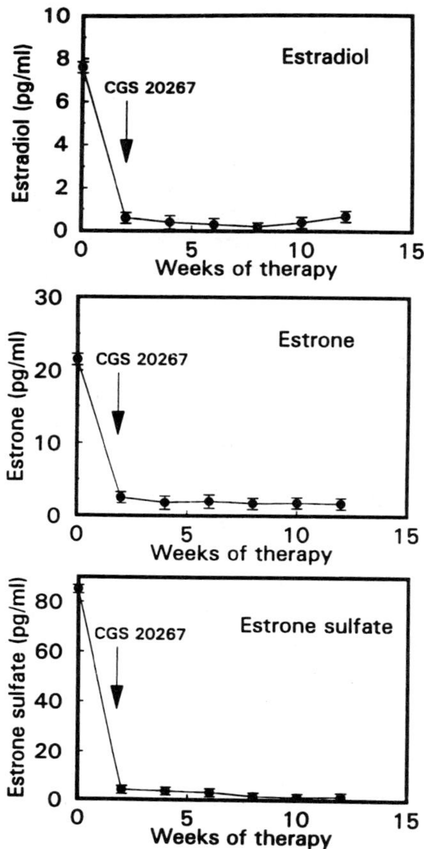

Figure 74.8. Effects of letrozole on plasma estradiol, estrone, and estrone sulfate in eight patients, at doses of 0.1 mg per day (first 6 weeks) and 0.25 mg per day (second 6 weeks), over 12 weeks of therapy. Results represent the mean plus or minus the standard deviation. (Data reproduced from Demers [14], with permission.)

have led to phase III clinical trials comparing letrozole to megestrol acetate in postmenopausal patients previously treated with tamoxifen.

Arimidex. Arimidex (ICI-D1033; 2,2′-[5-(1H-1,2,4-triazol-1-y-lmethyl)-1,3-phenylene]bis(2-methyl-propiononitrile) (Fig. 74.7) is another potent and selective benzyltriazole derivative. At a concentration of 15 nmol/L this compound inhibits aromatase enzyme activity by 50%. Maximal hormonal suppression was achieved with an oral dose of 0.1 mg/kg. In rats, this activity was assayed as inhibition of ovulation and androstenedione-induced uterine hypertrophy, and in monkeys, as suppression of plasma estradiol. The estimated elimination half-life is 32.2 hours.

In a phase I study, healthy postmenopausal women received 0.5, 1, 3, 5, or 10 mg arimidex once daily for 8 to 14 days. Doses of 1 to 10 mg caused maximal suppression of estradiol without altering either cortisol or aldosterone levels. There were no serious adverse drug reactions (44). Similarly, in men given single oral doses of arimidex ranging from 0.1 to 30 mg, serum estradiol levels fell below 80% of baseline values. Suppression was maximal at doses of at least 7.5 mg and greater. Gonadotropins were elevated in reflex fashion secondary to estrogen suppression, but treatment resulted in no other changes in hormone levels (17).

In another phase I study, 19 postmenopausal women with advanced breast cancer who had failed between two and five previous treatments received arimidex as a single 5-mg oral dose daily for 14 days, followed by 10 mg for 14 days. Seventeen of these patients went on to receive arimidex, 10 mg daily, in a compassionate open-label extension of the study. Although not designed as an efficacy trial, it is interesting to note that, in this group of heavily pretreated patients, the time to tumor progression is greater than 4 months in more than half the patients and approaches 2 years in 4 of them.

These encouraging results led to two large, phase III trials. Data from these pivotal studies indicate that arimidex is similar to megestrol in efficacy but causes less weight gain and fewer thromboembolic side effects. Arimidex is well tolerated and is the first aromatase inhibitor approved in the United States for treatment of women with advanced breast cancer. The recommended dose is 1 mg once daily.

Selection of Patients for Aromatase Inhibition Therapy

POSTMENOPAUSAL WOMEN

Endocrine therapy is usually offered to patients with metastatic disease who have estrogen or progesterone receptor–positive or receptor-unknown disease. In addition to the level of receptors, clinical features that might suggest a favorable response include a long disease-free interval after initial surgery or the presence of nodal, soft tissue, bone, pleural or nodular lung metastases. Patients with CNS involvement, extensive liver disease, lymphangitic spread of tumor in the lungs, or rapidly progressing and life-threatening disease are not ordinarily considered candidates for hormone therapy. Considerable clinical experience and data from the literature suggest that most endocrine therapies, with the possible exceptions of androgens and glucocorticoids, are equally efficacious. The decision to choose one endocrine therapy over another depends upon the menopausal status of the patient, considerations of efficacy, ease of administration, cost, and side effects. Historically, of all the endocrine therapies, tamoxifen was associated with the fewest side effects. This aspect still favors tamoxifen as the endocrine therapy of first choice. Aromatase inhibitors are then considered, as either second- or third-line endocrine approaches. More recently, however, the widespread use of tamoxifen as adjuvant therapy, frequently administered for long periods, presents the clinician with a new therapeutic dilemma. A practical approach is to rely on tamoxifen as first-line therapy for patients with metastatic disease who have not received this agent in the adjuvant setting or have discontinued tamoxifen for more than a year. For other patients who are still candidates for hormone therapy, the major choices at present are between progestins such as megestrol acetate or medroxyprogesterone acetate and aromatase inhibitors. It is probable that one (or even several) of the new generation aromatase inhibitors will become more widely available to clinicians. Given their potency and highly favorable therapeutic profile, the authors would favor choosing these agents over progestins as the next endocrine therapy (Fig. 74.9).

It has been speculated that the determination of the aromatase content of a particular tumor, by either biochemical measurement or immunohistochemistry, might aid in selecting patients who are likely to respond to therapy with aromatase inhibitors; however, this concept needs further clinical testing.

PREMENOPAUSAL PATIENTS

Considerations of efficacy, cost, toxicity, and ease of administration also dictate the choice of endocrine therapy in premenopausal patients. Based on these considerations, first-line therapy would include either tamoxifen or oophorectomy. Effective castration can be accomplished either by surgery, pelvic irradiation, or the use of LH-RH analogues. Because of the resistance of the ovary to aromatase inhibition (discussed above) (50), aromatase inhibitors have traditionally been tested in postmenopausal patients. On the other hand, the activity of the very potent third-generation inhibitors makes it likely that these compounds will also inhibit ovarian steroidogenesis and therefore may be of use in the treatment of premenopausal women, although supporting clinical studies have not yet been reported.

MALE BREAST CANCER

Male breast cancer, although a rare condition, is frequently an estrogen-dependent tumor. Only anecdotal reports are available concerning the activity of aromatase inhibitors in this setting.

Future Perspectives

As discussed above, a large number of aromatase inhibitors are being developed for the treatment of breast cancer (27). The goals of clinical research with these agents should be to obtain a drug that is convenient to administer at a dose that specifically inhibits aromatase without exerting other endocrine effects and does not cause significant clinical toxicity. Unlike the case with other antitumor agents, our ability to precisely assay hormonal levels in clinical subjects makes it possible to determine the specificity and the optimal dose of an aromatase inhibitor that causes maximal estrogen suppression.

Future clinical trials with these promising agents must address several questions, including their role in the treatment of premenopausal women as discussed above. Although presently tested as second-line therapies after tamoxifen failure, perhaps in the future, aromatase inhibitors might prove to be effective as first-line endocrine treatment for breast cancer. Coombes and associates have reported that 4-OHA prevents NMU-induced rat mammary carcinoma (11). Similar observations with other aromatase inhibitors and animal models suggest that inhibitors of estrogen biosynthesis can prevent breast cancer. Moreover, these agents would not be expected to induce endometrial carcinoma in women and, so, could be investigated both as adjuvant hormonal therapy and in the chemoprevention of human breast cancer.

A few clinical studies have attempted to combine different classes of endocrine agents, but there are no data to support this approach as being superior to the use of these agents in sequence to treat metastatic breast cancer (e.g., tamoxifen followed by an aromatase inhibitor, followed by a progestin). In clinical practice the sequential use of hor-

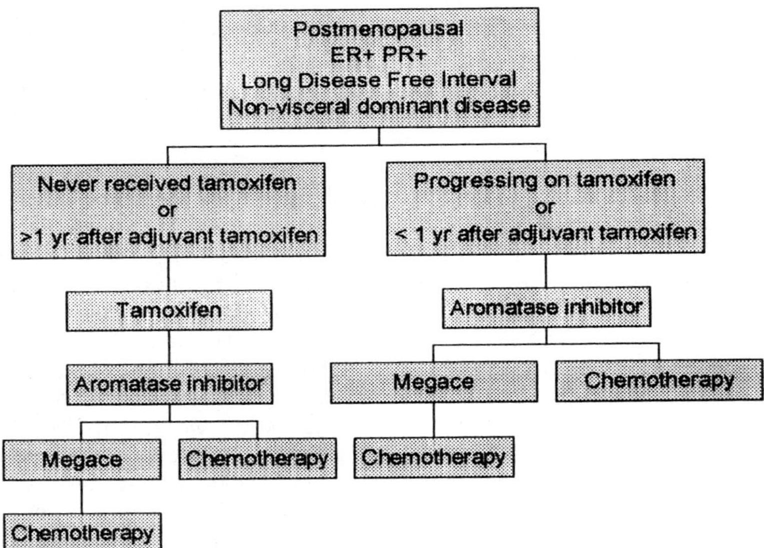

Figure 74.9. Selection of patients for therapy with aromatase inhibitors. Algorithm for integrating aromatase inhibitors into the management of metastatic hormone-dependent breast cancer.

monal agents can produce long-term palliation of hormone-dependent breast cancer. Eventually, however, the problem of hormone resistance is encountered. The mechanisms by which tumors become resistant to hormones in general are only partially understood. Refractoriness to therapy with aromatase inhibitors is related not to the failure of these agents to suppress estradiol levels but rather to some mechanism of hormone resistance.

The paracrine production of aromatase, specific growth factors, and cytokines within the microenvironment of a breast tumor requires further study. Greater understanding of the biologic interaction of these factors could lead, for example, to the development of new therapeutic strategies.

In summary, ongoing clinical studies of highly potent aromatase inhibitors have shown that it is possible to develop specific, nontoxic compounds which reduce serum estradiol concentrations to undetectable levels in breast cancer patients (13). These compounds are emerging as a valuable approach to the treatment of hormone-dependent breast cancer. Should the new aromatase inhibitors prove to effectively inhibit ovarian steroidogenesis as well as extraglandular and intratumor aromatase, then they may have a role in the treatment of other malignancies, such as endometrial cancer, granulosa cell tumors, melanoma, prostate cancer, and pancreatic carcinoma, as well as benign conditions such as precocious puberty, uterine leiomyoma, endometriosis, and other hyperestrogenic states.

References

1. Abul-Hajj YJ, Iverson R, Kiang DT. Aromatization of androgens by human breast cancer. Steroids 1979;33:205–222.
2. Bhatnagar AS, Hausler A, Schieweck K, Lang M, Bowman R. Highly selective inhibition of estrogen biosynthesis by CGS 20267, a new nonsteroidal aromatase inhibitor. J Steroid Biochem Molec Biol 1990;37:1021–1027.
3. Bradlow HL. A reassessment of the role of breast tumor aromatization. Cancer Res 1982;42:3382S–3386S.
4. Brodie AMH, Longcope C. Inhibition of peripheral aromatization by aromatase inhibitors, 4-hydroxy- and 4-acetoxy-androstene-3,17-dione. Endocrinology 1980;106:19–21.
5. Brodie AMH, Romanoff LD, Williams KIH. Metabolism of the aromatase inhibitor 4-hydroxy-4-androstene-3,17-dione by male rhesus monkeys. J Steroid Biochem 1981;14:693–696.
6. Brodie AMH, Santen RJ. Aromatase in breast cancer and the role of aminoglutethimide and other aromatase inhibitors. Crit Rev Oncol/Hematol 1986;5:361–396.
7. Bulun SE, Simpson ER. Regulation of aromatase expression in human tissues. Breast Cancer Res Treat 1994;30:19–29.
8. Cash R, Brough AJ, Cohen MNP, Satoh PS. Aminoglutethimide (Elipten-CIBA) as an inhibitor of adrenal steroidogenesis. Mechanism of action and therapeutic trial. J Clin Endocrinol Metab 1967;27:1239–1268.
9. Chakraborty J, Hopkins R, Parke D. Inhibition studies on the aromatization of androst-4ene-3,17-dione by human placental microsomes. Biochem J 1972;130:19P–20P.
10. Coombes RC, Goss PE, Dowsett M, Gazet JC, Brodie AMH. 4-Hydroxy-androstenedione in treatment of postmenopausal patients with advanced breast cancer. Lancet 1984;2:1237–1239.
11. Coombes RC, Wilkinson JR, Bliss JM, Shah P, Easton DF, Dowsett M. 4-Hydroxyandrostenedione in the prophylaxis of *N*-methyl-*N*-nitrosourea induced mammary tumourigenesis. Br J Cancer 1991;64:247–250.
12. DeCoster R, Wouters W, Bowden CR, Vanden Bossche H, Bruynseels J, Tuman RW, VanGinckel R, Snoeck E, VanPeer A, Janssen PA. New nonsteroidal aromatase inhibitors: focus on R76713. J Steroid Biochem Molec Biol 1990;37:335–341.
13. Demers LM. Effects of fadrozole (CGS 16949A) and Letrozole (CGS 20267) on the inhibition of aromatase activity in breast cancer patients. Breast Cancer Res Treatment 1994;30:95–102.
14. Demers LM, Lipton A, Harvey HA, Kambic KB, Grossberg H, Brady C, Santen RJ. The efficacy of CGS 20267 in suppressing estrogen biosynthesis in patients with advanced stage breast cancer. J Steroid Biochem Molec Biol 1993;44:687–691.
15. Dowsett M, Cunnigham DC, Stein RC, Evans S, Dehennin L, Hedley A, Coombes RC. Dose-related endocrine effects and pharmacokinetics of oral and intramuscular 4-hydroxyandrostenedione in postmenopausal breast cancer patients. Cancer Res 1989;49:1306–1312.
16. Dowsett M, MacNeill F, Mehta A, Newton C, Haynes B, Jones A, Jarman M, Lonning P, Powles TJ, Coombes RC. Endocrine, pharmacokinetic and clinical studies of the aromatase inhibitor 3-ethyl-3-(4-pyridyl)piperidine-2,6-dione ("pyridoglutethimide") in postmenopausal breast cancer patients. Br J Cancer 1991;64:887–894.
17. Dowsett M, Yates RA, Lindsay A, Dukes M. Endocrine effects of arimidex, a potent aromatase inhibitor, in men and postmenopausal women (Abstract 87). Breast Cancer Res Treat 1993;27:152.
18. Edery M, Goussard J, Dehennin L, Scholler R, Reiffsteck J, Drosdowsky MA. Endogenous oestradiol 17β concentration in breast tumors determined by mass fragmentography and radioimmunoassay: relationship to receptor content. Eur J Cancer 1951;17:115–120.
19. Esteban JM, Warsi Z, Haniu M, Hall P, Shively JE, Chen S. Detection of intratumoral aromatase in breast carcinomas. Am J Pathol 1992;140:337–343.
20. Evans CT, Corbin CJ, Saunders CT, Merrill JC, Simpson ER, Mendelson CR. Regulation of estrogen biosynthesis in human adipose stromal cells: effects of dibutyryl cyclic AMP, epidermal growth factor, and phorbol esters on the synthesis of aromatase cytochrome P_{450}. J Biol Chem 1987;262:6914–6920.
21. Evans TRJ, di Salle E, Ornati G, Lassus M, Benedetti MS, Pianezzola E, Coombes RC. Phase I and endocrine study of exemestane (FCE 24304), a new aromatase inhibitor, in postmenopausal women. Cancer Res 1992;52:5933–5939.
22. Fishman J, Nisselbaum JS, Menendez-Botet CJ, Schwartz MK. Estrone and estradiol content in human breast tumors. Relationship to estradiol receptors. J Steroid Biochem 1977;8:893–896.
23. Fishman J, Hahn EF. The nature of the final oxidative step in the aromatization sequence. Steroids 1987;50:339–345.
24. Foster AB, Jarman M, Leung C-S, Rowlands MG, Taylor GN, Plevey RG, Sampson P. Analogues of aminoglutethimide. Selective inhibition of aromatase. J Med Chem 1985;28:200–204.
25. Fox KR, Glick JH, MacDonald JS, Vogel CL, Cartwright T, Auerbach M, Schulz JJ, Ahlgren JD, Heim WJ, Demers L, Conner G, Keller M, Reynolds RD, Mitchell EP, Capizzi RL, Schein P. Randomized phase II trial of Rogletimide in advanced breast cancer: a preliminary report. Breast Cancer Res Treat (Abstract 85) 1993;27:152.
26. Goss PE, Powles TJ, Dowsett M, Hutchison G, Brodie AMH, Gazet J-C, Coombes RC. Treatment of advanced postmenopausal breast cancer with an aromatase inhibitor, 4-hydroxyandrostenedione: phase II report. Cancer Res 1986;46:4823–4826.
27. Goss PE, Gwyn KMEH. Current perspectives on aromatase inhibitors in breast cancer. J Clin Oncol 1994;12:2460–2470.
28. Goss PE, Clark RM, Ambus U, Weizel HA, Wadden NA, Crump M, Walde D, Tye LM, De Coster R, Bruynseels J. Phase II study of vorozole (R83842), a new aromatase inhibitor, in postmenopausal women with advanced breast cancer in progression on tamoxifen. Clin Cancer Res 1995;1:287–94.
29. Harnett AN, Canney P, Coombes RC, et al. A randomized phase II trial of rogletimide in hormone relapsed advanced breast cancer. Breast Cancer Res Treat 1993;27:152.
30. Harvey HA, Santen RJ, Osterman J, Samojlik E, White D, Lipton A. A comparative trial of transsphenoidal hypophysectomy and estrogen suppression with aminoglutethimide in advanced breast cancer. Cancer 1979;43:2207–2214.
31. Harvey HA, Lipton A, Santen RJ, Demers L, Henderson IC, Miller AA, Navari R, Mulagha MT, Hanagan J. Clinical trials with the aromatase inhibitor CGS16949A in advanced breast cancer: the US experience. In Aromatase Inhibition Present and Future. Edited by W Jonat, RJ Santen. New Jersey: Parthenon, 1991, pp 89–96.
32. Henderson D, Norbisrath G, Kerb U. 1-methyl-1,4-androstadiene-3,17-dione (SH 489) Characterization of an irreversible inhibitor of estrogen biosynthesis. J Steroid Biochem 1986;24:303–306.
33. Höffken K, Jonat W, Possinger K, Kolbe, M, Kunz TH, Wagner H, Becher R, Callies R, Friederich P, Willmanns W, Maass H, Schmidt CG. Aromatase inhibition with 4-hydroxyandrostenedione in the treatment of postmenopausal patients with advanced breast cancer: a phase II study. J Clin Oncol 1990;8:875–880.
34. Iveson TJ, Smith IE, Ahern J, Smithers DA, Trunet PF, Dowsett M. Phase I study of the oral nonsteroidal aromatase inhibitor CGS 20267 in postmenopausal patients with advanced breast cancer. Cancer Res 1993;53:266–270.
35. Judd HL, Judd GE, Lucas WE, Yen SSC. Endocrine function of the postmenopausal ovary: concentration of androgens and estrogens in ovarian and peripheral vein blood. J Clin Endocrinol Metab 1974;39:1020–1024.
36. Kirschner MA, Schneider G, Ertel NH, Worton E. Obesity, androgens, estrogens, and cancer risk (Abstract). Cancer Res 1982;42(suppl):3218s.
37. Koos RD, Banks PK, Inkster SE, Yue W, Brodie AMH. Detection of aromatase and keratinocyte growth factor expression in breast tumors using reverse transcription-polymerase chain reaction. J Steroid Biochem Molec Biol 1993;45:217–225.
38. Lipton A, Santner SJ, Santen RJ, Harvey HA, Feil PD, White-Hershey D, Bartholomew MJ, Antle CE. Aromatase activity in primary and metastatic human breast cancer. Cancer 1987;59:779–782.
39. Lipton A, Demers L, Harvey HA, Kambic K, Grossberg H, Brady C, Adlercruetz H, Trunet P, Santen RJ. Letrozole (CGS 20267)—Phase I study of a new potent oral aromatase inhibitor in breast cancer. Cancer 1995;75:2132–2138.
40. Mahendroo MS, Mendelson CR, Simpson ER. Tissue-specific and hormonally controlled alternative promoters regulate aromatase cytochrome P_{450} gene expression in human adipose tissue. J Biol Chem 1993;268:19463–19470.
41. Murray FT, Santner S, Samojlik E, Santen RJ. Serum aminoglutethimide levels: studies of serum half-life, clearance and patient compliance. J Clin Pharmacol 1979;19:704–711.
42. O'Neill JS, Miller WR. Aromatase activity in breast adipose tissue from women with benign and malignant breast diseases. Br J Cancer 1987;56:601–604.
43. Petru E, Schmahl D. On the role of additive hormone monotherapy with tamoxifen, medroxyprogesterone acetate and aminoglutethimide in advanced breast cancer. Klin Wochenschr 1987;65:959–966.
44. Plourde PV, Dyroff M, Dukes M. ARIMIDEX: a potent and selective fourth-generation aromatase inhibitor. Breast Cancer Res Treatment 1994;30:103–111.
45. Possinger K, Langecker P. The role of aromatase inhibition in the treatment of metastatic breast cancer. In Aromatase Inhibition Present and Future. Edited by W Jonat, RJ Santen. New Jersey: Parthenon, 1991, pp 29–34.
46. Raats JI, Falkson G, Falkson HC. A study of fadrozole. A new aromatase inhibitor on postmenopausal women with advanced breast cancer. J Clin Oncol 1992;10:111–116.
47. Santen RJ, Lipton A, Kendall J. Successful medical adrenalectomy with aminoglutethimide. Role of altered drug metabolism. JAMA 1974;230:1661–1665.
48. Santen RJ, Wells SA, Cohn N, Demers LM, Misbin R, Foltz EL. Compensatory increase

in TSH secretion without effect on prolactin secretion in patients treated with aminoglutethimide. J Clin Endocrinol Metab 1977;45:739–746.
49. Santen RJ, Santner SJ, Davis B, Veldhuis J, Samojilik E, Ruby E. Aminoglutethimide inhibits extraglandular estrogen production in postmenopausal women with breast carcinoma. J Clin Endocrinol Metab 1978;47:1257–1265.
50. Santen RJ, Samojilik E, Wells SA. Resistance of the ovary to blockade of aromatization with aminoglutethimide. J Clin Endocrinol Metab 1980;51:473–477.
51. Santen RJ, Worgul TJ, Samojlik E, Interrante A, Boucher AE, Lipton A, Harvey HA, White DS, Smart E, Cox C, Wells SA. A randomized trial comparing surgical adrenalectomy with aminoglutethimide plus hydrocortisone in women with advanced breast cancer. N Engl J Med 1981;305:545–551.
52. Santen RJ, Worgul TJ, Lipton A, Harvey HA, Boucher AE, Samojlik E, Wells SA. Aminoglutethimide as treatment of postmenopausal women with advanced breast carcinoma: correlation of clinical and hormonal responses. Ann Intern Med 1982;96: 94–101.
53. Santen RJ, Leszczynski D, Tilson-Mallet N, Fiel PD, Wright C, Manni A, Santner SJ. Enzymatic control of estrogen production in human breast cancer: relative significance of aromatase vs. sulfatase pathways. In Endocrinology of the Breast: Basic and Clinical Aspects. Edited by A Angeli, HL Bradlow, vol 464. New York: Academic, 1986, p 126.
54. Santen RJ, Demers LM, Adlercreutz H, Harvey HA, Santner S, Sanders S, Lipton A. Inhibition of aromatase with CGS-16949A in postmenopausal women. J Clin Endocrinol Metab 1989;68:99–106.
55. Santen RJ, Demers LM, Lynch J, Harvey H, Lipton A, Mulagha M, Hanagan J, Garber JE, Henderson IC, Navari RM, Miller AA. Specificity of low dose fadrozole hydrochloride (CGS 16949A) as an aromatase inhibitor. J Clin Endocrinol Metab 1991;73: 99–106.
56. Santen RJ, Martel J, Hoagland M, Naftolin F, Roa L, Harad N, Hafer L, Zaino R, Santner SJ. Stromal spindle cells contain aromatase in human breast tumors. J Clin Endocrinol Metab 1994;79:627–632.
57. Schieweck K, Bhatnagar AS, Matter A. CGS 16949A, a new nonsteroidal aromatase inhibitor: effects on hormone-dependent and -independent tumors in vivo. Cancer Res 1988;48:834–838.
58. Schieweck K, Bhatnagar AS, Batzl CH, Lang M. Anti-tumor and endocrine effects of non-steroidal aromatase inhibitors on estrogen-dependent rat mammary tumors. J Steroid Biochem Molec Biol 1993;44:633–636.
59. Simpson ER, Merrill JC, Hollub AJ, Graham-Lorence S, Mendelson CR. Regulation of estrogen biosynthesis by human adipose cells. Endocrinol Rev 1989;10:136–148.
60. Simpson ER, Mahendroo MS, Means GD, Kilgore MW, Corbin CJ, Mendelson CR. Tissue-specific promoters regulate aromatase cytochrome P_{450} expression. Clin Chem 1993;39:317–324.
61. Steele RE, Mellor LB, Sawyer WK, Wasvary JM, Browne LJ. In vitro and in vivo studies demonstrating potent and selective estrogen inhibition with the nonsteroidal aromatase inhibitor CGS 16949A. Steroids 1987;50:147–161.
62. Stuart-Harris R, Dowsett M, D'Souza A, Donaldson A, Harris AL, Jeffcoate SL, Smith IE. Endocrine effects of low dose aminoglutethimide as an aromatase inhibitor in the treatment of breast cancer. Clin Endocrinol 1985;22:219–226.
63. Thompson EA, Siiteri PK. The involvement of human placental microsomal cytochrome P_{450} in aromatization. J Biol Chem 1974;249:5373–5378.
64. Trunet P, Muller PH, Bhatnagar A, Chaudri N, Beh I, Monnet G. Phase I study in healthy male volunteers with the non-steroidal aromatase inhibitor GCS 20267 (Abstract 109). Eur J Cancer 1990;26:173.
65. Wouters W, DeCoster R, Goeminne N, Beerens D, Van Dun J. Aromatase inhibition by the antifungal ketoconazole. J Steroid Biochem 1988;30:387–389.
66. Wouters W, DeCoster R, Krekels M, Van Dun J, Beerens D, Haelterman C, Raeymaekers A, Freyne E, Van Gelder J, Venet M, Janssen PAJ. R76713. A new specific nonsteroidal aromatase inhibitor. J Steroid Biochem 1989;32:781–788.

CHAPTER 75

Progestins

KENNETH S. McCARTY, JR. AND KENNETH S. McCARTY, SR.

Introduction

Progestins are involved to some degree in differentiation in a broad spectrum of tissues. Examples included among the myriad effects of progesterone are profound changes in the breast and the uterus during the menstrual cycle as well as changes in glandular epithelium and smooth muscle in other sites. Evidence has implicated progesterone in the control of proliferation in the breast, contrasting to the predominant role of estrogen in proliferation in the uterus (1). In both of these organs, progestins effect a secretory differentiation after estrogen priming. The dominant naturally occurring progestin is progesterone, which in nongravid women is principally derived from the corpus luteum of the ovary. Progesterone is required for the development of a secretory endometrium in which the blastocyst can implant. After the eighth week of pregnancy the major source of progesterone becomes the placenta. While the trophoblast is the dominant cell responsible for progesterone production by the placenta after the eighth week of gestation, progesterone is also synthesized by the adrenals through conversion of pregnenolone. In the luteal phase of the menstrual cycle progesterone levels of 25 ng/ml are usual, while levels to 150 ng/ml are typical of pregnancy at term. Such high levels of progesterone as those seen in term pregnancy are associated with a number of effects that have implications for other conditions. Among these are progesterone-associated inhibition of T lymphocyte cell-mediated immune response, inhibition of prostaglandin formation, and inhibition of smooth muscle contractility through binding to receptors in the uterine smooth muscle.

Progestins have emerged as antineoplastic agents in uterine and breast cancer, have been tested with promising results in meningiomas and pulmonary lymphangiomyomatosis, and have been studied for antineoplastic effects against other neoplasms; however, the principal pharmacologic use of these hormones is in contraceptive preparations. Thus, the use of progestins or antiprogestins in contraceptive preparations is the area in which the greatest effort has been applied to understanding the pharmacology and mechanism of action of progesterone and the various synthetic progestins and antiprogestins. Recommendations for progestin addition to estrogen replacement therapy in the climacteric places new emphasis on understanding the mechanism of progesterone action in settings other than contraception, particularly in populations with a significant incidence of endometrial and breast cancer (16, 79).

Target cells not only must distinguish progesterone in the presence of other steroids present in small amounts but also must distinguish progesterone from other hydrophobic molecules that are frequently found in 100-fold or greater excess. Thus, while progesterone may affect a number of physiologic processes, such a high degree of discrimination is limited to differentiated cells that possess progesterone receptor proteins (PRs) and progesterone-responsive elements (PRE) in their genome (88).

PR is a prototypic member of a superfamily of transcriptional regulatory proteins (18). The target gene mRNA level regulation is primarily dependent on progesterone activation of PR that results in a complex series of events (50). As with other members of this superfamily, activated PR acquires the capacity to modulate the activity of specific target genes. Some target genes are under the regulation of both PR and glucocorticoid receptor (GR). Such genes include estrogen receptor (76), human metallothionein IIA (75), uteroglobin (19), vitellogenin (84), and human pregnancy-specific beta glycoprotein (74). The molecular mechanisms to provide discrimination are dependent on highly specific protein-DNA interactions that involve specific amino acid residues of the PR and nucleotide residues of the target genes. The amino acid residues of the PR are defined as the "DNA-binding domain" (DBD), and the DNA elements of these target genes as "progesterone-responsive elements" (PREs). The PRE sequences of a whole network of target genes are recognized by the *trans*-activated PR (3). These PRE gene sequences are further characterized as "enhancer-like" in that neither their precise orientation nor their position appear to be critical (82). The PREs that are recognized by the DBD are confined, however, to the 5′ "upstream" end of the genes, near the promoter regions of all progesterone-responsive target genes examined to date (23, 47).

The critical feature that determines the specificity of the progesterone/progesterone receptor is the precise protein-DNA interaction of the *trans*-activated PR with specific target genes. This feature of hormone induction is common to the whole superfamily of steroid receptors (32,88). The progesterone-PR complex (90) activates the positively charged cysteine-rich amino acid residues of the DBD (32), which in turn function to increase its binding affinity for specific PRE residues of target genes (70). This activation is often referred to as *trans*-activation, denoting that its function spans many amino acid residues (29). The response mechanism is dependent on the steps, beginning with hormone recognition, followed by activation of the DBD, and then interaction of the

DBD with chromosomal DNA target gene progesterone-responsive element sequences (3, 15, 46).

Analyses of the DNA sequences also demonstrate that most progesterone-responsive target genes have not only multiple PRE copies but also other hormone-responsive elements (HRE), including in particular, glucocorticoid-responsive elements (GRE). Many of these HREs have the capacity to modify the function of the PR. This knowledge of the existence of multiple PRE and HRE elements in combination provides for the first time a plausible mechanism to account for the clinical observation that both the dose and prior hormone history have a profound effect on the clinical response of patients' tumors to hormone manipulation. As a specific example, it is frequently observed that the administration of different levels of progesterone enhances the co-operative binding to HREs and that a number of hormone combinations both down- and up-regulate the progesterone-responsive gene (21, 23).

The chromosomal DNA target gene configuration is a critical factor in gene response that includes many proteins (RNA polymerase II enzyme complexes and specific proteins essential for RNA polymerase function) (8, 72, 77). Thus any inappropriate DNA hypermethylation and/or heterochromatin configuration is likely to exert a profound effect on the PR response and may in some tumors account for clinical failures. This failure to respond must also be passed to the metastatic tumor by maintenance methylase (77).

The structure and function that contribute to receptor-ligand interactions at the molecular level have been extensively studied and are the subject of a number of reviews (18, 36, 38, 59, 61, 64, 82, 88).

A cogent understanding of present knowledge of the significance of progestins in neoplasia begins with a presentation of the pharmacology of progestins, followed by a discussion of some of the functions of progesterone receptors in terms of genetic structure, differentiation, synthesis, postsynthetic modification, and intracellular location. Selected aspects of the clinical response to progestins of specific neoplasms, as in the discussion that follows, are principally empirical observations. Discussion of steroid hormone, including progesterone, induction of proto-oncogenes, and modulation of cell cycle activity is of significance (11, 27, 31) and is provided elsewhere in this volume.

Pharmacology

Progestins are properly classified as natural or synthetic. Progesterone occupies a position early in the scheme of the synthetic pathway involving the conversion of precursor cholesterol to the production of adrenal cortex–derived hormones, including androgens and estrogens. After menopause and in the absence of hormone replacement, the adrenal is the principal source of these sex steroids.

Progesterone is poorly absorbed when given orally, and when injected must be administered with an oil carrier. A number of synthetic progestins are available which are well absorbed in the gastrointestinal tract. Synthetic progestins are derivatives of the steroid structure of either progesterone or testosterone. Knowledge of this derivative relationship provides the basis for the classification of the synthetic progestins. The synthetic progestin steroids most often encountered include 17-hydroxyprogesterone, medroxyprogesterone (Provera), medroxyprogesterone acetate, megestrol acetate (Megace), norethindrone, norethindrone enanthate, norethindrone acetate, norethynodrel, norgestrol, desogestrel, and gestodene. In view of their importance in contraception as well as their therapeutic use in the climacteric and neoplastic disease, new synthetic progestational compounds are under continued development and evaluation.

Progesterone may be either administered intramuscularly or taken orally. Oral progesterone, however, as noted above, is associated with relatively poor bioavailability when compared to intramuscular administration of progesterone. The issue of bio-availability with oral agents has been overcome with some of the synthetic progestins, but at the cost of adverse effects on plasma lipid levels (66), and alternate administration routes have been sought (17). Medroxyprogesterone given as a single intramuscular injection of 25 to 50 mg shows an effect on estrogen-stimulated endometrium for just over 2 weeks, although increases in basal body temperature from such treatment may last 6 weeks or more. Depo-Provera has a period of action which is considerably longer. Oral medroxyprogesterone and oral megestrol acetate are well-absorbed. Medroxyprogesterone produces a luteal effect in anovulatory patients with an oral dose of 5 mg daily for 5 days. A dose of 5 to 10 mg/day for 5 days is typically recommended for anovulatory patients and in programs of cyclic estrogen-progesterone therapy for the climacteric.

The 19-norsteroid, RU 486 is a true antiprogesterone. This compound is effectively absorbed orally and appears to bind to the progesterone receptor with high affinity. RU 486 also has significant antiglucocorticoid activity as well as weak anti-androgen activity (7).

Quantitative increases in progesterone receptor concentration in target cells are induced by preovulatory estrogen surges. Target cells are thus primed to respond to the progesterone rise produced by the corpus luteum formed subsequent to ovulation. Loss of the function of the corpus luteum (luteolysis) is associated with a rapid decrease of progesterone and estradiol. Associated with this rapid decrease of progesterone and estrogen, there is disintegration of the endometrium. Since progesterone activity is dependent on intact functional progesterone receptor, one molecular mechanism proposed for RU 486 action is a modulation of PR function. This mechanism suggests that RU 486 facilitates the binding of a heat shock protein (Hsp-90) to the PR as a postsynthetic modification (6). The Hsp-90 when bound to the PR keeps it in an inactive configuration, preventing its interaction with the target genes. Some aspects of the Hsp-90 with hormone receptors will be discussed below under Postsynthetic Modifications.

Effects on bone metabolism, water retention, lipid metabolism and the central nervous system must all be considered in developing treatment strategies using progestins (17, 35, 81).

Progesterone Receptor Function

Progesterone response is dependent on the presence of functionally intact PR. Progestin-induced activity is only initiated when the steroid is bound to the carboxy terminal or progesterone-binding domain (PBD) to induce *trans*-activation at the DBD (76). An absence of hormone response will result from either the absence of the PR or its failure to bind the steroid-binding domain (SBD) and is the usual finding when progestin response is lost (91). Many tumors arising in progestin-responsive tissues which normally demonstrate functional PR lack PR, but there is also evidence of point mutations or total deletions in the SBD of the PR from some neoplasms.

If one considers the complexity of the multilevel controls to include defects at the level of recognition of the PRE in the selective transcription of the target gene heterogeneous nuclear RNA (hnRNA) (50), processing of this (mRNA) (91), transport from the nucleus to the cytoplasm of this mRNA (1), and/or modulation of the mRNA half-life (4), there is the potential for multiple defects to account for loss of responsivity to progestins.

Differentiation and Receptor Activation

Two Progesterone Receptors

In humans, PR is composed of two hormone-binding proteins, A and B. PR-B is slightly larger than PR-A (22). Both are synthesized from a single mRNA, where the PR-A corresponds to the smaller amino-terminally truncated form of the PR-B that is cleaved at an internal methionine residue. The amino terminal of PR specifies target gene activity. There appears to be a functional difference between PR-A and PR-B in the transcriptional activation of target genes.

Progesterone Receptor Synthesis

In breast epithelial tissue, differentiation is dependent on the synthesis and activation of both PR and estrogen receptor (ER). The synthesis of either PR or ER requires both a specific signal response and a permissive chromosomal configuration in the region of the steroid receptor gene. This permissive state requires that a number of nuclear events have occurred, including the synthesis of *trans*-activating nuclear proteins; demethylation of the DNA, estrogen modulation of PR, and postsynthetic modification of a number of specific nuclear proteins (78). PR and ER activation then are not only dependent on receptor synthesis and ligand-binding affinity but equally dependent on associations with at least five additional proteins, including a 45kd and a 35kd protein and two classes of tsps.

Modulation of Receptor Activity

The progesterone response mediated by *trans*-activated PR represents critical interactions with chromatin and its complement of associated proteins. Most abundant among these are the histones (40, 49, 83) and the HMG1 and HMG2 chromosomal proteins (14) which have been shown to interact directly with steroid receptors. These proteins are postsynthetically modified by both histone kinases and acetylases (60).

PR not only functions in its binding to *cis*-activating PRE elements at the 5′ upstream DNA sequences of a number of progesterone-responsive genes, it also has the capacity to function as a down-regulator of the synthesis of other HRs (e.g., ER) (62, 72). PR should be considered a target gene for estrogen response in that a functional ER is required to up-regulate the synthesis of PR (33). This mechanism may also account for the modulation of PR synthesis in response to glucocorticoid (61, 65, 86) modulating the binding affinity of PREs on PR target genes.

Postsynthetic modifications involve both subtle alterations in the PR structure and as *cis*- and *trans*-acting factors. Modifications include (*a*) phosphorylation and acetylation of chromosomal proteins such as histones HMG1 and HMG2; (*b*) postsynthetic modification of the binding of heat-shock proteins to PR; and (*c*) the phosphorylation of both of these proteins. In addition to the multiple *cis*-activating components described for HRE, *trans*-acting elements are also required for RNA transcription that is critical for the hormone response (21).

HORMONE AND DNA-BINDING RESIDUE STRUCTURE AND SEQUENCE

Progesterone Receptor as a Member of the Superfamily of Receptor Proteins

The superfamily of receptor proteins that interact with many lipophilic ligands have a number of features in common with PR (36). Early studies using proteolytic digestion of progesterone receptor proteins demonstrated a loss of DNA binding in spite of retention of the specific ligand binding (39). These proteolytic receptor digests were referred to as "mero receptor" fragments (39).

A number of highly conserved regions for the receptor protein genes have been observed through cloning of receptor proteins (30, 44, 87). The structures of the receptor proteins for progesterone (21, 26) estrogen (51, 55, 85), and glucocorticoid (86) show a striking homology with other hydrophobic signal proteins, including thyroid receptor, retinoic acid receptors, and vitamin D3 receptor (21, 88).

Structure of the DNA-Binding Domain

The DBD of all of the receptors that are known to respond to lipophilic signals is defined as a highly conserved sequence. The consensus sequence cores involved in DNA binding are composed of approximately 70 amino acids that include nine perfectly conserved cysteines. There are two zinc fingers, each of which has one zinc coordinated with four cysteines. One of these fingers appears to be involved in dimer formation, and the other is needed for recognition of PREs of the DNA of progesterone-responsive genes in a complex series of reactions (24, 28, 30, 37, 59, 68, 69). *Trans*-activation appears to be a positive modification that unmasks the DBD (42). Steroid receptors function as dimers, with one of the fingers interacting in the wide DNA groove while the other maintains the dimer configuration.

Progesterone-Responsive Elements and Target Genes

The DNA-binding mechanism of the PR resembles that of other steroid receptors. Therefore, the ability to discriminate between different HRE must depend on a limited number of subtle postsynthetic modifications or the presence of *trans*-acting elements. Perturbation of the amino acid sequence, postsynthetic modification of the amino acid sequence, interaction with other proteins, deletion or mutations in the PRE, changes in the open configuration of the chromatin, or ligand competition will alter the delicate balance that determines the affinity or specificity of DNA binding. Target genes can have at least two HREs with competitive binding for more than one type of activated receptor such as the competitive binding of ER and GR (30). The PREs of hormone-responsive genes must be maintained in an open chromatin configuration and are located 5′ to the DNA-promoter region of the progesterone-responsive genes.

Receptor Protein–Target Gene Interactions

PR is likely similar to GR where GR protein binds as a dimer to the DNA glucocorticoid-responsive elements (GREs). Definition of the mechanism of HR enhancer element interaction is primarily based on observations using solution nuclear magnetic resonance spectroscopy (NMR) and distance geometry (42). Specific amino acid residues are critical in the interaction of protein with DNA GRE elements and in dimer formation. (Figure 75.1). Protein-protein contacts appear to be essential for dimer formation and are likely to involve a segment of the receptor that is important for its co-operativity. This provides a plausible mechanism by which a limited, subtle conformational distortion of amino acid residues at one end of the receptor in the ligand-binding region could exert such a profound effect on the DBD. PR is a member of the HR superfamily and the mechanism of dimer formation is likely to resemble that of GR. For the GR, one of the zinc fingers is involved in dimer formation; the other (42) in the specificity of gene recognition and activation (Figure 75.1).

Intracellular Localization and Postsynthetic Modifications

Progesterone is a hydrophobic signal, and, so, is unrestricted by plasma or nuclear membranes, being free to diffuse through membranes to interact with specific proteins which are confined to humans. Whereas it is clear that the specificity attained by hydrophilic signals is dependent on its interaction with cell surface receptors, the precise intracellular localization of all hydrophobic steroid molecules is unresolved. The use of antireceptor antibodies to PR and ER demonstrates these proteins in the nucleus, whereas immunoreactive GR in the absence of ligand are found in the cytoplasm. All steroid receptors after complexing with their specific ligands are detected only in the nucleus. The presence of the specific ligand is a primary signal for nuclear translocation.

Prior to hormone activation, when receptors are isolated under low ionic conditions, steroids form large oligomeric complexes. Being large complexes, these receptors lack the capacity to bind DNA. Oligomers appear to be complexed with a specific protein detected immunologically as a 90-kd heat shock protein (Hsp-90). When the Hsp-90 is complexed to the PR, DNA binding is prevented. Hsp-90 binds as a dimer at the carboxy terminal of a single PR molecule. The Hsp dimer–PR complex may maintain an inactive configuration in the absence of progesterone. Such postsynthetic modifications function to modify both the initial activation of PR, the hormone receptor, and secondary hormone receptor–HRE interactions. Many of the enzymes involved in these postsynthetic modifications are also under hormone control. These include, for example, Hsps (5, 10, 34, 67, 71, 87), kinases (89), and RNA transcription factors (8).

Clinical Observations on Progestin Receptor– and Target Tissue Response to Progestins

Progesterone is associated with a number of biologic activities: a critical role in the support of the products of conception; the differentiation of the endometrium and the promotion of the secretory phase of the endometrium following the estrogen-induced proliferative phase; maturation and cornification of the vaginal mucosal epithelium; suppression of ovulation; inhibition of gonadotropin release; proliferation of breast epithelium; secretory activity in breast epithelium; and a natriuretic effect on the kidneys. A number of these biologic effects of progesterone are seen only in concert with priming of the target tissues with estrogen, whereas other effects appear to be interrelated with the actions of other steroid hormones, peptide hormones and/or growth factors. Both progesterone and estrogen influence the response when superpharmacologic doses are used. Possible interactions between progesterone, estrogen, and growth factors must be taken into account when constructing treatment strategies.

UTERUS

Normal Uterus

The cyclic response of the uterus to estrogen and progesterone is among the best-studied examples of hormonal modulation of tissue response. There is clear evidence for cyclic regulation of ER and PR proteins in the endometrial epithelium, the myometrium, and the endometrial stroma. The induction of PR by estrogen has been shown both in vitro and in vivo. An increase in PR at the end of the proliferative phase of the menstrual cycle occurs in the stromal/myometrial tissue 24 to 48 hr before the observed peak of PR levels in endometrial epithelial tissue (52). This cyclic change can be aborted by the administration of 10 mg of Provera for 5 to 10 days, associated with regression of the epithelium. Epithelial hyperplasia of the uterus exposed to

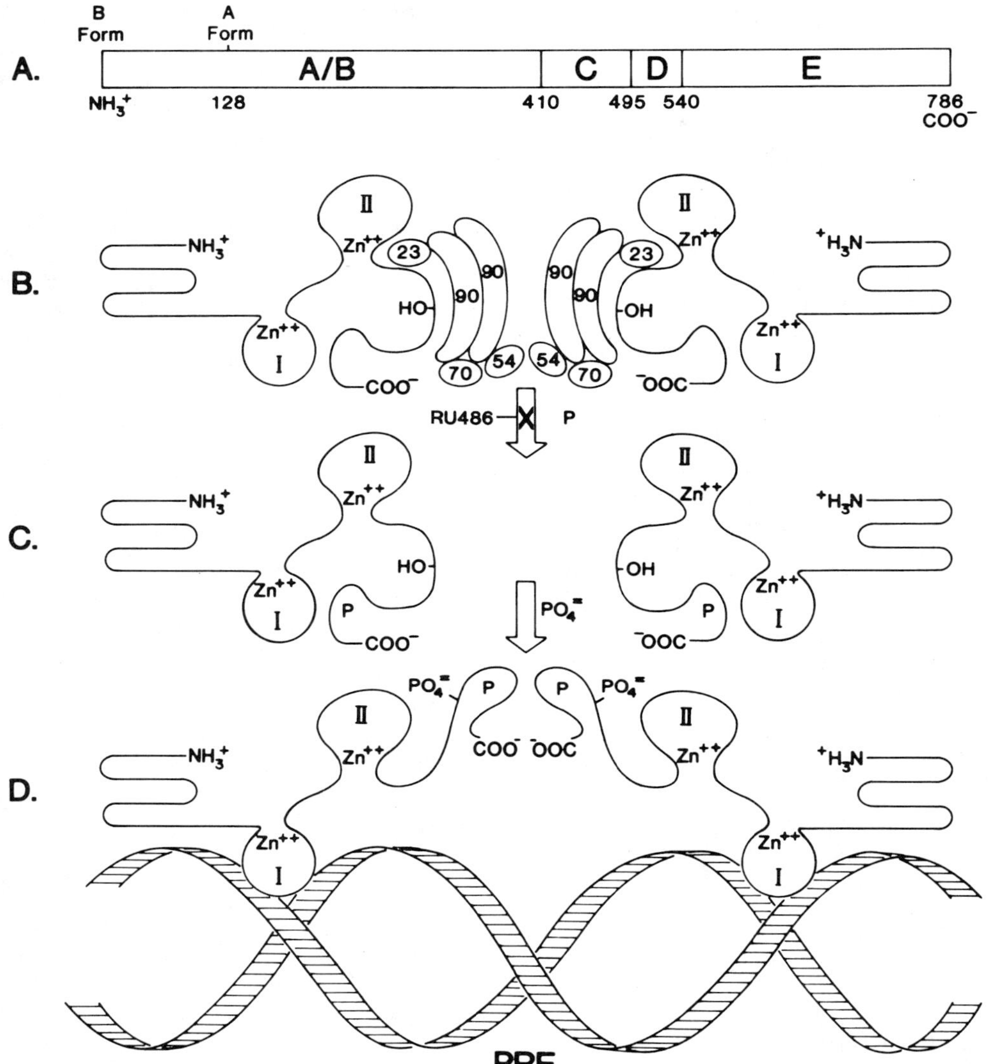

Figure 75.1. **A.** Linear amino acid sequence of progesterone receptor illustrating relation of functional domains. PR-B is composed of a total of 786 amino acids. PR-A consists of 658 amino acids representing a truncated form of the PR lacking 128 amino acids of the amino terminal of PR-B. Both PR-B and its truncated form, PR-A, are synthesized from the same mRNA as described in the text. A/B domain extends from the amino-terminal end to amino acid residue 410 and functions in tissue-cell specificity. C domain (residues 410 to 495) function as the DNA binding domain (DBD) required for recognition of the target gene progesterone responsive elements (PRE). D domain (residues 495 to 540) is often referred to as the "hinge" region to designate its functional interaction with heat shock protein (Hsp 90) and other proteins 23, 70, and 54. The function of the E domain or steroid-binding domain (SBD) (residues 540 to 786) is to bind PR and trans-activate the DBD. **B–D.** PR interaction with target gene PRE and DNA elements. Inactive form of the PR sediments is an inactive 8S complex, composed of Hsp-90 dimer, Hsp-70, and at least two other proteins of 23 and 70 kd. The present concept suggests that, in the absence of progesterone (P), the Hsp-90 dimer is associated with the D domain or hinge region. The function of this complex is to maintain the PR in its inactive configuration. The binding of P in the hinge or E domain induces the release of the Hsp-90 dimer (and possibly the 23, 70, and 54) as the first step in the *trans*-activation of the C region or DBD domain (**B**). When progesterone antagonist as RU486 binds to the SBD the Hsp-90 dimer fails to be released from the hinge region D and the inactive 8S PR complex fails to become *trans*-activated to the 4S PR configuration **C** and **D**. Evidence also implicates phosphorylation as an essential final step of *trans*-activation of the DBD. As diagramed in **D**, the progesterone bound *trans*-activated PR requires phosphorylation to assume its function as a protein–DNA–PRE complex. In its active configuration, the PR is maintained as a dimer, with the zinc finger region (I) interacting through a charge interaction with the DNA of the PRE in the major groove. The second zinc finger (II) appears to function to stabilize the PR dimer configuration, as described in the text.

progestins first shows acanthomatous changes (a change wherein the cells resemble squamous cells) followed by secretory differentiation and finally regression of the hyperplastic change with eventual atrophy after 10 to 14 days.

Uterine Carcinoma

Uterine carcinoma is a localized disease in the majority of cases. In clinical practice, there is an increased incidence of adenocarcinoma of the uterus when a woman is given unopposed estrogen in physiologic doses and this increased frequency is significantly reduced if progestins are also given. Progestins can be given for the last 10 days of the estrogen replacement cycle or at a lower dose throughout the cycle.

When diagnosed, adenocarcinoma of the uterus is cured by local therapy in 80% of cases. In the event of recurrence, exogenous progestin is an effective treatment in a significant fraction of cases: more than 30% of patients with recurrent disease demonstrate objective response to exogenous progestins. ER and PR can be measured in these tumors, and the presence of these receptors correlates with differentiation of the tumor, prognosis for the patient, and response to progestins. The duration of response is not predicted by the presence of receptor and varies from months to years. Tumors that lack ER and PR respond objectively to progestins in fewer than 10% of cases. Tumors that have been treated with radiotherapy have a greater tendency to be progesterone receptor negative than tumors that have not been treated with radiation. Because of the low toxicity of progestins, a trial of progestin therapy is often warranted, even if receptors have not been measured in the tumor or appear to be absent in recurrent or inoperable endometrial carcinoma.

The effective use of progestins in treating endometrial hyperplasia associated with "unopposed" estrogen and in patients with receptor-rich well-differentiated adenocarcinomas further supports the role of progestins in suppressing proliferation of the endometrium. The use of hormone therapy has readily demonstrable effects on endometrial histology (25).

Other Neoplasms of the Uterus

Pharmacologic progestin has a clearly beneficial effect on uterine leiomyomas, and significant levels of PR have been demonstrated in these proliferations of mesenchymal origin (54). Uterine sarcomas, including stromal sarcomas and leiomyosarcomas, have a variable response to progesterone (48). PR is not consistently observed in these tumors.

PR has been reported in some studies of squamous carcinoma of the uterine cervix (up to 41% of tumors) (45). Cervical epithelial maturation was correlated with progesterone secretion (ovulation). PR was not found in the majority of tumors in other studies, and no firm evidence for clinical or histologic correlation of the presence of PR has been shown (20).

BREAST

Normal Breast

Progestin response in the human breast is complex and influences both proliferation and differentiated function. The luteal phase of the menstrual cycle (progesterone dominant) is characterized both by active secretion and by the peak of proliferative activity in the normal breast (56). Epidemiologic data appear to implicate progestins in proliferative disorders and cancers of the breast in a more direct fashion than had been previously thought (56). It has been recognized from the earliest studies of ER and PR in breast epithelial systems that progesterone action, mediated through PR, resulted in down-regulation of the ER in breast epithelium. This observation suggested that the influence of estrogen would be to stimulate proliferation of the breast epithelium and that the effect of progesterone might be to inhibit proliferation, similar to the effect seen in the uterus. While the effect on regulation of ER appears to be similar, the effect of progestins—and specifically progesterone in physiologic amounts—is not similar. The assumption that progestins will act to reduce "estrogen-associated" proliferative change does not appear to be valid. This must be considered in recommending sex steroid replacement therapy in the climacteric. Thought should be given to the fact that adding progestin to estrogen replacement therapy does not reduce the risk of breast cancer and may actually increase it. Three factors support this consideration: (*a*) ovarian hormones are critical to breast cancer risk; (*b*) inclusion of progestin in combination oral contraceptive pills does not effectively oppose the risk of cancer; and (*c*) in women who have had surgical oophorectomy, even daily unopposed conjugated estrogens in a dose of 1.25 mg does not produce risk comparable to that associated with prolonged years of "normal" menstrual cycles or with replacement therapy with estrogen and progestin in the climacteric.

Breast Cancer

PRs have been studied extensively in cancerous human breast tissue. Patients whose tumors are PR positive have a higher probability of responding to endocrine therapy (not necessarily progestins) and in most series show a somewhat better prognosis, with respect to both survival and disease-free interval (11). Considerable controversy exists with respect to the effect of menstrual cycle phase at surgery on the evaluation of tissue for receptor, as well as to whether there is an effect of this timing on prognosis (9, 58, 63). PR, in contrast to ER, does not show increasing levels with increasing age of the population studied (57).

Progestin therapy for metastatic breast cancer has been used principally as a second-line therapy following tamoxifen. The principal progestin used has been megestrol acetate. The response of metastatic breast cancer to megestrol is predicted by the presence of ER and/or PR, but is best predicted by the observation of objective response to prior hormonal therapy (73). One of the more interesting aspects of progestin therapy for metastatic breast cancer is the observation of a dose-response increase in efficacy. Patients who have relapsed or progressed on conventional therapeutic doses of medroxyprogesterone (100 to 200 mg per day) or megestrol (160 mg per day) may show additional response with increased dose (to 2,000 mg per day for medroxyprogesterone or to 1,600 mg per day for megestrol). A beneficial side effect of the progestin is increased appetite and weight gain, although some of the weight gain can be associated with fluid retention (2). The mechanism of the increased appetite and actual weight gain is poorly understood, although this property of appetite enhancement has been used clinically to treat cancer-associated anorexia and cachexia. There are a number of other central nervous system effects of progestins which have been characterized, including beneficial effects on climacteric symptoms (53).

Other Tumors of the Breast

Progesterone receptors have been reported in fibroadenomas, cystosarcoma phylloides, and breast sarcomas. There is no convincing evidence for a biologic response to progestin manipulation of either cystosarcoma phylloides or stromal sarcoma of the breast.

OVARY

Epidemiologic data have shown an effect on the incidence of ovarian epithelial carcinoma in patients who have used estrogen-progesterone preparations to inhibit ovulation (80). PR is observed in 30 to 40% of ovarian carcinomas (43). While some studies have observed a trend toward better survival in patients with PR-positive carcinomas (38) no convincing data to indicate objective response to progestin therapy have been reported.

OTHER TISSUES

PR and response to progestins have been reported in meningiomas, pulmonary lymphangioleiomyomatosis, renal cell carcinomas, and squamous cell carcinoma of the head and neck. The presence of PRs in meningiomas is consistently observed and in some trials a response to progestin has been observed (41). In squamous cell carcinoma of the head and neck the presence of progestin receptors has been detected, but in these tumors, as in renal cell carcinoma, objective response to progestin treatment has not been observed (12). In contrast, progestin therapy has become a mainstay in the treatment of pulmonary lymphangioleiomyomatosis, which was a uniformly fatal condition before progestin-hormonal therapy was shown to be effective (13). In patients whose pulmonary lymphangiomyomatosis is treated early in the course of the disease, before extensive chylous effusion is present, objective response to continued progesterone therapy is noted in the majority of patients. This response continues only so long as the progestin is continued. Responses of greater than 5 years have been observed, although in some patients the disease progresses after a period of remission, despite continued progesterone.

Conclusion

Progesterone and the various synthetic progestins have a role in the treatment of a number of neoplasms, in particular tumors of the endometrium and breast. Study of the biochemistry of the PR and the cellular mechanisms of progesterone action are prototypes for the study of the sex steroid hormone receptors. Further such studies are prerequisite to understanding the relationship of these hormones to development, differentiation, and neoplasia in their target tissues.

References

1. Anderson T, Howell A, Williams G. Oral contraceptive use increases proliferation and decreases oestrogen receptor content of epithelial cells in the normal human breast. Int J Cancer 1991;48:206–210.
2. Aisner J, Simon T, Moody M, Tait N. High-dose megestrol acetate for the treatment of advanced breast cancer: dose and toxicities. Semin Hematol 1987;24:48.
3. Bagchi MK, Elliston JF, Tsai SY, Edwards DP, Tsai MJ, O'Malley BW. Steroid hormone–dependent interaction of human progesterone receptor with its target enhancer element. Mol Endocrinol 1988;2:1221.
4. Bagchi MK, Tsai SY, Weigel NL, Tsai MJ, O'Malley BW. Regulation of in vitro transcription by progesterone receptor characterization and kinetic studies. J Biol Chem 1990;265:5129.
5. Baulieu EE. RU486 (an anti-steroid hormone) receptor structure and heat shock protein mol. wt 90,000 (hsp 90). Hum Reprod 1988;3:541.
6. Baulieu EE. A novel approach to human fertility control: contragestion by the anti-progesterone RU 486. Eur J Obstet Gynecol Reprod Biol 1988;28:125.
7. Baulieu EE. Contragestion and other clinical applications of RU 486, an antiprogesterone at the receptor. Science 1989;245:1351.
8. Bautz KF, Petersen G. Eukaryotic RNA polymerases. In Molecular Biology of Chromosome Function. Edited by KW Adolph. New York: Springer-Verlag, 1989, pp 157–206.
9. Bawde RA, Gregory WM, Chaudary MA, et al. Timing of surgery during the menstrual cycle and survival of premenopausal women with operable breast cancer. Lancet 1991;337:1261–1264.
10. Ben-Ze'ev A, Amsterdam A. Regulation of heat shock protein synthesis by gonadotropins in cultured granulosa cells. Endocrinology 1989;124:2584.
11. Benner SE, Clark GM, McGuire WL. Steroid receptors, cellular kinetics, and lymph node status as prognostic factors in breast cancer. Am J Med Sci 1988;296:59.
12. Berg NJ, Colvard DS, Neel HB III, Weiland LH, Spelsberg TC. Progesterone receptors in carcinomas of the upper aerodigestive tract. Laryngol. Head Neck Surgery 1989;101:527.
13. Berger U, Khaghani A, Pomerance A, Yacoub MH, Coombes RC. Pulmonary lymphangioleiomyomatosis and steroid RE receptors. An immunocytochemical study. Am J Clin Pathol 1990;93:609.
14. Bernues J, Querol E. Non-random reconstitution of HMG1 and HMG2 in chromatin. Determination of the histone contacts. Biochim Biophys Acta 1989;1008:52.
15. Bocquel MT, Kumar V, Stricker C, Chambon P, Gronemeyer H. The contribution of the N- and C-terminal regions of steroid receptors to activation of transcription is both receptor and cell-specific. Nucleic Acids Res 1989;17:2581.
16. Brinton LA, Hoover RN. Estrogen replacement therapy and endometrial cancer risk. Unresolved issues. Obstet Gynecol 1993;81:265–271.
17. Crook D, Crust MP, Gangar, KF et al. Comparison of transdermal and oral estrogen-progestin replacement therapy: effects on serum lipids and lipoproteins. Am J Obstet Gynecol 1992;166:950–955.
18. Carson-Jurica MA, Schrader WT, O'Malley BW. Steroid receptor family: structure and functions. Endocr Rev 1990;11:201.
19. Chilton BS, Mani SK, Bullock DW. Servomechanism of prolactin and progesterone in regulating uterine gene expression. Mol Endocrinol 1988;2:1169.
20. Ciocca DR, Puy LA, Fasoli LC. Study of estrogen receptor, progesterone receptor, and the estrogen-regulated mr 24,000 protein in patients with carcinomas of the endometrium and cervix. Cancer Res 1989;49:4298.
21. Conneely OM, Dobson AD, Carson MA, Maxwell BL, Tsai MJ, Schrader WT, O'Malley BW. Structure-function relationships of the chicken progesterone receptor. Biochem Soc Trans 1988;16:683.
22. Conneely OM, Kettelberger DM, Tsai MJ, Schrader WT, O'Malley BW. The chicken progesterone receptor A and B isoforms are products of an alternate translation initiation event. J Biol Chem 1989;264:14062.
23. Dean DC, Knoll BJ, Riser ME, O'Malley BW. A 5′-flanking sequence essential for progesterone regulation of an ovalbumin fusion gene. Nature 1983;305:551.
24. Dobson AD, Conneely OM, Beattie W, Maxwell BL, Mak P, Tsai MJ, Schrader WT, O'-Malley BW. Mutational analysis of the chicken progesterone receptor. J Biol Chem 1989;264:4207.
25. Deligdisch L. Effects of hormone therapy on the endometrium. Mod Pathol 1993;6: 94–106.
26. Dufrene L, Pageaux JF, Fanidi A, Renoir JM, Laugier C, Baulieu EE. Biochemical characterization and subunit structure of quail oviduct progesterone receptor. J Steroid Biochem 1989;32:703.
27. Eilers M, Picard D, Yamamoto KR, Bishop JM. Chimaeras of myc oncoprotein and steroid receptors cause hormone-dependent transformation of cells foundation. Nature 1989;340:66.
28. Eul J, Meyer ME, Tora L, Bocquel MT, Quirin-Stricker C, Chambon P, Gronemeyer H. Expression of active hormone and DNA-binding domains of the chicken progesterone receptor in *E. coli*. EMBO J 1989;8:83.
29. Evans RM, Hollenberg SM. Cooperative and positional independent trans-activation domains of the human glucocorticoid receptor. Cold Spring Harbor Symp Quant Biol 1988;53:813.
30. Evans RM, Hollenberg SM. Zinc fingers: gilt by association. Cell 1988;52:1.
31. Fink KL, Wieben ED, Woloschak GE, Spelsberg TC. Rapid regulation of c-myc protooncogene expression by progesterone in the avian oviduct. Proc Natl Acad Sci USA 1988;85:1796.
32. Freedman LP, Yoshinaga SK, Vanderbilt JN, Yamamoto KR. In vitro transcription enhancement by purified derivatives of the glucocorticoid receptor. Science 1989;245: 298.
33. Gasc JM, Baulieu EE. Regulation by estradiol of the progesterone receptor in the hypothalamus and pituitary: an immunohistochemical study in the chicken. Endocrinology 1988;122:1357.
34. Gasc JM, Renoir JM, Faber LE, Delahaye F, Baulieu EE. Nuclear localization of two steroid receptor-associated proteins, hsp90 and p59. Exp Cell Res 1990;186:362.

35. Grady D, Rubin SM, Petitti DB, et al. Hormone therapy to prevent disease and prolong life in postmenopausal women. Ann Intern Med 1992;117:1016–1021.
36. Green S, Chambon P. A superfamily of potentially oncogenic hormone receptors. Nature 1986;324:615.
37. Green S, Chambon P. Oestradiol induction of a glucocorticoid-responsive gene by a chimaeric receptor. Nature 1987;325:75.
38. Green S, Chambon P. Nuclear receptors enhance our understanding of transcription regulation. TIG 1988;4:309.
39. Gronemeyer H. The chicken progesterone receptor. In Affinity Labelling and Cloning of Steroid and Thyroid Hormone Receptors. Edited by H Gronemeyer. Ellis Horwood, 1988, pp 55–67.
40. Grunstein M, Han M, Kim U, Schuster T, Kayne P. Histone and nucleosome function in yeast. In Molecular Biology of Chromosome Function. Edited by KW Adolph. New York: Springer-Verlag, 1989, pp 347–365.
41. Halper J, Colvard DS, Scheithauer BW, Jiang NS, Press MF, Graham ML, Riehl E, Laws ER, Spelsberg TC. Estrogen and progesterone receptors in meningiomas: comparison of nuclear binding, dextran-coated charcoal and immunoperoxidase staining assays. Neurosurgery 1989;25:546.
42. Hard T, Kellenbach E, Boelens R, Maler BA, Dahlman K, Freedman L, Carlstedt-Duke J, Yamamoto KR, Gustafsson J, Kaptein R. Solution structure of the glucocorticord receptor DNA-binding domain. Science 1990;249:157.
43. Harding M, Cowan S, Hole D, Cassidy L, Kitchener H, Davis J, Leake R. Estrogen and progesterone receptors in ovarian cancer. Cancer 1990;65:486.
44. Horwitz KB, Francis MD, Weill. Hormone dependent covalent modification and processing of human progesterone receptors in the nucleus. DNA 1985;4:451–460.
45. Hunter RE, Longcope C, Keough P. Steroid hormone receptors in carcinoma of the cervix. Cancer 1987;60:392.
46. Isola JJ. Distribution of estrogen and progesterone receptors and steroid-regulated gene products in the chick oviduct. Mol Cell Endocrinol 1990;69:235.
47. Kastner P, Krust A, Turcotte B, Stropp U, Tora L, Gronemeyer H, Chambon P. Two distinct estrogen-regulated promoters generate transcripts encoding the two functionally different human progesterone receptor forms A and B. EMBO J 1990;9:1603.
48. Keen CE, Philip G. Progestin-induced regression in low-grade endometrial stromal sarcoma. Case report and literature review. Br J Obstet Gynaecol 1989;96:1435.
49. Kelner DN, McCarty KS Sr. Porcine liver nuclear histone acetyltransferase: partial purification and basic properties. J Biol Chem 1984;259:3413.
50. Klein-Hitpass L, Tsai SY, Weigel NL, Allan GF, Riley D, Rodriguez R, Schrader WT, Tsai MJ, O'Malley BW. The progesterone receptor stimulates cell-free transcription by enhancing the formation of a stable preinitiation complex. Cell 1990;60:247.
51. Kumar V, Green S, Stack G, Berry M, Jin JR, Chambon P. Functional domains of the human estrogen receptor. Cell 1987;51:941.
52. Lessey BA, Metzger DA, Haney AF, McCarty KS Jr. Immunohistochemical analysis of estrogen and progesterone receptor in endometriosis: comparison with normal endometrium during the menstrual cycle and the effect of medical therapy. Fertil Steril 1989;51:409.
53. Lobo RA, Gibbons WE. The role of progestin therapy in breast disease and central nervous system function. J Reprod Med 1982;27:515.
54. Maheux R. Treatment of uterine leiomyomata: past, present and future. Hormone Res 1989;32:125.
55. Maxwell BL, McDonnell DP, Conneely OM, Schulz TZ, Greene GL, O'Malley BW. Structural organization and regulation of the chicken estrogen receptor. Mol Endocrinol 1987;1:25.
56. McCarty KS Jr. Proliferative stimuli in the normal breast: estrogens or progestins. Hum Pathol 1989;20:1137.
57. McCarty KS Jr, Silva JS, Cox EB, Leight GS Jr, Wells SA, McCarty KS Sr. Relationship of age and menopausal status to estrogen receptor content in primary carcinoma of the breast. Ann Surg 1983;197:123.
58. McGuire WL, Hilsenbeck S, Clark GM. Optimal mastectomy timing. JNCI 1992;84: 346–348.
59. Miesfeld RL. The structure and function of steroid receptor proteins. Crit Rev Biochem Mol Biol 1989;24:101.
60. Mold DE, McCarty KS Sr. A chinese hamster ovary cell histone deacetylase that is associated with a unique class of mononucleosomes. Biochemistry 1987;26:8257.
61. Moore DD. Promiscuous behaviour in the steroid hormone receptor superfamily. Trends Neurosci 1989;12:165.
62. Nardulli AM, Greene GL, O'Malley BW, Katzenellenbogen BS. Regulation of progesterone receptor messenger ribonucleic acid and protein levels in mcf-7 cells by estradiol: analysis of estrogen's effect on progesterone receptor synthesis and degradation. Endocrinology 1988;122:935.
63. Nathan B, Bates T, Anbazhagan R, et al. Timing of surgery for breast cancer in relation to the menstrual cycle and survival of premenopausal women. Br J Surg 1993;80:43.
64. O'Malley BW. The steroid receptor superfamily: more excitement predicted for the future. Mol Endocrinol 1990;4:353.
65. Oro AE, Hollenberg SM, Evans RM. Transcriptional inhibition by a glucocorticoid receptor-beta-galactosidase fusion protein studies. Cell 1988;55:1109.
66. Ottosson UB, Johansson BG, Shultz B. Subfraction of high density lipoprotein cholesterol during estrogen replacement therapy: a comparison between progestin and natural progesterone. Am J Obstet Gynecol 1985;6:746.
67. Picard D, Salser SJ, Yamamoto KR. A movable and regulable inactivation function within the steroid binding domain of the glucocorticoid receptor. Cell 1988;54:1073.
68. Pinney KG, Carlson KE, Katzenellenbogen JA. A high affinity ligand and novel photoaffinity labeling reagent for the progesterone receptor. J Steroid Biochem 1990;35: 179.
69. Power RF, Conneely OM, McDonnell DP, Clark JH, Butt TR, Schrader WT, O'Malley BW. High level expression of a truncated chicken progesterone receptor in Escherichia coli. J Biol Chem 1990;265:1419.
70. Pratt WB, Jolly DJ, Pratt DV, Hollenberg SM, Giguere V, Cadepond FM, Schweizer-Groyer G, Catelli MG, Evans RM, Baulieu EE. A region in the steroid binding domain determines formation of the non-DNA-binding, 9 S glucocorticoid receptor complex. J Biol Chem 1988;263:267.
71. Pratt WB, Redmond T, Sanchez ER, Bresnick EH, Meshinchi S, Welsh MJ. Speculations on the role of the 90 kDa heat shock protein in glucocorticoid receptor transport and function. In The Steroid/Thyroid Hormone Receptor Family and Gene Regulation. Edited by J Carlstedt-Duke, H Eriksson, and JA Gustafsson. Basel: Birkhauser Verlag, 1989, pp 109–126.
72. Ree AH, Landmark BF, Eskild W, Levy FO, Lahooti H, Jahnsen T, Aakvaag A, Hansson V. Autologous down-regulation of messenger ribonucleic acid protein levels for estrogen receptors in MCF-7 cells: an inverse correlation to progesterone receptor levels. Endocrinology 1989;124:2577.
73. Robertson, JFR, Williams MR, Todd J, Nicholson RI, Morgan DAI, Blamey RW. Factors predicting the response of patients with advanced breast cancer to endocrine (megace) therapy. Eur J Clin Oncol 1989;25:469.
74. Rye PD, Walker RA. Analysis of glycoproteins released from benign and malignant human breast: changes in size and fucosylation with malignancy. Eur J Cancer Clin Oncol 1989;25:65.
75. Slater EP, Cato AC, Karin M, Baxter JD, Beato M. Progesterone induction of metallothionein-IIA gene expression. Mol Endocrinol 1988;2:485.
76. Smanik EJ, Calderon JJ, Muldoon TG, Mahesh VB. Effect of progesterone on the activity of occupied nuclear estrogen receptor in vitro. Mol Biol 1989;64:111.
77. Spelsberg TC, Graham ML, Berg NJ, Umehara T, Riehl E, Coulam CB, Ingle JN. A nuclear binding assay to assess the biological activity of steroid receptors in isolated animal and human tissues. Endocrinology 1987;121:631.
78. Spelsberg TC, Rories C, Rejman JJ, Goldberger A, Fink K, Lau CK, Colvard DS, Wiseman G. Steroid action on gene expression: possible roles of regulatory genes and nuclear acceptor sites. Biol Reprod 1989;40:54.
79. Spicer DV, Pike MC. Sex steroids and breast cancer prevention. JNCI Monogr 1994;16:139–147.
80. Stanford JL, Thomas DB. Depot-medroxyprogesterone acetate (DMPA) and risk of epithelial ovarian cancer. Int J Cancer 1991;49:191–195.
81. Tremollieres F, Pouilles JM, Ribot C. Effect of long-term administration of progestogen on post menopausal bone loss: result of a two-year, controlled randomized study. Clin Endocrinol 1993;38(Oxf):627–631.
82. Tsai SY, Tsai MJ, O'Malley BW. Cooperative binding of steroid hormone receptors contributes to transcriptional synergism at target enhancer elements. Cell 1989;57:443.
83. Ueda K, Isohashi F, Okamoto K, Yoshikawa K, Sakamoto Y. Interaction of rat liver glucocorticoid receptor with histones. Endocrinology 1989;124:1042.
84. Wahli W. Evolution and expression of vitellogenin genes. Trends Genet 1988;4:227.
85. Walter P, Green S, Greene GL, Krust A, Bornert J, Jeltsch J, Staub A, Jensen E, Scrace G, Waterfield M, Chambon P. Cloning of the human estrogen receptor cDNA. Proc Natl Acad Sci USA 1985;82:7889.
86. Webster NJG, Green S, Jin JR, Chambon P. The hormone-binding domains of the estrogen and glucocorticoid receptors contain an inducible transcription activation function. Cell 1988;54:199.
87. Weigel NL, Schrader WT, O'Malley BW. Antibodies to chicken progesterone receptor peptide 523–536 recognize a site exposed in receptor-deoxyribonucleic acid complexes but not in receptor-heat shock protein-90 complexes. Endocrinology 1989;125: 2494.
88. Weinberger C, Bradley DJ. Gene regulation by receptors binding lipid-soluble substances. Ann Rev Physiol 1990;52:823.
89. Williams JA, Schlichter D, Wicks WD. Progesterone decreases DNA binding factor activity and the expression in xenopus oocytes of a cAMP responsive gene from rat liver. Second Messengers Phosphoproteins, 1989;12:261.
90. Yamamoto KR, Godowski PJ, Picard D. Ligand-regulated nonspecific inactivation of receptor function: a versatile mechanism for signal transduction. Cold Spring Harbor Symp Quant Biol 1988;53:803.
91. Zeitlin S, Parent A, Silverstein S, Efstratiadis A. Pre-mRNA splicing and the nuclear matrix. Mol Cell Biol 1987;7:111.

CHAPTER 76

Androgens and Antiandrogens

NICHOLAS BRUCHOVSKY

Introduction

The collective title for compounds which resemble testosterone in biologic action is the term *androgen*, derived from the Greek *andros*, genitive of *aner* (man) and *gennan* (to produce). The actual isolation and characterization of naturally occurring androgens in the 1930s was the crowning point of a process of observation and discovery which started early in history, when primitive man first became aware of the more obvious effects of removing the testes from animals, not excluding members of his own species. Castration is found in mythology and was a feature of certain religions, used as an instrument of punishment and revenge in many societies, and served to guarantee the supply of eunuchs for guard duty in harems and of male sopranos for the embellishment of sacred and secular music to the end of the 19th century (28, 38, 114). Aristotle was the first to make castration the subject of inquiry, describing its effect in considerable detail and recognizing that the testes were essential for the virility and fertility of an animal (114). The first experimental demonstration that the testes contributed an endocrine factor to the bloodstream was made by John Hunter in 1794, when he showed that the spur of a hen would undergo masculine development if transplanted into the leg of a cock (28). In 1849, Berthold reported that the secondary sexual characteristics of capons could be restored by transplantation of the testes from cocks (12). In 1889, at the age of 72 years, Brown-Sequard gave himself subcutaneous injections of extracts from the testes of dogs and guinea pigs and reported increased bodily and mental vigor, which he correctly hesitated to ascribe to his preparation (28).

The first objective evidence of a hormonal rejuvenating factor was provided by Pezard in 1911, who showed that simple extracts of porcine testes contained active material (28, 38). Two decades later the first androgen, androsterone, was purified from human urine by Butenandt (28, 38). In 1935, David and colleagues isolated an androgenic compound from fresh testicular tissue more potent than androsterone which they named testosterone (28). Shortly thereafter, the synthesis of testosterone from cholesterol by Ruzicka and Wettstein and Butenandt and Hanisch paved the way for the preparation of artificial androgens (28). These achievements were succeeded by a long period of vigorous investigation of many aspects of the production, excretion, relative biological activity, and clinical usefulness of androgenic compounds, including applications to the treatment of breast cancer (113).

Opportunities for studying the molecular action of androgens emerged in the 1960s, when radioactive compounds suitable for experimentation were initially introduced. In 1968, Bruchovsky and Wilson and Anderson and Liao reported that dihydrotestosterone is the active intracellular form of testosterone, and receptors for dihydrotestosterone were demonstrated for the first time (4, 18, 19). Subsequent attempts to purify the androgen receptor met with little or no success; however in 1988, Trapman and colleagues, Chang and colleagues, and Lubahn and colleagues cloned the androgen receptor complementary DNA and deduced the amino acid sequence of the receptor protein (30, 74, 124). Not only did these results confirm that the androgen receptor belongs to a superfamily of regulatory thyroid- and steroid-binding proteins, but also they set the stage for the discovery of numerous mutations in the androgen receptor gene which give rise to disorders of male sexual differentiation (88). Additionally, the identification of point mutations affecting the androgen receptor in malignant prostate cells drew attention to possible new mechanisms of tumor progression and androgen independence (47, 120).

With the development of bioassays to measure androgenic activity, a large number of compounds with inhibitory action were found. In 1962, Dorfman suggested that substances with antiandrogenic activity might be useful in the treatment of hirsutism and androgen-dependent prostatic tumors (39). Two years later, Lerner formalized the concept of hormone inhibition, specifying that "an antagonist is a compound that inhibits the activity of a hormone at one or more sites without regard to the route of administration or the dose employed," and noted that antiandrogenic substances might be employed clinically to alleviate a number of pathologic conditions (71). In the next decade, the prototype antiandrogens cyproterone acetate (81) and flutamide (79) were synthesized and, as predicted, have been successfully applied to the treatment of a variety of androgen-dependent conditions.

Androgens

MECHANISM OF ACTION

The basic steps of androgen action on a target cell are outlined in Figure 76.1. In the blood, testosterone, the principal male sex hormone secreted by the testes, circulates in association with two major plasma proteins, sex hormone-

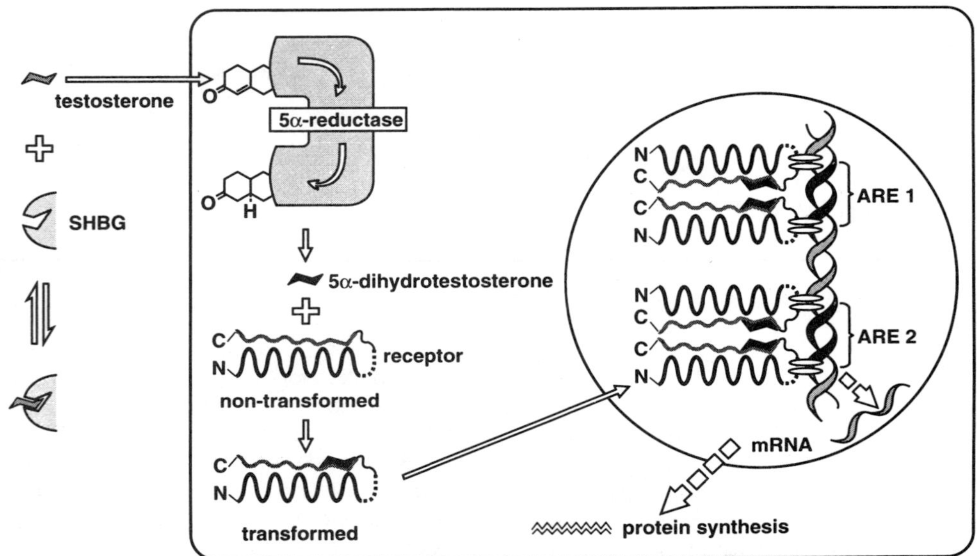

Figure 76.1. Mechanism of action of androgens.

binding globulin (SHBG) and albumin (41). Under equilibrium conditions, only 2% of the testosterone is unbound and available for diffusion into the target cell, where it is immediately converted to dihydrotestosterone by the enzyme 5α-reductase (18). Two isoforms of the enzyme have been identified (5, 83): type 1 is found in skin and prostatic epithelium and, to a lesser extent, in stroma, and type 2 predominates in prostatic stromal tissue. Dihydrotestosterone binds with high affinity and specificity to an androgen-receptor protein in the cytoplasm, causing its dissociation from heat shock proteins (transformation) and subsequent translocation into the target cell nucleus.

The androgen receptor itself is a transcription factor composed of 919 amino acids structurally organized into three major functional domains: a carboxy (C)-terminal steroid-binding domain, an amino (N)-terminal region involved in the activation of transcription, and an intermediate DNA-binding domain. The latter contains nine cysteine amino acids, eight of which contribute to the formation of two zinc finger motifs, each containing a molecule of zinc. The first zinc finger specifies the particular androgen response element located in genomic DNA adjacent to target genes to which the androgen receptor binds. The second zinc finger contains a receptor dimerization region of five amino acids between the first two cysteines. Specific gene activation by androgens depends upon the binding of a homodimer of two androgen receptor molecules to two asymmetric nucleotide sequences of six base pairs separated by a three base pair spacer. The resulting element is an imperfect "palindrome" and there is now evidence that at least two of these (eg., 5′-ATAGCAtctTGTTCT-3′ and 5′-AGTACTccaAGAACC-3′) are required for maximum gene induction by androgens (65). Carried to completion, this complex receptor-DNA–binding reaction triggers a cascade of transcriptional events underlying a given biologic response.

Under physiologic conditions, not only is most of the dihydrotestosterone in the cell concentrated in the nucleus (23), but also, in the presence of dihydrotestosterone, most of the androgen receptor in the cell is nuclear bound. The signal responsible for the nuclear import of the androgen receptor is in the hinge region between the steroid- and the DNA-binding domains and is encoded by two clusters of the basic amino acids, arginine and lysine, joined by a sequence of 10 amino acids (i.e., [n3] RK [n10] RKnKKn (64). Entry of dihydrotestosterone into the nucleus appears to depend largely on a non–receptor-mediated transport process since the accumulation of dihydrotestosterone is 10- to 30-fold greater than that of receptor (23, 24).

Following orchiectomy or equivalent androgen withdrawal therapy the intranuclear concentration of dihydrotestosterone drops by about 90%, and most of the androgen receptor appears to leave the nucleus (102). Although the native androgen receptor possesses a molecular weight of 117 kd, the principal form recovered from the nucleus is a proteolytic fragment with a molecular weight of about 33 kd which lacks the amino terminus but retains the steroid-binding properties of the native receptor (26). As yet, no functional role has been assigned to this fragment.

BIOLOGIC EFFECTS

The androgenic regulation of a target tissue is characterized by three broadly defined responses, as shown in Figure 76.2 for prostate (22). In the presence of androgen, undifferentiated or involuted cells initiate new rounds of DNA synthesis and cell proliferation; the DNA initiation response (i.e., androgen sensitivity) is an example of positive gene regulation by androgens (8). When the tissue becomes normal in size, an inhibitory mechanism comes into play which shuts down DNA synthesis and cell proliferation. This distinctive "wearing off" effect is a consequence of negative gene regulation by androgens (i.e., transcription is inhibited in the presence of a rising concentration of hormone) (8). Withdrawal of androgen induces apoptosis, a form of controlled cell death which decreases the size of the prostate by 50 to 80% largely through the elimination of epithelial cells. This

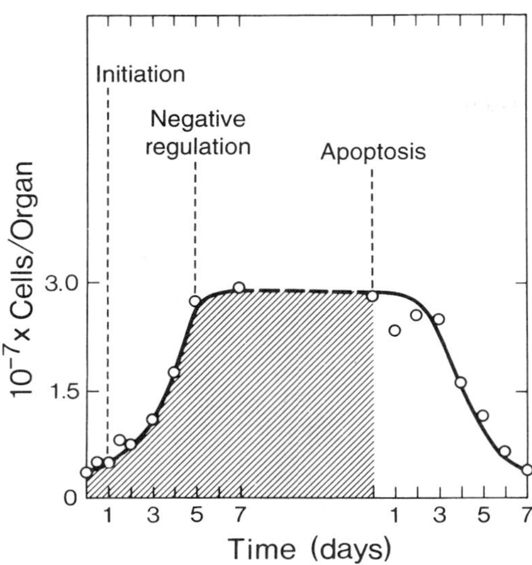

Figure 76.2. Androgenic regulation of the prostate: (*a*) initiation of DNA synthesis and cell proliferation by androgens; (*b*) negative regulation; (*c*) apoptosis.

manifestation of tissue atrophy (i.e., androgen dependence) involves a number of androgen-repressed genes (77, 101) which become active when androgens are withdrawn and inactive when replaced. A functional androgen receptor mechanism is clearly essential for each of the positive, negative, and androgen-repressed types of gene regulation. It is assumed that the complexity of such disparate receptor-mediated events is made possible by different hetero- and homodimeric combinations of androgen receptor interacting with multiple androgen response elements.

Malignant transformation of a target cell is associated with progressive stepwise loss of hormonal control over growth (20). Deletion of the negative type of gene regulation (i.e., the mechanism that limits the number of cells) results in an androgen-sensitive, androgen-dependent tumor. Deletion of both the negative and androgen-repressed types of gene regulation (i.e., those mechanisms responsible for cell number and apoptosis) produces an androgen-sensitive, androgen-independent tumor. With further progression, positive gene regulation (i.e., control over DNA initiation) disappears as well, and the tumor, now androgen insensitive and androgen independent, is characterized by completely autonomous growth. Since all androgen-dependent (and some androgen-independent) tumors retain androgen sensitivity, any treatment which elevates the concentration of plasma testosterone carries the risk of accelerated tumor growth and clinical manifestations of a flare reaction. Optimum therapeutic results will be observed when androgen withdrawal therapy has the double effect of arresting the initiation of DNA synthesis and inducing apoptotic cell death. Withdrawal-induced killing of cells follows zero-order kinetics (17); the one-time total cell kill is probably related, but not proportional, to the decrease in intranuclear concentration of dihydrotestosterone.

The system of androgen regulation described above for the prostate is also observed in male breast cancer, which responds to both orchiectomy and antiandrogens (43, 72) and is duplicated in the androgen-dependent Shionogi mouse mammary carcinoma (25). In contrast, since female breast cancer is brought into remission by the administration of androgens, it is highly unlikely that the same regulatory mechanisms apply. In fact, androgen-induced responses appear to be mediated by the estrogen receptor; prior aromatization to estrogen may be required for this action. Other less direct effects on growth factors, growth inhibitors, and differentiation of malignant stem cells are also possible.

DESCRIPTION OF AGENTS

A large number of androgens are available in potent forms for oral or parenteral administration; generally speaking, lower doses are anabolic, higher doses both anabolic and androgenic (50). In recent years, such agents have gained notoriety owing to sensational revelations of improper use in competitive sports, where it is often taken for granted, rightly or wrongly, that an athlete's level of performance is improved by androgenic steroids, sometimes taken in massive doses (133).

Ironically, as androgen misuse has become more prevalent, clinical interest in such compounds has waned. Once somewhat popular for the treatment of breast cancer, only a small number of androgens remain in use for this purpose. The most commonly used oral compounds are fluoxymesterone (10 to 20 mg/day) and methyltestosterone (50 to 100 mg/day); for intramuscular administration, nandrolone phenpropionate (25 to 50 mg/week) is sometimes tried. Agents are tolerated better if started in small doses and gradually increased until a clinical response is evident.

CLINICAL APPLICATIONS

Breast Cancer

In previous detailed studies on the therapeutic effects of androgenic compounds in breast cancer, an objective response was observed in about 20% of women, regardless of menopausal status, and patients with objective remissions survived significantly longer than patients who did not respond (3, 113). From the outset, however, the use of androgens for treating breast cancer was not strongly endorsed, owing to the distressing physiologic changes (i.e., deepening of the voice, hirsutism, acne and seborrhea, increased libido, clitoral hypertrophy, alopecia, and increased muscle mass) (3). In addition, treatment was sometimes complicated by hypercalcemia and symptomatic flareup of disease (125). Increasing use of tamoxifen, megestrol acetate, aminoglutethimide, and cytotoxic drugs further reduced the need for androgens, now considered suitable only for third- or fourth-line therapy (94).

Notwithstanding the disadvantages of androgens when administered in therapeutic doses, a more conservative regimen sometimes produces minor but beneficial results; these include reduction of bone pain, augmented energy, improved appetite, and increased hemoglobin. Occasionally there is evidence of healing of bone metastases, but in this respect androgens are probably no better than standard therapy (3, 118). Treatment can be started with a small

Table 76.1. Androgen Withdrawal Therapies

Type	How supplied	Administration	Dose
Standard			
Orchiectomy (58)			
Diethylstilbestrol (121)	Tablet	PO	1 mg t.i.d.
Steroidal antiandrogens			
Cyproterone acetate (Androcur) (89)	Tablet	PO	100 mg b.i.d.
Megestrol acetate (Megace) (49)	Tablet	PO	160 mg q.d.
Nonsteroidal antiandrogens			
Flutamide (Eulevin) (96)	Tablet	PO	250 mg t.i.d.
Nilutamide (Anandron) (10)	Tablet	PO	100 mg t.i.d.
Bicalutamide (Casodex) (129)	Tablet	PO	150 mg q.d.
LHRH agonists			
Leuprolide (Lupron) (121)	Aqueous solution	SC	1.0 mg q.d.
	Suspension of microcapsules	IM	7.5 mg q.4 w.
Goserelin (Zoladex) (35)	Cylindrical implant	SC	3.6 mg q.4 w.
Buserelin (Suprefact) (69)	Aqueous solution	SC	200 μg q.d.
		IN	400 μg t.i.d.
Nafarelin (Synarel) (93)	Aqueous solution	IN	200 μg b.i.d.
Tryptorelin (Decapeptyl) (54)	Suspension of microcapsules	IM	2.8 mg q.4 w.
5α-Reductase inhibitors			
Finasteride (Proscar) (130)		PO	5 mg q.d.
Adrenalectomy			
Medical (aminoglutethimide) (57)			
Surgical (55)			
Steroidogenesis inhibitors			
Aminoglutethimide (Cytadren) (57)	Tablet	PO	250 mg b.i.d.
Ketoconazole (Nizoral) (126)	Tablet	PO	400 mg t.i.d.
Combinations			
A. *Concurrent*			
Orchiectomy + cyproterone acetate (PO 50 mg b.i.d.) (111)			
Orchiectomy + nilutamide (PO 50 mg t.i.d.) (10)			
Cyproterone acetate (PO 100 mg b.i.d.) + low-dose DES (PO 0.1 mg/d) (53)			
Megestrol acetate (PO 120 mg/d) + low-dose DES (PO 0.1 mg/d) (128)			
Leuprolide (SC 1.0 mg/d) + flutamide (PO 250 mg t.i.d.) (32)			
Goserelin (SC 3.6 mg q.4w.) + flutamide (PO 250 mg t.i.d.) (62)			
Goserelin (SC 3.6 mg q.4w.) + bicalutamide (PO 50 mg/d) (105)			
Buserelin (SC 500 μg/d) + nilutamide (PO 100 mg q.d.) (70)			
Buserelin (SC 1.5 mg/d) + cyproterone acetate (50 mg t.i.d.) (107)			
B. *Sequential* (to eliminate flare reaction)			
DES (PO 1 mg t.i.d.) + leuprolide (SC 1 mg q.d.) (117)			
Cyproterone acetate (PO 100 mg t.i.d.) + buserelin (SC 1.5 mg/d) (13)			
Cyproterone acetate (PO 50 mg b.i.d.) + low-dose DES (PO 0.1 mg/d) + goserelin (SC 3.6 mg q.4 wk) (21)			

amount of androgen (fluoxymesterone, 5 mg per day) and gradually increased to a dose which restores the patient's sense of well-being but avoids virilization.

When fluoxymesterone (20 mg/day) and tamoxifen are given together, the objective response rate and time to progression are increased over to results obtained with tamoxifen alone (123); however, no significant differences between the two treatments with regard to duration of response or survival have been observed (60), and in one study monotherapy with tamoxifen was superior (131). Owing to the lack of demonstrable effect on survival and the increased incidence of side effects, the combination of tamoxifen plus fluoxymesterone (20 mg per day) is not recommended for routine use in the treatment of breast cancer (60); however, in certain situations the combination of low-dose fluoxymesterone (5 to 10 mg/day) with tamoxifen or megestrol acetate can be rationalized by the clinical value of the minor benefits related to the androgenic component of the treatment.

Androgenic agents, especially fluoxymesterone, have been included in multiple-drug chemotherapy regimens for advanced breast cancer. In studies by Tormey and colleagues, the addition of androgen was associated with maintenance of higher blood counts, better tolerance of chemotherapy, and a longer time to treatment failure (122). Thus, it may be possible to bring about a greater degree of cell kill if the bone marrow is supported by androgens. The dose of fluoxymesterone used in such protocols is usually 20 mg per day but lower doses might be tried to keep side effects to a minimum.

Prostate Cancer

In the past, testosterone was given occasionally as initial hormonal therapy of prostate cancer (15, 46, 95), and also as a form of "shock" therapy to reestablish the estrogen-responsiveness of a tumor (91). More recently, it has been used as a priming agent to increase the rate of proliferation of advanced (androgen-sensitive, androgen-independent) prostate cancer. In theory, since the uptake of lethal radioactive isotopes and cytotoxic drugs is greater in rapidly dividing cells than in slowly growing or resting ones, there should be a proportional increase in cell kill. Unfortunately, the high incidence of bone pain, urinary obstruction, spinal cord compression, and other adverse responses has discouraged acceptance of this approach (45, 76, 119).

It has been pointed out that androgen priming might be more beneficial if instituted 2 to 3 months after orchiectomy, when tumor burden has reached a nadir (76). Not only would there be less chance of major side effects, but, in theory, chemotherapy should be more effective in the presence of minimal disease (17). An attractive alternative to priming with exogenous androgen is self-priming (51), a stratagem which relies on the gradual recovery of testicular function after the interruption of certain types of androgen withdrawal therapy (Table 76.1) where the suppressive effects are completely reversible. It should be emphasized that the potential of such applications remains to be fully explored, and, as yet, there are no clear indications for the use of androgens in prostate cancer treatment.

Antiandrogens

DESCRIPTION OF AGENTS

According to Dorfman, "Antiandrogens are substances which prevent androgens from expressing their activity at target sites" (40). He suggested that the inhibitory effect of these substances should be differentiated from compounds which decrease the secretion of hypothalamic releasing factors and anterior pituitary hormones, particularly luteinizing hormone. He also excluded materials which act directly on the gonads to inhibit synthesis and secretion of androgens. From a practical point of view, it is difficult to adhere to this definition. On the one hand, antiandrogens with a progestin-like ring structure are both antigonadotropic and antiandrogenic and would not meet Dorfman's criteria. On the other hand, a 5α-reductase inhibitor might qualify under a liberal interpretation of the criteria, but in the mechanistic sense is not an antiandrogen. Since antiandrogens are frequently combined with luteinizing hormone–releasing-hormone (LHRH) agonists and other agents, their individual effects may be of little relevance in therapeutic situations.

Until recently, androgen withdrawal therapy was restricted to a choice between bilateral orchiectomy or estrogens, usually in the form of diethylstilbestrol. When these measures failed, adrenalectomy was occasionally tried, seldom yielding an objective response (55, 78). The advent of antiandrogens and LHRH agonists has greatly increased the number of options now available for suppressing the influence of androgens on the growth of prostate cancer (see Table 76.1).

MECHANISM OF ACTION

The effectiveness of an antiandrogen, either alone or in combination with other agents, is related to its ability to reduce the amount of functionally active androgen receptor in the nucleus of the target cell (Fig. 76.3) (102). This is ac-

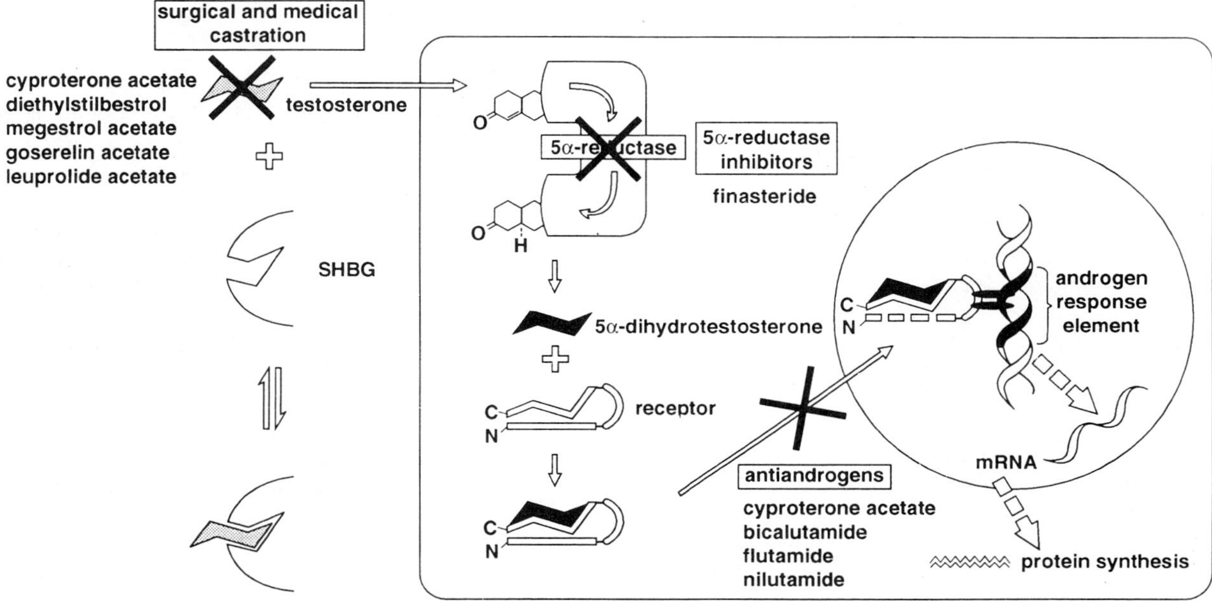

Figure 76.3. Types of androgen withdrawal therapy.

complished therapeutically to varying degrees by medical or surgical castration, the inhibition of 5α-reductase activity, and the blockade of receptor translocation into the nucleus by steroidal and nonsteroidal antiandrogens (64). Also, as demonstrated in the experimental LNCaP prostate tumor cell line, antiandrogens may affect the DNA-binding state of the androgen receptor and in some cases exhibit unexpected agonistic properties (127). The nuclear depletion of androgen receptor is thought to be more complete with those types of androgen withdrawal therapy that combine medical or surgical castration with a steroidal or nonsteroidal antiandrogen; however, there is no direct experimental evidence showing that this assumption is correct (110). Each particular type of treatment has both advantages and disadvantages, which are related to effects on both the target cell and the hypothalamic–pituitary–gonadal axis of the endocrine system. Some of the main changes for several representative treatments are described below.

NORMAL REGULATION

The normal pathways of the neuroendocrine control of gonadal function are summarized in Figure 76.4*A*. Testicular synthesis of testosterone accounts for 90% or more of the dihydrotestosterone formed in the prostate (102), the remainder being derived from the weak adrenal androgens androstenedione and dehydroepiandrosterone (27), and dietary sources. Testosterone provides a negative-feedback signal to the hypothalamus, regulating the secretion of LHRH and thereby of luteinizing hormone (LH). Negative feedback regulation of the hypothalamus by testosterone also involves the release of endogenous opioid peptides, which act as inhibitory factors to suppress the intrahypothalamic release of catecholamines (norepinephrine and dopamine); the amount of LHRH secreted is directly proportional to the concentration of catecholamines in the hypothalamus (98).

ORCHIECTOMY

The principal result of bilateral orchiectomy, as shown in Figure 76.4*B*, is the elimination of the testicular source of testosterone. Not only does this result in lowering of the concentration of dihydrotestosterone in the prostate but it also eliminates the negative-feedback regulation of the hypothalamus. Resultant increases in the circulating levels of LHRH and LH are probably without significance except for their indirect association with vasomotor symptoms. Since the concentration of testosterone-dependent opioid peptide decreases, catecholamine levels in the hypothalamus increase with consequent stimulation of the thermal regulatory center (98).

Radio-orchiectomy for the treatment of metastatic prostatic carcinoma was first described by Keyes and Ferguson in 1936 and surgical orchiectomy by Huggins and Hodges in 1941 (58, 115); the latter procedure has withstood the test of time and remains in widespread use for the treatment of advanced prostate cancer. No other treatment exists that equals or surpasses androgen ablation in checking the growth of prostate cancer in 60 to 80% of patients. All patients are rendered impotent, and hot flashes are experienced by many.

ESTROGENS

As depicted in Figure 76.4*C*, estrogenic compounds such as diethylstilbestrol substitute for testosterone in the negative-feedback inhibition of the hypothalamus. The resultant suppression of both LHRH and LH is accompanied by marked lowering of the concentration of plasma testosterone (radioimmunoassay measures total of bound and free) into the castrate range. Estrogens were used for the treatment of prostate cancer as early as 1935 (115), and diethylstilbestrol continues to be employed as a cost-effective drug for this condition. Loss of libido and potency, gynecomastia, breast tenderness, cardiovascular complications, edema, deep vein thrombosis, and pulmonary embolus are the chief side effects (29, 121).

CYPROTERONE ACETATE

Cyproterone acetate, derived from 17μ-hydroxyprogesterone, is characterized by progestin-like activity in addition to being a potent antiandrogen; the resultant dual mode of action (80, 81, 89) is illustrated in Figure 76.4*D*. Owing to its progestational antigonadotropic properties, cyproterone acetate imitates the negative feedback inhibition of the hypothalamus by testosterone; in addition to lowering the concentration of testosterone in the blood, it is antiandrogenic at the peripheral level, where it inhibits the translocation of androgen receptor from cytoplasm to nucleus in the prostate and other target tissues (102). Hot flashes are rarely experienced, since the antigonadotropic negative feedback of testosterone is replaced by that of cyproterone acetate. The most frequently recorded adverse effects of treatment are those related to hormone deprivation, namely loss of libido, impotence, reduced energy, and weakness. Drug-related effects include nipple tenderness, breast swelling, shortness of breath and thrombosis, but the complication rate is low relative to that observed with diethylstilbestrol (34, 53). Megestrol acetate (49) and chlormadinone acetate (1), other members of the large steroidal antiandrogen group of compounds (99), are similar in action to cyproterone acetate.

FLUTAMIDE

The action of nonsteroidal antiandrogens of the flutamide type (79, 108) is illustrated in Figure 76.4*E*. Flutamide inhibits the translocation of androgen receptor from cytoplasm to nucleus in target tissues, including both the prostate and the hypothalamus. Negative feedback signals provided by testosterone are no longer registered in the hypothalamus, with resultant increases in the secretion of LHRH and LH. The testis is stimulated to increase its production of testosterone, resulting in elevation of plasma testosterone (67, 75, 90). The mean concentration increases slowly, to a peak 50% above the mean normal value after 6 months of treatment; a gradual decline follows, such that, after 12 months, a normal baseline value is again observed (75). Corresponding fluctuations are likely to take place in the concentration of dihydrotestosterone in tissue (102) and there is some doubt whether the rising titers of testosterone and dihydrotestosterone are wholly offset by the peripheral antiandrogenic action of the drug (108). Indeed, the observation

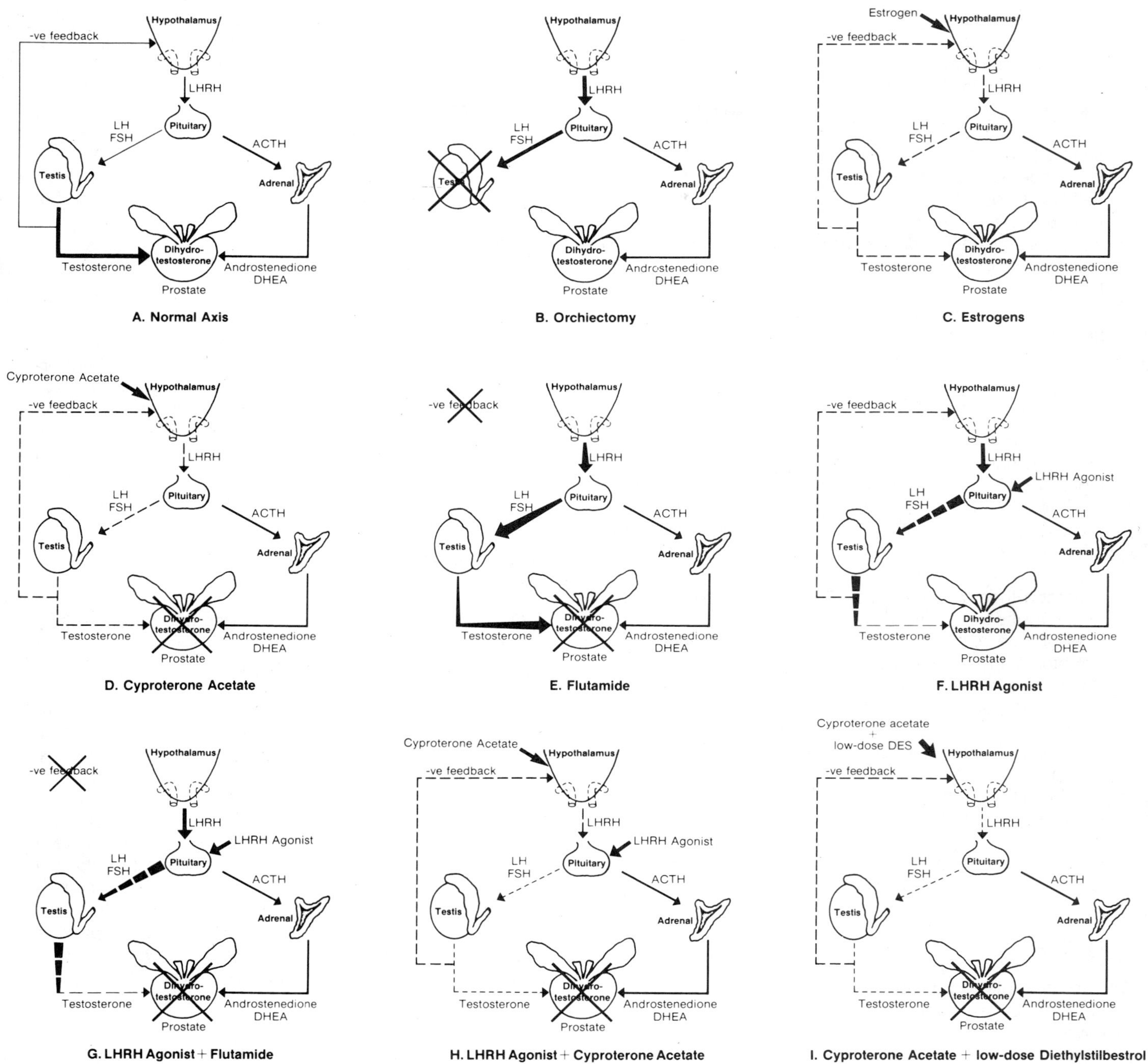

Figure 76.4. Effects of antiandrogens on hypothalamic-pituitary-gonadal axis of the endocrine system.

that the plasma testosterone level declines after 6 months implies that the negative feedback effect of testosterone on the hypothalamus is reestablished at this time, owing to diminished effectiveness of the flutamide-dependent receptor blockade. Persistence of normal or elevated levels of plasma testosterone probably account for the low incidence of hot flashes and the preservation of potency in 70 to 80% of men receiving the agent (90, 96, 116). About half of all patients are already impotent when they first require systemic therapy for metastatic prostate cancer; thus the benefit of flutamide in maintaining potency is limited to the other half, or about 40% of the total number.

Another consequence of the excessive production of testosterone is a higher level of estrogen in the bloodstream (67), with the attendant side effect of gynecomastia in 60 to 70% of patients (90, 96, 116). Occasionally severe and painful, the gynecomastia can be averted by prior irradiation of breast tissue. Other side effects, in order of importance, include diarrhea, nausea, vomiting, reversible abnormalities of liver enzymes, and neutropenia. Fatal hepatotoxicity has been reported (135). The related agent, nilutamide, in addition to gastrointestinal side effects, causes an impairment in light to dark visual adaptation, alcohol intolerance, and interstitial pneumonitis; all of which to some extent limit its usefulness (10). A new member of the group of non-steroidal antiandrogens, bicalutamide, is characterized by a long half-life of 6 days as compared with 5 hours for flutamide and 45 hours for nilutamide (129). Thus, bicalutamide can be administered in smaller daily doses improving patient compliance owing to fewer side effects and avoiding loss of antiandrogenic effect when the medication is not taken regularly. A high percentage of patients do develop gynecomastia, however.

LHRH AGONISTS

The inhibitory action of an LHRH agonist is characterized by many changes in the hypothalamic-pituitary-gonadal axis Figure 76.4*F*. The pituitary is normally stimulated by the pulsatile release of LHRH from the hypothalamus; when this periodicity is effaced by the continuous infusion of an exogenous LHRH agonist the pituitary becomes refractory to hypothalamic regulation. Gonadotropin secretion initially rises and then tapers off, as does the secretion of testosterone by the testis. Associated with the initial transient surge in plasma testosterone is an acute exacerbation of clinical symptoms and signs (flare reaction) in 5 to 10% of patients (125). In addition, transient prostate enlargement may occur in 30 to 50% of men (68, 93), and presumably tumor growth is temporarily stimulated with similar frequency. Thus, until it is definitely known whether or not an LHRH agonist causes early flare-related progression of disease, the assumption that LHRH agonist monotherapy is equivalent to conventional treatment of prostate cancer should be accepted with caution. LHRH agonists generally do not produce any side effects except for hot flashes in 60 to 70% of patients and loss of libido and potency in all patients.

LHRH AGONIST AND FLUTAMIDE

In attempts to cancel out the adverse features of nonsteroidal antiandrogens and LHRH agonists, the agents have been combined to achieve a better balance of control of testicular function as shown in Figure 76.4*G* (32). On the one hand, the LHRH agonist prevents the rise in the titer of plasma testosterone caused by flutamide or similar antiandrogen (i.e., nilutamide, bicalutamide). On the other hand, flutamide reduces the risk of a flare reaction that may occur during the surge in the concentration of plasma testosterone caused by the LHRH agonist.

Since adrenal androgens have yet to be implicated in the recurrent growth of prostate cancer (84, 110, 111) the strongest justification for combining an antiandrogen with an LHRH agonist is to avert symptoms, signs, and other untoward side effects of a flare reaction. Moreover, once the concentration of plasma testosterone is in the castrate range and the danger of a flare reaction has passed, continued administration of the antiandrogenic component of therapy is probably unnecessary, especially if there is a sustained decrease in serum prostate specific antigen (PSA) without it. This conclusion is supported indirectly by the failure of combined therapy with an LHRH agonist and flutamide (i.e., complete androgen blockade) to consistently improve survival over that observed with standard therapy of orchiectomy alone (36, 62, 104). Side effects associated with treatment are loss of libido and potency in all patients, and hot flashes in 60 to 70%.

LHRH AGONIST AND CYPROTERONE ACETATE

As shown in Figure 76.4*H*, the combination of an LHRH agonist and cyproterone acetate preserves the negative feedback mechanism in the hypothalamus, owing to the progestational action of cyproterone acetate (107). Furthermore, if cyproterone acetate is administered for several days prior to the first administration of LHRH agonist, the plasma concentrations of LH and testosterone will be suppressed, eliminating the risk of a biochemical or clinical flare reaction (13). Longer-term administration of cyproterone acetate (100 mg/day) reduces the incidence of hot flashes (98). All patients are rendered impotent by therapy.

CYPROTERONE ACETATE AND LOW-DOSE DIETHYLSTILBESTROL

One of the shortcomings of androgen withdrawal therapy with either cyproterone acetate or megestrol acetate is that the suppression of hypothalamic function is incomplete and the testis thus continues to synthesize a small amount of testosterone. In therapeutic situations, this may not be important, in view of the peripheral antiandrogenic action of these agents; nonetheless, in order to reinforce the central inhibitory action of the antiandrogens on the hypothalamus (Fig. 76.4*I*), they may be combined with a very small amount of an estrogen such as diethylstilbestrol (0.1 mg/day) if plasma testosterone is to be maintained in the castrate range (49, 53, 128). The cyproterone acetate (100 to 200 mg/day) and low-dose diethylstilbestrol (0.1 mg/day) combination has been shown to have a rapid onset of action, significantly lowering the concentration of plasma testosterone within 1 day, and down to the castrate range within 1 week (53). Side effects are similar to those reported for cyproterone acetate alone.

OTHER ACTIONS

In experimental situations, both steroidal and nonsteroidal antiandrogens sometimes demonstrate anomalous activity and appear to behave as weak androgens (7, 132). Cyproterone acetate is known to have virilizing effects during fetal development of some animal species, and at very high doses will delay the involution of the prostate in castrated rats (42). Since glucocorticoids in high doses will also retard the involution of prostatic tissue (100), the slowing action of cyproterone acetate is probably an indication of slight glucocorticoid activity related to its structural similarity to progesterone. Detailed information on such effects is available, and there are no findings indicative of a potential hazard or limitation with respect to the clinical use of steroidal antiandrogens such as cyproterone acetate in prostate cancer (56).

Both steroidal and nonsteroidal antiandrogens have also been found to stimulate the growth of prostatic cells in tissue culture (85, 132). The mechanism of this effect has not been entirely explained but appears to be related to a mutation in codon 877 (ACT to GCT, threonine to alanine) of the steroid-binding domain of the androgen receptor (47, 127), and possibly to a direct or indirect effect on negative gene regulation (see Fig. 76.2). Paradoxical agonistic activity also has been observed in hormone-refractory prostate cancer, revealed in the form of a clinical response to the withdrawal of antiandrogen (1, 82, 106). In the presence of depressed levels of testosterone and dihydrotestosterone, it appears that the DNA-binding affinity of the androgen receptor can be sufficiently increased by antiandrogen to elicit androgen-like activity. One such mechanism leading to the expression of an agonistic effect involves the formation of homodimers of androgen receptor when the concentration of the ligand, hydroxyflutamide, the active metabolite of flutamide, greatly exceeds that of dihydrotestosterone (134). Another is the codon 877 mutation in the androgen receptor, which broadens the specificity of ligand-mediated receptor binding to androgen response elements. The antiandrogen withdrawal response may occur in as many as one third of patients with progressive disease and is most often associated with a decline in serum PSA of short duration, sometimes accompanied by other objective signs of improvement (1, 33, 82, 106). Withdrawal responses so far have been observed with flutamide, nilutamide, bicalutamide, chlormadinone acetate and megestrol acetate.

CLINICAL APPLICATIONS

Breast Cancer

Experience with antiandrogens in the treatment of breast cancer in women is limited, but promising results have been obtained in male breast cancer. Responses were observed in 7 of 11 male patients with breast cancer who were treated with cyproterone acetate at a dose of 200 mg/day (72). In a study of 33 women with breast cancer, flutamide at a dose of 750 mg/day yielded only one brief partial response (92). Further studies are needed to determine if antiandrogens are as effective as antiestrogens in the treatment of the condition when it occurs in males. Until this point is clarified, sequential therapy with tamoxifen (87) followed by cyproterone acetate might be tried before proceeding to orchiectomy (9).

Prostate Cancer

There are several options for first-line therapy of stage D2 prostate cancer: orchiectomy, diethylstilbestrol, cyproterone acetate, cyproterone acetate plus low-dose diethylstilbestrol, megestrol acetate plus low-dose diethylstilbestrol, and LHRH agonist plus flutamide (or another antiandrogen). The choice of a procedure or an agent for first-line therapy will rest on a number of factors, including acceptance by the patient, preference of attending physician, availability, expense, and other concurrent health problems. Treatment is clinically indicated when evidence is found of (symptomatic or life-threatening) metastases to lymph nodes and/or bone in addition to local disease. With all first-line therapies the response rate is between 60 and 90%. Treatments that combine different modalities such as orchiectomy and antiandrogen, LHRH agonist and antiandrogen, or cyproterone acetate and low-dose diethylstilbestrol tend to yield a response rate at the high end of the range and a slight increase in time to progression. On the other hand, the rate of survival is approximately the same with all treatments (i.e., 80, 60, 40, and 20% after 1, 2, 3, and 5 years respectively (10, 11, 29, 51, 62, 89, 111)). A complete response is more likely to be observed when the initial tumor burden is relatively small and limited to prostate and lymph nodes, and this is a favorable prognostic sign. In contrast, extensive skeletal metastases are indicative of a poor prognosis (53).

The majority of men, especially elderly ones, will likely accept bilateral orchiectomy as initial therapy. Although the use of diethylstilbestrol at a conventional dose of 3 mg per day is associated with a high incidence of gynecomastia and an increased risk of cardiovascular complications, it is inexpensive, effective, and well-tolerated by some men.

Cyproterone acetate has been shown to be as effective as standard therapy and is associated with a lower incidence of side effects as compared to diethylstilbestrol. Owing to the uncertain effects of an elevated plasma testosterone level on the growth of prostate cancer, nonsteroidal antiandrogens such as flutamide should be used with caution, especially if the agent will be used over an extended period of time. If maintenance of libido and potency are major considerations, flutamide may have some appeal.

Monotherapy with an LHRH agonist carries the risk of a flare reaction and on rare occasions precipitates acute urinary retention, hydronephrosis, and spinal cord compression in patients with a large tumor burden. In addition, there is circumstantial evidence suggesting that earlier progression of disease may occur owing to the initial LHRH agonist-induced increase in plasma testosterone concentration. By combining an LHRH agonist with an antiandrogen (e.g., leuprolide and flutamide or cyproterone acetate), the risk of a flare reaction is reduced or eliminated. Few if any cardiovascular side effects are observed, so this option is indicated for patients with cardiovascular or peripheral vascular disease who are not candidates for surgical orchiectomy and for whom diethylstilbestrol is contraindicated.

There has been considerable interest in the possibility that the "complete androgen blockade" achieved by the combination of LHRH agonist and antiandrogen might prove superior to conventional androgen withdrawal therapy, which ignores the potential effect of adrenal androgens on growth of prostate cancer; however, a number of clinical trials testing this hypothesis have failed to produce any conclusive evidence for the involvement of adrenal androgens in prostate cancer (104). The main supportive results, provided by the U.S.A. National Cancer Institute Intergroup Study INT 0036 of leuprolide versus leuprolide plus flutamide are consistent with the conclusion that treatment with leuprolide and flutamide is superior to treatment with leuprolide alone when the end points of median progression-free survival and median overall survival are compared (32). No concurrent study was done to prove that leuprolide monotherapy was equiva-

Table 76.2. Comparison of Results of Clinical Trials on Combined Androgen Blockade

Trial	Treatments	*N*	Median TTP (mo)	Overall Median Survival (mo)
1. Intergroup 0036	Leuprolide + placebo	603	14	29
	Leuprolide + flutamide		17	35[a,b]
2. International Prostate Cancer Group	Goserelin	301	—	27
	Goserelin + flutamide		—	29[c]
3. EORTC 30853	Orchiectomy	327	21	27
	Goserelin + flutamide		33	34[a]
4. Danish Group	Orchiectomy	262	17	28
	Goserelin + flutamide		17	23[c]
5. EORTC 30845	Orchiectomy	353	—	24
	Buserelin + cyproterone acetate		—	24[c]
6. Canadian Group	Orchiectomy + placebo	208	12	19
	Orchiectomy + nilutamide		12	24[c]
7. International Anandron Group	Orchiectomy + placebo	457	15	24
	Orchiectomy + nilutamide		21	27[c]
8. Australian Group	Orchiectomy		—	31
	Orchiectomy + flutamide	222	—	23[c]
9. EORTC 30805	Orchiectomy		18	24
	Orchiectomy + cyproterone acetate	351	18	24[c]
	Diethylstilbestrol	351	24	26

[a] Statistically significant
[b] Initial log rank statistic has changed from significant to insignificant
[c] Not statistically significant

lent to standard therapy, however, leaving open the question of whether combination treatment is indeed superior to surgical orchiectomy or estrogen therapy. Also, the log rank statistic, which initially supported a median survival time estimate in favor of combined androgen blockade, is no longer significant.

A large number of similar studies have been conducted by other national and international groups Table 76.2(37). The overall median survival estimate is significantly different from that of control in only two of the nine studies listed, the Intergroup 0036 discussed above and the EORTC 308539. Notwithstanding the controversial issue of perceived weaknesses in clinical trial methods (16), no clear picture of extended survival with combined androgen blockade emerges from these results, nor from their meta-analysis (11, 37). It should be noted that patients in the control arm of two studies experience longer survival and that survival figures for the same compounds vary widely between studies. Consequently, survival time should not be the only consideration when deciding upon a particular androgen blockade regimen. Regardless of the treatment chosen, a better prognosis can be anticipated if the serum PSA falls to a stable or decreasing nadir in the normal range between 24 and 32 weeks of therapy (21).

The progestational antiandrogen, cyproterone acetate, produces a therapeutic effect similar to that of the combination of an LHRH agonist and a nonsteroidal antiandrogen. When it is combined with low-dose diethylstilbestrol (0.1 mg/day), castrate levels of plasma testosterone are uniformly achieved and long-term maintenance of plasma testosterone within the castrate range is more reliable. Owing to the synergistic action of low-dose diethylstilbestrol, cyproterone acetate can be used at a reduced dose of 100 mg/day, and the comparable agent megestrol acetate, at a dose of 120 mg/day, making these antiandrogens the most cost-effective after diethylstilbestrol.

Some of the androgen withdrawal therapies listed in Table 76.1 are not ideally suited for first-line therapy. The combination of orchiectomy and antiandrogen (flutamide, nilutamide, or cyproterone acetate) has not proven to be superior to orchiectomy alone (see Table 76.1); the supplement of antiandrogen might be reserved, therefore, for patients whose serum PSA does not respond adequately to orchiectomy. At the present time, there is no evidence that the 5α-reductase inhibitor finasteride (130) is effective against established prostate cancer (103). The combination of finasteride and flutamide has given rise to encouraging preliminary results (44); however, severe gynecomastia can be expected in some patients after long-term administration, owing to the reflex elevation of serum testosterone (Fig. 76.4*E*) and increased aromatization to 17β-estradiol. In the absence of a scientifically validated rationale for an adrenal contribution to the growth of prostate cancer, neither surgical (78) nor medical adrenalectomy procedures should be considered for first-line therapy (57). The steroidogenesis inhibitor ketoconazole (126), characterized by gastrointestinal side effects, skin reactions, gynecomastia, and severe asthenia, should be considered only for use in emergency situations requiring an acute reduction in the concentration of plasma testosterone.

Prevention of Flare Reaction

A flare reaction usually begins with symptoms of localized or low back pain which starts 1 to 3 days after the administration of an LHRH agonist and resolves after another 1 to 4 days. Biochemical manifestations include temporary increases in the plasma levels of LH, testosterone, prostatic acid phosphatase, and PSA lasting 7 to 14 days. Transient stimulation of tumor growth may also take place, leading to urinary and neurologic complications. The flare phenomenon has been implicated in the early progression of disease by the results of the Leuprolide Study Group Trial comparing leuprolide to diethylstilbestrol (121), and those of the N.C.I. INT 0036 study comparing leuprolide with, and without, flutamide (32). In the former clinical trial, treatment was considered to have failed at the 3-month point in ten patients receiving leuprolide, as compared with two receiving diethylstilbestrol because of early progression of disease. In the latter trial, a 2.6-month gain in median time to progression was observed in the group receiving leuprolide plus flutamide. This advantage was already evident at the 3-month point, implying that there was earlier progression of disease in the leuprolide monotherapy group.

The flare reaction can be avoided with any of several methods. Cyproterone acetate (preferably in combination with low-dose diethylstilbestrol) given as "lead-in" therapy for 3 to 4 weeks before the first dose of LHRH agonist presuppresses the pituitary and completely eliminates any possiblity of a flare reaction (21). Alternatively, flutamide, nilutamide (70), or cyproterone acetate (107) given concurrently with the first administration of LHRH agonist, safely blunts the reaction. Prior administration of diethylstilbestrol in doses of 1 mg or 3 mg daily for 1 week has proven to be less effective (117). Since the danger of a flare reaction abates in the second week following LHRH agonist administration, there is no compelling reason for continuing antiandrogens much beyond this time, and such antiflare treatment can safely be stopped after 1 month, provided that the plasma testosterone value is in the castrate range.

Second-Line Therapy

When a relapse follows a response to first-line therapy, the probability of an objective response to a second androgen withdrawal procedure is less than 10% (110). Before steps are taken to introduce second-line therapy, it is necessary to measure the plasma testosterone level to determine whether there has been an escape from primary therapy. The choice of a second-line option will be determined to some extent by the original treatment (Table 76.3).

Following orchiectomy, it is unlikely that the plasma testosterone concentration will be elevated, but, nevertheless, a trial of cyproterone acetate or flutamide for a period of 3 months is reasonable; the PSA level in the blood should be followed for any indication of a response. A common mistake is to administer LHRH agonist monotherapy after failure of orchiectomy; such treatment is totally ineffective in the absence of the testes.

An elevated plasma testosterone value is more likely to be seen with diethylstilbestrol, owing to incomplete absorption of tablet preparations or noncompliance. In this case the second-line treatment should be effective in lowering plasma testosterone and cyproterone acetate, LHRH agonist (alone or combined with antiandrogen), or orchiectomy suffices for this purpose.

Plasma testosterone may be incompletely suppressed if cyproterone acetate is used as monotherapy and thus the addition of low-dose diethylstilbestrol (0.1 mg/day) should be tried first, the other options being an LHRH agonist or orchiectomy. A patient who progresses while taking flutamide will invariably be found to have a normal or elevated level of plasma testosterone. The option selected for second-line therapy in this situation should result in a lowering of plasma testosterone to castrate levels; this can be achieved with cyproterone acetate, an LHRH agonist, or orchiectomy. If LHRH agonist monotherapy has been used as first-line therapy, antiandrogen should be tried in addition for a short period, followed by orchiectomy if no effect is observed.

Table 76.3. Options for Second-Line Therapy of Prostate Cancer

First-line option	Second-line options
Orchiectomy	Cyproterone acetate, flutamide
Diethylstilbestrol	Cyproterone acetate, LHRH agonist, orchiectomy
Cyproterone acetate	Cyproterone acetate + low-dose diethylstilbestrol, LHRH agonist, orchiectomy
Flutamide	Cyproterone acetate, LHRH agonist, orchiectomy
LHRH agonist	Cyproterone acetate, flutamide, orchiectomy
LHRH agonist + flutamide	Flutamide withdrawal, LHRH agonist + cyproterone acetate, orchiectomy
LHRH agonist + cyproterone acetate	LHRH agonist + flutamide, orchiectomy

In the event that a patient progresses while receiving the combination of LHRH agonist and flutamide as first-line therapy, discontinuation of flutamide may produce a response (106). A short trial of antiandrogen withdrawal monitored by serum PSA is worthwhile with other antiandrogenic medications as well (1, 33, 82). Changing the antiandrogen in the combination occasionally lowers the PSA tumor marker. Otherwise, the orchiectomy option is indicated. There is no evidence that second-line therapy increases the 6- to 12-month median survival time between progression and death (31, 63).

Management of Hormone-Resistant Disease

Advanced prostate cancer which has become refractory to primary androgen withdrawal therapy has a poor prognosis, and the question arises whether the patient would benefit from continuation of such treatment. Owing to the retained androgen sensitivity of androgen-independent malignancy (Fig. 76.2), there is a strong possibility that termination of medical castration therapy will result in an acceleration of tumor growth. This is particularly true where flutamide has been used as monotherapy, since the acceleration of growth may start very shortly after the drug has been discontinued. Two factors contribute to this acute complication: first, the 5- to 6-hour half-life of flutamide in plasma is quite short; second, with clearance of flutamide, the normal or elevated level of plasma testosterone is no longer countered by antiandrogen. Thus, in the face of progressive disease in patients who have not been surgically castrated, therapy with LHRH agonists and/or antiandrogens should probably be continued, recognizing however, that there is little evidence to support this practice (59).

Intermittent Therapy

The shortcomings of medical and surgical castration in the treatment of prostate cancer have been recognized for some time. For reasons that remain unknown, androgen ablation fails to eliminate the entire malignant cell population and it increases the rate of tumor progression to androgen independence and autonomous growth. In attempting to avert or delay progression, it has been hypothesized that, if the cells which survive androgen withdrawal are forced into a normal pathway of differentiation by androgen replacement (Fig. 76.5), then apoptotic potential might be restored, giving rise to another opportunity to induce regression of tumor by androgen withdrawal (2). Under experimental conditions apoptosis can indeed be induced multiple times in a tumor cell population by repeated cycles of androgen withdrawal and replacement (2). The results of preliminary clinical studies suggest that the repetitive induction of apoptosis is also achievable in prostate cancer with periodic interruption of androgen blockade therapy (2, 51, 52, 66).

The reversibility of the action of LHRH agonists and antiandrogens affords the potential advantage of a full recovery from therapy and allows a patient to alternate between periods of treatment and no treatment. Moreover, careful sequential monitoring of plasma testosterone and PSA make it possible to track successive periods of response and progression with considerable precision. Each cycle of intermittent therapy can be started with any treatment that reduces plasma testosterone into the castrate range and should be interrupted after 36 weeks only if the serum PSA has reached a stable or decreasing nadir in the normal range at 24 and 32 weeks of therapy (21) (Fig. 76.6). When the patient is off treatment, the function of the testes and the concentration of serum testosterone return to normal slowly over a period of 8 to 14 weeks (2). The second cycle of treatment is started when the serum PSA value increases to the level prescribed in Table 76.4.

In theory, this approach should be suitable for long-term management of inoperable, incompletely excised, or locally recurrent prostate cancer, especially after failure of external-beam radiation. The standard regimen developed for stage D2 prostate cancer (Fig. 76.6) has been adapted for use in the treatment of patients with initially localized prostate cancer whom radical prostatectomy, or irradiation, or radical prostatectomy and irradiation has failed as demonstrated by a rising serum PSA. The therapeutic strategy in each situation is guided by the serum PSA Table 76.4; however, until more information is obtained about PSA trigger points from clinical trials focussing on the subsets of patients specified above, the suggested upper and lower PSA limits should be regarded as tentative only.

Intermittent therapy provides improved quality of life, characterized by the recovery of sexual function and a greater sense of well-being during the off-treatment part of each cycle. Other potential benefits include the prolongation of the androgen-dependent condition of the tumor, a lower risk of antiandrogen-induced progression, and less cumulative drug toxicity. Survival appears to be in keeping with results obtained with continuous androgen blockade (52).

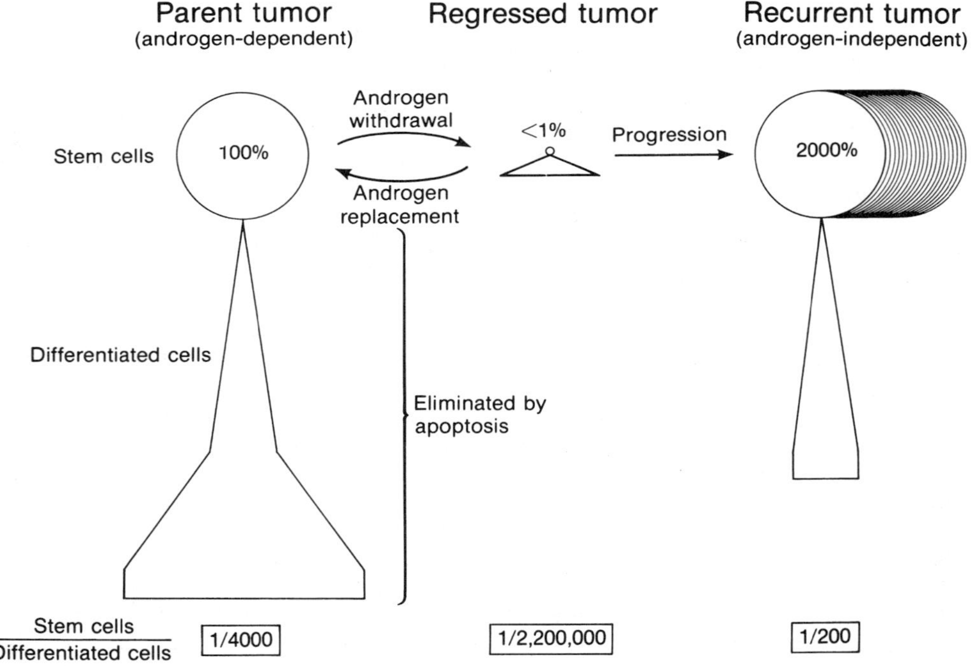

Figure 76.5. Model of stem cell composition of the androgen-dependent Shionogi carcinoma. Change in the ratio of stem cells to differentiated cells, which occurs after androgen withdrawal, is shown. Effect of androgen replacement in stimulating the differentiation of stem cells in the regressed tumor and the recovery of apoptotic potential also is illustrated. (From reference 2, with permission.)

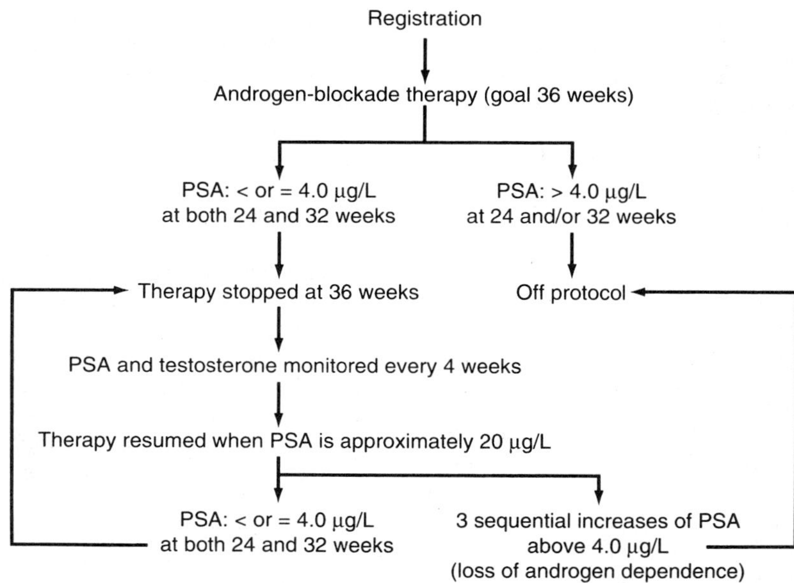

Figure 76.6. Schema for intermittent androgen suppression in the treatment of stage D2 prostate cancer.

Neoadjuvant Therapy

A better understanding of the biology of prostate cancer has highlighted the fact that the risk of systemic spread is already appreciable at the time of initial diagnosis. Under such conditions, the results of radical prostatectomy will be less than optimal, although it may still be indicated for control of local-regional disease. Preoperative treatment with a reversible androgen withdrawal agent affords the possibility of down-staging the primary tumor (112), reducing the incidence of positive surgical resection margins, and eradicating micrometastases. Preliminary evidence suggests that long-term treatment of 8 months (48) is superior to a shorter regimen of 3 months (6, 109). The same principle has been used in the cytoreduction of prostate cancer prior to external-beam irradiation, with beneficial effects (97).

Adjuvant Therapy

It is intuitively evident, but not proven, that adjuvant therapy in conjunction with radical prostatectomy should be beneficial when there is evidence of positive margins of resection, histologic evidence of lymph node involvement, or a failure of the PSA to fall to zero (14). Experimental data from studies on animal models of prostate cancer indicate that androgen withdrawal therapy is more effective when started early in the treatment history of a tumor (61). Although the clinical applications of adjuvant hormonal therapy are subject to controversy, nine men with pathologic stage C disease appeared to have a lower local recurrence rate with the combination of radical prostatectomy and simultaneous androgen withdrawal therapy (136). Furthermore, men with diploid prostate cancer (pathologic stage D1) who received early androgen withdrawal therapy following radical prostatectomy, survived longer than men with nondiploid or aneuploid cancer who received no early endocrine therapy (137). Such results suggest that both DNA ploidy pattern and response to androgen withdrawal therapy are major prognostic factors for patients with operable disease.

The optimum duration of adjuvant hormonal therapy has not been established. In advanced disease, regression of

Table 76.4. Serum PSA Guidelines in Intermittent Androgen Suppression

Stage	Condition	Serum PSA (ng/ml)				
		At start of cycle 1	24 wk	32 wk	To initiate cycle 2	Refractory disease 3 increases above
D1 or D2	Untreated	>20	4 or <4	4 or <4[a]	~20	4
B2 or C	Failed irradiation	>6	4 or <4	4 or <4[a]	~10	4
A2, B or C	Failed prostatectomy	1	0.2 or <0.2	0.2 or <0.2[a]	~1	0.2
A2, B or C	Failed prostatectomy Failed irradiation	>1	1 or <1	1 or <1[a]	~1	1

[a] Stable or decreasing value relative to result at 24 weeks.

soft tissue tumor and normalization of PSA are usually observed within 3 to 6 months of starting therapy, suggesting that 6 to 12 months of adjuvant treatment may be sufficient; this period is consistent with the observed rate of regression of prostate cancer after orchiectomy (68).

The reversibility of some types of androgen withdrawal therapy (see Table 76.1) adds to the appeal of adjuvant hormonal therapy, since, even if there is a recurrence of malignancy after therapy has been interrupted, the tumor is likely to be androgen dependent and to respond again to the first-line agent.

Treatment of Emergency Conditions

Urinary retention is a common presenting sign in patients with prostate cancer and is rapidly relieved by catheterization and subsequent transurethral resection. Androgen withdrawal therapy which results in a rapid decline of plasma testosterone may also be used to bring about regression of the obstructing lesion, especially in a high-risk surgical patient or a man with extensive local disease. If orchiectomy is not indicated, agents such as cyproterone acetate (200 mg/day), preferably with diethylstilbestrol (0.1 mg/day) or ketoconazole (1,200 mg/day) may be used as alternatives. In situations where there are signs of impending or early spinal cord compression, it is reasonable to add to conventional management with the administration of a steroidal or nonsteroidal antiandrogen. The use of an LHRH agonist is not advised, since any acute elevation of plasma testosterone may stimulate tumor growth and exacerbate the condition.

Treatment of Hot Flashes

Hot flashes can be blocked by the administration of central antiadrenergic medication (clonidine) (86) or steroids with central inhibitory action which reduce the concentration of catecholamines in the hypothalamus. Cyproterone acetate, owing to its partial progestational action, has been successful in significantly suppressing hot flashes with minimum side effects at a dose of 100 mg/day (98). Megestrol acetate (40 mg/day) is similarly active (73). Nonsteroidal antiandrogens which lack a central antigonadotropic action have no effect.

Summary

The history of androgens is old and prodigious, yet the hormonal nature of androgens was not discovered until the earlier part of this century. Clinical testing of testosterone and other androgenic compounds began soon after their isolation and synthesis. Although breast cancer proved responsive to such therapy, the virilization induced by androgens and the introduction of antiestrogens caused a marked decline in the use of androgens for this purpose. Additive therapy with androgens is not indicated in the treatment of prostate cancer. This is in contrast to various types of androgen withdrawal therapies, including orchiectomy, steroidal and nonsteroidal antiandrogens, LHRH agonists, and others, which have become increasingly accepted as conventional treatment for prostate cancer. Reversible androgen withdrawal therapies based on the use of antiandrogens and LHRH agonists have found a number of applications in the treatment of prostate cancer at different stages offering flexibility and many new potential approaches. Of considerable interest is the application of reversible androgen withdrawal therapy to conventional treatment-regimens which might be enhanced by neoadjuvant or adjuvant endocrine therapy. Intermittent therapy with reversible modalities based on antiandrogens and LHRH agonists offer potential for long-term control of prostate cancer while minimizing side effects, especially suppression of libido and potency, in younger men. Conceivably, the intermittent therapy option will become an alternative to radical prostatectomy or irradiation for the primary treatment of localized prostate in older men with a life expectancy of less than 10 years. Augmentation of intermittent therapy to increase the length and number of cycles might be accomplished by the administration of cytotoxic drugs, differentiation agents or gene therapies at specific times during a cycle of treatment when the modality of choice would have its maximum effect. In the near future, it is likely that the indications for the use of antiandrogens will expand in these directions and that the number of antiandrogenic agents available for treating prostate cancer will increase.

References

1. Akakura K, Akimoto S, Ohki T, Shimazaki J. Androgen withdrawal syndrome in prostate cancer after treatment with steroidal antiandrogen chlormadinone acetate. Urology 1995;45:700.
2. Akakura K, Bruchovsky N, Goldenberg SL, Rennie PS, Buckley AR, Sullivan LD. Effects of intermittent androgen suppression on androgen-dependent tumors. Apoptosis and serum prostate-specific antigen. Cancer 1993;71:2782.
3. American Medical Association Council on Drugs. Androgens and estrogens in the treatment of disseminated mammary carcinoma. JAMA 1960;172:1271.
4. Anderson KM, Liao S. Selective retention of dihydrotestosterone by prostatic nuclei. Nature 1968;219:277.
5. Andersson S, Bishop RW, Russell DW. Expression cloning and regulation of steroid 5μ-reductase, an enzyme essential for male sexual differentiation. J Biol Chem 1989;264:16249.
6. Aprikian AG, Fair WR, Reuter VE, Sogani P, Herr H, Russo P, Sheinfeld J. Experience with neoadjuvant diethylstilboestrol and radical prostatectomy in patients with locally advanced prostate cancer. Br J Urol 1994;74:630.
7. Bardin CW, Brown T, Isomaa VV, Janne O. A Progestins can mimic, inhibit and potentiate the actions of androgens. Pharmacol Ther 1984;23:443.
8. Beato M, Chalepakis G, Schauer M, Slater EP. DNA regulatory elements for steroid hormones. J Steroid Biochem 1989;32:737.
9. Becher R, Hoeffken K, Pape H, Schmidt C-G. Tamoxifen treatment before orchiectomy in advanced breast cancer in men. N Engl J Med 1981;305:169.
10. Beland G, Elhilali M, Fradet Y, Laroche B, Ramsey EW, Trachtenberg J, Tewari H, Venner P. A comparison of the treatment of metastatic prostate cancer by testicular ablation or total androgen blockade. In Therapy for Genitourinary Cancer. Edited by H Lepor, RK Lawson. Boston: Kluwer Academic Publishers, 1992, p 29.
11. Bertagna C, De Géry A, Hucher M, François JP, Zanirato J. Efficacy of the combination of nilutamide plus orchiectomy in patients with metastatic prostatic cancer. A meta-analysis of seven randomized double-blind trials (1056 patients). Br J Urol 1994;73:396.
12. Berthold AA. Uber Die Transplantation Der Hoden. In Male Reproduction. Edited by BP Setchell. New York: Van Nostrand Reinhold, 1984, p 225.
13. Boccon-Gibod L, Laudat MH, Dugue MA, Steg A. Cyproterone acetate lead-in prevents initial rise of serum testosterone induced by luteinizing hormone-releasing hormone analogs in the treatment of metastatic carcinoma of the prostate. Eur Urol 1986;12:400.
14. Bosch R, Schroeder FH. Radical prostatectomy and adjuvant endocrine treatment: a review. In EORTC Genitourinary Group Monograph 8: Treatment of Prostatic Cancer—Facts and Controversies. Edited by FH Schroeder. New York: Wiley-Liss, 1990, p 239.
15. Brendler H, Chase WE, Scott WW. Prostatic cancer, further investigation of hormonal relationships. Arch Surg 1950;61:433.
16. Blumenstein BA. Some statistical considerations for the interpretation of trials of combined androgen therapy. Cancer 1993;72(suppl):3834.
17. Bruchovsky N, Goldie JH. Basis for the use of drug and hormone combinations in the treatment of endocrine-related cancer. In Drug and Hormone Resistance in Neoplasia, Vol. II. Edited by N Bruchovsky, JH Goldie. Boca Raton, FL: CRC Press, 1983, p 129.
18. Bruchovsky N, Wilson JD. The conversion of testosterone to 5α-androstan-17β-ol-3-1 by rat prostate in vivo and in vitro. J Biol Chem 1968;243:2012.

19. Bruchovsky N, Wilson JD. The intranuclear binding of testosterone and 5α-androstan-17β-ol-3-1 by rat prostate. J Biol Chem 1968;243:5953.
20. Bruchovsky N, Brown EM, Coppin CM, Goldenberg SL, Le Riche JC, Murray NC, Rennie PS. The endocrinology and treatment of prostate tumor progression. In Current Concepts and Approaches to the Study of Prostate Cancer. Edited by DS Coffey, N Bruchovsky, WA Gardner Jr, MI Resnick, and JP Karr. New York: Alan R. Liss, 1987, p 347.
21. Bruchovsky N, Goldenberg SL, Akakura K, Rennie PS. Luteinizing hormone-releasing hormone agonists in prostate cancer. Elimination of flare reaction by pretreatment with cyproterone acetate and low-dose diethylstilbestrol. Cancer 1993;72:1685.
22. Bruchovsky N, Lesser B, Van Doorn E, Craven S. Hormonal effects on cell proliferation in rat prostate. Vitam Horm 1975;33:61.
23. Bruchovsky N, Rennie PS, Vanson A. Studies on the regulation of the concentration of androgens and androgen receptors in nuclei of prostatic cells. Biochim Biophys Acta 1975;394:248.
24. Bruchovsky N, Rennie PS, Wilkin RP. New aspects of androgen action in prostatic cells: stromal localization of 5α-reductase, nuclear abundance of androstanolone and binding of receptor to linker deoxyribonucleic acid. In Steroid Receptors, Metabolism and Prostatic Cancer. Edited by FH Schroeder, HJ de Voogt. Amsterdam: Excerpta Medica, 1980, p 57.
25. Bruchovsky N, Rennie PS, Coldman AJ, Goldenberg SL, To M, Lawson D. Effects of androgen withdrawal on the stem cell composition of the Shionogi carcinoma. Cancer Res 1990;50:2275.
26. Bruchovsky N, Rennie PS, To MP, Snoek R, Lefebvre YA, Golsteyn EJ. Chemical demonstration of nuclear androgen receptor following affinity chromatography with immobilized ligands. Prostate 1987;10:207.
27. Bruchovsky N. Comparison of the metabolites formed in rat prostate following the in vivo administration of seven natural androgens. Endocrinology 1971;89:1212.
28. Burrows H. Biological Actions of Sex Hormones. Cambridge: Cambridge University Press. 1949:p 176.
29. Byar DP, Corle DK. Hormone therapy for prostate cancer: results of the Veterans Administration cooperative urological research group studies. NCI Monogr 1988;7:165.
30. Chang C, Kokontis J, Liao S. Molecular cloning of human and rat complementary DNA encoding androgen receptors. Science 1988;240:324.
31. Collste LG. Second line treatment of hormone refractory prostatic cancer patients. In EORTC Genitourinary Group Monograph 7: Prostatic Cancer and Testicular Cancer. Edited by DWW Newling, WG Jones. New York: Wiley-Liss, 1990, p 29.
32. Crawford ED, Eisenberger MA, McLeod DG, Spaulding JT, Benson R, Dorr A, Blumenstein BA, Davis MA, Goodman PJ. A controlled trial of leuprolide with and without flutamide in prostatic carcinoma. N Engl J Med 1989;321:419.
33. Dawson NA, McLeod DG. Dramatic prostate specific antigen decrease in response to discontinuation of megestrol acetate in advanced prostate cancer: expansion of the antiandrogen withdrawal syndrome. J Urol 1995;153:1946;.
34. De Voogt HJ, Smith PH, Pavone-Macaluso M, De Pauw M, Suciu S, Members of the European Organization for Research on Treatment of Cancer Urological Group. Cardiovascular side effects of diethylstilbestrol, cyproterone acetate, medroxyprogesterone acetate and estramustine phosphate used for the treatment of advanced prostatic cancer: results from European Organization for Research on Treatment of Cancer trials 30761 and 30762. J Urol 1986;135:303.
35. Debruyne FMJ, Denis L, Lunglmayer G, Mahler C, Newling DWW, Richards B, Robinson MRG, Smith PH, Weil EHJ, Whelan P. Long-term therapy with a depot luteinizing hormone-releasing hormone analogue (Zoladex) in patients with advanced prostatic carcinoma. J Urol 1988;140:775.
36. Denis LJ, Carnelro-de-Moura JL, Bono A, Sylvester R, Whelan P, Newling D, Depauw M. Goserelin acetate and flutamide versus bilateral orchiectomy: a phase III EORTC trial (30853). Urology 1993;42:119.
37. Denis L, Murphy GP. Overview of phase III trials on combined androgen treatment in patients with metastatic prostate cancer. Cancer 1993;72(suppl):3888.
38. Dorfman RI, Shipley RA. Androgens, Biochemistry, Physiology, and Clinical Significance. New York: Wiley, 1956, p 5.
39. Dorfman RI. Anti-Androgenic Substances. In Methods in Hormone Research, Volume II. Edited by RI Dorfman. New York: Academic Press, 1962, p 315.
40. Dorfman RI. Biological activity of antiandrogens. Br J Derm 1970;82(suppl):6, 3.
41. Dunn JF, Nisula BC, Rodbard D. Transport of steroid hormones: binding of 21 endogenous steroids to both testosterone-binding globulin and corticosteroid-binding globulin in human plasma. J Clin Endocrinol Metab 1981;53:58.
42. El Etreby MF, Habenicht U-F, Louton T, Nishino Y, Schroeder HG. Effect of cyproterone acetate in comparison to flutamide and megestrol acetate on the ventral prostate, seminal vesicle, and adrenal glands of adult male rats. Prostate 1987;11: 361.
43. Everson RB, Lippman ME. Male Breast Cancer. In Breast Cancer 3, Advances in Research and Treatment. Edited by WL McGuire. New York: Plenum, 1979, p 239.
44. Fleshner NE, Trachtenberg J. Treatment of advanced prostate cancer with the combination of finasteride plus flutamide: early results. Eur Urol 1993;24(suppl 2):106.
45. Fowler JE Jr, Whitmore WF Jr. Considerations for the use of testosterone with systemic chemotherapy in prostatic cancer. Cancer 1982;49:1373.
46. Fowler JE Jr, Whitmore WF Jr. The response of metastatic adenocarcinoma of the prostate to exogenous testosterone. J Urol 1981;126:372.
47. Gaddipati JP, McLeod DG, Heidenberg HB, Sesterhenn IA, Finger MJ, Moul JW, Srivastava S. Frequent detection of codon 877 mutation in the androgen receptor gene in advanced prostate cancers. Cancer Res 1994;54:2861.
48. Gleave ME, Goldenberg SL, Jones EC, Bruchovsky N, Sullivan LD. Biochemical and pathological effects of eight months of neoadjuvant androgen withdrawal therapy prior to radical prostatectomy in clinically confined prostate cancer. J Urol 1996;155:213.
49. Geller J, Albert J, Yen SSC. Treatment of advanced cancer of prostate with megestrol acetate. Urology 1978;12:537.
50. Goldenberg IS, Segaloff A. Androgens. In Cancer Medicine, 2nd ed. Edited by JF Holland, E Frei III. Philadelphia: Lea & Febiger, 1982, p 990.
51. Goldenberg SL, Bruchovsky N. The use of cyproterone acetate in prostate cancer. Urol Clin North Am 1991;18:111.
52. Goldenberg SL, Bruchovsky N, Gleave ME, Sullivan LD, Akakura K. Intermittent androgen suppression in the treatment of prostate cancer: a preliminary report. Urology 1995;45:839.
53. Goldenberg SL, Bruchovsky N, Rennie PS, Coppin CM. The combination of cyproterone acetate and low dose diethylstilbestrol in the treatment of advanced prostatic carcinoma. J Urol 1988;140:1460.
54. Gonzalez-Barcena D, Perez-Sanchez PL, Graef A, Gomez AM, Berea H, Comaru-Schally AM, Schally AV. Inhibition of the pituitary-gonadal axis by a single intramuscular administration of d-trp-6-LH-RH (Decapeptyl) in a sustained-release formulation in patients with prostatic carcinoma. Prostate 1989;14:291.
55. Grayhack JT. Adrenalectomy and hypophysectomy for carcinoma of the prostate. JAMA 1969;210:1075.
56. Habenicht U-F, Schroeder FH, El Etreby MF, Neumann F. Advantages and disadvantages of pure antiandrogens and of antiandrogens of the cyproterone acetate-type in the treatment of prostatic cancer. In Management of Advanced Cancer of Prostate and Bladder. Edited by PH Smith, M Pavone-Macaluso. New York: Alan R. Liss, 1988, p 63.
57. Havlin KA, Trump DL. Aminoglutethimide. Theoretical considerations and clinical results in advanced prostate cancer. In Endocrine Therapies in Breast and Prostate Cancer. Edited by C Kent Osborne. Boston: Kluwer, 1988, p 83.
58. Huggins C, Hodges CV. Studies on prostate cancer: I. Effect of castration, estrogen, and androgen injection on serum phosphatases in metastatic carcinoma of the prostate. Cancer Res 1941;1:293.
59. Hussain M, Wolf M, Marshall E, Crawford ED, Eisenberger M. Effects of continued androgen-deprivation therapy and other prognostic factors on response and survival in phase II chemotherapy trials for hormone-refractory prostate cancer: a Southwest Oncology Group report. J Clin Oncol 1994;12:1868.
60. Ingle JN, Twito DI, Schaid DJ, Cullinan SA, Krook JE, Mailliard JA, Marschke RF, Long HJ, Gerstner JG, Windschitl HE, Everson LK, Pfeifle DM. Randomized clinical trial of tamoxifen alone or combined with fluoxymesterone in postmenopausal women with metastatic breast cancer. J Clin Oncol 1988;6:825.
61. Isaacs JT. The timing of androgen ablation therapy and/or chemotherapy in the treatment of prostatic cancer. Prostate 1984;5:1.
62. Iverson P, Rasmussen F, Klarskov P, Christensen IJ. Long-term results of Danish Prostatic Cancer Group Trial 86. Cancer 1993;72(suppl):3851.
63. Jacobi GH. Second-line endocrine treatment. In The Medical Management of Prostate Cancer. Edited by L Denis. Berlin: Springer-Verlag, 1988, p 73.
64. Jenster G, Trapman J, Brinkmann AO. Nuclear import of the human androgen receptor. Biochem J 1993;293:761.
65. Kasper S, Rennie PS, Bruchovsky N, Sheppard PC, Cheng H, Lin L, Shiu RPC, Snoek R, Matusik RJ. Cooperative binding of androgen receptors to two DNA sequences is required for androgen induction of the probasin gene. J Biol Chem 1994;269:31763.
66. Klotz LH, Herr HW, Morse MJ, Whitmore WF Jr. Intermittent endocrine therapy for advanced prostate cancer. Cancer 1986;58:2546.
67. Knuth UA, Hano R, Nieschlag E. Effect of flutamide or cyproterone acetate on pituitary and testicular hormones in normal men. J Clin Endocrinol Metabol 1984;59:963.
68. Kojima M, Watanabe H, Ohe H, Miyashita H, Inaba T. Kinetic evaluation of the effect of LHRH analog on prostatic cancer using transrectal ultrasonotomography. Prostate 1987;10:11.
69. Koutsilieris M, Faure N, Tolis G, Laroche B, Robert G, Ackman CFD. Objective response and disease outcome in 59 patients with Stage D2 prostatic cancer treated with either buserelin or orchiectomy. Urology 1986;27:221.
70. Kuhn J-M, Billebaud T, Navratil H, Moulonguet A, Fiet J, Grise P, Louis J-F, Costa P, Husson J-M, Dahan R, Bertagna C, Edelstein R. Prevention of the transient adverse effects of a gonadotropin-releasing hormone analogue (Buserelin) in metastatic prostatic carcinoma by administration of an antiandrogen (Nilutamide). N Engl J Med 1989;321:413.
71. Lerner LJ. Hormone antagonists. Inhibitors of specific activities of estrogen and androgen. Rec Prog Horm Res 1964;20:435.
72. Lopez M, Di Lauro L, Lazzaro B, Papaldo P. Hormonal treatment of disseminated male breast cancer. Oncology 1985;42:345.
73. Loprinzi CL, Michalak JC, Quella SK, Fallon JR, Hatfield AK, Nelimark RA, Dose AM, Fischer T, Johnson C, Klatt NE, Bate WW, Rospond RM, Oesterling JE. Megestrol acetate for the prevention of hot flashes. N Engl J Med 1994;331:347.
74. Lubahn DB, Joseph DR, Sullivan PM, Willard HF, French FS, Wilson EM. Cloning of human androgen receptor complementary DNA and localization to the X chromosome. Science 1988;240:327.
75. Lund F, Rasmussen F. Flutamide versus stilboestrol in the management of advanced prostatic cancer, a controlled prospective study. Br J Urol 1988;61:140.
76. Manni A, Santen RJ, Boucher AE, Lipton A, Harvey H, Simmonds M, White-Hershey D, Gordon RA, Rohner TJ, Drago J, Wettlaufer J, Glode LM. Androgen priming and response to chemotherapy in advanced prostatic cancer. J Urol 1986;136:1242.
77. Montpetit ML, Lawless KR, Tenniswood M. Androgen-repressed messages in the rat ventral prostate. Prostate 1986;8:25.
78. Morales PA, Brendler H, Hotchkiss RS. The role of the adrenal cortex in prostatic cancer. J Urol 1955;73:399.
79. Neri R, Florance K, Koziol P, Van Cleave S. A biological profile of a nonsteroidal antiandrogen, SCH 13521 (4′-nitro-3′-trifluoromethylisobutyranilide). Endocrinology 1972;91:427.
80. Neumann F, Humpel M, Senge T, Schenck B, Tunn U. Cyproterone acetate—biochemical and biological basis for treatment of prostatic cancer. In Prostate Cancer. Edited by GH Jacobi, R Hohenfellner. Baltimore: Williams & Wilkins, 1982:p 269.
81. Neumann F, von Berswordt-Wallrabe R, Elger W, Steinbeck H, Hahn JD, Kramer M. Aspects of androgen-dependent events as studied by antiandrogens. Rec Prog Horm Res 1970;26:337.
82. Nieh PT. Withdrawal phenomenon with the antiandrogen casodex. J Urol 1995;153: 1070.
83. Normington K, Russell DW. Tissue distribution and kinetic characteristics of rat steroid 5α-reductase isoenzymes. Evidence for distinct physiological functions. J Biol Chem 1992;267:19548.
84. Oesterling JE, Epstein JI, Walsh PC. The inability of adrenal androgens to stimulate the adult human prostate: an autopsy evaluation of men with hypogonadotropic hypogonadism and panhypopituitarism. J Urol 1986;136:1030.
85. Olea N, Sakabe K, Soto AM, Sonnenschein C. The proliferative effect of "anti-androgens" on the androgen-sensitive human prostate tumor cell line LNCaP. Endocrinology 1990;126:1457.
86. Parra RO, Gregory JG. Treatment of post-orchiectomy hot flashes with transdermal administration of clonidine. J Urol 1990;143:753.

87. Patterson JS, Battersby LA, Bach BK. Use of tamoxifen in advanced male breast cancer. Cancer Treat Rep 1980;64:801.
88. Patterson MN, Hughes IA, Gottlieb B, Pinsky L. The androgen receptor gene mutations database. Nucl Acids Res 1994;22:3560.
89. Pavone-Macaluso M, De Voogt HJ, Viggiano G, Barasolo E, Lardennois B, De Pauw M, Sylvester R. Comparison of diethylstilbestrol, cyproterone acetate and medroxyprogesterone acetate in the treatment of advanced prostatic cancer: final analysis of a randomized phase III trial of the European Organization for Research on Treatment of Cancer Urological Group. J Urol 1986;136:624.
90. Pavone-Macaluso M, Pavone C, Serretta V, Daricello G. Antiandrogens alone or in combination for treatment of prostate cancer: the European experience. Urology 1989;34(suppl):27.
91. Pedrotti R, Frizzi V. Treatment of prostatic carcinoma by hormonal shock as suggested by Mayor. Cancer Chemother Absr 1966;7:100.
92. Perrault DJ, Logan DM, Stewart DJ, Bramwell VHC, Paterson AHG, Eisenhauer EA. Phase II study of flutamide in patients with metastatic breast cancer. A National Cancer Institute of Canada Clinical Trials Group study. Invest New Drugs 1988;6:207.
93. Peters CA, Walsh PC. The effect of nafarelin acetate, a luteinizing-hormone-releasing hormone agonist, on benign prostatic hyperplasia. N Engl J Med 1987;317:599.
94. Pritchard KI, Sutherland DJ. The use of endocrine therapy. Hematol/Oncol Clin of North Am 1989;3:765.
95. Prout GR Jr, Brewer WR. Response of men with advanced prostatic carcinoma to exogenous administration of testosterone. Cancer 1967;20:1871.
96. Prout GR Jr, Keating MA, Griffin PP, Schiff SF. Long-term experience with flutamide in patients with prostatic carcinoma. Urology 1989;34(suppl):37.
97. Pilepich MV, Krall JM, Al-Sarraf M, John MJ, Doggett RLS, Sause WT, Lawton CA, Abrams RA, Rotman M, Rubin P, Shipley WU, Grignon D, Caplan R, Cox JD. Androgen deprivation with radiation therapy compared with radiation therapy alone for locally advanced prostatic carcinoma: a randomized comparative trial of the Radiation Therapy Oncology Group Urology 1995;45:616.
98. Radlmaier A, Bormacher K, Neumann F. Hot flushes: mechanism and prevention. In EORTC Genitourinary Group Monograph 8: Treatment of Prostatic Cancer—Facts and Controversies. Edited by FH Schroeder. New York: Wiley-Liss, 1990, p 131.
99. Raynaud J-P, Ojasoo T. The design and use of sex-steroid antagonists. J Steroid Biochem 1986;25:811.
100. Rennie PS, Bowden J-F, Freeman SN, Bruchovsky N, Cheng H, Lubahn DB, Wilson EM, French FS, Main L. Cortisol alters gene expression during involution of the rat ventral prostate. Molec Endocrinol 1989;3:703.
101. Rennie PS, Bruchovsky N, Buttyan R, Benson M, Cheng H. Gene expression during the early phases of regression of the androgen-dependent Shionogi mouse mammary carcinoma. Cancer Res 1988;48:6309.
102. Rennie PS, Bruchovsky N, Goldenberg SL, Lawson D, Fletcher T, Foekens JA. Relative effectiveness of alternative androgen withdrawal therapies in initiating regression of rat prostate. J Urol 1988;139:1337.
103. Rittmaster RS. Finasteride. N Engl J Med 1994;333:120.
104. Robinson MRG. Reasons against total androgen suppression. In EORTC Genitourinary Group Monograph 8: treatment of Prostatic Cancer—Facts and Controversies. Edited by FH Schroeder. New York: Wiley-Liss, 1990, p 117.
105. Schellhammer P, Sharifi R, Block N, Soloway M, Venner P, Patterson AL, Sarosdy M, Vogelzang N, Jones J, Kovenbag G. A controlled trial of bicalutamide versus flutamide, each in combination with luteinizing hormone-releasing hormone analogue therapy, in patients with advanced prostatic cancer. Urology 1995;45:745.
106. Scher HI, Kelly WK. Flutamide withdrawal syndrome: its impact on clinical trials in hormone-refractory prostate cancer. J Clin Oncol 1993;11:1566.
107. Schroeder FH, Lock TMTW, Chadha DR, Debruyne FMJ, Karthaus HFM, de Jong FH, Klijn JGM, Matroos AW, de Voogt HJ. Metastatic cancer of the prostate managed with buserelin versus buserelin plus cyproterone acetate. J Urol 1987;137:912.
108. Schroeder FH. Pure antiandrogens as monotherapy in prospective studies of prostatic carcinoma. In EORTC Genitourinary Group Monograph 8: Ttreatment of Prostatic Cancer—Facts and Controversies, New York: Wiley-Liss, 1990, p 93.
109. Schulman CC. Neoadjuvant androgen blockade prior to prostatectomy: a retrospective study and critical review. Prostate 1994;(suppl 5):9.
110. Schulze H, Oesterling JE, Isaacs JT, Coffey DS. Hormonal therapy of prostate cancer: limitations in the total androgen ablation concept. In A Multidisciplinary Analysis of Controversies in the Management of Prostate Cancer. Edited by DS Coffey, MI Resnick, FA Dorr, JP Karr. New York: Plenum, 1986, p 215.
111. Schulze H, Isaacs J, Senge T. Inability of complete androgen blockade to increase survival of patients with advanced prostatic cancer as compared to standard hormonal therapy. J Urol 1987;137:909.
112. Scott WW, Boyd HL. Combined hormone control therapy and radical prostatectomy in the treatment of selected cases of advanced carcinoma of the prostate: a retrospective study based upon 25 years of experience. J Urol 1969;101:86.
113. Segaloff A. Results of studies of the cooperative breast cancer group—1961–63. Cancer Chemother Rep 1964;41:1.
114. Setchell BP. Introduction. In Male Reproduction. Edited by BP Setchell. New York: Van Nostrand Reinhold, 1984, p 1.
115. Sharifi R, Kiefer J. History of endocrine manipulation in the treatment of carcinoma of the prostate—who was first? J Endocrinol Invest 1987;10(suppl 2):91.
116. Sogani PC, Vagaiwala MR, Whitmore WF Jr. Experience with flutamide in patients with advanced prostatic cancer without prior endocrine therapy. Cancer 1984;54:744.
117. Stein BS, Smith J. A DES lead-in to use of luteinizing hormone-releasing hormone analogs in treatment of metastatic carcinoma of prostate. Urology 1985;25:350.
118. Stoll BA. Hormonal therapy—pain relief and recalcification. In Bone Metastasis, Monitoring and Treatment. Edited by BA Stoll, S Parbhoo. New York: Raven, 1983, p 321.
119. Suarez AJ, Lamm DL, Radwin HM, Sarosdy M, Clark G, Osborne CK. Androgen priming and cytotoxic chemotherapy in advanced prostatic cancer. Cancer Chemother Pharmacol 1982;8:261.
120. Taplin M-E, Bubley GJ, Shuster TD, Frantz ME, Spooner AE, Ogata GK, Keer HN, Balk SP. Mutation of the androgen-receptor gene in metastatic androgen-independent prostate cancer. N Engl J Med 1995;332:1393.
121. The Leuprolide Study Group. Leuprolide versus diethylstilbestrol for metastatic prostate cancer. N Engl J Med 1984;311:1281.
122. Tormey DC, Gelman PR, Band PR, Sears M, Bauer M, Arseneau JC, Falkson G. A prospective evaluation of chemohormonal therapy remission maintenance in advanced breast cancer. Breast Cancer Res Treat 1981;1:111.
123. Tormey DC, Lippman ME, Edwards BK, Cassidy JG. Evaluation of tamoxifen doses with and without fluoxymesterone in advanced breast cancer. Ann Intern Med 1983;98:139.
124. Trapman J, Klaassen P, Kuiper GGJM, van der Korput JAGM, Faber PW, van Rooij HCJ, van Kessel AG, Voorhorst MM, Mulder E, Brinkmann AO. Cloning, structure and expression of a cDNA encoding the human androgen receptor. Biochem Biophys Res Commun 1988;153:241.
125. Vallis K, Waxman J. Tumour flare in hormonal therapy. In Endocrine Management of Cancer 2, Contemporary Therapy. Edited by BA Stoll. Basel: S Karger AG, 1988, p 144.
126. Vanuytsel L, Ang KK, Vantongelen K, Drochmans A, Baert L, Van Der Schueren E. Ketoconazole therapy for advanced prostatic cancer: feasibility and treatment results. J Urol 1987;137:905.
127. Veldscholte J, Berrevoets CA, Brinkmann AO, Grootegoed JA, Mulder E. Anti-androgens and the mutated androgen receptor of LNCaP cells: differential effects on binding affinity, heat-shock protein interaction, and transcription activation. Biochemistry 1992;31:2393.
128. Venner PM, Klotz PG, Klotz LH, Stewart DJ, Davis IR, Orovan WL, Ramsey EW. Megestrol acetate plus minidose diethylstilbestrol in the treatment of carcinoma of the prostate. Semin Oncol 1988;15(suppl 1):621988.
129. Verhelst J, Denis L, Van Vliet P, Van Poppel H, Braeckman J, Van Cangh P, Mattelaer J, D'Hulster D, Mahler Ch. Endocrine profiles during administration of the new non-steroidal anti-androgen Casodex in prostate cancer. Clin Endocrinol 1994;41:525.
130. Vermeulen A, Giagulli VA, De Schepper P, Buntinx A, Stoner E. Hormonal effects of an orally active 4-azasteroid inhibitor of 5α-reductase in humans. Prostate 1989;14:45.
131. Westerberg H. Tamoxifen and fluoxymesterone in advanced breast cancer: a controlled clinical trial. Cancer Treat Rep 1980;64:117.
132. Wilding G, Chen M, Gelmann EP. Aberrant reponse in vitro of hormone-responsive prostate cancer cells to antiandrogens. Prostate 1989;14:103.
133. Wilson JD. Androgen abuse by athletes. Endocrine Rev 1988;9:181.
134. Wong GI, Kelce WR, Sar M, Wilson EM. Androgen receptor antagonist versus agonist activities of the fungicide vindozolin relative to hydroxyflutamide. J Biol Chem 1995;270:19998.
135. Wysowski DK, Freiman JP, Tourtelot JB, Horton ML III. Fatal and nonfatal hepatoxicity associated with flutamide. Ann Intern Med 1993;118:860.
136. Zincke H. Bilateral pelvic lymphadenectomy and radical prostatectomy for stage C or D1 adenocarcinoma of the prostate: possible beneficial effect of adjuvant treatment. NCI Monogr 1988;7:109.
137. Zincke H. Extended experience with surgical treatment of stage D1 adenocarcinoma of prostate: significant influences of immediate adjuvant hormonal treatment (orchiectomy) on outcome. Urology 1989;33(suppl):27.

CHAPTER 77

Paraneoplastic Syndromes

WILLIAM D. ODELL

Introduction

In addition to producing symptoms by direct tissue invasion and tumor mass, neoplasms may produce abnormalities that are distant from the tumor itself. Symptoms caused by processes distant from the tumor have been termed *paraneoplastic syndromes.* When I first reviewed this subject some 30 years ago, it generally was believed that such syndromes were rare and caused by an unusual expression or "derepression" of genes not expressed by the noncancer tissues (1). As these syndromes were studied further and improved methods developed, however, it became apparent that many, or even all, neoplasms produced protein hormones or protein hormone precursors, and that the biologic activity of these precursors was smaller than that of the usual biologically active hormone. For example, data from our laboratory (2) showed that extracts from normal human tissues contained small amounts of immunoreactive chorionic gonadotropin, lipotropin, vasopressin, and ACTH. Extracts from carcinomas showed the same activities but generally in greater quantities. We postulated that so-called "ectopic" hormone production was a universal concomitant of neoplasia and probably was not "ectopic" but instead an increased expression of a normal cell function (2). Subsequently, it has been found that in addition to protein hormone materials, locally acting proteins (i.e., cytokines) may be produced by some neoplasms, in turn producing still other clinical syndromes. In addition to the production of protein hormones, their precursors, and cytokines, cancers also often cause striking neurologic disorders that cannot be explained by increased protein hormone or cytokine production. Within the past 10 years, the cause of these remote neurologic disorders has been clarified and related to tumor-antigen stimulation of antibody formation, wherein the antibody reacts with one or more neuronal antigens, thus damaging normal tissue. As might be implied by these several mechanisms, the range of symptoms and laboratory findings in patients with paraneoplastic neurologic syndromes is enormous, and the causes of this broad array of paraneoplastic syndromes are shown in Table 77.1.

TUMOR PRODUCTION OF PROTEIN HORMONES OR THEIR PRECURSORS

Four paraneoplastic syndromes are discussed in separate sections: sustained inappropriate antidiuretic hormone (SIADH) production, hypercalcemia as caused by parathormone-related peptide production, Cushing's syndrome as caused by precursor ACTH and ACTH production, and hypoglycemia as caused by production of insulin-like growth factors (IGFs). Each of these protein hormone paraneoplastic syndromes is now understood in terms of molecular genetics, control mechanisms for protein hormone gene expression, and intracellular processing of prohormones to hormones. These data as well as those from other syndromes related to protein hormone production indicate that hormone precursors generally possess less biologic activity than the mature hormone itself. For example, equilibrium-type radioimmunoassays may demonstrate strikingly elevated blood ACTH levels in many patients with carcinomas who do not have Cushing's syndrome, while measurement of ACTH by receptor assays or bioassays shows little or no elevation (2). Similarly, ACTH extracted from normal cells reacts in equilibrium assays for ACTH, but it possesses little or no biologic activity. This ACTH is a precursor molecule that can be converted enzymatically to bioactive ACTH (3, 4). Immunoactivity results from the reaction of these ACTH precursors in the equilibrium assay. Use of more structurally specific immunoradiometric assays demonstrates that in patients with cancers and Cushing's syndrome, both ACTH precursors and ACTH itself are increased (5). Thus, specific endoprotease activity is increased in those cancers that result in clinical Cushing's syndrome and largely is lacking in the bulk of cancers that do not produce this syndrome. In this context, the most common cancer to produce paraneoplastic Cushing's syndrome is small cell carcinoma of the lung (SCCL); however, only 1.6 to 2.8% of patients with SCCL have Cushing's syndrome (6).

Table 77.2 lists the protein hormones and related proteins that have been reported to be produced by cancers (most often carcinomas). Whereas each now can be discussed in terms of clinical symptoms, association with various tumor types, molecular pathogenesis, diagnosis, and treatment, that task is far too extensive for this review. General comments, however, may be summarized as follows: many normal, nonendocrine cells appear to produce small amounts of protein hormones or protein hormone precursors that presumably act in paracrine or autocrine functions. Cancers often produce increased quantities of such protein hormone precursors, which have less biologic activity than the most potent forms of the hormone. A small fraction of cancers either produce very large quantities of weakly bioactive protein hormone precursor or convert the precursor to a more

Table 77.1. Pathogenesis of Paraneoplastic Syndromes

Tumor production of protein hormones or their precursors
Metabolism of steroids by the tumor
Tumor production of enzymes or fetal proteins
Tumor production of cytokines
Tumor stimulation of antibody production
Not known

potent product to produce the clinical syndrome. It is in this context that *ectopic hormone production is not ectopic* (2, 4).

A separate section reviews the syndrome of hypercalcemia as produced by tumor production of excess parathormone-related peptide (PTH-RP). The most common cause of tumor-associated hypercalcemia is excess PTH-RP production; however, other causes of hypercalcemia may be associated with cancer, including: (1) increased hydroxylation of 25-hydroxyvitamin D by the neoplasm that produces vitamin D toxicity; (2) production of osteoclast-activating cytokines such as interleukin-1, transforming growth factor-alpha, and prostaglandins of the E series; (3) rarely, parathormone production by the cancer (7); and (4) widespread bony metastatic disease. The last also may be caused by cytokine-mediated increases in bone resorption.

METABOLISM OF STEROIDS

Metabolism of normally produced precursor steroids by a neoplasm to create biologically active products are rare. Two examples exist. First, increased aromatase activity of a neoplasm leading to increased estrogen formation and gynecomastia in male patients with hepatic cancers and large sarcomas has been reported. These neoplasms metabolize androgen precursors such as dehydroepiandrosterone (produced by the adrenal glands) or testosterone (produced by the testes) to estradiol. The increased estradiol produces gynecomastia. Second, increased vitamin D hydroxylase activity leading to increased 1,25-dihydroxyvitamin D formation and hypercalcemia also has been reported. For example, T-cell lymphomas may produce hypercalcemia by hydroxylating circulating 25-hydroxyvitamin D to the more potent 1,25-dihydroxyvitamin D. Other hematologic neoplasms as well as granulomatous diseases such as sarcoidosis and tuberculosis may produce hypercalcemia by a similar mechanism.

TUMOR PRODUCTION OF ENZYMES OR FETAL PROTEINS

A variety of fetal proteins may be produced by neoplasms. Generally, these produce no clinical symptoms but still may be useful as tumor markers. Examples include alpha-fetoprotein, carcinoembryonic antigen, and alkaline phosphatase isoenzymes.

TUMOR PRODUCTION OF CYTOKINES

Some paraneoplastic syndromes appear to be caused by tumor production of substances that under normal circumstances are locally acting paracrine or autocrine message proteins (i.e., cytokines). Table 77.3 lists some of these syndromes. These have not been studied or documented as extensively as the paraneoplastic protein hormone syndromes. Yoneda and colleagues (8) reviewed 225 patients with oral cancers to evaluate the frequency of paraneoplastic syndrome of hypercalcemia and leukocytosis. Ten (4.4%) of the 225 patients had hypercalcemia, 11 (4.9%) had leukocyto-

Table 77.2. Protein and Hormone Precursors Reportedly Produced by Neoplasms

Pro-opiomelanocortin and related peptides
Corticotropin-releasing hormone
Chorionic gonadotropin and its subunits (α and β)
Vasopressin
Cytokine growth factors (e.g., TGF-β, EGF, IGF-II)
Parathyroid hormone-related protein
Parathormone
Erythropoietin
Eosinophilopoietin
Growth hormone
Growth hormone–releasing hormone
Prolactin
Gastrin
Gastrin-releasing peptide (and bombesin)
Secretin
Glucagon
Calcitonin
Renin, prorenin
Vasoactive intestinal peptide
Somatostatin
Hypophosphatemia-producing factor
Endothelin-1

EGF—Epidermal growth factor; IGF-II—insulin-like growth factor II; TGF-β—transforming growth factor-beta.

Table 77.3. Pathophysiology of the Humoral Syndromes of Cancer

Endocrine syndromes
Tumor production of protein hormones or hormone precursors
Tumor metabolism of steroids
Neuromuscular syndromes
Tumor stimulation of antibody production
Antibody reacts with normal neuronal synaptic tissues
Dermatologic syndromes
Tumor stimulation of antibody formation; antibody reacts against skin component
Tumor production of cytokines
Glomerulonephritis
Deposition of tumor antigen–antibody complexes on renal mesangium
Hematologic syndromes
Tumor production of antibody that reacts against a cell line (e.g., thrombocytopenia)
Tumor production of hormone (e.g., erythropoietin)
Miscellaneous syndromes (probably caused by tumor cytokine production)
Anorexia/cachexia
Fever
Digital clubbing/pulmonary osteoarthropathy
Tumor production of other proteins
Fetal proteins (e.g., alpha-fetoprotein, carcinoembryonic antigen)
Enzymes (e.g., alkaline phosphatase, thymidine kinase)

sis, and 5 (2.2%) had both hypercalcemia and leukocytosis. The cause of the syndrome was not evaluated in their review. Wetzler and colleagues (9), however, evaluated a patient with transitional cell carcinoma of the bladder and leukocytosis, and they found that plasma granulocyte-macrophage colony-stimulating factor (GM-CSF) was elevated but granulocyte CSF and interleukin 3 were not. They postulated that increased tumor production of GM-CSF caused the leukocytosis, but whether GM-CSF is the cytokine causing leukocytosis in most or all patients with this paraneoplastic syndrome is unknown.

As discussed in the protein hormone section, local cytokine production with osteoclast-activated bone resorption appears to be the cause of hypercalcemia in multiple myeloma and of some additional hematologic neoplasms that may cause hypercalcemia.

TUMOR STIMULATION OF ANTIBODY PRODUCTION

Neoplasms may express immunoaccessible antigens that normally are not available to the immune system. Such antigens may lead to the production of antibodies, which in turn may produce striking symptoms if the normal tissue expressing those antigens is damaged. Table 77.4 lists the syndromes that have been described as being associated with cancer and that may be caused by antibody production.

It is tempting to postulate that a particular antibody causes a particular clinical syndrome, but this has not been proven. The most common type of cancer associated with neurologic syndromes is SCCL; however, other carcinomas also are associated with such neurologic syndromes. As was true for the protein hormone–related syndromes, only a small percentage of patients with a given neoplasm develop a neurologic syndrome. Thus, in a prospective study of 150 patients with SCCL, only 2 had Eaton-Lambert syndrome, and 1 had subacute sensory neuropathy (10). When patients with specific neurologic syndromes are studied, however, the incidence of cancer is high. Approximately 60% of patients with Eaton-Lambert syndrome and 50% of patients with subacute cerebellar degeneration have an associated cancer. When cerebellar degeneration is associated with breast or ovarian cancer, an antibody directed against the Purkinje cells usually is present. When cerebellar degeneration is associated with other cancers, anti-yo usually is absent. Patients with encephalomyelitis and SCCL almost always have antibodies against a neuronal nuclear antigen (anti-hu) (11).

Buchanovich and colleagues (12) recently reported that the circulating antibody in patients with breast and lung cancer or the paraneoplastic opsoclonus-ataxia syndrome is directed against a nuclear neuronal protein. This protein is highly homologous to the yeast-splicing protein MER 1. Opsoclonus-ataxia is a dramatic disturbance that is characterized by an abnormal ability or an inability to control the eyes, limbs, and trunk that occurs in women with breast or lung cancer.

MISCELLANEOUS SYNDROMES

A number of other indirect effects of neoplasms have been described for which the pathogenesis remains unknown. Some of these are listed in Table 77.5.

Table 77.5. Miscellaneous Paraneoplastic Syndromes of Unknown Cause

Sweet syndrome (acute febrile neutrophilia dermatosis)
Acute necrotizing myopathy
Fever
Pulmonary osteoarthropathy

Table 77.4. Paraneoplastic Syndromes that May Be Caused by Antibody Production

Syndrome	Possible antigen	Comment
Stiff-man	Synaptic neural protein[a]	Symptoms are progressive rigidity of body musculature
Visual	Photoreceptor protein (recoverin)	Retinal degeneration
Subacute cerebellar degeneration	Purkinje cell proteins (e.g., Yo)	Progressive cerebellar symptoms
Lambert-Eaton	Voltage-operated calcium-channel protein	Multifocal central nervous symptoms
Encephalomyelitis	Neuronal protein (homologous to *Drosophila* elav and sex-lethal protein)	Multifocal central nervous symptoms
Intestinal pseudo-obstruction	Antineuronal nuclear protein	Degeneration of the myenteric plexus gut dysmotility
Subacute sensory neuropathy	A pan-neuronal nuclear antigen	Painful sensory neuropathy
Opsoclonus-ataxia	DNA-binding protein (homologus to yeast-splicing protein, MER 1)	Abnormal motor control of eyes, trunk, and limbs
Glomerulonephritis	Multiple tumor antigens	Antigen–antibody complex deposition
Pemphigus	Desmoplakin I and II epithelial cell junction proteins	Acantholysis
Idiopathic thrombocytopenic purpura	Platelet antigens	Thrombocytopenia

[a] Most patients with stiff-man syndrome do not have cancer; 60% of these patients with noncancer-associated stiff-man syndrome have antibodies against the synaptic enzyme glutamic acid decarboxylase.

Endocrine Syndromes

With rare exceptions, paraneoplastic endocrine syndromes are caused by tumor production of protein hormones or hormone precursors. Such proteins generally are produced in small amounts by some, or many, normal tissues, and they presumably act in paracrine or autocrine functions. Thus, these endocrine syndromes are not strictly speaking ectopic humoral syndromes; rather, they represent the abnormal regulation of a normal cell function (13, 14).

A rare exception to this mechanism is tumor metabolism of a normal circulating steroid to produce a different biologic function. For example, Kew and colleagues (15) reported that hepatic cancer converted dehydroepiandrosterone to estrone and estradiol, and Herr and colleagues (16) reported a pelvic sarcoma that metabolized testosterone to estradiol to produce feminization. With the exception of neoplasms originating from adrenal glands, testes, or ovaries, which may retain steroid-synthesizing capabilities, cancers do not synthesize steroid hormones de novo.

Table 77.2 lists the protein hormones and hormone precursors that have been reported as being produced by cancers. This section discusses only a few selected hormones. The syndromes reviewed, which include cancer production of Cushing's syndrome, hypercalcemia, SIADH, hypoglycemia, cancer production of chorionic gonadotropin (CG), as well as growth hormone and growth hormone–releasing hormone, are exemplary of the endocrine syndromes of cancer and their pathophysiology.

CANCER PRODUCTION OF ACTH AND RELATED PEPTIDES

Cushing's syndrome associated with cancer was first described in 1928 and was only the second (after hypercalcemia) hormonal syndrome of cancer to be described. In the 1960s, Liddle and colleagues (17) published their study of 88 patients with cancer and Cushing's syndrome, which demonstrated that the primary cancer and its metastases contained large amounts of biologically active ACTH. Several hundred patients with this syndrome have now been reported, and the types of neoplasms that produce biologically active ACTH are listed in Table 77.6.

Table 77.6. Neoplasms Associated with "Ectopic" Cushing's Syndrome

Neoplasms	Approximate percentage of reported patients
Carcinoma of the lung (predominantly small or oat cell)	50
Carcinoma of the thymus	10
Carcinoma of the pancreas (including carcinoid and islet cell)	10
Pheochromocytoma, neuroblastoma, ganglioma, and paraganglioma	5
Medullary carcinoma of the thyroid	5
Bronchial adenoma and carcinoid	2
Miscellaneous carcinomas[a] or hematologic malignancies	18

[a] For example, carcinoma of the ovary, prostate, breast, thyroid, kidney, salivary glands, testes, stomach, colon, gallbladder, esophagus, appendix, and acute myeloblastic leukemia.
Adapted from Odell and Appleton (18).

The production of Cushing's syndrome by a cancer generally can be distinguished from a pituitary ACTH-producing adenoma or pituitary-dependent Cushing's disease by several findings: (1) hypokalemia is common in cancer-induced Cushing's syndrome but is unusual in Cushing's disease; (2) serum and urine cortisol concentrations usually are markedly elevated in cancer-induced Cushing's syndrome but in the high-normal range without diurnal variation or modestly above normal in Cushing's disease; (3) plasma ACTH level usually is very highly elevated in cancer-induced Cushing's syndrome, but it is "normal" or slightly elevated in Cushing's disease; (4) suppression of A.M. ACTH and cortisol levels by large doses of dexamethasone (e.g., 2 mg every 6 h for 2 days, or a single 8-mg dose at 10 P.M.) is unusual in cancer-induced Cushing's syndrome but expected in Cushing's disease; and (5) an increase in plasma ACTH/cortisol levels in response to corticotropin-releasing hormone (CRH) stimulation is present in Cushing's disease but usually is not seen in cancer-associated Cushing's syndrome (18–21). Occasionally, however, the cancer-ACTH syndrome is subtle and the tumor small. In such patients, diagnosis must be made by metabolic criteria and followed by a careful search. Computed tomography of the chest and abdomen or venous catheterization (at times including the petrosal veins) may be required to identify the tumor. Patients with bronchial carcinoid or carcinoma of the thymus (Table 77.6) causing Cushing's syndrome are particularly difficult to distinguish from those patients with Cushing's disease. Suppression of ACTH/cortisol with high-dose dexamethasone is seen in 40 to 50% of carcinoid-produced Cushing's syndrome and also is expected in Cushing's disease (18–22). Response to CRH is brisk in Cushing's disease and usually absent in Cushing's syndrome caused by bronchial carcinoid, although some patients with bronchial carcinoid do show CRH stimulation (21).

The precursor molecule of ACTH is a glycoprotein proopiomelanocortin (POMC). POMC contains the amino acid sequences of lipotropin, melanocyte-stimulating hormone, endorphins and enkephalins, and of ACTH itself (23). Odell and colleagues, both in 1977 (13) and 1979 (24, 25), reported that extracts from all carcinomas of several histological types from patients without signs of Cushing's syndrome (i.e., cancers not producing biologically active ACTH) contained large amounts of both ACTH and lipotropin as measured by immunoassay. Furthermore, prospective clinical studies showed that an immunoreactive, ACTH-like material was present in plasma in amounts greater than those found in patients without cancer (13, 24, 25). This ACTH-like material showed no biological activity as assessed by in vitro radioreceptor assay and had a size larger than the 4,500 d of biologically active ACTH. Subsequently, Odell and colleagues (14, 26, 27) showed that nonendocrine tissues from humans without cancer as well as normal tissues from rats contained a 26,000-d glycoprotein possessing both ACTH and lipotropin immunoactivities. This molecule contained no biologic ACTH activity as assessed by in vitro dispersed adrenal cell assays. However, a biologically active, 4,500-d ACTH was produced by treatment of the glycoprotein with trypsin in vitro. This precursor ACTH molecule resembled POMC. Odell and colleagues (14, 25–27) hypothesized that the same molecule was synthesized in greatly increased quantities by all carcinomas, and that a subset of carcinomas metabolized this ACTH precursor to biologically active ACTH to produce the so-called ectopic ACTH syndrome.

More recent data have given some insights into the molecular mechanisms of ectopic ACTH production. In humans a single POMC gene exists. This gene is unusual in that it contains three distinct promoter regions that control transcription: P1, P2, and P3. (For an excellent review, see White and Clark [28].) Promoter P2 is the one that is found in the normal pituitary gland. The upstream promoter, P1, produces a larger transcript than P2, but the protein product is identical to that produced by P2 as only one translation initiation site exists. In contrast, the downstream promoter, P3, is weakly active in a variety of peripheral tissues and produces a smaller transcript. In some tumors expressing the ectopic ACTH syndrome, the upstream promoter, P1, appears to be the dominant promoter (29, 30). As stated, this contrasts with the normal pituitary gland, where P2 is the dominant controller. Thus, normal peripheral tissues produce small amounts of ACTH-related molecules as controlled by P3, while cancers appear to have altered promoter control that increases transcription rates.

Treatment of cancer-associated Cushing's syndrome is best achieved by treating the causative tumor. Frequently, life expectancy is short in patients with untreatable tumors, and symptomatic treatment at times may not be selected. However, medical treatment with oral ketoconazole (i.e., an inhibitor of steroidogenesis) in doses adequate to suppress the 24-hour urinary cortisol level to normal may be elected. Use of ketoconazole as a treatment for Cushing's syndrome or Cushing's disease is not approved by the U.S. Food and Drug Administration, but it often is effective if adequate doses are employed. Bilateral adrenalectomy may be considered for some patients with long life expectancy and a very slow-growing neoplasm. Mitotane (o,p′-DDD) is an adrenolytic agent that also may be used to decrease cortisol production in selected patients.

CHORIONIC GONADOTROPIN PRODUCTION

Human CG is a glycoprotein comprised of single α and β chains linked by charge–charge interaction. The α chain of CG is identical in amino acid sequence to the α chain of three other human glycoprotein hormones: thyrotropin, luteinizing hormone (LH), and follicle-stimulating hormone (31). In the 1960s, it generally was believed that CG was produced solely by the trophoblast cell during normal pregnancy, by gestational trophoblastic neoplasms derived from these cells, or rarely, by teratomas containing trophoblast cells. Between 1949 and 1972, approximately eight patients were reported who had nontrophoblastic carcinomas (i.e., malignant melanoma, adrenocortical carcinoma, renal carcinoma, breast carcinoma, carcinoma of the lung) that appeared to produce a CG-like hormone (18). In 1972, Vaitukaitis and colleagues (32) reported the development of the beta CG assay, which has an increased ability to distinguish CG from its very close biochemical relative LH. Using this assay, Braunstein and colleagues (33) studied serum samples from a large number of patients with a wide variety of carcinomas, including carcinoma of the lung, stomach, colon, and pancreas; they found that 6 to 13% of these patients had increased blood CG concentrations.

Odell and colleagues (18, 34–36) reported that when extracts of carcinomas were studied, all contained a CG-like material as assessed by both the beta CG immunoassay and CG radioreceptor assays. In addition, these investigators showed that similar to the story for ACTH, a CG-like material also was extractable from normal human tissues (13, 34–36). This CG-like material bound to testicular LH/CG receptors, and judged by concanavalin A (CON-A), a plant lectin that binds glycoproteins containing mannose and glucopyranose sugars, this CG-like material was shown to have a strikingly different carbohydrate structure from that of placental CG. The normal tissue CG-like material showed little or no binding to CON-A, while placental CG was 95 to 100% bound to CON-A. Furthermore, the molecular weight of normal tissue CG-like material was less than that of placental CG and similar to carbohydrate-free placental CG (14, 18). The CG-like material in the blood of patients with carcinomas and in extracts of carcinomas had variable CON-A binding, ranging from 5% (i.e., similar to that of normal tissue CG) to 85% (i.e., similar to that of placental CG).

Alteration or removal of carbohydrate from placental CG alters biologic activity by changing the metabolic degradation rate. For example, desialated CG has a half-life of degradation ($t_{1/2}$) in humans of 3.6 minutes, whereas carbohydrate-rich CG has a $t_{1/2}$ of approximately 9 hours (37). In essence, degradation of carbohydrate-poor CG is so rapid that it is unlikely blood concentrations would be increased to detectable levels. Odell and colleagues (13, 14, 35) hypothesized that all carcinomas and normal human tissues produce CG. Those carcinomas associated with increased blood concentrations of CG either produced very large quantities of this normal tissue CG and/or glycosylated the CG, thus transforming it into a hormone with a longer half-life and increased biologic activity in vivo.

Employing monoclonal antibodies in immunoradiometric (sandwich) assays, entirely specific assays for CG subsequently were developed by Griffin and Odell (38) and by Stenman and colleagues (39). These assays made it possible to detect small amounts of CG in the blood of all normal men and women studied, to show that CG was secreted in parallel with LH, to show that CG was absent from the blood of hypopituitary subjects, and to show that the CG level was suppressed by estrogen treatment and gonadotropin-releasing hormone agonists in postmenopausal women and castrated men, respectively (39, 40). Odell and colleagues (41, 42) also showed that human pituitary cell cultures secreted CG in vitro and that a previously unknown pituitary cell type immunostained for CG but not LH or other anterior pituitary hormones. All of these data indicate that the source of the small amounts of CG in the blood of normal humans is the pituitary gland, not the nonendocrine tissues (e.g., liver, kidney). It is important to note that differences in the pres-

Table 77.7. Expected Ranges of Blood CG in Normal Subjects and Patients with Cancer

Patients	Range (mIU/mL)
Gestational trophoblastic neoplasms	20–>10,000
Carcinomas producing CG	4–25
Castrate or postmenopausal	1.0–3.5
Eugonadal subjects	0.04–0.65

CG—Chorionic gonadotropin.

ence of CG in the blood of patients with cancer versus normal humans without cancer are quantitative and not a question of the presence or absence of CG. Table 77.7 gives the expected ranges of CG in various conditions.

Treatment of excess CG production by cancer is not necessary. Symptoms that are produced by CG either are none or gynecomastia in males. CG may be useful as a diagnostic or a treatment tumor marker.

URINARY GONADOTROPIN PEPTIDE

A CG-related protein termed *urinary gonadotropin peptide* (UGP), or beta core fragment of the beta subunit of hCG (beta core), has more recently been described as a useful marker of neoplasia. Beta core initially was described as one of the components of pregnancy urine (42–45), and it is a major form of the hCG immunoreactivity in pregnancy urine, existing in concentrations as high as seven times greater than that of hCG itself (46). The IRMA assay used to identify sources of hCG in blood (47–50) does not react with purified beta core; therefore, these studies apply to intact holo hCG. Earlier studies using equilibrium assays and polyclonal anti-hCG and anti-beta subunit assays, however, cross-react well with both purified beta subunit and the beta core.

Birken and colleagues (51) as well as Blithe and colleagues (52) reported purification and characterization of the beta core fragment from pregnancy urine in 1988. Beta core is a disulfide-linked protein with a molecular weight of 10.5 kd. The primary amino acid sequence is identical to residues 6-40 and 55-92 of the beta subunit of hCG (51, 52). The carbohydrate composition differs from that of the beta subunit, and that of beta core from pregnancy urine is heterogeneous. There probably are two sources of beta core: (1) beta core is a degradation product produced in the kidney, and (2) beta core is secreted directly by trophoblastic tissue and some cancers. Cole and Birken (46) demonstrated that beta core was secreted directly into media by 24-hour organ cultures of trophoblastic tissue from first-, second-, and third-trimester pregnancies; the amount of beta core exceeded that of hCG. Wehmann and Nisula (53) reported that the amount of beta core present in urine greatly exceeded that in serum, thus suggesting beta core was a renal metabolic product produced from the beta subunit of hCG.

Beta core appears to be a potentially useful marker of normal pregnancy and also gynecologic malignancies. Walker and colleagues (54) measured beta core in 866 urines from normal women as well as women with benign or malignant gynecologic diseases. Quantitative differences were observed, and using a cutoff value for normal creatinine of 4 fmol/mg, 2% of normal premenopausal and nonpregnant women had elevated values, while 15% of postmenopausal women and 5% of women with ovarian cancer had elevated values. There was no correlation with any specific histologic type of cancer. The expression of beta core and another ovarian tumor antigen, CA125, also was not correlated, and use of both markers increased sensitivity. Postmenopausal women produce greater amounts of intact hCG than are found in premenopausal women, and the increased beta core in urine of postmenopausal women may derive from this increased production (47–50, 55).

HYPERCALCEMIA

Hypercalcemia is a relatively common manifestation of cancer. For example, hypercalcemia occurs in 20 to 40% of patients with multiple myeloma (56), in over 50% of patients with type C virus-induced T-cell lymphoma (57), and in 12.5% of patients with bronchogenic carcinoma (58). Among patients with bronchogenic carcinoma, the frequency of hypercalcemia varies with the histologic type: 23% with epidermoid carcinoma, 13% with large cell anaplastic carcinoma, and 2% with adenocarcinoma (58). The mechanisms producing hypercalcemia are several and can be divided into three major categories. Table 77.8 lists these categories along with the approximate percentage of total patients reported in the literature that each represents.

Hypercalcemia is associated with poor life expectancy in patients with cancer. Ralston and colleagues (59) reviewed their experience with 126 patients treated for hypercalcemia caused by cancer, and regardless of the response of serum calcium to treatment, the median survival was 30 days.

The pathophysiology of hypercalcemia is described in Table 77.8. Solid tumors without evidence of bony metastases or with minimal metastatic disease usually produce hypercalcemia by production of a protein that binds to the parathormone receptor (59–64). The syndrome of hypercal-

Table 77.8. Neoplasms Associated with Hypercalcemia

Neoplasm	Approximate percentage of cases
Carcinomas	
Carcinoma of the lung	35
Carcinoma of the kidney	24
Carcinoma of the ovary	8
Miscellaneous carcinomas[a]	<2 each
Hematologic malignant neoplasms	
Multiple myeloma	7
T-cell lymphoma	2
Other	1
Tumors with bony metastases	
Breast carcinoma	
Others not included in frequency estimates	

[a] This includes almost every type of carcinoma (e.g., pancreas, urinary bladder, colon, prostate, penis, esophagus, parotid glands, testes, liver, and stomach).

cemia associated with solid tumors was the earliest of the hormonal cancer syndromes to be reported, in 1924 (65). Albright (66) discussed such a patient in a 1941 clinical conference and first postulated that these tumors produced a parathormone-like substance. The patient had hypercalcemia and hypophosphatemia with normal parathyroid glands at autopsy. Several publications employing early generation parathormone radioimmunoassays reported increased parathormone levels in the blood of such patients (67–70). As assay methods improved, however, it became clear that parathormone per se rarely was produced by such tumors. Federman (71) reported a patient in 1971, also at a clinical pathologic conference, who had squamous cell carcinoma, hypercalcemia, and hypophosphatemia but no detectable plasma parathormone. In 1973, Powell and colleagues (72) studied 11 patients with cancer and no bony metastases who had hypercalcemia and hypophosphatemia; treatment of the tumor-restored calcium levels to normal in 9 patients. Using several parathormone immunoassays designed to react with fragments as well as intact parathormone, no parathormone was detectable in either tumor extracts or blood. In extracts of all 11 tumors, however, a substance was detected that caused the resorption of calcium from mouse calvaria incubated in vitro. In 1983, Simpson and colleagues (73) studied five human and three animal cancers producing hypercalcemia using a sensitive and specific hybridization assay from parathormone messenger RNA; no parathormone message was detected in these tumors. These studies all suggest that a substance with parathormone-like biologic properties was produced but that it was not structurally identical to parathormone.

Subsequently, several investigators purified the proteins that are responsible for tumor hypercalcemia, sequenced these proteins, and identified the responsible gene (60–64, 74–76). Their results show that a single gene appears to be expressed as two different proteins by alternative splicing (74, 75). The most abundant protein contains 139 amino acids, of which the amino terminal portion shows a 70% homology with parathormone (74). It is this amino acid sequence, however, that is required for binding to the parathormone receptor. The 139 amino-acid protein has biologic properties very similar to parathormone, but the potency relative to parathormone varies with the different tissues or assays employed (76). The gene for this protein, which has been called *parathyroid hormone–related protein* (PTH-RP), is expressed in normal, lactating mammary tissue (77) and probably in normal keratinocytes as well (78). Li and Drucker (79) confirmed that the gene encoding PTH-RP is expressed at low levels in normal tissues; however, cellular transformation by the EJ-Ha-*ras* or v-*src* oncogenes is associated with a dramatic increase in PTH-RP gene expression. These investigators showed that the PTH-RP gene is a downstream target for *ras* and *src,* thus providing a possible explanation for malignancy-associated hypercalcemia. Therefore, the ectopic hormone syndrome of hypercalcemia in carcinomas is another example of cancers expressing, in greater amounts, a function of normal tissues.

Recently, three groups of investigators (80–82) have developed equilibrium-type immunoassays as well as immunoradiometric assays for PTH-RP, and they have shown that PTH-RP concentrations increase in most patients with solid tumors and hypercalcemia. Increased PTH-RP concentrations correlate with increased urinary cyclic AMP excretion. Plasma from normal subjects contains low or undetectable concentrations of PTH-RP. Because the normal lactating breast produces large amounts of PTH-RP, the mechanism of hypercalcemia in patients with breast cancer has been reevaluated. Several groups have reported that the PTH-RP level is elevated in the blood of most patients with breast cancer and hypercalcemia (80–84). Ikeda and colleagues (85) detected messenger RNA for PTH-RP in breast cancer from a patient with hypercalcemia, and now is known that large quantities of PTH-RP are secreted in milk and that PTH-RP plays a major physiologic role in the normal lactation process (77, 86). Therefore, in summary, PTH-RP appears to be a product of the normal lactating breast and is produced by some breast cancers, creating hypercalcemia. It is curious that lactating mothers do not become hypercalcemic, however, thus suggesting either differences in the amounts of PTH-RP produced or some control or functional differences in the PTH-RP produced.

This discussion has been conducted along historical lines, starting with the (erroneous) postulate that parathormone per se was commonly produced by cancers to cause hypercalcemia and ending with the knowledge that PTH-RP was the cause of hypercalcemia associated with solid tumors. Recent data using current sandwich-type parathormone assays indicate that a cancer very rarely may produce hypercalcemia by the production of parathormone per se. Both Nussbaum and colleagues (87) and Rizzoli and colleagues (88) have reported two well-evaluated patients with hypercalcemia of cancer where parathormone production by the cancer appeared to be the cause.

Hematologic malignancies produce hypercalcemia by different mechanisms. In 1974, Mundy and colleagues (89) reported that a bone-resorbing substance produced by myeloma cells was similar to osteoclast-activating factor (OAF), a substance that also is produced by normal leukocytes activated in vitro. Subsequently, it has appeared that OAF likely is not a single substance but instead a group of substances that include lymphotoxin (produced by normal lymphocytes) and tumor necrosis factor (also called *cachectin,* produced by normal monocytes (90). Both substances are potent stimulators of bone resorption in vitro. Garrett and colleagues (91) reported that cultured myeloma cells secrete lymphotoxin and that this production relates to the hypercalcemia caused by myeloma.

Hypercalcemia caused by type C virus-induced T-cell lymphoma, and occasionally by other neoplasms, is caused by still another mechanism. Breslau and colleagues (92) as well as Rosenthal and colleagues (93) demonstrated that these patients have increased quantities of 1,25-dihydroxyvitamin D (1,25-D) in their blood. Helikson and colleagues (94) described a patient with a large plasma cell myeloma and hypercalcemia who had an increased blood 1,25-D level. Following tumor resection, 1,25-D concentrations returned to normal. The resected tumor was shown to convert 25-hydroxyvitamin D to 1,25-D. Hypercalcemia with increased 1,25-D in blood also has been reported in a patient with leiomyoblastoma and one with Hodgkin's disease. The patients' solid tumors and hypercalcemia (previously described) did not have elevated blood 1,25-D levels.

Treatment of hypercalcemia caused by cancer often is an emergency. Frequently, hypercalcemic patients are anorexic and hypovolemic, with decreased glomerular filtration. Some are immobilized by hypercalcemia-produced lethargy or somnolence or by pain related to the cancer. Volume expansion with normal saline, often in amounts up to 6 L/d, is a useful first treatment. Furosemide often is added, because it decreases calcium reabsorption and thus increases excretion. Complications include development of pulmonary edema, hypokalemia, and hypomagnesemia; careful monitoring of central venous pressure and/or urine volume and electrolytes reduces the likelihood of complications. Many additional agents have been used to treat hypercalcemia, including calcitonin, cisplatin, mithramycin, gallium nitrate, and biphosphonates. In my opinion, intravenous infusion of 90 mg of pamidronate over a 24-hour period following volume expansion is the best choice of treatment (94a). Lower doses (60 mg) of pamidronate given over 4 hours also have been reported to be effective (94b). Such single-dose therapy usually will keep calcium in the normal range for 7 days or longer. The other agents mentioned either are less effective, act for a shorter period, or are associated with greater toxicity. Side effcts of intravenous pamidronate are mild and include, in some patients, low-grade fever or asymptomatic hypocalcemia or hypophosphatemia.

VASOPRESSIN (ANTIDIURETIC HORMONE) PRODUCTION

In 1957, Schwartz and colleagues (95) first described the syndrome of hyponatremia, renal sodium loss, hypervolemia, and inappropriately high urine osmolality in association with cancer. They attributed this syndrome to vasopressin (i.e., antidiuretic hormone [ADH]) production by the cancer. Subsequently, several investigators verified that ADH could be extracted from cancers, and direct synthesis of ADH by a cancer was also reported (96, 97). ADH is split enzymatically from a larger, precursor molecule that also contains a second, larger protein; neurophysin. The neurophysin portion of the precursor molecule has been reported to be present in extracts from tumors associated with the syndrome of cancer ADH production (98). ADH production has been reported in a wide spectrum of histologic carcinoma types and in Hodgkin's disease as well, but not to our knowledge in sarcomas. The most common cancer that is associated with ADH production is lung carcinoma, predominantly small or oat cell carcinoma. Gilby and colleagues (99) reported that 40% of patients with oat cell carcinoma have inappropriate ADH production. Odell and colleagues (13) reported that 41% of patients with lung carcinoma of several histologic types had elevated plasma ADH levels, and North and colleagues (100) reported that 42% of unselected patients with small cell carcinoma have elevated blood neurophysin concentrations.

It is important to note in reference to the last two studies (13, 100) that not all patients were hyponatremic; however, they presumably would become hyponatremic if they were water loaded. The syndrome of hyponatremia, renal sodium loss, and hypervolemia depends not only on the presence of tumor ADH production but also on an associated and perhaps inappropriate thirst with excess water intake.

HYPOGLYCEMIA

The histologic types of neoplasms that cause hypoglycemia are quite different from those producing ACTH, CG, ADH, or hypercalcemia. Table 77.9 lists cancers that are associated with hypoglycemia and their approximate frequency. Approximately two-thirds of patients with this syndrome either have a mesenchymal tumor or a hepatic carcinoma. Etiology of the hypoglycemia is debated, but it probably is caused by tumor production of IGF-I and/or IGF-II.

In 1963, Field and colleagues (101) studied 25 cancers that were associated with hypoglycemia. Insulin, as measured by radioimmunoassay, was not present in tumor extracts, but an insulin-like substance was detected by bioassay in extracts of all 25 cancers. Using an IGF-radioreceptor assay employing rat liver membranes, Gordon and colleagues (102) found IGF concentrations to be increased in the plasma of 19 of 52 patients (37%) with cancer and hypoglycemia. In 1988, Daughaday and colleagues (103) reported that both extracts of a large leiomyosarcoma producing hypoglycemia and the patient's serum had markedly increased amounts of IGF-II. Levels of IGF-II messenger RNA also was increased in tumor extracts. IGF-I concentrations were low in tumor extracts and serum, and IGF-II concentrations decreased to normal when the tumor was removed. In contrast to these striking findings, Froesch and colleagues (104) as well as Widmer and colleagues (105) studied 22 patients with hypoglycemia and cancer and were unable to demonstrate elevated concentrations of either IGF-I or IGF-II in serum.

The reasons for the striking discrepancies among these studies is uncertain. IGFs possibly are labile in serum, and stored sera may not contain the same concentrations as fresh sera. Ron and colleagues (106) studied two additional patients with mesenchymal tumors and hypoglycemia, and they reported that IGF-II concentrations in blood were highly elevated. In addition, the serum growth hormone increase that is expected with hypoglycemia was blunted. Plasma IGF-I concentrations were low as well. They postulated that the combination of increased IGF-II and suppressed growth hormone led to hypoglycemia. Lowe and colleagues (107)

Table 77.9. Neoplasms Associated with Hypoglycemia

Tumor	Approximate percentage of cases
Mesenchymal[a]	45
Hepatic carcinoma	23
Adrenal carcinoma	10
Gastrointestinal carcinoma[b]	8
Hematologic neoplasms	6
Miscellaneous	8

[a] Includes fibrosarcomas, mesotheliomas, neurofibromas, neurofibrosarcomas, spindle cell carcinomas, rhabdomyosarcomas, and leiomyosarcomas.
[b] Includes cholangiomas, gastric carcinomas, colon carcinomas, pancreatic carcinomas, and carcinoid tumors.
Adapted from Odell and Appleton (18).

identified abundant messages for IGF-II in the extracts from four tumors that produced hypoglycemia, and Daughaday and colleagues (103) reported that circulating IGF-II has a larger molecular weight than the usual IGF-II. In a follow-up to this finding, Daughaday and Kapadia (108) studied two additional patients with elevated "big" IGF-II levels. Because IGF-binding proteins can modify IGF biologic activity, they characterized the binding proteins in patients with tumoral hypoglycemia. In contrast to normal subjects, these patients showed a smaller-molecular-weight binding protein. They hypothesized that this IGF-II-binding protein complex may transverse capillary membranes more easily than normal complexes can, and this might result in increased biologic potency in vivo.

Treatment of hypoglycemia caused by non-islet-cell cancers optimally is directed at the tumor itself. For a patient in whom this is no longer effective, frequent feedings with avoidance of fasting are necessary. Often, infusion of glucose in amounts that are adequate to prevent hypoglycemia also is necessary. Diazoxide, which is effective in treating malignant insulinomas, is not effective in this cancer hypoglycemia syndrome. Its mode of action is to inhibit insulin secretion, and as discussed, insulin is not the cause of the hypoglycemia in this syndrome. It may be worth attempting treatment with octreotide, which is a long-acting analogue of somatostatin, if other treatment is ineffective. To our knowledge, however, no reports of octreotide used for this purpose have been published.

GROWTH HORMONE AND GROWTH HORMONE-RELEASING HORMONE PRODUCTION

A growth hormone–like material, as defined by radioimmunoassay, has been extracted from several carcinomas of the lung (109–112), stomach (112), breast (113), and ovary (113). Kyle and colleagues (104) reported small amounts of a material that was identical to pituitary growth hormone (as assessed by radioimmunoassay, radioreceptor assay, and molecular weight) and were extractable from virtually all normal human tissues. Interestingly, only one case of acromegaly has been reported to be caused by tumor production of growth hormone (115).

In contrast, acromegaly has been reported to be caused by tumor production of GHRH in a small number of patients (116–119). GHRH normally is produced by hypothalamic neurons and is secreted into the pituitary portal vessels to stimulate growth hormone secretion. The tumors reported to have produced GHRH and acromegaly predominantly have been bronchial carcinoids and pancreatic islet cell tumors.

Treatment of growth hormone or GHRH production by cancers is best performed by surgical removal of the neoplasm. If this is not possible, treatment with octreotide (i.e., the long-acting somatostatin analogue) may be effective.

Paraneoplastic Syndromes of the Nervous System

Table 77.10 lists syndromes of the central nervous system that are associated with cancer. In contrast to the hormone syndromes, where cancer directly produces a substance that circulates in the blood to produce symptoms, the neurologic syndromes generally are produced through the stimulation of antibody production by cancer. This antibody initially may impair tumor growth, but it also circulates and cross-reacts with one or more antigens in normal tissues to produce symptoms.

Table 77.10. Paraneoplastic Syndromes Affecting the Nervous and Muscular Systems

Visual paraneoplastic syndrome
Central nervous system
  Cerebellar degeneration
  Encephalomyelitis (e.g., limbic, bulbar)
  Dementia
Peripheral nerves
  Subacute sensory neuropathy
Other
  Intestinal pseudo-obstruction
  Lambert-Eaton myasthenic syndrome

One or more of these syndromes (if carefully searched for) are common in patients with lung cancer. For example, Gomm and colleagues (120) prospectively evaluated 100 patients with lung cancer, of which 35 had SCCL and 65 non-SCCL, for paraneoplastic syndromes. Thirty-three patients had polymyopathy (18 with cachexia/myopathy), 15 proximal myopathy, 2 Lambert-Eaton myasthenia syndrome, 1 dermatomyositis, and 1 Cushing's syndrome. Muscle biopsies performed on all patients, however, that showed 99 patients had abnormal muscle histology, suggesting that more subtle manifestations of paraneoplastic neurologic/muscular syndromes may be present in most patients. Elrington and colleagues (121) prospectively studied 150 patients with SCCL, and neuromuscular or autonomic deficits were present in 44% of these patients. In contrast, more clear-cut syndromes (e.g., Lambert-Eaton syndrome) were present in two patients, and one patient had subacute sensory syndrome.

VISUAL PARANEOPLASTIC SYNDROME

Visual paraneoplastic syndrome has been described under several names, including visual paraneoplastic syndrome, photoreceptor degeneration, cancer-associated retinopathy, and paraneoplastic retinopathy. The first report (122) in 1976 described a woman with oat cell carcinoma who complained of night blindness and visual hallucinations that consisted of shimmering and flickering gold specks. Approximately 16 patients now have been described, most with SCLC (122–127) but also some with cervical, endometrial, and breast carcinoma; malignant melanoma; and non-SCCL (126, 128–131).

In 1985, Grunwald and colleagues (124) found that sera from two patients with this syndrome contained antibodies reacting with both the cancer tissue and normal retina. Kornguth and colleagues (123, 125) have reported seven patients with this syndrome, and they found serum antibodies reacting with retinal ganglia cells, photoreceptors, and with cells from the small cell carcinomas of the same patients. In addition, they reported that the antigens for these antibodies corresponded to three proteins composing a known neurofilament triplex that also has been identified in lung cancer. Crofts and colleagues (131) identified a woman with endometrial carcinoma and this syndrome whose serum had high titers (1:1000) of antibodies reacting with human retina and optic nerve. In 1992, Thirkill and colleagues (132) reported that the retinopathy antigen was a recoverin-like protein.

In summary, the visual paraneoplastic syndrome is believed to be caused by tumor stimulation of antibody production, with antibodies directed against the antigens shared by the tumor and the retina and/or optic nerve. Low titers of such antibodies now have been found in sera from subjects without cancer (133).

CEREBELLAR SYNDROMES

Cerebellar cortical degeneration most often is associated with carcinoma of the lung or ovary. However, this syndrome also has been associated with carcinoma of the fallopian tubes, larynx, colon, stomach, uterus, breast, and with malignant melanoma, chondrosarcoma, and Hodgkin's, non-Hodgkin's, and T-cell lymphomas. The symptoms of cerebellar degeneration often precede diagnosis of the responsible neoplasm. Trotter and colleagues (134) reported in 1976 a patient with Hodgkin's disease and cerebellar degeneration whose serum contained antibodies reacting with cerebellar Purkinje cells. Subsequently, three patients with ovarian carcinoma (135, 136) and cerebellar degeneration were described whose cerebrospinal fluid or sera contained antibodies reacting with Purkinje cells as well as cells in the deep cerebellum. Greenlee and Sun (137) tested sera from five patients with this syndrome against cerebellar tissue from a number of animal species. Reactions against cerebellum from monkey, pig, and rabbit were strong, while reactions against tissue from sheep, cat, or rat were weak and variable. Subsequently, a man with chondrosarcoma and a woman with fallopian tube carcinoma and cerebellar degeneration were described; these patients had regression of the cerebellar symptoms when the tumor was resected (138).

In 1987, Dropcho and colleagues (139) cloned a gene coding for a brain protein identified by antibodies obtained from a patient with adenocarcinoma (unknown primary) and cerebellar degeneration. Expression of this gene largely was restricted to brain tissue in normal subjects, but it also was expressed by cell lines derived from human cancers of neuroectodermal, renal, and pulmonary origin. The anti-Purkinje cell antibody was termed *anti-Yo.* In 1992, Peterson and colleagues (140) reviewed the clinical findings in 55 patients with cerebellar degeneration that was associated with the anti-Yo antibody. All of these patients were women aged 26 to 85 years. Fifty-two patients (95%) had a malignancy, almost exclusively breast cancer or gynecologic cancers that usually were confined to the involved organ and local nodes. One woman had carcinoma of the lung, while three had no malignancy identified. In 34 of 52 patients (65%) the neurologic syndrome preceded recognition of the cancer and, in many patients, led to suspicion that a cancer was present. Unfortunately, the cerebellar degeneration led to a disabling clinical state in most patients, with approximately 80% being unable to sit or walk unassisted. The cancer often was successfully treated, but the neurologic symptoms did not appear to improve.

Hammack and colleagues (141) reviewed the clinical findings of 18 men and three women with cerebellar degeneration associated with Hodgkin's disease. In contrast to those with breast and gynecologic cancers, the diagnosis of lymphoma preceded neurologic symptoms in these patients by 1 to 54 months, but tumor stage or activity did not correlate with the severity of neurologic disease. Strikingly, six patients developed cerebellar degeneration while in remission from Hodgkin's disease. Also, treatment with plasmapheresis or glucocorticoids did not appear to improve neurologic symptoms. One patient improved dramatically after treatment with clonazepam, but two improved spontaneously. Clinical neurologic symptoms usually were only those of cerebellar degeneration, but one patient also had encephalopathy, three had long tract signs, and two had sensory neuropathy.

In summary, cerebellar degeneration associated with anti-Yo antibody is a particularly disabling neurologic syndrome that almost always is associated with a neoplasm. Antibodies react with both the neoplasm and cerebellar Purkinje cells, but proof that this causes this clinical syndrome is lacking.

ENCEPHALOMYELITIS

Encephalomyelitis, either localized to certain anatomic areas of the nervous system such as limbus or bulbar areas or more generalized and associated with dementia, also occurs as a paraneoplastic syndrome of cancer. The neoplasm commonly is an SCCL. Dalmau and colleagues (142) evaluated 71 patients with encephalomyelitis, many of whom also had sensory neuropathy. Seventy-eight percent of these patients had an SCLC, but 9 patients (13%) had no detectable tumor. The cause of this degenerative disorder is not known, and it may be seen in patients with several antibodies, including anti-Hu, and anti-Yo (141, 143).

Sekido and colleagues (144) evaluated the HuD gene, which encodes for a neuronal antigen homologous to the *Drosophila elar* and *Sx1* genes involved in neuronal and sexual development. In the human, Hu was mapped to chromosome region 1p. Sekido and colleagues sequenced the gene in 26 patients with detectable anti-HuD out of 46 patients with cancer who were studied. The gene had no mutation and was identical to the normal HuD gene. In patients with cancer, however, this gene produces four messenger RNAs by alternative splicing, resulting in both full-length and truncated proteins.

SUBACUTE SENSORY NEUROPATHY

Subacute sensory neuropathy is a debilitating syndrome of sensory disorder that is characterized by loss of sensory function, areflexia, and sensory ataxia. Motor and other central nervous system functions often remain intact, but neuronal loss leads to degeneration of axons and demyelination in dorsal and posterior roots of the spinal cord.

Most patients with this syndrome have SCCL. Graus and colleagues (145) reported four patients with this syndrome and SCCL whose sera contained antibodies reacting with the nuclei of neurons. They identified the immunogen as a basic protein with a molecular weight of 38,000. A similar protein was identified in the carcinoma from one of these patients. Subsequently, a polyclonal IgG from some patients was characterized and termed *anti-Hu* (146, 147). These antibodies react with neuronal nuclei in the central nervous system, dorsal root, and trigeminal ganglia, but they do not react with nuclei from other normal, nonneuronal tissues.

Anti-Hu recognizes a group of nucleoprotein antigens with molecular weights from 35,000 to 40,000. The antibodies were not entirely specific for lung cancer tissue from patients with this syndrome, however. Dalmau and colleagues (143), employing a quantitative Western blot technique, evaluated the titers of anti-Hu in 50 normal subjects, 44 patients with SCCL and no paraneoplastic syndromes, and 25 patients with SCCL and paraneoplastic sensory neuropathy and/or encephalomyelitis. No detectable anti-Hu was present in the sera of normal subjects; 7 patients with SCCL without paraneoplastic syndromes had low titers of anti-Hu, averaging 76 U/mL; and titers in the 25 patients with SCCL and a paraneoplastic syndrome averaged 4592 U/mL. In 1992, Dalmau and colleagues (142) described 71 patients with circulating anti-Hu antibodies. Of these, 62 had SCCL, but 9 had no detectable tumor. Fifty-two had multifocal central nervous system lesions, with 28 in two distinct areas and 24 in three or more identifiable areas of the nervous system. These studies show that a small number of patients may develop anti-Hu-associated sensory neuropathy or encephalitis without an identifiable cancer, and also that anti-Hu titers may be associated not only with sensory neuropathy but with encephalomyelitis as well.

Chalk and colleagues (148) reviewed the clinical features of 26 patients with paraneoplastic sensory neuropathy. Twenty patients were female; 6 were male. Nineteen (73%) had SCCL, (15%) had breast carcinoma, and three (12%) had other types of cancers. Symptoms of the sensory neuropathy included pain, paresthesias, and sensory loss, and these symptoms often were asymmetric early in the disease course. Fifty percent of the patients had other neurologic symptoms in addition to the sensory neuropathy, including cerebellar degeneration, encephalomyelitis, or autonomic symptoms. In contrast to the previously discussed neurologic syndromes, successful treatment of the neoplasm seemed to halt progression of the sensory symptoms, at least in some patients; however, no neurologic symptoms improved.

INTESTINAL PSEUDO-OBSTRUCTION

Intestinal pseudo-obstruction is a paraneoplastic syndrome that also usually is associated with SCCL and presents as symptoms of intestinal obstruction. Neuron and nerve fiber loss are found, usually during postmortem examination, in the myenteric plexus. Lennon and colleagues (149) evaluated 34 patients with SCCL and identified 5 with chronic intestinal pseudo-obstruction. Four of these 5 (80%) had IgG antibodies that reacted with neurons of the myenteric and submucosal plexus of the jejunum and stomach. Antibodies of this type were not found in the 29 patients with SCCL and no gut dysmotility, nor were such antibodies found in 8 patients with chronic idiopathic intestinal pseudo-obstruction. Condom and colleagues (150), however, reported a patient with high titers of anti-Hu antibodies and this syndrome as the only neurologic paraneoplastic symptom of cancer. It would appear that antibodies other than anti-Hu, directed specifically to tumor antigen(s) also present in the myenteric and submucosal plexus of the gut, most likely are the cause of this recently described paraneoplastic syndrome.

LAMBERT-EATON MYASTHENIC SYNDROME

Lambert-Eaton myasthenic syndrome (LEMS) is a somewhat rare autoimmune neuromuscular syndrome that is characterized clinically by fluctuating muscle weakness, hyporeflexia, and autonomic dysfunction. While it often is associated with patients with malignancies, particularly with SCCL, it also is seen in patients without cancer.

Gutmann and colleagues (151) reviewed 28 patients with LEMS, 14 with cancer and 14 with no detectable cancer. LEMS also may be seen in patients with cancer who also have another paraneoplastic neurologic syndrome. At a neurophysiology level, LEMS is associated with a reduction in nerve-evoked release of acetylcholine at the neuromuscular junction. Hewett and Atchison (152) demonstrated in 1991 that serum from patients with LEMS inhibited calcium-channel activity in isolated nerve terminals of the central nervous system. Leys and colleagues (153) tested 36 patients with LEMS for serum antibodies to voltage-gated calcium channels using an immunoprecipitation assay, and 44% had elevated antibody levels. Interestingly, patients with LEMS without associated SCCL had a higher percentage of elevated antibody levels (61%) than patients with LEMS and SCCL (28%). Eight of 12 patients with rheumatoid arthritis or systemic lupus erythematosus had mildly elevated antibody titers compared with those of healthy controls.

Rosenfeld and colleagues (154) screened a human fetal-brain-expression library and isolated an antigen to the antibodies in sera from patients with LEMS. When cloned, the protein product of this expression showed a high degree of homology to the beta subunit of calcium channel complexes. The premessenger RNA is alternatively spliced to produce three forms of the protein. More recently David and colleagues (155) detected antibodies against the synaptic vesicle protein, synaptotagmin. Furthermore, a panel of SCCL tumor lines expressed several proteins of the secretory pathway, including synaptotagmin, syntaxin, and N-type calcium channels.

In summary, tumor protein production may provoke anti-calcium-channel-antibody production to produce LEMS. LEMS also may develop as an autoimmune syndrome in patients without cancer.

Dermatologic Syndromes of Cancer

Many skin disorders have been reported to be associated with cancer; however, a direct causal relationship only rarely has been supported by experimental data. Table 77.11 lists the cutaneous syndromes associated with cancers (156).

Table 77.11. Cutaneous Syndromes and Commonly Associated Neoplasms

Paraneoplastic syndrome	Commonly associated neoplasms
Erythema gyratum repens	Lungs, uterus, breast, upper GI tract
Sign of Leser-Trélat	Adenocarcinoma of the GI tract, usually the stomach
Hypertrichosis lanuginosa acquisita	Carcinoma of lung and colon
Subcutaneous fat necrosis	Acinar cell carcinoma of the pancreas
Sweet's syndrome	Acute myelogenous leukemia
Melanosis	Melanoma, ACTH-producing tumors
Pityriasis rotunda	Liver carcinoma, hematologic malignancies
Acrokeratosis paraneoplastica (Bazex's syndrome)	Squamous cell carcinoma of upper aerodigestive tract
Acanthosis nigricans	Adenocarcinoma of GI tract, usually the stomach
Keratosis palmaris et plantaris	GI tract
Keratosis palmaris	Bladder, lung
Acquired ichthyosis	Lymphoproliferative neoplasms, primarily Hodgkin's disease
Erythroderma	Lymphoma, leukemia
Necrolytic migratory erythema	Glucagonoma
Vasculitis	Leukemia, lymphoma
Flushing	Carcinoid syndrome, leukemia
Migratory thrombophlebitis (Trousseau's syndrome)	Pancreatic tumor
Cowden's disease	Breast, thyroid carcinoma
Nevoid basal cell carcinoma syndrome	Medulloblastoma
Gardner's syndrome	Carcinoma of the colon
Mucosal neuroma syndrome	Medullary thyroid carcinoma, pheochromocytoma
Peutz-Jeghers syndrome	GI tract, breast, genital system, pancreas
Dermatomyositis	Bronchial carcinoma (males) Genital tumors (females)
Pachydermoperiostosis	Bronchogenic carcinoma

GI—Gastrointestinal.
From Politi and colleagues (156).

As with other paraneoplastic syndromes, the cutaneous paraneoplastic syndrome may precede diagnosis or lead to diagnosis of an underlying cancer. Cutaneous paraneoplastic syndromes are estimated to occur in 7 to 15% of patients with cancer (157, 158). These cutaneous syndromes are not discussed in detail here because of limitations in space; the interested reader is referred to the review by Politi and colleagues (156). Three examples of syndromes, however, are discussed.

SIGN OF LESER-TRÉLAT

This clinical sign manifests by intense growth of seborrheic keratosis. Although its occurrence in patients with cancer may be co-incidental, possible direct relationships have been suggested by the simultaneous occurrence of seborrheic keratosis and cancer and, occasionally, by regression of the skin lesion after the cancer is treated (159–161). Grob and colleagues (162), however, conducted a case-control study of 82 patients with a recent diagnosis of solid tumors compared with 82 age- and sex-matched controls; no differences in the features or incidence of seborrheic keratosis were found.

PARANEOPLASTIC PEMPHIGUS

A variety of malignancies have been reported to be associated with pemphigus, including those derived from the thymus, lymphatic tissue, ovary, breast, uterus, stomach, esophagus, and bronchus. A direct cause has not been established; however, Anhalt and colleagues (163) described five patients with neoplasms who developed painful mucosal ulcerations and polymorphous skin lesions that progressed to blistering eruptions of the trunk and extremities. Immunofluorescence studies revealed atypical, pemphigus-like autoantibodies in perilesional epithelium and in the sera of all five patients. One antigen of the antibodies was shown to be a 250-kd protein that co-migrated with desmoplakin I, which is a protein found in the desmosomes of epithelial cells.

ACANTHOSIS NIGRICANS

These skin lesions usually are symmetric, hyperpigmented, velvety plaques typically affecting the axillae, neck, flexure areas, and anogenital area. Acanthosis nigricans often is associated with endocrine disorders or occurs as an inherited disorder; however, it also occurs in association with malignancies. While it has been postulated as resulting from tumor production of one or more growth factors, a direct cause and effect has not been established. Wilgenbus and colleagues (164) reported a single patient with gastric cancer and acanthosis nigricans and who showed increased expression of the epidermal growth factor (EGF) receptor, which is the binding receptor for both EGF and TGF-α. In 4 of 25 gastric carcinomas from patients without acanthosis, amplification of the EGF receptor was found as well. In 1987, Ellis and colleagues (165) also reported a patient with this syndrome, suggesting that increased TGF-α production was present.

POLYMYOSITIS AND DERMATOMYOSITIS

Polymyositis and dermatomyositis are two related skeletal muscle disorders that occur in patients either with cancer or without cancer. Both polymyositis and dermatomyositis are characterized by proximal muscle weakness and inflammatory myopathic changes with mononuclear cell infiltration. Association of this syndrome with cancer has been reported for a wide variety of carcinomas as well as histiocytic lymphoma and Hodgkin's disease. Barnes and Mawr (166) reviewed 258 cases selected as having dermatomyositis and a cancer. In 31%, the diagnosis of the neoplasm preceded the appearance of myopathy. In a second series from the Mayo Clinic, however, 115 patients were selected because they had dermatomyositis (167). The incidence of cancer in these patients was not greater than that in a similar, sex-matched population. Thus, the causal association of dermatomyositis with cancer remains uncertain. Most patients, however, do have circulating antibodies against myosin or myoglobin, but cross-reaction against a tumor antigen has not been proven.

Glomerulonephritis

Abnormalities in glomerular histology are found in many patients with malignant solid neoplasms. The most common lesion is membranous glomerulonephritis, which is present in approximately 75% of patients with glomerulonephropathy and a solid neoplasm (168–170). Crescentic glomerulonephritis is not commonly associated with cancer (169); Pascal (171) analyzed 314 patients with cancer and reported glomerulopathy (excluding amyloidosis) in only 1.6%. Neoplasms most commonly associated with membranous glomerulonephritis include carcinomas of the lung, gastrointestinal tract, and breast. Glomerulonephritis may occur before diagnosis of the neoplasm, be diagnosed at the same time, or may occur during the course of treatment. In two patients with prostate carcinoma and glomerulonephritis, renal disease occurred after treatment of the cancer (171, 172). The pathogenesis is similar to that described in experimental immune-complex renal disease. The source of the antigen is tumor-associated antigens or tumor expression of fetal antigens (168, 173).

Hematologic Syndromes

THROMBOCYTOPENIA

Idiopathic thrombocytopenic purpura (ITP), pure red-cell aplasia, and aplastic anemia all have been reported to be associated with a variety of carcinomas and lymphatic neoplasms. In 1979, Kim and Boggs (174) reviewed 10 patients with ITP and cancer. Four had lymphoid neoplasms, and in 7 patients, ITP occurred either when the cancer was diagnosed or following its recognition. Subsequently, 3 patients (2 with multiple myeloma, and 1 with endometrial carcinoma) were reported to have ITP and circulating antiplatelet antibodies (175, 176). It was not possible to prove that the tumor induced these antibodies. In 1987, however, Aghai and colleagues (177) reported a patient with ITP and hepatic lymphoma; removal of the hepatic lymphoma was the only effective way of treating the ITP and was associated with return of the platelet count to normal.

ERYTHROCYTOSIS

Erythrocytosis or polycythemia is associated with several neoplasms and appears to be caused by tumor production of erythropoietin (i.e., the hormone normally produced by kidney cells to modulate red-cell production). The most common types of neoplasms to produce erythrocytosis derive from renal tissue, so in a sense, this property of erythropoietin production is retained by the tumor and not developed as a new or "ectopic" property. Table 77.12 shows the types of tumors that are associated with erythrocytosis and their approximate distribution among reported cases (18, 178, 179).

Approximately 10% of patients with hepatocellular carcinoma have erythrocytosis (180, 181). Waldman and colleagues (182, 183) first reported that fluid from renal cysts and cerebellar cysts in patients with erythrocytosis contained an erythropoietin-like hormone as bioassayed in the polycythemic mouse. Later, Ljungberg and colleagues (184) measured erythropoietin by an enzyme immunoassay in 165 patients with renal carcinoma; 55 patients (33%) had elevated serum concentrations. Thorling (178) estimated that between 1 and 4% of patients with hypernephroma have erythrocytosis; thus, the frequency of erythropoietin overproduction is greater than that of erythrocytosis. In addition, the level of erythropoietin in patients with erythrocytosis correlates poorly with the degree of erythrocytosis (184).

Removal of the neoplasm has resulted in disappearance of the polycythemia in many patients with all types of neoplasms. Goldberg and colleagues (185) studied a hepatoma cell line that produced erythropoietin in vitro, and they found that increasing cell density and cell hypoxia greatly increased erythropoietin production. It is unknown whether increased erythropoietin production may occur in vivo by increasing tumor mass or tumor hypoxia. Rarely, some patients with hematologic malignancies may have erythrocytosis. For example, Ballard and Kouri (186) reported three patients with chronic lymphocytic leukemia and erythrocyto-

Table 77.12. Tumors Associated with Erythrocytosis

Neoplasm	Approximate percentage of reported cases
Renal carcinoma	40
Hepatocellular carcinoma	18
Cerebellar hemangioblastoma	16
Renal cystic disease and hydronephrosis	15
Uterine fibroids and leiomyosarcomas	8
Miscellaneous[a]	3

[a] Carcinomas of the adrenal gland, lung, prostate, breast, and thymus, virilizing ovarian neoplasms, pheochromocytoma, and Wilms' tumor.

sis. These likely are not humoral manifestations of these neoplasms but rather a disorder of a pluripotent stem cell with capacity to differentiate into lymphoid and erythroid pathways.

Other Syndromes

Table 77.3 lists a number of other syndromes that have been reported to be associated with cancer. These mostly are less well understood than the hormone or neurologic syndromes. Anorexia is a common symptom in patients with cancer, especially in those with lung carcinoma, hypernephroma, and carcinoma of the pancreas. This has been attributed to tumor production of the protein tumor necrosis factor (TNF), which also is called *cachectin*. This protein has a molecular weight of 17,000 (187–189), and it has been speculated that tumor induces TNF production by host cells. In 1985, Aderka and colleagues (190) reported that TNF was produced by peripheral blood mononuclear cells in patients with cancer. Balkwill and colleagues (191) reported in 1987 that 114 of 226 freshly obtained sera (50%) from patients with cancer had detectable TNF; in contrast, only 1 of 32 samples (3%) from normal controls and 7 of 39 samples (18%) from asymptomatic patients with cancer had detectable TNF. In contrast to these suggestive findings, four other groups (192–195) have reported that TNF is not detectable in the sera of patients with cancer and cachexia. The explanation for these differences is uncertain. Balkwill and colleagues (191) emphasized the importance of using freshly obtained serum samples, but Selby and colleagues (195) used fresh samples and still did not detect TNF.

While it is attractive to postulate that TNF/cachectin produced in response to a cancer is the cause of cancer-associated anorexia and weight loss, data do not support such a view.

FEVER AND CANCER

Fever may be seen in patients who have cancer but no evidence of infection. It is estimated, for example, that 18% of patients with renal adenocarcinoma have fever (196). Hodgkin's disease also can be associated with fever in the absence of infection. Fever could be produced either by tumor induction of pyrogen formation through host white cells or by direct tumor production of a pyrogen. Pyrogen production by human tumor cell lines grown in vitro also has been reported (197).

Tumor Production of Other Proteins

Many proteins are expressed in embryonic cells during fetal life that are not expressed by adult cells. A variety of cancers produce these fetal proteins, which often are discussed under the heading "tumor-associated antigens." These proteins include fetal isoenzymes (e.g., Regan alkaline phosphatase (198) and thymidine kinase) and other proteins of uncertain function but that may serve as tumor markers. Two examples are carcinoembryonic antigen (CEA) (199) and alpha-fetoprotein (AFP) (200). CEA is a 200-kd glycoprotein that commonly is produced by colon carcinoma but also by a wide array of carcinomas, and its level in blood is elevated in a number of benign disorders, such as inflammatory bowel disease, hepatic cirrhosis, and pulmonary infections. AFP is a 70-kd globulin normally produced by the liver and yolk sac in the fetus (200). AFP also is produced by hepatic carcinomas and germ cell tumors such as teratocarcinomas. Fetal proteins are not discussed here in detail as they are discussed separately in most oncology textbooks.

Conclusions

Cancers produce a wide array of symptoms or findings that manifest as humoral or paraneoplastic syndromes. Knowledge of this spectrum and associated pathophysiology is useful to the oncologist, endocrinologist, and generalists for three practical reasons: (1) to permit differentiation of cancer-associated syndromes from benign disorders that resemble paraneoplastic syndromes, (2) to permit earlier diagnosis of a neoplasm through paraneoplastic symptoms or findings, and (3) to permit use of the cancer-produced hormone or product as a tumor marker to follow a patient's response to antitumor therapy. Advances in our knowledge regarding the molecular mechanisms of these paraneoplastic syndromes also may lead to better means of diagnosing neoplasms or controlling their development or growth.

REFERENCES

1. Lipsett MB, Odell WD, Rosenberg LE, Waldmann TA. Humoral syndromes associated with non-endocrine tumors. Ann Intern Med 1964;61:733–756.
2. Odell WD, Wolfsen A, Yoshimoto Y, Weitzman R, Fisher D, Hirose F. Ectopic peptide synthesis: a universal concomitant of neoplasia. Trans Assoc Am Physicians 1997;15: 204–227.
3. Saito E, Iwasa S, Odell WD. Widespread presence of large molecular weight adrenocorticotropin-like substances in normal rat extrapituitary tissues. Endocrinology 1983; 113:1010–1019.
4. Odell WD, Saito E. Protein hormonelike materials from normal and cancer cells–"Ectopic" hormone production. In 13th Internationl Cancer Congress Part E; Cancer Management, New York: Liss 1983, pp 247–258.
5. Stewart PM, Gibson S, Crosby SR, Penn R, Holders R, Ferry D, Thatcher N, Phillips P, London DR, White A. ACTH precursors characterized the ectopic ACTH syndrome. Clin Endocrinol 1994;40:199–204.
6. Delisle L, Boyer MJ, Warr D, Killinger D, Payne D, Yeoh JL, Field R. Ectopic corticotropin syndrome and small-cell carcinoma of the lung. Clinical features, outcome, and complications. Arch Intern Med 1953;153:46–52.
7. Nussbaum SR, Gaz RD, Arnold A. Hypercalcemia and ectopic secretion of parathyroid hormone by an ovarian carcinoma with rearrangement of the gene for pocathormone. N Engl J Med 1990;323:1324–1328.
8. Yoneda T, Nishimura R, Kato I, Ohmae M, Tanita M, Sakuda M. Frequency of the hypercalcemia-leukocytosis syndrome in oral malignancies. Cancer 1991;68:617–622.
9. Wetzler M, Estrov Z, Talpaz M, Markowitz A, Gutterman JU. Granulocyte macrophage colony-stimulating factor as a cause of paraneoplastic leukemoid reaction in advanced transitional cell carcinoma. J Intern Med 1993;234:417–420.
10. Elmington GM, Murray NM, Spiro SG. Neurological paraneoplastic syndromes in patients with small cell lung cancer. A prospective survey of 150 patients. J Neurol Neurosurg Psychiatr 1991;54:764–767.
11. Graus F, Rene R. Clinical and pathological advances on central nervous paraneoplastic syndromes. Rev Neurol Paris 1992;148:496–501.
12. Buckanovich RJ, Posner JB, Darnell RB. Nova, the paraneoplastic Ri antigen, is homologous to an RNA-binding protein and is specifically expressed in the developing motor system. Neuron 1993;11:657–672.
13. Odell WD, Wolfsen A, Yoshimoto Y, Weitzman R, Fisher D, Hirose F. Ectopic peptide synthesis: a universal concomitant of neoplasia. Trans Assoc Am Physicians 1977;90: 204–227.
14. Odell WD, Saito E. Protein hormone-like materials from normal and cancer cells–"Ectopic" hormone production. In 13th International Cancer Congress Part E; Cancer Management Edited by EA Mirand, WB Hutchinson, E Mihich. New York: Liss, 1983, pp 247–248.
15. Kew MC, Kirschner MA, Abrahams GE, Katz M. Mechanism of feminization in primary liver cancer. N Engl J Med 1977;296:1084–1088.
16. Herr HW, Hennessy WT, Kantor A. Pelvic sarcoma causing gynecomastia. J Urol 1990;143:1008–1009.
17. Liddle GW, Nicholson WE, Island DP, Orth DN, Abe K, Lowder SC. Clinical Labora-

tory studies of "ectopic" hormonal syndromes. Rec Prog Horm Res 1969;25: 283–314.
18. Odell WD, Appleton WS. Humoral manifestations of cancer. In Williams Textbook of Endocrinology, 8th ed. Edited by JD Wilson, DW Foster. Orlando: Saunders, 1992, pp 1599–1617.
19. Nieman LK, Chrousos GP, Oldfield EH, Avgerinos PC, Cutler GB Jr, Loriaux DL. The ovine corticotropin-releasing hormone stimulation test and the dexamethasone suppression test on the differential diagnosis of Cushing's syndrome. Ann Intern Med 1986;105:862–867.
20. Howlett TA, Drury PL, Perry L, Doniach I, Rees LH, Besser GM. Diagnosis and management of ACTH-dependent Cushing's syndrome: comparison on the features in ectopic and pituitary ACTH Production. Clin Endocrinol (Oxford). 1986;24:699–713.
21. Malchoff CD, Orth DN, Abhoud C, Carney JA, Pairolero PC, Carey RM. Ectopic ACTH syndrome caused by a bronchial carcinoid tumor responsive to dexamethasone, metyrapone and corticotropin-releasing factor. Am J Med 1988;84:760–764.
22. Pass HI, Doppman JL, Nieman L, et al. Management of the ectopic ACTH syndrome due to thoracic carcinoids: The NIH experience and review of the world literature. Ann Thoracic Surg 1990;50:52–57.
23. Nakanishi S, Inoue A, Kita T, et al. Nuclectide sequence of a cloned cDNA for bovine corticotropin-β-lipotropin precursor. Nature 1979;278:423–427.
24. Odell WD, Wolfsen AR, Bachelot I, Hirose FM. Ectopic production of lipotropin by cancer. Am J Med 1979;66:631–638.
25. Wolfsen AR, Odell WD. ProACTH: use for early detection of lung cancer. Am J Med 1979;66:765–772.
26. Saito E, Odell WD. Corticotropin/lipotropin common precursor-like material in normal rat extrapituitary tissues. Proc Natl Acad Sci USA 1983;80:3792–3796.
27. Saito E, Iwasa S, Odell WD. Widespread presence of large molecular weight adrenocorticotropin-like substances in normal rat extrapituitary tissues. Endocrinology 1983; 113:1010–1019.
28. White A, Clark AJL. The cellular and molecular basis of the ectopic ACTH syndrome. Clin Endocrinol (Oxford) 1993;39:131–141.
29. DeKeyzer Y, Bertagna X, Lenne F, Girard F, Luton J, Kahn A. Altered pro-opiomelanocortin gene expression in ACTH-producing non-pituitary tumors. J Clin Invest 1985;76:1892–1898.
30. Clark AJL, Lavender PM, Besser GM, Rees LH. Proopiomelanocortin mRNA size heterogeneity in ACTH-dependent Cushing's syndrome. J Mol Endocrinol 1989;2:3–9.
31. Pierce JG, Parsons TF. Glycoprotein hormones: structure and function. Ann Rev Biochem 1981;50:465–495.
32. Vaitukaitis JL, Braunstein GD, Ross GT. A radioimmunoassay which specifically measures human chorionic gonadotropin in the presence of human luteinizing hormone. Am J Obstet Gynecol 1972;113:751–758.
33. Braunstein GD, Vaitukaitis JL, Carbone PP, Ross GT. Ectopic production of human chorionic gonadotropin by neoplasms. Ann Intern Med 1973;78:39–45.
34. Yoshimoto Y, Wolfsen AR, Odell WD. Human chorionic gonadotropin-like substance in non-endocrine tissues of normal subjects. Science 1977;197:575–577.
35. Yoshimoto Y, Wolfsen AR, Odell WD. Glycosylation, a variable in the production of hCG by cancers. Am J Med 1979;67:414–420.
36. Yoshimoto Y, Wolfsen AR, Hirose F, Odell WD. Human chorionic gonadotropin-like material: presence in normal human tissue. Am J Obstet Gynecol 1979;134:729–733.
37. Rosa C, Amr S, Birken S, Wehmann R, Nisula B. Effect of desialylation of human chorionic gonadotropin on its metabolic clearance rate in humans. J Clin Endocrinol Metab 1984;59:1215–1219.
38. Griffin J, Odell WD. Ultrasensitive immunoradiometric assay for chorionic gonadotropin which does not cross react with luteinizing hormone nor free beta chain of hCG and which detects hCG in blood of nonpregnant humans. J Immunol Meth 1987; 103:276–283.
39. Stenman U-H, Alfthan H, Ranta T, Vartianinen E, Jalkanen J, Seppälä M. Serum levels of human chorionic gonadotropin in nonpregnant women and men are modulated by gonadotropin-releasing hormone and sex steroids. J Clin Endocrinol Metab 1987; 64:730–736.
40. Odell WD, Griffin J. Pulsatile secretion of human chorionic gonadotropin in normal adults. N Engl J Med 1987;317:1688–1691.
41. Odell WD, Griffin J, Bashey HM, Snyder PJ. Secretion of chorionic gonadotropin by cultured human pituitary cells. J Clin Endocrinol Metab 1990;71:1318–1321.
42. Hammond E, Griffin J, Odell WD. A chorionic gonadotropin-secreting human pituitary cell. J Clin Endocrinol Metab 1991;72:747–754.
43. Franchimont P, Gaspard U, Reuter A, Heynen G. Polymorphism of protein and polypeptide hormones. Clin Endocrinol 1972;1:315–336.
44. Good A, Ramos-Uribe M, Ryan R, Kempers RD. Molecular forms of human chorionic gonadotropin in serum, urine and placental extracts. Fertil Steril 1977;28:846–850.
45. Kato Y, Braunstein GD. Beta-core fragment is a major form of immunoreactive urinary chorionic gonadotropin in human pregnancy. J Clin Endocrinol Metab 1988;66: 1197–1201.
46. Cole LA, Birken S. Origin and occurrence of human chorionic gonadotropin beta-subunit core fragment. Mol Endocrinol 1988;2:825–830.
47. Hammond CB, Hertz R, Lipsett MB, Odell WD. Chemotherapy of metastatic and nonmetastatic gestational trophoblastic neoplasms. Texas Rep Biol Med 1966; 24(Suppl):.
48. Hammond CB, Hertz R, Ross GT, Lipsett MB, Odell WD. Diagnostic problems of choriocarcinoma and related trophoblastic neoplasms. Obstet Gynecol 1967;29: 224–229.
49. Kohler PO, O'Malley BW, Rayford L, Lipsett MB, Odell WD. Effect of pyrogen on blood levels of pituitary trophic hormones. Observations of the usefulness of the growth hormone response in the detection of pituitary disease. J Clin Endocrinol Metab 1967; 27:219–226.
50. Ross GT, Odell WD, Rayford PL. LH activity in plasma during the menstrual cycle. Science 1967;155:1679–1680.
51. Birken S, Armstrong EG, Kolks MAG, Cole LA. The structure of the human chorionic gonadotropin beta core fragment from pregnancy urine. Endocrinology 1988;123: 572–583.
52. Blithe DL, Akar AH, Wehmann RE, Nisula BC. Purification of beta core fragment from pregnancy urine and demonstration that its carbohydrate moieties differ from those of native human chorionic gonadotropin. Endocrinology 1988;122:173–180.
53. Wehmann RE, Nisula BC. Characterization of a discrete degradation product of human chorionic gonadotropin β-subunit in humans. J Clin Endocrinol Metab 1990;51: 101–105.
54. Walker R, Crebbin V, Stern J, Scudder S, Schwartz P. Urinary gonadotropin peptide (UGP) as a marker of gynecologic malignancies. Anticancer Res 1994;14: 1703–1710.
55. Stenman U-H, Alfthan H, Ranta T, Vartianinen E, Jalkanen J, Seppälä M. Serum levels of human chorionic gonadotropin in nonpregnant women and men are modulated by gonadotropin-releasing hormone and sex steroids. J Clin Endocrinol Metab 1987; 64:730–736.
56. Mundy GR. Pathogenesis of hypercalcemia of malignancy. Clin Endocrinol (Oxford). 1985;23:705–714.
57. Bunn PA Jr, Schechter GP, Jaffe E, et al. Clinical course of retrovirus-associated adult T-cell lymphoma in the United States. N Engl J Med 1983;309:257–264.
58. Bender RA, Hansen H. Hypercalcemia in bronchogenic carcinoma. A prospective study of 200 patients. Ann Intern Med 1974;80:205–208.
59. Ralston SH, Gallacher SJ, Patel U, Campbell J, Boyle IT. Cancer-associated hypercalcemia: morbidity and mortality. Clinical experience in 126 treated patients. Ann Intern Med 1990;112:499–504.
60. Burtis WJ, Wu T, Bunch C, et al. Identification of a novel 17,000-dalton parathyroid hormone-like adenylate cyclase-stimulating protein from a tumor associated with humoral hypercalcemia of malignancy. J Biol Chem 1987;262:7151–7156.
61. Moseley JM, Kubota M, Diefenbach-Jagger H, et al. Parathyroid hormone-related protein purified from a human lung cancer cell line. Proc Natl Acad Sci USA 1987;84: 5048–5052.
62. Strewler GJ, Stern PH, Jacobs JW, et al. Parathyroid hormone-like protein from human renal carcinoma cells. Structural and functional homology with parathyroid hormone. J Clin Invest 1987;80:1803–1807.
63. Suva LJ, Winslow GA, Wettenhall RE, et al. A parathyroid hormone-related protein implicated in malignant hypercalcemia: cloning and expression. Science 1987;237: 893–896.
64. Mangin M, Webb AC, Dreyer BE, et al. Identification of a cDNA encoding a parathyroid hormone-like peptide from a human tumor associated with humoral hypercalcemia of malignancy. Proc Natl Acad Sci USA 1988;85:597–601.
65. Zondek H, Petow H, Siebert W. Die Bedeutungder Calcium Best Immung in Blute fur die Diagnose der Niereninsuffizienz. Ztshr f. Klin Med Berl 1924;99:129–138.
66. Albright F. Case records of the Massachusetts General Hospital; Case 27461. N Engl J Med 1941;225:789–791.
67. Tashjian AH Jr, Levine L, Munson PL. Immunochemical identification of parathyroid hormone in non-parathyroid neoplasms associated with hypercalcemia. J Exp Med 1964;119:467–484.
68. Berson SA, Yalow RS. Parathyroid hormone in plasma in adenomatous hyperparathyroidism, uremia, and bronchogenic carcinoma. Science 1966;154:907–909.
69. Sherwood LM, O'Riordan JLH, Aurbach GD, Potts JT Jr. Production of parathyroid hormone by nonparathyroid tumors. J Clin Endocrinol Metab 1967;27:140–146.
70. Buckle RM, McMillan M, Mallinson C. Ectopic secretion of parathyroid hormone by a renal adenocarcinoma in a patient with hypercalcemia. BMJ 1970;4:724–726.
71. Federman DD. Case records of the Massachusetts General Hospital; Case 15-1971. N Engl J Med 1971;284:839–847.
72. Powell D, Singer FR, Murray TM, Minkin C, Potts JT Jr. Non-parathyroid humoral hypercalcemia in patients with neoplastic diseases. N Engl J Med 1973;289:176–181.
73. Simpson EL, Mundy GR, D'Souza SM, Ibbotson KJ, Bockman R, Jacobs JW. Absence of parathyroid hormone messenger RNA in non-parathyroid tumor associated with hypercalcemia. N Engl J Med 1983;309:325–330.
74. Thiede MA, Strewler GJ, Nissenson RA, Rosenblatt M, Rodan GA. Human renal carcinoma expresses two messages encoding a parathyroid hormone-like peptide: evidence for the alternative splicing of a single-copy gene. Proc Natl Acad Sci USA 1988;85:4605–4609.
75. Mangin M, Ikeda K, Dreyer BE, Milstone L, Broadus AE. Two distinct tumor-derived, parathyroid hormone-like peptides result from alternative ribonucleic acid splicing. Mol Endocrinol 1988;2:1049–1055.
76. Thorikay M, Kramer S, Reynolds FH, et al. Synthesis of a gene encoding parathyroid hormone-like protein-(1-141): Purification and biological characterization of the expressed protein. Endocrinology 1989;124:111–118.
77. Thiede MA, Rodan GA. Expression of a calcium-mobilizing parathyroid hormone-like peptide in lactating mammary tissue. Science. 1988;242:278–280.
78. Merendino JJ Jr, Insogna KL, Milstone LM, Broadus AE, Stewart AF. A parathyroid hormone-like protein from cultured human keratinocytes. Science 1986;231: 388–390.
79. Li X, Drucker DJ. Parathyroid hormone-related peptide is a downstream target for ras and src activation. J Biol Chem 1994;269:6263–6266.
80. Burtis WJ, Brady TG, Orloff JJ, et al. Immunochemical characterization of circulating parathyroid hormone-related protein in patients with humoral hypercalcemia of cancer. N Engl J Med 1990;322:1106–1112.
81. Budayr AA, Nissenson RA, Klein RF, et al. Increased serum levels of a parathyroid hormone-like protein in malignancy-associated hypercalcemia. Ann Intern Med 1989; 111:807–812.
82. Henderson JE, Shustik C, Kremer R, Rabbani SA, Hendy GN, Goltzman D. Circulating concentrations of parathyroid hormone-like peptide in malignancy and in hyperparathyroidism. J Bone Miner Res 1990;5:105–113.
83. Kao PC, Klee GG, Taylor RL, Heath H III. Parathyroid hormone-related peptide in plasma of patients with hypercalcemia and malignant lesions. Mayo Clin Proc 1990; 65:1399–1407.
84. Bundred NJ, Ratcliffe WA, Walker RA, Coley S, Morrison JM, Ratcliffe JG. Parathyroid hormone related protein and hypercalcemia in breast cancer. BMJ 1991;303: 1506–1509.
85. Ikeda K, Mangin M, Dreyer BE, et al. Identification of transcripts encoding a parathyroid hormone-like peptide in messenger RNAs from a variety of human and animal tumors associated with humoral hypercalcemia of malignancy. J Clin Invest 1988;81: 2010–2014.
86. Grill V, Hillary J, Ho PMW, et al. Parathyroid hormone-related protein: A possible endocrine function in lactation. Clin Endocrinol (Oxford) 1992;37:405–410.
87. Nussbaum SR, Gaz RD, Arnold A. Hypercalcemia and ectopic secretion of parathyroid hormone by an ovarian carcinoma with rearrangement of the gene for parathyroid hormone. N Engl J Med 1990;323:1324–1325. Brief report.

88. Rizzoli R, Pache J-C, Didierjean L, Bäurger A, Bonjour J-P. A thymoma as a cause of true ectopic hyperparathyroidism. J Clin Endocrinol Metab 1994;79:912–915.
89. Mundy GR, Raisz LG, Cooper RA, Schechter GP, Salmon SE. Evidence for the secretion of an osteoclast stimulating factor in myeloma. N Engl J Med 1974;291: 1041–1046.
90. Aggarwal BB, Henzel WJ, Moffat B, Kohr WJ, Harkins RN. Primary structure of human lymphotoxin derived from 1788 lymphoblastoid cell line. J Biol Chem 1985;260: 2334–2344.
91. Garrett IR, Durie BG, Nedwin GE, et al. Production of lymphotoxin, a bone-resorbing cytokine, by cultured human myeloma cells. N Engl J Med 1987;317:526–532.
92. Breslau NA, McGuire JL, Zerwekh JE, Frenkel EP, Pak CY. Hypercalcemia associated with increased serum calcitriol levels in three patients with lymphoma. Ann Intern Med 1984;100:1–6.
93. Rosenthal N, Insogna KL, Godsall JW, Smaldone L, Waldron JA, Stewart AF. Elevations in circulating 1,25-dihydroxyvitamin D in three patients with lymphoma-associated hypercalcemia. J Clin Endocrinol Metab 1985;60:29–33.
94. Helikson MA, Havey AD, Zerwekh JE, Breslau NA, Gardner DW. Plasma-cell granuloma producing calcitriol and hypercalcemia. Ann Intern Med. 1986;105:379–381.
94a. Nussbaum SR, VandePol CJ, Gagel RF, et al. Single-dose intravenous therapy with pamidronate for the treatment of hypercalcemia of malignancy: Comparison of 30-, 60-, and 90-mg dosages. Am J Med 1993;95:297–304.
94b. Gucalp R, Theriault R, Gill I, et al. Treatment of cancer-associated hypercalcemia. Double-blind comparison of rapid and slow intravenous infusion regimens of pamidronate disodium and saline alone. Arch Intern Med 1994;154:1935–1944.
95. Schwartz WB, Bennett W, Curelop S, et al. A syndrome of renal sodium loss and hyponatremia probably resulting from inappropirate secretion of antidiuretic hormone. Am J Med 1957;23:529–542.
96. Vorherr H, Massry SG, Utiger RD, Kleeman CR. Anti-diuretic principle in malignant tumor extracts from patients with inappropriate ADH syndrome. J Clin Endocrinol Metab 1968;28:162–168.
97. George JM, Capen CC, Phillips AS. Biosynthesis of vasopressin in vitro and ultrastructure of a bronchogenic carcinoma. Patient with the syndrome of inappropriate secretion of antidiuretic hormone. J Clin Invest 1972;51:141–148.
98. Hamilton BP, Upton GV, Amatruda TT Jr. Evidence for the presence of neurophysin in tumors producing the syndrome of inappropriate antidiuresis. J Clin Endocrinol Metab 1972;35:764–767.
99. Gilby ED, Rees LH, Bondy PK. Ectopic hormones as markers of response to therapy in cancer. In Advances in Tumour Prevention, Detection and Characterization. Vol. 3: Proceedings of the 6th International Symposium on Biological Characterization of Human Tumors. Edited by W Davis, C. Maltoni. New York: Elsevier, 1976, p. 132.
100. North WG, LaRochelle FT Jr, Melton J, et al. Human neurophysins (HNPs) as potential tumor markers for small-cell carcinoma (SCC). Clin Res. 1978;26:536A, Abstract.
101. Field JB, Keen H, Johnson P, et al. Insulin-like activity of non-pancreatic tumors associated with hypoglycemia. J Clin Endocrinol Metab 1963;23:1229–1236.
102. Gorden P, Hendricks CM, Kahn CR, Megyesi K, Roth J. Hypoglycemia associated with non-islet-cell tumor and insulin-like growth factors. A study of the tumor types. N Engl J Med 1981;305:1452–1455.
103. Daughaday WH, Emanuele MA, Brooks MH, Barbato AL, Kapadia M, Rotwein P. Synthesis and secretion of insulin-like growth factor II by a leiomyosarcoma with associated hypoglycemia. N Engl J Med 1988;319:1434–1440.
104. Froesch ER, Zapf J, Widmer U. Hypoglycemia associated with non-islet-cell tumor and insulin-like growth factors. N Engl J Med 1982;306:1178–1179.
105. Widmer U, Zapf J, Froesch ER. Is extrapancreatic tumor hypoglycemia associated with elevated levels of insulin-like growth factor II? J Clin Endocrinol Metab 1982;55: 833–839.
106. Ron D, Powers AC, Pandian MR, Godine JE, Axelrod L. Increased insulin-like growth factor II production and consequent suppression of growth hormone secretion: a dual mechanism for tumor-induced hypoglycemia. J Clin Endocrinol Metab 1989;68: 701–706.
107. Lowe WL Jr, Roberts CT Jr, Roith D, et al. Insulin-like growth factor-II in nonislet cell tumors associated with hypoglycemia: increased levels of messenger ribonucleic acid. 1989;69:1153–1159.
108. Daughaday WH, Kapadia M. Significance of abnormal serum binding of insulin-like growth factor II in the development of hypoglycemia in patients with non-islet-cell tumors. Proc Natl Acad Sci U S A 1989;86:6778–6782.
109. Cameron DP, Burger HG, DeKretzer DM, Catt KJ, Best JB. On the presence of immunoreactive growth hormone in a bronchogenic carcinoma. Australas Ann Med 1969;18:143–146.
110. Steiner H, Dahlback O, Waldenstrom J. Ectopic growth-hormone production and osteoarthropathy in carcinoma of the bronchus. Lancet 1968;i:783–785.
111. Sparagana M, Phillips G, Hoffman C, Kucera L. Ectopic growth hormone syndrome associated with lung cancer. Metabolism 1971;20:730–736.
112. Beck C, Burger HG. Evidence for the presence of immunoreactive growth hormone in cancers of the lung and stomach. Cancer 1972;30:75–79.
113. Kaganowicz A, Farkouh H, Frantz AG, Blaustein AU. Ectopic human growth hormone in ovaries and breast cancer. J Clin Endocrinol Metab 1979;48:5–8.
114. Kyle CV, Evans MC, Odell WD. Growth hormone-like material in normal human tissues. J Clin Endocrinol Metab 1981;53:1138–1144.
115. Melmed S, Ezrin C, Kovacs K, Goodman RS, Frohman LA. Acromegaly due to secretion of growth hormone by an ectopic pancreatic islet-cell tumor. N Engl J Med 1985;312:9–17.
116. Dabek JT. Bronchial carcinoid tumour with acromegaly in two patients. J Clin Endocrinol Metab 1974;38:329–333.
117. Saeed uz Zafar M, Mellinger RC, Fine G, Szabo M, Frohman LA. Acromegaly associated with a bronchial carcinoid tumor: Evidence for ectopic production of growth hormone-releasing activity. J Clin Endocrinol Metab 1979;48:66–71.
118. Frohman LA, Szabo M, Berelowitz M, Stachura ME. Partial purification and characterization of a peptide with growth hormone-releasing activity from extrapituitary tumors in patients with acromegaly. J Clin Invest 1980;65:43–54.
119. Barkan AL, Shenker Y, Grekin RJ, Vale WW, Lloyd RV, Beals TF. Acromegaly due to ectopic growth hormone (GH)-releasing hormone (GHRH) production: dynamic studies of GH and ectopic GHRH secretion. J Clin Endocrinol Metab 1986;63:1057–1064.
120. Gomm SA, Thatcher N, Barber PV, Cumming WJ. A clinicopathological study of the paraneoplastic neuromuscular syndromes associated with lung cancer. Q J Med 1990;75:577–595.
121. Elrington GM, Murray NM, Spiro SG, Newsom-Davis J. Neurological paraneoplastic syndromes in patients with small cell lung cancer. A prospective survey of 150 patients. J Neurol Neurosurg Psychiatry 1991;54:764–767.
122. Sawyer RA, Selhorst JB, Zimmerman LE, Hoyt WF. Blindness caused by photoreceptor degeneration as a remote effect of cancer. Am J Ophthalmol 1976;81: 606–613.
123. Kornguth SE, Klein R, Appen R, Choate J. Occurrence of antiretinal ganglion cell antibodies in patients with small cell carcinoma of the lung. Cancer 1982;50: 1289–1293.
124. Grunwald GB, Klein R, Simmonds MA, Kornguth SE. Autoimmune basis for visual paraneoplastic syndrome in patients with small-cell lung carcinoma. Lancet 1985;i: 658–661.
125. Kornguth SE, Kalinke T, Grunwald BG, Schutta H, Dahl D. Antineurofilament antibodies in the sera of patients with small cell carcinoma of the lung and with visual paraneoplastic syndrome. Cancer Res 1986;46:2588–2595.
126. Thirkill CE, Roth AM, Keltner JL. Cancer-associated retinopathy. Arch Ophthalmol 1987;105:372–375.
127. Buchanan TA, Gardiner TA, Archer DB. An ultrastructural study of retinal photoreceptor degeneration associated with bronchial carcinoma. Am J Ophthalmol 1984; 97:277–287.
128. Keltner JL, Roth AM, Chang RS. Photoreceptor degeneration. Possible autoimmune disorder. Arch Ophthalmol 1983;101:564–569.
129. Klingele TG, Burde RM, Rappazzo JA, Isserman MJ, Burgess D, Kantor O. Paraneoplastic retinopathy. J Clin Neurol Ophthalmol 1984;4:239–245.
130. Berson EL, Lessell S. Paraneoplastic night blindness with malignant melanoma. Am J Ophthalmol 1988;106:307–311.
131. Crofts JW, Bachynski BN, Odel JG. Visual paraneoplastic syndrome associated with undifferentiated endometrial carcinoma. Can J Ophthalmol 1988;23:128–132.
132. Thirkill CE, Tait RC, Tyler NK, Roth AM, Keltner JL. The cancer-associated retinopathy antigen is a recoverin-like protein. Invest Ophthalmol Vis Sci 1992;33:2768–2772.
133. Stefansson K, Marton LS, Dieperink ME, Molnar GK, Schlaepfer WW, Helgason CM. Circulating autoantibodies to the 200,000-dalton protein of neurofilaments in the serum of healthy individuals. Science 1985;228:1117–1119.
134. Trotter JL, Hendin BA, Osterland CK. Cerebellar degeneration with Hodgkin's disease. An immunological study. Arch Neurol 1976;33:660–661.
135. Steven MM, Mackay IR, Carnegie PR, Bhathal PS, Anderson RM. Cerebellar cortical degeneration with ovarian carcinoma. Postgrad Med J 1982;58:47–51.
136. Greenlee JE, Brashear HR. Antibodies to cerebellar Purkinje cells in patients with paraneoplastic cerebellar degeneration and ovarian carcinoma. Ann Neurol 1983;14: 609–613.
137. Greenlee JE, Sun M. Immunofluorescent labeling of non-human cerebellar tissue with sera from patients with systemic cancer and paraneoplastic cerebellar degeneration. Acta Neuropathol (Berlin) 1985;67:226–229.
138. Kearsley JH, Johnson P, Halmagyi GM. Paraneoplastic cerebellar disease. Remission with excision of the primary tumor. Arch Neurol 1985;42:1208–1210.
139. Dropcho EJ, Chen YT, Posner JB, Old LJ. Cloning of a brain protein identified by autoantibodies from a patient with paraneoplastic cerebellar degeneration. Proc Natl Acad Sci USA 1987;84:4552–4556.
140. Peterson K, Rosenblum MK, Kotanides H, Posner JB. Paraneoplastic cerebellar degeneration. I. A clinical analysis of 55 anti-Yo antibody-positive patients. Neurology. 1992;42:1931–1937.
141. Hammack J, Kotanides H, Rosenblum MK, Posner JB. Paraneoplastic cerebellar degeneration. II. Clinical and immunologic findings in 21 patients with Hodgkin's disease. Neurology 1992;42:1938–1943.
142. Dalmau J, Graus F, Rosenblum MK, Posner JB. Anti-Hu associated paraneoplastic encephalomyelitis/sensory neuronopathy. A clinical study of 71 patients. Medicine (Baltimore) 1992;71:59–72.
143. Dalmau J, Furneaux HM, Gralla RJ, Kris MG, Posner JB. Detection of the anti-Hu antibody in the serum of patients with small cell lung cancer–A quantitative Western blot analysis. Ann Neurol 1990;27:544–552.
144. Sekido Y, Bader SA, Carbone DP, Johnson BE, Minna JD. Molecular analysis of the HuD gene encoding a paraneoplastic encephalomyelitis antigen in human lung cancer cell lines. Cancer Res 1994;54:4988–4992.
145. Graus F, Elkon KB, Cordon-Cardo C, Posner JB. Sensory neuronopathy and small cell lung cancer. Antineuronal antibody that also reacts with the tumor. Am J Med 1986;80:45–52.
146. Graus F, Cordon-Cardo C, Posner JB. Neuronal anti-nuclear antibody in sensory neuronopathy from lung cancer. Neurology 1985;35:538–543.
147. Graus F, Elkon KB, Lloberes P, et al. Neuronal anti-nuclear anti-body (anti-Hu) in paraneoplastic encephalomyelitis simulating acute polyneuritis. Acta Neurol Scand 1987;75:249–252.
148. Chalk CH, Windebank AJ, Kimmel DW, McManis PG. The distinctive clinical features of paraneoplastic sensory neuronopathy. Can J Neurol Sci 1992;19:346–351.
149. Lennon VA, Sas DF, Busk MF, et al. Enteric neuronal autoantibodies in pseudoobstruction with small-cell lung carcinoma. Gastroenterology 1991;100:137–142.
150. Condom E, Vidal A, Rota R, Graus F, Dalmau J, Ferrer I. Paraneoplastic intestinal pseudoobstruction associated with high titres of Hu autoantibodies. Virchows Arch A Pathol Anat Histopathol 1993;423:507–511.
151. Gutmann L, Phillips LH II, Gutmann L. Trends in the association of Lambert-Eaton myasthenic syndrome with carcinoma. Neurology 1992;42:848–850.
152. Hewett SJ, Atchison WD. Serum and plasma from patients with Lambert-Eaton myasthenic syndrome reduce depolarization-dependent uptake of 45Ca2+ into rat cortical synaptosomes. Brain Res 1991;566:320–324.
153. Leys K, Lang B, Johnston I, Newsom-Davis J. Calcium channel autoantibodies in the Lambert-Eaton myasthenic syndrome. Ann Neurol 1991;29:307–314.
154. Rosenfeld MR, Wong E, Dalmau J, et al. Cloning and characterization of a Lambert-Eaton myasthenic syndrome antigen. Ann Neurol 1993;33:113–120.
155. David P, Martin-Moutot N, Leveque C, el-Far O, Takahashi M, Seagar MJ. Interaction of synaptotagmin with voltage gated calcium channels: a role in Lambert-Eaton myasthenic syndrome? Neuromusc Disord 1993;3:451–454.
156. Politi Y, Ophir J, Brenner S. Cutaneous paraneoplastic syndromes. Acta Derm Venereol (Stockh) 1993;73:161–170.
157. Abeloff MD. Paraneoplastic syndromes: A window on the biology of cancer. N Engl J Med 1987;317:1598–1600. Editorial.
158. Ihde DC. Paraneoplastic syndromes. Hosp Prac Off Ed. 1987;22:105–124.

159. Venencie PY, Perry HO. Sign of Leser-Trélat: Report of two cases and review of the literature. J Am Acad Dermatol 1984;10:83–88.
160. Sperry K, Wall J. Adenocarcinoma of the stomach with eruptive seborrheic keratoses: The sign of Leser-Trélat. Cancer 1980;45:2434–2437.
161. Berman A, Winkelmann RK. Seborrheic keratoses: appearance in course of oxfoliative erythroderma and regression associated with histologic mononuclear cell inflammation. Arch Dermatol 1982;118:615–618.
162. Grob JJ, Rava MC, Gouvernet J, et al. The relation between seborrheic keratoses and malignant solid tumours. A case control study. Acta Derm Venereol Stockh 1991;71:166–169.
163 Anhalt GJ, Kim SC, Stanley JR, et al. Paraneoplastic pemphigus. An autoimmune mucocutaneous disease associated with neoplasia. N Engl J Med 1990;323:1729–1735.
164. Wilgenbus K, Lentner A, Kuckelkorn R, Handt S, Mittermayer C. Further evidence that acanthosis nigricans maligna is linked to enhanced secretion by the tumour of transforming growth factor alpha. Arch Dermatol Res 1992;284:266–270.
165. Ellis DL, Kafka SP, Chow JC, et al. Melanoma, growth factors, acanthosis nigricans, the sign of Leser-Trelat, and multiple acrochordons. A possible role for alpha-transforming growth factor in cutaneous paraneoplastic syndromes. N Engl J Med 1987;317:1582–1587.
166. Barnes BE, Mawr B. Dermatomyositis and malignancy. A review of the literature. Ann Intern Med 1976;84:68–76.
167. Lakhanpal S, Bunch TW, Ilstrup DM, Melton LJ III. Polymyositis-dermatomyositis and malignant lesions: does an association exist? Mayo Clin Proc 1986;61:645–653.
168. Kaplan BS, Klassen J, Gault MH. Glomerular injury in patients with neoplasia. Annu Rev Med 1977;27:117–125.
169. Zimmerman SW, Vishnu Moorthy A, Burkholder PM, et al. Glomerulopathies associated with neoplastic disease. In Cancer and the Kidney. Edited by RE Rieselbach, MB Garnick. Philadelphia: Lea & Febiger, 1982, pp. 306–378.
170. Martinez-Maldonado M, Baez-Diaz L, Benabe JE. Nonrenal neoplasms and the kidney. In Disease of the Kidney. Edited by R Schrier, JE Benabe. Boston: Little, Brown, 1988, pp. 2511–2532.
171. Pascal RR. Renal manifestations of extrarenal neoplasms. Hum Pathol. 1980;11:7–15.
172. Haskell LP, Fusco MJ, Wadler S, Sablay LB, Mennemeyer RP. Crescentic glomerulonephritis associated with prostatic carcinoma: evidence of immune-mediated glomerular injury. Am J Med 1990;88:189–192.
173. Eagen JW, Lewis EJ. Glomerulopathies of neoplasia. Kidney Int. 1977;11:297–306.
174. Kim HD, Boggs DR. A syndrome resembling idiopathic thrombocytopenic purpura in 10 patients with diverse forms of cancer. Am J Med 1979;67:371–377.
175. Verdirame JD, Feagler JR, Commers JR. Multiple myeloma associated with immune thrombocytopenic purpura. Cancer 1985;56:1199–1200.
176. Furie B. Case records of the Massachusetts General Hospital: Case 8-1988. N Engl J Med 1988;318:500–508.
177. Aghai E, Quitt M, Lurie M, et al. Primary hepatic lymphoma presenting as symptomatic immune thrombocytopenic purpura. Cancer 1987;60:2308–2011.
178. Thorling EB. Paraneoplastic erythrocytosis and inappropriate erythropoietin production. Scand J Haematol Suppl 1972;17:1–166.
179. Athens JW, Lee GR. Polycythemia: Erythrocytosis. In Wintrobe's Clinical Hematology. Edited by GR Lee, TC Bithell, J Foerster, JW Athens, JW Lukens. Philadelphia: Lea & Febiger, 1993, pp. 1245–1261.
180. McFadzean AJS, et al. Polycythemia in primary carcinoma of the liver. Blood 1958;13:427.
181. Brownstein MH, Ballard HS. Hepatoma associated with erythrocytosis. Am J Med 1966;40:204–210.
182. Waldmann TA, Levin EH, Baldwin M. The association of polycythemia with a cerebellar hemangioblastoma. Am J Med 1961;31:318–324.
183. Lipsett MP, Odell WD, Rosenberg LE, Waldmann TA. Humoral syndromes associated with nonendocrine tumors. Ann Intern Med 1964;61:733–756.
184. Ljungberg B, Rasmuson T, Grankvist K. Erythropoietin in renal cell carcinoma: Evaluation of its usefulness as a tumor marker. Eur Urol 1992;21:160–163.
185. Goldberg MA, Glass GA, Cunningham JM, Bunn HF. The regulated expression of erythropoietin by two human hepatoma cell lines. Proc Natl Acad Sci U S A 1987;84:7972–7976.
186. Ballard HS, Kouri Y. The association of erythrocytosis and chronic lymphocytic leukemia. Cancer 1992;70:2431–2435.
187. Shear MJ, Turner FC, Perrault A, et al. Chemical treatment of tumors. V. Isolation of the hemorrhage-producing fraction from Serratia marcescens (Bacillus prodigiosus) culture filtrate. HNCI 1943;4:81–97.
188. Beutler B, Cerami A. Cachectin: more than a tumor necrosis factor. N Engl J Med. 1987;316:379–385.
189. Cerami A, Tracey KJ, Lowry SF, Beutler B. Cachectin: A pluripotent hormone released during the host response to invasion. Rec Prog Horm Res 1987;43:99–112.
190. Aderka D, Fisher S, Levo Y, Holtmann H, Hahn T, Wallach D. Cachectin/tumor-necrosis-factor production by cancer patients. Lancet 1985;ii:1190.
191. Balkwill F, Osborne R, Burke F, et al. Evidence for tumour necrosis factor/cachectin production in cancer. Lancet 1987;ii:1229–1232
192. Socher SH, Martinez D, Craig JB, Kuhn JG, Oliff A. Tumor necrosis factor not detectable in patients with clinical cancer cachexia. J Natl Cancer Inst 1988;80:595–598.
193. Scuderi P, Sterling KE, Lam KS, et al. Raised serum levels of tumour necrosis factor in parasitic infections. Lancet 1986;ii:1364–1365.
194. Waage A, Espevik T, Lamvik J. Detection of tumour necrosis factor-like cytotoxicity in serum from patients with septicaemia but not from untreated cancer patients. Scand J Immunol 1986;24:739–743.
195. Selby P, Hobbs S, Viner C, et al. Tumour necrosis factor in man: clinical and biological observations. Br J Cancer 1987:803–808.
196. Laski ME, Vugrin D. Paraneoplastic syndromes in hypernephroma. Semin Nephrol 1987;7:123–130.
197. Bernheim HA, Block LH, Atkins E. Fever, pathogenesis, pathophysiology, and purpose. Ann Intern Med 1979;91:261–270.
198. Stolbach LL, Krant MJ, Fishman WH. Ectopic production of an alkaline phosphatase isoenzyme in patients with cancer. N Engl J Med 1969;281:757–761.
199. Krupey J, Gold P, Freedman SO. Purification and characterization of carcinoembryonic antigens of the human digestive system. Nature 1967;215:67–68.
200. Waldmann TA, McIntire KR. The use of a radioimmunoassay for alpha-fetoprotein in the diagnosis of malignancy. Cancer 1974;34(Suppl):1510–1515.

SECTION XVIII

PRINCIPLES OF BIOTHERAPEUTICS

CHAPTER 78

Immunostimulants

ROBERT C. BAST, JR. AND DONALD L. MORTON

Introduction

Bacteria and their products have been used to treat cancer patients for more than a hundred years. During the last two decades of the 19th century, physicians and surgeons in Europe and in the United States had observed tumor regression associated with successful resolution of erysipelas (1). Based on these observations, William B. Coley had utilized culture supernatants from *Micrococcus pyogenes* and *Serratia marcescens* to treat cancer patients, with impressive if anecdotal responses (2). Coley's mixed bacterial vaccine (MBV) was given to several hundred patients and activity was observed against a variety of human cancers (3). A formal clinical trial of MBV was undertaken more recently in patients with nodular non-Hodgkin's lymphoma to compare chemotherapy with and without the addition of the bacterial immunostimulants. In an early analysis, MBV appeared to enhance the results of conventional chemotherapy (4), but improvement was not maintained during subsequent follow-up (5). A carefully controlled trial in hepatocellular carcinoma has also been reported in which MBV appeared to improve the survival of patients who received cisplatin chemotherapy, but the differences between the immunochemotherapy and the chemotherapy groups did not achieve statistical significance (6).

Many different immunostimulants and immunomodulators have been evaluated in preclinical studies and in clinical trials. Contact allergens, bacillus Calmette-Guérin, muramyl dipeptide, *Corynebacterium parvum*, and levamisole have received particular attention. In addition, certain cancer chemotherapeutic agents thought to act by direct cytotoxicity have been shown to modulate the immune response (7). Notable among these are 6-mercaptopurine (8), doxorubicin (9), cisplatin (10), and cyclophosphamide (11, 12). When given in high doses, cyclophosphamide can inhibit both T-cell– and B-cell–mediated reactions, but in low doses this agent can eliminate suppressor cells and act as an immunostimulant in a fraction of trials (11, 12). This chapter focuses on those immunostimulants for which reproducible antitumor activity against human cancer has been documented, although a number of other immunopotentiators have been evaluated (13–16).

Contact Allergens

The intense delayed hypersensitivity evoked by contact allergens has been used to treat cutaneous neoplasms (17, 18). Primary squamous and basal cell carcinomas have regressed following application of contact allergens such as dinitrochlorobenzene (DNCB) or triethyleneiminobenzoquinone. Patients with multiple basal and squamous cell carcinomas have been sensitized to contact allergens. Dilutions of the contact allergens were then found that would not produce reactivity on normal skin. When these were applied to tumor-bearing areas, both neoplastic and preneoplastic lesions developed marked erythema and regressed. Complete control of tumor growth has been obtained in some patients for more than 4 years. In dermatologic practice, topical application of Efudex (5-fluorouracil; 5-FU) has proved as effective (see Chapter 137). Here, direct cytotoxic activity as well as contact allergy is probably important.

Contact allergens have also been used to treat gynecologic neoplasms. Topical application of DNCB or 5-FU has been evaluated in patients with vulvar, vaginal, and cervical carcinomas (19–25). DNCB induced regression of vulvar carcinoma in situ in as many as 60% of patients in early studies, although lower response rates have been observed in more recent series. Topical application of DNCB produced long-term control of disease in 26% of 180 patients with positive cervical cytologies in the absence of demonstrably invasive cancer (20). Use of DNCB has, however, been associated with marked vulvar discomfort, and 5-FU may be somewhat better tolerated (21). In small series, topical 5-FU has eradicated vaginal carcinoma in situ or cervical intraepithelial neoplasia in a majority of cases (24, 25). In light of the efficacy of alternative methods for managing these lesions, contact allergens are still not sufficiently reliable to be the treatment of choice for many patients. Studies with contact allergens in dermatologic and gynecologic practice have, however, provided excellent examples of the antitumor activity of delayed cutaneous reactivity when it can be focused on tumor tissue.

Bacillus Calmette-Guérin (BCG)

BCG is an attenuated strain of *Mycobacterium bovis* that has been widely used as a tuberculosis vaccine (26, 27). Vaccination with BCG induces intense and prolonged reactivity to purified protein derivative (PPD), precluding the use of tuberculin skin tests to document exposure to virulent mycobacteria. With the development of effective antituberculous chemotherapy, BCG has been used less frequently for the prevention of tuberculosis in the United States.

In animals, BCG can delay or prevent the development of

cancers induced with chemical carcinogens, oncogenic viruses, or radiation (28). Treatment with BCG can also delay the onset of leukemias (29) and mammary cancers (30) in animals genetically predisposed to the development of these neoplasms.

The incidence of acute leukemia appeared to be decreased in children who received BCG vaccination (31, 32). Prospective confirmatory trials were discouraged by the results of other retrospective trials that suggested that BCG vaccination in Puerto Rico was associated with a slight excess of lymphomas (33, 34).

In tumor transplant models, pretreatment with BCG has inhibited or suppressed progressive tumor growth when tumor cells were subsequently injected (35). Growth of established tumor transplants could also be inhibited. Systemic treatment with BCG has been most effective when treatment with the immunostimulant has been combined with more conventional modalities such as surgical excision, cytotoxic chemotherapy, hormonal manipulation, or radiotherapy (28). In animal models and in the clinic, the most dramatic effects have been obtained with direct intralesional injection of BCG (36, 37). The efficacy of intralesional therapy has related to contact between tumor cells and microorganisms, the size of the tumor, the dose of BCG, the immunocompetence of the host, and, possibly, the immunogenicity of the tumor cells (28). Intralesional injection of BCG has eliminated regional lymph node metastases of a poorly immunogenic guinea pig hepatoma and has established systemic immunity (37).

Several mechanisms have been proposed for the activity of BCG in animal models. Tumor cells can be eliminated by the development of a specific T-cell–mediated response to tumor associated antigens (see Chapter 79) or can be killed as "bystanders" at the site of an intense host response to the mycobacteria. Chronic macrophage-mediated cytotoxicity may be particularly important for bystander killing. Activated histiocytes have been found in close association with degenerating tumor cells (38). Antigenic mycobacterial products such as PPD can specifically stimulate T lymphocytes that can attract, arrest, and activate macrophages through the release of different cytokines, including interferon gamma (INF-γ). Once activated, macrophages can control the growth of phagocytized microorganisms and can kill adjacent tumor cells (39). Tumor necrosis factor (TNF) (40), reactive oxygen species, and nitric oxide (41) may all be important mediators of macrophage cytotoxicity in different systems. INF-γ and interleukin-2 (IL-2) produced by BCG-activated TH1-like T cells (42) can stimulate BCG-activated killer (BAK) cells that are $CD8^+$ $CD56^+$ lymphocytes which can kill NK-resistant tumor cell lines (43) without restriction by MHC antigens. NK cells (44), lymphotoxin (45), antibodies (36), and microvascular damage (28) may also contribute to the antitumor activity of BCG. Production of cytokines such as IL-2 that augment inducer function is likely to facilitate the development of T-cell–mediated immunity against tumor-associated antigens. Suppressor cells can, however, also be induced by treatment with BCG.

Cutaneous metastases from malignant melanoma have regressed following intralesional injection of BCG (36). In patients who are immunocompetent, more than 90% of cutaneous melanoma metastases have regressed after direct intralesional injection. Overall, more than 60% of cutaneous lesions have responded (28). In addition, 15% of noninjected lesions have also regressed, consistent with a systemic antitumor effect (28, 36). Cutaneous lesions have responded most frequently, regional node metastases have been controlled less often, and visceral metastases have regressed only on rare occasions. In the absence of BCG therapy, the median survival of patients with cutaneous recurrence of melanoma has been approximately 13.3 months (46). Survival in excess of 5 years was observed in 27% of patients who responded completely to BCG and in 10% of 57 patients treated with the mycobacterial vaccine (47).

A large number of studies have been undertaken to demonstrate the systemic impact of cutaneous administration of BCG on a variety of human cancers. Despite promising early reports of BCG used with or without tumor cells as a vaccine (48, 49), most carefully controlled studies have failed to document a therapeutic effect following the systemic administration of BCG (1, 28, 50, 51). Possible exceptions include intravenous administration of BCG to patients with acute myeloid leukemia (52) and the intralesional administration of BCG to patients with primary melanoma prior to resection (53). Intratumoral injection of BCG was associated with a significant fraction of long-term survivors. An initial observation that intrapleural administration of BCG prolonged the survival of patients with resectable lung cancer (54, 55) was not confirmed in a larger subsequent trial (56).

Local complications of BCG administration have included erythema, induration, pruritus, and ulceration at injection sites, associated with regional lymphadenopathy (28). Systemic reactions have been observed more frequently after intralesional injection than after intradermal administration of the vaccine. Chills, fever, and malaise have been observed after repeated injections (57). Rarely, erythema nodosum, granulomatous hepatitis, anaphylaxis, and shock associated with DIC have been observed. Progressive BCG infection has occurred in a small number of profoundly immunosuppressed patients. When recognized, BCG infection has responded to treatment with multiple antituberculous drugs. In a comparison of intralesional treatment of melanoma metastases with BCG and DNCB, the two agents were similarly effective in controlling injected lesions, but the contact allergen was significantly less toxic (58).

The major clinical application of BCG has been in the treatment of bladder cancer by intravesical administration of the agent (59–61). Regional administration of BCG permits direct contact between the microorganisms and superficial lesions on the bladder mucosa. BCG may bind selectively to fibronectin exposed on disrupted urothelial surfaces (62). Direct attachment of BCG to tumor cells can also occur independent of fibronectin (63). In collected series, BCG administered therapeutically has produced complete regression of Ta, T1, or Tis lesions in approximately 70% of cases (64). Moreover, intravesical BCG administered prophylactically has significantly delayed disease progression, prolonged the period of bladder preservation, and increased overall survival in a randomized, concurrently controlled study (65). In five randomized studies with follow-up of 12 to 60 months, 70% of patients at high risk for recurrence remained tumor free after intravesical BCG administration, compared to 31% of patients managed by repeated transurethral resection (64). In direct comparisons and in a meta-analysis of studies of intravesical therapy, BCG has proved superior to cytotoxic drugs, including thiotepa, doxorubicin, and mitomycin C (64, 66). In addition, BCG has produced a complete response in up to 50% of patients in whom intravesical thiotepa or mitomycin C therapy has failed (67). Intravesical delivery of BCG has been essential in that systemic administration was ineffective, and a combination of systemic and intravesical therapy was no more effective than intravesical therapy alone. Maintenance of therapy with monthly BCG administration for 2 years was no more effective than induction therapy alone but did increase dysuria, frequency, and urgency (68). When relapse occurred after 1 or more years, patients were likely to respond to reinduction with BCG (64). In one recent randomized study, the addition of oral megadose vitamins, (B_6, C, and E, plus zinc) to intravesical BCG decreased recurrences at 5 years from 91% to 41% (69).

The intense inflammation evoked by the intravesical administration of BCG can produce dysuria, frequency, urgency, and hematuria, but severe cystitis has occurred in less than 10% of patients in large series (64, 70). Systemic reactions have generally been mild, with fever above 103° F in less than 4% of patients. Less than 1% of those treated with intravesical BCG have experienced pneumonitis, hepatitis, arthralgia, arthritis, skin rash, ureteral obstruction, epididymoorchitis, or bladder contracture (71).

Following intravesical administration of BCG, several cytokines, including IL-1, IL-2, and TNF, can be detected in the urine (72). Urinary levels of IL-2 and of an IL-2 inhibitor have both correlated with a favorable response to BCG (73). As the inhibitor can neutralize IL-2 activity, correlation of both markers with prognosis calls into question the importance of urinary IL-2 in controlling tumor growth. Both markers might, however, reflect the intensity of local inflammation.

Chemically Defined Components of Mycobacterial Immunostimulants

Much of the local antitumor and systemic adjuvant activity of BCG is maintained in the mycobacterial cell walls when they are presented to the host on the surface of oil droplets. Intralesional injection of such preparations can produce local regression of guinea pig hepatoma transplants or primary autochthonous tumors of the lid and conjunctiva in cattle (74, 75). Muramyl dipeptide (MDP) and trehalose dimycolate (TDM) are components of mycobacteria that have been analyzed in greatest depth (76). MDP is the smallest compound identified to date that retains the adjuvant properties of whole mycobacteria in Freund's complete adjuvant. MDP can activate macrophages, stimulate NK cells, and modify T- and B-cell reactivity to unrelated antigens. MDP has stimulated the expression of IL-6 (77), membrane-associated IL-1 (78, 79), and paf-Acether (79) by macrophages. Oral administration of MDP has primed mice for the release of tumor necrosis factor (80). MDP has augmented the effect of INF-γ on macrophages (81, 82), as well as the effects of IL-2 and IL-4 on B cells (83). TDM is closely related to the "cord factor" of virulent mycobacteria that prevents fusion of lysosomes with endosomal vacuoles (84). A combination of MDP and TDM is required to produce regression of guinea pig hepatoma transplants after intralesional injection (85, 86). Following parenteral administration, MDP is cleared from the circulation within 60 minutes, an interval that does not permit systemic activation of macrophages (87, 88). When contained in negatively charged liposomes, MDP is preferentially localized in macrophages and released slowly (89). MDP in liposomes can produce regression of pulmonary metastases in several murine models.

Greater antitumor activity has been obtained with muramyl tripeptide phosphatidylethanolamine (MTP-PE), a lipophilic derivative of water-soluble MDP that can associate more effectively with liposomes. MTP-PE in liposomes has activated macrophages in T-cell–deficient hosts (90). Additional macrophage activation was achieved when MTP-PE and INF-γ were combined within liposomes. The combination of MTP-PE and INF-γ has proved particularly effective for eradicating pulmonary metastases in a murine melanoma model (89).

In a concurrently controlled trial of liposome-encapsulated MTP-PE following resection of primary autochthonous canine osteosarcomas, MTP-PE prolonged median survival from 77 to 222 days and produced disease-free survivors at 1 year (89). Phase I trials in human cancer patients have demonstrated that the optimal dose of MTP-PE for stimulating macrophage function is several fold lower than the maximum tolerated dose, a property that is shared with several other biological response modifiers (91, 92). In a phase II trial, liposomal MTP-PE was administered for 12 to 24 weeks to osteosarcoma patients whose pulmonary metastases had been resected. Among 16 patients who had been treated for 24 weeks, disease-free survival was prolonged from 4.5 to 9 months ($P < .03$), compared to an historical control (93).

Corynebacterium parvum (*Propionobacterium acnes*)

C. parvum is an anaerobic, gram-positive bacillus that can modulate a number of host immune functions. Nonviable *C. parvum* can exert antitumor activity, avoiding the possibility of progressive growth of the bacteria in immunocompromised patients. Both local and systemic effects have been observed in experimental systems. Systemic administration of the agent has produced regression of established murine tumor transplants (94–96). Intraperitoneal treatment with *C. parvum* has cured mice bearing more than 10^5 syngeneic ovarian carcinoma cells (97, 98). Intralesional injection has been particularly effective in producing regression of well-established tumor transplants and in inducing systemic antitumor immunity (99–102).

C. parvum can affect T-cell, B-cell, NK cell, macrophage, and granulocyte function (103–107). T-cell–mediated reactions can be stimulated or suppressed. Incubation of *C. parvum* with human peripheral blood mononuclear cells can induce INF-γ (108, 109), and TNF-α (110). As in the case of BCG, *C. parvum* is thought to kill tumor cells as bystanders at sites of intense local inflammation and also to induce specific T-cell–mediated immunity that can be expressed systemically. Macrophages, granulocytes, and NK cells may be most important as effectors of local bystander killing by *C. parvum*. In contrast to BCG, the antitumor activity of *C. parvum* is only partially reduced in T-cell–deficient hosts (102, 111). *C. parvum* can induce tumoricidal activity in different macrophage populations by T-cell–dependent (112) or –independent (104) mechanisms. Contact between *C. parvum* and tumor cells can also induce specific immunity toward tumor-associated antigens mediated by T-cells (113, 114). Potentiation of B-cell activity has also been observed (107). Treatment with *C. parvum* restored the impaired accessory cell function of adherent splenocytes from mice bearing transplants of EL4 lymphoma and partially restored the ability of tumor-bearing mice to produce antibodies against exogenous antigens (115).

In the clinic, the systemic administration of *C. parvum* has failed to affect tumor growth reproducibly in advanced disease or in adjuvant trials (1, 116–121). One possible exception to this generalization has been raised by the long-term analysis of two concurrently controlled, randomized trials that had compared subcutaneous injection of *C. parvum* and intradermal injection of BCG as adjuvant immunotherapy for stage II melanoma (122). When data from the two trials were pooled, patients treated with *C. parvum* enjoyed significantly greater disease-free survival and overall survival than those treated with BCG. Subcutaneous injection of *C. parvum* has produced local inflammation, swelling, low-grade fever, and chills. Intravenous administration has been associated with more severe side effects, including high fever, rigors, headache, cyanosis, blanching, mild hypertension, more severe hypotension, nausea, and vomiting (123–126).

The most convincing clinical activity of *C. parvum* has been observed after regional administration of the agent into the pleura or peritoneum to control malignant effusions (127–131). In one study of lung and breast cancer patients, three weekly intrapleural injections of *C. parvum* produced total resolution in 50 of 53 malignant pleural effusions (127). Toxicity was limited to fever, pleuritic pain, and cough judged less intense than that produced by other agents (127). Sequential studies of pleural fluid have been performed in a limited number of patients (127, 130). At 6 to 72 hours after treatment, granulocytes, lymphocytes, and macrophages appeared in increased numbers associated with tumor necrosis (127). By 1 week, decreased fluid accumulation was associated with a decrease in the concentration of leukocytes in the pleural fluid (130). On a percentage basis, granulocytes were persistently elevated, whereas lymphocytes and macrophages had decreased. At this late interval, NK activity and interferon levels did not differ from baseline.

Consistent with earlier studies in a murine model (97, 98), intraperitoneal injection of *C. parvum* produced regression of small tumor nodules (<1 cm) in 30% of ovarian cancer patients (132, 133). Intraperitoneal injection of the agent attracted and activated macrophages and NK cells capable of more effective tumor cell killing in the absence or presence of antibodies against tumor-associated antigens (132–134). Intense inflammation and formation of adhesions has, however, limited the use of *C. parvum* for the treatment of ovarian cancer. More recent phase I studies of intraperitoneal immunotherapy have tested purified cytokines including the interferons (135) and IL-2 (136, 137). Intraperitoneal injection of INF-γ has, in general, been well tolerated and has been substantially more effective than systemic injection of the same agent in controlling ovarian tumor growth (138). Use of IL-2 in this setting may be limited by the same regional toxicity observed with *C. parvum*.

Other Bacterial Vaccines

NOCARDIA RUBRA CELL WALL SKELETONS

Systemic administration of *Nocardia rubra* cell wall skeletons (N-CWS) has suppressed the growth of murine leukemia transplants (139). Intralesional injection of N-CWS produced regression of autochthonous bovine lymphosarcomas (140). Administration of N-CWS induced tumoricidal macrophages (141, 142) and augmented the production of several cytokines by peritoneal cells, including IL-1 (143), TNF (144), and INF-α, β, and γ (145). N-CWS has also induced the local accumulation of NK cells (146) as well as precursors for lymphokine-activated killer (LAK) cells, which may contribute to synergistic interactions with IL-2 (147). Intratumor injection of murine and rat fibrosarcomas has augmented specific concomitant immunity that is apparently mediated through T cells (148) or macrophages (149).

In clinical studies, N-CWS has augmented human NK cell activity (150), ADCC effector function (150), interferon production (150), IL-1, and TNF release (151), as well as granulocyte cytostatic activity (152). N-CWS has also activated human pleural macrophages to inhibit lung cancer cells (153) and potentiated the production of human LAK cells in the presence of suboptimal concentrations of IL-2 (154). During a concurrently controlled adjuvant trial in patients with operable lung cancer, intrapleural injection of N-CWS prolonged remission, decreased the incidence of systemic or local recurrence, and prolonged survival in a subset of patients (155). In lung cancer patients with malignant pleural effusions, regional administration of N-CWS and doxorubicin produced better local control than did doxorubicin alone (156). A concurrently controlled clinical trial has also been conducted in 213 patients with gastric cancer treated with gastrectomy to compare immunochemotherapy with N-CWS and tegafur to chemotherapy alone (157). Survival was significantly prolonged by immunochemotherapy. Treatment with N-CWS has also been reported to reduce the incidence of cancer in workers occupationally exposed to sulfur mustard (158). Administration of N-CWS has been well tolerated, with fever most frequently observed after intratumoral and intrapleural injection (159). Erythema, induration, and sterile abscesses have occurred at intradermal injection sites (159).

OK-432

OK-432 (picibanil) has been prepared from a strain of Group A *Streptococcus pyogenes* by treatment with heat and penicillin. The preparation has activated NK effectors and high-density T cells that kill both autologous tumor cells (160–163) and drug-resistant allogeneic tumor cells (164). OK-432 has also activated macrophages (165, 166), stimulated polymorphonuclear leukocytes (167), and potentiated the effect of IL-2 for generating LAK cells from human peritoneal precursors (168). Treatment of lymphoid populations with OK-432 has induced the production of INF-γ and IL-2 (169). The latter cytokines may be particularly important for the activation of NK cells by OK-432 (170). In vivo, OK-432 has inhibited the growth of several murine tumors (165).

Clinical application of OK-432 has emphasized local injection of the immunostimulant to achieve contact with tumor cells and to attract cytotoxic effector cells. Intralesional injection of OK-432 produced complete regression of benign lymphangiomas in 23 of 46 patients (171). Intracavitary injection of OK-432 produced regression of malignant effusions in 7 of 13 patients (172). Response correlated with the induction of ICAM-1 in tumor cells. Intralesional injection of human hepatomas with OK-432 increased the levels of peripheral blood LAK cells in 7 of 12 patients. Among the 7 patients with enhanced LAK activity, 3 partial responses and 1 complete response were observed (173). Intralesional injection of OK-432 into bladder cancers increased the number of NK cells and T cells infiltrating tumor nodules (174). Local injection of OK-432 in fibronectin gel produced local regression in 3 of 15 head and neck cancers (175).

OK-432 has been combined with radiotherapy or chemotherapy in several large trials. Seventy patients with esophageal cancer were treated with intralesional OK-432 and radiotherapy, which produced a 70% complete response rate and a 30% partial response rate (176). The 5-year survival rate among the complete responders was a remarkable 45%. In a concurrently controlled trial with 382 cervical cancer patients, repeated intradermal injection of OK-432 significantly prolonged the recurrence-free interval in patients with stage II disease, but not in those with stage III disease. In those stage II patients who had undergone radical hysterectomy and pelvic lymphadenectomy in addition to radiotherapy, treatment with OK-432 significantly prolonged survival (177). Overall, addition of intraperitoneal OK-432 to chemotherapy failed to affect the survival of patients with intraperitoneal dissemination of gastric cancer (178). A subset of patients with stage III gastric cancer benefited from the addition of OK-432 to a chemotherapeutic regimen of mitomycin and tegafur (179). In a separate study, the addition of intraperitoneal and subcutaneous OK-432 to mitomycin C and tegafur prolonged the survival of patients with gastric cancer (180). Intrapleural injection of OK-432 did not, however, improve survival in patients with non-small cell lung cancer (181). Despite the demonstration of biologic activity in several settings, the precise role of OK-432 in the management of cancer remains to be defined.

LENTINAN

Lentinan is a beta (1–3) glucan with beta (1–6) branches. Both T cell and macrophage function have been stimulated by lentinan, as was the production of several cytokines such as IL-1, IL-3, IL-6, TNF, and INF-γ (182–186). In murine systems, endogenous production of LAK cells by IL-2 was potentiated by treatment with lentinan in vivo, but not in vitro (187). Human LAK activity can, however, be augmented when lentinan is added to IL-2 in cell culture (188). Lentinan can prime macrophages for tumor cell killing (189) and for more effective ADCC mediated by monoclonal antibodies (190). Growth of syngeneic tumor transplants in mice (191) and rats (192) was suppressed by the administration of lentinan.

In the clinic, intracavitary administration of lentinan controlled pleural effusion or ascites in 16 of 20 patients (193). A randomized clinical trial in patients with advanced or recurrent gastric cancer compared chemoimmunotherapy with lentinan and tegafur to chemotherapy with tegafur alone (194). Significant prolongation of survival was observed in the chemoimmunotherapy group. Similarly, the addition of lentinan to 5-FU and mitomycin C significantly prolonged the survival of patients with advanced gastric and colorectal cancer (195). The results of these trials await further confirmation.

Levamisole

Levamisole is a low molecular weight anthelmintic agent with immunomodulatory activity (196, 197). Levamisole has affected T-cell, macrophage, and granulocyte function in some reports (198, 199). Suboptimal immune function has been restored more often than normal function has been stimulated. Many studies were performed more than a decade ago, antedating our current understanding of lymphocyte phenotype, immunoregulation, cytokine production, and intracellular signaling. A more recent attempt failed to demonstrate the immunostimulatory or immunorestorative activity of levamisole in vitro over a broad range of concentrations using a comprehensive battery of phenotypic and functional studies (200). In clinical trials, a maximally tolerated dose of 5 mg/kg in vivo raised serum neopterin and soluble T-cell receptor levels. Phenotypic evidence of monocyte activation was detected, with less consistent evidence of T-cell activation (201). In animal models, limited activity against tumor transplants has been detected. In some models, antitumor activity has been critically dependent on dosage (202). The most effective approaches have combined levamisole with chemotherapy or radiotherapy.

In cancer patients, levamisole has augmented or restored delayed cutaneous hypersensitivity (203, 204). The maximally tolerated dose of levamisole (150 mg/d) has produced blood levels of 1 μg/mL or less (199). When observed, the optimal modulation of immune function has been achieved in vitro with levels of 20 to 400 μg/mL. Several potential explanations have been suggested for this discrepancy, including induction of an endogenous immunostimulant, transformation to a more potent metabolite, inhibition of an endogenous immunosuppressant, or modulation of cholinergic receptors (199).

In clinical trials, conflicting results have been obtained when levamisole was added to other modalities for the treatment of melanoma (197, 205–208), breast cancer (209–215), lung cancer (216–223), and colon cancer (224–226). Among these studies, the most reproducible activity appears to have been obtained in patients with Duke's C colon cancer (226), where three of four randomized clinical trials demonstrated that adjuvant treatment with 5-FU and levamisole for 1 year significantly prolonged survival (227–230). In one of the four trials, subgroup analysis was required to demonstrate an effect (227, 231). In previous adjuvant trials, 5-FU alone or levamisole alone generally failed to affect the survival of patients with resected colorectal cancer. Whether the more intensive 5-FU regimens used in combination with levamisole would have impacted on survival cannot be determined. Although 5-FU is an immunosuppressive agent, it is not certain that immunomodulation is responsible for the antitumor activity observed. Direct toxic effects of levamisole on colon cancer cell lines have, however, been found only with suprapharmacologic concentrations of the drug (232). Levamisole can inhibit thymidylate synthase and tyrosine phosphatase activities (233).

In malignant melanoma, one of four randomized adjuvant studies demonstrated a decreased risk of recurrence and death in patients treated with levamisole (206, 208, 234, 235). The single positive study had administered levamisole at the highest dosage.

Levamisole has been well tolerated with gastrointestinal distress and fatigue reported most frequently. The most significant toxic effect associated with levamisole has been granulocytopenia, in 2 to 13% of patients, which has usually resolved when the drug was discontinued (236). IgM antibodies against human granulocytes have been detected in sera from patients who developed granulocytopenia after treatment with levamisole (237).

Conclusion

Immunostimulants and immunorestorative agents have demonstrated significant antitumor activity when used locally and regionally. Application to clinical practice has, however, generally been limited to the treatment of cutaneous neoplasms, superficial bladder cancers, and malignant effusions. Local or regional control of cancer can usually be achieved with more conventional agents, but elimination of systemic metastases remains the major barrier to the cure of many epithelial neoplasms. Recent results with levamisole and 5-FU could contribute to the control of visceral metastases from a frequently occurring human cancer.

Because of the complex interactions of cells and factors that regulate the immune response to specific tumor-associated antigens, "stimulating" immunity nonspecifically might even amplify inappropriate signals that could suppress a response to tumor-associated antigens. On the other hand, intralesional injection of BCG, mycobacterial products, or *C. parvum* has stimulated systemic tumor-specific immunity in a number of animal models. Regression of noninjected lesions has been observed in patients treated with BCG for metastatic melanoma, consistent with the stimulation of specific immunity to tumor-associated antigens. In the past, a major obstacle to more specific active immunotherapy was the difficulty in identification and isolation of relevant antigens. Using techniques of molecular biology it is now possible to characterize and clone several tumor-associated antigens. With these molecular targets identified, vaccines can now be prepared. Appropriate regulation of the immune response to these vaccines must still be achieved, and immunostimulants may well have a role as adjuvants in this setting.

References

1. Oettgen HF, Old LJ. The history of cancer immunotherapy. In Biologic Therapy of Cancer. Edited by VT DeVita Jr, S Hellman, and SA Rosenberg. Philadelphia: Lippincott, 1991, p 87.
2. Coley WB. Treatment of inoperable malignant tumors with the toxins of erysipelas and the bacillus prodigiosus. Trans Am Surg Assoc 1894;12:183.
3. Nauts HC. The beneficial effects of bacterial infections of host resistance to cancer. End results in 449 cases. Cancer Res Inst Monogr 8, 1980.
4. Kempin S, Cirrincione C, Straus DS, Gee TS, Arlin Z, Koziner B, Pinsky C, Nisce L, Myers J, Lee BJ III, Clarkson BD, Old LJ, Oettgen HF. Improved remission rate and duration in nodular non-Hodgkin lymphoma (NNHL) with the use of mixed bacterial vaccine (MBV). Proc Am Soc Clin Oncol 1981;22:514.
5. Kempin S, Cirrincione C, Myers J, Lee B III, Straus D, Koziner B, Arlin Z, Gee T, Mertelsmann R, Pinsky C, Comacho E, Nisce L, Old L, Clarkson B, Oettgen H. Combined modality therapy of advanced nodular lymphomas (NL): the role of nonspecific immunotherapy (MBV) as an important determinant of response and survival. Proc Am Soc Clin Oncol 1983;24:56.
6. Tang ZY, Zhou HY, Zhao G, Chai LM, Zhou M, Lu JZ, Liu KD, Havas HF, Nauts HC. Preliminary results of mixed bacterial vaccine as adjuvant treatment of hepatocellular carcinoma. Med Oncol Tumor Pharmacother 1991;8:23.
7. Ehrke MJ, Mihich E. Immunoregulation by cancer chemotherapeutic agents. In The Reticuloendothelial System: A Comprehensive Treatise. Vol 8, Pharmacology. Edited by JW Hadden, A Szentivanyi. New York: Plenum, 1985:p 309.
8. Schwartz RS. Immunosuppressive drugs. Prog Allergy 1965;9:246.
9. Ehrke MJ, Tomazic V, Ryoyama K, Cohen SA, Mihich E. Adriamycin induced immunomodulation: dependence upon time of administration. Int J Immunopharmacol 1983;5:43.
10. Lichtenstein AK, Pende D. Enhancement of natural killer cytotoxicity by cis-diamminedichloroplatinum (II) in vivo and in vitro. Cancer Res 1986;46:639.
11. Hoon DS, Foshag LJ, Nizze AS, Bohman R, Morton DL. Suppressor cell activity in a randomized trial of patients receiving active specific immunotherapy with melanoma cell vaccine and low dosages of cyclophosphamide. Cancer Res 1990;50:5358.
12. Oratz R, Dugan M, Roses DF, Harris MN, Speyer JL, Hochster H, Weissman J, Henn M, Bystryn JC. Lack of effect of cyclophosphamide on the immunogenicity of a melanoma antigen vaccine. Cancer Res 1991;51:3643.
13. Fudenberg HH, Whitten HD. Immunostimulation-Synthetic and biological modulators of immunity. Ann Rev Pharmacol Toxicol 1984;24:147.
14. Oates KK, Sztein MB, Goldstein AL. Mechanism of action of the thymosins: modulation of lymphokines, receptors, and T-cell differentiation antigens. In Cell Surface Antigen Thy-1: Immunology, Neurology, and Therapeutic Applications. Edited by AE Reif, M Schlesinger. New York: Marcel Dekker, 1989, p 273.
15. Ruszala-Mallon V, Linn Y-I, Durr FE, Wang BS. Low molecular weight immunopotentiators. Int J Immunopharmacol 1988;10:497.
16. Smalley RV, Oldham RK. Chemical inducers of lymphokines. In Principles of Cancer Biotherapy. Edited by RK Oldham. New York: Raven, 1987, p 223.
17. Klein E. Hypersensitivity reactions at tumor sites. Cancer Res 1969;29:2351.
18. Klein E. Immunotherapy of cancer in man, a reality. Natl Cancer Inst Monogr 1973;39: 139.
19. Guthrie D, Way S. Immunotherapy of non-clinical vaginal cancer. Lancet 1975;2: 1242.
20. Guthrie D, Way S. Failure of topical DNCB immunotherapy in most patients with non-clinical carcinoma of the cervix. Br J Cancer 1979;39:445.
21. Hull MG, Bowen-Simpkins P, Paintin DB. 5-Fluorouracil versus immunotherapy for non-clinical vaginal cancer. Lancet 1976;1:588.
22. Krupp PJ, Bohm JW. 5-Fluorouracil topical treatment of in situ vulvar cancer. A preliminary report. Obstet Gynecol 1978;51:702.
23. Mansell PW, Litwin MS, Ichinose H, Krementz ET. Delayed hypersensitivity to 5-fluorouracil following topical chemotherapy of cutaneous cancers. Cancer Res 1975;35: 1288.
24. Piver MS, Barlow JJ, Tsukada Y, Gamarra M, Sandecki A. Postirradiation squamous cell carcinoma in situ of the vagina: treatment by topical 20 percent 5-fluorouracil cream. Am J Obstet Gynecol 1979;135:377.
25. Pride GL, Chuprevich TW. Topical 5-fluorouracil treatment of transformation zone intraepithelial neoplasia of cervix and vagina. Obstet Gynecol 1982;60:467.
26. Guerin C. The history of BCG. In BCG Vaccination Against Tuberculosis. Edited by SR Rosenthal. Boston: Little, Brown, 1957, p 48.
27. Mande R. BCG Vaccination. London: Dowsons, 1968.
28. Bast RC Jr. Zbar B, Borsos T, Rapp HJ. BCG and cancer. N Engl J Med 1974;290: 1413.
29. Lemonde P, Dubreuil R, Guindon A, Lussier G. Stimulating influence of Bacillus Calmette-Guérin on immunity to polyoma tumors and spontaneous leukemia. JNCI 1971;47:1013.
30. Weiss DW, Lavrin DH, Dezfulian M, Vaage J, Blair PB. Studies on the immunology of spontaneous mammary carcinomas of mice. In Viruses Inducing Cancer. Edited by WJ Burdette. Salt Lake City: University of Utah Press, 1966, p 138.

31. Davignon L, Robillard P, Lemonde P, Frappier A. BCG vaccination and leukemia mortality. Lancet 1970;2:638.
32. Rosenthal SR, Crispen RG, Thorne MG, Piekarski N, Raisys N, Rettig PG. BCG vaccination and leukemia mortality. JAMA 1972;222:1543.
33. Comstock GW, Martinez I, Livesay VT. Efficacy of BCG vaccination in prevention of cancer. JNCI 1975;54:835.
34. Snider DE, Comstock GW, Martinez I, Caras GJ. Efficacy of BCG vaccination in prevention of cancer: an update. JNCI 1978;60:785.
35. Old LJ, Benacerraf B, Clarke DA, Carswell EA, Stockert E. The role of the reticuloendothelial system in the host reaction to neoplasia. Cancer Res 1961;21:1281.
36. Morton DL, Eilber FR, Malmgren RA, Wood WC. Immunological factors which influence response to immunotherapy in malignant melanoma. Surgery 1970;68:158.
37. Zbar B, Bernstein ID, Bartlett GL, Hanna MG Jr, Rapp HJ. Immunotherapy of cancer: regression of intradermal tumors and prevention of growth of lymph node metastases after intralesional injection of living *Mycobacterium bovis*. JNCI 1972;49:119.
38. Hanna MG Jr, Zbar B, Rapp HJ. Histopathology of tumor regression after intralesional injection of *Mycobacterium bovis*. I. Tumor growth and metastasis. JNCI 1972;48: 1441.
39. Meltzer MS, Nacy CA. Delayed-type hypersensitivity and the induction of activated, cytotoxic macrophages. In Fundamental Immunology, 2nd ed. Edited by WE Paul. New York: Raven, 1989, p 765.
40. Kim CI, Shin JS, Kim HI, Lee JM, Kim SJ. Production of tumor necrosis factor by intravesical administration of bacillus Calmette Guérin in patients with superficial bladder cancer. Yonsei Med J 1993;34:356–364.
41. Farias-Eisner R, Sherman MP, Aeberhard E, Chaudhuri G. Nitric oxide is an important mediator for tumoricidal activity in vivo. Proc Natl Acad Sci USA 1994;91:9407–9411
42. Thanhauser A, Bohle A, Schneider B, Reiling N, Mattern R, Ernst M, Flad HD, Ulmer AJ. The induction of bacillus-Calmette-Guérin-activated killer cells requires the presence of monocytes and T-helper type-1 cells. Cancer Immunol Immunother 1995;40: 103–108.
43. Bohle A, Thanhauser A, Ulmer AJ, Mattern T, Ernst M, Flad HD, Jocham D. On the mode of action of intravesical bacillus Calmette-Guérin: In vitro characterization of BCG-activated killer cells. Urol Res 1994;22:185–190.
44. Mandeville R, Sombo F-M, Rocheleau N. Natural cell-mediated cytotoxicity in normal human peripheral blood lymphocytes and its in vitro boosting with BCG. Cancer Immunol Immunother 1983;15:17.
45. Parr IB, Jackson LE, Alexander P. Role of "lymphotoxin" in the local anti-tumor action associated with inflammation caused by delayed hypersensitivity responses or intralesional BCG. I. Variations in response of different syngeneic mouse tumours. Br J Cancer 1983;48:385.
46. Nathanson L, Schoenfeld D, Regelson W, et al. Prospective comparison of intralesional and multipuncture BCG in recurrent intradermal melanoma. Cancer 1979;43: 1630–1635.
47. Morton DL, Barth A. Local therapy with biologic agents. In Biologic Therapy of Cancer, 2nd ed. Edited by VT DeVita Jr, S Hellman, SA Rosenberg. Philadelphia: Lippincott, 1995, pp 691–704.
48. Gutterman JU, Mavligit G, McBride C, Frei E, III, Freireich EJ, Hersh EM. Active immunotherapy with BCG for recurrent malignant melanoma. Lancet 1973;1:1208.
49. Mathé G, Amiel JL, Schwarzenberg L, Schneider M, Cattan A, Schlumberger JR, Hayat M, De Vassal F. Active immunotherapy for acute lymphoblastic leukaemia. Lancet 1969;1:697.
50. Heyn R, Borges W, Joo P, Karon M, Nesbit M, Shore N, Breslow N, Hammond D. BCG in the treatment of acute lymphocytic leukemia (ALL). Proc Am Assoc Cancer Res 1973;14:45.
51. Treatment of acute lymphoblastic leukaemia. Comparison of immunotherapy (BCG), intermittent methotrexate, and no therapy after a five-month intensive cytotoxic regimen (Concord trial). Preliminary report to the Medical Research Council by the Leukaemia Committee and the Working Party on Leukaemia in Childhood. Br Med J 1971;4:189.
52. Whittaker JA, Bailey-Wood R, Hutchins S. Active Immunotherapy for the treatment of acute myelogenous leukemia: the use of intravenous BCG and a comparison between BCG and irradiated leukemic blast cells. In Immunotherapy of Human Cancer. Edited by WD Terry, SA Rosenberg. New York: Excerpta Medica 1982, p 23.
53. Rosenberg SA, Rapp H, Terry W, Zbar B, Costa J, Seipp C, Simon R. Intralesional BCG therapy of patients with primary stage I melanoma. In Immunotherapy of Human Cancer. Edited by WD Terry, SA Rosenberg. New York: Excerpta Medica 1982, p 239.
54. McKneally MF, Maver C, Kausel HW. Regional immunotherapy of lung cancer with intrapleural BCG. Lancet 1976;1:377.
55. McKneally MF, Maver C, Lininger L, Kausel HW, McIlduff JB, Older TM, Foster ED, Alley RD. Four-year follow-up of the Albany experience with intrapleural BCG in lung cancer. J Thorac Cardiovasc Surg 1981;81:485.
56. Ludwig Lung Cancer Study Group (LLCSG). Immunostimulation with intrapleural BCG as adjuvant therapy in resected non-small cell lung cancer. Cancer 1986;58: 2411.
57. Sparks FC, Silverstein MJ, Hunt JS, Haskell CM, Pilch YH, Morton DL. Complications of BCG immunotherapy in patients with cancer. N Engl J Med 1973;289:827.
58. Cohen MH, Jessup JM, Felix EL, Weese JL, Herberman RB. Intralesional treatment of recurrent metastatic cutaneous malignant melanoma: a randomized prospective study of intralesional Bacillus Calmette-Guérin versus intralesional dinitrochlorobenzene. Cancer 1978;41:2456.
59. Lamm DL, Thor DE, Harris SC, et al. Intravesical and percutaneous BCG immunotherapy of recurrent superficial bladder cancer. In Immunotherapy of Human Cancer. Edited by WD Terry, SA Rosenberg. New York: Elsevier/North Holland 1982, p 315.
60. Morales A, Eidenger D, Bruce AW. Intracavitary Bacillus Calmette-Guérin in the treatment of superficial bladder tumors. J Urol 1976;116:180.
61. Pinsky CM, Camacho FJ, Kerr D, Braun DW Jr, Whitmore WF Jr, Oettgen HF. Treatment of superficial bladder cancer with intravesical BCG. In Immunotherapy of Human Cancer. Edited by WD Terry, SA Rosenberg. New York: Elsevier/North Holland, 1982, p 309.
62. Hudson MLA, Brown EJ, Ritchey JK, Ratliff TL. Modulation of fibronectin-mediated Bacillus Calmette-Guérin attachment to murine bladder mucosa by drugs influencing the coagulation pathways. Cancer Res 1991;51:3726.
63. Schneider B, Thanhauser A, Jocham D, Loppnow H, Vollmer E, Galle J, Flad HD, Ulmer AJ, Bohle A. Specific binding of bacillus Calmette-Guerin to urothelial tumor cells in vitro. World J Urol 1994;12:337–344.
64. Herr HW, Laudone VP. Intravesical therapy for superficial bladder cancer. In Cancer: principles & Practice of Oncology: updates 2. Edited by VT DeVita Jr, S Hellman, SA Rosenberg. New York: Lippincott, 1988a, p 1.
65. Herr HW, Laudone VP, Badalament RA, Oettgen HF, Sogani PC, Freedman BD, Melamed MR, Whitmore WF Jr. Bacillus Calmette-Guérin therapy alters the progression of superficial bladder cancer. J Clin Oncol 1988b;6:1450.
66. Lamm DL, Blumenstein BA, Crawford ED, Montie JE, Scardino P, Grossman HB, Stanisic TH, Smith JA Jr., Sullivan J, Sarosdy MF, et al. A randomized trial of intravesical doxorubicin and immunotherapy with bacille Calmette-Guérin for transitional-cell carcinoma of the bladder. N Engl J Med 1991;325:1205–1209.
67. Soloway MS, Perry A. Bacillus Calmette-Guérin for treatment of superficial transitional cell carcinoma of the bladder in patients who have failed thiotepa and/or mitomycin C. J Urol 1987;137:871.
68. Badalament RA, Herr HW, Wong GY, Gnecco C, Pinsky CM, Whitmore WF Jr, Fair WR, Oettgen HF. A prospective randomized trial of maintenance versus nonmaintenance intravesical Bacillus Calmette-Guérin therapy of superficial bladder cancer. J Clin Oncol 1987;5:441–449.
69. Lamm DL, Riggs DR, Shriver JS, et al. Mega-dose vitamins in bladder cancer: a double-blind clinical trial. J Urol 1994;151:21–26.
70. Orihuela E, Herr NW, Pinsky CM, Whitmore WF Jr. Toxicity of intravesical BCG and its management in patients with superficial bladder tumors. Cancer 1987;60:326.
71. Lamm DL, Thor DE, Winters WD, Stogdill VD, Radwin HM. BCG immunotherapy of bladder cancer: inhibition of tumor recurrence and associated immune responses. Cancer 1985;48:82.
72. Bauohle A, Nowc C, Ulmer AJ, Musehold J, Gerdes J, Hofstetter AG, Flad HD. Detection of urinary TNF, IL 1, and IL 2 after local BCG immunotherapy for bladder carcinoma. Cytokine 1990;2:175.
73. Fleischmann JD, Toossi Z, Ellner JJ, Wentworth DB, Ratliff TL, Imbembo AL. Urinary interleukins in patients receiving intravesical Bacillus Calmette-Guérin therapy for superficial bladder cancer. Cancer 1989;64:1447.
74. Gray GR, Ribi E, Granger D, Parker R, Azuma I, Yamamoto K. Immunotherapy of cancer: tumor suppression and regression by cell walls of Mycobacterium phlei attached to oil droplets. JNCI 1975;55:727.
75. Klein WR, Ruitenberg EJ, Steerenberg PA, De Jong WH, Kruizinga W, Misdorp W, Bier J, Tiesjema RH, Kreeftenberg JG, Teppema JS, Rapp HJ. Immunotherapy by intralesional injection of BCG cell walls or live BCG in bovine ocular squamous cell carcinoma: a preliminary report. JNCI 1982;69:1095.
76. Lederer E, Chedid L. Immunomodulation by synthetic muramyl peptides and trehalose diesters. In Immunological Approaches to Cancer Therapeutics. Edited by E Mihich. New York: Wiley, 1982, p 107.
77. Sancúaeau J, Falcoff R, Beranger F, Carter DB, Wietzerbin J. Secretion of interleukin-6 (IL-6) by human monocytes stimulated by muramyl dipeptide and tumour necrosis factor alpha. Immunology 1990;69:52.
78. Bahr GM, Chedid LA, Behbehani K. Induction, in vivo and in vitro, of macrophage membrane interleukin-1 by adjuvant-active synthetic muramyl peptides. Cell Immunol 1987;107:443.
79. Salem P, Deryckx S, Dulioust A, Vivier E, Denizot Y, Damais C, Dinarello CA, Thomas Y. Immunoregulatory functions of paf-Acether. IV. Enhancement of IL-1 production of muramyl dipeptide-stimulated monocytes. J Immunol 1990;144:1338.
80. Noso Y, Parant M, Parant F, Chedid L. Production of tumor necrosis factor in nude mice by muramyl peptides associated with bacterial vaccines. Cancer Res 1988;48: 5766.
81. Sone S, Lopez-Berestein G, Fidler IJ. Potentiation of direct antitumor cytotoxicity and production of tumor cytolytic factors in human blood monocytes by human recombinant interferon-gamma and muramyl dipeptide derivatives. Cancer Immunol Immunother 1986;21:93.
82. Utsugi T, Sone S. Comparative analysis of the priming effect of human interferon-μ, β, and γ on synergism with muramyl dipeptide analog for anti-tumor expression of human blood monocytes. J Immunol 1986;136:1117.
83. Souvannavong V, Brown S, Adam A. Muramyl dipeptide (MDP) synergizes with interleukin 2 and interleukin 4 to stimulate, respectively, the differentiation and proliferation of B cells. Cell Immunol 1990;126:106.
84. Spargo BJ, Crowe LM, Ioneda T, Beaman BL, Crowe JH. Cord factor (μ, μ-trehalose 6, 6′-dimycolate) inhibits fusion between phospholipid vesicles. Proc Natl Acad Sci USA 1991;88:737.
85. McLaughlin CA, Schwartzman SM, Horner BL, Jones GH, Moffatt JG, Nestor JJ Jr, Tegg D. Regression of tumors in guinea pigs after treatment with synthetic muramyl dipeptides and trehalose dimycolate. Science 1980;208:415.
86. Yarkoni E, Lederer E, Rapp HJ. Immunotherapy of experimental cancer with a mixture of synthetic muramyl dipeptide and trehalose dimycolate. Infect Immun 1981;32: 273.
87. Fogler WE, Wade R, Brundish DE, Fidler IJ. Distribution and fate of free and liposome-encapsulated (^{3}H)nor-muramyl dipeptide and (^{3}H) muramyl tripeptide phosphatidylethanolamine in mice. J Immunol 1985;135:1372.
88. Parant M, Parant F, Chedid L, Yapo A, Petit JF, Lederer E. Fate of the synthetic immunoadjuvant, muramyl dipeptide (^{14}C-labeled) in the mouse. Int J Immunopharmacol 1979;1:35.
89. Pak CC, Fidler IJ. Liposomal delivery of biological response modifiers to macrophages. Biotherapy 1991;3:55.
90. Key ME, Talmadge JE, Fogler WE, Bucana C, Fidler IJ. Isolation of tumoricidal macrophages from lung melanoma metastases of mice treated systemically with liposomes containing a lipophilic derivative of muramyl dipeptide. JNCI 1982;69: 1189.
91. Kleinerman ES, Murray JL, Snyder JS, Cunningham JE, Fidler IJ. Activation of tumoricidal properties in monocytes from cancer patients following intravenous administration of liposomes containing muramyl tripeptide phosphatidylethanolamine. Cancer Res 1989;49:4665.
92. Urba WJ, Hartmann LC, Longo DL, Steis RG, Smith JW II, Kedar I, Creekmore S, Sznol M, Conlon K, Kopp WC, Huber C, Herold M, Alvord WG, Snow S, Clark JW. Phase I and immunomodulatory study of a muramyl peptide, muramyl tripeptide phosphatidylethanolamine. Cancer Res 1990;50:2979.
93. Kleinerman ES, Fidler IJ. Systemic activation of macrophages by liposomes contain-

ing immunomodulators. In Biologic Therapy of Cancer, 2nd ed, Edited by VT DeVita Jr, S Hellman, SA Rosenberg. Philadelphia: Lippincott, 1995, pp 829–839.

94. Halpern BN, Biozzi G, Stiffel C, Mouton D. Inhibition of tumour growth by administration of killed *Corynebacterium parvum*. Nature 1966;212:853.
95. Milas L, Hunter N, Basic I, Withers HR. Complete regression of an established murine fibrosarcoma induced by systemic application of *Corynebacterium granulosum*. Cancer Res 1974;34:2470.
96. Woodruff MFA, Boak JL. Inhibitory effect of injection of *Corynebacterium parvum* on the growth of tumour transplants in isogenic hosts. Br J Cancer 1966;20:345.
97. Bast RC Jr, Knapp RC, Mitchell AK, Thurston JG, Tucker RW, Schlossman SF. Immunotherapy of a murine ovarian carcinoma with *Corynebacterium parvum* and specific heteroantiserum. I. Activation of peritoneal cells to mediate antibody-dependent cytotoxicity. J Immunol 1979;123:1945.
98. Knapp RC, Berkowitz RS. *Corynebacterium parvum* as an immunotherapeutic agent in an ovarian cancer model. Am J Obstet Gynecol 1977;128:782.
99. Kreider JW, Bartlett GL, Purnell DM, Webb S. Immunotherapy of an established rat mammary adenocarcinma (13762A) with intratumor injection of *Corynebacterium parvum*. Cancer Res 1978;38:689.
100. Likhite VV. Rejection of tumors and metastases in Fischer 344 rats following intratumor administration of killed *Corynebacterium parvum*. Int J Cancer 1974a;14:684.
101. Likhite VV, Halpern BN. Lasting rejection of mammary adenocarcinoma cell tumors in DBA-2 mice with intratumor injection of killed *Corynebacterium parvum*. Cancer Res 1974b;34:341.
102. Scott MT. *Corynebacterium parvum* as a therapeutic antitumor agent in mice. II. Local injection. JNCI 1975;53:861.
103. Bast RC Jr, Bast BS. Critical review of previous reported animal studies of tumor immunotherapy with nonspecific immunostimulants. Ann NY Acad Sci 1976;227:60.
104. Keller R, Keist R, Van der Meide PH, Groscurth P, Aguet M, Leist TP. Induction, maintenance, and reinduction of tumoricidal activity in bone marrow-derived mononuclear phagocytes by *Corynebacterium parvum*. Evidence for the involvement of a T cell- and interferon–independent pathway of macrophage activation. J Immunol 1987;138: 2366.
105. Lichtenstein A, Bick A, Cantrell J, Zighelboim J. Augmentation of NK activity by *Corynebacterium parvum* fractions in vivo and in vitro. Int J Immunopharmacol 1983;5:137.
106. Lichtenstein A, Seelig M, Berek J, Zighelboim J. Human neutrophil-mediated lysis of ovarian cancer cells. Blood 1989;74:805.
107. Oettgen HF, Pinsky CM, Delmonte L. Treatment of cancer with immunomodulators. *Corynebacterium parvum* and levamisole. Med Clin North Am 1976;60:511.
108. Hertzog PJ, Cheetham BF, Sexton JL, Linnane AW. Characterization of interferons produced by peripheral blood mononuclear cells from healthy subjects in response to *Corynebacterium parvum* or poly I: poly C. Biochem Int 1989;19:1427.
109. Hirt HM, Schwenteck M, Becker H, Kirchner H. Interferon production and lymphocyte stimulation in human leucocyte cultures stimulated by *Corynebacterium parvum*. Clin Exp Immunol 1978;32:471.
110. Rossol S, Voth R, Brunner S, Mauuller WEG, Buttner M, Gallati H, Meyer zum Bauschenfelde K-H, Hess G. *Corynebacterium parvum* (*Propionibacterium acnes*): an inducer of tumor necrosis factor-α in human peripheral blood mononuclear cells and monocytes in vitro. Eur J Immunol 1990;20:1761.
111. Woodruff M, Dunbar N, Ghaffar A. The growth of tumours in T-cell deprived mice and their response to treatment with *Corynebacterium parvum*. Proc R Soc Lond Biol 1973;184:97.
112. Christie GH, Bomford R. Mechanisms of macrophage activation by *Corynebacterium parvum*. I. In vitro experiments. Cell Immunol 1975;17:141.
113. Tuttle RL, North RJ. Mechanisms of antitumor action of *Corynebacterium parvum*: the generation of cell-mediated tumor specific immunity. J Reticuloendothel Soc 1976;20:197.
114. Tuttle RL, North RJ. Mechanisms of antitumor action of *Corynebacterium parvum* replicating short-lived T cells as the mediators of potentiated tumor-specific immunity. J Reticuloendothel Soc 1976;20:209.
115. Okuda S, Taniguchi K, Kubo C, Nomoto K. Accessory cell function in tumor-bearing mice and effects of *Corynebacterium parvum*. JNCI 1982;69:1293.
116. DiSaia PJ, Bundy BN, Curry SL, Schlaerth J, Thigpen JT. Phase III study on the treatment of women with cervical cancer, Stage IIB, IIIB, and IVA (confined to the pelvis and/or periaortic nodes), with radiotherapy alone versus radiotherapy plus immunotherapy with intravenous *Corynebacterium parvum*. A Gynecologic Oncology Group study. Gynecol Oncol 1987;26:386.
117. Fisher B, Brown A, Wolmark N, Fisher ER, Redmond C, Wickerham L, Margolese R, Dimitrov N, Pilch Y, Glass A, Sutherland C, Foster R. Evaluation of the worth of *Corynebacterium parvum* in conjunction with chemotherapy as adjuvant treatment for primary breast cancer. Cancer 1990;66:220.
118. Hilal EY, Pinsky CM, Hirshaut Y, Wanebo HJ, Hansen JA, Braun DW Jr, Fortner JG, Oettgen HF. Surgical adjuvant therapy of malignant melanoma with *Corynebacterium parvum*. Cancer 1981;48:245.
119. Petersen E, Hokland P, Ellegaard J. Adjuvant immune stimulation with *Corynebacterium parvum* during maintenance chemotherapy of acute myeloid leukemia. A prospective randomized study. Cancer Immunol Immunother 1983;16:88.
120. Vogl SE, Schoenfeld DA, Kaplan BH, Lerner HJ, Horton J, Creech RH, Barnes LE. Methotrexate alone or with regional subcutaneous *Corynebacterium parvum* in the treatment of recurrent and metastatic squamous cancer of the head and neck. Cancer 1982;50:2295.
121. Woodruff M, Walbaum P. A phase-II trial of *Corynebacterium parvum* as adjuvant to surgery in the treatment of operable lung cancer. Cancer Immunol Immunother 1983;16:114.
122. Lipton A, Harvey HA, Balch CM, Antle CE, Heckard R, Bartolucci AA. *Corynebacterium parvum* versus Bacille Calmette-Guérin adjuvant immunotherapy of Stage II malignant melanoma. J Clin Oncol 1919;9:1151.
123. Cheng VST, Suit HD, Wang CC, Cummings C. Nonspecific immunotherapy by *Corynebacterium parvum*. Phase I toxicity study in 12 patients with advanced cancer. Cancer 1976;37:1687.
124. Fisher B, Rubin H, Sartiano G, Ennis L, Wolmark N. Observations following *Corynebacterium parvum* administration to patients with advanced malignancy. A phase I study. Cancer 1976;38:119.
125. Gall SA, DiSaia PJ, Schmidt H, Mittelstaedt L, Newman P, Creasman W. Toxicity manifestations following intravenous *Corynebacterium parvum* administration to patients with ovarian and cervical carcinoma. Am J Obstet Gynecol 1978;132:555.
126. Gill PG, Morris PJ, Kettlewell M. The complications of intravenous *Corynebacterium parvum* infusion. Clin Exp Immunol 1977;30:229.
127. Casali A, Gionfra T, Rinaldi M, Tonachella R, Tropea F, Venturo I, De Martino C, Curcio CG. Treatment of malignant pleural effusions with intracavitary *Corynebacterium parvum*. Cancer 1988;62:806.
128. Mantovani A, Sessa C, Peri G, Allavena P, Introna M, Polentarutti N, Mangioni C. Intraperitoneal administration of *Corynebacterium parvum* in patients with ascitic ovarian tumors resistant to chemotherapy: effects on cytotoxicity of tumor-associated macrophages and NK cells. Int J Cancer 1981;27:437.
129. Millar JW, Hunter AM, Horne NW. Intrapleural immunotherapy with *Corynebacterium parvum* in recurrent malignant pleural effusions. Thorax 1980;35:856.
130. Rossi GA, Felletti R, Balbi B, Sacco O, Cosulich E, Risso A, Melioli G, Ravazzoni C. Symptomatic treatment of recurrent malignant pleural effusions with intrapleurally administered *Corynebacterium parvum*. Clinical response is not associated with evidence of enhancement of local cellular-mediated immunity. Am Rev Respir Dis 1987;135:885.
131. Webb HE, Oaten SW, Pike CP. Treatment of malignant ascitic and pleural effusion with *Corynebacterium parvum*. Br Med J 1978;1:338.
132. Bast RC Jr, Berek JS, Obrist R, Griffiths CT, Berkowitz RS, Hacker NF, Parker L, Lagasse LD, Knapp RC. Intraperitoneal immunotherapy of human ovarian carcinoma with *Corynebacterium parvum*. Cancer Res 1983;43:1395.
133. Berek JS, Knapp RC, Hacker NF, Lichtenstein A, Jung T, Spina C, Obrist R, Griffiths CT, Berkowitz RS, Parker L, Zighelboim J, Bast RC Jr. Intraperitoneal immunotherapy of epithelial ovarian carcinoma with *Corynebacterium parvum*. Am J Obstet Gynecol 1985;152:1003.
134. Lichtenstein A, Berek J, Bast R, Spina C, Hacker N, Knapp RC, Zighelboim J. Activation of peritoneal lymphocyte cytotoxicity in patients with ovarian cancer by intraperitoneal treatment with *Corynebacterium parvum*. J Biol Response Mod 1984;3: 371.
135. Berek JS, Hacker NF, Lichtenstein A, Jung T, Spina C, Knox RM, Brady J, Greene T, Ettinger LM, Logasse LD, Bonnem EM, Spiegel RJ, Zighelboim J. Intraperitoneal recombinant alfa-interferon for "salvage" immunotherapy in stage III epithelial ovarian cancer: a Gynecologic Oncology Group study. Cancer Res 1985;45:4447.
136. Steis RG, Urba WJ, VanderMolen LA, Bookman MA, Smith JW, Clark JW, Miller RL, Crum ED, Beckner SK, McKnight JE, Ozols RF, Stevenson HC, Young RC, Longo DL. Intraperitoneal lymphokine-activated killer-cell and interleukin-2 therapy for malignancies limited to the peritoneal cavity. J Clin Oncol 1990;8:1618.
137. Urba WJ, Clark JW, Steis RG, Bookman MA, Smith JW II, Beckner S, Maluish AE, Rossio JL, Rager H, Ortaldo JR, Longo DL. Intraperitoneal lymphokine-activated killer cell-interleukin-2 therapy in patients with intra-abdominal cancer: immunologic considerations. JNCI 1989;81:602.
138. Bookman MA, Bast RC Jr. The immunobiology and immunotherapy of ovarian cancer. Semin Oncol 1991;18:270.
139. Izumi S, Ogawa T, Miyauchi M, Fujie K, Okuhara M, Kohsaka M. Antitumor effect of *Nocardia rubra* cell wall skeleton on syngeneically transplanted P388 tumors. Cancer Res 1991;51:4038.
140. Onuma M, Yamamoto M, Yasutomi Y, Takahashi K, Kawakami Y, Azuma I. Regression of bovine lymphosarcoma by treatment with cell-wall skeleton of *Nocardia rubra*. Vaccine 1989;7:121.
141. Inamura N, Fujitsu T, Nakahara K, Abiko M, Horii Y, Hashimoto S, Aoki H. Potentiation of tumoricidal properties of murine macrophages by *Nocardia rubra* cell wall skeleton (N-CWS). J Antibiot 1984;37:244.
142. Ito M, Iizuka H, Masuno T, Yasunami R, Ogura T, Yamamura Y, Azuma I. Killing of tumor cells in vitro by macrophages from mice given injections of squalene-treated cell wall skeleton of *Nocardia rubra*. Cancer Res 1981;41:2925.
143. Inamura N, Nakahara K, Kuroda Y, Yamaguchi I, Aoki H, Kohsaka M. Effect of *Nocardia rubra* cell wall skeleton on interleukin-1 production from mouse peritoneal macrophages. Int J Immunopharmacol 1988;10:547.
144. Izumi S, Hirai O, Hayashi K, Konishi Y, Okuhara M, Kohsaka M, Aoki H, Yamamura Y. Induction of a tumor necrosis factor-like activity by *Nocardia rubra* cell wall skeleton. Cancer Res 1987;47:1785.
145. Izumi S, Ueda H, Okuhara M, Aoki H, Yamamura Y. Effect of *Nocardia rubra* cell wall skeleton on murine interferon production in vitro. Cancer Res 1986;46:1960.
146. Saijo N, Ozaki A, Beppu Y, Irimajiri N, Shibuya M, Shimizu E, Takizawa T, Taniguchi T, Hoshi A. In vivo and in vitro effects of *Nocardia rubra* cell wall skeleton on natural killer activity in mice. Gann 1983;74:137.
147. Miyazaki K, Yasumoto K, Yano T, Matsuzaki G, Sugimachi K, Nomoto K. Synergistic effect of *Nocardia rubra* cell wall skeleton and recombinant interleukin 2 for in vivo induction of lymphokine-activated killer cells. Cancer Res 1991;51:5261.
148. Kawase I, Uemiya M, Yoshimoto T, Ogura T, Hirao F, Yamamura Y. Effect of *Nocardia rubra* cell wall skeleton on T-cell-mediated cytotoxicity in mice bearing syngeneic sarcoma. Cancer Res 1981;41:660.
149. Ogura T, Hara H, Yokota S, Hosoe S, Kawase I, Kishimoto S, Yamamura Y. Effector mechanism in concomitant immunity potentiated by intratumoral injection of *Nocardia rubra* cell wall skeleton. Cancer Res 1985;45:6371.
150. Yamakido M, Ishioka S, Onari K, Matsuzaka S, Yanagida J, Nishimoto Y. Changes in natural killer cell, antibody-dependent cell-mediated cytotoxicity and interferon activities with administration of *Nocardia rubra* cell wall skeleton to subjects with high risk of lung cancer. Gann 1983;74:896.
151. Inamura N, Sone S, Ogawa T, Nishio M, Ogura T. Human blood monocyte activation by *Nocardia rubra* cell wall skeleton for production of interleukin 1 and tumor necrosis factor-alpha. Biotherapy 1992;4:155–163.
152. Shimizu E, Saijo N, Shibuya M, Takizawa T, Hoshi A. The analysis of cytostatic activity of human peripheral blood granulocytes and its augmentation with *Nocardia rubra* cell wall skeleton (N-CWS). J Cancer Res Clin Oncol 1983;106:130.
153. Sakatani M, Ogura T, Masuno T, Kishimoto S, Yamamura Y. Effect of *Nocardia rubra* cell wall skeleton on augmentation of cytotoxicity function in human pleural macrophages. Cancer Immunol Immunother 1987;25:119.
154. Shirasaka T, Kawase I, Okada M, Kitahara M, Ikeda T, Komuta K, Hosoe S, Yokota S, Masuno T, Kishimoto S. Augmentative effect of *Nocardia rubra* cell-wall skeleton on the induction of human lymphokine-activated killer (LAK) cells by the production of LAK cell helper factor(s). Cancer Immunol Immunother 1989;30:195.

155. Yamamura Y, Ogura T, Sakatani M, Hirao F, Kishimoto S, Fukuoka M, Takada M, Kawahara M, Furuse K, Kuwahara O, Ikegama H, Ogawa N. Randomized controlled study of adjuvant immunotherapy with *Nocardia rubra* cell wall skeleton for inoperable lung cancer. Cancer Res 1983;43:5575.
156. Ogura T, Sakatani M. Randomized controlled study on adjuvant immunotherapy for unresectable lung cancer with *Nocardia rubra* cell wall skeleton. Nippon Kyobu Shikkan Gakkai Zasshi 1985;23:62.
157. Koyama S, Ozaki A, Iwasaki Y, Sakita T, Osuga T, Watanabe A, Suzuki M, Kawasaki T, Soma T, Tabuchi T, Nakayama M, Koizumi S, Yokoyama K, Uchida T, Orii K, Tanaka T. Randomized controlled study of postoperative adjuvant immunotherapy with *Nocardia rubra* cell wall skeleton (N-CWS) and Tegafur for gastric carcinoma. Cancer Immunol Immunother 1986;22:148.
158. Yamakido M, Ishioka S, Hozawa S, Matsuzaka S, Yanagida J, Shigenobu T, Otake M, Nishimoto Y. Effect of *Nocardia rubra* cell-wall skeleton on cancer prevention in humans. Cancer Immunol Immunother 1992;34:389–392.
159. Yamamura Y, Ogura T, Hirao F, Yasumoto K, Sawamura K, Hattori S, Hayata Y, Kishimoto S, Yamada K, Niitani H, Masaoka T. Phase I study with cell wall skeleton of *Nocardia rubra*. Cancer Treat Rep 1981;65:707.
160. Colotta F, Rambaldi A, Colombo N, Tabacchi L, Introna M, Mantovani A. Effect of a streptococcal preparation (OK432) on natural killer activity of tumour-associated lymphoid cells in human ovarian carcinoma and on lysis of fresh ovarian tumour cells. Br J Cancer 1983;48:515.
161. Uchida A, Micksche M, Hoshino T. Cancer patients: augmentation of autologous tumor killing activity of tumor-associated large granular lymphocytes. Cancer Immunol Immunother 1984;18:5.
162. Uchida A. Augmentation of autologous tumor killing activity of tumor-associated large granular lymphocytes by the streptococcal preparation OK432. Methods Find Exp Clin Pharmacol 1986;8:81.
163. Vanky F, Uchida A, Klein E, Willems J. Lysis of autologous tumor cells by high-density lymphocytes is potentiated by the streptococcal preparation OK432 (Picibanil). Int J Cancer 1986;37:531.
164. Allavena P, Peccatori F, Maggioni D, Pirovano P, Mantovani A. Killing of tumor cells with pleiotropic drug resistance by OK432-activated effector cells. Immunopharmacol Immunotoxicol 1989;11:257.
165. Chirigos MA, Saito T, Talmadge JE, Budzynski W, Gruys E. Cell regulatory and immunorestorative activity of picibanil (OK432). Cancer Detect Prev 1987;1(suppl):317.
166. Yanagawa E, Uchida A, Moore M, Micksche M. Autologous tumor killing and natural cytotoxic activity of tumor-associated macrophages in cancer patients. Cancer Immunol Immunother 1985;19:163.
167. Ueta E, Umazume M, Yamamoto T, Osaki T. Enhancement of polymorphonuclear leukocyte (PMN) function by OK-432. Int J Immunopharmacol 1994;16:7–17.
168. Boyer PJ, Berek JS, Zighelboim J. Lymphocyte activation by recombinant interleukin-2 in ovarian cancer patients. Obstet Gynecol 1989;73:793.
169. Christmas SE, Meager A, Moore M. Studies of the enhancement of natural cytotoxicity by the streptococcal immunopotentiator OK432. Int J Immunopharmacol 1986;8:83.
170. Yamaue H, Tanimura H, Iwahashi M, Tani M, Tsunoda T, Tabuse K, Kuribayashi K, Saito K. Role of interleukin-2 and interferon-gamma in induction of activated natural killer cells from mice primed in vivo and subsequently challenged in vitro with the streptococcal preparation OK432. Cancer Immunol Immunother 1989;29:79.
171. Ogita S, Tsuto T, Nakamura K, Deguchi E, Iwai N. OK-432 therapy in 64 patients with lymphangioma. J Pediatr Surg 1994;29:784–785.
172. Kitsuki H, Uchiyama A, Yoshida T, Torisu M. OK-432-induced enhancement of ICAM-1 expression on tumor cells positively correlates to therapeutic effects for malignant effusion. Clin Immunol Immunopathol 1994;71:89–95.
173. Shirai M, Watanabe S, Nishioka, M Intratumoral injection of OK432 and lymphokine-activated killer activity in peripheral blood of patients with hepatocellular carcinoma. Eur J Cancer 1990;26:965.
174. Tsujihashi H, Matsuda H, Uejima S, Akiyama T, Kurita T. Immunocompetence of tissue infiltrating lymphocytes in bladder tumors. J Urol 1988;140:890.
175. Kumazawa H, Yamashita T, Tachikawa T, Minamino M, Nakata Y. Local injection of OK-432/fibrinogen gel into head and neck carcinomas. Eur J Cancer 1994;30A:1741–1744.
176. Mukai M, Kubota S, Morita S, Akanuma A. A pilot study of combination therapy of radiation and local administration of OK-432 for esophageal cancer. Five-year survival and local control rate. Cancer 1995;75:2276–2280.
177. Noda K, Teshima K, Tekeuti K, Hasegawa K, Inoue K-Y, Yamashita K, Sawaragi I, Nakajima T, Takashima E, Ikeuchi M, Sekiba K, Okuda H, Ichijo J, Saito T, Ozawa M, Tamura H, Chihara T, Kuzuya K, Ozaki M, Inagaki M, Tominaga S. Immunotherapy using the streptococcal preparation OK-432 for the treatment of uterine cervical cancer. Gynecol Oncol 1989;35:367.
178. Sugimachi K, Maehara Y, Akazawa K, Kondo Y, Kunil Y, Kitamura M, Yamaoka H, Takahashi Y, Kito T, Katou M, et al. Postoperative chemotherapy including intraperitoneal and intradermal administration of the streptococcal preparation OK-432 for patients with gastric cancer and peritoneal dissemination: a prospective randomized study. Cancer Chemother & Pharmacol 1994;33:366–370.
179. Tanaka N, Gouchi A, Ohara T, Mannami T, Konaga E, Fuchimoto S, Okamura S, Sato K, Orita K. Intratumoral injection of a streptococcal preparation, OK-432, before surgery for gastric cancer. A randomized trial. Cooperative Study Group of Preoperative Intratumoral Immunotherapy for Cancer. Cancer 1994;74:3097–3103.
180. Maehara Y, Okuyama T, Kakeji Y, Baba H, Furusawa M, Sugimachi K. Postoperative immunochemotherapy including streptococcal lysate OK-432 is effective for patients with gastric cancer and serosal invasion. Am J Surg 1994;168:36–40.
181. Lee YC, Luh Sp, Wu RM, Lee CJ. Adjuvant immunotherapy with intrapleural *Streptococcus pyogenes* (OK-432) in lung cancer patients after resection. Cancer Immunol Immunother 1994;39:269–274.
182. Chihara G, Hamuro J, Maeda Y, Shiio T, Suga T, Takasuka N, Sasaki T. Antitumor and metastasis-inhibitory activities of lentinan as an immunomodulator: an overview. Cancer Detect Prev (suppl) 1987;1:423.
183. Fruehauf JP, Bonnard GD, Herberman RB. The effect of lentinan on production of interleukin-1 by human monocytes. Immunopharmacology 1982;5:65.
184. Miyakoshi H, Aoki T. Acting mechanisms of lentinan in human-II. Enhancement of non-specific cell-mediated cytotoxicity as an interferon inducer. Int J Immunopharmacol 1984;6:373.
185. Sakamaki S, Kohgo Y, Suzuki M, Ogiwara R, Suga T, Kondo N, Izawa M, Kanisawa Y, Niitsu Y. Individual diversity of IL-6 generation by human monocytes with lentinan administration. Int J Immunopharmacol 1993;15:751–756.
186. Arinaga S, Karimine N, Takamuku K, Nanbara S, Nagamatsu M, Ueo H, Akiyoshi T. Enhanced production of interleukin 1 and tumor necrosis factor by peripheral monocytes after lentinan administration in patients with gastric carcinoma. Int J Immunopharmacol 1992;14:43–47.
187. Suzuki M, Higuchi S, Taki Y, Taki S, Miwa K, Hamuro J. Induction of endogenous lymphokine-activated killer activity by combined administration of lentinan and interleukin 2. Int J Immunopharmacol 1990;12:613.
188. Tani M, Tanimura H, Yamaue H, Tsunoda T, Iwahashi M, Noguchi K, Tamai M, Hotta T, Mizobata S. Augmentation of lymphokine-activated killer cell activity by lentinan. Anticancer Res 1993;13:1773–1776.
189. Ladanyi A, Timar J, Lapis K. Effect of lentinan on macrophage cytotoxicity against metastatic tumor cells. Cancer Immunol Immunother 1993;36:123–126.
190. Herlyn D, Kaneko Y, Powe J, Aoki T, Koprowski H. Monoclonal antibody-dependent murine macrophage-mediated cytotoxicity against human tumors is stimulated by lentinan. Jpn J Cancer Res 1985;76:37.
191. Suga T, Shiio T, Maeda YY, Chihara G. Antitumor activity of lentinan in murine syngeneic and autochthonous hosts and its suppressive effect on 3-methylcholanthrene-induced carcinogenesis. Cancer Res 1984;44:5132.
192. Jeannin JF, Lagadec P, Pelletier H, Reisser D, Olsson NO, Chihara G, Martin F. Regression induced by lentinan of peritoneal carcinomatoses in a model of colon cancer in rat. Int J Immunopharmacol 1988;10:855.
193. Oka M, Yoshino S, Hazama S, Shimoda K, Suzuki T. Immunological analysis and clinical effects of intraabdominal and intrapleural injection of lentinan for malignant ascites and pleural effusion. Biotherapy 1992;5:107–112.
194. Taguchi T. Clinical efficacy of lentinan on patients with stomach cancer: end point results of a four-year follow-up survey. Cancer Detect Prev 1987;1(suppl):333.
195. Wakui A, Kasai M, Konno K, Abe R, Kanamura R, Takahashi K, Nakai Y, Yoshida Y, Koie H, Masuda H. Randomized study of lentinan on patients with advanced gastric and colorectal cancer. Gan To Kagaku Ryoho 1986;13:1050.
196. Chirigos MA, Mastrangelo MJ. Immunorestoration by chemicals. In Immunological Approaches to Cancer Therapeutics. Edited by E Mihich. New York: Wiley, 1982, p 191.
197. Janssen PAJ. Levamisole as an adjuvant in cancer treatment. J Clin Pharmacol 1991;31:396.
198. Stevenson HC, Green I, Hamilton JM, Calabro BA, Parkinson DR. Levamisole: Known effects on the immune system, clinical results and future applications to the treatment of cancer. J Clin Oncol 1991;9:2052.
199. Van Wauwe J, Janssen PAJ. Review article on the biochemical mode of action of levamisole: an update. Int J Immunopharmacol 1991;13:3.
200. Schiller JH, Lindstrom M, Witt PL, Hank JA, Mahvi D, Wagner RJ, Sondel P, Borden EC. Immunological effects of levamisole in vitro. J Immunother 1991;10:297.
201. Janik J, Kopp WC, Smith JW, et al. Dose-related immunologic effects of levamisole in patients with cancer. J Clin Oncol 1993;11:125–135.
202. Sampson D, Peters TG, Lewis JD, Metzig J, Kurtz BE. Dose dependence of immunopotentiation and tumor regression induced by levamisole. Cancer Res 1977;37:3526.
203. Lewinski UH, Mavligit GM, Hersh EM. Cellular immune modulation after a single high dose of levamisole in patients with carcinoma. Cancer 1980;46:2185.
204. Tripodi D, Parks LC, Brugmans J. Drug-induced restoration of cutaneous delayed hypersensitivity in anergic patients with cancer. N Engl J Med 1973;289:354.
205. Gonzalez RL, Spitler LE, Sagebiel RW. Effect of levamisole as a surgical adjuvant therapy for malignant melanoma. Cancer Treat Rep 1978;62:1703–1707.
206. Loutfi A, Shakr A, Jerry M, Hanley J, Shibata HR. Double blind randomized prospective trial of levamisole/placebo in stage I cutaneous malignant melanoma. Clin Invest Med 1987;10:325–328.
207. Quirt IC, Shelley WE, Pater JL, Bodurtha AJ, McCulloch PB, McPherson TA, Paterson AHG, Prentice R, Silver HKB, Willan AR, Wilson K, Zee B. Improved survival in patients with poor-prognosis malignant melanoma treated with adjuvant levamisole: a phase III study by the National Cancer Institute of Canada Clinical Trials Group. J Clin Oncol 1991;9:729.
208. Spitler LE. A randomized trial of levamisole versus placebo as adjuvant therapy in malignant melanoma. J Clin Oncol 1991;9:736–740.
209. Hortobagyi GN, Gutterman JU, Blumenschein GR, Tashima CK, Buzdar AU, Hersch EM. Levamisole in the treatment of breast cancer. Prog Cancer Res Ther 1978;7:131.
210. Klefstrauom P. Combination of levamisole immunotherapy and polychemotherapy in advanced breast cancer. Cancer Treat Rep 1980;64:65.
211. Klefstrauom P, Grauohn P, Heinonen E, Holsti L, Holsti P. Adjuvant postoperative radiotherapy, chemotherapy, and immunotherapy in stage III breast cancer. II. 5-year results and influence of levamisole. Cancer 1987;60:936.
212. Klefstrauom P, Nuortio L. Levamisole in the treatment of advanced breast cancer. A ten-year follow-up of a randomized study. Acta Oncol 1991;30:347.
213. Rojas AF, Feierstein JN, Glait HM, Olivari AJ. Levamisole action in breast cancer stage III. In Immunotherapy of Cancer: Present Status of Trials in Man. Edited by WD Terry, D Windhorst. Prog Cancer Res Ther 1978, p 696.
214. Stephens EJW, Wood HF, Mason B. The influence of levamisole on the survival of patients with disseminated mammary carcinoma treated with chemotherapy. In Immunotherapy of Human Cancer. Edited by WD Terry, SA Rosenberg. New York: Elsevier/North Holland, 1982, p 199.
215. Treurniet-Donker AD, Meischke-De Jongh ML, van Putten WLJ. Levamisole as adjuvant immunotherapy in breast cancer. Cancer 1987;59:1590.
216. Amery WK. Final results of a multicenter placebo-controlled levamisole study of resectable lung cancer. Cancer Treat Rep 1978;62:1677.
217. Chahinian AP, Goldberg J, Holland JF, Reisman A, Jaffrey IS, Mandel EM. Chemotherapy versus chemoimmunotherapy with levamisole or *Corynebacterium parvum* in advanced lung cancer. Cancer Treat Rep 1982;66:1291.
218. Davis S, Mietlowski W, Rohwedder JJ, Griffin JP, Neshat AA. Levamisole as an adjuvant to chemotherapy in extensive bronchogenic carcinoma: a Veterans Administration Lung Cancer Group study. Cancer 1982;50:646.
219. Herskovic A, Bauer M, Seydel HG, Yesner R, Doggett RLS, Perez CA, Durbin LM, Zinninger M. Post-operative thoracic irradiation with or without levamisole in non-small

cell lung cancer: Results of a Radiation Therapy Oncology Group study. Int J Radiat Oncol Biol Phys 1988;14:37.

220. Perez CA, Bauer M, Emami BN, Byhardt R, Brady LW, Doggett RLS, Gardner P, Zinninger M. Thoracic irradiation with or without levamisole (NSC #177023) in unresectable non-small cell carcinoma of the lung: a phase III randomized trial of the RTOG. Int J Radiat Oncol Biol Phys 1988;15:1337.
221. Pines A. BCG plus levamisole following irradiation of advanced squamous bronchial carcinoma. Int J Radiat Oncol Biol Phys 1980;6:1041.
222. White JE, Chen T, Reed R, Mira J, Stuckey WJ, Weatherall T, O'Bryan R, Samson MK, Seydel HG. Limited squamous cell carcinoma of the lung: a Southwest Oncology Group randomized study of radiation with or without doxorubicin chemotherapy and with or without levamisole immunotherapy. Cancer Treat Rep 1982;66:1113.
223. Wright PW, Hill LD, Peterson AV Jr, Pinkham R, Johnson L, Ivey T, Bernstein I, Bagley C, Anderson R. Preliminary results of combined surgery and adjuvant Bacillus Calmette-Guérin plus levamisole treatment of resectable lung cancer. Cancer Treat Rep 1978;62:1671.
224. Borden EC, Davis TE, Crowley JJ, Wolberg WH, McKnight B, Chirigos MA. Interim analysis of a trial of levamisole and 5-fluorouracil in metastatic colorectal carcinoma. In Immunotherapy of Human Cancer. Edited by W Terry and SA Rosenburg. New York: Elsevier, 1982, p 231–235.
225. Davis TE, Borden EC, Wolberg WH, Crowley JJ. Levamisole and 5-fluorouracil in metastatic colorectal carcinoma. Proc Am Soc Clin Oncol 1982;1:102.
226. Grem JL. Levamisole as a therapeutic agent for colorectal carcinoma. Cancer Cells 1990;2:131.
227. Laurie JA, Moertel CG, Fleming TR, Wieand HS, Leigh JE, Rubin J, McCormack GW, Gerstner JB, Krook JE, Malliard J, Twito DI, Morton RF, Tschetter LK, Barlow JF. Surgical adjuvant therapy of large-bowel carcinoma: an evaluation of levamisole and the combination of levamisole and fluorouracil. J Clin Oncol 1989;7:1447–1456.
228. Moertel CG, Fleming TR, MacDonald JS, Haller DG, Laurie JA, Goodman PJ, Ungerleider JS, Emerson WA, Tormey DC, Glick JH, Veeder MH, Mailliard JA. Levamisole and fluorouracil for adjuvant therapy of resected colon carcinoma. N Engl J Med 1990;322:352–358.
229. Windle R, Bell PRF, Shaw D. Five year results of a randomized trial of adjuvant 5-fluorouracil and levamisole in colorectal cancer. Br J Surg 1987;74:569.
230. Sarker SK, Choudhary R, Subhas P, et al. Follow-up study of adjuvant chemoimmunotherapy in colorectal carcinoma after definitive surgery. Indian J Cancer 1985;22:113–120.
231. Skillings JR, Levine M, Rayner HL, Eisenhauer E, Erlichman C, Germond C, Kerr I, Lofters W, Maroun J, Yoshida S. Levamisole and 5-fluorouracil therapy for resected colon cancer. A new indication. Can Med Assoc J 1991;144:297.
232. Grem JL, Allegra CJ. Toxicity of levamisole and 5-fluorouracil in human colon carcinoma cells. JNCI 1989;81:1413.
233. Kovach JS, Svingen PA, Schaid DJ. Levamisole potentiation of fluorouracil antiproliferative activity mimicked by orthovanadate, an inhibitor of tyrosine phosphatase. JNCI 1992;84:515–519.
234. Lejeune FJ, Macher E, Kleeber U, et al. An assessment of DTIC versus levamisole or placebo in the treatment of high risk stage 1 patients after surgical removal of a primary melanoma of the skin. A phase III adjuvant study EORTC protocol 18761. Eur J Cancer Clin Oncol 1988;24(suppl 2):S81–S90.
235. Quirt IC, Shelley WE, Bodurtha MB, et al. A phase 3 study demonstrating improved survival in patients with poor prognosis malignant melanoma treated with adjuvant levamisole. J Clin Oncol 1991;9:729–735.
236. Ruuskanen O, Remes M, Makela AL, Isomaki H, Toivanen A. Levamisole and agranulocytosis. Lancet 1976;2:958.
237. Thompson JS, Herbick JM, Klassen LW, Severson CD, Overlin VL, Blaschke JW, Silverman MA, Vogel CL. Studies on levamisole-induced agranulocytosis. Blood 1980;56:388.

CHAPTER 79

Active Specific Immunotherapy with Vaccines

MEPUR H. RAVINDRANATH AND DONALD L. MORTON

The clinical use of cancer vaccines was initiated at the turn of the century, prompted by the success of vaccines against infectious disease. However, unlike vaccines against infectious disease, which are administered prophylactically, cancer vaccines are generally administered after the advent of disease. Both types of vaccines utilize attenuated whole cells, cell walls, specific antigens, or nonpathogenic strains of living organisms to stimulate the patient's immune system to fight the disease (70). The specific goals of active immunotherapy with cancer vaccines are to overcome the immunosuppression produced by tumor-derived factors, to stimulate specific immunity that will destroy tumor cells, and to enhance the immunogenicity of tumor-associated antigens (TAA).

Several observations support the potential value of active specific immunotherapy for the treatment of cancer. These include 1) vaccine-induced immunity against cancer in animal models, 2) the regression and eradication of tumors injected directly with immunostimulants (19, 167, 223, 224, 254), 3) occasional regression of noninjected tumors after the intralesional injection of bacillus Calmette-Guerin (BCG) (143, 150, 151, 161, 163, 168, 173, 203), and 4) the development of antitumor antibodies. This chapter will discuss theoretical requirements for tumor vaccines and review the outcome of vaccine trials.

Tumor–Host Interactions

TAA AS TARGETS FOR IMMUNOTHERAPY

Tumor cells express potentially immunogenic molecules commonly referred to as TAA. TAA systems can be grouped into four categories. The first includes neoantigens (202) not expressed by the normal cells from which cancer cells are derived but found in other normal tissues. For example, the human melanoma-associated ganglioside GD_2, which is expressed on the surface of human melanomas (24, 196) but not on normal melanocytes (24), is found in human brain and spinal cord. *O*-acetylated GD_3 is also expressed on the surface of melanoma cells (194, 196) but not biochemically documented on normal melanocytes; however, it has been recognized on human T-lymphocytes (114A, 198A). Recently identified melanoma-associated protein antigens MAGE-1 and MAGE-3 are not expressed in normal melanocytes but can be found in testes tissues (233A). A second group of TAA systems includes oncofetal antigens such as carcinoembryonic antigen (CEA), which are not expressed by any normal tissues but may be expressed on fetal tissues. Third is a small group of apparently tumor-specific antigens not found in normal adult or fetal tissues. Examples include gangliosides containing *N*-glycolylneuraminic acid in human gastric, liver, and colon cancers as well as lymphoma (110). Finally, there is accruing evidence that tumor antigens recognized by T-cells may also be found in normal progenitors. Because of their ability to recognize peptides derived from either intracellular or cell-membrane antigens, T-cells can specifically recognize mutations in neoplastic cells. In melanoma, these peptide antigen systems include MUC-1 (commonly expressed in pancreatic and breast tumors), Melan-A/MART-1, tyrosinase (the product of the *c* or *albino* locus), and pMel 17 (the product of *silver* locus) (96A). Under appropriate conditions, all TAA systems can serve as targets for active immunotherapy with cancer vaccines.

If TAA are found in normal cells, why are they not recognized by the host's immune system (102)? TAA may be cryptic on the normal cell due to the orientation or physical conformation of the antigen on the cell surface, a physical separation by cell membranes, or masking by other normal cell surface components. The density of the antigen on a normal cell my be lower than a threshold level required for recognition by the immune system (246). The surface distribution of the antigen may differ between normal and tumor cells (28, 29). Immunorecognition of tumor antigens (*N*-glycolylneuraminic acid-containing gangliosides) may also involve secondary recognition of neoantigens. Thus, antibodies produced against *O*-AcGD_3 in melanoma patients after active specific immunotherapy selectively cross-react with the progenitor of the antigen, namely, GD_3 (195).

HOST IMMUNOSUPPRESSION BY SHED TAA

One common explanation for a host's failure to reject tumors is that TAA may be continuously shed from the tumor cell surface (22, 39, 87, 88, 89, 119, 120, 158, 188, 192) and bind to reticuloendothelial cells and antibodies, causing immunosuppression (14, 39, 93, 94, 119, 187). Thus, repeated washing of the peripheral blood lymphocytes from cancer patients restored and enhanced lymphocyte killing of tumor cells (39).

In contrast to peripheral blood lymphocytes, tumor-infiltrating lymphocytes proliferate less readily in response to interleukin-2 (IL-2) or mitogens (248). Similarly, peripheral blood lymphocytes exposed to tumor cells or to their shed products show significantly reduced proliferation (150). A gradient of suppression in the lymph node lymphocytes of melanoma patients correlates inversely with distance from the tumor mass (32). Although further characterization of the immunosuppressive substances produced by tumors is needed, there is impressive evidence that shed tumor-associated gangliosides are involved in blocking the functions of lymphocytes (14, 93, 94, 187).

The degree to which immune recognition is suppressed correlates with the stage of disease and overall tumor burden (50, 78, 250). The presence of circulating TAA-antibody complexes in cancer patients who have not received immunotherapy suggests that an antibody response against some TAA is initiated early during tumor growth (43, 81). Such antitumor antibodies may be masked by shed antigens during tumor progression (126). Such suppression may be reversed by removing the growing neoplasm (159). When serum samples were analyzed for antitumor antibodies before and after surgery for primary sarcoma (50), successful resection of tumor was associated with a 4-fold rise in antitumor antibody titer. In contrast, most patients who had no antitumor antibodies before or after surgery developed recurrences within 6 months. Patients who had developed pulmonary metastasis postoperatively showed a progressive decline in their antitumor antibody titers. Studies of complement-fixing antibody titers in patients with sarcomas (50) and melanomas (78, 236, 250) have shown that complement-fixing antibodies are masked by the shed TAA, neutralizing antitumor activity.

ANTIGEN ALTERATION AND IMMUNOLOGICAL HETEROGENEITY

Although a malignant neoplasm usually evolves from a single transformed cell, most cancers are composed of genetically unstable populations of proliferating cells that become heterogeneous over time (86, 176). Heterogeneity enables subsets of the tumor cell population to evade the host's immune response and resist chemical, physical, and biological therapies (151, 176). Tumors recurring at the resection site of a primary neoplasm can differ antigenically from the primary tumor (182). This is consistent with the possibility that antigenic variants have been selected for their ability to escape immune surveillance.

The biochemical profile of gangliosides in human melanoma is a classic example of heterogeneic antigen expression (196). GM_3 constitutes >95% of the gangliosides on melanocytes, the progenitors of human melanoma (24). During the early, radial phase of migration, neoplastically transformed melanocytes express more GD_3, a derivative of GM_3, than do normal progenitors (89, 194). After the appearance of GD_3, the tumor cells begin to migrate vertically. Subsequently, levels of GD_3 continue to increase (89, 194) and other derivatives of GD_3, namely, GD_2 and *O*-AcGD_3, begin to appear (195, 196, 197). These alterations in gangliosides correlate with and may facilitate invasion and metastasis. During the progression of melanoma, there are similar alterations in MHC antigens (HLA-DR), cell adhesion molecules (ICAM-I), and mucins (MUC18) (220).

HLA class I antigens are important molecules that contribute to interactions between cytotoxic T-lymphocytes (CTL) and their TAA targets. Defects in or loss of HLA class I antigen expression may therefore impair recognition of tumor cells by CTL and minimize the efficacy of active specific immunotherapy. The absence of HLA class I antigen expression in nevi and in many melanoma lesions has been well documented and related to the clinical course of disease (16b, 205a, 234c). In murine tumor systems, loss of HLA class I antigen expression is associated with failure of the host to reject a tumor challenge (43A, 55A).

Cell-surface sialic acid can mask TAA (128, 130, 132, 207). Sialylated TAA are only weakly immunogenic. Removal of sialic acid with neuraminidase can enhance immune recognition and tumor cell destruction (7, 91, 227). *Vibrio cholera* neuraminidase (VCN) has been used to remove cell-surface sialic acids from autologous and allogeneic tumor cells before immunization (58, 91, 215, 230).

Heterogeneity in the expression of TAA within a given tumor poses a significant obstacle to vaccine therapy. Elimination of cells that bear a single major antigen can still permit the survival of a subpopulation that expresses a minor antigenic variant (67, 234b). Antigenic heterogeneity may reflect the selective elimination of immunogenic cells, leading to the outgrowth of less immunogenic subpopulations. To compensate for heterogeneic antigen expression, several antigenetically distinct tumor cell lines can be combined within a single tumor cell vaccine (TCV), or combinations of purified antigens can be used, so that the vaccine collectively expresses all the TAA contained within a given neoplasm (157, 158).

STRATEGIES FOR INCREASING THE IMMUNOGENICITY OF VACCINES

The goals of active immunotherapy are to combat the decreasing immunocompetence that results from interaction of tumor-related products with components of the immune system and to eliminate the diverse clones within a tumor cell population by augmenting cellular and/or humoral immunity. Thus, a tumor vaccine should be able to clear immunosuppressive TAA from the circulation (14, 93, 94, 187, 188) minimize the immunosuppressive activity of suppressor T cells and suppressor inducer cells (8–10, 12, 155, 164, 167), and activate the antigen-presenting function of macrophages, monocytes, histiocytes, and dendritic cells (1, 82–84). It should also be able to elicit an antibody response against TAA on the tumor cell surface (164, 167), not only to clear the shed TAA but also to kill tumor cells. Finally, it should be able to stimulate the generation of newly activated T-cells capable of killing tumor cells (37) and direct migration of these lymphocytes into metastatic tumors (10, 179) that rarely contain lymphocytes (10, 17).

Several strategies have been utilized to augment tumor cell immunogenicity.

Modify the Composition of Allogeneic Tumor Cell Vaccines

By exposing the patient's immune system to diverse TAA from different tumor cell lines, Morton and colleagues (164, 167, 170) nearly doubled the fraction of patients who developed a humoral response to tumor cell vaccines.

Diminish Generation of Suppressor T Cells

Suppressor T cells interfere with B-cell production of antibodies and with other immunoregulatory functions. Cyclophosphamide can reduce suppressor cell functions and enhance the antibody response leading to immunity to TAA (8–13, 20, 21, 155, 164, 167).

Combine Adjuvants with Tumor Cell Vaccines

Adjuvants used in clinical trials have included live vaccinia virus, *Salmonella* extracts, and viable BCG and BCG derivatives (156, 239, 240) such as cell wall skeleton, trehalose dimycolate, muramyl dipeptide, and glycolipids. Table 79.1 lists the tumor vaccines and immunopotentiators used in clinical trials for different cancers. Data obtained in clinical trials and in animal models underline the importance of the ratio of tumor cells to adjuvant as well as the sequence and site of administration of the tumor cell preparation and the adjuvant.

Table 79.1. Different Kinds of Tumor-Specific Vaccines Used in Clinical Trials to Promote Immunogenicity of Tumor-associated Antigens

Autologous tumor cells
- Whole cells alone (238)
- Whole cells + BCG (11, 95, 121, 122, 123)
- Whole cells + *C. parvum* (118, 148, 206)
- Whole cells + PPD + *C. albicans* (191, 228, 233)
- Whole cells-cholesterol hemisuccinate (CHS) (213, 214)
- Whole cells-muramyl dipeptide and TDM (46)
- Whole cells-neuraminidase treated + Freund's (C) (227)
- Cell extract + PPD (228, 237)
- Oncolysate-VSV (129)

Allogeneic tumor cells
- Whole cells alone (30, 80, 157)
- Whole cells + BCG (133, 162, 198, 199, 249)
- Whole cells + *C. parvum* (64, 131, 152)
- Whole cells + BCG-CWS (251)
- Whole cells + cholesteryl hemisuccinate (208, 209)
- Whole cells + muramyl dipeptide and TDM (46)
- Whole cells-neuraminidase treated + BCG (7, 58, 215, 229)
- Cell extract (201)
- Cell extract + Fc (92, 222, 227)
- Cell extract + BCG-CWS + TDM-MPL (155)
- Oncolysate-NDV (25, 26)
- Oncolysate-vaccinia (90, 209, 241–244)

Purified tumor-associated antigens
- Gangliosides-*S. minnesota* R595 (128)
- Gangliosides-BCG (129,130)
- Gangliosides-MPL (130)

BCG, bacillus Calmette-Guérin; FC, Freund's complete adjuvant; PPD, purified protein derivative (tuberculin) from *M. tuberculosis;* CWS, mycobacteria cell wall skeleton; TDM, trehalose dimycocholate; MPL, monophosphoryl lipic A extracted from *S. minnesota* R595; VSV, vesicular stomatitis virus; NDV, Newcastle disease virus.

Protein Adjuvants. Addition of a highly antigenic carrier protein to an otherwise nonantigenic substance can often evoke an immune response. The antibodies formed against this complex are specifically directed against the previously nonantigenic substance, as well as against the foreign protein in the complex. Early reports (36, 42) using rabbit gamma globulin attached to proteins of autologous tumor cells reported some therapeutic benefit, but the efficacy of this type of treatment has not been confirmed. Recently, administration of keyhole limpet hemocyanin (KLH) attached to melanoma-associated ganglioside GD_3 was shown to elicit a persistent anti-GD_3 IgM antibody response in melanoma patients (85b).

Viral Adjuvants. There is convincing evidence in animal models that infection of tumor cells by certain viruses augments the immunogenicity of tumor antigens (4, 90, 115). Based on animal models, randomized clinical trials have been undertaken with allogeneic or autologous tumor cells infected with Newcastle disease virus (25, 26), vesicular stomatitis virus (129), and vaccinia virus (90, 209, 241–244) in patients with melanoma and osteosarcoma (76). Tumor vaccines of viral etiology are the focus of several investigations (77b). Wallack and Sivanandham updated the results of clinical trials using vaccinia-melanoma oncolysate (VMO vaccine) in 250 patients with stage II melanoma (244A). Those patients who had the highest anti-melanoma titers after vaccination sustained the longest survival. Gissmann and co-workers recently discussed the prospects for development of a papilloma viral vaccine (67a) based on a report that papilloma viral extracts stimulate immunity against existing tumors in women with cervical cancer (22a).

Bacterial Adjuvants. Whole bacteria (BCG, *Corynebacterium parvum, Salmonella minnesota*) and bacterial components including cell wall skeleton, trehalose dimycolate, monophosphoryl lipid A, MER (methanol extractable residue of tubercle bacillus), and Freund's adjuvant are potent immunostimulants. These bacterial adjuvants can evoke tumor-specific cellular (44, 45, 55, 68, 69, 239, 240, 255) and humoral (78, 195, 250) immune responses.

Chemical Adjuvants. TAA in human cells can also be modified chemicals such as iodoacetate and cholesteryl hemisuccinate (208, 209, 213, 214), which increase the immunogenicity of tumor cells. Certain enzymes, such as neuraminidase, enhance the immunoresponse to neoplasms by chemically altering the surface glycoconjugates (7, 58, 211, 215, 227, 230). Repeated intradermal immunization with neuraminidase-treated allogeneic acute myeloid leukemic cells prolonged disease-free survival in patients treated with chemotherapy (91).

Genetically Altered Tumor Cells. Transduction of murine tumor cells with the genes for cytokines such as IL-2 (55a) and IL-4 (69a) has led to rejection of the genetically altered tumor cells by the syngeneic host. Immunized mice withstood challenge by native homologous tumor cells but not by dissimilar tumor cells, indicating tumor specificity. In the case of IL-4, nontransduced subcutaneously transplanted renal carcinoma cells regressed following innoculation in the opposite leg with IL-4 transduced cells. Dranoff and colleagues found that when ten genes for cytokines or immunogenic cell-surface molecules were transduced into B16 murine melanoma cells, only granulocyte-macrophage colony-stimulating factor (GM-CSF) was effective in preventing growth of challenge tumors (43A). Irradiated B16 melanoma cells protected only 1 of 19 C57 BL/6 mice from a challenge dose of B16 cells, whereas the irradiated GM-CSF transduced cells protected 16 of 20. In another experiment, 100% of mice immunized with irradiated GM-CSF transduced cells survived a challenge of a million cells, whereas no more than 50% immunized with other cytokine-transduced cells survived a tumor challenge. In addition, administration of GM-CSF transduced cells several days after a tumor challenge was associated with prolonged survival and complete regression of tumor. Selective depletion experiments with antibodies showed that both CD4+ and CD8+ cells were necessary, whereas NK cells were not (43a). These impressive results have already led to an exploratory randomized phase I trial of GM-CSF gene transduction in renal carcinoma (180a). The success of this and other trials of active specific immunotherapy using genetically altered tumor cells will require a stable method of gene transfer, sufficient number of transduced tumor cells, a cytokine concentration high enough to evoke an antitumor response, and an intradermal route of vaccine administration. The documented superiority of the intradermal route (157–167a) may reflect the presence of Langerhans' cells that differentiate into potent antigen-presenting cells. In addition, the genetically altered tumor cells must be viable but unable to replicate in the host.

Whole Cell Tumor Vaccines

Many vaccines have been prepared from whole tumor cells. In animal models, injection of living autologous tumor cells in numbers too small to cause progressive tumor growth has generally provided the most effective immunogen (77a). For the treatment of certain tumors that share common TAA, such as melanomas, one patient could be immunized with an allogeneic vaccine of living tumor cells from another patient (133, 156a, 157, 158, 165). An immune response should develop against the foreign major histocompatibility complex antigens on the transplanted tumor cells, causing their rejection. In addition, the foreign MHC antigens may induce a strong immune response against the common cross-reacting TAA.

There is a debate between those who advocate a whole living cell vaccine and those who believe that vaccines based on highly defined components or highly defined, purified tumor antigens or peptides are better for cancer immunotherapy. Recent experimental studies in animal models clearly document that a whole cell vaccine is superior to soluble vaccines or oncolysates in eliciting cytotoxic T-cell (CTL) responses (207a) or humoral responses leading to antitumor activity (193a, 195a). An investigation to augment antiganglioside antibody response in a mouse model revealed that a whole cell or liposome vaccine was superior to purified or mixed vaccines (193a, 195a). Although it is possible to envisage a liposome universal vaccine (assuming identification of all important immunogenic melanoma-associated antigens), this study shows that whole cell vaccines elicited better humoral responses, even when liposomes contained a 27-fold higher level of TAA than the intact tumor cells (195a). Recently, Schirrmacher and Hoegen have demonstrated that irradiated trypan blue-excluding live tumor cells are superior to dead cells or crude membrane preparations (oncolysates) administered in equivalent or greater amounts, in eliciting a syngeneic MHC class I-restricted tumor-specific CTL response (207a). When comparing T-cell stimulatory capacity of a whole cell vaccine with that of a vaccine consisting of a glutaraldehyde-fixed polyvalent ultrasonicated tumor extract, in the absence or presence of IL-2, only the whole cell vaccine was able to trigger a specific CTL response in vitro. Furthermore, these investors have demonstrated that disruption of tumor cells by freeze-thawing led to a complete loss of CTL stimulatory capacity. Also, viral oncolysates did not stimulate a tumor-specific CTL response in tumor-bearing animals, whereas whole cell vaccines did. All these observations clearly indicate that tumor cell membrane integrity (as revealed by trypan blue exclusion) is required in this tumor model for stimulating a tumor-specific class I MHC-restricted CD8+ CTL response.

The possibility that viable autologous tumor cells could result in tumor growth at the inoculation site has precluded their clinical use in cancer vaccines. Viable tumor cells are inactivated by a variety of different methods, including irradiation, mitomycin C, freezing and thawing, or heat treatment. Such treatments may, however, chemically alter tumor antigens and diminish the effectiveness of the vaccine.

AUTOLOGOUS VERSUS ALLOGENEIC VACCINES

Because autologous tumor cells express the same blood group and histocompatibility antigens as the host, they are considered ideal for tumor cell vaccines. However, the restricted availability of autologous tumor tissues limits the amount of vaccine and, thus, the number of immunizations. Moreover, antigen expression may vary from site to site; cells isolated from nodules at one site may not have the same TAA profile as autologous cells from another metastatic site.

Allogeneic tumor grown in cell culture can provide sufficient vaccine for multiple injections. Mixtures of cells from different tumors can provide a spectrum of TAA. On the other hand, passage of tumor cells in culture may introduce contaminants and favor the growth of subpopulations that diverge from the antigenic phenotype of the original cancer. Fetal bovine serum (FBS), for example, is widely used in culture media. Often the proteins and glycolipids in FBS are incorporated into tumor cells and function as xenogeneic antigens (63). Patients who receive tumor cells grown in FBS develop an antibody response against FBS components (21, 137, 138). Serum-free media or media that contain human serum are considered ideal for the preparation of tumor cell vaccines. Tumor cells grown in culture may also undergo antigenic alterations similar to those documented for ganglioside profiles of human melanoma (194, 232) and glioma (61). In some cases, these alterations have been used to advantage by mixing different cell lines with increased TAA expression to prepare allogeneic tumor cell vaccines (164, 167).

Clinical Trials of Tumor Vaccines

The history of vaccine therapy can be divided into early and late phases, reflecting different levels of understanding of the immune response (37).

EARLY VACCINE TRIALS

Therapy with tumor cell vaccines was first described in 1902 by von Leyden and Blumenthal (238), followed shortly thereafter by other reports (31, 237). Coca and colleagues attributed several instances of tumor regression (5/48) to the repeated administration of viable autologous and allogeneic tumor cells in large numbers at 14-day intervals (30, 31). Risley immunized tumor-bearing patients with large volumes of autologous or allogeneic tumor cell extract every 14 days without apparent benefit (201). Vaughan administered tumor extracts intraperitoneally and recognized that "the best results were obtained in cases in which the amount of tumor tissue present was small, and in which the differential leucocyte count of the patient show[ed] a decided reaction following administration of the cancer protein" (235). Kellock and co-workers irradiated the site of live tumor-cell immunization in an attempt to reduce the risk of tumor growth at the implantation site (111). Later, irradiated tumor cells were used in patients with malignant melanoma (73). Graham and Graham reported that the administration of a tumor cell vaccine to patients from whom tumor had been removed "appeared to radiosensitize the residual disease" (73).

LATER VACCINE TRIALS

Since 1960, greater emphasis has been given to tumor cell antigens in various forms and to the use of different adjuvants mixed with tumor cell vaccine. Finney and co-workers (57) administered a tumor cell homogenate admixed with complete Freund's adjuvant (containing components of *Mycobacterium bovis*) intramuscularly to patients with a variety of malignant tumors and found that all treated patients developed antibodies against tumor cells. Injecting these antibodies after purification into subcutaneous nodules produced dramatic, albeit temporary, regression of tumor.

Czajkowski and colleagues chemically coupled rabbit gamma globulin to human tumor cells and found that it enhanced the immunogenicity of the tumor cell vaccine (42). Cunningham and co-workers treated 42 cancer patients with autologous TCV-rabbit gamma globulin vaccine (36). In another study, responders showed delayed-type hypersensitvity (DTH) responses to the TCV-adjuvant complex, suggesting that the vaccine had evoked cell-mediated immunity (99).

Table 79.2. Response to Intralesional Administration of BCG in Melanoma Patients

Strain of BCG	Patients (*n*)	Responders complete + partial	Regression at non-injected sites	References
Glaxo	8	5	2/5	156A
	1	0	0	124
	22	11	0/11	208
	8	3	0/3	109
Tice	9	2 + 5	2/7	173
	19	5	na	16
	7	3	1/3	216
	2	1	0/1	5
	36	6 + 9	6/25	161
	22 (intratumor)	3 + 7	3/10	174
	22 (intraderm)	0 + 2	0/2	174
	25	6 + 15	0/21	33
	15	2 + 3	na	141
Tice/Glaxo	29	2 + 13	2/15	184
	6	3 + 1	2/4	127
Connaught	3	2	1/2	112
Pasteur	11	7	0/7	104
Not specified	4	1	1/4	116
	8	2	0/8	154
	50	19	2/19	59
	19	4 + 14	na	218
	13	3 + 4	na	200
Methanol extract	18	8 + 4	na	117
	101	61	na	210
	6	2 + 2	na	135
	19	14 + 1	5/15	185

There have been conflicting reports regarding the value of vaccine therapy. Frequent immunization with allogeneic tumor cells did prolong the period of remission and the survival times of patients with acute lymphoblastic leukemia (144). Autoimmunization was also found to augment both circulating antibodies and, specifically, cytotoxic lymphocytes (40, 100). The first report (163) on the regression of cutaneous metastases of melanoma following intralesional injection of live BCG not only redirected the course of immunotherapy trials (143) (Table 79.2) but also rekindled interest in combining tumor cell vaccines with extrinsic adjuvants such as BCG for active specific therapy.

Goodnight and Morton have addressed this area in detail and identified several factors that limit interpretation of trials with tumor vaccines (70, 71). These include 1) the variability of human cancer and thus the need for precise definitions of the patient population chosen for a clinical trial and 2) the need for appropriate randomly selected controls. The problems of experimental design and performance of clinical trials for immunotherapy are not fundamentally different from those encountered more generally in cancer clinical trials. The principles and approaches to designing clinical trials are presented in Chapter 26.

Current Status of Vaccine Therapy for Different Human Cancers

The current status of active immunotherapy is best understood by examining the results of past clinical trials for different cancers (160). Table 79.5 condenses the results of immunotherapy trials classified according to Goodnight and Morton (70, 71). Patients with malignant melanoma seem to benefit the most from active immunotherapy, as shown by tumor regression and increased disease-free survival. Some of the results for other cancers are also encouraging. However, all of these trials must be interpreted according to the source of vaccine, its method of preparation and schedule of administration, and the patient's tumor burden prior to therapy. Reducing the tumor burden enhances the success of immunotherapy. Trial results also vary with the quality, quantity, and route of administration of immunopotentiators such as BCG or *C. parvum.* Other variables affecting the success of vaccine therapy include the patient's disease status and duration of treatment, effects of other therapies, and degree of immunological impairment.

MALIGNANT MELANOMA

Active specific immunotherapy is a reasonable modality of treatment for patients with metastatic malignant melanoma, and its evolution in melanoma is of considerable interest. Morton and co-investigators were the first to demonstrate complete regression of metastatic tumor nodules after intralesional injection of living BCG: 90% of 184 melanoma metastases in eight patients regressed (163). Many clinical trials have subsequently confirmed this observation (Table 79.2). Contact between tumor cells and BCG appears to have produced systemic immunity evidenced by 1) regression of noninjected nodules at sites distant from intralesional injections (143, 255) (Table 79.2), 2) the relationship between the clinical course of disease and the in vitro cytotoxicity of the patient's lymphocytes in the presence of the patient's serum (16), and 3) the regression of a pulmonary metastasis in a patient treated for multiple intradermal metastases (141). The interaction of BCG with tumor cells may facilitate the infiltration of antigen-presenting cells and lymphocytes into tumor nodules. Antibodies may be directed against antigenic determinants shared by BCG and tumor cells (153, 163), or the administration of BCG may enable the patient's immune system to recognize the TAA on tumor cells more effectively.

In animal models, Hanna and co-workers observed that histiocytes infiltrated lesions in response to BCG infection (82–84). Barlett and Zbar tested this possibility by mixing irradiated tumor cells with BCG before administration and confirmed that the mixture evoked a better antitumor response than did either component alone (6). Similarly, Morton and colleagues admixed TCV with BCG and administered it intradermally to melanoma patients (Tables 79.3 and 79.4). They noted an increase in the number of disease-free survivors and a lengthening of disease-free intervals, but found no striking difference from BCG alone (161, 165, 170). Observations of Ratliff and co-workers have shown that tumor cells that are able to fuse with BCG in the presence of fibronectin (98) elicit better immune responses than do tumor cells that are not capable of fusing with BCG (193). After Zbar and co-workers administered irradiated tumor cells admixed with BCG intradermally to animals and showed antigen specificity of the therapeutic effect of tumor cell-BCG vaccine, a number of investigators (Table 79.4) undertook clinical trials with tumor cell vaccines (6, 252–254).

The design of a melanoma vaccine must consider intraindividual and interindividual tumor heterogeneity, factors augmenting immunogenicity of melanoma-associated antigens (MAA), unfavorable immunological responses, tumor-derived or host-derived circulating immunosuppressive factors causing general immunosuppression (as well as specific immunosuppression caused by tumor antigens), tumor infiltration of immune effector cells such as lymphocytes and macrophages, and in vivo fixation of antibodies to tumor cells. Early melanoma vaccines consisted of whole autologous or allogeneic tumor cells or cell extracts/lysates, with or without an immunostimulant such as BCG (58, 80, 121, 122, 149C, 157, 166, 169, 171), Freund's complete adjuvant (93), Newcastle disease virus (25, 26), vaccinia virus (91, 244), vesicular stomatitis virus (129), alum (21), purified protein derivative from *Mycobacterium tuberculosis* (228), or DETOX (a combination of mycobacterial cell wall with trehalose dimycolate and monophosphoryl lipid A derived from *Salmonella)* (155, 155a). Their usual route of administration was intradermal, although subcutaneous administration was not uncommon (25, 215), and some investigators observed a clinical response after intralymphatic administration (245). Several trials have administered cyclophosphamide, an immunosuppressive drug, prior to the vaccine to induce cell-mediated immunity, since a subset of T lymphocytes can specifically suppress immunological responses to the tumor antigens (9, 21, 155, 155a, 170).

Melanoma vaccines administered in recent clinical trials

Table 79.3. Disease-free Survival of Melanoma Patients after Administration of BCG

Route	No. of patients			Disease-free survivors			References
	Control	BCG	BCG + TCV	Control	BCG	BCG + TCV	
Intralesional	13	13	na	3	8	na	204
Intradermal	46	45	49	19	19	26	165

na, not applicable; TCV, tumor cell vaccine.

Table 79.4. A Survey of Clinical Trials Involving Active Specific Immunotherapy of Metastatic Melanoma with Vaccines

Stage	Nature of vaccine	Adjuvant	Route	No. of patients	Percent response	Percent survival (yrs)	References
II	Allo/whole	BCG	i.d.	28		60 (1)	80
	Asialo-allo/whole[a]	BCG	i.d.	166		45 (3)	58
	Asialo-allo/whole[a]	BCG	s.c.	846		(Control) 33 (3)	215
						(1 node) 53 (5)	
						(<4 node) 43 (5)	
						(>4 node) 25 (5)	
	Allo/whole (Cy)		i.d.	68		52 (<2)	161
	Allo/extract	FC	i.d.	16	69		92
	Allo/lysate	NDV	s.c.	32		88 (3)	25
	Allo/lysate	NDV	s.c.	21		71 (<3)	26
	Allo/lysate	VV	i.d.	38		55 (1)	244
				39		(Hist Contl) 25 (1)	
	Allo/lysate	VV	i.d.	90		75 (2)	90
				56		(Control) 47 (2)	
	Allo/extract (Cy)	CWS/TDM/MPL	i.d.	5			155
	Allo/subcell (Cy)	alum	i.d.	36			21
	Allo/subcell (Cy)	alum	i.d.	63		(23 DTH+) 52 (5)	21
						(40 DTH−) 26 (5)	
	Auto/extract	PPD	s.c.	5			228
III	Auto/whole	BCG	i.d.	18	22		121
	Auto/whole	BCG	i.d.	5			122
	Auto/whole	BCG	i.d.	13	0		134
	Auto/whole (Cy)	BCG	i.d.	33	12		12
	Allo/whole	BCG	i.d.	22	0		133
	Allo/whole		i.l.	34	26		245
	Allo/whole	BCG	i.d.	139		(Control) 41 (5)	170
						(BCG) 53 (5)	
						(BCG-TCV) 52 (5)	
	Allo/extract	FC	i.d.	23	35		92
	Auto/lysate	VSV	s.c.	11	0		129
	Allo/lysate	VSV	s.c.	13	0		
	Allo/extract (Cy)	CWS/TDM/MPL	i.d.	17	29		155

[a] *Vibrio cholerae* neuraminidase-treated tumor cells.
BCG, bacillus Calmette-Guérin; FC, Freund's complete adjuvant; PPD, purified protein derivative (tuberculin) from *M. tuberculosis;* CWS, mycobacterial cell wall skeleton; TDM, trehalose dimycolate, a diglucose containing glycolipid extracted from CWS; MPL, monophosphoryl lipid A extracted from *S. minnesota* R595; TCV, tumor cell vaccine; VSV, vesicular stomatitis virus; NDV, Newcastle disease virus; VV, vaccinia virus; i.d., intradermal; i.l., intralymphatic; s.c., subcutaneous; DTH, delayed-type hypersensitivity response; Hist Contl, historical control; response refers to clinical response; Cy, cyclophosphamide.

may broadly be classified into purified vaccines, cell lysate vaccines, and whole cell vaccines, as discussed below.

Purified Melanoma Vaccines

These may include fully or partially purified TAA. Purification eliminates HLA antigens. Among the purified melanoma vaccines are ganglioside vaccines, recombinant protein vaccines, anti-idiotypic antibody vaccines, and polyvalent shed antigen vaccines. These vaccines are reasonably well characterized, reproducible, and do not induce anti-HLA class I and II antibodies, which may confound measurement of cellular immune functions involved in vaccine responses.

Ganglioside Vaccines. The concept that purified vaccines are superior to whole cell vaccines was proposed by Livingston and co-investigators (128, 131). These investigators noticed only "occasional" responses to MAA such as gangliosides in recipients of ten different cell vaccines consisting of irradiated autologous (134) or allogeneic (129, 133) melanoma cell lines mixed with adjuvants such as BCG or *C. parvum* or vesicular stomatitis virus (129), or treated with neuraminidase or trypsin or glutaraldehyde (131). They noticed that humoral responses were often directed against HLA, viral antigens, bovine proteins used in culture of melanoma cells, and several nonspecific antigens. Further analysis of serum antibodies revealed that melanoma-associated gangliosides GM_2 and GD_2 were immunogenic. These observations led Livingston to initiate a clinical trial of purified GM_2 (127A, 127B). One hundred twenty-two patients with resected regional melanoma (American Joint Committee on Cancer [AJCC] stage III disease) were treated with low-dose cyclophosphamide followed by BCG with or without GM_2. After a median follow-up of 63 months, the increases in disease-free survival (DFS) and overall survival were insignificant (18 and 11%, respectively). However, exclusion of patients with elevated prestudy anti-GM_2 antibody levels significantly increased DFS ($P = .02$). These investigators recently tested the immunogenicity of gangliosides coupled to KLH and administered with QS-21 adjuvant in melanoma patients (85b, 85e).

Immune responses to univalent ganglioside vaccines may have severe limitations (234b). Although all tumor cells expressing the targeted ganglioside can be eliminated, residual tumor cells with no or low levels of the ganglioside antigen may proliferate and create a tumor that is resistant to therapy. The heterogeneity of melanoma-associated gangliosides can be the major impediment to success of therapies with univalent ganglioside antigens. Portoukalian and co-workers administered autoclaved polyvalent purified melanoma ganglioside vaccine (188a). Patient response was assessed by titers of IgM and IgG antibodies against all the melanoma gangliosides. Responders had significantly fewer recurrences (11 out of 17) than did patients without elevated IgG antibody titers (13 out of 15) ($P < .001$). The median DFI was 71 weeks for responders versus 26 weeks for nonresponders.

Purified Protein or Peptide Vaccines. Morton's group reported that sera of melanoma patients immunized with an allogeneic whole cell vaccine show cellular immune responses against autologous melanoma cells (163a). These investigators also reported that MAA shared by vaccine and host tumor cells may be presented to the host by distinct HLA-A antigens that are recognized by host CTL. CTL clones derived from these melanoma patients recognized a variety of melanoma-associated peptide sequences. These findings support the concept of purified proteins or peptides as a melanoma vaccine.

Van der Bruggen and co-workers identified a gene called *MAGE-1* that directs expression of an MAA recognized by CTL derived from patients with melanoma (233a). The MAGE-1 protein, a nine-amino acid epitope sequence restricted by HLA-A1, has been identified in fresh tumor tissues from some patients with melanoma, small cell lung cancer, and breast cancer but not in normal tissue (except testis) from patients without malignancy. Recent reports of Coulie et al. (34a) and Kawakami et al. (110a, 110b) describe an antigen called Melan-A or melanoma antigen recognized by T cells (MART-1). These antigens are also expressed by melanocytes and pigmented retinal cells but not other normal tissues. This melanocyte differentiation antigen was presented to CTL of at least 11 different persons through class I MHC HLA-A2.1 molecules expressed by melanoma, thus constituting an additional species of shared MAA. A recent study reported that CTL clones of a melanoma patient recognized a normal melanocyte constituent, tyrosinase, presented by HLA-A2.1 (16a). Recently, Morioka et al. (155b) at the John Wayne Cancer Institute found that CTL from melanoma patients recognized a decapeptide sequence in a 43-kd protein associated with a human melanoma cell line. This antigen may be presented to CTL through class I MHC HLA-A2 and -A11 molecules expressed by melanoma.

Most of these peptide antigens are expressed by the tumor cell and by its normal precursor cell (melanocyte) grown in culture. It has therefore been suggested that humoral and cell-mediated responses to these purified antigens may represent an autoimmune reaction not to the tumor but to tissue injury or some other event in the host (96a).

Anti-idiotypic Antibody Vaccines. Anti-idiotypic antibodies (anti-ids) are considered a potent melanoma vaccine since they mimic MAA. Ferrone and Kagashita administered intradermally (0.5–4 mg) a monoclonal anti-id mimicking the epitope of a high molecular weight MAA (HMW-MAA) to 24 patients with AJCC stage IV melanoma (56a, 56b). One patient showed a partial response and 8 others had minor responses or stabilization of disease. Disease progression was observed in 10 patients.

Shed Antigen Vaccines. Within 3 hours, melanoma cells in culture release almost half of the material expressed on their external surface but only a fraction of their internal molecules (22). The shed material comprises highly enriched cell surface macromolecules and antigens in a fairly purified form. The polyvalent nature of the vaccine increases its chances of stimulating protective immunity. Bystryn's group harvested polyvalent shed antigens from four melanoma cell lines (three human and one hamster), purified these antigens to deplete their HLA component, and then tested the HLA-depleted antigens as a vaccine in a phase I clinical trial. The vaccine caused complete regression of cutaneous metastases in one patient (1 out of 13 AJCC stage IV patients) who had no evidence of disease for more than 60 months (20). The vaccine stimulated both humoral and cellular responses to melanoma in approximately 50% of 94 evaluable sequential patients with surgically resected regional (AJCC stage III) disease (21a, 21b). There was a relation between antimelanoma cellular immune responses and favorable clinical outcome; median DFS was 4.7 years longer, and overall survival was 3.7 years longer in patients with a strong vaccine-induced DTH response. Three years after the onset of treatment, 70% of patients with a strong DTH response but only 31% of nonresponders were still disease-free. A similar correlation was observed between vaccine-induced antimelanoma antibodies and improved survival. Overall median DFS was 30 months for vaccine recipients versus 18 months for historical controls; overall, 5-year survival was 50% for vaccine recipients versus 33% for historical controls.

Cell Lysate Vaccines

Kobayashi proposed that immune and antitumor responses can be augmented by attaching a foreign component (a virus or a bacterial derivative) to vaccines (115). Viral melanoma oncolysate vaccine and bacterial melanoma lysate vaccine are based on this principle.

Viral Melanoma Oncolysate Vaccine. Wallack and co-workers (244, 244d) used vaccinia virus to prepare a viral melanoma oncolysate (VMO) from cell lines established from four patients with primary and metastatic melanoma. Each cell line was infected with vaccinia virus at a ratio of 1 cell to 10 $TCID_{50}$ (50% tissue culture infectious dose). The four nucleus-free cell lysates were pooled at equal concentrations (in terms of total cell count) to obtain a polyvalent VMO vaccine.

VMO is polyvalent and allogeneic, which is an advantage with respect to melanoma's heterogeneity, and it reportedly can be produced without significant batch-to-batch variation. Only 4 of 25 vaccine recipients produced antibodies to polymorphic MHC antigens, suggesting a possible down-regulation of MHC antigens consequent to vaccinia virus infection (244a). Most VMO recipients developed DTH reactions; in addition, sera of patients who were negative for anti-MAA antibodies before treatment developed antibodies after vaccine treatment. Statistical comparison of VMO recipients with 39 matched controls (patients treated with BCG or *C. parvum*) revealed a significant ($P \geq .04$) increase in the DFS of VMO recipients (242). In a separate phase II study of VMO vaccine, Hersey and co-workers also reported improved survival (90). VMO recipients with the highest antimelanoma IgM and IgG antibody titers had better survival than did patients with low titers. The results of this trial led to a phase III randomized, multi-institutional prospective, double-blind trial of VMO versus vaccinia virus in 215 evaluable patients with high-risk stage II melanoma. Thus far, this trial has not shown a significant therapeutic benefit for VMO. Similarly, a recent report by Wallack's group failed to show a significant difference in DFI or overall survival between recipients of VMO and recipients of vaccinia virus only (244b, 244c).

A French study documents a humoral immune response after immunizing melanoma patients with a different VMO (43b). Lymphocytes from vaccine recipients responded in vitro to VMO stimulation in the presence of low concentrations of IL-2, and this response was greater than that of lymphocytes from normal individuals. Berthier-Vergnes and co-workers recently reported that sera of VMO vaccine recipients contain IgG antibodies which react with a 31-kd melanoma antigen and are not found in preimmune sera (14a). Western blot immunostaining revealed that this protein is not in the allogeneic melanoma cell lines used to prepare VMO vaccine, in the vaccinia virus preparation, or in the fetal calf serum used to culture the tumor cells; however, it is in tumor metastases. Interestingly, this antigen disappears within 5 days after culturing the tumor cells in vitro but is synthesized after exposure to vaccinia virus. Expression of this antigen in tumor metastases and induction of IgG antibodies against this protein antigen in patients immunized with VMO vaccine indicate the possible therapeutic benefit of VMO vaccine in human melanoma. These findings are remarkably parallel to those of Savage and co-workers (206a, 219), who reported antibody development in six melanoma patients following 6 weeks of immunization with allogeneic melanoma oncolysates prepared from three Newcastle virus-infected melanoma cell lines.

Bacterial DETOX-coupled Lysate Vaccine. Mitchell and co-workers prepared bacterial cell wall derivatives to tumor cell membranes by mixing tumor cell lysate with DETOX, which contains nontoxic lipid A (monophosphoryl lipid A from *S. minnesota*) and cell wall skeletons of *Mycobacterium phlei* in squalene oil and Tween 80 (155, 155a). The mixed lysate is referred to as melanoma Theracine, and a lyophilized preparation (Melacine) was made by Ribi Immunochemical Research, Inc. The immunization dose was about 2×10^7 tumor cell equivalents of allogeneic melanoma cell lysate with DETOX, and treatment was restricted to patients with measurable lesions of metastatic melanoma. Melanoma Theracine was administered on days 1, 8, 15, 22, and 36. In several patients cyclophosphamide was given 5 to 7 days before the first Theracine injection to inhibit possible suppressor T cells. The reported response rate was approximately 20%, 20 of 106 evaluable patients. Approximately 5% of the patients had complete remission, and 15% had partial remission. The median duration of response was 17 months, and the median duration of complete remission was 21 months. Median survival was approximately 6 to 12 months after the appearance of metastatic disease.

Data from phase II multicenter trials of Melacine appeared to confirm Mitchell's results and also suggested that the DETOX-melanoma lysate vaccine contributed to improved survival (52a, 52b). However, a recent phase III randomized trial failed to confirm the earlier phase II results. The strongest correlate of clinical response was an increase in CTL precursors (155A). Before immunization, patients had 1 CTL in 10,000 to 50,000 lymphocytes. Three to six weeks after immunization, this ratio increased to 1 CTL in 2,500 to 5,000 lymphocytes. There was no clinical response in patients who failed to generate CTL against at least one component of the vaccine. Of those who generated CTL, 30% had objective remission or long-term stability.

In a separate study, clones of T cells were derived from the tumor tissues of immunized patients (84a). Of the 117 clones produced, 64 were CD4+ CD8− phenotype and 53 were CD8+. Intensive analysis of specificity and HLA-restricted studies utilizing matched lymphoblastoid cell lines proved that CTL reactivity was specific to melanoma. Analysis of the first 77 patients treated with Theracine revealed an association between three HLA class I alleles and clinical response to therapy. HLA-A2/A28 and HLA-B12/44/45 are strong presenting molecules for melanoma-associated epitopes (42a, 250a) and may permit CTLs from patients sharing these alleles to recognize and kill melanoma cells most efficiently after immunization with the allogeneic Theracine. It is not clear whether the similarity in alleles from the immunizing melanomas and the autologous tumors accounted for their improved effectiveness in eliciting a tumor response. However, autologous (fully matched) immunization has thus far been less successful than allogeneic vaccine therapy. This study emphasizes the need to determine whether the HLA class I antigens of an allogeneic vaccine must match those of the cancer patient for efficient induction of CTL.

Whole Cell Vaccines

Among this group are autologous, allogeneic, and hapten-conjugated melanoma cell vaccines.

Hapten-attached Cell Vaccines. The need to induce better T-cell responses to melanoma antigens led several investigators to develop hapten-conjugated tumor antigens. One such hapten-conjugated tumor vaccine was used to immunize patients with surgically incurable metastatic melanoma. Berd and co-workers immunized melanoma patients with dinitrophenyl (DNP)-conjugated autologous irradiated melanoma cells (10–25 $\times 10^6$ cells) mixed with BCG (10). Forty-six patients were sensitized to DNP by topical application of 1% dinitrofluorobenzene (DNFB) in acetone-corn oil on 2 consecutive days. Cyclophosphamide was administered 3 days before the sensitization. Two weeks later, patients were again given cyclophosphamide, followed 3 days later by injection of DNP-conjugated melanoma vaccine. Administration of cyclophosphamide plus DNP-conjugated vaccine was repeated every 28 days. The development of DTH was tested with DNP-conjugated autologous peripheral blood mononuclear cells; a DTH response was induced in all patients by DNFB sensitization. Twenty of 46 patients had clinically evident inflammatory responses in metastatic tumors 2 to 4 months after initiation of treatment. The tumors were infiltrated with CD8+ T cells, in contrast to tumors derived from control subjects not treated with vaccine. In a panel of 14 subcutaneous melanoma metastases from untreated patients, T cells (CD3+) constituted approximately 10% of the total viable cells, compared with 40% in DNFB vaccine-treated patients. The CD8 : CD4 ratio of T cells in treated patients was about 5 : 1. T-cell clones were generated from the tumor metastases of vaccine recipients. Of 140 clones generated, 70 killed cultured autologous melanoma cells but failed to kill a panel of four allogeneic melanoma cell lines.

The clinical impact of DNP-conjugated vaccine in patients with a lower tumor burden (i.e., surgically curable regional metastases) was examined in a separate study. Forty-one patients with large (>3 cm), clinically palpable lymph nodes received the vaccine as adjuvant therapy following regional lymph node dissection. Eight injections of DNP-conjugated vaccine were administered at 4-week intervals. Cyclophosphamide was administered 3 days before the first two vaccine treatments. Of 27 disease-free patients, 22 survived more than 1 year after surgery and 11 survived 2 years. This clinical outcome is reportedly better than that of a similar group of 22 patients previously treated with the nonhapten vaccine. However, the small number of patients and the use of selected historical controls prohibit any conclusions regarding therapeutic effectiveness.

Polyvalent Antigen-adjusted Melanoma Cell Vaccine. The observation that injecting BCG into the cutaneous metastases of melanoma patients produced a systemic enhancement of active immunity, remarkable tumor infiltration, and distinct clinical regression led to intradermal or intralymphatic injection of randomly selected irradiated autologous and allogeneic irradiated whole cells mixed with BCG (157, 166, 169, 171). These investigations had limited success; only 35% of immunized patients produced antibodies to cell surface antigens (159). Consequently, Morton and co-workers developed a polyvalent melanoma cell vaccine (MCV) consisting of three allogeneic melanoma cell lines selected for their high levels of six immunogenic glycoprotein, lipoprotein, or ganglioside MAA. All six MAA were expressed on the cell surface, which is considered a prerequisite for effective immune response.

In late 1984, a phase II trial was initiated to evaluate MCV in melanoma patients with regional soft tissue metastases (AJCC stage IIIA disease) or distant metastases (AJCC stage IV disease). MCV was produced in large batches and analyzed for MAA expression to determine variance between lots. An outside laboratory screened MCV for viral, bacterial, and fungal infectious organisms. Before cryopreserving the vaccine, the cells were irradiated to 100 to 150 Gy. MCV was injected intradermally in axillary and inguinal regions on a schedule of every 2 weeks for 4 weeks, then monthly for 1 year. For the first two treatments, MCV was mixed with BCG (Glaxo, England) (24×10^6 organisms/vial). After 1 year, the immunization interval was increased to every 3 months ×4, and then every 6 months. One of the following biological response modifiers known to down-regulate suppressor cell activity was administered: cimetidine, indomethacin, or cyclophosphamide. Survival after MCV immunization correlated significantly with DTH (P = .0066) and antibody response to MCV (P = .0117). Of 40 AJCC stage IV patients with evaluable disease, 9 (23%) had regression (3 complete). MCV increased the median and 5-year survival of stage IIIA patients 2-fold (P = .00024) and stage IV patients 3-fold (P = .0001), compared with non-MCV immunotherapy and other treatments. Of particular interest were the following observations.

1. IgM antibodies to cell surface antigens correlated best with survival (163a, 167a); there was no significant correlation between survival and IgG antibody to melanoma cell surface antigens. Patients developing high IgM titers (immunofluorescence index >50%) had almost a 3-fold increase in 5-year survival (9.6–26.8%) and a 2-fold increase in median survival (16–30 months). IgM antibodies were directed against a variety of melanoma-associated gangliosides (193a, 195, 197).
2. A highly significant correlation (P = .0066) exists between survival and DTH response (163a, 167a). Median survival was 30 months for those whose DTH reaction exceeded 10 mm and only 17 months for those whose DTH was less than 10 mm. Respective 5-year survival rates were 27.7 and 10.0%. A significant association between survival and DTH was also noted after immunization with HLA-depleted polyvalent melanoma shed antigen (21b) and autologous whole cell vaccine (10).
3. A significant positive correlation (P = .013) exists between in vivo DTH response and in vitro mixed lymphocyte tumor reaction (MLTR) (163a, 167a). Of the 40 patients for whom these data were available, 82% showed significantly (P = .005) enhanced stimulation to one or more MCV cell lines at either week 4 or 16 compared with week 0. Of these, 91% showed sensitization to at least two MCV lines.
4. Autologous MLTR studies revealed that immunization with allogeneic MCV enhanced the response to autologous melanoma cells, confirming the existence of cross-reacting antigens demonstrated by antibodies to membrane-associated antigens (163a, 167a).
5. MLTR responses correlated with survival. Two-year DFS was 53% for patients responding to one or more MCV lines in the MLTR, compared with 20% for patients who showed no response (P = .055).
6. MCV immunization changed the profile of tumor-infiltrating lymphocytes; activated T and B cells (CD25) and NK cells (CD56) were significantly enhanced, and the CD4:CD8 ratio was markedly elevated (163a).
7. In our recent study of 135 AJCC stage III melanoma patients, 83% responded by a positive DTH reaction (>6 mm) during the first 4 months of MCV therapy (5a). Sixteen of 33 developed more than a 50% increase in CTL activity against one of the MCV cell lines during this period. Overall survival was significantly prolonged in patients with a positive DTH (P = .0054) and/or increased CTL activity (P = .02), suggesting that MCV induces specific T-cell responses that are correlated with clinical course.

8. In a separate study of 53 melanoma patients immunized with MCV, 57% had significantly elevated anti-MAGE-1 IgG serum levels after immunization with MCV (94b).

Five lines of evidence indicate that MCV can enhance the immune response to autologous melanoma cells: 1) the strong correlation between humoral and cell-mediated immune responses and survival (163a, 167a); 2) the complete and partial regressions in patients with evaluable disease (163a, 167a); 3) the concomitant increase in CTL activity, MLTR, and humoral antibodies to allogeneic and autologous melanoma cells (5a, 163a, 167a); 4) the changes in tumor-infiltrating lymphocytes in melanoma metastases (163a); and 5) the ability of allogeneic melanoma cells to induce sensitization to autologous melanomas that share HLA class I antigens, and thereby render the autologous cells susceptible to in vitro killing by CTL (85a).

MHC class I or II restriction has been raised as an argument against the use of allogeneic vaccines. However, there is significant loss of HLA class I antigen expression in melanocytic nevi and melanoma lesions (108a, 108b, 135a, 205a), and the expression of HLA class I also decreases with the progression of disease (234). Approximately 16% of primary melanoma lesions and 58% of metastatic melanoma lesions are not detected by monoclonal antibodies against HLA class I antigens (23a). Moreover, the allogeneic melanoma cells of MCV share MHC class I cross-reactive antigens with more than 90% of melanomas. MCV enhances the T-cell response in vitro to autologous melanoma cells (5a) possibly by direct recognition of MAA presented by shared or cross-reactive HLA molecules on MCV lines (5b, 85c, 85d). It is also possible that MAA recognition occurs through antigen processing and presentation of MCV's MAA by antigen-presenting cells. The allogeneic HLA antigens on the vaccine may stimulate alloreactive T-cells that infiltrate the site of MCV injection, resulting in production of cytokines to attract nearby antigen-presenting cells. Approximately 20% of patients did not show a T-cell response to MCV (5a), which could be due to T-cell anergy or to T-cell-specific immunosuppression. Nabel and co-workers recently demonstrated that in vivo transfection of the gene for an allogeneic HLA class I antigen into a patient's melanoma induced specific systemic T-cell immunity (172a).

Genetically Altered Cytokine-producing Tumor Cell Vaccines. Encouraged by studies involving immunization of tumor-bearing animals with genetically altered cytokine-producing tumor cell vaccines (IL-2 [18a, 64a, 64b, 125]; IL-4 [126a, 229]; gamma interferon [64b, 244e]; alpha tumor necrosis factor [14b], investigators at the John Wayne Cancer Institute developed a preclinical model to determine whether transfection of *IL-2* gene into human melanoma cells would augment the response of autologous and allogeneic peripheral blood lymphocytes (PBL) from melanoma patients (234a). *IL-2* gene was transfected into three human melanoma cell lines, and the secretion of IL-2 from stable transfected cells was confirmed by enzyme-linked immunosorbent assay (ELISA). The PBL response to these melanoma cells was then examined in an MLTR using PBL from eight melanoma patients. The PBL response was significantly higher to autologous (P = .01) or HLA-A cross-reacting (P = .05) transfected melanoma cells than to nontransfected melanoma cells. These data suggest that *IL-2* gene transfection may be an important strategy for enhancing specific immune responses induced by a polyvalent melanoma cell vaccine. These investigators have also observed that IL-4, gamma interferon, and tumor necrosis factor augment the expression of HLA class I and HLA-DR antigens. IL-4 alone or in combination with interferon or tumor necrosis factor also increases GD_2 expression (94, 94a).

LEUKEMIA

Mathe and co-workers administered BCG plus allogeneic leukemic cells to 20 children with acute lymphoblastic leukemia (144). Long-term follow-up revealed that 8 were alive in remission, with 7 in their first complete remission (145). Mathe and colleagues reported an approximately 50% overall rate of 5-year survival for a larger group of 100 patients undergoing the same treatment (146). Unfortunately, several similar clinical trials could not confirm these findings, possibly because of differences in treatment protocols (172). Immunotherapy with BCG and allogeneic leukemic cells has also been used for the maintenance of patients with acute myeloid leukemia (AML) (35, 52). Patients who received BCG plus irradiated tumor cells had longer remissions than did those maintained on either BCG or tumor cells, but this difference was not statistically significant. Powles and colleagues reported that the 45 of 107 leukemic patients who received BCG plus irradiated tumor cells achieved complete remission with a median duration of 70 weeks (190). A long-term follow-up of the trial, which closed in 1973 (189), reported that the actual median duration of remission for patients receiving maintenance chemotherapy was 191 days, versus 305 days for those receiving chemoimmunotherapy (not statistically significant). However, the median survival was significantly prolonged by active specific immunotherapy (270 days versus 510 days (p = .03)). In a similar study involving irradiated allogeneic AML blast cells and BCG, therapy was most successful in patients with a low tumor burden (Table 79.5) (62).

In another study, 191 adults with AML received combination chemotherapy consisting of daunorubicin and cytosine arabinoside (85). Sixty-three patients achieved remission and were admitted to one of the three arms of an active immunotherapy trial: immunotherapy alone, immunotherapy with maintenance chemotherapy, or no treatment. Unlike immunotherapy plus chemotherapy, immunotherapy alone was associated with easy and repeated reinduction of remission and marked prolongation of survival after first relapse. In a study of 182 patients, Whittaker and co-workers found that BCG alone was as effective as BCG plus allogeneic blast cells (249). Reizenstein and colleagues reported that 57% of 195 patients with acute myeloid leukemia entered complete remission after treatment with chemotherapy and BCG plus tumor cells (199). After remission, patients received maintenance chemotherapy with or without active specific immunotherapy involving weekly administration of frozen, nonirradiated allogeneic blast cells with BCG. The median survival was 690 days in the 40 chemoimmunotherapy patients versus 408 days in 36 chemotherapy patients ($P < .01$). Immunotherapy for AML using allogeneic cells with *C. parvum* showed no detectable impact on the rate of remission or the duration of survival (64). Table 79.5 surveys other clinical trials of immunotherapy for patients with AML and ALL.

Neuraminidase removes sialic acids from tumor cells, thereby increasing their immunogenicity (7, 41, 91). A randomized clinical trial compared the efficacy of chemotherapy alone, neuraminidase-treated allogeneic myeloblasts alone, and neuraminidase-treated myeloblasts plus methanol extract of BCG (MER) (41, 91). Patients received 10^{10} asialo-myeloblasts injected at 50 sites draining into node-bearing regions at one session. A total dose of 1 mg of MER was distributed in five equal injections. All immunotherapy was given midway between courses of chemotherapy. The median duration of remission for patients in each immunotherapy arm was >78 weeks, compared with only 20 weeks for patients in the chemotherapy arm. There were 27 survivors among the 32 immunotherapy patients, compared with only 4 survivors among the 21 chemotherapy patients. In other trials of active specific immunotherapy, BCG and cultured cell lines were administered intradermally to 15 patients with uncomplicated Philadelphia chromosome-positive chronic myeloid leukemia (CML) (217). CML patients who received immunotherapy survived twice as long as historical controls treated in the same institution.

Kwak and co-workers used a tumor-specific antigen for active specific immunotherapy in B-cell lymphoma (118A). Nine patients with minimal residual disease or complete remission after chemotherapy received a series of subcutaneous injections of immunoglobulin derived from autologous tumor cells (immunoglobulin-idiotype protein), conjugated to KLH and admixed with the immunologic adjuvant SAF-1. Seven of the nine patients showed idiotype-specific humoral

Table 79.5. Results of Some of the Clinical Trials Using Immunotherapy as a Modality of Cancer Treatment (Melanoma Excluded)

Kinds of tumor	Type of vaccine	Route	Outcome	References
Brain	TCV			72
	TCV			56
	TCV (autologous)	i.d.	nil	15
	TCV			137
	TCV (mitomycin + auto + allo + MDP + TDM)	s.c.	+ cell response	46
Colorectal	TCV (auto) + BCG	i.d.	DTH + (16/24)	95, 96
Gynecologic	TCV (allo)	i.d.	no response	73
	TCV (allo) + BCG	i.d.	+ response	101
	TC antigen + BCG + Chemo.	i.d.	no response	181
	TCV + BCG + Chemo.	i.d.	+ response	97
Genitourinary	TCV (auto)	i.d.	+ response	191
	TCV (auto) + *C. parvum*	i.d.	25% response	147, 148
	TCV (auto) + *C. parvum*	i.d.	+ response	206
	TCV (auto/allo) + *C. parvum*	i.d.	24% response	118
	TCV (auto/allo) + PPD + *Candida albicans*	i.d.	+ response	227
	TCV (auto) + PPD + *C. albicans*	i.d.	+ response	228
	TCV + PPD + PHA	i.d.	+ response	175
Leukemia (ALL)	TCV (allo) + BCG	i.d.	+ survival	144–146
	TCV (allo) + BCG-MetOH extract	i.d.	no response	123
	TCV (allo) + BCG + Chemo.	i.d.	no response	186
	TCV (allo) + BCG	i.d.	− response	180
(AML)	TCV (allo) + BCG + Chemo.	i.d.	Signf. surv.	189
	TCV (allo) + BCG	i.d.	Signf. surv.	190
	TCV (allo) + BCG	i.d.	+ response	62
	TCV (allo) + BCG + Chemo.	i.d.	Signf. surv.	247
	TCV (asialo-allo) + BCG	i.d.	Signf. response	41, 91
	TCV (allo) + BCG	i.d.	Signf. response	85
	TCV (allo) + BCG	i.d.	Signf. surv.	249
	TCV (allo) + BCG	i.d.	Signf. surv.	199
	TCV (allo) + *C. parvum*	i.d.	no response	64
Lung	TC antigen + Chemo.	i.d.	+ surv.	22
	TCV (asialo-allo)	i.d.	+ surv.	226–227
	TCV extract	i.d.	no response	2
	TCV + BCG	i.d.	no response	198
Sarcoma (osteo)	TCV (allo-extract)	i.d.	+ response	140
	TCV (allo) + BCG	i.d.	no response	51
	TCV (allo) + BCG	i.d.	+ surv.	157
	TCV (allo) + BCG	i.d.	+ response	217
	TCV (allo) + BCG	i.d.	+ response	231
	TCV (allo) + BCG + viral oreolysate + Chemo.	i.d.	+ response	212
	Viral oncolysate	i.d.	no response	76

TCV, tumor cell vaccine; TCV-asialo, neuraminidase-treated TCV free of sialic acids; MDP, muramyl dipeptide; TDM, trehalose dimycolate; BCG-MetOH ext, methanol extract of BCG; Chemo, chemotherapy; i.d., intradermal; s.c., subcutaneous; nil, no effect; surv, survival; PHA, phytohemagglutinin. (For further details see Refs. 70 and 71.)

and/or cellular immunologic responses. The induced antibodies bound specifically to autologous immunoglobulin idiotypes and autologous tumor cells. Cell-mediated responses were demonstrated by the in vitro proliferation of PBL in response to the soluble immunoglobulin-idiotype protein. The tumors of patients with measurable disease regressed completely. These results provide the basis for design of a large-scale clinical trial.

LUNG CANCER

More than 35% of lung cancer patients undergoing pulmonary resection harbor residual tumor cells within the thorax or at distant sites. Most lung cancer patients experience immunosuppression accompanying tumor growth and surgical intervention. In the postoperative interval, Stewart and colleagues injected intracutaneously a vaccine composed of purified antigenic extracts from autochthonous lung cancer cells in combination with complete Freund's adjuvant (222). Survival in stage I patients treated with immunotherapy was superior to that in nonrandomized controls. DTH responses in the skin showed increases in cell-mediated immunity to antigenic tumor preparations. Takita and co-workers treated 15 stage III lung cancer patients with complete Freund's adjuvant in combination with antigens extracted from autochthonous tumor (227). The survival rate for this group increased to 63% at 2 years (Table 79.5). Reid and colleagues randomized 45 stage I and 6 stage II patients with operable non-small-cell lung cancer to receive 1) no further therapy after resection, 2) BCG alone, or 3) BCG plus allogeneic tumor cells administered intradermally twice monthly for 2 years (198). They found that BCG with or without tumor cells was of marginal benefit in patients with resected lung cancer.

Another study investigated the effects of 1) methotrexate alone ($n = 8$), 2) immunotherapy with a homogenate of soluble tumor cell vaccine admixed with Freund's complete adjuvant ($n = 15$), and 3) chemoimmunotherapy ($n = 13$). Survival in immunized patients was significantly prolonged ($P <$ .01). Takita and colleagues randomized postoperative patients into three different therapy groups: no treatment, tumor antigens admixed with Freund's adjuvant intradermally three times, and Freund's adjuvant (226). Estimated 3-year survival rates were 34, 84, and 89%, respectively. The difference in survival rates between the control arm and the immunotherapy arms was statistically significant ($P < .05$). These studies, together with those reviewed in Table 79.5, suggest that immunopotentiation using adjuvant with or without tumor cells may be beneficial. Further studies are indicated.

SARCOMA

Evidence of immunogenic TAA in human and animal sarcomas prompted clinical trials with tumor vaccines. Morton and colleagues administered an admixture of BCG with 5 to 75×10^6 irradiated autologous tumor cells to 15 sarcoma patients (48, 49, 157). Vaccine recipients had an increase in complement fixing and cytotoxic antibodies concomitant with a slowing of tumor progression. A year later, Morton and colleagues reported encouraging results in patients receiving immunotherapy after surgical resection of pulmonary nodules (169). The eight vaccine recipients had a modest prolongation of survival compared to the nine patients who received surgery alone. Most patients with slowly growing tumors (doubling time over 40 days) did well after surgery, with no apparent benefit from immunotherapy.

Currie described the recovery of immunological competence in a patient treated monthly with BCG plus irradiated autologous cells (38). Similarly, Green and co-workers observed higher titers of antitumor cytotoxic antibodies and improved in vitro cellular immunity in osteosarcoma patients treated with irradiated autologous or allogeneic cells infected with influenza virus (76). No clinical benefit was derived from the irradiated whole cell vaccine or cell lysates (139). Sokal and Aungst treated patients who had undergone resection of primary osteosarcoma with vaccines that contained autologous or allogeneic tumor cells and BCG; two were free of disease at 13 and 18 months and a third developed pulmonary metastases shortly after initiation of therapy (217). Townsend and colleagues used tine-administered Tice BCG and cultured allogeneic sarcoma cells injected intradermally at five separate sites in patients who had undergone surgery for localized soft-tissue sarcoma (231). With follow-up as long as 3.5 years, 11 of 18 patients (61%) receiving active specific immunotherapy remained disease-free, compared with only 5 of 15 patients (33%) treated by surgery alone. Immunotherapy doubled the median disease-free interval in patients who experienced recurrence.

BREAST CANCER

Intralesional injection of BCG has produced regression of skin metastases from breast carcinoma (79). Complete regression was observed in 7 of 8 patients in one study (216) and in 7 of 14 patients in another (113). However, other investigators have been unsuccessful (65). Giuliano et al. reported no statistically significant benefit of adjuvant BCG therapy with or without an allogeneic tumor cell vaccine in patients with stage II breast carcinoma (67b). In another study, the administration of an autologous tumor vaccine after radical mastectomy for breast carcinoma showed no therapeutic benefit (3). Several clinical trials have attempted combination immunotherapy and chemotherapy (67b, 103, 183). Springer and colleagues recently summarized the results of a clinical trial initiated in 1974 to examine the potential of T/Tn antigens (carbohydrate precursors of MN blood group antigens) as vaccines for breast cancer (219a). T/Tn antigen (10 mg) was admixed with 0.5 units of typhoid vaccine, USP *(Salmonella typhi)* and injected intradermally in 16 patients with stage II, III, or IV breast cancer. Mean survival exceeded 5 years; the 10 patients who survived more than 10 years included three stage III and three stage IV patients. MacLean and co-workers (149b) have undertaken a pilot study to determine whether human breast carcinoma patients immunized with a second carbohydrate epitope (sialyl-Tn-KLH plus DETOX) produce specific anti-sialyl-Tn antibody responses. Following immunization, all 12 patients developed increased titers of complement-mediated cytotoxic antibodies specific for sialyl-Tn. Five patients were alive 12 or more months after entry and another 4 patients were alive 6 or more months after entry into the study.

GENITOURINARY CANCER

Active immunotherapy of renal cell carcinoma has been thoroughly reviewed (47, 74, 225, 234). Tumor cell vaccines with or without adjuvants have been administered in renal cell carcinoma (108, 148, 233). McCune and colleagues administered weekly intracutaneous injections of autologous irradiated tumor cells admixed with *C. parvum* in 5 patients with residual renal carcinoma (148). In another study, autologous tumor cell vaccine with *C. parvum* was administered to 14 patients with metastatic renal carcinoma; 4 of the 14 patients had objective responses and a fifth had prolonged stabilization.

Tykka demonstrated a significant increase in survival of stage IV renal cell carcinoma patients treated with a vaccine containing autologous tumor polymerized with ethylchlorformate and PPD or *Candida albicans* (233). Tallberg and colleagues used polymerized autologous tumor cell vaccine to treat 71 patients with advanced renal adenocarcinoma; after at least 3 years of follow-up, 13 vaccine patients remained alive, compared with only 3 of 56 patients treated by the best conventional measures (228). Prager and colleagues also observed a significant increase in survival among recipients of autologous tumor cell vaccine (191). Neidhart reported two complete responses and two partial responses among 30 patients treated with autologous tumor cells plus tuberculin or phytohemagglutinin as an adjuvant (175).

In an attempt to increase immunogenicity by abrogating the T-suppressor cell activity, Sahasrabudhi and co-workers administered cyclophosphamide to 20 patients before vaccination with an admixture of tumor cells and *C. parvum* (206). One patient had a complete response and 4 patients had partial responses. Four of 15 patients developed DTH responses to autologous renal carcinoma cells. Of these 4, 3 had clinical responses. Of the 11 patients who failed to develop DTH, only 1 had a clinical response. The results of this study are consistent with the possibility that inhibiting suppressor function during active specific immunotherapy can enhance T-helper function, induce a DTH response to autologous tumor cells, and induce objective regression of metastases.

More recently, Kurth and colleagues reported on 33 renal cell carcinoma patients who underwent palliative nephrectomy or excision of metastases followed by monthly intradermal injections of an autologous or allogeneic irradiated tumor cell preparation mixed with *C. parvum* (118). Antitumor activity was evident in eight vaccine recipients (one complete, four partial, and three minor responses). The median survival was 32 months for responding patients versus 17 months for all patients. In summary, most trials of active specific immunotherapy for renal cancer have demonstrated low toxicity, reasonable responses, and prolonged survival.

Carpinto and colleagues used autopheresis combined with cimetidine to abrogate suppressor cell activity in 16 patients (23). Autopheresis involves the pheresis of lymphocytes from a patient, incubation of the cells with autologous or heterologous tumor antigens, and reinfusion of the cells. In theory, the incubated cells will be specifically activated by TAA and will be further stimulated by endogenous lymphokines to destroy antigenic tumor cells in vivo. Treatment can be performed in outpatient facilities and toxicity is minimal. The study of Carpinto's group reported an objective response rate of 19% (3/16) (23). In a later series of patients with renal cell carcinoma, the survival rate was 25% at 24 months compared with an historical survival rate of 5 to 10% at 24 months (74).

GYNECOLOGICAL CANCERS

A preliminary report indicated that administration of tumor cell vaccine admixed with BCG, but not with tumor cells alone (73), may have benefited patients with ovarian carcinoma (101). Hudson and co-workers found that patients with advanced ovarian carcinoma who received a combination of BCG, tumor cell vaccine, and chemotherapy lived longer than patients who received chemotherapy alone (97). MacLean and co-workers (149a) reported limited success for immunization of ovarian cancer patients with KLH-conjugated common carcinoma (Thomsen-Friedenreich) determinant admixed with DETOX.

COLORECTAL CANCER

One of the most interesting and well-designed clinical studies of active specific immunotherapy is the prospectively randomized, controlled trial undertaken by Hoover and colleagues (96). Following standard surgical resection of Dukes' stage B and C colon or rectal cancer, patients at high risk for recurrence were randomly assigned to receive no immunotherapy (control) or active specific immunotherapy using 10^7 irradiated, autologous tumor cells mixed with 10^7 BCG organisms and administered weekly for 3 weeks. DTH to the autologous tumor cells developed in 67% of immunotherapy patients but in no control patients (95). After a mean follow-up of 28 months, immunotherapy patients had fewer recurrences and deaths than control patients (96). In a recent update of this study, these investigators reported that the apparent advantage of immunotherapy was limited to patients with colon cancer (94c). In a separate report, they noted that expression of HLA-Dr and ICAM-1 by tumor cells in the vaccine was predictive of disease-free survival (81a). Immunized patients developed a DTH response and an in vitro T-cell proliferative response to a 32-kd protein antigen; the authors suggest that this soluble antigen could replace the cellular vaccine.

GLIOBLASTOMA

There recently has been increased interest in the evaluation of immunotherapy for glioma and glioblastomas. In a phase I pilot study, 19 patients with anaplastic gliomas were immunized with allogeneic human glioma cell lines (137, 138). One patient showed antibody against glioma antigen after absorption with FBS, human platelets, and other allogeneic glioma cell lines (137, 138). In another study, Eggers and co-workers immunized a glioblastoma patient with a mixture of autologous and allogeneic cells inactivated with mitomycin and coupled to muramyl dipeptide and trehalose dimycolate (TDM) (46). Immune activity of peripheral blood lymphocytes against autologous tumor target cells was measured in a short-term chromium-release assay. The patient developed cell-mediated cytotoxicity against TAA.

Future Directions

PROBLEMS ASSOCIATED WITH VACCINE THERAPY

A large tumor burden significantly compromises immunotherapy and should be reduced before this therapeutic modality is undertaken. Animal models indicate an inverse relationship between tumor burden and therapeutic outcome. A tolerable tumor burden in a mouse generally does not exceed one million cells. If results in murine models can be extrapolated to humans (142), a tolerable tumor burden for a 70-kg man would be 3.5×10^9 tumor cells with a spherical tumor volume of about 2.5 cm^3 and a diameter of about 1.5 cm. The human immune response should be capable of rejecting this small but clinically evident tumor.

Spontaneous regression of large visceral metastases of malignant melanoma and of accidentally transplanted allogeneic tumors suggests that the human immune response may sometimes be capable of eliminating larger tumor nodules. Mastrangelo and colleagues argue that, given the proper circumstances, such as depletion of suppressor T cells, tumor-specific immunity can cope with much larger tumor burdens than is generally appreciated (142). Combining vaccines with more conventional modes of therapy could enable tumor-specific immunity to cope with greater numbers of tumor cells. Thus, immunotherapy in combination with chemotherapy has shown promise for the treatment of leukemia, lung cancer, and melanoma (230).

NEW APPROACHES

Future directions in the active specific immunotherapy of cancer depend on understanding the modus operandi of adjuvants administered with tumor cell vaccines. While BCG has proven to be an excellent nonspecific immunopotentiator, immunoregulation and trafficking of cells within the immune system are not well understood. The role of various components of BCG and other mycobacteria, such as BCG cell walls, trehalose dimycolate, muramyl dipeptide, and nontoxic derivatives from lipopolysaccharides of Gram-negative bacteria, in augmenting immunogenicity of tumor-cell vaccines requires further study.

Melanoma patients can be classified into different groups based on the distribution of four biosynthetically related tumor-associated glycolipids (197). Vaccine treatment can be adjusted depending upon antigenic profile of biopsied tumor cells. Different combinations of tumor cell vaccines may prove optimal for different groups of patients. A similar strategy has been utilized to choose appropriate monoclonal antibodies for serotherapy in melanoma (10). In the future, the ultimate success of immunotherapy depends on a better understanding of TAA heterogeneity with respect to preparation of tumor cell vaccines, as well as the role of immunopotentiators in rectifying the immunodeficiency encountered in patients with different kinds of cancers.

Infiltration with T cells may be required for immunologically mediated regression of human cancer. Factors favoring T-cell infiltration must be identified (180a). The absence of infiltrating T cells in metastatic tumors excised from cancer patients (171) and their presence in metastatic tumors after immunotherapy (10, 179) suggest that vaccines may have a role in potentiating the appropriate migration of cytotoxic effectors.

The use of genetically altered tumor vaccines is a promising approach currently under study. Transfection of autologous or allogeneic tumor cells with genes encoding different cytokines should increase vaccine potency. For example, IL-4 participates in the regulation, growth, and differentiation of B cells and T cells and in the generation of cytotoxic lymphocytes. Transfection of a renal cell carcinoma with the *IL-4* gene causes the tumor cells to secrete large amounts of this cytokine. The rejection of IL-4 transfected tumor cells by the host is associated with development of tumor-specific immunity mediated primarily by CD8+ T cells; this immunity is also effective against tumor cells that do not express IL-4 (69a). Several studies have documented an increase in cytolytic T-cell killing of tumor cells following transfection with the *IL-2* gene (55a, 207b, 234a, 251a). Tumor cells transfected with GM-CSF have also been associated with specific, long-lasting antitumor immunity (43a) and are under clinical investigation (180a). Related approaches involve the genetic engineering of tumor-infiltrating lymphocytes with cytokine-producing genes such as tumor necrosis factor (204a, 204b).

Conclusions

The present status of cancer vaccines can be best summarized by stating that we are at the end of the beginning. Despite 25 years of efforts toward effective active specific immunotherapy, there is no neoplasm for which cancer vaccines can be considered standard therapy. However, many reports from phase I or II trials indicate that partial and complete responses are observed, with little or no toxicity, in a small proportion of vaccine recipients, particularly those with metastatic melanoma or renal cell cancer. The striking aspect of such responses is that they are often durable and may continue for many years. Thus, the underlying concept of clinically useful responses is no longer in question.

The challenge for the future will be to apply advances in basic knowledge of immunogenic tumor antigens to vaccine adjuvants and delivery systems that will allow the cancer patient to develop an immune response capable of inducing tumor regression. This may require better methods of selecting candidates for vaccine therapy. Most phase I/II trials have used patients with advanced disease who are not ideal candidates for vaccine therapy. Future trials should focus on cancer patients with minimal subclinical microscopic disease.

Cancer vaccines are again a "hot topic" for research. Several are now entering phase III trials, and we look forward to the time when active immunotherapy becomes a standard approved treatment for neoplastic disease.

References

1. Alexander P. Activated macrophages and the antitumor action of BCG. Natl Cancer Inst Monogr 1973;39:127.
2. Alth G, Denck H, Fischer M, Karrer K, Kokron O, Korizek E, Micksche M, Ogris E, Reider C, Titscher R, Wrba H. Aspects of the immunologic treatment of lung cancer. Cancer Chemother Rep 1973;4:271.
3. Anderson JM, Kelly F, Wood SE, Holnan KE. Stimulatory immunotherapy in mammary cancer. Br J Surg 1974;61:778.
4. Austin FC, Boone CW. Virus augmentation of the antigenicity of tumor cell extracts. Adv Cancer Res 1979;30:301.
5. Baker MA, Taub RN. BCG in malignant melanoma. Lancet 1973;1:1117.
5a. Barth A, Hoon DSB, Foshag LJ, Nizze JA, Famatiga E, Okun E, Morton DL. Polyvalent melanoma cell vaccine induces delayed-type hypersensitivity and in vitro cellular immune response. Cancer Res 1994;54:3342–3345.
5b. Barth AM, Irie RF, Morton DL. Update on immunotherapy for advanced melanoma. Contemp Oncol 1994;4:52.
6. Bartlett GL, Zbar B. Tumor-specific vaccine containing *Mycobacterium bovis* and tumor cells: safety and efficacy. JNCI 1972;46:1709.
7. Bekesi JG, St. Arneault G, Walter L, Holland JF. Immunogenicity of leukemia L1210 cells after neuraminidase treatment. JNCI 1972;49:107.
8. Berd D, Herlyn M, Koprowski H, Mastrangelo MJ. Flow cytometric determination of the frequency and heterogeneity of expression of human melanoma-associated antigens. Cancer Res 1989;49:6840.
9. Berd D, Maguire HC Jr, Mastrangelo MJ. Induction of cell-mediated immunity to autologous melanoma cells and regression of metastases after treatment with a melanoma cell vaccine preceded by cyclophosphamide. Cancer Res 1986;46:2572.
9a. Berd D, Maguire HC Jr, Mastrangelo MJ. Treatment of human melanoma with a hapten modified autologous vaccine. Ann NY Acad Sci 1993;690:147.
10. Berd D, Maguire HC Jr, McCue P, Mastrangelo MJ. Treatment of metastatic melanoma with an autologous tumor-cell vaccine: clinical and immunological results in 64 patients. J Clin Oncol 1990;8:1858.
11. Berd D, Mastrangelo MJ. Effect of low dose cyclophosphamide on the immune system of cancer patients: reduction of T suppressor function without depletion of the CD8+ subset. Cancer Res 1987;47:3317.
12. Berd D, Mastrangelo MJ. Active immunotherapy of human melanoma exploiting the immuno-potentiating effects of cyclophosphamide. Cancer Invest 1988;6:335.
13. Berd D, Mastrangelo MJ. Effective of low dose cyclophosphamide on the immune system of cancer patients: depletion of CD4+2H4+ suppressor-inducer T-cells. Cancer Res 1988;48:1671.
14. Bergelson LD, Dyatlovitzkaya EV. Gangliosides and antitumor immunity. J Cancer Res Clin Oncol 1990;116 (suppl.):1159.
14a. Berthier-Vergnes O, Portoukalian J, Lefheriotis E, Dore JF. Induction of IgG antibodies directed to a M_r 31,000 melanoma antigen in patients immunized with vaccinia virus melanoma oncolysates. Cancer Res 1994;54:2433.
14b. Blankenstein T, Qin Z, Uberla K, Muller W, Rosen H, Volk H, Diamanstein T. Tumor suppression after tumor cell-targeted tumor necrosis factor α gene transfer. J Exp Med 1991;173:1047.
15. Bloom WH, Peckham MJ, Richardson AE, Alexander PA, Payne PM. Glioblastoma multiforme: a controlled trial to assess the value of specific active immunotherapy in patients treated by radical surgery and radiotherapy. Br J Cancer 1973;27:253.
16. Bornstein RS, Mastrangelo MJ, Sulit H. Immunotherapy of melanoma with intralesional BCG. Cancer Inst Monogr 1973;39:213.
16a. Brichard V, Van Pel A, Wolfel T, Wolfel C, De Plaen E, Lethe B, Coulie P, Boon T. The tyrosinase gene codes for an antigen recognized by autologous cytolytic T lymphocytes on HLA-A2 melanomas. J Exp Med 1993;178:489.
16b. Brocker EB, Suter L, Bruggen J, Ruiter DJ, Macher E, Sorg C. Phenotypic dynamics of tumor progression in human malignant melanoma. Int J Cancer 1985;36:29.
17. Brocker EB, Zwaldo G, Holzmann B, Macher E, Sorg C. Inflammatory cell infiltration in human melanoma at different stages of tumor progression. Int J Cancer 1989;41:562.
18a. Bubenick J, Simova J, Jandlova T. Immunotherapy of cancer using local administration of lymphoid cells transformed by cDNA and constitutively producing IL2. Immunol Lett 1990;23:287.
19. Burdick JF, Wells SA, Herberman RB. Immunologic evaluation of patients with cancer by delayed hypersensitivity reaction. Collective review. Surg Gynecol Obstet 1975;141:779.
20. Bystryn J-C, Jacobsen S, Harris M, Roses D, Speyer J, Levin M. Preparation and characterization of a polyvalent human melanoma antigen vaccine. J Biol Response Mod 1986;5:211.
21. Bystryn J-C, Oratz R, Harris MN, Roses DF, Golomb FM, Speyer JC. Immunogenicity of a polyvalent melanoma antigen vaccine in humans. Cancer 1988;61:1065.
21a. Bystryn J-C, Oratz R, Roses DF, Harris MN, Henn M, Lew R. Improved survival of melanoma patients with delayed hypersensitivity response to melanoma vaccine immunization. Clin Res 1991;39:503A.
21b. Bystryn J-C, Oratz R, Henn M, Adler A, Harris MN, Roses DF. Relationship between immune response to melanoma vaccine and clinical outcome in stage II malignant melanoma. Cancer 1992;69:1157.
22. Bystryn J-C, Tedholm CA, Heaney-Kieras J. Release of surface macromolecules by human melanoma and normal cells. Cancer Res 1981;41:91.
22a. Campo MS. Towards vaccines against papillomavirus. In Human Papillomaviruses and Cervical Cancer. Edited by P Stern, M Stanley. New York: Oxford, 1993.
23. Carpinto GA, Levine S, Hamilton H, Krane RJ, Osband ME. Successful adoptive immunotherapy of cancer using in vitro immunized autologous lymphocytes and cimetidine. Surg Forum 1986;37:418.
23a. Carrel S, Dore JF, Ruiter DJ, Prade M, Lejeune FJ, Kleeberg UR, Rumke P, Brocker EB. The EORTC Melanoma Group exchange program: evaluation of a multicenter monoclonal antibody study. Int J Cancer 1991;48:836.
24. Carubia JM, Yu RK, Macala LJ, Kirkwood JM, Varga JM. Gangliosides of normal and neoplastic human melanocytes. Biochem Biophys Res Commun 1984;120:500.
25. Cassel WA, Murray DR, Phillips HS. A phase II study on the postsurgical management of stage II malignant melanoma with a Newcastle disease virus oncolysate. Cancer 1983;52:856.
26. Cassel WA, Weidenheim KM, Campbell WG, Murray DR. Malignant melanoma: inflammatory mononuclear cell infiltrates in cerebral metastases during concurrent therapy with viral oncolysate. Cancer 1986;57:1302.
27. Chassot PG, Guttmann RD, Beaudoin JG, Morehouse DD, Gonda A, MacLean LD. Cancer in renal allograft recipients. Prog Exp Tumor Res 1974;19:91.
28. Cheung NK, Lazarus H, Miraldi FD, Abramowsky CR, Kallick S, Saarinen UM, Spitzer T, Strandojord SE, Coccia PF, Berger NA. Ganglioside GD2 specific monoclonal antibody 3F8: a phase I study in patients with neuroblastoma and malignant melanoma. J Clin Oncol 1987;5:1430.
29. Cheung NK, Miraldi FD. Iodine 132 labelled GD2 monoclonal antibody in the diagnosis and therapy of human neuroblastoma. Prog Clin Biol Res 1988;27:595.
30. Coca AF, Dorrance GM, Lebredo MG. Vaccination in cancer: a report of the results of vaccination therapy as applied to seventy-nine cases of human cancer. Z Immun Exp Ther 1912;13:543.
31. Coca AF, Gilman G. The specific treatment of carcinoma. Phil J Sci Med 1909;4:381.
32. Cochran AJ, Pihl E, Wen D-R, Hoon DBS, Korn L. Zoned immune suppression of lymph nodes draining malignant melanoma. Histologic and immunohistologic studies. JNCI 1987;78:399.
33. Cohen MH, Jessup JM, Felix EL, Wesse JL, Herberman RB. Intralesional treatment of recurrent metastatic cutaneous malignant melanoma: a randomized prospective study of intralesional bacillus Calmette-Guerin versus intralesional dinitrochlorobenzene. Cancer 1978;41:2456.
34. Cole WH. Spontaneous regression of cancer: the metabolic triumph of the host. Ann NY Acad Sci 1974;230:111.
34a. Coulie PG, Brichard V, Van Pel A, Wolfel J, Szikora JP, Renauld JC, Boon T. A new gene coding for a differentiation antigen recognized by autologous cytolytic T lymphocytes on HLA-A2 melanomas. J Exp Med 1994;180:35.
35. Crowther D, Powles RL, Bateman CJJ, Beard MEJ, Gauci CL, Wrigley PFM, Malpas JS, Fairley GH, Scott RB. Management of adult acute myelogenous leukemia. Br Med J 1973;1:131.
36. Cunningham TJ, Olson KB, Laffin R, Horton J, Sullivan J. Treatment of advanced cancer with active immunization. Cancer 1969;24:932.
37. Currie GA. Eighty years of immunotherapy: a review of immunological methods used for the treatment of human cancer. Br J Cancer 1972;26:141.
38. Currie GA. Effect of active immunization with irradiated tumor cells on specific serum inhibition of cell-mediated immunity in patients with disseminated cancer. Br J Cancer 1973;28:25.
39. Currie GA, Basham S. Serum mediated inhibition of the immunological reactions of the patient to his own tumor: a possible role of circulating antigen. Br J Cancer 1972; 26:427.
40. Currie GA, Lejeune F, Fairley GH. Immunization with irradiated tumor cells and specific lymphocyte cytotoxicity in malignant melanoma. Br Med J 1971;2:305.
41. Cuttner J, Glidewell O, Holland JF. A controlled trial of chemoimmunotherapy of acute myelogenous leukemia with the methanol extraction residue of tubercle bacilli (MER). In Immunotherapy of Human Cancer. Edited by WD Terry, SA Rosenberg. New York: Excerpta Medica, 1982, p 33.
42. Czajkowski NP, Rosenblatt M, Wolf PL, Vasquez J. A new method of active immunization to autologous human tumour tissue. Lancet 1967;2:905.
42a. Darrow TL, Slingluff CL Jr, Seigler HF. The role of HLA class I antigens in recognition of melanoma cells by tumor-specific cytotoxic T lymphocytes: evidence for shared tumor antigens. J Immunol 1989;142:3329.
43. de Kernion JB, Ramming KP, Gupta RK. The detection and clinical significance of antibodies to tumor associated antigens in patients with renal cell carcinoma. J Urol 1974;111:330.
43a. Dranoff G, Jaffee E, Lazenby A, Golumbek P, Levitsky H, Brose K, Jackson V, Hamada H, Pardoll D, Mulligan RC. Vaccination with irradiated tumor cells engineered to secrete murine granulocyte-macrophage colony-stimulating factor stimulates potent, specific, and long-lasting anti-tumor immunity. Proc Natl Acad Sci USA 1993;90:3539.
43b. Dore JF, Portoukalian J, Berthier-Vergnes O, Jacubovich R, Geneve J, Bailly M, Lefheriotis E, Weissbrod A, Mayer M. Responses de malades atteints de melanome a l'immunisation par oncolysats de melanomes au virus de la vaccine. Bull Cancer (Paris) 1990;77:881.
44. Dufour FD, Morton DL. Induction of melanoma specific monocyte cytotoxicity in patients receiving BCG immunotherapy. Surg Forum 1977;28:165.
45. Edwards FR, Whitwell F. Use of BCG as an immunostimulant in the surgical treatment of carcinoma of the lung. Thorax 1974;29:654.
46. Eggers AE, Tarmin L, Gamboa ET. In vivo immunization against autologous glioblastoma-associated antigens. Cancer Immunol Immunother 1985;19:43.
47. Eidinger D. Genitourinary cancer. In Clinical Immunotherapy. Edited by AF Lobuglio. New York: Marcel Dekker, 1980, p 243.
48. Eilber FR, Holmes EC, Morton DL. Immunotherapy experiments with a methylcholanthrene-induced guinea pig liposarcoma. JNCI 1971;46:803.
49. Eilber FR, Morton DL. Impaired immunologic reactivity and recurrence following cancer surgery. Cancer 1970;25:362.
50. Eilber FR, Nizze A, Morton DL. Sequential evaluation of general immune competence in cancer patients: correlation with clinical course. Cancer 1975;35:660.
51. Eilber FR, Townsend CM Jr, Morton DL. Osteosarcoma: results of treatment employing adjuvant immunotherapy. Clin Orthop 1975;111:94.
52. Ekert H, Jose DG. Chemotherapy and BCG in acute lymphocytic leukemia. Lancet 1975;2:713.
52a. Elliott GT, Perez J, McLeod RA, Von Eschen KB. A potential surrogate marker of efficacy for a therapeutic melanoma vaccine. Ann NY Acad Sci 1993;690:147.
52b. Elliott GT, McLeod RA, Perez J, Von Eschen KB. Results of phase II multicenter trial evaluating the activity of melacine melanoma theraccine in the treatment of disseminated melanoma. Proc Am Assoc Cancer Res 1992;33:332.
53. Everson TC, Cole WH. Spontaneous Regression of Cancer. Philadelphia: Saunders, 1966, p 11.
54. Fairlamb DJ. Spontaneous regression of metastases of renal cancer: a report of two

cases including the first recorded regression following irradiation of a dominant metastasis and review of the world literature. Cancer 1981;47:2102.
55. Falk RE, MacGregor AB, Landi S, Ambus U, Langer B. Immunostimulation with intraperitoneally administered bacillus Calmette-Guerin for advanced malignant tumors of the gastrointestinal tract. Surg Gynecol Obstet 1976;142:363.
55a. Fearon ER, Pardoll DM, Itaya T, Golumbek P, Levitsky HI, Simons JW, Karasuyama H, Vogelstein B, Frost P. Interleukin-2 production by tumor cells bypasses T helper function in the generation of an antitumor response. Cell 1990;60:397.
56. Febvre H, Maunoury R, Constans JP, Trouillas P. Reactions d'hypersensibilite retardee avec des lignees de cellules tumorales humaines cultivees in vitro chez des malades porteurs de tumeurs cerebrales malignes. Int J Cancer 1972;10:221.
56a. Ferrone S. Human tumor-associated antigen mimicry by anti-idiotypic antibodies: immunogenicity and clinical trials in patients with solid tumors. Ann NY Acad Sci 1993; 690:214.
56b. Ferrone S, Kagashita T. Human high molecular weight–melanoma associated antigen as a target for active specific immunotherapy: a phase I clinical trial with murine monoclonal antibodies. J Dermatol 1988;15:457.
57. Finney JW, Byers EH, Wilson RH. Studies in tumour auto-immunity. Cancer Res 1960; 20:351.
58. Fisher RI, Terry WD, Nodes RJ. Rosenberg SA, Makuch R, Gordon HG, Fisher SG. Adjuvant immunotherapy or chemotherapy for malignant melanoma. Surg Clin N Am 1981;61:1267.
59. Fortner JG, Booker RJ, Pack GT. Results of groin dissection for malignant melanoma in 200 patients. Surgery 1964;55:485.
60. Fortner JG, Shiu MH. Organ transplantation and cancer. Surg Clin North Am 1974;54: 871.
61. Fredman P, von Holst H, Collins VP, Ammar A, Delheden B, Wahren B, Granholm L, Svennerholm L. Potential ganglioside antigens associated with human gliomas. Neurol Res 1986;8:123.
62. Freeman CB, Harris RG, Colin G, Leyland MJ, MaCiver JE, Delamore IW. Active immunotherapy used alone for the maintenance of patients with acute myeloid leukaemia. Br Med J 1973;4:571.
63. Furukawa K, Yamaguchi H, Oettgen HF, Old LJ, Lloyd KO. Analysis of the expression of *N*-glycolylneuraminic acid-containing gangliosides in cells and tissues using two human monoclonal antibodies. J Biol Chem 1988;263:18507-18512.
64. Gale RP, Foon KA, Yale C, Zighelboim J. Immunotherapy of acute myelogenous leukemia using *Corynebacterium parvum* and allogeneic cells. In Immunotherapy of Human Cancer. Edited by WD Terry, SA Rosenberg. New York: Excerpta Medica, 1982, p 40.
64a. Gansbacher B, Zier K, Daniels B, Cronin K, Bannerji R, Gilboa E. Interleukin-2 gene transfer into tumor cells abrogates tumorigenicity and induces protective immunity. J Exp Med 1990;172:1217.
64b. Gansbacher B, Bannerji R, Daniels B, Zier K, Cronin K, Gilboa E. Retroviral vector-mediated gamma-interferon gene transfer into tumor cells generates potent and long lasting antitumor immunity. Cancer Res 1990;50:7820.
65. Garas J, Besbeas S, Papmatheakis J, Gropas G, Maragoudakis S, Katsenis A, Kiparissiadis P, Konstadakos P, Georgaka A. Attempt with immunotherapy to control metastatic skin nodules from breast cancer by BCG. Panminerva Med 1975;17:193.
66. Gatti RA, Good RA. Occurrence of malignancy in immunodeficiency diseases: a literature review. Cancer 1971;28:89.
67. Ghosh S, White LM, Ghosh R, Bankert RB. Vaccination with membrane associated idiotype provides greater and more prolonged protection of animals from tumor challenge than the soluble form of idiotype. J Immunol 1990;145:365.
67a. Gissmann L, Jochmus I, Nindl I, Muller M. Immune response to genital papillomavirus infections in women: prospects for the development of a vaccine against cervical cancer. Ann NY Acad Sci 1993;690:80.
67b. Giuliano AE, Sparks FC, Patterson K, Spears I, Morton DL. Adjuvant chemo-immunotherapy in stage II carcinoma of the breast. J Surg Oncol 1986;31:255.
68. Golub SH, Forsythe AB, Morton DL. Sequential examination of lymphocyte proliferative capacity in patients with malignant melanoma receiving BCG immunotherapy. Int J Cancer 1977;19:18.
69. Golub SH, Roth JA, Forsythe A, Morton DL. In vitro monitoring of cellular function during BCG immunotherapy. Bibl Haematol 1976;43:270.
69a. Golumbek PT, Lazenby AJ, Levitsky HI, Jaffee LM, Karasuyama H, Baker M, Pardoll DM. Treatment of established renal cancer by tumor cells engineered to secrete interleukin-4. Science 1991;254:713.
70. Goodnight JE, Morton DL. Immunotherapy for malignant disease. Annu Rev Med 1978;29:231.
71. Goodnight JE, Morton DL. Immunotherapy of cancer: current status. Prog Exp Tumor Res 1980;25:61.
72. Grace JT Jr, Perese DM, Metzgar RS, Sasabe T, Holdridge B. Tumor autograft responses in patients with glioblastoma multiforme. J Neurosurg 1961;18:159.
73. Graham JB, Graham RM. Autologous vaccine in cancer patients. Surg Gynecol Obstet 1962;109:121.
74. Graham SD Jr. Immunotherapy of renal cell carcinoma. Semin Urol 1989;7:215.
75. Grant RM, Mackie R, Cochran AJ, Murray EL, Hoyle D, Ross C. Results of administering BCG to patients with melanoma. Lancet 1974;2:1096.
76. Green AA, Pratt C, Webster RG, Smith K. Immunotherapy of osteosarcoma patients with virus-modified tumor cells. Ann NY Acad Sci 1976;277:396.
77. Greene MH, Young TI, Clark WH Jr. Malignant melanoma in renal transplant recipients. Lancet 1981;1:1196.
77a. Gross L. Intradermal immunization of C3H mice against a sarcoma that originated in an animal of the same line. Cancer Res 1943;3:326.
77b. Gruber J, Cole JC III. Vaccines for human cancers of viral etiology. Ann NY Acad Sci 1993;690:311.
78. Gupta RK, Golub SH, Morton DL. Correlation between tumor burden and anticomplementary activity in sera from patients. Cancer Immunol Immunother 1979;6:63.
79. Gutterman JU, Mavligit TJ, Burgess MA, Cardenas JO, Blumenschein GR, Gottlieb JA, McBride CM, McCredie KB, Bodey GP, Rodriquez V, Freireich EJ, Hersh EM. Immunotherapy of breast cancer, malignant melanoma, and acute leukemia with BCG: prolongation of disease-free interval and survival. Cancer Immunol Immunother 1976; 1:99.
80. Hadley DW, McElwain TJ, Currie GA. Specific active immunotherapy does not prolong survival in surgically treated patients with stage IIB malignant melanoma and may promote early recurrence. Br J Cancer 1978;37:491.
81. Hakansson L, Fredman P, Svennerholm L. Gangliosides in serum immune complexes from tumor-bearing patients. J Biochem 1985;98:843.
81a. Hanna MG Jr, Ransom JH, Pomato N, Peters L, Bloemena E, Vermorken JB, Hoover HC Jr. Active specific immunotherapy of human colorectal carcinoma with an autologous tumor cell/Bacillus Calmette-Guerin vaccine. Ann NY Acad Sci 1993;690:135.
82. Hanna MG Jr, Snodgrass MJ, Zbar B, Rapp H. Histopathology of tumor regression after intralesional injection of *mycobacterium bovis:* IV. Development of immunity to tumor cells and BCG. JNCI 1973;51:1897.
83. Hanna MG Jr, Zbar B, Rapp HJ. Histopathology of tumor regression and intralesional injection of *Mycobacterium bovis:* I. Tumor growth and metatasis. JNCI 1972;48: 1441.
84. Hanna MG Jr, Zbar B, Rapp HJ. Histopathology of tumor regression after intralesional injection of *mycobacterium bovis:* II. Comparative effects of vaccinia virus, oxazolone, and turpentine. J Natl Cancer Inst 1972;48:1697.
84a. Harel W, Goedegebuure PS, LeMay LG, Huang XQ, Kan-Mitchell J, Mitchell MS. Melanoma-specific lysis by cloned CD4+ and CD8+ T cells from actively immunized melanoma patients. Vaccine Res (In press).
85. Harris R, Zuhrie SZ, Freeman CB, Read AP, MacIver JE, Geary CG, Delamore IW, Tooth JA. A successful randomized trial of immunotherapy alone versus no maintenance treatment in acute myelogenous leukemia. In Immunotherapy of Human Cancer. Edited by WD Terry and SA Rosenberg. New York: Excerpta Medica, 1982, p 11.
85a. Hayashi Y, Hoon DSB, Foshag LJ, Park MS, Terasaki PI, Morton DL. A preclinical model to assess the antigenicity of an HLA-A2 melanoma cell vaccine. Cancer 1993; 72:750.
85b. Helling F, Calves M, Shang H, Oettgen HF, Livingston PO. Construction of immunogenic GD3-conjugate vaccines. Ann NY Acad Sci 1993;690:396.
85c. Hayashi Y, Hoon DSB, Park MS, Terasaki PI, Foshag LJ, Morton DL. Induction of CD4+ cytotoxic T cells by sensitization with allogeneic melanomas bearing shared or cross-reactive HLA-A. Cell Immunol 1992;139:411.
85d. Hayashi Y, Hoon DSB, Park MS, Terasaki PI, Morton DL. Cytotoxic T cell lines recognize autologous and allogeneic melanomas with shared or cross-reactive HLA-A. Int Arch Allergy Immunol 1992;97:8.
85e. Helling F, Shang A, Calves M, Zhang S, Ren S, Yu RK, Oettgen HF, Livingston PO. GD_3 vaccines for melanoma: superior immunogenicity of keyhole limpet hemocyanin conjugate vaccines. Cancer Res 1994;54:197.
86. Heppner GH. Tumor heterogeneity. Cancer Res 1984;44:2259.
87. Herlyn M, Guerry D, Koprowski H. Recombinant gamma-interferon induces changes in expression and shedding of antigens associated with normal human melanocytes, nevus cells and primary and metastatic melanoma. J Immunol 1985;134:4226.
88. Herlyn M, Rodeck U, Koprowski H. Shedding of human tumor associated antigens in vitro and in vivo. Adv Cancer Res 1987;49:189.
89. Herlyn M, Thurin J, Balaban G, Bennicelli JL, Herlyn D, Elder DE, Bondi E, Guerry D, Nowell P, Clark WH, Koprowski H. Characteristics of cultured human melanocytes isolated from different stages of tumor progression. Cancer Res 1985;45:5670.
90. Hersey P, Edwards A, Coates A, Shaw H, McCarthy WH, Milton GW. Evidence that treatment with vaccinia melanoma cell lysates (VMCL) may improve survival of patients with stage II melanoma. Cancer Immunol Immunother 1987;25:257.
91. Holland JF, Bekesi JG, Cuttner J. Chemoimmunotherapy for acute myelocytic leukemia. In Immunotherapy of Human Cancer. New York: Raven Press, 1978, p 237.
92. Hollinshead A, Arlen M, Yonemoto R, Cohen M, Janner K, Kundin WD, Scherrer J. Pilot studies using melanoma tumor-associated antigens (TAA) in specific active immunochemotherapy of malignant melanoma. Cancer 1982;49:1387.
93. Hoon DSB, Irie RF, Cochran AJ. Gangliosides from melanoma immunomodulate response of T-cells to interleukin-2. Cell Immunol 1988;111:1.
94. Hoon DSB, Banez M, Okun E, Morton DL, Irie RF. Modulation of human melanoma cells by interleukin-4 and in combination with gamma-interferon or a-tumor necrosis factor. Cancer Res 1991;51:2002.
94a. Hoon DSB, Hayashi Y, Morisaki T, Foshag LJ, Morton DL. Interleukin-4 plus tumor necrosis factor α augments the antigenicity of melanoma cells. Cancer Immunol Immunother 1993;37:378.
94b. Hoon DSB, Yuzuki D, Hayashida M, Morton DL. Melanoma patients immunized with melanoma cell vaccine induce antibody responses to recombinant MAGE-1 antigen. J Immunol 1995;154:730-737.
94c. Hoover HC Jr, Brandhorst JS, Peters LC, Surdyke MG, Takeshita Y, Madariaga J, Muenz LR, Hanna MG Jr. Adjuvant active specific immunotherapy for human colorectal cancer: 6.5-year median follow-up of a phase III prospectively randomized trial. J Clin Oncol 1993;11:390.
95. Hoover HC Jr, Surdyke M, Dangel RB, Peter LC, Hanna MG Jr. Delayed cutaneous hypersensitivity to autologous tumor cells in colorectal cancer patients immunized with an autologous tumor cell: Bacillus Calmette-Guerin vaccine. Cancer Res 1984; 44:1671.
96. Hoover HC Jr, Surdyke MG, Dangel RB, Peters LC, Hanna MG Jr. Prospectively randomized trial of adjuvant active-specific immunotherapy for human colorectal cancer. Cancer 1985;55:1236.
96a. Houghton AN. Cancer antigens: immune recognition of self and altered self. J Exp Med 1994;180:1.
97. Hudson CN, McHardy JE, Curling OM, English PE, Levin L, Poulton TA, Crowther M, Leighton M. Active specific immunotherapy for ovarian cancer. Lancet 1976;2:877.
98. Hudson MA, Richey JK, Catalona WJ, Brown EJ, Ratliff TL. Comparison of the fibronectin-binding ability and antitumor efficacy of various mycobacteria. Cancer Res 1990;50:3843.
99. Hughes LF, Kearney R, Tully M. A study in clinical cancer immunotherapy. Cancer 1970;26:269.
100. Ikonopisov RL, Lewis MG, Hunter-Craig ID, Bodenham DC, Phillips TM, Cooling CI, Proctor J, Hamilton-Fairley G, Alexander P. Autoimmunization with irradiated tumor cells in human malignant melanoma. Br Med J 1970;2:752.
101. Imperato S, Rossi R, Ermiglia G, De Marini M, Cassolino A. Active specific immunotherapy with immunological monitoring in late stage ovarian cancers. Acta Eur Fertil 1974;5:25.
102. Irie RF, Ravindranath MH. Gangliosides as targets for monoclonal antibody therapy of cancer. In Therapeutic Monoclonal Antibodies. Edited by CAK Borrebaeck and JW Larrick. New York: Stockton Press, 1990, p 75.

103. Israel L. Report on 414 cases of human tumors treated with *Corynebacteria*. In *Corynebacterium parvum:* Applications in Experimental and Clinical Oncology. Edited by B Halpern. New York: Plenum Press, 1975, p 389.
104. Israel L, de Pierre A, Edelstein R. Effect of intranodal BCG in 22 melanoma patients. Proc IVth Int Symp Locoregional Treatment of Tumors. Turin, Italy: IUCC, 1973.
105. Israel L, Edelstein R, de Pierre A, Dimitrov N. Daily infusions of *Corynbacterium parvum* in twenty patients with disseminated cancer: a preliminary report of clinical and biological findings. J Natl Cancer Inst 1975;55:29.
106. Janik P. Cell proliferation during the course of immunological rejection of Ehrlich ascites tumor cells. Cell Tissue Kinet 1971;4:69.
107. Janik P, Steel GG. Cell proliferation during immunological perturbation in three transplanted tumours. Br J Cancer 1972;26:108.
108. Juillard GJK, Boyer PJJ, Yamashiro CH. A phase I study of active specific intralymphatic immunotherapy (ASILI). Cancer 1978;41:2215.
108a. Kageshita T, Nakamura T, Yamada M, Kuriya N, Arao T, Ferrone S. Differential expression of melanoma associated antigens in acral lentiginous melanoma and in nodular melanoma lesions. Cancer Res 1991;51:1726.
108b. Kageshita T, Kimura T, Yoshi A, Hirai S, Ono T, Ferrone S. Antigenic profile of mucosal melanoma lesions. Int J Cancer 1994;56:370.
109. Karakousis CP, Douglass HO, Yeracaris PM, Holyoke ED. BCG immunotherapy in patients with malignant melanoma. Arch Surg 1976;111:716.
110. Kawai T, Kato A, Higashi H, Kato S, Naiki M. Quantitative determination of *N*-glycolylneuraminic acid expression in human cancerous tissues and avian lymphoma cell lines as a tumor associated sialic acid by gas chromatography-mass spectrometry. Cancer Res 1991;51:1242.
110a. Kawakami YS, Eliyanu CH, Delgado PF, Robbins L, Rivoltini SL, Topalian T, Miki T, Rosenberg SA. Cloning of the gene coding for a shared human melanoma antigen recognized by autologous T cells infiltrating into tumor. Proc Natl Acad Sci USA 1994; 91:3515.
110b. Kawakami YS, Eliyanu S, Sakaguchi K, Robbins PF, Rivoltini L, Yannelli JR, Appella E, Rosenberg SA. Identification of the immunodominant peptides of the MART-1 human melanoma antigen recognized by the majority of HLA-A2 restricted tumor infiltrating lymphocytes. J Exp Med 1994;180:347.
111. Kellock TH, Chambers H, Russ S. An attempt to procure immunity to malignant disease in man. Lancet 1922;1:217.
112. Klein E, Holterman OA. Immunotherapeutic approaches to the management of neoplasms. NCI Monogr 1972;35:379.
113. Klein E, Holterman O, Milgrom H, Case RW, Klein D, Rosner D, Djerassi I. Immunotherapy for accessible tumors utilizing delayed hypersensitivity reactions and separated components of the immune system. Med Clin North Am 1976;60:389.
114. Kleinschuster SJ, Rapp HJ, Lueker DC, Kainer RA. Regression of bovine ocular carcinoma by treatment with mycobacterial vaccine. JNCI 1977;58:1805.
114a. Kneip B, Peter-Katalinic J, Flegel W, Northorff H, Rieber EP. CDw 60 antibodies bind to acetylated forms of ganglioside GD3. Biochem Biophys Res Commun 1992;187: 1343.
115. Kobayashi H. Immunological xenogeneration of tumor cells. Tokyo: Japan Scientific Societies, 1979.
116. Krementz ET, Samuels MS, Wallace JH, Benes EN. Clinical experiences in immunotherapy of cancer. Surg Gynecol Obstet 1971;133:209.
117. Krown SE, Hilal EY, Pinsky CM, Hirshaut Y, Wanebo HJ, Hansen JA, Huvos AG, Oettgen HF. Intralesional injection of the methanol extraction residue of bacillus Calmette-Guerin (MER) into cutaneous metastases of malignant melanoma. Cancer 1978;42:2648.
118. Kurth KH, Marquet R, Zwartendijk J, Warnar SO. Autologous anticancer antigen preparation for specific immunotherapy in advanced renal cell carcinoma. Eur Urol 1987;13:103.
118a. Kwak LW, Campbell MJ, Czerwinski BS, Hart S, Miller RA, Levy R. Induction of immune responses in patients with B-cell lymphoma against the surface-immunoglobulin idiotype expressed by their tumors. N Engl J Med 1992;327:1209.
119. Ladisch S. Tumor gangliosides: shedding, structural characterization and immunosuppressive activity. In Gangliosides and Cancer. Edited by HF Oettgen. New York: VCH Publishers, 1989, p 219.
120. Ladisch S, Wu ZL, Feig S, Ulsh L, Schwartz E, Floutsis G, Wiley F, Lenarsky C, Seeger R. Shedding of GD2 gangliosides by human neuroblastoma. Int J Cancer 1987;39: 73.
121. Laucius JF, Bodurtha AJ, Mastrangelo MJ, Bellet RE. A phase II study of autologous irradiated tumor cells plus BCG in patients with metastatic malignant melanoma. Cancer 1977;40:2091.
122. Leong SPL. Detection of human malignant melanoma antigens by immunofluorescence and autologous postimmune antimelamona sera. Ann NY Acad Sci 1983;420: 237.
123. Leventhal BG, LePourheit A, Halterman RH, Henderson ES, Herberman RB. Immunotherapy in previously treated acute lymphatic leukemia. NCI Monogr 1973;39: 177.
124. Levy NL, Mahaley MS Jr, Day ED. Serum-mediated blocking of cell-mediated antitumor immunity in a melanoma patient: association with BCG immunotherapy and clinical deterioration. Int J Cancer 1972;10:244.
125. Levitsky JW, Simmons H, Vogelstein B, Frost P. Interleukin-2 production by tumor cell bypasses T helper function in the generation of an antitumor response. Cell 1990;60: 397.
126. Lewis MG, Phillips TM, Cook KB, Blake J. Possible explanation for loss of detectable antibody in patients with disseminated malignant melanoma. Nature (Lond) 1971; 232:52.
126a. Li J, Henn M, Oratz RF, Bystryn JC. The antibody response to immunization to a polyvalent melanoma antigen vaccine. J Clin Res 1990;38:660A.
127. Lieberman R, Wybran J, Epstein W. The immunologic and histopathologic changes of BCG-mediated tumor regression in patients with malignant melanoma. Cancer 1975;35:756.
127a. Livingston P. Active specific immunotherapy in the treatment of patients with cancer. Immunol Allergy Clin North Am 1991;11:401.
127b. Livingston PO. Approaches to augmenting the IgG antibody response to melanoma ganglioside vaccines. Ann NY Acad Sci 1993;690:204.
128. Livingston PO. The basis for ganglioside vaccines in melanoma. In Human Tumor Antigens and Specific Tumor Therapy: UCLA Symposia on Molecular and Cellular Biology, vol 99. Edited by RS Metzgar and MS Mitchell. New York: Alan Liss, 1989, p 287.
129. Livingston PO, Albino AP, Chung TJC, Real FX, Houghton AN, Oettgen HF, Old LJ. Serological response of melanoma patients to vaccines prepared from VSV lysates of autologous and allogeneic cultured melanoma cells. Cancer 1985;55:713.
130. Livingston PO, Calves MJ, Natoli EJ. Approaches to augmenting the immunogenicity of the ganglioside GM2 in mice: purified GM2 is superior to whole cells. J Immunol 1987;138:1524.
131. Livingston PO, Kaelin K, Pinsky CM, Oettgen HR, Old LJ. The serological response of patients with stage II melanoma to allogeneic melanoma cell vaccines. Cancer 1985; 56:2194.
132. Livingston PO, Natoli EJ, Calves MJ, Stockert E, Oettgen HF, Old LJ. Vaccines containing purified GM2 ganglioside elicit GM2 antibodies in melanoma patients. Proc Natl Acad Sci USA 1987;84:2911.
133. Livingston PO, Takeyama H, Pollack MS, Houghton A, Albino A, Oettgen HF, Old LJ. Serological responses of melanoma patients to vaccines derived from allogeneic cultured melanoma cells. Int J Cancer 1983;31:567.
134. Livingston PO, Watanabe T, Shiku H, Houghton AN, Albino A, Takahashi T, Resnick LA, Pinsky CM, Oettgen HF, Old LJ. Serological response of melanoma patients receiving melanoma cell vaccines: 1. Autologous cultured melanoma cells. Int J Cancer 1982;30:413.
135. Lokich JJ, Garnick MB, Legg M. Intralesional immune therapy: methanol extraction residue of BCG or purified protein derivative. Oncology 1979;36:236.
135a. Lopez-Nevot MA, Garcia E, Romero C, Oliva MR, Serrano S, Garrido F. Phenotypic and genetic analysis of HLA class I and HLA-DR antigen expression on human melanomas. Exp Clin Immunogenet 1988;5:203.
136. Ludwig G, Jentzsch R, Nuri M. Spontanregression von Lungenmetastasen beim Hypernephroma Med Klin 1978;21:173.
137. Mahaley MS Jr, Bigner DD, Dudka LF, Wilds PR, Williams DH, Bouldin TW, Whitaker JN, Bynum JM. Immunobiology of primary intracranial tumors. Part 7: Active immunization of patients with anaplastic human glioma cells: a pilot study. J Neurosurg 1983;59:201.
138. Mahaley MS Jr, Gillespie GY, Gillespie RP, Watkins PJ, Bigner DD, Wikstrand CJ, MacQueen JM, Sanfilippo F. Immunobiology of primary intracranial tumors. Part 8: Serological responses to active immunization of patients with anaplastic gliomas. J Neurosurg 1983;59:208.
139. Marcove RC. A clinical trial of autogenous vaccines in the treatment of osteogenic sarcoma. In Investigation and Stimulation of Immunity in Cancer Patients. Edited by G Mathe and R Weiner. New York: Springer-Verlag, 1974, p 488.
140. Marcove RC, Southam CM, Levin A, Mike V, Huvos A. A clinical trial of autogenous vaccine in osteogenic sarcoma in patients under the age of twenty-five. Surg Forum 1971;22:434.
141. Mastrangelo MJ, Bellet RE, Berkelhammer J, Clark WH Jr. Regression of pulmonary metastatic disease associated with intra-lesional BCG therapy of intracutaneous melanoma metastases. Cancer 1975;36:1305.
142. Mastrangelo MJ, Berd D, Maguire HC. Current condition and prognosis of tumor immunotherapy: a second opinion. Cancer Treat Rep 1984;68:207.
143. Mastrangelo MJ, Sulit HL, Prehn LM, Bornstein RS, Yarbo JW, Prehn RT. Intralesional BCG in the treatment of metastatic malignant melanoma. Cancer 1976;37:684.
144. Mathe G, Amiel JL, Schwarzenberg L. Active immunotherapy for acute lymphoblastic leukaemia. Lancet 1969;1:697.
145. Mathe G, Pouillart P, Schwarzenberg L, Amiel JL, Schneider M, Hayat M, De Vassal F, Jasmin C, Rosenfeld C, Weiner R, Rappaport H. Attempts at immunotherapy of 100 patients with acute lymphoid leukemia: Some factors influencing results. NCI Monogr 1972;35:361.
146. Mathe G, Schwarzenberg L, de Vassal F, Delgado M, Pena-Angulo J, Belpomme D, Pouillart P, Machover D, Misset JL, Pico JL, Jasmin C, Hayat M, Schneider M, Cattan A, Amiel JL, Musset M, Rosenfeld C. Chemotherapy followed by active immunotherapy (A.I.) in the treatment of acute lymphoid leukemias (A.L.L.) for patients of all ages. In Immunotherapy of Cancer: Present Status of Trials in Man. Edited by WD Terry and E Windhorst. New York: Raven, 1978, p 451.
147. McCune CS, Marquis DM. Interleukin I as an adjuvant for active specific immunotherapy in a murine tumor model. Cancer Res 1990;50:1212.
148. McCune CS, Patterson WB, Henshaw EC. Active specific immunotherapy with tumor cells and *Corynebacterium parvum:* a phase I study. Cancer 1979;43:1619.
149. McCune CS, Schapira DV, Henshaw EC. Specific immunotherapy of advanced renal carcinoma: evidence for polyclonality of metastases. Cancer 1981;47:1984.
149a. MacLean GD, Bowen-Yacyshyn MB, Samuel J, Meikle A, Stuart G, Nation J, Poppema S, Jerry M, Koganty R, Wong T, Longenecker BM. Active immunization of human ovarian cancer patients against a common carcinoma (Thomsen-Friedenreich) determinant using a synthetic carbohydrate antigen. J Immunother 1992;11: 292.
149b. MacLean GD, Reddish M, Koganty RR, Wong T, Gandhi S, Smolenski M, Samuel J, Nabholtz JM, Longenecker BM. Immunization of breast cancer patients using a synthetic sialyl-Tn glycoconjugate plus DETOX adjuvant. Cancer Immunol Immunother 1993;36:215.
149c. Mehigan JT, Gray BK, Morton DL. Serum cytotoxic antibody in human sarcoma following autologous cellular immunotherapy. Surg Forum 1971;22:108.
150. Miescher S, Whiteside TL, Carrel S, von Fliedner V. Functional properties of tumor-infiltrating and blood lymphocytes in patients with solid tumors: effect of tumor cells and their supernatants on proliferative responses of lymphocytes. J Immunol 1986; 136:1899.
151. Miller BE, Miller FR, Leith J, Heppner GH. Growth interaction in vivo between tumor subpopulations derived from a single mouse mammary tumor. Cancer Res 1980;40: 3977.
152. Miller GA, Pontes JE, Huber RP, Goldrosen MH. Humoral immune response of patients receiving specific active immunotherapy for renal cell carcinoma. Cancer Res 1985;45:4478.
153. Minden P. Shared antigens between animal and human tumors and microorganisms. In BCG in Cancer Immunotherapy. Edited by G Lamoureux, R Turcotte and V Portelance. New York: Grune & Stratton, 1976, p 73.
154. Minten JP. Mumps virus and BCG vaccine in metastatic melanoma. Arch Surg 1973; 106:503.
155. Mitchell MS, Kan-Mitchell J, Kempf RA, Harel W, Shau H, Lind S. Active specific im-

munotherapy for melanoma: phase I trial of allogeneic lysates and a novel adjuvant. Cancer Res 1988;48:5883.
155a. Mitchell MS, Harel W, Kan-Mitchell J, LeMay LG, Goedegebuure P, Huang XQ, Hofman F, Groshen S. Active specific immunotherapy of melanoma with allogeneic cell lysates: rationale, results and possible mechanisms of action. Ann NY Acad Sci 1993; 690:153.
155b. Morioka N, Kikumoto Y, Hoon DSB, Morton DL, Irie RF. Cytotoxic T cell recognition of a human melanoma derived peptide with a carboxyl-terminal alanine-proline sequence. Mol Immunol 1995;32:573-581.
156. Moertel CG, Ritts RE Jr, Schutt AJ, Hahn RG. Clinical studies of methanol extraction residue fraction of bacillus Calmette-Guerin as an immunostimulant in patients with advanced cancer. Cancer Res 1975;35:3075.
156a. Moore GE, Germen RE. Cancer immunity—hypothesis and clinical trial of lymphocytotherapy for malignant diseases. Ann Surg 1970;172:733.
157. Morton DL. Immunotherapy of human melanomas and sarcomas. JNCI 1972;35:375.
158. Morton DL. Cancer immunotherapy: an overview. Semin Oncol 1974;1:297.
159. Morton DL. Changing concepts of cancer surgery: surgery as immunotherapy. Am J Surg 1978;135:367.
160. Morton DL. Active immunotherapy against cancer: present status. Semin Oncol 1986; 13:180.
161. Morton DL, Eilber FR, Holmes EC, Hunt JS, Ketcham AS, Silverstein MJ, Sparks FC. BCG immunotherapy of malignant melanoma: summary of a seven year experience. Ann Surg 1974;180:635.
162. Morton DL, Eilber FR, Holmes EC, Sparks FC, Ramming KP. Present status of BCG immunotherapy of malignant melanoma. Cancer Immunol Immunother 1976;1:93.
163. Morton DL, Eilber FR, Malmgren RA, Wood WC. Immunological factors which influence response to immunotherapy in malignant melanoma. Surgery 1970;68:158.
163a. Morton DL, Foshag LJ, Hoon DSB, Nizze A, Famatiga E, Wanek LA, Chang C, Davtyan DG, Gupta RG, Elashoff R, Irie RF. Prolongation of survival in metastatic melanoma after active specific immunotherapy with a new polyvalent melanoma vaccine. Ann Surg 1992;216:463.
164. Morton DL, Foshag LJ, Nizze JA, Gupta RK, Famatiga E, Hoon DSB, Irie RF. Active specific immunotherapy in malignant melanoma. Semin Surg Oncol 1989;5:420.
165. Morton DL, Holmes EC, Eilber FR, Ramming KP. Adjuvant immunotherapy of malignant melanoma: results of a randomized trial in patients with lymph node metastases. In Immunotherapy of Human Cancer. Edited by WD Terry and SA Rosenberg. New York: Excerpta Medica, 1982, p 245.
166. Morton DL, Holmes EC, Eilber FR, Wood WC. Immunological aspects of neoplasia: a rational basis for immunotherapy. Ann Intern Med 1971;74:587.
167. Morton DL, Hoon DSB, Gupta RG, Nizze AJ, Famatiga E, Foshag LJ, Furutani S, Irie RF. Treatment of malignant melanoma by active specific immunotherapy in combination with biological response modifiers. In New Horizons of Tumor Immunotherapy. Edited by M Torisu and T Yoshida. New York: Elsevier, 1989, p 665.
167a. Morton DL, Hoon DSB, Nizze JA, Foshag LJ, Famatiga E, Wanek LA, Chang C, Irie RF, Gupta RK, Elashoff R. Polyvalent melanoma vaccine improves survival of patients with metastatic melanoma. Ann NY Acad Sci 1993;690:120.
168. Morton DL, Hunt KK, Bauer RL, Lee JD. Immunotherapy by active immunization of the host using mono-specific agents. In Biologic Therapy of Cancer. Edited by VT DeVita, Jr, S Hellman, and SA Rosenberg. Philadelphia: JB Lippincott, 1991, p 627.
169. Morton DL, Joseph WL, Ketcham AS, Geedhold GW, Adkins PC. Surgical resection and adjunctive immunotherapy for selected patients with pulmonary metastasis. Ann Surg 1973;178:1118.
170. Morton DL, Nizze JA, Gupta RK, Famatiga E, Hoon DSB, Irie RF. Active specific immunotherapy of malignant melanoma. In Current Status of Cancer Control and Immunobiology Edited by JP Kim, BS Kim, and JG Park. Seoul: 1987, p 152.
171. Morton DL, Wells SA Jr. Immunobiology of neoplastic disease. In Christopher's Text Book of Surgery. Edited by DC Sabiston. Philadelphia: Saunders, 1972, p 542.
172. Murphy S, Hersh E. Human leukemia. In Clinical Immunotherapy. Edited by AF LuBuglio. New York: Marcel Dekker, 1980, p 73.
172a. Nabel GJ, Nabel EG, Yang ZY, Fox BA, Plautz GE, Gao X, Huang L, Shu S, Gordon D, Chang AE. Direct gene transfer with DNA-liposome complexes in melanoma: expression, biologic activity, and lack of toxicity in humans. Proc Natl Acad Sci USA 1993;90:11307.
173. Nathanson L. Regression of intradermal malignant melanoma after intralesional injection of *Mycobacterium bovis* strain BCG. Cancer Chemother Rep 1972;56:659.
174. Nathanson L, Schoenfeld D, Regelson W, Colsky J, Mittelman A. Prospective comparison of intralesional and multipuncture BCG in recurrent intradermal melanoma. Cancer 1979;46:1640.
175. Neidhart JA, Murphy SG, Hennick LA, Wise HA. Active specific immunotherapy of stage IV renal carcinoma with aggregated tumor antigen adjuvant. Cancer 1980;46: 1126.
176. Nowell PC. Mechanisms of tumor progression. Cancer Res 1986;46:2203.
177. Oettgen HF. Immunotherapy of cancer. N Engl J Med 1977;297:484.
178. Oldham RK. Biologicals and biological response modifiers: fourth modality of cancer treatment. Cancer Treat Rep 1984;68:221.
179. Oratz R, Cockrell C, Speyer JL, Harris M, Roses D, Bystryn J-C. Induction of tumor-infiltrating lymphocytes in human malignant melanoma metastases by immunization to melanoma antigen vaccine. J Biol Response Mod 1989;8:355.
180. Otten J. Immunotherapy of Cancer: Present Status of Trials in Man. Edited by WD Terry and D Windhorst. New York: Raven, 1977.
180a. Pardoll DM. Paracrine cytokine adjuvants in cancer immunotherapy. Ann Rev Immunol 1995;13:399.
181. Patillo RA. Immunotherapy and chemotherapy of gynecologic cancers. Am J Obstet Gynecol 1976;124:808.
182. Pimm MV, Baldwin RW. Antigenic differences between primary methylcholanthrene-induced rat sarcoma and post-surgical recurrences. Int J Cancer 1977;20:37.
183. Pinsky CM, DeJager RL, Whittes RE, Wong PP, Kaufman RJ, Mike V, Hansen JA, Oettgen HF, Krakoff IH. *Corynebacterium parvum* as adjuvant to combination chemotherapy in patients with advanced breast cancer: preliminary results of a prospective randomized trial. In Immunotherapy of Cancer: Present Status of Trials in Man. Edited by WD Terry and D Windhorst. New York: Raven, 1978, p 647.
184. Pinsky CM, Hirshaut Y, Oettgen HF. Treatment of malignant melanoma by intratumoral injection of BCG. NCI Monogr 1973;39:225.
185. Plesnicar S, Rudolf Z. Combined BCG and irradiation treatment of skin metastases originating from malignant melanoma. Cancer 1982;50:1100.
186. Poplack DG, Graw RG, Pomeroy TC, Henderson ES, Leventhal BG. Chemotherapy (CT) versus chemotherapy and immunotherapy (CT + IMT) in childhood acute lymphatic leukemia (ALL). Proc Am Soc Clin Oncol 1975;16:230.
187. Portoukalian J. Immunoregulatory activity of gangliosides shed by melanoma tumors. In Gangliosides and Cancer. Edited by HF Oettgen. New York: VCH Publishers, 1989, p 209.
188. Portoukalian J, Zwinglestein G, Abdul-Malek N, Dore JF. Alteration of gangliosides in plasma and red cells of human bearing melanoma tumors. Biochem Biophys Res Commun 1978;85:916.
188a. Portoukalian J, Carrel S, Dore JF, Rumke P. Humoral immune response in disease-free advanced melanoma patients after vaccination with melanoma-associated gangliosides: EORTC Cooperative Melanoma Group. Int J Cancer 1991;49:893.
189. Powles RL. Immunologic maneuvers in the management of acute leukemia. Med Clin North Am 1976;60:463.
190. Powles RL, Crowther D, Bateman CJT, Beard MEJ, McElwain TJ, Russel J, Lister TA, Whitehouse JMA, Wrigley PFM, Pike M, Alexander P, Hamilton-Fairley G. Immunotherapy for acute myelogenous leukaemia. Br J Cancer 1973;28:365.
191. Prager MD, Baechtel FS, Peters PC, Brown GL, Greene CL. Specific immunotherapy of human metastatic renal cell carcinoma. Proc Am Assoc Cancer Res 1981;22:163.
192. Rahman AFR, Liao SK, Dent P. Characterization of human malignant melanoma cell lines: VII. Glycoprotein synthesis and shedding as revealed by (3H) glucosamine labelling. In Vitro. 1977;13:580.
193. Ratliff TL, Kavoussi LR, Catalona WJ. Role of fibronectin in intravesical BCG therapy for superficial bladder cancer. J Urol 1988;139:410.
193a. Ravindranath MH, Brazeau SM, Morton DL. Efficacy of tumor cell vaccine after incorporating monophosphoryl lipid A (MPL) in tumor cell membranes containing tumor-associated ganglioside. Experientia 1994;50:648–653.
193b. Ravindranath MH, Guenther M, Kunnath S, Nizze A, Famatiga E, Morton DL. Anti-ganglioside IgM responses to a new melanoma cell vaccine (MCV) in melanoma patients. Proc Am Assoc Cancer Res 1993;84:2915.
194. Ravindranath MH, Irie RF. Gangliosides as antigens of human melanoma. In Malignant Melanoma: Biology, Diagnosis and Therapy. Edited by L Nathanson. Boston: Kluwer Academic, 1988, p 14.
195. Ravindranath MH, Morton DL, Irie RF. An epitope common to gangliosides O-AcGD3 and GD3 recognized by antibodies in melanoma patients after active specific immunotherapy. Cancer Res 1989;49:3891.
195a. Ravindranath MH, Morton DL, Irie RF. Attachment of monophosphoryl lipid A (MPL) to cells and liposomes augments antibody response to membrane-bound gangliosides. J Autoimmun 1994;7:803.
196. Ravindranath MH, Paulson JC, Irie RF. Human melanoma associated antigen *O*-acetylganglioside GD3 is recognized by cancer antennarius lectin. J Biol Chem 1985; 260:8838.
197. Ravindranath MH, Tsuchida T, Morton DL, Irie RF. Gangliosides GM3 : GD3 ratio as an index for management of melanoma. Cancer 1991;67:1.
198. Reid JW, Perlin E, Oldham RK, Weese JL, Heim W, Mills M, Miller C, Blom J, Green D, Ballinger S, Cannon GB, Law I, Connor R, Herberman RB. Immunotherapy of carcinoma of the lung with intradermal BCG and allogeneic tumor cells. In Immunotherapy of Human Cancer. Edited by WD Terry and SA Rosenberg. New York: Excerpta Medica, 1982, p 147.
198a. Reivinen J, Holthofer H, Miettinen A. *O*-acetyl GD_3 ganglioside in human peripheral blood T-lymphocytes. Int Immunol 1994;6:1409.
199. Reizenstein P, Anderssorn B, Bjorkholm M, Brenning G, Engstedt L, Gahrton G, Hat R, Holm G, Hornsten P, Killander A, Lantz B, Lindemalm Ch, Lockner D, Lonnqvist B, Mellstedt H, Palmblad J, Paul C, Simonsson B, Sjogren A-M, Stalfelt A-M, Uden A-M, Wadman B, Oberg G, Osby E. BCG plus leukemic cell therapy in patients with acute nonlymphoblastic leukemia: effect in groups with high and low remission rates. In Immunotherapy of Human Cancer. Edited by WD Terry and SA Rosenberg. New York: Excerpta Medica, 1982, p 17.
200. Richman SP, Gutterman JU, Hersh EM, Ribi EE. Phase I-II study of intratumor immunotherapy with BCG cell wall skeleton plus P3. Cancer Immunol Immunother 1978; 5:41.
201. Risley EH. The Gilman-Coca vaccine emulsion treatment of cancer. Boston Med Surg J 1911;165:784.
202. Roitt I, Brostoff J, Male D. Immunology. St. Louis: CV Mosby, 1985.
203. Rosenberg SA, Rapp HJ. Intralesional immunotherapy of melanoma with BCG. Med Clin North Am 1976;60:419.
204. Rosenberg SA, Rapp H, Terry WD, Zbar B, Costa J, Seipp C, Simon R. Intralesional BCG therapy of patients with primary stage I melanoma. In Immunotherapy of Human Cancer. Edited by WD Terry and SA Rosenberg. New York: Excerpta Medica, 1982, p 239.
204a. Rosenberg SA. Adoptive immunotherapy for cancer using lymphokine activated killer cells and IL2. In Important Advances in Oncology. Edited by H DeVita and SA Rosenberg. Philadelphia: Lippincott, 1986, p 55.
204b. Rosenberg SA, Spiess P, Lutuvenieve RA. A new approach to the adoptive immunotherapy of cancer with tumor infiltrating lymphocytes. Science 1986;233:1318.
205. Rudowski W. Two cases of spontaneous neoplasm regression extending over many years. Nowotwory 1978;28:173.
205a. Ruiter DJ, Mattijssen V, Broecker EB, Ferrone S. MHC antigens in human melanomas. Semin Cancer Biol 1991;2:35.
206. Sahasrabudhi DM, de Kernion JB, Pontes JE, Ryan DM, O'Donnell RW, Marquis DM, Mudholkar GS, McCune CS. Specific immunotherapy with suppressor function inhibition for metastatic renal cell carcinoma. J Biol Response Mod 1986;5:581.
206a. Savage HE, Rossen RD, Hersh EM, Freedman RS, Bowen JM, Plager C. Antibody development to viral and allogeneic tumor cell-associated antigens in patients with malignant melanoma and ovarian carcinoma treated with lysates of virus-infected cells. Cancer Res 1986;46:2127.
207. Schauer R. Sialic acids. Adv Carbohydr Chem Biochem 1982;40:131.
207a. Schirrmacher V, Hoegen PL. Importance of tumor cell membrane integrity and viability for cytotoxic T lymphocyte activation by cancer vaccines. Vaccine Res 1993;2: 183.
207b. Schmidt W, Schweighoffer T, Herbst E, Maass G, Berger M, Schilcher F, Schaffner G,

Birnstiel ML. Cancer vaccines: the interleukin 2 dosage effect. Proc Natl Acad Sci USA 1995;92:4711.

208. Seigler HF, Buckley CE, Sheppard LD, Horne BJ, Shingleton WW. Adoptive transfer and specific active immunization of patients with malignant melanoma. Ann NY Acad Sci 1976;277:522.
209. Seigler HF, Shingleton WW, Metzgar RS, Buckley CE, Bergoc PM, Miller DS, Fetter BG, Phaup MD. Nonspecific and specific immunotherapy in patients with melanoma. Surgery 1972;72:162.
210. Seigler HF, Shingleton WW, Pickrell KI. Intralesional BCG, intravenous immune lymphocytes and immunization with neuraminidase-treated tumor cells to manage melanoma: a clinical assessment. Plast Reconstr Surg 1975;55:294.
211. Simmons RL, Rios A, Ray PR, Lundgren G. Effect of neuraminidase on growth of a 3-methylcholanthrene-induced fibrosarcoma in normal and immunosuppressed syngeneic mice. JNCI 1971;47:1087.
212. Sinkovics JG. Immunotherapy with viral oncolysates for sarcoma. JAMA 1977;237:869.
213. Skornick Y, Danciger E, Rozin RR, Shinitzky M. Positive skin tests with autologous tumor cells of increased membrane viscosity: first report. Cancer Immunol Immunother 1981;11:93.
214. Skornick YG, Rong GH, Sindelar WF, Richert L, Klausner JM, Rozin RR, Shinitzky M. Active immunotherapy of human solid tumor with autologous cells treated with cholesteryl hemisuccinate: a phase I study. Cancer 1986;58:650.
215. Slingluff CL, Vollmer R, Seigler HF. Stage II malignant melanoma: presentation of a prognostic model and assessment of specific active immunotherapy in 1,273 patients. J Surg Oncol 1988;39:139.
216. Smith GV, Morse PA, Deraps GD, Raju S, Hardy JD. Immunotherapy of patients with cancer. Surgery 1973;74:59.
217. Sokal JE, Aungst CW. Immunization with cultured cell-BCG mixtures. In Investigation of Immunity of Cancer Patients. Edited by G Mathe and R Weiner. New York: Springer Verlag, 1974, p 488.
218. Sopkova B, Kolar V. Intralesional BCG application in malignant melanoma. Neoplasma 1976;23:421.
219. Sorg C, Bruggen J, Seibert E, Macher E. Membrane-associated antigens of human malignant melanoma VI: changes in expression of antigens on cultured melanoma cells. Cancer Immunol Immunother 1978;3:259.
219a. Springer GF, Desai PR, Tegtmeyer H, Spencer BD, Scanion EF. Pancarcinoma T/Tn antigen detects human carcinoma long before biopsy does and its vaccine prevents breast carcinoma recurrence. Ann NY Acad Sci 1993;690:355.
220. Stade BG, Lehmann J, Riethmoller G, Johnson JP. Markers for melanoma progression. J Cancer Res Clin Oncol 1990;166 (suppl.):784.
221. Steel GG. Cell loss from experimental tumours. Cell Tissue Kinet 1968;1:193.
222. Stewart THM, Hollinshead AC, Harris JE, Raman S. Specific active immunotherapy of Stage II lung cancer patients. In Immunotherapy of Cancer. Edited by WD Terry and SA Rosenberg. New York: Excerpta Medica, 1982, p 153.
223. Steward THM, Orizaga M. The presence of delayed hypersensitivity reactions in patients toward cellular extracts of their malignant tissues: 3. The frequency, duration and cross-reactivity of this phenomenon in patients with breast cancer, and its correlation with survival. Cancer 1971;28:1472.
224. Stjernsward J, Levin A. Delayed hypersensitivity-induced regression of human neoplasms. Cancer 1971;28:628.
225. Swanson DA. Systemic treatment for renal cell carcinoma: An overview. In Uro-oncology: Current Status and Future Trends. New York: Wiley-Liss, 1990, p 201.
226. Takita H, Hollinshead AC, Bhayana JN, Edgerton F, Conway D, Moskowitz RM, Adler RH, Ramundo M, Han T, Rao U, Vincent RG, Federico A, Takita L, Smith R. Specific active immunotherapy of squamous cell lung carcinoma. In Immunotherapy of Human Cancer. Edited by WD Terry and SA Rosenberg. New York: Excerpta Medica, 1982, p 159.
227. Takita H, Takada M, Minowada J, Han T, Edgerton F. Adjuvant immunotherapy of stage III lung carcinoma. In Immunotherapy of Cancer: Present Status of Trials in Man. Edited by WD Terry and D Windhorst. New York: Raven, 1978, p 217.
228. Tallberg T, Kalimo T, Halttunen P, Tykka H, Mahlberg K, Matous B, Sundell B. Post-operative active specific immunotherapy with supportive measures in patients suffering from recurrent metastasized melanoma: case reports of six patients. J Surg Oncol 1986;33:115.
229. Tepper RI, Pattengale PK, Leder P. Murine interleukin-4 displays potent anti-tumor activity in vivo. Cell 1989;57:503.
230. Terry WD, Hodes RJ, Rosenberg SA, Fisher RI, Makuch R, Gordon HG, Fisher SG. Treatment of stage I and II malignant melanoma with adjuvant immunotherapy or chemotherapy: preliminary analysis of a prospective randomized trial. In Immunotherapy of Human Cancer. Edited by WD Terry and SA Rosenberg. New York: Excerpta Medica, 1982, p 251.
231. Townsend CM, Eilber FR, Morton DL. Skeletal and soft tissue sarcomas. JAMA 1976;236:2187.
232. Tsuchida T, Ravindranath MH, Saxton RE, Irie RF. Gangliosides of human melanoma: altered expression in vivo and in vitro. Cancer Res 1987;47:1278.
233. Tykka H. Active specific immunotherapy with supportive measures in the treatment of advanced palliatively nephrectomized renal adenocarcinoma: a controlled clinical study. Scand J Urol Nephrol 1981;63:1.
233a. Van der Bruggen P, Traversari C, Chomex P, Lurquin C, De Plaen E, Van den Eynde B, Knuth A, Boon T. A gene encoding an antigen recognized by cytolytic T-lymphocytes on a human melanoma. Science 1991;254:1643.
234. van der Meijden APM, Debruyne FMJ, Steerenberg PA, de Jong WH. Aspects of non-specific immunotherapy with BCG in superficial bladder cancer: an overview. In EORTC Genitourinary Group Monograph 6: BCG in Superficial Bladder Cancer. New York: Alan R. Liss, 1989, p 11.
234a. Uchiyama A, Hoon DSB, Morisaki T, Kaneda Y, Yuzuki DH, Morton DL. Transfection of interleukin 2 gene into human melanoma cells augments cellular immune response. Cancer Res 1993;53:949.
234b. Vadhan-Raj S, Cordon-Cardo C, Carswell E, Mintzer D, Dantis L, Duteau C, Templeton MA, Oettgen HF, Old LJ, Houghton AN. Phase I trial of a mouse monoclonal antibody against GD_3 ganglioside in patients with melanoma: induction of inflammatory responses at the tumor sites. J Clin Oncol 1986;6:1636.
234c. van Duinen SG, Ruiter DJ, Broecker EB, van der Velde EA, Sorg C, Welvaart K, Ferrone S. Level of HLA antigens in locoregional metastases and clinical course of the disease in patients with melanoma. Cancer Res 1988;48:1019.
235. Vaughan JW. Cancer vaccine and anti-cancer globulin as an aid in the surgical treatment of malignancy. JAMA 1914;63:1258.
236. Vlock DR, Kirkwood JM. Serial studies of autologous antibody reactivity to melanoma: relationship to clinical course and circulating immune complexes. J Clin Invest 1985;76:849.
237. von Dungren E. Über Immunitat gegen Geschwulst. Munch Med Wschr 1909;56:1099.
238. von Leyden VE, Blumenthal F. Vorlautige Mitteilungen ubber einige Ergebnisse der Krebsforschung auf der 1. medizinischen Klinik Dt Med Wschr 1902;28:637.
239. Vosika GJ. Clinical immunotherapy trials of bacterial components derived from Mycobacteria and Nocardia. J Biol Res Mod 1983;2:321.
240. Vosika GJ, Schmidtke JR, Goldman A, Parker R, Gray GR. Intralesional immunotherapy of malignant melanoma with *Mycobacterium smegmatis* cell wall skeleton combined with trehalose dimycolate (P3). Cancer 1979;44:495.
241. Wallack MK. Specific immunotherapy with vaccinia oncolysates. Cancer Immunol Immunother 1981;12:1.
242. Wallack MK, Bash J, Leftheriotis E, Seigler H, Bland K, Wanebo H, Balch C, Bartolucci AA. Positive relationship of clinical and serologic responses to vaccinia melanoma oncolysate. Arch Surg 1987;122:1460.
243. Wallack MK, McNally K, Leftheriotis E, Seigler H, Balch C, Wanebo H, Bartolucci AA, Bash JA. A Southeastern Cancer Study Group phase I/II trial with vaccinia melanoma oncolysates. Cancer 1986;57:649.
244. Wallack MK, Meyer M, Bourgoin A, Dore JF, Leftheriotis E, Carcagne J, Koprowski H. A preliminary trial of vaccinia oncolysates in the treatment of recurrent melanoma with serologic responses to the treatment. J Biol Response Mod 1983;2:586.
244a. Wallack MK, Sivanandham M. Clinical trials with VMO for melanoma. Ann NY Acad Sci 1993;690:178.
244b. Wallack M, Sivanandham M, Balch C, Urist M, Murray D, Bartolucci A, Rosen L. A phase III randomized multi-institutional double blind adjuvant study of vaccinia melanoma oncolysate (VMO) versus vaccinia (V) alone in stage II melanoma. Proc Am Soc Clin Oncol 1994;13:1352.
244c. Wallack M, Sivanandham M, Balch CM, Urist MM, Bland KI, Murray D, Robinson WA, Flaherty LE, Richards WA, Bartolucci AA, Rosen L. A phase III randomized, double-blind multi-institutional trial of vaccinia melanoma oncolysate-active specific immunotherapy for patients with stage II melanoma. Cancer 1995;75:34.
244d. Wallack MK, Steplewski Z, Koprowski H, Rosato E, George J, Hulihan B, Johanson J. A new approach in specific, active immunotherapy. Cancer 1977;39:560.
244e. Watanabe Y, Kuribayashi K, Miyatake S, Nishihara K, Nakayama E, Taniyama T, Sakata T. Exogenous expression of mouse interferon-gamma cDNA in mouse neuroblastoma C1300 cells results in reduced tumorigenicity by augmented anti-tumor immunity. Proc Natl Acad Sci USA 1989;86:9456.
245. Weisenburger TH, Jones PC, Ahn SC, Irie RF, Juillard GJF. Active specific intralymphatic immunotherapy in metastatic malignant melanoma: evidence of clinical response. J Biol Response Mod 1982;1:57.
246. Welt S, Carswell EA, Vogel CW, Oettgen HF, Old LJ. Immune and nonimmune effector functions of IgG_3 mouse monoclonal antibody R24 detecting the disialoganglioside GD_3 on the surface of melanoma cells. Clin Immunol Immunopathol 1987;45:214.
247. Whiteside MG, Cauchi MN, Paton C, Stone J. Chemoimmunotherapy for maintenance in acute myeloblastic leukemia. Cancer 1976;38:1581.
248. Whiteside TL, Miescher S, Hurlimann J, Moretta L, von Fliedner V. Separation, phenotyping and limiting dilution analysis of lymphocytes infiltrating human solid tumors. Int J Cancer 1986;37:803.
249. Whittaker JA, Bailey-Wood R, Hutchins S. Active immunotherapy for the treatment of acute myelogenous leukemia: the use of intravenous BCG and a comparison between BCG and irradiated leukemic blast cells. In Immunotherapy of Human Cancer. Edited by WD Terry and SA Rosenberg. New York: Excerpta Medica, 1982, p 23.
250. Wile AG, Sparks FC, Morton DL. Monitoring immunotherapy with bacillus Calmette-Guerin by antibody titer. Cancer Res 1977;37:2251.
250a. Wolfel T, Klehmann E, Muller C, Schutt KH, Bucschenfelde MZ, Knuth A. Lysis of human melanoma cells by autologous cytolytic T cell clones: identification of human histocompatibility leukocyte antigen A2 as a restriction element for three different antigens. J Exp Med 1989;170:787.
251. Yamamura Y, Yoshizaki K, Azuma I, Yagura T, Watanabe T. Immunotherapy of human malignant melanoma with oil-attached BCG cell-wall skeleton. Gann 1975;66:355.
251a. Zatloukal K, Schneeberger A, Berger M, Schmidt W, Koszik F, Kutil R, Cotten M, Wagner E, Buschle M, Maass G. et al. Elicitation of a systemic and protective anti-melanoma immune response by an IL-2-based vaccine. Assessment of critical cellular and molecular parameters. J Immunol 1995;154:3406.
252. Zbar B. Tumor regression mediated by *Mycobacterium bovis* (strain BCG). NCI Monogr 1972;35:341.
253. Zbar B, Bernstein ID, Bartlett GL, Hanna MG Jr, Rapp HJ. Immunotherapy of cancer: regression of intradermal tumors and prevention of growth of lymph node metastases after intralesional injection of living *Mycobacterium bovis*. JNCI 1972;49:119.
254. Zbar B, Ribi E, Rapp HJ. An experimental model for immunotherapy for cancer. NCI Monogr 1973;39:3.
255. Zbar B, Tanaka T. Immunotherapy of cancer: regression of tumors after intralesional injection of living *Mycobacterium bovis*. Science 1971;172:271.

CHAPTER 80

Interferons

ERNEST C. BORDEN

Introduction

Interferons (IFNs) are now licensed worldwide as therapeutic agents for cancer and also as antivirals and for multiple sclerosis. IFNs have been a prototype for dissecting biologic and clinical effects of cytokines. Like other cytokines, IFNs are a family of molecules that includes more than 20 different proteins coded on human chromosome 9 (except IFN-γ on chromosome 12). Cellular action follows binding to a relatively small (<2000/cell) number of high affinity receptors. Positive and negative nuclear regulatory proteins that modulate gene expression, resulting in production of induced proteins, have been identified. Cellular proteins induced by IFNs underlie the pleiotropic biologic effects, which include virus inhibition, immunomodulation, slowing of cell proliferation, oncogene suppression, angiogenesis inhibition, and alterations in differentiation. However, which cellular proteins result in the various biologic and therapeutic effects remain undefined as do cellular mechanisms of antitumor action.

In more than a dozen cancers, IFNs result in regression or control of disease process (Table 80.1). As part of combinations, IFNs are now establishing their roles as curative therapies. The spectrum of single-agent activity of IFNs compares favorably with other systemic antitumor modalities. Like many other drugs, IFNs are more active against hematologic malignancies than solid tumors. Antitumor effects of IFNs can be enhanced in experimental tumor models when given with cytotoxic compounds, radiation, and other biologicals.

Molecules: Their Induction, Receptors, and Gene Regulation

IFNs are a family of proteins, each residing at a specific genetic locus. Three major classes of IFNs (α, β, γ) were initially defined on the basis of chemical, antigenic, and biologic differences. These have now been confirmed to result from significant differences in primary amino acid sequence. With the advances in molecular biology and sequencing technology, complete nucleotide sequences for more than 15 human IFNs have been defined (142, 159, 203). Human IFN-α and IFN-β are structurally similar and located on chromosome 9. Both IFN-α and IFN-β are 166 amino acids in length with an additional 20-amino acid secretory peptide present on the amino-terminal end. Comparison of the sequences of IFN-α and IFN-β has defined approximately 45% homology of nucleotides and 29% homology of amino acids. Each of the nonallelic human IFN-α genes differ by approximately 10% in nucleotide sequence and 15 to 25% in amino acid sequence (Table 80.2). IFN-γ, 143 amino acids in length, is located on chromosome 12 and also contains a 20-amino acid secretory peptide (68). IFN-γ has only minimal sequence homology with IFN-α or IFN-β (Table 80.2). A fourth IFN class, Ω, has recently been defined (1, 31). Although IFN-β and IFN-γ, produced by eukaryotic cells, are glycosylated, biologic differences from the unglycosylated proteins produced in *E. coli* have not yet been identified. All IFNs have the defining biologic effect of induction of cellular resistance to replication of both RNA and DNA viruses.

IFN INDUCTION

Conceptually, it is important to distinguish IFN production and action (Fig. 80.1) Viruses remain the prototypic producer of IFN-α and IFN-β. All body cells probably have the capacity to produce IFN-α and IFN-β. IFN-γ was identified after exposure of lymphocytes to mitogens or sensitized lymphocytes to specific antigens. Interleukin-2 (IL-2), TNF, and IL-12, a 15-kd protein induced by IFN-α and IFN-β, are also potent inducers of IFN-γ, under some circumstances resulting in substantial IFN titers (33, 93, 125, 172, 234). Production of IFNs are part of host defense mechanisms for response to pathogens and neoplasia. Experimental suppression of IFN production in mice results in increased lethality from both tumors and viruses (72, 74).

Molecular mechanisms underlying cellular production of IFNs have been partially dissected by use of a series of promoter sequence mutations. Positive and negative nuclear regulatory proteins have been identified (131, 213). The codon sequences for control of production of IFN-β consist of two separable positive domains and an overlapping negative control sequence. In uninduced cells, the IFN-β gene is suppressed by a protein repressor, which blocks interaction with one of two positive IFN regulatory elements. Virus exposure results in inactivation or displacement of the repressor and subsequent binding of activated transcriptional regulatory proteins to both positive regulatory domains.

The first chemically defined inducer of IFNs were double-stranded polyribonucleotides, which are potent IFN inducers

Table 80.1. Interferons: Current Status

- Pivotol regulation of gene transcription
- Biologic response modulatory effects defined in man
- Phase II antitumor activity confirmed in more than 12 human cancers
- Phase III trials demonstrate improved survival with combined modality therapies

Table 80.2. The Family of Interferon Molecules

Family	Interferon families			
	Chr (Hu)	Types (n)	Amino acids	
			N	Homology[a] %
Alpha[b]	9	>14	165–166	75–85
Beta	9	1	166	30
Gamma	12	1	143	1
Omega	9	>1	173	50

[a] Compared to IFNα.
[b] The IFN, licensed for clinical use and produced by recombinant DNA technology, is IFN α2. IFN α2a (Hoffmann LaRoche) differs from IFN α2b (Schering-Plough) by a single amino acid at amino acid 23 (lysine in IFN α2a; arginine in IFN α2b). IFN α2 is 165 amino acids, with a deletion at amino acid 44 of an aspartate residue. Chv (Hu) = Human chromosome on which gene is found.

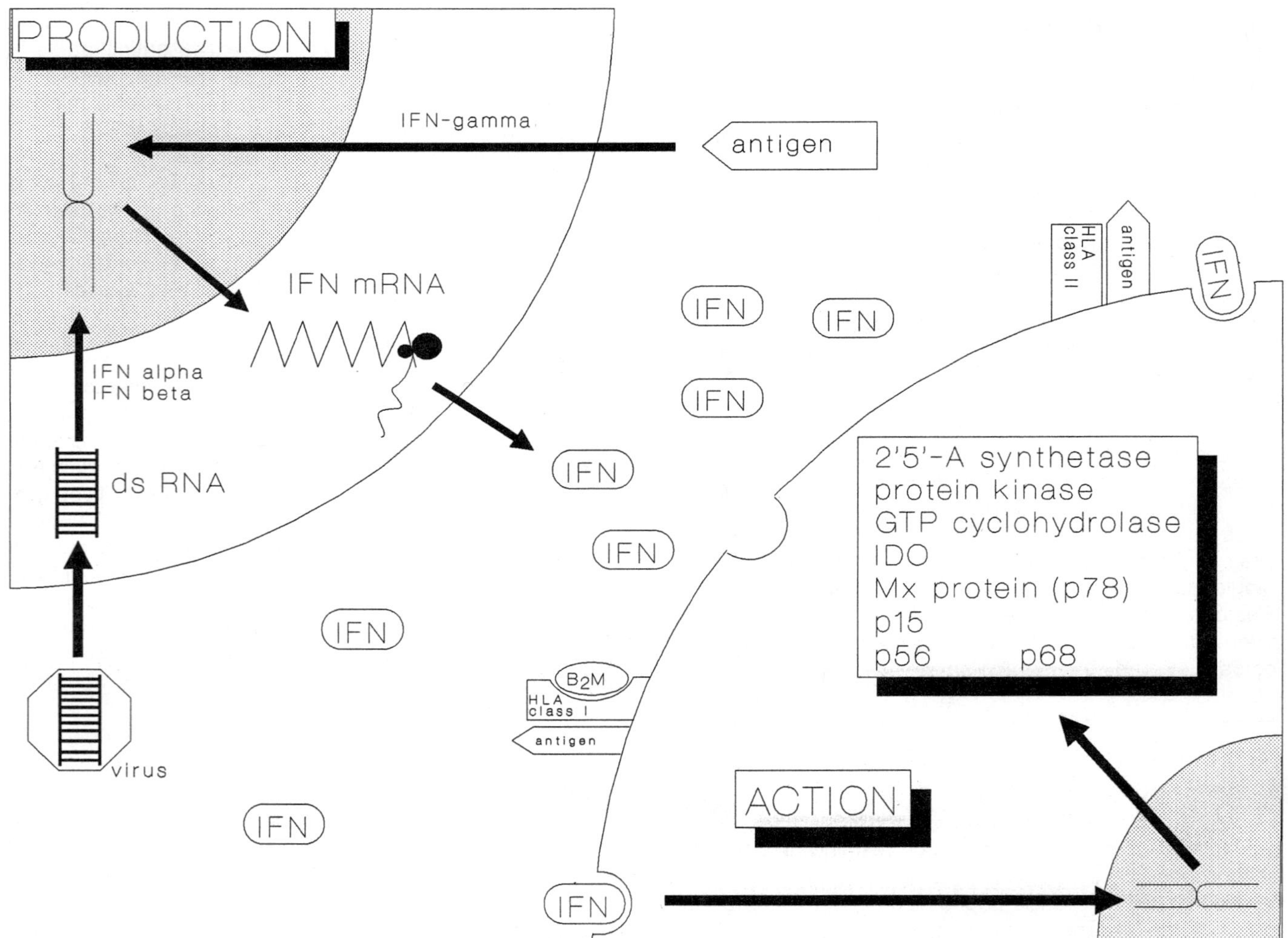

Figure 80.1. Production of IFN α or IFN β is stimulated by viruses through a final common pathway of double-stranded RNA or, in the case of IFN-γ, exposure to specific antigens. Action of IFNs is mediated via binding to a specific receptor on the cell surface with induction of cell surface (HLA classes I and II, β2 microglobulin, tumor-associated antigens) and intracellular (2–5A synthetase, protein kinase, GTP cyclohydrolase, indoleamine dioxygenase, and other proteins of unidentified function) proteins that mediate biologic effects.

and immunomodulators in mice. Polyriboadenylate:polyribouridylic acid may have a clinically useful therapeutic index (20, 114, 233). Low molecular weight organic inducers of IFNs, which include tilorone, halopyrimidinones, acridines, substituted quinolines, and flavone acetic acid, have been identified in different animal species. In addition to IFN production, these molecules are also immunomodulators. Several low molecular weight inducers have been introduced into clinical trial (44, 124, 178, 217). Orally active inducers, such as the acridines, halopyrimidinones, or substituted quinolines, would be convenient and useful not only for therapeutic purposes but also as chemopreventive agents (20). Clinical effectiveness of halopyrimidinones has begun to be established for low grade transitional carcinomas of the bladder (185).

RECEPTORS

The cellular response to IFNs only requires the interaction of a small number of molecules with high affinity, species-specific multimeric cell surface receptors. Interferon receptors (usually 2×10^2 to 2×10^3 high affinity sites/cell) have been found on the surface of most cells, although cell lines without receptors have been identified. IFN-α and IFN-β share and compete for the same receptor, although IFN-β binds with higher affinity (4, 22, 182). One or more species-specific protein components cooperate with IFN receptors to confer species restrictions and mediate biologic effects (146, 194, 218). Binding of IFN-β to the nuclear membrane has also been observed (111). The gene for the receptor for human IFN-α and IFN-β is on chromosome 21, while chromosome 6 codes for the human IFN-γ receptor (2, 169, 212). Receptors for IFN-α and IFN-β and for IFN-γ have been cloned and sequenced (2, 219). Although down-regulation of receptors occurs with IFN-α2 administration, neither this event nor receptor number has clearly correlated with therapeutic effects in hematologic malignancies (13, 50).

SIGNAL TRANSDUCTION

Dissecting the pathways leading to activation of genes stimulated by IFNs should lead to greater understanding of the diverse effects of IFNs (virus inhibition, immunomodulation, and oncogene suppression). Over the past 3 years, a

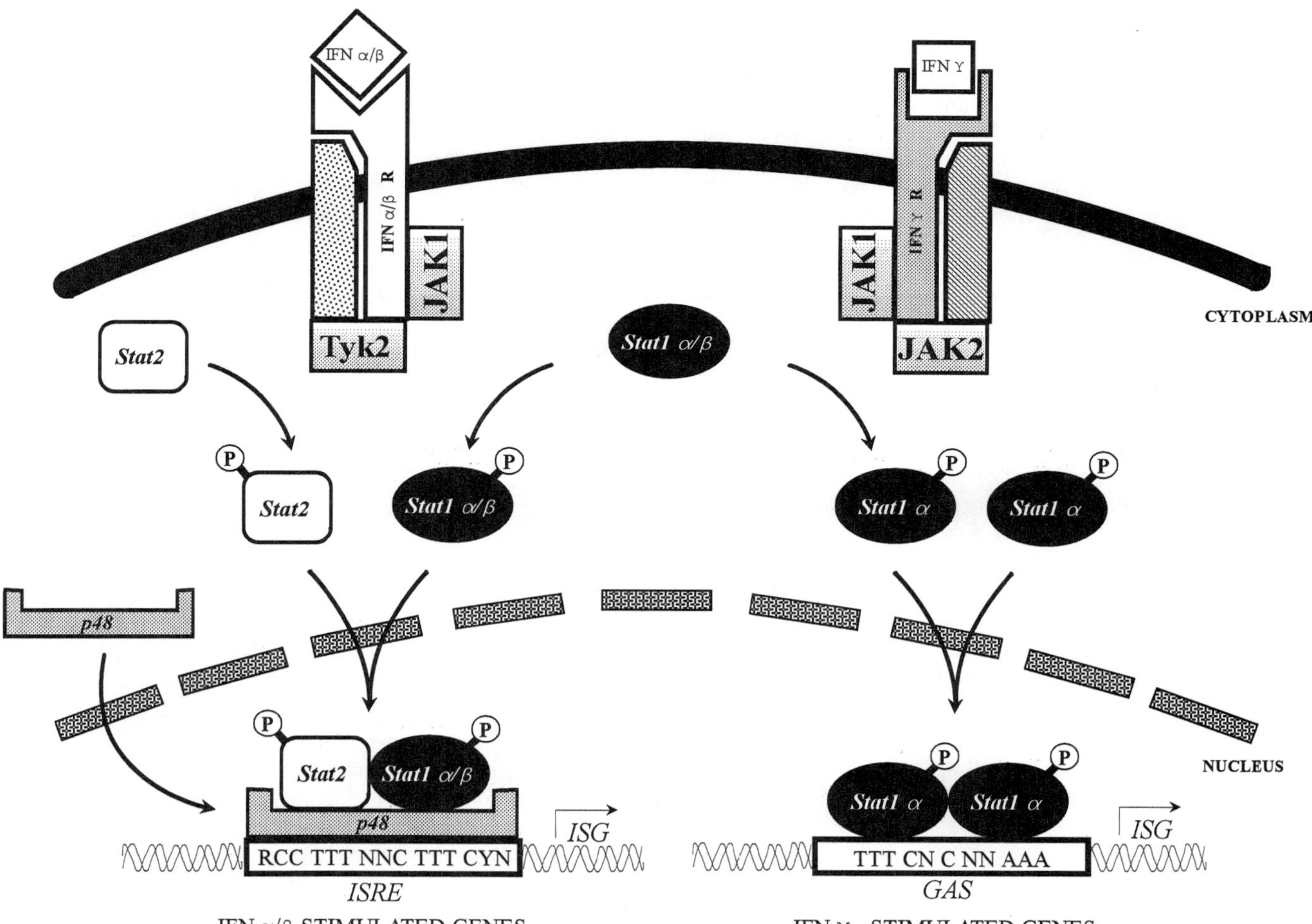

Figure 80.2. Pathway of signal transduction by IFNs. After binding to specific receptors, tyrosine kinase (JAK-1, JAK-2, tyk2) are activated. These tyrosine kinases phosphorylate inactive transcription factors (STAT 1α, STAT 1β, STAT), which form a transcriptional factor, ISGF-3, or STAT 1α dimer. The interferon-stimulated response element (ISRF) or gamma activation site (GAS) has shared nucleotides for all IFN-stimulated genes. N, nucleotide; R, purine; Y, pyrimidine.

combination of biochemical and genetic approaches has led to the identification of a new cellular signal transduction pathway for gene activation. In identifying this novel signal transduction pathway, IFNs have again served as a prototype for probing the action of other cytokines.

After receptor binding specific tyrosine kinases, tyk2 (which is not part of the receptor structure per se), together with one or more additional tyrosine kinases, JAK-1 and JAK-2, is phosphorylated. These activated tyrosine kinases activate the single transducing peptides (58, 158, 228) (Fig. 80.2) and induce the formation of a complex that consists of three protein subunits of a complex (ISGF-3α), ISGF-α is translocated to the nucleus (40, 59, 60, 76, 98, 119). ISGF-3 consists of three proteins (STAT—signed transducers and activators of transcription) 1α, STAT 1β, and STAT 2. The proteins STAT 1α and STAT 1β are alternatively spliced products of the same gene. The STAT 1α protein contains at its carboxyl end 39 additional amino acids to which specific antibodies have been targeted (188). Once phosphorylated, the ISGF-3α complex is translated to the nucleus and forms (with the addition of a fourth subunit, ISGF-3γ) a DNA binding complex specific for the IFN-stimulated response element ISRE, resulting in the activation of IFN-specific genes (40, 59, 60, 76, 98, 119).

The STAT 1α component of the IFN signal transduction pathway is a component of activation of other cytokine genes, epidermal growth factor, and interleukin-6. With receptor activation by ligands, different patterns of factors with distinct DNA binding specificities are induced. Through the differential use of the cytoplasmic protein components, receptors regulate both common and unique sets of genes (116).

Mechanisms of Antitumor Action

IFNs are pleiotropic cellular modulators (Table 80.3). Antitumor effects are postulated to result from either a direct effect on functional capacity or antigenic composition of tumor cells or from an indirect effect on modulation of immune effector cell populations with tumor cell specificities. IFNs regulate gene expression, modulate expression of proteins on the cell surface, and induce synthesis of new enzymes. The alterations in gene expression result in modulation of levels of receptors for other cytokines, concentration of regulatory proteins on the surface of immune effector cells, and activities of enzymes that modulate cellular growth and function. On a cellular basis, these effects translate into alterations of the state of differentiation, rate of proliferation, and functional activity of many cell types.

Table 80.3. Pleiotropic Biologic Effects of Interferons

Microbial inhibition	Immunomodulatory
RNA viruses	Cytotoxicity
DNA viruses	T cell
Intracellular pathogens	NK/LAK cell
Protein induction	Monocytes
Adhesion proteins	Antibody dependent
Enzyme induction	Antigen processing
Cytokines	Vascular
Cell modulation	Angiogenesis inhibition
Ongogene depression	Lipoprotein reduction
Slow mitotic cycle	Antitumor
Differentiation	Mouse
Trophoblastic implantations	Man

BIOLOGIC RESPONSE MODULATION

In probing mechanisms of antitumor action, particular attention has been paid to the immunomodulatory effects of IFNs. IFNs augment the effectiveness of all immune effector cell types that have the potential to kill tumor target cells. These include cytotoxic T-cells, non-major histocompatibility complex (MHC) restricted cytotoxic cells, and monocytes (Table 80.3). Antibody-dependent, cell-mediated cytotoxicity, mediated by subpopulations of these effectors, can also be boosted by IFNs. The ability of IFNs to augment NK cell activity and monocyte function has been demonstrated both in vitro and in vivo (42, 43, 85, 86, 101, 128, 144). Addition of IFNs to NK cells, even those of depressed lytic activity, can result in augmented tumor cell cytotoxicity. Patients given IFNs demonstrate augmented NK cell and monocyte activity 24 to 72 hours after IFN administration. Doses of IFNs lower than that maximally tolerated, indeed as much as 30 to 100-fold lower, have demonstrated maximal NK cell and monocyte augmentation.

In experimental systems, equivalent antitumor effectiveness of IFNs in vivo has been identified for tumor cells sensitive or resistant to antiproliferative effects of IFNs in vitro (11, 175). Additional evidence, supporting a role for host immune effector cell response to IFNs, comes from studies in which mice with Friend leukemia, syngenec tumor, or human prostate and HeLa tumor xenografts received antibody to murine IFN (174). These mice, in the absence of exogenous IFN, experienced enhanced tumor growth and transplantability, suggesting that neutralization of endogenous IFN removes aspects of host defense to tumor (174). However, studies in nude mice with human tumor xenografts have also demonstrated antitumor effects of human IFNs, which demonstrate, in view of the strict species specificity of IFNs, that the direct antiproliferative effects can also limit tumor growth (9, 179).

Host modulatory effects of IFNs are part of the network of cytokine and cellular interactions. Induced gene modulation with subsequent production of specific proteins must underlie immune regulatory effects of IFNs (Table 80.4). IFNs enhance cell surface expression of MHC antigens, tumor-associated antigens (TAA), and Fc receptors. All IFNs augment MHC class I expression, and IFN-γ enhances MHC class II expression on tumor cells as well (10, 19, 51, 99, 157). IFN-β and IFN-γ also increase MHC class I and II expression on monocytes. Increase in MHC expression may enhance monocyte/macrophage antigen-presenting functions. Following IFN-γ, respiratory activity in macrophages has increased with production of toxic oxygen intermediates, such as hydrogen peroxide and superoxide anion (143). Monocytes stimulated by IFNs secrete monokines including colony-stimulating factor, tumor necrosis factor, and IL-1 as well as plasminogen activator, complement, and a

Table 80.4. Modulation of Gene Expression by Interferons

Induced Proteins	
Cell surface proteins	Enzymes and other proteins
Antigen processing	2–5A synthetase[a]
Ring 4	Protein kinase R
Ring 12	Indoleamine dioxygenase[a]
HLA complex	Guanylate-binding proteins[a]
Class I (A, B, C)[a]	Mx protein (p78)[a]
Class II (DR, DP, DQ)[a]	GTP cyclohydrolase[a]
β_2-Microglobulin[a]	Metallothionein II
Invariant chain	Mn^{2+} superoxide dismutase
Tumor-associated antigens	IL-16 (ISG15)
TAB 72	p56
CEA[a]	Transcriptional factors
Adhesion proteins	IRF-1 (ISGF-2)
ICAM-1	IRF2
p16 (Leu-13)	ICSBP
p56	
Depressed functional activities	
Ornithine decarboxylase	
Oncogenes	
c-*myc*, c-Ha-*ras*, c-*fos*, c-*mos*	
p450 microsomal enzymes	

[a] Modulation demonstrated after IFNs in patients in vitro and in vivo.

variety of enzymes and other cytotoxic mediators (5, 199). A maximally tolerated dose of IFNs is not required for all biologic modulatory effects and induction of IFN-induced proteins (19, 129, 231). Clinical investigations are beginning to correlate therapeutic response with induction of these immune response proteins (6, 139).

Enhancement of expression of TAA, such as TAG72 and carcinoembryonic antigens, has both diagnostic and therapeutic implications (15, 70). In vitro and in vivo increase in TAA follows treatment of breast, colon, ovarian, and melanoma cell lines with IFN-α, IFN-β, and IFN-γ (Table 80.4). No increase in TAA occurs on normal cells. Enhanced expression of TAA and HLA classes I and II antigens may lead to improved tumor cell recognition by host immune cells, with resultant enhancement of killing. In addition, accurate localization of primary and metastatic tumor by monoclonal antibodies directed against appropriate TAAs may allow more directed therapy by utilizing monoclonal antibodies as a carrier for radionuclides or cytotoxic agents.

The enzymes 2–5′ oligoadenylate synthetase (2–5A synthetase), a protein kinase (PKR), and indoleamine 2,3-dioxygenase (IDO) are induced by IFNs (Table 80.3) (160, 176). 2–5A synthetase has been shown to transfer a nucleoside 5′ monophosphate to the 2′ position of an accepting chain. 2–5A synthetase is a relatively specific marker of IFN system activation. A latent ribonuclease is activated by 2–5A; the result of induction of these enzymes is in part inhibition of DNA and protein synthesis. The level of the ribonuclease (RNAase L) increased in growth-arrested cells and during cellular differentiation (81, 104). Expression in cells of an enzymatically inactive RNAase L resulted in inhibition of the antiviral and antiproliferative effects of IFNs (81).

A dormant protein kinase with a unique requirement for double-stranded RNA (dsRNA) (PKR) undergoes induction and activation by IFNs (78, 88, 109). The activated enzyme phosphorylates several cellular proteins including protein synthesis initiation factor 2a, which results in cessation of peptide chain initiation (34, 102, 137). The major function of this kinase is growth control; it can also induce apoptosis (34, 118). Cells expressing PKR mutants form colonies in soft agar and upon injection into nude mice produce large tumors (102).

PKR expression may be controlled by an IFN-induced transcriptional factor, IRF-1. Since IRF-1 increased rapidly in growth-arrested cells (80), it may influence expression of genes involved in negative control of cell growth and may mediate antiproliferative effects of IFNs. A second transcription factor, IRF-2, identified in murine cells, has sequence hematology to IRF-1 and is a functional antagonist of IRF-1 (79). Upon constitutive expression, IRF-2 can result in cell transformation, which is inhibited by IRF-1 (80).

The degradation of tryptophan to kynurenine by IDO has been implicated in protein synthesis inhibition and antiproliferative effects as a result of depletion of tryptophan (30, 155, 205, 209, 232). Low tryptophan levels and increased kynurenine excretion have occurred in patients treated with IFNs. Depletion of this essential amino acid may be related to both IFN action and side effects of treatment. Production of neopterin, a metabolite of GTP, is increased in serum following IFNs and is catalyzed by an induced enzyme GTP cyclohydrolase I (89, 113).

Induced proteins and their products can be identified on cells and in serum of treated patients (Table 80.4). Their measurement or the quantitation of immune effector cell function can be used to define biologically active molecules, doses, schedules, and routes of administration. Most biologic response modulatory effects peak at 24 to 48 hours, which contrasts with maximal serum levels in pharmacokinetic studies (65, 136). After intravenous bolus administration, the *t*[u12] of IFN-α2 is short (<60 minutes); mean terminal half-life is 4 to 5 hours with no serum levels measurable at 12 hours. After intramuscular or subcutaneous administration, peak levels are 6 to 10 hours (77, 230). The pharmacologic hallmark of IFN-β is virtual absence of serum levels with subcutaneous or intramuscular administration; yet, biologic response modulatory and therapeutic effects occur (65, 84). These findings suggest that traditional measurements of serum levels may not be the best guide for clinical trial design with IFNs.

ANTIPROLIFERATIVE AND DIFFERENTIATIVE EFFECTS

In addition to immune effector cells, IFNs regulate function and proliferation of somatic cells (Table 80.3). IFNs retard growth and proliferation of tumor cells and normal cells by prolonging the cell cycle. Diploid cells are somewhat less sensitive to the antiproliferative effects of IFNs than are aneuploid cells. Substantial differences exist among normal as well as tumor cells in their sensitivity to direct antiproliferative actions, with some being extremely sensitive and others completely resistant (187, 191, 216). For example, the human lymphoblastoid β-cell lines transformed by Epstein-Barr virus (EBV) are extraordinarily sensitive to the antiproliferative action of IFN-α and IFN-β but not IFN-γ. Another EBV-transformed lymphoblastoid cell line (Namalwa), a vigorous producer of IFN-α subtypes, is essentially resistant to the action of IFNs. IFN-resistant mutant cells can be isolated from IFN-sensitive cell lines. Since the resistant mutants can sometimes retain their antiviral sensitivity (121), resistance is not necessarily due to the reduced number or absence of IFN receptors but points to some other mechanism of resistance.

IFN-α and IFN-β can affect all phases of the cell cycle: M, G_1, and G_2. When fibroblasts are stimulated to grow by serum, epidermal growth factor, insulin, or vasopressin, IFNs cause a prolongation of the G_1 phase, a reduced rate of entry into the S phase and a lengthening of the S and the G_2 phases (8, 195, 198). The cumulative effects of prolongation of the cell cycle of both normal and tumor cells by IFNs results in cytostasis, increase in cell size, and occasionally cell death (62, 161).

IFNs alter differentiation of many cell types. IFN-α, IFN-β, and IFN-γ induced B-cell blast transformation as well as plasmacytoid differentiation in chronic lymphocytic leukemic cells (45, 154). IFN-α and IFN-β induce differentiation of multilineage colony-forming cells in hairy cell leukemia (138), and IFN-γ induces differentiation of monocytes (184). Treatment of HL-60 promyelocytic leukemia cells with IFN-α alone or in combination with retinoic acid resulted in enhancement of differentiation (120). Melanoma cells were differentiated by IFN-β, an effect that did not correlate directly with an antiproliferative effect (53). Human IFN-α, given to nude mice bearing xenografts of human osteosarcoma, inhibited tumor growth. In some cases, the sarcoma was replaced by normal bone and marrow, an effect possibly explained by tumor differentiation (23).

Other observations have raised the possibility that IFNs may progressively cause reversion of the transformed phenotype. When radiation-transformed mouse fibroblasts were cultivated and passaged in the continuous presence of mouse IFN-α/β, the cells no longer produced tumors in nude mice, and their morphology changed from fibroblastic to epithelioid. When IFN treatment ceased, cells reverted to the transformed phenotype and became tumorigenic (25). Mouse 3T3 cells transformed with the human HA-*ras*-1 gene and cultured continuously in the presence of murine IFN-α/β produced revertant colonies in which transcription of the *ras* gene was inhibited. Most cells retained the revertant phenotype during many cell generations despite renewed high levels of transcription of the *ras* gene and of p21 Ras protein (183). However, one line of bladder tumor cells seemed to become more tumorigenic in nude mice than cells not treated with IFN (24). Thus, it has not yet been possible to predict what change in phenotype may occur by long-term in vitro exposure to interferon.

Antitumor Activity in Humans

IFNs as single agents are active in inducing regressions in more than a dozen different malignancies (Table 80.5). IFN-α2 was the first previously unlicensed therapeutic, produced by recombinant DNA technology, to be approved for marketing by the U.S. Food and Drug Administration (16, 64, 106). Large-scale trials of IFNs as treatment for malignancies began in 1979 with the American Cancer Society program. The IFN-α used in that program, produced from buffy coat leukocytes by the pioneering program of Cantell of the Finnish State Serum Institute and National Red Cross, was only a partially purified preparation, which by today's standards was quite crude. The American Cancer Society program did, however, confirm the activity of this IFN-α preparation in inducing disease regression in multi-institutional studies. With this evidence in hand, the infant biotechnology industry was willing to make the commitment to cloning and large-scale production of recombinant IFNs. A substantially expanded therapeutic role for IFN-α2 in human malignancy has occurred over the past decade.

Table 80.5. Antitumor Effectiveness of Interferon Alpha in Phase II Trials

Chronic leukemias	Malignant melanoma
Myeloid[a]	Mid-gut carcinoids
Hairy cell[a]	Gliomas
Lymphocytic	Kaposi's sarcomas[a]
Lymphomas	Ovarian carcinomas[a]
Follicular[a]	Basal cell carcinomas[b]
T-cell[a]	Bladder carcinomas[b]
Large cell	
Multiple myeloma	
Renal carcinoma	

[a] Response rates >40%.
[b] Intralesional or regional administration.

HEMATOLOGIC MALIGNANCIES

The degree of activity and improvement in quality of life of patients with hairy cell leukemia resulted in the first licensed approval for an IFN in the United States. More than 85% of patients have objective evidence of partial or complete hematologic response to IFN-α2 (54, 163). Following IFNs, there is a gradual decrease in bone marrow infiltration with malignant cells as well as a normalization of peripheral hematologic parameters. This has resulted in reduced morbidity from the disease process, a reduction in red cell and platelet transfusion requirements, and a decreased frequency of infection (66). Reduction of hairy cells in peripheral blood may occur in <1 month, but improvement in peripheral cytopenias may take much longer (from 2 to 8 months in marrow and peripheral blood). Responses may occur at doses as low as 0.2×10^6 units/m^2 but more slowly than at the more conventional dose of 2×10^6 units/m^2. Although duration of optimal treatment remains uncertain, the time required to induce objective response and persistence of hairy cells in the bone marrow even after 6 months suggests a need for relatively continuous treatment (170). Some evidence suggests that with the exquisite sensitivity of hairy cell leukemia to IFNs, maintenance treatment can be given as infrequently as one or two times per week.

In chronic myelogenous leukemia, IFN-α results in sustained therapeutic response in a majority (>75%) of patients (3, 96, 156, 206, 207). Untreated patients or patients with disease lasting less than 1 year are more likely to respond (207). A higher dose (5×10^6 units/m^2) than required for hairy cell leukemia is needed to achieve the best therapeutic control. Frequency of administration for optimal clinical effect has not been critically examined, but higher response rates have been reported with daily rather than 3 times per week subcutaneous administration. In addition to reduction in leukemic cell mass, a gradual reduction has occurred in frequency of cells bearing the underlying 9 to 22 chromosomal translocations. The best data in chronic myelogenous leukemia have demonstrated sustained clinical and cytogenetic responses with IFN-α2 (96). With continued treatment, approximately 25% of patients will develop cytogenetic complete response with loss of expression of the Ph chromosome. The median survival for responding patients who show some evidence, although not complete, of cytogenetic response is approximately 6 years. Over 90% of cytogenetic complete responders will be in remission at 10 years.

The equivalence and/or superiority of IFN-α2 to busulfan and hydroxyurea has been demonstrated (82, 90). Possibly as a result of the lower, less frequent dose of IFN-α2 used, the cytogenetic complete response rate was only 7%. Survival in this series for IFN-treated patients will, however, exceed 5 years. Median survival of hydroxyurea-treated patients was approximately 4 years. Suppression of these clones of cells suggests a profound change in the neoplastic process, which may in part result in augmentation in adhesion of CML progenitors to bone marrow stroma (220). To sustain hematologic and cytogenetic response in myeloproliferative disorders, continued treatment seems to be required. IFN-γ can also result in complete and partial responses in CML (110). Thrombocytosis associated with myeloproliferative disorders, whether Philadelphia chromosome positive or negative, can be effectively controlled by IFN-α2 (126, 209). The clonal, life-threatening hypereosinophilic syndrome can also be effectively controlled (29). In 5 of 6 patients refractory to other therapies, eosinophils decreased from a median of 15,000/μL to about 1,000/μL.

Response rates of 10 to 20% occur in patients with advanced multiple myeloma treated with various schedules (35, 162, 226). When patients who received 12×10^6 units/m^2 of IFN-α2a intramuscularly daily were analyzed according to prior therapy, 50% of previously untreated patients had responded (162). Similarly, patients who had received only phenylalanine mustard and prednisone had a 40% response rate (35). In patients who had a tumor response, levels of serum immunoglobulins were restored, an effect infrequently seen with chemotherapy (162). Complete responses can be sustained for more than 2 years, an unusual event in myeloma. Thus, IFNs will probably eventually become part of the treatment of various stages of multiple myeloma (17).

In chronic lymphocytic leukemia, previously treated patients received either 50×10^6 units/m^2 or 5×10^6 units/m^2 of IFN-α2a, a dose based upon pretreatment platelet count (55). Of patients at the higher dose, 2 of 12 responded versus 0 of 6 at the lower dose. However, in other trials, 30 to 35% of patients receiving 2 to 5×10^6 units/m^2, three times a week or daily responded (210, 226). Of possible importance is schedule; response in two patients could not be sustained on a weekly schedule (151). Intensive treatment with IFNs in chronic lymphocytic leukemia merits further evaluation.

In lymphomas of various histologies and of both B- and T-cell phenotypes, IFN-α may have a therapeutic role (17). IFN-α2a, 50×10^6 units three times a week, was effective in 45% of patients with advanced cutaneous T-cell lymphoma (26); responses lasted from 3 months to >25 months (median, 5 months). Partial response to IFN-β occurs in T-cell leukemias (211). IFNs may prove to be more effective for cutaneous T-cell lymphomas and leukemias than any other reported agent. In nodular, poorly differentiated B-cell lymphomas, a greater than 45% response frequency has occurred with IFN-α2 (56, 151, 226). Many responding patients have been pretreated with combination chemotherapy. Responses can persist for >6 months after cessation of therapy. Patients who have relapsed after IFN was discontinued have subsequently responded to second courses. Doses of 50×10^6 units/m^2 intramuscularly three times weekly, a dose that required at least 50% reduction within 4 weeks in all patients, and a much lower dose, 2×10^6 units/m^2 three times weekly, have been effective. Thus, as in hairy cell leukemia, objective response can be achieved at lower doses.

SOLID TUMORS

For some solid tumors, IFN-α has resulted in response rates in metastatic disease equivalent to the best chemotherapeutic approaches. Response rates of melanoma to IFN-α have ranged from 2 to 29%; the cumulative response totaled from three series of 124 patients involving patients utilizing recombinant IFN-α2 was 15% (10% partial and 5% complete), a level comparable to results with cytotoxic agents (36, 38, 180). Response has been correlated with better performance status, no prior chemotherapy, and low volume of visceral disease. Response has not yet been clearly correlated with dose. For example, IFN-α2a at 50×10^6 units/m^2 intramuscularly three times a week resulted in partial or complete responses in 7 of 31 (23%) patients. This dose resulted in >80% of patients developing deterioration in performance status. A lower dose (12×10^6 units/m^2 given three times a week) was used in a subsequent trial. Although fewer complete responses occurred, results were statistically indistinguishable (6 of 30 responses) from the prior trial (36, 38). Response rates to IFN-γ have been reported between 6 and 11% (37, 48).

Metastatic renal cell carcinoma has a response rate to cytotoxic agents of less than 10%. Response rates from 4 to 26% have been reported in trials of recombinant IFN-α2 in this disease, with a mean response of 15% in cumulative summary of several trials (145). In one of the initial trials, either 2 or 20×10^6 units/m^2 was administered daily (165). No objective responses occurred at the lower dose, but at the high dose, 4 of 15 patients responded. Subsequently, 26 additional patients were treated at 20×10^6 units/m^2 with 8 of 26 responses; median duration of response was 3 months, and dose reduction was required in more than half the patients (166). To ameliorate toxicity, IFN-α2 was evaluated in a schedule of gradual dose escalation from 3 to 36×10^6

units intramuscularly over a 10-day period (105). Patients were maintained at 36×10^6 units daily for 9 weeks, after which responding and stable patients continued on a thrice-weekly schedule. In 62 evaluable patients, 7 partial responses were observed. By gradually increasing the dose, the acute toxicity of fever and chills was lessened, with <10% of patients developing fever greater than 38.5°C. However, dose reduction to 18×10^6 units was required in many patients for granulocytopenia, fatigue, and anorexia. A more favorable response has been observed in patients who have had resection of bulky primary disease; lung metastases appear to respond better than disease at other sites. Two studies of IFN-γ or combinations of IFN-α and -γ have had response rates of 9 to 30% (complete plus partial response, CR plus PR) in renal cell carcinoma (6, 164, 173). The response rate of 30% occurred in patients receiving IFN-γ at a biologically effective but low dose (1×10^6 units weekly) (6).

Response rates for recombinant IFN-α2 in Kaposi's sarcoma have had a mean of 33% (41, 75, 108, 115, 171, 177, 222). A dose-response effect has been identified, and responses have been seen in patients with visceral and nodal disease. Responses occur in the skin, nodes, and gastrointestinal tract with a mean duration of 13 months. In Kaposi's sarcoma patients who respond, the rates of opportunistic infection have been fewer after IFN-α administration, but no overall decrease in infection frequency has been identified (75, 108).

Clinical trials of IFN-α in endocrine pancreatic tumors have reported a high objective rate (>75%) of response (decrease in tumor-produced peptides) (47, 148). In addition, a partial response has occurred in approximately one-third of patients. IFN-α has also been useful in decreasing the severe diarrhea common in pancreatic endocrine tumors. Midgut carcinoid tumors, although often behaving in an indolent fashion, produce symptoms such as flushing and diarrhea, which may interfere with daily activities. In trials of recombinant IFN-α, a mean response rate (improvement in symptoms or decrease in 5 hydroxyindoleacetic acid (5HIAA)) of approximately 50% has been reported (140, 149, 150). The decrease in 5HIAA has been correlated with lessened symptoms; rebound of 5HIAA levels frequently occurred when IFN was discontinued or with development of antibodies to the administered IFN-α2 (149). Objective tumor regression occurs less frequently, being observed in approximately 20% of patients, but can include both primary tumors and hepatic metastases.

Other solid tumors, such as gliomas, ovarian, bladder, and basal cell carcinomas, have responded to IFN-α administered regionally. Trials have defined an objective response rate of up to 40% for IFN-β given by combined intratumor and/or systemic administration (141, 235). Systemic injection of IFN-α has also resulted in partial responses in patients with malignant gliomas (127). Recurrent and persistent ovarian carcinoma presents an opportunity for local therapy because of its predilection for intra-abdominal serosal surfaces. To reach IFN levels that are inhibitory for ovarian carcinoma cell proliferation in vitro, trials with all three IFN types have been conducted with intraperitoneal (i.p.) administration (227). In 14 patients with persistent disease at second-look laparotomy, who received weekly i.p. IFN-α2 postoperatively, 4 complete responses and 1 partial response were documented in the 11 patients who underwent laparotomy following IFN treatment (12). An additional patient was considered a complete responder on the basis of physical examination alone. In eight patients receiving intraperitoneal IFN-β, four experienced resolution of ascites (168). IFN-γ was administered intraperitoneally to 27 patients with residual carcinoma following combination chemotherapy; no responses occurred (39). Thus, in ovarian cancer, effectiveness has been greater in minimal residual disease. In superficial bladder carcinoma (carcinoma in situ or noninvasive, low grade transitional cell carcinoma), IFN-α2 gave a greater than 40% objective response and was effective in patients with large disease volumes. A dose-response correlation and higher response rates with intraepithelial neoplasia than with frank bladder carcinoma were identified (215, 229). Intralesional treatment for another intraepithelial neoplasm, basal cell carcinoma, has also been effective in yielding a high (>75% CR) objective response frequency (69).

A new perspective on IFNs as antitumor proteins has resulted from clinical observations on effectiveness of IFN-α2 in life-threatening hemangiomas of infancy (49). IFN-α2 was beneficial in leading to angioma regression in more than 80% of children treated. Not only did hemangiomas regress, but their life-threatening complications, including consumptive coagulopathy and high output cardiac failure, were controlled. Effectiveness of IFNs as an antiangiogenic agent is further suggested by their clinical efficacy in two other vascular proliferative disorders: Kaposi's sarcoma (108) and subretinal neovascular proliferation (61). Inhibition of experimental angiogenesis by IFNs has been demonstrated in mouse tumor models as has inhibition of expression of mRNA and protein of basic fibroblast growth factor (63, 192). Thus, in addition to augmenting expression of specific genes, inhibiting cellular proliferation, and augmenting immune effector cell function, IFNs have an additional physiological effect that may yield the antitumor activity.

COMBINATIONS

Greater effectiveness of IFNs with tumor cell burden first reduced by surgery or chemotherapy has been demonstrated for established murine tumors (73). Immunomodulatory effects may be greater when tumor cell mass is reduced (92). The pioneering studies of IFNs in osteosarcoma involved this clinical setting (202). Randomized trials are currently underway in the U.S. with IFN-α being used as adjuncts to surgery in melanoma and renal carcinoma. Prolongation of disease-free survival and impact on overall survival may emerge in use of IFN-α2 as an adjuvant to surgery for high risk patients with primary melanoma (32, 100). Thus, international randomized trials with comparison to standard treatment (observation) continue to explore this application. In a World Health Organization Melanoma Program trial of cutaneous malignant melanoma with nodal metastases, the 2-year disease-free survival was 46 percent for patients given IFN-α (3 million units subcutaneously three times/week for 3 years) after surgical excision of nodes, compared to 27 percent in patients receiving surgery alone. IFN-α therapy, sex, and number of nodes involved with tumor were all independent determinants of disease-free survival. In the Eastern Cooperative Oncology Group (ECOG) trial, median disease-free survival of all entered patients (T_4 or N_1) was 8 months longer ($P < .05$) than controls. However, the high dose IFN regimen used resulted in grade 3 or 4 toxicity in more than 60% of patients, suggesting a potentially important biologic effect that may or may not be of clinical advantage. Together with a similar ongoing study in renal carcinoma, these trials should begin to establish whether IFN-α is effective in the minimal tumor burden setting.

Trials in myeloma are prototypes for the approaches being used for combination of IFNs with chemotherapy (17). In phase II trials of the ECOG, both complete response and 2-year survival with the IFN-α2a and chemotherapy are better than historical controls (152). This IFN combination, which involves alternate cycles of IFN-α2 and chemotherapy, is currently being compared in prospectively randomized trials to chemotherapy alone by ECOG. A similar alternating therapy program in hairy cell leukemia shows promise of resulting in sustained responses (133). An Italian multi-institutional study has identified prolonged survival when 3×10^6 units/m^2, three times weekly of IFN-α2b was used as maintenance therapy for patients stable or responding to 1 year of induction chemotherapy. Median duration of response for the IFN-α2b-treated patients was 26 months (compared to 14 months for the untreated patients, $P = .0002$), and median survival was 52 months for treated patients and 39 months for controls ($P = .05$) (130). For myeloma, randomized studies have suggested that either for induction or maintenance, IFN-α2 will add to effectiveness (130, 153). For example, IFN-α with melphalan and prednisone was compared to melphalan and prednisone alone. IFN increased the response rate to 68% from 42% ($P < .0001$) (153). However, because significant impact on maintenance has not been confirmed in all trials (90, 96), whether IFN will ultimately be used in this disease for induction, maintenance, or both continues under study.

For B-cell lymphomas, the significant single agent activity of IFN-α2 is being integrated into effective combined modality treatments for both low and intermediate grade non-Hodgkin's lymphoma (17, 193, 196). Combination with a doxorubicin-based regimen has been identified as prolonging both disease-free survival and overall survival in two prospectively randomized trials. Despite careful design to ensure that effective chemotherapy doses would not be compromised, total cytotoxic chemotherapy doses were reduced by participating investigators in the chemotherapy-alone arm on one of these phase III trials; despite this, a positive therapeutic impact of IFN-α2 was evident (193). In the other, although 11% of patients had to have IFN-α2 stopped for toxicity, it resulted in significant gains in event-free survival ($P < .001$) and overall survival ($P = .02$) for follicular lymphoma ($P = .02$).

IFN-α and IFN-β have potentiated 5-fluorouracil (5-FU) in preclinical, antiproliferative, and antitumor experimental models (46, 200, 201). Some responses have been sustained for more than a year. IFNs used in mice not only increased therapeutic effectiveness but also protected them from lethal toxicities of 5-FU (201). Initial and recent phase II studies of IFN in combination with 5-FU suggested a high objective response rate for patients with metastatic colorectal and other gastrointestinal malignancies (71, 224, 225). However, phase III trials have failed to confirm any benefit when doses of IFN and 5-FU, which together yielded moderate toxicity, were utilized. The possible role of more intense chemotherapy in conjunction with 5-FU continues to be explored in both the metastatic and adjuvant settings (28). It may augment activity of 5-FU for squamous and renal cell carcinomas in addition to adenocarcinomas (95, 221).

For rational pharmacology, complementary mechanisms can be used to develop effective combination therapies (14, 18). Because of their pleiotropic regulatory effects on cell function, IFN combinations may have potent inhibitory effects in both viral and neoplastic diseases. For example, the differing mechanisms of inhibition of HIV replication may result in greater therapeutic effectiveness when combined with zidovudine for AIDS (103, 107). Further, the complication of thrombocytopenia induced by zidovudine may also be ameliorated (132). Not only do IFNs potentiate cytotoxic drugs, they also potentiate radiation and the effects of other cytokines (67, 186). In conjunction with radiation, a role of IFN-β as a radiosensitizer has been suggested (135). A response rate of 90% has been reported for T-cell lymphomas treated with IFN-α2 and phototherapy (112). Whether these results will be confirmed in randomized phase III trials remains to be determined. To dissect logical strategies for biochemical or cellular inhibition with other molecules, expanded preclinical research will be required. Dose, route, and schedule will become increasingly important considerations.

Combination with IL-2 has not yet yielded any substantial advance in the single-agent activity of these two cytokines individually in renal carcinoma or melanoma (52, 197). A low dose of IFN-γ may yield objective responses in renal carcinoma (6). This could result in a regimen of modest effectiveness and very low morbidity. This is being explored in controlled phase II and phase III trials. Because graft versus host disease may be associated with improved outcomes in allogenic bone marrow transplantation, IFN-α together with cyclosporine has been used to induce graft versus host disease after autologous bone marrow transplantation for breast cancer (97). In combination with retinoids, substantial regressions have been observed with IFN-α2 in squamous carcinomas of the skin and cervix (122, 123). This combination has not yet proved effective in other squamous cell carcinomas and remains under evaluation for other malignancies. Cells resistant to biological effects in vitro can be induced to respond and become sensitive with retinoids (94). Like retinoids, IFNs have the potential to be effective chemopreventive agents (19). These innovative approaches suggest the therapeutic potential of IFNs has just begun to be exploited and that the spectrum of therapeutic applications for malignancies will substantially broaden over the next decade.

SIDE EFFECTS

Like other potent physiologic products such as glucocorticoids, IFNs have toxicities when administered with pharmacologic intent (Table 80.6). Side effects with the initial dose are predominantly constitutional. These are dominated by malaise, fever, and chills, which begin a few hours after the commonly used subcutaneous route and last for 2 to 8 hours. These influenza-like symptoms occur uniformly following the initial injection with subsequent development of tachyphylaxis with subsequent daily injections. The rapidity of tachyphylaxis is dependent upon type of IFN, dose, route, and schedule. Flu-like symptoms that occur despite increases in endogenous glucocorticoids (147, 189) can be partially controlled with aspirin or acetaminophen. The chronic fatigue may necessitate dose reduction; tolerance can be improved with lower doses and intermittent scheduling. Fatigue and anorexia are the dose-limiting toxicities with chronic administration; weight loss occurs and may be significant (>10%). Any nausea and vomiting have usually been mild and of short duration. The most frequent neurologic side effect (other than the possible relationship of the fatigue) is somnolence and confusion, which may result from a diffuse slowing seen on EEG. In general, older patients tolerate these side effects less well than younger patients.

Hematologic effects include mild granulocytopenia with a reduction in counts by 40 to 60% followed by rapid rebound to normal after discontinuation of therapy. No increase in infectious sequelae has occurred during IFN-induced leukopenia, and granulocytopenia is rarely dose limiting. Anemia occurs with chronic therapy but is rarely severe. This may reflect an influence on the erythropoiesis because recovery of normal hematocrit has often required weeks or months. Mild thrombocytopenia has been reported in 5 to 50% of patients and is influenced by marrow infiltration with tumor.

Elevation of transaminases, usually mild, has occurred more commonly in the presence of pretreatment hepatic abnormalities and is dose related. Cholesterol levels decrease, often accompanied by a rise in triglycerides. LDL commonly declines, and HDL both increases and decreases, depending on dose and type of IFN (134, 181). A statistically significant, though rarely clinically important, hypocalcemic effect occurs. The decrease in calcium is out of proportion to mild declines in albumin. Creatinine does not change. The most common renal toxicity described has been mild proteinuria, but nephrotic syndrome and acute renal insufficiency have been rarely reported (7, 190). Although little or no IFN can be identified in urine, nephrectomy in the rat reduces but does not eliminate clearance, suggesting catabolism by renal tubular cells is one degradation pathway (204, 214). Although occasional patients may develop alterations in thyroid function (27), in general, no residual toxicities in parenchymal organ function have been identified (167). With improved understanding of mechanism of action and clinical introduction of other members of the IFN-α family (83, 87), it can be anticipated that the therapeutic index of IFNs will improve.

With chronic administration, a minority of patients develop neutralizing antibody to the administered IFN-α2 and IFN (91, 117, 223). Antibody development is a function of dose, schedule, route, and possibly underlying disease. Antibodies have rarely been identified with <4 months of IFN administration. Particularly when present in high titer, they may be correlated with disease progression (57, 168).

Perspective

IFNs have improved therapeutic approaches for viral diseases and malignancies. They are the first human proteins to be effective as a cancer treatment modality. The full spectrum of actions and interactions, mechanism of antitumor effects, and optimal dose, schedule, and type of IFN for specific clinical indications has not yet been fully delineated (Table 80.7). IFNs, both themselves and as a prototype for other biologic response modifiers, have opened a new era in oncologic treatment. The groundwork has been laid for the use of IFNs to modulate specific gene regulation, oncogene expression, cell proliferation and differentiation, and immunologic function. This must be complemented by studies dissecting other aspects of IFN cellular and clinical actions (Table 80.7). In combination with other lymphokines, monoclonal antibodies, and cytoreductive approaches, IFNs will continue to reduce morbidity and mortality from cancer.

ACKNOWLEDGMENT

Terri Joneckis and Jon D'Cunha contributed valuable assistance in manuscript completion.

Table 80.6. Clinical Side Effects of Interferons

Acute	Chronic
Fever	Fatigue
Chills	Anorexia
Malaise	Weight loss
Myalgias	Mild neutropenia
Headache	Transaminase elevations
Nausea	Diarrhea
	Depression
	Less common: mental slowing, confusion, hair shedding, thrombocytopenia, diarrhea, nausea, and vomiting

Summarized in greater detail in Ref. 167.

Table 80.7. Studies Resulting in More Effective Use of Interferons in Cancer

Molecules	Mechanism of action
Inducers	Protein modulation
Structure-function relationships	Immunomodulatory effects
Effects of new types	Antiproliferative/ differentiation effects
Cellular activation mechanisms	Angiogenesis inhibition
Receptors	Clinical Strategies
Transcriptional regulation	Dose/schedule optimization
Function-induced proteins	Combination therapies
	New disease targets
	Minimizing side effects

References

1. Adolf GR. Antigenic structure of human interferon omega1 (interferon alpha II1): comparison with other human interferons. J Gen Virol 1987;68:1669.
2. Aguet M, Dembic Z, Merlin G. Molecular cloning and expression of the human interferon-γ receptor. Cell 1988;55:273.
3. Alimena G, Morra E, Lazzarino M, et al. Interferon alpha-2b as therapy for pH-positive chronic myelogenous leukemia: a study of 82 patients treated with intermittent or daily administration. Blood 1988;72:642.
4. Anderson P, Yip YK, Vilcek J. Specific binding of ^{125}I-human interferon-gamma to high affinity receptors on human fibroblasts. J Biol Chem 1982;257:11301.
5. Arenzana-Seisdedos F, Virelizier JL, Fiers W. Interferons as macrophage-activating factors III: preferential effects of interferon-gamma on the interleukin 1 secretory potential of fresh or aged human monocytes. J Immunol 1985;134:2444.
6. Aulitzky W, Gastl G, Aulitzky WE, et al. Successful treatment of metastatic renal cell carcinoma with a biologically active dose of recombinant interferon-gamma. J Clin Oncol 1989;7:1875.
7. Averbach SD, Austin HA III, Sherwin SA, et al. Acute interstitial nephritis with nephrotic syndrome following recombinant leukocyte A IFN therapy for mycosis fungoides. N Engl J Med 1984;310:32.
8. Balkwill F, Taylor-Papadimitriou J. Interferon affects both G_1 and $S + G_2$ in cells stimulated from quiescence to growth. Nature 1978;274:798.
9. Balkwill FR, Moodie EM, Freedman V, Fantes KH. Human interferon inhibits the growth of established human breast tumors in the nude mouse. Int J Cancer 1982;30:231.
10. Basham TY, Bourgeade MF, Creasey AA, Merigan I. Interferon increases HLA synthesis in melanoma cells: interferon-resistant and sensitive cell lines. Proc Natl Acad Sci USA 1982;79:3625.
11. Belardelli F, Gresser I, Maury C, Maunoury MT. Antitumor effects of interferon in mice injected with interferon-sensitive and interferon-resistant Friend leukemia cells: II. Role of host mechanisms. Int J Cancer 1982;30:821.
12. Berek JS, Hacker NF, Lichtenstein A, et al. Intraperitoneal recombinant alpha-interferon for "salvage" immunotherapy in stage III epithelial ovarian cancer: a Gynecologic Oncology Group study. Cancer Res 1985;45:4447.
13. Billard C, Sigaux F, Castaigne S, et al. Treatment of hairy cell leukemia with recombinant alpha IFN: II. In vivo down-regulation of alpha IFN receptors on tumor cells. Blood 1986;67:821.
14. Borden EC. Interferons and cancer: how the promise is being kept. In Interferons, Vol. 5. Edited by I Gresser. London: Academic Press, 1984, p 43.
15. Borden EC. Augmented tumor-associated antigen expression by interferons. JNCI 1988;80:148.
16. Borden EC. Effects of interferons in neoplastic diseases of man. Pharmacol Ther 1088;37:213.
17. Borden EC. Innovative treatment strategies for non-Hodgkin's lymphoma and multiple myeloma. Semin Oncol 1994;21(suppl 14):14.
18. Borden EC, Hawkins MJ. Biologic response modifiers as adjuncts to other therapeutic modalities. Semin Oncol 1986;13:144.
19. Borden EC, Hawkins MJ, Sielaff KM, Storer BM, Schiesel JD, Smalley RV. Clinical and biological effects of recombinant interferon-beta administered intravenously daily in phase I trial. J Interferon Res 1988;8:357.
20. Borden EC, Sidky Y, Erturk E, Wierenga W, Bryan GT. Protection from carcinogen-induced murine bladder carcinoma by interferons and an oral interferon-inducing pyrimidinone, bropirimine. Cancer Res 1990;50:1071.
21. Borden EC, Verma AJ, Wolberg WH. Potential role of polyribonucleotides in human neoplastic diseases. J Biol Response Mod 1985;4:676.
22. Branca AA, Baglioni C. Evidence that types I and II interferons have different receptors. Nature 1981;294:768.
23. Brosjo O, Bauer HCF, Brostrom LA, Nilsson OS, Reinholt FP, Tribukait B. Growth inhibition of human osteosarcomas in nude mice by human interferon-α: significance of dose and tumor differentiation. Cancer Res 1987;47:258.
24. Brouty-Boye D. Interferon and the tumour cell phenotype. In Interferon, Vol. 7. Edited by I. Gresser. London: Academic, 1986, p 145.
25. Brouty-Boye D, Gresser I. Reversibility of the transformed and neoplastic phenotype: I. Progressive reversion of the phenotype x-ray-transformed C3H/10T[u12] cells under prolonged treatment with interferon. Int J Cancer 1981;28:165.
26. Bunn PA, Foon KA, Ihde DC, et al. Recombinant leukocyte A interferon: an active agent in advanced cutaneous T-cell lymphomas. Ann Intern Med 1984;101:484.
27. Burman P, Totterman TH, Oberg K, Karlsson KA. Thyroid autoimmunity in patients on long-term therapy with leukocyte-derived interferon. J Clin Endocrinol Metab 1986;63:1086.
28. Buter J, Sinnige H, Sleiffer D, et al. 5-fluorouracil/leucovorin/interferon alpha 2a in patients with advanced colorectal cancer. Cancer 1995;75:1072.
29. Butterfield JH, Gleich GJ. Interferon-α treatment of six patients with the idiopathic hypereosinophilic syndrome. Ann Intern Med 1994;121:648.
30. Byrne GI, Lehmann LK, Kirschbaum JG, Borden EC, Lee CM, Brown RR. Induction of tryptophan degradation in vitro and in vivo: a gamma-interferon-stimulated activity. J Interferon Res 1986;6:389.
31. Capon DJ, Shepard HM, Goeddel DV. Two distinct families of human and bovine interferon-alpha genes are coordinately expressed and encode functional polypeptides. Mol Cell Biol 1985;5:768.
32. Cascinelli N, Buffalino R, Morabito A, Mackie R. Results of adjuvant interferon study in WHO melanoma programme. Lancet 1994;343:913.
33. Chan SH, Kobayashi M, Santoli D, et al. Mechanisms of IFN-gamma induction by natural killer cells stimulatory factor (NKSF/IL-12): role of transcription and mRNA stability in the synergistic interaction between NKSF and IL-2. J Immunol 1992;148:92.
34. Chong KL, Feng L, Schappert K, et al. Human p68 kinase exhibits growth suppression in yeast and homology to the translational regulator GCN2. EMBO J 1992;11:1553.
35. Costanzi JJ, Cooper MR, Scarffe JH, et al. Phase II study of recombinant alpha-2 interferon in resistant multiple myeloma. J Clin Oncol 1985;3:654.
36. Creagan ET, Ahmann DL, Green SJ. Phase II study of recombinant leukocyte A interferon (RIFN-alpha-A) in disseminated malignant melanoma. Cancer 1984;54:2844.
37. Creagan ET, Ahmann DL, Long HJ, Frytak S, Sherwin SA, Chang MN. Phase II study of recombinant interferon-gamma in patients with disseminated malignant melanoma. Cancer Treat Rep 1987;71:843.
38. Creagan ET, Kovach JS, Long HJ, Richardson RL. Phase I study of recombinant leukocyte A human interferon combined with BCNU in selected patients with advanced cancer. J Clin Oncol 1986;4:408.
39. D'Acquisto R, Markman M, Hakes T, et al. A phase I trial of intraperitoneal recombinant gamma-interferon in advanced ovarian carcinoma. J Clin Oncol 1988;6:689.
40. David M, Romero G, Zhang ZY, Dixon JE, Larner AC. In vitro activation of the transcription factor ISGF3 by interferon alpha involves a membrane-associated tyrosine phosphatase and tyrosine kinase. J Biol Chem 1993;268:6593.
41. DeWit R, Boucher CAB, Veenhof KHN, Schattenkerk JKME, Bakker PJM, Danner SA. Clinical and virological effects of high dose recombinant interferon α in disseminated AIDS-related Kaposi's sarcoma. Lancet 1988;2:1214.
42. Edwards BS, Hawkins MJ, Borden EC. Correlation between in vitro and systemic effects of native and recombinant interferons alpha upon human NK cell cytotoxicity. J Biol Response Mod 1983;2:409.
43. Edwards BS, Merritt JA, Fuhlbrigge RC, Borden EC. Low doses of interferon alpha result in more effective clinical natural killer cell activation. J Clin Invest 1985;75:1908.
44. Eggermont AMM, Sugarbaker PH, Marquet RL, Jeekel J. In vivo generation of lymphokine activated killer cell activity by ABPP and interleukin-2 and their antitumor effects against immunogenic and nonimmunogenic tumors in murine tumor models. Cancer Immunol Immunother 1988;26:23.
45. Einhorn S, Robert KH, Ostlund L, Juliusson G, Biberfeld P. Interferon induces proliferation and differentiation in primary chronic lymphocytic leukemia cells. In The Biology of the Interferon System. Edited by H Kirchner, H Schellekens. Amsterdam: Elsevier, 1985, p 293.
46. Elias L, Sandoval JM. Interferon effects upon fluorouracil metabolism by HL-60 cells. Biochem Biophys Res Commun 1989;163:867.
47. Eriksson B, Oberg K, Alm G, et al. Treatment of malignant endocrine pancreatic tumors with human leukocyte interferon. Cancer Treat Rep 1987;71:31.
48. Ernstoff MS, Trautman T, Davis CA, et al. A randomized phase I/II study of continuous versus intermittent intravenous interferon gamma in patients with metastatic melanoma. J Clin Oncol 1987;5:1804.
49. Ezekowitz RAB, Mulliken JB, Folkman J. Interferon alpha-2a therapy for life-threatening hemangiomas of infancy. N Engl J Med 1992;326:1456.
50. Faltynek CR, Princler GL, Rossio JL, et al. Relationship of the clinical response and binding of recombinant IFN-α in patients with lymphoproliferative diseases. Blood 1986;67:1077.
51. Fellous M, Nir U, Wallach D, Merlin G, Rubinstein M, Revel M. Interferon-dependent induction of mRNA for the major histocompatibility antigens in human fibroblasts and lymphoblastoid cells. Proc Natl Acad Sci USA 1982;79:3082.
52. Figlin RA, Belldegrun A, Moldawer N, Zeffren J, deKernion J. Concomitant administration of recombinant human interleukin-2 and recombinant interferon alpha-2a: an active outpatient regimen in metastatic renal cell carcinoma. J Clin Oncol 1992;10:414.
53. Fisher PB, Prignoli DR, Hermo H Jr, Weinstein IB, Pestka S. Effects of combined treatment with interferon and mezerein on melanogenesis and growth in human melanoma cells. J Interferon Res 1985;5:11.
54. Foon K, Maluish AE, Abrams PG, et al. Recombinant leukocyte A interferon therapy for advanced hairy cell leukemia: therapeutic and immunologic results. Am J Med 1986;80:351.
55. Foon KA, Bottino GC, Abrams PG, et al. Phase II trial of recombinant leukocyte A interferon in patients with advanced chronic lymphocytic leukemia. Am J Med 1985;78:216.
56. Foon KA, Sherwin SA, Abrams PB. Treatment of advanced non-Hodgkin's lymphoma with recombinant leukocyte A interferon. N Engl J Med 1984;311:1148.
57. Freund M, von Wussow P, Diedrich H. Recombinant human IFN-alpha-2b in chronic myelogenous leukaemia: dose dependency of response and frequency of neutralizing anti-IFN antibodies. Br J Haematol 1989;72:350.
58. Fu XY. A transcription factor with SH2 and SH3 domains is directly activated by an interferon alpha-induced cytoplasmic protein tyrosine kinase(s). Cell 1992;70:323.
59. Fu XY, Kessler DS, Veals SA, Levy DE, Darnell JE Jr. ISGF3, the transcriptional activator induced by interferon alpha, consists of multiple interacting polypeptide chains. Proc Natl Acad Sci USA 1990;87:8555.
60. Fu XY, Schindler C, Improta T, Aebersold R, Darnell JE Jr. The proteins of ISGF-3, the interferon alpha-induced transcriptional activator, define a gene family involved in signal transduction. Proc Natl Acad Sci USA 1992;89:7840.
61. Fung WE. Interferon alpha 2a for treatment of age-related macular degeneration. Am J Ophthalmol 1991;112:349.
62. Gewert DR, Moore G, Tilleray VJ, Clemens MJ. Inhibition of cell proliferation by interferons: 1. Effects on cell division and DNA synthesis in human lymphoblasts (Daudi) cells. Eur J Biochem 1984;139:619.
63. Gohji K, Nakajima M, Fabra A, et al. Regulation of gelatinase production in metastatic renal cell carcinoma by organ-specific fibroblasts. Jpn J Cancer Res 1994;85:152.
64. Goldstein D, Laszlo J. Interferon therapy in cancer: from imaginon to interferon. Cancer Res 1986;46:4315.
65. Goldstein D, Sielaff KM, Storer BE, et al. Human biologic response modification by IFN in the absence of measurable serum concentrations: a comparative trial of subcutaneous and intravenous IFN-betaser. JNCI 1989;81:1061.
66. Golomb HM, Jacobs A, Fefer A, et al. Alpha-2 IFN therapy of hairy-cell leukemia: a multicenter study of 64 patients. J Clin Oncol 1986;4:900.
67. Gould MN, Kakria RC, Olson S, Borden EC. Radiosensitization of human bronchogenic carcinoma cells by interferon beta. J Interferon Res 1984;4:123.
68. Gray PW, Goeddel DV. Structure of the human immune interferon gene. Nature 1982;298:859.
69. Greenway HT, Cornell RC, Tanner DJ, Peets E, Bordin GM, Nagi C. Treatment of basal cell carcinoma with intralesional interferon. J Acad Dermatol 1986;15:437.
70. Greiner JW, Schlom J, Pestka S, et al. Modulation of tumor-associated antigen expression and shedding by recombinant human leukocyte and fibroblast interferons. Pharmacol Ther 1987;31:209.
71. Grem JL, McAtee N, Murphy RF, et al. A pilot study of interferon alpha-2a in combination with fluorouracil plus high-dose leucovorin in metastatic gastrointestinal carcinoma. J Clin Oncol 1991;9:1811.

72. Gresser I, Belardelli F, Maury C, Maunoury MT, Tovey MG. Injection of mice with antibody to interferon enhances the growth of transplantable murine tumors. J Exp Med 1983;158:2095.
73. Gresser I, Maury C, Belardelli F. Anti-tumor effects of IFN in mice injected with IFN-sensitive and IFN-resistant Friend leukemia cells: VI. Adjuvant therapy after surgery in the inhibition of liver and spleen metastases. Int J Cancer 1987;39:789.
74. Gresser I, Tovey MG, Maury C, Bandu MT. Role of interferon in the pathogenesis of virus diseases in mice as demonstrated by the use of anti-interferon serum: II. Studies with herpes simplex, Moloney sarcoma, vesicular stomatitis, Newcastle disease, and influenza viruses. J Exp Med 1976;144:1316.
75. Groopman JE, Gottlieb MS, Goodman J, et al. Recombinant alpha-2 interferon therapy for Kaposi's sarcoma associated with the acquired immunodeficiency syndrome. Ann Intern Med 1984;100:671.
76. Gutch MJ, Daly C, Reich NC. Tyrosine phosphorylation is required for activation of an alpha interferon-stimulated transcription factor. Proc Natl Acad Sci USA 1992;89: 11411.
77. Gutterman JU, Fine S, Quesada J. Recombinant leukocyte A IFN: pharmacokinetics, single-dose tolerance, and biologic effects in cancer patients. Ann Intern Med 1982;96:549.
78. Haines DS, Strauss KI, Gillespie DH. Cellular response to double-stranded RNA. J Cell Biochem 1991;46:9.
79. Harada H, Fujita T, Miyamoto M. Structurally similar but functionally distinct factors, IRF-1 and IRF-2, bind to the same regulatory elements of IFN and IFN-inducible genes. Cell 1989;58:729.
80. Harada H, Kitagawa M, Tanaka N, et al. Antioncogenic and oncogenic potentials of interferon regulatory factors-1 and -2. Science 1993;259:971.
81. Hassel BA, Zhou A. Sotomayor C, et al. A dominant negative mutant of 2–5A-dependent RNase suppresses antiproliferative and antiviral effects of interferon. EMBO J 1993;12:3297.
82. Hehlmann R, Heimpel H, Hasford J. Randomized comparison of interferon-α with busulfan and hydroxyurea in chronic myelogenous leukemia. Blood 1994;84:4064.
83. Hawkins MJ, Borden EC, Merritt JA, et al. Comparison of the biologic effects of two recombinant human interferons alpha (rA and rD) in humans. J Clin Oncol 1984;2: 221.
84. Hawkins MJ, Krown SE, Borden EC, et al. American Cancer Society phase I trial of naturally produced interferon beta. Cancer Res 1984;44:5934.
85. Herberman RB, Djeu JY, Ortaldo JR, Holden HT, West WH, Bonnard GD. Role of interferon in augmentation of natural and antibody-dependent cell-mediated cytotoxicity. Cancer Treat Rep 1978;62:1893.
86. Herberman RB, Ortaldo JR, Mantovani A, Hobbs DS, Kung HF, Pestka S. Effect of human recombinant interferon on cytotoxic activity of natural killer (NK) cells and monocytes. Cell Immunol 1982;67:160.
87. Horisberger MA, deStaritzky K. A recombinant human IFN-α B/D hybrid with a broad host range. J Gen Virol 1987;68:945.
88. Hovanessian A. Interferon-induced and double-stranded RNA-activated enzymes: a specific protein kinase and 2′-5′ oligoadenylate synthetases. J Interferon Res 1991;11:199.
89. Huber C, Batchelor JR, Fuchs D. Immune response-associated production of neopterin: release from macrophages primarily under control of interferon-gamma. J Exp Med 1984;160:310.
90. The Italian Cooperative Study Group on Chronic Myeloid Leukemia. Interferon alpha-2a as compared with conventional chemotherapy for the treatment of chronic myeloid leukemia. N Engl J Med 1994;330:820.
91. Itri LM, Sherman MI, Palleroni AV, et al. Incidence and clinical significance of neutralizing antibodies in patients receiving recombinant IFN-α2a. J Interferon Res 1989;9:S9.
92. Jaffe HS, Herberman RB. Rationale for recombinant human interferon-gamma adjuvant immunotherapy for cancer. JNCI 1988;80:616.
93. Johnson HM, Torres BA. Peptide growth factors PDGF, EGF, and FGF regulate interferon-gamma. J Immunol 1985;134:2824.
94. Kalvakolanu DV, Sen GC. Differentiation-dependent activation of interferon-stimulated gene factors and transcription factor NF-kappa B in mouse embryonal carcinoma cells. Proc Natl Acad Sci USA 1993;90:3167.
95. Kelsen D, Lovett D, Wong J, et al. Interferon alpha-2a and fluorouracil in the treatment of patients with advanced esophageal cancer. J Clin Oncol 1992;10:269.
96. Kantarjian HM, Deisseroth A, Kurzrock R, Estrov Z, Talpaz M. Chronic myelogenous leukemia: a concise update. Blood 1993;82:691.
97. Kennedy MJ, Vogelsang GB, Jones RJ. Phase I trial of interferon gamma to potentiate cyclosporine-induced graft-versus-host disease in women undergoing autologous bone marrow transplantation for breast cancer. J Clin Oncol 1994;12:249.
98. Kessler DS, Veals SA, Fu XY, Levy DE. Interferon-alpha regulates nuclear translocation and DNA-binding affinity of ISGF3, a multimeric transcriptional activator. Genes Dev 1990;4:1753.
99. King DP, Jones PP. Induction of IA and H-2 antigens on a macrophage cell line by immune interferon. J Immunol 1983;131:315.
100. Kirkwood J, Hunt M, Smith T, Ernstoff M, Borden E, Blum R. A randomized controlled trial of high-dose IFN-alpha-2b for high-risk melanoma. J Clin Oncol 1995, in press.
101. Kleinerman ES, Kurzrock R, Wyatt D, Quesada JR, Gutterman JU, Fidler IJ. Activation or suppression of the tumoricidal properties of monocytes from cancer patients following treatment with human recombinant gamma-interferon. Cancer Res 1986;46:5401.
102. Koromilas AE, Roy S, Barber GN, et al. Malignant transformation by a mutant of the IFN-inducible dsRNA dependent protein kinase. Science 1992;257:1685.
103. Kovacs JA, Deyton L, Davey R. Combined zidovudine and interferon-alpha therapy in patients with Kaposi sarcoma and the acquired immunodeficiency syndrome (AIDS). Ann Intern Med 1989;111:280.
104. Krause D, Silverman RH, Jacobsen H, et al. Regulation of ppp(A2′*p*)*n*-dependent RNase levels during interferon treatment and cell differentiation. Eur J Biochem 1985;146:611.
105. Krown SE. Therapeutic options in renal cell carcinoma. Semin Oncol 1985;12:13.
106. Krown SE. Interferons and interferon inducers in cancer treatment. Semin Oncol 1986;13:207.
107. Krown SE, Gold JWM, Niedzwiecki D, et al. Interferon alpha with zidovudine: safety, tolerance and clinical and virological effects in patients with Kaposi sarcoma associated with the acquired immunodeficiency syndrome. Ann Intern Med 1990;112:812.
108. Krown SE, Real FX, Cunningham-Rundles S, et al. Preliminary observations on the effect of recombinant leukocyte A interferon in homosexual men with Kaposi's sarcoma. N Engl J Med 1983;308:1071.
109. Kumar A, Haque J, Lacoste J, et al. Double-stranded RNA-dependent protein kinase activates transcription factor NF-κB by phosphorylating IκB. Proc Natl Acad Sci USA 1994;91:6288.
110. Kurzrock R, Talpaz M, Kantarjian H, et al. Therapy of chronic myelogenous leukemia with recombinant IFN-γ. Blood 1987;70:943.
111. Kushnaryov VM, MacDonald HS, Sedmak JJ, Grossberg SE. Murine interferon-beta receptor-mediated endocytosis and nuclear membrane binding. Proc Natl Acad Sci USA 1985;82:3281.
112. Kuzel TM, Roenigk HH, Samuelson E, et al. Effectiveness of interferon alpha-2a combined with phototherapy for mycosis fungoides and the Sezary syndrome. J Clin Oncol 1995;13:257.
113. Kuzmits R, Ludwig H, Kratzik C, et al. Neopterin as tumor marker: serum and urinary neopterin concentrations in malignant diseases. J Clin Chem Biochem 1986;24:119.
114. Lacour J, Laplanche A, Delozier, et al. Polyadenylic-polyuridylic acid plus locoregional and pelvic radiotherapy versus chemotherapy with CMF as adjuvants in operable breast cancer. Breast Cancer Res Treat 1991;19:15.
115. Lane HC, Kovacs JA, Feinberg J. Anti-retroviral effects of interferon-α in AIDS-associated Kaposi's sarcoma. Lancet 1988;2:1218.
116. Larner AC, David M, Feldman GM. Tyrosine phosphorylation of DNA binding proteins by multiple cytokines. Science 1993;261:1730.
117. Larocca AP, Leung SC, Marcus SG, Colby CB, Borden EC. Evaluation of neutralizing antibodies in patients treated with recombinant IFN-beta$_{ser}$. J Interferon Res 1989;9:S51.
118. Lee SB, Esteban M. The interferon-induced double-stranded RNA-activated protein kinase induces apoptosis. Virology 1994;199:491.
119. Levy D, Darnell JE Jr. Interferon-dependent transcriptional activation: signal transduction without second messenger involvement? New Biol 1990;2:923.
120. Lin J, Sartorelli AC. Stimulation by interferon of the differentiation of human promyelocytic leukemia (HL-60) cells produced by retinoic acid and actinomycin D. J Interferon Res 1987;7:379.
121. Lin SL, Greene JJ, Ts'o POP, Carter WA. Sensitivity and resistance of human tumor cells to interferon and rIn·rCn. Nature 1982;297:417.
122. Lippman SM, Kavanagh JJ, Paredes-Espinoza M, Delgadillo-Madrueno F et al. 13-cis-retinoic acid plus interferon α-2a: highly active systemic therapy for squamous cell carcinoma of the cervix. JNCI 1992;84:241.
123. Lippman SM, Parkinson DR, Itri LM, Weber RS, Schantz SP, et al. 13-cis-retinoic acid and interferon α-2a: effective combination therapy for advanced squamous cell carcinoma of the cervix. JNCI 1992;84:235.
124. Litton GJ, Hong R, Grossberg SE, Vechlekar D, Goodavish CN, Borden EC. Biological and clinical effects of the oral immunomodulator 3,6-bis (2-piperidinoethoxy)acridine trihydrochloride in patients with malignancy. J Biol Response Mod 1990;9:61.
125. Lotze MT, Frana LW, Sharrow SO, Robb RJ, Rosenberg SA. In vivo administration of purified human interleukin 2: half-life and immunologic effects of the Jurkat cell line-derived interleukin 2. J Immunol 1985;134:157.
126. Ludwig H, Cortelezzi A, van Camp BGK, et al. Treatment with recombinant IFN-α-2C: multiple myeloma and thrombocythaemia in myeloproliferative diseases. Oncology 1985;42:19.
127. Mahaley MS, Urso MB, Whaley RA. Immunobiology of primary intracranial tumors. Part 10: therapeutic efficacy of interferon in the treatment of recurrent gliomas. J Neurosurg 1985;63:719.
128. Maluish AE, Leavitt R, Sherwin SA, Oldham RK, Herberman RB. Effects of recombinant interferon-alpha on immune function in cancer patients. J Biol Response Mod 1983;2:470.
129. Maluish AE, Urba WJ, Longo DL, et al. The determination of an immunologically active dose of interferon-gamma in patients with melanoma. J Clin Oncol 1988;6:434.
130. Mandelli F, Avvisati G, Amadori S, et al. Maintenance treatment with recombinant interferon alpha-2b in patients with multiple myeloma responding to conventional induction chemotherapy. N Engl J Med 1990;322:1430.
131. Maniatis T. Mechanisms of human beta-interferon gene regulation. Harvey Lect 1988;82:71.
132. Marroni M, Gresele P, Landonio G, et al. Interferon-α is effective in the treatment of HIV-1-related, severe, zidovudine-resistant thrombocytopenia. Ann Intern Med 1994;121:423.
133. Martin A, Nerenstone S, Urba WJ, et al. Treatment of hairy cell leukemia with alternating cycles of pentostatin and recombinant leukocyte A interferon: results of a phase II study. J Clin Oncol 1990;8:721.
134. Massaro ER, Borden EC, Hawkins MJ, Wiebe DA, Shrago E. Effects of recombinant interferon-alpha-2 treatment upon lipid concentrations and lipoprotein composition. J Interferon Res 1986;6:655.
135. McDonald S, Chang AY, Rubin P, Wallenberg J, Kim IS, et al. Combined Betaseron R (recombinant human interferon β) and radiation for inoperable non-small cell lung cancer. Int J Radiat Oncol Biol Phys 1993;27:613.
136. Merritt JA, Ball LA, Sielaff KM, Meltzer DM, Borden EC. Modulation of 2′,5′-oligoadenylate synthetase in patients treated with alpha-interferon: effects of dose, schedule, and route of administration. J Interferon Res 1986;6:189.
137. Meurs EF, Galabru J, Barber GN, et al. Tumor suppressor function of the interferon-induced double-stranded RNA-activated protein kinase. Proc Natl Acad Sci USA 1993;90:232.
138. Michaelvicz R, Revel M. IFNs regulate the in vivo differentiation of multilineage lympho-myeloid stem cells in hairy cell leukemia. Proc Natl Acad Sci USA 1987;84:2307.
139. Miles SA, Wang H, Cortes E, Carden J, Marcus S, Mitsuyasu RT. Beta-interferon therapy in patients with poor-prognosis Kaposi sarcoma related to the acquired immunodeficiency syndrome (AIDS). Ann Intern Med 1990;112:582.
140. Moertel CG, Rubin J, Kvols LK. Therapy of metastatic carcinoid tumor and the malignant carcinoid syndrome with recombinant leukocyte A IFN. J Clin Oncol 1089;7:865.
141. Nagai M, Arai T. Clinical effect of interferon in malignant brain tumours. Neurosurg Rev 1984;7:55.
142. Nagata S, Mantei N, Weissmann C. The structure of the eight or more distinct chromosomal genes for human interferon-alpha. Nature 1980;287:401.
143. Nathan CF. Secretory products of macrophage. J Clin Invest 1987;79:319.

144. Nathan CF, Prendergast TJ, Wiebe ME. Activation of human macrophages comparison of other cytokines with interferon-alpha. J Exp Med 1984;160:600.
145. Nelson BE, Borden EC. Interferons: biological and clinical effects. Semin Surg Oncol 1989;5:391.
146. Novick D, Cohen B, Rubinstein M. The human interferon α/β receptor: characterization and molecular cloning. Cell 1994;77:391.
147. Nolten WE, Goldstein D, Lindstrom M, et al. Effects of cytokines on the pituitary adrenal axis in humans. J Inf Res 1993;13:349.
148. Oberg K, Alm G, Lindstrom H, Lundqvist G. Successful treatment of therapy-resistant pancreatic cholera with human leukocyte interferon. Lancet 1985;1:725.
149. Oberg K, Alm G, Magnusson A, et al. Treatment of malignant carcinoid tumors with recombinant interferon alpha-2b: development of neutralizing IFN antibodies and possible loss of antitumor activity. JNCI 1989;81:531.
150. Oberg K, Norheim I, Lind E, et al. Treatment of malignant carcinoid tumors with human leukocyte interferon: long-term results. Cancer Treat Rep 1986;70:1297.
151. O'Connell MJ, Colgan JP, Oken MM, Ritts RE Jr, Kay NE, Itri LM. Clinical trial of recombinant leukocyte A interferons as initial therapy for favorable histology non-Hodgkin's lymphoma and chronic lymphocytic leukemia: an ECOG pilot study. J Clin Oncol 1986;4:128.
152. Oken MM, Kyle RA, Greipp PR, Kay NE, Tsiatis A, O'Connell MJ. Chemotherapy plus IFN in the treatment of multiple myeloma. Proc ASCO 1990;9:288.
153. Osterborg A, Björkholm M, Björeman M, et al. Natural interferon-alpha in combination with melphalan/prednisone (MP/IFN) versus melphalan/prednisone (MP) in the treatment of multiple myeloma stages II and III: a randomized study from the Myeloma Group of Central Sweden (MGCS). Blood 1993;81:1428.
154. Ostlund L, Einhorn S, Robert KH, Juliusson G, Biberfeld P. Chronic B-lymphocytic leukemia cells proliferate and differentiate following exposure to interferon in vitro. Blood 1986;67:152.
155. Ozaki Y, Edelstein MP, Duch DS. Induction of indoleamine 2,3-dioxygenase: a mechanism of the antitumor activity of IFN-γ. Proc Natl Acad Sci USA 1988;85:1242.
156. Ozer H. Biotherapy of chronic myelogenous leukemia with IFN. Semin Oncol 1988;15:14.
157. Paulnock DM, Havlin KA, Storer BM, Spear GT, Sielaff KM, Borden EC. Induced proteins in human peripheral mononuclear cells over a range of clinically tolerable doses of interferon-gamma. J Interferon Res 1989;9:457.
158. Pellegrini S, John J, Shearer M, Kerr IM, Stark GR. Use of a selectable marker regulated by alpha interferon to obtain mutations in the signaling pathway. Mol Cell Biol 1989;9:4605.
159. Pestka S. The purification and manufacture of human interferon. Sci Am 1983;249:37.
160. Pestka S, Langer JA, Zoon KC, Samuel CE. IFNs and their actions. Annu Rev Biochem 1987;56:727.
161. Pfeffer LM, Tamm I. Comparison of the effects of α and β interferons on the proliferation and volume of human tumor cells (HeLa-S3, Daudi, P3HR-1). J Interferon Res 1983;3:395.
162. Quesada JR, Alexanian R, Hawkins MJ, Barlogie B, Borden EC, Gutterman J. Treatment of multiple myeloma with recombinant alpha interferon. Blood 1986;67:275.
163. Quesada JR, Hersh EM, Manning J, Reuben J, Keating M, Schnipper E, Itri L, Gutterman JU. Treatment of hairy cell leukemia with recombinant alpha-interferon. Blood 1986;68:493.
164. Quesada JR, Kurzrock R, Sherwin SA, Guttermann JU. Phase II studies of recombinant human interferon γ in metastatic renal cell carcinoma. J Biol Res Mod 1987;6:20.
165. Quesada JR, Swanson DA, Gutterman JU. Phase II study of alpha interferon in metastatic rena cell carcinoma: a progress report. J Clin Oncol 1985;3:1086.
166. Quesada JR, Rios A, Swanson D, Trown P, Gutterman JU. Antitumor activity of recombinant derived interferon alpha in metastatic renal carcinoma. J Clin Oncol 1985;3:1522.
167. Quesada JR, Talpaz M, Rios A, Kurzrock R, Gutterman JU. Clinical toxicity of interferons in cancer patients: a review. J Clin Oncol 1986;4:234.
168. Rambaldi A, Introna M, Colotta F, et al. Intraperitoneal administration of interferon β in ovarian cancer patients. Cancer 1985;56:294.
169. Rashidbaigi A, Langer JA, Jung V. The gene for the human immune interferon receptor is located on chromosome 6. Proc Natl Acad Sci USA 1986;83:384.
170. Ratain MJ, Golomb HM, Bardawil RG, et al. Durability of responses to interferon alpha-2B in advanced hairy cell leukemia. Blood 1987;69:872.
171. Real FX, Oettgen HF, Krown SE. Kaposi's sarcoma and the acquired immunodeficiency syndrome: treatment with high and low doses of recombinant leukocyte A interferon. J Clin Oncol 1986;4:544.
172. Recht M, Borden EC, Knight E Jr. A human 15-kDa IFN-induced protein induces the secretion of IFN-gamma. J Immunol 1991;147:2617
173. Recombinant Human Interferon Gamma (S-6810) Research Group on Renal Cell Carcinoma. Phase II study of recombinant human interferon gamma (S-6810) on renal cell carcinoma: summary of two collaborative studies. Cancer 1987;60:929.
174. Reid LM, Minato N, Gresser I, Holland J, Kadish AR, Bloom BR. Influence of antimouse interferon serum on the growth and metastasis of tumor cells persistently infected with virus and of human prostatic tumors in athymic mice. Proc Natl Acad Sci USA 1981;78:1171.
175. Reid TR, Race ER, Wolff BH, Friedman RM, Merigan TC, Basham TY. Enhanced in vivo therapeutic response to interferon in mice with an in vitro interferon-resistant B-cell lymphoma. Cancer Res 1989;49:4163.
176. Revel M, Chebath J. IFN-activated genes. Trends Biochem Sci 1986;11:166.
177. Rios A, Mansell PWA, Newell GR, Reuben JM, Hersh EM, Guttermann JU. Treatment of acquired immunodeficiency syndrome-related Kaposi's sarcoma with lymphoblastoid interferon. J Clin Oncol 1985;3:506.
178. Rios A, Stringfellow DA, Fitzpatrick FA, Reele SB, Gutknecht GD, Hersh EM. Phase I study of 2-amino-5-bromo-6-phenyl-4(3H)-pyrimidinone (ABPP), an oral interferon inducer, in cancer patients. J Biol Response Mod 986;5:330.
179. Riviere Y, Hovanessian AG. Direct action of interferon and inducers of interferon on tumor cells in athymic nude mice. Cancer Res 1983;43:4596.
180. Robinson WA, Mughal TI, Thomas MR, Johnson M, Spiegel RJ. Treatment of metastatic melanoma with recombinant interferon alpha 2. Immunobiology 1986;172:275.
181. Rosenzweig IB, Wiebe DA, Borden EC, Storer B, Shrago ES. Plasma lipoprotein changes in humans induced by beta interferon. Atherosclerosis 1987;67:261.
182. Ruzicka FJ, Jach ME, Borden EC. Binding of recombinant-produced interferon betaser to human lymphoblastoid cells: evidence of two binding domains. J Biol Chem 1987;262:16142.
183. Samid D, Flessate DM, Greene JJ, Chang EH, Friedman RM. Persisting revertants after interferon treatment of oncogene-transformed cells. In The Biology of the Interferon System. Edited by WE Stewart III, H Schellekens. Amsterdam: Elsevier, 1986, p 327.
184. Sariban E, Mitchell T, Griffin J, Kufe DW. Effects of interferon-γ on proto-oncogene expression during induction of human monocytic differentiation. J Immunol 1987;138:1954.
185. Sarosdy MF, Lamm DL, Williams RD, et al. Phase I trial of oral bropirimine in superficial bladder cancer. J Urol 1992;147:31.
186. Schiller JH, Bittner G, Storer B, Willson JKV. Synergistic antitumor effects of tumor necrosis factor and gamma-interferon on human colon carcinoma cell lines. Cancer Res 1987;47:2809.
187. Schiller JH, Groveman DS, Schmid SM, Willson JKV, Cummings KB, Borden EC. Synergistic antiproliferative effects of human recombinant α54- or βser interferon with γ interferon on human cell lines of various histogenesis. Cancer Res 1986;46:483.
188. Schindler C, Fu XY, Improta T, Aebersold R, Darnell JE Jr. Proteins of transcription factor ISGF-3: one gene encodes the 91- and 84-kDa ISGF-3 proteins that are activated by interferon alpha. Proc Natl Acad Sci USA 1992;89:7836.
189. Scott GM, Ward RJ, Wright DJ, Robinson JA, Onwubalili JK, Gauci CL. Effects of cloned IFN-α2 in normal volunteers: febrile reactions and changes in circulating corticosteroids and trace metals. Antimicrob Agents Chemother 1983;23:589.
190. Selby P, Kohn J, Raymond J, Judson I, McElwain T. Nephrotic syndrome during treatment with IFN. Br Med J 1985;290:1180.
191. Shearer M, Taylor-Papadimitriou J. Regulation of cell growth by interferon. Cancer Metastasis Rev 1987;6:199.
192. Sidky YA, Borden EC. Inhibition of angiogenesis by interferons: effects on tumor- and lymphocyte-induced vascular responses. Cancer Res 1987;47:5155.
193. Smalley VM, Anderson JW, Hawkins MJ, et al. Interferon alpha combined with cytotoxic chemotherapy for patients with non-Hodgkin's lymphoma. N Engl J Med 1992;327:1336.
194. Soh J, Donnelly RJ, Kotenko S, et al. Identification and sequence of an accessory factor required for activation of the human interferon γ receptor. Cell 1994;76:793.
195. Sokawa Y, Watanabe Y, Kawade Y. Interferon suppresses the transition of quiescent 3T3 cells to a growing state. Nature 1977;268:236.
196. Solal-Celigny P, Lepage E, Brousse N, et al. Recombinant interferon alpha-2b combined with advanced follicular lymphoma. N Engl J Med 1993;329:1608.
197. Sparano JA, Fisher RI, Sunderland M, et al. Randomized phase III trial of treatment with high-dose interleukin-2 either alone or in combination with interferon alpha-2a in patients with advanced melanoma. J Clin Oncol 1993;11:1969.
198. Sreevalsan T, Taylor-Papadimitriou J, Rozengurt E. Selective inhibition by interferon of serum-stimulated biochemical events in 3T3 cells. Biochem Biophys Res Commun 1979;87:679.
199. Stevenson HC, Dekaban GA, Miller PJ, Benyajati C, Pearson ML. Analysis of human blood monocyte activation at the level of gene expression. J Exp Med 1985;161:503.
200. Stolfi RL, Martin DS. Modulation of chemotherapeutic drug activity with polyribonucleotides or with interferon. J Biol Response Mod 1985;4:634.
201. Stolfi RL, Martin DS, Sawyer RC, Spiegelman S. Modulation of 5-fluorouracil-induced toxicity in mice with interferon or with the interferon inducer, polyinosinic-polycytidylic acid. Cancer Res 1983;43:561.
202. Strander H, Adamson U, Aparisi T. Adjuvant interferon treatment of human osteosarcoma. Recent Results Cancer Res 1978;68:40.
203. Streuli M, Nagata S, Weissmann C. At least three human type alpha interferons: structure of alpha 2. Science 1980;209:1343.
204. Sumpio BE, Ernstoff MS, Kirkwood JM. Urinary excretion of IFN, albumin and β2-microglobulin during IFN treatment. Cancer Res 1984;44:3599.
205. Takikawa O, Kuroiwa T, Yamazaki F, Kido R. Mechanism of interferon γ action: characterization of indoleamine 2,3-dioxygenase in cultured human cells induced by interferon gamma and evaluation of the enzyme-mediated tryptophan degradation in its anticellular activity. J Biol Chem 1988;263:2041.
206. Talpaz M. Use of interferons in the treatment of chronic myelogenous leukemia. Semin Oncol 1994;21(suppl 14):3.
207. Talpaz M, Kantarjian HM, McCredie KB, Keating MJ, Trujillo J, Gutterman J. Clinical investigation of human alpha IFN in chronic myelogenous leukemia. Blood 1987;69:1280.
208. Talpaz M, Kantarjian HM, McCredie K, Trujillo JM, Keating MJ, Gutterman JU. Hematologic remission and cytogenetic improvement induced by recombinant human interferon alpha (A) in chronic myelogenous leukemia. N Engl J Med 1986;314:1065.
209. Talpaz M, Kurzrock R, Kantarjian H, O'Brien S, Gutterman JU. Recombinant IFN-α therapy of Philadelphia: chromosome-negative myeloproliferative disorders with thrombocytosis. Am J Med 1989;86:554.
210. Talpaz M, Rosenblum M, Kurzrock R, Reuben J, Kantarjian H, Gutterman J. Clinical and laboratory changes induced by alpha IFN in chronic lymphocytic leukemia: a pilot study. Am J Hematol 1987;24:341.
211. Tamura K, Makino S, Araki Y, Imamura T, Seita M. Recombinant IFN-β and γ in the treatment of adult T-cell leukemia. Cancer 1987;59:1059.
212. Tan YH. Chromosome 21 and the cell growth inhibitory effect of human interferon preparations. Nature 1976;260:141.
213. Taniguchi T. Regulation of interferon-beta gene: structure and function of cis-elements and trans-acting factors. J Interferon Res 1989;9:633.
214. Tokazewski-chen SA, Marafino BJ Jr, Stebbing N. Effects of nephrectomy on the pharmacokinetics of various cloned human IFNs in the rat. J Pharmacol Exp Ther 1983;227:9.
215. Torti FM, Shortliffe LD, Williams RD. Alpha interferon in superficial bladder cancer: a Northern California Oncology Group study. J Clin Oncol 1988;6:476.
216. Tsuruo T, Iida H, Tsukagoshi S, Oku T, Kishida T. Different susceptibilities of cultured mouse cell lines to mouse interferon. Gann 1982;73:42.
217. Urba WJ, Longo DL, Weiss RB. Enhancement of natural killer activity in human peripheral blood by flavone acetic acid. JNCI 1988;80:521.
218. Uze G, Lutfalla G, Bandu MT, Proudhon D, Mogensen KE. Behavior of a cloned murine interferon alpha/beta receptor expressed in homospecific or heterospecific background. Proc Natl Acad Sci USA 1992;89:4774.

219. Uze G, Lutfalla G, Gresser I. Genetic transfer of a functional human IFNα receptor into mouse cells: cloning and expression of its DNA. Cell 1990;60:225.
220. Verfaialle CM. Soluble factor(s) produced by human bone marrow stroma increase cytokine-induced proliferation and maturation of primitive hematopoietic progenitors while preventing their terminal differentiation. Blood 1993;82:2045.
221. Vokes EE, Ratain MJ, Mick R, et al. Cisplatin, fluorouracil, and leucovorin augmented by interferon alpha-2b in head and neck cancer: a clinical and pharmacologic analysis. J Clin Oncol 1993;11:360.
222. Volberding PA, Mitsuyasu RT, Golando JP, Spiegel RJ. Treatment of Kaposi's sarcoma interferon alpha-2b (Intron A). Cancer 1987;59:620.
223. Von Wussow P, Jakschies D, Freund M, Deicher H. Humoral response to recombinant IFN-α2b in patients receiving recombinant IFN-α2b. J Interferon Res 1989;9:S25.
224. Wadler S, Lembersky B, Atkins M, Kirkwood J, Petrelli N. Phase II trial of fluorouracil and recombinant interferon alpha-2a in patients with advanced colorectal carcinoma: an Eastern Cooperative Oncology Group Study. J Clin Oncol 1991;9:1806.
225. Wadler S, Schwartz EL, Goldman M, et al. Fluorouracil and recombinant alpha-2A interferon: an active regimen against advanced colorectal carcinoma. J Clin Oncol 1989;7:1769.
226. Wagstaff J, Scarffe JH, Crowther D. Interferon in the treatment of multiple myeloma and the non-Hodgkin's lymphomas. Cancer Treat Rep 1985;12B:39.
227. Welander CE. IFN in the treatment of ovarian cancer. Semin Oncol 1988;15:26.
228. Wilks AF, Harpur AG, Kurban RR, Ralph SJ, Zurcher G, Ziemiecki A. Two novel protein-tyrosine kinases, each with a second phosphotransferase-related catalytic domain, define a new class of protein kinase. Mol Cell Biol 1991;11:2057.
229. Williams RD. Intravesical IFN-α in the treatment of superficial bladder cancer. Semin Oncol 1988;15:10.
230. Wills RJ, Dennis S, Spiegel HE, Gibson DM, Nadler PI. IFN kinetics and adverse reactions after intravenous, intramuscular, and subcutaneous injection. Clin Pharmacol Ther 1984;35:722.
231. Witt PL, Storer BE, Bryan GT, et al. Pharmacodynamics of biological response in vivo after single and multiple doses of interferon-β. J Immunother 1993;13:191.
232. Yasui H, Takai K, Yoshida R, Hayaishi O. Interferon enhances tryptophan metabolism by inducing indoleamine 2,3-dioxygenase: its possible occurrence in cancer patients. Proc Natl Acad Sci USA 1986;83:6622.
233. Youn JK, Kim BS, Min JS, et al. Adjuvant treatment of operable stomach cancer with polyadenylic-polyuridylic acid in addition to chemotherapeutic agents: a preliminary report. Int J Immunopharmacol 1990;12:289.
234. Young HA, Ortaldo JR. One-signal requirement for interferon-gamma production by human large granular lymphocytes. J Immunol 1987;139:724.
235. Yung WKA, Castellanos A, Van Tassel T, Moser R, Marcus S. A pilot study of recombinant IFN betaser in patients with recurrent gliomas. J Neurooncol 1990;9:29.

CHAPTER 81

Cytokines: Biology and Applications in Cancer Medicine

DAVID R. PARKINSON AND ELIZABETH A. GRIMM

Introduction

From an immunologic perspective, the very fact that metastatic human cancers exist suggests that they are not significantly immunogenic, they have suppressed the immune response, or both. The availability of recombinant human interleukins has provided material in quantities sufficient for clinical trials of pharmacologic manipulation of the immune antitumor response, and the reproducible observations that regression of metastatic cancer in humans can be achieved using these agents provides a compelling impetus for their continued study. The biologic characterizations of the various interleukins, the rationales for their use in therapy of patients with cancer, and the accumulated clinical experience represent the subjects of this chapter.

The term *interleukin* has been used to designate any soluble protein or glycoprotein product of leukocytes that regulates the responses of other leukocytes. While the term emphasizes the roles these polypeptides play in coordination of the immune system, its distinction from the term *growth factors* is arbitrary and misleading, because most interleukins are growth factors and vice versa. As hormones of the immune response, interleukins produce their effects through endocrine, autocrine, and paracrine interactions. The cascades of interleukins that are generated by both pathogen exposure and antigen-specific interactions are primarily secreted and act locally, with the functions of individual interleukins mediated by interaction with specific receptors expressed differentially on different cell types, including hematopoietic and immunologic cells but also including endothelial and many other cells not part of the immune system. The paracrine effects of these interleukins include the initiation, amplification, maintenance, and termination of various phases of the immune response. Potent systemic effects are also observed with the interleukins through their interactions with cells of the vascular endothelium, fibroblasts, keratinocytes, adipocytes, and the central nervous system. The challenge of clinical oncologists and immunobiologists is to harness this biology for improved therapy of human cancer.

Interleukin-2

BIOLOGY

Interleukin-2 (IL-2) was originally described in 1976 as "T-cell growth factor" for its ability to support the growth of T lymphocytes (138). IL-2, together with interferon-γ represent the major cytokine products of the Th1 helper cells induced by antigen and IL-12 and counterregulated by the cytokines IL-4 and IL-10 (164, 243). IL-2 is a 133–amino acid glycoprotein of 15-kd molecular weight and contains an intrachain disulfide bond. Through interaction with a specific receptor located on T cells, B cells, macrophages, and natural killer (NK) cells, IL-2 plays a central role in the maturation and development of T cells.

The IL-2 receptor complex is composed of at least three subunits, an α chain (p55, Tac), a β chain (p75), and the more recently described γ chain (p64), this last being a common component of receptors for numerous other cytokines (108, 208). The different subunits have different functions, with the α chain being responsible for the rapid association with IL-2 and the β-γ complex responsible for the long dissociation time; the net result is a highly specific, trimeric receptor of high affinity (kd, 10^{-11}) for IL-2 expressed on a narrow range of cell types (228). Following interaction of IL-2 with the trimeric receptor complex, internalization occurs and cell cycle progression from G1 to the S phase is induced in association with the expression of a defined series of genes (201). A second functional response occurs through the IL-2 receptor β-γ dimeric receptor, also known as the "intermediate affinity" dimeric complex (kd, 10^{-9}) and involves the differentiation of several subclasses of lymphocytes into "lymphokine-activated killers" (LAK). This response occurs in patients with cancer who receive IL-2 (239, 240) and was originally considered to be part of the anticancer effect of IL-2, because the major histocompatibility complex (MHC)-unrestricted cytotoxicity expressed by LAK includes all fresh human tumor cells tested (79). More recently, IL-2-induced secondary cytokine elaboration (135, 155) and monocyte tumoricidal activity have been appreciated.

In summary, the multiple biologic effects of IL-2 on immune cells include the induced proliferation of antigen-stimulated T cells and induction of cytotoxicity in MHC-restricted, antigen-specific T lymphocytes, in the large granular lymphocyte NK cells leading to non-MHC-restricted LAK activity, and in monocytes. Which of these cytotoxic activities, as well as the contributions of the induced cytokines, are responsible for the occasional antitumor effect is yet to be resolved.

PRECLINICAL RATIONALE FOR USE IN CANCER THERAPY

As noted earlier, the incubation of both cytotoxic T lymphocytes and large granular lymphocytes results in the induction of in vitro lytic activity for autologous as well as allogeneic tumor cells, and to a lesser extent, nontransformed cells (80). Numerous studies have documented the therapeutic benefits of IL-2-activated effector cells, IL-2 alone, or optimally, a combination of both in the therapy of murine tumors (177). These models suggest that the intensity of IL-2 treatment, the degree of intrinsic immunogenicity of the tumor, the host's immune status, and the tumor burden all may affect the responsiveness of IL-2 therapy (118). Studies also suggest that in addition to the activated lymphoid cell populations, secondary cytokines induced during IL-2 therapy contribute to the antitumor activity. The reproducible observations that virtually all malignant cells can be lysed by IL-2 stimulated lymphocytes in a manner directly related to the intensity of IL-2 administration encouraged the pursuit of aggressive, intensive clinical trials involving IL-2 in patients with cancer.

CLINICAL APPLICATIONS

Renal Cell Carcinoma

IL-2 (Aldesleukin, Proleukin) is approved by the U.S. Food and Drug Administration and by regulatory authorities in Canada and the European Community for the treatment of patients with metastatic renal cell carcinoma of good performance status. The database for approval in the United States included 255 patients treated in seven separate clinical studies that used a treatment regimen developed in the Surgery Branch of the National Cancer Institute (NCI); recombinant IL-2 administered at a dose of 600,000 or 720,000 Iu/kg by 15-minute bolus infusion every 8 hours to tolerance from days 1 to 5 and repeated on days 15 to 19 (1, 6, 130, 178–182). As summarized in this database, the overall response rate among patients with renal cell carcinoma was 14%, with 4% of patients achieving complete regression (63). Although these response rates are modest, the prolonged median duration of all responses (approximately 20 months) and the apparent permanence of most complete responses in a population of patients with advanced progressive renal cell carcinoma were felt to represent evidence for significant benefit to patients. Responses occurred at all treated sites, including the liver, adrenal glands, and the renal primary and renal bed recurrences, although most responses occurred in patients with lung or lymph node metastatic disease.

The toxicity of the high-dose bolus regimen, or the high-dose continuous infusion regimens used more commonly in Europe, is significant, as discussed later (70, 162). By selecting patients with renal cell carcinoma more likely to respond to this cytokine, patients who are unlikely to benefit would be spared the toxicity and costs associated with this therapy. However, beyond the observations that patients with a Karnofsky performance status of 90 to 100 tolerated therapy better and were more likely to respond, no other pretreatment patient characteristics, including multiple laboratory studies, time from diagnosis to therapy, and involved sites, have proven to be prognostic (17). In a group of 327 patients with advanced renal cell carcinoma treated in Europe by continuous infusion of IL-2, baseline performance status, the time from diagnosis to treatment (greater or less than 24 months) and the number of metastatic sites (one versus two or more) were prognostically important (156). In a smaller group of patients treated with this same regimen, patients who continued to produce elevated serum levels of tumor necrosis factor (TNF) in the days following completion of IL-2 administration were more likely to respond (15).

Management of the bulky renal primary in patients who present with metastatic disease remains an issue for discussion. In 93 such patients who underwent surgery, 40% ultimately could not be treated with immunotherapy. These patients generally had low performance scores (Eastern Cooperative Oncology Group ≥2) at presentation. In the 56 patients who were able to undergo IL-2 therapy, the response rate was 27% (227). On the other hand, long, progression-free intervals have been documented in a number of patients whose residual primary tumor was removed only after response of metastatic sites to IL-2 therapy (56).

An important issue relates to the IL-2 treatment regimen itself. Modifications of the original regimen developed at the NCI have attempted to maintain or increase the antitumor effects of this treatment while reducing its toxicity. However, despite a large number of published trials conducted in this field involving therapy with IL-2 administered in a wide variety of doses, schedules, and combinations with other agents, and despite the difficulties in a comparative analysis of multiple small trials, it would appear that none of these manipulations has led to dramatic increases in response rates (205).

Similarly, the toxicities of the high-dose bolus and continuous infusion IL-2 regimens approved by regulatory authorities in the United States and Europe, respectively, and the fact that many patients with limitations of cardiac, pulmonary, or other organ systems are not appropriate candidates for aggressive IL-2 treatment regimens have led to widespread use of less aggressive, more chronic approaches to IL-2 therapy, usually by subcutaneous daily therapy. The published experience with this approach in renal carcinoma is limited, and although it is clear that objective responses can be achieved with this approach, the central questions of response duration and net clinical benefit have not been answered (194). Comparative data with the high-dose regimen is even more limited, but a preliminary analysis of the results of a randomized clinical trial with high-dose bolus IL-2 on a similar schedule using 10% of the normal dose suggests that similar response rates can be achieved (238).

Based on the promising preclinical findings, investigators

have also performed extensive studies of IL-2 combined with other cytokines in renal cell carcinoma (206, 226). The most extensively studied combination is with interferon-α, where Phase II results give little suggestion of a dramatically enhanced benefit from the combination (169, 188, 225). Therefore, despite the preclinical predictions of dramatic improvement in the therapeutic efficacy of IL-2 with the addition of other cytokines, these combinations, on the basis of Phase II studies, have not produced dramatic enough changes in either response rate or quality to be declared as being clearly superior.

Malignant Melanoma

Although still considered to be investigational in the United States for its use in this cancer, IL-2 has clear antitumor activity in melanoma (46). Three large, Phase II trials using the NCI Surgery Branch high-dose regimen have been published, with 5 complete (4%) and 22 partial (16%) responses reported among 134 patients treated (130, 160, 178). Despite the clear activity, the relatively brief duration of many responses has led to the investigation of IL-2 administered with combination chemotherapy for melanoma to develop a therapy with greater benefit to patients. Lower-dose regimens of IL-2, used either alone or with cyclophosphamide, have also yielded objective responses, although these have been generally partial and of short duration (120). High response rates for combination chemoimmunotherapy regimens have been reported by several investigators, with a number of these regimens combining interferon-α with IL-2. Response rates have routinely been 45 to 55% in these reports, with complete response rates as high as 20% (5, 23, 104, 113, 172). Both the duration of these responses and net benefit to the patients who undergo this demanding therapy, are under study in ongoing, Phase III clinical trials.

Other Cancers

Possible roles exist for IL-2 in other cancers as well as nonmalignant conditions (97, 173, 210, 211, 236). Responses have been reported in individual patients with ovarian cancer (with both systemic and intraperitoneal cavity therapy), non-small-cell lung cancer, head and neck cancer (with IL-2 administered regionally), colon cancer, breast cancer, bladder cancer (via intracavitary administration), and leptomeningeal metastases (via intraventricular injection) (125, 139, 204, 205). For the most part, however, these are anecdotal responses, and formal Phase II evaluation of IL-2 in these malignancies has been limited.

One strategy to integrate IL-2 therapy with best conventional treatment includes IL-2 administered after optimal debulking of disease with chemotherapy to induce an immune response against residual tumor. A limited amount of information suggests this might be a useful strategy with some solid tumors. For example, following the administration of IL-2 to 24 patients with metastatic small-cell lung cancer who had completed four cycles of combination chemotherapy, further tumor regression developed in 5 patients (34). While such results are intriguing, delayed responses to chemotherapy may account for this finding, and true confirmation of an IL-2-associated benefit in this setting would require Phase III clinical trials.

There have been a number of reports involving the administration of IL-2, either alone or with LAK cells in patients with malignant glioma. Generally, this approach has involved surgical resection of recurrent tumor and either direct instillation of IL-2 at surgery or placement of an Ommaya reservoir to allow therapy with cytokine either alone or with IL-2-activated lymphocytes. While clinical responses have been reported, the clinical benefit of such an approach to treatment remains to be established (82).

A promising clinical role for IL-2 is following high-dose chemotherapy associated with bone marrow transplantation for hematologic malignancies. Several clinical reports have been published involving the use of IL-2 in patients with relapsed acute leukemia, with objective responses reported (57, 122). In addition, preliminary studies have suggested clinical benefits, in comparison to matched controls, for patients receiving IL-2 following high-dose therapy and bone marrow transplantation for acute myeloid leukemia in first or second relapse (13, 50); it has been suggested that following bone marrow transplantation IL-2 might amplify the graft-versus-leukemia effect and decrease the graft-versus-host effect (203). Phase III investigations of this approach in acute myeloid leukemia are underway, and a similar approach is being used after high-dose chemotherapy in non-Hodgkin's lymphoma.

IL-2 with Adoptive Cellular Immunotherapy

As noted earlier, preclinical studies suggest enhanced antitumor activity when IL-2 is used together with ex vivo activated and expanded antitumor lymphocytes. The first objective responses with high-dose bolus IL-2 therapy were noted in patients receiving IL-2 together with LAK cells prepared through in vitro activation of autologous peripheral blood lymphocytes that were harvested by lymphopheresis, and initially, it appeared that the combination of IL-2/LAK was more active than IL-2 alone (5). Major IL-2/LAK clinical trials in patients with renal cell carcinoma have been conducted by several groups, including the NCI Surgery Branch, the IL-2/LAK Working Group, and the NCI-sponsored Modified Group C centers (53, 130, 178, 182). A subset of the NCI Surgery Branch's patients with renal cell carcinoma and with all patients entered into the Modified Group C trials were randomized to receive IL-2 alone or together with LAK cells. Response rates to IL-2 used alone and together with LAK cells as well as durability of responses did not differ substantially, and at present, the data do not support a major contribution of ex vivo activated and adoptively transferred LAK cells to the efficacy of high-dose bolus IL-2 in patients with renal cell carcinoma (182, 231).

A similar conclusion can be reached regarding the adoptive transfer of LAK cells in patients with melanoma treated with high-dose bolus IL-2. Among 136 patients with metastatic melanoma treated with this regimen in three separate trials, there were 8 complete (6%) and 14 partial (10%) responses (130, 175). A hybrid regimen involving both bolus and continuous infusion IL-2 together with intravenous administration of LAK cells had a 14% response rate, although large clinical studies of IL-2 administered entirely by continuous infusion together with LAK cells revealed little activity (12, 40, 41, 45). While response rates with IL-2/LAK are not different from those observed with high-dose IL-2 alone, the 4 to 5% of patients with melanoma who achieve durable response with this approach represent a qualitative difference from results with IL-2 alone (205). IL-2/LAK therapy in other solid tumors has been disappointing (125, 204).

Perhaps of greatest interest with respect to its implications for the future use of IL-2 in cancer therapy have been the clinical trials conducted with IL-2 used with tumor infiltrating lymphocytes (TIL) (178, 183). These lymphocytes are produced by placing digested, fresh tumor biopsies into an in vitro culture with IL-2. Over a period of 3 to 4 weeks, expanded populations of antigen-specific, MHC-restricted T cells (often CD8+ cytotoxic T cells) can be generated for administration together with IL-2 in treatment in approximately half of patients with melanoma whose tumor was obtained surgically. Although response rates using TIL cells together with IL-2 in the 30 to 40% range have been reported (178, 183), comparative response data with TIL cells compared with IL-2 alone do not exist; however, some patients who failed to respond to high-dose IL-2 alone have responded to their autologous TIL cells. The recent identification of many epitopes recognized by cytotoxic T cells on human melanoma has permitted characterization of the antigen specificities of TIL cells cultured from patients, and this will be useful in the design of vaccine strategies for the development of antigen-specific T cells (19, 98–101, 174, 221). In this context, IL-2 may prove useful either as a vaccine adjuvant or in the in vitro culture of antigen-specific T cells harvested from patients who have received vaccines (242).

TOXICITIES

The substantial toxicity of high-dose bolus IL-2 treatment has represented the major concern regarding clinical use of this regimen (192). The unique spectrum of toxicities encountered is quite different from the myelosuppression and related problems that are encountered with most chemotherapeutic agents. The acute toxicities resemble acute sepsis physiologically, and include hypotension, which may require pressor support, a vascular leak syndrome, and respiratory insufficiency related to replacement fluid therapy in the setting of both phenomena (124, 233). While the mechanism of the vascular leak remains unclear, it may involve the activation of endothelial cell antigens as well as the induction of secondary cytokines such as TNF-α. In addition, confusion, renal dysfunction, hepatic dysfunction, anemia, and thrombocytopenia can all be encountered. Toxicities that are less life-threatening but nevertheless may be treatment-limiting include nausea, emesis, diarrhea, myalgias and arthralgias, skin erythema, and pruritus. Other less common toxicities include myocardial infarction, myocarditis, cardiac dysrhythmias, infection, renal failure, bowel infarction, and death.

In the initial experience there was a 4% mortality rate among patients treated with the high-dose bolus IL-2 regimen (180); this has been greatly decreased with further patient management experience, careful screening of patients for underlying cardiac and pulmonary disease using cardiac stress treadmill examination and pulmonary function tests, and routine use of prophylactic antibiotics in patients receiving high-dose IL-2 who have indwelling central venous lines (165). There may be a genetic predisposition to greater IL-2 toxicity, linked with particular MHC-linked Class II alleles (127).

The mechanism of IL-2-induced hypotension has been studied in detail and appears related to the induction by IL-2 of TNF-α, which in turn causes the release of nitric oxide (NO) from endothelial cells. NO is a powerful regulator of vascular tone, and patients treated with IL-2 have been shown to produce high levels of NO (152).

A number of strategies have been adopted to decrease IL-2 toxicity (134). The use of alternative IL-2 doses and schedules has already been discussed and agents such as pentoxifylline, which block IL-2-induced TNF-α production, are under clinical trial in combination with IL-2 (47). Other agents such as *N*-monomethyl-arginine, which inhibits the TNF-induced production of NO by endothelial cells, are also under study (105, 106). Development of second-generation IL-2 analogues that do not induce the same high levels of secondary cytokines is also proceeding (83).

Interleukin-12

BIOLOGY AND PRECLINICAL RATIONALE FOR USE IN CANCER THERAPY

Human IL-12 was originally described under the terms *natural killer stimulatory factor* and *cytotoxic lymphocyte maturation factor* (107, 200, 216). This cytokine, which appears to be a product of activated monocytes, was recognized through its distinct structure and biologic properties. It is a heterodimeric glycoprotein of approximately 70-kd molecular weight and is composed of two unrelated glycoproteins of 40 and 35kd, respectively, which are linked covalently by a single disulfide bond (236). This structure makes IL-12 unique among cytokines. The 40-kd subunit has homology with the extracellular domain of the hematopoietic cytokine receptor family (69, 133), particularly the IL-6 receptor; the 35-kd subunit, on the other hand, has homologies with other cytokines, particularly IL-6 and granulocyte colony-stimulating factor (G-CSF) (133). Therefore, the complete molecule has characteristics of a complex of both cytokine and cytokine receptor, which may account for some of its unique properties, including its rather long plasma half-life of 6 to 7 hours compared with the several-minute half-lives of cytokines such as IL-2. A receptor for IL-12 has been described only on activated T cells, NK cells, and bone marrow progenitors, thus suggesting that this agent has direct biologic effects restricted to the immune and hematopoietic systems (33, 94).

Interleukin-12 exhibits a unique spectrum of biologic activities on the immune system (87). The molecule is a powerful inducer of interferon-γ from both T and NK cells (27, 28, 107). Induction of other cytokines such as TNF and granulocyte-macrophage colony-stimulating factors from these same cells is quite limited, however, distinguishing it in this regard from IL-2 (148, 149). IL-12 is capable of enhancing NK activity, generating LAK activity, and facilitating both the proliferation and cytolytic activity of human CD8+ T lymphocytes (132, 176). These in vitro observations also extend to the in vivo administration of IL-12. Mice treated with murine IL-12 exhibit a dose-dependent increase in both NK cell numbers and activity, and can be demonstrated to have enhanced CD8+ MHC-restricted T-cell cytolytic activity (66). The depressed spontaneous NK-cell activity of peripheral blood mononuclear cells from cancer patients could be enhanced in vitro with IL-12 (197).

A major biologic characteristic of IL-12 is its ability to promote the differentiation of progenitor T cells into Th1 cells, which is the helper-cell population distinguished by their production of IL-2 and interferon-γ. In contrast to the Th2 helper-cell population, which produces the cytokines IL-4 and IL-10 and mediates the humoral immune response, the Th1 helper subset is critical in the development of inflammatory and cellular immune response and is therefore considered to be critical to development of the antitumor response (38).

In summary, it would appear that the key immunobiologic role of IL-12 is to stimulate innate immunity through such functions as the stimulation of interferon-γ production and NK cell activity while also promoting the development of acquired cellular immunity through the promotion of Th1 T-lymphocyte differentiation. IL-12 also has been found to have effects on the hematopoietic stem cells, enhancing myelopoiesis and supporting the growth of B-cell progenitors. While in these studies IL-12 by itself had no effects on colony formation, synergism was demonstrated when it was used in combination with stem cell factor and IL-3 in the promotion of multilineage hematopoietic colony formation, although the effects were less than those observed with IL-6 or IL-11 (2, 5).

Based on these immunoregulatory properties, IL-12 has been studied for its potential antitumor properties. In a range of murine tumor models, including the B16F10 melanoma, the M5076 reticulum cell sarcoma, and the Renca renal cell adenocarcinoma, IL-12 exhibited potent antitumor and antimetastatic activity (21). IL-12 had no direct effect on these tumor cells in vitro, however. In these studies, activity was dose dependent, and mediated at least partly through a CD8+ T-cell mechanism, with interferon-γ production also being very important to the antitumor effect (20, 147). NK-mediated mechanisms did not seem to contribute to this therapeutic effect. An additional biologic mechanism also may contribute to the antitumor activity observed with this cytokine, however, because while diminished, the antitumor activity of IL-12 was not completely absent in studies involving T-cell-deficient mice. IL-12 was demonstrated to be a potent suppressor of angiogenesis, an effect that apparently is mediated through its ability to induce interferon-γ (103, 224). In these studies, the use of IL-12 with another inhibitor of angiogenesis, the fumagillin analogue TNP-470, resulted in increased antitumor efficacy. In mice receiving IL-12, a reversible dose- and time-dependent anemia, lymphopenia, and neutropenia were noted (66). Dose-limiting toxicities in early human clinical trials have included mucositis and transient reversible, hepatotoxicity.

POSSIBLE CLINICAL APPLICATIONS

The apparent central role of IL-12 in the differentiation of Th1 helper cells and the induction of interferon-γ suggest that this cytokine could play an important role, either directly or in conjunction with vaccine strategies, as a therapeutic agent designed to enhance the cellular immune response against cancer cells or a wide variety of intracellular pathogens. As noted earlier, this induction of interferon-γ appears to be critical both to the demonstrated antitumor and antimicrobial activities of IL-12. Initial clinical development strategies in cancer include the study of this agent alone in Phase I trials, followed by Phase II trials in renal cell carcinoma and other malignancies, and combination trials of IL-12 administered with cancer vaccines. Based on the ability of this agent to enhance the cytolytic activity of peripheral blood mononuclear cells from HIV-infected patients, trials of IL-12 in patients with AIDS are also being conducted (31). Preclinical data also exist to support the use of IL-12 in clinical studies of patients with leishmaniasis, toxoplasmosis, cryptococcidiosis, and tuberculoid leprosy (68, 84, 235).

Tumor Necrosis Factor-α

BIOLOGY

A nonglycosylated, 17-kd polypeptide, TNF-α, is expressed in both secreted and membrane-bound forms, with the secreted form circulating as a homotrimer. TNF binds to either of two distinct cell surface receptors of 55- and 75-kd molecular weight, respectively; these different receptor forms are independently expressed on different cell types (117). The lack of homology between the intracellular domains of these two receptor proteins suggests that they may subserve distinct cellular responses (75). Some information exists concerning these differential functions, particularly for the p55 receptor, which is important in the mediation of TNF-induced cytolytic activity, antiviral activity, IL-6 induction, and other biologic effects. A distinct role of the p75 receptor beyond facilitating the binding of TNF to p55, was less clear until the recent observation that p75 is critical to the inflammatory skin reaction noted with TNF-α.

The cytokine studied in human clinical trials to date is TNF-α. A second cytokine, termed TNF-β, or *lymphotoxin*, is produced by a distinct gene closely linked within the MHC complex on the short arm of chromosome 6; a 28% amino acid homology exists between the two cytokines (163). While activated monocytes and macrophages represent a major cellular source of TNF-α, TNF-α also is produced by activated T and NK cells and a wide variety of other cells. Depending on the cell type, TNF production can be stimulated by a number of signals, including lipopolysaccharide (monocytes), anti-CD3 monoclonal antibody (T cells), and other cytokines, including IL-2 (T cells). IL-4 is a potent downregulator of TNF production, similar to its effects on the production of interferon-γ and IL-6 (48).

Although the name *tumor necrosis factor* is still used for this interleukin, it merely reflects one of the first functional, in vivo effects attributed to this cytokine. In mice, it was observed that sera from BCG-injected mice would cause hemorrhagic necrosis of some, but not all, tumors (25). Further studies revealed that the effect was on the tumor vasculature and not on normal vasculature, thus suggesting differences in these two vascular beds. Subsequent purification of TNF-α has led to the identification of multiple roles for the cytokine, including direct tumor cell cytotoxicity, support of the growth and proliferation of immune system cells, induction of cachexia, and amplication of the human immune system via synergy with IL-2 (42, 43, 168). Induction of NO and subsequent hypotension is the dose-limiting toxicity of TNF in humans (105). The extreme toxicity of this agent in humans was not apparent in preclinical mouse studies; the mouse response to human TNF is incomplete, with recent findings indicating that at least one of the TNF receptors is species specific in the mouse and does not respond to human TNF (115, 168). Therefore, other functions described in preclinical models also may be irrelevant to humans, and further research is needed for an accurate description of the clinically important responses.

PRECLINICAL RATIONALE FOR USE IN CANCER TREATMENT

Tumor necrosis factor has direct, in vitro antitumor cytotoxicity on 30 to 50% of tumor cell lines, and it has been demonstrated to be active in vivo against both murine tumors and human tumor xenografts, particularly when they have reached a size of at least 5 mm in diameter (4, 10, 184, 191, 202). Which of the pleiotropic biologic activities of TNF contributes primarily to its antitumor effects is unclear. Subcutaneous tumors undergo hemorrhagic necrosis after TNF administration, which suggests that interference with tumor neovasculature is important. Indeed, TNF affects endothelial cells directly, resulting in the appearance on the tumor vessel endothelial cell surface of procoagulant activity and leading to fibrin formation, leukocyte infiltration, defective perfusion, and hemorrhagic necrosis. Immunogenic tumors are most responsive to the effects of this cytokine, however, suggesting that other events also are involved in the mechanism (191).

Considerable rationale exists for the use of TNF with chemotherapy. In vitro, enhanced cell killing is noted when TNF is combined with chemotherapeutic agents that inhibit DNA topoisomerases I and II, including agents such as doxorubicin, teniposide, etoposide, and actinomycin D (2, 219). The apparent mechanism involves TNF-mediated increases in DNA strand breakage. This enhanced effect also was observed in preclinical in vivo models, where enhanced antitumor activity was observed when TNF was combined with doxorubicin or etoposide (22, 109).

CLINICAL APPLICATIONS

Systemic Therapy

Based on the preclinical information described earlier, a series of Phase I clinical trials were performed involving the systemic administration of TNF-α. These trials involved recombinant TNF-α's from several different pharmaceutical sources; nevertheless, the results have been rather consistent among studies (29, 51, 199). The maximum tolerated dose (MTD) of bolus TNF in patients has consistently been in the range of 200 to 400 $\mu g/m^2$, 5- to 10-fold lower than the doses achievable in rodents that were active against tumors. The single-dose MTD was quite similar regardless of whether TNF was administered as a single dose, three times weekly, or five days a week. Shortly after TNF infusion, rigors, hypertension, and tachycardia develop, followed within 1 to 2 hours by fever and several hours later by hypotension. The dose-limiting toxicity has consistently been hypotension, which responds to therapy with fluid and vasopressors, although patients also develop a variety of constitutional symptoms. In studies where continuous infusion TNF has been administered, side effects of reversible thrombocytopenia, leukopenia, and hepatotoxicity, in addition to constitutional symptoms including fatigue, malaise, diarrhea, headache, and confusion, have been observed.

Minimal antitumor activity was observed in patients who were treated with systemically administered TNF, either in the Phase I studies or in a series of Phase II trials performed across the spectrum of common solid tumors, including renal cell carcinoma, melanoma, sarcomas, and adenocarcinomas of the colon, stomach, and pancreas. Phase I clinical trials involving TNF in combination with either chemotherapeutic agents or other biologic agents have also been conducted. Several clinical trials of TNF combined with IL-2 have been conducted based on compelling preclinical evidence for synergy, particularly when TNF was administered before IL-2 (11, 244). These trials show no evidence for an increased clinical benefit to the combination but do show evidence for an increased toxicity when TNF is administered either together with or following IL-2, which is not surprising given that IL-2 is a powerful inducer of TNF in patients (135, 150, 239, 240). Similarly, despite some preclinical data suggesting an interaction, no apparent clinical benefit, or increased immunologic stimulation has been observed in clinical trials of TNF and combined with interferon-γ (10, 53, 187, 195).

To date, results with TNF used together with chemotherapy have also been disappointing given the impressive evidence from in vitro and animal studies. Myelosuppression was dose-limiting when using a combination of TNF and etoposide (154). In a randomized, Phase II trial of carmustine (BCNU) administered either alone or with TNF, no apparent benefit, but increased toxicity, was observed with the combination (96).

One explanation for the discrepant results between the antitumor activity observed in rodent models and human trials involving TNF alone or in combination is the large difference in the tolerability of systemic doses of human TNF between different species and the fact that only limited systemic doses of TNF (considerably lower than the active doses in rodents) can be administered safely to patients. As noted later, the development of isolation-perfusion limb therapy with TNF has allowed exploration of therapeutic activity of levels of the cytokine similar to those that are achievable in preclinical models (114).

The role of TNF-α as well as other cytokines such as IL-1, and IL-6 in the wasting syndrome or cachexia, which is observed in many patients with cancer, has been investigated

(119). A "cachectin" isolated from animals with cancer was shown to be identical to TNF-α (14), and it has also been observed that athymic mice bearing TNF-secreting tumors become progressively more wasted compared with mice bearing non-TNF-secreting tumors (153). Because many patients with cancer have elevated plasma TNF levels, therapeutic strategies to decrease TNF production have been developed to interrupt this wasting syndrome. One such strategy involves the administration of pentoxifylline, which lowers TNF expression at both the RNA and protein levels (47). In preliminary studies, lowered TNF levels, associated with an improved sense of well-being and improved appetite, were observed (39).

REGIONAL PERFUSION THERAPY

The paradox between the remarkable antitumor activity of high-dose TNF in animal systems and its lack of clinical utility when administered systemically at tolerable doses in humans has led to extensive clinical study of TNF administered locoregionally (58–60, 114, 212). TNF has been administered intratumorally, intraperitoneally, and by intravesical or intra-arterial infusion. The most interesting and clinically beneficial results, however, have followed isolated limb perfusion of TNF together with melphalan, interferon-γ, and hyperthermia in patients with regionally recurrent melanoma or primary limb sarcomas. This strategy allows the achievement of high peak TNF concentrations, while greatly limiting systemic exposure. One complete response was noted among three patients treated using isolated limb perfusion with TNF alone (116); all other patients have been treated with one or another variant of the biologic-chemotherapeutic combination therapy. The origin of the combination infusion approach with melphalan, interferon-γ, and hyperthermia was the demonstrated synergy between TNF and each of these agents or modalities (10, 121). Systemic leakage is monitored continuously during the perfusion procedure by using radioactive serum albumin and a gamma detector placed above the heart (89). Clinical results using this approach are dramatic, with objective response rates of 100% in patients with regional extremity melanoma metastases and complete response rates in several studies exceeding 70%. Systemic toxicities are minimal, with hypotension managed by fluid supplement and administration of vasoactive amines. Regional toxicities appear to be similar to those observed with hyperthermic melphalan perfusion alone (see Chapter 55). Responses appear to be durable, and although this locoregional approach in melanoma in unlikely to affect median survival, the palliative effects can be significant in individual patients (see Chapter 138). Angiographic and immunohistologic studies show rapid elimination of tumor hypervascularization and endothelial cell destruction, suggesting that the interruption of tumor blood supply is an important mechanism of this approach, which is consistent with the biologic properties of TNF (171). Randomized trials in Europe and the United States are examining the relative contributions of each biologic constituent to the baseline activity observed with melphalan and hyperthermia alone. Similar regional treatment strategies are being attempted in isolated lung and liver perfusions (61).

Interleukin-1

BIOLOGY

Produced primarily by activated monocytes and macrophages, IL-1 is a cytokine with diverse immunologic, physiologic, and hematopoietic effects. Two forms of IL-1 (α and β) exist. Although these two glycoproteins of 17-kd molecular weight are distinct gene products and despite only a 26% homology, they bind to the same receptors and have similar biologic activities (42, 43, 123). IL-1 appears to be primarily involved in inflammation, having direct effects on endothelial cells as well as on both B and T cells. Through induction of other cytokines, including TNF, a cascade of biologic events are affected by IL-1. This cytokine has direct antitumor activity both in vitro and in vivo, and the in vivo effects are characterized by acute hemorrhagic necrosis associated with microvascular injury, decreased tumor blood flow, and significant clonogenic tumor cell kill (18).

Interleukin-1 also has a number of effects on the hematopoietic system, inducing bone marrow stromal cells to produce IL-6 in addition to a range of colony-stimulating factors (8, 193, 245). Furthermore, IL-1 synergizes with these colony-stimulating factors in vitro to promote the differentiation and proliferation of hematopoietic progenitor cells, is myeloprotective if administered before radiation or chemotherapy in preclinical studies, and can accelerate the recovery of both neutrophils and platelets after chemotherapy or sublethal radiation (26, 52, 62, 137, 151).

Additionally, the use of IL-1 with chemotherapy has resulted in improved antitumor efficacy through a variety of possible mechanisms, which include chemotherapy-induced upregulation of IL-1 receptors on the surface of tumor cells and IL-1-induced alterations in tumor blood flow (145, 217). The diverse mechanisms by which IL-1 may exert a beneficial antitumor effect, including through direct cytotoxicity, induction of tumor hemorrhagic necrosis, activation of immune effector cells, and enhancement of chemotherapy effect together with attenuation of chemotherapy-induced hematopoietic effects, have made it an attractive candidate for clinical trials in patients with cancer.

CLINIAL TRIALS

Interleukin-1 also has been studied for its myelorestorative functions. Platelet counts increased 1 to 2 weeks following therapy with IL-1 in the Phase I trials of both IL-1 β and IL-1 α, in association with increases in bone marrow megakaryocytes and serum levels of the thrombopoietin IL-6. In clinical trials, IL-1 was shown to accelerate the recovery of platelets and to shorten the duration of carboplatin-induced thrombocytopenia (196).

Interleukin-6

Interleukin-6, as well as IL-3 and IL-11, are important regulatory proteins for hematopoiesis, and their greatest relevance to clinical oncology probably relates to their use as growth factors for chemotherapy-associated myelosuppression, as discussed in Chapter 82. In addition to its properties as a thrombopoietin, however, IL-6 has a wide variety of biologic effects, which have led to its use in cancer treatment (93, 129, 222). IL-6 is produced by a range of cells, including T cells, monocytes and macrophages, fibroblasts, keratinocytes, and endothelial cells, and its variety of biologic effects led to its initial, independent characterizations as a B-cell growth factor and T-cell differentiation factor, a plasmacytoma growth factor (see Chapter 152), and a hepatocyte-stimulating factor (9, 67, 214, 215, 218, 220). IL-6 is a 21- to 30-kd glycoprotein of 212 amino acids that binds to a specific receptor that requires the same 130-kd membrane glycoprotein for mediation of signal transduction, as has been described for several cytokines, including IL-2 (207, 237). The biologic effects of IL-6 include those on the synthesis of acute phase reactants in the liver, on the hypothalamic-pituitary axis, on bone resorption, and on both the humoral and cellular arms of the immune system (71, 85, 95, 198, 214). As a major inducer of the acute phase response, the cytokine may play a role in the pathogenesis of sepsis. The ability of IL-6 to induce the differentiation of cytotoxic T cells through IL-2-independent mechanisms led to its study in preclinical models, where it has been active against a variety of murine tumors by mechanisms involving both CD4+ and CD8+ T cells (140, 141).

Phase I trials of both intravenous and subcutaneous IL-6 have been conducted in patients with advanced cancer (229, 230). All patients experienced constitutional symptoms, including fever, chills, and fatigue. Significant increases in C-reactive protein, fibrinogen, platelet counts, and soluble lymphocyte IL-2 receptor levels were observed at doses greater than 3 μg/kg. These increases in inflammation-associated proteins were accompanied by a fall both in serum albumin and hemoglobin levels. In general, the cytokine was well tolerated, although both hyperbilirubinemia and atrial fibrillation were observed at 10 μg/kg.

Interleukin-4

BIOLOGY

Interleukin-4 is the product of a subset of activated T-helper cells and was originally characterized by its ability to stimulate the proliferation of activated B cells. IL-4 has been reported to exhibit many other biologic activities as well, including induction of Class II MHC expression on B cells, regulation of IgE and IgG1 secretion, as well as the expression of specific receptors of IgE. In addition to B cell regulation, IL-4 possesses the ability to directly stimulate as well as inhibit various subclasses of T cells. Additional reports indicate that IL-4 activates the connective-tissue-type mast cells. The various functions of IL-4 are not resolved, but its apparent ability to inhibit lymphocyte reponse to IL-2 while promoting antigen-specific interactions may prove to be applicable to tumor regulation, especially in melanoma, where tumor-specific, tumor-infiltrating lymphocytes are reported to maintain tumor specificity in response to IL-4 and lose specificity when cultured in IL-2.

Human IL-4 is expressed in a single form, as evidenced by one major peak of activity on immunoelectrophoresis gels (85). The apparent molecular weight is 12 to 15 kd as determined by SDS-polyacrylamide gel electropheresis. Similar to IL-2, the one interchain disulfide bond is required for biologic activity. IL-4 apparently exerts its biologic activity through a single class of high-affinity receptors found on both hematopoietic and nonhematopoietic lineage cells. IL-4 receptor-positive cells include resting T and B cells, macrophages, myeloid progenitors, stromal cells, fibroblasts, and liver cells. In addition to potentiating antigen-specific immune responses, potential clinical applications are suggested by its anti-inflammatory effects (81).

PRECLINICAL RATIONALE FOR CLINICAL TRIALS

Interleukin-4 is a pleiotropic B- and T-cell growth and differentiation factor. Unlike IL-2 but similar to TNF, it is species specific, and the differences between the immunologic activities of murine and human IL-4 as well as the absence of predictive tumor models for human IL-4 have made the preclinical study of recombinant human IL-4 difficult. Because IL-4 can augment antigen-specific cytolytic T cells and induce differentiation of human B lymphocytes, including some leukemic B lymphocytes, clinical trials have been initiated to assess its clinical activity in patients with solid and hematologic malignancies.

A series of Phase I and II clinical trials have been conducted with recombinant IL-4 administered by both the subcutaneous and intravenous routes (7, 73, 166). At higher doses, side effects that have been associated with cytokine treatment include diarrhea, gastric ulceration, headache with nasal congestion, fluid retention, and arthralgia in addition to constitutional symptoms such as fatigue, anorexia, nausea, and vomiting. Interestingly, intravenous IL-4 therapy was associated with no increase in TNF levels, and the observed increase in the levels of IL-1 receptor antagonist (in contrast to IL-2 therapy) is consistent with predictions from the preclinical studies (7). Multi-institutional, Phase II trials of intravenously administered IL-4 were conducted in both renal cell carcinoma and melanoma, with only a single response, in a patient with melanoma (126). Clinical trials of IL-4 continue, particularly in patients with hematologic malignancies, including chronic lymphocytic leukemia and refractory Hodgkin's disease.

Macrophage Colony-Stimulating Factor

Macrophage colony-stimulating factor (M-CSF) is a bone marrow–derived glycoprotein that is capable of supporting the proliferation, maturation, and activation of cells of the mononuclear phagocyte lineage (167, 190). M-CSF binds to a specific, high-affinity tissue receptor that is expressed on monocytes and macrophages and is encoded by the c-*fms* oncogene (189). M-CSF-activated monocytes and macrophages have enhanced in vitro tumoricidal as well as antimicrobial activity which form the basis of the interest in this agent for both its potential anticancer and antiinfectious properties (16, 143, 213, 234). M-CSF has antitumor activity in preclinical studies, with reduced number of metastases and prolonged survival noted in B16 melanoma, although apparently greater activity was observed when the cytokine was used in therapy with an antitumor monoclonal antibody (92, 142).

Based on this rationale, recombinant human M-CSF has been used in early clinical trials in patients with cancer. Significant biologic and clinical effects have been observed with two different recombinant M-CSFs as well as with a urine-derived human M-CSF studied in Japan, with relatively little toxicity except at the very highest doses (9, 35, 170, 186, 241). Dose- and schedule-dependent monocytosis were observed and associated with reciprocal changes in the peripheral blood platelet count (35). Decreases in serum cholesterol and low-density lipoproteins, similar to observations made in preclinical studies, also were observed. In association with the monocytosis, evidence for monocyte activation was observed, as well as increases in the in vitro measurements of antibody-dependent monocyte cytotoxicity (B[9]). Although only Phase I studies with two different recombinant M-CSFs have been performed to date, clinical responses in patients with melanoma, renal cell carcinoma, and leiomyosarcoma have been observed. Potential uses for M-CSF in clinical oncology include its administration with monoclonal antitumor antibodies or other cytokines in cancer therapy or following bone marrow transplantation, where its monocyte-activating properties might be useful for both antitumor and antifungal effects (112, 128).

Interleukin-7

First described as a bone marrow stromal cell–derived growth factor involved in early B-lymphocyte development, IL-7 is now known to be produced in addition by fetal liver, thymus, and keratinocytes as well as by a number of lymphoid tumor cell lines (76, 146). The biologic activities subserved by IL-7 have also expanded following additional study; in addition to its effects on pre-B cells, it serves as a thymocyte growth factor, pre-T-cell differentiation factor, and activation factor for NK cells, cytotoxic T lymphocytes, monocytes, and macrophages (232). IL-7 has been successfully used in the long-term culture of antigen-specific cytotoxic T-lymphocytes. Both lymphoid and myeloid recovery are accelerated in mice when IL-7 is administered after bone marrow transplant, but IL-7 was effective in a human colon carcinoma xenograft model in immunodeficient mice only when human T cells also were administered (145). These properties have suggested clinical roles for IL-7 either directly as an antitumor agent when used with cytoreductive therapy, as an in vitro growth factor for the long-term culture of antigen-specific T cells, or as an immunorestorative agent following bone marrow transplantation. IL-7 has not yet been introduced into clinical trial.

Interleukin-10

Interleukin-10 is a relatively recently defined, important immunoregulatory cytokine whose principal biologic function appears to involve the suppression of cytokine synthesis in the Th1 subset of CD4 + T helper cells. Originally described as "cytokine synthesis inhibitory factor," this 35-kd noncovalently linked homodimeric peptide is produced by both Th1 and Th2 T cells, monocytes, B lymphocytes, and keratinocytes (90, 223). The suppression by IL-10 of IL-2 and interferon-γ production by Th1 CD4+ cells—and of IL-1, TNF, IL-6, IL-8, and colony-stimulating factors by monocytes, coupled with its ability to stimulate B-cell growth and immunoglobulin production—suggest that IL-10 could find a therapeutic use in sepsis and a number of autoimmune diseases that are associated with inflammation. Indeed, therapy with this cytokine in animal models of sepsis results in improved survival (72, 89, 91). The suppressive effects of IL-10 on cell-mediated immunity suggest that it might find a role in transplant rejection or the treatment of graft-versus-host disease (77). In a Phase I trial of a single bolus, intravenous dose of recombinant IL-10 administered to normal volunteers, no adverse side effects were noted, and a transient neutrophilia and monocytosis associated with significant lymphopenia, inhibition of T-cell proliferation, and dose-dependent inhibition of TNF-α and IL-1-β production were also noted (32).

Interleukin-13

Like IL-4 and IL-10, IL-13 is another cytokine that is produced by activated T cells that shares the capacity to inhibit cytokine synthesis by activated monocytes and modulates B-cell responses through its effects on the activation, proliferation, and differentiation of B cells (37, 136).

Interleukin-15

Interleukin-15 is a recently defined, novel cytokine that, despite having no sequence homology with IL-2, binds with the β and γ components of the IL-2 receptor (74, 78). IL-15 is expressed in a much wider range of tissues than IL-2, including activated monocytes and macrophages and skeletal muscle, kidney, and placenta. Similar to IL-2, IL-15 has been demonstrated to potentiate NK-cell cytokine production and cytotoxic activity; together with its production by monocytes and macrophages, these observations suggest that it may play a role in normal host immunity (24). Potential uses for IL-15 in cancer therapeutics are still being considered.

Transforming Growth Factor-β

Transforming growth factor-β is a family of proteins thought to play critical roles in the regulation of tissue development and repair (175). Three isoforms, termed β-1, β-2, and β-3, have been identified; all three forms appear to have similar biologic actions. TGF-β is produced by most cells, and receptors for TGF-β is present on most cells. A wide variety of biologic effects, depending on the cell types involved and the concentration of TGF-β used, are observed following exposure to TGF-β. One important effect that may apply to a cancer-related clinical application is its powerful effect on tissue healing. Endogenous TGF-β has been demonstrated at sites of repair in wound-healing models, including those where healing has been compromised by the administration of chemotherapeutic agents. Application of exogenous TGF-β leads to increased numbers of inflammatory cells and fibroblasts at the repair site and increased accumulation of new connective tissue (36, 111, 185). For these reasons, topical TGF-β has been introduced into clinical trials for the prophylaxis and treatment of chemotherapy-associated mucositis. In preclinical models, TGF-β also can protect against chemotherapy- and radiation therapy–associated myelosuppression; however, this potential clinical application will need to be balanced against the known and powerful immunosuppressive effects of this cytokine.

Gene Therapy with Cytokines

The clinical applications using cytokines that have been described in this chapter largely involve regional or systemic administration of genetically engineered, recombinant protein. A significantly different strategy, based on the paracrine physiology common to the biology of many cytokines, relates to the insertion of cytokine genes into autologous tumors, or autologous or allogeneic fibroblasts subsequently introduced in proximity to autologous tumor, to increase the immunogenicity of the tumors (157). Experimentally, this approach has been used successfully in a wide range of animal models using a broad spectrum of cytokines, including IL-2, IL-4, IL-7, IL-12, TNF-α, interferon-γ, and GM-CSF (3, 11, 64, 65, 88, 209). A common principle is local production of very high concentrations of cytokine, although the actual biologic mechanisms involved in the induction of immunity appear to differ significantly with different cytokines. Presumably, this alteration in the local environment of the tumor cell results in enhanced presentation of tumor-specific antigens and increased activation of tumor-specific lymphocytes as well as nonspecific responses. With some cytokines, such as GM-CSF and IL-4, extensive local inflammation is induced, following which the genetically modified tumor cells are rejected and long-term T-cell-mediated tumor-specific immunity against parental nonengineered tumor cells develops (44, 158). In contrast, the infiltrate observed with IL-2-transfected tumor cells is largely lymphocytic (49). Regardless of which cytokine is used, this approach represents another strategy for the induction of T-cell immunity. Clinical trials using these approaches have been initiated with a number of different cytokine genes.

Conclusions

Much has been learned after a decade of clinical investigation involving recombinant cytokines. In general, clinical studies have proceeded in parallel with basic investigations concerning the biology of these regulatory proteins and their interactions with the spectrum of lymphoid- effector cells, and in many cases, clinical observations have led to further preclinical study. Despite the wide clinical experience with these agents and the optimistic predictions from the preclinical studies, defined areas of meaningful therapeutic utility for these agents still remain modest. Seeking an explanation for this apparent discrepancy is a valid exercise. One apparent possibility is that while useful in defining biologic mechanisms and establishing general principles related to dose, schedule, and other variables, the preclinical models do not define the immunobiologic heterogeneity of the patient populations under treatment. In some cases, it is now appreciated that the pattern of cytokine response in murine models does not parallel that observed in humans. In contrast to the contrived homogeneity of preclinical models which often use tumor cell lines in homozygous animal systems, the biologically heterogeneous tumors developing in a genetically diverse patient population challenge attempts to dissect the value of a single therapeutic manipulation during an individual trial. Determination of simple response rates in the setting of the limited numbers of biologically dissimilar patients entered into the classic Phase II trial may not provide an accurate test of therapeutic hypotheses. It would seem, therefore, that more rapid therapeutic advances will follow our improved ability to define the biology of the tumors and patients under therapy and correlation with clinical outcome. Better characterization of groups of patients who are more likely to respond will lead to an improved therapeutic benefit ratio for individual patients and greater efficiency in the conduct of clinical trials (159).

References

1. Abrams JS, Rayner AA, Wiernik PH, et al. High-dose recombinant interleukin-2 alone. JNCI 1990;82:1202–1206.
2. Alexander RB, Nelson WG, Coffey DS. Synergistic enhancement by tumor necrosis factor of in vitro cytotoxicity from chemotherapeutic drugs targted at DNA topoisomerase II. Cancer Res 1987;47:2403–2406.
3. Asher A, Mule J, Kasid A, et al. Murine tumor cells transduced with the gene for tumor necrosis factor-alpha. J Immunol 1991;146:3227.
4. Asher A, Mule JJ, Reichert CM, et al. Studies on the antitumor efficacy of systemically administered recombinant tumor necrosis factor against several murine tumors in vivo. J Immunol 1987;138:963–974.
5. Atkins MB, O'Boyle K, Sosman J, et al. A multi-institutional phase II trial of intensive combination chemoimmunotherapy for metastatic melanoma. Proc Am Soc Clin Oncol 1993;12:394.
6. Atkins MB, Sparano J, Fisher RI, et al. Randomized phase II trial of high-dose interleukin-2 either alone or in combination with interferon alfa-2b in advanced renal cell carcinoma. J Clin Oncol 1993;11:661–670.
7. Atkins MB, Vachino G, Tilg HJ, et al. Phase I evaluation of thrice daily intravenous bolus interleukin-4 in patients with refractory malignancy. J Clin Oncol 1992;10:1802–1809.
8. Bagby GC Jr, Dinnarello CA, Wallace P, et al. Interleukin 1 stimulates granulocyte macrophage colony-stimulating activity release by vascular endothelial cells. J Clin Invest 1986;78:1316–1323.
9. Bajorin DF, Jakubowski A, Cody B, et al. Recombinant macrophage colony stimulating factor: a Phase I trial in patients with metastatic melanoma. Proc Am Soc Clin Oncol 1990;9:183 (Abstract).
10. Balkwill FR, Lee A, Aldam G, et al. Human tumor xenografts treated with recombinant human tumor necrosis factor alone or in combination with interferons. Cancer Res 1986;46:3990–3993.
11. Bannerji R, Arroyo CD, Cordon-Cordo C, et al. The role of IL-2 secreted from genetically modified tumor cells in the establishment of antitumor immunity. J Immunol 1994;152:2324.
12. Bar MH, Sznol M, Atkins MB, et al. Metastatic malignant melanoma treated with combined bolus and continuous infusion interleukin-2 and lymphokine-activated killer cells. J Clin Oncol 1990;8:1138–1147.
13. Benyunes MC, Fefer A. IL-2 in the treatment of hematologic malignancies. In Therapeutic Applications of Interleukin. Edited by M Atkins, J Mier. New York: Marcel Dekker, 1993, pp 163–175.
14. Beutler B, Cerami A. Cachectin, more than a tumor necrosis factor. N Engl J Med 1987;316:379–385.
15. Blay JY, Favrot MC, Negrier S, et al. Correlation between clinical response to interleukin-2 therapy and sustained production of tumor necrosis factor. Cancer Res 1990;50:2371.

16. Bock SN, Cameron RB, Kragel P, et al. Biologic and antitumor effects of recombinant human macrophage colony-stimulating factor in mice. Cancer Res 1991;51: 2649–2654.
17. Boldt DH, Mills BJ, Gemlo BT, et al. Laboratory correlates of adoptive immunotherapy with recombinant interleukin-2 and lymphokine-activated killer cells in humans. Cancer Res 1988;48:4409–4416.
18. Braunschweiger PG, Johnson CS, Kumar N, et al. Antitumor effects of recombinant human interleukin-1 alpha on RIF-1 and Panc02 solid tumors. Cancer Res 1988;48: 6011–6016.
19. Brichard V, Van Pel A, Wolfel T, Wolfel C, De Plaen E, Lethe B, Coulie P, Boon T. The tyrosinase gene codes for an antigen recognized by autologous cytolytic T-lymphocytes on HLA-A2 melanomas. J Exp Med 1993;178:489–495.
20. Brunda MJ, Luistro L, Warrier RR, et al. Antitumor and antimetastatic activity of interleukin-12 against murine tumors. J Exp Med 1993;178:1223–1230.
21. Brunda MJ, Luistro L, Warrier RR, Wright RB, Hubbard BR, Murphy M, Wolf SF, Gately MK. Antitumor and antimetastatic activity of interleukin-12 against murine tumors. J Exp Med 1993;178:1223–1230.
22. Burgers JK, Marshall FF, Isaacs JT. Enhanced antitumor effects of recombinant human tumor necrosis factor plus VP-16 on metastatic renal cell carcinoma in a xenograft model. J Urol 1989;142:160–164.
23. Buzaid AC, Legha SS. Combination of chemotherapy with interleukin-2 and interferon-alpha for the treatment of advanced melanoma. Semin Oncol 1994;21:23–28.
24. Carson WE, Giri JG, Lindemann MJ, et al. Interleukin (IL) 15 is a novel cytokine that activates human natural killer cells via components of the IL-2 receptor. J Exp Med 1994;180:1395–1403.
25. Carswell EA, Old LJ, Kassel RC, Green S, Fiore N, Williamson B. An endotoxin-induced serum factor that causes necrosis of tumors. Proc Natl Acad Sci USA 1975;72: 3666.
26. Castelli MP, Black PL, Schneider M, et al. Protective, restorative, and therapeutic properties of recombinant human IL-1 in rodent models. J Immunol 1988;140: 3380–3387.
27. Chan SH, Kobayashi M, Santoli D, Perussia B, Trincheiri G. Mechanism of IFN-γ induction by natural killer cell stimulatory factor (NKSF/IL-12). J Immunol 1992;148: 92–98.
28. Chan SH, Perussia B, Gupta JW, Kobayashi M, Pospisil M, Young HA, Wolf SF, Young D, Clark SC, Trinchieri G. Induction of interferon gamma production by natural killer cell stimulatory factor: characterization of the responder cells and synergy with other inducers. J Exp Med 1991;173:869–879.
29. Chapman PB, Lester TJ, Casper ES, et al. Clinical pharmacology of recombinant human tumor necrosis factor in patients with advanced cancer. J Clin Oncol 1987;5: 1942–1951.
30. Chehimi J, Starr, Frank I, Rengaraju M, Jackson SJ, Llanes C, Kobayashi M, Perussia B, Young D, Nickbarg E, Wolf SF, Trinchieri G. Natural killer cell stimulatory factor (NKSF) increases the cytotoxic activity of NK cells from both healthy donors and HIV-infected patients. J Exp Med 1992;175:789–796.
31. Chehimi J, Trinchieri G. Interleukin-12: a bridge between innate resistance and adaptive immunity with a role in infection and acquired immunodeficiency. J Clin Immunol 1994;14:149–161.
32. Chernoff AE, Granowitz EV, Shapiro L, et al. A randomized, controlled trial of IL-10 in humans. Am Assoc Immunologists 1995:95:1722–1767.
33. Chizzonite R, Truitt T, Desai B, Nunes P, Podlaski F, Stern A, Gately M. IL-12 receptor: I. Characterization of the receptor on phytohemagglutinin-activated human lymphoblasts. J Immunol 1992;148:3117–3124.
34. Clamon G, Herndon J, Perry MC, et al. Interleukin-2 activity in patients with extensive small-cell lung cancer: a phase II trial of Cancer and Leukemia Group B. JNCI 1993;85:316–320.
35. Cole DJ, Sanda MG, Yang JC, et al. Phase I trial of recombinant human macrophage colony-stimulating factor administered by continuous intravenous infusion in patients with metastatic cancer. JNCI 1994;86:39–45.
36. Curtsinger LL, Pietsch MJD, Brown GL, et al. Reversal of Adriamycin-impaired wound healing by transforming growth factor-beta. Surg Gynecol Obstet 1989;517–522.
37. DeFrance T, Carayon P, Gisele B, et al. Interleukin 13 is a B cell stimulating factor. J Exp Med 1994;179:135–143.
38. Del Prete GF, DeCarli M, Mastromauro C, Biagiotti R, Macchia D, Falagiani P, Ricci M, Romagnani S. Purified protein derivative of *Mycobacterium tuberculosis* and excretory-secretory antigen(s) of *Toxocara canis* expand in vitro human T cells with stable and opposite (type 1 T helper or type 2 T helper) profile of cytokine production. J Clin Invest 1991;88:346–350.
39. Dezube BJ, Sherman ML, Fridovich-Keil JL, Allen-Ryan J, Pardee AB. Down-regulation of tumor necrosis factor expression by pentoxifylline in cancer patients: a pilot study. Cancer Immunol Immunother 1993;36:57–60.
40. Dillman RO, Oldham RK, Barth NM, et al. Continuous interleukin-2 and tumor-infiltrating lymphocytes as treatment of advanced melanoma: a National Biotherapy Study Group trial. Cancer 1991;68:1–8.
41. Dillman RO, Oldham RK, Tauer KW, et al. Continuous interleukin-2 and lymphokine-activated killer cells for advanced cancer: a National Biotherapy Study Group trial. J Clin Oncol 1991;9:1233–1240.
42. Dinarello CA. Biology of interleukin 1. FASEB J 1988;2:108–115.
43. Dinarello CA. Interleukin-1 and interleukin-1 antagonism. Blood 1991;77:1627–1652.
44. Dranoff G, Jaffee E, Lazenby A, Golumbek P, Levitsky H, Brose K, Jackson V, Hamada H, Pardoll D, Mulligan RC. Vaccination with irradiated tumor cells engineered to secrete murine granulocyte-macrophage colony-stimulating factor stimulates potent, specific, and long-lasting antitumor immunity. Proc Natl Acad Sci USA 1993;90:3539.
45. Dutcher JP, Creekmore S, Weiss GR. A phase II study of interleukin-2 and lymphokine-activated killer cells in patients with metastatic malignant melanoma. J Clin Oncol 1989;7:477–485.
46. Dutcher JP, Gaynor ER, Boldt DH, et al. A phase II study of high-dose continuous infusion interleukin-2 with lymphokine-activated killer cells in patients with metastatic melanoma. J Clin Oncol 1991;9:641–648.
47. Edwards MJ, Heniford TB, Klar EA, Doak KW, Miller F. Pentoxifylline inhibits interleukin-2-induced toxicity in C57BL/76 mice but preserves antitumor efficacy. J Clin Invest 1992;90:637–641.
48. Essner R, Rhoades K, McBride WH, et al. IL-4 downregulates IL-1 and TNF gene expression in human monocytes. J Immunol 1989;142:3857.
49. Fearon ER, Pardoll DM, Itaya T, Golumbek P, Levitsky HI, Simons JW, Karasuyama H, Vogelstein B, Frost P. Interleukin-2 production by tumor cells bypasses T helper function in the generation of an antitumor response. Cell 1990;60:397.
50. Fefer A, Benyunes MC. Interleukin-2 as consolidative immunotherapy: clinical follow-up of patients treated with autologous bone marrow transplantation/interleukin-2 or interleukin-2/lymphokine-activated killer for acute myeloid leukemia 52. In Immunotherapy and Bone Marrow Transplantation. Edited by TR Spitzer, A Mazumder. Mount Kisco NY: Futura, 1995, pp 111–120.
51. Feinberg B, Kurzock R, Talpaz M, et al. A phase I trial of intravenously-administered recombinant tumor necrosis factor-alpha in cancer patients. J Clin Oncol 1988;6: 1328–1334.
52. Fibbe WE, van der Meer JWM, Falkenburg JHF, et al. A single low dose of human recombinant interleukin 1 accelerates the recovery of neutrophils in mice with cyclophosphamide-induced neutropenia. Exp Hematol 1989;17:805–808.
53. Fiedler W, Zeller W, Peimann C-J, et al. A phase II combination trial with recombinant human tumor necrosis factor and gamma interferon in patients with colorectal cancer. Klin Wochenschr 1991;69:261–268.
54. Fiorentino DF, Bond MW, Mosmann TR. Two types of mouse T helper cell. IV. TH2 clones secrete a factor that inhibits cytokine production by TH1 clines. J Exp Med 1989;170:2081.
55. Fisher RI, Coltman CA, Doroshow JH, et al. Metastatic renal cancer treated with interleukin-2 and lymphokine-activated killer cells. Ann Intern Med 1988;108:518–523.
56. Fleischmann JD, Kim B. Interleukin-2 immunotherapy followed by resection of residual renal cell carcinoma. J Urol 1991;145:938–941.
57. Foa R, Meloni G, Tosti S, et al. Treatment of anti myeloid leukemia patients with recombinant interleukin-2: a pilot study. Br J Haematol 1991;77:491–496.
58. Fraker DL, Alexander RH. Isolated limb perfusion with high-dose tumor necrosis factor for extremity melanoma and sarcoma. Adv Oncol 1994;179–192.
59. Fraker DL, Alexander RH, Andrich M, Rosenberg SA. Palliation of regional symptoms of advanced extremity melanoma by isolated limb perfusion with melphalan and high-dose tumor necrosis factor. Cancer J Sci Am 1995;1:1081–4442.
60. Fraker DL, Alexander RH, Andrich M, Rosenberg SA. Treatment of patients with melanoma of the extremity using hyperthermic isolated limb perfusion with melphalen, tumor necrosis factor, and interferon-gamma: results of a TNF dose escalation study. J Clin Oncol 1995.
61. Fraker DL, Alexander RH, Thom AK. Use of tumor necrosis factor in isolated hepatic perfusion. Circulatory Shock 1994;44:45–50.
62. Futami H, Jansen R, MacPhee MJ, et al. Chemoprotective effects of recombinant human IL-1 alpha in cyclophosphamide-treated normal and tumor-bearing mice: protection from acute toxicity, hematologic effects, development of late mortality, and enhanced therapeutic efficacy. J Immunol 1990;145:4121–4130.
63. Fyfe G, Fisher R, Rosenberg SA, Sznol M, Parkinson D, Louie A. Results of treatment of 255 patients with metastatic renal cell carcinoma who received high-dose recombinant interleukin-2 therapy. J Clin Oncol 1995;13:688–696.
64. Gansbacher B, Bannerji R, Daniels B, et al. Retroviral vector-mediated gamma-interferon gene transfer into tumor cells generates potent and long lasting antitumor immunity. Cancer Res 1990;50:7820.
65. Gansbacher B, Zier K, Daniels B, et al. Interleukin-2 gene transfer into tumor cells abrogates tumorigenicity and induces protective immunity. J Exp Med 1990;172:1217.
66. Gately MK, Warrier RR, Honasoge S, et al. Administration of recombinant IL-12 to normal mice enhances cytolytic lymphocyte activity and induces production of IFN-gamma in vivo. Int Immunol 1994;6:157–167.
67. Gauldie J, Richards C, Harnish D, et al. Interferon B_2/BSF-2 shares identity with monocyte-derived hepatocyte stimulating factor (HSF) and regulates the major acute phase protein response in liver cells. Proc Natl Acad Sci USA 1987;84:7251–7255.
68. Gazzinelli S, Hieny TA, Wynn SF, Wolf SF, Sher A. Interleukin-12 is required for the T-lymphocyte-independent induction of interferon by an intracellular parasite and induces resistance in T-cell-deficient hosts. Proc Natl Acad Sci USA 1993;90: 6115–6119.
69. Gearing DP, Cosman D. Homology of the p40 subunit of natural killer cell stimulatory factor (NKSF) with the extracellular domain of the interleukin-6 receptor. Cell 1991;66: 9–10.
70. Geertsen PF, Hermann GG, von der Maase H, et al. Treatment of metastatic renal cell carcinoma by continuous intravenous infusion of recombinant interleukin-2: a single-center phase II study. J Clin Oncol 1992;10:753–759.
71. Geiger T, Andus T, Klapproth J, et al. Induction of rat acute phase proteins by interleukin-6 in vivo. Eur J Immunol 1988;18:717–721.
72. Gerard C, Bruyns C, Marchant A, et al. Interleukin 10 reduces the release of tumor necrosis factor and prevents lethality in experimental endotoxemia. J Exp Med 1993;177:547.
73. Gilleece MH, Scarffe JH, Ghosh A, et al. Recombinant human interleukin 4 (IL-4) given as daily subcutaneous injections—a phase I dose toxicity trial. Br J Cancer 1992;66:204–210.
74. Giri JG, Ahdieh M, Eisenman J, et al. Utilization of the beta and gamma chains of the IL-2 receptor by the novel cytokine IL-15. EMBO J 1994;13:2822.
75. Goodwin RG, Anderson D, Jerzy R, et al. Molecular cloning and expression of the type 1 and type 2 murine receptors for tumor necrosis factor. Molec Cell Biol 1991;11: 3020–3026.
76. Goodwin RG, Lupton S, Schmierer A, et al. Human interleukin 7: molecular cloning and growth factor activity on human and murine B-lineage cells. Proc Natl Acad Sci USA 1989;86:302–306.
77. Gorczynski RM, Wojcik D. A role for nonspecific (cyclosporin A) or specific (monoclonal antibodies to ICAM-1, LFA-1 and IL-10) immunomodulation in the prolongation of skin allografts after antigen-specific pretransplant immunization or transfusion. J Immunol 1994;152:2011.
78. Grabstein KH, Eisenman J, Shanebeck C, et al. Cloning of a T cell growth factor that interacts with the B chain of the interleukin-2 receptor. Science 1994;264:965.
79. Grimm EA, Mazumder, Zhang HZ, Rosenberg SA. The lymphokine activated killer cell phenomenon: lysis of NK-resistant fresh solid tumor cells by IL-2 activated autologous human peripheral blood lymphocytes. J Exp Med 1982;155:1823–1841.
80. Grimm EA, Ransey K, Mazumder A, et al. Lymphokine activated killer cell phenomenon: II. Precurser phenotype is serologically distinct from peripheral T lympho-

cytes, memory cytotoxic thymus-derived lymphocytes, and natural killer cells. J Exp Med 1983;157:884–897.
81. Hart PH, Vitti DR, Burgess GA, Whitty DS, Piccoli DS, Hamilton JA. Potential anti-inflammatory effects of interleukin-4: suppression of human monocyte tumor necrosis factor alpha, interleukin-1, and prostaglandin E2. Proc Natl Acad Sci USA 1989;86: 3803.
82. Hayes RL. The cellular immunotherapy of primary brain tumors. Rev Neurol 1992;148: 454–466.
83. Heaton K, Ju G, Grimm EA. Human interleukin-2 analogs that preferentially bind the intermediate-affinity IL-2 receptor lead to reduced secondary cytokine secretion. Cancer Res 1993;53:2597–2602.
84. Heinzel FP, Schoenhaut DS, Rerko RM, Rosser LE, Gately MK. Recombinant interleukin-12 cures mice infected with *Leishmania major*. J Exp Med 1993;177: 1505–1509.
85. Hirano T, Kishimoto T. Purification to homogeneity and characterization of human B-cell differentiation factor (BCDF or BSF p-2). Proc Natl Acad Sci USA 1985;82: 5490–5494.
86. Hirano T, Yasukawa K, Harada H, et al. Complementary DNA for a novel human interleukin (BSF-2) that induces B lymphocytes to produce immunoglobin. Nature 1986;324:73–76.
87. Hirayama F, Katayama N, Neben S, Donaldson D, Nickbarg EB, Clark SC, Ogawa M. Synergistic interaction between interleukin-12 and steel factor in support of proliferation of murine lymphohemopoietic progenitors in culture. Blood 1994;83:92–98.
88. Hock H, Dorsch M, Dramanstein T, et al. Interleukin-7 induces CD4+ T cell-dependent tumor rejection. J Exp Med 1991;174:1291.
89. Hoekstra HJ, Naujocks T, Schrafford Koops H, et al. Continuous leakage monitoring during hyperthermic isolated regional perfusion of the lower limb: technique and results. Reg Cancer Treat 1992;4:301–304.
90. Howard M, Farrar J, Hilfiker H, Johnson B, Takatsu K, Hamoka T, Paul WE. Identification of T cell derived B-cell growth factor distinct from interleukin-4. J Exp Med 1982;155:914–923.
91. Howard M, Muchamuel T, Andrade S, et al. Interleukin 10 protects mice from lethal endotoxemia. J Exp Med 1993;177:1205.
92. Hume DA, Donahue RE, Fidler IJ. The therapeutic effect of human recombinant macrophage colony stimulating factor in experimental murine metastatic melanoma. Lymphokine Res 1989;8:69–77.
93. Ishibashi T, Kimura H, Shikama Y, et al. Interleukin-6 is a potent thrombopoietic factor in vivo in mice. Blood 1988;74:1241.
94. Jacobsen SEW, Veiby OP, Smeland EB. Cytotoxic lymphocyte maturation factor (interleukin 12) is a synergistic growth factor for hematopoietic stem cells. J Exp Med 1993;178:413–418.
95. Jilka RL, Hangoc G, Grasole G, et al. Increase osteoclast development after estrogen loss: mediation by interleukin-6. Science 1992;257:88–91.
96. Jones AL, O'Brien MER, Lorentzos A, et al. A randomized phase II study of carmustine alone or in combination with tumour necrosis factor in patients with advanced melanoma. Cancer Chemother Pharmacol 1992;30:73–76.
97. Kaplan G, Britton WJ, Hancock GE, et al. The systemic influence of recombinant interleukin-2 on the manifestations of lepromatous leprosy. J Exp Med 1991;173: 993–1006.
98. Kawakami Y, Eliyahu S, Delgado C, et al. Cloning of the gene coding for a shared human melanoma antigen recognized by autologous T cells infiltrating into tumor. Proc Natl Acad Sci USA 1994;91:3515–3519.
99. Deleted in proof.
100. Kawakami Y, Eliyahu S, Delgado CH, et al. Identification of a human melanoma antigen recognized by tumor-infiltrating lymphocytes associated with in vivo tumor rejection. Proc Natl Acad Sci USA 1994;91:6458–6462.
101. Kawakami Y, Eliyahu S, Sakaguchi K, et al. Identification of the immunodominant peptides of the MART-1 human melanoma antigen recognized by the majority of HLA-A2 restricted tumor-infiltrating lymphocytes. J Exp Med 1994;180:347–352.
102. Kawakami Y, Nishimura MI, Restifo NP, Topalian SL, O'Neil BH, Shilyansky J, Yannelli JR, Rosenberg SA. T-cell recognition of human melanoma antigens. J Immunother 1993;14:88–93.
103. Kerbel RS, Hawley RG. Interleukin-12: newest member of the antiangiogenesis club. JNCI 1995;87:557–559.
104. Khayat D, Borel C, Tourani JM, et al. Sequential chemoimmunotherapy with cisplatin, interleukin-2, and interferon alpha-2 for metastatic melanoma. J Clin Oncol 1993;11: 2173–2180.
105. Kilbourn RG, Gross SS, Jubran A, Adams J, Griffith OW, Levi R, Lodato RF. N^G-Methyl-L-arginine inhibits tumor necrosis factor-induced hypotension: implications for the involvement of nitric oxide. Proc Natl Acad Sci USA 1990;87:3629–3632.
106. Kilbourn RG, Owen-Schaub LB, Cromeens DM, Gross SS, Flaherty MJ, Santee SM, Alak AM, Griffith OW. N^G-methyl-L-arginine, an inhibitor of nitric oxide formation, reverses IL-2-mediated hypotension in dogs. J Appl Physiol 1994;76(3):1130–1137.
107. Kobayashi M, Fitz L, Ryan M, Hewick RM, Clark SC, Chan S, Loudon R, Sherman F, Perussia B, Trinchieri G. Identification and purification of natural killer cell stimulatory factor (NKSF), a cytokine with multiple biologic effects on human lymphocytes. J Exp Med 1989;170:827–845.
108. Kondo M, Takeshita T, Ishii N, et al. Sharing of the interleukin-2 (IL-2) receptor gamma chain between receptors for IL-2 and IL-4. Science 1993;262:1874–1877.
109. Krosnick JA, Mule JJ, McIntosh JK, Rosenberg SA. Augmentation of antitumor efficacy by the combination of recombinant tumor necrosis factor and chemotherapeutic agents in vivo. Cancer Res 1989;49:3729–3733.
110. Kyle RA, Beard CM, O'Fallen WM, et al. Incidence of multiple myeloma in Olmstead County, Minnesota: 1978 through 1990, with a review of the trend since 1945. J Clin Oncol 1994;12:1577–1583.
111. Lawrence WT, Sporn MB, Gorschboth C, et al. The reversal of an Adriamycin induced healing impairment with chemoattractants and growth factors. Ann Surg 1986;203: 142–147.
112. Lee M-T, Warren MK. CSF-induced resistance to viral infection in murine macrophages. J Immunol 1987;138:3019–3022.
113. Legha S, Plager C, Ring S, et al. A phase II study of biochemotherapy using interleukin-2 (IL-2) + interferon alpha-1A (IFN) in combination with cisplatin (C), vinblastine (V), and DTIC (D) in patients with metastatic melanoma. Proc Am Soc Clin Oncol 1992;11:343.
114. Lejeune FJ. High-dose recombinant tumour necrosis factor (rTNFa) administered by isolation perfusion for advanced tumours of the limbs: a model for biochemotherapy of cancer. Eur J Cancer 1995;31A:1009–1016.
115. Lewis M, Tartaglia LA, Lee A, Bennett GL, Rice GC, Wong GH, Chen, EY, Goddel DV. Cloning and expression of cDNA-s for two distinct murine tumor necrosis factor receptors demonstrate one receptor is species specific. Proc Natl Acad Sci USA 1991;88:2830–2834.
116. Lienard D, Ewalenko P, Delmotti JJ, et al. High-dose recombinant tumor necrosis factor alpha in combination with interferon gamma and melphalan in isolation perfusion of the limbs for melanoma and sarcoma. J Clin Oncol 1992;10:52–60.
117. Loetscher H, Steinmetz M, Lesslauer W. Tumor necrosis factor: receptors and inhibitors. Cancer Cells 1991;3:221–226.
118. Lotze MT. Biologic therapy with interleukin-2: preclinical studies. In Biologic Therapy of Cancer. Edited by VT Devita, A Hellman, SA Rosenberg. Philadelphia: Lippincott, 1995, pp 207–234.
119. Lowry SF, Moldawer LL. Tumor necrosis factor and other cytokines in the pathogenesis of cancer cachexia. Principles Pract Oncol Updates 1990;4:1–12.
120. Malksova V, Sosman JA, Hank J, et al. Low-dose IL-2 in cancer therapy. In Therapeutic Applications of IL-2. Edited by MB Atkins, JW Mier. New York: Marcel Dekker, 1993.
121. Manusama ER, Durante NMC, Marquet RL, et al. Isolated limb perfusion with tumor necrosis factors and melphalan for fibrosarcoma in brown Norway rats. Proc Am Assoc Cancer Res 1994;35:524.
122. Maraninchi D, Blaise D, Viens P, et al. High-dose recombinant interleukin-2 and acute myeloid leukemias in relapse. Blood 1991;78:2182–2187.
123. March CJ, Mosley B, Larsen A, et al. Cloning, sequence and expression of two distinct human interleukin-1 complementary DNAs. Nature 1985;315:641–647.
124. Margolin K. The clinical toxicities of high-dose interleukin-2. In Therapeutics Applications of Interleukin-2. Edited by MB Atkins, JW Mier. New York: Marcel Dekker, 1993, pp 331–362.
125. Margolin KA, Rayner AA, Hawkins MJ, et al. Interleukin-2 and lymphokine-activated killer cell therapy of solid tumors. J Clin Oncol 1989;7:486–498.
126. Margolin R, Aronson FR, Sznol M, et al. Phase II studies of recombinant human IL-4 in advanced renal cancer and malignant melanoma. J Immunother 1994;15:147–153.
127. Marincola FM, Venzon D, White D, et al. HLA association with response and toxicity in melanoma patients treated with IL-2-based immunotherapy. Cancer Res 1992;52: 6561–6566.
128. Masaoka T, Shibata H, Ohno R, et al. Double blind test of human urinary macrophage colony stimulating factor for allogeneic and syngeneic bone marrow transplantation: effectiveness of treatment and 2 year follow up for relapse of leukemia. Br J Haematol 1990;76:501–505.
129. Matsuda T, Hirano T. Interleukin-6 (IL-6). Biotherapy 1990;363–373.
130. McCabe MS, Stablein D, Hawkins MJ. The Modified Group C experience—phase III randomized trials of IL-2 vs IL-2/LAK in advanced renal cell carcinoma and advanced melanoma. Proc Am Soc Clin Oncol 1991;10:213.
131. McIntosh JK, Mule JJ, Merino MJ, Rosenberg SA. Synergistic antitumor effects of immunotherapy with recombinant interleukin-2 and recombinant tumor necrosis factor. Cancer Res 1988;48:4011–4017.
132. Mehrotra PT, Wu D, Crim JA, Mostowski HS, Stegel JP. Effects of IL-12 on the generation of cytotoxic activity in human CD8+ T lymphocytes. J Immunol 1993;151: 2444–2452.
133. Merberg D, Wolf S, Clark S. Sequence similarity between NKSF and the IL-6/G-CSF family. Immunol Today 1992;13:77–78.
134. Mier JW. Abrogation of interleukin-2 toxicity. In Therapeutic Applications of Interleukin-2. Edited by MB Atkins, JW Mier. New York: Marcel Dekker, 1993, pp 455–475.
135. Mier JW, Vachino G, Van Der Meer JWM, et al. Induction of circulating tumor necrosis factor (TNF alpha) as the mechanism for the febrile response to interleukin-2 (IL-2) in cancer patients. J Clin Immunol 1988;8:426–436.
136. Minty A, Chalon P, Derocq M, et al. Interleukin 13 is a new human lymphokine regulating inflammatory and immune responses. Nature 1992;362:248.
137. Moore MAS, Warren DJ. Synergy of interleukin 1 and granulocyte colony-stimulating factor: in vivo stimulation of stem-cell recovery and hematopoietic regeneration following 5-fluorouracil treatment of mice. Proc Natl Acad Sci USA 1987;84:7134–7138.
138. Morgan DA, Ruscetti FW, Gallo RG. Selective in vitro growth of T-lymphocytes from normal bone marrows. Science 1976;193:1007–1008.
139. Moser RP, Bruner JM, Grimm EA. Biological therapy of brain tumors. Cancer Bull 1991;43:117–126.
140. Mule JJ, Custer MC, Travis WD, et al. Cellular mechanisms of the antitumor activity of recombinant IL-6 in mice. J Immunol 1992;148:2622–2626.
141. Mule JJ, Marcus SG, Yang JC, et al. Clinical applications of IL-6 in cancer therapy. Res Immuol 1992;143:777–779.
142. Munn DH, Cheung NK. Antibody dependent antitumor cytotoxicity by human monocytes cultured with recombinant macrophage colony stimulating factor. J Exp Med 1989;170:511–526.
143. Munn DH, Cheung N-KV. Phagocytosis of tumor cells by human monocytes cultured in recombinant macrophage colony stimulating factor. J Exp Med 1990;172: 231–237.
144. Murphy WJ, Back T, Conlon K, et al. Antitumor effects of interleukin-7 and adoptive immunotherapy on human colon carcinoma xenografts. J Clin Invest 1993;92: 1918–1924.
145. Nakamura S, Kashimoto S, Kajikawa F, et al. Combination effect of recombinant human interleukin 1 alpha with antitumor drugs on syngeneic tumors in mice. Cancer Res 1991;51:215–221.
146. Namen AE, Lupton S, Hjerrild K, et al. Stimulation on B-cell progenitors by cloned murine interleukin-7. Nature 1988;333:571–573.
147. Nastala CL, Edington HD, McKinney TG, Tahara H, Nalesnik MA, Brunda MJ, Gately MK, Wolf SF, Schreiber RD, Storkus WJ, Lotze MT. Recombinant IL-12 administration induces tumor regression in association with IFN-gamma production. Am Assoc Immunologists 1994;153:1697.
148. Naume B, Gately M, Espevik TA. A comparative study of IL-12 (cytotoxic lymphocyte maturation factor), IL-12, and IL-7 induced effects on immunomagnetically purified CD56+ NK cells. J Immunol 1992;148:2429–2436.
149. Naume B, Gately MK, Desai BB, Sundan A, Espevik T. Synergistic effects of interleukin 4 and interleukin 12 on NK cell proliferation. Cytokine 1993;5:38–46.

150. Negrier MS, Pourreau CN, Palmer PA, et al. Phase-I trial of recombinant interleukin-2 followed by recombinant tumor necrosis factor in patients with metastatic cancer. J Immunother 1992;11:93–102.
151. Neta R, Douches S, Oppenheim JJ. Interleukin 1 is a radioprotector. J Immunol 1986;136:2483–2485.
152. Ochoa JB, Carti B, Peitzman AB, et al. Increased circulating nitrogen oxides after human tumor immunotherapy: correlation with toxic hemodynamic changes. JNCI 1992;84:864–867.
153. Oliff A, Defeo-Jones D, Boyer M, et al. Tumors secreting human TNF/cachectin induce cachexia in mice. Cell 1987;50:555–563.
154. Orr D, Oldham R, Lewis M, et al. Phase I study of the sequenced administration of etoposide (VP-16) and recombinant tumor necrosis factor (rTNF; Cetus) in patients with advanced malignancy. Proc Am Soc Clin Oncol 1989;8:A741.
155. Owen-Schaub LB, de Mars M, Murphy EO Jr, Grimm EA. IL-2 dose regulates TNF-a mRNA transcription and protein secretion in human peripheral blood lymphocytes. Cell Immunol 1991;132:193–200.
156. Palmer PA, Vinke J, Philip T, et al. Prognostic factors for survival in patients with advanced renal cell carcinoma treated with recombinant interleukin-2. Ann Oncol 1992;3:475–480.
157. Pardoll DM. New strategies for enhancing the immunogenicity of tumors. Curr Opin Immunol 1993;5:719.
158. Pardoll DM. Paracrine cytokine adjuvants in cancer immunotherapy. Annu Rev Immunolo 1995;13:399.
159. Parkinson DR. Interleukin-2: further progress through greater understanding. JNCI 1990;82:1374.
160. Parkinson DR, Abrams JS, Wiernik PH, et al. Interleukin-2 therapy in patients with metastatic malignant melanoma: a phase II study. J Clin Oncol 1990;8:1650–1656.
161. Parkinson DR. Interleukin-2 therapy: future directions. Enhancement of the antineoplastic activity of interleukin-2. In Therapeutic Applications of Interleukin-2. Edited by MB Atkins, JW Mier. New York: Marcel Dekker, 1993, pp 439–454.
162. Parkinson DR, Sznol M. High-dose interleukin-2 in the therapy of metastatic renal-cell carcinoma. Semin Oncol 1995;22:61–66.
163. Paul NL, Ruddle NH. Lymphotoxin. Annu Rev Immunol 1988;6:407–438.
164. Paul WE, Seder RA. Lymphocyte responses and cytokines. Cell 1994;76:241–251.
165. Pockaj BA, Topalian SL, Steinberg SM, White DR, Rosenberg SA. Infectious complications associated with interleukin-2 administration: a retrospective review of 935 treatment courses. J Clin Immunol 1993;11:136–147.
166. Prendiville J, Thatcher N, Lind M, et al. Recombinant human interleukin-4 (rhu IL-4) administered by the intravenous and subcutaneous routes in patients with advanced cancer—a phase I toxicity study and pharmacokinetic analysis. Eur J Cancer 1993;29A:1700–1707.
167. Ralph P, Sampson-Johannes A. Macrophage growth and stimulating factor, M-CSF. Prog Clin Biol Res 1990;338:43–63.
168. Ranges GE, Bombara MP, Aiyer RA, Rice GG, Palladino MA. Tumor necrosis factor-alpha as a proliferative signal for an IL-2 dependent T cell line: strict species specificity of action. J Immunol 1989;142:1203–1208.
169. Ravaud A, Negrier S, Cany L, et al. Subcutaneous low-dose recombinant interferon-2 and alpha-interferon in patients with metastatic renal cell carcinoma. Br J Cancer 1994;69:1111–1114.
170. Redman BG, Flaherty L, Chou TH, et al. Phase I trial of recombinant macrophage colony-stimulating factor by rapid intravenous infusion in patients with cancer. J Immunother 1992;12:50–54.
171. Renard N, Lienard D, Lespagnard L, et al. Early endothelium activation and polymorphonuclear cell invasion precede specific necrosis of human melanoma and sarcoma treated by intravascular high-dose tumor necrosis factor alpha. Int J Cancer 1994;57:656–663.
172. Richards JM, Mehta N, Ramming K, et al. Sequential chemoimmunotherapy in the treatment of metastatic melanoma. J Clin Oncol 1992;10:1338–1343.
173. Riddell SR, Watanabe KS, Goodrich JM, et al. Restoration of viral immunity in immunodeficient humans by the adoptive transfer of T cell clones. Science 1992;257: 238–242.
174. Robbins PF, El-Gamil, Kawakami Y, Rosenberg SA. Recognition of tyrosinase by tumor-infiltrating lymphocytes from a patient responding to immunotherapy. Cancer Res 1994;54:3124–3126.
175. Roberts AB, Sporn MB. Physiological actions and clinical applications of transforming growth factor-β (TGF-β). Growth Factors 1993;8:1–9.
176. Robertson MJ, Soiffer RJ, Wolf SF, Manley TJ, Donahue C, Young D, Herrmann SH, Ritz J. Response of human natural killer cells to natural killer cell stimulatory factor: cytolytic activity and proliferation of NK cells are differentially regulated by NKSF. J Exp Med 1992;175:779–788.
177. Rosenberg SA. Adoptive immunotherapy of cancer using lymphokine activated killer cells and recombinant interleukin-2. In Important Advances in Oncology. Philadelphia: Lippincott, 1986.
178. Rosenberg SA. Karnofsky Memorial Lecture: the immunotherapy and gene therapy of cancer. J Clin Oncol 1992;10:180–199.
179. Rosenberg SA, Lotze MT, Muul LM, et al. A progress report on the treatment of 157 patients with advanced cancer using lymphokine-activated killer cells and interleukin-2 or high-dose, interleukin-2 alone. N Engl J Med 1987;316:889–897.
180. Rosenberg SA, Lotze MT, Muul LM, et al. Observations on the systemic administration of autologous lymphokine-activated killer cells and recombinant interleukin-2 to patients with metastatic cancer. N Engl J Med 1985;313:1485–1492.
181. Rosenberg SA, Lotze MT, Yang JC, et al. Experience with the use of high-dose interleukin-2 in the treatment of 652 cancer patients. Ann Surg 1989;210:474–485.
182. Rosenberg SA, Lotze MT, Yang JC, et al. Prospective randomized trial of high-dose interleukin-2 alone or in conjunction with lymphokine-activated killer cells for the treatment of patients with advanced cancer. JNCI 1993;85:622–632.
183. Rosenberg SA, Packard BS, Aebersold PM, et al. Use of tumor-infiltrating lymphocytes and interleukin-2 in the immunotherapy of patients with metastatic melanoma. N Engl J Med 1988;319:1676–1680.
184. Salmon SE, Young L, Scuderi P, et al. Antineoplastic effects of tumor necrosis factor alone and in combination with gamma-interferon on tumor biopsies in clonogenic assay. J Clin Oncol 1987;5:1816–1821.
185. Salomen GD, Kasid A, Bernstein E, et al. Gene expression in normal and doxorubicin-impaired wounds: importance of transforming growth factor-beta. Surgery 1990;108: 318–323.
186. Sanda MG, Yang JC, Topalian SL, et al. Intravenous administration of recombinant human macrophage colony-stimulating factor to patients with metastatic cancer: a phase I study. J Clin Oncol 1992;10:1643–1649.
187. Schiller JH, Witt PL, Storer B, et al. Clinical and biologic effects of combination therapy with gamma-interferon and tumor necrosis factor. Cancer 1992;69:562–571.
188. Sella A, Kilbourn RG, Gray I, et al. Phase I study of interleukin-2 combined with interferon-alpha and 5-fluorouracil in patients with metastatic renal cell cancer. Cancer Biotherapy 1994;9:103–111.
189. Sherr CJ. Colony-stimulating factor-1 receptor. Blood 1990;75:1–12.
190. Sherr CJ. Regulation of mononuclear phagocyte proliferation by colony-stimulating factor-1. Int J Cell Cloning 1990;8:46–60.
191. Sidhu RS, Bollon AP. Tumor necrosis factor activities and cancer therapy—a perspective. Pharmacol Ther 1993;57:79–128.
192. Siegel JP, Puri RK. Interleukin-2 toxicity. J Clin Oncol 1991;9:694–704.
193. Sironi M, Breviario F, Prosperio P, et al. IL-1 stimulates IL-6 production in endothelial cells. J Immunol 1989;142:549–553.
194. Sleijfer DTH, Janssen RAJ, Buter J, et al. Phase II study of subcutaneous interleukin-2 in unselected patients with advanced renal cell cancer on an outpatient basis. J Clin Oncol 1993;10:1119–1123.
195. Smith JW, Urba WJ, Clark JW, et al. Phase I evaluation of recombinant tumor necrosis factor given in combination with recombinant interferon-gamma. J Immunother 1991;10:355–362.
196. Smith JW II, Longo DL, Alvord WG, et al. The effects of treatment with interleukin-1 alpha on platelet recovery after high-dose carboplatin. 1993;328:756–761.
197. Soiffer RJ, Robertson MJ, Murray C, Cochran K, Ritz J. Interleukin-12 augments cytolytic activity of peripheral blood lymphocytes from patients with hematologic and solid malignancies. Blood 1993;82:2790–2796.
198. Spangelo BL, Judd AM, Isakson PC, et al. Interleukin-6 stimulates anterior pituitary hormone release in vivo. Endocrinology 1989;125:575–577.
199. Spriggs DR, Sherman ML, Michie H, et al. Recombinant human tumor necrosis factor administered as a 24-hour intravenous infusion: a phase I and pharmacologic study. JNCI 1988;80:1039–1044.
200. Stern AS, Podlaski FJ, Hulmes JD, Pan YE, Quinn PM, Wolitzy AG, Familletti PC, Stremlo CL, Truitt T, Chizzonite R, Gately MK. Purification to homogeneity and partial characterization of cytotoxic lymphocyte maturation factor from human B-lymphoblastoid cells. Proc Natl Acad Sci USA 1990;87:6808–6812.
201. Stern JB, Smith KA. Interleukin-2 induction of T-cell G_1 progression and c-*myb* expression. Science 1986;233:203–206.
202. Sugarman BJ, Aggarwal BB, Hass PE, et al. Recombinant human tumor necrosis factor-alpha: effects on proliferation of normal and transformed cells in vitro. Science 1985:230:943–945.
203. Sykes M, Harty MW, Szot GL, et al. IL-2 inhibits graft-versus-host-disease-promoting activity of CD4+ cells while preserving CD4- and CD8-mediated graft-vs-leukemia effects. Blood 1994;83:2560–2569.
204. Sznol M, Hawkins MJ. Interleukin-2 in malignancies other than melanoma and renal cell carcinoma. In Therapeutic Applications of IL-2. Edited by MB Atkins, JW Mier. New York: Marcel Dekker, 1993, p 177.
205. Sznol M, Parkinson D. Clinical applications of IL-12. Oncology 1994;8:61–67.
206. Sznol M, Thurn A, Parkinson DR. Overview of interleukin-2 trials in patients with renal cell carcinoma. In Immunobiology of Renal Carcinoma. Edited by R Bukowski. New York: Marcel Dekker, 1993.
207. Tagga T, Hibi M, Hirata Y, et al. Interleukin-6 triggers the association of its receptor with a possible signal transducer gp 130. Cell 1989;58:573–581.
208. Takeshita T, Asao H, Ohtani K, Ishii N, et al. Cloning of the gamma chain of the human IL-2 receptor. Science 1992;257:379–382.
209. Tepper R, Pattengale P, Leder P. Murine interleukin-4 displays potent antitumor activity in vivo. Cell 1989;57:503.
210. Teppler H, Kaplan G, Smith K, et al. Efficacy of low doses of the polyethylene glycol derivative of interleukin-2 in modulating the immune response of patients with human immunodeficiency virus type 1 infection. J Infect Dis 1993;167:291–298.
211. Teppler H, Kaplan G, Smith KA, et al. Prolonged immunostimulatory effect of low-dose polyethylene glycol interleukin-2 in patients with human immunodeficiency virus type 1 infection. J Exp Med 1993;177:483–492.
212. Thom AK, Alexander RH, Andrich MP, et al. Cytokine levels and systemic toxicity in patients undergoing isolated limb perfusion with high-dose tumor necrosis factor, interferon-gamma, and melphalan. J Clin Oncol 1995;13:264–273.
213. Thomassen MJ, Barna BP, Weidman HP, et al. Modulation of human alveolar macrophage tumoricidal activity by recombinant macrophage colony-stimulating factor. J Biol Response Mod 1990;9:87–91.
214. Tosato G, Pike S. Interferon B2/interleukin-6 is a costimulant for human T lymphocytes. J Immunol 1988;141:1556–1562.
215. Tosato G, Seamon KB, Goldman ND, et al. Monocyte derived human B-cell growth factor identified as interferon-B_2 (BSF-3, IL-6). Science 1988;239:502–504.
216. Trinchieri G. Interleukin-12: a cytokine produced by antigen-presenting cells with immunoregulatory functions in the generation of T-helper cells type 1 and cytotoxic lymphocytes. Blood 1994;84:4008–4027.
217. Usui N, Mimnaugh EG, Sinha BK. A role for the interleukin 1 receptor in the synergistic antitumor effects of human interleukin 1 alpha and etoposide against human melanoma cells. Cancer Res 1991;51:769–774.
218. Uyttenhove C, Coulie PG, Van Snick J. T cell growth and differentiation induced by interleukin-HP1/IL-6, the murine hybridoma/plasmacytoma growth factor. J Exp Med 1988;167:1417–1427.
219. Valenti M, Cimoli G, Parodi S, et al. Potentiation of tumor necrosis factor-mediated cell killing by VP16 on human ovarian cancer cell lines. In vitro results and clinical implications. Eur J Cancer 1993;29A:1157–1161.
220. Van Damme J, Opdenakker G, Simpson RJ. Identification of the human 26-kd protein, interferon beta-2 (IFN b2) as a B cell hybridoma/plasmacytoma growth factor induced by interleukin and tumor necrosis factor. J Exp Med 1987;165:914–920.
221. van der Bruggen P, Traversari C, Chomez P, et al. A gene encoding an antigen recognized by cytotoxic T lymphocytes on a human melanoma. Science 1991;254: 1643–1647.
222. Van Snick J. Interleukin-6: an overview. Annu Rev Immun 1990;8:253–278.

223. Viera P, De Waal Malefyt R, Dang MN, et al. Isolation and expression of human cytokine synthesis inhibitory factor cDNA clones: homology to Epstein-Barr virus open reading frame BCRFI. Proc Natl Acad Sci USA 1991;88:1172.
224. Voest EE, Kenyon BM, O'Reilly MS, Truitt G, D'Amato RJ, Folkman J. Inhibition of angiogenesis in vivo by interleukin 12. JNCI 1995;87:581–586.
225. Vuoristo M, Jantunen I, Pyrhonen S, et al. A combination of subcutaneous recombinant interleukin-2 and recombinant interferon-alpha in the treatment of advanced renal cell carcinoma or melanoma. Eur J Cancer 1994;30A:530–532.
226. Wagstaff J, Baars JW, Wolbink GJ, et al. Renal cell carcinoma and interleukin-2: a review. Eur J Cancer 1995;31A:401–408.
227. Walther MM, Alexander RB, Weiss GH, et al. Cytoreductive surgery prior to interleukin-2-based therapy in patients with metastatic renal cell carcinoma. Urology 1993;42:250–258.
228. Wang H-M, Smith KA. The interleukin-2 receptor. Functional consequences of its bimolecular structure. J Exp Med 1987;166:1055–1069.
229. Weber J, Gunn H, Yang J, et al. A phase I trial of intravenous interleukin-6 in patients with advanced cancer. J Immunotherapy 1994;15:292–302.
230. Weber J, Yang JC, Topalian SL, et al. Phase I trial of subcutaneous interleukin-6 in patients with advanced malignancies. J Clin Oncol 1993;11:499–506.
231. Weiss GR, Margolin KA, Aronson FR, et al. A randomized phase II trial of continuous infusion interleukin-2 or bolus injection interleukin-2 plus lymphokine-activated killer cells for advanced renal cell carcinoma. J Clin Oncol 1992;10:275–281.
232. Welch PA, Namen AE, Goodwin RG, et al. Human IL-7: a novel T cell growth factor. J Immunol 1989;143:3562–3567.
233. White RL, Schwartzentruber DJ, Guleria A, et al. Cardiopulmonary toxicity of treatment with high-dose interleukin-2 in 199 consecutive patients with metastatic melanoma or renal cell carcinoma. Cancer 1994;74:3212–3222.
234. Wing EJ, Waheed A, Shadduck RK, et al. Effect of colony stimulating factor on murine macrophages. Induction of antitumor activity. J Clin Invest 1982;69:270–276.
235. Wolf SF, Sieburth D, Sypek J. Interleukin 12: a key modulator of immune function. Stem Cells 1994;12:154–168.
236. Wood R, Montoya JG, Kundu SK, et al. Safety and efficacy of polyethylene glycol-modified interleukin-2 and zidovudine in human immunodeficiency virus type 1 infection: a phase I/II study. J Infect Dis 1993;167:519–525.
237. Yanasaki K, Taga T, Hirata Y, et al. Cloning and expression of the human interleukin-6 (BSF-2/IFNB2) receptor. Science 1988;241:825–828.
238. Yang JC, Topalian SL, Parkinson DR, et al. Randomized comparison of high-dose and low-dose intravenous interleukin-2 for the therapy of metastatic renal cell carcinoma: an interim report. J Clin Oncol 1994;12:1572–1576.
239. Yang SC, Grimm EA, Parkinson DR, et al. Clinical and immunomodulatory effects of combination immunotherapy with low-dose interleukin 2 and tumor necrosis factor alpha in patients with advanced non-small cell lung cancer: a phase I trial. Cancer Res 1991;51:3669–3676.
240. Yang SC, Owen-Schaub LB, Grimm EA, Roth JA. Induction of lymphokine activated killer cytotoxicity with interleukin-2 and tumor necrosis factor alpha against primary lung cancer target. Cancer Immunol Immunother 1989;29:193–196.
241. Zamkoff DW, Hudson J, Groves ES, et al. A phase I trial of recombinant human macrophage colony-stimulating factor by rapid intravenous infusion in patients with refractory malignancy. J Immunother 1992;11:103–110.
242. Zatloukal K, Schneeberger A, Berger M, et al. Elicitation of a systemic and protective anti-melanoma immune response by an IL-2-based vaccine. J Immunol 1995;154:3406–3419.
243. Zeh HJ, Hurd S, Storkus WJ, et al. Interleukin 12 promotes the proliferation and cytolytic maturation of immune effectors: implications for the immunotherapy of cancer. J Immunother 1993;14:155–161.
244. Zimmerman RJ, Gauny S, Chan A, Landry P, et al. Sequence dependence of administration of human recombinant tumor necrosis factor and interleukin-2 in murine tumor therapy. JNCI 1989;81:227–231.
245. Zucali JR, Dinarello CA, Oblon DJ, et al. Interleukin 1 stimulates fibroblasts to produce granulocyte-macrophage colony-stimulating activity and prostaglandin E_2. J Clin Invest 1986;77:1857–1863.

CHAPTER 82

Hematopoietic Growth Factors

GEORGE D. DEMETRI

Introduction

Hematopoiesis, the process by which the formed elements of blood are produced, is a complex and tightly regulated physiologic function that is critical to survival. Since inhibition of hematopoiesis (i.e., myelosuppression) represents the most common serious toxicity associated with the cytotoxic therapy of cancer, research that improves our understanding of hematopoiesis has direct relevance to improving the therapeutic index of most cancer treatments. Remarkable progress has been made in the past 2 decades in understanding the regulatory mechanisms that control hematopoiesis, particularly in the characterization and clinical development of hematopoietic cytokines. The hematopoietic cytokines are glycoprotein regulators of blood production that control the survival, proliferation, and differentiation of hematopoietic precursor cells; additionally, many of these regulatory molecules stimulate functional activities of mature blood cells (1). The introduction of hematopoietic cytokines into clinical oncology and the treatment of hematologic malignancies have provided demonstrable advances in the supportive care of patients undergoing myelosuppressive therapy (2). The basic biologic, technologic, and clinical research efforts that form the foundation upon which hematopoietic cytokines were developed as therapeutic agents are a paradigm of "translational research" and serve as important examples of practical benefits that may accrue from the application of fundamental research. Research in hematopoietic cytokines, transferring observations, knowledge, and technology from the bench to the bedside and back again, continues to proceed rapidly; research in mechanisms of hematopoiesis and hematopoietic support is yielding an abundance of new data, novel agents with clinical promise, and important clinical controversies related to the appropriate clinical applications of hematopoietic cytokines in cancer medicine. Hematopoietic cytokines, produced through biotechnology and administered in pharmacologic doses, can modify the production of human blood elements in vivo in an attempt to optimize physiology beyond the endogenous host response. Additionally, careful observations by clinical investigators utilizing hematopoietic cytokines may provide important insights to the mechanisms of blood production and cell trafficking in normal individuals and in various abnormal physiologic states (such as recovery from high-dose chemoradiotherapy with stem cell transplantation). This chapter summarizes important aspects of the control of hematopoiesis by regulatory cytokines and interprets these data in the context of clinical cancer medicine.

Hematopoiesis: History and Scientific Background

HUMORAL REGULATION OF HEMATOPOIESIS: HYPOTHESIS

Hematopoiesis research has progressed rapidly in the 20th century, with tools ranging from (1) in vivo assays in animals to (2) clonogenic assays of distinct cellular subtypes to (3) the molecular dissection of subcellular events fundamental to the survival, growth, and differentiation of blood cells and their precursors. With such increasingly precise and sophisticated laboratory tools, investigators have been able to evaluate the regulatory mechanisms that control hematopoiesis with progressively more detail. Hematopoiesis offers an outstanding model system for the study of cellular growth and differentiation, as well as for the regulatory mechanisms of cellular receptors and their soluble ligands.

The control of blood cell production by soluble mediators was a theory that was postulated for the red blood cell lineage by Carnot at the turn of the 20th century. In 1906, these investigators bled rabbits until they were anemic and maintained them at a lower-than-normal hemoglobin level. Injection of serum obtained from these anemic animals into normal rabbits stimulated the production of erythrocytes (3). This simple but elegant in vivo experiment demonstrated the presence of a circulating "humoral factor" in the blood of the anemic rabbits that could stimulate supraphysiologic red blood cell production when passively transferred into normal animals. This very early experimental model provided a crude bioassay for the high endogenous levels of erythropoietin (EPO) present in the serum of the anemic animals. However, it then took the better part of the 20th century for the techniques of protein chemistry and molecular biology to advance so that scientists could prove that EPO as a single molecular regulator was sufficient to induce the stimulation of erythropoiesis associated with the anemic rabbit serum. EPO was the first hematopoietic cytokine to be identified, both in animal systems and in humans (4–7). EPO was also among the first of the hematopoietic cytokines to be purified (8, 9) and to have its gene isolated and cloned (10, 11).

HIERARCHICAL NATURE OF HEMATOPOIESIS

In the middle of the 20th century, other significant developments in hematopoiesis research occurred that would ultimately provide both the conceptual framework for assessing hematopoiesis and the technical assays that would make possible the identification of other hematopoietic cytokines. The hierarchical model of hematopoiesis was an important conceptual development. In this model, the expansion, maturation, and differentiation of hematopoietic precursor cells lead to the trilineage production of the formed elements of the blood (myeloid, lymphoid, erythroid). A central concept of this hypothesis is the existence of a single, most primitive class of precursor cell known as the totipotent stem cell, which possesses the capacity to give rise to all blood elements (12). A corollary hypothesis in this schema of hematopoiesis is that blood production over multiple lineages may be clonal in origin. Many lines of experimental evidence have provided objective support to these hypotheses (13, 14). These concepts evolved from the development of useful in vivo assays for marrow-repopulating multilineage stem cells, such as the spleen colony-forming unit (CFU-S), which would form clonal and macroscopic foci of extramedullary multilineage hematopoiesis in the spleens of lethally irradiated animals. Although more recent research has identified that the CFU-S is not a true stem cell, the CFU-S assay nevertheless remains an important tool with which to quantify relatively primitive levels of the hematopoietic hierarchy.

Further elucidation of the hematopoietic hierarchy followed the development of culture techniques that allowed the ex vivo growth of blood progenitor cells. Two groups of investigators nearly simultaneously developed in vitro culture systems that permitted the growth and differentiation of bone marrow cells into mature blood elements by using semisolid media and optimal culture conditions, which included rich sources of humoral regulators of hematopoiesis, such as serum from endotoxin-treated mice. In this manner, the groups of Pluznik and Sachs in Israel (15) and Bradley and Metcalf in Australia (16) provided important new tools for the laboratory evaluation of blood production that were absolutely necessary for defining the complex network of hematopoietic cytokines that regulate blood production. In these culture systems, individual cells were noted to give rise to clonal "colonies" made up of either single or multiple cell lineages, and the ill-defined factors that regulated this process of cell growth and lineage-specific differentiation could be assayed, purified, and eventually cloned by molecular genetic techniques.

DISTINCT SUBSETS OF HEMATOPOIETIC PRECURSOR CELLS

Culture assays of hematopoietic precursor cells may distinguish different levels of the hematopoietic hierarchy by functional growth characteristics, not by morphologic or cell surface marker characteristics. Hematopoietic progenitor cells have been operationally defined by their ability to form specific types of colonies (e.g., single lineage versus multilineage), as well as by their ability to give rise to further colonies if serially replated. The most mature subset of hematopoietic precursor cells are mature progenitor cells that exhibit lineage-restricted colony growth. Such cells have essentially no self-renewal capacity and a very limited secondary plating efficiency. Examples of these relatively mature progenitor cells include the CFU-GM, the BFU-e, and the CFU-mega.

A somewhat more primitive level of hematopoietic progenitor cell has the potential to give rise to several lineages. An example of such a multipotent myeloid progenitor is the CFU-GEMM, which gives rise to colonies composed of granulocytic, erythroid, monocytic, and megakaryocytic lineages. Like their more differentiated progeny the CFU-GM, CFU-GEMMs have essentially no self-renewal capacity and a low secondary plating efficiency. It has been thought that the majority of the normal physiologic requirements of basal hematopoiesis are met by the proliferative activity of multipotent and lineage-restricted progenitor cells, essentially sparing the quiescent pool of true stem cells and very primitive precursor cells.

The most primitive levels of the hematopoietic hierarchy still represent a relative "black box," which is only beginning to be understood. Adequate assays for true stem cells are lacking, and the available assays (such as serial transplantation and competitive repopulation of marrow) are cumbersome and only semiquantitative. The current status of research involving hematopoietic stem cells has been reviewed in detail (12, 17). The stem cell pool appears to be relatively resistant to cytotoxic treatments, compared with the actively cycling and more mature progenitor cell pools. Much current research aims to define regulatory molecules with beneficial stimulatory effects on stem cells, potentially by expanding the number of true stem cells without losing the "stemness" (i.e., totipotent differentiation and engraftable self-replication potential). It remains unclear whether cell divisions within the true stem cell pool can be fully isolated from some degree of lineage commitment and loss of replication potential.

IDENTIFICATION OF DISTINCT HEMATOPOIETIC CYTOKINES

The soluble factors required for the in vitro survival, growth, and differentiation of hematopoietic precursor cells have been identified based on the in vitro assays of hematopoiesis noted above. Progressive technical advances have allowed the definition of a number of different gene products that account for the colony-stimulating activities (CSA) present in various crude sources, such as endotoxin-treated mouse sera or tumor-cell conditioned media. It is now clear that the regulation of hematopoiesis is accomplished by a complex network of hematopoietic cytokines with overlapping activities, often with synergistic interactions (Table 82.1) (1). The physiologic roles of individual cytokines and the endogenous mechanisms for coordination of cytokine activities are just beginning to be understood. Highly sophisticated models, such as gene knockout mouse models, are proving invaluable in the study of how individual cy-

Table 82.1. Summary of Selected Hematopoietic Cytokines

Cytokine	Year cloned	Chromosomal site	U.S. clinical availability	Indication(s)
Cytokines that stimulate leukocyte production				
G-CSF	1986	17q11-22	Commercial	(1) Infectious prophylaxis with myelosuppressive chemoRx (2) Recovery from ABMT (3) Treatment of severe chronic neutropenic states (4) Mobilization of PBPCs (not FDA approved)
GM-CSF	1985	5q23-31	Commercial	Same as above
IL-3/GM-CSF Fusion molecule (PIXY321)	Developed 1989	Not applicable	In clinical trials (phase III)	Same as above
M-CSF	1985	5q23	In clinical trials (phase III)	Immunologic augmentation (antifungal)
Cytokines that stimulate erythropoiesis				
EPO	1985	7q11-22	Commercial	Treatment of anemia of cancer or AIDS
Cytokines that stimulate thrombopoiesis				
TPO	1994	3q26-27	In clinical trials (phase I/II)	Mitigation of chemotherapy-induced thrombocytopenia
IL-3	1986	5q23-32	In clinical trials (phase III)	Same as above
IL-6	1986	7q15	In clinical trials (phase III)	Same as above
IL-11	1990	24	In clinical trials (phase II)	Same as above
IL-1	1984	2q14	In clinical trials (phase II)	Same as above
Cytokines with activity on primitive hematopoiesis				
SCF	1990	4q	In clinical trials (phase III)	Mobilization of PBPCs
flt3 ligand	1993		Preclinical	Not applicable as yet

tokines act to regulate different aspects of hematopoiesis and host physiology.

The nomenclature of hematopoietic cytokines has proved confusing and remains somewhat arcane. Certain molecules were named colony-stimulating factors (CSFs), while others, which might also exhibit some induction of progenitor cell colony growth in vitro, were deemed interleukins (e.g., interleukin-3, or IL-3). Still other cytokines have been named outside of the CSF or interleukin nomenclature (e.g., EPO, stem cell factor, flt3-ligand). Most cytokines with hematopoietic activity are multifunctional molecules, often inducing a range of other effects on both hematologic and nonhematologic cells (see Table 82.3). Additionally, the lineage-restricted distinctions between hematopoietic cytokines blur as one studies early-acting factors that affect the more primitive levels of hematopoietic cells, since these tend to affect multiple lineages and include activities on both myeloid and lymphoid precursor cells.

Specific Individual Hematopoietic Growth Factors

More than 25 cytokines have now been identified that exhibit some sort of hematopoietic activity (Table 82.1). These may be grouped by a variety of criteria, such as the lineage upon which the cytokine has activity or the level(s) of hematopoiesis affected by an individual cytokine. A matrix

Table 82.2.

Level of hematopoiesis affected	Lineage activity	Example
Early	Multiple	SCF *flt3* ligand IL-6
Middle	Multiple	SCF IL-3 IL-6 TPO
Late	Multiple	GM-CSF TPO
	Single	G-CSF EPO SCF (mast cells)

may also be constructed for conceptual analysis of the hematopoietic cytokine network, relating the lineages to the levels of the hematopoietic hierarchy, such as in Figure 82.1.

As noted in Table 82.2, cytokines often exhibit activities on more than one lineage. Additionally, cytokines may affect cells in various levels of the hematopoietic hierarchy; for example, stem cell factor (SCF) will enhance the survival of multilineage early hematopoietic precursor cells (18), increase the peripheralization of cells with the ability to reconstitute hematopoiesis (19–21), and stimulate the mature mast cell lineage with a relative lineage restriction (22).

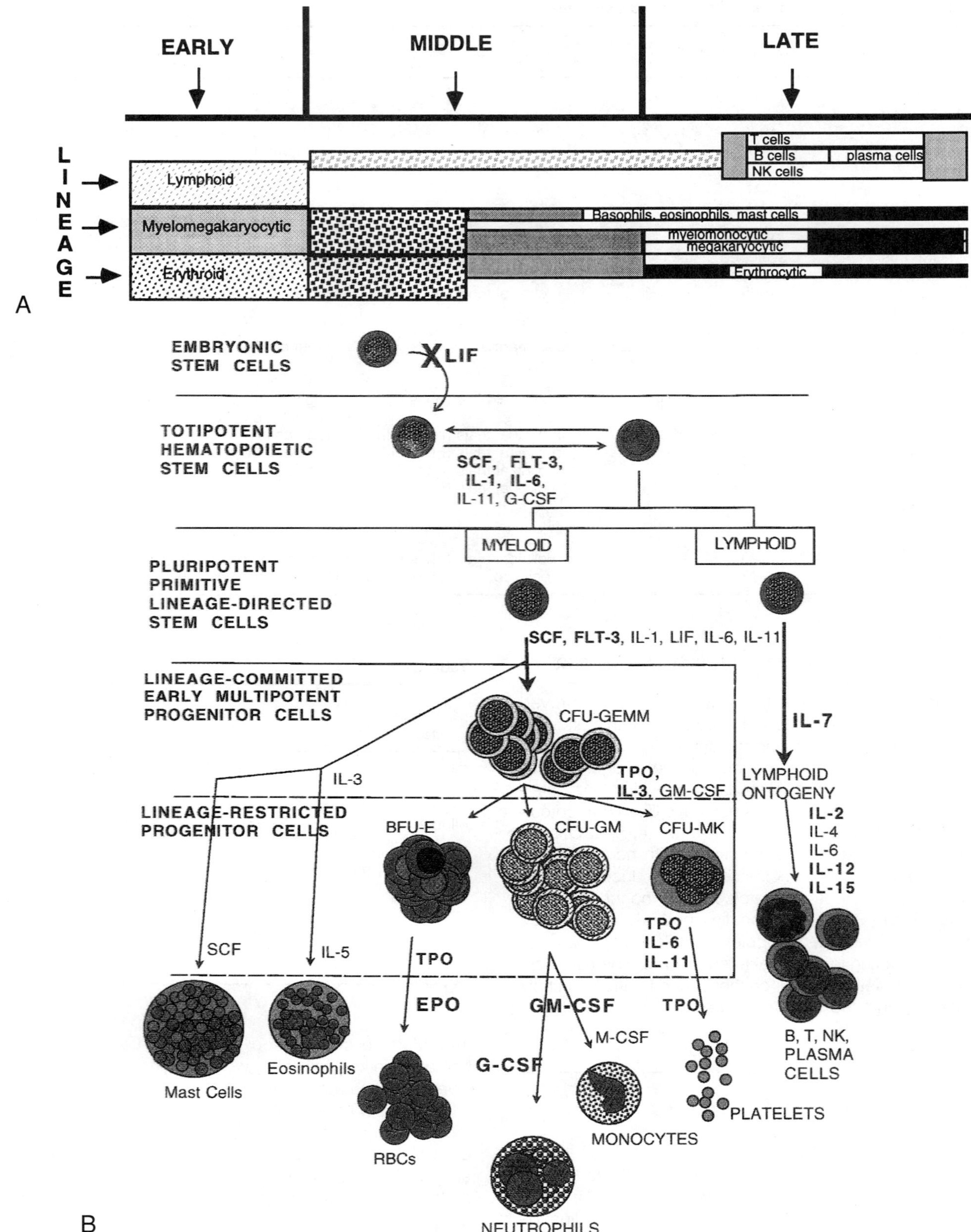

Figure 82.1. **A.** Matrix analysis of hematopoiesis by lineage and hierarchical level. **B.** Mature cellular elements of blood. *Source:* Demetri GD. Curr Prob Cancer 1992;4:184. Adapted and updated with permission.

HEMATOPOIETIC CYTOKINES ACTIVE ON LEUKOCYTES

As shown in Table 82.2, hematopoietic cytokines active on the most mature progenitor cells tend to exhibit lineage-restricted activities, stimulating proliferation, the final stages of lineage-specific differentiation, and effector cell functions in the fully differentiated progeny cells. However, even for factors such as EPO and G-CSF, which are considered relatively lineage specific, multilineage effects can be demonstrated under certain experimental conditions. For example, EPO has been shown to promote megakaryocyte differentiation under certain conditions and to stimulate platelet production in animal models (23–25). G-CSF has also been shown to enhance the response of immature multipotent progenitor cells to other early-acting cytokines (such as IL-1 or IL-3) (26, 27).

GRANULOCYTE COLONY-STIMULATING FACTOR

Granulocyte colony-stimulating factor (G-CSF) was first identified as a hematopoietic regulatory activity, present in the serum of endotoxin-treated mice, which could induce terminal differentiation in a mouse leukemia cell line (28, 29). This murine differentiation factor copurified with a colony-stimulating activity (CSA) that stimulated marrow progenitor cells to form granulocytic colonies in vitro. It was important that effects on differentiation and cell proliferation were linked and represented different biologic activities of a single factor, which was named G-CSF (30). A human glycoprotein with the activities attributable to G-CSF was purified in 1985 (31), and in 1986, the gene encoding G-CSF was cloned (32). The molecular and cell biologies of G-CSF have been reviewed (33). The gene, present in a single copy on chromosome 17, encodes a protein of 174 amino acids with an apparent molecular weight of approximately 18,000 dalton.

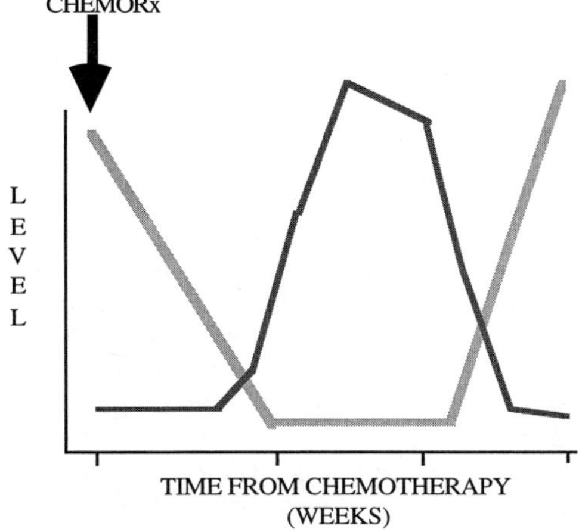

Figure 82.2. Inverse relationship between circulating levels of G-CSF and blood neutrophil counts. Following administration of myelosuppressive chemotherapy (*arrow*), there is a later decline in the levels of neutrophils, to which the host responds by increasing the levels of circulating G-CSF. High levels of circulating G-CSF decline following neutrophil recovery. *Gray line*, neutrophil counts; *black line*, G-CSF levels.

Physiologically, G-CSF appears to be the primary control mechanism by which the host regulates the circulating levels of neutrophilic granulocytes, both in the basal state and under stress conditions, such as bacterial infection. Dogs that express neutralizing antibodies against G-CSF exhibit chronic neutropenia (34). Endogenous levels of circulating G-CSF in normal human volunteers are generally near the detection limits of immunoassays (10 pg/mL or more) (35, 36). However, in certain stress conditions, such as infection or during the recovery from cytotoxic chemotherapy, G-CSF serum levels rise, peaking just prior to recovery from the neutrophil nadir and decreasing as the circulating neutrophil count increases (35), as schematized in Figure 82.2.

Similar fluctuations in the circulating levels of G-CSF have been reported in certain patients with cyclic neutropenia (35), and elevated levels of G-CSF have also been observed in patients with chronic neutropenic states (37). This reciprocal relationship between the circulating levels of G-CSF and the peripheral neutrophilic granulocyte counts strongly supports the hypothesis that G-CSF regulates the level of circulating neutrophils. Additional support for this hypothesis comes from murine studies in which the gene encoding G-CSF is inactivated ("G-CSF knockout" mice). G-CSF knockout mice exhibit chronic neutropenia with circulating neutrophil counts only 30% those of control mice, although they are otherwise without evident physiologic impairments (38). These mice lacking endogenous G-CSF could mount a neutrophilic response when pharmacologic doses of G-CSF were administered, demonstrating the presence of G-CSF–responsive progenitor cells. The lack of absolute lineage restriction in the activity of G-CSF is also suggested by these experiments, since the G-CSF knock-out mice exhibit low levels of monocytes and monocyte precursor cells and are particularly susceptible to infection with *Listeria monocytogenes* (38).

The temporal pattern of endogenous G-CSF production by the myelosuppressed host (Fig. 82.2) suggests that exogenous administration of G-CSF might offer a kinetic advantage to neutrophil recovery following myelotoxic chemotherapy. Thus, it appears that the host must first "sense" the presence of neutropenia, and then react to it by producing high levels of G-CSF (although the physiologic "neutrostat" by which levels of neutrophils are "sensed" remains unknown). It is reasonable to hypothesize that, in situations where one can predict that administration of a cytotoxic agent will lead to clinically relevant neutropenia, there may be a pharmacologic rationale for dosing G-CSF to stimulate hematopoietic activity before the host "senses" the abnormal physiologic state (Fig. 82.3). As shown in the schematic of Figure 82.3*A*, a temporal shift to the left of increased G-CSF levels is associated with exogenous dosing of G-CSF following chemotherapy, depending on the schedule of G-CSF administration; if G-CSF dosing begins 24 hours after chemotherapy, the G-CSF levels will be elevated before the endogenous host response would have occurred. Such a dosing strategy is correlated with a more rapid recovery of circulating neutrophil counts following the period of myelosuppression, as shown in Figure 82.3*B*. This pattern of enhanced neutrophil recovery is characteristic of the results of many preclinical and clinical trials in which pharmacologic

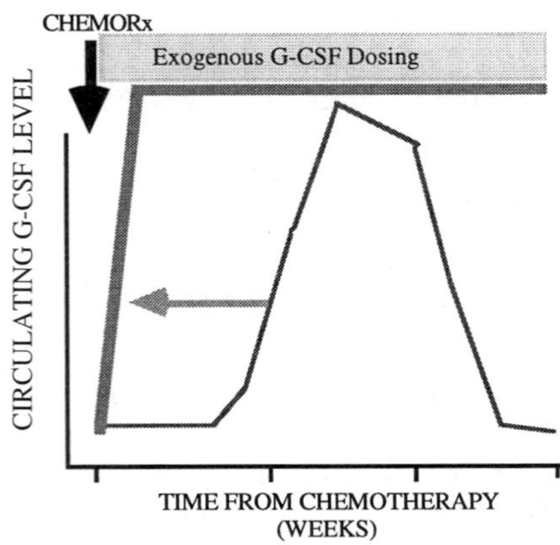

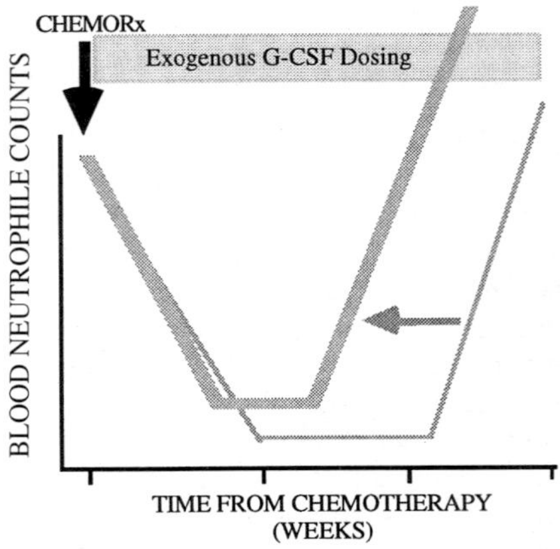

Figure 82.3. Effects of pharmacologic supplementation of exogenous G-CSF on circulating G-CSF levels (*left*) and on neutrophil recovery (*right*) following myelosuppressive chemotherapy. Thick line denotes patterns with pharmacologic dosing of G-CSF, while thin line represents pattern of native host response following chemotherapy.

doses of G-CSF are used to mitigate chemotherapy-induced myelotoxicity.

GRANULOCYTE-MACROPHAGE COLONY-STIMULATING FACTOR

Granulocyte-Macrophage Colony-Stimulating Factor (GM-CSF), purified to homogeneity in 1977 from medium conditioned by cultured mouse lung tissues (39), was one of the first hematopoietic cytokines identified with defined activity on cells of the myeloid lineage. GM-CSF stimulates the formation of colonies containing both neutrophilic and monocyte/macrophage lineages. The human GM-CSF protein was isolated and purified in 1984 (40) and was noted to be identical to a soluble activator of mature neutrophil function derived from T lymphocytes. The gene encoding human GM-CSF was cloned in 1985 (41). This gene is localized to the long arm of chromosome 5 and encodes a glycoprotein of 127 amino acids with a core protein molecular weight of approximately 14,000 daltons. While GM-CSF alone can induce both proliferation and terminal differentiation of granulocytes, monocytes, and eosinophils, other late-acting differentiation factors appear to be necessary to induce complete terminal differentiation of other lineages (particularly of erythroid and megakaryocytic precursor cells) (1, 17, 42).

Circulating levels of GM-CSF are generally not detectable, except in certain pathophysiologic conditions (e.g., paraneoplastic syndromes associated with malignancies) (43). The inference from this finding is that endogenous GM-CSF probably does not serve as the primary regulator of leukocyte production, but rather functions as a locally active factor within the microenvironment of the bone marrow (for stimulation of hematopoiesis) or at sites of inflammation (for activation of mature effector cell functions). The physiologic roles of GM-CSF are beginning to be elucidated by inactivating the GM-CSF gene in mice and studying the resulting "GM-CSF knockout" mice. Basal hematopoietic activity appears to be normal in such mice lacking production of GM-CSF, indicating that GM-CSF is not absolutely necessary as a regulator of leukocyte production (44, 45). However, the GM-CSF knockout mice developed a pathologic accumulation of surfactant lipids and protein within the alveolar spaces, analogous to an unusual human disorder known as pulmonary alveolar proteinosis. This syndrome of alveolar proteinosis is present also in mice genetically deficient in the production of both GM-CSF and M-CSF (46). In summary, these data indicate that the normal processing of pulmonary alveolar materials is dependent on GM-CSF, possibly through effects on mature alveolar macrophage function. The primary physiologic role of GM-CSF in stimulating hematopoiesis seems less clear than for G-CSF on the basis of these genetic "knockout" studies in mice.

Table 82.3. Activities of G-CSF and GM-CSF

Activity	Reference
Antagonism of apoptosis in progenitor cells	47, 48
Stimulation of proliferation and differentiation	Reviewed in 33, 49
Enhanced cellular cytotoxicity of mature effector cells	50–55
Mobilization of hematopoietic progenitor cells into the circulation	56–58
Stimulation of migration and proliferation of vascular endothelial cells	59, 60

ACTIVITIES OF G-CSF AND GM-CSF

Both G-CSF and GM-CSF are multifunctional regulators of hematopoiesis and hematopoietic cells, and they have rather overlapping biological activities. A listing of the activities of these molecules appears in Table 82.3. Although there are numerous demonstrable biologic activities associated with both GM-CSF and G-CSF, the primary clinical activities that have been studied are (1) the stimulation of hematopoietic precursor cell growth and differentiation into mature leukocytes and (2) the mobilization of hematopoietic progenitor cells into the peripheral blood to serve as cellular support in place of bone marrow transplantation.

CLINICAL TRIALS OF G-CSF AND GM-CSF

Preclinical studies of G-CSF and GM-CSF, both in vitro and in nonhuman in vivo testing, suggested that these

Table 82.4.

Cytokine	Generic name	Biosynthetic source	Glycosylation status	Availability as of 1995
G-CSF	Filgrastim	*E coli*	−	Worldwide
G-CSF	Lenograstim	CHO cells (mammalian)	+	Not in North America
GM-CSF	Sargramostim	Yeast	+	Worldwide
GM-CSF	Molgramostim	*E coli*	−	Not in North America
GM-CSF	Regramostim	CHO cells	+	No longer under development
GM-CSF	Ecogramostim	*E coli*	−	No longer under development

Table 82.5. Adverse Effects of GM-CSF and G-CSF (Incidence)

	GM-CSF	G-CSF
Common	Bone pain (20%)	Bone pain (24%)
	Fever/chills (25%)	Reversible elevations in LDH, alkaline phosphatase, and/or uric acid (50%)
	Headache (25%)	
	Myalgias (18%)	
Uncommon	Rash (2%)	Rash (2%)
	Allergic reaction (0.01%)	Allergic reaction (0.01%)
	First-dose syndrome of hypoxemia (<5%)	Cutaneous vasculitis (e.g., Sweet's syndrome) (<0.01%)
	Pericardial effusion (3%)	Flare of preexisting psoriasis (<1%)
	Edema/capillary leak (4%)	Splenomegaly with chronic administration (>2 years)
	Supraventricular cardiac arrhythmias (<5%)	

molecules would be clinically useful in stimulating host leukocyte production. Interpretation of data from clinical trials in this field is complicated by the somewhat overlapping activity of GM-CSF and G-CSF on myelopoiesis and the occasional study in which these agents are used interchangeably. Additionally, different recombinant moieties exist for both G-CSF and GM-CSF, as noted. For example, the clinical research literature regarding GM-CSF has reported studies using two different recombinant preparations of G-CSF and four different recombinant versions of GM-CSF, as noted in Table 82.4.

Although differences between these versions of the same cytokine (for either cytokine-associated toxicities or therapeutic efficacy) are not evident from the research literature, it is not possible to determine this with certainty. For example, most of the clinical trials with Lenograstim have been done using doses in the range of 2 to 5 μg/kg/d, while studies with Filgrastim have generally been performed using 5 to 10 μg/kg/d. Similarly, toxicity differences have been postulated to exist between glycosylated and nonglycosylated preparations of GM-CSF, but these are impossible to assess without a properly controlled concurrent comparative study.

The clinical effects of both G-CSF and GM-CSF were striking even in the earliest phase I trials (60–66). Administration of either cytokine can increase circulating leukocyte counts in a dose-dependent manner. Overall, both cytokines have been adequately well tolerated in vivo, with the primary toxicity being bone pains, primarily in marrow-rich bony areas (e.g., the pelvis) (see Table 82.5). Toxicities of both molecules are also, to a large degree, dose related, so that early phase I toxicity data (using GM-CSF, for example, at doses greater than 20 μg/kg/d) may not directly apply to current clinical practice in which either cytokine is generally dosed in the range of 5 μg/kg/d.

The incidence of fever associated with GM-CSF may relate to the physiologic role of this agent as a proinflammatory mediator that is generally produced locally at a site of inflammation (humans, even under stress conditions of infection or recovery from myelosuppressive chemotherapy, do not produce detectable endogenous GM-CSF levels in the circulation). Pharmacologic dosing with exogenous GM-CSF so that elevated GM-CSF levels circulate may thus represent a more abnormal physiologic state than for G-CSF.

Besides the differences in side-effect profiles, GM-CSF and G-CSF are clearly both quite active in stimulating host hematopoiesis. The mechanisms by which these agents stimulate peripheral leukocytosis differ somewhat. G-CSF stimulates more rapid differentiation of immature progenitor cells into mature neutrophils (66). GM-CSF diminishes the time required for cells to traverse the cell cycle and allows faster proliferation of committed progenitor cells (67). The clinical activity of either molecule is apparent within 1 to 2 days of dosing. The appearance of neutrophilia induced by G-CSF may be somewhat more rapid than the host response to GM-CSF, possibly due to the activity of G-CSF on the most mature lineage-restricted progenitor cell pool. GM-CSF induces a leukocytosis over days in the absence of a myelosuppressive stimulus, and this response may be somewhat more sustained following discontinuation of GM-CSF dosing than would be seen with G-CSF because of the stimulation and expansion of a more immature multilineage pool of progenitor cells. These clinical activities of G-CSF and GM-CSF are thus quite consistent with their documented in vitro biologic activities on hematopoiesis.

DEFINITIVE RANDOMIZED STUDIES OF HEMATOPOIETIC CYTOKINES

Based on the activity seen in the phase I trials of G-CSF and GM-CSF, pivotal randomized phase III trials were designed. Relatively few phase II studies were performed with these molecules to define the optimal doses, routes, and schedules of administration, or to study potential differences in efficacy of these agents in association with various myelotoxic drugs with different modes of inhibiting hematopoiesis (e.g., cycle-specific agents, true stem cell poisons). This fact has continued to plague the field, with relatively little definitive data available on these important aspects concerning the use of GM-CSF and G-CSF. Nevertheless, both molecules exhibit a relatively broad therapeutic index of activity, and it has proved possible to estimate doses and schedules for each agent to demonstrate clinical benefits for patients undergoing myelosuppressive therapies.

Severe myelosuppression has been the sine qua non for clinical trials that have demonstrated beneficial effects of G-CSF and GM-CSF in randomized studies. It is crucial that clinicians recognize that cytokine trials are designed to give the test agent a chance to mitigate myelotoxicity: thus, myelosuppression must be consistent and result in clinically unfavorable outcomes for the cytokine to have a beneficial effect. It is, therefore, crucial to distinguish cancers for which a chemotherapy dose–response effect exists, so that higher doses (with the resulting more severe myelosuppression) are not administered without reason simply because the addition of hematopoietic cytokine support now renders them equitoxic to lower doses without cytokine support.

The majority of the initial clinical research studies tested the ability of either G-CSF or GM-CSF to prevent infectious complications of myelosuppressive therapy prior to the development of any complications. Such a preemptive strategy for use of hematopoietic growth factors has become known as primary prophylaxis of infectious complications (such as fever with neutropenia).

Randomized Studies of G-CSF in Primary Prophylaxis

The pivotal study of G-CSF was a prospective multicenter, randomized, double-blinded, placebo-controlled clinical trial. This study combined relatively myelotoxic doses of three commonly used chemotherapeutic agents (cyclophosphamide (C), doxorubicin (A), etoposide (E); in patients with previously untreated small cell lung cancer. All study patients were treated with CAE, and the groups were randomized only in their supportive care regimen: placebo versus G-CSF as primary prophylaxis. One multicenter study was conducted in the United States (68) and a second study was performed in Europe (69). The data from both studies showed that patients myelosuppressed by CAE experienced a median of 6 days of severe neutropenia if the chemotherapy was given with placebo, while the group randomized to receive adjunctive G-CSF experienced half as much toxicity (i.e., 3 days of similarly severe neutropenia). The surrogate laboratory end point (neutropenia) was closely correlated with beneficial effects on other clinical outcomes. In both studies, the patients suffered exceptionally high rates of infectious complications, prompting admission to the hospital (57% of placebo-treated patients receiving these doses of CAE in the first cycle); these toxicity rates appear much higher than standard incidences of comparable toxicities, perhaps because of the intensive doses of chemotherapy employed, or because of the intensive monitoring of patients for adverse events. The addition of G-CSF as an adjunct to the supportive care of these patients decreased the incidence of infectious complications by 50% (i.e., a 28% incidence of fever with neutropenia in the group receiving G-CSF). A decreased incidence of hospitalization for toxicities, shorter durations of inpatient hospitalizations, and lower requirements for parenteral antibiotics were also reported. Therefore, it is clear that adjunctive G-CSF can diminish certain clinically relevant toxicities of aggressive myelotoxic chemotherapy. This is taken as a proof of principle that the increased levels of circulating neutrophils associated with the exogenous dosing of recombinant G-CSF function as immunologic effector cells. On the basis of these randomized data and prior pilot studies, one recombinant version of G-CSF (Filgrastim) was approved for commercial distribution by the U.S. Food and Drug Administration (FDA) in February 1991. The FDA approval was remarkably broad in scope, allowing the use of G-CSF as an adjunct to any myelosuppressive chemotherapies used in the treatment of all types of non-myeloid malignancies.

RANDOMIZED TRIAL OF GM-CSF IN ABMT AS PRIMARY PROPHYLAXIS

The definitive study of GM-CSF was a prospective randomized, double-blinded, placebo-controlled clinical trial performed at three academic transplant centers using patients with lymphoid malignancies undergoing high-dose chemoradiotherapy and autologous bone marrow transplantation (ABMT) (70). Given the aggressive nature of ABMT compared with nonablative chemotherapy, infectious complications are essentially universal; nevertheless, since the GM-CSF was administered before complications occurred, this should be considered a test of GM-CSF as primary prophylaxis. In this trial, the group randomized to receive adjunctive GM-CSF following ABMT exhibited significantly more rapid leukocyte recovery than the group receiving placebo. This was correlated with a modest reduction in duration of inpatient hospitalization (of the order of 1 week earlier than the placebo group) and a lower requirement for parenteral antibiotics in the group receiving adjunctive GM-CSF. Fewer documented infections and fewer fungal infections were noted in the group receiving adjunctive GM-CSF. This trial, along with other supportive pilot data, formed the foundation for the decision by the FDA to approve one recombinant version of GM-CSF (Sargramostim) in February 1991. However, the FDA approval was far more limited than that granted for G-CSF, allowing the use of this molecule only as an adjunct to ABMT for patients with nonmyeloid malignancies. Although occasionally physicians will administer GM-CSF "off-label" as an adjunct to routine nontransplant chemotherapy, data remain nondefinitive regarding whether GM-CSF improves clinical outcomes in such patients. Randomized trials reporting both positive (71) and negative (72) results have been published, suggesting that the role of GM-CSF as an adjunct to nonablative chemotherapy remains controversial.

Other Clinical Indications for G-CSF and GM-CSF

Many patients may benefit from chemotherapy that does not routinely lead to severe myelosuppression or clinical sequelae of myelosuppression. In such patients, it may not be optimal to use G-CSF or GM-CSF as primary prophylaxis. However, if the patient suffers unexpectedly severe myelotoxicity and a complication of therapy, it may be reasonable to offer hematopoietic support. For example, G-CSF or GM-CSF may be used as secondary prophylaxis. This may be defined as the use of a cytokine to prevent recurrence of an infectious complication in subsequent treatment cycles following an initial adverse event. Although no prospective randomized study has been conducted to evaluate the efficacy of either G-CSF or GM-CSF as secondary prophylaxis, certain data support the hypothesis that benefit may be obtained if the agents are used with this intent (68, 73).

G-CSF has also been used with therapeutic intent, rather than as prophylaxis, for patients experiencing active infectious complications of cancer therapy. One randomized trial demonstrated a decreased risk of prolonged hospitalization (e.g., more than 10 days) and a lower requirement for antifungal therapy in a large, heterogeneous group of patients presenting with fever and neutropenia and randomized between G-CSF with standard supportive care (e.g., parenteral antibiotics, standard inpatient nursing care) versus supportive care alone. This supports the hypothesis that adjunctive hematopoietic support may provide clinical benefit to patients with very severe myelosuppression, and these results are consistent with the results of trials using these agents as prophylaxis. However, it is then critical to define prognostic factors that allow the identification of patients at presentation who are destined to exhibit prolonged myelosuppression, and this has proved to be challenging (74). In summary, more intensive evaluation of the clinical activities of G-CSF or GM-CSF in the management of patients with active infectious complications of cancer therapy is necessary.

Mobilization of Progenitor/Stem Cells into the Circulation

Both G-CSF and GM-CSF exhibit an activity that is reshaping the field of cellular support for high-dose therapy of cancer. Early trials of these agents showed that early progenitor cells are induced to migrate from the bone marrow into the peripheral blood during the administration of pharmacologic doses of either G-CSF or GM-CSF, and that this mobilization stimulus is far more potent when the cytokine is dosed during recovery from myelosuppressive chemotherapy (56, 57). Peripheral blood progenitor cells (PBPCs) appear to be in active cell cycle status, since they are exceptionally avid targets for retrovirally mediated gene transfer (75). Gene-marking studies have demonstrated that such PBPCs have the capacity to contribute to long-term hematopoietic recovery of the myelosuppressed host (76). Following high-dose, ablative therapy, cellular support with PBPCs results in more rapid trilineage hematopoietic reconstitution as compared with bone marrow–derived cells (77–79). The hematopoietic recovery associated with PBPC support is so rapid that it has been difficult to demonstrate much benefit to adding adjunctive hematopoietic cytokines to the posttransplant regimen, as long as sufficient numbers of PBPCs are collected and infused (80–83). Much current research is attempting to define optimal methods and cytokines for PBPC mobilization, but already many transplant centers have switched from bone marrow to PBPCs as cellular support for high-dose chemotherapy. Allogeneic PBPC transplantation is also possible and appears to be associated with far less graft-versus-host disease than one might expect, based on the high concentration of functional T cells that would be collected in a PBPC-based allograft (84).

ERYTHROPOIETIN: A SPECIFIC STIMULUS TO ERYTHROPOIESIS

Human EPO was among the first of the human hematopoietic cytokines to be purified and to have its gene cloned (10, 11). The human EPO gene encodes a protein of 193 amino acids, which is processed into a mature protein with a molecular weight of approximately 18,400 daltons. However, as is true for most of the hematopoietic cytokines, the protein then undergoes extensive posttranslational modification through glycosylation, and the final circulating EPO molecule exhibits a molecular weight in the range of 30,000 daltons. Glycosylation of EPO appears critical for full biologic activity in vivo, perhaps due to an increased clearance rate of the nonglycosylated protein (85).

EPO is one of the hematopoietic cytokines that is true hormone. Physiologic levels of EPO are easily detectable in the circulation by immunoassays, usually with a normal range of 4 to 30 mU/mL of serum. It has long been known that hypoxia is probably the most potent stimulus to EPO production (6), although the molecular biologic mechanisms that regulate EPO gene expression and protein production remain somewhat obscure. Patients with active cancer exhibit circulating EPO levels that are significantly lower than those noted in non–tumor-bearing patients with iron-deficiency anemia (86). The mechanisms responsible for this inappropriate blunting of the endogenous EPO response to anemia in patients with cancer are poorly understood, but this suggests that pharmacologic dosing of EPO to supraphysiologic levels might stimulate erythropoiesis in cancer patients. Based on positive results of replacing EPO by exogenous dosing in patients with chronic renal failure (87), randomized trials of EPO as adjunctive hematopoietic support have been conducted in other groups of patients with anemia. EPO dosing can ameliorate anemia associated with multiple myeloma (88) and AIDS-related therapy (89). Randomized trials in cancer patients have also demonstrated a decrease in transfusion requirements associated with EPO supplementation, with associated increases in certain quality-of-life measures (90). Certain prognostic algorithms have attempted to predict which cancer patients might respond optimally to EPO (90). Overall, the cost–benefit ratio will likely determine the clinical use of EPO in cancer medicine, since transfusional support of red blood cells remains common and easily accessible. Rigorous studies of transfusional support, full cost analyses (including indirect costs such as time lost from work), and patient preferences have not been ascertained. Thus, the appropriate utilization of EPO support for cancer patients remains poorly defined.

HEMATOPOIETIC CYTOKINES THAT STIMULATE PLATELET PRODUCTION

In the late 1950s, investigators hypothesized the existence of soluble factor(s) that regulate platelet production, and termed the as-yet-uncharacterized substance "thrombopoietin" (92, 93). The mechanisms that control platelet production are now being elucidated by the same laboratory techniques by which leukopoiesis and erythropoiesis have been studied so successfully. Several hematopoietic cytokines have been identified with stimulatory activity on platelet production, including IL-1, IL-3, IL-6, and IL-11 (94). However, the most critical physiologic regulator of platelet production remained unknown until the recent studies that identified the ligand for the c-*mpl* proto-oncogene receptor as the long-sought thrombopoietin (TPO) (95). Although other cytokines, such as IL-3 and IL-6, have been more thoroughly tested in clinical trials, preclinical trials of TPO offer compelling support to the hypothesis that the primary control of thrombopoiesis is directed by TPO. Nevertheless, other molecules have interesting activities that may prove clinically useful, and these are discussed in this section as well.

THE C-*MPL* LIGAND (THROMBOPOIETIN), MEGAKARYOCYTE GROWTH AND DEVELOPMENT FACTOR

The c-*mpl* proto-oncogene is the normal analogue of the transforming activity of the myeloproliferative leukemia virus (96). The role of c-*mpl* in megakaryopoiesis was strongly suggested by experiments in which antisense oligonucleotides were introduced into primitive hematopoietic precursor cells to block c-*mpl* expression: megakaryopoiesis was specifically inhibited, without inhibition of erythropoiesis or leukopoiesis in vitro (97). The ligand for the c-*mpl* cell surface receptor was, therefore, a prime candidate to be an important regulator of thrombopoiesis. Using different strategies, four groups virtually simultaneously reported the isolation and cloning of TPO, the ligand for c-*mpl* (98–101). The human gene for TPO, localized to the long arm of chromosome 3, encodes approximately 350 amino acids with a predicted molecular weight of 35,000 daltons before glycosylation, which is a relatively large molecule in comparison with other hematopoietic cytokines. The amino terminal domain of human TPO shows a high degree of sequence conservation with erythropoietin (nearly 50%, with 23% sequence homology). The carboxy-terminal domain of TPO has a high concentration of glycosylation sites.

An important physiologic role of TPO in regulating thrombopoiesis is supported by several lines of experimental evidence. Mice deficient in the c-*mpl* genes (c-*mpl* "knockouts") exhibit chronic thrombocytopenia, with an 85% reduction in the level of circulating platelets as compared to normals (102). Interestingly, a low level of basal thrombopoiesis was noted in these mice, indicating that alternative thrombopoietic mechanisms exist to allow platelet production even in the absence of TPO. Administration of TPO to mice can increase the number of marrow megakaryocytes, expand the pool of megakaryocytic progenitor cells by 20-fold, and elevate circulating platelet counts by 400% (100, 103). TPO appears to act both as a proliferative and differentiative stimulus to megakaryocytes and their precursor cells (104). Early preclinical studies suggest that TPO may accelerate platelet recovery following a myelosuppressive insult (105), and the results from clinical testing of TPO are eagerly anticipated but not yet available.

Interleukin-3

A factor known initially as multi-CSF and subsequently renamed interleukin-3 was identified in the early 1980s; this factor could enhance colony formation by multiple hematopoietic lineages, including granulocytes, monocytes, erythroid cells, and megakaryocytic cells. In 1981, mouse IL-3 became the first hematopoietic cytokine for which the gene was identified and cloned (106), and the human IL-3 gene, located on the long arm of chromosome 5, was cloned in 1986 (107). The gene for IL-3 encodes a mature core protein of 133 amino acids with a molecular weight of approximately 14,000 daltons. The human IL-3 gene is closely linked at the genetic locus with the gene for GM-CSF. Like GM-CSF, IL-3 does not circulate in detectable concentrations in the blood.

Interleukin-3 is a true multilineage hematopoietic growth factor in vitro, supporting the proliferation of more primitive progenitor cells than those affected by GM-CSF. It stimulates the growth and differentiation of relatively early stages of megakaryocytic progenitor cells, and recent data suggest that IL-3 does not act on the most mature megakaryocytic cells to enhance platelet formation (104). It appears to have unique properties in stimulating proliferation of early megakaryocyte precursor cells and its effects may be additive to those of TPO (108).

In preclinical trials, the in vivo stimulatory effects of IL-3 on leukopoiesis were noted to be slower in onset and to reach a more moderate peak, in contrast to the more rapid kinetics of GM-CSF (109). In clinical trials, IL-3 induces moderate increases in circulating levels of leukocytes, platelets, and, occasionally, certain erythroid elements, such as reticulocytes (110, 111). The clinical toxicities associated with IL-3 administration at high doses (more than 10 μg/kg/d by daily subcutaneous bolus injection) have generally included low-grade fevers, constitutional symptoms (severe fatigue, malaise, myalgias), and headaches (111, 112).

The use of IL-3 as a single agent to mitigate the multilineage myelosuppression induced by cytotoxic chemotherapy has been investigated, although the results of prospective randomized, placebo-controlled trials are not yet available. Overall, any effects of IL-3 in stimulating more rapid platelet recovery from myelosuppressive chemotherapy have been modest (113, 114). Given the in vitro synergism between IL-3 and other cytokines, such as GM-CSF, there is a sound rationale for studies in which these cytokines are administered together. One clever biosynthetic approach has been to link the genes encoding IL-3 and GM-CSF as a fusion molecule. This fusion protein, known as PIXY321 and currently in clinical trials, appears to exhibit the activities of GM-CSF, but the important clinical activity of platelet stimulation remains poorly defined (115). Alternatively, other investigators have chosen to explore the sequential administration of IL-3 followed by GM-CSF (116). Randomized trials are necessary to demonstrate whether IL-3 adds any significant clinical benefit to GM-CSF.

Interleukin-6

Interleukin-6 exhibits an exceptionally broad range of biologic activities (117). The human gene for IL-6, localized to the short arm of chromosome 7, encodes a protein of 212 amino acids with a predicted molecular weight of the nonglycosylated protein core of approximately 18,000 daltons. Circulating levels of IL-6 may be detectable in humans, both in health and disease (117). The autocrine production of IL-6 by myeloma cells has been shown to stimulate proliferation of these malignant cells (118). Such aberrant IL-6 production may play an important role in the generation, maintenance, and progression of the malignant phenotype of myeloma cells, and novel therapeutic strategies are being developed to block IL-6 action as treatment for myeloma. It has also been implicated as a pathophysiologic mechanism involved in the etiology of the lymph node hyperplastic disorder known as Castleman's disease (119). It has immunomodulatory activities on effector cells, and systemic administration of exogenous IL-6 was associated with antitumor activity in vivo in one study (120).

Interleukin-6 enhances megakaryocyte colony formation, primarily through inducing polyploidization and maturation of megakaryocytes; this is associated with increased production of platelets in preclinical testing (121–123). Clinical trials of IL-6 in humans have demonstrated that it is relatively specific in stimulating thrombopoiesis, but that constitutional toxicities, such as fever, headache, and myalgias, accompanied IL-6 administration (124–126). Tolerance of IL-6 seems much worse in the setting of ABMT and myelodysplastic syndromes, with hepatic dysfunction and severe constitutional symptoms as the respective dose-limiting toxicities (127, 128). Prospective randomized trials are ongoing to determine the efficacy of IL-6 in accelerating platelet recovery from nonablative myelosuppression.

Interleukin-11

A molecule cloned from bone marrow stromal cells (129), IL-11 has significant similarities to IL-6 due to a common signal transduction mechanism through the gp130 cell-surface–associated molecule. Interleukin-11 stimulates hematopoietic activity at a very primitive level of early progenitor cells and also functions as a maturation factor in megakaryocytopoiesis (130). Preclinical models of myelosuppression suggest that IL-11 stimulates multilineage hematopoietic recovery (131). Clinical trials have been conducted with IL-11 as an adjunct to both nonablative chemotherapy (132) and bone marrow transplantation (133). The toxicity profile of IL-11 appears related but nonoverlapping with that of IL-6. While constitutional symptoms, such as malaise, are common to both IL-6 and IL-11, fevers, which appear with great frequency in association with IL-6, have not been reported as a prominent toxicity with IL-11. Conversely, pleuropericardial effusions have been reported with IL-11, and these have not been commonly reported with IL-6. Both IL-6 and IL-11 are associated with a transient increase in circulating plasma volume that leads to a dilutional anemia during the period of cytokine administration (132, 134). Randomized trials are ongoing to determine the clinical activities and toxicities of IL-11 with greater precision.

IL-1

One of the earliest pleiotropic humoral regulators identified, IL-1 was described as endogenous pyrogen in the 1940s (135). The IL-1 activity represents the aggregate effects of two separate gene products, IL-1-α and IL-1-β, both of which act on the same receptors. Interleukin-1 can occasionally be detected in the circulation of healthy humans, and elevated IL-1 levels appear in the circulation under a variety of stress conditions, such as infection or inflammation. It is able to stimulate a very primitive hematopoietic compartment, potentially even affecting the true pluripotent stem cell pool (17). Human clinical trials with IL-1 have demonstrated the impressive toxicities of this molecule, which is not unexpected based on its role as a proinflammatory mediator and possible inducer of septic shock. Doses greater than 0.3 μg/kg have induced unacceptably severe hypotension, renal dysfunction, cardiac arrhythmias, fever, and cognitive changes (136). Although IL-1 administration is associated with increases in circulating platelet counts (136), the toxicities appear unacceptable for an adjunctive agent of supportive care, especially with the availability of other, less toxic thrombopoietic regulators.

HEMATOPOIETIC CYTOKINES ACTIVE ON PRIMITIVE MULTILINEAGE PRECURSORS

Several cytokines with activities on very primitive hematopoietic precursor cells have been identified. Clinical applications for such early-acting cytokines range from the expansion of target cells for later-acting, lineage-restricted cytokines (such as G-CSF) to the potential of shifting into active cell cycle an early population of hematopoietic cells with long-term reconstituting capacity so that gene transfer can occur with greater efficiency (137, 138). Although these cytokines in many ways are the most poorly understood, they represent the most exciting prospects for future research in applied hematopoiesis.

c-*kit* Ligand (Stem Cell Factor, *Steel* Factor, Mast Cell Growth Factor)

The ligand for the c-*kit* proto-oncogene cell surface receptor has numerous unique activities to support and enhance early cells in the hematopoietic hierarchy. Deficiency in the c-*kit* ligand is responsible for the hematopoietic defects noted in the *Steel* mutant mouse strain, denoted as Sl/Sl^d, which exhibits a severe macrocytic anemia and mast cell defects in addition to dyspigmentation. Sl/Sl^d mice have a defect in the bone marrow microenvironment that is not curable with marrow transplantation, and it is now established that this lesion represents the defective presentation of c-*kit* ligand by marrow stromal cells. The mouse mutant strain, W/W^v, which exhibits another pigmentation defect (the white spotting locus), also has a hematopoietic stem cell deficiency unrelated to microenvironmental problems. Mutations in the c-*kit* proto-oncogene represent the molecular etiology for the W locus deficiency. Thus, c-*kit* and its ligand are crucial for hematopoiesis at a very early stage and are also related to pigmentation in mice. The gene encoding the stem cell factor (CSF), a ligand for the c-*kit* receptor was cloned by several groups (139–141), resides on the long arm of chromosome 4 and produces a 248-amino-acid precursor molecule that is cleaved in posttranslational processing to a mature protein of 165 amino acids and 18,500 daltons. However, native human SCF exists as a homodimeric glycoprotein with a molecular weight in the range of 50,000 to 70,000 daltons. Membrane-bound and soluble forms exist for both SCF (141) and the c-*kit* receptor (143), and a form of SCF has been shown to circulate in normal humans in relatively high concentrations (approximately 3 ng/mL of serum). The surface expression of SCF by marrow stromal cells may be a critical element underlying the ability of the microenvironment to support normal hematopoietic activity. SCF may also function as an adhesion molecule retaining stem and progenitor cells in the marrow microenvironment, since c-*kit* receptors are lost from the surface of most hematopoietic cells during maturation. While mature neutrophils and lymphocytes do not express the c-*kit* receptor, mature mast cells and melanocytes do express c-*kit* into their terminally differentiated state.

Although SCF does not stimulate formation of hematopoietic colonies by itself, it markedly enhances multilineage hematopoietic activity in vitro in the presence of other cytokines, including G-CSF, EPO, GM-CSF, and IL-3 (17). Clinical trials of SCF have reported subtle changes in early hematopoiesis, but no alterations in more mature cell populations (144–146). Additionally, increased numbers of dermal mast cells have been observed in patients treated with SCF, and the dose-limiting toxicities of SCF have included generalized urticaria and an anaphylactoid syndrome of upper airway constriction (22). Sustained hyperpigmentation has also been observed in patients at the local sites of SCF injection due to melanocyte proliferation (147). More recent studies are evaluating the potential of SCF to synergize with G-CSF in the mobilization of hematopoietic progenitor/stem cells into the circulation (19, 148). A randomized trial is planned to study whether SCF increases the yield, quality, or clinical impact of PBPCs compared with G-CSF alone as the mobilizing stimulus.

flt3 Ligand

Another hematopoietic regulator, the ligand for the cell-surface tyrosine kinase receptor known as *flt3* or *flk2*, has been identified as stimulating survival and expansion of early lymphohematopoietic progenitor cells (149, 150). Screening for ligands of so-called orphan receptors may identify other important cytokines active on primitive hematopoiesis. The gene for human *flt3* ligand encodes a transmembrane protein that consists of 235 amino acids. Like SCF, the molecular structure of the *flt3* ligand suggests that it may exist in both cell-bound and soluble forms; the distinctive physiologic functions of such different forms remain obscure. Early studies demonstrate a synergism between the *flt3* ligand and other hematopoietic cytokines in vitro. In striking contrast to SCF, the *flt3* ligand has no specific action on mast cells or their precursors, and thus this agent may have a very different toxicity profile. Clinical testing of the ligand for *flt3* has not yet begun.

SELECTED IMMUNOREGULATORY HEMATOPOIETIC CYTOKINES

Many other hematopoietic regulators have been identified, several of which may have clinical applicability as biologic response modifying agents. These are briefly enumerated here.

Macrophage Colony-Stimulating Factor

First identified in 1977, macrophage colony-stimulating factor (M-CSF) is a relatively pure stimulator of monocyte/macrophage colony formation in vitro. It is crucial for bone physiology, and the absence of functional M-CSF leads to osteopetrosis (46). Like EPO, M-CSF circulates in normal humans at levels of 2 to 7 ng/mL, although the physiologic role of M-CSF in the circulation remains unclear. In vitro, M-CSF acts as a potent activator of effector cell function for cells of the monocyte/macrophage lineage, and this activity is being studied in the clinic. Clinical trials of M-CSF have demonstrated that this cytokine induces the appearance of large, vacuolated monocytic cells; thrombocytopenia has emerged as the dose-limiting toxicity (151). The efficacy of this agent in invasive fungal disorders has been explored.

Interleukin-2

Although IL-2 acts as a T-cell growth factor, it also is an important regulator of natural killer (NK) cells. It has been approved by the FDA as an immunomodulator with activity against renal cell carcinoma and is discussed in Chapter 52.

Interleukin-4

Pleiotropic immunomodulatory activities (152), including certain anti-inflammatory properties, are exhibited by IL-4. Cellular expression of high levels of IL-4 has been shown to have antitumor activity (153, 154). Clinical dose-finding trials with rHu-IL-4 have been conducted. Doses up to 1,290 μg/m (2)/d by intravenous bolus have been relatively well tolerated. The toxicities of intravenous bolus administration have included a flulike syndrome (fever, chills, headache, constitutional symptoms, such as malaise, fatigue) and a mild vascular leak syndrome consisting of edema and oliguria (155). Clinical trials continue to evaluate whether pharmacologic doses of IL-4 might exhibit antineoplastic activity.

Interleukin-5

First identified as eosinophil differentiation factor, aberrant expression of IL-5 has been noted in Reed-Sternberg cells of Hodgkin's disease and may be pathophysiologically related to the eosinophilia associated with that neoplasm. No clinical tests have been conducted with IL-5, but IL-5 antagonists are being explored for allergic disorders.

Interleukin-7

Potent stimulator of lymphocyte growth and differentiation, recent studies indicate that IL-7 also may possess a significant ability to stimulate early hematopoietic progenitors in addition to SCF (156). No clinical trials of IL-7 have yet begun.

Interleukin-8

A potent activator of neutrophil killing and a chemotactic molecule, IL-8 has also been reported to be active in mobilizing PBPCs in preclinical modeling (157). There is no clinical experience with IL-8.

Interleukin-9

IL-9 enhances the proliferation of early erythroid progenitor cells, particularly in association with SCF (158), and also acts as a lymphoid immunomodulatory agent. It has not yet entered clinical trials.

Interleukin-10

IL-10 inhibits the production of cytokines, such as IL-1, IL-6, G-CSF, and TNF, from activated monocytes and may be the critical "off switch" for cytokine production. It may be an interesting anti-inflammatory cytokine, although overproduction of IL-10 has been associated with lymphomagenesis in a murine model (159). No clinical trials have been conducted with IL-10.

Interleukin-12

Also known as natural killer cell stimulatory factor (NKSF), IL-12 is a critical regulator of cell-mediated immunity (160). It is in active phase II clinical trials as a biologic response modifier.

Interleukin-13

IL-13 appears to share anti-inflammatory activities with IL-4 and IL-10 (161), and it can stimulate macrophage production from primitive hematopoietic precursor cells. No clinical trials have been reported with IL-13.

Interleukin-15

IL-15 appears to be an important physiologic regulator of lymphoid cell activation and proliferation. It binds to subunits of the IL-2 receptor (162).

NEGATIVE REGULATORS OF HEMATOPOIESIS

To balance the effects of cytokines that stimulate blood production, there appear to be regulatory molecules that function to inhibit hematopoiesis. Negative regulators include tumor necrosis factor (TNF), transforming growth factor beta (TGF-beta), and macrophage inflammatory protein 1-alpha (MIP-1-α). Such negative regulators remain poorly understood, although they may play a protective role for cells at the earliest levels of the hematopoietic hierarchy (163, 164).

Summary: How Should Hematopoietic Cytokines be Used in Cancer Medicine?

Many controversies remain when discussing the optimal utilization of hematopoietic cytokines in cancer medicine. Important to note there is a clear consensus that chemotherapy-induced myelosuppression can be mitigated by such agents as G-CSF or GM-CSF. The unanswered question is whether dose reduction represents an equally valid strategy for the treatment of cancer, or whether improvements in clinical outcomes will result from the delivery of dose-intensive chemotherapy (165). In many ways, the approach to this problem will determine the utilization of hematopoietic cytokines to a large degree.

With the sophisticated technology responsible for the bench-to-bedside translational research of hematopoietic cytokine development has come an economic impact. While use of G-CSF or GM-CSF can certainly diminish the frequency and length of inpatient hospitalizations, overuse of these agents when they are not required (e.g., as adjuncts to minimally myelosuppressive chemotherapy) can waste limited resources (166). Alternatively, patient preferences may drive important decisions in the choice of supportive care, and the economic impact has not been well studied for secondary end points, such as return to work or days of symptomatic treatment-related toxicities.

It is clear that there is not one definitive correct way to use hematopoietic cytokines as support of cytotoxic chemotherapy. Figure 82.4 represents a treatment algorithm that may be useful in making decisions about the utilization of these agents. Recognizing the importance of offering clinicians reasonable interpretations of this rapidly evolving data set, the American Society of Clinical Oncology (ASCO) sponsored the development of evidence-based practice guidelines concerning the appropriate clinical use of hematopoietic cytokines (167). Certain areas have evolved rapidly (such as the safety of CSFs as supportive care for patients with myeloid leukemia), and the ASCO CSF Practice Guidelines will be updated periodically based on new information from ongoing studies. It is also clear that more practice-based clinical trials will be needed to define aspects of CSF use that are important determinants of the costs of care (such as the optimal dose and schedule of CSF to use with nonablative chemotherapy).

Hematopoietic cytokines offer new potential for innovative

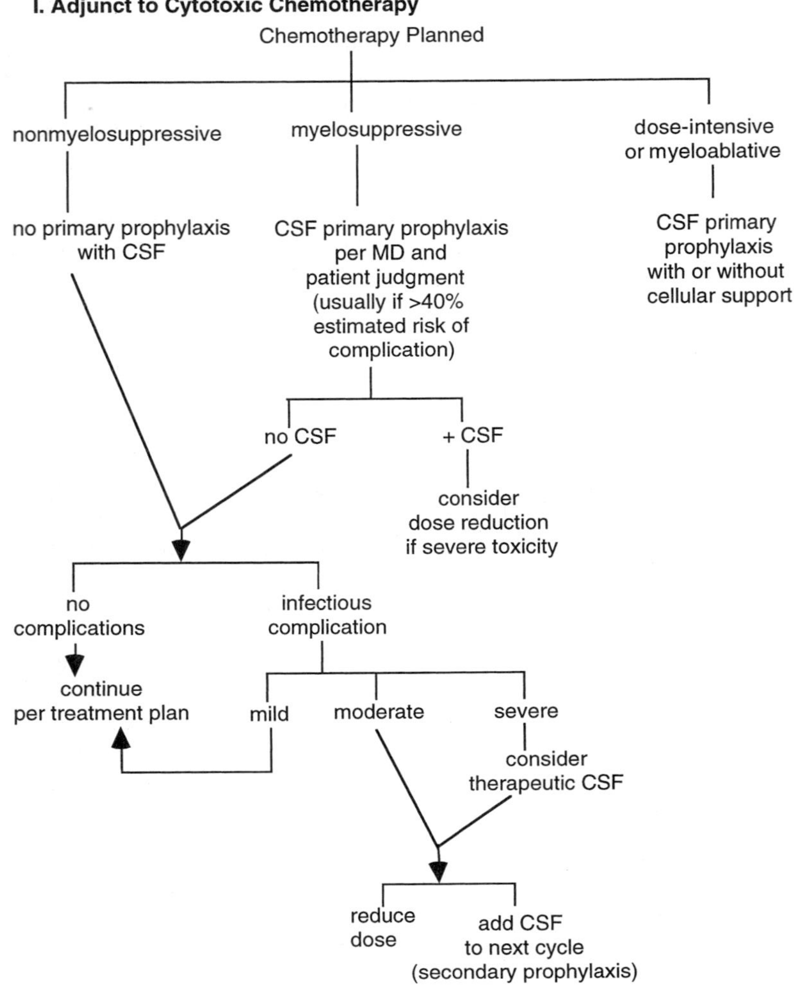

Figure 82.4. Algorithm for use of hematopoietic cytokines.

clinical initiatives, as well. Gene therapy studies in the clinic will be modeled on experiments using gene transfer into hematopoietic cells stimulated by cytokines (75, 76, 137, 138). Antitumor vaccinations may take advantage of the immunomodulatory effects of certain hematopoietic cytokines, and pharmacologic doses of exogenous cytokines may be able to stimulate significant immunoreactivity to cancer if the proper antigenic targets are identified. Correction of stem cell deficits may be possible with ex vivo expanded populations of primitive hematopoietic precursors maintained in a cytokine milieu that maintains the undifferentiated state of "stemness." Finally, differentiation therapy of hematologic neoplasms may be possible using the proper sequence and combination of cytokines to trigger differentiative signal transduction pathways. While the current generation of clinical research in hematopoietic cytokines has focused on the supportive care of cancer patients receiving cytotoxic chemotherapy, future research directions with these molecules are broad and exciting.

References

1. Metcalf D. Review: hematopoietic regulators. Redundancy or subtlety? Blood 1993;82:3515–3523.
2. Vose J, Armitage JO. Clinical applications of hematopoietic growth factors. J Clin Onc 1995;13:1023–1035.
3. Carnot P, Deflandre C. Sur l'activite hemopoietique des differents organeau au cours de la regeneration du sang. CR Searces Acad Sci 1906;143:432–435.
4. Reissmann KR. Studies on the mechanisms of erythropoietic stimulation in parabiotic rats during hypoxia. Blood 1950;5:372–376.
5. Erslev A. Humoral regulation of red cell production. Blood 1953;8:349–352.
6. Stohlman FJ, Rath CE, Rose JC. Evidence for a humoral regulation of erythropoiesis: studies on a patient with polycythemia secondary to regional hypoxia. Blood 1954;9: 721–725.
7. Jacobson LO, Goldwasser E, Fried W, Plzak L. Studies on erythropoiesis, VII. The role of the kidney in the production of erythropoietin. Trans Assoc Am Physicians 1957;70: 305.
8. Goldwasser E, Kung CKH. Purification of erythropoietin. Proc Natl Acad Sci USA 1971;68:697–701.
9. Miyake T, Kung CKH, Goldwasser E. Purification of human erythropoietin. J Biol Chem 1977;252:5558.
10. Lin FK, Suggs S, Lin CH, et al. Cloning and expression of the human erythropoietin gene. Proc Natl Acad Sci USA 1985;82:7580–7584.
11. Jacobs K, Shoemaker C, Rudersdorf R, et al. Isolation and characterization of genomic and cDNA clones of human erythropoietin. Nature 1985;313:806.
12. Spangrude GJ, Smith L, Uchida N, Ikuta K, Heimfeld S, Friedman J, Weissman IL. Mouse hematopoietic stem cells. Blood 1991;78:1395–1402.
13. Ford CE, Hamerton JL, Barnes DWH, Loutit JF. Cytological identification of radiation chimeras. Nature 1956;177:452.

14. Till JE, McCullough EA. Direct measurement of the radiation sensitivity of normal mouse bone marrow cells. Radiat Res 1961;14:213.
15. Pluznik DH, Sachs L. The cloning of normal "mast" cells in tissue culture. J Cell Physiol 1965;66:319–324.
16. Bradley TR, Metcalf D. The growth of mouse bone marrow cells in vitro. Aust J Exp Biol Med Sci 1966;44:287–300.
17. Moore MAS. Clinical implications of positive and negative hematopoietic stem cell regulators. Blood 1991;78:1–19.
18. Li CL, Johnson GR. Stem cell factor enhances the survival but not the self-renewal of murine hematopoietic long-term repopulating cells. Blood 1994;84:408–414.
19. Andrews RG, Briddell RA, Knitter GH, Opie T, Bronsden M, Myerson D, Appelbaum FR, McNiece I. In vivo synergy between recombinant human stem cell factor and recombinant human granulocyte colony-stimulating factor in baboons: enhanced circulation of progenitor cells. Blood 1994;84:800–810.
20. Yan XQ, Briddell R, Hartley C, Stoney G, Samal B, McNiece I. Mobilization of long-term hematopoietic reconstituting cells in mice by the combination of stem cell factor plus granulocyte colony-stimulating factor. Blood 1994;84:795–799.
21. Yan XQ, Hartley C, McElroy P, Chang A, McCrea C, McNiece I. Peripheral blood progenitor cells mobilized by recombinant human granulocyte colony-stimulating factor plus recombinant rat stem cell factor contain long-term engrafting cells capable of cellular proliferation for more than two years as shown by serial transplantation in mice. Blood 1995;85:2303–2307.
22. Costa JJ, Demetri GD, Hayes DF, Merica EA, Menchaca DM, Galli SJ. Increased skin mast cells and urine methylhistamine in patients receiving recombinant methionyl human stem cell factor (abstract). Proc AACR 1993;34:211
23. McDonald TIP, Cottrell MB, Clift RE, Cullen WC, Lin FK. High doses of recombinant erythropoietin stimulate platelet production in mice. Exp Hematol 1987;15:719–721.
24. Berridge MV, Fraser JK, Carter JM, Lin FK. Effects of recombinant human erythropoietin on megakaryocytes and on platelet production in the rat. Blood 1988;72: 970–977.
25. Ishibashi T, Koziol JA, Burstein SA. Human recombinant erythropoietin promotes differentiation of murine megakaryocytes in vitro. J Clin Invest 1987;79:286.
26. Ikebuchi K, Ihle JN, Hirai Y, Wong GG, Clark SC, Ogawa M. Synergistic factors for stem cell proliferation: Further studies of the target stem cells and the mechanism of stimulation by interleukin-1, interleukin-6, and granulocyte colony-stimulating factor. Blood 1988;72:2007–2014.
27. Ikebuchi K, Clark SC, Ihle JN, Souza LM, Ogawa M. Granulocyte colony-stimulating factor enhances interleukin 3-dependent proliferation of multipotential hemopoietic progenitors. Proc Natl Acad Sci USA 1988;85:3445–3449.
28. Burgess A, Metcalf D. Characterization of a serum factor stimulating the differentiation of myelomonocytic leukemia cells. Int J Cancer 1980;26:647–654.
29. Metcalf D. Clonal extinction of myelomonocytic leukemia cells by serum from mice injected with endotoxin. Int J Cancer 1980;25:225–233.
30. Nicola NA, Metcalf D, Matsumoto M, Johnson GR. Purification of a factor inducing differentiation in murine myelomonocytic leukemia cells. Identification as granulocyte colony-stimulating factor. J Biol Chem 1983;258:9017–9023.
31. Nicola NA, Begley CG, Metcalf D. Identification of the human analogue of a regulator that induces differentiation in murine leukaemic cells. Nature 1985;314:625–628.
32. Souza LM, Boone TC, Gabrilove J, Lai PH, Zsebo KM, Murdock DC, Chazin VR, Bruszewski J, Lu H, Chen KK, et al. Recombinant human granulocyte colony-stimulating factor: effects on normal and leukemic myeloid cells. Science 1986;232:61–65.
33. Demetri GD, Griffin JD. Granulocyte colony-stimulating factor and its receptor. Blood 1991;78:2791–2808.
34. Hammond WP, Csiba E, Canin A, Hockman H, Souza LM, Layton JE, Dale DC. Chronic neutropenia: a new canine model induced by human granulocyte colony-stimulating factor. J Clin Invest 1991;87:704–710.
35. Watari K, Asano S, Shirafuji N, Kodo H, Ozawa K, Takaku F, Kamachi S. Serum granulocyte colony-stimulating factor levels in healthy volunteers and patients with various disorders as estimated by enzyme immunoassay. Blood 1989;73:117–122.
36. Kawakami M, Tsutsumi H, Kumakawa T, Abe H, Hirai M, Kurosawa S, Mori M, Fukushima M. Levels of serum granulocyte colony-stimulating factor in patients with infections. Blood 1990;76:1962–1964.
37. Mempel K, Pietsch T, Menzel T, Zeidler C, Welte K. Increased serum levels of granulocyte colony-stimulating factor in patients with severe congenital neutropenia. Blood 1991;11:1919.
38. Lieschke GJ, Grail D, Hodgson G, Metcalf D, Stanley E, Cheerts C, Fowler KJ, Basu S, Zhan YF, Dunn AR. Mice lacking granulocyte colony-stimulating factor have chronic neutropenia, granulocyte and macrophage progenitor cell deficiency, and impaired neutrophil mobilization. Blood 1994;84:1737–1746.
39. Burgess AW, Camakaris J, Metcalf D. Purification and properties of colony-stimulating factor from mouse lung conditioned medium. J Biol Chem 1977;252:1998.
40. Gasson JC, Weisbart RH, Kaufman SE, Clark SC, Hewick RM, Wong GG, Golde DW. Purified human granulocyte-macrophage colony-stimulating factor: direct action on neutrophils. Science 1984;226:1339–1342.
41. Wong GG, Witek JS, Temple PA, Wilkens KM, Leary AC, Luxenberg DP, Jones SS, Brown EL, Kay RM, Orr EC, Shoemaker C, Golde DW, Kaufman RJ, Hewick RM, Wang EA, Clark SC. Human GM-CSF molecular cloning of the complementary DNA and purification of the natural and recombinant proteins. Science 1985;228:810–815.
42. Metcalf D. The molecular biology and functions of the granulocyte-macrophage colony-stimulating factors. Blood 1986;67:257–267.
43. Cebon J, Dempsey P, Fox R, et al. Pharmacokinetics of human granulocyte-macrophage colony-stimulating factor using a sensitive immunoassay. Blood 1988;72:1340–1347.
44. Dranoff G, Crawford AD, Sadelain M, Ream B, Rashid A, Bronson RT, Dickersin GR, Bachurski CJ, Mark EL, Whitsett JA, Mulligan RC. Involvement of granulocyte-macrophage colony-stimulating factor in pulmonary homeostasis. Science 1994;264: 713–716.
45. Stanley E, Lieschke GJ, Grail D, Metcalf D, Hodgson G, Gall JAM, Maher DW, Cebon J, Sinickas V, Dunn AR. Granulocyte-macrophage colony-stimulating factor-deficient mice show no major perturbation of hematopoiesis but develop a characteristic pulmonary pathology. Proc Natl Acad Sci USA 1994;91:5592.
46. Lieschke GJ, Stanley E, Grail D, Hodgson G, Sinickas V, Gall JAM, Sinclair RA, Dunn AR. Mice lacking both macrophage- and granulocyte-macrophage colony-stimulating factor have macrophages and coexistent osteoporosis and severe lung disease. Blood 1994;84:27–35.
47. Han JH, Gileadi C, Rajapaksa R, Kosek J, Greenberg PL. Modulation of apoptosis in human myeloid leukemic cells by GM-CSF. Exp Hematol 1995;23:265–272.
48. Williams GT, Smith CA, Spooncer E, Dexter TM, Taylor DR. Haemopoietic colony stimulating factors promote cell survival by suppressing apoptosis. Nature 1990;343: 76–79.
49. Lieschke GJ, Burgess AW. Granulocyte colony-stimulating factor and granulocyte-macrophage colony-stimulating factor (parts I and II). N Engl J Med 1992;327:28–35, 99–106.
50. Grabstein KH, Urdal DL, Tushinski RJ, Mochizuki DY, Price VL, Cantrell MA, Gillis S, Conlon PJ. Induction of macrophage tumoricidal activity by granulocyte-macrophage colony-stimulating factor. Science 1986;232:506–508.
51. Weisbart RH, Kacena A, Schuh A, Golde DW GM-CSF induces human neutrophil IgA-mediated phagocytosis by an IgA Fc receptor activation mechanism. Nature 1988;332:647–648.
52. Weisbart RH, Kwan L, Golde DW, Gasson JC. Human GM-CSF primes neutrophils for enhanced oxidative metabolism in response to the major physiological chemoattractants. Blood 1987;69:18–21.
53. Cannistra S, Vellenga E, Groshek P, Rambaldi A, Griffin J. Human granulocyte-monocyte colony-stimulating factor and interleukin-3 stimulate monocyte cytotoxicity through tumor necrosis factor-dependent mechanisms. Blood 1988;71:672–676.
54. Nathan CF. Respiratory burst in adherent human neutrophils: Triggering by colony-stimulating factors CSF-GM and CSF-G. Blood 1989;73:301–306.
55. Rose RM. The role of colony-stimulating factors in infectious disease: Current status, future challenges. Semin Oncol 1992;19:415–421.
56. Socinski MA, Cannistra SA, Elias A, Antman KH, Schnipper L, Griffin JD. Granulocyte-macrophage colony-stimulating factor expands the circulating haemopoietic progenitor cell compartment in man. Lancet 1988:1194–1198.
57. Duhrsen U, Villeval JL, Boyd J, Kannourakis G, Morstyn G, Metcalf D. Effects of recombinant human granulocyte colony-stimulating factor on hematopoietic progenitor cells in cancer patients. Blood 1988;72:2074–81.
58. Goldman J. Peripheral blood stem cells for allografts. (Editorial) Blood 1995;85: 1413–1415.
59. Bussolino F, Wang JM, Defilippi P, et al. Granulocyte- and granulocyte-macrophage-colony stimulating factors induce human endothelial cells to migrate and proliferate. Nature 1989;337:471–473.
60. Bussolino F, Ziche M, Wang JM, Alessi D, Mobidelli L, Cremona O, Bosai A, Marchisio PC, Mantovani A. In vitro and in vivo activation of endothelial cells by colony-stimulating factors. J Clin Invest 1991;87:986–995.
61. Bronchud MH, Scarffe JH, Thatcher N, Crowther D, Souza LM, Alton NK, Testa NG, Dexter TM. Phase I/II study of recombinant human granulocyte colony-stimulating factor in patients receiving intensive chemotherapy for small cell lung cancer. Br J Cancer 1987;56:809–13.
62. Gabrilove JL, Jakubowski A, Fain K, Grous J, Scher H, Sternberg C, Yagoda A, Clarkson B, Bonilla MA, Oettgen HF, Alton K, Boone T, Altrock B, Welte K, Souza L. Phase I study of granulocyte colony-stimulating factor in patients with transitional cell carcinoma of the urothelium. J Clin Invest 1988;82:1454–61.
63. Morstyn G, Campbell L, Souza LM, Alton NK, Keech J, Green M, Sheridan W, Metcalf D, Fox R. Effect of granulocyte colony stimulating factor on neutropenia induced by cytotoxic chemotherapy. Lancet 1988;1:667–672.
64. Groopman JE, Mitsuyasu RT, DeLeo MJ, Oette DH, Golde DW. Effect of recombinant human granulocyte-macrophage colony-stimulating factor on myelopoiesis in the acquired immunodeficiency syndrome. N Engl J Med 1987;317:593–598.
65. Antman K, Griffin J, Elias A, Socinski M, Ryna L, Cannistra S, Oette D, Whitley M, Frei E, Schnipper L. Effect of recombinant human granulocyte-macrophage colony-stimulating factor on chemotherapy-induced myelosuppression. N Engl J Med 1988;319: 593–598.
66. Brandt SJ, Peters WP, Atwater SK, Kurtzberg J, Borowitz MJ, Jones RB, Shpall EJ, Bast RCJ, Gilbert CJ, Oette DH. Effect of recombinant human granulocyte-macrophage colony-stimulating factor on hematopoietic reconstitution after high-dose chemotherapy and autologous bone marrow transplantation. N Engl J Med 1988;318:869–876.
67. Lord BI, Bronchud MH, Owens S, Chang J, Howell A, Souza L, Dexter TM. The kinetics of human granulopoiesis following treatment with granulocyte colony-stimulating factor in vivo. Proc Natl Acad Sci USA 1989;86:9499–9503.
68. Aglietta M, Piacibello W, Sanavio F, Stacchini A, Apra F, Schena M, Mossetti C, Carnino F, Caligaris-Cappio F, Gavosto F. Kinetics of human hemopoietic cells after in vivo administration of granulocyte-macrophage colony-stimulating factor. J Clin Invest 1989;83:551–557.
69. Crawford J, Ozer H, Stoller R, Johnson D, Lyman G, Tabbara I, Kris M, Grous J, Picozzi V, Rausch G, Smith R, Gradishar W, Yahanda A, Vincent M, Stewart M, Glaspy J. Reduction by granulocyte colony-stimulating factor of fever and neutropenia induced by chemotherapy in patients with small-cell lung cancer. N Engl J Med 1991;325:164–170.
70. Trillet-Lenoir V, Green J, Manegold C, Von Pawel J, Gatzemeier U, Lebeau B, Depierre A, Johnson P, Decoster G, Tomita D, Ewen C. Recombinant granulocyte colony stimulating factor reduces the infectious complications of cytotoxic chemotherapy. Eur J Cancer 1993;29A:319–324.
71. Nemunaitis J, Rabinowe SN, Singer JW, Bierman PJ, Vose JM, Freedman AS, Onetto N, Gillis S, Oette D, Gold M, Buckner CD, Hansen JA, Ritz J, Appelbaum FR, Armitage JO, Nadler LM. Recombinant granulocyte-macrophage colony-stimulating factor after autologous bone marrow transplantation for lymphopid cancer. N Engl J Med 1991;324:1773–1778.
72. Gerhartz HH, Engelhard M, Meusers P, et al. Randomized, double-blind, placebo-controlled, phase III study of recombinant human granulocyte-macrophage colony-stimulating factor (rhGM-CSF) as adjunct to induction treatment of high-grade malignant non-Hodgkin's lymphomas. Blood 1993;82:2329–2339.
73. Bajorin DF, Nichols CR, Schmoll H-J, Kantoff PW, Bokemeyer C, Demetri GD, Einhorn

LH, Bosl GJ. Recombinant human granulocyte-macrophage colony-stimulating factor as as adjunct to conventional-dose ifosfamide-based chemotherapy for patients with advanced or relapsed germ cell tumors: a randomized trial. J Clin Oncol 1994;13:79–86.
74. Vadhan-Raj S, Broxmeyer HE, Hittelman WN, et al. Abrogating chemotherapy-induced myelosuppression by recombinant granulocyte-macrophage colony-stimulating factor in patients with sarcoma: protection at the progenitor cell level. J Clin Oncol 1992;10:1266–1277.
75. Talcott JA, Siegel RD, Finberg R, Goldman L. Risk assessment in cancer patients with fever and neutropenia: a prospective, two-center validation of a prediction rule. J Clin Oncol 1992;10:316–322.
76. Bregni M, Magni M, Siena S, Di Nicola M, Bonadonna G, Gianni AM. Human peripheral blood hematopoietic progenitors are optimal targets of retroviral-mediated gene transfer. Blood 1992;80:1418–1422.
77. Dunbar CE, Cottler-Fox M, O'Shaughnessy JA, Doren S, Carter C, Berenson R, Brown S, Moen RC, Greenblatt J, Stewart FM, Leitman SF, Wilson WH, Cowan K, Young NS, Nienhuis AW. Retrovirally marked CD-34 enriched peripheral blood and bone marrow cells contribute to long-term engraftment after autologous transplantation. Blood 1995;85:3048–3057.
78. Sheridan WP, Begley CG, Juttner CA, Szer J, To LB, Maher D, McGrath KM, Morstyn G, Fox RM. Effect of peripheral-blood progenitor cells mobilised by filgrastim (G-CSF) on platelet recovery after high-dose chemotherapy. Lancet 1992;339:640–644.
79. Elias AD, Ayash L, Anderson KC, Hunt M, Wheeler C, Schwartz G, Tepler I, Mazanet R, Lynch C, Pap S, Pelaez J, Reich E, Critchlow J, Demetri G, Bibbo J, Schnipper L, Griffin JD, Frei E, Antman KH. Mobilization of peripheral blood progenitor cells by chemotherapy and granulocyte-macrophage colony-stimulating factor for hematologic support after high-dose intensification for breast cancer. Blood 1992;79: 3036–3044.
80. Beyer J, Schwella N, Zingsem J, Strohscheer I, Schwaner I, Oettle H, Serke S, Huhn D, Siegert W. Hematopoietic rescue after high-dose chemotherapy using autologous peripheral-blood progenitor cells or bone marrow: A randomized comparison. J Clin Oncol 1995;13:1328–1335.
81. Spitzer G, Adkins DR, Spencer V, Dunphy FR, Petruska PJ, Velasquea WS, Bowers CE, Kronmueller N, Niemeyer R, McIntyre W. Randomized study of growth factors post-peripheral-blood stem-cell transplant: neutrophil recovery is improved with modest clinical benefit. J Clin Oncol 1994;12:661–670.
82. Cortelazzo S, Viero P, Bellavita P, Rossi A, Buelli M, Borleri GM, Marziali S, Bassan R, Comotti B, Rambaldi A, Barbui T. Granulocyte colony-stimulating factor following peripheral-blood progenitor-cell transplant in non-Hodgkin's lymphoma. J Clin Oncol 1995;13:935–941.
83. Klumpp TR, Mangan KF, Goldberg SL, Pearlman ES, Macdonald JS. Granulocyte colony-stimulating factor accelerates neutrophil engraftment following peripheral-blood stem-cell transplantation: a prospective, randomized trial. J Clin Oncol 1995;13:1323–1327.
84. Bensinger WI, Weaver CH, Appelbaum FR, Rowley S, Demirer T, Sanders J, Storb R, Buckner CD. Transplantation of allogeneic peripheral blood stem cells mobilized by recombinant human granulocyte colony-stimulating factor. Blood 1995;85: 1655–1658.
85. Zanjani ED, Ascensao JL. Erythropoietin. Transfusion 1989;29:46–57.
86. Miller CB, Jones RJ, Piantadose S, et al. Decreased erythropoietin response in patients with the anemia of cancer. N Engl J Med 1990;322:1689–1692.
87. Eschbach JW, Egrie JC, Downing MR, et al. Correction of the anemia of end-stage renal disease with recombinant human erythropoietin. N Engl J Med 1987;316:73–78.
88. Ludwig H, Fritz E, Kotzmann H, Hoecker P, Gisslinger H, Barnas U. Erythropoietin treatment of anemia associated with multiple myeloma. N Engl J Med 1990;322: 1693–1699.
89. Fischl M, Galpin JE, Levine JD, et al. Recombinant human erythropoietin for patients with AIDS treated with zidovudine. N Engl J Med 1990;322:1488–1493.
90. Abels RI. Use of recombinant human erythropoietin in the treatment of anemia in patients who have cancer. Semin Oncol 1992;19(suppl 8):29–35.
91. Ludwig H, Fritz E, Leitgeb C, Pecherstorfer M, Samonigg H, Schuster J. Prediction of response to erythropoietin treatment in chronic anemia of cancer. Blood 1994;84: 1056–1063.
92. Yamamoto S. Mechanism of the development of thrombocytosis due to bleeding. Acta Haematol Jpn 1957;20:163–178.
93. Kelemen E, Cserhati I, Tanos B. Demonstration and some properties of human thrombopoietin in thrombocythemic sera. Acta Haematolo (Basel) 1958;20:350–355.
94. Gordon MS, Hoffman R. Growth factors affecting human thrombopoiesis: potential agents for the treatment of thrombocytopenia. Blood 1992;80:302–307.
95. Metcalf D. Thrombopoietin—at last (editorial). Nature 1994;369:519–520.
96. Vigon I, Mornon JP, Cocault L, Mitjavila MT, Tambourn P, Gisselbrecht S, Souyri M. Molecular cloning and characterization of MPL, the human homolog of the v-mpl oncogene: identification of a member of the hematopoietic growth factor receptor family. Proc Natl Acad Sci USA 1992;89:5640–5644.
97. Methia N, Louache F, Vainchenker W, Wendling F. Oligodeoxynucleotides antisense to the proto-oncogene c-mpl specifically inhibit in vitro megakaryocytopoiesis. Blood 1993;82:1395–1401.
98. De Sauvage FJ, Hass PE, Spencer SD, Malloy BE, Gurney AL, Spencer SA, Darbonne WC, Henzel WJ, Wong SC, Kuang WJ, Oles KJ, Hultgren B, Solberg LA, Goeddel DV, Eaton DL. Stimulation of megakaryocytopoiesis and thrombopoiesis by the c-Mpl ligand. Nature 1994;369:533–538.
99. Bartley TD, Bogenberger J, Hunt P, Li Y-S, Lu HS, Martin F, Chang MS, Samal B, Nichol JL, Swift S, Johnson MJ, Hsu RY, Parker VP, Suggs S, Skrine JD, Merewether LA, Clogston C, Hsu E, Hokom MM, Hornkol A, Choi E, Pangelinan M, Sun Y, Mar V, McNich J, et al. Identification and cloning of a megakaryocyte growth and development factor that is a ligand for the cytokine receptor mpl. Cell 1994;77:1117–1124.
100. Lok S, Kaushansky K, Holly R, Kuijper JL, Lofton-Day C, Oort P, Grant F, Helpel MD, Burkhead SK, Kramer JM, Bell LA, Sprecher CA, Blumberg H, Johnson R, Prunkard D, Ching AFT, Mathewes SL, Bailey MC, Forstrom JW, Buddle MM, Osboprn SG, Evans SJ, Sheppard PO, Presnell SR, O'Hara PJ, Hagen FS, Roth GJ, Foster DC. Cloning and expression of murine thrombopoietin cDNA and stimulation of platelet production in vivo. Nature 1994;369:565–568.
101. Miyazaki H, Kato T, Ogami K, Iwamatsu A, Shimada Y, Souma Y, Akahori H, Horie K, Kokubo A, Kudo Y, Maedo E, Kawamura K, Sudo T. Isolation and cloning of a novel human thrombopoietic factor (abstract). Exp Hematol 1994;22:838.
102. Gurney AL, Carver-Moore K, de Sauvage FJ, Moore MW. Thrombocytopenia in c-*mpl*-deficient mice. Science 1994;265:1445–1447.
103. Kaushansky K, Lok S, Holly RD, Broudy VC, Lin N, Bailey MC, Forstrom JW, Buddle MM, Oort PJ, Hagen FS, Roth GJ, Papayannopoulou T, Foster DC. Promotion of megakaryocyte progenitor expansion and differentiation by the c-*mpl* ligand thrombopoietin. Nature 1994;369:568–571.
104. Kaushansky K, Broudy VC, Lin N, Jorgensen MJ, McCarty J, Fox N, Zucker-Franklin D, Lofton-Day C. Thrombopoietin, the *mpl* ligand, is essential for full megakaryocyte development. Cell Biol 1995;92:3234–3238.
105. Sprugel KH, Humes JM, Grossmann A, Ren HP, Kaushansky K. Recombinant thrombopoietin stimulates rapid platelet recovery in thrombocytopenic mice (abstract 952). Blood 1994;84.
106. Yokota T, Lee F, Rennick D, et al. Isolation and characterization of a mouse cDNA clone that expresses mast-cell growth factor activity in monkey cells. Proc Natl Acad Sci USA 1981;81:1070–1073.
107. Yang Y-C, Ciarletta AB, Temple PA, Chung MP, Kovacic S, Witek-Giannotti JS, Leary AC, Kriz R, Donahue RE, Wong GG, Clark SC. Human IL-3 (Multi-CSF) Identification by expression cloning of a novel hematopoietic growth factor related to murine IL-3. Cell 1986;47:3–10.
108. Broudy VC, Lin NL, Kaushansky K. Thrombopoietin (c-mpl ligand) acts synergistically with erythropoietin, stem cell factor, and interleukin-11 to enhance murine megakaryocyte colony growth and increases megakaryocyte ploidy in vitro. Blood 1995;85: 1719–1726.
109. Donahue RE, Seehra J, Metzger M, Lefebvre D, Rock B, Carbone S, Nathan DG, Garnick M, Sehgal PK, Laston D, et al. Human IL-3 and GM-CSF act synergistically in stimulating hematopoiesis in primates. Science 1988;241:1820–1823.
110. Ganser A, Lindemann A, Seipelt G, Ottmann OG, Herrmann F, Eder M, Frisch J, Schulz G, Mertelsmann R, Hoelzer D. Effects of recombinant human interleukin-3 in patients with normal hematopoiesis and in patients with bone marrow failure. Blood 1990;76:666–676.
111. Kurzrock R, Talpaz M, Estrov Z, Rosenblum MG, Gutterman JU. Phase I study of recombinant human interleukin-3 in patients with bone marrow failure. J Clin Oncol 1991;9:1241–1250.
112. Demetri GD, Young DC, Merica E, Edwards R, Pratt ES, Oldham F, Nadler P, Antman K, Griffin JD. Clinical effects of interleukin-3 (IL-3) in patients with advanced sarcomas: a phase I/II trial. Blood 1991;78(suppl 1):12.
113. Postmus PE, Gietema JA, Damsma O, Biesma B, Limburg PC, Vellenga E, de Vries EGE. Effects of recombinant human interleukin-3 in patients with relapsed small-cell lung cancer treated with chemotherapy: a dose-finding study. J Clin Oncol 1992;10: 1131–1140.
114. Tepler I, Elias A, Kalish L, Shulman L, Strauss G, Skarin A, Lynch T, Levitt D, Resta D, Demetri G, Gaynes L, Schnipper L. Effect of recombinant human interleukin-3 on haematological recovery from chemotherapy-induced myelosuppression. Br J Haematol 1994;87:678–686.
115. Vadhan-Raj S, Papadopoulos NE, Burgess MA, Linke KA, Patel SR, Hays C, Arcenas A, Plager C, Kudelka AP, Hittelman WN, Broxmeyer HE, Williams DE, Garrison L, Benjamin RS. Effects of PIXY321, a granulocyte-macrophage colony-stimulating factor/interleukin-3 fusion protein, on chemotherapy-induced multilineage myelosuppression in patients with sarcoma. J Clin Oncol 1994;12:715–724.
116. Fay JW, Lazarus H, Herzig R, Saez R, Stevens DA, Collins RH, Pineiro LA, Cooper BW, DiCesare J, Campion M, Felser JM, Herzig G, Bernstein SH. Sequential administration of recombinant human interleukin-3 and granulocyte-macrophage colony-stimulating factor after autologous bone marrow transplantation for malignant lymphoma: a phase I/II multicenter study. Blood 1994;84:2151–2157.
117. Kishimoto T. The biology of interleukin-6. Blood 1989;74:1–10.
118. Kawano M, Hirano T, Matsuda T, et al. Autocrine generation and requirement of BSF-2/IL-6 for human multiple myelomas. Nature 1988;332:83–85.
119. Leger-Ravet MB, Peuchmaur M, Devergne O, et al. Interleukin-6 gene expression in Castleman's disease. Blood 1991;78:2923–2930.
120. Mule JJ, McIntosh JK, Jablons DM, Rosenberg SA. Antitumor activity of recombinant interleukin 6 in mice. J Exp Med 1991;171:629–636.
121. Ishibashi T, Kimura H, Shikama Y, et al. Interleukin-6 is a potent thrombopoietic factor in vivo in mice. Blood 1989;74:1241.
122. Asano S, Okano A, Ozawa K, et al. In vivo effects of recombinant human interleukin-6 in primates: stimulated production of platelets. Blood 1990;75:1602.
123. Carrington PA, Hill RJ, Stenberg PE, et al. Multiple in vivo effects of interleukin-3 and interleukin-6 on murine megakaryopoiesis. Blood 1991;77:34.
124. Demetri GD, Bukowski RM, Samuels B, Gordon M, Antman K, Merica EA, Samuel S, Campion M, Levitt D, Isaacs R. Stimulation of thrombopoiesis by recombinant human interleukin-6 (IL-6) pre- and post-chemotherapy in previously untreated sarcoma patients with normal hematopoiesis. Blood 1993;82(suppl 1):367a.
125. Demetri GD, Hayes DF, Merica EA, Cap B, Sparano J. Concurrent IL-6 plus G-CSF to support dose-intensified cyclophosphamide/doxorubicin (CD) possible acceleration of hematologic recovery from chemotherapy-induced thrombocytopenia. Blood 1994;84(suppl 1):580a.
126. D'Hondt V, Humblet Y, Guillaume T, Baatout S, Chatelain C, Berliere M, Longueville J, Feyens AM, De Greve J, Van Osterom A, Von Graffenried B, Donnez J, Symann M. Thrombopoietic effects and toxicity of interleukin-6 in patients with ovarian cancer before and after chemotherapy: a multicentric placebo-controlled, randomized Phase Ib study. Blood 1995;85:2347–2353.
127. Lazarus HM, Winton EF, Williams SF, et al. Phase I study of recombinant human Interleukin-6 after ABMT in patients with poor-prognosis breast cancer (abstract 677). Blood 82 1993;(suppl 1):173a.
128. Gordon MS, Nemunaitis J, Hoffman R, Paquette RL, Rosenfeld C, Manfreda S, Isaacs R, Nimer SD. A phase I trial of recombinant human interleukin-6 in patients with myelodysplastic syndromes and thrombocytopenia. Blood 1995;85:3066–3076.
129. Paul SR, Bennett F, Calvetti JA, Kelleher K, Wood CR, O'Hara RM, Leary AC, Sibley B, Clark SC, Williams DA, Yang Y-C. Molecular cloning of a cDNA encoding interleukin 11, a stromal cell-derived lymphopoietic and hematopoietic cytokine. Proc Natl Acad Sci USA 1990;87:7512–7516.

130. Du XX, Williams DA. Review: interleukin-11. A multifunctional growth factor derived from the hematopoietic microenvironment. Blood 1994;83:2023–2030.
131. Leonard JP, Quinto CM, Kozitza MK, Neben TY, Goldman SJ. Recombinant human interleukin-11 stimulates multilineage hematopoietic recovery in mice after a myelosuppressive regimen of sublethal irradiation and carboplatin. Blood 1994;83:1499–1506.
132. Gordon MS, Hoffman R, Battiato L, et al. Recombinant Human Interleukin-11 prevents severe thrombocytopenia in breast cancer patients receiving multiple cycles of cyclophosphamide and doxorubicin chemotherapy (abstract 326). Proc ASCO 1994;13:133.
133. Champlin R, Mehra R, Kaye J, et al. Phase I study of recombinant human Interleukin-11 following autologous BMT in patients with breast cancer (abstract 201). Proc ASCO 1994;13:100.
134. Atkins MB, Kappler K, Mier JW, Isaacs RE, Berkman EM. Interleukin-6 associated anemia: determination of the underlying mechanism. Proc Am Soc Clin Oncol 1994;13:295.
135. Dinarello CA. Interleukin-1 and Interleukin-1 antagonism. Blood 1991;77:1627–1652.
136. Smith II JA, Longo DL, Alvord WG, Janik JE, Sharfman WH, Gause BL, et al. The effects of treatment with interleukin-1alpha on platelet recovery after high-dose carboplatin. N Engl J Med 1993;328:756–761.
137. Brenner MK, Rill DR, Moen RC, et al. Gene-marking to trace origin of relapse after autologous bone marrow transplantation. Lancet 1993;341:85.
138. Rill DR, Santans VM, Roberts WM, Nilson T, Bowman LC, Krance RA, Heslop HE, Moen RC, Ihle JN, Brenner MK. Direct demonstration that autologous bone marrow transplantation for solid tumors can return a multiplicity of tumorigenic cells. Blood 1994;84:380–383.
139. Zsebo KM, Wypych J, McNiece IK, Lu HS, Smith KA, Karkare SB, Sachdev RK, Yuschenkoff VN, Birkett NC, Williams LR, Satyagal VN, Tung W, Bosselman RA, Mendiaz EA, Langley KE. Identification, purification, and biological characterization of hematopoietic stem cell factor from Buffalo rat liver-conditioned medium. Cell 1990;63:195–201.
140. Williams DE, Eisenman J, Baird A, et al. Identification of a ligand for the c-*kit* proto-oncogene. Cell 1990;63:167.
141. Huang E, Nocka K, Beler DR, et al. The hematopoietic growth factor KL is encoded by the Sl locus and is the ligand of the c-*kit* receptor, the gene product of the W locus. Cell 1990;63:225.
142. Langley KE, Bennett LG, Wypych J, Yancik SA, Liu XD, Westcott KR, Chang DG, Smith KA, Zsebo KM. Soluble stem cell factor in human serum. Blood 1993;81:656.
143. Broudy VC, Bartley TD, Parker VP, Langley KE. Soluble kit receptor in human serum. Blood 1995;85:66–73.
144. Demetri GD, Costa J, Hayes DF. Phase I trial of recombinant methionyl human stem cell factor (SCF) in patients with advanced breast cancer pre- and post-chemotherapy (chemo) with cyclophosphamide (C) and doxorubicin (A) (abstract 367). Proc Am Soc Clin Oncol 1993;12:142.
145. Demetri GD, Gordon M, Hoffman R, Hayes DF, Sledge GSS, Edwards R, Merica E, Battiato L, Griffin JD. Effects of recombinant methionyl human stem cell factor on hematopoietic progenitor cells in vivo: preliminary results from a phase I trial. Proc AACR 1993;34:217.
146. Crawford J, Lau D, Erwin R, et al. A phase I trial of recombinant methionyl human stem cell factor (SCF) in patients (pts) with advanced non-small cell lung carcinoma (NSCLC) (abstract 338). Proc Am Soc Clin Oncol 1993;12:135.
147. Costa JJ, Demetri GD, Harrist TJ, Dvorak AM, Hayes DF, Merica EA, Menchaca DM, Gringeri AJ, Schwartz LB, Galli SJ. Recombinant human stem cell factor (*kit* ligand) promotes human mast cell and melanocyte hyperplasia and functional activation in vivo. J Exp Med 1996 (in press).
148. Glaspy J, McNiece I, LeMaistre F, et al. Effects of stem cell factor and filgrastim on mobilization of PBPCs and on hematological recovery posttransplant.early results from a phase I/II study (abstract 76). Proc ASCO 1994;13:68.
149. Lyman SD, James L, Johnson L, Brasel K, de Vries P, Escobar SS, Downey H, Splett RR, Beckmann MP, McKenna HJ. Cloning of human homologue of the murine flt3 ligand: a growth factor for early hematopoietic progenitor cells. Blood 1994;83:2795–2801.
150. Hirayama F, Lyman SD, Clark SC, Ogawa M. The flt3 ligand supports proliferation of lymphohematopoetic progenitors and early B-lymphoid progenitors. Blood 1995;85:1762–1768.
151. Nemunaitis J, Shannon-Dorcy K, Appelbaum FR, et al. Long-term follow-up of patients with invasive fungal disease who received adjunctive therapy with recombinant human macrophage colony-stimulating factor. Blood 1993;82:1422–1427.
152. Paul WE. Interleukin-4: a prototype immunoregulatory lymphokine. Blood 1991;77:1859–1870.
153. Golumbek PT, Lazenby AJ, Levitsky HI, Jaffee LM, Karasuyama H, Baker M, Pardoll MD. Treatment of established renal cancer by tumor cells engineered to secrete interleukin-4. Science 1991;254:713–716.
154. Tepper RI, Coffman RL, Leder P. An eosinophil-dependent mechanism for the antitumor effect of interleukin-4. Science 1992;257:548.
155. Atkins MB, Vachino G, Tilg HJ, Karp DD, Robert NJ, Kappler K, Mier JW. Phase I evaluation of thrice-daily intravenous bolus Interleukin-4 in patients with refractory malignancy. J Clin Oncol 1992;10:1802–1809.
156. Blomhoff HK, Veiby OP, McNiece IK, Jacobsen SEW. Stem cell factor and interleukin-7 synergize to enhance early myelopoiesis. Blood 1994;84:1450–1456.
157. Laterveer L, Lindley IJD, Hamilton MS, Willemze R, Fibbe WE. Interleukin-8 induces rapid mobilization of hematopoietic stem cells with radioprotective capacity and long-term myelolymphoid repopulating ability. Blood 1995;85:2269–2275.
158. Lemoli RM, Fortuna A, Fogli M, Motta M, Rizzi S, Benini C, Tura S. Stem cell factor (c-*kit* ligand) enhances the interleukin-9 dependent proliferation of human CD34+ and CD34+CD33-DR-cells. Exp Hematol 1994;22:919–923.
159. Baiocchi RA, Ross ME, Tan JC, et al. Lymphomagenesis in the SCID-hu mouse involves abundant production of interleukin-10. Blood 1995;85:1063–1074.
160. Allavena P, Paganin C, Zhou D, Bianchi G, Soazzani S, Mantovani A. Interleukin-12. Blood 1994;84:2261–2268.
161. Zurawski G, de Vries JE. Interleukin 13 elicits a subset of the activities of its close relative interleukin-4. Stem Cells 1994;12:169–174.
162. Carson WE, Grabstein K, Giri JG, et al. Interleukin-15 is a novel cytokine which activates human natural killer cells using components of the interleukin-2 receptor. Proc ASCO 1994;13:296.
163. Hornung RL, Longo DL. Hematopoietic stem cell depletion by restorative growth factor regimens during repeated high-dose cyclophosphamide therapy. Blood 1992;80:77–83.
164. Moore MAS. Does stem cell exhaustion result from combining hematopoietic growth factors with chemotherapy? If so, how do we prevent it? Blood 1992;80:3–7.
165. Demetri GD. The use of hematopoietic growth factors to support cytotoxic chemotherapy for patients with breast cancer. Hematol/Oncol Clin N Am 1994;8:233–249.
166. Nichols CR, Fox EP, Roth BJ, Williams SD, Loehrer PJ, Einhorn LH. Incidence of neutropenic fever in patients treated with standard-dose combination chemotherapy for small-cell lung cancer and the cost impact of treatment with granulocyte colony-stimulating factor. J Clin Oncol 1994;12:1245–1250.
167. Ozer H. Factors AAHCoHG. Recommendations for the clinical use of hematopoietic colony-stimulating factors (CSFs): evidence-based guidelines recommended by the American Society of Clinical Oncology. J Clin Oncol 1994;12:2471–2508.

CHAPTER 83

Monoclonal Serotherapy

ROBERT C. BAST, JR, MICHAEL R. ZALUTSKY, AND ARTHUR EDWARD FRANKEL

Introduction

Following the initial report of Kohler and Milstein (1), monoclonal antibody technology has exerted a prompt and substantial impact on laboratory investigation. Over the past 2 decades, the availability of monoclonal reagents has permitted the development of novel markers for in vitro applications, including monitoring response to treatment, detecting malignant cells histochemically, identifying subsets of patients with particularly favorable or unfavorable prognoses, and distinguishing some tumors of unknown origin. Progress in the use of monoclonal antibodies for the in vivo diagnosis and treatment of human cancer has, however, been less dramatic. Serotherapy with unmodified monoclonal antibodies has produced tumor regression in lymphomas, melanomas, and breast cancer, but has yielded more equivocal results in leukemias and gastrointestinal neoplasms (2, 3).

Obstacles to effective serotherapy include shed tumor-associated antigen, antigenic modulation, heterogeneity of antigen expression, potency of effector mechanisms, and the immune response to foreign immunoglobulin (4–8). Several of these obstacles have been avoided in ex vivo applications, such as the positive selection of stem cells and the elimination of malignant cells from human bone marrow prior to autologous transplantation in patients with lymphoreticular and solid neoplasms.

In an attempt to exert greater antitumor activity in situ, monoclonal antibodies have been linked to cytotoxic drugs, radionuclides, and immunotoxins. Extensive preclinical studies have been carried out and phase I and II clinical trials have now been performed with each type of immunoconjugate. This chapter considers some of the possibilities for, and limitations of, monoclonal reagents for the treatment of cancer patients.

Therapy with Unmodified Monoclonal Antibodies

TREATMENT IN VIVO

With rare exceptions, murine monoclonal antibodies raised against human neoplasms recognize tumor-associated antigens, which are also expressed by normal adult or fetal tissues. Some antigens, however, are expressed by only a small number of normal cells that may not be essential to the patient's well-being. One of the most promising reports remains that of Miller and colleagues, who prepared tumor-specific murine monoclonal antibodies against the unique idiotopes associated with the cell surface membrane immunoglobulin present on human B-cell lymphomas (9). The original patient treated with a specific anti-idiotypic antibody remained in complete remission for 72 months. Overall, treatment of 14 lymphoma patients with anti-idiotypic antibodies produced an objective response rate of 57% (10). Genes encoding the cell surface membrane immunoglobulin continue to undergo point mutations, resulting in the loss of idiotypic determinants (11). The use of multiple monoclonal antibodies has provided one approach to eliminating tumor cells that lack particular idiotypic determinants. Another approach combined serotherapy with other forms of biologic response modification. In a subsequent trial, 11 patients were treated with anti-idiotypic antibody and interferon alfa (INF-α). Nine of the 11 patients responded objectively and one response was complete, lasting more than a year. Most of the antibodies that produced responses in vivo were of the IgG1 isotype, which is generally least efficient in fixing complement or participating in antibody-dependent cell-mediated cytotoxicity (ADCC).

Monoclonal antibodies against differentiation antigens have been used to treat patients with non-Hodgkin's lymphoma, as well as acute and chronic leukemias. Repeated administration of a chimeric anti-CD20 antibody produced a 42% response rate in 26 patients with relapsed non-Hodgkin's lymphoma, with 10 of 11 responses lasting over 2 to more than 6 months (12). In the case of CD 10–positive acute lymphoblastic leukemia, anti-CD10 antibody induced prompt modulation of the common acute lymphoblastic leukemia antigen, preventing effective therapy (13). Intravenous infusion of anti-CD5 also produced antigenic modulation and only transient, partial regression in a fraction of patients with T-cell leukemia/lymphoma and chronic lymphocytic leukemia (14). In one of the first studies of serotherapy with monoclonal reagents, a serum blocking factor was demonstrated that prevented binding of monoclonal antibody to circulating lymphosarcoma cells, consistent with the presence of shed tumor antigen (15).

Unmodified murine monoclonal antibodies have produced regression of metastases from malignant melanoma. Intravenous administration of antibodies against GD3, a prominent ganglioside on the surface of melanoma cells, produced objective responses in 7 of 51 patients (16). Inflammatory reactions were noted around tumor sites. Biopsies demonstrated infiltration with lymphocytes and mast cells, degranulation of the mast cells, and deposition of complement components. Studies ex vivo suggest that a threshold level of GD3 expression may be required for susceptibility to host effector mechanisms (17). Antibodies capable of mediating ADCC and complement cytotoxicity were most effective (16). Recent trials have attempted to combine anti-GD3 antibodies with different cytokines that might enhance effector function for ADCC (18). Administration of R24 anti-GD3 antibody prior to interleukin-2 (IL-2) produced only 1 response in 20, whereas administration of R24 2 weeks after the initiation of IL-2 treatment produced 10 responses in 32 patients (19). Combination of R24 with INF-γ, GM-CSF, or M-CSF was ineffective (16), but a tumor lysis syndrome was observed in one melanoma patient treated with TNF-α and R24 (20).

The ability of monoclonal antibodies to reach tumor cells can be limited by abnormal vascularity, elevated interstitial pressure, and relatively large distances for transport of immunoglobulins through the interstitium (21, 22). Intravenous injection of an IgG2a murine monoclonal antibody against a 250 kilodalton (kd) melanoma-associated chondroitin sulfate proteoglycan core protein resulted in selective localization of antibody in metastatic nodules of malignant melanoma (23). The greater the amount of antibody administered, the greater was the accumulation of murine immunoglobulin that could be demonstrated immunohistochemically in biopsied material (23). Even after the infusion of 500 mg of antibody, however, complete saturation of antigenic sites was not achieved in all patients, consistent with limited access of antibody to tumor cells outside the vascular compartment. Intravenous administration of different antibodies against GD_2 ganglioside produced responses in only 2 of 42 patients with melanoma.

Contact of antibodies with tumor cells can be enhanced by direct intratumoral injection. Intratumoral injection of a human IgM monoclonal antibody reactive with the GD2 ganglioside produced partial and complete regression of injected cutaneous melanoma nodules in 4 of 8 patients (24) (Figs. 83.1 and 83.2). Tumor nodules that failed to respond to repeated injection had relatively lower levels of antigen than did nodules that regressed. A mononuclear infiltrate was observed at the sites of antibody injection.

Several clinical trials have utilized the 17-1A murine IgG2a antibody, which reacts with human gastrointestinal carcinomas (25–28). Responses have been reported in colorectal and pancreatic carcinoma, although evidence of tumor regression has often been equivocal and the role of antibody difficult to define. In one study, however, 6 of 22 patients (27%) experienced an objective response to prolonged treatment (27). Injection of 17-1A has evoked a human anti-murine immunoglobulin response and some of the patient's antibodies have had anti-idiotypic specificity. Development of anti-murine immunoglobulin antibodies has generally been regarded as an undesirable consequence of injecting a foreign protein because they shorten the circulating half-life of the monoclonal antibody. Anti-idiotypic antibodies can, however, bear the internal image of the antigen and stimulate endogenous immunity in recipients (29–35). Development of specific immunity may be one of the factors contributing to the outcome of a prospective concurrently controlled trial of 17-1A adjuvant therapy in patients with resected Duke's C colon cancer. Treatment with unconjugated 17-1A antibody decreased recurrence by 27% and increased 5-year survival by 30% (36).

Substantial effort has been expended on the development of human monoclonal antibodies that should be less immunogenic, but their titer, specificity, isotype, and affinity continue to limit the clinical utility of these reagents (37). Immunization of patients with autologous tumor cells and bacillus Calmette-Guérin has produced one method for expanding relevant human B cells prior to fusion (38). An alter-

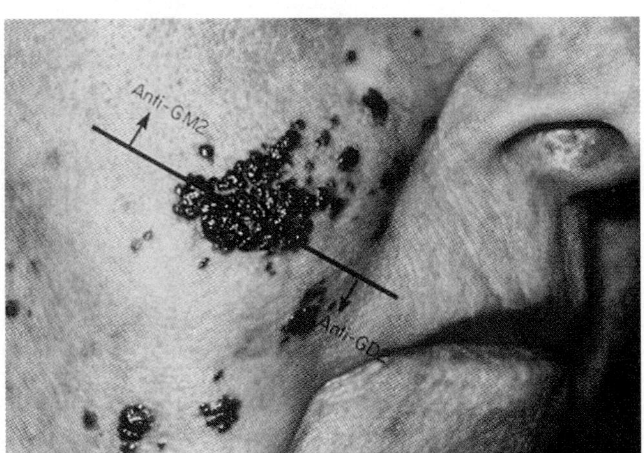

Figure 83.1. Recurrent melanoma, unresponsive to radiotherapy, prior to immunotherapy with intralesional injections of human monoclonal antibody to GM_2 or GD_2.

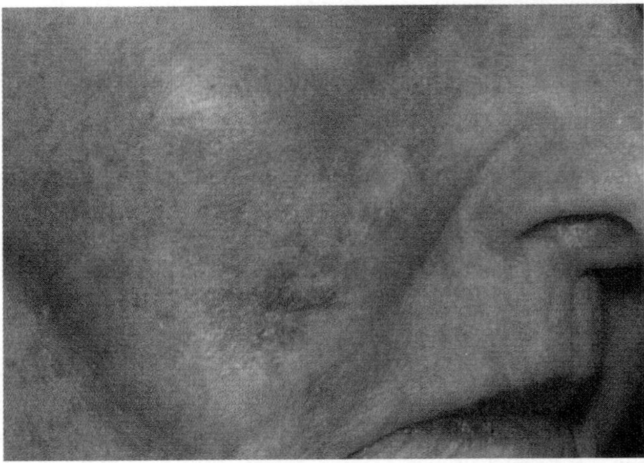

Figure 83.2. The same patient 2 1/2 years later following complete regression of all disease.

native approach involves the molecular engineering of murine and human immunoglobulin genes to produce chimeric antibodies with human constant and mouse variable domains (39–42). The hypervariable complementarity-determining region (CDR) of the human heavy chain can be replaced with the CDR of a murine monoclonal immunoglobulin (43). Although the immunogenicity of such antibodies can be substantially reduced, their injection can still evoke an anti-idiotypic response. Genetic engineering has also been utilized to produce single-chain antigen binding proteins that may have more favorable pharmacokinetic properties than intact immunoglobulin or Fab fragments (44).

To the extent that unmodified monoclonal antibodies inhibit tumor growth, several mechanisms may be important for antitumor activity, including direct growth inhibition, complement dependent lysis, and ADCC, in addition to possible intervention in the specific immunoregulatory network of the host. Antibodies that react with the epidermal growth factor receptor (EGFR) can inhibit the growth of tumor cells ex vivo in the absence of complement components or host effector cells (45–47). Antibodies that block EGF binding to EGFR affect growth more readily than do antibodies that bind to other sites on the receptor. Antibodies that react with the extracellular domain of the c-*erb*B-2 (HER-2/neu) proto-oncogene product also inhibit tumor cell growth in the absence of complement or cellular effectors (48, 49). Inhibition of ligand binding appears important for the inhibition of anchorage-dependent, but not anchorage-independent, growth (49). A phase II study of recombinant human anti-HER-2 monoclonal antibody produced objective responses in 12% of 46 patients with stage IV breast cancer (50). Recently, antibodies have been described that produce apoptosis (i.e., programmed cell death) in some lymphoid cell lines and activated T cells (51).

Murine antibodies of the IgM, IgG2a, and IgG3 isotypes can fix human complement, but often rather poorly. The rat monoclonal antibody CAMPATH 1 is an important exception to this generalization in that the antibody can mediate lysis of human cells that bear the appropriate antigen in the presence of human complement components (52). Murine antibodies of IgG3, IgG2a, and IgG2b have been reported to mediate ADCC in which large granular lymphocytes (LGL), monocytes, macrophages, or polymorphonuclear leukocytes are bound to tumor cells through Fc receptors after antibody has bound to specific antigenic determinants on the tumor cell surface. IgG3 appears to be particularly important for ADCC with LGL, whereas IgG2a may interact more effectively with human monocytes (53). In some instances, it has been possible to arm mononuclear leukocytes with antibody prior to interaction with tumor targets. In vivo, ADCC may be compromised in cancer patients due to a paucity of appropriate effector cells or to the presence of circulating immune complexes that occupy or downregulate Fc receptors. Antibodies that react against GD3 on melanoma cells can also bind to GD3 on the surface of T cells, enhancing their cytotoxic and proliferative responses (54). Hybrid antibodies have been generated with one binding site for T-cell–associated antigens and one binding site for tumor-associated antigens (55). Such hybrid antibodies enhance tumor cell killing by IL-2–activated T cells (56), possibly by encouraging contact between effector cells and tumor targets.

Whatever the mechanism of tumor killing, cells that lack the relevant antigen are likely to escape elimination. Substantial heterogeneity has been observed within and between neoplasms, particularly in the case of solid tumors. When the expression of 11 distinct antigen families was studied in a panel of breast carcinomas using biotin-avidin immunoperoxidase, 16 of 18 of the tumors exhibited a distinct phenotype (57). Similar heterogeneity was observed in epithelial ovarian carcinomas. Important to note, use of five antibodies in combination apparently can compensate for this heterogeneity.

ELIMINATION OF MALIGNANT CELLS FROM BONE MARROW EX VIVO

Autologous bone marrow transplantation is likely to be most effective in those instances where tumors respond dramatically to primarily myelotoxic chemoradiotherapy and for those patients whose marrow is free of clonogenic tumor cells or can be freed from tumor by treatment ex vivo. Murine monoclonal antibodies have proved useful for the selective elimination of tumor cells while sparing clonogenic precursors. In this setting, the clinician can avoid several of the usual obstacles to serotherapy in vivo. Shed antigen can be washed from the system. Marrow can be chilled, minimizing antigenic modulation. Rabbit complement can be utilized that interacts effectively with a wide range of murine antibodies. Alternatively, immunomagnetic beads may eliminate the need for complement altogether. Multiple monoclonal antibodies can be incubated with bone marrow ex vivo and immunization with foreign protein is generally not an issue. In model systems, up to 99.9% of clonogenic lymphoma cells can be eliminated from mixtures with normal human bone marrow using multiple murine monoclonal antibodies and rabbit complement (58) with or without 4-hydroperoxycyclophosphamide (4-HC) (59). Treatment with antibodies of appropriate specificity spares normal marrow precursors, although 4-HC destroys mature CFU-GM.

Phase I trials in patients with acute lymphoblastic leukemia (60–62), acute nonlymphocytic leukemia (63), and neuroblastoma (64) have confirmed that reconstitution can occur in vivo after purging of malignant cells using antibody and complement or using immunomagnetic separation mediated by magnetite-laden beads that are coated with an antimurine immunoglobulin. In two very similar trials, 25 to 30% of children with acute lymphoblastic leukemia who had failed conventional treatment enjoyed long-term disease-free survival after receiving myeloblative chemoradiotherapy and an infusion of autologous bone marrow that had been treated ex vivo in the presence of rabbit complement with murine monoclonal anti-CD9 and anti-CD10 with or without anti-CD24 (60, 62). Antibody and complement have also been used to purge marrow from lymphoma patients. Among 49 patients with relapsed non-Hodgkin's lymphoma, 34 remained disease-free a median of over 11 months (range more than 2 to more than 52 months) after receiving transplant doses of cyclophosphamide, total body irradiation (TBI), and autologous bone marrow that had been treated with anti-CD20 and rabbit complement (65). Recent studies have permitted the removal of neuroblastomas and breast cancer cells from human bone marrow using multiple monoclonal antibodies and immunomagnetic beads with or without cytotoxic drugs (66, 67).

Whether or not purging of marrow is necessary has been debated. Controlled trials have been difficult to perform. When residual lymphoma cells were detected by PCR techniques, the inability to eliminate tumor cells from marrow was the single most important prognostic indicator in predicting relapse after autologous transplantation (68). This outcome is consistent with the usefulness of ex vivo purging of marrow, at least in this setting. As many, if not all, of the pluripotent stem cells bear CD34 determinants, anti-CD34 antibodies have been used to select stem cells. Gene-marking studies have suggested that positive selection of $CD34^+$ cells does not completely eliminate precursors for CML cells in that genes introduced after separation ex vivo have been found in leukemic cells at relapse (69).

Improvement of autologous bone marrow transplantation depends critically on the effective removal of tumor cells from the patient, as well as from the bone marrow. More effective treatment of residual disease could result from the use of fractionated TBI, use of multiple alkylating agents, treatment of disease at an earlier stage, and use of adjunctive modalities, such as immunotherapy. To the extent that these techniques improve the control of tumor in vivo, complete elimination of tumor cells from harvested bone marrow to be reinfused will become more important. More effective purging of marrow has been achieved with several models using both immunoseparation and chemoseparation with such agents as 4-HC. Cells that evade immunoseparation are still susceptible to cytotoxic drugs. Chemoseparation appears to compensate, in part, for heterogeneity in antigenic phenotype.

THERAPY WITH DRUG–MONOCLONAL ANTIBODY CONJUGATES

Murine monoclonal antibodies have been coupled to a variety of conventional cytotoxic agents (70, 71), including antifoles, anthracyclines, vinca alkyloids, alkylating agents, and neocarzinostatin (72–85). Prepolymerization of some drugs, such as doxorubicin, prior to conjugation can achieve higher ratios of drug to antibody (86). Drugs can be bound to the amino side chains of lysine residues, provided that the most reactive residues are not found in the antibody binding site. Linkage of drugs to antibody through the carbohydrate moieties of the murine immunoglobulin has provided site-specific conjugation that generally does not impair antibody binding (87, 88).

One concern raised by some investigators is based on the observation that many cell surface antigens have fewer than 10^5 copies per cell. Release of 1 to 3 times 10^6 drug molecules at the cell surface might or might not be sufficient to eliminate tumor. Another concern relates to the ability of large immunoglobulin carrier complexes to translocate across tumor capillaries. In recent preclinical studies, however, drug–monoclonal antibody conjugates proved substantially more effective than the free drug. Only some of these conjugates are more potent, but many are less toxic, providing an improved therapeutic index. Therapeutic advantage may relate to different rates or patterns of drug uptake when linked with monoclonal reagents. In some instances, novel linkages have been devised that would release drug at low pH or only in the presence of lysosomal proteases. Not all drug–antibody conjugates, however, must enter cells to provide effective antitumor therapy in nude mouse heterograft models (89). One of the most promising immunoconjugates in preclinical studies, BR96-DOX, utilizes an anti-Le^Y antibody linked to multiple doxorubicin molecules with an acid labile bond (90, 91). In phase I studies, upper gastrointestinal toxicity was noted consistent with the known distribution of Le^Y determinants.

Other investigators have explored the use of drug-containing liposomes coated with monoclonal antibodies to deliver larger aliquots of drug (92, 93). Because of their size, liposomes are likely to lodge in normal liver, spleen, and lung after intravenous injection. Thus, antibody-coated liposomes may be more useful for intracavitary therapy.

Radiolabeled Monoclonal Antibodies

Monoclonal antibodies directed against human cancer–associated antigens also have been exploited as carrier molecules for the selective delivery of radionuclides to malignant cell populations. The feasibility of using antibodies to target radioactivity to tumors was demonstrated more than 40 years ago (94). Some years later, Spar and colleagues (95) reported that a variety of tumors could be visualized in patients by gamma-camera imaging following injection with ^{131}I-labeled polyclonal antibodies reactive with fibrinogen. Although these studies confirmed the conceptual appeal of using labeled antibodies for the diagnosis and treatment of cancer, methodological limitations in antibody production and characterization, as well as in nuclear imaging and labeling technology, inhibited progress in this area for more than a decade.

The development of hybridoma technology, in concert with advances in the field of nuclear medicine instrumentation, offered the prospect of utilizing monoclonal antibodies labeled with gamma-emitting radionuclides for the detection of tumor sites in a noninvasive fashion. Although radioimmunoscintigraphy may never have the impact on diagnostic oncology that was originally anticipated, labeled antibody imaging, particularly with tomographic methods, provides information that complements that obtained by more anatomically rigorous modalities, such as computed tomography (CT) and magnetic resonance imaging (MRI).

The most promising application of radioimmunoscintigraphy is as a prelude for a therapeutic study using the same antibody labeled with a more cytotoxic nuclide, such as a beta- or an alpha-emitter. Unlike conventional external beam radiotherapy, radioimmunotherapy offers the possibility of selectively targeting radiation to malignant cell populations while minimizing the destruction of neighboring normal cells that are antigen negative. Antibody imaging adds to the appeal of this approach since one can calculate tumor and normal tissue dosimetry, and thus determine whether an adequate therapeutic index would be achievable in each patient prior to initiation of therapy. The use of positron emission tomography (PET) is particularly attractive for this application because of the superior quantitative capabilities of this imaging modality.

Unrealistic expectations for the application of radiolabeled monoclonal antibodies in clinical oncology were generated by the results of multiple investigations in athymic rodent models that demonstrated high uptake ratios between human tumor xenograft and normal rodent tissues (96–98) and the ability to achieve tumor regression, and even cures, in these model systems (99, 100). Unfortunately, after intravenous injection of these and similar antibodies into patients, only $1–10 \times 10^{-3}$ percent of the injected dose can generally be found per gram tumor (101–106), levels that are at least 10,000 times lower than those observed in rodent models. Nonetheless, the successful imaging and treatment of a variety of cancers have been accomplished in patients despite the low degree of antibody accumulation in tumor.

In evaluating the potential impact of labeled antibodies in clinical oncology, it is important to consider the broad range of factors that can profoundly influence the ability to achieve selective targeting in vivo. Tumor hemodynamic characteristics, such as blood flow, permeability, and interstitial pressure, can act as impediments to homogeneous uptake of antibody in tumor (107, 108), as can the "binding-site barrier" (109). Other considerations are specific for a given antibody-antigen system, and include antibody specificity and affinity, the fraction of tumor cells that are antigen positive, the average number of antigen copies per cell, and the presence or absence of circulating antigen. The following sections focus on some of the factors that influence the effectiveness of radiolabeled antibodies, including type and quality of radiative emissions, as well as selection of the radionuclide, labeling approach, and imaging method.

RADIOIMMUNOSCINTIGRAPHY

Selection of the Radionuclide

Iodine 131 was the first radionuclide used for imaging with radiolabeled antibodies, and it remains in frequent use for this purpose. Its advantages include its low cost, the ready availability of protein radioiodination methodology, and the fact that its beta emissions allow its use for radioimmunotherapy. These beta emissions detract from its merit for diagnostic screening applications because they increase the radiation-absorbed dose received by the patient. In addition, the 364-keV gamma ray of ^{131}I is not ideal for either conventional planar imaging or single photon emission computed tomography (SPECT) because of low count rate per unit dose, high scatter background, and collimator penetration. These characteristics all contribute to the suboptimal spatial resolution in images obtained with this radionuclide. However, ^{131}I is particularly attractive when imaging is being used as a prelude to therapy, since the same radionuclide can be used for both applications, thus facilitating meaningful estimation of tumor and normal tissue radiation dosimetry (110).

From an imaging perspective, it would be ideal if the radionuclide decayed by the emission of gamma rays with an energy of between 120 and 200 keV and had a physical half-life compatible with the pharmacokinetics of antibody localization in tumor. This led to a considerable effort in both the academic and industrial sectors to develop monoclonal antibody imaging agents utilizing 2.8-day half-life ^{111}In as the radiolabel. Indeed, the first antibody-based radiopharmaceutical, Onco-scint, approved for use by the United States Food and Drug Administration is a ^{111}In-labeled anti-TAG72 antibody for imaging colorectal cancer (111).

Two radionuclides considered to have optimal physical properties for external imaging are 6-hour half-life ^{99m}Tc, which emits 140-keV gamma rays, and 13-hour half-life ^{123}I, which emits 159-keV gamma rays. Technetium-99m, the most frequently used radionuclide in nuclear medicine, is routinely available at low cost, while ^{123}I is considerably more expensive. On the other hand, the longer half-life of ^{123}I permits imaging at later times after injection, when contrast between tumor and surrounding normal tissues is generally more favorable.

The gamma rays emitted by ^{123}I and ^{99m}Tc are superior to those of ^{131}I and ^{111}In for both conventional gamma-camera imaging and SPECT, particularly for applications where rigorous quantitation of activity distributions is required. The tomographic nature of SPECT also is advantageous because it facilitates identification of tumor in the presence of background activity in overlying or underlying image planes. In addition, with the development of image registration techniques, the superior anatomic images obtainable with CT or MRI can be used in combination with SPECT antibody scans (112). In this way, functional and anatomic data can be used in tandem to better define both the location and nature of suspected abnormalities.

The idea of combining monoclonal antibodies with tomographic imaging techniques has led a number of laboratories to pursue the use of positron emission tomography (PET) to augment the clinical utility of radioimmunoscintigraphy. PET is the modality of choice for quantification of tracer distribution in vivo, and is generally considered to be the best method for physiologic and metabolic imaging. Improved capabilities in the quantification of antibody distribution in patients could be valuable for radioimmunotherapy, not only for patient selection, but also better to define normal-tissue maximum tolerated dose and tumor dose–response relationships. Selective tumor uptake in human tumor xenografts in athymic mice using antibodies radiolabeled with the positron-emitting nuclides ^{124}I (113) and ^{64}Cu (114) has been reported. Recently, PET imaging of both primary and metastatic osteosarcoma has been accomplished in dogs with spontaneous tumors using an ^{18}F-labeled monoclonal antibody Fab fragment (115).

Clinical Imaging Studies

Some of the first experiences in patients evaluating the potential utility of radioimmunoscintigraphy involved the use of affinity-purified, polyclonal goat antibodies reactive with carcinoembryonic antigen (CEA) labeled with ^{131}I. In one study, a lesion-detection rate of 91% was reported in patients with a variety of CEA-secreting tumors (116), whereas in another, a sensitivity of only 39% was observed (117). The dissimilarity of these results could have been related to differences in circulating CEA levels or other variables, such as tumor size and location, as well as the subjective nature of the blood pool background techniques that had been utilized. While they differ in terms of detection rate, both trials were critical in that they demonstrated the feasibility of imaging tumors with radiolabeled antibodies, resurrecting interest in this area.

A recent review article has estimated that nearly 200 clinical radioimmunodetection trials have been performed using radiolabeled antibodies (118). Most of these investigations have been carried out with murine monoclonal antibodies labeled with either ^{131}I or ^{111}In. A wide variety of patient populations have been studied, including those with melanoma (105, 119), neuroblastoma (120), glioma (121, 122), and lymphoma (123, 124), as well as ovarian (125), colorectal (126), and breast (127) carcinomas. These and similar studies reported a wide range of sensitivities and specificities, with overall lesion-detection rates of greater than 70% generally observed. With ^{111}In-labeled antibodies, high levels of accumulation of activity in normal liver and spleen complicate the detection of hepatic metastases. For example, in a recent multicenter study, only 53% of hepatic metastases were detected in patients with colorectal cancer imaged with ^{111}In-labeled C110 monoclonal antibody (126).

Efforts to improve the sensitivity and specificity of tumor detection have been directed at multiple facets of antibody imaging methodology. For example, combinations of antibodies reactive with distinct tumor-associated antigens have been explored as an approach to compensate for heterogeneities in antigen expression within a given type of cancer (128). With certain antibodies, particularly those cross-reactive with normal tissues, optimization of antibody protein dose has been a valuable strategy. This is illustrated by a study using ^{111}In-labeled anti-gp240 antibody that reported that increasing the protein dose from 5 to 20 mg increased the detection rate of metastatic melanomas from 23 to 87% (129). Lower-molecular-weight Fab and $F(ab')_2$ monoclonal antibody fragments, which clear more rapidly from the blood pool, have also been used to improve image contrast between tumor and surrounding normal tissues (102).

The fact that antibody fragments permit much more rapid achievement of reasonable tumor-to-normal-tissue uptake ratios has greatly facilitated the use of the radionuclides with optimal imaging characteristics, ^{123}I and ^{99m}Tc, despite their relatively short half-lives. In a retrospective study of patients with colorectal cancer, 82% and 89% of tumor sites could be detected using SPECT imaging with ^{123}I-labeled $F(ab')_2$ and Fab fragments of an anti-CEA antibody, respectively (130). A key aspect of this study, confirmed in a subsequent prospective investigation (131), is that tumor sites could be detected that either were not observed or were detected more than 1 month later by other imaging modalities.

Prospective trials with ^{123}I-labeled antibody fragments have been critical to the field of radioimmunoscintigraphy since they have demonstrated the potential role of this imaging method in the management of cancer patients. However, the cost and inconvenience of labeling antibodies with ^{123}I have impeded the widespread application of this methodology. With the development of straightforward, direct methods for labeling monoclonal antibodies with ^{99m}Tc via their sulfhydryl groups (132, 133), radioimmunoscintigraphy has become a practical imaging modality for use at nearly every hospital.

Clinical investigations using ^{99m}Tc-labeled antibodies, primarily in fragmented form, have been performed in a number of patient populations and the results generally have been promising. In a multicenter study evaluating ^{99m}Tc-labeled antibody fragments in melanoma patients, 70% of lesions were visualized, including 92 that were previously occult but later confirmed (134). Recently, a sensitivity of 94% and a specificity of 100% were observed in 15 patients with neck lymph node metastases from a squamous-cell carcinoma of the head and neck (135). In a preliminary study, imaging with ^{99m}Tc-labeled Fab fragments of LL2 antibody was found to be valuable in the staging of non-Hodgkin's B-cell lymphoma, resulting in an alteration of disease stage in 27% of patients (136).

Although direct ^{99m}Tc-labeling methods have made a major impact on the direction of clinical imaging trials of radiolabeled monoclonal antibodies, loss of ^{99m}Tc from the antibody in vivo (137) can be problematic, particularly when imaging is to be used as a prelude to radioimmunotherapy with either ^{188}Re or ^{186}Re. To circumvent this problem, several groups have developed indirect methods for labeling antibodies that involve reaction of the ^{99m}Tc with a chelator (138, 139). Although more complex, these labeling methods improve in vivo stability, and also avoid exposure of the antibody to reducing agents, which, in some cases, can compromise immunoreactivity.

RADIOIMMUNOTHERAPY

Selection of the Radionuclide

In developing radioimmunotherapeutic strategies, it is important to bear in mind that this type of therapy will probably be utilized as an adjuvant to less specific treatment modalities, such as chemotherapy and external beam radiation therapy. An advantage of antibody-mediated radiotherapy that is distinct from immunotoxins is the wide variation in toxicity and range of action that potentially can be achieved through the use of radionuclides decaying by the emission of radiation of differing qualities. Irradiation of volumes approximating subcellular, cellular, and multicellular dimensions could be accomplished using radionuclides emitting Auger electrons, alpha-particles and beta-particles, respectively. Thus, it should be possible to select a radionuclide with physical properties that are compatible with the treatment of a tumor with a particular size, location, and radiosensitivity.

With the exception of a single study using an internalizing antibody labeled with ^{125}I (140), clinical radioimmunotherapeutic trials have been performed with antibodies labeled

Table 83.1. Some Radionuclides of Potential Utility for Radioimmunotherapy

Radionuclide	Half-life	Emmission Tyee[a]	Decay Energy E_{max} (keV)[b]
^{131}I	8.1 d	β	336,**606**
^{90}Y	64.1 hr	β	2288
^{186}Re	90.6 hr	β	934,**1072**
^{188}Re	16.9 hr	β	1973
^{177}Lu	6.7 hr	β	175,384,**497**
^{67}Cu	61.9 hr	β	395,**484**,577
^{211}At	7.2 hr	α	5866,**7450**
^{212}Bi	1.0 hr	α	6051,**6090**
^{125}I	60.1 d	Auger	>5

[a] Type of emission relevant to therapeutic use; other emissions, primarily gamma rays, are often present.
[b] Principal emission in bold.

with beta-emitters, with ^{131}I being by far the most frequently used radionuclide. Since beta particles have a range in tissue of the order of 1 to 10 mm, they should be well suited for the treatment of larger tumors. The relatively long range of beta particles, particularly those of higher energy, such as those emitted by ^{90}Y (Table 83.1), facilitate the destruction of adjacent antigen-negative or poorly perfused tumor cells through radiative cross-fire. From a theoretic perspective, the ideal beta emitter for labeling an antibody would depend on the size of the tumor, with those of shorter range, such as ^{131}I and ^{67}Cu (Table 83.1), preferred for micrometastatic disease since they would deposit a greater fraction of their decay energy in the tumor (141).

For some applications of radiolabeled antibody therapy, such as the treatment of intracavitary disease, micrometastases, or tumors of the circulatory system, other types of radiation, such as alpha particles or low-energy electrons, might be preferable to beta-emitters (Table 83.1). Alpha-particles, such as those emitted by ^{211}. At have a range in tissue of only 55 to 80 μm and are radiation of high linear energy transfer (LET). As a result, their relative biologic effectiveness is much higher than that of beta-emitters; indeed, only 1 to 10 alpha-particle traversals per cell are required to achieve effective cell kill (142, 143). An additional advantage of high LET radiation for radioimmunotherapy is that cytotoxic effectiveness does not require the presence of oxygen, nor is it dependent on dose rate. When localized in the cell nucleus, low-energy electrons, such as those emitted by ^{125}I, act as high LET radiation and might be valuable for use with antibodies that are internalized into the tumor cell after binding to their antigenic targets (140).

Clinical Treatment Studies

The first extensive investigations in patients of the feasibility of radioimmunotherapy were performed using ^{131}I-labeled polyclonal anti-ferritin antibodies (144). Hepatoma patients received doses of up to 150 mCi of ^{131}I with only limited toxicity observed. In a multidose protocol using one to four doses of 20 to 30 mCi of ^{131}I-labeled antiferritin derived from different animal species, complete responses were observed in 7% and partial responses in 43% of patients with hepatoma (145).

The therapeutic efficacy of a variety of monoclonal antibodies labeled with ^{131}I has now been evaluated in several patient populations. Not surprisingly, the most encouraging results reported to date were observed in patients with relatively radiation-sensitive malignancies such as B-cell lymphoma (146, 110). A critical aspect of these trials was the use of imaging at different antibody protein doses in order to determine the best strategy for compensating for the reactivity of these antibodies with normal B-cell populations. In one study performed on nine patients receiving one or two doses of 34 to 66 mCi of ^{131}I-labeled anti-CD20 antibody, four complete responses (one patient remained in remission for 8 months) and two partial responses were seen (146). A second trial involved the use of considerably higher radiation doses (234 to 777 mCi of ^{131}I) followed by autologous marrow reinfusion (110). Of the 19 patients so treated, complete remissions were observed in 16, with 9 of those remaining in continuous complete remission for periods ranging from 3 to 53 months.

Radioimmunotherapy has also been performed in patients with melanoma and cutaneous T-cell lymphoma using ^{131}I-labeled antibodies; however, with considerably less effectiveness (147, 148). More recently, two phase II radioimmunotherapy trials of ^{131}I-labeled monoclonal antibodies in patients with colorectal cancer were reported. The first study utilized monoclonal antibody A33, which reacts with a high-molecular-weight glycoprotein that is rapidly internalized (149). A maximum tolerated dose of 75 mCi/m^2 and no major clinical responses were observed in a heavily pretreated population of patients with advanced colon cancer. In the second trial, 15 patients received 75 mCi/m^2 of ^{131}I-labeled CC49, an antibody reactive with the TAG72 antigen (150). Although tumor uptake could be demonstrated on gamma-camera images, only limited therapeutic efficacy was seen. Iodine 131–labeled CC49 has also been investigated for the treatment of prostate carcinoma (151). Again, no significant radiographic or objective responses were observed.

The lack of efficacy of ^{131}I-labeled antibodies in most patient populations can be attributed to multiple factors, including the physical properties of this radionuclide. This has led to the clinical investigation of antibodies labeled with other beta-emitters, most notably ^{90}Y. Advantages of this radionuclide include its higher beta-energy and longer retention on tumor as compared with antibodies radioiodinated using conventional methods. A disadvantage is the higher accumulation of ^{90}Y in normal tissues, an observation that contributes to the fact that at equitoxic doses of ^{90}Y and ^{131}I in animals, a considerably higher radiation dose could be delivered to tumor using ^{131}I (152, 153). Only limited data concerning clinical trials with ^{90}Y-labeled antibodies have been published. In patients with end-stage Hodgkin's disease given 20 to 50 mCi of ^{90}Y-labeled polyclonal anti-ferritin, a 62% response rate, with complete responses lasting 2 to 26 months, was reported; however, significant hematologic toxicities were observed (154). A preliminary study investigating the pharmacokinetics and toxicity of ^{90}Y-labeled HMFG1 given intraperitoneally to patients with ovarian cancer suggests that the appropriate dose for treatment will be

18.5 mCi/m^2, with bone marrow toxicity being the dose-limiting factor (155). Using ^{90}Y-labeled HMFG1, 21 patients with ovarian cancer were treated in an adjuvant setting. Relative to historic controls, survival was significantly prolonged (156). Concurrently, controlled trials are under way.

STRATEGIES FOR ENHANCING THE EFFICACY OF RADIOLABELED ANTIBODIES

Introduction

Most tumor biopsies obtained from patients injected intravenously with radiolabeled antibodies contain only about 0.005% of the injected dose per gram of tumor (102). This low level of uptake is probably the major cause for the limited efficacy of radioimmunotherapy that has been observed in most clinical trials. This has led to the investigation of a wide variety of strategies for increasing tumor dose, as well as tumor-to-normal-tissue radiation absorbed dose ratios. Among these approaches are improving radiolabeling chemistry, altering tumor hemodynamics, administering antibody by nonintravenous routes, and utilizing molecular constructs designed via recombinant DNA technology.

Radiolabeling Chemistry

The development of improved methods for labeling proteins by chelation with radiometals and radiohalogenation remains an active area of research. In both cases, the goal has been to increase retention of the radiolabel on the antibody after in vivo administration and to minimize accumulation of labeled catabolites in normal tissues. The principal problem encountered with ^{90}Y has been the rapid release of the radiometal from most chelates, resulting in unacceptable accumulation of activity in the bone (157). Recent studies in animal models have demonstrated that bone uptake can be reduced considerably through the use of macrocyclic ligands, such as DOTA to complex ^{90}Y to the antibody (158, 159).

When conventional protein radiohalogenation methods are used to label antibodies with ^{131}I, dehalogenation can decrease radioactivity levels in tumor and increase uptake in those tissues accumulating free iodide, such as the stomach and thyroid. By decreasing the structural similarity of the labeled site on the antibody to iodotyrosine, a compound recognized by multiple deiodinases, it has been possible to lower protein deiodination rates considerably. For example, radioiodination of an antibody using *N*-succinimidyl-3-[^{131}I]iodobenzoate has been demonstrated to decrease thyroid uptake by 100-fold, to increase tumor xenograft accumulation by more than a factor of 3, and to increase therapeutic efficacy significantly as compared with the same antibody labeled using a conventional method (101, 160).

Alteration of Tumor Hemodynamics

Heterogeneities in tumor blood flow and permeability and interstitial pressure can have a major impact on the homogeneity and level of accumulation of macromolecules in tumor (107). Manipulation of tumor hemodynamics has been attempted using external beam irradiation, hyperthermia, vasoactive substances, and biologic response modifiers.

Although some investigators have claimed that irradiation of tumor prior to the administration of radiolabeled antibodies enhanced tumor uptake (161, 162), more recent studies have reported that external beam irradiation did not significantly increase tumor accumulation (163, 164). Interpretation of these experiments is complicated by the fact that external beam irradiation can decrease tumor size, an effect that itself can increase antibody accumulation on a percent-per-gram basis.

The potential of local hyperthermia for increasing the uptake of radiolabeled antibodies and fragments in tumor xenograft models has also been investigated. Significant increase in tumor uptake with minimal alteration in normal tissue levels has been observed in several studies (165–167). Consensus with regard to the optimal temperature and duration for maximizing the effects of hyperthermia on tumor uptake has not been reached; however, dosimetric calculations suggest that hyperthermia might be best exploited with radionuclides of short half-lives (168).

Vasoactive compounds, such as norepinephrine, vasopressin, and histamine, have been used in an attempt to improve tumor uptake of antibody by increasing tumor blood flow, but with only limited success (169). A more fruitful approach has been to enhance tumor uptake through the use of antibodies coupled to vasoactive biologic response modifiers or other compounds. Administration of an antibody–IL-2 conjugate prior to the radiolabeled antibody resulted in a significantly higher tumor accumulation with little alteration in normal tissue levels (170). Other antibody conjugates, including those with IFN-γ, IL-1β, and TNF, exerted similar effects, but of a lower magnitude than seen with IL-2 (171).

Nonintravenous Routes

Another strategy for increasing the rate and magnitude of tumor uptake applicable to some types of malignancies is to administer the radiolabeled antibody by a nonintravenous route. Intraperitoneal administration has been shown to increase antibody uptake in peritoneal colorectal lesions (104) and ovarian carcinoma (125), and treatment of ovarian carcinoma via this route has also been investigated (172, 155).

Encouraging results have been reported for the treatment of tumors of the central nervous system by the nonintravenous administration of ^{131}I-labeled antibodies. Glioma patients with cystic lesions and surgically created resection cavities have been treated with single or multiple doses of radioiodinated antibody given intracystically (173–175). Prolonged retention of radioactivity in the injection site was observed, and significant objective and radiographic responses were seen in many patients.

Iodine 131–labeled monoclonal antibodies administered intrathecally also have been investigated for the treatment of neoplastic meningitis. Significant clinical responses have been observed in a number of patients with a variety of leptomeningeal tumors, including breast carcinoma, melanoma, lymphoma, and pineoblastoma (175–177). Because of their short range, alpha-emitters, such as ^{211}At, might be even better suited for the treatment of neoplastic meningitis than the beta-particles emitted by ^{131}I. This hypothesis is supported by a recent report demonstrating significant survival prolongation and, in some animals, cures, after the treatment of neoplastic meningitis in the rat using ^{211}At-labeled monoclonal antibody 81C6 (178).

Recombinant Antibody Constructs

The development of an immune response frequently occurs in immunocompetent patients who have received murine monoclonal antibodies (179). These human antimurine antibodies, commonly referred to as HAMA, can alter the pharmacokinetics of subsequent doses of radiolabeled antibodies through the formation of labeled immune complexes that are rapidly removed from the circulation before they can be delivered to tumor. One approach to circumventing this problem is to use recombinant DNA technology to generate human/mouse chimeric antibodies, which consist of a murine variable region linked to a human constant region.

Several chimeric antibodies have been radiolabeled and their properties evaluated in animal models and in patients. The pharmacokinetics of chimeric MOv18, an IgG_1, have been reported to be similar to those of its murine parent in ovarian cancer patients (180). In contrast, the blood clearance of the chimeric versions of B72.3 and 17-1A antibodies was prolonged as compared with that of their murine counterparts (181, 182). This behavior resulted in bone marrow suppression at therapeutic levels, a problem that could be significantly reduced by administering the antibody in multiple doses (183). The ability to utilize multidose treatment radioimmunotherapy protocols is one of the potential advantages of human/murine chimeric constructs that, it is hoped, will be confirmed in future clinical trials.

Another class of recombinant molecules that has emerged as candidates for radiolabeled approaches is that of single-chain Fv (sFv) fragments (184, 185). These sFv molecules consist of heavy-chain and light-chain variable-region amino-acid sequences linked together by a peptide designed to maintain the immunoreactivity of the intact antibody parent. Several sFv molecules and sFv dimers have been radiolabeled and evaluated as potential diagnostic and therapeutic agents.

The results of these studies suggest that, compared with intact antibodies and $F(ab')_2$ and Fab fragments, sFv molecules could offer several advantages for selectively delivering radionuclides to tumors. First, the washout kinetics of sFv from the blood and normal tissues is much faster than observed with intact IgG, $F(ab')_2$, or Fab fragments (186, 187). This offers the possibility of imaging at earlier times with radionuclides with shorter– half-lives, and for therapy, reducing the radiation absorbed dose received by normal tissues. Although sFv offer superior tumor-to-normal-tissue ratios, the absolute magnitude uptake of sFv in tumor is lower than that seen with intact IgG and large antibody fragments. This suggests that therapeutic applications of radiolabeled sFv will probably require multidose protocols.

Autoradiographic measurements have shown that penetration of sFv into tumor occurs much more rapidly than with intact antibodies and larger antibody fragments (188). This is important for radioimmunotherapeutic applications because it should increase the homogeneity of radiation dose deposition within the tumor. Recently, the construction of an sFv dimer that retained the specificity of its parent antibody, anti-c-*erb*B-2 741F8, was reported (189). Accumulation of the radioiodinated $(sFv)_2$ in tumor was higher than that of the monomer, suggesting that the dimer may offer advantages for therapeutic applications.

Immunotoxins

Immunotoxins or fusion toxins consist of monoclonal antibodies or other peptide ligands covalently attached to peptide toxins. The antibody or other polypeptide ligand targets the molecule to the tumor cell surface; the toxin moiety then enters the cell and induces apoptosis by inactivating protein synthesis. Extremely potent catalytic toxins that can kill cells with as few as one molecule per cell are found in plants, bacteria, and fungi. The atomic three-dimensional structures of a number of toxins used clinically and in the laboratory have been defined (190–193).

TOXIN STRUCTURE

Diphtheria toxin (DT) produced by *Corynebacterium diphtheriae* is a 58-kd protein with an *N*-terminal ADP-ribosylation catalytic domain (194), a furin-sensitive RVRR peptide within a disulfide loop (195) followed by a hydrophobic middle domain responsible for translocation of the ADP-ribosylation domain to the cytosol (196), and a C-terminal cell binding domain capable of binding cell-associated heparin-binding EGF (Fig. 83.3*A*) (197). The *N*-terminal first 10 amino acid residues of DT are also required for translocation of the catalytic domain to the cytosol (198). One or more pairs of apo-

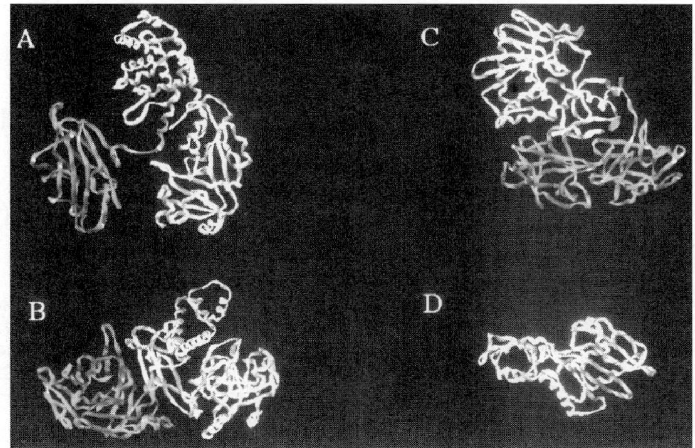

Figure 83.3. All molecules depicted are based on coordinates read from Protein Data Bank files. The PDB abbreviations are **A.** 1ddt-diphtheria toxin, **B.** 1dma-Pseudomonas exotoxin, **C.** 2aa1-ricin, **D.** 1paf-pokeweed. The MUSC BioMolecular Computing ResourceÕs SYBYL molecular modeling software was used to render the toxins as shaded ribbons derived from cubic spline fits to the C-alpha backbone.The translocation domains are yellow, the catalytic domains are white, and the lectin binding domains are red.

lar alpha helices in the transmembrane middle domain of DT are involved in membrane insertion and channel formation (199).

Pseudomonas exotoxin (PE), a product of *Pseudomonas aeruginosa*, is a 68-kd protein with an *N*-terminal domain that binds the alpha^2-macroglobulin receptor/low-density lipoproteinlike receptor protein (200), a furin-sensitive RQPR sequence (195), a transmembrane domain with amphipathic helices that participates in membrane translocation (201), a RDEL sequence recognized by the KDEL receptor, and a C-terminal lysine sensitive to intracellular carboxypeptidase (Fig. 83.3*B*) (202).

Ricin toxin from *Ricinus communis* plant seeds has two separate polypeptide chains linked by a disulfide bond (Fig. 83.3*C*). The B chain (RTB) is a 33-kd glycoprotein lectin that binds two or more galactose-terminated oligosaccharides on cell surfaces (203). The A chain (RTA) is a 32-kd glycoprotein possessing an active site cleft with RNA N-glycosidase activity (204), and a C-terminal membrane insertion signal, ILIPIIALMVY (205).

Pokeweed antiviral protein (PAP) and saporin (SAP) are type I ribosome-inactivating proteins isolated from the leaves and seeds of *Phytolacca americana* and *Saponaria officinalis*, respectively. The three-dimensional structures of these 28-kd proteins closely resemble RTA, and the proteins have similar enzymatic activity (Fig. 83.3*C*).

TOXIN PHYSIOLOGY

Intoxication of mammalian cell by peptide toxins requires a number of discrete steps mediated by different portions of the molecules (Fig. 83.4). The first step is cell surface binding. Diphtheria toxin binds a membrane form of heparin-binding EGF (197). Pseudomonas exotoxin-binds the alpha^2-macroglobulin/low density lipoprotein-like receptor protein (200). Ricin is a lectin with specificity for galactosyl pyranoside groups on cell surface glycoproteins and glycolipids (203). The plant hemitoxins or type I RIPs, PAP and SAP, lack cell-binding domains. The second step is internalization into endosomes (206). The third step is transfer to a compartment for membrane translocation. In the case of diphtheria toxin, the acidic environment of the endosomes triggers alterations in the structure of the translocation domain of DT (196). In the case of Pseudomonas exotoxin and ricin, toxins pass to the transreticular Golgi and then travel by retrograde pathways to the endoplasmic reticulum (207). The fourth step is membrane translocation. The enzymatic domain of DT passes through channels created by the transmembrane domain (208). In the case of ricin and Pseudomonas exotoxin, the enzymatic domains may use the translocon to reach the cytosol (209). The third and fourth steps taken by type I RIPs are unknown. The final step is inactivation of protein synthesis. Diphtheria toxin and Pseudomonas exotoxin ADP-ribosylate EF-2 at its diphthamide residue prevent ribosome binding (194). Ricin and the type I RIPs remove an adenine base from a conserved rRNA loop, irreversibly modifying the EF-2 binding site (210).

TOXIN MODIFICATION

For synthesis of immunotoxins or fusion toxins, the normal cell binding site(s) of the toxin must be removed and replaced with a tumor-selective ligand (Fig. 83.5). The C-terminal amino-acid residues 386 to 535 of diphtheria toxin

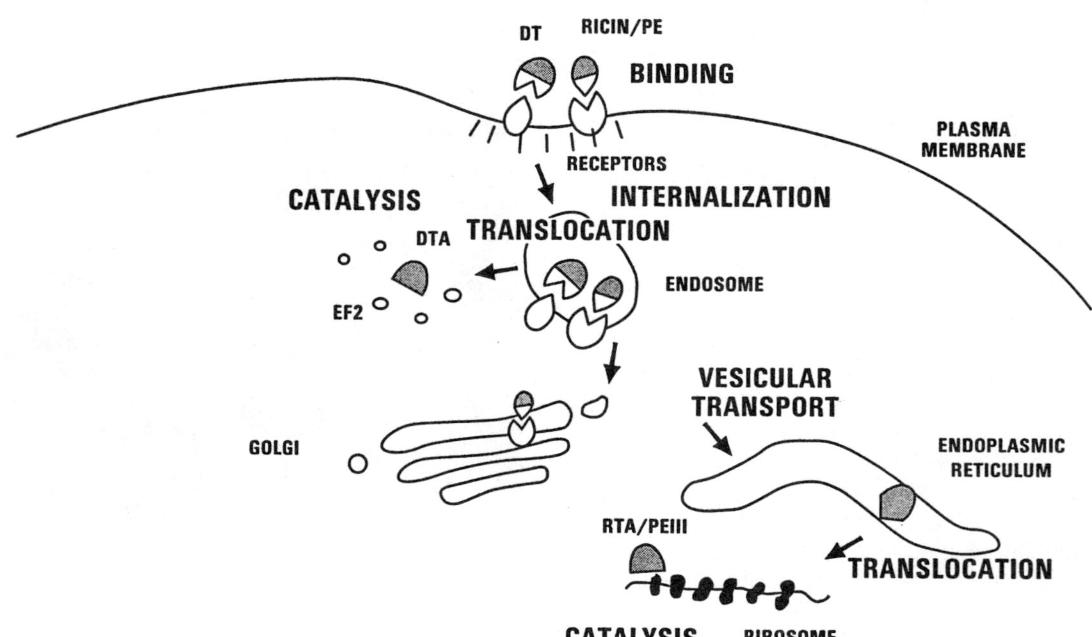

Figure 83.4. Mechanism of cell intoxication by toxins. Toxins bind to cell surface receptors; the complex internalizes to endosomes; the toxin reaches a translocation-competent compartment (endosomes for diphtheria toxin and endoplasmic reticulum for PE and ricin); the catalytic domain of the toxin crosses the membrane to the cytosol; cytosolic toxin inactivates protein synthesis.

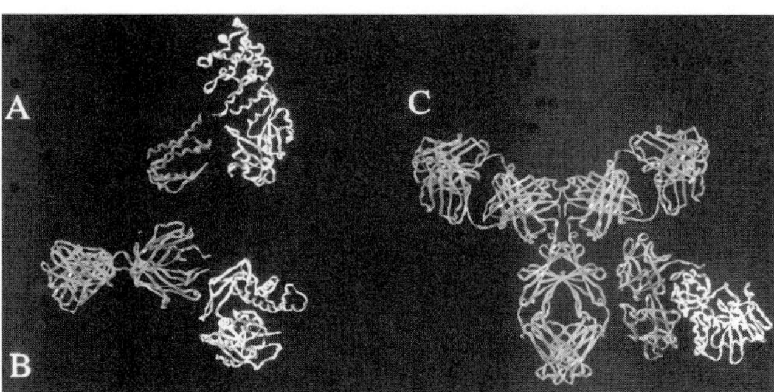

Figure 83.5. All molecules depicted are based on coordinates read from Protein Data Bank files. The PDB abbreviations are **A.** 1ddt-diphtheria toxin and 3ink-interleukein 2, **B.** 2ig2-FAB and 1dma-Pseudomonas exotoxin, **C.** 2ig2 and 1fc2-immunoglobulin and 2aa1-ricin. The MUSC BioMolecular Computing ResourceÕs SYBYL molecular modeling software was used to modify and arrange the molecules in their respective positions to clearly represent the fusion proteins. The models are rendered as shaded ribbons derived from cubic spline fits to the C-alpha backbone. The targeting subunits are green. The translocation domains are yellow and the catalytic domains are white. The lectin binding domain is red. This figure and Figure 83.3 were prepared by Dr. Starr Hazard.

containing the normal cell binding site were replaced by genetic engineering with the amino-acid sequence for IL-2 or EGF (211, 212). Domain Ia of Pseudomonas exotoxin (amino acids 1 to 252), containing its normal cell binding domain was deleted again by genetic engineering and replaced with TGF-α or a single-chain Fv reactive with Lewis^y antigen (213, 214). The cell binding sites in ricin have been removed in one of three ways. Ricin was reduced and RTB discarded. RTA was then coupled through its available thiol group to thiolated monoclonal antibodies reactive with CD5, CD7, CD19, CD22, CD25, proteoglycan, or gp72 (215–221). RTA was expressed alone in bacteria and the recombinant RTA coupled through its thiol group to thiolated monoclonal antibodies to gp55 and transferrin receptor (222, 223). Alternatively, the lectin binding sites of ricin were blocked with oligosaccharides containing a reactive dichlorotriazine group. The blocking reagent also provided a maleimide group for coupling to thiolated monoclonal antibodies to CD19, CD56, and CD33 (224–226). PAP and SAP, which lack normal tissue binding sites, were thiolated and coupled to thiolated or partially reduced anti-CD19 and anti-CD30 monoclonal antibodies (227–229).

Initial efforts were focused on identifying tumor-selective antigens for targeting. Differentiation antigens on melanoma cells (220), colorectal carcinoma cells (221), ovarian carcinoma cells (230), breast carcinoma cells (222, 223), acute myelogenous leukemia (226), small-cell lung cancer (225), and B and T leukemias and lymphomas (215–219) were identified and mouse monoclonal antibodies prepared reactive with epitopes on these antigens. In no case were the target antigens tumor specific, but different antigen densities or cell surface distribution afforded the hope for a useful therapeutic index. After conjugation to toxins, only a subset of immunotoxins exhibited tumor cell cytotoxicity (231). Subsequent work showed that cell intoxication required internalization of the toxin conjugate–antigen complex (232). A number of immunotoxins showing selective in vitro tumor cell killing at nanomolar–picomolar concentrations were selected for development.

CLINICAL TRIALS

Based on the extreme potency of these hybrid proteins (approximately 1 million times more active than current cytotoxic drugs), 10 clinical trials were conducted with these molecules between 1985 and 1990. The small number of the protocols was attributable to complexities in the manufacture and safety assurance of these drugs.

Patients with advanced refractory neoplasms were treated with a short course of daily systemic infusions of immunotoxins (Table 83.2). Twenty-two patients with melanoma received antiproteoglycan-RTA conjugate (220); 16 patients with metastatic colon carcinoma received anti-gp72-RTA conjugate (221); 18 patients with chronic lymphocytic leukemia (215, 233) and 14 patients with cutaneous T-cell lymphoma (CTCL) (234) received anti-CD5-RTA. Four patients with adult T-cell leukemia were given one to two doses of anti-CD25-PE (235), and 9 patients with refractory metastatic breast carcinoma were given anti-gp55-recombinant RTA (222, 236). Three clinical trials were conducted using intracavitary treatment to expose local tumor deposits to high concentrations of immunotoxins (Table 83.1). Twenty-three patients with refractory stage III ovarian cancer received several intraperitoneal infusions of anti-adenocarcinoma antigen–Pseudomonas exotoxin conjugate (230). Twenty patients with metastatic adenocarcinoma on the peritoneal wall were given intraperitoneal infusions of anti-transferrin receptor antibody coupled to recombinant RTA (223). The same anti-transferrin receptor–recombinant RTA conjugate was given intrathecally to 8 patients with leptomeningeal neoplasms (237).

In each of these studies, the large size of the molecules (around 200 kd) led to high intravascular drug concentrations but low concentrations in the tumor interstitia. Consequently, toxicities to accessible normal tissues (vascular endothelium, platelets, liver) were high and rapid humoral immune responses were evoked, but efficacy was poor. Even the intracavitary treatments were ineffective, as most of the malignancy was deeply embedded in the peritoneal wall, inaccessible to drug. In several cases, the antibody reacted with neural tissue antigens and produced serious, and sometimes fatal, nervous system toxicities.

A series of second-generation clinical studies was initiated between 1990 and 1995 with improved immunotoxins in settings more likely to produce clinical efficacy. Ten systemic trials and two regional/cavitary treatment trials were performed (Table 83.2). Anti-CD22 antibody (intact or Fab) conjugated to deglycosylated RTA was used to treat 25 and 16 patients, respectively, with refractory B-cell non-Hodgkin's lymphoma (NHL) (218, 238). Anti-CD19 antibody conjugated to blocked ricin was given either by bolus or continuous infusion to 25 and 34 patients, respectively, with non-Hodgkin's lymphoma (213, 247). Anti-CD19-PAP was given to 30 patients with B-ALL (227). Anti-CD30-SAP was administered as one or two infusions lasting 3 hours to 12 patients

Table 83.2. Systemic Immunotoxin Trials[a]

Conjugate	Disease	Specific toxicity	Response rate	Reference
Anti-proteog-RTA	Melanoma	VLS	1/22	220
Anti-gp72-RTA	Colorectal cancer	VLS	2/16	221
Anti-CD5-RTA	CLL	VLS	2/18	215,223
Anti-CD5-RTA	CTCL	VLS	4/14	234
Anti-CD25-PE	ATL	Hepatic	0/4	235
Anti-gp55-rRTA	Breast cancer	Schwann, VLS	1/9	222,236
Anti-ov.ant.-PE	Ovarian carcinoma	CNS	0/23	230
Anti-TfR-rRTA	Adenocarcinoma	CNS	0/20	223
Anti-TfR-rRTA	Leptomeningeal cancer	Arachnoid	0/8	237
Anti-CD22-dgRTA	NHL	VLS	5/24	218
Anti-CD22-dgRTA	HIV-NHL	VLS	3/6	217
Anti-CD22Fab-dgRTA	NHL	VLS	4/16	238
Anti-CD19-bR	NHL	Hepatic	8/59	224,239
Anti-CD30-SAP	Hodgkin's disease	VLS	5/12	229
DAB_{486}IL2	CD25+malignancy	None	5/40	211,240
DAB_{389}IL2	CTCL	None	12/34	241
DAB_{389}IL2	NHL	None	3/17	241
DAB_{389}IL2	Hodgkin's disease	None	0/21	241
Anti-CD19-PAP	B-ALL	VLS	9/19	227
LMB1	Carcinomas	VLS	0/30	242
Anti-CD56-bR	SCLC	VLS	1/21	225
Tf-CRM107	Brain	None	8/15	243
TP40	Bladder	None	8/43	213

[a] Response rate is (CR + PR)/total. VLS = vascular leak syndrome; RTA = ricin toxin A chain; PE = Pseudomonas exotoxin; rRTA = recombinant ricin toxin A chain; dgRTA = deglycosylated ricin toxin A chain; bR = blocked ricin; Leptomen. cancer = leptomeningeal neoplasms; SAP = saporin; PAP = pokeweed antiviral protein; Tf = human transferrin; CRM107 = mutant DT with binding site inactive; TP40 = TGF-α fused to a 40-kd fragment of PE; LMB1 = anti-Lewis y conjugated to a 38-kd fragment of PE with a single Lys at the N-terminus for derivatization; SCLC = small cell lung cancer; CD25+ malig. = hematopoietic malignancies with IL-2 receptor, including chronic lymphocytic leukemia, cutaneous T-cell lymphoma, non-Hodgkin's lymphoma, and Hodgkin's disease; B-ALL = B-cell acute lymphoblastic leukemia; CTCL = cutaneous T-cell lymphoma; NHL = non-Hodgkin's lymphoma; TfR = transferrin receptor.

with refractory Hodgkin's disease (229). IL-2 was fused to fragments of diphtheria toxin (DAB_{486}IL-2 and DAB_{389}IL-2) and used to treat 40 and 73 patients, respectively, with IL-2 receptor positive hematopoietic malignancies (211, 240, 241). Antibody to Lewis^y antigen coupled to a 38-Kd fragment of PE (LMB-1) was used to treat 32 patients with Lewis^y antigen positive metastatic carcinomas (242). Anti-CD56-blocked ricin was administered by a 7-day continuous infusion to 30 patients with small-cell lung carcinoma (225). Two regional/cavitary protocols were used to treat patients with bladder carcinoma and brain tumors (Table 83.1). TGF-α growth factor peptide was fused to a 40-Kd fragment of PE (TP40) and repeatedly instilled into the bladder of 43 patients with refractory superficial bladder carcinoma (213). Human transferrin coupled to a binding defective mutant of diphtheria toxin, CRM107, was inoculated into the lesions of 15 patients with refractory brain tumors (243).

Most of these clinical experiments were phase I and had interpatient dose escalation. Thus, the observed 20 to 40% partial and complete response rates were encouraging. The improved therapeutic indices were attributed to better access of immunotoxin and fusion toxin to leukemia/lymphoma cells and bladder/brain tumor cells in vivo and higher-potency reagents. However, few of the clinical responses were durable.

In 1995, a number of third-generation phase II studies were initiated to find the optimal setting for immunotoxin/fusion toxin therapy (Table 83.3). Based on observations from the second-generation studies of higher response rates in

Table 83.3. Ongoing Immunotoxin Trials[a]

Conjugate	Disease	Setting	Reference
Antii-CD19-bR	NHL	Post-autoBMT	54
Anti-CD19-bR	HIV-NHL	With chemo	55
Anti-CD56-bR	SCLC	With chemo	36
DAB_{389}IL-2	CTCL	Stages I and II	50
DAB_{389}IL-2	Psoriasis	Refractory	56
Anti-CD19-PAP	B-ALL, NHL	With chemo	38
Tf-CRM107	Brain tumors	Few lesions	53
Anti-CD7-dgRTA	T-ALL	Refractory	27
Anti-CD25-dgRTA	Hodgkin's	Refractory	30
Anti-CD19-SAP	B-ALL	Refractory	39
αCD19&22-dgRTA	NHL	Refractory	28
DAB_{389}EGF	Carcinomas	Refractory	23
LMB-7	Carcinomas	Refractory	25

[a] Abbreviations as in Table 83.2. and HIV-NHL = HIV-positive patients with NHL; T-ALL = T-cell acute lymphoblastic leukemia; DAB_{389}EGF = EGF fused to 389 amino acid fragment of DT; LMB-7 = Anti-Lewis^{y}Fv-PE38KDEL. AutoBMT = autologous bone marrow transplantation; chemo = combination chemotherapy; αCD19&22-dgRTA = cocktail of both immunotoxins.

patients with minimal disease and in vitro synergy of immunotoxins and chemotherapy, the latest immunotoxin trials treat patients earlier in their natural history. Anti-CD19–blocked ricin is given immediately post autologous bone marrow transplantation to patients with refractory B-cell NHL (244). The same drug is given concurrently with combination chemotherapy in HIV-positive patients with NHL (245). Anti-CD56–blocked ricin is being administered by 7-day continuous infusion immediately after induction chemotherapy in patients with limited small-cell lung carcinoma (225). IL-2 fused to a 389-amino-acid fragment of DT (DAB_{389}IL-2) is being administered to patients with stage I or II CTCL and psoriasis (241, 246). Anti-CD19-PAP is infused intravenously concurrently with chemotherapy in patients with B-cell ALL and NHL (227). Transferrin-CRM107 will be given intratumorally to a large number of patients with early recurrence of brain tumors (243). Dose-escalation studies of anti-CD7-deglycosylated RTA for refractory T-cell ALL (216); anti-CD25-deglycosylated RTA for refractory Hodgkin's disease (219); anti-CD19-SAP for B-cell ALL (228); a cocktail of anti-CD22-deglycosylated RTA and anti-CD19-deglycosylated RTA as an 8-day continous infusion in patients with B-cell NHL (217); EGF fused to the 389-amino-acid fragment of DT (DAB_{389}EGF) for patients with metastatic carcinomas (212); and single-chain Fv anti-Lewis^{y} fused to a 38-kd PE fragment with C-terminal KDEL (LMB-7) for patients with metastatic adenocarcinomas (214) are continuing. In each study, smaller, more potent immunotoxins with better pharmacodynamics are being administered in settings with either minimal tumor burden or concurrent cytotoxic chemotherapy.

TOXICITIES

Vascular leak syndrome (VLS) has been the major dose-limiting toxicity during treatment of cancer with antibody-RTA conjugates (218), antibody-blocked ricin conjugates (225), and an antibody-PE conjugate (242). VLS is characterized by weight gain, increased vascular permeability, hypoalbuminemia, myalgias, and, in some cases, aphasias and pulmonary edema. The degree of toxicity has been correlated with peak serum concentrations of immunotoxin, but not with levels of cytokines or nitrates (217). In vitro human endothelial cell cultures were intoxicated by concentrations of RTA and PE fragment (PE38) achieved after systemic administration (247, 248). Endothelial cell apoptosis and increased monolayer permeability have been observed. Endothelial cells may be uniquely sensitive due to exposure to high concentrations of toxin in the bloodstream, alveoli, low bcl-2 expression, and high levels of KDEL receptor in the Golgi. Prolonged exposure enhances cytotoxicity. Thus, use of smaller fusion toxins with shorter circulating half-lives may avoid VLS. In support of this hypothesis, no VLS has been seen with diphtheria fusion toxins, which have short circulating half-lives in vivo. These molecules are able, however, to damage human endothelial cells in vitro. While no animal model reproduces human VLS, a syndrome of hydrothorax, hypoalbuminemia, hemoconcentration, and neutrophilia developed in rats after intravenous injection of anti-Lewis^{y} Fv-PE40 (249). Interestingly, the syndrome was prevented by prophylaxis with steroids or nonsteroidal anti-inflammatory drugs (NSAIDs) (250). No molecular mechanism was demonstrated. Nevertheless, small molecular weight endothelial cell protectants may be feasible in the future, although no such agent has been shown to be protective either for endothelial cell cultures or for patients in immunotoxin clinical trials.

PHARMACOLOGY

The poor tumor localization and significant immunogenicity of immunotoxins and fusion toxins limit their clinical utility. While an initial study with antimelanoma immunotoxin showed some conjugate localized to skin tumor nodules (220), no extravascular immunotoxin was found after systemic administration of anti-CD5-RTA and anti-gp55-recombinant RTA in patients with chronic lymphocytic leukemia and breast carcinoma, respectively (215, 222). No clinical protocol has been reported that comprehensively correlated percent of extravascular tumor cell saturation with dose of immunotoxin. The assumption has been that toxicities, including VLS, hepatotoxicity, or neurotoxicities, prevented sufficient doses to saturate extravascular tumor sites. In vitro studies with multicellular tumor spheroids and mathematic models using data from other proteins suggest that smaller-sized fusion toxin and permeability enhancers—such as cisplatinum or hyaluronidase—may improve tumor uptake (251, 252). Clinical responses with immunotoxins in lymphomas and leukemias may be due in part to a significant fraction of circulating malignant stem cells in these diseases. One approach to overcoming the capillary barrier is to direct toxins to tumor endothelium. Antitumor vascular immunotoxins have shown dramatic activity in animal models, but immunotoxins to human tumor endothelial antigens are only beginning to be synthesized (261).

Immunotoxins and fusion toxins generated humoral immune responses in all patients, except those with chronic lymphocytic leukemia. Although antitoxin may not block the killing of circulating tumor cells, the immune complexes likely inhibit extravascular tumor uptake and limit effective treatment periods for nonhematologic malignancies. Immunodominant neutralizing epitopes have been identified for both PE (253) and ricin (254) and may serve as targets for genetic engineering. 15-Deoxyspergualin and CTLA4Ig given systemically reduce humoral immune responses to foreign proteins in animals and patients, and may permit repeated treatment schedules with immunotoxins and fusion toxins (255, 256). Finally, the use of human ribonucleases as the toxophore may be an additional method for reducing conjugate immunogenicity (257).

EFFICACY

The first-generation studies of immunotoxin produced few responses. There were no complete responses in 102 patients with metastatic melanoma treated with antiproteoglycan-RTA (220, 258, 239), 16 patients with metastatic colorectal carcinoma treated with anti-gp72-RTA (221), 18 patients with CLL receiving anti-CD5-RTA (215, 233), 14 patients with CTCL given anti-CD5-RTA (234), 4 adult T-cell leukemia patients treated with anti-CD25-PE (235), 9 metastatic breast cancer patients given anti-gp55-recombinant RTA (222, 236), 23 ovarian cancer patients who received intraperitoneal antiovarian cancer antigen-PE (230), 20 patients with metastatic intraperitoneal adenocarcinoma given intraperitoneal antitransferrin receptor–recombinant RTA (223), nor 8 patients with leptomeningeal cancer given intrathecal antitransferrin receptor–recombinant RTA (237).

The pharmacologic problems described above lowered the therapeutic index. Further, whenever tested, fresh tumor cells appeared less sensitive than established tumor cell lines to toxin conjugates (215, 258).

In the second-generation protocols, response rates approached 40%, with most of these partial responses and a few complete responses. Anti-CD22-deglycosylated RTA yielded 5 of 24 partial responses and anti-CD22 Fab-deglycosylated RTA produced 4 of 16 partial responses in evaluable patients with refractory B-cell NHL (218, 238). When using anti-CD22-deglycosylated RTA in HIV-positive patients with NHL, there were 3 complete responses among 6 evaluable patients (217). Anti-CD19–blocked ricin given as a bolus daily infusion to 25 patients with B-cell NHL produced 1 complete response lasting 21 months and 2 partial responses (224). The same drug continuously infused over 7 days in 34 B-cell NHL patients produced 2 complete responses lasting 16 and 33 months and 3 partial responses lasting 1 to 3 months (239). Anti-CD30-SAP produced partial remissions lasting 2 to 4 months in 5 of 12 patients with advanced refractory Hodgkin's disease (229). DAB_{486}IL-2 was given by bolus infusion in several schedules to 40 patients with CD25-positive lymphoid malignancies, and there were 1 complete response and 4 partial responses (211, 240). After modification of the drug, DAB_{389}IL-2 was given to 73 patients with CD25 expressing lymphomas (17 NHL, 21 Hodgkin's disease, and 34 CTCL) (229). There were 5 complete responses and 7 partial responses in the 34 patients with CTCL. There were 1 complete response lasting 19 months and 2 partial responses of 2 and 9 months' duration in 17 patients with B-cell NHL, and no responses in 21 patients with Hodgkin's disease. Anti-CD19-PAP yielded 6 complete responses and 3 partial responses among 19 evaluable patients with B-cell ALL (227). Two phase I studies in solid tumor malignancies were less successful. LMB1 produced no responses in 30 patients with refractory Lewis^y positive solid tumors (242). Anti-CD56–blocked ricin given to 21 small cell lung cancer patients led to 1 partial response (225). Regional/cavitary therapy appears active only in the former case. In 15 patients with refractory brain tumors treated with local instillation of transferrin-CRM107, there were 8 partial responses (243). In contrast, intravesical instillation of TP40 yielded no responses in 11 patients with visible Ta or T1 superficial bladder carcinomas and partial responses in 8 of 9 patients with carcinoma in situ (213). While conclusions about efficacy are premature from phase I dose-escalation studies, the observations suggest the best disease targets are leukemia and lymphomas for systemic therapy, and regional therapy rather than cavitary treatment for local disease. Closer analysis of the subset of patients showing responses revealed that these individuals had lower tumor burden than did nonresponders.

These results fit with the Schipper model of fractional or log cell kill by targeted toxins similar in nature to cytotoxic chemoradiotherapy (259). Since toxins kill cells by a mechanism independent of that of chemoradiotherapy and have different toxicity profiles, the logical extension of these studies is to combine standard chemoradiotherapy with targeted toxins. Cytoreduction by 5 to 6 logs may lead to prolonged remissisons even if residual clonogenic tumor cells are present in vivo (260). The third-generation phase II studies are too immature to permit us to draw conclusions. However, preliminary results are striking. Twelve patients with B-cell NHL were treated with both anti-CD19–blocked ricin and autologous bone marrow transplantation. Eleven of 12 patients remain in complete remission 2 years posttransplant (244). Six of 8 patients with stage I or II CTCL have shown complete responses to DAB_{389}IL-2 (241).

A role for systemic immunotoxins and fusion toxins in the treatment of minimal residual disease leukemias and lymphomas is being established. Similarly, small-volume residual brain tumors are palliated in most cases by locally infused toxin conjugates. New advances in genetic engineering of fusion toxins should lead to improvements in clinical activity in solid tumors. Correlations of three-dimensional molecular structures for toxins and ligands with in vivo pharmacodynamics, immunogenicity, and cell cytotoxicity should further aid in drug design over the next decade.

References

1. Kohler G, Milstein C. Continuous cultures of fused cells secreting antibody of predefined specificity. Nature 1975;256:495.
2. Badger CC, Anasetti C, Davis J, Bernstein ID. Treatment of malignancy with unmodified antibody. Pathol Immunopathol Res 1987;6:419.
3. Waldmann TA. Monoclonal antibodies in diagnosis and therapy. Science 1991;252: 1657.
4. Dillman RO. Monoclonal antibodies for treating cancer. Ann Intern Med 1989;111: 592.
5. Dillman RO. Human antimouse and antiglobulin responses to monoclonal antibodies. Antibody Immunocon Radiopharm 1990;3:1.
6. Foon KA. Biological response modifiers: the new immunotherapy. Cancer Res 1989;49:1621.
7. Goldenberg DM. Challenges to the therapy of cancer with monoclonal antibodies. JNCI 1991;83:78.
8. Harris DT, Mastrangelo MJ. Serotherapy of cancer. Semin Oncol 1989;16:180.
9. Miller RA, Maloney DG, Warnke R, Levy R. Treatment of B-cell lymphoma with monoclonal anti-idiotype antibody. N Engl J Med 1982;306:517.
10. Levy R, Miller RA. Therapy of lymphoma directed at idiotypes. NCI Monogr 1990;10: 61.
11. Raffeld M, Neckers L, Longo DL, Cossman J. Spontaneous alteration of idiotype in a monoclonal B-cell lymphoma. Escape from detection by anti-idiotype. N Engl J Med 1985;312:1653.
12. Maloney DG, Bodkin D, Grillo-Lopez AJ, White C, Foon K, Schilder R, Neidhart J, Janakiraman N, Waldichuk C, Varns C, Royston I, Levy R. IDEC-C2B8 Final report on a phase II trial in relapsed non-Hodgkin's lymphoma. Blood 1994;(10 suppl 1):1692.
13. Ritz J, Pesando JM, Notis-McConarty J, Clavell LA, Sallan SE, Schlossman SF. Use of monoclonal antibodies as diagnostic and therapeutic reagents in acute lymphoblastic leukemia. Cancer Res 1981;41:4771.
14. Dillman RO, Shawler DL, Dillman JB, Royston I. Therapy of chronic lymphocytic leukemia and cutaneous T-cell lymphoma with T101 monoclonal antibody. J Clin Oncol 1984;2:881.
15. Nadler LM, Stashenko P, Hardy R, Kaplan WD, Button LN, Kufe DW, Antman KH, Schlossman SF. Serotherapy of a patient with a monoclonal antibody directed against a human lymphoma-associated antigen. Cancer Res 1980;40:3147.
16. Houghton AN, Chapman PB. Melanoma. In Biologic Therapy of Cancer. Edited by VT DeVita, S Hellman, SA Rosenberg. Philadelphia: Lippincott, 1995, p 576.
17. Cheresh DA, Honsik CJ, Staffileno LK, Jung G, Reisfeld RA. Disialoganglioside GD3 on human melanoma serves as a relevant target antigen for monoclonal antibody-mediated tumor cytolysis. Proc Natl Acad Sci USA 1985;82:5155.
18. Bajorin DF, Chapman PB, Dimaggio J, et al. Phase I evaluation of a combination of monoclonal antibody R24 and interleukin 2 in patients with metastatic melanoma. Cancer Res 1990;50:7490.
19. Creekmore S, Urba W, Koop W, et al. Phase IB/II trial of R24 antibody and interleukin-2 (IL2) in melanoma. Proc Am Soc Clin Oncol 1992;186:345.
20. Minasian LM, Szatrowski TP, Rosenblum M, et al. Hemorrhagic tumor necrosis during a pilot trial of tumor necrosis factor-α and anti-GD3 ganglioside monoclonal antibody in patients with metastatic melanoma. Blood 1993;83:56.
21. Jain RK. Transport of molecules in the tumor interstitium: a review. Cancer Res 1987;47:3039.
22. Jain RK. Physiological barriers to delivery of monoclonal antibodies and other macromolecules in tumors. Cancer Res 1990;50:814.
23. Schroff RW, Woodhouse CS, Foon KA, Oldham RK, Farrell MM, Klein RA, Morgan AC Jr. Intratumor localization of monoclonal antibody in patients with melanoma treated with antibody to a 250,000-dalton melanoma-associated antigen. JNCI 1985;74:299.
24. Irie RF, Morton DL. Regression of cutaneous metastatic melanoma by intralesional injection with human monoclonal antibody to ganglioside GD2. Proc Natl Acad Sci USA 1986;83:8694.
25. Blottiere HM, Maurel C, Douillard JY. Immune function of patients with gastrointestinal carcinoma after treatment with multiple infusions of monoclonal antibody 17.1A. Cancer Res 1987;47:5238.

26. LoBuglio AF, Saleh M, Peterson L, Wheeler R, Carrano R, Huster W, Khazaeli MB. Phase I clinical trial of CO17-1A monoclonal antibody. Hybridoma (suppl) 1986;5: 117.
27. Mellstedt H, Frauodin JE, Ragnhammar P, Masucci G, Shetye J, Christensson B, Biberfeld P, Makower J, Pihlstedt P, Cedermark B, Harmenberg U, Wahren B, Rieger A, Magnusson I, Nathansson J, Erwald R. The clinical use of monoclonal antibodies MAb 17-1A in the treatment of patients with metastatic colorectal carcinoma. Med Oncol Tumor Pharmacol 1989;6:99.
28. Sears HF, Herlyn D, Steplewski Z, Koprowski H. Effects of monoclonal antibody immunotherapy on patients with gastrointestinal adenocarcinoma. J Biol Response Mod 1984;3:138.
29. Herlyn D, Ross AH, Koprowski H. Anti-idiotypic antibodies bear the internal image of a human tumor antigen. Science 1986;232:100.
30. Herlyn D, Wettendorff M, Schmoll E, Iliopoulos D, Schedel I, Dreikhausen U, Raab R, Ross AH, Jaksche H, Scriba M, Koprowski H. Anti-idiotype immunization of cancer patients: modulation of the immune response. Proc Natl Acad Sci USA 1987;84:8055.
31. Koprowski H, Herlyn D, Lubeck M, DeFreitas E, Sears HF. Human anti-idiotype antibodies in cancer patients. Is the modulation of the immune response beneficial for the patient? Proc Natl Acad Sci USA 1984;81:216.
32. Mittelman A, Chen ZJ, Kageshita T, Yang H, Yamada M, Baskind P, Goldberg N, Puccio C, Ahmed T, Arlin Z, Ferrone S. Active specific immunotherapy in patients with melanoma: a clinical trial with mouse antiidiotypic monoclonal antibodies elicited with syngeneic anti-high-molecular-weight-melanoma-associated antigen monoclonal antibodies. J Clin Invest 1990;86:2136.
33. Nepom GT, Hellström K. E Anti-idiotypic antibodies and the induction of specific tumor immunity. Cancer Metast Rev 1987;6:489.
34. Wettendorff M, Iliopoulos D, Tempero M, Kay D, DeFreitas E, Koprowski H, Herlyn D. Idiotypic cascades in cancer patients treated with monoclonal antibody CO17-1A. Proc Natl Acad Sci USA 1989;86:3787.
35. Yamamoto S, Yamamoto T, Saxton RE, Hoon DS, Irie RF. Anti-idiotype monoclonal antibody carrying the internal image of ganglioside GM3. JNCI 1990;82:1757.
36. Riethmüller G, Schlimok G, Schneider-Gädicke E, Schmiegel W, Raab R, Höffken K, Gruber R, Pichlmaier H, Hirche H, Pichlmayr R. University of Munich, Dept. Immunology and German 17-1A study group. Monoclonal antibody (MAB) treatment of resected Dukes C colorectal carcinoma (CRC): a prospective randomized trial. Proc ASCO 1994;13:199.
37. James K, Bell GT. Human monoclonal antibody production. Current status and future prospects. J Immunol Meth 1987;100:5.
38. Haspel MV, McCabe RP, Pomato N, Janesch NJ, Knowlton JV, Peters LC, Hoover HC Jr, Hanna MG Jr. Generation of tumor cell-reactive human monoclonal antibodies using peripheral blood lymphocytes from actively immunized colorectal carcinoma patients. Cancer Res 1985;45:3951.
39. Boulianne GL, Hozumi N, Shulman MJ. Production of functional chimaeric mouse/human antibody. Nature 1984;312:643.
40. Morrison SL, Johnson MJ, Herzenberg LA, Oi VT. Chimeric human antibody molecules: mouse antigen-binding domains with human constant region domains. Proc Natl Acad Sci USA 1984;81:6851.
41. Morrison SL. Transfectomas provide novel chimeric antibodies. Science 1985;229: 1202.
42. Morrison SL, OI VT. Genetically engineered antibody molecules. Adv Immunol 1989;44:65.
43. Jones PT, Dear PH, Foote J, Neuberger MS, Winter G. Replacing the complementarity-determining regions in a human antibody with those from a mouse. Nature 1986;321:522.
44. Colcher D, Bird R, Roselli M, Hardman KD, Johnson S, Pope S, Dodd SW, Pantoliano MW, Milenic DE, Schlom J. In vivo tumor targeting of a recombinant single-chain antigen-binding protein. JNCI 1990;82:1–191.
45. Masui H, Moroyama T, Mendelsohn J. Mechanism of antitumor activity in mice for anti-epidermal growth factor receptor monoclonal antibodies with different isotypes. Cancer Res 1986;46:5592.
46. Mendelsohn J. Growth factor receptors as targets for antitumor therapy with monoclonal antibodies. Prog Allergy 1988;45:147.
47. Rodeck U, Herlyn M, Herlyn D, Molthoff C, Atkinson B, Varello M, Steplewski Z, Koprowski H. Tumor growth modulation by a monoclonal antibody to the epidermal growth factor receptor: immunologically mediated and effector cell-independent effects. Cancer Res 1987;47:3692.
48. Drebin JA, Link VC, Greene MI. Monoclonal antibodies specific for the neu oncogene product directly mediate anti-tumor effects in vivo. Oncogene 1988;2:387.
49. Xu FJ, Rodriguez GC, Whitaker R, Boente M, Berchuck A, McKenzie S, Houston L, Boyer CM, Bast RC Jr. Antibodies against immunochemically distinct epitopes on the extracellular domain of HER-2/neu (c-erbB-2) inhibit growth of breast and ovarian cancer cell lines. Int J Cancer 1993;53:401.
50. Baselga J, Tripath D, Mendelsohn J, Benz C, Dantis L, Moore J, Rosen PP, Henderson IC, Baughman S, Twaddel T, Norton L. Phase II study of recombinant human anti-HER2 monoclonal antibody (rhuMAb HER2) in stage IV breast cancer (BC) HER2-shedding dependent pharmacokinetics and antitumor activity. Proc ASCO 1994;13: 103.
51. Debatin KM, Goldmann CK, Bamford R, Waldmann TA, Krammer PH. Monoclonal-antibody-mediated apoptosis in adult T-cell leukaemia. Lancet 1990;335:497.
52. Waldmann H, Cobbold S, Wilson A, Clark M, Watt S, Hale G, Tighe H. Rat monoclonal antibodies for bone marrow transplantation–the CAMPATH series. Adv Exp Med Biol 1985;186:869.
53. Steplewski Z, Lubeck MD, Koprowski H. Human macrophages armed with murine immunoglobulin G2a antibodies to tumors destroy human cancer cells. Science 1983;221:865.
54. Hersey P, MacDonald M, Burns C, Cheresh DA. Enhancement of cytotoxic and proliferative responses of lymphocytes from melanoma patients by incubation with monoclonal antibodies against ganglioside GD3. Cancer Immunol Immunother 1987;24: 144.
55. Clark M, Gilliland L, Waldmann H. Hybrid antibodies for therapy. Prog Allergy 1988;45:31.
56. Mezzanzanica D, Canevari S, Menard S, Pupa SM, Tagliabue E, Lanzavecchia A, Colnaghi MI. Human ovarian carcinoma lysis by cytotoxic T cells targeted by bispecific monoclonal antibodies: analysis of the antibody components. Int J Cancer 1988;41:609.
57. Boyer CM, Borowitz MJ, McCarty KS Jr, Kinney RB, Everitt L, Dawson DV, Ring D, Bast RC Jr. Heterogeneity of antigen expression in benign and malignant breast and ovarian epithelial cells. Int J Cancer 1989;43:55.
58. Bast RC Jr, De Fabritiis P, Lipton J, Gelber R, Maver C, Nadler L, Sallan S, Ritz J. Elimination of malignant clonogenic cells from human bone marrow using multiple monoclonal antibodies and complement. Cancer Res 1985;45:499.
59. DeFabritiis P, Bregni M, Lipton J, Reynolds C, Nadler L, Ritz J, Bast RC Jr. Antigenic heterogeneity among Burkitt's lymphoma cells surviving treatment with monoclonal antibody and complement. Leuk Res 1986;10:35.
60. Ramsay N, LeBien T, Nesbit M, McGlave P, Weisdorf D, Kenyon P, Hurd D, Goldman A, Kim T, Kersey J. Autologous bone marrow transplantation for patients with acute lymphoblastic leukemia in second or subsequent remission: results of bone marrow treated with monoclonal antibodies BA-1, BA-2, and BA-3 plus complement. Blood 1985;66:508.
61. Ritz J, Bast RC, Clavell LA, Hercend T, Sallan SE, Lipton JM, Feeney M, Nathan DG, Schlossman SF. Autologous bone-marrow transplantation in CALLA-positive acute lymphoblastic leukemia after in vitro treatment with J5 monoclonal antibody and complement. Lancet 1982;2:60.
62. Sallan SE, Niemeyer CM, Billett AL, Lipton JM, Tarbell NJ, Gelber RD, Murray C, Pittinger TP, Wolfe LC, Bast RC Jr, Ritz J. Autologous bone marrow transplantation for acute lymphoblastic leukemia. J Clin Oncol 1989;7:1594.
63. Ball ED, Mills LE, Coughlin CT, Beck JR, Cornwell GG III. Autologous bone marrow transplantation in acute myelogenous leukemia: in vitro treatment with myeloid cell-specific monoclonal antibodies. Blood 1986;68:1311.
64. Kemshead JT, Heath L, Gibson FM, Katz F, Richmond F, Treleaven J, Ugelstad J. Magnetic microspheres and monoclonal antibodies for the depletion of neuroblastoma cells from bone marrow: experiences, improvements and observations. Br J Cancer 1986;54:771.
65. Takvorian T, Canellos GP, Ritz J, Freedman AS, Anderson KC, Mauch P, Tarbell N, Coral F, Daley H, Yeap B. Prolonged disease-free survival after autologous bone marrow transplantation in patients with non-Hodgkin's lymphoma with a poor prognosis. N Engl J Med 1987;316:1499.
66. Anderson IC, Shpall EJ, Leslie DS, Nustad K, Ugelstad J, Peters WP, Bast RC Jr. Elimination of malignant clonogenic breast cancer cells from human bone marrow. Cancer Res 1989;49:4659.
67. Shpall EJ, Jones RB, Bast RC Jr, Rosner GL, Vandermark R, Ross M, Affronti ML, Johnston C, Eggleston S, Tepperburg M, Coniglio D, Peters WP. 4-Hydroperoxycyclophosphamide purging of breast cancer from the mononuclear cell fraction of bone marrow in patients receiving high-dose chemotherapy and autologous marrow support. A phase I trial. J Clin Oncol 1991;9:85.
68. Gribben JG, Freedman AS, Neuberg D, Roy DC, Blake KW, Woo SD, Grossbard ML, Rabinowe SN, Coral F, Freeman GJ, Ritz J, Nadler LM. Immunologic purging of marrow assessed by PCR before autologous bone marrow transplantation for B-cell lymphoma. N Engl J Med 1991;325:1525.
69. Deisseroth AD, Zu Z, Claxton D, Hanania EG, Fu F, Ellerson D, Goldberg L, Thomas M, Janicek K, Anderson WF, Hester J, Korbling M, Durett A, Moen R, Berenson R, Heimfeld S, Hamer J, Calvert L, Tibbets P, Talpaz M, Kantarjian H, Champlin R, Reading C. Genetic marking shows that Ph^+ cells present in autologous transplants of chronic myelongenous leukemia contribute to relapse after autologous bone marrow in CML. Blood 1994;83:3068.
70. Ghose T, Blair AH. The design of cytotoxic-agent-antibody conjugates. Crit Rev Ther Drug Carrier Syst 1987;3:263.
71. Pimm M. V Drug-monoclonal antibody conjugates for cancer therapy: potentials and limitations. Crit Rev Ther Drug Carrier Syst 1988;5:189.
72. Baldwin RW, Embleton MJ, Gallego J, Garnett M, Pimm MV, Price MR. Monoclonal antibody drug conjugates for cancer therapy. In Monoclonal Antibodies in Cancer. Advances in Diagnosis and Treatment. Edited by JA Roth. New York: Futura, 1986, p 215.
73. Baldwin RW, Embleton MJ, Garnett MC, Pimm MV. Conjugates of monoclonal antibody 791T/36 with methotrexate in cancer therapy. NCI Monogr 1987;3:95.
74. Bumol TF, Laguzza BC, Baker AL, Todd GC, Pohland RC, Apelgren LD. Studies on 9.2.27–4-desacetyl vinblastine-3-carboxyhydrazide (9.2.27-DAVLB-hydrazide). Preclinical pharmacology and toxicology profiles for human melanoma therapy. Proc Annu Meet Am Assoc Cancer Res 1988;29:A1667.
75. Kanellos J, Pietersz GA, Cunningham Z, McKenzie IFC. Anti-tumor activity of aminopterin-monoclonal antibody conjugates; in vitro and in vivo comparison with methotrexate-monoclonal antibody conjugates. Immunol Cell Biol 1987;65:483.
76. Luders G, Kohnlein W, Sorg C, Bruggen J. Selective toxicity of neocarzinostatin-monoclonal antibody conjugates to the antigen-bearing human melanoma cell line in vitro. Cancer Immunol Immunother 1985;20:85.
77. Peitersz GA, Smyth MJ, Tjandra JJ, McKenzie IF. Preclinical and clinical studies with n-acetyl melphalan (N-AcMEL) immunoconjugates and tumor necrosis factor alpha (TNF-α). Presented at Third International Conference on Monoclonal Antibody Immunoconjugates for Cancer USCD Cancer Center, San Diego, 1988, p 20.
78. Shawler DL, Johnson DE, Sweet MD, Myers LJ, Tudor SD, Beidler DE, Koziol JA, Dillman RO. Preclinical trials using an immunoconjugate of T101 and methotrexate in an athymic mouse/human T-cell tumor model. J Biol Response Mod 1988;7:608.
79. Sheldon K, Marks A, Baumal R. Sensitivity of multidrug resistant KB-C1 cells to an antibody-Dextran-Adriamycin conjugate. Anticancer Res 1989;9:637.
80. Shouval D, Adler R, Wands JR, Hurwitz E, Isselbacher KJ, Sela M. Doxorubicin conjugates of monoclonal antibodies to hepatoma-associated antigens. Proc Natl Acad Sci USA 1988;85:8276.
81. Smyth MJ, Pietersz GA, McKenzie IF. The mode of action of methotrexate-monoclonal antibody conjugates. Immunol Cell Biol 1987;65:189.
82. Smyth MJ, Pietersz GA, McKenzie IF. The cellular uptake and cytotoxicity of chlorambucil-monoclonal antibody conjugates. Immunol Cell Biol 1987;65:315.
83. Smyth MJ, Bogdanovski M, McKenzie IFC, Pietersz GA. Antitumor activity of idarubicin-monoclonal antibody conjugates in a disseminated thymic lymphoma model. Cancer Res 1991;51:310.
84. Spearman ME, Goodwin RM, Apelgren LD, Bumol TF. Disposition of the monoclonal antibody-vinca alkaloid conjugate KS1/4-DAVLB (LY256787) and free r-desacetylvinblastine in tumor-bearing nude mice. J Pharmacol Exp Ther 1987;241:695.

85. Takahashi T, Yamaguchi T, Kitamura K, Suzuyama H, Honda M, Yokota T, Kotanagi H, Takahashi M, Hashimoto Y. Clinical application of monoclonal antibody-drug conjugates for immunotargeting chemotherapy of colorectal carcinoma. Cancer 1988;61:881.
86. Wrasidlo W, Muller B, Yang H-M, Reisfeld RA. Oligomerization of doxorubicin results in improved cytotoxicity of antibody-drug conjugates. Presented at Third International Conference on Monoclonal Antibody Immunoconjugates for Cancer USCD Cancer Center, San Diego, 1988, p 64.
87. McKearn TJ, Lopes AD, Radcliffe RD. In vivo efficacy of site-specific anti-folate monoclonal antibody conjugates. Presented at Third International Conference on Monoclonal Antibody Immunoconjugates for Cancer UCSD Cancer Center, San Diego, 1988, p 17.
88. Rodwell JD, Alvarez VL, Lee C, Lopes AD, Goers JW, King HD, Powsner HJ, McKearn TJ. Site-specific covalent modification of monoclonal antibodies: in vitro and in vivo evaluations. Proc Natl Acad Sci USA 1986;83:2632.
89. Starling J, Hinson A, Marder P. Rapid internalization of antigen-immunoconjugate complexes is not required for anti-tumor activity of monoclonal antibody-drug conjugates. Presented at Third International Conference on Monoclonal Antibody Immunoconjugates for Cancer USCD Cancer Center, San Diego, 1988, p 23.
90. Sugerman S, Murray JL, Saleh M, LoBuglio AF, Jones D, Daniel C, LeBherz D, Brewer H, Healy D, Kelley S, Hellström KE, Onetto N. A phase I study of BR96-doxorubicin (BR96-DOX) in patients with advanced carcinoma expressing the Lewis^Y antigen. Am Soc Clin Oncol Edu Book 1995;14:423.
91. Trail PA, Willner D, Lasch SJ, Henderson AJ, Hofstead S, Casazza AM, Firestone RA, Hellström I, Hellström KE. Cure of xenografted human carcinomas by BR96-doxorubicin immunoconjugates. Science 1993;261:212.
92. Connor J, Sullivan S, Huang L. Monoclonal antibody and liposomes. Pharmacol Ther 1985;28:341.
93. Matthay KK, Heath TD, Badger CC, Bernstein ID, Papahadjopoulos D. Antibody-directed liposomes: comparison of various ligands for association, endocytosis, and drug delivery. Cancer Res 1986;46:4904.
94. Pressman D, Korngold L. The in vivo localization of anti-Wagner osteogenic sarcoma antibodies. Cancer 1953;6:7619.
95. Spar IL, Bale WF, Marrack D, Dewey WC, McCardle RJ, Harper PV. I-131 labeled antibodies to human fibrinogen: diagnostic studies and therapeutic trials. Cancer 1967;20:865.
96. Colcher D, Zalutsky M, Kaplan W, Kufe D, Austin F, Schlom J. Radiolocalization of human mammary tumors in athymic mice by a monoclonal antibody. Cancer Res 1983;43:736.
97. Vacca A, Buchegger F, Carrel S, Mach J-P. Imaging of human leukemic T-cell xenografts in nude mice by radiolabeled monoclonal antibodies and $F(ab')_2$ fragments. Cancer 1988;61:58.
98. Wahl RL, Parker CW, Philpott GW. Improved radioimaging and tumor localization with monoclonal $F(ab')_2$. J Nucl Med 1983;24:316.
99. Cheung NV, Landmeier B, Nealy J, Nelson AD, Abramowsky C, Ellery S, Adams RB, Miraldi F. Complete tumor ablation with iodine-131radiolabeled disialoganglioside G_{D2}-specific monoclonal antibody against human neuroblastoma xenografted in nude mice. JNCI 1986;77:739.
100. Lee Y, Bullard DE, Humphrey PA, Colapinto DV, Friedman HS, Zalutsky MR, Coleman RE, Bigner DD. Treatment of intracranial human glioma xenografts with ^{131}I-labeled antitenascin monoclonal antibodies 81C6. Cancer Res 1988;48:2904–2910.
101. Zalutsky MR, Moseley RP, Coakham HB, Coleman RE, Bigner DD. Pharmacokinetics and tumor localization of ^{131}I-labeled anti-tenascin monoclonal antibody 81C6 in patients with gliomas and other intracranial malignancies. Cancer Res 1989;49:2807.
102. Carrasquillo, JA, Radioimmunoscintigraphy with polyclonal or monoclonal antibodies. In Antibodies in Radiodiagnosis and Therapy. Edited by MR Zalutsky. Boca Raton, FL: CRC 1989, p 169.
103. Colcher D, Esteban JM, Carrasquillo JA, Sugarbaker P, Reynolds JC, Bryant G, Larson SM, Schlom J. Quantitative analyses of selective radiolabeled monclonal antibody localization in metastatic lesions of colorectal cancer patients. Cancer Res 1987;47:1185.
104. Colcher D, Esteban J, Carrasquillo JA, Sugarbaker P, Reynolds JC, Bryant G, Larson SM, Schlom J. Complementation of intracavitary and intravenous administration of a monoclonal antibody (B72.3) in patients with carcinoma. Cancer Res 1987;47:4218.
105. Halpern SE, Dillman RO, Witztum KF, Shega JF, Hagan PL, Burrows WM, Dillman JB, Clutter ML, Sobol RE, Frincke JM, Bartholomew RM, David GS, Carlo D. Radioimmunodetection of melanoma utilizing ^{111}In-96.5 monoclonal antibody: a preliminary report. Radiology 1985;155:493.
106. Larson, SM. Clinical radioimmunodetection: overview and suggestions for standardization of clinical trials. Cancer Res (suppl) 1990;50:829s.
107. Boucher Y, Baxter LT, Jain RK. Interstitial pressure gradients in tissue-isolated and subcutaneous tumors: implications for therapy. Cancer Res 1990;50:4478.
108. Baxter LT, Jain RK. Transport of fluid and macromolecules in tumors. III. Role of binding and metabolism. Microvascular Res 1991;41:5.
109. van Osdol W, Fujimori K, Weinstein JN. An analysis of monoclonal antibody distribution in microscopic tumor nodules: consequences of a "binding site barrier." Cancer Res 1991;51:4776.
110. Press OW, Eary JF, Appelbaum FR, Martin PJ, Badger CC, Nelp WB, Glenn S, Butchko G, Fisher D, Porter B, Matthews DC, Fisher LD, Bernstein ID. Radiolabeled-antibody therapy of B-cell lymphoma with autologous bone marrow support. N Engl J Med 1993;329:1219.
111. Nabi HA, Doerr RJ. Radiolabeled monoclonal antibody imaging (immunoscintigraphy) of colorectal cancers: current status and future directions. Am J Surg 1992;163:448.
112. Scott AM, Macapinlac H, Zhang JJ, Kalaigian H, Graham MC, Divgi CR, Sgouros G, Goldsmith SJ, Larson SM. Clinical applications of fusion imaging in oncology. Nucl Med Biol 1994;21:775.
113. Bakir MA, Eccles SA, Babich JW, Aftab N, Styles JM, Dean CJ, Ott, RJ. c-erbB2 protein overexpression in breast cancer as a target for PET using iodine-124-labeled monoclonal antibodies. J Nucl Med 1992;33:2154.
114. Anderson CJ, Connett JM, Schwarz SW, Rocque PA, Guo LW, Philpott GW, Zinn KR, Meares CF, Welch MJ. Copper-64-labeled antibodies for PET imaging. J Nucl Med 1992;33:1685.
115. Page RL, Garg PK, Garg S, Archer GE, Bruland OS, Zalutsky MR. PET imaging of osteosarcoma in dogs using a fluorine-18-labeled monoclonal antibody Fab fragment. J Nucl Med 1994;35:1506.
116. Goldenberg DM, DeLand FH, Kim E, Bennett S, Primus FJ. Van Nagell JR, Estes N, DeSimone P, Rayburn P. Use of radiolabeled antibodies to carcinoembryonic antigen for the detection and localization of diverse cancers by external photoscanning. N Engl J Med 1978;298:1384.
117. Mach J-P, Carrel S, Forni M, Ritschard J, Donath A, Alberto P. Tumor localization of radiolabeled antibodies against carcinoembryonic antigen in patients with carcinoma. N Engl J Med 1980;303:5.
118. Larson SM, Macapinlac HA, Scott AM, Divgi CR. Recent achievements in the development of radiolabeled monoclonal antibodies for diagnosis, therapy and biologic characterization of human tumors. Acta Oncol 1993;32:709.
119. Carrasquillo JA, Abrams PG, Schroff RW, Reynolds JC, Woodhouse CS, Morgan AC, Keenan AM, Foon KA, Perentesis P, Marshall S, Horowitz M, Szymendera J, Enlert J, Oldham RK, Larson SM. Effect of antibody dose on the imaging and biodistribution of indium-111 9.2.27 anti-melanoma monoclonal antibody. J Nucl Med 1988;29:39.
120. Miraldi FK, Nelson AD, Kraly C, Ellery S, Landmeir B, Coccia PF, Strandjord SE, Cheung NKV. Diagnostic imaging of human neuroblastoma with radiolabeled antitumor antibody. Radiology 1986;161:413.
121. Zalutsky MR, Noska MA, Colapinto EV, Garg PK, Bigner DD. Enhanced tumor localization and in vivo stability of a monoclonal antibody radioiodinated using N-succinimidyl-3-(tri-n-butyl-stannyl)benzoate. Cancer Res 1989;49:5543.
122. Dadparvar S, Krishna L, Miyamoto C, Brady LW, Brown SJ, Bender H, Slizofski WJ, Eshleman J, Chevres A, Woo DV. Indium-111-labeled anti-EGFr-425 scintigraphy in the detection of malignant gliomas. Cancer 1994;73:884.
123. Carrasquillo JA, Bunn, PA, Keenan AM, Reynolds JC, Schroff RW, Foon KA, Su M-H, Gazdar AF, Mulshine JL, Oldham RK, Perentesis P, Horowitz M, Eddy J, James P, Larson SM. Radioimmunodetection of cutaneous T-cell lymphoma with ^{111}In-labeled T101 monoclonal antibody. N Engl J Med 1986;315:673.
124. Carrasquillo JA, Mulshine JL, Bunn PA Jr, Reynolds JC, Foon KA, Schroff RW, Perentesis P, Steis RG, Keenan AM, Horowitz M, Larson SM. Indium-111 T101 monoclonal antibody is superior to iodine-131 T101 in imaging of cutaneous T-cell lymphoma. J Nucl Med 1987;28:281.
125. Ward BG, Mather SJ, Hawkins LR, Crowther ME, Shepherd JH, Granowska M, Britton KE, Slevin ML. Localization of radioiodine conjugated to the monoclonal antibody HMFG2 in human ovarian carcinoma: assessment of intravenous and intraperitoneal routes of administration. Cancer Res 1987;47:4719.
126. Divgi CR, McDermott K, Griffin TW, Johnson DK, Schnobrich KE, Fallone PS, Scott AM, Hilton S, Cohen AM, Larson SM. Lesion-by-lesion comparison of computerized tomography and indium-111-labeled monoclonal antibody C110 radioimmunoscintigraphy in colorectal carcinoma: a multicenter trial. J Nucl Med 1993;34:1656.
127. Kramer EL, DeNardo SJ, Liebes L, Kroger LA, Noz ME, Mizrachi H, Salako QA, Furmanski P, Glenn SD, DeNardo GL, Ceriani R. Radioimmunolocalization of metastatic breast carcinoma using indium-111-methyl benzyl DTPA BrE-3 monoclonal antibody: phase I study. J Nucl Med 1993;34:1067.
128. Chatal JF, Saccavini JC, Funoleau P, Douillard JY, Curtet C, Kremer M, Le Mervel B, Koprowski H. Immunoscintigraphy of colon carcinoma. J Nucl Med 1984;25:307.
129. Kirkwood JM, Neumann RD, Zoghbi SS, Ernstoff MS, Cornelius EA, Shaw C, Ziyadeh T, Fine JA, Unger MW. Scintigraphic detection of metastatic melanoma using indium 111/DTPA conjugated anti-gp240 antibody (ZME-018). J Clin Oncol 1987;5:1247.
130. Delaloye B, Bischof-Delaloye A, Buchegger F, von Fliedner V, Grob J-P, Volant J-C, Pettavel J, Mach J-P. Detection of colorectal carcinoma by emission-computerized tomography after injection of ^{123}I-labeled Fab or $F(ab')_2$ fragments from monoclonal anti-carcinoembryonic antigen antibodies. J Clin Invest 1986;77:301.
131. Bischof-Delaloye A, Delaloye B, Buchegger F, Gilgien W, Studer A, Curchod S, Givel, J-C, Mosimann F, Pettavel J, Mach J-P. Clinical value of immunoscintigraphy in colorectal carcinoma patients: a prospective study. J Nucl Med 1989;30:1646.
132. Schwarz A, Steinsträsser AA. A novel approach to Tc-99m-labeled monoclonal antibodies [abstract]. J Nucl Med 1987;28:721.
133. Thakur ML, DeFulvio J, Richard MD, Park CH. Technetium-99m labeled monoclonal antibodies: evaluation of reducing agents. Nucl Med Biol 1991;18:227.
134. Siccardi AG. Tumor immunoscintigraphy by means of radiolabeled monoclonal antibodies: multicenter studies of the Italian National Research Council–special project "Biomedical Engineering." Cancer Res (suppl) 1990;50:899.
135. De Bree R, Roos JC, Quak JJ, den Hollander W, van den Brekel MWM, van der Wal JE, Tobi H, Snow GB, van Dongen GA. Clinical imaging of head and neck cancer with technetium-99m labeled monoclonal antibody E48 IgG or $F(ab')_2$. J Nucl Med 1994;35:775.
136. Baum RP, Niesen A, Hertel A, Adams S, Kojouharoff G, Goldenberg DM, Hör G. Initial clinical results with technetium-99m-labeled LL2 monoclonal antibody fragment in the radioimmunodetection of B-cell lymphomas. Cancer 1994;73:896.
137. Hnatowich DJ, Mardirossian G, Rusckowski M, Fogarasi M, Virzi F, Winnard P Jr. Directly and indirectly technetium-99m-labeled antibodies: a comparison of in vitro and animal in vivo properties. J Nucl Med 1994;34:109.
138. Fritzberg AR, Abrams PG, Beaumier PL, Kasina S, Morgan AC, Rao TN, Reno JM, Sanderson JA, Srinivasan A, Wilbur DS. Specific and stable labeling of antibodies with technetium-99m with a diamide dithiolate chelating agent. Proc Natl Acad Sci USA 1988;85:4025.
139. Abrams MJ, Juweid M, tenKate CI, Schwartz DA, Hauser MM, Gaul FE, Fuccello AJ, Rubin RH, Strauss HW, Fischman AJ. Technetium-99m-human polyclonal IgG radiolabeled via the hydrazine nicotinamide derivative for imaging focal sites of infection in rats. J Nucl Med 1990;31:2022.
140. Brady LW, Mymoto C, Woo DV, Rackover M, Emrich J, Bender H, Dadparvar S, Steplewski Z, Koprowski H, Black P, Lazzaro B, Nair S, McCormack T, Nieves J, Morabito M, Eshleman J. Malignant astrocytomas treated with iodine-125 labeled monoclonal antibody 425 against epidermal growth factor receptor: a phase II trial. Int J Radiat Oncol Biol Phys 1992;22:225.
141. Wheldon TE, O'Donoghue JA, Barrett A, Michalowski AS. The curability of tumours of differing size by targeted radiotherapy using ^{131}I or ^{90}Y. Radiother Oncol 1991;21:91.
142. Brown I. Astatine-211: its possible applications in cancer therapy. Int J Appl Radiat Isot 1986;37:789.

143. Strickland DK, Vaidyanathan G, Zalutsky MR. Cytotoxicity of α-particle-emitting m (211At)astatobenzylguanidine on human neuroblastoma cells. Cancer Res 1994;54: 5414.
144. Order SE, Klein JL, Ettinger D, Alderson P, Siegelman S, Leichner P. Phase I-II study of radiolabeled antibody integrated n the treatment of primary hepatic malignancies. Int J Radiat Oncol Biol Phys 1980;6:703.
145. Order SE, Stillwagon GB, Klein JL, Leichner PK, Siegelman SS, Fishman EK, Ettinger DS, Haulk T, Kopher K, Finney K, Surdyke M, Self S, Leibel S. Iodine 131 antiferritin, a new treatment modality in hepatoma. A radiation therapy oncology group study. J Clin Oncol 1985;3:1573.
146. Kaminski MS, Zasadny KR, Francis IR, Milik AW, Ross CW, Moon SD, Crawford SM, Burgess JM, Petry NA, Butchko GM, Glenn SD, Wahl RL. Radioimmunotherapy of B-cell lymphoma with [^{131}I] anti-B1(anti-CD20) antibody. N Engl J Med 1993;329:459.
147. Carrasquillo JA, Krohn KA, Beaumier P, McGuffin RW, Brown JP, Hellstrom KE, Hellstrom I, Larson SM. Diagnosis of and therapy for solid tumors with radiolabeled antibodies and immune fragments. Cancer Treat Rep 1984;68:317.
148. Rosen ST, Zimmer M, Goldman-Leikin R, Gordon LI, Kazikiewicz JM, Kaplan EH, Variakojis D, Marder RJ, Dykewicz MS, Piergies A, Silverstein EA, Roenigk HH Jr, Spies SM. Radioimmunodetection and racioimmunotherapy of cutaneous T cell lymphomas using an ^{131}I-labeled monoclonal antibody: an Illinois Cancer Council Study. J Clin Oncol 1987;5:562.
149. Welt S, Divgi CR, Kemeny N, Finn RD, Scott AM, Graham M, St. Germain J, Richards EC, Larson SM, Oettgen HF, Old LJ. Phase I/II study of iodine 131-labeled monoclonal antibody A33 in patients with advanced colon cancer. J Clin Oncol 1994;12: 1561.
150. Murray JL, Macey DJ, Kasi LP, Rieger P, Cunningham J, Bhadkamkar V, Zhang H-Z, Schlom J, Rosenblum MG, Podoloff DA. Phase II radioimmunotherapy trial with 131I-CC49 in colorectal cancer. Cancer 1994;73:1057.
151. Meredith RF, Bueschen AJ, Khazaeli MB, Plott WE, Grizzle WE, Wheeler RH, Schlom J, Russell CD, Liu T, LoBuglio AF. Treatment of metastatic prostate carcinoma with radiolabeled antibody CC49. J Nucl Med 1994;35:1017.
152. Sharkey RM, Motta-Hennessy C, Pawlyk D, Siegel JA, Goldenberg DM. Biodistribution and radiation dose estimates for yttrium- and iodine-labeled monoclonal antibody IgG and fragments in nude mice bearing human colonic tumor xenografts. Cancer Res 1990;50:2330.
153. Buchsbaum DJ, Lawrence TS, Roberson PL, Heidorn DB, Ten Haken RK, Steplewski Z. Comparison of ^{131}I- and ^{90}Y-labeled monoclonal antibody 17-1A for treatment of human colon cancer xenografts. Int J Radiat Oncol Biol Phys 1993;25:629.
154. Vriesendorp HM, Herpst JM, Germack MA, Klein JL, Leichner PK, Loudenslager DM, Order SE. Phase I-II studies of yttrium-labeled antiferritin treatment for end-stage Hodgkin's disease, including Radiation Therapy Oncology Group 87-01. J Clin Oncol 1991;9:918.
155. Maraveyas A, Snook D, Hird V, Kosmas C, Meares CF, Lambert HE, Epenetos AA. Pharmacokinetics and toxicity of an yttrium-90-CITC-DTPA-HMFG1 radioimmunoconjugate for intraperitoneal radioimmunotherapy of ovarian cancer. Cancer 1994;73:1067.
156. Hird V, Maraveyas A, Snook D, Dhokia B, Soutter WP, Meares CF, Stewart JSW, Mason P, Lambert HE, Epenetos AA. Adjuvant therapy of ovarian cancer with radioactive monoclonal antibody. Br J Cancer 1993;68:403.
157. Roseli M, Schlom J, Gansow OA, Raubitschek A, Mirzadeh S, Brechbiel MW, Colcher D. Comparative biodistribution of yttrium- and indium-labeled monoclonal antibody B72.3 in athymic mice bearing human colon carcinoma xenografts. J Nucl Med 1989;30:672.
158. Camera L, Kinuya S, Garmestani K, Wu C, Brechbiel MW, Pai LH, McMurry TJ, Gansow OA, Pastan I, Paik CH, Carrasquillo JA. Evaluation of the serum stability and in vivo biodistribution of CHX-DTPA and other ligands for yttrium labeling of monoclonal antibodies. J Nucl Med 1994;35:882.
159. DeNardo GL, Kroger LA, DeNardo SJ, Miers LA, Salako Q, Kukis DL, Fand I, Shen S, Renn O, Meares CF. Comparative toxicity studies of yttrium-90 MX-DTPA and 2-IT-BAD conjugated monoclonal antibody (BrE-3). Cancer 1994;73:1012.
160. Schuster JM, Garg PK, Bigner DD, Zalutsky MR. Improved therapeutic efficacy of a monoclonal antibody radioiodinated using N-succinimidyl-3-(tri-n-butylstannyl)benzoate. Cancer Res 1991;51:4164.
161. Msirikale JS, Klein JL, Schroeder J, Order SE. Radiation enhancement of radiolabeled antibody deposition in tumors. J Radiat Oncol 1987;13:1839.
162. Stickney DR, Gridley DS, Kirk GA, Slater JM. Enhancement of monoclonal antibody binding to melanoma with single dose radiation or hyperthermia. NCI Monogr 1987;3: 47.
163. Shrivastav S, Schlom J, Raubitschek A, Molinolo A, Simpson J, Hand PH. Studies concerning the effect of external irradiation on localization of radiolabeled monoclonal antibody B72.3 to human colon carcinoma xenografts. J Radiat Oncol Biol Phys 1989;16:721.
164. Wong JYC, Williams LE, Hill LR, Paxton RJ, Beatty BG, Shively JE, Beaty JD. The effects of tumor mass, tumor age, and external beam radiation on tumor-specific antibody uptake. Int J Radiat Oncol Biol Phys 1989;16:715.
165. Cope DA, Dewhirst MW, Friedman HS, Bigner DD, Zalutsky MR. Enhanced delivery of a monoclonal antibody F(ab')$_2$ fragment to subcutaneous human glioma xenografts using local hyperthermia. Cancer Res 1990;50:1803.
166. Mittal BB, Zimmer AM, Sathiaseelan V, Rosen ST, Radosevich JA, Rademaker AW, Saini A, Pierce MC, Webber DI, Spies SM. Effects of hyperthermia and iodine-131-labeled anti-carcinoembryonic antigen monoclonal antibody on human tumor xenografts in nude mice. Cancer 1992;70:2785.
167. Wilder RB, Langmuir VK, Mendonca HL, Goris ML, Knox SJ. Local hyperthermia and SR 4233 enhance the antitumor effects of radioimmunotherapy in nude mice with human colonic adenocarcinoma xenografts. Cancer Res 1993;53:3022.
168. Schuster JM, Zalutsky MR, Noska MA, Dodge R, Friedman HS, Bigner DD, Dewhirst MW. Hyperthermic modulation of radiolabelled antibody uptake in a human glioma xenograft and normal tissues. Int J Hyperther 1994; In press.
169. Peterson H-I. Modification of tumour blood flow—a review. Int J Radiat Biol 1991;60: 201.
170. LeBerthon B, Khawli LA, Alauddin M, Miller GK, Charak BS, Mazumder A, Epstein AL. Enhanced tumor uptake of macromolecules induced by a novel vasoactive interleukin 2 immunoconjugate. Cancer Res 1991;51:2694.
171. Khawli LA, Miller GK, Epstein AL. Effect of seven new vasoactive immunoconjugates on the enhancement of monoclonal antibody uptake in tumors. Cancer 1994;73:824.
172. Epenetos AA, Munro AJ, Stewart S, Rampling R, Lambert HE, McKenzie CG, Soutter PA, Rahemtulla G, Hooker G, Sivolapenko GB, Snook D, Courtenay-Luck N, Dhokia B, Krausz T, Taylor-Papadimitriou J, Durbin H, Bodmer WF. Antibody-guided irradiation of advanced ovarian cancer with intraperitoneally administered radiolabeled monoclonal antibodies. J Clin Oncol 1987;5:1890.
173. Papanastassiou V, Pizer BL, Coakham HB, Bullimore J, Zananiri T, Kemshead JT. Treatment of recurrent and cystic malignant gliomas by a single intracavity injection of ^{131}I monoclonal antibody: feasibility, pharmacokinetics and dosimetry. Br J Cancer 1993;67:144.
174. Riva P, Arista A, Tison V, Sturiale C, Franceschi G, Spinelli A, Riva N, Casi M, Moscatelli G, Frattarelli M. Intralesional radioimmunotherapy of malignant gliomas. Cancer 1994;73:1076.
175. Bigner DD, Brown M, Coleman RE, Friedman AH, Friedman HS, McLendon RE, Bigner SH, Wikstrand CJ, Pegram CN, Kerby T, Zalutsky MR. Phase I studies of treatment of malignant gliomas and neoplastic meningitis with ^{131}I-radiolabeled monoclonal antibodies anti-tenascin 81C6 and anti-chondroitin proteoglycan sulfate Mel-14 F(ab')2—a preliminary report. J Neuro-Oncol 1994 (in press).
176. Lashford LS, Davies AG, Richardson RB, Bourne SP, Bullimore JA, Eckhert H, Kemshead JT, Coakham HB. A pilot study of ^{131}I monoclonal antibodies in the therapy of leptomeningeal tumors. Cancer 1988;61:857.
177. Moseley RP, Benjamin JC, Ashpole RD, Sullivan NM, Bullimore JA, Coakham HB, Kemshead JT. Carcinomatous meningitis: antibody-guided therapy with I-131 HMFG1. J Neurol Neurosurg Psych 1991;54:260.
178. Zalutsky MR, McLendon RE, Garg PK, Archer GE, Schuster JM, Bigner DD. Radioimmunotherapy of neoplastic meningitis in rats using an α-particle-emitting immunoconjugate. Cancer Res 1994;54:4719.
179. Shawler DL, Bartholomew RM, Smith LM, Dillman RO. Human immune response to multiple injections of murine IgG1. J Immunol 1985;135:1530.
180. Buist MR, Kenemans P, Hollander WD, Vermorken JB, Molthoff CJM, Burger CW, Helmerhorst TJM, Baak JPA, Roos JC. Kinetics and tissue distribution of the radiolabeled chimeric monoclonal antibody MOv18 IgG and F(ab')$_2$ fragments in ovarian carcinoma patients. Cancer Res 1993;53:5413.
181. Meredith RF, LoBuglio AF, Plott WE, Orr RA, Brezovich IA, Russell CD, Harvey EB, Yester MV, Wagner AJ, Spencer SA, Wheeler RH, Saleh MN, Rogers KJ, Plansky A, Salter MM, Khazaeli MB. Pharmacokinetics, immune response, and biodistribution of iodine-131-labeled chimeric mouse/human IgG 1.k 17-1A monoclonal antibody. J Nucl Med 1991;32:1162.
182. Meredith RF, Khazaeli MB, Plott WE, Saleh MN, Liu T, Allen LF, Russell C, Colcher D, Schlom J, Shochat D, LoBuglio AF. Phase I trial of iodine-131-chimeric B72.3 (human IgG4) in metastatic colorectal cancer. J Nucl Med 1992a;33:23.
183. Meredith RF, Khazaeli MB, Liu T, Plott G, Wheeler RH, Russell C, Colcher D, Schlom J, Shochat D, LoBuglio AF. Dose fractionation of radiolabeled antibodies in patients with metastatic colon cancer. J Nucl Med 1992b;33:1648.
184. Bird RE, Hardman KD, Jacobson JW, Johnson S, Kaufman BM, Lee S-M, Lee T, Pope S, Riordan GS, Whitlow M. Single-chain antigen-binding proteins. Science 1988;242: 423.
185. Huston JS, Levinson D, Mudgett-Hunter M, Tai M-S, Novotny J, Margolies MN, Ridge RJ, Bruccoleri RE, Haber E, Crea R, Oppermann H. Protein engineering of antibody binding sites: recovery of specific activity in an anti-digoxin single-chain F_v analogue produced in *Escherichia coli*. Proc Natl Acad Sci USA 1988;85:5879.
186. Colcher D, Bird R, Roselli M, Hardman KD, Johnson S, Pope S, Dodd SW, Pantoliano MW, Milenic DE, Schlom J. In vivo tumor targeting of a recombinant single-chain antigen-binding protein. JNCI 1990;82:1-191.
187. Milenic DE, Yokota T, Filpula DR, Finkelman MAJ, Dodd SW, Wood JF, Whitlow M, Snoy P, Schlom J. Construction, binding properties, metabolism, and tumor targeting of a single-chain F_v derived from the pancarcinoma monoclonal antibody CC49. Cancer Res 1991;51:6363.
188. Yokota T, Milenic DE, Whitlow M, Schlom J. Rapid tumor penetration of a single-chain F_v and comparison with other immunoglobulin forms. Cancer Res 1992;52:3402.
189. Adams GP, McCartney JE, Tai M-S, Oppermann H, Huston JS, Stafford WF III, Bookman MAFI, Houston LL, Weiner LM. Highly specific in vivo tumor targeting by monovalent and divalent forms of 741F8 anti-c-erbB-2 single-chain Fv. Cancer Res 1993;53:4026.
190. Choe S, Bennett M, Fujii G, Curmi P, Kantardjieff K, Collier R, Eisenberg D. The crystal structure of diphtheria toxin. Nature 1992;357:216.
191. Brandhuber B, Allured V, Falbel T, McKay D. Mapping the enzymatic active site of *Pseudomonas aeruginosa* exotoxin A. Proteins 1988;3:146.
192. Montfort W, Villafranca J, Monzingo A, Ernst S, Katzin B, Rutenber E, Xuong N, Hamlin R, Robertus J. The three-dimensional structure of ricin at 2.8 angstroms. J Biol Chem 1987;262:5398.
193. Monzingo A, Collins E, Ernst S, Irvin J, Robertus J. The 2.5 Angstrom structure of pokeweed antiviral protein. J Mol Biol 1993;233:705.
194. Middlebrook J, Dorland R. Bacterial toxins: cellular mechanisms of action. Microbiol Rev 1984;48:199.
195. Chiron M, Fryling C, FitzGerald D. Cleavage of Pseudomonas exotoxin and diphtheria toxin by a furin-like enzyme prepared from beef liver. J Biol Chem 1994;269:18167.
196. Madshus I. The N-terminal alpha-helix of fragment B of diphtheria toxin promotes translocation of fragment A into the cytoplasm of eukaryotic cells. J Biol Chem 1994;269:17723.
197. Hooper K, Eidels L. Localization of a critical diphtheria toxin-binding domain to the C-terminus of the mature heparin-binding EGF-like growth factor region of the diphtheria toxin receptor. Biochem Biophys Res Commun 1995;206:710.
198. Abrol S, Chaudhary V. A new role of the ADP-ribosylation domain in the cytotoxicity of diphtheria toxin and its fusion proteins. Proceedings, Fourth International Symposium Immunotoxins, Myrtle Beach, 1995, p 1.
199. Mindell J, Zhan H, Huynh P, Collier R, Finkelstein A. Reaction of diphtheria toxin channels with sulfhydryl-specific reagents: observation of chemical reactions at the single molecule level. Proc Natl Acad Sci USA 1994;91:5272.
200. Kounnas M, Morris R, Thompson M, FitzGerald D, Strickland D, Saelinger C. The alpha 2-macroglobulin receptor/low density lipoprotein receptor-related protein binds and internalizes *Pseudomonas* exotoxin A. J Biol Chem 1992;267:12420.

201. Hwang J, FitzGerald D, Adhya S, Pastan I. Functional domains of *Pseudomonas* exotoxin identified by deletion analysis of the gene expressed in *E. coli.* Cell 1987;48: 129.
202. Seetharam S, Chaudhary V, FitzGerald D, Pastan I. Increased cytotoxic activity of Pseudomonas exotoxin and two chimeric toxins ending in KDEL. J Biol Chem 1991;266:17376.
203. Baenziger J, Fiete D. Structural determinants of *Ricinus communis* agglutinin and toxin specificity for oligosaccharides. J Biol Chem 1979;254:9795.
204. Endo Y, Mitsui K, Motizuki M, Tsurugi K. The mechanism of action of ricin and related toxic lectins on eukaryotic ribosomes. J Biol Chem 1987;262:5908.
205. Robertus J, Steighardt J, Svinth M, Day P, Kelly C, Hernandez R. Structural analysis of membrane translocation by ricin. Proceedings, Fourth International Symposium on Immunotoxins, Myrtle Beach, 1995, p 5.
206. Sandvig K, Olsnes S. Entry of the toxic proteins abrin, modeccin, ricin and diphtheria toxin into cells. II. Effect of pH, metabolic inhibitors and ionophores and evidence for penetration from endocytotic vesicles. J Biol Chem 1982;257:7504.
207. Wales R, Roberts L, Lord J. Addition of an endoplasmic reticulum retrieval sequence to ricin A chain significantly increases its cytotoxicity to mammalian cells. J Biol Chem 1993;268:23986.
208. Kagan B, Finkelstein A, Colombini M. Diphtheria toxin fragment forms large pores in phospholipid bilayer membranes. Proc Natl Acad Sci USA 1981;78:4950.
209. Pelham H, Roberts L, Lord J. Toxin entry: how reversible is the secretory pathway? Trends Cell Biol 1992;2:183.
210. Moazed D, Robertson J, Noller H. Interaction of elongation factors EF-G and EF-Tu with a conserved loop in 23 S rRNA. Nature 1989;334:362.
211. Foss F, Borkowski T, Gilliom M, Stetler-Stevenson M, Jaffe E, Figg W, Tompkins A, Bastian A, Nylen P, Woodworth Chimeric fusion protein toxin DAB486IL-2 in advanced mycosis fungoides and the Sezary syndrome: correlation of activity and interleukin-2 receptor expression in a phase II study. Blood 1994;84:1765.
212. Bacha P, Shaw J, Baselga J, Marshal M, Osborne C, Eder J, von Hoff D, Estis L, Nichols J. Phase I dose-escalation studies of the safety and tolerability of DAB389EGF in patients with epidermal growth factor receptor (EGF-R) expressing solid tumors. Proceedings, Fourth International Symposium on Immunotoxins, Myrtle Beach, 1995, p 138.
213. Goldberg M, Heimbrook D, Russo P, Sarosdy M, Greenberg R, Giantonio B, Linehan W, Walther M, Fisher H, Messing E, Crawford E, Oliff A, Pastan I. Phase I clinical study of the recombinant oncotoxin TP40 in superficial bladder cancer. Clin Cancer Res 1995;1:57.
214. Brinkmann U, Lee B, Pastan I. Recombinant immunotoxins containing the V_H or V_L domain of monoclonal antibody B3 fused to Pseudomonas exotoxin. J Immunol 1993;150:2774.
215. Hertler A, Schlossman D, Borowitz M, Blythman H, Casellas P, Frankel A. An anti-CD5 immunotoxin for chronic lymphocytic leukemia: enhancement of cytotoxicity with human serum albumin-monensin. Int J Cancer 1989;43:215.
216. Jansen B, Vallera D, Jaszcz W, Nguyen D, Kersey J. Successful treatment of human acute T-cell leukemia in SCID mice using the anti-CD7-deglycosylated ricin A-chain immunotoxin DA7. Cancer Res 1992;52:1314.
217. Sausville E, Headlee D, Stetler-Stevenson M, Jaffe E, Figg W, Amlot P, Kaplan L, Stone M, Wittes R, Ghetie V, Schindler J, Uhr J, Vitetta E. Deglycosylated ricin-A chain immunotoxins in the treatment of B-cell non-Hodgkin's lymphoma. Proceedings, Fourth International Symposium on Immunotoxins, Myrtle Beach, 1995, p 122.
218. Amlot P, Stone M, Cunningham D, Fay J, Newman J, Collins R, May R, McCarthy M, Richardson J, Ghetie V, Ramilo O, Thorpe P, Uhr J, Vitetta E. A phase I study of an anti-CD22-deglycosylated ricin A chain immunotoxin in the treatment of B-cell lymphomas resistant to conventional therapy. Blood 1993;82:2625.
219. Schnell R, Hatwig M, Radszuhn A, Cebe F, Drillich S, Schon G, Bohlen H, Tesch H, Hansmann M, Schindler J, Ghetie V, Uhr J, Diehl V, Vitetta E, Engert A. A clinical phase I study of an anti-CD25-deglycosylated ricin A-chain immunotoxin (RFT5-SMPT-dgA) in patients with refractory Hodgkin's disease. Proceedings, Fourth International Symposium on Immunotoxins, Myrtle Beach, 1995, p 126.
220. Spitler L, del Rio M, Khentigan A, Wedel N, Brophy N, Miller L, Harkonen W, Rosendorf L, Lee H, Mischak R, Kawahata R, Stoudemire J, Fradkin L, Bautista E, Scannon P. Therapy of patients with malignant melanoma using a monoclonal antimelanoma antibody-ricin A chain immunotoxin. Cancer Res 1987;47:1717.
221. Byers V, Rodvien R, Grant K, Durrant L, Hudson K, Baldwin R, Scannon P. Phase I study of monoclonal antibody ricin A chain immunotoxin XOMAZYME-791 in patients with metastatic colon cancer. Cancer Res 1989;47:6153.
222. Gould B, Borowitz M, Groves E, Carter P, Anthony D, Weiner J, Frankel A. A phase I study of a continuous infusion anti-breast cancer immunotoxin: report of a targeted toxicity not predicted by animal studies. JNCI 1989;81:775.
223. Bookman M, Godfrey S, Padavic K, Griffin T, Corda J, Hamilton T, Ozols R, Groves E. Anti-transferrin receptor immunotoxin (IT) therapy: phase I intraperitoneal (i.p.) trial. Proc Am Soc Clin Oncol 1990;9:187.
224. Grossbard M, Freedman A, Ritz J, Coral F, Goldmacher V, Eliseo L, Spector N, Dear K, Lambert J, Blattler W, Taylor J, Nadler L. Serotherapy of B-cell neoplasms with anti-B4-blocked ricin. A phase I trial of daily bolus infusion. Blood 1992;79:576.
225. Epstein C, Lynch T, Shefner J, Wen P, Maxted D, Braman V, Ariniello P, Coral F, Ritz J. Use of the immunotoxin N901-blocked ricin in patients with small-cell lung cancer. Int J Cancer suppl 1994;8:57.
226. Roy D, Griffin J, Belvin M, Blattler W, Lambert J, Ritz J. Anti-My9-blocked ricin: an immunotoxin for selective targeting of acute myeloid leukemia cells. Blood 1991;77: 2404.
227. Uckun F. B43-pokeweed antiviral protein (B43-PAP) immunotoxin. Proceedings, Fourth International Symposium on Immunotoxins, Myrtle Beach, 1995, p 134.
228. Flavell D, Boehm D, Noss A, Emery L, Flavell S. Therapy of human B-cell lymphoma bearing SCID mice is more effective with anti-CD19 and anti-CD38-saporin immunotoxins used in combination than with either immunotoxin used alone. Proceedings, Fourth International Symposium on Immunotoxins, Myrtle Beach, 1995, p 98.
229. Falini B, Bolognesi A, Flenghi L, Tazzari P, Broe M, Stein H, Durkop H, Aversa F, Corneli P, Pizzolo G, Barbabietola G, Sabattini E, Pileri S, Martelli M, Stirpe F. Response of refractory Hodgkin's disease to monoclonal anti-CD30 immunotoxin. Lancet 1992;339:1–195.
230. Pai L, Bookman M, Ozols R, Young R, Smith J, Longo D, Gould B, Frankel A, McClay E, Howell S, Reed E, Willingham M, FitzGerald D, Pastan I. Clinical evaluation of intraperitoneal Pseudomonas exotoxin immunoconjugate OVB3-PE in patients with ovarian cancer. J Clin Oncol 1991;9:2095.
231. Bjorn M, Ring D, Frankel A. Evaluation of monoclonal antibodies for the development of breast cancer immunotoxins. Cancer Res 1985;45:1214.
232. Preijers F, Tax W, DeWitte T, Janssen A, Heijden H, Vidal H, Wessels J, Capel P. Relationship between internalization and cytotoxicity of ricin A-chain immunotoxins. Br J Haematol 1988;70:289.
233. LeMaistre CF, Deisseroth A, Fogel B, Meneghetti C, Ma J, Anderson J, Saria E, Lomen P, Byers V. Phase I trial of H65-RTA in patients with chronic lymphocytic leukemia. Blood 76 (suppl) 1990;1:295a.
234. LeMaistre C, Rosen S, Frankel A, Kornfeld S, Saria E, Meneghetti C, Drajesk J, Fishwild D, Scannon P, Byers V. Phase I trial of H65-RTA immunoconjugate in patients with cutaneous T-cell lymphoma. Blood 1991;76:1173.
235. Waldman T, Pastan I, Gansow O, Junghans R. The multichain interleukin-2 receptor: a target for immunotherapy. Ann Intern Med 1992;116:148.
236. Weiner L, O'Dwyer J, Kitson J, Comis R, Frankel A, Bauer R, Konrad M, Groves E. Phase I evaluation of an anti-breast ca monoclonal antibody 260F9-recombinant ricin A chain immunoconjugate. Cancer Res 1989;49:4062.
237. Laske D, Muraszko K, Oldfield E, DeVroom H, Sung C, Dedrick R, Simon T, Solomon D, Copeland C, Katz D, Groves E, Greenfield L, Houston L, Youle R. Intraventricular immunotoxin therapy for leptomeningeal neoplasia. Third International Symposium on Immunotoxins, Orlando, 1992, p 124.
238. Vitetta E, Stone M, Amlot P, Fay J, May R, Till M, Newman J, Clark P, Collins R, Cunningham D, Ghetie V, Uhr J, Thorpe P. Phase I immunotoxin trial in patients with B-cell lymphoma. Cancer Res 1991;51:4052.
239. Spitler L, Mishak R, Scannon P. Therapy of metastatic melanoma with Xomazyme Mel, a murine monoclonal antibody -ricin A chain immunotoxin. Nucl Med Bul 1989;16:625.
240. LeMaistre CF, Craig F, Meneghetti C, McMullin B, Parker K, Reuben J, Boldt D, Rosenblum M, Woodworth T. Phase I trial of a 90-minute infusion of the fusion toxin DAB486IL-2 in hematological cancers. Cancer Res 1993;53:3930.
241. Foss F, Nichols J, Parker K. Seragen Lymphoma Study Group. Phase I/II trial of DAB_{389}IL-2 in patients with NHL, HD and CTCL. Proceedings, Fourth International Symposium on Immunotoxins, Myrtle Beach, 1995, p 140.
242. Pai L, Wittes R, Setser A, Goldspiel B, FitzGerald D, Willingham M, Pastan I. Phase I and pharmacokinetic study of the immunotoxin LMB-1 (B3-LysPE38). Proceedings, Fourth International Symposium on Immunotoxins, Myrtle Beach, 1995, p 128.
243. Laske D, Oldfield E, Youle R. Immunotoxins for brain tumor therapy. Proceedings, Fourth International Symposium on Immunotoxins, Myrtle Beach, 1995, p 127.
244. Grossbard M, Gribben J, Freedman A, Lambert J, Kinsella J, Rabinowe S, Eliseo L, Taylor J, Blattler W, Epstein C, Nadler L. Adjuvant immunotoxin therapy with anti-B4-blocked ricin after autologous bone marrow transplantation for patients with B-cell non-Hodgkin's lymphoma. Blood 1993;81:2263.
245. Esseltine D, Braman G, Lambert J, Blattler W. Clinical studies using anti-B4-blocked ricin (anti-B4-bR) in leukemias and lymphomas. Proceedings, Fourth International Symposium on Immunotoxins, Myrtle Beach, 1995, p 124.
246. Estis L, Krueger J, Nichols J, Parker K. Psoriasis: a potential target for DAB_{389}IL-2. Proceedings, Fourth International Symposium on Immunotoxins, Myrtle Beach, 1995, p 136.
247. Soler-Rodriguez A, Ghetie M, Oppenheimer-Marks N, Uhr J, Vitetta E. Ricin A-chain and ricin A-chain immunotoxins rapidly damage human endothelial cells: implications for vascular leak syndrome. Exp Cell Res 1993;206:227.
248. Willingham M, Tagge D, Brothers T, Frankel A. Apoptosis of endothelial cells: a potential mechanism for the vascular leak syndrome associated with immunotoxin therapy. Proceedings, Fourth International Symposium on Immunotoxins, Myrtle Beach, 1995, p 99.
249. Chace D, Siegall C. Characterization of immunotoxin-induced vascular leak syndrome in rats. Proceedings, Fourth International Symposium on Immunotoxins, Myrtle Beach, 1995, p 105.
250. Siegall C, Liggitt D, Chace D, Tepper M, Fell H. Prevention of immunotoxin-mediated vascular leak syndrome in rats with retention of antitumor activity. Proc Natl Acad Sci USA 1994;91:9514.
251. Ohnuma T, Kikuchi T, Kohno N, Spitler L, Holland J. Penetration of immunotoxin and cytotoxic agents into multicellular tumor spheroids and their cell kill effects. Proceedings, Fourth International Symposium on Immunotoxins, Myrtle Beach, 1995, p 109.
252. Sung C, van Osdol W. Effects of molecular weight and intracellular processing on tumor penetration of immunotoxins. Proceedings, Fourth International Symposium on Immunotoxins, Myrtle Beach, 1995, p 107.
253. Roscoe D, Jung S, Benhar I, Pai L, Lee B, Pastan I. Primate antibody response to immunotoxin: serological and computer-aided analysis of epitopes on a truncated form of Pseudomonas exotoxin. Infect Immun 1994;62:5055.
254. Lemley P, Amanatides P, Wright D. Identification and characterization of a monoclonal antibody that neutralizes ricin toxicity in vitro and in vivo. Hybridoma 1994;13: 417.
255. Pai L, FitzGerald D, Tepper M, Schacter B, Spitalny G, Pastan I. Inhibition of antibody response to Pseudomonas exotoxin and an immunotoxin containing Pseudomonas exotoxin by 15-deoxyspergualin in mice. Cancer Res 1990;50:7750.
256. Linsley P, Ledbetter J. The role of CD28 receptor during T cell responses to antigen. Ann Rev Immunol 1993;11:191.
257. Rybak S, Hoogenboom H, Meade H, Youle R. Humanization of immunotoxins. Proc Natl Acad Sci USA 1992;89:3165.
258. Oratz R, Speyer J, Wernz J, Hochster H, Meyers M, Mischak R, Spitler L. Anti-melanoma monoclonal antibody-ricin A chain immunoconjugate (XMMME-001-RTA) plus cyclophosphamide in the treatment of metastatic malignant melanoma: results of a phase II trial. J Biol Respir Mod 1990;9:345.
259. Schipper H, Perry S. Kinetics of normal and leukemic leucocyte populations and relevance to chemotherapy. Cancer Res 1970;30:1883.
260. Schipper H, Goh C, Wang T. Shifting the cancer paradigm: must we kill to cure? J Clin Oncol 1995;13:801.
261. Burrows F, Thorpe P. Eradication of large solid tumors in mice with an immunotoxin directed against tumor vasculature. Proc Natl Acad Sci USA 1993;90:8996.

SECTION XIX

PRINCIPLES OF GENE THERAPY

CHAPTER 84

Cancer Gene Therapy

HOWARD A. FINE AND DONALD W. KUFE

Advances in our understanding of the molecular and cellular biology of cancer have led to improved tools for the diagnosis of cancer and cancer risk. Advances have also led to the identification and pharmaceutical development of a number of biologics, such as interleukin-2 (IL-2) and interferon alpha (INF-α), that have limited usefulness in the treatment of a number of malignancies. Additionally, several cytokines, such as granulocyte colony-stimulating factor (G-CSF), granulocyte-monocyte colony-stimulating factor (GM-CSF), and erythropoeitin, have been approved for use in the supportive care of patients undergoing chemotherapy and radiotherapy. Despite all the advances made in molecular biology thus far, only a few have translated into significant advances in cancer therapy. Gene therapy represents another attempt to take lessons learned in the laboratory and apply them directly to the development of novel cancer therapies. The excitement over the potential power of gene therapy has stimulated collaboration between scientists and clinicians, and between academic and the private sector, in unprecedented ways. The enthusiasm for gene therapy is represented by the rapidly growing number of journals and biotechnology companies devoted to the science and business of therapeutic gene transfer. In this chapter we define basic terminology and the principles that underlie the science behind gene transfer. We also describe gene therapy strategies that are currently being employed for the treatment of cancer.

Gene therapy can be loosely defined as the transfer of nucleic acids into target cells for the purpose of perturbing or correcting some pathophysiologic process. Gene transfer is generally divided into two major categories: (*a*) in vitro gene therapy, in which genes are transferred (or transduced) into target cells ex vivo and those cells are then placed back into the animal or patient, and (*b*) in vivo gene therapy, in which the gene is directly transduced into target cells in vivo. The strategy behind therapeutic gene transfer involves at least two separate but interrelated components: the therapeutic nucleic acid or gene, and the delivery system. The mechanism of action of the gene product, its size, the need for stability of expression, and the expected effect on the transduced cell and organism are all important variables in selecting an appropriate therapeutic gene. The second component of therapeutic gene transfer involves the delivery of the therapeutic gene to the intended target cell, which expresses the transgene. The delivery system, or vector, is generally made up of a "minigene cassette" consisting of a nucleic acid sequence or element (promoter) that drives transcription of the target gene (or "transgene") and a polyadenylation signal that stabilizes the transcribed messenger RNA (mRNA). The minigene cassette is usually located within a larger nucleic acid backbone that consists of sequences as simple as those found in bacteriophage (thereby allowing in vitro propagation of the vector in bacteria) or as complicated as large DNA viruses. Finally, the minigene cassette within the DNA backbone is often encapsulated by other macromolecules, such as proteins and carbohydrates, that perform specific functions in the stabilization, targeting, and expression of the transgene.

The number of genes identified as having potential value for gene therapy is increasing rapidly. However, the selective and efficient delivery as well as expression of these genes present great challenges to the successful application of therapeutic gene transfer in humans. Thus, much of the current emphasis in the basic science of gene therapy is being placed on the development of better vectors.

Gene Transfer Systems

Gene delivery systems can be divided into two major categories, viral-based and non-viral-based vectors. Viral vectors are presently more efficient, and the vast majority of animal and clinical trials are using these systems. Therefore, the following section is devoted primarily to viral-based vectors.

VIRAL VECTORS

The basic premise behind the use of viral-based vectors is the attempt to use the inherent ability of these obligate intracellular organisms to carry foreign genetic material into eukaryotic cells and to exploit the cellular machinery to encode viral genes. An understanding of vector function requires knowledge of the biology of RNA and DNA viruses. The reader is referred to the appropriate chapters in this book and to several excellent reviews (1, 2).

Retroviral Vectors

The most common vectors currently in use for gene therapy are recombinant retroviruses. These small, single-stranded RNA viruses were originally discovered because of their propensity to cause tumors in animals. The most common retroviral vectors are based on Moloney murine leukemia retrovirus (MoMULV). These simple viruses consist of the 5′ and 3′ long terminal repeats (LTRs) and the three *gag*, *pol*, and *env* structural genes. *Gag* encodes preproteins that are eventually cleaved into the three proteins that form the shell of the virion. *Pol* encodes the enzymes, including reverse transcriptase (RT), integrase, and RNase H, the last of which is necessary for viral integration into host chromosomal DNA. The *env* gene encodes the envelope glycoprotein that protrudes from the lipid membrane surrounding the virion and that functions as the ligand for the cellular viral receptor. Several years ago it was shown that viruses deleted of one or more of their structural genes (e.g., *env*) are still fully infectious as long as the missing gene is supplied by the viral producer cell (3). A foreign gene, or "transgene," can then be placed into the deleted virus. When this deleted virus infects a target cell it integrates into the host genome and mediates expression of viral genes as well as the transgene. Following infection (or transduction) of the target cell, however, the viral vector is incapable of undergoing another round of infection because the gene necessary for viral replication has been deleted and is not expressed in the target cell. In this way the vector allows transfer and expression of the transgene but avoids induction of active infection in the host.

Since these initial observations were made, it has been demonstrated that both the 5′ and 3′ LTRs and a short sequence just 5′ to the initiation codon of *gag* (the "packaging sequence") are sufficient to allow packaging of this minimal vector, as long as all of the structural genes are supplied by the producer cell. To accomplish this, a number of cell lines have been created that stably express structural genes of different retroviruses but do not express packageable RNA transcripts. One can then transfect these packaging cell lines (now making them "producer cell lines") with a minimal vector containing the transgene of interest, and use the harvested recombinant viruses to transduce target cells.

The advantages of these vectors include their relative simplicity, which makes construction of different vectors relatively simple. This simplicity also means that vectors can be created that express no viral genes at all, thereby minimizing the chance for the development of significant antiviral immune responses. Retroviruses integrate into target cell DNA, thus achieving stable integration of the transgene. Theoretically, stable integration should allow for long-term transgene expression, although in reality expression usually falls off with time because of methylation of the LTR (4). Another potential advantage of MoMULV-based vectors is that the specific envelope receptor is found on almost all human cell types. Thus, cell type is not a limiting factor for vector transduction. On the other hand, a potential disadvantage to retrovirus-based vectors is the ubiquitous distribution of the receptor and thereby little target cell selectivity. Recently, however, hybrid envelope proteins have been constructed as a result of fusing a portion of the natural *env* gene to a DNA sequence that encodes a ligand for a specific cell surface receptor, thereby targeting only cells that express that receptor. An example of such an approach is fusion of the binding domain of erythropoietin to the envelope glycoprotein, thus creating recombinant retroviral vectors that selectively target cells which express the erythropoietin receptor.

Another important limitation of retrovirus-based vectors is that MoMULV-based vectors can only infect and integrate into actively dividing cells. This property is important, because most solid tumors have relatively low growth fractions in vivo (<20% of cells are in active cell cycle at any given time), thus making it unlikely that retroviral vectors would be capable of transducing a significant proportion of the tumor. Further, cell-free infection with retroviruses is very inefficient; generally, direct cell-to-cell contact is required for optimal transduction efficiency. Finally, there are biosafety concerns based on the potential for retroviral vector–mediated insertional mutagenesis that could result in malignant transformation of the target cell. Although this seems highly unlikely, and no murine retrovirus has ever been demonstrated to be pathogenic in humans, a recent study in nonhuman primates demonstrated the development of lymphomas/leukemias following treatment of monkeys with high doses of retroviral vectors contaminated by helper viruses (replication-competent virus) (5). For many of these reasons, retroviruses are best suited for in vitro transduction, in which specific target cells can be isolated and induced to divide, and are thereby transduced with efficiency and selectivity. For strategies that require in vivo gene transduction, the ultimate utility of retroviral vectors appears less certain.

Adenoviral Vectors

Adenoviruses contain linear, double-stranded DNA complexed with core proteins surrounded by capsid proteins (6). There are nearly 50 distinct serotypes of adenovirus. The prototype adenovirus vector is based on adenovirus type 5 (Ad5), a common serotype belonging to the subgroup C (6). By convention, the 36-kilobase (kb) of adenovirus DNA is divided into 100 map units (mu; 360 base pairs [bp]/mu). The structure of the adenovirus is described on the basis of the timing of the adenovirus genes expressed following infection of human cells. The viral genome is transcribed in two major stages, an early (E) phase, which precedes viral DNA replication, and a late (L) phase, which starts 6 to 8 hours later. Among the early-phase genes the E1A and E1B products are the first adenovirus proteins generated after infection and are critical for viral replication. Other early region genes encode regulatory proteins or genes necessary for viral replication and late gene transcription. The late region genes are mostly related to production of the structural proteins required for assembly of the nucleoprotein core and the capsid forming the outer shell of the virus (6, 7).

Adenovirus vectors have been constructed based on the observation that deletion of the E1A and part of the E1B genes renders virus replication deficient. Vector propagation can be achieved by transfection of the E1A-deleted adenoviral vector DNA into 293 cells. These cells harbor a stably integrated segment of a defective adenoviral genome, and thus can provide E1 gene function in trans. Recent data suggest that adenoviruses can efficiently package up to approximately 105% of their total genomic DNA content. Thus, E1A-deleted viruses can generally accommodate inserts of 5 to 6 kb. An additional 2 kb of space can be made for foreign gene insertion by deleting the E3 portion of the adenoviral genome (8). Although E3 may have an important role in the interaction of the virus with the host immune system, E3 has not been shown to be important for adenovirus growth in vitro, and E3-deleted viruses appear to be fully infectious.

Adenoviral vectors have a number of potential advantages over retroviral vectors, including high-efficiency cell-free infection of most human cell types (9, 10). Additionally, adenoviral vectors can transduce nondividing as well as dividing cells (11). Because adenoviral virions are relatively stable and resistant to physical manipulation, vectors can be concentrated to high titers and frozen for use at later times (something that is not generally possible with retroviruses because of their fragility under physical stresses like freezing). A promoter of choice can be used to drive the inserted transgene, thereby a mechanism of tissue-selective expression or inducibility. In contrast, the use of heterologous promoters in retroviral vectors is much more problematic because promoter-mediated selectivity is often overridden by the strong constitutive promoter activity of the LTR. Another advantage of adenoviral vectors is that since they exist within the target cell as episomal DNA, insertional mutagenesis is much less of a concern than it is for retroviral vectors.

The major disadvantage of the current generation of adenoviral vectors is that they provoke a significant host immune response (12). A cellular host response against adenoviral-transduced cells causes a local inflammatory reaction that can potentially result in damage to the target tissue (13). As demonstrated in animal models, local inflammation results in relatively short duration of adenoviral vector–mediated transgene expression because of destruction of the transduced cells. The major stimulus for this cellular response may be low-level production of late adenoviral structural proteins. Thus, a current theme in adenoviral vector development is to create vectors that express few or no viral proteins and thereby lessen target tissue inflammation and extend transgene expression. Another potential concern in using adenoviral vectors in vivo is the development of virus-neutralizing antibodies. Attempts at rechallenging immunocompetent animals with multiple administrations of adenoviral vectors have resulted in greatly diminished transgene expression. Lack of effectiveness of these subsequent vector challenges correlates with the development of neutralizing antibodies to adenovirus. Antiviral antibodies may prove to be an even greater problem in clinical trials because most people have been previously exposed to wild-type adenovirus and thus may already have neutralizing antibodies.

Herpes Simplex Virus–Based Vectors

HSV-based vectors, although initially developed for gene transfer into the central nervous system, may eventually be useful for cancer gene therapy (25). HSV is a large (150-kb) double-stranded DNA virus that is naturally neurotropic but highly infectious to many types of epithelial cells. HSV can follow a replicative or latency life cycle after infection. The replicative life cycle is typically cytopathic. Infected cells release high titers of virus, which eventually result in cell lysis (14). In contrast to the burst of viral activity in the lytic life cycle, the latency life cycle is associated with little viral gene transcription and normal host cell function. The two major types of HSV vectors are plasmid-derived vectors and recombinant vectors. Plasmid-derived vectors require a wild-type helper virus and therefore are not useful for most in vivo studies (15). Recombinant vectors are constructed by homologous recombination between wild-type HSV and cloning vectors that carry homologous flanking sequences (in the same way that adenovirus vectors are constructed) (16). Through the use of these cloning vectors it is possible to mutate specific viral genes and thereby make it theoretically possible to control the degree of vector toxicity, replication, and neurovirulence. In theory, HSV vectors offer a number of potential advantages for gene transfer, including their ability to accommodate at least 30 kb of foreign DNA, a high efficiency of cell transduction in a wide host range, and the potential for establishing latency with long-term transgene expression.

A number of difficulties have arisen with the current generation of HSV vectors. It has been difficult to generate stocks of replication-incompetent virus because of the complexity of the herpes genome and the lack of a complete understanding of the function of many of the viral genes. Even though replication-incompetent herpes vectors have been recently described, vector-mediated cytotoxicity may still be a problem because of the expression of a number of ill-defined viral genes. Expression of these genes in vivo also contributes to the potential for a significant antiviral immune response, as is the case for adenoviral vectors. The high predilection of herpes infection for neuronal cells raises concern over the development of neuropathic effects following in vivo vector transduction. In addition, HSV disrupts normal cellular macromolecule synthesis during replicative infection, and many vector-based promoters may not be active during latent infection (17). Thus, despite many potential advantages to the use of HSV vectors, much in vitro work is required before a safe and reliable vector is available for widespread clinical use.

Adeno-Associated Virus

AAV is a parvovirus with a small, single-stranded DNA genome of approximately 5,000 bp. AAV is dependent for its replication on factors provided by helper viruses such as adenovirus, herpesvirus, and vaccinia virus (18, 19). Genotoxic stress may also induce factors permissive for AAV replication (20, 21). AAV has a number of characteristics that make it attractive for vector development. The genome is small and relatively simple, so that it would be easy to manipulate genetically. Like retroviruses, a minimal vector devoid of all structural genes except for only the inverted terminal repeats (ITRs) and a small packaging signal is sufficient for vector packaging and transfer as long as the replicative (rep) and structural (cap) genes are supplied in trans (22). Additionally, AAV stably integrates into the host genome, with a special predilection for a small region on chromosome 19 (23). Whether site-specific integration offers an advantage over the random integration found with retroviral vectors relative to transgene expression and the potential for insertional mutagenesis remains uncertain. Finally, AAV is reportedly capable of infecting and integrating into nondividing cells, a property that would be important and distinguish it from other available viral vectors. To date, however, the data remain inconclusive as to whether this really occurs, particularly in the context of a deleted AAV vector. As promising as AAV appears, the widespread use of these vectors is currently limited by low vector titers secondary to difficulty in constructing high-efficiency packaging cell lines. Another practical and major limitation of AAV vectors is the relatively small size constraint (approximately 4,000 bp) that can be packaged into AAV virions.

Other Viruses

As our understanding of molecular virology increases, a number of additional viruses will undoubtedly be utilized as genetic vectors. Vectors based on vaccinia and polio have already been developed for cancer vaccine purposes (see below), while vectors based on the Epstein-Barr virus have been shown to be capable of transiently expressing transgenes at high levels.

NONVIRAL VECTORS

There are a number of strategies to deliver foreign genes to cells without using virally based vectors. These methods generally rely on normal cellular mechanisms for uptake of macromolecules. The oldest of these methods is calcium phosphate (Ca_2PO_4) precipitation, whereby DNA is complexed to Ca_2PO_4 crystals with subsequent entry of the complex through the cell membrane by an ill-defined mechanism. Electroporation is another common laboratory technique for gene transfer: passage of an electrical current across the cell leads to transient opening of unidentified channels in the cellular membrane and the entry of foreign DNA. Both Ca_2PO_4 precipitation and electroporation are rather inefficient processes that generally allow transduction of no more than 0.1 to 10% of all cells, and both are limited to transduction of cells in vitro.

The simplest method of gene transfer is the injection of naked DNA (24). Such transfer can be accomplished in vitro using microinjection techniques to introduce DNA into individual cells. Needless to say, this is a tedious process that allows transduction of only a few cells, in contrast to the millions of cells that can be transduced using virally based vectors. Nevertheless, this technique is useful for the transduction of highly selected cells such as oocytes and embryonic cells. Likewise, direct injection of naked DNA into tissue (e.g., cardiac and skeletal muscle, liver) results in low-level transient gene expression (25). Expression can be improved by techniques that allow DNA to be injected with greater force. An example of such a strategy is the "gene gun:" naked DNA is coated onto microprojectiles (often minute gold pellets) and injected into the target tissue by means of a burst of air. This approach may prove important, in light of recent observations that plasmid injection into muscle is an efficient means of generating an immune response to the plasmid-encoded transgene (26). Thus, the use of plasmid DNA may still be an important method for vaccine gene therapy strategies (see below). A somewhat surprising finding is that naked plasmid DNA injected intravenously into animals results in diffuse, multiorgan, transient expression of a transgene. Although this use of plasmid DNA is theoretically attractive because of its relative safety and poor immunogenicity, intravenous administration of plasmid DNA will probably prove far too nonspecific and inefficient to be useful for most gene therapy applications.

Liposomes represent a widely used, non-viral-vector-based gene transfer approach. In their simplest form, liposomes are bilipid membranes surrounding an aqueous center. Hydrophilic substances such as drugs or nucleic acids can be stably maintained within the aqueous milieu of the liposome. Contact and fusion of the surrounding lipid membrane with cell membranes enhance the efficiency of DNA entry into the cell cytoplasm. Liposome-mediated DNA transduction in vitro is significantly more efficient than Ca_2PO_4 transfection or electroporation, and more efficient than plasmid DNA transduction in vivo (27). Like plasmid DNA, however, liposomes lack target cell specificity and in general are much less efficient for overall gene transduction than most viral vectors.

Recent efforts to improve non-viral-vector-mediated gene transduction have centered on attempts to exploit the receptor-mediated endocytic pathway. These strategies involve the generation of complexes consisting of plasmid DNA with specific polypeptide ligands (28). One of the first examples of such a strategy was the targeting of the asialoglycoprotein receptor on hepatocytes by conjugating the polypeptide ligand for this receptor to a complex of poly-L-lysine and plasmid DNA. A similar strategy was used to target cells that expressed the transferrin receptor (29, 30). Of relevance for cancer gene therapy is the finding that the concentration of transferrin receptors on cells correlates with their proliferative potential, and thus many cancer cells overexpress the receptor. Thus, transferrin-based ligand-DNA complexes may be selectively targeted to tumor cells, particularly when the tumor cells reside in tissues with low concentrations of transferrin receptors.

Although the initial work with DNA-polypeptide ligand complexes demonstrated the ability to achieve target cell selectivity, the level of transgene expression was disappointingly low and the duration of expression short. Following binding of the polypeptide ligand to its cell surface receptor the complex is internalized by way of the endocytic pathway. Much of the DNA internalized within the endosome is then degraded or damaged by the intraendosomal acidic environment or by nucleases. Recent efforts to improve the level and duration of transgene expression following DNA-ligand complex transduction have focused on methods of disrupting the endocytic pathway. Disruption has been achieved by binding inactivated adenoviral virions to the DNA-ligand complex (31, 32); the complex-containing endosome is rapidly disrupted secondary to the ability of a portion of the adenoviral virion to fuse with, and disrupt the endosomal lipid membrane (33). As specific "fusogenic" peptides, such as the influenza hemagglutinating antigen (HA) peptide and the penton base (one of the viral core proteins) of adenovirus, are identified, more refined strategies are being developed to incorporate these peptides into the DNA-polypeptide ligand complexes (34).

Non-virus-based delivery systems represent a potentially safer method of in vivo gene transfer than the use of viral vectors. These approaches are also less likely to induce a significant antivector immune response than that associated with viral vectors. With the recent advances in ligand targeting, nonviral delivery systems also offer the promise of improved target cell selectivity. Nevertheless, non-viral-vector-mediated in vivo gene transduction is presently at least an order of magnitude less efficient than viral vector gene transfer. Thus, although it is likely that nonviral delivery systems will ultimately replace viral vectors, virus-based vectors will continue to be the principal method of in vivo gene transduction for the foreseeable future.

SELECTIVE GENE EXPRESSION

One of the major limiting factors of standard chemotherapy and radiotherapy is toxicity to normal tissue secondary to nonselective DNA damage. Gene therapy strategies aimed at transferring cytotoxic genes to tumor cells will ultimately face a similar problem of nonselectivity. There are several potential ways to make gene transduction more selective. The natural tropism of some viral vectors for specific cell types based on the presence or absence of the appropriate viral receptor theoretically might allow for some level of selectivity. Unfortunately, receptors for the amphotropic murine retroviruses, the adenoviral receptor, and the herpes virus receptor all appear to be ubiquitously expressed on most human cell types. As discussed, alternative strategies are being developed with hybrid envelope glycoproteins that target specific target cell receptors (e.g., erythropoietin receptor). Other vectors are also being constructed based on retroviruses that use different envelopes, and thus different receptors, than those used by MoMULV. Such examples include retroviral vectors based on the human immunodeficiency virus (HIV) that specifically target cells that express CD4. MoMULV-based vector retroviruses have some level of target cell selectivity in that viral integration and expression only occur in cells that are actively dividing. To date, however, both adenovirus-, AAV-, and herpes-based vectors remain almost totally nonselective in host range.

If viral vector host range cannot be made substantially more restrictive, gene transfer can potentially still be made more selective by constructing vectors with genetic elements that are activated in only certain cell types. Thus, it is possible to construct retroviral and adenoviral vectors that transduce a wide spectrum of cell types but only express the transgene in selected cells. Such selective gene expression is achieved through the construction of viral vectors with promoter and/or enhancer elements that mediate tissue-selective transcription. Examples of vectors with tissue-selective expression include those the α-1 antitrypsin and albumin promoters (liver selective), tyrosine hydroxylase promoter (melanocytes), villin promoter (intestinal epithelium), glial fibrillary acidic protein promoter (astrocytes), myelin basic protein promoter (glial cells), immunoglobulin gene enhancer (B lymphocytes), and the globin gene enhancer/promoter (erythroid precursors), to name just a few (35–37). Potentially more exciting has been the recent identification and cloning of promoter/enhancer sequences that appear to be up-regulated in specific cancer cell types. Construction of viral vectors with these sequences has led to vectors that can mediate tumor-selective gene expression. Examples include viral vectors expressing their transgene from the prostate-specific antigen (PSA) promoter (prostate-selective gene expression), DF3/MUC-1 enhancer/promoter (breast carcinoma selective), α-fetoprotein (AFP) promoter (hepatoma selective), and the carcinoembryonic antigen (CEA) (colon cancer selective) (38, 39).

Another strategy for developing better control over transgene expression is through the use of inducible promoters. Such promoters include the metalloproteinase promoter, which can be induced to increase gene expression several hundredfold on exposure to cationic heavy metals such as cadmium or lithium. Whether this promoter will ultimately be useful in vivo remains to be seen, because of the potential toxicity from the heavy metals. The LTR from the mouse mammary tumor virus (MMTV) is inducible by a number of steroid hormones, although the usefulness of this system in vivo may be limited by a relatively high basal level of promoter activity in the noninduced state. Another system that has been useful in transgenic mice utilizes the bacterial lac operon to repress transcription from a heterologous promoter. Transcriptional repression is released following systemic administration of IPTG. Again, toxicity from IPTG administration may not allow use of this strategy in humans.

The tetracycline repressor and radiation-inducible systems are two particularly exciting approaches to transcriptional induction because of their high potential for human application. In the tetracycline system, minigene cassettes are constructed that include the bacterial tet operon mediating transcriptional repression of a heterologous promoter in the presence of the tet repressor (tet^R) protein that is expressed either from another vector or on another coding sequence from the same vector. Transcriptional repression is relieved following exposure to tetracycline, which binds to tet^R and thereby prevents its interaction with the tet operon (40). Not only does this system allow tight control of transgene expression, but release from transcription repression in mammals can be achieved at doses of tetracycline significantly lower than those used for antimicrobial purposes (41). Another strategy for inducible transgene expression with potential human application is the use of radiotherapy-inducible promoters. The promoter from the early growth response gene-1 (*EGR1*) can be induced severalfold on exposure to ionizing radiation in vivo (42). The *EGR1* system demonstrates that it may be possible in the future to have widely distributed viral vectors induced to express transgenes in distinct anatomic locations at distinct times (genetic radiotherapy).

Therapeutic Genes

CHEMOSENSITIZATION GENES

The general strategy behind the transfer of chemosensitization genes is to directly transduce tumor cells with a transgene that encodes a protein that converts an otherwise nontoxic prodrug into a cytotoxic substance. The prototype for chemosensitization genes is the herpes simplex thymidine kinase gene (*tk*).

Herpes Simplex Thymidine Kinase Gene (*tk*)

The mechanism of action of the *tk* gene is based on its ability to phosphorylate a number of nucleoside analogues such as acyclovir and ganciclovir. Once phosphorylated, the nucleotide analogue is incorporated into replicating DNA by DNA polymerase. The incorporated analogue terminates DNA strand and elongation and results in cell death. Eukaryotic cells do not normally possess a *tk* gene and therefore cannot efficiently phosphorylate acyclovir or ganciclovir, which is why these nucleosides are relatively nontoxic to nontransduced cells. The potential success of this strategy is supported by the demonstration that *tk*-transduced experimental animal tumors can be eradicated following treatment of animals with ganciclovir (43).

An example of this strategy can be found in the experiments by Culver and co-workers. When mouse fibroblasts, genetically engineered to produce retroviruses that carry the *tk* gene (producer cells), were injected into established experimental gliomas in vivo, animals were cured of their tumor by systemic treatment with ganciclovir. This finding was considered surprising because of the expectation that every tumor cell would need to be transduced by the *tk* gene in order to eradicate the entire tumor—an unlikely occurrence, given the inefficiency of retrovirus-mediated gene transduction in vivo. Indeed, similar experiments with a retrovirus that transduces the β-galactosidase marker gene revealed that only 10 to 70% of all tumor cells within the established gliomas were directly transduced by the retrovirus. These findings indicated that not every cell within the tumor has to be transduced by *tk* in order to completely eradicate the tumor. This phenomenon has been referred to as the "bystander effect" (44). The mechanism responsible for the bystander effect remains unknown, although it is generally believed that it involves passive transfer of phosphorylated ganciclovir from the *tk*-transduced cell to adjacent nontransduced cells via intracellular connections such as gap junctions. This mechanism would explain the in vitro observation that direct cell-to-cell contact is necessary for the bystander effect. Others have suggested that the bystander effect is secondary to a more complex mechanism whereby nontransduced cells are induced to undergo programmed cell death (apoptosis) by signals from adjacent dying *tk*-transduced cells. Whatever the mechanism, the bystander effect is important for the successful utilization of the *tk*-ganciclovir system despite the inability of most currently utilized vectors to transduce every tumor cell in vivo.

Cytosine Deaminase (*cd*)

The *cd* gene is another example of a chemosensitization, or suicide, gene that may be potentially useful for therapeutic gene transfer. Cytosine deaminase is found in a number of organisms, including bacteria and fungi, but not in mammalian cells. Cytosine deaminase has the ability to deaminate a number of pyrimidine analogues including 5-fluorocytosine (5-FC). Deamination of 5-FC results in the formation of the cytotoxic molecule, 5-fluorouracil (5-FU). Recently the *Escherichia coli cd* gene has been cloned and demonstrated to be capable of sensitizing tumor cells to 5-FC (45, 46). In addition to being capable of destroying 5-FU–sensitive tumors such as colon carcinoma, the *cd*-5-FC system can also mediate a powerful cytotoxic effect on tumor cells not usually thought to be 5-FU responsive (e.g., gliomas) (47). The effectiveness of the *cd* system is a result of the extraordinarily high intracellular concentrations of 5-FU that are not obtainable following systemic administration of 5-FU without causing severe toxicity.

Cytosine deaminase has several potential advantages over *tk*, including the fact that 5-FC can be given at very high doses to humans with little toxicity. As with *tk*, *cd*-induced cytotoxicity is associated with a bystander effect. Unlike what occurs with *tk*, however, this bystander effect does not appear to be dependent on direct cell-to-cell contact. The *cd* bystander effect may result from passive transfer of the intracellularly generated 5-FU through the cell membrane into the interstitial space. Thus, any cell in that local area, whether or not in direct contact with the transduced cell, will be exposed to high concentrations of 5-FU. The potential drawback of this bystander effect is that there is little tumor specificity. However, since 5-FU is preferentially toxic to dividing cells, the *cd* system could be utilized for tumors that reside in mitotically quiescent tissues such as the brain (gliomas), liver (breast and colon metastases, hepatoma), and muscle (sarcomas).

Additional Suicide Genes

A number of other genes show promise for chemosensitization gene therapy but are less well characterized than *tk* or *cd* (47a). Among these is the mammalian gene that encodes the cytochrome P-450 2B1 isoenzyme. Cytochrome P-450 2B1 is the specific isoenzyme responsible for converting the frequently utilized chemotherapeutic agent cyclophosphamide to its active metabolite, 4-hydroxycyclophosphamide. Most normal cells but few tumor cells express cytochrome P-450 (48). Thus, introduction of the cDNA encoding cytochrome P-450 2B1 into tumor cells potentially sensitizes them to the cytotoxic effects of cyclophosphamide. C6 rat glioma cells stably transfected with the P-450 2B1 gene become highly sensitive to cyclophosphamide both in vitro and in vivo (49). This cytotoxicity is also associated with a bystander effect.

Other potential chemosensitization genes include the *E. coli gpt* gene, which encodes the xanthine-guanine phosphoribosyl transferase (XGPRT) enzyme. XGPRT, which is usually not found in mammalian cells, can convert the xanthine analogue, 6-thioxanthine to 6-thioxanthine monophosphate by the addition of a ribose phosphate. 6-Thioxanthine monophosphate is then converted by demethylation within the cell to 6-thioguanine monophosphate, a potent inhibitor of nucleic acid synthesis (50). Another *E. coli* gene that may be useful in chemosensitization is DeoD, which encodes a purine nucleoside phosphorylase (PNP) (51). In contrast to mammalian PNP, *E. coli* PNP can hydrolyze the nontoxic drug 6-methylpurine-2′-deoxyribonucleoside to the toxic purine analogue 6-methylpurine. Transduction of DeoD, followed by administration of the prodrug, causes marked cytotoxicity with a pronounced bystander effect that may be secondary to the ability of 6-methylpurine to diffuse across cell membranes.

Transduction of chemosensitization genes is an effective approach to eradicating tumor cells in vitro and experimental tumors in vivo. Successful use of chemosensitization genes in clinical trials, however, will require specific and efficient vector delivery of these genes. Inefficient vector delivery will result in low tumor cell transduction and suboptimal tumor destruction, while nonspecific gene expression will result in normal tissue toxicity (much as occurs with standard chemotherapy). Thus, as promising as the chemosensitization approach appears, the ultimate usefulness of these genes will be closely linked to the development of better vectors.

IMMUNOMODULATORY GENES

For years, investigators have attempted to modulate the immune system to generate an effective antitumor response. Lack of success led to a period of pessimism for immunotherapy. The recent identification of an increasing number of the molecular components of the immune response and development of gene transduction techniques, however, have led to a resurgence of interest in immunotherapy of cancer. The two assumptions underlying gene transduction–based immunotherapy are that tumor-specific antigens exist and that the host immune system is potentially capable of recognizing these antigens and eradicating the tumor cells. The natural host immune response is thought to be incapable of eradicating developing tumors, either because tumor antigens are not recognized and/or presented in the correct context to antigen-presenting cells or because the immune response is not appropriately or efficiently primed to allow the generation of a sufficient effector cell response. Gene therapy strategies are being developed to address each of these potential problems. Several approaches that exemplify the current direction of laboratory and clinical investigation are cited below.

Cytokine Gene-Modified Tumor Cells

Following the cloning of various cytokine genes and characterization of their pleiotropic effects on immune and inflammatory cells, it became apparent to many investigators that local tumor growth and possibly systemic antitumor immunity could be enhanced by one or several of these factors. Accordingly, an approach increasingly used to enhance antitumor immunity in animal tumor models is to transduce tumor cells ex vivo with a specific cytokine gene, irradiate the cells, and transplant them back into the host animal. By means of such an approach, a number of cytokine genes have been shown to reduce tumorigenicity and enhance systemic immunity. Such genes include IL-2, IL-4, IL-1, IL-6, IL-7, IL-12, TNF-α, G-CSF, GM-CSF, JE/MCP-1, and INF-γ, just to name a few (52–61). This strategy does not require sophisticated or efficient vectors since gene transduction is occurring ex vivo. The action of some cytokines, such as IL-4 and G-CSF, results in potent killing of a number of tumor types by inducing local infiltration of effector cells. For IL-4, the most important effector cells appear to be eosinophils, while for G-CSF, granulocytes appear to be the primary antitumor mediator. However, it is generally believed that cytotoxic T-cell responses must be generated for systemic tumor immunity. This assumption may explain the observation that neither IL-4 nor G-CSF induces an effective systemic antitumor response. In contrast, tumor cells transduced by GM-CSF are still directly tumorigenic; however, if these cells are irradiated and used as a vaccine, a systemic antitumor immunity is generated (54). Finally, tumor cells engineered to secrete IL-2 lead to local infiltration by various cytotoxic T-cell and natural killer cell populations and result in both direct tumor cell destruction and the establishment of systemic immunity. As promising as these experiments appear for inducing an effective immune response that is protective against tumor rechallenge, few of these studies have convincingly demonstrated the capability of eradicating large established tumors. Thus, the ultimate usefulness of this approach as a clinical therapeutic strategy remains unproved.

Modulation of Tumor Cell Antigen Presentation

The underlying hypothesis behind the cytokine-transduced tumor cell approach is that an effective immune response can be generated against the tumor cell if the necessary immune effector cells can be appropriately recruited and stimulated. An alternate hypothesis, however, for the lack of an effective antitumor immune response is that tumor antigens are not appropriately presented to T cells or they do not exist. In the generation of an effective cytotoxic T-cell response, the T-cell receptor (TCR) must be presented with the specific antigen complexed to a major histocompatibility complex (MHC) type I molecule by an antigen-presenting cell (APC). Why tumor cells that express MHC molecules on their surface, and presumably tumor-specific antigens, fail to elicit an effective T-cell response remains a fundamental question in tumor immunology. One possible explanation comes from recent observations that additional "co-stimulatory" (i.e., B7) molecules must be present on the APC to fully activate cytotoxic T cells following interaction of the antigen-MHC complex with the TCR. Because only professional APCs generally express these co-stimulatory molecules, tumor cells may not be capable of eliciting an efficient T-cell response. Recent studies in animals have shown that when B7 is transfected into a highly malignant melanoma cell line and then implanted into an immunocompetent mouse, tumors initially grow and then completely regress over 3 to 4 weeks (62). Further, these animals are protected against subsequent rechallenge with the parental (non-B7-expressing cells) cell line. This has led to a strategy whereby a patient's tumor cells are transduced ex vivo with B7, irradiated, and then reimplanted back into the patient. Whether such a simplistic approach will be sufficient for generating antitumor immunity is unknown. Indeed, one group of investigators working with the same melanoma animal model system found that B7 transduction is not sufficient to elicit antitumor immunity unless the tumor cells are also transduced with a viral antigen known to be capable of eliciting a strong cytotoxic response (63). The explanation for these discrepant results remains unclear, but emphasizes the complexity of the immune response and our lack of a complete understanding of all the signals necessary for inducing antitumor immunity.

A similar approach currently being explored is based on

the assumption that although tumor antigens exist, tumor cells are unable to present antigens because they lack functional MHC class I expression (64). This concept is supported by the demonstration that an effective T-cell–mediated antitumor response is generated when tumor cells lacking functional MHC molecules are transduced in vitro with genes encoding the HLA-B7 MHC molecule and are then implanted into the host. Immune responses can also be elicited following in vivo transduction of tumor cells by HLA-B7 (65). The observation in the initial pilot study that one of five melanoma patients responded to transduction of HLA-B7 has led to a multi-institutional trial of direct intralesional injection of HLA-B7 plasmid DNA.

Although strategies aimed at transducing tumor cells with certain membrane proteins to more efficiently present antigens to T cells are under investigation, it must be appreciated that the generation of an effective T-cell response requires a complex interaction of a number of cell types, cytokines, and cellular signals. Thus, it seems unlikely that transduction of tumor cells by a single molecule will be sufficient for generating an effective antitumor response. As we learn more about the necessary stimuli for eliciting such a response, we will probably see the development of vectors that transduce a number of different molecules necessary for effective antigen presentation and T-cell activation.

Tumor Vaccines

Effective immunization against viruses is achieved through the expression of viral proteins in infected cells and the subsequent breakdown of these proteins in the cytoplasm. These peptide fragments are transported to the endoplasmic reticulum, where they associate with MHC class I molecules for eventual display on the cell surface. The peptide-MHC I complex mediates activation of a $CD8^+$ cytotoxic T-cell response. The recent demonstration that inoculation of different DNA expression plasmids into animals can lead to the generation of a T-cell response to the expressed protein, presumably by the same mechanism as the antiviral response, has led to enthusiasm for the possibility of DNA vaccination for the treatment of tumors. It was demonstrated more than a decade ago that direct DNA injection into the peritoneal cavity of rats resulted in expression of the encoded genes in the livers of the treated animals (66). More recently it has been shown that direct injection of nucleic acids into skeletal muscle results in expression of the encoded proteins in a small percentage of muscle cells (26). Although muscle is not the only tissue capable of expressing naked DNA following direct injection, it appears to be the most efficient. The mechanism of DNA uptake remains obscure but may be an energy-dependent process that involves the caveolae pathway. Uptake is more efficient in regenerating muscle than in mature muscle (67, 68). To exploit higher expression in regenerating muscle, a number of strategies are currently being evaluated for optimizing expression of naked DNA by damaging muscle. These strategies include the local injection of substances toxic to muscle (e.g., bipuvacaine) or the use of physical trauma such as the "gene gun," whereby the muscle is bombarded by gene-coated gold particles (69).

Studies have clearly demonstrated that animals inoculated intramuscularly with plasmid DNA generate an immune response to the encoded antigen (70). Effective antiviral immune responses in animals have been achieved against herpesvirus, hepatitis B, and influenza following the injection of plasmids that encode virus-specific proteins (5–21). The reason why the intramuscular route of injection is so effective at generating an immune response remains unclear. Further, the mechanism of antigen presentation within the muscle remains unknown. Although it is clear that myocytes express plasmid-encoded genes following intramuscular injection, whether these cells actually function as APCs is not known. Insofar as myocytes express variably low levels of MHC class I molecules under normal conditions and apparently do not possess co-stimulatory molecules, it is quite possible that the myocyte is not the responsible APC. Other possibilities include dendritic cells, known to be potent APCs, that reside within the muscle. Another possibility is that following trauma to the muscle, infiltrating inflammatory cells phagocytize damaged myocytes that are expressing the transgene. The transgene product is then processed intracellularly by the inflammatory cell and presented as a foreign antigen to T cells. This mechanism could explain the observation that damaged muscle tends to induce a greater immune response.

Choosing the appropriate antigen remains the principal challenge for the strategy of DNA vaccination. The optimal antigen to target for an immune response is one that is exclusively expressed on tumor cells or on tumor cells and nonessential normal tissue. Examples of such antigens include carcinoembryonic antigen (CEA) and prostate-specific antigen (PSA) (71). Other strategies include attempting to generate anti-idiotypic antibodies and cellular responses to the variable region of surface immunoglobulin on malignant B-cell lymphoma cells. Similar strategies could be envisioned for the induction of an anti-idiotypic response against specific T-cell receptors in T-cell lymphomas and leukemias. Finally, it may be possible to target new epitopes formed by the mutation of normal cellular molecules, such as p53 and $p21^{ras}$. One potential concern about this strategy is that autoimmunity could be generated if an immune response is generated against an antigen found in normal tissue. Similarly, injection of DNA into an animal raises the theoretical concern of generating anti-nucleic acid antibodies and thereby inducing a disease similar to systemic lupus erythematosis.

The successful application of gene transfer-mediated antitumor immunotherapy rests on several fundamental assumptions, the most important of which is that tumor antigens do exist. Although such antigens are clearly present in a number of tumors (e.g., melanoma, chronic myelogenous leukemia) it is not clear that they exist for all tumors and all tumor types. Further, the induction of an effective immune response against a specific tumor antigen could lead to the selection of tumor cells that do not express these antigens. The second important assumption is that the immune system in cancer patients can be perturbed by transduction of the appropriate genes to generate antitumor immunity. However, it is possible that cancer patients develop immunologic tolerance to their tumor antigens, and it is unclear whether such tolerance can be broken by any approach. Finally, even if a tumor-specific immunologic response can be induced, it remains to be seen whether the immune system of patients with advanced cancer will be capable of eradicating a substantial systemic tumor burden. Although it has been relatively easy to demonstrate effective immunity against tumor rechallenge in various animal models using a number of different immunologic approaches, few studies have demonstrated eradication of large established tumors. Thus, although gene therapy–mediated immunotherapy theoretically remains an exciting novel approach to cancer treatment, its eventual effectiveness remains to be proved.

REPLACEMENT AND KNOCKOUT GENE THERAPY

Therapeutic gene transfer was initially envisioned as a method for replacing missing or mutated genes for single-gene metabolic disorders such as adenosine deaminase (ADA) deficiency and familial hypercholesterolemia. With our growing understanding of the molecular mechanisms leading to the malignant transformation of cells, it has been proposed that replacement gene therapy may have a role in cancer therapy. For example, it is known that the p53 tumor suppressor gene is mutated in at least half of all human cancers. Transduction of a wild-type p53 gene can partially revert the malignant phenotype of p53-mutated tumor cells and substantially slow their growth (72, 73). Similar experiments have been performed with the gene that encodes the retinoblastoma tumor suppressor gene.

An alternative strategy is based on attempting to target molecules such as oncogenes that induce cellular proliferation. There are a number of potential ways to inactivate these molecules through gene transfer. One such strategy employs the transduction of a dominant negative mutant of the oncogene. Another strategy is to inhibit translation of the oncogene by transduction of a DNA molecule that encodes a specific ribozyme molecule. Ribozymes are RNA molecules that possess an RNA recognition site and enzymatic activity such that the specific ribozyme-target RNA is cleaved and destroyed. Another strategy developed to destroy specific intracellular proteins is transduction of a gene that encodes the single-chain variable region of an antibody specific to the target molecule. Following intracellular binding of this single-chain antibody to the target, the molecule is usually inactivated and then destroyed by intracellular proteases.

The strategy best developed for down-regulation of intracellular targets is the use of antisense nucleic acids (74). Short (15–40 bp) oligonucleotides that are complementary to mRNA sequences can result in partial or complete down-regulation of the encoded protein. The mechanism responsible for this effect remains unclear but probably involves several processes. The simplest mechanism for antisense inhibition of protein synthesis is direct interference with translation from mRNAs to its complementary antisense strands. A second effect is that double-stranded RNA molecules appear to be recognized by the cellular machinery as foreign (possibly viral) and are rapidly cleaved by cytoplasmic nucleases such as RNase H. Finally, antisense oligonucleotides can directly bind to the DNA template, interfere with the transcriptional machinery and thereby prevent mRNA synthesis. One of the major advantages to strategies utilizing antisense technology is the specificity of the approach. Expression of only the specific target gene will be affected by the antisense oligonucleotide. However, since most antisense strategies require prolonged duration of gene down-regulation, a major disadvantage of the current antisense technology is the difficulty in delivering oligonucleotides in vivo, and their relatively rapid degradation. Gene therapy offers a possible solution to these problems by the creation of vectors that can stably express antisense mRNA transcripts over prolonged periods of time (i.e., retroviral vectors).

An example of a potential target for antisense approaches is the activated *ras* proto-oncogene. Activated or mutated (oncogenic) *ras* is found in 20 to 30% of all cancers, including more than 50% of colon cancers and more than 90% of pancreatic cancers. Inhibition of *ras* activity by inhibiting posttranslational modification of the protein by farnesyltransferase inhibitors results in diminished tumor growth. Once administration of the farnesyltransferase inhibitor is terminated, the tumors begin to grow again. Thus, chronic suppression of *ras* activity is necessary. Gene transduction of antisense oligonucleotides, or dominant negative mutants, to either *ras* itself or farnesyltransferase may be an effective approach to chronic tumor growth inhibition (75). Since such strategies will probably not be associated with a bystander effect (as is true for delivery of cytotoxic genes), the use of vector-mediated transduction of antisense transcripts for cancer therapy, however, will still require the development of better vectors with more efficient gene transduction.

Replacement gene therapy employing all of the above-mentioned technologies has been successfully used in vitro for slowing the growth of malignant cells and occasionally for demonstrating reversion of the malignant phenotype. Nevertheless, malignant transformation is thought to be a process that involves multiple genetic aberrations, and thus the chances of completely abolishing the transformed phenotype with the addition or inactivation of a single molecule seems unlikely. Ultimately, multiple corrections will probably be required to fully convert the neoplastic cells to either a normal or at least a benign phenotype. Possibly the greatest obstacle to the successful use of replacement gene therapy for cancer will be the need to transduce every malignant cell with the therapeutic gene in order to cure the cancer. We are currently many years away from a safe vector that is efficient enough to achieve this task. Thus, although replacement therapy remains an interesting and theoretically attractive strategy for gene therapy, it will probably be years before this approach can be effectively tested in the clinic.

OTHER USES OF GENE THERAPY IN CANCER

Along with strategies that are intended to be directly antitumor, gene transfer offers a number of additional opportunities for supportive care of patients and the study of cancer biology in patients. Examples of where gene transfer may offer supportive care to cancer patients can be found in a growing number of animal and clinical studies where drug-resistance genes, such as MDR1, are being transduced into hematopoietic stem cells ex vivo. The transduced stem cells are then reimplanted into the host for the purpose of allowing greater dose-intensive chemotherapy with less hematologic toxicity (76).

Another use of gene transfer technology is to help answer key biologic questions concerning cancer biology in humans. The most common of these studies are termed "marker" studies: the cell of interest is transduced ex vivo with a marker gene (i.e., neomycin-resistance gene) and then the cell is transferred back into the patient for the purpose of eventually determining its fate. Examples of such studies include the genetic marking of harvested bone marrow cells prior to their reimplantation in children undergoing autologous bone marrow transplantation for leukemia. The goal of the first of these trials was to determine whether patients who eventually experienced relapse did so secondary to inefficient induction chemotherapy or to contamination of the reinfused bone marrow with leukemic cells. The finding that a population of the relapsed leukemic cells contained the genetic marker demonstrated that these leukemic cells contaminated the transplanted bone marrow (77). Other marker studies include the ex vivo transduction of immunologic effector cells (e.g., tumor-infiltrating and lymphokine-activated killer cells) with subsequent reinfusion back into the patient. Cells are subsequently harvested from different anatomic locations, such as the lymph nodes, bone marrow, and tumor, and assayed for the presence of the marker in order to track migration of the marked effector cells (78). Given the inefficient delivery systems currently available, marker studies (which do not require highly efficient vectors, since transduction is accomplished ex vivo and transduced cells are selected) may prove to be the most informative gene therapy trials for the next several years.

References

1. McLauchlin JR, Cornetta K, Eglistis MA, Anderson WF. Retroviral-mediated gene transfer. Prog Nucleic Acid Re Mol Biol 1990;38:91–135.
2. Ali M, Lemoine NR, Ring CJA. The use of DNA viruses as vectors for gene therapy. Gene Ther 1994;1:367–384.
3. Miller AD. Retroviral vectors. Curr Top Microbiol Immunol 1993;158.
4. Challita P-M, Kohn DB. Lack of expression from a retroviral vector after transduction of murine hematopoietic stem cells is associated with methylation in vivo. Proc Natl Acad Sci USA 1994;91:2567–2571.
5. Donahue RE, Kessler SW, Bodine D, McDonagh K, Dunbar C, Goodman S, Agricola B, Byrne E, Raffeld M, Moen R, Bacher J, Zsebo KM, Nienhuis AW. Helper virus induced T cell lymphoma in nonhuman primates after retroviral mediated gene transfer. J Exp Med 1992;176:1125–1135.
6. Horowitz MS. Adenoviridae and their replication. In Fundamental Virology, 2nd ed. Edited by BN Fields, DM Knipe, et al. 1991, pp 771–813.
7. Ginsberg HS. The Adenoviruses. New York: Plenum Press, 1984.
8. Fejer G, Gyory I, Tufariello J, Horwitz MS. Characterization of transgenic mice containing adenovirus early region 3 genomic DNA. J Virol 1994;68:5871–5881.
9. Berkner KL. Expression of heterologous sequences in adenviral vectors. Curr Top Microbiol Immunol 1992;158:39–66.
10. Quantin B, Perricaudet LD, Tajbakhsh S, Mandel JL. Adenovirus as an expression vector in muscle cells in vivo. Proc Natl Acad Sci USA 1992;89:2581–2584.
11. Rosenfeld MA, Yoshimura K, Trapnell BC, et al. In vivo transfer of the human cystic fibrosis transmembrane conductance regulator gene to the airway epithelium. Cell 1992;68:143–155.
12. Yang Y, Nunes FA, Berencsi K, Furth EE, Gonczol E, Wilson JM. Cellular immunity to viral antigens limits E1-deleted adenoviruses for gene therapy. Proc Natl Acad Sci USA 1994;91:4407–4411.
13. Engelhardt JF, Ye X, Doranz B, Wilson JM. Ablation of E2A in recombinant adenoviruses improves transgene persistence and decreases inflammatory response in mouse liver. Proc Natl Acad Sci USA 1994;91:6196–6200.
14. Roizman B, Sears AE. Herpes virus and their replication. In Virology. Edited by BN Fields, DM Knipe. New York: Raven, 1991, pp 1795–1842.
15. Spaete RR, Frenkel N. The Herpes Simplex Virus Amplicon: A New Eucaryotic Defective-Virus Cloning-Amplifying Vector. Cell 1982;30:295–304.
16. Roizman B, Batterson W. Herpes Viruses and Their Replication. In: Edited by Fields BN, Virology. New York: Raven, 1985, pp 497–526.
17. Kwong AD, Frenkel N. The herpes simplex virus virion host shutoff function. J Virol 1989;63:4834–4839.
18. Schlehofer JR, Ehrbar M, Hausen H. Vaccinia virus, herpes simplex virus and carcinogens induce DNA amplification in a human cell line and support replication of a helper virus dependent parvovirus. Virology 1986;152:110–117.
19. Siegl G, Bates RC, Berns KI, Carter BJ, Kelly DC, Kurstak E, Tattersall P. Characteristics and taxonomy of Parvoviridae. Intervirology 1985;23:61–73.
20. Yalkinoglu AO, Heilbronn R, Burkle A, Schlehofer JR, Hausen H. DNA amplification of adeno-associated virus as a response to cellular genotoxic stress. Cancer Res 1988;48:3123–3129.
21. Heilbronn R, Schlehofer JR, Yalkinoglu AO, Hausen H. Selective DNA amplication induced by carcinogens (initiators): evidence for a role of proteases and DNA polymerase alpha. Int J Cancer 1985;36:85–91.
22. Samulski RJ, Chang, L-S, Shenk T. Helper-free stocks of recombinant adeno-associated viruses: normal integration does not require viral gene expression. J Virol 1989;63:3822–3828.
23. Kotin RM, Linden RM, Berns KI. Characterization of a preferred site on human chromosome 19q for integration of adeno-associated virus by non-homologous recombination. EMBO J 1992;11:5071–5078.
24. Wolff JA, Lederberg J. An early history of gene transfer and therapy. Hum Gene Ther 1994;5:469–480.
25. Manthorpe M, Cornefert-Jensen FJ, Hartikka, Felgner J, Rundell A, Margalith M, Dwarki V. Gene therapy by intramuscular injection of plasmid DNA: studies on firefly luciferase gene expression in mice. Hum Gene Ther 1993;4:419–431.
26. Wolff JA, Malone RW, Williams P, et al. Direct gene transfer into mouse muscle in vivo. Science 1990;247:1465–1468.
27. Nicolau C, et al. In vivo expression of rat insulin after intravenous administration of the liposome-entrapped gene for rat insulin 1. Proc Natl Acad Sci USA 1983;80: 1068–1072.
28. Wu, GY, Wilson JM, Shalaby F, Grossman M, Shafritz DA, Wu CH. Receptor-mediated gene delivery in vivo. J Biol Chem 1991;266:14338–14342.
29. Wagner E, Zenke M, Cotten M, Beug H, Birnstiel ML. Transferrin-polycation conjugates as carriers for DNA uptake into cells. Proc Natl Acad Sci USA 1990;87:3410–3414.
30. Zenke M, Steinlein P, Wagner E, Cotten M, Beug H, Birnstiel ML. Receptor-mediated endocytosis of transferrin-polycation conjugates: an efficient way to introduce DNA into hematopoietic cells. Proc Natl Acad Sci USA 1990;87:3655–3659.
31. Curiel DT, Agarwal S, Wagner E, Cotten M. Adenovirus enhacement of transferrin-polylysine-mediated gene delivery. Proc Natl Acad Sci USA 1991;88:8850–8854.
32. Wagner E, Zatloukal K, Cotten M, Kirlappos H, Mechtler K, Curiel DT, Birnstiel ML. Coupling of adenovirus to transferrin-polylysine/DNA complexes greatly enhances receptor-mediated gene delivery and expression of transfected genes. Proc Natl Acad Sci USA 1992;89:6099–6103.
33. Cristiano RJ, Smith LC, Woo SL. Hepatic gene therapy: adenovirus enhancement of receptor-mediated gene delivery and expression in primary hepatocytes. Proc Natl Acad Sci USA 1993;90:2122–2126.
34. Wagner E, Plank C, Zatloukal K, Cotten M, Birnstiel ML. Influenza virus hemagglutinin HA-2 N-terminal fusogenic peptides augment gene transfer by transferrin-polylysine-DNA complexes: toward a synthetic virus-like gene-transfer vehicle. Proc Natl Acad Sci USA 1992;89:7934–7938.
35. Robine S, Sahuquillo-Merino C, Louvard D, Pringault E. Regulatory sequences on the human villin gene trigger the expression of a reporter gene in a differentiating HT29 intestinal cell line. J Biol Chem 1993;268:11426–11434.
36. Miller AD, Bender MA, Harris EAS, Kaleko M, Gelinas RE. Design of retrovirus vectors for transfer and expression of the human β-globin gene. J Virol 1988;62:4337–4345.
37. Rettinger SD, Kennedy SC, Wu X, Saylors RL, Hafenrichter DG, Flye MW, Ponder KP. Liver-directed gene therapy: quantitative evaluation of promoter elements by using in vivo retroviral transduction. Proc Natl Acad Sci USA 1994;91:1460–1464.
38. Wen P, Crawford N, Locker J. A promoter-linked coupling region required for stimulation of α-fetoprotein transcription by distant enhancers. Nucleic Acids Res 1993;21: 1911–1918.
39. Manome Y, Abe M, Hagen MF, Fine HA, Kufe DW. Enhancer sequences of the DF3 gene regulate expression of the herpes simplex virus thymidine kinase gene and confer sensitivity of human breast cancer cells to ganciclovir. Cancer Res 1994;54: 5408–5413.
40. Gossen M, Bujard H. Tight control of gene expression in mammalian cells by tetracycline-responsive promoters. Proc Natl Acad Sci USA 1992;89:5547–5551.
41. Fishman GI, Kaplan ML, Buttrick PM. Tetracycline-regulated cardiac gene expression in vivo. J Clin Invest 1994;93:1864–1869.
42. Hallahan DE, Mauceri HJ, Seung LP, Dunphy EJ, Wayne JD, Hanna NN, Toledano A, Hellman S, Kufe DW, Weichselbaum RR. Spatial and temporal control of gene therapy using ionizing radiation. Nature Med 1995;1:786–791.
43. Smythe WR, Hwang HC, Amin KM, Eck SL, Davidson BL, Wilson JM, Kaiser LR, Albelda SM. Use of recombinant adenovirus to transfer the herpes simplex virus thymidine kinase (HSVtk) gene to thoracic neoplasms: an effective in vitro drug sensitization system. Cancer Res 1994;54:2055–2059.
44. Freeman SM, Abboud CN, Whartenby KA, Packman CH, Koeplin DS, Moolten FL, Abraham GN. The "bystander effect": tumor regression with a fraction of the tumor mass is genetically modified. Cancer Res 1993;53:5274–5283.
45. Austin EA, Huber BE. A first step in development of gene therapy for colorectal carcinoma: cloning, sequencing, and expression of *Escherichia coli* cytosine deaminase. Mol Pharmacol 1993;43:380–387.
46. Huber BE, Austin EA, Good SS, Knick VC, Tibbels S, Richards CA. In vivo antitumor activity of 5-fluorocytosine on human colorectal carcinoma cells genetically modified to express cytosine deaminase. Cancer Res 1993;53:4619–4626.
47. Dong Y, Wen P, Manome Y, Parr M, Hirshowitz A, Chen L, Hirschowitz EA, Crystal R, Weichselbaum R, Kufe DW, Fine HA. In vivo replication-defective adenovirus vector-mediated transduction of the cytosine deaminase gene sensitizes glioma cells to 5-fluorocytosine. Hum Gene Ther 1996; 7:713–720.

47a. Manome Y, Wen PY, Dong Y, Tanaka T, Mitchell BS, Kufe DW, Fine HA: Viral vector transduction of the human deoxycytidine kinase cDNA sensitizes glioma cells to the cytotoxic effects of cytosine arabinoside. Nature Med 1996; 2:567–573.

48. Chang TKH, Waxman DJ. Cyclophosphamide modulates rat hepatic cytochrome P450 2C11 and steroid 5α-reductase activity and messenger RNA levels through the combined action of acrolein and phosphoramide mustard. Cancer Res 1993;53: 2490–2497.

49. Wei MX, Tamiya T, Chase M, Boviatsis EJ, Chang TKH, Kowall NW, Hochberg FH, Waxman DJ, Breakfield XO, Chiocca A. Experimental tumor therapy in mice using the cyclophosphamide-activating cytochrome P450 2B1 gene. Hum Gene Ther 1994;5: 969–978.
50. Mroz PJ, Moolten FL. Retrovirally transduced *Escherichia coli* gpt genes combine selectability with chemosensitivity capable of mediating tumor eradication. Hum Gene Ther 1993;4:589–595.
51. Sorscher EJ, et al. Tumor cell bystander killing in colonic carcinoma utilising the *Escherichia coli* DeoD gene to generate toxic purine. Gene Ther 1994;1:233–238.
52. Zitvogel L, Tahara H, Cai Q, Storkus WJ, Muller G, Wolf SF, Gately M, Robbins PD, Lotze MT. Construction and characterization of retroviral vectors expressing biologically active human interleukin 12. Hum Gene Ther 1994;5:1493–1506.
53. Manome Y, Wen PY, Hershowitz A, Tanaka T, Rollins BJ, Kufe D, Fine HA. Monocyte chemoattractant protein-1 (MCP-1) gene transduction: an effective tumor vaccine strategy for non-intracranial tumors. Cancer Immunol Immunother 1995;41:227-235.
54. Dranoff G, Jaffee E, Lazenby A, Golumbek P, Levitsky H, Brose K, Jackson V, Hamada H, Pardoll D, Mulligan RC. Vaccination with irradiated tumor cells engineered to secrete murine granulocyte-macrophage colony-stimulating factor stimulates potent, specific, and long-lasting antitumor immunity. Proc Natl Acad Sci USA 1993;90: 3539–3543.
55. Rice CD, Merchant RE. Systemic treatment with murine recombinant interleukin-1β inhabits the growth and progression of malignant glioma in the rat. J Neurooncol 1992;13:43–55.
56. Wei MX, Tamiya TRK, Hurford J, Boviatis EJ, Tepper RI, Chiocca EA. Enhancement of interleukin-4 mediated tumor regression in athymic mice by in situ retroviral gene transfer. Hum Gene Ther 1995;6:437–443.
57. Ogasawara M, Rosenberg SA. Enhanced expression of HLA molecules and stimulation of autologous human tumor infiltrating lymphocytes following transduction of melanoma cells with γ-interferon genes. Cancer Res 1993;53:3561–3568.
58. Tepper RI, Pattengale PK, Leder P. Murine interleukin-4 displays potent antitumor activity in vivo. Cell 1989;57:503–512.
59. Hock H, Dorsch M, Diamantstein T, Blankenstein T. Interleukin 7 induces CD4$^+$ T cell-dependent tumor rejection. J Exp Med 1991;174:1291–1298.
60. Fearon ER, Pardoll DM, Itaya T, Golumbek P, Levitsky HI, Simons JW, Karasuyama H, Vogelstein B, Frost P. Interleukin-2 production by tumor cells nypasses T helper function in the generation of an antitumor response. Cell 1990;60:397–403.
61. Dalgleish AG. The role of IL-2 in gene therapy. Gene Ther 1994;1:83–87.
62. Townsend SE, Allison JP. Tumor rejection after direct costimulation of CD8$^+$ T cells by B7-transfected melanoma cells. Science 1993;259:368–370.
63. Chen L, Ashe S, Brady WA, Hellstrom I, Hellstrom KE, Ledbetter JA, McGowan P, Linsley PS. Costimulation of antitumor immunity by the B7 counterreceptor for the T lymphocyte molecules CD28 and CTLA-4. Cell 1994.
64. Plautz GE, Yang ZY, Wu BY, Gao X, Huang L, Nabel GJ. Immunotherapy of malignancy by in vivo gene transfer into tumors. Proc Natl Acad Sci USA 1993;90:4645–4649.
65. Nabel GJ, Nabel EG, Yang Z-Y, Fox BA, Plautz GE, Gao X, Huang L, Shu S, Gordon D, Chang AE. Direct gene transfer with DNA-liposome complexes in melanoma: expression, biologic activity, and lack of toxicity in humans. Proc Natl Acad Sci USA 1993;90: 11307–11311.
66. Benvensity N, Reshef L. Direct introduction of genes into rats and expression of the genes. Proc Natl Acad Sci USA 1986;83:9551–9555.
67. Wells DJ. Improved gene transfer by direct plasmid injection associated with regeneration in mouse skeletal muscle. FEBS Lett 1993, 332:179–182.
68. Wolff JA, et al. Expression of naked plasmids by cultured myotubes and entry of plasmids into T tubules and caveolae of mammalian skeletal muscle. J Cell Sci 1992;103: 1249–1259.
69. Williams RS, et al. Introducion of foreign genes into tissues of living mice by DNA-coated microprojectiles. Proc Natl Acad Sci USA 1991;88:2726–2730.
70. Wang B, Merva M, Dang K, Ugen KE, Williams WV, Weiner DB. Immunization by direct DNA inoculation induces rejection of tumor cell challenge. Hum Gene Ther 1995;6: 407–418.
71. Conry RM, LoBuglio AF, Kantor J, Schlom J, Loechel F, Moore SE, Sumerel LA, Barlow DL, Abrams S, Curiel DT. Immune response to a carcinoembryonic antigen polynucleotide vaccine. Cancer Res 1994;54:1164–1168.
72. Clayman GL, El-Naggar AK, Roth JA, Zhang WW, Goepfert H, Taylor DL, Liu TA. In vivo molecular therapy with p53 adenovirus for microscopic residual head and neck squamous carcinoma. Cancer Res 1995;55:1–6.
73. Wills KN, Maneval DC, Menzel P, Harris MP, Sutjipto S, Vaillancourt MT, Huang WM, Johnson DE, Anderson SC, Wen SF, Bookstein R, Shepard HM, Gregory RJ. Development and characterization of recombinant adenoviruses encoding human p53 for gene therapy of cancer. Hum Gene Ther 1994;5:1079–1088.
74. Stein CA, Cheng YC. Antisense oligonucleotides as therapeutic agents: is the bullet really magical? Science 1993;261:1004–1012.
75. Ogiso Y, Sakai N, Watari H, Yokoyama T, Kuzumaki N. Suppression of various human tumor cell lines by a dominant negative H-ras mutant. Gene Ther 1994;1:403–407.
76. Podda S, Ward M, Himelstein A, Richardson C, Flor-Weiss EDL, Smith L, Gottesman M, Pastan I, Bank A. Transfer and expression of the human multiple drug resistance gene into live mice. Proc Natl Acad Sci USA 1992;89:9676–9680.
77. Rill DR, Santana VM, Roberts WM, Nilson T, Bowman LC, Krance RA, Heslop HE, Moen RC, Ihle JN, Brenner MK. Direct demonstration that autologous bone marrow transplantation for solid tumors can return a multiplicity of tumorigenic cells. Blood 1994;84: 280–283.
78. Hwu P, Rosenberg SA. The genetic modification of T cells for cancer therapy: an overview of laboratory and clinical trials. Cancer Detect Prev 1994;18:43–50.

SECTION XX

PRINCIPLES OF BONE MARROW TRANSPLANTATION

CHAPTER 85

Autologous Bone Marrow Transplantation

WILLIAM P. PETERS

Successful treatment of many cancers is often prevented by intrinsic tumor resistance or by tumor volume. In some cases, increasing dose intensity may overcome these constraints (67), but this approach is often limited by bone marrow or other organ tolerance. The success of allogeneic bone marrow transplantation in the treatment of relapsed acute leukemia and in certain lymphomas has demonstrated that dose intensification can, in certain circumstances, produce curative results when for similar patients standard dose therapy is not curative (218). Allogeneic marrow transplantation is, however, complicated by substantial morbidity and mortality related to graft- versus-host disease or complications associated with chronic immunosuppression (219). Availability of an appropriate donor of allogeneic bone marrow has limited its application even in the setting of the leukemias and lymphomas, since only 35 to 40% of patients have an HLA-identical sibling although the use of matched unrelated donors has expanded the options for allogeneic transplantation to some extent. Nonetheless, there has been increasing interest over the past decade in the development of autologous bone marrow transplantation for leukemias, lymphomas, and for solid tumors. This is a field in rapid evolution.

Rationale and Requirements for Autologous Bone Marrow Transplantation

Requirements for successful autologous bone marrow transplantation (ABMT) are listed in Table 85.1. The cancer being treated must be responsive to intensive cytoreductive therapy but not be curable by conventional-dose therapy. A source of cells capable of producing complete trilineage hematopoietic engraftment must also be available (105, 220). Bone marrow has most frequently provided these cells, but other sources of hematopoietic progenitors, such as leukopheresed peripheral blood collections, are increasingly being used (106). The requirement for freedom from malignant involvement may be critical. It is not certain, however, that the marrow needs to be completely free of limited numbers of tumor cells. Experience from the treatment of myeloma (23), as well as the lymphomas (17), suggests that limited marrow involvement may not preclude successful ABMT. To limit the amount of tumor cell contamination in marrow used for ABMT, strategies have been developed to remove malignant cells from the marrow, termed "purging," and have been studied in the leukemias and lymphomas, and more recently in the solid tumors (7).

Principles

The principles which underlie the use of ABMT and other methods for supportive care depend upon the disease which is being treated. Modifications of the general therapeutic strategy of dose intensification are, of necessity, targeted at the particular disease. In contrast to allogeneic transplantation, in which the administration of immunosuppressive agents is required to assure the engraftment of the transplanted bone marrow, the use of cytotoxic drugs prior to ABMT can be directed entirely toward cytoreduction of tumor, since engraftment readily occurs.

Although there may be differences between therapeutic strategies targeted at different diseases, a number of features appear to be common among therapeutic regimens. These features are outlined in Table 85.2.

Dose Intensity

The dose-response relationship for many antitumor agents is steep, both for therapeutic and for toxic effects (67). Even for resistant experimental system tumors such relationships can be shown to be linear-log (207). As shown in Figure 85.1, cellular kill is a first-order function of dose of administered cyclophosphamide for several solid animal malignancies, even for the most resistant cell lines such as the B-16 melanoma. For more sensitive tumors, a doubling of the administered dose leads to a two- to five-log increase in tumor cell kill in these experimental tumors. Moreover, the dose-response curve does not appear to plateau. This does not apply, however, to all antineoplastic agents. While the primary limitation for many agents is toxicity in the bone marrow, other drugs are toxic for other organs at or near the myelotoxic dose. The use of high-dose chemotherapy relies on an ability to escalate dose substantially before toxicity occurs in nonhematopoietic organs (Table 85.3). In ABMT, it is the difference between the response curves for tumor and for normal tissues that must be exploited. In practice, this difference between the myelotoxic dose and the dose that produces unacceptable damage to other organs is usually less than tenfold (90).

Table 85.1. Requirements for Autologous Bone Marrow Transplantation

Malignancy is responsive to intensive cytoreductive therapy and not curable by marrow-tolerable doses.
Tumor burden does not exceed therapeutic capability of cytoreductive regimen.
Source of marrow progenitor cells capable of restoring hematopoiesis and free of clonogenic tumor cells is available.

Table 85.2. Commonly Applied Principles in Autologous Bone Marrow Transplantation

Dose is a critical factor in treatment, and even minor compromises of administered dose can result in reduction of therapeutic efficacy.
Combination chemotherapy is generally required for the successful treatment of most cancers to overcome intrinsic resistance or tumor burden.
Alkylating agents have properties which are particularly appropriate to use in high-dose treatment settings.
- Alkylating agents are broadly active in many cancers.
- The common dose-limiting side effect is myelosuppression.
- At higher doses, selected alkylating agents differ in their non-myelosuppressive dose-limiting toxicities.
- Alkylating agents in general possess a steep dose-response effect which in certain settings appears linear-log and non-saturable at clinically attainable doses.
- Laboratory investigations demonstrate substantial non–cross resistance among selected agents of this class.

Treatment in the clinical setting of minimal disease and early stage is more likely to be associated with a valuable therapeutic outcome.

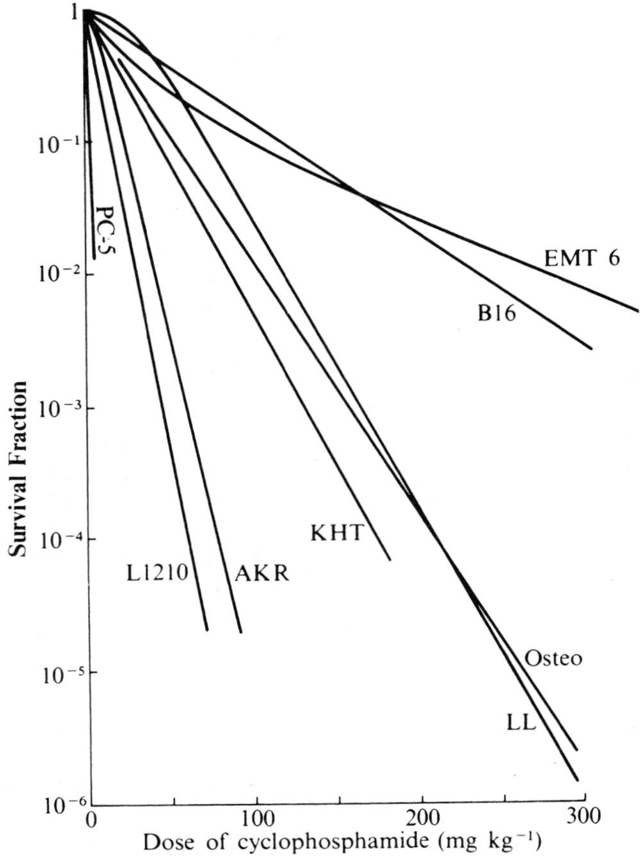

Figure 85.1. First-order kinetics in cell killing of several transplanted animal tumors with cyclophosphamide. *Source:* Steel (207).

Combination Chemotherapy

Both radiation therapy and chemotherapy have been used in ABMT. The probable occurrence of drug resistance to any single agent generally mandates the use of multiple drugs, with or without radiation therapy. Agents selected should have activity against the neoplasm being treated. Many myelosuppressive agents have not, however, been tested adequately at high doses against most cancers because myelosuppression has limited the usefulness of these drugs in the absence of bone marrow support. While total body radiation has a major role in transplantation for acute leukemias and lymphomas, total body radiation is of limited value in breast cancer and other localized solid tumors where doses required for elimination of macroscopic and even microscopic disease often exceed the tolerable limits that can be administered.

Many agents are not amenable to dose escalation or do not have a linear dose-response effect (see Chapter 54). For example, antimetabolites such as 5-fluorouracil and methotrexate plateau in their dose-response after only a small dose escalation (Fig. 85.2). Other agents which appear to possess a dose-response effect, such as doxorubicin, while limited predominantly by myelosuppression, have non-hematopoietic toxicities which quickly limit further dose escalation (39). Cardiotoxicity and mucosal and epithelial toxicity do not permit substantial dose escalation for

Table 85.3. Non-hematopoietic Dose-Limiting Toxicities of Various Antineoplastic Agents

Drug	Standard tolerated dose (mg/m^2)	Maximum tolerated dose (mg/m^2)	With bone marrow support: Target organ or side effects
Doxorubicin	60–75	150	Hand-foot syndrome
Nitrogen mustard		33	CNS
Cyclophosphamide	750	7,500	Hemorrhagic myocarditis
Mitolactol (Dibromodulcitol)	300	ND	
Mitomycin C	20	60	Venoocclusive disease
Methotrexate		NA	
Melphalan	40	180–220	Enterocolitis
Carmustine	200	1,000	Pulmonary fibrosis, toxic hepatitis
Thiotepa	30	1,500	CNS syndrome
Cisplatin	120	180	Renal, neuropathy
Busulfan	2–4	1,100	Anorexia

Key: ND, not done; NA, not achieved

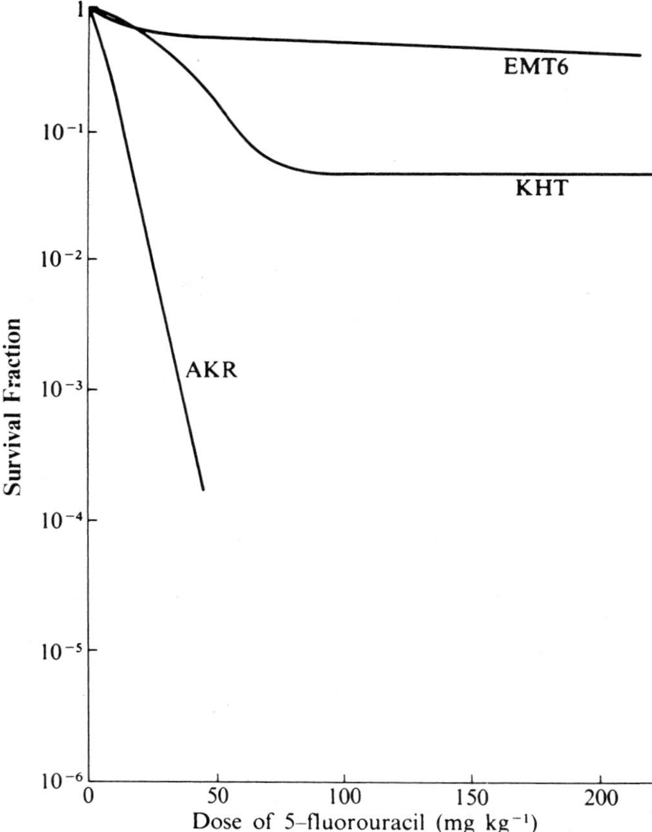

Figure 85.2. Plateau in cell killing of two transplanted animal tumors using fluorouracil. *Source:* Steel (207).

doxorubicin and several other agents. It is unlikely that such compounds will play a major role in high-dose therapeutic regimens, although synergy with other active agents could provide a role for these agents in high-dose programs.

Volume of Disease

Disease volume will limit the potential of intensive therapy. As tumors begin to exceed a certain volume, even high-dose therapeutic approaches may be unable to produce complete tumor regression, let alone tumor eradication. Consolidative radiation therapy or surgical approaches to areas of pretreatment bulk disease may be useful.

Principles of tumor kinetic modeling should be considered in the development of therapeutic regimens using ABMT. The Golde-Coldman hypothesis suggests that spontaneous development of resistance occurs relatively early in neoplastic evolution and, so, treatment in early stage of disease is more likely to be effective than later treatment (73). Whether or not the dose escalation afforded by marrow protection techniques will allow sufficient increase in therapeutic effect to overcome such resistance, particularly in combination regimens, is at present uncertain for most tumors and will need to be evaluated carefully. Norton-Simon kinetic theory would predict that the application of intensive therapy after cytoreduction would provide the most useful place in which to utilize dose intensification (157–159). Formal testing of these hypotheses has not been evaluated at high doses.

Procedure

SELECTION OF PATIENT

ABMT can be utilized in older patients than can allogeneic marrow transplantation, where complications preclude use in most patients over age 55, owing to the increasing severity of graft-versus-host disease. Successful autografting has been performed into the seventh decade, though such attempts in this age group are uncommon. Complicating concomitant illness and medical disability may be expected to increase the morbidity of patients of advanced age. Patient performance status at the start of therapy appears to be a major predictor of toxicity in ABMT.

Further evaluation of quality of life attributes need to be undertaken to evaluate the short-term and long-term effects of transplantation. Patients who have failed multiple therapies for their malignancy may not be good candidates for intensive therapy, as resistant tumor cells may have been selected and patient tolerance will be reduced, compromising the therapeutic efficacy of intensive therapy and resulting in greater treatment-related toxicity (14).

MARROW HARVESTING TECHNIQUE AND COMPLICATIONS

Bulk aspiration of bone marrow is generally performed under regional or general anesthesia from the posterior or anterior iliac crests (220), the most attractive areas for bulk marrow collection. Patients who have received extensive pelvic irradiation may require aspiration of marrow from the sternum, or the harvest of hematopoietic progenitor cells from the peripheral blood (see below). Approximately 1 to 3 $\times$ 10^8 nucleated cells/kg is collected, using needle aspiration from multiple sites in the iliac crests. Small aspirations (<10 ml) from multiple sites are obtained to try to minimize contamination with peripheral blood. Marrow is generally anticoagulated using heparin. After an adequate volume of marrow has been obtained, cells are usually passed through stainless steel screens to remove bone chips and to create a single cell suspension. There is disagreement about the use of screening because large cells such as megakaryocytes, other hematopoietic progenitors, or malignant cells may be removed by this technique. Nonetheless, most practitioners continue to use screens in the preparation of marrow.

Bulk marrow obtained in this way is generally concentrated by centrifugation and a buffy coat preparation obtained. The marrow is generally mixed with 10% dimethylsulfoxide or other cryoprotectants and autologous plasma, and is cryopreserved at control rate in liquid nitrogen. Some authors have reported that the characteristics of the freezing process are important to marrow viability and hematopoietic reconstitution (59, 125), although others have disputed this (86, 210). Once frozen, cryopreserved marrow retains viability in liquid nitrogen for extended periods of time (18).

Marrow harvest is associated with few complications, which are mainly related to anesthesia. Pain in the harvest area is the most common but is generally short-lived and controlled by simple analgesia. Local infection, bleeding, bone injury, nerve damage, and even air embolism have been rarely reported during marrow harvesting (132). Efforts to perform outpatient marrow harvest procedures have been undertaken (36).

At the time of administration, the marrow is rapidly thawed at 37°C and infused intravenously without further treatment. In some early reports, marrow was treated with enzymes followed by washing, but such processing generally is not necessary and is associated with increased febrile reactions at the time of marrow reinfusion (66). Infused marrow stem cells circulate through the pulmonary circulation and "home" to marrow cavities. The molecular mechanism underlying this homing to marrow sites has recently been reviewed and appears related to the presence of unique antigens present on early marrow progenitor cells. The administration of bone marrow can be associated with hypertension and bradycardia, presumably related to the dimethylsulfoxide used as a cryoprotectant (56). Hemolyzed red cells contaminating bulk marrow preparations produce hemoglobinuria, of which the patient should be warned; it has been associated with renal dysfunction in the early posttransplant setting (85, 204). Other side effects of marrow infusion include acute anaphylaxis to infusion of autologous bone marrow, apparently mediated through an IgE antibody to bovine serum albumin (116).

PERIPHERAL BLOOD STEM CELL AND PROGENITOR CELL COLLECTION

An alternative method for collecting cells capable of hematopoietic reconstitution involves leukopheresis to collect peripheral blood mononuclear cells. Levels of peripheral blood progenitor cells, or stem cells, increase during the recovery phase from chemotherapy, and after priming with hematopoietic colony-stimulating factors (CSFs) such as G-CSF or GM-CSF (69, 205). Approximately 9 to 10 L of peripheral blood is processed on multiple occasions using a continuous-flow centrifuge (105). Mononuclear cells collected in this fashion are concentrated and cryopreserved as described above with marrow. Satisfactory hematopoietic reconstitution appears to correlate with the number of progenitor cells measured in the CFU-GM assay (100). Studies in murine systems suggested that peripheral stem cells were not likely to be effective for autotransplantation, since their capacity for cell renewal was limited as compared with that of bone marrow (142). Transplantation experiments in dogs, however, did demonstrate that these circulating stem cells could rescue animals from supralethal radiation therapy (45, 111). The numbers of peripheral blood stem cells could be increased by exercise, ACTH, dextran, or the administration of hematopoietic CFSs (206). Higher levels of CFU-GM have also been observed during the period of recovery from chemotherapy (70).

During the late 1970s, Goldman and his colleagues demonstrated that circulating mononuclear cells could produce complete and sustained hematopoietic engraftment in patients with chronic myeloid leukemia after high-dose chemotherapy (74, 87). Subsequent studies have attempted to use peripheral blood progenitor cells to reconstitute patients with acute myeloid leukemia (182), Burkitt's lymphoma (112), Hodgkin's disease (113), breast cancer (107), and non-Hodgkin's lymphoma (27, 114). In these studies, rapid hematopoietic reconstitution could be consistently obtained at relatively low doses of progenitor cells measured by CFU-GM. In other studies, however, such rapid engraftment did not occur and platelet recovery was extremely slow (44), especially in settings where the CFU-GM was low. Some patients did not attain sustained hematopoietic reconstitution (89).

Some have claimed that peripheral blood progenitor collections have fewer contaminating malignant cells, even in patients with acute myeloid leukemia, chronic myelogenous leukemia (115), lymphoma (108), or solid tumors in which bone marrow contamination is evident. The level of tumor cell contamination has not been adequately measured. Recent data suggest that peripheral blood progenitor collections do contain tumor cells in neuroblastoma (120, 146, 147, 192).

MARROW PROCESSING

Ex Vivo Purging

ABMT is limited to patients from whom marrow progenitors can be obtained without contaminating clonogenic malignant cells. Many cancers involve the marrow, and in the

Table 85.4. Methods of Ex Vivo Purging of Bone Marrow

- Tumoricidal Methods
  - Pharmacologic
    - Cyclophosphamide derivatives
      - 4-hydroperoxycyclophosphamide
      - ASTA-Z 7557 (Mafosphamide)
    - Cytosine arabinoside analogues
    - Cisplatin and analogues
    - Deoxynucleosides
    - Deoxycoformycin
    - Doxorubicin
    - Verapamil
    - Glucocorticoids
    - Alkyl-lysophospholipids
    - Etoposide
  - Biophysical
    - Photoradiation
      - Merocyanin-540 (MC-540)
      - Dihematoporphyrin ether (DHE)
    - Radioisotopes
  - Immunologic
    - Monoclonal antibodies and complement
    - Monoclonal antibodies and ricin or other toxins
    - IL-2 leukocyte activated killer cells (LAK cells)
    - Alpha 2b interferon
- Tumor Removal Methods
  - Immunologic
    - Immunomagnetic beads and monoclonal antibodies
    - Immunorosettes
  - Physical
    - Counterflow Elutriation
    - Centrifugation
    - Immunoabsorption

leukemias, the primary site for disease is the marrow. A variety of methods to remove malignant cells from marrow have been utilized. Table 85.4 lists various methods of ex vivo purging of bone marrow, using either direct cytotoxic activity against tumor or tumor removal methods. Randomized comparative trials establishing the efficacy of these purging methods have not yet been completed, although some trials are currently under way. Infusion of marrows contaminated with malignant cells have been suggested to result in unusual patterns of recurrence (80). With the development of monoclonal antibodies that recognize antigens present on early hematopoietic "stem" cells, column, bead, and cell sorting techniques have been devised to select these early cells specifically.

Chemical

A variety of antineoplastic agents have been employed to remove malignant cells from marrow. The most common method has involved a short-term exposure ex vivo to cytotoxic agents such as 4-hydroperoxycyclophosphamide (4-HC) or mafosphamide (ASTA-Z), cyclophosphamide derivatives that do not require hepatic activation and that show antitumor activity in animal models, etoposide, cisplatin, cytosine arabinoside, and others. Several considerations, including the number of malignant cells contaminating the marrow, may limit the efficacy of this approach. Some clinical trials suggest an advantage for purged versus unpurged marrows (77). Exposure to 4-HC or other chemotherapeutic agents does not appear to exhibit major selectivity with respect to normal and leukemic clonogenic cells, nor do these agents completely inhibit the self-renewal capacity of leukemic myeloblasts in culture. In addition, the antileukemic–and, particularly, antisolid tumor— effect of 4-HC may be limited, with only modest reduction in tumor cell numbers. The use of 4-HC in acute myelocytic leukemia in second or greater complete remission has demonstrated long-term outcome superior to that expected using non-purged marrow (189, 193, 239). Comparative trials of 4-HC purging technology are currently under way. The use of methods to differentially protect hematopoietic progenitors from toxic chemotherapy effects in vitro via the use of amiofostine (140) has been advocated.

The use of chemical purging has limited the use of certain hematopoietic CSFs such as GM-CSF, which is then ineffective in stimulating recovery (33). This is due to a lack of the progenitors bearing receptors capable of responding to the late CSFs. Other factors, such as interleukin-3, which act on an earlier progenitor, may be effective in this setting (143).

Antibody

The ability of monoclonal antibodies to identify specific tumor-associated antigens has been exploited in technologies to remove malignant cells. The use of anti-CALLA antibodies and complement have been used to purge leukemic cells in acute lymphocytic leukemia in childhood (186, 187), and similar technologies have been applied to lymphomas and other diseases (8, 152). Attachment of toxins such as ricin or *Pseudomonas* toxin to monoclonal antibodies (22, 55, 59, 72, 145, 151, 179, 180, 194, 211, 212), or coupling the antibodies to immunomagnetic beads (31, 50, 130, 178, 191, 199, 200, 231, 232) produces enhanced tumor cell kill. Superior survival in children with neuroblastoma receiving marrows purged with a panel of antibodies and a magnetic separation technique has been reported (118).

Antibody-mediated purging may be limited by antigenic heterogeneity of the tumor cells (57, 134), as heterogeneity in drug sensitivity among tumor clones may limit its usefulness. It is likely that combination modalities may be complementary (58, 145, 223–225) and lead to enhanced tumor removal.

Other Separation Techniques

Multiple other techniques for removing malignant cells from marrow have been reported, including immunorosetting (203), countercurrent elutriation (103), and the use of lymphokine-activated killer cells (1, 2, 3, 91, 129, 222, 227). Nevertheless, despite the variety, logic, and availability of techniques, the importance and utility of removal of malignant cells has yet to be demonstrated. Some have even claimed that leukemia cells do not cryopreserve as well as normal hematopoietic cells (6).

Long-Term Culture

Recently, hematopoietic reconstitution of patients with chronic myeloid leukemia and acute myeloid leukemia has been reported using autologous marrow that had been cultured long term in vitro. After patient preparation for marrow transplantation has been performed using busulfan and cyclophosphamide (46, 47, 53), the cultured autologous transplant has been reported to result in sustained normalization of disease-specific karyotypic abnormalities. Culture of CML marrow appears to yield terminally differentiated malignant cells and the outgrowth of a normal population in the in vitro setting. Expansion and collection of these cells and their subsequent reengraftment appears to argue that two clones of cells are present in CML-affected marrow and that reconstitution with an unaffected clone may occur.

Stem Cell Collection and Expansion

The identification of the CD34 antigen on early hematopoietic progenitors has led to attempts to isolate and expand these progenitors with subsequent use for hematopoietic reconstitution (215). Positive selection of a stem cell may enable the elimination of most neoplastic cells and lead to sustained reconstitution. Studies in dogs (28), primates (29), and, more recently, in humans (30) have demonstrated that sustained engraftment can be achieved with positive selection of marrow for CD34-positive–CD33-negative hematopoietic progenitors. The importance of these observations, coupled with the recent molecular cloning of c-kit ligand (41, 51, 240) offers the potential for ex vivo expansion of early hematopoietic progenitors and reconstitution (233).

CYTOREDUCTIVE THERAPY: ADMINISTRATION AND SUPPORTIVE CARE

After satisfactory collection and storage of hematopoietic progenitors, high-dose chemotherapy and/or total body irradiation is used to treat the neoplasm. Following intensive chemoradiation therapy, rapid and profound myelosuppression ensues. Hematopoietic reconstitution to a neutrophil count greater than 500/μ3 usually requires 15 to 19 days; thrombocytopenia generally persists longer. Supportive care techniques vary from center to center, but generally include reverse isolation, transfusion therapy, and empiric and therapeutic antibacterial and antifungal therapy. Radiation of blood products is performed to eliminate the potential for graft-versus-host disease resulting from transfused blood products. Parenteral nutrition has frequently been utilized, since many patients, particularly those treated with total body radiation, experience severe mucositis. Studies in nontransplant patients have demonstrated the value of low–bacterial content diets, and reduced risk of systemic *Aspergillus* infections have been documented in patients treated in high efficiency particulate air (HEPA)-filtered air environments (197). Recommendations for hospital facilities and for transplant team capabilities have been developed by the American Society of Clinical Oncology and the American Society of Hematology (12).

Specific Diseases

ACUTE MYELOCYTIC LEUKEMIA

ABMT has been used as consolidation in patients with acute myelocytic leukemia in first, second, or subsequent remission, and studies have been performed using both purged and unpurged bone marrow. Interpretation of the available studies is complicated by differences in therapeutic regimens, differences in the interval between complete remission and autografting, and inadequate descriptions of the patient populations. Results in advanced resistant disease indicate that although complete responses occurred in more than 50% of patients, relapse was nearly universal. More recent efforts have concentrated on patients in first or second complete remission using purged or nonpurged bone marrow. Most series have involved only small numbers of patients with relatively short follow-up. A recent analysis of 263 patients with acute myelocytic leukemia, autografted in first complete remission between 1982 and 1987, has been reported (77). Leukemia-free survival at 3 years was 39%; among those patients whose marrow was purged with mafosphamide, who were autografted within 6 months of complete remission, relapse-free survival was significantly improved (Fig. 85.3). There is a profound influence of the time from achievement of the first complete remission to ABMT upon the probability of relapse and leukemia-free survival (Fig. 85.4). This relationship is most likely explained by time-censoring selection bias, in which patients transplanted late after complete remission is achieved, when others in the cohort have already relapsed and thus do not present for transplant, are more likely to have been cured by their chemotherapy than were patients treated early in their remission. These data are consistent with earlier data of Yeager and colleagues using 4-HC (239) to purge marrow involved by acute myelocytic leukemia during a second complete remission. Randomized comparative data in first

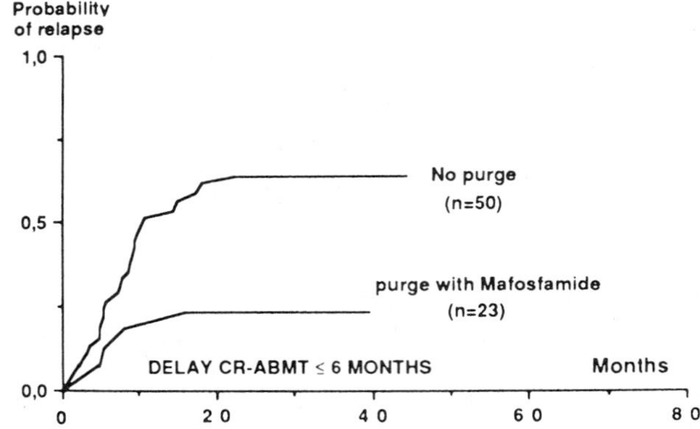

Figure 85.3. Autologous bone marrow transplant in acute myeloid leukemia within six months of achieving complete remission. Patients whose marrows underwent purging with Mafosfamide had significantly fewer relapses. *Source:* Gorin et al. (77).

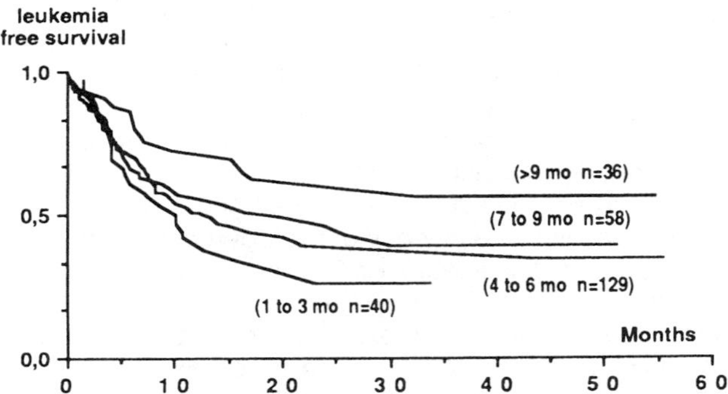

Figure 85.4. Autologous bone marrow transplantation in acute myeloid leukemia appears to be more successful the later it is undertaken after attaining complete remission. This is artifactual. See text. *Source:* Gorin et al. (77).

complete remission have not been undertaken, nor have comparative trials been performed in which high-dose consolidation was not used (see Chapter 142).

ACUTE LYMPHOCYTIC LEUKEMIA

Results of ABMT in patients with acute lymphocytic lymphoblastic leukemia (ALL) have been less satisfactory. In a comparison of autografting to allografting in 91 patients with acute lymphocytic leukemia in first through fourth remission, 20% of autografted, and 27% of allografted patients became long-term disease-free survivors (104). Although several series have demonstrated prolonged disease-free survival in some transplanted patients with high-risk ALL who failed conventional chemotherapy, the degree of success is less than that in AML. The major reason for treatment failure is relapse. Some authors have suggested that allograft recipients without graft-versus-host disease and autograft recipients have indistinguishable relapse curves, suggesting that the source of relapse in those patients is residual leukemia cells in the patient and not residual leukemia cells in the transplanted bone marrow.

Purging of ALL using monoclonal antibodies has been evaluated in several studies. A recent analysis of 47 patients comparing relapse frequency in allogeneic- versus ABMT indicated that the probability of relapse was 9% for patients receiving an allogeneic bone marrow transplant and 52% for patients receiving ABMT (32). Graft-versus host leukemia or -tumor effect of autologous marrow may be responsible for the difference in relapse frequency. In vitro treatment with monoclonal antibodies and complement, immunotoxins, and 4-HC has been performed. The impact of purging remains less clear at present from these studies (26, 78, 79). None of the data permit a conclusion that there is a benefit derived from purging bone marrow in ALL.

NON-HODGKIN'S LYMPHOMA

The therapeutic results of ABMT in patients with non-Hodgkin's lymphoma appears to be related to the grade and extent of disease and its resistance to previous chemotherapy. In advanced-stage intermediate and high-grade lymphoma, 3-year progression-free survival ranges from 20 to 60%, reflecting small study numbers and selection effects. In general, results appear superior in patients with smaller volume disease and in patients who respond to induction therapy (68, 82). A recent randomized trial in patients with slow response to initial first-line chemotherapy for non-Hodgkin's lymphoma compared ABMT with continued CHOP chemotherapy. At 4 years in this study, there was no significant difference in survival (230a). However, in patients who relapse after primary therapy for non-Hodgkin's lymphoma and respond to second-line therapy, a recent prospective randomized study from the Parma group comparing ABMT to conventional-dose therapy demonstrated a highly significant advantage to the use of transplantation—in both disease-free and survival overall (176a).

Multiple conditioning regimens have been used in ABMT for lymphomas, but few comparative trials between regimens have been performed. In patients with relapsed lymphoma who have a good performance status and minimal disease following conventional induction therapy, the probability of disease-free survival on an actuarial basis is 50% at 38 months (Fig. 85.5). This therapeutic outcome is achieved with minimal treatment-related mortality (66). Patients in resistant relapse who have not responded to a second induction chemotherapy program fare poorly following ABMT, and few remain alive (174). The role of purging in this setting remains controversial.

The nature of the preparative regimen may be very important with regard to both therapeutic benefit and toxicity. Dose escalations of the same drugs have resulted in frequencies of complete remission varying from 47 to 80% (19). Regimens containing total body irradiation (TBI) have a higher incidence of diffuse alveolar hemorrhage than do regimens without TBI (48, 148, 188).

Studies with an early combination chemotherapy regimen, carmustine, cytarabine, cyclophosphamide, 6-thioguanine (BACT), used in the treatment of non-Hodgkin's lymphoma revealed that few patients with advanced bulky disease achieved extended disease-free survival. Canellos and his colleagues, in a survey of published reports, showed only 16 of 112 long-term disease-free survivors when ABMT was used for refractory relapse of lymphoma, as opposed to 33 of 53 patients transplanted in second or subsequent remission or in first partial remission (43).

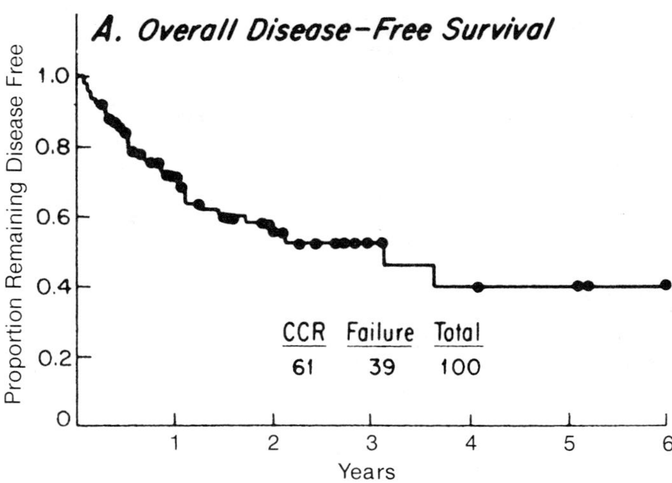

Figure 85.5. Non-Hodgkin's lymphoma disease-free survival after autologous bone marrow transplant. CCR, complete clinical remission. *Source:* Freedman et al. (66).

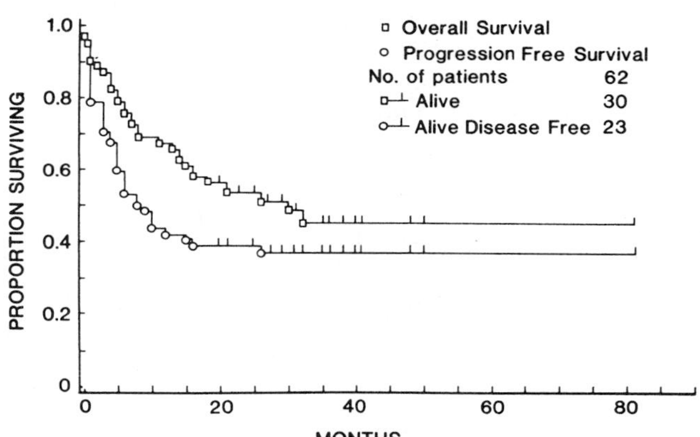

Figure 85.6. Intensive chemotherapy and autologous bone marrow transplantation in relapsed Hodgkin's disease.

HODGKIN'S DISEASE

High-dose combination chemotherapy using high-dose cyclophosphamide and BCNU/VP-16 can result in a 45% overall survival for more than six years in patients who have failed a MOPP-like regimen and adriamycin therapy for relapsed Hodgkin's disease (Fig. 85.6) (95). Outcome of ABMT was affected by performance status, by having received more than two chemotherapy regimens, by high tumor burden, and by the recurrence of disease irradiated within a previous radiation field. Any of these features reduce the probability of long-term survival and help to identify patients who are poor candidates for utilizing this therapeutic approach. Local radiation therapy may improve the outcome in patients with bulky disease prior to ABMT (37). Other authors have reported similar results (4, 5, 37, 75, 83, 84).

Similar treatment results have been reported from ABMT and allogeneic transplantation for Hodgkin's disease (128). While relapses are slightly higher in autologous transplants, there is an absence of graft-versus-host (and graft-versus-lymphoma) disease. Given the difficulties often associated with allogeneic transplantation, this suggests that ABMT may represent the preferable approach for Hodgkin's relapse.

BREAST CANCER

Increasing interest has been focused over the past decade on the role of dose intensity in the treatment of breast cancer. Retrospective analysis and prospective clinical trials have demonstrated a dose-response relationship in terms of objective response, duration of remission, and quality of life. Responsiveness of breast cancer to high-dose combination chemotherapy regimens has been demonstrated; most studies show a higher complete and total response rate (165). Most studies are small, and include heterogeneous patient populations, making interpretation of data difficult (13, 14, 92, 93). Early regimens were associated with substantial toxicity and when applied to patients who have failed a standard dose regimen for metastatic cancer, the responses are not durable (139, 166). Patients in this setting do not appear to benefit from regimens tested thus far. Selection of patients at high risk for relapse and poorly responsive to standard therapies can be assisted by certain pretreatment characteristics; appropriate patients would include premenopausal women with hormone receptor-negative or hormone-insensitive metastatic disease (141) in whom prior chemotherapy for metastases has not failed. More recent studies, using high-dose combination alkylating agents in patients meeting these characteristics, either with no prior chemotherapy for metastases or as part of a program involving induction chemotherapy followed by high-dose consolidation, have demonstrated that between 15 and 25% of patients can achieve durable extended remissions from 3 to more than 6 years (15, 60, 61, 167–169). Patients with limited disease volume and less prior chemotherapy respond better. Durable remissions after a single high-dose therapy and no other intervention extending beyond 10 years have been observed, and several studies now have found extended disease-free survival even in poor prognosis patients. Recent survey of ABMTs performed in North America found an overall survival at 5 years in over 25% of patients receiving high-dose consolidation and ABMT for metastatic breast cancer.

In the setting of high-risk primary breast cancer involving 10 or more axillary lymph nodes, high-dose consolidation with the combination of autologous bone marrow and peripheral blood progenitor cell support has been studied. Results from this sequential trial are intriguing (Fig. 85.7). Apparent benefit has derived from this approach compared with contemporary and historical series (170, 171). Recent analyses with follow-up beyond a median 5 years have demonstrated a 15 to 25% improvement in disease-free survival for patients receiving high-dose therapy compared with matched controls (173b). Survey data reporting experience of the North American transplant groups demonstrated an overall survival rate of 79% for 662 patients with high-risk primary breast cancer receiving autologous bone marrow– or peripheral blood cell–supported transplants (173a). Prospective, randomized, comparative trials are in progress, but full results are not expected until near year 2000. While purging of bone marrow has been undertaken using chemi-

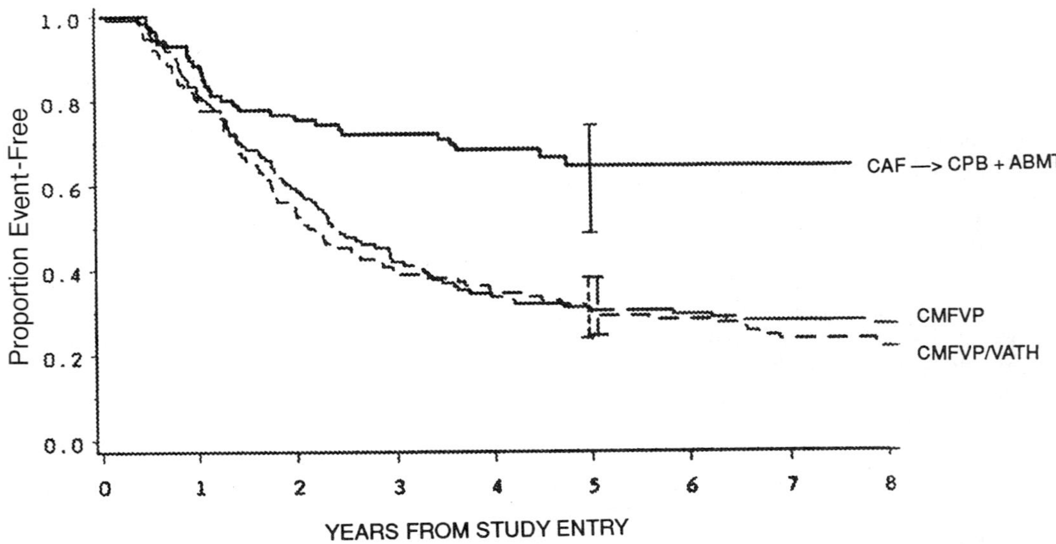

Figure 85.7. Chemotherapy with ABMS for breast cancer: event-free survival. Figure shows the event-free survival time for 85 patients with breast cancer and metastatic nodes treated with four cycles of CAF (cyclophosphamide, adriamycin, fluorourcil) followed by consolidation with cyclophosphamide, cisplatin, and carmustine with ABMT and peripheral progenitor cell support (*solid line*) and compared to age- and disease-matched controls selected from two CALGB trials, 7581 (CMFVP) and 8082 (CMFVP/VATH). Vertical bars indicates 95% confidence intervals determined at 5-years follow-up. Follow-up is 6 years median, minimum follow-up for all patients is 4 years, with lead follow-up of 8 years.

cal and monoclonal methods (see Purging, above) early results do not differ from those obtained without purging techniques.

Two recently completed studies provide support for the use of high-dose chemotherapy with autologous cellular support in the treatment of poor prognosis metastatic breast cancer. In a study from South Africa (30a), 90 patients with metastatic breast cancer were randomized to receive either two cycles of high cyclophosphamide, mitoxantrone and etoposide with autologous cellular support, versus 6 to 8 cycles of conventional dose of cyclophosphamide, mitoxantrone and vincristine. The study was well conducted and balanced, and demonstrated a significantly higher frequency of complete remission (51% versus 4%) in favor of high-dose chemotherapy. Disease-free survival for patients treated with high-dose therapy was twice that of patients on the conventional dose arm, and overall survival was extended a median 1 year by the use of high-dose chemotherapy in this direct comparison. Further, while all but one patient relapsed with conventional dose therapy, 20% of patients treated with high-dose chemotherapy were alive and disease-free at lead follow-up beyond 3 years. These data are consistent with multiple Phase II trials in which high-dose chemotherapy is utilized in patients with metastatic breast cancer.

In a second study which has been reported in abstract form(173c), patients with hormone-insensitive metastatic breast cancer who achieved a complete remission after an intensive doxorubicin based induction chemotherapy regimen were randomized either to be treated with high-dose cyclophosphamide, cisplatin, and BCNU with autologous cellular support versus observation, and at time of recurrence treated with high-dose consolidation at that point. The study allowed the evaluation of the effectiveness of consolidation with high-dose therapy, as well as the importance of the timing of high-dose therapy. The data indicated a threefold increase in the median disease-free survival (0.3 to 0.9 years). For the patients treated with immediate high-dose consolidation overall event free survival at five years was 20%. Interestingly, the strategy of utilizing high-dose therapy at the time of recurrence after induction of complete remission using standard dose chemotherapy resulted in an overall survival that was nearly double that of the median transplant. These data indicate the value of high-dose therapy in improving disease-free survival. The timing of high-dose therapy may be an important variable in the overall treatment plan for patients with metastatic breast cancer.

The toxicity of these treatment programs appears to be influenced by several factors, including extent of disease, performance status, the induction chemotherapy used prior to particular high-dose regimens, and the regimens themselves. Modification of treatment-associated toxicity appears to be possible using hematopoietic colony-stimulating factors and particularly with the use of colony stimulating factor primed peripheral blood progenitor cells. Widespread application of this technology will depend on the ability to achieve substantial cost reductions given the number of potential patients whom it might benefit.

At the present time, the use of high-dose approaches should be restricted to centers possessing the expertise and facilities to safely utilize this approach and only in the context of clinical trials. Very few regimens have been sufficiently tested to provide reliable information about outcome.

SMALL-CELL LUNG CANCER

Several series have examined the role of high-dose intensification in the treatment of small-cell lung cancer, and, in general, the results have been disappointing. Clearly, in advanced, resistant disease, high-dose consolidation appears to offer few durable remissions. Two series have reported that, of patients with minimal disease treated in complete remission, approximately 15% can achieve sustained remissions in excess of 2 years. The technique is limited in this patient population, usually because of generally poor performance, extent of disease, and age of the patients who present with this disease. A randomized trial in small-cell lung cancer showed a significant increase in disease-free survival but did not improve overall survival (94).

OVARIAN CANCER

Ovarian carcinoma has been demonstrated to display a dose-response relationship to several chemotherapy agents. Because of the poor prognosis of patients for whom initial chemotherapy for this disease fails, the use of high-dose chemotherapy with ABMT is attractive. Several studies have demonstrated high response rates in ovarian cancer, but the durability of these remissions has, in general, been brief (49, 54, 149, 156, 201). While several different therapeutic regimens have been tested, long-term results and comparative effects have not been studied in detail.

MELANOMA AND COLON CANCER

A small series of patients have been treated with high-dose chemotherapy regimens for metastatic melanoma (52, 88, 109, 119, 121, 196, 216, 217, 221, 235), and colon cancer (208). In general, therapeutic results in these diseases indicate that the complete response rate has not been changed substantially by the use of high-dose intensification with myelotoxic drugs and that the application of these techniques has not, as yet, changed the ultimate outcome. Evaluation, however, has been done predominantly in the setting of advanced resistant disease, and testing in earlier settings may be valuable.

MYELOMA

Many myeloma patients are elderly, and often frail, and for these reasons have not generally been considered for high-dose therapy approaches requiring bone marrow or stem cell support. However, there is apparently a steep dose-response effect to alkylating agents in patients with disease refractory to standard doses. Melphalan appears preferable to cyclophosphamide in small uncontrolled observations (24). Several large pilot studies have been reported in which high-dose melphalan or thiotepa, with or without total body radiation (TBI) has been used in previously treated patients (25, 76, 96). Complete responses (as defined by the disappearance of monoclonal gammopathy on standard protein electrophoresis) occur in 25 to 50%, and projected 3- to 4-year survival rates are 26 to 80%, depending on response to induction therapy. Bone marrow purging of myeloma cells using anti–B cell monoclonal antibodies (9, 10, 72) or 4-HC (181) has been presented, but small samples and uncontrolled design do not permit conclusions to be drawn about efficacy. Peripheral blood cell collections have also been utilized as support after high-dose therapy (62, 183). Again, small and heterogeneous patient populations, varying treatment programs, numbers, and short follow-up do not allow adequate assessment. In general, responses are higher, and more readily achieved in patients with lower tumor burden and when secondary resistance has not yet been developed. But there is no evidence of a plateau for disease-free survival after ABMT in myeloma patients as there appears to be after allogeneic bone marrow transplantation (42). Further evaluation is required.

CHRONIC MYELOID LEUKEMIA

Based upon the hypothesis that there may exist normal clones within CML marrow, ABMT in patients with CML has been undertaken using either CML remission marrow or peripheral blood stem cell collections. Remissions of short duration were achieved, but relapse of chronic-phase leukemia has been the rule. More recently, the long-term in vitro cultured bone marrows of patients with CML from which the Philadelphia chromosome has been lost have been used in these patients. Further evaluation is required (see Chapter 143).

GLIOMAS

Despite in vitro evidence for a dose-response effect for cytotoxic drugs in glioblastoma multiforme, high-dose chemotherapy has, in general, been disappointing (110, 209). To a large extent, trials have employed single agents, most commonly BCNU or other alkylating agents, and have produced only brief remissions with significant toxicity (71, 98, 153, 155, 190, 236, 238). In uncontrolled trials with this agent, no significant prolongation of survival has been achieved in either the advanced disease or in the adjuvant setting. Three studies suggested a small prolongation of survival for high-grade malignant gliomas with adjuvant high-dose BCNU and ABMT (98, 138, 236). Some remissions among the patients treated in these series appear to be prolonged (237). More recently, experience in pediatric brain tumors has suggested that a limited number of children with gliomas treated with multidrug regimens may achieve extended survival (63) (see Chapter 166).

TESTICULAR CANCER

The prognosis for patients with advanced resistant testicular cancer is poor. Recently, the use of high-dose therapy, including autologous bone marrow support, has resulted in greater than 1-year disease-free survival in 40% of completely responding patients (10% of all treated) with recurrent testicular cancer (40). Such results suggest that a fraction of these patients can be salvaged using high-dose intensification, even when prior chemotherapy has failed (154, 162) (see Chapter 128).

NEUROBLASTOMA AND EWING'S SARCOMA

The prognosis for children older than 1 year with neuroblastoma is poor: most suffer relapse and die of disease within 2 years. The use of phenylalanine mustard and total body irradiation in patients with neuroblastoma, with or without marrow purging, has been explored and demonstrates that about 25 to 35% of children with stage 3 or 4 neuroblastoma can remain continuously disease free after this treatment (65, 117, 120, 175, 177). Relapses after 21 months have not been observed in most series. Because of the high frequency of marrow involvement in neuroblastoma, several different approaches to purging have been applied in uncontrolled studies (101, 102, 130, 137a, 176, 184, 202, 226) (see Chapter 167).

Ewing's sarcoma has also attracted interest as a tumor which is potentially treatable by high-dose therapy and ABMT (133). The low frequency of this disease has not permitted controlled trials to be undertaken.

TOXICITIES

ABMT is frequently associated with both morbidity and mortality, depending on the nature and extent of the cancer, patient performance status, prior chemotherapy, conditioning regimen, and other factors. While most of the early toxicity is associated with the conditioning regimen, complications may result from the antibiotic and antifungal regimens associated with treatment of presumed or actual infection or from other supportive treatments such as CSFs. The timing of the toxicities associated with ABMT are usually characteristic, and valuable differential diagnostic information can be derived from these considerations (Fig. 85.8).

MYELOSUPPRESSION, COLONY-STIMULATING FACTORS, AND PERIPHERAL STEM CELLS

The use of high-dose chemotherapy has been associated with significant periods of myelosuppression. The average time to achievement of a neutrophil count greater than $500/\mu L^3$ in most studies ranges between 15 and 25 days; thrombocytopenia lasts somewhat longer. In some cases, particularly when patients have received extensive prior

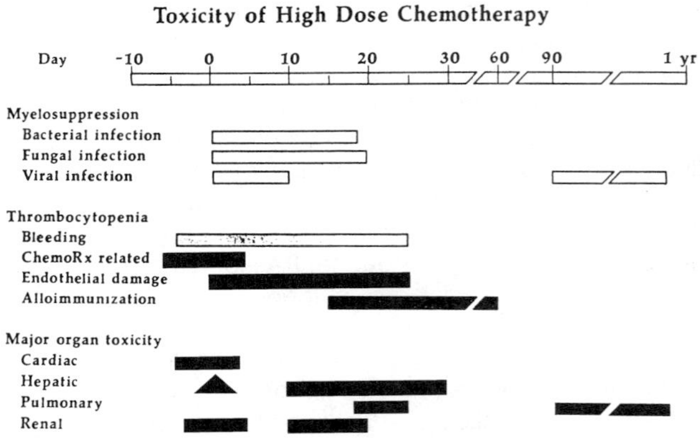

Toxicity of High Dose Chemotherapy

Day -10 0 10 20 30 60 90 1 yr

Myelosuppression
Bacterial infection
Fungal infection
Viral infection

Thrombocytopenia
Bleeding
ChemoRx related
Endothelial damage
Alloimmunization

Major organ toxicity
Cardiac
Hepatic
Pulmonary
Renal

Figure 85.8. Toxicities and the times they usually are most prominent after the procedure of intensive chemotherapy and autologous bone marrow transplantation.

chemotherapy, persistent thrombocytopenia can be a major problem, and some patients remain platelet dependent for more than 100 days. Various explanations have been put forth for extended periods of thrombocytopenia, including reduced tolerance of megakaryocyte to cryopreservation and removal of megakaryocytic precursors by the filtration process in which large cells are retained preferentially on the steel mesh filters used to process bone marrow.

Hematopoietic CSFs, such as GM- and G-CSF, have been utilized more recently to accelerate hematopoietic recovery (16, 35, 38, 172, 198). Several groups have now used CSFs as adjuncts in the bone marrow transplant setting and have reported remarkably consistent results. In each case, use of the hematopoietin accelerated myeloid recovery after high-dose therapy with bone marrow support. Platelet reconstitution was variably improved; however, always, there remained a period of absolute leukopenia which was not correctable by CSF alone at any dose utilized. This is presumed to be related to a relative deficiency in cryopreserved marrow of the committed progenitors bearing responsive receptors for the late-acting CSFs. In addition, the utilization of these compounds, either directly or indirectly, has led to a reduction of the organ system toxicity associated with high-dose chemotherapy.

The addition of hematopoietic progenitors derived from peripheral blood after chemotherapy, with or without CSF priming, has, in uncontrolled studies, resulted in a profound reduction in both the duration of absolute leukopenia and in the toxicity of transplantation (69, 70, 173). Studies have demonstrated an accelerated rate of hematopoietic recovery after a period of absolute leukopenia and a reduction in the infectious complications seen in these settings. Some studies have noted a reduction in the need for platelet transfusions, and of red cell transfusions.

The major consequence of myelosuppression continues to be infectious complications. Bacterial and fungal infections are the major problems associated with ABMT although viral infections, especially reactivated infections of herpes simplex virus (150), adenovirus-related hemophagocytic syndrome (124), and transfusion-associated cytomegalovirus (185, 229, 230, 234) may all occur with ABMT.

Immune Function Posttransplant

Recovery of immune function after ABMT appears to depend on the preparation regimen (busulfan) and ex vivo treatment, if any, of the graft marrow (11, 164). In addition, there are poorly understood effects, such as persistently inverted CD4–CD8 ratios (160) and disappearance of CD4 lymphocyte circadian cycles (135), perhaps related to differential repopulation kinetics of hematopoietic progenitors (228).

Organ Toxicity

Organ system toxicity follows high-dose chemotherapy in the marrow transplant setting, generally as a direct effect on organ systems of the chemotherapy and radiation therapy. It is likely that infectious complications, as well as the need for supportive care, such as antibacterial and antifungal medication, contribute to these injuries.

During administration of chemotherapy multiple complications have been described, including acute fluid imbalance, syndrome of inappropriate antidiuretic hormone secretion, hemorrhagic myocarditis, nephrogenic diabetes insipidus after cyclophosphamide therapy (64), hypertension with combination alkylating agents (81), disseminated intravascular coagulopathy (DIC) (85), metabolic abnormalities such as idiopathic hyperammonemia (144), an acquired platelet secretion defect (161), interstitial pneumonitis (163), and late vasculitis with pulmonary hemorrhage (195). All have been reported as complications of high-dose therapy where autologous bone marrow support has been used. In addition, failure to provide adequate bladder irrigation or to administer protective compounds such as mesna, has been associated with the development of hemorrhagic cystitis.

Mucositis and enterocolitis are major side effects of many, though not all, regimens. TBI, etoposide, melphalan, thiotepa, and regimens containing significant doses of these agents often produce severe mucositis. Tissue breakdown results in a higher risk of systemic infection, and often in nutritional imbalances. The possibility of fungal or viral causes of mucositis and esophagitis should not be overlooked. Diarrhea in patients undergoing ABMT may result from many causes, including the conditioning regimen, *Clostridium difficile* toxin, various medications, or fungal or viral infections.

Veno-occlusive disease (VOD) of the liver, reflecting endothelial damage and subsequent clot formation or fibrosis in the small hepatic venules associated with endothelial toxicity and centrolobular hemorrhage, occurs in as many as 20 to 40% of patients who undergo ABMT with some chemotherapy regimens. The mechanism of injury presumably reflects the deposition of activated drug metabolites into the hepatic venules after activation in the liver and subsequent injury to endothelial cells. The syndrome is generally manifested by right upper quadrant pain, hepatomegaly, ascites, jaundice, and veno-occlusive disease. No specific therapy is known, but various supportive efforts have been reported. Efforts to utilize prostaglandin synthetase inhibitors or heparin to prevent clot formation during the period of chemotherapy, diagnosis of VOD by ultrasonography (137), or treatment by tissue plasminogen activator (21) have been studied, with some success reported in uncontrolled trials.

Nephrotoxicity in the setting of ABMT can result from many causes, including specific chemotherapeutic agents known to influence kidney function (cisplatin, nitrosoureas, phenylalanine mustard), coupled with nephrotoxic effects of antibiotics generally used during supportive care. Late renal dysfunction (214) probably related to radiation therapy can occur.

Pulmonary drug toxicity has been reported in the post-transplant setting (97, 127). Cyclophosphamide produces pulmonary alveolitis which has been characterized in animal systems (34) and probably is expressed in humans in a combined injury resulting from radiation therapy and cyclophosphamide as part of the preparative regimen. Pulmonary drug toxicity is commonly associated with carmustine when the acute or chronic dose exceeds 1200 mg/m^2 of body surface. The clinical syndrome is generally manifested by fever, interstitial infiltrates, and dyspnea. It is characterized pathologically by type II pneumocyte proliferation, fibrosis, and alveolar inflammation. Pulmonary insufficiency can be rapidly progressive, and diagnostic efforts should be instituted promptly. The clinical syndrome is often confused with an infectious disease because of the complicating fever, and delay in making a specific diagnosis can lead to rapid progression of the toxicity. While no controlled trials have been undertaken, empirical observations suggest that chemoradiation injury is worsened by exposure to high concentrations of oxygen. The use of corticosteroids in large doses is often useful in ameliorating this toxicity (4) (see Chapter 182).

The most frequent serious cardiac complication associated with ABMT is hemorrhagic myocarditis, generally due to cyclophosphamide administration, alone or in combination with other drugs. The pathology suggests that the lesion is due to endothelial injury and subsequent bleeding into the myocardium. Prior radiation therapy or extensive adriamycin therapy may predispose children to this injury. Other reported cardiac complications include nonbacterial thrombotic endocarditis and catheter associated right-sided endocarditis (136) hypertension, both during marrow infusion (213) and after chemotherapy, perhaps mediated through atrial natriuretic factor (81).

The use of high-dose agents has resulted in a variety of central nervous system complications, including organic brain syndrome from thiotepa (235) and etoposide (122), infectious complications (123), and an encephalopathy like Wernicke's (131).

Cutaneous toxicity is frequently noted during ABMT from drug allergies manifested as a variety of rashes, cutaneous toxicity of chemotherapy (126), and a macular erythematous eruption called "host-versus-host syndrome" or "autologous graft-versus-host disease" (99), felt to be related to a type of graft-versus-host disease, though the mechanism is unclear.

Future Directions

Current therapeutic interventions in neoplastic diseases using high-dose therapy and ABMT do not appear to have reached their limit. CSFs and peripheral blood progenitor cells appear to offer the potential to further increase the dose intensity of treatment programs. It appears that major decrease in toxicity is possible and, thus, simplification of the treatment approach should yield a more cost-effective treatment. The first efforts toward reducing the hospitalization required for this approach have been undertaken (36).

Interpretation of the outcomes in most of the diseases for which ABMT is undertaken is hampered by the lack of randomized trial designs. Primary response and outcome variables are most frequently compared to historical or contemporary results. There is little information on the relative efficacy of various high-dose regimens; however, large controlled studies are hampered by the high cost of the procedure, resulting in third-party reimbursement difficulty for patients receiving high-dose procedures. Considerable controversy remains regarding the importance, if any, of purging in all disease settings, and resolution of this issue will require completion of randomized comparative trials.

Retroviral vector–mediated gene transfer into pluripotent stem cells uses autologous transplantation techniques and may extend the application of this treatment approach to other nonmalignant conditions. The technique remains limited owing to difficulties of gene packaging and expression, though early clinical trials placing new genetic material into cytotoxic T cells have been undertaken.

References

1. Ades EW, Peacocke N, Sabio H. Lymphokine-activated killer cell lysis of human neuroblastoma cells: a model for purging tumor cells from bone marrow. Clin Immunol Immunopathol 1988;46:150.
2. Agah R, Malloy B, Kerner M, Girgis E, Bean P, Twomey P, Mazumder A. Potent graft antitumor effect in natural killer–resistant disseminated tumors by transplantation of interleukin 2-activated syngeneic bone marrow in mice. Cancer Res 1989;49:5959.
3. Agah R, Malloy B, Kerner M, Mazumder A. Generation and characterization of IL-2-activated bone marrow cells as a potent graft vs tumor effector in transplantation. J Immunol 1989;143:3093.
4. Ahmed T. Autologous marrow transplantation for Hodgkin's disease: current techniques and prospects. Cancer Invest 1990;8:99.
5. Ahmed T, Ciavarella D, Feldman E, Ascensao J, Hussain F, Engelking C, Gingrich S, Mittelman A, Coleman M, Arlin ZA. High-dose, potentially myeloablative chemotherapy and ABMT for patients with advanced Hodgkin's disease. Leukemia 1989;3:19.
6. Allieri MA, Lopez M, Douay, et al. Intrinsic leukemic progenitor cell sensitivity to cryopreservation: incidence for autologous bone marrow transplantation. In Autologous Bone Marrow Transplantation: Proceedings of the Fourth International Symposium. Edited by KA Dicke, G Spitzer, S Jagannath, Houston: MD Anderson Hospital, 1988, pp 35–39.
7. Anderson IC, Shpall EJ, Leslie DS, Nustad K, Ugelstad J, Peters W, Bast RC Jr. Elimination of malignant clonogenic breast cancer cells from human bone marrow. Cancer Res 1989;49:4659.
8. Anderson KC, Ritz J, Takvorian T, Coral F, Daley H, Gorgone BC, Freedman AS, Canellos GP, Schlossman SF, Nadler LM. Hematologic engraftment and immune reconstitution post transplantation with anti-B1 purged autologous bone marrow. Blood 1987;69:597.
9. Anderson K, Barut B, Takvorian T, Freedman A, Mauch P, Ritz J, Nadler L. Monoclonal antibody (MoAb) purged ABMT for multiple myeloma (MM) (abstract). Blood 1989;74:202a.
10. Anderson KC, Barut BA, Ritz J, Freedman AS, Takvorian T, Rabinowe SN, Soiffer R, Heflin L, Coral F, Dear K, Mauch P, Nadler LM. Monoclonal antibody-purged autologous bone marrow transplantation therapy for multiple myeloma. Blood 1991;77:712.
11. Anderson KC, Soiffer R, DeLage R, Takvorian T, Freedman AS, Rabinowe SL, Nadler LM, Dear K, Heflin L, Mauch P, Ritz J. T-cell-depleted autologous bone marrow transplantation therapy: analysis of immune deficiency and late complications. Blood 1990;76:235.
12. Anonymous. The American Society of Clinical Oncology and American Society of Hematology recommended criteria for the performance of bone marrow transplantation. J Clin Oncol 1990;8:563.
13. Anonymous. Autologous bone marrow transplantation for advanced breast cancer. Med Lett 1991;33:39.
14. Antman K, Bearman SI, Davidson N, et al. Dose intensive therapy in breast cancer: current status. In New Strategies in Bone Marrow Transplantation. Edited by RP Gale, RE Champlin. New York: Alan R Liss, 1990, pp 423–436.
15. Antman K, Eder J, Elias A, Ayash L, Wheeler C, Schnipper L, Frei E III. High-dose cyclophosphamide, thiotepa, and carboplatin intensification with autologous bone marrow support in patients with breast cancer responding to standard dose induction therapy. Proc Am Soc Clin Oncol 1990;9:10(33a).
16. Antman KH. G-CSF and GM-CSF in clinical trials. Yale J Biol Med 1990;63:387.
17. Appelbaum FR, Deisseroth AB, Graw RG Jr, Herzig GP, Levine AS, Magrath IT, Pizzo PA, Poplack DG, Ziegler JL. Prolonged complete remission following high-dose chemotherapy of Burkitt's lymphoma in relapse. Cancer 1978;41:1059.
18. Areman EM, Sacher RA, Deeg HJ. Cryopreservation and storage of human bone marrow: a survey of current practices. In Bone Marrow Purging and Processing. Edited by S Gross, AP Gee, DA Worthington-White. New York: Alan R Liss, 1990, pp 415–433.
19. Armitage JO, Bearman PJ. Is there an optimal conditioning regimen for patients with lymphoma undergoing autologous bone marrow transplantation? In Autologous Bone Marrow Transplantation: Proceedings of the Fourth International Symposium. Edited by KA Dicke, G Spitzer, S Jagganath, MJ Evinger-Hodges. Houston: MD Anderson Hospital, 1988, pp 299–303.
20. August CS, Auble B. Autologous bone marrow transplantation for advanced neuroblastoma at the Children's Hospital of Philadelphia: an update. In Autologous Bone Marrow Transplantation: Proceedings of the Fourth International Symposium. Houston: MD Anderson Hospital, 1989, pp 567–573.
21. Baglin TP, Harper P, Marcus RE. Veno-occlusive disease of the liver complicating ABMT successfully treated with recombinant tissue plasminogen activator (rt-PA). Bone Marrow Transplant 1990;5:439.
22. Barbieri L, Dinota A, Gobbi M, Tazzari PL, Rizzi S, Bontadini A, Lemoli RM, Tura S, Stirpe F. Immunotoxins containing saporin 6 and monoclonal antibodies recognizing plasma cell-associated antigens: effects on target cells and on normal myeloid precursors (CFU-GM). Eur J Haematol 1989;42:238.
23. Barlogie B, Hall R, Zander A, Dicke K, Alexanian R. High-dose melphalan with autologous bone marrow transplantation for multiple myeloma. Blood 1986;67:1298.
24. Barlogie B, Alexanian R, Smallwood L, Cheson B, Dixon D, Dicke K, Cabanillas F. Prognostic factors with high dose melphalan for refractory multiple myeloma. Blood 1988;72:2015.
25. Barlogie B, Gahrton G. Bone marrow transplantation in multiple myeloma. Bone Marrow Transplant 1991;7:71.

26. Bast RC Jr, Sallen RE, Reynolds C, et al. Autologous bone marrow transplantation with CALLA positive ALL: update. In Proceedings of the First International Symposium of autologous bone marrow transplantation. Edited by KA Dicke, G Spitzer, A Zander, et al. Houston: University of Texas, 1985, pp 3–6.
27. Bell AJ, Figes A, Oscier DG, Hamblin TJ. Peripheral blood stem cell autografting. Lancet 1986;1:1027.
28. Berenson RJ, Bensinger WI, Kalamasz D, Schuening F, Deeg HJ, Graham T, Storb R. Engraftment of dogs with la-positive marrow cells isolated by avidinbiotin immunoadsorption. Blood 1987;69:1363.
29. Berenson RJ, Andrews RG, Bensinger WI, Kalamasz D, Knitter G, Buckner CD, Bernstein ID. Antigen CD34+ marrow cells engraft lethally irradiated baboons. J Clin Invest 1988;81:951.
30. Berenson RJ, Bensinger WI, Hill RS, Andrews RG, Garcia-Lopez J, Kalamasz DF, Still BJ, Spitzer G, Buckner CD, Bernstein ID, Thomas ED. Engraftment after infusion of CD34+ marrow cells in patients with breast cancer or neuroblastoma. Blood 1991;77: 1717.
30a. Bezwoda WR, Seymour L, Dansey RD. High-dose chemotherapy with hematopoietic rescue as primary treatment for metastatic breast cancer: A randomized trial. J of Clin Oncol 1995;13:10, 2483–2489.
31. Bieva CJ, Vander Brugghen FJ, Stryckmans PA. Malignant leukemic cell separation by iron colloid immunomagnetic adsorption. Exp Hematol 1989;17:914.
32. Blaze D, Gaspard MH, Stoppa AM, Michel G, Gastaut JA, Lepeu G, Tubiana N, Blanc AP, Rossi JF, Novakovitch G, Mannoni P, Mawas C, Maraninchi D, Caccassonne Y. Allogeneic or autologous bone marrow transplantation for acute lymphoblastic leukemia in first complete remission. Bone Marrow Transplant 1990;5:7.
33. Blazer BR, Widmer MB, Kersey JH, Ramsay NK, McGlave PB, Urdal DL, Gillis S, Henney C, Vallera DA. Recombinant granulocyte-macrophage colony stimulating factor in human and murine bone marrow transplantation. Behring Inst Mitt 1988;83:170.
34. Blumenstock DA, Cannon FD, Hales CA, Vlahovic VL, Alpern H, Kazemi H. Pulmonary function of DLA-nonidentical lung allografts in dogs treated with lethal total-body irradiation, autologous bone marrow transplantation, and methotrexate. Transplantation 1979;28:223.
35. Brandt SJ, Peters WP, Atwater SK, Kurtzberg J, Borowitz MJ, Jones RB, Shpall EJ, Gilbert C, Bast RC Jr, Oette DH. Effect of recombinant human granulocyte-macrophage colony stimulating factor on hematopoietic reconstitution following high-dose chemotherapy and autologous bone marrow transplantation. N Engl J Med 1988;318:869.
36. Brandwein JM, Callum J, Rubinger M, Scott JG, Keating A. An evaluation of outpatient bone marrow harvesting. J Clin Oncol 1989;7:648.
37. Brandwein J, Callum J, Sutcliffe SB, Scott JG, Keating A. The evaluation of cytoreductive therapy prior to high-dose treatment with autologous bone marrow transplantation, relapsed and refractory Hodgkin's disease. Bone Marrow Transplant 1990;5:99.
38. Brandwein JM, Nayar R, Baker MA, Sutton DM, Scott JG, Sutcliffe SB, Heating A. GM-CSF therapy for delayed engraftment after autologous bone marrow transplantation. Exp Hematol 1991;19:191.
39. Bronchud MH, Howell A, Crowther D, Hopwood P, Souza L, Dexter TM. The use of granulocyte colony-stimulating factor to increase the intensity of treatment with doxorubicin in patients with advanced breast and ovarian cancer. Br J Cancer 1989;60: 121.
40. Broun ER, Nichols CR, Tricot G, Loehrer PJ, Williams SD, Einhorn LH. High dose carboplatin/VP16 plus ifosfamide with autologous bone marrow support in the treatment of refractory germ cell tumors. Bone Marrow Transplant 1991;7:53.
41. Broxmeyer HE, Cooper S, Lu L, Hangoc G, Anderson D, Cosman D, Lyman SD, Williams DE. Effect of murine mast cell growth factor (c-kit proto-oncogene ligand) on colony formation by human marrow hematopoietic progenitor cells. Blood 1991;77: 2142.
42. Buckner CD, Fefer A, Bensinger W, Storb R, Durie BG, Appelbaum FR, Petersen FB, Weiden P, Clift RA, Sanders JE, Sullivan KM, Witherspoon RP, Hill R, Martin P, Thomas ED. Marrow transplantation for malignant plasma cell disorders: summary of the Seattle experience. Eur J Hematol (suppl) 1989;43:186.
43. Canellos GP, Nadler L, Takvorian T. Autologous bone marrow transplantation in the treatment of malignant lymphoma and Hodgkin's disease. Semin Hematol 1988;25: 58.
44. Castaigne S, Calvo F, Douay L, Thomas F, Benbunan M, Gerota J, Degos L. Successful haematopoietic reconstitution using autologous peripheral blood mononuclear cells in a patient with acute promyelocytic leukemia. Br J Hematol 1986;63:209.
45. Cavins JA, Kasakura S, Thomas ED, Ferrebee JW. Recovery of lethally irradiated dogs following infusion of autologous marrow stored at low temperature in dimethylsulfoxide. Blood 1962;20:730.
46. Chang J, Morgenstern GR, Coutinho LH, Scarffe JH, Carr T, Deakin DP, Testa NG, Dexter TM. The use of bone marrow cells grown in long-term culture for autologous bone marrow transplantation in acute myeloid leukaemia: an update. Bone Marrow Transplant 1989;4:5.
47. Chang J, Morgenstern GR, Testa NG, Dexter TM. Marrow grown in long-term culture can be used for autologous transplantation in the treatment of acute myeloid leukaemia. Folia Haematol (Leipz) 1989;116:597.
48. Chao NJ, Duncan SR, Long GD, Horning SJ, Blume KG. Corticosteroid therapy for diffuse alveolar hemorrhage in autologous bone marrow transplant recipients. Ann Intern Med 1991;114:145.
49. Ciobanu N, Bunowicz CD, Wiernik PH, Strauman T, Sheridan C, Bast RC Jr. Ca^{125} levels in patients with ovarian carcinoma undergoing autologous bone marrow transplantation. Am J Obstet Gynecol 1989;160:354.
50. Combaret V, Favrot MC, Chauvin F, Bouffet E, Philip I, Philip T. Immunomagnetic depletion of malignant cells from autologous bone marrow graft: from experimental models to clinical trials. J Immunogenet 1989;16:125.
51. Copeland NG, Gilbert DJ, Cho BC, Donovan PJ, Jenkins NA, Cosman D, Anderson D, Lyman SD, Williams DE. Mast cell growth factor maps near the steel locus on mouse chromosome 10 and is deleted in a number of steel alleles. Cell 1990;63:175.
52. Cornbleet MA, McElwain TJ, Kuman PJ, Filshie J, Selby P, Carter RL, Hedley DW, Clark ML, Millar JL. Treatment of advanced malignant melanoma with high-dose melphalan and autologous bone marrow transplantation. Br J Cancer 1983;48:329.
53. Coutinho LH, Testa NG, Chang J, Morgenstern G, Harrison C, Dexter TM. The use of cultured bone marrow cells in autologous transplantation. In Bone Marrow Purging and Processing. Edited by S Gross, AP Gee, DA Worthington-White. New York: Alan R Liss, 1990, pp 415–433.
54. Dauplat J, Legros M, Condat P, Ferriere JP, Ben Ahmed S, Plagne R. High-dose melphalan and autologous bone marrow support for treatment of ovarian carcinoma with positive second-look operation. Gynecol Oncol 1989;34:294.
55. Davis BH, Bigelow NC. Flow cytometric reticulocyte quantification using thiazole orange provides clinically useful reticulocyte maturity index. Arch Pathol Lab Med 1989;113:684.
56. Davis J, Rowley SD, Santos GW. Toxicity of autologous bone marrow graft infusion. Prog Clin Biol Res 1990;333:531.
57. De Fabritiis P, Bregni M, Lipton J, Reynolds C, Nadler L, Ritz J, Bast RC Jr. Antigenic heterogeneity among Burkitt's lymphoma cells surviving treatment with monoclonal antibody and complement. Leuk Res 1986;10:35.
58. De Fabritiis P, Bregni M, Lipton J, Greenberger J, Nadler L, Rothstein L, Korbling M, Ritz J, Bast RC Jr. Elimination of clonogenic Burkitt's lymphoma cells from human bone marrow using 4-hydroperoxycyclophosphamide in combination with monoclonal antibodies and complement. Blood 1985;65:1064.
59. Douay L, Gorin NC, Mary JY, Lemarie E, Lopez M, Najman A, Stachowiak J, Giarratana MC, Baillou C, Salmon C, Duhamel G. Recovery of CFU-GM from cryopreserved marrow and in vivo evaluation after autologous bone marrow transplantation are predictive of engraftment. Exp Hematol 1986;14:358–365.
60. Dunphy FR, Spitzer G, Buzdar AU, Hortobagyi GN, Horwitz LJ, Yau JC, Spinolo JA, Jagannath S, Holmes F, Wallerstein RO, Bohannan PO, Dicke KA. Treatment of estrogen receptor-negative or hormonally refractory breast cancer with double high-dose chemotherapy intensification and bone marrow support. J Clin Oncol 1990;8: 1207.
61. Dunphy FR, Spitzer G. Long-term complete remission of stage IV breast cancer after high-dose chemotherapy and autologous bone marrow transplantation. Am J Clin Oncol 1990;13:364.
62. Fermand JP, Levy Y, Gerota J, Benbunan M, Cosset JM, Castaigne S, Seligmann M, Brouet JC. Treatment of aggressive multiple myeloma by high-dose chemotherapy and total body irradiation followed by blood stem cells autologous graft. Blood 1989;73:20.
63. Finley JL, August C, Packer R, Zimmerman R, Sutton L, Fried A, Rorke L, Bayever E, Kamani N, Kramer E, Cohen B, Sturgill B, Nachman J, Strandjord S, Turski P, Freirdich S, Steeves R, Javid M. High-dose multi-agent chemotherapy followed by bone marrow "rescue" for malignant astrocytomas of childhood and adolescence. J Neurooncol 1990;9:239.
64. Finn G, Denning D. Transient nephrogenic diabetes insipidus following high-dose cyclophosphamide chemotherapy and autologous bone marrow transplantation. Cancer Treat Rep 1987;71:220.
65. Franzone P, Scarpati D, Vitale V, Corvio R, Barra S, Guenzi M, Orsatti M, Dini G. Chemo-radiotherapy and autologous bone marrow transplantation in poor prognosis neuroblastoma. Radiother Oncol 1990;18:102.
66. Freedman AS, Takvorian T, Anderson KC, Mauch P, Rabinowe SN, Blake K, Yeap B, Soiffer R, Coral F, Heflin L, Ritz J, Nadler LM. Autologous bone marrow transplantation in B-cell non-Hodgkin's lymphoma: very low treatment-related mortality in 100 patients in sensitive relapse. J Clin Oncol 1990;8:784.
67. Frei E III, Canellos GP. Dose, a critical factor in cancer chemotherapy. Am J Med 1986;69:585.
68. Gale RP, Armitage JO, Dicke KA. Autotransplants: now and in the future. Bone Marrow Transplant 1991;7:153.
69. Gianni AM, Siena S, Bregni M, Tarella C, Stern AC, Pileri A, Bonadonna G. Granulocyte-macrophage colony-stimulating factor to harvest circulating haemopoietic stem cells for autotransplantation. Lancet 1989;II:580.
70. Gianni AM, Bregni M, Siena S, Villa S, Sciorelli GA, Ravagnani F, Pellegris G, Bonadonna G. Rapid and complete hemopoietic reconstitution following combined transplantation of autologous blood and bone marrow cells. A changing role for high dose chemo-radiotherapy? Hematol Oncol 1989;7:139.
70a. Gianni AM, Siena S, Bregin M, Di Nicola M, Dodero R, Zambetti M, Orefice S, Salvadori B, Luini A, Breco M, Zucali R, Valagossa P, Bonadonna G. 5-Year results of high-dose sequential (HDS) adjuvant chemotherapy in breast cancer with ≥10 positive nodes. Proc Am Soc Clin Oncol 1995;14:90.
71. Giannone L, Wolff SN. Phase II treatment of central nervous system gliomas with high-dose etoposide and autologous bone marrow transplantation. Cancer Treat Rep 1987;71:759.
72. Gobbi M, Cavo M, Tazzari PL, Dinota A, Tassi C, Bontadini A, Albertazzi L, Miggiano C, Rizzi S, Rosti G, Bolognesi A, Stirpe F, Tura S. Autologous bone marrow transplantation with immunotoxin-purged marrow for advanced multiple myeloma. Eur J Haematol 1989;43:176.
73. Goldie JH, Goldman AJ. A mathematic model for relating the drug sensitivity of tumors to the spontaneous mutation rate. Cancer Treat Rep 1979;63:1727.
74. Goldman JM, Catovsky D, Hows J, Spiers ASD, Galton DAG. Cryopreserved peripheral blood cells functioning as autografts in patients with chronic granulocytic leukemia in transformation. Brit Med J 1979;11:1310.
75. Goldstone AH, Gribben JG. The role of autologous bone marrow transplantation in the treatment of malignant disease. Blood Rev 1987;1:193.
76. Gore ME, Selby PJ, Viner C, Clark PI, Meldrum M, Millar B, Bell J, Maitland JA, Milan S, Judson IR, Zuiable A, Tillyer C, Slevin M, Malpas JS, McElwain TJ. Intensive treatment of multiple myeloma and criteria for complete remission. Lancet 1989;2:879.
77. Gorin NC, Aegerter P, Auvert B, Meloni G, Goldstone AH, Burnett A, Carella A, Korbling M, Herve P, Maraninchi D, Löwenberg R, Verdonck LF, de Planque M, Hermans J, Helbig W, Porcellini A, Rizzoli V, Alesandrino EP, Franklin IM, Reiffers J, Colleselli P, Goldman JM. Autologous bone marrow transplantation for acute myelocytic leukemia in first remission: a European survey of the role of marrow purging. Blood 1990;75:1606.
78. Gorin NC, Herve P, Aegerter P, Goldstone A, Linch D, Maraninchi D, Burnett A, Helbig W, Meloni G, Verdonck LF, De Witte T, Rizzoli V, Carella A, Parlier Y, Auvert B, Goldman J. Autologous bone marrow transplantation for acute leukemia in remission. Br J Haematol 1986;64:385.
79. Gorin NC, Caegerter P, Auvert B. Autologous bone marrow transplantation for acute leukemia in remission: an analysis of 1322 cases. Bone Marrow Transplant 1989;4:3.
80. Graeve JL, de Alarcon PA, Sato Y, Pringle K, Helson L. Miliary pulmonary neuroblastoma. A risk of autologous bone marrow transplantation? Cancer 1988;62:2125.

81. Graves SW, Eder JP, Schryber SM, Sharma K, Brena A, Antman KH, Peters WP. Endogenous digoxin-like immunoreactive factor and digitalis-like factor associated with the hypertension of patients receiving multiple alkylating agents as part of autologous bone marrow transplantation. Clin Sci 1989;77:501.
82. Gribben JG, Goldstone AH, Linch DC, Taghipour G, McMillan AK, Souhami RL, Earl H, Richard JD. Effectiveness of high-dose combination chemotherapy and autologous bone marrow transplantation for patients with non-Hodgkin's lymphomas who are still responsive to conventional-dose therapy. J Clin Oncol 1989;7:1621.
83. Gribben JG, Lynch DC, Singerl CR, McMillan AK, Jarrett M, Goldstone AH. Successful treatment of refractory Hodgkin's disease by high-dose combination chemotherapy and autologous bone marrow transplantation. Blood 1989;73:340.
84. Gribben JG, Goldstone AH, Linch DC. Preliminary results of autologous bone marrow transplantation in the management of resistant Hodgkin's disease: experience of the Bloomsbury Transplant Group at University College, London. Recent Results Cancer Res 1989;117:242.
85. Guinan EC, Tarbell NJ, Niemeyer CM, Sallan SE, Weinstein HJ. Intravascular hemolysis and renal insufficiency after bone marrow transplantation. Blood 1988;72:451.
86. Gulati S, Shank B, Yahalom J, et al. Autologous BMT for patients with poor-prognosis lymphoma and Hodgkin's disease. In Autologous Bone Marrow Transplantation: Proceedings of the Fourth International Symposium. Edited by KA Dicke, G Spitzer, S Jagannath. Houston: MD Anderson Hospital, 1988, pp 231–239.
87. Hanes MA, Goldman JM, Worsley AM, McCarthy DM, Wyeth SE, Dowding C, Kerney L, Th'ng KH, Wareham NH, Pollock A, Galvin MC, Samson D, Geary CG, Davotsky D, Dalton DAG. Chemotherapy and autografting for chronic granulocytic leukemia in transformation, probable prolongation of survival for some patients. Br J Hematol 1984;58:711.
88. Hartmann DW, Robinson WA, Morton NJ, Mangalik A, Glode LM. High-dose nitrogen mustard (HN2) with autologous nonfrozen bone marrow transplantation in advanced malignant melanoma. A phase I trial. Blut 1981;42:209.
89. Hershko C, Ho WG, Gale RP, Cline MJ. Cure of aplastic anemia in paroxysmal nocturnal haemoglobinuria by marrow transfusion from identical twins: failure of peripheral-leukocyte transfusion to correct marrow aplasia. Lancet 1979;1:945.
90. Herzig G. Autologous marrow transplantation in cancer therapy. In Progress in Hematology. Edited by EB Brown. New York: Grune & Stratton, 1981, pp 1–23.
91. Higuchi CM, Thompson JA, Cox T, Lindgren CG, Buckner CD, Fefer A. Lymphokine-activated killer function following autologous bone marrow transplantation for refractory hematological malignancies. Cancer Res 1989;49:5509.
92. Hortobagyi GN. The role of high-dose chemotherapy with autologous bone marrow transplantation in the treatment of breast cancer. Bone Marrow Transplant 1988;3: 525.
93. Hortobagyi GN, Dunphy F, Buzdar AU, Spitzer G. Dose intensity studies in breast cancer—autologous bone marrow transplantation. Prog Clin Biol Res 1990;354:195.
94. Humblet Y, Symann M, Bosly A, Delaunois L, Francis C, Machiels J, Beauduin M, Doyen C, Weynants P, Longueville J, Prignot J. Late intensification chemotherapy with autologous bone marrow transplantation in selected small-cell carcinoma of the lung: a randomized study. J Clin Oncol 1987;5:1864.
95. Jagannath S, Armitage JO, Dicke KA, Tucker SL, Valasquez WS, Smith K, Vaughan WP, Kessinger A, Horwitz LJ, Hagemeister FB, Cabanillas F, Spitzer G. Timing of high dose CBV and autologous bone marrow transplantation in the management of relapsed or refractory Hodgkin's disease. In Autologous Bone Marrow Transplantation: Proceedings of the Fourth International Symposium. Edited by KA Dicke, G Spitzer, S Jagannath. Houston: MD Anderson Hospital, 1988, pp 275–283.
96. Jagannath S, Barlogie B, Dicke K, Alexarian R, Zagars C, Cheson B, Lemaistre FC, Smallwood L, Pruitt K, Dixon DO. Autologous bone marrow transplantation in multiple myeloma: identification of prognostic factors. Blood 1990;76:1860.
97. Jochelson M, Tarbell NJ, Freedman AS, Rabinowe SN, Takvorian T, Soiffer R, Anderson K, Ritz J, Nadler LM. Acute and chronic pulmonary complications following autologous bone marrow transplantation in non-Hodgkin's lymphoma. Bone Marrow Transplant 1990;6:329.
98. Johnson DB, Thompson JM, Corwin JA, Mosley KR, Smith MT, de los Reyes RA, Daly MB, Petty AM, Lamaster D, Pierson WP, Ruxer RL Jr, Leff RS, Messerschmidt GL. Prolongation of survival for high-grade malignant gliomas with adjuvant high-dose BCNU and autologous bone marrow transplantation. J Clin Oncol 1987;5:783.
99. Jones RJ, Vogelsang GB, Hess AD, Farmer ER, Mann RB, Geller RB, Piantadosi S, Santos GW. Induction of graft-versus-host disease after autologous bone marrow transplantation. Lancet 1989;1:754.
100. Juttner CA, To LB, Haylock DN, Dyson PG. Peripheral blood stem cell selection, collection, and autotransplantation. In Bone Marrow Purging and Processing. Edited by S Gross, AP Gee, DA Worthington-White. New York: Alan R Liss, 1990, pp 447–460.
101. Kemshead JT, Black J. Developments in the biology of neuroblastoma: implications for diagnosis and treatment. Dev Med Child Neurol 1980;22:816.
102. Kemshead JT, Walsh F, Pritchard J, Greaves M. Monoclonal antibody to ganglioside GQ discriminates between haemopoietic cells and infiltrating neuroblastoma tumour cells in bone marrow. Int J Cancer 1981;27:447.
103. Keng PC, Rubin P, Constine LS, Frantz C, Nakissa N, Gregory P. Characterization of the biophysical properties of human tumor and bone marrow cells as a preliminary step to the use of centrifugal elutriation in autologous bone marrow transplantation. Int J Radiat Oncol Biol Phys 1984;10: 1913.
104. Kersey JH, Weisdorf D, Nevitt ME, LeBien TW, Woods WG, McLave PB, Kim T, Vallera DA, Goldman AI, Bostrom B, Perd D, Ramsey N. Comparison of autologous and allogeneic bone marrow transplantation for treatment of high-risk refractory acute lymphoblastic leukemia. N Engl J Med 1987;317:461.
105. Kessinger A, Armitage JO. Harvesting marrow for autologous transplantation from patients with malignancies. Bone Marrow Transplant 1987;2:15.
106. Kessinger A, Armitage JO, Smith DM, Landmark JD, Bierman PJ, Weisenburger DD. High-dose therapy and autologous peripheral blood stem cell transplantation for patients with lymphoma. Blood 1989;74:1260.
107. Kessinger A, Armitage JO, Landmark JD, Weisenburger DD. Reconstitution of human hematopoietic function with autologous cryopreserved circulating stem cells. Exp Hematol 1986;114:192.
108. Kessinger A, Bierman P, Armitage J. Refractory intermediate grade non-Hodgkin's lymphoma (NHL) treated with high dose therapy and autologous peripheral stem cell transplantation (PSCT): response and survival. Proc ASCO 1990;9:255.
109. Kessinger A. High-dose chemotherapy with autologous marrow transplantation for malignant melanoma. Case reports and literature review. J Am Acad Dermatol 1985;12:337.
110. Kessinger A. High dose chemotherapy with autologous bone marrow rescue for high grade gliomas of the brain: a potential for improvement in therapeutic results. Neurosurgery 1984;15:747.
111. Korbling M, Fliedner TM, Calvo W, Ross WM, Northdurft W, Steinbach I. Albumin density gradient purification of canine hematopoietic stem cells (HBSC): long-term allogeneic engraftment without graft vs. host reaction. Exp Hematol 1979;7:277.
112. Korbling M, Dorken B, Ho AD, Pezzutto A, Hunsttein W, Gliedner TM. Autologous transplantation of blood-derived hemopoietic stem cells after myeloablative therapy in a patient with Burkitt's lymphoma. Blood 1986;67:529.
113. Korbling M, Martin H, Gliedner TM. Autologous blood stem cell transplantation. In Proceedings of the Keystone Meeting on Bone Marrow Transplantation. Edited by RP Gale, RE Champlin. New York: Alan R Liss, 1986, pp 1–12.
114. Korbling M, Hess AD, Tutschka PJ, Kaizer H, Colvin MO, Santos GW. 4-Hydroperoxycyclophosphamide. A model for eliminating residual human tumour cells and T lymphocytes from the bone marrow graft. Br J Haematol 1982;52:89.
115. Korbling M, Burke P, Braine H, Elfenbein G, Santos G, Kaizer H. Successful engraftment of blood-derived hemopoietic stem cells in chronic myelogenous leukemia. Exp Hematol 1981;9:684.
116. Kubel M, Helbig W, Schwenke H, Wotzel M, Thierbach V, Standke E, Hoffmann FA. Autologous bone marrow transplantation (ABMT) using unpurged marrow as intensification for first complete remission in acute leukaemia (AL). Folia Haematol (Leipz) 1989;116:493.
117. Kushner BH, O'Reilly RJ, Mandell LR, Gulati SC, LaQuaglia M, Cheung NK. Myeloablative combination chemotherapy without total body irradiation for neuroblastoma. J Clin Oncol 1991;9:274.
118. Kvalheim G, Fodstad O, Pihl A, Nustad K, Pharo A, Ugelstad J, Funderud S. Elimination of B-lymphoma cells from human bone marrow model experiments using monodisperse magnetic particles coated with primary monoclonal antibodies. Cancer Res 1987;47:846.
119. Lakhani S, Selby P, Bliss JM, Perren TJ, Gore ME, McElwain TJ. Chemotherapy for malignant melanoma: combinations and high doses produce more responses without survival benefit. Br J Cancer 1990;61:330.
120. Lanino E, Melodia A, Casalaro A, Cornaglia-Gerraris P. Neuroblastoma cells circulate in peripheral blood. Ped Hematol Oncol 1989;6:193.
121. Lazarus HM, Herzig RH, Wolff SN, Phillips GL, Spitzer TR, Fay JW, Herzig GP. Treatment of metastatic malignant melanoma with intensive melphalan and autologous bone marrow transplantation. Cancer Treat Rep 1985;69:473.
122. Leff RS, Thompson JM, Daly MB, Johnson DB, Harden EA, Mercier RJ, Messerschmidt GL. Acute neurologic dysfunction after high-dose etoposide therapy for malignant glioma. Cancer 1988;62:32.
123. Leff RS, Martino RL, Pollock WJ, Knight WA III. Pituitary abscess after autologous bone marrow transplantation. Am J Hematol 1989;31:62.
124. Levy J, Wodell RA, August CS, Bayever E. Adenovirus-related hemophagocytic syndrome after bone marrow transplantation. Bone Marrow Transplant 1990;6:349.
125. Leibo SP, Farrant J, Mazur P, Hanna MG Jr, Smith LH. Effects of freezing on marrow stem cell suspension: interaction of cooling and warming rates in the presence of PVP, sucrose, or glycerol. Cryobiology 1970;6:315.
126. Linassier C, Colombat P, Reisenleiter M, Haillot O, Chazard M, Binet C, Desbois I, Lamagnere JP. Cutaneous toxicity of autologous bone marrow transplantation in nonseminomatous germ cell tumors. Cancer 1990;65:1143.
127. Litam JP, Dail DH, Spitzer G, Vellekoop L, Verma DS, Zander AR, Dicke KA. Early pulmonary toxicity after administration of high-dose BCNU. Cancer Treat Rep 1981;65: 39.
128. Litzow MR, Peterson FB, Appelbaum FR, Buckner CD. Autologous versus allogeneic bone marrow transplantation (BMT) for Hodgkin's disease. Blood 1990;76:550a.
129. Long GS, Cramer DV, Harnaha JB, Hiserodt JC. Lymphokine-activated killer (LAK) cell purging of leukemic bone marrow. Range of activity against different hematopoietic neoplasms. Bone Marrow Transplant 1990;6:169.
130. Lopez M, Zucker JM, Urresola R, Douay L, Quintana E, Kemshead J, Gorin NC, Vilcoq JR. Influence of single and double immunomagnetic depletion on the hemopoietic capacity of marrow in patients with advanced neuroblastoma submitted to autologous bone marrow transplantation. Bone Marrow Transplant 1987;2:413.
131. Majolino I, Caponetto A, Scimie R, Vasta S, Fabbiano F, Caronia F. Wernicke-like encephalopathy after autologous bone marrow transplantation. Haematologica 1990;75:282.
132. Mangan KF, Boucek C, Powers D, Shadduck RK. Rapid detection of venous air embolism by mass spectrometry during bone marrow harvesting. Exp Hematol 1985;13: 639.
133. Marcus RB Jr, Graham Pole JR, Springfield DS, Fort JA, Gross S, Mendenhall NP, Elfenbein GJ, Weiner RS, Enneking WF, Million RR. High-risk Ewing's sarcoma: end-intensification using autologous bone marrow transplantation. Int J Radiat Oncol Biol Phys 1988;15:53.
134. Marder RJ, Winter J, Epstein A. Heterogeneity of phenotypic expression in normal and neoplastic B-cell proliferations detected by monoclonal antibodies LN-1 and DLC-48. Am J Clin Pathol 1988;90:149.
135. Martini E, Gorin NC, Gastal C, Doinel C, Roquin H, Najman A, Salmon C. Disappearance of CD4 lymphocyte circadian cycles after autologous bone marrow transplantation. Biomed Pharmacother 1988;42:357.
136. Martino P, Micozzi A, Venditti M, Gentile G, Girmenia C, Raccah R, Santilli S, Alessandri N, Mandelli F. Catheter-related right-sided endocarditis in bone marrow transplant recipients. Rev Infec Dis 1990;12:250.
137. Matsuishi E, Anzai K, Dohmen K, Taniguchi S, Gondo H, Kudo J, Shibuya T, Ishibashi H, Harada M, Niho Y. Sonographic diagnosis of venoocclusive disease of the liver and danazol therapy for autoimmune thrombocytopenia in an autologous marrow transplant patient. Jpn J Clin Oncol 1990;20:188.
137a. Matthay KK, Seeger RC, Reynolds CP, Stram DO. Allogeneic versus autologous purged bone marrow transplantation for neuroblastoma: a report from the Children's Cancer Group. J Clin Oncol 1994;12:2382–2389.
138. Mbidde EK, Selby PJ, Perren TJ, Dearnaley DP, Whitton A, Ashley S, Workman P, Bloom HJ, McElwain TJ. High dose BCNU chemotherapy with autologous bone marrow transplantation and full dose radiotherapy for grade IV astrocytoma. Br J Cancer 1988;58:779.

139. McGuire WL, Herzig RH, Lemaistre CF, Peters WP. Autologous bone marrow transplantation in breast cancer. A panel discussion. Breast Cancer Res Treat 1988;11:7.
140. Meagher RC, Rothman SA, Paul P, Koberna P, Willmer C, Baucco PA. Purging of small cell lung cancer cells from human bone marrow using ethiofos (WR-2721) and light-activated merocyanine 540 phototreatment. Cancer Res 1989;49:3637.
141. Mick R, Begg CB, Antman KH, Korzun AH, Frei E III. Diverse prognosis in metastatic breast cancer: who should be offered alternative initial therapies? Breast Cancer Res Treat 1989;13:33.
142. Micklem HS, Anderson N, Ross E. Limited potential circulating hematopoietic stem cells. Nature 1975;256:41.
143. Minegishi N, Minegishi M, Tuchiya S, Konno T. Preservation of immature hematopoietic progenitor cells responding to interleukin 3 in marrow treated with 4-hydroperoxycyclophosphamide. Tohoku J Exp Med 1989;159:113.
144. Mitchell RB, Wagner JE, Karp JE, Watson AJ, Brusilow SW, Przepiorka D, Storb R, Santos GW, Burke PJ, Saral R. Syndrome of idiopathic hyperammonemia after high-dose chemotherapy: review of nine cases. Am J Med 1988;85:662.
145. Montgomery RB, Kurtzberg J, Rhinehardt-Clark A, Haleen A, Ramakrishnan S, Olsen GA, Peters WP, Smith CA, Haynes BF, Houston LL, Bast RC Jr. Elimination of malignant clonogenic T cells from human bone marrow using chemoimmunoseparation with 2'-deoxycoformycin, deoxyadenosine and an immunotoxin. Bone Marrow Transplant 1990;5:395.
146. Moss TJ, Sanders DG, Lasky LC, Bostrom B. Contamination of peripheral blood stem cell harvests by circulating neuroblastoma cells. Blood 1990;76:1879.
147. Moss TJ, Sanders DG. Detection of neuroblastoma cells in blood. J Clin Oncol 1990;8:736.
148. Mulder PO, Meinesz AF, deVries EG, Mulder NH. Diffuse alveolar hemorrhage in autologous bone marrow transplant recipients [Letter]. Am J Med 1991;90:278.
149. Mulder PO, Willemse PH, Aalders JG, deVries EG, Sleijfer DT, Sibinga CT, Mulder NH. High-dose chemotherapy with autologous bone marrow transplantation in patients with refractory ovarian cancer. Eur J Cancer Clin Oncol 1989;25:645.
150. Mulder PO, Schroder P, deVries EG, Hospers HG, van der Geest S, Sleijfer DT, Mulder NH. Incidence and effects of herpes simplex virus infection after autologous bone marrow transplantation for solid tumours. Neth J Med 1989;34:126.
151. Myers DE, Uckun FM, Ball ED, Vallera DA. Immunotoxins for ex vivo marrow purging in autologous bone marrow transplantation for acute nonlymphocytic leukemia. Transplantation 1988;46:240.
152. Nadler LM, Takvorian T, Botnick L, Bast RC Jr, Finberg R, Hellman S, Canellos GP, Schlossman SF. Anti-B1 monoclonal antibody and complement treatment in autologous bone-marrow transplantation for relapsed B-cell non-Hodgkin's lymphoma. Lancet 1984;II:427.
153. Nakagawa H, Murasawa A, Taki T, Nakajima S, Niiyama K, Furuta Y, Nakamura H, Shibata H, Masaoka T. Treatment of malignant gliomas with high-dose ACNU and autologous bone marrow transplantation [Jpn]. Gan To Kagaku Ryoho 1988;15:3153.
154. NIchols CR, Tricot G, Williams SD, van Besien K, Loehrer PJ, Roth BJ, Akard L, Hoffman R, Goulet R, Wolff SN, Giannone L, Greer J, Einhorn LH, Jansen J. Dose-intensive chemotherapy in refractory germ cell cancer: a phase I/II trial of high dose carboplatin and etoposide with autologous bone marrow transplantation. J Clin Oncol 1989;7:932.
155. Nomura K, Watanabe T, Nakamura O, Ohira M, Shibui S, Takakura K, Miki Y. Intensive chemotherapy with autologous bone marrow rescue for recurrent malignant gliomas. Neurosurg Rev 1984;7:13.
156. Nor'es JM, Dalayeun JF, Otmezguine Y, Folgoas C, Nenna AD. High-dose chemotherapy, total abdomen irradiation and autologous bone marrow infusion in ovarian cancer: an observation. Gynecol Obstet Invest 1989;27:55.
157. Norton L, Simon R. Tumor size, sensitivity to therapy, and the design of treatment schedules. Cancer Treat Rep 1977;61:1307.
158. Norton L, Simon R. The Norton-Simon hypothesis revisted. Cancer Treat Rep 1986;70:163.
159. Norton L, Day R. Potential innovation in scheduling of cancer chemotherapy. In Important Advances in Oncology. Edited by VT DeVita, S Hellman, SA Rosenberg. Philadelphia: Lippincott, 1991, pp 57–72.
160. Olsen GA, Gockerman JP, Bast RC Jr, Borowitz M, Peters WP. Altered immunologic reconstitution after standard-dose chemotherapy or high-dose chemotherapy with autologous bone marrow support. Transplantation 1988;46:57.
161. Panella TJ, Peters W, White JG, Hannun YA, Greenberg CS. Platelets acquire a secretion defect after high-dose chemotherapy. Cancer 1009;65:1711.
162. Pcio JL, Droz JP, Ostronoff M, et al. High dose chemotherapy and autologous bone marrow transplantation for poor prognosis non-seminomatous germ cell tumors. In Autologous Bone Marrow Transplantation: Proceedings of the Fourth International Symposium. Houston: MD Anderson Hospital, 1989, pp 469–476.
163. Pecego R, Hill R, Appelbaum FR, Amos D, Buckner CD, Fefer A, Thomas ED. Interstitial pneumonitis following autologous bone marrow transplantation. Transplantation 1986;42:515.
164. Pedrazzini A, Freedman AS, Andersen J, Heflin L, Anderson K, Takvorian T, Canellos GP, Whitman J, Coral F, Ritz J, Nadler LM. Anti-B-cell monoclonal antibody-purged autologous bone marrow transplantation for B-cell non-Hodgkin's lymphoma: phenotypic reconstitution and B-cell function. Blood 1989;74:2203.
165. Peters WP. Dose intensification using high-dose combination alkylating agents and autologous bone marrow support in the treatment of primary and metastatic breast cancer: a review of the Duke Bone Marrow Transplantation Program experience. In High-Risk Breast Cancer. Edited by J Ragaz, IM Ariel. Berlin: Springer-Verlag, 1991, pp 437–446.
166. Peters WP. Dose intensification using combination alkylating agents and autologous bone marrow support in the treatment of primary and metastatic breast cancer: a review of the Duke Bone Marrow Transplantation Program experience. Prog Clin Biol Res 1990;354:185.
167. Peters WP, Shpall EJ, Jones RB, Olsen GA, Gockerman JP, Bast RC Jr, Moore JO. High dose combination alkylating agents with bone marrow support as initial treatment for metastatic breast cancer. J Clin Oncol 1988;6:1368.
168. Peters WP, Shpall EJ, Jones RB, Ross M. High dose combination cyclophosphamide, cisplatin, and carmustine with bone marrow support as initial treatment for metastatic breast cancer: three to six year follow-up. Proc Am Soc Clin Oncol 1990;9:10a.
169. Peters WP, Jones RB, Shpall EJ, Gockerman J, Kurtzberg J, et al. Strategies in the treatment of breast cancer with intensive chemotherapy and autologous bone marrow support. In Autologous Bone Marrow Transplantation: Proceedings of the Fourth International Symposium. Edited by KA Dicke, G Spitzer, S Jagannath. Houston: MD Anderson Hospital, 1987, pp 465–474.
170. Peters WP, Davis R, Shpall EJ, Jones R, Ross M, Marks L, Norton L, Hurd D. Adjuvant chemotherapy involving high dose combination cyclophosphamide, cisplatin and carmustine, and autologous bone marrow support for stage II/III breast cancer involving ten or more lymph nodes (CALGB 8782): a preliminary report. Proc Am Soc Clin Oncol 1990;9:22(80a).
171. Peters WP. High-dose chemotherapy and autologous bone marrow support for breast cancer. In Important Advances in Oncology, 1991. Edited by VT DeVita, S Hellman, SA Rosenberg. Philadelphia: Lippincott, 1991, pp 135–150.
172. Peters WP, Kurtzberg J, Atwater S, Borowitz M, Gilbert C, Rao M, Currie M, Shogan J, Jones RB, Shpall EJ, Souza L. Comparative effects of rHuG-CSF and rHuGM-CSF on hematopoietic reconstitution and granulocyte function following high dose chemotherapy and autologous bone marrow transplantation (ABMT). Blood 1988;71:130a.
173. Peters WP, Kurtzberg J, Kirkpatrick G, Atwater S, Gilbert C, Borowitz M, Shpall E, Jones R, Ross M, Affronti M, Coniglio D, Mathias B, Oette D. GM-CSF primed peripheral blood progenitor cells (PBPC) coupled with autologous bone marrow transplantation (ABMT) will eliminate absolute leukopenia following high dose chemotherapy (HDC). Blood 1989;74:178.
173a. Peters WP. Unpublished data.
173b. Peters WP, Berry D, Vredenburgh JJ, Hussein R, Rubin P, Zrkordy M, Ross M, Henderson IC, Budman D, Norton L, Weiss R, Hurd D. Five-year follow-up of high-dose combination alkylating agents with ABMT as consolidation after standard dose AF for primary breast cancer involving axillary lymph nodes (Duke/CALGB 8782). Proc Am Soc Clin Oncol 1995;14:317.
173c. Peters WP, Jones RB, Bredenburgh J, Shpall EJ, Hussein A, Elkordy M, Rubin P, Ross M, Affronti ML, Moore S, Berry D. A large, prospective, randomized trial of high-dose combination alkylating agents (CPB) with autologous cellular support (ABMS) as consolidation for patients with metastatic breast cancer achieving complete remission after intensive doxorubicin-based induction therapy (AFM). Submitted to *19th Annual San Antonio Breast Cancer Symposium*, 1995.
174. Philip T, Armitage O, Spitzer G, Chauvin F, Jagannath S, Cahn JY, Colombat P, Goldstone AH, Gorin NC, Flesh M, Laporte JP, Maraninchi D, Pico J, Bosly A, Anderson C, Schots R, Biron P, Cabanillas F, Dicke K. High Dose Therapy and autologous bone marrow transplantation after failure of conventional chemotherapy in adults with intermediate-grade or high-grade non-Hodgkin's lymphoma. N Engl J Med 1987;316:1493.
175. Philip T, Bernard JL, Zucker JM, Pinkerton R, Lutz P, Bordigoni P, Plouvier E, Robert A, Carton R, Philippe N, Philip I, Chauvin F, Favrot M. High-dose chemoradiotherapy with bone marrow transplantation as consolidation treatment in neuroblastoma: an unselected group of stage IV patients over 1 year of age. J Clin Oncol 1987;5:266.
176. Philip T, Bernard JL, Zucker JM, Souillet G, Favrot M, Philip I, Bordigoni P, Lutz JP, Plouvier E, Carton P, Robert A, Kemshead J. Purged autologous bone marrow transplantation in 25 cases of very poor prognosis neuroblastoma [letter]. Lancet 1985;I:576.
176a. Philip T, Guglielmi C, Chauvin F, Hazenbeck A, Van Der Lely J, Bron D, Sonneveld P, Gisselbrecht C, Cahn JY, Harousseau JL, Coiffier B, Biron P, Somers R. Autologous bone marrow transplantation (ABMT) versus conventional chemotherapy (DHAP) in relapsed non-Hodgkin's lymphoma (NHL): final analysis of the Parma randomized study (216 patients). Proc Am Soc Clin Oncol 1995;14:340.
177. Pinkerton CR, Hartmann O, Dini G, Philip T. High dose chemo-radiotherapy with bone marrow rescue in stage IV neuroblastoma: EBMT Survey 1988. In Autologous Bone Marrow Transplantation: Proceedings of the Fourth International Symposium. Edited by KA Dicke, G Spitzer, S Jagganath, MJ Evinger-Hodges. Houston: MD Anderson Hospital, 1989, pp 543–548.
178. Pole JG, Gee A, Janssen W, Lee C, Gross S. Immunomagnetic purging of bone marrow: a model for negative cell selection. Am J Pediatr Hematol Oncol 1990;12:257.
179. Preijers FW, De Witte T, Wessels JM, De Gast GC, Van Leeuwen E, Capel PJ, and Haanen C. Autologous transplantation of bone marrow purged in vitro with anti-CD7-(WT1-) ricin A immunotoxin in T-cell lymphoblastic leukemia and lymphoma. Blood 1989;74:1152.
180. Ramakrishnan S, Uckun FM, Houston LL. Anti-T cell immunotoxins containing pokeweed anti-viral protein: potential purging agents for human autologous bone marrow transplantation. J Immunol 1985;135:3616.
181. Reece DE, Barnett MJ, Connors JM, Klingemann HG, O'Reilly SE, Shepherd JD, Phillips GL. Intensive therapy with busulfan, cyclophosphamide and melphalan (bucy + mel) and 4-hydroperoxycyclophosphamide (4HC) purged autologous bone marrow transplantation (AUTOBMT) for multiple myeloma (MM) (Abstract). Blood 1989;74:754a.
182. Reiffers J, Bernard P, David B, Vezon G, Sarrat A, Marit G, Moulinier J, Broustet A. Successful autologous transplantation with peripheral blood hemopoietic cells in a patient with acute leukemia. Exp Hematol 1986;114:312.
183. Reiffers J, Marit G, Boiron JM. Autologous blood stem cell transplantation in high-risk multiple myeloma. Br J Hematol 1989;72:296.
184. Reisner Y. Differential agglutination by soybean agglutinin of human leukemia and neuroblastoma cell lines: potential application to autologous bone marrow transplantation. Proc Natl Acad Sci USA 1983;80:6657.
185. Reusser P, Fisher LD, Buckner CD, Thomas ED, Meyers JD. Cytomegalovirus infection after autologous bone marrow transplantation: occurrence of cytomegalovirus disease and effect on engraftment. Blood 1990;75:1888.
186. Ritz J, Sallan SE, Bast RC Jr, Lipton JM, Clavell LA, Feeney M, Hercend T, Nathan DG, Schlossman SF. Autologous bone-marrow transplantation in CALLA-positive acute lymphoblastic leukemia after in-vitro treatment with J5 monoclonal antibody and complement. Lancet 1982;II:60.
187. Ritz J, Sallan SE, Bast RC Jr, Lipton JM, Nathan DG, Schlossman SF. In vitro treatment with monoclonal antibody prior to autologous bone marrow transplantation in acute lymphoblastic leukemia. Hamatol Bluttransfus 1983;28:117.
188. Robbins RA, Linder J, Stahl MG, Thompson AB, Haire W, Kessinger A, Armitage JO, Arneson M, Woods G, Vaughan WP, Rennard SI. Diffuse alveolar hemorrhage in autologous bone marrow transplant recipients. Am J Med 1989;87:511.
189. Rowley SD, Jones RJ, Piantadosi S, Braine HG, Colvin OM, Davis J, Saral R, Sharkis S, Wingard J, Yeager AM, Santos GW. Efficacy of ex vivo purging for autologous bone

marrow transplantation in the treatment of acute nonlymphoblastic leukemia. Blood 1989;74:501.
190. Saarinen UM, Pihko H, Makipernaa A. High-dose thiotepa with autologous bone marrow rescue in recurrent malignant oligodendroglioma: a case report. J Neurooncol 1990;9:57.
191. Saleh RA, Gross S, Cassano W, Gee A. Metastatic retinoblastoma successfully treated with immunomagnetic purged autologous bone marrow transplantation. Cancer 1988;62:2301.
192. Sanders DG, Wiley FM, Moss TJ. Serial immunocytologic analysis of blood for tumor cells in two patients with neuroblastoma. Cancer 1991;67:1423.
193. Santos GW, Yeager AM, Jones RJ. Autologous bone marrow transplantation. Ann Rev Med 1989;40:99.
194. Schmidberger H, King L, Lasky LC, Vallera DA. Antitumor activity of L6-ricin immunotoxin against the H2981-T3 lung adenocarcinoma cell line in vitro and in vivo. Cancer Res 1990;50:3249.
195. Seiden MV, O'Donnell WJ, Weinblatt M, Licht J. Vasculitis with recurrent pulmonary hemorrhage in a long-term survivor after autologous bone marrow transplantation. Bone Marrow Transplant 1990;6:345.
196. Shea TC, Antman KH, Eder JP, Elias A, Peters WP, Schryber S, Henner WD, Schoenfeld DA, Schnipper LE, Frei E III. Malignant melanoma. Treatment with high-dose combination alkylating agent chemotherapy and autologous bone marrow support. Arch Dermatol 1988;124:878.
197. Sherertz RJ, Belani A, Kramer BS, Elfenbein GJ, Weiner RS, Sullivan ML, Thomas RG, Samsa GP. Impact of air filtration on nosocomial *Aspergillus* infections. Unique risk of bone marrow transplant recipients. Am J Med 1987;83:709.
198. Sheridan WP, Morstyn G, Wolf M, Dodds A, Lusk J, Maher D, Layton JE, Green MD, Souza L, Fox RM. Granulocyte colony-stimulating factor and neutrophil recovery after high-dose chemotherapy and autologous bone marrow transplantation. Lancet 1989;II:891.
199. Shpall EJ, Bast RC Jr, Joines WT, Jones RB, Anderson I, Johnston C, Eggleston S, Tepperberg M, Edwards S, Peters WP. Immunomagnetic purging of breast cancer from cancer marrow for autologous transplantation. Bone Marrow Transplant 1991;7:145.
200. Shpall EJ, Anderson IC, Bast RC Jr, Joines WT, Jones RB, Ross M, Edwards S, Eggleston S, Johnston C, Tepperberg M, et al. Immunopharmacologic purging of breast cancer from bone marrow for autologous bone marrow transplantation. Prog Clin Biol Res 1990;333:321.
201. Shpall EJ, Clarke-Pearson D, Soper JT, Berchuck A, Jones RB, Bast RC Jr, Ross M, Lidor Y, Vanecek K, Tyler T, Peters WP. High-dose alkylating agent chemotherapy with autologous bone marrow support in patients with stage III/IV epithelial ovarian cancer. Gynecol Oncol 1990;38:386.
202. Sieber F, Rao S, Rowley SD, Blum M. Dye-mediated photolysis of human neuroblastoma cells: implications for autologous bone marrow transplantation. Blood 1986;68:32.
203. Slaper-Cortenbach IC, Admiraal LG, van Leeuwen EF, Kerr JM, von dem Borne AE, Tetteroo PA. Effective purging of bone marrow by a combination of immunorosette depletion and complement lysis. Exp Hematol 1990;18:49.
204. Smith DM, Weisenburger DD, Bierman P, Kessinger A, Vaughan WP, Armitage JO. Acute renal failure associated with autologous bone marrow transplantation. Bone Marrow Transplant 1987;2:195.
205. Socinski MA, Cannistra SA, Elias A, et al. The in vivo effect of granulocyte-macrophage colony-stimulating factor on circulating progenitor cells in man. In Autologous Bone Marrow Transplantation: Proceedings of the Fourth International Symposium. Edited by KA Dicke, G Spitzer, S Jagannath, MJ Evinger-Hodges. Houston: MD Anderson Hospital, 1989, pp 677–683.
206. Socinski MA, Cannistra SA, Elias A, Antman KH, Schnipper L, Griffin JD. Granulocyte-macrophage colony stimulating factor expands the circulating haemopoietic progenitor cell compartment in man. Lancet 1988;I:1194.
207. Steel GG. Growth and survival of tumor stem cells. In Growth Kinetics of Tumors. Edited by GG Steel. Oxford: Clarendon, 1977, pp 244–267.
208. Steward WP, Scarffe JH, Dirix LY, Chang J, Radford JA, Bonnem E, Crowther D. Granulocyte-macrophage colony-stimulating factor (GM-CSF) after high-dose melphalan in patients with advanced colon cancer. Br J Cancer 1990;61:749.
209. Stewart DJ. The role of chemotherapy in the treatment of gliomas in adults. Cancer Treat Rev 1989;16:129.
210. Stiff PJ, DeRisi MF, Langleben A, Gulati S, Koester A, Lanzotti V, Clarkson BD. Autologous bone marrow transplantation using unfractionated cells without rate-controlled freezing in hydroxyethyl starch and dimethyl sulfoxide. Ann NY Acad Sci 1983;411:378.
211. Stong RC, Uckun F, Youle RJ, Kersey JH, Vallera DA. Use of multiple T cell-directed intact ricin immunotoxins for autologous bone marrow transplantation. Blood 1985;66:627.
212. Stong RC, Youle RJ, Vallera DA. Elimination of clonogenic T-leukemic cells from human bone marrow using anti-Mr 65,000 protein immunotoxins. Cancer Res 1984;44:3000.
213. Sugarman J, Bashore TM, Ohman EM, Jones R, Peters WP. Hypertension and reversible myocardial depression associated with autologous bone marrow transplantation. Am J Med 1990;88:52N.
214. Tarbell NJ, Guinan EC, Niemeyer C, Mauch P, Sallan SE, Weinstein HJ. Late onset of renal dysfunction in survivors of bone marrow transplantation. Int J Radiat Oncol Biol Phys 1988;15:99.
215. Tarella C, Ferrero D, Bregni M, Siena S, Gallo E, Pileri A, Gianni AM. Peripheral blood expansion of early progenitor cells after high-dose cyclophosphamide and rhGM-CSF. Eur J Cancer 1991;27:22.
216. Tchekmedyian NS, Tait N, Van Echo D, Aisner J. High-dose chemotherapy without autologous bone marrow transplantation in melanoma. J Clin Oncol 1986;4:1811.
217. Thatcher D, Lind M, Morgenstern G, Carr T, Chadwick G, Jones R, Craig P. High-dose, double alkylating agent chemotherapy with DTIC, melphalan, or ifosfamide and marrow rescue for metastatic malignant melanoma. Cancer 1989;63:1296.
218. Thomas ED, Storb R, Clift RA, Fefer A, Johnson L, Neiman PE, Lerner KG, Glucksberg H, Buckner CD. Bone marrow transplantation. N Engl J Med 1975;292:832.
219. Thomas ED, Buckner CD, Clift RA, Fefer A, Johnson FL, Neiman PE, Sale GE, Sanders JE, Singer JW, Shulman H, Storb R, Weiden PL. Marrow transplantation for acute nonlymphoblastic leukemia in first remission. N Engl J Med 1979;301:597.
220. Thomas ED, Storb R. Technique for human marrow grafting. Blood 1970;36:507.
221. Thomas MR, Robinson WA, Glode LM, Dantas ME, Koeppler H, Morton N, Sutherland J. Treatment of advanced malignant melanoma with high-dose chemotherapy and autologous bone marrow transplantation. Preliminary results—Phase I study. Am J Clin Oncol 1982;5:611.
222. Tzeng CH, Chuang MW, Wang SY, Hsieh RK, Liu CJ, Fan S, Chen PM. Generation of lymphokine-activated killer (LAK) cells and possible implications in autologous bone marrow transplantation—a preliminary report. Proc Natl Sci Counc Repub China 1990;14:47.
223. Uckun FM, Gajl-Peczalska K, Meyers DE, Ramsay NC, Kersey JH, Colvin M, Vallera DA. Marrow purging in autologous bone marrow transplantation for T-lineage acute lymphoblastic leukemia: efficacy of ex vivo treatment with immunotoxins and 4-hydroperoxycyclophosphamide against fresh leukemic marrow progenitor cells. Blood 1987;69:361.
224. Uckun FM, Stong RC, Youle RJ, Vallera DA. Combined ex vivo treatment with immunotoxins and mafosfamid: a novel immunochemotherapeutic approach for elimination of neoplastic T cells from autologous marrow grafts. J Immunol 1985;134:3504.
225. Uckun FM, Kersey JH, Vallera DA, Ledbetter JA, Weisdorf D, Myers DE, Haake R, Ramsay NK. Autologous bone marrow transplantation in high-risk remission T-lineage acute lymphoblastic leukemia using immunotoxins plus 4-hydroperoxycyclophosphamide for marrow purging. Blood 1990;76:1723.
226. Urban C, Slace I, Kaulfersch W, Greinix H, Hocker P. Treatment of stage IV neuroblastoma with high-dose melphalan and autologous bone marrow transplantation following in vitro preliminary treatment of the bone marrow with the active cyclophosphamide derivative Asta Z-7654. Pediatr Padol 1986;21:275.
227. van den Brink MR, Voogt PJ, Marijt WA, van Luxenburg Heys SA, van Rood JJ, Brand A. Lymphokine-activated killer cells selectively kill tumor cells in bone marrow without compromising bone marrow stem cell function in vitro. Blood 1989;74:354.
228. Vellenga E, Sizoo W, Hagenbeek A, Lowenberg B. Different repopulation kinetics of erythroid (BFU-E), myeloid (CFU-GM) and T lymphocyte (TC-CFU) progenitor cells after autologous and allogeneic bone marrow transplantation. Br J Haematol 1987;65:137.
229. Verdonck LF, de Graan Hentzen YC, Dekker AW, Mudde GC, de Gast GC. Cytomegalovirus seronegative platelets and leukocyte-poor red blood cells from random donors can prevent primary cytomegalovirus infection after bone marrow transplantation. Bone Marrow Transplant 1987;2:7.
230. Verdonck LF, de Gast GC. Is cytomegalovirus infection a major cause of T cell alterations after (autologous) bone-marrow transplantation? Lancet 1984;I:932.
230a. Verdonck LF, van Putten WL, Hagenbeek A, Schouten HC, Sonneveld P, van Imhoff GW, Kluin-Nelemans HC, Raemaekers JM, van Oers RH, Haak HL, et al. Comparison of CHOP chemotherapy with autologous bone marrow transplantation for slowly responding patients with aggressive non-Hodgkin's lymphoma. N Engl J Med 1995;332:1045–1051.
231. Vredenburgh JJ, Ball ED. Elimination of small cell carcinoma of the lung from human bone marrow by monoclonal antibodies and immunomagnetic beads. Cancer Res 1990;50:7216.
232. Vredenburgh JJ, Simpson W, Memoli VA, Ball ED. Reactivity of anti-CD15 monoclonal antibody PM-81 with breast cancer and elimination of breast cancer cells from human bone marrow by PM-81 and immunomagnetic beads. Cancer Res 1991;51:2451.
233. Welham MJ, Schrader JW. Modulation of c-kit mRNA and protein by hemopoietic growth factors. Mol Cell Biol 1991;11:2901.
234. Wingard JR, Chen DY, Burns WH, Fuller DJ, Braine HG, Yeager AM, Kaiser H, Burke PJ, Graham JL, Santos GW, Saral R. Cytomegalovirus infection after autologous bone marrow transplantation with comparison to infection after allogeneic bone marrow transplantation. Blood 1988;71:1432.
235. Wolff SN, Herzig RH, Fay JW, LeMaistre CF, Frei E III, Lahr D, Lowder J, Bolwell B, Giannone L, Herzig GP. High-dose thiotepa with autologous bone marrow transplantation for metastatic malignant melanoma: results of phase I and II studies of the North American Bone Marrow Transplantation Group. J Clin Oncol 1989;7:245.
236. Wolff SN, Phillips GL, Herzig GP. High-dose carmustine with autologous bone marrow transplantation for the adjuvant treatment of high-grade gliomas of the central nervous system. Cancer Treat Rep 1987;71:183.
237. Wolff SN, Phillips GL, Fay JW, Giannone L, LeMaistre CF, Herzig RH, Herzig GP. High-dose chemotherapy with autologous marrow transplantation for gliomas of the central nervous system. In Autologous Bone Marrow Transplantation: Proceedings of the Third International Symposium. Houston: MD Anderson Hospital, 1987, pp 557–563.
238. Yamashita J, Kawamura T, Shoin K. High dose chemotherapy in malignant gliomas using autologous bone marrow transplantation and GM-CSF: granulocyte-macrophage colony stimulating factors [Jpn]. No Shinkei Geka. Neurological Surgery 1990;18:329.
239. Yeager AM, Kaizer H, Santos GW, Saral R, Colvin OM, Stuart RK, Braine HG, Burke PJ, Ambinder RF, Burns WH, Fuller DJ, Davis JM, Karp JE, Stratford W, Rowley SD, Sensenbrenner LL, Vogelsang GB, Wingard JR. Autologous bone marrow transplantation in patients with acute nonlymphocytic leukemia, using ex vivo marrow treatment with 4-hydroperoxycyclophosphamide. N Engl J Med 1986;315:141.
240. Zsebo KM, Wypych J, McNiece IK, Lu HS, Smith KA, Karkare SB, Sachdev RK, Yuschenkoff VN, Birkett NC, Williams LR, Satyagal VN, Tung W, Bosselman RA, Mendiaz EA, Langley KE. Identification, purification, and biological characterization of hematopoietic stem cell factor from buffalo rat liver–conditioned medium. Cell 199063:195.

CHAPTER 86

Allogeneic Transplantation

RICHARD J. O'REILLY AND ESPERANZA B. PAPADOPOULOS

Introduction

In the 27 years since human leukocyte antigen (HLA)-compatible sibling marrow grafts were first successfully applied to the curative treatment of lethal congenital immune deficiencies (32, 160), allogeneic marrow transplantation has evolved as a treatment of choice for patients with aplastic anemia (83, 350), acute leukemias relapsing early after induction of first remission (76), chronic myelogenous leukemia (171, 366), and several lethal congenital disorders of hematopoiesis and immunity (278). Allogeneic marrow grafts have also achieved impressive successes in the treatment of myelodysplastic syndromes (15, 268), myelofibrosis, non-Hodgkin's lymphoma (17, 269), and myeloma (78, 375). They are also being applied on a large scale for the curative treatment of the hemoglobinopathies, particularly thalassemia (235), and are currently being explored as a method for introducing self-renewing populations of enzymatically normal progenitors of tissue macrophages for the treatment of several lethal genetic disorders of metabolism (228).

Improvements in transplantation results over the past 10 years reflect significant advances in our understanding of the immunogenetics of histocompatibility and the cellular events contributing to graft rejection and graft-vs.-host disease (GvHD). There also have been advances in the development of new and more effective methods for ensuring engraftment and abrogating GvHD, and in the discovery and application of new agents for the treatment or prevention of the infectious complications to which transplant recipients are particularly susceptible. These advances will be reviewed and an attempt made to assess their impact on current clinical applications of allogeneic marrow transplants in the treatment of malignant neoplastic diseases. Subsequently, new advances will be discussed that have extended the application of marrow grafts to an increasing proportion of individuals who do not have an HLA-matched sibling donor.

Biology of Allogeneic Marrow Transplants Applied to the Treatment of Hematologic Neoplasia

HLA GENE PRODUCTS: MAJOR DETERMINANTS OF HISTOCOMPATIBILITY IN HUMAN MARROW TRANSPLANTATION

Recognition of the importance of matching for the determinants of the major histocompatibility complex (MHC) in the prevention of lethal GvH reactions in rodent models (58) led to the initial successful applications of HLA-matched marrow grafts in humans (32, 160). The HLA gene complex, the major histocompatibility region in humans, is located on the short arm of chromosome 6 and is composed of a series of genes, each possessing an extraordinary degree of allelic polymorphism (Fig. 86.1) (66). The HLA complex is divided into class I genes (HLA-A, -B, -C), which encode proteins expressed on the surface of all nucleated cells; class II genes (HLA-DR, -Dq, -Dp), which encode surface proteins on a more restricted group of cell types, including early hematopoietic cells, mature macrophages and monocytes, dendritic cells, endothelial cells, B cells, and activated T cells; and class III genes, which encode other functional proteins such as the complement proteins C2 and C4 (66, 398). The HLA genes are codominantly expressed, permitting identification of haplotypes inherited from each parent by serologic typing of HLA-A, -B, -C, and -DR determinants. Histocompatibility for determinants within the entire HLA-D region is defined by mutual unresponsiveness in mixed lymphocyte culture (MLC) (415). HLA haplotypes are usually inherited en bloc from each parent. Thus, the likelihood that any two siblings will receive the same parental haplotypes is 1:4. Because of variations in the size of families, in practice, HLA-identical siblings can be identified for 35 to 40% of patients.

HLA phenotypically matched or partially matched related donors can be identified for an additional 5 to 10% of subjects if the parents of the subject share one or more HLA alleles that are inherited on one of the subject's HLA haplotypes, or if the subject inherits one HLA haplotype that includes HLA alleles known to be genetically linked. In the family pedigree illustrated in Figure 86.2, the parents share HLA-A10 and HLA-B35 on one haplotype. As a result, individual A could receive a single-HLA-allele-disparate graft from her father. In this pairing, the donor possesses a unique HLA-DR4 and the recipient an HLA-DR7. On the other hand, individual B could receive an HLA-DR–disparate graft from either parent or from her sibling. In this case, each donor would possess a unique HLA-A and HLA-B allele that could serve as a target for graft rejection. Cells of individual B, however, would possess only one HLA-DR determinant as a target for GvHD.

The family illustrated in Figure 86.2 also presents a different basis for donor identification. Note that individual A inherits HLA-A3, -B7, and -DR2 as a haplotype from her father.

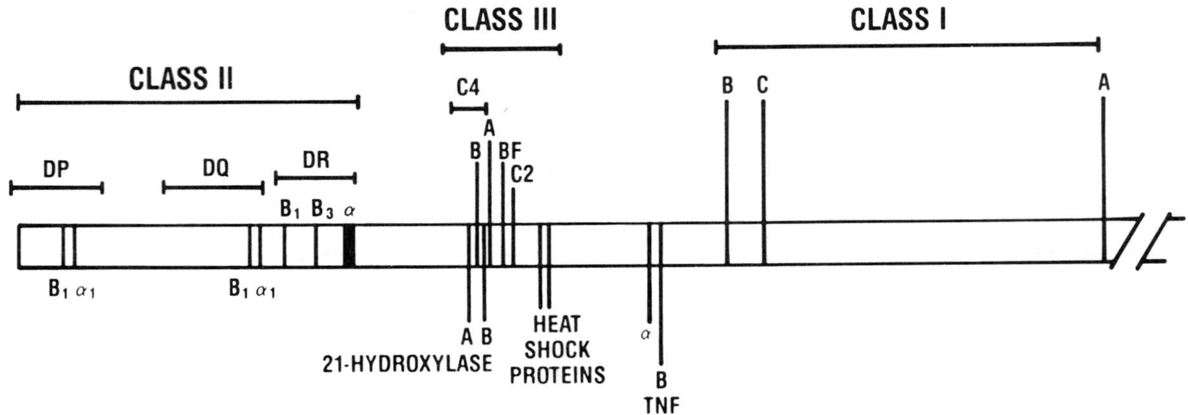

Figure 86.1. A map of expressed genes of the HLA region on the short arm of chromosome 6.

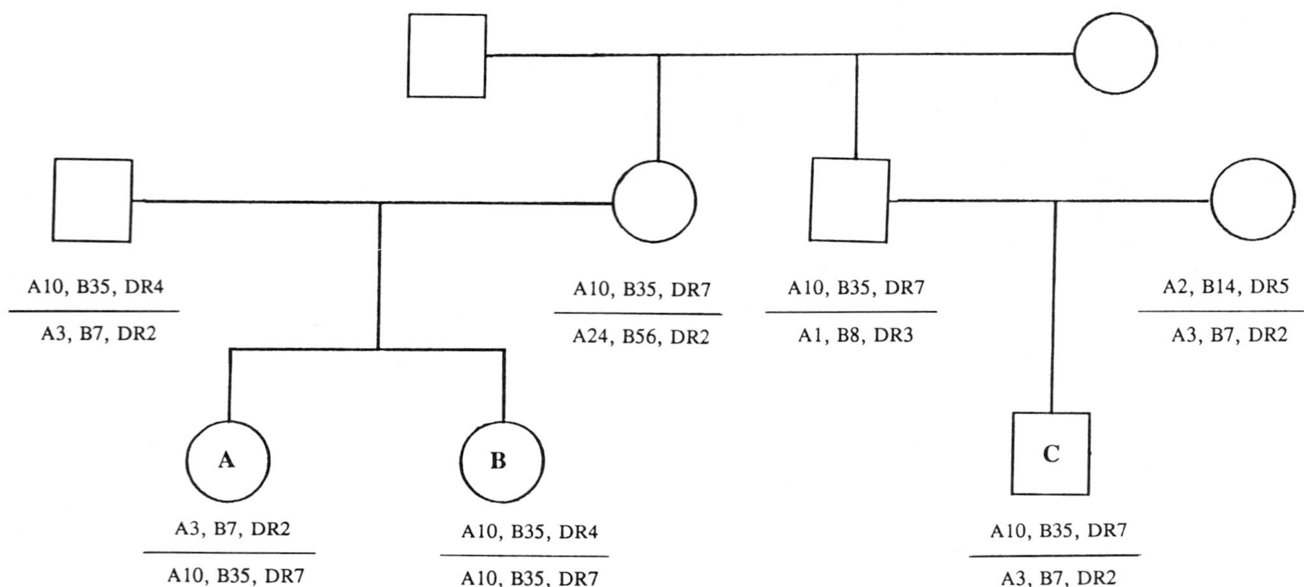

Figure 86.2. An example of genetics of histocompatability. See text.

The HLA alleles in this haplotype are known to be in strong linkage dysequilibrium, which means that the frequency with which they are co-associated on a haplotype is far greater than would be predicted by the product of each allele's frequency in the general population. Examples of full HLA-A, -B, -D haplotypes that are detected at significantly increased frequency among individuals of caucasian background are presented in Table 86.1 (43). In the family in Figure 86.2, if the father and sibling were not living, a search could be made among the offspring of maternal relatives sharing with the patient the uncommon and nonlinked haplotype HLA-A10, -B35, -D7. In such cases, a cousin, such as individual C, could be found who derives the HLA-A3, -B7, -DR2 haplotype from a totally different pedigree and the HLA-A10, -B35, -DR7 haplotype from a relative of the mother.

Unrelated donors who are phenotypically matched may also be identified for a proportion of patients. Over the past 9 years, a National Bone Marrow Donor Registry has been established in St. Paul, Minnesota. It is connected to several donor registries and most of the major marrow transplantation centers (252). The national registry currently maintains a computerized bank of over 1.7 million typed donors. The Anthony Nolan Foundation, a registry of over 265,000 donors based in London, is now computer-linked to this registry. Other European registries and the Canadian registry are also joined to this network. Currently, these registries can identify serologically HLA-A, -B, -DR matched donors for up to 20 to 30% of patients who are of a European caucasian background, and particularly for patients inheriting two common HLA-A, -B, -DR haplotypes (53, 338). However, the proportion of successful searches for patients who are black, Asian, or Native American is still low.

Despite matching for HLA-A, -B, and -DR, the incidence of graft rejection and severe GvHD in recipients of HLA serologically matched unrelated marrow is markedly higher than that observed in recipients of HLA-matched sibling marrow

Table 86.1. HLA-A, HLA-B, and HLA-DR Haplotypes: Caucasoids

HLA-A	HLA-B	HLA-DR
1	8	3
3	7	2
2 or 24	7	2
29	44	7
23	44	7
2	44	4
2	44	2 or 11
30 or 31	18	3
2	18	11
3 or 11	35	1
—	35	2,4,11,13,14
2	62	4 or 11
1 or 24	61	2 or 8
2 or 30	13	7
2	51	2 or 11
1	57	7
1	41	8

(5, 52). Indeed, such transplants carry a risk of severe GvHD equivalent to that associated with transplantation of marrow from a related, genotypically HLA-haplotype-identical donor differing from the recipient by two HLA alleles on the unshared haplotype (6). This suggests that within the HLA region, genetic disparities exist between unrelated HLA-matched individuals that cannot be detected by conventional typing methods. The use of newer, more discriminatory techniques such as isoelectric focusing of class I HLA proteins (413) has, in fact, demonstrated multiple molecular variants of several HLA class I antigens. Several of these microvariants can be distinguished by microvariant-disparate alloreactive T cells in vitro. Recent reports have demonstrated that these microvariant-specific T cells can also contribute to graft rejection and GvHD (151, 213). Analysis of DNA restriction fragment length polymorphisms of HLA class II determinants have documented a high frequency of HLA-DP disparities among "matched" unrelated donors, reflecting the absence of genetic linkage between HLA-DR and DP (285). Further, molecular disparities of DRB_1 alleles have been associated with a higher frequency of severe GvHD and posttransplantation mortality (286).

MINOR ALLOANTIGEN SYSTEMS CONTRIBUTING TO GRAFT REJECTION AND GRAFT-VS.-HOST DISEASE AFTER MARROW TRANSPLANTATION IN HUMANS

Although the products of the HLA gene complex are the major determinants of histocompatibility in humans, other alloantigenic systems also affect the growth of a marrow transplant in a nonsyngeneic host and tolerance of it by the transplant recipient. Indeed, despite intensive pretransplantation immunosuppression and posttransplantation drug prophylaxis for GvHD, marrow allografts between HLA genotypically identical siblings are still associated with significant frequencies of both graft rejection and GvHD (see below). These alloreactions have been ascribed to the responses of host or donor T cells against minor alloantigens unique to hematopoietic cells of the graft or the tissues of the host, respectively. Although several polymorphic minor alloantigenic systems, such as the MLS, H-Y, and QA-1 alloantigens, have been identified as potential targets of allointeractions in rodents (113, 227), the minor alloantigens targeted during human marrow allograft rejections or GvHD remain poorly defined. The human Y chromosome encodes a minor alloantigen, termed H-Y, which is expressed on the human male hematopoietic cells and can be targeted by cytotoxic T cells (177, 178, 387). The decreased risk of rejection and the increased likelihood of GvHD associated with marrow allografts from female donors administered to male recipients may reflect in vivo responses to this minor alloantigen (152, 157, 219, 348). Goulmy et al. (177, 322) have also generated a series of T-cell clones from marrow allograft recipients that are HLA restricted and recognize at least four antigens on hematopoietic cells (HA-1 to HA-4) that appear to be the products of single nonallelic genes that segregate in a mendelian pattern of inheritance. HA-1 and HA-2 are uniquely expressed by cells derived from the hematopoietic system, while HA-3 and HA-4 are also expressed by other types of cells (114, 322). Disparities of HA-3 have been implicated in GvHD (177). Minor alloantigen–reactive HLA-restricted T cells have also been implicated in graft rejections (241, 389).

Until recently, the nature of the minor HA alloantigens targeted was completely unknown. However, in 1995 den Haan et al. (117) succeeded in isolating the HA-2 peptide antigen from its HLA-restricting element and thereafter sequencing it. The approach to peptide isolation utilized reverse-phase high performance liquid chromatography to distinguish peptides eluted from the HLA-restricting element. To identify the relevant peptide antigen, target cells expressing the HLA-restricting element were pulsed with the different isolated peptide fractions and exposed to the minor alloantigen–specific cytolytic T cells. HA-2 was found to be a member of the nonfilamentous class I myosin family of proteins, which contributes to cell locomotion. Studies are in progress to determine whether this protein exhibits allelic polymorphisms. Similar approaches are also being used to isolate and characterize other minor alloantigens.

PREPARATIVE CYTOREDUCTION FOR ALLOGENEIC MARROW GRAFTS

Hematopoietic and lymphoid cells are considerably more susceptible to growth inhibition or rejection by host resistance systems than are solid organs such as the kidney or the liver. As a consequence, durable engraftment and expansion of marrow cells within an allogeneic environment can only be achieved if the host's immune system is ablated. Only patients with severe combined immune deficiency (SCID) are sufficiently compromised to permit the regular engraftment of unmanipulated HLA-matched marrow grafts. Transplants for all other conditions require intensive immunosuppressive therapy in the immediate pretransplantation period. Of the agents currently available, only total body irradiation (TBI) and the alkylating agents cyclophosphamide and nitrogen mustard, administered in high doses, have been demonstrated to be sufficiently immunosuppressive to permit engraftment of foreign hematopoietic cells (315, 354, 364). Total body irradiation at doses of at least 9.0 to 10.0 Gy induces a degree of myeloablation and immunosuppression sufficient to permit durable engraftment of an allogeneic marrow transplant and expansion of donor progenitors in all hematopoietic lineages. Of the chemotherapeutic agents, cyclophosphamide (50 mg/kg/d times 4) is the most immunosuppressive, but it provides effective preparation only for patients with aplastic anemia (349). For disorders that do not affect the overall cellularity of a patient's marrow, cyclophosphamide must be used in combination with a myeloablative agent such as TBI, busulfan, dimethylmyleran, or thiotepa so that adequate space can be created for the establishment of donor hematopoietic elements within the host marrow microenvironment (212, 283).

Cytoreductive regimens developed for patients undergoing transplantation for leukemia are designed primarily to eliminate leukemia clones but must also be sufficiently immunosuppressive and myeloablative to ensure engraftment of allogeneic hematopoietic cells. Initially, TBI administered in single doses of 10 Gy was used in combination with cyclophosphamide for this purpose (364). However, in the past 7 to 10 years, alternative cytoreductive regimens have been introduced that incorporate higher doses of fractionated TBI (76, 125) and other chemotherapeutic agents such as etoposide (64, 320), cytosine arabinoside (94, 104), L-PAM (187), or thiotepa (30, 280, 281) in addition to or as substitutes for cyclophosphamide. A regimen employing high doses of busulfan and cyclophosphamide has also been developed (376) to circumvent the use of TBI. Results achieved with several of these approaches will be discussed in later sections.

PREENGRAFTMENT PERIOD

Following infusion of the marrow allograft, the hematopoietic progenitor cells migrate to sites in the marrow and spleen. The cellularity of the marrow begins to recover 10 to 14 days following transplantation and by 14 to 21 days after grafting, neutrophils of donor origin can be detected in the circulation. However, from the time the myeloablative preparative regimen is completed to the time that donor hematopoietic function begins to recover, the patients are profoundly pancytopenic, requiring intensive support with platelets and red cells and aggressive treatment with antibiotics for presumed or documented infectious complications. Blood products used to support transplant recipients must be irradiated, since they contain allogeneic lymphocytes that can induce lethal GvH reactions (8).

The spectrum of organisms causing infections in this period of marrow aplasia predominantly includes the constituents of the microflora of the skin and gastrointestinal tract. Because of the mucositis and ulcerations of the intestinal mucosa induced by radiation and the high doses of chemotherapeutic agents used to induce myeloablation and immunosuppression, gram-negative bacteria in the gut, including *E. coli*, *Pseudomonas*, *Klebsiella*, and other enteric bacteria, are particularly common isolates. Similarly, enterococci and other streptococcal organisms in the mouth may gain access to the bloodstream through damaged tissues. The most common gram-positive organisms, however, are staphylococci, particularly *S. epidermidis*, which may gain access to the bloodstream via a contaminated venous catheter (403). Fungal pathogens, particularly *Candida albicans* and *C. tropicalis* account for 5 to 20% of systemic infections in this period (399). *Aspergillus*, *Mucor*, *Cryptosporidium*, and *Fusarium* may also cause severe infections of the lung, sinuses, and oropharyngeal structures that are difficult to treat despite the aggressive use of antifungal agents.

Viral infections common in this period principally include recurrences of herpes simplex labialis and progenitalis. These infections may cause significant morbidity but are particularly of concern as portals of entry for bacterial superinfection. Susceptibility to severe herpes simplex infections usually resolves by days 18 to 21, coincident with the development of functional donor-derived natural killer (NK) cells. Herpes zoster infections may occur at any time in the posttransplantation period. Indeed, the cumulative risk of reactivation of herpes zoster in the first 2 to 3 years post-transplantation has been estimated to be as high as 50% (233, 259). However, when such infections occur prior to engraftment, they are commonly disseminated and may cause lethal pneumonias, meningoencephalitis, or hepatitis (233). The papovavirus BK is also commonly activated during this period and has been implicated in the pathogenesis of encephalopathies, hepatitis, and hemorrhagic cystitis (23, 276). Adenovirus and rotavirus may cause severe enteritis in this period (371). Adenovirus has also been implicated as a cause of hepatitis and hemorrhagic cystitis (3). Another recently described agent, herpes simplex virus type 6 (HSV-6), may also be activated in this period and has been implicated as a cause of marrow suppression and graft failure (81, 85).

Several approaches have been developed to reduce the incidence of serious microbial infections and their associated mortality early in the posttransplantation period. The use of laminar flow isolation with skin and mucosal decontamination constitutes one such measure which, in prospective randomized trials, has been found to be effective, particularly for patients who have undergone transplantation for aplasia (346). Oral decontamination with chlorhexidine may significantly reduce the oral microflora and ameliorate mucositis, thereby reducing the prevalence of systemic infections (147). Another approach useful in reducing the frequency of candidemia has been the prophylactic administration of low-dose amphotericin (266). Recently, newer strategies have employed liposomal forms of amphotericin B, as well as the new antifungal triazoles, fluconazole and itraconazole, in the prevention and treatment of systemic fungal infections (172, 368, 377). Prophylactic treatment with acyclovir reduces the frequency of genital and labial herpes infections as well as herpes zoster infections (316, 324). HSV-6 infections, on the other hand, have often been resistant to acyclovir but have been responsive to foscarnet. Case reports also suggest that ribavirin may be effective in the treatment of adenovirus infections causing hemorrhagic cystitis (87) or pneumonia (298).

Total body irradiation and the intensive chemotherapy administered prior to transplantation each cause severe toxic effects that particularly affect rapidly dividing cells. These effects, when superimposed, may lead to significant morbidity and mortality. Alkylating agents and TBI can induce severe mucositis and enteritis. In addition, up to 10% of patients who have undergone transplantation for leukemia may develop clinical signs and symptoms of venoocclusive disease of the liver (158, 208, 253). This disorder is caused by damage to the endothelial lining of the hepatic sinusoids that initially induces edema and obstruction to the flow of blood through the capillaries and hepatic venules, thereby causing hepatomegaly, massive ascites, and jaundice. This process may be mild and transient. However, in its severe form, the endothelial damage leads to intrahepatic hemostasis and subsequently extensive centrilobular necrosis of the liver, which results in impaired hepatic detoxification and conjugation and markedly reduced synthesis of coagulation factors and albumin. Obstruction of the portal circulation may lead to hemorrhage from gastric and esophageal varices as well as a marked reduction in the central venous blood volume. The resultant low output state reduces perfusion of the kidneys and induces prerenal azotemia, which may progress to overt renal failure.

Treatment of veno-occlusive disease involves careful replacement of albumin and coagulation factors; maintenance of central venous pressure, renal output, and electrolyte balance; and treatment of the vascular complications and respiratory compromise induced by massive ascites and severe portal hypertension. In addition, treatment with tissue plasminogen activator (tPA) has been reported to induce clinical improvement in a proportion of cases (45, 46, 231). Although studies have been performed examining the role of various agents in the prophylaxis of veno-occlusive disease, including heparin, ursodeoxycholic acid, and prostaglandin E_1, results have been contradictory (26, 46, 153, 168).

Certain of the chemotherapeutic agents used to prepare patients for marrow allografts also cause unique early toxic effects that require careful monitoring and preventative measures. Cyclophosphamide may induce an acute cardiomyopathy, resulting in a marked reduction in cardiac output. This complication is a particular risk for a patient who has received prior treatment with anthracyclines and other cardiotoxic agents (16, 176). Cyclophosphamide may also induce severe hemorrhagic cystitis, a complication that may be prevented by the administration of mesna (59, 77, 203, 331). Busulfan administered in high doses may be neurotoxic and result in seizures. Dilantin administered prophylactically before and during treatment with high doses of busulfan effectively prevents this complication. The alkylating agents busulfan, melphalan, thiotepa, and TBI may induce pulmonary microvascular injury, with interstitial infiltrates or diffuse hemorrhages (109). Cytosine arabinoside, when administered in high doses, may induce cerebellar toxicity and often causes a severe conjunctivitis requiring topical steroids for prevention and treatment (386).

CLINICAL AND BIOLOGIC DETERMINANTS OF ENGRAFTMENT OR GRAFT FAILURE

Early engraftment is signalled by the development of myelogenous and erythroid progenitors of donor origin in the marrow and the emergence of neutrophils in the blood 14 to 21 days posttransplantation. By day 28 to 35, the cellularity of the marrow may be normal and peripheral blood neutrophil and platelet counts may be stable at levels above 1,000/μL and 20,000/μL, respectively. In a proportion of cases, full recovery of peripheral blood counts may be impaired (68), and boost infusions of donor marrow may be necessary. Persistent thrombocytopenia and leukopenia are also common in patients developing intercurrent infections with viruses such as cytomegalovirus (CMV) and HSV-6, as well as in those who develop GvHD (44). However, proof of engraftment can be ascertained by demonstration of donor cells in T-lymphocyte and hematopoietic lineages using any one of several techniques, including cytogenetics (341), detection of donor-specific restriction fragment length polymorphisms (RFLPs) (62) or minisatellite allelic polymorphisms, or in sex-mismatched cases, detection of X and Y probes using fluorescence in situ hybridization techniques (206).

Graft failure is empirically defined either as failure of marrow function to recover after transplantation or a reversion to marrow aplasia after initial hematopoietic reconstitution. Graft failure is also indicated by the loss of donor-type lymphoid and hematopoietic cells in the marrow and blood. Most instances of graft failure occur within the first 60 days posttransplantation but they have been documented as late as 4 to 5 months posttransplantation.

The type of cytoreduction used to prepare the patient, the type of transplant administered, and the degree of HLA disparity existing between donor and recipient each contribute to the incidence of graft failure in the posttransplantation period. For example, the frequency of graft failure ranges from 10 to 30% for patients with aplastic anemia who are prepared with cyclophosphamide alone, with the likelihood depending on the patient's prior transfusion history (89, 345, 348). Although unmodified, HLA-matched marrow grafts induce consistent engraftment in leukemic patients prepared with TBI and cyclophosphamide (124, 125, 364), unmodified grafts from HLA-nonidentical donors remain at increased risk of failure, with the probability of this complication ranging from 6 to 28%, depending on the number and type of HLA allodisparities unique to the donor (1). In addition, depletion of T cells from a marrow allograft renders the transplant more susceptible to graft failure and rejection even when the graft is HLA matched with the recipient (184, 246, 275). The rate of graft failure has been reported to be as high as 10 to 30% in leukemic recipients of T-cell–depleted HLA-matched marrow (184, 219, 245) and as high as 40 to 50% in recipients of two- to three-allele-HLA-disparate grafts (272).

Graft failures complicating allogeneic marrow transplants usually reflect active rejection of the donor cells by host resistance systems. In murine models, two types of marrow graft resistance have been identified: the resistance to parental marrow grafts exhibited by irradiated nonsensitized F_1 hybrids of specific genetic backgrounds, which has been ascribed to the activity of NK cells (215), and the resistance of hosts presensitized to donor cells by transfusion, which is mediated by alloreactive cytotoxic host T cells (118).

NK-cell–mediated resistance to HLA-haplotype-disparate, T-cell–depleted marrow transplants has been implicated as the basis for graft failure in a proportion of patients with SCID who undergo transplantation without preparatory cytoreduction (271). However, for individuals treated with cyclophosphamide or fractionated TBI which abrogate NK-cell–mediated resistance, host NK cells likely play little or no role in the pathogenesis of graft failures. Indeed, the development of functional donor-type NK cells, which occurs as early as 18 days after transplantation, is the hallmark of engraftment (221).

The fact that animals and humans sensitized by transfusion are more susceptible to marrow graft rejection provided early evidence suggesting an immunologic basis for the failures observed (345, 347, 349). Recently, evidence directly implicating host T cells has been developed, through a series of studies documenting the emergence of host-type $CD3^+$, $CD8^+$, $CD56^-$ T cells exhibiting specific reactivity against donor marrow cells at the time of rejection of an unmodified (387) or a T-cell–depleted marrow graft (69, 133). Following HLA-disparate, T-cell–depleted marrow grafts, cytotoxic, $CD3^+$, $CD8^+$ host T cells exhibiting specificity for single class I HLA alleles unique to the donor have been detected (69, 133). In addition, in a smaller proportion of cases, $CD3^+$, $CD4^+$ cytolytic T cells of host origin exhibiting specific reactivity against donor-unique HLA-DR and -DQ disparities have been identified (125). T cells detected in the circulation of patients rejecting HLA-matched marrow grafts are $CD3^+$, $CD8^+$, and $Leu7^+$ and have been shown to specifically inhibit donor colony-forming hematopoietic cells in vitro (69). Although these $CD8^+$ T cells have been found to be donor reactive and HLA restricted (241), the nature of the minor alloantigens targeted by these cells is still unclear. Two recently isolated antigens, the H-Y antigen expressed on male cells (178, 387) and the HA-3 antigen, an autosomal antigen expressed on hematopoietic cells, have been implicated (177).

Other factors may also contribute to suppress hematopoietic reconstitution in the posttransplantation period. Several antimicrobials, such as vancomycin and the antiviral ganciclovir (173), may suppress hematopoiesis. In addition, viruses, particularly CMV and HSV-6, have been implicated as inducers of graft suppression or failure in some cases (224, 259). In rare instances, cumulative damage to the marrow microenvironment of the host has been suggested to result in inability of the host to support donor hematopoietic progenitor growth (244).

As the factors contributing to rejection or graft failure have been identified, strategies for the reversal or prevention of this complication have been developed and applied in preclinical and clinical trials. These strategies have included intensification of preparative immunosuppressive regimens, additional treatment of the host with T-cell–specific monoclonal and heteroantibodies (28, 74, 83, 219), and the use of cytokines such as granulocyte-macrophage colony-stimulating factor (GM-CSF) and granulocyte colony-stimulating factor (G-CSF) to induce early recovery of hematopoiesis after transplantation (122, 249, 265). Early detection of infections with CMV and HSV-6 and treatment of these infections with ganciclovir or foscarnet coupled with hyperimmune globulin have also reversed graft failures in a proportion of cases (133).

GRAFT-VS.-HOST DISEASE

Graft-vs.-host disease is a pathologic process initiated by the response of engrafted immunocompetent donor T lymphocytes against alloantigens expressed on host cells. The principal targets thought to stimulate this reaction are cells derived from the host's lymphohematopoietic system (351). Of the many cells in this system, the most potent stimulants appear to be dendritic cells (342). In response to host alloantigens, donor T lymphocytes proliferate and mature to form both cytotoxic T cells and helper cells, which can either directly injure targeted host tissues or recruit other cells, particularly NK cells and macrophages, to destroy host cell targets (143, 412). These T cells may also generate cytokines such as tumor necrosis factor (TNF), which may further contribute to the pathology observed (288).

The principal clinical manifestations of acute GvHD are a maculopapular skin rash that may be focal or generalized, hepatitis, enteritis, particularly affecting the colon and small bowel, and a delayed reconstitution of hematopoietic and lymphoid function (169, 385, 408). Pathologic changes in the skin are distinctive but not pathognomonic and include infiltration of the perivascular spaces in the dermis and of the dermoepidermal junction with $CD8^+$ cytotoxic T lymphocytes and NK cells, associated with piecemeal necrosis of the overlying epidermis (333). This mononuclear cell infiltration is also seen in the epithelium of the oropharynx and esophagus, at the bases of the intestinal crypts of the small and large bowel, and in the periportal areas of the liver (333), but in these areas the pathologic features are difficult to discriminate from those of an acute viral infection.

The incidence and severity of acute GvHD are principally determined by the type and degree of allodisparity existing between donor and recipient. They are also strongly influenced by other host factors such as the patient's age, sex, the intensity of the cytoreductive regimen used to prepare the patient for transplantation, the presence or absence of intercurrent infection, and the type of resident microflora, as well as donor features such as sex, prior sensitization to host minor alloantigens by pregnancy, and the number of T cells inoculated in the marrow allograft (152, 157, 348).

Chronic GvHD is a complex disorder that is pathologically distinct from acute GvHD. Although it usually develops in patients with antecedent acute GvHD, it may evolve spontaneously late after transplantation in association with an intercurrent infection. Clinically, chronic GvHD manifests with localized or widespread scleroderma-like changes of the skin with hypo- and hyperpigmentation, focal lichen planus lesions, and, in severe cases, recurrent, shallow skin ulcerations, debilitating scars, and contractures of joints. Systemic manifestations include xerostomia, xerophthalmia, biliary cirrhosis, malabsorption, and failure to thrive (356). The pathologic features of chronic GvHD are strikingly different from those of acute GvHD. Infiltration with mononuclear cells is sparse, if seen. Rather, marked sclerosis is observed in the dermis, lamina propria of the intestinal tract, and biliary triads, as well as around the ducts of the salivary and lacrimal glands. With this sclerosis, superficial ulcers of the skin may be observed, as well as marked blunting of the papillae of the tongue and villi of the intestinal tract. At least 20% of patients with chronic GvHD may also develop an obliterative bronchiolitis that may progress to a chronic obstructive pulmonary disease with subsequent death due to respiratory failure or intercurrent pulmonary infection (198).

Chronic GvHD impairs and delays full reconstitution of hematopoiesis and immune function. Among patients with chronic GvHD, persistent thrombocytopenia is a particularly ominous sign (355). Prolonged immune deficiencies, particularly of the humoral immune system, result in markedly enhanced susceptibility and recurrent pyogenic infections caused by *S. pneumoniae*, *H. influenzae*, and other encapsulated organisms, a spectrum of infections that is similar to that observed in individuals with agammaglobulinemia (27, 28).

Detailed studies of the immunopathologic events precipitated by acute and chronic forms of GvHD have uncovered distinctive features of each process. In murine models (282), acute GvHD is usually marked by the development of donor-derived T cells that are specifically cytotoxic to host lymphohematopoietic cells. In contrast, T cells cloned from animals with chronic GvHD express a helper phenotype and, in response to either donor or host IA+ cells, proliferate and generate factors that stimulate collagen synthesis, the hallmark of chronic GvHD pathology. In humans with chronic GvHD, T lymphocytes and monocytes capable of nonspecific suppression of antigen-specific T-cell immunity and B-cell immunoglobulin production are regularly observed (236, 373). As in the murine model, these T cells also generate cytokines that stimulate fibroblast proliferation and collagen secretion. In normal individuals, such broadly reactive, potentially autocytotoxic cells can be detected at significant frequency in the blood by limiting dilution analyses (168). However, such cells are usually limited in their activity by specific suppressor cells also detected in the circulation. In patients with chronic GvHD, such specific suppressor cells are either absent or markedly reduced in number (306). Taken together, these findings suggest that chronic GvHD may reflect ineffectively controlled immunosuppressive and potentially autoreactive clones of cells, possibly generated in response to populations of host-reactive donor T cells participating in acute GvHD reactions.

As will be discussed below, several strategies have been used to prevent acute GvHD. Patients who have received a marrow graft from an HLA genotypically matched sibling and who have been treated with low-dose methotrexate as prophylaxis against GvHD have a 50 to 70% risk of developing this complication. Over half of these patients will develop more serious forms of the disease (grades II–IV) and require immunosuppressive treatment with glucocorticoid steroids (126, 216). Responses, reflected by stabilization and improvement of the skin rash and hepatic and gastrointestinal abnormalities, are usually manifested within 5 to 7 days of initiating treatment. For patients with severe (grades III–IV) GvHD and those with moderate (grade II) forms of the disease refractory to initial steroid treatment, the prognosis has been poor (247). Additional treatment with antithymocyte globulin, CD5-specific immunotoxins, or other unmodified T-cell–specific monoclonal antibodies has cleared skin manifestations in a proportion of patients but has had little effect on GvHD involving the liver and intestines (7, 82, 247). Promising results with an antibody to the interleukin-2 (IL-2) receptor have recently been reported (191). However, in prior experience, 70 to 80% of patients with steroid-refractory GvHD have ultimately succumbed to sequelae of GvHD or associated infections, particularly interstitial pneumonias caused by CMV (126, 127, 216, 247).

Chronic GvHD is reversible in a significant proportion of patients, but responses to treatment must be measured over months to years. Without systemic immunosuppressive treatment, only 18 to 23% of patients have survived more than 18 months (356). Chronic treatment with prednisone coupled with either azathioprine or Cyclosporine can induce slow reversals of pathology in up to 76% of cases (356–358). Treatment of the skin with methoxypsoralen and ultraviolet irradiation may also help reverse changes (136). In steroid-refractory cases, treatment with other immunosuppressive agents, such as thalidomide, clofazimine, or low-dose total lymphoid irradiation, has been proposed, based on promising results in small reported series (334, 384, 393).

PREVENTION OF GRAFT-VS.-HOST DISEASE BY PROPHYLACTIC USE OF DRUGS OR ANTIBODIES AFTER TRANSPLANTATION

The high mortality associated with severe forms of acute and chronic GvHD observed, particularly in older adult recipients of HLA-matched sibling marrow grafts and in patients receiving transplants from matched unrelated donors, has continuously underscored the need for more effective methods of preventing this complication or abrogating its clinical expression. Recognition of the essential role of donor T cells in the initiation of GvHD (351) has focused attention on two principal approaches: (1) administration of combinations of immunosuppressive agents in the immediate post-transplantation period to prevent or inhibit the proliferation and function of host-reactive donor T cells following engraftment of unmodified marrow, and (2) treatment of the marrow graft to remove alloreactive T cells capable of inducing GvHD.

Early studies in canine models led to the recognition that low-dose methotrexate could significantly reduce both the incidence and severity of acute GvHD following DLA identical marrow grafts. This standard approach was adopted in clinical trials in the 1970s. However, despite methotrexate prophylaxis, 50 to 70% of individuals receiving HLA-matched marrow grafts developed acute GvHD, and 30% ultimately developed chronic GvHD. An alternative approach, the administration of a combination of antithymocyte globulin (ATG) and prednisone, has been reported to reduce the severity of GvHD but has also been associated with a higher incidence of death from infection (294). As a result, long-term disease-free survival is not affected. In randomized trials, Cyclosporine has been found to be equivalent to methotrexate in the prevention of GvHD (344). The combination of these two agents is significantly more effective than either alone in preventing the development of severe acute GvHD (343). Further, this combination significantly improves survival in prospective trials (343). However, this combination has had little effect on either the incidence or the severity of chronic GvHD and has not been effective in preventing severe GvH reaction in 70 to 80% of recipients of HLA-disparate related or HLA-matched unrelated marrow grafts. A recent report suggests that the combination of prednisone, Cyclosporine, and short-course methotrexate can reduce the incidence of grade II to IV acute GvHD in good-risk patients who receive transplants of HLA-matched sibling marrow to as low as 9% (95). However, this regimen is also associated with an increased incidence of chronic GvHD (65%). Further, the prolonged administration of steroids has been associated with a markedly high incidence (20%) of culture-proven invasive fungal infections (267). Although prophylactic administration of low-dose amphotericin B reduces this risk, for unclear reasons, such prophylaxis is associated with a higher incidence of GvHD (267). Thus, it remains unclear whether this triple regimen provides a significant long-term advantage. Randomized trials are in progress to resolve this issue.

Prophylaxis with the monoclonal antibody OKT3, which has been successful in preventing kidney allograft rejection, has not proved effective in preventing GvHD (291). In animal models and in preliminary clinical trials, monoclonal antibodies to the IL-2 receptor have been shown to inhibit the expansion of alloreactive T cells and thereby to reduce the incidence of GvHD (4, 144, 195). However, prospective randomized clinical trials in humans have failed to demonstrate an advantage (61). Similarly, clinical trials of prophylaxis with other T-cell–reactive monoclonal antibodies such as the humanized monoclonal antibody Campath 1G and the immunotoxin Xomaxyme H65, a CD5-specific mouse monoclonal antibody conjugated to the toxin A chain of ricin, have thus far shown no significant reductions in the incidence or severity of GvHD (397). In addition to these studies, strategies aimed at neutralizing the effects of cytokines generated by T cells participating in GvHD are also being explored. Antibodies to tumor necrosis factor and the IL-1 receptor (145, 199, 288), have been found to be effective in preventing lethal GvHD in mice when administered in the early post-transplantation period and are now in clinical trials. Several other immunosuppressive agents, including tacrolimus (FK506), rapamicin, thalidomide, and deoxycoformycin (Pentostatin), have also achieved promising results in animal models of marrow transplantation and clinically in the maintenance of immunosuppression following organ allografts (384). However, these agents are only now in clinical trials as adjuncts to marrow transplantation.

PREVENTION OF GRAFT-VS.-HOST DISEASE BY T-CELL–DEPLETED MARROW TRANSPLANTS

Although no combination of agents administered to recipients of an unmodified marrow graft has prevented the development of GvHD in HLA-nonidentical recipients, GvHD can be prevented in both HLA-matched and HLA-disparate recipients through the use of marrow grafts suitably depleted of T lymphocytes prior to administration. The most extensively studied techniques for T-cell depletion include lectin agglutination and E-rosette depletion, as described by Reisner et al. (275, 300): treatment with CamPATH 1M, a rat monoclonal antibody that binds human complement derived from the donor's own plasma (184); treatment of the bone marrow with one or more T-cell–specific mouse monoclonal antibodies and rabbit complement (24, 245, 291, 293); treatment with T-cell–specific immunotoxins (148); and immunoadsorption of T cells to monoclonal antibodies bound to immunomagnetic beads or polystyrene membranes (277, 382) and positive selection of $CD34^+$ progenitor cells by immunoadsorption (125). In addition, less selective techniques capable of reducing T cells by 1 to 1.5 log, such as the use of elutriation, are also being explored (149). As summarized in Table 86.2, these techniques may differ by 1 to 2 log_{10}–fold in the level of T-cell depletion achieved (153). Since the dose of clonable T cells administered in the human marrow graft has been strongly correlated with the risk of developing GvHD in recipients of HLA-matched marrow (220), it is not surprising that the incidence of moderate to severe acute and chronic GvHD recorded in results from large series tend to reflect the efficiency of the T-cell depletion techniques used. This trend is even more striking among recipients of HLA-disparate marrow grafts. For such patients, only techniques that reduce the dose of clonable T cells to less than 10^5/kg have regularly prevented the development of severe acute GvHD (274).

Although several series have demonstrated that T-cell-depleted marrow grafts may reduce the incidence and severity of acute GvHD and, with certain techniques, chronic GvHD, a clear advantage of such transplants over unmodified marrow grafts translating into a significant improvement in long-term disease-free survival has thus far been documented only in patients with lethal congenital immune deficiencies who received transplants from HLA-nonidentical donors (274). In such cases, T-cell–depleted transplants from HLA-A, -B, -D haplotype parental donors may produce

Table 86.2. Methods of T-Cell Depletion in Clinical Trials

Method of T-cell depletion	Cells removed	T-cell depletion ($\times$ log_{10} by LDA)
SBA lectin and E-rosette depletion	T, B, M, N	2.5–3.0
Multiple E-rosette depletions	T	2.0
Mouse MoAb (anti-CD2, CD8) + rabbit C	T	2.0
Rat MoAb (Campath-1) + human C	T, B, M	2.5
Anti-CD5 immunotoxin—ricin A	T	1.5–2.0
Immunomagnetic separation (anti-CD3, CD8)	T	2.0
SBA lectin + immunomagnetic separation	T, B, M, N	3.1
SBA lectin + CD5/CD8 AIS collector	T, B, M, N	3.0
Elutriation	T, B, M, N	1.5

Abbreviations: SBA, soybean agglutinin; MoAb, monoclonal antibody; T, T lymphocytes; B, B lymphoctes; M, monocytes; N, neutrophils; LDA, limiting dilution analysis.

rates of long-term disease-free survival with immunologic reconstitution that are comparable to those achieved with unmodified HLA-matched marrow grafts. However, among patients undergoing transplantation for leukemia and aplastic anemia, reductions in GvHD and GvH-associated mortality through the use of T-cell–depleted grafts have, until recently, been largely counterbalanced by the sensitivity of such transplants to graft failure or rejection and by the increased risk of leukemic relapse, particularly observed among patients who have received HLA-matched T-cell–depleted grafts as treatment for CML (171, 179, 243).

This situation is now changing rapidly. With the introduction of tolerable, more effectively immunosuppressive preparatory regimens, the risk of graft failure following transplantation of T-cell–depleted marrow has been dramatically reduced (30), resulting in a significant improvement in survival and in 1- to 2-year disease-free survival rates, particularly among older recipients of matched sibling grafts and recipients of marrow transplants from unrelated donors (280). As T-cell–depleted marrow grafts have become more widely applied, it has also become clear that the increased risk for leukemic relapse ascribed to T-cell–depleted transplants is not observed in all leukemic groups. Although patients undergoing transplantation for CML are clearly at increased risk, patients undergoing transplantation for AML are not (13, 171, 185, 200, 243, 416). These observations, coupled with demonstrations of the potential of infusions of donor peripheral blood mononuclear cells to induce durable remissions of CML in patients whose disease relapsed after transplantation, have fostered a reexamination of the basis of the enhanced resistance to leukemia conferred by a marrow graft, a phenomenon termed the graft-vs.-leukemia effect.

GRAFT-VS.-LEUKEMIA EFFECT: ENHANCED RESISTANCE TO LEUKEMIA CONFERRED BY A MARROW ALLOGRAFT AND ITS AUGMENTATION BY ADOPTIVE CELL TRANSFER IN THE POSTTRANSPLANTATION PERIOD

An enhanced resistance to leukemia incurred as a result of an allogeneic marrow transplant in humans was first suggested by comparisons of the actuarial risks of leukemic relapse following HLA-matched allogeneic as compared to syngeneic unmodified marrow grafts applied to the treatment of AML in first remission (156). Subsequently, Weiden et al. (394) analyzed a large series of patients who underwent transplantation for leukemia and found that the risk of relapse was lower among patients who developed grade II to IV acute GvHD or chronic GvHD. These data spawned the hypothesis that the antileukemic effect of a marrow allograft is largely or exclusively based on the activity of alloreactive T cells participating in GvHD.

Early surveys of results of T-cell–depleted marrow grafts applied to patients with leukemia supported this general hypothesis, since the incidence of relapse following such transplants was higher than that reported for unmodified grafts (200). The increment in relapse risk was not consistently detected among patients who underwent transplantation for acute leukemias (275). However, in several studies the use of T-cell–depleted HLA-matched sibling grafts was repeatedly demonstrated to be associated with an increment in the incidence of leukemic relapse posttransplantation in patients who received grafts for CML (71, 141, 200, 243), suggesting that T cells exert a critical role not only in securing engraftment of the donor marrow but also in eliminating residual leukemic cells known to survive the myeloablative preparative regimens.

Direct evidence that donor-derived lymphoid cells contribute to resistance against CML has recently been provided by the demonstrations by Kolb et al. (225), confirmed by several others (34, 130, 165, 188, 193, 226, 238, 289, 381), that infusions of donor-derived peripheral blood mononuclear cells can induce durable remissions in over 75% of patients with relapse of CML following transplantation of allogeneic unmodified or T-cell–depleted marrow grafts (Table 86.3). Doses of T cells in the mononuclear cells administered have generally ranged from 1 to 10 times 10^8/kg. Such infusions have been associated with a significant incidence of acute GvHD. However, approximately 25% of the patients who have achieved remission have exhibited no evidence of GvHD (226). Studies of stepwise escalations of T-cell doses administered to patients with relapsing CML in chronic phase more than 9 months after receipt of a T-cell–depleted marrow graft have also shown that remissions can be regularly induced with T-cell doses as low as 10^7/kg (238). At the time of transplantation, such doses of T cells

Table 86.3. Donor Leukocyte Therapy for Posttransplantation Relapsed CML

Study	Patients	Cell dose ($\times 10^8$/kg)	Remission	GvHD/CR	Aplasia
Kolb et al. (225)	3	4.4–7.4	3/3	2/3	3
Bar et al. (34)	6	0.34–5.2	5/6	5/5	5
Helg et al. (188)	3	3.8–12.3	3/3	3/3	3
Hertenstein et al. (193)	8	3.0–5.5	6/8	5/6	6
Drobyski et al. (130)	8	2.5–5.0	7/8	7/7	7
Porter et al. (289)	11	0.9–7.9	7/11	7/7	7
van Rhee et al. (381)	14	0.6–10.1	10/14	8/10	2
Giralt et al. (165)	7	0.23–0.7	3/7	0/3	—
Mackinnon et al. (238)	22	0.1–5.0	19/22	8/19	4

Abbreviations: GvHD/CR, graft-vs.-host disease/complete recovery.

would induce GvHD in 60 to 70% of cases, but after 9 to 12 months posttransplantation, these doses induce mild GvHD in fewer than 10% of HLA-matched recipients (220, 238).

The identity and target cell specificities of the effector cells that induce regressions of CML are still unknown. These cells are unlikely to be leukemia specific since presumably normal, host-type, Philadelphia chromosome–negative (Ph−) T cells, which are commonly detected in the mixed chimeric states that often develop following administration of a T-cell–depleted graft, are also consistently eradicated in those patients who achieve a remission (238). However, while this observation is consistent with the hypothesis that alloreactive T cells recognizing minor alloantigens expressed on hematopoietic cells are the major effectors of the antileukemic response, it does not rule out the possibility that other effector cells, such as NK cells, which have been shown to have cytotoxic and colony-inhibiting activity against CML cells (186, 236, 388), contribute to this process.

Among patients who undergo transplantation for AML while in early remission, the risk of relapse following receipt of a T-cell–depleted marrow graft has not been increased in several series (13, 185, 416). However, the graft-vs.-leukemia (GvL) effect derived from an allograft in the treatment of ALL is controversial. Although patients with ALL who receive a T-cell–depleted HLA-matched transplant without developing GvHD have a relapse rate no higher than that of recipients of unmodified grafts who do not develop GvHD or recipients of syngeneic transplants, the presence of acute GvHD significantly reduces the relapse rate as compared to recipients of unmodified grafts without any GvHD (200). These findings suggested that, in ALL, GvL might not be separable from GvHD in the majority of cases (39). On the other hand, when donor leukocytes have been given to patients with ALL in relapse or in second or subsequent remission at the time of transplantation, to promote GvHD and its hypothesized antileukemic effect, no reduction in relapse rate has been observed, despite an increase in the incidence and severity of GvHD. Similarly, donor leukocyte infusions have been relatively ineffective in the treatment of posttransplantation relapses of acute leukemia. In a recent compendium of the experience of the European Group for Blood and Marrow Transplantation, Kolb et al. (226) found that donor leukocyte infusions induced remissions in only 29% of transplant recipients with relapsed AML and in 0% of patients treated for relapsed ALL, compared to a 78% incidence of remission for patients treated for relapsed CML. Taken together, these findings suggest the possibility that the enhanced leukemia resistance conferred by a marrow allograft for AML or ALL may not be as dependent on alloreactive T cells for its expression as it apparently is for CML.

Of the non-T-cell-effector cells that might contribute to an antileukemic effect, the NK cells may be of particular importance. In murine models, Truitt et al. (372) have shown that infusions of IL-2-preactivated LAK cells can confer significant leukemic resistance to H_2 compatible, minor alloantigen–disparate hosts bearing AKR leukemia without inducing GvHD. Similarly, Warner and Dennert (392) have shown that infusion of IL-2-activated NK cell clones can confer marked resistance to recurrence in animals bearing the AKR thymoma.

Analysis of donor cells arising in the posttransplantation period that exhibit reactivity against host AML or ALL have also revealed a predominance of cells with an NK cell rather than a T-cell phenotype (192). Based on these observations, Soiffer et al. (336) are conducting clinical trials testing whether chronic administration of low-dose IL-2 or IL-12, which stimulates the activity of NK cells but not alloreactive T cells, can reduce the incidence of relapse posttransplantation.

Mixed leukocyte cultures between engrafted donor human T cells emerging early posttransplantation and normal or transformed lymphoblasts derived from an HLA-matched host have also led to the generation of several HLA-restricted T-cell lines and clones specific for minor alloantigens of the host (141). When these T-cell lines have been tested, they have been found to be capable of inducing cytotoxicity or clonal inhibition of host leukemic cells. However, the reactivity of these cells against leukemic clonogenic populations has usually been equivalent to or lower than their reactivity against normal hematopoietic progenitor cells expressing these antigens (141).

Recently, an alternative strategy for the generation of leukemia-reactive T cells has been explored in which HLA-matched or partially matched T lymphocytes are continuously sensitized to host leukemic cells in vitro. Lines and clones of T cells derived by this approach have been assessed for their capacity to discriminate between leukemic cells and nonleukemic targets such as phytohemagglutinin (PHA)-stimulated T lymphoblasts and Epstein-Barr virus (EBV)-transformed normal B cells obtained from the same host during remission. Using this approach, Sosman et al. (339, 340) have been able to generate $CD3^+$, $CD4^+$ T-cell lines and HLA-DR and -DP restricted $CD4^+$ T-cell clones exhibiting selective, proliferative, and cytotoxic responses against ALL cells derived from an HLA-ABD mismatched patient. Faber et al. (139) have also generated leukemia-specific HLA-restricted $CD8^+$ cytotoxic T cells from the peripheral blood lymphocytes of an HLA-matched sibling of a patient with AML. Although the frequency of such clones has been low when compared with the frequency of clones exhibiting reactivity against both normal and leukemic cells of the host, this latter study clearly indicates the possibility of generating leukemia-selective cytotoxic T cells potentially lacking GvHD-inducing alloreactivity, even from HLA-matched donors.

From these studies, it is increasingly clear that several effector systems can contribute to the antileukemic effect of a marrow allograft, including alloreactive, potentially GvHD-inducing T cells, T cells reactive against major and minor alloantigens expressed on both normal and leukemic cells, T cells reactive against differentiation antigens preferentially expressed on leukemic cells, and both nonspecific cytotoxic T cells and activated NK cells that may preferentially lyse leukemic cell blasts. Following an unmodified marrow graft, the expression of both GvHD and GvL may reflect the summation not only of the major and minor allodisparities between donor and host recognizable by donor T cells, but also the genetically regulated capacity of donor T cells to respond to these allodisparities. It may also reflect the capacity of these cells to recruit other effector cells such as T cells and NK cells, as well as the genetically controlled capacity of the T and NK effector cells to bind to and inhibit or kill leukemic versus normal targets. In recipients of T-cell–depleted marrow grafts, the number of alloreactive T cells transferred to the host is markedly reduced, preventing or blunting the clinical expression of GvHD and its contribution to leukemic resistance. However, the NK cell system, which is functionally intact by 21 days posttransplantation (214), could, if activated and of a resistant genotype, still confer resistance to leukemias sensitive to their activity. Similarly, both MHC-restricted leukemia-reactive T cells and broadly cytotoxic MHC-nonrestricted $CD8^+$, $CD28^-$, $CD3^+$ T cells exhibiting relatively selective cytotoxicity against leukemic cells could be generated from donor lymphoid elements developing in the host environment.

INFECTIOUS COMPLICATIONS IN THE INTERVAL BETWEEN ENGRAFTMENT AND EARLY IMMUNOLOGIC RECONSTITUTION

Following initial engraftment and recovery of neutrophil counts, the spectrum of infections complicating a marrow allograft changes significantly. Infections in this period, which usually comprises the interval between 1 and 6 months posttransplantation, principally reflect severe deficiencies of T-cell immune responses. Certain of these infections, such as CMV-induced pneumonias, may also be fostered by allointeractions between donor and host and are, therefore, frequent and severe in patients with active GvHD.

Interstitial pneumonias still constitute the most common cause of death in the first 3 months following a marrow allograft. Overall, 25 to 35% of patients who undergo transplantation for leukemia develop this process. Over 50% of cases can be ascribed to CMV (402). However, other viruses, particularly adenovirus and respiratory syncytial virus, have recently gained prominence as prophylactic or preemptive therapy of CMV infection has become standard (87, 194). *Pneumocystis carinii* is now an uncommon cause of interstitial pneumonia because of the widespread use of cotrimoxazole prophylaxis both before and after transplantation. However, more intensive and prolonged use of steroids, either for prophylaxis or for treatment of GvHD, has led to a significant increase in the incidence of *Aspergillus* pneumonias (267). Despite the increased use of diagnostic bronchoalveolar lavage and transbronchial or open lung biopsies, and despite the development of rapid, highly sensitive immunologic and molecular techniques for detection of CMV and other viruses (97, 134), at least 40% of cases cannot be ascribed to a pathogen and may represent processes caused by aberrant inflammatory responses induced by the combined effects of infection and/or GvHD on a lung parenchyma and supporting vasculature already damaged by radiation and chemotherapy.

Of the known pathogens, CMV has been particularly problematic. Overall, 70 to 90% of transplant recipients who are seropositive, or who receive grafts from seropositive donors, become viremic posttransplantation, usually after engraftment has been detected (18, 261). Of those who develop viremia, 30 to 40% develop interstitial pneumonia. In contrast, the risk of this complication among seronegative recipients of a marrow graft who receive blood cell support from seronegative donors is low (18). These data, coupled with molecular analyses of CMV isolates, suggest that the CMV infections observed are usually due to reactivations of virus latent in the host or the donor graft (405). Alloreactions between donor and host potentiate the risk of CMV infection and interstitial pneumonia. Thus, patients with moderate to severe GvHD have a high incidence of this complication (261, 264, 395), whereas recipients of syngeneic or autologous marrow grafts are at low risk (400). The intensity of cytoreductive therapy also increases this risk (260, 395).

In the past 5 to 7 years a number of advances have been made that are reducing the incidence of CMV-induced interstitial pneumonias and improving the prognosis of affected patients. For seronegative transplant recipients, the risk of developing CMV pneumonia may be drastically reduced by restricting their exposure to the virus through the exclusive use of platelets and other blood components from CMV-seronegative donors for transfusion support (239). Seroprophylaxis with CMV-antibody-containing γ-globulin is also effective in reducing the incidence of CMV pneumonia (42, 353) in seropositive adult recipients of unmodified marrow allografts. However, recent studies have raised a question as to whether the infusions of γ-globulin achieve this result by interfering with the growth or spread of CMV or by reducing the intensity of the allointeraction between donor and host, manifested by GvHD that promotes CMV infection (353). Indeed, in another prospective trial of seroprophylaxis conducted in recipients of T-cell–depleted marrow grafts who rarely developed GvHD, the incidence of CMV disease was equivalently low in both the prophylaxis and the control groups (135).

In 1988, a series of trials demonstrated that CMV interstitial pneumonias could be effectively treated and reversed in 50 to 70% of cases with a combination of the antiviral agent ganciclovir and CMV-antibody-containing preparations of intravenous γ-globulin (75, 132, 299). Results with this combined regimen were particularly striking since neither agent, used alone, had had any significant effect on the course of CMV interstitial pneumonia. Subsequent case reports have further indicated that for patients who cannot tolerate ganciclovir (e.g., because of drug-induced myelosuppression), foscarnet may also be effective (20).

Several groups have also been evaluating the effectiveness of ganciclovir alone when used either for the preemptive treatment of patients with detectable virus in their body fluids who have not developed CMV disease or for general prophylaxis of seropositive patients or recipients of marrow allografts from seropositive donors, since they are at high risk for developing disease. Two randomized trials have demonstrated that early treatment of patients with detectable virus in body fluids can significantly reduce the frequency of CMV interstitial pneumonia, thereby reducing transplant-associated mortality (174, 319). However, the overall adequacy of this approach rests on the ability of the transplant physician to detect virus before the onset of disease. Although new techniques, including shell vial cultures, and sensitive tests for the pp65 antigen of CMV or for polymerase chain reacton (PCR)-amplifiable CMV DNA in body fluids have improved early diagnosis (67, 131, 166), their impact depends on the type, practicability, and timeliness of the surveillance schedules employed. Prophylactic administration of ganciclovir to all seropositive transplant recipients at risk has also been shown to be effective (406). However, in the same study, up to 30% of patients developed neutropenia severe enough to warrant discontinuation of treatment. In such patients, the incidence of other infections was increased. As a result, overall survival at 6 months posttransplantation was not improved. Thus, at this time, close surveillance and early treatment of CMV infection with ganciclovir is likely preferred until more tolerable but equally effective prophylactic regimens employing ganciclovir or another antiviral agent are developed.

Another approach to prophylaxis, namely, the administration of marrow donor-derived, in vitro selected and expanded, CMV-specific T-cell clones has recently been introduced. Preliminary results in clinical trials have been highly promising (303). The adoptive transfer of 3 to 10 $\times$ 10^7 CMV-specific T cells/kg has induced significant levels of T cells exhibiting CMV-specific cytotoxicity in the blood of transplant recipients, and those levels have been sustained for periods of at least 8 weeks following infusion. Repeated doses can be administered without risk of toxicity or GvHD. None of the first five patients so treated developed CMV disease (303). Larger trials of this approach have confirmed and extended these promising results (391) and suggest that the use of adoptive cell transfer strategies to restore virus-specific T-cell immunity early after transplantation may radically reduce the risk of such infections without increasing the risk of other processes that contribute to posttransplantation mortality.

Late Complications of Marrow Transplantation

There are several late complications of marrow transplantation that occur at significant frequency. These can be divided into those resulting from delays in immune reconstitution, particularly those induced by GvHD and its treatment, and those attributable to the toxic and oncogenic sequelae of the drugs and radiation used to prepare patients for receipt of transplants.

Redevelopment of a competent donor-derived immune system following a marrow allograft is a protracted process. T-cell populations begin to redevelop within the first 2 months, but responses to mitogens and antigens may be severely depressed for at least 6 to 9 months posttransplantation (214, 408). The risk of infections with HSV, CMV, and *Candida* falls off rapidly after the first 3 to 6 months after transplantation. The risk of *Aspergillus* infections extends further into the posttransplantation period, particularly for patients receiving steroids for the prevention or treatment of GvHD. The risk of reactivation and dissemination of varicella zoster virus infections also persists through the first 1 to 2 years (233). Treatment with intravenous acyclovir effectively eradicates varicella zoster infections, with low mortality (327). Long-term prophylaxis with acyclovir may also prevent this complication (284).

During the periods of profound T-cell deficiency between engraftment and 6 to 8 months after transplantation, BMT recipients are also susceptible to polyclonal or oligoclonal B-cell lymphoproliferative disorders and monoclonal lymphomas induced by Epstein-Barr virus (407). Such lymphomas are rare following transplantation of HLA-matched unmodified marrow (0.6%) or when marrow grafts depleted of both T and B lymphocytes by lectin agglutination or CamPATH 1M have been used as the sole approach for GvHD prevention (<2%) (184, 274, 407). On the other hand, an estimated risk of 6.4% has been observed following transplantation of HLA-matched grafts depleted of T cells with T-cell–specific mouse monoclonal antibodies (419). The risk has been reported to be as high as 8 to 24% in patients treated with HLA-nonidentical grafts depleted of T cells with T-cell–specific monoclonal antibodies (149) and in recipients of unmodified marrow transplants receiving infusions of certain T-cell–specific monoclonal antibodies for the treatment of GvHD (248). Usually the lymphomas have been of donor rather than host origin (248). The basis for susceptibility to such B-cell transformations is unclear but in part reflects an inability of such patients to generate T cells capable of regulating donor B-cell expansions early in the posttransplantation period (234).

Until recently, treatment of EBV-induced lymphoproliferative disorders (LPD) in marrow transplant recipients was discouraging, for these processes are refractory to classic chemotherapy and radiation. Polyclonal EBV LPDs have been reversed in some cases with interferon or following infusion of B-cell–specific monoclonal antibodies (246, 326). However, monoclonal disease has failed to respond. Recently, our group has shown that infusions of small doses (10^6 $CD3^+$ T cells/kg) of donor T lymphocytes induce complete and durable remissions of EBV LPDs in a high proportion of cases (279). The efficacy of this therapeutic approach likely reflects the high frequency of EBV-specific cytotoxic T-cell precursors in the circulation of normal seropositive marrow donors (72). Indeed, Rooney et al. (305) and Servida et al. (325) have confirmed our findings, demonstrating sustained remissions following infusion of small numbers of genetically marked EBV-specific T cells generated in vitro.

Recovery of B-cell function is more protracted, with antibody deficiency states persisting for 12 to 18 months (15, 214, 408). In patients with chronic GvHD, severe humoral immune deficiencies may persist for 3 to 5 years. As a result, patients with chronic GvHD are particularly susceptible to infections, such as recurrent sinusitis, otitis media, pneumonia, and sepsis, caused by the same spectrum of pyogenic bacteria that affect children with agammaglobulinemia, such as pneumococci, streptococci, and *Hemophilus influenzae* (29, 404).

The late sequelae of radiation and other alkylating agents used to prepare patients for transplantation may be mild or severe, depending on the types of agents used and their dose intensity, the treatment received by the patient prior to referral for transplantation, and the age of the patient at the time of transplantation. In general, patients prepared with cyclophosphamide alone sustain limited and generally transient damage, while injury induced by total body irradiation tends to be more profound and enduring. Similarly, radiation administered in a single large dose tends to be more damaging than if this dose is administered in multiple fractions (115, 312).

The most devastating of late complications resulting from damage induced by TBI and chemotherapy is leukoencephalopathy (367). This complication occurs almost exclusively in patients who have undergone transplantation for leukemia and who received cranial irradiation or extended courses of intrathecal methotrexate as treatment or prophylaxis for CNS leukemia prior to referral for transplantation. In such patients, the risk of leukoencephalopathy has been reported to be 7% (367). This complication usually induces severe symptoms, including slurred speech, confusion, ataxia, seizures, and spasticity, which may progress to coma and death. Less severe CNS toxic reactions may also be observed in the form of neuropsychological dysfunctions and varying degrees of retardation (419). However, the incidence of the latter complications has not been established. Transient neurologic toxic reactions, including tremors, seizures, and paresis, may also complicate the use of Cyclosporine for prophylaxis of GvHD (390).

Endocrine deficiencies are common sequelae of the cytoreductive regimens used for allogeneic marrow transplants. Thyroid failure requiring supplementation has been detected in 10% (232, 329), and compensated hypothyroidism in an additional 34 to 36% of patients transplanted for leukemia. Among younger women prepared for transplantation with cyclophosphamide alone, deficiencies of ovarian function usually recover over the first year after transplantation (median, 6 months), but in over 35% of older women (>27 years of age), sustained ovarian failure is observed. The incidence of this complication increases to 55% for young and 74% for older women who undergo transplantation for leukemia after preparation with TBI and cyclophosphamide (309). Pregnancies and normal births have occurred among women who underwent transplantation for aplasia after cyclophosphamide pretreatment alone, but have been rare in patients who underwent transplantation for leukemia. Among male transplant recipients prepared with cyclophosphamide alone, Leydig cell dysfunction is uncommon. Even among leukemic male transplant recipients treated with TBI, deficiencies of testosterone are rare, although 76% may have compensatory elevations of follicle-stimulating hormone. However, sustained reduction or eradication of spermatogenesis has been recorded in at least 75% of patients treated with TBI and in up to a third of patients prepared with cyclophosphamide alone (330).

The linear growth of children prepared for transplantation with TBI is often limited. In part, this reflects injury to the hypothalamus, resulting in decreased production of growth hormone–releasing factor (GHRF) and consequently abnormal growth hormone secretion (232, 312). However, TBI also affects growing bone, reducing, to a variable degree, the ultimate growth potential of young transplant recipients. The use of fractionated TBI is associated with less stunting of growth than are single-dose regimens (204). Whether and to what degree treatment with growth hormone or GHRF can partially correct short stature in these cases is under study.

Radiation may also induce cataract formation in the lens late in the posttransplantation period. In patients treated with single, high doses of TBI, the incidence of cataracts is 50%. This frequency is lower in patients treated with fractionated TBI (10–20%) (115).

Treatment with alkylating agents also predisposes to secondary malignancies other than the EBV-associated lymphomas previously described. To date, such neoplasms have been recorded in only a relatively small proportion of marrow transplant recipients, and predominantly among patients who underwent transplantation for leukemia (116, 407). Solid tumors, including basal cell carcinomas, squamous cell carcinomas of the skin, adenocarcinomas of the stomach, osteosarcomas, and glioblastomas, have developed in a small proportion (1–2%) of cases followed for 1 to 10 years post transplantation (407). Again, the incidence of these cancers appears to be lower than that recorded in patients given comparable or lower localized doses of radiation and chemotherapy for other neoplasms such as Hodgkin's disease. More prolonged follow-up is still needed, however, before full assessments can be made of the incidence of such tumors in transplant recipients.

HLA-MATCHED MARROW TRANSPLANTATION FOR LEUKEMIA

Between 1968 and 1978, marrow transplants were almost exclusively applied to the treatment of patients with leukemia refractory to chemotherapy. Overall, 13 to 18% of such patients achieved durable disease-free survival (362). However, for patients who underwent transplantation when in good physical condition, the probability of extended disease-free survival was 25%. Based on these results, transplants were then applied to patients in good clinical condition, at a stage in the disease when the leukemic cell burden was low and the residual leukemic cells were likely to be still sensitive to the cytoreduction employed (363). In 1979, the Seattle group reported a series of patients with AML who underwent transplantation in first remission, of whom 63% achieved long-term disease-free survival. In this series, the risk of relapse was only 12%. This study was quickly confirmed by several transplant centers (270) and led to the widespread exploration of HLA-matched marrow grafts in the treatment of acute leukemias in first or second remission and of CML in the first chronic phase. Approximately 15 years of this experience can now be evaluated. Results can also be compared with those achieved with current chemotherapy and with autologous marrow grafts at different stages in the disease course.

Marrow Transplantation for Acute Myelogenous Leukemia

TRANSPLANTATION AFTER FIRST RELAPSE OF AML

For patients with AML in second or later remission or relapse, an allogeneic HLA-matched marrow graft is generally regarded as the treatment of choice. Few if any patients with AML in whom an initial remission proved not durable survive disease free if treated with chemotherapy alone (91). In contrast, cytoreduction with TBI or busulfan, together with cyclophosphamide, followed by transplantation of HLA-matched marrow has led to extended disease-free survival for 20 to 30% of adults and 30 to 51% of children who receive grafts in a second remission (76, 91, 100, 124). An alternative strategy is to proceed directly to allogeneic BMT during the first relapse. This approach has been associated with a 23% relapse-free survival rate (101). Results recently reported also indicate that similar cytoreduction followed by administration of an autologous, drug-purged marrow graft obtained during second remission may lead to long-term (5-year) disease-free survival in 30% of cases (175, 414). Although such autologous grafts carry a higher risk of post-transplantation relapse (>50%) than HLA-matched marrow grafts (20–25%) and a somewhat lower probability of extended disease-free survival, they are, at present, the treatment of choice for patients in second remission lacking an HLA-matched donor, and superior to other chemotherapeutic approaches (see Chapter 85).

TRANSPLANTATION IN FIRST REMISSION OF AML

The role of allogeneic marrow transplantation in the treatment of patients with AML in first remission is considerably more controversial. Results of published prospective trials evaluating this issue are discussed in Table 86.4. Four prospective clinical trials performed in the 1980s attempted to address this question by comparing results following transplantation of HLA-matched marrow grafts with results of chemotherapy for the treatment of AML in first remission in young adults (<45 years of age) (14, 93, 105, 417). In each of these trials the incidence of posttreatment relapse was significantly lower among transplant patients (9–40%) than among patients treated with chemotherapy alone (71–88%). However, non-relapse-related mortality in the transplant arms of each of these studies was significantly higher than in the chemotherapy controls. The 3- to 5-year disease-free survival rates were superior in the transplant arms in each study. However, these differences reached statistical significance in only two of the studies (14, 105). Concerns regarding selection bias and the adequacy of the treatment and support administered to the chemotherapy control group have also been raised (251). Although the postinduction therapies in the chemotherapy control arms varied from study to study, they were representative of standard consolidation or intensification regimens of the time.

In order to address some of the issues raised by these earlier trials, two large randomized studies have been performed. These trials compared the results of transplantation, either allogeneic or autologous, with the results of chemotherapy in the treatment of AML. A preliminary analysis of the first study, the MRC AML-10 Trial, which enrolled over 1,800 patients, has now been reported (80). Patients in this study were treated with four courses of chemotherapy, two induction and two consolidation courses, and were then randomized to the allogeneic transplant arm or autologous versus observation arm, based on availability of an HLA-identical sibling and age of the recipient less than 45 years. Data were analyzed on an intent-to-treat basis in this study. Overall survival at 5 years was no different among the three groups: 58%, 54%, and 52% for the allogeneic transplant, autologous transplant, and observation arms, respectively. However, the risk of relapse was significantly lower in the group of patients with an HLA-identical donor, 33%, whereas it was 50% for those without an HLA-identical donor. Good-risk patients, which this group defined as patients with t(8;21), t(15;17), inv(16) abnormalities, had a 71% survival rate at 5 years, whereas those patients considered standard risk had a 46% survival rate at 5 years. Poor-risk patients, defined as those with more than 20% blasts in the "course one" bone marrow, had a 16% survival at 5 years. The presence or absence of a donor affected only the standard-risk group, in which survival at 5 years was 64% and 48%, respectively. Having a donor made no difference in the good-risk or poor-risk groups. Based on an intent-to-treat analysis, there were no detectable differences between any of the arms at the time of this analysis.

In a second trial, Zittoun and colleagues performed a similar study comparing allogeneic and autologous transplantation to intensive chemotherapy (418). In this study, patients achieving and maintaining a complete remission after stan-

Table 86.4. Results of Prospective Trials Comparing Bone Marrow Transplantation (BMT) and Chemotherapy for the Treatment of AML in First Remission

Center	BMT		Chemotherapy		Study
	DFS (%)	Rate of relapse (%)	DFS (%)	Rate of relapse (%)	
Fred Hutchinson	49**	15	20	74	Appelbaum et al. (14)
UCLA	40	40	27	71	Champlin et al. (93, 94)
Univ. of Cantabria	70**	10	10	88	Conde et al. (105)
M. D. Anderson	36	9	15	85	Zander et al. (417)
EORTC/GI MEMA[a]	55	24	30 (OS)	57	Zittoun et al. (418)
MRC AML-10 trial[a]	58[b] (OS)	33	52[b] (OS)	54	Burnett et al. (80)

Abbreviations: DFS, disease-free survival; OS, overall survival.
** Statistically significant difference.
[a] Analyzed on an intent-to-treat basis.
[b] Reported only overall survival.

dard induction therapy (daunorubicin and Ara-C) and a single course of intensive consolidation therapy (intermediate-dose Ara-C, 500–1,000mg/m (2) every 12 hours × 12 doses, and amsacrine, 120 mg/m (2)/d × 3 doses) were randomized to allogeneic transplantation, if they had an HLA-identical sibling, or to autologous transplantation versus a second course of intensive chemotherapy. The intensification regimen consisted of high-dose Ara-C, 2 g/m (2) every 12 hours × 8 doses, and daunorubicin, 45 mg/m (2)/d × 3 doses. Again, no patient above the age of 45 years was randomized to the allogeneic arm. At 4 years, the projected rate of disease-free survival was 55% for the allogeneic arm vs. 48% for the autologous arm vs. 30% for the intensive chemotherapy arm. The difference between the results in the autologous arm and the chemotherapy arm reached statistical significance at $p = .05$. The difference between the allogeneic arm and the chemotherapy arm was also statistically significant at $p = .04$. Relapse was noted to be lower in the allogeneic arm, 25%, whereas it was 41% and 57% in the autologous and chemotherapy arms, respectively. However, when overall survival at 4 years was compared among the three groups on an intent-to-treat analysis, no significant difference could be appreciated.

As was seen in earlier trials comparing transplantation and chemotherapy, benefits from lower relapse rates in the allogeneic arm were offset by higher non-relapse-related mortality. In addition, questions have been raised as to whether the chemotherapy control arm in the latter study received optimal therapy. A recent report from the Cancer and Leukemia Group B (CALGB) examined the efficacy of sequential low-, intermediate-, or high-dose Ara-C as postremission intensification therapy in patients less than 60 years old with AML. Their report demonstrated a 44% probability of remaining in continuous remission at 4 years for the group of patients receiving the high-dose Ara-C regimen (3 g/m (2) every 12 hours × 6 doses) (251). These results are not dissimilar from those achieved in the autologous transplant arm of the Zittoun study. In addition, a follow-up study from the CALGB demonstrated that certain "good"-risk cytogenetic abnormalities such as t(8;21)(q22;q22) and inv(16)(p13q22), predict responsiveness to intensive chemotherapy with high-dose cytarabine. In this study, patients with these abnormalities who received four courses of high-dose cytarabine as postinduction consolidation therapy (63) achieved a 51% disease-free survival. Future trials in the treatment of AML will likely require incorporation of cytogenetic information in the treatment strategy.

Although the results of more intensive chemotherapeutic regimens over the past decade have improved the outcomes of patients with AML, novel approaches to allogeneic transplantation using T-cell–depleted techniques have also been developed that result in a lower non-relapse-related mortality and diminish the incidence and severity of GvHD (79, 281, 335). A recent report from our own group (281) demonstrated a 79% disease-free survival at 2 years for adult patients with AML who underwent transplantation while in first remission. The regimen consisted of a T-cell–depleted allograft following cytoreduction with TBI/thiotepa/cyclophosphamide, a regimen that has been associated with a 10 to 15% regimen-related mortality and a 7% incidence of relapse. T-cell depletion with soybean lectin agglutination followed by sheep red blood cell rosetting resulted in a 2.5 to 3.0 log depletion of T cells, resulting in near eradication of acute and chronic GvHD. Recently, transplant teams from the Dana Farber Cancer Center (335) and Ulm University Hospital in Germany (79) reported similar findings, with a 65% and 80% disease-free survival, respectively, for patients with AML who underwent transplantation while in first remission. These groups also employed T-cell depletion techniques involving either CD6 depletion or CamPATH 1M, respectively. Therefore, although intensive postremission chemotherapy regimens have improved results in patients with AML, comparable advances in allogeneic transplantation techniques have led to a reduction in regimen-related mortality and improved disease-free survival. In light of these developments, selection of an optimal approach for the treatment of adults with AML must await the results of planned or active protocols comparing these second-generation chemotherapy and transplantation regimens.

The role of marrow transplantation in the treatment of children with AML is particularly controversial since new chemotherapeutic regimens have significantly increased the proportion of children who achieve and remain in first remission. Currently, 40 to 50% of children treated with such regimens who achieve a first remission are alive and in sustained remission 5 years later (110, 396). However, HLA-matched marrow grafts administered to children with AML in first remission have also achieved impressive results: 49 to 67% of such patients are alive and disease free 3 to 5 years post transplantation (76, 311). In a recent prospective trial conducted by the Children's Cancer Study Group, 49% of children who underwent transplantation for AML while in primary remission were alive and in sustained remission 3 years after treatment, compared to 40% for patients treated with chemotherapy alone ($P < .05$) (142). Thus, for children with AML in first remission, HLA-matched marrow grafts appear to be superior to chemotherapy alone (see Chapter 165).

The relative efficacy of autologous marrow grafts when compared with allogeneic marrow grafts in the treatment of patients with AML in first remission is not yet established. Several studies in which either drug-purged or untreated autologous marrow grafts, obtained in first remission, were administered after cytoreductive regimens consisting of either TBI or busulfan together with cyclophosphamide, have been conducted in the treatment of adults. Disease-free survival rates of 45 to 50% have been reported (175, 258). However, these results may be skewed by the particularly good results achieved in a proportion of patients who underwent transplantation more than 12 months after initial remission induction—patients who, with chemotherapy alone, are likely to have an improved prognosis. For patients who underwent transplantation within 6 months of achieving first remission, relapse rates following autologous transplants are 40 to 45%, with overall disease-free survivals ranging from 30 to 45% at 2 to 3 years (175).

Marrow Transplantation for Acute Lymphoblastic Leukemia

TRANSPLANTATION FOR ALL IN FIRST REMISSION

Current multidrug chemotherapeutic regimens combining systemic treatment and CNS prophylaxis regimens are able to induce sustained remissions or cures in 70 to 80% of children with ALL presenting with standard risk features (374). Further, more intensive regimens applied to children at high risk for relapse have increased their probability of sustained disease-free survival to 60 to 70% (99, 342). Because of these results, it has been difficult to identify pediatric patients with ALL in first remission for whom an allogeneic transplant clearly affords an improved probability of cure. Indeed, allogeneic marrow grafts in children and adolescents with high- risk features have been associated with long-term disease-free survival rates of 56 to 84%, which are not superior to those that can now be achieved with chemotherapy alone (38, 40, 70).

The place of allogeneic marrow grafts in the treatment of adults with ALL who have achieved an initial remission is only somewhat less controversial (90). Current chemotherapeutic regimens induce remissions in 70 to 85% of adults, but these remissions are sustained in only 20 to 43% of cases (161, 197, 292). For patients who, at initial diagnosis, present with disease features associated with a high risk of relapse, such as a high initial white blood cell count (>20,000/mm^3), older age (>60 years), CNS involvement, chromosomal translocations t(4:11), t(8:14), or t(9:22), null or B-cell phenotype, or a failure to achieve remission within 5 weeks of initiation of induction therapy, sustained remission is seen in only 10 to 20% of patients. However, in several series evaluating the role of HLA-matched marrow transplants applied to the treatment of high-risk young adults less than 40 years old and in first remission, such transplants have led to 3- to 5-year disease-free survival rates of 30 to 71%, with relapse rates after transplantation of 9 to 36%, depending on the type of cytoreductive regimen used (60, 65, 127, 128, 196, 401) and the method of GvHD prophylaxis incorporated into the transplantation regimen (38). These promising results suggest that allogeneic marrow grafts may offer a significant advantage for the adult with ALL who presents with high-risk features.

Recently, two prospective randomized trials attempted to define the optimal postremission therapy in adult patients with ALL. In the first of these trials, patients younger than 40 were "naturally" randomized to the allogeneic arm of the study if they had an HLA-identical sibling. Patients younger than 40 without a donor and those between the ages of 40 and 50 were randomized to chemotherapy versus autologous transplantation (323).

In an intent-to-treat analysis, the 5-year survival rates were not statistically different between the patients randomized to the allogeneic arm and those randomized to the autologous BMT or chemotherapy arm. Allogeneic transplantation did not offer any benefit to adult patients with standard-risk ALL. However, when patients with high-risk features were considered, there was a significant difference in overall and disease-free survival, favoring the allogeneic BMT arm, 44% vs. 20%, respectively.

In the second prospective study, following induction therapy, patients achieving complete remission were "randomized" either to allogeneic transplantation if they had an HLA-identical sibling, or to autologous transplantation with or without interleukin-2 (25). This study did not have a chemotherapy control arm. In this study, which included patients through the age of 55, the 3-year probability of disease-free survival was significantly higher in the HLA-identical sibling group than in the non-HLA-identical sibling group, 68% vs. 26%. The use of IL-2 after autologous BMT did not alter the 3-year probability of continuous complete remission in the autologous transplant group, 29% vs. 27%. Once again, relapse was the primary cause of failure in the autologous transplantation arm. These studies demonstrate that there is a role for allogeneic transplantation in certain subsets of patients with adult ALL in first remission. In particular, allogeneic marrow grafts may offer a significant advantage to the adult with ALL who presents with high-risk features.

TRANSPLANTATION FOR ALL IN SECOND OR SUBSEQUENT REMISSION OR RELAPSE

Results reported for series of children who have received HLA-matched marrow grafts for ALL when in second remission vary considerably both in the incidence of relapse post-transplantation and in the proportion of patients achieving long-term disease-free survival. Transplants administered after cytoreduction with variations of the Seattle regimen of single-dose TBI and cyclophosphamide have been associated with relapse rates ranging from 30 to 57% at 2 years and with disease-free survival rates of 33 to 50% (313, 411). In contrast, newer approaches incorporating higher doses of hyperfractionated TBI followed by cyclophosphamide (76), or fractionated TBI administered with high-dose cytosine arabinoside (104), etoposide (65), or altered doses of cyclophosphamide (401), have reduced the incidence of relapse after transplantation to 5 to 16% and have concurrently improved long-term disease-free survival to 59 to 64% at 5 years.

For meaningful comparisons between results of transplantation and the results achievable with chemotherapy alone, it is critical to compare characteristics of the patient populations treated, particularly the duration of the first remission prior to relapse. Children with ALL whose disease relapses early in the course of their initial chemotherapy (e.g., in the first 18 months) may be induced into a second remission with chemotherapy, but they are unlikely to survive free of disease for more than 6 to 12 months. In contrast, chemotherapy alone may secure long-term remission or cure for up to 40% of patients with ALL whose disease relapses after they have completed 18 to 24 months of chemotherapy (see Chapter 164) (304). Given these statistics, it has been argued that while transplantation is indicated for children whose disease relapses early, it may not be an appropriate option for patients with relapse after a prolonged initial remission.

To address this issue, we and others have conducted retrospective analyses of single-center and multicenter experiences from this point of view (76). In these studies, children with ALL in second remission whose initial relapse occurred while they were on chemotherapy in the first 2 years postdiagnosis fared significantly better if they received an allogeneic marrow transplant than if they were treated with chemotherapy alone. For these patients, 5-year disease-free survival rates for children who received transplants ranged from 30 to 56% while, for patients treated with chemotherapy those rates ranged from 6 to 22%. In each comparative analysis, the results of transplantation were significantly better than those achieved with chemotherapy. These results strongly suggest that an allogeneic marrow graft is superior to chemotherapy for children with ALL whose disease relapses within 1 to 2 years of first remission. In our own series (72) and in those reported by Chessels et al. (96) and Barrett et al. (41), transplantation may also be superior to chemotherapy when applied to patients with ALL who experience a relapse late in their first remission. In our own single-center series, patients whose first remissions lasted longer than 24 months and who were treated by transplantation have had a 10-year disease-free survival rate of 81% vs. 31% for patients treated with chemotherapy alone. In the multicenter analysis conducted by Chessels et al. (96) and in the large matched pair study of children reported to the International Bone Marrow Transplant Registry and the Pediatric Oncology Group by Barrett et al. (41), the 5-year leukemia-free survival rates for children who received transplants were 47% and 55%, respectively, compared to leukemia-free survival rates of 18% and 32% for children treated with chemotherapy alone. Prospective trials comparing these two approaches are still needed to explore this issue.

For adults with ALL who have failed an initial remission, an HLA-matched marrow graft is the treatment of choice and the only therapy with curative potential. For adults treated by transplantation in a second remission, different groups have reported extended disease-free survival rates ranging from 22 to 43%, with posttransplantation relapse the cause of failure in 26 to 56% of cases (38, 125, 196, 401). For children and adults who undergo transplantation in later remissions or during a relapse, the probability of extended disease-free survival is more limited, ranging from 8 to 25% at 3 to 5 years after grafting (40, 125, 310).

Marrow Transplantation for Chronic Myelogenous Leukemia

Allogeneic bone marrow transplantation is clearly the treatment of choice for patients with chronic myelogenous leukemia (CML) who are less than 60 years old and have an HLA-compatible donor (102). Single-agent chemotherapy applied to the treatment of CML has been only palliative and has not been shown to significantly prolong survival (337). Further, although intensive combination chemotherapies have been used in an attempt to eradicate the Ph+ clone, suppression of Ph+ cells has been transient at best. As a result, these regimens, which are associated with significant morbidity secondary to myelosuppression, have not resulted in a significant improvement in median survival (359). In contrast to the results achieved with chemotherapy, INF-α, used as first-line therapy in CML, has induced hematologic remissions in as many as 70% of patients. However, complete cytogenetic remissions have been less common, occurring in no more than 20% of patients so treated (360). However, a large multi-institutional study from the Italian Cooperative Study Group recently reported a statistically significant improvement in overall survival for patients treated with INF-α compared to conventional therapy with hydroxyurea or busulfan, with median survival rates of 72 months vs. 52 months, respectively (207). In addition, other investigators have demonstrated a significant improvement in overall survival for those patients achieving either a complete, major, or minor cytogenetic response versus those not achieving a cytogenetic response or versus historical controls treated with standard chemotherapy (see Chapter 143) (210, 321).

In contrast to the results achieved with chemotherapy or interferon, HLA-matched allogeneic marrow transplants have induced durable eradications of Ph+ cells and extended disease-free survival in a significant proportion of patients, depending on the phase of disease at the time of transplantation. Long-term survival rates ranging from 50 to 60% in multicenter studies to as high as 70 to 90% in single-institution trials have been achieved when patients received transplants in chronic phase (19, 102, 103, 170). For patients who received transplants in later stages of CML, eradication of disease has been less consistent. The long-term disease-free survival rate has been 10 to 40% in patients who received transplants when in the accelerated phase of disease and 10 to 20% in patients who received transplants when in blast crisis (92, 106).

Various factors have been analyzed for their effect on relapse- and non-relapse-related mortality. Status of disease at the time of transplantation is unanimously viewed as a significant predictor of subsequent relapse and survival (120, 255, 366). In the three largest series reported to date (171, 254, 366), patients who received transplants in the first chronic phase of CML had a 5 to 30% probability of relapse, whereas those who received transplants in the accelerated phase of disease had a 40% risk, and patients who received transplants while in blast crisis had a 60 to 80% probability of relapse.

Non-relapse-related mortality appears to be influenced by various other factors. The time between diagnosis and transplantation is an important prognosticator of the non-relapse-related mortality. An early report from the team at the Fred Hutchinson Cancer Research Center (365) demonstrated a statistically significant difference in actuarial survival between patients who received transplants within the first 17 months from diagnosis and those who received transplants more than 17 months after diagnosis—73% vs. 54%, respectively. A more recent Seattle analysis suggests that this difference is significant only when transplantation is delayed more than 2 years from diagnosis (102). However, an extra year of delay exposes the chronic-phase patient to the risk of acceleration or blastic transformation, which would then lower the probability of disease-free survival following a bone marrow transplantation. A recent report from the International Bone Marrow Transplant Registry (IBMTR) also addressed this issue and demonstrated that chronic-phase patients who underwent transplantation within 1 year of diagnosis experienced a significantly lower regimen-related mortality and relapse rate, resulting in significantly higher disease-free and overall survival rates than achieved by patients who underwent transplantation after the first year (170). These reports are important for assessing the optimal timing of transplantation in view of the recent data regarding the efficacy of INF-α in the treatment of patients with CML. Patients treated with INF often are not fully evaluable until after 12 to 18 months of treatment. This may result in a detrimental delay for patients with related, HLA-identical donors who do not respond to INF treatment and who receive transplants later than the first 1 to 2 years after diagnosis. It will be important to analyze currently available data for the possible impact that such a delay might have on the outcome of transplantation for patients who do or do not respond to INF. Identification of variables that predict response to INF would also greatly facilitate selection of treatment options. At this time, few physicians would question the role of allogeneic transplantation as first-line treatment for younger patients (<40 years) with newly diagnosed CML. However, controversy still exists regarding the timing and use of transplantation in older patients with CML. Randomized trials comparing results of transplantation performed early after diagnosis versus after an extended course of INF treatment will be required in this patient population to resolve this issue.

Controversy also exists as to the impact of pretransplant treatment with INF on the outcome of transplantation. One study recently demonstrated that patients who received INF prior to transplantation had a 2.5-fold higher risk of transplantation-related mortality than patients treated with either hydroxyurea or busulfan (54). This increased mortality was primarily ascribed to a 3-fold higher incidence of fatal posttransplantation infections after prolonged INF treatment prior to transplantation. In sharp contrast to this study, a study conducted by the group at the M. D. Anderson Cancer Center failed to show any adverse effect of prior INF therapy on transplantation outcome (164).

The type of chemotherapy used prior to transplantation also affects transplantation results. The IBMTR compared outcomes for patients previously treated with hydroxyurea or busulfan and found a significantly lower disease-free survival rate and overall survival rate in the group of patients treated with busulfan (170). The lower survival rate was directly related to a significantly higher regimen-related mortality. When both the time to transplantation and the pretransplantation treatment were considered in a multivariate analysis, both were found to be independent predictors of outcome. Therefore, prior treatment with busulfan had a negative impact on transplantation outcome, regardless of the time to transplantation. This finding is presumably attributable to the additional toxic burden on host tissues induced by the cumulative toxicity of this drug. This study suggests that treatment with busulfan should be avoided in patients with HLA-identical donors who are likely to undergo an allogeneic bone marrow transplantation.

Acute or chronic GvHD can also impact significantly on the outcome of transplantation in patients with CML. Although moderate to severe forms of acute GvHD can have a negative impact on overall survival (35% at 4 years in patients with moderate to severe acute GvHD, vs. 74% in those with no or mild acute GvHD (171), the development of GvHD is also associated with a lower relapse rate, the so-called, graft-vs-leukemia phenomenon. Indeed, there appears to be an inverse correlation between the grade of acute GvHD and the incidence of relapse (180), as well as a lower risk of relapse in patients who develop only chronic GvHD (200).

As discussed earlier in this chapter, direct evidence of a GvL effect has recently been provided by the numerous reports demonstrating the efficacy of donor-derived leukocytes in producing complete hematologic and cytogenetic remissions in CML patients who have experienced relapse after a marrow allograft (34, 130, 165, 188, 193, 225, 226, 238, 289, 381). These findings have led some investigators to reexamine strategies incorporating T-cell–depleted transplants in the treatment of CML. In the past, the use of T-cell–depleted transplants for CML was criticized because of their association with high relapse rates. However, T-cell depletion, by reducing both the incidence and severity of acute and in some cases chronic GvHD, has reduced peritransplant morbidity and mortality, particularly among the older patients most frequently afflicted with CML (19, 171). A new strategy currently under investigation is the use of T-cell–depleted transplants for the older patient with CML, followed by an infusion of donor cells 9 to 12 months after transplantation, when the dose of T cells required to induce GvHD is higher, either for the treatment of early relapse or for persistence of molecular evidence of disease. This strategy is particularly practicable in patients who undergo transplantation for CML, since most relapses do not occur until after 6 months posttransplantation and are usually associated with a subsequent prolonged and relatively stable chronic phase of disease (20). Recent studies have demonstrated that detecting the emergence or persistence of *bcr abl* in mRNA transcripts by polymerase chain reaction (PCR)-amplified assays in the marrow of patients after transplantation is highly predictive of the subsequent development of clinical relapse (307). In view of this, patients with persistently positive PCR assays can be treated with donor leukocytes prophylactically, before either cytogenetic or hematologic relapse occurs. Ongoing studies are currently examining this approach for the treatment of CML.

Marrow Transplantation for Myelodysplastic Syndromes

The myelodysplastic syndromes are a heterogeneous series of disorders marked by peripheral cytopenias associated with normal to increased marrow cellularity and abnormal maturation of the myelogenous series. In over 70% of cases, clonal cytogenetic abnormalities are observed, particularly single deletions of 5q, monosomy 7, and trisomy 8.

Based on the percentage of blast cells in the marrow or blood, the presence of Auer rods in myelogenous precursors, and the presence of ringed sideroblasts, five categories of MDS have been described: refractory anemia (RA), refractory anemia with ringed sideroblasts (RARS), refractory anemia with excess blasts (RAEB), refractory anemia with excess blasts in transformation (RAEB-t), and chronic myelomonocytic leukemia (CMMOL) (see Chapter 141) (56). There also appears to be a subgroup of patients who exhibit a "hypoplastic MDS" characterized by a hypocellular bone marrow with dysplastic features (250). This latter entity is often confused with aplastic anemia (AA), but the presence of well-recognized MDS-associated cytogenetic abnormalities in addition to the dysplastic features separates this entity from AA. In addition, although idiopathic myelofibrosis is categorized as a myeloproliferative disorder, studies evaluating transplantation in patients with MDS often include patients with myelofibrosis. Therefore, this discussion will include patients with this entity (see Chapter 144).

Treatment for most patients with MDS continues to be supportive therapy. Intensive chemotherapeutic regimens have yielded only short-term remissions and have been associated with significant morbidity and mortality (211). Although certain subgroups of patients may respond to treatments with danazol (205), low-dose cytosine arabinoside (189), azacitidine (328), and supportive measures such as the use of G-CSF or GM-CSF to induce production of mature neutrophils (12, 263), these strategies have failed to produce sustained complete remissions in the majority of patients.

In contrast to these results, allogeneic marrow grafts administered to patients prepared with TBI or busulfan and cyclophosphamide have led to sustained remissions of disease in 40 to 50% of cases (15, 22, 121, 183, 268). Accumulated experience suggests that patients who undergo transplantation for RA or RARS enjoy better prospects for disease-free survival (53–61%) than patients with RAEB (20–32%) or RAEB-t (14–27%). This difference reflects the extremely low rate of disease relapse among patients who undergo transplantation for RA or RARS (0–6%), in contrast to the high relapse rates (45–50%) associated with transplantation for RAEB or RAEB-t (15, 123). Because of these findings, new strategies are being explored that either intensify the pretransplantation cytoreductive regimen (297) or attempt to induce a complete remission or return to an "RA-like" state with intensive chemotherapy prior to transplantation (121).

Patients treated with HLA-matched marrow transplants for severe myelofibrosis and malignant myelosclerosis, once engrafted, may recover normal hematopoiesis and achieve complete resolution of fibrosis with sustained disease-free survival (295, 410). However, the presence of marrow fibrosis may be associated with a delay in engraftment and with graft rejection (15). Experience with bone marrow transplantation for this group of patients remains limited.

Marrow Transplantation for Lymphoma

Current regimens employing multiple chemotherapeutic agents in dose-intensive protocols induce durable curative remissions in approximately 50% of adults and over 70% of children with intermediate- and high-grade lymphomas (see Chapter 150). Similarly, primary treatment of Hodgkin's disease is now curative in over 70% of cases (see Chapter 149). As a result, transplantation of either allogeneic or autologous marrow, performed after administration of myeloablative doses of TBI or alkylating agents together with cyclophosphamide, has largely been applied to patients who fail to attain or sustain a primary remission of disease. Although experience with allogeneic marrow transplants applied to the treatment of non-Hodgkin's lymphoma remains limited (21), it strongly indicates that disease status at the time of transplantation and sensitivity to prior chemotherapy, rather than initial stage or type of lymphoma, are the most important prognostic indicators of long-term disease-free survival. For patients with chemotherapy-refractory non-Hodgkin's lymphoma, prospects for extended disease-free survival range from 10 to 23% (107, 137, 287) compared with 25 to 44% for patients who receive grafts during a second remission and 88% for those who receive grafts during a first remission (85, 235). Although prior studies comparing results of allogeneic transplants to autologous transplants for patients with non-Hodgkin's lymphoma failed to demonstrate a survival advantage for allograft recipients (17, 182, 209), more recent studies have shown a significant progression-free survival advantage for recipients of allogeneic transplants (296). In addition, although most trials have examined the role of allogeneic marrow transplants in patients with recurrent or refractory, intermediate-, or high-grade lymphomas, recent evidence suggests that this treatment modality may also be applicable to patients with advanced low-grade lymphomas (379). Clearly, there appear to be subsets of patients with Hodgkin's disease or non-Hodgkin's lymphoma who may benefit from an allogeneic transplant. However, further studies are needed to define prognostic factors that accurately identify patients who would be most likely to benefit from this aggressive therapy.

Marrow Transplantation for Multiple Myeloma

Until recently, the treatment of multiple myeloma has been limited to combination chemotherapy, either alone or with INF-α (see Chapter 152) (181, 241). Despite initial response rates of 50 to 60%, the median survival time of patients with multiple myeloma is only 3 years (36). Thus, attention has focused on the use of highly intensive chemoradiotherapy regimens with hematopoietic support, in the form of either autologous marrow or peripheral blood stem cells (11, 35, 317). Several hundred patients have now been treated by this approach. Unfortunately, relapse remains a major obstacle in the use of autologous bone marrow or peripheral blood stem cell transplantation to treat multiple myeloma (57, 369).

Recent advances in transplantation approaches and supportive care have extended the use of allogeneic bone marrow transplantation to older patients. Thus, this treatment modality has now become available to selected patients with multiple myeloma, a disease characterized by a peak incidence between the ages of 50 and 70. However, the experience with allogeneic BMT preceded by high-dose chemotherapy regimens with or without TBI remains limited (78, 108, 154, 375).

At the present time, 3-year survival rates for allografted patients with multiple myeloma receiving transplants at different stages of disease ranges from 30 to 60% (37, 154). A recent update from the European Group for Blood and Marrow Transplantation (EBMT) revealed an overall survival rate of 32% at 4 years and of 28% at 7 years for patients treated with allografts following TBI and intensive chemotherapy or high-dose chemotherapy alone (154). The overall relapse-free survival rate of those patients who were in complete remission after BMT was 34% at 6 years. This study aimed to identify favorable pretransplantation prognostic factors that would predict for improved survival following transplantation. They identified female sex, stage I disease at diagnosis, one line of previous treatment, and being in complete remission before pretransplantation conditioning as favorable prognostic factors. The presence of a low β^2 microglobulin concentration as well as IgA myeloma also predicted a favorable outcome. Of posttransplantation factors, only attainment of a complete remission after transplantation predicted an improved transplantation outcome. These authors concluded that patients with a low tumor burden who respond to treatment before transplantation and receive transplants early in their disease course have the best prognosis following allogeneic BMT. Relapse, regimen-related mortality, and complications from GvHD remain major obstacles to an improved transplantation outcome in patients with multiple myeloma.

Recently, there has been increasing evidence that a graft-vs.-myeloma effect exists, similar to that seen in chronic myelogenous leukemia. Vesole and colleagues were able to demonstrate marked tumor reduction after donor leukocyte infusions in patients with relapsed or persistent multiple myeloma following allografting (383). In addition, Kwak et al. were able to demonstrate the transfer of myeloma idiotype-specific immunity from an actively immunized marrow donor (229), thereby potentially enhancing the antimyeloma effect of the allogeneic graft.

Although these recent developments in the use of allogeneic BMT for the treatment of multiple myeloma are promising, further improvements in the results will depend on better selection of patients most likely to benefit from this intensive approach and on initiating this form of treatment earlier in the course of disease. In addition, improved conditioning regimens and posttransplantation treatment of infection and GvHD will be required if improved disease-free survival rates are to be achieved.

Marrow Transplantation for Patients Lacking an HLA-Identical Sibling Donor

As recognition of the curative potential of allogeneic marrow transplants has grown, the need to develop approaches that would permit transplantation of normal marrow in the 60 to 70% of patients who lack an HLA-matched sibling has increased markedly. Several approaches to such patients are being actively explored, particularly the use of unmodified or T-cell–depleted marrow grafts from partially matched related or HLA-compatible unrelated donors. Each of these approaches has shown considerable promise, but each is also associated with an increased risk of either graft rejection or severe GvHD.

UNMODIFIED MARROW GRAFTS FROM PARTIALLY MATCHED RELATED DONORS

Since the early 1970s, several groups have conducted limited explorations of the use of HLA partially matched related donors in an attempt to identify tolerable histoincompatibilities within the HLA region. These early studies concentrated on the use of HLA-haplotype-identical but MLC-compatible related donors because of results in murine transplantation models indicating that marrow grafts from MHC class II–disparate donors were most likely to induce lethal GvHD (223). Initial studies, which were conducted in patients with SCID, tended to support this approach to donor selection, since disparities for HLA-A and/or -B on one haplotype were tolerated without lethal GvHD. In a review of 10 such cases (217), 8 developed GvHD, but it was severe in only 2 patients. However, 5 of these patients died of infections early after transplantation, which prevented an assessment of the incidence or severity of chronic GvHD. Of 3 patients grafted with HLA-D-incompatible marrow, none survived long enough for GvH reactions to be assessed. Patients with SCID who received transplants from donors incompatible for both class I and class II determinants had a poor outcome. Of 19 evaluable patients, 3 experienced failure of engraftment and 10 developed severe GvHD. None of these patients survived.

Experience with partially matched related donor marrow grafts in the treatment of aplastic anemia underscores the incremental risk of marrow graft rejection when HLA-disparate grafts are used. In one large series of patients prepared with cyclophosphamide alone, HLA phenotypically matched nonsibling donor transplants were associated with consistent engraftment, while 7 of 11 grafts from one-locus-disparate donors and 3 of 3 transplants from two HLA-locus-disparate donors were rejected (49). Among the 13 patients who ultimately achieved sustained engraftment, 5 of 8 phenotypically matched and each of 5 one HLA-allele-disparate recipients developed grade II to IV GvHD.

In 1985, Beatty et al. (52) reported that transplants administered to leukemic patients differing from their donors at a single HLA allele resulted in grade II to IV GvHD in over 75% of cases. However, long-term disease-free survival was comparable to that observed following HLA-matched sibling marrow transplantation. In this series, no one allelic disparity (i.e., HLA-A, -B, or -D) could be identified that placed the patient at greater risk for severe GvHD. Graft rejections were observed in 9% of such cases, an increase in incidence over that seen following HLA-matched sibling grafts. Leukemia patients who received transplants from donors differing at more than one HLA allele on the unshared haplotype were even more prone to experience graft rejection (21%) or to develop severe acute and chronic GvHD (80–85%). The overall survival of such patients (<15%) was markedly inferior to that observed following HLA phenotypically matched or HLA-single-allele-disparate marrow transplantation (40–45%). Taken together, these data indicate that engraftment of unmodified bone marrow from a donor exhibiting unique HLA disparities requires a level of pretransplantation immunosuppression at least comparable to that induced by the combination of cyclophosphamide and supralethal TBI, and that even with such immunosuppression, the incidence of graft rejection following receipt of transplants from donors disparate for more than one HLA allele is prohibitive. Further, such transplants are associated with a significantly higher incidence of severe acute and chronic GvHD. However, the complications of single-allele-disparate marrow grafts, at least in patients receiving transplants for leukemia, are tolerable and may be associated with long-term disease-free survival rates comparable to those achieved with HLA-matched sibling grafts.

TRANSPLANTATION OF UNMODIFIED MARROW FROM UNRELATED DONORS

In 1977, our group reported successful reconstitution of immunologic function in a child with SCID engrafted with marrow from an HLA-compatible unrelated donor (273). Subsequent case reports demonstrated that unrelated marrow grafts could also reconstitute hematopoiesis in patients who received transplants for leukemia and aplastic anemia. In 1988, a series of 40 patients was reported with refractory forms of leukemia and aplastic anemia who had received marrow grafts from unrelated, HLA-matched, or partially mismatched donors obtained from a statewide registry developed in Iowa (163). Of these patients, 15% survived disease free for periods of more than a year. Acute severe GvHD was observed in 67%, and all but one of the surviving patients also had chronic GvHD. Consistent engraftment was observed in leukemic patients prepared with TBI and cyclophosphamide. However, of 4 patients who underwent transplantation for aplastic anemia, 2 suffered graft failures despite preparation with total lymphoid irradiation (TLI) and cyclophosphamide (163). Of 5 aplastic patients reported by Gajewski et al. (155), 1 also experienced graft rejection after preparation with TLI and cyclophosphamide. These early experiences thus indicated an increased risk of both GvHD and graft failure following unrelated marrow transplantation.

The early results of unrelated marrow grafts used in the treatment of CML were considerably more encouraging. In a series of 102 recipients of unrelated marrow grafts who underwent transplantation at four centers for CML, 29% achieved extended disease-free survival (257). In this series, patients receiving transplants from unrelated HLA phenotypically matched donors achieved a somewhat better long-term disease-free survival (39%) than those who received marrow transplants from single-allele-disparate donors (27%). Among recipients of unmodified HLA-matched unrelated marrow grafts, the incidence of grade II to IV GvHD was 80%. In this series, recipients of T-cell–depleted marrow transplants developed severe GvHD less frequently without an increased risk of graft failure. However, long-term disease-free survival was comparable to that observed following transplantation of unmodified marrow. In a subsequent report from Seattle, 52 patients were described who had undergone transplants with HLA phenotypically matched unrelated marrow as treatment for leukemia (50). The incidence of grade II to IV acute GvHD was 79%, compared to 36% for patients who received transplants from HLA-matched siblings. This incidence of severe acute GvHD is comparable to that seen following transplantation of marrow from one- or two-HLA-allele-disparate related donors (52).

The cumulative results of the first 462 transplantations that used donors identified by the National Marrow Donor Program were recently summarized (218). Of these patients, 352 received transplants for leukemia, 38 for myelodysplastic or lymphoid malignancies, and 72 for aplasias and congenital disorders of immunity or metabolism. In this series, early or late graft failures were observed in 14% of cases. Acute GvHD of grade II or greater severity was observed in 64% of cases; in 47%, grade III or IV acute GvHD was observed. Severe grade III or IV acute GvHD was significantly increased among recipients of unmodified marrow grafts (60%) when compared to the group that received T-cell–depleted marrow (30%). Limited or extensive chronic GvHD was observed in 55% of cases, again particularly among recipients of unmodified marrow grafts. Despite the increased incidence of graft failure and severe acute or chronic GvHD, patients with acute leukemia in first or second remission and patients with CML in first chronic phase achieved overall 2-year disease-free survival rates of 45% and 37%, respectively. Results were particularly encouraging for younger transplant recipients (<18 years old) with these "good-risk" leukemias (53% disease-free survival at 2 years vs. 37% for older patients). A separate detailed analysis of the results of these grafts applied to 196 patients with CML (266) recorded a 2-year disease-free survival rate of 45% for patients in first chronic phase who received grafts within 1 year of diagnosis (vs. 36% for patients in chronic phase who received grafts more than 1 year after diagnosis). Results of unrelated marrow grafts applied to patients with aplastic anemia and myelodysplasia were poor, with 2-year disease-free survival rates of only 29% and 18%, respectively (218).

The basis for the marked increase in the incidence of severe acute GvHD in recipients of HLA phenotypically matched unrelated marrow when compared with that observed in recipients of HLA genotypically matched sibling marrow is still poorly understood. It may reflect alloreactions generated against molecular differences in class I and II alleles that can be detected only by more discriminatory molecular approaches such as isoelectric focusing or hybridization with HLA-microvariant sequence-specific oligonucleotides. In recent studies, up to 30% of HLA serologically matched MLC-compatible unrelated individuals selected as potential donors were found to differ from their intended recipient by one or two alleles distinguishable by isoelectric focusing (222) and over 60% by sequence analyses of HLA class I determinants (314). Preliminary evidence suggests that microvariant disparities for class II determinants also occur with significant frequency among HLA-matched unrelated donor-recipient pairs (2, 201). These molecular differences in HLA class I and II alleles likely also explain the increased frequency of allocytotoxic T cells that can be generated in mixed lymphocyte cultures between HLA phenotypically matched unrelated donor-recipient pairs, in comparison with the low frequency of such cells generated in mixed lymphocyte cultures between HLA matched siblings (51).

A series of recent retrospective analyses strongly suggests that molecular matching for HLA determinants may improve the results of transplantation of unmodified marrow from unrelated donors. For example, Petersdorf et al. (286) demonstrated severe GvHD in 48% of recipients of HLA-A, -B, -DR serologically matched unrelated marrow that were also matched by sequence-specific oligonucleotide probe hybridization for DRB1 alleles vs. 70% among recipients with DRB1 mismatches. Similarly, results from two centers have documented an increase in the severity of acute GvHD in recipients of unrelated marrow mismatched for one HLA-A or HLA-B allele (47, 112). Although overall survival was not significantly affected by the single HLA-A or HLA-B disparity in young patients, it was markedly decreased among adults (19–49 years) (112). When unrelated donors are selected using serologic matching for HLA-A and -B and molecular matching for DRB and DQB, Nademanee et al. (262) suggest that GvHD and disease-free survival rates comparable to those obtainable with transplantation of unmodified marrow from HLA-matched siblings may be achieved.

T-Cell–Depleted HLA-Nonidentical Related and HLA-Compatible Unrelated Marrow Grafts

A central limitation to the use of single-HLA-allele-disparate related donors and suitably matched unrelated donors is that realistically, such donors are available only for 20 to 30% of individuals lacking an HLA-matched sibling. Further, it is already clear that restricted donor availability persists, even though registries in excess of 1 million unrelated donors have been recruited (338). The development of more sensitive techniques for the selection of donors matched for HLA class I and class II microvariants, while important to our understanding of incompatibilities contributing to graft rejection, GvHD, and impaired immunologic reconstitution posttransplantation, will nevertheless only serve to further restrict the proportion of patients for whom an adequately compatible donor will be identified. Thus, there is a continuing need for the development of transplantation approaches whereby consistent engraftment and functional reconstitution can be achieved in HLA-disparate recipients without severe or lethal GvHD.

The development of techniques for depleting T lymphocytes from a marrow allograft has provided one such approach to this dilemma. In 1981, our group showed that transplants of HLA-A, -B, DR HLA-haplotype-disparate parental marrow depleted of T cells by agglutination with a soybean lectin followed by E-rosette depletion could reconstitute hematopoietic and lymphoid function in children with leukemia or SCID (301) without GvHD. In our series of over 50 patients with SCID who have received transplants of T-cell–depleted, HLA-haplotype-disparate parental marrow over the past 15 years, 74% currently survive with reconstitution of immunity and stable donor lymphoid chimerism. In this series, only 3 patients have developed grade I acute GvH reactions. The actuarial disease-free survival at 6 years for this group is not different from that achieved following the use of unmodified HLA-matched grafts in SCID. Other centers incorporating this and other approaches to T-cell depletion have reported similar results (274). These studies of T-cell–depleted, HLA-disparate marrow grafts used in children with SCID demonstrate the potential of this approach and illustrate the feasibility of broad application of marrow grafting to patients lacking a matched sibling donor. Unfortunately, when T-cell–depleted, HLA-nonidentical marrow grafts have been used for the treatment of other genetic and acquired diseases of hematopoiesis or leukemia, they have been considerably less effective. Although techniques of T-cell depletion achieving a 3 $\log_{10}$ depletion of clonable T-cells can consistently prevent severe acute and chronic GvHD in both HLA-matched and HLA-disparate recipients, such transplants are associated with a high incidence of graft rejection. In 23 children with genetic immune deficiencies other than SCID who underwent transplantation with T-cell–depleted HLA-nonidentical marrow, reported from the EORTC, 11 experienced failure of engraftment despite conditioning with busulfan and cyclophosphamide (150). For these patients, 2–4 year disease-free survival was 29%, compared to 47% for recipients of HLA-matched grafts. Among leukemic recipients of HLA-nonidentical T-cell–depleted marrow administered after cytoreduction with TBI and cyclophosphamide, the incidence of graft failures or rejection has ranged from 10 to 50%, depending on the number of disparate HLA alleles unique to the donor, the efficiency of the T-cell depletion technique used, and the intensity of the preparative cytoreduction administered before and immediately after transplantation.

Recently, new techniques employing more intensive cytoreductive measures, coupled with less stringent or more selective T-cell depletion methods and the administration of T-cell–specific immunotoxins or antithymocyte globulin in the early posttransplantation period have reduced the frequency of rejection following transplants of T-cell–depleted marrow from HLA-matched unrelated donors without unduly increasing the risk of severe GvHD. For example, in a series of patients who underwent transplantation of T-cell–depleted marrow from unrelated donors for hematologic malignancies (24), those who received transplants for acute leukemia in early remission or chronic phase CML achieved a 48% extended disease-free survival. In this series, employing a technique achieving a $2 \times \log_{10}$ level of T-cell depletion, HLA-matched unrelated marrow grafts were associated with a 20% frequency of grade II to IV GvHD, a rate markedly lower than that observed among recipients of unmodified marrow transplants. A similarly low frequency of grade II to IV GvHD was observed among recipients of HLA phenotypically matched, T-cell–depleted unrelated marrow grafts in the four-center study of unrelated marrow transplants applied to the treatment of CML (257). In a compilation of the results of unrelated marrow transplants from four centers in the United Kingdom reported by Howard et al. (202), the use of such novel preparative regimens resulted in a frequency of engraftment comparable to that observed following transplantation of unmodified marrow. As a result, the T-cell–depleted grafts, which were associated with a markedly reduced frequency of acute GvHD, were also associated with significant improvement in disease-free survival (60% vs. 29% at 3 months), a difference that was not observed among recipients of HLA-matched sibling marrow grafts. Similarly, in a review of results of marrow grafts from donors identified by the National Marrow Donor Program applied to patients with CML, McGlave et al. (256) found that prevalence of durable engraftment following transplantation of T-cell–depleted grafts (94%) did not differ from that following transplantation of unmodified grafts (88%), reflecting improvements in the cytoreductive regimens used for these transplants. As expected, the frequencies of severe (grades II–IV) acute GvHD and chronic GvHD were significantly reduced in recipients of T-cell–depleted grafts. Strikingly, the rate of relapse following a transplantation of T-cell–depleted unrelated graft—16% at 2 years—did not differ significantly from that observed following transplantation of an unmodified graft—10% at 2 years. The finding of a low relapse rate following transplantation of unrelated T-cell–depleted grafts in patients with CML stands in striking contrast to the markedly increased incidence of relapse of CML observed following transplantation of T-cell–depleted grafts obtained from matched siblings. As a result, T-cell–depleted grafts were again shown to be associated with a significant improvement in long-term disease-free survival.

The results of T-cell–depleted, partially matched related and HLA phenotypically compatible unrelated marrow transplants in children have yielded particularly promising results. In a series of 10 children with aplastic anemia who received marrow transplants from a related partially matched or unrelated matched donor, reported by Camitta et al. (84), 5 achieved long-term reconstitution. Similarly, in a report by Casper et al. of 50 children with leukemia who received transplants of HLA-matched or one-antigen disparate unrelated T-cell–depleted marrow, 44% were able to secure extended disease-free survival (86). In addition, a 50% extended disease-free survival rate has been reported in patients who underwent transplantation for leukemia with partially T-cell–depleted marrow from HLA-one-to-three-antigen-disparate related donors after more intensive cytoreduction and treatment posttransplantation with a T-cell–specific ricin A immunotoxin (190). In these series, results of T-cell–depleted transplants from related, one-to-two-HLA-allele-disparate donors and unrelated HLA-matched donors have been similar.

While the use of HLA-A, -B, -D haplotype–disparate marrow, if suitably depleted of T cells, can induce full hematologic and immune reconstitution without GvHD, as shown in large series of patients who underwent transplantation for SCID (274), the high risk of graft rejection associated with such transplants has limited their use for patients with leukemia. As previously discussed, several recent studies in animal models and in clinical trials have clarified the mechanisms of graft rejection and the host effector cells contributing to this process (69, 133, 387). Furthermore, tolerable, more immunosuppressive cytoreductive regimens combining high-dose thiotepa or cytosine arabinoside and T-cell–specific antibodies with TBI and cyclophosphamide have been developed that have eliminated the risk of graft rejection following transplantation of T-cell–depleted grafts from matched related or unrelated donors (74, 361) without increasing the low risk of GvHD associated with such transplants. Recently, Reisner et al. (129, 146, 302, 378) demonstrated in murine models that the incidence and quality of engraftment of T-cell–depleted MHC-disparate grafts could be strikingly increased by increasing the dose of marrow cells 10- to 100-fold. Acting on this lead, Aversa et al. (31) have explored the use of combined transplants of marrow and G-CSF–stimulated peripheral blood progenitor cells that have been depleted of T cells by lectin agglutination and E-rosette depletion (275, 300). The use of T-cell–depleted, G-CSF–stimulated peripheral blood stem cells increases by 5- to 10-fold the number of $CD34^+$ progenitors transplanted. Of the initial 17 patients with advanced or refractory leukemia who received transplants of T-cell–depleted marrow and G-CSF–stimulated peripheral blood stem cells from HLA -A, -B, -D haplotype–mismatched related donors after cytoreduction with TBI, thiotepa, cyclophosphamide, and antithymocyte globulin, 16 achieved durable, full engraftment and hematopoietic reconstitution. Only 1 patient developed grade III to IV GvHD (31). Subsequently, Aversa et al. have used this approach to administer transplants to an additional 27 leukemia patients with marrow and purified blood stem cells from HLA-A, -B, -DR haplotype–disparate donors. Graft failure has been observed in 7%, an incidence comparable to that observed following transplantation of one-allele-disparate unmodified grafts. Grade II GvHD has been observed in 8%. Although follow-up is short, 55% survive disease free up to 15 months after transplantation.

These studies, if confirmed in larger series, would ensure the possibility of allogeneic transplantation in almost all patients with types of leukemia for which a transplant is currently recognized as a treatment of choice, and would likely eliminate the need for protracted and expensive searches among large registries of unrelated donors for patients with uncommon HLA haplotypes. At that point, the choice between an unrelated matched and an HLA genotypically matched related T-cell–depleted graft will likely rest on the relative capacity of each type of transplant to induce durable and complete hematopoietic and immunologic reconstitution and the relative potential of each type of graft to confer on the transplant recipient-enhanced resistance to leukemia.

Although the results of trials incorporating techniques that permit more consistent engraftment together with a low frequency of severe GvHD are encouraging, HLA partially matched related or HLA-matched unrelated marrow grafts have thus far not attained rates of extended disease-free survival comparable to those achieved following HLA-matched sibling grafts. In most of these series, the difference is due to a disturbingly high frequency of infectious complications following transplantation of HLA partially matched related or unrelated marrow grafts, complications that may reflect the relatively profound and protracted state of immunodeficiency observed following these marrow transplantations (242). The basis for these immunodeficiencies is not clear but may indicate limitations to the redevelopment or reeducation of donor cells in a partially HLA-disparate environment. Research in this critical area is urgently needed to identify and potentially circumvent such limitations to immune reconstitution. On the positive side, however, the rate of relapse following such transplantations, when performed in the treatment of patients with acute and chronic leukemias, has been strikingly low, possibly reflecting advantages of increased genetic disparity between donor and host for the expression of the antileukemic effects of a marrow allograft.

References

1. Abraham LD, Muir H, Olsen I, Winchester B. Direct enzyme transfer from lymphocytes corrects a lysosomal storage. Biochem Biophys Res Commun 1985;129:415–417.
2. Al-Daccak R, Loiseau P, Rabian C, et al. HLA-DR, DQ and/or genotypic mismatches between recipient-donor pairs in unrelated bone marrow transplantation and transplant clinical outcome. Transplantation 1990;50:960.
3. Ambinder RF, Burns W, Forman M, et al. Hemorrhagic cystitis associated with adenovirus infection in bone marrow transplantation. Arch Intern Med 1986;146: 1400–1401.
4. Anasetti C, Martin PJ, Hansen JA, et al. A phase I-II study evaluating the murine anti-IL-2 receptor antibody 2A3 for treatment of acute graft-versus-host disease. Transplantation 1990;50:49–54.
5. Anasetti C, Amos D, Beatty PG, et al. Effect of HLA compatibility of engraftment of bone marrow transplants in patients with leukemia or lymphoma. N Engl J Med 1989;320:197–204.
6. Anasetti C, Beatty PG, Storb R, et al. Effect of HLA incompatibility on graft versus host disease, relapse and survival after marrow transplantation for patients with leukemia or lymphoma. Hum Immunol 1989;29:79–91.
7. Anasetti A, Martin PJ, Storb R, et al. Treatment of acute graft-versus-host disease with a non-mitogenic anti-CD3 monoclonal antibody. Transplantation 1992;54:844–851.
8. Anderson KC, Weinstein HJ. Transfusion-associated graft-versus-host disease. N Engl J Med 1990;323:315–321.
9. Anderson KC, Barut BA, Ritz J, Freedman AS, Nadler LM. Autologous bone marrow transplantation therapy for multiple myeloma. Eur J Haematol 1989;53(suppl 51):157–163.
10. Anderson KC, Barut BA, Ritz J, et al. Monoclonal antibody-purged autologous bone marrow transplantation therapy for multiple myeloma. Blood 1991;77:712–720.
11. Anderson KC, Anderson J, Soiffer R, et al. Monoclonal antibody purged bone marrow transplantation therapy for multiple myeloma. Blood 1993;82:2568–2576.
12. Antin JH, Smith BR, Holmes W, Rosenthal DS. Phase I/II study of recombinant human granulocyte macrophage colony-stimulating factor in aplastic anemia and myelodysplastic syndrome. Blood 1988;72:705–713.
13. Antin JH, Bierer BE, Smith BR, et al. Selective depletion of bone marrow T-lymphocytes with anti-CD5 monoclonal antibodies: effective prophylaxis for graft-versus-host disease in patients with hematologic malignancies. Blood 1991;78:2139–2149.
14. Appelbaum FR, Dahlberg S, Thomas ED, et al. Bone marrow transplantation or chemotherapy after remission induction for adults with acute nonlymphoblastic leukemia: a prospective comparison. Ann Intern Med 1984;101:581–588.
15. Appelbaum FR, Barrall J, Storb R, et al. Bone marrow transplantation for patients with myelodysplasia: pretreatment variables and outcome. Ann Intern Med 1990;112: 590–597.
16. Appelbaum FR, Strauchen JA, Graw RG. Acute lethal carditis caused by high-dose combination chemotherapy: a unique clinical and pathological entity. Lancet 1976;1: 58–65.
17. Appelbaum FR, Sullivan KM, Buckner CD, et al. Treatment of malignant lymphoma in 100 patients with chemotherapy, total body irradiation, and marrow transplantation. J Clin Oncol 1987;5:1340–1347.
18. Apperley JF, Goldman JM. Cytomegalovirus: biology, clinical features and methods for diagnosis. Bone Marrow Transplant 1988;3:253–264.
19. Apperley JF, Jones L, Hale G, et al. Bone marrow transplantation for patients with chronic myeloid leukaemia: t-cell depletion with Campath-1 reduces the incidence of graft-versus-host disease but may increase the risk of leukaemic relapse. Bone Marrow Transplant 1986;1:53–60.
20. Apperley JF, et al. Foscarnet for CMV pneumonitis. Lancet 1985;1151.
20a. Arcese W, Goldman JM, D'arcangelo E, et al. Outcome for patients who relapse after allogeneic bone marrow transplantation for chronic myeloid leukemia. Blood 1993;82: 3211–3219.
21. Armitage JO. Bone marrow transplantation in the treatment of patients with lymphoma. Blood 1989;73:1749.
22. Arnold R, Heimpel H. Allogeneic bone marrow transplantation for myelodysplastic syndromes (MDS). Bone Marrow Transplant 1989;4(suppl 4):101–103.
23. Arthur RR, Shah KV, Baust SJ, Santos GW, Saral R. Association of BK viruria with hemorrhagic cystitis in recipients of bone marrow transplants. N Engl J Med 1986;315:230–234.
24. Ash RC, Casper JT, Chitambar CR, et al. Successful allogeneic transplantation of T-cell depleted bone marrow from closely HLA-matched unrelated donors. N Engl J Med 1990;322:485–494.
25. Attal M, Blasie D, Marit G, et al. Consolidation treatment of adult acute lymphoblastic leukemia: a prospective, randomized trial comparing allogeneic versus autologous bone marrow transplantation and testing the impact of recombinant interleukin-2 after autologous bone marrow transplantation. Blood 1995;86:1619–1628.
26. Attal H, Huguet F, Rubie H, et al. Prevention of hepatic veno-occlusive disease after bone marrow transplantation by continuous infusion of low dose heparin: a prospective randomized trial. Blood 1992;79:2834–2840.
27. Atkinson K, Norrie S, Chan P, Zehnwirth B, Downs K, Biggs J. Hematopoietic progenitor cell function after HLA-identical sibling bone marrow transplantation: influence of chronic graft-versus-host disease. Int J Cell Cloning 1986;4:203–220.
28. Atkinson K, Storb R, Prentice RL, et al. Analysis of late infections in 89 long-term survivors of bone marrow transplantation. Blood 1979;53:720–731.
29. Atkinson K, Farewell V, Storb R, et al. Analysis of late infections after human bone marrow transplantation: role of non-specific suppressor cells in patients with chronic graft-versus-host disease and genotypic non-identity between marrow donor and recipient. Blood 1982;60:714–719.
30. Aversa F, Terenzi A, Carrotti, et al. Addition of thiotepa improves results in T-cell depleted bone marrow transplant for advanced leukemia. Blood 1993;82(suppl 1):81a. Abstract.
31. Aversa F, Tabilio A, Terenzi A, et al. Successful engraftment of T-cell-depleted haploidentical "three-loci" incompatible transplants in leukemia patients by addition of recombinant human granulocyte colony-stimulating factor-mobilized peripheral blood progenitor cells to bone marrow inoculum. Blood 1994;84:3948–3955.
32. Bach FH, Albertini RJ, Joo P, Anderson JL, Bortin MM. Bone marrow transplantation in a patient with the Wiskott-Aldrich syndrome. Lancet 1968;2:1364–1366.
33. Baglin TP, Harper P, Marcus RE. Veno-occlusive disease of the liver complicating ABMT successfully treated with recombinant tissue plasminogen activator (rt-PA). Bone Marrow Transplant 1990;5:439–441.
34. Bar B, Schattenberg A, Mensink EJBM, et al. Donor leukocyte infusions for chronic myeloid leukemia relapsed after allogeneic bone marrow transplantation. J Clin Oncol 1993;11:513–519.
35. Barlogie B, Alexanian, Dicke KA, et al. High-dose chemoradiotherapy and autologous bone marrow transplantation for resistant myeloma. Blood 1987;70:869–872.
36. Barlogie B, Epstein J, Selvanayagam P, Alexanian R. Plasma cell myeloma: new biological insights and advances in therapy. Blood 1989;73:865–879.
37. Barlogie B, Gahrton G. Bone marrow transplantation in multiple myeloma. Bone Marrow Transplant 1991;7:71–79.
38. Barrett AJ, Horowitz MM, Gale RP, et al. Marrow transplantation for acute lymphoblastic leukemia: factors affecting relapse and survival. Blood 1989;74:862–871.
39. Barrett AJ, Horowitz MM. Transplants in ALL. Bone Marrow Transplant 1992;10(suppl 1):30–36.
40. Barrett AJ, Joshi R, Kendra JR, et al. Prediction and prevention of relapse of acute lymphoblastic leukaemia after bone marrow transplantation. Br J Haematol 1986;64: 179–186.
41. Barrett AJ, Horowitz MM, Pollock BH, et al. Bone marrow transplants from HLA identical siblings as compared with chemotherapy for children with acute lymphoblastic leukemia in a second remission. N Engl J Med 1994;331:1253–1258.
42. Bass EB, Powe NR, Graziano SL, et al. Efficacy of intravenous immune globulin in preventing complications of bone marrow transplantation: a meta-analysis. Bone Marrow Transplant 1993;12:273.
43. Dupont B, Yang SY. Histocompatibility. In Bone Marrow Transplantation. Edited by S Foreman, K Blume, ED Thomas. Cambridge, MA: Blackwell, 1994, pp 22–40.
44. Baughan AS, Worsley AM, McCarthy DM, et al. Haematological reconstitution and severity of graft-versus-host disease after bone marrow transplantation for chronic granulocytic leukaemia: the influence of previous splenectomy. Br J Haematol 1984;56:445–454.
45. Bearman SI, Shuhart MC, Hinds MS, McDonald GB. Recombinant human tissue plasminogen activator for the treatment of established severe veno-occlusive disease of the liver after bone marrow transplantation. Blood 1992;80:2458–2462.
46. Bearman SI. The syndrome of hepatic veno-occlusive disease after marrow transplantation. Blood 1995;85:3005–3020.
47. Beatty PG, Anasetti C, Hansen JA, et al. Marrow transplantation from unrelated donors for treatment of hematologic malignancies: effect of mismatching for one HLA locus. Blood 1993;81:249–253.
48. Beatty PG, Ash R, Hows JM, McGlave PB. The use of unrelated bone marrow donors in the treatment of patients with chronic myelogenous leukemia: experience of four marrow transplant centers. Bone Marrow Transplant 1989;4:287–290.
49. Beatty PG, Bartolomeo P, Storb R, et al. Treatment of aplastic anemia with marrow grafts from related donors other than HLA genotypically matched siblings. Clin Transplant 1987;1:117–124.
50. Beatty PG, Hansen JA, Longton GM, et al. Marrow transplantation from HLA-matched unrelated donors for treatment of hematologic malignancies. Transplantation 1991;51:443–447.
51. Beatty PG, Hansen JA, Anasetti C, et al. Significance of different levels of histocompatibility in patients receiving marrow grafts from unrelated donors. Exp Hematol 1990;15:509a.
52. Beatty PG, Clift RA, Michelson EM, et al. Marrow transplantation from related donors other than HLA-identical siblings. N Engl J Med 1985;313:765–771.
53. Beatty PG, Dahlberg S, Mickelson EM, et al. Probability of finding HLA-matched unrelated marrow donors. Transplant Proc 1988;45:714–718.
54. Beelen DW, Graeven U, Elmaagacli AH, et al. Prolonged administration of interferon-alpha in patients with chronic phase Philadelphia: chromosome-positive chronic myelogenous leukemia before allogeneic bone marrow transplantation may adversely affect transplant outcome. Blood 1995;85:2918–2990.
55. Begg CB, McGlave PB, Bennett JM, Cassileth PA, Oken MM. A critical comparison of allogeneic bone marrow transplantation and conventional chemotherapy as treatment for acute lymphocytic leukemia. J Clin Oncol 1984;2:369.
56. Bennett JM, Catovsky D, Daniel MT, Flandrin G, Galton DAG, Gralnick HR, Sultan C. (FAB Cooperative Group) Proposals for the classification of the myelodysplastic syndromes. Br J Haematol 1982;51:189–199.

57. Billadeau D, Quam L, Thomas W, et al. Detection and quantitation of malignant cells in the peripheral blood of multiple myeloma patients. Blood 1992;80:1818–1824.
58. Billingham RE. The biology of graft-versus-host reactions. Harvey Lect 1966–67;62:22.
59. Blacklock H, Ball L, Knight C, Schey S, Prentice G. Experience with mesna in patients receiving allogeneic bone marrow transplants for poor prognostic leukaemia. Cancer Treat Rev 1983;10(suppl A):45–52.
60. Blaise D, Gaspard MH, Stoppa AM, et al. Allogeneic or autologous bone marrow transplantation for acute lymphoblastic leukemia in first complete remission. Bone Marrow Transplant 1990;5:7–12.
61. Blaise D, Olive D, Michallet M, et al. Impairment of leukemia-free survival by addition of Interleukin-2 receptor antibody to standard graft-vs-host prophylaxis. Lancet 1995;345:1144–1146.
62. Blazar BR, Orr HT, Arthur DC, Kersey JH, Filipovich AH. Restriction fragment length polymorphisms as markers of engraftment in allogeneic marrow transplantation. Blood 1985;66:1436–1444.
63. Bloomfield CD, Lawrence D, Arthur CD, Berg DT, Schiffer CA, Mayer RJ. Cancer and Leukemia Group B. Curative impact of intensification with high-dose cytarabine (HiDAC) in acute myeloid leukemia varies by cytogenetic group. Blood 1994;84(suppl 1):111a. Abstract.
64. Blume KG, Forman SJ, O'Donnell MR, et al. Total body irradiation and high-dose etoposide: a new preparatory regimen for bone marrow transplantation in patients with advanced hematologic malignancies. Blood 1987;69:1015–1020.
65. Blume KG, Forman SJ, Snyder DS, et al. Allogeneic bone marrow transplantation for acute lymphoblastic leukemia during first complete remission. Transplant Proc 1987;43:389–392.
66. Bodmer WF. HLA 1987. In Immunobiology of HLA, vol II: Immunogenetics and Histocompatibility. Edited by B Dupont. New York: Springer-Verlag, 1989, pp 1–9.
67. Boeckh M, Bowden RA, Goodrich JM, Pettinger M, Meyers JD. Cytomegalovirus antigen detection in peripheral blood leukocytes after allogeneic marrow transplantation. Blood 1992;80:1358.
68. Bolger GB, Sullivan KM, Storb R, et al. Second marrow infusion for poor graft function after allogeneic marrow transplantation. Bone Marrow Transplant 1986;1:21–30.
69. Bordignon C, Keever CA, Small TN, Flomenberg N, Dupont B, O'Reilly RJ. Graft failure after T-cell depleted human leukocyte antigen identical marrow transplants for leukemia: in vitro analyses of host effector mechanisms. Blood 1989;74:2227–2236.
70. Bordigoni P, Vernant JP, Souillet G, et al. Allogeneic bone marrow transplantation for children with acute lymphoblastic leukemia in first remission: a cooperative study of the groupe d'etude de la greffe de moelle osseuse. J Clin Oncol 1989;7:747–753.
71. Borgna-Pignatti C, Zxurlo MG, Destefano P, et al. In Advances and Controversies in Thalassemia Therapy. Edited by CD Buckner, RP Gale, G Lucarelli. New York: Alan R Liss, 1988, pp 27–33.
72. Boulad F, Steinherz P, Reyes B, Gillio A, Small T, Kernan NA, O'Reilly RJ. Allogeneic bone marrow transplantation (BMT) versus chemotherapy for the treatment of childhood acute lymphoblastic leukemia (ALL) in second remission (CR2): the MSKCC experience. Blood 1994;84(suppl 1):251a. Abstract.
73. Bourgault I, Gomez A, Gomard E, Levy JP. Limiting-dilution analysis of the HLA restriction of anti-Epstein-Barr virus-specific cytolytic T lymphocytes. Clin Exp Immunol 1991;84:501–507.
74. Bozdech MJ, Sondel PM, Trigg ME, et al. Transplantation of HLA-haploidentical T-cell depleted marrow for leukemia: addition of cytosine arabinoside to the pretransplant conditioning prevents rejection. Exp Hematol 1985;13:1201–1210.
75. Bratanow NC, Ash RC, Turner PA, et al. Successful treatment of serious cytomegalovirus disease with 9(1,3-dihydroxy-2-propoxymethyl)-guanine and intravenous immunoglobulin in bone marrow transplant patients. Exp Hematol 1987;15:541.
76. Brochstein JA, Kernan NA, Groshen S, et al. Allogeneic bone marrow transplantation after hyperfractionated total-body irradiation and cyclophosphamide in children with acute leukemia. N Engl J Med 1987;317:1618–1624.
77. Brugieres L, Hartmann O, Travagli, et al. Hemorrhagic cystitis following high-dose chemotherapy and bone marrow transplantation in children with malignancies: incidence, clinical course and outcome. J Clin Oncol 1989;7:194–199.
78. Buckner CD, Fefer A, Bensinger WI, et al. Marrow transplantation for malignant plasma cell disorders: summary of the Seattle experience. Eur J Haematol 1989;43(suppl 51):186–190.
79. Bunjes D, Hertenstein B, Wiesneth M, et al. In vivo/ex vivo T cell depletion reduces the morbidity of allogeneic bone marrow transplantation in patients with acute leukemias in first remission without increasing the risk of treatment failure: comparison with cyclosporin/methotrexate. Bone Marrow Transplant 1995;15:563–568.
80. Burnett AK, Goldstone AH, Stevens RF, et al. The role of BMT in addition to intensive chemotherapy in AML in first CR: Results of the MRC AML-10 trial. Blood 1994;84(suppl 1):252a. Abstract.
81. Burns WH, Sandford GR. Susceptibility of human herpesvirus 6 to antivirals in vitro. J Infect Dis 1990;162:634–637.
82. Byers VS, Henslee PJ, Kernan NA, et al. Use of an anti-pan T-lymphocyte ricin A chain immunotoxin in steroid-resistant acute graft-versus-host disease. Blood 1990;75:1426–1432.
83. Camitta B, O'Reilly RJ, Sensenbrenner L, et al. Antithoracic duct lymphocyte globulin therapy of severe aplastic anemia. Blood 1983;62:883–888.
84. Camitta B, Ash R, Menitove J, Murray K, Lawton C, Hunter J, Casper J. Bone marrow transplantation for children with severe aplastic anemia: use of donors other than HLA-identical siblings. Blood 1989;74:1852–1857.
85. Carrigan DR, Drobyski WR, Russler SK, et al. Interstitial pneumonitis associated with human herpesvirus 6 infection after marrow transplantation. Lancet 1991;2:147–149.
86. Casper J, Camitta B, Truitt R, et al. Unrelated bone marrow donor transplants for children with leukemia or myelodysplasia. Blood 1995;85:2354–2363.
87. Cassano WF. Intravenous ribavirin therapy for adenovirus cystitis after allogeneic bone marrow transplantation. Bone Marrow Transplant 1991;7:247–248.
88. Cavo M, Tura S, Rosti G, et al. Allogeneic bone marrow transplantation for multiple myeloma. The Italian experience. Bone Marrow Transplant 1991;7:31.
89. Champlin RE, Horowitz MM, van Bekkum DW, et al. Graft failure following bone marrow transplantation for severe aplastic anemia: risk factors and treatment results. Blood 1989;73:606–613.
90. Champlin RE, Gale RP. Acute lymphoblastic leukemia: recent advances in biology and therapy. Blood 1989;73:2051–2066.
91. Champlin RE, Gale RP. Acute myelogenous leukemia: recent advances in therapy. Blood 1987;69:1551–1562.
92. Champlin RE, Goldman JM, Gale RP. Bone marrow transplantation in chronic myelogenous leukemia. Semin Hematol 1988;25:74–80.
93. Champlin RE, Ho WG, Gale RP, et al. Treatment of acute myelogenous leukemia: a prospective controlled trial of bone marrow transplantation versus consolidation chemotherapy. Ann Intern Med 1985;102:285–291.
94. Champlin R, Jacobs A, Gale RP, et al. High-dose cytarabine in consolidation chemotherapy or with bone marrow transplantation for patients with acute leukemia: preliminary results. Semin Oncol 1985;12(suppl 3):190–195.
95. Chao NJ, Schmidt GM, Niland JC, et al. Cyclosporine, methotrexate and prednisone compared with cyclosporine and prednisone for prophylaxis of acute graft-versus-host disease. N Engl J Med 1993;329:1225–1230.
96. Chessels JM, Leiper AD, Richards SM, et al. A second course of treatment for childhood acute lymphoblastic leukemia: long-term followup is needed to assess results. Br J Haematol 1994;86:48–54.
97. Churchill MA, Zaia JA, Forman SJ, Sheibani K, Azumi N, Blume KG. Quantitation of human cytomegalovirus DNA in lungs from bone marrow transplant recipients with interstitial pneumonia. J Infect Dis 1987;155:501–509.
98. Clarkson B, Berman E, Little C, et al. Update on clinical trials of chemotherapy and bone marrow transplantation in acute myelogenous leukemia in adults at Memorial Sloan-Kettering Cancer Center 1966–1989. In Acute Myelogenous Leukemia: Progress and Controversies. New York: Wiley-Liss, 1990, pp 239–272.
99. Clavell LA, Gelber RD, Cohen JH, et al. Four-agent induction and intensive asparaginase therapy for treatment of childhood acute lymphoblastic leukemia. N Engl J Med 1986;315:657.
100. Clift RA, Buckner CD, Thomas ED, et al. The treatment of acute non-lymphoblastic leukemia by allogeneic marrow transplantation. Bone Marrow Transplant 1987;2:243–258.
101. Clift RA, Buckner CD, Appelbaum FR, et al. Allogeneic marrow transplantation during untreated first relapse of acute myeloid leukemia. J Clin Oncol 1992;10:1723–1729.
102. Clift RA, Appelbaum FR, Thomas ED. Treatment of chronic myeloid leukemia by marrow transplantation. Blood 1993;82:1954–1956.
103. Clift RA, Buckner CD, Thomas ED, et al. Marrow transplantation for chronic myeloid leukemia: a randomized study comparing cyclophosphamide and total body irradiation with busulfan and total body irradiation with busulfan and cyclosphosphamide. Blood 1994;84:2036–2043.
104. Coccia PF, Strandjord SE, Warkentin PI, et al. High-dose cytosine arabinoside and fractionated total-body irradiation: an improved preparative regimen for bone marrow transplantation of children with acute lymphoblastic leukemia in remission. Blood 1988;71:888–893.
105. Conde E, Iriondo A, Rayon C, et al. Allogeneic bone marrow transplantation versus intensification chemotherapy for acute myelogenous leukaemia in first remission: a prospective controlled trial. Br J Haematol 1988;68:219–226.
106. Copelan EA, Grever MR, Kapoor N, Tutschka PJ. Marrow transplantation following busulfan and cyclophosphamide for chronic myelogenous leukaemia in accelerated or blastic phase. Br J Haematol 1989;71:487–491.
107. Copelan EA, Kapoor N, Gibbons B, Tutschka PJ. Allogeneic marrow transplantation in non-Hodgkin's lymphoma. Bone Marrow Transplant 1990;5:47.
108. Copelan EA, Tutschka PJ. Marrow transplantation following busulfan and cyclophosphamide in multiple myeloma. Bone Marrow Transplant 1988;3:363–365.
109. Crawford SW, Hackman RC, Clark JG. Open lung biopsy diagnosis of diffuse pulmonary infiltrates after marrow transplantation. Chest 1988;94:949–953.
110. Creutzig V, Ritter J, Riehm H, et al. Improved treatment results in childhood acute myelogenous leukemia: a report of the German Cooperative Study AML-BFM 78. Blood 1985;65:298–304.
111. Cullis JO, Jiang YZ, Schwarer, et al. Donor leukocyte infusions for chronic myeloid leukemia in relapse after allogeneic bone marrow transplantation. Blood 1992;79:1379–1381.
112. Davies SM, Shu XO, Blazar BR, et al. Unrelated donor bone marrow transplantation: influence of HLA A and B incompatibility on outcome. Blood 1995;86:1636–1642.
113. Davis AP, Roopenian DC. Complexity at the mouse minor histocompatibility locus H-4. Immunogenetics 1990;31:7.
114. deBueger M, Bakker A, van Rood JJ, van der Woude F, Goulmy E. Tissue distribution of human minor histocompatibility antigens: ubiquitous versus restricted tissue distribution indicates heterogeneity among human cytotoxic T lymphocyte-defined non-MHC antigens. J Immunol 1992;149:1788–1794.
115. Deeg HJ, Flournoy N, Sullivan KM, et al. Cataracts after total body irradiation and marrow transplantation: a sparing effect of dose fractionation. Int J Radiat Oncol Biol Phys 1984;10:957–964.
116. Deeg HJ, Sanders JE, Martin P, et al. Secondary malignancies after marrow transplantation. Exp Hematol 1984;12:660–666.
117. den Haan JMM, Sherman NE, Blokland E, et al. Identification of a graft versus host disease-associated human minor histocompatibility antigen. Science 1995;268:1476–1480.
118. Dennert G, Anderson CG, Warner J. T killer cells play a role in allogeneic bone marrow graft rejection but not in hybrid resistance. J Immunol 1985;135:3729–3734.
119. Devergie A, Blaise D, Attal M, et al. Allogeneic bone marrow transplantation for chronic myeloid leukemia in first chronic phase: a randomized trial of busulfan-cytoxan versus cytoxan-total body irradiation as preparative regimen: a report from the French Society of Bone Marrow Graft (SFGM) Blood 1995;85:2264–2268.
120. Devergie A, Reiffers J, Vernant JP, et al. Long-term follow-up after bone marrow transplantation for chronic myelogenous leukemia: factors associated with relapse. Bone Marrow Transplant 1990;5:379–386.
121. DeWitte T, Zwaan F, Hermans J, et al. Allogeneic bone marrow transplantation for secondary leukaemia and myelodysplastic syndrome: a survey by the Leukaemia Working Party of the European Bone Marrow Transplantation Group (EMBTG). Br J Haematol 1990;74:151–155.
122. DeWitte T, Gratwohl A, Van der Lely N, et al. Recombinant human granulocyte-macrophage colony-stimulating factor (rhGM-CSF) reduces infection-related mortal-

ity after allogeneic T-depleted bone marrow transplantation. Bone Marrow Transplant 1991;7(suppl 2):83.
123. DeWitte T, Hermans J, et al. Prognostic variables in bone marrow transplantation for secondary leukaemia and myelodysplastic syndromes: a survey of the working party on leukaemia. Bone Marrow Transplant 1991;8(suppl 1):40.
124. Dinsmore R, Kirkpatrick D, Flomenberg N, et al. Allogeneic bone marrow transplantation for patients with acute nonlymphocytic leukemia. Blood 1984;63:649–656.
125. Dinsmore R, Kirkpatrick D, Flomenberg N, et al. Allogeneic bone marrow transplantation for patients with acute lymphoblastic leukemia. Blood 1983;62:381–388.
125. DiPersio J, Martin B, Abboud C, Ryan D, Berenson R. Allogeneic BMT using bone marrow and CD34-selected mobilized PBSC; comparison to BM alone and mobilized PBSC alone. Blood 1994;84(suppl 1):91a. Abstract.
125. Donahue J, Homge M, Kernan NA. Characterization of cells emerging at the time of graft failure following bone marrow transplantation from an unrelated marrow donor. Blood 1993;82:1023–1029.
126. Doney KC, Weiden PL, Storb R, Thomas ED. Treatment of graft-versus-host disease in human allogeneic graft recipients: a randomized trial comparing antithymocyte globulin and corticosteroids. Am J Hematol 1981;11:1–8.
127. Doney KC, Buckner CD, Kopecky KJ, et al. Marrow transplantation for patients with acute lymphoblastic leukemia in first marrow remission. Bone Marrow Transplant 1987;2:355–363.
128. Doney K, Fisher LD, Appelbaum FR, et al. Treatment of adult acute lymphoblastic leukemia with allogeneic bone marrow transplantation. Multivariate analysis of factors affecting acute graft-versus-host disease, relapse, and relapse-free survival. Bone Marrow Transplant 1991;7:453–459.
129. Drizlikh G, Schmidt-Sole J, Yankelevich B. Involvement of the K and I regions of the H-2 complex in resistance to hemopoietic allografts. J Exp Med 1984;159:1070.
130. Drobyski WR, Keever CA, Roth MS, et al. Salvage immunotherapy using donor leukocyte infusions as treatment for relapsed chronic myelogenous leukemia after allogeneic bone marrow transplantation: efficacy and toxicity of a defined T-cell dose. Blood 1993;82:2310–2318.
131. Einsele H, Steidle M, Vallbracht A, Saal JG, Ehninger G, Muller CA. Early occurrence of human cytomegalovirus infection after bone marrow transplantation as demonstrated by the polymerase chain reaction technique. Blood 1991;77:1104.
132. Emanuel D, Cunningham I, Jules-Elysee K, et al. Cytomegalovirus pneumonia after bone marrow transplantation successfully treated with the combination of ganciclovir and high-dose intravenous immune globulin. Ann Intern Med 1988;109(12):777–782.
133. Emanuel D, Kernan NA, Castro-Malaspina H, et al. Cytomegalovirus-associated bone marrow failure after allogeneic bone marrow transplantation successfully treated with the combination of ganciclovir and high dose CMV immune globulin. Blood 1989;74(suppl 1):905a. Abstract.
134. Emanuel D, Peppard J, Stover D, Gold J, Armstrong F, Hammerling U. Rapid immunodiagnosis of cytomegalovirus pneumonia by bronchoalveolar lavage using human and murine monoclonal antibodies. Ann Intern Med 1986;104:476–481.
135. Emanuel D, Taylor J, Brochstein J, et al. The use of intravenous immune globulin as prophylaxis for the infectious complications of allogeneic marrow transplantation. Blood 1992;80(suppl 1):271a.
136. Eppinger T, Ehninger G, Steinhert M, Niethammer D, Dopfer R. 8-Methoxypsoralen and ultraviolet. A therapy for cutaneous manifestations of graft-versus-host disease. Transplantation 1990;50:807–811.
137. Ernst P, Maraninchi D, Jacobsen N, et al. Marrow transplantation for non-Hodgkin's lymphoma: a multi-centre study from the European Co-operative Bone Marrow Transplant Group. Bone Marrow Transplant 1986;1:81.
138. Essel HJ, Thompson MM, Harman GS, et al. Pilot trial of prophylactic ursodiol to decrease the incidence of veno-occlusive disease of the liver in allogeneic bone marrow transplant patients. Bone Marrow Transplant 1992;10:367–372.
139. Faber LM, Luxemburg-Heijs SAB, Willemze R, Falkenburg JHF. Generation of leukemia-reactive cytotoxic T lymphocyte clones from the HLA-identical bone marrow of a patient with leukemia. J Exp Med 176:1283–1289.
141. Falkenburg JHF, Goselink HM, Van der Harst D, et al. Growth inhibition of clonogenic leukemic precursor cells by minor histocompatibility antigen-specific cytotoxic T-lymphocytes. J Exp Med 1991;174:27–33.
142. Feig S, Nesbit M, Buckley, et al. Superiority of allogeneic bone marrow transplantation over conventional maintenance chemotherapy in children with acute non-lymphocytic leukemia. Exp Hematol 1987;15:373a.
143. Ferrara JL, Guillen FJ, Dijken PJ, Marion A, Murphy GF, Burakoff SJ. Evidence that large granular lymphocytes of donor origin mediate acute graft-versus-host disease. Transplantation 1989;47:50–54.
144. Ferrara J, Marion A, McIntyre JF, Murphy GF, Burakoff SJ. Amelioration of acute graft-versus-host disease due to minor histocompatibility antigens by in vitro administration of anti-interleukin-2 receptor antibody. J Immunol 1986;137:1874–1877.
145. Ferrara JLM, Weinstein HJ, Guinan EC, et al. Phase I/II trial of recombinant human IL-1 receptor antagonist (IL-IRA) for steroid resistant GVHD. Blood 1992;80(suppl 1):270a. Abstract.
146. Ferrara J, Lipton J, Hellman S, Burakoff S, Mauch P. Engraftment following T-cell -depleted marrow transplantation. I. The role of major and minor histocompatibility barriers. Transplantation 1987;43:461.
147. Ferretti GA, Ash RC, Brown AT, Parr MD, Romond EH, Lillich TT. Control of oral mucositis and candidiasis in marrow transplantation: a prospective, double-blind trial of chlorhexidine digluconate oral rinse. Bone Marrow Transplant 1988;3:483–493.
148. Filipovich AH, Vallera DA, Youle RJ, et al. Graft-versus-host disease prevention in allogeneic bone marrow transplantation from histocompatible siblings. Transplantation 1987;44:62–69.
149. Fischer A. Bone marrow transplantation in immunodeficiency and osteopetrosis. Bone Marrow Transplant 1989;4(suppl 14):12–14. Abstract.
150. Fischer A, Griscelli C, Friedrich W, et al. Bone marrow transplantation for immunodeficiencies and osteopetrosis: European Survey 1968–1985. Lancet 1986;2:1080–1084.
151. Fleischhauer K, Kernan NA, O'Reilly RJ, et al. Bone marrow allograft rejection by T lymphocytes recognizing a single amino acid difference in HLA-B44. N Engl J Med 1990;323:1818–1822.
152. Flowers MED, Pepe MS, Longton G, et al. Previous donor pregnancy as a risk factor for acute graft-versus-host disease in patients with aplastic anaemia treated by allogeneic marrow transplantation. Br J Haematol 1990;74:492–496.
153. Frame J, Collins NH, Cartagena T, Waldmann H, O'Reilly RJ, Kernan NA. T-cell depletion of human bone marrow: comparison of Campath-1 plus complement, anti-T-cell ricin A chain immunotoxin and soybean agglutinin alone or in combination with sheep erythrocytes or immunomagnetic beads. Transplantation 1989;47:984–988.
154. Gahrton G, Tura S, Ljungman P, et al. Prognostic factors in allogeneic bone marrow transplantation for multiple myeloma. J Clin Oncol 1995;13:1312–1322.
155. Gajewski J, Ho WG, Feig SA, Hunt L, Kaufman N, Champlin RE. Bone marrow transplantation using unrelated donors for patients with advanced leukemia or bone marrow failure. Transplantation 1990;50:244–249.
156. Gale R, Champlin R. How does bone marrow transplantation cure leukaemia? Lancet 1984;2:28–30.
157. Gale RP, Bortin MM, van Bekkum DW, et al. Risk factors for acute graft-versus-host disease. Br J Haematol 1987;67:397–406.
158. Ganem G, Giarardin M, Kuentz M, et al. Veno-occlusive disease of the liver after allogeneic bone marrow transplantation in man. Int J Radiat Oncol Biol Phys 1988;14:879–884.
159. Garicochea B, Chase A, Lazaridou A, Goldman JM. T-lymphocytes in CML. No evidence of the BCR/ABL fusion gene detected by fluorescence in situ hybridization in 143 patients. Leukemia 1994;8:1197.
160. Gatti RA, Meuwiissen HJ, Allen HD, Hong R, Good RA. Immunological reconstitution of sex-linked lymphopenic immunological deficiency. Lancet 1968;2:1366–1369.
161. Gaynor J, Chapmann D, Little C, et al. A cause-specific hazard rate analysis of prognostic factors among 199 adults with acute lymphoblastic leukemia: the Memorial Hospital experience since 1969. J Clin Oncol 1988;6:1014–1030.
162. Gharton G, Tura S, Belanger C, et al. For the European Group for Bone Marrow Transplantation. Allogeneic bone marrow transplantation in patients with multiple myeloma. Eur J Haematol 1989;43(suppl 51):182–185.
163. Gingrich RD, Ginder GD, Goeken D, et al. Allogeneic marrow grafting with partially mismatched, unrelated donors. Blood 1988;71:1375–1381.
164. Giralt SA, Kantarjian HM, Talpaz M, et al. Effect of prior interferon-alfa therapy on the outcome of allogeneic bone marrow transplantation for chronic myelogenous leukemia. J Clin Oncol 1993;11:1055–1061.
165. Giralt SA, Hester J, Hugh Y, et al. CD8+ depleted donor lymphocyte infusion as treatment for relapsed chronic myelogenous leukemia after allogeneic bone marrow transplantation: Graft vs leukemia without graft vs host disease. Blood 1994;84(suppl:1):538. Abstract.
166. Gleaves CA, Smith TF, Shuster EA, Pearson GR. Rapid detection of cytomegalovirus in MRC-5 cells innoculated with urine specimens by using low-speed centrifugation and monoclonal antibody to an early antigen. J Clin Microbiol 1984;19:917.
167. Gluckman E. Bone marrow transplantation for Fanconi anemia. In Aplastic Anemia and Other Bone Marrow Failure Syndromes. Edited by NT Shahid. New York: Springer-Verlag, 1990, p. 134–144.
168. Gluckman E, Joliver I, Scrobohaci ML, et al. Use of prostaglandin E_1 for prevention of liver veno-occlusive disease in leukaemic patients treated by allogeneic bone marrow transplantation. Br J Haematol 1990;74:277–281.
169. Glucksberg H, Storb R, Fefer A, et al. Clinical manifestations of GvHD in human recipients of marrow from HLA-matched sibling donors. Transplantation 1974;18:295–304.
170. Goldman JM, Szydlo R, Horowitz MM, et al. Choice of pretransplant treatment and timing of transplants for chronic myelogenous leukemia in chronic phase. Blood 1993;82:2235–2238.
171. Goldman JM, Gale RP, Horowitz MM, et al. Bone marrow transplantation for chronic myelogenous leukemia in chronic phase: increased risk for relapse associated with T-cell depletion. Ann Intern Med 1988;108:806–814.
172. Goodman JL, Drew MD, Winston MD, et al. A controlled trial of fluconazole to prevent fungal infections in patients undergoing bone marrow transplantation. N Engl J Med 1992;326:845–851.
173. Goodrich JM, Bowden RA, Fisher L, Keller C, Schoch BA, Meyers JD. Prevention of cytomegalovirus disease after allogeneic marrow transplant by ganciclovir prophylaxis. Ann Intern Med 1993;118:173–178.
174. Goodrich JM, Mori M, Gleaves CA, et al. Early treatment with ganciclovir to prevent cytomegalovirus disease after allogeneic bone marrow transplantation. N Engl J Med 1991;325:1601.
175. Gorin NC, Aegerter P, Auvert B. Autologous bone marrow transplantation (ABMT) for acute leukemia in remission: fifth European Survey. Evidence in favour of marrow purging. Bone Marrow Transplant 1989;4(suppl 1):206.
176. Gottdiener JS, Appelbaum FR, Ferrans VJ, Deisseroth A, Ziegler J. Cardiotoxicity associated with high-dose cyclophosphamide therapy. Arch Intern Med 1981;141:758–763.
177. Goulmy E. Minor histocompatibility antigens in man and their role in transplantation. Transplant Rev 1988;2:29.
178. Goulmy E, Termijtzlen A, Bradley BA, van Rood JJ. Y-antigen killing by T-cells of woman restricted by HLA. Nature 1977;226:544–545.
179. Gratwohl A, Hermans J, Niederwieser D, et al. Bone marrow transplantation for chronic myeloid leukemia: long term results. Bone Marrow Transplant 1993;12:509–516.
180. Gratwohl A, Hermans J, Apperley J. Acute graft-versus-host disease: grade and outcome in patients with chronic myelogenous leukemia. Blood 1995;86:813–818.
181. Gregory WM, Richards MA, Malpas JS. Combination chemotherapy versus melphalan and prednisone in the treatment of multiple myeloma: an overview of published trials. J Clin Oncol 1992;10:334–342.
182. Gribben J, Goldstone AH, Ernst P, et al. Bone marrow transplantation for non-Hodgkin's lymphoma in remission-allogeneic versus autologous. Bone Marrow Transplant 1987;2(suppl s):204.
183. Guinan EC, Tarbell NJ, Tantravahi R, Weinstein HJ. Bone marrow transplantation for children with myelodysplastic syndromes. Blood 1989;73:619–622.
184. Hale G, Cobbold S, Waldmann H. T-cell depletion with Campath-1 in allogeneic bone marrow transplantation. Transplantation 1988;45:753–759.
185. Hale G, Waldmann H. Campath-1 for prevention of graft-versus-host disease and graft rejection. Summary of results from a multi-centre study. Bone Marrow Transplant 1988;3:11–14.

186. Hauch M, Gazzola MV, Small T, et al. Anti-leukemia potential of interleukin-2 activated natural killer cells after bone marrow transplantation for chronic myelogenous leukemia. Blood 1990;75:2250–2262.
187. Helenglass G, Powles RL, McElwain TJ, et al. Melphelan and total body irradiation (TBI) versus cyclophosphamide and TBI as conditioning for allogeneic matched sibling bone marrow transplants for acute myeloblastic leukemia in first remission. Bone Marrow Transplant 1988;3:21–29.
188. Helg C, Roux E, Beris P, et al. Adoptive immunotherapy for recurrent CML after BMT. Bone Marrow Transplant 1993:12:125–129.
189. Hellstrom-Lindberg E, Rober K-H, Gahrton G, et al. Predictive model for the clinical response to low dose Ara-C: a study of 102 patients with myelodysplastic syndromes or acute leukaemia. Br J Haematol 1992;81:503–511.
190. Henslee PJ, MacDonald JS, Messino MJ. Freedom from relapse following histoincompatible marrow transplantation in patients with high risk acute lymphoblastic leukemia. Exp Haematol 1989;17:547a.
191. Herbelin C, Stephan J-L, Donadieu J, LeDeist F, Racadot E, Wijdenes J, Fischer A. Treatment of steroid-resistant acute graft-versus-host disease with an anti-IL-2 receptor monoclonal antibody (BT 563) in children who received T cell-depleted, partially matched, related bone marrow transplants. Bone Marrow Transplant 1994;13: 563–569.
192. Hercend T, Takvorian T, Nowill A, et al. Characterization of natural killer cells with antileukemia activity following allogeneic bone marrow transplantation. Blood 1986;67(3):722–728.
193. Hertenstein B, Wiesneth M, Novotny J, et al. Interferon-α and donor buffy coat transfusions for treatment of relapsed chronic myeloid leukemia after allogeneic bone marrow transplantation. Transplantation 1993;56:1114–1118.
194. Hertz MI, Englund JA, Snover D, Bitterman PB, McGlave PB. Respiratory syncytial virus-induced acute lung injury in adult patients with bone marrow transplants: a clinical approach and review of the literature. Medicine 1989;68:269–281.
195. Herve P, Wijdenes J, Bergerat JP, et al. Treatment of corticosteroid resistant acute graft-versus-host disease by in vivo administration of anti-interleukin-2 receptor monoclonal antibody (B-B10). Blood 1990;75:1017–1023.
196. Herzig RH, Bortin MM, Barrett AJ, et al. Bone marrow transplantation in high-risk acute lymphoblastic leukaemia in first and second remission. Lancet 1987;1: 786–789.
197. Hoelzer D, Gale RP. Acute lymphoblastic leukemia in adults: recent progress, future directions. Semin Hematol 1987;24:27–39.
198. Holland K, Wingard JR, Beschorner WE, Saral R, Santos GW. Bronchiolitis obliterans after bone marrow transplantation: relationship to chronic graft-versus-host disease and serum IgG. Blood 1988;72:621–627.
199. Holler E, Kolb HJ, Moller A, et al. Increased serum levels of tumor necrosis factor α precede major complications of bone marrow transplantation. Blood 1990;75: 1011–1016.
200. Horowitz MM, Gale RP, Sondel PM, et al. Graft versus leukemia reactions after bone marrow transplantation. Blood 1990;75:555–562.
201. Howard MR, Brookes P, Bidwell JL, et al. HLA-DR and DQ matching by DNA restriction fragment length polymorphism methods and the outcome of mixed lymphocyte reaction tests in unrelated bone marrow donor searches. Bone Marrow Transplant 1992;9:161–166.
202. Howard MR, Hows JM, Gore SM, et al. Unrelated donor marrow transplantation between 1977 and 1987 at four centers in the United Kingdom. Transplantation 1990;49(3):547–553.
203. Hows JM, Mehta A, Ward L, et al. Comparison of mesna with forced diuresis to prevent cyclophosphamide induced haemorrhagic cystitis in marrow transplantation: a prospective randomized study. Br J Cancer 1984;50:753–756.
204. Huma Z, Boulad F, Black P, Heller G, Sklar C. Growth in children after bone marrow transplantation for acute leukemia. Blood 1995;86(2):819–824.
205. Hurtado RM, Sosa RC, Majjuf AC, et al. Refactory anaemia type I FAB treated with oxymethalone: long-term results. Br J Haematol 1993;85:235–236.
206. Hutchinson RM, Pringle JH, Potter L, Patel I, Jeffreys AJ. Rapid identification of donor and recipient cells after allogeneic bone marrow transplantation using specific genetic markers. Br J Haematol 1989;72:133–140.
207. Italian Cooperative Study Group on Chronic Myeloid Leukemia. Interferon alfa-a as compared with conventional chemotherapy for the treatment of chronic myeloid leukemia. N Engl J Med 1994;330:820–825.
208. Jones RJ, Lee KS, Beschorner WE, et al. Veno-occlussive disease of the liver following bone marrow transplantation. Transplantation 1987;44:778–783.
209. Jones RJ, Ambinder RF, Piantadosi S, Santos GW. Evidence of a graft-versus-lymphoma effect associated with allogeneic bone marrow transplantation. Blood 1991;77:649–653.
210. Kantarjian HM, Smith TL, O'Brien S, et al. Prolonged survival in chronic myelogenous leukemia after cytogenetic response to Interferon-alpha therapy. Ann Intern Med 1995;122:254–261.
211. Kantarjian HM, Keating MJ, Walters RS, Smith TL, Cork A, McCredie KM, Freireich EJ. Therapy-related leukemia and myelodysplastic syndrome: clinical, cytogenetic and prognostic features. J Clin Oncol 1986;4:1748–1757.
212. Kapoor N, Kirkpatrick D, Blaese RM, et al. Reconstitution of normal megakaryocytopoiesis and immunologic functions in Wiscott-Aldrich Syndrome by marrow transplantation following myeloablation and immunosuppression with busulfan and cyclophosphamide. Blood 1981;57:692–696.
213. Keever CA, Leong N, Cunningham I, et al. HLA-B-44-directed cytotoxic T cells associated with acute graft-versus-host disease following unrelated bone marrow transplantation. Bone Marrow Transplant 1994;14:137–145.
214. Keever CA, Small TN, Flomenberg N, et al. Comparison of recipients of T-cell depleted marrow with recipients of conventional marrow grafts. Blood 1989;73: 1340–1350.
215. Keissling R, Hochman PS, Haller O, Shearer GM, Wigzell H, Cudkowicz G. Evidence for a similar or common mechanism for natural killer activity and resistance to hemopoietic grafts. Eur J Immunol 1977;7:655.
216. Kennedy MS, Deeg HJ, Storb R, et al. Treatment of acute graft-versus-host disease after allogeneic marrow transplantation: randomized study comparing corticosteroids and cyclosporine. Am J Med 1985;78:978–983.
217. Kenny AB, Hitzig WH. Bone marrow transplantation for severe combined immunodeficiency. Reported from 1968 to 1977. Eur J Pediatr 1979;131:155–177.
218. Kernan NA, Barsch G, Ash RC, et al. Analysis of 462 transplantations from unrelated donors facilitated by the national marrow donor program. N Engl J Med 1993;328: 593–602.
219. Kernan NA, Bordignon C, Heller G, et al. Graft failure after T-cell-depleted human leukocyte antigen identical marrow transplants for leukemia: I. Analysis of risk factors and results of secondary transplants. Blood 1989;74:2227–2236.
220. Kernan NA, Collins NH, Juliano I, Cartagena BS, Dupont B, O'Reilly RJ. Clonable T-lymphocytes in T-cell depleted bone marrow transplants correlate with development of graft-versus-host disease. Blood 1986;68:770–773.
221. Kernan NA, Flomenberg N, Dupont B, O'Reilly RJ. Graft rejection in recipients of T-cell depleted HLA-non-identical marrow transplants for leukemia. Transplantation 1987;43:842–847.
222. Kernan NA, Khan R, Landrey C, O'Reilly RJ, Dupont B, Yang SY. Identification of unrelated bone marrow donors based on matching for class I IEF subtypes. Blood 1990;76:548a.
223. Klein J, Park JM. Graft-versus-host reaction across different regions of the H-2 complex of the mouse. J Exp Med 1973;137:1213–1225.
224. Knox K, Carrigan DR. In vitro suppression of bone marrow progenitor cell differentiation by human herpesvirus 6 infection. J Infect Dis 1992;165:925–929.
225. Kolb HJ, Mittermuller J, Clemm CH, et al. Donor leukocyte transfusions for treatment of recurrent chronic myelogenous leukemia in marrow transplant patients. Blood 1990;76:2462–2465.
226. Kolb HJ, Schattenberg A, Goldman JM, et al. Graft-versus-leukemia effect of donor lymphocyte transfusions in marrow grafted patients. Blood 1995;86:2041–2050.
227. Korngold R, Sprent J. Lethal GvHD across minor H barriers. Nature of the effector cells and of the role of the H-2. Immunology 1983;71:5.
228. Krivit W, Whitley CB, Chang PN, Belani KG, Snover D, Summers CG, Blazar BR. Lysomal storage diseases treated by bone marrow transplantation: review of 21 patients. In Bone Marrow Transplantation in Children. Edited by C Pochedly and L Johnson. New York: Raven, 1990, pp 261–287.
229. Kwak LW, Taub DD, Duffey PL, Bensinger WI, Bryant EM, Reynolds CW, Longon DL. Transfer of myeloma idiotype-specific immunity from an actively immunized marrow donor. Lancet 1995;345:1016–1020.
230. Kyle RA. Multiple myeloma. An update on diagnosis and management. Acta Oncol 29 1990;1:1.
231. Laporte JP, Lesage S, Tilleul P, Majman A, Gorin NC. Alteplase for hepatic veno-occlusive disease complicating bone marrow transplantation. Lancet 1992;339:1057.
232. Leiper AD, Stanhope R, Lau T, et al. The effect of total body irradiation and bone marrow transplantation during childhood and adolescence on growth and endocrine function. Br J Haematol 1987;67:419–426.
233. Locksley RM, Flournoy N, Sullivan KM, Meyers JD. Infection with varicella-zoster virus after marrow transplantation. J Infect Dis 1985;152:1172–1178.
234. Lucas K, Small T, O'Reilly RJ, Dupont B. The development of Epstein-Barr virus specific cellular immunity following allogeneic marrow transplantation. Blood 1994;84:98.
235. Luccarelli G, Galimberti M, Polchi P, et al. Bone marrow transplantation in patients with thalassemia. N Engl J Med 1990;322:417–421.
236. Lum LG. The kinetics of immune reconstitution after human marrow transplantation. Blood 1987;69:369–380.
237. Mackinnon S, Hows JM, Goldman JM. Induction of in vitro graft-versus-leukemia activity following bone marrow transplantation for chronic myeloid leukemia. Blood 1990;76:2037–2045.
238. Mackinnon S, Papadoupoulos EB, Carabasi MH, et al. Adoptive immunotherapy evaluating escalating doses of donor leukocytes for relapse of chronic myeloid leukemia following bone marrow transplantation: separation of graft-versus-host leukemia responses from graft-versus-host disease. Blood 1995;86:1261–1268.
239. Mackinnon S, Burnett AK, Crawford RJ, Cameron S, Leask BGS, Somerville RG. Seronegative blood products prevent primary cytomegalovirus infection after bone marrow transplantation. J Clin Pathol 1988;41:948.
240. Mandelli F, Avvisati G, Amadori S, et al. Maintenance treatment with recombinant interferon alfa-2b in patients with multiple myeloma responding to conventional induction chemotherapy. N Engl J Med 1990;322:1430–1434.
241. Marijt WAF, Kernan NA, Diaz-Barrientos T, Veenhof WFJ, O'Reilly RJ, Willemze R, Falkenburg JHF. Multiple minor histocompatibility antigen-specific cytotoxic T lymphocyte clones can be generated during graft rejection after HLA-identical bone marrow transplantation. Bone Marrow Transplant 1995;16:125–132.
242. Marks DI, Cullis JO, Ward KN, et al. Allogeneic bone marrow transplantation for chronic myeloid leukemia using sibling and volunteer unrelated donors: a comparison of complications in the first 2 years. Ann Intern Med 1993;119:207–214.
243. Marmont AM, Gale RP, Butturini A, et al. T-cell depletion in allogeneic bone marrow transplantation: progress and problems. Haematologica 1989;74:235–248.
244. Marsh JC, Harhalakis N, Dowding C, Laffan M, Gordon-Smith EC, Hows JM. Recurrent graft failure following syngeneic bone marrow transplantation for aplastic anemia. Bone Marrow Transplant 1989;4:581–585.
245. Martin PJ, Hansen JA, Buckner CD, et al. Effects of in vitro depletion of T-cells in HLA-identical allogeneic marrow grafts. Blood 1985;66:664–672.
246. Martin PJ, Hansen JA, Torok-Storb B, et al. Graft failure in patients receiving T-cell depleted HLA-identical allogeneic marrow transplants. Bone Marrow Transplant 1988;3: 345–356.
247. Martin PJ, Schoch G, Fisher, et al. A retrospective analysis of therapy for acute graft-versus-host disease: initial treatment. Blood 1990;76:1464–1472.
248. Martin PJ, Shulman HM, Schubach WH, et al. Fatal Epstein-Barr-virus-associated proliferation of donor B-cells after treatment of acute graft-versus-host disease with a murine anti-T-cell antibody. Ann Intern Med 1984;101:310–315.
249. Masaoka T, Takafu F, Kato S, et al. Recombinant human granulocyte colony-stimulating factor in allogeneic bone marrow transplantation. Exp Hematol 1989;17: 1047–1050.
250. Maschek H, Kaloutsi V, Rodriguez-Kaiser M, et al. Hypoplastic myelodysplastic syndrome: incidence, morphology, cytogenetics and prognosis. Ann Hematol 1993;66: 117–122.
251. Mayer RJ. Current chemotherapeutic treatment approaches to the management of

previously untreated adults with de novo acute myelogenous leukemia. Semin Oncol 1987;14:385–396.
251a. Mayer RJ, Davis RB, Schiffer CA, et al. Intensive postremission chemotherapy in adults with acute myeloid leukemia. N Engl J Med 1994;331:896–903.
252. McCullough J, Hansen JA, Perkins H, Stroncek D, Bartsch G. The national marrow donor program: how it works, accomplishments to date. Oncology 1989;3:63.
253. McDonald GB, Sharma P, Mattews DE, Schulman HM, Thomas ED. Veno-occlusive disease of the liver after bone marrow transplantation: diagnosis, incidence and predisposing factors. Hepatology 1984;4:116–122.
254. McGlave P, Arthur D, Haake R, et al. Therapy of chronic myelogenous leukemia with allogeneic bone marrow transplantation. J Clin Oncol 1987;5:1033–1040.
255. McGlave PB, Arthur DC, Kim TH, Ramsay NKC, Hurd DD, Kersey J. Successful allogeneic bone marrow transplantation for patients in the accelerated phase of chronic granulocytic leukaemia. Lancet 1982;2:625–627.
256. McGlave P, Bartsch G, Anasetti C, Ash R, Beatty P, Gajewski J, Kernan NA. Unrelated donor marrow transplantation therapy for chronic myelogenous leukemia: initial experience of the national marrow donor program. Blood 1993;81:543–550.
257. McGlave PB, Beatty PG, Ash R, Hows JM. Therapy for chronic myelogenous leukemia and unrelated donor bone marrow transplantation: results in 102 cases. Blood 1990;75:1728–1732.
258. Meloni G, DeFabritiis P, Carella AM, et al. Autologous bone marrow transplantation in patients with AML in first complete remission. Results of two different conditioning regimens after the same induction and consolidation therapy. Bone Marrow Transplant 1990;5:29–32.
259. Meyers JD, Thomas ED. Infection complicating bone marrow transplantation. In Clinical Approach to Infection in the Compromised Host, ed 2. Edited by RJ Rubin and LS Young. New York: Plenum, 1981, pp 525–556.
260. Meyers JD, Flucrnoy N, Thomas ED. Nonbacterial pneumonia after allogeneic marrow transplantation. A review of ten years' experience. Rev Infect Dis 1982;4:1119–1132.
261. Meyers JD, Flucrnoy N, Thomas ED. Risk factors for cytomegalovirus infection after human marrow transplantation. J Infect Dis 1986;153:478–488.
262. Nademanee A, Schmidt GM, Parker P, et al. The outcome of matched unrelated donor bone marrow transplantation in patients with hematologic malignancies using molecular typing for donor selection and graft-versus-host disease prophylaxis regimen of cyclosporine, methotrexate, and prednisone. Blood 1995;86:1228–1234.
263. Negrin RS, Haeuber DH, Nagler A, et al. Maintenance treatment of patients with myelodysplastic syndromes using recombinant human granulocyte colony-stimulating factor. Blood 1990;76:36–43.
264. Neiman PE, Reeves W, Ray G, et al. A prospective analysis of interstitial pneumonia and opportunistic viral infection among recipients of allogeneic bone marrow grafts. J Infect Dis 1977;136:754–767.
265. Nemunaitis J, Anasetti C, Storb R, et al. Phase II trial of recombinant human granulocyte-macrphage colony stimulating factor (rhGM-CSF) in patients undergoing allogeneic bone marrow transplantation from unrelated donors. Blood 1992;79:2572–2577.
266. O'Donnell MR, Schmidt GM, Tegtmeier B, et al. Prophylactic low dose amphotericin B (AM-B) decreases systemic fungal infection (SFT) in allogeneic bone marrow transplant (BMT) recipients. Blood 1990;76(suppl 1):558. Abstract.
267. O'Donnell MR, Schmidt GM, Tegtmeier BR, et al. Prediction of systemic fungal infection in allogeneic marrow recipients: impact of amphotericin prophylaxis in high-risk patients. J Clin Oncol 1994;12(4):827–834.
268. O'Donnell MR, Nademanee AP, Snyder DS, et al. Bone marrow transplantation for myelodysplastic and myeloproliferative syndromes. J Clin Oncol 1987;5:1822–1826.
269. O'Leary M, Ramsay NKC, Nesbit ME, et al. Bone marrow transplantation for non-Hodgkin's lymphoma in children and young adults. Am J Med 1983;74:497.
270. O'Reilly RJ. Allogeneic bone marrow transplantation: current status and future directions. Blood 1983;62:941–964.
271. O'Reilly RJ, Brochstein J, Collins N, et al. Evaluation of HLA-haplotype disparate parental marrow grafts depleted of T lymphocytes by differential agglutination with a soybean lectin and E-rosette depletion for the treatment of severe combined immunodeficiency. Vox Sang 1986;51:81–86.
272. O'Reilly RJ, Collins NH, Kernan NA, et al. Transplantation of marrow depleted of T-cells by soybean lectin agglutination and E-rosette depletion: major histocompatibility complex-related graft resistance in leukemia transplant patients. Transplant Proc 1985;17:455–459.
273. O'Reilly RJ, Dupont B, Pahwa S, et al. Reconstitution in severe combined immunodeficiency by transplantation of marrow from an unrelated donor. N Engl J Med 1977;297:1311–1318.
274. O'Reilly RJ, Keever CA, Small T, Brochstein JA. The use of HLA-non-identical T-cell depleted marrow transplants for correction of severe combined immunodeficiency disease. Immunodefic Rev 1989;1:273–309.
275. O'Reilly RJ, Kernan NA, Cunningham I, et al. Allogeneic transplants depleted of T-cells by soybean lectin agglutination and E-rosette depletion. Bone Marrow Transplant 1988;3:3–6.
276. O'Reilly RJ, Lee FK, Grossbard E, et al. Papovavirus excretion following marrow transplantation: incidence and association with hepatic dysfunction. Transplant Proc 1981;13:262–266.
277. O'Reilly RJ, Carabasi MH, Collins NH, et al. T-cell depletion and allogeneic bone marrow transplantation. Semin Hematol 1992;29:20–26.
278. O'Reilly R J, Brochstein J, Dinsmore R, Kirkpatrick D. Marrow transplantation for congenital disorders. Semin Hematol 1984;21:188–221.
279. Papadopoulos E, Ladanyi M, Emanuel D, et al. Infusions of donor leukocytes as treatment of Epstein-Barr virus associated lymphoproliferative disorders complicating allogeneic marrow transplantation. N Engl J Med 1993;330:1185–1191.
280. Papadopoulos E, Carabasi M, Young JW, et al. Results of T-cell depleted (TCD) allogeneic BMT after TBI, thiotepa and cyclosphosphamide in patients with leukemia. Blood 1992;80:170a. Abstract.
281. Papadopoulos EB, Boulad F, Carabasi MH, et al. Improved disease-free survival in recipients of T cell depleted bone marrow allografts for acute non-lymphocytic leukemia in first remission. Blood 1994;84(suppl 1):331a. Abstract.
282. Parkman R. Clonal analysis of murine graft-versus-host disease. I. Phenotypic and functional analysis of T-lymphocyte clones. J Immunol 1986;136:3543–3548.
283. Parkman R, Rappaport J, Geha R, et al. Complete correction of the Wiskott-Aldrich syndrome by allogeneic bone marrow transplantation. N Engl J Med 1978;298:921–927.
284. Perren TJ, Powles RL, Easton D, Stolle K, Selby PJ. Prevention of herpes zoster in patients by long-term oral acyclovir after allogeneic bone marrow transplantation. Am J Med 1988;85(suppl 2A):99. Abstract.
285. Petersdorf EW, Smith AG, Mickelson EM, et al. The role of HLA-DPB1 disparity in the development of acute graft-versus-host disease following unrelated donor marrow transplantation. Blood 1993;81:1923–1932.
286. Petersdorf EW, Longton GM, Anasetti C, et al. The significance of HLA-DRB1 matching on clinical outcome after HLA-A, B, DR identical unrelated donor marrow transplantation. Blood 1995;86:1606–1613.
287. Phillips GL, Herzig RH, Lazarus HM, et al. High-dose chemotherapy, fractionated total-body irradiation, and allogeneic marrow transplantation for malignant lymphoma. J Clin Oncol 1986;4:480.
288. Piguet PF, Grau GE, Allet B, Vassali P. Tumor necrosis factor/cachectin is an effector of skin and gut lesions of the acute phase of graft-versus-host disease. J Exp Med 1987;166:1280–1289.
289. Porter DL, Roth MS, McGarigle C, Ferrara JLM, Antin JH. Induction of graft-versus-host disease as immunotherapy for relapsed chronic myeloid leukemia. N Engl J Med 1994;330:100.
290. Powles RL, Morgenstern G, Clink HM, et al. The place of bone-marrow transplantation in acute myelogenous leukaemia. Lancet 1980;1:1047–1050.
291. Prentice HG, Bradstock KF, Janossy G, et al. Use of anti-T-cell monoclonal antibody OKT3 to prevent acute graft-versus-host disease in allogeneic bone marrow transplantation for acute leukemia. Lancet 1982;1:700–703.
292. Preti A, Kantarjian HM. Management of adult acute lymphocytic leukemia: present issues and key challenges. J Clin Oncol 1994;12:1312–1322.
293. Racadot E, Herve P, Beaujean F, et al. Prevention of graft-versus-host disease in HLA-matched bone marrow transplantation for malignant disease: a multicentric study of 62 patients using 3 pan-T monoclonal antibodies and rabbit complement. J Clin Oncol 1987;5:426–435.
294. Ramsay NKC, Kersey JH, Robinson LL, et al. A randomized study of the prevention of acute graft-versus-host disease. N Engl J Med 1982;306:392–397.
295. Rappeport J, Parkman R, Belli J, Levey R, Rosen F, Nathan D. Reversibility of myelofibrosis (MF) after bone marrow transplantation. Blood 1978;52:589a. Abstract.
296. Ratanatharathorn V, Uberti J, Karanes C, et al. Prospective comparative trial of autologous versus allogeneic bone marrow transplantation in patients with non-Hodgkin's lymphoma. Blood 1994;84:1050–1055.
297. Ratanatharathorn V, Karanes C, Uberti J, et al. Busulfan-based regimens and allogeneic bone marrow transplantation in patients with myelodysplastic syndromes. Blood 1993;81:2194–2199.
298. Ray CG. Respiratory viruses. In Medical Microbiology: An Introduction to Infectious Diseases. Edited by JC Sherris. New York: Elsevier, 1990, pp 499–516.
299. Reed EC, Bowden RA, Dandliker PS, Lilleby KE, Meyers JD. Treatment of cytomegalovirus pneumonia with ganciclovir and intravenous cytomegalovirus immunoglobulin in patients with bone marrow transplants. Ann Intern Med 1988;109:783–788.
300. Reisner Y, Kapoor N, Kirkpatrick D, et al. Transplantation for severe combined immunodeficiency with HLA-A,B,DR incompatible parental marrow fractionated by soybean agglutin and sheep red blood cells. Blood 1983;61:341–348.
301. Reisner Y, Kapoor N, Kirkpatrick D, et al. Transplantation for acute leukemia with HLA-A and B non-identical parental marrow cells fractionated with soybean agglutinin and sheep blood cells. Lancet 1981;2:327–331.
302. Reisner Y, Itzicovitch L, Meshorer A, Sharon N. Hematopoietic stem cell transplantation using mouse bone-marrow and spleen cells fractionated by lectins. Proc Natl Acad Sci USA 1978;75:2933.
303. Riddell SR, Watanabe KS, Goodrich JM, Li CR, Agha ME, Greenberg PD. Restoration of viral immunity in immunodeficient humans by the adoptive transfer of T cell clones. Science 1992;257:238.
304. Rivera GK, Buchanan G, Boyett JM, et al. Intensive retreatment of childhood acute lymphoblastic leukemia in first bone marrow relapse: a pediatric oncology group study. N Engl J Med 1986;315:273.
305. Rooney CM, Smith CA, Ng CYC, et al. Use of gene-modified virus-specific T lymphocytes to control Epstein-Barr-virus-related lymphoproliferation. Lancet 1995;345:9.
306. Rosenkrantz K, Keever C, Kirsch J, et al. In vitro correlates of graft-host tolerance after HLA-matched and mismatched marrow transplants: suggestions from limiting dilution analysis. Transplant Proc 1987;196:98–103.
307. Roth MS, Antin JH, Ash R, et al. Prognostic significance of Philadelphia: chromosome-positive cells detected by the polymerase chain reaction after allogeneic bone marrow transplant for chronic myelogenous leukemia. Blood 1992;79:276–282.
308. Rotzschke O, Falk K, Hans-Joachim W, Faath S, Rammensee HG. Characterization of naturally occurring minor histocompatibility peptides including H-4 and H-Y. Science 1990;249:283–250.
309. Sanders JE, Buckner CD, Amos D, et al. Ovarian function following marrow transplantation for aplastic anemia or leukemia. J Clin Oncol 1988;6:813–818.
310. Sanders JE, Fluornoy N, Thomas ED, et al. Marrow transplant experience in children with acute lymphoblastic leukemia: an analysis of factors associated with survival, relapse and graft-versus-host disease. Med Pediatr Oncol 1985;13:165.
311. Sanders JE, Thomas ED, Buckner CD, et al. Marrow transplantation for children in first remission of acute nonlymphoblastic leukemia: an update. Blood 1985;66:460.
312. Sanders JE, Pritchard S, Mahoney P, et al. Growth and development following marrow transplantation for leukemia. Blood 1986;68:1129–1135.
313. Sanders JE, Thomas ED, Buckner CD, Doney K. Marrow transplantation for children with acute lymphoblastic leukemia in second remission. Blood 1987;70:324.
314. Santamaria P, Reinsmoen NL, Lindstrom AL, et al. Frequent HLA class I and DP sequence mismatches in serologically (HLA-A, HLA-B, HLA-DR) and molecularly (HLA-DRB1, HLA-DQA1, HLA-DQB1) HLA-identical unrelated bone marrow transplant pairs. Blood 1994;83:280–287.
315. Santos G W. Immunosuppression for clinical marrow transplantation. Semin Hematol 1974;11:341–351.
316. Saral R, Burns WH, Laskin OL, Santos GW, Leitman PS. Acyclovir prophylaxis of

herpes-simplex-virus infections. A randomized, double-blind, controlled trial in bone marrow transplant recipients. N Engl J Med 1981;305:63–67.
317. Schiller G, Vescio R, Freytes C, et al. Transplantation of CD34+ peripheral blood progenitor cells after high-dose chemotherapy for patients with advanced multiple myeloma. Blood 1995;86:390–397.
318. Schmidt GM, Kovacs A, Zaia JA, Horak DA, et al. Ganciclovir/immunoglobulin combination therapy for the treatment of human cytomegalovirus-associated interstitial pneumonia in bone marrow allograft recipients. Transplantation 1988;46:905–907.
319. Schmidt GM, Horak DA, Niland JC, Duncan SR, Forman SJ, Zaia JA. City of Hope-Stanford-Syntex CMV Study Group. a randomized controlled trial of prophylactic ganciclovir for cytomegalovirus pulmonary infection in recipients of allogeneic bone marrow transplants. N Engl J Med 1991;324:1005–1011.
320. Schmitz N, Gassmann W, Rister M, et al. Fractionated total body irradiation and high-dose VP 16–213 followed by allogeneic bone marrow transplantation in advanced leukemias. Blood 1988;72:1567–1573.
321. Schofield JR, Robinson WA, Murphy JR, Rovira DK. Low doses of interferon-alpha are as effective as higher doses in inducing remissions and prolonging survival in chronic myeloid leukemia. Ann Intern Med 1994;121:736–744.
322. Schreuder I, Pool J, Blokland E, van Els C, Bakker A, van Rood JJ, Goulmy E. A genetic analysis of human minor histocompatibility antigens demonstrates Mendelian segregation independent of HLA. Immunogenetics 1993;38:98–105.
323. Sebban C, Lepage E, Vernan J, et al. Allogeneic bone marrow transplantation in adult acute lymphoblastic leukemia in first complete remission: a comparative study. J Clin Oncol 1994;12:2580–2587.
324. Selby P, Jameson B, Watson J, et al. Parenteral acyclovir for herpes virus infections of man. Lancet 1979;2:1267–1270.
325. Servida P, Rossini S, Traversari C, et al. Gene transfer into peripheral blood lymphocytes for in vivo immunomodulation of donor anti-tumor immunity in a patient affected by EBV-induced lymphoma. Blood 1993;82:214a.
326. Shapiro R, Chauvenet A, McGuire W, et al. Treatment of B-cell lymphoproliferative disorders with interferon alfa and intravenous gammaglobulin. N Engl J Med 1988;318:1334.
327. Shepp DH, Dandiliker PS, Meyers JD. Treatment of varicella-zoster virus infection in severely immunocompromised patients–a randomized comparison of acyclovir and citarabine. N Engl J Med 1986;314:208–212.
328. Silverman LR, Holland JF, Nelson D, et al. Trilineage response of myelodysplastic syndromes to subcutaneous azacytidine. Proc Am Soc Clin Oncol 1991;10:747.
329. Sklar CA, Kim TH, Ramsay NK. Thyroid dysfunction among long-term survivors of bone marrow transplantation. Am J Med 1982;73:688–694.
330. Sklar CA, Kim TH, Ramsay NK. Testicular function following bone marrow transplantation performed during or after puberty. Cancer 1984;53:1498–1501.
331. Sladek NE, Smith PC, Bratt PM, et al. Influence of diuretics on urinary general base catalytic activity and cyclosphosphamide-induced bladder toxicity. Cancer Treat Rep 1982;66:1889–1900.
332. Slavin S, Ackerstein A, Naparstek E, Or R, Weiss L. The graft-versus-leukemia (GVL) phenomenon: is GVL separable from GVHD? Bone Marrow Transplant 1990;6: 155–161.
333. Slavin RE, Woodruff JM. The pathology of bone marrow transplantation. Pathol Annu 1974;91:291–344.
334. Socie G, Devergie A, Cosset JM, et al. Low-dose (one gray) total-lymphoid irradiation for extensive, drug-resistant chronic graft-versus-host disease. Transplantation 1990;49:657–658.
335. Soiffer R, Murray C, Fairclough D, et al. CD6-depleted allogeneic BMT for adults with acute leukemia. Blood 1994;84(suppl 1):332a. Abstract.
336. Soiffer RJ, Murray C, Cochran K, et al. Clinical and immunologic effects of prolonged infusion of low-dose recombinant interleukin-2 after autologous and T-cell-depleted allogeneic bone marrow transplantation. Blood 1992;79:517–526.
337. Sokal JE, Baccarani M, Russo D, Tura S. Staging and prognosis in chronic myelogenous leukemia. Semin Hematol 1988;25:49–61.
338. Sonnenberg FA, Eckman MH, Pauker SG. Bone marrow donor registries: the relation between registry size and probability of finding complete and partial matches. Blood 1989;74:2569–2578.
339. Sosman JA, Oettel KR, Hank JA, Fisch P, Sondel PM. Specific recognition of human leukemic cells by allogeneic T-cell lines. Transplantation 1989;48:486–495.
340. Sosman JA, Oettel KR, Smith SD, Hank JA, Fisch P, Sondel PM. Specific recognition of human leukemic cells by allogeneic T-cells: II. Evidence for HLA-D restricted determinants on leukemic cells that are crossreactive with determinants present on unrelated nonleukemic cells. Blood 1990;75:2005–2016.
341. Sparks RS. Cytogenetic analysis in human bone marrow transplantation. Cancer Genet Cytogenet 1981;4:345–352.
342. Steinherz PG, Gaynon P, Miller DR, et al. Improved disease free survival of children with acute lymphoblastic leukemia at high risk for early relapse with the "New York: regimen–a new intensive therapy protocol: a report from the Children's Cancer Study Group. J Clin Oncol 1986;4:744–752.
342. Steinman RM. The dendritic cell system and its role in immunogenicity. Annu Rev Immunol 1991;9:271.
343. Storb R, Deeg HJ, Farewell V, et al. Marrow transplantation for severe aplastic anemia: methotrexate alone compared with a combination of methotrexate and cyclosporine for prevention of acute graft-versus-host disease. Blood 1986;68: 119–125.
344. Storb R, Deeg HJ, Thomas ED, et al. Marrow transplantation for chronic myelocytic leukemia: a controlled trial of cyclosporine versus methotrexate for prophylaxis of graft-versus-host disease. Blood 1985;66:698–702.
345. Storb R, Epstein RB, Rudolph RH, Thomas ED. The effect of prior transfusion on marrow grafts between histocompatible canine siblings. J Imunol 1970;107:409–413.
346. Storb R, Prentice RL, Buckner CD, et al. Graft vs. host disease and survival in patients with aplastic anaemia treated by marrow grafts from HLA-identical siblings. N Engl J Med 1983;308:302–307.
347. Storb R, Prentice RL, Thomas ED. Marrow transplantation for treatment of aplastic anemia: an analysis of factors associated with graft rejection. N Engl J Med 1977;296: 61–66.
348. Storb R, Prentice RL, Thomas ED. Treatment of aplastic anemia by marrow transplantation from HLA identical siblings. J Clin Invest 1977;59:625–632.
349. Storb R, Prentice RL, Thomas ED, et al. Factors associated with graft rejection after HLA-identical marrow transplantation for aplastic anaemia. Br J Haematol 1983;55: 573–585.
350. Storb R, Thomas ED, Weiden PL, et al. Aplastic anemia treated by allogeneic bone marrow transplantation: a report of 49 new cases from Seattle. Blood 1976;48: 817–841.
351. Steilein WJ, Billingham RE. An analysis of graft-versus-host disease in Syrian hamsters. J Exp Med 1970;132:163–180.
353. Sullivan KM, Kopecky KJ, Jocom J, et al. Immunomodulatory and antimicrobial efficacy of intravenous immunoglobulin in bone marrow transplantation. N Engl J Med 1990;323:705–712.
354. Sullivan KM, Storb R, Shulman HR, et al. Immediate and delayed neurotoxicity after mechlorethamine preparation for bone marrow transplantation. Ann Intern Med 1982;97:182–189.
355. Sullivan KM, Mori M, Witherspoon R, et al. Alternating-day cyclosporine and prednisone (CSP/PRED) treatment of chronic graft-vs-host disease (GVHD): predictors of survival. Blood 1990;76(suppl 1):568a. Abstract.
356. Sullivan KM, Shulman HM, Storb R, et al. Chronic graft-versus-host disease in 52 patients: adverse natural course and successful treatment with combination immunosuppression. Blood 1981;57:267–276.
357. Sullivan KM, Witherspoon RP, Storb R, et al. Alternating day cyclosporine and prednisone for treatment for high risk chronic graft-versus-host disease. Blood 1988;72: 555–561.
358. Sullivan KM, Witherspoon RP, Storb R, et al. Prednisone and azathioprine compared with prednisone and placebo for treatment of chronic graft-versus-host disease: prognostic influence of prolonged thrombocytopenia after allogeneic marrow transplantation. Blood 1988;72:546–554.
359. Talpaz M, Kantarjian H, Kurzrock R, Gutterman J. Therapy of chronic myelogenous leukemia: chemotherapy and interferons. Semin Hematol 1988;25:62.
360. Talpaz M, Kantarjian H, Kurzrock R, Trugillo JM, Gutterman JU. Interferon-alpha produces sustained cytogenetic responses in chronic myelogenous leukemia. Ann Intern Med 1991;114:532–538.
361. Terenzi A, Lubin I, Lapidot T, et al. Enhancement of T-cell depleted bone marrow allografts in mice by thiotepa. Transplantation 1990;50:717.
362. Thomas ED, Buckner CD, Banaji M, et al. One hundred patients with acute leukemia treated by chemotherapy, total body irradiation and allogeneic marrow transplantation. Blood 1977;49:511–533.
363. Thomas ED, Buckner CD, Clift RA, et al. Marrow transplantation for acute nonlymphoblastic leukemia in first remission. N Engl J Med 1979;301:597–599.
364. Thomas ED, Buckner CD, Rudolph RH, et al. Allogeneic marrow grafting for hematologic malignancy using HLA matched donor recipient sibling pairs. Blood 1971;38: 267–287.
365. Thomas ED, Clift RA. Indications for marrow transplantation in chronic myelogenous leukemia. Blood 1989;73:861–864.
366. Thomas ED, Clift RA, Fefer A, et al. Marrow transplantation for the treatment of myelogenous leukemia. Ann Intern Med 1986;104:155–163.
367. Thompson CB, Sanders JE, Flournoy N, Buchner CD, Thomas ED. The risks of central nervous system relapse and leukoencephalopathy in patients receiving marrow transplants for acute leukemia. Blood 1986;67:195–199.
368. Tollemar J, Ringden O, Tyden G. Liposomal amphotericin -B (AmBisome)[R] treatment in solid organ and bone marrow transplant recipients. Efficacy and safety evaluation. Clin Transplant 1990;4:167–175.
369. Tricot G, Jagannath S, Vesole DH, Croley J, Barlogie B. Relapse of multiple myeloma after autologous transplantation: survival after salvage therapy. Bone Marrow Transplant 1995;16:7–11.
370. Trigg ME, Gingrich R, Goeken N, et al. Low rejection rate when using unrelated or haploidentical donors for children with leukemia undergoing marrow transplantation. Bone Marrow Transplant 1989;4:431–437.
371. Troussard X, Bauduer F, Galler E, et al. Virus recovery from stools of patients undergoing bone marrow transplantation. Bone Marrow Transplant 1993;12:573–576.
372. Truitt RL, LeFever AV, Charles CY, Jeske JM, Martin TM. Clonal basis of the graft-versus-leukemia effect induced by alloimmunization and its relationship to graft-versus-host disease. In Cellular Immunotherapy of Cancer. Edited by S Burakoff, J Deeg, J Ferrara, K Atkinson. New York: Alan R Liss, 1987, p 401–408.
373. Tsoi MS, Storb R, Dobbs S, et al. Non-specific suppressor cells in patients with chronic graft-versus-host disease after marrow grafting. J Immunol 1979;123:1970.
374. Tubergen D, Gilchest G, Coccia P, et al. The role of intensified chemotherapy in intermediate risk acute lymphoblastic leukemia (ALL) of childhood. Proc Am Soc Clin Oncol 1990;9:216.
375. Tura S, Cavo J, Gobbi M, et al. High-dose chemoradiotherapy and allogeneic bone marrow transplantation in multiple myeloma. Eur J Haematol 1989;43(suppl 51):191–195.
376. Tutschka PJ, Copelan EA, Klein JP. Bone marrow transplantation for leukemia following a new busulfan and cyclophosphamide regimen. Blood 1987;70:1382–1389.
377. Uzun O, Anaissie EJ. Antifungal prophylaxis in patients with hematologic malignancies: a reappraisal. Blood 1995;86:2063–2072.
378. van Bekkum DW, Lowenberg B. Bone Marrow Transplantation: Biological Mechanisms and Clinical Practice. New York: Dekker, 1985.
379. van Besien KW, Khouri IF, Giralt SA, et al. Allogeneic bone marrow transplantation for refractory and recurrent low-grade lymphoma: the case for aggressive management. J Clin Oncol 1995;13:1096–1102.
380. van Els CACM, D'Amaro J, Pool J, et al. Immunogenetics of human minor histocompatibility antigens: their polymorphism and immunodominance. Immunogenetics 1992;35:161–165.
381. van Rhee F, Lin F, Cullis JO, et al. Relapse of chronic myeloid leukemia after allogeneic bone marrow transplant: the case for giving donor leukocyte transfusions before the onset of hematologic relapse. Blood 1994;83:3377.
382. Vartdal F, Albrechtsen D, Ringden O, et al. Immunomagnetic treatment of bone marrow allografts. Bone Marrow Transplant 1987;2(suppl 2):94.
383. Vesole D, Tricot G, Jagannath S. Induction of graft-versus myeloma effect following allogeneic bone marrow transplantation. Blood 1994;84:331a.
384. Vogelsang GV, Farmer EB, Hess AD, et al. Thalidomide for the treatment of chronic graft versus host disease. N Engl J Med 1992;326:1055–1058.

385. Vogelsan GB, Hess AD, Santos GW. Acute graft-versus-host disease: clinical characteristics in the cyclosporine era. Medicine 1988;67:163–174.
386. Vogler WR, Winton EF, Heffner LT, et al. Ophthalmological and other toxicities related to cytosine arabinoside and total body irradiation as preparatory regimen for bone marrow transplantation. Bone Marrow Transplant 1990;6:405–409.
387. Voogt PJ, Goulmy WE, Fibbe WE, Veenhof WJF, Brand A, Falkenberg JHF. Minor histocompatibility antigen H-Y is expressed on human hematopoietic progenitor cells. J Clin Invest 1988;82:906–912.
388. Voogt PJ, Falkenburg JHF, Fibbe WE, et al. Normal hematopoietic progenitor cells and malignant lymphohematopoietic cells show different susceptibility to direct cell-mediated MHC-non-restricted lysis by T cell receptor $^-$/CD3$^-$ T cell receptor $\gamma\delta^+$/CD3$^+$ and T cell receptor-$\alpha\beta$/CD3$^+$ lymphocytes. J Immunol 1989;142:1774–1780.
389. Voogt PJ, Fibbe WE, Marijt WAF, et al. Rejection of bone marrow graft by recipient-derived cytotoxic T lymphocytes against minor histocompatibility antigens. Lancet 1990;335:131–134.
390. Walker RW, Brochstein JA. Neurologic complications of immunosuppressive agents. Neurol Clin 1988;6:261–278.
391. Walter EA, Greenberg PD, Gilbert MJ, et al. Reconstitution of cellular immunity against cytomegalovirus in recipients of allogeneic bone marrow by transfer of T-cell clones from the donor. N Engl J Med 1995;333:1038–1044.
392. Warner JF, Dennert G. Effects of a cloned cell line with NK activity on bone marrow transplants, tumour development and metastasis in vivo. Nature 1982;300:31–34.
393. Wegner SA, Laughlin C, McGarigle C, Bierer BE, Antin JH. Clofazimine therapy of chronic graft-v-host disease. Blood 1992;80(suppl 1):135a. Abstract.
394. Weiden PL, Flournoy N, Thomas ED, et al. Antileukemic effects of graft versus host disease in human recipients of allogeneic marrow grafts. N Engl J Med 1979;300:1068–1073.
395. Weiner RS, Bortin MB, Gale RP, et al. Interstitial pneumonitis after bone marrow transplantation: assessment of risk factors. Ann Intern Med 1986;104:168–175.
396. Weinstein HJ, Mayer RL, Rosenthal DS, Coral FS, Camitta BM, Gelber RD. Chemotherapy for acute myelogenous leukemia in children and adults: VAPA update. Blood 1983;62:315.
397. Weisdorf D, Filipovich A, McGlave P, et al. Combination graft-versus-host disease prophylaxis using immunotoxin (anti-CD5-RTA [Xomazyme-CD5]) plus methotrexate and cyclosporine or prednisone after unrelated donor marrow transplantation. Bone Marrow Transplant 1993;12:531–536.
398. White PC. Molecular genetics of the class III region of the HLA complex. Immunobiology of HLA, vol 2: In Immunogenetics and Histocompatibility. Edited by B Dupont. New York: Springer-Verlag, 1989, pp 62–69.
399. Wingard JR, Merz WG, Saral R. Candida tropicalis: a major pathogen in immunocompromised patients. Ann Intern Med 1979;91:539.
400. Wingard JR, Chen DY, Burns WH, et al. Cytomegalovirus infection after autologous bone marrow transplantation with comparison to infection after allogeneic bone marrow transplantation. Blood 1988;71:1432.
401. Wingard JR, Piantadosi S, Santos GW, et al. Allogeneic bone marrow transplantation for patients with high-risk acute lymphoblastic leukemia. J Clin Oncol 1990;8:820–830.
402. Wingard JRED, Mellitis MB, Sostrin DY-H, et al. Interstitial pneumonitis after allogeneic bone marrow transplantation. Nine-year experience at a single institution. Medicine 1988;67:175–186.
403. Winston DJ, Gale RP, Meyers DV, et al. Infectious complications of human bone marrow transplantation. Medicine 1979;58:1–31.
404. Winston DJ, Schiffman G, Wang DC, et al. Pneumococcal infections after human bone marrow transplantation. Ann Intern Med 1979;91:835–841.
405. Winston DJ, Huang E, Miller MJ, et al. Molecular epidemiology of cytomegalovirus infections associated with bone marrow transplantation. Ann Intern Med 1985;102:16–20.
406. Winston DJ, Ho WG, Bartoni K, DuMond C, Ebeling DF, Buhles WC, Champlin RE. Ganciclovir prophylaxis of cytomegalovirus infection and disease in allogeneic bone marrow transplant recipients. Ann Intern Med 1993;118:179.
407. Witherspoon RP, Fisher LD, Schoch G, et al. Secondary cancers after bone marrow transplantation for leukemia or aplastic anemia. N Engl J Med 1989:321:784–789.
408. Witherspoon RP, Lum LG, Storb R. Immunologic reconstitution after human marrow grafting. Semin Hematol 1984;21:2–10.
409. Wiznitzer M, Packer RJ, August CS, Burkey PA. Neurological complications of bone marrow transplantation in childhood. Ann Neurol 1984;15:569–576.
410. Wolf JL, Spruce WE, Bearman RM, et al. Reversal of acute ("malignant") myelosclerosis by allogeneic bone marrow transplantation. Blood 1982;59:191–193.
411. Woods WG, Nesbit ME, Ransay NKC, et al. Intensive therapy followed by bone marrow transplantation for patients with acute lymphocytic leukemia in second or subsequent remission: determination of prognostic factors (report from the University of Minnesota Bone Marrow Transplantation Team). Blood 1983;61:1182–1189.
412. Xun C, Brown SA, Jennings CD, Henslee-Downey PJ, Thompson JS. Acute graft-versus-host-like disease induced by transplanation of human activated natural killer cells into SCID mice. Transplantation 1993;56:409–417.
413. Yang SY, Morishima Y, Collins NH, et al. Comparison of one-dimensional IEF patterns for serologically detectable HLA-A and -B allotypes. Immunogenetics 1994;19:217.
414. Yeager A, Kaizer H, Santos GW, et al. Autologous bone marrow transplantation in patients with acute nonlymphocytic leukemia, using ex-vivo marrow treatment with 4-hydroperoxycyclophosphamide. N Engl J Med 1986;315:141–147.
415. Yunis EJ, Amos DB. Three closely linked genetic systems relevant to transplantation. Proc Natl Acad Sci USA 1971;68:3031.
416. Young JW, Papadopoulos E, Cunningham I, et al. T-cell-depleted allogeneic bone marrow transplanation in adults with acute nonlymphocytic leukemia in first remission. Blood 1992;79:3380–3387.
417. Zander AR, Keating M, Dicke K, et al. A comparison of marrow transplantation with chemotherapy for adults with acute leukemia of poor prognosis in first complete remission. J Clin Oncol 1988;6:1548–1557.
418. Zittoun RA, Mandelli F, Willemze R, et al. Autologous or allogeneic bone marrow transplantation compared with intensive chemotherapy in acute myelogenous leukemia. N Engl J Med 1995;332:217–223.
419. Zutter MM, Martin PJ, Sale GE, et al. Epstein-Barr virus lymphoproliferation after bone marrow transplantation. Blood 1988;72:520–529.

SECTION XXI

PRINCIPLES OF PSYCHO-ONCOLOGY

CHAPTER 87

Principles of Psycho-Oncology

JIMMIE C. HOLLAND

Introduction

Quality of life for patients at all stages of cancer has received increasing attention in recent years. More concern also has been directed toward understanding the stresses on families and the staff who care for patients with cancer. Research is more actively exploring social, behavioral, and psychologic contributions to cancer risk, detection, and survival. Psycho-oncology, which has emerged over the past two decades as a subspecialty of oncology, focuses on these areas and now has its own body of information, training, and research (46).

Psycho-oncology addresses the two major psychologic dimensions of cancer: the psychologic response of patients to cancer at all stages of disease as well as that of their families and their caretakers (i.e., psychosocial aspect); and the psychologic, behavioral, and social factors that influence risk, detection, and survival (i.e., psychobiologic aspect). To develop these aspects of oncology, several efforts are currently being pursued: training of a group of clinicians and investigators as psycho-oncologists; developing a psychologic component in the clinical training of all oncologic disciplines; encouraging research in the psychologic, humanistic, ethical, and spiritual aspects of patient care; incorporating quality-of-life concepts in clinical care and as an outcome variable in clinical trials; and an active exploration of brain, immune, and endocrine links through the new field of psychoneuroimmunology.

These psychologic dimensions impact on all aspects of oncology and the care of all patients. The clinical oncologic specialties (medical oncology, surgical, radiologic, gynecologic, orthopedic, urologic, pediatric, and neuro-oncology) are all affected. Epidemiology, cancer control and prevention, bioethics, palliative and supportive care, and both clinical trial research and decision-making have psychosocial and behavioral issues. Psychologic, social, and quality-of-life questions are now being added to research studies in these areas which traditionally have not included such inquiry (57).

To address psychologic issues, most cancer centers or oncology divisions in community hospitals now have programs to assist patients with psychologic distress and provide support for families and staff (34). The disciplines most often represented in these programs are nursing, social work, psychology, psychiatry, and chaplaincy. Trained volunteers, particularly those who have experienced cancer either personally or in their families, play an increasingly important role as well. Only a few centers have programs that include research and training. This chapter is an overview of present knowledge about the psychologic and social aspects of patient care and about the most significant psychiatric complications. The bibliography serves as a guide for seeking information in these separate areas, each of which has a rapidly expanding base of clinical and research information.

Historical Perspective

The stigma that cancer equals death, which has been attached to the disease for centuries, led to the long respected dictum that doctors should not tell patients that they had cancer (Table 87.1). The first effective treatment for cancer was surgery, beginning in Egypt over 500 years ago with amputations. The use of ether in 1847 and the advent of antisepsis led to the successful surgical removal of some tumors in the last half of the nineteenth century. By 1912, radiotherapy was becoming recognized as a potentially powerful additional treatment; by 1950, chemotherapy was added. Education of the public about the warning signals of cancer became more important to encourage early detection of curable cancer, but influencing patients' fatalistic attitudes was difficult. By the 1960s, multimodality therapy, combining surgery, radiation, and chemotherapy, along with immunotherapy, began to impact significantly on the grim survival statistics, especially in children and young adults.

By the early 1970s, as survival improved and U.S. society questioned all authority in the post-Vietnam War era, the diagnosis of cancer began to be more frequently revealed to patients. At about the same time, concern for more humane care of patients dying from cancer appeared in England with the beginning of the hospice movement. This spread to the United States slowly, however greater openness in revealing the diagnosis, increased concern for the dying, and enhanced concern about quality of life and the rights of patients led to more attention for the supportive and psychologic aspects of care. Evidence for the link of environmental exposures to cancer, particularly cigarette smoking, gave new impetus to examining the role of psychologic and behavioral factors in cancer prevention (49).

By 1970, the stage was set for greater interest in psychologic issues; however, tools to assess these variables were few. Early investigators were forced to develop new instruments or modify those originally developed to assess psychiatric patients, and investigators with knowledge of both

Table 87.1. Key Events in Cancer and Psycho-Oncology from 1850 to 1970

Year	Cancer	Behavioral/psychosocial
1850–1900	Anesthesia (1847) Antisepsis First cancer surgery	Cancer = death; word not used
1900–1936	Surgical excision Radiation = palliative American Cancer Society founded (1913)	Education about early detection
1937	National Cancer Institute founded	Enthusiasm for research Education for public
1940s	Nitrogen mustards First remission of leukemia by chemotherapy Radical surgery	Optimism about care Psychosomatic concepts Grief studied
1950s	First cure by drug alone (choriocarcinoma, 1956) Combination chemotherapy	First psychologic studies of cancer patients[a]
1960s	Prolonged survival from combined modalities	Debate about informing patient of diagnosis Peer support Consultation-liaison psychiatry

[a] Massachusetts General Hospital and Memorial Sloan-Kettering Cancer Center.

Table 87.2. Key Events In Psycho-Oncology from 1970 to 1995

Year	Behavior/psychosocial
1972	National Cancer Program National Cancer Plan: Control and Rehabilitation (first NCI-supported psycho-oncology studies)
1975	First National Psychosocial Research Conference
1976	First Psychiatry Committee in a Cooperative Group (CALGB)
1977–1984	Psychosocial Collaborative Group (PSYCOG) (five centers)
1977–1987	Project Omega (MGH) Child studies Pain research Breast cancer studies
1977	Psychiatry Service, Memorial Sloan-Kettering Clinical and Research Training Program Biennial Symposia on Current Concepts (6) First Chair of Psychiatric Oncology (1989)
1980	American Cancer Society Peer Review Committee for Psychosocial Review
1980s	Research Methodology Conferences (4)
1984	International Psycho-Oncology Society
1988	American Society for Psychiatric Oncology/AIDS
1990s	Use of Quality of Life Assessment as an outcome variable in cancer clinical trials Trials of psychosocial Interventions Studies of individuals at high genetic risk of cancer

NCI—National Cancer Institute.

cancer and social science research methods were few. During the 1970s and 1980s, remarkable progress was made, particularly in Europe and North America, in drawing attention to some behavioral and psychosocial issues in patient care, particularly delay, treatment compliance, and environmental exposures to tobacco.

In the early 1980s, as more clinicians and researchers began to share these interests, several national and regional groups devoted to psychosocial issues were created to provide a means of education and communication. The International Psychooncology Society (IPOS) was formed in 1984, and in 1988, the American Society for Psychiatric Oncology/AIDS. The National Cancer Institute and the American Cancer Society also began to encourage development of the field (Table 87.2). In addition, the psychiatric group at Memorial Sloan-Kettering Cancer Center, which was begun as the first psychiatric effort in a cancer hospital in 1950 by Sutherland, was reactivated in 1977 by Holland and colleagues, developing clinical and research training, publishing the first textbook of psycho-oncology and establishing an academic chair of psychiatric oncology. This brief history underscores the relative youth of this subspecialty of oncology compared to the mature fields of surgery, radiation, and chemotherapy. The major progress has been made in the past 20 years, and most of that, since the early 1980s. Areas reviewed in this chapter reflect the rapid development of diagnostic and treatment guidelines for common psychologic problems (e.g., depression and anxiety) that previously were poorly defined and therefore underdiagnosed and undertreated. These advances have been paralleled by those in pain management, which also is much better recognized and treated today.

Normal Adaptation to Cancer

REACTION TO DIAGNOSIS

Learning that one has cancer, or that a close relative has it, is a catastrophic event. Information of such import is processed mentally like any news of a personal loss (36, 43). The information has greater import, however, because of the meaning that individuals and society attach to cancer: death, disability, disfigurement, dependence, and disruption of relationships to others. These five easy-to-recall "Ds" reflect fears of death, of the uncertain future, and of possible physical changes and their impact on others. This period of crisis is an expected and normal emotional upheaval (Table 87.3) (49). The initial period usually is one of disbelief and denial that the news is true. During phase I, patients often

Table 87.3. Normal Response to Crises Encountered with Cancer

Phase	Symptoms	Time interval
Phase I: Initial response	Disbelief or denial or despair ("I knew it all along")	Usually less than 1 week
Phase II: Dysphoria	Anxiety, depressed mood, anorexia, insomnia, poor concentration, inability to function	Usually 1 to 2 weeks, but varies
Phase III: Adaptation	Accepts validity of information and begins dealing with the options available. Finds reasons for optimism and resumes usual activities	Usually by 2 weeks, but adaptation continues over months; may or may not be successful

seek to prove that the diagnosis is not true ("they must have mixed up the slides"). Feeling "numb" and appearing not to understand the import are common reactions, but this usually lasts less than a week. Some patients (a much smaller group) experience despair instead of denial; these are individuals who always feared or expected to develop cancer.

Phase II follows, which is characterized by a period of emotional turmoil and dysphoria in which reality is slowly recognized. The patient often becomes anxious and depressed, has poor concentration and diminished appetite, is unable to sleep, and is unable to maintain his or her daily routine. Thoughts of illness and death frequently recur and cannot be dispelled. This period may last 1 to 2 weeks, usually dissipating as the person begins treatment and to sense that all is not lost. A therapeutic alliance with the doctor encourages a return of optimism through co-operation with a treatment plan. Some patients, at times prompted by a family member, seek second or multiple opinions until they find the oncologic plan that best fits their concepts.

Phase III represents the longer-term adaptation, lasting from weeks to months, in which the patient adjusts to the diagnosis and treatment, finds reason for compartmentalized optimism, and returns to normal routines and ways of coping that were characteristic and successful in the past. The quality of this adaptation depends on the patient's prior level of adjustment and emotional maturity. It is important that family, friends, and staff be aware that there is no single way to cope (42, 77). Individuals have their own coping styles that, for better or worse, have gotten them through prior life crises. There is a strong tendency in today's society to demand that individuals with cancer have a positive attitude to "beat it.". They are made to feel guilty if they do not, and they often are told that the absence of a positive attitude leads to faster tumor growth. While these strategies work well for some individuals, they do not for others (42). Respect for each individual's way of coping is critically important.

This sequence of disbelief, dysphoria, and adaptation may reappear with each new crisis that occurs in the course of illness. Depression becomes more prominent when the news is progressive disease or treatment failure.

FACTORS IN ADAPTATION

While the acute response to catastrophic news is similar in most patients at the time of diagnosis, individuals vary widely in how well or how poorly they adapt to cancer. Therefore, it is, important to recognize factors that predict good or poor adjustment, thereby enabling early identification of particularly vulnerable individuals (44). Factors that contribute to adaptation derive from three areas: (*a*) society derived, which are the social attitudes and beliefs about cancer that impact on the patient; (*b*) patient derived, which are the personal attributes the person brings to illness; and, (*c*) the cancer derived, which represent the clinical reality of the illness to which the patient must adapt (Table 87.4.)

Table 87.4. Factors that Determine Psychologic Adjustment to Cancer

- Society derived
  - Open discussion of diagnosis vs. unrevealed secret
  - Knowledge of treatment options, prognosis, and participation as partner
  - Popular beliefs (stress causes cancer)
- Patient derived
  - Intrapersonal
    - Coping ability; emotional maturity at time of cancer; philosophic, spiritual, or religious beliefs that influence coping
    - Developmental stage at time of cancer and meaning of curtailed goals (e.g., marriage, children)
  - Interpersonal
    - Spouse, family, friends (social support)
- Cancer derived
  - Site, stage, symptoms (especially pain) and prognosis
  - Treatment required (surgery, radiation, chemotherapy) and sequelae (immediate and delayed)
  - Altered body structure or function, rehabilitation/restoration available
  - Psychologic management by the treating staff

Society-derived Factors

The society-derived factors are dynamic, changing as people change their perceptions of medicine, illness, and cancer. Long feared and stigmatized, cancer is somewhat less fearsome today. The diagnosis is more routinely given and the public justifiably becomes more optimistic about the outcome, particularly among those in the prime of life. Coupled with society's demands for informed consent and for knowledge of treatment options, better communication between doctor and patient has been a positive spin-off. This has resulted, however, in an added burden for the patient because of the fuller knowledge of the realistic prognosis that is associated with each treatment option. Uncertainty about the future thus is far greater today. An additional burden is the widely popularized belief that stress causes cancer. Some patients mistakenly feel that they themselves, by some stressful event or events they did not manage properly, caused their cancer to develop.

Patient-derived Factors

The patient-derived factors come from three sources that affect adaptation: developmental stage at which cancer occurs; intrapersonal factors, and interpersonal social resources. The developmental stage of the person at the time that cancer develops, in relation to biologic, personal, and social life tasks and goals, determines the meaning of certain losses, such as fertility and altered appearance. Actual and potential losses have different meaning at different stages of life.

An awareness of the individual's developmental stage and its expected psychologic and social tasks permits a better understanding of the meaning of cancer to that individual. Because of this insight, strategies for successful intervention often can be deduced. Each age has its particular life tasks that must be taken into account by the clinician. Table 87.5 outlines developmental stages, giving the normal tasks that must be achieved at each age, the disruption that cancer produces, and the interventions that can be employed to minimize the deleterious effects of illness on development. These are particularly important in childhood and adolescence to maintain normal developmental milestones. Detailed developmental tables of the life cycle have been published elsewhere (67).

The intrapersonal resources a person brings to the illness are those derived by way of personality, emotional maturity, coping strategies, and prior experiences (68). A prior psychiatric disturbance usually means greater vulnerability during physical illness (44). The patient's social environment provides the interpersonal resources of family, friends, and social support that materially contribute, positively or negatively. Each variable contributes to the strength and weakness of resources that are central to adaptation, and they should be assessed in each patient. With this knowledge, an individualized plan for psychosocial support and intervention can be developed.

Much has been written on coping with cancer. Serious illness calls on coping abilities to accomplish several goals: (*a*) *to keep distress within manageable levels;* (*b*) to maintain a sense of personal worth; (*c*) to restore or maintain relations with significant others; (*d*) to enhance recovery and physical function; and (*e*) to work out a socially acceptable post illness status with maximal physical function (43). Taken overall, good coping strategies appear to be important in main-

Table 87.5. Developmental Stages and Cancer

Stage	Tasks	Disruption	Intervention
Children			
Childhood (early)	Motor	Developmental	Physical/social
	Speech	Slowing	Stimulation
	Cognition	Regression	Structured play
	Family Bonding	Separation anxiety	Increasing family contact
	Socialization	Withdrawal	Continuity of staff
	Confidence	Increasing fears (pain)	Trust of staff
Childhood (late)	Prepubertal	Being "different"	Maintain appearance
	Peer relations	School phobia	Minimize absences
	Intellectual and physical prowess	Death fears	Discuss illness and monitor responses
Adolescents and Adults			
Adolescence	Menarche/puberty	Alopecia/amputation "Differentness"	Maintain appearance
	Peer acceptance	Decreasing school/physical performance	Maintain peer contact
	Increasing independence	Increasing dependence	Support independence
	Sexual experimentation	Conflicts about self and sexuality	Counseling
	Formation of identity	Impact of illness	Counseling
Adult (young)	Intimacy	Decreasing attractiveness	Maintain appearance
	Marriage	Sterility/impotence	Sex counseling
	Parental role	Decreasing family role	Homemaker
			Support children
	Work role	Disruption of job performance	Decreasing job interruptions
Adult (middle)	Changing hormonal status/menopause	Altered appearance	Maintain appearance
	Older children	Disrupted marital/family role	Counseling (patient and family)
	"Empty nest"	Disrupted achievements	Financial planning
	Peak of career		
Adult (old)	Aging changes	Increasing physical/emotional	Health related
	Physical limitations	Services to maintain	Care of self
	Adjustment to increasing losses	Increasing dependence on others	Social support system
	Increasing social support needed	Increasing isolation	Promote social/familial network
	Retirement	Decreasing financial security	Financial planning

Table 87.6. Predictors of Poor Coping with Cancer

Social isolation
Low socioeconomic status
Alcohol or drug abuse
Prior psychiatric history
Prior experience with cancer (e.g., death of a relative)
Recent losses/bereavement
Inflexibility and rigidity of coping
Pessimistic philosophy of life
Absence of a belief/value system
Multiple obligations

Adapted from Holland and Rowland (49).

taining a sense of control, optimism, and acceptance of the facts while seeking constructive, positive approaches to illness and treatment as well as sharing information and obtaining support from others. Coping ability is influenced by personality, level of illness, and other factors, such as spiritual and religious beliefs. For many individuals, religion supplies an existential view of life, death, and illness, a Supreme Being from whom help can be requested; and a supportive social community. For others, philosophic or spiritual beliefs provide the meaning to illness, life, and death that helps in coping.

Prior experience with cancer often is a negative factor, especially when it relates to childhood memories regarding the death of a parent or sibling from cancer. Chronic hypochondriasis and cancerophobia appear to be more common following such early experiences. The death of a relative from the same tumor adds a particularly heavy burden. Table 87.6 outlines the major predictors of poor coping that can readily be elicited in a standard medical history, thus identifying those patients who would benefit most from early intervention (74). In addition, these individuals who have survived extreme experiences (e.g., Holocaust survivors) may have more distress in coping with cancer (63).

Cancer-derived Factors

The cancer-derived factors that contribute to adaptation constitute the clinical facts of stage of disease at diagnosis, site of the cancer, symptoms (especially pain), and prognosis; the type(s) of treatment required and their impact on function, both immediate and long-term; and the extent of rehabilitation that is possible and the psychologic management by the health-care team. The wise and sensitive physician often becomes an important source of interpersonal support, offering concern and "caring" in the context of professional ministrations (36). Absence of such a relationship is a negative factor that must be addressed by providing added support from other members of the team, such as the nurse, social worker, or mental-health professional.

PSYCHOSOCIAL PROBLEMS

Psychosocial problems of patients are quite different depending on the stage of their illness. Interventions to reduce distress must take the stage, treatment, and prognosis into account. The four categories that require different approaches are: (*a*) patients receiving active treatment with cure as a goal; (*b*) patients receiving palliative care with control or comfort as a goal; (*c*) patients who have completed active treatment and who are survivors, although outcome remains uncertain; and (*d*) presymptomatic, healthy individuals who have a known genetic risk of cancer.

Adaptation to Active Treatment

In patients undergoing active treatment, the goal of psychosocial care is to support their ability to cope with the stresses of treatment and to reduce their distress, which can be viewed from the perspective of "short-term loss, long-term gain." (55) The goal of cure encourages most individuals to tolerate the temporary discomfort and side effects of surgery, chemotherapy, and radiation, and to adapt to the permanent losses or organ-preserving procedures that may be necessary to achieve successful antineoplastic treatment (64). Many clinical trials today measure quality of life as an outcome variable in determining the efficacy of a new agent (see the discussion of quality-of-life-assessment later) (23). Control of anxiety, depression, delirium, nausea and vomiting, and encouraging adherence to treatment are examples of the symptom control and support needed (see the discussion of interventions later). Counseling, self-help groups, cognitive-behavioral interventions, and psychopharmacologic agents all represent interventions available to control psychologic symptoms and distress. Most symptoms can be controlled with careful evaluation and thoughtful intervention (12).

Adaptation to Palliative Care

The transition from a curative approach to a palliative one is extremely difficult for the patient, family, and the physician who has worked with the patient through months of arduous treatment. This transition constitutes a crisis that carries greater anguish than that experienced at the time of initial diagnosis (21). A transient period of distress, however, is followed by adaptation to the new reality and a new therapeutic goal, consonant with the individual's way of coping before illness. The patient who senses a physician's commitment to continued care and maximal quality of life has an easier adjustment. Issues such as appointing a health proxy and discussion of wishes about resuscitation and life-sustaining measures are best discussed early rather than late. Decisions about where care will be given need to be discussed, as well as assessing whether the family can manage the patient at home. Patients appear to do better when care can be given at home; the grieving relative also benefits from the closeness of the last days. Increasing availability of support to help families manage at home, using nurse clinicians with expertise in pain and psychiatric management in home-care programs is an encouraging sign (69). Considerable information exists today about symptom control and comfort care in advanced stages of illness, with better control of pain, anorexia, constipation, dyspnea, weakness, weight loss, and psychologic distress. There are growing numbers of controlled trials for medication, behavioral, and psychologic interventions for better palliation, which suggests a greater concern for quality of life. Many studies are being done in programs of hospice and home care, which increasingly collaborate with cancer centers (13).

A mental-health professional may be requested when it is difficult for the family or patient to confront the reality that treatment now aims at containment and comfort rather than cure. The patient, family, and physician have been allied in a course of treatment with the hope for cure or, at least, control of the disease. The transition is accompanied by a confrontation with death that may largely have been denied to this point. A sense of hopelessness may be countered by participation in experimental programs that offer some hope and from which information may be gleaned to help other patients in the future, as in phase I and II trials. This more aggressive approach is preferred by some patients who do not find it acceptable to give up "fighting."

Other decisions follow rapidly, including where care is to be given and how aggressive life-sustaining efforts should be. Ideally, both patients and families are better off emotionally if the patient can be managed at home. Home care often requires active professional support to see the family through it, and preexisting psychiatric disorders in the patient or family will require special, and often intensive, management during this time. A special Home Care Program within the Psychiatry Service at Memorial Sloan-Kettering Cancer Center addresses those patients whose psychiatric difficulties complicate their care (69).

Symptom control becomes critical and often benefits from a psychiatric consultation. Evaluation of mental status and mood to recognize changes indicative of delirium, anxiety, or depression is frequent in advanced disease (discussed later). Comfort care must focus on control of pain, psychologic distress, and suffering, as well as fatigue, weakness, nausea, vomiting, pain, hiccough, anorexia, and insomnia. Portenoy and colleagues measured symptom type and prevalence in patients with cancer and identified the most common to be fatigue, weakness, pain, and emotional distress (64).

Adaptation to Being a Survivor

One of the growing and increasingly vocal group of patients are those who have completed active treatment and, on returning to their lives and routine, find it helpful to share their experience with others. The National Coalition of Cancer Survivors is an advocacy group providing a voice in health policy and care. It publishes practical and sensitive "how-to" books for survivors. Concern about delayed physical effects, risk of recurrent or second cancers, and sterility are common. The negative dose-related effects of cranial radiation in children have been found to result in underachievement in school and significant neuropsychologic impairment (16). Remediation research has been slow to start, but it is beginning.

Studies of young adult survivors of Hodgkin's disease, acute leukemia, and testicular cancer reveal some psychosocial characteristics that appear to apply to survivors across tumor sites (Table 87.7) (56). First, there is an early, positive effect of a greater appreciation of life and often a search for the meaning of life and worthwhile goals. Importantly, even psychologically healthy individuals emerge from cancer treatment without serious psychologic sequelae or serious psychiatric disorders. Subtle and sometimes significantly increased levels of anxiety are present, however, which focus on possible recurrence and death (i.e., Damocles syndrome), as well as a greater sense of vulnerability and lower self-esteem. This uncertainty becomes frank anxiety at times of follow-up evaluations and development of minor symptoms when blood tests and imaging studies are performed. Even when no treatment-related gonadal toxicity is present, there often is lower sexual desire and poorer sexual satisfaction and performance. These sexual problems likely reflect the lower self-confidence of the patient in intimate relationships.

Table 87.7. Psychosocial Sequelae in Cancer Survivors

Positive effect of appreciating life more
Major psychiatric disorders are uncommon
Subtle psychologic distress is common
Anxiety about recurrence/illness/death (Damocles syndrome)
Greater sense of vulnerability (less control, lower self-esteem)
Reminders (smells, sights) of chemotherapy produce anxiety and nausea
Marital and sexual problems (not treatment related); less sense of attractiveness, lower sexual desire, poorer sexual performance
Career goals altered negatively (fewer risks, less ability to change jobs)
Job and health insurance problems

Career goals suffer from difficulty in changing jobs and pursuing career goals with the same vigor, based in part on realistic concerns about health insurance and prejudice about having had cancer. Chemotherapy results in longlasting, conditioned, Pavlovian responses to reminders of the treatment situation where nausea and vomiting occurred with cyclic chemotherapy. Conditioned anxiety was seen by Jacobsen and colleagues (52) as a part of the outcome. The finding of posttraumatic stress disorder (PTSD) in patients after cancer treatment raises the question of the relation of learned responses and the development of PTSD. Cella and colleagues (20) found that smells, tastes, and sights that were reminders of treatment, even as long as 11 years later, resulted in a sudden sense of unexplained anxiety and nausea (but rarely vomiting) that only, on reflection was recognized as a reminder of prior treatment (20). Anxiety diminishes over time, especially after the first 5 years associated with maximal risk of recurrence, but it continues to be exacerbated at times of periodic medical examinations or appearance of minor symptoms.

Adaptation to Increased Genetic Risk of Cancer

Healthy individuals increasingly recognize that they are at risk of cancer by virtue of others in their family having it. They are informed today about the increased risk of breast, colon, ovarian, and prostate cancer among first-degree relatives as well as of melanoma and endocrine tumors (MENS I and II). The psychologic impact of this knowledge results in a new and increasing number of individuals who are healthy and fearful of disease. They constitute the "worried well" who must deal with knowledge of enhanced risk despite present good health. Some perceive themselves as "walking time bombs." In a study by Kash and colleagues of women with two or more first-degree relatives with breast cancer (54, 58) those most anxious were least able to carry out regular breast self-examination or have mammograms, despite their importance because of the higher risk. How to counsel these women is being actively studied. Women usually overestimate their actual risk, and genetic counseling is helpful. They need support in carrying out breast self-examination and in regular physicals and mammograms. Factors that may reduce risk, such as diet, tamoxifen, and prophylactic mastectomy, must be explained. Many questions arise about whether replacement hormones raise the risk of breast cancer (9, 58).

The public regularly receives news of each new cancer gene as it is discovered. They assume that germline DNA testing is "just around the corner." Linkage studies have provided some background for understanding individuals' responses to learning their gene-carrier status. Biesecker and colleagues (9) outlined the issues that have emerged in families with the BRCAI mutation. Before germline testing becomes feasible clinically, it is important to develop guidelines for several aspects: pretesting information and counseling; post testing counseling about the meaning of the results, follow-up and options; and identification of those who are psychologically vulnerable. The impact within a family also is apt to be significant: who to tell, how to tell family members, and what to do about minors.

Results of gene testing have great potential for social harm. Discrimination in the workplace, for health and life insurance, and breach of privacy regarding the information all are areas of major potential effects. The potential harm to minors is particularly worrisome. The Institute of Medicine and the Human Genome Project have examined the social policy issues, suggesting that there must be federal oversight of laboratories for the quality of their work, assurances of confidentiality, and availability of guidelines for counseling those tested. A major educational effort for the public also will be needed (4).

PSYCHIATRIC DISORDERS

When patients cope with serious illness, responses of fear, worry, and sadness are expected and normal. Usually, they are transient and dissipate as a crisis passes. When these normal emotions become persistent, pervasive, and distressing, however, they may become a deterrent to treatment. At this point, worry and sadness that exceed normal become identifiable as anxiety or depression. Such "symptoms" should be evaluated and, if significant, treated. Sensitivity to this dimension of care requires the ability to evaluate a psychologic symptom, recognizes the clusters of symptoms that represent a psychiatric disorder, and be able to identify treatment options and resources (7, 34). There is considerable interest in finding self-report measures that could be filled out in clinics and would identify and "red flag" those who are most vulnerable to developing significant distress (74).

The most common form of distress in patients with cancer is anxiety, and the next most common is depression. They are often seen together. Anxiety is best considered as a symptom that exists on a continuum, ranging from normal fears to situational anxiety and, finally, to a disabling anxiety disorder. Depression is on a continuum from sadness, which increases to reactive depression and, finally, to its most severe form, major depression. Prior vulnerability to depressions or bipolar disorder predicts a recurrence during physical illness.

A prevalence study at three cancer centers of psychiatric disorders in patients with cancer (60% inpatients and 40% outpatients) but uncontrolled for stage of disease (28), found that 53% were coping adequately despite the stresses they were encountering. However, 47% had levels of distress that reached diagnostic criteria for a psychiatric disorder; among these patients, 32% showed a mixture of reactive depression and anxiety (adjustment disorder with depressed anxious mood, in the DSM-III classification of psychiatric disorders). Six percent had major depression; 4% organic mental disorders; 3% personality disorder and/or alcohol abuse; and 2% anxiety disorders. Data support the premise that most psychiatric disturbances in patients with cancer directly relate to illness. Indeed, the predominant symptoms seen in one-third of all patients were combined reactive anxiety and depression, with one or the other predominating. Farber and colleagues (30) and Stefanek and colleagues (74), studying outpatients in oncology clinics, independently found that one-third had significantly high levels of distress. Using a form of the SCL-90, they found that between 20 and 30% of patients had clinically relevant levels of distress. The percentage of distressed patients rises in hospitalized patients because of greater disability, pain, and treatments that produce confusional states (14). These forms of distress from depression or anxiety and confusional states (organic mental disorders) constitute by far the most likely psychiatric diagnoses encountered.

Anxiety Disorders

Anxiety is the most common form of psychologic distress in patients with cancer. It occurs from four sources: (*a*) situational (functional) anxiety in response to a frightening aspect of illness or treatment, (*b*) as a manifestation of disease, (*c*) as a symptom resulting from treatment, and (*d*) as an exacerbation of a preexisting anxiety disorder (Table 87.8). Situational anxiety occurs at the time of diagnosis, with anticipation of a procedure or new treatment, at transitional points in illness, after treatment is finished, and as a recurrent concern, even years later, about exacerbation of disease. Fears of recurrence appear to be present to some degree in all cancer survivors (Table 87.7); however, in some individuals the level of anxiety can be so pervasive that it interferes with their ability to function and requires treatment.

Anxiety related to medical problems most often is seen as an accompaniment to poorly controlled pain; it usually disappears when pain is adequately controlled (Table 87.9). Anxiety also occurs with abnormal metabolic states such as hypoxia, pulmonary embolus, sepsis, delirium, bleeding, cardiac arrhythmia, and hypoglycemia. Hormone-secreting tumors that produce anxiety are pheochromocytoma, thyroid adenoma or carcinoma, parathyroid adenoma, ACTH-producing tumors, and insulinoma.

Table 87.8. Causes of Anxiety in Patients with Cancer

Situational
- Diagnosis of cancer, prognosis discussion
- Crisis, illness/treatment
- Conflicts with family or staff
- Anticipating a frightening procedure
- Awaiting results of tests
- Fears of recurrence

Disease related
- Poorly controlled pain
- Abnormal metabolic states
- Hormone secreting tumors
- Paraneoplastic syndromes (remote CNS effects)

Treatment related
- Frightening or painful procedures (MRI, scans, wound debridement)
- Anxiety-producing drugs (antiemetic neuroleptics, bronchodilators)
- Withdrawal states (opioids, benzodiazepines, alcohol)
- Conditioned (anticipatory) anxiety, nausea, and vomiting with cyclic chemotherapy

Exacerbation of preexisting anxiety disorder
- Phobias (needles, claustrophobia)
- Panic or generalized anxiety disorders
- Posttraumatic stress disorder (Holocaust survivors, Vietnam veterans, recall of the death of a relative with cancer)

CNS–Central nervous system.

Table 87.9. Anxiety Related to Common Medical Problems in Cancer

Medical problems	Examples
Poorly controlled pain	Unresponsive or undertreated pain
Abnormal metabolic states	Hypoxia, pulmonary embolus, sepsis, fever, delirium, hypoglycemia, bleeding, coronary occlusion and heart failure, cardiac arrhythmia
Hormone-secreting tumors	Pheochromocytoma, thyroid adenoma or carcinoma, parathyroid adenoma, ACTH-producing tumors, insulinoma
Anxiety-producing drugs	Corticosteroids, neuroleptics used as antiemetics, thyroxine, bronchodilators, β-adrenergic stimulants, antihistamines, (paradoxic reactions), withdrawal states (alcohol, narcotic analgesics, sedative-hypnotics)
Side effects of treatment	Allergic skin rash to antibiotics, unexpected toxicity (e.g., diarrhea)

Among cancer treatment–related causes of anxiety, the most common are: anxiety related to frightening or painful procedures, especially those occurring repeatedly, such as wound debridement. Approximately 20% of patients have trouble tolerating imaging procedures such as the MRI or CT because of the small, enclosed space, which triggers claustrophobic fears. Approximately 5% are unable to undergo it. Several drugs frequently used in cancer also produce symptoms of anxiety: corticosteroids, neuroleptics used as antiemetics, bronchodilators, thyroxine, and stimulants. Unexplained restlessness, anxiety, and agitation often develop in patients who receive large doses of metoclopramide or other neuroleptics during chemotherapy for the control of nausea and vomiting as part of the extrapyramidal symptoms of akathesias and dystonias. Withdrawal states from alcohol, narcotic analgesics, and sedative-hypnotics produce anxiety as a prominent symptom and must be kept in mind. Unexpected effects of treatment or toxicity also lead to heightened anxiety, especially when the etiology is unclear.

Some patients undergoing cyclic chemotherapy using an emetogenic regimen begin to develop anticipatory anxiety, nausea, and vomiting by about the third cycle, a few days to hours in advance of receiving the next cycle of treatment (5, 52, 66). This is a learned, conditioned, Pavlovian autonomic response to the repeated experience of nausea and vomiting. In fact, two-thirds of women receiving adjuvant chemotherapy for breast cancer develop conditioned anxiety and nausea, although not usually vomiting. The response has been seen as long as 12 years later on encountering smells or tastes that reminded the person of the chemotherapy received for Hodgkin's disease (20). Behavioral interventions and antianxiety medication are effective in controlling symptoms. The response does not develop when nausea and vomiting during chemotherapy are controlled, as is the case with the increasingly effective antiemetic regimens.

Patients who have preexisting phobias, panic attacks, generalized anxiety, or posttraumatic stress disorders are at risk of exacerbating their symptoms during cancer treatment (Table 87.8) (59). Phobias of needles, blood, hospitals, claustrophobia, or agoraphobia sometimes are troublesome symptoms during treatment. Panic attacks and generalized anxiety symptoms must be controlled to enable the patient to tolerate anxiety-provoking medical treatments. Patients who experienced the Holocaust or have traumatic memories of war or frightening events may recall these painful memories during illness and treatment (63). Individuals who recall the death of a relative from cancer, especially when it was the same neoplasm, have more anxiety.

The treatment of simple situational anxiety usually is handled adequately by the physician, who reassures the patient, reviews frightening anticipated events, allows the person to "rehearse" them, and engenders confidence that the person can cope with the feared treatment or procedure (Table 87.10). The oncology nurse or social worker often is helpful in reviewing circumstances more fully and adding reassurance. For persistent or distressing anxiety, three means of treatment are available: counseling (by individual or group means and by professional or peer counseling), behavioral, and pharmacologic means. Counseling or formal psychotherapy using a supportive crisis intervention model is helpful (15, 32, 61). Fawzy and colleagues (34) outlined the range of psychosocial interventions that have been proven efficacious in controlled trials. There are several forms being tried: psychoeducational, interpersonal psychotherapy (IPT), supportive, and cognitive-behavioral. Several behavioral interventions are effective: relaxation exercises with guided imagery and hypnosis most frequently are employed. These methods are particularly helpful to patients who wish to maintain and enhance their beleaguered sense of control over their emotions and body. Relaxation is a useful adjunct to pain control and for control of conditioned chemotherapy-related nausea and vomiting (66).

Significant anxiety symptoms most often are treated pharmacologically by sedative-hypnotics from the benzodiazepine class of drugs, but other types also are effective, such as antihistamines, β-blockers, and neuroleptics in low dose (Table 87.10). Many patients feel it is a sign of weakness to accept medication and must be encouraged to use them during a crisis period. The benzodiazepine is chosen by the desired half-life and route of administration, with knowledge of its metabolism and active metabolites (Table 87.11). A shorter half-life provides better control and less likelihood of poor elimination and oversedation. Patients whose anxiety manifests as insomnia respond to a bedtime dose of temazepam, 15 mg; triazolam, 25 mg; or clonazepam, 1 mg; or zolpidem, 5 mg. Daytime anxiety responds to lorazepam, .5 mg or alprazolam, .25-.50 mg tid or qid or clonazepam, .5 mg bid, which is longer acting, as well as to diazepam. It is important to taper these medications to prevent a mild increase in anxiety or withdrawal symptoms. Buspirone is useful, because it has no sedating effects and no addictive qualities. The neuroleptic, thioridazine is useful in low dose (10 mg qid) when a benzodiazepine is contraindicated, as in older individuals. Haloperidol, .5 to 1.0 mg bid, and chlorpromazine, 25 to 50 mg also are useful (59).

Table 87.10. Treatment of Anxiety Disorders

Treatment modality	Components
Supportive psychotherapy	Providing information, rehearsal of feared events, reassurance
Behavioral	Relaxation
	Hypnosis
	Systematic desensitization
Psycho-pharmacologic	Benzodiazepines
	Short acting (alprazolam, lorazepam, oxazepam)
	Long acting (diazepam, clorazepate, clonazepam)
	β-Blockers (propranolol)
	Tricyclic antidepressants (amitriptyline, doxepin, nortriptyline)
	Monoamine oxidase inhibitors (phenelzine, isocarboxazid)
	Antihistamines
	Neuroleptics (thioridazine, trifluperazine, haloperidol)
	Buspirone
Combinations of the above	

Adapted from Massie (59).

Table 87.11. Commonly Prescribed Benzodiazepines in Cancer Patients

Drug	Approximate dose equivalent	Initial dosage po (mg)	Half-life (h)
Short to intermediate half-life			
Alprazolam	0.5	0.25–0.50 tid	10–15
Chlordiazepoxide	10.0	10–25 tid	5–30
Clonazepam	1.0	0.5 bid	18–50
Lorazepam[a]	1.0	0.5–2.0 tid	10–20
Oxazepam	10.0	10–15 tid	5–15
Temazepam[b]	15.0	15–30 qhs	10–15
Triazolam[b]	0.25	0.125–0.250 qhs	1.5
Zolpidem[b]	5.0	5.0–10.0 qhs	2–4
Long half–life			
Chlorazepate	7.5	7.5–15.0 bid	30–200
Diazepam	5.0	5–10	20–70

[a] Lorazepam also can be administered intramuscularly; other benzodiazepines are erratically absorbed when given intramuscularly.
[b] Hypnotic agents.

Depression

While it is expected and normal for a patient to feel sad on learning a diagnosis of cancer or hearing news that another crisis related to illness has occurred, some individuals experience far greater distress, at a level that is abnormal and constitutes a diagnosable depressive disorder. It is important to keep in mind that depression does respond to treatment and should not be left untreated because it is "based on current reality." A recent review by McDaniel and colleagues (60) provided prevalence, biology, and treatment data.

Depression is difficult to diagnose in patients with cancer, because the neoplastic disease itself may produce fatigue, weakness, loss of libido, loss of interest or concentration, and of motivation. Most depressive disorders are reactive to illness (called *adjustment disorders*) and are seen in approximately 25% of oncology patients in the clinic; the percentage is higher in hospitalized patients (14). Symptoms of depression are dysphoric mood, insomnia, restlessness, psychomotor slowing, a sense of hopelessness and helplessness, and suicidal ideation. Psychotic depressive symptoms such as delusions of guilt are rare. Table 87.12 outlines

Table 87.12. Evaluation of Depression and Predisposing Factors

Evaluative category	Findings
Family history	Depression
	Suicide
Personal history	Previous psychiatric illness (depression or manic episodes, alcoholism, drug abuse)
	Suicide attempt
Signs and symptoms	Psychologic
	Dysphoric mood (e.g., sad, depressed, anxious, crying, diurnal mood change)
	Feelings of hopelessness; helplessness
	Loss of interest and pleasure
	Guilt, burden on others, worthlessness
	Poor concentration
	Mood incongruent to disease outlook
	Suicidal thoughts or plans
	Delusional thoughts (psychotic symptoms rare, except in organic affective syndrome)
	Somatic (less interpretable in more physically impaired patients)
	Insomnia
	Anorexia and weight loss
	Fatigue
	Psychomotor retardation or agitation
	Constipation
	Decreased libido

the history and symptoms that are relevant to making a diagnosis of major depression. A family history of depression or bipolar illness and prior personal psychiatric disorder or substance abuse should be explored. Evaluation should explore mental status, signs and symptoms of mood, hopelessness, feeling of being a burden, and suicidal ideation. Insomnia, anorexia, fatigue, agitation, or psychomotor retardation may relate to illness and must be interpreted in light of that fact; they also serve as symptoms that can be monitored for treatment effect.

Table 87.13 outlines the major risk factors that predict which individuals are most likely to develop significant depression during cancer. A history of depression or attempted suicide, substance abuse, poor social supports, or recent bereavement is important. In terms of illness, greater levels of debilitation, advanced disease and presence of another chronic illness or disability predict depression. Several medications contribute: steroids, some chemotherapeutic agents (interferon, vincristine), and medications given for other reasons. Depression appears as a part of the metabolic picture of organ failure and with some nutritional, endocrine, and neurologic complications of cancer. It is a common symptom of pancreatic cancer, which has led to speculation about a tumor-induced mood change.

Depression is managed first by maintaining good rapport with the patient and assuring support from available family or friends. Supportive psychotherapeutic as well as behavioral interventions and psychotropic agents are important resources for the treatment of depression. Behavioral interventions are effective in depression using cognitive-behavioral methods, which encourage the patient to reframe the problems more constructively and to approach each aspect intellectually, with a planned response that reduces uncontrolled distressing emotions. This has been particularly helpful in coping with the meaning of pain, which is so frightening in cancer when viewed as evidence of tumor progression. Cognitive approaches also can alter distressing sensations and responses to them (12).

Psychotropic drugs have been shown in clinical trials to be effective in controlling depressive symptoms with medical illness, including cancer. Table 87.14 lists the most frequently used antidepressant medications in patients with cancer and their starting and maintenance dose (25). The antidepressants commonly used are the tricyclics, second-generation antidepressants, heterocyclics, selective serotonin-reuptake inhibitors (SSRIs), monoamine oxidase inhibitors, psychostimulants, lithium carbonate, and benzodiazepines. The SSRIs are first line now because of their efficacy and low side-effects profile. Fluoxetine has been widely used, as well as paroxetine and sertraline. Venlafaxine has become available, representing a serotonin and norepinephrine-reuptake inhibitor. Nefazodone, which is similar in effect to trazodone, offers a safe, new, and effective antidepressant. Tricyclics

Table 87.13. Risk Factors for Developing Depressive Symptoms in Patients with Cancer

Category	Influence
Personal	History of depression (patient or family)
	History of alcoholism or substance abuse
	Prior suicide attempt
	Poor social supports
	Recent loss (bereavement)
Illness and treatment	Advanced stages of cancer
	Poorly controlled pain
	Other chronic disease/disability
	Medications
	Corticosteroids
	Prednisone, dexamethasone
	Other chemotherapeutic agents
	Vincristine, vinblastine, procarbazine, L-asparaginase, interferon, amphotericin B
	Other medications
	Cimetidine
	Diazepam
	Indomethacin
	Levodopa
	Methyldopa
	Pentazocine
	Phenmetrazine
	Phenobarbital
	Propranolol
	Rauwolfia alkaloids
	Estrogens
	Other medical conditions
	Metabolic
	Nutritional
	Endocrine
	Neurologic

Table 87.14. Commonly Used Antidepressants in Cancer

Drug	Starting daily dosage po (mg)	Therapeutic daily dosage po (mg)
Tricyclic antidepressants		
Amitriptyline	25	75–100
Doxepin	25	75–100
Imipramine	25	75–100
Desipramine	25	75–100
Nortriptyline	25	50–100
Second-generation antidepressants		
Bupropion	15	200–450
Trazodone	50	150–200
Selective serotonin-reuptake inhibitors		
Fluoxetine	20	20–60
Paroxetine	20	20–50
Sertraline	50	50–150
Serotonin- and norepinephrine-reuptake inhibitor		
Venlafaxine	25	75–100
Heterocyclic antidepressants		
Maprotiline	25	50–75
Amoxapine	25	100–150
Monoamine oxidase inhibitors		
Isocarboxazid	10	24–40
Phenelzine	15	30–60
Tranylcypromine	10	20–40
Lithium carbonate	300	600–1200
Psychostimulants		
Dextroamphetamine	2.5 at 8 AM and noon	5–30
Methylphenidate	2.5 at 8 AM and noon	5–30
Pemoline	18.75 in AM and noon	37.5–150.0
Benzodiazepines		
Alprazolam	0.25–1.00	0.75–6.00

are the next most commonly used, started at low dose (10 to 25 mg at bedtime) and slowly increased by 10 to 25 mg increments over 4- to 7-day intervals. Patients usually are maintained 4 to 6 months on a tricyclic, chosen in part by its side-effects profile. A tricyclic with sedating effects, such as amitriptyline or doxepin, is best for agitation and insomnia; psychomotor slowing is better treated with desipramine. Nortriptyline and desipramine should be used for patients in whom minimal anticholinergic effects are desired. The tricyclics also are helpful in controlling chemotherapy-related peripheral neuropathy pain and discomfort.

Maprotiline, amoxapine, bupropion, and trazodone are useful. In general, they have side effects similar to the tricyclics. Maprotiline can lower the seizure threshold. Antidepressant effects may take 2 to 3 weeks to become evident with the drugs discussed above, and maximal benefit usually is obtained by 4 weeks.

Among the other antidepressants, psychostimulants are most widely used to promote well-being and counteract the fatigue from advanced illness. Drowsiness associated with opioids often is diminished by dextroamphetamine, methylphenidate, or pemoline, which is a non-controlled stimulant with no addicting potential. Alprazolam has the advantage of being effective against anxiety and depression, and it is useful when stronger antidepressants are contraindicated (48).

Suicide and Cancer

The incidence of suicide is increased in patients with cancer compared to the general population, but it is not as high as often is assumed (10, 11). It is likely, however, that suicide by overdose at home during the terminal stages of cancer is underdiagnosed and underreported. Suicide is more likely to occur in advanced disease, when depression, hopelessness, and the presence of poorly controlled symptoms (especially pain) increase. Table 87.15 outlines risk factors that predict the acting out of suicidal thoughts. They are similar to factors predicting depression (Table 87.12), must be assessed when evaluating a patient for suicidal risk and the strengths to be identified for support (Table 87.16). Evaluation of the patient with suicidal ideation should query the nature of suicidal thoughts (passive or active), past history of psychiatric problems, recent loss or bereavement, poor prior adjustment or suicidal attempt, family history of depression or suicide, present symptoms that the patient feels are poorly controlled, and the patient's understanding of disease and prognosis.

Table 87.15. Risk Factors for Suicide in Cancer

Personal
Prior history of suicide (personal or family)
Prior psychiatric disorder
Prior alcohol or drug abuse
Depression and hopelessness
Recent loss/bereavement
Medical
Pain
Delirium
Advanced illness
Debilitation, exhaustion, fatigue

Table 87.16. Evaluation of Suicidal Risk

Establish rapport
Ask about symptoms (pain, discomfort, and adequacy of their control)
Ask about depression and suicidal thoughts at present or in the past
Ask about suicidal thoughts (Are they passive ["I wish I could die"] or active ["I am thinking of ways to do it"])
Ask about family or friends and sense of support from others
Ask about any recent loss of close person, especially if by cancer
Ask about understanding of illness, presence of confusion, fatigue
Asking does not cause suicidal thoughts; the patient is usually relieved to express them

Table 87.17. Suicide in Relation to Stage of Disease

Patients at all stages of cancer
Suicidal thoughts are common and serve as a means to maintain a sense of control over the disease
Carrying out the act is viewed as for "the future when I need to do it"
Some maintain a means of suicide (e.g., drugs) to assure ultimate control over feared intolerable symptoms
Patients in remission, with good prognosis
Serious suicidal thoughts represent underlying psychiatric disorder (depression, substance abuse)
Unlikely to appear "rational"; treat aggressively, including hospitalization
Patients with poor prognosis and poorly controlled symptoms
Thoughts of suicide often appear "rational"
May request advice about physician-assisted suicide
Need evaluation for presence of treatable depression
Need attention to quality-of-life issues and comfort
Suicidal wishes usually diminish with control of distressing symptoms
Adequate symptom control by physician may hasten death (dual effect) but is not actual physician-assisted suicide
Patients in terminal stage
May request euthanasia by lethal injection from physician
Request often reflects poor quality of life, hopelessness, and depression
Need for control of symptoms, even when hastens death
Physicians and public need more education about available palliative-care options
Legalize assisted death or euthanasia in United States? Public and professional debate needed

It is not possible to consider suicidal thoughts and actual acts without taking into account disease stage and prognosis. Issues and management vary greatly with these factors. Table 87.17 outlines the range of issues in relation to the stage of disease. To consider suicide in cancer, it is helpful to consider the issue from four perspectives: (*a*) suicidal thoughts in patients at all stages of disease, (*b*) suicidal thoughts in patients who are in remission with a good prognosis, (*c*) suicidal thoughts in patients with poor prognosis/poor symptom control, and (*d*) patients in terminal stages.

First, almost all patients who receive a diagnosis of cancer, even when the prognosis is good, carry a "secret," rarely acknowledged, thought that says "I won't die in pain with advanced cancer—I'll kill myself first." This may include having a secret supply of drugs, which is kept for this purpose and usually serves as a "steam valve" with which the person is able to maintain a sense of ultimate control over the disease and an intolerable future. The thought actually serves as a protective coping device that must be recognized by the physician and the psychiatrist as a normal, healthy means of maintaining control. For most patients, the time never comes to take the pills, and life becomes dearer as death approaches. The intensity of suicidal thoughts is greater among patients who have seen a relative die with poor control of pain, as was more typical of earlier times, and especially if they had the same tumor as the patient. It is important that the physician listen to these fears and concerns and even answer questions about what constitutes a lethal dose of sedative. The rapid climb to the top of the U.S. best-seller list of *Final Exit* by Derek Humphry of the Hemlock Society shows the degree to which people fear the loss of control over death and the desire to avoid meaningless life and protracted dying (51).

Serious ruminating about suicide in a patient for whom the disease is in remission or in whom a good prognosis exists, is not rational. In fact, careful evaluation very likely will elicit the presence of major depression, a history of substance abuse, or recent bereavement. A study by Hietanin and Lonquist (45) of all suicides in Finland in 1987 found that 4.3% had cancer. Surprisingly, half of these patients with cancer were in remission at the time of the suicide; they had greater prior psychiatric problems, particularly substance abuse, than those who suicided in advanced stages of cancer. It is important that these patients be recognized and aggressively treated for depression and suicidal risk, including psychiatric hospitalization if necessary.

Patients with a poor prognosis, advanced disease, and poorly controlled symptoms often have thoughts of suicide that are more likely to be viewed as rational (24). They may request help from a physician for assistance in committing suicide. Many of these patients experience reduction of the suicidal wish when their desperation is countered by good control of their symptoms and distress, especially control of pain and depression. Chochinov and colleagues (22) found that the persistent desire for death in the terminally ill is closely associated with the diagnosis of depression. Adequate pain control by the physician actually also may have the dual effect of hastening death, but few physicians have difficulty in carrying out such a treatment aimed at comfort when it reflects the patient's and family's wishes. Most physicians do not regard this as assisted suicide but as appropriate treatment geared to maximal comfort.

Patients who are in the terminal stages and too weak to carry out a suicidal act are those most likely to request euthanasia by a lethal injection from the physician. U.S. health care, with its emphasis on tertiary care and the frequent absence of a long, preexisting relationship with patients, makes this a more difficult issue than in The Netherlands. Of the 2,000 to 3,000 acts of euthanasia carried out each year there, almost all are done in patients' homes by physicians who have known them for many years and have informed the local magistrate of the plan. Few are done in hospitals or nursing homes.

Physicians in the United States are being drawn into a public debate about the right of patients who are mentally competent to request euthanasia by a lethal injection from a physician. This is in contrast to the painstaking development of legislation to assure that patients have an opportunity to provide advance directions about life-sustaining treatments by identification of a proxy who can make decisions when they are no longer competent. The legislative agenda on euthanasia in several states is occurring without adequate attention to the issue of the frequency of depression in patients with advanced cancer and that suicidal wishes may reflect unrecognized depression, uncontrolled pain, or the sense that "my family will be better off because my care costs too much." Quill and colleagues (85) proposed clinical criteria for physician-assisted suicide, outlining the evaluation, including capacity to make decisions and presence of depression, that would be necessary to consider the request in an appropriate manner. They support legislation for assisted suicide, but not euthanasia. Thoughtful debate about euthanasia must weigh the rights of individuals to demand euthanasia carried out by a physician, taking into account that recognition and control of symptoms for many terminally ill patients is woefully inadequate. Identification and treatment of depression and hopelessness, which may be at the heart of the request for euthanasia, may remain unrecognized. Until supportive care and symptom control are more clearly acknowledged by the public and health-care policy makers, legislative efforts to legalize euthanasia may represent a slippery slope on which physicians will be required by law to make medical judgments without an adequate opportunity for attention to the complex psychiatric, medical, and ethical issues involved.

Delirium

In patients with cancer, especially those in advanced stages of disease, it is prudent to consider a sudden change in mood or behavior for its possible relationship to a change in neurologic, vascular, or metabolic status; a functional basis is far less likely. In fact, in advanced and terminal illness, 75% of hospitalized patients may be found to develop a confusional state (delirium) during the period before death. Common causes of delirium in cancer are outlined in Table 87.18 (35). A change in behavior in which the person becomes irritable, uncooperative, agitated or somnolent, and misinterprets sounds or objects is apt to represent common signs of early delirium. This picture may be followed by delusions, usually paranoid ("there are people here trying to hurt me"), frank hallucinations, and difficulty in being maintained in their bed and hospital room because of mental aberrations (Table 87.19). It is important to have a familiar person present who can interpret what is happening while also limiting the number of new faces and experiences. Older patients are most prone to become confused, and delirium may be superimposed on dementia. Physical restraints should be used with caution to avoid falls; chemical restraint may be helpful. Low-dose haloperidol, .5 to 1.0 mg doses bid to qid, often reduces confusion. Lorazepam reduces agitation in doses of .5 to 1.0 mg tid to qid. Haloperidol and lorazepam often are given together to reduce confusion and diminish agitation. Correcting the underlying metabolic or neurologic

Table 87.18. Common Causes of Delirium in Cancer

Causes	Examples
Metabolic encephalopathy because of vital organ failure	Liver, kidney, lung (hypoxia), thyroid, adrenal
Electrolyte imbalance	Sodium, potassium, calcium, glucose
Treatment side effects	Narcotics Anticholinergics Phenothiazines Antihistamines Chemotherapeutic agents Steroids Radiation therapy
Infection	Septicemia
Hematologic abnormalities	Microcytic and macrocytic anemias, coagulopathies
Nutritional	General malnutrition, thiamine, folic acid, vitamin B_{12}
Paraneoplastic syndromes	Remote effects of tumors Hormone-producing tumors

Table 87.19. Behavioral Symptoms of Delirium in Patients with Cancer

State	Symptom
Early, mild	Change in sleep pattern with restlessness, attempts to get out of bed, transient periods of disorientation Unexplained anxiety and sense of dread Increased irritability, anger, temper outbursts Withdrawal, refusal to talk to staff or relatives Forgetfulness, not previously present
Late, severe with behavioral changes	Refusal to cooperate with reasonable requests Angry, swearing, shouting, abusive Demanding to go home, pacing corridor Illusions (misidentifies staff, visual and sensory clues) Delusions (misinterprets events, usually paranoid, fears of being harmed) Hallucinations (visual and auditory)

problem is not always possible, however, and comfort for the patient and family may depend materially on being able to control the symptoms of confusion and agitation.

Behavioral and Psychosocial Variables in Cancer Morbidity and Mortality

Many questions have been raised about the role of behavioral, psychologic, and social variables in cancer morbidity and mortality (Table 87.20). There are five areas in which factors have been explored for their contribution: lifestyle and behaviors, social environment and social support, personality and coping, affective states/life events, and effects of psychosocial and behavioral interventions (37).

In terms of life-style and behaviors, reduced exposures to carcinogens through change in habits (e.g., smoking cessation, sunburn avoidance, dietary guidelines) has the greatest potential for reducing cancer mortality. Behaviors associated with an individual's assuring early detection of cancer is important (e.g., breast self-examination, cervical cytology, mammography), and adherence to the prescribed treatment regimen clearly affects outcome. Attention to attitudes and behaviors that reduce exposure to carcinogens, and assure early diagnosis as well as treatment adherence is critically important.

Aspects of the social environment have been increasingly identified as contributing to cancer morbidity and mortality (50). A study by Cella and colleagues (19) of 2,400 patients treated by randomized protocols in the Cancer and Leukemia Group B (CALGB) found, that after known predictors of outcome were considered, lowest education and income correlated with shortest survival. Ability to understand and comply with treatment regimens may need special attention in those with the lowest educational level. Individuals who are economically disadvantaged suffer from poor access to health care and, in addition, have such factors as nutritional deficiencies, greater presence of other medical illnesses, and chronic stress of poverty. A recent study by Adler and colleagues (3), however, found a stepwise gradient by each lower social class and lower income group. These data suggest that the issue is not just a break at the poverty line indicating poor access to services, but that some higher-order factor may account for it.

Data from a meta-analysis of six studies done in three countries showed that poor or absent social ties had an impact on the overall age-adjusted morbidity and mortality from a range of diseases, including cancer (50). Similar findings found in married versus single individuals suggest that better lifestyle, habits, and earlier seeking of health care may be the factors that account for better survival. Looking at studies overall, there may be a relative risk of 1.1 or 1.2 associated with lower social support, and this low order would produce the mixed results of studies reported (37).

Exploration for a personality type associated with cancer, similar to the Type A personality and cardiovascular disease, has not been successful. Characteristics of a Type C personality associated with cancer have been postulated as outwardly controlled but with repressed emotions. "Fighting spirit" has been associated with better survival, but overall, the association of personality with incidence or survival is not proven by present data.

Bereavement and depression have been most extensively studied for a role in cancer morbidity and mortality. They also

Table 87.20. Primary Behaviors and Psychosocial Factors that Impact on Cancer Morbidity and Mortality

Lifestyle/behaviors associated with carcinogenic exposures (tobacco, sun)
Poor socioeconomic status, poor education
Early detection and treatment compliance
Availability of social supports

have been examined for an impact on immune function in physically healthy individuals. As bereavement studies have been more carefully controlled, they have failed to confirm a relationship with either cancer morbidity or mortality. Likewise, depression has shown less likelihood of a correlation with mortality. The large prospective study by Zonderman and colleagues (82) of a nationally representative sample studied for the prevalence of depression found no increased cancer mortality 10 years later. That immune changes have accompanied depressive and grieving symptoms has been of great interest; however, questions have been raised about the interpretation of psychoimmune data in terms of how clinically relevant small changes in function that occur with emotional states may be.

Many studies have identified the nature and frequency of distress in patients with cancer (74). They have led to intervention studies aimed at improving coping and well being, with an interest in whether they also might affect length of survival. Over 20 studies, using a range of interventions and often combining support and behavioral methods, have shown enhanced well-being and improved quality of life (52, 78, 80). A positive effect on disease outcome and survival has been reported only by Spiegel and colleagues (72), but this report has had a major impact on this area of research. They found that women with advanced breast cancer who were randomized to a weekly group psychiatric intervention for 1 year survived significantly longer than those who had been assigned to the control arm. A 10-year follow-up of their "exceptional cancer patients," however, found no difference in the survival of these patients compared with matched nonparticipants (40, 62). Similar results were found at the Bristol Clinic (6); however, Fawzy and colleagues (31, 33) found a survival advantage at 5 years for patients with stage I and II malignant melanoma who were randomized to psychosocial intervention in a controlled trial.

In summary, four areas clearly show the impact of behavior and social factors on cancer morbidity and mortality: lifestyle and behaviors, low socioeconomic and educational status, early detection and treatment compliance, and, availability of social supports (perhaps mediated through early detection and treatment compliance) (Table 87.20). Of great interest, but still awaiting confirmation, is whether psychosocial intervention may have a salutary effect not only on well-being, but on survival as well.

Alternative Cancer Treatments

Any group of disease with largely unknown cause, high likelihood of fatality, and uncertain cure, causes great fear in the public. Cancer and mental illness have been most feared historically, and for the same reasons, AIDS has now been added. Diseases for which traditional medicine cannot provide a cure always elicit an array of nontraditional treatments (81). The history of cancer quackery is of great psychologic interest, because these therapies have flourished over centuries. They have only changed in type and nature. In general, the popular unconventional treatments of a particular period reflect the public's perception of cancer and medicine at that time (17). Thus, balms, tonics, and electrical waves were popular early in this century, giving way to krebiozen in the 1960s, laetrile in 1970s and most recently, natural holistic approaches using diet, immune-enhancement therapies, and psychologic interventions with imagery for anti-tumor effects. All are proposed to work by enhancing the body's defenses. The alternative therapy community tends to exist separately from mainstream medicine, with considerable hostility between the two worlds, causing patients to be confused.

There has been a recent effort to bridge this gap by preparing a thoughtful and comprehensive report (which should be read by anyone interested in the area) on alternative therapies in the United States, undertaken by the Office of Technological Assessment at the request of the U.S. Congress (79). This report elucidates the present status of these treatments, outlining the four major areas of alternative therapies: psychologic and behavioral approaches, nutritional, herbal, and pharmacologic/biologic. Many therapies, such as those of Gerson and of Kelly, combine several of these approaches and include a spiritual or religious context as well. The best-known psychologic approaches are Simonton's visualization methods to enhance immune function, and Spiegel's Exceptional Cancer Patients approach to improve survival by positive emotional expression. Commonweal, where Lerner combines group discussion, yoga, touch, relaxation, and visualization in a week-long therapeutic experience, provides these activities as complementary therapies, to be used in conjunction with traditional treatment. The fear that patients will leave their medical treatment for an alternative appears to be less of a threat today, although it still occurs (17).

It is important to understand these issues clearly, because some of the psychologic and behavioral methods that are used in mainstream medicine (psychologic support, visual imagery, relaxation) for enhancing quality of life and symptom control also are included in alternative therapies, with the promise of curing cancer through visualizing the immune system's attack on cancer cells in the body. This gray zone grows even broader in view of psychoimmune studies that show an impact of stress in healthy subjects on immune function, and of studies that have reported greater survival both among women with advanced breast cancer who received weekly psychotherapeutic group meetings and patients with melanoma treated following initial surgery (33, 72). It is hard for frightened individuals to view these findings only as early research data that warrant further study.

Many psychologic alternative therapies suggest that the patient had a role in developing cancer, either because of stress or personality. They also exhort the patient to be "positive," and "fight—outcome depends largely on attitude." Some patients grow fearful when they become depressed, because their mental state "may make the cancer grow faster." These deleterious aspects of the present era of alternative therapies, with its emphasis on psychologic and "mind-over-matter" approaches, has been examined from a sociologic view (42). Society tends to use myths to understand frightening phenomena. Often, the cancer patient is portrayed as the heroic warrior fighting the dragon of cancer. Some individuals gain strength by assuming the warrior stance and should be encouraged to maintain it. They find cancer self-help books, visualization, and mental attitude methods to be helpful and should be encouraged to use them. There are other patients, however, for whom the warrior myth is distressing. They feel guilty, because they believe they cannot fight hard enough. Sometimes, a distraught family blames the patient for not fighting hard enough. These individuals need to know that there are many ways of coping effectively with cancer; there is no single "right" way for all individuals. In fact, most patients do best when they rely on their own self-validated, effective means of coping developed over years by trial-and-error. They also can be told that several studies have not supported longer survival in patients using unconventional therapies (6, 40).

Several key points have emerged from research on alternative therapies, and their use is helpful as a guide. Patients who use alternative therapies today usually are not poorly educated individuals with advanced disease who are grasping at straws. They tend to be educated individuals who are seeking all information, many at the time of diagnosis; they may be entranced by the mind-body relationship that is proposed by the alternative approaches. Many assume a posture of "what harm can it do." Most receive conventional therapies at the same time. Internationally, approximately 10 to 20% of patients with cancer use alternative treatments in Western countries; among them, only a small percent appear to stop conventional therapy (17). Patients who are told "there is nothing more I can do for you" by their doctor, however, are highly vulnerable, because they feel both abandoned and rejected. A sensitive presentation of palliative care, symptom control, and attempts to continue controlling the tumor are important for these patients and their families. There is never nothing that can be done; only the goals have changed.

It is helpful to stay informed about current local alternative therapies, so as to be able to advise patients. It also is important to provide support for patients' psychologic needs, which nontraditional therapies provide extremely well. In addition, it is important to encourage patients to discuss their thoughts about alternative therapies (47). Angry responses from oncologists place the patient in an untenable situation, which encourages lack of disclosure. A therapy that is harmful should be condemned; a therapy that is aimed at quality of life and is to be used as an adjunct to conventional therapy should be condoned if it helps the patient cope, and has no deleterious effect. Patients should be warned, however, that if a psychologic alternative approach makes them feel distressed (e.g., "you caused the cancer and now it is up to you to cure it"), they should discontinue it.

Quality-of-Life Assessment

The definition of quality of life as used in oncology is the level of performance in the major domains of life function (physical, work, psychologic, social, and sexual) compared with the normal level for that individual. In the last decade, clinical trials have increasingly included the assessment of quality of life in its outcome variables (25, 26, 76). Interest in quality of life grew after 1984, when the U.S. Food and Drug Administration demanded that the efficacy of new anticancer agents be demonstrated by improved survival or evidence of enhanced quality of life. Coupled with increased patient involvement in their treatment decisions and concerns about informed consent, issues regarding quality of life with one treatment versus another led to heightened interest in finding ways to measure this variable (29). Karnofsky and Burchenal (53) actually described in 1949 that, in addition to survival, subjective improvement was equally important to the evaluation of patients' responses to treatment. Despite that early observation, however, less than 5% of clinical trials had included a quality-of-life variable in 1990 (1).

Today, six domains of function generally are included in multidimensional quality-of-life measures: physical, functional, psychologic, social, sexual, and work (Table 87.21). No "gold standard" of measurement, however, currently exists to assess quality of life, but there are several frequently used scales that can be employed to monitor function and the effects of treatment. Initially, the most widely used was the Functional Living Index-Cancer (FLIC) (71). A 22-item scale with physical well-being and emotional subscales, the FLIC has largely been replaced by scales that provide broader information specifically for use with cancer. The Cancer Rehabilitation Evaluation System (CARES) is a scale that consists of 139 items concerning cancer problems across the six quality-of-life domains (70). A series of new quality-of-life measures has been carefully developed and tested by the European Organization for Research and Treatment of Cancer (EORTC) (2). The scales have a core of questions that are applicable to the quality of life for all patients with cancer and modules that query the specific issues related to a disease site (e.g., prostate, breast, lung cancer). This approach also has been used by Cella and colleagues (18) in development of the Functional Assessment of Cancer Therapy (FACT), which adds an aspect of patient assessment regarding the discrepancy between prior and present functions. Aside from the Karnofsky rating scale, Spitzer and colleagues' Quality of Life Index (QL-index) is the only observer-rated measure of quality of life that is used with some frequency (73).

Additional scales, not developed specifically for cancer but widely used, are the Psychosocial Adjustment to Illness Scale (PAIS) and the Sickness Impact Profile (SIP) (8, 27). The PAIS in particular has been used extensively with several chronic illnesses, including cancer. The SIP scale is similar in format to CARES in that it lists 136 problems that can result from illness that affect quality of life.

Table 87.21. Quality-of-Life Measurement: Functional Areas of Living Assessed

Physical	Symptoms of disease and treatment of side effects
Functional	Ability to perform usual activities
Psychologic	Mood, sense of well-being
Sexual	Desire, performance
Social	Family, friends, leisure
Work	Usual level of activity

Most quality-of-life scales presently being developed are designed for self-report or to be completed in response to structured interview questions (23, 75). Traditionally, such forms were administered at the time of clinic visits; however, use of trained telephone interviewers in co-operative group trials in the CALGB has found this approach not only more practicable but more effective, because it takes the collection of quality-of-life data away from the hectic clinic setting. The method ensures consistency in terms of evaluation and promotes better compliance as well as patient satisfaction. There are fewer missing data points, because questions can be clarified with the patient by the interviewer. Using this type of telephone approach, in which the patient has the written questions and responds to them at the interviewer's request, findings were comparable to those attained using a face-to-face interview.

Recent efforts in quality-of-life research have concentrated on development of a unitary measure that might combine length of survival and quality of life, referred to as "quality-adjusted life years" or QALYS. "TWIST," or time without symptoms or toxicity, is another QALY method developed by Goldhirsch and colleagues (39, 41). In this method, the number of months in which the patient experienced symptoms (weighted as to toxicity) or was in relapse is subtracted from overall survival time, yielding a QALY score. In QALY research, weights, which are either empirically derived or chosen arbitrarily, are assigned equally to disabilities and symptoms in the two treatment arms. In this manner, the effects on quality of life of difference between symptoms can be mathematically taken into account.

This area of inquiry is only now emerging. It offers intriguing new opportunities to evaluate treatment effectiveness through the combination of physical and subjective information. Information derived from quality-of-life studies will be helpful both to physicians and patients in the future in weighing treatment options (38, 39).

Summary

The subspecialty of psycho-oncology is a recent development within oncology, reflecting the increased interest in behavioral, psychologic, ethical, and social factors in cancer prevention and the quality of life for patients with cancer at all stages. Quality-of-life issues are different in respect to patients under active treatment, during palliative care, for survivors, and for healthy individuals who are at known increased risk. Early identification of patients who are not coping well with the diagnosis and treatment is important, both for treatment compliance and control of distress. It is important to recognize and diagnose the common psychiatric disorders and psychologic problems, primarily anxiety and depressive symptoms, that occur in cancer patients and the altered mental states caused by drugs and disease. The modalities available to treat these symptoms that impact on the quality of life are psychotherapeutic, behavioral, and pharmacologic. Referral to a mental-health professional familiar with the care of patients with cancer often is important. Knowledge of alternative therapies is necessary to discuss them thoughtfully with patients and their families. Behavioral, psychologic, and social factors play a role in cancer morbidity and mortality, by lifestyle and habits leading to exposures (e.g., sun, cigarettes); through the environment, related to poor socioeconomic conditions and poor education; behaviors resulting in late detection and poor compliance with therapy; and by the presence of social support, which likely contributes to better health behaviors. The measurement of quality of life that assesses patients' functioning in the major domains of their lives has been a valuable addition to clinical trials research, emphasizing not only quantity of life, but its quality as well. This merger of medical and social science data augurs well for future research initiatives.

References

1. Aaronson NK. Methodologic issues in assessing the quality of life of cancer patients. Cancer 1991;67:844.
2. Aaronson NK, Bakker W, Stewart AL, et al. Multidimensional approach to the measurement of quality of life in lung cancer clinical trials. In The Quality of Life of Cancer Patients. New York: Raven, 1987, p 63.
3. Adler NE, Boyce T, Chesney M. Socioeconomic status and health: the challenge of the gradient. Am Psychologist 1994;9:15–24.
4. Andrews LB, Fullarton JE, Holtzman NA, Motulsky AG. Assessing Genetic Risk: Implications for Health and Social Policy. Washington, DC: National Academy Press, 1994.
5. Andrykowski MA, Redd WH. Longitudinal analysis of the development of anticipatory nausea. J Consult Clin Psychol 1987;55:36.
6. Bagenal FS, Easton D F, Harris E, Chilvers CED, McElwain TJ. Survival of patients with breast cancer attending Bristol Cancer Help Centre. Lancet 1990;336:606.
7. Barg FK, Cooley M, Pasacrita J, Senay B, McCorkle R. Development of a self-administered psychosocial cancer screening tool. Cancer Pract 1994;2:288–296.
8. Bergner M, Bobbitt RA, Carter WB, Gilson BS. The Sickness Impact Profile: development and final revision of a health status measure. Med Care 1981;19:787.
9. Biesecker BB, Boenike M, Calzone K, et al. Genetic counseling for families with inherited susceptibility to breast and ovarian cancer. JAMA 1993;269:1970.
10. Bolund C. Suicide and cancer. I: Demographical and suicidological description of suicides among cancer patients in Sweden. J Psychosoc Oncol 1985;3:17.
11. Bolund C. Suicide and cancer. II: Medical and care factors in suicide by cancer patients in Sweden, 1973–1976. J Psychosoc Oncol 1986;3:31.
12. Breitbart W, Holland JC. Psychiatric Aspects of Symptom Management in Cancer Patients. Washington, DC: American Psychiatric Press, 1993.
13. Breitbart W, Passik S. Psychiatric aspects of palliative care. In: Oxford Textbook of Palliative Care. Edited by D Doyle, G Hanks, N MacDonald. Oxford: Oxford Medical Publications, 1993, p 607.
14. Bukberg J, Penman D, Holland JC. Depression in hospitalized cancer patients. Psychosom Med 1984;46:199.
15. Burton MV, Parker RW, Farrell A, et al. A randomized controlled trial of preoperative psychological preparation for mastectomy. Psycho-oncology 1995;4:1–19.
16. Butler RW, Hill JM, Steinherz P, Meyers PA, Finlay JL. Neuropsychologic effects of cranial irradiation, intrathecal, methotrexate and systemic methotrexate in childhood cancer. J Clin Oncol 1994;12:2621–2629.
17. Cassileth BR, Brown H. Unorthodox cancer medicine. CA 1988;38:176.
18. Cella D, Tulsky D, Gray G, et al. The functional assessment of cancer therapy scale: development and validation of the general measurement. J Clin Oncol 1993;11:570.
19. Cella DF, Orav E, Kornblith AB, et al. (for the Cancer and Leukemia Group B). Socioeconomic status and cancer survival. J Clin Oncol 1991;9:1500.
20. Cella DF, Pratt A, Holland JC. Persistent anticipatory nausea, vomiting, and anxiety in cured Hodgkin's disease patients after completion of chemotherapy. Am J Psychiatry 1986;143:641.
21. Cherny NI, Coyle N, Foley KM. Suffering in the advanced cancer patient: a definition and a toxonomy. J Palliat Care 1994;10:57–70.
22. Chochinov HM, Wilson KG, Enns M. Desire for death in the terminally ill. Am J Psychiatry 1995;152:1185–1192.
23. Coates A, Gebski V, Bishop JF, et al. Improving the quality of life during chemotherapy for advanced breast cancer: a comparison of intermittent and continuous treatment strategies. N Engl J Med 1987;317:1490.
24. Conwell Y, Caine ED. Rational suicide and the right to die: reality and myth. N Engl J Med 1991;325:1100.
25. de Haes JCJM, van Knippenberg FCE. The quality of life of cancer patients: a review of the literature. Soc Sci Med 1985;20:809.
26. de Haes JCJM, van Oostrom MA, Welvaart K. Quality of life after breast cancer surgery. J Surg Oncol 1985;28:123.
27. Derogatis LR, Lopez M. PAIS and PAIS-SR: administration, scoring and procedures manual. I: Baltimore. In Clinical Psychometric Research, 1983.
28. Derogatis LR, Morrow GR, Fetting D, et al. The prevalence of psychiatric disorders among cancer patients. JAMA 1983;249:751.
29. Deyo RA, Patrick DL. Barriers to the use of health status measures in clinical investigation, patient care, and policy research. Med Care 1989;27(suppl):S54.
30. Farber DM, Wienerman BH, Kuypers JA. Psychosocial distress in oncology outpatients. J Psychosoc Oncol 1984;2:109.
31. Fawzy FI, Cousins N, Fawzy NW, Kemeny ME, Elashoff R, Morton D. A structured intervention for cancer patients. I: Changes over time in methods of coding and affective disturbance. Arch Gen Psychiatry 1990;47:720.
32. Fawzy FI, Fawzy NW. A structured psychoeducational intervention for cancer patients. Gen Hosp Psychiatry 1994;16:149–192.

33. Fawzy FI, Fawzy NW, Hyun CS, et al. Malignant melanoma: effects of early structured psychiatric intervention coping and affective state of recurrence and survival 6 years later. Arch Gen Psychiatry 1993;50:681.
34. Fawzy FI, Fawzy NW, Pasnau RO. Critical review of psychosocial interventions in cancer care. Arch Gen Psychiatry 1995;52:100–113.
35. Fleishman SB, Lesko LM. Delirium and Dementia. In Handbook of Psychooncology: Psychological Care of the Patient with Cancer. Edited by JC Holland, JH Rowland. New York: Oxford, 1989, p 342.
36. Ford S, Fallowfield L, Lewis S. Can oncologists detect distress in their out-patients and how satisfied are they with their performance during bad news consultations? Br J Cancer 1994;767–770.
37. Fox B. The role of psychological factors in cancer incidence and prognosis oncology. Oncology 1995;9:245–255.
38. Ganz PA, Haskell CM, Figlin RA, La Soto N, Siau J. Estimating the quality of life in a clinical trial of patients with metastatic lung cancer using the Karnofsky Performance Status and the Functional Living Index-Cancer. Cancer 1988;61:849.
39. Gelber RD, Goldhirsch A. A new endpoint for the assessment of adjuvant therapy in postmenopausal women with operable breast cancer. J Clin Oncol 1986;4:1772.
40. Gellert GA, Maxwell RM, Siegel BS. Survival of breast cancer patients receiving adjunctive psychosocial support therapy: a 10-year follow-up study. J Clin Oncol 1993;11:66.
41. Goldhirsch A, Gelber RD, Simes RJ, Glasziou P, Coates AS. Costs and benefits of adjuvant therapy in breast cancer: a quality-adjusted survival analysis. J Clin Oncol 1989;7:36.
42. Gray RE, Doan BD. Heroic self-healing and cancer: clinical issues for the health professions. J Palliat Care 1990;6:32.
43. Hamburg DA, Adams JE. A perspective on coping behavior: seeking and utilizing information in major transitions. Arch Gen Psychiatry 1967;17:277.
44. Harrison J, Maquire P. Predictors of psychiatric morbidity in cancer patients. Br J Psychiatry 1994;165:593–598.
45. Hietanen P, Lonnqvist J. Cancer and suicide. Ann Oncol 1991;2:19.
46. Holland JC. Psycho-oncology Overview, obstacles and opportunities. Psycho-oncology 1992;1:1–13.
47. Holland JC, Geary N, Furman A. Alternative cancer therapies. In Handbook of Psychooncology: Psychological Care of the Patient with Cancer. New York: Oxford, 1989, p 508.
48. Holland JC, Morrow GR, Schmale A, et al. A randomized clinical trial of alprazolam versus progressive muscle relaxation in cancer patients with anxiety and depressive symptoms. J Clin Oncol 1991;9:1004.
49. Holland JC, Rowland JH. Handbook of Psychooncology: Psychological Care of the Patient with Cancer. New York: Oxford, 1989.
50. House JS, Landis KR, Umberson D. Social relationships and health. Science 1988;241:540.
51. Humphry D. Final Exit: The Practicalities of Self-Deliverance and Assisted Suicide for the Dying. Eugene, OR: Hemlock Society, 1991.
52. Jacobsen PB, Bovbjerg DH, Schwartz M, Hudis CA, Gilewski TA, Norton L. Conditioned emotional distress in women receiving chemotherapy for breast cancer. J Consult Clin Psychol 1995;63:108–114.
53. Karnofsky DA, Burchenal JH. The clinical evaluation of chemotherapeutic agents in cancer. In Evaluation of Chemotherapeutic Agents. Edited by CM McLeod. New York: Columbia University Press, 1949, p 191.
54. Kash KM, Holland JC, Halper S, Miller DG. Psychological distress and surveillance behaviors of women with a family history of breast cancer. JNCI 1992;84:24–30.
55. Kemeny MM, Wellisch DK, Schain WS. Psychosocial outcome in a randomized surgical trial for treatment of primary breast cancer. Cancer 1988;62:1231.
56. Kornblith AB, Anderson J, Cella DF, et al. Quality of life assessment of Hodgkin's Disease survivors: a model for cooperative clinical trials. Oncology 1990;4:93.
57. Lederberg MS, Holland JC. Psycho-Oncology. In Comprehensive Textbook of Psychiatry. Edited by H Kaplan, B Sadock. Baltimore: Williams & Wilkins, 1995, pp 1570–1592.
58. Lerman C, Kash K, Stefanek M. Younger women and increased risk for breast cancer: perceived risk, psychological well-being and surveillance behaviors. Monogr Natl Cancer Inst 1994;16:171–177.
59. Massie MJ. Anxiety panic and phobias. In Handbook of Psychooncology: Psychological Care of the Patient with Cancer. Edited by JC Holland, JH Rowland. New York: Oxford, 1989, p 302.
60. McDaniel JS, Musselman DL, Porter MR. Depression in cancer: diagnosis, biology and treatment. Gen Psych 1995;52:89–99.
61. Moorey S, Greer S, Watson M, et al. Adjuvant psychological therapy for patients with cancer: outcome at one year. Psycho-oncology 1994;3:1–10.
62. Morgenstern H, Gellert GA, Walter SD, Ostfeld AM, Seigel BS. The impact of a psychosocial support program on survival with breast cancer: the importance of selection bias in program evaluation. J Chronic Dis 1984;37:273.
63. Peretz T, Baider L, Ever-Hadani P, De-Nows AK. Psychological distress in female cancer patients with Holocaust experience. Gen Hosp Psychiatry 1994;16:413–418.
64. Portenoy RK, Thaler HT, Kornblith AB, et al. Symptom prevalence, characteristics and distress in a cancer population. Qual Life Res 1994;3:189–194.
65. Quill T, Cassel E, Meyer D. Care of the hopelessly ill. Proposed clinical criteria for physician assisted suicide. N Engl J Med 1992;327:1380.
66. Redd WH, Jacobsen PB, Die-Trill M, Dermatis H, McEvoy M, Holland JC. Cognitive/attentional distraction in the control of conditioned nausea in pediatric oncology patients receiving chemotherapy. J Consult Clin Psychol 1987;55:391.
67. Rowland JH. Developmental stage and adaptation: Adult model. In Handbook of Psychooncology: Psychological Care of the Patient with Cancer. Edited by JC Holland, JH Rowland. New York: Oxford, 1989, p 25.
68. Rowland JH. Intrapersonal resources: Coping. In Handbook of Psychooncology: Psychological Care of the Patient with Cancer. Edited by JC Holland, JH Rowland. New York: Oxford, 1989, p 44.
69. Schachter S. Quality of life for families in the management of home care patients with advanced cancer. J Palliat Care 1992;8:61–66.
70. Schag CC, Heinrich RL. CARES. Cancer Rehabilitation Evaluation System. 1988.
71. Schipper H, Clinch J, McMurray A, Levitt M. Measuring the quality of life of cancer patients: the Functional Living Index-Cancer Development and validation. J Clin Oncol 1984;2:472.
72. Spiegel D, Kraemer H, Bloom JR, Gottheil D. Effect of psychosocial treatment on survival of patients with metastatic breast cancer. Lancet 1989;2:88.
73. Spitzer WO, Dobson AJ, Hall J, et al. Measuring the quality of life of cancer patients: a concise QL-index for use by physicians. J Chronic Dis 1981;34:585.
74. Stefanek ME, Derogatis LP, Shaw A. Psychological distress among oncology outpatients. Psychosomatics 1987;28:530.
75. Stewart AL, Hays RD, Ware JE. The MOS Short-form General Health Survey: reliability and validity in a patient population. Med Care 1988;26:724.
76. Sugarbaker PH, Barofsky I, Rosenberg SA, Gianola FJ. Quality of life assessment of patients in extremity sarcoma clinical trials. Surgery 1982;91:17.
77. Taylor SE, Aspinwall LG. Psychosocial aspects of chronic illness. In Psychological Aspects of Serious Illness: Chronic Conditions Fatal Diseases and Clinical Care. Edited by PT Costa Jr, GR VandenBos. Washington, DC: American Psychological Association, 1990, p 7.
78. Toseland RW, Blanchard CG, McCalleon P. A problem solving intervention for caregivers of cancer patients. Soc Sci Med 1995;40:517–528.
79. US Congress Report. Unconventional Cancer Treatments (OTA-H-405). 1990.
80. Watson M. Cancer Patient Care: Psychosocial Treatment Methods. Cambridge, England: Cambridge University Press, 1991.
81. Wharton JC. Traditions of folk medicine in America. JAMA 1987;257:1632.
82. Zonderman AB, Costa PT, McCrae RR. Depression as a risk for cancer morbidity and mortality in a nationally representative sample. JAMA 1989;262:1191.

SECTION XXII

PRINCIPLES OF ONCOLOGY NURSING

CHAPTER 88

Principles of Oncology Nursing

CONNIE HENKE YARBRO

Introduction

Any text on cancer medicine would be incomplete without a discussion of oncology nursing. Cancer management is a multidisciplinary endeavor, and understanding the principles of oncology nursing is fundamental to the effective practice of all other oncologic subspecialties.

Oncology nurses are engaged in a collaborative practice with all members of the care team to provide optimal management of patients with cancer. Their professional practice requires detailed knowledge of the biologic and psychosocial dimensions of the cancer problem. They have key roles not only as caregivers but in patient and family education and clinical cancer research. Cancer nurses also are continuously involved in the enhancement of nursing practice through research, continuing education, and advanced education.

Oncology Nursing as a Specialty

Historically, nurses have had a special role in the care of patients with cancer, a role that was especially significant in those few institutions devoted exclusively to cancer care before the National Cancer Act of 1971. However, the expanded research and treatment program against cancer that has occurred during the past quarter century has been a catalyst for the development of oncology nursing as a separate specialty (32, 35, 37, 88). The recognition of cancer as a major national health problem was key to formally establishing the specialty of oncology nursing. This increased attention to cancer coincided with and complemented a major new emphasis in the nursing profession toward expanded roles in comprehensive patient care. Many oncology nurses first worked both as nurses and data managers for cancer research studies. As oncology called for increasingly more complex therapy, the collaborative relationship between nurse and physician became the best way to provide uniquely comprehensive patient care (3, 33, 78).

The Oncology Nursing Society (ONS) was established by a small group of nurses working primarily in research settings with medical oncologists involved in clinical research (88, 90). Their initial goals were to provide a forum for discussing practice issues in cancer nursing and to develop mechanisms for nurses to contribute to this new and evolving specialty area. There was a need to promote the advanced practice of oncology nurses in different care settings and develop national as well as local networking and continuing education programs. Research in cancer nursing subsequently became a high priority of the society. The success of this national (and international) organization has contributed to the recognition of oncology nursing as a valued specialty.

Today, the ONS has a membership of over 25,000 and 181 chapters across the United States. The majority of members (72%) provide direct patient care (59). Educational conferences, publications, legislative activities, and research initiatives are just a few of the concentrated areas of effort. The Oncology Nursing Foundation, which was established by the ONS in 1981, awarded more than $250 million dollars in research grants, scholarships, and awards in 1994 alone.

The ONS and the American Nurses' Association have developed Professional Practice Standards (Table 88.1) (2, 67), and the ONS has developed Advanced Practice Standards (Table 88.2) (64). These standards serve as a legal definition of the highest quality of oncology nursing practice.

CERTIFICATION

In 1985, the ONS established the Oncology Nursing Certification Corporation to provide an examination for the formal certification of oncology nurses. Certification in oncology nursing promotes continuing education and communicates to the public and other professionals that an oncology nurse has specialized knowledge and expertise. Nurses who pass the generalist certification examination may use the OCN (oncology certified nurse) credential with their signature. Recertification is required every 4 years by examination. As of 1995, there are a total of 13,711 oncology nurses who have been certified.

The ONCC has finalized plans for an advanced certification examination, and the first examination of this type was given in April 1995. The ONS is the first nursing specialty organization to provide certification for advanced practice nurses. Unique to the advanced examination is the requirement that an oncology nurse must have at least a master's degree. Nurses who pass the advanced examination may use the ACON (advanced certified oncology nurse) credential with their signature. Table 88.3 describes the eligibility criteria for oncology nursing certification at both the generalist and advanced levels (58).

Table 88.1. Professional Practice Standards

Standard I. Theory

The oncology nurse applies theoretic concepts as a basis for decisions in practice.

Standard II. Data Collection

The oncology nurse systematically and continually collects data regarding the health status of the client. The data are recorded, accessible, and communicated to appropriate members of the multidisciplinary team.

Standard III. Nursing Diagnoses

The oncology nurse analyzes assessment data to formulate nursing diagnoses.

Standard IV. Planning

The oncology nurse develops an outcome-oriented care plan that is individualized and holistic. This plan is based on nursing diagnoses and incorporates preventive, therapeutic, rehabilitative, palliative, and comforting nursing actions.

Standard V. Intervention

The oncology nurse implements the nursing care plan to achieve the identified outcomes for the client.

Standard VI. Evaluation

The oncology nurse regularly and systematically evaluates the client's responses to interventions to determine progress toward achievement of outcomes and to revise the data base, nursing diagnoses, and the plan of care.

Standard VII. Professional Development

The oncology nurse assumes responsibility for professional development and continuing education and contributes to the professional growth of others.

Standard X. Ethics

The oncology nurse uses the code for nurses and the Patient's Bill of Rights as guides for ethical decision making in practice.

Standard XI. Research

The oncology nurse contributes to the scientific base of nurse practice and the field of oncology through the review and application of research.

From American Nurses Association and Oncology Nursing Society (2).

ONCOLOGY NURSING EDUCATION

Educational curricula have been developed and implemented to provide oncology nurses with an appropriate understanding of cancer biology, epidemiology, prevention, treatment, nursing practice issues, and trends in cancer care. Table 88.4 summarizes a curriculum for oncology nurses at both the generalist and advanced practice levels (13).

Several cancer nursing texts and journals are published that deal with these topics in appropriate formats (4, 6, 10–13, 18, 20, 26–28, 44, 54, 55, 68, 92, 93). Cancer nursing is part of the general undergraduate and graduate nursing educational curriculum. In addition, doctoral programs and oncology nursing professorships have been established.

The usual educational level of the oncology nurse at the time of entry into practice is a bachelor's degree in nursing. Figure 88.1, which is based on the membership demographics of the ONS, shows the highest educational de-

Table 88.2. Professional Advanced Practice Standards

Standard I. Direct Caregiver Function

The advanced practice oncology nurse who functions as a direct caregiver provides, guides, directs, and evaluates the nursing practice delivered to clients with actual or potential diagnoses of cancer.

Standard II. Co-ordinator Function

The advanced practice oncology nurse who functions as a co-ordinator uses systems theory and the change process with the interdisciplinary oncology team to determine and achieve realistic health care goals for the client, the community, and/or the health care system.

Standard III. Consultant Function

The advanced practice oncology nurse who functions as a consultant provides expert knowledge about oncology to colleagues, health professionals, allied health personnel, health care consumers, and professional/public organizations.

Standard IV. Educator Function

The advanced practice oncology nurse who functions as an educator assesses the learning needs of the client, health professionals and/or the community, and then designs, implements, and evaluates educational activities.

Standard V. Researcher Function

The advanced practice oncology nurse who functions as a researcher identifies current researchable problems in oncology nursing, tests relevant theories related to oncology nursing, collaborates in research, and evaluates and implements research findings that have an impact on cancer care and cancer nursing.

Standard VI. Administrator Function

The advanced practice oncology nurse who functions as an administrator uses management theory to create an environment that provides quality care to the client and/or the community and that promotes professional nursing practice.

Standard VII. Professional Development

The advanced practice oncology nurse assumes responsibility for individual professional development and continuing education and serves as a role model and mentor to other health professionals.

Standard VIII. Ethics

The advanced practice oncology nurse applies the American Nurses' Association Code for Nurses and the Patient's Bill of Rights to ethical decision making in cancer nursing practice.

Standard IX. Legal Issues

The advanced practice oncology nurse demonstrates knowledge of the legal issues in cancer nursing practice.

Standard X. Quality Assurance

The advanced practice oncology nurse monitors and evaluates oncology nursing practice to ensure that high-quality care is provided to clients and/or the community.

Standard XI. Health Care Policy

The advanced practice oncology nurse demonstrates knowledge of the political process as a mechanism to address health care policy and issues to improve health care.

Reprinted with permission from the Oncology Nursing Society (65).

Table 88.3. **Eligibility Criteria for Oncology Nursing Certification**

Generalist	Advanced
Current RN license Minimum of 2.5 years (30 months) of oncology nursing practice within 5 years before application Minimum of 1000 hours of oncology nursing practice within 2.5 years before application	Current RN license Minimum of 2.5 years (30 months) experience as an RN within 5 years before application Minimum of 2000 hours of oncology nursing practice within 5 years before application Master's degree or higher in nursing

Table 88.4. **Core Curriculum for Oncology Nursing**

Cancer nursing practice
- Standards of oncology nursing practice
- Standards of oncology education
- Factors affecting responses to the risk of cancer
- Primary prevention
- Secondary prevention
- Patient and public education
- Nursing management of responses to the cancer experience
- Structural oncological emergencies
- Metabolic and physiologic oncologic emergencies

Issues and trends in cancer care
- Sociodemographic and attitudinal changes affecting cancer care
- Changes in oncology health care settings
- Professional issues in cancer care
- Selected ethical issues in cancer care
- Legal issues influencing cancer care
- Cancer survivorship issues

Pathophysiology of cancer

Cancer epidemiology

Treatment of cancer
- Diagnosis and staging of treatment goals and strategies
- Surgical treatment
- Radiation therapy
- Antineoplastic therapy
- Principles of preparation, administration, and disposal of antineoplastic agents
- Biologic response modifier therapy
- Bone marrow transplantation
- Unproven methods
- Supportive therapies in cancer care
- Supportive procedures in cancer care

Nursing principles specific to the major cancers
- Lung cancer
- Breast cancer
- Genitourinary cancers
- Reproductive cancers
- Colorectal cancers
- Leukemias
- Skin cancer
- Head and neck cancers
- Neurologic cancers
- Human immunodeficiency virus–related cancers
- Lymphomas

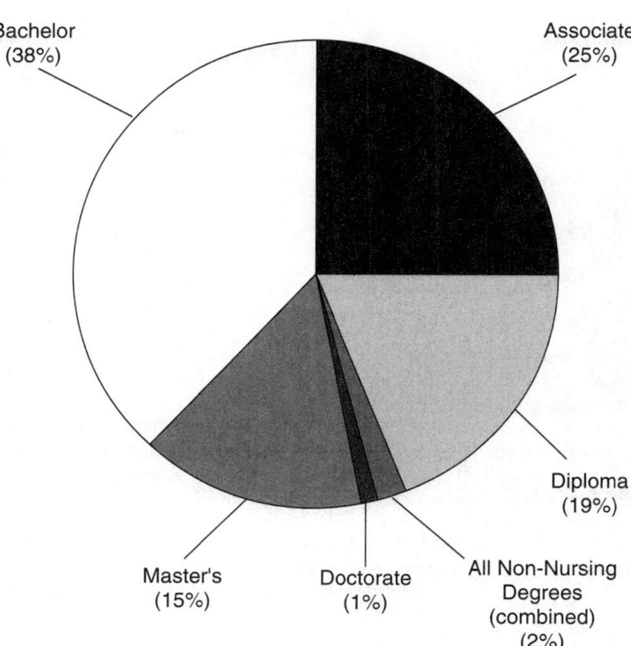

Figure 88.1. Highest educational degrees in nursing of Oncology Nursing Society members. *Source:* Oncology Nursing Society (59).

grees in nursing of ONS members. Membership in the ONS offers opportunities for the study and education necessary to qualify for the OCN credential by passing the certification examination. Increasingly master's level preparation is specified in many oncology job descriptions. For example, a master's degree is required for oncology clinical nurse specialists and nurse practitioners. Currently, 62% of the ONS members are pursuing graduate education, and 14% are doctoral students.

Role of the Oncology Nurse

Oncology nurses practice in a variety of settings: acute care hospitals, ambulatory care clinics, private oncologists' offices, radiation therapy facilities, home health care agencies, and community agencies. They practice in association with a number of oncologic disciplines: surgical oncology, radiation oncology, gynecologic oncology, pediatric oncology, and medical oncology. Figure 88.2 shows the primary areas of practice of the ONS members (59). Fifty percent of ONS members describe their positions as staff nurses, 7% as clinical nurse specialists, and 1% as nurse practitioners. Approximately 16.5% work in the outpatient/ambulatory care setting, 5.2% in physician offices, and 5% in home care. Positions in the outpatient and home care setting are increasing at a tremendous rate, however, as progressively more patients are being moved out of the hospital setting (6, 46). Their roles vary from the intensive care focus of bone marrow transplantation to the community focus of cancer screening, detection, and prevention. The advanced practice of oncology nursing includes participation as principal investigators in nursing research studies, serving as patient care consul-

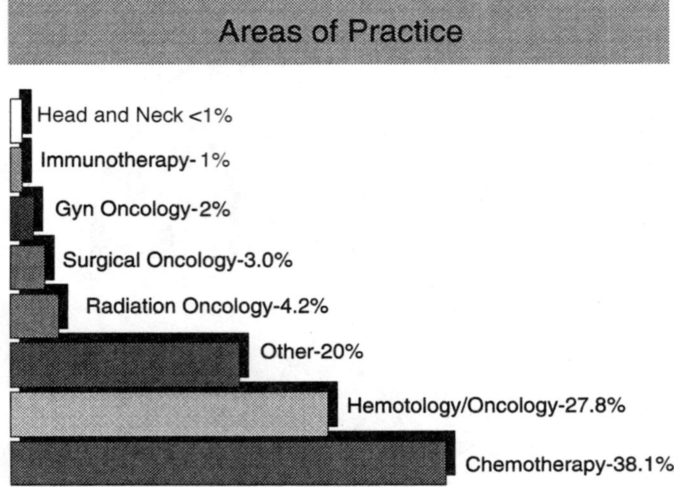

Percents do not total 100 because of rounding and because all members did not respond to all questions. Statistcs as of July 1, 1995

Figure 88.2. Primary areas of practice of the Oncology Nursing Society members. *Source:* Oncology Nursing Society (59).

tants, designing educational curricula, and performing executive functions. In all of these roles, there is an emphasis on providing nursing care to patients and families by efficient use of the nursing process, including assessment and data collection, nursing diagnosis, planning, intervention, and evaluation. This process allows for an organized and systematic approach to nursing care.

The following discussion on the role of the oncology nurse focuses on patient assessment, patient education, and coordination of care. This is followed by a specific discussion on nursing care related to surgery, radiation therapy, chemotherapy, biotherapy and supportive care aspects of pain management, unconventional therapy and survivorship issues.

PATIENT ASSESSMENT

Nurses are expected to be expert in assessing patients' physical and emotional status, past health history, health practices, and both patients' and families' knowledge of the disease and its treatment. It is essential that a detailed nursing history and physical examination be completed. An oncology nurse is expected to be aware of the results and general implications of all relevant laboratory, pathology, and imaging studies.

PATIENT EDUCATION

The nurse often has a better opportunity than any other member of the health care team to spend the necessary time with patients and their families to develop the required rapport for effective educational efforts. Such education has been described as a "series of structured and unstructured experiences which are designed to assist patients cope voluntarily with the immediate crisis response to their diagnosis, with long-term adjustments and with symptoms; gain needed information about sources of prevention, diagnosis and care; develop needed skills, knowledge and attitudes to maintain or regain health status" (40). The ONS has enhanced this definition by recommending the following patient education outcome criteria (66). The patient and/or family will be able to (*a*) describe the state of the disease and therapy at a level consistent with his or her educational and emotional status; (*b*) participate in the decision-making process pertaining to the plan of care and life activities; (*c*) identify appropriate community resources that provide information and services; (*d*) describe appropriate actions for highly predictable problems, oncologic emergencies, and major side effects of the disease and/or therapy; and (*e*) describe the schedule when ongoing therapy is predicted.

There are a variety of teaching tools and methods available, the choice of which is based on individual patient needs and abilities. Printed, visual, and audiovisual educational materials are used in conjunction with discussion and continued reinforcement. Numerous patient educational materials also are available that relate to cancer, cancer therapy, and the management of side effects (19, 27, 57, 76, 79, 80).

Patients should be encouraged to keep personal, written, daily diaries that record treatment dates, symptoms, test dates, and questions. A personal diary provides additional written documentation of the onset of specific phenomena and accurate dates of therapy in case the patient's medical record is not available.

COORDINATION OF CARE

The oncology nurse plays a vital role in coordinating the multiple and complex technologies now common in cancer diagnosis and treatment. This coordination encompasses direct patient care, documentation in the medical record, participation in therapy, symptom management, and both patient and family education as well as counseling throughout diagnosis, therapy, and follow-up. The nurse should serve as the patient's first line of communication. Ideally, the patient and family should feel free to contact the oncology nurse by phone during the entire treatment program. Many patients travel long distances, so the importance of the telephone must be emphasized. It allows continuous patient communication, early recognition of emergencies, and regular emotional support.

Camp-Sorrell (9) noted that most patient problems can be managed without the patient being seen in the office or emergency room. However, it is important for the nurse to gather sufficient information to determine patient management. She developed a telephone triage flow sheet (Fig. 88.3) that identifies the basic steps that are helpful in identifying patient problems over the phone before consulting with the physician and relaying specific instructions for follow-up care (9). This format can be used with difficult problem areas, and several specific examples are included below in the discussion on chemotherapy.

Modern cancer care is performed at multiple sites by a variety of personnel at a pace that is accelerated by a cost-conscious staff. Communication between personnel at different facilities may be suboptimal, and the communication and coordination that the oncology nurse can provide represents an invaluable service to patients who may be confused and frightened.

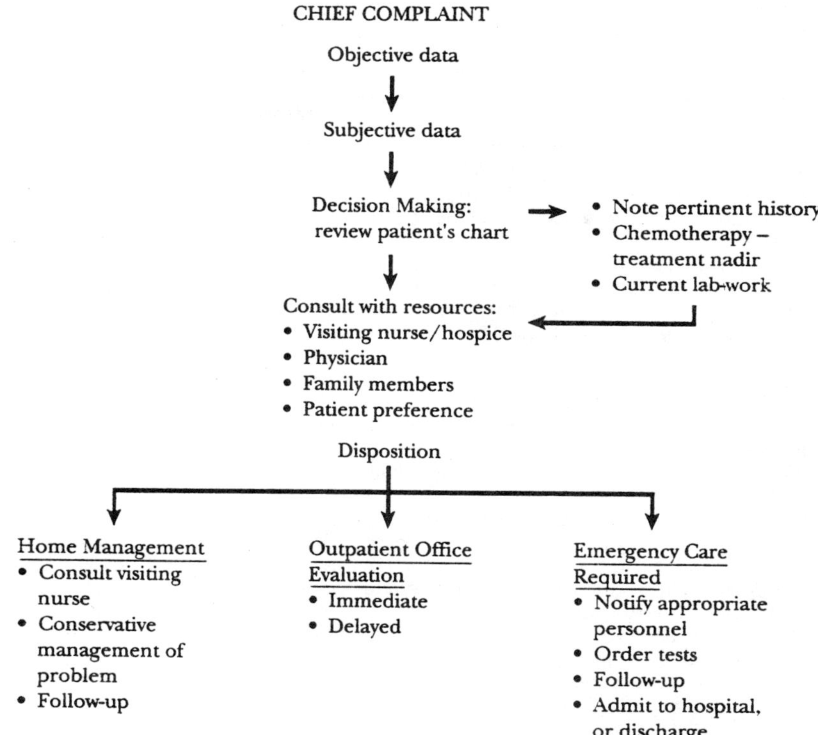

Figure 88.3. Telephone triage flow sheet of the basic steps to identify patient problems. *Source:* Camp-Sorrell (9).

Nursing Care Related to Specific Cancer Therapies

Nursing care of a patient receiving surgery, radiotherapy, chemotherapy, or biologic therapy begins with preparing the patient physically and psychologically for treatment. The oncology nurse should review the treatment plan with the responsible oncologist, and the nurse should be aware of any expected complications and required patient follow-up before the therapy is administered. The nurse should independently assess the patient's general physical, psychologic, and nutritional status.

Assessment of the patient's understanding of the disease and proposed therapy is fundamental to allaying the normal anxiety related to any procedure. The nurse should assess what the patient has been told by others about the disease and treatment to avoid misunderstanding and confused expectations. Anticipated side effects should be explained, along with recommendations to prevent, minimize, or alleviate these effects. Proper patient preparation improves compliance with instructions and treatment schedules. The nurse should be sure that the patient is familiar with the personnel who will be delivering the therapy. In many cases the oncology nurse will administer the chemotherapy or biotherapy and be present to monitor its acute effects.

A nursing care plan must be developed in response to the particular needs that are identified as the patient is prepared for treatment (7). This plan should at a minimum (*a*) promote the patient's understanding of therapy goals, treatment time schedules, and related side effects of therapy; (*b*) promote physical and psychological preparation for therapy; (*c*) promote physical comfort; and (*d*) promote compliance with instructions, treatment schedules, and symptom reporting. Both the patient and the family must be prepared for the upcoming treatment.

Table 88.5 identifies the assessment factors and interventions for common problems associated with chemotherapy, radiation therapy, and biologic therapy; these will be discussed in more detail later. The nurse should always review the treatment plan with the physician to ensure its consistency with any research study or institutional protocol. Teaching commences before therapy begins and continues during and after treatment. It may be reinforced with appropriate written and visual learning materials. When indicated, patients and families can be referred to other professionals, community programs, and agencies.

Special Considerations Related to Surgery

Surgery is the oldest and most frequently used treatment for cancer. Because a definitive diagnosis requires a biopsy, most patients undergo some type of surgical procedure early in the course of cancer treatment. Beyond diagnosis, surgery is the definitive means of cure for most solid tumors and has many other applications in cancer management. Surgical procedures are performed for cancer prevention, primary tumor removal, disease staging, tumor debulking, hormonal ablation, disease palliation, and reconstruction.

Table 88.5. Oncology Nursing Care for Common Problems Related to Cancer Therapies

Nausea and vomiting

Assessment: Assess the patient's general appearance, skin color and turgor, activity intolerance, anxiety, and environmental factors. Evaluate vital signs, time, frequency, amount and character of emesis, and serum electrolytes and chemistries for hypercalcemia, hyponatremia, uremia, and dehydration. Examine abdomen and auscultate for bowel sounds (intestinal obstruction). Obtain a diet history, medication schedules, and past patient measures that may have provided relief. Grade frequency and severity of emesis from 1 (minimal) to 4 (maximal).

Intervention: Advise the patient to eat dry foods such as toast or crackers; take clear, cool liquids; and eat small portions of low-fat foods and foods high in nutritional value. Consult a dietician as necessary. Patients should report symptoms and severity. Administer antiemetics as prescribed, and suggest using antiemetics in suppository form, taking antiemetics before receiving therapy. Offer support by explaining that nausea and vomiting are expected side effects, suggesting relaxation techniques and diversionary activity, and being available for questions and follow-up.

Mucositis

Assessment: Inspect oral cavity for moisture; color; ulceration; inflammation; quality, color and amount of saliva; and condition of teeth. Ascertain patient symptoms, including pain, dysphagia, ability to open mouth, ability to eat and take fluids, and taste and voice changes. Grade extent and severity of mucositis from 1 to 4.

Intervention: Implement measures to alleviate symptoms by teaching mouth care, including mouth rinsing with alkaline solutions every hour (1 tsp of baking soda in 8 oz of warm water) or a mouthwash containing sodium bicarbonate, diphenhydramine, and lidocaine; use soft sponge or gauze instead of toothbrush, removing thick, ropey saliva with gauze; irrigate mouth with sodium bicarbonate solution. Remove dentures for cleaning, and keep dentures in mouth only if comfortable and not causing irritation. Suggest and evaluate effects of topical analgesics, artificial saliva, and lip lubricant. Have the patient avoid alcohol, smoking, commercial mouthwashes, and hot, spicy, and acidic foods and fluids. Encourage fluids, popsicles, a soft and bland diet, and use of a straw to sip soups and beverages. Confer with physician regarding the need for systemic antibiotic, antifungal agents, and analgesics.

Evaluation: Based on the outcome of all therapeutic measures.

Diarrhea

Assessment: Assess frequency, character, and approximate volume of bowel movements, usual elimination patterns, nutrition history, height, weight, vital signs, hydration status, tissue turgor, condition of mucous membranes, and serum electrolyte values. Ascertain patient's knowledge and symptoms related to diarrhea and patient-initiated measures to control diarrhea.

Intervention: Implement measures to control and prevent diarrhea. Avoid irritating foods, gas-forming foods, fatty foods, lactose- and caffeine-containing products, smoking, and foods that are too hot or cold. Suggest a diet low in residue, high in protein and carbohydrates, and small, frequent meals.

Teach perianal hygiene: Cleanse with water and mild soap after bowel movement, use sitz baths if indicated, and use topical anesthetics to anal area if indicated. Administer and monitor the effects of ordered medications to control diarrhea. Evaluate patient and family for causes of diarrhea. Evaluate dietary modifications, medication schedules, symptom reporting, and measures implemented to alleviate diarrhea.

Constipation

Assessment: History of defecation, food or dietary fiber intake, and any changes in lifestyle. Assess patient symptoms of cramping, pain, diarrhea, anorexia, abdominal distention, and hemorrhoids. Also assess abdominal appearance, tenderness, bowel sound patterns, and usual bowel habits. Ascertain patient's knowledge related to constipation. Obtain schedule of all medications, previous medications, and interventions used to treat constipation.

Intervention: Implement measures to alleviate and prevent constipation. Suggest a diet high in fiber, roughage, and fluid. Drink warm fluids to stimulate intestinal motility. Use toilet or bedside commode instead of bedpan. If patient has a past history of constipation and will receive vinca alkaloid agents, suggest all of the above to start with the first chemotherapy dose. Avoid using enemas or suppositories without consulting the physician. Administer and monitor the effects of medications prescribed to relieve constipation:

Stool softeners: docusate sodium, mineral oil.

Bulk producers: psyllium, hydrophilic mucilloid, methylcellulose.

Osmotic and saline laxatives: lactulose (especially effective for constipation caused by vinca alkaloids), sorbitol, sodium biphosphate, magnesium citrate, magnesium hydroxide.

Cathartics: senna, cascara, bisacodyl.

Evaluation: Patient understanding of the causes of constipation, dietary modifications, medication schedules, and symptom reporting.

Hyperpigmentation/photosensitivity

Assessment: Inspect skin for increased pigmentation and relationship to clothed body areas, dark veins near chemotherapy injection sites, areas of increased pigmentation in mouth and nailbeds, sunburn, and rashes.

Intervention: Teach patient to avoid rays of the direct sun, wear protective clothing, and apply sunscreen (SPF 15 or higher) if exposure to the sun is unavoidable. Report signs and symptoms. Follow topical medication schedules if prescribed by a physician. Explain to the patient that skin reactions are expected and related to therapy, nail growth may be slowed, and that skin changes as well as vein and nail darkening are usually temporary.

Leukopenia

Assessment: Observe for signs and symptoms of infection. Be aware that patients with a low white-blood-cell count may not exhibit the normal signs of infection, such as productive cough, elevated body temperature, redness of skin, edema, or pain, because of the absence of neutrophils. Monitor the white-blood-cell count, calculate the absolute neutrophil count, and obtain vital signs. Inspect all body orifices, including the perianal area and skin, for infection. Inspect all venous access sites. Ascertain patient complaints along with emotional status. Obtain specimens for culture if indicated (e.g., blood, urine, stool, skin, sputum, vaginal, rectal). Obtain history of medication schedule. Monitor fluid balance (intake and output, daily weight).

Intervention: Implement measures to prevent infection by protecting the patient from people with known infections; provide a separate room if possible; and teach the patient, family, and visitors good handwashing technique. Encourage fluids if not contraindicated by other medical disorders. Administer colony-stimulating factor as prescribed by a physician. Suggest a low-bacteria diet that excludes fresh fruits and vegetables; all foods should be cooked. Maintain skin integrity by bathing daily with antiseptic soap and include nail care. Change intravenous tubing every 24 hours. Avoid injections and skin breakdown. Monitor exit sites of central venous catheters, intravenous site, or other venous access devices. Prevent respiratory infection by encouraging ambulation, coughing, and deep breathing. Prevent urinary infections by avoiding indwelling urinary catheters, providing adequate fluid intake and good hygienic measures. Prevent rectal abscess by avoiding enemas, rectal suppositories, and rectal temperatures, avoiding constipation. Inspect perianal area for fissures and hemorrhoids. Have patient report any rectal pain and/or discomfort. Administer antibiotics and antifungal agents as prescribed by the physician. Provide comfort measures to control fever by administering antipyretics if prescribed and providing tepid sponge bath and increased fluids. Teach the patient and family signs and symptoms of infection. Explain to the patient and family how to notify medical personnel if signs of infection appear.

Evaluation: Based on the patient's knowledge related to signs and symptoms of infection and understanding of interventions required to reduce the risk of infection.

Thrombocytopenia/anemia

Assessment: Inspect patient for signs and symptoms of bleeding; inspect skin for petechiae, ecchymoses, and hematomas. Observe neurologic status for changes associated with intracranial bleeding. Inspect for bleeding into joints, and test all body secretions and excreta for blood. Assessment includes monitoring vital signs and blood pressure in reclining, sitting, and standing position to assess for postural hypotension. Obtain hemoglobin, hematocrit, and platelet levels. Ascertain symptoms of fatigue, syncope, drowsiness, dyspnea, diaphoresis, chest pain, and edema. Auscultate lungs for rales, and assess abdominal girth weight. Ascertain if the patient is currently taking steroids or products that contain aspirin. Monitor all intravenous sites for bleeding.

Intervention: Implement measures to prevent and control bleeding by limiting injections and venipunctures. Use small-gauge needles, and apply pressure after all skin punctures. Avoid shaving with a razor blade, using a toothbrush or dental floss, straining during bowel movements, taking any medications that contain aspirin, nasotracheal suctioning, and bladder catheterization. Eliminate objects in patient's environment that may cause falls or bruising. Suggest mouth care with sponges or gauze. Increase fluid intake and stool softeners if indicated. For menstruating females, estrogen-progesterone agents can be given to stop menses if indicated. Encourage a soft diet high in fiber and protein. Limit physical activity; if indicated, pad side rails of the bed and prevent falls. Use a humidifier if oxygen therapy is indicated to prevent mucosal drying. For nosebleed, place patient in high Fowler's position, apply ice packs and pressure to upper lip, and notify a physician. Administer and monitor platelet and/or red-blood-cell transfusions if prescribed by a physician. Administer antacids and ice-water lavages for gastric bleeding if prescribed by a physician.

Evaluation: Based on patient's ability to recognize and report signs and symptoms of anemia and bleeding and the effectiveness of all interventions in preventing and controlling anemia and/or bleeding.

Sexual dysfunction

Assessment: Inform patient and his or her partner that there may be side effects from the cancer therapies that will affect sexual functioning. Ascertain questions and concerns related to sexual function and fertility concerns, and determine current methods of birth control if any.

Intervention: Inform females of possible amenorrhea, onset of early menopause with symptoms of "hot flashes," vaginal dryness, and possible dyspareunia related to decreased lubrication of vaginal walls. Use water-soluble lubricant or steroid cream if indicated. Explain that a decreased libido may be related to fatigue and hormonal changes. Use birth control methods if premenopausal. Inform males of possible temporary or permanent sterility and possible impotence related to therapy, which often is temporary. If indicated, suggest sperm banking before therapy begins. Refer patients and partners to appropriate professionals as indicated. Allow time for discussion of sexual dysfunction. Provide written information regarding contraception methods.

Evaluation: Based on the patient's understanding of possible sexual dysfunction related to therapy and the patient's ability to identify personal strategies to assist with alterations in sexual functioning. Patient reports symptoms and concerns related to sexual dysfunction.

Adapted from Bushkin (7).

Surgical procedures also are required to insert central venous access devices for the administration of cancer therapies.

The psychologic impact of cancer surgery cannot be overemphasized. Both the patient and family may experience a wide range of emotions and reactions to the diagnosis of cancer and the need for surgery. The diagnosis often has been made only a few days before a major procedure is scheduled. The nurse plays a key role in assessing the patient's understanding of possible surgical outcomes, such as change or loss of body function, limitations of mobility, and change in physical appearance. Based on this assessment, attention must be directed to promoting the patient's understanding of the surgical procedure and its outcome. Nursing care of the patient undergoing surgery for cancer includes fostering the patient's understanding of the specific procedure and expected outcome, preparing the patient physically and psychologically for the surgery, reducing anxiety, supporting the patient's postoperative physiologic stability, relieving pain, preventing complications, and promoting compliance with postoperative instructions.

Patient teaching should begin with a discussion of the type and purpose of the surgical procedure. This should be coordinated with the surgeon so that the patient is presented with complete and consistent information and instructions. The oncology nurse should reinforce and interpret surgical information to the patient and family. Surgical terms must be defined, and possible physical outcomes must be explained. Details such as dressing placements and postoperative devices (e.g., chest tubes, nasogastric tubes, central venous catheters) should be discussed. The routine preoperative and postoperative procedures, schedules, deep breathing and coughing exercises, and the like also must be explained.

Special attention must be devoted to issues such as the loss of body function and change in body appearance (21). There may be an incomplete understanding or a denial by the patient of these aspects of treatment. Additionally, progress in cancer surgery and prior exposure to cancer therapies have increased the risk for postsurgical problems as well as the numbers of surgical oncology patients who are critically ill (69). Risks for infection and bleeding; cardiopulmonary dysfunction; nutritional deficiencies; fluid, electrolyte, and metabolic abnormalities; and renal and liver dysfunction in the surgical oncology patient challenge the nurse in providing highly specialized care.

The nurse has a responsibility for coordinating early discharge planning and home care as indicated. Referrals to appropriate professionals and community support services should be considered. Other professional referrals include clinical nurse specialists, social workers, as well as physical and occupational therapists as indicated.

Special Considerations Related to Radiation Therapy

Like surgery, radiation therapy often is the initial definitive cancer treatment delivered shortly after the diagnosis is made. Thus, the patient may not have had time to fully adjust to the diagnosis. Nursing care of the patient receiving teletherapy or brachytherapy must focus on preparing the patient both physically and psychologically for therapy (20, 34). This requires an assessment of the patient's understanding of the therapy and the disease. There will be anxiety related to the procedure, especially with the first treatment. Many people have an irrational fear of radiation in all forms, and they may be especially disturbed by the idea of receiving a large dose. Acute and late side effects must be reviewed with the patient and family to ensure compliance with instructions and treatment schedules (20, 73, 93).

Unlike surgery which is delivered to an anesthetized patient, radiation is given to an awake and often anxious patient. Furthermore, there are many technical terms and treatment variations that must be explained to allay anxiety. Teletherapy is radiation therapy that is administered externally, and patient understanding of the machinery and isolation is necessary. Brachytherapy involves implanting a radioactive isotope into or adjacent to tumors, and it may occur in an operating room or the radiation oncology department. Patient understanding of the isolation and precautions exercised by the personnel will reduce anxiety.

When teletherapy is planned, patients must realize that during the procedure, they will be alone in the room while the radiation is administered and must lie still on the radiation-machine table but will be seen and heard by the technician at all times. They must understand that during the administration, they will not feel the radiation. The patient must be instructed not to remove skin markings that designate the treatment port.

When brachytherapy is planned, it may be delivered as high-dose brachytherapy through an afterloading device for a short time in the radiation oncology department or it may be given at a lower dose for a longer time, requiring that the patient be confined to a special, shielded hospital room. The patient must understand both the procedure and the necessary radiation precautions. The nurse should explain principles of time, distance, and shielding to the patient, family, visitors, and other hospital staff. For patients receiving brachytherapy in a hospital room, the nurse should promote self-care and implement measures to improve comfort by encouraging change of positions in bed and supporting body parts with pillows. The nurse should encourage patient communication and suggest diversionary activities such as reading, watching television, listening to music, and/or relaxation exercises. The nurse should assess the patient for complaints of muscle aches and pain at the implant site and, if indicated, obtain a physician's order for muscle relaxants and analgesics. Special precautions may be required for the disposal of body wastes and removal of linen and equipment.

Afterloading refers to first placing receivers for isotopes within the tissues to allow roentgenographic confirmation of proper arrangement and avoid exposure of personnel before inserting the radioactive material. The procedure is done under local or general anesthesia in the operating room. If low-dose brachytherapy is used, the radioactive pellet or wire is later inserted into the tubes in the patient's hospital room. The patient requires a separate room during the time a gamma radiation source is in use, and staff and visitors must maintain suitable radiation precautions, particularly distance from the source. The radioactive implant may remain in place for several days. In some cases, if removal of the isotope would be difficult and the half life of the isotope is short, the implant may remain permanently.

The isotopes used for brachytherapy can deliver very intensive local therapy; these isotopes include radium, iridium, and cesium. Most are sealed in tubes, needles, capsules, wires, or seeds. The sealed radioisotope is then placed in the affected tissue, such as needles in the tongue, a tube or capsule in the endocervical canal, or wires in the breast. These are usually removable, but seeds sometimes may be placed in the depths of a dissection for carcinoma or sarcoma and remain permanently.

Unsealed isotopes are contained in solution and may enter into the metabolic pathway of the tumor to be treated, such as radioactive iodine for thyroid cancer or radioactive phosphorus for polycythemia vera. Alternately, intracavitary suspensions of isotopes may be used in the pleura or peritoneum for the treatment of malignant pleural effusion or ovarian cancer.

SAFETY PRECAUTIONS

The Nuclear Regulatory Commission has developed guidelines for occupational exposure to radiation that concern all health professionals, particularly oncology nurses and others working in radiation oncology. Every hospital has a radiation safety officer who is responsible for assuring compliance with federal and state standards. Hospital personnel who care for patients receiving radiation are given special dosimetry badges to wear; these badges contain a film that measures radiation exposure. The badges are regularly measured, and a permanent record of radiation exposure is kept for all personnel. Federal regulations stipulate the maximum permissible annual radiation exposure.

Radiation precautions must be followed when caring for a patient with a radioactive implant. Radiation safety is based on three important factors: time, distance, and shielding (20, 34). Actual time spent in the patient's room should be minimized and limited to a total of 30 minutes every 8 hours (31). The amount of radiation exposure decreases by the inverse square of the distance from the source; working twice as far from the radiation source reduces the amount of radiation to one-fourth. Thus, it is important to maintain maximum physical distance from the patient whenever possible. Lead shielding provides additional protection, although lead shields and aprons have significant disadvantages. They are cumbersome to use and actually may induce a nurse to remain in the room for longer periods of time. The nurse should consistently adhere to principles of time and distance while caring for the patient. Patient self-care must be encouraged and all procedures and necessary precautions explained.

SIDE EFFECTS OF RADIATION THERAPY

During radiation therapy, cells of normal tissue in the radiation port that are subjected to ionizing radiation can be damaged. Some side effects are acute and temporary, while others may be irreversible.

Skin Toxicity

External radiation must pass through the skin to reach the tumor. The most common effect of this is a change in skin color within the radiation port. Erythema is caused by dermal capillary engorgement and may cause varying degrees of itching. Tanning is caused by the increased production of pigment. Dry desquamation with flaking of the skin is caused by the accumulation of dead skin cells. In cases where the basal skin cells are destroyed, moist desquamation may lead to serum leakage. Skin reactions usually are temporary, but if severe, they may lead to long-term effects, including scarring, changes in skin texture, and telangiectasis (i.e., dilatation of small skin venules). Necrosis requiring skin grafting is extremely rare and suggests improper technique. In patients who have received or later receive certain drugs (e.g., doxorubicin, actinomycin), these skin changes may be exaggerated and quite severe, in a reaction referred to as *radiation recall.*

Patients should be informed of the possible skin side effects in skin of radiation therapy. The nurse should observe the radiation sites for changes in color as well as the presence of dry or moist desquamation and be prepared to explain the cause of the skin reactions. In conjunction with the radiation oncologist, the nurse should also be prepared to offer suggestions and interventions to alleviate and control these side effects (73). Nursing care is planned to promote the patient's understanding of possible skin toxicities and the interventions required, to prevent and alleviate impairment of the skin integrity, and to promote comfort. Patient teaching includes instructing the patient to wear loose-fitting cotton clothing, gently washing the area with a mild soap, avoiding pressure and rubbing of the area, and avoiding the use of lotion, perfumes, and deodorants. Men receiving radiation to the head and neck area should use an electric razor and avoid aftershave colognes. Sun exposure and swimming in salt or chlorinated water should be avoided until the skin is completely healed. After healing is complete, an SPF 15 sunscreen should be used. Only water-based lubricants should be used for dry desquamation, and the patient should be cautioned against the application of heat and cold to irritated areas of the skin. Cool, moist compresses may relieve itching, and oral antihistamines and topical antipruritic lotions may be prescribed. Moist desquamation is kept clean, dry and exposed to air without dressings. The patient should be instructed to report promptly any signs and symptoms of infection.

Mucositis/Stomatitis

Inflammation of the mucous membranes with stomatitis in the mouth or vulvovaginitis of the genital tract may complicate radiotherapy. Whereas mild stomatitis may be transient and easily managed, severe stomatitis can cause extraordinary oral pain, infection, and further complicate the nutritional and hydration status of the patient. Injury to the salivary glands can cause a decreased production of saliva, resulting in xerostomia with severe dryness of the mouth. Saliva is important for lubricating and cleansing the oral cavity and keeping an alkaline environment that limits bacterial growth. Salivary secretions may become thick and expectoration difficult. Teeth can be indirectly affected by radiation because of periodontal membrane damage and the presence of less saliva, and of different composition, which allows for a change in the type and number of oral bacteria.

Hypogeusia (i.e., alteration or loss of taste sensation) can relate to the effect of radiation on the patient's taste buds. Dysgeusia (i.e., the presence of unpleasant tastes sometimes described as metallic) may occur from radiotherapy or chemotherapy. Ageusia (i.e., the absence of taste sensation) rarely is seen. The oral toxicities of radiation therapy can potentially undermine the hydration and nutritional status of the patient.

The nurse should coordinate a dental evaluation before any radiation that will encompass the oropharyngeal region. Appropriate oral preventive care may include the extraction of teeth. Before the initiation of radiation therapy, the nurse should encourage oral hygiene measures after meals and before sleep. These measures include use of a soft toothbrush and nonabrasive toothpaste as well as frequent oral rinsing with water, saline solution, or a nonalcohol–oral care preparation. An elixir of a 1:16 solution of diphenhydramine (Benadryl) and water is a soothing agent for individuals with mucositis (34). Daily oral self-examination should be taught, with report of changes in oral status to the health care provider. The nurse should encourage fluid intake and discourage smoking.

If stomatitis occurs, the patient should be instructed in (*a*) the maintenance of nutrition with frequent liquid, high-caloric drinks or blenderized foods; (*b*) avoidance of acids such as citrus juices or vinegar; (*c*) avoidance of retaining food residues in the mouth; (*d*) the use of alkaline anesthetic mouthwashes after eating (a mixture of bicarbonate, diphenhydramine, and lidocaine is helpful); and (*e*) realistic dialog with the physician about prescriptions of analgesics, up to and including narcotic drugs for the duration of painful stomatitis. If hydration or nutrition become deficient or pain control inadequate, the oncology nurse must be certain that these problems are appropriately addressed by the radiation oncologist.

For xerostomia, the nurse should encourage good oral hygiene and frequent rinsing with water. Commercially available artificial saliva and lip lubricants may provide temporary relief. The patient should be instructed to avoid the use of commercial mouthwash products that contain drying agents such as alcohol. Breathing through the mouth should be discouraged, and if fluid overload is not a problem, a fluid intake of at least 3000 mL/d should be encouraged. Sour, hard candies can be helpful in stimulating saliva production and in providing oral lubrication as well as creating a pleasant taste.

For thick oral secretions, the oncology nurse should encourage frequent rinsing with water or saline solution. The patient should be taught to remove thick mucus with a swab and to use an oral gavage bag to irrigate the mouth. In severe cases, oral suction equipment may be required.

Alopecia

Hair follicles are damaged or destroyed by radiation, and patients receiving radiation to the head will experience hair loss. This may be temporary or permanent, depending on the amount of radiation received. Patient teaching related to alopecia is discussed in the section on chemotherapy.

Complications of Chest Radiation

Side effects of radiation to the chest include esophagitis, pneumonitis, and delayed pulmonary fibrosis. Esophagitis can result in difficulty swallowing, severe chest pain, and superinfection, often with *Candida* sp. Esophagitis also compromises the patient's nutritional and hydration status.

Nursing care includes teaching the patient and family about the anticipated signs and symptoms (e.g., sore throat, dyspnea, dry cough, dysphagia, hemoptysis) and the rationale for maintaining hydration and nutrition. For esophagitis, a liquid or blenderized diet that includes protein and high calories served at room temperature is desirable, with the avoidance of irritation from spices or mechanical trauma (e.g., toast). If experiencing toxicity from chest radiation, the patient should be monitored for the need for supplemental oxygen, cough suppressant, analgesics, and nutritional supplements.

Complications of Abdominal Radiation

Radiation can damage the rapidly growing cells of the gastrointestinal tract leading to nausea and vomiting. With radiation to the lower gastrointestinal tract, the patient may experience diarrhea and abdominal cramping. Nursing care for these side effects is similar to care for those caused by chemotherapy, which are discussed later.

Complications of Pelvic Radiation

Cancers of the cervix, endometrium, prostate, bladder, and rectum often are treated with external radiation therapy and sometimes internal implants. Patients may experience side effects that include diarrhea, cystitis, vaginitis, late mucosal atrophy, and sometimes stenosis. Sexual dysfunction can result from effects on the gonads, prostate, and other male secretory glands as well as the vagina and its secretory glands.

Sexual dysfunction may result from narrowing of the walls of the vagina, decreased vaginal secretion during sexual arousal, and inflammation and scarring of the vaginal tissues. Patients should be informed of these possible side effects, shown how to use a vaginal dilator, and/or encouraged to continue sexual intercourse to keep the vaginal walls open and flexible. Artificial lubrication can be provided through use of commercially available creams and lubricants. Impotence may be seen in men after radiotherapy for prostate cancer, though less frequently than after surgical management. Patients should be aware of this complication and the availability of effective therapeutic approaches such as intrapenile injection of vasodilators to cause erection.

Ovarian function can be totally eradicated when high levels of radiation are given to the ovaries, leading to premature menopause. When possible, the reproductive organs may be shielded from radiation, but patients must be informed of the possibility of temporary or permanent sterility. Radiation can result in partial or permanent sterility in males, and men should be aware of the existence of sperm banks. Sexual function often is altered in both sexes by fatigue and weakness during the actual therapy along with the multiple physical and psychologic effects of the disease and side effects of therapy. Sexual dysfunction may persist as well.

Special Considerations Related to Chemotherapy and Biotherapy

Chemotherapy is a major treatment intervention that can cure several types of cancer, particularly in children, and palliate many others. Chemotherapy drugs are cytotoxic, because they have the ability to disrupt the metabolism of cells in a variety of ways. The major limiting factor in use of chemotherapy is the toxicity to normal tissue. The multiple side effects of chemotherapy range from minor patient discomfort to life-threatening toxicity. This treatment modality has become exceedingly complex as new drugs are developed and new combinations of drugs are formulated and tested. Over 50 different chemotherapy and biotherapy agents have been approved by the U.S. Food and Drug Administration for the treatment of cancer.

Chemotherapy may be used alone or combined with the other treatment modalities of radiation, surgery, and biotherapy. It may be used before surgery (sometimes called *neoadjuvant therapy*) or after surgery (*adjuvant therapy*). It may be used alone as curative therapy for some neoplasms. Chemotherapy most often is used in patients with metastatic cancer for its palliative effects. Thus, the treatment goals of chemotherapy may be cure, control, or palliation of cancer.

The mechanism of cell kill by drugs, relationship of drugs to the cell cycle, pharmacologic target molecules and cellular receptors, and drug side effects are all part of the educational preparation of the oncology nurse. These topics are covered in depth elsewhere in this text. As is the case with surgery and radiation, educating the patient and family is a key role played by the nurse to supplement and reinforce the physician's explanation.

Biologic therapy may alter immune response to the tumor or be primarily aimed at reconstituting normal host functions such as granulocyte repopulation. On occasion, the precise function of a noncytotoxic pharmacologic agent may be unknown, as in the case of levamisole. Biologic agents include the interferons, interleukins, vaccines, and colony-stimulating factors. These often are used in conjunction with other forms of cancer therapies, such as chemotherapy, radiotherapy, and surgery.

SAFE HANDLING OF CHEMOTHERAPY

In some settings, chemotherapeutic agents are prepared for administration by a central pharmacy; in others, the oncology nurse may have primary responsibility for this function. In either case, the cytotoxic nature of chemotherapeutic agents requires that personnel who prepare and administer the drugs take precautions to protect themselves from contact with or inhalation of these agents (29, 64, 81). Protective gloves, gowns, and masks are worn to guard against accidental skin contact and airborne droplets. In areas where large volumes of chemotherapy are prepared, a biologic vertical laminar air-flow hood is now standard. Table 88.6 describes precautions for the preparation, administration, and disposal of chemotherapy agents (64).

DOSAGE, SCHEDULING, AND ADMINISTRATION

The amount of chemotherapy and biotherapy that is prescribed for a patient is based on the type of tumor to be treated, previous chemotherapy and radiotherapy, bone marrow and other organ function, age, weight, physical status, and concomitant medical illnesses. Total dosage of most agents is calculated from total body surface area. It is an important responsibility of the oncology nurse to double check all such calculations, because the margin between a therapeutic and a toxic dose is very small for most agents.

Oncology nurses have taken a primary role in the safe administration of chemotherapy and biologic response modifiers (39, 44, 61, 62, 70, 77, 89). Over one-third of the ONS membership list their practice roles as being related to chemotherapy. Chemotherapy usually is given orally or intravenously, but it also may be given topically, intramuscularly, subcutaneously, intraperitoneally, intrathecally, intraarterially, intravesically, and intrapleurally. Nurses often are responsible for all but the last four routes, and particularly for the administration of oral and intravenous chemotherapy. Several of the chemotherapeutic agents known as *vesicants* may be seriously irritating to veins and surrounding tissues; these agents must be closely monitored for tissue infiltration when administered through a peripheral vein. Recommendations for the treatment of tissue infiltration of chemotherapy vary, but the major actions that are universally accepted include stopping the intravenous infusion, elevating the extremity, and except for the vinca alkaloids, applying ice to the skin infiltrate. The ONS has developed guidelines for the management of vesicant extravasation (63). The problem of tissue infiltration and vein damage from chemotherapy led to the development of alternative venous access devices. These include several versions of the central venous catheter and the implantable venous port. Infusion pumps, both stationary and portable, can be connected to venous access devices for the continuous administration of chemotherapy. A central venous catheter may be inserted into the subclavian vein through a trochar on a temporary basis or a semipermanent basis after surgical placement. The catheter tip is advanced into the superior vena cava near the right atrium. The tube then is tunneled under the skin of the chest and exits with an external catheter that is anchored to the skin. The external catheter can be used to obtain blood specimens; administer chemotherapy or other intravenous medications, blood, and blood products; and if it has a double lumen, parenteral nutrition, which requires a specific lumen that is not subject to contamination from frequent manipulation. Practice guidelines are available for access devices, implanted ports, and infusion pumps (60). These approaches are discussed in Chapter 46.

Nursing care focuses on patient education as well as placement and care of the catheter. Preventive measures, recognition of early signs and symptoms of complications and regular care also are important (24, 71, 84). Care includes periodic instillation of a heparinized solution to maintain the catheter's patency, dressing changes over the entrance and exit sites, and inspection of the incisions.

Table 88.6. Guidelines for Safe Handling and Disposal of Antineoplastic Agents

A. Preparation and Handling
1. All antineoplastic drugs should be prepared by specially trained individuals in a separate quiet area.
2. Drugs are prepared in a laminar air flow, class II biologic safety cabinet with vents to the outside, if possible. The blower is left on 24 hours a day, 7 days a week. The hood is serviced regularly according to the institutional and manufacturer's recommendations.
3. A thermoplastic face shield or goggles and a powered air-purifying respirator should be used if a biologic safety cabinet is not available.
4. The work surface is covered with an absorbent pad to minimize contamination; the pad is changed in the event of contamination and at the completion of drug preparation each day or shift.
5. Disposable surgical latex unpowdered gloves (0.007–0.009 inch thick) are used at all times when handling the drugs. Gloves should be changed every 30 to 60 minutes or if contaminated.
6. A disposable long-sleeved, cuffed gown made of lint-free nonabsorbent fabric with a closed front is worn during drug preparation.
7. Precautions are taken to avoid contamination and spills when removing air from the syringe or infusion line and when priming intravenous tubing. All procedures are carried out under the protection of the hood.
8. Avoid drug leakage during drug preparation by venting the vial and using large-bore needles, locking fittings for needles and syringes, and sterile gauze or sponge around the neck of the vial during needle withdrawal.
9. Aerosolization also may be minimized by attaching an aerosol protection device to the vial of drug before adding the diluent.
10. Once reconstituted, the drug is labeled according to institutional policies and procedures. The label should include an antineoplastic drug warning. The warning should state that the syringe or intravenous solution contains chemotherapy and should be handled with gloves and disposed of properly.
11. Antineoplastic drugs are transported in an impervious packing material.

B. Drug Administration
1. All physician orders are reviewed, including drug and drug dosage, route of administration, and pretreatment requirements.
2. The nurse ensures that informed consent has been completed and clarifies any questions that the patient might have regarding the drugs and their side effects.
3. Appropriate laboratory data are reviewed before the drugs are administered.
4. The drug(s) are administered according to established institutional policies and procedures.
5. Documentation of drug administration, including any adverse reaction, is made in the patient's medical record.

C. Accidental Exposure
1. In the event of accidental exposure, remove contaminated gloves or gown immediately and discard according to official procedures.
2. Wash the contaminated skin with soap and water.
3. Wash an eye that is accidentally exposed to chemotherapy with water or isotonic eye wash for at least 5 minutes.
4. Obtain a medical evaluation as soon as possible after exposure, and document the incident according to institutional policies and procedures.
5. In the event of a spill, personnel should don double surgical latex gloves; eye protection; and a disposable gown made of a lint-free, low-permeability fabric with a closed front, long sleeves, and elastic or knit closed cuffs.
6. Small amounts of liquids are cleaned up with gauze pads, whereas larger spills (> 5 mL) are cleaned up with absorbent pads.
7. The spill area is cleaned three times with a detergent followed by clean water.
8. Broken glassware and disposable contaminated materials are placed in a leak-proof, puncture-proof container and then placed in a sealable 4-mil polyethylene or 2-mil polypropylene bag and marked with a distinctive warning label.

D. Drug and Equipment Disposal
1. All equipment and unused drugs are treated as hazardous and are disposed of according to the institution's policies and procedures.
2. All contaminated equipment including needles are disposed of intact.
3. All contaminated materials used in drug preparation and administration are disposed of in a leak-proof, puncture-proof container with a distinctive warning label and are placed in a sealable 4-mil polyethylene or 2-mil polypropylene bag with appropriate labeling.
4. Linen contaminated with bodily secretions of patients who have received chemotherapy within the previous 48 hours is placed in a specially marked laundry bag, which then is placed in an impervious bag that is marked with a distinctive warning label.

E. Institutional Policies
1. Personnel who prepare and administer antineoplastic agents should receive specialized training.
2. Policies should provide for separate labeling and disposal of cytotoxic waste. This includes needles, syringes, glassware, intravenous tubing, and contaminated linen.
3. Smoking, eating, or drinking, and application of cosmetics should be prohibited in the preparation area.
4. Policies related to drug handling should be established, reviewed, and accessible.
5. Employee Health Services should be able to identify all employees who handle cytotoxic agents.

Data from Oncology Nursing Society (64) and U.S. Department of Labor (81).

Although institutional care protocols differ, the patient generally is taught to change the dressing daily for the first 2 weeks, using sterile technique, and then twice weekly until healed. The catheter is anchored onto the skin with tape, and patients are instructed to observe the incision sites for swelling, erythema, and drainage. Patients are further instructed in how to instill a heparinized flush solution into the catheter on a precise time schedule.

The nurse explains and demonstrates aseptic technique, sterile dressing changes, site inspection, and the method to flush the catheter. Occasional patients are taught to self-administer medication. In addition, the nurse provides the patient and family with written instructions, encourages symptom reporting, and indicates the symptoms or findings that require immediate attention. Patients must understand how to contact the nurse and physician 24 hours a day in an emergency.

An implanted venous port provides both a reservoir and a central venous catheter without an external device. A metallic chamber with a plastic resealing port is implanted under the skin; dressing changes and frequent heparinization are not required. The port is flushed with a heparin solution either after use or monthly. Although patients can be taught to access the port for self-administration of medications and heparinization, these tasks usually are performed by the oncology nurse. This provides an opportunity for overall assessment. The risk of infection is reduced significantly by the implanted venous port. The Ommaya reservoir is a subcutaneous port that is implanted under the scalp over a small surgical hole in the skull, which allows a catheter that is attached to the reservoir to be threaded into the lateral ventricle for administering chemotherapy into the cerebrospinal fluid.

Continuous intravenous administration of chemotherapy can be given over time intervals from several hours to several weeks. To provide continuous infusion therapy, specialized pumps have been developed. Some are portable and can be attached to a waist belt; the patient can be fully ambulatory and active while receiving continuous chemotherapy. The pump is filled with a solution containing the chemotherapeutic agent and is attached to a central venous line. Some pumps are implanted under the skin and externally filled with chemotherapy. The pumps then can be programmed to deliver small amounts of drug continuously over a given time period. More sophisticated pumps can deliver several drugs at variable rates in different time periods.

SIDE EFFECTS OF CHEMOTHERAPY

While the chemotherapy drugs are attacking malignant tumor cells, normal rapidly growing cells also are temporarily or permanently damaged. Chemotherapeutic agents lack the ability to differentiate malignant cells from rapidly growing normal body cells, which results in damage to normal cells that manifests as side effects. These can range from minor annoyances to life-threatening toxicities.

GASTROINTESTINAL

The lining of the gastrointestinal tract is composed of rapidly growing cells that are renewed as a mechanism to protect and maintain the integrity of the tract. Any part of the gastrointestinal tract can be affected by chemotherapy, resulting in nausea, vomiting, mucositis, taste alterations, diarrhea, and constipation.

Nausea and vomiting are the most common early side effects of many chemotherapy drugs. The chemoreceptor trigger zone of the medulla is located near the emetic center, and it is stimulated by the presence of chemicals in the blood. It is believed that chemotherapy stimulates the emetic center. Some drugs, such as cisplatin and the nitrosoureas, cause severe vomiting. In addition, dose intensification of chemotherapeutic agents intensifies the problem. Nausea and vomiting also may result from actual irritation of the lining of the gastrointestinal tract. Nausea and vomiting are classified as acute (i.e., usually occurs 1 to 6 hours after chemotherapy), delayed (i.e., persists or develops 24 hours after chemotherapy), or anticipatory (i.e., before chemotherapy).

Several antiemetic drugs are used to minimize nausea and vomiting with varying results. The antiemetic agents in the phenothiazine class, such as prochlorperazine, are used because they depress stimulation of the emetic center and the chemoreceptor trigger zone. Phenothiazines offer only mild relief, and when the more emetic types of chemotherapy are used, their effectiveness is minimal. Because the phenothiazines cause sedation, extrapyramidal symptoms, and orthostatic hypotension, the oncology nurse must be concerned about patient safety (87).

Metoclopramide, which is a derivative of the procainamide class of drugs, is an effective antiemetic agent against highly emetogenic therapy. It blocks the chemoreceptor trigger zone, increases gastrointestinal motility, and causes gastric emptying. In high intravenous doses, metoclopramide is effective against nausea and vomiting, but adverse side effects ascribed to this drug limit its usefulness. However, antihistamines can be given with the drug to eliminate these side effects. Antihistamines and intravenous steroids have some antiemetic action and also are used to enhance the effectiveness of other antiemetic agents. Anxiolytic drugs, such as lorazepam, have been used both alone or in combination with other antiemetics for their amnesic and sedative affect.

Serotonin inhibitors such as ondansetron and granisetron recently have proven to be highly effective antiemetics (17, 82). These agents, arguably the most potent antiemetics available, are particularly valuable in management of the severe emesis induced by cisplatin (22, 30) (see Chapter 174).

The psychogenic aspects of nausea, vomiting, and behavioral interventions continue to be studied. Many patients benefit from relaxation exercises (15, 72); biofeedback tapes; self-hypnosis (14), diversionary activities such as music (23, 45), reading, or television; aerobic exercises (85); and mental imagery (23). Behavioral therapies provide the patient with something that allows their active participation in care. Any of these techniques can be used in conjunction with the administration of pharmacologic antiemetics.

It is important to obtain an in-depth emetic history and develop an action plan to prevent nausea and vomiting. The patient and family must be informed of the potential occurrence of nausea and vomiting and what to do if they occur. Because most patients receive their therapy on an outpatient basis, telephone follow-up at 24 to 48 hours after treatment is of utmost importance to check on the patient's compliance with the antiemetic regimen prescribed and his or her well-being. Figure 88.4 shows a telephone triage flow sheet for nausea and vomiting.

Anorexia may occur along with nausea and vomiting, as a side effect of chemotherapeutic or biologic agents, or because of the cancer itself. A nutritional history should be obtained early in the course of therapy, and the patient should be taught the importance of adequate nutritional intake (see Chapter 173). Consultation with a registered dietician may be necessary. Oral nutritional supplements, hyperalimentation, or enteral nutrition may be required to provide adequate nutritional intake. For severe anorexia-cachexia, megestrol acetate may be indicated (47) (see Chapter 75).

Mucositis

The rapidly growing cells of the mucous membrane provide a protective lining throughout the oral cavity, gastrointestinal tract, and genital tract. The cytotoxic action of

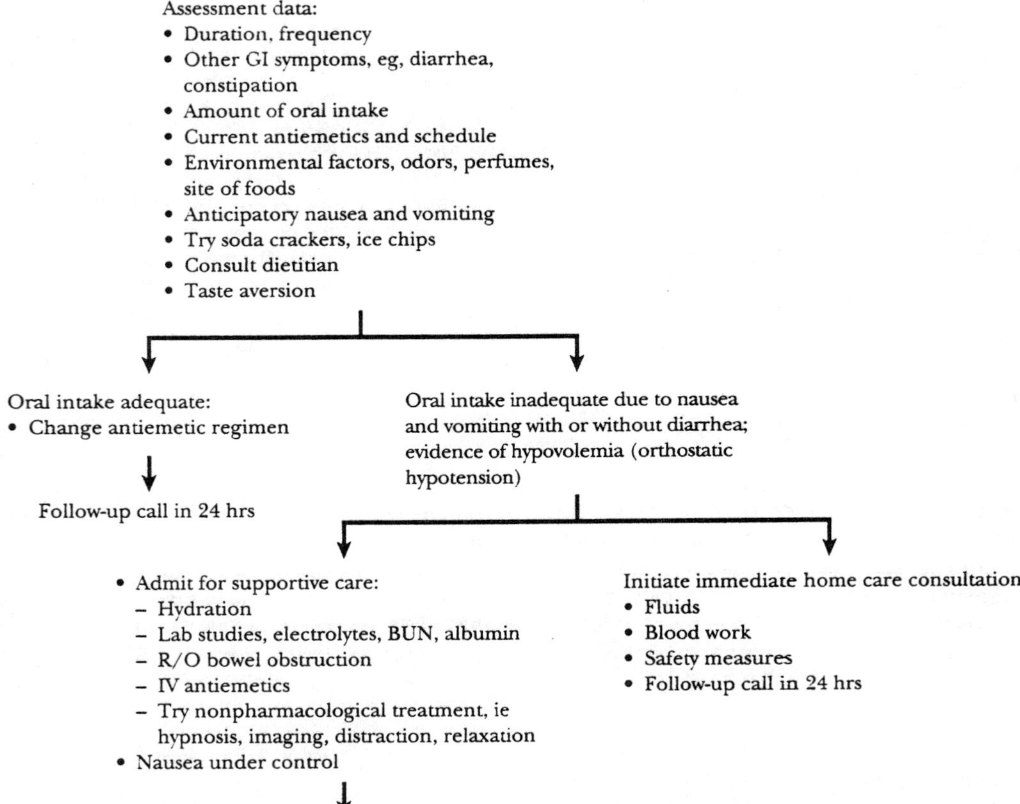

Assessment data:
• Duration, frequency
• Other GI symptoms, eg, diarrhea, constipation
• Amount of oral intake
• Current antiemetics and schedule
• Environmental factors, odors, perfumes, site of foods
• Anticipatory nausea and vomiting
• Try soda crackers, ice chips
• Consult dietitian
• Taste aversion
Oral intake adequate:
• Change antiemetic regimen
Follow-up call in 24 hrs
Oral intake inadequate due to nausea and vomiting with or without diarrhea; evidence of hypovolemia (orthostatic hypotension)
• Admit for supportive care:
– Hydration
– Lab studies, electrolytes, BUN, albumin
– R/O bowel obstruction
– IV antiemetics
– Try nonpharmacological treatment, ie hypnosis, imaging, distraction, relaxation
• Nausea under control
Follow-up for home antiemetic regimen in 24 hrs
Initiate immediate home care consultation:
• Fluids
• Blood work
• Safety measures
• Follow-up call in 24 hrs

Figure 88.4. Telephone triage flow sheet for nausea and vomiting. *Source:* Camp-Sorrell (9).

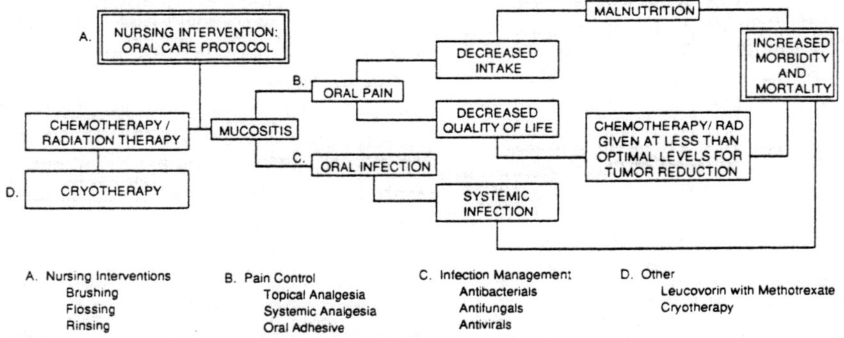

Figure 88.5. Process of stomatitis development with proposed sites for intervention. *Source:* Wujcik (87).

chemotherapy can damage or destroy these cells lining the oral cavity, resulting in bacterial invasion and varying degrees of inflammation. The necrosis of mucosal cells and exposure of underlying tissues to the outside environment ordinarily excluded by the mucosa lead to stomatitis, esophagitis, and vulvovaginitis.

Patients may develop painful oral and esophageal ulcers as the cells of the mucosa are damaged and cellular repair is decreased. Stomatitis and esophagitis may be exaggerated if the patient is immunosuppressed from the disease or treatment or is depleted from malnutrition or dehydration. Mucositis also can alter the patient's nutritional and hydration status as a result of inhibiting his or her consumption of food and fluids. Mucositis predisposes to the development of infection in the mouth or esophagus, predominantly due to candidiasis, herpes simplex, or mouth organisms. The intensity and degree of inflammation varies, depending on the physical status of the patient as well as the type, dosage, and scheduling of the chemotherapy and/or radiotherapy and concomitant cytopenias. Oral topical analgesics, parenteral analgesics including narcotics, antibiotics, and both antiviral and antifungal agents may be prescribed by the physician. Vulvovaginitis may accompany stomatitis when drug toxicity is severe. Figure 88.5 identifies the process of stomatitis development and proposed sites for therapeutic interventions (87).

Xerostomia and Taste Alterations

The cytotoxic effects of chemotherapy on the salivary glands can decrease production of saliva, resulting in xerostomia or mouth dryness. Injury to the taste buds causes alterations in taste: hypogeusia, a decrease in taste sensation; dysgeusia, the presence of unpleasant tastes sometimes described as metallic; and ageusia, the absence of taste. These side effects can further compromise the patient's nutritional and hydration status.

Diarrhea

Injury of the intestinal lining by chemotherapy results in inflammation and impaired production of digestive enzymes. Intestinal motility may be stimulated, which results in diarrhea. Along with frequent loose bowel movements, patients also can experience abdominal cramping, flatulence, bloating, and irritation of the anus. Diarrhea also may relate to the patient's anxieties and fears. The incidence of chemotherapy-related diarrhea is high, occurring with many of the antimetabolites and antitumor antibiotics. Potential alterations in nutritional status can result from inadequate digestion, a decrease in nutrient absorption, and a loss of water and electrolytes. Pharmacologic agents, such as diphenoxylate with atropine (Lomotil), loperamide (Imodium), or morphine may be indicated along with nutritional interventions to slow intestinal peristalsis. The somatostatin analogue, octreotide acetate, may be beneficial for patients with chemotherapy- or radiotherapy-related diarrhea (42) (see Chapters 71, 184).

Constipation

Chemotherapy-related constipation is a side effect of the vinca alkaloid drugs and a major toxicity of opioids given for pain relief. The autonomic neurotoxicity of vincristine and vinblastine can decrease intestinal peristalsis, causing constipation. Bowel status must be assessed before and during treatment to avoid constipation and possible adynamic ileus. Older patients are especially susceptible to constipation caused by the vinca alkaloids. Constipation may be further aggravated by decreased fluid intake and physical activity. Ample fluid intake, fiber, stool softeners, laxatives, and if necessary, enemas should be used to ensure against obstipation. Because opioids, particularly morphine and its derivatives, cause smooth muscle contraction and constipation, patients must be placed on a prophylactic regimen to avoid or diminish this complication.

Integumentary Changes

Skin side effects include hyperpigmentation, photosensitivity, erythematous skin rashes, radiation recall, alopecia, and chemical tissue infiltration.

Hyperpigmentation of the skin and nail beds is caused by an increased stimulation of melanin-producing cells in the basal level of the dermis. Skin darkening can be localized in small areas, such as over the veins, or be more widespread, such as over the face and trunk. Several agents cause photosensitivity, which is an acceleration of the tanning process caused by the sun's ultraviolet rays, resulting in marked hyperpigmentation and deeply tanned skin or, in fair-skinned patients, severe sunburn. Hyperpigmentation and photosensitivity are known side effects of fluorouracil, methotrexate, and bleomycin.

Skin rashes may take many guises. Among the most important, folliculitis, which is a fine, papular erythematous rash that occurs around hair roots on the body surface, is thought to be caused by drug effects on the epithelial lining of the hair follicles. A maculopapular, erythematous, and often pruritic rash often is caused by medications, but this results more commonly from antibiotics, allopurinol, or other drugs rather than the chemotherapeutic agents. A hypersensitivity reaction is serious, and the offending agent must be stopped immediately. Antimetabolites and anthracyclines can cause allergic skin reactions.

Radiation recall is a term describing the effect that chemotherapy may have on areas of the skin previously or concomitantly exposed to radiation therapy. This can result in erythema, ulceration, wet desquamation, and permanent hyperpigmentation.

Alopecia can be an extremely devastating side effect, because hair is a significant part of an individual's self-image. Chemotherapy causes alopecia by damaging the rapidly growing and renewing hair follicles. Hair is weakened at the shaft and is easily removed from the scalp. The amount of hair loss depends on the drug, the dosage, and the treatment duration; however, not all chemotherapeutic agents cause alopecia. Hair loss can range from mild thinning on the scalp to total loss of all scalp hair.

Facial and body hair are less frequently affected by chemotherapy, because their growth and renewal rate is slower. Nevertheless, patients may experience a loss of facial and body hair, including eyebrows, lashes, axillary, and pubic hair. Despite their normally slower growth, brows and lashes ordinarily regrow before scalp hair. Alopecia may cause the scalp to become irritated and sensitive, along with producing dry and flaking skin, for which a mild shampoo should be used. Hair loss is almost always temporary (except after heavy irradiation) and complete regrowth can be expected after the treatment is stopped. Hair loss usually starts approximately 14 to 21 days after treatment.

Patient preparation must be emphasized as an important component of adaptation to alopecia. Wigs, scarves, hairpieces, and hats can be suggested, and an insightful oncology nurse has a ready list of reliable and sensitive salespersons for wigs. Hair sometimes grows back while still on treatment but then falls out again. Hair starts to grow after treatment is withdrawn, and the new hair may be different in color and texture (often darker and curlier). Purchasing a wig or hairpiece before alopecia begins allows the choice of a wig to preserve a nearly normal appearance. Cutting long hair after chemotherapy is initiated, decreases the anxiety associated with losing large amounts of hair and provides a transitional stage. Methods to reduce the rate of hair loss include limiting brushing, avoiding harsh shampoos, and wearing a hair net to sleep at night. The patient should be informed that the cost of a wig or hairpiece is covered by most health insurance companies. Local units of the American Cancer Society often will lend patients wigs free of charge as well.

Scalp hypothermia describes application of ice to the scalp to decrease the circulation of drug-containing blood during chemotherapy administration. This technique has been studied as a means to minimize hair loss. Its use remains controversial, however, because reducing chemotherapy distribution to the scalp could theoretically create a safe area for cancer cells. Scalp hypothermia is contraindicated in cancers that are known to spread to the brain and soft tissues of the scalp. Furthermore, scalp hypothermia is relatively ineffective for high-dose combination chemotherapy.

Hematologic Toxicities

Chemotherapy can directly affect the blood-producing mechanism, with a potential for the most lethal complications. Myelosuppression induced by chemotherapy is the most common dose-limiting side effect, with a potential for hemorrhagic and infectious complications as the major concerns. Blood components (i.e., red blood cells, white blood cells, platelets) are continually being made by the rapidly growing cells of the bone marrow. The cytotoxic action of chemotherapy inhibits this production, and anemia is seen after prolonged treatment. White blood cells are an integral component of the immune system, and neutropenia leads to an increased susceptibility to infection. A decrease in the number of circulating platelets causes an increased susceptibility to bleeding. Three major factors that affect the magnitude of the myelosuppression are the various life cycles of the blood cells, the pharmacokinetic characteristics of the particular chemotherapeutic agents, and patient characteristics (e.g., age, health, bone marrow reserve) (48).

Peripheral blood counts are monitored regularly and always evaluated individually by both the oncology nurse and the medical oncologist before beginning a chemotherapy treatment cycle. Based on these blood counts, therapy is modified or delayed. Hematologic status also can be compromised by invasion of the primary tumor into the bone marrow or by malnutrition.

Nursing care of the patient with myelosuppression cannot be overemphasized. Prevention and early detection of potential bleeding problems and sepsis are primary goals of the oncology nurse, and guidelines for nursing care and patient education exist for the patient with thrombocytopenia. Figure 88.6 shows an example of a telephone triage flow sheet that the oncology nurse can use with such a patient.

During episodes of neutropenia, hematopoietic growth factors may be prescribed. Nurses must be knowledgeable of the various colony stimulating factors, aspects of administration, and potential toxicities. Additionally, patients must be instructed on the signs of infections and measures for preventing this complication. Figure 88.7 shows a telephone triage sheet for the assessment and management of fever, an indication of infection.

Renal Toxicity

Renal toxicity is a less common side effect, but it can be seen after the administration of cisplatin, nitrosoureas, methotrexate, or mitomycin-C. With appropriate preparation, which requires careful attention to hydration, renal toxicity can be minimized. Renal damage also can result from rapid tumor destruction with liberation of large amounts of various metabolites that may precipitate in the renal tubules, or from the use of very high-dose methotrexate, which also may precipitate in the kidney. Premedication with allopurinol, alkalinization of the urine with sodium bicarbonate, and fluids to induce a brisk urine flow are used to minimize toxicity.

Bladder Toxicity

Hemorrhagic cystitis is caused by mucosal irritation in the bladder induced by the breakdown products of cyclophosphamide and ifosfamide, which are excreted in the urine after high-dose therapy. Proper attention to hydration and neutralization with sodium methyl ethane sulfonate (Mesna) are critical to dilute and inactivate the toxic metabolites.

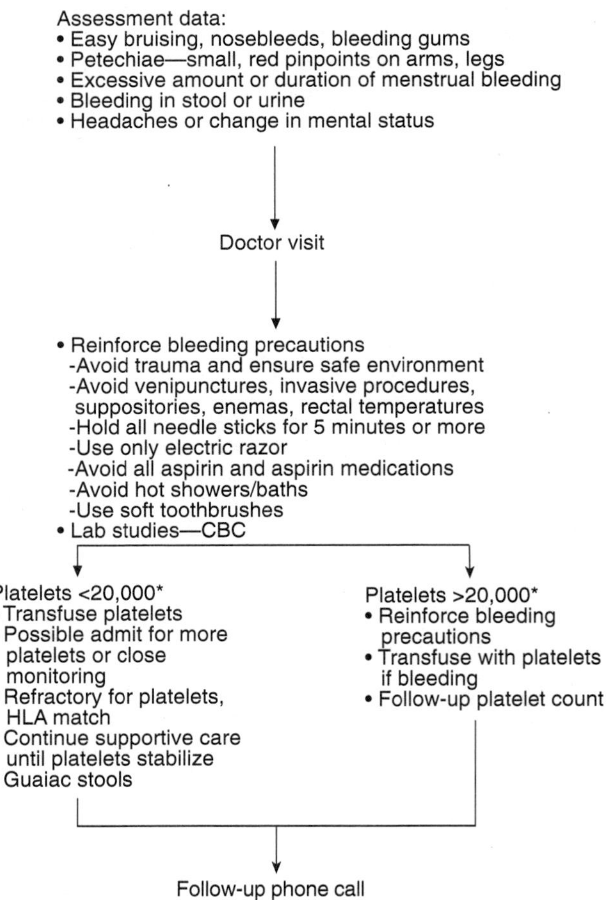

Figure 88.6. Telephone triage flow sheet for the patients with thrombocytopenia. *Threshold (5) may be 5,000–10,000 for many diseases. *Source:* Camp-Sorrell (9).

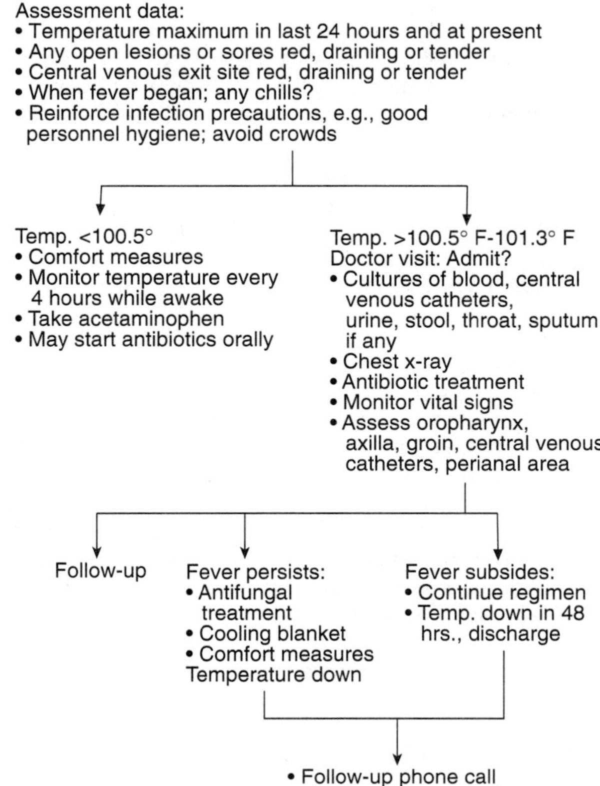

Assessment data:
• Temperature maximum in last 24 hours and at present
• Any open lesions or sores red, draining or tender
• Central venous exit site red, draining or tender
• When fever began; any chills?
• Reinforce infection precautions, e.g., good personnel hygiene; avoid crowds
Temp. <100.5°
• Comfort measures
• Monitor temperature every 4 hours while awake
• Take acetaminophen
• May start antibiotics orally
Temp. >100.5° F-101.3° F
Doctor visit: Admit?
• Cultures of blood, central venous catheters, urine, stool, throat, sputum if any
• Chest x-ray
• Antibiotic treatment
• Monitor vital signs
• Assess oropharynx, axilla, groin, central venous catheters, perianal area
Follow-up
Fever persists:
• Antifungal treatment
• Cooling blanket
• Comfort measures
Temperature down
Fever subsides:
• Continue regimen
• Temp. down in 48 hrs., discharge
• Follow-up phone call
• Monitor culture result

Figure 88.7. Telephone triage flow sheet for the assessment and management of fever. *Source:* Camp-Sorrell (9).

Pulmonary Toxicity

Pulmonary toxicity manifested as inflammation and fibrosis has been associated with bleomycin, methotrexate, mitomycin-C, alkylating agents, and the nitrosoureas. Assessment of risk factors and symptoms of pulmonary toxicity as well as monitoring the cumulative doses of toxic agents may prevent damage to pulmonary tissue. Baseline and follow-up pulmonary function tests may be ordered in patients receiving these toxic agents.

Cardiotoxicity

Cardiotoxicity is a major dose-limiting factor for the antitumor agents doxorubicin, daunorubicin, and idarubicin, and, to a lesser degree, mitoxantrone, high-dose cyclophosphamide, and paclitaxel. Cardiotoxicity results from cumulative drug exposure and often can be anticipated based on the total dose. The ventricular ejection fraction is the best clinical tool to determine whether damage has been sustained. A careful history of exercise and other activities is useful as well. Cardiotoxic effects include arrhythmias and congestive heart failure. Prevention is only possible by limiting the total dose of drug delivered or, in part, by use of a cardioprotective agent such as dexrazoxane (Zinecard).

Neurotoxicity

Sensory and perceptual alterations result from the effects of chemotherapy on nerve conduction fibers. Neurotoxicity most often is associated with the vinca alkaloids (vincristine, vinblastine), cisplatin, and paclitaxel. It usually manifests by peripheral neuropathy. Symptoms are feelings of numbness and tingling in the hands and feet (i.e., paresthesias), loss of deep tendon reflexes, generalized motor weakness, and in severe cases, atonia of the bowel and bladder. Cisplatin can cause motor and sensory neuropathy, tinnitus, and hearing loss. Procarbazine causes peripheral neuropathy and altered levels of consciousness. Ifosfamide also may cause neurotoxicity in the form of somnolence.

SIDE EFFECTS OF BIOLOGIC THERAPY

The two most common side effects associated with biotherapy are flu-like syndrome and fatigue. Intradermal, subcutaneous, and intralesional vaccines can cause localized skin inflammation and the systemic side effects of elevated body temperature, chills, diaphoresis, and fatigue. Intravenous administration of immunomodulators has a wider range of systemic side effects including fever, chills, diaphoresis, fluid retention, dyspnea, nausea, vomiting, and fatigue.

A detailed description of chemotherapy and biotherapy as well as their toxicities can be found in Chapters 58 to 68 and 78 to 83 of this text, and elsewhere in the cancer literature (39, 43, 89).

Pain Control

Cancer pain is a complex multidimensional phenomenon. The International Association for the Study of Pain has defined pain as "an unpleasant sensory and emotional experience associated with actual or potential tissue damage or described in terms of such damage" (56). It is a subjective experience evidenced by the unique psychologic and physiologic responses by the patient to pain. Six major components affect the patient's interpretation and perception of the pain experience (1, 51): (*a*) physiologic; (*b*) sensory; (*c*) affective; (*d*) cognitive; (*e*) behavioral; and (*f*) sociocultural.

More than 4 million people in the world suffer from cancer-related pain each day (86). Because pain is a significant problem in patients with cancer and the numerous barriers interfere with adequate pain management, agencies, organizations, and researchers have taken great strides in addressing this major problem and improving the management of cancer pain. The U.S. Agency for Health Care Policy and Research has developed guidelines for the management of cancer pain (38). These guidelines provide assistance to the practitioner to improve the assessment and management of such pain. They stress the importance of controlling cancer pain to promote the quality of life and prevent loss of control and unnecessary suffering. Barriers to effective pain management that relate to legal regulation of opioids as well as cost and reimbursement issues are discussed. The guidelines also review pain assessment and both pharmacologic and nonpharmacologic interventions for pain control.

Cancer pain most often is associated with tissue damage and infiltration from the growing, malignant neoplasm. As tumors grow they stretch normal boundaries of the organ, causing pain. Adjacent organs and structures also are affected. This can result in nerve compression, obstruction of hollow organs, and stretching of capsules and tissue membranes, periosteal irritation, and pathologic fractures. Pain may be an acute or a chronic event. Unrelieved pain affects a patient's lifestyle, treatment compliance, and ability to cope with the disease.

The primary way to relieve tumor-related pain is to destroy the tumor that is the cause. Surgical removal of a tumor mass sometimes is an option. More often, however, radiation therapy can be directed to painful, localized areas of tissue infiltration, particularly for metastatic lesions of bone. Chemotherapy sometimes may shrink a tumor mass and relieve pain. Often, however, destruction of the tumor is not possible, and pharmacologic relief is the only alternative. Even so, inadequate knowledge of analgesic drugs is one of the most commonly cited reasons for the undertreatment of cancer pain (16).

PHARMACOLOGICAL MANAGEMENT

Nonsteroidal anti-inflammatory drugs (NSAIDs) and acetaminophen, opioid analgesic agents, and adjuvant analgesic agents are used either alone or in combination for the treatment of pain. These agents control the symptom, with the goal of improving the patient's comfort. NSAIDs, aspirin, and acetaminophen are effective for the relief of mild pain. Opioids control pain by acting on the central nervous system and include codeine, morphine, hydromorphone, meperidine, and oxycodone. Adjuvant analgesic drugs are valuable during all phases of pain management and may enhance pain relief. These agents include corticosteroids, anticonvulsants, antidepressants, neuroleptics, antihistamines, local anesthetics, and psychostimulants.

Side effects from opioids include drowsiness, constipation, nausea and vomiting, and drying of the oral mucosa. Aspirin and NSAIDs can cause gastrointestinal bleeding and interfere with platelet function.

Agents such as steroids, psychotropics, muscle relaxants, and sedatives also are used to control pain-related symptoms. Pharmacologic agents can be given orally or parenterally and on intermittent or continuous dosing schedules. Careful attention to the dosing schedule is particularly important for effective pain control. The objective of pain control is to prevent pain, not allow it to periodically reappear so that it can be relieved again. The patient should be enlisted as a partner in this effort. Research continues in the area of self-administration and self-dose titration of parenteral and oral narcotics. Selection of pharmacologic agents should be based on patient pain-control history, preference, and response (see Chapter 172).

The side effects of pharmacologic agents also must be considered. Opioids can depress the function of the central nervous system so much that enjoyable social activity becomes impossible. Stimulants may then be of value without impairing pain relief.

NONPHARMACOLOGIC MANAGEMENT

Nondrug methods to alleviate cancer pain are important components of a comprehensive, multidisciplinary approach to the management of cancer pain. These methods do not take the place of adequate analgesic medications, but they can serve as important adjuvants. The reader is referred elsewhere for an excellent review by Spross and Burke (75) of the nonpharmacologic management of cancer pain.

Behavioral Therapies

Behavioral therapies can be used in conjunction with pharmacologic therapies to promote patient participation. Behavioral therapies, which vary in approach, are intended to decrease tension and increase muscle relaxation. These therapies may assist with pain control while ameliorating nausea and vomiting related to radiation or chemotherapy. General anxiety can be reduced as well. Diversionary activities such as exercise, hobbies, or reading assist in the redirection of pain sensations and perceptions. Relaxation therapy includes exercises and progressive muscle relaxation; advanced relaxation techniques can be achieved through hypnosis and guided imagery. These therapies can be learned and self-induced as a means of achieving deep relaxation.

Physical Interventions

Cutaneous therapies such as skin massage or the application of heat, cold, lotions, and transcutaneous electronic nerve stimulation can offer additional temporary pain relief. Breathing exercises, movement, positioning, acupressure, and acupuncture also are used to reduce pain.

Transcutaneous electronic nerve stimulation is accomplished through a small electrical device, powered by a battery pack, that provides electrical stimulation to the skin. The large fibers of the peripheral nervous system are stimulated to override pain stimuli and close the gate that controls pain perception.

ROLE OF THE NURSE IN PAIN MANAGEMENT

Because nurses spend more time with a patient experiencing pain than any other health professional, it is of utmost importance that the nurse be knowledgeable about pain assessment and both pharmacologic and nonpharmacologic management of pain in order to provide good pain control as well as patient and family education. However, barriers to providing effective pain control have not eluded the nursing profession. Misconceptions and fears about addiction, drug tolerance, sedation, and respiratory depression; lack of knowledge about pain assessment and analgesics; and undertreatment with analgesics are major problems (52). This is understandable when one considers the minimal curriculum content that is devoted to pain control. Fortunately, these problems are now being addressed, and the education programs and resources available have much improved (25). State cancer pain initiatives, guidelines, and organizational position statements have been excellent efforts toward improving pain management. The ONS developed a position paper on cancer pain that delineated the scope of practice for nurses with different levels of expertise (52). Even the Joint Commission for Accreditation for Healthcare Organizations has recognized the problem of inadequate pain management and changed their standards of care to emphasize appropriate management (41).

Nursing care should be planned to promote patient comfort, provide patients and their families with information related to pain control, provide information about and assistance with behavioral and physical interventions, prevent and alleviate side effects of pharmacologic therapies, and promote patient compliance with therapy and required follow-up. The nurse should explain the rationale of interventions and provide time for patient and family questions. Patient education should include the names of the pharmacologic agents, dosage schedules, side effects, interventions to alleviate nausea and vomiting, antiemetics, and interventions to alleviate constipation (Table 88.5). The nurse should monitor the effectiveness and side effects of pharmacologic interventions, respiratory status, bowel functioning, as well as mental and cognitive functioning. The patient and family must know how to contact medical personnel in case of an emergency and should feel free to do so. The topic of pain control is discussed in detail in Chapter 172 and in medical and oncology nursing literature (50–53).

Unconventional Therapies

The very success of medical research and treatment in eradicating such diseases as polio and smallpox has inculcated a public expectation of a definitive "cure" for cancer. The search for such a "miracle cure" has led patients to investigate and participate in a wide range of therapies such as special diets, megavitamins, unproven and potentially unsafe biologic vaccines, and many others. Meditation and mental imaging also have been "sold" to patients who are led to believe that mental conditioning can stop the growth and spread of tumor cells. Such unconventional methods are costly and prevent timely treatment and restoration of health when they are used instead of the generally accepted treatments. When used in addition to standard therapy, these remedies can complicate or compromise otherwise effective therapy.

Questionable or unconventional methods of cancer treatment may be eagerly sought by patients and their families (36, 91). Patients may request information related to alternative therapies to ensure they are reviewing all treatment alternatives. The oncology nurse's primary response to such requests is to provide whatever accurate information is known relating to these therapies while listening and exploring the reasons for seeking such unproven methods. If this is unsatisfactory to the patient, the nurse should provide referrals to educational materials or other professionals who can provide additional current information regarding the hazards and risks of questionable treatments. Such sources include publications by the U.S. Food and Drug Administration, the National Cancer Institute, and the American Cancer Society. These agencies have literature that reviews and assesses questionable drugs, substances, and treatment centers (see Chapter 96).

The oncology nurse must be sensitive to the fact that many patients and families seeking unconventional therapy have exhausted all conventional therapy without achieving control of their disease. A patient's inclination to explore unproven approaches to complex problems may be a typical life pattern, but it also may be founded in desperation rather than logical reason. The nurse should remain objective and present the information to patients that will assist in their understanding of the risks and implications of questionable cancer therapies. The nurse must accept the patient's right to choose whatever therapy seems most desirable, even if in the nurse's judgment it is not the correct choice. The nurse should apprise the physician of the interview.

This ethical dilemma is most difficult when the patient has curable disease but inclines toward an unproven remedy out of fear and ignorance. In such a situation, support and negotiation, often most influentially by the oncology nurse, may persuade the patient to adhere to a potentially curative regimen.

Survivorship

Over 50% of individuals who are diagnosed with invasive cancer will live beyond 5 years, and most will be considered cured. Thus, issues of survivorship and living with the effects of cancer and its treatment are a significant concern. This is evidenced by the emphasis on rehabilitation. The ONS was the first professional group to provide a practical definition of cancer rehabilitation as a "process by which individuals within their environments are assisted to achieve optimal functioning within the limits imposed by cancer" (49).

The National Coalition of Cancer Survivors and the American Cancer Society have brought survivorship issues to the public and are promoting rehabilitation as the first phase in preparing cancer survivors to lead fulfilling lives (83). Bushkin (8), the previous author of this chapter, died of cancer in 1993. She said "surviving a chronic illness is a hard fight." She also provided insight and understanding into the process of being a cancer survivor through her teaching, caring, and conceptualization of the process of survival, best expressed in her lecture entitled "Signposts of Survivorship" (8). She provided by word and example a mechanism to combine the challenges of life into a cohesive plan for living.

Summary

The progress of professional oncology nursing parallels the progress made in the surgical, radiologic, and medical approaches to the treatment of cancer. The oncology nurse has become an integral component of the cancer care team. Oncology nurses have earned the respect of physicians, other health care professionals, and most importantly, of patients and their families. Oncology nursing will continue to develop as a dynamic element within the health care delivery process as the number of these nurses increases and their levels of knowledge, experience, and expertise advance.

References

1. Ahles TA, Blanchard EB, Ruckdeschel JC. The multidimensional nature of cancer-related pain. Pain 1983;17:277–288.
2. American Nurses Association and the Oncology Nursing Society. Standards of Oncology Nursing Practice. Washington, DC: American Nurses Association, 1987.
3. Baird SB. Nursing roles in continuing care: home care and hospice. Semin Oncol 1980;7:28–38.
4. Baird SB, McCorkle R, Grant M. Cancer Nursing. Philadelphia, PA: Saunders, 1991.
5. Beutler E. Platelet transfusions: the 20,000 μL trigger. Blood 1993;81:1411–1413.
6. Buchsel PC, Yarbro CH, eds. Oncology Nursing in the Ambulatory Setting. Boston: Jones and Bartlett, 1993.
7. Bushkin E. Principles of oncology nursing. In Cancer Medicine, 3rd ed. Edited by JF Holland, E Frei, RC Bast, DW Kufe, DL Morton, RR Weichselbaum. 1993, pp 1034–1053.
8. Bushkin E. Signposts for survivorship: a universal travel guide. Oncol Nurs Forum 1993;20:869–875.
9. Camp-Sorrell D. Chemotherapy: toxicity management. In Cancer Nursing: Principles and Practice, 3rd ed. Edited by SL Groenwald, MH Frogge, M Goodman, CH Yarbro. Boston: Jones and Bartlett, 1993, 331–365.
10. Carnevali DL, Reiner CA, eds. The Cancer Experience: Nursing Diagnosis and Management. Philadelphia: Lippincott, 1990.
11. Carrieri VK, Lindsey AM, West CM (eds). Pathophysiological Phenomena in Nursing. Human Response to Illness. Philadelphia: Saunders, 1986.
12. Chernecky CC, Ramsey PW, eds. Critical Nursing Care of the Client with Cancer. Norwalk, CT: Appleton-Century-Crofts, 1984.
13. Clark JC, McGee R, eds. Core Curriculum for Oncology Nursing, 2nd ed. Philadelphia: Saunders, 1992.
14. Cotanch P, Hockenberry M, Herman S. Self-hypnosis as antiemetic therapy in children receiving chemotherapy. Oncol Nurs Forum 1985;12:41–46.
15. Cotanch P, Strum S. Progressive muscle relaxation as antiemetic therapy for cancer patients. Oncol Nurs Forum 1987;14:33–37.
16. Coyle N, Cherny N, Portenoy RK. Pharmacologic management of cancer pain. In Cancer Pain Management, 2nd ed. Edited by DB McGuire, CH Yarbro, BR Ferrell. Boston, MA: Jones and Bartlett, 1995, pp 89–130.
17. Cubbedau LX, Hoffman IS, Guenmayor NT, et al. Efficacy of ondansetron (GR 38032F) and the role of serotonin in cisplatin-induced nausea and vomiting. N Engl J Med 1990;322:810–816.
18. Daeffler RJ, Petrosino B, eds. Manual of Oncology Nursing Practice. Rockville, MD: Aspen Publishing, 1990.
19. Dodd MJ. Managing Side Effects of Chemotherapy and Radiation Therapy: A Guide for Patients and Nurses. Norwalk, CT: Appleton & Lange, 1987.
20. Dow KH, Hilderley LJ, eds. Nursing Care in Radiation Oncology. Philadelphia PA: Saunders, 1992.
21. Dudas S. Altered body image and sexuality. In Cancer Nursing Principles and Practice. 3rd ed. Edited by SL Groenwald, MH Frogge, M Goodman, CH Yarbro. Boston, MA: Jones and Bartlett, 1993, pp 719–733.
22. Einhorn LH, Nagy C, Werner K, et al. Ondansetron: a new antiemetic for patients receiving cisplatin chemotherapy. J Clin Oncol 1990;8:731–735.
23. Frank JM. The effects of music therapy and guided visual imagery on chemotherapy-induced nausea and vomiting. Oncol Nurs Forum 1985;12:47–52.
24. Goodman M, Wickham R. Vascular access devices: an overview. Oncol Nurs Forum 1984;11:16–23.
25. Grant MM, Rivera LM. Pain education for nurses, patients, and families. In Cancer Pain Management, 2nd ed. Edited by DB McGuire, CH Yarbro, BR Ferrell. Boston, MA: Jones and Bartlett, 1995, pp 289–320.
26. Groenwald SL, Frogge MH, Goodman M, Yarbro CH, eds. Cancer Nursing: Principles and Practice, 3rd ed. Boston, MA: Jones and Bartlett, 1993.
27. Groenwald SL, Frogge MH, Goodman M, Yarbro CH, eds. Cancer Symptom Management. Boston, MA: Jones and Bartlett (in press).
28. Gross J, Johnson BL, eds. Handbook of Oncology Nursing, 2nd ed. Boston, MA: Jones and Bartlett, 1994.
29. Gullo SM. Safe handling of antineoplastic drugs: translating the recommendations into practice. Oncol Nurs Forum 1988;15:595–601.
30. Hainsworth J, Harvey W, Pendergrass K, et al. A single-blind comparison of intravenous ondansetron, a selective serotonin antagonist, with intravenous metoclopramide in the prevention of nausea and vomiting associated with high-dose cisplatin chemotherapy. J Clin Oncol 1991;9:721–728.
31. Hassey K. Principles of radiation safety and protection. Semin Oncol Nurs 1987;3:23–29.
32. Henke C. Emerging roles of the nurse in oncology. Semin Oncol 1980;7:4–8.
33. Hilderley LJ. The role of the nurse in radiation oncology. Semin Oncol 1980;7:39–47.
34. Hilderley LJ. Radiotherapy. In Cancer Nursing Principles and Practice, 3rd ed. Edited by SL Groenwald, MH Frogge, M Goodman, CH Yarbro. Boston, MA: Jones and Bartlett, 1993, pp 235–269.
35. Hilkemeyer R. A historical perspective in cancer nursing. Oncol Nurs Forum 1985;12(suppl.):6–15.
36. Holland JC, Rowland JH (eds). Handbook of Psychooncology: Psychological Care of the Patient with Cancer. New York: Oxford, 1989.
37. Hubbard SM, Donehower MG. The nurse in a cancer research setting. Semin Oncol 1980;7:9–17.
38. Jacox A, Carr DB, Payne R, et al. Management of cancer pain. Clinical Practice Guideline, No. 9. AHCPR Pub. No. 94-0592, Rockville, MD: Agency for Health Care Policy and Research, USDHHS, PHS, March 1994.
39. Jassak P. Biotherapy. In Cancer Nursing: Principles and Practice, 3rd ed. Edited by SL Groenwald, MH Frogge, M Goodman, CH Yarbro. Boston, MA: Jones and Bartlett, 1993, pp 366–392.
40. Johnson JL, Blumberg BD. A commentary on cancer patient education. Health Education Q 1984;10:7.
41. Joint Commission on Accreditation of Healthcare Organizations. Accreditation Manual for Hospitals. Oak Brook Terrace, IL: JCAHO, 1993.
42. Kennedy P. Sandostatin (s) therapy for chemotherapy (CT) and radiotherapy (RT) related diarrhea. Proc Am Soc Clin Oncol 1990;9:324. Abstract.
43. Knobf MK, Durivage HJ. Chemotherapy: Principles of Therapy. In Cancer Nursing: Principles and Practice, 3rd ed. Edited by SL Groenwald, MH Frogge, M Goodman, CH Yarbro. Boston, MA: Jones and Bartlett, 1993, pp 270–292
44. Knobf MK, Fischer DS (eds). Cancer chemotherapy treatment and care, 3rd ed. Boston, MA: Hall, 1989.
45. Lane D. Music therapy: a gift beyond measure. Oncol Nurs Forum1992;19:863–867.
46. Linn EM, Martin VR. Ambulatory cancer care. Semin Oncol Nurs 1994;10:227–305.
47. Loprinzi CL, Ellison NM, Schain DJ, et al. A controlled trial of megestrol acetate for the treatment of anorexia-cachexia. JNCI 1990;82:1127–1132.
48. Maxwell MB, Maher KE. Chemotherapy-induced myelosuppression. Semin Oncol Nurs 1992;8:113–123.
49. Mayer D, O'Connor L. Rehabilitation of persons with cancer: an ONS position statement. Oncol Nurs Forum 1989;16:433.
50. McCaffery M, Beebe A. Pain: Clinical Manual for Nursing Practice. St. Louis: Mosby, 1989.
51. McGuire DB. The multiple dimensions of cancer pain: a framework for assessment and management. In Cancer Pain Management, 2nd ed. Edited by DB McGuire, CH Yarbro, BR Ferrell. Boston, MA: Jones and Bartlett, 1995, pp 1–18.
52. McGuire DB, Sheidler VR. Pain. In Cancer Nursing: Principles and Practice, 3rd ed. Edited by SL Groenwald, MH Frogge, M Goodman, CH Yarbro. Boston, MA: Jones and Bartlett, 1993, pp 499–556.
53. McGuire DB, Yarbro CH, Ferrell BR, eds. Cancer Pain Management, 2nd ed. Boston, MA: Jones and Bartlett, 1995.
54. McIntire S, Cioppa AN. Cancer Nursing—A Developmental Approach. New York: Wiley, 1984.
55. McNally JC, Somerville ET, Miaskowski C, Rostad M, eds. Guidelines for Oncology Nursing Practice, 2nd ed. Philadelphia, PA: Saunders, 1991.
56. Mersky H, Albe-Fessard DG, Bonica JJ, et al. Pain terms: a list with definitions and notes on usage. Pain 1979;6:249–252.
57. National Cancer Institute: Chemotherapy and You: A Guide to Self Help During Treatment. NIH Publication #92–1136. Bethesda, MD: U.S. Department of Health and Human Services, 1991.
58. Oncology Nursing Certification Corporation. Test Bulletin. Pittsburgh, PA: ONCC, 1995.
59. Oncology Nursing Society. 1994/1995 Annual Report. ONS News 1995;10(suppl):8.
60. Oncology Nursing Society. Access Device Guidelines, Modules I-III. Pittsburgh, PA: Oncology Nursing Press, 1989–1990.
61. Oncology Nursing Society. Biological Response Modifier Guidelines. Pittsburgh, PA: Oncology Nursing Press, 1989.
62. Oncology Nursing Society. Cancer Chemotherapy: Guidelines and Recommendations for Nursing Education and Practice. Pittsburgh, PA: Oncology Nursing Press, 1989.
63. Oncology Nursing Society. Recommendations for the Management of Vesicant Extravasation, Hypersensitivity, and Anaphylaxis. Pittsburgh, PA: Oncology Nursing Press, 1992.
64. Oncology Nursing Society. Safe Handling of Cytotoxic Drugs. Independent Study Module. Pittsburgh, PA: Oncology Nursing Press, 1989.
65. Oncology Nursing Society. Standards of Advanced Practice in Oncology Nursing. Pittsburgh, PA: Oncology Nursing Press, 1990.
66. Oncology Nursing Society. Standards on Oncology Education: Patient/Family and Public. Pittsburgh, PA: Oncology Nursing Press, 1989.
67. Oncology Nursing Society and American Nurses Association Division of Medical Surgical Nursing Practice. Outcome Standards for Cancer Nursing Practice. Kansas City, MO: American Nurses Association, 1989.
68. Oppenheimer SB. Cancer. A Biological and Clinical Introduction, 2nd ed. Boston, MA: Jones and Bartlett, 1990.
69. Polomano R, Weintraub FN, Wurster A. Surgical critical care for cancer patients. Semin Oncol Nurs 1994;10:165–176.
70. Reiger PT, ed. Biotherapy: A Comprehensive Overview. Boston, MA: Jones and Bartlett, 1995.
71. Reymann PE. Chemotherapy: Principles of administration. In Cancer Nursing Principles and Practice, 3rd ed. Edited by SL Groenwald, MH Frogge, M Goodman, CH Yarbro. Boston, MA: Jones and Bartlett, 1993, pp 293–330.
72. Scott DW, Donahue DC, Mastrovito RC, et al. Comparative trial of clinical relaxation and an antiemetic drug regimen reducing chemotherapy induced nausea and vomiting. Cancer Nurs 1986;9:178–197.
73. Sitton E. Early and late radiation-induced skin alterations. Part II: Nursing care of irradiated skin. Oncol Nurs Forum 1992;19:907–912.
74. Spross JA, Burke MW. Nonpharmacological management of cancer pain. In Cancer Pain Management, 2nd ed. Edited by DB McGuire, CH Yarbro, BR Ferrell. Boston, MA: Jones and Bartlett, 1995, pp 159–206.
75. Spross J, McGuire DB, Schmitt R. Oncology Nursing Society Position Paper on Cancer Pain. Pittsburgh, PA: Oncology Nursing Press, 199[illegible].
76. Stevenson E, Crosson K. Patient education: history, development, and current directions of the American Cancer Society and National Cancer Institute. Semin Oncol Nurs 1991;7:135-142.
77. Tennebaum L, ed. Cancer Chemotherapy and Biotherapy, 2nd ed. Philadelphia, PA: Saunders, 1994.
78. Thaney KM. The nurse in a community hospital setting. Semin Oncol 1980;7:18–27.
79. U.S. Department of Health and Human Services, Public Health Service, National Institutes of Health. Eating Hints, Recipes and Tips for Better Nutrition During Cancer Treatment. NIH Publication No. 92-2079, 1992.
80. U.S. Department of Health and Human Services, Public Health Service, National Institutes of Health. Radiation Therapy and You. A Guide to Self-Help During Treatment. NIH Publication No. 92-2227, 1992.
81. U. S. Department of Labor, Office of Occupational Medicine, Occupational Safety and Health Administration. Work Practice Guidelines for Personnel Dealing with Cytotoxic (Antineoplastic) Drugs. Publication No. 8.1.1, 1986.
82. Warr D, Willan SF, Wilson K, et al. Superiority of granisetron to dexamethasone plus prochlorperazine in the prevention of chemotherapy induced emesis. JNCI 1991;83:1169–1173.
83. Watson PG. Cancer rehabilitation: an overview. Semin Oncol Nurs 1992;8:167-173.
84. Wickham R, Purl S, Welker D. Long-term central venous catheters. Issues for care. Semin Oncol Nurs 1992;8:133–147.
85. Winningham ML, MacVicar MG. The effect of aerobic exercise on patient reports of nausea. Oncol Nurs Forum 1988;15:447–450.

86. World Health Organization. Cancer Pain Relief and Palliative Care. Geneva: World Health Organization, 1990.
87. Wujcik D. Current research in side effects of high-dose chemotherapy. Semin Oncol Nurs 1992;8:102–112.
88. Yarbro CH. The history of cancer nursing. In Cancer Nursing. Edited by SB Baird, R McCorkle, M Grant. Philadelphia, PA: Saunders, 1991, pp 10–20.
89. Yarbro CH. Nursing implications in the administration of cancer chemotherapy. In The Chemotherapy Source Book. Edited by MC Perry. Baltimore, MD: Williams and Wilkins, 1991, pp 873–883.
90. Yarbro CH. ONS the early days: four smiles and a post office box. Oncol Nurs Forum 1984;11:79–85.
91. Yarbro CH. Questionable methods of cancer therapy. In Cancer Nursing: Principles and Practice, 3rd ed. Edited by SL Groenwald, MH Frogge, M Goodman, Yarbro CH. Boston: Jones and Bartlett, 1993, pp 1536–1552.
92. Yasko JM. Care of the Client Receiving External Radiation Therapy. Reston, VA: Reston, 1982.
93. Yasko JM. Guidelines for Cancer Care: Symptom Management. Reston, VA: Reston, 1983.

SECTION XXIII

PRINCIPLES OF REHABILITATION MEDICINE

CHAPTER 89

Principles of Cancer Rehabilitation Medicine

KRISTJAN T. RAGNARSSON

Introduction

Medical advances in the diagnosis and management of cancer have markedly increased survival rates. While the treatment for some patients may now result in complete cure and no perceived physical deficits, for others an aggressive definitive treatment may result in significant physical impairment or disability. To ensure quick restoration of optimal function, early and continued aggressive rehabilitation interventions should be provided, including physical and occupational therapy, prosthetic and orthotic devices, and assistive equipment. Application of rehabilitation techniques frequently results in a swift functional improvement and a reduction of subjective complaints, even when the prognosis for life is considered poor. It has always been difficult to predict with a degree of certainty the life expectancy of an individual with cancer. Modern diagnostic techniques and effective treatment of malignant neoplastic disease have invalidated old statistics and dogmas regarding life expectancy and thus made accurate prognostication even more difficult for the clinician. No cancer patient, even one with widespread metastases, should be denied the benefits of aggressive treatment, including appropriate surgical intervention, chemotherapy, radiation, and comprehensive rehabilitation. These interventions, when offered in an integrated and timely fashion, prolong life, protect organs and residual healthy tissue, reduce pain, and maximize self-care and mobility skills, and thereby help to reduce the stigma of cancer and physical impairment while providing dignity and a better quality of life for the cancer patient.

Early referral for rehabilitation services and good communication among the oncologist, the surgeon, the physiatrist, and the other members of the cancer rehabilitation team are essential to a successful return to optimal function. Every effort should be made to coordinate the rehabilitation treatment with other types of intervention. A comprehensive and well-coordinated rehabilitation approach that concurrently deals with the physical, psychologic, and social problems caused by the malignancy and the consequent disability usually yields the best results. Most important for success, however, is the patient's personal interest and ability to participate in the rehabilitation program and to pursue the established functional goals supported by family and friends.

Application of Rehabilitation Concepts

Many persons afflicted by cancer develop some form of functional impairment or disability that will interfere with self-care, mobility, and a smooth transition to their former lifestyle. These patients should be identified early and referred for rehabilitation treatment. Cancer rehabilitation can be broadly defined as the maximum restoration of physical, psychologic, social, vocational, recreational, and economic function within the limits imposed by the malignancy and its treatment. To make a significant and timely impact on such a wide variety of functions and needs, the efforts of a well-coordinated and goal-oriented multidisciplinary cancer rehabilitation team are required (Table 89.1). Because of the cancer's often uncertain prognosis, most cancer rehabilitation programs focus on quick gains in mobility and self-care skills, and the provision of psychosocial support to the patient and family. Flexibility in goal setting is unavoidable because of the patient's changing needs, stamina, and medical status.

Despite the potential benefits, referrals of cancer patients for rehabilitation services are often made needlessly late or not made at all. This may reflect a reluctance on the part of the oncologist. Many physicians are unfamiliar with the concepts of rehabilitation treatment and its potential impact. Clinical problems amenable to rehabilitation interventions are often identified too late or not at all. Pessimistic prognostication by the oncologist and the rehabilitation specialist may hinder rehabilitation referrals as cancer patients are inappropriately compared with patients disabled by trauma or other relatively static medical disorders. Fortunately, the prognosis for most types of cancers has improved, and consequently the demand for rehabilitation services for cancer patients with disabilities has grown.

Several studies have shown that cancer rehabilitation programs result in measurable benefits when individualized, specific, and realistic goals are set (16). Comprehensive inpatient rehabilitation services may be economically provided for disabled cancer patients who are considered "cured or controlled," but precise short-term rehabilitation interventions may enable even those with a poor prognosis to gain the mobility and self-care skills that facilitate early hospital discharge.

Table 89.1. Multidisciplinary Cancer Rehabilitation Team

Physician (physiatrist)	Speech pathologist
Rehabilitation oncology nurse	Social worker
Physical therapist	Psychologist
Occupational therapist	Chaplain
Prosthetist/orthotist	Vocational counselor
Nutritionist	Recreational therapist

Table 89.2. Activities of Daily Living[a]

Eating and drinking	Moving in bed
Dressing and undressing	Changing position
Bathing and grooming	Walking
Toileting	Climbing stairs
Managing bladder and bowel functions	General wheelchair skills
Manipulating small objects	Using a manual wheelchair
Caring for health and fitness	Using an electric wheelchair

[a] Rehabilitation indicators: skill indicators.

The physical impairment experienced by cancer patients may result from tissue destruction caused by the cancer itself, prolonged bed rest, or inactivity, or from definitive treatment, such as surgery, radiation, or chemotherapy. The exact nature of the impairment may vary, but in essence it is no different from impairment caused by trauma or noncancerous disease, and is customarily managed by the rehabilitation team. A specific rehabilitation goal must be established for each patient, and an individualized program prescribed that is designed to obtain measurable early results. The main rehabilitation goals for all people with physical disabilities are, first, to develop maximum skills in the activities of daily living (ADL) (Table 89.2) allowed by the disability and, second, to obtain independent ambulation with or without assistive devices, such as wheelchairs, prostheses, orthoses, walkers, crutches, or canes. To reach these goals, the therapist will utilize physical exercise to improve muscle strength, endurance, joint flexibility, and self-care skills, as well as apply physical modalities to decrease pain and swelling. Prescription, fabrication, and fitting of prosthetic and orthotic devices and other assistive equipment, followed by training in their use, is essential for amputees and individuals with significant muscle weakness, paralysis, or unstable skeletal structures.

It is essential to provide rehabilitation interventions that also aim at the often profound psychologic, sexual, social, and vocational consequences of the cancer and the physical impairment. Preferably, the anticipated psychosocial difficulties should be addressed when the initial diagnosis is made and when treatment is begun. The goal of cancer care is not just to eradicate or control the malignancy and extend the patient's life, but to maintain or reestablish a life of quality. While fatal or physically disabling consequences of cancer are quickly recognized and usually well managed by the hospital staff, the psychosocial effects of cancer, which frequently become manifest after hospital discharge, may be unnoticed and therefore go untreated. As a result, they may become more disabling than the physical impairment.

The rehabilitation goals of cancer patients may be broadly classified according to the different stages of the disease. (*a*) Preventive rehabilitation therapy is started early after the diagnosis of cancer is made, that is, before or immediately after surgery, radiotherapy, and or chemotherapy. At this stage no significant physical impairment exists, but therapy is started to prevent functional loss. (*b*) Restorative rehabilitation therapy is directed at the comprehensive restoration of maximum function for patients considered "cured or controlled" but who have a residual physical impairment and disability. (*c*) Supportive rehabilitation therapy attempts to increase the self-care skills and mobility of the cancer patient with growing cancer and progressive impairment and disability by the application of quick, effective methods, for example, providing appropriate assistive devices and the teaching of simple techniques for self-care (47). Supportive rehabilitation therapy also includes physical exercises to prevent the effects of immobilization, such as joint contractures, muscle atrophy, weakness, and pressure sores. (*d*) Palliative rehabilitation therapy aims to increase or maintain the comfort and function of patients with terminal cancer by utilizing physical modalities, simple orthotic devices, and assistive equipment to manage pain, joint contractures, and pressure sores, and to provide at least partial self-sufficiency (47).

Cancer Rehabilitation and Adaptation Team

Organized cancer rehabilitation programs can significantly improve a patient's physical function and community reintegration (16, 44). An integral part of such programs is a multidisciplinary cancer rehabilitation and adaptation team (Table 89.1). The exact composition of the team may vary considerably depending on the program's philosophy and size, the type of institution, and the range of disabilities encountered. The team is led by a physician who is either an oncologist or, more commonly, a physiatrist (44). An oncology nurse, social worker, psychologist, physical therapist, occupational therapist, vocational counselor, chaplain, and nutritionist are present on most teams (44). Other rehabilitation professionals may contribute to the rehabilitation of cancer patients, depending on each patient's specific physical impairment, including prosthetist, orthotist, speech pathologist, driver's trainer, and recreational therapist. The roles of the various team members are described in the following.

The *physiatrist*, the medical specialist who usually directs the cancer rehabilitation team, needs to be knowledgeable in oncology in addition to having expertise in the field of physical medicine and rehabilitation. The physiatrist is the team's primary link with other treating physicians. To establish realistic goals and prescribe an appropriate rehabilitation program, the physiatrist needs to know (*a*) details of the cancer diagnosis with respect to organ site, histology, and grade of anaplasia, (*b*) the cancer's anatomic staging (primary site only, involvement of regional nodes or metastases), (*c*) the patient's life expectancy, that is, whether the patient is "cured or controlled," and if not, the anticipated rapidity of the cancer's progression, and (*d*) the definitive treatment plan for the cancer, that is, the timing of surgery, chemotherapy, or radiation, and its anticipated efficacy and potential side effects. The physiatrist discusses this information with the rehabilitation team as the basis for developing a specific and realistic plan of preventive, restorative, supportive, and palliative therapy. The physiatrist introduces the patient and family to the goals of the cancer rehabilitation team and meets regularly with the team, as well as with the patient and family, to direct and coordinate their efforts while taking into account the patient's progress and changing needs.

The *rehabilitation oncology nurse* serves primarily as an easily accessible resource to the nursing staff that gives care to the cancer patient, as well as to the patient and the family. The nurse evaluates the patient's specific nursing needs; plans the patient's care; helps to obtain nursing supplies; educates other nurses, the patient, and his or her family about nursing techniques and the principles of cancer treatment; facilitates patient and family self-management; and monitors discharge plans and assists in the discharge process. After discharge, the nurse may provide advice for the caregivers in the home on the management of the different and complex treatment problems that may arise.

The *physical therapist* teaches the patient to perform specific exercises to strengthen muscles, to increase stamina, and to maintain or improve joint range of motion and trunk flexibility. When indicated, training is provided to improve balance and coordination, as well as functional skills: transfers into and out of bed, wheelchair locomotion, and ambulation with or without assistive devices. Instructions are provided on how to normalize gait patterns and to safely ascend and descend stairs and curbs. Various physical modalities may be used by the therapist to reduce pain, such as superficial and deep heat, cold, transcutaneous electrostimulation (TENS), and massage, but the clinician needs to stipulate that heat modalities and massage should not be applied directly over or immediately adjacent to a site of cancer. Physical exercise is perhaps the most important therapeutic modality in the rehabilitation management of physical disabilities. Muscle-strengthening exercises may be either isometric, isotonic, or isokinetic. Isometric exercise does not involve joint motion, and so is prescribed for painful or unstable body parts, whereas isotonic exercise involves joint motion against variable resistance. Isokinetic exercise, a most effective strengthening exercise, involves the use of specific devices (e.g., the Cybex apparatus) to maintain constant speed of motion independent from the force applied (81). Passive stretching exercises are done by the therapist without the patient's direct participation to maintain or increase joint mobility. Task-oriented exercises, such as ambulation or training in self-care, may improve function and safety by repetition and prolonged therapy.

The *occupational therapist* focuses in on upper-extremity exercises and training in self-care activities. The exercises are designed to improve strength, coordination, and skills in the various ADL (Table 89.2). Different adaptive equipment may be provided to make the patient more proficient in self-care and activities related to work and recreation. When indicated, the therapist fabricates simple orthotic devices, such as hand splints for immobilization or to compensate for weak muscles. When brain dysfunction is present, a gross assessment of cognitive and visual perceptual skills is performed, and therapy is initiated to compensate for deficits in these areas. The home and workplace are evaluated and recommendations are offered to make these sites more accessible and more conducive to complete self-sufficiency and greater productivity. Working independently, or with a recreational therapist, the occupational therapist strives to make a resumption of leisure time activities easier for the patient.

The *prosthetist/orthotist* is called on to make artificial limbs (prostheses) or special braces (orthoses) for patients in need of such devices. The prosthetist/orthotist should evaluate the patient with the physiatrist and the therapist and help to select the proper components and materials for the device, as well as determine its general design and methods of fabrication based on the pathology and biomechanics involved. After delivery, the physiatrist checks out the device for comfort and fit, but it is the duty of the prosthetist/orthotist to modify and service the equipment as long as it remains in use.

The *nutritionist* evaluates the patient's nutritional condition, predicts the additional metabolic demands that the cancer places on the body, and recommends the optimal diet with respect to specific clinical condition, caloric intake, food ingredients of choice, optimal consistency for easy swallowing, and the individual's tastes. The nutritionist judges total food intake by closely monitoring the patient's weight and counting calories and, if nutrition is inadequate, may recommend interventions to facilitate adequate intake in the presence of poor appetite and swallowing disorders. The nutritionist should teach the patient and family general and specific dietary principles and consult with the clinical staff on the optimal parenteral nutrition when the need for that arises.

The *speech pathologist* evaluates and provides therapy for impaired oral communication and works closely with the occupational therapist and nutritionist in the assessment and care of swallowing disorders.

The *social worker* has many important roles in the rehabilitation of the cancer patient, but especially with respect to discharge planning, facilitating a smooth transition from the hospital to the community, ensuring continuity of care, and securing appropriate follow-up services after discharge. The social worker helps the patient to secure financial resources, including health insurance coverage, and Social Security and disability compensation, as well as to obtain authorization and payment for necessary devices and home help. Before hospital discharge, arrangements need to be made for transportation, attendant, or nursing care, home modifications, and other appropriate posthospital services. This may involve transfer to and placement in other health institutions. The social worker often acts as a liaison among the patient, the family members, and the various health care professionals.

The *rehabilitation psychologist* assesses the patient's psychologic functions, including intelligence, personality (i.e., ideational, emotional, behavioral, and character patterns), personal history, motivation, reaction to the illness, and coping skills. Following the diagnosis of cancer and the development of a disability, both the patient and family members may experience reactive depression or grief, which often is expressed in diverse ways, including denial, anger, anxiety, panic, fear, dependent behavior, depression, and the unmasking of previously controlled psychopathology. The primary role of the psychologist is to assist the patient and the family in coping, as well as to counsel and consult with the rehabilitation team members in managing the emotional reactions. The effectiveness of psychosocial intervention has been successfully demonstrated with cancer patients (36, 48).

A *chaplain* or religious counselor is often included in the cancer rehabilitation team. This professional may be able to relate to the patient and the family in a way that can help them use their faith to adjust to the illness and disability.

A *vocational counselor* should participate in the care of physically impaired cancer patients who have any potential of returning to work. An initial interview should be conducted at the hospital and vocational services continued after discharge. These services may include detailed evaluation, counseling, testing, career exploration, and educational planning. The counselor will have to proceed to the extent and at a pace that are sensitive to the patient's need and readiness to resume vocational activities, whether education or employment. At the proper time, the counselor may make visits to work or school sites and consult with employers and teachers to facilitate transition from disability to productivity as a worker or student. For school-age children, home tutoring may have to be arranged. Patients who are unemployed may be taught skills to seek jobs successfully. The Office of Vocational Rehabilitation (OVR) in each state can be a source of funding for various vocational rehabilitation services, that is, certain aspects of rehabilitation, education, training, job placement, and equipment and environmental modifications, if these will enable the disabled person eventually to return to school or work. The counselor makes the initial referral to OVR and maintains a close cooperative and effective relationship with the OVR representatives.

The *recreational therapist* offers activities to meet the different needs and interests of disabled individuals both in and out of the hospital, such as art therapy, music therapy, attending art shows and sports events, going to theaters, eating at restaurants, and shopping. Family and friends may join in these recreational activities, which serve to enhance socialization, leisure-time activities, and positive attitudes. The trips into the community may facilitate the institutional discharge for the physically disabled person and reintegration into community life.

Functional Assessment

A medical intervention should not be offered unless measurable benefits will result. Unlike other fields of medicine, the outcome of rehabilitation interventions cannot be measured by survival or by the disappearance of symptoms. The effectiveness of rehabilitation interventions is judged by the patient's degree of functional independence. The terms *impairment*, *disability*, and *handicap* have been carefully defined by the World Health Organization to clarify the impact of a physical deficit (87). Impairment is "any loss or abnormality of psychological, physical, or anatomical structure of function," for example, paralysis. Disability is "any restriction or lack (resulting from an impairment) of an ability to perform an activity in a manner within the range considered normal for a human being," for example, paralysis resulting in an inability to walk. Handicap is "a disadvantage for a given individual resulting from an impairment or disability that limits or prevents the fulfillment of a role that is normal (depending on age, sex, and social and cultural factors) for that individual," for example, the person is paralyzed and unable to walk and thus is unable to meet the requirements of the job and so cannot return to work.

To assess and monitor function accurately, the performance in different activities of self-care, mobility, and communication must be numerically rated according to the patient's level of independence: completely independent; independent with devices; requires assistance (supervision, "spotting," reminding, physical help); or completely depen-

Table 89.3. Functioning Independence Measure (FIM)

	Levels	
L	7 Complete independence (Timely, Safely)	NO
E	6 Modified independence (Device)	HELPER
V	Modified Dependence	
E	5 Supervision	
L	4 Minimal Assist (Subject = 75%+)	
S	3 Moderate Assist (Subject = 50%+)	HELPER
	Complete Dependence	
	2 Maximal Assist (Subject = 25%+)	
	1 Total Assist (Subject = 0%+)	

	ADMIT	DISCHG	FOL-UP
Self Care			
A. Eating			
B. Grooming			
C. Bathing			
D. Dressing-Upper Body			
E. Dressing-Lower Body			
F. Toileting			
Sphincter Control			
G. Bladder Management			
H. Bowel Management			
Mobility			
Transfer:			
I. Bed, Chair, Wheelchair			
J. Toilet			
K. Tub, Shower			
Locomotion			
L. Walk/wheel Chair	W / C	W / C	W / C
M. Stairs			
Communication			
N. Comprehension	a / v	a / v	a / v
O. Expression	v / n	v / n	v / n
P. Social Interaction			
Q. Problem Solving			
R. Memory			
Total FIM			

NOTE: Leave no blanks: enter 1 if patient not testable due to risk.

Table 89.4. Karnofsky Performance Status Index

General category	Index	Specific criteria
Able to carry on normal activity, no special care needed	100	Normal, no complaints, no evidence of disease
	90	Able to carry on normal activity, minor signs or symptoms of disease
	80	Normal activity with effort, some signs or symptoms of disease
Unable to work, able to live at home and care for most personal needs, varying amount of assistance needed	70	Able to care for self, unable to carry on normal activity or do work
	60	Requires occasional assistance from others; frequent medical care
	50	Requires considerable assistance from others; frequent medical care
Unable to care for self, requires institutional or hospital care or equivalent, disease may be rapidly progressing	40	Disabled, requires special care and assistance
	30	Severely disabled, hospitalization indicated; death not imminent
	20	Very sick, hospitalization necessary; active supportive treatment necessary
	10	Moribund
	0	Dead

dent. This requires the collection of numerous diverse data by various means, including physical examination, observation, and a review of records and reports from the various rehabilitation team members, as well as the gathering of information directly from the patient and family. Several evaluation scales exist. Some are simple and easy to use, but provide incomplete information, whereas others are detailed but time-consuming, as they address a whole range of quality-of-life factors, which include mobility, self-care, employment, income, education, family activities, living arrangements, and transportation. Computer technology has made the gathering, analysis, and plotting of data easier and has enabled clinicians to document the patient's progress numerically, during inpatient and outpatient rehabilitation care. The functional evaluation scale that currently is gaining the widest acceptance by rehabilitation professionals is the Functional Independence Measure (FIM) (Table 89.3) (19, 42, 46), but for cancer patients, the Karnofsky Performance Status Scale has been most widely used (Table 89.4) (60).

A new scale developed specifically to measure quality of life and functional outcome for patients with cancer, the Cancer Rehabilitation Evaluation System (CARES), has been shown to be valid, reliable, and sensitive to changes in status (69, 70).

The Rehabilitation Process

Rehabilitation services are frequently requested too late in the care of the cancer patient. The physiatrist should be consulted as soon as it may be anticipated that the cancer will result in a physical disability. The rehabilitation interventions may thus be planned and explained to the patient before, during, or immediately following definitive treatment. Physical and occupational therapy is initially provided at the bedside, but the patient should be mobilized out of bed as soon as possible and escorted to the rehabilitation area, where facilities and equipment are conducive to better performance. Other members of the rehabilitation team become involved in the care of the disabled cancer patient as deemed appropriate by the physiatrist. If these interventions allow the patient to become self-sufficient and ambulatory, he or she should be discharged home directly from the acute service, when medically indicated, having received proper instructions, equipment, and referrals for specific nursing interventions.

A more comprehensive and intensive rehabilitation program on an inpatient rehabilitation service is provided for physically disabled cancer patients who do not gain independence in ADL and mobility with 1 or 2 weeks of daily therapy on the acute service, whose life expectancy is greater than 1 year, who are medically capable of actively participating in the program for at least 3 hours daily, and who are motivated and mentally capable of following instructions and learning the different tasks.

The inpatient rehabilitation unit should be in a hospital with an in-house physician on call and the various medical and surgical consultation services available at all times. Here the disabled cancer patient is reevaluated by the physiatrist, who obtains a detailed medical and social history and performs a careful physical examination to assess the general medical and the precise musculoskeletal and neurologic condition, as well as the current functional ability. The physiatrist writes the routine medical orders, as for nursing care, medications, and disability-specific diagnostic tests, including radiologic studies, urologic evaluation, pulmonary function tests, electrodiagnostic studies, and blood and urine analyses. The physiatrist at this time sets the general rehabilitation goals for the patient and prescribes evaluation and interventions to be undertaken by the members of the multidisciplinary rehabilitation team. The physiatrist prescribes the specific exercises and training methods to be given by the physical and occupational therapists, as well as interventions by the psychologist, speech pathologist, vocational and recreational counselors, and others when they are needed.

The rehabilitation program begins promptly after transfer to the inpatient rehabilitation service. Initially, the actual participation of patients on the program may be impeded by the physical deconditioning or by special evaluations and tests, but after the first few days, 4 to 6 hours each day are spent in an active therapy program in addition to different ward activities, such as self-care training, management of bowel and bladder dysfunction, and educational and recreational activities. When serious medical complications arise during the course of rehabilitation and interfere with the patient's ability to attend the rehabilitation program for at least 3 hours a day for more than 3 consecutive days, the patient should be transferred to the appropriate medical or surgical services for definitive care.

Within 1 week of admission, an initial team conference is held at which the patient's medical, functional, psychologic, social, vocational, and recreational status, as well as the rehabilitation potential and prognosis, are presented and discussed. More specific rehabilitation goals are set, needs for equipment and personal assistance are assessed, and a discharge date is predicted. Soon after this conference, the physiatrist meets with the patient and the family, together or separately, to discuss these issues and answer questions regarding the patient's medical condition and rehabilitation program. Team rehabilitation conferences are held biweekly to discuss the patient's progress and plans for discharge. While the patient is making continuous and measurable progress toward the set functional goals of independence in ADL and mobility, continued inpatient stay may be justified. Communication among members of the rehabilitation team, a most critical component, is facilitated through informal meetings during which specific concerns that any member of the team may have about any patient are shared and discussed. When a patient is discharged to home, it is most important to ensure that needed equipment and supplies have been obtained, family members or home health aides have been instructed and trained in the patient's care, follow-up by the visiting nurse service has been arranged, and referrals have been made for continued therapy and visits with various physicians, including the oncologist, surgeon, physiatrist, and family doctor.

CANCER OF THE BRAIN

Brain damage may result from primary tumors of the brain, from metastatic disease, or from treatment of the cancer—surgery, radiation, or, more rarely, chemotherapy. The symptoms and disability that may result vary extensively, but in essence are similar to those that are seen in patients who have sustained traumatic brain injury or a stroke involving different parts of the brain (Table 89.5). The main difference here is the potentially progressive or recurrent nature of the brain cancer and its uncertain prognosis. The greatest deficits are frequently seen immediately after surgery or during radiation and chemotherapy, after which remarkable improvement may occur. Late brain injury from radiation with infarction or necrosis also may occur, but the resulting disability has a less favorable prognosis for recovery. All patients with brain cancer and impaired function in mobility or ADL should be referred for rehabilitation services. The majority can be helped with simple rehabilitation measures whereas others may require comprehensive inpatient rehabilitation, which should be provided when longer life expectancy allows. Following definitive treatment of primary brain tumors in children, it has been shown that rehabilitation significantly improves outcome in self-care activities, transfers into and out of bed, and locomotion by a wheelchair or walking (63).

Table 89.5. Rehabilitation Problems Associated with Cancer of the Brain

Paralysis	Dysarthria
Spasticity	Aprosodia
Joint contractures	Dysphagia
Pain	Ataxia
Sensory deficits	Visual-perceptual deficits
Visual field deficits	Cognitive and behavioral deficits
Diplopia	Psychosocial-vocational problems
Aphasia	

Most commonly, the rehabilitation intervention starts after surgical resection or removal of the brain tumor. When medically stable the patient should be helped to sit up, get out of bed, and start on active restoration program that is designed according to the patient's general condition. The location and size of the cerebral lesion clearly determine the clinical symptoms encountered. The variability of the symptoms precludes a standard rehabilitation approach, but demands an individual evaluation and treatment plan. Broadly, the problems of patients with cancer of the brain are physical, psychologic, social, and vocational. Table 89.5 gives a detailed list of problems that are most commonly found, and are briefly discussed below.

Paralysis, often in the form of hemiplegia or hemiparesis, can be a conspicuous consequence of brain cancer. While the paralysis is most profound just after the brain surgery, a certain return of motor power is common and may continue for several weeks or months. As a rule, the earlier this return, the greater the recovery. However, muscles that are still totally paralyzed 4 to 8 weeks postoperatively generally remain so. At this point, functional improvement can still occur through physical training and provision of appropriate assistive devices, (orthoses or canes). While the medical condition is unstable, the patient is kept in bed, resting on a firm mattress with a soft surface, such as sheepskin, to prevent pressure sores. He or she should usually lie in the extended position with the affected arm abducted, externally rotated, and slightly elevated. Joint range-of-motion exercises should be applied to the paralyzed parts and active exercises to the uninvolved parts twice a day.

Mobilization training starts when the patient is ready to be transferred out of bed. Depending on the extent of the paralysis, the patient may be taught to ambulate with assistive devices or to maneuver a wheelchair. When the motor dysfunction is severe, the patient is first placed on a tilt table to decrease orthostatic hypotension and fear of the upright position, to stimulate antigravity muscles, and to improve body balance. Upon regaining some degree of body balance and lower-extremity strength, the patient is stood up between parallel bars for balancing exercises and early ambulation training. At this stage, the knee extensors on the affected side may be weak and require stabilization with a temporary knee-ankle-foot orthosis (KAFO), which locks the knee in extension for weight bearing. As the body balance improves and the patient has learned to lean consistently to his or her good side, ambulation outside of parallel bars can begin, with the patient supporting himself or herself on a broad-based cane carried in the unaffected upper extremity. Usually some knee extensor strength returns, allowing the patient adequate knee support, but the ankle dorsiflexors and invertors still may be weak. Here a plastic ankle-foot orthosis (AFO) may be prescribed to prevent foot dragging during the swing phase of gait. This orthosis is easily inserted into most shoes. It is cosmetically superior to the old metal orthoses and usually provides equal or better function. If knee extensor strength does not return, fabrication of a KAFO may be considered, but the prognosis for functional ambulation with such a device is poor.

Training and elevation activities, such as climbing and descending stairs, ramps, or curbs, are started when a good gait pattern on level ground has been achieved. Patients with severe neurologic deficits may require a wheelchair, either for mobility at all times or only when ambulation endurance or safety is impaired.

The major goal in the rehabilitation of the patient with cancer of the brain is independence in ADL, which may be obtained through training, prescription of proper assistive devices, and possibly modification of the patient's clothing and the architecture of the patient's home.

Spasticity frequently interferes with mobility and performance of ADL. Factors that may aggravate the spasticity (e.g., skin lesions, infections, and anxiety) need to be identified and treated. Thorough stretching of all joints should be performed daily. Medications—dantrolene sodium, baclofen, or diazepam—may be of some benefit, but should be used sparingly in view of their potential side effects. Selected nerve blocks with dilute solutions of phenol or concentrated alcohol are usually effective in reducing spasticity in the distribution of the nerve, but surgical procedures for reduction of spasticity in patients with cancer of the brain are rarely indicated.

Joint contractures, whether due to muscle imbalance, spasticity, poor nursing care, improper bed positioning or an inadequate exercise program, may change the rehabilitation prognosis significantly. A 10-degree flexion contracture of the knee, for example, will greatly increase oxygen consumption during ambulation and thus markedly reduce endurance. Knee contractures that exceed 15 degrees will usually make functional ambulation impossible for the patient with brain cancer and hemiplegia. Development of a frozen shoulder may make independent dressing impossible. Prevention of contractures by proper joint range-of-motion exercises is imperative from the onset of the disability, since treatment of contracture is relatively ineffective.

Pain in different parts of the body may be experienced in patients with neurologic deficits caused by cancer of the brain. Dysesthetic thalamic pain is notably refractive to treatment, although various centrally acting agents may be helpful. Pain with motion of the hemiplegic shoulder is common, perhaps due to muscle imbalance at the shoulder girdle and recurrent minor trauma to the periarticular structures. Shoulder support by an arm sling or a lap board, administration of analgesics, application of heat or cold modalities, and gentle range-of-motion and strengthening exercises may all help to reduce the pain and improve shoulder function. Reflex sympathetic dystrophy (shoulder-hand syndrome) may occur and requires similar treatment, but more effective relief may be obtained by simply administering oral steroids, for example, prednisone 5 mg four times a day for 2 to 3 weeks (14). Serial stellate ganglion blocks may be performed when symptoms are more persistent.

Sensory deficits of varying degrees are commonly seen in patients with brain cancer, either in the distribution of the cranial nerves or on one or both sides of the body. Cancer affecting the parietal lobes of the brain may cause severe sensory loss with little muscle weakness. This may interfere with balance and mobility since the patient who cannot feel motion is unable to control it. Although physical exercise cannot decrease the sensory loss, training with adaptive gait aids (i.e., canes, crutches, or a walker, and wearing of proper shoes) may help the patient to ambulate functionally again.

Visual deficits, such as double vision or visual field deficits, are commonly seen as a result of cancer in the lower brain or above the tentorium, respectively. While double vision may improve spontaneously, the wearing of alternating or unilateral eye patches or special prism glasses may be helpful. The value of exercises for retraining the eye muscles is uncertain. Homonymous hemianopsia—that is, blindness to the affected side of the body due to a contralateral brain tumor—rarely resolves spontaneously. While a patient with a left brain lesion usually learns easily to compensate for hemianopsia through scanning of the environment, the patient with right brain lesion may experience severe difficulties owing to accompanying anosognosia, or lack of awareness of the affected left side of the body and of the surroundings. However, specialized programs of cognitive remediation have been found to be effective with these patients (37).

Aphasia may be seen in patients with cancer in the left dominant hemisphere of the brain. This is an impairment of the central language process, with reduced capacity for interpretation and formulation of the symbols for communication. Although all components of language—listening, speaking, reading, and writing—are usually affected, they are not affected to an equal extent and thus several types of aphasia are recognized (2, 32). Expressive or nonfluent aphasia is caused by lesions in the Broca area of the brain and is characterized by reduced language production, vocabulary and use of grammar. The patient is well aware of these difficulties and becomes very frustrated. Less well known is receptive or fluent aphasia, which is caused by lesions in the Wernicke area of the brain. Here the patient primarily has difficulty in understanding language, both his or her own, and that of others. The patient thus may be able to speak continuously at normal speed and with normal melody without giving any pertinent information and be unaware of the errors. Most aphasic patients, however, understand nonverbal sounds and enjoy listening to music, and frequently some automatic speech is retained.

Different objective tests can be performed to assess the patient's language and communication skills, but many patients perform better during a conversation than on such tests, since they may be able to grasp certain key words and successfully make guesses, as well as understand gesticulations, facial expressions, the tone of voice, and other situational clues. The efficiency of speech therapy is debated since most patients will have a degree of spontaneous improvement. Nonetheless, speech therapy is indicated, whenever available, not only for psychologic support but also to provide the necessary stimulation for the patient to utilize his or her maximum speech ability, to adjust to new circumstances, and to instruct the family in proper communication with the patient by such means as using short simple sentences at a normal voice volume and utilizing gestures and facial expressions while widening respect, optimism, patience, and encouragement.

Dysarthria is a motor disturbance of speech, which implies weakness, slowness, or incoordination of the muscles that produce speech. Understanding of written or spoken language is, therefore, never a problem. Articulation is usually the main problem, but speed, rhythm, sound, and intonation may also be disturbed. Mild dysarthria accompanies many brain cancers that involve cranial nerves and cerebrum and affect the facial musculature, but it is particularly prominent in brainstem tumors. Management, which is often successful, emphasizes teaching the patient to use the remaining speech muscles more effectively or to bypass the effects of disturbed function. First, the patient is guided in producing sounds, then words, and finally whole sentences. If speech still remains completely unintelligible, other communication methods are introduced, such as writing, typing, sign language, or pictures.

Aprosopia is a little-known communication disorder that is seen with lesions of the nondominant right hemisphere (66). This condition relates to the inability to express and comprehend variations in pitch, rhythm, and stress, which give emotional meaning to speech. These patients may speak in a relatively flat voice and are often unable to recognize the emotional tones of speech, including the meaning of nonlanguage speech sounds, such as grunts or sighs. It is important for the clinician and the family to understand this deficit and communicate with the patient strictly by words, since specific therapy does not exist. Considerable improvement usually occurs with time.

Dysphagia, or impaired swallowing, is frequently seen in patients with brain cancer, especially when the brain stem is involved. In its most severe form, the patient may be totally unable to swallow, but in milder cases, there may only be difficulty with the swallowing of liquids. Aspiration with resulting pneumonia may occur, thus demanding careful evaluation of the condition and proper intervention. Serial radiographic swallowing studies should be done for proper monitoring of the condition until it is resolved or other and safer means of nutrition are established. A swallowing training program may be instituted by the speech or occupational therapist where the patient attempts to swallow food of different consistency using different techniques and positions. While a nasogastric tube can be used for several weeks while waiting for spontaneous recovery, a more persistent dysphagia warrants insertion of a gastrostomy tube for prolonged feeding.

Neuropsychologic changes may be prominent when cancer affects the cerebral hemispheres. Reduced memory and judgment frequently make successful rehabilitation impossible as the patient may be unable to remember instructions. Severe agitation may need treatment with a major tranquilizer, such as chlorpromazine or haloperidol. Visual perceptual deficits, caused by a central disturbance in organizing visual stimuli from the environment, frequently accompany *right* brain damage even when visual field and acuity are normal. These patients may experience difficulty in recognizing the three dimensions: depth and distances, the relationship of lines and objects, and vertical and horizontal lines. This may, in turn, affect different functions, including reading, understanding maps, recognizing familiar objects, and driving vehicles safely. Similarly, these patients may be unable to recognize the emotional significance of facial expressions, adding to the communication problems caused by the frequently accompanying aprosopia. There is a tendency to be impulsive and careless, to minimize or even ignore the problems in functioning, to make frequent mistakes, and often to neglect the left environment (anosognosia). Patients with lesions in the *left* hemisphere, on the other hand, usually act and learn slowly, make few mistakes, and are aware of their deficits, which frustrate them severely. In recent years, neuropsychologic training programs designed to help patients overcome the visual, perceptual, and cognitive deficits have been reported as being successful (38). In addition, repeated neuropsychologic evaluations have been found to be sensitive indicators of recurrence (58).

CANCER OF THE SPINE

While primary tumors of the vertebrae (e.g., multiple myeloma) are uncommon, metastases to the spine are frequent. The spine is the most common site for skeletal metastases (1). At autopsy, 70% of patients who die from cancer demonstrate vertebral metastases (43) and more than 5% have evidence of metastatic compression of the spinal cord (4). This is usually an extradural anterior mass that involves bone. Intradural extramedullary tumors are usually histologically benign meningiomas or neurofibromas. Gliomas (i.e., ependymomas, astrocytomas, and medulloblastomas) are usually intramedullary, although occasionally they also are found in an extramedullary site. Although the histology and response to treatment are quite different for all of these tumors, the neurologic symptoms, signs, and rehabilitation interventions are quite similar, which permits the clinical findings and therapy for these conditions to be addressed simultaneously in this chapter.

Injury to the spinal cord and peripheral nerves is a recognized risk of therapeutic radiation that may not become manifest for many months, or even years (30). A transient radiation myelopathy involving primarily sensory neurons may occur in 10 to 15% of patients receiving mantle radiation for Hodgkin's disease (86). This condition is usually associated only with sensory symptoms, such as paresthesias and Lhermitte's sign, and resolves in 1 to 9 months (86). Delayed radiation myelopathy is an irreversible and progressive neurological condition that may affect motor, sensory, and sphincter functions, and has a reported incidence of 1 to 12% (20).

Clinical Presentation

By far the most frequent presenting symptom of a tumor of the spine is pain. The pain may be localized, diffuse, or radicular in nature. It is characteristically made worse by activity and by straining. Different from more benign back pain, the pain caused by tumors tends to be persistent, to be present or even worse at night, and is not relieved by rest. Additional symptoms at presentation may be weakness of the legs, difficulty in walking, and urinary sphincteric problems leading to overflow symptomatology or incontinence.

Neurologic deficits may develop insidiously or occur suddenly, depending on the tumor's rate of growth and location, or on the occurrence of a sudden pathologic fracture. Slowly progressive neurologic dysfunction is often seen with tumors of the lower spine that encroach on the cauda equina, whereas tumors of the thoracic spine may cause the sudden collapse of a vertebral body with direct compression of the spinal cord or of its blood supply. Although only half of all tumors of the spine are located in the thoracic region, these cause 70% of all spinal cord compressions that result in paraplegia. Such paraplegia may be neurologically complete, that is, with total paralysis and sensory loss below the level of the lesion. More frequently, however, the neurologic lesion is incomplete, with sensation and motor function preserved to a varying degree, as may be rated by the Frankel Classification Scale or the ASIA Impairment Scale (18), which is a modified version of the Frankel Scale (17, 27). Impaired bladder and bowel control at first may present clinically as urinary urgency or hesitancy, but with progressive cord compression, urinary retention or bowel and bladder incontinence may occur.

Treatment

Proper rehabilitation management plan and intervention depend on an accurate diagnosis and staging of the tumor, just as does the medical and surgical management. Most patients with spinal metastases can and should be managed nonsurgically with radiation, chemotherapy, and orthotic stabilization of the spine, since it has been demonstrated that radiation alone provides results that are similar to those of surgery followed by radiation (33). In general, laminectomy with decompression has been found to be of limited use as compared with radiation, since the compressive lesion is usually located anteriorly to the cord and the surgical procedure itself contributes to spinal instability. However, profound neurologic deficits, especially when occurring rapidly, may warrant surgical decompression, which preferably should be done by an anterior approach followed by surgical stabilization of the spine. Surgical decompression of the spinal cord is not very effective once the patient has become completely paraplegic. Surgical stabilization may often be indicated when gross spinal instability is present, as two of the three "columns" (anterior, middle, and posterior) of the spine have been destroyed by the tumor (24). The extent of surgical stabilization varies, depending on the patient's anticipated life expectancy. Patients with short life expectancy (less than 1 year) benefit most from a relatively simple procedure employing methylmethacrylate, which allows immediate spinal stability and rapid mobilization of the patient, whereas patients with a more favorable prognosis may be better served by vertebrectomy, spinal instrumentation, and bony fusion in conjunction with methylmethacrylate (24).

Spinal metastases and myelomatous lesions, even when accompanied by compression fractures and minor or modest spinal instability, can be successfully managed by spinal orthotic support and radiation. Both modalities may significantly decrease pain. Lesions in the cervical spine are most rigidly immobilized by a halo brace (Fig. 89.1), but also may be adequately supported by a SOMI brace (sternal-occipital-mandibular immobilizer) (Fig. 89.2). When such lesions are present in the upper thoracic spine, spinal orthoses may not be necessary, as this part of the spine is stabilized inherently by the rib cage. Lesions in the more mobile lower thoracic and lumbar spine are often associated with severe pain. An adjustable thoracolumbar sacral (TLS) orthosis (Fig. 89.3) with posterior stays may provide sufficient support for less severe lesions, decrease pain, and allow greater mobility. The soft anterior portion of the corset, the apron, should fit snugly over the entire abdomen for optimal support. Larger lesions and postoperative conditions may require fabrication of a custom-molded plastic TLS brace, a

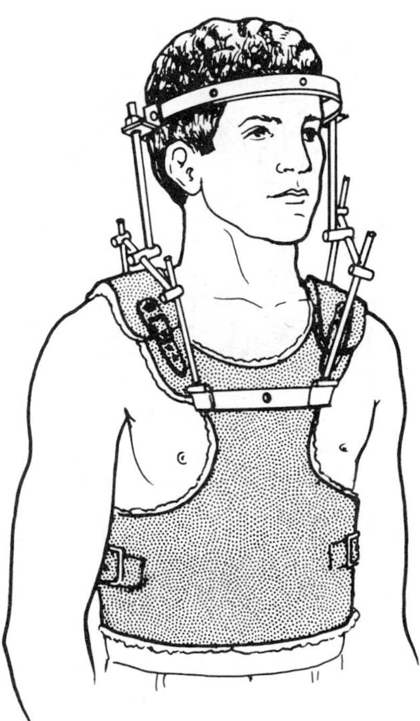

Figure 89.1. Halo-orthosis. *Source:* Ragnarsson KT: Orthotics and shoes. In Rehabilitation Medicine: Principles and Practice. Edited by JA DeLisa. Philadelphia: Lippincott, 1988.

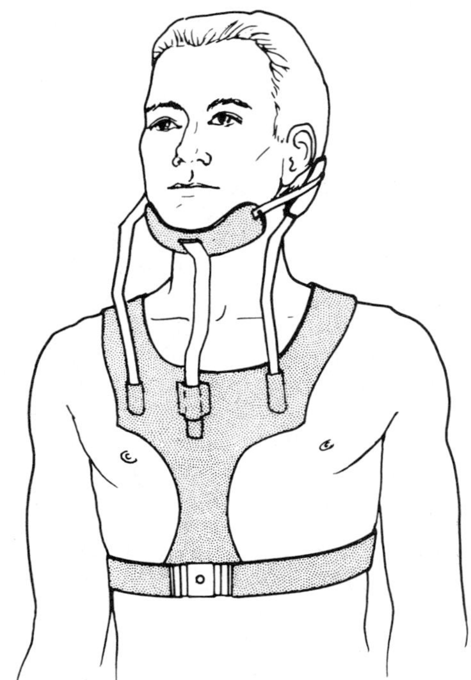

Figure 89.2. Sternal-occipital-mandibular immobilizer (SOMI orthosis). *Source:* Ragnarsson KT. Orthotics and shoes. In Rehabilitation Medicine: Principles and Practice. Edited by JA DeLisa, Philadelphia: Lippincott, 1988.

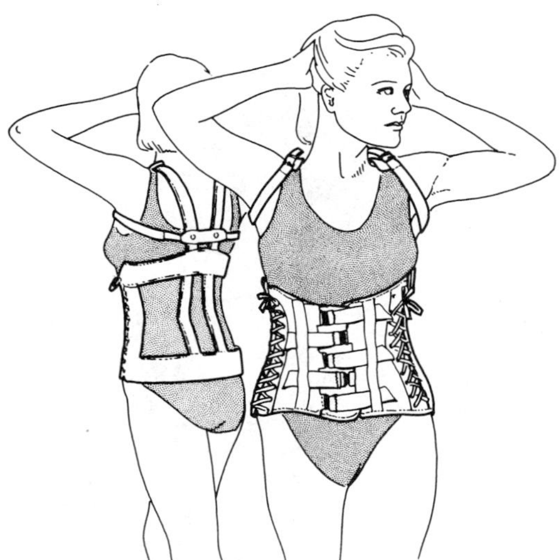

Figure 89.3. Thoracolumbar-sacral orthosis (TLSO, Knight-Taylor brace). *Source:* Ragnarsson, KJ: Rehabilitation of patients with physical disabilities caused by tumors of the musculoskeletal system. In Tumors of the Musculoskeletal System. Edited by MM Lewis. New York: Saunders, 1991.

two-piece removable orthosis (Fig. 89.4) that firmly grabs the pelvis below and the chest above.

When neurologic loss has occurred, the rehabilitation therapy must be carefully individualized, based on the extent of the neurologic dysfunction, the medical/surgical condition, and the patient's life expectancy. Spinal cord dysfunction

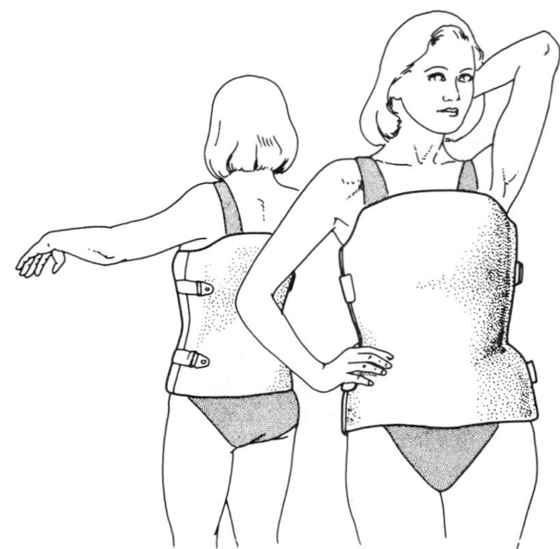

Figure 89.4. Custom-molded thoracolumbar-sacral orthosis (TLSO), a two-piece removable plastic orthosis (body jacket). *Source:* Ragnarsson, KT: Rehabilitation of patients with physical disabilities caused by tumors of the musculoskeletal system. In Tumors of the Musculoskeletal System. Edited by MM Lewis. New York: Saunders, 1991.

Table 89.6. Conditions and Complications Associated with Spinal Cord Dysfunction

Loss of motor power	Metabolic disturbances
Loss of sensation	a. Negative calcium balance
Pressure sores	b. Negative nitrogen balance
Urinary dysfunction	c. Hormonal imbalance
Bowel dysfunction	Circulatory disturbances
Sexual dysfunction	a. Orthostatic hypotension
Autonomic hyperreflexia	b. Edema
Pain	c. Deep vein thrombosis
Spasticity	Respiratory disturbances
Joint contractures	Psychological problems
Heterotopic ossifications	Social problems
	Vocational problems

with severe or complete paralysis and sensory loss, and perhaps bladder and bowel dysfunction, warrants a comprehensive but relatively short-term rehabilitation program involving as many members of the rehabilitation team as judged appropriate by the physiatrist. The rehabilitation programs should be designed to address each of the many clinical complications and conditions that may be seen in individuals with spinal cord dysfunction of traumatic origin (Table 89.6). Early intervention should include bedside physical and occupational therapy, establishment of bowel and bladder training programs, and the application of nursing principles to prevent complications, such as pressure sores and joint contractures, that increase morbidity, worsen the functional prognosis, and prolong the rehabilitation phase. Proper positioning of the patient in bed and turning at least every 2 hours is of paramount importance in this regard. The patient and family are given emotional support and are educated in the medical aspects of spinal cord dysfunction and management. If the prognosis is poor (i.e., less than 6 months) the patient is instructed early in the ADL skills, which he or she can quickly learn to perform, and provided with the necessary assistive devices, such as a wheelchair, nursing supplies, and personal assistance. As soon as medically appropriate, discharge from the hospital to the home or a nursing facility can be accomplished. When life expectancy is greater and the general criteria for admission to the inpatient rehabilitation service are met, the patient may be transferred there for a more comprehensive and intensive rehabilitation program.

CANCER OF THE HEAD AND NECK

Definitive treatment of cancer that arises from the skin of the face and neck or tissues of the nose, mouth, throat, and larynx may result in impairments in cosmesis, oral communication, feeding, and respiration, as well as affect the senses of sight, hearing, taste, and smell. These functional deficits may have major psychologic, social, and vocational consequences if not adequately addressed early and managed properly. Surgical excision and reconstruction are frequently followed by radiation, which by itself may produce clinical problems, including skin erythema, blistering and peeling, edema, delayed wound healing, muscle atrophy and fibrosis with reduced mobility, nerve damage with weak muscles and sensory deficits, dry mouth, and bad or lost taste. Sensory deficits and radiation-induced skin changes require careful grooming and hygiene to prevent further skin damage, by using nonirritating soaps and cosmetic products, an electric razor instead of a blade, lukewarm water for washing, loose-fitting garments, and similar measures. Meticulous oral hygiene is essential, and the patient should frequently use diluted mouthwash with 3% hydrogen peroxide but avoid all irritating agents (i.e., alcohol, tobacco, and astringent toothpaste) and should limit denture wear. A sense of noxious taste and dry mouth may be reduced by the use of artificial saliva and by increasing fluid intake. Mobilizing exercises for the mouth, jaw, neck, and shoulders should be emphasized to prevent adhesions and contractures.

Cosmetic defects of the face are primarily treated by surgical reconstruction, but different types of maxillofacial prostheses may be custom-made from plastic materials to closely match the facial contours and complexion. Surgical resection of cancer involving the mouth, pharynx, and larynx may result in impaired functions of chewing, swallowing, and speaking in different proportions. Following resection of the tongue and mandible, physical exercise of the residual muscles may improve chewing and swallowing, and special tubes or utensils may help to place the food into the pharynx or esophagus and thus ease the swallowing process. Defects in the palate may be corrected by a prosthetic device, an obturator, placed between the oral and nasal cavities.

Total laryngectomy results in a complete loss of voice and a permanently open tracheostomy (53). Preoperatively, a speech pathologist should meet with the patient to explain ways to communicate postoperatively. Communication is initiated postoperatively by using writing materials, communication boards, or electronic typing gadgets, but as early as possible the patient is instructed in the use of an artificial electrolarynx. Here a hand-held battery powered "diaphragm" is placed firmly against the neck to transmit sound waves through the tissues into the mouth, where it resonates and may be articulated with relative ease as comprehensible speech. Greater training, however, is required to become proficient in so-called esophageal speech, which is generated by trapping air in the upper esophagus by the tongue and releasing it suddenly into the pharynx, thus producing a "burplike" low-pitched sound that may be articulated into words. Other patients may prefer pharyngeal speech, which is produced by capturing air within the mouth or pharynx. In some cases, a tracheopharyngeal shunt may be surgically reconstructed to restore a more normal voice (50). Due to the open tracheostomy, the laryngectomized patient is unable to strain during lifting, pushing, or defecation, except by manually closing the stoma. The permanent tracheostomy requires not only good local care, but also inhalation of humidified air through a stoma cover made of a piece of gauze that acts as a sieve for dust and other foreign materials.

Certain laryngeal cancers may be treated with partial resection of the larynx, that is, hemilaryngectomy or supraglottic laryngectomy. Hemilaryngectomy removes one vocal cord, while supraglottic resection removes the epiglottis. The former is associated with a voice change that may be improved with voice therapy, whereas the latter is associated with impaired deglutition, which is restored with appropriate therapy.

Radical neck dissection may involve the removal of several neck muscles and temporary or permanent damage of the spinal accessory nerve that supplies the sternocleidomastoid and the trapezius muscles. This is likely to result in gross asymmetry of the neck and shoulders, restriction of motion, overstretching of remaining muscles, and persistent pain if not treated early. During the rehabilitation of these patients, it is of primary importance to unload the shoulder immediately postoperatively, reduce shoulder and neck pain, and prevent stretch fibrosis of the trapezius and contracture of the unopposed pectoralis muscles, as well as to provide strengthening exercises for the residual muscles in the neck and shoulder girdle to compensate for lost muscles (84). The patient is instructed to maintain good posture, both while sitting and standing, and to pull back the shoulders frequently. Sleeping on the back is preferable, with proper support provided by pillows placed between the scapulae and under the posterior neck. Lying on the affected side is to be avoided, and when lying on the unaffected side, the affected arm should be slightly raised and supported on a pillow. Occasionally, it may be helpful to wear a sling, or even a shoulder orthosis, to compensate for trapezius paralysis. Therapeutic exercises are initially passive, but gradually progress to active-assistive and eventually resistive exercises as tolerated by the patient. Strenuous physical activities should initially be avoided, such as lifting, carrying, pulling, and pushing, but may be resumed in the course of time as the physical condition improves.

CANCER OF THE LUNG

The physical disabilities associated with lung cancer and its treatment include respiratory insufficiency, shoulder pain and stiffness, scoliosis, and the remote effects of certain lung cancers that cause a neuromuscular disorder that becomes manifest as weakness and incoordination. However, the functional limitations associated with lung cancer frequently do not receive adequate attention and intervention because of the heretofore high mortality and short life expectancy associated with the disease.

Reduced respiratory capacity after lung resection or pneumonectomy, especially when combined with preexisting chronic bronchitis, may result in respiratory complications and insufficiency during both the postoperative period and long-term follow-up. These may best be prevented by preoperatively teaching the patient deep-breathing exercises, segmental breathing, effective means of coughing, and the principles of postural drainage. On the first postoperative day, these activities are resumed with a physical or respiratory therapist to eliminate mucus, which otherwise might plug the bronchi and cause atelectasis and pneumonia. As the patient recuperates and becomes ambulatory, shoulder range-of-motion, general strengthening, and endurance exercises, as well as postural training, are added to the therapy program to increase strength and stamina and to prevent postthoracotomy scoliosis and scapulohumeral displacement (77).

CANCER OF THE BREAST

Breast cancer is usually treated with mastectomy, or with surgically conservative lumpectomy followed by radiation and often chemotherapy. This treatment not only may result in considerable physical disability, but the women's self-image and emotional well-being may be adversely affected. The cosmetic impact of the loss of the breast, a symbol of femininity, is profound and adds to the emotional turmoil created by the cancer diagnosis and the uncertain prognosis of the disease. Radical mastectomy with removal of the pectoralis muscles, although now rarely performed, may cause shoulder weakness and, together with axillary node dissection, may produce swelling of the ipsilateral arm. Stiffness of the shoulder and hand may limit reach and manual dexterity. Fortunately, the recent trend to performing modified radical mastectomies or lumpectomies and routinely providing proper postoperative rehabilitation therapy has reduced the frequency and severity of these problems.

Postoperative rehabilitation has three main goals: prevention of physical disability, restoration of cosmetic appearance, and psychosocial and vocational readjustment. Physical rehabilitation aims at improving muscle strength and mobility at the shoulder, minimizing arm swelling, and facilitating resumption of all functional activities—ADL, recreation, and work. Following radical mastectomy, the arm should be kept slightly elevated with the shoulder abducted to 80 to 90 degrees and externally rotated, keeping the elbow free (15). The entire arm is compressed by a well-wrapped elastic Ace bandage, which is reapplied every 8 hours to reduce the swelling. Substantially less physical rehabilitation is necessary following modified radical mastectomy and axillary dissection, an operation that spares the pectoralis major and usually the pectoralis minor. Lumpectomy with axillary dissection requires even less physical and psychologic rehabilitation, which may proceed at a more rapid pace. Depending on the extent of the mastectomy, physical exercises may be started within 2 to 5 days postoperatively. The nurse or therapist first instructs the patient in deep-breathing and relaxation exercises, and in how to move about in bed comfortably, to get up and perform light self-care tasks using primarily the unaffected arm. Gentle exercises are started at this time, with the patient actively moving all the unaffected limbs, as well as the elbow, wrist, and hand on the affected side, and isometrically contracting the distal muscles (hand squeezing) while supine and with the affected arm elevated. When the drains have been removed from the surgical site, the exercises may become more demanding. The patient starts performing gentle active exercises of the affected shoulder while still in a supine position. Approximately 10 days postoperatively, when the sutures are removed, active or active assistive shoulder exercises in the upright position are begun, that is, "wall climbing" exercises using the uninvolved arm or an overhead pulley system to ease the task. Upon discharge, the patient receives a series of exercises to perform at home to ensure that full shoulder mobility and maximum strength will be regained.

Cosmetic restoration following mastectomy involves either surgical reconstruction of the breast or provision of a prosthesis. During the initial postmastectomy period, a temporary Dacron-filled prosthesis may be provided, but a more definitive prosthesis can be furnished when the surgical incision is well healed, usually 1 or 2 months following the surgery (56). Reconstruction is usually done several months after surgery, following the completion of chemotherapy and radiation, although immediate reconstruction at the same operation after mastectomy and axillary dissection has many advocates. Reconstruction is particularly indicated in younger women who have good life expectancy but whose self-image has suffered due to the mastectomy, although neither age nor an uncertain prognosis should be a contraindication to this procedure. Simple and temporary fillings of soft materials may be inserted into the brassiere initially for cosmetic effect, but a permanent prosthesis is ordered 2 to 3 months postoperatively, or after completion of the radiation therapy.

Lymphedema of the arm after radical mastectomy is seen in approximately 10 to 15% of patients, although relatively mild or moderate arm swelling is much more common, especially in the early postoperative days. Lymphedema is rare after modified radical mastectomy, and virtually unknown after lumpectomy, even though both procedures do have axillary dissection. When lymphedema is severe, it may result in both a significant disability and a disfigurement. While surgical removal of lymph nodes and lymph vessels or their destruction by radiation undoubtedly is the major etiologic factor, a number of other contributing factors may play a role, including infection, inflammation, scar formation, obesity, thrombophlebitis, arm dominance, and habitual dependent position of the arm. The greatest incidence of lymphedema has been noted among those who received high-dose radiation or had a history of one or more infections (74). Prevention of lymphedema with proper postoperative care and initiation of an exercise program, as outlined above, is most important because treatment of persisting lymphedema is relatively ineffective. Such treatment usually involves different physical interventions: performing several times a day sets of isometric exercises of all the arm muscles while the arm is maintained in an elevated position, and using sequential pneumatic compression with a multicompartmental inflatable sleeve (65). These modalities help to pump the fluid from the hand and distal arm toward the body. Many hours of pump use may be required each day to reduce the edema significantly. Compression therapy by manual massage of both the edematous (22) and the contralateral arm (26) has also been advocated but is considered by some to be time-consuming and inefficient (41). Between periods of use, the arm should be carefully wrapped with elastic bandages, and when maximum reduction of the edema has been obtained, a custom pressure-gradiated elastic sleeve should be fabricated and worn continuously. The entire limb should be guarded against even trivial trauma, which may be caused by constricting garments and excessive heat, or exercise, to minimize swelling. Treatment with these physical modalities has been shown to benefit the majority of patients with postoperative lymphedema and is more effective than diuretics, salt-restriction diets, benzopyrones, or surgical procedures (26, 41, 89). Recently, benzopyrone is shown to cause a slow but safe reduction of high-protein lymphedema of the extremities by stimulating proteolysis by macrophages (11).

CANCER OF THE GASTROINTESTINAL TRACT

The cancer rehabilitation team is involved in the care of the patient who has cancer limited to the gastrointestinal tract when the definitive surgical treatment has resulted in an ostomy. The enterostomal therapist (ET nurse) plays a major role in helping the cancer patient with an ostomy (i.e., colostomy, ileostomy, or urostomy) to understand the principles of ostomy care, to learn the different aspects of ostomy management, and to adjust to the altered self-image.

Colostomy

The surgical treatment of cancer of the rectum usually mandates the creation of a colostomy, using the sigmoid colon. A cancer higher in the colon can frequently be resected and the bowel reconnected by anastomosis. Before undergoing a surgical procedure for cancer that will result in a colostomy, the surgeon needs to discuss the plans carefully with the patient. Subsequently, the ET nurse should meet with the patient and family members to explain in simple but clear terms the nature of the colostomy, for example, where the stoma will be located on the abdominal wall, how it will look, what coverings and collection appliances will be needed, how evacuation will occur, and so on. A positive attitude on the part of the medical and nursing staff is important at this time, although the patient's fears and concerns regarding function, appearance, and sexual activity need to be acknowledged and discussed. Excessive and explicit explanations, particularly regarding the details of the surgical procedure and subsequent care, should be based on a patient's individual needs. Too much information that the patient is not ready to absorb may do little but increase anxiety. A visit by a person who is successfully managing his or her colostomy may be very helpful. Good preoperative preparation reduces the patient's fears and builds confidence, both of which will facilitate postoperative rehabilitation.

Postoperatively, protecting the skin and collecting the drainage should be the primary goals. This is accomplished by a properly fitted appliance. Modern appliances with protective skin barriers cut to fit the exact size of the stoma will avoid postoperative peristomal skin excoriation and keep the patient dry and odor-free. A person with a colostomy has a choice of allowing the bowels to function normally or to irrigate as a method of attempting to control bowel movements. Often the bowel habits return to normal patterns and a well-fitting appliance may be emptied or changed as needed. Proper fit of an appliance by an ET nurse allows the patient to make an informed choice, as the appliances are odorproof and disposable, and have protective pectin skin barriers attached to keep peristomal skin healthy and free of irritating discharge.

If the patient chooses to learn irrigation techniques, these cannot always be taught in the hospital setting given current reimbursement regulations (diagnostic related groups, or DRGs) and pressure for early discharge. Outpatient ET services and/or visiting nurses often teach or continue to teach the irrigation in the home after discharge. The purpose of the irrigation is to establish a bowel routine, with the goal of evacuating only after the irrigation, rather than spontaneously or at inopportune moments. However, this is not always possible. Therefore, the patient should always be instructed in the care and use of a properly fitted appliance. This may help the patient to avoid the frustrations that usually are experienced when bowel discharge continues between the irrigations. Irrigation of the colostomy may be done daily, every other day, or even every third day, and usually either in the morning or in the evening, depending on the patient's preferences. Initially, a full hour should be allocated for the irrigation and evacuation, although later 30 minutes may suffice to complete the task. The first irrigation is an important event that requires both sensitivity and technical skills on the part of the ET nurse. The irrigation should be done in private, preferably with the patient sitting by the toilet on a comfortable soft chair. A lubricated cone is gently inserted into the stoma and 1 liter of lukewarm tap water is instilled over a period of approximately 10 minutes from an enema bag placed no higher than at the shoulder level, similar to administering an enema. The water distends the bowel, causing peristalsis and expulsion of the stools. Following evacuation, the skin is cleansed with warm water and patted dry. The pouch is reapplied. A family member may want instructions in colostomy care, both to understand the patient's plight and to be able to assist or take over the care during periods of illness. The patient and the family are provided with information on the United Ostomy Association, and its local chapters and publications, as a resource for further information. After surgery, the patient is placed on a diet of clear liquids, which is followed by full fluids, and later solid food. What constitutes a well-balanced diet and the importance of a high-fiber, low-fat diet are discussed. It is best to increase the diet's fiber content gradually to avoid gas formation and bloating by adding fruits, vegetables, and wholegrain food in slowly increasing amounts.

Numerous clinical problems may arise at any time after the creation of a colostomy. Constipation is often due to inadequate intake of fluids or dietary fiber, but may be successfully managed by increasing dietary fiber (Fiber-all) and increasing fluid intake. Diarrhea may be caused by different foods (spicy, greasy, or fried foods; certain vegetables, fruits, and juices), but small amounts of liquid stools may indicate incomplete evacuation or the presence of impacted feces. Excessive gas formation also may result from the ingestion of certain foods (baked beans, onions, greasy food), anxiety, and other factors, which need to be identified and treated appropriately. Noxious odor may be increased by various foods and liquids (cabbage, eggs, onions, garlic, beer, coffee). Each person must experiment with different foods. What may adversely affect one person may not affect another. Deodorant tablets placed in the disposable colostomy pouch may help to diminish odors. Skin excoriation and maceration will usually respond to appropriate local care by gentle washing with soap and water and applying a properly fitted appliance. Skin infections may be caused by fungi or bacteria. Fungal infections should be treated with mycostatin (Nystatin) powder and bacterial infections by administering topical or, occasionally, oral antibiotics. Stomal bleeding in small amounts is usually of little concern, but if persistent, mixed with stools, or in large amounts, it will require proper diagnostic evaluation and intervention. Sexual dysfunction after colostomy is not common, but when impotence does occur, it is primarily due to damage to the autonomic nerves in the pelvis sustained during extensive abdominal perineal resection of the cancerous bowel. The altered self-image often associated with the colostomy can cause temporary dysfunction. Men may become impotent and women anorgasmic, while sexual desire is not lessened (39). Sexual counseling for both partners, good communication, and the learning of new techniques for mutual satisfaction can do much to restore successful sexual activity. The colostomy patient will normally experience a reactive depression or grief, and subsequently go through the different stages of adaptation that are associated with any kind of major personal loss. The colostomy's negative influence on the patient's self-image is best counteracted by the physician and the ET nurse when they are able to make an accurate assessment of the patient's complaints and condition, plan experiences and interventions accordingly, and provide supportive counseling on an individual basis (5).

Ileostomy

This surgical treatment for cancer is performed in some chronic cases of ulcerative colitis. The principles and techniques of stoma care are similar to those of colostomy. The stools are of a loose consistency and drain continuously from the ileostomy. It is, therefore, necessary that the collecting pouch be worn at all times and that it be properly fitted by an ET nurse. Small bowel contents contain active digestive enzymes, which can cause severe peristomal skin excoriation if leakage occurs. The collecting pouch must be emptied as needed, usually every 3 to 6 hours, by releasing the clamp from the bottom of the pouch and emptying the contents directly into the toilet. Since the fluid loss through ileostomy is greater than with colostomy, fluid intake must be increased to prevent dehydration. There are no dietary restrictions except to avoid corn and peanuts, but the food should be eaten slowly and chewed well to prevent food blockage. A greater loss of electrolytes and certain vitamins, especially B-12, may also be experienced, thus requiring regular monitoring and supplementation. Certain coated medications and time-release capsules may pass through the gut without being digested, a fact to be considered whenever physicians prescribe medications for individuals with ileostomy. In general, the psychosocial adjustment and rehabilitation outcome for an individual with ileostomy are similar to those after any surgery that requires alteration of elimination habits and results in living with a stoma.

CANCER OF THE GENITO-URINARY SYSTEM

Invasive cancer of the bladder frequently requires radical cystectomy and a urinary diversion, that is, the creation of a new outlet for urine. More than 40 years ago, Bricker developed the ileal conduit procedure by connecting the ureters to an isolated section of ileum, which is surgically closed at one end but opens at the other as a stoma on the abdominal wall, allowing free elimination of the urine. This procedure has become the traditional form of long-term urinary diversion. The management principles of ileal conduit stoma care are similar to those of colostomy and ileostomy. Since urine flows continuously from the stoma, the collecting system must be well fitted and watertight to prevent leakage. The collecting pouch must have a drain valve for easy emptying and for connecting to a nighttime urine collection bag. Skin or stoma problems from the urine are not uncommon and may be caused by alkaline urine. Many physicians prescribe vitamin C, 1,000 mg daily, to keep urine slightly acid. The intake of 8 to 10 glasses of fluid daily is very important. In recent years, the continent urostomy has gained considerable popularity when used with compliant patients. The Kock pouch and the Indiana pouch, with several modifications of both procedures, result in an internal reservoir (6, 10, 55, 67, 68, 78). The patient inserts a catheter into the stoma every 4 to 6 hours to empty the internal pouch contents. This procedure eliminates the need for external devices.

Genital Cancer

Members of the cancer rehabilitation team may occasionally be asked to provide care for a patient with cancer involving the genital organs, or when the cancer and its treatment have caused sexual dysfunction. Rehabilitation interventions usually involve carefully planned reconstructive surgery and psychologic and sexual counseling. The form of surgical reconstruction varies, depending on the type of the cancer and the extent of the surgical resection, but also on the specific needs of the patient. The woman who has undergone radical gynecologic surgery with resection of the vagina may benefit from vaginal reconstruction that allows resumption of sexual intercourse (21). The male who is unable to achieve penile erection can be taught intrapenile injection of vasodilating drugs to cause erection when desired or can have a penile prosthesis implanted. The choice of prosthesis is between semirigid silicone rod implants and a system of inflatable cylinders implanted into the shaft of the penis with scrotal pump and fluid reservoir placed in the abdominal wall (25, 62, 73). The implantation of the semirigid rod is a relatively simple surgical procedure that incurs relatively few mechanical problems, but the penis stays semierect permanently. The inflatable prosthesis provides a more normal appearance of the penis when both flaccid and erect, but mechanical problems with the system arise quite often.

Cancer of the testes is usually treated with prompt surgical excision of one or both of the testicles followed by radiation and/or chemotherapy. Surgical implantation of a prosthetic testicle at a later date may be very gratifying for many patients concerned about their appearance and self-image.

Sexual rehabilitation obviously is not limited to those who have cancer affecting the genital organs, but should be available for anyone who experiences sexual dysfunction for physical or psychologic reasons due to the cancer and its treatment. Different members of the rehabilitation team collaborate in providing sexual counseling for patients with different forms of cancer, both on an individual basis and by organizing courses and seminars on the physiology and anatomy of sexual function, on human sexuality, and on ways of adjusting to sexual dysfunction. Male sexual impotence compounds the reactive depression associated with the cancer diagnosis and adds to the stigma of any physical disability. This condition is frequently met with prejudice and poor understanding, on the part of both the patient and his sexual partner. Sexual rehabilitation emphasizes that sexuality is considered part of the whole person and cannot be lost due to an illness or injury. Physical disability, in contrast to a physical illness, does not decrease sexual drive, although it may affect sexual function both physically and psychologically. The anatomy and physiology of sexual function should be carefully explained to the disabled patients and their spouses or partners and general guidelines for success given. Good communication and strengthening of relationships between sexual partners are emphasized. The different physical aspects of sexual performance are clarified in order to make expectations compatible with performance capability. For most cancer patients with a physical disability, impairment of mobility, sensation, continence, and erection should not interfere with building a solid personal relationship, with having sensitivity to the partner's desires, or with being able to please and enjoy. Sexual rehabilitation is built on the concept that if sexual comfort is taught, sexual competence may result (12). No treatment or rehabilitation of the patient with cancer can be considered complete until the clinician has adequately addressed the impact of the condition on sexual function. Sexual health cannot be separated from total health. The extra time spent considering sexual adequacy and providing guidelines for help can benefit the patient for years.

CANCER OF THE LIMBS

Primary malignant tumors of the limbs require surgical treatment. The main surgical goal is to remove the tumor, either by an excision with wide margins through a site well clear of any malignant growth, or by a radical resection, that is, removal of the entire bone or the compartment afflicted by the tumor. A subsequent surgical goal is to reconstruct the resulting defect for optimal function and cosmesis. The customary and most accepted surgical treatment is limb amputation, although in recent years limb preservation by extended local or regional excision and reconstruction has been advocated. The survival rate and period of disease-free life after both types of surgical approaches are similar and have been improved in recent years by the use of chemotherapy, radiation, or both. The return to optimal function can best be assured by a multidisciplinary rehabilitation team approach that includes the surgeon, the medical and radiation oncologists, the physiatrist, and all the members of the rehabilitation team (64).

Skeletal metastases are more common than primary bone tumors (61). Metastases to the limb bones are less common than those to the spine. While some patients may complain of localized pain, others are essentially asymptomatic until a pathologic fracture occurs. Such fractures occur in approximately 10 to 15% of patients who have radiographic evidence of skeletal metastasis. Pathologic fractures are most debilitating and often result in diminished survival for otherwise stable patients (1). At particular risk are women with metastatic breast cancer, patients with advanced metastatic disease, and those with a large single lytic lesion eroding the bony cortex (7). Active rehabilitation and physical mobilization do not seem to increase the fracture risk significantly. When prognosis allows many months of anticipated function, prophylactic surgery for impending fracture of the femoral neck or shaft often diminishes the total disability consequent to pathologic fracture and more difficult surgical repair. Open surgical treatment of a pathologic fracture with adequate internal fixation and conjunctive use of methylmethacrylate may be employed successfully to relieve pain, increase mobility, ease nursing care, and provide psychologic reassurance (75). Postoperative immobilization should be brief, and aggressive physical therapy should be started early to return the patient swiftly to previous function, as well as to minimize hospitalization. Prophylactic surgery is otherwise generally not warranted but radiation may have some effect in reducing pain and limiting tumor growth (71).

Preoperative Rehabilitation

Rehabilitation care should start immediately after the diagnosis of primary cancer of a limb is established, regardless of whether amputation or limb-sparing reconstructive surgery is planned for cancer removal, or whether chemotherapy and radiation are to be instituted pre- or postoperatively. The implications of surgery and the postoperative course should be discussed at this time with the patient and family. Simultaneously, an appropriate physical exercise program should begin. These interventions during the emotionally stressful preoperative days may ease the patient's adjustment and reaction to the postoperative course. Emotional support is best given by recognizing the patient's fear and anxiety and by providing in a positive way some practical information and explicit factual instructions that can be easily understood and followed. While it is important that the positive aspects of the surgical treatment be explained (i.e., that it is a swift, lifesaving technique, and that modern technology and training allow significant restoration of function), it is best for the physician to resist overly optimistic predictions and to discourage unrealistic hopes until postoperative rehabilitation success has been ensured. On the other hand, pessimistic statements as to what the patient will never be able to do are needless and are usually inaccurate. A time frame is provided for postoperative rehabilitation efforts and possible return to various functional activities, taking into consideration the extent of reconstruction, level of amputation, general physical and mental status, age, athletic ability, and lifestyle. Peer counseling by a successful rehabilitated amputee may further help the patient to anticipate postoperative events and function.

When amputation or limb-sparing surgery is planned, the exact level of amputation and the surgical approach should be thoughtfully chosen, taking into account not only the location and the type of cancer, but also the probability of good wound healing and the successful fitting of a prosthesis when required. It may be helpful for the surgeon to consult with the physiatrist and prosthetist for this purpose. Preoperatively, strengthening exercises should be started for muscles in the uninvolved extremities and the trunk, as well as for muscles to be spared in the affected limb. Specifically, the patient should learn to perform isometric exercises for the quadriceps and gluteal muscles. Strengthening exercises for the unaffected limbs should focus specifically on shoulder depressors and elbow extensors, which are critical for ambulation with crutches or walkers. Trunk-strengthening and balancing exercises may further ensure postoperative ambulation success. Ambulation with a walker or a pair of crutches, non–weight bearing on the affected limb, should be practiced preoperatively while the patient has no fear of falling because of lack of limb support and is not impaired by incisional pain, medications, or postoperative complications. Such preoperative therapy not only will help the patient succeed swiftly postoperatively in ambulation and self-care activities, but a quick restoration of function will ease the emotional adjustment to the disability, whether it be amputation or limb sparing with an internal prosthesis.

Limb Amputation

Limb amputation for cancer at one time was discouraged as the prevailing opinion was that poor life expectancy did not justify the expense of surgery and prosthetic fitting. However, the 5-year survival for patients who have undergone amputations for limb cancer (49%) compares favorably with the survival of patients with amputations for limb ischemia (81), and the functional skills of cancer amputees are reportedly better than the skills of those patients who have had amputations for other reasons (52).

Until recently, amputations for cancer were done in a radical fashion and left little, if any, residual limb (stump), except when amputating for very distal limb tumors, since the basic clinical rule was to amputate proximally to the joint next above the tumor site. Lower-limb amputations for cancer involving the knee joint or thigh thus were frequently performed by a hip disarticulation or hemipelvectomy, and upper-limb amputations by shoulder disarticulation or interscapulothoracic (forequarter) amputations. These radical limb operations were believed to be mandatory due to the high risk of metastasis, especially metastasis to the lungs. Modern diagnostic techniques now can demonstrate the presence or absence of metastases with a high degree of accuracy. According to a recent survey, since the use of adjuvant chemotherapy, sarcomatous metastases are not as common as was previously thought (31). Thus, less extensive amputation techniques can now be employed, such as cross-bone amputations with 3 to 4 inches of normal bone left as the margin. Greater residual limb length thus results and functional outcome is better for most patients. Accordingly, primary cancer in the distal femur now permits an amputation through the proximal femur, a cancer in the proximal tibia permits amputation in the mid or distal femur, and cancer in the distal tibia allows a below-knee amputation. Analogous amputation levels may be appropriately considered for cancer of the upper limbs.

While maximum preservation of stump length compatible with eradication of the cancer is desirable, certain amputation levels may result in stumps that are difficult to fit and, therefore, best avoided, such as the hind foot, the distal third of the leg, and the femoral supracondylar region. It is critical to preserve the knee joint if possible to ensure smoothness of gait, lower energy cost, and better function. Whenever possible, 12 to 18 cm of tibia should be retained for optimal prosthetic fitting, but even a very short below-knee amputation (BKA) that retains the tibial tubercle will preserve knee extension by the quadriceps muscle, and preservation of the knee joint will provide needed position sense. This amputation level is, therefore, better than amputating above the knee. When the fibula is retained, it should be cut slightly shorter than the tibia. Disarticulation at the knee is also preferable to above-knee amputation (AKA) as it provides a wide weight-bearing surface, long lever arm, and proprioception. Unfortunately, this level often cannot be chosen due to intra-articular spread of cancer located in the mid or proximal tibia. It is preferable to have the AKA stump as long as possible to preserve maximal adduction power. Prosthetic knee joints can accommodate any length of femur. A femoral stump length that is less than 8 cm from the greater trochanter to the tip functions poorly. As a rule, hip disarticulation is preferred to an amputation level above the lesser trochanter. Hip disarticulation and hemipelvectomy need reconstruction with a long posterior flap in order to create a proper sitting area on the prosthesis (23). When provided with a well-fitting plastic laminated socket and an endoskeletal modular-design prosthesis, persons with hip disarticulation are able to stand, walk, and sit quite comfortably (Fig. 89.5). Hemicorporectomy (translumbar amputation) has been performed on rare occasions on patients with widespread cancer of the pelvis, but without metastases elsewhere. This procedure is a challenging alternative to the nonsurgical approach and has been shown to have a good rehabilitation outcome (28). Cancers in the upper limbs unfortunately are primarily found in the proximal humerus and require shoulder disarticulation or interscapulothoracic amputation. Here it is important to retain quality skin and maximum muscle mass for padding the shoulder, but retention of the humeral head, if possible, will result in better prosthetic fitting.

Successful prosthetic use depends to a large extent on proper surgical techniques of amputation (9). It is not adequate only to provide a long stump, although this is important for both leverage and large total contact area for weight bearing. Optimally, the stump should be firm, tapered or cylindrical in shape, with all bone ends well padded. The skin must have good innervation and vascular supply, and not be adherent to bone or have sensitive scars.

Postoperative care should ensure optimal wound healing, minimize stump swelling, prevent joint contractures, and improve muscle strength and function. Application of appropriate dressing and external pressure on the stump is very important (51). Stump wrapping with the customary elastic bandages must be done skillfully with frequent reapplications to maintain maximum sustained pressure and to avoid a tourniquet effect. Different forms of semirigid dressings have been used, such as Unna paste dressings, custom-made elastic stump socks, plastic films, and inflatable air splints, each of which has different advantages and disadvantages. Inflatable and removable air splints, recently popularized, are made of clear plastic and have a zipper, which allows easy inspection, attachments, and removal.

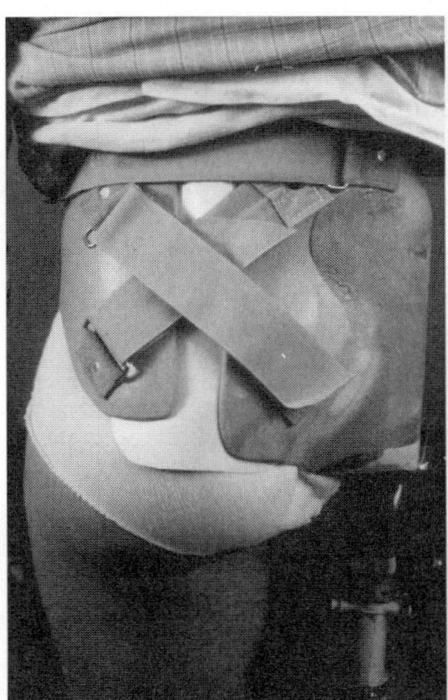

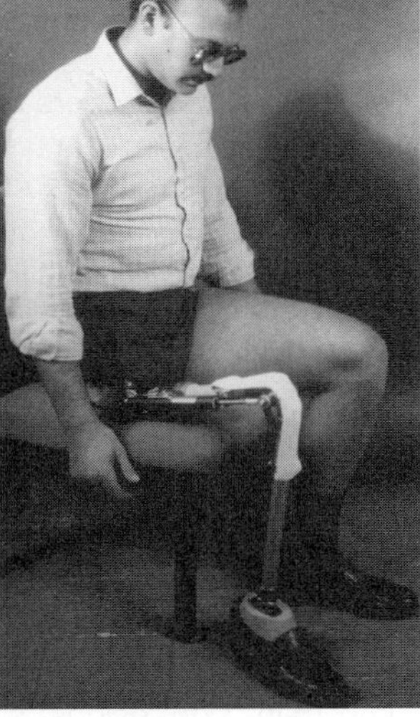

Figure 89.5. Custom-molded, plastic laminated socket, endoskeletal, and modular prosthesis with hip and knee joints and hydropneumatic control for hemipelvectomy. *Source:* H. Richard Lehneis, Roslyn, NY.

An elastic plaster bandage may be applied to the stump immediately after the amputation. This technique, referred to as immediate postsurgical fitting, is a rigid form of dressing that can effectively reduce edema and postoperative pain. A prosthetic pylon and foot can be attached directly to the plaster to allow standing within 2 days postoperatively. Initially, only minimal weight bearing is allowed, but progressive ambulation is continued and full weight bearing may be possible in 3 to 4 weeks (8). Several disadvantages of this technique have made it difficult to implement. A removable rigid dressing provides for easier stump inspection, dressing change, and adjustment for progressive stump shrinkage, and may even allow attachment of a temporary adjustable prosthesis (40, 88).

Postoperative Exercise Program

Physical and occupational therapy should be initiated within 2 days after the amputation. The preoperative exercise program is resumed for muscle strengthening and joint mobilization. Knee flexion contractures may easily develop after BKA, whereas hip flexion and abduction contractures are frequently seen with short AKA. Mobilization is started at bedside, but within a few days, the patient is taken by wheelchair to the therapy area and ambulation in parallel bars or with a walker is started. The skillful amputee is subsequently provided with a pair of crutches, but when prosthetic fitting has been completed, a single cane will usually suffice. Different types of ready-made or prefabricated temporary prosthetic devices exist for the earliest ambulation efforts, but a custom-fitted provisional prosthesis should be provided as soon as the surgical incision has healed. The amputee, however, may be discharged from the hospital even without a prosthesis, if the patient is ambulating safely with assistive gait devices and is independent in ADL. Transfer to the inpatient rehabilitation unit for more intensive therapy may be advisable at any time before these two goals are reached if the amputee is otherwise medically stable.

Prescription of an Artificial Limb

The physician needs to consider multiple factors when prescribing a limb prosthesis. The amputation level and stump condition clearly are of primary importance, but prosthetic candidacy may be affected by numerous other factors, including associated medical conditions, other physical disabilities, life expectancy, muscle strength and coordination, stamina, various psychological factors (i.e., motivation, emotional adjustment, and cognition), and individual lifestyle factors (i.e., age, weight, family support, recreational interest, environment, and type of work). The extent of prosthetic usage is to some degree predictable, since each symptomatic medical problem adversely affects functional prognosis. The ability of the patient to ambulate with a walker or a pair of crutches, but without a prosthesis, strongly suggests prosthetic candidacy. After carefully considering these different factors, the physiatrist may have to choose between a prosthesis that provides relatively greater safety with stability and one with greater function and mobility, between durability and low prosthetic weight, besides considering differences in cost and cosmesis. When new or advanced designs are chosen, the skill and expertise of the prosthetist are crucial factors, and the prosthetist must be easily accessible to the patient as well.

Most prostheses are currently fabricated from metals and plastics. The customary below-knee (BK) prosthesis consists of a socket, shank, and ankle-foot components, as well as a suspension system. The socket usually has a patellar tendon-bearing (PTB) design and a total stump contact for maximum pressure distribution. Soft liners inside the socket add comfort by absorbing shocks. Several layers of stump socks may need to be worn to accommodate a shrinking stump. The shank is either of an endoskeletal design with an internal metal pylon or an exoskeletal structure made from laminated plastic. The solid ankle cushioned heel (SACH) foot is simple, durable, lightweight, and cosmetic, and is still most commonly prescribed despite the arrival of a variety of new energy-storing prosthetic feet, such as the Seattle and the FLEX feet designs. The prosthesis is usually attached to the residual limb by a supracondylar cuff, although several other alternatives exist. The AK amputee traditionally obtains a prosthesis with a rigid quadrilateral socket and a posterior ischial seat for additional weight bearing. More modern socket designs promise greater comfort in sitting and better control during ambulation (72). The popular single-axis knee joint with constant friction is simple and durable, whereas the more costly and complex polycentric or hydraulic knee units can provide better function for young, physically active amputees. Stability of the knee joint during stance may be increased by posterior placement of the knee axis, but for maximum safety, manual or automatic knee locks may be added. The AK prosthesis optimally is suspended by total suction, or by partial suction and a Silesian bandage or a pelvic band. An endoskeletal pylon connects the knee unit above to the prosthetic foot below. After a hip disarticulation, the amputee receives the Canadian-type prostheses, which has a plastic laminated socket encircling the pelvis. This provides a resting surface for the ischial tuberosity for weight bearing. With proper molding, it is suspended from the iliac crest. A similar prosthesis is worn after hemipelvectomy, with the rib cage providing the weight-bearing surface.

Cancer in the upper limb frequently requires shoulder disarticulation or interscapular thoracic amputation, both of which make fitting the patient with a functional body-powered prosthesis difficult or impossible. Myoelectrically controlled and externally powered prostheses, however, may provide some gross function, but such prostheses are relatively expensive, are heavy, and require repair more often than a body-powered prostheses.

In recent years, prosthetic techniques for all types of amputations have advanced significantly, especially with respect to evaluation methods, socket design, ankle-foot components, and cosmesis (80).

Prosthetic Fitting and Training

Before completion of the prosthesis, the amputee needs to visit the prosthetist several times to ensure optimal fit, function, and comfort. When fabrication has been completed, the prescribing physician checks the prosthesis for fit and comfort, socket stability, joint motions, appearance, and function. The lower-limb amputee receives gait training, with or without gait aids, depending on motor skills, instructions in attachment and removal techniques, and exercises to increase muscle strength, joint range of motion, balance, and posture. The upper-limb amputee learns to open and close the terminal device, position the arm, manipulate objects, and perform self-care tasks. Initially, a prosthesis may not be worn comfortably for more than 15 to 30 minutes at a time. The amputee thus requires frequent rest periods and short therapy sessions. After each wear, the stump skin must be examined for signs of excessive pressure or poor socket fit.

At the beginning of prosthetic wear, confrontational situations may develop between the amputee and the health professional, especially when the patient's expectations do not match the actual situation. New and increased demands may produce discomfort at the prosthesis–user interface and in other body parts. Disappointment with the final appearance, weight, ease of wear, level of comfort, and functional limitations of the prosthesis is common. The health professional needs to understand the adjustment process and assist the amputee by paying attention to legitimate complaints, providing encouragement, and making judicious adjustment to the prosthesis. Poor communication may force the amputee to obtain a new, but often no better, prosthesis elsewhere. Various deviations of gait occur with lower-limb prosthetic use due to stump problems, inadequate prosthetic fit, psychological reactions, and improper training. These need to be carefully analyzed and proper intervention offered.

Lower-limb amputees ambulate at greater energy costs than do nondisabled persons (35, 83). The BK amputee expends 23 to 68% more energy per unit distance than does an able-bodied person, and the AK amputee expends 52 to 124% more (34). However, to save energy, most amputees decrease their speed of ambulation, which is approximately 2.0 to 2.5 mph for BK and 1.0 to 1.5 mph for AK amputees, as compared with a normal speed of 3 to 4 mph for nondisabled persons. The lower energy cost and greater speed of ambulation for the BK amputee clearly show the importance of sparing the knee joint whenever possible. Patients with hip disarticulation or hemipelvectomy ambulate with lower energy expenditure if they use axillary crutches without a prosthesis, as compared with prosthetic use (34).

Various clinical problems may occur as the result of the amputation and consequent prosthetic wear, including stump pain, skin lesions, swelling, joint contractures, and mental depression. Most amputees experience phantom sensation, which is a painless awareness of the amputated part. In contrast, phantom pain may be described as burning, crushing, cramping, or shooting sensations in the amputated phantom limb. The reported incidence of phantom pain has varied between 10 and 85% (13). This variation may be due to differences in classification of the types of pain (85), the fear of presumed mental illness if a phantom pain is reported (13), and the time delay since surgery (49). The pain may be aggravated by stump contact and different physical activities, but the exact cause remains unknown as no detectable stump pathology or premorbid emotional problems are usually discovered. Phantom pain (45) may be preventable or effectively managed by careful preoperative explanations of the nature of the phantom phenomenon, good surgical techniques, regular examinations postoperatively, and frequent manual handling and good care of the stump, as well as by effective treatment of stump infections and early provision of a functional prosthesis. Definitive treatment, however, is difficult, but symptoms usually improve when a relatively normal situation has been restored, for example, ambulation with a prosthesis. Other beneficial interventions include desensitization by frequent self-inspection and manipulation of the stump, application of superficial heat or cold, deep heating with diathermy, massage, vibration, TENS, imaginary exercises of the phantom limb, active exercises of the entire body, local anesthesia of the stump, and psychologic interventions. Analgesic medications are relatively ineffective, but agents acting on the central nervous system may be helpful.

Actual and localized stump pain occurs frequently after amputation for various pathologic reasons, such as infection, scar adhesion, muscle spasm, or poor socket fit. Skin reactions occur frequently over the stump and require meticulous care. The stump should be gently washed with soap and water and thoroughly dried each evening rather than in the morning. The prosthetic socket should be cleansed with a moist soapy cloth, and stump socks should be washed immediately after removal and thoroughly dried before they are worn again. The stump should be kept dry and free of trauma to prevent maceration. Talcum powder is often used to make the skin dry and smooth, but cocoa butter may be applied to lubricate the scar. During early prosthetic wear, the amputee may frequently experience skin maceration, abrasions, blisters, and infections of hair follicles and sweat glands, each of which requires specific treatment. Open, draining, or painful skin lesions require that prosthetic wear be discontinued until healing has occurred. Gradually, the skin will toughen with regular prosthetic use and skin problems become fewer in the course of time.

Reactive depression and grieving the limb loss may be anticipated, but these reactions are compounded by the cancer's uncertain prognosis. Early restoration of function and psychologic support provided by the entire health care team may be the best intervention, although psychiatric treatment may occasionally be indicated (see Chapter 87).

Limb-Sparing Surgical Reconstruction

Local resection of cancer with limb-sparing reconstruction may result in survival and a disease-free period equal to those for amputation, and function that is superior (76). Amputation, however, is still a primary treatment for many limb tumors since it may, at times, be impossible to perform a proper resection while preserving key nerves and vessels, and to reconstruct a functional limb.

Limb-sparing reconstructive surgery obviously is an attractive alternative to amputation for both cosmetic and emotional reasons, but it should only be undertaken if it will restore better and longer-lasting function than amputation with subsequent prosthetic fitting (57). Depending on the location and size of the tumor, it may be a difficult procedure where muscles, bone, and even joints are removed with the tumor. The cancerous bone may be replaced by transplanting a fresh frozen cadaveric bone allograft or an autologous graft, but more commonly by installing a synthetic metallic prosthetic implant (3, 54, 59). An expandable and adjustable prosthesis may now be installed in growing children, who formerly were felt to fare better with an amputation (29). Just as when amputation is planned, all patients should be carefully told preoperatively what degree of function to expect after the operation.

Rehabilitation interventions preferably should begin preoperatively when physical and/or occupational therapists should first teach the patient the muscle-strengthening, range-of-motion, and ambulation exercises that will be resumed postoperatively. Following lower-limb-sparing surgery, the patient may begin, on the first postoperative day, exercising the uninvolved limbs, but the initiation, pace, and intensity of exercises and the amount of weight bearing for the affected limb depend on the exact mode of reconstruction and the postoperative course. In general, continuous passive motion (CPM), active-assistive exercises, and weight bearing as tolerated may be allowed 6 to 10 days postoperatively if no surgical complications occur and no specific contraindications exist. During rehabilitation and a 2.5-year follow-up of 17 children who underwent resection of malignant bone tumors in the lower limbs with insertion of expandable prostheses, 7 of these children walked without any assistive devices, but 10 required knee orthoses, crutches, or both for ambulation (29). Following upper-limb-saving surgery, active hand and isometric shoulder muscle exercises are started on the first postoperative day, but if humeral resection was performed, active elbow and shoulder exercises should not begin for 2 or 8 weeks postoperatively, depending on whether a metallic implant or allo-/autografts, respectively, were used. It is thus of primary importance that the rehabilitation staff know exactly which muscles, nerves, and bones were resected, and what the reconstruction entailed, to plan a safe and effective rehabilitation program. Training in ADL is initiated approximately 1 week postoperatively. Prior to discharge, a decision is made as to whether the patient requires a permanent orthosis or other assistive devices to compensate for lost function. Following discharge, most patients are referred for continued therapy and are given specific instructions for exercise and other activities at home.

Conclusion

Management of cancer appropriately focuses on prevention, early diagnosis, and cure, but following effective treatment most cancer patients experience some physical impairment that results in a physical disability or a handicap. As the prognosis for most types of cancers improves, it becomes more important to ensure that all cancer patients regain maximum function in the broadest sense to ensure return to all former roles. Multidisciplinary rehabilitation, therefore, is an integral part of the total management of the cancer patient. The exact functional deficits need to be identified for each patient and proper rehabilitation interventions started promptly or at the same time as other treatments.

References

1. Aaron AD. The management of cancer metastatic to bone. JAMA 1994;272: 1206–1209.
2. Albert ML, Helm-Estabrooks N. Diagnosis and treatment of aphasia. Part I & Part II. JAMA 1988;259:1043, 1205.
3. Barbera C, Lewis MM. Surgical considerations in tumors about the knee. In Musculoskeletal Oncology: a Multidisciplinary Approach. Edited by MM Lewis. Philadelphia: Saunders, 1992, pp 327–342.
4. Barron KD, Hirano A, Araki S, Ferry RD. Experiences with metastatic neoplasms involving the spinal cord. Neurology 1959;9:91.
5. Brogna L. Self concept and rehabilitation of the person with an ostomy. J Enterostomal Ther 1985;12:205.
6. Brogna L, Lakaszawski M. Nursing management. The continent urostomy. J Enterostomal Therapy 1986;13:139.
7. Bunting R, Lamont-Havers W, Schweon D, Kliman A. Pathologic fracture risk in rehabilitation of patients with bony metastases. Clin Orthop 1985;192:222.
8. Burgess EM, Romano RL. Management of lower extremity amputees using immediate post surgical prostheses. Clin Orthop 1968;57:137.
9. Burgess EM, Zettl JH. Amputations below the knee. Artif Limbs 1969;13:1.
10. Carroll PR, Presti JC Jr, McAninch JW, Tanagho EA. Functional characteristics of the continent ileocecal urinary reservoir: mechanisms of urinary continence. J Urol 1989;142:1032.
11. Casley-Smith JR, Morgan RG, Piller NB. Treatment of lymphedema of the arms and legs with 5, 6-benzo-[(α)-pyrone. N Engl J Med 1993;329:1158.
12. Comfort A. Sexual Consequences of Disability. Philadelphia: Stickley, 1978.
13. Davis RW. Phantom sensation, phantom pain, and stump pain. Arch Phys Med Rehab 1993;74:79–91.
14. Davis SW, Petrillo CR, Eichberg RD, Chu DS. Shoulder hand syndrome in a hemiplegic population: a five year retrospective study. Arch Phys Med Rehab 1977;58:353.
15. Degenshein GA. Mobility of the arm following radical mastectomy. Surg Gynecol Obstet 1977;145:77.
16. Dietz JH. Rehabilitation Oncology. New York: Wiley, 1981, pp 69–75.
17. Ditunno JF, Young WS, Donovan WH, Bracken MB, Brown M, Creasey G, Ducker TB, Maynard FM, Stover SL, Tator CH, Waters RL, Wilberger JE. Standards for Neurological Classification of Spinal Injury Patients. Chicago: American Spinal Injury Association, 1992.
18. Ditunno JF, Young W, Donovan WH, Creasey G. The International Neurological Standards booklet for neurological and functional classification of spinal cord injury. Paraplegia 1994;32:70–80.
19. Dodds TA, Martin DP, Stolow WC, Deyo RA. A validation of the functional independence measurement and its performance among rehabilitation inpatients. Arch Phys Med Rehab 1993;74:531.
20. Dropcho EJ. Central nervous system injury by therapeutic irradiation. Neurol Clin 1991;9:969–988.
21. Edwards CL, Loeffler M, Rutledge F N. Vaginal reconstruction. In Sexual Rehabilitation of the Urologic Cancer Patient. Edited by AC VonEschenbach and DB Rodriguez. Boston: Hall, 1981, pp 250–265.
22. Elkins E. Effect of various procedures on the flow of lymph. Arch Phys Med Rehabil 1953;34:31–39.
23. Enneking WF, Dunham WK. Resection and reconstruction of a primary neoplasm involving the innominate bone. J Bone Joint Surg 1978;60:731.
24. Errico TJ, Kostuik JP. Diagnosis and treatment of metastatic disease of the spinal column: a review. Contemp Ortho 1986;13:15.
25. Finney RP. The treatment of erectile impotence with semi-rigid penile prosthesis. In Sexual Rehabilitation of the Urologic Cancer Patient. Edited by AC VonEschenbach and DB Rodriquez. Boston: Hall, 1981, pp 228–229.
26. Foldi E, Foldi M, Clodius L. The lymphadema chaos: a lancet. Ann Plast Surg 1989;22: 505–515.
27. Frankel H, Hancock D, Hyslop G, Melzak J, Michaelis L, Ungar G, Vernon J, Walsh J. The value of postural reduction in the initial management of closed injuries to the spine with paraplegia and tetraplegia. Paraplegia 1969;7:179.
28. Frieden FH, Gertler M, Tosberg W, Rusk HA. Rehabilitation after hemicorporectomy. Arch Phys Med Rehabil 1969;50:259.
29. Frieden RA, Ryniker D, Kenan S, Lewis MM. Assessment of patient function after limb sparing surgery. Arch Phys Med Rehab 1993;74:38–43.
30. Garden FH. Radiation injuries to the spinal cord and peripheral nerves. Phys Med Rehab State Art Rev 1994;8:405–411.
31. Gebhardt MC, Mankin HJ. Osteosarcomas: the treatment controversy, Part II. Surgi Rounds Orthopa, 1988, pp 25–42.
32. Geschwind N. Aphasia, current concepts. N Engl J Med 1971;284:654.
33. Gilbert RW, Kim JH, Posner JB. Epidural spinal cord compression from metastatic tumor: diagnosis and treatment. Ann Neurol 1978;3:40.
34. Gonzalez EG, Corcoran PJ. Energy expenditure during ambulation. In The Physiological Basis of Rehabilitation Medicine. Edited by AJ Downey, SJ Myers, EG Gonzalez, JS Lieverman. Boston: Butterworth-Heinemann, 1994.
35. Gonzalez EG, Corcoran PJ, Reyes RL. Energy expenditure in below knee amputees: correlation with stump length. Arch Phys Med Rehabil 1974;55:111.
36. Gordon WA, Freidenbergs I, Diller L, Hibbard M, Wolf C, Levine L, Lipkins R, Ezrachi O, Lucido D. The efficacy of psychosocial intervention with cancer patients. J Consult Clin Psychol 1980;48:743.
37. Gordon WA, Hibbard M, Egelko S, Diller L, Shaver MS, Lieberman A, Ragnarsson KT. Perceptual remediation in patients with right brain damage: a comprehensive program. Arch Phys Med Rehab 1985;66:353.
38. Gordon WA, Hibbard MR, Kreutzer J. Cognitive remediation Issues in research and practice. J Head Trauma Rehab 1989;4:76.
39. Gottesman JE. Male sexual dysfunction. Ostomy Q 1981;19:18.
40. Gottschalk F, Mooney V, McClellan B, Carlton A. Early fitting of the amputee with plastic temporary adjustable below knee prosthesis. Contemp Orthop 1986;13:15.
41. Grabois M. Breast cancer: post-mastectomy lymphedema. Phys Med Rehab State Art Rev 1994:8:267–277.
42. Grenger, CV, Hamilton BB, Shriver SF. Guide for the Use of the Uniform Data System for Medical Rehabilitation. Buffalo: State University of New York at Buffalo, 1986.
43. Harrington KD. Metastatic disease of the spine. J Bone Joint Surg Am 1986;68: 1110–1115.
44. Harvey RF, Jellinek HM, Habeck RV. Cancer rehabilitation: an analysis of 36 program approaches. JAMA 1982;247:2127.
45. Harwood DD, Hanumanthu S, Stoudemire A. Pathophysiology and management of phantom limb pain. Gen Hosp Psychiatry 1992;14:107–118.
46. Heinemann AW, Linacre JM, Wright BD, Hamilton BB, Granger C. Relationship between impairment and physical disability as measured by the functional independence measure. Arch Phys Med Rehab 1993;74:566.
47. Hinterbuchner C. Rehabilitation of the disability in cancer. NY State J Med 1978;1066.
48. Holland JC, Rowland JH. Handbook of Psychooncology. Psychological Care of the Patient with Cancer. New York: Oxford, 1989.
49. Houghton AD, Nicholls G, Houghton AL, Saadah E, McColl L. Phantom pain: natural history and association with rehabilitation. Ann R Coll Surg Engl 1994;76:22–45.
50. Juarbe C, Shemen L, Eberle R, Klatsky I, Fox M. Primary tracheoesophageal puncture for voice restoration. Am J Surg 1986;152:464.
51. Katz RT, Wu Y. Postoperative and pre-prosthetic management of the below knee amputee. Contemp Orthop 1985;10:53.
52. Kegel B, Carpenter ML, Burgess EM. Functional capabilities of lower extremity amputees. Arch Phys Med Rehabil 1978;59:109.
53. Keith RL, Darley FL. Laryngectomee Rehabilitation. Boston: College Hill Press, 1986.
54. Kenan S, Kleinbart FA, Lewis M. Tumors and tumor like conditions of the shoulder girdle. In Musculoskeletal Oncology: A Multidisciplinary Approach. Edited by MM Lewis. Philadelphia: Saunders, 1992, pp 283–306.
55. Kock NG, Nilson AE, Nilsson LO, Norlen LJ, Philpson BM. Urinary diversion via continent ileal reservoir: clinical results in twelve patients. Urology 1982;128:469.
56. Levinson SF. Rehabilitation of the patient with cancer or human immunodeficiency virus. In Rehabilitation Medicine: Principles and Practice, 2nd ed. Edited by J DeLisa. Philadelphia: Lippincott, 1993, pp 916–933.
57. Lewis MM. Bone Tumor Surgery. Limb Sparing Techniques. Philadelphia: Lippincott, 1988.
58. Lieberman AN, Foo SH, Ransohoff J, Wise A, George A, Gordon W, Walker R. Long-term survival among patients with malignant brain tumors. Neurosurgery 1982;10:450.
59. Mankin HJ, Gebhardt MC. Allografts in the management of bone tumors: part II. Surg Rounds Orthop 1988:24–40.
60. Mor V, Laliberte L, Morris JN, Wiemann M. The Karnofsky Performance Status Scale: an examination of its reliability and validity in a research setting. Cancer 1984;53:2002.
61. Neff JR. Metastatic disease to bone. In Musculoskeletal Oncology A Multidisciplinary Approach. Edited by MM Lewis. Philadelphia: Saunders, 1992, pp 377–399.
62. Pearman RO. Treatment of organic impotence by implantation of a penile prosthesis. J Urol 1976;97:716.
63. Philip PA, Ayyangar R, Vanderbilt J, Gaebler-Spira DJ. Rehabilitation outcome in children after treatment of primary brain tumor. Arch Phys Med Rehab 1994;75:36–39.
64. Ragnarsson KT. Rehabilitation of patients with physical disabilities caused by tumors of the musculoskeletal system. In Musculoskeletal Oncology—A Multidisciplinary Approach. Edited by MM Lewis. Philadelphia: Saunders, 1992, pp 429–448.
65. Richmand DM, O'Donnell TF, Jr, Zelikovski A. Sequential pneumatic compression for lymphedema. A controlled study. Arch Surg 1985;120:1116.
66. Ross ED, Mesulam MM. Dominant language functions of the right hemisphere. Prosody and emotional gesturing. Arch Neurol 1979;36:144.
67. Rowland RG, Mitchell ME, Bihrle R. The cecoiled continent urinary reservoir. World J Urol 1985;3:185.
68. Rowland RG, Mitchell ME, Bihrle R, Kahnoski RJ, Piser JE. Indiana continent reservoir. J Urol 1987;137:1136.
69. Schag CA, Ganz BA, Heinrich RL. Cancer rehabilitation evaluation system—short form (CARES-SF). A cancer specific rehabilitation and quality of life instrument. Cancer 1991;68:1406–1413.
70. Schag CA, Heinrich RL. Development of a comprehensive quality of life measurement tool: CARES. Oncology 1990;4:135–138.
71. Schocker JD, Brady LW. Radiation therapy for metastasis. Clin Orthop 1982;169: 38–43.
72. Schuch CM. Transfemoral amputation: prosthetic management. In Atlas of Limb Prosthetics: Surgical, Prosthetic and Rehabilitation Principles. Edited by JH Bowker, JW Michael. St. Louis: Mosby, 1992.
73. Scott FB, Bradley WE, Timm GW. Management of erectile impotence: use of implantable inflatable prosthesis. Urology 1973;2:80.
74. Segerstrom K, Bjerle P, Graffman S, Nystrom A. Factors that influence the incidence of brachial edema after treatment of breast cancer. Scand J Plast Reconstr Surg Hand Surg 1992;26:223–227.
75. Sherry HS, Levy RN, Siffert RS. Metastatic disease of bone in orthopaedic surgery. Clin Orthop 1982;8:44.

76. Simon MA, Aschliman MA, Thomas N, Mankin HJ. Limb salvage treatment versus amputation for osteosarcoma of the distal end of the femur. J Bone Joint Surg Am 1986;68:1331.
77. Sinclair JD. Exercise in pulmonary disease. In Therapeutic Exercise, 3rd ed. Edited by JW Basnajian. Baltimore: Williams & Wilkins, 1978.
78. Skinner D, Boyd SD, Lieskovsky G. Clinical Experience with a Kock continent ileal reservoir for urinary diversion. J Urol 1984;132:1101.
79. Sparwasser C, Drescher P, Pust RA, Madsen PO. Long term results of therapy with intracaverousal injections and penile venous surgery in chronic erectile dysfunction. Scand J Urol Nephrol. 1994;157(suppl):107–112.
80. Staats TB. Advanced prosthetic techniques for below knee amputations. Orthopaedics 1985;8:249.
81. Subbarao JV, McPhee MC. Prosthetic rehabilitation. Comparison of the outcome in patients with cancer and vascular amputations of the extremities. Orthop Rev 1982;11:43.
82. Thistle HG, Hislop HJ, Moffroid M, Lowman EW. Isolinetic contraction. A new concept of resistive exercises. Arch Phys Med Rehabil 1967;48:279.
83. Traugh GH, Corcoran PJ, Reyes RL. Energy expenditure of ambulation in patients with above knee amputations. Arch Phys Med Rehabil 1975;56:67.
84. Villanueva R, Ajmani C. The role of rehabilitation medicine in physical restoration of patients with head and neck cancer. Cancer Bull 1977;29:46.
85. Weinstein SM. Phantom pain. Oncology (Huntington) 1994;8:65–70.
86. Word JA, Kalokhe UP, Aron BS, et al. Transient radiation myelopathy (Lhermitte's sign) in patients with Hodgkin's disease treated by mantle irradiation. Int J Radiat Oncol Biol Phys 1980;6:1731–1740.
87. World Health Organization International Classification of Impairment, Disabilities and Handicaps. A Manual or Classification Relating to Consequences of Disease, Geneva: World Health Organization, 1980.
88. Wu Y, Keagy RD, Krick HJ, Stratigos JS, Betts HB. An innovative removable rigid dressing technique for below the knee amputation. J Bone Joint Surg 1979;61A:724.
89. Zeissler RH, Rose GB, Nelson PA. Post mastectomy lymphedema: late results of treatment in 385 patients. Arch Phys Med Rehab 1972;53:159.

SECTION XXIV

PRINCIPLES OF MULTIDISCIPLINARY MANAGEMENT

CHAPTER 90

Principles of Multidisciplinary Management

JAMES F. HOLLAND, EMIL FREI III, DONALD W. KUFE, ROBERT C. BAST, JR., DONALD L. MORTON, AND RALPH R. WEICHSELBAUM

The cancer patient, and society in general, would like to think that the entire team of doctors, nurses, and scientists are cooperatively involved in solving each cancer patient's problems. Those who are ill have little understanding of turf battles, professional egos, personal animosities, or fads in medicine, and if they knew of their existence would have even less tolerance for them. Happily, oncologists of all disciplines and other physicians who interact with them are human, and not unemotional automatons. The energies invested in the picayune and counterproductive activities cited above are small compared with the constructive and positive activities of individuals who practice the full scope of their particular professions with pride, and if necessary, determination, and are consistently seeking improved (not just new) approaches to cancer.

The keystone for building a successful interdisciplinary management team is humility. None of us is so skilled that he or she can be as expert in every discipline as a highly competent exponent of that particular specialty. Possessing all the intellectual resources required for the earliest possible diagnosis and best possible management of all cancers is beyond the reach of ordinary mortals. No one individual can simultaneously be the best roentgenologist, endoscopist, pathologist, surgeon, radiotherapist, and physician, even after years of commitment solely to cancer. Thus we are, and must be, interdependent.

It is important to work with individuals who are trustworthy and friendly. More failures of interdisciplinary management appear to occur because of personality conflicts than because of intellectual disagreements. In the heat of confrontational oratory, emotional preferences may win out over reasoned accord. Resorting to the literature should be a mechanism that sheds more light on a problem, rather than more heat. Not surprisingly, a selective literature survey can usually be construed to support either side of an acrimonious dispute. Where factual answers are sparse, opinions proliferate luxuriantly.

In actual clinical practice, controversies are usually settled by the first oncologist to encounter the patient. A better way is to work with trusted colleagues and consultants whose opinions, where appropriate, are solicited before the first irreversible step is taken. "Where appropriate" could be the excuse for a multitude of arbitrary undisciplined actions. A formal tumor conference serves the purpose of institutionalizing a forum for discussion, thereby diminishing the impact of bias and prior anecdotal experience. It serves the additional function of allowing oncologists of several disciplines to recognize individuals of other disciplines whose opinions and consultations appear to be most learned and whose personalities are compatible. A tumor conference occasionally alters the primary oncologist's opinions and plans, and thus the therapeutic approach to a specific patient. It makes its most important contribution, however, in the dialogue established, which impacts on the future disposition of similar clinical problems.

Most interdisciplinary actions should occur before any other action, not after. The second oncology specialist who initially encounters a patient after the first discipline has already changed the tumor and the patient may rightly point out a better approach for the future. A medical oncologist or radiation oncologist can better know, and eventually better treat, a patient seen before definitive surgical treatment rather than after. A surgical oncologist (and the patient) would be ill-treated if a patient were prepared for surgery by chemotherapy or radiation therapy without the surgeon's examining the tumor and the patient beforehand. In diseases where radiotherapy and chemotherapy both play a role, joint planning is mandatory.

In the absence of absolute oncologic truths, there is much room for diverse opinions. Multidisciplinary oncology implies that each discipline performs a complementary function, an estate much to be desired. The best analogy is to a symphony: each instrument is played harmoniously, rather than all on the same note or with abandon and cacophony.

Primary Physician

No universal blood or urine tests exist that can diagnose asymptomatic cancer. Isolated patients may present abnormal protein patterns or marker alterations, but such tests are not sufficiently sensitive or specific to justify them as screening tests. Until a reasonable approximation of such a desirable test is discovered, probably tumor by tumor, the most important diagnostic tool is the history. Many cancers can be found in asymptomatic status, justifying screening for cancers of the skin, oral cavity, thyroid, nodes, breast, gynecologic tract, testes, anus, prostate, and rectum and colon. Many of these can be found by careful periodic physical examination. Some cancers are announced asymptomatically by a simple laboratory test: leukocytosis, microscopic hematuria, occult fecal blood, cervical cytology, or prostatic-specific antigen. Regrettably, these diagnoses, when asymptomatic, are uncommon.

Most cancers are discovered when the patient exhausts other simple explanations and remedies for a new significant symptom and finally seeks medical attention. Most early symptoms of cancer are protean. The family physician has the greatest opportunity to make an early diagnosis of cancer. By attentive consideration of every minor symptom, a good doctor must sift the symptom that could be cancer from that which is not likely to be. Indeed, early symptoms that later turn out to be representations of cancer are difficult to distinguish from the vagaries of ordinary dysfunctions. It is the constellation of symptoms, their duration, and associated findings that provoke the alert physician to consider cancer in the differential diagnosis. Cough, gastritis, anorexia, hoarseness, constipation, diarrhea, weight loss, fever, fatigue, or pain which has existed unexplained for two weeks requires considering cancer in the differential diagnosis. Indeed, other more obvious possible causes may exist and lead to other diagnoses, but cancer that is not thought of is always diagnosed later than necessary. Cancer need not be characterized by symptoms that are so severe that the diagnosis becomes obvious. Cancer symptoms can be remittent. Pain at the outset is most often not constant, and when present may be poorly localized or even migratory. Early systemic dysfunction may be so mild as not to lead to spontaneous complaint. Histories that are given are less valuable than histories that are taken.

Upon suspecting cancer, the primary physician is often able to order the appropriate tests to confirm that suspicion and to arrange for histologic or cytologic confirmation. It is at this point that the multidisciplinary process should start. Studies that do not establish a diagnosis of cancer could be the wrong studies. Oncologic consultation might suggest other procedures of value. The primary physician often sends a patient to a surgeon for biopsy, which when positive may be followed by resection without further consultation. We believe that after a diagnosis is suspected, or after it is proved, but before the inauguration of surgical therapy is the proper time for discussion with representatives from the many disciplines that might eventually become involved. Psycho-oncologic consultation and formal rehabilitation may not be necessary for every patient, but when needed should be arranged before the definitive therapeutic program is initiated. Pathology consultation is always needed, and all oncologic specialists who will be engaged in care should avail themselves of the pathologist's interpretation; surgical, radiation, and medical oncologists should see the tissue with their own eyes, as well.

The surgeon, medical oncologist, and radiation oncologist should, in many cases, have protocols for therapy of common cancers. Where possible these programs should be part of designed studies that will accumulate sufficient numbers so that conclusions can be drawn. Sometimes this involves single-institution (or even single-practice) endeavors; whenever possible it should be part of institutional or national protocols designed to answer fundamental questions concerning the management of cancer. Where no protocol exists, agreement should be sought ahead of time that defines the procedures and sequence for this particular patient. The family physician should be a full partner in all of these decisions.

Radiologist

Imaging specialties are essential in the discovery and staging of prospective cancer patients. Every oncologist should review relevant imaging studies with the appropriate radiologist, sonographer, or specialist in nuclear medicine. No written report compares with having personally seen the films, report in hand, or better still, with the radiologist at the viewbox. Although it is commonplace to order standard menus (computed tomography [CT] or magnetic resonance imaging [MRI]), considerably greater efficiency and some economy attends the oncologist who seeks advance expert consultation concerning the problem to be imaged. Special CT scans at much closer distances can provide better definition of small lesions, or special MRI views (axial, coronal, sagittal, with or without gadolinium) may provide optimal visualization. Follow-up examinations using single photon–emission CT (SPECT), sonographic or CT-guided needle aspiration, dynamic flow scanning, and similar procedures require professional imaging input. (See Chapters 32 to 42.)

Oncologists can require, however, that the specialist in imaging not give an interpretation directly to the patient. Thoughtless reporting of radiologic findings to patients before they are known by the responsible oncologist causes significant difficulty in management, not only for the oncologist but usually for the patient. Information given out of context to an individual whose personality the radiologist has not fathomed provides none of the benefits that advocates of complete disclosure maintain. The compact lies between the oncologist and the imaging specialist. The radiologist is a consultant to the oncologist, not to the patient. The responsibility for interpretation of findings to the patient, and the support that often must go with it, rests on the oncologist.

Pathologist

The pathologist is arguably the indispensable member of every interdisciplinary team. That we are all dependent on the proper diagnosis establishes pathology as a defining control. When a pathologist is not sure, it is not a disgrace. Other local pathologists render opinions, and the Armed Forces Institute of Pathology and several prominent universities and cancer centers are justly famed for their consultations by which pathologists, with humility but not shame, accept advice.

The ready access of the entire gastrointestinal tract to endoscopic inspection and biopsy, similar access to the external genitalia of both sexes, the accessibility of many bronchogenic carcinomas by fiberoptic bronchoscopy, and the safe intraoperative biopsy of central nervous system, pulmonary, ovarian, skeletal, and soft tissue neoplasms mean that preoperative or intraoperative pathologic confirmation of diagnosis should be available for nearly every tumor. Renal and testicular masses are typically removed without first establishing histologic proof, based on characteristic physical examination, sonography, other imaging techniques, and tumor-associated markers. This is justified by the disadvantage of tumor spillage and the characteristic clinical picture. For other diseases, radical surgery without pathologic basis is unnecessary and dangerous. Similarly, an inadequate surgical procedure performed because the nature of the pathologic process was not appreciated suggests insufficient or mistaken intraoperative consultation. Amputation of a breast or extremity without pathologic diagnosis in advance or intraoperatively is malpractice. A surgeon may conscientiously and competently sacrifice an adjacent dispensable normal organ which appears to be involved with cancer, such as spleen, kidney, adrenal, a segment of gut, diaphragm, bladder wall, or vaginal wall without histologically establishing invasion, based on surgical judgment. In other circumstances, the pathologist's imprimatur is necessary to justify cancer therapies. The same restrictions apply to radiation therapy or chemotherapy unless one stipulates and documents that the therapeutic procedure is intended "prophylactically," for subclinical disease that may exist.

The pathologist is responsible for giving as definitive a description of the tumor as determined effort can guarantee: its extent, its relationship to surgical margins, normal structures, and the involvement of lymph nodes, lymphatics, and blood vessels. Wherever possible, a specimen of fresh tissue should be kept frozen, since increasingly, new molecular biologic and biochemical techniques allow classification of tumors for receptors, oncogenes, tumor suppressor genes, and viral antigens that may someday provide prognostic information of great value. In selected circumstances, fresh tissue can be utilized for assays that predict chemotherapeutic sensitivity.

In addition to tissue preservation for more sophisticated studies if needed, pathology now allows better classification of tumors whose type and origin are somewhat uncertain. Immunopathology and cytochemistry should be able to distinguish among most anaplastic neoplasms by study with leukocyte common antigen, cytokeratin, vimentin, mucin, neuron-specific enolase, and S100 protein, whether the tumor is a lymphoma, squamous carcinoma, sarcoma, adenocarcinoma, neuroectodermal tumor, or melanoma, all of which in their anaplastic state may resemble one another in hematoxylin and eosin staining. A small fresh sample of representative neoplasm should be placed in glutaraldehyde fixative in the operating room for eventual electron microscopy if any suggestion exists that pathologic classification might be complex. Today's research classifications may well become tomorrow's standard rubric and nomenclature. Oncologists should encourage the most discriminating description and classification of tumors.

When uncertainty exists concerning the nature of a neoplasm, additional opinions are always appropriate. Pathologic confusion is a shaky foundation on which to build therapeutic strategy. (See Chapter 31.)

Surgical Oncologist

The surgical oncologist is most often likely to see a patient before other oncology specialists. The family physician or internist most commonly seeks a diagnosis, and in circumstances where this requires biopsy, the surgeon is usually consulted. For decades, any surgeon was considered wholly competent to exercise all surgical skills, including cancer surgery. Indeed, while most surgeons may be acceptably competent, the specialty of surgical oncology is increasingly recognized by other oncologists. Surgical oncologists are surgeons with knowledge of and experience in cancer surgery that comes from additional training, limitation of the scope of general surgical practice, and familiarity with the natural history of cancers and the role of the other oncologic specialties in their diagnosis and management. Until surgical oncology becomes recognized by the proper accrediting agencies, other oncologists must exercise their judgment about the oncologic qualifications of their surgical confreres. Membership in the Society of Surgical Oncology, postgraduate training in a cancer institute or university program with a mentor known for cancer surgical expertise, limitation of surgical practice to cancer and related diseases, publications, and a personal assessment of the depth of interest and knowledge are some of the appropriate criteria. (See Chapter 45.)

Because a general surgeon may perform the biopsy, it is uncommon for a surgical oncologist to be called to supersede the first surgeon on the case. Herein lies some of the problem, because the primary cancer operation is of utmost importance for determining cure. In this regard, any mass to be biopsied should be considered in the context of whether the operating surgeon will be the one to perform eventual definitive surgical therapy. Since a considerable portion of their activity deals with neoplasms, thoracic surgeons, urologic surgeons, and neurosurgeons must be chosen for their general expertise, because there is not likely to be an oncologic subspecialty in the near future for those specific organ systems. Conversely, gynecologic oncology, orthopedic oncology, otorhinolaryngologic oncology, and surgical oncology are well defined, and the general gynecologist, orthopedist, otorhinolaryngologist, or surgeon is unlikely to be as well qualified as the oncologist within the specialty.

Because the implications for a proven neoplasm, potentially resectable, entail many other considerations to optimize curability, the prudent surgical oncologist surveys the potential contributions of medical oncology, radiation oncology, and other specialties before proceeding with operation.

Where appropriate and possible, patients should be entered into clinical investigative trials. There is so much that is unknown about cancer that investigative activities should still be of prime concern to all oncologists. In institutions where investigative programs are not employed, sober consideration of joining in this effort through a community oncology program or in alliance with some other active institution may be possible. In the absence of a structured protocol, joint assessment is appropriate to determine whether chemotherapy or radiotherapy before surgery may improve outcome. Most often this entails direct consultation with the medical and radiation oncologists. An opportunity for the three specialties to see the patient in the native state is of great value for subsequent planning. Confidence building makes for easy consultation over the years with colleagues who share mutual trust. The treatment of breast cancer, rectal cancer, head and neck cancer, and soft tissue sarcoma, for example, is most often best approached by multidisciplinary components from all three specialties. Whereas specific diseases may be treated well by single-modality approaches, bidisciplinary or tridisciplinary opinion is usually valuable.

Surgical oncologists must also be available for surgical aspects of management later in the course of disease. End-staging laparotomy in many instances may make more sense than earlier operation, so that the medical oncologist may be certain that a complete clinical remission is pathologically confirmed rather than waiting expectantly for a lymphoma or ovarian cancer to relapse. Minimally invasive surgical procedures will enjoy greater use for these purposes. (See Chapter 47.) Intestinal obstruction in the course of cancer may require operative surgical management. The surgeon may be obliged to obtain long-term or permanent venous access. A medical or radiation oncologist may discover a suspicious mass or infiltration that needs biopsy and pathologic assessment.

Palliative surgery is an area where medical and radiation oncologists often present problems to the surgeon in hopes of potential operative remedy. Debulking, diverting, and pain-relieving operations are all appropriate procedures in the proper circumstance.

Surgical oncologists also have legitimate interests in adjuvant chemotherapy and immunotherapy. For those willing to devote the time required for this undertaking, use of established drugs in adjuvant programs can be an improvement over surgical procedures alone. Indeed, the National Surgical Adjuvant Breast and Bowel Project has contributed significantly to our knowledge of adjuvant therapy for these diseases. (See Chapters 121 and 136.) Surgical oncologic investigators have also been among the pioneers of immunological cancer research. The rarity of surgical oncologists in practice, however, ordinarily precludes these activities for surgeons, since so much of their time is ordinarily invested in pre- and postoperative care and in actual surgery. Medical oncologists must stand ready to assume primary responsibility for subsequent oncologic management. Orthopedic oncologists, otorhinolaryngologic oncologists, and neurosurgical oncologists ordinarily ally themselves with a medical oncologist with specialized interests and expertise in neoplasms of their particular discipline.

Anesthesiologist

Few patients get to choose their anesthesiologist. Intraoperative management of a cancer patient is similar to that for any serious surgery. Since anesthesiologists often run the recovery room and even the intensive care units, however, their interaction with patients who may be awake can be consequential. The description of operative findings should be reserved for the surgeon. Assurance of effective pain control in the immediate postoperative period is important to avoid the exaggeration of anxiety and depression that may come with pain when the patient first learns the significance of the operation and its findings. Patient-controlled analgesia in the immediate postoperative period, and at other times for efficient pain control, is a technique of importance to all branches of oncology and not one that should be considered a proprietary anesthesiologic exclusive.

Medical Oncologist

The medical oncologist usually serves the traditional role of internist in the multidisciplinary management of cancer. Whereas the surgical procedure, or even the radiotherapeutic treatment course, is of short duration, the medical oncologist has continuing responsibility that may stretch over months or years of therapy, and decades of follow-up, depending on the neoplasm (see Chapter 51).

There is an understandable but regrettable tendency for each specialty that has interacted with a patient to schedule follow-up appointments, which may entail many more visits and much greater expense than is necessary or prudent. Each therapist is entitled to see the results of the particular treatment regimen that was applied. Absence of disease in the region subjected to surgery or radiotherapy is in the purview of the treating specialist, but that is only a portion of the patient's overall health concerns. The more cogent question is the search for remediable disease in regional and distant areas and a continuing assessment of the impact of the disease and its treatment on the patient as a whole, tasks ordinarily considered medical. A useful technique is dictation by the medical oncologist of the findings at a follow-up visit, including laboratory and radiologic results, so that the surgeon and radiologist (or other appropriate specialist) does not feel excluded from what is going on. The medical oncologist may superintend the medical activities of the patient that are not addressed by a family physician or internist, together with oncologic assessment that would be of importance to surgeon, radiotherapist, and medical oncologist alike. In circumstances where the patient has not received adjuvant therapy by a medical oncologist and is not undergoing treatment for metastatic disease, the involvement of a medical oncologist is discretionary on the part of the family physician or internist and other oncology specialists already engaged.

The medical oncologist should partake in the decisions of therapeutic choice and in the clinical staging, which may determine operability. The medical oncologist should be the one to address the potential for induction or neoadjuvant chemotherapy and the choice of regimen for postoperative chemotherapeutic or immunotherapeutic management. With few exceptions, most notable of which are the brilliant works in breast cancer done by Fisher and colleagues and by Veronesi and colleagues, surgeons may be remote from recent research achievements and from the best chemotherapeutic and immunotherapeutic approaches to cancers which are appropriately treated with these therapies. A substantial portion of this treatise is devoted to activities of the medical oncologist in his or her diagnostic and therapeutic responsibilities.

The medical oncologist is most often the physician to reassure the patient when there is no evident cancer. Although absent tumor may only be an eclipse, the medical oncologist must keep the patient from dwelling incessantly and anxiously on imminent relapse. Indeed, the medical oncologist may need to encourage a return to normal living when the cancer is not manifest. This should never involve a lie, just a reasoned basis for hope that relapse will not occur. Osler's admonition to live life in day-tight packages is helpful.

Radiation Oncologist

Radiation oncology is the only specialty devoted entirely to the study of cancer. The radiation oncologist must therefore be in a position to make an overall oncologic evaluation, as well as specific recommendations for radiotherapy.

When radiotherapy can effect curative treatment, as for localized lymphomas, cancer of the tongue and oral cavity, and cancer of the cervix, the radiation oncologist must have equal early access to the patient to set forth the possible indications for and accomplishments of radiation therapy for such tumors. Cordial interactive liaison with surgical and medical oncologists is crucial to allow this delineation of options before the patient is changed by another treatment approach. (See Chapter 48.)

Controversy exists over the relative debilities and late toxicities of surgery and radiotherapy. Where equal curative potential exists, there is reason to assess the disruption of anatomy and the dysfunction that might occur from either surgery or radiotherapy. This assessment produces little consensus in head and neck, early cervical, prostate, and bladder cancers. The major improvement in immediate reconstructive techniques has made surgery around the oral cavity less disfiguring. Surgeons cite the dry mouth and sometimes diminished taste as late and undesirable toxicities of radiation, while radiotherapists decry the cosmetic and physiologic distortions of surgery. Similar controversy attends the dysfunction of vaginal secretions after radiation treatment for early carcinoma of the cervix, with many male gynecologic oncologists attesting the lesser implications for sexual function of total hysterectomy. With carcinomas of the bladder and prostate the discordance is even greater, because total cystectomy is admittedly debilitating and American urologists question whether radiation therapy is ever equivalent, stage for stage. Thus, although radiotherapy for T1 and T2 bladder cancers is reportedly highly effective in Europe, there has been relatively little clinical investigation of this in the United States. Radical surgery for carcinoma of the prostate, until recently nearly always associated with impotence, offered sound basis for trials of interstitial radiotherapy. For tumors too locally advanced for surgery, radiotherapeutic consultation concerning teletherapy is usually sought. The definitive comparison of earlier-stage prostatic cancer therapies has not been made, nor is there consensus about which patients do not need immediate treatment at all.

In the area of operable oral, pharyngeal, cervical, bladder, and prostatic cancer, closer cooperation of radiation oncologist and surgeon before decisions are put into action might, if therapy is equivalent stage for stage, provide for greater organ preservation and less dysfunction. The great problem, however, is to overcome the prejudice that the results will not be the same, with each exponent nearly equally persuaded and equally unpersuasive. Definitive clinical trials are sorely needed but may never be done because of the evolution of the combined-modality approaches.

In combined-modality approaches, chemotherapy is a major component together with radiotherapy and surgery. Data abound that indicate that chemotherapy can induce major regressions when used as primary therapy for head and neck cancer and bladder cancer, as well as for breast cancer, pediatric sarcomas, and lymphomas. There is as yet no consensus about primary chemotherapy, with its major theoretical advantage of decreasing the number of cells to be killed by radiation or to be removed by surgery. For the present, prudence supports the proposition that radiation field size and surgical boundaries cannot be importantly reduced below the original extent of the tumor, where residual cells after chemotherapy may remain. One advantage of primary chemotherapy, in addition to a decrease in primary tumor burden, is an early attack against undetected micrometastatic disease. Furthermore, when the tumor vasculature is intact, unimpaired by radiation angiopathy and fibrosis or surgical disruption, there is a greater chance of delivering a chemotherapeutically effective dose. Last, the regression of tumor seen in the primary neoplasm reinforces the confidence in using the same chemotherapeutic regimen for presumed micrometastases during the adjuvant period.

Much of the interrelation among radiation, chemotherapy, and surgery is still evolving, hampered by the absence of solid data and the paucity of attempts to compare modern multimodality regimens.

For tumors regionally beyond surgical compass, in the pharynx, parametria, pelvis, and periprostatic tissues, radiation is usually employed as primary therapy. The dismal results that often attend these advanced tumors erroneously color the potential contributions of radiation oncology for earlier tumors, because nonparticipating observers ordinarily see only the failures. Substantial opportunity exists here for pilot efforts within an institution to fashion combined-modality approaches for tumors which are regionally inoperable at first encounter but which might become resectable after chemotherapy and/or radiation therapy; or which might not require surgery at all after their use. Esophageal cancer and localized pancreatic cancer appear to fit this category.

Primary brain tumors are usually best treated by primary surgery and radiotherapy, often with chemotherapy. When surgery is unfeasible, new techniques of radiosurgery, delivering precisely localized therapy from several angles so as to spare normal brain, offer some promise.

Radiotherapy can cure localized and regionalized lymphomas of certain types. The advantages and disadvantages of combined-modality therapy or of chemotherapy alone are presented in detail for the specific diseases. There continues to be a clear indication for combined chemotherapy and radiotherapy in patients whose lymphomas are massive and where confidence in tumor eradication by either modality alone is ill-founded. Radiotherapy may be a critical component in salvage regimens for relapsed leukemias and lymphomas, where maximal chemotherapy together with autologous or allogeneic marrow or stem-cell transplantation is undertaken.

For palliation and pain relief, radiation therapy is indispensable to the practice of oncology. Radiotherapy can usually offer relief from the pain of tumor infiltration in bone, regardless of tumor type. Although the extent of tumor regression (as a measure of radiosensitivity) varies, this may determine length of remission rather than initial pain relief.

Gynecologic Oncologist

Gynecologic oncologists as a class may belong to the most integrated oncologic specialty. Gynecologic oncologists are fully qualified to diagnose and treat neoplasia of the female genital organs by surgery and chemotherapy and to share in radiotherapeutic planning and execution to a considerable degree, particularly for brachytherapy. Highly skilled gynecologic oncologists are divided on whether gastrointestinal complications of ovarian or other cancers should be handled by surgical oncologists, general surgeons, or gynecologic oncologists. Much of this depends on local custom rather than expertise at performing lysis of adhesions or enteroenterostomies. The preoperative preparation for and execution of procedures that involve urinary tract manipulation are almost invariably conducted cooperatively with urologists.

Many medical oncologists treat gynecologic neoplasms with chemotherapy in investigational and clinical settings. This is true for adjuvant therapy as well as treatment of manifest clinical metastasis. In many academic institutions medical and gynecologic oncologists have collaborated to develop new treatment programs and to study the biology of gynecologic cancers. Local custom, the surgical obligations of gynecological oncologists, and collaborative undertakings involving both specialties determine the allocation of work. A prime instance where medical oncologists should be active is when a gynecologist without specific oncologic expertise or interest has undertaken the surgery. (See Chapters 129 to 135.)

Pediatric Oncologist

Pediatric oncologists generally remain aloof from adult oncologic specialties. Radiotherapists and surgeons in major centers subspecialize in pediatric neoplasms. Some gynecologists and urologists have particular interests in pediatric diseases. Orthopedic oncologists devote much of their best time to pediatric sarcomas, and thus there is no specialized subset for pediatric neoplasms. The replication in major centers of pediatric counterparts to all the medical oncologic resources, such as pediatric neurologists, radiologists, and even pathologists, illustrates the specificity of pediatric oncologic information. Nearly every child in the United States can have access to programs of the Children's Cancer Group or the Pediatric Oncology Group. The dramatic progress in cancer therapeutics in children derives in part from the universal recognition that childhood cancer is a tragedy and that every effort must be made to derive all possible information from every case. This allows the child to benefit from all the information that has gone before, and creates a new data base for those who will come after. (See Chapters 157–171.)

Psycho-Oncologist

The mind is the only organ function that is affected in every patient with cancer. Nonetheless, all patients do not need formal psychiatric help. General psychiatrists often lack full understanding of the organic aspects of cancers and the therapeutic procedures that are commonly employed; their effectiveness in dealing with these real life problems is thus diminished. Psycho-oncologists have, by dint of special education and experience, a better foundation from which to undertake supervision of those patients too difficult for oncologists of other disciplines to manage. Psycho-oncologists implement much of their influence by interaction with staff rather than patients. "Sensitivity training" has been trivialized by its use in describing lesser activities. Helping oncologists to deal sensitively and gently with their own patients is a continuing task for psycho-oncologists. Some oncologists seem to overlook the fact that a patient's cancer is usually the greatest challenge in life that he or she has ever faced. Staring into the abyss, often for the first time, requires more equanimity and fortitude than many patients can muster. Teaching doctors how to handle their own inadequacies, how to tolerate their own frustrations and failures, and how to convey a humanitarian dimension to the grim reality of their cancer therapeutics is one of psycho-oncology's best offerings. Not all the medicine comes in a bottle. (See Chapter 87.)

Rehabilitation Specialist

Rehabilitation specialists provide patients the opportunity for self-reliance. Cutting the bonds of dependency can be the best of all remedies. Whether the challenge is speech, ambulation, ostomy care, physical appearance, occupational rehabilitation, or sexual expression, oncologists must maintain the goal that patients should lead pain-free lives with minimal if any deficits in normal function. Early and vigorous rehabilitation efforts can make life more worth living. Oncologists could and should consult rehabilitation medicine specialists earlier and more often. (See Chapter 89.)

Nurse-Oncologist

The oncology nurse has become an indispensable specialist. An oncologist's nightmare is to have a complex cancer patient admitted to a general service floor. The unique medications, procedures, and tests for oncology patients are themselves adequate justification for the specialty of oncology nursing. Two other attributes are critical. Oncology nurses have a greater than ordinary understanding of cancer pain and of the psychic stresses that cancer patients may suffer. These two precious insights allow much more aggressive advocacy for pain control and humanistic yet realistic support of patients and families during their crises. Oncology nurses in ambulatory settings become telephone specialists in patient management, to the great advantage and comfort of cancer patients and to the great advantage and security of oncologists.

Nurse oncologists have become the prime movers in home care, rendering active therapy or supervision of palliative measures. As this movement gains momentum, it is probable that home hospice care will become more common and more economical. The regulatory hand of government will likely soon extend to the companies organized to provide oncology nursing at home, in an attempt to modulate the expense of the end stages of cancer. (See Chapter 88.)

Other Support Personnel

A few additional people are crucial in the oncologic approach to advanced cancer at home. A social worker familiar with the great stresses of cancer on every member of the family is a treasured asset. The complexities in social, economic, and service spheres can be greatly simplified by the kindly professional interest of an oncology social worker. Additional community resources such as the American Cancer Society, Cancer Care, various support groups, Meals on Wheels, companion visits, and home health care aides, often critical factors, may seem to be effortlessly mobilized by a social worker.

For those who have been guided by religious tenets and who have practiced their religion, the clergy can be extremely helpful and religious practice a strengthening act. Deathbed conversions are uncommon, however. For those who have not made religion a significant portion of their lives, visits of the clergy or allusions to afterlife provide little comfort.

The principal support throughout the cancer experience comes from a loving family. All else good may pale in comparison to the radiant affection of a spouse or other close family member. The loved one who recognizes that all the good that can be done must be done, rather than be left undone, will create the palpable substance of love for the patient. In addition to the benefit for the patient, such behavior creates comforting memories for the doer and the satisfaction that, in the ultimate crisis, he or she was steadfast.

SECTION XXV

PRINCIPLES OF SOCIETAL ONCOLOGY

CHAPTER 91

Ethical Aspects of Caring for Patients with Cancer

EZEKIEL J. EMANUEL AND FREDERIC C. KASS

Introduction

During the past three decades, concern over medical ethical issues has risen dramatically. Many believe this has been driven by the proliferation of medical technology (106, 159). Others believe that most medical ethical issues are inherent in medical practice and have long been with us (149). In this view, the current preoccupation with medical ethical issues stems less from technology than from changes in political values, especially heightened concern for individual rights. Whatever the reason, physicians, generally, and oncologists, in particular, are now both more aware of and more frequently confronted by medical ethical issues. Indeed, medical ethical issues seem to pervade almost all decisions regarding the care of cancer patients, from selecting patients for bone marrow transplantation to obtaining informed consent for experimental protocols to making routine decisions about pain management. Yet the maze of legal requirements and regulations governing medical decisions generally provides oncologists little guidance in the day-to-day practice of medicine. Hence, there is a need for a review of medical ethical issues as they relate to the practice of oncology.

Medical ethical issues can be divided into five broad types (Table 91.1). To review these issues comprehensively as they affect oncologic decisions and practice is beyond the scope of this chapter. Instead, we shall try to clarify the prevailing ethical and legal standards for the three commonly encountered medical ethical issues: informed consent, terminating medical care, and conflict of interest. In addition we shall consider several clinical cases raising common ethical and legal dilemmas and the responses that are consistent with prevailing ethical and legal standards. Excellent books and reviews are available on other medical ethical issues, from the methods of medical ethics (11, 56, 91, 177) to the allocation of scarce resources (1, 20–22, 44, 139) to genetic engineering (49, 140, 186).

Informed Consent

HISTORICAL PERSPECTIVE

The first reported legal case in the English language involving informed consent was the English case of *Slater v Baker & Stapelton* decided in 1767 (161). A patient sued two surgeons for rebreaking a partially healed leg fracture in an effort to improve its alignment. Relying on the statements of physicians who testified on behalf of the patient, the court ruled that it is "the usage and law of surgeons" to obtain the patient's consent before embarking on an operation; it held that the two practitioners had violated the well-known and accepted rules of consent. While the substance of this consent and the process by which it is obtained have since evolved, the obligation to obtain patient consent prior to initiating interventions has been recognized over the centuries. Although physicians have often fulfilled this traditional requirement with perfunctory disclosures and few formalities, the historical record demonstrates an awareness by physicians of the ethical and legal obligation to inform patients of their intentions and obtain their prior consent (58).

In the United States, the modern era of informed consent began in the early 20th century with a series of legal cases, including most notably *Schloendorff v Society of New York Hospitals* (152). Interestingly, the actual term "informed consent" first appeared in the 1957 case of *Salgo v Leland Stanford Jr. University Board of Trustees* (150). This and subsequent cases began the long effort to specify information physicians are obligated to provide. We shall review the ethical and legal principles of informed consent and conclude with an examination of common problems confronted in clinical practice (3, 58).

ETHICAL STANDARDS GOVERNING INFORMED CONSENT

The physician's obligation to obtain informed consent arises out of respect for the patient's autonomy (3, 11, 47, 56, 58, 177). Directly translated from the Greek, *autonomy* means "self-rule." Although originally a term used to characterize the self-governing Greek city-states, the concept now encompasses a wide variety of ideas relating to individuals, including self-governance, liberty rights, privacy, individual choice, liberty to follow one's will, liberty to cause one's own behavior, and liberty to be one's own person (11).

Lying at the heart of autonomy is the idea that the person is a free moral agent who can (*a*) establish, modify, or change goals and objectives for his or her life and (*b*) have the opportunity to pursue these goals and objectives through actions and decisions.

The current emphasis in medical ethics on autonomy is a

Table 91.1. A Typology of Medical Ethical Issues

Medical ethical issues	Examples
1) The relationship between the physician and the patient	Truth telling Confidentiality Informed consent
2) The selection of medical interventions	Terminating care "Baby Doe" cases Euthanasia
3) The allocation of medical resources	Just health care Patient selection criteria for scarce resources
4) The application of personally transforming technologies	Genetic engineering Brain tissue transplants Psychosurgery
5) The conduct of biomedical research	Fraud, fabrication, and plagiarism Conflict of interest

recent phenomenon. Traditionally, there has been more concern about the risks of sharing knowledge with patients than about the benefits. Physicians have been motivated more by the principle of beneficence, the duty to promote the welfare of the patient, and by the principle of nonmalfeasance, the duty to avoid doing harm, than by concern for patient autonomy (11, 56, 177). Such an approach emphasized patient care rather than patient wishes, patient needs rather than patient "rights," and physician discretion rather than patient autonomy and self-determination (158).

This concern for the patient's welfare over his or her autonomy has been prominent in cancer medicine. Faced with limited therapeutic options, physicians have in the past freely utilized secrecy and deception to maintain the comfort and serenity of their patients. Donald Oken began his landmark study "What to Tell Cancer Patients" (129) with the observation that "no problem is more vexing than the decision about what to tell the cancer patient." In 1961 he surveyed 219 physicians to determine whether or not they told their patients they had cancer. Almost 90% of the physicians reported that their "usual policy" was to withhold this information. Moreover, the majority of physicians admitted that they "very rarely, if ever" informed their patients of the diagnosis. Where information was given, euphemisms were used (129). In Oken's study, physicians almost unanimously agreed on one particular goal: the maintenance of hope. Physicians appeared to have devised a means of communicating "the possibility, even the likelihood of recovery" (129).

In the decades after Oken's study attitudes began to change. Scholars began emphasizing the importance of truthfulness in the physician-patient relationship (91, 177), the studies of Kubler-Ross emphasized the importance of communication in the care of dying patients (96), and leading physicians argued that excessive paternalism undermined the welfare of patients (92–94). Much of this view has now been widely accepted. Indeed, when Oken's study was repeated in 1977, 98% of the physicians stated that it was their usual policy to tell patients that they had cancer (126). Moreover, 68% of those physicians added that they very rarely, if ever, made exceptions to that practice. All of the physicians agreed that patients had a "right to know" their diagnosis.

Strict adherence to patient autonomy has been criticized by those who believe that the physician's involvement in medical decisions should not be restricted to providing information and options to the patient. Dr. Franz Ingelfinger eloquently expressed this perspective when reflecting on his personal battle with cancer.

I received from physician friends throughout the country a barrage of well-intentioned but contradictory advice . . . As a result, not only I but my wife, my son and daughter-in-law (both doctors), and other family members became increasingly confused and emotionally distraught. Finally, when the pangs of indecision had become nearly intolerable, one wise physician friend said, "What you need is a doctor." He was telling me . . . to seek . . . a person who would dominate, who would tell me what to do, who would in a paternalistic manner assume responsibility for my care (86).

Ingelfinger argued that paternalism not "accentuated by insolence, vanity, arbitrariness, or a lack of empathy" could serve a noble purpose.

In oncology, where illness can be both severe and catastrophic, the physician has an obligation to respect patient autonomy without hiding behind it. As one observer noted:

> [T]he fears of encroachment on patient autonomy may have caused many physicians to become noncommittal. Instead of providing advice based on years of clinical experience, they may simply present a mass of medical facts and figures that leave the patient adrift . . . Physicians should be willing to answer the often asked question "what would you do if you were I?" (107).

In elucidating how patient autonomy can be achieved in health care decision making without paternalism on the one hand or abandonment on the other, ethicists have emphasized four factors should be fulfilled. Patients need relevant information on the proposed intervention. Second, they need to understand this information. Third, they need to make a decision voluntarily (i.e., without coercion). Finally, patients need a recommendation by the physician. All these factors must be fulfilled simultaneously for patients to act autonomously and for their decisions to satisfy the ethical standards of informed consent.

LEGAL STANDARDS GOVERNING INFORMED CONSENT

In the United States, the legal principles governing informed consent evolved from a series of cases in the early part of this century. In these cases, the physician's failure to obtain consent was viewed as a battery, that is, contact which was both intentional and unpermitted. It was held that this civil wrong could be redressed through the award of monetary damages. Among the most prominent statements of this position was that of Justice Cardozo in the 1914 case of *Schloendorff v. Society of New York Hospitals*: "Every human being of adult years and sound mind has a right to determine what shall be done with his own body; and a surgeon who performs an operation without his patient's consent commits an assault, for which he is liable in damages."

Over the next 50 years two changes occurred in the standards of informed consent (3, 58). First, many courts abandoned the role of battery in informed consent and began viewing the physician's disclosure of information to the patient as a professional duty. Physicians who failed to fulfill that duty were deemed negligent and therefore liable for malpractice.

Second, courts began delineating the requirements necessary for a valid informed consent. In general, however, courts have focused on the information requirements for informed consent; there has been much less litigation and fewer rulings delineating what constitutes valid understanding and voluntariness. One of the most important legal precedents was the 1960 case of *Natanson v Kline* (125). In this case a woman with resectable breast cancer underwent adjuvant cobalt radiation therapy that was complicated by severe radiation burns. The patient charged her physician with negligence in the administration of the radiation and in the failure to warn her of its potential risks. The court found for the patient, ruling that mere consent to radiation therapy was insufficient. Full disclosure required the physician to inform the patient about the nature of her ailment, the proposed treatment, the treatment's probability of success, the treatment's potential adverse effects, and the availability of alternative treatments. In the absence of such full disclosure of information, the patient's consent was invalid and the physician was guilty of malpractice.

Drawing on malpractice law, the Natanson court established what came to be known as the "professional" or "physician-based" standard of informed consent. According to this standard, physicians must convey the information "which a reasonable medical practitioner would [disclose] under the same or similar circumstances" (125).

Subsequently this professional standard has been severely criticized. Critics claim that there are few, if any, shared standards for disclosure. Furthermore, they argue, physician-based standards are unlikely to provide for the disclosure of all the information the Natanson court delineated as essential (157).

Coeval with the general ascendancy of patient autonomy was a call to replace the physician-based standard with a patient-based standard that would require the physician to provide the patient with all the medical information that a rational patient would want to know. This standard was first articulated in 1972 in the case of *Canterbury v Spence* (25). The patient underwent a laminectomy and suffered paralysis. He sued the physician, claiming that the complication had not been mentioned prior to surgery. In response, the physician claimed that the incidence of paralysis was about 1% and that the professional standard did not require disclosure of this information. The court held that disclosure should reflect what the "average, reasonable patient" would want to know before submitting to surgery (3, 58).

Recently, this patient-based standard has been criticized because it fails to offer prospective guidelines for the physician. Determination of what a reasonable patient would want to know occurs retrospectively in a court by the jury and therefore, it is argued, is an "unpredictable" and unhelpful standard in guiding physicians at the bedside (42).

Since Canterbury, the tension between the professional- and the patient-based standards of informed consent has persisted. Individual states determine what their standard of informed consent will be, and different states have enacted different standards, with most relying on the professional standard (3, 58). In addition, different states have initiated diverse efforts to specify further disclosure requirements. Four such efforts are worth noting. In a recent case, *Arato v Avedon* (5), the question arose whether physicians had to disclose the precise survival rates or statistical life expectancy data to a patient considering a therapy. Mr. Arato was a 43-year-old man who had pancreatic cancer incidentally discovered during a nephrectomy. The cancer was resected. His oncologists told him there was a high risk of recurrence and offered and recommended experimental therapy with radiation and chemotherapy; they noted, however, that the therapy might provide Mr. Arato absolutely no benefit. During therapy, the cancer recurred. After Mr. Arato died, his family sued, claiming he would not have consented to the chemotherapy had he known the statistical mortality rates of pancreatic cancer. The oncologists noted that they told Mr. Arato if the pancreatic cancer recurred it was incurable and that his situation was very serious and that Mr. Arato had never asked for further clarification with specific percentages or statistics in more than 70 office visits. The California Supreme Court unanimously rejected the family's claim requiring disclosure of statistical survival rates. The court argued that the physician-patient relationship is filled with judgments about what precise information should be provided and when and that there could not be a requirement for disclosing a specific piece of information (5). Furthermore, the court noted that statistical morbidity values derived from the experience of population groups are inherently unreliable and offer little assurance regarding the fate of the individual patient.

Indeed, in Mr. Arato's case his cancer was discovered incidentally and was completely resected, which is not typical of cases reported in studies providing statistical mortality data. However, it should also be noted that recent studies have suggested that oncologists do tend to overestimate benefits (as well as risks) from their therapies. For instance, Tannock and colleagues (143) have shown that oncologists "overestimate the therapeutic gain from use of adjuvant chemotherapy for breast cancer." In preliminary studies, others have shown that oncologists overestimate the benefits of phase I trials. Thus, while oncologists may not have an obligation to provide statistical survival or response data, they need to be careful that they do not overstate in a qualitative manner the benefits of chemotherapy, otherwise patients will be ill-informed and unable to fulfill the requirements of informed consent.

Second, California courts have extended the physician's legal duty to inform patients not only about situations in which a procedure occurs but also about those situations where no procedure or intervention is made. In *Truman v Thomas* (172), a patient repeatedly refused a Pap smear. She subsequently died of cervical cancer. Her children brought suit, alleging that her physician failed to disclose the risks of refusing the pap smear. The court held that physicians can be subject to suit for inadequate disclosure even if no procedure is performed. The justices maintained that physicians are obligated to explain the risks of doing nothing as diligently as they explain the risks of intervening.

Other states have mandated disclosure of specific medical information to patients. Massachusetts, for instance, requires physicians to inform women with resectable breast cancer of "all alternative treatments which are medically viable" (108). California requires physicians to advise patients scheduled for elective surgery of the alternatives for avoiding transfusion of nondirected blood collected from volunteer donors.

In an effort to formulate regulations governing the disclosure of information, Texas established the Medical Disclosure Panel. Composed of both physicians and lawyers, the panel was charged with generating two lists of medical procedures, one itemizing procedures requiring full disclosure and one listing actions requiring no advance disclosure. For procedures requiring full consent, a standard consent form with a mandatory list of risks was provided. This system has fared better than expected.

Finally, it should be mentioned that there are four generally recognized exceptions to the legal requirements for informed consent (111). In an emergency, a patient's consent is said to be implied. Although the courts vary in their definitions of an emergency, the exception is to facilitate treatment where delay for informed consent would subject the patient to irreversible harm (3, 58). The second exception allows patients to waive their right to informed consent. This waiver must be arrived at freely and rationally by the patient. The third exception applies to incompetent patients. When a patient is incapable of understanding the treatment issues, a proxy must be identified to act on his or her behalf (185).

Finally there is the exception granted for therapeutic privilege. This stipulates that physicians can withhold information that would be harmful to the patient (110). It permits the physician to withhold information that would, if communicated, clearly subvert the patient's ability to participate in medical decision making. However, it does not generally provide a vehicle for obtaining consent from difficult or hesitant patients: "The privilege does not accept the paternalistic notion that the physician may remain silent simply because divulgence might prompt the patient to forgo therapy the physician feels the patient really needs" (25).

PERSISTENT PROBLEMS IN INFORMED CONSENT

Most observers agree that the legal rules of informed consent have not achieved their objectives (28, 119, 124). Often, patients are not actively involved in the medical decision-making process. Studies by Lidz and co-workers (102) have shown that many patients leave treatment decisions entirely to their physicians. In these studies only about 10% of patients interviewed saw themselves as having an active role in the decision-making process. In addition, many physicians viewed informed consent solely as a legal requirement rather than as an element of good patient care. In this regard, physicians often see consent as a task to be accomplished by obtaining a signature on a form rather than as an integral part of the physician-patient relationship.

At the other extreme, many oncology patients have made decisions about the therapy they want before they actually meet with the treating oncologist (131). For instance, recent studies indicate that families of patients referred for bone marrow transplantation have generally decided to undergo the therapy prior to arriving at the transplant center and becoming informed about the procedure's risks and benefits.

With the understanding that eventual death from disease is a virtual certainty in many clinical situations, families often grasp at marrow transplantation as a life-saving alternative, regardless of how poor the statistical outcome may be or the complications that may result from the transplant procedure. The referring pediatric oncologist and staff at transplant institutions must be aware of this and provide balanced information that clearly outlines the negative aspects of bone marrow transplantation. However, too negative an approach may dissuade a family from the only option that may prove curative for their child (30).

Most transplant centers have established a comprehensive patient education and evaluation program, designed to provide families with a balanced, current assessment of the risks and benefits of the therapy. However, these studies show that this education process will not influence the family that comes to the transplant center with a "real determination to proceed with transplantation. . . . [Consequently] the real obligation to obtain consent rests with the referring pediatric physician" (30).

This new role for referring physicians is not restricted to transplant situations. General practitioners and oncologists in the community now frequently investigate appropriate experimental therapies on behalf of their patients. Often, the treating physicians are in cities distant from the patient's home and most of the informed consent occurs in discussion with physicians who ultimately will have little or no role in the patient's care.

In this regard, it should be noted that the value of informed consent documents continues to be a source of significant controversy (134, 188). These documents could serve as valuable educational tools but are infrequently used for that purpose. Most physicians and patients view these forms solely as perfunctory legal documents to be completed.

Federal regulations require that written consent be obtained from patients enrolled in clinical trials. However, there is no requirement in common law or in state statutes that consent to medical treatment must be in writing. A number of state statutes appear to encourage the use of informed consent documents and a number of court decisions have upheld their validity (41, 109). Physicians probably overestimate the legal protection afforded by written consent documents. Patients who sign them may still contest their validity by questioning the consent process. In particular, patients have claimed that they were not accorded an opportunity to read the document or were misinformed as to the document's significance.

The complexities of many cancer therapies and the patient's frequent hope of receiving the most current, innovative treatments have combined to undermine the process of informed consent in contemporary oncology practice. Patients frequently present to their oncologists with news clippings from the lay press and request specific therapies. Consequently, legally defined informed consent procedures that focus on the particular physician-patient interaction may protect patients less than regulations that require scientific and human subjects to have protection reviews of clinical trials and chemotherapeutic treatments that occur before any treatments are given in the clinic.

RECOMMENDATIONS FOR THE PRACTICING ONCOLOGIST

Having reviewed the legal and ethical principles governing informed consent, the practicing oncologist may feel bewildered and uncertain of what constitutes a valid informed consent process. In part, this is because many of the ethical and legal standards are contested among ethicists, lawyers, and physicians and therefore are in a state of evolution. Furthermore, the law governing informed consent varies from state to state making it impossible to provide a uniform set of disclosure rules applicable to all locales. None of this is helpful to the physician who must discuss medical treatments with patients.

The best practical advice to offer physicians probably comes from the general requirements of informed consent delineated in the federal regulations for the protection of human subjects (192). These regulations establish standards applicable to all participants in research conducted or funded by the Department of Health and Human Services. As such they address a number of matters restricted to informed consent for research including the provisions for confidentiality, the availability of compensation for injuries, and the procedures for withdrawing from the research protocol. Importantly, however, the regulations also concisely describe essential elements of informed consent that are applicable to all medical decisions. They represent the only set of rules that could be considered a national standard for informed consent. As such they constitute minimum standards rather than ideals that should be aspired to.

First, the regulations require that informed consent be obtained under circumstances that provide the patient sufficient opportunity to consider whether or not to participate and that minimize the possibility of coercion or undue influence (192).

Second, the regulations recognize three basic information components to proper disclosure: (*a*) the risks or discomforts that can be reasonably anticipated, (*b*) the benefits from the therapy that can be reasonably anticipated, and (*c*) the alternative treatments that are appropriate and might be advantageous. All three components are given equal weight in the regulations, even though it is the element of risk that is emphasized in statutes and case law.

In addressing the risks of medical interventions, the regulations emphasize the probability that the injury will occur and the nature of the injury. They imply that risks need not be disclosed if the likelihood of their occurrences is remote and the magnitude of the risk is low; however, risks that are very severe—life-threatening or causing significant permanent damage, such as paralysis—must be disclosed even if very unlikely. Thus, prevailing standards of disclosure usually emphasize the nature, magnitude, and imminence of the risk, and physicians should take these factors into account in their discussions with patients.

The regulations note that there will be disclosure of anticipated benefits. They imply that patients will also understand the limitations of the medical intervention. In oncology it is especially important to distinguish for patients the difference between curative, adjuvant, and palliative treatments.

In addition, the regulations emphasize the disclosure of alternative therapies, even though this is infrequently recognized in statutes and case law. In part this is because the federal regulations usually apply to informed consent for experimental treatments where there may be a standard alternative treatment for the patient's condition. According to the regulations, patients are entitled to choose among those "appropriate" therapies that "might be advantageous" and physicians must be prepared to implement choices that, in their view, are less than optimal. Informed consent is more than the acceptance or rejection of the medically recommended treatment; it includes selecting among a range of reasonable therapeutic options.

These standards should help practicing oncologists secure valid informed consent. But as the debate over informed consent procedures and requirements continues, these standards are likely to evolve.

Terminating Medical Care

HISTORICAL PERSPECTIVE

The first suggestion that physicians withhold medical interventions from terminally ill patients probably dates to Hippocrates. In *The Art* (75), he urged physicians "to refuse to treat those [patients] who are overmastered by their disease realizing that in such cases medicine is powerless." Many centuries later, in 1835, Jacob Bigelow urged members of the Massachusetts Medical Society to withhold interventions—cathartics, emetics, and other "therapies"—from hopelessly and terminally ill patients (89). In 1848, John Warren, the surgeon who performed the first operation with ether anesthesia, urged that ether should be used "in mitigating the agonies of death" (53). In 1958, Pope Pius XII responded to questions about resuscitating patients and maintaining comatose patients on respirators by stating that physicians had no obligation to use such extraordinary means to forestall death (136).

In 1976, however, the *Quinlan* case dramatically changed the nature and content of terminating care discussions. One of the enduring legacies of the *Quinlan* decision is the recognition of the right to refuse medical care. In *Quinlan* (180), the New Jersey Supreme Court ruled that patients have a right to refuse medical care based on the unstated but implicit constitutional right of privacy. Thereafter, physicians, ethicists, and the courts began to focus on constitutional rights, do-not-resuscitate orders, living wills, and health care proxies. And it is in these terms that terminating care issues are currently discussed. Therefore, for physicians to understand acceptable practices for the termination of care it is most useful to consider four topics: (*a*) resuscitation and DNR orders; (*b*) legal standards governing the termination of medical care; (*c*) advance care documents; and (*d*) assisted suicide and euthanasia.

RESUSCITATION AND DNR ORDERS

In 1960, Kouwenhoven and colleagues (95) described closed-chest cardiac massage, the essence of cardiopulmonary resuscitation (CPR). Their study involved 20 patients, most of whom suffered cardiac arrest during anesthesia induction. They reported a 70% long-term survival rate. Subsequent to this report the techniques of cardiopulmonary resuscitation were both refined and utilized in other settings. By 1970, resuscitation was attempted on almost every patient in the hospital who arrested. This prompted empirical studies of the efficacy of CPR, formal procedures for withholding resuscitation from patients, and a reexamination of the criteria for offering patients CPR.

Over the past three decades there have been more than 100 empirical studies of both out-of-hospital and in-hospital arrests (7, 10, 12, 29, 62, 64, 68, 70, 76, 90, 98, 100, 101, 103, 112, 122, 132, 148, 151, 154, 169, 179). Cumulatively these studies suggest three important conclusions. First, approximately 25 to 50% of patients may initially survive CPR; however, a much lower proportion, between 5 and 25%, actually live long enough—and recover enough function—to be discharged from the hospital. Second, between 2 and 3% of patients resuscitated suffer severe, permanent neurological damage (12).

Third, the highest rates of successful resuscitation occur in patients who suffer cardiac arrest during anesthesia induction, acute myocardial infarctions, and tachyarrhythmias. Conversely, patients with chronic organ failure, such as renal failure or cirrhosis, do poorly, with survival-to-discharge rates after CPR of between 0 and 3% (12). In three of these studies, none of the patients with malignancies survived cardiopulmonary resuscitation to be discharged from the hospital (90, 123, 132, 169). However, the generalizability of these data has been questioned since they rely on rather small numbers with wide confidence limits. In addition, a recent study from Memorial Sloan-Kettering (179) demonstrated a 10.5% survival-to-discharge rate for patients with cancer.

As early as 1974 the AMA suggested that there be a mechanism to record in the hospital charts decisions not to resuscitate patients (163). In 1976, following the *Quinlan* decision, the Beth Israel Hospital of Boston became the first hospital to announce and implement a do-not-resuscitate (DNR) policy (141). The policy acknowledged that "it is the general policy of hospitals to act affirmatively to preserve the life of all patients," including terminally ill ones, but went on to state that competent patients may refuse medical treatment including cardiopulmonary resuscitation. Thus the DNR policy was an attempt to protect the rights of patients to refuse medical care. Following the lead of the Beth Israel Hospital many other hospitals adopted similar policies (115). In 1988, the Joint Commission on Accreditation of Healthcare Organizations (JCAHO) required all hospitals to institute DNR policies for accreditation.

The published empirical studies of DNR orders and patients' resuscitation preferences suggest five conclusions. First, DNR orders are inconsistently interpreted and implemented by health care personnel. Some interpret DNR orders as limited to the withholding of chest compressions; others interpret DNR orders to include the withholding or withdrawing of almost any medical treatment, from dialysis to blood transfusions to intravenous fluids (99, 175). This expansive understanding has led many physicians to refrain from using DNR orders because they worry terminally ill patients will not receive proper care. Second, discussions of resuscitation and DNR orders are often left until very late in a patient's clinical course. Frequently, discussions are postponed so that patients who were competent to discuss resuscitation status become incompetent before the issue is addressed. In one study, only 22% of patients given a DNR status were actually involved in the discussion regarding resuscitation (13, 57, 190).

Third, and of particular importance for oncologists, discussions of resuscitation and DNR status are not held uniformly with patients. Oncology patients are much more likely to have discussed CPR and to be designated DNR than patients with other diseases that have the same overall prognosis. In one study, 47% of patients with non–small cell lung cancer were DNR, while only 16% of patients with cirrhosis and esophageal varices and 5% of patients with severe congestive heart failure were DNR (180). Other studies suggest most patients would like to discuss DNR status with their physicians although few actually have had such discussions (59, 60, 156, 167, 181). Importantly, recent data have suggested that there is a significant "framing effect" in relation to patients' desires for CPR, making these discussions essential. In one study, 41% of elderly patients wanted CPR but only 22% wanted it when told that survival was only 10 to 17%. This means that a significant responsibility rests on physicians to provide patients with information—if not precise statistical survival rates—because this is important to their decision-making processes.

Fourth, physicians are unable to predict which patients will suffer cardiac or pulmonary arrest (12). Finally, physicians are unable to predict accurately their patients' resuscitation preferences. In one study, physicians failed to predict patients who would arrest 50% of the time, and they were no better than chance when predicting what their patients' resuscitation preferences would be (13). More importantly, there is a "framing effect"—patients' preferences for resuscitation change depending upon how much information they are provided and how the question is posed. Thus, the ineffectiveness of resuscitation efforts in many patients and the inadequacy of DNR policies in most institutions have led some to reassess resuscitation and DNR policies (14, 171). Some physicians maintain that resuscitation should not even be offered to patients in certain situations—including metastatic cancer—where empirical studies have demonstrated that patients do not survive to discharge following CPR. It is suggested that in such situations physicians should enter DNR orders on the chart without the need for a discussion with the patient. This approach reflects the view that physicians should not provide patients with futile treatments, ones that have no hope of offering any benefits (14, 139).

When resuscitation offers no medical benefit, the physician can make a reasoned determination that a DNR order should be written without any knowledge of the patient's values in the matter. The decision that CPR is unjustified because it is futile is a judgment that falls entirely within the physician's technical expertise (17).

Such a policy has not been widely adopted in large measure because of questions about its legality. While there are no federal or state laws requiring that patients be resuscitated, no legal case has endorsed the notion that physicians may enter DNR orders based on medical futility without con-

Table 91.2. Selected Legal Cases Involving the Termination of Life-Sustaining Medical Care

Case and citation	Year	State	Facts	Decision
Superintendent of Belchertown v Saikewicz 373 Mass 728	1977	Mass.	67-year-old retarded man with a mental age of 2 years 8 months who has always lived in a state institution develops AMMoL. The institution inquires whether he should require chemotherapy.	All persons including incompetent persons have the right to refuse medical treatment. Using substituted judgment, the court determined that the patient would not want chemotherapy.
In re Eichner (Brother Fox) 52 NY 2d 262	1981	N.Y.	83-year-old priest who had a cardiac arrest during a herniorrhaphy that left him vegetative and respirator-dependent. Prior to the event he had publicly discussed the Quinlan case and stated that he would not want to be respirator-dependent if he were vegetative.	Patients have the right to determine the course of their own medical care. Brother Fox's wishes were known even if not expressed in writing, and they should determine whether his respirator is disconnected.
In re Conroy 98 N.J. 321	1985	N.J.	84-year-old bedridden, totally impaired woman with organic brain syndrome living in a nursing home being fed by a nasogastric tube. Her nephew requests removal of the tube.	Nasogastric tube feedings are medical interventions that can be withdrawn. In addition, the court outlines a "pure objective test" for determining when to terminate medical care from incompetent patients who have left no indication of their wishes. According to this test care can be terminated when it causes "recurring, unavoidable and severe pain" rendering life "inhumane."
Brophy v New England Sinai Hospital 398 Mass. 417	1986	Mass.	49-year-old man in persistent vegetative state after a ruptured aneurysm maintained by gastric tube feedings. While he had no written living will, he had explicitly stated that he would never want to live on life support systems. After having rescued a man from a burning truck who lived for some time with severe burns before dying, he stated that he regretted his actions and requested that if he were ever in a similar situation the plug should be pulled.	Common law and the constitutional right of privacy give a person the right to refuse medical treatment. The patient's wishes are clearly known from explicit conversations. Thus, by using substituted judgment the gastric tube can be withdrawn.
Bouvia v Superior Court 225 Cal Rptr 297	1986	Calif.	29-year-old woman with cerebral palsy that left her almost completely immobile and totally unable to care for herself is receiving morphine by pump for painful degenerative arthritis. Physicians insert a nasogastric tube to supplement her inadequate oral intake. She requests that the nasogastric tube be removed.	The patient has the "right to refuse any medical treatment even that which may save or prolong her life."
In re Jobes 108 N.J. 394	1987	N.J.	32-year-old woman who is in a permanent vegetative state and receiving J-tube feedings. Her husband and parents request termination of the feedings. She left no clear written or verbal indication of her wishes on such care.	Incompetent patients have the right to refuse medical care even if they have left no clear indication of their wishes. This right can be exercised by the incompetent patient's family. Using substituted judgment the family is permitted to terminate the J-tube feedings.
Cruzan v Director of Missouri Department of Health 110 S. Ct. 2841	1990	U.S.	33-year-old woman left in a persistent vegetative state after suffering anoxic brain damage in a car accident. She was maintained by gastric tube nutrition and hydration. Her parents requested that these tube feedings be terminated.	By 8 to 1, the court ruled that patients have a constitutional right to refuse medical care and that this applies to artificial nutrition and hydration. The majority argued that states could regulate the family's ability to exercise an incompetent patient's right to refuse treatment if there was no clear and convincing written or verbal statement of the patient's wishes. Since the state of Missouri felt that families should not be permitted to terminate care from patients without explicit prior statements by the patient, Cruzan's feedings continued. Other states could permit families to exercise the incompetent's right to refuse care in the absence of explicit directives.

(continued)

Table 91.2. *(continued)*

Case and Citation	Year	State	Facts	Decision
In re Helga Wangie Fourth judicial district (Dist. Ct., Probate Ct. Div.) PX-91-283. Minnesota Hennepin Country	1991	Minn.	85-year-old woman admitted for dyspnea and is emergently intubated. After 5 months on the respirator she was discharged to a chronic care facility. After 1 week at the facility, she had a cardiac arrest but was resuscitated and taken to an intensive care unit. After several weeks, physicians concluded that she was in a persistent vegetative state. Physicians suggested withdrawing life-sustaining treatment because the patient was receiving no benefit. The family refused to have any life-sustaining treatments withdrawn. No other facility would accept the patient in transfer. After 7 months the hospital went to court hoping to have the respirator discontinued.	A trial court ruled the husband should represent the patient's interests, and he refused to discontinue the respirator.

sulting the patient. Indeed, there is now a case in Massachusetts in which a patient was made DNR based on futility over the objections of her family. In addition to the legal uncertainty, there is residual empirical uncertainty about such a position. The data on the success of resuscitation for patients with co-morbid conditions, such as metastatic cancer, rely on relatively small numbers and are not without dissenting studies (64, 179). In addition, the standards of "futility" physicians use to withhold treatments, including CPR, are quite variable. Indeed, one study found that futility was invoked to justify withholding CPR in 63% of patients, but that some physicians defined futility as greater than 5% survival, and some even claimed CPR could be futile even with higher than 20% survival. Thus there is no established consensus about making DNR decisions in the absence of discussions with patients (8, 43).

Others have suggested additional reforms of CPR and DNR policies including the routine inquiry into patients' DNR preferences at the time of nonemergency admissions to the hospital. Such policies have not been widely adopted. Nevertheless, over the next few years it is likely that there will be significant revisions of DNR policies to identify patients for whom resuscitation is futile and to increase the frequency of physician-patient discussion of DNR.

LEGAL STANDARDS GOVERNING THE TERMINATION OF MEDICAL CARE

Prior to 1976, legal cases involving the refusal of life-sustaining medical care usually involved Jehovah's Witnesses who refused blood transfusions. Judgments in these cases were justified by balancing the patient's well-being and the First Amendment's right of religious freedom (4, 83).

In 1976, the *Quinlan* case changed the focus of discussions regarding terminating care from a matter of religious freedom to one of patient control over medical care. It established the ethical and legal framework guiding all subsequent discussions concerning the termination of medical interventions. This framework involves addressing four basic questions: (*a*) Do patients have a right to refuse medical care? (*b*) What types of care can be terminated? (*c*) Who can make terminating care decisions? and (*d*) what criteria should guide such terminating care decisions (80)?

In June 1990, the U.S. Supreme Court addressed for the first time the issue of terminating medical care in the *Cruzan* case (see Table 91.2) (40). In this landmark case, the Court settled some of the questions, but left some important unresolved issues.

There have been recent reviews of the general area of terminating care (50, 69, 128) as well as the more particular area of terminating care for incompetent patients (52, 187).

Is There a Right to Refuse Medical Care?

In *Cruzan*, by 8 to 1 the U.S. Supreme Court agreed that patients have a constitutional right to refuse medical care; the Court maintained that this right came from the Fourteenth Amendment's guarantee "that no State shall 'deprive any person of life, liberty, or property, without due process of law'" (40). By identifying the basis of this right on a constitutional amendment, the Supreme Court has strengthened it, making it a national standard, and ensured that it will no longer be subject to the vagaries of individual state laws or court rulings. This right has been recognized not just for competent patients but for incompetent patients as well (50, 79, 168).

Patients need not be terminally or hopelessly ill to exercise this right to refuse care; it can be invoked by any patient regardless of health status (16). Moreover, the right to refuse treatment applies equally to withholding treatments and to discontinuing treatments already initiated. Finally, the right to refuse medical care does not imply a correlative right to demand treatment. A patient cannot demand therapy the physician deems useless or "countertherapeutic" (138).

In theory, this right to refuse medical therapy can be limited by four countervailing interests: (*a*) preservation of life; (*b*) prevention of suicide; (*c*) protection of third parties such as children; and (*d*) preserving the integrity of the medical profession (50, 168). In practice, these interests almost never override the right of competent patients and incompetent patients who have left explicit advance care documents. However, for incompetent patients who have not left advance care documents one of these interests, especially the state's interest in preserving life, may override their rights (40).

What Types of Medical Interventions May Be Terminated?

The *Quinlan* case focused on the withdrawal of mechanical respirators. Subsequently legal cases have sanctioned the withholding or withdrawal of chemotherapy, blood transfusions (78), hemodialysis (33, 85), and major surgical operations (97) (see Table 91.2) (50).

In the early 1980s physicians and ethicists began discussing the ethics of withholding or withdrawing artificial fluid and nutrition. Do artificial nutrition and hydration constitute medical interventions that can be terminated like all other interventions? In the *Cruzan* case (40), the U.S. Supreme Court definitively stated that artificial nutrition and hydration are medical interventions, not basic nursing care, and can be withheld or withdrawn under the guidelines that apply to other medical treatments. In the words of Justice O'Connor: "The liberty guaranteed by the Due Process Clause must protect, if it protects anything, an individual's deeply personal decision to reject medical treatment, including the artificial delivery of food and water."

Who Decides Whether Care Can Be Terminated?

There is general agreement that competent patients have the exclusive right to refuse medical care. Even in cases where the patient's wishes may conflict with those of his or her family, the patient's right to refuse care is determinative (97). For incompetent patients who left living wills or other advance care documents, the wishes in these directives are determinative. Indeed, courts have utilized well-considered, explicit, but unrecorded conversations with family, friends, and others in justifying decisions to terminate care (see Table 91.2) (19).

For incompetent patients who did not leave advance care documents or other explicit indications of their views on terminating care, the situation is more uncertain. Many physicians (184), medical organizations (36), ethicists, the President's Commission (138), and state courts have maintained that the incompetent patient's family is the most appropriate surrogate decision maker and should make terminating care decisions for the patient. However, there have been legal, ethical, and empirical objections to this position. For instance, in other areas of medical care, families are not necessarily permitted to make decisions for incompetent patients (6, 52). In addition, empirical studies suggest that spouses and other family members generally do not know the preferences of patients regarding the termination of life-sustaining treatments; therefore they may not reach the same decision that the patient would have reached (175, 191).

This was the very issue that confronted the U.S. Supreme Court in the *Cruzan* case. After suffering anoxic brain damage after a car accident, Nancy Cruzan remained in a persistent vegetative state maintained by artificial nutrition and hydration (see Table 91.2). Her parents asked that the feedings be discontinued. The State of Missouri agreed that the patient had a right to refuse medical care but argued that without a living will or explicit statement of Nancy Cruzan's views on terminating life-sustaining care, her parents were not entitled to exercise her right to terminate the artificial nutrition and hydration. The U.S. Supreme Court held that there is no constitutional requirement that families be permitted to exercise the right of incompetent patients to terminate care when the patients have not left explicit statements of their preferences. Importantly, however, the Court did not delineate uniform national rules regarding who should decide for incompetent patients. Instead the Court permitted each individual state to make the rules it deemed best regarding who will decide for incompetent patients in the absence of living wills or designated proxies. Thus some states may emulate New Jersey and California and permit families to exercise the incompetent patient's right to refuse medical care even in the absence of explicit advance care documents (35, 82). Conversely, other states may follow Oklahoma and New York and prohibit families from exercising the incompetent patient's right to terminate care in the absence of explicit advance care documents. In the *Cruzan* case, the Missouri courts terminated her artificial nutrition and hydration, relying on the recollection of a conversation with a friend many years before. (Ironically, such casual conversations made in youth without specific references to medical treatments and conditions have been ruled in other cases as insufficient evidence of the patient's wishes.)

For the moment, policies on who may decide for incompetent individuals vary among the states. One problem that seems to be arising with increasing frequency is that families want patients in a coma, in a persistent vegetative state, or with anencephaly maintained with life-sustaining treatments, while the treating physicians object to providing such care. In the *Wanglie* case, for instance, the family of an elderly woman in a persistent vegetative state wanted her respirator continued. Her physicians objected and went to court to have her feedings terminated, arguing that they were not providing a benefit to the patient (Table 91.2). The court ruled that the family had a right to decide what treatments the patient should receive (114). As physicians become more comfortable in terminating life-sustaining treatments and see this as appropriate care, these conflicts between physicians who want to terminate treatment and families demanding life-sustaining treatment will become more common (114).

What Criteria Should Guide Decisions to Terminate Care?

Competent patients have the right to refuse medical care and can use whatever criteria they deem acceptable; it is their values, whatever they are, that guide the choice. In the words of the California Supreme Court: "The right to refuse medical treatment is basic and fundamental... Its exercise requires no one's approval. It is not merely one vote subject to being overridden by medical opinion... The controlling decision belongs to a competent informed patient... It is a moral and philosophical decision that, being a competent adult, is the [patient's] alone" (16).

For incompetent patients, this question has been subject to extensive and, as yet, unresolved controversy (50, 52). Traditionally, three guiding criteria have been identified: (*a*) the ordinary/extraordinary care distinction; (*b*) substituted judgment; and (*c*) best interests.

First, some advocate a distinction between ordinary/extraordinary care, which holds that ordinary care should be administered but extraordinary care may be withheld. Many ethicists and courts have concluded that this distinction is too vague and has "too many conflicting meanings" to be helpful in guiding surrogate decision makers and physicians (79).

Second, many courts have advocated using the substituted judgment criterion, which holds that the surrogate should try to imagine what the patient would do if he or she were competent. The problem with this criterion is that most surrogates, even close family members, cannot accurately predict what the patient would have wanted (175, 191). Therefore, substituted judgment becomes more of a guessing game than a way of fulfilling the patient's wishes. Many have now acknowledged this standard to be a fiction.

Third, the best interests criterion holds that the surrogate should evaluate treatments by balancing their benefits and risks and select those treatments in which the benefits maximally outweigh the burdens of treatment. This criterion has been criticized because there is no objective way of determining the balance between benefits and burdens; it depends upon a patient's personal values (50, 82).

Unfortunately, in the *Cruzan* case the U.S. Supreme Court avoided discussing what criteria should help guide surrogate decision makers when they consider whether to terminate medical care from incompetent patients who left no indication of their wishes. The justices relegated this question to the individual states. But state legislatures and courts have been less than enlightening on this question. Consequently, physicians, patients, and families await the development of sound criteria to guide surrogate decision makers when the patient has not left explicit wishes.

Summary

Physicians should recognize that both competent and incompetent patients have a constitutional right to refuse medical care. This right applies both to the withholding and to the withdrawal of any and all interventions, including artificial nutrition and hydration. Competent patients have the right to make these terminating decisions themselves, and their wishes must be respected even if they conflict with their family's wishes. For incompetent patients there is no national rule on who should act as the incompetent's surrogate. In some states, courts have recognized the family, but the U.S. Supreme Court has permitted other states to refuse to grant the family the opportunity to exercise the incompetent's right. Finally it remains unclear what criteria should guide decision making in the absence of an incompetent's explicit wishes (40, 52).

ADVANCE CARE DOCUMENTS AND DURABLE POWERS OF ATTORNEY

Since the *Cruzan* decision there has been renewed interest in advance care documents and durable powers of attorney. To understand the role of advance care documents and durable powers of attorney it is helpful to review (*a*) their legal status, (*b*) their advantages and disadvantages, and (*c*) the future directions of these documents.

The living will was first proposed in 1967. The next year a Florida physician and state legislator introduced a bill to recognize this living will. It was defeated (162). Over the next several years similar living will bills were defeated in many state legislatures. In the wake of the *Quinlan* decision, however, the states finally began to act. In 1976 the California legislature adopted the first living will law, the California Natural Death Act. By 1995, 48 states and the District of Columbia had adopted such laws. Moreover, in other states, such as Massachusetts, where the legislature has not enacted living will statutes, the courts have recognized living will documents as legally enforceable expressions of patients' wishes.

Verbal statements by patients that are clearly stated and are well considered are also legally binding (see Table 91.2) (19, 82). This is the precedent established in the *Brother Fox* case, in which an 83-year-old priest suffered a cardiac arrest during a herniorrhaphy and remained in a persistent vegetative state. Prior to the operation he had participated in a teaching session on the *Quinlan* case and had clearly stated that he would never want to be maintained by mechanical respirator if he became vegetative. The New York court permitted the withdrawal of the respirator because Brother Fox had clearly expressed his considered opinion even if only verbally (81). Similarly in the *Brophy* case, a fireman suffered a ruptured aneurysm of the basilar artery, leaving him in a persistent vegetative state. Prior to this, he had stated to his wife and children that he did not want to be sustained if he became comatose. The Massachusetts Supreme Judicial Court stated that Brophy's wishes must be respected even if they were not written down as long as they were clearly expressed and reiterated over time (19). Thus, it seems that any written advance care document and even well considered and clearly expressed oral statements are legally binding whether or not they conform to specific state living will language, because they are expressions of patients' preferences and must be honored.

In 1984 California passed the first law recognizing the appointment of a designated proxy for health care decisions (165). By 1995, 46 states and the District of Columbia had enacted statutes recognizing durable power of attorney for health care decisions. Importantly, in 1987 the New Jersey Supreme Court ruled that a proxy designated under a regular durable power of attorney law that does not specifically mention health care decisions still may make decisions regarding the termination of medical care (84). Other states have also explicitly adopted this position. Although this position has not been explicitly tested, it now appears that any properly filled out advance care documents or durable power of attorney designation, whether it conforms to a state's specific document or not, is probably protected by the U.S. Constitution and must be honored.

Despite this legal endorsement of advance care documents and proxy decision makers, these mechanisms remain problematic. First, few people have advance care documents. Current surveys reveal that despite widespread public support for living wills only 20 to 25% of the population actually have one (164), although it should be noted that oncology patients have completed advance care directives at much higher rates. One study found that over 40% of oncology patients had an advance care directive. In addition, preliminary data indicate that the federal Patient Self-Determination Act, which requires hospitals (and other health care institutions) receiving Medicare funds to enquire whether admitted patients have advance care documents, to distribute forms to patients who do not have such documents, and to include them in the patient's hospital record, has not had a significant impact in increasing the use of advance care documents (54). Second, the language of many predrafted living will forms is both restrictive and vague (48). For instance, the living will in the Uniform Rights of the Terminally Ill Act sanctions the termination of medical care only if the patient has "an incurable or irreversible condition that will cause . . . death within a relatively short time."

Third, these forms only permit patients to refuse medical interventions, leaving no place for patients who might want some interventions under selected circumstances. Finally, some studies are beginning to demonstrate that living wills are not available when needed and not invoked when available. However, there is need for significantly more empirical study of the effectiveness of living will forms in directing physicians or surrogate decision makers. We simply do not know how well they work as guides in difficult terminating care situations.

These problems with living will forms have led many to endorse proxy decision makers because people who are cognizant of the nuances of each individual case are better guides than abstract and imprecise documents (144). Proxy decision making, however, is also fraught with difficulty. Most importantly, as noted above, empirical studies suggest that even when proxy decision makers are closely related to patients they often do not know the wishes of patients (175, 191). Further, even if a proxy had discussed terminating care with the patient, the patient's views were likely to have been expressed in the same vague terms that plague living wills. In addition, surveys suggest that relatives of patients are often unwilling to accept responsibility for terminating care to their relatives (164). Finally, there are very few empirical data on how well proxy decision makers work. The one study of proxy decision makers for AIDS patients shows that patients frequently change their minds about who should act as their proxy (166).

Despite these difficulties with advance care documents and proxies there remains significant interest in such documents. Indeed, the federal government is exploring additional legislation on advance care documents. In addition there have been efforts to improve the documents to eliminate their disadvantages. One recent proposal has been *The Medical Directive* (51), which combines into one six-page document a specific living will, a place to designate a durable power of attorney, and a place to express preferences on organ donation. The living will section is more specific than other living wills because it solicits the patient's wishes on nine life-sustaining interventions in seven commonly encountered clinical scenarios. *The Medical Directive* has been shown to be valid and reliable.

Finally and most importantly, there will soon be more empirical research on the use of advance care documents and proxy decision makers. Until now there has been woefully little understanding of what factors impede the use of advance care documents, patients' preferences on life-sustaining treatments, and what format and setting are best for soliciting patient preferences. Data on these issues are essential if advance care documents and durable powers of attorney are to be used more often and are to be helpful in the clinical setting.

ASSISTED SUICIDE AND EUTHANASIA

The widespread acceptance of terminating life-sustaining medical care, the permissibility of euthanasia in The Netherlands, the Kevorkian suicide machine, and the "It's over, Debbie" article in JAMA (88) have sparked increased debate on the ethics and legality of assisted suicide and euthanasia. In reviewing these topics it is important first to define terms and then to consider the arguments for and against assisted suicide and euthanasia. Finally, the positions adopted in various countries on assisted suicide and euthanasia will be reviewed.

Much confusion has surrounded the issues of assisted

Table 91.3. Definitions of Assisted Suicide and Euthanasia

Term	Definition
Voluntary active euthanasia	Intentionally administering medications or other interventions to cause the patient's death with the patient's informed consent.
Involuntary active euthanasia	Intentionally administering medications or other interventions to cause the patient's death when the patient was competent to consent but did not—e.g., the patient may not have been asked.
Nonvoluntary active euthanasia	Intentionally administering medications or other interventions to cause the patient's death when the patient was incompetent and was mentally incapable of consenting—e.g., the patient might have been in a coma.
Passive euthanasia (terminating life-sustaining treatments)	Withholding or withdrawing life-sustaining medical treatments from a patient to let him or her die.
Indirect euthanasia	Administering narcotics or other medications to relieve pain with the incidental consequence of causing sufficient respiratory depression to result in the patient's death.
Physician-assisted suicide	A physician provides medications or other interventions to a patient with the understanding that the patient can use them to commit suicide.

suicide and euthanasia because of imprecise terminology. Table 91.3 summarizes the essential definitions. It is important to notice that passive euthanasia is the withdrawal or withholding of life-sustaining medical interventions and is widely accepted as both ethical and legal. In addition, indirect euthanasia, increasing narcotics to ease a patient's pain even if this has the consequence of hastening the patient's death, has generally been deemed both ethical and legal (138). Almost all commentators agree that involuntary, active euthanasia is unethical because it is imposed on a competent patient who has not consented. Consequently, the focus of debate in the United States is on physician-assisted suicide and voluntary, active euthanasia. To avoid confusion, use of the term *euthanasia* should be—and will in this chapter be—restricted to voluntary, active euthanasia.

Frequently, the endorsement of assisted suicide or euthanasia is made without any reasons offered as justification (183). However, proponents typically cite four reasons to justify assisted suicide or euthanasia (142). First, it is claimed that euthanasia ensures patients' autonomy. Individuals have different values and goals in life; we protect patient autonomy by permitting patients to pursue their goals. A proper death is as essential to a person's goals and values as any other choice. Hence, to respect patients' autonomy, we must respect patients' wishes regarding the manner and timing of their death through euthanasia and physician-assisted suicide. Second, it is argued that for some patients the dying process inflicts significant pain and suffering and that euthanasia may relieve them of these burdens. Hence euthanasia furthers beneficence or the well-being of sick patients. Indeed, for some people just knowing there is the possibility of having euthanasia or assisted suicide may be psychologically beneficial even if they ultimately never use these interventions. Third, proponents argue euthanasia is morally indistinguishable from the accepted practices of withholding and withdrawing life-sustaining care. This is because the final result, the death of a patient, is the same in either scenario and because there is no moral difference between acts of omission and acts of commission. From a moral standpoint there is no difference between merely letting nature take its course and actively killing a patient if the patient consciously and knowingly requests his or her life be terminated. Finally, it is argued that the adverse practical consequences of legalizing euthanasia are too speculative and hypothetical to determine whether to permit euthanasia. Indeed permitting euthanasia should enhance the physician-patient relationship since it means physicians will provide whatever care—including euthanasia—that is necessary for dying patients.

Opponents to euthanasia offer four parallel arguments. First, opponents claim that autonomy does not justify euthanasia. Autonomy does not mean a person should be permitted to do anything he or she wishes. On this basis we do not permit voluntary duelling or voluntary enslavement. In addition, even if a person wants to commit suicide it is another issue entirely to permit others to help; having a right to commit suicide does not imply a right to have others participate. Second, beneficence may not justify euthanasia. Many terminally ill patients experience inadequately treated pain, fatigue, and depression. If we treated these symptoms adequately few people would have extreme pain and suffering that would justify euthanasia. Third, it is argued that there is an ethical distinction between acts of omission and acts of commission. Evaluating the ethics of an act does not only depend on its final result, we also must evaluate how that result was produced and the intention of the actors. We recognize in the law of murder differences between cases in which a person was killed by mistake and cases in which the killing was premeditated. Similarly, there is a difference between stopping a medical treatment and letting a patient die and intentionally and actively injecting the patient with a medication to cause his or her death. Finally, opponents note

Table 91.4. Physician Attitudes and Practices Regarding Euthanasia

	Percent receiving requests for euthanasia	Percent committing euthanasia	Percent willing to commit euthanasia	Response rate	Sample question
Washington State Medical Association	39.1%	NA	29.7%	55.2%	Has a terminal patient ever asked you to hasten his or her death?
Physician's Management	19.0%	9.4%	NA	24.9%	Have you ever deliberately taken clinical action(s) that would directly cause a patient's death?
American Society of Internal Medicine	24.1%	19.9%	NA	40.2%	Have you ever taken a deliberate action that would directly cause a patient's death?
Caralis and Hammond (26)	43.8%	NA	NA	66.0%	NA
Fried et al. (61)	13.2%	1.3%	28.0%	65.3%	Have you ever been approached by a patient to administer an injection which would result in his or her death?
Shapiro et al. (155)	35.2%	2.2%	30.0%	33.0%	
Cohen et al. (32)	NA	NA	33.0%	69.0%	
Bachman et al. (9)	NA	NA	25.0%	63.0%	

a variety of adverse consequences that might result from legalizing euthanasia, including disruption of the physician-patient relationship, intrusion of the courts into terminating care decisions, coercion of terminally ill patients to commit euthanasia, and extension of euthanasia to children, mentally incompetent patients, and others (160, 189).

In the United States, interest in euthanasia and assisted suicide has extended beyond ethics to the law. Referenda to legalize euthanasia were defeated in Washington State in 1991 and in California in 1992 by 54 to 46% votes. While more than 10 state legislatures have considered laws to either legalize or explicitly prohibit euthanasia or assisted suicide, no state legislature has passed a bill legalizing either intervention. In 1994, Oregonians voted 51.3 to 48.7% to legalize physician-assisted suicide, although court challenges have prevented implementation. The Oregon law is restricted to assisted suicide and does not permit euthanasia. It requires that eligible patients be over 18 and have "an incurable and irreversible disease that . . . will, within reasonable medical judgment, produce death within six months."[129a] In addition, the physician must obtain a consultation from another physician who concurs in the diagnosis and prognosis. However, there is no requirement for a psychiatric evaluation. There is a 15-day waiting period between the initial request and when the prescription can be written. At some point in the process the patient must put the request in a written form. Finally, physicians who find assisted suicide unacceptable are not required to carry out the patient's request and cannot be censured or otherwise disciplined for their refusal. Many objections have been raised against the Oregon law, including that the physician who prescribes the medication need not know the patient for more than 15 days, that without mandatory psychiatric evaluations patients who have reversible depression may be permitted to commit suicide, and that such a momentous social policy change will not be adequately evaluated (32, 53, 130).

There is also growing empirical study of euthanasia and assisted suicide. Surveys of the public have indicated that 64% believe a "physician should be legally permitted to give a terminally ill patient in pain a lethal injection to aid in dying" and that 20% would ask their physician for euthanasia if they had a terminal illness and were suffering pain. However, only 14% would be willing to help a terminally ill relative or friend commit suicide. There have been many studies of physicians' attitudes and practices regarding euthanasia (Table 91.4). Although these studies have several methodological flaws, including low response rates and poorly worded questions, they indicate that many physicians (13.2–43.8%) have received requests for euthanasia. In addition, in the best studies 1 to 2% of physicians have participated in euthanasia. There is also a consistent third of physicians who would be willing to participate in euthanasia if it were legalized.

The Netherlands is the only Western country that permits euthanasia. Technically, euthanasia is not legal in the Netherlands (46, 99, 133). There had been some well-publicized cases of euthanasia in Holland in the late 1970s and early 1980s that prompted the formation of a State Commission on Euthanasia. In 1985 this commission voted 13 to 2 to recommend exempting voluntary, active euthanasia from criminal prosecution. Due to opposition mainly by religious groups, this recommendation has still not been enacted into law. Indeed, Article 293 of the Dutch criminal code still makes terminating a life a crime punishable by up to 12 years' imprisonment. Instead, Dutch state prosecutors and judges have agreed not to prosecute physicians for terminating the life of patients if three conditions are simultaneously met: (*a*) the patient has unbearable pain and suffering that cannot be medically relieved, (*b*) the patient is competent and repeatedly makes a request to be killed, and (*c*) the physician consults a second physician (46, 99, 133). Over 50% of Dutch physicians have participated in euthanasia, 24% within the previous 2 years. Studies indicate that there are 2,500 to 3,000 cases of euthanasia each year in The Netherlands, totaling 1.8% of all deaths. Importantly, almost 70% of these cases involve patients with cancer (46). Finally, participating in euthanasia is not without adverse consequences for the physician. According to investigators, "many physicians who had practiced euthanasia mentioned that they would be most reluctant to do so again." This is a limited result in need of additional study.

Conflict of Interest

HISTORICAL PERSPECTIVE

Conflicts of interest are inherent in any profession; the professional must render service for another person and yet earn an income from rendering the service. Recognition and debate about conflicts of interest are not new. At the turn of the century the most common conflicts of interest arose over fee splitting—the practice in which the physician who referred a patient to a specialist or surgeon would expect a payment, or "commission," and there was concern about the ethics of such practices. For instance, in 1899 a physician surveyed Chicago area surgeons to see if they would pay him 50% commission for surgical referrals. Other conflicts, such as physicians receiving payments from diagnostic laboratories based on the number of patients they referred, ophthalmologists selling glasses, or physicians dispensing pharmaceuticals, were recognized and debated for many decades. However, the response of physicians and organized medicine to such conflicts has been inconsistent, and enforcement of prohibitions on such conflicts was lax under most circumstances. Given the tremendous increase in the financial power of medicine and the sheer dollars flowing through it, there has been more attention paid to conflicts of interest within the last two decades, especially the last 10 years.

TYPES OF CONFLICTS OF INTEREST

Conflicts of interest occur when some factor can excessively influence or undermine a primary interest. In the context of medicine, it is commonly argued that the physician's primary interest is in promoting his or her patient's well-being and health. Typically, physicians will have other medical interests, such as interests in biomedical research and teaching, as well as nonmedical interests, such as interests in money, fame, family, or the pursuit of other avocational activities. A conflict of mission or commitment occurs when a medical interest can—or can appear to—undermine or compromise the physician's commitment to his or her patient's interest. For instance, a well-recognized conflict of mission occurs for clinical researchers who are committed to enrolling patients in their own research protocols and providing optimal care for their individual patients. To prevent or mitigate these conflicts of missions, American society has developed procedures, such as IRB review of research protocols and signed informed consent for research. A conflict of interest occurs when a nonmedical interest, such as financial gain, can—or can appear to—undermine or compromise the physician's commitment to his or her patient's interest.

Broadly speaking, it is possible to distinguish two different types of conflicts of interest. There are conflicts of interest by commission in which physicians have a financial or other incentive to provide more care than is deemed appropriate. Conflicts of interest by commission occur in fee-for-service medicine, when physicians receive payment for services provided to their patients. They also occur when physicians have an investment in medical facilities, refer their patients to those facilities and, thereby, realize a profit when the patients receive medical services from the facilities. There are conflicts of interest by omission in which physicians have a financial or other incentive to provide less care than is deemed appropriate. Conflicts of interest by omission occur in capitated health care reimbursement. They also occur when physicians receive salary bonuses or other payments for withholding tests, consultations, hospitalizations, or other medical care services.

STUDIES OF CONFLICTS OF INTEREST

There have been a number of studies documenting conflicts of interest of commission in which physicians receive financial gain for providing services. For instance, it has been found that in Florida, radiation therapy facilities that are joint ventures, in which physicians own the facilities and therefore receive financial gains from greater use of radiation facilities, had provided more services when compared with national averages and had higher costs per service provided. Others have also found greater use of radiological, laboratory, physical therapy, and other medical services when physicians participate in joint ventures (66, 74, 116–118).

There are fewer empirical studies documenting conflicts of interest of omission, in large part because the practice circumstances in which these arise are relatively new. However, recent studies have shown that more than 60% of managed care plans withhold a portion of physicians' salaries to cover expenditures that exceed target projections for use of specialists or hospital admissions. The data indicate that most plans withhold more than 11% of physicians' salaries and that some even withhold more than 30% of physicians' salaries. In addition, more than 35% of managed care plans provide physicians a bonus based on personal practice productivity. More importantly, markets with high penetration of managed care are more likely to use capitation payments and other financial incentives. Thus, as competition increases and managed care spreads we can expect greater use of financial incentives. Data on how these financial incentives affect physicians' patient care decisions and patient outcomes are limited. Hillman and colleagues (71–74) did determine that managed care plans that placed physicians financially at risk for referrals had fewer out-patient visits and that managed care plans that paid physicians on a capitated basis had fewer hospitalizations. Over the next several years more detailed studies linking financial incentives in managed care plans to physicians' decisions and patient outcomes should be forthcoming (71, 72, 73, 74, 77, 116–118, 121, 135, 145–147).

ETHICAL STANDARDS GOVERNING CONFLICTS OF INTEREST

The ethical standards related to conflicts of interest are fairly clear. Since ancient times, it has been claimed that the physician's primary commitment is to his or her patients' well-being. Of course, we recognize that in some circumstances physicians can override their patients' interests. In some circumstances, such as infectious diseases, physicians should place the interests of third parties over the interests of their own patients. However, this standard means that physicians' personal financial and other interests should not distort or undermine care of their personal patients. At various points in history, this standard has been recognized more by its breech than by compliance. Nevertheless, it remains the acknowledged ethical norm.

This ethical norm has been implemented in laws and policies. An exhaustive list of such laws and policies is beyond the scope of this chapter. Moreover, with increasing attention being paid to financial conflicts of interest, the laws and rules regulating them are likely to change rapidly over the next few years. Nevertheless, it is worthwhile reviewing some of the laws and policies that prohibit some financial conflicts, require disclosure of others, and mandate oversight of still others (127). For instance, the ethical standards on conflicts of interest have led to the recommendation by the American Medical Association, the Pharmaceutical Research and Manufacturers of America, and others on gifts to physicians. The recommendation states that physicians may accept gifts of "minimal value" but should refuse substantial gifts from drug companies, such as "the costs of travel, lodging, or other personal expenses . . . for] attending conferences or meetings" (38). In addition, under the so-called Stark rules, physicians are prohibited from profiting by sending patients to facilities in which they have an ownership stake. Ethical standards on conflict of interest have also prompted medical journals to require authors to disclose any financial interests that might affect their research results. In addition, some courts have ruled that researchers need to disclose financial interests in obtaining informed consent from patients for research. Some medical schools and universities require oversight of certain financial arrangements in which physicians receive payments for research. Harvard Medical School, for instance, requires disclosure, review, and approval by an oversight committee when a faculty member participates in clinical research on a technology owned by a company in which the faculty member or a member of his of her family "has a consulting relationship, holds stock or similar ownership interest" (37, 38, 55).

Finally, it is worth noting an important distinction between policies for the conflicts of interest of commission and of omission. Personal investments in medical facilities or gifts from drug companies are optional; the ethical physician can, therefore, avoid most serious conflicts of interest of commission at relatively small cost by a personal decision. One of the disturbing characteristics of these new financial incentives, however, is that they are not optional. They are dictated by those paying for patient care, and their use is likely to grow. Consequently, in the absence of rules restricting their use, it may be hard for physicians in some health care markets to earn a living without participating in contracts that contain these incentives. This means that avoiding conflicts of interest of omission may not be a personal decision. Conflicts of interest of omission are becoming institutionalized. Preventing or minimizing them is less a personal act but rather requires organized institutional action, which is much harder (55, 71–73).

CLINICAL CASES

Case 1

A recently married 38-year-old female with newly diagnosed breast cancer presents to her oncologist for a discussion of further therapy. Axillary node dissection revealed 7 of 10 lymph nodes positive for metastatic carcinoma. In the general discussion about breast cancer the patient makes clear that she is fearful of the side effects of chemotherapy. She implies, although she does not explicitly state, that she will refuse any suggested therapy that risks permanent loss of reproductive fertility.

Should the oncologist provide the patient with a full recitation of the risks of treatment with the consequence that the patient will refuse chemotherapy? Even if the physician is extraordinarily sensitive to the patient's fears, tries to reassure her, and clarifies the potential benefits of therapy, the patient may still refuse life-prolonging therapy. In such situations the physician has an obligation to provide the patient with the relevant information. Indeed, the Canterbury court stated that a physician may not hide information from the patient "simply because divulgence might prompt the patient to forgo therapy the physician feels the patient really needs." But other decisions, in particular *Truman v Thomas*, have stated that physicians must explain to patients the risks of doing nothing as carefully as they explain the risks of therapy. Consequently, the physician should advise the patient, perhaps in writing, that her refusal is against medical advice because it will reduce her overall survival. However, in such cases the ultimate choice to accept or refuse therapy remains with the patient (25, 172).

Case 2

A 54-year-old male has recently been diagnosed with Dukes C adenocarcinoma of the colon. He is eager for chemotherapy and is referred by his surgeon to a medical oncologist. At a recent meeting, the oncologist learned that there have been therapy-related deaths as a result of such treatment, although the frequency is less than 1%.

In providing informed consent to chemotherapy should the physician reveal this relatively low risk? While the risk of therapy-related mortality is low, the implications are grave. The Canterbury court confronted a case in which a patient undergoing a laminectomy suffered paralysis. The risk of paralysis was about 1%. The court was unequivocal in its determination that disclosure of such a grave, although remote risk should occur (25). Similarly, in *Cobbs v Grant*, a case involving ulcer surgery, the court stated that physicians must disclose "all significant perils," which it defined as those involving "the risk of death or bodily harm, and problems of recuperation" (31). Although both these decisions come from courts that adopt the patient-based standard of informed consent, which remains the minority view, the risk of death from treatment in the adjuvant setting probably would require disclosure under the physician-based standard as well. It seems that physicians do disclose low-incidence life-threatening or fatal toxicities of therapy.

Case 3

A 46-year-old male with extensive small cell lung cancer, including bone metastases, has discussed issues surrounding the termination of care with his physician. On several occasions the patient explicitly stated to his physician that he did not want to be maintained on a respirator, given artificial nutrition and hydration, or any further chemotherapy. The patient had never completed a living will document or appointed a proxy decision maker. The patient is admitted to the hospital for pain control. A DNR order is not entered in the chart, and the patient has a cardiopulmonary arrest and is successfully resuscitated. He remains unconscious on a respirator.

What should the physician do? The respirator should be withdrawn and the patient be permitted to die. Competent and incompetent patients have a constitutional right to refuse medical care, including life-sustaining medical treatments. This patient has clearly expressed his wishes regarding the termination of life-sustaining medical treatment to his physician. Even though he never completed a written document, his wishes regarding terminating care were clearly expressed and therefore are ethically and legally binding. Furthermore, the physician should have no hesitation in withdrawing an intervention already begun. Both philosophers and judges clearly recognize that there is no ethical or legal distinction between withholding a particular intervention and withdrawing the same intervention. Thus, while it is unfortunate that a patient who requested not to be placed on a respirator was resuscitated, once it becomes clear that he had previously expressed his wishes, these wishes should be honored (8, 12, 19, 57, 141).

Case 4

At the conclusion of her first office visit a 33-year-old woman with breast cancer tells her physician that she knows in the near future she will die of breast cancer. The patient asks her physician to promise that when her condition "gets bad" he will give her "something" to end her life quickly.

How should the physician respond? Initially the physician should inquire for the reasons that the patient anticipates the need for assisted suicide or euthanasia. Frequently such requests are based on the patient's fear of unrelieved pain. If this patient has such a fear, the physician should reassure the patient that unremitting pain and suffering can be controlled with medications in almost all cases. The physician should also emphasize that it is ethical for him to provide whatever medications are necessary to relieve the patient's pain even if they should have the consequence of hastening her death. Thus he will not withhold pain medications if she is suffering pain. Finally, he should state that while some commentators, including physicians, have endorsed physician-assisted suicide, the ethics of assisted suicide and euthanasia are highly controversial and both remain illegal (15, 17, 27).

Case 5

A bone marrow biopsy confirms that a 65-year-old woman without any previous medical problems has the diagnosis of acute myelogenous leukemia, M1 type. The oncologist presents her with the diagnosis and describes the treatment options and attendant risks. While recognizing that patients over age 60 do worse with induction chemotherapy, the physician notes that the patient has no comorbid conditions and suggests that she begin standard chemotherapy with 3 days of daunorubicin and 7 days of continuous infusion cytarabine. The patient's husband agrees. The patient, however, refuses chemotherapy, stating that she has lived a full life and would rather die quickly of her disease than suffer through the chemotherapy with a risk of dying during the induction process. The husband tries to persuade the patient to begin chemotherapy. At the husband's request a psychiatric consultation is called which confirms that the woman is competent and not clinically depressed. The husband then approaches the physician and demands that his wife be treated with the standard chemotherapy.

What should the physician tell the husband? Clearly the physician should reassure the husband that different people can have different views on the appropriateness of chemotherapy for AML in patients over 60 years old where there is a higher mortality and complication rate with induction therapy. Ultimately the physician must state that it is the competent patient's choice whether to undergo or forgo chemotherapy. Further, in disputes among family members regarding the use of life-sustaining therapies the competent patient has the final decision. This position has been reaffirmed in legal precedents. Consequently, regardless of the strength and depth of the husband's wishes and regardless of his good intentions, the physician cannot force the patient to receive chemotherapy if she is competent and refuses it (40, 47, 80).

References

1. Aaron HJ, Schwartz WB. The Painful Prescription. Washington DC: Brookings Institution, 1984.
2. Annas GJ. Informed Consent, Cancer, and Truth in Prognosis. N Engl J Med 1994;330:223.
3. Appelbaum PS, Lidz CW, Meisel A. Informed consent: legal theory and clinical practice. New York: Oxford University Press, 1987.
4. Application of President and Directors of Georgetown College, 331 R2d 1000 (D.C. cir) cert denied 377 U.S. 978 (1964).
5. Arato v Avedon, 11 Cal Rptr 2d 169 (1992).
6. Areen J. The legal status of consent obtained from families of adult patients to withhold or withdraw treatment. JAMA 1987;258:229.
7. Arena FP, Perlin M, Turnbull AD. Initial experience with a "code-no-code" resuscitation system in cancer patients. Crit Care Med 1980;8:733.
8. Asch DA, Hansen-Flaschen J, Lanken PN. Decisions to limit or continue life-sustaining treatment by critical care physicians in the United States: conflicts between physicians' practices and patients' wishes. Am J Respir Crit Care Med 1995;151:288.
9. Bachman JG, Doukas DJ, Lichtenstein RL, Alcsers KH. Assisted suicide and euthanasia in Michigan. N Engl J Med 1994;331:812.
10. Bayer AJ, Ang BC, Pathy MS. Cardiac arrests in a geriatric unit. Age Aging 1985;14:271.
11. Beauchamp TL, Childress JF. Principles of Biomedical Ethics, 4th ed. New York: Oxford University Press, 1994.
12. Bedell SE, Delbanco TL, Cook EF, Epstein FH. Survival after cardiopulmonary resuscitation in the hospital. N Engl J Med 1983;309:569.
13. Bedell SE, Delbanco TL. Choices about cardiopulmonary resuscitation in the hospital: when do physicians talk with patients? N Engl J Med 1984;310:1089.
14. Blackhall LJ. Must we always use CPR? N Engl J Med 1987;317:1281.
15. Blendon RJ, Szalay US, Knox RA. Should physicians aid their patients in dying? JAMA 1992;267:2658.
16. Bouvia v Superior Court, 225 Cal Rptr 297 (1986).
17. Brett AS, McCullough LB. When patients request specific interventions: defining the limits of the physician's obligation. N Engl J Med 1986;315:1347.
18. Brock DW. Voluntary active euthanasia. Hastings Cent Rep 1992;22:10.
19. Brophy v New England Sinai Hospital, 398 Mass 417 (1986).
20. Calabresi G, Bobbitt P. Tragic Choices. New York: Norton, 1978.
21. Callahan D. Setting Limits. New York: Simon & Schuster, 1987.
22. Callahan D. What Kind of Life. New York: Simon & Schuster, 1990.
23. Callahan D. When self determination runs amok. Hastings Cent Rep 1992;22:52.
24. Canellos GP. Who should pay for clinical research? J Clin Oncol 1990;8:1775.
25. Canterbury v Spence, 464 F.2d 772 (D.C. Cir 1972) 1987;17:24.
26. Caralis PV, Hammond JS. Attitudes of medical students, housestaff, and faculty physicians toward euthanasia and termination of life-sustaining treatment. Crit Care Med 1992;20:683.
27. Cassel CK, Meier DE. Morals and moralism in the debate over euthanasia and assisted suicide. N Engl J Med 1990;323:750.
28. Cassileth BR, Zupris RV, Sutton-Smith K, March V. Informed consent—why are its goals imperfectly realized? N Engl J Med 1980;302:896.
29. Charlson ME, Sax FL, MacKenzie R, Fields SD, Braham RL, Douglas RG. Resuscitation: how do we decide? JAMA 1986;255:1316.
30. Chauvenet AR, Smith NM. Referral of pediatric oncology patients for marrow transplantation and the process of informed consent. Med Pediatr Oncol 1988;16:40.
31. Cobbs v Grant, 104 Cal. Rptr. 505 (1972).
32. Cohen JS, Fihn SD, Boyko EJ, Jonsen AR, Wood RW. Attitudes toward assisted suicide and euthanasia among physicians in Washington state. N Engl J Med 1994;331:89.
33. Commissioner of Correction v Myers, 379 Mass 255 (1979).
34. Conn. Blues offers primary care bonus. American Medical News, April 1994;18:25.
35. Conservatorship of Drabick, 200 Cal. App 3d 185, 245 Cal Rptr 840 (1988).
36. Council on Ethical and Judicial Affairs. Current Opinions of the Council on Ethical and Judicial Affairs of the American Medical Association. Chicago: American Medical Association, 1995.
37. Council on Ethical and Judicial Affairs, American Medical Association conflicts of interest: physician ownership of medical facilities. JAMA 1992;267:2366.
38. Council on Ethical and Judicial Affairs, American Medical Association: gifts to physicians from industry. JAMA 1991;265:501.
39. Crosby C. Internists grapple with how they should respond to requests for aid in dying. Internist 1992;33:10.
40. Cruzan v Director of Missouri Department of Health, U.S.
41. Curran WJ. Informed consent and blanket consent forms. Am J Public Health 1971;61:1245.
42. Curran WJ. The first mechanical heart transplant: informed consent and clinical experimentation. N Engl J Med 1984;291:1015.
43. Curtis JR, Park DR, Krone MR, Pearlman RA. Use of the medical futility rationale in do-not-attempt-resuscitation orders. JAMA 1995;273:124.
44. Daniels N. Just Health Care. New York: Cambridge University Press, 1985.
45. Danis M, Southerland LI, Garrett JM, et al. A prospective study of advance directives for life-sustaining care. N Engl J Med 1991;324:882.
46. de Wachter MAM. Active euthanasia in The Netherlands. JAMA 1989;262:3316.
47. Dworkin G. The Theory and Practice of Autonomy. New York: Cambridge University Press, 1988.
48. Eisendrath SJ, Jonsen AR. The living will: help or hindrance? JAMA 1983;249:1054.
49. Elias S, Annas G. Reproductive Genetics and the Law. Chicago: Year Book, 1987.
50. Emanuel EJ. A review of the ethical and legal aspects of terminating medical care. Am J Med 1988;84:291.
51. Emanuel LL, Emanuel EJ. The medical directive: a new comprehensive advance care document. JAMA 1989;261:3288.
52. Emanuel EJ, Emanuel LL. Proxy decision making for incompetent patients. JAMA 1992;267:2067.
53. Emanuel EJ. Euthanasia: historical, ethical and empiric perspectives. Arch Intern Med 1994;154:1890.
54. Emanuel EJ, Weinberg DS, Gonin R, Hummel LR, Emanuel LL. How well is the patient self-determination act working?: an early assessment. Am J Med 1993;95:619.
55. Emanuel EJ, Steiner D. Institutional conflict of interest. N Engl J Med 1995;332:262.
56. Engelhardt HT. The Foundations of Bioethics. New York: Oxford University Press, 1986.
57. Evans AL, Brody BA. The do-not-resuscitate order in teaching hospitals. JAMA 1985;253:2236.
58. Faden RR, Beauchamp TL. A History and Theory of Informed Consent. New York: Oxford University Press, 1986.
59. Finucane TE, Shumway JM, Powers RL, D'Alessandri RM. Planning with elderly out-

patients for contingencies of severe illness: a survey and clinical trial. J Gen Intern Med 1988;3:322.
60. Frankl D, Oye RK, Bellamy PE. Attitudes of hospitalized patients toward life support: a survey of 200 medical inpatients. Am J Med 1989;86:645.
61. Fried TR, Stein MD, O'Sullivan PS, Brock DW, Novack DH. The limits of patient autonomy: physician attitudes and practices regarding life-sustaining treatments and euthanasia. Arch Intern Med 1993;153:722.
62. Fusgen I, Summa JD. How much sense is there in an attempt to resuscitate an aged person? Gerontology 1978;24:37.
63. Gaylin W, Kass LR, Pellegrino ED, Siegler M. Doctors must not kill. JAMA 1988;259: 2139.
64. George AL, Folk BP, Crecelius PL, Campbell WB. Pre-hospital morbidity and other correlates of survival after in-hospital cardiopulmonary arrest. Am J Med 1989;87:28.
65. Giving death a hand: rending issue. New York Times, June 14 1990:A6.
66. Green RM. Medical joint-venturing. Hastings Cent Rep 1990;20:22.
67. Greenhouse L. Hospital Appeals Decision Ordering Treatment for Baby Missing a Brain. New York Times, Sept 24 1993:A10.
68. Gulati RS, Bhan GL, Horan MA. Cardiopulmonary resuscitation of old people. Lancet 1983;ii:267.
69. Hastings Center Guidelines on the Termination of Life-Sustaining Treatment and the Care of the Dying. Bloomington IN: Indiana University Press, 1987.
70. Hershey CO, Fisher L. Why outcome of cardiopulmonary resuscitation in general wards is poor. Lancet 1982;ii:31.
71. Hillman AL. Managing the physician: rules versus incentives. Health Affairs 1991;10: 138.
72. Hillman AL. Financial incentives for physicians in HMOs: is there a conflict of interest? N Engl J Med 1987;317:1743.
73. Hillman AL, Pauly MV, Kerstein JJ. How do financial incentives affect physicians' clinical decisions and the financial performance of health maintenance organizations? N Engl J Med 1989;321:86.
74. Hillman BJ, Joseph CA, Mabry MR, Sunshine JH, Kennedy SD, Noether M. Frequency and cost of diagnostic imaging in office practice—a comparison of self-referring and radiologist-referring physicians. N Engl J Med 1990;323:1604.
75. Hippocrates. The art. In Hippocrates: The Loeb Classical Library. Edited by WHS Jones. Cambridge: Harvard University Press, 1923.
76. Hollingsworth JH. The results of cardiopulmonary resuscitation: a three year university hospital experience. Ann Intern Med 1969;71:459.
77. Iglehart JK. Efforts to address the problem of physician self-referral. N Engl J Med 1991;325:1820.
78. In re Brown, 478 So. 2d 1033 (1985).
79. In re Conroy, 98 NJ 321 (1985).
80. In re Quinlan, 70 NJ 10 (1976).
81. In re Eichner (Brother Fox), 52 NY2d 262 (1981).
82. In re Jobes, 108 N.J. 394 (1987).
83. In re Osborne, 294 A 2d 372 (1972).
84. In re Peter, 108 N.J. 365 (1987).
85. In re Spring, 380 Mass. 629 (1980).
86. Ingelfinger FJ. Arrogance. N Engl J Med 1980;303:1507.
87. Institute of Medical Ethics Working Party on the Ethics of Prolonging Life and Assisting Death. Assisted death. Lancet 1990;ii:610.
88. A piece of my mind. It's over, Debbie. JAMA 1988;259:272.
89. Bigelow J. Self limited disease: address to the Massachusetts Medical Society, May 27, 1835. In Nature in Disease. Boston: Ticknor and Fields, 1854.
90. Johnson AL, Tanser PH, Ulan RA, Wood TE. Results of cardiac resuscitation in 552 patients. Am J Cardiol 1967;20:831.
91. Kass LR. Toward a More Natural Science. New York: Free Press, 1985.
92. Kassirer JP. Adding insult to injury: usurping patients' prerogatives. N Engl J Med 1983;308:898.
93. Katz J. Informed consent—a fairy tale? Law's vision. Univ Pitt L Rev 1977;39:137.
94. Katz J. The Silent World of Doctor and Patient. New York: Free Press, 1984.
95. Kouwenhoven WB, Jude JR, Knickerbocker GG. Closed-chest cardiac massage. JAMA 1960;173:1064.
96. Kubler-Ross E. On Death and Dying. New York: Macmillan, 1970.
97. Lane v Candura, 6 Mass. App 377 (1978).
98. LaPuma J, Silverstein MD, Stocking CB, Roland D, Siegler M. Life-sustaining treatment: a prospective study of patients with DNR orders in a teaching hospital. Arch Intern Med 1988;148:2193.
99. Leenen HJJ. Euthanasia, assistance to suicide and the law: developments in The Netherlands. Health Policy 1987;8:197.
100. Lemire JG, Johnson AL. Is cardiac resuscitation worthwhile? A decade of experience. N Engl J Med 1972;286:970.
101. Liberthson RR, Nagel EL, Hirschman JC, Nussenfeld SR. Prehospital ventricular defibrillation: prognosis and follow-up course. N Engl J Med 1974;291:317.
102. Lidz CW, Meisel A, Osterweis M, et al. Barriers to informed consent. Ann Intern Med 1983;99:539.
103. Logstreth WT, Cobb LA, Fahrenbruch CE, Copass MK. Does age affect outcomes of out-of-hospital cardiopulmonary resuscitation? JAMA 1990;264:2109.
104. Lydston GF. The surgical commission man and surgical canvassing. Philadelphia Med J 1899;4:837.
105. Lynn J, Childress JF. Must patients always be given food and water? Hastings Cent Rep 1983;13:17.
106. Macklin R. Mortal Choices. New York: Pantheon, 1987.
107. Marzuk PM. The right kind of paternalism. N Engl J Med 1985;313:1474.
108. Mass Gen Stat, Ch III. Section 70E (1979).
109. Meisel A, Kabnick LD. Informed consent to medical treatment: an analysis of recent legislation. Univ Pitt L Rev 1980;41:407.
110. Meisel A, Roth LH. Toward an informed discussion of informed consent: a review and critique of the empirical studies. Ariz L Rev 1983;25:265.
111. Meisel A. The "exceptions" to the informed consent doctrine: striking a balance between competing values in medical decision making. Wisc L Rev 1979;2:413.
112. Messert B, Quaglieri CE. Cardiopulmonary resuscitation: perspectives and problems. Lancet 1976;ii:410.
113. Micetich KC, Steinecker PH, Thomasma DC. Are intravenous fluids morally required for dying patients? Arch Intern Med 1983;143:975.
114. Miles SH. Informed demand for "non-beneficial" medical treatment. N Engl J Med 1991;325:512.
115. Miles SH, Cranford R, Schultz AL. The do-not-resuscitate order in a teaching hospital: considerations and a suggested policy. Ann Intern Med 1982;96:660.
116. Mitchell JM, Sunshine JH. Consequences of physicians' ownership of health care facilities—joint ventures in radiation therapy. N Engl J Med 1992;327:1497.
117. Mitchell JM, Scott E. New evidence of the prevalence and scope of physician joint ventures. JAMA 1992;268:80.
118. Mitchell JM, Scott E. Physician ownership of physical therapy services: effects on charges, utilization, profits, and service characteristics. JAMA 1992;268:2055.
119. Monaco GP. Informed consent: does the consent process reflect the realities of current treatment, procedures, and side effects? Am J Pediatr Hematol Oncol 1983;5: 401.
120. Morreim EH. Balancing act: the new medical ethics of medicine's economics. Boston: Kluwer, 1991.
121. Morreim EH. Conflicts of interest: profits and problems in physician referrals. JAMA 1989;262:390.
122. Murphy DJ, Murray AM, Robinson BE, Campion EW. Outcomes of cardiopulmonary resuscitation in the elderly. Ann Intern Med 1989;111:199.
123. Murphy DJ, Burrows D, Santilli S, Kemp AW, Tenner S, Kreling B, Teno J. The influence of the probability of survival on patients' preferences regarding cardiopulmonary resuscitation. N Engl J Med 1994;330:545.
124. Muss HB, White DR, Michielutte R, et al. Written informed consent in patients with breast cancer. Cancer 1979;43:1549.
125. Natanson v Kline, 186 Kan. 393 (1960).
126. Novack DH, Plumer R, Smith RL, et al. Changes in physicians' attitudes toward telling the cancer patient. JAMA 1979;241:897.
127. Office of Inspector General. Financial arrangements between physicians and health care businesses. Washington DC: Department of Health and Human Services, 1989.
128. Office of Technology Assessment. Life-sustaining technologies and the elderly. Washington DC: Government Printing Office, July 1987.
129. Oken D. What to tell cancer patients: a study of medical attitudes. JAMA 1961;175: 1120.
129a. Oregon Death with Dignity Act, 1994.
130. Overmyer M. National Survey: physicians' views on the right to die. Physicians Management 1991;31:40.
131. Patenaude AF, Rappeport JM, Smith BR. The physician's influence on informed consent for bone marrow transplantation. Theoret Med 1986;7:165.
132. Peatfield RC, Taylor D, Sillett RW, McNicol MW. Survival after cardiac arrest in hospital. Lancet 1977;i:1223.
133. Pence GE. Do not go slowly into that dark night: mercy killing in Holland. Am J Med 1988;84:139.
134. Penman DT, Holland JC, Bahna GF, et al. Informed consent for investigational chemotherapy: patients' and physicians' perceptions. J Clin Oncol 1984;2:849.
135. Physician Payment Review Commission Arrangements between Managed Care Plans and Physicians: Results from a 1994 Survey of Managed Care Plans. Washington DC: PPRC, Feb 7, 1995.
136. Pope Pius XII. The Prolongation of Life. Reprinted in Ethics in Medicine. Edited by SJ Reiser, AJ Dyck, WJ Curran. Cambridge: MIT Press, 1977, pp 501–504.
137. Poses RM, Bekes C, Copare FJ, Scott WE. The answer to "What are my chances, doctor?" depends on whom is asked: prognostic disagreement and inaccuracy for critically ill patients. Crit Care Med 1989;17:827.
138. President's Commission for the Study of Ethical Problems in Medicine and Biomedical and Behavioral Research. Deciding to forego life-sustaining treatment. Washington DC: Government Printing Office, 1983.
139. President's Commission for the Study of Ethical Problems in Medicine and Biomedical and Behavioral Research. Securing access to health care. Washington DC: Government Printing Office, 1983.
140. President's Commission for the Study of Ethical Problems in Medicine and Biomedical and Behavioral Research. Splicing life. Washington DC: Government Printing Office, 1982.
141. Rabkin MT, Gillerman G, Rice NR. Orders not to resuscitate. N Engl J Med 1976;295: 364.
142. Rachels J. The End of Life: Euthanasia and Morality. New York: Oxford University Press, 1986.
143. Rajagopal S, Goodman PJ, Tannock IF. Adjuvant chemotherapy for breast cancer: discordance between physicians' perception of benefit and the results of clinical trials. J Clin Oncol 1994;12:1296.
144. Relman AS. Michigan's sensible "living will." N Engl J Med 1979;300:1270.
145. Relman AS. Dealing with conflicts of interest. N Engl J Med 1984;310:1182.
146. Relman AS. The new medical-industrial complex. N Engl J Med 1980;303:963.
147. Rodwin M. Medicine, Money and Morals. New York: Oxford University Press, 1993.
148. Rosenberg M, Wang C, Hoffman-Wilde S, Hickham D. Results of cardiopulmonary resuscitation: failure to predict survival in two community hospitals. Arch Intern Med 1993;153:1370.
149. Ryan KJ. Tradition and change in the teaching of bioethics: observations from the field. Harvard Medical Alumni Bulletin 1986;60:25.
150. Salgo v Leland Stanford Jr, University Board of Trustees 317 P.2d 170 (1957).
151. Saphir R. External cardiac massage: prospective analysis of 123 cases and review of the literature. Medicine (Balt) 1968;47:73.
152. Schloendorff v Society of New York Hospitals, 211 N.Y. 125 (1914).
153. Schwartz R, Grubb A. Why Britain can't afford informed consent. Hastings Center Rep 1985;15:19.
154. Scott RPF. Cardiopulmonary resuscitation in a teaching hospital: a survey of cardiac arrests occurring outside intensive care units and emergency rooms. Anaesthesia 1981;36:526.
155. Shapiro RS, Derse AR, Gottlieb M, Schiedermayer D, Olson M. Willingness to perform euthanasia:a survey of physician attitudes. Arch Intern Med 1994;154:575.
156. Shmerling RH, Bedell SE, Lillienfeld A, Delbanco TL. Discussing cardiopulmonary resuscitation: a study of elderly outpatients. J Gen Intern Med 1988;3:317.
157. Shultz M. Informed consent: a symbol analyzed. Hastings Center Rep.
158. Siegler M. The progression of medicine from patient paternalism to patient autonomy to bureaucratic parsimony. Arch Intern Med 1985;145:713.
159. Silber TJ. Introduction: bioethics and the pediatrician. Pediatr Ann 1981;10:381.

160. Singer PA, Siegler M. Euthanasia—A critique. N Engl J Med 1990;322:1881.
161. Slater v Baker & Stapelton, 95 Eng. Rep. 860 (K.B. 1767).
162. Society for the Right to Die. The First Fifty Years: 1938–1988. New York: Society for the Right to Die, 1988.
163. Standards for cardiopulmonary resuscitation and emergency cardiac care V. Medicolegal considerations and recommendations. JAMA 1974;227(suppl):864.
164. Steiber SR. Right to die: public balks at deciding for others. Hospitals 1987;61:72.
165. Steinbrook R, Lo B. Decision making for incompetent patients by designated proxy: California's new law. N Engl J Med 1984;310:1598.
166. Steinbrook R, Lo B, Moulton J, Saika G, Hollander H, Volberding PA. Preferences of homosexual men with AIDS for life-sustaining treatment. N Engl J Med 1986;314:457.
167. Stolman CJ, Gregory JJ, Cunn D, Levine JL. Evaluation of patient, physician, nurse, and family attitudes toward do not resuscitate orders. Arch Intern Med 1990;150:653.
168. Superintendent of Belchertown v Saikewicz, 373 Mass. 728 (1977).
169. Taffet GE, Teasdale TA, Luchi RJ. In-hospital cardiopulmonary resuscitation. JAMA 1988;260:2069.
170. Thompson DF. Understanding financial conflicts of interest. N Engl J Med 1993;329:573.
171. Tomlinson T, Brody H. Ethics and communication in do-not-resuscitate orders. N Engl J Med 1988;318:43.
172. Truman v Thomas, 165 Cal Rptr 308 (1980).
173. Twycross RG. Assisted death: a reply. Lancet 1990;ii:796.
174. Uhlmann RF, Cassel CK, McDonald WJ. Some treatment-withholding implications of no-code orders in an academic hospital. Crit Care Med 1984;12:879.
175. Uhlmann RF, Pearlman RA, Cain KC. Physicians and spouses' predictions of elderly patients' resuscitation preferences. J Gerontol 1988;43:m115.
176. Van der Maas PJ, van Delden JJM, Pinjnenborg L, Looman CWN. Euthanasia and other medical decisions concerning the end of life. Lancet 1991;338:669.
177. Veatch RMA. Theory of Medical Ethics. New York: Basic Books, 1981.
178. Veatch RM. DRGs and the ethical reallocation of resources. Hastings Center Rep 1986;16:32.
179. Vitelli CE, Cooper K, Rogatoko A, Brennan MF. Cardiopulmonary resuscitation and the patient with cancer. J Clin Oncol 1991;9:111.
180. Wachter RM, Luce JM, Hearst N, Lo B. Decisions about resuscitation: inequities among patients with different diseases but similar prognoses. Ann Intern Med 1989;111:525.
181. Wagner A. Cardiopulmonary resuscitation in the aged: a prospective survey. N Engl J Med 1984;310:1129.
182. Waldholz M. Warm bodies: doctor-owned labs earn lavish profits in a captive market. Wall Street Journal, March 1989;1:A1,6.
183. Wanzer SH, Adelstein SJ, Cranford RE, et al. The physician's responsibility toward hopelessly ill patients. N Engl J Med 1984;310:955.
184. Wanzer SH, Federman DD, Adelstein SJ, et al. The physician's responsibility toward hopelessly ill patients: a second look. N Engl J Med 1989;320:844.
185. Warren JW, Sobal J, Tenney JH, et al. Informed consent by proxy: an issue in research with elderly patients. N Engl J Med 1986;315:1124.
186. Weatherall DJ. The New Genetics and Clinical Practice, 2nd ed. New York: Oxford University Press, 1985.
187. Weir RF, Gostin L. Decisions to abate life-sustaining treatment for nonautonomous patients. JAMA 1990;264:1846.
188. White DR, Muss HB, Michielutte R, et al. Informed consent: patient information forms in chemotherapy trials. Am J Clin Oncol 1984;7:183.
189. Wolf SM. Holding the line on euthanasia. Hastings Center Rep 1989;19:13.
190. Youngner SJ, Lewandowski W, McClish DK, Juknialis BW, Coulton C, Bartlett ET. "Do not resuscitate" orders: incidence and implications in a medical intensive care unit. JAMA 1985;253:54.
191. Zweibel NR, Cassel CK. Treatment choices at the end of life: a comparison of decisions by older patients and their physician-selected proxies. Gerontologist 1989;29:615.
192. 45 CFR section 46.116 (1983).

CHAPTER 92

Legal Aspects of Cancer

JOSEPH TARASKA

Introduction

Today, the physician who works with the diagnosis or treatment of cancer has a difficult dilemma. On the one hand, a patient's expectations regarding the discovery and cure of his or her disease often are at odds with the realities of cancer (1). These expectations are fueled by communications suggesting that early detection means cure. This perception combines with society's general belief that modern technology provides all of the answers. Patients are familiar with such wondrous advances as mammography, CTs, MRIs, chemotherapy, and radiation/oncology. As a result, they come to the physician with the hope, and often the expectation, that he or she will be able to save them. Despite progress in the detection and treatment of cancer, this disease unfortunately often still is beyond medicine's reach. This "box" around the physician is further aggravated by the movement of medicine to the managed-care setting. Physicians are caught in a struggle to provide each patient with as much time and attention as possible while also facing the realities of cost, care, reimbursement schedules, and a system that seems to discourage participation and follow-up by the specialist.

Nowhere is this dilemma reflected more clearly than in the statistics relating to medical malpractice claims brought against physicians. One reliable source of such statistics is the Physician Insurers Association of America, an organization that is comprised of professional liability insurers owned or managed by physicians. This association has been engaged in a data-sharing project through which it has collected such statistics since 1985; as of the early 1990s, they had evaluated over 70,000 claims (2). Of particular interest is that when determining which patient conditions lead to the most claims being filed, cancer of the breast, of the bronchus or lung, and of the colon or large intestine made the Top 20 list. As might be expected, these, along with cancer of the rectum or anus, also were in the Top 20 conditions resulting in the largest pay-outs by malpractice insurers (3). In fact, according to these studies, the top five misdiagnosed conditions were: (*a*) breast cancer, (*b*) cancer of the bronchus and lung, (*c*) appendicitis, (*d*) acute myocardial infarction, and (*e*) ectopic pregnancy (4).

The statistics are not all bad, however. Fully two-thirds of all malpractice claims brought against physicians are resolved without payment of any indemnity by the physician or carrier. Unfortunately, the other one-third result in significant indemnities and disruption to the life and practice of the physician. This chapter is designed to assist the physician whose practice involves the diagnosis and treatment of cancer to gain an understanding of the legal process as it relates to the commonly encountered problems in this field. With this understanding, it is hoped that the physician will be better able to avoid entanglements in the legal system and so devote him- or herself more fully to the patients.

This chapter begins by discussing the elements of a medical malpractice claim. It continues with a section on preventing the most commonly encountered problems for physicians who deal with cancer, and it concludes with sections on managed care as it affects the cancer specialist and the developing law regarding euthanasia.

The Elements of Liability

In the U.S. judicial system, the same elements must be proven to establish a right to recovery, regardless of the nature of the claim. These are: (*a*) a duty existed which was breached, (*b*) the breach caused an injury, and (*c*) an injury, in fact, resulted. Despite the fact that these elements are the same for all claims, however, the necessary proof to establish these elements in cases involving cancer may vary because of the particular characteristics of this area of medicine.

THE STANDARD OF CARE

The first element, breach of duty, more commonly is referred to as failure to abide by the applicable "standard of care." In most jurisdictions, instructions are given to the jury against which they measure the facts and determine if a breach occurred (5).

The first question this instruction raises is: Who establishes the standard of care? Because of the complexity of medicine, it is almost universally held that jurors may not create the standard to which doctors are held; rather, jurors must apply the standard that is recognized by the medical profession. This standard generally is established through expert testimony. Unfortunately, litigation often is seen as a battle of experts, wherein the jury is left to measure the credibility of two competing viewpoints. As might be expected, this at times leads to confusion in a juror's mind. Medicine is not static, and the overlap between competing schools of thought or evolution from a prior practice to a more current approach creates a gray zone wherein most litigation of this nature occurs. The only remedy for the physician is to stay constantly informed about developing practice parameters and understand when to refer patients to those with greater expertise. If the physician elects to provide treatment in an area not usually managed by those with his or her training, the physician may be held to the standard of the specialist whose role has been assumed.

The question of who is qualified to act as an expert often creates intense argument at trial. It seems logical that an oncologist should be called to testify against an oncologist or a radiologist against a radiologist; however, this is not the norm. In most jurisdictions, if an expert can demonstrate an understanding of the appropriate standard of care, either through training, practice, or association with those in the field, he or she often is given the latitude to testify. It then is up to opposing counsel to assist the jury in weighing the credibility of this testimony by demonstrating any shortfalls that individual may have in his or her understanding of the relevant medical practice. This general practice is illustrated by a recently litigated case in Florida (6). In that circumstance, a surgeon was charged with failure to diagnose breast cancer in a timely manner. The expert called against him was an oncologist, who testified that he was involved in breast cancer screening as well as teaching breast self-examination to patients. He also noted that he regularly referred patients to surgeons and was knowledgeable about when a surgeon should perform a biopsy. Even though this expert conceded that the surgeon made the ultimate decision, the appellate court held that he had sufficient knowledge to qualify as an "expert" on the standard of care that is expected from the surgeon.

In addition to the use of expert testimony, counsel often attempts to establish the standard of care by referring to general medical literature and practice parameters. For example, a joint effort by the American Colleges of Radiology, Surgeons, Pathologists, and the Society of Surgical Oncology has resulted in a practice guideline for breast conservation treatment against which one's actual practice may be measured (7). Although most jurisdictions currently hold that such literature and guidelines, if established as authoritative, may be introduced as evidence for the standard of care, they are not considered to be dispositive of that issue. The usual practice is to preclude the introduction of such parameters to establish the standard but to allow it in cross-examination and impeachment of the opposing side's expert. In this fashion, the jury has the benefit of the standards when measuring the testimony of an expert and may consider them as they deem appropriate (8).

There is, however, a concerted effort to expand the use of such guidelines in the defense of malpractice cases. Maine, for example, has established an experimental project to analyze whether practice parameters are useful in resolving such claims (9). Under the Maine statute, patients would not be allowed to use practice parameters as proof of their claim; however, the physician would be allowed to introduce the guidelines as a defense in such actions. The rationale for allowing their use in what at first appears to be an inequitable balance between the patient and physician is that doing otherwise would inhibit the development of such standards. Understanding that these standards are static, physicians would be unlikely to promote them if they were applied against them. For the foreseeable future, practitioners can expect that literature and practice guidelines will continue to be used as evidence of, but not in and of themselves, the appropriate standard. Therefore, it is imperative that physicians remain current on the literature in their field, including practice guidelines. This does not mean they should blindly follow such guidelines, however. Rather, they should rely, as they always have, on their training, experience, interaction with peers, and knowledge of the literature in determining the appropriate care for each patient.

A final point to consider is whether the standard of care is that of the physician's own community or a more broadly based standard. In earlier times, the standard was that of each physician's local community. This was necessitated by the often significant difference in facilities and equipment from one community to another and the rather laborious dissemination of medical information. With the advent of mass communication and educational techniques as well as the proliferation of technology to some of the most remote U.S. communities, the local standard recently has given way to a national standard of care. This is best evidenced by Board examinations, which are national in scope. As a result, physicians can expect that the standard to which they must adhere will be that normally accepted in the country.

CAUSATION

As stated previously, not only must there be a breach of the appropriate standard of care to impose liability, that breach must be causally related to an injury. In legal terminology, the words *proximate cause* generally are used. This was discussed most eloquently by a prominent legal scholar who wrote:

> In a philosophic sense, the consequences of an act go forward to eternity, and the causes of an event go back to the dawn of human events and beyond. But any attempt to impose responsibility on such a basis would result in infinite liability for all wrongful acts, and would "set society on edge and fill the courts with endless litigation." As a practical matter, legal responsibility must be limited to those causes which are so closely connected with the result and with such significance that the law is justified in imposing liability. Some boundary must be set to liability for the consequences of an act, upon the basis of some social idea of justice or policy (10).

In applying this concept, most jurisdictions now require proof that "but for" the act, the injury would not have occurred. This test is explained most clearly in jury instructions such as the following:

> Negligence is a legal cause of injury if it directly in a natural and continuous sequence produces or contributes substantially to producing such injury, so that it can reasonably be said that but for the negligence, the injury would not have occurred (11).

When following this instruction, a jury could not impose liability in most instances, unless it determined that the act had probably (interpreted as a greater than 50% chance) caused the injury. Cancer cases, however, present a complicating factor that recently led to the application by some courts of a more inclusive test; this has occurred because of the nature of the disease itself. In many cases, a patient may have started out with a less than 50% chance of survival. Although negligence may have occurred, there was never a greater than 50% chance that the patient would survive. That now has been reduced to less than 50%. As a result, some jurisdictions have allowed recovery for a "lost chance of survival," regardless of how small the chance was initially (12). Courts that continue to follow the traditional approach opine that lowering the standard would require health-care providers to defend claims arising out of inevitably unfavorable results. Those that follow the more expansive approach rationalize their view by asserting that recovery is not based on the fact that the act caused death but rather that it caused a decreased opportunity for survival. An example of the application of this expanded rule occurred in 1988 (13), in which a man sought medical therapy for gastric difficulties. Although he was suffering from gastric cancer at the time, it was not diagnosed, and he ultimately died 18 months later. The testimony at trial was that he had only a 30% chance of cure at the outset. In considering this, the court noted that

> medical science has given patients real chances to recover, sometimes only a small chance, but still a chance, in circumstances that used to be hopeless. When patients go to the doctor with serious illnesses, they expect to have those chances that medical science has provided (14).

Even though it could not be said in this circumstance that the failure to diagnose caused the death it did in the court's opinion decrease the chance of survival, which was compensatable.

Regardless of the rule that is applied, cancer cases have become a statistic battleground. To properly defend him- or herself, the physician must seek out and present a statistical analysis that most accurately reflects the state of medical knowledge.

DAMAGES

The final element establishing liability is damages. In other words, if the act fell below the acceptable standards, it must have resulted in an injury or loss. Such damages are uniformly divided into compensatory and punitive. Compensatory damages are those meant to compensate an individual for a loss and are measured by the value of that loss. Punitive damages, however, have no relationship to the loss but are intended simply to punish or deter conduct that society deems to be outrageous. As might be expected, the type of act that is necessary to support this form of compensation is significantly greater than simple negligence, and it generally requires that the act be so wanton or reckless as to be considered intentional. Such is seldom seen in these cases.

Compensatory damages, on the other hand, have seen expanded application in litigation involving cancer. One example is the recovery that was allowed for "lost chance of survival" discussed earlier. Fortunately, a number of courts adopting this more inclusive test tend to ameliorate the rather harsh result that occurs when compensation is allowed and there was never a probability of survival. They accomplish this by limiting the amount recovered to less than the value of all damages that flowed from the death. For example, if a 30% loss in the chance for survival occurred, the injured party may only be entitled to recover 30% of all damages related to his death (15).

Some courts also have expanded the traditional concept of mental anguish in cancer cases. One example occurred in a case where a patient was referred to an oncologist to discuss chemotherapy after a mastectomy to remove a breast cancer (16). A recommendation was made to use chemotherapy, thereby increasing her chances of avoiding a recurrence of the cancer. The patient agreed, and a dosage of Cytoxan calculated by the physician's nurse was administered. The calculation turned out to be in error and, in fact, called for five times the appropriate dose. Although the calculation was checked by the physician, the error was not caught. On a return visit to the physician's office, the patient explained that she had become extremely ill and did not wish to continue the chemotherapy. The overdose was discovered at that time. Unfortunately, the medication had damaged the patient's bone marrow. The cancer ultimately did return and, because of the bone marrow impairment, could not be treated by chemotherapy. At trial, the patient was unable to demonstrate that the Cytoxan was related in any way to the recurrence of the cancer. She did, however, demonstrate an injury to her bone marrow. The court found that her mental anguish could reasonably have been increased by the knowledge that her plight was now hopeless in that she could no longer be treated with chemotherapy for this condition.

In most circumstances, there must be some physical injury or impact from which mental anguish arises before a court will allow a claim for mental anguish, however it is described. This helps to discourage fraudulent claims. In the case discussed here, there was a physical injury (i.e., damage to the bone marrow) from which the emotional stress arose. There have, however, been exceptions to this general rule. Although not universally recognized, one such exception has been noted where a diagnosis of cancer is made and no cancer actually existed, thus causing emotional distress. A case where a dentist observed a lesion on the roof of a patient's mouth is illustrative (9). He performed a biopsy; although no cancer was noted in the specimen, the dentist referred the patient to an oral surgeon. The oral surgeon advised the patient there was a 50% chance that she was suffering from lethal midline granuloma, which is a rapidly growing form of cancer that may result in death. Ultimately, it was determined that no cancer existed. The patient sought recovery for "cancer phobia." The court noted there had been expert testimony that the dentist deviated from acceptable standards in telling the patient she had cancer when his own test results were negative. It then was reasoned that it was foreseeable to expect that a mistaken diagnosis of cancer would result in emotional harm to the patient.

Such cases place the physician in an awkward circumstance. The physician cannot avoid the responsibility of communicating his or her opinion to the patient. If that communication is not based on sufficient information, however, it may be the basis for a cause of action and damages. The lesson is that when imparting the diagnosis of cancer, the physician should take reasonable steps to ensure that the diagnosis has a medical basis and include this in the discussion.

Preventing Legal Complications

A physician's time is best spent in medical endeavors and time taken away from these activities can only operate to the detriment of the public. Unfortunately, physicians today find themselves embroiled with the law to the extent that it often absorbs an inordinate amount of time and saps their enthusiasm for interaction with patients. For this reason, a physician should endeavor to understand the interface between the law and his or her practice. Once this is accomplished, especially in those areas that most commonly produce difficulties, the physician will find that time spent on the legal ramifications of medicine is sharply reduced. This section discusses the most commonly occurring difficulties for physicians whose practice includes cancer medicine.

THE DOCTOR/PATIENT RELATIONSHIP

It generally is acknowledged that a physician has no duty, absent constitutional or statutory requirements, to render care unless he or she has agreed to do so. This premise was brought to us through the common law and serves as a foundation of U.S. jurisprudence. A physician may find, however, that he or she has created a doctor/patient relationship and thus is obligated to care for the patient even when the physician had not thought that he or she had done so.

The most common manner in which the doctor/patient relationship is created is by express agreement. The physician simply agrees to render medical care and attention, and the patient consents to that relationship. Traditionally, this occurs when the patient presents him- or herself to the physician's office or the physician consults on the patient while in a medical facility. This relationship also can arise, however, where a physician has contracted with an entity that provides medical care to a group of patients. For example, hospital by-laws often provide that a staff physician cover the emergency room on an on-call basis. This often is considered a contract between the physician and the hospital and patients are considered to be third-party beneficiaries of this contract. As such, a patient who presents to the emergency room may claim the benefit of that contract. In other words, because the on-call physician has been contacted, he or she generally is responsible to make a determination as to whether further evaluation is required and, if so, to provide that evaluation until the patient either is stable or referred to another physician or entity. Without the contractual arrangement (in this instance, the by-laws) the duty does not exist.

A question that often arises with specialists is whether an appointment made by a patient to see the physician in and of itself creates a doctor/patient relationship. Generally, such a call only implies that the doctor has agreed the patient may come to the office so that he or she can determine whether they will enter into such a relationship. This can be altered, however, depending on the manner in which the appointment is made. Such a circumstance may arise where the patient provides his or her clinical history by phone to the doctor's office and it is apparent he or she has an acute illness that requires urgent care. If an appointment is made in this circumstance, the lines blur as to whether there was an agreement to treat that illness. As such, it is better to go forward and commence the relationship, using a legally sufficient manner to terminate the relationship when appropriate. Of course, the one exception to this is if the requested therapy is beyond the capabilities of the physician. In this circumstance, there is no obligation to treat, but the physician should assist in making arrangements for follow-up care with another physician.

Casual encounters are fraught with potential difficulties. Every physician has been in a situation where a friend or acquaintance asks for medical advice in an informal setting. This may be as innocent as asking the physician to look at an unusual mole or listen to a particularly bothersome cough. Although it is difficult to disengage from such conversations, this is the more prudent course. If one listens to such complaints and gives advice, it may be assumed that a doctor/patient relationship has been created; it is not necessary that compensation change hands. The better course in such circumstances is to advise the patient that perhaps he or she should come to your office, or that of another physician, for a full medical evaluation of the difficulty.

Informal conversations with a patient generally are not considered in the same light as an informal conversation with another physician. Generally, when one physician informally discusses his or her patient with a second physician, and there is no agreement for the second physician to undertake care of the patient or provide a formal consult, no doctor/patient relationship has been created (18). To hold otherwise would severely hamper the free flow of information between physicians. Each must have the opportunity to discuss with peers the conduct of their profession. This same circumstance applies when various cases are presented for educational reasons, whether in a school environment or hospital meeting (e.g., tumor boards) (19). This, however, must be clearly distinguished from a formal consultation. Such can occur face to face, through a note in the hospital chart, or by phone. The distinguishing line is where the physician consulted understands that he or she is being engaged to provide a professional opinion for the medical care and attention of a patient.

Another question that often is encountered by those who specialize in cancer therapy is whether the patient who once was seen by the physician can claim the benefit of that doctor/patient relationship for all time. In other words, does a relationship, once started, continue in perpetuity? In most areas of medical practice, the line is fairly clear. Once a patient begins treatment for an acute illness, the relationship between patient and physician continues until the illness subsides or one party withdraws from the arrangement in a legally sufficient manner. This line may not, however, be as clear when treating cancer, which has the potential for long-term therapy, follow-up, and recurrence. For this reason, it is imperative that the physician clarify his or her expected role with the patient. In the event there has been no understanding with regard to future care and the patient seeks care from the physician, the physician should make a determination regarding whether an acute or unstable situation exists. If the patient is unstable, the appropriate course is to assist the patient in stabilizing and then to assure that he or she is transferred to another physician if one does not wish to continue care.

TERMINATING THE DOCTOR/PATIENT RELATIONSHIP

Once the doctor/patient relationship has begun, a physician may not abandon the patient without incurring liability. Terminating the relationship usually requires either a mutual agreement of the parties, the patient deciding to withdraw from the physician's care, or the physician making a unilateral decision to withdraw in a manner that complies with legal requirements.

When making this determination, the circumstance that created the relationship must first be analyzed. If there was a contract to render care, the physician may not be able to withdraw. For example, as noted earlier, hospital staff by-laws create an obligation for an on-call specialist to attend when called by the emergency-room physician. Unless the by-laws provide a method in which this relationship may be avoided, the physician may have no choice but to attend. This does not, however, require that he or she continue to care for the patient. In such circumstances, the physician's only obligation generally is to attend during the immediate and unstable condition. The patient then may be referred to another physician for follow-up care. Similarly, in the case of managed-care contracts, the physician may not be allowed to terminate the relationship with a patient unless he or she follows the prerequisites of those contracts.

In most circumstances, the physician may elect to terminate for any reason that does not violate federal or state laws, such as those that prohibit discrimination. In doing so, however, there are general tenets that should be followed:

1. The physician should determine whether the patient's condition requires immediate attention. If so, the patient should be stabilized before terminating the relationship.
2. The patient should be made aware of the nature of his or her illness and, if required, that follow-up care is necessary.
3. The patient should be notified by the physician of his or her intent to withdraw from care as of a specific date.
4. The patient should be made aware that the physician will cover the patient for emergencies up to the date set out in the previous tenet.
5. If the physician wishes to provide a specific referral, that may be accomplished. He or she is under no obligation to do so, however, and may instead refer the patient to the general medical community. In this circumstance, the physician should make the patient aware of the type of medical specialist to be sought and cover the patient for a reasonable time.
6. The patient also should be informed that he or she is entitled to a copy of his or her medical records and that such will be provided or, if the patient prefers, to a subsequent treating physician on request (20).

These instructions may be made orally, but they should be followed up in writing. Perhaps the most practical method of documentation is simply to post a letter to the patient with this information at his or her last known address. As with all medical communications, the documents should be marked as personal and confidential and a copy kept with the chart.

Consent

It is axiomatic that touching an individual without consent is battery. If battery results, it is actionable. This theory of law generally has been applicable to the medical profession since the early 1900s (21); however, in the field of cancer, there has been increasing confusion with regard to obtaining informed consent. In part, this results from the nature of the disease itself, the evolving therapies that are available, and the role of the physician both as a treater of the disease and a researcher. In this regard, many questions have arisen, such as how much information patients with incurable diseases really wish to know, and whether it is counterproductive to disclose dismal prognoses; whether statistic data on morbidity or mortality are irrelevant to the individual patient's course; and whether the physician's personal interest, either through research or otherwise, should be disclosed to the patient. This section discusses these and other questions and, hopefully, will be instructive to the physician in avoiding the pitfalls that have been led to increased litigation.

As a starting point, it is necessary to understand that the basis for informed consent springs from four primary assumptions. These have been cogently outlined by an appellate court of California as follows:

1. ... patients are generally persons unlearned in the medical sciences and therefore, except in rare cases, courts may safely assume the knowledge of patient and physician are not in parity.
2. ... a person of adult years and in sound mind has the right, in the exercise of control over his own body, to determine whether or not to submit to lawful medical treatment.
3. ... the patient's consent to treatment, to be effective, must be an informed consent.
4. ... the patient being unlearned in medical sciences, has an abject dependence upon and trust in his physician for the information upon which he relies during the decisional process, thus raising an obligation in the physician that transcends arms' length transactions (22).

Applying these four assumptions requires an analysis of the following questions: who has the duty to obtain the consent of the patient, who has the right to give consent, what information must be imparted to form a basis on which consent may be predicated, and what exceptions exist to obtaining consent? Regarding the first question, it generally is accepted that the physician who performs the diagnostic procedure or therapy has the duty to obtain consent. Physicians may delegate this responsibility to others, but they cannot avoid the responsibility itself. For example, a physician may allow a resident or office personnel to explain a procedure and its risks to the patient; however, if information is incorrectly imparted, the physician will bear the responsibility for failing to obtain informed consent. This does not suggest that physicians should not use assistants in the technical aspects of consent, such as having the forms signed. However, the physician should participate in the direct communication with the patient when the essential information is imparted.

Another area of concern is whether a referring physician or the referred physician has the duty to obtain the party's consent. This may occur, for example, when a family-practice doctor sends a patient to a surgeon or oncologist for treatment of cancer. Courts that have reviewed this issue generally find that the obligation to obtain informed consent rests with the specialist who is to perform the procedure or render the care (23). This does not suggest that the referring physician should avoid discussion with the patient before referral. Rather, the referring physician should keep in mind that too detailed a discussion may confuse the patient if conflicting information is provided by the specialist who is to render the care.

The second question in obtaining informed consent is who has the right to give the consent. As a general rule, the competent adult whose health is at risk has the right to receive the information and provide consent. If this individual is not competent, however, then the physician must look to another. In those circumstances where a court has declared the individual to be incompetent and appointed another, this process is relatively easy. If the physician is unsure in this regard, he may contact the clerk of the local court, who will determine whether a guardian has been appointed. If the individual has not been declared to be incompetent but the physician nonetheless believes this may be the case, he or she has several options. The first, when time is not of the essence, is to advise the family that a judicial determination may need to be made and have them seek counsel for the appointment of an appropriate guardian. The second is to rely on consent of the next of kin; however, this is not universally accepted in that jurisdictions vary regarding who may consent under various circumstances. As a result, it is appropriate for the physician to consult legal counsel in this circumstance.

Another question often raised in the diagnosis and treatment of cancer is who has the authority to consent for a child. Parents generally hold this right, and the physician is justified in relying on them. As with other areas of the law, however, confusion may exist in certain circumstances. This most often occurs when the child (i.e., an individual under 18 years of age in most states) is mature. With greater frequency, courts are beginning to require that mature minors be involved in the decision-making process (24). Unfortunately, no bright line exists by which a physician can judge this circumstance. Rather, if he or she believes the minor is mature enough to understand the nature of the illness, the risks of providing or withholding therapy, and the likely results, then that minor should be involved in the process. Most cases that have addressed this area of the law have done so regarding children in their teenage years. Closely related to the circumstance of the mature minor is that of the emancipated minor. This generally is thought of as someone who is below the statutory age of adulthood but who, nonetheless, is living on his or her own and is self-sufficient. These minors usually are thought of as having the right to consent to their own care.

Once it has been determined which physician will obtain the consent and who has the right to give consent, the next concern is what information must be imparted. The consensus of most jurisdictions is that the following information should be included in discussion with the patient:

1. Nature of the patient's illness,
2. Nature of the proposed therapy,
3. Reasonable alternative therapies,
4. Chance of success with the proposed therapies,
5. Substantial risks inherent in the therapies, and
6. Risk of failing to undergo therapy for the illness (25).

When considering the quantum of information to be contained in these categories, courts have divided along two tracks. The first is to measure the quantum of information that reasonable physicians would provide to their patients under the same or similar circumstances. The second is to consider what a reasonable patient would want to know in making his or her determination (26). Regardless of which test is used, the best rule is for physicians to understand the information generally imparted by their peers and, additionally, to consider what they would like to know if in the patient's position attempting to make the decision. This combination of considerations generally will lead to an appropriate disclosure.

In considering the required disclosure, physicians who work in this area should be aware of a developing line of cases that may expand the quantum of information to be disclosed. This is illustrated by a recent Florida case, where the question was whether a duty existed on the part of a surgeon to advise a husband and wife that the wife's condition (medullary thyroid carcinoma) could be inherited by her children (27). Those courts that require such disclosures follow the line of cases imposing on psychiatrists a duty to warn certain individuals about a danger of harm from their patient (28) or to protect others from infectious diseases (29). Although in the Florida case, the court declined to hold the physician liable for failing to inform the parents, the better rule would be to advise if such risks of inheritability exist. In deciding such questions, courts generally seek to determine whether an injury was foreseeable and the injured person was in the zone of risk. In the case of inheritable diseases, the risk would seem to be foreseeable, and the children certainly would seem to be in the zone of danger.

There are, of course, exceptions to obtaining consent. In the realm of diagnosis and treatment for cancer, however, these are less common. The first is the emergency circumstance. Obviously, the law allows one to act in an emergency, if time would not permit obtaining an appropriate consent; it is presumed that the patient would consent. The second, which occurs in the rarest of circumstances, is the therapeutic privilege. As one court explained:

> ... patients occasionally become so ill or emotionally distraught on disclosure as to foreclose a rational decision, or complicate or hinder the treatment, or perhaps even pose psychological damage to the patient. Where that is so, the cases have generally held that the physician is armed with a privilege to keep the information from the patient, and we think it clear

> that portents of that type may justify the physician in action he deems medically warranted (30).

Even in this circumstance, however, the best rule to follow is that if the patient is not to be provided information for therapeutic reasons, then his or her next of kin should be given the information and provide consent for therapy.

Another line of cases examined whether physicians must disclose a personal interest when obtaining informed consent. Such interests may occur with research protocols, grants, and patents. The Supreme Court of California most recently addressed this issue (31); in that circumstance, a patient was undergoing treatment for hairy-cell leukemia. Because of the patient's particular blood type, the physicians were able, over a period of time, to develop a cell line from his blood that ultimately was patented by them. Unfortunately, they had neglected to tell the patient they were drawing blood for this purpose. In reviewing the matter, the court held that:

1. A physician must disclose personal interests unrelated to the patient's health, whether research or economic that may affect the physician's professional judgment; and
2. A physician's failure to disclose such interests may give rise to a cause of action for performing medical procedures without informed consent or breach of fiduciary duty (32).

In reaching this conclusion, the court noted that there may be conflicting loyalties under these circumstances. Physicians who add their own economic or research interests to the balance

> ... may be tempted to order a scientifically useful procedure or test that offers marginal, or no, benefit to the patient. The possibility that an interest extraneous to the patient's health has affected the physician's judgment is something that a reasonable patient would want to know in deciding whether to consent to a proposed course of treatment. It is material to the patient's decision and thus a prerequisite to informed consent (33).

Finally, a question also has been raised as to the proper role of statistical data in describing to a patient risks that are inherent in his or her disease and the success of proposed therapies. Most recently, this was considered by the Supreme Court of California (34); in this case, the patient was suffering from pancreatic cancer. Discussions were held with the patient concerning the use of a chemotherapy known as FAM (5-fluorouracil, Adriamycin, and mitomycin C) and radiation therapy. Apparently, this combination had shown some promise in treating pancreatic cancer in experimental trials at that time. (The patient's care was rendered in 1980.) Neither the operating surgeon nor the treating oncologist, however, disclosed to the patient the high statistical mortality rate that was associated with pancreatic cancer. The patient later testified that had he known, he would have chosen to forgo this therapy and, thus, improve the quality of his life over the time remaining. In considering the matter, the court noted that statistics are inherently unreliable in predicting the fate of an individual patient. As such, the court refused to mandate that statistical data regarding the mortality rate of a given cancer, be provided to a patient. In doing so, it did not preclude the physician from using this information; rather, it indicated that this question should be decided on a case-by-case basis, which might include statistical data depending on the circumstance (35). Considering the state of the law, no specific rule can be fashioned. Rather, as noted, the physician must consider this for each patient. It would seem, however, that caution is warranted, because such statistical data would seem to be relevant to most lay individuals.

As might be expected, some of the more traditional concepts of informed consent (e.g., which physician has the duty to obtain consent and which individual may provide consent) are remaining relatively static. With the development of new therapies, methods for measuring the success of those therapies, and participation of physicians in research, however, an evolution is occurring in the quantum of information that is expected to be imparted to the patient. As a result, legal counsel should be sought if confusion exists in the mind of the practitioner.

Documentation

A physician may practice medicine that is above reproach. If it is not appropriately documented, however, the patient may suffer if subsequent physicians are unable to understand the previous therapies. Additionally, the physician may find him- or herself in an untenable circumstance years later, unable to recall pertinent events and, thus, unable to defend his or her medical judgment.

Information must be recorded accurately and in a fashion that can be read. A simple mechanism for ensuring accuracy is to dictate notes, where possible, in front of the patient. If the note is incorrect, the patient is there, has heard the dictation, and may make the appropriate correction. There are, of course, circumstances when this is not advisable because of the sensitivity of the patient at that time.

A second significant problem area in accuracy concerns notes made by rounding nurses, interns, and residents on behalf of the responsible physician. Often, these are simply countersigned by the physician without reading and information contained therein becomes the reality at a subsequent time, regardless of its foundation in fact. It is nearly impossible for the physician to rebut this information when he or she has countersigned the note. The only remedy is to read notes before signing to ensure their accuracy.

The method of documenting medical information also should be reconsidered. Handwritten notes are susceptible to misinterpretation by others and, interestingly, often are unreadable even by the individual who made the notes. Printed notes, whether taken from handwritten copies or dictation, are preferable. This obviously is not possible on a hospital chart, but it is a recommended practice for the physician's own office notes.

The next consideration in documentation is what information should be maintained by a physician. You might think that only the record itself is relevant; however, if the physician is subsequently called to defend his actions, other source documents may be of assistance. These include office calendars, which frequently demonstrate appointment times, appointment cancellations, and other activities on critical dates. In addition, telephone logs recording long distance calls may provide immeasurable assistance, demonstrating that a call was in fact made, who originated the call, and the length of the call. It is not necessary to maintain all scratch pads and message information pads as long as the pertinent information has been transcribed into the medical record. It may be particularly helpful for a physician to maintain a message pad in his home, however, and, in today's world, in his car. A brief note as to the nature of the patient's complaint and the recommended course of action, including any prescriptions, can be jotted down at the time the phone call is made. These notes should be taken into the office on a routine basis and transcribed into the physician's office chart. Finally, in this age of computer-generated information, back-up disks should be preserved for all computer-generated medical records. The American Medical Association has provided a set of comprehensive guidelines that can be used by the physician to assist in ensuring the integrity of a computer system (36). Many physicians provide published material for their patients, and this may come from various journals, texts, or a manufacturer. Whatever the source, at least one copy should be maintained in a central file if these types of documents are provided to patients. Whether such information is provided also should be noted in the patient's chart. In this fashion, one will always be able to reconstruct information given to the patient. Finally, all information relating to any protocol in which the physician has participated should be maintained; these include the protocols themselves, interaction with the Institutional Review Board, and statistical compilations from those protocols made by the physician.

The next issue to be considered is how long a record must be maintained. Most jurisdictions have either statutes or regulatory guidelines on this matter; however, these time limits always should be considered as minimums. The driving rationale for the appropriate length of time actually should be based on two other considerations, the first of which is medical. The needs of the patient and subsequent treating physicians is of paramount importance. This does not suggest that records must be kept in perpetuity; rather, the physician will have to use reasonable judgment in making this determination. The second consideration is more susceptible to a defined time. Records should be kept at least for the length of time set out in the statute of limitations (i.e., the time limit during which suit may be brought against the physician). This will vary from one jurisdiction to another, but as noted, it is defined in each state. When calculating this time, the wisest starting point is the date of the last patient contact (37).

For Whose Acts Must the Physician Respond?

It generally is appreciated that physicians are responsible for their own acts and must answer if these are not within the acceptable standard of care. In this age of increased specialization and use of allied health professionals, however, physicians may find themselves responsible for the acts of numerous others. The first such category is the physicians' or their professional associations' employees and agents. The law has taken note of the fact that employees may not be able to respond adequately in damages for professional acts; as a result, the burden has been shifted to the employer, for public reasons. This does not mean that the employee escapes liability, only that the employer shares in that liability and may be held accountable.

This general rule of liability has been expanded to several other circumstances. A parent agency has been found to exist where there was no actual employment or agency relationship but the physician created a circumstance in which it appeared that such existed. For this to occur, it must appear to the public that the physician has held out that individual so that a patient could reasonably believe that individual was the agent or employee of the physician and that the patient relied to his or her detriment on that representation. This theory most frequently has been applied to hospitals, where it often is held that they are responsible for the acts of emergency room physicians, pathologists, and radiologists who the public believed were employees of the hospital. Regarding physicians, there are circumstances where independent laboratory, pharmaceutic, or other medical services may be performed on the physician's premises. In this circumstance, the public may reasonably believe that these are employees or agents of the physician, and responsibility may be established. To avoid this circumstance, the physician must make it clear, through signs and other disclosures, that these services are not being rendered by his or her employees or agents but are independent of the physician's practice.

Another expansion of the physician's or the professional association's liability has been brought under the theories of "Borrowed Servant" and "Captain of the Ship." Under the borrowed servant theory, it generally is held that if a physician uses the employee of another, such as a hospital nurse, intern, or resident, that person may become his or her servant for the purpose of the endeavor. This generally requires that the physician directly supervise the other individual in the manner in which the act is to be performed. For example, when a physician uses a rounding nurse or surgical assistant and, in detail, directs the acts of that individual, responsibility may attach. It generally would not cover, however, the circumstance where orders are left for nurses, residents, or interns, which they then carry out on their own with the medical training available to them (38). In that this line often is gray, the only advice for the practicing physician is to understand that a borrowed servant relationship may be found to exist and to exercise prudence when directing the acts of those working with him or her.

The captain of the ship doctrine really is an expansion of the borrowed servant rule. It was first enunciated in Pennsylvania in 1949 (39), and it has been fairly restricted to operating room circumstances, where it has been held in various states that the surgeon is responsible for everyone within the room. Fortunately, with the advent of various specialties, each specialist has come to be responsible for his or her own acts, and the doctrine has seen decreasing popularity in application by the courts (40). In its place, the court now looks to determine whether the individual practicing with the surgeon is an independently trained professional or is in fact acting under the direct supervision and guidance of the surgeon, thus making the individual a borrowed servant.

Another circumstance in which physicians who practice cancer medicine may find themselves is whether they are responsible for the acts of other specialists to whom they refer patients for consult or therapy. In this regard, it generally has been held that once a referral is made, and if there has not been negligence in selecting of the other physician (i.e., selecting someone when it is known that he is incompetent) then the initial physician will not be responsible for the acts of the other specialist. An example would be the question of whether an oncologist is liable for the side effects of chemotherapy when his or her decision to prescribe the medication was based on an inaccurate pathologic diagnosis. If no other information suggested to the oncologist that the diagnosis was incorrect, then one could expect in this circumstance that he or she would not be liable for the other in that the pathologist operates within a separate specialty (41). This same rationale is applicable to the interaction between radiologists, internists, and surgeons; each is responsible for his own acts. The only caveat is that if one does not use a consultant but rather takes on duties that normally are deemed to be part of another specialist's practice, then the initial physician may be judged by the standard of care applicable to the specialist. This does not imply that there cannot be overlap between the acts of two physicians in different medical specialties. Where overlap does occur, the rule has no application (42). It is only where the acts performed generally are not taken on by the physician that charges are brought. The obvious lesson from such cases is that physicians must be aware of their own capabilities and limitations and use consultants when the condition under consideration falls out of their own training. In fact, one of the leading causes of litigation in cancer medicine is delayed diagnosis. In many circumstances, this has been brought on by failure of an initial treating physician to refer the patient for consultation and further diagnostic studies by appropriate specialists.

The Physician as an Expert Witness

The system of U.S. jurisprudence that currently is used to resolve disputes in medical management is adversarial. Each side presents its point of view, supported by those with experience in the appropriate medical endeavor. These experts may, and often do, have opposite views. It then is within the province of the jury to attempt to resolve the dispute.

For as long as this system continues, it is essential that physicians who do qualify as having sufficient training and experience agree to review these matters and provide testimony where appropriate. If this does not occur, data may be presented to the jury which is not correct, thus resulting in an unjust result. This discussion focuses on the physician's role in this crucible of competing viewpoints.

A common question is whether a treating physician can be compelled to provide testimony. The judicial system allows either side to subpoena treating physicians to render their thoughts regarding the medical aspects of the case. The American Medical Association Council on Ethical and Judicial Affairs has in its Code of Medical Ethics supported this view. In so doing, the Council notes that although a physician should not become an advocate or partisan in legal proceedings, he or she has an ethical obligation to assist in the administration of justice by providing testimony regarding a patient when requested (43). This does not, however, open the floodgate to any question an attorney may seek to ask of the treating physician. Rather, physicians generally are allowed to limit their testimony to their own care and treatment as well as their thoughts regarding the prognosis of the patient. In most circumstances, they are not compelled to render expert opinions on hypothetical facts presented by either side, nor are they compelled to render testimony as to whether another physician deviated from the acceptable standards of care. They may elect to participate in this fashion but, as noted, generally are not compelled to do so.

The hypothetical expert is in a different category. This individual usually is retained by one side or the other because of a special expertise to comment on one or more aspects of the litigation (i.e., standard of care, proximate cause to injury, injuries suffered by the patient). If the physician elects to participate in this fashion, it should be with the full understanding that absent some advanced limitation, he or she will be expected to review the materials submitted as well as render testimony in discovery depositions and subsequently in a court proceeding. This is a significant commitment, and it should not be undertaken unless the physician is willing to complete the work once accepted. Otherwise, an unjust result may occur, because one side or the other is deprived of necessary testimony.

Once a physician has elected to participate, it is incumbent on him or her to request of the attorney submitting materials those documents that are required for testimony. The treating physician may need no more than his or her own records; however, the hypothetical expert is in a different circumstance. In most instances the expert's review should consist of the medical records of the treating physicians, hospitalization records, and deposition testimony of the various treating physicians and the patient. Although some physicians elect to forgo the testimony and base their opinions solely on the records, they should nonetheless review this testimony before appearing in court. Failing to do so subjects their opinion to an attack on credibility in that they may not have considered all of the relevant facts. In addition to a review of pertinent medical records and depositions, an expert should review his or her own medical literature on the subject in question. In today's arena of computer-assisted litigation, both sides may avail themselves of Med-line searches and often start with a search of all published literature by experts retained in the matter. This does not suggest that a physician's opinions may never change once published. However, the physician should be aware of his or her prior thoughts so that an adequate explanation of his or her current thinking, aside from the literature, can be given. Most experts who are adequately trained and experienced may not find it necessary to conduct a general review of all literature. This is a matter of personal preference and usually will not affect the case one way or the other. The only exception is that if a physician does consider a particular author, text, or journal article as being authoritative on a point, then that physician should review the same and be prepared to explain his or her own opinions if they diverge from those contained in that literature.

Managed Care

As the transition to managed care continues, there is an increased risk that patients may not receive the care they had expected or that is required, and that this disenchantment will be directed at the physicians who are tasked with providing the care. This is especially problematic for specialists. Managed care has the basic tenet that primary-care physicians screen patients, render care when possible, and make the decision as to whether a specialty referral is required. This limits referrals to specialists and deprives them of the opportunity for long-term follow-up, where they can establish a rapport with their patients and continually evaluate the course of therapy. Therefore, it is incumbent on the physician, whether primary care or specialist, to understand the most commonly occurring problems that are evolving so as to avoid being involved in the legal system while providing care.

Physicians always have been required to exercise independent medical judgment within the appropriate standards for their specialty. Payment on a fee-for-service basis has not significantly affected this working relationship; however, managed care offers reimbursement through capitation and distribution of funds when risk pools have not been depleted. This gives the appearance that avoiding the use of hospitalizations, specialists, or expensive diagnostic tests benefits the provider in a tangible way, but to date, attacks on this financial reimbursement system have not been successful (44). Rather, it has been noted that these types of plans have been favored by legislatures as a method to reduce costs and, therefore, benefit the public (45). In fact, it has been held by at least one appellate court that physicians do not have to disclose the existence of risk pools and reimbursement policies to their patients (46). Nonetheless, the appearance of impropriety may be sufficient to sway a jury when the issue is whether a physician should have used a specialty referral or diagnostic procedure. The plaintiff's argument would be that the physician's motive was to increase his or her income. There is no golden rule to assist the physician in avoiding this difficulty other than to be steadfast in exercising appropriate medical judgment. In other words, the physician must be vigilant in ensuring that he or she continues to use the health-care system as appropriate and not distinguish between those patients who are part of a managed-care program and those who are not.

This issue of referrals creates an additional difficulty. In most circumstances, physicians have established a referral pattern based on their comfort with the experience of the physicians to whom they refer patients. Under many managed-care programs, the choice of referrals is limited. In fact, the physician may not be acquainted with those listed by the managed-care entity. The preferred course for physicians to avoid difficulty is to become familiar with at least some of the physicians listed on the provider panel. If this is not possible, the physician should tell the patient before a referral that he or she does not know the qualifications of a panel member. In this circumstance, the patient then can make personal determination whether to rely on the managed-care entity's certification of these physicians or to seek further advice.

Another common difficulty that managed care exacerbates is the potential for misunderstanding who is to follow the patient. Managed-care entities using the "gatekeeper" system create a circumstance where patients are referred back and forth between physicians as authorization is required for further diagnostic studies or care. To avoid patients falling through the proverbial "crack," it is incumbent on both the primary-care physician and the specialist to ensure that the patient is being followed by one or the other. The best mechanism is for the physicians to correspond and, in that correspondence, set out their understanding with regard to who has the responsibility for follow-up. In addition, patients should be made aware of how the referral system works and instructed regarding their obligation to return to whichever physician is mandated under the system if they require further care. This conversation should be documented in the physician's medical record.

Recently, litigation also has focused on the the physician's duty to advocate on behalf of the patient (49). Although this area of the law is evolving, there already has been discussion suggesting that physicians will be under an increasing duty to seek approval for the medical attention they think is appropriate when the managed-care entity initially denies coverage. Of course, the extent to which a physician must go will vary under the circumstances; however, it seems clear that if coverage is denied and the physician believes this is inappropriate, he or she should at least follow the appellate procedure of the managed-care plan. Whether this is simply a phone conversation with a medical director or further written documentation on the need for care, as noted, depends on the circumstances. Most plans understand their own liability for refusing to authorize care that is strenuously recommended by a physician. As a result, advocacy often will inure to the patient's benefit. This most recently was seen in litigation involving high-dose chemotherapy with autologous bone marrow transplant for stage 4 metastatic breast cancer. A number of managed-care plans throughout the country have routinely denied this coverage, stating that it was experimental and, therefore, not authorized. There have, however, been a number of court decisions indicating this is not experimental therapy but rather is within the mainstream of cancer treatment (48). Such advocacy on behalf of the patient cannot help but to inure to the patient's benefit and, perhaps, change industry-wide perceptions as to what care is covered.

Withdrawing Life Support/Physician-Assisted Suicide and Euthanasia

Tracing the origin of laws pertaining to suicide is not an easy task; however, it does appear that some of the earliest writings on the subject appeared in Roman law. That body of law did not prohibit suicide, but it did enact a forfeiture of property by those who committed suicide to avoid criminal punishment (49). This seems to have been picked up in early English law. The early writings by Bracton in the 1200s summarized the law as follows:

1. If a man has slain himself after having committed a felony, and for the purpose of evading the punishment therefore, his lands escheat and his chattels are forfeited.
2. If he has brought death on himself "without any cause, through anger or ill will, as when he wished to hurt another, and could not fulfill what he wished," he is likewise to be punished with escheat of lands and forfeiture of goods.
3. If he commits suicide from "weariness of life or impatience of pain" his lands descend to his heir and his chattels only are to be confiscated.
4. If he was insane when he did the act that caused his death, or if he did it by accident he is to be held guiltless and forfeits nothing (50).

U.S. law has its roots in the early English common law; as a result, this history of the treatment of suicide also has found its way into the criminal law of this country. As noted by a more current scholar and author on the subject, it is the criminal treatment of suicide that is the basis for criminal sanctions against one who aids in the commission of suicide (51).

Since the early 1970s, there has been a great deal of judicial and legislative attention focused on how to deal with the patient, and those who assist the patient, in the withdrawal and/or withholding of life support. The seminal case was that of the New Jersey Supreme Court involving Karen Quinlan (52). This started a line of decisions that most recently brought us to the U.S. Supreme Court decision in *Cruzan* (53). The effect of these decisions has been to recognize the right of patients to refuse medical treatment even to the extent of withholding and/or withdrawing life support, including artificial nutrition and hydration. Additionally, the courts that have considered the matter have held that as the right exists, it should not be diminished upon the incompetence of the individual; therefore, substitute decision makers are allowed under various circumstances.

A distinction, however, has been drawn between the withdrawal/withholding of life support and physician-assisted suicide and euthanasia. The prior are considered to be as passive in nature, in that they simply allow nature to take its course. The latter two categories, however, are considered to be more active, in that they involve the participation of a physician either in prescribing medication or using medical devices to cause death.

These distinctions have been challenged most recently by Dr. Jack Kevorkian, who was convinced that Michigan had no laws that prohibited assisted suicide by a physician (54). Dr. Kevorkian initially used an IV line attached to a device that delivered saline solution, followed by the sedative thiopental, followed by potassium chloride. He eventually replaced this mechanism with the administration of carbon monoxide. His activities and those of Dr. Thomas Quill, a New York physician who prescribed sufficient barbiturates to cause death in his patient with the intent of reducing pain and allowing her to end her life, have increased public awareness and attempts at legislative change (55). The primary thrust of legislative change has come from the Hemlock Society, which has attempted through the initiative process, to have legislation voted on by the public. The first two such attempts were Washington State's Initiative 119 and California's Proposition 161. Neither was successful but they did form the basis of the subsequently successful Oregon Initiative. These two public initiatives used the phrase "physician aid-in-dying." In California, aid-in-dying was defined as

> a medical procedure that will terminate the lives of the qualified patient in a painless, humane and dignified manner, whether administered by the physician of the patient's choice or direction or whether the physician provides means to the patient for self-administration.

The Oregon Initiative probably was successful because of its more limited scope. Like Washington's, it applied to patients with less than 6 months to live, but it was further limited in that it allowed only prescriptions of lethal drugs. It was stated as follows:

> An adult who is capable, is a resident of Oregon, has been determined by the attending physician and consulting physician to be suffering from a terminal disease, and who has voluntarily expressed his or her wish to die, may make a written request for medication for the purpose of ending his or her life in a humane and dignified manner in accordance with this Act.

Some of the safeguards included the following:

1. The initial request for drug prescriptions had to be in writing and witnessed by two individuals concurring that the patient was competent.
2. At least two physicians had to concur that the patient was suffering from a terminal illness and was likely to die within 6 months.
3. In the event the patient was thought to be suffering from a psychiatric disorder, the patient would have to be referred for counseling.
4. Records had to be maintained and submitted annually to the Health Division of the state for review.
5. Two oral requests were required, separated by at least 15 days before a physician could accept the written request. Once accepted, the prescription could not be filled for 48 hours after the written request (56).

The constitutionality of the Oregon Initiative has been challenged, and until that is determined, it is being held in abeyance by an injunction issued by the court. Interestingly, statutes prohibiting physician-assisted suicide likewise are being challenged based on their constitutionality (57). Ultimately, the validity of these enactments either allowing or disallowing physician-assisted suicide will be determined by the courts. The most likely basis for the determination will be whether a constitutionally protected right to suicide and to assist in the suicide of a terminally ill patient exists. Those courts that favor such enactments see no distinction between refusals of treatment resulting in the withdrawing or withholding of life support, which has been protected by the courts, and physician-assisted suicide. Those opposed suggest that a distinction lies in the active/passive characterization of the acts. If such enactments are held to be constitutional, it can safely be assumed that safeguards such as those included in the legislation of most states allowing withdrawal and withholding of life support will be built in to protect against abuse. It also may be that a further distinction will be drawn between a physician providing the means for the patient to end his or her own life and the physician actually using those means on behalf of the patient. For example, the Oregon Initiative allows the prescription of medication that the patient would take; this is thought by some to be distinguishable from a physician actually injecting a lethal medication or using other devices to cause death.

In the event that physician-assisted suicide is held to be constitutional, one can anticipate that the laws of each state will vary regarding the appropriate safeguards. This would be consistent with the manner in which withdrawal and withholding of life support has evolved. For this reason, and because the law is quickly changing, physicians are encouraged to consult legal counsel in their individual jurisdictions.

References

1. Spratt J, Spratt S. Medical and legal implications of screening and follow-up procedures for breast cancer. Cancer 1990;66:1362.
2. Data Sharing Project, Physician Insurers Association of America, 65 S. Main Street, Building D, Pennington, NJ 08534–2827.
3. Id.
4. Id.; See also, Kern K. Causes of breast cancer malpractice litigation: a 20-Year Civil Court Review, Arch Surg 1992;127:542; and Kern K., Medical malpractice involving colon and rectal disease: a 20-Year Review of United States Civil Court Litigation, Dis Colon Rectum 1993;36:531.
5. Florida Standard Jury Instructions, 4.2(a), p 1.
6. Green v Goldberg, 630 So 2d 606 (Fla App 4th Dist. 1993).
7. Winchester D, Cox J. Standards for breast conservation treatment. Cancer J Clin 1992;42:134.
8. Hirschfield E. Should practice parameters be the standard of care in malpractice litigation. JAMA 1991;266:2886.
9. 24 ME Rev. Stat. §2906–2978; see also Garnick D, Hendricks A, Toryen B, Can practice guidelines reduce the number and costs of malpractice claims. JAMA 1991;266: 2856.
10. Prosser W, Keeton W. The Law of Torts, 264, 5th Ed. (1984) (footnote omitted).
11. Florida Standard Jury Instructions, 5.1(a), p 1.
12. Kilpatrick v Bryant, 868 SW 2d 594 (Tenn Sup Ct, Dec 22, 1993).
13. Wollen v DePaul Health Center, 828 SW 2d 681 (Mo 1992).
14. Supra at 684.
15. Proving causation in medical malpractice actions alleging loss of a chance of survival or cure. Med Liability Rep 1990:197; Cause of action for loss of survival or cure: recent developments. 1991:177.
16. Duarte v Zachariah, 22 Cal App 4th 1652, 28 Cal Rptr. 2d 88 (Cal App 1994).
17. Rodriguez v Calman, NYLJ Sept. 18, 1992 at 22 (NY County Sup Ct, Sept. 1992).
18. Oliver v Brock, 342 So 2d 1 (Ala 1977).
19. Raynor v Grossman, 31 Cal App 3d 539, 107 Cal Rptr 469 (1973).
20. Taraska J. Legal Guide for Physicians, AHAB Press, New York, N.Y. 2.04(1), 1987.
21. Schloendorff v Society of New York Hospital, 211 NY 125, 105 N.E. 92, 93 (1914);Canterbury v Spence, 464 Fed 2d 772, 780 (DC Cir), cert denied 409 U.S. 1064 (1972).
22. Cobbs v Grant, 104 Cal Rptr 505 at 513 (Cal 1972), 502 P.2d 1; see also Schloendorff v The Society of New York Hospital, 211 NY 125, 105 NE 92, 93 (1914).
23. Johnson v Whithurst, 652 SW 2d 441 (Tex Civ App 1983).
24. Belcher v Charleston Area Medical Center, 188 W Va 105, 422 S.E.2d 827 (W Va. 1992).
25. Taraska Joseph M., Legal Guide for Physicians, π6.02 (1987).
26. Culbertson v Mernitz, 602 NE 2d 98 (Ind. 1992).
27. Pate v Threlkel, 640 So 2d 183 (Fla App 1st Dist, 1994).
28. Tarasoff v Regents of the University of California, 141 Cal Rptr 14, 551 P 2d 334 (Cal. 1976)
29. Hofmann v Blackman, 241 So 2d 752 (Fla. 4th DCA 1970) cert denied, 245 So 2d 257 (Fla. 1971).
30. Canterbury v Spence, 464 Fed 2d 772, 789 (DC Cir) cert denied 409 U.S. 1064 (1972); Nishi v Hartwell, 473 P 2d 116 (Hawaii 1970).
31. Moore v Regents of the University of California, 271 Cal Rptr 146, 793 P 2d 479 (Cal. 1990).
32. Id. at 483.
33. Id. at 484; see also Annas G. Informed consent, cancer and truth in prognosis. N Engl J Med 1994;330:223; but see, Pulvers v Kaiser Foundation Health Plan, 99 Cal App 3rd 650, 160 Cal Rptr. 392 (1979).
34. Arato v Avedum, 5 Cal 4th 1172, 23 Cal Rptr 2d 131, 858 P.2d 598 (Cal 1993).
35. But see Annas G. Informed consent, cancer and truth in prognosis. N Engl J Med 1994;330:223.
36. American Medical Association, Council on Ethical and Judicial Affairs, Code of Medical Ethics, §5.07 (1994).
37. For additional guidelines, see Id. at §7.04.
38. Variety Children's Hospital, Inc v Perkins, 382 So 2d 331 (Fla Dist Ct App 1980).
39. McConnell v Williams, 361 Pa 355, 65 A 2d 243 (1949).
40. Sparger v Worley Hospital Inc, 547 SW 2d 582 (Tex 1977).
41. Hiers v Lemley, No. 56379 (Mo Ct App, E Dist, Div 4, Oct 1, 1991).
42. Hobbs v Tierney, 495 NE 2d 217 (Ind Ct App 1986).
43. American Medical Association, Council on Ethical and Judicial Affairs, Code of Medical Ethics §9.07 (1994 Ed.).
44. Pulver v Keiser Foundation Health Plan, 99 Cal App 3rd 560, 160 Cal Rptr 392 (1979).
45. See 42 U.S.C. §300(e)–300(e)–17.
46. Pulvers v Kaiser Foundation Health Plan, 99 Cal App 3rd 560, 160 Cal Rptr 392 (1979).
47. Wickline v State, 192 Cal App 3rd 1630, 239 Cal Rptr 810 (1986); Wilson v Blue Cross, 222 Cal Rptr 876 (1990).
48. Fuja v Benefit Trust Life Insurance Co, 809 F Supp 1333 (N D Ill 1992); Pirozzi v Blue Cross Blue Shield of Virginia, 741 F Supp 586 (E D Va 1990); but see Boland v King County Medical Blue Shield, 798 F Supp. 638 (W D Wash 1992).
49. Williams G. The sanctity of life in the criminal law at 254. (1957).
50. As reported by Mikell WE. Is suicide murder? 3 Colum L Rev 379 (1903).
51. Alesandro JA. Physician-assisted suicide and New York law, Albany Law Rev 1994;57: 827.
52. In Re: Quinlan, 70 NJ 10, 355 A 2d 647 (1976) cert denied 429 US 922 (1976).
53. Cruzan v Director, Mo Dept of Health, 497 US 261 (1990).
54. Kevorkian J. Prescription: Medicine. New York: Prometheus Books, 1991; see also, Annas G. Physician-assisted suicide—Michigan's temporary solution. N Engl J Med 1993;328:1573.
55. Quill T. Death and dignity. N Engl J Med 1991;234:691.
56. Annas G. Death by prescription. N Engl J Med 1994;331:1240–1241.
57. Compassion in dying v Washington. 850 F. Supp. 1454, (DC Wash 1994); People v Kevorkian, 205 Mich App 194, 518 NW 2d 487 (1994).

CHAPTER 93

Government and Cancer Medicine

JOHN E. ULTMANN, MARGUERITE DONOGHUE, AND TERRY L. LIERMAN

Introduction

The cooperation between government and medicine is crucial to cancer research and treatment. This chapter describes how the alliance between government and medical research was formed and discusses some of the forces that have eroded its effectiveness. We conclude by suggesting how members of the research community can work to rebuild the alliance. The inclusion of information on cancer legislation in a work such as this is unique in and of itself. It reflects an understanding, and perhaps an acceptance, by the medical and research communities that comingling the roles of government and science is crucial for the future of cancer research and care in this country.

Legislative History of the National Cancer Institute

NATIONAL CANCER INSTITUTE ACT

On August 5, 1937, President Franklin D. Roosevelt signed into law the National Cancer Institute Act, Public Law (P.L.) 244, which mandated that the Institute "provide for, foster, and aid in coordinating research relating to cancer" (2). Thus began a research effort entirely devoted to cancer, an effort whose roots went back to 1887, to a small laboratory at Marine Hospital on Staten Island, New York, site of the government's first commitment to medical research. This small facility, known as the Hygienic Laboratory, evolved into the National Institutes of Health (NIH), an institution with worldwide preeminence that is devoted to health research in its broadest context, emphasizing prevention, care, and the fundamental understanding of the process of human disease.

NATIONAL CANCER ACT

On December 23, 1971, as a result of substantial pressure from research advocates and the Congress, President Richard M. Nixon signed into law P.L. 92-218, the National Cancer Act, a bill that codified the recommendations of the National Panel of Consultants on the Conquest of Cancer, better known as the Yarborough Panel (2). Choosing to preserve the National Cancer Institute (NCI) as an integral component of the NIH, the bill created special authorities that accelerated and enhanced the basic biomedical research efforts already under way, and "war" was declared on cancer. These authorities have been "reauthorized" and expanded five times since the original legislation was passed.

Early in the panel's consideration of what was necessary to revitalize our cancer research efforts, opposition to any alteration of the NCI mounted within the scientific community. The opposition was based on the concerns that changes in the authorities of the NCI would weaken the rest of the NIH, the increase in the cancer budget would be at the expense of other science programs, the changes would mandate a program outside the integrity of the peer review system, increased funding for cancer research would result in mediocrity, and increased research in this area would create false optimism within the general public (3).

Changes were made despite the opposition, and the scientific community's concerns did not prove valid. The integrity of the peer review system has been maintained. The authorities have not weakened the NIH; in fact, several of the authorities have been adopted throughout the NIH. Increased resources for cancer research have caused an explosion of knowledge and resulted in dramatic research advances, not the predicted mediocrity. Further, research funding has grown in all other programs at the NIH over the past decade, with the NCI receiving the smallest percent increase of any NIH Institute (Fig. 93.1).

SPECIAL AUTHORITIES

The National Cancer Act established a National Cancer Program and provided the NCI with specific and unique authorities to accelerate cancer research, and to apply the fruits of research to persons afflicted with cancer. The legislation removed administrative impediments that were believed to be hampering the ability to carry out research initiatives. The original statutes, together with later amendments, provide for improving access to the president of the United States, expediting research conducted in the National Cancer Program, and expanding program responsibilities.

Access to the president was improved through several provisions in the original legislation. The three-member President's Cancer Panel oversees the National Cancer Program and is mandated by law to inform the president of impediments to an effective program. The 1971 law also established a presidentially appointed National Cancer Advisory Board (NCAB), with representatives from the scientific and lay communities, which provides independent and objective

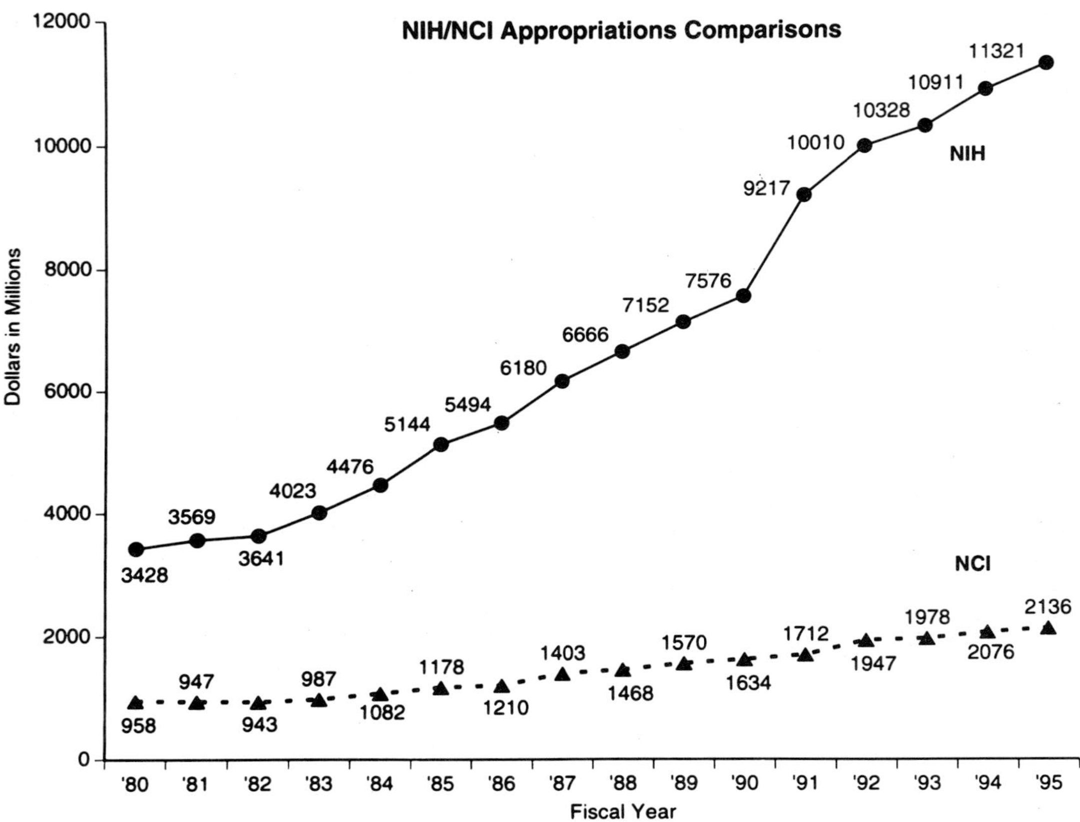

Figure 93.1. National Cancer Institute (*dashed line*) and National Institutes of Health (*solid line*) appropriations in millions of dollars for fiscal years 1980 to 1995.

advice on all aspects of our National Cancer Program. The original legislation made the directorship of the NCI a presidential appointment. The arrangement was intended to provide special autonomy, as well as to indicate the national priority given to this area of research. In order to preserve the relationship of the NCI to the NIH, the law mandated that the director of the NCI report to the director of the NIH in all matters except budget, and the NIH director was also made a presidential appointment.

Unique to the NCI was the establishment of the by pass budget, frequently referred to as a research-needs budget. The director of the NCI is mandated to provide a budget that represents the optimal support for the research needs of the NCI. The law requires that this budget be submitted to the president and the Congress without modification at other levels of the executive branch. In addition, the Department of Health and Human Services (DHHS) requires the NCI to submit an "operating" budget through the standard budget process that is subject to (downward) adjustments and is suboptimal.

Expediting research conducted in the National Cancer Program was achieved through several approaches described in the original law and subsequent amendments. Many of these authorities have been expanded NIH-wide as they have proven effective in facilitating research efforts. Included are

1. The authority to appoint advisory committees, such as the Boards of Scientific Counselors and ad hoc committees as needed.
2. The authority to appoint Committees for peer review by the director of the NCI, instead of by the director of the NIH and the NCAB, and the authority, both intramural and extramural, for basic and clinical research facility construction, including biohazard and animal facilities. Subsequently, similar extramural construction authority was provided to the National Heart, Lung and Blood Institute and the National Eye Institute.
3. The authority to enter into contracts, which the National Panel of Consultants believed was unnecessarily delayed because of multiple layers of review at the level of the Secretary, DHHS. All other NIH Institutes, except the National Heart, Lung and Blood Institute, are still required to enter into contracts through the Secretary.
4. The authority to hire expert consultants without regard to Civil Service requirements or employment ceilings imposed by the administration.
5. The mandate to expand, intensify, and coordinate federal and nonfederal cancer research, including that in other NIH institutes and federal agencies.
6. The mandate to collaborate with industry. This contributed to an expanded and productive drug development program for cancer, which was readily adapted for

use in some aspects of the human immunodeficiency virus (HIV) infection.
7. The mandate to develop and update a National Cancer Plan to meet emerging priorities.
8. The authority to accept unconditional gifts, such as money and property, as well as voluntary and uncompensated services.

Expanded program responsibilities were achieved in the original legislation, when the Institute was provided with authority to conduct cancer control activities; to establish national research and demonstration centers; to expand information-dissemination activities; to collect, catalog, store, and disseminate cancer research information internationally; to provide special training authority for health professionals; and to engage in foreign research and training.

Funding for Cancer Research

The most important sponsor of medical research in this country has been, and must continue to be, the federal government. This embodies the concept that a nation's greatest treasure is the health of its people. Although its partners in discovery in the private sector—business, academia, and voluntary health organizations—have made valuable contributions in the battle against disease, disability, and death, medical research is a high-risk enterprise that demands a large-scale, societal commitment best led by the federal government.

America's medical researchers have achieved their impressive track record because of their adherence to the principle that scientific explorations will yield the most fruitful results if research is concentrated on basic science. However, in recent years, policy makers have been forced to seek a balance between basic and applied science and the economic constraints of a federal deficit that is ballooning. In August 1994, the Clinton administration released a report, "Science in the National Interest," which highlighted the administration's priorities in seeking to maintain this delicate balance. Those priorities include: "Improving human health, creating breakthrough technologies that lead to new industries and high quality jobs, enhancing productivity with information technologies and improved understanding of human interactions, meeting our national security needs, protecting and restoring the global environment, and feeding and providing energy for a growing population" (4).

To appreciate the challenges of this mandate and identify an effective course of action, an understanding of the budget process and the recent political changes in the U.S. House of Representatives and the U.S. Senate is important.

Federal Budget Process

The Constitution entrusts to the Congress most of the power necessary to govern the nation, including the powers to tax, regulate, engage in commerce, declare war, approve treaties, and raise and maintain armies. In this array of responsibilities, perhaps the most important are the fiscal powers, the ability to alter the spending plans and policy of the nation.

BUDGET COMMITTEE

In 1974, Congress integrated its tax and spending powers in the Congressional Budget and Impoundment Control Act, mandating that Congress set an overall fiscal agenda and then use the agreed-upon agenda in framing national priorities. The law's purpose was to create an orderly procedure for developing and executing a budget, and it established budget committees in both the House and the Senate to reign over this legislative process.

However, by the mid-1980s, differing fiscal policy within the Democrat-controlled Congress and the Republican White House, coupled with weak fiscal restraint in both the executive and legislative branches, caused the deficit to balloon. In 1985, a drastic measure was passed by the Congress and signed into law by the president, the Balanced Budget and Emergency Deficit Reduction Act of 1985, more commonly referred to as "Gramm-Rudman-Hollings," referencing its congressional sponsors. This legislation established requirements, or targets, to meet in reducing the deficit. Further, it created a new method of fiscal constraint, called sequestration, that would implement automatic spending cuts in the event that the Congress and the White House could not agree on spending cuts or sources of revenue. Sequestration provided an incentive to meet the deficit targets, as half of the mandatory cuts would come from the military; the remaining half would come from domestic programs, excluding Medicare, Medicaid, and Social Security.

To illustrate the point, in any given fiscal year, if congressional leaders and the White House could not meet the deficit targets by September 30, sequestration, or automatic cuts of 34% in domestic programs, would be put into effect by the president. At the NCI, this would necessitate substantial reductions in the number of funded grants, research trainees, cancer centers, and clinical trials, as well as in NCI personnel.

The House and Senate budget committees have traditionally carried out their responsibilities with little input from outside advocates. Their work begins the day that the president submits a budget to the Congress, generally sometime during the third week of January, initiating the congressional budget process and usually consuming an entire legislative session. By mid-April (although the target date is rarely met), these committees are required by law to present a joint budget to the House and Senate for approval. This budget then acts as the fiscal policy guideline for the Congress to proceed with funding of domestic and defense programs through the appropriations process.

Since 1974, members of the medical and cancer research communities have not had great success in shaping the priorities of the budget committees (5, 11). This changed in 1990, however, when the House Budget Committee held its first oversight hearing on medical research. Of the four witnesses who appeared, two were representatives of the cancer research community. On April 23, 1990, the House passed the Concurrent Resolution on the Budget—Fiscal Year 1991. In the committee report that accompanied the budget resolution, a discussion of cancer research as a national priority accounted for one of the three paragraphs included on the NIH. Of note is the following excerpt: "The Committee is especially concerned that the Nation's commitment to eradicating cancer is not adequately funded . . . it is the intention of the Committee to give attention to this area in the future" (6).

This presents a challenge to the cancer research community, inviting greater efforts, and, it is hoped, producing greater results in the future.

On September 27, 1994, more than 300 Republican candidates and members of the House of Representatives signed what is known as the "Contract with America." The contract was an attempt to dispel the doubts and lack of confidence overwhelming the American people and their attitudes toward Congress. It was a partisan attempt to make a clear distinction between the unfulfilled promise of the Democratic party and the unbreachable contractual commitment of the Republican party to make government more accountable. The Contract with America outlined 10 legislative proposals that the Republicans, if elected into the majority, would bring to the House floor for a vote within the first 100 days of the new Congress. These proposals were an ambitious attempt to replace the Democratic agenda and restructure the role of government in America.

One key component of the contract deals with the fiscal responsibility act, which sets out a plan to cut spending, not increase taxes, as the most effective way to reduce the deficit and balance the budget. The bill provides institutional reforms that would pressure Congress to decrease spending, including a balanced budget amendment, a line item veto authority, and a supra-majority approval for tax increases. Passage of the balanced budget amendment, which would be an amendment to the Constitution of the United States, would require a balanced budget by the year 2002 or the second year after ratification by the states. The amendment also calls for a three-fifths approval by the Congress for all tax increases. Balancing the budget by the year 2002 would mean holding federal spending growth to 3.2% a year, instead of the projected 5.4%. In addition, a line item veto, the authority to delete any single item in an appropriations bill, gives permanent line-item veto authority to the president.

On election day in 1994, the contract caught the eye of the voting public. For the first time in over 40 years, the electorate voted a Republican majority into the House of Representatives. In addition, the Senate, which had had a Republican majority rule from 1981 to 1986, again had a Republican majority.

APPROPRIATIONS COMMITTEE

The appropriations committees in the House and Senate are the committees responsible for funding federal programs. There are 13 appropriations committees in the House and 13 appropriations committees in the Senate that annually review all federal programs and make decisions about

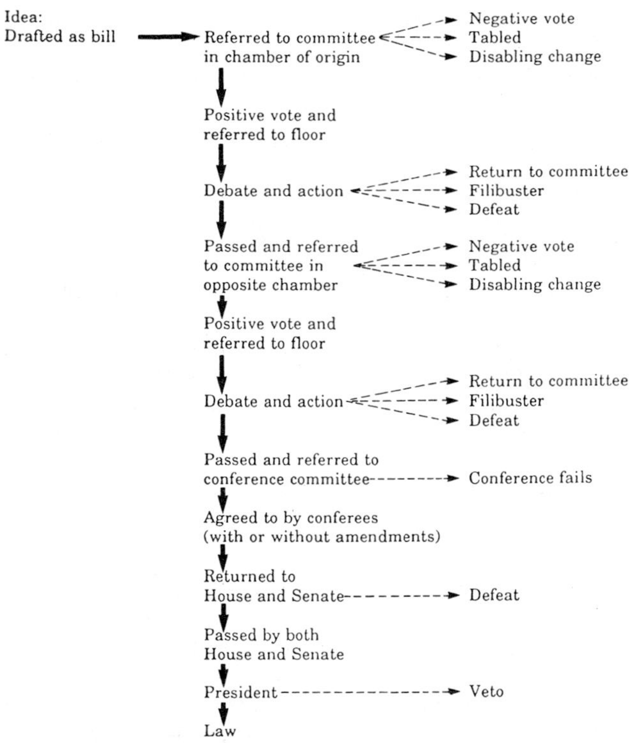

Figure 93.2. How a bill becomes law.

actual funding priorities within the guidelines established by the Budget Committee.

Once a program has been authorized, through such legislation as the National Cancer Institute Act or the National Cancer Act, it can be funded. By custom and tradition, appropriations measures originate in the House of Representatives, and once the process is completed in the House, it is referred to the Senate for action.

The first step in this process is departmental testimony, when all agency heads, including the director of the NCI, must appear before the Congress in defense of the president's budget request. Whether they agree with the priorities or not, as employees of the president they are required to present and support the administration's budget request at these hearings. Once this testimony is received, participation by the general public is invited. A seemingly endless stream of testimony from special-interest advocates is presented before the House and Senate committees. While this testimony may make an impact, it is no secret that the crucial impact on this process is the number of constituents of any given member of Congress who contacts him or her, personally or through correspondence, urging the representative's support of a specific issue.

When public witness testimony is completed, the committee members and staff enter a closed room for "mark-up," and begin the arduous task of determining what programs will receive increases and what programs will be cut. Once their deliberations are completed, the bill is referred to the full Appropriations Committee, where it can be amended. If approved, it is sent to the floor of the House, where it can be further amended. When the bill passes by a vote of the full

House, it is sent to the Senate, where a similar process begins. After the Senate has approved its own version of the bill, a conference committee of members of the House and of the Senate meet to work out the differences in the two versions. After the conferees agree to a combined package, it is sent to the floor of each chamber, and voted on. If passed by both chambers, the bill is then forwarded to the president for signature into law (Fig. 93.2).

Accompanying the very technical appropriations bill is a committee report, which describes in lay, nonbinding terms the programs being funded and how the committee directs that the funds be used. While not legally binding, the committee reports are viewed as directives from the Congress that provide guidance for agency officials in the expenditure of funds.

Research Funding Trends

The overall effect of congressional budgetary actions in recent years has been to limit the growth of expenditures for cancer research; this has occurred at a time when research opportunities are expanding. In the initial years after the "war on cancer" was declared, funding for cancer research doubled in inflation-adjusted dollars, and increased threefold in actual dollars. Since 1976, there has been little real growth in the cancer research budget, and, in fact, a sharp drop in funding was seen in the early 1980s. In 1980, the NCI's budget was $985 million. In 1995, it was $2.1 billion. However, the 1995 appropriation reflects a funding level of $972 million in 1980 inflation-adjusted dollars, and only a 1.4% increase over the 1980 purchasing power (Fig. 93.3).

On January 20, 1993, President William J. Clinton was sworn into office; on April 8, 1993, President Clinton presented his first budget to the U.S. Congress. Included in his first budget proposal were cuts in 9 of the 13 Institutes at the NIH. In addition, to mask the cuts in the remaining Institutes, the president "forward-funded" programs. In essence, he calculated increases that the Institutes were to receive in fiscal years 1995, 1996, and 1997 into the figures for fiscal year 1994 so that it appeared that increases to select Institutes were provided.

With regard to the NCI, the president proposed increased spending in two specific areas: breast cancer and HIV infection. The recommended increase in these critically important funding areas was $206 million. The administration's proposed increase for the NCI was only a total of $163 million. As a result, the president's budget assumed that cuts in existing cancer research programs would be necessary. The programs in which budgetary cuts were assumed to be necessary in 1994 are shown in Table 93.1.

Congress restored the cuts proposed by the president and provided a 5.2% increase for the NCI. However, as a result of the Omnibus Budget Agreement of 1993, the outlook for the next 4 years appears dim with regard to medical re-

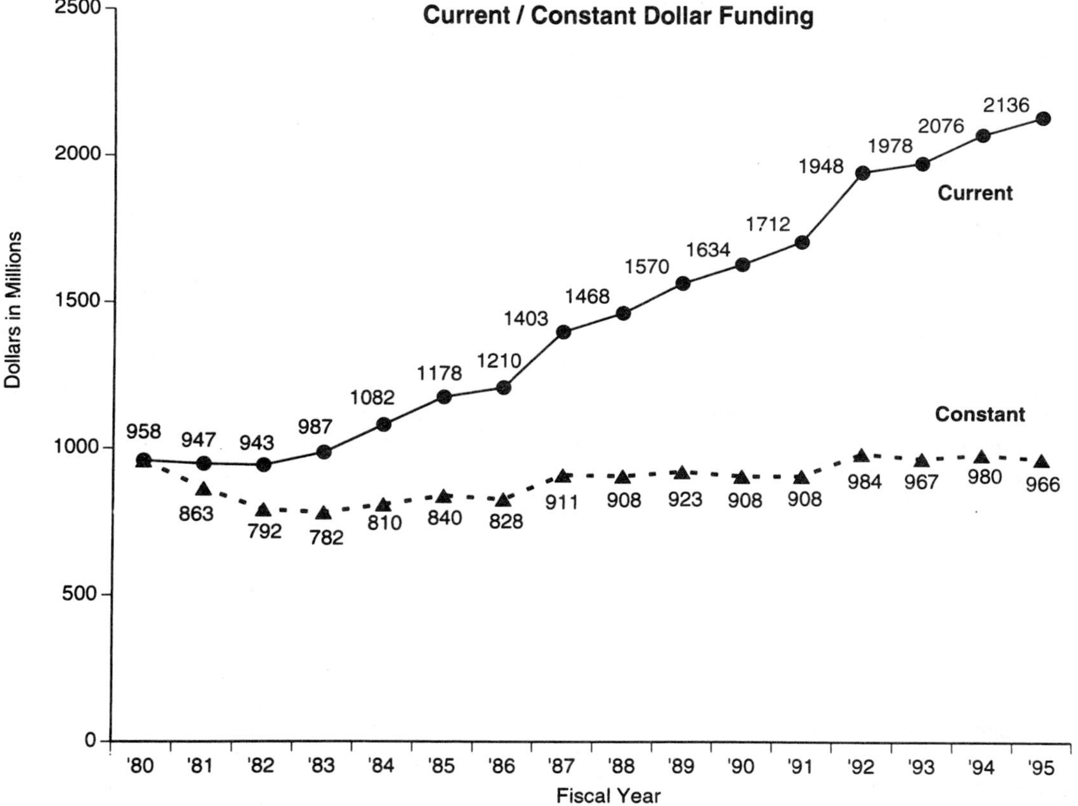

Figure 93.3. Funding for the National Cancer Institute in millions of dollars for fiscal years 1980 to 1995. *Solid line*, absolute amounts; *dashed line*, inflation-adjusted amounts.

Table 93.1. Cuts in 1994 Cancer Programs

- Basic research not relevant to breast cancer and HIV infection
- Detection, prevention, and treatment research related to leukemia and cancer of the lung, colon, rectum, brain, kidney, and bladder
- Psychosocial and behavioral research
- Antismoking research and outreach
- Outreach to minorities, the underserved, the elderly, and low literacy populations
- Innovative research on gene therapy, cancer vaccines, clinical trials, and prevention

Table 93.2. National Cancer Institute Success Rates

Fiscal year	Awarded	Received	Success rate[a]
1987	1,061	2,939	36.1%
1988	979	3,133	31.2%
1989	728	3,127	23.3%
1990	728	3,057	23.8%
1991	840	3,040	27.6%
1992	1,079	3,346	32.2%
1993	991	4,139	23.9%
1994	969	4,598	21.1%

[a] The success rate is the ratio of awarded to received RO1 applications.

search funding. Based on this budget agreement, a $10 billion reduction in domestic programs will need to be realized as a result of a 5-year freeze on domestic and defense spending. While some in Washington circles are calling this a "hard freeze" on spending, the reality is that significant cuts in programs will need to occur if President Clinton is to obtain funding for any of his new initiatives. Further, there is a disposition in Congress to deepen these spendings cuts to address the $4.4 trillion debt. It is widely believed that additional cuts in domestic spending will be made.

The federal deficit and push toward controlling spending have led to a crisis in cancer research. The crisis is not in the laboratory where creative scientists continue their important work. The problem is in funding the work and training of young scientists in cancer research who will eventually take over for today's investigators. And this problem is not confined to cancer research. In the current fiscal climate, funding for cancer research is not keeping pace with research opportunities. In fact, the percent change in 1980 constant dollars for the NCI is only 1%, as compared with the NIH, which is 15%. Further, the 1995 appropriation is $1.6 billion below the recommended funding level for the NCI in the bypass budget. The viability of a number of research laboratories and clinical investigative groups is threatened. The effects of inadequate funding are particularly evident in three types of research support: individual investigator-initiated awards, training grants, and cancer centers.

PROJECT GRANTS

In the past decade, funding for NIH programs, based on inflation-adjusted data, has increased, mainly because funding for research project grants has increased. On the other hand, funding for research centers, training, and research contracts has leveled off or decreased. While this may appear to be rosy on the surface, most researchers would argue that substantial constraint has seriously disrupted research in laboratories across the country and that quality science is going unfunded. The funding increases have not been adequate to meet the escalating costs of research or to allow pursuit of the tremendous scientific opportunities that exist.

Several major policy decisions made in 1985 by the NIH have had a significant impact on funding for research grants in the 1990s. The NIH extended the funding period by increasing the number of 5- and 7-year grants awarded. This decision was made for sound scientific reasons: extending the award period improved the maturation of research data prior to resubmission. When senior scientists with a proven track record are not required to resubmit a grant application every 18 months, they can devote more of their expertise to scientific exploration. On the other hand, this grant restructuring necessitated increases in continuation funds in the additional years to guarantee support, and the increases were not included in the funding base of the NIH. A funding shortfall was thus "inadvertently" created.

The NIH had traditionally managed most of its grants on a 3-year funding cycle. Continuation costs for many grants suddenly required funding beyond that traditionally planned or provided. In order to meet those requirements, it was necessary to decrease the approval of new grants at the NIH. In addition, Congress stopped mandating a specified number of new grant awards, which in turn decreased opportunities for young investigators to obtain funding. New and competing grant awards at the NIH dropped from 6,446 in 1987 to an estimated 6,031 in 1995. Furthermore, any additional resources appropriated by Congress were directed to the shortfalls in research grants, necessitating virtually no-growth budgets in practically every other funding mechanism throughout the NIH.

Additionally, the NIH was forced to implement a policy of "downward negotiations" or mandated cuts in new and noncompeting grants in order to meet its fiscal commitments. These reductions typically range from 10 to 20% below the level approved by the peer review groups. Since their inception in the mid-1980s, they have become a standard component of the administration's proposed budget.

The net result is that the number of new and competing grants awarded by the NIH is significantly decreased. What is the overall impact in cancer research? In 1971, when the National Cancer Act was passed, one of every two approved grants was funded. Under the 1995 appropriation, NCI will only be able to fund one out of every five approved competing grants (Table 93.2).

TRAINING GRANTS

In 1988, the NIH decided to increase the stipends for research trainees without requesting an increase in the appropriation from the Congress. As a result, the number of trainees funded under the 1989 budget was cut by approximately 1,000.

The increase in stipends was justifiable and long overdue, and brought the average postdoctorate NIH stipend to

$17,000 a year, below the salary level for cab drivers or secretaries in our nation's capital. In order to diminish the effects of this reduction, Congress approved a reprogramming request in mid-1989 partially to restore the number of research trainees cut in fiscal year 1989. In the 1990 appropriation, Congress fully restored the level of research training. Based on funding levels available in the 1995 budget, the NIH will support 14,388 research trainees; the NCI will support 1,388 of those trainees. The NIH level is 2,368 fewer than the number supported in 1969 when research training supported by the NIH was at its peak. In the early 1970s, approximately 13% of the overall NIH budget was devoted to research training. Today, less than 5% of the budget is so allocated.

CANCER CENTERS

The National Cancer Act provided a clear mandate to strengthen existing cancer centers and create additional ones. The Cancer Centers Program had been established by the NCI in the late 1960s, and in the subsequent years became a productive and valuable national resource. Many other programs at the NIH have modeled their basic and applied research centers after the cancer centers model.

The congressional intent in endorsing the Cancer Centers Program in 1971, and subsequent reauthorizations, is clear. The National Cancer Act mandates that cancer centers provide for (*a*) a multidisciplinary effort in basic research, clinical research, prevention, improved delivery of patient care, and provision of community resources through outreach and education; (*b*) a focus for a critical mass of scientists and physicians to address crucial issues in cancer research cooperatively and collaboratively; and (*c*) appropriate geographic distribution, lending support and assistance to clinics and community medical centers.

In essence, the National Panel of Consultants believed that the Cancer Centers Program would be one of the most vital components of the National Cancer Program. Today, there are 57 federally funded cancer centers throughout the United States, which have been categorized as basic science, clinical, consortium, and comprehensive centers because of the varying degree to which they pursue fundamental research, applied research, education, prevention, cancer control, or community outreach programs.

The effectiveness of cancer centers requires a multipronged approach to funding; in addition to federal research grants and core support, cancer centers have sought funding from many other sources, including the American Cancer Society, drug companies, foundations, and individual donors. The American Cancer Society spends almost $100 million per year in support of cancer research. Although it is known that drug companies spend a total of $6.5 billion on research and development, no data are available about how much of this is devoted to cancer. Similarly, information about total foundation funding for cancer research cannot be obtained.

Although nonfederal sources provide substantial funding, the federal sources are larger and far outweigh all other sources. Thus, the stability of the Cancer Centers Program was threatened as a result of the severe budgetary constraints in medical research at the end of the 1980s. The resources to fund cancer centers have been level for the past 5 years, necessitating a reduction in the total number of centers, as well as a downward negotiation of about 15% below the peer-reviewed recommended levels. Over the past decade, the number of NCI-supported cancer centers has decreased from 64 to 54. Further, if funding were provided to the cancer centers at the recommended level, the NCI budget would only provide for the funding of 46 centers.

Public Policy Factors Affecting Medical Research

Several major trends have hampered the funding and conduct of cancer research over the past several years. If these trends are left unaltered, their impact is expected to increase and to have a detrimental effect on the future of investigator-initiated research.

BIG SCIENCE PROJECTS

What has become apparent in the allocation of resources during times of fiscal constraint is that funding of targeted research initiatives is growing while new funding has decreased for nontargeted research, including program grants, cancer centers, and investigator-initiated research. The Congressional Research Service recently completed an inventory of "big science" projects worldwide (Fig. 93.4). The report shows that the federal government has embarked on an ambitious program of funding big projects. This approach poses a tremendous threat to future scientific efforts because it is the nontargeted approaches that have been the lifeline to most research advances in the past two decades.

The 1980s saw a major increase in several special or targeted scientific initiatives whose costs many believe may cripple vital components of our scientific efforts (Fig. 93.4).

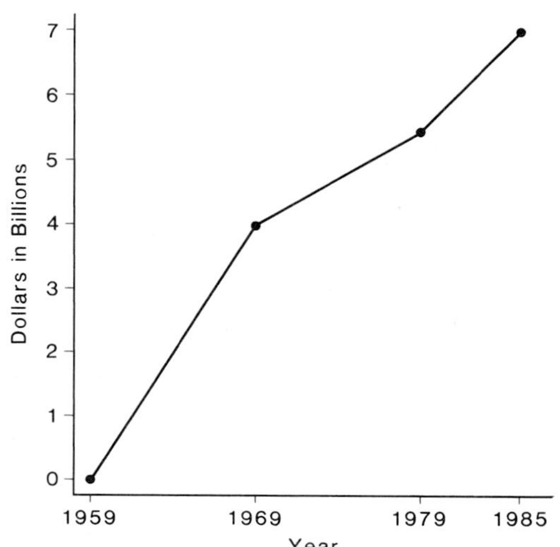

Figure 93.4. Expenditures in billions of dollars for targeted scientific initiatives, 1959 to 1985. *Source:* World Inventory of Big Science Research Instruments and Facilities, Congressional Research Service.

These efforts included the Superconductor Super Collider, Hubble Space Telescope, mapping of the human genome, research on the acquired immune deficiency syndrome (AIDS), and Star Wars. While these scientific issues represent important national priorities, the decision to increase their funding does not depend entirely on scientific significance. All of these projects had champions, either in the Congress or the White House, that raised their visibility and ensured a strong funding base from year to year. Cancer research needs more champions, not only in science and among the public, but also in government.

ANIMALS IN RESEARCH

Funding for cancer research is not the only issue to have a detrimental effect on our ability to make progress against cancer. The 1980s will be remembered as the decade in which the animal rights debate became strident. The number of animal rights activists and proponents grew rapidly, and the membership in animal rights organizations is estimated now to be more than 10 million, with a combined total budget of $50 million. Activists have engaged in a variety of tactics, ranging from legislative initiatives to curb the use of animals in medical research, to acts of vandalism, burglary, and arson. The National Association for Biomedical Research, a nonprofit organization that actively works with Congress to support the responsible conduct of research with animals, reports that there have been over 56 terrorist attacks since 1982.

Major legislative victories have been realized on both sides of the issue. In fact, the first legislative milestone in animal rights was in 1986 when a bill was introduced to regulate the use of animals in research in the District of Columbia. The bill was eventually defeated, but the advocates of animal rights were not deterred. Their efforts have continued, and many legislators and scientists have expressed concern that animal rights extremists may achieve a legislative victory that will seriously impede the future of medical research.

The use of animals in medical research has dramatically altered human existence. Medical research involving animals has led to great changes in public health and patient care, including the development of antibiotics, insulin, drugs for the mentally ill, cardiac surgery, vaccines, and cancer therapies. Animal research has even benefited animals by producing advances in veterinary medicine itself. The National Association for Biomedical Research estimates that medical advances made possible through the use of animals in research have extended life expectancy by over 20 years. Researchers must not be deterred from using this indispensable component of research resources because of a lack of understanding or the emotionally exaggerated and often untrue assertions of a vocal group. Scientific researchers should bear in mind that, with enough clamor, a small minority can pass itself off as the majority. Furthermore, the voices of an emotional minority may seem more persuasive to unsuspecting legislators than the reasoned arguments of the scientific community.

While the majority of the members in Congress continue to support animal research, the activists have embarked on a strategy to increase the costs of research by having federal statutes enacted that mandate expensive, unnecessary, and unproved programs for the care and housing of the animals used in research. Amendments to the Animal Welfare Act, which were passed in 1985, are expected to cost somewhere between $1 and $2 billion to implement.

With over 10 million supporters calling for a halt to the use of animals in medical research, it is critical that the research community counter their effect. Failure to educate legislators and the American public on the imperatives of animal research could contribute to the transfer of physiologic discovery and development out of the United States. This would lead to disintegration of the finest biomedical research programs the world has known.

TARGETING RESEARCH

The early 1990s gave rise to a strong grassroots movement by women advocating for breast cancer research. The National Breast Cancer Coalition (NBCC) led an effort to enlist women throughout America in advocating for increased funding for breast cancer research. In 1992, when Congress was considering fiscal year 1993 spending priorities, all 435 members of the House of Representatives and one third of the Senate were running for reelection in what was dubbed "the year of the woman," and many candidates were looking for the support of women voters. It was in this political climate that the breast cancer advocates put forth their efforts.

Clearly, they achieved results. Congress directed the NCI to increase efforts in breast cancer research, as well as prostate and ovarian cancer, by $100 million. Unfortunately, an increase of only $30 million was provided to the NCI, and cuts in existing cancer research programs were thus necessary in order to address the new mandates from Congress. This was the first time that cuts in ongoing cancer research programs were mandated to provide increases for other cancer research initiatives. The programs that were cut are shown in Table 93.1.

This congressional directive brought breast cancer research spending to $196 million at the NCI, which was less than the $365 million urged by the NBCC. As a result, many members of the cancer research and advocacy communities, scientists and lay advocates alike, worked with congressional supporters to identify new funds further to reduce the need to cut existing cancer research programs. During consideration of the 1993 Department of Defense (DOD) Appropriations bill on the Senate floor, Senator Tom Harkin (D-Iowa) put forward an amendment to increase funding for breast cancer research within the DOD by $185 million, to bring the total breast cancer research program in DOD to $210 million. Known as the "Harkin Amendment for Breast Cancer," it was passed in the Senate by a vote of 89 to 4.

In the debate during consideration of this amendment, Senator Harkin clearly outlined his intent to have these funds made available to the cancer research community by the Department of the Army in collaboration with the NCI and the NIH.

Subsequent to the passage of the amendment, the Department of the Army contracted with the Institute of Medicine (IOM) to make recommendations on how the DOD should manage its $210 million breast cancer research program. The report recommended that a two-tiered peer review process be established by the DOD for scientific and technical review and Advisory Council review to determine program relevance. In addition, the following program investments were recommended: training and recruitment, $27 million; infrastructure enhancement, $21 million; and investigator-initiated research, $151 million.

As fiscal constraints continue to grow, it is imperative to present a united front with regard to advocacy for cancer research priorities. Gains may be illusory and counterproductive when cuts are forced in existing programs or increases are targeted in only one area over all others in cancer research. Many would argue that real breakthroughs are not likely to come from targeted initiatives, but rather from basic research, as they have in the past.

Public Policy Factors Affecting Costs of Treating and Preventing Cancer

The escalating cost of health care in this country is having a staggering effect on cancer care. Health care costs account for over 13% of the gross national product (GNP), the highest for any developed nation. Expenditures for cancer care account for more than 5% of the GNP. The overall economic cost of cancer in the United States (including lost wages and the like) is still higher, and that does not take into consideration the human costs, which are incalculable.

Efforts to control costs have been and will continue to be scrutinized by legislators and policy analysts. In 1983, a prospective payment system (PPS) was put in place by the Medicare program in an effort to provide economic incentives that would encourage cost-effective patterns of care. This shift, from a cost-based system to a cost-reimbursement system, has been a fundamental change within our health care system, as it provides for a fixed reimbursement for services rendered under Medicare. The PPS was established to meet several critical goals of the Health Care Financing Administration to address escalating health care costs—chiefly, the establishment of an incentive-based system to manage health care expenditures in individual hospitals and the implementation of a cost-efficient system that would not detrimentally affect access to care.

The PPS altered economic incentives for hospitals providing care to persons with cancer. In order to stay within the reimbursement levels of the PPS, a variety of changes in the delivery of care were necessary, including decreased length of stay; increased use of outpatient services and day hospitals for chemotherapy and surgical procedures; shifting in staffing patterns, both nursing and medical, to accommodate sicker patients in the outpatient setting; and increased acuity in home care programs.

Unfortunately, the advent of a PPS brought to the forefront many complex issues related to the delivery of care that it was attempting to ameliorate. Implementation brought with it greater public scrutiny and interest, greater congressional interest and oversight, and more concern about quality of care than had previously existed.

Further, the PPS created several major policy issues with regard to cancer care, research, and prevention—specifically, access to clinical trials and prevention services. Each of these remains an ongoing subject of debate in the 1990s, and it will be imperative that effective solutions be found, as these issues stand to threaten the integrity of cancer care as we know it today.

Innovative cancer therapies are available through the clinical trials mechanism that has been put in place in cancer centers, community clinical oncology programs (CCOPs), and cooperative groups across the United States. Further, it is through the clinical trials mechanism that new therapies are evaluated and proved. This approach has given us cures for such illnesses as Hodgkin's disease, testicular cancer, and childhood leukemia. Traditionally, Medicare and other insurers have paid for the costs associated with clinical trials, but not for the experimental therapy itself. Recent trends indicate that third party reimbursement for clinical trials is being denied, albeit intermittently. Several studies are under way to determine the breadth of this issue. If the data bear out the early indications, we will be well on the way to supporting a system where only the rich can have access to clinical trials and, therefore, innovative therapies.

Two decades of intensive cancer research have produced significant knowledge about cancer prevention and early detection. At the present time, there are numerous prevention and screening services which, when implemented in the appropriate manner, allow for diagnosis and intervention at a much earlier stage. Such methods include mammography, screening for occult blood in stool, proctoscopic examinations, Papanicolaou (PAP) tests, and the prostate-specific antigen (PSA). In addition, recent research progress will soon provide more sophisticated tools, such as blood screening assays.

With the inauguration of President Clinton came his expressed intent to reform the health care delivery system. He designated Hillary Rodham Clinton to chair the White House Health Care Reform Task Force and to develop the administration's blueprint for health care reform. In November 1993, the administration presented to Congress a conceptual package that included some of the most fundamental reforms of health care delivery ever envisioned.

The Health Security Act would place increased emphasis on prevention initiatives, authorizing an additional $400 million for research in this area at the NIH. It would make support for patient care costs associated with clinical trials discretionary in the basic benefit package. Specific criteria addressed the parameters of this coverage if offered. Only "qualifying investigational therapies" were to be covered. Qualifying was defined as any investigational treatment whose effectiveness has not yet been determined that is under clinical investigation as part of an approved research trial. An "approved research trial" was defined as one "approved by the secretary of the Department of Health and Human Services, the director of the National Institutes of Health, the commissioner of the Food and Drug Administration, the secretary of Veterans' Affairs, the secretary of Defense, or a qualified nongovernmental research entity as defined in guidelines of the National Institutes of Health, or a peer-reviewed and approved research program as defined by the secretary of Health and Human Services, conducted for the primary purpose of determining whether or not a treatment is safe, efficacious, or having any other characteristic of a treatment which must be demonstrated in order for the treatment to be medically necessary or appropriate."

In the second session of the 103rd Congress, health care reform legislation was proposed and considered over a 12-month period by no less than seven committees in the U.S. House of Representatives and the U.S. Senate. Owing to the complexities of the administration's proposal and the variety of proposals introduced on both sides of the aisle in the House and Senate, the following major committees ended up with jurisdiction over health care reform:

House of Representatives—Ways and Means Committee, Energy and Commerce Committee, Health and the Environment Subcommittee, Education and Labor Committee, Judiciary Committee;

U.S. Senate—Finance Committee, Labor and Human Resource Committee, Judiciary Committee.

To deal effectively with the potential impact that health care reform would have on the delivery of cancer care, the cancer research community developed and advocated for a Statement of Principles that supported cancer research. Under the umbrella of the National Coalition for Cancer Research, a national coalition of 20 research, professional, and lay organizations, the cancer research community worked with Congress to urge consideration of the following principles as key to any reform measure: (*a*) access to and the right to choose appropriately trained specialists in cancer management; (*b*) support for an expanded basic and applied research effort; (*c*) coverage of investigational therapies as a basic benefit; and (*d*) support for the unique costs of cancer treatment in a research setting

While many aspects of the bills introduced and considered by the Congress were of major importance to the delivery of cancer care in this country, the two key components directly affecting the ability to support research were reimbursement for investigational therapy and the Health Research Fund. These legislative initiatives were included in all of the major bills considered, including S.2351; S.2296; H.R. 3600, Ways and Means; H.R. 3600, House Leadership Substitute; Admt. 2560, Senate Leadership Proposal.

Because of the broad nature of the administration's proposal to completely alter the delivery system, and the various interests of the congressional committees and subcommittees in different aspects of health care reform, compromise on a final package and floor consideration of a final health care reform bill never materialized.

Analysis

Annually, over 1.2 million people in the United States are diagnosed with cancer (excluding the common skin cancers), and it is expected that one out of every three Americans will be diagnosed as having cancer at some point in life. One person dies of cancer every 58 seconds (7). That equates to 1,490 deaths every day and 538,000 deaths annually—the equivalent of the population of one congressional district. Another way to understand the impact of the disease is to compare the number of Americans who die of cancer with the number of American service personnel killed in battle. In all our nation's wars combined (from the American Revolution to the war in the Persian Gulf), a total of 652,799 battle deaths have been recorded. Thus, the number of Americans killed in battle during all of our 215-year history is 114,799 more than the number killed every year by cancer. These data reflect the grim statistics of cancer, and create compelling evidence that cancer research efforts are as important today as they were 20 years ago, or at any other time in the past.

In 1971, with the passage of the National Cancer Act, it was widely believed by the American public, as well as by many in Congress, that with a little extra effort and money, cancer could be eliminated. In fact, in the fanfare associated with its passage, the Congress unanimously passed a resolution calling for an end to cancer by 1976 as an "appropriate commemoration of the two-hundredth anniversary of the independence of our country" (8). Congress's commitment to eradicate cancer was genuine; its expectations were unrealistic.

In the years that have followed the passage of this landmark legislation, it has widely been recognized that the "war" has not been won. That cancer was not cured by this nation's 200th birthday is stating the obvious. Many believe that this has diminished, albeit unconsciously, a willingness to commit fiscal resources for our National Cancer Program. Because of the inability to claim total victory against cancer, the public and the Congress have been less willing, and at times altogether unable, to recognize the tremendous successes derived from this landmark legislation. Two decades after the passage of the National Cancer Act, one can make a compelling argument that the act strengthened all of biomedical research, gave birth to the burgeoning new industry of biotechnology, and unlocked many secrets of the workings of the cancer cell. Most important, it has enabled tremendous lifesaving advances with positive impact on the lives of millions, in this and future generations.

The resources directed to the act have had a direct impact on the lives of over 8 million cancer survivors. Many cancers, such as leukemia, lymphoma, Hodgkin's disease, cervical cancer, and childhood malignancies, that were almost always fatal are now most often curable. The NCI-supported research in testicular cancer has led to a 91% cure rate. Adjuvant chemotherapy, a direct result of the innovative drug research supported under the National Cancer Act, has decreased the recurrence rate and the mortality associated with many cancers, such as breast cancer and osteogenic sarcoma.

The importance of the ability to cure many cancers is matched by the equally important success in maintaining the highest quality of life for those afflicted with the disease. Surgical procedures, which in the past compromised the ability of cancer patients to return to active, productive lives, and which often led to severe psychologic problems due to disfigurement, have been modified significantly. Today, multimodality therapy, incorporating surgery, radiation therapy, and chemotherapy, is often the standard treatment. Women with breast cancer and their physicians now have a choice of effective procedures and, in many cases, may select treatments that conserve the breast. Children and young adults afflicted with soft tissue sarcomas are now spared removal of their affected limb through advanced surgical techniques used in conjunction with radiation and chemotherapy.

Furthermore, research has improved the quality of life for those undergoing treatment for many cancers, by controlling more effectively nausea and vomiting, as well as other side effects. Because of innovative techniques in pain management, patients no longer need fear the pain that once seemed an inevitable consequence of cancer.

Perhaps then the flaw in the war against cancer was declaring it a war in the first place. Addressing the rising incidence of cancer, advancing our understanding of the disease, and establishing a network to ensure access to innovative therapy for all Americans afflicted with cancer were moral responsibilities that the government properly undertook to combat the disease its citizens fear most. Those responsibilities have not diminished.

When the National Cancer Act was passed, the National Panel of Consultants highlighted the inadequacy of funding for cancer research. In 1969, for every man, woman, and child in the United States, $410 was spent on national defense and 89 cents for cancer research. Today, we are spending $1,200 per person on national defense and $7.41 per person for cancer research.

In their 1971 report, the National Panel of Consultants questioned the allocation of national priorities. In 1996, that question remains on the table. Priorities today, as in 1971, are out of balance. Thirteen percent of the GNP, over $900 billion, is spent on health care costs, such as medication, syringes, and hospitalizations, while only 0.3% of the GNP is spent on medical research. From 1980 to 1989, research and development in the DOD increased 89% in real dollars. In contrast, research and development in domestic programs, including medical research, decreased by 9% in real dollars (9).

To reverse this trend, it is imperative to understand how the process of allocating dollars works and where the scientific and medical community must make an impact. It has been stated that "to stimulate federal support of medical research and education . . . requires voluntary expenditures of time and energy, cultivating Senators and [members of] Congress, educating them and creating forceful advocates for medical progress" (8).

The past decade of fiscal constraint has placed the biomedical research community in a false dilemma by seeming to pit science against science. This degrades the segments of the scientific community that deem one area of science less worthy than another. The idea of pitting one disease or institute against another is counterproductive and shortsighted, and the medical research community should avoid being caught in this trap. Medical research, including cancer research, is crucial for the advancement of the biologic sciences and for the hope that those advances will prevent or cure diseases and disabilities. On that merit alone, funding should be a national priority.

In recent years, the principal target of much of this debate has been AIDS research. Since 1984 when the first congressional appropriation for AIDS was provided, total U.S. funding to meet the demands of this epidemic has grown in excess of 2000%. Whether or not this funding would have been provided to other biomedical research programs is irrelevant, although many believe that the NIH would not have received so large an increment for any other reason. What is important to learn from this is that when Congress and the administration are forced by public sentiment to find the resources to meet a crucial need, the resources are found.

Annually, over 100,000 AIDS activists have taken to the streets in Washington, D.C., drawing public, congressional, and media attention to funding needs of the HIV epidemic. This is not unlike the scenario that occurred when the National Cancer Act was passed in 1971. The Citizens Committee for the Conquest of Cancer, established by Mary Woodard Lasker, took out full-page advertisements in the *New York Times*. In bold print, the ads declared, "Mr. Nixon, you can cure cancer," and then went on to describe how that could be achieved. Visibility, media, attention, and public sentiment can influence fiscal priorities. When legislators are made to understand that an issue is important to their constituents, it becomes their priority also.

Members of the cancer research community need to apply the lessons learned from the successes of the Citizens Committee for the Conquest of Cancer and from the AIDS activists. One important way to start is by urging Congress to increase support for the NIH. Dr. Lewis Thomas once stated, "If you are looking about for examples of things that government can do, and do beautifully well, rest your eyes on the NIH. The existence of this institution in its present form owes much to the political leaders, in and out of Congress, whose wisdom and statecraft put it in place" (11).

During the past 10 years, disastrous years for most domestic programs, the NIH was relatively unscathed in comparison with many other federally funded programs. Congress has always been an ardent supporter of medical research. There has never been a time since the inception of the NIH that the Congress has provided less funding for the NIH than was requested by the president. However, in the past 2 years, the NCI's final operating budget has been below the recommended appropriation because of "taps" on the NCI budget to pay for emerging and high-priority initiatives important to programs in the Public Health Service, but outside of the jurisdiction of the NIH.

Why have the increases for cancer research not been substantial over the past decade? While the fiscal concerns regarding our ballooning deficit have played a role, fiscal issues have not been the primary factor. If they had been, funding for the "big science" projects would not have been possible.

At the present time, there is little institutional memory within the Congress regarding the importance of providing adequate funding for cancer research. We have relied for far too long on too few champions in Congress, many of whom now are departed. A new generation of devoted legislators determined to contribute to the fight against cancer has not emerged. While many, many factors could be cited, the authors contend that one is of paramount importance: the need to provide increased funding for cancer research is not being presented persuasively, intensively, or passionately enough. That cancer can be cured is rarely mentioned. As a result, no one is listening to the few individuals who have taken the case to Congress. It is time for researchers, physicians, patients, families, and survivors to join together in greater numbers and in more active ways. It is time for those who deal with cancer in their daily lives to offer more persuasive arguments. They must convey the message that additional resources are vital if our society is to address the full spectrum of these diseases. Legislators, and the general public, need to be persuaded that cancer research warrants strong support and that such support is more than justified by the achievements of the past 2 decades.

A Call to Action

Each and every person involved in research has a responsibility to educate the community and its elected officials about the important benefits and goals of research. Recent articles in the scientific press have urged the research community to take its case to the policy makers and the general public, to broaden the base of support for research. The day is long gone when the research community can stay within the confines of the laboratory and expect that the resources will automatically be available to pursue crucial scientific quests. And the responsibility goes beyond this. It is a moral imperative that health professionals involved in cancer care act as resources to elected officials in health policy development.

One of the classic examples of where the cancer community has failed to use its skill and expertise to alter public policy is with tobacco use. The "Year 2000 Goals" for the NCI have indicted tobacco use as the culprit responsible for approximately 35% of the incidence of cancer in this country. And yet public relations firms continue their advertising; in many states, children legally purchase tobacco and even smoke in schools; and the Bush administration adopted trade policies facilitating tobacco exports to developing nations that have continued under the Clinton administration. What will be needed to persuade the cancer community to take its research data on the link between tobacco and cancer to legislators so as to influence and direct health policy in the area of tobacco?

The impetus for enacting the National Cancer Act was the desire of a diverse group of people, including scientists, philanthropists, legislators, and media representatives, who had joined forces in a common cause, to call a halt to the further progression of cancer. Distinguished leaders worked hard and well to persuade the Congress that the National Cancer Act was good public policy. The people needed little persuasion.

The cancer community must learn from these precedents, and carry on the legacy. It involves taking responsibility to educate the community and elected officials about the important benefit of cancer research. In doing so, it is advisable to develop both short- and long-term strategies to make a sustained and effective impact. A few questions: (*a*) What have you done to educate your local community, through radio, television, or speeches at local organizations, on the benefits of cancer research? (*b*) When did you last solicit the support of your patients, colleagues, and neighbors to gain the backing from elected officials for cancer research and affordable and accessible care? (*c*) When was the last time that your hospital, cancer center, or research laboratory held an open house for the press or the community, if ever? (*d*) Can you name your two senators and your representatives? When was the last time you met with them in Washington, or at home in your district? When did you last invite them to tour your research laboratory, patient unit, or medical facility? (*e*) When was the last time you wrote your legislators expressing concern on a specific issue, requesting their support, and providing the necessary follow-up to ensure a sustained commitment?

Epilogue

In 1971, momentum existed to make cancer research a national priority. Those involved had both a personal and professional commitment to the cause. Some had personal experiences with cancer prior to enacting the National Cancer Act; others lost loved ones or their own lives to cancer subsequent to its passage. Given that we are dealing with a group of diseases that will affect one in three Americans, any of us may similarly be emotionally, as well as intellectually, motivated to regenerate the legislative momentum to assure a vigorous program of cancer research and an efficient and humane program of cancer care. This is an agenda that is truly worthy of the United States and its citizens.

References

1. P.L. 244, 75th Congress, 2d Session. The National Cancer Institute Act of 1937. S. 2607, 1937.
2. P.L. 92-218, 92nd Congress, 2d Session. The National Cancer Act of 1971. S. 1828, 1971.
3. Schmidt BC. Remarks on the 15th anniversary of the National Cancer Act of 1971. JNCI 1987;78:1040.
4. Budget of the United States Government, Fiscal Year 1991. Washington DC: Government Printing Office, 1990.
5. Science in the National Interest, President William J. Clinton, Vice President Albert Gore, Jr. Executive Office of the President, Office of Science and Technology Policy, August 1994.
6. Committee on the Budget, U.S. House of Representatives. Report from the Committee on Budget, Fiscal Year 1991.
7. National Cancer Institute. Epidemiology and Biostatistics Program. SEER Data, 1990.
8. Langone J. Cautious optimism. Discover, p 47, 1986.
9. Committee on Appropriations, HUD and Independent Agencies, U.S. Senate. Report from the Committee on Fiscal Year 1990.
10. Rettig RA. Cancer Crusade. The Story of the National Cancer Act of 1971. Princeton, 1977.
11. Thomas L. Remarks upon acceptance of the Albert Lasker Medical Research Award, September 1986.

CHAPTER 94

Clinical Oncology in a Reforming Health Care Environment

MARTIN N. RABER AND JOSEPH S. BAILES

Introduction

It is impossible to practice medicine today without being affected by changes in the health care delivery system. Driven by a market-based reform movement of unprecedented force, a new health care system is forming. While these changes have implications for all physicians, the unique aspects of oncology suggest that while the role of those physicians who treat patients with cancer will change, the changes may be different from those in other specialty areas. These unique aspects include the following facts.

IDENTIFICATION OF THE CANCER PATIENT

Unlike many other diseases, once the diagnosis of cancer is made on a histologic basis it is not in doubt. Thus, the patient with cancer is easily identified for treatment.

NEED FOR SPECIALIZED TREATMENT

Although the training of general internists provides experience with cancer patients, after the diagnosis is made, most primary care physicians feel uncomfortable making therapeutic decisions and administering treatment. While the role of the general internist and family practitioner in the prevention, screening, and diagnosis of cancer remains paramount, the treatment of cancer patients remains the domain of specialists.

MULTIDISCIPLINARY TREATMENT OF CANCER

Unlike many other illnesses, the treatment of patients with cancer often requires a prospectively designed multidisciplinary treatment plan. This requires the collaboration of a team of specialists. The organization of such a team is beyond the expertise of general practitioners and internists.

CHANGING NATURE OF CANCER THERAPY

Given the overall poor results of systemic therapy for patients with metastatic cancer, it is not surprising that oncologists are quick to incorporate new strategies and new therapies into treatment plans. Keeping current in oncology demands a significant commitment beyond the scope of most primary care physicians.

DEMANDS OF PATIENTS FACING TERMINAL ILLNESSES

When faced with terminal disease, the American patient is particularly demanding in searching for information and treatment options. This need is met best by specialists broadly knowledgeable in the natural history and therapeutic options available. These specialists must be current in the latest results of clinical trials and must serve as a counselor and a reference standard for patients who wish to pursue alternative treatment. They also must be expert in the ethical and social issues surrounding management of patients with fatal illnesses and the resources required for such care.

At the same time, it is important to understand the forces driving change in health care. The impetus to control the rate of increase in health care spending comes from the true purchasers of care, private industry, and government. Industry believes health care costs must be reduced to remain competitive, while federal and state governments have identified health care costs as a major, if not the major, contributor to budgetary deficits.

Attempts to rein in health care spending have focused on "managed care" as the strategy of choice in controlling costs. At its essence, *managed care* is a term that implies that the insurer (or payer) will exert financial management over the delivery of health care. In the "managed" system, providers are contractually linked to insurers. This management linkage may take many forms, and at any given time different patients in a physician's practice, and different physicians in the same city, may be working under substantially different reimbursement formulas.

While the first goal of health care reform is the control of health care costs, from the perspective of the major purchasers (corporate employers) quality is also a high priority. Unfortunately, medicine has not clearly defined quality in health care. While we struggle for true measures of quality and outcome, we are forced to adopt by default an industrial perspective that focuses on the process of health care delivery as a surrogate for the outcome.

Current Strategies for the Delivery of Cancer Care

The training and development of a cadre of cancer specialists over the past two decades, coupled with significant scientific advancement, has resulted in the current era of high quality, multidisciplinary cancer care. While it can be argued that the system of unrestricted reimbursement resulted in the overuse of medical resources and in some cases the overtreatment of some patients, it also allowed physicians to focus on the individual patient's needs and provide the maximum treatment available.

In changing the reimbursement philosophy, the physician is now increasingly rewarded for providing less service, and the needs and desires of the individual patient are increasingly placed in a position subservient to the perceived needs of the community as a whole. In this environment, oncologists must develop a comprehensive approach that provides appropriate care for all patients at what the community considers acceptable costs and what the physician considers adequate reimbursement. This requires strategies that result in predictable costs and predictable outcomes, in a setting in which evaluation of outcome is feasible. It also requires a plan that allows for multidisciplinary care and the incorporation of new, effective therapies as they become available.

GUIDELINES AND PATHWAYS

The ability to deliver high quality health care in an environment where cost is a primary consideration will depend on broad agreement among specialists about the management of the common cancers. Guidelines are an overview of cancer treatments, appropriately sequenced for the management of specific clinical presentations. These guidelines must include the common presentations of cancer patients and detail the multidisciplinary approach. Such a consensus approach allows some uniformity of pretreatment evaluation, treatment planning, and follow-up for patients across the country and allows the providers to better estimate the costs of therapy. This approach also has the advantage of protecting the providers against accusations of negligence or concerns that the pressures to reduce cost have unreasonably affected treatment planning.

Guidelines as defined above are being developed across the country through large specialty societies, cancer centers, and groups of providers, and they are becoming standard practices in many communities. The same approach must also be taken for cancer prevention and screening, where the guidelines will be applied by primary care physicians with potentially tremendous impact on the cancer problem as a whole. However, guidelines are not a complete answer to the problem of providing high quality cancer treatment in a managed environment.

"Clinical pathways" provide a more detailed approach to patient management and allow the individual groups of providers to detail their specific resource utilization (e.g., specific chemotherapy regimens, drug doses and schedules, schedules for imaging studies, follow-up parameters). While there seems to be some uniformity in the guidelines under preparation, there is more diversity in the specifics of the clinical pathways being developed. At the same time that these standardized approaches to care are being developed, providers must also develop case management systems to ensure that the approaches agreed upon are being followed and to deal with patients whose clinical situations do not fit a clear pathway. At the moment, case management is centered on hospitalized patients, since the inpatient arena still encompasses a large portion of the expense of treating patients. However, to truly control costs and outcomes, this approach will need to be integrated into the outpatient setting and be extended to the management of the entire course of the disease.

Strategies for the Integration of Clinical Research

The costs of patient care in clinical trials are coming under increased scrutiny by third party payers. The potential chilling effect on drug development cannot be underestimated. The recognition that a clinical trial in a cancer patient may be "state of the art" therapy and not an "experiment" is not widespread. One of the apparent messages that employers and legislators have given the medical profession is that clinical research will not be paid for through charges for clinical care. Historically, clinical investigators have cost-shifted their hospital and professional charges to support research. While the costs of specific investigational drugs and the costs related to data management are often paid by the sponsor of a study, patient care–related costs have usually been paid by a third party payer. In the new paradigm, clinical costs associated with clinical investigations are not reimbursed. It is felt by insurers and employers that these charges should be paid by the study sponsor. Given the high costs of clinical care and pressures to keep pharmaceutical costs down, it is likely that fewer new drugs will be developed. In oncology, where many major advances have been made by academic investigators in unsponsored studies conducted after FDA drug approval, the problem is already significant. Since there is no effective therapy for many cancer patients, pressure to pursue experimental treatments is intense, and the patient and physician often find themselves in a situation where approved therapies known to be ineffective are reimbursed, while promising experimental treatments will not be paid for.

The resolution of this problem will no doubt take many forms and stretch over a period of years as the public becomes increasingly aware of the limitations intrinsic to a heavily managed medical environment. One way the marketplace itself is dealing in part with the issue is through its move to "capitation," or risk shifting. In the capitated system, cancer care may be "carved out" of the usual provider system and given to the specialty provider and center, who assume the financial risk for the delivery of care. Here, the provider chooses the appropriate therapy, ideally basing it on consensus-developed guidelines and pathways. The therapeutic choice and the decision regarding participation in a clinical trial is no longer dependent on specific approval from the insurer. A comprehensive solution will most likely involve some requirement that insurers provide access to investigational therapy if it meets accepted criteria such as those developed by the American Society of Clinical Oncology (ASCO) or the National Cancer Institute.

While these issues will not be resolved immediately, oncologists need to have a responsible approach to the treatment of patients with today's incurable cancers. The concept that care will not be reimbursed if it is given in the context of a clinical trial regardless of the agents used is not tenable. Patients who receive drugs for FDA-approved indications at the approved dose and schedule should have their care reimbursed, regardless of participation in a trial, particularly if the costs are similar to those of conventional therapy. The "off-label" use of anticancer drugs is an important issue since many of our most active drugs are used for indications that are not specifically approved. Oncologists are known for the speed with which they integrate new therapies into clinical practice. Thus, it is reasonable that patients receiving drugs used for off-label indications in diseases in which their efficacy has been demonstrated should be reimbursed under the same conditions outlined above. This applies as well to changes of dose, schedule, and route of administration. While there may be argument over what constitutes demonstrated efficacy, a listing of an indication in one or more of the pharmaceutical compendia (Compendia-based drug bulletin, Association of Community Cancer Centers, Rockville, MD. Spring 1995) or a reference in the peer-reviewed literature is a clear sign of support. In the same context, care given in conjunction with FDA "group C" drugs, in which there is FDA support for the indication prior to the formal approval process, should be reimbursed. These are all situations in which patients and physicians expect to be able to use what are considered effective agents. The Medicare and Medicaid programs are currently required by law to cover off-label use of anti-cancer drugs if they are listed as active drugs in one of the accepted pharmaceutical compendia or the peer-reviewed literature.

A more difficult situation arises with drugs that are of unproven benefit. Most current insurance policies exclude "investigational" therapy, and the use of these agents is often not reimbursed or reimbursable. When the experimental agent is given along with drugs approved for treatment of the disease, insurers should be willing to pay the charges associated with the standard treatment. In those cases where the experimental drugs are given alone for disease states in which there is no known effective therapy, the investigational nature of the treatment must be acknowledged and a source of support identified.

Another impact of the changing reimbursement system more directly affects investigators. As the reimbursement for care decreases, physicians must work harder to maintain their income level. This decreases the time available for clinical trials, which are often more time consuming from the physician's perspective. Furthermore, as profits decrease, hospitals are less willing to support the infrastructure required to maintain an active clinical trials program.

It is too early to assess the effects of health care reform on the entry into clinical trials. The risks are great that access will be significantly reduced and that community programs will flounder. On the other hand, the new emphasis on outcomes measurement suggests that the clinical trials model developed in oncology may in fact be an excellent resource for outcomes-directed clinical research. Oncologists are well trained in following research protocols and may in fact find themselves in a good position to take the lead in developing treatment guidelines and pathways and conducting the research necessary to improve them.

Conclusions

Market-driven health care reform is proceeding rapidly across the United States. It is taking on different formats in different parts of the country, but in all cases it is focused on decreasing health care costs. In the most mature markets it is succeeding in significantly decreasing hospitalization, length of stay, resource utilization, and referral to specialists. Driven by large employers, as it reduces overall costs and charges become similar among providers, health care reform will hopefully focus on quality as a differentiating factor. Without good measures of quality, the medical profession is obliged to standardize the process of delivery of care and develop acceptable measurements of outcome. This standardization will allow predictable costs, prices, and outcomes. At the same time, it allows physicians to set standards of care that will prevent a price-driven decrease in quality and afford some protection against litigation.

Oncology, unlike most other specialties, is potentially amenable to being "carved out" of many insurance policies. This may allow the oncologist to become the "gatekeeper" for cancer care, a role to which the medical oncologist is particularly well suited. A "carve out" may also foster the delivery of multidisciplinary care and allow the physician to decide, based on value, the therapeutic strategy to employ, eliminating the frustrating and time-consuming problems associated with the current process for obtaining approval and reapproval of services. It will also address some of the problems associated with off-label use of therapeutic agents and access to clinical trials. Nevertheless, the effect of health care reform on clinical research and drug development remains unclear, as does its effect on the number of oncologists the country will need.

CHAPTER 95

Outcomes Assessment

JANE WEEKS

Over the past decade there has been an explosion of interest in measuring the outcomes of medical care. The science of measuring outcomes and of integrating that process into the routine care of patients has come to be known as the "outcomes movement." "Outcomes" is an imprecise term that has different meanings in different contexts. In the narrowest sense, outcomes are what patients experience as a result of disease and its treatment. Often, the discipline of outcomes assessment is interpreted more broadly and encompasses, in addition, the study of how patients are treated, the determinants of treatment choice, the costs of delivering medical care under various conditions, and the proper allocation of society's and individual institutions' limited health care resources. This blending of clinical and policy perspectives is the hallmark of outcomes assessment.

Historical Perspective

In the classic paradigm of quality assessment in health care, three types of information can be considered: structure, process, and outcome. *Structure* describes the environment, including the physical plant and resources available; *process* is what is done for patients; and *outcome* is what is accomplished for patients (1). There were early proponents of measurement of outcomes as the primary indicator of quality, most notably Ernest Codman, a Boston surgeon and zealous advocate of the "end results idea" of relating specific interventions to their effects on patients (2). However, until recently, measures of structure and process were the dominant methods of assessing the quality of medical care.

In the 1980s two important observations rekindled interest in the assessment of outcomes. First, efforts at health care cost containment that focused on reimbursement mechanisms were failing to produce the hoped-for decreases in the escalating proportion of the gross domestic product spent on health care. It was recognized that the primary cause of the cost crisis was not so much the price of health care, but rather the increasing volume and intensity of medical services (3). Second, a number of investigators examined large, administrative data bases and found substantial geographic variability in the use of various medical interventions, without associated differences in medical outcomes (4–6). These observations laid the groundwork for what Arnold Relman labeled the "third revolution in medical care," namely, the "era of assessment and accountability" (7).

The most tangible effect of this revolution was the creation in 1989 of the federal Agency for Health Care Policy and Research. The mission of the AHCPR is to generate and disseminate information to improve the delivery of health care (8). The primary funding mechanism of the AHCPR, the Patient Outcome Research Teams (PORTs) are large-scale, 3- to 5-year clinical studies designed to evaluate the effectiveness, in clinical settings, of health care interventions (8). Of the 21 PORTs funded as of April, 1995, only one, which studies breast cancer in the elderly, is focused primarily on cancer therapy (9). Similarly, of the 16 guidelines produced by AHCPR, only one, management of cancer pain (10), addresses cancer treatment.

Several factors may account for AHCPR's inattention to cancer outcomes assessment, including the relatively low proportion of total inpatient hospital days attributable to cancer treatment and the complexity of the problem. Cancer is a heterogeneous group of diseases, and the available cancer therapies are not routinely used by investigators in general medicine, who have led the study of outcomes in other common conditions.

The recognition of the importance of outcomes in determining the value of medical treatments has not been limited to the federal government. Insurers also use outcome data in making decisions about what treatments to include in benefit packages. Increasingly, managed care organizations are also taking institutional outcomes into account in contracting decisions with hospitals and other providers.

Outcome Measures

DISEASE OUTCOMES

In outcomes research as well as in clinical trials, the effectiveness of cancer therapy is judged primarily in terms of its impact on the course of the disease. The most important outcome to consider in evaluating a cancer treatment in a clinical trial or clinical practice setting is survival. Disease-free survival may also be a useful end point to consider, especially in the adjuvant setting. In its position paper on outcomes of cancer therapy for technology assessment and cancer treatment guidelines, the American Society of Clinical Oncology (11) distinguishes between *patient outcomes*, such as survival, and *cancer outcomes*, such as tumor response and biomarker measurements. The report concludes that whereas cancer outcomes may be useful in the drug development process, technology assessments and guidelines should be based primarily on evaluations of the impact of treatment on patient outcomes.

QUALITY OF LIFE

A full assessment of the outcomes of cancer treatment involves a consideration of its impact on not only length of life, but also quality of life. As discussed in detail in Chapter 87, quality of life is a multidimensional concept that includes physical, social, and psychological functioning. It is particularly important to consider quality of life outcomes when treatment is given with palliative intent or when toxic therapy is likely to yield only a modest survival benefit. In treatment decisions involving trade-offs between length and quality of life, it may be useful to measure quality-adjusted survival, a single outcome that incorporates both length and quality of life (Fig. 95.1). Calculation of quality-adjusted survival requires that quality of life be measured in such a way that the product of length times quality of life is meaningful, e.g., that 1 year of life at a quality of x is as desirable as 6 months of life at a quality of $2x$. Measures of quality of life that have this property are called *utilities* (12). Utilities are defined as the quantitative measure of the strength of a person's preference for an outcome (13). By convention, utilities are measured on a scale of 0 to 1, in which 0 represents death and 1 represents excellent health. Utilities differ from more familiar measures of quality of life in that they reflect how a patient *values* a state of health, not just the characteristics of the health state. The terms "utilities," "values," and "preferences" are sometimes used interchangeably.

COST AND COST-EFFECTIVENESS

The goal of any health economic analysis is to determine whether the cost of a particular intervention is justified by the health benefits it produces. The question is usually framed by asking not how much it costs to deliver a particular treatment, but how much *more* it costs to provide that treatment than the most reasonable alternative (14). This alternative may be a "no-treatment" strategy, but it is not necessarily a "no-cost" strategy.

All economic analyses examine the difference in cost between alternative strategies; they differ in how they measure the benefits resulting from those strategies (Table 95.1) (14–16). The four basic types of economic analysis measure these benefits in four different ways. A *cost minimization* study simply assesses the additional cost of one strategy in comparison with another and therefore implicitly assumes that the two treatments produce comparable benefits. Because alternative medical interventions rarely produce truly equivalent outcomes, this type of analysis generally does not suffice as a complete economic evaluation of competing interventions. Usually, one wants to know whether the additional benefit conferred by the more expensive treatment is sufficient to justify the additional cost.

Cost-benefit analyses answer this question by assigning a dollar value to the health outcome in order to determine whether the incremental benefit of one treatment over another, measured in monetary terms, is greater than or equal to the incremental cost. *Cost-effectiveness* analyses, in contrast, measure the benefits of health care interventions in units of medical effect. For example, the cost-effectiveness of combination chemotherapy compared to single-agent therapy for a given disease could be assessed by calculating the additional cost (in dollars) per additional patient reaching the 5-year disease-free survival mark. However, one of the goals of cost-effectiveness analysis is to facilitate resource allocation decisions between interventions to treat or prevent different diseases. Cost-effectiveness data are much more useful if health benefits are measured in units that are common across diseases. Years of life saved is the most frequently used measure. Cost-effectiveness ratios are therefore usually expressed in terms of dollars per year of life saved.

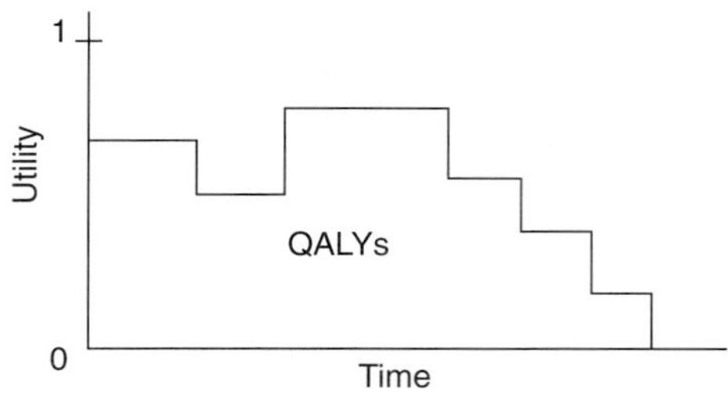

Figure 95.1. Quality-adjusted survival, measured in quality-adjusted life years (QALYs), is represented by the area under the curve of survival versus quality of life, measured in utilities.

Table 95.1. Types of Economic Analysis

Analysis	Measurement of cost	Measurement of benefits	Units of ratio
Cost minimization	Dollars	Assumed to be identical	Dollars
Cost-benefit	Dollars	Dollars	Unitless
Cost-effectiveness	Dollars	Effect of interest	Dollars/unit of effect
Cost-utility	Dollars	QALYs	Dollars/QALY

Abbreviation: QALY, quality-adjusted life year.

Medical interventions, however, affect not only length of life but also quality of life. A cancer cure may be bought at the expense of substantial treatment-related morbidity. Conversely, palliative therapy may bring marked relief of symptoms even if it does not lengthen life dramatically. *Cost-utility* analysis, a specific type of cost-effectiveness analysis, takes into account the impact of a health intervention on quality of life as well as length of life. Most commonly, this is done by assessing health benefits in terms of quality-adjusted survival, measured in quality-adjusted life years (QALYs) (Fig. 95.1). The units of a cost-utility ratio are thus dollars per QALY.

Study Designs

COHORT STUDIES

Outcomes research emphasizes the effectiveness rather than the efficacy of medical interventions. *Efficacy*, defined as the results of an intervention in carefully selected patients treated under controlled conditions, is best measured by a phase III trial. *Effectiveness*, in contrast, is a measure of the impact of routine medical interventions in all patients. It is assessed by observing the outcomes of care, typically in a cohort study design.

In a cohort study, subjects are not assigned to a particular treatment or intervention by the investigator, as they are in a randomized trial. Instead, treatment is chosen in the course of routine care, and subjects are then followed to determine outcomes (17). The advantages of a cohort study design include its comparatively low cost, the ability to evaluate the effects of treatments in types of patients who are underrepresented in clinical trials, such as the elderly or patients with comorbid disease, and the opportunity to evaluate the effectiveness of a treatment when it is given under routine conditions. The major disadvantage of the cohort study design is confounding—the influence of factors that affect both treatment choice and outcome. For example, if patients with extensive comorbid disease are consistently treated with a less aggressive regimen and have a poorer outcome, one might mistakenly conclude that the regimen is less effective when in fact those patients fared poorly simply because of a higher burden of comorbidity. Prospective enrollment of patients with careful attention to pretreatment measurement of potential confounding factors and the use of techniques such as multivariable analysis to control for them enhance the validity of a cohort study.

One particular type of cohort study that deserves specific mention is the large data base study. Data bases amassed for administrative purposes, such as the Health Care Financing Administration's Medicare billing data, may contain fairly extensive clinical data. These data bases have been used effectively to study the outcomes associated with common medical treatments in huge cohorts of patients treated in the community. They have been especially useful in detecting the influence of factors such as geographic location, race, and age on treatment choice and outcome. Large data base studies have been less useful in studying cancer than in studying other diseases, however, because they do not contain a sufficient level of detail about either the known predictors of outcome, such as disease stage, or the specific treatment regimens administered to allow meaningful conclusions to be drawn about the relationship between treatment and outcome.

CLINICAL TRIALS

Phase I and II trials, while an essential component of the drug development process, are not particularly helpful in evaluating the outcomes of new or established therapies. Phase III trials, in contrast, are an essential source of information on the outcomes of alternative treatments. If the trial is sufficiently large, randomization eliminates the problem of confounding by distributing equally among arms all known and unknown factors that may influence outcomes. The primary limitation of randomized controlled trials as a source of outcome data is that the results may not be generalizable. It is well documented that the tiny proportion of patients who participate in clinical trials are not representative of the population as a whole in terms of race, socioeconomic factors, or level of comorbidity (18, 19). In addition, clinical trials often dictate procedures for staging, treatment, and evaluation of outcomes that differ dramatically from practices that would be adopted in routine clinical care. "Large simple trials" are one solution to enhancing the generalizability of outcome data from clinical trials (20, 21). Oncology has lagged behind other disciplines such as cardiology in incorporating such trials into its clinical research portfolio.

The value of randomized trials in generating outcome data may also be augmented by broadening the array of end points to include quality of life and costs. Randomization enhances the validity of conclusions regarding the effects of treatment on these outcomes, just as it does for survival and other biologic outcomes. If costs, for example, are related to pretreatment characteristics and those characteristics also influence treatment choice, then it may be difficult or impossible to determine the independent impact of treatment choice on cost in a cohort study design. In addition, surveys to elicit quality-of-life and economic data are expensive, and it may be more efficient to piggyback them onto clinical trials than to collect data through another mechanism. The medical record reviews, audits, data management, and follow-up that occur in a clinical trial may be used to collect information on economic end points, for example, at relatively little additional cost.

DECISION ANALYSIS

For many medical decisions, some empirical data on the effectiveness of alternative therapies are available but the definitive experimental and observational studies have not been done. Decision-analytic models may be very helpful in aggregating the available data under these circumstances and in pinpointing areas where additional research is needed (22, 23). The first step in performing a decision analysis is to construct a computer model in the form of a decision tree that diagrams all the possible downstream outcomes of a particular treatment choice (Fig. 95.2). Probabilities are then assigned to each branch of this tree. These probabilities come from relevant clinical trials or cohort studies; when no data are available, expert judgment may be used. Outcomes are then assigned to each branch of the tree. A variety of outcomes may be used in decision analysis, including survival, quality-adjusted survival, and cost. The model is then analyzed to determine which treatment yields the best overall outcome. The most important step in decision-analytic modeling is sensitivity analysis. Each estimate in the model is varied, singly and in combination, to determine how sensitive the results are to any particular estimate. Sensitivity analysis is analogous to tests of significance in empirical studies in that it indicates how much confidence one should have in the conclusions.

COST-EFFECTIVENESS ANALYSIS

A comprehensive cost-effectiveness analysis requires data on how the alternative treatments being compared affect (*a*) length of life, (*b*) quality of life (measured in utilities), and (*c*) costs. Often, cost is determined by measuring resource use (e.g., hospital days, drugs) and multiplying each unit of resource by an estimate of its cost. Ideally, costs

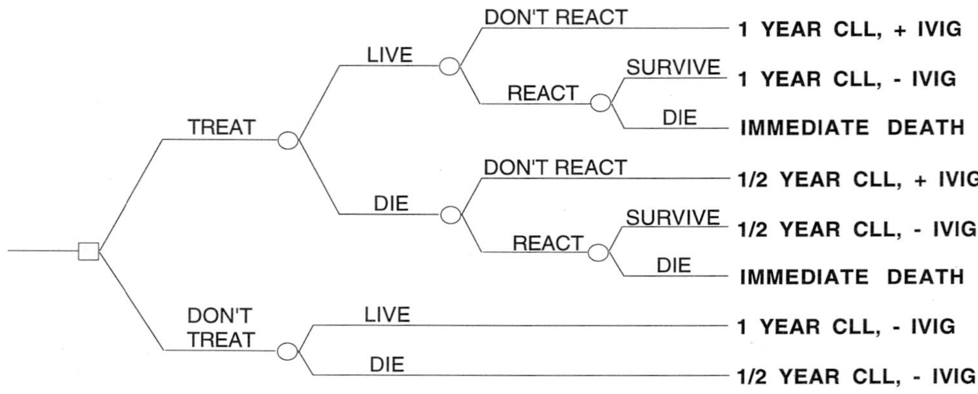

Value of One Year Outcomes:

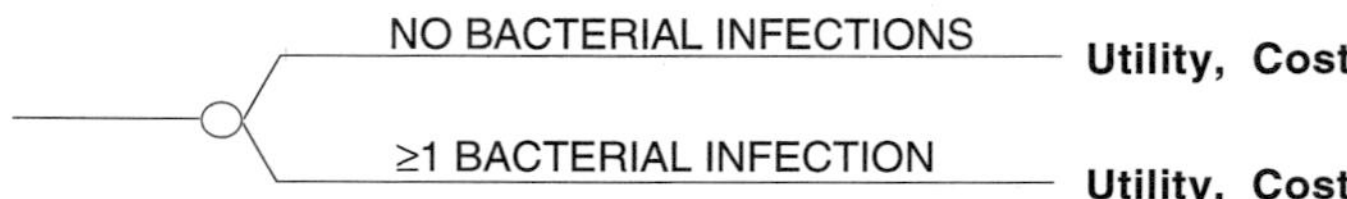

Figure 95.2. Example of a simple decision tree. The tree models the choice, represented by a square decision node, between treatment with prophylactic intravenous immune globulin (IVIG) in chronic lymphocytic leukemia (CLL) versus no prophylactic IVIG. Subsequent chance events, represented by round chance nodes, include death from CLL, adverse reactions to IVIG, and death from an adverse reaction. Outcomes are assessed at 1 year and include both quality-adjusted life years (QALYs) and costs. QALYs are calculated by multiplying the proportion of the year survived by the quality of life. The quality of life, measured in utilities, depends on the number of bacterial infections. As described by Weeks et al. (46), the probabilities of death, adverse reactions, and infection were derived from a randomized controlled trial. Utilities and costs were based on expert judgment. *Source*: Adapted from Weeks et al. (46), with permission.

$$\Delta C = \Delta C_{Rx} + \Delta C_{SE} - \Delta C_{Morb} + \Delta C_{Rx/LE}$$

where

Δ is difference between treatment and alternative strategy

ΔC is net health care cost of an intervention

ΔC_{Rx} is net direct medical care cost of the intervention

ΔC_{SE} is net cost of caring for the side effects attributable to the intervention

ΔC_{Morb} is net savings in direct medical costs, rehabilitation, etc., due to prevention or alleviation of disease

$\Delta C_{Rx/LE}$ is net cost of treating diseases that would not have occurred if patient had not lived longer as a result of the intervention

Figure 95.3. Net health care costs of an intervention. *Source*: Weinstein (25). Reproduced with permission.

rather than charges are used. In economic terms, costs are a measure of the resources consumed to provide a service. Charges may include some degree of profit and also are influenced by regulation and cost shifting between departments, and therefore are poor proxies for costs (24). A full accounting of the direct medical costs of a particular medical intervention includes not only the drugs, physicians' fees, and hospital days required to deliver that intervention but also the downstream cost consequences of treatment side effects, the morbidity avoided if the disease is successfully treated, and the additional diseases and medical problems that occur in patients who live longer as a result of the original treatment (Fig. 95.3). Depending on the perspective of the analysis, direct nonmedical costs for items such as transportation to the hospital and family care, as well as indirect costs in the form of wages gained or lost because of disease and its treatment, may also be included (14, 15).

A variety of sources may be used to generate each of the categories of data involved in estimating cost-effectiveness (Table 95.2). In the past, most cost-effectiveness analyses were done using decision-analytic techniques to combine data on effectiveness, drawn from published studies or expert judgement, with cost data, often estimated from a single institution's experience in treating similar patients. Increasingly, data for cost-effectiveness analyses are being collected prospectively alongside cancer clinical trials. The pharmaceutical industry has taken the lead in these studies, spurred by Australia's requirement that evidence of cost-effectiveness be included in requests to the public health service to add new drugs to the list of medications approved for payment, and by the practice of regulators in many European countries of relying on economic data to set drug prices (26). Several of the cooperative groups, including the Cancer and Leukemia Group B (CALGB), Eastern Cooperative Oncology Group, and Pediatric Oncology Group, are following suit and have opened or are soon to open phase III trials in which resource use data and bills of study patients are collected prospectively (27). These data will be used to estimate how much more it costs to treat patients in one arm of the study than the other and will be combined with clinical data from the trials to generate estimates of the cost-effectiveness of one treatment in comparison with the other.

Table 95.2. Potential Sources of Data for Cost-Effectiveness Analysis

Efficacy
- collected prospectively during clinical trial
- published data on a single trial
- published data on multiple trials, cohort studies

Resource use
- collected prospectively during clinical trial
- collected after trial by chart review
- expert estimates

Costs
- bills collected prospectively during clinical trial
- insurance billing data
- resource use units priced out after trial completed

Utilities
- collected prospectively during clinical trial
- health state specific utilities collected independent of trial from patients or surrogates
- expert estimates

Outcomes Studies in Oncology

PATTERNS OF CARE

Although not outcomes studies in the narrowest sense, analyses of the nature and determinants of treatment choice among patients with a particular diagnosis are fundamental to the outcomes movement. Using administrative billing data collected by the federal government and other payers, as well as data from the Surveillance, Epidemiology, and End Results (SEER) registry and other tumor registries, a number of investigators have shown that geographic location, hospital type and size, and nonmedical patient characteristics may influence cancer treatment choice (28). For example, recent large data base studies have found that the proportion of women with breast cancer who receive mastectomy rather than breast-conserving surgery is up to three times higher in the central United States than on the coasts (29–31). In addition, women who are younger and who are treated in large, urban, university-affiliated hospitals are more likely to undergo breast-conserving surgery (31–35). One particularly disturbing study found that patients' health insurance status predicted for stage at diagnosis and survival, stage for stage, in breast cancer (36). Similarly, rates of radical prostatectomy for early prostate cancer show wide geographic variation (37), and several studies have demonstrated that older and non-Caucasian men receive less aggressive therapy, differences that persist after controlling for stage, comorbidity, and treatment site (38, 39).

These studies relied on secondary data sources and therefore were unable to examine whether these differences reflect unmeasured clinical characteristics, physician prejudices, or patient preferences. In-depth studies of the decision-making process have suggested that the primary determinant of cancer treatment choice is physicians' recommendations (40). These recommendations, in turn, may be heavily influenced by physicians' specialties. For example, in a study in which physicians were presented with hypothetical scenarios describing patients with prostate cancer, respondents generally favored the modality in which they were trained, with urologists opting for surgery, radiotherapists favoring radiotherapy, and medical oncologists dividing their votes equally between the two treatments (41).

EFFECTIVENESS STUDIES

Little systematic research on the effectiveness of alternative cancer therapies in the community setting have been performed. Several large-scale prospective cohort studies are now in progress, however, that should help elucidate not only the determinants of treatment choice, but also the outcomes of treatment in the routine care setting for two common cancers. These include a PORT study of breast cancer in the elderly and an AHCPR-funded study of treatment choice and outcomes in early prostate cancer being conducted by investigators at the Dana-Farber Cancer Institute. The results of the study of prostate cancer may be particularly enlightening since efforts to mount randomized trials in this disease have been marked by very poor accrual. Preliminary findings from this study demonstrate higher rates of treatment-related morbidity than have been reported in case series from single institutions or surgeons (42, 43). For example, among the first 150 patients studied, 77% of those treated with radical prostatectomy reported impotence 1 year after treatment, compared with 41% of patients treated with radiotherapy, despite equivalent pretreatment impotence rates of approximately 15% (44).

COST-EFFECTIVENESS STUDIES

Until recently, the majority of cost-effectiveness studies in cancer were economic studies of screening. In the past few years, a number of studies of the cost-effectiveness of various treatments for cancer have appeared in the literature. This literature has been summarized in a recent comprehensive review (45); the cost-effectiveness ratios for a subset of those studies are given in Table 95.3 (46–57). There is no absolute standard for what constitutes a reasonable number of dollars per year of life saved. A range for this threshold has been established by examining cost-effectiveness ratios for interventions that are generally regarded by society as reasonable and those that are generally regarded as inordinately expensive for the degree of benefit produced. The conclusion is that interventions costing under approximately $50,000 per year of life saved are cost-effective and those costing over $100,000 are cost-ineffective. Cost-effectiveness ratios falling between these levels are in a gray zone. Applying this standard to the results shown in Table 95.3, it is evident that cost-effectiveness ratios for cancer treatment are much more sensitive to the magnitude of the benefit produced than to the price tag of the therapy. In general, cancer therapies that result in clinically meaningful improvements in patient outcomes have been shown to be cost-effective regardless of the cost of the treatment.

What is the relevance of cost-effectiveness analyses to the practicing clinician? In the United States, though not necessarily in all developed countries, it is generally believed that the physician should function as the patient's advocate in these discussions and should offer any treatment likely to be

Table 95.3. Examples of Published Cost-Effectiveness Analysis in Cancer

Therapy	Alternative	Cost-effectivenss ratio
Intravenous immune globulin in chronic lymphocytic leukemia (46)	No infection prophylaxis	$6,000,000[a]
Diagnosis and therapy of carcinoma of unknown primary (47)	Supportive care	$2,400,000
Autologous bone marrow transplant in metastatic breast cancer (48)	Conventional chemotherapy	$116,000
Chemotherapy in node-negative breast cancer (49)	No chemotherapy	$50,000[a]
Adjuvant CMF in 75-year-old women with breast cancer (50)	No chemotherapy	$44,000[a]
Hemodialysis (51)	No dialysis	$35,000
Propranolol for moderate hypertension (52)	No therapy	$33,000[a]
Autologous bone marrow transplant for Hodgkin's disease in second complete remission (53)	Conventional chemotherapy	$26,000
Tamoxifen and chemotherapy in premenopausal, node-positive, estrogen receptor-positive breast cancer (54)	Chemotherapy alone	$15,000[a]
Vindesine/cisplatin for non-small cell lung cancer (55)	Best supportive care	$15,000
Bone marrow transplant for acute myelogenous leukemia (56)	Conventional chemotherapy	$10,000
Etoposide/cisplatin alternating with cytoxan/Adriamycin/vincristine for small cell lung cancer (57)	Cytoxan/Adriamycin/vincristine	$4,500[a]

[a] Quality adjusted.

of net benefit, regardless of the cost to society. But some clinicians serve other roles as well, as administrators and policymakers, jobs in which they need to consider whether the costs of various health care services are justified by the benefits they produce. And all practitioners must have some understanding of issues of cost and cost-effectiveness if they are to have any voice in the debate over allocation of health care dollars and other resources.

Outcomes Management

Outcomes management describes the process by which studies of the outcomes of care are used to improve the delivery of medical services. Paul Ellwood has characterized outcomes management as a way "to help patients, payers, and providers make rational medical care-related choices based on better insight into the effect of these choices on the patient's life" (58). To accomplish this goal, he argues, outcomes management requires four components: (*a*) guidelines that physicians can use in selecting appropriate interventions; (*b*) systematic measurement of the functioning and well-being of patients; (*c*) pooling of clinical and outcome data on a massive scale; and (*d*) analysis and dissemination of the results of the data base.

Clinical practice guidelines are at the heart of outcomes management. These standards, referred to by some as "cookbook" medicine, specify how patients in particular clinical circumstances should be treated (59–63). Guidelines dictate what the treatment should be; "critical paths," in contrast, specify how that therapy should be delivered, including the frequency of follow-up visits and testing, the tasks to be assumed by physicians and nurses, and so forth. Guidelines are designed to eliminate variation in patterns of care that represent deviations from what is believed to be the most effective and cost-effective therapy for a given disease. How much emphasis to place on consideration of cost in the development of guidelines is an area of great controversy. The Institute of Medicine has laid out criteria for selecting topics for guidelines that take into account the prevalence of the problem, the burden of illness imposed by the condition, cost, variability in practice, the potential to improve health outcomes, and the potential to reduce costs (64). Clearly, many cancer diagnoses fulfill these criteria. Therefore, it is not surprising that cancer clinical practice guidelines are proliferating.

Although AHCPR has published only one guideline directed toward cancer treatment, on the management of cancer pain, other groups have been more active in developing guidelines for cancer care. After each of its consensus development conferences, the NIH issues statements distilling the presentations of experts to identify areas of consensus, emerging trends in the clinical literature, and areas requiring further investigation. These reports include both definitive statements about what constitutes optimal care in areas where consensus was reached and recommendations regarding therapeutic approaches to be considered in other areas. Recently, the trend has been away from such consensus-based guidelines to an evidence-based approach in which guidelines are explicitly grounded in a comprehensive review of the relevant literature graded for the quality of the evidence presented. ASCO has charged a Health Services Research Committee with producing such evidence-based guidelines. The first ASCO guideline addressed the use of hematopoietic colony-stimulating factors (65); guidelines on the use of tumor markers in breast and colon cancer, treatment of metastatic non-small cell lung cancer, and follow-up after treatment for breast cancer and colon cancer are currently under development. Other national societies are also in the process of writing clinical practice guidelines. For example, the American Urological Society is developing guidelines for the treatment of renal cell carcinoma, the management of superficial bladder cancer, and the management of localized prostate cancer (66).

Under pressure to control costs and minimize unwarranted variability in care, many institutions are developing their own guidelines for the treatment of common cancers. To be successful, such an effort requires a substantial commitment of time and money, an investment that may be beyond the resources of some institutions. However, the involvement of the ultimate users of a guideline in its development and the tailoring of the guideline to local conditions help ensure buy-in by clinicians. Proponents of institutional guidelines argue that as a result, these guidelines may produce more sustained effects on practice patterns than guidelines promulgated by national bodies have been able to achieve (67).

Summary

At the heart of the outcomes movement is a very simple idea: The value of the health care we deliver should be determined by a systematic examination of patient outcomes. The novelty of this approach lies largely in its emphasis on how patients fare in routine clinical care, not just clinical trials, and in broadening the array of outcomes to include quality of life and costs as well as biologic end points. To accomplish this goal, methods are required that are relatively unfamiliar to cancer clinical researchers and practitioners, including observational cohort studies, decision analysis, and cost-effectiveness analysis. In comparison to the finely honed, sophisticated study design and statistical methods that have been developed for use in clinical trials, many of these techniques are relatively untested. Further methodologic work is clearly needed. However, there is a more fundamental challenge that must be met if the outcomes movement is to deliver on the grandiose promises made by many of its proponents. Physicians, patients, and health care institutions must agree to participate in data collection efforts on a massive scale. Assessments of outcomes must be integrated into the daily routine of caring for cancer patients. The resulting data must be shared and continuously analyzed to create a feedback loop that produces continuous modification of, and improvement in, clinical practice guidelines. In the short term, interest in outcomes assessment and management is being driven largely by a desire to control health care costs. If this "third revolution in medical care" is successful, however, the real pay-off will be higher quality medical care for cancer patients.

References

1. Donabedian A. The role of outcomes in quality assessment and assurance. Quality Rev Bull 1992;356–360.
2. Codman EA. The Shoulder: Rupture of the Supraspinatus Tendon and Other Lesions in or about the Subacromial Bursa. Boston: Thomas Todd, 1934.
3. Roper WL. Perspectives on physician-payment reform: the resource-based relative value scale in context. N Engl J Med 1988;319:865–867.
4. Wennberg JE, Freeman JL, Culp WJ. Are hospital services rationed in New Haven or overutilized in Boston? Lancet 1987:1185–1187.
5. Wennberg JE, Freeman JL, Shelton RA, Bubolz TA. Hospital use and mortality among Medicare beneficiaries in Boston and New Haven. N Engl J Med 1989;321:1168–1173.
6. Wennberg JE, Mulley AG, Hanley D, Timothy RP, Fowler FJ, Roos NP, et al. An assessment of prostatectomy for benign urinary obstruction: geographic variations and the evaluations of medical care outcomes. JAMA 1988;259:3027–3030.
7. Relman AM. Assessment and accountability: the third revolution in medical care. N Engl J Med 1988;319:1220–1222.
8. Agency for Health Care Policy and Research. AHCPR Profile: The 1996 Medical Outcomes and Guidelines Sourcebook. Edited by MT Youngs, L Wingerson. New York: Faulkner & Gray, 1995.
9. Federal medical treatment effectiveness. In AHCPR Profile: The 1996 Medical Outcomes and Guidelines Sourcebook. Edited by MT Youngs, L Wingerson. New York: Faulkner & Gray, 1995.
10. Management of Cancer Pain. Washington: Agency for Health Care Policy and Research, 1994, no. 9.
11. Outcomes Working Group, Health Services Research Committee, American Society of Clinical Oncology. Outcomes of cancer treatment for technology assessment and cancer treatment guidelines. J Clin Oncol 1996;14:671–679.
12. Tsevat J, Weeks JC, Guadagnoli E, Tosteson ANA, Mangione CM, Pliskin JS, Weinstein MC, Cleary PD. Using health-related quality of life information: clinical encounters, clinical trials, and health policy. J Gen Intern Med 1994;9:576–582.
13. Torrance GW. Measurement of health state utilities for economic appraisal: a review. J Health Econ 1985;5:1–30.
14. Detsky AS, Naglie IG. A clinician's guide to cost-effectiveness analysis. Ann Intern Med 1990;113:147–154.
15. Eisenberg JM. Clinical economics. JAMA 1989;262:2879–2886.
16. Weeks JC. Taking quality of life into account in health economic analyses. JNCI (in press).
17. Hennekens CH, Buring JE. Epidemiology in Medicine. Boston: Little, Brown, 1987.
18. Svensson CK. Representation of American blacks in clinical trials of new drugs. JAMA 1989;261:263–265.
19. Hunninghake DB, Darby CA, Probstfield JL. Recruitment experience in clinical trials: literature summary and annotated bibliography. Controlled Clin Trials 1987;8:6S–30S.
20. Yusuf S, Collins R, Peto R. Why do we need large, simple randomized trials? Stat Med 1984;3:409–422.
21. Peto R, Collins R, Gray R. Large scale randomized evidence: large, simple trials and overviews of trials. J Clin Epidemiol 1995;48:23–40.
22. Richardson WS, Detsky AS. Users' guides to the medical literature: VII. How to use a clinical decision analysis. JAMA 1995;273:1610–1613.
23. Weinstein MC, Fineberg HV. Clinical Decision Analysis. Philadelphia: Saunders, 1980.
24. Finkler SA. The distinction between costs and charges. Ann Intern Med 1982;96: 102–109.
25. Weinstein MC, Stason WB. Foundations of cost-effectiveness analysis for health and medical practices. N Engl J Med 1977;296:716–721.
26. Bloom BS. Issues in mandatory economic assessment of pharmaceuticals. Health Affairs 1994;Winter:197–201.
27. Nelson H, Weeks JC, Weiand HS. Proposed phase III prospective randomized trial comparing laparoscopic-assisted colectomy versus open colectomy for colon cancer. Monogr Natl Cancer Inst 1995;19:51–56.
28. Desch CE, Johantgen M, Smith TJ, Hillner BE, Retchin SM. Practice variation in oncology: cause, effects, and treatments. JNCI (in press).
29. Nattinger AB, Gottlieb MS, Veum J, et al. Geographic variation in the use of breast-conserving treatment for breast cancer. N Engl J Med 1992;326:1102–1107.
30. Osteen RT, Steele GD, Menck HR, Winchester DP. Regional differences in surgical management of breast cancer. CA 1992;42:39–43.
31. Farrow DC, Hunt WC, Samet JM. Geographic variation in the treatment of localized breast cancer. N Engl J Med 1992;324:1097–1101.
32. Lazovich D, White E, Thomas DB, Moe RE. Underutilization of breast-conserving surgery and radiation therapy among women with stage I or II breast cancer. JAMA 1991;266:3433–3488.
33. Hand R, Sener S, Imperato J, et al. Hospital variables associated with quality of care for breast cancer patients. JAMA 1991;266:3429–3432.
34. Hynes DM. The quality of breast cancer care in local communities: implications for health care reform. Med Care 1994;32:328–340.
35. Greenfield S, Blanco DM, Elashoff R, Ganz PA. Patterns of care related to age of breast cancer patients. JAMA 1987;257:2766–2770.
36. Ayanian JZ, Kohler BA, Abe T, Epstein AM. The relation between health insurance coverage and clinical outcomes among women with breast cancer. N Engl J Med 1993;329:326–331.
37. Lu-Yao GL, McLerran D, Wasson J, Wennberg JE. An assessment of radical prostatectomy time trends, geographic variation and outcomes. JAMA 1993;269:2633–2636.
38. Bennett CL, Greenfield S, Aronow H, Ganz P, et al. Patterns of care related to prostate cancer. Cancer 1991;67:2633–2641.
39. Schapira MM, McAuliffe TL, Nattinger AB. Treatment of localized prostate cancer in African-American compared to caucasian men: less use of aggressive therapy for comparable disease. Med Care 1995;33:1079–1088.
40. Siminoff LA, Fetting JH, Abeloff MD. Doctor-patient communication about breast cancer adjuvant therapy. J Clin Oncol 1989;7:1192–1200.
41. Moore MJ, O'Sullivan B, Tannock IF. How expert physicians would wish to be treated if they had genitourinary cancer. J Clin Oncol 1988;6:1739–1745.
42. Walsh PC. Radical prostatectomy, preservation of sexual function, cancer control: the controversy. Urol Clin North Am 1987;14:663–673.
43. Catalona WJ, Bigg SW. Nerve-sparing radical prostatectomy: evaluation of results after 250 patients. J Urol 1990:143:538–543.
44. Talcott JA, Rieker P, Propert K, Kalish L, Clark J, Weeks JC, Kantoff P. Complications of the treatment for early prostate cancer: a prospective multi-institutional outcomes study. Proc Am Soc Clin Oncol 1994;13:231A.
45. Smith TJ, Hillner BE, Desch CE. Efficacy and cost-effectiveness of cancer treatment: rational allocation of resources based on decision analysis. JNCI 1993;85:1460–1474.
46. Weeks JC, Tierney MR, Weinstein MC. Cost effectiveness of prophylactic intravenous immunoglobulin in chronic lymphocytic leukemia. N Engl J Med 1991;325:81–86.
47. Levine MN, Drummond MF, Labelle RJ. Cost-effectiveness in the diagnosis and treatment of carcinoma of unknown primary origin. Can Med Assoc J 1985;133:977–983.
48. Hillner BE, Smith TJ, Desch CE. Efficacy and cost-effectiveness of autologous bone marrow transplantation in metastatic breast cancer. JAMA 1992;267:2055–2061.
49. Hillner BE, Smith TJ. Efficacy and cost effectiveness of adjuvant chemotherapy in women with node-negative breast cancer. N Engl J Med 1991;324:160–168.
50. Desch CE, Hillner BE, Smith TJ, et al. Should the elderly receive chemotherapy for node-negative breast cancer? J Clin Oncol 1993;11:777–782.
51. Churchill DN, Lemon BC, Torrance GW. A cost-effectiveness analysis of continuous ambulatory peritoneal dialysis and hospital hemodialysis. Med Decis Making 1984;4: 439–500.
52. Edelson JT, Weinstein MC, Tosteson ANA, et al. Long-term cost-effectiveness of various initial monotherapies for mild to moderate hypertension. JAMA 1990;263:407–413.
53. Desch CE, Lasala MR, Smith TJ, Hillner BE. The optimal timing of autologous bone marrow transplantation in Hodgkin's disease after chemotherapy relapse. J Clin Oncol 1992;10:200–209.
54. Smith TJ, Hillner BE. The efficacy and cost-effectiveness of adjuvant therapy of early breast cancer in premenopausal women. J Clin Oncol 1993;11:771–776.
55. Jaakkimainen L, Goodwin PJ, Pater J, et al. Counting the costs of chemotherapy in a National Cancer Institute of Canada trial in nonsmall-cell lung cancer. J Clin Oncol 1990;8:1301–1309.

56. Welch HG, Larson EB. Cost-effectiveness of bone marrow transplantation in acute nonlymphocytic leukemia. N Engl J Med 1989;321:807–812.
57. Goodwin PJ, Feld R, Evans WK, Pater J. Cost-effectiveness of cancer chemotherapy: an economic evaluation of a randomized trial in small-cell lung cancer. J Clin Oncol 1988;6:1537–1547.
58. Ellwood PM. Shattuck lecture. Outcomes management: a technology of patient experience. N Engl J Med 1988;318:1549–1556.
59. Cook DJ, Guyatt GH, Laupacis A, Sackett DL. Rules of evidence and clinical recommendations on the use of antithrombotic agents. Chest 1992;103:305S–311S.
60. GAO/PEMD-91-11. Practice Guidelines: The Experience of Medical Specialty Studies. Washington, DC: General Accounting Office, Feb 1991.
61. Woolf SH. Practice guidelines, a new reality in medicine. Arch Intern Med 1992;152: 946–952.
62. Committee to Advise the Public Health Service on Clinical and Practice Guidelines. Clinical Practice Guidelines: Directions for a New Program. Edited by MJ Field, KN Lohr. Washington DC: National Academy Press.
63. Kapp MB. "Cookbook" medicine: a legal perspective. Arch Intern Med 1990;150: 496–500.
64. Institute of Medicine. Setting Priorities for Clinical Practice Guidelines. Washington DC: National Academy Press, 1995.
65. American Society of Clinical Oncology. Recommendations for the use of hematopoietic colony-stimulating factors: evidence-based, clinical practice guidelines. J Clin Oncol 1994;12:2471–2508.
66. American Medical Association. Practice Parameters Update, November 1994. Chicago: American Medical Association, 1994.
67. Browman GP, Levine MN, Mohide EA, Hayward RS, Pritchard KI, Gafni A, Laupacis A. The practice guideline development cycle: a conceptual tool for practice guidelines development and implementation. J Clin Oncol 1995;13:502–512.

CHAPTER 96

Questionable Cancer Therapies

STEPHEN BARRETT AND VICTOR D. HERBERT

What Are "Questionable Methods"?

The American Cancer Society (ACS) defines questionable methods as life-style practices, clinical tests, or therapeutic modalities that are promoted for *general* use for the prevention, diagnosis, or treatment of cancer, and that are, on the basis of careful review by scientists and/or clinicians, deemed to have no real evidence of value (1). Under the rules of science (and federal law), proponents who make health claims bear the burden of proof. It is their responsibility to conduct suitable studies and report them in sufficient detail to permit evaluation and confirmation by others. The ACS's Committee on Questionable Methods of Cancer Management evaluates methods by asking three questions: (*a*) Has the method been objectively demonstrated in the peer-reviewed scientific literature to be effective? (*b*) Has the method shown potential for benefit that clearly exceeds the potential for harm? (*c*) Have objective studies been correctly conducted under appropriate peer review to answer these questions?

Wallace F. Janssen, historian for the Food and Drug Administration (FDA), has noted that in every decade since 1940, a questionable cancer remedy has attracted a large following and become a national issue (2). It was Koch antitoxins in the 1940s, Hoxsey treatment in the 1950s (3), Krebiozen in the 1960s (4), laetrile in the 1970s (5), and immunoaugmentative therapy in the 1980s (6). Today's questionable methods include corrosive agents, plant products, special diets and "dietary supplements," drugs, correction of "imbalances," biologic methods, devices, miscellaneous concoctions, psychologic approaches, and worthless diagnostic tests. Many promoters combine methods to make themselves more marketable. A 1987 ACS investigation found that 452 (9%) of 5,047 cancer patients identified through a telephone survey had used questionable treatments. Of these, 49% had used "mind therapies" (mental imagery, hypnosis, or psychic therapy) and 38% had used diets (7). The dangers of using questionable treatments include a delay in getting appropriate treatment, decreased quality of life, direct physical harm, interference with proved treatments, a waste of valuable time, financial harm, and psychological damage.

Typical Misrepresentations

Proponents of questionable methods typically claim that marketplace demand and testimonials from satisfied customers are proof that their remedies work. However, these proponents almost never keep score or reveal what percentage of their cases end in failure. Cancer cures attributed to questionable methods usually fall into one or more of five categories: (*a*) the patient never had cancer; (*b*) a cancer was cured or put into remission by proved therapy, but questionable therapy was also used and erroneously credited for the beneficial result; (*c*) the cancer is progressing, but is erroneously represented as slowed or cured (example: Fig. 96.1); (*d*) the patient has died as a result of the cancer (or is lost to follow-up) but is represented as cured; or (*e*) the patient had a spontaneous remission (very rare) or a slow-growing cancer that is publicized as a cure.

Promoters of questionable methods often misrepresent their methods as "alternatives." *Genuine* alternatives are comparable methods that have met the criteria for safety and effectiveness. *Experimental* alternatives are unproved but have a plausible rationale and are undergoing responsible investigation. *Questionable* "alternatives" are unproved and lack a scientifically plausible rationale. When referring to the last, we use quotation marks because they are not true alternatives. Some promoters of "alternative" methods are physicians or other highly educated scientists who have strayed from scientific thought. Their motivation can include delusional thinking, misinterpretation of personal experience, financial considerations, and pleasure derived from notoriety and/or patient adulation.

Misinformation about questionable cancer therapies is spread through books, articles, audiotapes, videotapes, talk shows, news reports, lectures, health expositions, "alternative" practitioners, information and referral services, and word of mouth. Promoters typically explain their approach in common sense terms and appear to offer patients an active role in their care: (*a*) cancer is a symptom, not a disease; (*b*) symptoms are caused by diet, stress, or environment; (*c*) proper fitness, nutrition, and mental attitude allow biologic and mental defense against cancer; and (*d*) conventional therapy weakens the body's reserves, treating the symptoms rather than the disease (8). Questionable therapies are portrayed as natural and nontoxic, while standard (responsible) therapies are portrayed as highly dangerous (example: Fig. 96.2).

During the past few years, the news media have publicized "alternative" methods in ways that are causing great public confusion. Most of these reports have contained no critical evaluation and have featured the views of proponents and their satisfied clients. Many have exaggerated the significance of the National Institutes of Health's (NIH) recently opened Office of Alternative Medicine (OAM). Creation of this office was spearheaded by promoters of questionable cancer therapies who wanted more attention paid to their methods. Most of its advisory panel members have been promoters of "alternative" therapies. In 1994, the OAM's first director resigned, charging that political interference had hampered his ability to carry out OAM's mission in a scientific manner (9). The OAM has funded several dozen studies related to "alternative" methods, including a few related to cancer treatment. However, it remains to be seen whether such research will yield useful results. Even if it does, the benefit is unlikely to outweigh the publicity bonanza given to questionable methods (10). Some of today's "alternative" methods are described below in alphabetical order.

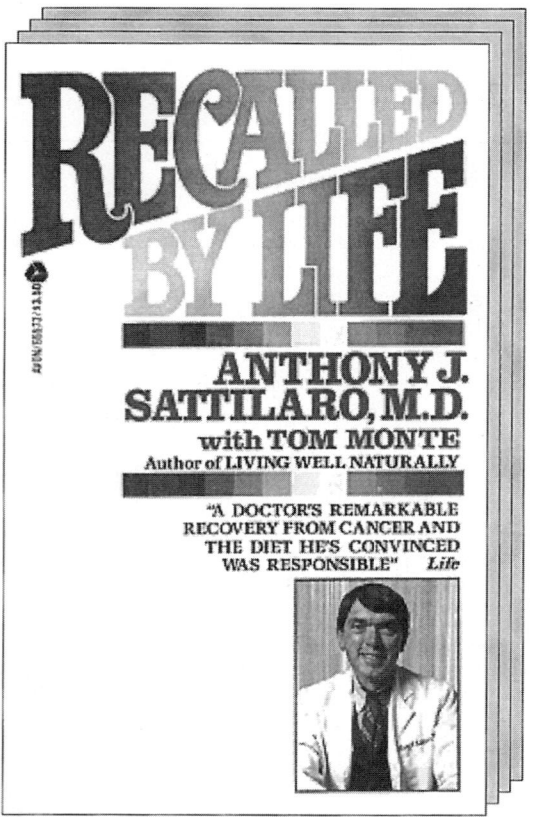

Figure 96.1. The author of this 1982 book underwent responsible treatment for prostate cancer but credited macrobiotics for placing him in "permanent remission." He died of his disease in 1989.

ANTINEOPLASTONS

Stanislaw R. Burzynski, M.D., has given the name "antineoplastons" to substances he claims can "normalize" cancer cells that are constantly being produced within the body. He has published many papers stating that antineoplastons extracted from urine or synthesized in his laboratory have been proved to be effective against cancer in laboratory experiments. He also claims to have helped many people with cancer get well. A recent analysis concluded that none of Burzynski's "antineoplastons" has been proved to normalize tumor cells (11). In 1995, a federal grand jury indicted Burzynski for mail fraud and marketing an unapproved drug. The indictment charged that he had fraudulently billed insurance companies using procedure codes for chemotherapy.

In 1988, Burzynski got a tremendous boost when talk-show hostess Sally Jesse Raphael featured four "miracles," patients of Burzynski, who, she said, were cancer-free. The patients stated that Burzynski had cured them when conventional methods had failed. In 1992, *Inside Edition* reported that two of the four patients had died and a third was

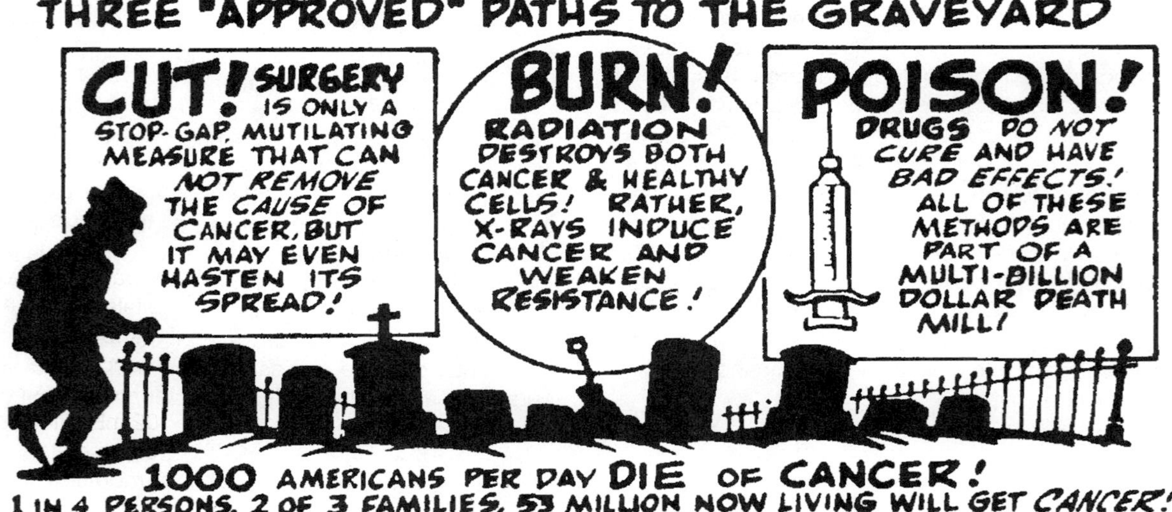

Figure 96.2. Cartoon from comic book circulated by an organization promoting questionable cancer therapies.

having a recurrence of her cancer. (The fourth patient had bladder cancer, which has a good prognosis.) The widow of one of Raphael's guests stated that her husband and five others from the same city had sought treatment after learning about Burzynski from a television broadcast—and that all had died of their disease.

CANCELL

CanCell, originally called Entelev, is a liquid claimed to cure cancer by "lowering the voltage of the cell structure by about 20%," causing cancer cells to "digest" and be replaced with normal cells. Accompanying directions have warned that bottles of CanCell should not be allowed to touch each other or be placed near any electrical appliance or outlet. CanCell has also been promoted for the treatment of AIDS, amyotrophic lateral sclerosis, multiple sclerosis, Alzheimer's disease, "extreme cases of emphysema and diabetes," and several other diseases. In 1989, the FDA reported that CanCell contained inositol, nitric acid, sodium sulfite, potassium hydroxide, sulfuric acid, and catechol (12). Subsequently, its promoters claimed to be modifying the formulation to make it more effective. They have also claimed that CanCell cannot be analyzed because it varies with atmospheric vibrations and keeps changing its energy (13). Laboratory tests conducted between 1978 and 1991 by the NCI found no evidence that CanCell was effective against cancer. The FDA has obtained an injunction forbidding its distribution to patients.

DEVICES

Many types of devices are used with unfounded claims that they are effective against cancer (14). These include devices that pass low-voltage electric current through tumors or the body, "electroacupuncture" devices purported to measure the electrical resistance of "acupuncture points," electrical devices claimed to "charge" blood samples taken from patients and later reinjected, negative ion generators claimed to have an effect against tumors, radionics devices claimed to diagnose and cure cancer by analyzing and emitting radio waves at the correct frequencies, magnets claimed capable of curing cancers by "improving circulation" or by intracellular effects, and projectors of colored light claimed to exert healing effects.

ESSIAC

Essiac is an herbal remedy that was prescribed and promoted for about 50 years by Rene M. Caisse, a Canadian nurse who died in 1978. Shortly before her death, she turned over the formula and manufacturing rights to the Resperin Corporation, a Canadian company that has provided it to patients under a special agreement with Canadian health officials. Several reports state that the formula contains burdock, Indian rhubarb, sorrel, and slippery elm, but there may be additional ingredients. Essiac tea claimed to be Caisse's original formulation is also marketed in the United States. Several animal tests using samples of Essiac have shown no antitumor activity (15)—nor did a review of data on 86 patients conducted by the Canadian federal health department during the early 1980s.

FRESH CELL THERAPY

Fresh cell therapy, also called live cell therapy or cellular therapy, involves injections of fresh embryonic animal cells taken from the organ or tissue that corresponds to the unhealthy organ or tissue in the patient. Proponents claim that the recipient's body automatically transports the injected cells to the target organ, where they repair and rejuvenate the ailing cells. The ACS states that fresh cell therapy has no proved benefit, and has caused serious side effects (infections and immunologic reactions to the injected protein) and death (16).

GERSON METHOD

Proponents of the Gerson diet claim that cancer can be cured only if toxins are eliminated from the body. They recommend "detoxification" with frequent coffee enemas and a low-sodium diet that includes more than a gallon a day of juices made from fruits, vegetables, and raw calf's liver. This method was developed by Max Gerson, a German-born physician who emigrated to the United States in 1936 and practiced in New York City until his death in 1959. Still available at a clinic near Tijuana, Mexico, Gerson therapy is actively promoted by his daughter, Charlotte Gerson, through lectures, talk show appearances, and publications of the Gerson Institute in Bonita, California. Gerson protocols have included liver extract injections, ozone enemas, "live cell therapy," thyroid tablets, royal jelly capsules, linseed oil, castor oil enemas, clay packs, laetrile, and vaccines made from influenza virus and killed *Staphylococcus aureus* bacteria.

In 1947, the NCI reviewed 10 cases selected by Dr. Gerson and found his report unconvincing. That same year, a committee appointed by the New York County Medical Society reviewed records of 86 patients, examined 10 patients, and found no evidence that the Gerson method had value in treating cancer. An NCI analysis of Dr. Gerson's book *A Cancer Therapy: Results of Fifty Cases* concluded in 1959 that most of the cases failed to meet the criteria (such as histologic verification of cancer) for proper evaluation of a cancer case (17). A recent review of the Gerson treatment rationale concluded: (*a*) the "poisons" Gerson claimed to be present in processed foods have never been identified, (*b*) frequent coffee enemas have never been shown to mobilize and remove poisons from the liver and intestines of cancer patients, (*c*) there is no evidence that any such poisons are related to the onset of cancer, (*d*) there is no evidence that a "healing" inflammatory reaction exists that can seek out and kill cancer cells (18).

Between 1980 and 1986, at least 13 patients treated with Gerson therapy were admitted to hospitals in the San Diego area with *Campylobacter fetus* sepsis attributable to the liver injections. None of the patients was cancer-free, and one died of his malignancy within a week. Five were comatose due to low serum sodium (as low as 102 mEq/liter), presumably as a result of the "no sodium" Gerson dietary regimen (19). As a result, Gerson personnel modified their techniques for handling raw liver products and biologicals. However, the Gerson approach still has considerable potential for harm. Deaths also have been attributed to the coffee enemas administered in the Tijuana clinic.

Charlotte Gerson claims that treatment at the clinic has produced high cure rates for many cancers. In 1986, however, investigators learned that patients were not monitored after they left the facility (20). Although clinic personnel later said they would follow their patients systematically, there is no published evidence that they have done so. A naturopath who visited the Gerson clinic in 1983 was able to track 21 patients over a 5-year period (or until death) through annual letters or phone calls. At the 5-year mark, only 1 was still alive (but not cancer-free); the rest had succumbed to their cancer (21).

GREEK CANCER CURE

The principal proponent of the Greek cancer cure was microbiologist Dr. Hariton-Tzannis Alivizatos, of Athens, Greece, who died in 1991. He claimed to have a blood test that could determine the type, location, and severity of any cancer. He also asserted that his "serum" enabled the patient's immune system to destroy cancer cells, and helped the body to rejuvenate parts destroyed by cancer. Knowledgeable observers believe that the principal ingredient of the so-called Greek cancer cure was niacin. The ACS and the NCI asked Alivizatos several times for detailed information on his methods, but he never replied (22).

HOXSEY TREATMENT

Naturopath Harry Hoxsey promoted an herbal treatment consisting of an externally used paste or powder and a tonic taken orally. The external preparations contained corrosive agents, such as arsenic sulfide. The internal medicine, said to be adjusted on a case-by-case basis, contained potassium iodide and such things as red clover, licorice, burdock root, Stillingia root, Berberis root, pokeroot, cascara, prickly ash bark, and buckthorn bark. Hoxsey said that the formulas were developed in 1840 by his great grandfather and passed on to him by his father while the latter was dying of cancer.

Hoxsey's treatment was offered at clinics in the United States from 1924 until repeated clashes with the FDA led him to close his main clinic in Dallas in the late 1950s. Since 1963, it has been available only at a clinic in Tijuana, Mexico, operated by Hoxsey's former chief nurse, Mildred Nelson (23). Hoxsey himself contracted prostate cancer in 1967 and underwent surgery after treating himself unsuccessfully with his tonic. Most of the herbs in the tonic have been tested for antitumor activity in cancer, with negligible results for a few and no results for the others. Some of these herbs, most notably pokeroot, have toxic side effects. The NCI evaluated case reports submitted by Hoxsey and concluded that no assessment was possible because the records did not contain adequate information (15). Hoxsey died in 1974.

HYDRAZINE SULFATE

In the mid-1970s, hydrazine sulfate was proposed for treating the progressive weight loss and debilitation characteristic of advanced cancer. Based on animal data and preliminary human studies, it has also been claimed to cause tumor regression and subjective improvement in patients. However, three recent placebo-controlled trials sponsored by the NCI demonstrated no benefit attributable to hydrazine sulfate. The trials involved 243 patients with newly diagnosed non–small cell lung cancer (24), 266 patients with advanced non–small cell lung cancer (25), and 127 patients with advanced colorectal cancer (26). The largest of these studies found that sensory and motor neuropathy occurred more often and that quality of life was significantly worse in the hydrazine sulfate group.

"HYPEROXYGENATION" THERAPIES

"Hyperoxygenation" therapy—also called bio-oxidative therapy and oxidative therapy—is based on the erroneous concept that cancer is caused by oxygen deficiency and can be cured by exposing cancer cells to more oxygen than they can tolerate. The most touted agents are hydrogen peroxide, germanium sesquioxide, and ozone. Although these compounds have been the subject of legitimate research, there is little or no evidence that they are effective for the treatment of any serious disease, and each has demonstrated potential for harm (27). Germanium products have caused irreversible kidney damage and death (28). The FDA has banned their importation and has seized products from several U.S. manufacturers.

IMMUNOAUGMENTATIVE THERAPY

Immunoaugmentative therapy (IAT) was developed by Lawrence Burton, Ph.D., a zoologist who claimed to treat cancer patients by manipulating an immune defense system that he postulated. He claimed to accomplish this by injecting protein extracts isolated with processes he had patented. However, experts believe that the substances Burton claimed to use cannot be produced by these procedures and have not been demonstrated to exist in the human body. The NCI scientists who analyzed treatment materials given to several patients concluded that the materials were dilute solutions of ordinary blood proteins, primarily albumin. None was electrophoretically pure, and none contained Burton's postulated components (29). Burton did not publish detailed clinical reports, divulge to the scientific community the details of his methods, publish meaningful statistics, conduct a controlled trial, or provide independent investigators with specimens of his treatment materials for analysis (6). During the mid-1980s, several of his patients developed serious infections following IAT.

In 1979, CBS-TV's *60 Minutes* gave Burton a tremendous publicity boost when a prominent physician stated that one of his patients appeared to have recovered miraculously with Burton's treatment. Although the patient died of his cancer 12 days after the program was shown, *60 Minutes* refused to inform viewers of this fact. In 1986, the Congressional Office of Technology Assessment assembled a group of technical experts and representatives of Burton to design a clinical trial to evaluate IAT. However, communication between Burton and U.S. government authorities broke down after he insisted that a "pretest" be conducted at his clinic (15). Burton died in 1993, but the clinic is still operating.

ISCADOR

Iscador is an extract of mistletoe first proposed for the treatment of cancer in 1920 by Rudolph Steiner, a Swiss physician who espoused occult beliefs. Steiner founded the Society for Cancer Research to promote mistletoe extracts and occult-based practices he called anthroposophical medicine. A 1962 report by the society claimed that the time of picking the plants was important because they react to the influences of the sun, moon, and planets. Various mistletoe juice preparations have been studied with the hope of finding an effective anticancer agent. However, in 1984, the expert working group of the Swiss Society for Oncology concluded that there was no evidence that Iscador was effective against human cancers (30).

KELLEY METABOLIC THERAPY

In the 1960s, William Donald Kelley, D.D.S., developed a program for cancer patients that involved dietary measures, vitamin and enzyme supplements, and computerized "metabolic typing." Kelley classified people as "sympathetic dominant," "parasympathetic dominant," or metabolically "balanced," and made dietary recommendations for each type. He claimed that his Protein Metabolism Evaluation Index could diagnose cancer before it was clinically apparent and that his Kelley Malignancy Index could detect "the presence or absence of cancer, the growth rate of the tumor, the location of the tumor mass, prognosis of the treatment, age of the tumor and the regulation of medication for treatment."

In 1970, Kelley was convicted of practicing medicine without a license after witnesses testified that he had diagnosed lung cancer on the basis of blood from a patient's finger and prescribed dietary supplements, enzymes, and a diet as treatment (31). In 1976, following court appeals, his dental license was suspended for 5 years. However, he continued to promote his methods until the mid-1980s through his Dallas-based International Health Institute. Under the institute's umbrella, licensed professionals and "certified metabolic technicians" throughout the United States would administer a 3,200-item questionnaire and send the answers to Dallas. The resultant computer printout provided a lengthy report on "metabolic status" plus detailed instructions covering foods, supplements (typically 100 to 200 pills per day), "detoxification" techniques, and life-style changes (15).

Treatment said to be similar is still provided by Nicholas Gonzales, M.D., of New York City, who claims to have analyzed Kelley's records and drafted a book about his findings. The manuscript was never published, but experts who evaluated its chapter on 50 cases found no evidence of benefit (15). Gonzales says that he offers "10 basic diets with 90 variations" and typically prescibes coffee enemas and "up to 150 pills a day in 10 to 12 divided doses."

LAETRILE

Laetrile, which achieved great notoriety during the 1970s and early 1980s, is the trade name for a synthetic relative of amygdalin, a chemical in the kernels of apricot pits, apple seeds, bitter almonds, and some other stone fruits and nuts. Many laetrile promoters have called it "vitamin B_{17}" and falsely claimed that cancer is a vitamin deficiency disease that laetrile can cure. Claims for laetrile's efficacy have varied considerably (32). First it was claimed to prevent and cure cancer. Then it was claimed not to cure, but to "control" cancer while giving patients an increased feeling of well-being. More recently, laetrile has been claimed to be effective, not by itself, but as one component of "metabolic therapy" (described below).

Laetrile was first used to treat cancer patients in California in the 1950s. According to proponents, it kills tumor cells selectively while leaving normal cells alone. Although laetrile has been promoted as safe and effective, clinical evidence indicates that it is neither (33). When subjected to enzymatic breakdown in the body, it forms glucose, benzaldehyde, and hydrogen cyanide (34). Some cancer patients treated with laetrile have suffered nausea, vomiting, headache, and dizziness, and a few have died of cyanide poisoning. Laetrile has been tested in at least 20 animal tumor models and found to have no benefit, either alone or with other substances. Several case reviews have found no benefit for the treatment of cancer in humans.

In response to political pressure, a clinical trial was begun in 1982 by the Mayo Clinic and three other U.S. cancer centers under NCI sponsorship. Laetrile and "metabolic therapy" were administered as recommended by their promoters. The patients had advanced cancer for which no proven treatment was known. Of 178 patients, not one was cured or stabilized, and none had any lessening of any cancer-related symptoms. The median survival rate was about 5 months from the start of therapy. In those still alive after 7 months, tumor size had increased. Several patients experienced symptoms of cyanide toxicity or had blood levels of cyanide approaching the lethal range (35).

In 1975, a class action suit was filed to stop the FDA from interfering with the sale and distribution of laetrile. Early in the case, a federal district court judge in Oklahoma issued orders allowing cancer patients to import a 6-month supply of laetrile for their personal use if they could obtain a physician's affidavit that they were "terminal." In 1979, the U.S. Supreme Court ruled that it is not possible to be certain who is terminal, and that even if it were possible to do so, both terminally ill patients and the general public deserve protection from fraudulent cures. In 1987, after further appeals were denied, the district judge (a strong proponent of laetrile) finally yielded to the higher courts and terminated the affidavit system. Few sources of laetrile are now available in the United States, but it still is utilized at several Mexican clinics.

LIVINGSTON-WHEELER REGIMEN

Virginia C. Livingston, M.D., who died in 1990, postulated that cancer is caused by a bacterium she called *Progenitor cryptocides*, which invades the body when "immunity is stressed or weakened." She claimed to combat this by strengthening the body's immune system with vaccines (including one made from the patient's urine); "detoxification" with enemas; digestive enzymes; a vegetarian diet that avoided chicken, eggs, and sugar; vitamin and mineral supplements; visualization; and stress reduction. She claimed to have a very high recovery rate, but published no clinical data to support this. Attempts by scientists to isolate the organism Livingston postulated were not successful. Researchers at the University of Pennsylvania Cancer Center compared 78 of its patients with similar patients treated at the Livingston-Wheeler Clinic. All had advanced cancers for which no proven treatment was known. As expected, the study found no difference in average survival time of the two groups. However, Livingston-Wheeler patients reported more appetite difficulties and pain (36).

MACROBIOTICS

Macrobiotics is a quasireligious philosophical system that advocates a semivegetarian diet. (*Macrobiotic* means "way of long life.") Macrobiotic diets have been promoted for maintaining general health and for preventing and "relieving" cancer and other diseases. The optimal diet is said to balance "yin" and "yang" foods. It is composed of whole grains (50 to 60% of each meal), vegetables (25 to 30% of each meal), whole beans or soybean-based products (5 to 10% of daily food), nuts and seeds (small amounts as snacks), miso soup, herbal teas, and small amounts of white meat or seafood once or twice weekly. Some macrobiotic diets contain adequate amounts of nutrients, but others do not.

Macrobiotic practitioners may base their recommendations on "pulse diagnosis" and other unscientific procedures related to Chinese medicine. Pulse diagnosis supposedly involves six pulses at each wrist that correspond to 12 internal spheres of bodily function. Other diagnostic methods include "ancestral diagnosis," "astrological diagnosis," "aura and vibrational diagnosis," "environmental diagnosis" (including consideration of celestial influences and tidal motions), and "spiritual diagnosis" (evaluation of "atmospheric vibrational conditions" to identify spiritual influences, including "visions of the future").

Today's leading proponent is Michio Kushi, founder and president of the Kushi Institute in Brookline, Massachusetts. According to institute publications, the macrobiotic way of life should include chewing food at least 50 times per mouthful (or until it becomes liquid), not wearing synthetic or woolen clothing next to the skin, avoiding long hot baths or showers, having large green plants in the house to enrich the oxygen content of the air, and singing a happy song every day. Kushi claims that cancer is largely due to improper diet, thinking, and way of life and can be influenced by changing these factors. He recommends yin foods for cancers due to excess yang, and yang foods for tumors that are predominantly yin. His books contain case histories of people whose cancers supposedly disappeared after they adopted macrobiotic eating. However, the only reports of efficacy are testimonials by patients, many of whom also received responsible therapy (37). The diet itself can cause cancer patients to undergo serious weight loss.

METABOLIC THERAPY

Proponents of "metabolic therapy" claim to diagnose abnormalities at the cellular level and correct them by normalizing the patient's metabolism. They regard cancer, arthritis, multiple sclerosis, and other "degenerative" diseases as the result of metabolic imbalance caused by a buildup of "toxic substances" in the body. They claim that scientific practitioners merely treat the symptoms of the disease while they treat the cause by removing toxins and strengthening the immune system so the body can heal itself. The toxins are neither defined nor objectively measurable. Metabolic treatment regimens vary from practitioner to practitioner, and may include a "natural food" diet, coffee enemas, vitamins, minerals, glandulars, enzymes, laetrile, and various other nostrums that are not legally marketable in the United States. No scientific study has ever shown that "metabolic therapy" or any of its components is effective against cancer or any other serious disease.

The most visible proponent of "metabolic therapy" was Harold Manner, Ph.D., a biology professor who, in 1977, announced that he had cured cancer in mice with injections of laetrile, enzymes, and vitamin A. (Actually, he digested the tumors by injecting them with digestive enzymes, which cannot cure cancers that have metastasized.) During the early 1980s, Manner left his teaching position and became affiliated with a clinic in Tijuana, Mexico (Fig. 96.3). Although he claimed a 74% success rate in treating cancers, there is no evidence that he kept track of patients after they left his clinic (38). He died in 1988, but the clinic is still operating.

PAU D'ARCO

Pau d'Arco tea, sold in health food stores and by mail, is also called taheebo, lapacho, lapacho morado, ipe roxo, or ipes. The tea is claimed to be an ancient Incan remedy prepared from the inner bark of various species of *Tabebuia,* an evergreen tree native to the West Indies and Central and South America. However, stories about its origins contain geographic and botanic errors (39). Proponents claim that pau d'arco tea is effective against cancer and many other ailments. *Tabebuia* wood contains lapachol, which has been demonstrated to have antitumor activity in a few animal tumor models. However, no published study has shown a significant effect on cancer in humans (40). Studies during the early 1970s found that lapachol is not as readily absorbed by humans as by rats, and that plasma levels high enough to influence tumors would be accompanied by anticoagulant effects. Even low doses can cause nausea and vomiting and can interfere with blood clotting. Some researchers believe that lapachol should be studied further, using vitamin K to inhibit its anticoagulant activity (15).

PSYCHIC SURGERY

Psychic surgery is claimed to remove tumors without leaving a skin wound. Actually, its practitioners use sleight-of-hand to create the illusion that surgery is being performed. A false finger or thumb may be used to store a red dye that appears as blood when the skin is "cut." Animal parts or cotton wads soaked in the dye are palmed and then exhibited as diseased organs supposedly removed from the patient's body. The ACS has concluded that "all demonstrations to date of psychic surgery have been done by various forms of trickery" (41). Most "psychic surgeons" practice in the Philippines or Brazil, but some have toured the United States. A

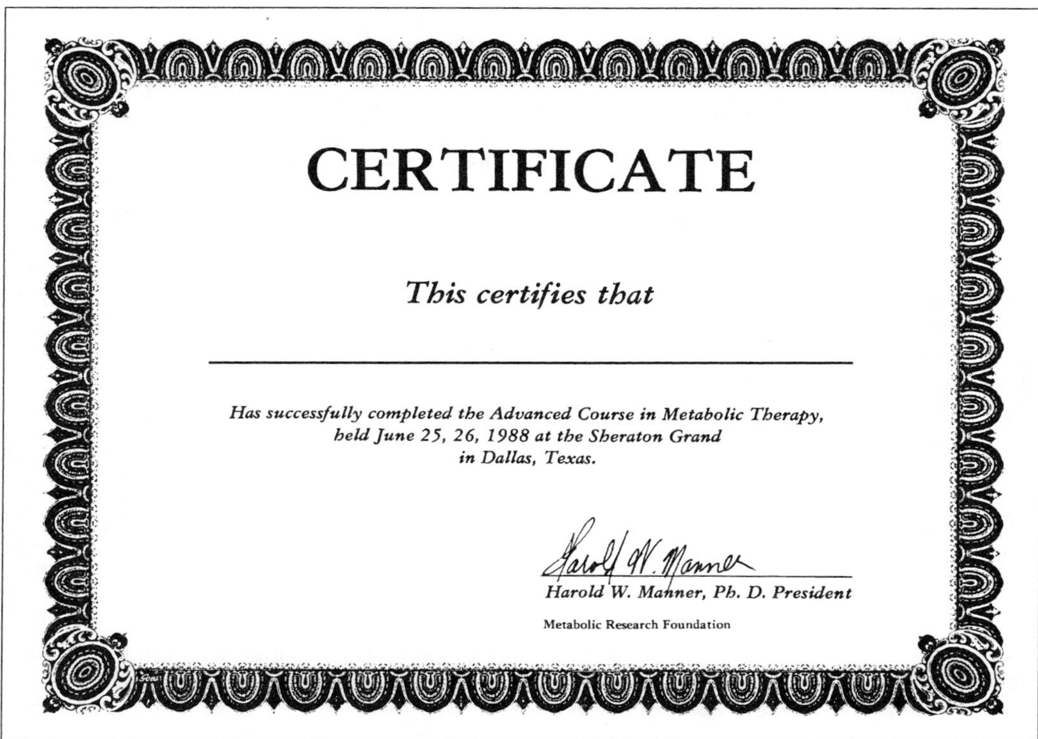
CERTIFICATE

This certifies that

Has successfully completed the Advanced Course in Metabolic Therapy, held June 25, 26, 1988 at the Sheraton Grand in Dallas, Texas.

Harold W. Manner, Ph. D. President

Metabolic Research Foundation

Figure 96.3. This certificate was obtained by a reporter who gained admission to Harold Manner's "Advanced Course in Metabolic Therapy" by pretending to be a chiropractor. Attendees who joined the Manner Metabolic Foundation were promised a $200 "referral fee" for each patient they referred to Manner's Mexican clinic. One speaker described how his company collected money for "alternative health care facilities" by submitting claim forms with code numbers for standard treatment. In 1994, he and two associates were indicted for wire fraud and conspiring to defraud insurance companies.

few have been prosecuted for theft and/or practicing medicine without a license.

PSYCHOLOGIC METHODS

Various psychologic methods are being promoted to cancer patients as cures or adjuncts to other treatment. The techniques include imagery, visualization, meditation, progressive muscle relaxation, and various forms of psychotherapy. These techniques may reduce stress, alleviate depression, help control pain, and enhance patients' feelings of mastery and control. Individual and group support can have a positive impact on quality of life and overall attitude. A positive attitude may increase a patient's chance of surviving cancer by increasing compliance with proven treatment. However, it has not been demonstrated that emotions directly influence the course of the disease.

Bernie Siegel, M.D., author of *Love, Medicine & Miracles* and *Peace, Love & Healing*, claims that "happy people generally don't get sick" and that "one's attitude toward oneself is the single most important factor in healing or staying well." Siegel also states that "a vigorous immune system can overcome cancer if it is not interfered with, and emotional growth toward greater self-acceptance and fulfillment helps keep the immune system strong." However, no scientific study supports these claims. A 10-year study found that 34 breast cancer patients participating in Siegel's Exceptional Cancer Patients program did not live longer after diagnosis than did comparable nonparticipants. The program consisted of weekly peer support and family therapy, individual counseling, and the use of positive imagery (42).

O. Carl Simonton, M.D., claims that cancers can be affected by relaxation and visualization techniques. He claims that this approach can lessen fears and tension, strengthen the patient's will to live, increase optimism, and alter the course of a malignancy by strengthening the immune system. However, he has not published the results of any well-designed study testing his ideas. Simonton theorizes that the brain can stimulate endocrine glands to inspire the immune system to attack cancer cells. He and his wife, Stephanie (a psychotherapist), taught cancer patients to imagine their cancer being destroyed by their white blood cells. However, there is no evidence that white cells actually attack cancer cells in this manner or that "immune suppression" is a factor in the development of common cancers.

Simonton's book *Getting Well Again* included reports on patients who got better after using his methods. However, an analysis of five of the reports that might seem most impressive to laypersons noted that two of the patients had undergone standard treatment, one had a slow-growing tumor, and one probably did not have cancer. The fifth patient's tumor was treatable by standard means (43).

Some people suggest that programs such as that of Siegel or Simonton may have positive psychologic effects that help people to relax and to feel that they are "doing something" positive. Although the methods are physically harmless, they can waste people's time and money and encourage some patients to abandon effective care. They can also cause people to feel ashamed or guilty that some inner inadequacy caused them to develop cancer and is interfering with their recovery.

A British study has disclosed how evangelical zeal can lead people to misjudge the effectiveness of psychologic approaches to cancer. In 1986, personnel at the Bristol Cancer Help Center felt a need to validate their program of counseling, "healing," a vegetarian diet, homeopathy, acupuncture, and various other therapies believed to enhance the quality of life and to help develop a positive attitude. They invited a research team, which compared the course of 334 of the center's breast cancer patients and 461 similar patients treated at conventional hospitals during a 16-month period. Survival times and metastasis-free periods were significantly shorter among the center's patients. The study demonstrated how people who believe in a treatment can overestimate its effectiveness (44).

REVICI CANCER CONTROL

Revici cancer control (also called lipid therapy and "biologically guided chemotherapy") is based on the notion that cancer is caused by an imbalance between constructive ("anabolic") and destructive ("catabolic") body processes. Its main proponent, Emanuel Revici, M.D., prescribed lipid alcohols, zinc, iron, and caffeine, which he classified as anabolic; and fatty acids, sulfur, selenium, and magnesium, which he classified as catabolic. His formulations were based on his interpretation of the specific gravity, pH (acidity), and surface tension of single samples of the patient's urine. Scientists who offered to evaluate Revici's methods were unable to reach an agreement with him on procedures to ensure a valid test (45). However, his method of urinary interpretation is obviously not valid. The specific gravity of urine reflects the concentration of dissolved substances and depends largely on the amount of fluid a person consumes. The acidity depends mainly on diet, but varies considerably throughout the day. Thus, even when these values are useful for a metabolic determination, information from a single urine sample would be meaningless. The surface tension of urine has no medically recognized diagnostic value. Recently, following a lengthy struggle with New York State licensing authorities, Revici's medical license was permanently revoked.

SHARK CARTILAGE

Powdered shark cartilage is purported to contain a protein that inhibits the growth of new blood vessels needed for the spread of cancer. Although a modest antiangiogenic effect has been observed in laboratory experiments (3), it has not been demonstrated that feeding shark cartilage to humans significantly inhibits angiogenesis in patients with cancer. Even if direct applications were effective, oral administration would not work because the protein would be digested rather than absorbed intact into the body.

Nevertheless, in the spring of 1993, *60 Minutes* aired a program promoting the claims of biochemist/entrepreneur William I. Lane, Ph.D., author of the book *Sharks Don't Get Cancer*. The program highlighted a Cuban study of 29 "terminal" cancer patients who received shark-cartilage preparations. Narrator Mike Wallace filmed several of the patients doing exercise and reported that most of them felt better several weeks after the treatment had begun. The fact that "feeling better" does not indicate whether a cancer treatment is effective was not mentioned—nor was the fact that sharks do get cancer, even of their cartilage (10). NCI officials subsequently reviewed the Cuban data and concluded that they were "incomplete and unimpressive" (46).

VITAMIN C

The claim that vitamin C is useful in the treatment of cancer is largely attributable to Linus Pauling, Ph.D. During the mid-1970s, Pauling began claiming that high doses of vitamin C are effective in preventing and curing cancer. In 1976 and 1978, he and a Scottish physician, Ewan Cameron, reported that a group of 100 terminal cancer patients treated with 10,000 mg of vitamin C daily had survived three to four times longer than had historically matched patients who did not receive vitamin C supplements (47, 48). However, Dr. William DeWys, chief of clinical investigations at the NCI, found that the patient groups were not comparable (49). The vitamin C patients were Cameron's, while the other patients were managed by other physicians. Cameron's patients were started on vitamin C when he labeled them "untreatable" by other methods, and their subsequent survival was compared with the survival of the "control" patients after they were labeled untreatable by their doctors. DeWys found that Cameron's patients were labeled untreatable much earlier in the course of their disease—which meant that they entered the hospital before they were as sick as the other doctors' patients and would naturally be expected to live longer. Nevertheless, to test whether Pauling might be correct, the Mayo Clinic conducted three double-blind studies involving a total of 367 patients with advanced cancer. All three studies found that patients given 10 g of vitamin C daily did no better than those given a placebo (50–52). Despite many years of taking huge daily amounts of vitamin C, both Pauling and his wife, Ava, died of cancer—she in 1981 and he in 1994.

COUNSELING PATIENTS

How can responsible clinicians help protect cancer patients from being exploited by questionable methods? Psychiatrist Jimmie C. Holland, M.D., advises that "if patients feel cared for in the most humanistic way by health professionals who are trying to minimize the side effects of their treatments, far fewer patients will seek unproven methods" (53). Open communication is vital (54). Some physicians fear that discussing questionable cancer treatments with their patients will plant seeds of suggestion in their minds. However, it is better to assume that patients will hear about these treatments regardless. Patients should be asked whether they are using or considering the use of any questionable methods, and their underlying reasons for doing so should be uncovered and dealt with. Discussion of the myths and fallacies used to promote questionable methods may be helpful (55). Explaining why testimonials are unreliable may decrease their allure. Patients using a questionable method should be asked periodically how their therapy is progressing. If standard treatment modalities have been exhausted, participation in a clinical trial may be an option. Holland further suggests that at least one person at each medical center should make a special effort to investigate questionable methods that are available nearby.

The ACS (800-227-2345 or a local office) can supply position papers on many questionable methods. Direct advice can be obtained from the Candlelighters Childhood Cancer Foundation Ombudsman's program (301-657-8401), the Consumer Health Information Research Institute (816-228-4595), and the National Council Against Health Fraud (909-824-4690). The Council's recommended antiquackery publications list can be obtained by sending a self-addressed, stamped envelope to NCAHF Books, P.O. Box 1747, Allentown, PA 18105.

The NCI's Information Service (1-800-4-CANCER) answers questions and provides literature about the latest cancer treatments, clinical trials, and community services for patients and their families. Physicians can obtain information on treatment protocols, results, and clinical trials through NCI's Physician Data Query (PDQ), a computerized database that is updated monthly. This enables most cancer patients to benefit from the latest scientific knowledge without having to travel far. Neither the Cancer Information Service nor the NIH Office of Alternative Medicine provides detailed information on the safety or efficacy of questionable methods.

References

1. American Cancer Society. Questionable Methods of Cancer Treatment. Atlanta: American Cancer Society, 1993.
2. Janssen WF. Cancer quackery—past and present. FDA Consumer 1977;11(6):27–32.
3. Young JH. The Medical Messiahs. Princeton, NJ: Princeton University Press, 1992, pp 360–389.
4. Holland JF. The Krebiozen story: is cancer quackery dead? JAMA 1967;200:213–218.
5. Young JH. Laetrile in historical perspective. In Politics, Science and Cancer: The Laetrile Phenomenon. Boulder CO: Westview Press, 1980, pp 11–60.
6. American Cancer Society. Questionable methods of cancer management: immunoaugmentative therapy (IAT). CA 1991;41:357–363.
7. Lerner IJ, Kennedy BJ. The prevalence of questionable methods of cancer treatment in the United States. CA 1992;42:181–191.
8. Brigden ML. Unorthodox therapy and your cancer patient. Postgrad Med 1987;81:271–280.
9. Marshall E. The politics of alternative medicine. Science 1994;265:2000–2002.
10. Barrett S, Herbert V. The Vitamin Pushers: How the "Health Food" Industry Is Selling America a Bill of Goods. Amherst, NY: Prometheus Books, 1994, pp 370–375.
11. Green S. "Antineoplastons." An unproved cancer therapy. JAMA 1992;267:2924–2928.
12. Gelb L. Unproven cancer treatments: help or hoax? FDA Consumer 1992;26(2):10–15.
13. Trull L. The CanCell Controversy. Norfolk VA: Hampton Roads Publishing, 1993.
14. American Cancer Society. Questionable methods of cancer management: electronic devices. CA 1994;44:115–127.
15. Congress, Office of Technology Assessment. Unconventional cancer treatments, OTA-H-405. Washington DC: Government Printing Office, 1990.
16. American Cancer Society. Unproven methods of cancer management: fresh cell therapy. CA 1991;41:126–128.
17. American Cancer Society. Unproven methods of cancer management: Gerson method. CA 1990;40:252–256.
18. Green S. A critique of the rationale for cancer treatment with coffee enemas and diet. JAMA 1992;268:3224–3227.
19. Ginsberg MM, Thompson MA, Peter CR, et al. Campylobacter sepsis associated with "nutritional therapy"—California. MMWR 1981;30:294–295.
20. Lowell J. The Gerson clinic. Nutr Forum 1986;3:9–12.
21. Austin S. Cited in Walters R. Options: The Alternative Cancer Therapy Book. Garden City Park NY: Avery, 1993, p 94.
22. American Cancer Society. Unproven methods of cancer management: Greek cancer cure. CA 1990;40:368–371.
23. Lowell J. Hoxsey treatment still available. Nutr Forum 1987;4:89–91.
24. Loprinzi CL, Goldberg RM, Su JQ, et al. Placebo-controlled trial of hydrazine sulfate in patients with newly diagnosed non-small cell lung cancer. J Clin Oncol 1994;12:1126–1129.
25. Kosty MP, Fleishman SB, Herndon JE II, et al. Cisplatin, vinblastine, and hydrazine sulfate in advanced, non-small cell lung cancer: a randomized placebo-controlled, double-blind phase III study of the Cancer and Leukemia Group B. J Clin Oncol 1994;12:1113–1120.
26. Loprinzi CL, Kuross SA, O'Fallon JR, et al. Randomized placebo-controlled evaluation of hydrazine sulfate in patients with advanced colorectal cancer. J Clin Oncol 1994;12:1121–1125.
27. American Cancer Society. Questionable methods of cancer management: hydrogen peroxide and other "hyperoxygenation" therapies. CA 1993;43:47–55.
28. Obara K, Saito T, Sato H, et al. Germanium poisoning: clinical symptoms and renal damage caused by long-term intake of germanium. Jpn J Med 1991;30:67–72.
29. Curt GA, Katterhagen G, Mahaney F. Immunoaugmentative therapy—a primer on the perils of unproved treatments. JAMA 1986;255:505–507.
30. Working Group on Unproven Methods in Oncology. Iscador. File No. 10E. Bern: Swiss Cancer League, 1984.
31. Dentist directed McQueen therapy. ADA News, Nov 17, 1980.
32. Wilson B. The rise and fall of laetrile. Nutr Forum 1988;5:33–40.
33. American Cancer Society. Unproven methods of cancer management: laetrile. CA 1991;1:187–192.
34. Herbert VD. Pseudovitamins. In Modern Nutrition in Health and Disease, 7th ed. Edited by ME Shils, VR Young. Philadelphia: Lea & Febiger 1988, pp 471–477.
35. Moertel C, Fleming TR, Rubin J, et al. A clinical trial of amygdalin (laetrile) in the treatment of human cancer. N Engl J Med 1982;306:201–206.
36. Cassileth BR, Lusk EJ, Guerry D, et al. Survival and quality of life among patients receiving unproven as compared with conventional cancer therapy. N Engl J Med 1991;324:1180–1185.
37. American Cancer Society. Unproven methods of cancer management: macrobiotic diets for the treatment of cancer. CA 1989;39:248–251.
38. South J. The manner clinic. Nutr Forum 1988;5:61–67.
39. Tyler VE. Pau d'Arco. Nutr Forum 1985;2:8.
40. American Cancer Society. Questionable methods of cancer management: "nutritional therapies." CA 1993;309–319.
41. American Cancer Society. Unproven methods of cancer management: "psychic surgery." CA 1990;40:184–188.
42. Gellert G, Maxwell RM, Siegel BS. Survival of breast cancer patients receiving adjunctive psychosocial support therapy: a 10-year follow-up study. J Clin Oncol 1993;11:66–69.
43. Friedlander ER. Mental imagery. In Dubious Cancer Treatment. Edited by S Barrett, B Cassileth. Tampa, FL: American Cancer Society, Florida Division, 1991, pp 73–78.
44. Baginal FS, Easton DF, Harris E, et al. Survival of patients with breast cancer attending Bristol Cancer Help Center. Lancet 1990;336:606–610.
45. American Cancer Society. Unproven methods of cancer management: Revici method. CA 1989: 39:119–122.
46. Mathews J. Media feeds frenzy over shark cartilage as cancer treatment. JNCI 1993;85:1190–1191.
47. Cameron E, Pauling L. Supplemental ascorbate in the supportive treatment of cancer: prolongation of survival times in terminal human cancer. Proc Natl Acad Sci USA 1976;73:3685–3689.
48. Cameron E, Pauling L. Supplemental ascorbate in the supportive treatment of cancer: reevaluation of prolongation of survival times in terminal human cancer. Proc Natl Acad Sci USA 1978;75:4538–4542.
49. DeWys WD. How to evaluate a new treatment for cancer. Your Patient and Cancer 1982;2:31–36.
50. Creagan ET, Moertel CG, O'Fallon JR, et al. Failure of high-dose vitamin C (ascorbic acid) therapy to benefit patients with advanced cancer, a controlled trial. N Engl J Med 1979;301:687–690.
51. Moertel CG, Fleming TR, Creagan E, et al. High-dose vitamin C versus placebo in the treatment of patients with advanced cancer who have had no prior chemotherapy. N Engl J Med 1985;312:137–141.
52. Tschetter L, Creagan ET, O'Fallon JR, et al. A community-based study of vitamin C (ascorbic acid) in patients with advanced cancer. Proc ASCO 1983;2:92.
53. Holland JC. Why dubious treatment is chosen. In Dubious Cancer Treatment. Edited by S Barrett, B Cassileth. Tampa, FL: American Cancer Society, Florida Division, 1991, pp 73–78.
54. Jarvis WT. Your cancer patient wants to try an alternative treatment. Physician's Mt 1994;March:36.
55. Jarvis WT. Helping your patients deal with questionable cancer treatments. CA 1990;36:293–301.

SECTION XXVI

NEOPLASMS OF THE CENTRAL NERVOUS SYSTEM

CHAPTER 97

Neoplasms of the Central Nervous System

MICHAEL D. PRADOS AND CHARLES B. WILSON

Introduction

Tumors of the central nervous system (CNS) account for approximately 1.4% of all tumors and 2.3% of cancer-related deaths. These often highly malignant tumors affect more elderly adults (18 per 100,000 population per year at age 70) than adolescents and young adults (2 per 100,000 population annually) and slightly more males than females (93, 259, 284). It is estimated that at least 17,500 new cases of primary brain and CNS malignant neoplasms (7.3 per 100,000 population) are diagnosed each year in the United States. The majority of these tumors is either glioblastoma multiforme or anaplastic astrocytoma, and few of these patients will ultimately be cured of their disease (259, 284). If neoplasms metastatic to the CNS were included, these numbers would be much higher.

Despite the relatively small numbers of malignant CNS tumors overall, the morbidity and mortality they cause are significant. Among children younger than age 15 years, CNS tumors rank next to leukemia as the second leading cause of death from cancer. Among men 15 to 54 years old, they are the third leading cause of cancer-related mortality, and in women 15 to 34 years of age, they are the fourth leading cause of death (259).

For children with primary tumors of the nervous system, the past two decades have shown an important trend toward improved survival, largely because of better therapies developed for medulloblastoma and primitive neuroectodermal tumor. During the same period, survival rates for patients with glioblastoma multiforme, the most common malignant tumor in adults, have shown only modest improvement (259). Nonetheless, new or refined techniques of surgery, radiation therapy, and systemic chemotherapy, together with intensive research efforts into molecular genetics and the immunologic aspects of the disease, give reason for optimism.

As a consequence of the therapeutic achievements made so far, a new approach to the management of malignant CNS neoplasms has developed. The truly multidisciplinary strategy includes neurosurgeons, radiation oncologists, medical and pediatric oncologists, and neuro-oncologists, all working in close collaboration in the care of the patient. A number of medical centers have adopted this multidisciplinary approach to treating patients who take part in clinical research trials of new drugs and therapies for CNS tumors. These trials are developed with consultation to ensure proper statistical design and interpretation, and with direct input from scientists doing basic research in the fields of immunology, molecular biology and genetics, radiobiology, biochemistry, research pharmacology, and organic chemistry. Rapid completion and statistical accuracy of the trials are assured through a referral system based on a cooperative group mechanism of patient accrual among participating centers. Since the last edition of this book, three new multi-institutional consortia have been funded by the National Cancer Institute to investigate new agents in the treatment of patients with recurrent malignant glioma. These new cooperative groups will facilitate phase I and phase II drug development and allow rapid clinical research to take place.

There is compelling evidence that, in certain disease states, survival can be improved through this multimodality approach. In a survey of national trends in the care of patients with malignant brain tumors, for example, patients with glioblastoma multiforme who were treated in investigational protocols had an almost threefold higher 5-year survival rate (12%) than did patients who were not (4.5%) (170). Although patients increasingly are referred to centers engaged in such studies, at present less than about 10% of eligible patients are actually entered into clinical research trials each year. During this decade, while changes occur as rapidly as our technology expands, every effort must be made to maximize applications of our gains in the management of neoplastic CNS disease. There must be greater attention to attracting more patients to clinical trials and, as survival times increase, a greater emphasis on further reducing the toxicity of therapies and on issues related to patients' quality of life.

Tumors of Glial Origin

In a review of nine registries in the United States National Cancer Institute's Surveillance, Epidemiology and End Results (SEER) Program, 1983–1985, glioblastoma multiforme was the most common malignant CNS tumor type in patients, both male and female, aged 35 to 64 years; among men in this age range in the San Francisco registry, for example, glioblastoma multiforme accounted for 52% and astrocytoma for 34%, of the primary malignant CNS tumors diagnosed (259, 283). The mean age of patients with glioblastoma is 52 years; of those with astrocytoma and anaplastic astrocytoma, 48 years; and of those with oligodendroglioma, 42 years. For glioblastoma more than for other glial neoplasms, however, the incidence increases with increasing age, suggesting a different mechanism of oncogenesis. Since 1973, SEER data for primary CNS tumors have revealed an increased incidence of approximately 1.2% per year, with an increased incidence in advancing age. Greig and colleagues, in reviewing this SEER data, found that incidence rates in 1985 were 187% higher for patients aged 75 to 79 years as compared with 1973 (97). The higher incidence rates are not fully accounted for by improved diagnostic techniques, yet the reasons for the increase are not known.

ETIOLOGY AND EPIDEMIOLOGY

Chromosomal abnormalities have been identified in some patients harboring gliomas; and glial neoplasms are associated with neurofibromatosis (NF), tuberous sclerosis, and, in rare cases, other genetically inherited diseases. NF types 1 and 2 are autosomal-dominant diseases characterized by cutaneous neurofibromas, café au lait spots, bone abnormalities, and a variety of intracranial and/or intraspinal tumors. Reviewing 121 cases of NF1 and NF2 in children under 18 years of age, Blatt and colleagues identified 17 patients (14%) who developed brain tumors, three of them anaplastic astrocytomas (30). The gene responsible for classic NF1 is located on chromosome 17. Using various DNA probes, Barker and colleagues have further identified the location of NF1 to be near the centromere of chromosome 17 (17). The location of the NF1 gene was recently further isolated to the q11.2 region of chromosome 17. The gene encodes a protein of 2,818 amino acids that has significant homology to the catalytic domain of mammalian guanosine triphosphatase (GTPase)–activating proteins (GAP). This GAP-related domain of the NF1 gene product has been shown to stimulate *ras* GTPase and consequently to inactivate *ras* protein. The NF1 gene product may be important in signal transduction pathways by interacting with *ras* and thus may be related to cell growth and differentiation (298).

Recent evidence has linked abnormalities on chromosome 22 with NF2, previously called *central NF* (177). Patients with NF2 have bilateral eighth-nerve tumors and may have other CNS tumors, as well, including malignant glioma, meningioma, and/or schwannoma. The location of the NF2 gene has also been identified recently, lying between the Ewing sarcoma region and the leukemia inhibitory factor locus; the gene product or products may soon be identified as well (292).

Abnormalities of chromosome 17 may also be involved in malignant gliomas not associated with NF. For example, a loss of constitutional heterozygosity suggesting chromosomal losses or deletions has been identified on chromosomes 1, 10, and 17 in patients who have anaplastic astrocytoma (119). In 50% of cases in one series, which included both low-grade and high-grade astrocytomas, the loss was on the short arm of chromosome 17 (66). This area on chromosome 17 is distinct from the abnormality seen in patients with NF1, which is located on the proximal long arm.

Other chromosomal abnormalities have been described in astrocytomas, including anomalies on chromosomes 17, 10, 1, 19, 22, 7, and are likely to be found at other loci, as well. Indeed, glioblastoma tends to occur frequently in patients showing changes on chromosome 10. Fujimoto and colleagues studied 13 patients with glioblastoma, screening with polymorphic markers localized to chromosome 10 (86). In 10 of the 13 cases, loss of heterozygosity for these markers was found on chromosome 10; the smallest and most common region of loss of heterozygosity was between 10q23.3 and the middle of 10p. This finding strongly suggests that a gene or genes important in tumor development may exist on this chromosome. It seems evident that the genesis of a glial tumor can involve many genetic aberrations and a complex etiologic process involving multiple steps, including chromosome deletions, gene amplification, chromosome rearrangement, and overexpression of oncogenes.

There is speculation that certain gene products may be antioncogene protein products. Fearon and colleagues have described abnormalities on chromosome 17 in patients with colon cancer, as well as the related gene product designated p53 (76). They suggested that the gene may be an antioncogene, or tumor suppressor gene, that codes for the protein product. One common denominator of p53 and brain tumors is the association of Turcot's syndrome with both malignant lesions of the colon and, rarely, with malignant astrocytoma and medulloblastoma. It may be that the oncogenesis of colon and brain tumors is related in part to chromosomal deletions on 17 (21, 66). Losses in the p53 region of chromosome 17 have frequently been seen in cases of malignant astrocytoma, in some series in as many as 60% (88). Glioblastoma cells that have the wild-type p53 gene replaced revealed that expression of p53 had antiproliferative effects (179). Although p53 gene mutations are found in all grades of astrocytoma, they are more frequent in the higher-grade lesions such as glioblastoma multiforme, suggesting an early genetic event with clonal expansion (257). Recently, the Li-Fraumeni syndrome was more fully characterized as an association of multiple cancers within families. There is a germline mutation of one allele of the p53 gene in this syndrome. Malkin and colleagues reviewed 43 families with the Li-Fraumeni syndrome and identified 231 tumors, of which 28 were brain tumors (172). Only breast cancer and soft-tissue sarcomas occurred more frequently. Mutations of the p53 gene appear to be one of the most common genetic abnormalities in human cancer. Further research into the function of this gene and its protein products will, hopefully, offer important clues to the pathogenesis of malignant gliomas and ultimately allow more specific therapeutic stategies to be developed for clinical use.

Other genetic abnormalities may be important in brain tumor development. Cavenee noted a loss of heterozygosity as measured from loci on chromosome 17p (locus D17S5) in differentiated low-grade astrocytomas, attributing the abnormality to a chromosomal loss and either duplication of the remaining homologue or mitotic recombination (41). Similar changes were seen in anaplastic astrocytoma and glioblastoma. All patients with glioblastoma who were evaluated using probes for three loci on chromosome 10 showed a deletion at one or more of these loci, but no patient with a lower-grade astrocytoma showed similar changes on chromosome (10). These findings suggest that glioblastomas may arise from tumor cells partially deficient on both chromosomes 10 and 17 and that they may have transformed from lower-grade lesions showing changes only on 17. Genotypic analysis of this kind may be useful in predicting transformations and perhaps ultimately in therapeutic decision making.

Also affecting the development and/or growth of astrocytomas may be genes encoding growth factors, peptides that act by binding to surface receptors on normal and neoplastic cells. Binding of the growth factor to specific receptors on cells elicits intracellular responses that modify growth and development, often signaling intracellular events such as increased protein synthesis and mitogenesis, which, when disturbed, may result in neoplastic growth. Autocrine and paracrine factors that have been identified in human gliomas include transforming growth factors alpha (TGF-α) and beta (TGF-β), bombesin, platelet-derived growth factor (PDGF), epidermal growth factor (EGF), and insulin-like growth factors I and II, as well as fibroblastic growth factor and endothelial cell growth factor. These growth factors are related to oncogenes, normal cellular genes that, when altered through mutation, amplification, or loss of control, may cause transformation. Many known oncogenes are thought to be related to the development of human brain tumors, several of which encode for either growth factors or receptors, establishing the link governing the genetic control of abnormal growth.

Neoplastic transformation is a multistep process that appears to include activation of proto-oncogenes and subsequent amplification or overexpression of growth factors or receptors. EGF receptor (EGF-R) is often overexpressed in glial neoplasms, and the EGF-R gene has been mapped to chromosome 7. Sang and colleagues, studying the tumorigenicity of several glioblastoma cell lines, noted the amplification and enhanced expression of the EGF-R gene in most glioblastoma cells, although there did not appear to be a good correlate with these events and tumorigenicity in nude mice (279). Their study of proto-oncogene abnormalities in several neuronal and glial tumors showed extensive amplification and expression of the oncogene N-*myc* in neuroblastomas and retinoblastomas, and amplification of the EGF-R gene in glioblastomas. It appears, from this work, that neuronal and glial malignant changes occur from separate pathways. The exact role of EGF-R in glial oncogenesis is still undefined, but conceivably the EGF-R gene acts together with one or several oncogenes to cause cellular transformation. The EGF receptor consists of 1,186 amino acids, with the protein kinase domain possessing a 85% homology with the v-*erb* oncogene product (67). Mutations of the EGF-R appear to uncouple the tyrosine kinase activity of the receptor from the binding of the external ligand, whereby the mutated receptor stimulates cell proliferation in the absence of appropriate stimuli. EGF-R amplification may thus be another event associated with anaplastic transformation of the astrocyte. Fujimoto and colleagues examined the accumulation and amplification of four proto-oncogenes—c-*myc*, N-*myc*, v-*sis*, and v-*fos*—in messenger ribonucleic acid (mRNA) in 10 primary human brain tumors (87). Amplification of v-*fos* was seen in both glioblastoma and low-grade glioma, as well as in ependymoma and medulloblastoma. The proto-oncogene c-*myc* was amplified in some of the low-grade and high-grade gliomas and was strongly increased in a medulloblastoma that did not show increases in N-*myc* or v-*sis*. The amplification of two oncogenes in one tumor suggests a complicated process that may involve regulation of one oncogene by another.

PDGF, a polypeptide mitogen, is often seen in patients with glioblastoma or other gliomas. The PDGF gene has been identified in a primate retrovirus, simian sarcoma virus (SSV), as the gene involved in transformation to neoplastic growth; SSV produces glioblastoma when injected into the brain of newborn marmoset monkeys. The PDGF gene encodes for either polypeptide chain A or B, which corresponds to an A-type or B-type receptor mRNA, the latter having an intracellular tyrosine kinase domain. Amino acid analysis of the B chain shows a resemblance to the protein product of the v-*sis* transforming gene of SSV. Human glioblastomas and other human malignant tumors express the PDGF gene, and glioblastomas express both the A-type and B-type receptor mRNA. PDGF B-chain and B-type receptor mRNA are also seen in proliferating endothelial cells. While the exact role of these entities in the development of glial neoplasms is unknown, the possible relation of PDGF to endothelial hyperplasia suggests autocrine growth stimulation.

Inhibitory factors may also be important in tumor growth or maintenance. Human glioblastomas produce a factor that inhibits T-cell proliferation and interferes with interleukin 2 (IL-2)–dependent T-cell growth (297). Now thought to be TGF-β, the inhibitor may prevent or modify antigen-induced immune response, in effect isolating the tumor from immune surveillance and control. TGF-β may also regulate or partially control other growth factors, including c-*sis*–encoded PDGF. In their study of regulation of c-*sis* oncogene expression in glioma cell lines, Press and colleagues found enhanced expression of the c-*sis* mRNA by phorbol ester, diacylglycerol, and TGF-β (223). The TGF-β–induced c-*sis* expression was thought to result from an increase in transcription in the nucleus of the cell. As compared with the phorbol ester protein kinase C pathway, the signaling pathway of TGF-β has a different mechanism, probably a different protein kinase. Other oncogenes and their products found in glioblastoma include *neu*, n-*ras*, *src*, *ros*, and *GLI*, all of which may potentially help to explain malignant transformation and may provide clues for improving treatment (27, 69, 91, 133).

Tuberous sclerosis is inherited as an autosomal-dominant disorder with a frequency of 1 in 30,000 population annually. Patients are born with ash-leaf unpigmented nevi and later develop adenoma sebaceum as well as other deformities. The intracranial lesions that may develop are usually benign and most often are giant cell astrocytomas.

Other than these few instances of a genetic predisposition, currently there are only sparse data to support a primary inherited genetic basis for the development of malignant glial neoplasms. Several families with a larger than expected aggregation of brain tumors are being investigated in an attempt to identify any chromosome or DNA abnormalities (230).

Occupational exposure has also been investigated as a potential cause of gliomas. The tumors may be produced experimentally in rats with several chemicals, including N-nitroso compounds, aromatic hydrocarbons, triazenes, and hydrazines, or by exposure to vinyl chloride through inhalation (173, 174). Epidemiologic evidence from the National Institute for Occupational Safety and Health (NIOSH), in a study of vinyl chloride–induced angiosarcoma of the liver, has suggested that workers exposed to vinyl chloride also have an increased incidence of brain tumors, supporting its role as an oncogen; most of the 10 brain tumors noted in that study were glioblastomas, 9 of which were fatal (292). Currently there are few data to suggest that other chemical agents may be responsible for the development of malignant gliomas, and often those data are conflicting.

Virally induced brain tumors include the Rous sarcoma virus canine gliosarcoma, the avian sarcoma virus rat glioma, and the human Jakob-Creutzfeldt (JC) virus, which can produce brain tumors in monkeys (52, 117, 208). Adenoviruses have been documented to produce neuroblastoma and retinoblastoma in rats and hamsters. Human brain tumors have not been shown to have a viral origin, with the possible exception of primary CNS lymphoma, which has a strong association with Epstein-Barr virus (EBV), discussed later in this chapter.

Tumors of the CNS may be a delayed consequence of radiation therapy, although rarely. Generally, these tumors develop after the patient undergoes cranial irradiation for other neoplastic diseases, such as acute leukemia, and often they are sarcomas or meningiomas (175, 225, 239, 264, 265). Because patients with diseases such as childhood leukemia are now living longer, owing to more effective therapy, usually including cranial irradiation, it is likely that more cases of secondary astrocytoma will be identified in the future. During the past few years at the University of California, San Francisco (UCSF), we have seen several cases in which malignant gliomas developed following such therapies (46, 220).

PATHOLOGY GRADING SYSTEMS

In 1926, Bailey and Cushing classified glial neoplasms using a three-tiered system: astrocytoma, astroblastoma, and spongioblastoma multiforme (16). Since that time, many grading systems have been used. Kernohan and colleagues of the Mayo Clinic used a four-tiered system: the better-differentiated tumors were grades I and II, and grades III and IV corresponded to glioblastoma multiforme (130). Ringertz introduced a three-tiered system: astrocytoma, anaplastic astrocytoma, and glioblastoma multiforme (227). In this classification, which is used by several cooperative groups, glioblastoma multiforme is defined as an anaplastic astrocytoma that has vascular endothelial proliferation and necrosis, whereas the anaplastic astrocytomas lack necrosis and are more differentiated than the glioblastoma multiforme. The previous World Health Organization (WHO) classification of glial neoplasms was similar to these schemes, but, in an important variation from other systems, it omitted glioblastoma multiforme from the classification of astrocytomas and included it in the group of poorly differentiated and embryonal tumors (305). In this older WHO classification, the grade III astrocytoma was considered a malignant astrocytoma, not a glioblastoma multiforme (305). At UCSF, we previously used a four-tiered system: differentiated astrocytoma, moderately anaplastic astrocytoma, highly anaplastic astrocytoma, and glioblastoma multiforme. We now classify tumors according to the revised WHO classification system (see below) (134).

At present, a generally acknowledged three-tiered grading system exists, although modified varieties of this type of scheme are still used. The variations among the systems make it extremely difficult to compile a comparative review of published clinical trials. To add to the confusion, different pathologists using the same system may disagree, one pathologist classifying a lesion as a grade II tumor while another classifies the same tumor as grade III. As judged on the basis of survival data, however, there tends to be general agreement among the various grading systems on the tumors classified as glioblastoma multiforme or the grade III and grade IV astrocytomas of the system devised by Kernohan and colleagues (130). Unfortunately, the anaplastic astrocytomas other than glioblastoma multiforme are more difficult to delimit, and criteria vary considerably with respect to the proportion of mildly and moderately anaplastic astrocytomas included in a designation.

Fortunately, a recent consensus panel of neuropathologists was convened by the WHO with the express goal of specifically defining a unified system of classification. Based upon this meeting in 1990 and subsequent meetings, a revised WHO classification system was agreed upon (134). This system identifies astrocytic tumors as being either astrocytoma, anaplastic astrocytoma, or glioblastoma. Separate descriptions are given for juvenile pilocytic astrocytoma, pleomorphic xanthoastrocytoma, and subependymal giant cell astrocytomas. A specific description of the pathology of each tumor appears in the sections that follow. For this purpose, a three-tiered system is used based upon the revised WHO classification: astrocytoma, anaplastic astrocytoma, and glioblastoma multiforme.

PROLIFERATIVE POTENTIAL

Recent efforts have been directed toward finding markers that provide biologic correlates with tumor histopathology and are predictive of a tumor's clinical behavior. These markers include molecular probes and biologic labels introduced into tumors to permit assessment of their cellular proliferative potential. The two most commonly used markers provide a bromodeoxyuridine (BUdR) or a monoclonal antibody Ki-67-labeling index.

BUdR, a thymidine analog that incorporates into DNA during cell synthesis, is given to patients through intravenous infusion 1 hour before surgery. When tumor cells obtained during surgery are exposed to a monoclonal antibody against BUdR, the cells with the greatest proliferative potential are labeled by the marker and stain brown. Counting those cells, a labeling index can be calculated that correlates strongly, although imprecisely, with the tumor's histopathology. Cells from glioblastoma multiforme have the highest mean BudR-labeling index, those from anaplastic astrocytomas have an intermediate BudR-labeling index, and cells from lower-grade astrocytomas have a low BudR-labeling index (112). Within tumor grades, the BudR-labeling index appears to have predictive potential, particularly in the prognosis of lower-grade lesions; in terms of statistical probabilities, low-grade astrocytomas showing a high BudR-labeling index are more likely than those with a lower labeling index to behave in a malignant fashion. For this reason, patients treated at UCSF are routinely given an intravenous bolus injection of BUdR before surgery and the tissue removed during surgery is processed to obtain the BudR-labeling index as an estimate of the malignant proliferative potential of the tumor.

The BudR-labeling technique is relatively easily performed and because of its proven accuracy in predicting a tumor's behavior, the BudR-labeling index provides important information for the planning of treatment. In assessing lower-grade lesions, Hoshino and colleagues have shown the impact of the BUdR labeling index on patients' survival rates (Table 97.1) (114). Among patients with a low-grade astrocytoma, for example, the 3-year survival rate was 85% for the 60% of patients who had a labeling index of less than 1%, whereas the 40% of patients with a labeling index greater than 1% had only a 10% survival rate 3 years after surgery.

The monoclonal antibody Ki-67 index can be used in a similar fashion to the BudR-labeling index (303). This immunohistochemical technique detects a nuclear antigen in cells in all phases of the cell cycle except the G_0 phase. The number obtained using this technique differs from the BudR-labeling index, yet it provides similar information and affords clinicians an assessment of a tumor's growth rate. Nishizaki and colleagues, assessing cell proliferation in human brain tumors using Ki-67, BUdR, and DNA content with flow cytometry, showed that both the Ki-67-labeling index and the BudR-labeling index correlated with degree of malignancy, the average Ki-67-labeling index being 1.7 times greater than the BudR-labeling index in individual tumors (196). They also showed a direct correlation between aneuploidy and high Ki-67- and BudR-labeling indexes. All aneuploid tumors were malignant, although all malignant tumors did not show DNA aneuploidy. Assuming no sampling error, these correlations were not infallibly predictive, either in this study or in our own experience. Some tumors with a high labeling index followed a benign course and others with a relatively low labeling index have behaved aggressively. Indeed, of 78 gliomas which Jimenez and colleagues studied for DNA aneuploidy with flow cytometry, 63% were diploid and 37% aneuploid (125). Except for two oligodendrogliomas that were aneuploid, the rest of the aneuploid lesions were astrocytomas. They found no correlation between DNA ploidy and histology or between DNA ploidy and survival. The factors that were most important in determining survival were age and vascular endothelial proliferation.

IMMUNOPATHOLOGY

Although circulating antiglioma antibodies have been shown to participate in complement-dependent and antibody-dependent reactions, further testing has proved that the antibody response is not specific, showing cross-reactivity to other tumors and to connective tissue (28). Nonetheless, further testing in this area is warranted.

Immune cellular responses are depressed in patients with gliomas. Peripheral blood lymphocytes have reduced mitogenic activity, and recent work has suggested a possible concomitant increase in suppressor T cells (238). The reduction in T-cell function may be a consequence of glioma-linked factors and may account for other immunologic abnormalities observed in patients with such tumors.

Many studies have evaluated the mononuclear cell infiltration observed in malignant gliomas. Rossi and colleagues evaluated 65 malignant astrocytomas for the presence of macrophages, lymphocytes, and natural killer cells (237). Using immunoperoxidase staining with various monoclonal antibodies, they demonstrated macrophage infiltration in more than 85% of tumors; 88% contained T cells, the majority being cytotoxic suppressor T cells. Natural killer cells were observed in 9% of tumors tested; B cells were absent in 88% of the tumors. An important finding was that human leukocyte antigen (HLA-DR) class II antigens existed not only in 100% of the tissue macrophages tested but also in the tumor cells in 40% of these malignant astrocytomas. The

Table 97.1. BUdR Labeling Indices of 227 Neuroectodermal Tumors Treated at the University of California, San Francisco Up to 1988

Tumor type	Cases (No.)	Labeling index (%)		Cases of LI (No.)		
		Median	Range	<1%	1–5%	>5%
Medulloblastoma	13	9.8	<1.0–38.2	1	1	11
Glioblastoma multiforme	78	7.3	<1.0–30.5	0	17	61
Highly anaplastic astrocytoma	36	2.7	<1.0–21.2	5	21	10
Moderately anaplastic astrocytoma	48	<1.0	<1.0–9.3	29	16	3
Ependymoma	20	<1.0	<1.0–18.9	15	4	1
Juvenile pilocytic astrocytoma	14	<1.0	<1.0–4.3	7	7	0
Mixed glioma	12	1.7	<1.0–8.0	5	5	2
Ganglioglioma	6	<1.0	<1.0–2.4	4	2	0
Total	227	——	——	66	73	88

Courtesy of Dr. Takao Hoshino, University of California, San Francisco, unpublished data, 1990.

detection of HLA-DR class II antigens on tumor cells is highly suggestive of a specific immune-response capability, those cells possibly serving as the antigen-presenting cell. Class II antigens are necessary for macrophage-antigen interactions to take place after antigen presentation. T cells then become activated, after which a cascade of events can take place, including the production of interferon-gamma, IL-2, and subsequently natural killer cells and tumor necrosis factor. Despite this host response, tumor-related factors are known to exist that have the ability to suppress IL-2–dependent T-cell proliferation. One of these factors is thought to be TGF-β (297).

Host-tumor interactions are complex, yet they have potential for therapeutic immunologic interventions and suggest a possibility that the interactions might be detectable and analyzed with imaging modalities, as discussed later in this chapter. Intensive research into these events has as its goal the development of treatment strategies that are specific and not toxic to normal tissues.

CLINICAL PRESENTATION

Patients with tumors of glial origin often present with either general, nonfocal signs and symptoms or with focal manifestations related to the specific area of the brain occupied by the lesion. General signs include headache, nausea, vomiting, generalized seizures, and/or changes in level of consciousness. Although headache accompanies many brain tumors, few patients with headache have a brain tumor. The headaches associated with tumors may be intermittent, moderate to severe, more prominent in the early morning, or aggravated by maneuvers that can increase intracranial pressure, such as coughing. The pain is caused by pressure on nerve endings in the dura and blood vessels throughout the cranium. Headache associated with an increase in intracranial pressure, as occurs in most cases, is generalized and nonfocal and does not lateralize to the site of the tumor. Conversely, headaches not associated with increased intracranial pressure may truly localize a tumor: tumors in the anterior and/or middle cranial fossa may present with frontal, often supraorbital, headaches; those in the posterior fossa may present with suboccipital pain.

Seizures may be the initial manifestation of a brain tumor, and eventually as many as 30% of patients with brain tumors develop seizures. Typically, seizures occur in conjunction with slower-growing, superficial tumors that involve the sensorimotor cortex. Rapidly growing tumors, such as glioblastoma multiforme, may not cause seizures as a presenting sign but may do so in time. In an adult, the new onset of seizure requires that tumor be excluded as the cause; as many as 10% of patients with generalized seizures are found to harbor a tumor. Focal seizures and partial complex seizures are more likely to reflect a tumor than is a grand mal seizure with no focal component. Neuroimaging should be performed, and if there is a lesion, it should be subjected to histologic diagnosis. In children, seizures are due to intracranial tumors in less than 1% of cases; however, a child with seizures that are difficult to control, especially partial complex seizures, should be assessed using magnetic resonance imaging (MRI). A lesion or abnormality on the image may represent a neoplastic growth, often a slow-growing tumor such as a ganglioglioma. In one series of patients who were to undergo surgery for the control of seizures, 15% had a mass, and in 70% of those, the mass was a tumor (266). At UCSF, patients with long-standing seizures often are referred for an operation to provide control and, during surgery, are found to have a tumor, a management issue discussed shortly in the section on low-grade gliomas.

Vomiting by a patient with a glial tumor may be related to a rise of intracranial pressure or, rarely, may reflect a tumor's invasion of the area postrema or vagal nucleus in the posterior fossa. Usually, the vomiting is related to increases in intracranial pressure and is accompanied by nausea. Projectile vomiting is not usually a presenting symptom but may occur with rapid rises in intracranial pressure. Disequilibrium and even true vertigo may occur as a consequence of the increased pressure on medullary nuclei and vestibular apparatus.

Signs of intracranial glial tumors include papilledema, diplopia, cranial nerve palsies, motor and sensory abnormalities, and changes in level of consciousness. Most patients exhibit some focal sign or symptom, either at presentation or later during treatment. In following patients during treatment, the neurologic examination often provides the first clue to a change in status. Defining the etiology of a change may pose difficulties, however, requiring confirmatory neuroimaging to distinguish change caused by the tumor from change caused by edema or change as a complication of therapy. Acute changes may be related to events independent of the tumor, to irradiation and/or chemotherapy, to infections, to seizures or medications for seizure control, or to depression, hormone imbalances such as hypothyroidism, or other medical conditions. A systematic search should be undertaken for the underlying cause of change, because a change does not necessarily mean tumor progression. Acute changes caused by tumor that may be reversible with surgery include hydrocephalus due to shunt failure, hemorrhage related to tumor growth, necrosis related to irradiation, and cyst formation that may or may not be related to tumor progression.

Tumors of the frontal lobes often cause changes in mental status, including impaired intellect, reduced attention span, poor judgment, labile behavior, or dulled thought processes to the point of inability to communicate with any consistent or logical train of thought. Often, patients show losses of social inhibition alternating between vulgarity and bouts of crying. Both frontal lobes are usually affected to produce these changes, but unilateral frontal lobe tumors may produce the same effects. Lesions that affect the premotor area may produce apraxia and mild rigidity but no loss of strength, whereas those that affect the motor cortex produce contralateral weakness. Dominant hemispheric lesions may produce motor (expressive) aphasia, often with agraphia. Patients' ability to repeat words spoken to them may be preserved, even if there is loss of volitional speech. There may be reflex changes, including abnormal grasp, suck, snout, and palmomental reflexes.

Tumors of the temporal lobes may cause abnormalities in speech, hearing, memory, and vision. Dominant temporal lobe syndromes include auditory hallucinations, dysnomia, receptive aphasia, impairment of recent memory, and homonymous quadrantanopia. Nondominant temporal lobe findings may include spatial disorientation and problems with perception of taste, hearing, vision, or movement, as well as difficulty in memory retention. Seizures may accompany tumors in either temporal lobe and often are complex partial seizures that may cause disorders of awareness and abnormal perceptions including those of the senses just described.

Lesions in the parietal lobes may cause abnormalities of sensation, including patients' inability to localize parts of their body, defects in two-point discrimination, and inability to recognize letters or numbers traced on the skin or objects placed in the hand. Neglect syndromes may occur contralateral to the side of the lesion, including lack of awareness of objects in the contralateral visual field or of movement or position of the body on the opposite side. Gerstmann's syndrome, a dominant parietal lobe disorder, includes agraphia, acalculia, finger agnosia, and right-left disorientation. Difficulty in performing complex tasks of motor function when instructed to do so may also occur. Visual field testing may reveal an inferior quadrantanopia or hemianopia.

Occipital lobe tumors cause deficits in almost all cases, including visual field defects, visual hallucinations occurring with or without seizures, and failure to recognize familiar faces or objects. Complete destruction of the occipital lobe causes contralateral homonymous hemianopia; bilateral lesions cause blindness. Visual hallucinations without seizures are strongly suggestive of an occipital lesion.

Glial tumors of the thalamus often manifest with increases in intracranial pressure, hemisensory loss or hemiparesis, and pain syndromes. Choreoathetosis may occur. Lesions of the hypothalamus produce endocrine dysfunction and visual pathway abnormalities. Patients may present with retarded growth, obesity, anorexia, and in infants, the diencephalic syndrome of cachexia, euphoria, hyperkinesia, and nystagmus. Endocrine manifestations may include acromegaly, Cushing's disease, precocious puberty, infertility, loss of libido, amenorrhea, and galactorrhea. Diabetes insipidus and the syndrome of inappropriate antidiuretic hormone secretion may also occur. Tumors that extend into the chiasm cause visual field defects, loss of visual acuity, papilledema, and optic atrophy. Lesions in the region of the third ventricle usually manifest as a consequence of obstructive hydrocephalus, with headache, nausea, and papilledema.

Tumors of the cerebellum cause patients to show ipsilateral signs when the hemisphere is involved, including ataxia, hypotonia, nystagmus, and a tendency to fall to the affected side. They have coordination abnormalities during voluntary movement. Midline cerebellar lesions produce a wide-based unsteady gait (truncal ataxia) and nystagmus. Patients often have hydrocephalus from obstruction of the fourth ventricle and the resulting nausea, headache, and papilledema.

Lesions of the brainstem cause cranial-nerve and long-tract signs, and possibly hydrocephalus when the upper midbrain is involved or compression of the fourth ventricle occurs. Bilateral facial-nerve and abducens-nerve palsies frequently occur, as well as hemiparesis, hemiplegia, or limb and gait ataxia.

While these highlights reflect some of the more common findings associated with brain tumors, it is important to be aware that most patients who ultimately are diagnosed as having a malignant brain tumor have had signs and symptoms of their disease for weeks, months, or sometimes years before a histologic diagnosis is made. For any adult who has a new-onset seizure, personality change, or new focal neurologic findings, the suspicion of a brain neoplasm should at least be considered in the differential diagnosis and the patient should be referred for neurologic evaluation.

DIAGNOSTIC NEUROIMAGING

Patients with signs and symptoms that suggest an intracranial mass should undergo neuroimaging studies, and if they show a lesion it should be subjected to histologic diagnosis.

Computed Tomography

Contrast-enhanced computed tomography (CT) is almost 95 to 97% sensitive in detecting a lesion and rarely shows false-negative results. Tumors less than 1 cm in diameter can be detected with third- and fourth-generation CT scanners. Contrast agents must be used in order to fully characterize an abnormality; a noncontrast CT scan is not sufficient to make the diagnosis and should never be relied on to exclude a CNS lesion.

Despite the decisive superiority of contrast-enhanced CT to all forms of neuroimaging except MRI, several limitations exist. Generally, CT is done only in the axial plane, and computer reconstructions in other planes, such as coronal images, have some loss of detail. In addition, bone-hardening artifacts make the evaluation of lesions in the posterior fossa difficult to interpret; this particular problem makes CT a less desirable modality for evaluating lesions in this area. Despite these limitations, contrast-enhanced CT is a valuable tool for both the initial evaluation and follow-up studies of many malignant brain tumors.

Magnetic Resonance Imaging

MRI is now the neuroimaging technique most frequently used in the evaluation and follow-up review of patients with malignant brain tumors. MRI has several advantages over contrast-enhanced CT. The patient is not exposed to radiation. Multiple planar images are available with no loss of detail. Lesions of the spine or posterior fossa are seen in more detail than with CT, and different sequences are available to characterize the tumor. Moreover, patients are not exposed to iodinated contrast agents, obviating possible allergic reactions. The new paramagnetic agent, gadolinium (Gd) with the agent diethylenetriamine-penta-acetic acid (DTPA), permits contrast-enhanced MRI with an essentially minimal risk of allergic reactions and it shows enhancement in areas of disrupted or abnormal blood-brain barrier.

Comparison of CT and MR Imaging

In a review of the role of Gd-DTPA–enhanced MR imaging (MRI-Gd), Stack and colleagues compared such images with contrast-enhanced CT scans in patients with intracranial pathology (267). MRI sequences were obtained with T1 and T2 weighting and with T1 weighting and Gd. In all cases of high-grade gliomas, the T2-weighted (T2-W) image revealed a lesion. However, the T2-W sequence was not reliable in differentiating solid tumor from surrounding peritumoral edema. Even with (T1-W) sequences done without Gd, lesions were identified, but demarcation of the tumor from surrounding normal brain was not optimally clear. When Gd was used with T1-W sequences, contrast enhancement was seen in most of the tumors, distinguishing gross tumor margin from surrounding edema. Not all high-grade gliomas enhance on either CT or MRI-Gd, and the presence or absence of enhancement cannot be relied on to predict the tumor histology.

In a comparison of MRI-Gd with contrast-enhanced CT in cases of low-grade tumors, the primary advantage of MRI-Gd was the ability to view the lesions in more than one plane, even when enhancement was similar with both techniques (267). In many cases of low-grade lesions, no enhancement is seen on either CT or MRI; however, there are tumors identifiable with MRI-Gd that do not show enhancement on CT. Some tumors are seen better on CT, mostly because of the extent of calcification in the lesion, a feature not easily demonstrated with MRI, with or without Gd. In fact, CT is more desirable for following patients with calcified lesions because CT defines the anatomy more clearly.

Cases in which MRI may be more useful than CT include dural lesions. Although contrast-enhanced CT clearly defines dura-based meningiomas well, the advantage of MRI-Gd is its ability to view the lesion in multiple planes and to image the extent of dural involvement and en plaque lesions. All intracranial meningiomas enhance on MRI-Gd, making the tumor's anatomy easily identifiable for the surgeon. MRI-Gd also may reveal additional or multiple lesions not appreciated with contrast-enhanced CT.

In cases of metastatic disease to the brain, MRI-Gd is the technique of choice because of its sensitivity. The apparently single lesion shown on contrast-enhanced CT may actually represent multiple intracranial lesions that are more accurately identified with MRI-Gd. Lesions of the brainstem, spinal cord, and leptomeninges are also identified more easily with MRI-Gd, and for brainstem tumors MRI-Gd is preferred. Tumors that involve intramedullary spinal cord often have MRI signal characteristics that are different from those of a normal spinal cord, mainly because of prolonged T1 and T2 relaxation times. Tumor nodules within cysts are easily visualized with MRI-Gd, affording valuable information for the surgeon. In most cases, MRI-Gd can replace myelography, or it at least complements it after an initial myelogram is made, to the extent that lesions may be followed sequentially without the need for additional myelography.

In some cases, MRI-Gd should replace CT, but, as yet, few prospective trials have evaluated both of these techniques for specific tumor types. Although contrast-enhanced CT is a valuable diagnostic tool for the most common tumor types followed in our clinic, most patients are followed with sequential MRI-Gd studies. This includes patients with supratentorial and infratentorial tumors and all patients with spinal cord lesions.

The disadvantages of MRI are its cost and its inability to detect calcium or the bone changes that present with some tumors. In such cases, CT and MRI may be complementary, CT showing the margins of bone erosion and MRI, the mass within the area of bone involvement. In any case, a specific diagnosis is not possible based on CT or MRI alone. The diagnosis must depend on a histopathologic analysis of surgical material.

Other Imaging Techniques

Although proton MRI has much improved our ability to detect and follow tumors in patients with malignant gliomas, it still lacks diagnostic specificity. New MRI techniques are being developed to investigate the biochemical basis of tumors. One such tool is phosphorus 31 MR spectroscopy (^{31}P-MRS), which is being used to evaluate such points as its applicability in assessing the response to therapy, the analysis of differences in the phosphorus spectrum between normal and abnormal brain tissue, and the correlation, if any, of this spectrum with specific tumor types. ^{31}P-MRS is performed using conventional MRI techniques, changing the field strengths for specific spectral imaging.

Heindel and colleagues, who studied 35 patients with ^{31}P-MRS, could monitor different phosphorus signals, including phosphomonoester (PME), phosphodiester (PDE), phosphocreatine (PCr), inorganic phosphate (Pi), and adenosine triphosphate (ATP); tissue pH could be calculated from a chemical shift of Pi and PCr (104). Their patients with meningiomas showed markedly reduced PCr peak levels, diminished PDE levels, and occasional increases in PME, whereas those with glioblastoma multiforme had variable changes that included reduced PME and PCr. Low-grade tumors, as compared with normal brain in the same patient, often did not show changes. Hubesch and colleagues observed reductions in PCr, PME, PDE, and decreased ratios of PCr to Pi in patients with malignant glioma (116). Measurements of tissue pH have shown inconsistent results, with a suggestion that tumors are alkaline relative to normal brain (116).

Among other investigators using ^{31}P-MRS to study patients during treatment, Arnold and colleagues evaluated a patient before and after administration of intra-arterial therapy with 1,3,bis(2-chloroethyl)-1-nitrosourea (carmustine, also BCNU) (14). As compared to the phosphorus spectrum before therapy, ^{31}P-MRS showed a decrease in PCr and PDE just after treatment and an increase in tissue pH 8 hours later. By 32 hours after treatment, the PCr and PDE had begun to increase again, with a still greater increase in tissue pH. No changes were seen by concurrent MRI or CT. Sagebarth and colleagues studied 12 patients with ^{31}P-MRS before and after therapy (247). In one patient with an astrocytoma, a comparison of ^{31}P-MRS images made before and after radiation therapy showed changes in the postirradiation PME and Pi peaks. In a patient with lymphoma, ^{31}P-MRS images before radiation therapy showed high concentrations of PME and a low PCr-ATP ratio, and in the images made after irradiation, the spectrum was indistinguishable from normal brain. The patient had improved clinically and proton MRI also showed significant improvement. Other investigators similarly have assessed changes with therapy using ^{31}P-MRS as a potential noninvasive method for studying the biochemical characteristics of the lesion seen on proton MRI. One useful application of such an analysis would be to distinguish radiation-induced tissue necrosis from tumor regrowth, which at present is difficult to do using standard imaging techniques, particularly in patients treated with interstitial brachytherapy.

^{31}P-MRS is a noninvasive diagnostic and monitoring technique potentially available wherever MRI is used. An established means of demonstrating metabolic changes, it may become a useful tool for studying biochemical events within tumors and for following them during therapy. Proton MRS is also being developed for the same indications as ^{31}P-MRS. This imaging modality may actually be easier to perform than ^{31}P-MRS (275).

Thallium 201 (^{201}Tl) single photon–emission CT (SPECT) has been used in the evaluation of many tumors, recently including primary brain tumors. There is very little uptake of thallium in normal brain, and its distribution is similar to that of potassium, depending on blood flow, blood-brain barrier permeability, and active pumping of this analog into malignant cells. It has been proposed that thallium is taken up preferentially by tumor cells, as opposed to necrotic tissue, and that the rate of uptake correlates with the tumor growth rate (126). Mountz and colleagues calculated a tumor-cardiac ^{201}Tl-uptake ratio to distinguish residual tumor from post-therapeutic changes such as necrosis in patients with brain tumors (187). Their study suggested that an increased ratio of tumor to cardiac uptake correctly identified residual tumor, even in some cases when contrast-enhanced CT did not. The ^{201}Tl uptake ratio was also helpful in distinguishing necrosis from viable tumor in a contrast-enhancing lesion. Black and colleagues also used this method to compare ^{201}Tl uptake in brain tumor with that in noninvolved normal brain tissue (29). A lesion with an index greater than 1.5 was shown to be highly suggestive of a high-grade lesion.

Positron emission tomography (PET) using rubidium 82 (^{82}Rb) or fluorine 18-fluorodeoxyglucose (18-FDG) has shown promise in differentiating viable tumor from necrosis related to various forms of radiation therapy. Valk and colleagues followed 34 patients with high-grade malignant gliomas who had been treated with external and interstitial irradiation (281). When a patient's CT scans and clinical history suggested either tumor recurrence or radiation necrosis, impossible to distinguish on CT alone, ^{82}Rb was used to define the area of blood-brain barrier breakdown and the 18-FDG images were used to evaluate this area. Whenever the 18-FDG uptake was greater in the lesion than in adjacent tissue, a diagnosis of tumor recurrence was made. As determined on the basis of the patient's clinical course and the results of subsequent surgery, the PET diagnosis was accurate in 15 of 17 patients with active regrowth of tumor and in 17 of 21 with radiation injury. Francavilla and colleagues, comparing 18-FDG PET scans made at early and later phases of development of the same lesion, showed changes in metabolism, the tumor's becoming hypermetabolic during malignant degeneration of a low-grade to a higher-grade glioma (81). This work suggests that PET can be used in follow-up evaluations of patients with low-grade malignancies, to correctly diagnose malignant degeneration and thus guide subsequent management.

The hope for all of these experimental neuroimaging studies is that they may offer clinicians relatively noninvasive tools to evaluate patients, to further characterize the biochemical makeup of tumors, to help in predicting response to therapy, and to aid in quickly making a differential diagnosis, allowing for more precise treatment decisions.

SURGICAL DIAGNOSIS AND RESECTION

Despite the significant improvements in neuroimaging and its usefulness in deciding on surgical approaches, a specific diagnosis cannot be established through imaging alone (103, 231). A tissue diagnosis is necessary for prognostic reasons, and a precise tumor diagnosis is absolutely necessary to plan therapy effectively.

Surgery is undertaken in most cases with the intention of doing a biopsy for histologic diagnosis of the tumor type followed by a craniotomy and an appropriate tumor resection. Neurosurgical morbidity and mortality rates have improved to such a degree over the past several decades that a decision not to operate on an operable brain tumor is rare. At present, virtually the only reason not to operate on an otherwise healthy brain tumor patient is MRI indicating that any diagnosis other than a diffuse brainstem lesion is extremely unlikely, that the histologic diagnosis is not necessarily of prognostic value, and that surgery has a significant risk of complications. For almost every other intracranial lesion, tissue can be obtained for histologic diagnosis either by craniotomy and biopsy or resection or by ultrasound-guided or stereotactic-guided biopsy.

From a purely oncologic point of view, surgery is still the most rapid method of tumor cell removal. Apart from diagnostic accuracy, there are several other reasons for a surgical approach to the management of malignant brain tumors. Surgery potentially increases patients' survival period, during which they may receive other therapies. Moreover, surgery reduces the tumor cell population, leaving fewer tumor cells to be eradicated with irradiation and chemotherapy. Surgery also produces partial or complete resolution of symptoms and may delay the onset of new symptoms. By changing the kinetics of tumor growth, surgery perhaps enhances the effectiveness of sequential therapies, such as irradiation and chemotherapy.

Decision making in the neurosurgical management of a patient thought to have an intracranial neoplasm entails an understanding of the anatomy and vascularity of the tumor, its relation to adjacent structures and the neurologic function of the area, the implications of the patient's age and medical condition, and the desires of the patient and family regarding the possible outcome of treatment. Variables that affect the overall outcome must also be understood in order to plan surgery most effectively. Many slow-growing, low-grade astrocytic lesions are difficult to treat surgically, for instance, because they are diffusely infiltrative, having indistinct margins and minimal mass effect. For patients with a very large hemispheric lesion, surgery would be used not to relieve symptoms, but rather to make a diagnosis. If extensive tumor removal is virtually certain to improve overall survival, then the risk of neurologic deterioration should be discussed with the patient and weighed against the benefit of longer life.

Because the quality of patients' lives can be defined only by each patient individually, choices affecting quality of life must be decided by patients themselves if at all possible, after they are provided with the best information available concerning the risks of surgical resection in their particular case. In the case of large, diffuse hemispheric lesions, the impact of extensive tumor removal in improving survival is still debatable, a fact the patient must clearly understand. In other situations, the impact of surgery is more definable. A lesion causing severe mass effect with the potential for herniation urgently requires surgery. In a patient over 50 years of age, the most common tumor causing severe mass effect is a malignant glioma, most likely a glioblastoma multiforme. Such cases require more than simply a diagnostic biopsy: extensive tumor resection makes the diagnosis, relieves symptoms, improves survival, and affords time to discuss and implement further therapies. The benefit of initial, extensive resection to improve survival in such situations has been documented (170). The recommended approach is to perform as nearly total a resection as is possible while preserving function. In our experience, most of the long-term survivors of malignant gliomas have had nearly total or gross-total removal of tumor.

Patients who are in poor physical health and harbor a deep-seated lesion may be treated best with stereotactic biopsy under local anesthesia to document the tumor histology before more extensive surgery is undertaken. If the histologic diagnosis is primary CNS lymphoma, for instance, then attempts at extensive tumor resection are unwarranted because they would not change the prognosis for survival; however, if the lesion is an astrocytoma, then a more definitive surgical resection is indicated.

The extent of surgical resection depends on the medical and anesthesia risks to the patient and the location and histology of the tumor. Although a tumor that is resected completely requires no further therapy, total resection is seldom an attainable goal with gliomas, the only exceptions being among such childhood tumors as hemispheric astrocytomas. For this reason, even if a lesion appears to have well-defined margins, the likelihood that some tumor cells remain after surgery is adequate reason for additional therapy to eliminate residual tumor.

Protection of normal brain is the consideration limiting aggressive tumor removal, but within that restriction the possibility of increasing survival has renewed surgeons' interest in pursuing extensive tumor removal, even in the knowledge that total resection is impossible and that further therapy is anticipated (296). As opposed to a large residual tumor burden, which often has hypoxic or poorly vascularized areas that make the lesion less responsive to radiation therapy and chemotherapy, the reduced tumor burden afforded by extensive resection is more easily managed with adjuvant therapies. Particularly in young children, the negative effects of wide-field radiation therapy required to treat a large residual tumor burden are sufficient reason to aspire to total tumor removal and improvement in severe seizures refractory to medical treatment that may accompany residual and regrowing lesions.

CORTICAL MAPPING

In light of the potential advantages of extensive resection in both children and adults, cerebral cortical mapping with neurophysiologic monitoring is an important surgical adjunct. Cortical mapping during surgery permits more complete resection of tumor with a higher probability of retaining function and minimizing neurologic morbidity. It permits a physiologic representation to be drawn in relation to the gross anatomy of the brain, giving the surgeon a more precise knowledge of the probable effects of operating in the area of the tumor. Subcortical stimulation permits more extensive resection of lesions deep within the white matter as well.

The technique entails stimulation of excitable cortex. The cortical loci of eloquent faculties, such as language, appear to be variable and peculiar to individual patients (198). Identification of the appropriate cortical loci permits more or less extensive resection of intervening tumor while preserving eloquent function. Motor cortex can be defined with the patient under general anesthesia, but only local anesthesia can be given when localizing language functions. Nonetheless, with the patient's cooperation the process is easily managed in older children and adults.

With its other possible benefits, cortical mapping can also provide seizure control with simultaneous resection of the seizure foci, although often the focus of seizure activity is adjacent to, rather than in the area of, the tumor (26). In some cases, a better outcome is obtained by monitoring the focus of seizure activity while tumor resection is under way. Difficulties of the technique are that a longer perioperative period is often required and that patients must be awake during the mapping of eloquent brain (which is impracticable in young children). Also, patients who have complex language disturbances cannot comprehend or sufficiently cooperate to make the procedure worthwhile.

Cortical mapping with neurophysiologic monitoring requires a knowledgeable and specialized team consisting of a surgeon, anesthesiologist, neurologist, and neurophysiologist. The potential for longer survival and improved quality of life makes this technique very attractive in efforts to achieve the maximum safe resection of tumor. If properly done, it is an extremely useful and valuable surgical tool deserving wider application.

POSTOPERATIVE IMAGING

Contrast enhancement on the postoperative CT or MRI-Gd image may be attributable to residual tumor volume as well as to events related to surgery, such as gliosis and revascularization. In canine models, the contrast changes attributable to surgery are not evident on CT until at least 1 week after surgery, suggesting that CT scans made soon after surgery demonstrate residual tumor rather than changes related to surgical resection and healing (120). Cairncross and colleagues studied postoperative contrast enhancement in 10 patients with gliomas, noting that enhancement in the margin of resection did not occur until later than 5 days after surgery (39). For these reasons, at UCSF, we obtain the initial postoperative CT or MR images within 72 hours after surgery to assess accurately the residual tumor volume and the extent of resection.

CLINICAL TRIALS

Patients entered into clinical trials are routinely followed with neuroimaging studies based on their specific diagnosis. For patients with glioblastoma multiforme or anaplastic astrocytoma, a postoperative contrast-enhanced CT scan or MRI-Gd image should be obtained first within 72 hours after surgery, once again after the completion of radiation therapy, and then usually between each cycle of systemic chemotherapy. Sequential images or scans are analyzed for changes and, based on both the serial scans and the patient's neurologic status, the response to treatment is designated according to standardized response criteria.

In conducting clinical trials, a designation of response or no response is important to assess the impact of specific therapies. It is crucial to recognize, however, that there are no pathognomonic neurologic findings that document tumor progression with absolute certainty. Patients who have tumor progression may show no clinical signs or symptoms whatever, whereas those who show changes in clinical status may not have tumor progression but rather may exhibit complications of treatment, such as infection, cyst formation, hemorrhage, injury related to irradiation, or hydrocephalus. Only serial scans and images can be relied on to portray reliably the status or progression of tumor.

The new imaging techniques, such as MRI-Gd and PET, may make it possible to document changes related to treatment or tumor progression earlier than has been possible. In terms of managing a recurrent tumor, multiple therapies, in sequence, including techniques such as interstitial brachytherapy, have increased survival rates, perhaps because the amount of tumor regrowth that must be treated is smaller as a result of earlier detection with MRI-Gd or PET.

Some tumors require surveillance more frequently than others, whether because of their estimated growth potential or because of a need to assess their response to experimental therapies independent of their growth potential. The hazards of frequent imaging are minimal, particularly with MRI. Cost is an important issue, however, and the clinician must weigh the information to be gained from a scan or image against the expense involved. It is difficult to place a cost factor into the formula for treatment of malignant glioma. Clearly, with more effective therapies, patients may live longer and in better health, and thus earlier intervention and closer follow-up review may actually reduce overall medical costs. In addition to the intangible benefits of improved quality of life and a sense of well-being for the patient, factors such as a patient's continued ability to work are also important to consider in assessing the cost-benefit ratio.

The discussion of individual glial tumor types that follows adds specificity to the general information about tumors of glial origin just described.

Glioblastoma Multiforme and Anaplastic Astrocytoma

These two astrocytic tumor types have been treated similarly in the past. Most series that have been reported include both tumor types, the majority being glioblastoma multiforme, but the results can be difficult to interpret because of the different classification schemes used. In addition, the survival expectations and response to therapy differ for these two malignant gliomas. Since 1990, patients at UCSF have been treated according to disease-specific protocols, with different treatment strategies developed for patients with newly diagnosed glioblastoma and anaplastic astrocytoma. New studies from the Radiation Therapy Oncology Group (RTOG) have also adopted this strategy, and all new studies from this cooperative group will also be disease specific.

Most of the grading systems for malignant astrocytomas described earlier and the older UCSF system show similar survival rates within the category of glioblastoma multiforme or, according to Kernohan and colleagues, grade III or IV (130, 227). Nelson and colleagues reviewed a large series of patients classified according to a three-tiered system (glioblastoma multiforme, anaplastic astrocytoma, and astrocytoma) and the system of Kernohan and colleagues (130, 193). For patients with glioblastoma multiforme and those in grades III and IV, the median survival times were 8, 9, and 10 months, respectively. At UCSF, the median survival time for patients with glioblastoma multiforme is 12.5 to 15 months overall (164). In a strict comparison of survival data, however, survival must take into account such very important factors as the patient's age and the extent of resection, as well as the histologic variable. On that basis, patients with glioblastoma multiforme have a median survival of 10 to 12 months overall.

Patients with anaplastic astrocytoma, depending on the specific classification used, have widely differing reported median survival times. The median survival at UCSF ranges from 36 to 44 months, whereas the joint RTOG/Eastern Cooperative Oncology Group (ECOG) trial shows a median survival of 28 months (43). Comparatively, the 2-year survival rate for these patients graded according to the UCSF and RTOG systems is close to 70%, but it is only 50% for patients classified according to the system of Kernohan and colleagues and 35% using the European Organisation for Research on Treatment of Cancer (EORTC) system (36, 37, 130, 227). Daumas-Duport and co-workers have described another grading system for the diffuse astrocytic tumors, and it uses a four-tiered grading schema (55). This system grades tumors based upon the presence or absence of nuclear atypia, mitosis, endothelial proliferation, and necrosis.

If the tumor has none of these features it is called a grade 1 lesion; tumors with one feature are grade 2, those with two features are grade 3, and those with three features are grade 4. The three highest grades in this system correspond roughly to astrocytoma, anaplastic astrocytoma, and glioblastoma in the three-tiered systems. A Daumas-Duport grade 1 tumor is so rare as to be essentially nonexistent; thus, this system is actually a three-tiered system. Clinical-pathological correlations have been shown closely to approximate patient survival. One of the major advantages of this system is the ease and reproducibility of the schema among individual pathologists. Until a classification system is agreed upon and adopted worldwide, such as the revised WHO system, there will be confusion about response and survival data, at least within this category of tumors.

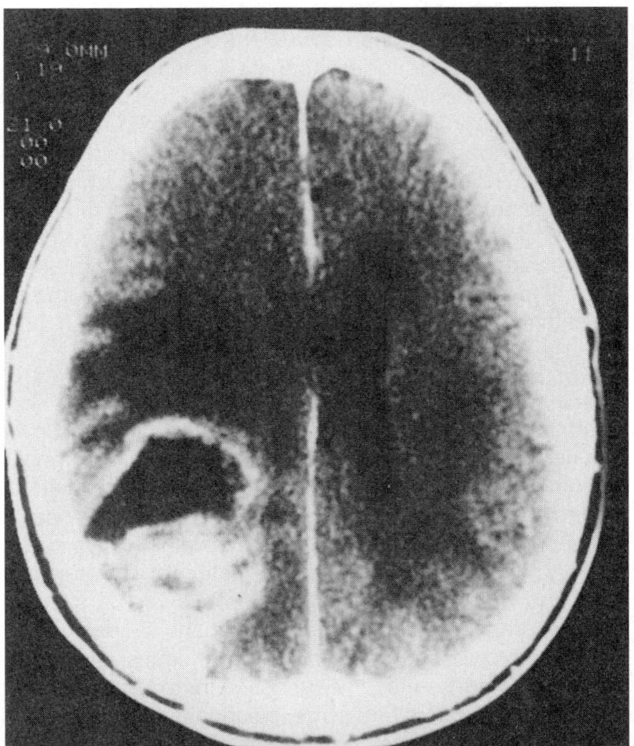

Figure 97.1. Contrast-enhanced computed tomography (CT) scan of a primary glioblastoma multiforme.

EPIDEMIOLOGY

Patients with glioblastoma multiforme (mean age, 54 years) are generally older than those with anaplastic astrocytoma (mean age, 45 years) and have a shorter median survival time.

PATHOLOGY

For the purposes of this chapter, the diagnosis of glioblastoma multiforme requires a histologic pattern consisting of a highly cellular astrocytic tumor with nuclear and cellular pleomorphism, vascular proliferation, and mitotic figures. Necrosis frequently is present, and, although necrosis is requisite for a diagnosis of glioblastoma multiforme in most grading systems, it is not a requirement according to the revised WHO schema. Most glioblastomas multiforme are microscopically infiltrative lesions and have a high labeling index. In contrast, anaplastic astrocytomas, which are highly cellular astrocytic neoplasms with moderate nuclear and cytoplasmic pleomorphism, may have mitotic figures and do not have necrosis. They are infiltrative with a high labeling index, although typically the labeling index is lower than that in glioblastoma multiforme.

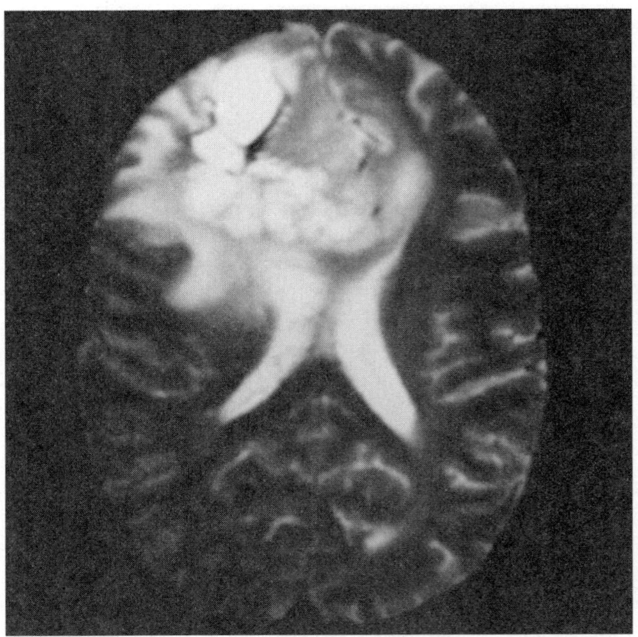

Figure 97.2. T2-W axial MRI of a glioblastoma multiforme.

DIAGNOSTIC NEUROIMAGING

The usual appearance of a glioblastoma multiforme or an anaplastic astrocytoma on MRI and CT is that of a single, contrast-enhancing lesion, frequently showing mass effect (Figs. 97.1 through 97.4). Kelly and colleagues, from multiple stereotactic biopsies, showed that the contrast-enhancing lesion on CT represents proliferative malignant cells, the central low-density region is true necrosis, and the region of low attenuation surrounding the contrast margins harbors infiltrating cells; there may also be active tumor cells within the larger area of abnormality seen on a T2-W image, although the margin at which tumor cells cease to exist and only edema is present may be indistinct (129).

SURGICAL DIAGNOSIS AND TREATMENT

Surgery for patients with malignant glioma, whether a glioblastoma multiforme or an anaplastic astrocytoma, is designed to make a diagnosis, to preserve life, to alleviate symptoms, and to remove as much tumor as is safely possible. It is impossible to remove all microscopic disease, even if, on postoperative images, removal appears to be total, because of the infiltrative character of these lesions. In patients with glioblastoma multiforme, surgery without adjuvant ther-

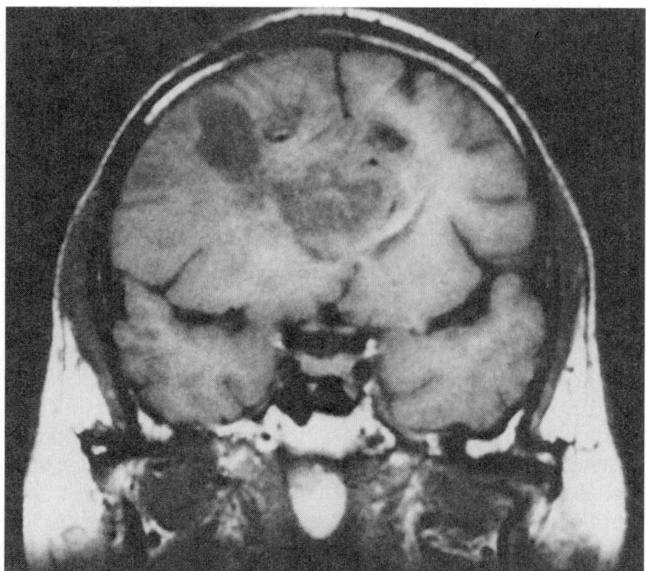

Figure 97.3. T1-W coronal MRI of the same glioblastoma multiforme as shown in Figure 97.2.

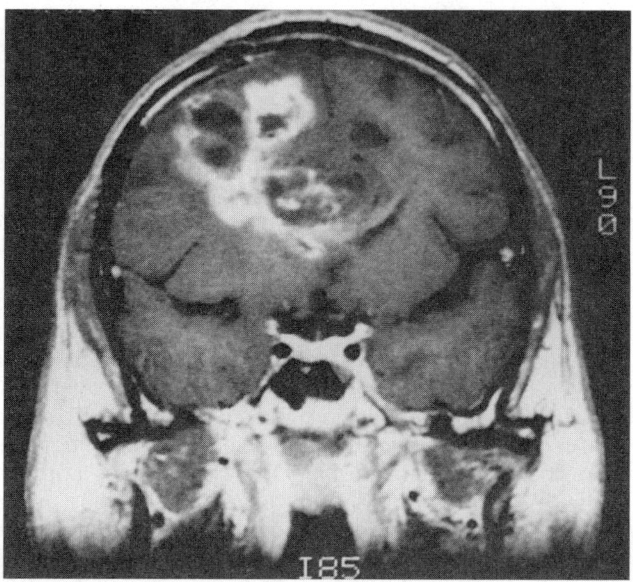

Figure 97.4. T1-W coronal MRI of the same glioblastoma multiforme as shown in Figure 97.2 made with Gd as contrast agent.

apies can control the disease no longer than a few months, as proved in the initial trials comparing surgery alone with the combination of surgery and irradiation for glioblastoma multiforme. The extent of surgery achieved may have an impact on overall survival.

A recent study from the Brain Tumor Cooperative Group (BTCG) showed that a greater extent of residual tumor volume after surgery correlates directly with a shorter period of survival, but there is no such relation based on preoperative tumor volume (296). This relation of residual tumor volume to survival was independent of age, Karnofsky performance status (KPS), and tumor histology (128). There was a similar relation between survival and the extent of residual tumor volume after radiation therapy. Other trials have suggested that the greater the extent of surgery, the more favorable may be its impact on functional survival; that is, the maintenance or improvement of neurologic status or KPS (10, 12, 191). Andreou and colleagues correlated the amount of residual tumor burden after surgery with both the length and quality of survival (KPS greater than 30) (12). A residual tumor volume of less than 45 mm was associated with a 70% chance of the patient's surviving more than 700 days. With smaller tumor volumes, the possible survival time increased. Other studies have confirmed this correlation. Ammirati and colleagues showed an improvement in patients' postoperative functional status after gross total tumor removal, with a median survival of 90 weeks, as compared with 43 weeks for patients who had a subtotal removal; both groups received radiation therapy. In a study from the RTOG, patients with a malignant astrocytoma who were treated with radiation survived a median of 47 months after subtotal removal but only 15 months after undergoing only biopsy (10, 191). Finally, combining patients from various studies, the RTOG analyzed outcome for 645 patients and found that the extent of resection was a signficant variable that influenced survival, along with age and performance status (261). Unless there are significant medical reasons for not performing a craniotomy, performing only a biopsy is not justified in a patient who is thought to harbor a surgically accessible malignant astrocytoma.

Radiation Therapy and Chemotherapy

After surgery, patients with glioblastoma multiforme or anaplastic astrocytoma are treated with radiation therapy. Irradiation is an effective adjuvant to surgery for malignant gliomas and in prospective studies has afforded better survival than either surgery alone or surgery plus chemotherapy. Indeed, after surgical resection, radiation therapy is the single most effective treatment for both of these tumor types.

Chemotherapy is used adjuvantly with surgery and radiation therapy. The early studies of chemotherapy involved the nitrosoureas, chosen for their lipophilic characteristics and in vitro sensitivity. These drugs include carmustine, 1-(2-chloroethyl)-3-cyclohexyl-1-nitrosourea (lomustine, also CCNU), 1-(2-chloroethyl)-3-(2, 6-dioxo-3-piperidyl)-1-nitrosourea (PCNU), (1-4-amino-2-methyl-5-pyrimidinyl)-methyl-3-(2-chloroethyl)-3-nitrosourea (ACNU), methyl-CCNU (semustine, also MeCCNU), and streptozotocin. Other agents known to have antitumor activity include procarbazine, dibromodulcitol, etoposide and teniposide, vincristine, aziridinylbenzoquinone (AZQ), cisplatin, carboplatin, tamoxifen, taxol, and temozolomide.

The initial studies of irradiation and chemotherapy adjuvant to surgery were conducted by the BTSG in 1969 (285). In this landmark study, patients who had undergone surgery were randomized into four different treatment groups: (1) supportive care only; (2) carmustine (80 mg/m^2) given on three successive days every 6 weeks for 1 year; (3) whole-brain irradiation to a total of 50 to 60 Gy; and (4) whole-brain irradiation to a total of 50 to 60 Gy and carmustine (80 mg/m^2) given on three successive days every 6 weeks for 1 year. Patients with glioblastoma multiforme constituted 90% of the treated groups. The median survival periods in the four groups were 14, 19, 36, and 35 weeks, respectively. The 12-month survival rates were 3, 12, 24, and 32%, respectively. Comparison of the survival rates showed that surgery plus radiation therapy offered a significantly improved survival time over that afforded by either surgery alone or surgery plus chemotherapy ($P < .05$), documenting the advantage of adjuvant irradiation in increasing survival for patients with glioblastoma multiforme. The 12-month survival rates for patients treated with radiation plus carmustine were only slightly higher than those for patients receiving radiation only.

After this study, a series of trials undertaken by the BTSG reaffirmed the survival advantage afforded by radiation therapy after surgery and suggested a further advantage in some subsets of patients with the addition of adjuvant nitrosourea chemotherapy (94, 286). For example, in one study comparing the results of irradiation plus either carmustine or semustine to those of irradiation or semustine alone, patients receiving carmustine plus radiation had a longer survival than those receiving semustine alone, but the survival rates with carmustine plus radiation were not significantly longer than those for people treated with radiation alone or with radiation plus semustine (286). In trials attempting to enhance the survival advantage with postoperative irradiation, higher doses of radiation were investigated initially as investigators sought the optimal dose using single fractions. Evaluating data from more than 600 patients treated with median doses of 50 Gy, 55 Gy, and 60 Gy, for whom the median survival times were 28, 36, and 42 weeks, respectively, the BTSG noted a significant difference in favor of the higher dose (287). The next trials evaluated postoperative irradiation plus carmustine, or procarbazine or high-dose methylprednisolone, either alone or with carmustine (95). Survival was longer in the groups receiving carmustine or procarbazine adjuvant to irradiation than in the methylprednisolone group, and no advantage was obtained by adding methylprednisolone to carmustine. No control group treated with radiation alone was used in this trial.

A four-arm trial conducted jointly by the RTOG and the ECOG compared whole-brain irradiation to (1) a total dose of 60 Gy, (2) whole-brain irradiation to 60 Gy plus a boost of 10 Gy to the tumor bed, (3) whole-brain irradiation to 60 Gy plus carmustine alone, (4) and whole-brain irradiation to 60 Gy plus semustine and imidazole carboxamide (DTIC) (41). There were no differences in survival between the patients treated with 60-Gy whole-brain irradiation and those receiving whole-brain irradiation to 60 Gy with a 10-Gy boost to the tumor bed. The chemotherapy plus irradiation arms showed longer survival than either irradiation-only arm, but only in patients 40 to 60 years old; no advantage was seen in patients younger than 40 years or older than 60 years. More patients survived 2 years or longer in the chemotherapy arms. The DTIC plus semustine combination was more toxic than the carmustine treatment.

Salazar and colleagues, reviewing patients treated with whole-brain irradiation in increasing doses from 50 y to 60 Gy and up to 75 Gy, noted increasing survival in patients receiving the higher doses; however, the consequence of the highest dose was a steady decline in KPS to a state of general debilitation by 18 to 24 months (223). Peritumoral necrosis was often seen on CT. It appears from these and later trials that 60 Gy is the optimal dose when single-dose radiation fractions are used (43, 242).

The Northern California Oncology Group (NCOG) evaluated the results obtained in a three-drug regimen of procarbazine, lomustine, and vincristine (PCV) with results in patients receiving carmustine alone after radiation therapy (157). Patients with anaplastic astrocytoma had a survival advantage when treated with PCV as compared with carmustine alone, median survivals being 157 weeks versus 82 weeks, respectively ($P = .021$). The three-drug combination offered no survival advantage over survival obtained with carmustine alone in patients with glioblastoma multiforme.

Whole-Brain Irradiation. In a large prospective trial from the BTCG comparing various forms of irradiation and chemotherapy, the three chemotherapy regimens included carmustine alone, carmustine alternating with procarbazine, and carmustine plus hydroxyurea alternating with procarbazine plus teniposide (250). All patients, 80% of whom had a glioblastoma multiforme, were treated with radiation according to two regimens, either with whole-brain treatment to 60.2 Gy or with whole-brain irradiation to 43 Gy plus a 17.2-Gy boost to the local tumor bed. The results were similar in all groups and no significant survival advantage was found with any of the forms of chemotherapy or irradiation. The median survival ranged from 11.3 to 13.8 months. The group receiving the higher dose of whole-brain irradiation showed no survival advantage. The BTCG concluded that giving the radiation partly as a coned-down boost plus carmustine is as effective as whole-brain irradiation plus any of the other combinations of chemotherapy.

Although the earliest trials of radiation therapy treated whole-brain fields, recent studies with limited-field irradiation have shown survival times comparable to those obtained with whole-brain therapy. At UCSF, the treatment volume includes the contrast-enhancing lesion observed on CT plus a margin of 2 to 3 cm surrounding this edge. If MR imaging is used, the volume includes the T2-W signal plus approximately a 1-cm margin. Sheline, using limited fields in patients with malignant gliomas, reported a median survival time of 10 months, which was identical to that in BTSG trials using whole-brain fields (94, 95, 253, 285, 286). Later studies from the RTOG, BTSG/BTCG, and NCOG using smaller than whole-brain fields have shown equivalent or better survival data than the results with whole-brain irradiation (59, 157, 159, 188, 250).

Hochberg and Pruitt compared postmortem findings in patients with glioblastoma multiforme compared with antemortem CT scans (108). In 80% of cases, the CT contrast-enhancing lesion included the tumor and microscopic margins within a 2-cm margin. Wallner and colleagues reviewed the patterns of glioblastoma multiforme and anaplastic astrocytoma regrowth, comparing the initial CT appearance at the original diagnosis with the CT appearance at recurrence as documented by surgical resection: 78% of tumors recurred within 2 cm, and 56% within 1 cm, of the presurgical initial tumor margin (288). No unifocal tumors recurred as multifocal tumors.

Our experience at UCSF shows that, in 90% of cases, the tumor recurs within a 2-cm margin of the primary lesion (46). Until local tumor control can be achieved for prolonged periods of time, there appears to be no survival advantage for the use of whole-brain irradiation.

Hyperfractionation. In standard fractionated radiation therapy, doses of 1.8 to 2.0 Gy are given daily until the prescribed total dose is reached. Different fractionation schemes and total delivered doses have been evaluated by the RTOG (188, 192). In hyperfractionated radiation therapy, more than one fraction of the total dose is given each day, generally in smaller doses of radiation per fraction. The rationale for hyperfractionation is to reduce late effects of radiation, especially necrosis, and to prevent tumor repopulation by using more than one treatment each day (13, 68, 256). Late injury effects of hyperfractionation depend more on the size of the fraction than on the intertreatment interval. Administering smaller doses minimizes the amount of sublethal radiation injury to normal brain and maximizes cellular repair. Small doses given more than once a day, usually at intervals of 4 to 8 hours, produce a redistribution of proliferating tumor cells: some cells enter a radiation-sensitive stage. Nonproliferating tissue or dose-limiting tissue such as normal brain is spared this effect of redistribution, or sensitization.

Douglas used a fraction scheme with 1.0-Gy doses administered three times daily, ultimately to a whole-brain radiation dose of 54 Gy, with a tumor boost of another 10 Gy (62). The survival curves for patients with glioblastoma multiforme showed better results than did those for historical controls, with a 1-year survival rate of 44%. However, in a series of trials from the BTSG, BTCG, and RTOG that evaluated hyperfractionated irradiation, with or without radiation sensitizers and adjuvant chemotherapies, there was no significant difference in median survival between groups undergoing hyperfractionated irradiation to a total dose as high as 76.8 Gy and those receiving standard single-fraction radiation doses to 60 Gy (59, 94, 188). Urtasun and colleagues treated patients with malignant glioma three times daily to a total dose of 61.41, 71.20, or 80.00 Gy, and, when a tumor recurred, the patient received single-agent lomustine (280). Median survival times were 45.8, 37.2, and 60.5 weeks, respectively, using this approach—again, no better than the data for historical controls. The RTOG studies evaluated doses of 64.8, 72, and 76.8 Gy and found median survival to be better in the 72-Gy arm (190). A second randomization compared 72 Gy with 81.6 Gy, and, again, found better median survival in the 72-Gy arm (189). A current randomized trial compares 72 Gy to the conventional dose of 60 Gy, to try to determine if there is any advantage to the higher dose. There is a concern that the worse survival rate seen with higher doses may be related to increased toxicity.

From the current data, it appears that higher doses of radiation therapy for supratentorial glioblastoma multiforme and anaplastic astrocytoma, whether in single or multiple daily fractions, do not significantly improve median survival times over those achieved with standard single-fraction 60-Gy irradiation. Newer schemes using even higher doses per fraction, termed accelerated hyperfractionation, are being investigated, but the results are preliminary.

Radiation-Enhancing Agents. Because radiation is thought to be less cytocidal under hypoxic conditions, and because malignant astrocytomas are presumed to contain hypoxic tumor cells, tolerated radiation doses now used for therapy may produce poor local tumor control; increasing the radiation dose increases the risk of radiation necrosis. Studies to improve the efficacy of radiation given in the conventional dosage include investigations of hypoxic cell sensitizers. The two nitroimidazoles, misonidazole and metronidazole, given during irradiation, are electronaffinic and, under conditions of hypoxia, are taken up by cells and substitute for oxygen in producing radiation-induced DNA damage (31, 192). Unfortunately, neither agent has been successful in improving survival, and both have significant toxicity in clinical use. Although other imidazole compounds with—potentially—less toxicity, such as etanidazole, are being investigated in the hope of improving efficacy; studies thus far show no hypoxic cell sensitizers that conclusively improve survival of patients with malignant glioma.

Radiation sensitizers such as the halogenated pyrimidines have been investigated in several studies. BUdR and 5-iodo-2-deoxyuridine (IUdR), two nonhypoxic cell-sensitizing agents, are given through constant infusion. They incorporate into the DNA of dividing cells in place of thymidine. Nondividing cells, such as those in normal glial and neuronal tissue, do not take up these agents. Hoshino treated 107 patients with a continuous intra-arterial infusion of BUdR concurrently with irradiation and found that more than 50% survived 18 months or longer (111). The study was not repeated because of technical difficulties with intra-arterial delivery system. Greenberg and colleagues also studied intra-arterial BUdR, using a simplified delivery system, and, as compared with historical control subjects, found a survival advantage in a small group of patients with grades III and IV malignant gliomas (96). Data from the NCOG phase II trials suggest a survival advantage with BUdR administered intravenously to patients with anaplastic astrocytoma, but not to patients with glioblastoma multiforme (159). The data for anaplastic astrocytoma are particularly encouraging: median survival is 190 weeks. These data require confirmation by a prospective randomized phase III trial that is currently ongoing. The new study treats only patients with newly diagnosed anaplastic astrocytoma, and requires central neuropathology review for entry into the study. It is the first disease-specific trial of its kind, and emphasizes the fact that patients with anaplastic astrocytoma have different response and survival expectations than patients with glioblastoma.

IUdR is in clinical trials for use in primary and metastatic tumors. In a phase I study, continuous intravenous IUdR was delivered concurrently with hyperfractionated irradiation in a dose-escalating scheme (132). The results suggest that IUdR is less toxic than BUdR and that the kinetics of the drug are linear at doses between 250 and 1,200 mg/m^2, reaching steady state within 1 hour. The results of these investigations are preliminary but suggestive of increased local control rates with IUdR. The main adverse effects of these agents are myelosuppression, photosensitization, changes in the skin and nail bed, allergic reactions, and hepatic injury. However, the toxicities have been mild and generally well tolerated and further trials are planned.

High–Linear Energy Transfer (LET) Irradiation. Other forms of radiation therapy less dependent on cellular oxygen include neutron and heavy-ion therapy and are called *high-LET irradiation.* The RTOG has conducted a randomized dose-finding study of neutrons given as a boost to conventional external-beam photon therapy (138). Patients were treated initially using whole-brain irradiation with photons to a dose of 45 Gy, then boosted with fast neutrons using six different dose levels. There was no difference, between the doses, in the survival obtained overall, but, in patients with tumors other than glioblastoma multiforme, there was a suggestion that neutrons contributed to poorer survival with the higher doses.

Two trials performed with fast neutrons and one using three different schemes and the other study combining misonidazole with neutron therapy, both yielded negative results (136, 244). Other ions, including helium and neon ions, have been studied, and negative pi mesons have been considered because of the theoretical advantage of less resistance from hypoxic cells and more general cell-cycle-specific activity. The NCOG conducted a trial using neon irradiation at two dose levels in patients with glioblastoma multiforme, and the preliminary results suggest no benefit in terms of median survival in this patient group.

Interstitial Brachytherapy. Interstitial brachytherapy, the implantation of high-activity radioactive sources, or "seeds," within a tumor, has been used to treat highly anaplastic tumors and recurrent primary and metastatic tumors. Stereotactic technique and local anesthesia ensure accurate neurosurgical placement of catheters into the tumor bed, into which the radioactive seeds are after-loaded. The seeds remain in place within the tumor until the desired dose is delivered, and, then, in a simple maneuver done in the patient's room, the catheters and sources are removed. Patients tolerate the procedure well: the major complications are seizures during source placement and, rarely, infection. Because of its risks and the precision required for proper placement of the radioactive sources, careful selection of patients for brachytherapy is imperative. A dedicated radiation physics and oncology staff ensure the proper dosimetry.

Several radiation sources have been investigated for interstitial use, but the one most commonly used is iodine 125 (^{125}I). Gutin and colleagues have reviewed their experience at UCSF using high-activity ^{125}I interstitial brachytherapy in 45 patients with recurrent glioblastoma multiforme and 50 patients with recurrent anaplastic astrocytoma (145). The minimum dose delivered to the tumor ranged from 50 to 120 Gy. Median survival time was 54 weeks for patients with recurrent glioblastoma multiforme and 87 weeks for those with anaplastic astrocytoma, measured from the date of implantation. These encouraging survival data show interstitial brachytherapy to be one of the best techniques available for therapy for patients with recurrent tumors. Toxicity, however, is significant. In this series, 46% of the patients underwent reoperation for clinical deterioration caused by an increasing mass of radiation necrosis, although long-term maintenance of quality survival was achieved with an average KPS of 80 (145).

Although the results have been quite impressive, it is necessary to reduce the incidence of clinically significant necrosis with this technique. In a trial also conducted at UCSF, hyperthermia was used in conjunction with brachytherapy in an attempt to increase local control, to reduce the radiation dose because heat enhances the effects of radiation therapy, and to lessen the risk of radiation necrosis (262). This pilot phase II trial documented that hyperthermia was both technically feasible and that it added only minor toxicity over that seen with brachytherapy alone. It also demonstrated that efficient heating was crucial to local control. Because of this favorable phase II data, a new phase III study is currently ongoing that randomizes patients with newly diagnosed glioblastoma multiforme to receive brachytherapy alone versus brachytherapy with hyperthermia following conventional external beam radiotherapy. The results of the phase III trial are not known at this time.

Based on the success of brachytherapy in treating patients with recurrent gliomas, several investigators have begun to evaluate this technique in patients at the time of initial diagnosis. In a recently completed trial from the NCOG, interstitial brachytherapy was used after conventional external-beam radiotherapy for the initial treatment of newly diagnosed malignant gliomas. The interstitial brachytherapy was followed by adjuvant chemotherapy. The results revealed a median survival time of 88 weeks for patients with glioblastoma multiforme (101). Among a similar group of patients treated in a pilot study using the same strategy, median survival was 87 weeks in patients with newly diagnosed glioblastoma multiforme (217).

Unfortunately, many patients are not candidates for brachytherapy. The tumor volume that can be safely implanted is generally less than 5 cm in any dimension; lesions in eloquent areas (corpus callosum, thalamus, and other midline deep-seated areas) of the brain are not implanted. The typical lesion treated is superficial, small, and in an area where necrosis produced by the procedure can be tolerated. Given these limitations, most patients with glioblastoma multiforme, malignant astrocytoma, or even recurrent tumor, are ineligible for brachytherapy, but for those who have a smaller tumor volume it is a technique that, with further investigation, could, overall, add to the length and quality of survival.

Radiosurgery. While more commonly used for arteriovenous malformations, radiosurgery has recently been evaluated as a possible treatment for gliomas. So far, it has been used most in patients with recurrent gliomas, including metastatic lesions, that have not responded to standard radiation therapy (166). In this technique, an external beam of radiation is precisely collimated and directed to a small volume in a single large fraction. Several radiation sources have been investigated for use with radiosurgery, including heavy particles, cobalt 60 (^{60}Co), and the conventional linear accelerator. The radiation beam is directed using coordinates on a standard stereotactic head frame or using a gamma unit, a device with a sophisticated head frame that permits precise assignment of coordinates along concentric arcs to cause a convergence of the ^{60}Co source (168). The objective of radiosurgery is to deliver a finely focused radiation beam precisely to the target. Critical evaluation in recently opened trials must address issues about dose and tumor volume and identify specific criteria for selecting tumors that would benefit from this therapy. There are now some preliminary data from the RTOG on the use of this technique in recurrent malignant gliomas and metastatic tumors of the brain. Important dose-volume parameters have been identified, and recommended doses of radiation based upon the volume of the target lesion have been suggested. Further phase II testing will now take place to evaluate radiosurgery given with various radiosensitizers, such as etanidazole. Ultimately, phase III studies will be required to define the role of radiosurgery both in recurrent tumors and newly diagnosed disease. It is possible that radiosurgery may become as effective as interstitial brachytherapy for these indications, at least for lesions that can be treated with either modality. This question will also need to be studied in carefully conducted phase III studies. Brachytherapy may still have a preferred role in larger lesions, since radiosurgery has a tumor volume limit that is smaller than that of brachytherapy.

Multimodality Therapy

Attempts to improve the survival advantage obtained with adjuvant chemotherapy include trials of intra-arterial drug delivery with the nitrosoureas and platinum compounds and high-dose chemotherapy with autologous bone marrow transplantation (ABMT). The theoretical advantage of intra-arterial therapy over intravenous infusion is in the increased uptake of drug during its first pass through the tumor capillary bed; however, while systemic toxicity may be less than that associated with conventional chemotherapy, the local and regional toxicity is greater: it substitutes one toxicity for another, with no obvious therapeutic advantage.

The BTCG, in a prospective randomized study comparing intra-arterial with intravenous carmustine administered concurrently with radiation therapy, showed no survival advantage for patients treated through the intra-arterial route, but 8% of patients developed leukoencephalopathy and 16% developed unilateral blindness (249). In a trial by Bashir and colleagues of intra-arterial carmustine preceding irradiation, a high incidence of leukoencephalopathy (7%) led them to recommend that this regimen not be used in phase III studies (18).

Mahaley and colleagues gave 40 patients cisplatin monthly as an intra-arterial infusion at the time of tumor recurrence (169). The median survival time for the patients who could be evaluated in this group was 27.5 weeks. Adverse effects included renal, otologic, and neural toxicity. Newton and colleagues used cisplatin in 12 patients at the time of tumor recurrence and found that only 1 patient had a partial response; all the others had progressive disease or severe toxicity including seizures, weakness, coma, and visual deterioration (195). In another recently reported trial in which 23 patients received intra-arterial carboplatin monthly, 10 patients achieved either a partial response or stabilization of their disease (79). The investigators proposed that this agent was less toxic than intra-arterial cisplatin and that it warrants further trial.

Other nitrosoureas that have been investigated include ACNU and PCNU, and other cytotoxic agents such as teniposide are undergoing trial (269, 270, 299). There is no convincing evidence that these agents improve overall survival, and their toxicity is significant. Intra-arterial administration of drugs should be used only in the setting of a controlled clinical trial designed to overcome toxicity and improve efficacy.

High-dose chemotherapy with ABMT has also shown only limited success. The difficulty with this approach is the end-organ toxicity of agents such as carmustine or platinum compounds, as well as the paucity of agents with activity against malignant gliomas. Carmustine has been given in large doses, resulting in pulmonary, hepatic, and infectious complications; for 11 patients treated at recurrence, the median survival was 7 months (107). Other alkylating agents investigated include thiotepa, etoposide, and busulfan. One preliminary trial that combined high-dose thiotepa and etoposide with ABMT for treatment of pediatric high-grade astrocytoma showed encouraging results (77). Because of these results, a second phase II study was conducted using high-dose carboplatin with thiotepa and etoposide, the results of which are still pending full review. Currently, a study being conducted by the Children's Cancer Group (CCG) treats patients with newly diagnosed glioblastoma multiforme and incompletely resected anaplastic astrocytoma with high-dose BCNU, thiotepa, and etoposide. Currently, no ongoing phase III trials randomize patients to standard-dose chemotherapy versus high-dose chemotherapy with bone marrow or stem cell support.

Recommendation for Adjuvant Therapy

From the studies of various combinations of radiation therapy and adjuvant chemotherapy reported thus far, the standard treatment to which other therapies should be compared is still single daily fraction irradiation to a total dose of 60 Gy plus adjuvant carmustine. For patients with glioblastoma multiforme, there is no survival advantage in using whole-brain radiation therapy or other forms of chemotherapy. Adjuvant chemotherapy improves 2-year survival rates, but not the median survival, in glioblastoma patients and clearly improves median and long-term survival in patients with anaplastic astrocytoma. At least one study supports PCV chemotherapy over therapy with only carmustine in this group. In a select group of patients with glioblastoma, interstitial brachytherapy appears to improve survival, but further trials are needed to confirm these early results. The role of stereotactic radiosurgery is currently being tested in clinical trials.

RECURRENCE

The precarious character of brain tumor therapy is illustrated by recurrence of astrocytomas after irradiation, for which the latency period from irradiation to diagnosis may be as short as 3 years or longer than 20 years (304). The diagnosis of tumor recurrence requires, at the minimum, an increase in tumor volume demonstrated on sequential contrast-enhanced CT scans or on MR images. While seemingly straightforward, neuroimaging studies may be difficult to interpret in the light of previous treatment, or the changes seen on the image may be only slightly worse in the case of a clinically stable patient. Changes seen on CT scans or MRI after interstitial brachytherapy are, in particular, very difficult to interpret and may represent tumor recurrence, radiation necrosis, or a combination of both. ^{201}Tl-SPECT or PET studies can be helpful in differentiating these events, but neither is 100% accurate or specific.

New forms of radiation therapy, including accelerated hyperfractionation techniques and radiosurgery, have created yet another set of uncertainties similar to those attending brachytherapy. MRI-Gd is very sensitive to changes associated with radiation injury. Although the tumor volume may remain the same, the internal enhancing characteristics may vary over several images. The significance of these changes continues to be investigated; they may not represent tumor progression.

Clinical neurologic examinations are done concurrently with the neuroimaging assessment and an assessment of the patient's steroid requirements. All three factors are important in the determination of the tumor's status, but the neuroimaging study is the most important indicator of response or progression.

Once it is determined that a tumor has progressed, further treatment may include palliative care, another surgical resection, reirradiation (including brachytherapy or radiosurgery), and chemotherapy. Several factors are important in the assessment of further treatment, including the patient's age and KPS, the tumor's histology, the expected outcome of additional therapies weighed against specific risks, and the needs and expectations of the patient and family. Elderly patients with poor KPS and recurrent glioblastoma multiforme have a poor prognosis and little chance of increasing their survival longer than an additional 2 to 3 months with further therapy. In the clinical situation of a bedridden patient with little remaining cognitive function, even maintenance of the status quo may be undesirable. Conversely, for a younger patient who is neurologically intact and has a small tumor regrowth, there is a greater chance of achieving tumor control with little risk of a negative impact on quality of life. In such a case, it may be possible to achieve a median survival time of greater than a year, as measured from recurrence, in selected patient groups.

Patients with recurrent malignant gliomas who are treated on research protocol studies generally live longer than those who are not; this reflects both an institutional referral bias and the benefit of further interventions that often occur in sequential treatment regimens. Patients on aggressive treatment programs are often well motivated, young, and in relatively good neurologic condition. For these reasons, the individual characteristics of groups tested should be weighed carefully and critically when interpreting the results of trials in patients with tumor recurrence.

When tumor recurrence is diagnosed, often the first decision to be made is Is further surgery recommended? Several studies have addressed the impact of reoperation on quality of survival. Ammirati and colleagues reviewed 55 patients with recurrent malignant astrocytoma who underwent a second resection and reported median survival of 36 weeks, which is similar to the reported survival of other groups (9). In reviewing the data from 70 consecutive patients who underwent reoperation for recurrent glioblastoma multiforme and anaplastic astrocytoma, Harsh and colleagues reported a median survival of 36 weeks for patients with glioblastoma multiforme, and of 83 weeks for those with anaplastic astrocytoma measured from the date of the second operation (102). Age and preoperative KPS were important in predicting the quality of survival based on the KPS. Because the patients had additional therapies following their second operation, the impact of surgery must be considered in the context of multimodality treatment at recurrence. Salcman and colleagues achieved a median survival of 36 weeks in patients with recurrent glioblastoma multiforme who were treated initially with a second resection; in the group of 15 patients who survived at least 36 months from the initial diagnosis of their original tumor, each patient had undergone an average of almost three craniotomies (243). It appears evident that a repeat surgical resection is an option with the potential for improved survival in at least some groups of patients. Appropriate selection of patients for reoperation is important, as is the use of additional therapies following surgery.

As discussed earlier, interstitial brachytherapy or stereotactic radiosurgery are important salvage techniques for the small group of patients who have a recurrent malignant glioma of sufficiently small size in an appropriate location to permit accurate and safe placement of the interstitial catheters or treatment planning for radiosurgery (145). Unfortunately, most patients with recurrent tumors are not eligible for either procedure, primarily because of the size and location of their recurrence.

In patients who are not eligible for brachytherapy or radiosurgery, treatment with chemotherapy is a reasonable alternative. The nitrosoureas are still the most active agents for the treatment of recurrent tumors. In patients who have never received adjuvant chemotherapy with these drugs, their use in treating recurrence often produces high response or stabilization rates. Many trials using carmustine, alone or in combination, with other agents show median survival times of 20 to 50 weeks, depending on tumor histology, glioblastoma multiforme being more rapidly lethal than anaplastic astrocytoma (147, 294). Combination therapies, including lomustine (such as with the PCV regimen), are also effective secondary therapies (153).

Investigations of new agents continue in structured phase I and phase II studies, including trials with AZQ, dibromodulcitol, the biologicals (such as interferons and IL-2), as well as other cytotoxic agents, including cisplatin, carboplatin, etoposide, cyclophosphamide, methotrexate, thiotepa, vincristine, and, recently, the polyamine inhibitors α-difluoromethylornithine (DFMO) and mitoguazone, methylglyoxyl *bis*(guanylhydrazone) (MGBG) (135, 148). Trials of drugs for recurrent tumors are often aimed at identifying new agents, or combinations of agents, that eventually may be used in phase III trials, but none can be assumed to be advantageous.

New approaches to therapy for tumor recurrence, all of which are still investigational, include intratumoral injections, intra-arterial therapy, high-dose chemotherapy with ABMT, and the use of biologicals, including monoclonal antibody therapy. Other avenues of treatment include methods to overcome tumor cell resistance to the nitrosoureas, whether inherent or acquired. Studies with the interferons, IL-2, and the polyamine inhibitors are assessing novel therapies for brain tumors. New studies that use gene transfer are also beginning as well, which, potentially, open a new era of therapeutic strategies, given the number of potential molecular targets being defined in the laboratory.

Each of the interferons has been evaluated in trials of tumors at recurrence. Both α-interferon and β-interferon have shown activity; generally less activity is seen with α-interferon. Most of the trials that have been done using intrathecal, intratumoral, and systemic therapy suggest therapeutic activity. Of the 19 patients treated at recurrence with α-interferon by Mahaley and his colleagues, 7 had either a response or stabilization (171). Median survival time for this group was 511 days; the patients who did not respond to the therapy survived (median) 147 days. Tumors of smaller volume were more likely to show response than were larger lesions. Most recently β-interferon has been given intravenously in studies of both adult and childhood gliomas and high response or stabilization rates of up to 50% were observed when it was used at recurrence (5, 301). Unfortunately, the duration of these responses was short lived. It is possible that these agents may be useful in combination with other agents. One ongoing trial is evaluating the use of α-interferon with carmustine as an adjuvant to surgery and irradiation. Another trial is randomizing patients to receive lomustine, either alone or with α-interferon for therapy of recurrent tumor. The adverse effects of interferons include malaise, fever, weight loss, hepatotoxicity, and mild myelosuppression; one serious neurotoxic effect is an only partially reversible dementia-like state, the pathogenesis of which is uncertain.

The regimen of IL-2 plus activated lymphocytes has recently been subjected to clinical trials. Merchant and colleagues treated 24 patients with intracerebral IL-2 and lymphokine-activated killer cells (LAK) at the time of recurrence (181). During subsequent craniotomy, previously harvested cells and IL-2–activated LAK cells were injected into areas of brain up to 2 cm surrounding the surgical cavity. Subsequently, IL-2 was given through a reservoir into the tumor cavity. Among these 24 patients, the median time to tumor progression was 5 months and median survival was 9 months. Adverse effects of the therapy included increased intracranial pressure (related to an increased amount of edema surrounding the tumor). Other trials have shown similar toxicity and tumor responses. Ongoing trials evaluating this approach include trials of IL-2 with LAK in combination with interferons (180).

The polyamines influence many cellular processes and are associated with growth regulation in particular. Blockade of polyamine accumulation in cells can prevent cellular proliferation in a variety of cell systems, including neoplastic growth. Polyamine inhibitors have been used in the treatment of brain tumors, because of this property of growth inhibition and because they are relatively nontoxic. One trial investigated the use of DFMO, an irreversible inhibitor of ornithine decarboxylase, in combination with MGBG, an inhibitor of S-adenosylmethionine decarboxylase, for the treatment of recurrent gliomas (150). The response and stabilization rate in 33 patients with recurrent anaplastic astrocytoma was 74%, and the median time to tumor progression was 52 weeks. A second trial, also in patients with recurrent gliomas, combined DFMO with carmustine (219). Of 21 patients with recurrent anaplastic astrocytomas, 57% had either a response or stabilization; the median survival time was 119 weeks in this group. Both trials with the polyamine inhibitors showed little activity in patients with recurrent glioblastoma multiforme. Toxicity was mild, and myelosuppression was minimal. Finally, a phase II study evaluated the response of single-agent DFMO in recurrent malignant gliomas, and reported minimal benefit in patients with glioblastoma multiforme. However, patients with recurrent anaplastic astrocytoma had a 45% response/stabilization rate, with a median time to tumor progression of 49 weeks (155). Trials to investigate these agents are ongoing, as is laboratory research to identify other polyamine analogs and inhibitors.

Trials investigating monoclonal antibodies alone or conjugated to radiopharmaceuticals, toxins, or drugs are inconclusive as yet, but show promise. Methods to overcome resistance to the nitrosoureas are also being investigated, as are trials of other mechanisms of resistance to therapy, including hypoxia-related resistance to drugs and radiation and multidrug resistance related to *p*-glycoprotein. Finally, new strategies to develop gene therapies are rapidly being developed, both clinically and in the laboratory. Based on the potential of studies such as these, it is anticipated that research during the next decade will change the face of therapy for recurrent gliomas.

Low-Grade Astrocytoma

The low-grade astrocytomas include the lesions designated astrocytoma in the three-tiered systems, including the revised WHO classification, those in grades I and II of the classification of Kernohan and colleagues, the moderately anaplastic astrocytoma in the old UCSF system, as well as the mixed tumors with low-grade components of astrocytoma and oligodendroglioma (16, 130, 227, 305). Astrocytomas may be further classified as pilocytic, protoplasmic, or fibrillary, based on their histologic appearance. The term *low-grade* suggests slow biologic growth that, on one hand, would account for the appearance of a lesion in a patient with a seizure disorder that remains unchanged for many years, or, on the other hand, a lesion that may be surgically cured with total resection.

The childhood cerebellar juvenile pilocytic astrocytoma is one of the most common of these lesions and is unique, and somewhat distinct from, the other low-grade lesions, because it has characteristic appearances on CT and MRI, characteristic clinical presentations, and a characteristic response to therapy.

ETIOLOGY AND EPIDEMIOLOGY

Low-grade astrocytomas may occur in any of many areas of the brain, including the optic nerve, cerebellum, hypothalamus, cerebral hemispheres, or brainstem. The mean age at diagnosis for patients with low-grade astrocytoma, other than juvenile pilocytic astrocytoma, is 35 years, and for those with juvenile pilocytic astrocytoma, 14 years. In children, the incidence of glial neoplasms is 2 to 5 cases in each 100,000 population per year, and approximately 70% of those neoplasms are low-grade astrocytomas (74, 300). Patients with NF1 or NF2 are at increased risk for these lesions, especially for low-grade astrocytomas of the optic pathways.

PATHOLOGY

Pathologically, low-grade astrocytomas are infiltrative lesions with a population of regular, uniform cells, a slight increase in cellularity, and minimal pleomorphism. Most often, there is no clear border between the tumor and surrounding normal brain parenchyma. The astrocytes may show a fibrillary or protoplasmic morphology, or they may be mixed with abnormal oligodendrocytes or ependymal cells. Cerebellar juvenile pilocytic astrocytomas consist of spongy tissue and microcysts interlaced with bundles of neoplastic cells, and they may have vascular endothelial proliferation. Lesions in the hypothalamus and optic pathways may appear identical. Biologic growth is slow, both in the infiltrative fibrillary astrocytomas and juvenile pilocytic astrocytomas.

The BudR-labeling index of infiltrative low-grade astrocytomas is usually less than 1% (a figure consistent with its low proliferative potential), but some low-grade astrocytomas have a greater labeling index and greater biologic potential (112). Those are often the lesions that recur quickly, despite a treatment course identical to that for a similar lesion that does not regrow.

The neuroimaging studies of low-grade astrocytomas show no contrast enhancement in most cases, with the exception of juvenile pilocytic astrocytoma, which uniformly shows an enhancing nodule associated with a cystic lesion. Even in lesions other than juvenile pilocytic astrocytoma, exceptions occur with respect to the presence or extent of enhancement. Some infiltrative astrocytomas enhance with both CT contrast agents and MRI-Gd. It is not possible, therefore, to predict the histology of a lesion accurately based on enhancement, and for this reason errors are made in evaluating both the low-grade and the higher-grade tumors. Tissue must be obtained in order to verify the diagnosis, and, if at all possible, additional biopsy material should be submitted for proliferative studies, as with BUdR or Ki-67. MR imaging may be more sensitive than CT in showing the extent of the lesion. The work of Kelly and colleagues using stereotactic biopsies demonstrated that the area of increased signal intensity on T2-W MRI reflects infiltrating tumor cells within otherwise normal brain tissue; this is also true of the low-density areas on CT, consistent with the truly infiltrative nature of these lesions (129).

CLINICAL PRESENTATION

Patients often present with seizures that may have been present for many years before the diagnosis. In most series, seizures are the most common presenting symptom, followed by headache and, finally, focal neurologic findings. The interval from the onset of symptoms to diagnosis may be as long as 10 years, in part because of the relative insensitivity of CT to detection of small low-grade lesions. Cerebellar juvenile pilocytic astrocytomas in children present with symptoms of clumsiness, ataxia, head tilt, and intermittent headaches and vomiting. Pilocytic astrocytomas of the optic nerve, chiasm, tract, and hypothalamus may present with eye movement disorders, visual field defects, and, in older children, precocious puberty. Cerebral lesions show signs and symptoms associated with the specific location of the lesion.

DIAGNOSTIC NEUROIMAGING

Neuroimaging studies include CT and MRI, the latter being more sensitive technique. In general, CT often shows a cystic or solid tumor of low density and variable amounts of contrast enhancement. Pilocytic astrocytomas reveal a cystic mass with intense contrast enhancement. Classically, the cerebellar juvenile pilocytic astrocytoma appears as a large, smooth-walled cyst with a small enhancing mural nodule (143). In adults, the diffuse infiltrative cerebral lesions often appear solid and hypodense and may or may not enhance. Often the lesion involves an entire lobe but has indistinct margins and causes minimal mass effect. MRI reveals either a hypointense or isointense lesion on T1-W images, with a larger area of T2 shortening very hyperintense in appearance. Gd enhancement is variably present. MRI may show abnormalities, though the CT scan appears normal, so MRI should be ordered if a tumor is suspected clinically but not seen with CT.

TREATMENT

The treatment of low-grade astrocytomas depends on the location of the tumor, the age of the patient, the extent of resection possible, and evaluations based on an understanding of the biology of these lesions. Childhood cerebellar juvenile pilocytic astrocytomas, for instance, are manageable in most cases with surgical resection alone (90, 274). Only in very unusual cases do juvenile pilocytic astrocytomas recur following gross total resection, and even the rare patient with recurrence may still enjoy a good outcome with repeat surgical interventions, with or without adjuvant radiation therapy. In contrast, infiltrative astrocytomas in adults often are not amenable to gross total surgical resection, usually require additional radiation therapy and possibly chemotherapy, and have a significantly worse prognosis with increasing age of the patient (214).

No prospective randomized trials have established how the extent of surgery relates to survival in patients with low-grade astrocytomas. The surgical options include stereotactic biopsy, limited resections, and an attempt at total removal. The results of surgery alone suggest excellent survival for patients with such tumors as pilocytic astrocytomas that are grossly resected: more than 80% of patients remain alive after 10 years (90). Most pediatric neurosurgeons attempt gross resection of a cerebellar cystic astrocytoma because of the potential for a surgical cure. Many supratentorial juvenile pilocytic astrocytomas are deep midline lesions, however, that cannot be totally resected, in which case the surgical approach is to remove as much tumor as can be removed safely, expecting to leave residual tumor.

Cerebral lesions are often large and in eloquent areas of the brain, creating the risk of neurologic defects if radical resection is attempted, even with cortical mapping. Leibel and colleagues, in a retrospective review of cases preceding the availability of MRI reported 100% survival at 10 years following gross total resection in patients with low-grade gliomas, and no survivors following biopsy alone (146). In a review of 194 cases, Gol reported a very short median survival (8 months) after biopsy, with or without radiation therapy, and a longer survival (34 months) following subtotal resection, with or without irradiation (92). Laws and colleagues showed progressively improved survival in patients undergoing radical partial or gross total removal, as compared with those who had biopsy and/or subtotal removal (140). A recent review by Berger and colleagues suggests that the extent of resection based upon pre- and postoperative measured tumor volumes, as well as the pre- and postoperative tumor volume independent of resection, is predictive of progression-free survival and subsequent malignant relapse (24). This latter review is compelling, because patients with lesions smaller than 10 cm^3 have significantly fewer relapses or episodes of malignant transformation. In fact, those tumors that were completely resected in this series have yet to relapse. These data strongly suggest that extensive resection, if possible to conduct safely, is the appropriate surgical option. Further studies are needed to confirm this option for low-grade glioma surgery.

Additional therapy after surgery includes radiation therapy or chemotherapy. Laws and colleagues, reviewing a large retrospective series, concluded that radiation therapy in doses over 40 Gy was beneficial in patients over age 40 who had undergone subtotal resection (141). Shaw and colleagues suggested that patients receiving more than 53 Gy did better (68% 5-year survival) than those receiving a lower dose (only 47% survival at 5 years) (251). Based on the relevant literature, Leibel suggested that postoperative irradiation increases 5-year survival, a rate of 46% with therapy but only 19% without (146). In contrast, Fazekas did not find a benefit to radiation in the subset of patients who underwent complete resection (75). In reviews by Shaw and colleagues and Piepmeier, patients had similar survival times as long as radiation therapy was given, regardless of the degree of surgery and even if only a biopsy was done (214, 251).

It would appear from these data that postoperative irradiation improves survival but that the extent of surgical resection needed is debatable. In general, low-grade lesions that are totally removed may be followed with no further therapy as long as the patient is well motivated and returns for frequent follow-up neuroimaging. Patients who have residual disease after surgery should probably receive postoperative irradiation to a limited field in a dose of at least 50 Gy.

Treatment of Young Children

In treating infants or young children, radiation therapy to the brain has been associated with intellectual deterioration, developmental delay, endocrine dysfunctions, and the long-term risk of secondary malignancy (204). Several trials have documented the benefit of chemotherapy as primary therapy following partial surgical resection for low-grade gliomas in children, especially in the group with juvenile pilocytic astrocytoma (205, 234). Among the regimens investigated are the use of actinomycin D with vincristine according to a protocol developed at Children's Hospital in Philadelphia (205), and a multiagent nitrosourea-based regimen used at UCSF that includes lomustine, procarbazine, 6-thioguanine, dibromodulcitol, and vincristine (213). The significance of these studies is that each has shown up to a 75% response or stabilization rate with chemotherapy alone, in some cases with years of disease-free survival. Ultimately, up to about one third or one half of patients require irradiation for tumor regrowth. Additional phase II data document that carboplatin alone or carboplatin with vincristine also may achieve high response rates and long progression-free survival intervals in children with both newly diagnosed and recurrent low-grade glioma (84, 201). In children under the age of 3 or 4 years, the use of chemotherapy remains a viable option for incompletely resected or symptomatic progressive low-grade tumors.

RECURRENCE

Assessments of the proliferative potential of tumors may be helpful in decisions about the use of irradiation or chemotherapy after surgery. Hoshino and colleagues, reviewing 47 patients with low-grade astrocytomas who received BUdR before surgery, reported 18 patients who had a BudR-labeling index greater than 1% (114). Among them, 12 had tumor recurrence within 3 years after surgery, of whom 9 died. In contrast, only 3 of the 29 patients with a BudR-labeling index less than 1% had a recurrence during the same time period. Similar analyses substantiate the impact of proliferative potential determinations in predicting biologic growth and their importance to our understanding of these low-grade lesions and their management (113).

RECOMMENDATION

Low-grade astrocytomas that can be removed totally may be managed with surgery alone. Incompletely resected tumors may be managed with surgery and irradiation. In infants and young children, primary chemotherapy may be useful in controlling the lesion while deferring irradiation until the child is over the age of 4 or 5 years. At UCSF, our policy is to attempt as extensive a resection as is safe, using cortical mapping as needed. Patients with incompletely resected low-grade gliomas receive 54 Gy using single daily dose fractions to the tumor volume and a small margin surrounding it.

Despite the optimism associated with the treatment of lower-grade lesions, many patients still die of this disease. New approaches are needed in the management of these tumors, with clinical research trials designed to answer questions concerning the optimal extent of resection, the timing and dose of radiation therapy, the use of chemotherapy, and the role, if any, of biologic or immunologic agents.

Oligodendroglioma

ETIOLOGY AND EPIDEMIOLOGY

Constituting less than 5% of the total number of gliomas, oligodendrogliomas most often occur in young and middle-aged adults and account for only 5 to 6% of CNS tumors in children (183). Oligodendrogliomas most often arise in hemispheric white matter but may be located wherever oligodendroglia cells occur in the CNS. Frequent locations are the frontal lobe (over 40%), parietal lobe (30%), and temporal lobe (20%). They may be pure tumors or mixed, with elements of astrocytoma or ependymoma. Most often, the mixed tumors are of a low grade and the principles of treatment are those described earlier for low-grade astrocytomas. This discussion concerns only aspects of the pure oligodendrogliomas

PATHOLOGY

Oligodendrogliomas appear as small, round cells in a monotonous pattern. The cytoplasm has distinct borders, the nuclei are dark and round, and an artifact of fixation often causes individual cells to look like fried eggs. The histologic appearance is that of a low-grade lesion with minimal anaplasia or pleomorphism; however, some oligodendrogliomas have anaplastic features with pleomorphism, in the extreme case even resembling glioblastoma multiforme. Others have intermediate features. Attempts to classify oligodendrogliomas using a grading system of A to D, from the least to the most anaplastic, have shown that survival data appear to be different only for the most anaplastic tumors (167). It may only be important, therefore, to grade oligodendrogliomas as either anaplastic or not.

CLINICAL PRESENTATION

Most patients with oligodendroglioma have a history of symptoms extending over many years. Seizures are common, occurring in as many as 50% of patients before diagnosis and eventually, during the course of the disease, in over 80% (45). Other focal findings depend on the location and rate of growth of the lesion. Occasionally, sudden onset of symptoms manifests as a consequence of hemorrhage into the tumor.

DIAGNOSTIC NEUROIMAGING

The CT appearance of oligodendroglioma is a hypodense or isodense lesion that may or may not enhance. Many oligodendrogliomas have calcifications scattered within the lesion, reflecting the mineralization seen histologically within blood vessel walls. There is little peritumoral edema. In some cases, the tumor appears to arise from the fourth ventricle. MRI reflects the CT lesion, with a hypointense or isointense lesion on T1-W images, a hyperintense lesion on T2-W images, and areas of signal void where calcifications arise. Enhancement with Gd is variable. Spread beyond the central lesion along the leptomeninges or into the spine is unusual but may occur, especially with lesions of the fourth ventricle.

TREATMENT

The treatment of choice is surgery, with the goal of gross total removal if possible. The 5-year survival rate varies from 30 to 80% with surgery alone (45, 255). Interpreting the retrospective series, it is difficult to say with certainty that surgery alone is adequate. Lindegaard and colleagues reported an 83-month median survival for patients with grossly resected tumors and a 26-month survival with subtotal resection (161). Earnest and colleagues, comparing results with subtotal or total removal, showed no difference in mean survival (63). There have been no prospective, randomized trials to compare the results of surgery alone as primary therapy with those of surgery and adjuvant irradiation or chemotherapy.

Most of the reported trials of radiation therapy support its use as a treatment for oligodendrogliomas. Chin and colleagues reported a 100% 5-year survival rate in a series of 24 patients who received radiation doses from 53 to 70 Gy following surgery; all were alive and 79% were disease-free in that group, whereas the group who did not receive radiation had an 82% 5-year survival and only 45% were disease-free (45).

Our experience at UCSF also supports the use of adjuvant irradiation. In a review of 32 patients, the 5-year survival rate was 85% for those who underwent irradiation but only 31% for those who did not (255). The recently compiled 10-year survival rate in that series was 56% in patients who received radiation to a dose greater than 45 Gy, but was 18% in those receiving no radiation therapy (289). Based on this experience, we give radiation therapy to all patients who have residual disease after surgery, using a dose of 54 Gy to a local field. Patients who have had a gross total resection and do not have anaplastic lesions may be observed carefully with serial CT or MRI; because this strategy has not been studied in controlled trials, patients are offered the option of foregoing irradiation if they are motivated and available for the frequent follow-up studies. All patients with an anaplastic lesion are treated with radiation to 60 Gy after surgery and are given adjuvant chemotherapy. The rationale for this aggressive treatment is the poor survival rates for anaplastic lesions (grade D): no long-term survivors 5 years after surgery. Patients with mixed tumors showing anaplastic elements, either in the astrocytic or oligodendroglioma components, are treated in the same fashion. Recent clinical trials were completed (see below) that strongly suggested that both low-grade and high-grade oligodendroglioma are chemosensitive, particularly to procarbazine, lomustine, and vincristine.

The RTOG is currently conducting a randomized phase III study in patients with high-grade oligodendroglioma in which one group of patients is treated first with chemotherapy and then with radiotherapy. The control group for this study gets radiotherapy only.

RECURRENCE

A recurrent oligodendroglioma may exhibit more aggressive histology than the original growth and frequently may behave like a recurrent anaplastic astrocytoma or glioblastoma multiforme. Pure anaplastic oligodendrogliomas may be very chemosensitive, particularly to nitrosourea-based combinations (38). The polyamine inhibitors, AZQ, and thiotepa have also been active. Survival following treatment is poor, approximately 1.5 to 2 years from the time of recurrence (149). If a recurrent tumor is small and in a favorable location, the treatment with first priority at UCSF is brachytherapy. Otherwise patients are treated with high-dose procarbazine, lomustine, and vincristine (PCV).

Ependymoma

EPIDEMIOLOGY

Ependymomas constitute about 5% of adult intracranial gliomas and up to 10% of childhood CNS tumors (61). There is a peak incidence at age 5 years and then again at age 34 years.

PATHOLOGY

Ependymomas have cells that resemble ependymal cells and tend to occur along the surfaces of the ventricles. Alternatively, they may occur in the parenchyma adjacent to the ventricle, or anywhere along the entire length of the spinal canal and the filum terminale (240). Over 60% of ependymomas occur below the tentorium, and most of those are in the posterior fossa, predominantly in the fourth ventricle. Supratentorial tumors most commonly arise from the lateral ventricles or parenchymal areas adjacent to or separate from the ventricular wall. Tumor extension may occur along the leptomeninges, around the medulla and upper cervical cord to the conus, and along nerve roots, and cells may be found in the cerebrospinal fluid (CSF).

Ependymomas are classified as either differentiated (low-grade) or anaplastic (malignant) tumors. Most are cellular tumors consisting of uniform polygonal cells in a collagenous background with well-defined cytoplasmic borders. Some groups of cells form clusters around a circumscribed central space, a configuration known as an ependymal rosette. Myxopapillary ependymomas have mucoid areas within the papillary structure and are found exclusively on the spinal cord at the cauda equina. Sometimes ependymomas are very anaplastic with features that resemble glioblastoma multiforme. Those lesions may have high mitotic activity, endothelial proliferation, and necrosis. In the WHO terminology, they are classified as anaplastic ependymomas, and in other systems as either anaplastic or malignant ependymomas (305).

A very highly cellular, embryonal form of ependymal tumor occurring in infants and children younger than age 5 years has been termed ependymoblastoma (184). This tumor is distinct from the other types of ependymomas just described, both biologically and pathologically. The ependymoblastoma often disseminates along the CSF pathways and requires irradiation of the craniospinal axis. Children with this tumor rarely live more than 2 to 3 years. Ependymoblastomas are most likely a form of primitive neuroectodermal tumor with ependymal differentiation and are treated in the same fashion as medulloblastoma. This variant of ependymoma should be regarded as distinct from malignant (anaplastic) ependymoma, in terms of treatment.

There are conflicting data concerning the prognostic implications of anaplasia in these tumors. Ross and Rubinstein reviewed a series of 15 patients classified as having anaplastic ependymomas (excluding cases of ependymoblastoma) in an attempt to correlate pathology with survival (236). In general, postoperative survival did not correlate with anaplastic histology. The median survival for 10 patients with malignant tumors was 8.8 years; 5 patients who had tumor recurrence died within 13 months to 6 years (median 2.5 years). Afra and colleagues reviewed 80 cases of supratentorial ependymoma with an overall 5-year survival of 34% (1). They classified these lesions into a low grade, an intermediate grade, or a highly anaplastic grade similar in appearance to glioblastoma. The 5-year survival rates were 41.5, 28.5, and 27.2%, respectively. Ernestus and colleagues, reviewing 128 cases of intracranial ependymoma, classified the tumors into grades I to IV: grade I was called subependymoma; grade II, a typical ependymoma; grade III, a malignant ependymoma; and grade IV, identical to glioblastoma (72). The 5-year survival rate without recurrence was 57.4% for patients with grade II but only 24.1% for those with grade III lesions. The mean survival was 83 months for the less malignant tumors and only 18 months for the more rapidly growing ependymomas.

CLINICAL PRESENTATION

Clinically, patients may present with subtle signs and symptoms for years before the diagnosis is made or may present abruptly with obstructive hydrocephalus or an expanding ependymoma of the spinal cord. Other focal findings include visual field defects, focal seizures, headache, or nausea and vomiting.

DIAGNOSTIC NEUROIMAGING

The neuroimaging of ependymomas is nonspecific, but some findings are useful to suggest the diagnosis, including calcification associated with a fourth ventricular tumor. Because many lesions may be confused with ependymomas, treatment should not proceed without histologic verification of the tumor and an assessment of the degree of anaplasia. The imaging studies and treatment for tumors of the spinal cord in general are covered more fully later.

TREATMENT

The goal of surgery for ependymoma should be removal of as much tumor as possible. Unfortunately, extensive resection is often impossible, particularly for lesions of the posterior fossa or for spinal cord ependymomas involving the cauda equina. Supratentorial lesions are more amenable to total resection, and every attempt should be made to accomplish gross removal.

In the series reported by Ernestus and colleagues, the addition of radiation therapy was particularly important in improving survival (72). In patients with grade II tumors treated with radiation, the median survival was 185 months. The benefit of postoperative irradiation was even more striking in patients who underwent only a partial resection: the median disease-free survival was 9 months in patients undergoing surgery only but was more than 108 months in those who received postoperative radiation therapy. Survival was only 21 months for those with grade III tumors, despite irradiation.

Other trials have documented the radiosensitivity of ependymomas. The literature does not identify, however, the optimal perimeters of the radiation field for treating ependymomas in specified locations or whether the craniospinal axis should always be included in the field. The risk of spinal subarachnoid metastasis is greatest with infratentorial anaplastic ependymomas (approximately 30%) and least likely with supratentorial typical ependymomas (5 to 10%). There is also a risk of intraventricular and intracranial spread from a malignant supratentorial lesion. For such reasons, the extent of the irradiated field is an important issue.

Salazar and colleagues reported a local control rate of 12% using small-volume fields, as compared to 78% control with whole-brain irradiation in a group of patients with low-grade ependymomas (241). The 5-year survival rate was 12% with partial-brain and 67% with whole-brain treatment. Sheline and colleagues showed similar results but a higher intracranial recurrence rate in patients receiving partial, as compared with whole-brain, irradiation, although all recurrences except one were in the original site (254). Read, however, comparing whole-brain to local-field irradiation, showed no difference in survival between the two groups (226). Because the primary site of recurrence of low-grade ependymomas is usually within the local radiation field, whole-brain irradiation for supratentorial ependymoma is not indicated. One rational approach to low-grade ependymomas would be to treat with local irradiation, provided that accurate staging procedures to assess the extent of disease are followed, including MRI of the spine as well as CSF cytology for infratentorial lesions.

In the case of an anaplastic or malignant ependymoma, irradiation of the entire craniospinal axis has been suggested by many groups. Salazar and colleagues reported a 47% survival rate at 5 years when craniospinal irradiation was given, as compared with only 8% survival for patients treated only with whole-brain irradiation (241). Other authors have not documented increased survival rates with craniospinal irradiation as compared with local treatment, and in most of those series, the site of tumor recurrence was most frequently in the immediate region of the original tumor (252). For these reasons, we believe anaplastic ependymomas should be staged carefully, including spinal MRI-Gd and CSF cytology examination, and the entire craniospinal axis should be irradiated if any evidence of disease distant from the primary site is detected. At UCSF, the dose directed to the tumor bed is 54 Gy, and 24 Gy is directed to the rest of the brain and spine if there is evidence of disseminated disease; boosts are given to known metastatic sites of disease. Even with this schema, most recurrences occupy the primary site. An alternative to this approach may be to increase the dose of radiation to the primary site, using hyperfractionation techniques. We are now investigating the use of craniospinal hyperfractionated radiation to a dose of 72 Gy directed to the primary site and 30 Gy to the rest of the craniospinal axis. In patients with malignant tumors showing such poor-risk features as positive cytology or disseminated disease, chemotherapy is added to this protocol, the current regimen including nitrosourea therapy with cisplatin.

Chemotherapy may be useful in treating recurrent ependymoma and perhaps as an adjuvant to radiation therapy in a newly diagnosed malignant ependymoma. These tumors are sensitive to several agents, including the nitrosoureas, the platinum compounds, procarbazine, and dibromodulcitol. In a UCSF trial involving recurrent ependymomas, the median time from initiation of therapy to tumor progression was 56 weeks for patients treated with dibromodulcitol and 67 weeks for those receiving carmustine (151). Carboplatin and cisplatin are also active agents that may be considered for use in patients who do not respond to treatment (85, 248). The role of adjuvant chemotherapy after radiation therapy in patients with primary malignant ependymomas has not been established; to date, the overall survival rates have been no better than those obtained with irradiation alone (32, 78). Certain subsets of patients may prove to be helped with chemotherapy, including those who have tumors with anaplastic features and less than a complete resection. The number of patients evaluated in prospective randomized studies is too small to permit conclusions concerning the role of adjuvant chemotherapy in the treatment of ependymoma.

Brainstem Glioma

EPIDEMIOLOGY

Brainstem gliomas account for 20% of childhood tumors and just short of 5% of adult tumors (50). They are seen most frequently in children between the ages of 3 and 10 years.

PATHOLOGY

Brainstem gliomas range from well-differentiated astrocytomas, including juvenile pilocytic astrocytomas, to anaplastic astrocytomas and glioblastoma multiforme (163). Neurosurgeons often do not biopsy a brainstem lesion when they judge that the risks of the procedure exceed the benefit of an exact diagnosis. Even with a biopsy specimen there is a risk of sampling error and underestimation of the grade of malignancy. In most series reported, 60 to 80% of patients do not have a histologic diagnosis, and the diagnosis of brainstem glioma is based only on clinical and radiographic findings (3).

CLINICAL PRESENTATION

The presenting neurologic findings and symptoms in patients with brainstem glioma follow one of two patterns. In one group, the insidious onset of symptoms may precede the diagnosis by as much as a year. In another group, an abrupt onset of signs and symptoms leads quickly to an evaluation. The duration of symptoms relates to outcome, the better survival rates accruing to the patients who have symptoms for a longer period before their diagnosis, because a rapid onset of symptoms and signs tends to relate to more rapidly growing tumors. Symptoms may include nausea, headache, speech and balance abnormalities, difficulty with swallowing, and weakness or numbness of the extremities. Signs include multiple cranial nerve palsies and cerebellar and long tract signs. Signs of increased intracranial pressure may occur in association with hydrocephalus from a tumor that compresses the fourth ventricle or aqueduct. Most patients, at some point in their clinical course, manifest cranial nerve palsies of the sixth and seventh nerves.

DIAGNOSTIC NEUROIMAGING

Brainstem gliomas are best evaluated by MRI-Gd (207). CT in many cases does not give the information necessary for evaluating the extent of the lesion and does not afford the spatial orientation provided by MRI. MRI can portray a diffuse lesion involving the pons and medulla, occasionally with extension down to the upper cervical cord or, less frequently, up into the thalamus. CT, in contrast, may miss these extensions because of a bone artifact at the base of the skull or may not be sensitive enough to visualize the true extent of tumor. Compression of the fourth ventricle may occur, as well as involvement of the parapontine cisterns, cerebellopontine angles, or the leptomeninges. Another characteristic appearance is that of more focal brainstem lesions, some with exophytic extension into the fourth ventricle or surrounding cisterns or extending inferiorly down to the cervicomedullary junction. Such lesions are more often found to be lower-grade astrocytomas, including juvenile pilocytic astrocytoma, and have a more favorable prognosis than other brainstem gliomas. The MRI appearance is that of a nonenhancing tumor, most commonly isointense or hypointense on T1-W images and hyperintense on T2-W images. Cystic areas may be present. Dissemination along the spinal axis is possible late in the course of the illness. Staging of the spine is not suggested at the time of the primary diagnosis.

SURGICAL DIAGNOSIS AND TREATMENT

Neuroimaging of brainstem lesions provides information sufficiently characteristic to make a diagnosis in most cases. The need for a histologic diagnosis might be questioned, especially because survival is determined more by location than by tumor grade. In the case of a diffuse, expansive pontine or pontomedullary tumor in a child who has had a rapid onset of symptoms, the outcome after therapy is at present the same, whatever of the tumor's histologic features. A biopsy sample actually may not reflect the histologic features of the most aggressive area of the lesion. Many brainstem lesions judged to be low-grade tumors based on a biopsy later prove to be anaplastic. In the case of a focal or exophytic lesion in the cervicomedullary junction, however, surgery may both establish the diagnosis and permit resection of some portion of the tumor. The outcome in such a case is better if the tumor is histologically verified as a low-grade lesion rather than an anaplastic glioma or a glioblastoma.

Epstein and Wisoff reviewed a series of 92 patients who underwent radical resection of a brainstem tumor, classifying the lesions as diffuse, focal, cystic (often with a mural nodule), exophytic (dorsal or posterolateral and anterolateral), and cervicomedullary (71). All patients had surgery with the goal of reduction of the tumor burden. All tumors that appeared as diffuse lesions on MRI were found to be histologically malignant. Two diffuse tumors were classified as grade II based on surgical findings, but at autopsy less than 1 month later both proved to be disseminated glioblastomas. All tumors that appeared as focal tumors based on MRI and clinical findings were found to be low-grade lesions. Tumors that appeared as focal lesions on CT, or as focal lesions on MRI with bilateral neurologic findings, were found to behave like a diffuse lesion. It proved possible to resect totally all cystic lesions in which the mural nodule enhanced on MRI-Gd and the cyst wall did not, whereas cyst walls that enhanced indicated more malignant potential. Cervicomedullary tumors were either low-grade astrocytomas or gangliogliomas in 80% of cases. Epstein and Wisoff concluded that surgical approaches should be guided by the appearance of the lesion on MRI as well as the clinical findings, and that surgery affords potential benefit in some cases of brainstem lesion (71). There appeared to be no survival benefit from attempted resection of diffuse lesions, or even of focal pontine lesions that showed bilateral neurologic findings.

RADIATION THERAPY, CHEMOTHERAPY, AND OTHER MODALITIES

Treatment options other than surgery for brainstem gliomas include irradiation and chemotherapy. The overall prognosis for the diffuse malignant tumor is poor, despite treatment (2, 25). Radiation therapy is the treatment of choice, and adjuvant chemotherapy appears to offer no benefit. The overall 5-year survival after irradiation is 20 to 30%, and prognosis relates to the duration of symptoms and the MRI appearance of the lesion. For patients with rapid onset of symptoms whose brainstem glioma appears as a diffuse lesion on MRI, the projected median survival is a year or less. Efforts to improve on these poor survival rates, including adjuvant multiagent chemotherapy, have provided no advantage (152).

One additional strategy in the treatment of brainstem gliomas is the use of hyperfractionated radiation therapy with treatments given twice a day. On such a schedule, higher total doses can be delivered. Treatment regimens using doses from 66 to 72 Gy, and more recently doses of 78 Gy, have now been evaluated (65, 82, 202, 222). Although the results are preliminary, it appears that these hyperfractionated higher doses are tolerable in terms of the associated radiation injury. It is uncertain if survival can be improved in certain groups of patients. Unfortunately, children with diffuse pontomedullary brainstem gliomas with a short clinical history often fail treatment within the first year after diagnosis, even with these higher doses of radiation.

One trial evaluating the use of interferon in children who had failed primary radiation therapy produced some objective responders, suggesting a possible role for this biologic agent (4). To date, nitrosourea-based regimens have not prolonged survival or achieved any beneficial response once a tumor has recurred. In a more recent study, high-dose chemotherapy with ABMT was used for recurrent tumors, with a plan to use the technique at the time of primary diagnosis as well (77). Preliminary data from these studies show no benefit with higher doses of chemotherapy thus far. Clearly, new treatment strategies are needed for these tumors.

Spinal Cord Tumors

ETIOLOGY AND EPIDEMIOLOGY

The most common spinal tumor is an extradural metastasis from another primary site. The most common primary spinal tumor is a spinal intradural lesion, either extramedullary or intramedullary. Primary spinal cord tumors constitute 10 to 15% of all primary CNS lesions (127). The spectrum of lesions in the adult population differs from that in the pediatric age groups. In children, the most common location of the spinal lesion is intramedullary and the most frequent tumor is an astrocytoma (224). In adults, extramedullary intradural tumors are more common, and the most common are neurofibromas and meningiomas. The most frequent intramedullary tumors in adults are ependymomas and astrocytomas. In unusual cases, adult ependymomas and astrocytomas may be exophytic and extramedullary.

CLINICAL PRESENTATION

Clinical symptoms of spinal cord lesions include pain, motor and sensory disturbances, and bowel, bladder, and sexual dysfunction. Extramedullary tumors grow in relation to nerve roots and produce radicular pain that frequently is worse at night and is aggravated by maneuvers that increase the intracranial pressure, such as straining or coughing. Intramedullary lesions frequently do not present with pain as the initial symptom but rather produce signs of central cord destruction, including reduced sensation to pain and extreme temperatures, long-tract signs, weakness, bowel and bladder incontinence, and sexual dysfunction. Ependymomas are frequently situated at the cauda equina and produce sphincter weakness and peripheral lower-extremity weakness.

DIAGNOSTIC NEUROIMAGING

MRI is rapidly becoming the radiographic technique of choice in the evaluation of spinal cord tumors, particularly since Gd became available several years ago. The ability of MRI to depict the extent of the lesion and its specific location in relation to other structures, as well as its definition of cysts associated with tumors, make it preferable to other techniques. MRI permits an accurate prediction of the histology of the lesion in many cases; for instance, astrocytomas often show heterogeneous enhancement in an asymmetric fashion, whereas ependymomas frequently enhance uniformly with smooth edges (246, 277, 302). Tumor nodules associated with cysts are easily visualized, providing valuable information for surgical planning. Indeed, the extent of cysts above or below the lesion defines the level of the laminectomy and the extent of exposure needed. In order to eliminate artifacts caused by cardiac pulsations, respiration, and CSF flow, cardiac gating and other flow-compensatory mechanisms are used. For young children, sedation is often required because the acquisition of data requires that they remain motionless for a long time.

SURGICAL DIAGNOSIS AND TREATMENT

The goal of surgery for spinal cord lesions is to remove tumor as well as to make a diagnosis. In the case of an ependymoma, meningioma, and neurofibroma, total removal is the treatment of choice. For an astrocytoma, especially a diffuse lesion occupying large areas of the spinal cord, only a biopsy and partial removal can be accomplished, although recently, some surgeons have emphasized a more aggressive approach to total removal, even with astrocytomas. Epstein, reviewing his surgical experience with 152 children with spinal cord astrocytomas, divided the lesions from a neurodiagnostic standpoint into two groups: holocord astrocytomas and focal astrocytomas (70). The holocord astrocytoma was a solid lesion surrounded by a cystic component that expanded the cord caudally and rostrally and extended the entire length of the spinal cord. The focal astrocytoma usually occupied 4 to 8 segments of the cord, often causing total blockage of the spinal subarachnoid space. Surgery was directed at the solid component of the lesion, with drainage of the cystic components. The tumor was removed, starting from the center of the lesion, using an ultrasonic dissector and a carbon dioxide laser and dissecting outward until a tumor-glia interface was encountered. Physiologic monitoring was obtained by measuring evoked potentials. Postoperatively, transient increases in weakness or sensory loss were common but resolved quickly, and only one patient in this series had a significant increase in neurologic deficit. Other reports have shown that, in some cases even a diffuse infiltrative astrocytoma of the spinal cord can be totally removed (268). There now appears to be an increasingly widespread enthusiasm for pursuing more extensive surgical resection of intramedullary astrocytomas.

More frequently than for spinal astrocytomas, spinal ependymomas can be approached with the intention of complete surgical removal. Complete removal is potentially curative with no need for further therapy. Cooper reviewed the results obtained in 51 adults with a variety of intramedullary tumors who were treated with radical surgical resection (51). In this series, of the 24 patients with ependymoma, only two died (one a suicide, one from a progressive tumor). In comparison, 12 of 18 patients with astrocytomas died. All patients with ependymoma who had residual tumor after surgery were treated with radiation therapy, as were all patients with an astrocytoma. The extent of surgery was considered important to outcome in the case of ependymomas, as only 1 of the 11 patients believed to have had total removal had a recurrence whereas tumor recurred in 5 of the 13 patients who had had incomplete resection. All of the patients with high-grade anaplastic astrocytomas eventually died of their tumor.

Radiation Therapy and Chemotherapy

Linstadt and colleagues reviewed the results of 42 patients with primary spinal cord tumors treated at UCSF with radiation therapy: 21 patients had ependymoma, 12 had low-grade astrocytoma, 3 had anaplastic astrocytoma, and 6 had tumors of uncertain histology (162). The radiation dose was in the range of 45 to 54.7 Gy. The projected actuarial 10-year disease-free survival for patients with localized ependymomas was 93%. Three patients had ependymoma diffusely involving the cord, one of whom died from a cerebral metastasis. The other two are alive and disease free. The corresponding 10-year survival rate for the 12 patients with low-grade astrocytoma was 91%, and no patient who had an anaplastic astrocytoma survived longer than 8 months. In both the ependymoma and low-grade astrocytoma groups, most patients who had a treatment failure had tumor regrowth in the original site of disease. One patient developed radiation myelitis following irradiation to a total dose of 50.4 Gy.

It is difficult to save a patient who has an anaplastic astrocytoma of the spinal cord. Most patients die of this disease despite extensive surgical resections and irradiation to the limit of cord tolerance. Other approaches to these lesions are needed. Chemotherapy only delays the inevitable. Various combinations of chemotherapy, primarily nitrosourea-based, have produced no long-term survivors, and other agents, including platinum compounds, thiotepa, and cyclophosphamide, have had only limited and transient benefit. No studies of spinal anaplastic astrocytoma have evaluated hyperfractionated irradiation or radiosensitizers. These might increase the therapeutic index of radiation therapy, which is the most beneficial form of treatment. Therapeutic attempts involving high-dose chemotherapy with ABMT, just beginning in the United States, may provide further insight into the potential for treatment of these refractory tumors.

RECURRENCE

The recurrent spinal cord ependymoma is more amenable to therapy, including repeat surgical resections, reirradiation using hyperfractionated techniques (especially for lesions of the conus), and chemotherapy with the nitrosoureas or platinum agents. When an ependymoma recurs in the spinal cord, we routinely scan the entire neuraxis to be certain of the extent of the disease, because occasionally even a histologically benign ependymoma disseminates. Using sequential therapies, it is possible to control this lesion for years.

Primary Central Nervous System Lymphoma

Primary CNS lymphoma accounts for less than 1% of all lymphomas not related to Hodgkin's disease and for less than 1% of all primary brain tumors. Termed non-Hodgkin's lymphoma of the CNS (NHL-CNS), this rare cancer has increased in incidence during the past several decades. While the acquired immunodeficiency syndrome (AIDS) epidemic has added substantially to this increased incidence, it cannot be attributed to AIDS alone. According to Eby and colleagues, the incidence of NHL-CNS increased from 2.7 cases per 10 million to 7.5 per 10 million population during the years between 1973 to 1975 and 1982 to 1984 (64). This increase, which antedated the AIDS epidemic, comprised younger as well as older populations and men as well as women. Other than lesions caused by immunocompromise of recognized forms, the reason for the change is uncertain. Among patients with AIDS, NHL-CNS has been reported in 1.9 to 2.6% (160). It is estimated that, with the increasing numbers of patients with AIDS, more than 1,800 new cases of NHL-CNS may be diagnosed in the United States in 1991 (232). This incidence would exceed that of newly diagnosed low-grade astrocytomas and approximate the numbers of newly diagnosed meningiomas.

ETIOLOGY AND EPIDEMIOLOGY

Patients at risk for NHL-CNS include immunocompromised patients and organ transplant recipients. In the AIDS population, there is some evidence that the Epstein-Barr virus (EBV) may be implicated in the development of this lesion. Most patients with NHL-CNS have elevated EBV antibodies. Studying NHL-CNS tissue with in situ hybridization techniques, Bashir and colleagues documented EBV sequences in four patients with immunodeficiency (19). Four other cases of NHL-CNS not associated with immunodeficiency did not show these same sequences. In a similar review from UCSF by Baumgartner and colleagues, all cases of AIDS-related NHL-CNS studied were positive for EBV sequences (22). Also supporting this link is the observation that, among people not in the AIDS population who have the X-linked lymphoproliferative syndrome (Duncan's syndrome), EBV-related disease is common, as is the development of NHL-CNS (211). The association of this virus with NHL-CNS is speculative but, if proven, potential interventions with antiviral agents might be helpful in its treatment. Other syndromes associated with a high incidence of NHL-CNS include Wiskott-Aldrich syndrome and severe combined immunodeficiency syndrome (SCID). Cases of NHL-CNS have also been described in association with sarcoidosis, rheumatoid arthritis, systemic lupus erythematosus, and the vasculitic syndromes. Organ transplant patients, especially those awaiting renal or cardiac transplants, account for as many as 30% of cases of NHL-CNS (105).

Most cases of NHL-CNS are not associated with any known risk factor, however, and patients are not immunosuppressed. The etiology of this illness is clearly multifactorial and at present is ill understood.

PATHOLOGY

The pathology of NHL-CNS resembles that of systemic NHL. The tumors are most commonly large-cell immunoblastic lymphomas, as classified according to the International Working Formulation (197). Small cleaved-cell lymphoma and large noncleaved-cell lymphoma are the next most common cell types, but others have been described as well. There may be some correlation between the tumor's histology and the prognosis for survival, longer survival being associated with the small cleaved- and noncleaved-cell lymphoma types (33). However, survival depends on many factors, including the patient's age and the type of therapy, and the association of tumor type to survival may change over time.

Histologically, the lesions are often diffusely infiltrative and advance along perivascular spaces, invading blood vessel walls. There are no nodular or follicular patterns. Most NHL-CNS tumors are of B-cell origin, although rare cases of T-cell NHL-CNS have been described (176).

CLINICAL PRESENTATION

Patients with AIDS-related NHL-CNS most often present with confusion, memory loss, focal neurologic deficits, seizures, and lethargy. Most patients with AIDS have other concurrent manifestations of AIDS, including systemic infections and other CNS pathology. In 10 to 15% of cases NHL-CNS is the first presentation of AIDS, and any patient with NHL-CNS should be evaluated for HIV infection. The usual age range in this population is 35 to 40 years. The most common CNS mass lesion seen in AIDS patients is toxoplasmosis, NHL-CNS being the second most common (233). These two illnesses may coexist in more than 10% of cases and are difficult to distinguish radiographically. Frequently, the diagnosis of NHL-CNS in patients with AIDS is made after treatment of CNS toxoplasmosis has failed (233).

For patients with NHL-CNS who do not have AIDS, the clinical presentation differs somewhat and the patients are, on the average, older at presentation (median age, 55 years). The clinical findings include headache, focal weakness, and personality changes. There may be visual findings as well as cerebellar findings, depending on the location of the tumor. Occasionally, such patients present with clinical features of dementia or encephalitis.

DIAGNOSTIC NEUROIMAGING

Neuroimaging studies in the AIDS population often reveal multiple contrast-enhancing lesions, but as many as 35% may be unifocal (263). Spinal cord dissemination of NHL-CNS has not been described frequently in AIDS, nor has the presence of leptomeningeal disease or positive CSF cytology. Among patients with NHL-CNS who do not have AIDS, lesions are frequently multifocal, CSF is positive in as many as 10%, and involvement of the vitreous occurs in 10 to 20%. The appearance on MRI is that of an isointense central area on T1-W images, with hyperintense regions on T2-W images. The tumor often enhances on MRI-Gd. CT scans reveal a hypointense lesion that enhances with contrast. NHL-CNS has a predilection for involvement of the basal ganglia, thalami, corpus callosum, the periventricular system, and the vermis of the cerebellum. None of these findings is pathognomonic, however, and the diagnosis must be verified by biopsy.

SURGICAL DIAGNOSIS AND TREATMENT

The role of surgery is to make a diagnosis, usually by means of a stereotactic biopsy or craniotomy with sampling of the tumor. No survival advantage has been observed from attempts to totally resect the lesions (194). In AIDS patients, because of the chance that multiple neuropathologic processes may be present, a negative biopsy evaluation for lymphoma should not exclude this diagnosis, especially if multiple lesions are present. If they are clinically suspicious, several lesions may need to be sampled.

Radiation Therapy

The treatment of choice in patients with AIDS-related NHL-CNS is radiation therapy. Whole-brain irradiation to 40 Gy over a period of 3 weeks provides good control of the tumor. Survival data from the NHL-CNS series treated at UCSF reveal a median survival of 134 days if radiation was used, but only 42 days in patients treated solely with surgery; patients with AIDS NHL-CNS frequently die of other manifestations of AIDS rather than of the lymphoma (22). Neuroimaging after irradiation documented a complete or partial response in 70% of AIDS patients treated for NHL-CNS and stable disease in another 22%. Formenti and colleagues treated 10 patients with various doses of radiation, obtaining a median survival of 5.5 months overall (80). Patients receiving a higher dose of radiation (to 50 Gy) survived more than 12 months. The longest survivals in both series were in patients who also received chemotherapy.

For patients without AIDS, radiation therapy is also a very effective modality. High response rates are achievable using whole-brain irradiation. The RTOG treated patients using whole-brain irradiation to a dose of 54 Gy, obtaining a median survival of 7.5 months in patients over 60 years old and a median of 32 months in younger patients. Hochberg and Miller, treating 44 patients with 50 to 60 Gy to the whole brain, achieved a 79% complete-plus-partial response rate and a median survival of 21.5 months in the patients who could be evaluated (106).

Regardless of AIDS, a cure is rarely achieved in patients with NHL-CNS, and survival is particularly poor for older patients. Systemic spread of the disease occurs in as many as 10% of patients, and a higher percentage have dissemination within the CNS.

Chemotherapy

In an attempt to improve overall survival, systemic chemotherapy has been used, either adjuvantly or primarily, in patients with NHL-CNS who do not have AIDS. Combination therapy using standard lymphoma regimens has proved effective in achieving objective responses with a variety of agents, including the nitrosoureas, methotrexate, doxorubicin, cyclophosphamide, vincristine, cytosine arabinoside, and procarbazine (56, 89, 178, 215). At UCSF, we have treated patients after surgery with a combination of irradiation and chemotherapy using the combined PCV regimen of procarbazine, lomustine (CCNU), and vincristine in the same schedule used for malignant gliomas. Median survival has been in the range of 30 months. Other groups have used adjuvant therapies such as the CHOP regimen (consisting of cyclophosphamide, doxorubicin [hydroxydaunomycin], vincristine [Oncovin], and prednisone), the M-BACOP regimen (consisting of methotrexate/citrovorum factor-bleomycin, doxorubicin [Adriamycin], cyclophosphamide, vincristine, and prednisone), or single-agent high-dose methotrexate. When chemotherapy is used as the only therapy given at tumor recurrence, patients may in some cases remain in remission for years and often have a complete response. In view of these responses to chemotherapy alone, these drugs have been used before and/or after radiation therapy. One current regimen is to administer CHOP together with high-dose methotrexate for three cycles before whole-brain irradiation to 45 Gy with a boost to 60 Gy to tumor areas. A regimen used at Memorial Sloan-Kettering Cancer Center, reported by DeAngelis and colleagues, includes high-dose systemic methotrexate as well as intrathecal methotrexate given before, and high-dose AraC given after, radiation therapy (56). A recent update of this study revealed a median time to recurrence of 41 months in the 31 patients who completed therapy (57). Unfortunately, there have been no randomized trials to compare the results of chemotherapy and irradiation with those obtained using radiation therapy alone. Because of the rarity of NHL-CNS and the different schedules and treatment regimens being evaluated, it is difficult to establish what may be the most effective strategy against the tumor. The current RTOG study is a single-arm phase II study for treating patients with non–AIDS-related NHL of the CNS using preradiotherapy chemotherapy (high-dose methotrexate, vincristine, procarbazine, and intra-Ommaya methotrexate), followed by whole-brain radiotherapy (45 Gy with no boost to known disease), and postradiotherapy cytosine arabinoside (ara-C). This study just opened groupwide, and no results are available at this time.

In cases of AIDS-related NHL-CNS, several investigators have included chemotherapy with irradiation. Despite the fear that chemotherapy in AIDS patients may cause the underlying disease process to progress more rapidly or may produce many infectious complications, some patients have completed complicated combination chemotherapy regimens successfully. Systemic chemotherapy has been used in only a small number of cases of AIDS-related NHL-CNS. Three of the patients with the longest survival in the UCSF series just mentioned had received high-dose methotrexate, and the one with the longest survival from the series reported by Formenti and colleagues had received the BACOD regimen (consisting of bleomycin, Adriamycin, Cytoxan, Oncovin, dexamethasone) (80). It may be possible to use systemic chemotherapy even in AIDS patients, if screening includes such careful selection criteria as admission only of patients who have no other manifestation of AIDS or those who have high CD4 lymphocyte counts.

Medulloblastoma and Primitive Neuroectodermal Tumors

ETIOLOGY AND EPIDEMIOLOGY

Medulloblastoma, the most common primary malignant intracranial tumor of childhood, is not common in adults. The lesion accounts for more than 30% of all posterior fossa tumors, and approximately 250 new cases are diagnosed each year in the United States. More than 80% of medulloblastomas are diagnosed in children during the first 15 years of life, the median age at diagnosis being 5 years. Medulloblastomas arise from the midline cerebellum, but histologically similar lesions may occur in the cerebral hemispheres and the pineal region.

PATHOLOGY

There is controversy about the proper nomenclature to assign to several histologically similar tumors that occur within the cerebellum, cerebrum, and pineal region, among them primitive neuroectodermal tumor and medulloblastoma (229). For lack of a conclusive histogenesis, proposals to explain these lesions range from one speculating a single primitive cell of origin that exhibits different degrees of differentiation along astrocytic, oligodendroglial, ependymal, neuronal, melanocytic, and mesenchymal cell lines, to one at the opposite extreme describing a previously mature tumor that undergoes neoplastic "dedifferentiation" to a primitive state. Pending resolution of the debate, some pathologists and clinicians use the terms primitive neuroectodermal tumor and medulloblastoma interchangeably (PNET/MB). In fact, these tumors do have features in common and they share similar biologic properties, including the ability to disseminate throughout the nervous system and, in some cases, systemically. Until the nosology is resolved, we prefer to restrict the use of the term medulloblastoma to the characteristic lesion seen in the cerebellum and to use the term primitive neuroectodermal tumor for similar lesions found elsewhere in the CNS. Because, however, the treatment and biology of these lesions are similar, both terms are used collectively as PNET/MB for the rest of this section.

Histologically, about half of these tumors have recognizable cell lines combined with undifferentiated components. A relation between prognosis and the degree of cellular differentiation has been proposed, but while some reports suggest that the more undifferentiated tumors are associated with a better outcome than those with predominant differentiation along astrocytic lines, others suggest that differentiation imparts a better prognosis (40, 206). Clearly, there is no consensus concerning prognosis as it relates to histology. Cytogenic studies show frequent karyotypic abnormalities, both numerical and structural, most often involving chromosomes 1, 6, and 17 (98). Recent work suggests that the lesion on chromosome 17 represents a deletion resulting from a loss of heterozygosity and may play a role in the control of oncogene expression (49). The area on 17 is in the same region as a known tumor suppressor gene, p53. Conceivably, mutations in this area may be responsible for the development of PNET/MB; however, this early work must be confirmed.

Dissemination exists in as many as 30% of patients at the time of primary diagnosis (47, 58). Disease may exist outside the primary site as nodular lesions anywhere within the neuraxis, including the spine and supratentorial fossa, or it may involve the CSF as indicated by positive cytology results. Occasionally, there may be disease beyond the CNS at the time of the original diagnosis, most often in the bone and/or soft tissue structures, including the lymph nodes. The prognosis is directly related to the presence and extent of disease beyond the primary tumor site.

CLINICAL PRESENTATION

Most PNET/MB lesions arise from the posterior fossa in children younger than age 5 years (200). Frequently, the tumor produces hydrocephalus and symptoms of increased intracranial pressure, including nausea, emesis, headache, diplopia, and unsteadiness. Papilledema is often found on examination. In infants less than 1 year old, increasing lethargy and enlarging head circumference are seen, together with developmental delays.

DIAGNOSTIC NEUROIMAGING

Neroimaging reveals a contrast-enhancing lesion in the cerebellum (115, 200). The CT appearance is that of a hypointense or isointense lesion that enhances homogeneously. MRI shows low signal intensity on T1-W images and high signal intensity on T2-W images; Gd produces enhancement. Because of the extent of PNET/MB lesions and their relation to adjacent structures, MRI-Gd is the neuroimaging technique of choice.

STAGING

Postoperative staging, assessment of the extent of disease, is required to treat PNET/MB properly. It should include an evaluation of the entire craniospinal axis using MRI-Gd of the brain and spinal cord, as well as a CSF sample obtained by lumbar puncture to assess the presence of malignant cells in the spinal CSF. The presence of any disease outside the primary site of the lesion adversely influences survival. In a large series reported from the Children's Cancer Group (CCG) and the International Society for Pediatric Oncology (SIOP), the risk of a poor outcome is determined by the extent of disease (6, 47, 58). In the CCG trials, 58% of children without dissemination, as opposed to only 32% of those with metastatic disease, survived disease-free at 54 months.

The timing of staging is somewhat controversial. At most centers, including our own, spinal staging is done approximately 2 weeks after surgery, to obviate misleading results caused by PNET/MB cells remaining in the CSF; it seems probable that many are nonclonogenic cells dispersed during resection. Blood within the CSF or spinal canal may produce filling defects or abnormal enhancement on myelography and MRI of the spine. Although such contamination should be resolved by 2 weeks postoperatively, both noncontrast and contrast MRI should be done during this evaluation to maximize the likelihood of distinguishing true tumor from postoperative artifact. If the first CSF cytology shows malignant tumor cells, then another examination should be performed 1 week later. If the results are still positive, they most likely represent true dissemination. If the results of the second examination are negative, then the initial result can be considered a false-positive finding.

Other prognostic variables include the patient's age and the extent of surgical resection. Young children (those under 4 years of age) tend to have a worse outcome than older ones, in some part because younger children often have disseminated disease and infants cannot be treated as aggressively with radiation therapy owing to the morbidity high-dose irradiation causes to the developing nervous system.

The size of the tumor has also been considered important, regardless of the extent to which it is resected. According to a staging system developed by Chang and colleagues, tumors are classified according to size at the time of surgery: tumors classified as T1 or T2 lesions were less than 3 cm in diameter and did not fill the fourth ventricle completely; larger tumors, T3 or T4 lesions, filled the fourth ventricle and caused hydrocephalus (T3a lesions) or invaded the brainstem (T3b lesions) or the upper cervical cord (T4 lesions) (44). Larger lesions were considered to have a worse prognosis, but significantly so only when they were associated with dissemination, according to the CCG and SIOP trials (6, 47, 58). The impact of surgical resection on outcome, as related to tumor size, has not been fully appreciated. It would seem that even a patient with a large lesion that is totally or almost completely removed would do as well as one treated similarly who had a smaller lesion at diagnosis, assuming that there was no evidence of dissemination. In fact, the most recent study from the CCSG seems to suggest that the size of the lesion alone has no impact on survival (73). The strongest predictors of a poor outcome are the presence of dissemination and young age. Current clinical trials of the CCG and Pediatric Oncology Group (POG) no longer use preoperative or intraoperative staging to assign risk status. Rather, the extent of residual disease is assessed using postoperative MRI. If residual tumor is larger than 1.5 cm^3, the patient is felt to represent a poor-risk status and is treated accordingly.

SURGICAL DIAGNOSIS AND TREATMENT

The goal of surgery for PNET/MB is to remove all visible tumor. Survival rates as high as 80% at 5 years after surgery have been reported following total removal, as compared to rates of 40 to 50% in patients who have only subtotal removal

(278). Patients undergoing biopsy only are unlikely to survive, even if they receive appropriate radiation therapy (278). Other studies have not documented increased survival rates after total, as opposed to subtotal, resection but showed significantly similar survival rates in both cases (73). In some trials, the documented extent of resection may have been underestimated or overestimated because it was based on the operative report and not on postoperative imaging studies (58, 199). Conversely, some residual disease may not be detected with postoperative imaging, including small-volume residual tumor that may extend into the brainstem. Thus, even postoperative imaging may not show the extent of resection completely accurately. There appears to be consensus, however, that total removal, whenever possible, is the goal of surgical therapy.

Some controversy also remains regarding hydrocephalus, whether resection should be performed before or after a shunting procedure. The proponents of immediate surgery without shunting argue that a significant number of children do not require permanent shunting after resection and that surgery eliminates the risk of intraperitoneal spread of tumor by way of the shunt. Immediate surgery also lessens the risk of upward herniation, obviating a second procedure under anesthesia. Proponents of primary shunting suggest that the subsequent surgery is easier because the brain is relaxed, resulting in less distortion of the posterior fossa, thus permitting more complete resection. At UCSF, we favor an immediate surgical approach with the goal of total removal.

Radiation Therapy

Radiation therapy is the basis of curative treatment. Before the introduction of craniospinal axis irradiation, few patients survived 5 years after a diagnosis of PNET/MB. Landberg and colleagues reported a 10-year survival rate of 5% for patients irradiated to the posterior fossa alone, as compared with 53% when irradiation of the craniospinal axis was used (137). Other reports have verified the improved survival obtained with this approach, and currently all patients diagnosed with PNET/MB are treated with irradiation of the craniospinal axis (6, 47, 58).

The most common sites for recurrence are the original tumor site and spinal cord metastasis. Control rates are higher, and the risk of dissemination is less when a dose of 50 Gy or more is delivered to the posterior fossa. Therapy with less than 50 Gy is associated with higher local failure rates, more spinal cord metastases, and reduced survival. The question of the optimal dose to the craniospinal axis has not been completely resolved, as some uncertainty remains about the most effective dose in clinically uninvolved areas of the CNS.

Because most patients with this disease are children, concern about the delayed effects of radiation has prompted speculation about lowering the dose to the brain and spine. Late effects include hormone abnormalities such as reduced growth hormone levels, cognitive defects such as lowered IQ score with learning disabilities, and spinal abnormalities such as reduced vertebral body height, shortened stature, and kyphoscoliosis. Standard radiation doses to the craniospinal axis have included 35 to 45 Gy to the brain and 30 to 40 Gy to the spine. Recently, several groups have reported survival outcomes similar to those in the CCG and SIOP trials with irradiation in lowered doses to the craniospinal axis (6, 47, 58). At UCSF, patients considered good-risk candidates were treated with 54 Gy to the posterior fossa and 24 to 30 Gy to the rest of the craniospinal axis (156). Their survival rate at 5 years was 66%, which is comparable to survival rates from the CCG and SIOP trials; most recurrences were in the posterior fossa (6, 47, 58). Tomita and McLone also reported good survival rates when patients were treated with 25 Gy to the craniospinal axis; most of their patients had had total surgical removal of tumor (278). Despite good local control rates, however, as many as 30 to 40% of patients have recurrence, either within or outside the CNS. A recently closed study of the CCG and POG randomized children with good-risk features to receive either 24 or 36 Gy to the cranioaxis, with a standard dose of 54 Gy to the posterior fossa. This study was closed prior to full accrual because of the excess number of failures in the spine in the group treated with the lower spine dose. The impact of the excessive spine metastases on survival is not known for the entire group at this time, but the concern of reducing overall survival prompted the early closure of this study. A new study by the CCG and POG has now opened that randomizes children with good-risk features into two groups. The control group is treated with conventional radiotherapy to a dose of 54 Gy to the posterior fossa and 36 Gy to the cranioaxis. The experimental group is treated with the same posterior fossa dose, but a lower dose of 24 Gy to the cranioaxis is given. In this study, however, the patients treated with lower cranioaxis radiotherapy are also treated with adjuvant chemotherapy, in the hope that chemotherapy will reduce the risk of spine relapse (or other relapse) in the lower-dose radiotherapy-treated group.

Chemotherapy and Multimodality Therapy

In an attempt to increase survival rates, adjuvant chemotherapy has been used, with variable success, in some groups of patients. In two large trials conducted by the CCG and the SIOP, patients were randomized to receive radiation therapy, either alone or with adjuvant chemotherapy (6, 73). In the CCG trial, lomustine, vincristine, and prednisone were used; the SIOP study omitted prednisone but was otherwise similar (6, 73). A marginal benefit was suggested overall in the group receiving chemotherapy but was significant only in patients with larger tumors and with metastatic disease (CSG and SIOP trials) or in those with brainstem invasion (SIOP trial only).

Overall, there is no survival advantage when chemotherapy is added to radiation therapy for patients with a newly diagnosed PNET/MB, but for certain subsets of patients there is clearly an advantage. A recent updated report of the SIOP trial revealed 45% overall survival at 10 years, documenting patients who had a relapse after 5 years (276). This result reaffirms the benefit of adjuvant chemotherapy in patients who have had either partial tumor removal only or brainstem involvement and disease at stage T3 or T4. In the CCG study, patients with relatively large tumors who also had evidence of dissemination had a clear survival advantage if they received adjuvant chemotherapy (73). Survival at 5 years in patients who had advanced tumors (T3, T4) with dissemination was 46% after irradiation and chemotherapy but 0% after radiation therapy alone. Conversely, in a group of 124 patients with T3 or T4 tumors without evidence of dissemination, the 5-year disease-free survival was 61% after combined therapy and 51% after irradiation alone, a statistically insignificant difference (73). It appears from this large randomized trial that chemotherapy is primarily beneficial in the case of metastatic disease and that the extent of surgical resection does not confer a survival advantage between patients with total removal and those with partial removal. Children younger than 4 years of age did less well, having a 5-year survival rate of only 32%. Other ongoing studies are evaluating a variety of agents, including a combination of lomustine, cisplatin, and vincristine.

RECURRENCE

In the CCG trial and other studies of PNET/MB, there remains a high rate of local recurrence (73). Attempts to improve on those rates now focus on increasing the dose of radiation using hyperfractionation techniques, a strategy that proved to be successful in the treatment of brainstem gliomas. Several studies have used hyperfractionated irradiation to doses of 72 Gy to the posterior fossa as well as hyperfractionated irradiation of the craniospinal axis. These trials began treating patients in the early 1990s, and the final results will not be fully analyzed for several more years. At UCSF, good-risk patients were treated with radiation only, using hyperfractionation to 72 Gy to the posterior fossa and 30 Gy to the rest of the craniospinal axis. When poor-risk factors were found, adjuvant chemotherapy was added to this regimen. Preliminary data suggest that the regimens are tolerable with minimal risk of radionecrosis seen thus far (221). Higher doses are given to the cranioaxis in other institutional studies, also recently completed (4). Because of this favorable toxicity experience, a new study by the CCG has recently begun to treat children with high-risk disease using neoadjuvant chemotherapy followed by cranioaxis hyperfractionated radiotherapy. In this new study, the dose to be delivered to the posterior fossa is 72 Gy and the rest of the neuroaxis is treated with 44 Gy. Results of this study are not available at this time.

It is difficult to save patients with PNET/MB once they have failed initial therapies; however, if they have not had chemotherapy previously, there is a role for it. The most active agents against recurrent PNET/MB include the nitrosoureas, cyclophosphamide, melphalan, thiotepa, vincristine, procarbazine, cisplatin, and carboplatin (83). Combination therapy with lomustine, cisplatin, and vincristine is also being evaluated (203); others include the MOPP regimen (consisting of Mustargen, Oncovin, procarbazine, and prednisone) as used for the treatment of Hodgkin's disease (282), PCV therapy similar to that used for malignant gliomas(158), and a regimen called 8 in 1, in which eight drugs are delivered over a 24-hour period (212). Unfortunately, even if the patient's initial response is good, long-term control is unlikely. In the CCSG trial described earlier, patients who were therapeutic failures of irradiation and adjuvant chemotherapy had a median survival after recurrence of only 3.9 months (73). Patients who had undergone only irradiation could be salvaged for a median of 10.4 months. There are several options other than chemotherapy alone, such as repeat irradiation using hyperfractionation therapy combined with combination chemotherapy, and more recently the use of high-dose chemotherapy with ABMT.

We strongly recommend that patients with PNET/MB be referred to regional institutions for entry into clinical research trials, both at the time of original diagnosis and at the time of tumor recurrence.

Other Primary Tumors of the Central Nervous System

PRIMARY GERM-CELL TUMORS

Etiology and Epidemiology

Primary intracranial germ-cell tumors are a rare group of diverse tumors that account for less than 5% of childhood tumors and less than 1% of adult tumors. In the United States, fewer than 50 cases are diagnosed each year (245). Most germ-cell tumors occur during the second and third decades of life. For unknown reasons, their incidence is higher in Japan (123). The most common histologic type is germinoma, believed to be the most primitive form, and the spectrum of other tumors includes embryonal carcinoma, choriocarcinoma, endodermal sinus tumor, and malignant or immature teratoma (121). In general, these lesions are grouped together as either germinoma or nongerminoma because the former are very radiation-sensitive and the latter are not. Except for the benign teratoma, all germ-cell tumors are malignant neoplasms with the potential to disseminate throughout the neuraxis.

Pathology

Intracranial germ-cell tumors are histologically identical to gonadal germ-cell tumors, the only difference in terminology being that the term germinoma is used for the same tumor as a seminoma of the testis or dysgerminoma of the ovary. The germ-cell tumor may be a mixture of several elements or may exhibit only one element. It has been suggested that germ-cell tumors arise from developmental nests of primitive germ cells in midline structures, including the pineal and suprasellar regions of the brain (124). Germinoma accounts for 65% of CNS germ-cell tumors; teratoma is the next most frequent at 18%; and choriocarcinoma is the rarest. Embryonal carcinoma and endodermal sinus tumors are intermediate in frequency. Germinomas consist of two cell populations: large round cells and a lymphocytic infiltrate. In rare cases, syncytiotrophoblasts may be present that stain positively for β-human chorionic gonadotrophin (β-HCG). Germinoma also stains positively for alkaline phosphatase. The nongerminomas, including teratomas, usually have mixtures of many cellular elements. Immunoperoxidase staining reveals β-HCG and/or α-fetoprotein in embryonal carcinoma and choriocarcinoma, as well as in endodermal sinus tumors (123).

Two thirds of the germ-cell tumors in the pineal region occur in male patients, whereas two thirds of suprasellar tumors affect females. Most nongerminomas arise from the pineal region, whereas germinomas may present either there or in the suprasellar region, or in both areas; 10% of germ-cell tumors arise elsewhere in the brain, for example, the thalamus.

Clinical Presentation

Patients present with acute findings related to obstructive hydrocephalus and increased intracranial pressure. Other findings include abnormalities of eye movement, including upward gaze paresis, retraction nystagmus, and diminished pupillary responses. For patients with suprasellar lesions, hypothalamic and pituitary dysfunction dominate, including growth failure, precocious puberty, and diabetes insipidus. Neuroimaging studies reveal a contrast-enhancing lesion, occasionally with calcification.

Surgical Diagnosis and Treatment

Surgery is strongly recommended to determine the histology of a lesion in the pineal region. The differential diagnosis of lesions in this area includes germinoma, nongerminoma, teratoma, pineocytoma, pineoblastoma, astrocytoma, and in rare instances metastatic tumor. The therapeutic options depend on the tumor type. A negative β-HCG orga-fetoprotein finding in the CSF or serum does not exclude a nongerminoma, although the presence of these markers is indicative of these tumors (8). A slight elevation of β-HCG may be present with germinomas as well. Modern surgical techniques make sampling or partial removal of tumors in this area safe and appropriate. In the past, because of the risks of surgery, such tumors were treated without tissue diagnosis, as if they were germinomas. If the lesion disappeared after a short course of irradiation it was believed to be a germinoma, but if it did not disappear the puzzle of its exact etiology could not be resolved. A regimen of chemotherapy for pineoblastoma, for instance, might be different from that for a mixed germ-cell tumor, as would be the decision on craniospinal axis irradiation.

Radiation Therapy

Radiation is directed to localized germinomas using the involved field as well as encompassing the ventricular system; 25 Gy is directed to the larger field, with a boost of an additional 20 to 25 Gy to the tumor bed. The field of irradiation and the dose are topics of controversy. Some authors advocate irradiation of the craniospinal axis for all patients with germinomas, especially if a biopsy has been done, because of the risk of dissemination. Wara and colleagues found that only 8.3% of 109 patients with pineal tumors developed spinal metastasis if no spinal irradiation was given (290). The issue of craniospinal axis irradiation has not been resolved with germinomas. Jenkin and colleagues found that two of five cases of germinoma spread to the spinal subarachnoid space when spinal irradiation was not used, but no instance of spread occurred in 5 patients who had spinal irradiation (122). Currently, if CSF markers are negative and staging of the spine, including cytology and MRI-Gd or myelography, is negative, then wide-field irradiation, including the ventricular volume, is used. Germinomas are very radiation sensitive. The survival rate for patients with biopsy-proven germinoma is as high as 70% in some series, and as high as 90% when whole-brain irradiation to at least 50 Gy was used (273). There is some concern that the 50-Gy dose of radiation is too high, and for this reason lesser doses comparable to those used for testicular seminoma (30 Gy or less) have been suggested (122, 273).

Chemotherapy

Nongerminomas are less responsive to radiation and frequently are treated initially with chemotherapy. The drugs used are similar to those used for gonadal tumors, including cisplatin, etoposide, vinblastine, bleomycin, and cyclophosphamide (7). As many as six courses of chemotherapy with a combination of agents has been used, followed by restaging. Residual disease is then treated with radiation therapy. At UCSF, a combination of cisplatin, etoposide, bleomycin, and vinblastine or a three-drug combination of carboplatin, etoposide, and bleomycin has been used. There are other reports which document high objective response rates with the two-drug combinations of cisplatin and etoposide or of carboplatin and etoposide. Shorter-course therapy of only four cycles has also been used. Considering the rarity of these tumors, a consensus has not developed concerning the optimal regimen and duration of therapy. Unfortunately, the survival rate is much less with nongerminomas than with most germ cell tumors. Of 11 patients treated by Bruce and Stein, only 33% were alive 2 years after diagnosis (35).

In the case of disseminated germinomas, primary treatment with chemotherapy is also reasonable in order to defer or omit the use of craniospinal axis irradiation. All cases are routinely staged before treatment, to define what therapy is to be used.

CRANIOPHARYNGIOMAS

Etiology and Epidemiology

Craniopharyngiomas are histologically benign tumors that arise from remnants of Rathke's pouch. They are generally found in children and young adults but exhibit a second peak incidence late in adult life. They account for as many as 4% of all brain tumors and are most often situated at the junction of the infundibular stalk and the pituitary gland. Because of their proximity to the stalk, the pituitary gland, the optic apparatus, and the third ventricle, they pose significant risks to these structures.

Pathology and Diagnosis

Most craniopharyngiomas are cystic, although some are solid or both cystic and solid. The cyst contains cholesterol-laden fluid. Calcifications are also common. These tumors may be entirely intrasellar and expand the sella turcica, may extend into the suprasellar space, or may exist primarily in the prechiasmatic cisterns and encroach on the chiasm and optic nerves, obstructing the third ventricle (109). Patients present with hydrocephalus and/or endocrine dysfunction and visual symptoms. Neuroimaging studies reveal a cystic or mixed cystic and solid tumor, occasionally with calcifications. MRI is very helpful in defining the relation of the tumor to surrounding structures.

Treatment

Complete surgical removal is possible in some cases, although extensive resections involve a risk of hemorrhage, visual deterioration (including loss of vision), memory deficits, diabetes insipidus, and the need for cortisol, thyroid, or growth hormone replacement therapy. In contrast, the risk of recurrence is greater than 50% with only a partial resection, and even after a presumed total resection, tumor may still recur in 20 to 25% of cases (110). As many as 40% of these tumors cannot be removed. The dilemma concerning this "benign tumor" is therefore evident. A partial resection may avoid some neuroendocrine or visual disturbances, but frequently the tumor recurs. Extensive resection may cause deficits requiring long-term hormone therapy, and still the tumor may recur. If possible, and if risks are thought to be minimal, an attempt at total resection should be considered for children with this disease. If postoperative neuroimaging documents total removal, radiation therapy may be deferred for years. Close follow-up review with imaging studies is required. In the case of residual disease or a less than complete removal, postoperative irradiation is recommended.

Postoperative irradiation can produce excellent long-term results. In 74 patients treated at UCSF with partial resection and postoperative irradiation, a 91% remission rate was obtained over a mean follow-up period of 4 years (20). Of those patients with preoperative visual disturbances, 93% improved and 33% gained normal vision. The most common radiation dose used was higher than 50 Gy. Other series have documented the benefit of irradiation after a less than complete resection. Irradiation entails some hazard, however, especially in children, and the potential for long-term negative effects on cognition, for endocrine deficits, and rarely for induced secondary tumors must be considered (54). The treatment of recurrence after surgery alone, or surgery combined with irradiation, is difficult, mostly because of the effects of previous surgery and radiation therapy.

Cystic portions of craniopharyngiomas may become refractory to usual methods of control, including repeated cyst aspirations, multiple surgeries, and radiation therapy. Several trials have documented control with the instillation of radiation isotopes into the cyst cavity; phosphorus, gold, and yttrium isotopes have been used (48). This technique requires careful attention to placement of the isotope, which is often done through a reservoir or using stereotactic technique. The consistency of the cyst fluid also is important, because some cavities have fluid that is very thick or sludge-like, precluding adequate distribution of the isotope within the cavity. Multicystic lesions are difficult if not impossible to treat in this manner. There are other problems with this technique as well, including the risk of further radiation damage to vision when the cyst wall is very thin, allowing penetration into adjacent neural structures.

Another method of treatment for craniopharyngioma includes stereotactic radiosurgery, which permits precise localization of a radiation dose to a small field in one treatment setting (15, 48). Special units, including the focused gamma irradiation device called the gamma unit, have become available, as have specially designed linear accelerators with collimators. Although too few patients have been treated with this form of therapy to permit generalizations about results, it appears that it may prove a useful therapeutic tool. One strategy involves radiosurgery at the time of recurrence, or perhaps its use as primary therapy after partial surgical resections. The ability to localize the target precisely with radiosurgery could minimize the exposure of sensitive areas of the brain, including the pituitary gland and optic chiasm, nerves, and tracts.

MENINGIOMA

Epidemiology

Meningiomas account for 13 to 17% of intracranial brain tumors. They most often occur during the fourth through the sixth decades of life with a peak at about 45 years of age. About 65% of all meningiomas occur in women (99).

Pathology

Meningiomas are classified as malignant, either on the basis of histologic criteria or invasiveness. Histologically malignant or anaplastic features include the presence of frequent mitotic figures (more than one or two per 10 high-power fields), atypical mitoses, papillary structures, high cellularity, and necrosis (118). Invasiveness is itself thought to represent malignant potential, as are the variant subtypes of hemangiopericytoma and other forms of angioblastic meningiomas. According to these criteria, malignant meningiomas constitute 2 to 10% of all meningiomas. There is debate over the specific features that determine malignancy because some benign meningiomas have several characteristically malignant features, yet behave in a typically benign fashion. Conversely, in rare cases, meningiomas that appear benign metastasize both within the CNS and outside the cranium to the lymph nodes and lung. At UCSF, we use the criterion of invasiveness as well as the histologic criteria of increased mitoses, anaplastic features such as pleomorphism, necrosis, and a high labeling index (greater than 1%) to assign malignancy to meningiomas.

Treatment

Most meningiomas are benign tumors that are treated successfully with surgical resection alone. The goal of surgery is to remove the tumor and its dural attachment with any involved bone. Incompletely resected tumors are treated with radiation therapy.

The treatment of malignant meningiomas is as extensive a resection as possible followed by irradiation to a dose of 60 Gy using single daily fractions. We previously included adjuvant chemotherapy with cyclophosphamide, Adriamycin, and vincristine with this treatment in the hope of reducing the high recurrence rate, but compared with historical controls, there is no evidence that any form of chemotherapy is useful for primary management of malignant meningiomas.

Options in the treatment of malignant or invasive meningioma, other than surgery and conventional radiation therapy, include the use of interstitial brachytherapy and/or stereotactic radiosurgery. High-activity or low-activity brachytherapy sources can be used to obtain good local control rates. The technique appears to confer a survival advantage. Leibel and colleagues reviewed the UCSF data obtained with brachytherapy for recurrent newly diagnosed malignant meningiomas; 13 patients were treated, 2 with high-activity sources, and 11 with permanent low-activity radioactive iodine sources (144). Of the patients treated with low-activity sources, 8 of 9 with malignant meningiomas and 1 of 2 with recurrent meningioma had stable disease ranging from 2 to 77 months; the two recurrences were at 8 and 22 months. One of these malignant tumors was treated with interstitial brachytherapy before the patient underwent external radiation therapy. Of the 2 patients treated with high-activity sources, 1 had recurrence after 58 months and one remains stable at 58 months. Both required reoperation for radiation necrosis, 1 at 12 months and 1 at 35 months. None of the patients with permanent implants developed symptomatic necrosis.

Aggressive surgery may also be possible if embolism of the feeding vessels is performed before surgery, to reduce the risk of bleeding during extensive resection. The most aggressive approach to these tumors would include preoperative embolization and extensive resection, followed by interstitial brachytherapy and possibly adjuvant chemotherapy. None of these approaches has been evaluated in a randomized study but because of the relative rarity of the tumor, there have been very few clinical trials in the treatment of malignant meningioma.

Recurrence

The recurrence rate for presumably completely removed meningiomas is low, generally less than 10%, but it can be as high as 40 to 50% in patients with gross residual disease remaining postoperatively (182). In patients who had undergone a partial resection, Wara and colleagues found recurrence in 75% of a nonirradiated group but in only 29% of the group undergoing irradiation after surgery (291). Others do not advocate irradiation routinely for residual benign meningiomas, rather relying on a repeat surgical resection at the time of recurrence (42, 131).

Disease Metastatic to the Central Nervous System

ETIOLOGY AND EPIDEMIOLOGY

As many as 25% of all patients with cancer develop metastasis to the brain or spinal cord, and the disease becomes clinically significant in most patients. As the population in general lives longer and as other therapies become more successful in controlling disease outside the CNS, it is likely that the incidence of CNS metastases will increase. The AIDS epidemic has produced an increasing incidence of unusual metastatic tumors, including CNS lymphoma. In the 1986 data compiled by the American Cancer Society, the number of cancer deaths from intracranial metastases was estimated at 124,000 cases, and the number of deaths from primary CNS neoplasms at 10,200 cases (258). Clearly, metastatic tumors are an important clinical problem and a frequent cause of death.

PATHOLOGY

The most common primary sites of metastases to the CNS are the lung and breast, metastases from the lung being more frequent overall because of the larger numbers of patients with this malignancy. Other common primary sites include melanoma from any site, leukemia and lymphoma, and renal cancers. Virtually any primary cancer may spread to the CNS with involvement of brain and spinal cord parenchyma, leptomeninges, dura, and pituitary gland (216).

Lung cancer is the most common primary source of brain parenchymal metastases, and of the various forms of lung cancer, small-cell tumors are the most likely to metastasize. Metastasis to the dura, in contrast, arises more frequently from cancer of the breast or prostate or lymphoma. Leptomeningeal disease occurs frequently as a consequence of cancer of the breast, lung, and melanoma, as well as lymphoma and leukemia. Breast cancer is the most frequent tumor to metastasize to the pituitary gland.

CLINICAL PRESENTATION

The signs and symptoms of intracranial metastases are identical to those of primary brain tumors and are thus indistinguishable. Patients present with signs and symptoms related to the location of the lesion or with more generalized signs such as personality changes, headache, generalized seizures, or weakness; dexamethasone is useful for diminishing peritumoral edema that may contribute greatly to the symptoms. An initial manifestation as a brain tumor is common for lung cancer but rare for other cancers. Every adult with symptoms of a brain tumor should have a CT scan of the lungs because plain x-ray films of the chest may not reveal small pulmonary lesions that could be the primary neoplasm. Acute findings may be the result of hemorrhage into the tumor and may be caused by hydrocephalus or by acute increases in intracranial pressure. Leptomeningeal findings include more general symptoms, such as headache and nausea, or more specific signs and symptoms related to the area most affected, such as lower cranial nerve involvement (oculomotor or facial nerve) or lower spinal nerve invasion causing weakness, reflex changes, and bowel and bladder dysfunction. Dissemination of the tumor into the CSF (carcinomatous, lymphomatous, or leukemic meningitis) may produce hydrocephalus and may cause nuchal rigidity. Involvement of the dura may produce symptoms of pain and specific nerve root compression. Pain over the site of the metastasis or pain radiating in a nerve root pattern is the most common clinical finding associated with epidural spinal metastasis.

DIAGNOSIS

Of the parenchymal lesions, approximately 50% are solitary metastases (216). In the absence of a recognized primary tumor, the diagnosis must be verified histologically. With a known primary tumor, either before or after it is treated and in the absence of obvious systemic dissemination, we do not assume a metastatic origin but rather advocate stereotactic needle biopsy of a solitary brain tumor. In cases of a known systemic primary lesion, multiple lesions in the brain almost certainly are due to metastatic disease, and a presumptive diagnosis of metastatic tumor to the brain would be warranted.

Radiographic findings of intracranial metastases include contrast-enhancing single or multiple lesions (Figs. 97.5 and 97.6). In general, metastatic brain tumors are surrounded by a large area of edema. Hemorrhage may occur and, if extensive, can obscure the tumor. Some tumors have central areas of necrosis that do not enhance, or the entire lesion may enhance uniformly with sharply demarcated borders. MRI-Gd may be more sensitive than CT because it can visualize smaller lesions and view the posterior fossa free of the bone artifacts observed with CT (34). Areas of abnormal enhancement along the dura or leptomeninges are also better visualized with MRI-Gd (228). If contrast-enhanced CT reveals one lesion, we routinely follow CT with MRI-Gd to exclude other lesions. MRI of the spine, with and without Gd, is the first diagnostic test used to assess the spinal compartment.

In patients known to have a primary tumor, specific restaging may be done after a metastatic brain or spinal tumor has been documented, to assess the overall extent of tumor and to coordinate treatment strategies based on that information. At times, the site of origin of a systemic primary lesion is determined only after CNS metastasis has been documented. Although in some cases the primary site is not determined despite extensive searches, a CNS metastasis usually is diagnosed in association with a known primary site, and usually within the first year after diagnosis of the primary lesion. Other primary tumors may not manifest a CNS recurrence for many years after the initial diagnosis, most notably in patients with breast, colon, and renal cancer. Because of the wide diversity and overall frequency of CNS spread, a high index of suspicion is needed in evaluating predisposed patients.

Differential Diagnosis

The differential diagnosis of a space-occupying lesion or lesions in the CNS includes other primary CNS tumors, such as glioblastoma (most often found as a single enhancing tumor) or meningioma. In patients with AIDS or other causes of immunocompromise, infectious processes must be included. Clinically significant intraparenchymal hemorrhage may occur in association with chemotherapy-induced thrombocytopenia or disseminated coagulopathies and may add confusion to the etiology of secondary bleeding. Cere-

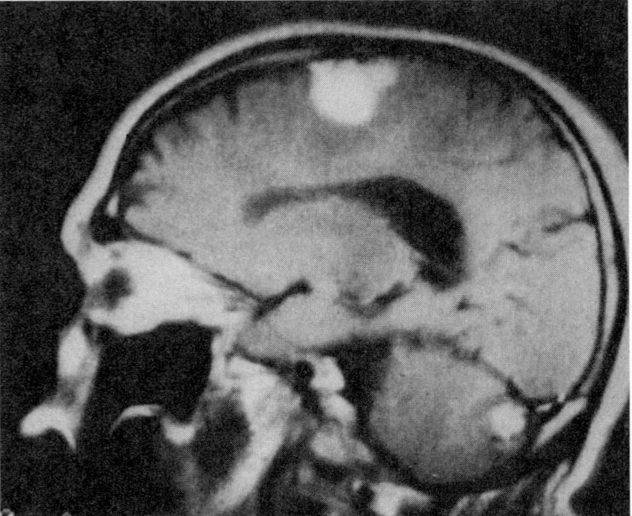

Figure 97.5. T1-W MRI made with Gd in the sagittal plane shows multiple intracranial lesions metastatic from the kidney.

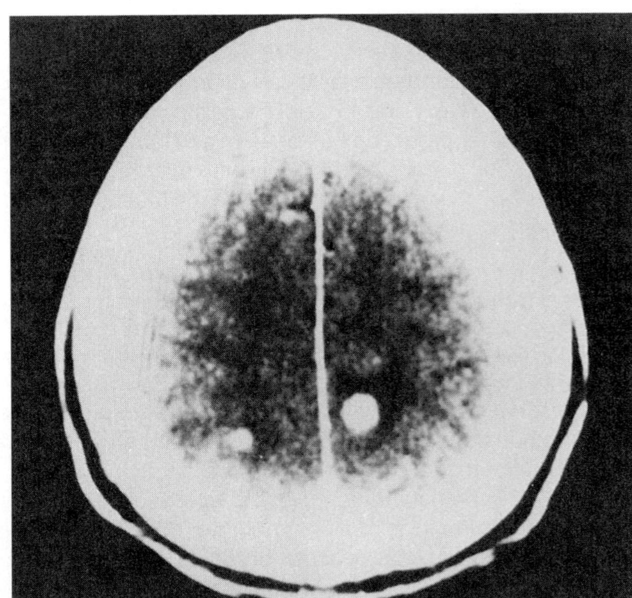

Figure 97.6. Contrast-enhanced CT scan of multiple metastases from a malignant melanoma.

brovascular disease can cause variable enhancing lesions that may be confused with tumor, but such lesions resolve over time. The clinical setting in which the lesion exists and the patient's physical and laboratory findings should be helpful in differentiating other causes. When doubt exists regarding diagnosis and appropriate therapy, surgical biopsy or resection should be done to establish the diagnosis.

SURGERY AND RADIATION THERAPY

Brain Metastases

A decision to operate for metastatic brain tumor depends in large part on the patient's neurologic status, the extent of disease in the CNS, and most importantly, the extent of systemic disease. Certainly, a decision to resect a lesion or lesions in the CNS must take into account the nature of the primary disease as well as expectations for its control. A craniotomy is seldom of benefit to a patient with melanoma that is widely disseminated both systemically and intracranially. However, a patient with controlled primary lung cancer and no other evidence of disease except a single brain metastasis is a candidate for surgical intervention. The rationale for resecting a solitary metastasis to the CNS is based partly on retrospective, uncontrolled studies comparing outcome after surgery plus irradiation with that after irradiation alone. All of those studies suggest that combined surgery and irradiation are of benefit in treating controlled primary disease and single metastases to brain. Of 125 patients treated by Sundaresen and Galicich at Memorial Sloan-Kettering Cancer Center from 1978 to 1982, for example, all had metastatic tumors resected either before or after undergoing irradiation (271). Failure to respond to whole-brain irradiation prompted surgery in 31 cases, and 81 patients had symptomatic metastases resected and received radiation therapy postoperatively. All but 6 patients had single metastatic lesions; the most common primary site was the lung, followed by melanoma, kidney, and then less common primary sites such as colon, sarcoma, and breast. The median survival for the series was 12 months, with 12% of the patients surviving for more than 5 years. Patients who had only CNS disease with a controlled primary site showed a distinct therapeutic advantage, with their median survival being 22 months as compared with only 5 months for patients with active extracranial disease.

The period of survival after radiation therapy alone is generally shorter than that after surgery plus irradiation. In a retrospective study matching patients with lung cancer, Patchell and colleagues compared survival in those with metastatic brain tumors treated with radiation alone and those having surgery plus irradiation (209). The median survival was 19 months in the combined treatment group but only 9 months in the group receiving radiation therapy alone. Several similar reports show survival of only 6 to 12 months after radiation therapy alone. Patchell and colleagues more recently reported a prospective controlled trial comparing irradiation plus surgical resection or biopsy in patients with single brain metastases (210). The local recurrence rate was significantly greater in the group undergoing biopsy only (52%) than in the group having resection (20%), and median survival was better in the resection group (40 weeks) than in the group that had biopsy (15 weeks). They concluded that surgical resection followed by irradiation is indicated for patients with a single metastatic lesion.

There is also a role for surgical resection in treating symptomatic lesions that do not respond to irradiation, for both palliation and the possibility of improved survival. Some metastatic tumors are conspicuously less responsive to irradiation, and local recurrence is common. Complete removal of a single lesion, when possible, may be the best form of local control in this situation and potentially provides long-term survival.

Spinal Metastases

A decision to use surgery for spinal metastases is based largely on the status of the patient both systemically and neurologically, the extent of the lesion, and the advantages offered by other forms of treatment such as irradiation, chemotherapy, or hormonal therapy. The ideal candidate for surgical resection has a single lesion and minimal neurologic deficit. The goal of surgery is removal of the lesion, preservation of function, and maintenance of spinal integrity (260). Extradural tumors may quickly cause irreversible deficits by compression of the spinal cord, but how long complete paralysis may exist before it becomes irreversible is not fully known. As a general guideline, complete paralysis lasting longer than 24 hours is most likely irreversible. Partial deficits may be completely reversible with rapid therapy, including high-dose corticosteriods to diminish peritumoral edema, surgery, and irradiation. If radiation therapy has not been used as primary therapy before surgery, then it should be used after surgery in most patients who have symptomatic spinal metastases.

The availability of new techniques that help achieve decompression with spinal stabilization has influenced surgeons to treat more of the patients who may benefit from surgery (272). Nonetheless, a comparison of surgery and irradiation with regard to potential benefits still favors irradiation in most cases (11, 260, 272). Appropriate indications for surgical resection include cases in which the diagnosis cannot be defined, in which spinal cord compression is progressive despite maximum radiation therapy, and, rarely, when palliation of pain is required. Ominus and colleagues achieved excellent pain relief in most of 57 patients treated surgically for spinal metastases, and 65% of those who had been bedridden before surgery recovered the ability to walk (199). Indications for surgery further include progressive neurologic decline due to cord compression produced by a collapsed vertebral body, improvement being attributable to vertebral body resection and stabilization of the spine with methacrylate and metal or bone internal splinting.

RADIATION THERAPY ALONE

Radiation therapy is used in most cases of intracranial and spinal metastases. The RTOG recently reviewed their data on dose and fractionation schedules for patients with metastatic intracranial lesions (60). No difference in outcome was observed in one series of sequential trials evaluating several regimens, including whole-brain irradiation given to a total dose of either 20 Gy within 1 week, or up to 40 Gy within 4 weeks; or in a second trial evaluating irradiation to 30 Gy within 2 weeks as compared with 50 Gy within 4 weeks. Further studies compared two other fractionation schemes: 30 Gy given in 10 fractions over 2 weeks and 30 Gy given in six fractions over 3 weeks. Misonidazole was also evaluated in these arms in a randomized fashion, and, in general, there was no significant difference in survival favoring either misonidazole or a hypofractionated scheme.

The misonidazole trials distinguished subgroups of patients destined for poor survival from those subgroups who could be expected to survive more than 200 days. Favorable factors were patient age 60 years or less plus a single brain metastasis, a Karnofsky Performance Score (KPS) of 70 or above, and primary sites that were either not identifiable or controlled. The median survival for the group in the more favorable condition was 7.4 months, but it was only 2 months for patients in the less favorable group. Other studies now evaluating the role of hyperfractionated irradiation in this disease state suggest that higher doses are more effective in controlling local disease when given more often than once a day, but the final results are pending (295).

Interstitial brachytherapy, with or without hyperthermia, and radiosurgery are also useful for brain metastases. A series reported by Prados and colleagues included several cases of long-term survival and good local control in patients treated with high-activity radioactive iodine brachytherapy (218). Fourteen patients with metastatic tumor who either had just completed radiation therapy or had not responded to whole-brain irradiation underwent interstitial brachytherapy to boost irradiation of the immediate tumor area. Eight of the 14 were alive a median of 63 weeks later (range 52 to 239 weeks) and median survival of the entire group was weeks. This was a select group of patients whose lesions were of a favorable size and location to permit brachytherapy. Similarly eligible patients are now being treated with a combination of interstitial brachytherapy and hyperthermia, in an attempt to further improve on these results.

Radiosurgery, precisely focused irradiation of tumor, has also been used in similar groups of patients. Loeffler and colleagues treated 18 patients with stereotactic radiosurgery for recurrent or persistent brain metastases; the selection criteria included a KPS of 70 or greater and stable systemic disease (165). All patients had previously had conventional radiation therapy. Single doses of radiation of 9 to 25 Gy were used. Within a median follow-up period of 9 months, all tumors had been controlled in the field and two did not respond outside the margin of the field. Now with even further clinical evaluation, it is clear that radiosurgery is an appropriate option to consider in patients with single or even multiple metastatic tumors to the brain. In most cases, there is continual local control of the lesions treated and minimal morbidity. Local control rates are greater than 80% with careful selection based upon volume and location of tumors. Death frequently occurs because of uncontrolled systemic disease or other metastatic lesions that subsequently develop within the brain or spinal cord. Many patients with metastatic tumors are now routinely being treated with radiosurgery. Clinical trials are being developed by the RTOG to clarify the specific instances where stereotactic radiosurgery should be used, and most importantly, to identify guidelines for specific dosing requirements. Ultimately, it is anticipated that clinical trials will be developed that compare the outcome of patients treated with surgery or radiosurgery, either at the time of initial diagnosis of a single metastatic lesion or at the time of relapse after whole-brain radiotherapy. Finally, as local control improves for these tumors, the role of whole-brain radiotherapy will be evaluated. It is possible that in some tumor types, the use of stereotactic radiosurgery alone, rather than whole-brain radiotherapy, may be sufficient to control CNS disease. These clinical research trials are eagerly awaited.

In cases of spinal cord compression, irradiation is effective in controlling pain and preventing disease progression—not only in patients who show only radiographic evidence of spinal metastasis but are normal on neurologic examination, but also in those with irreversible cord compression causing paralysis and loss of bowel and bladder control. Ampil reviewed 20 patients who had paraplegia caused by epidural cord compression, most of whom received at least 30 Gy to the tumor site; the tumors principally were metastatic from a lung or prostatic primary lesion (11). Of this group, 78% achieved symptomatic pain relief, although none showed improvement in neurologic function and the overall median survival was only 2.5 months.

In patients with progressive neurologic decline short of complete paralysis, radiation therapy is as effective as surgery, particularly for highly radiation-sensitive tumors, including lymphomas and leukemia, oat cell tumors, breast and colon cancer, and prostatic tumors. For other tumors that are not as responsive to radiation, such as melanoma and renal cell cancers, surgical resection using new approaches may be beneficial. Radiation therapy may then be useful for small residual tumors. If the tumor can be identified by MR imaging as arising from the vertebral body, laminectomy may not be sufficient and vertebrectomy through an exterior approach may be necessary to decompress the spinal cord. Surgical resection is indicated, both for decompression and diagnosis, in cases of progressive neurologic decline when the nature of a tumor is unknown. It is also indicated for progressive neurologic decline that does not respond to radiation therapy and for pain control when other measures are ineffective.

CHEMOTHERAPY

Corticosteroids should be used routinely in the urgent treatment of epidural cord compression. Their effect is to reduce vasogenic edema secondary to tumor and to relieve pain as well as neurologic symptoms in many cases. Short courses of high-dose dexamethasone—up to 100 mg administered as a bolus and given in divided doses on a daily basis—are given concurrently with definitive therapy such as surgery and irradiation. Following a 3- to 4-day course, the dose may be tapered to the lowest dose that maintains good control of symptoms. Dexamethasone is also helpful in controlling symptoms related to intracranial tumors, which frequently present with significant mass effect as a result of peritumoral edema. If the clinical situation is severe, doses similar to those used for cord compression may be used. In most cases, however, much smaller doses are required. The dose should be tapered to the lowest dose that sustains a response while more definitive therapy is given. The response to steroids is dose dependent and may be short lived in the case of cord compression unless definitive therapy is given.

In some cases, metastatic brain tumors may be treated with systemic chemotherapy. At UCSF, a multiagent chemotherapy regimen including lomustine, 6-thioguanine (6-TG), dibromodulcitol, procarbazine, 5-fluorouracil (5-FU), and hydroxyurea has been used for tumors that have recurred despite surgery and/or irradiation. Although the results are preliminary in this ongoing trial, this regimen controls metastatic disease in the brain and causes objective reductions in tumor size in some cases of CNS lesions metastatic from breast and lung cancer as well as melanoma (154). Other investigators have shown objective responses in the brain using a variety of drugs. Lee and colleagues, reporting from the University of Texas M. D. Anderson Hospital, showed that among 11 evaluable patients with small-cell lung cancer metastatic to the brain who received a chemotherapy regimen including doxorubicin, cyclophosphamide, etoposide, and vincristine, 8 achieved at least a partial response; median survival for the group was 34 weeks (142). Rosner and colleagues also documented objective responses in patients with metastatic breast carcinoma to brain using various combinations of cyclophosphamide, 5-FU, methotrexate, doxorubicin, and prednisone (235). Objective responses and stable disease can be achieved with these and other drug regimens that should be considered as a therapeutic strategy against metastatic brain tumors.

Leptomeningeal Disease

The treatment of diffuse leptomeningeal disease, or neoplastic meningitis, is difficult and offers few options. Traditionally, treatment has included chemotherapy, given intrathecally or through an Ommaya reservoir, with agents such as methotrexate, ara-C, and thiotepa. Combination therapy using two or three drugs, with or without steroids, has also been tried. In general, responses to treatment have been short lived except in the case of very sensitive tumors such as leukemia, some lymphomas, and CSF spread of medulloblastoma and primitive neuroectodermal tumor. Irradiation of the craniospinal axis may be helpful but can severely compromise the bone marrow reserve if systemic chemotherapy is given. New approaches to this disease are needed.

Benjamin and colleagues reported one patient who received intrathecal monoclonal antibody therapy conjugated to iodine 131 for carcinomatous meningitis secondary to bladder cancer (23). The monoclonal antibody was raised against human milk fat globulin (HMFG1). The patient died within 4 days of treatment. At autopsy, the leptomeninges showed infiltration by carcinoma cells, which stained positively with HMFG1. Autoradiographic examination of the brain revealed isotope that had concentrated within the periventricular white matter and leptomeningeal layers. It appeared that labeled antibody diffused into white matter wherever contact occurred with CSF. Lashford and colleagues treated five patients who had leptomeningeal tumors with radiolabeled antibody given intrathecally, using antibodies selected for the specific tumor type from a panel of available antibodies (139). Minimal toxicity was observed, and four of the five patients achieved an objective response varying from 7 months to 2 years. The tumor types included pineoblastoma, lymphoma, teratoma, primitive neuroectodermal tumor, and melanoma. Moseley and colleagues found that the HMFG1 antigen could be detected in 18 of 20 cases of carcinomatous meningitis from a variety of epithelial primary tumors that included ovary, bladder, lung, breast, and stomach (186). It was also detected in two cases of neoplastic meningitis from lymphoma and medulloblastoma. Evidently this antigen could be a target for monoclonal antibody therapy for a number of tumors that invade this compartment. Moseley and colleagues also used a panel of monoclonal antibodies successfully to identify melanoma cells in cases of neoplastic meningitis. The use of specific monoclonal antibodies conjugated to radioisotopes is appealing as a therapeutic strategy for leptomeningeal disease when other therapies are not successful (185).

Future Directions

Gene therapy for brain tumors represents the newest treatment strategy being developed in the laboratory. Early phase I and II studies in patients with recurrent malignant gliomas have begun. The first studies have used the herpes simplex–thymidine kinase gene (Hs-tk gene) for in vivo gene transfer experiments (53). This gene is transferred into a retroviral vector, packaged in a mouse fibroblast, and injected directly into the tumor. Tumor cells that are transduced with the Hs-tk gene become susceptible to the antiviral drug ganciclovir. An in vivo intracranial rat brain tumor model using the 9L rat gliosarcoma was used to test whether gene transfer could take place and if tumor destruction occurred following administration of ganciclovir. In these experiments, rats treated in this fashion survived significantly longer than control rats. Rats sacrificed to evaluate extent of tumor were found to have complete macroscopic and, in most cases, microscopic elimination of tumor. Because of this laboratory research, a phase I study of gene therapy was begun in 1993 at the National Institutes of Health, and a phase II study was begun in 1994. Results are preliminary, but some patients have shown what appears to be an antitumor response, and the studies are currently ongoing.

Neuro-oncology is making significant progress through such laboratory investigations into the molecular biology and genetics of CNS neoplasms. Clues to the etiology and pathogenesis of malignant brain tumors are being detected at a rapid pace, and with the fundamental understanding of the nature of these tumors that this information provides, it is likely that a greater number of rationally designed, specific, nontoxic therapies may be forthcoming.

Investigations into the control of growth and oncogene expression, or the lack of controlling mechanisms, afford particularly exciting avenues of research. The potential of monoclonal antibody therapies is encouraging, as are the trials of gene therapy being developed. Radiation therapy has contributed greatly to the multidisciplinary approach to treatment, affording new fractionation schemes, interstitial brachytherapy, radiosurgery, and radiation-enhancing agents. The ability to overcome a tumor's resistance to certain drugs may additionally enhance response rates, as may new agents such as the polyamine inhibitors and *temozolomide*. Growth stimulators such as granulocyte-monocyte–colony-stimulating factor should permit greater dose intensity and provide additional support for high-dose chemotherapy with ABMT. Surgical techniques now permit more extensive resection with less risk than at any time in the history of neurosurgery. Perhaps the single most important ingredient in this new era of neuro-oncology is a willingness to abolish the pessimism of the past, replacing it with acceptance that CNS tumors should and will be treated as successfully as are tumors elsewhere in the body.

References

1. Afra D, Müller I, Slowik F, Wilcke A, Budka H, Turoczy L. Supratentorial lobar ependymomas: reports on the grading and survival periods in 80 cases, including 46 recurrences. Acta Neurochir (Wien) 1983;69:243.
2. Albright AL, Guthkelch AN, Packer RJ, Price RA, Rourke LB. Prognostic factors in pediatric brain-stem gliomas. J Neurosurg 1986;65:751.
3. Albright AL, Price RA, Guthkelch AN. Brain stem gliomas of children. A clinicopathological study. Cancer 1983;52:2313.
4. Allen J, Nirenberg A, Donahue B. A phase I/II pilot study employing hyperfractionated radiotherapy and adjuvant chemotherapy for high-risk primitive neuroectodermal tumors. Ann Neurol 1991;30:457–458.
5. Allen J, Packer R, Bleyer A, Zeltzer P, Prados M, Nirenberg A, Etcubanas E. Recombinant β-interferon A phase I/II dose finding trial in pediatric brain tumor patients (abstract). J Neurooncol 1989;7:S4.
6. Allen JC, Bloom J, Ertel I, Evans A, Hammond D, Jones H, Levin V, Jenkin D, Sposto R, Wara W. Brain tumors in children: current cooperative and institutional chemotherapy trials in newly diagnosed and recurrent disease. Semin Oncol 1986;13:110.
7. Allen JC, Bosl G, Walker R. Chemotherapy trials in recurrent primary intracranial germ cell tumors. J Neurooncol 1985;3:147.
8. Allen JC, Nisselbaum J, Epstein F, Rosen G, Schwartz MK. Alphafetoprotein and human chorionic gonadotropin determination in cerebrospinal fluid. An aid to the diagnosis and management of intracranial germ-cell tumors. J Neurosurg 1979;51:368.
9. Ammirati M, Galicich J, Arbit E, Liao Y. Reoperation in the treatment of recurrent intracranial malignant gliomas. Neurosurgery 1987;21:607.
10. Ammirati M, Vick N, Liao YL, Ciric I, Mikhael M. Effect of the extent of surgical resection on survival and quality of life in patients with supratentorial glioblastomas and anaplastic astrocytomas. Neurosurgery 1987;21:201.
11. Ampil FL. Epidural compression from metastatic tumor with resultant paralysis. J Neurooncol 1989;7:129.
12. Andreou J, George AE, Wise A, de Leon A, Kricheff II, Ransohoff J, Foo SH. CT prognostic criteria of survival after malignant glioma surgery. AJNR 1983;4:488.
13. Arcangeli G, Munro R, Morelli B. Multiple daily fractionation in radiotherapy: biological rationale and preliminary clinical experience. Eur J Cancer 1979;15:1077.
14. Arnold DL, Shoubridge EA, Feindel W, Villemure JG. Metabolic changes in cerebral gliomas within hours of treatment with intra-arterial BCNU demonstrated by phosphorus magnetic resonance spectroscopy. Can J Neurol Sci 1987;14:570.
15. Backlund E. Solid craniopharyngioma treated by stereotactic radiosurgery. In Stereotactic Cerebral Irradiation, INSERM Symposium, No. 12. Edited by G. Szilka. New York: Elsevier/North Holland, 1979, p 271.
16. Bailey P, Cushing H. A Classification of the Tumors of the Glioma Group on a Histogenetic Basis with a Correlated Study of Prognosis. Philadelphia: Lippincott, 1926.
17. Barker D, Wright E, Nguyen N, Cannon L, Fain P, Goldgar D, Bishop DT, Carey J, Baty J, Kivlin J, Willard H, Waye JS, Greig G, Leinwand L, Nakamura Y, O'Connell P, Leppert M, Lalouel JM, White R, Skolnick M. Gene for von Recklinghausen neurofibromatosis is in the pericentromeric region of chromosome 17. Science 1987;236:1100.
18. Bashir R, Hochberg FH, Linggood RM, Hottleman K. Pre-irradiation internal carotid artery BCNU in treatment of glioblastoma multiforme. J Neurosurg 1988;68:917.
19. Bashir RM, Harris NL, Hochberg FH, Singer RM. Detection of Epstein-Barr virus in CNS lymphomas by in-situ hybridization. Neurology 1989;39:813.
20. Baskin DS, Wilson CB. Surgical management of craniopharyngiomas. A review of 74 cases. J Neurosurg 1986;65:22.
21. Baughman FA, JA, List CF, Williams JR, Muldoon JP, Segarra JM, Volkel JS. The glioma-polyposis syndrome. N Engl J Med 1969;281:1345.
22. Baumgartner JE, Rachlin JR, Beckstead JH, Meeker TC, Levy RM, Wara WM, Rosenblum ML. Primary central nervous system lymphomas: natural history and response to radiation therapy in 55 patients with acquired immunodeficiency syndrome. J Neurosurg 1990;73:206.
23. Benjamin JC, Moss T, Moseley RP, Maxwell R, Coakham HB. Cerebral distribution of immunoconjugate after treatment for neoplastic meningitis using an intrathecal radiolabeled monoclonal antibody. Neurosurgery 1989;25:253.
24. Berger MS, Deliganis AV, Dobbins J, Keles GE. The effect of extent of resection on recurrence in patients with low grade cerebral hemisphere glioma. Cancer 1994;74: 1784–1791.
25. Berger MS, Edwards MS, LaMasters D, Davis RL, Wilson CB. Pediatric brain stem tumors: radiographic, pathological, and clinical correlations. Neurosurgery 1983;12: 298.
26. Berger MS, Kincaid J, Ojemann GA, Lettich E. Brain mapping techniques to maximize resection, safety, and seizure control in children with brain tumors. Neurosurgery 1989;25:786.
27. Birchmeier C, Sharma S, Wigler M. Expression and rearrangement of the ROS1 gene in human glioblastoma cells. Proc Natl Acad Sci USA 1987;84:9270.
28. Birkmayer GD, Stass HP. Humoral immune response in glioma patients: a solubilized glioma-associated membrane antigen as a tool for detecting circulating antibodies. Int J Cancer 1980;25:445.
29. Black KL, Hawkins RA, Kim KT, Becker DP, Lerner C, Marciano D. Use of thallium-201 SPECT to quantitate malignancy grade of gliomas. J Neurosurg 1989;71:342.
30. Blatt J, Jaffe R, Deutsch M, Adkins JC. Neurofibromatosis and childhood tumors. Cancer 1986;57:1225.
31. Bleehen NM, Wiltshire CR, Plowman PN, Watson JV, Gleave JR, Holmes AE, Lewin WS, Triep CS, Hawkins TD. A randomized study of misonidazole and radiotherapy for grade 3 and 4 cerebral astrocytoma. Br J Cancer 1981;43:436.
32. Bloom, H. Intracranial tumors. Response and resistance to therapeutic endeavors 1970–1980. Int J Radiat Oncol Biol Phys 1982;8:1083.
33. Bogdahn U, Bogdahn S, Mertens HG, Dommasch D, Wodarz R, Wauunsch PA, Kauuhl P, Richter E. Primary non-Hodgkin's lymphoma of the CNS. Acta Neurol Scand 1986;73:602.
34. Brant-Zawadzki M, Berry I, Osaki L, Brasch R, Murovic J, Norman D. Gd-DPTA in clinical MR of the brain. 1. Intraaxial lesions. AJR 1986;147:1223.
35. Bruce J, Stein B. Pineal region tumors. In Current Therapy in Neurological Surgery. Edited by D. Long. Toronto: Decker, 1989, p 73.
36. Brauucher JA, Dalesio O, Solbu G. Prospective analysis of Grade III and IV gliomas, with consideration of histologic classification (an EORTC Brain Tumor Group study). In Brain Oncology. Edited by M Chatel, F Darcel, J Pecker. Dordrecht: Martinus Nijhoff, 1987, p 237.
37. Burger PC. Malignant astrocytic neoplasms: classification, pathologic anatomy, and response to treatment. Semin Oncol 1986;13:16.
38. Cairncross JG, MacDonald DR. Successful chemotherapy for recurrent malignant oligodendroglioma. Ann Neurol 1988;23:360.
39. Cairncross JG, Pexman JH, Rathbone MP, DelMaestro RF. Postoperative contrast enhancement in patients with brain tumor. Ann Neurol 1985;17:570.
40. Caputy AJ, McCullough D, Manz HJ, Patterson K, Hammock MK. A review of the factors influencing the prognosis of medulloblastoma. The importance of cell differentiation. J Neurosurg 1987;66:80.
41. Cavenee WK. Loss of heterozygosity in stages of malignancy. Clin Chem 1989;35(suppl 7):B48.
42. Chan RC, Thompson GB. Morbidity, mortality, and quality of life following surgery for intracranial meningiomas. A retrospective study in 257 cases. J Neurosurg 1984;60: 52.
43. Chang CH, Horton J, Schoenfeld D, Salazer O, Perez-Tamayo R, Kramer S, Weinstein A, Nelson JS, Tsukada Y. Comparison of postoperative radiotherapy and combined postoperative radiotherapy and chemotherapy in the multidisciplinary management of malignant gliomas. A Joint Radiation Therapy Oncology Group and Eastern Cooperative Oncology Group study. Cancer 1983;52:997.
44. Chang CH, Housepian EM, Herbert C Jr. An operative staging system and a megavoltage radiotherapeutic technic for cerebellar medulloblastomas. Radiology 1969;93:1351.
45. Chin HW, Hazel JJ, Kim TH, Webster JH. Oligodendrogliomas. I. A clinical study of cerebral oligodendrogliomas. Cancer 1980;45:1458.
46. Choucair AK, Levin VA, Gutin PH, Davis RL, Silver P, Edwards MS, Wilson CB. Development of multiple lesions during radiation therapy and chemotherapy in patients with gliomas. J Neurosurg 1986;65:654.
47. Choux M, Lena G, Hassoun J. Prognosis and long-term follow-up in patients with medulloblastoma. Clin Neurosurg 1983;30:246.
48. Coffey RJ, Lunsford DL. The role of stereotactic techniques in the management of craniopharyngiomas. Neurosurg Clin North Am 1990;1:161.
49. Cogen PH, Daneshvar L, Metzger AK, Edwards MS. Deletion mapping of the medulloblastoma locus on chromosome 17p. Genomics 1990;8:279.
50. Cohen ME, Duffner PK. Brain Tumors in Children: Principles of Diagnosis and Treatment. International Review of Child Neurology series. New York: Raven, 1984, p 1.
51. Cooper PR. Outcome after operative treatment of intramedullary spinal cord tumors in adults: intermediate and long-term results in 51 patients. Neurosurgery 1989;25: 855.
52. Copeland DD, Bigner DD. Glial-mesenchymal tropism of in vivo avian sarcoma virus neuro-oncogenesis in rats. Acta Neuropathol (Berl) 1978;41:23.
53. Culver KW, Ram Z, Wallbridge S, Ishii H, Oldfield EH, Blaese RM. In vivo gene transfer with retroviral vector-producer cells for treatment of experimental brain tumors. Science 1992;256:1550–1552.
54. Danoff BF, Cowchock FS, Kramer S. Childhood craniopharyngioma: survival, local control, endocrine and neurologic function following radiotherapy. Int J Radiat Oncol Biol Phys 1983;9:171.
55. Daumas-Duport C, Scheithauer B, O'Fallon J, Kelly P. Grading of astrocytomas. A simple and reproducible method. Cancer 1988;62:2152.
56. DeAngelis LM, Yahalom J, Heinemann MH, Cirrincione C, Thaler HT, Krol, G. Primary CNS lymphoma. Combined treatment with chemotherapy and radiotherapy. Neurology 1990;40:80.

57. DeAngelis LM, Yahalom J, Thaler HT, Kher U. Combined modality therapy for primary central nervous system lymphoma. J Clin Oncol 1992;10:635.
58. Deutsch M. Medulloblastoma staging and treatment outcome. Int J Radiat Oncol Biol Phys 1988;14:1103.
59. Deutsch M, Green SB, Strike TA, Burger PC, Robertson JT, Selker RG, Shapiro WR, Mealey J Jr, Ransohoff J Jr, Paoletti P, Smith K, Odom G, Hunt W, Young B, Alexander E, Walker M, Pistenmaa D. Results of a randomized trial comparing BCNU plus radiotherapy, streptozotocin plus radiotherapy, BCNU plus hyperfractionated radiotherapy, and BCNU following misonidazole plus radiotherapy in the postoperative treatment of malignant glioma. Int J Radiat Oncol Biol Phys 1989;16:1389.
60. Diener-West M, Dobbins TW, Phillips TL, Nelson DF. Identification of an optimal subgroup for treatment evaluation of patients with brain metastases using RTOG study 7916. Int J Radiat Oncol Biol Phys 1989;16:669.
61. Dohrmann G. Ependymomas. In Neurosurgery, Vol. 1. Edited by RH Wilkins and SS Rengachary. New York: McGraw Hill, 1985, p 767.
62. Douglas BG. Preliminary results using superfractionation in the treatment of glioblastoma multiforme. J Can Assoc Radiol 1977;28:106.
63. Earnest F, Kernohan J, Craig W. Oligodendroglioma. A review of two hundred cases. Arch Neurol Psychiatry 1950;63:964.
64. Eby NL, Grufferman S, Flannelly CM, Schold SC, JA, Vogel FS, Burger PC. Increasing incidence of primary brain lymphoma in the US. Cancer 1988;62:2461.
65. Edwards MS, Wara WM, Urtasun RC, Prados M, Levin VA, Fulton D, Wilson CB, Hannigan J, Silver P. Hyperfractionated radiation therapy for brain-stem glioma: a phase I-II trial. J Neurosurg 1989;70:691.
66. el-Azouzi M, Chung RY, Farmer GE, Martuza RL, Black PM, Rouleau GA, Hettlich C, Hedley-Whyte ET, Zervas NT, Panagopoulos K, Nakamura Y, Gusella J, Seizinger B. Loss of distinct regions on the short arm of chromosome 17 associated with tumorigenesis of human astrocytomas. Proc Natl Acad Sci USA 1989;86:7186.
67. Ekstrand AJ, James CD, Cavenee WK, Seliger B, Pettersson RF, Collins VP. Genes for epidermal growth factor receptor, transforming growth factor alpha, and epidermal growth factor and their expression in human gliomas. Cancer Res 1991;51:2164.
68. Ellis F. Dose, time and fractionation: a clinical hypothesis. Clin Radiol 1969;20:1.
69. Engelhard HH III, Butler AB IV, Bauer KD. Quantification of the c-*myc* oncoprotein in human glioblastoma cells and tumor tissue. J Neurosurg 1989;71:224.
70. Epstein F. Spinal cord astrocytomas of childhood. Prog Exp Tumor Res 1987;30:135.
71. Epstein F, Wisoff J. Surgical management of brain stem tumors of childhood and adolescence. Neurosurg Clin North Am 1990;1:111.
72. Ernestus RI, Wilcke O, Schroder R. Intracranial ependymomas: prognostic aspects. Neurosurg Rev 1989;12:157.
73. Evans AE, Jenkin RDT, Sposto R, Ortega JA, Wilson CB, Wara W, Ertel IJ, Kramer S, Chang CH, Leiken SL, Hammond GD. The treatment of medulloblastoma. Results of a prospective randomized trial of radiation therapy with and without CCNU, vincristine, and prednisone. J Neurosurg 1990;72:572.
74. Farwell JR, Dohrmann GJ, Flannery JT. Central nervous system tumors in children. Cancer 1977;40:3123.
75. Fazekas JT. Treatment of grades I and II brain astrocytomas. The role of radiotherapy. Int J Radiat Oncol Biol Phys 1977;2:661.
76. Fearon ER, Hamilton SR, Vogelstein B. Clonal analysis of human colorectal tumors. Science 1987;238:193.
77. Finlay J, August C, Packer R, Zimmerman R, Sutton L, Nachman J, Levin A, Turski P, Steeves R, Longo W, Javid M. High-dose chemotherapy with autologous marrow rescue in children with recurrent brain tumor. In Autologous Bone Marrow Transplantation. Proceedings of the Fourth International Symposium. Edited by KA Dicke, G Spitzer, S Jagannath, and MJ Eringer-Hodges. Houston: University of Texas MD Anderson Cancer Center, 1989, p 449.
78. Finlay JL, Goins SC. Brain tumors in children. III. Advances in chemotherapy. Am J Pediatr Hematol Oncol 1987;9:264.
79. Follezou J, Fauchon F, Chiras J. Intra-arterial infusion of carboplatin in the treatment of malignant gliomas: a phase II study. Neoplasma 1989;36:349.
80. Formenti SC, Gill PS, Lean E, Rarick M, Meyer PR, Boswell W, Petrovich Z, Chak L, Levine AM. Primary central nervous system lymphoma in AIDS. Results of radiation therapy. Cancer 1989;63:1101.
81. Francavilla TL, Miletich RS, Di Chiro G, Patronas NJ, Rizzoli HV, Wright DC. Positron emission tomography in the detection of malignant degeneration of low-grade gliomas. Neurosurgery 1989;24:1.
82. Freeman CR, Krischer J, Sanford RA, Burger PC, Cohen M, Norris D. Hyperfractionated radiotherapy in brain stem tumors: results of a Pediatric Oncology Group study. Int J Radiat Oncol Biol Phys 1988;15:311.
83. Friedman HS, Colvin OM, Skapek SX, Ludeman SM, Elion GB, Schold SC Jr, Jacobsen PF, Muhlbaier LH, Bigner DD. Experimental chemotherapy of human medulloblastoma cell lines and transplantable xenografts with bifunctional alkylating agents. Cancer Res 1988;48:4189.
84. Friedman HS, Krischer JP, Burger P, Oakes WJ, Hockenberger B, Weiner MD, Falletta JM, Norris D, Ragab AH, Mahoney DH Jr, et al. Treatment of children with progressive or recurrent brain tumors with carboplatin or iproplatin: a Pediatric Oncology Group randomized phase II study. J Clin Oncol 1992;10:249.
85. Friedman HS, Oakes WJ. The chemotherapy of posterior fossa tumors in childhood. J Neurooncol 1987;5:217.
86. Fujimoto M, Fults DW, Thomas GA, Nakamura Y, Heilbrun MP, White R, Story JL, Naylor SL, Kagan-Hallet KS, Sheridan PJ. Loss of heterozygosity on chromosome 10 in human glioblastoma multiforme. Genomics 1989;4:210.
87. Fujimoto M, Sheridan PJ, Sharp ZD, Weaker FJ, Kagan-Hallet S, Story JL. Proto-oncogene analyses in brain tumors. J Neurosurg 1989;70:910.
88. Fults D, Tippets R, Thomas A, Nakamura Y, White R. Loss of heterozygosity for loci on chromosome 17p in human malignant astrocytoma. Cancer Res 1989;49:6572.
89. Gabbai AA, Hochberg FH, Linggood RM, Bashir R, Hotleman K. High-dose methotrexate for non-AIDS primary central nervous system lymphoma. Report of 13 cases. J Neurosurg 1989;70:190.
90. Garcia DM, Latifi HR, Simpson JR, Picker S. Astrocytomas of the cerebellum in children. J Neurosurg 1989;71:661.
91. Gerosa MA, Talarico D, Fognani C, Raimondi E, Colombatti M, Tridente G, De Carli L, Della Valle G. Overexpression on N-ras oncogene and epidermal growth factor receptor gene in human glioblastomas. JNCI 1989;81:63.
92. Gol A. The relatively benign astrocytomas of the cerebrum. J Neurosurg 1961;18:501.
93. Green JR, Waggener JD, Kriegsfeld BA. Classification and incidence of neoplasms of the central nervous system. Adv Neurol 1976;15:51.
94. Green S, Byar D, Strike T. Randomized comparisons of BCNU, streptozotocin, radiosensitizer, and fractionation in the postoperative treatment of malignant glioma (study 77–02) (abstract). Proc Am Soc Clin Oncol 1984;3:260.
95. Green SB, Byar DP, Walker MD, Pistenmaa DA, Alexander E Jr, Batzdorf U, Brooks WH, Hunt WE, Mealey J Jr, Odom GL, Paoletti P, Ransohoff J Jr, Robertson JT, Selker RG, Shapiro WR, Smith KR Jr, Wilson CB, Strike TA. Comparisons of carmustine, procarbazine, and high-dose methylprednisolone as additions to surgery and radiotherapy for the treatment of malignant glioma. Cancer Treat Rep 1983;67:121.
96. Greenberg HS, Chandler WF, Diaz RF, Ensminger WD, Junck L, Page MA, Gebarski SS, McKeever P, Hood TW, Stetson PL, Litchter AS, Tankanow R. Intra-arterial bromodeoxyuridine radiosensitization and radiation in treatment of malignant astrocytomas. J Neurosurg 1988;69:500.
97. Greig NH, Ries LG, Yancik R, Rapoport SI. Increasing annual incidence of primary malignant brain tumors in the elderly. JNCI 1990;82:1621.
98. Griffin CA, Hawkins AL, Packer RJ, Rorke LB, Emanuel BS. Chromosome abnormalities in pediatric brain tumors. Cancer Res 1988;48:175.
99. Gutherie BL, Ebersold MJ, Scheithaner BW. Neoplasms of the intracranial meninges. In Neurological Surgery: A Comprehensive Reference Guide to the Diagnosis and Treatment of Neurosurgical Problems, 3rd Edition. Edited by JR Youmans. Philadelphia: Saunders, 1990, p 3263.
100. Gutin PH. Personal communication 1990.
101. Gutin PH, Prados MD, Phillips TL, Wara WM, Larson DA, Leibel SA, Sneed PK, Levin VA, Weaver KA, Silver P, Lamborn K, Lamb S, Ham B. External irradiation followed by an interstitial high activity iodine-125 implant "boost" in the initial treatment of malignant gliomas: NCOG study 6G-82–2. Int J Radiat Oncol Biol Phys 1991;21:601.
102. Harsh GR IV, Levin VA, Gutin PH, Seager M, Silver P, Wilson CB. Reoperation for recurrent glioblastoma and anaplastic astrocytoma. Neurosurgery 1987;21:615.
103. Harsh GR IV, Wilson CB. Neuroepithelial tumors of the adult brain. In Neurological Surgery: A Comprehensive Reference Guide to the Diagnosis and Treatment of Neurosurgical Problems, 3rd Edition. Edited by JR Youmans. Philadelphia: Saunders, 1990, p 3040.
104. Heindel W, Bunke J, Glathe S, Steinbrich W, Mollevanger L. Combined 1H-MR imaging and localized 31P-spectroscopy of intracranial tumors in 43 patients. J Comput Assist Tomogr 1988;12:907.
105. Helle TL, Britt RH, Colby TV. Primary lymphoma of the central nervous system. Clinicopathological study of experience at Stanford. J Neurosurg 1984;60:94.
106. Hochberg FH, Miller DC. Primary central nervous system lymphoma. J Neurosurg 1988;68:835.
107. Hochberg FH, Parker LM, Takvorian T, Canellos GP, Zervas NT. High-dose BCNU with autologous bone marrow rescue for recurrent glioblastoma multiforme. J Neurosurg 1981;54:455.
108. Hochberg FH, Pruitt A. Assumptions in the radiotherapy of glioblastoma. Neurology 1980;30:907.
109. Hoffman HJ. Craniopharyngiomas. Can J Neurol Sci 1985;12:348.
110. Hoffman HJ. Craniopharyngiomas: the role for resection. Neurosurg Clin North Am 1990;1:173.
111. Hoshino T. Radiosensitization of brain tumors. In Central Nervous System Tumors. Modern Radiotherapy and Oncology series. Edited by TJ Deeley. London: Butterworth, 1974, p 170.
112. Hoshino TA. Commentary on the biology and growth kinetics of low-grade and high-grade gliomas. J Neurosurg 1984;61:895.
113. Hoshino T, Prados M, Wilson CB, Cho KG, Lee KS, Davis RL. Prognostic implications of the bromodeoxyuridine labeling index of human gliomas. J Neurosurg 1989;71:335.
114. Hoshino T, Rodriquez LA, Cho KG, Lee KS, Wilson CB, Edwards MS, Levin VA, Davis RL. Prognostic implications of the proliferative potential of low-grade astrocytomas. J Neurosurg 1988;69:839.
115. Hubbard JL, Scheithauer BW, Kispert DB, Carpenter SM, Wick MR, Laws ER Jr. Adult cerebellar medulloblastomas: the pathological, radiographic, and clinical disease spectrum. J Neurosurg 1989;70:536.
116. Hubesch B, Sappey-Marinier D, Roth K, Meyerhoff DJ, Matson GB, Weiner MW. $_{31}$P NMR spectroscopy of normal brain and brain tumors. Radiology 1990;174:401.
117. Ibelgaufts H. DNA viruses and brain tumors. Trends Neurosci 1982;5:16.
118. Inoue H, Tamura M, Koizumi H, Nakamura M, Naganuma H, Ohye C. Clinical pathology of malignant meningiomas. Acta Neurochir (Wien) 1984;73:179.
119. James CD, Carlbom E, Dumanski JP, Hansen M, Nordenskjold M, Collins VP, Cavenee WK. Clonal genomic alterations in glioma malignancy stages. Cancer Res 1988;48:5546.
120. Jeffries BF, Kishore PR, Singh KS, Ghatak NR, Krempa J. Contrast enhancement in the postoperative brain. Radiology 1981;139:409.
121. Jellinger K. Primary intracranial germ cell tumours. Acta Neuropathol (Berl) 1973;25:291.
122. Jenkin RD, Simpson WJ, Keen CW. Pineal and suprasellar germinomas. Results of radiation treatment. J Neurosurg 1978;48:99.
123. Jennings M, Gelman R, Hochberg F. Intracranial germ-cell tumors: natural history and pathogenesis. In Diagnosis and Treatment of Pineal Region Tumors. Edited by EA Neuwelt. Baltimore: Williams & Wilkins, 1984, p 166.
124. Jennings MT, Gelman R, Hochberg F. Intracranial germ-cell tumors: natural history and pathogenesis. J Neurosurg 1985;63:155.
125. Jimenez O, Timms A, Quirke P, McLaughlin JE. Prognosis in malignant glioma: a retrospective study of biopsy specimens by flow cytometry. Neuropathol Appl Neurobiol 1989;15:331.
126. Kaplan WD, Takvorian T, Morris JH, Rumbaugh CL, Connolly BT, Atkins HL. Thallium-201 brain tumor imaging: a comparative study with pathologic correlation. J Nucl Med 1987;28:47.
127. Karlsson U, Brady L. Tumors of the spinal cord and canal. In Principles and Practice of Radiation Oncology. Edited by CA Perez, LW Brady. Philadelphia: Lippincott, 1987, p 437.
128. Karnofsky DA, Burchenal JH. The clinical evaluation of chemotherapeutic agents in

cancer. In Evaluation of Chemotherapeutic Agents. Edited by CM MacLeod. New York: Columbia University, 1949, p 122.
129. Kelly PJ, Daumas-Duport C, Scheithauer BW, Kall BA, Kispert DB. Stereotactic histologic correlations of computed tomography- and magnetic resonance imaging-defined abnormalities in patients with glial neoplasms. Mayo Clin Proc 1987;62:450.
130. Kernohan J, Mabon R, Svien H, Adson A. A simplified classification of gliomas. Proc Staff Mayo Clin 1949;24:71.
131. King DL, Chang CH, Pool JL. Radiotherapy in the management of meningiomas. Acta Radiol Ther Phys Biol 1966;5:26.
132. Kinsella TJ, Russo A, Mitchell JB, Collins JM, Rowland J, Wright D, Glatstein E. A phase I study of intravenous iododeoxyuridine as a clinical radiosensitizer. Int J Radiat Oncol Biol Phys 1985;11:1941.
133. Kinzler KW, Ruppert JM, Bigner SH, Vogelstein B. The GLI gene is a member of the Kruppel family of zinc finger proteins. Nature 1988;332:371.
134. Kleihues P, Burger PC, Scheithauer BW. Histological Typing of Tumours of the Central Nervous System. World Health Organization International Histological Classification of Tumors, 2nd Edition. Berlin: Springer-Verlag, 1993, pp 11–16.
135. Kornblith PL, Walker M. Chemotherapy for malignant brain tumors. J Neurosurg 1988;68:1, J Neurosurg 1988;69:645 (erratum).
136. Kurup PD, Pajak TF, Hendrickson FR, Nelson JS, Mansell J, Cohen L, Awschalom M, Rosenberg I, Ten Haken RK. Fast neutrons and misonidazole for malignant astrocytomas. Int J Radiat Oncol Biol Phys 1985;2:679.
137. Landberg TG, Lindgren ML, Cavallin-Stahl EK, Svahn-Tapper GO, Sundbarg G, Garwicz S, Lagergren JA, Gunnesson VL, Brun AE, Cronqvist SE. Improvements in the radiotherapy of medulloblastoma 1946–1975. Cancer 1980;45:670.
138. Laramore GE, Diener-West M, Griffin TW, Nelson JS, Griem ML, Thomas FJ, Hendrickson FR, Griffin BR, Myrianthopoulos LC, Saxton J. Randomized neutron dose searching study for malignant gliomas of the brain: results of an RTOG study. Radiation Therapy Oncology Group. Int J Radiat Oncol Biol Phys 1988;14:1093.
139. Lashford LS, Davies AG, Richardson RB, Bourne SP, Bullimore JA, Eckert H, Kemshead JT, Coakham HB. A pilot study of 131-I monoclonal antibodies in the therapy of leptomeningeal tumors. Cancer 1988;61:857.
140. Laws ER Jr, Taylor WF, Bergstralh EJ, Okazaki H, Clifton MB. The neurosurgical management of low-grade astrocytoma. Clin Neurosurg 1986;33:575.
141. Laws ER Jr, Taylor WF, Clifton MB, Okazaki H. Neurosurgical management of low-grade astrocytoma of the cerebral hemispheres. J Neurosurg 1984;61:665.
142. Lee JS, Murphy WK, Glisson BS, Dhingra HM, Holoye PY, Hong WK. Primary chemotherapy of brain metastases in small-cell lung cancer. J Clin Oncol 1989;7:916.
143. Lee YY, Van Tassel P, Bruner JM, Moser RP, Share JC. Juvenile pilocytic astrocytomas: CT and MR characteristics. AJR 1989;152:1263.
144. Leibel SA, Gutin PH, Sneed PK, Prados M, Levin VA, Larson DA, Wara WM, Weaver KA, Phillips TL. Interstitial irradiation for the treatment of primary and metastatic brain tumors. Principles and Practice of Oncology Update Series 1989;3:1.
145. Leibel SA, Gutin PH, Wara WM, Silver PS, Larson DA, Edwards MS, Lamb SA, Ham B, Weaver KA, Barnett C, Phillips TL. Survival and quality of life after interstitial implantation of removable high-activity iodine-125 sources for the treatment of patients with recurrent malignant gliomas. Int J Radiat Oncol Biol Phys 1989;17:1129.
146. Leibel SA, Sheline GE, Wara WM, Boldrey EB, Nielsen SL. The role of radiation therapy in the treatment of astrocytomas. Cancer 1975;35:1551.
147. Levin VA. Chemotherapy of recurrent brain tumors. In Nitrosoureas: Current Status and New Developments. Edited by AW Prestayko and ST Crooke. New York: Academic, 1981, p 159.
148. Levin VA. Chemotherapy of primary brain tumors. Neurol Clin 1985;3:855.
149. Levin VA. Personal communication 1990.
150. Levin VA, Chamberlain MC, Prados MD, Choucair AK, Berger MS, Silver P, Seager M, Gutin PH, Davis RL, Wilson CB. Phase I-II study of eflornithine and mitoguazone combined in the treatment of recurrent primary brain tumors. Cancer Treat Rep 1987;71:459.
151. Levin VA, Edwards MS, Gutin PH, Vestnys P, Fulton D, Seager M, Wilson CB. Phase II evaluation of dibromodulcitol in the treatment of recurrent medulloblastoma, ependymoma, and malignant astrocytoma. J Neurosurg 1984;61:1063.
152. Levin VA, Edwards MS, Wara WM, Allen J, Ortega J, Vestnys P. 5-Fluorouracil and 1-(2-chloroethyl)-3-cyclohexyl-1-nitrosourea (CCNU) followed by hydroxyurea, misonidazole, and irradiation for brain stem gliomas. A pilot study of the Brain Tumor Research Center and the Childrens Cancer Group. Neurosurgery 1984;14:679.
153. Levin VA, Edwards MS, Wright DC, Seager ML, Schimberg TP, Townsend JJ, Wilson CB. Modified procarbazine, CCNU, and vincristine (PCV 3) combination chemotherapy in the treatment of malignant brain tumors. Cancer Treat Rep 1980;64:237.
154. Levin VA, Prados MD, et al. Unpublished data 1990.
155. Levin VA, Prados MD, Yung WKA, Gleason MJ, Ictech S, Malec M. Treatment of recurrent glioma with eflornithine. JNCI 1992;84:1432.
156. Levin VA, Rodriguez LA, Edwards MS, Wara W, Liu H-C, Fulton D, Davis RL, Wilson CB, Silver P. Treatment of medulloblastoma with procarbazine, hydroxyurea, and reduced radiation doses to whole brain and spine. J Neurosurg 1988;68:383.
157. Levin VA, Silver P, Hannigan J, Wara WM, Gutin PH, Davis RL, Wilson CB. Superiority of post-radiotherapy adjuvant chemotherapy with CCNU, procarbazine, and vincristine (PCV) over BCNU for anaplastic gliomas: NCOG 6G61 final report. Int J Radiat Oncol Biol Phys 1990;18:321.
158. Levin VA, Vestnys PS, Edwards MS, Wara WM, Fulton D, Barger G, Seager M, Wilson CB. Improvement in survival produced by sequential therapies in the treatment of recurrent medulloblastoma. Cancer 1983;51:1364.
159. Levin VA, Wara WM, Gutin PH, Wilson CB, Phillips TL, Prados MD, Flam MS, Ahn D. Initial analysis of NCOG 6G-82–1: bromodeoxyuridine (BUdR) during irradiation followed by CCNU, procarbazine, and vincristine (PCV) chemotherapy for malignant gliomas (abstract). Proc Am Soc Clin Oncol 1990;9:91.
160. Levy RM, Bredesen DE, Rosenblum ML. Neurological manifestations of the acquired immunodeficiency syndrome (AIDS): Experience at UCSF and review of the literature. J Neurosurg 1985;62:475.
161. Lindegaard KF, Mtork SJ, Eide GE, Halvorsen TB, Hatlevoll R, Solgaard T, Dahl O, Ganz J. Statistical analysis of clinicopathological features, radiotherapy, and survival in 170 cases of oligodendroglioma. J Neurosurg 1987;67:224.
162. Linstadt DE, Wara WM, Leibel SA, Gutin PH, Wilson CB, Sheline GE. Postoperative radiotherapy of primary spinal cord tumors. Int J Radiat Oncol Biol Phys 1989;16:1397.
163. Littman P, Jarret P, Bilanuik LT, Rorke LB, Zimmerman RA, Bruce DA, Carabell SC, Schut L. Pediatric brain stem gliomas. Cancer 1980;45:2787.
164. Liu H, Davis R, Vestnys P, Resser K, Levin V. Correlation of survival and diagnosis in supratentorial malignant gliomas. J Neurooncol 1984;2:268.
165. Loeffler JS, Kooy HM, Wen PY, Fine HA, Cheng CW, Mannarino EG, Tsai JS, Alexander E III. The treatment of recurrent brain metastases with stereotactic radiosurgery. J Clin Oncol 1990;8:576, J Clin Oncol 1990;8:571 (comment).
166. Loeffler JS, Wen P, Fine H, Alexander E. The treatment of recurrent brain metastasis with stereotactic radiosurgery (abstract). Proc Am Soc Clin Oncol 1990;9:91.
167. Ludwig CL, Smith MT, Godfrey AD, Armbrustmacher VW. A clinicopathological study of 323 patients with oligodendrogliomas. Ann Neurol 1986;19:15.
168. Lunsford LD, Flickinger J, Lindner G, Maitz A. Stereotactic radiosurgery of the brain using the first United States 201 cobalt-60 source gamma knife. Neurosurgery 1989;24:151.
169. Mahaley MS Jr, Hipp SW, Dropcho EJ, Bertsch L, Cush S, Tirey T, Gillespie GY. Intracarotid cisplatin chemotherapy for recurrent gliomas. J Neurosurg 1989;70:371.
170. Mahaley MS Jr, Mettlin C, Natarajan N, Laws ER Jr, Peace BB. National survey of patterns of care for brain-tumor patients. J Neurosurg 1989;71:826.
171. Mahaley MS Jr, Urso MB, Whaley RA, Blue M, Williams TE, Guaspari A, Selker RG. Immunobiology of primary intracranial tumors. Part 10: therapeutic efficacy of interferon in the treatment of recurrent gliomas. J Neurosurg 1985;63:719.
172. Malkin D, Li FP, Strong LC, Fraumeni JF Jr, Nelson CE, Kim DH, Kassel J, Gryka MA, Bischoff FZ, Tainsky MA. Germ line p53 mutations in a familial syndrome of breast cancer, sarcomas, and other neoplasms. Science 1990;250:1233.
173. Maltoni C. Occupational carcinogenesis Predictive value of carcinogenesis bioassays. Ann NY Acad Sci 1976;271:431.
174. Maltoni C, Ciliberti A, Caretti D. Experimental contributions in identifying brain potential carcinogens in the petrochemical industry. Ann NY Acad Sci 1982;381:216.
175. Malone M, Lumley H, Erdohazi M. Astrocytoma as a second malignancy in patients with acute lymphoblastic leukemia. Cancer 1979;57:1986.
176. Marsh WL Jr, Stevenson DR, Long HJ III. Primary leptomeningeal presentation of T-cell lymphoma. Report of a patient and review of the literature. Cancer 1983;51:1125.
177. Martuza RL, Eldridge R. Neurofibromatosis 2 (bilateral acoustic neurofibromatosis). N Engl J Med 1988;318:684.
178. McLaughlin P, Velasquez WS, Redman JR, Yung WK, Hagemeister FB, Rodriguez MA, Cabanillas F. Chemotherapy with dexamethasone, high-dose cytarabine, and cisplatin for parenchymal brain lymphoma. JNCI 1988;80:1408.
179. Mercer WE, Shields MT, Amin M, Sauve GJ, Apella E, Romano JW, Ullrich SJ. Negative growth regulation in a glioblastoma cell line that conditionally expresses human wild-type p53. Proc Natl Acad Sci USA 1990;87:6166.
180. Merchant R, McVicar D, Merchant L, Young H. Treatment of patients with recurrent glioblastoma by repeated intralesional injections of recombinant interleukin-2 alone or in combination with systemic interferon-alpha (abstract). J Neurooncol 1989;7:S19.
181. Merchant RE, Ellison MD, Young HF. Immunotherapy for malignant glioma using human recombinant interleukin-2 and activated autologous lymphocytes. A review of pre-clinical and clinical investigations. J Neurooncol 1990;8:173.
182. Mirimanoff RO, Dosoretz DE, Linggood RM, Ojemann RG, Martuza RL. Meningioma analysis of recurrence and progression following neurosurgical resection. J Neurosurg 1985;62:18.
183. Mtork SJ, Lindegaard KF, Halvorsen TB, Lehmann EH, Solgaard T, Hatlevoll R, Harvei S, Ganz J. Oligodendroglioma. Incidence and biological behavior in a defined population. J Neurosurg 1985;63:881.
184. Mtork SJ, Rubinstein LJ. Ependymoblastoma. A reappraisal of a rare embryonal tumor. Cancer 1985;55:1536.
185. Moseley RP, Davies AG, Bourne SP, Popham C, Carrel S, Monro P, Coakham HB. Neoplastic meningitis in malignant melanoma: diagnosis with monoclonal antibodies. J Neurol Neurosurg Psychiatry 1989;52:881.
186. Moseley RP, Oge K, Shafqat S, Moseley CM, Sullivan NM, Badley RA, Burchell J, Taylor-Papadimitriou J, Coakham HB. HFMG1 antigen. A new marker for carcinomatous meningitis. Int J Cancer 1989;44:440.
187. Mountz JM, Stafford-Schuck K, McKeever PE, Taren J, Beierwaltes WH. Thallium-201 tumor/cardiac ratio estimation of residual astrocytoma. J Neurosurg 1988;68:705.
188. Nelson D, Curran E, Nelson J, Weinstein A, Martz K, Ahmad K, Keller J, Murray K, Hanks G. Hyperfractionation in malignant glioma. Report on a dose searching phase I/II protocol of the Radiation Therapy Oncology Group (RTOG) (abstract). Proc Am Soc Clin Oncol 1990;9:90.
189. Nelson DF, Curran WJ Jr, Scott C, Nelson JS, Weinstein AS, Ahmad K, Constine LS, Murray K, Powlis WD, Mohiuddin M, et al. Hyperfractionated radiation therapy and bis-chlorethyl nitrosourea in the treatment of malignant glioma—possible advantage observed at 72.0 Gy on 1.2 Gy B.I.D. fractions: report of the Radiation Therapy Oncology Group protocol 8302. Int J Radiat Oncol Biol Phys 1991;25:193.
190. Nelson DF, Diener-West M, Horton J, Chang CH, Schoenfeld D, Nelson JS. Combined modality approach to treatment of malignant gliomas—re-evaluation of RTOG 7401/ECOG 1374 with long-term follow-up: a joint study of the Radiation Therapy Oncology Group and the Eastern Cooperative Oncology Group. NCI Monogr 1988;6:279–284.
191. Nelson DF, Nelson JS, Davis DR, Chang CH, Griffin TW, Pajak TF. Survival and prognosis of patients with astrocytoma with atypical or anaplastic features. J Neurooncol 1985;3:99.
192. Nelson DF, Schoenfeld D, Weinstein AS, Nelson JS, Wasserman T, Goodman RL, Carabell S. A randomized comparison of misonidazole sensitized radiotherapy plus BCNU and radiotherapy plus BCNU for treatment of malignant glioma after surgery: preliminary results of an RTOG study. Int J Radiat Oncol Biol Phys 1983;9:1143.
193. Nelson JS, Tsukada Y, Schoenfield D, Fulling K, Lamarche J, Peress N. Necrosis as a prognostic criterion in malignant supratentorial, astrocytic gliomas. Cancer 1983;52:550.
194. Neuwelt EA, Frenkel EP, Gumerlock M, Braziel R, Dana B, Hill SA. Developments in the diagnosis and treatment of primary CNS lymphoma. A prospective series. Cancer 1986;58:1609.
195. Newton HB, Page MA, Junck L, Greenberg HS. Intra-arterial cisplatin for the treatment of malignant gliomas. J Neurooncol 1989;7:39.
196. Nishizaki T, Orita T, Furutani Y, Ikeyama Y, Aoki H, Sasaki K. Flow-cytometric DNA

analysis and immunohistochemical measurement of Ki-67 and BUdR labeling indices in human brain tumors. J Neurosurg 1989;70:379.
197. Non-Hodgkin's Lymphoma Pathologic Classification Project. National Cancer Institute sponsored study of classifications of non-Hodgkin's lymphomas: summary and description of a working formulation for clinical usage. Cancer 1982;49:2112.
198. Ojemann G, Ojemann J, Lettich E, Berger M. Cortical language localization in left, dominant hemisphere. An electrical stimulation mapping investigation in 117 patients. J Neurosurg 1989;71:316.
199. Onimus M, Schraub S, Bertin D, Bosset JF, Guidet M. Surgical treatment of vertebral metastasis. Spine 1986;11:883.
200. Packer R, Finlay J. Medulloblastoma presentation, diagnosis, and management. Oncology 1988;2:35.
201. Packer RJ, Lange B, Ater J, Nicolson HS, Allen J, Walker R, Prados M, Jakacki R, Reaman G, Needles MN, Phillips PC, Ryan J, Boyett JM, Geyer R, Finlay J. Carboplatin and vincristine for recurrent and newly diagnosed low-grade gliomas of childhood. J Clin Oncol 1993;11:850–856.
202. Packer RJ, Littman PA, Sposto RM, D'Angio G, Priest JR, Heideman RL, Bruce DA, Nelson DF. Results of a pilot study of hyperfractionated radiation therapy for children with brain stem gliomas. Int J Radiat Oncol Biol Phys 1987;13:1647.
203. Packer RJ, Siegel KR, Sutton LN, Evans AE, D'Angio G, Rorke LB, Bunin GR, Schut L. Efficacy of adjuvant chemotherapy for patients with poor-risk medulloblastoma: a preliminary report. Ann Neurol 1988;24:503.
204. Packer RJ, Sposto R, Atkins TE, Sutton LN, Bruce DA, Siegel KR, Rorke LB, Littman PA, Schut L. Quality of life in children with primitive neuroectodermal tumors (medulloblastoma) of the posterior fossa. Pediatr Neurosci 1987;13:169.
205. Packer RJ, Sutton LN, Bilaniuk LT, Radcliffe J, Rosenstock JG, Siegel KR, Bunin GR, Savino PJ, Bruce DA, Schut L. Treatment of chiasmatic/hypothalamic gliomas of childhood with chemotherapy: an update. Ann Neurol 1988;23:79.
206. Packer RJ, Sutton LN, Rorke LB, Littman PA, Sposto R, Rosenstock JG, Bruce DA, Schut L. Prognostic importance of cellular differentiation in medulloblastoma of childhood. J Neurosurg 1984;61:296.
207. Packer RJ, Zimmerman RA, Luerssen TG, Sutton LN, Bilaniuk LT, Bruce DA, Schut L. Brainstem gliomas of childhood: magnetic resonance imaging. Neurology 1985;35: 397.
208. Palmiter RD, Brinster RL. Transgenic mice. Cell 1985;41:343.
209. Patchell RA, Cirrincione C, Thaler HT, Galicich JH, Kim JH, Posner JB. Single brain metastases: surgery plus radiation or radiation alone. Neurology 1986;36:447.
210. Patchell RA, Tibbs PA, Walsh JW, Dempsey RJ, Maruyama Y, Kryscio RJ, Markesbery WR, MacDonald JS, Young BA. Randomized trial of surgery in the treatment of single brain metastases to the brain. N Engl J Med 1990;322:494, N Engl J Med 1990;322:544 (comment)
211. Pattengale PK, Taylor CR, Panke T, Tatter D, McCormick RA, Rawlinson DG, Davis RL. Selective immunodeficiency and malignant lymphoma of the central nervous system. Possible relationship to the Epstein-Barr virus. Acta Neuropathol (Berl) 1979;48: 165.
212. Pendergrass TW, Milstein JM, Geyer JR, Mulne AF, Kosnik EJ, Morris JD, Heideman RL, Ruymann FB, Stuntz JT, Bleyer WA. Eight drugs in one day chemotherapy for brain tumors: experience in 107 children and rationale for preirradiation chemotherapy. J Clin Oncol 1987;5:1221.
213. Petronio J, Edwards MS, Prados M, Freyberger S, Rabbitt J, Silver P, Levin VA. Management of chiasmal and hypothalamic gliomas of infancy and childhood with chemotherapy. J Neurosurg 1991;74:701.
214. Piepmeier JM. Observations on the current treatment of low-grade astrocytic tumors of the cerebral hemispheres. J Neurosurg 1987;67:177.
215. Pollack IF, Lunsford LD, Flickinger JC, Dameshek HL. Prognostic factors in the diagnosis and treatment of primary central nervous system lymphoma. Cancer 1989;63: 939.
216. Posner JB, Chernik NL. Intracranial metastases from systemic cancer. Adv Neurol 1978;19:579.
217. Prados MD, Gutin PH, Phillips TL, Wara WM, Sneed PK, Larson DA, Lamb SA, Ham B, Malec M, Wilson CB. Interstitial brachytherapy for newly diagnosed patients with malignant gliomas: the UCSF experience. Int J Radiat Oncol Biol Phys 1992;24:593.
218. Prados M, Leibel S, Barnett CM, Gutin P. Interstitial brachytherapy for metastatic brain tumors. Cancer 1989;63:657.
219. Prados M, Rodriguez L, Chamberlain M, Silver P, Levin V. Treatment of recurrent gliomas with 1, 3-bis(2-chloroethyl)1-nitrosourea and alpha-difluoromethylornithine. Neurosurgery 1989;24:806.
220. Prados MD. Unpublished data 1990.
221. Prados MD, Wara WM, Edwards MSB, Cogen PH. Hyperfractionated craniospinal radiation therapy for primitive neuroectodermal tumors: early results of a pilot study. Int J Radiat Oncol Biol Phys 1994;28:431–438.
222. Prados MD, Wara WM, Edwards MSB, Larson DA, Lamborn K, Lavin VA. The treatment of brain stem and thalamic gliomas with 78 Gy of hyperfractionated radiation therapy. Int J Radiat Oncol Biol Phys 1995;32:85–91.
223. Press RD, Misra A, Gillaspy G, Samols D, Goldthwait DA. Control of the expression of *c-sis* mRNA in human glioblastoma cells by phorbol ester and transforming growth factor beta 1. Cancer Res 1989;49:2914.
224. Raffel C, Edwards MS. Intraspinal tumors in children. In Neurological Surgery: A Comprehensive Reference Guide to the Diagnosis and Treatment of Neurosurgical Problems, 3rd Edition. Edited by JR Youmans. Philadelphia: Saunders 1990, p 3574.
225. Raffel C, Edwards MS, Davis RL, Ablin AR. Postirradiation cerebellar glioma. Case report. J Neurosurg 1985;62:300.
226. Read G. The treatment of ependymoma of the brain or spinal canal by radiotherapy: a report of 79 cases. Clin Radiol 1984;35:163.
227. Ringertz N. Grading of gliomas. Acta Pathol Microbiol Scand 1950;27:51.
228. Rodesch G, Van Bogaert P, Mavroudakis N, Parizel PM, Martin JJ, Segebarth C, Van Vyve M, Baleriaux D, Hildebrand J. Neuroradiologic findings in leptomeningeal carcinomatosis: the value interest of gadolinium-enhanced MRI. Neuroradiology 1990;32:26.
229. Rorke LB. The cerebellar medulloblastoma and its relationship to primitive neuroectodermal tumors. J Neuropathol Exp Neurol 1983;42:1.
230. Rosenblum ML. Personal communication 1990.
231. Rosenblum ML. The role of surgery in brain tumor management. Neurosurg Clin North Am 1990;1:1.
232. Rosenblum ML, Levy RM, Bredesen DE. Overview of AIDS and the nervous system. In AIDS and the Nervous System. Edited by MA Rosenblum, RM Levy, DE Bredesen. New York: Raven, 1988, p 1.
233. Rosenblum ML, Levy RM, Bredesen DE, So YT, Wara W, Ziegler JL. Primary central nervous system lymphoma in patients with AIDS. Ann Neurol 1988;23:S13.
234. Rosenstock JG, Packer RJ, Bilaniuk L, Bruce DA, Radcliffe JL, Savino P. Chiasmatic optic glioma treated with chemotherapy. A preliminary report. J Neurosurg 1985;63: 862.
235. Rosner D, Nemoto T, Lane WW. Chemotherapy induces regression of brain metastases in breast carcinoma. Cancer 1986;58:832.
236. Ross GW, Rubinstein LJ. Lack of histopathological correlation of malignant ependymomas with postoperative survival. J Neurosurg 1989;70:31.
237. Rossi ML, Hughes JT, Esiri MM, Coakham HB, Brownwell DB. Immunohistological study of mononuclear cell infiltrate in malignant gliomas. Acta Neuropathol (Berl) 1987;74:269.
238. Roszman TL, Brooks WH, Elliott LH. Inhibition of lymphocyte responsiveness by a glial tumor cell-derived suppressive factor. J Neurosurg 1987;67:874.
239. Rubinstein AB, Shalit MN, Cohen ML, Zandbank U, Reichenthal E. Radiation-induced cerebral meningioma: a recognizable entity. J Neurosurg 1984;61:966.
240. Russell DS, Rubinstein LJ. Pathology of Tumours of the Nervous System, 4th ed. Baltimore: Williams & Wilkins, 1977.
241. Salazar OM, Castro-Vita H, VanHoutte P, Rubin P, Aygun C. Improved survival in cases of intracranial ependymoma after radiation therapy. Late report and recommendations. J Neurosurg 1983;59:652.
242. Salazar OM, Rubin P, Feldstein ML, Pizzutiello R. High dose radiation therapy in the treatment of malignant gliomas: final report. Int J Radiat Oncol Biol Phys 1979;5:1733.
243. Salcman M, Kaplan RS, Ducker TB, Abdo H, Montgomery E. Effect of age and reoperation on survival in the combined modality treatment of malignant astrocytoma. Neurosurgery 1982;10:454.
244. Saroja KR, Mansell J, Hendrickson FR, Cohen L, Lennox A. Failure of accelerated neutron therapy to control high grade astrocytomas. Int J Radiat Oncol Biol Phys 1989;17:1295.
245. Schmidek HH. Surgical management of pineal region tumors. In Pineal Tumors. Edited by HH Schmidek. New York: Masson, 1977 p 99.
246. Scotti G, Scialfa G, Colombo N, Landoni L. Magnetic resonance diagnosis of intramedullary tumors of the spinal cord. Neuroradiology 1987;29:130.
247. Segebarth CM, Baleriaux DF, Arnold DL, Luyten PR, den Hollander JA. MR image-guided P-31 MR spectroscopy in the evaluation of brain tumor treatment. Radiology 1987;165:215.
248. Sexauer CL, Khan A, Berger PC, Krischer JP, van Eys J, Vats T, Ragab AH. Cisplatin in recurrent pediatric brain tumors. A POG Phase II study. A Pediatric Oncology Group Study. Cancer 1985;56:1497.
249. Shapiro WR, Green SB. Reevaluating the efficacy of intra-arterial BCNU (letter). J Neurosurg 1987;66:313.
250. Shapiro WR, Green SB, Burger PC, Mahaley MS Jr, Selker RG, VanGilder JC, Robertson JT, Ransohoff J, Mealey J Jr, Strike TA, Pistenmaa DA. Randomized trial of three chemotherapy regimens and two radiotherapy regimens in postoperative treatment of malignant glioma. Brain Tumor Cooperative Group Trial 8001. J Neurosurg 1989;71:1.
251. Shaw EG, Daumas-Duport C, Scheithauer BW, Gilbertson DT, O'Fallon JR, Earle JD, Laws ER Jr, Okazaki H. Radiation therapy in the management of low-grade supratentorial astrocytomas. J Neurosurg 1989;70:853.
252. Shaw EG, Evans RG, Scheithauer BW, Ilstrup DM, Earle JD. Postoperative radiotherapy of intracranial ependymoma in pediatric and adult patients. Int J Radiat Oncol Biol Phys 1987;13:1457.
253. Sheline GE. Radiation therapy of primary tumors. Semin Oncol 1975;2:29.
254. Sheline GE, et al. Unpublished data 1990.
255. Sheline GE, Boldrey EB, Karlsberg P, Phillips TL. Therapeutic considerations in tumors affecting the central nervous system: oligodendrogliomas. Radiology 1964;82: 84.
256. Sheline GE, Wara WM, Smith V. Therapeutic irradiation and brain injury. Int J Radiat Oncol Biol Phys 1980;6:1215.
257. Sidransky D, Mikkelsen T, Schwechheimer K, Rosenblum ML, Cavanee W, Vogelstein B. Clonal expansion of p53 mutant cells is associated with brain tumor progression. Nature 1992;355:846.
258. Silverberg E. Cancer statistics 1986. CA 1986;36:9.
259. Silverberg E, Lubera JA. Cancer statistics 1989. CA 1989;39:3, CA 1989;39:254 (comment), CA 1989;39:399(comment).
260. Simeone F. Spinal cord tumors in adults. In Neurological Surgery: A Comprehensive Reference Guide to the Diagnosis and Treatment of Neurosurgical Problems, 3rd ed. Edited by JR Youmans. Philadelphia: Saunders, 1990, p 3531.
261. Simpson JR, Horton J, Scott C, Curran WJ, Rubin P, Fischbach J, Issacson S, Rotman M, Asbell SO, Nelson JS, et al. Influence of location and extent of surgical resection on survival of patients with glioblastoma multiforme: results of three consecutive Radiation Therapy Oncology Group (RTOG) clinical trials. Int J Radiat Oncol Biol Phys 1993;26:239–244.
262. Sneed PK, Gutin PH, Stauffer PR, Phillips TL, Prados MD, Weaver KA, Suen S, Lamb SA, Ham B, Ahn DK, Lamborn K, Larson DA, Wara WM. Thermoradiotherapy of recurrent malignant brain tumors. Int J Radiat Oncol Biol Phys 1992;23:853–861.
263. So YT, Choucair A, Davis RL, Wara WM, Ziegler JL, Sheline GE, Beckstead JH. Neoplasms of the central nervous system in acquired immunodeficiency syndrome. In AIDS and the Nervous System. Edited by ML Rosenblum, RL Levy, DE Bredesen. New York: Raven, 1988, p 285.
264. Sogg RL, Donaldson SS, Yorke CH. Malignant astrocytoma following radiotherapy of a craniopharyngioma. Case report. J Neurosurg 1978;48:622.
265. Spallone A, Gagliardi FM, Vagnozzi R. Intracranial meningiomas related to external cranial irradiation. Surg Neurol 1979;12:153.
266. Spencer DD, Spencer SS, Matson RH, Williamson PD. Intracerebral masses in patients with intractable partial epilepsy. Neurology 1984;34:432.
267. Stack JP, Antoun NM, Jenkins JP, Metcalf R, Isherwood I. Gadolinium-DPTA as a contrast agent in magnetic resonance imaging of the brain. Neuroradiology 1988;30:145.

268. Stein BM. Intramedullary spinal cord tumors. Clin Neurosurg 1983;30:717.
269. Stewart D, Grahovac Z, Hugenholtz H, Russell N, Richard M, Benoit B. Combined intraarterial and systemic chemotherapy for intracerebral tumors. Neurosurgery 1987;21:207.
270. Stewart D, Grahovac Z, Riding M. Intracarotid PCNU: an NCI Canada study (abstract). Proc Am Soc Clin Oncol 1986;5:A136.
271. Sundaresan N, Galicich JH. Surgical treatment of brain metastases. Clinical and computed tomography evaluation of the results of treatment. Cancer 1985;55:1382.
272. Sundaresan N, Galicich JH, Lane JM, Bains MS, McCormack P. Treatment of neoplastic epidural cord compression by vertebral body resection and stabilization. J Neurosurg 1985;63:676.
273. Sung DI, Harisliadis L, Chang CH. Midline pineal tumors and suprasellar germinomas: highly curable by irradiation. Radiology 1978;128:745.
274. Sutton L. Current management of low-grade astrocytomas of childhood. Pediatr Neurosci 1987;13:98.
275. Sutton LN, Wang Z, Gusnard D, Lange B, Perilongo G, Bogdan AR, Detre JA, Rorke L, Zimmerman RA. Proton magnetic resonance spectroscopy of pediatric brain tumors. Neurosurgery 1992;31:195.
276. Tait DM, Thornton-Jones H, Bloom HJ, Lemerle J, Morris-Jones P. Adjuvant chemotherapy for medulloblastoma: the first multi-centre control trial of the International Society of Paediatric Oncology (SIOP I). Eur J Cancer 1990;26:464.
277. Takemoto K, Matsumura Y, Hashimoto H, Inoue Y, Fukuda T, Shakudo M, Nemoto Y, Onoyama Y, Yasui T, Hakuba A, Nishimura S, Ban S. MR imaging of intraspinal tumors–capability in histological differentiation and compartmentalization of extramedullary tumors. Neuroradiology 1988;30:303.
278. Tomita T, McLone DG. Medulloblastoma in childhood: results of radical resection and low-dose neuraxis radiation therapy. J Neurosurg 1986;64:238.
279. U HS, Kelley PY, Hatton JD, Shew JY. Proto-oncogene abnormalities and their relationship to tumorigenicity in some human glioblastomas. J Neurosurg 1989;71: 83.
280. Urtasun R, Fulton D, Huyser-Wierenga D, Scott-Brown I, Shin K, Geggie P, Hanson J. Dose intensity in radiotherapy: "is more better" for patients with malignant gliomas (abstract)? Proc Am Soc Clin Oncol 1989;8:84.
281. Valk PE, Budinger TF, Levin VA, Silver P, Gutin PH, Doyle WK. PET of malignant cerebral tumors after interstitial brachytherapy. Demonstration of metabolic activity and correlation with clinical outcome. J Neurosurg 1988;69:830.
282. van Eys J, Baram TZ, Cangir A, Bruner JM, Martinez-Prietro J. Salvage chemotherapy for recurrent primary brain tumors in children. J Pediatr 1988;113:601.
283. Velema JP, Percy CL. Age curves of central nervous system tumor incidence in adults: variation of shape by histologic type. JNCI 1987;79:623.
284. Walker AE, Robins M, Weinfeld FD. Epidemiology of brain tumors: the national survey of intracranial neoplasms. Neurology 1985;35:219.
285. Walker MD, Alexander E Jr, Hunt WE, MacCarty CS, Mahaley MS Jr, Mealey J Jr, Norrell HA, Owens G, Ransohoff J, Wilson CB, Gehan EA, Strike TA. Evaluation of BCNU and/or radiotherapy in the treatment of anaplastic gliomas. A cooperative clinical trial. J Neurosurg 1978;49:333.
286. Walker MD, Green SB, Byar DP, Alexander E Jr, Batzdorf U, Brooks WH, Hunt WE, MacCarty CS, Mahaley MS Jr, Mealey J Jr, Owens G, Ransohoff J Jr, Robertson JT, Shapiro WR, Smith KR Jr, Wilson CB, Strike TA. Randomized comparisons of radiotherapy and nitrosoureas for the treatment of malignant glioma after surgery. N Engl J Med 1980;303:1323.
287. Walker MD, Strike TA, Sheline GE. An analysis of dose-effect relationship in the radiotherapy of malignant gliomas. Int J Radiat Oncol Biol Phys 1979;5:1725.
288. Wallner KE, Galicich JH, Krol G, Arbit E, Malkin MG. Patterns of failure following treatment for glioblastoma multiforme and anaplastic astrocytoma. Int J Radiat Oncol Biol Phys 1989;16:1405.
289. Wallner KE, Gonzales M, Sheline GE. Treatment of oligodendrogliomas with or without postoperative irradiation. J Neurosurg 1988;68:684.
290. Wara WM, Jenkin RD, Evans A, Ertel I, Hittle R, Ortega J, Wilson CB, Hammond D. Tumors of the pineal and suprasellar region. Children's Cancer Study Group treatment results 1960–1975: a report from the Children's Cancer Study Group. Cancer 1979;43:698.
291. Wara WM, Sheline GE, Newman H, Townsend JJ, Boldrey EB. Radiation therapy of meningiomas. Am J Roentgenol Radium Ther Nucl Med 1975;123:453.
292. Watson CJ, Gaunt L, Evans G, Patel K, Harris R, Strachan T. A disease-associated germline deletion maps the type 2 neurofibromatosis (NF2) gene between the Ewing sarcoma region and the leukaemia inhibitory factor locus. Hum Mol Genet 1993;2:701.
293. Waxweiler RJ, Alexander V, Leffingwell SS, Haring M, Lloyd JW. Mortality from brain tumor and other causes in a cohort of petrochemical workers. JNCI 1983;70:75.
294. Wilson CB, Gutin P, Boldrey EB, Crafts D, Levin VA, Enot KJ. Single-agent chemotherapy of brain tumors. A five-year review. Arch Neurol 1976;33:739.
295. Withers HR. Biologic basis for altered fractionation schemes. Cancer 1985;55(Suppl.):2086.
296. Wood JR, Green SB, Shapiro WR. The prognostic importance of tumor size in malignant gliomas: a computed tomographic scan study by the Brain Tumor Cooperative Group. J Clin Oncol 1988;6:338.
297. Wrann M, Bodmer S, de Martin R, Siepl C, Hofer-Warbinek R, Frei K, Hofer E, Fontana A. T cell suppressor factor from human glioblastoma cells is a 12.5-kd protein closely related to transforming growth factor-beta. EMBO J 1987;6:1633.
298. Xu G, O'Connell P, Viskochil D, Cawthon R, Robertson M, Culver M, Dunn D, Stevens J, Gesteland R, White R, Weiss R. The neurofibromatosis type 1 gene encodes a protein related to GAP. Cell 1990;62:599.
299. Yamashita J, Handa H, Tokuriki Y, Ha YS, Otsuka SI, Suda K, Taki W. Intra-arterial ACNU therapy for malignant brain tumors Experimental studies and preliminary clinical results. J Neurosurg 1983;59:424.
300. Young JL Jr, Miller RW. Incidence of malignant tumors in U.S. children. J Pediatr 1975;86:254.
301. Yung W, Prados M, Levin V, Fetell M, Bennett J, Mahaley S, Salcman M, Etcubanas E. Recombinant beta interferon in patients with recurrent malignant gliomas (abstract). J Neurooncol 1989;7:S32.
302. Zimmerman RA, Bilaniuk LT. Imaging of tumors of the spinal canal and cord. Radiol Clin North Am 1988;26:965.
303. Zuber P, Hamou M, de Tribolet N. Identification of proliferating cells in human gliomas using the monoclonal antibody Ki-67. Neurosurgery 1988;22:364.
304. Zuccarello M, Sawaya R, deCourten-Meyers G. Glioblastoma occurring after radiation therapy for meningioma: case report and review of the literature. Neurosurgery 1986;19:114.
305. Zauulch KJ. Histological Typing of Tumors of the Central Nervous System. International Histological Classification of Tumors, No. 21. Geneva: World Health Organization, 1979, p.15.

SECTION XXVII

NEOPLASMS OF THE EYE

CHAPTER 98

Neoplasms of the Eye

DAVID H. ABRAMSON, IRA J. DUNKEL, AND BERYL McCORMICK

Introduction

Ophthalmic oncology is foreign to most adult and pediatric oncologists. It is a subspecialty dominated by ophthalmologists who frequently work out of Eye Institutes, publish their findings in the ophthalmic literature, diagnose and treat diseases that are unfamiliar to most oncologists, and use a vocabulary unlike most others involved in cancer medicine. The anatomy, specialized imaging techniques, and methods of examination are ophthalmic-based. Most striking is the fact that the major intraocular malignancies—retinoblastoma in children and uveal melanomas in adults—are routinely diagnosed and treated without pathologic confirmation. Systemic chemotherapy, ocular irradiation, and removal of one or both eyes are routinely performed throughout the world without needle biopsies, incisional biopsies, or pretreatment cytologic study of any form. Furthermore, the evaluation of local control is based on ophthalmic techniques with which most oncologists are unfamiliar: indirect ophthalmoscopy under anesthesia aided by fundus photography, fluorescein angiography, and ocular ultrasonography, all of which are performed by the ophthalmologist.

When pathologic specimens are available they are usually interpreted by ophthalmic pathologists. Even expert pathologists working in large cancer centers are usually unfamiliar with ocular anatomy, pathology, and artifacts. In some cases, such as the interpretation of ocular melanomas, ocular pathologists have evolved their own classification schemes, cell type terminology, and descriptions that at times are at odds with traditional oncologic pathology.

Finally, the eye is a common site for metastasis, and it may be the general ophthalmologist who first detects that a patient has a metastatic tumor and needs to be referred to an oncologist.

Because the appropriate management of many ophthalmic malignancies routinely requires surgery, chemotherapy, radiation (external beam and brachytherapy), lasers, and cryotherapy, and because retinoblastoma has such a strong genetic pattern, successful management of these patients requires a well-integrated team of ophthalmologists, radiation oncologists, and radiation physicists, and often of pediatric oncologists, pediatricians, nurses, ophthalmic pathologists, genetic counselors, social workers, and diagnostic radiologists.

This chapter reviews benign and malignant ocular, orbital, and lid tumors in both children and adults. The most common of these are listed in Table 98.1.

Ophthalmic Oncology in Children

OCULAR DISEASE

Benign

Benign tumors of children's eyes are very rare. Choroidal nevi, which are present in more than 10% of the adult population, are rare before puberty and are never seen in the infant. If choroidal nevi are thought to be present in the first year of life they are probably choroidal neurofibroma and frequently part of neurofibromatosis.

Conjunctival nevi are also extremely rare in prepubertal children, as are iris nevi. Iris nevi in children may represent Lisch nodules, a manifestation of neurofibromatosis type 2. Benign retinal tumors are also rare. When found they are usually astrocytic hamartomas and frequently part of the tuberous sclerosis syndrome. Astrocytic hamartomas usually look like ill-defined transparent plastic-wrap overlying the retina and obscuring retinal blood vessels. They may enlarge and calcify with time. They may be confused with myelinated nerve fibers; the latter are usually fan-shaped, white, and may characteristically fan out to be broader the more distant from the optic nerve, follow the distribution of the nerve fiber layer, and often obscure retinal vessels. Hamartomas of the retinal pigment epithelium are rare in children. They are frequently near the optic disc and pigmented, with distortion of retinal vessels and a crinkled, slightly opaque appearance. They have no malignant potential.

Malignant (Retinoblastoma)

The most common primary ocular malignancy of childhood is retinoblastoma (1). The second most common is ocular involvement from leukemias. Retinoblastoma is a true neoplasm of the retina. Although relatively rare it has been the subject of great interest because of its well-established genetic pattern and because of the well-studied molecular mechanisms that characterize this tumor (2).

Retinoblastoma occurs in one in 18,000 to 30,000 live births worldwide. Surveys suggest a relatively constant occurrence in this century (3). The incidence in the United States is relatively low, at 3.58 cases for each million children under the age of 15, and is closely correlated with age. For ages 1 to 4 years the incidence is 10.6 per million; for 5 to 9 years, 1.53 per million; and for 10 to 14 years, 0.27 per mil-

Table 98.1. Commonly Occurring Ophthalmic Neoplasms

Site	Benign	Malignant	
		Primary	Secondary
Children			
Ocular	—	Retinoblastoma	Leukemia
Orbital	Hemangioma (Capillary)	Rhabdomyosarcoma	Leukemia
Adult			
Ocular	Choroid nevus	Uveal melanoma	Metastasis
Orbital	Hemangioma (Cavernous)	Lymphoma	Sinus cancer

lion. It is the seventh most common pediatric cancer, and in some countries (e.g., Mexico) it is the most common solid tumor in childhood.

There is no difference in incidence by sex or by right or left eye. Some data suggest clustering, but convincing evidence is lacking. Retinoblastoma appears to occur more commonly in poor patients worldwide.

In the United States there are approximately 350 cases per year. One-third of these occur bilaterally and two-thirds unilaterally. Bilateral patients are diagnosed at an earlier age, 13 months versus 24 months for the unilaterally affected (4). While it is true that the recognition of a family history partially explains the difference in age of detection, even without a family history of retinoblastoma the disease is detected at an earlier age in bilateral patients. It is this observation that led Knudson (5) to calculate that germinal retinoblastoma must be formed by a minimum of two events, called hits, now recognized to be a primary inherited loss of homozygosity at the 1.4 locus of the long arm of chromosome 13 followed by a second hit on the opposite allele.

Retinoblastoma occurs in two forms, germinal and nongerminal. In germinal cases both eyes are usually affected and the mean number of tumors distributed between the two eyes is 5. Inheritance usually follows an autosomal dominant pattern with 90% penetrance. All patients with bilateral retinoblastoma have a germinal mutation on chromosome 13 although only 8% have an antecedent family history of the disease. About 15% of patients with germinal retinoblastoma have only one eye involved. When patients with germinal retinoblastoma have unilateral disease it is almost always multifocal.

Nongerminal retinoblastoma is always unilateral and unifocal, although seeding of the tumor, as it breaks apart because of a lack of cohesiveness may cause hundreds of tiny intraocular seeds to appear. Genetic counseling based on these factors is schematically presented in Figure 98.1

Molecular Biology of Retinoblastoma. Retinoblastoma is one of the prototypical models demonstrating the genetic etiology of cancer. Knudson proposed the now classic "two hit" model in 1971 after noting that the timing of tumor development (earlier diagnosis of bilateral tumors than of unilateral tumors) suggested a mechanism in which at least two events would be responsible for the development of the tumor (5). Patients with multifocal bilateral disease are germline carriers for the first hit, with only one second hit necessary to develop retinoblastoma. Unilateral, unifocal patients usually have a normal germline genome, but develop both hits in the progenitor tumor cell.

The nature of these hits was suggested by karyotypic abnormalities on the long arm of chromosome 13 in rare patients and tumors. In 1986, Friend et al. isolated the RB1 gene, located on the long arm of chromosome 13, band 14.2 (6). Further characterization of the gene revealed that it spans 200 kb and is composed of 27 exons. The gene encodes a 4.7 kb transcript which is expressed in all adult tissues. The 110 kD nuclear phosphoprotein consists of 928 amino acids.

The protein seems to be a regulator at the cell cycle checkpoint between G1 and the entry into S phase. The phosphorylation pattern of p110 RB varies during the cell cycle and the current model (see Figure 98.2) suggests that the un-

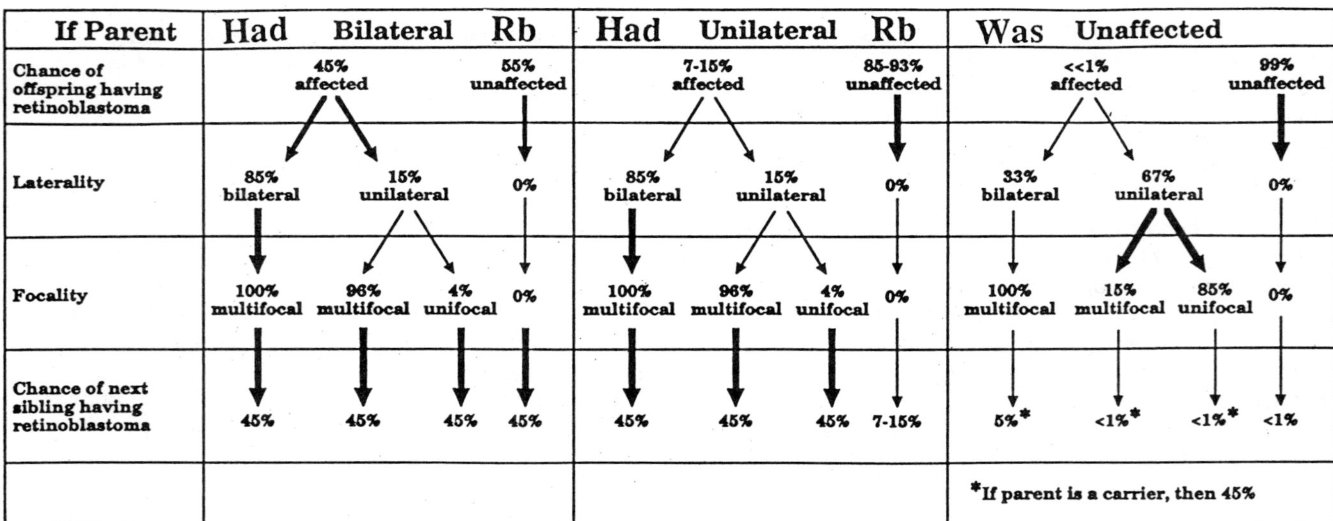

Figure 98.1. Genetic counseling considerations in retinoblastoma.

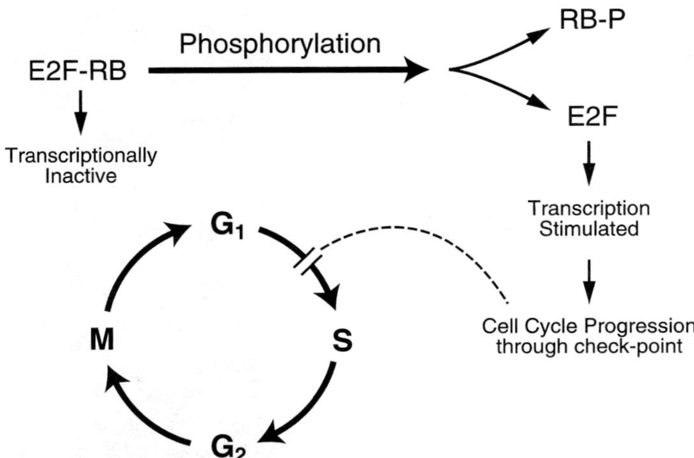

Figure 98.2. Molecular mechanism of retinoblastoma gene action.

phosphorylated normal RB1 protein binds transcriptional regulators that promote entry into S phase. When the normal RB1 protein is phosphorylated, it dissociates from E2F (one of these transcription factors) freeing it to bind to DNA and stimulate transcription of as yet unknown downstream genes that promote progression through the cell cycle. Loss of normal RB1 function, as in the case of the tumors, presumably allows for the uncontrolled entry into S phase, more rapid cell cycling, and therefore rapid cell division.

Because it is the loss of function of the RB1 gene that provides the impetus toward malignant transformation, the gene falls into the category of tumor suppressor genes. Retinoblastoma research has provided much of the initial understanding of this class of oncogenes. Whether replacement of normal RB1 into a fully transformed tumor cell is sufficient to reverse the malignant state is still controversial (7), and failure to do so would be consistent with the concept that while RB1 gene mutations are a necessary first step in tumorigenesis, they are not sufficient, and that additional steps are necessary to cause retinoblastoma.

Additional studies designed to better understand the function of the normal RB1 protein have included the creation of "knock-out mice" which have been genetically engineered to lack the normal RB1 gene in their germline (8). Heterozygotes are normal at birth, but have a propensity to develop pituitary tumors. Notably, these animals do not develop retinoblastomas. Animals homozygously lacking RB1 do not survive to birth, dying by embryonic day 16 due to hematopoietic and nervous system abnormalities.

Several groups of investigators have begun to use single-stranded conformational polymorphism analysis and DNA sequencing to identify specific mutations found in the RB1 gene in retinoblastoma tumors and in the germline of patients with the hereditary form. In cells with a single mutation (germline cells that carry the mutated gene), transcription of the abnormal allele cannot be detected, and it has been hypothesized that the normal allele somehow inhibits the expression of the abnormal mutant allele. This means that detection of the germline mutation in normal cells of potential carriers must be done at the DNA level, not on RNA.

While only limited amounts of data have been published to date, it seems that the majority of first hits are point mutations, with most of the remainder being small deletions, and only about 2–3% karyotypically visible larger deletions of material in the 13q14 band. Some of the children with this cytogenetic abnormality in their germline have a constitutional disease, with severe developmental delay and dysmorphic features, while others are phenotypically normal other than their retinoblastoma. The second hit usually consists of loss of the normal allele ("loss of heterozygosity"), though a minority of patients may have a second independent point mutation, and an even smaller fraction, a second independent small deletion.

Mutations in the RB1 gene seem to occur throughout the gene, without any "hot spots" being recognized thus far. The majority of the mutations are nonsense, introducing a premature stop codon and therefore producing a truncated and presumably non-functional protein. Yandell has described a series of tumors that have had the mutations characterized at the molecular level (9). Of 92 germline mutations, 86% were nonsense, while 9% were missense and 5% were in the promoter region. Similarly, in 44 tumors from patients without germline mutations, 98% of the mutations were nonsense and only 2% missense. Additionally, 9 patients who had developed "trilateral" disease (development of a pineal tumor in addition to bilateral retinoblastoma) were studied, and no specific mutation seemed to be associated with the development of this unusual presentation.

While much work has focused on the RB1 gene mutations, it seems that retinoblastomas, like other cancers such as colon carcinomas and glial brain tumors, require other genetic abnormalities to occur prior to full transformation and development of the tumor. A rare benign clinical entity called a retinoma is thought to be the result of the loss of the RB1 gene without the subsequent acquisition of other mutations that allow progression to the full blown malignant state. It is unclear what these subsequent steps in the development of the retinoblastoma tumor are, but cytogenetic studies have revealed some consistent abnormalities that provide clues. Squire noted gross aneuploidy of chromosome 1q (1q+)

was present in 21/27 tumors studied (10). Additionally, a cytogenetic abnormality specific to the retinoblastoma tumor was noted, isochromosome 6p, or 6p+, in 15/27 cases. Which genes present at these loci are responsible for malignant transformation is at present unclear.

Other known oncogenes have been investigated in retinoblastoma tumors. Yandell noted that 0/57 retinoblastoma tumor specimens had p53 mutations, but did note an abnormality in a retinoblastoma cell line, providing a reminder of the danger of extrapolating cell line data to tumors without direct tumor tissue confirmation (9). Doz et al. were stimulated by the histologic similarity between retinoblastoma and neuroblastoma to investigate whether 2 genetic abnormalities common in stage 4 neuroblastoma (N-myc amplification and loss of material from the short arm of chromosome 1) are also common in retinoblastoma (11). They determined that only 1/45 retinoblastoma tumors had amplification of the N-myc protooncogene, but did note that while only 3/35 primary retinoblastoma tumors had loss of heterozygosity of 1p, 4/8 distant metastases did, suggesting that a tumor suppressor gene on this arm may contribute to the metastatic potential of retinoblastomas.

While the amount of progress in our understanding of the molecular mechanisms underlying retinoblastoma development is impressive (12, 13), it is important to put this into perspective and remember that the question that the patient's family asks the physician is, "Why does my child have this disease?" In the 90% of the cases without an antecedent family history, the reason for the RB1 gene mutation is still unclear, and therefore future discoveries that may explain the mechanisms responsible for the gene mutations are eagerly awaited.

Presenting Signs and Symptoms of Retinoblastoma. The presenting signs and symptoms of retinoblastoma vary depending on where in the world a child with retinoblastoma is seen. In developing countries children often present with extraocular disease; proptosis and orbital mass when the retinoblastoma has grown within the eye causing rupture of the globe and direct extension into the orbit (Figure 98.3). Regional node metastasis may be found in the pre-auricular or submandibular nodes. These children are older (age 4–6 years) and few survive. In the United States most children present with signs rather than symptoms.

The most common sign (60% of cases) is leukocoria, the term applied to a white pupillary reflex or cat's eye reflex (Figure 98.4) (14). The reflex is caused by tumor itself in the vitreous or by the retinal detachment caused by the underlying tumor.

The second most common sign is strabismus or misalignment of the two eyes. Of the 22% of patients that so present, half have eyes crossed in (esotropia) and half out (exotropia). Esotropia in children in general is more common than exotropia so that an infant with exotropia must be feared to have retinoblastoma until proven otherwise. The crossed eyes are caused by tumor or retinal detachment in the area of central vision, the macula.

The next most common sign is painful glaucoma with inflammatory eye signs. These children may present to the pediatric emergency room with a picture like orbital cellulitis;

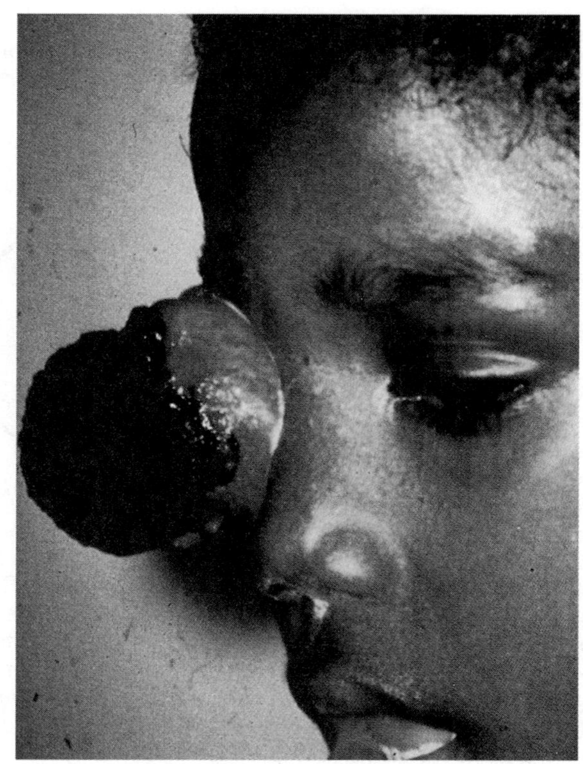

Figure 98.3. Advanced orbital presentation of retinoblastoma. (Courtesy of A. Wachtel, M.D., Lima, Peru.)

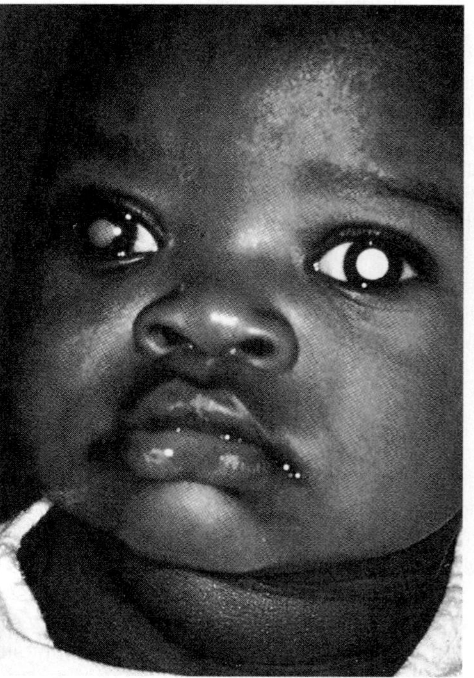

Figure 98.4. Leukocoria (white pupillary reflex) caused by retinoblastoma. The tumor can be seen in the vitreous. There are seeds in the anterior chamber, anterior to the iris.

they appear systematically ill with irritability, failure to eat and even low grade fever. Although the clinical exam and diagnostic imaging may suggest extraocular disease it is curious that these children usually have only intraocular disease, frequently with massive necrosis.

Other symptoms in the United States include anisocoria (different sized pupils), heterochromia (different colored irides), hyphema (blood in the anterior chamber), tumor hypopyon (tumor in the anterior chamber) and nystagmus. Less than 5% of our patients were detected on routine pediatric screening by a pediatrician. More than 90% of cases are detected by the mother.

When retinoblastoma is detected in the first 6 months of life the patterns are different (15). Sixty percent of such patients have no signs or symptoms; they are examined because of a family history of retinoblastoma. In those retinoblastomas we have discovered in the first 3 months of life none were referred with strabismus or inflammation and only 30% had leukocoria.

The anatomic location within the retina and the age at which these tumors are found has been well studied (Figure 98.5). Retinoblastoma may be present anywhere in the retina at birth, but clear patterns were seen in time and location. By age 9 months 50% of bilateral tumors were identified. By 2 years 89% were diagnosed. There is a direct relationship between the age at tumor diagnosis and retinal topography. This relationship follows a central to peripheral distribution with macular tumors presenting earliest and peripheral, anterior tumors appearing later. While the average macular tumor was diagnosed at 5.6 months and one never presented after 15.5 months, peripheral tumors were diagnosed at an average of 16.4 months and as late as 8 years.

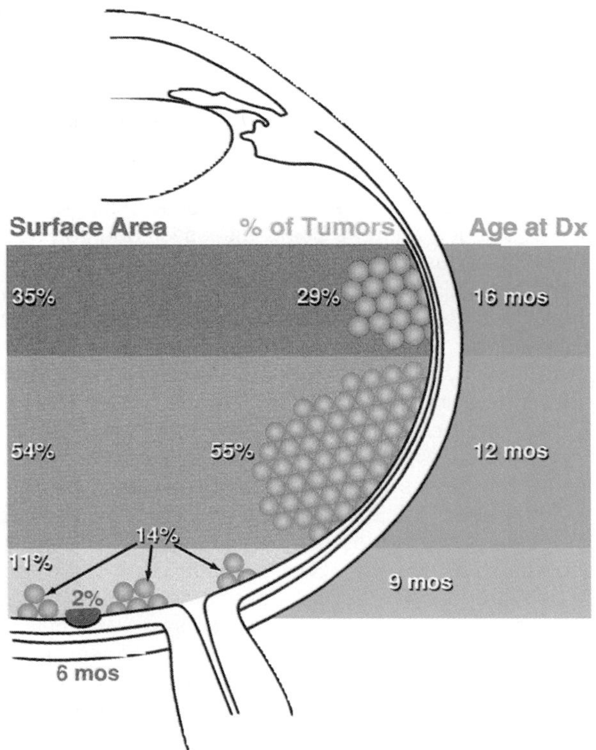

Figure 98.5. Relationship between age at diagnosis, surface area of involved retina, and location of intraocular foci of retinoblastoma.

The Reese-Ellsworth Classification scheme is the most commonly used for describing intraocular tumor (16). It is not a true staging scheme, for untreated patients do not progress from Group I to higher groups but it has served as an excellent ocular reference for comparison of different series and treatment schemes. Since that scheme does not deal with extraocular disease we have created another extraocular classification. Both schemes are outlined in Table 98.2.

The diagnosis of retinoblastoma is usually made on examination of a child with the indirect ophthalmoscope with scleral indentation, under anesthesia if necessary (17). The tumor begins as a glassy hemisphere in one or multiple sites bulging from the retina. With time the tumor becomes pink and vascularized and grows. As it grows it may detach the retina and/or break apart causing characteristic "seeds"

Table 98.2. Intraocular and Extraocular Classification of Retinoblastoma

Reese-Ellsworth scheme for intraocular retinoblastoma[a]

Group I
- a. Solitary tumor, less than 4 disc diameters in size, at or behind the equator
- b. Multiple tumors, none over 4 disc diameters in size, all at or behind the equator

Group II
- a. Solitary tumor, 4 to 10 disc diameters in size, at or behind the equator
- b. Multiple tumors, 4 to 10 disc diameters in size, behind the equator

Group III
- a. Any lesion anterior to the equator
- b. Solitary tumors larger than 10 disc diameters behind the equator

Group IV
- a. Multiple tumors, some larger than 10 disc diameters
- b. Any lesion extending anteriorly to the ora seratta

Group V
- a. Massive tumors involving over half the retina
- b. Vitreous seeding

Abramson classification for extraocular retinoblastoma

Stage I Intraocular disease
- a. Retinal tumor(s)
- b. Extension into choroid
- c. Extension up to lamina cribrosa
- d. Extension into sclerae

Stage II Orbital disease
- a. Orbital tumor
  - Suspicious (pathology of scattered episcleral tumor cells)
  - Proved (biopsy-proved orbital tumor)
- b. Regional nodes

Stage III Optic nerve disease
- a. Tumor beyond lamina but not up to cut section
- b. Tumor at cut section of optic nerve

Stage IV Intracranial metastases
- a. Positive cerebrospinal fluid
- b. Retinoblastoma mass in central nervous system

Stage V Hematogenous metastasis
- a. Positive marrow/bone lesions
- b. Other organ involvement

[a] From Reese (16).

within the vitreous and beneath the retina. Depending on the stage of disease progression it may look similar to other ophthalmic conditions that are not malignant. Extensive lists of these simulating lesions, called "pseudoglioma" in ophthalmic texts are presented elsewhere (18). The most common and difficult ones are presented in Table 98.3 and are discussed below.

Lesions Simulating Retinoblastoma. Astrocytic hamartomas may be seen in children with the syndrome of tuberous sclerosis or as "incidental" findings. If they have the syndrome the children may have intracranial calcifications, seizures, delayed development, mental retardation, dermal adenoma sebaceum and characteristic "ash leaf" skin findings. With time astrocytic hamartomas become more defined, may increase in number and calcify in part or completely. They require no ocular treatment.

The lesions of toxocara canis represent the retinal eosinophilic abscess(es) of presumably dead, migrated second stage larvae of toxocara canis, the same round worm that causes the clinical syndrome of visceral larval migrans. Curiously, intraocular lesions are usually not found in the patients who have the full blown syndrome. Children are diagnosed at an average age of 6 years (later than retinoblastoma) and get the disease by ingesting feces from puppies who are in the first year of life. It is a congenital infection of dogs and more prevalent in warmer parts of the United States.

Coats' disease is a purely ocular condition that mostly mimics retinoblastoma. It represents a unilateral (90%) retinal vascular anomaly of boys (80%) characterized in early stages by localized retinal vascular "light bulb like" telangetasia. With time these vessels leak an exudate that becomes rich in cholesterol crystals, macrophage laden, that detaches the retina simulating retinoblastoma. While it is not a malignancy it usually blinds the affected eye and may be very difficult to differentiate clinically from retinoblastoma.

Retinopathy of prematurity (ROP), formerly called retrolental fibroplasia (RLF) is a cicitricial disease of the vitreous and retina seen in low birth weight children who received oxygen at birth. It has also been seen in term babies who required no oxygen. It is usually bilateral, both eyes are small (microphthalmic) and myopic.

PHPV may simulate retinoblastoma. It refers to "persistent hyperplastic primary vitreous," the term given to congenital findings of one eye that is smaller, contains a membrane that is vascularized behind the lens simulating a cataract, and usually has many other anomalies including abnormal iris blood vessels, a vascular stalk extending from the optic nerve to the back of the retrolental membrane and anomalous formation of some of the layers of the retina. Though congenital it is not heritable.

Table 98.3. Some Common Lesions Simulating Retinoblastoma

Solitary ocular tumor
Astrocytic hamartoma
Toxocara canis
Total retinal detachment
Coats' disease
Retinopathy of prematurity
Persistent hyperplastic primary vitreous (PHPV)

Needle biopsies are rarely, if ever indicated in retinoblastoma. More than 50 years ago it was demonstrated that planned or unplanned puncturing of the eye allowed tumor cells to seep out of the eye, cause orbital invasion and death. As a result of this many ancillary tests have been pursued to help the clinician make a correct diagnosis. While these tests may be helpful in some cases, in some institutions they are not considered routine. As recently as 15 years ago it was reported from some centers that as many as 20% of eyes enucleated for retinoblastoma did not contain this tumor. In our institution there have been no eyes enucleated for retinoblastoma in more than 20 years that did not have retinoblastoma.

Skull x-rays demonstrate intraocular calcification in 75% of cases of retinoblastoma. They have been supplanted by modern CT scans where more than 90% of retinoblastoma patients will demonstrate intraocular calcification. Unfortunately the following conditions in the pediatric age group also demonstrate CT calcifications: Coats' disease, toxocara canis, retinopathy of prematurity, astrocytic hamartomas, PHPV, intraocular hemorrhage and phthisis after trauma, infection or surgery. Fortunately experienced radiologists can usually differentiate these lesions based on topography, laterality, size of the globe and associated findings. It should be emphasized that not all intraocular retinoblastomas demonstrate intraocular calcification but we have never seen an eye with complete replacement of the vitreous cavity that did not have retinoblastoma. The CT scan is unreliable for determining extension of the tumor into the choroid, optic nerve or transsclerally.

MR imaging for retinoblastoma has distinct disadvantages and advantages. Because it is difficult to detect calcification by MRI the most diagnostic feature of retinoblastoma can not be demonstrated. On the other hand MRI has been the test that clinches the difficult clinical differentiation of retinoblastoma from Coats' disease. Retinoblastoma is darker on T2 weighted images whereas Coats' disease is brighter, due to the proteinaceous exudate.

Ophthalmic ultrasound, performed by the ophthalmologist at the same time as the examination without anesthesia is extensively and routinely used. It demonstrates masses with high reflectivity that block sound, causing characteristic shadowing behind the tumor.

There has been great interest in aqueous taps for retinoblastoma (19). We no longer use this test because it is invasive and carries with it the risk of spreading the tumor. Many enzymes of the Embden-Myerhof pathways are in very high levels in the aqueous and vitreous of patients with retinoblastoma, however. Enzymes studied include lactic acid dehydrogenase, phosoglucoseisomerase and gamma-gamma enolase (or neuron-specific enolase). We have recently demonstrated high levels of other substances, including uric acid, Vandylmandelic acid (VMA), homovanillic acid (HVA) and 3-methoxy, 4-hydroxyphenyl-glycol (MHPG).

Treatment of Retinoblastoma. The treatment of retinoblastoma can be divided into treatment of the intraocular disease (21) and treatment of extraocular disease (22).

Intraocular Disease

EXENTERATION. Exenteration refers to the surgical removal of the eye and lids, orbital portion of the optic nerve, and all orbital tissue including extraocular muscles, fat, nerves, and muscles. It is rarely, if ever used for retinoblastoma nowadays. Disease that is extensively within the orbit will not be cured by this technique and excellent local control in cases like that can be obtained with external beam radiation and/or systemic chemotherapy. In cases of superimposed life threatening orbital infection or bleeding, however, it may still be appropriate.

ENUCLEATION. Enucleation refers to the surgical removal of the eye, leaving behind the lids, extraocular muscles, but removing as long a portion of the optic nerve within the orbit as possible. In children the procedure is done under general anesthesia, though the children do not require overnight hospitalization. In adults the procedure can be done under local anesthesia.

Clear consent must be obtained. Rather than having a distressed family sign permission for "enucleation OD" we write "surgical removal of the complete right eye" and add "with permission to remove or biopsy any suspicious tissue behind the eye." We always dilate both eyes of the patient on whom we are operating to inspect and confirm which eye is to be removed. Enucleation must be done with skill, getting a long stump of optic nerve and making sure not to perforate the globe (22). A ball is placed where the eye was (silicone, plastic), and 3 weeks later a thin contact like "prosthesis" is molded and painted by an ocularist to match the fellow eye.

EXTERNAL BEAM IRRADIATION. Radiation therapy for retinoblastoma is designed and prescribed to encompass the entire globe and at least 1 cm of optic nerve while avoiding as much normal tissue as possible, including the very radiosensitive lens (and lacrimal gland, if possible). For children with bilateral disease, the conventional parallel opposing fields from left and right are designed with a "D" shaped block (23). Using plain films taken in the radiation therapy simulator unit, and information in terms of globe size and lens position derived from a head CT or MRI study, the field is designed with the straight edge of the "D" the posterior pole of the lens. The curved portion of the "D" is shaped to encompass the eye as described above, with a margin of about 5 mm in all directions. For children with bilateral disease where one eye has been enucleated, we use similar field arrangement involving a single or bilateral fields, with the empty orbit receiving some exit dose of radiation. For patients with unilateral disease, we have designed a technique described in detail elsewhere, which employs two lateral oblique photon fields and one lateral electron field, to spare the contralateral globe (24).

The dose prescribed to the retinal target volume ranges from 4200 to 4600 cGy, with the lower dose reserved for children under the age of 6 months, and the higher doses for children with advanced bilateral disease. Children are treated 5 days/week, with daily fractions of 180 to 300 cGy per day. Although occasionally sedation is necessary for these children, we have successfully employed the use of a Plaster of Paris case mold to a restraining board which swaddles the child's body and for younger patients, may actually induce a sense of security and sleep.

Post-radiation, frequent follow-up visits for examinations under anesthesia with the ophthalmologist are scheduled to assess a tumor regression. Regression patterns have been described elsewhere in detail.

Of note, even after treatment, some scarring and residual calcification are the rule in these children's eyes, rather than the exception. After 10 years 90% of treated tumors still have visible intraocular material when viewed with the ophthalmoscope, ultrasound or CT scan.

PHOTOCOAGULATION. Since the late 1950s, thanks to the pioneering work of G. Meyer-Schwickerath (25) we have been able to photocoagulate retinoblastoma successfully. A comprehensive review of the subject is presented elsewhere (3). Traditionally we focus light through the dilated pupil under anesthesia and burn the tiny blood vessels that supply the retinal tumors. By destroying the blood supply the tumor involutes and is permanently cured. Photocoagulation has few side effects and causes complete remissions of treated tumors when they are no larger than 3 mm in diameter. Most tumors require more than one session to be cured. In recent years we have been able to use lasers both in the visible (argon) or invisible wave length (diode, infrared laser) with success.

CRYOTHERAPY. In the late 1960s Lincoff demonstrated that cryotherapy could effectively destroy small retinoblastomas (26). There has since been extensive experience with this technique (27). Under anesthesia a pencil like blunted probe is precisely placed on the outside of the sclera directly behind an intraocular focus of retinoblastoma. Rapid freezing (faster than −90°C a minute) causes intracellular ice crystals to form. These crystals cause rupture of tumor cells in addition to vascular occlusion and are locally successful in more than 90% of tumors when the tumor is smaller than 3 mm in diameter.

BRACHYTHERAPY. Brachytherapy for retinoblastoma has been in use since the 1930s when it was devised and refined by the legendary British ophthalmologist Mr. Henry Stallard (28). Though the technique has remained similar there has been an evolution of isotopes in recent years. Stallard used ^{60}Co plaques but in recent years ^{125}I plaques have been employed. Ruthenium plaques, gold plaques, palladium plaques and strontium plaques have all been used with success. The plaques are sutured on the outside of the sclera overlying the intraocular tumor. They deliver localized radiation of 4000 to 4500 cGy at a dose rate of approximately 1000 cGy per day. In a second operation the plaque is removed. The tumor usually disappears and forms a Type IV regression pattern (29). When plaques are used after failure of all other conservative measures, success rates of 50% are still attainable (30).

SYSTEMIC CHEMOTHERAPY. Systemic chemotherapy for intraocular disease was introduced in the 1950s. Over the years there have been waves of enthusiasm for different agents. It has been recognized that single or multiple agents cause dramatic reduction in size of intraocular tumors but not permanent responses. As a result of this chemotherapy is presently being investigated to cause chemoreduction of tumors, and when the tumor shrinks it is then treated with an additional modality, such as photocoagulation, hyperthermia, cryotherapy or radioactive plaques which appear to cause permanent inactivation of the tumor. This is an area of active clinical and research interest in the hope of replacing external beam radiation, and because of the hope that eyes that might previously have been enucleated could be locally cured with this newer approach.

EXTRAOCULAR DISEASE. While chemotherapy is the mainstay of treatment for most pediatric malignancies, its use has been much more limited in retinoblastoma. Historically, chemotherapy has been reserved for the treatment of extraocular disease, but precisely which patients deserve treatment is still controversial (see Table 98.4) and the optimal agents and regimens to use are not well established. In the developed world, extraocular disease occurs only in a small minority of patients. It is seen in both unilateral and bilateral cases, but presents sooner after diagnosis in patients with unilateral disease (2.7 ± 3.2 months) than in patients with bilateral disease (11.4 ± 11.7 months) (31).

The literature regarding efficacy of various chemotherapeutic agents against retinoblastoma is relatively sparse. Alkylating agents are felt to be the most active agents (31). Nitrogen mustard and TEM were frequently used in the past, and cyclophosphamide and ifosfamide are currently thought to be the most active single agents. Other reportedly active single agents include vincristine, doxorubicin and cytarabine. Trials utilizing single-agent carboplatin have not been reported, but our unpublished experience clearly shows this to be an active agent in the context of intraocular disease. Most reports of multi-agent regimens have utilized cyclophosphamide and vincristine. Other agents used in multiple-drug regimens include cisplatin and etoposide.

Extraocular disease can be divided according to the sites of involvement (Table 98.2). The natural course of untreated retinoblastoma is one of progressive, localized ocular involvement with eventual extension into the brain along the optic nerve or extension into the overlying conjunctiva with spread to regional nodes. This pattern is still common in underdeveloped countries but treatment of the intraocular disease significantly alters this pattern. Since unilateral patients and bilateral patients, before and after intraocular treatments have different patterns and timing of spread it is impossible to develop a useful staging system for extraocular disease and we have therefore utilized a classification scheme as a guide for treatment (Table 98.2). Retinoblastoma can spread via several routes. It may grow contiguously through the choroid and into the sclera (Stage I) and then into the orbit (Stage II), or may grow back through the optic nerve and then invade the brain (Stage III). It may enter the subarachnoid space and then spread throughout the leptomeninges via the cerebrospinal fluid (Stage IV). It may also spread hematogenously, causing metastatic disease in the bone marrow, bone, and organs such as the liver and spleen (Stage V). Rarely retinoblastoma may spread through the lymphatics to produce cervical node disease (Stage IIb), but of note, the eye only has lymphatic drainage through the conjunctiva. An algorithm for the management of extraocular retinoblastoma is shown in Figure 98.6.

OPTIC NERVE/CHOROID INVASION. When eyes containing retinoblastoma are enucleated, the extent of disease present in the pathologic specimen has been used to determine the need for chemotherapy (32, 33). There are a number of such analyses in the literature and some lack of agreement regarding which criteria indicate a high risk of micrometastases and the need for presumptive treatment with chemotherapy. Two factors extensively discussed are whether optic nerve invasion is present and whether choroidal invasion is present. If optic nerve disease is present at the cut end (positive margin), then there is little controversy that central nervous system spread is likely and that treatment is indicated. More commonly, however, invasion of the nerve is noted with a surgical margin free of tumor. An important landmark used to define the extent of optic nerve invasion is the lamina cribrosa, which is the extension of sclera at the site of the optic nerve. Data suggest that 30–40% of patients with optic nerve invasion beyond the lamina cribrosa, but with a negative surgical margin, will later

Table 98.4. Summary of Recent Reports of Chemotherapy for Extraocular Retinoblastoma[a]

References	Drugs[b]	IT[c]	Site	Patients with disease-free survival (range mo.)
Grabowski and Abramson (32)	VDC	MA	Orbit	3/4 (11–105)
	VDC	MA	CNS	5/5 (50–105)
	VDCPE	MA	Bone/BM	4/6 (2–58)
Goble et al. (33)	Unclear	M	Orbit	5/5 (8–84)
Zelter et al. (34)	VDC		Orbit	4/4
	VDC		CNS (micro)	6/13
	CDPE	MAX	CNS (macro)	0/3
	CDPE	MAX	Bone	0/4
Doz et al. (35)	Various		Orbit (± nodes)	9/22 (2–149)
			CNS (± bone)	0/7
			Bone	3/4 (13–137)

[a] Most patients also received radiation therapy.
[b] V, vincristine; D, doxorubicin; C, cyclophosphamide; P, cisplatin; E, etoposide.
[c] IT, intrathecal; M, methotrexate; A, cytarabine; X, dexamethasone.

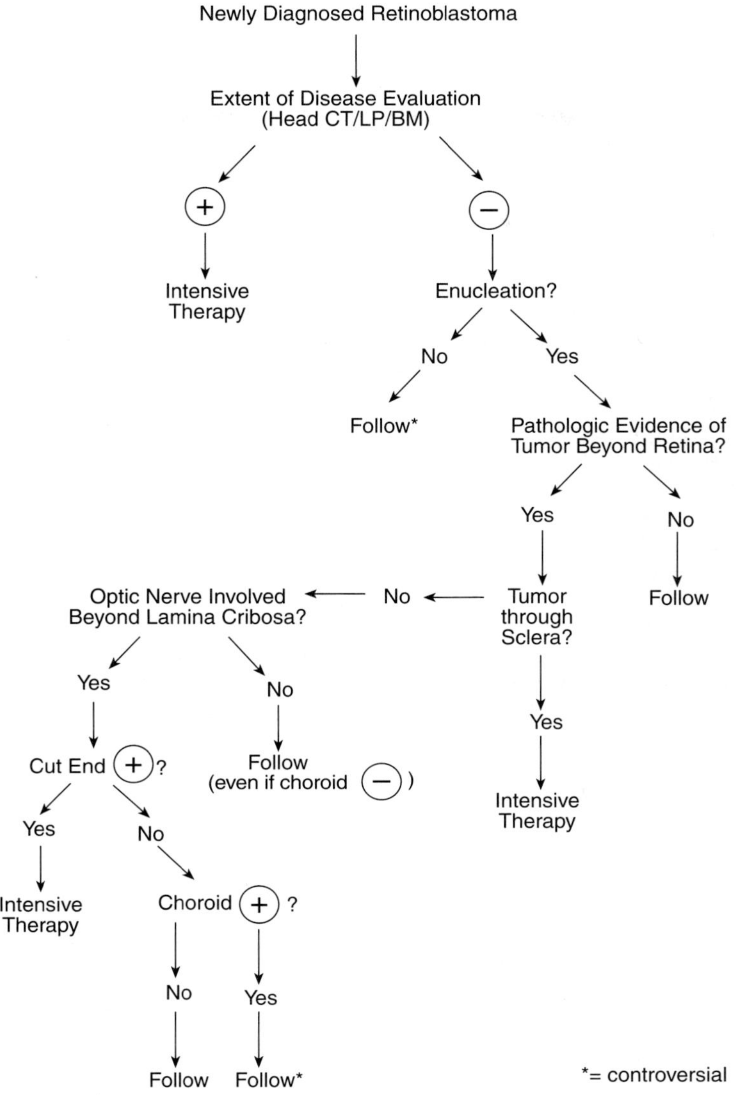

Figure 98.6. Algorithm for management of extraocular retinoblastoma.

develop metastatic disease (32, 33, 34). Invasion of the choroid only, without associated optic nerve disease is questionable as a prognostic factor for metastatic disease. It has been suggested that patients with both invasion of the optic nerve beyond the lamina cribrosa and with massive choroidal involvement are those deserve to be treated with chemotherapy, and that this be investigated on a multi-institutional basis.

Whether a 30–40% risk of metastasis justifies treating the 60–70% of patients who would not develop metastases is a difficult question. The toxicity, expense, and success of treating presumptively needs to be considered in conjunction with the efficacy of treatment designed to retrieve patients once overt metastatic disease is detected. If a significant proportion of patients with recurrent or metastatic disease can be salvaged with contemporary therapies, then it may be reasonable to closely follow patients with optic nerve invasion beyond the lamina cribrosa, but with a negative surgical margin, and to reserve aggressive chemotherapy for the minority whose disease recurs.

ORBITAL DISEASE. Until recently, disease extending into the orbit was uniformly fatal despite aggressive surgery and radiation therapy. In the past few years, however, reports of the successful use of aggressive systemic chemotherapy in conjunction with radiation therapy have appeared in the literature (35). Doz et al. reported on 33 patients with histologically proven orbital disease treated between 1977 and 1991. Twenty patients had isolated orbital disease, while 7 also had CNS metastases and 6 had metastatic disease outside of the CNS. Most patients received both intensive chemotherapy and orbital radiation. Several chemotherapeutic regimens were used, and the agents included cyclophosphamide, platinum compounds, etoposide, doxorubicin and vincristine. An overall survival of 34% (±8%) was noted, with most recurrences occurring within the first year following diagnosis of the orbital disease. Patients without CNS disease fared better, and there was a trend toward improvement in the outcome of the more recently treated patients (post-1985). While survival is clearly possible, orbital disease still carries a high risk of mortality, and aggressive multimodality therapy, including the possible use of high-dose chemotherapy regimens in conjunction with autologous stem cell rescue, is warranted. It is also important to note that several groups have reported good outcomes for patients with local nodal disease extension, and it appears that these patients should not be analyzed together with patients with CNS or hematogenously spread distant metastases.

CENTRAL NERVOUS SYSTEM/DISTANT METASTASES. Likewise, metastatic disease to the central nervous system or to distant sites was considered incurable until fairly recently. Grabowski described 16 children with CNS or hematogenous metastases and showed that aggressive treatment with chemotherapy and radiation could cure a substantial proportion of these patients (37). Of the patients who received treatment at New York Hospital, all 5 with intracranial disease were disease-free survivors, as were 4/6 patients with bone and bone marrow disease. Treatment included systemic chemotherapy with cyclophosphamide, doxorubicin, and vincristine, intrathecal methotrexate and cytarabine, and, in patients at least 1 year-old, whole brain radiation (1800 cGy) plus involved field boosts to a total of 4500–5500 cGy. In contrast, however, Doz reported that all 7 of their patients with CNS involvement in addition to orbital disease died despite aggressive therapy.

Even if the promising results of Grabowski are replicated, the young age of most of these patients makes the use of craniospinal radiation extremely toxic to normal development and severe developmental delay and intellectual impairment is a frequent sequelae. This same problem has been addressed by pediatric oncologists for the treatment of young children with primary brain tumors, and a strategy of utilizing high-dose chemotherapeutic agents that penetrate the blood-brain barrier has been employed to delay or avoid the use of radiation. Evaluation of the use of high-dose systemic chemotherapy in conjunction with autologous stem cell rescue for patients with CNS or metastatic retinoblastoma is underway at our and other centers. This strategy (without intrathecal medications) has been used to treat brain tumors that have a propensity to disseminate along the leptomeninges (such as medulloblastoma), and therefore the need for intrathecal therapy for retinoblastoma is unclear. Additionally, the role of intrathecal therapy must be questioned because of the in vitro data that suggest that retinoblastoma cell lines are invariably resistant to methotrexate, though some were sensitive to cytarabine (38).

Second Malignancies. Since the first report of the successful treatment of bilateral retinoblastoma with combinations of surgery and irradiation (39), it has been recognized that some retinoblastoma patients develop second non-ocular cancers years after the successful treatment for the eye neoplasm. Our center has repeatedly published on the largest such experience with the longest follow-up; we will emphasize the highlights of our findings here, but those interested in more details are encouraged to review the primary references (40–42).

Only retinoblastoma patients with the germinal form of the disease are at risk for the development of these second tumors. Unilateral retinoblastoma patients without the constitutional mutation of one allele are at no higher risk for developing cancer, even if treated exactly as a germinal retinoblastoma. In particular, unilateral patients without the mutation are at no higher risk than background if they receive external beam irradiation, brachytherapy, photocoagulation, cryotherapy or enucleation.

Patients with the germinal mutation are at risk for the development of second cancers. This represents *any* bilateral patient, whether or not that patient has a family history of the disease. It also represents virtually all of the unilateral patients who have a family history of the disease.The risk also attends any unilateral retinoblastoma patient who has been demonstrated with molecular techniques to have a germinal mutation. On clinical grounds we have found that unilateral patients who are diagnosed at a young age (under 6 months) and those who present with multifocal unilateral tumors (not multiple tumors from seeding) are at a high risk of having the germinal mutation and most of these are at risk for the development of second cancers.

Although all patients with the germinal mutation are thought to be at risk for the development of second cancers, there may be other factors, as yet unknown, that also govern their development since 100% have not yet developed second neoplasms.

Patients with the germinal mutation for retinoblastoma develop second cancers more often than do patients with any other cancer of childhood or adult life. Because the initial cancer, retinoblastoma, is successfully cured in the United States in more than 90% of cases, and because there are few other complications from the initial treatment that might compromise survival, many patients are available for study.

When we studied the incidence of second tumors we found that for as long as the patients were followed their incidence of second cancers increased. By 32 years 90% of the survivors of germinal mutation retinoblastoma had developed second malignancies. The possible error at 32 years was up to 20%, but even a figure of 70% second neoplasms by 32 years was startling. When we subdivided the germinal cases into those that received irradiation and those that did not, there was an obvious difference. Without radiation 50% had developed a second malignancy by 32 years. There were other differences in the two groups. In the radiated patients the second malignancies were "in the radiation field" two-thirds of the time and out of the field one-third of the time. In the non-radiated patients the tumors were out of what would have been the field two-thirds of the time and in the field one-third of the time. Thus, some patients developed second malignancies "in the field of radiation" who had not been treated with radiation.

Survival was worse for the patients who received irradiation for three reasons. The latent period until the second cancer was shorter for those who received irradiation. The incidence for those who received irradiation was higher. The success in treating the second cancers that arose in the radiation field was less. The predominant tumor, both in and out of the radiation field, was osteogenic sarcoma.

A recent long term analysis of our experience has been published and merged with the experience at Harvard (43). Overall the relative risk for death from second primary tumors was 30 fold, with excess mortality from second primary neoplasms of bone and connective tissue, cutaneous melanoma and benign and malignant neoplasms of the brain and meninges. The cumulative probability of death from second neoplasms was 26% at 40 years; death was more frequent in females (RR = 39) than males (RR = 22). The risk in germinal cases increased by irradiation was also apparent in unilateral retinoblastoma patients with the germinal mutation. Although the children with the germinal form of retinoblastoma appear to be at risk for their entire lives the second cancers they develop and when they develop them do not appear random. For example, retinoblastoma patients do not subsequently develop the most common pediatric cancer, leukemia. The cancers which are at higher incidence are listed in the Table 98.5. Osteogenic sarcoma of the skull occurs more than 2,000 times as commonly in this group as in the general age matched population and osteogenic sarcoma of the extremities occurs hundreds of time more commonly. The second cancers seem to occur in tissues during expansive growth. For example, osteogenic sarcoma of the skull develops in the first 10 years of life whereas osteogenic sarcoma of the extremity develops during the teenage years.

An important and curious second cancer is now recognized. It has been referred to as trilateral retinoblastoma because it occurs in the primitive third eye, the pineal gland, in patients who have bilateral retinoblastoma. Typically it has occurred in patients with bilateral retinoblastoma who have a family history of the disease, who have been diagnosed early in life (within the first 6 months) and who have been treated with radiation. All such children have died from their pinealblastoma with leptomeningeal spread despite a variety of attempts to cure the tumor.

The most common cause of death of a retinoblastoma patient with the germinal mutation is not retinoblastoma but a second cancer. While retinoblastoma is the most common cause of death in these children within the first 5 years of life, pinealblastoma is the most common cause of death in the 5- to 10-year period (10%). In the next 10 years sarcomas of the extremity predominate. The retinoblastoma gene is the cause of these second cancers but we now recognize that treatment with external beam radiation further increases the incidence.

Table 98.5. Second Cancers in Retinoblastoma Patients

Osteogenic sarcoma
Sarcomas
Brain tumors
Pinealomas ("Trilateral retinoblastoma")
Cutaneous melanomas
Hodgkin's disease

Leukemia. Childhood leukemia, particularly acute lymphocytic leukemia (ALL) are the most common malignant tumors that involve the eyes of children. Leukemic infiltrates involve the eye in three distinct presentations of leukemia. In all cases the site of involvement appears the same. Leukemic involvement primarily involves the uveal tract; the iris, ciliary body and/or choroid. Leukemic infiltration is virtually impossible to detect ophthalmoscopically in the choroid or ciliary body, but when present in the iris, the child may have iris infiltrates causing heterochromia (different color of the two irides), cells in the anterior chamber (mimicking and in some cases treated as idiopathic iritis), bleeding in the anterior chamber (hyphema) that may be associated with glaucoma with a painful, photophobic, red, sensitive eye.

Tumor in the choroid has been identified in 90% of eyes at autopsy after death from leukemia, but there are no good clinical descriptions of its appearance in the choroid. Tumor in the choroid is not seen because ALL diffusely invades the choroidal blood channels and even with extravasation beneath these vessels the only effect is that the choroid is thicker. Fortunately B-scan ultrasound examination by an ophthalmologist, frequently performed at the bedside, reveals thickening of the choroid (43). Retinal involvement, which is rare, has been described: Roth's spots and white patches are seen.

The three situations when leukemia is seen within the eye follow.

1. Simultaneous with the first presentation of leukemia. The majority of eyes demonstrate ultrasonic findings. Occasionally the effect of thrombocytopenia or sludging is noted with hemorrhages, infarcts and dilated vessels. When leukemia is treated the choroidal involvement disappears within days.
2. As a recurrence following induction treatment and CNS radiation prophylaxis. In these children the CNS has been treated with radiation but the eye has been spared treatment and a sanctuary site is created. Although this is rare, treatment of the eye alone in such cases may be justified.
3. As a sign of CNS recurrence. This is by far the most important presentation because ocular recurrence is a marker for CNS recurrence whether or not CNS tumor can be identified. These patients frequently develop cells near the posterior pole of the eye. At times the cells appear to be coming directly from the optic nerve into the vitreous clouding the appearance of the optic nerve itself. It was formerly thought that ocular recurrence indicated systemic hematogenous recurrence, but recent evidence (44) suggests that the eye itself recurs because it is seeded by the CNS directly through the optic nerve. This is important because if ocular recurrence occurs without apparent systemic or CNS recurrence the brain should be treated. The traditional treatment for ocular recurrence of leukemia has been radiation with 800 to 1800 cGy, but we have found that treating the eye via a CNS route (ventricular methotrexate, through an Ommaya reservoir) quickly and effectively eliminates ocular recurrence.

ORBITAL TUMORS

Benign

Benign tumors of the orbit in children are frequently incidental problems detected on CT scan or because lid or orbital asymmetry is observed. Many require no treatment.

The most common benign orbital tumor of childhood is the capillary hemangioma (unlike the most common benign orbital tumor of adults which is a cavernous hemangioma) (45). Capillary hemangiomas are highly cellular, angioblastic and rarely encapsulated. As many as 25% may not be apparent at birth, but they grow so rapidly and frequently bleed that they may be mistaken for a rhabdomyosarcoma. Biopsy of rhabdomyosarcomas is always done so diagnostic imaging may be able to differentiate capillary hemangiomas from rhabdomyosarcomas. On CT scanning capillary hemangiomas are usually associated with congenitally enlarged orbits while rhabdomyosarcomas are not. Despite growth that may appear explosive their natural course is to stop growing after 6 to 12 months when they will slowly involute (over 2 to 5 years) and largely regress. They may be associated with strawberry hemangiomas of the nearby skin.

These tumors usually cause profound and permanent visual loss if left untreated. The mechanism of visual loss is not simply ptosis with occlusion of the pupil and consequent development of "deprivation amblyopia." The mass displaces the eye and causes strabismus with strabismic amblyopia. The mass usually presses on the eye itself causing significant astigmatism with the development of anisometropic amblyopia. Rarely hemangiomas cause corneal damage by proptosis and exposure, and they may press on the optic nerve and cause optic atrophy. If they sequester platelets they may cause thrombocytopenia and high output cardiac failure.

Treatment of these hemangiomas is difficult. Surgery, either conventional or with the KTP (532 nm potassium titanyl phosphate) laser rarely removes enough of the lesion to prevent the ocular complications. The tumors respond to low dose radiation and we have used fractionated doses up to 800 cGy with success. There have been reports of injecting sclerosing solutions into the lesions or even occluding them with interventional radiological techniques but experience is limited.

Fortunately these tumors respond to local or systemic steroids. Hemangiomas have responded to systemic steroids, but all have recurred when the steroids were discontinued after a few weeks. Systemic treatment must continue for months, and with the doses recommended for the young children (20 mg/day) systemic toxicity is common and worrisome. Local injections of short and long acting steroids are probably the treatment of choice when mandated by visual or overwhelming cosmetic reasons.

Dermoid Cysts. Dermoid cysts are among the most common orbital tumors of childhood. They are benign and represent congenital ectodermal rests. They are congenital, usually in the anterior portion of the superior orbit and cause a characteristic hollowed out appearance of bone. Occasionally the dermoids have calcification and even aberrant tooth formation within the mass. Treatment is surgical but utmost care must be taken because many have dumbbell shaped posterior orbital extensions sometimes intracranially. When the cysts rupture, either from trauma or from incomplete surgical removal a violent orbital inflammation may ensue.

Lymphangioma. Despite the fact that lymphatics do not exist in the orbit, benign lymphangiomas do (46). These tumors are thought to be congenital, have no malignant potential but in contrast to hemangiomas are rarely present at birth. They are most commonly seen at age 6 with explosive proptosis cased by bleeding of the tumor into the cystic spaces referred to as "chocolate cysts." These lesions consist of primitive lymphatic channels with lymphoid hyperplasia and may enlarge during upper respiratory infections. Differentiation from rhabdomyosarcomas is important. As many as 20% of lymphangiomas have lymphangioma tissue on the palate and many have anterior, visible orbital extensions. Their diffuseness on imaging techniques is unlike the typical more localized rhabdomyosarcoma.

Treatment is difficult. They do not respond to steroids or radiation and they are impossible to remove completely by surgery. Surgery with electrocautery, which may have to be repeated many times, with or without the KTP laser is the treatment of choice. Satisfactory cosmetic results are difficult to attain.

Malignant

The most common primary malignant orbital tumor of childhood is rhabdomyosarcoma. The average age at diagnosis is 6 years and the sexes are equally affected as are the two orbits. Although the hallmark of an orbital rhabdomyosarcoma is rapid, progressive, painless proptosis, the next most common finding is ptosis followed by a sub-conjunctival fleshy mass (47). The most common location in the orbit is a mass superonasally and the most common histologic type is an embryonal rhabdomyosarcoma. When rhabdomyosarcomas present in the inferior orbit they are usually histologically alveolar type. Interestingly, these malignancies do not originate from extraocular muscles but from skeletal rests within the orbit. CT scans may reveal extension into the sinuses. Rhabdomyosarcomas can originate from the sinuses and extend into the orbits or they may extend into the sinuses from the orbit. In both cases if there is sinus involvement prognosis for survival is poorer.

Early biopsy is mandatory. All attempts should be made to biopsy the lesion directly without going through the sinuses or skull because of the possibility of tracking tumor.

Local excision of these tumors is rarely effective. In 1959 Jones reported that exenteration offered a 3-year cure rate of 47% (48). External beam irradiation was started in the 1960s, and it was subsequently shown that irradiation combined with chemotherapy not only produced excellent local cures but better than 90% long term survival (late metastases in orbital rhabdomyosarcoma do not occur). Radiation doses of 6,000 cGy were employed. The chemotherapy that was originally used, vincristine, cyclophosphamide and doxorubicin has changed as results of various Intergroup Rhab-

Table 98.6. Causes of Rapid Proptosis in Childhood

Orbital rhabdomyosarcoma
Orbital lymphanigioma
Orbital hemangioma (capillary)
Metastatic neuroblastoma
Encephalocele
Inflammatory disease
Orbital cellulitis (infectious, following rupture of dermoid; teratoma)
Benign reactive lymphoid hyperplasia
Leukemia

domyosarcoma studies have demonstrated that the most effective combination for disease localized to the orbit is vincristine, actinomycin-D and radiation (49). In giving radiation, the eye is not spared nor shielded. Within 5 years one-third of such eyes have been enucleated. Only 19% of such patients retain useful vision after 10 years but the majority do keep their minimally sighted eyes (52).

We recently reviewed the long term experience in patients treated in the 1960s and 1970s with external beam irradiation alone (50). Their survival was similar to those patients treated with irradiation and chemotherapy. Interestingly second non-ocular tumors have occurred in rhabdomyosarcoma patients who received adjunctive chemotherapy but not in those patients who received irradiation alone.

Recurrent rhabdomyosarcoma following irradiation and chemotherapy occurs (though infrequently) 1 year after completion of therapy with the same local signs (proptosis, ptosis, mass) and symptoms (diplopia, decreased vision) and poses a special problem for treatment. No long term survivors have been reported after recurrence but since 1988 we have used a system that is promising. To date each of the 5 patients treated is alive and free of disease following exenteration and specialized brachytherapy. A mold of the orbit (59) is made from an algae based dental material which is then exactly replicated in plastic ^{125}I seeds are placed in holes drilled in the mold which is left in situ until a total dose to the remaining microscopic tumor of 6,000 cGy is attained without significant reirradiation of the brain. Though healing has been slow all orbits are reepithelializing (51).

While distant metastases from rhabdomyosarcoma are traditionally to the lungs it is the absence of local spread to the sinuses that predicts success of treatment. If no sinus involvement is found at diagnosis, overall success is more than 90%; with sinus involvement (primary or secondary) success is almost halved. Metastasis from orbital rhabdomyosarcoma always occurs within 5 years from diagnosis.

The diagnosis of rhabdomyosarcoma should be considered whenever rapid progressive proptosis occurs in the first twenty years of life. Other conditions must be considered in the differential diagnosis and they are listed in Table 98.6.

Adult Ocular Tumors

BENIGN

Benign tumors of the lid, conjunctiva, iris and choroid are common while those of the retina and cornea are rare. Benign tumors of the lens and vitreous do not exist. The most important benign tumors of the eye are the choroidal nevi.

Choroidal Nevi

Choroidal nevi are never present at birth. Pigmentation that looks like choroidal nevi in infancy is usually from choroidal neurofibroma, seen as a part of systemic neurofibromatosis. Nevi of the choroid can be seen before puberty but they are unusual. With puberty they become visible. In the U.S. population 10 to 13% of the adult population have choroidal nevi. They are racially related; choroidal nevi in blacks are very rare.

Choroidal nevi are flat, pigmented benign lesions with edges that can be feathered and irregular or rounded (Fig. 98.7). They are usually slate gray to light chocolate in color. With time (months to years) there may be associated findings with the nevi. Many demonstrate changes on their surface such as drusen or sub-retinal fluid and may cause overlying visual field defects and can even be associated with overlying neovascular membranes. Since 10% of the adult population have choroidal nevi and there are only 1500 choroidal melanomas in the United States yearly it is assumed that the chance of a choroidal nevus becoming a melanoma is less than one in a thousand. A number of studies have now demonstrated which nevi change into melanomas. The predictive factors are shown in Table 98.7.

The diagnosis of a nevus is straightforward and can be made with ophthalmoscopy alone. The development of retinal detachment over and around the tumor can be treated medically or with lasers. Many ophthalmologists treat symptomatic fluid with systemic acetazolamide. There are no controlled studies proving that the treatment works.

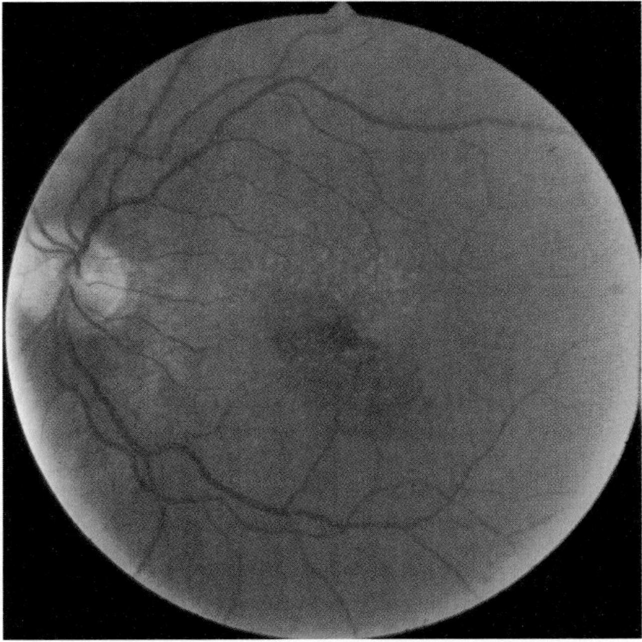

Figure 98.7. Choroidal nevus.

Table 98.7. Predictive Factors in Transformation of Nevus to Melanoma

Size	The greater the thickness of a choroidal nevus, the greater the chance of its becoming a melanoma About 1% per month of nevi 2.5 mm thick become melanomas
Location	Nevi at the posterior portion of the eye more commonly become melanomas than those situated anteriorly
Orange pigment	Development of orange pigment on surface of choroidal nevi greatly increases the chance of development into melanoma
Serous fluid	Serous fluid in the form of an overlying retinal detachment can be seen with nevi, but such nevi more likely become melanomas
Hot spots	On fluorescein angiography
Symptoms	Decreased vision or visual field defect

Photocoagulation with lasers of the leaking areas over the nevi has been done. While the fluid usually resorbs and leakage stops within days to weeks it has been suggested that photocoagulation itself somehow weakens the layer between the retina and choroid (Bruch's membrane) and in some way may stimulate transformation to malignancy.

A special type of nevus that is not flat has been described in the choroid. It is a melanocytoma, or pathologically a magnocellular nevus with jet black pigmentation. This consists of large cells in darker skinned whites who are frequently of Mediterranean origin. These lesions originate in cells within the optic nerve itself and may obscure a view of the nerve. The lesions may be several millimeters high, grow slowly and can affect the visual field or visual acuity. While these lesions are benign, rare cases of transformation to malignancy have been recorded.

The differential diagnosis of a nevus is straightforward. Other flat lesions in the choroid that have been confused with nevi and melanoma include: hyperplasia of the retinal pigment epithelium (that lesion, also flat, is darker, almost black in coloration, frequently with bare spots devoid of pigment within the lesion with very sharp edges and usually circular in shape), hamartomas of the retinal pigment epithelium, and hemorrhages within the retina (especially hemorrhages beneath the retinal pigment epithelium as part of macular degeneration). The differentiation of these lesions from melanoma is made by size, thickness, fluorescein patterns and ultrasonography.

Iris Nevi

Iris nevi are, by definition, pigmented and flat. They are common, may be multiple and occur more often in blue eyed individuals. Iris nevi are also rarely present at birth and like all other ocular nevi become apparent around puberty. They are always benign and of no real consequence for the eye or for life. Confusion exists however in the use of the term "iris melanoma." Ophthalmologists have traditionally described elevated pigmented lesions of the iris as "iris melanomas" to differentiate them from the flat nevi. This has been further confused by pathologic interpretation of elevated pigmented iris masses that were excised (or enucleated!) which were described as malignant. Elevated iris pigmented masses may grow, may shed cells into the angle, clogging the trabecular meshwork and causing a severe secondary glaucoma that can blind the eye; but iris melanomas metastasize extremely rarely, if ever. Lack of metastasis may be a function of size. An iris melanoma that filled the anterior chamber would, if in the back of the eye (in the choroid) be small enough never to cause metastasis. Management of iris melanoma is based on what is best for the eye and the glaucoma and is not a decision about life. Ciliary body melanomas that present as iris lesions do metastasize.

MALIGNANT

The most common primary malignant tumor of the eye of adults is malignant melanoma, also referred to as "melanosarcoma of the choroid" (52). There are about 1500 new cases of choroidal malignant melanoma yearly in the U.S. The average age at diagnosis is 55 to 65 years with men and women equally affected and the two eyes equally susceptible. In the U.S. 99% of choroidal melanomas originate in whites. The most common reason for detection of the tumor is a routine exam (41%) (53). Men more often present with symptoms and when there are symptoms the right eye is more often found to have the tumor. The most common symptom is a decrease in the peripheral visual field followed by decreased vision. The lesion is not painful, unlike metastatic tumors to the eye where pain is not unusual.

The visual field defect is characteristic. There is an absolute scotoma overlying the tumor associated with a surrounding relative field defect that does not obey the horizontal meridian (as most ocular defects do) and does not observe the vertical meridian (as many CNS defects do) (54).

Melanomas of the choroid originate in melanocytes that normally lie within the choroid. The choroid, that layer between the sclera and retina is a rich, high flow, syncytium of vascular lobules that not only supply blood to the photoreceptors (rods and cones) of the retina but also serve as a heat sink to dissipate heat energy liberated by absorbed visible light.

Whether melanomas of the choroid originate in nevi alone is not known, but patients with flat pigmented, untreated nevi followed for more than 20 years have developed melanomas arising from the previously dormant lesion. The cause of choroidal melanomas is unknown but sunlight has not been proven to play a role.

The diagnosis of choroidal melanoma can usually be made on ophthalmoscopic grounds alone. With the direct ophthalmoscope it may be difficult to appreciate the three dimensional shape but with dilated pupils and the indirect ophthalmoscope the tumor is easily identified. The tumor can have many shapes. A flat, diffuse type may be difficult to detect ophthalmoscopically but most tumors are elevated, frequently dome shaped (the height of the tumor being half the base diameter) and occasionally multilobed. The tumor is held back by Bruch's membrane but when it ruptures this taut, transparent plastic layer develops a rounded "top" on the surface of a domed shaped mass; this is referred to as "mushroom shaped."

Pigmentation of choroidal melanomas varies from patient to patient and frequently from area to area within the tumor. 40% of the tumors have no pigment clinically. When pigmented they are frequently a dusky gray to charcoal in color but occasionally they are deep brown. Black lesions within the eye are rarely melanomas.

All choroidal melanomas have associated retinal detachments. At times it may be difficult to detect ophthalmoscopically while at other times the retinal detachment may be so extensive that the melanoma is not seen (or suspected) clinically.

Since there are no lymphatics in the eye or within the orbit melanomas of the choroid metastasize through vascular channels. More than 75% of such metastases are first identified within the liver. Treatment strategies for metastatic melanoma are covered elsewhere (see Chapter 12). Fewer than 1% of patients with metastasis survive 5 years.

The diagnosis of melanoma is aided by fundus photography (Fig. 98.8) and fluorescein angiography but the most commonly performed test is ocular ultrasonography. Typically the B-scan demonstrates an elevated solid tumor (55) and the A-scan demonstrates medium to low reflectivity (56). As recently as 1974, 20% of eyes enucleated for melanoma did not have a melanoma. In recent years with standardization of criteria and careful attention to ocular ultrasound the diagnosis has been shown to be accurate, without biopsy, in more than 99.5% of cases.

Since clinical accuracy is so high needle biopsy is rarely needed. Some centers have had large experience with needle biopsy and report high accuracy and few problems but there has always been the concern that tumor cells might exit through the biopsy site, seed and spread. It has been shown that when a needle is inadvertently placed through the sclera of cases of choroidal melanoma that seeding and death may occur. We rarely use needle biopsy but look forward to careful analysis of the merits and risks from other centers as more data are gained.

A number of clinical and pathological features have been shown to correlate with patient survival (57).

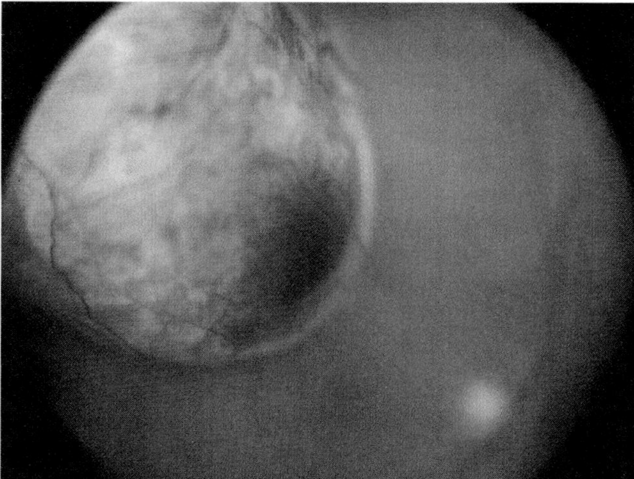

Figure 98.8. Malignant melanoma of the choroid.

- **Size.** The greater the size of the tumor, measured clinically using the height, and/or greatest base diameter to volume, the greater the incidence of metastasis.
- **Location.** Iris melanomas, as previously discussed, have the best prognosis. Ciliary body melanomas have a threefold mortality compared with choroidal melanomas.
- **Age.** Patients younger than 60 have better survival than those older than 60.
- **Extraocular extension.** Patients with extraocular extension have mortality rates many times those who do not. The greater the amount of local extension into the orbit the poorer the prognosis.
- **Pathologic features.** Many pathologic features (only available in cases where the eye has been removed) correlate with survival and are covered extensively elsewhere (61). The best known of these is cell type. Ocular melanomas that contain plumper so-called epithelioid cells have a poorer prognosis.

The treatment of choroidal melanoma has received wide coverage in the ophthalmic literature (58, 59). Most authors have classified choroidal melanomas as small, medium and large. The actual definitions of these sizes vary despite the words, which makes it difficult to generalize about prior studies. The Collaborative Ocular Melanoma Study definition is seen in Table 98.8.

Meta analysis reveals that patients with "small melanomas" have a 5 year survival of over 90% (60). Patients with "medium sized melanomas" sustain a 5-year survival of 67% (60). Patients with "large sized melanomas" have a 5-year survival of only 50% (60).

A number of treatment options exist for choroidal melanomas (59, 61). Although the best treatment is not known, the treatment options depend on the size of the tumor. Melanomas under 1.5 mm in height are not treated and probably have no metastasis nor mortality untreated (if they stay that size). Melanomas between 1.5 mm and 10 mm in height have been treated with local excision, enucleation or radiation with external photons, external protons or brachytherapy. Melanomas larger than 10 mm in height are usually treated by enucleation, although in exceptional cases (e.g., patients with only one eye) radiation may be considered. Because patients with "large" melanomas have such a poor prognosis, pre-operative external beam radiation (2,000 cGy) has also been used.

Radiation therapy for ocular melanomas has a long history. Brachytherapy for melanomas was first conceived 60

Table 98.8. Classification of Choroidal Melanomas

Small melanomas
Height <2.5 mm
Base diameter <16 mm
Medium melanomas
Height 2.5 to 10 mm
Base diameter ≤16 mm
Large melanomas
Height >10 mm, or <2.5 mm if base diameter >16 mm

From the Collaborative Ocular Melanoma Study.

years ago by Mr. Henry Stallard (62). His original plaques utilized cobalt-60, and he reported that the "majority of the tumors became flat." In recent years cobalt has been largely abandoned because of safety issues, and several beta emitting (strontium, ruthenium) or gamma emitting plaques (iodine, palladium, iridium) have become available. In recent years brachytherapy has been combined with concurrent hyperthermia. External photons have been used and there has also been a large experience with helium ions/protons (63). Some general conclusions about radiation therapy can now be made (64). About 70% of irradiated tumors decrease in size and there is a correlation between local control and survival. Tumors that continue to grow after treatment more commonly metastasize. Doses of 7,500 cGy to 10,000 cGy are used. The fractionation schemes vary markedly without an apparent effect on either local control, metastasis or complications. All radiation techniques have radiation complications (66). External irradiation is more commonly associated with anterior segment complications: dry eye, corneal complications, iritis and cataract. Plaque therapy is more commonly associated with posterior complications, namely radiation retinopathy and optic neuropathy.

There has been intense interest in which of the therapeutic techniques is best for patient survival in the medium sized tumor group (65). Presently a 44 institution, prospective, randomized clinical trial (the Collaborative Ocular Melanoma Study) is in progress in the United States and Canada. Started in the mid 1980s the trial has two arms. Medium-sized-tumor patients are randomly assigned to enucleation or brachytherapy with (125)I plaques at a tumor dose of 10,000 cGy. Large sized tumors are randomized to enucleation or enucleation preceded immediately by 5 fractions of 200 cGy daily within 72 hours of the enucleation. Recruitment for the large tumor study (1,003 patients reached before Jan 1, 1995) has been attained but recruitment for the medium trial continues.

Metastatic Ocular Cancer (Adult)

The most common malignant neoplasm in the eye or orbit, in children or adults, is metastatic carcinoma to the choroid. For example, there are 350 cases of retinoblastoma yearly in the United States, 1500 cases of choroidal melanoma, and over 100,000 cases of metastasis to the eye.

Metastasis to the eye most commonly occurs in adults between 55 and 65 (the same distribution as ocular melanomas). The pattern in men and women is different. When men present with ocular metastasis they are usually unaware of a primary neoplasm. The decreased vision caused by the metastasis is their first sign of cancer. In women the diagnosis of cancer is usually well known and they may even be aware of other metastases besides the eye. To a large part this has been because the metastases in men are usually from lung cancer while in women they have usually been from carcinoma of the breast. As lung cancer has now surpassed breast cancer as a cause of cancer deaths in women, it is anticipated that their pattern will become more similar to that of men. Many other cancers metastasize to the eye, including G.I., prostate (though more commonly to orbital bones), thyroid, ovarian, cutaneous melanoma and sweat gland cancers to mention a few. Virtually all cancers have been found capable of metastasizing to the eye.

Most cancers metastasize to the uveal tract, but metastasis to the lids, conjunctiva, optic nerve, orbit, extraocular muscles and orbital bones are well known. Metastasis to the retina is rare. While metastasis to the iris and ciliary body is not unusual, it is metastasis to the choroid that represents most of the metastases to the eye.

Choroidal metastases are usually amelanotic (whereas ocular melanomas are usually pigmented), multiple (whereas ocular melanomas are solitary in more than 99% of cases), bilateral (whereas bilateral ocular melanomas are extremely rare), minimally elevated (whereas most ocular melanomas are many millimeters high) and when situated around the optic nerve or invading the sclera they are painful (whereas ocular melanomas are painless in nearly all cases). Metastatic tumors, like melanomas always have an, associated serous detachment but the amount of detachment is proportionally greater in cases of metastasis. Ultrasonographically most metastases have high reflectivity on ultrasound in contrast to melanomas which usually have low to medium reflectivity.

In melanomas most patients are detected as a result of routine exams; in metastases the serous detachment causes decreased visual field and diminished acuity so patients are usually seen because of symptoms. Metastases can be detected on routine exams in asymptomatic patients, however.

The most striking feature of metastatic ocular lesions is their association with concurrent CNS metastases. While the true concordance of these two is unknown, it has been our experience that more than 75% of cases of ocular metastasis have concurrent, though frequently difficult to demonstrate, CNS metastases. It has been speculated therefore that some ocular metastases do not arrive through blood borne routes but that CNS metastases may actually seed the choroid via the sub-arachnoid space as it does in childhood leukemia.

Treatment for ocular metastasis is considered when symptoms of diminished vision, pain or diplopia demand it. Treating the ocular lesion rarely has an impact on survival, except in carcinoid metastases but may significantly alter the quality of life. Many ocular metastases respond to chemotherapy the way other metastases respond. Chemotherapy and/or hormonal manipulation may cause rapid regression of the tumor and of sub-retinal fluid. Patients with undiagnosed ocular metastases occasionally demonstrate coarse brown pigmentation on the surface of a regressed choroidal metastases following successful chemotherapy. External beam irradiation is also used frequently for ocular metastases. Choroidal metastases are treated with lateral photons to a dose of 3000 cGy in 10 fractions over 2 weeks, sparing the lens and anterior segment. Complications other than transient skin erythema are rare. When metastases involve the anterior segment, anterior irradiation is necessary, and if they survive for long, patients would have to face the complications of dry eye, cataract, and red uncomfortable eyes. Except for carcinoid and breast cancer, however, median survival in patients with metastatic choroidal lesions is just over 6 months.

Ocular Lymphoid Tumors

Intraocular lymphomas are increasing in incidence because of their association with AIDS. Both benign and malignant types occur. Benign reactive hyperplasia may diffusely involve the uvea and be difficult to diagnosis without biopsy. It is not associated with systemic findings.

Primary malignant lymphomas of the eye also called reticulum cell sarcoma or microgliomatosis, usually present with cells in the vitreous and may have associated retinal and optic nerve involvement. These patients frequently have CNS disease but rarely systemic disease. Diagnosis is made by vitrectomy. Treatment is accomplished with systemic steroids and radiation therapy of 2,400 cGy to the affected eye and/or chemotherapy as if for intermediate grade systemic lymphoma. There is controversy about whether to treat the brain in these cases when diagnostic spinal tap and MRI studies show no cancer. Eventual CNS involvement is very common, as is bilateral ocular disease. Median survival is 3.5 years and usually determined by the brain involvement. Cure is rare, as is systemic spread.

Malignant lymphomas of the uvea present as diffuse uveal involvement and are usually associated with systemic disease with involvement of lymph nodes and viscera but rarely with CNS involvement.

Orbital Tumors

The diagnosis of orbital tumors has undergone a revolution in the past 20 years as a result of the widespread use of ultrasonography, CT scans, and MRI. Prior to that virtually all cases of proptosis required biopsy and it was not unusual to be unable to find a tumor. The number of orbits that require biopsy has decreased, and the chance of finding the diseased area has become much higher as a result of noninvasive imaging. Fortunately, malignant tumors of the orbit are unusual. In most cases they come from adjacent sinuses or from the overlying skin. Biopsy is rarely needed for definitive diagnosis, even in cases of metastatic disease, as in metastasis of breast cancer to the orbit. Malignant primary cancers of the orbit that do require biopsy and surgical management arise almost exclusively from the lacrimal gland. Finally, lymphomatous lesions of the orbit are common; definitive biopsy may be necessary and at times is the easiest way to establish pathologically the type of lymphoma. The clinical findings suggestive of an orbital tumor are listed in Table 98.9.

All cases of suspected orbital tumor should have imaging: ophthalmic ultrasound, CT scans with or without contrast material, and MRI with or without contrast. Any of these techniques alone, and two of them in combination, will lead to the anatomic location of the tumor. An algorithm for differential diagnosis and treatment of orbital tumors is shown in Figure 98.9.

Bone Lesions

CT scanning best delineates bony lesions causing proptosis. Primary bony lesions include osteomas, osteogenic sarcomas, and fibrous dysplasia. Secondary lesions include metastases, especially from prostate, thyroid, lung, breast, and kidney cancers. The radiologic appearances of these are detailed elsewhere (66).

Lacrimal Gland Tumors

Lacrimal gland tumors can be easily found with ophthalmic B-scan at ultrasonography. The complete extent, especially bony involvement, is best demonstrated with CT scans. When lacrimal gland tumors are bilateral patients have either inflammatory lesions (sarcoid, pseudotumor) or lymphomas. Inflammatory lesions tend to be somewhat tender and represent the overwhelming majority of such lesions. Many clinicians treat painful bilateral lacrimal gland tumors without biopsy with high-dose aspirin, nonsteroidal anti-inflammatory agents, or systemic prednisone.

Unilateral lacrimal gland masses almost always require biopsy, although their clinical presentations may be distinct. Benign mixed tumors are painless, slowly (over years!) enlarging masses of the gland in patients 30 to 40 years old causing infradisplacement of the globe. They present a rounded or globular soft tissue mass in the lacrimal gland that may even have formed a fossa within bone. Treatment is surgical.

Adenoid cystic carcinoma, the most common malignant epithelial tumor of the lacrimal gland, may also present at

Table 98.9. Findings Suggestive of Orbital Tumor

Proptosis/exophthalmos	Anterior displacement of globe
Globe displacement	Masses in the inferior orbit cause vertical displacement of the globe; superior masses cause infra displacement
Limitation of motility	Globe motility limited by simple mass effect, direct involvement of extraocular muscle(s), direct or indirect effect on the nerves to extraocular muscles, adhesions of tumor to globe
Orbital pain	Especially in rapidly progressing tumors
Increased retropulsion	Digitally pushing back the globe gives more resistance on the side of the tumor
Foreshortened globe	Mass effect flattens globe with increased hyperopia/decreased myopia
Periocular paresthesias/anesthesia	Effect on sensory nerves
Ptosis	Droopy lid caused by proptosis
Palpable mass	Possible in anteriorly placed tumors only
Visual field defects	Defect limited to one eye
Lid edema	May indicate obstruction of venous flow
Papilledema	From mass effect on the retrobulbar optic nerve

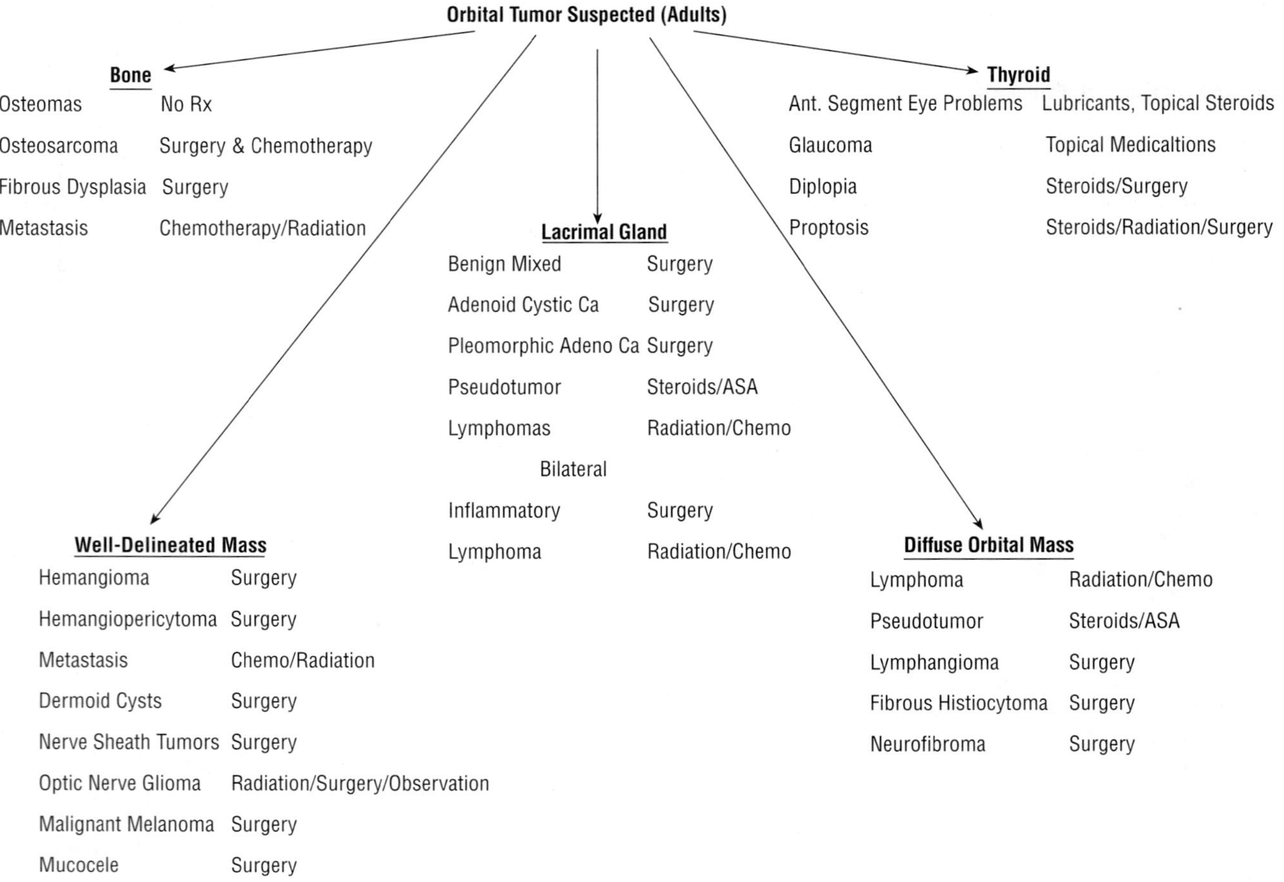

Figure 98.9. Algorithm for diagnosis and treatment of orbital tumors in adults.

age 30 to 40 with infradisplacement of the globe. Frequently there is pain, numbness, diplopia, and visual disturbance. Symptoms are less than 1 year in duration, and CT scan shows a circumscribed lacrimal gland mass, frequently with ragged, infiltrating edges into bone. Treatment is surgical. Recurrences may take many years to appear. Nonetheless, 90% of patients develop metastases and die within 15 years.

Pleomorphic adenocarcinomas (malignant mixed tumors) occur in older patients (50 to 60) in three distinct clinical patterns. Patients may present with a painless mass de novo. They may have a history of years of a painless lacrimal gland mass (probably representing a pleomorphic adenoma) with sudden (3–6 month) increase in size. Finally they may have a history of a prior biopsy of a benign mixed tumor that was incompletely excised many years before. Treatment is surgical. More than three-quarters die of metastases within 5 years.

Benign mixed tumors and carcinomas represent only 25% of lacrimal gland tumors. Nonepithelial lesions account for 75% of lacrimal gland tumors. Of these, 80% are inflammatory; previously called orbital pseudotumor now they are lumped together as benign reactive lymphoid hyperplasia. These lesions can be slow growing or sudden, painful or painless, and may be associated with any of the earlier mentioned signs and symptoms. They are treated with systemic high-dose aspirin, steroids, or in rare cases with low-dose irradiation. Their cause is unknown.

The remainder of the lacrimal gland tumors are lymphomas. As with all lymphomas careful pathologic analysis, aided by fresh tissue with appropriate marker studies and systemic staging, help to define the disease and guide treatment with chemotherapy alone, local radiation alone, or a combination of both. There is much controversy about the clinical course and prognosis of periocular lymphoid lesions, but it appears that histology, stage at diagnosis, and anatomic site of involvement are predictive (67). One-third to two-thirds of patients will develop systemic disease (if not already present at the time of orbital biopsy), and almost all of these do so within 2.5 years of orbital biopsy. The higher the grade lymphoma the greater the chance of widespread disease (which is the opposite of nodal disease). Of patients with localized, extranodal disease 86% were disease-free a median of 51 months after radiation treatment; 32% of patients who had disseminated disease had died (68).

Some studies suggest that patients with bilateral orbital involvement have a poorer prognosis. Conjunctival lesions have the lowest chance (20%) of developing systemic disease. Eyelid lymphomas have the highest chance (67%), with orbital lesions in between (35%) (69).

Thyroid Ophthalmopathy

Thyroid-related orbital disease represents the most common cause of both bilateral and of unilateral proptosis. The eye findings may be associated with clinical or laboratory evidence of hyperthyroidism, hypothyroidism, or euthyroidism. The disease is 4 to 5 times more common in women, usually those in middle age. While the eye findings in this disease may be subtle and varied, in cases of mistaken diagnosis of orbital tumor proptosis is always present. A straightforward clinical examination of the patient with thyroid eye disease will usually differentiate it from a true orbital tumor. In both cases there may be proptosis. In the case of a tumor the eye is displaced forward, which causes stretching of the upper lid, and the distance between the eyelid and the lid fold is increased. In cases of thyroid disease, because of "retraction" attributed to overactivity of the levator muscle, the displaced eye is associated with a shorter distance between the lid margin and the lid fold.

The signs and symptoms of thyroid eye disease include lid retraction, lid lag, lid edema, inability to fully close the eye with corneal drying, infection, and ulcers. Because of the muscle involvement there may be limitation of ocular movement with diplopia. Elevated intraorbital pressure, especially on looking up, may cause a severe, blinding glaucoma. CT and/or MRI may demonstrate the proptosis, enlargement of one (usually the inferior rectus) or any combination of extraocular muscles, with increased fat in the orbit but no clear masses.

Laboratory testing for thyroid ophthalmopathy is frequently confusing. Among the tests used are T_4 (thyroxine) and TSH (thyroid-stimulating hormone). T_3 (triiodothyronine), T_3 uptake (a measure of the relative saturation of thyroid-binding globulin), and radioactive iodine uptake are sometimes used. In cases of autoimmune thyroid disease microsomal antibodies and thyroid stimulating immunoglobulin are also used. The thyroid-releasing hormone (TRH) stimulation test may be useful in cases of so-called euthyroid Graves' disease.

Treatment is directed at cosmetics, vision, double vision, and problems related to corneal exposure. Glaucoma may have to be treated in one eye only. Treatment includes systemic steroids, irradiation (2,000 cGy), and surgical decompression. Systemic diuretics, cyclophosphamide, azathioprine, and cyclosporin have also been used with some success.

Well-Defined Orbital Masses

The most common benign orbital tumor of adults is the cavernous hemangioma (in contrast to the capillary hemangioma for children). Patients have slowly progressive painless proptosis with a mass indenting the globe showing striae in the retina and a flattened globe on imaging studies. Treatment is surgical, and complete removal is possible.

A mucocele is a cystic, encapsulated mass originating in a paranasal sinus (usually the frontal sinus) that follows repeated bouts of sinusitis often leading to recurrent orbital cellulitis. The bony wall is not intact on imaging studies. Treatment involves excision of the mucocele and surgical attention to the involved sinus.

Diffuse Orbital Mass

Diffuse orbital masses usually require a biopsy and include lymphoma, benign reactive lymphoid hyperplasia ("orbital pseudotumor"), orbital cellulitis, fibrous histiocytoma (benign and malignant), neurofibromas, and sarcomas. Their management is presented in Figure 98.9.

References

1. Abramson DH. Retinoblastoma. Pediatr Emerg Casebook 1985;3:3–15.
2. Abramson DH. Retinoblastoma: diagnosis and management. CA 1982;32:130–140.
3. Abramson DH. The focal treatment of retinoblastoma with emphasis on xenon arc photocoagulation. Acta Ophthalmol 1989;67:1–63.
4. Abramson DH, Ellsworth RM, Grumbach N, Kitchin FD. Retinoblastoma: survival, age at detection and comparison 1914–1958, 1958–1983. J Pediatr Ophthalmol Strabismus 1985;22:246–250.
5. Knudson AG. Mutation and cancer: statistical study of retinoblastoma. Proc Natl Acad Sci USA 1971;68:820–823.
6. Friend SH, Bernards R, Rogelj S, Weinberg RA, Rapaport JM, Albert DM, Dryja TP. A human DNA segment with properties of the gene that predisposes to retinoblastoma and osteosarcoma. Nature 1986;323:643–646.
7. Muncaster MM, Cohen BL, Philips RA, Gallie BL. Failure of RB1 to reverse the malignant phenotype of human tumor cell lines. Cancer Res 1992;52:654–661.
8. Harlow E. Retinoblastoma: for our eyes only. Nature 1992;359:270–271.
9. Yandell DW. Presented at the Third International Conference on Long-Term Complications of Treatment of Children and Adolescents for Cancer, Jun 1994, Niagara Falls, NY.
10. Squire J, Gallie BL, Philips RA. A detailed analysis of chromosomal changes in heritable and non-heritable retinoblastoma. Hum Genet 1985;70:291–301.
11. Doz F. N-*myc* amplification, loss of heterozygosity in 1p and DNA index in tumor specimens of 45 patients with retinoblastoma. Presented at the Seventh International Retinoblastoma Symposium; Jun 1994, Ontario, Canada.
12. Bookstein R, Lee WH. Molecular genetics of the retinoblastoma suppressor gene. Crit Rev Oncogenesis 1991;2:211–227.
13. Schubert EL, Hansen MF, String LC. The retinoblastoma gene and its significance. Ann Med 1994;26:177–184.
14. Ellsworth RM. The practical management of retinoblastoma. Trans Am Ophthalmol Soc 1969;67:462–533.
15. Abramson DH, Servodidio CA. Retinoblastoma in the first year of life. In The Eye in Infancy, 2nd ed. Edited by SJ Eisenberg. St. Louis: Mosby, 1994, pp 426–436.
16. Reese AB. Tumors of the Eye, 3rd ed. New York: Harper & Row, 1976.
17. Abramson DH. The diagnosis of retinoblastoma. Bull NY Acad Med 1988;64:282–317.
18. Shields JA. Diagnosis and Management of Intraocular Tumors. St. Louis: Mosby, 1983.
19. Abramson DH. Lactate dehydrogenase and retinoblastoma. In Ocular and Adnexal Tumors. Edited by FA Jakobiec. Birmingham AL: Aesculaoius, 1978, pp 454–459.
20. Abramson DH. The surgical management of retinoblastoma. Ophthalmic Surg 1980;11:556–558.
21. Grabowski E, Abramson DH. Intraocular and extraocular retinoblastoma. Hematol Oncol Clin North Am 1987;1:721–735.
22. Abramson DH. Treatment of retinoblastoma. In Retinoblastoma (Contemporary Issues in Ophthalmology). Edited by FC Blodi. New York: Churchill Livingstone, 1985, pp 63–93.
23. Abramson DH, Jereb B. External beam radiation for retinoblastoma. Bull NY Acad Med 1981;57:787–803.
24. McCormick B, Ellsworth RM, Abramson DH, Lo Sasso T, Grabowski E. Results of external beam radiation for children with retinoblastoma: a comparison of two techniques. J Pediatr Ophthalmol Strabismus 1989;26:239–243.
25. Meyer-Schwickerath G; Drance SM, trans. Light Coagulation. St. Louis: Mosby, 1960.
26. Lincoff H, McLean J, Long R. The cryosurgical treatment of intraocular tumors. Am J Ophthalmol 1967;63:389.
27. Abramson DH. Cryotherapy in retinoblastoma. In Advanced Techniques in Ocular Surgery. Edited by F Jakobiec. Philadelphia: Saunders, 1984, pp 433–437.
28. Stallard HB. The conservative treatment of retinoblastoma. Highlights Ophthalmol 1963;6:129–130.
29. Buys R, Abramson DH, Ellsworth RM, Haik BG. Radiation regression patterns after cobalt plaque insertion for retinoblastoma. Arch Ophthalmol 1983;101:1206–1208.
30. Abramson DH, Ellsworth RM, Haik BG. Cobalt plaques in advanced retinoblastoma. Retina 1983;3:12–15.
31. White L. Chemotherapy in retinoblastoma: current status and future directions. Am J Pediatr Hematol Oncol 1991;13:189–201.
32. Magramm I, Abramson DH, Ellsworth RM. Optic nerve involvement in retinoblastoma. Ophthalmology 1989;96:217–222.
33. Shields CL, Shields JA, Baez K, Cater JR, DePotter P. Optic nerve invasion of retinoblastoma: metastatic potential and clinical risk factors. Cancer 1994;73:692–698.
34. Zelter M, Damel A, Gonzalez G, Schwartz L. A prospective study on the treatment of retinoblastoma in 72 patients. Cancer 1991;68:1685–1690.
35. Doz F, Khelfaoui F, Mosseri V, Validire P, Quintana E, Michon J, Desjardins L, Schlienger P, Neuenschwander S, Vielh P, Putterman M, Dufier JL, Zucker JM. The role of chemotherapy in orbital involvement of retinoblastoma. Cancer 1994;74:722–732.
36. Goble RR, McKenzie J, Kingston JE, Plowman PN, Hungerford JL. Orbital recurrence of retinoblastoma successfully treated by combined therapy. Br J Ophthalmol 1990;74:97–98.

37. Grabowski EF, Abramson DH. Retinoblastoma. In Clinical Pediatric Oncology, 4th ed. Edited by DJ Fernbach, TJ Vietti. St. Louis: Mosby, 1991, pp 427–435.
38. Chan HSL, Canton MD, Gallie BL. Chemosensitivity and multidrug resistance to antineoplastic drugs in retinoblastoma cell lines. Anticancer Res 1989;9:469–474.
39. Reese AB, Merriam GR, Martin HE. Treatment of bilateral retinoblastoma by irradiation and surgery. Report on 15-year results. Am J Ophthalmol 1949;32:175–190.
40. Abramson DH, Ellsworth RM, Zimmerman LE. Non-ocular cancer in retinoblastoma survivors. Trans Am Acad Ophthalmol Otolaryngol 1976;81:454–458.
41. Abramson DH, Ellsworth RM, Kitchin FD, Teung G. Second nonocular tumors in retinoblastoma survivors: Are they radiation-induced? Ophthalmology 1984;91: 1351–1355.
42. Eng C, Li FP, Abramson DH, Ellsworth RM, Wong L, Goldman MB, Seddon J, Tarbell N, Boice JD. Mortality from second tumors among long-term survivors of retinoblastoma. JNCI 1993;85:1121–1128.
43. Abramson DH, Jereb B, Wollner N, Murphy L, Ellsworth RM. Leukemic ophthalmopathy detected by ultrasound. J Pediatr Ophthalmol Strabismus 1983;20:92–97.
44. Gomez DG, Manzo RP, Fenstermacher JD, Potts DG. Cerebrospinal fluid absorption in the rabbit. Optic pathways. Graefe's Arch Exp Ophthalmol 1988;226:1–7.
45. Haik BG. Vascular tumors of the orbit. In Ophthalmic and Orbital Plastic Reconstructive Surgery. Edited by A Hornblass. Baltimore: Williams & Wilkins, 1989, pp 509–517.
46. Jones IS. Lymphangiomas of the ocular adnexae: an analysis of 62 cases. Am J Ophthalmol 1961;51:481–509.
47. Abramson DH, Ellsworth RM, Tretter P, Wolff JA, Kitchin FD. The treatment of orbital rhabdomyosarcoma with irradiation and chemotherapy. Ophthalmology 1979;86: 1330–1335.
48. Jones IS, Reese AB, Kraut J. Orbital rhabdomyosarcoma: an analysis of 62 cases. Am J Ophthalmol 1966;61:721–735.
49. Wharam M, Beltangady M, Hays D, Heyn R, Ragab A, Soule E, Tefft M, Maurer H. Localized orbital rhabdomyosarcoma. An interim report of the Intergroup Rhabdomyosarcoma Study Committee. Ophthalmology 1987;94:251–254.
50. Abramson DH, Notis C. Visual acuity after radiation for orbital rhabdomyosarcoma. Am J Ophthalmol 1994;6:808–809.
51. Abramson DH. Orbital rhabdomyosarcoma. Clin Decisions Ophthalmol 1990;14:6–10.
52. Johnson RN. Choroidal and Ciliary Body Malignant Melanoma: Diagnosis and Management. Korea: Retina Research Fund, 1993.
53. Servodidio CA, Abramson DH. Presenting signs and symptoms of choroidal melanoma: what do they mean? Ann Ophthalmol 1992;24:190–194.
54. Abramson DH. Computerized visual defects of choroidal melanomas. Glaucoma 1988;10:39–44.
55. Coleman DJ, Abramson DH, et al. Ultrasonic diagnosis of tumors of the choroid. Arch Ophthalmol 1974;91:344–355.
56. Byrne SF, Green WL. Ultrasound of the Eye and Orbit. St. Louis: Mosby, 1992.
57. Shields J, Shields CL, Donoso LA. Management of posterior uveal melanomas. Survey Ophthalmol 1991;36:161–195.
58. Shammas H, Blodi FC. Prognostic factors in choroidal and ciliary body melanomas. Arch Ophthalmol 1977;95:63–69.
59. Shields JA. Diagnosis and Management of Intraocular Tumors. St Louis: Mosby, 1983.
60. Diener-West M, Hawkins B, et al. A review of mortality from choroidal melanoma. II. A meta-analysis of 5-year mortality rates following enucleation 1966 through 1988. Arch Ophthalmol 1992;110:245–250.
61. Char D. Clinical Ocular Oncology, New York: Churchill Livingstone, 1988.
62. Stallard HB. Radiotherapy of malignant intraocular neoplasms. Br J Ophthalmol 1948;32:618–639.
63. Char D, et al. Helium ion therapy for choroidal melanoma. Ophthalmology 1983;90: 1219–1225.
64. Abramson DH, Servodidio CA. Ocular complications due to cancer treatment. In Survivors of Childhood Cancer: Assessment and Management. St. Louis: Mosby, 1994, pp 111–132.
65. Fine S. Do I take the eye out or leave it in? Arch Ophthalmol 1986;104:653–654.
66. Henderson JH. Orbital Tumors, 2nd ed. New York: Georg Thieme, 1980.
67. Knowles DM, et al. Lymphoid hyperplasia and malignant lymphoma occurring in the ocular adnexa (orbit, conjunctiva and eyelids). Hum Pathol 1987;31:959.
68. McNally L, Jakobiec F, Knowles DM. Clinical, morphologic, immunophenotypic, and molecular genetic analysis of bilateral ocular adnexal lymphoid neoplasms in 17 patients. Am J Ophthalmol 1987;103:555–568.

SECTION XXVIII

NEOPLASMS OF THE ENDOCRINE GLANDS

CHAPTER 99

Pituitary Neoplasms

CHARLES B. WILSON AND THOMAS MINDERMANN

Introduction

The classic histologic designation of pituitary adenomas as acidophilic, basophilic, or chromophobic based on their histologic appearance as seen with light microscopy has been superseded by a system derived from the work of Landolt (74) and Kovacs and colleagues (66, 67), in which adenomas are classified according to the hormone(s) they secrete (66, 67, 74, 140). More recent work has shown that pituitary adenomas may be classified at three levels: origin, morphology, and endocrine function (Table 99.1). Northern blot and in situ hybridization reveal the adenoma's cell line of origin by determining its genetic structure and its messenger RNA (mRNA) for hormone synthesis. Electron microscopy reveals the adenoma's cell line of origin and, indirectly, the adenoma's hormone synthesis by showing the cellular ultrastructure and the type of hormone stored as determined by the size of secretory granules. Immunostaining indirectly reveals the adenoma's hormone synthesis by showing the type of hormone stored as determined by binding of specific antibodies. Endocrine function is defined by the adenoma's clinical endocrine activity, which depends on the release of hormone(s) into the bloodstream. Pituitary adenomas are generally considered either endocrine-active or endocrine-inactive. They are endocrine-active only if they secrete enough biologically active hormone to exceed normal levels in the blood and become clinically evident. Endocrine inactive adenomas, in contrast, have secretory granules and the cellular constituents for hormone production (67, 74), but either they produce normal hormones or hormonal compounds (52, 108) that do not cause clinically detectable symptoms or signs or, alternatively, they have lost the ability to produce hormone through degeneration or dedifferentiation. Molecular biologic studies ultimately will provide an even more informative classification of pituitary adenomas.

Early evidence has shown a monoclonal origin for most adenomas, implying that somatic mutation of a single cell is likely to be the event initiating hormone hypersecretion and neoplastic transformation (47, 60). The adenomatous transformation of the cell not only affects its growth and secretory characteristics, but also seems to alter the ability of the adenomatous pituitary cell to respond to feedback from the hypothalamus and pituitary-dependent endocrine glands. For example, an absence of thyrotropin-releasing hormone (TRH) receptors has been demonstrated in thyroid-stimulating hormone (TSH)-releasing adenomas associated with hyperthyroidism (21). The cell kinetics of an adenoma may be determined by proliferative indices obtained by using the monoclonal antibody Ki-67 or the bromodeoxyuridine technique, which reflects the tumor's growth potential. These indices are generally low in pituitary adenomas, regardless of cell line, and so far have not been of any therapeutic consequence (19, 51, 63, 77, 100). The occurrence of oncogene mutations seems to offer a more promising basis on which to identify subsets of clinically aggressive pituitary adenomas, however. The expression of the c-myc protein seems to correlate with an adenoma's clinical aggressiveness (51). Ras oncogene mutations are infrequent in pituitary adenomas, but, if present, they may be a marker indicating an invasive tumor (56). G protein oncogene mutations have been found in a subset of growth hormone (GH)-releasing adenomas (73, 86, 122, 132). A large percentage of patients with acromegaly have somatic mutations in the α chain of the G protein (Gs) regulating the hormone-stimulatory activity of adenylyl cyclase. The adenomas with these Gs protein mutations are significantly smaller than those without mutations, and they are more sensitive to inhibitory factors such as somatostatin or dopamine—a characteristic that may prove to have therapeutic as well as diagnostic importance.

The adenoma's local growth characteristics and size, irrespective of endocrine activity, predict its nonendocrine clinical presentation (45, 139). Wilson's anatomic (radiographic and operative) scheme (139, 141, 142), derived from Hardy's (42, 45), classifying pituitary adenomas by the degree of sellar destruction (grade) and extrasellar extension (stage) is valuable in establishing a prognosis and helpful in designing therapy. The following generalizations provide a framework for discussion of the more prevalent pituitary neoplasms.

For patients suspected of or known to be harboring a pituitary adenoma, the diagnostic neuroimaging procedure of choice is magnetic resonance (MR) imaging. While gadolinium enhancement should be used for microadenomas (less than 10 mm in diameter) (101), its use for macroadenomas is optional. The image is preferably obtained using a 1.5-tesla MR imager with thin sections in coronal and sagittal planes (142). A preoperative diagnosis that relies only on imaging techniques and clinical data is of limited accuracy, however. The production, suppression, or release of one or more anterior-lobe hormones or hormonal compounds by adenomatous or nonadenomatous cells can occur in any of a variety of combinations (93). Classic clinical symptoms

Table 99.1. Classification of Pituitary Adenomas According to . . .[a]

Cell line(s) (hormone synthesis[b])	Immunophenotype (hormone storage[c])	Clinical phenotype (hormone release[d])
Clinically endocrine-active pituitary adenomas[e]		
Mammotropic cell	PRL	Prolactinoma
Corticotropic cell	ACTH	Cushing's disease
Corticotropic cell	ACTH	Nelson's syndrome
Somatotropic cell	GH, or GH and PRL	Acromegaly, prolactinoma, or both
Acidophil stem cell	GH and PRL	Prolactinoma, acromegaly, or both
Thyrotropic cell	TSH	TSH-secreting PA
Unclassified plurihormonal cell(s)	Any combination of PRL, GH, ACTH, LH, FSH, TSH, and αSU	Plurihormonal PA of one dominant clinical phenotype[f]
Clinically endocrine-inactive ("nonsecreting") pituitary adenomas[g]		
Null cell	Nonreactive	Null cell adenoma
Oncocytic cell	Nonreactive	Oncocytoma
Gonadotropic cell[e]	LH, FSH, or LH and FSH	Gonadotropic PA
Corticotropic cell[e]	ACTH	Silent corticotropic PA
Somatotropic cell	GH	Silent somatotropic PA
Acidophil stem cell	GH and PRL	Nonsecreting acidophil stem cell PA
Thyrotropic cell	TSH	Silent thyrotropic PA
Unclassified pure αSU cell	αSU	Pure αSU-secreting PA
Unclassified plurihormonal cell(s)	Any combination of PRL, GH, ACTH, LH, FSH, TSH, and αSU	Nonsecreting plurihormonal PA

[a] PRL = prolactin; ACTH = adrenocorticotropic hormone; GH = growth hormone; TSH = thyroid-stimulating hormone (thyrotropin); LH = luteinizing hormone; FSH = follicle-stimulating hormone; αSU = α subunit.
[b] As determined by in situ hybridization and electron microscopy.
[c] As determined by electron microscopy and immunostaining.
[d] As determined clinically by symptoms, signs, and serum hormone levels.
[e] Cosynthesis of the clinically inactive αSU and its release into the bloodstream is possible.
[f] LH and FSH are clinically inactive; their release into the bloodstream can be measured.
[g] May present clinically as prolactinoma when stalk effect or raised intrasellar pressure leads to an increased release of prolactin by nonadenomatous cells or when PRL is cosynthesized by tumorous cells.

and signs are not necessarily diagnostic of the clinically expected adenoma type (50, 94, 96, 114, 145) and, moreover, adenomas can change their immunophenotype (93).

The transsphenoidal approach is the preferred surgical technique for almost all pituitary adenomas and the treatment of choice for those secreting GH (acromegaly) or ACTH (Cushing's disease or Nelson's syndrome) as well as for certain nonsecreting tumors that extend out of the sella to compress adjacent structures and produce clinical manifestations, usually impaired vision. The operative approaches to pituitary adenomas have been described (78, 141, 142). The objectives of surgery are to eliminate any mass effect of the tumor, to halt endocrine hyperactivity, to retain or improve existing pituitary function (4), to achieve these goals immediately and with minimal morbidity (63), and to predict accurately the need for adjuvant therapy (110).

It is debated whether the initial treatment for prolactin-secreting adenomas should be medical or surgical, with bromocriptine or irradiation reserved for surgical failures. For the rare and aggressive tumors secreting thyroid-stimulating hormone, the role and timing of surgery are unclear. An endocrine-inactive tumor in an asymptomatic patient with unimpaired pituitary function should, with some exceptions, be left alone and its course observed with serial MR images. Less well defined is the most effective management for pituitary apoplexy, the symptom complex that evolves acutely or subacutely as a consequence of hemorrhage and necrosis within an adenoma. At the University of California, San Francisco (UCSF), we tend to prepare the patient quickly and proceed directly with transsphenoidal surgery. If hypopituitarism is treated with suitable replacement therapy, but no surgery, the compressive symptoms may resolve in time, but the tumor will almost certainly require treatment at a later date. Medical management does not spare the patient an operation—it merely postpones it. The only exceptions are in some cases of prolactin(PRL)-secreting adenomas (142).

Prolactinomas

Prolactinomas and clinically endocrine-inactive adenomas are the most prevalent pituitary adenomas treated surgically at UCSF (93). The occurrence of prolactinomas varies greatly with gender and age (95). In children experiencing puberty, adolescents, and women of childbearing age, prolactinoma is the most frequent adenoma type (96). The vast majority of prolactinomas occur in women of childbearing age, resulting in a female-to-male ratio of 14.5:1 during the third decade of life (95). After the third decade, the number of women affected declines, and the female-to-male ratio equalizes during the fifth decade. Among patients older than 50 years of age, prolactinomas are 2 to 3 times more common in men (95). Of all pituitary adenomas treated surgically at UCSF, prolactinomas have the lowest postoperative recurrence rate (2%) (93). The behavior and benign clinical manifestations of small prolactinomas distinguish them from the adenomas that produce Cushing's disease and acromegaly, two distinct metabolic entities that have severe and eventually fatal consequences independent of their effects as a mass. Unlike those lesions, prolactinomas manifest differently in men and women. Whereas large prolactinomas are slightly more prevalent in women than men, men rarely present with microadenomas.

PATHOLOGY

The level of PRL in blood, taken as an index of secretory activity, correlates directly with the size of the prolactinoma, exclusive of bulk contributed by necrosis and cysts. Necrosis is a common surgical finding in prolactinomas of all sizes. Prolactinomas, with relatively rare exceptions, grow slowly (142).

CLINICAL PRESENTATION

Prolactinomas may produce primary (37), or secondary amenorrhea, and galactorrhea. The frequency of hyperprolactinemia in amenorrheic women is now well recognized. Equally evident is that prolactinoma is a common cause of hyperprolactinemia. Among women with prolactinomas treated at UCSF over two decades (142), 80% had secondary amenorrhea and spontaneous or expressible galactorrhea; 10% had primary amenorrhea, one-half of whom also had galactorrhea; and 10% had oligomenorrhea with galactorrhea, secondary amenorrhea without galactorrhea, or secondary amenorrhea only. In men, a prolactinoma usually goes undetected during the initial phase of hyperprolactinemia, and the diagnosis may be established only after the adenoma has become large and caused significant hypopituitarism or compressed and invaded parasellar structures; a history of lessened libido, and eventually impotence, often precedes clinical manifestations of a large mass.

Hyperprolactinemia may have extragonadal manifestations, although possibly only in patients predisposed to these disorders. A recent, rapid, often excessive, and unwanted weight gain is reported by hyperprolactinemic women with a frequency that suggests a relation. Correction of hyperprolactinemia through surgery or bromocriptine therapy is in some cases followed by impressive weight loss despite no change in dietary habits. Equally impressive is the incidence of emotional lability and its reversal after correction of hyperprolactinemia (16, 109, 120, 121). Obesity and emotional instability may reflect multiple nonendocrine factors, but hyperprolactinemia that is neither extreme nor long-standing also causes significant demineralization of bone, with its potential morbidity (62, 115).

DIAGNOSIS

A preoperative diagnosis of prolactinoma should be made with great caution. Stalk effect and raised intrasellar pressure, which may be caused by any other adenoma type or by cosynthesis of prolactin (PRL) in a plurihormonal adenoma or in PRL-and GH-producing adenomas, can clinically mimic a prolactinoma with symptoms and signs, including elevated serum PRL levels, menstrual irregularities, and galactorrhea (50, 81, 82, 96, 114, 133, 145). Even with unequivocal radiographic demonstration of a pathologic abnormality in the pituitary gland, transsphenoidal explorations have in some cases revealed either a diffusely enlarged anterior lobe (pituitary "hyperplasia") or a nonneoplastic cyst, usually in the pars intermedia (142). Attempts to distinguish functional or nonneoplastic hyperprolactinemia from the hyperprolactinemia produced by prolactinomas on the basis of laboratory values alone have yielded conflicting conclusions. No single test or combination of tests is infallible. In men with basal PRL values over 100 ng/ml, a prolactinoma is almost always the cause of hyperprolactinemia. In women, hyperprolactinemia and basal values over 200 ng/ml almost always indicate a prolactinoma; with some exceptions, basal values of 100 to 200 ng/mL have nearly the same significance. Women with basal levels of 50 to 100 ng/mL, for which the term moderate hyperprolactinemia seems appropriate, present a quandary. Values in this range may have no recognized cause, and a confident prediction of a prolactinoma cannot be based solely on laboratory values in women whose moderate hyperprolactinemia is unrelated to medication, pregnancy, or hypothyroidism. In a few patients, moderate hyperprolactinemia is the result of a stalk section effect produced by a readily identified pathologic intrasellar or suprasellar lesion, usually an endocrine-inactive adenoma or infrequently a suprasellar tumor such as a craniopharyngioma (55) that interferes with downward blood flow through the pituitary stalk.

TREATMENT

Unlike long-term medical therapy for Cushing's disease and acromegaly, which is relatively ineffective, bromocriptine corrects the biochemical pathology of prolactinomas and reduces their size, at times dramatically. One view is that medical therapy should be used for all patients except the 30% or so who have unacceptable side effects from the medication. In contrast is the opinion that surgery should be the initial treatment, bromocriptine or irradiation being reserved for patients who are not cured (9). Although some clinicians question the wisdom of treating these patients at all, the potential for adverse systemic and psychological effects from hyperprolactinemia and the potential for invasive behavior of the tumor provide compelling arguments for treatment, whether surgical or nonsurgical. The middle ground seems preferable. Surgery does not predictably cure these adenomas, and the higher the patient's PRL level, the greater is the potential for therapeutic failure. Moreover, serious surgical complications may occur, although with an experienced surgeon the likelihood is no more than 1%. Medical management is hardly a perfect solution, however. It appears that medication must be a lifetime commitment for most if not all of the patients, a significant portion of whom have unpleasant and sometimes unacceptable side effects at effective dose levels. A few tumors are relatively resistant to bromocriptine as judged by insufficiently lowered PRL levels and, in some cases, continued tumor growth (69). Finally, patients with macroadenomas who become pregnant may develop complications from accelerated tumor growth. Although treatment with bromocriptine usually resolves the problem, it may not (107).

The low morbidity rates, the low incidence of recurrence, and the high likelihood of cure associated with selective transsphenoidal microsurgery support its use as the treatment of choice for patients with microprolactinomas. In patients with large, invasive tumors and extremely high PRL levels, the administration of a dopamine agonist, such as bromocriptine, either alone or in combination with surgery, pituitary irradiation, or both appears to be the appropriate mode of therapy (137). Unless an MR image shows unquestioned invasion of the cavernous sinus, surgical cure is a reasonable expectation in any patient with a PRL level of 500 ng/mL or less (7). The lower the PRL level, the greater the likelihood of cure. The younger the patient, the clearer are the advantages of surgery and the less desirable is medical management. Patients who cannot tolerate medication become surgical candidates, with varying expectations of cure. Irradiation sterilizes but does not inactivate prolactinomas and is reserved for patients who are not cured with surgery and cannot tolerate medication (10).

RECOMMENDATION

The policies currently determining recommended management at UCSF reflect our favorable experience with the microsurgical approach, the assumption that most prolactinomas grow relatively slowly, and the evidence that surgical treatment is less successful in older patients, patients with a longer duration of amenorrhea, and patients with higher PRL values and larger tumors. These recommendations apply for the cases in which the clinical presentation, laboratory data, and MR images eliminate any reasonable doubt that the patient harbors a prolactinoma.

Operative removal is recommended for most macroadenomas, virtually all of which are accompanied by PRL values greater than 100 ng/mL. For tumors smaller than 2 cm, a surgical cure is likely. For noninvasive tumors larger than 2 cm, preliminary treatment with bromocriptine should reduce tumor volume and increase the likelihood of surgical cure. Residual tumor is managed medically. Irradiation is indicated for patients who cannot tolerate bromocriptine or have tumor progression despite treatment. For macroadenomas of a size or invasiveness precluding surgical cure, an initial trial of bromocriptine is appropriate (136). The management of microadenomas is more controversial. At UCSF, our indications for operative removal are (141, 142) a desire for pregnancy, the presence of primary amenorrhea, the patient's being male, and the patient's personal choice. For other patients, bromocriptine is prescribed, and the tumor is monitored at regular intervals with basal PRL measurements and periodic MR images; these tumors rarely expand without a concomitant rise in PRL levels. In patients electing nonoperative management initially, two subsequent developments indicate surgery: progressive elevation of PRL levels approaching 200 ng/mL in an untreated patient or a progressive elevation of PRL values in a patient taking bromocriptine; and enlargement of the tumor as determined by serial MR images.

Pregnancy

Induced pregnancy in a patient who has a prolactinoma carries a small but serious risk of complications related to rapid expansion of the tumor (11, 119). Prophylactic pituitary irradiation has been used in patients who desire pregnancy. If a tumor becomes symptomatic during pregnancy, bromocriptine can be given. We advise against pregnancy for patients known to have a prolactinoma and recommend that bromocriptine therapy be accompanied with contraception by mechanical means. As the risk of a serious complication during pregnancy seems significantly larger than the risk of transsphenoidal surgery, we advise surgical treatment when pregnancy is desired.

Growth Hormone-Releasing Adenomas

CLINICAL PRESENTATION

GH-secreting pituitary adenomas produce acromegaly and gigantism with their classic presentation marked by progressive enlargement of the hands, feet, and face. Although they progress slowly, these adenomas cause crippling cosmetic and orthopedic deformities and life-threatening metabolic effects, with 50% of untreated patients dead by the age of 50 years (33) and a death rate twice that of the general population (143). GH-releasing adenomas are slightly more prevalent in patients aged 31 to 70 years than in younger or older patients (95). They are 2 to 3 times more common in men before the female-to-male ratio equalizes at about age 45; thereafter, they occur twice as often in women (95).

DIAGNOSIS

With considerable accuracy, the diagnosis of acromegaly and gigantism can be made by history and physical examination. Evaluations of GH dynamics, including tests of glucose suppression, thyrotrophin-releasing hormone stimulation, and/or insulin-tolerance, may be performed. Patients with GH levels greater than 10 ng/mL have active disease (5), and a fasting growth hormone level in serum of less than 5 ng/mL is the benchmark normal value (6, 80, 126, 129–131). MR imaging is used to define the anatomical extent of the tumor.

TREATMENT

Although various surgical approaches have been used in the past, the treatment of choice is selective transsphenoidal removal of the adenoma. Although promising, somatostatin analogs to date do not provide a long-term alternative to operation (105, 123). Irradiation, used in the treatment of acromegaly since 1909 (40), still provides an alternative to surgery, although its efficacy is compromised by the delay in its therapeutic effect and its significant failure rate when used primarily (3, 44, 59, 71, 111, 112).

Despite the significance of clinical improvement as a measure of therapeutic success, the primary factor determining a cure is the restoration of normal GH production. Radioimmunoassays for GH and somatomedin C for the documentation of disease activity have provided quantitative information from which to assess the relative efficacy of particular forms of therapy. Based on these quantitations, transsphenoidal surgery is at present the preferable therapy in virtually every case of acromegaly. The results of transsphenoidal surgery for acromegaly at UCSF over a period of 14 years have been good (8,110), with long-term follow-up review showing GH levels of less than 5 ng/mL in 79.4%, and less than 10 ng/mL in 92.7%, of patients operated. The rates of recurrence after an apparent surgical cure (4.3%) and complications—i.e., new anterior pituitary hypofunction in 5%, cerebrospinal fluid (CSF) leak in 2.2%, and postoperative meningitis in 1.8%–are low, with no cases of permanent diabetes insipidus or death. Because the transsphenoidal procedure is short and postoperative stress minimal, the patient's age or medical status is rarely a contraindication (141). The surgical strategy is tailored to the size, shape, location, and consistency of the individual tumor (44). Factors predictive of a poor prognosis are high preoperative basal serum GH levels, high preoperative somatomedin C levels, tumor size greater than 10 mm, extrasellar extension of the tumor, failure of oral glucose to induce suppression of serum GH levels shortly after surgery, and high postoperative basal serum GH levels within 1 to 5 days after surgery (15, 28, 96, 128). For incompletely removed tumors, postoperative irradiation has a high probability (approaching 95%) of preventing future growth, but the risk of radiation-induced hypopituitarism is very high and there is a rare, but unequivocal, possibility of catastrophic complications (110).

Recently, there have been reports that medical therapy with the long-acting somatostatin analogue octreotide may result in a reduction of tumor size, reduction of left ventricular hypertrophy, and decrease of serum GH levels in patients with a clinical diagnosis of acromegaly, although the diagnosis was not confirmed histologically (34, 84). A side effect of long-term therapy was the development of cholelithiasis (34). In the absence of contraindications, we advocate transsphenoidal surgery as the treatment of choice for GH-releasing adenomas and consider the option of sellar irradiation or medical therapy only if a sustained postoperative remission cannot be achieved. Patients with acromegaly have a decreased life expectancy probably related to cardiovascular complications. Progression-free survival times are shorter for patients with macroadenomas that stain for GH than for patients with other macroadenomas (68). In addition, patients with acromegaly have an increased risk for colonic adenomas (135).

PITUITARY ADENOMAS PRODUCING PROLACTIN AND GROWTH HORMONE

Patients with adenomas co-producing PRL and GH may present with the symptoms and signs of prolactinoma, acromegaly, or both. There is good evidence that the well-differentiated somatotrophic cell adenomas, well-differentiated mixed mammotropic and somatotropic cell adenomas, and well-differentiated mammosomatotropic cell adenomas represent one basic tumor type belonging to the somatotropic cell line. These adenomas have mRNA for both PRL and GH (83). All PRL- and GH-producing adenomas may present clinically as prolactinomas, as adenomas causing acromegaly, or with the symptoms of both clinical phenotypes. We classify these adenomas as belonging to the somatotrophic cell line (see Table 99.1). There is evidence that the adenomas co-producing PRL and GH in patients with acromegaly are clinically distinct from the purely GH-producing adenomas (102), and postoperative serum GH is higher in those patients as well.

The immature acidophil stem-cell adenomas that also produce PRL and GH seem to be more closely related to the mammotropic cell line, but not closely enough to justify their classification together with the well-differentiated mammotropic cell adenomas (83). Acidophil stem cell adenomas may present with the symptoms of prolactinomas, acromegaly, or both. They may also present as endocrine-inactive pituitary adenomas, particularly in men. Acidophil stem-cell adenomas occur infrequently (4% of surgically treated pituitary adenomas) (66), and, in contrast to adenomas of the somatotrophic cell line, they seem to grow quickly and invasively into the adjacent tissue (49). Serum PRL levels do not necessarily correspond with tumor size, and women seem to be affected at a younger age than men (49). Transsphenoidal adenomectomy is the preferred treatment for patients with adenomas producing PRL and GH.

ADRENOCORTICOTROPIC HORMONE-RELEASING PITUITARY ADENOMAS

Hypersecretion of adrenocorticotropic hormone (ACTH) by a pituitary adenoma causes Cushing's disease and Nelson's syndrome. Cushing's disease is the subset of Cushing's syndrome caused by excessive ACTH secretion by the pituitary adenoma that produces bilateral adrenal hyperplasia and hypercortisolism. Nelson's syndrome is the result of ACTH hypersecretion by a pituitary adenoma that occurs in certain patients with Cushing's syndrome following adrenalectomy, and its mechanism is thought to be an absence of the negative feedback effect of cortisol on the hypothalamus, which leads to chronic overstimulation of the pituitary gland by corticotrophin-releasing factor (87).

CUSHING'S DISEASE

Cushing's disease is a serious endocrinopathy that occurs predominantly in women and has its peak incidence during the second through sixth decades of life (95). In prepubescent children, pituitary adenomas causing Cushing's disease are the most common type of adenoma (96).

Clinical Presentation

The classic features of Cushing's disease are centripetal obesity, moon facies, buffalo hump, purple abdominal striae, ecchymoses, acne, and hirsutism. Diabetes mellitus, hypertension, and osteoporosis are features that can cause significant morbidity. Weakness in the form of a proximal myopathy is often one of the most prominent findings. Mental disturbance in a patient with Cushing's disease should not be underestimated because, to the patient and family, it may be the most distressing feature of the disease (87).

Diagnosis

The diagnosis of Cushing's disease and subsequent therapeutic decision making are based on endocrinologic criteria. After verification of sustained hypercortisolism with loss of diurnal variation through the measurement of 17-OH corticosteroids and free cortisol in urine, the diagnosis is established by demonstrating nonsuppressibility of serum or urinary corticoids by the low-dose dexamethasone test (8 times 0.5 mg by mouth every 6 hours), less than 50% suppressibility by the high-dose dexamethasone test (4 times 2.0 mg by mouth every 6 hours), and normal or slightly elevated plasma ACTH levels (41). Low or undetectable ACTH levels suggest Cushing's syndrome caused by an adrenal neoplasm, whereas extremely high ACTH levels suggest that the cause is an ectopic ACTH-producing tumor (87).

Neuroimaging studies are only to provide anatomic localization after the diagnosis of Cushing's disease is established. MR imaging is the preferred neuroimaging test for localization, although it has a significant incidence of false-negative and false-positive results. If a high-quality MR image does not document an adenoma unequivocally in the case of a biochemical and clinical diagnosis, bilateral simultaneous selective venous sampling of ACTH from the cavernous sinuses is done. A central-to-peripheral ACTH gradient of greater than 2.0:1 identifies pituitary-dependent Cushing's disease, and a lateralized ACTH gradient of greater than 1.4:1 predicts an adenoma's localization correctly in most (70–80%) cases (14, 41, 103).

Treatment

The decision to operate relies solely on the clinical and endocrinologic data. Transsphenoidal surgery is the initial treatment of choice (87, 88, 142). Selective adenomectomy is a successful and safe treatment for Cushing's disease. The presence or absence of extrasellar extension of the adenoma is the principal determinant of the prognosis (87). During the early postoperative period, a low-dose dexamethasone suppression test confirms a probable surgical cure. Postoperative hypoadrenalism and prolonged suppression of the pituitary-adrenal axis are noted routinely among patients who experience remission of disease after surgery. All patients are maintained on replacement hydrocortisone as long as evidence of hypoadrenalism persists.

Results in our series treated at UCSF (13, 87) resemble others (18, 20, 43, 79) in terms of the patient population and its overall results (17–20, 43, 125). Remission of disease was achieved in 76% of our 216 patients, and the percentage remission was significantly higher ($p < 0.001$) among patients with microadenomas than in those with macroadenomas, and also higher ($p < 0.001$) among patients with intrasellar adenomas than among those with extrasellar extension of their adenoma or perforation of the sellar floor by adenoma. Five of 6 patients in whom no grossly abnormal tissue was found during the exploration were cured by surgery. Two patients had diffuse pituitary hyperplasia. Operative mortality and morbidity were minimal. Complications occurred in 9.3% of patients, including persistent diabetes insipidus in 2.8% of patients, and visual deficits, CSF leak, and persistent sinusitis in fewer than 2% each. Adults and children do not differ in their response to transsphenoidal microsurgery (142), and transsphenoidal adenomectomy is as effective therapeutically in children as in adults. Our results, like those in other large series (18, 113), refute the notion that diffuse pituitary hyperplasia might constitute up to 25% of the cases of Cushing's disease (72, 92).

Pituitary irradiation can be used as primary or adjuvant therapy for Cushing's disease. Heavy-particle irradiation has a high cure rate and usually can be given as a single treatment with multiple ports, but it is available at only two centers in the United States and has a higher rate of complications than conventional irradiation. Because of high cure rates reported with conventional irradiation for children with Cushing's disease, some institutions use pituitary irradiation as the standard therapy for children. However, the lag period between treatment and remission of disease is typically several months. In adults, pituitary irradiation has been much less effective.

Pharmacological therapy can afford palliation for patients with Cushing's disease or Nelson's syndrome who have tumors that are resistant to surgery and radiation therapy. Various drugs (87) are used in order to reduce the secretion of ACTH by the pituitary or to block steroidogenesis by the adrenal glands. Pharmacologic agents that inhibit secretion of ACTH and corticotrophin-releasing hormone include cyproheptadine and bromocriptine; drugs that inhibit cortisol synthesis include aminoglutethimide, metyrapone, ketoconazole, and mitotane; and those that block the action of cortisol at the glucocorticoid receptor level include RU-486 (116). Except for mitotane, whose use is limited by its toxicity, the action of these drugs ceases almost immediately with discontinuation of treatment (116). They can be used as a temporary measure, to improve a patient's condition in preparation for surgery or concurrently with pituitary irradiation, or after both surgery and irradiation have failed to produce remission (see XXVI-3).

Recommendation

Selective adenomectomy is a successful and safe treatment for Cushing's disease and is preferable to bilateral adrenalectomy, pituitary irradiation, or total hypophysectomy as the primary treatment (87). It provides a likely selective removal of the ACTH-secreting adenoma, immediate cure of the hypercortisolism, preservation of pituitary function, and minimal morbidity. The overall percentage of remissions compares favorably with the approximately 80% obtained with primary total hypophysectomy, and adenomectomy does not entail the inevitable hypopituitarism of that procedure (127). Because bilateral adrenalectomy is associated with a greater perioperative mortality (up to 5%), with an occasional persistence of hypercortisolism due to incomplete adrenalectomy, and frequently (8–35%) with the development of Nelson's syndrome, it should be used only as a last resort after pituitary surgery, irradiation, and pharmacological therapy have all failed (18). Although primary irradiation of the pituitary gland can eventually produce remission in 50 to 80% of patients with Cushing's disease, hypercortisolism may not resolve for many months after pituitary irradiation (2, 85, 118). In contrast, selective adenomectomy corrects the condition immediately (2, 18). We recommend transsphenoidal pituitary exploration as the treatment of first choice for most patients with Cushing's disease, reserving radiation therapy for patients who either are at extremely high surgical risk or harbor residual adenoma after transsphenoidal surgery. In consenting adults, if no adenoma is observed during surgical exploration, then total hypophysectomy can be performed because the result is usually a cure. For children in whom exploration shows no evidence of an adenoma, postoperative irradiation, drug therapy, or adrenalectomy is recommended (87).

Recurrence

Because patients can develop recurrence of Cushing's disease as late as 8 years after surgery, patients in clinical remission should have periodic endocrinologic reevaluations. Anatomic reasons for failure of initial operations are related to the size of the tumors, which usually are small; the extreme variability of their location within or on the surface of the gland; our inability to predict the adenoma's site accurately in every case; the extrasellar extension of tumor and invasion of the cavernous sinus; a possible tendency of the adenomatous pituitary gland to form multiple coexisting tumors; and the possibility that ACTH-releasing adenomas develop within the cavernous sinus without a continuous connection to the pituitary gland (97). Postoperative recurrence rates at UCSF are 9.3% (93). Reoperation is safe and effective therapy for many recurrent or persistent tumors, as the initial operation's failure permits the surgeon to tailor the approach accordingly at reoperation. The majority of patients derive benefit and many are cured (87), sometimes with the addition of chemotherapy. Medical management of recurrent tumors is effective in the long term only in patients with prolactinomas who tolerate, and whose tumors are sensitive to, bromocriptine mesylate.

NELSON'S SYNDROME

Nelson's syndrome occurs in 20 to 40% of patients who undergo bilateral adrenalectomy, once the major treatment for Cushing's disease despite its significant drawbacks. The tumors causing Nelson's syndrome are much more likely to be large and invasive than are those causing Cushing's disease (142), and while in many patients the tumor is indolent, in a significant minority it is aggressive or frankly malignant and directly causes death (142). The intervals between adrenalectomy and transsphenoidal surgery for Nelson's syndrome range from a few months to more than two decades, reflecting the unpredictable behavior of these tumors.

Clinical Presentation

Because of the large size and invasiveness of tumors causing Nelson's syndrome, headaches and visual disturbances are more common than in association with Cushing's disease. The documentation of extremely high plasma ACTH values, often several thousand picograms per milliliter, is sufficient to make the diagnosis, which can be corroborated by MR imaging of the sella. Hyperpigmentation is the hallmark of Nelson's syndrome (142).

Diagnosis

The diagnosis of Nelson's syndrome is straightforward. The loss of cortisol inhibition caused by adrenalectomy allows the pituitary gland to secrete very large amounts of ACTH and may promote rapid growth of the adenoma. Cutaneous melanocytes are stimulated by the high levels of ACTH to produce the characteristic hyperpigmentation of Nelson's syndrome. The development of hyperpigmentation in a patient known to have undergone adrenalectomy for Cushing's syndrome is diagnostic of Nelson's syndrome (142).

Treatment

In cases of Nelson's syndrome, the prognosis is guarded and generally unfavorable (88), but transsphenoidal surgery offers the best hope of controlling the disease. Craniotomy should be used only for patients in whom large parasellar or suprasellar extension or an unusually small sella turcica precludes adequate transsphenoidal access. Radiation therapy and drug therapy are important adjuvant therapies because most patients who develop the syndrome usually have large and invasive tumors with extrasellar extension by the time they come for treatment, and complete removal of the tumor is possible in fewer than 30%. Heavy-particle irradiation is more effective than conventional irradiation, but heavy-particle irradiation is suitable only for adenomas confined to the sella. Fortunately, there has been a profound reduction in the incidence of Nelson's syndrome as transsphenoidal microsurgery has replaced bilateral adrenalectomy as the primary treatment for Cushing's disease (140).

THYROTROPIN-RELEASING PITUITARY ADENOMAS

TSH-secreting adenomas are rare, accounting for 1.2 to 2.8% of all pituitary adenomas treated surgically in our series at UCSF (93, 94). They occur too infrequently to establish an age- or gender-related pattern of occurrence. A history of some form of thyroid ablation (surgical ablation, radiation therapy, or Hashimoto's disease) is common in patients who later develop TSH-secreting pituitary adenomas (94). As with ACTH-secreting adenomas, there is clinical and experimental evidence that these tumors develop in response to low serum levels of the hormone secreted by the gland affected (94).

Patients with a TSH-secreting adenoma may present with hyperthyroidism, with hypothyroidism, or in a euthyroid state; other endocrine symptoms are menstrual irregularities, impotence or decreased libido, acromegaly, galactorrhea, and hypogonadism (94, 114). Focal neurologic deficits, caused by the tumor's compression of cranial nerves, are common (37%) (94). For a pituitary mass lesion, a preoperative diagnosis is based on increased basal serum TSH levels, the detectability of serum TSH in hyperthyroid patients, or the unresponsiveness of TSH after TRH administration; this unresponsiveness is probably related to the loss of TRH receptors on the surface of adenomatous thyrotrophic cells (21).

Typically, TSH-producing pituitary adenomas are aggressive macroadenomas with a high rate of tissue invasion (63%) and a relatively high rate of tumor recurrence (8.4–10.5%) after surgical removal (93, 94). More than other adenomas, they seem to have a tendency to change immunophenotype at tumor recurrence (8.4%) (36, 93). In addition, and in contrast to other pituitary adenomas, they are associated with potentially life-threatening cardiovascular and neurological complications (58, 94, 138). Women tend to develop these tumors at a younger age after a longer history of symptoms, yet they have smaller and less often invasive tumors than men (94). In our series, 50% have been purely TSH-producing and 50% have been plurihormonal (94).

Unless contraindicated, surgical resection of these locally aggressive tumors, which have a tendency toward producing potentially life-threatening cardiovascular and neurologic complications, is the treatment of choice. At least in men, whose tumors seem to grow faster and more aggressively, routine postoperative sellar irradiation might be indicated. Medical treatment with the long-acting somatostatin analogue octreotide appears to be beneficial (22, 23, 26), although it should probably be reserved for patients in whom surgery is contraindicated and in cases of tumor recurrence.

Clinically Endocrine-Inactive Pituitary Adenomas

ETIOLOGY AND EPIDEMIOLOGY

Clinically endocrine-inactive pituitary adenomas account for about one-third of all surgically treated pituitary adenomas at UCSF (93). Endocrine-inactive adenomas are an inhomogeneous group of adenomas deriving from various cell lines (see Table 99.1). Either they do not produce anterior lobe hormones or they produce clinically silent hormones or hormonal compounds like the α subunit (52, 108). As a group, these adenomas have a unique epidemiology in that they have a peak occurrence at an older age; most of these adenomas occur during the sixth through ninth decades of life (95). Before the fourth decade of life, they are 2 to 3 times more common in women, and thereafter they are 2 to 3 times more common in men (95). Their postoperative recurrence rate, as a group, is 8.7% at UCSF (93).

PATHOLOGY

Endocrine-inactive adenomas were formerly classified as chromophobic adenomas, but this term is not useful because the agranular light microscopic appearance of the tumors is misleading: ultrastructural studies show secretory granules in "chromophobic" adenomas, and sensitive radioimmunoassays show that as many as 50% of them produce a hormone (91, 139). The pituitary glycoprotein hormone α subunit has been demonstrated in many endocrine-inactive, undifferentiated pituitary adenomas (46, 75, 76, 104). It now appears likely that endocrine-inactive pituitary adenomas that are not clinically evident release small quantities of hormones, primarily gonadotrophins, and it is possible that the hormone release occurs from only a small percentage of the tumor cells (144). Excessive secretion of gonadotrophins and/or their subunits by these adenomas is rare and may occur primarily in men. Women, however, may show an elevated ratio of α subunit to luteinizing hormone and follicle-stimulating hormone, which may be useful in making a diagnosis (70). The null cell adenoma and the oncocytoma, both characterized by Kovacs and colleagues (67), are nonsecreting, as determined by immunostaining. A few scattered cells may stain positively for follicle-stimulating hormone (FSH), luteinizing hormone (LH), or the α subunit in a small fraction of null cell adenomas (67). Northern and in situ hybridization show that null cell adenomas and oncocytomas have the potential to secrete FSH, LH, chromogranin A, and secretogranin (30, 53).

CLINICAL PRESENTATION

Endocrine-inactive adenomas have an insidious clinical progression (31), and by the time patients present for a diagnosis the tumor is usually a macroadenoma producing symptoms caused by mass effect or hypopituitarism (61). The most frequent symptoms are headache and visual disturbances caused by the adenoma's encroachment on the visual pathway (32, 39).

DIAGNOSIS

Both thin-section MR imaging and high-resolution computed tomography detect the macroadenomas accurately (124), but MR imaging is the superior technique because of the greater soft-tissue contrast it provides, permitting clear visualization of the optic chiasm, optic nerves, cavernous sinuses, and carotid arteries (54, 124). Visual evoked potential evaluations reliably assess the function of the intracranial visual pathways and can be more sensitive than conventional methods of examination (48).

Patients suspected of having an endocrine-inactive adenoma should undergo MR imaging, assessment of pituitary hormone function, and a determination of the pituitary glycoprotein hormone α serum (61). Elevated or high-normal gonadotrophin levels suggest an underlying gonadotrophic adenoma, although pituitary adenomas secreting gonadotrophins are often diagnosed as endocrine-inactive adenomas because of the clinical findings; for example, a middle-aged woman experiencing visual disturbances (27). Some patients have a tumor producing no hormone or a tumor with defects in hormone biosynthesis or processing that prevent detectable hormone hypersecretion. In a few patients, the endocrine-inactive pituitary adenoma interferes with the pituitary stalk and produces a moderate hyperprolactinemia (basal levels 50–100 ng/mL) as a result of a "stalk section effect."

TREATMENT

An endocrine-inactive tumor in an asymptomatic elderly patient with unimpaired pituitary function should, with some exceptions, be left alone and its course followed with serial MR images (142). For patients with symptomatic endocrine-inactive adenomas, transsphenoidal surgery with microscopic surgical technique is the preferred treatment. In some patients, transsphenoidal surgery improves pituitary function (1, 4, 61, 142), but even in patients with very large or giant adenomas, it permits rapid and satisfactory decompression of the optic nerves and chiasm, averts significant pituitary insufficiency in the majority of cases (98), is well-tolerated by elderly patients (25), and is associated with low morbidity, mortality (98), and recurrence rates.

Conventional radiation therapy is often recommended when there is evidence of residual tumor postoperatively and/or extensive extrasellar extension preoperatively (61), but an increasing proportion of endocrine-inactive tumors is being followed, rather than referred for irradiation, after surgery because of gross total removal and potential cure.

Medical treatment of endocrine-inactive adenomas with bromocriptine, whether preoperatively or as primary therapy, is a matter of controversy. Both the long-acting synthetic somatostatin analog octreotide (29, 57) and the dopamine agonist bromocriptine (27, 38, 134) have been used for the medical treatment of endocrine-inactive pituitary adenomas. Octreotide seems to decrease tumor size, visual field deficits, and serum α SU levels in some patients with gonadotrophic or pure α SU-secreting pituitary adenomas (29, 57); some of these tumors were shown to have somatostatin receptors (29). There are also isolated cases in which bromocriptine is well tolerated and produces good to impressive results (27, 38). The consensus is at present, however, that with the possible exception of pituitary adenomas showing recent growth, bromocriptine is unlikely to cause growth arrest or reduce the size of endocrine-inactive pituitary adenomas (12, 134). An obstacle in the evaluation of medical therapy for endocrine-inactive adenomas is that they constitute a heterogenous group of adenomas deriving from different cell lines.

A CHANGE IN IMMUNOPHENOTYPE AT RECURRENCE

Pituitary adenomas may change immunophenotype at recurrence (35, 93); the first such case was reported by the Kovacs group (35). Of all pituitary adenomas that recurred after surgery at UCSF (overall recurrence rate 6.3%), 7.7% changed immunophenotype (93). Typically, these changes occur in clinically active plurihormonal adenomas, the clinical phenotypes of ACTH and TSH secretion seemingly more commonly involved (35, 36, 93). Usually, such a change occurs in such malignancies as those of the gastrointestinal tract and not in benign tumors. The ability of these pituitary adenomas to change immunophenotype, together with the high incidence of macroadenomas, of invasive behavior, and of hemorrhage among them, suggest that they might be a distinct, aggressive subgroup of pituitary adenomas. Until it is known whether this subgroup of pituitary adenomas is indeed more aggressive than other recurring pituitary adenomas, we recommend complete immunostaining for PRL, GH, ACTH, TSH, and α SU in all pituitary adenomas, including those that recur, to detect and further characterize these tumors.

MULTIPLE COEXISTING PITUITARY ADENOMAS

The occurrence of multiple coexisting pituitary adenomas has been estimated to be 0.37% in series of surgically removed adenomatous pituitaries (65), 1.5% in surgically removed pediatric adenomatous pituitaries (96), 4.8% in surgically removed pediatric adenomatous pituitaries causing Cushing's disease (98), 0.9% in unselected autopsy pituitaries, and 8.9% in adenomatous pituitaries observed at autopsy (64). Their occurrence may be underestimated in series of surgically treated adenomas because their diagnosis depends on the neurosurgeon's and the pathologist's awareness of their existence and an appropriate reconstruction of fragmented tissue. Their existence is easier to prove if they differ in immunophenotype, which is probably why most of the multiple coexisting pituitary adenomas that have been diagnosed are of differing immunophenotypes. If our observation about pediatric pituitary adenomas is correct, that adenomatous pituitaries in patients with Cushing's disease have a tendency to harbor multiple adenomas (96), it has clinical implications—among them, that a failed cure after surgical removal of an adenoma might indicate that a second adenoma was overlooked during surgery.

Pituitary Adenomas in Childhood and the Elderly

CLINICALLY RELEVANT ANATOMICAL ASPECTS OF PITUITARY ADENOMAS

Several anatomical aspects of pituitary adenomas may cause problems in detecting the adenoma both preoperatively and intraoperatively. (1) Adenomas causing Cushing's disease are small (typically 2 mm in diameter), are of a watery consistency, and vary greatly in their location in and on the pituitary gland. (2) Adenomas may occur ectopically in the parasellar region, such as in the sphenoid sinus, sphenoid bone, cavernous sinus, or above the diaphragma sellae. Usually, these adenomas are in close proximity to, but without direct contact with, the pituitary gland. (3) Pituitary adenomas may occur multiply. These purely anatomical factors may be responsible for an adenoma's being overlooked during preoperative assessment or surgery. Coincidentally, the very same anatomical factors can be the reason that reoperation by an experienced surgeon has a good chance of achieving a cure, if the surgeon is aware of the specific difficulties. Preoperatively, the site of adenomas causing Cushing's disease that are difficult to detect may be determined by simultaneous bilateral petrosal sampling of ACTH. Appropriate imaging techniques with MRI and sometimes cavernous venography may detect ectopic parasellar adenomas, and careful intraoperative exploration may detect multiple coexisting pituitary adenomas and small adenomas causing Cushing's disease.

Microscopic invasion of sellar dura occurs in 85% of cases of pituitary adenoma (117). Invasiveness is greatly underestimated by surgeons: in the same series (117), invasive growth was suspected in only 40% of cases. Even microprolactinomas, which are considered the least aggressive form of pituitary adenoma, are invasive in 62.5% of cases (117). This aspect of tumor biology should be considered when advising patients whether or not to undergo surgery for pituitary adenoma. The tendency of the adenoma to invade adjacent tissue is of special interest if the adenoma is located laterally in close proximity to, or in contact with, the wall of the cavernous sinus. Once the adenoma begins to invade the cavernous sinus wall, the operation becomes technically more difficult and the patient bears the risk of subtotal tumor resection that will leave residual tumor in place.

There are a few characteristics that distinguish pituitary adenomas occurring in childhood and those in elderly patients from pituitary adenomas in other age groups. The distribution of the several adenoma types varies depending on age. In prepubescent children, the pituitary adenomas causing Cushing's disease are the most common type (96). During puberty and adolescence, prolactinomas are the most common (96). Whereas clinically endocrine-inactive pituitary adenomas rarely occur in children (96), in elderly patients they are the most common adenoma type. The older the patient, the less likely is an endocrine-active tumor (94).

Endocrine symptoms, in addition to the typical symptoms of the clinically predominant adenoma type, may be observed in children (96). Growth arrest is common for all adenoma types except for GH-releasing tumors. Menstrual irregularities are common for all adenoma types except for the tumors that cause Nelson's syndrome (96).

MALIGNANT PITUITARY NEOPLASMS

There are three types of malignant pituitary tumors: primary pituitary adenocarcinomas, intrasellar metastasis, and postirradiation sarcomatous transformation of the sellar contents. All three forms of intrasellar malignancy are rare. The diagnosis of a primary pituitary adenocarcinoma should only be made in a patient who has remote metastasis (66). The occurrence of such tumors is extremely rare; at UCSF they account for about 0.1% of primary tumors deriving from the pituitary gland (unpublished data). Syndromes of hormonal hypersecretion seem to be present in almost half of the cases (99). One case has been reported in which a metastatic primary pituitary carcinoma developed during medical treatment of a recurrent prolactinoma with bromocriptine (89).

Tumors metastatic to the pituitary gland are infrequent, occurring in 1 to 3.8% of autopsies of patients with known malignancies (90). Most commonly, the tumors metastasize to the posterior lobe (50%); in one-third of cases, the metastasis is to both the posterior and anterior lobe, and rarely is there spread to the anterior lobe (15%) (90). Accordingly, diabetes insipidus is a common symptom (24). In a review of 220 metastases to the pituitary, the primary neoplasms were most commonly of the breast (50%) and lung (20%) (90). Pituitary metastasis may occur in an early or a later stage of malignancy. Surgical removal of the metastatic lesion at the earliest possible stage in the development of the primary disease is recommended and may improve survival time (24); however, surgery for the metastasis is contraindicated if the primary disease is advanced.

Postirradiation sarcomatous transformation of the sellar contents is a rare condition that typically occurs after a long latent interval of about 20 years following irradiation of a pituitary adenoma. The tumors grow very large and do not metastasize (106).

References

1. Adams CB. The management of pituitary tumours and post-operative visual deterioration. Acta Neurochir (Wien) 1988;94:103.
2. Ahmed SR, Shalet SM, Beardwell CG, Sutton M L. Treatment of Cushing's disease with low dose radiation therapy. Br Med J 1984;289:643.
3. Aloia JF, Field RA, Kramer S. Treatment of acromegaly. Arch Intern Med 1973;131:509.
4. Arafah BM. Reversible hypopituitarism in patients with large nonfunctioning pituitary adenomas. J Clin Endocrinol Metab 1986;62:1173.
5. Arosio M, Giovanelli MA, Riva E, Nava C, Ambrosi B, Faglia G. Clinical use of pre- and postsurgical evaluation of abnormal GH responses in acromegaly. J Neurosurg 1983;59:402.
6. Balagura S, Derome P, Guiot G. Acromegaly: analysis of 132 cases treated surgically. Neurosurgery 1981;8:413.
7. Barrow DL, Mizuno J, Tindall GT. Management of prolactinomas associated with very high serum prolactin levels. J Neurosurg 1988;68:554.
8. Baskin DS, Boggan JE, Wilson CB. Transsphenoidal microsurgical removal of growth hormone-secreting pituitary adenomas. A review of 137 cases. J Neurosurg 1982;56:634.
9. Baskin DS, Wilson CB. Bromocriptine treatment of pituitary adenomas. Neurosurgery 1981;8:741.
10. Belchetz PE, Carty A, Clearkin LG, Davis JC, Jeffreys RV, Rae PG. Failure of prophylactic surgery to avert massive pituitary expansion in pregnancy. Clin Endocrinol 1986;25:325.
11. Bergh T, Nillius SJ, Wide L. Clinical course and outcome of pregnancies in amenorrhoeic women with hyperprolactinaemia and pituitary tumors. Br Med J 1978;1:875.
12. Bevan JS, Adams CB, Burke CW, Morton KE, Molyneux AJ, Moore RA, Esiri MM. Factors in the outcome of transsphenoidal surgery for prolactinoma and non-functioning pituitary tumour, including pre-operative bromocriptine therapy. Clin Endocrinol 1987;26:541.
13. Boggan JE, Tyrrell JB, Wilson CB. Transsphenoidal microsurgical management of Cushing's disease. Report of 100 cases. J Neurosurg 59:195;1983.
14. Boolell M, Gilford E, Arnott R, McNeill P, Cummins J, Alford F. An overview of bilateral synchronous inferior petrosal sinus sampling (BSIPSS) in the pre-operative assessment of Cushing's disease. Aust N Z J Med 1990;20:765.
15. Buchfelder M, Brockmeier S, Fahlbusch R, Honegger Pichl J, Manzl M. Recurrence following transphenoidal surgery for acromegaly. Horm Res 1991;35:113.
16. Buckman MT, Kellner R. Reduction of distress in hyperprolactinemia with bromocriptine. Am J Psychiatry 1985;142:242.
17. Burch W. A survey of results with transsphenoidal surgery in Cushing's disease (letter). N Engl J Med 1983;308:103.
18. Burch WM. Cushing's disease. A review. Arch Intern Med 1985;145:1106.
19. Carboni P Jr, Detta A, Hitchcock ER, Postans R. Pituitary adenoma proliferative indices and risk of recurrence. Br J Neurosurg 1992;6:33.
20. Chandler WF, Schteingart DE, Lloyd RV, McKeever PE, Ibarra-Perez G. Surgical treatment of Cushing's disease. J Neurosurg 1987;66:204.
21. Chanson P, Li JY, Le Dafniet M, Derome P, Kujas M, Murat M, Charpentier G, Racadot J, Peillon F. Absence of receptors for thyrotropin (TSH)-releasing hormone in human TSH-secreting pituitary adenomas associated with hyperthyroidism. J Clin Endocrinol Metab 1988;66:447.
22. Chanson P, Weintraub BD, Harris AG. Octreotide therapy for thyroid-stimulating hormone-secreting pituitary adenomas. A follow-up of 52 patients. Ann Intern Med 1993;119:236.
23. Chayen SD, Gross D, Makhoul O, Glaser B. TSH producing pituitary tumor: biochemical diagnosis, and long-term medical management with octreotide. Horm Metab Res 1992;24:34.
24. Chiang MF, Brock M, Patt S. Pituitary metastases. Neurochirurgia (Stuttg) 1990;33:127.
25. Cohen DL, Bevan JS, Adams CB. The presentation and management of pituitary tumours in the elderly. Age Ageing 1989;18:247.
26. Comi RJ, Gesundheit N, Murray L, Gorden P, Weintraub BD. Response of thyrotropin-secreting pituitary adenomas to a long-acting somatostatin analogue. N Engl J Med 1987;317:12.
27. Comtois R, Bouchard J, Robert F. Hypersecretion of gonadotropins by a pituitary adenoma: pituitary dynamic studies and treatment with bromocriptine in one patient. Fertil Steril 1989;52:569.
28. Davis DH, Laws ER Jr, Ilstrup DM, Speed JK, Caruso M, Shaw EG, Abboud CF, Scheithauer BW, Root LM, Schleck C. Results of surgical treatment for growth hormone-secreting pituitary adenomas. J Neurosurg 1993;79:70.
29. de Bruin TW, Kwekkeboom DJ, Van't Verlaat JW, Reubi JC, Krenning EP, Lamberts SW, Croughs RJ. Clinically nonfunctioning pituitary adenoma and octreotide response to long term high dose treatment, and studies in vitro. J Clin Endocrinol Metab 1992;75:1310.
30. Deftos LJ, O'Connor DT, Wilson CB, Fitzgerald PA. Human pituitary tumors secrete chromogranin-A. J Clin Endocrinol Metab 1989;68:869.

31. Dietel P, Heberling HJ, Lohmann D, Brachmann J. [Clinical symptoms and duration of anamnesis in patients with hypophyseal tumors.] Z Gesamte Inn Med 1989;44:293.
32. Eitel B. [Ambulatory diagnosis and outpatient management of patients with hypophyseal adenomas.] Z Gesamte Inn Med 1987;42:321.
33. Evans HM, Briggs JH, Dixon JS. The physiology and chemistry of growth hormone. In The Pituitary Gland. Edited by GW Harris and BT Donovan. Berkeley/Los Angeles: University of California, 1966, vol 1, p 439.
34. Ezzat S, Snyder PJ, Young WF, Boyajy LD, Newman C, Klibanski A, Molitch ME, Boyd AE, Sheeler L, Cook DM, Malarkey WB, Jackson I, Vance ML, Thorner MO, Barkan A, Frohman LA, Melmed S. Octreotide treatment of acromegaly. A randomized, multicenter study. Ann Intern Med 1992;117:711.
35. Felix I, Asa SL, Kovacs K, Horvath E. Changes in hormone production of a recurrent silent corticotroph adenoma of the pituitary: a histologic, immunohistochemical, ultrastructural, and tissue culture study. Hum Pathol 1991;22:719.
36. Felix I, Asa SL, Kovacs K, Horvath E, Smyth HS. Recurrent plurihormonal bimorphous pituitary adenoma producing growth hormone, thyrotropin and prolactin. Arch Pathol Lab Med 1994;118:66.
37. Forbes AP, Henneman PH, Griswold GC, et al. Syndrome characterized by galactorrhea, amenorrhea and low urinary FSH: comparison with acromegaly and normal lactation. J Clin Endocrinol Metab 1954;14:265.
38. Garcia-Luna PO, Leal-Cerro A, Pereira JL, Montero C, Acosta D, Trujillo F, Mazuelos C, Astorga R. Rapid improvement of visual defects with parenteral depot-bromocriptine in a patient with a non-functioning pituitary adenoma. Horm Res 1989;32:183.
39. Giorgis B, Campiche R, Burckhardt P, Gomez F. [Diagnosis, treatment and course of hypophyseal tumors.] Retrospective study of 123 cases. Schweiz Med Wochenschr 1986;116:1431.
40. Gramegna AG. Un cas d'acromégalie traité par la radiothérapie. Rev Neurol 1909;17:15.
41. Grua JR, Nelson DH. ACTH-producing pituitary tumors. Endocrinol Metab Clin North Am 1991;20:319.
42. Hardy J. Transsphenoidal surgery of hypersecreting pituitary tumors. In Diagnosis and Treatment of Pituitary Tumors. Proceedings of a conference sponsored jointly by the National Institute of Child Health and Human Development and the National Cancer Institute, January 1973:15–17. International Congress Series, No. 303. Edited by PO Kohler and GT Ross. Amsterdam: Excerpta Medica, 1973, pp 179–194.
43. Hardy J. Microsurgery of pituitary disorders. In Functioning Pituitary Adenoma and Bromocriptine: Proceedings of the Second Workshop on Pituitary Tumors. Edited by K Sano, K Takakura, T Fukushima, et al. Tokyo: Sandoz Pharmaceuticals 1981, pp 41–46.
44. Hardy J, Somma M, Vezina JL. Treatment of acromegaly: radiation or surgery? In Current Controversies in Neurosurgery. Edited by TP Morley. Philadelphia: Saunders, 1976, pp 377–391.
45. Hardy J, Vezina JL. Transsphenoidal neurosurgery of intracranial neoplasm. In Neoplasia in the Nervous System. Advances in Neurology series, Vol 15. Edited by RA Thompson and JR Green. New York: Raven, 1976, pp 261–274.
46. Heitz PU, Landolt AM, Zenklusen HR, Kasper M, Reubi JC, Oberholzer M, Roth J. Immunocytochemistry of pituitary tumors. J Histochem Cytochem 1987;35:1005.
47. Herman V, Fagin J, Gonsky R, Kovacs K, Melmed S. Clonal origin of pituitary adenomas. J Clin Endocrinol Metab 1990;71:1427.
48. Holder GE, Bullock PR. Visual evoked potentials in the assessment of patients with non-functioning chromophobe adenomas. J Neurol Neurosurg Psychiatry 1989;52:31.
49. Horvath E, Kovacs K, Singer W, Smyth HS, Killinger DW, Erzin C, Weiss MH. Acidophil stem cell adenoma of the human pituitary: clinicopathologic analysis of 15 cases. Cancer 1981;47:761.
50. Hyperprolactinaemia. When is a prolactinoma not a prolactinoma? Lancet 1987;2:1002.
51. Ikeda H, Yoshimoto T. The relationship between c-myc protein expression, the bromodeoxyuridine labeling index and the biological behavior of pituitary adenomas. Acta Neuropathol (Berl) 1992;83:361.
52. Jautzke G. Simultaneous production of the alpha-subunit of glycoprotein hormones and other hormones in pituitary adenomas. Pathol Res Pract 1988;183:601.
53. Jin L, Chandler WF, Smart JB, England BG, Lloyd RV. Differentiation of human pituitary adenomas determines the pattern of chromogranin/secretoranin messenger ribonucleic acid expression. J Clin Endocrinol Metab 1993;76:728.
54. Juliani G, Avataneo T, Potenzoni F, Sorrentino T. [CT and MR compared in the study of hypophysis.] Radiol Med (Torino) 1989;77:51.
55. Kapcala LP, Molitch ME, Post KD, Biller BJ, Prager RJ, Jackson IM, Reichlin S. Galactorrhea, oligo/amenorrhea, and hyperprolactinemia in patients with craniopharyngiomas. J Clin Endocrinol Metab 1980;51:798.
56. Karga HJ, Alexander JM, Hedley-Whyte ET, Klibanski A, Jameson L. Ras mutations in human pituitary tumors. J Clin Endocrinol Metab 1992;74:914.
57. Katznelson L, Oppenheim DS, Coughlin JF, Kliman B, Schoenfeld DA, Klibanski A. Chronic somatostatin analog administration in patients with alpha-subunit-secreting pituitary tumors. J Clin Endocrinol Metab 1992;75:1318.
58. Kiso Y, Yoshida K, Kaise K, Kaise N, Masuda T, Ando N, Kameyama M, Yamamoto M, Sakurada T, Yoshinaga K. A case of thyrotropin (TSH)-secreting tumor complicated by periodic paralysis. Jpn J Med 1990;29:399.
59. Kjellberg RN, Shintani A, Frantz AG, Kliman B. Proton-beam therapy in acromegaly. N Engl J Med 1968;278:689.
60. Klibanski A. Editorial: further evidence for a somatic mutation theory in the pathogenesis of human pituitary tumors. J Clin Endocrinol Metab 1990;71:1415A.
61. Klibanski A. Nonsecreting pituitary tumors. Endocrinol Metab Clin North Am 1987;16:793.
62. Klibanski A, Neer RM, Beitinis IZ, Ridgeway EC, Zervas NT, McArthur JW. Decreased bone density in hyperprolactinemic women. N Engl J Med 1980;303:1511.
63. Knosp E, Kitz K, Perneczky A. Proliferation activity in pituitary adenomas: measurement by monoclonal antibody Ki-67. Neurosurgery 1989;25:927.
64. Kontogeorgos G, Kovacs K, Horvath E, Scheithauer BW. Multiple adenomas of the human pituitary. A retrospective autopsy study with clinical implications. J Neurosurg 1991;74:243.
65. Kontogeorgos G, Scheithauer BW, Horvath E, Kovacs K, Lloyd RV, Smyth HS, Rologis D. Double adenomas of the pituitary: a clinicopathological study of 11 tumors. Neurosurgery 1992;31:840.
66. Kovacs K, Horvath E. Tumors of the pituitary gland. Atlas of Tumor Pathology, Series 2, Fascicle 21. Washington DC: Armed Forces Institute of Pathology, 1986, p 269.
67. Kovacs K, Horvath E, Ryan N, Ezrin C. Null cell adenoma of the human pituitary. Virchows Arch (A) 1980;387:165.
68. Kovalic JJ, Mazoujian G, McKeel DW, Fineberg BB, Grigsby PW. Immunohistochemistry as a predictor of clinical outcome in patients given postoperative radiation for subtotally resected pituitary adenomas. J Neurooncol 1993;16:227.
69. Kupersmith MJ, Kleinberg D, Warren FA, Budzilovitch G, Cooper P. Growth of prolactinoma despite lowering of serum prolactin by bromocriptine. Neurosurgery 1989;24:417.
70. Kwekkeboom DJ, de Jong FH, Lamberts SW. Gonadotropin release by clinically nonfunctioning and gonadotroph pituitary adenomas in vivo and in vitro: relation to sex and effects of thyrotropin-releasing hormone, gonadotropin-releasing hormone, and bromocriptine. J Clin Endocrinol Metab 1989;68:1128.
71. Lamberg BA, Kivikangas V, Vartianen J, Raitta C, Pelkonen R. Conventional pituitary irradiation in acromegaly. Effect on growth hormone and TSH secretion. Acta Endocrinol (Copenh) 1976;82:267.
72. Lamberts SW, de Lange SA, Stefanko SZ. Adrenocorticotropin-secreting pituitary adenomas originate from the anterior or the intermediate lobe in Cushing's disease. Differences in the regulation of hormone secretion. J Clin Endocrinol Metab 1982;54:286.
73. Landis CA, Harsh G, Lyons J, Davis RL, McCormick F, Bourne HR. Clinical characteristics of acromegalic patients whose pituitary tumors contain mutant Gs protein. J Clin Endocrinol Metab 1990;71:1416–1420.
74. Landolt AM. Ultrastructure of human sella tumors. Correlations of clinical findings and morphology. Acta Neurochir (Wien) 1975;22(suppl):1.
75. Landolt AM, Heitz PU. Alpha-subunit-producing pituitary adenomas. Immunocytochemical and ultrastructural studies. Virchows Arch A 1986;409:417.
76. Landolt AM, Heitz PU, Zenklusen HR. Production of the alpha-subunit of glycoprotein hormones by pituitary adenomas. Pathol Res Pract 1988;183:610.
77. Landolt AM, Shibata T, Kleihues P. Growth rate of human pituitary adenomas. J Neurosurg 1987;67:803.
78. Landolt AM, Wilson CB. Tumors of the sella and parasellar area in adults. In Neurological Surgery: A Comprehensive Reference Guide to the Diagnosis and Treatment of Neurosurgical Problems, 2nd Edition. Edited by JR Youmans. Philadelphia: Saunders, 1982, vol 5, pp 3107–3162.
79. Laws ER, Ebersold MJ, Piepgras DG, et al. The results of transsphenoidal surgery in specific clinical entities. In Management of Pituitary Adenomas and Related Lesions with Emphasis on Transsphenoidal Microsurgery. Edited by ER Laws, RV Randall, EB Kern, et al. New York: Appleton-Century-Crofts, 1982, pp 277–305.
80. Laws ER Jr, Piepgras DG, Randall RV, Abboud CF. Neurosurgical management of acromegaly. Results in 82 patients treated between 1972 and 1977. J Neurosurg 1979;50:454.
81. Lees PD. Intrasellar pressure. Acta Neurochir Suppl (Wien) 1990;47:68.
82. Lees PD, Pickard JD. Hyperprolactinemia, intrasellar pituitary tissue pressure, and the pituitary stalk compression syndrome. J Neurosurg 1987;67:192.
83. Li J, Stefaneanu L, Kovacs K, Horvath E, Smyth HS. Growth hormone (GH) and prolactin (PRL) gene expression and immunoreactivity in GH- and PRL-producing human pituitary adenomas. Virchows Arch A 1993;422:193.
84. Lim MJ, Barkan AL, Buda AJ. Rapid reduction of left ventricular hypertrophy in acromegaly after suppression of growth hormone hypersecretion. Ann Intern Med 1992;117:719.
85. Linfoot JA. Heavy ion therapy: alpha particle therapy of pituitary tumors. In Recent Advances in the Diagnosis and Treatment of Pituitary Tumors. Edited by JA Linfoot. New York: Raven, 1979, pp 245–267.
86. Lyons J, Landis CA, Harsh G, Vallar L, Grünewald K, Feichtinger H, Duh QY, Clark OH, Kawasaki E, Bourne HR, McCormick F. Two G protein oncogenes in human endocrine tumors. Science 1990;249:655.
87. Mampalam TJ, Tyrrell JB, Wilson CB. Transsphenoidal microsurgery for Cushing disease. A report of 216 cases. Ann Intern Med 1988;109:487.
88. Mampalam TJ, Wilson CB. ACTH-secreting tumors, cushing's disease, and Nelson's syndrome. In Current Therapy in Neurological Surgery—2. Edited by DM Long. Toronto/Philadelphia: BC Decker, 1989, pp 131–135.
89. Martin NA, Hales M, Wilson CB. Cerebellar metastasis from a prolactinoma during treatment with bromocriptine. J Neurosurg 1981;55:615.
90. McCormick PC, Post KD, Kandji AD, Hays AP. Metastatic carcinoma to the pituitary gland. Br J Neurosurg 1989;3:71.
91. McCormick WF, Halmi NS. Absence of chromophobe adenomas from a large series of pituitary tumors. Arch Pathol 1971;92:231.
92. McKeever PE, Koppleman MC, Metcalf D, Quindlen E, Kornblith PL, Strott CA, Howard R, Smith BH. Refractory Cushing's disease caused by multinodular ACTH-cell hyperplasia. J Neuropatol Exp Neurol 1982;41:490.
93. Mindermann T, Kovacs K, Wilson CB. Changes in immunophenotype of recurrent pituitary adenomas. Neurosurgery 1994;35:39.
94. Mindermann T, Wilson CB. Thyrotropin-producing pituitary adenomas. J Neurosurg 1993;79:521.
95. Mindermann T, Wilson CB. Age- and gender-related occurrence of pituitary adenomas. J Clin Endocrinol 1994;41:359.
96. Mindermann T, Wilson CB. Pediatric pituitary adenomas. Neurosurgery 1995;36:259.
97. Wilson CB, Mindermann T, Tyrell JB. Extrasellar, intracavernous sinus adrenocorticotropin-releasing adenoma causing Cushing's disease. J Clin Endocrinol Metab 1995;80:1774.
98. Mohr G, Hardy J, Comtois R, Beauregard H. Surgical management of giant pituitary adenomas. Can J Neurol Sci 1990;17:62.
99. Mountcastle RB, Roof BS, Mayfield RK, Mordes DB, Sagel J, Biggs PJ, Rawe SE. Pituitary adenocarcinoma in an acromegalic patient: response to bromocriptine and pituitary testing: a review of the literature on 36 cases of pituitary carcinoma. Am J Med Sci 1989;298:109.
100. Nagashima T, Murovic JA, Hoshino T, Wilson CB, DeArmond SJ. The proliferative potential of human pituitary tumors in situ. J Neurosurg 1986;64:588.

101. Newton DR, Dillon WP, Norman D, Newton TH, Wilson CB. gd-DTPA-enhanced MR imaging of pituitary adenomas. AJNR 1989;10:949.
102. Nyquist P, Laws ER, Elliott E. Novel features of tumors that secrete both growth hormone and prolactin in acromegaly. Neurosurgery 1994;35:179.
103. Oldfield EH, Doppman JL, Nieman LK, Chrousos GP, Miller DL, Katz DA, Cutler GB, Loriaux DL. Petrosal sinus sampling with and without corticotropin-releasing hormone for the differential diagnosis of Cushing's syndrome. N Engl J Med 1991;325:897.
104. Oppenheim DS, Kana AR, Sangha JS, Klibanski A. Prevalence of alpha-subunit hypersecretion in patients with pituitary tumors: clinically nonfunctioning and somatotroph adenomas. J Clin Endocrinol Metab 1990;70:859.
105. Oppizzi G, Petroncini MM, Dallabonzana D, Cozzi R, Verde G, Chiodini PG, Luizzi A. Relationship between somatomedin-C and growth hormone levels in acromegaly: basal and dynamic evaluation. J Clin Endocrinol Metab 1986;63:1348.
106. Pieterse S, Dinning TA, Blumbergs PC. Postirradiation sarcomatous transformation of a pituitary adenoma: a combined pituitary tumor. Case report. J Neurosurg 1982;56:283.
107. Richards AM, Bullock MR, Teasdale GM, Thomson JA, Khan MI. Fertility and pregnancy after operation for a prolactinoma. Br J Obstet Gynaecol 1986;93:495.
108. Ridgway EC, Klibanski A, Ladenson PW, Clemmons D, Beitins IZ, McArthur JW, Martorana MA, Zervas NT. Pure alpha-secreting pituitary adenomas. N Engl J Med 1981;304:1254.
109. Roncoroni D. Relations between psychotic symptoms and serum prolactin levels. Pharmacopsychiatry 1989;22:71.
110. Ross DA, Wilson CB. Results of transsphenoidal microsurgery for growth hormone-secreting pituitary adenoma in a series of 214 patients. J Neurosurg 1988;68:854.
111. Roth J, Glick SM, Cuatrecasas P, Hollander CS. Acromegaly and other disorders of growth hormone secretion. Combined clinical staff conference at the National Institutes of Health. Ann Intern Med 1967;66:760.
112. Roth J, Gorden P, Brace K. Efficacy of conventional pituitary irradiation in acromegaly. N Engl J Med 1970;282:1385.
113. Salassa RM, Laws ER Jr, Carpenter PC, Northcutt RC. Transsphenoidal removal of pituitary microadenoma in Cushing's disease. Mayo Clin Proc 1978;53:24.
114. Scanlon MF, Howells S, Peters JR, Williams ED, Richards S, Hall R, Thomas JP. Hyperprolactinaemia, amenorrhoea and galactorrhoea due to a pituitary thyrotroph adenoma. Clin Endocrinol (Oxf) 1985;23:35.
115. Schlechte J, el-Khoury G, Kathol M, Walkner L. Forearm and vertebral bone mineral in treated and untreated hyperprolactinemic amenorrhea. J Clin Endocrinol Metab 1987;64:1021.
116. Schteingart DE. Cushing's syndrome. Endocrinol Metab Clin North Am 1989;18:311.
117. Selman WR, Laws ER, Scheithauer BW, Carpenter SM. The occurrence of dural invasion in pituitary adenomas. J Neurosurg 1986;64:402–407.
118. Sheline GE. Conventional Radiation Therapy in the Treatment of Pituitary Tumors. In Clinical Management of Pituitary Disorders. Seminars in Neurological Surgery series. Edited by GT Tindall, and WF Collins. New York: Raven, 1979, pp 287–314.
119. Shewchuk AB, Adamson GD, Lessard P, Ezrin C. The effect of pregnancy on suspected pituitary adenomas after conservative management of ovulation defects associated with galactorrhea. Am J Obstet Gynecol 1980;136:659.
120. Sobrinho LG. Neuropsychiatry of prolactin: causes and effects. Baillière's Clin Endocrinol Metab 1991;5:119.
121. Sobrinho LG. The psychogenic effects of prolactin. Acta Endocrinol (Copenh) 1993;129(suppl):38.
122. Spada A, Arosio M, Bochicchio D, Bazzoni N, Vallar L, Bassetti M, Faglia G. Clinical, biochemical, and morphological correlates in patients bearing growth hormone-secreting pituitary tumors with or without constitutively active adenylyl cyclase. J Clin Endocrinol Metab 1990;71:1421.
123. Spinas GA, Zapf J, Landolt AM, Stuckmann G, Froesch ER. Pre-operative treatment of 5 acromegalics with a somatostatin analogue: endocrine and clinical observations. Acta Endocrinol (Copenh) 1987;114:249.
124. Stein AL, Levenick MN, Kletzky OA. Computed tomography versus magnetic resonance imaging for the evaluation of suspected pituitary adenomas. Obstet Gynecol 1989;73:996.
125. Tagliaferri M, Berselli ME, Loli P. Transsphenoidal microsurgery for Cushing's disease. Acta Endocrinol (Copenh) 1986;113:5.
126. Teasdale G. Surgical management of pituitary adenoma. Clin Endocrinol Metab 1983;12:789.
127. Thomas JP, Richards SH. Long term results of radical hypophysectomy for Cushing's disease. Clin Endocrinol (Oxf) 1983;19:629.
128. Tindall GT, Oyesiku NM, Watts NB, Clark RV, Christy JH, Adams DA. Transsphenoidal adenomectomy for growth hormone-secreting pituitary adenomas in acromegaly: outcome analysis and determinants of failure. J Neurosurg 1993;78:205.
129. Tindall GT, Tindall SC. Transsphenoidal surgery for acromegaly: long-term results in 50 patients. In Secretory Tumors of the Pituitary Gland: Progress in Endocrine Research and Therapy, Vol. 1. Edited by P McL Black, NT Zervas, EC Ridgway, and JB Martin. New York: Raven, 1984, pp 175–178.
130. Tucker HS, Grubb SR, Wigand JP, Watlington CO, Blackard WG, Becker DP. The treatment of acromegaly by transsphenoidal surgery. Arch Intern Med 1980;140:795.
131. U HS, Wilson CB, Tyrrell JB. Transsphenoidal microhypophysectomy in acromegaly. J Neurosurg 1977;47:840.
132. Vallar L, Spada A, Giannattasio G. Altered Gs and adenylate cyclase activity in human GH-secreting pituitary adenomas. Nature 1987;330:566–568.
133. Vance ML, Thorner MO. Prolactinomas. Endocrinol Metab Clin North Am 1987;16:731.
134. van Schaardenburg D, Roelfsema F, van Seters AP, Vielvoye GJ. Bromocriptine therapy for non-functioning pituitary adenoma. Clin Endocrinol (Oxf) 1989;30:475.
135. Vasen HFA, van Erpecum KJ, Roelfsema F, Raue F, Koppeschaar H, Griffioen G, van Berge Honegouwen GP. Increased prevalence of colonic adenomas in patients with acromegaly. Eur J Endocrinol 1994;131:235–237.
136. Wang C, Lam KS, Ma JT, Chan T, Liu MY, Yeung RT. Long-term treatment of hyperprolactinaemia with bromocriptine: effect of drug withdrawal. Clin Endocrinol (Oxf) 1987;27:363.
137. Weiss MH, Wycoff RR, Yadley R, Gott P, Feldon S. Bromocriptine treatment of prolactin-secreting tumors: surgical implications. Neurosurgery 1983;12:640.
138. Werner SC, Stewart WB. Hyperthyroidism in a patient with a pituitary chromophobe adenoma and fragment of normal pituitary. J Clin Endocrinol Metab 1958;18:266.
139. Wilson CB. Neurosurgical management of large and invasive pituitary tumors. In Clinical Management of Pituitary Disorders. Seminars in Neurological Surgery series. Edited by GT Tindall, and WF Collins. New York: Raven, 1979, pp 335–342.
140. Wilson CB. Surgical management of endocrine-active pituitary adenomas. In Oncology of the Nervous System. Edited by MD Walker (series volume in Cancer Treatment and Research. Edited by WL McGuire). Boston: Martinus Nijhoff, 1983, pp 117–150.
141. Wilson CB. A decade of pituitary microsurgery. The Herbert Olivecrona Lecture. J Neurosurg 1984;61:814.
142. Wilson CB. Role of surgery in the management of pituitary tumors. Neurosurg Clin North Am 1990;1:139.
143. Wright AD, Hill DM, Lowy C, Fraser TR. Mortality in acromegaly. Q J Med 1970;39:1.
144. Yamada S, Asa SL, Kovacs K, Muller P, Smyth HS. Analysis of hormone secretion by clinically nonfunctioning human pituitary adenomas using the reverse hemolytic plaque assay. J Clin Endocrinol Metab 1989;68:73.
145. Yamada S, Horvath E, Kovacs K, Aiba T, Shimizu T, Shishiba Y, Hara M. Gonadotroph adenoma of the pituitary mimicking a prolactinoma. Neurosurgery 1991;28:444.

CHAPTER 100

Neoplasms of the Thyroid

BLAKE CADY AND ARTURO R. ROLLA

Introduction

Thyroid cancer has always elicited concern beyond its relative incidence and death rate because of its occurrence in children and young adults and the vagaries of its clinical behavior in different age groups. In 1995, there were expected to be only 15,600 cases in the United States of which only 1,210 will involve persons who will die of the disease. Like many endocrine gland cancers, various types of thyroid carcinomas have extremely variable time courses and biologic patterns and various separate pathologic forms, which have led to difficulty in defining common themes in the disease.

Incidence

Autopsy studies of the thyroid gland worldwide demonstrate high incidences of microscopic foci of papillary carcinoma, but also occasionally other pathologic varieties ranging from less than a millimeter to a centimeter in size. This incidence is partly related to the number of sections taken through the thyroid gland at pathologic study; whole organ sections taken at frequent intervals throughout the gland illustrate an incidence of such occult cancers that ranges from 6 to over 30%. In survivors of the atomic bomb explosions in Japan, the incidence in the exposed population is even higher. In other countries, studies have shown a high rate without known exposure to atomic radiation. In the United States, the incidence of these microscopically defined occult cancers has ranged from 6 to 15% in various reports. This would indicate that there are at least 15 million to more than 30 million Americans with such microscopic cancer. The enormous gap between that figure and the 15,600 cases of cancer reported each year provides yet another source of confusion about the biologic behavior of differentiated thyroid carcinoma. Furthermore, it should be recognized that a significant proportion of the 15,600 cases of thyroid cancer reported in tumor registries actually are incidentally discovered microscopic foci of papillary carcinoma in thyroid glands that were resected for benign conditions, but with a pathology report of cancer. Thus, the actual number of clinical thyroid cancers each year in the United States is probably less than 10,000.

Epidemiology and Etiology

Up to the 1950s, it was common practice in this country to give low-dose radiation therapy to children for a variety of benign head and neck conditions, such as enlarged tonsils or adenoids, cutaneous acne, or an enlarged thymus seen on chest x-ray in infants with respiratory symptoms. These children, when followed, were found to have an increased incidence of thyroid carcinoma in glands removed because of nodules detected by clinical examination or radioactive iodine (RAI) scan (7). In those patients who underwent operation, 30% or more had a thyroid cancer, but less than one half of those were clinical cancers (palpable nodule), while the remainder were small or microscopic lesions similar to those discovered on routine autopsy studies. Thus, in this group of patients who received small amounts of radiation exposure to the immature thyroid gland, an increased incidence of both occult and clinical thyroid cancers apparently occurred. Such clinical cancers associated with radiation exhibit exactly the same clinical or biologic behavior as do other differentiated thyroid cancers in young adults and children. The use of radiation therapy for benign conditions in childhood has disappeared in the past 30 years. As a result, radiation-associated cancers due to these exposures have virtually disappeared, as well, since the median interval of about 20 years from the use of radiation to the appearance of the thyroid carcinoma has now been exceeded. Recent reports of cancers arising in children downwind of the Chernobyl nuclear accident are being analyzed, but definitive conclusions are difficult to reach owing to inadequate baseline population data and the brief time interval since the event (18, 22).

Researchers throughout the world have noted a relationship between iodine deficiency and the incidence of thyroid carcinoma. Areas in which there is a relative iodine deficiency have an increased number of thyroid cancers, an increased relative proportion of follicular carcinomas, and a larger number of giant and spindle cell undifferentiated carcinomas of the thyroid gland. Thus, geographic regions subject to endemic goiter may well have increased incidences of thyroid carcinoma with a different pattern of pathologic varieties at presentation than found in the United States. The changes in the pattern of thyroid cancers in the United States may well have dated to the 1930s when the iodination of salt was instituted. The proportion of follicular carcinoma has decreased, whereas papillary cancers have increased. Furthermore, anaplastic cancers, which accounted for over 15% of cases in the 1930s, have virtually disappeared.

Only a few carcinomas of the thyroid following RAI administration have been reported. This probably relates to the larger dose of radiation with RAI in contrast to the low dose of radiation given externally for benign childhood conditions. Although at extremely low doses there seems to be a linear relationship between the incidence of thyroid carcinoma and the radiation dose, it is known that a peak risk of cancer induction seems to occur at about 1,200 cGy, above which associated carcinomas seem to appear much less often. Because of the extremely high doses given when therapeutic RAI is used (i.e., Graves disease), there is little induction of clinical cancer in such patients. Also there seems to be no increased risk of thyroid cancer after diagnostic radioactive scans.

Whether the use of large oral doses of iodine following nuclear accidents that release radioactive isotopes of iodine prevents thyroid cancer is unproved and conjectural. The major radioisotope contamination after the Three-Mile Island accident was RAI, but the doses were not high and no cases of induced thyroid cancer have yet been reported. The practicality of having iodine solutions stored in geographic areas around nuclear plants, when it cannot be predicted that radioiodine isotopes will be the primary contaminant, seems unnecessary, considering the low risk of eventual thyroid carcinoma, the nearly benign behavior of low-risk thyroid cancer, and the fact that infants and children are the only ones apparently at risk for radiation induction by low-dose radiation exposure. Nevertheless, administration of iodine to entire populations has been proposed.

Pathology

Thyroid carcinoma falls into two general types, differentiated and undifferentiated, and several uncommon specific types. Essentially all thyroid carcinomas in the United States today are differentiated, consisting of pure papillary, mixed papillary and follicular (with varying proportions of each), pure follicular (with some Hürthle cell variants), and some poorly differentiated follicular forms. Undifferentiated carcinomas generally consist of spindle and giant cell anaplastic forms, but small cell varieties do occur. Thyroid lymphoma of the non-Hodgkin's type is an uncommon but well-recognized entity. Some small cell thyroid cancers seen in past decades, when studied by newer immunohistochemical techniques, have been shown to be thyroid lymphomas.

Some rare types, such as squamous cell carcinoma and sarcoma of the thyroid, also are seen. Metastatic cancers to the thyroid are uncommon, with the most likely primary sites being renal, lung, or breast carcinomas, or melanoma. A variety of other primary cancers can metastasize to the thyroid gland, however. Finally, medullary carcinoma of the thyroid is not of thyroid follicle cell origin, but arises from the parafollicular C cells (derived from the ultimobranchial body), which migrate embryologically to lie in the anatomic thyroid gland. Medullary carcinoma makes up approximately 4% of thyroid gland cancers and is found in both sporadic and familial forms. These can be distinguished not only by family histories, but also by pathologic features (see Chapter 102). Eighty percent of medullary cancers are of the sporadic type.

DIFFERENTIATED THYROID CARCINOMA

Papillary and Mixed Papillary and Follicular Forms

Studies by us (6) and by others (10) have demonstrated similar clinical behavior of thyroid carcinomas that have any papillary histologic features (Fig. 100.1). This is in contradistinction to those differentiated thyroid carcinomas that are of pure follicular type (Fig. 100.2). The clinical features of all forms of papillary carcinomas include a high incidence of multifocality within the thyroid gland, an extremely high incidence of metastases in the regional lymph nodes, infrequent distant metastatic disease, younger age, and a better survival. Papillary carcinomas are characterized by (*a*) papillae with a fibrovascular stalk, (*b*) nuclei that are large and clear (Orphan Annie eye) with grooves or pseudoinclusions attributable to cytoplasmic invaginations, (*c*) concentric whorls of squamous metaplasia, (*d*) psammoma bodies made of concentric calcific laminations around necrotic cells that may also be seen in benign thyroid tumors, follicular car-

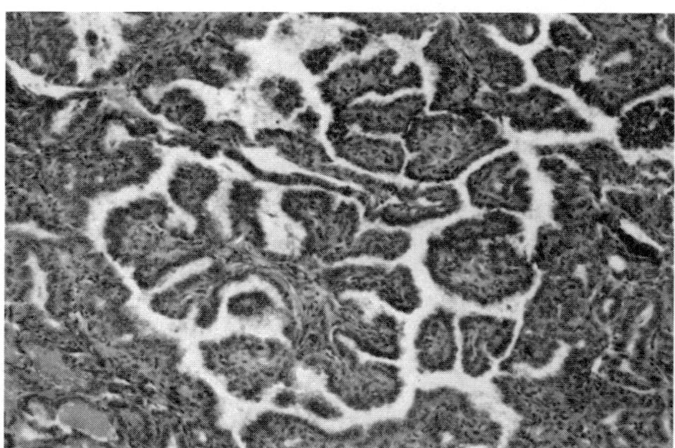

Figure 100.1. Papillary carcinoma.

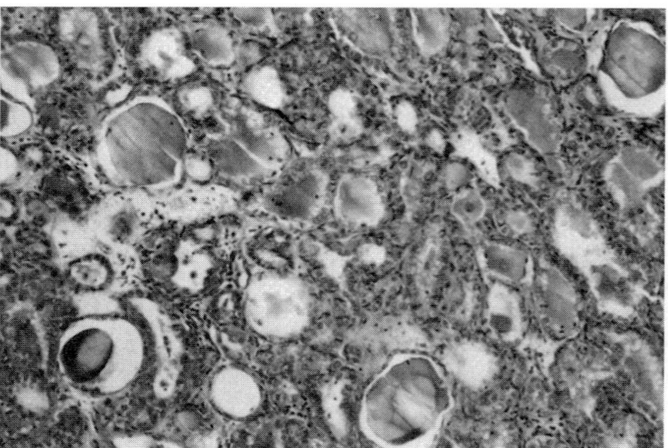

Figure 100.2. Follicular carcinoma.

cinomas of the thyroid, metastatic tumors to the thyroid, and papillary tumors from other organs, such as the ovaries.

Papillary thyroid cancers may penetrate the thyroid gland capsule and invade adjacent structures, including the trachea, larynx, esophagus, recurrent laryngeal nerves, muscles, and soft tissue. Studies show that lymph node metastases occur in up to 80% of cases in young patients. The lymph node metastases are not indicators of poor outcome as they are in every other human cancer, but seem to be irrelevant in evaluating prognosis. In the 1930s, an entity known as lateral aberrant thyroid was described, since young patients frequently presented with a palpable mass in the neck that, on excision, showed relatively benign-appearing thyroid tissue, and when treated by local nodal excision, seldom led to any serious outcome. More recently, of course, these cases (with rare exceptions) are assumed to reflect lymph node metastases from occult papillary carcinoma of the thyroid. Twenty-five percent of young patients present because of such palpable lymph nodes in the neck, frequently without a palpable thyroid mass. It can be regarded as a truism that lymph node metastases of thyroid carcinoma discovered in the neck always have a primary tumor in the thyroid gland, even if it cannot be discovered by preoperative imaging techniques. Sometimes it is even difficult for the operating surgeon to find the tiny focus of primary papillary carcinoma in the thyroid gland accompanying lymph node metastases, but usually the primaries can be palpated as a small, or even tiny, hard, fibrotic nodule in the ipsilateral thyroid gland.

Follicular carcinoma consists of only follicular cells without any papillary features (Fig. 100.2). These lesions are usually surrounded by a pseudocapsule of compressed normal thyroid and fibrous tissue. Follicular adenocarcinomas are presumed to arise from follicular adenomas, since the incidence of follicular thyroid adenocarcinoma increases as a function of size of the follicular lesion. Thus, large follicular lesions are frequently follicular adenocarcinomas; most follicular adenomas less than 2 cm in diameter do not show penetration of the capsule or blood vessel invasion. As in many endocrine cancers, the histologic appearance of the cells does not define the difference between adenoma and adenocarcinoma. Follicular adenocarcinoma is defined by the demonstration of follicular cells penetrating the pseudocapsule (Fig. 100.3) or within the lumen of blood vessels. Needle biopsies of the thyroid cannot distinguish a follicular adenoma from a follicular carcinoma. The extent of the tumor pseudocapsule involvement by follicular cells separates follicular adenocarcinoma into the two general subcategories of minor capsular involvement and major capsular involvement.

Follicular adenocarcinoma with minor capsular involvement (Fig. 100.3) has a prognosis not different from that for an age-adjusted normal population. Thus, although some tumor cells may be seen in the pseudocapsule of the tumor, or to a small extent, in some blood vessels, the biologic behavior of these lesions technically called cancer is not different from that of follicular adenomas. The demonstration of minor tumor pseudocapsular invasion by tumor cells is critically dependent on the sampling of the entire spherical tumor by the pathologist. Thus, some cases of metastatic follicular

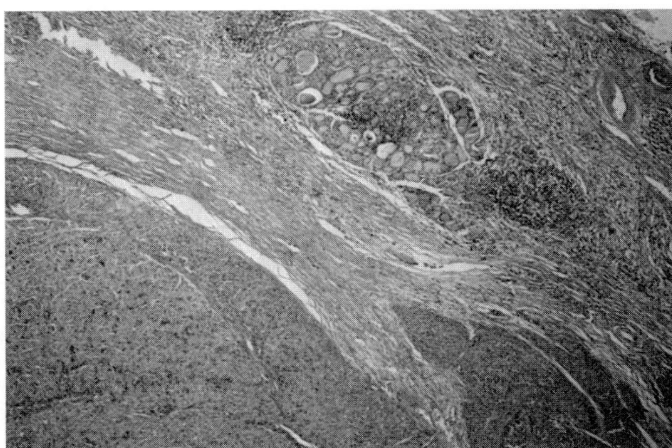

Figure 100.3. Follicular adenocarcinoma with capsular invasion.

adenocarcinoma of the thyroid may have been mistakenly labeled follicular adenoma on the original thyroid pathology because sampling limitations failed to detect the area of capsular penetration. Such "benign metastasizing follicular adenomas" obviously were follicular adenocarcinomas with capsular invasion that was not detected on initial capsule sampling. The metastatic rate of such follicular adenocarcinomas with minor capsular invasion is extremely low, which contributes to an overall excellent prognosis that is similar to that of the normal population.

The pathologic diagnosis of follicular adenocarcinoma with major capsular invasion, therefore, implies gross breaching of the tumor pseudocapsule by follicular cells or extensive involvement of blood vessels. Such follicular adenocarcinoma has a significant risk of metastatic disease, whether in young or old patients. Metastases are most common in the lung, but may also affect bone, brain, liver, and other sites in descending order of frequency. Since metastatic potential is generally a function of the primary tumor size, metastasis without obvious thyroid pathology by clinical examination or scans is seldom encountered with follicular thyroid carcinomas. The ability to do histochemical staining for thyroglobulin offers the additional ability to confirm or deny the primary thyroid origin of the rare distant metastases from an occult primary lesion.

Follicular adenocarcinomas uncommonly metastasize to lymph nodes in the regional area, and when cervical lymph node metastases are described as follicular adenocarcinoma, one should assume that they arose from a mixed papillary and follicular carcinoma. Hürthle cell variants of follicular adenocarcinoma have been an area of controversy (Fig. 100.4). Some authors consider them to be distinct entities with worse prognoses than other follicular adenocarcinomas. We and most authors consider oxyphilic Hürthle cell carcinomas to be variants of follicular adenocarcinoma with similar general prognostic features and similar local growth and metastatic patterns.

Follicular thyroid carcinomas can be classified as well differentiated or poorly differentiated according to their pathologic characteristics. Poorly differentiated follicular adenocarcinomas have a poor prognosis even though undifferentiated elements are not seen.

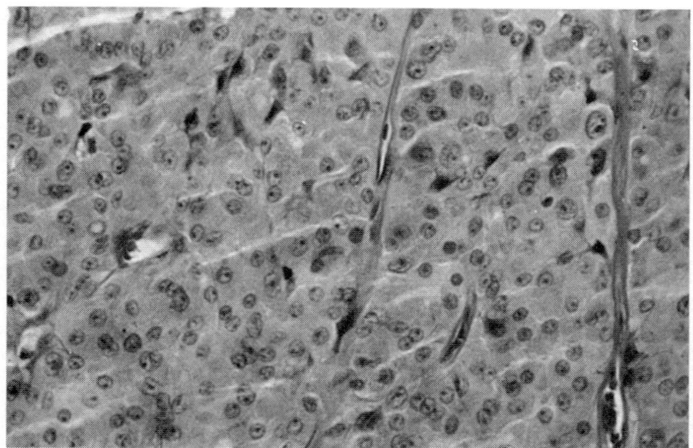

Figure 100.4. Hürthle cell variant of follicular adenocarcinoma.

UNDIFFERENTIATED CARCINOMAS

Undifferentiated carcinomas are usually of the spindle and giant cell anaplastic variety. These cancers are extremely aggressive, resulting in a median survival of less than 6 months. Long-term survival does not exceed 10%, and in most series it is zero. Such anaplastic carcinomas frequently cause compression of the trachea and esophagus and directly invade all the structures surrounding the thyroid. They can metastasize widely and are relatively resistant to treatment. They seldom can be removed surgically, and most therapy is purely palliative. These cancers were common in the United States in the 1930s and 1940s but have gradually decreased over the past 50 years to the point that they now represent less than 1 to 2% of thyroid carcinomas, possibly owing to to the iodization of table salt. Spindle and giant cell undifferentiated thyroid carcinomas sometimes arise against the background of an apparently longstanding quiescent or recurrent papillary carcinoma of the thyroid, and such lesions may have surrounding areas in the thyroid of multifocal papillary carcinoma. It has been postulated that the radiation therapy utilized to treat papillary carcinoma of the thyroid is the stimulus that creates the conversion to anaplastic carcinoma.

THYROID LYMPHOMA

The thyroid is a recognized extranodal site of non-Hodgkin's lymphoma, usually of B cells. These lesions appear as rapidly growing masses in the thyroid with frequent involvement of surrounding structures and compression of the trachea and esophagus. They may arise from the lymphoid elements of Hashimoto's thyroiditis. Small lesions of the thyroid diagnosed as lymphoma need to be differentiated from the lymphoid infiltrate of Hashimoto's thyroiditis. Lymphomas can be accurately diagnosed by immunohistochemical staining, electron microscopy, and other special pathologic techniques. Patients with lymphomas of the thyroid must be diagnostically staged to distinguish between a localized primary lymphoma and more widespread disease.

SQUAMOUS CELL CARCINOMA OF THE THYROID

Squamous cell carcinoma of the thyroid is rare and needs to be differentiated from direct involvement of the thyroid by squamous cell carcinoma arising in the upper aerodigestive tract. The pathogenesis is uncertain. Therapy is radical surgery and adjuvant radiotherapy. The prognosis is very poor.

METASTASES TO THE THYROID

Masses in the thyroid with progressive growth that are seen in patients with other known primary cancers should always be suspected of being metastatic disease. Needle biopsy techniques will usually be sufficient to confirm this diagnosis.

MEDULLARY CARCINOMA OF THE THYROID

Medullary carcinoma of the thyroid (MCT) accounts for about 4% of all thyroid carcinomas and arises in the parafollicular C cells normally scattered in between the follicles throughout the thyroid lobes, particularly the upper portions. Pathologically, the small, uniform, round cells, which resemble neuroendocrine cells, and the amyloid stroma are diagnostic of MCT. MCTs secrete calcitonin, which helps in their histochemical diagnosis by staining, and the elevated serum calcitonin levels are useful for both clinical diagnosis and follow-up. Carcinoembryonic antigen (CEA) may also be elevated in the sera of these patients. Over 80% of MCTs occur sporadically, while the rest are part of three autosomal dominant syndromes: (*a*) familial MCT; (*b*) multiple endocrine neoplasia (MEN) type 2A with MCT, pheochromocytoma, and primary hyperparathyroidism; (*c*) MEN type 2B with MCT, pheochromocytoma, and mucosal neuromas. (See Chapter 102.) Patients with the familial syndromes have a germ cell mutation of the *RET* proto-oncogene on chromosome 10 (27).

Patients with sporadic MCT are usually in their 40s and 50s when they present with a thyroid nodule and lymph node metastases in 50% of cases. Their tumors are unifocal and there is no C-cell hyperplasia in the rest of the gland. Multifocal and bilateral MCT with C-cell hyperplasia in the rest of the gland should immediately suggest the possibility of one of the familial syndromes, even in persons without an apparent positive family history. Poor prognosis factors in sporadic and familial MCT are older age, male sex, large tumor, more extensive disease with lymph node involvement, and inadequate initial surgery. The behavior of these cancers may be quite indolent, however, and patients may have a very prolonged clinical course, even though eventually they may die of the disease. Distant metastases may occur, particularly in mediastinal nodes, lungs, and bones, and serum levels of calcitonin may be used to follow these patients. The penetrance of the familial syndromes is about 50% by age 15 and almost 100% by age 30. The familial forms of MCT are preceded by diffuse, bilateral C-cell hyperplasia with increased levels of serum calcitonin, particularly supranormal responses to pentagastrin and calcium infusion. Total thyroidectomy is completely curative at this stage. Unfortunately, there are false-positive calcitonin stimulation tests, but DNA analysis may eliminate the need for periodic calcitonin stimulation tests of family members. All the relatives with the *RET* proto-oncogene mutation will develop MCT and require an early prophylactic thyroidectomy. What is not known is the age at which this surgery should be done.

Clinical Presentation

The majority of thyroid carcinomas and benign thyroid neoplasms present as a painless thyroid nodule. In young patients, 25% of cases present initially as a palpable lymph node metastasis in the cervical area. Thus, marked lymphadenopathy in young adults and children should arouse suspicion of thyroid carcinoma even when a mass in the thyroid itself is not palpable. In only about 10% of older patients is the first manifestation a regional lymph node metastasis. Uncommonly, a distant metastasis is the first presentation of the disease. While thyroid carcinoma usually presents as a solitary thyroid mass, a multinodular goiter with a dominant nodule or a nodule that grows rapidly on a background of an enlarged gland may be a clinical presentation.

In the past, 75% of thyroid carcinomas in older adults were found in women, but the proportion in men has steadily increased so that in older patients, 50% of thyroid cancers are now found in men. Younger patients and children continue to display a marked female predominance of roughly 4:1. Because of the frequency of benign thyroid nodules in the population and the rarity of clinical thyroid cancers, the vast majority of thyroid nodules detected either clinically or with radiologic techniques proves to be benign. Those lesions that arouse concern about cancer clinically display progressive growth, unusual hardness, fixation, accompanying hoarseness, concomitant lymph node metastases, or symptoms of dysphagia or stridor. Any solitary nodule, any nodule displaying the above characteristics, or any prominent nodule deserves a needle biopsy if any concern about cancer is present.

Anaplastic carcinomas tend to occur in older patients, frequently with a background of a chronically enlarged thyroid presumed to be an adenomatous goiter. Lymphomas are seldom seen in patients under the age of 40. Both of these lesions display rapid growth and unusually large size.

Diagnostic Studies

The most valuable initial diagnostic study of thyroid gland nodules or lymph node metastases in the neck is a fine-needle aspiration for cytology. The results of thyroid aspiration cytology improve with increasing experience on the part of both the person performing the aspiration and the cytologist reading the slides. Needle aspiration cytology separates benign, suspicious, and malignant lesions with an extremely high degree of accuracy. All suspicious or malignant masses should undergo operative removal. Hashimoto's thyroiditis, nonspecific thyroiditis, or adenomatous goiters are accurately portrayed as benign by aspiration cytology combined with clinical examination. Of nodules subjected to aspiration cytology, 10 to 15% produce insufficient material to make a histologic diagnosis and should lead to a repeat needle biopsy or excision. In the largest and most thoroughly analyzed series of needle cytologies of thyroid masses, Mayo Clinic authors (12) reported only three cases of cancer in over 400 patients with nodules diagnosed as benign by needle aspiration and excised. Thus, the false-negative rate of needle aspiration cytology was less than 1%.

Histologic and cellular details of many endocrine tumors do not establish the diagnosis of carcinoma. A cancer diagnosis is made by finding pseudocapsule and/or blood vessel invasion, not by cellular morphology. Thus, aspiration cytology of the thyroid that reveals follicular cells cannot accurately separate follicular adenomas from follicular adenocarcinomas, or even from follicular nodules in an adenomatous goiter. Extensive pathologic sampling of the pseudocapsule around a follicular lesion may be required to discover invasion by follicular cells, the definition of follicular adenocarcinoma. Reports in the literature that allude to the accurate separation of follicular adenoma from follicular adenocarcinoma by needle aspiration should be viewed with skepticism. Cytology that is read as "microfollicular pattern," "follicular neoplasm," or "suspicious" should be operated on for final definition of the follicular lesion. In contrast, most papillary carcinomas can be accurately diagnosed as malignant by fine-needle aspiration cytology because of the characteristic Orphan Annie (Fig. 100.5) nuclei and other features. Anaplastic, metastatic, and medullary carcinomas of the thyroid are also accurately diagnosed by needle aspiration. Needle aspiration cytology of a neck node is highly accurate in diagnosing thyroid carcinoma of either papillary or follicular variants. Open biopsy of a lymph node in the neck of a patient suspect for thyroid cancer should never be performed without first attempting needle aspiration cytology.

The technique of fine-needle aspiration of thyroid nodules is simple, uncomplicated, virtually devoid of complications, and relatively easily taught and mastered. The thyroid nodule is held with the fingers of the left hand and a needle is introduced through a tiny skin wheal of anesthesia and into the thyroid nodule with the right hand. The location of the tip of

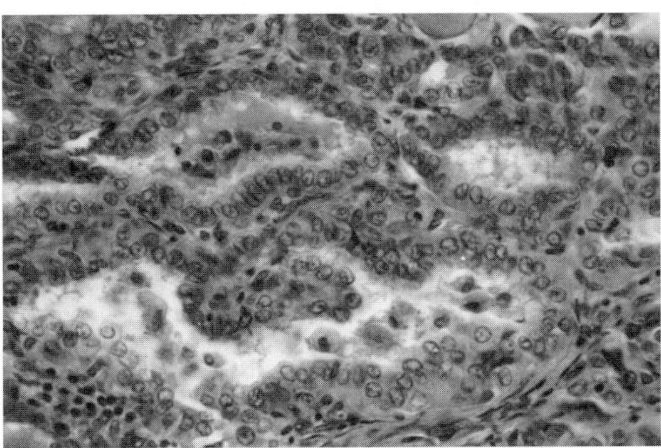

Figure 100.5. Orphan Annie nuclei.

the needle can be accurately surmised by the palpating fingers of the left hand. Once in place, a vigorous vacuum is created by a one-handed syringe holder and the needle moved back and forth over a range of 1 cm or so within the palpable nodule. Before withdrawing the needle, the syringe plunger is released, eliminating the vacuum. The cellular material is then squirted onto slides, smeared as a hematology preparation, and dropped promptly into fixative, or fixative is aspirated into the syringe and the contents squirted into a centrifuge tube. In evaluating thyroid nodules, a cytology report of insufficient material should lead to repeated aspiration, and a malignant or suspicious cytology should lead to thyroid surgery (12). A cytology diagnosis of benign cells might then inspire further studies of anatomy or function of the thyroid gland, with reassurance that the nodule is not cancer. If the repeat aspiration is inconclusive, a third attempt under ultrasound guidance is indicated. When a thyroid nodule is the clinical presentation and a differential diagnosis of cancer one of the primary concerns, aspiration should be the initial step. Since a thyroid cyst is diagnosed by initial needle aspiration, ultrasound has little to offer initially and is far more expensive. Thyroid cyst aspiration fluid should always be submitted to cytologic evaluation, however, since papillary carcinoma of the thyroid occasionally presents as a cystic lesion.

Ultrasound may be utilized after thyroid needle aspiration to help diagnose a multinodular gland. Radioactive iodine and technetium scans of the thyroid gland are generally not helpful, since benign nodules are frequently cold. Separation of suspicious from nonsuspicious nodules in the thyroid by a course of thyroid hormone administration for suppression of thyroid-stimulating hormone (TSH) with evaluation of shrinkage of the nodule is not as reliable as aspiration. Since some cancers respond to TSH suppression and thyroid hormone used in this way has been found to be no more effective than placebo in achieving a reduction of solitary nodule size, this management generally should not be utilized initially (14). There may be a role for thyroid suppression once a needle aspiration cytology has proved the nodule not to be suspicious of cancer, but the nodule continues to grow and the patient wishes to avoid removal.

Thyroid function tests are of no use in evaluating thyroid nodules for suspicion of carcinoma since thyroid carcinoma does not alter thyroid hormone secretion. Only in the situation of extensive thyroid gland destruction from anaplastic carcinoma or lymphoma is thyroid insufficiency found as a manifestation of thyroid carcinoma.

Magnetic resonance imaging (MRI) or computed tomographic (CT) scans of the thyroid gland itself are of no help in the ordinary differentiated thyroid carcinoma. These studies may provide invaluable assistance, however, in evaluating the unlikely possibility of resection in an anaplastic carcinoma or lymphoma or rare forms of thyroid carcinoma. All other thyroid carcinomas require exploration and resection, if at all possible, regardless of findings by imaging techniques. In the presence of metastatic disease to the thyroid, other diagnostic studies are usually necessary to assess the extent of metastasis elsewhere.

Biologic Behavior of Differentiated Thyroid Carcinoma

Many studies have documented the critical biologic features of differentiated thyroid carcinoma and defined the multifactorial clinical risk assessments based on age, size, grade, presence of metastases, and extent of the primary thyroid carcinoma (3, 15, 16, 24). These prognostic scoring systems clearly illustrate that the vast majority of differentiated thyroid carcinomas fall into a low-risk group with a mortality expectation of less than 2%. This low risk applies whether the cancers are papillary or mixed papillary and follicular or pure follicular as to pathologic type. Follicular adenocarcinoma and papillary adenocarcinoma of the thyroid have distinctive and separable patterns of metastases, but their overall prognosis is not governed as much by that pathologic distinction as it is by the clinical risk group, accentuating age, size, and extent of disease. In our risk group definition, low-risk patients are men 40 years of age and younger, women 50 years of age and younger without distant metastases, and older patients whose carcinoma, if follicular, does not extend beyond the thyroid gland capsule, and is less than 5 cm in diameter. This AMES categorization (3) (age, metastases, extent, and size) corresponds closely to the AGES risk category (13) (age, grade, extent, and size) previously developed by the Mayo Clinic. In our AMES prognostic scoring system, regardless of pathologic type, 89% of patients are in the low-risk group, with a death rate of only 1.8% at a median follow-up of 13 years (3). The high risk AMES patients constituted 11% of the series, but had a death rate of 46%. The ratio of death rates of 1:26 illustrates the power of this AMES prognostic scoring system to separate low risk from high risk. Thus, an easily definable clinical prognostic scoring system enables the surgeon at the operating table readily to categorize the patient as at low risk or high risk of death. This assessment is critical in selecting an appropriate operative procedure, in counseling the patient, in advising on overall risk, in developing an overall therapeutic plan, and in organizing a follow-up scheme after initial treatment.

An updated multifactorial prognostic scoring system was recently published by the Mayo Clinic group, the MACIS system (16) (metastasis, age, completeness of surgery, extrathyroid invasion, and size). The lowest-risk group makes up 84% of all cases of papillary carcinoma, and these patients have only a 1% 20-year mortality and a 3% 10-year recurrence, largely of cervical lymph node metastases. This death rate is no higher than that for an age-adjusted normal population. The highest-risk population consists of only a small proportion of cases, but carries a 70% mortality rate at 20 years (16). The AMES prognostic scoring system applies without regard for the presence of lymph node metastases since they do not influence overall prognosis, as is also true with nearly all of the prognostic scoring systems.

Recent studies of the use of DNA histograms in evaluating the biologic behavior and aggressiveness of thyroid carcinomas also have been reported (8). This field is still under investigation and no reliance should be placed on these histograms at the present time. The DNA histograms reported are not as accurate in predicting outcome and aggressiveness of disease as the clinical scoring systems, and, therefore, further work needs to be done in this area. In particular, reports of differential DNA histograms in benign follicular adenoma and follicular adenocarcinomas need to be viewed with skepticism, since it is difficult even under the microscope to predict and define the technical separation of benign follicular adenoma from minor capsular invasion follicular adenocarcinoma.

TREATMENT OF DIFFERENTIATED THYROID CARCINOMA

Surgical removal is essential in the treatment of differentiated thyroid carcinoma. In the past several decades, the median diameter of thyroid carcinomas at presentation has fallen to 2 cm or less in almost two thirds of cases (5). Therefore, bilateral thyroid operations are seldom necessary for the sake of removing the presenting mass of the differentiated thyroid carcinoma itself. The standard operation today is total unilateral thyroid lobectomy with isthmus removal. Less than a total thyroid lobectomy may be performed in certain situations, such as small anterior or medially placed or isthmus thyroid carcinomas.

The major controversy regarding surgery for differentiated thyroid carcinoma involves the debate between the proponents of total thyroidectomy and those who recommend less than a total thyroidectomy as standard surgical treatment. This controversy centers around the alleged advantages of the total removal of the thyroid gland, including the frequent multifocality of papillary carcinoma of the thyroid, the reduced need for RAI therapy to eliminate normal residual thyroid gland when less than a total thyroidectomy is performed, the inability to use thyroglobulin as a tumor marker postoperatively when any normal thyroid tissue remains, and the conversion of longstanding unresected papillary carcinoma of the thyroid to anaplastic disease. These four arguments for the use of total thyroidectomy are balanced by the universal reports of the higher risk of permanent hypoparathyroidism and recurrent laryngeal nerve injury when total thyroidectomy is performed in contrast to less than total thyroidectomy (9, 13). The American College of Surgeons' survey of total thyroidectomy in this country indicates a risk of permanent hypoparathyroidism of 8% or more (9). The Mayo Clinic reports a rate of hypoparathyroidism of nearly 20%, but very low rates of recurrent laryngeal nerve injury (13). The Lahey Clinic, on the other hand, reports less than a 1% rate of hypoparathyroidism in over 2,000 cases that did not involve total thyroidectomy (4). Individual surgeons with unusual skills at thyroid surgery have reported rates of permanent hypoparathyroidism of 1% or less with total thyroidectomy (1).

The proponents of less than total thyroidectomy make several points.

(*a*) While papillary carcinoma is frequently multifocal, the multifocality is almost always in the form of microscopic disease that is clinically insignificant. During exploration of the thyroid at surgery, the opposite thyroid lobe is palpated, and if clinically apparent multifocal papillary carcinoma is detected, the opposite lobe should be removed with a bilateral thyroid operation.

(*b*) Radioactive iodine postoperatively is seldom necessary since nearly 90% of the patients are at extremely low risk of recurrence or death and rarely need RAI for either diagnosis or therapy on a routine basis after surgery.

(*c*) Thyroglobulin as a tumor marker used to follow patients seems hardly necessary when over 98% of patients in the low-risk group will never die of the disease and therefore do not need vigorous follow-up. Furthermore, high-risk patients are accurately separated by clinical criteria, and when so defined, can have more extensive initial thyroid surgery. In addition, almost all high-risk patients who develop metastases eventually die of the disease, so early detection of metastases by tumor markers does not materially influence therapy or outcome.

(*d*) The incidence of true conversion from papillary carcinoma to anaplastic carcinoma is extremely low; in the major reported series such conversions amount to much less than 1% of cases (20). The striking decline in the incidence of giant and spindle cell undifferentiated carcinoma makes this estimate of risk out of date and far too high (3).

Thus, with few substantial gains and major risks, advocating total thyroidectomy for all thyroid cancers both is unnecessary and creates extra morbidity. Thyroid surgery is extremely well tolerated with extremely few deaths after surgery and few major complications if the surgical procedure is conservative in extent. In the absence of bilateral thyroid gland dissection, hypoparathyroidism does not occur and recurrent laryngeal nerve paralysis, usually temporary, is seen in less than 1% of cases. If a vocal cord is paralyzed preoperatively, the recurrent laryngeal nerve may be deliberately sacrificed; however, all functioning recurrent laryngeal nerves should be preserved, if possible, even if that requires dissecting the nerve out of surrounding thyroid carcinoma or metastatic nodes. If the local extent of disease at initial lobectomy indicates that the patient is in a high-risk group or would be a candidate for postoperative RAI (i.e., extraglandular involvement, extensive pseudocapsular invasion by follicular carcinoma, greater than 5 cm diameter, older age), the surgeon should perform either a total or subtotal contralateral lobectomy. Even in low-risk patients, if suspicious nodules of multicentric papillary carcinoma are palpated in the opposite lobe, a contralateral thyroid lobectomy should be performed. By selective application of surgical removal based on risk group and disease extent, only a small minority of patients need be subjected to the increased risk of a total thyroidectomy. There is no justification for routine total thyroidectomy as a surgical approach to any benign thyroid condition.

If the primary thyroid carcinoma extends outside the thyroid gland and extensively involves adjacent vital structures, such as trachea, larynx, or esophagus, these should be preserved at the initial operative approach. Thus, direct involvement of the tracheal wall should be handled by sharply excising the tumor from the tracheal cartilages; the larynx or esophagus or a functioning recurrent laryngeal nerve should be preserved where such cases are in the low-risk group since, despite the extent of residual disease initially, such patients seldom die of the disease (21).

Sacrifice of surrounding soft tissue and strap muscles or of small areas of trachea or esophagus is justified, of course, whenever they are directly involved in the differentiated thyroid carcinoma and are easily and locally resectable. Direct extensions of thyroid cancer into trachea, esophagus, and surrounding tissues in low-risk, younger patients are usually treated successfully by RAI, external beam therapy, and thyroid hormone suppression of TSH to provide permanent control of the disease. We have demonstrated extremely low mortality rates (11%) for such patients who technically are surgically incurable, illustrating the unique biologic behavior of low-risk differentiated thyroid carcinoma (21). Such patients are uncommon currently because of the early diagnosis of disease. Less than 10% of patients currently have primary thyroid cancers larger than 3 cm in diameter.

For high-risk patients with extraglandular extension of cancer, however, the prognosis is almost uniformly fatal. Extensive resections, such as concomitant laryngectomy or tracheal resection, are not justified initially since the outcome is seemingly not altered by such an aggressive approach, at least as the initial operative procedure. On rare occasions, when such initially unresectable disease recurs as a symptomatic or clinical problem, radical surgery, such as laryngectomy, may be required in unusual circumstances for palliation, particularly of airway obstruction.

Metastatic lymph nodes in differentiated thyroid carcinoma can be resected with conservative function-preserving and tissue-sparing neck dissections, since these cancers essentially never implant in surgical wounds. The spinal accessory nerve should be preserved in every case, and the internal jugular vein and sternocleidomastoid muscle can frequently be preserved as well. The submandibular area need not be resected since metastases seldom occur there. Whether the modified dissections are "berry picking," limited resections of lymph nodes, or functional neck dissections, a logical schema of surgical treatment of lymph node metastases is as follows: (*a*) lymph node metastases palpable before initial thyroid surgery should be treated by modified or functional neck dissection through an upward extension of the thyroid collar incision; (*b*) if lymph node metastases are not palpable preoperatively but are discovered at the time of the thyroid lobectomy, lymph node dissection within the confines of the collar incision and in the central compartment of the neck should be performed, and this is possible only in piecemeal fashion; (*c*) if obvious lymph node metastases are not palpable, preoperatively or at the time of surgery, no formal lymph node dissection need be performed.

Two thirds of cases of recurrent cancer in low-risk patients with papillary carcinoma of the thyroid are cervical lymph node metastases. Recognizing the lack of a relationship of lymph node metastases to prognosis indicates that the treatment of such lymph node metastases should be conservative and usually is best accomplished by a modified neck dissection that preserves all the anatomic structures previously mentioned. Radioactive iodine treatment of cervical lymph node metastases can be avoided since these present a straightforward surgical problem in the vast majority of cases.

THYROID SCANNING

Thyroid scanning in patients with well-differentiated thyroid carcinoma is usually done with RAI. Preoperatively, it has seldom been necessary since the advent of needle aspiration biopsy. However, postoperative total-body RAI scanning is recommended for high-risk patients 4 to 6 weeks after the thyroidectomy, having left them without thyroxine replacement so that serum TSH will be elevated. The postoperative scan may show uptake in the thyroid bed or in local lymph nodes, even after "total" thyroidectomies. If there is significant thyroidal uptake, a prophylactic ablative dose of RAI (30 mCi) may be given on an outpatient basis. If the total-body scan shows distant metastasis, the patient should be treated with a higher dose of RAI (100 to 200 mCi). Abnormal RAI uptake areas should be further studied with other modalities of imaging because false-positive uptakes may be seen with periodontal surgery, esophageal strictures, hiatal hernia, Zenker's diverticulum, abdominal neurilemoma, rectal teratoma, ectopic kidney, lung carcinoma, pericardial effusion, struma ovarii, and external contamination.

There is a potential risk of decreasing the effectiveness of the therapeutic dose by giving a previous diagnostic dose of RAI (2 to 5 mCI). This phenomenon, called stunning of the thyroid tissue, tended to occur more with the larger diagnostic doses of RAI used in the past.

Postradiotherapy total-body scanning takes advantage of the larger RAI dose delivered, increasing the possibilities of visualizing metastasis with low uptake or volume. Obtaining a total-body scan is always recommended after each therapeutic dose of RAI. About a week after the dose has been administered, the patient is placed on full thyroxine suppression.

Follow-up total-body scans may be used in high-risk patients during the first years after the thyroidectomy to search for local recurrences and distant metastasis. Unfortunately, the patient has to discontinue thyroxine administration 4 to 6 weeks before the scan to allow serum TSH to increase over 40 mIU/mL and maximize the uptake of radioactive tracer. Patients all develop hypothyroid symptoms during that time. The period without thyroid replacement may be shortened by utilization of 50 to 75 μg triiodothyronine (T_3) for 4 weeks. The half-life of T_3 is much shorter, so that it allows scanning in 2 to 4 weeks after discontinuation of the hormone. Administration of recombinant human TSH may eliminate the need for thyroid hormone discontinuation to obtain a scan in the future. Scanning with radioactive thallium (T201) may be used in certain patients with differentiated thyroid tumors with RAI uptake but elevated serum thyroglobulin levels (28).

RADIOACTIVE IODINE TREATMENT

The use of RAI for therapy of distant metastatic or unresectable local differentiated thyroid carcinoma is a unique demonstration (and the first historically) of an idealized cancer treatment, since iodine is metabolized almost exclusively by thyroid tissue with only minor amounts taken up in salivary glands and gastric mucosa. Therefore, RAI is a uniquely specific agent that can seek out and destroy functioning thyroid tissue wherever it occurs in the body. In actual practice, however, thyroid carcinoma is never as efficient in iodine uptake as is normal thyroid tissue, and thus normal thyroid tissue must be completely removed surgically or ablated radiotherapeutically before the thyroid tumor can be induced to take up RAI.

The major controversy regarding the use of RAI is whether

it should be used routinely as an adjuvant to surgery or in a highly selective fashion. With the definition of risk groups, such as the AMES, AGES, and MACIS systems (3, 15, 16), the routine use of RAI for postoperative scanning and ablation can be limited to the very selective small minority of patients at high risk (10 to 15% of patients) or the few low-risk patients (1% or less) who develop metastases.

Postoperative RAI ablation of thyroid remnants is indicated in high-risk patients because (*a*) even after total thyroidectomies, some thyroid tissue is found in the neck; (*b*) the thyroid tumor may be multifocal, particularly the papillary carcinomas; (*c*) remnant thyroid tissue competes with the thyroid tumor of RAI uptake; (*d*) secretion of thyroglobulin by normal thyroid tissue decreases its specificity as a tumor marker; (*e*) there is a possibility of carcinomas appearing in the thyroid tissue left (de novo or recurrent tumor); (*f*) the prognosis of these patients may improve by decreasing recurrences (29, 30).

FOLLOW-UP OF PATIENTS WITH HIGH-RISK DIFFERENTIATED THYROID CARCINOMA AFTER INITIAL SURGERY

Every 6 months for the first 3 years, these patients should have careful examinations of the neck looking for recurrence and lymphadenopathy. A serum TSH determination by an ultrasensitive technique should be between 0.1 and 0.4 mIU/mL, indicating appropriate thyroxine suppression; otherwise the dose should be adjusted. Excessive TSH suppression (to less than 0.1 mIU/mL) is not necessary and may lead to accelerated bone loss, especially in women. Serum thyroglobulin level should be less than 10 ng/mL in patients with surgical and RAI ablation while they are on suppressive doses of triiodothyronine. A chest x-ray or CT scan may detect pulmonary metastasis but the usual technetium bone scans unfortunately are unreliable in trying to detect skeletal metastasis in thyroid carcinomas. If all of these tests are normal, after 3 years the patient may be seen at annual intervals.

Serum thyroglobulin is a sensitive and economic marker of residual or recurrent disease. In patients with antithyroglobulin antibodies, thyroglobulin determinations are not reliable, however. Thyroid hormone withdrawal with subsequent elevation of serum TSH tends to increase the levels of thyroglobulin. Most patients (96%) with a positive total body RAI scan have elevated serum thyroglobulin levels. For that reason, it is not necessary to do routine total-body RAI scans on patients with suppressed thyroglobulin levels, unless there are other clinical indications of recurrence (abnormal chest x-ray or CT scan, palpable cervical lymphadenopathy, or symptoms). False-negative levels of serum thyroglobulin are rarely seen with cervical adenopathy in the absence of distant metastasis or in tumors that do not secrete thyroglobulin de novo or after subsequent dedifferentiation.

Most patients with significant elevations of serum thyroglobulin have a positive total-body RAI scan and should be treated with 100 to 250 mCi of RAI. The RAI treatment should be repeated at 6-month intervals to allow enough time for the bone marrow to recover. RAI treatments are followed with posttherapy RAI total-body scans and are repeated until there is no uptake in the areas of metastasis or to a total dose of 500 mCi in children or 800 to 1,000 mCi in adults. With successful eradication of metastasis, the thyroglobulin usually returns to suppressed levels. Aggressive and repeated RAI treatments may decrease recurrences and mortality in patients with metastatic thyroid carcinoma, particularly patients in the low-risk group. High-risk patients, however, usually develop metastases (31).

There is a significant proportion of patients with elevated serum thyroglobulin levels but negative total-body RAI scans. If a chest x-ray or CT scan and skeletal x-rays find metastases that were not shown on the RAI scan, the patients should be treated with RAI as above. If the radiologic studies are also normal, the solitary elevation of serum thyroglobulin may be a strong indication to utilize therapeutic RAI. A posttherapy total-body scan usually reveals metastases not previously found with the regular diagnostic scan (32).

The efficacy of the RAI treatment depends heavily on the uptake by the thyroid tumors and basic risk-group determination. Approximately 50% of differentiated thyroid carcinomas show significant iodine uptake, although much less than does any normal thyroid tissue. This is the reason they appear as "cold" nodules in thyroid scanning. In general, follicular tumors have better uptake than papillary carcinomas. But the fact that a thyroid tumor has a lower uptake does not mean that it cannot be treated effectively with RAI. Adequate radiation of these tumors may still be obtained by increasing the dose. The site of metastasis also changes the response to RAI treatment. Cervical lymphadenopathy and pulmonary metastasis respond better than do brain and bone metastases.

Complications of RAI treatment are: (*a*) radiation thyroiditis with local tenderness and transient thyrotoxicosis are more common in patients with unilateral surgical excision; (*b*) sialoadenitis results since RAI is also taken up by the salivary glands; (*c*) radiation sickness with malaise, nausea, anorexia, and headache is quite uncommon; (*d*) pulmonary fibrosis is seen in patients with extensive lung metastasis; (*e*) brain edema can result in patients with intracranial metastasis, which may be prevented with prophylactic glucocorticoids; (*f*) permanent sterility may be seen with cumulative doses over 800 mCi, whereas lower doses may cause transient oligospermia or menstrual irregularities; (*g*) as teratogenesis and spontaneous abortions may occur, pregnancies should be delayed for at least 1 year after the RAI administration; (*h*) there is a small increase in the risk of leukemias and carcinomas of the breast and bladder.

External beam radiotherapy should be used for the treatment of unresectable or recurrent local neck disease if RAI cannot be utilized. External beam radiotherapy can also be used in specific metastatic sites (bone metastases) for palliation when RAI is not effective. The other adjuvant therapy employed universally is the suppression of TSH by exogenous ingestion of thyroid hormone. While this has been standard practice since the first demonstration of regression of metastatic disease by TSH suppression in 1957 by Crile, patients in low-risk groups with small or "occult" papillary carcinomas probably do not need such treatment as long as they are euthyroid. Patients with obvious clinical cancer should receive adjuvant thyroid hormone for TSH suppression, but whether that actually reduces the death rate is open to some question (2).

There is no standard protocol for the chemotherapeutic management of metastatic differentiated thyroid carcinoma. Adriamycin- and platinum-containing multiple drug programs have produced temporary palliation in a small percentage of patients.

Therapy of Undifferentiated Thyroid Carcinoma

Numerous articles cite the advantages of multidisciplinary management combining radiotherapy and chemotherapy with Adriamycin-containing regimens for the local and systemic treatment of anaplastic thyroid carcinoma (17, 25). Radiotherapeutic techniques sometimes include hyperfractionation. Because of the few cases currently seen, it is difficult to know which program should be preferred, but Adriamycin should be a component of any multidrug protocol. It has been reported that local neck disease can be controlled without the need for surgery or tracheostomy for airway obstruction in a significant proportion of patients whereas formerly tracheostomy was frequently required. Despite encouraging temporary responses to such combined treatments, few long-term survivors are reported.

Therapy of Thyroid Lymphoma

Non-Hodgkin's lymphoma of the thyroid should be treated as are other extranodal lymphomas. If the disease can be totally removed surgically, is of limited extent, and has not penetrated the thyroid capsule, it may be that no systemic therapy is required since cure and control rates are extremely high with or without adjuvant radiotherapy (11). However, if the lymphoma has penetrated the thyroid capsule, is extensive in the neck, or cannot be totally removed, multidrug chemotherapy programs, usually with radiotherapy, are essential to provide long-term control.

Metastatic Disease to the Thyroid Gland

Metastases to the thyroid seldom need complicated or unusual therapy. If the metastasis is symptomatic and isolated, a resection might be considered. If it is but one component of widespread metastases, it usually need not be treated separately unless airway obstruction occurs, in which case an attempt at removal or a tracheostomy may be required, or local radiotherapy given.

Medullary Carcinoma of the Thyroid

Medullary carcinoma of the thyroid has a unique biology and requires distinctive therapeutic planning. With needle aspiration of thyroid nodules, a specific diagnosis of medullary carcinoma can almost always be made as the neuroendocrine cells are typical. Thus, preliminary screening for calcitonin should not be performed routinely before surgery in all cases of thyroid nodules, but only in those patients in whom medullary carcinoma has been actually proved by needle aspiration cytology. Since most patients who present with medullary carcinoma of the thyroid do not have an adequate family history available prior to surgery, a total thyroidectomy should be the treatment of choice. Individual patients with clinical medullary carcinoma of the thyroid may be the index cases for a familial cluster yet to be discovered. In familial medullary thyroid carcinoma, total thyroidectomy is necessitated by both the multifocal nature of the medullary carcinoma and the C-cell hyperplasia discovered uniformly bilaterally in such cases.

Medullary carcinoma that presents clinically should have an ipsilateral functional neck dissection performed as part of initial surgical therapy, including the central compartment of the neck. This reflects the extremely high incidence of nodal metastases in both sporadic and familial forms. However, in the familial medullary cancer that is detected by calcitonin screening without clinical signs, the incidence of lymph node metastases is extremely low. While such patients should have total thyroidectomy, lymph node resections can be more selectively applied. If the medullary carcinoma is occult or only C-cell hyperplasia exists, lymph node resection need not be performed. If the medullary carcinoma is palpable but intraglandular, it is probably wise to perform a functional neck dissection on the ipsilateral side for both prognostic and therapeutic purposes (see Chapter 102).

The ability to screen family members at risk of medullary thyroid carcinoma syndromes by either basal detection or stimulated calcitonin diagnostic studies permits totally curative treatment to be performed in a preclinical stage at a young age. Thus, patients with MEN type 2A or 2B or the more restricted familial medullary thyroid cancer syndrome represent the ideal screening population in which patients at risk can now be detected by genetic markers, a disease precursor (C-cell hyperplasia) can be detected at a totally curable preclinical stage by serum markers, and curative therapy can be applied (total thyroidectomy). Every patient with medullary thyroid carcinoma should have extensive family screening to diagnose new familial clusters. It should be recognized, however, that the vast majority of medullary thyroid carcinoma (80% or more) appears in a sporadic form without implication of other family members (19). Calcitonin and CEA serum markers are used postoperatively following complete local and regional surgery (total thyroidectomy and neck dissection) for prognostic purposes (23). Because of the extremely long natural history of medullary carcinoma, however, it is probably not useful to pursue extensive metastatic workups for patients with elevated levels of CEA or calcitonin should they be asymptomatic. Whether extensive microdissection of regional lymph node areas by surgery to achieve normalization of calcitonin and CEA will actually improve cure rates is at present only conjectural (26).

The curative treatment of metastatic medullary carcinoma is not yet possible and no standard therapeutic programs have been described in the literature. Radiotherapy can be utilized with some success as medullary thyroid carcinoma is sometimes moderately radiosensitive. Obviously, systemic therapy could be considered for systemic manifestations of metastatic disease, but there is little guidance about particular drugs or programs to be offered. Occasional surgical resection for palliation of localized symptomatic disease can be attempted.

Future Directions in Thyroid Carcinoma

It has proved impossible to mount prospective trials in differentiated thyroid carcinoma because even several institutions cannot provide a sufficient number of cases. Attempts at multiinstitutional protocols have failed to generate research support, and thus therapeutic programs are developed by derivation from relatively small numbers of patients. The most important new research in thyroid cancer is that of identifying specific genetic markers for familial clusters of medullary carcinoma in the MEN (2) and familial cases. Such specific genetic markers will enable still more refined selection of patients for preventive surgery in these genetic varieties.

Finally, the ability clinically to separate high-risk and low-risk cases of thyroid cancer with a high degree of accuracy and reliability has been a major step forward in rationalizing therapy and follow-up procedures, but still needs to be more widely appreciated and applied in therapeutic planning.

References

1. Attie JN, Moskowitz GW, Margouleff D, Levy LM. Feasibility of total thyroidectomy in the treatment of thyroid carcinoma: postoperative radioactive iodine evaluation of 140 cases. Am J Surg 1979;138:555.
2. Cady B, Cohn K, Rossi RL, Sedgwick CE, Meissner WA, Werber J, Gelman RS. The effect of thyroid hormone administration upon survival in patients with differentiated thyroid carcinoma. Surgery 1983;94:978.
3. Cady B, Rossi RL. An expanded view of risk-group definition in differentiated thyroid carcinoma. Surgery 1988;104:947.
4. Cady B, Rossi RL. Surgery of the Thyroid and Parathyroid Glands, 3rd ed. Philadelphia: Saunders, 1990, p 150.
5. Cady B, Rossi RL, Silverman ML, Wool M. Further evidence of the validity of risk group definition in differentiated thyroid carcinoma. Surgery 1985;98:1171.
6. Cady B, Sedgwick CE, Meissner WA, Bookwalter JR, Romagosa V, Werber J. Changing clinical, pathologic, therapeutic, and survival patterns in differentiated thyroid carcinoma. Ann Surg 1976;184:541.
7. Cerletty JM, Guansing AR, Engbring NH, et al. Radiation-related thyroid carcinoma. Arch Surg 1978;113:1072–1076.
8. Cohn K, Backdahl M, Forsslund G, Auer G, Zetterberg A, Lundell G, Granberg PO, Lowhagen T, Willems JS, Cady B. Biologic considerations and operative strategy in papillary thyroid carcinoma: arguments against the routine performance of total thyroidectomy. Surgery.3 1984;96:957.
9. Foster RS. Morbidity and mortality after thyroidectomy. Surg Gynecol Obstet 1978;146:423.
10. Franssila KO. Prognosis in thyroid carcinoma. Cancer 1975;36:1138.
11. Friedberg MH, Coburn MC, Monchik JM. The role of surgery in stage 1-E non-Hodgkin's lymphoma of the thyroid. Surgery 1994;116:1061–1067.
12. Grant C, Hay I, Gough IR, Bergstralh EJ. Local recurrence in papillary thyroid carcinoma: is extent of surgical resection important? Surgery. 1988;104:954.
13. Grant CS, Hay ID, Gough IR, McCarthy PM. Long-term follow-up of patients with benign thyroid fine-needle aspiration cytologic diagnoses. Surgery 1989;106:980.
14. Gharib H, James M, Charboneau JW, et al. Suppressive therapy with levothyroxine for solitary thyroid nodules: a double-blind controlled clinical study. N Engl J Med 1987;317:70–75.
15. Hay I, Taylor WF, McConhey WM. A prognostic score for predicting outcome in papillary thyroid carcinoma. Endocrinology 1986;119(suppl):T15.
16. Hay ID, Bergstralh EJ, Goellner JR, et al. Predicting outcome in papillary thyroid carcinoma: development of a reliable prognostic scoring system in a cohort of 1779 patients surgically treated at one institution during 1940 through 1989. Surgery 1993;114:1050–1057.
17. Kim JH, Leeper RD. Treatment of anaplastic giant and spindle cell carcinoma of the thyroid gland with combination Adriamycin and radiation therapy: a new approach. Cancer 1983;52:954.
18. Nagataki S, Shibata Y, Iuoue S, Izumi, Shimacka K. Thyroid diseases among atomic bomb survivors in Nagasaki. JAMA 1994;272:364–370.
19. Rossi RL, Cady B, Meissner WA, Wool MS, Sedgwick CE, Werber J. Nonfamilial medullary thyroid carcinoma. Am J Surg 1980;139:554.
20. Rossi RL, Cady B, Silverman ML, Wool MS. Current results of conservative surgery for differentiated thyroid carcinoma. World J Surg 1986;10:612.
21. Rossi RL, Cady B, Silverman ML, Wool M. Surgically incurable well-differentiated thyroid carcinoma. Prognostic factors and results of therapy. Arch Surg 1988;123:569.
22. Rojas-Burke J. Scientists report surprised findings of thyroid cancer following chernobyl (new section) J Nuclear Med 1992;11:23_N–24_N;33_N–34_n.
23. Rougier P, Calmettes C, Laplanche A, Travagli JP, Lefevre M, Parmentier C, Milhaud G, Tubiana M. The value of calcitonin and carcinoembryonic antigen in the treatment and management of nonfamilial medullary thyroid carcinoma. Cancer 1983:51–855.
24. Shah JP, Loree TR, Dharker D, et al. Prognostic factors in differentiated carcinoma of the thyroid gland. Am J Surg 1992;164:658–661.
25. Tennvall J, Lundell G, Hallquist A, et al. Combined doxorubicin, hyperfractionated radiotherapy and surgery in anaplastic thyroid carcinoma. Report on two protocols. Cancer 1994;74:1348–1354.
26. Tisell LE, Hansson G, Jansson S, Salander H. Reoperation in the treatment of asymptomatic metastasizing medullary thyroid carcinoma. Surgery 1986;99:60–66.
27. Lips CJM, Landsvater RM, Höppener JWM, Geerdink RA, Blijham G, et al. Clinical screening as compared with DNA analysis in families with multiple endocrine neoplasia type 2A. N Engl J Med 1994;331:828–835.
28. Dadparvar S, Krishna L, Brady LW, Slizofski WJ, Brown SJ, Cheverest A, Micaily B. The role of iodine-131 and thallium-201 imaging and serum thyroglobulin in the management of differentiated thyroid carcinoma. Cancer 1994;71:3767–3773.
29. DeGroot LJ, Kaplan EL, McCormick M, Strauss FH. Natural history, treatment, and course of papillary thyroid carcinoma. J Clin Endocrinol Metab 1990;71:414–424.
30. Mazzaferri EL, Jhiang SM. Long term impact of initial surgical and medical therapy on papillary and follicular thyroid cancers. Am J Med 1994;97:418–428.
31. Samaan NA, Schultz PN, Hickey RC, Goepfert H, Johnston DA, Ordonez NG. The results of various modalities of treatment of well differentiated thyroid carcinoma: a retrospective review of 1599 patients. J Clin Endocrinol Metab 75:714–720.
32. Pineda JD, Lee T, Ain K, Renolds JC, Robbins J. Iodine-131 therapy for thyroid cancer patients with elevated thyroglobulin and negative diagnostic scan. J Clin Endocrinol Metab 1995;88:1488–1492.

CHAPTER 101

Neoplasms of the Adrenal Cortex

MARY R. FLACK AND GEORGE P. CHROUSOS

Historical Perspective

Eustachius first described the "suprarenal" glands in 1563. It was not until the 19th century, however, that Cuvier isolated the adrenal cortex from the medulla (1805) and Arnold defined the various histologic zones of the adrenal cortex (1866) (1). The importance of the adrenal cortex for sustaining life was suggested by Addison in 1855 (2) and confirmed the following year in animal studies by Brown-Séquard (3). In 1927, Hartman showed that purified adrenal cortical extract could be used to treat adrenal insufficiency. The active substances in these adrenal extracts would later be identified as cortisol, in 1949, and aldosterone, in 1952 (1).

Harvey Cushing first described the clinical syndrome associated with excess adrenal secretion in 1910. He attributed the syndrome to basophilic adenomas of the pituitary gland, but in 1934 Walters described this same syndrome in patients with adrenal tumors. In 1811, Rolleston noted the association of adrenal tumors with virilization, and in 1890 Thompson demonstrated decreased virilization in a woman following resection of an adrenal tumor (1). In 1952, Rapaport reported 188 cases of malignant adrenal tumors occurring between 1930 and 1949 associated with excess secretion of cortisol, androgens, and estrogens (4).

Natural History and Staging

The natural history of adrenal cancer is generally dismal. The survival of patients with untreated disease is usually less than 2 to 3 years after diagnosis (5–9). Macfarlane reported a mean survival time of only 2.9 months in 20 patients with surgically unresectable disease (9). Most patients have either locally invasive disease or distant metastases at the time of diagnosis (5–12). Even with surgical and medical treatment the prognosis is generally poor, with a mean survival time of approximately 4 years (5, 13–15). It should be noted, however, that younger patients with stage I or II disease have a better prognosis after complete surgical resection, and there are anecdotal reports of patients with adrenocortical carcinoma living up to 20 years after diagnosis (16). Children, particularly those under the age of 2 years, also have an improved survival, up to 82%, after complete resection (17).

The staging system for adrenal cancer (Table 101.1) depends on tumor size, nodal involvement, invasion of adjacent organs, and distant metastases (8, 9, 18). Stage I disease is defined as a tumor less than 5 cm in diameter that is confined to the adrenal gland. Stage I adrenal cancer is rare, accounting for 5% or less of adrenal cancers (8), and can be difficult to distinguish from a benign adrenal adenoma (16, 19). When it occurs and there is complete resection, the prognosis is relatively good, and long-term remissions have been reported (9, 18, 20–22). Because of the difficulty of distinguishing adenomas from carcinomas on the basis of pathologic criteria alone, however, some tumors classified as stage I carcinomas may actually be adrenal adenomas, which have an excellent prognosis after resection.

Stage II disease is defined as a tumor greater than 5 cm in diameter that is confined to the adrenal gland. Most patients with stage II disease will eventually have recurrent or metastatic disease, half of them within 2 years of tumor resection (5). The likelihood of metastases is higher in patients with larger tumors, pathologic evidence of necrosis, vascular invasion, and increased mitotic activity. There is no single pathologic criterion, however, that accurately predicts recurrence in a given patient, except unambiguous lymphatic or blood vessel invasion (9, 16, 19). The overall 5-year survival rate for patients with stage II disease is 30 to 40% when all visible tumor is resected. There have been reports, however, of patients living 10 years or more after a complete resection (12, 18, 20–24).

Seventy percent or more of patients with adrenal cancer have either stage III or IV disease at the time of diagnosis (5–12). Stage III disease is defined as a tumor greater than 5 cm in diameter that is confined to the adrenal gland with involvement of adjacent nodes, or as locally invasive disease without spread to adjacent organs. Despite complete resection, virtually 100% of patients with stage III disease have recurrent or metastatic disease within 5 years of tumor resection (4, 5, 10, 18). Tumor necrosis, vascular invasion, nuclear mitoses, pleomorphism, and involvement of the zona reticularis have been reported to be poor prognostic signs. The overall 5-year survival rate for patients with stage III adrenal cancer is generally less than 30% (5–7, 15, 22).

Stage IV disease is defined as a tumor greater than 5 cm in diameter with invasion of adjacent organs and/or distant metastases. Adrenal cancer can spread directly to adjacent organs, including the kidney, mesentery, posterior abdominal wall, pancreas, diaphragm, renal vein, and inferior vena cava (9, 12, 21). Adrenal cancer can spread via the lymphatics to regional and para-aortic lymph nodes, but more commonly it spreads by the hematogenous route to distant

Table 101.1. Staging of Adrenocortical Carcinoma

Stage	T, N, M	Description
I	T1, N0, M0	Tumor < 5 cm, confined to the adrenal gland
II	T2, N0, M0	Tumor > 5 cm, confined to the adrenal gland
III	T1 or T2, N1, M0	Tumor confined to the adrenal gland with involvement of local nodes or
	T3, N0, M0	Tumor extending beyond adrenal gland, but not invading adjacent organs
IV	T3 or T4, N1, M0; any T, M1	Tumor extending beyond adrenal, plus invasion of adjacent organs or local node involvement; or any tumor with metastases

Adapted from Macfarlane (9).

organs. The most frequent sites of metastasis are the lymph nodes (25–46%), lung (47–97%), liver (53–68%), abdomen (33–43%), and bone (11–33%). Metastases have been reported in the ovary, spleen, thyroid, pharyngeal tonsils, pleura, mediastinum, pericardium, myocardium, brain, spinal cord, skin, and subcutaneous tissues (5, 9, 13, 25–29). The survival for patients with stage IV disease is extremely poor. The 5-year survival rate is generally less than 15% if not all of the tumor can be resected (4–6, 8, 9, 17, 30). Luton and colleagues reported a mean 5-year survival rate of 22% in their patients with metastatic disease despite medical and surgical therapy; it was 25% for patients under age 40 and 15% for patients over age 40 (15).

Epidemiology

Adrenal carcinoma accounts for 0.05 to 0.2% of all cancers, with an annual incidence of two per million. A bimodal age distribution has been reported, with one peak occurring before age 5 years and the second occurring in the fourth to fifth decades. Adrenal cancer, however, occurs at all ages from several months to the seventh and eighth decades (4, 6, 9, 13, 24). In large cancer registries, there is a slight male predominance (30–32), while in large clinical series there is a female predominance (4, 13, 24). This is most likely due to the fact that secretory tumors, which are highly represented in clinical series, are diagnosed more commonly in women, while most adrenal cancers in men appear to be nonsecretory (9).

Pathogenesis

There are no known causative agents for adrenocortical carcinoma. There does not appear to be a strong association between chronic adrenal hyperplasia and the development of adrenal cancer, although cases of malignant transformation have been described. The majority of adrenal cancers occur sporadically, but occasionally they occur in familial cancer syndromes such as the Li-Fraumeni hereditary cancer syndrome (breast cancer, soft tissue sarcomas, gliomas), primary pigmented nodular adrenocortical disease (PPNAD) or the Carney complex (PPNAD, atrial myxomas, skin and mucosal schwannomas, spotty pigmentation of the skin and mucosae), familial adenomatous polyposis (FAP), and in patients with the Beckwith-Wiedemann syndrome (33–37).

Germ-line mutations of the p53 gene have been described in the Li-Fraumeni syndrome (38). Somatic mutations of this gene were also recently described in 25 to 30% of sporadic adrenocortical carcinomas examined, and in both of the two existing adrenocortical carcinoma cell lines (39). Also, overexpression of the IGF-2 gene has been shown in adrenocortical tumors. A recent study identified loss of heterozygosity in the region near the gene for adenomatous polyposis coli in a patient with FAP and adrenal cancer (40). In one study, a small percentage of sporadic adrenocortical carcinomas had mutations of the inhibitory G protein leading to constitutive activation of adenyl cyclase (41). This was not found in a second study of G-protein gene structure in patients with adrenal carcinoma (42). Interestingly, no activating mutations of the adrenocorticotropic hormone (ACTH) receptor were shown in a large series of malignant and benign adrenocortical neoplasms recently studied (43).

Clonality studies have shown that adrenocortical carcinomas are of monoclonal origin (44). Cytogenetic studies of adrenocortical tumors have shown abnormalities in chromosomes 17 and 11. The former are deletions possibly causing loss of heterozygosity of the p53 gene; the latter may represent amplification of the IGF-2 gene or may be related to changes in the gene for multiple endocrine neoplasia type. Overexpression of the IGF-2 gene has been suggested as the mechanism of adrenal and other tumorigenesis in the Beckwith-Wiedemann syndrome.

Diagnosis

Despite the frequent association of adrenocortical carcinoma with endocrine hypersecretion, nearly half the patients with adrenal cancer have no recognizable endocrine syndrome (5, 6, 9). These patients present either with abdominal pain or fullness or with the incidental finding of an adrenal mass on radiologic studies done for other reasons (8, 45, 46). Rarely, patients with adrenal cancer present with anorexia, weight loss, or fever of unknown origin, all of which are poor prognostic signs (5, 45, 46). Although these patients have no identifiable endocrine syndrome, there may be elevation in levels of urine or plasma steroids in 10 to 20% (12, 15, 18, 47).

Over 50% of patients with adrenal cancer have an associated endocrine syndrome such as Cushing's syndrome, virilization, Cushing's syndrome plus virilization, feminization, or hyperaldosteronism. These syndromes result from the secretion of cortisol and its precursors, adrenal androgens and their precursors, or, rarely, estrogen and aldosterone. Adrenal cancers are inefficient in their production of steroids. This results in the secretion of large amounts of

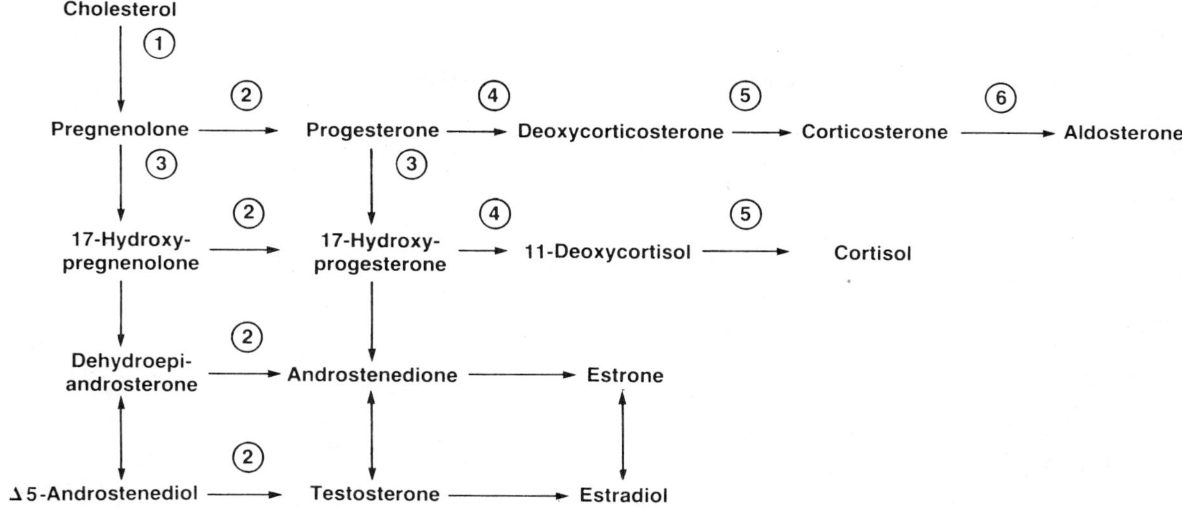

Figure 101.1. Biosynthetic pathway for production of steroids in adrenal cortex.

steroid precursors relative to the amount of end product (48). Furthermore, the amount of steroid produced is often lower than expected for the large size of these tumors. Recently, it has been shown that the amount and activity of the synthetic enzymes 3β-hydroxysteroid dehydrogenase and 21-hydroxylase are low in adrenal cancers, while the amount and activity of 17α-hydroxylase are relatively preserved (49). This leads to the disproportionate secretion of androgenic precursors compared to other steroids. Thus, the finding of high levels of androgenic precursors in relation to other steroid precursors is suggestive for adrenocortical carcinoma (Fig. 101.1).

A specific diagnosis of adrenal cancer depends on the identification of an adrenal mass on computed tomography (CT) or magnetic resonance imaging (MRI). The CT finding of a large unilateral adrenal mass with irregular borders is virtually diagnostic of adrenal cancer. If a smaller mass is present, it is more difficult to distinguish an adrenal cancer from an adrenal adenoma (see Differential Diagnosis below). On MRI, malignant adrenal lesions have an intermediate to high signal intensity on T2-weighted images, while nonfunctional adenomas have a low signal intensity and pheochromocytomas have an extremely high signal intensity (Fig. 101.2 (50, 51). In addition, MRI may be useful in detailing vena caval involvement prior to surgical resection (52). Iodocholesterol scanning shows poor adrenal uptake in adrenal cancer compared with the enhanced uptake that may be seen in adrenal adenomas or hyperplasia. This study is rarely indicated, however, given the accuracy of CT and MRI. Occasionally, angiography may be required to determine the site of tumor origin and for vascular mapping prior to surgery (53).

The most common syndrome associated with adrenal cancer is Cushing's syndrome, caused by the excess secretion of cortisol and its precursors. It accounts for 30 to 40% of patients with a clinical syndrome (13, 22, 28). Some of the typical signs and symptoms of Cushing's syndrome (Table 101.2) may be more subtle in patients with adrenal cancer, because of the inefficient steroidogenesis by many of these neoplasms. In women, hirsutism and amenorrhea may be seen more frequently than with benign adrenal conditions due to the propensity for these tumors to secrete androgenic steroid precursors. Children rarely present with the classic clinical features of Cushing's syndrome; growth retardation and a weight gain that is inappropriate for their height are more common (26, 48, 54).

Virilization is seen in 20 to 30% of those patients with an endocrine syndrome (4, 8, 13, 24). Virilization is rarely due to the secretion of testosterone itself but is primarily associated with secretion of androgenic steroid precursors such as androstenedione, dehydroepiandrosterone (DHEA), and 17-hydroxyprogesterone (13, 24). The signs and symptoms of excess androgen secretion in females include increased libido, excessive muscle mass, temporal balding, clitoromegaly, and heterosexual precocious puberty in girls. In males, the clinical manifestations of excess androgen secretion are obscured, except for isosexual precocious puberty in boys (Table 101.2).

The combination of Cushing's syndrome and virilization occurs in 10 to 30% of those patients with an endocrine syndrome (4, 13, 24). This combined syndrome is associated with the secretion of multiple steroids and their precursors, including cortisol, androstenedione, 17-hydroxyprogesterone and DHEA. The diagnosis can only be made in women when clitoromegaly, temporal balding, or increased muscle mass are present, because amenorrhea and hirsutism can be seen in Cushing's syndrome alone.

Feminization occurs in 5 to 10% of men with adrenal cancer (8, 13, 24, 55, 56) and manifests as decreased libido, impotence, gynecomastia, and testicular atrophy. Persistent questioning and careful examination may be required to elicit these findings, but they may be the only key to an early diagnosis in males, who generally have more clinically silent tumors.

Pure hyperaldosteronism is rare in adrenal cancer and accounts for 5% or less of patients with an endocrine syndrome

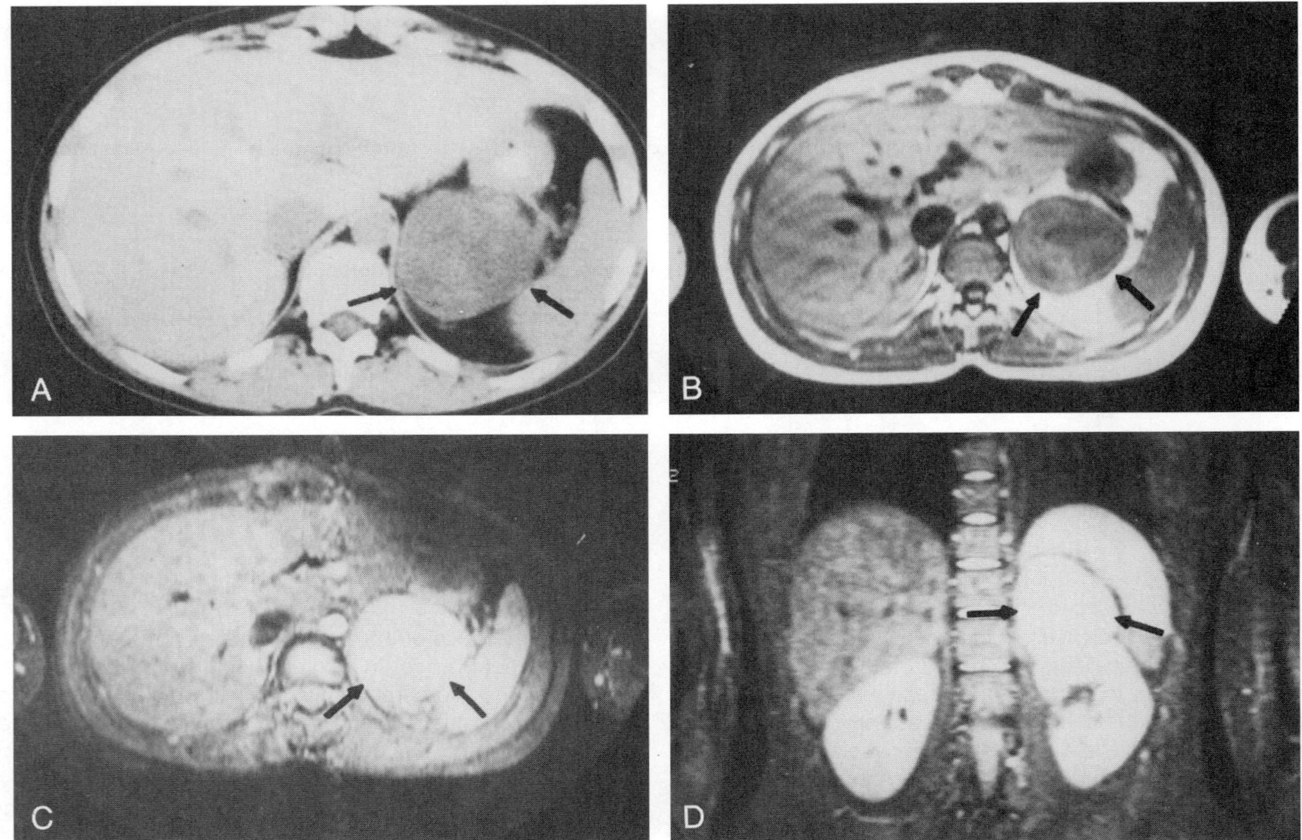

Figure 101.2. Adrenocortical carcinoma shown by computed tomography (**A**), T1-weighted MRI (TR 300 ms TE 26 ms) showing signal intensity equal to liver tissue (**B**), T2-weighted MRI (TR 1500 ms T1 100 ms) showing high signal intensity compared with liver (**C**), and T2-weighted MRI (TR 1510 ms T1 100 ms) showing mass in relation to upper pole of kidney (**D**). (Courtesy of J. Doppman.)

Table 101.2. Clinical and Laboratory Findings in Patients with Secretory Adrenal Cancers

Endocrine syndrome (%)	Clinical findings	Laboratory studies
Cushing's (30%)	Weight gain (truncal, dorsocervical, and supraclavicular); moon facies, plethora, hypertension, striae, hirsutism, peripheral wasting and weakness, glucose intolerance, amenorrhea, acne, mental changes, osteoporosis, edema, hypokalemia (54)	*Urine:* 17-ketosteroids = 30–200 mg/d (>100 μmol/d) 17-hydroxysteroids > 15 mg/g creatinine (>30 μmol/d) Free cortisol (UFC) > 200 μg/d (>400 nmol/d) Increased tetrahydro-compound S *Plasma:* ACTH suppressed < 11 pg/mL (<3 pmol/L) by RIA or < 5 pg/mL (<1.2 pmol/L) by IRMA DHEA-S > 3,500 ng/ml (>10 mmol/L)
Virilization (20%)	Temporal balding, increased muscle mass, clitoromegaly, deepening of the voice in women; heterosexual precocious puberty in girls; isosexual precocious puberty in boys	*Urine:* 17-ketosteroids = 30–200 mg/24 h (>100 μmol/d) Increased urinary pregnenolone *Plasma (females):* Testosterone > 200 ng/dL (>4 nmol/L) Androstenedione > 3.5 μg/L (>12 nmol/L)
Cushing's and virilization (30%)	Combination of above. The finding of virilization or precocious puberty in the setting of Cushing's syndrome is highly suggestive of adrenal carcinoma	Combination of above
Feminization (15%)	Impotence, loss of libido, testicular atrophy, fatigue, inability to concentrate in men	*Plasma (males):* Estrone > 100 pg/ml (>300 pmol/L) Estradiol > 50 pg/ml (>180 pmol/L)
Hyperaldosteronism (5%)	Hypertension, hypokalemia, metabolic alkalosis	*Plasma (normal salt intake):* Aldosterone > 30 ng/dL (>800 pmol/L)

(10, 13, 20, 24, 57, 58). When it does occur, it presents with hypertension, hypokalemia, and a metabolic alkalosis. Hypertension and hypokalemia, however, can occur with other syndromes in adrenal cancer owing to the excess secretion of mineralocorticoid precursors, such as 11-deoxycorticosterone and corticosterone. Even more unusual presentations of adrenal cancer that have been reported include hypoglycemia, insulin resistance, and polycythemia (59).

Several laboratory studies are useful in confirming excessive steroid secretion in patients with suspected adrenal cancer. Hypercortisolism is most often confirmed by measuring the urine free cortisol (UFC) or 17-hydroxysteroids in an aliquot from a 24-hour urine collection. Over 90% of patients with Cushing's syndrome have UFC values greater than 200 μg/24 h, while 97% of normal individuals have UFC values less than 100 μg/24 h. Values between 100 and 200 μg/24 h can be seen in patients with obesity, depression, stress, or alcoholism. In patients with ambiguous UFC results, an overnight dexamethasone suppression test may be helpful. This test involves the oral administration of 1 mg of dexamethasone at midnight and measurement of plasma cortisol levels the following morning at 8 A.M. Normal individuals have cortisol values less than 5 μg/dL following dexamethasone administration, while patients with Cushing's syndrome generally have values greater than 5 μg/dL (26).

Additionally, an aliquot from a 24-hour urine collection can be sent for measurement of 17-hydroxysteroids, 17-ketosteroids, and creatinine levels. Sixty percent of patients with adrenal cancer have elevated 17-hydroxysteroid excretion and over 70% of patients have elevated 17-ketosteroid excretion. Fifty percent of patients with adrenal cancer have increased levels of both 17-hydroxysteroids and 17-ketosteroids. Extreme elevations in urinary 17-ketosteroids are often seen in patients with adrenal cancer (up to 200 mg/dL). An unusually high level of urinary ketosteroids in a patient with hypercortisolism may be a clue to the presence of malignant adrenal disease, as opposed to a benign adrenal process (12, 13, 24, 29, 48, 54, 60, 61).

There are several other tests for the differential diagnosis of Cushing's syndrome once hypercortisolism has been established. A plasma ACTH level determined using a reliable radioimmunoassay (usually a two-site or "sandwich" assay) can distinguish patients with ACTH-dependent Cushing's syndrome (pituitary tumors or ectopic ACTH secretion) from those with ACTH-independent Cushing's syndrome (adrenal tumors or micronodular adrenal disease). Patients with pituitary disease or ectopic ACTH secretion have normal or elevated ACTH levels, while patients with primary adrenal disease, including adrenal carcinoma, generally have suppressed ACTH levels (26, 48, 54). An undetectable ACTH level with the appropriate findings of a large irregular adrenal mass on CT is virtually diagnostic of adrenocortical carcinoma.

The classic test for Cushing's syndrome is the high-dose dexamethasone suppression test. This test involves obtaining 24-hour urine collections for 6 consecutive days. Following 2 baseline days, dexamethasone is given orally: 0.5 mg every 6 hours for 48 hours, then 2.0 mg every 6 hours for 48 hours. Traditionally, a decline in 17-hydroxysteroid excretion to less than 50% of basal values indicates pituitary disease, while lack of suppression indicates primary adrenal diseases, such as adrenocortical carcinoma (26, 54). Updated criteria for this test require 64% suppression of 17-hydroxysteroids or 90% suppression of UFC (62). The high-dose dexamethasone test and other tests recommended for the differential diagnosis of Cushing's syndrome, such as ovine corticotropin-releasing hormone (CRH) stimulation and inferior petrosal sinus sampling, are not essential in the diagnosis of adrenal cancer, however, if the imaging studies are diagnostic and the ACTH level is suppressed.

Several other plasma and urinary steroids are elevated in patients with adrenal cancer. They include DHEA and its sulfated derivative (DHEA-S), pregnenolone, 17-hydroxypregnenolone and 11-deoxycortisol in the plasma, and the tetrahydro conjugate of 11-deoxycortisol (tetrahydro-compound S) in the urine (Fig. 101.1) (24, 29, 61). While these are generally not essential in the workup of hypercortisolism, they may occasionally be a clue to the presence of adrenal malignancy in a patient with Cushing's syndrome.

The clinical diagnosis of virilization can be confirmed by measurement of plasma androstenedione, testosterone, sex hormone–binding globulin, and urinary 17-ketosteroids. Plasma levels of DHEA and DHEA-S are elevated in the majority of patients with adrenal cancer, whether or not they have the clinical manifestations of virilization or Cushing's syndrome (24, 29, 60, 61). In contrast, patients with secretory adrenal adenomas have suppressed DHEA-S levels (see "Differential Diagnosis").

The clinical diagnosis of feminization can be confirmed by measurement of elevated plasma estradiol or estrone levels. Hyperaldosteronism can be confirmed by measurement of elevated plasma and urinary aldosterone levels. Although usually not needed clinically, plasma levels of corticosterone and deoxycorticosterone are frequently elevated in patients with adrenal cancer and the clinical appearance of hyperaldosteronism (57, 58).

Differential Diagnosis

"INCIDENTALOMAS"

There is a 0.5 to 1.0% incidence of unexpected adrenal lesions found on CT or MRI of the upper abdomen in patients older than age 40. These lesions can represent benign adrenal adenomas, adrenal carcinomas, metastases from an unknown primary cancer, cysts, or, rarely, myelolipomas (51, 63, 64). The incidental finding of these lesions has led to the diagnostic problem of distinguishing benign lesions from early adrenal cancer. With the increasing resolution of CT and MRI, adrenal cancers as small as 3.5 cm have been identified. Resection of these small lesions will no doubt have a better prognosis, so the question of the malignant potential of these incidentally discovered lesions is important. Copeland has suggested that lesions greater than 6 cm should be considered to have high malignant potential (64). Belldegrun and colleagues also found that most malignant lesions were greater than 6 cm in diameter, while nearly all lesions less than 6 cm were benign. However, they recommended that, because of the rare finding of small adrenal cancers, all lesions greater than 3 cm should be removed if there is no contraindication to surgery (63).

The issue of how to proceed when an incidentaloma is discovered is controversial. The consensus of most studies is that patients found to have an incidental adrenal lesion should undergo a preliminary screen for endocrine hypersecretion, including a complete history and physical examination and, if warranted based on the history and physical, a 24-hour urine assay for free cortisol, 17-hydroxysteroids, 17-ketosteroids, and creatinine. If flushing or hypertension are present, urine metanephrines and catecholamines should also be included. If signs and symptoms of virilization, feminization, or hyperaldosteronism are present, plasma levels of testosterone, estradiol, or aldosterone, respectively, can be obtained. If there is biochemical evidence of endocrine hypersecretion, the lesion should be resected.

If no endocrine hypersecretion is found, some would recommend MRI of the adrenals (50, 51). In general, nonfunctioning adenomas have a low signal intensity on T2-weighted MRI, carcinomas and adrenal metastases have an intermediate to high signal intensity, and pheochromocytomas have an extremely high signal intensity. Identification of a pheochromocytoma on MRI would be extremely important if manipulations such as fine-needle biopsy were being considered. The absence of hypertension or the lack of elevated levels of urine metanephrines does not rule out a pheochromocytoma in all cases. If the lesion is of intermediate to high signal intensity on T2-weighted MRI, it could still represent an adrenal metastasis from an unknown primary cancer. A reasonable effort should be made to exclude common adenocarcinomas (i.e., those of the breast, lung, and gastrointestinal tract).

If no endocrine syndrome or occult primary cancer is found and the lesion is less than 3 cm in diameter, the patient can be reassured with perhaps one follow-up CT scan. If the lesion is 3 to 6 cm, there are several reasonable courses of action. If the CT appearance of the lesion is suggestive of a cyst, fine-needle aspiration can be done with careful follow-up. If the patient is elderly or there are contraindications to surgery, observation and careful follow-up are reasonable. In these cases, periodic assessment of the secretory status and the size of the mass should be performed, since many tumors become secretory long before they lead to a clearly recognizable endocrine syndrome. If the patient is young and there are no contraindications, surgical resection should be undertaken for lesions greater than 5 to 6 cm or lesions greater than 3 to 4 cm that have suspicious features such as intermediate to high signal intensity on T2-weighted MRI, irregular borders or patchy contrast uptake on CT, or failure to take up iodocholesterol (50, 51, 63, 64).

ADRENAL ADENOMA

In general, adrenal adenomas are highly efficient steroid secretors and tend to produce a single end product, such as cortisol, testosterone, or aldosterone, rather than multiple steroid precursors as in adrenal carcinoma (24, 45, 48). A small lesion on CT that avidly takes up iodocholesterol in the setting of high levels of steroid secretion is highly suggestive of an adrenal adenoma. Following resection of an adrenal tumor, it may still be difficult to distinguish benign from malignant lesions using pathologic criteria. Hough and colleagues have suggested that the presence of a diffuse growth pattern, broad fibrous bands, tumor necrosis, frequent mitoses, or vascular invasion is highly correlated with malignancy (19). Others have emphasized the correlation between the size and weight of the lesion and the potential for malignancy (9, 16, 65–67). However, there is no single criterion that distinguishes a malignant from a benign lesion in a given patient other than local invasion or metastatic disease. Thus, lesions that have a number of suspicious features on pathologic examination should be followed up every 3 months initially to search for evidence of recurrence.

Therapy

Surgical resection is the only therapy that has been demonstrated to prolong survival in adrenal cancer (9, 17, 18, 22, 68, 69). Stage I and stage II disease should be treated by complete resection and careful follow-up (every 3 months initially, then every 6–12 months). Stage III disease should be treated by resection of all visible tumor and careful follow-up. Early recognition of recurrent or metastatic disease is important, since resection of isolated metastatic lesions has prolonged survival in some patients (22, 68). Stage IV disease should be treated by removal of as much tumor as possible, including resection of isolated metastases. Some centers recommend adjuvant medical treatment with ortho-para′-DDD (mitotane [Cytadren]) following complete resection of stage III and IV disease to increase the duration between recurrences (7, 15, 69–71), although this has not been tested in a randomized, placebo-controlled study. A recent study of 53 patients, 10 of whom received mitotane after surgical resection, showed no effect on either the recurrence rate or the length of the disease-free interval (72).

Medical therapy is generally recommended when all the tumor cannot be removed. While partial responses have been reported with medical therapy, it is generally ineffective in prolonging overall survival in adrenal cancer. Mitotane given orally in high doses (up to 15 g/d) causes remission of hypercortisolism in 50 to 60% of patients with adrenal cancer and Cushing's syndrome (14). Tumor responses, however, occur much less frequently. Initially, a 20 to 40% partial tumor response rate was reported with mitotane treatment, and there were several anecdotal reports of complete tumor responses (14, 23, 27, 69–71). Subsequent studies, however, involving large numbers of patients and more objective criteria for response indicated a partial response rate of less than 20% (15, 67). These responses are short-lived, lasting 6–10 months. Two recent studies, however, suggested that mitotane given after disease recurrence may have a beneficial effect on survival independent of surgical resection, but only when serum levels greater than 14 mg/mL were achieved (8, 72). Prolonged high-dose administration of mitotane causes adrenal insufficiency that may require temporary or even permanent replacement therapy with hydrocortisone and fludrocortisone (Florinef). Unfortunately, high-dose mitotane can also cause nausea, vomiting, anorexia, blood dyscrasias, lethargy, fatigue, dizziness, and other disturbing CNS effects.

Various conventional chemotherapeutic regimens have been used for the treatment of metastatic adrenal cancer. These have included agents such as cisplatin, etoposide, 5-fluorouracil, doxorubicin, and melphalan. In general, the response rates are less than 20% and are short-lived (73–78). Radiation therapy can be used in combination with chemotherapy for palliation, particularly with bone metastases (79).

In addition to mitotane, there are a number of other agents that can be used to treat hypercortisolism, including metyrapone (250 mg QID), aminoglutethimide (250 mg QID), and ketoconazole (10 mg/kg/d). In some patients, particularly with mitotane treatment, hydrocortisone (15 mg/m^2/d) or Florinef (100–400 μg/d) may be required to prevent adrenal insufficiency. Mineralocorticoid antagonists, such as spironolactone, or androgen antagonists, such as flutamide, may aid in controlling the signs and symptoms of mineralocorticoid or androgen excess (26, 53).

Perspectives

We need to continue our studies on the mechanisms of adrenal tumorigenesis. Receptors for agents that stimulate adrenocortical function, such as those for gastric inhibitory peptide, adenosine, α-MSH, and angiotensin II, should be examined for the presence of activating mutations. Major oncogenes and tumor suppressor genes should also be studied, starting with candidate genes of known importance for adrenal growth and function. Such an approach may illuminate the paths that lead to adrenocortical oncogenesis and suggest rational approaches for therapy.

One of the major problems with chemotherapy for adrenal cancer is the development of drug resistance. A surface glycoprotein (p-glycoprotein or MDR-glycoprotein) has been identified that may shuttle chemotherapeutic agents out of tumor cells. This protein is expressed at high levels in normal adrenals and in adrenal cancers (80–83). It may contribute to the development of resistance to drugs that are transported by this glycoprotein. Agents such as verapamil and amiodarone, and particularly mitotane, competitively inhibit this glycoprotein and may prolong the action of the other chemotherapeutic agents. There are anecdotal reports of increased tumor responses with a combination of mitotane and chemotherapy (73).

Experimental therapies such as suramin, a reverse transcriptase inhibitor, and gossypol, a plant toxin, are currently being tested. Suramin produced remissions in four of 16 patients with adrenal cancer in the United States and three of nine patients in Germany (84, 85). Suramin therapy was associated with considerable toxicity, however, including allergic skin reactions, coagulopathy, thrombocytopenia, and polyneuropathy. Gossypol produced partial remissions in three of 21 patients with adrenal cancer unresponsive to other therapies but was considerably less toxic than the other chemotherapeutic agents tested. (86).

References

1. Medvei VC. A History of Endocrinology. Hingham, MA: MTP Press, 1982.
2. Addison T. On the Constitutional and Local Effects of Disease of the Suprarenal Capsules. London: S Highley, 1855.
3. Brown-Séquard CE. Recherches experimentales sur la physiologie et la pathologie des capsules surrenales. C R Acad Sci Paris l856;43:422–425.
4. Rapaport E, Goldberg MB, Gordan, GS, Hinman F. Mortality in surgically treated adrenocortical tumors. Postgrad Med 1952;11:325.
5. Cohn D, Gottesman L, Brennan M. Adrenocortical carcinoma. Surgery 1986;100: 1170–1177.
6. Samaan NA, Hickey RC. Adrenal cortical carcinoma. Semin Oncol 1987;14:292–296.
7. Thompson NW, Cheung PS. Diagnosis and treatment of functioning and nonfunctioning adrenocortical neoplasms including incidentalomas. Surg Clin North Am l987;67: 423–436.
8. Icard P, Louvel A, Chapuis Y. Survival rates and prognostic factors in adrenocortical carcinoma. World J Surg 1992;16:753–758.
9. Macfarlane DA. Cancer of the adrenal cortex: the natural history, prognosis and treatment in a study of fifty-five cases. Ann R Coll Surg Engl 1958;23:155–186.
10. Brennan MF. Adrenocortical carcinoma. CA 1987;37:348–365.
11. Van Slooten H, Moolenaar AJ, Van Seters AP, Smeenk D. The treatment of adrenocortical carcinoma with *o,p'*-DDD: prognostic implications of serum level monitoring. Eur J Cancer Clin Oncol 1984;20:47–53.
12. Didolkar MS, Bescher RA, Elias EG, Moore RH. Natural history of adrenal cortical carcinoma: a clinicopathologic study of 42 patients. Cancer 1981;47:2153–2161.
13. Hutter AM, Kayhoe DE. Adrenal cortical carcinoma: clinical features of 138 patients. Am J Med 1966;41:572–580.
14. Hutter AM, Kayhoe DE. Adrenal cortical carcinoma; results of treatment with *o,p'*-DDD in 138 patients. Am J Med 1966;41:581–592.
15. Luton JP, Cerdas S, Billaud L, et al. Clinical features of adrenocortical carcinoma, prognostic factors, and the effect of mitotane therapy. N Engl J Med 1990;322: 1195–1201.
16. Van Slooten H, Schaberg A, Smeenk K, Moolenaar AJ. Morphologic characteristics of benign and malignant adrenocortical tumors. Cancer 1985;55:766–773.
17. Sabbaga CC, Avilla SG, Schulz C, Garbers JC, Blucher D. Adrenocortical carcinoma in children: clinical aspects and prognosis. J Pediatr Surg 1993;28:841–843.
18. Sullivan M, Boileau M, Hodges CV. Adrenal cortical carcinoma. J Urol 1978;120: 660–665.
19. Hough AJ, Hollifield JW, Page DL, Hartmann WH. Prognostic factors in adrenal cortical tumors. Am J Clin Pathol 1979;72:390–399.
20. Bertagna C, Orth DN. Clinical and laboratory findings and results of therapy in 58 patients with adrenocortical tumors admitted to a single medical center (1951 to 1978). Am J Med 1981;71:855–875.
21. Hajjar RA, Hickey RC, Samaan NA. Adrenal cortical carcinoma: a study of 32 patients. Cancer 1975;35:549–556.
22. Icard P, Chapuis Y, Andreassian B, Bernard A Proye C. Adrenocortical carcinoma in surgically treated patients: a retrospective study on 156 cases by the French Association of Endocrine Surgery. Surgery 1992;112:972–979.
23. Boven E, Vermorken JB, van Slooten H, Pinedo HM. Complete response of metastasized adrenal cortical carcinoma with *o,p'*-DDD. Cancer 1984;53:26–29.
24. Lipsett MB, Hertz R, Ross GT. Clinical and pathophysiologic aspects of adrenocortical carcinoma. Am J Med 1963;35:374–383.
25. Kelly WF, Barnes AJ, Cassar J, et al. Cushing's syndrome due to adrenocortical carcinoma: a comprehensive clinical and biochemical study of patients treated by surgery and chemotherapy. Acta Endocrinol 1979;91:303–318.
26. Loriaux DL, Cutler GB. Diseases of the adrenal glands. In Clinical Endocrinology. Edited by PO Kohler. New York: Wiley, 1986, pp 167–238.
27. Nakata A, Yagi S, Oyama K, Kida H, Sugioka G. Adrenocortical carcinoma with a giant pericardial mass. Intern Med 1993;32:438–440.
28. Lipsett MB, Wilson H. Adrenocortical cancer: steroid biosynthesis and metabolism evaluated by urinary metabolites. J Clin Endocrinol Metab 1962;22:906–915.
29. Lubitz JA. Mitotane use in inoperable adrenal cortical carcinoma. JAMA 1973;223: 1109–1112.
30. Clemmesen J. Statistical studies in the aetiology of malignant neoplasms. Munksgaard, Copenhagen: Danish Cancer Registry, National Anti-Cancer League, 1965.
31. Ferber B, Hardy VH, Gerhardt PR. Cancer in New York State, exclusive of New York City, 1941–l960. Albany: Bureau of Cancer Control, New York State Department of Health, 1962.
32. Griswold MH, Wilder CS, Cutler SJ, Pollack ES. Cancer in Connecticut, 1935–1951. Hartford: Connecticut State Department of Health, 1955.
33. Li FP, Fraumeni JF. Soft-tissue sarcomas, breast cancer, and other neoplasms: a family syndrome? Ann Intern Med 1969;71:747–752.
34. Li FP, Fraumeni JF. Prospective study of a family cancer syndrome. JAMA 1982;247: 2692–2694.
35. Lynch HT, Mulcahy GM, Harris RE, et al. Genetic and pathologic findings in a kindred with hereditary sarcoma, breast cancer, brain tumors, leukemia, lung, laryngeal, and adrenal cortical carcinoma. Cancer 1978;14:2055–2064.
36. Lynch HT, Katz DA, Bogard PJ, Lynch JF. The sarcoma, breast cancer, lung cancer, and adrenocortical carcinoma syndrome revisited. Am J Dis Child 1985;139:134–136.
37. Tsukamoto T, Kumamoto Y, Takahashi A, et al. Adrenocortical carcinoma in a child with specific pedigree of family associated with cancer aggregation. J Urol 1992;147: 104–106.
38. Sameshima Y, Tsunematsu Y, Watanabe S, et al. Detection of novel germ-line p53 mutations in diverse cancer-prone families identified by selecting patients with childhood adrenocortical carcinoma. JNCI 1992;84:703–707.
39. Reincke M, Karl M, Travis WH, et al. p53 mutations in human adrenocortical neoplasms: immunohistochemical and molecular studies. J Clin Endocrinol Metab 1994;78:790–794.
40. Seki M, Tanaka K, Kikuchi YR, et al. Loss of normal allele of the APC gene in an adrenocortical carcinoma from a patient with familial adenomatous polyposis. Hum Genet 1992;89:298–300.
41. Lyons J, Landis C, Harsh G, et al. Two G protein oncogenes in human endocrine tumors. Science 1990;249:655–658.

42. Reinke M, Karl M, Travis W, Chrousos GP. No evidence for oncogenic mutations in quanine nucleotide-binding proteins of human adrenocortical neoplasms. J Clin Endocrinol Metab 1993;77:1419–1422.
43. Latronico AC, Reincke M, Mendonca BB, et al. No evidence for oncogenic mutations in the adrenocorticotropin receptor (ACTH-R) gene in human adrenocortical neoplasms. J Clin Endocrinol Metab 1995. (in press)
44. Yano T, Linehan M, Angland P, et al. Genetic changes in human adrenocortical carcinoma. JNCI 1989;81:518–523.
45. Heinbecker P, O'Neal LW, Ackerman LV. Functional and nonfunctioning adrenal cortical tumors. Surg Gynecol Obstet 1957;105:21–30.
46. Lewinsky BS, Grigor KM, Symington T, Neville AM. The clinical and pathologic features of "non-hormonal" adrenocortical tumors. Cancer 1974;33:778–790.
47. Fukushima DK, Gallagher TF. Steroid production in "nonfunctioning" adrenal cortical tumor. J Clin Endocrinol Metab 1963;23:923–927.
48. Chrousos GP. Endocrine tumors. In Principles and Practice of Pediatric Oncology. Edited by PA Pizzo, DG Poplack. Philadelphia: Lippincott, 1988, pp 733–755.
49. Sakai Y, Yanase T, Hara T, et al. Mechanism of abnormal production of adrenal androgen in patients with adrenocortical adenomas and carcinomas. J Clin Endocrinol Metab 1994;78:36–40.
50. Doppman JL, Reinig JW, Dwyer AJ, Frank JP, Norton J, Loriaux DL, Kaiser H. Differentiation of adrenal masses by magnetic resonance imaging. Surgery 1987;102: 1018–1026.
51. Reinig JW, Doppman JL, Dwyer AJ, Frank J. MRI of indeterminate adrenal masses. AJR 1986;147:493–496.
52. Seigelbaum MH, Moulsdale JE, Murphy JB, McDonald GR. Use of magnetic resonance imaging scanning in adrenocortical carcinoma with vena caval involvement. Urology 1994;43:869–873.
53. Kolmannskog F, Kolbenstvedt A, Brekke IB. CT and angiography in adrenocortical carcinoma. Acta Radiology 1992;33:45–49.
54. Kamilaris TC, Chrousos GP. Adrenal diseases. In Diagnostic Endocrinology. Edited by T Moore, R Eastman. Toronto: BC Decker, 1990, pp 79–104.
55. Lanigan D, Choa RG, Evans J. A feminizing adrenocortical carcinoma presenting with gynaecomastia. Postgrad Med J 1993;69:481–483.
56. Zayed A, Stock JL, Liepman MK, Wollin M, Longcope C. Feminization as a result of both peripheral conversion of androgens and direct estrogen production from an adrenocortical carcinoma. J Endocrinol Invest 1994;17:275–278.
57. Arteaga E, Biglieri EG, Kater CE, Lopez JM, Schambelan M. Aldosterone-producing adrenocortical carcinoma. Ann Intern Med 1984;101:316–321.
58. Touitou Y, Boissonnas A, Bogdan A, Auzeby A. Concurrent adrenocortical carcinoma and Conn's adenoma in a man with primary hyperaldosteronism: in vivo and in vitro studies. Acta Endocrinol (Copenh) 1992;127:189–192.
59. Nader S, Hickey RC, Sellin RV, Samaan NA. Adrenal cortical carcinoma: a study of 77 cases. Cancer 1983;52:707–711.
60. Forbes AP, Albright F. A comparison of the 17-ketosteroid excretion in Cushing's syndrome associated with adrenal tumor and with adrenal hyperplasia. J Clin Endocrinol Metab 1951;11:926–933.
61. McKenna TJ, Miller RB, Liddle GW. Plasma pregnenolone and 17-OH-pregnenolone in patients with adrenal tumors, ACTH excess, or idiopathic hirsutism. J Clin Endocrinol Metab 1977;44:231–236.
62. Flack MR, Oldfield EH, Cutler GB, et al. Urine free cortisol in the high-dose dexamethasone suppression test for the differential diagnosis of Cushing syndrome. Ann Intern Med 1992;116:211–217.
63. Belldegrun A, Hussain S, Seltzer SE, Loughlin KR, Gittes RF, Richie JP. Incidentally discovered mass of the adrenal gland. Surg Gynecol Obstet 1986;163:203–208.
64. Copeland PM. The incidentally discovered adrenal mass. Ann Intern Med 1983;98: 940–945.
65. Richie JP, Gittes RF. Carcinoma of the adrenal cortex. Cancer 1980;45:1957–1964.
66. Tang CK Gray GF. Adrenocortical neoplasms: prognosis and morphology. Urology 1975;5:691–695.
67. Henley DJ, van Heerden JA, Grant CS, Carney JA Carpenter PC. Adrenal cortical carcinoma: a continuing challenge. Surgery 1983;94:926.
68. Appelquist P, Kostianinen S. Multiple thoracotomy combined with chemotherapy in metastatic adrenal cortical carcinoma: a case report and review of the literature. J Surg Oncol 1983;24:1–4.
69. Jarabak J, Rice K. Metastatic adrenal cortical carcinoma; prolonged regression with mitotane therapy. JAMA 1981;246:1706–1707.
70. Downing V, Eule J, Huseby RA. Regression of an adrenal cortical carcinoma and its neovascular bed following mitotane therapy: a case report. Cancer 1974;34: 1882–1887.
71. Hogan TF, Citrin DL, Johnson MB, Nakamura S, Davis TE, Borden EC. *o,p'*-DDD (mitotane) therapy of adrenal cortical carcinoma. Cancer 1978;42:2177–2181.
72. Pommier RF, Brennan MF. An eleven-year experience with adrenocortical carcinoma. Surgery 1992;112:963–970.
73. Berruti A, Terzolo M, Paccotti P, et al. Favorable response of metastatic adrenocortical carcinoma to etoposide, Adriamycin, and cisplatin (EAP) chemotherapy: report of two cases. Tumori 1992;78:345–348.
74. Haq MM, Legha, SS, Samaan NA, Bodey GP, Burgess MA. Cytotoxic chemotherapy in adrenal cortical carcinoma. Cancer Treat Rep 1980;64:909–913.
75. Hesketh PJ, McCaffrey RP, Finkel HE, Larmon SS, Griffing GT, Melby JC. Cisplatin-based treatment of adrenocortical carcinoma. Cancer Treat Rep 1987;71:222–224.
76. Johnson DH, Greco FA. Treatment of metastatic adrenal cortical carcinoma with cisplatin and etoposide (VP-16). Cancer 1986;58:2198–2202.
77. Schlumberger M, Ostronoff M, Bellaiche M, Rougier P, Droz JP, Parmentier C.5-Fluorouracil, doxorubicin, and cisplatin regimen in adrenal cortical carcinoma. Cancer 1988;61:1492–1494.
78. van Slooten H, van Oosterom AT. CAP (cyclophosphamide, doxorubicin, and cisplatin) regimen in adrenal cortical carcinoma. Cancer Treat Rep 1983;67:377–379.
79. Percarpio B, Knowlton A. Radiation therapy of adrenal carcinoma. Acta Radiat Ther Phys Biol 1976;15:288.
80. Flynn SD, Murren JR, Kirby WM, et al. P-glycoprotein expression and multidrug resistance in adrenocortical carcinoma. Surgery 1992;112:981–986.
81. Fojo AT, Akiyama SI, Gottesman MM, Pastan I. Reduced drug accumulation in multiple drug-resistant human KB carcinoma cell lines. Cancer Res 1985;45: 3002–3007.
82. Fojo AT, Ueda K, Slamon DJ, Poplack DG, Gottesman MM, Pastan I. Expression of a multidrug resistant gene in human tumors and tissues. Proc Natl Acad Sci USA 1986;00:000–000.
83. Fridborg H, Larsson R, Juhlin C, et al. P-glycoprotein expression and activity of resistance modifying agents in primary cultures of human renal and adrenocortical carcinoma cells. Anticancer Res 1994;14:1009–1016.
84. Arlt W, Reincke M, Siedmann L, Winkelmann W, Allolio B. Suramin in adrenocortical cancer: limited efficacy and serious toxicity. Clin Endocrinol (Oxf) 1994;41: 299–307.
85. LaRocca RV, Stein CA, Danesi R, et al. Suramin in adrenal cancer: modulation of steroid hormone production, cytotoxicity in vitro, and clinical antitumor effect. J Clin Endocrinol Metab 1990;71:497.
86. Flack M, Pyle R, Mullen N, et al. Oral gossypol in the treatment of metastatic adrenal cancer. J Clin Endocrinol Metab 1993;76:1019.

CHAPTER 102

Neoplasms of the Neuroendocrine System

LI-TEH WU, A. PHILIPPE CHAHINIAN, STEPHEN B. BAYLIN, NORMAN W. THOMPSON, AND STEVEN D. AVERBUCH

Introduction

This chapter focuses upon three neoplasms of endocrine organs (parathyroid carcinoma, medullary thyroid carcinoma, and pheochromocytoma) and three endocrine neoplastic syndromes that are linked together by at least two major considerations. First, each of the neoplasms has histological and biochemical features that are common to all normal and neoplastic endocrine cells of the body. Histologically, these cells contain the cytoplasmic neurosecretory granules, which store either small polypeptide hormones and/or biogenic amines. These secretory products reflect the specific endocrine function of the normal cells from which the neoplasms derive (Table 102.1). In terms of biochemical features, the tumors arise from the so-called group of "amine precursor uptake and decarboxylation" (APUD) cells, which constitute the diffuse system of neuroendocrine cells distributed throughout the body (209, 211). The "APUD" acronym denotes the capacity of these cells to synthesize and/or secrete biogenic amines formed through activity of the enzyme L-dopa decarboxylase (85).

The second feature linking these particular neoplasms and syndromes is that they can occur in individual patients as a consequence of autosomally dominant genetically transmitted disorders. Inherited genetic defects affect different groups of APUD cells and lead to neoplastic development of related cell types in diverse anatomical regions (19). It is essential to consider these genetic disorders when approaching patients with these tumors or syndromes.

Historically, each of the three neoplasms was initially identified as independent pathological entities. Parathyroid carcinoma was first described in 1935 by Hall and Chaffin (100), although parathyroid adenomas and hyperplasia had been recognized as early as 1903 (10). Hazard and coworkers first recognized medullary thyroid carcinoma as a distinct entity in 1959 (105). In 1886, Frankel's postmortem discovery of bilateral adrenal tumors in a young woman following sudden death was the first report of pheochromocytoma (78). Subsequently, complete descriptions of pheochromocytoma were made, and the surgical cure of the disease was demonstrated in the 1920s (175).

Although the first description of multiple endocrine tumors in a single individual was reported in 1903 (69), it wasn't until the 1950s that neoplasms of multiple endocrine glands in affected individuals and their families came to be recognized as three distinct syndromes, multiple endocrine neoplasia (MEN) types 1, 2a, and 2b. Wermer first described the autosomal dominant association of parathyroid adenoma or hyperplasia, pancreatic islet cell adenoma or carcinoma, and pituitary adenoma (MEN 1) in 1954 (309); Sipple first described the association of parathyroid adenoma or hyperplasia, medullary thyroid carcinoma, and familial pheochromocytoma (MEN 2a) in 1961 (265); and Williams and Pollock first described the association of medullary thyroid carcinoma, pheochromocytoma, and mucosal neuromas (MEN 2b) in 1966 (312). From these early descriptions up to the present, a number of other investigators have contributed their observations to establish these three MEN syndromes (58, 135, 168, 196, 244, 245). In addition, it is now recognized that medullary thyroid carcinoma can occur as an inherited tumor in families without other associated endocrine lesions (non-MEN familial medullary thyroid carcinoma) (72).

Based on morphological criteria, Pearse first proposed the APUD diffuse neuroendocrine system in 1968 (209). Subsequent experimental evidence has challenged the notion of a common embryologic origin of APUD cells as originally proposed by Pearse (7, 19, 124, 151). Thus, a neuroectodermal origin for the cells involved in the genetic medullary thyroid carcinoma syndromes separate from the endodermal origin of those in the MEN 1 syndrome is now considered likely. Nonetheless, the APUD concept as proposed by Pearse has been pivotal to exploring how single genetic defects may cause simultaneous neoplasms in the same individual, and it still provides an extremely useful framework in which these closely linked neoplasms and their syndromes may be considered.

Parathyroid Carcinoma

The vast majority (>95%) of parathyroid tumors are benign and produce signs of primary hyperparathyroidism. The emphasis in this chapter will be on parathyroid carcinoma and its differential features with the more common benign tumors (adenomas and hyperplasia).

EMBRYOLOGY AND ANATOMY

Embryology is the key to understand the normal and ectopic locations of the parathyroid glands. The upper glands are derived from the 4th pharyngeal pouch together with the

Table 102.1. Common Features of Amine Precursor, Uptake, and Decarboxylation (APUD) Cell

Biogenic amine synthesis
Amine precursor uptake
Amine (DOPA) decarboxylase
Small polypeptide hormone synthesis
Membrane-bound neurosecretory granules

lateral thyroid, whereas the lower glands are derived from the 3rd pharyngeal pouch together with the thymus (399, 456). In the majority of cases, the upper parathyroid glands are found at the cricothyroid junction posteriorly (77%), less commonly behind the upper pole of the thyroid underneath its capsule (22%), and exceptionally in a retropharyngeal or retroesophageal location (1%) (456). The lower parathyroid glands are located anywhere between the lower pole of the thyroid and the thymus, 42% being at the lower pole of the thyroid, 39% within the thymic tongue in the lower neck, and 2% being in the mediastinal thymus. Other ectopic locations are usually in the neck (15% juxtathyroidal, 2% in other locations) (456). In addition, supernumerary glands have been found in 2 to 6% of individuals (417). Therefore, parathyroid tumors, including carcinomas, may arise in ectopic (often mediastinal) locations or even from a fifth gland (417, 426).

PATHOLOGY

The normal parathyroid gland contains mainly chief cells, which are polyhedral, rich in glycogen (giving sometimes the appearance of clear cells) and fat, and secrete parathyroid hormone (PTH). Oxyphil cells appear later and increase in number with advancing age. They have a pyknotic nucleus and a granular eosinophilic cytoplasm packed with mitochondria (399). They are thought to represent senescent cells, whereas the water-clear cells are thought to represent transitional cells (444). In addition, fat cells and adipose tissue also increase with age (399).

The distribution of parathyroid tumors in 1,200 cases of hyperparathyroidism seen at the Massachusetts General Hospital from 1932 to 1983 was as follows (457): benign single adenoma = 83% (double adenomas < 1%), hyperplasia of all 4 glands = 14% (chief cell hyperplasia = 2%, clear cell hyperplasia = 12%), and carcinoma = 2%. The majority of cases of hyperplasia occur in patients with MEN, either type 1 or type 2.

It is often histologically difficult to differentiate these tumors, particularly to ascertain their benign or malignant nature. Parathyroid carcinoma appears as a grayish, hard, lobulated tumor, compared to the soft, reddish brown adenoma (399, 414, 457). It is surrounded by a dense fibrotic capsule. Its adherence to and invasion of surrounding structures reported in 50% of cases is an important sign of malignancy and should alert the surgeon (399, 414). The average size of carcinomas is 3 cm, with a mean weight of 6 to 12 g (399,440). Microscopically, the carcinoma cells resemble "watermelon seeds" (399) and are larger, better defined than adenomatous cells. The cells are bland and uniform, however, and cellular atypia is rare, surprisingly in contrast to adenomas. Criteria for malignancy as described by Castleman and Roth (399) include a trabecular pattern with thick fibrous bands, nuclear palisading, mitotic figures, and capsular and blood vessel invasion. These features are not absolutely conclusive nor constant, however, and even mitotic activity has been challenged as being "the single most valuable criterion" (399) since it was also found in 12 out of 17 benign adenomas and in 8 out of 10 parathyroid hyperplasias (447). An important corollary is that when a carcinoma is suspected on clinical grounds and/or gross appearance, the surgeon should resect the tumor "en bloc" without relying on biopsy or frozen section (442).

The use of flow cytometric DNA analysis to determine aneuploidy, S-phase fraction, and proliferation index values in an attempt to distinguish parathyroid carcinoma from adenoma or hyperplasia has yielded conflicting results (428, 429). Tumor markers such as opioid peptides (389) and chromogranin A (430) have been described in benign parathyroid tumors. Production of human chorionic gonadotropin (hCG) subunits alpha and beta has been observed in parathyroid carcinoma and apparently not in benign tumors (450).

EPIDEMIOLOGY AND ETIOLOGY

In contrast to benign parathyroid tumors, which have been diagnosed increasingly since the introduction of automated multi-channel analyzers in the 1970's, with an annual age-adjusted incidence of 28 per 100,000 (411), parathyroid carcinoma remains rare. Only about 200 cases have been reported (442). Its etiology is unknown. Usually, parathyroid carcinomas do not arise from adenoma or hyperplasia, and familial cases are exceptional (404, 442). Prior exposure to radiation in the neck is a well-known risk factor for thyroid carcinoma and has also been reported in 9 to 30% of patients with hyperparathyroidism and benign parathyroid tumors, with an average latency period of 37 years (418). Up to 79% of these patients also have associated thyroid tumors, mainly non-medullary carcinoma or adenoma. A history of prior radiation, however, has been reported in very few cases of parathyroid carcinoma (442). Chronic renal failure, which leads to secondary hyperparathyroidism, has been implicated in a patient with coexisting parathyroid carcinoma, adenoma, and hyperplasia (384). Another patient with parathyroid carcinoma had both chronic renal failure and a history of prior radiation to the neck (416).

A plasma factor with a very high mitogenic activity for bovine parathyroid glands in vitro has recently been isolated from patients with MEN-1 (390). Genetic studies have so far been largely limited to MEN syndromes. MEN type 1, where parathyroid hyperplasia is the rule, has been associated with loss of heterozygosity (indicating loss of a possible suppressor gene) on chromosome 11q (433, 454), as compared to chromosome 1p (together with a predisposing gene on chromosome 10) in MEN type 2 (433, 438). Despite earlier conflicting results, it appears that parathyroid adenomas, as well as hyperplasia in MEN type 1, are monoclonal neoplasms (378, 406). The relevance of these findings for parathyroid carcinoma has not yet been evaluated. Abnormal genes regulating the cell cycle have been observed in some benign parathyroid adenomas (PRAD1 or cyclin D1), whereas the retinoblastoma tumor-suppressor gene was completely inactivated in most specimens from nine patients with parathyroid carcinoma but not in those with parathyroid adenoma (402).

CLINICAL FEATURES

Parathyroid carcinomas are usually slow-growing tumors with a tendency to recur locally and metastasize late (399). The great majority of them (>95%) are functioning and produce a more severe picture of primary hyperparathyroidism as compared to parathyroid adenomas or hyperplasia (Table 102.2). The major distinguishing features of malignant hyperparathyroidism are equal incidence in men and women, younger mean age by more than a decade, presence of a palpable neck mass, and severe hypercalcemia, often >14 mg/dl. Hoarseness with recurrent nerve involvement is rare, occurring in less than 10% of patients (414, 457). Metastases are seen in 36% of patients with parathyroid carcinoma, including involvement of cervical nodes in 21%, and distant metastases to lungs, bone, liver, and other organs in 16% (414, 440, 441, 457). Almost all patients with malignant hyperparathyroidism are symptomatic at diagnosis, compared to only half of those with benign tumors. Symptoms are usually severe and include a range of classic manifestations (377, 381, 395, 401, 410, 411, 420, 423, 431): (1) renal involvement with polyuria, polydipsia, urolithiasis (calcium oxalate or calcium phosphate stones), nephrocalcinosis, and decreased function; (2) bone involvement with classic osteitis fibrosa cystica (subperiostal resorption of distal phalanges, salt and pepper appearance of the skull, disappearance of the lamina dura of the teeth, bone cysts, and "brown" tumors) and/or osteopenia, pathologic fractures, bone pain; concomitant renal and bone involvement, exceptional in benign hyperparathyroidism, is seen in up to 39% of patients with parathyroid carcinoma (437, 457); (3) neuromuscular symptoms with proximal muscle weakness, easy fatigability, muscle aches, paresthesias, mental disturbances (decreased recent memory, irritability, depression, somnolence), headaches, and pruritus; (4) rheumatologic symptoms with joint pains, gout, pseudo-gout (deposition of calcium pyrophosphate crystals), chondrocalcinosis, and calcific tendinitis; (5) gastrointestinal symptoms with anorexia, nausea, vomiting, constipation, peptic ulcer, and pancreatitis; (6) cardiovascular manifestations with decreased Q-T interval, arrhythmias, and possibly hypertension; and (7) calcifications of the cornea (classic band keratopathy) and other soft tissues (skin, lungs).

Table 102.2. Clinical Features of Primary Hyperparathyroidism Due to Parathyroid Carcinoma and Benign Tumors

	Cancer[a]	Benign[b]
Incidence	2–4%	96–98%
Female:Male	1:1	3:1
Age (years)		
Mean	45	58
Range	12–84	17–83
Palpable neck mass	42%	Rare
Serum calcium		
Mean mg/dl (mmol/l)	15 (3.75)	11–12 (2.75–3.0)
>14 mg/dl (3.5 mmol/l)	64%	<10%
Renal disease	56%	20%
Lithiasis	49%	20%
Nephrocalcinosis	23%	Rare
Decreased function	51%	14%
Bone disease	63%	6%
Osteitis fibrosa cystica	36%	4%
Renal and bone disease	39%	Rare
Gastrointestinal disease		
Peptic ulcer	11%	8%
Pancreatitis	11%	Rare
Asymptomatic	3%	47%

[a] From references 112, 236, 249, 301.
[b] From references 46, 77, 107, 144, 208.

About 73 cases of hyperparathyroidism have been reported during pregnancy (435), including two cases of parathyroid carcinoma (432). Hypercalcemia can have serious consequences on the fetus, and both maternal and fetal complication rates are high, including abortion, perinatal death, or neonatal tetany. Surgical treatment prior to delivery has been recommended, usually during the 2nd and 3rd trimester of pregnancy (413).

LABORATORY TESTS

Hypercalcemia, the hallmark of hyperparathyroidism, is usually severe in patients with parathyroid carcinoma. The serum calcium level is above 14 mg/dl in about two-thirds of the patients, compared to less than 10% of patients with benign hyperparathyroidism (Table 102.2). The total serum calcium, however, may be affected by several factors. Hypoalbuminemia lowers bound calcium and an emprical correction formula can be used short of measuring the physiologically important portion, i.e. the ionized calcium level (add 0.8 mg/dl of calcium for every g/dl of reduction of serum albumin) (386). Renal insufficiency lowers ionized calcium and can also mask the degree of hypercalcemia. Ionized calcium may also be lowered by the tumor lysis syndrome, severe hypomagnesemia, acute pancreatitis, vitamin D deficiency, and hypothyroidism (401). Drugs such as thiazide diuretics and lithium carbonate can increase serum calcium and should be avoided. Other laboratory features include hypophosphatemia, hypercalciuria (>250 mg/d in about 1/4 of patients), hyperphosphaturia, and in some cases hypomagnesemia, hypokalemia, and hyperuricemia (381, 383, 386). Increased serum chloride and decreased bicarbonate can lead to metabolic acidosis, which aggravates hypercalcemia by decreasing the binding of calcium to albumin and increasing the dissolution of bone mineral (377).

Urinary cyclic AMP is elevated as a result of PTH binding to renal receptors. Excessive PTH and hypophosphatemia also increase the renal production of 1,25-dihydroxyvitamin D, which is usually elevated in the serum. In cases of metabolic bone disease (without metastases), the serum alkaline phosphatase level is increased as well as the urinary excretion of hydroxyyproline, an amino acid unique to collagen. Recently, elevated serum levels of osteocalcin, a major noncollagenous protein of bone, have been reported in hyperparathyroidism (407).

Two features may be useful in differentiating parathyroid carcinoma versus benign tumors. Anemia is more common in carcinoma (up to 80% versus less than 10%, respectively) (420, 441) and serum levels of subunits of hCG as mentioned above.

By far the most important test to diagnose primary hyperparathyroidism is the serum level of immunoreactive PTH (iPTH) (377, 386). Different radioimmunoassays are now available directed either at the intact molecule or the active fragments (amino- or N-terminal) or at inactive fragments (mid-region, carboxyl- or C-terminal region). Elevated levels of iPTH are virtually diagnostic and can be very high in cases of functioning parathyroid carcinoma. Ectopic production of PTH is exceptional and has been documented in very few cases of non-parathyroid carcinomas (see below).

IMAGING TECHNIQUES

In benign hyperparathyroidism, first-time exploration of the neck by an experienced surgeon will successfully detect the tumor(s) in more than 90% of cases (460). Imaging techniques are most useful in cases of recurrent or persistent hyperparathyroidism after initial surgery. They are also useful before initial surgery whenever a carcinoma is suspected on clinical grounds, allowing evaluation of the local extent of the tumor particularly with regard to the thyroid, trachea, and esophagus, as well as possible metastases to cervical nodes and other organs.

Noninvasive Techniques

Esophagograms with careful evaluation of the cervical esophagus can indirectly visualize parathyroid tumors (448). Ultrasonography with high resolution, real-time technology is an excellent noninvasive technique, although its overall results are operator dependent (460). Also the retroesophageal, retrotracheal, and mediastinal areas cannot usually be well assessed (460). Computed tomography (CT) scanning can readily visualize these areas and also evaluate the extent of disease in patients with parathyroid carcinoma. Scintigraphy, formerly using radionuclides as selenomethionine-75 or gallium-67 citrate, has been improved by computer subtraction techniques. The sequential use of thallium-201, which concentrates both in para-thyroid and thyroid, and of technetium-99m, which concentrates in the thyroid, followed by subtraction allows imaging of the parathyroid tumors (460). It has good sensitivity, but its specificity can be affected by concomitant thyroid diseases, including adenomas and carcinomas (sometimes associated with parathyroid carcinoma). Thallium-201 can also accumulate in metastatic cancer to lymph nodes. Magnetic resonance imaging (MRI) is improving but at this time does not appear superior to CT. In a prospective comparison based on 100 patients with benign parathyroid tumors before surgery (419), overall sensitivities were as follows: scintigraphy = 73%, CT = 68%, MRI = 57%, sonography = 55%, with respective specificities of 94, 92, 87, and 95%. None of these imaging techniques had a sensitivity of more than 50% for small (<250 mg) tumors, and sensitivity also decreases in patients who had previous surgery to the neck.

For patients with parathyroid carcinoma, CT scanning appears most useful at this time since it has a good sensitivity in detecting the primary tumor and allows evaluation of its local extent and metastases. Technetium-99m-sestamibi scanning, previously used for myocardial perfusion studies, has been recently introduced for parathyroid imaging (455). A high sensitivity of up to 80 to 90% has been observed in detecting abnormal glands. Its evaluation in parathyroid carcinoma is in progress.

Invasive Techniques

They require highly skilled personnel and are currently indicated for difficult cases only. Venography with venous samplings for iPTH remains one of the most sensitive techniques (460). It measures PTH from the venous effluents (thyroid veins) before the hormone is degraded in the peripheral blood. A unilateral gradient is in favor of a single adenoma or carcinoma, whereas a bilateral gradient usually indicates diffuse hyperplasia. Multiple venous samples are usually taken, including the vertebral, thymic, and internal mammary veins in addition to the thyroid veins. It is a time-consuming but relativity safe procedure.

Angiographic studies have been obtained with a number of techniques and are rarely indicated today. Selective or superselective angiography necessitates experienced personnel. Nonectopic parathyroid glands are supplied by branches of the inferior thyroid artery, which originates from the thyrocervical trunk. Instances of severe neurologic complications, quadriplegia, and even death can occur by inadvertent injection of contrast material into spinal branches of the thyrocervical trunk or the costocervical trunk (451). Safer but less sensitive techniques include nonselective intra-arterial or intravenous digital subtraction angiography (460). Angiography has also been used to ablate functioning parathyroid tumors by direct injection of contrast material (451).

Sonography or CT can also guide percutaneous fine needle biopsy for diagnostic purposes, and some authors have even ablated functional tissue by direct injection of ethanol. The possible risks of these biopsies is spillage of cells, which in the case of carcinoma can lead to recurrent tumors (442). Even in cases of benign parathyroid adenomas, recurrent adenomas ("parathyromatosis") have been described following spillage. The diagnosis of primary hyperparathyroidism is clinical and biochemical. Biopsy is not necessary in the majority of cases before definitive surgery for either benign or malignant parathyroid tumors and is in fact generally contraindicated.

NONFUNCTIONING PARATHYROID CARCINOMA

The existence of nonfunctioning parathyroid carcinoma has long been controversial because of the difficulties in differentiating them from thyroid carcinomas. Nonfunctioning tumors, however, do occur throughout the endocrine system. We have reported a case in a 69-year-old woman with multiple recurrences in the neck, a large anterior mediastinal mass, and a malignant left pleural effusion (400). A total of 11 such cases including one of their own has been collected in the English literature by Murphy et al. (425), indicating that they represent about 5% of parathyroid carcinomas. There were six women and five men, with a median age of 50 years (range 27–71 years) and a median survival of 2 years (range 9 months to 5 years), a pattern similar to functioning carcinomas. These patients had no hypercalcemia, and serum iPTH levels were within normal limits (382, 400).

Electron microscopy is important to confirm the diagnosis by showing lipid, glycogen, and neurosecretory granules in the cytoplasm, thus distinguishing these tumors from thyroid carcinoma or metastatic renal cell carcinoma (400, 403). Three possible hypotheses may explain the absence of hyperparathyroidism: lack of hormone synthesis, impairment or decrease of hormone secretion, and synthesis of an abnormal hormone. The second hypothesis seems most likely in view of the presence of secretory granules by electron microscopy, the demonstration of immunoreactivity for PTH in the tumor tissue in one case (425) and the demonstration of mRNA coding for pre-pro-PTH, the cellular precursor of PTH, in the tumor tissue of another case (382). These investigations further support the parathyroid origin of these nonfunctioning carcinomas. These tumors should be distinguished from other nonfunctional parathyroid neoplasms, including oxyphil adenomas, parathyroid cysts, and metastatic carcinomas (most often from breast, lung, and renal carcinomas) (399).

DIFFERENTIAL DIAGNOSIS OF HYPERCALCEMIA

The major differential diagnosis of parathyroid carcinoma, besides benign parathyroid adenoma, is to rule out other causes of cancer-related hypercalcemia. In addition to the presence of lytic bone metastasis, hypercalcemia can result from humoral factors secreted by the tumor itself (humoral hypercalcemia of malignancy or HHM). This was hypothesized in 1941 by Fuller Albright who said "I suspect that the tumor might be producing parathyroid hormone" while discussing a patient with renal cell carcinoma and a lytic metastasis to the ilium (398). In addition to hypercalcemia, the patient also had hypophosphatemia, whereas most patients with hypercalcemia from bone metastasis have a normal serum phosphate level. Urinary cyclic AMP, an important marker, is increased in patients with HHM or primary hyperparathyroidism, whereas it is low in hypercalcemia related to lytic bone metastases (391, 415). Ectopic production of PTH by non-parathyroid tumors, however, is exceptional and was demonstrated only in a few cases, such as ovarian or small cell lung carcinomas (427). Most often, serum levels of iPTH are low in HHM, and PTH mRNA is not expressed by these tumors (445, 452).

Great progress has recently been accomplished in elucidating this syndrome. In 1987, isolation of a novel PTH-related protein (PTHrP) and cloning of its gene were reported (415, 452). That protein contains 141 amino acids, compared to 84 for PTH (Table 102.3), and 8 of the 13 amino acids of the biologically active N-terminal fragment are identical to PTH. Thereafter, the two molecules are totally different. The corresponding gene has been mapped to the short arm of human chromosome 12, compared to the short arm of chromosome 11 for PTH (391, 424). This similarity and proximity suggested that both genes derived from a common ancestral gene, which duplicated and separated during evolution (424, 452). There are now at least three forms of PTHrP mRNAs known. Homology at the N-terminal region may explain similarities in biologic activities of the two proteins, and the binding of PTHrP to PTH receptors. PTHrP increases bone resorption (but not bone formation), increases tubular calcium reabsorption (although less than PTH), and inhibits tubular phosphate reabsorption. Distinguishing features with primary hyperparathyroidism, however, include decreased production of 1,25-dihydroxyvitamin D, due to the limited capacity of PTHrP to stimulate 1-hydroxylase in the proximal tubule, and alkalosis rather than hyperchloremic acidosis (Table 102.3). In HHM, serum chloride levels are usually low or normal, and bicarbonate levels are normal or high (383). In contrast, bicarbonaturia is increased in primary hyperparathyroidism (377, 383). Hypokalemia is common in HHM (50%) and rare in primary hyperparathyroidism (17%) (383). Increased plasma levels of PTHrP have been found in about half the patients with HHM by assays using an antiserum against synthetic human PTHrP [1-34] (392). More sensitive radioimmunoassays directed at other fragments have been described (394). The primary tumors producing PTHrP are mainly squamous carcinomas (lung, esophagus, head, and neck) although a wide range of other tumors can also cause HMM, including renal, bladder, breast, and ovarian carcinomas. This syndrome can also occur in patients with bone metastasis as well (387). Of interest is that at the difference of PTH, which is restricted to the parathyroid cells, PTHrP has also been found in a wide range of normal tissues, such as keratinocytes, breast tissue, milk, placenta, central nervous system, adrenals, mesothelium, and even parathyroid glands, suggesting a widespread physiologic role (387, 422). Since PTHrP is not elevated in some patients with HHM and since some tumors producing PTHrP do not cause hypercalcemia, other factors that could act independently or synergistically with PTHrP may be implicated in HHM (387). These may include other bone resorbing factors such as transforming growth factor alpha (TGF alpha), interleukin-1 (IL-1), and tumor necrosis factor (TNF) (424).

In patients with multiple myeloma, the osteoclast-activating factors produced by the malignant plasma cells are thought to be cytokines, particularly lymphotoxin or TNF beta (424). In patients with lymphomas, production of 1,25-dihydroxyvitamin D by the neoplastic cells themselves has been implicated (391, 424). The urinary cAMP is depressed (391). A similar mechanism was proposed to account for the hypercalcemia of adult T-cell leukemias caused by HTLV-1, but it appears that these patients have classic HHM as described above, with increased urinary cAMP and decreased 1,25-dihydroxyvitamin D (391).

Prostaglandins, particularly of the E series, have been also implicated based on in vitro experiments in cases of

Table 102.3. Biologic Characteristics and Effects of Parathyroid Hormone (PTH) and Related Peptide (PTHrP)[a]

	PTH	PTHrP
No. of amino acids*	84	141
Chromosome location*	11p	12p
Serum calcium	High	High
Urinary calcium*	High (25%)	Higher
Serum phosphate	Low	Low
Urinary phosphate	High	High
Serum pH*	Acidosis	Alkalosis
Nephrogenous cAMP	High	High
1,25-Dihydroxyvitamin D*	High	Low
Bone resorption	Increased	Increased
Bone formation*	Increased	Decreased
Immunoreactive PTH*	Positive	Negative
Immunoreactive PTHrP*	Negative	Positive

[a] From references 39, 120, 185.
*Differentiating features.

metastatic breast cancer, particularly after administration of antiestrogens (424). Indomethacin and other prostaglandin inhibitors, however, have been rarely effective in treating hypercalcemia of malignancy.

Other causes of hypercalcemia are usually easy to rule out (386). Endocrine disorders include hyperthyroidism, adrenal insufficiency, pheochromocytoma, and VIPomas. The last two might coexist with hyperparathyroidism as part of MEN syndromes (386). It has been recently suggested that pheochromocytoma may also produce HHM as described above (449). Vitamin D excess can be seen in granulomatous disorders (sarcoidosis, tuberculosis, histoplasmosis, etcetera) or some lymphomas as mentioned above. Medications inducing hypercalcemia include thiazide diuretics and lithium carbonate. Estrogen and antiestrogen therapy (tamoxifen) can induce hypercalcemia in patients with breast cancer and bone metastasis. Vitamin A toxicity, milk-alkali syndrome, and immobilization are well-known causes of hypercalcemia. Familial hypocalciuric hypercalcemia can mimic primary hyperparathyroidism (386, 421). This autosomal dominant disease starts in childhood and follows a benign course with mild symptoms. Its etiology is unknown. PTH levels are normal or slightly elevated, and the parathyroid glands are normal or mildly hyperplastic.

A normal serum calcium with hypophosphatemia and hyperphosphaturia could raise the possibility of oncogenic osteomalacia, a rare paraneoplastic syndrome seen in benign mesenchymal tumors and sometimes in carcinomas (prostate, small cell lung) and characterized by low serum levels of 1,25-dihydroxyvitamin D (453). It may be caused by ectopic secretion of a factor that inhibits renal tubular reabsorption of phosphate (396).

TREATMENT

Surgery

Surgery is the major and only curative treatment of parathyroid carcinoma. It requires an impeccable technique, and the initial operation is the most important one (442). Removal of the tumor en bloc, with all involved surrounding structures and without violating its capsule is mandatory. For Wang and Gaz (457), all cases where the tumor capsule was violated had local tumor recurrence. Often, the surgeon will rely on the gross appearance to suspect a carcinoma: presence of a thick fibrous capsule with local adherences, gray-white color, and hard consistency, as opposed to the soft reddish brown appearance of adenomas. Simple biopsy with frozen sections should not be attempted in view of its unreliability in distinguishing benign from malignant lesions and its risk of tumor seeding (388, 442). The surgical specimen should include all areas of local adherence such as the ipsilateral thyroid lobe and isthmus, involved strap muscles, and blood vessels. If the recurrent laryngeal nerve is involved, it should be sacrificed as well, since attempts to dissect it from the tumor carry the risk of local recurrence (414). Occasionally, the trachea and/or esophagus may be involved as well. Biopsy of the lymph nodes of the tracheoesophageal groove should be performed. Lymph node metastasis is uncommon during initial surgery (457) and if not present most authors do not recommend a prophylactic radical neck dissection (442). When the gross distinction with a benign enlargement is in doubt, the other ipsilateral parathyroid should be removed as well to rule out the possibility of diffuse hyperplasia.

Close monitoring after surgery is essential to detect hypocalcemia ("hungry bone" syndrome), which is usually temporary but may require supplements of calcium and vitamin D (408).

The 5-year survival is about 50% (including 30% without recurrence) and the 10-year survival varies from 13 to 35% (414, 440, 441). Parathyroid carcinomas tend to grow slowly and metastasize late. The presence of mitosis or vascular invasion has not been useful in predicting prognosis (440). Early recurrence, however, seems to be an unfavorable factor. Most recurrences occur within 2 to 3 years following initial surgery. Since the disease grows slowly, and most patients die from metabolic complications of hyperparathyroidism rather than tumor burden, an aggressive surgical approach for recurrent or metastic disease is advisable (414, 440). Patients may survive many years despite repeated recurrences and metastasis (441). Local recurrences are common (30%), as well as metastases to cervical lymph nodes (30–40%). Distant metastases involve most commonly lungs (20–40%) but also other sites, including mediastinum, bone, pleura, pericardium, and pancreas (414, 441, 457).

Systemic Therapy

Parathyroid carcinomas are resistant to radiotherapy, although it can occasionally be useful for palliation of pain from bone metastasis (439). There is little experience with systemic therapy (400). Partial and temporary remissions were observed with hormonal therapy, including estrogens and testosterone. A partial remission of 10 months duration was reported with "Hexestrol," a synthetic estrogen compound (phenol, 4,4′-(1,2-diethylethylene) (405). Glucocorticoids do not appear active (405). One patient was treated with auto-immunotherapy (portion of resected parathyroid carcinoma emulsified with Freund's adjuvant and reinjected) without response (405).

Experience with chemotherapy is anecdotal. Nitrogen mustard was given to two patients without response (400). We described in 1981 the first successful combination chemotherapy in a patient with metastatic nonfunctioning parathyroid carcinoma (400). The "MACC" combination (methotrexate, doxorubicin, cyclophosphamide, and CCNU) produced a dramatic regression of a large metastatic mediastinal mass and malignant pleural effusion lasting 18 months. Cisplatin given once (50 mg/m^2) at relapse produced no response. A combination of cyclophosphamide, 5-fluorouracil, and DTIC produced complete regression of pulmonary metastases and a partial biochemical response of 13 months duration in a patient with a functioning carcinoma (393). DTIC alone has produced a partial response with marked decrease of serum calcium and iPTH but of short duration (<2 months) in a patient with functioning carcinoma (397). Another case of nonfunctioning carcinoma was treated with a modification of the MACC protocol (mitoxantrone substituted for doxorubicin) and had a partial response for 10+ months (425).

Treatment of Hypercalcemia

The treatment of hypercalcemia in patients with parathyroid carcinoma follows the same general methods used in other forms of hypercalcemia except that the calcium levels may be persistently elevated and more difficult to control by medical treatment, justifying attempts at palliative surgery as mentioned before. Whereas mild hypercalcemia (between 11 and 13 mg/dl) produces variable symptoms, levels higher than 13 mg/dl are usually poorly tolerated (379). Severe hypercalcemia (≥15 mg/dl) is life threatening and constitutes a medical emergency. Serum calcium levels as high as 24 mg/dl have been reported in parathyroid carcinoma (441). Hydration with normal saline, the fluid of choice, is the first step (385), since dehydration secondary to polyuria, anorexia, and nausea is often present. It also promotes renal calcium excretion by increasing the glomerular filtration rate and by reducing reabsorption of calcium and sodium, which are linked in the proximal tubule (379, 386). The volume of fluid should be carefully adjusted to avoid fluid overload. Loop diuretics (furosemide, ethacrynic acid) should be added to further increase urinary excretion of calcium and decrease the risk of fluid overload, but only after adequate hydration first. Thiazide diuretics are contraindicated since they may aggravate hypercalcemia. Care should also be given to correct other electrolyte disturbances (potassium, magnesium). It is unlikely that hydration and diuretics alone will normalize serum calcium or even decrease it to safe levels. The role of a calcium-poor diet is minimal in this setting. Mobilization may help but to a small extent.

Mithramycin is one of the most effective agents available (379, 386). It inhibits osteoclast function. The starting dose is usually 25 μg/kg as a single intravenous dose given by slow infusion of 4 hours or by IV bolus (the drug is a vesicant). This corresponds to one-tenth the antineoplastic dose. Serum calcium usually starts to decrease within 12–24 hours. The peak effect is seen in 48 to 72 hours, and serum calcium may remain low for variable periods of time, usually 3 to 9 days. Doses can be repeated either daily for 3 to 4 days (up to 7 days) or intermittently, depending on the effects on calcium levels. Repeated doses of mithramycin carry the risk of toxic effects, which may limit the usefulness of this agent in the chronic long-term treatment of hypercalcemia and may necessitate dose reductions. Side effects include nausea and vomiting, bone-marrow depression (particularly thrombocytopenia), bleeding diathesis, as well as hepatic, renal, and dermatologic (flushing, skin rash) toxicity.

Calcitonin inhibits osteoclastic bone resorption and also increases urinary excretion of calcium with relatively few side effects. It appears, therefore, to be an ideal agent, but unfortunately its effect is very limited, lasting less than 24 hours, and it loses its efficacy after repeated administration (386). This "escape" effect may be somewhat corrected by the addition of glucocorticoids as observed in a patient with parathyroid carcinoma (380).

Bisphosphonates (formerly diphosphonates) are analogs of the natural substance pyrophosphate. They bind to hydroxyapatite and inhibit bone crystal dissolution and also osteoclastic resorption (379, 436, 446). Clodronate has shown effectiveness in parathyroid carcinoma (443) but is no longer available in the United States because of potential leukemogenicity (436, 446). Etidronate is available in the United States. It is given intravenously at a dose of 7.5 mg/kg/day in 250 ml of normal saline infused over 2 hours during 1 to 4 consecutive days. Maintenance with oral etidronate may prolong the therapeutic effect, although oral bisphosphonates are poorly absorbed. Newer compounds in this class, such as pamidronate, hold promise because of increased effectiveness by both the intravenous and oral routes. The recommended dose of pamidronate is 60 to 90 mg as a single dose by 24-hour intravenous infusion or 60 mg as a single dose by 4-hour intravenous infusion. The effect on serum calcium is gradual, with a nadir occurring within 1 week. Addition of calcitonin may hasten its effect (434). Bisphosphonates also have less acute toxic effects than mithramycin and may even be useful in patients with various metastatic bone disease to limit the invasion and destruction of bone and alleviate pain in addition to controlling hypercalcemia (379). Alendronate, newly available, is orally active in osteoporosis and Paget's disease and will likely find a role in the treatment of hypercalcemia.

Neutral phosphates are modestly effective orally in mild to moderate hypercalcemia and indicated particularly when hypophosphatemia is present. The most common side effect is diarrhea, which is rare at doses below 3 g per day. The potential risk of ectopic calcifications by precipitation of calcium phosphates in soft tissues, however, limits its usefulness, particularly if intravenous phosphate is given. The latter is reserved for extreme, life-threatening hypercalcemia refractory to all other modalities (386).

Other agents such as glucocorticoids are of little value here, except occasionally in combination with calcitonin. They are effective in hypercalcemia secondary to abnormal production of 1,25-dihydroxyvitamin D such as lymphomas (see above). Prostaglandin synthesis inhibitors (indomethacin) have been disappointing in treating hypercalcemia of malignancy. Other less established drugs include beta-adrenergic inhibitors (propranolol), cimetidine, and estrogens (385). Cisplatin may have antihypercalcemic activity, distinct or not from its antineoplastic activity (436).

Gallium nitrate is an antineoplastic drug, which was found to produce hypocalcemia during phase I trials. It inhibits bone resorption and can control hypercalcemia mediated by PTH or related peptide (458, 459). At a dose of 200 mg/m^2 day for 5 to 7 days by continuous infusion, it has been effective and shown to be superior to calcitonin in treating hypercalcemia from various cancers (458) and from parathyroid carcinoma as well (459). Nephrotoxicity is a potential serious side effect. WR 2721 (amifostine) is an organic thiophosphate compound that is concentrated in normal tissues (except the central nervous system) and much less in most neoplastic tissues (409, 436). It has been used as a protective agent against the toxicity of radiation and chemotherapy. Phase I trials revealed that WR 2721 can cause hypocalcemia, which appears related not only to inhibition of bone resorption but also to inhibition of PTH secretion and increased urinary calcium excretion (386, 436). It has shown activity in parathyroid carcinoma (412).

Although mithramycin remains currently the most effective agent for hypercalcemia in patients with parathyroid carcinoma, the development of new drugs (bisphosphonates, gallium nitrate, WR 2721 (amfostine)) and perhaps in the future of peptide hormone antagonists (437) will significantly add to the therapeutic armamentarium to treat this most ominous metabolic complication.

Medullary Thyroid Carcinoma (MTC)

EPIDEMIOLOGY

MTC is an uncommon tumor representing 5 to 10% of all thyroid cancers (2). The only known etiologic factors for occurrence of this neoplasm are the autosomal dominant genetic disorders MEN 2a, MEN 2b, and familial non-MEN syndromes, which account for 20% of patients with MTC. Otherwise, MTC arises as a sporadic tumor with an equal frequency between men and women and among different ethnic groups. The peak onset of the sporadic form of MTC is in the fifth or sixth decade of life, while this tumor appears much earlier in the MEN syndromes discussed below (233).

NATURAL HISTORY

Pathologic Considerations

MTC is a neoplasm of the calcitonin-secreting C-cells, which are sparsely distributed in the thyroid gland (310). In approximately 80% of patients, MTC occurs as a sporadic tumor with a unilateral origin in the thyroid. In 20% of patients, however, the neoplasm occurs in an autosomal dominant genetic syndome, of which there are three or more that may involve other endocrine and neural lesions. In these inherited forms, MTC arises as multifocal, bilateral tumors in the thyroid.

Patients with the sporadic form of MTC present with palpable thyroid nodules and almost always have cervical lymph node involvement. MTCs are well-demarcated, whitish, firm nodules that, microscopically, consist of sheets or nests of polygonal cells separated by variable amounts of fibrous stroma (Fig. 102.1). Often the tumors stain positive for amyloid. The hallmark histologic feature of MTC, however, is positive immunostaining for the peptide hormone, calcitonin, which is the major biochemical product of normal thyroid C-cells. The presence of calcitonin can help make the diagnosis of MTC when patients present with one of the several variant histologic forms that have been described (182). Immunostaining for calcitonin is also necessary for the diagnosis of the precursor lesions for MTC, which occur bilaterally in the genetic forms of this tumor discussed in more detail below.

Biologic Characteristics

By far the most striking biologic characteristic of MTC is the occurrence of this neoplasm in a multifocal pattern in autosomal dominant genetic syndromes (315). The molecular basis for these genetic forms of MTC is not yet understood, but the known chromosomal changes and stages for development of the tumors are discussed below in the section on inherited MTC.

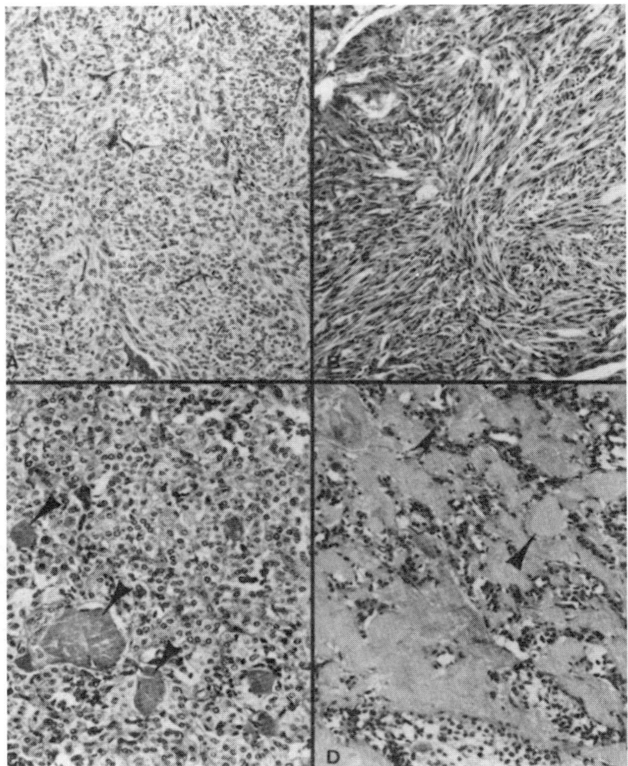

Figure 102.1. Histologic features of medullary thyroid cancer. **A.** Nests of polygonal cells. **B.** Spindle-shaped cells. **C.** Amyloid deposits (*arrows*). **D.** Large amount of fibrous stroma with sparse cells and amyloid nodules (*arrows*) (reproduced with permission from Mendelsohn et al. (181)).

The molecular basis for the loss of differentiation in the aggressive forms of MTC is not yet fully established. In contrast to many solid tumors, chromosomal changes in MTC, such as frequent allelic deletions, are not common (148, 192). Although several investigators have implicated chromosome 10 (145, 171, 188, 261, 262) the only consistent abnormalities appear to be deletions on the short arm of chromosome 1 (172), and these could be involved with tumor progression rather than initiation.

Studies of cultured MTC cells from a patient with virulent MTC indicate that whatever chromosome regions are involved, a deficient activation of one or more cellular signal transduction pathways may be a key step in progression of MTC. Activation of either the protein kinase C or protein kinase A pathways can partially differentiate cultured MTC cells as manifested by an increase in transcription of the calcitonin gene and slowing of cell growth (191). A virtually complete differentiation response can be elicited in these same cells by insertion of a mutated Harvey *ras* oncogene (191). In this situation, not only is there an increase in calcitonin gene expression, but the mRNA splicing for the resultant transcripts resembles the pattern of mRNA splicing in the normal thyroid C-cell. In addition, the cells acquire the typical mature neurosecretory granules of APUD cells, which are lacking in the control cultured cells. The final mediators of this response to an inserted *ras* gene are being investigated, but a coordinated increase in the protein kinase A and C pathways, plus other signal transduction input, is probably involved. A marked increase in expression of the c-*jun* oncogene (191), which is known to participate in multiple protein kinase C mediated events, accompanies the *ras* gene induced differentiation of the MTC cells. Presumably, the increase in this transcription factor activates a series of other transcription factors that mediate maturation of the cells.

Clinical Features

The most common clinical features are a local neck mass and, less commonly, morbid signs or symptoms from distant metastases. In general, the production of secretory peptides is of no clinical significance, although occasionally, apparent manifestations of MTC endocrine activity may be observed. For example, patients with MTC can develop Cushing's syndrome due to ACTH production (180). More often, serotonin, prostaglandins, and perhaps other hormones produced by the tumor may be implicated in the secretory diarrhea seen in up to 30% of patients with advanced MTC (56). Although a physiologic role for calcitonin gene-related peptide (CGRP) has not been established, it is possible that, as a powerful peripheral vasodilator, CGRP, together with substance P, may play a role in the flushing observed in certain patients with advanced MTC.

Another important feature of MTC is the variable clinical behavior of this cancer. Although MTC metastasizes early, especially to cervical lymph nodes and mediastinal structures, it behaves in a relatively indolent manner in approximately 70 to 80% of patients (2, 233, 239). Some patients, even with well-documented hepatic and pulmonary metastases, also take an indolent course. In another group of patients, however, MTC can behave aggressively, and patients die from widespread bony and visceral metastases to lung, liver, and adrenals (195). The overall survival rates for individuals with MTC are 80% for 5 years and 60% for 10 years (Fig. 102.2, *A* and *B*) (233).

The complete basis for the variable clinical behavior of MTC is not known. Inability of neoplastic C cells to attain a fully differentiated phenotype appears to be important (191). This deficiency in maturation is manifest as a marked decrease in the immunoreactive calcitonin and amyloid content of the tumor cells in patients with aggressive MTC (23, 191). Immunostaining of such tumors reveals large areas of calcitonin positive cells that can coexist with areas of negative staining (156, 191). This heterogeneous calcitonin staining pattern or lack of amyloid, when found in primary MTC lesions, is associated with a virulent course and poor survival at 5 years (Figure 102.2C and D) (23, 156, 232).

Biochemical Features

The distinguishing biochemical features of MTC relate primarily to the origin of this cancer in the calcitonin-producing C-cells of the thyroid (310) and from the general characteristics of the group of neuroendocrine cells to which these C-cells belong.

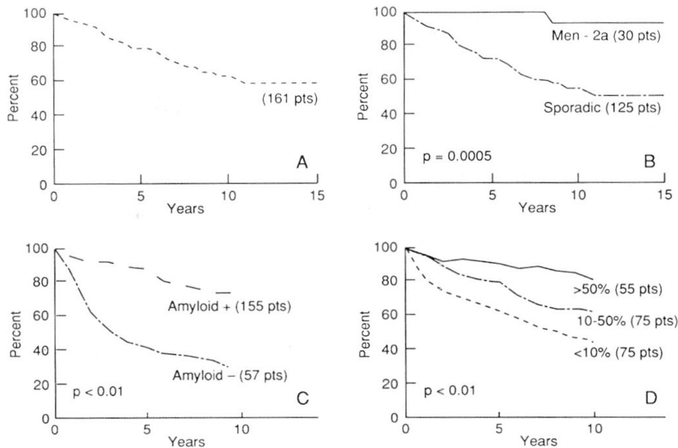

Figure 102.2. Survival of patients with medullary thyroid carcinoma (MTC). **A.** Adjusted survival of all patients with MTC. **B.** Survival of patients with sporadic MTC compared to patients with MEN 2a. **C.** Relative survival of patients according to amyloid positive (+) or negative (−) tumor-staining characteristics. **D.** Relative survival of MTC patients according to percentage of tumor cells positive for calcitonin immunoreactivity (reproduced with permission from Saad et al. (233) and Bergholm et al. (23)).

The main secretory product of the C-cells and the biochemical marker of most clinical utility in patients with MTC is the 32-amino acid peptide calcitonin. Calcitonin is encoded by a multiexonic gene, which by alternative processing of a primary RNA transcript generates two mRNAs. One codes for calcitonin itself and, another, for a 37-amino acid peptide called CGRP (4). The calcitonin mRNA predominates in normal thyroid C-cells but in MTC, both CGRP and calcitonin mRAs are often found in high quantities. Both peptides may circulate at high levels in the blood of patients with MTC, but CGRP levels are much more variable and are usually lower than calcitonin levels (170, 243). During provocative diagnostic testing, as discussed below, calcitonin levels increase briskly in response to calcium and/or pentagastrin stimulation, whereas CGRP responses have been variable (170, 243).

MTC cells also express several biochemical markers that relate to the APUD features of these neuroendocrine cells, including small polypeptide hormones such as somatostatin (226), adrenocorticotropic hormone (ACTH) (180), and gastrin-releasing peptide (GRP) (125). Like other neuroendocrine cells MTC contains the enzyme L-dopa decarboxylase (20), prostaglandins (311), chromogranin A (60), and neuron-specific enolase (NSE) (138, 258). High levels of the histamine-metabolizing enzyme, histaminase or diamine oxidase, are also characteristic of MTC (20). Furthermore, these biochemical markers may occasionally be of diagnostic utility. Immunostaining of chromogranin A is positive in a very high percentage of MTC tumors and thus may help make the diagnosis of MTC in tumors that stain poorly for calcitonin (60, 138, 258).

Another biochemical marker frequently expressed by MTC is carcinoembryonic antigen (CEA). This protein is synthesized by the tumor cells at all stages of disease (228, 231). Even in the aggressive forms of MTC, where the tumor tissue becomes heterogeneous for calcitonin staining, CEA remains present. In fact, a rising blood CEA level in the face of a stable or declining calcitonin level indicates a poor prognosis in patients with MTC (231).

DIAGNOSTIC TESTS

The majority of patients with sporadic MTC present with palpable thyroid nodules, which are manifested as cold nodules on ^{131}I radionuclide imaging and as solid masses on echography. Occasionally, plain x-rays of the neck reveal a dense pattern of calcifications that is characteristic of MTC, different from the fine calcification pattern observed with papillary carcinoma. In most patients, the diagnosis of MTC is made unexpectedly from examination of frozen or permanent sections of a thyroid mass removed at the time of initial surgery.

Even though virtually all patients with palpable MTC have elevated basal serum levels of calcitonin, the relative rarity of MTC makes it impractical to use this test to screen all patients who have thyroid nodules. Stimulated calcitonin secretion, as described in the section on MEN 2 below, should be reserved for testing patients suspected of having MEN 2 or familial non-MEN MTC and for screening their immediate family members (216, 307). A more practical approach involves use of fine needle aspiration (FNA) biopsy to assess any patient with a suspicious thyroid nodule (Fig. 102.3). The cytologic evaluation of such specimens, especially when combined with immunostaining for calcitonin, may suggest MTC and serum calcitonin immunoassays can be employed to confirm the diagnosis.

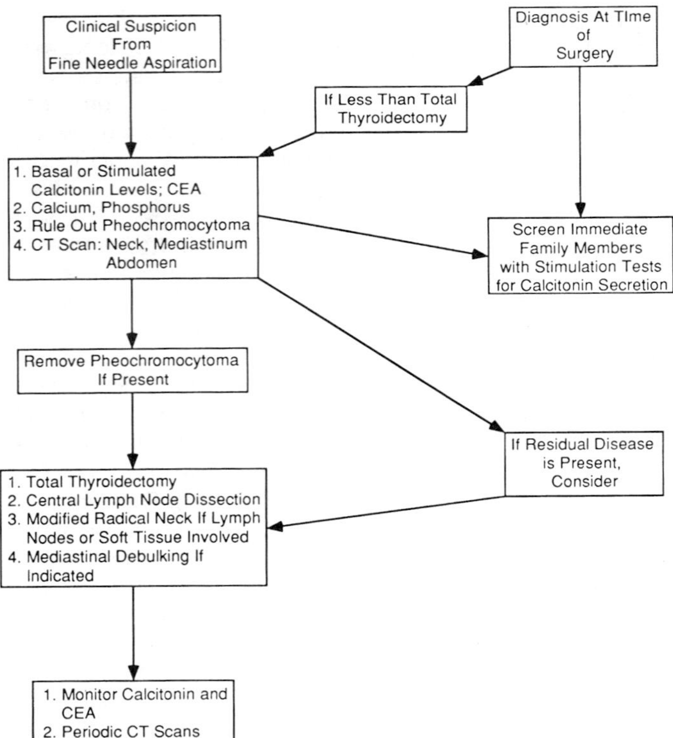

Figure 102.3. Algorithm for the diagnosis and management of medullary thyroid carcinoma.

In all patients documented to have MTC, a prime consideration is the possibility that the patient may represent the index case for one of the familial forms of the disease. In the rare genetic syndrome, MEN 2b, an associated Marfan-like habitus, and the presence of neuromas over the eyelids, lips, and tongue should make the diagnosis obvious. For the other forms of genetic MTC, however, there are no particular physical stigmata. The possibility of familial disease then must be ruled out in virtually every patient with MTC. One extremely helpful criterion for the diagnosis of familial MTC is the presence of bilateral tumors and/or C-cell hyperplasia. Occurrence of MTC in patients younger than 40 years of age also suggests familial disease. Screening of first degree relatives with calcitonin determinations is, however, the only definitive way to exclude genetic disease. Recent studies suggest that the genetic form of MTC is found in 10 to 15% of cases when evaluating relatives of patients with apparently sporadic MTC (216). The most effective approach, if possible, is first to screen the parents of a newly diagnosed MTC patient. A single negative test in the parents dramatically reduces the probability of familial disease. If the parents are not available, screening of as many siblings and offspring as possible is mandatory.

THERAPEUTIC CONSIDERATIONS

Surgical Management

Sporadic MCT usually presents as a solitary nodule in the upper half of the lateral lobe on either side, although in some cases, a metastatic lymph node may be detected first while the primary tumor remains occult to clinical examination. Currently, the diagnosis is frequently established before operation by FNA cytology, after which a basal serum calcitonin can be obtained to confirm the diagnosis (Figure 102.3). The calcitonin level may be of value in predicting the amount of tumor present and whether lymph nodes are likely to be involved. Urinary catecholamine levels must be obtained to rule out pheochromocytoma, even when the history is negative for MEN 2a and there are no physical findings to suggest MEN 2b before a thyroidectomy is undertaken (Figure 102.3). If present, the pheochromocytoma should always be removed prior to the thyroidectomy.

The minimal treatment of MTC is total thyroidectomy (102). In sporadic disease, this allows for excision of any intraglandular lymphatic spread and careful immunohistopathologic study of the contralateral lobe for possible C-cell hyperplasia. Even in some patients with metastases, given the fact that MTC is often slow growing, minimal treatment is a total thyroidectomy. Although not curative, this may prevent tumor growth that can impinge on major structures such as the trachea and esophagus. Most patients with sporadic disease have lymph node metastases when first diagnosed. A central lymph node compartment dissection, preserving the parathyroid glands and recurrent laryngeal nerves, is indicated. Dissection of the nodes includes the Delphian group, those around the upper pole of the thyroid lobe, those in the tracheo-esophageal groove along the recurrent laryngeal nerve and the anterior mediastinal lymph nodes to the level of the innominate artery. Some nodes contain metastases in nearly all patients with a palpable primary tumor within the thyroid gland at operation. If lateral lymph nodes are involved, a modified radical neck dissection should be done (230). Occasionally, because of invasion through the lymph node capsule and involvement of contiguous structures, a formal radical dissection may be required.

In patients with MTC, discovered by calcitonin screening and no palpable tumor, central compartment lymph nodes may be tumor free. Nevertheless, even normal-sized nodes should be sampled for frozen section examination to determine whether a complete and thorough central compartment dissection is required (Figure 102.3). Lateral lymph node involvement is treated by modified neck dissection, which may be bilateral, performed in one or two stages. When the lateral lymph nodes are involved with MCT, a biochemical cure, as determined by calcitonin testing, is unlikely (<20%). As a result, a formal (modified) radical neck dissection has been considered by many to be futile (230). Occasionally, this is still indicated if the procedure is required to excise all areas of gross disease because of lymph node invasion of local tissues. For this reason, when possible prior to initial surgery, or following surgery, computerized tomography or magnetic resonance image scans of the cervical, mediastinum, and abdominal regions should be done to document areas of discernible metastases. When calcitonin levels remain elevated despite lack of clinically evident disease after a total thyroidectomy and central compartment dissection, controversy continues as to whether a neck dissection on one, or both sides, should be done. Tissel favors a meticulous radical neck dissection and has achieved a biochemical cure in about half of a relatively small group of patients treated this way (288). Alternatively, others have favored regional excision of any palpable nodes or those suspected on the basis of a positive thallium scan or cervical ultrasound when the disease has been limited to the lateral neck or anterior mediastinum. One of the causes of failure after performing a radical neck dissection based entirely on an elevated calcitonin level is that clinically occult MTC already may have spread hematogenously to involve the liver, lungs, or bone. Therefore, it is reasonable to perform selective venous sampling for calcitonin to rule out disseminated disease before considering any extensive additional neck procedures.

Treatment of Recurrent or Metastatic Disease

When persistent, recurrent, or disseminated disease is present, MTC usually progresses slowly. Since effective radiation therapy or chemotherapy is not well established, it is important to consider several prognostic factors when deciding if chemotherapy is indicated. As discussed previously, tumors that have poor immunocytochemical staining for calcitonin tend to have a more aggressive course (23, 156, 232). Although the serum calcitonin level correlates with the extent of disease, it does not help in identifying patients with a poorer prognosis. Rapidly rising, high serum CEA is more predictive of a rapid disease course (231).

Recurrent tumors may be amenable to repeated surgical resection, especially for palliation of symptoms due to local tissue invasion or due to a syndrome of hormonal excess. Radiation therapy does not have an established role in the treatment of locally advanced MTC (239). In selected cases of patients with symptomatic bone metastases, a trial of radiation may offer transient palliative benefit.

Although most reports of chemotherapy for MTC are anecdotal, the experience provides some guidelines for therapeutic approaches. Since MTC belongs to the APUD family of neoplasms, a number of single agent and combination chemotherapy treatments that show activity in other "APUDomas" have been used in advanced MTC.

Gottlieb and colleagues reported three partial remissions and resolution of disease-related diarrhea in six patients with advanced MTC following treatment with doxorubicin (93). Additional reports by others suggest an overall partial reponse rate of 30% in 46 patients with MTC treated with doxorubicin as a single agent (118, 229, 256, 263). The combination of streptozocin and doxorubicin was not active in a small trial of patients (140, 306). Reports of the combination of 5-fluorouracil and dacarbazine (including a complete response) (212), doxorubicin and cisplatin (272), or dacarbazine (133), 5-fluorouracil (76), or etoposide (76, 115) used as single agents suggest limited activity for these drugs (256, 313). The combination of cyclophosphamide, vincristine, and dacarbazine found to be effective in malignant pheochromocytoma (14), has been studied in three patients by us (13, 59a). Two of these patients had a partial response demonstrated by reduced serum calcitonin and/or CEA and objective regression of radiologically demonstrated masses. The other patient had stable disease for more than 17 months. Until prospective multiinstitutional studies of combination chemotherapy regimens for patients with metastatic MTC are undertaken, dacarbazine or cisplatin and doxorubicin containing regimens should be considered for individual patients with progressive, symptomatic disease.

Since biologic response modifiers, such as the somatostatin analog, octreotide acetate, have been shown to reduce circulating hormones, halt progression, and occasionally reduce tumor size in various neuroendocrine tumors (92), this agent may have a role in patients with MTC (92, 183). Long term subcutaneous injection of octreotide acetate to 21 patients with MTC reduced serum calcitonin in 11, but CEA did not change (161, 183). Flushing and diarrhea improved in some, and several patients reportedly had objective tumor response. Additional clinical studies are required to determine the activity of somatostatin analogs in patients with metastatic MTC.

Pheochromocytoma

Pheochromocytoma and paraganglioma are terms describing a neoplasm of chromaffin cells found in the adrenal medulla or elsewhere within the sympathetic paraganglionic axis. The adrenal tumors are usually referred to as pheochromocytomas, while an extra-adrenal tumor is often termed either extra-adrenal pheochromocytoma or paraganglioma, the latter usually reserved for a nonfunctional (i.e. noncatecholamine secreting) neoplasm. This terminology is based on historical histopathological techniques, and since these neoplasms are otherwise indistinguishable, the terminology may be confusing. Therefore, all of these neoplasms considered here will be referred to as pheochromocytomas. Additional descriptions, e.g. nonfunctional, extra-adrenal, or malignant, should be included in the terminology as appropriate. Rare chromaffin neoplasms arising from special structures in the neck may be referred to as chemodectomas, glomus jugulare, or carotid body tumors (211, 255).

EPIDEMIOLOGY

Pheochromocytomas occur infrequently and are found in approximately 0.1 to 0.5% of hypertensive patients (21, 165, 292). Autopsy series suggest that up to one-third of pheochromocytomas may not be diagnosed pre-mortem (184, 247, 273). From the Mayo Clinic data, it is estimated that approximately 800 cases of pheochromocytoma are diagnosed in the US each year (21). The average annual incidence of pheochromocytoma in Sweden and Denmark is 2.1 and 1.9 cases per million population, respectively (6, 274).

Ninety percent of pheochromocytomas are sporadic neoplasms. Thus, when considering the diagnosis and management of this disease it is important also to consider the "rough rule of 10s." That is, 10% of neoplasms occur in children, 10% are associated with familial syndromes, 10% of sporadic cases are bilateral, 10% are extra-adrenal, and 10% are malignant. There is a higher chance of extra-adrenal disease in children (166, 224, 273, 292). This mnemonic provides only an estimate of these presentations, and there is overlap within the pediatric, familial, and bilateral groups (48, 157). The most common familial syndromes that include pheochromocytoma as an element are the autosomal dominant MEN syndrome types 2a and 2b and Von Hippel-Lindau (VHL) disease (131, 252, 292, 327). MEN 2a is characterized by parathyroid adenoma and MEN 2b by ganglioneuromatosis and Marfanoid-like body habitus. Medullary thyroid carcinoma and pheochromocytoma are common to both syndromes. VHL can have associated retinal angioma, hemangioblastoma of the central nervous system, renal cysts and carcinoma, and pancreatic cysts. Carriers of these familial syndromes can have pheochromocytoma as the only or the first manifestation of their inheritance. Hartmut et al. reported 23% of unselected patients with pheochromocytoma are carriers of either MEN 2 or VHL disease (327). Therefore, all patients with pheochromocytoma should have screening tests for these familial disorders. Conversely, all carriers of these familial syndromes should be screened for pheochromocytoma because of high prevalence (up to 80%). Many such patients discovered by screening are normotensive and asymptomatic. Pheochromocytomas have also been seen in neurofibromatosis as a component of Carney's triad and in families unassociated with other tumors or syndromes (48, 113, 141, 159, 187). Familial pheochromocytomas occur at younger age and very often involve both adrenal glands, either synchronously or metachronously. It typically follows a benign course, but because of their potential for causing significant morbidity or mortality, this tumor must be diagnosed and removed prior to any surgical management of thyroid or parathyroid disease.

Malignant pheochromocytoma is a rare entity among malignant diseases, and its exact incidence is not known. Multiple series have estimated the frequency of malignancy among pheochromocytomas from 5 to 46% (26, 99, 122, 127, 179, 247, 291), although the latter figure is probably inflated since it comes from a very selective referral patient population (26). Overall, a figure of 13% of all pheochromocytomas probably represents a reliable incidence for malignant pheochromocytoma (14). A review of SEER data for 1973 to 1985 suggests that the yearly age-adjusted rate of malignant pheochromocytoma is 0.04 per 100,000 population or approximately 100 cases per year in the US (14a). Extra-adrenal pheochromocytoma has been associated with a higher frequency of malignancy (30%) (122, 142, 179, 255, 292), although this has been recently challenged (89).

NATURAL HISTORY

Embryology and Anatomy

Chromaffin tissue constitutes one component of the diffuse neuroendocrine (APUD) system, thought to be derived from the embryonic neuroectodermal crest (210, 211). Although this embryologic origin of APUD tumors is now disputed (7, 19, 124, 151), the common genetic and clinicopathologic characteristics of pheochromocytoma and APUD tumors justify their consideration as entities of a common neuroendocrine system. In the fetus and in infancy, diffuse paraganglionic chromaffin tissue is prominent but later regresses, aside from that found within the adrenal medulla (143). Because of this, pheochromocytomas may arise from chromaffin remnants virtually anywhere, but the vast majority (90%) are found in the adrenal medulla (141, 179). The most common extra-adrenal sites are the region where the left renal vein crosses the aorta, renal hilus, and the origin of the inferior mesenteric artery (organ of Zuckerkandl).

Pathologic Characteristics

The typical adrenal pheochromocytoma is a sporadically occurring neoplasm, arising from either gland. When detected, it is approximately 5 cm in diameter and weighs 50 to 100 g (141). The adrenal mass is often pseudoencapsulated, and it is highly vascularized with a beefy appearance and consistency. Larger tumors frequently contain areas of hemorrhage or empty or fluid-filled cysts surrounded by connective tissue and calcifications (Fig. 102.4*A*). The microscopic appearance of a pheochromocytoma is similar to the architecture and morphology of normal chromaffin tissue. The cells are usually round or polygonal with abundant eosinophilic or basophilic fine granular cytoplasm and are frequently arranged in cords or clusters (Fig. 102.4*B*) (141). Nuclear pleomorphism and hyperchromasia are common. Mitotic figures are often seen in adrenal hyperplasia and in pheochromocytoma, but they are not necessarily prominent histological features. Chromaffin cells and pheochromocytomas show a characteristic brown staining following application of chromium salts (hence, chromaffin), although this method has largely been replaced by the Grimelius argyrophile stain (95). The demonstration of a wide array of neuroendocrine products by immunocytochemical analysis

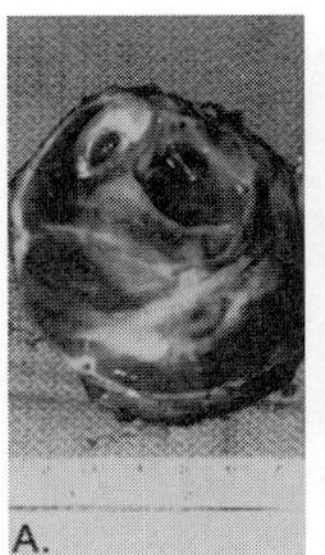

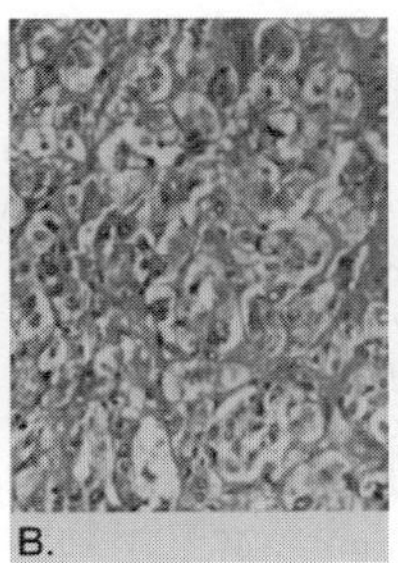

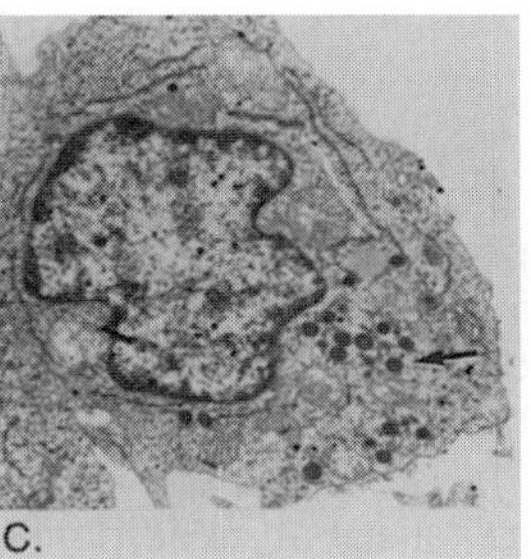

Figure 102.4. Pheochromocytoma. **A.** Gross appearance of a surgically removed hemisected extra-adrenal pheochromocytoma. **B.** Histopathologic appearance of a pheochromocytoma showing typical cords of glandular cells separated by bands of stroma (hematoxylin and eosin, 25 ×). **C.** Ultrastructural appearance of a single pheochromocytoma cell showing dense neurosecretory granules (*arrow*) (6,000 ×).

reflects the content of dense intracytoplasmic neurosecretory granules, which are apparent by electron microscopic examination (Fig. 102.4*C*) (141). Commonly identified products include biogenic amines, neuron-specific enzymes, and neuropeptides (Table 102.4) (55, 86, 104, 131, 141, 155, 158, 166, 198–200, 227, 240, 242, 296, 297, 305).

There are no pathognomonic criteria for malignancy of a pheochromocytoma other than the natural history of an individual's tumor that manifests chromaffin cell invasion or dissemination at sites where chromaffin tissue is normally not present. Malignant tumors have a predilection for spreading to bone (predominantly to spine, ribs, and skull) (160), lung, liver, and retroperitoneal and mediastinal lymph nodes (14, 64, 255). A number of studies have attempted to identify characteristics that can discriminate malignant from benign tumors (141, 178). Among these, nuclear pleomorphism, mitotic figures, vascular invasion, cortical extension, necrosis, and immunocytochemical characteristics are not particularly useful. Some authors have shown that increased tumor size and extra-adrenal location are associated with a malignant phenotype (178, 179, 292). Investigations of tumor DNA ploidy by flow cytometry have demonstrated the potential utility of this technique for defining a malignant subset (114, 136, 154). Of 62 tumors studied, approximately one-third of tumors containing aneuploid, polyploid, or tetraploid DNA were malignant, while all 18 that were diploid followed a benign course, a statistically significant difference (114). However, DNA ploidy is not discriminant for malignancy since this study and others demonstrated a high prevalence of aneuploidy in benign pheochromocytomas as well (5, 206, 207). Sustentacular cells are dendritic cells stained positive for S-100. These cells are found in normal paraganglionic tissue and benign pheochromocytomas. Absence of these cells suggests malignancy in several studies (340).

Table 102.4. Biologic Markers in Pheochromocytoma

	Blood	Immunocyto-chemistry	Molecular
Probe biogenic amines			
Norepinephrine	X		
Epinephrine	X		
Dopamine	X		
DOPA	X		
Serotonin	X		
Enzymes			
Neuron-specific enolase	X	X	
Dopa decarboxylase		X	
Dopamine-β-hydroxylase	X	X	
Peptides			
Chromogranin A	X	X	X
Neuropeptide Y	X	X	X
Enkephalins		X	
Corticotropin-releasing factor	X	X	
Somatotrophin-releasing factor	X	X	
Vasoactive intestinal polypeptide (VIP)	X	X	
Somatostatin	X	X	
PTH-related peptide	X		X
Pancreatic polypeptide		X	
Calcitonin	X	X	
Calcitonin gene-related peptide		X	
Substance P	X	X	
Gastrin-releasing peptide		X	
Neurotensin		X	
Insulin-like growth factor II			X
Gastrin		X	
Cholecystokinin		X	
Somatostatin receptor		X	

Biologic Characteristics

Germ line mutations of the *ret* oncogene have been found in lymphocytes, medullary thyroid carcinoma, and pheochromocytoma in carriers of MEN 2a and 2b (324, 328, 343, 344). *ret* oncogene encodes a transmembrane tyrosine kinase, but this mutation was rarely found in sporadic pheochromocytomas. Loss of heterozygosity, which suggests loss of a tumor suppressor gene at chromosomes 1p, 3p, 17p and 22q is common in both familial and sporadic pheochromocytomas (329, 332, 333). These molecular and cytogenetic findings suggest the development of pheochromocytoma follows the model of multistage carcinogenesis exemplified in colon cancer.

Clinical Features

There is no correlation between the amount of catecholamines produced and the severity of blood pressure changes (166, 321). Thus, patients may present anywhere in the spectrum from normotensive and asymptomatic to a severe, life-threatening hypertensive crisis causing cerebral hemorrhage, myocardial infarction, or cardiac failure (184, 241). In fact, many patients can be quite asymptomatic during their lifetime, specifically in the elderly, so that up to one-third of patients in autopsy series were not diagnosed before death (323). In clinically diagnosed patients, hypertension can be either sustained or episodic, and each occurs in approximately one-half of patients with pheochromocytoma. Five percent are normotensive. In rare cases, episodic hypotension is the main symptom due to secretion of predominantly epinephrine or dopamine. Hypertensive episodes may be precipitated by physical stress, an increase in intra-abdominal pressure, or by certain drugs including phenothiazine, a tricyclic antidepressant, metoclopramide, naloxone, and droperodol (131, 336). Characteristically, symptoms occur paroxysmally even in patients with sustained hypertension. The most common symptoms are headache, sweating, and palpitation; each occurs in about 60% of patients. Almost all patients have at least one or two of these three symptoms. But the positive predictive value of this triad is low because only 5.9% of hypertensive patients with this entire triad have pheochromocytoma. Other common symptoms, in decreasing frequency, are pallor, nausea, anxiety, weakness, dyspnea, visual disturbance, abdominal pain, tremor, and weight loss (326). Tachycardia, tremor, and anxiety are prominent in pheochromocytomas secreting a lot of epinephrine. Attacks of symptoms happen abruptly and usually do not last more than 15 minutes. An important feature that distinguishes hypertension of pheochromocytoma from essential hypertension (in the absence of pharmacologic therapy) is the presence of postural hypotension, manifested as a significant drop in systolic pressure in the upright position, but it happens in less than 50% of patients (22, 166, 184, 322). Because of chronic vasoconstriction, the down-regulation of peripheral alpha receptors, and the presence of vasodilatory biogenic amines or peptides, such as VIP and enkephalins, patients with pheochromocytoma are commonly hypovolemic, accounting for postural blood pressure changes (22, 131, 252). Cardiomyopathy and congestive heart failure due to persistently high circulating catecholamines have been reported. Pheochromocytomas in MEN patients are frequently asymptomatic, but these patients can go into hypertensive crises during surgery for hyperparathyroidism or medullary thyroid carcinoma. Therefore, all patients with MEN 2 should be carefully screened for the presence of pheochromocytoma before any surgery or invasive procedure.

Biochemical Features

Along with other neoplasms of the diffuse neuroendocrine (APUD, amine precursor uptake and decarboxylation) system, pheochromocytomas are specialized neoplasms that can synthesize, store, and secrete biological amines and

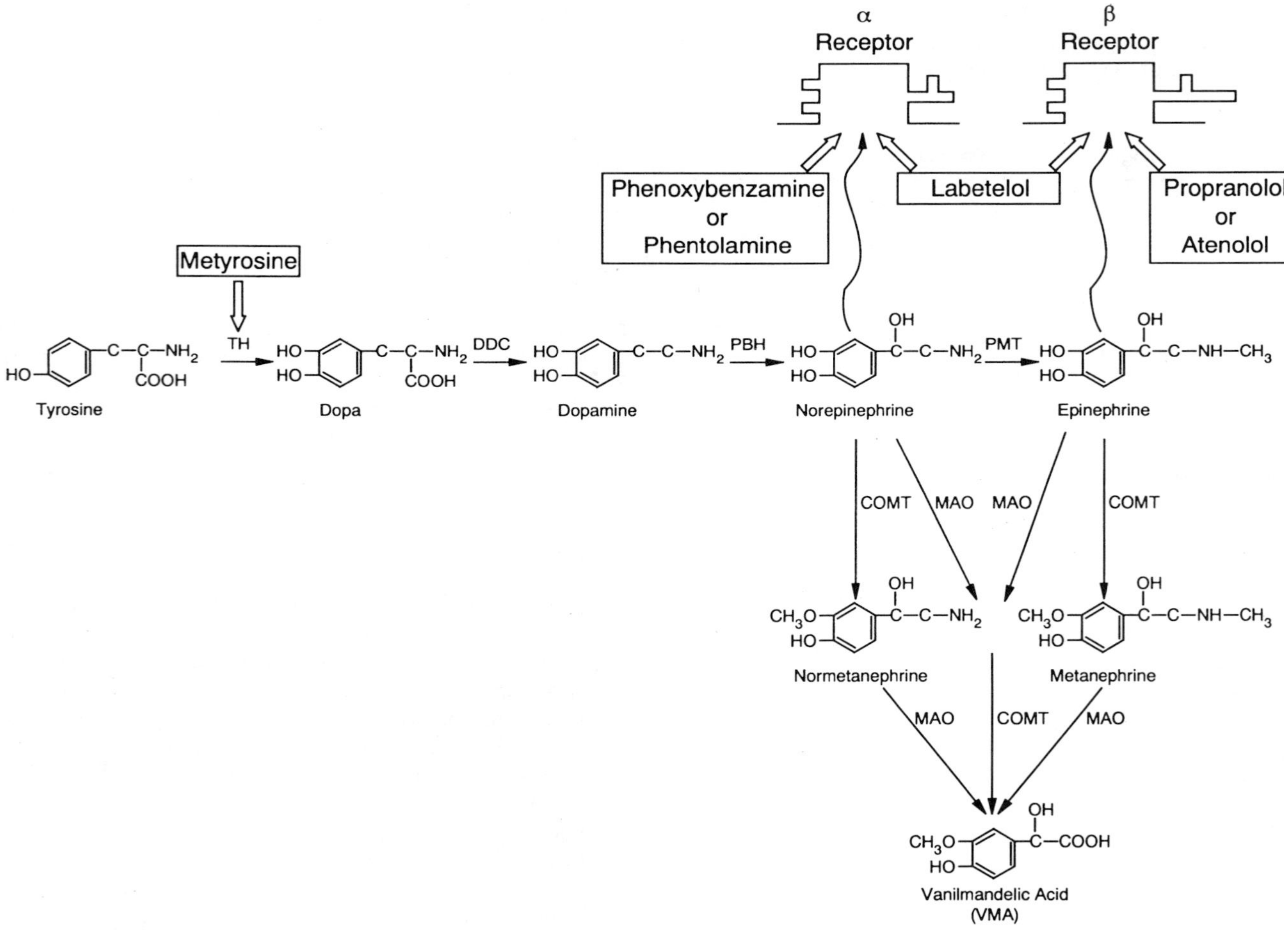

Figure 102.5. Synthetic and metabolic pathways for the catecholamines, norepinephrine and epinephrine, which are stored and secreted by chromaffin cells and pheochromocytomas. *Curved arrows*, physiologic agonist—receptor interaction. *Boxed arrows*, competitive antagonism at the rate-limiting step of synthesis or at receptor sites by therapeutic agents (see text). TH, tyrosine hydroxylase; DDC, dopa decarboxylase; PBH, phenylamine-β-hydroxylase; PMT, phenylethanolamine-*N*-methyltransferase; COMT, catechol-*O*-methyltransferase; MAO, monoamine oxidase.

peptides. A large number of these substances have been associated with pheochromocytoma, and they are often capable of producing specific clinical syndromes (Table 102.4) (55, 86, 104, 131, 166, 227, 240, 242, 296, 297, 305). Chromogranin A is a soluble binding protein found in the neurosecretory granule; it is the most prevalent biologic marker for pheochromocytoma (198). This marker is not specific, however, since it is also expressed in other neuroendocrine and non-endocrine neoplasms as well (109, 199, 269).

Neuropeptide Y is a peptide with potent vasoconstrictor activity. High neuropeptide Y immunoreactivity has been found in both benign and malignant pheochromocytomas (3, 97, 98, 108, 201); by far, the most important secretory products of pheochromocytomas are the biogenic amines (Fig. 102.5) (Table 102.4). The majority of these neoplasms secrete excess norepinephrine that results in sporadic or sustained hypertension (165). Epinephrine is the major catecholamine secreted by normal adrenal medulla, and it is frequently elevated in pheochromocytoma, especially in familial cases, but norepinephrine predominates in most tumors (35). Dopamine and the catecholamine precursor, dihydroxyphenylalanine (dopa), are also secreted by pheochromocytomas, and there is some evidence that high circulating levels of these norepinephrine precursors are more commonly associated with a malignant phenotype (90, 220).

DIAGNOSTIC TESTS

The fundamental basis for the diagnosis of pheochromocytoma is a high index of clinical suspicion with confirmation by biochemical determinations for catecholamines or catecholamine metabolites in blood or urine (22). The most common and reliable tests are the measurements of 24-hour urinary excretion for catecholamines, metanephrines, or vanillylmandelic acid (VMA) (Fig. 102.5) (35, 237). Urinary free catecholamine and metanephrines have higher sensitivity, but many medications can interfere with the measurements. More than 80% of patients with pheochromocytoma have urinary excretion of free catecholamines or metanephrines higher than twice the upper limit of normal. From 2 to 12% of all hypertensive patients have elevated urinary excretion, but patients without pheochromocytoma almost always have values less than twice the upper limit of normal (338). Spot (2-hour) urine specimens for metanephrines or plasma anorepinephrine are preferred by some authors, although these tests may be associated with a higher number of false positive and false negative outcomes (35, 214, 326, 338). Physiologic and pathologic fluctuations, such as anxiety and alcohol withdraw, can cause transient elevation of catecholamines. Conversely, blood taken during normotensive period in a patient with episodic hypertension may show normal or borderline levels of catecholamines. More sophisticated catecholamine metabolite assays have been proposed to increase the specificity of urinary determinations (36, 65, 126, 165, 319).

Bravo has suggested when the biochemical tests are diagnostically high, such as urinary metanephrines >3.0 mg/24 hours or plasma catecholamines >2000 pg/ml in hypertensive patients with typical symptoms, anatomical localization of the tumor should be carried out. In patients with borderline results, such as urinary metanephrines between 1.4 and 3.0 mg/24 hours or plasma catecholamines between 400 and 2000 pg/ml, pharmacological tests can be used to confirm the diagnosis. If patients are hypertensive and plasma catecholamines are more than 1000 pg/ml, a clonidine suppression test is preferred. Plasma catecholamines are sampled before and 3 hours after an oral dose of 0.3 mg of clonidine. Plasma catecholamines will fall below 500 pg/ml in patients with essential hypertension, but they do not fall in pheochromocytoma. Overnight urinary catecholamine determination after clonidine has also been used (339). Blood pressure needs to be monitored during the testing. Blood pressure will drop in both groups. For patients with mild hypertension or normotension and plasma catecholamines between 400 and 1000 pg/ml, a glucagon provocative test is preferred. Plasma catecholamines are sampled before and 1 to 3 minutes after injection of 1.0 to 2.0 mg of glucagon. A 3-fold increase in plasma catecholamines or values over 2000 pg/ml is diagnostic for pheochromocytoma. The rise of blood pressure can be prevented by prazocin or nifedipine given 1 hour before the glucagon injection (326).

For anatomic localization, angiography, selective venography, and intravenous pyelography now rarely have a role in the localization of pheochromocytoma because 90% of pheochromocytoma are located in the adrenal gland. CT scanning can visualize nearly all adrenal pheochromocytomas. Therefore, a CT scan should be conducted in all patients with a biochemical diagnosis of pheochromocytoma (336). Methyl-iodobenzylguanidine (MIBG) is a structural analogue of guanethidine and, as such, is readily taken up by the chromaffin cell and stored in neurosecretory granules (266). Experience reported in over 1,000 patients uniformly shows a sensitivity of approximately 90% and a specificity of

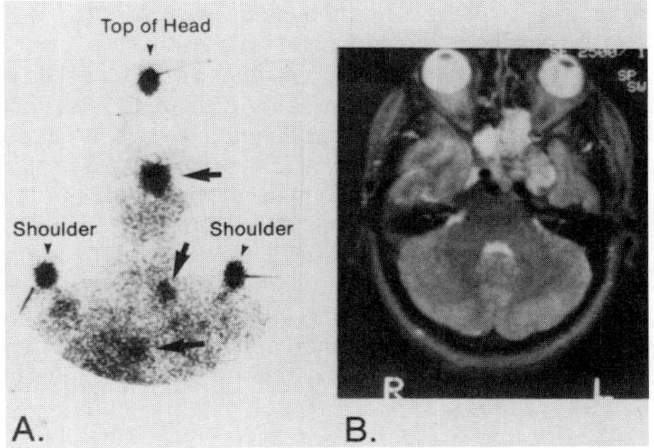

Figure 102.6. Diagnostic imaging in metastatic pheochromocytoma. **A.** Gamma camera image of the upper body of a patient 48 hours following injection of ^{131}I-metaiodobenzylguanidine. Areas of abnormal isotope uptake are noted at the base of the brain, the cervical region, and the mid-thoracic spine (*arrows*). **B.** T2-weighted magnetic resonance image of the same patient demonstrating a signal-intensive mass encroaching the circle of Willis, the left temporal lobe, and the left optic nerve.

nearly 100% (Fig.102.6*A*) (111, 237, 253, 254). As compared to CT and MRI, MIBG is at least as good as the other two modalities (294, 320). All patients should have an MIBG scan to confirm that the tumor seen in CT scan is a pheochromocytoma. In addition, extra-adrenal tumors, which are not well visualized in CT scans, can be picked up in an MIBG scan. The sensitivity of MIBG scanning may be considerably less in malignant pheochromocytoma, and its specificity is limited by the fact that MIBG is readily accumulated by other neuroendocrine tumors (111, 253, 298). Certain drugs (e.g., labetalol) may reduce the uptake of MIBG into the tumor's catecholamine storage vesicles, causing a false negative test (134, 253). Occasionally, the CT characteristics of size, contrast enhancement, and consistency may provide clues regarding the probability of malignancy (119). Because of the risk of catastrophic hemorrhage or hypertensive complications, fine-needle aspiration should not be attempted for cytologic diagnosis.

Although not possessing the resolution of CT, MRI may have a special role in the localization of pheochromocytomas. These tumors have a particularly intense detectable signal on T2-weighted magnetic resonance images, appearing as very bright spots compared to normal tissue (Fig. 102.6*B*) (67, 223). In addition, MRI reconstruction to demonstrate coronal or sagittal views of the tumor provide important preoperative anatomic information (74, 294). The MRI is probably not necessary for routine pheochromocytomas, but it should be used for localization in the case of malignant or extra-adrenal tumors, especially in the neck, mediastinum, liver, and retroperitoneum (246). Because of the high prevalence of bone metastases, a bone scan should be performed in patients thought to have metastatic disease, since this test has a higher sensitivity than MIBG for bone metastases (160). If the bone scan detects lesions in the axial skeleton, a spinal MRI may be considered to rule out early spinal cord compression.

Most pheochromocytomas express somatostatin receptors on the cell surface; therefore, these tumors can be shown in a ^{123}I-labeled octreotide scan (334). Like MIBG scan, many other neuroendocrine tumors also show positive uptake in an octreotide scan and thus limit its specificity. [^{11}C]Hydroxyepinephrine is a newly developed radiotracer that concentrates in adrenergic nerve terminals. Ninty percent of pheochromocytomas can be localized by a positron emission tomography (PET) scan using this agent (337). Malignant pheochromocytoma has also been reported to show up in thallium and gallium scans. The role of these new scans in clinical practice is undetermined. In summary, each of the methods for localization of pheochromocytoma described above are complementary; they should be employed in selective combination depending on individual circumstances (294).

DIFFERENTIAL DIAGNOSIS

There are many clinical situations and drugs that can alter catecholamine secretion and catabolism. Hypertension and elevated levels of catecholamines and their metabolites can be seen in anxiety, panic state, intracranial lesions, autonomic hyperreflexia, diencephalic seizure, eclampsia, use of monoamine oxidase inhibitors, decongestants, caffeine, diazoxide, vasodilators, theophylline, appetite suppressants, carcinoid, hypoglycemia, neuroblastoma, acute abdomen, alcohol or colonidine withdrawal, and acute coronary ischemia (326, 336).

THERAPEUTIC CONSIDERATIONS

Medical Management

The mainstay of preoperative pharmacological management is α-adrenergic blockade with phenoxybenzamine in doses ranging from 10 mg twice daily up to tolerable doses that will control blood pressure, allow for restitution of normal blood volume, and block catecholamine-induced gut hypomotility (Fig. 102.7) (35, 131, 184, 237, 274, 292). The major side effect is orthostatic hypotension, and reflex supraventricular tachycardias or arrhythmias may occur. The latter may be controlled with the addition of β-blocking agents such as propranolol, atenolol, or esmolol only after adequate α-blockade is established since unopposed β-blockade may worsen vasoconstriction and hypertension. Additional agents may need to be added or substituted for optimal management (22). These include α-blockers prazosin or terazosin (193), the combined α- and β-blocker labetolol (190), calcium channel antagonists (nifedipine or verapamil) (221), and the angiotensin-converting enzyme inhibitors (captopril or enalapril) (31). None of these agents has any particular advantages, and some have disadvantages, so their use depends on individual circumstances and the experience of the clinician. In severe hypertension, α-adrenergic blockade with intravenous phentolamine or vasodilation with nitroprusside may be used (117).

Metyrosine (α-methyl-paratyrosine) is a competitive inhibitor of the rate-limiting hydroxylation step of catecholamine synthesis, and it is used in addition to α- and β-adrenergic active agents to deplete tumor catecholamines and further reduce blood pressure before surgery or in patients who have failed standard treatment or whose tumor cannot be resected (Fig. 102.5) (22, 40). The starting dose is 250 mg four times daily, and it may be titrated up to 4 g per day. The central nervous system side effects of sedation, irritability, nightmares, sleep disturbance, and hallucinations are, however, often dose-limiting.

Surgical Management of Benign or Recurrent Resectable Disease

Nearly all benign pheochromocytomas can be cured by surgical resection. Because of its slow growth rate and accompanying significant morbidity, complete resection of local recurrence or limited metastases of malignant pheochromocytoma should be attempted. But the value of debulking surgery for patients whose tumor cannot be completely resected is not established (162, 248, 252, 255). Most soft tissue spread including some liver metastases is amenable to resection; the majority of patients with malignant pheochromocytoma also have bone metastases as well (14, 160).

Traditionally, all patients, regardless of blood pressure readings, would be prepared with an α-blocking agent or calcium channel blocker (221) as described above to con-

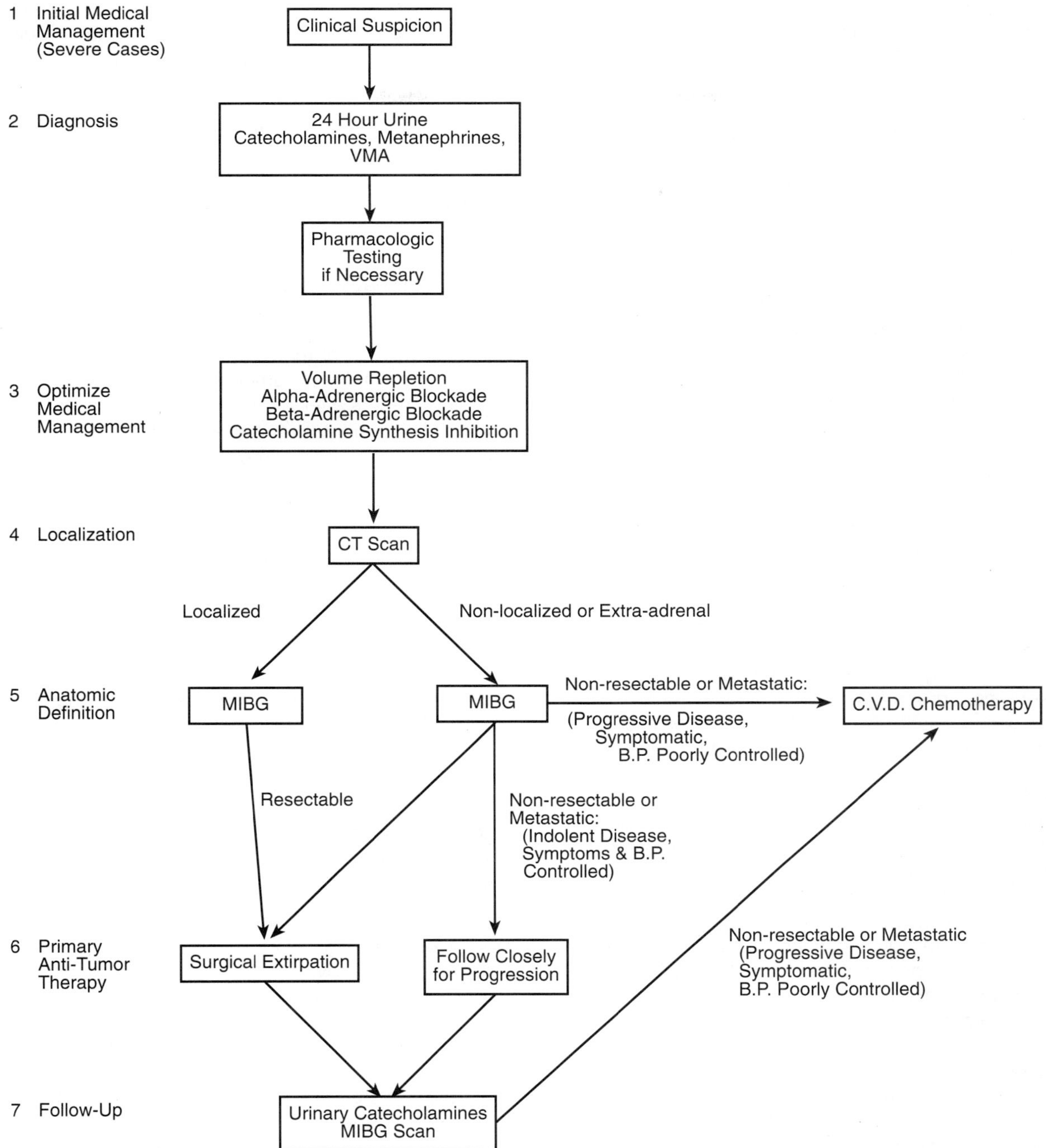

Figure 102.7. Algorithm for the diagnosis and management of pheochromocytoma.

trol blood pressure preoperatively. Induction of general anesthesia and manipulation of the tumor may provoke a release of massive amounts of catecholamines, making prior receptor blockade important. In addition, most patients have significant reduction of intravascular fluid volume, and α-blockade permits volume reexpansion. The administration of a β-blocker may not always be necessary but clearly should be given if the patient has tachycardia, arrhythmia, or a catecholamine profile showing a preponderance of epinephrine secretion. One approach is to give propranolol to most patients for 48 hours preoperatively, beginning with a dose of 10 mg four times a day. Propranolol and phenoxybenzamine may be given with a sip of water early on the morning of operation. The caveat of this approach is that it will be more difficult for surgeons to find other occult pheochromocytomas, because the clues of residual tumor, i.e. persistent hypertension after resection and hypertensive response during exploration of the abdomen after tumor removal, are abolished by pre-operative preparation. With advancement in anesthesiology and intra-operative monitoring, some surgeons prefer not to prepare patients for operation with an α-adrenergic blocker. The morbidity and mortality seem to be comparable in a major center (342).

The operative approach is determined by the location of the tumor(s) as determined by preoperative imaging investigations. For intra-abdominal pheochromocytomas, an anterior approach through a bucket handle or chevron upper abdominal approach is used to permit exploration of both adrenal glands and a thorough examination of the retroperitoneum for possible occult extra-adrenal pheochromocytomas with the least amount of manipulation (35, 50, 94, 131, 184, 248, 292). For MEN 2 patients, bilateral disease is common. Bilateral total adrenalectomy is associated with a lifelong requirement to manage adrenal insufficiency. In addition, malignant pheochromocytoma is very rare in MEN 2. Therefore, unilateral or bilateral subtotal resection with preservation of adrenocortical function can be considered in this population. For the control of hypertension intraoperatively, the rapidly acting direct vasodilating agent, sodium nitroprusside, nitroglycerin, phentolamine, nicardipine, or labetalol may be used intravenously as a drip when the systolic blood pressure exceeds 160 mm of Hg. The rate of infusion can be readily titrated to maintain the pressure at this level or lower. For cardiac arrhythmia or tachycardia, short acting esmolol or lidocaine is preferred. After the removal of the tumor, there may be an increase in the intravascular capacity and an acute fall in blood pressure that is best managed by intravenous fluid replacement rather than vasopressor drugs (24, 50, 252). Rarely, if the patient has been well prepared, an intravenous infusion of norepinephrine may be required while volume is being restored. Transient hypoglycemia can occur after surgery because of increased insulin secretion secondary to high circulating catecholamines. Blood sugar should be monitored postoperatively.

During operative manipulation of a pheochromocytoma, great care and gentleness are required not only to avoid episodes of severe hypertension but to avoid disruption of the tumor capsule. Malignancy cannot be determined either by the gross appearance or by histopathologic studies of the primary tumor in most cases. Some patients with proven malignant pheochromoctyoma as determined by bone, liver, or lung metastases have had well-encapsulated tumors without evidence of invasion or lymph node involvement. Capsular disruption by application of instruments or rough handling can result in implantation of tumor cells even when the neoplasm is considered benign.

Most patients become normotensive after resection of pheochromocytoma, but some remain hypertensive. Urinary or plasma catecholamines or metabolites should be checked 2 weeks after surgery. If test results are normal, these patients may have concurrent essential hypertension. Otherwise, residual tumors are likely to be present (326). The median time for recurrence following primary resection of malignant pheochromocytoma is approximately 6 years and may be as long as 20 years (26, 160, 224, 247). The lack of discriminating features of malignancy makes lifetime follow-up necessary for all patients (291). The follow-up consists of clinical and biochemical assessment several times during the first year and then a yearly test of urine catecholamines (26, 35, 162, 184, 247, 252, 271, 291). Patients with extra-adrenal primaries or non-diploid tumors may require more frequent follow-up with urine catecholamines and perhaps an MIBG scan (255).

Pheochromocytoma during pregnancy requires special considerations (68, 103). In general, if diagnosed in the first or second trimester, surgical removal of the tumor is indicated following medical preoperative preparation. If diagnosed in the third trimester, medical management is indicated, combined with Cesarean delivery of the mature fetus.

Medical Treatment of Recurrent or Metastatic Disease

The diagnosis of malignant pheochromocytoma can be made only when the tumor is locally invasive and unresectable, recurs after primary extirpation, or is found to be metastatic. Although the natural history of the disease in each of these situations may be variable and somewhat unpredictable, advanced malignant pheochromocytoma is associated with a high morbidity and mortality (14, 99, 142, 153, 224, 248, 292). These cancers also secrete catecholamines and often produce biogenic amines at a level much higher than benign neoplasms. Thus, the blood pressure elevations, cardiac effects, decreased bowel motility, and other clinical complications of catecholamine excess may be severe and unrelenting. The management of these problems utilizes the same principles of pharmacologic adrenergic blockade and inhibition of catecholamine synthesis described previously.

The rarity and highly variable natural history of malignant pheochromocytoma preclude determining accurate survival estimates. Analysis of SEER data demonstrated a 5-year relative survival rate of 52% with a median survival time of 4 years (14a). Three retrospective analyses with a long duration of patient follow-up reported a 5-year survival rate of 60, 32, and 44%, respectively (99, 122, 224). A recent series of 22 patients treated at the National Institutes of Health and the Mount Sinai Medical Center had a 5-year survival rate of 66% with a median survival time of 74 months from the time of initial diagnosis of pheochromocytoma (Fig. 102.8) (14a). All of these studies demonstrate that a significant number of patients with disseminated disease may live for long periods without specific antineoplastic therapy (38, 255). Overall, it appears that there are two distinct subsets within the population of patients with malignant pheochromocytoma: a group with aggressive disease that leads to early death (within 3 or 4 years) and a group with indolent disease that is compatible with long-term survival (up to 20 or more years) (Fig. 102.8) (224, 292).

From the Mayo Clinic series, it appears that survival has not changed over the past several decades despite advances in diagnosis, localization, and pharmacotherapy of catecholamine excess (224, 292). Surgical debulking of malignant pheochromocytomas that cannot be completely extirpated is controversial and carries a certain operative risk without clear benefit (162, 248, 252, 255). The results of standard external beam radiation therapy for malignant pheochromocytoma have been limited to reports from a small series of selected patients treated with a variety of

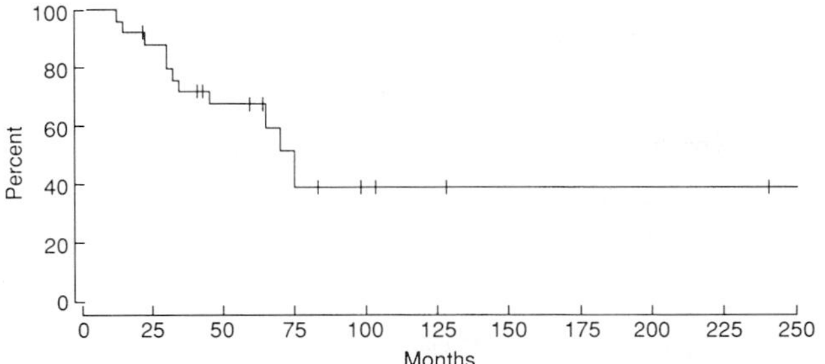

Figure 102.8. Actuarial survival of 22 patients with malignant pheochromocytoma from the time of surgical diagnosis.

techniques (Table 102.5) (64, 248, 257). In general, these data do not support the use of this modality except for palliation of painful bony metastases or spinal cord compression.

Targeted radiotherapy using high specific activity MIBG has been extensively investigated at the University of Michigan (252). Because of the specificity of MIBG uptake by chromaffin tumors, this novel therapeutic approach initially generated much interest; in practice it was found that the majority of patients with malignant pheochromocytoma do not take up and retain sufficient MIBG to deliver an effective radiation dose to the tumor (132, 164, 255). In their initial 63 patients screened with a tracer dose of MIBG, only 18 had sufficient uptake to permit therapeutic dosing, i.e. where between 100 and 250 mCi of MIBG will deliver 20 Gy to the tumor (254). Out of a total of 28 patients treated by the Michigan group, 8 patients had tumor and biochemical responses, with most responses requiring several months and repeated dosing to become manifest. The duration of benefit has been short (252, 253). Other investigators have reported similar results in highly selected patients (Table 102.5) (91, 111, 283, 289, 295, 330). The cause for the insufficient uptake of MIBG for therapy by malignant chromaffin neoplasms is not fully understood, but it may be due to the fact that these neoplasms may have a less differentiated amine uptake and storage phenotype compared to benign and normal chromaffin cells (90). Methods for accurate calculation of absorbed radiation dose are under development (137), and experimental models may provide new approaches to modulating tumor cell uptake of MIBG (30); but until such time as this and other difficulties are overcome, high dose MIBG for the treatment of pheochromocytoma has little clinical utility.

Until 1985, the data regarding standard systemic chemotherapy was limited to reports of empirically chosen single agents or combinations in small retrospective series and in anecdotal cases (64, 248). Because of its activity against gastroenteropancreatic tumors, streptozotocin was given to patients with metastatic pheochromocytoma with documented responses in some (73) but not others (Table 102.5) (101). Based on the premise that malignant pheochromocytoma and neuroblastoma are two APUD neoplasms that have many clinicopathologic features in common (90, 299), a regimen highly effective in children with advanced neuroblastoma (75, 132), was adapted for use in malignant pheochromocytoma. This regimen, a combination of cyclophosphamide, vincristine, and dacarbazine (CVD) was used in treatment of 23 patients with advanced, progressive and symptomatic pheochromocytoma at the National Cancer Institute and Mount Sinai Medical Center (13, 14). There were 2 (9%) complete and 12 (52%) partial tumor remissions for a median duration of more than 22 months. Improvement in hypertension, reduction in requirement for antihypertensive medication, and improvement in overall performance status correlated well with complete and partial biochemical responses in 17 (74%) of the patients. Toxicity included moderate nausea and vomiting, myelosuppression, and mild neurotoxicity. Some moderate degree of postural hypotension developed that responded promptly to volume replacement therapy (14). Major hemodynamic side effects from chemotherapy were observed in two patients with paroxysmal hypertension. The lack of hypertensive events in most patients is probably due to the fact that patients were prepared with adequate volume repletion and pharmacologic adrenergic blockade prior to initiating chemotherapy. Since hypertensive episodes with release of stored catecholamine have been observed following chemotherapy (14a, 59, 279), patients need to be prepared as if for surgery, and they require close monitoring during their initial chemotherapy treatment. Patients with paroxysmal hypertension often present with unique problems because they cannot tolerate a full dose of antihypertensives. These antihypertensives lower their base-line blood pressure and worsen their orthostatic hypotension. Two patients in our series developed hypertensive crises and severe ileus after CVD treatment. This problem resolved after optimizing

Table 102.5. Treatment of Malignant Pheochromocytoma

	No. patients	Tumor response	Biochemical response	Palliation	Reference
Radiation therapy					
External beam	42	—	—	19	37, 52, 64, 91, 99, 111, 247
Targets ^{131}I-MIBG	78	23	31	4	253, 283, 289, 295, 330
Chemotherapy					
Streptozotocin ± misc. agents	7	1	1	1	73, 101, 153, 248
Cyclophosphamide + vincristine + dacarbazine	23	14	17	—	13, 14, 235, 257
Cyclophosphamide ± misc. agents	19	2	2	7	43, 64, 153, 248, 257
Platinum analogs ± doxorubicin	4	0	0	—	123, 272

the antihypertensive regimens and adding metyrosine to deplete catecholamine storage (341).

The CVD study is the largest prospectively studied chemotherapy series in malignant pheochromocytoma. The results have been confirmed by additional clinical experience (13, 235, 257). Thus, CVD should be the treatment of choice for symptomatic, disseminated pheochromocytoma. With the introduction of colony-stimulating factors and newer antiemetics, dose escalation of CVD can be explored. Recent experience in neuroblastoma, where CVD has been replaced by the use of new agents and more intensive regimens (219), provides a basis for possible extrapolation to pheochromocytoma in future clinical trials.

There is no information regarding the activity of interferon in malignant pheochromocytoma despite its reported activity in other neuroendocrine tumors (204). The somatostatin analogue, octreotide acetate, has been reported to produce symptomatic response in patients with endocrine syndromes caused by peptide-secreting pheochromocytomas (104).

Multiple Endocrine Neoplasia (MEN) Syndromes

There are three distinct MEN syndromes and non-MEN familial medullary thyroid carcinoma (Table 102.6) that share two characteristics common to neuroendocrine neoplasms: (1) the tumors comprising MEN syndromes arise from amine precursor uptake and decarboxylation (APUD) neuroendocrine cells and (2) the syndromes are each inherited as an autosomal dominant trait. This second feature provides for a molecular diagnosis of affected individuals, and it has led to the recent recognition of specific genetic defects that will enable a fundamental understanding of the pathogenesis of these tumors.

MULTIPLE ENDOCRINE NEOPLASIA TYPE 1

Epidemiology

MEN 1 syndrome is quite rare, with an estimated prevalence of between 0.02 and 0.2 per thousand and an incidence of 0.25% as determined from randomly chosen postmortem studies (33, 66, 282). However, the importance of this syndrome is related to its autosomal dominant hereditary pattern with high penetrance (Fig. 102.9). Approximately one-third of patients with gastrinomas are associated with MEN 1 (see Chapter 103) (70, 80, 146, 285). In contrast, insulinomas are usually sporadic, and fewer than 5% are found in MEN 1 patients (116).

Table 102.6. Multiple Endocrine Neoplasia Syndromes

Type	Affected organs or tumor	Genetic loci
1	Pituitary Parathyroid Endocrine pancreas	11q13
2a	Parathyroid Medullary thyroid Pheochromocytoma	10
2b	Medullary thyroid Pheochromocytoma Mucosal ganglioneuromas	10
Non-MEN familial medullary thyroid cancer	Medullary thyroid	10

Pathologic Characteristics

MEN 1 is characterized by hyperplasia and/or neoplasms of the pituitary, parathyroid, and pancreatic islets. Hyperparathyroidism occurs in 90% of patients, pituitary adenomas in 40% of patients, and endocrine pancreatic tumors in 60% of patients (66, 205, 238).

Although the parathyroid glands are the most frequently involved organs (90%) (282) and hyperparathyroidism is usually the first manifestation of the syndrome, its presence may not be detected until clinical disease of the pituitary or pancreas has brought the patient to medical attention. Hyperparathyroidism is often found during the second decade of life when screening immediate family members of those with proven MEN 1. In adults first suspected of the MEN 1 syndrome because of manifestations of gastrinoma, hyperparathyroidism is often diagnosed after obtaining serum calcium and parathyroid hormone levels, even though such patients may have had a decade-long history of renal stones.

MEN 1 patients characteristically have multiglandular nodular hyperplasia as the cause of their hyperparathyroidism. Often, the individual gland involvement is variable and is best described as asymmetrical hyperplasia, resulting in enlargement of only one or two glands, particularly in younger patients. This disease usually takes a slow but progressive course, and eventually all glands are involved.

The most frequent manifestation of MEN 1 pancreatic involvement is gastrinoma, usually developing during the third or fourth decade of life. With biochemical screening of MEN 1 kindreds, pancreatic abnormalities have been found at a much earlier age and often become the first manifestation of the syndrome (346, 359). Gastrinomas in the MEN 1 syndrome are typically small, multiple adenomas of the endocrine pancreas or duodenum (213) that produce excess gastrin, causing gastric hyperacidity and multiple peptic ulcerations, classically known as the Zollinger-Ellison syndrome (see Chapter 103) (318). The malignant potential of MEN 1-associated gastrinomas is probably less than sporadic tumors. Additional tumors found are vasoactive intestinal polypeptidomas (VIPomas), glucagonomas, somatostatinomas, and pancreatic polypeptidomas (PPomas) (317).In some MEN 1 patients, tumors may develop and even metastasize to lymph nodes or liver with no clinical manifestations whatsoever. In others, more than one clinical functional syndrome may develop in the same patient either synchronously or more often metachronously.

Immunohistochemical studies of the pancreas from MEN 1 patients have shown that most tumors that stain positively for gastrin are in the head, uncinate process, or duodenum (285). Many of the larger tumors in the body or tail of the pancreas in gastrinoma patients stain positively only for hor-

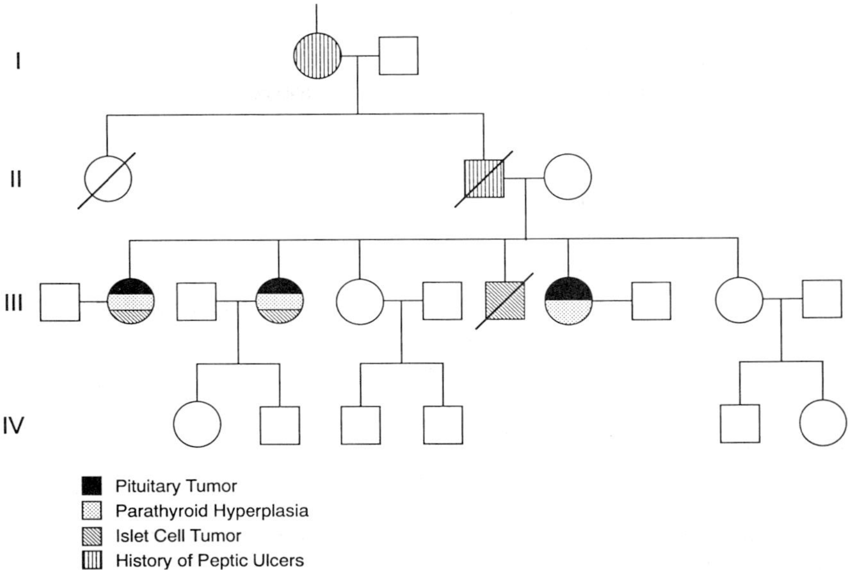

Figure 102.9. Pedigree of a typical kindred with MEN type 1 (reproduced with permission from Samaan et al. (238)).

mones such as pancreatic polypeptide and somatostatin. Furthermore, even though islet-cell dysplasia (nesidioblastosis, hyperplasia, microadenomas) was found in all cases, these cells failed to stain positively for either gastrin or insulin. Therefore, when serum gastrin is elevated, the disease is in a more advanced stage, and at least 50% of patients have metastases already (359). Discrete tumors rather than diffuse islet-cell disease are usually present in patients with clinical syndromes (194, 293). The subsequent use of selective venous sampling for gastrin, insulin, or other hormones in MEN 1 patients has supported this thesis (88). It has also become apparent that gastrinomas are most likely to develop in the duodenum in MEN 1 patients (213). These tumors may be multiple, and in some cases they may be associated with pancreatic gastrinomas.

Micro- or macroadenomas of the pituitary gland are commonly detected in MEN 1 patients when biochemical and imaging studies have been performed (33, 66). Most tumors are functionally active and secrete prolactin (352). Less frequently, MEN 1 patients may develop tumor-secreting ACTH or growth hormone and present with Cushing's syndrome or acromegaly. In the MEN 1 patient it is especially important to establish that the Cushing's syndrome is pituitary dependent (Cushing's disease) rather than caused by an adrenal adenoma or the ectopic secretion of ACTH or corticotropin-releasing factor (CRF) from islet-cell tumors or a bronchial carcinoid tumor.

Patients with MEN 1 syndrome have an increased frequency of both functional and non-functional adrenal cortical hyperplasia or adenomas (18, 116, 173, 244). Furthermore, there may be an increased frequency of adrenal cortical carcinoma in MEN 1 patients, although only five cases have been well documented.

Carcinoid tumors have been reported more frequently in MEN 1 patients than would be expected (71). Male patients appear to have a predilection for developing carcinoid tumors within the thymus, whereas bronchial carcinoids occur almost exclusively in women. Gastric carcinoids can develop in MEN 1 patients with Zollinger-Ellison syndrome who are on long-term H2 blocker or omeprazole (347).

Biologic Characteristics

The MEN 1 gene locus has been mapped to the long arm of chromosome 11 (11q13) (149). By using restriction fragment length polymorphism (RFLPs) and microsatellite polymorphisms from affected kindreds, MEN 1 gene carriers in the family can be identified with a predictive accuracy of 99.5%. When compared with leukocyte DNA, endocrine tumors from MEN 1 patients have loss of heterozygosity (LOH) at the region of chromosome 11q13 (17, 33, 45, 79, 281, 345, 347). The allele lost is always from the normal chromosome belonging to the unaffected parent. This is analogous to the second hit in retinoblastoma. The gene involved in MEN 1, although not identified yet, is most likely a tumor suppressor gene. Adrenal adenomas are exceptions because they do not have LOH at chromosome 11q13. Furthermore, they occur only in patients with pancreatic endocrine tumors. This suggests adrenal hyperplasia and adenoma are secondary to other endocrine abnormalities (359). Deletion at chromosome 11q13 has also been found in a significant portion of sporadic adenomas of parathyroid gland, pancreas, and pituitary gland (345, 353). The gene or genes in this region certainly play an important role in endocrine tumorigenesis, either familial or sporadic. In addition to chromosome 11, other chromosomes and genetic changes may also be involved, such as PRAD 1 in parathyroid adenoma and G_s α-chain gene in pituitary adenoma (345, 353).

Clinical Features

The clinical features of patients with MEN 1 depend entirely upon expression of the natural history of the individual tumor and endocrine hyperfunction. Most patients with MEN

1 pancreatic disease requiring surgical intervention present with a syndrome caused by hypersecretion of a specific hormone such as gastrin, insulin, VIP, or glucagon (205, 238). However, in some patients a tumor may be detected by imaging studies obtained after serum laboratory studies have shown an elevation of one or more hormones such as pancreatic polypeptide or somatostatin. Overall, patients with familial MEN 1 neoplasms have long survival that is significantly better than that for patients with sporadic endocrine pancreatic tumors (205, 238).

Diagnostic and Screening Tests

A patient presenting with hyperparathyroidism or with hypergastrinemia should be questioned carefully regarding a family history of MEN 1 syndrome (169). In patients without family history, the diagnosis of MEN 1 can be made only by repeated biochemical testing to screen for other endocrine abnormalities. DNA analysis cannot be applied because it requires DNA from at least two affected family members to conclude which allele of the marker is inherited with the MEN 1 gene. But this limitation will no longer exist when the gene is cloned in the future. Once MEN 1 is diagnosed in a proband, all family members should undergo biochemical screening. Because endocrine abnormalities occur at different time points in different carriers, biochemical screening needs to be repeated for many years. Depending on the extensiveness of the screening program, the yield can be quite different. In one program, only 44% of gene carriers are identified at age 20 (360). With more extensive screening, 100% of gene carriers can be identified at age 25 (358), whereas in known MEN 1 kindreds, genetic screening with restriction fragment length polymorphisms (RFLPs) detects 99.5% of gene carriers at birth (359, 360). Only those who carry the mutated allele need to undergo yearly biochemical screening from childhood and continue for life. Peptic ulcer, renal complications, and malignant tumors are the common causes of death in MEN 1 patients (363). Early detection and early treatment of endocrine abnormalities as the result of screening will reduce morbidity and possibly mortality from endocrinopathy.

The biochemical screening program that gives the highest yield includes PTH, albumin-corrected total serum calcium, prolactin, somatomedin C, blood glucose, insulin, proinsulin, gastrin, pancreatic polypeptide (PP), glucagon, and a meal test with PP and gastrin analysis. Radiologic examination of pituitary gland and upper abdomen can be done once every 3 to 5 years (359). The diagnostic approach to MEN 1 patients is determined by a clinical syndrome or clearly elevated hormone level. Hyperparathyroidism is diagnosed by hypercalcemia with elevated or non-suppressible PTH value. Pituitary adenomas usually have elevated serum prolactin or somatomedin C. The tumors are best visualized by MRI. Gastrinoma can be confirmed by measurements of basal and stimulated gastric acid output and provocative test with calcium or secretin. Insulinoma can be diagnosed by increased insulin and proinsulin level in the presence of hypoglycemia.

Localization procedures (see Chapter 103) for pancreatic endocrine tumors in MEN 1 syndrome present a special challenge due to their small size, multiplicity, and tendency to be malignant. However, this procedure is particularly important since complete excision of all tumors and cure are achievable (184, 284, 293). Sonography, CT scan, and arteriography are successful in less than 50% of patients (348). Endoscopic ultrasound has been shown to be much more sensitive and specific. Tumors as small as 0.5 cm can be identified (357). Calcium and secretin angiography and transhepatic venous sampling can be used for occult tumors not imaged with other modalities (350). ^{123}I-Octreotide scan may be helpful (351). Intraoperative ultrasound of the pancreas should be used to locate nonpalpable tumors. Gastrinomas commonly occur in the duodenum, which can elude all imaging studies (361). Intraoperative transduodenal endoscopic illumination may help to identify the tumor during exploration.

Therapeutic Considerations

Generally, the management of patients with MEN 1 is the same as for each sporadic tumor comprising the syndrome. Even when distant metastases are present, systemic chemotherapy is rarely indicated in this syndrome. The elements of the management of patients with MEN 1 may include surgical removal of all four parathyroid glands (transplanting a portion of one of the glands to the forearm), subtotal pancreatectomy (removing as many multifocal tumors as possible in patients with endocrine pancreatic tumors), and medical management of pituitary adenomas with bromocriptine for prolactinomas and octreotide for acromegaly.

The surgical treatment of the MEN 1 syndrome is dependent on the genetic expression in the individual patient. Because components of the syndrome may be metachronous, surgical procedures involving different endocrine organs may be required over a period of many years. Regardless of initial findings, MEN 1 patients must be followed for life for involvement of the pituitary gland, the parathryoid glands, the endocrine pancreas or duodenum, the adrenal glands, the thymus, and the lungs (bronchial carcinoids). Hypercalcemia in MEN 1 usually is subtle and nonaggressive; early intervention is not necessary except in patients with gastrinoma because calcium increases gastrin secretion and worsens peptic ulcer disease. A source of persistent or recurrent disease is an overlooked supernumerary parathyroid gland, which is found most commonly in the upper thymus in 6 to 15%. Because of this, cervical thymectomy is considered an essential component of an adequate neck exploration in the MEN 1 patient (57). A common approach is subtotal parathyroidectomy, which leaves only a small remnant gland in place. Transient hypocalcemia is the desired result of these procedures, and if it does not occur, it usually means a supernumerary gland has been overlooked and recurrence is likely. If properly performed, oral calcium and vitamin D therapy can usually be tapered and discontinued within weeks. If performed correctly, permanent hypocalcemia should not develop. Although recurrent hypercalcemia may occur in patients after 10 years, successful surgical management is accomplished by trimming the hypertrophied remnant back to 50 mg (53).

An alternative treatment, strongly advocated by some authors because of a recurrence rate as high as 40% after subtotal parathyroidectomy, is total parathyroidectomy, cervical thymectomy, forearm muscle autografting, and cryopreservation of parathyroid tissue for possible future need (218, 308). This operation requires just as thorough a cervical-mediastinal exploration as in subtotal parathyroidectomy to prevent cervical recurrence. Its advantage is that should recurrence develop from arm graft overgrowth, trimming back the implanted tissue can be performed under a local anesthesia. Its disadvantage is that all patients will require complete replacement therapy (vitamin D and oral calcium) for 3 months or longer, and some may be rendered permanently hypoparathyroid unless a subsequent thawed, cryopreserved transplant is successful. Both of these procedures are currently widely used in managing MEN 1 patients with hyperparathyroidism.

The surgical treatment of MEN 1 pancreatic disease is controversial (194, 293, 362). One of the major issues centers on the fact that virtually all patients with pancreatic disease have a diffuse islet-cell dysplasia expressed as nesidioblastosis, islet-cell hyperplasia, microadenomatosis, and/or benign or malignant islet-cell tumors. As a result, it can be concluded that a cure of the pancreatic disease can only be achieved by a total pancreatectomy. However, the malignant potential of MEN 1 islet-cell neoplasm is relatively low, and with current medical therapy, there is little justification for total pancreatectomy either because of hormone hypersecretion or potential malignancy. In contrast, there is accumulating evidence that the majority of duodenal gastrinomas are malignant and lymph node and/or hepatic metastases from them develop in most patients if followed for a long enough period (356, 361). Similarly, other functional and non-functional gastroenteropancreatic neuroendocrine neoplasms may have malignant potential (See Chapter 103).

By a combination of preoperative localization and thorough exploration of both the pancreas and the duodenum, selected MEN 1 patients with hypergastrinemia can be rendered eugastrinemic, avoiding the necessity for either long-term drug therapy or total gastrectomy (194, 284, 293). In patients with either insulinomas or gastrinomas, a distal pancreatectomy is performed, in most cases preserving the spleen, followed by a complete exploration of the remaining pancreatic head, uncinate process, and peri-pancreatic lymph nodes (284). Any tumor found in the head or uncinate process by palpation or intraoperative ultrasound is enucleated. In all patients with gastrinoma, a longitudinal duodenotomy is made, and the mucosa from the pylorus to the third portion is evaginated into the incision and carefully palpated for submucosal tumors, which may be as small as 1 to 2 mm. When present, they are locally excised as are any lymph nodes in their drainage area (286). Using this approach, we have been able to achieve eugastrinemia in 12 patients with gastrinoma since 1978 (284). Of significance is the fact that more than one-half have had at least one peri-pancreatic lymph node involved with metastases, although primary tumors were as small as 2 mm in diameter. Even though some of these patients have subsequently shown a positive response to secretin stimulation, they have not required drug therapy or gastric operations. For patients with persistent, symptomatic hypergastrinemia from unresectable or metastatic gastrinoma, medical therapy with histamine-2 blockers or proton-pump inhibitors is indicated (174).

MEN 1 patients with hyperinsulinism usually have had more than one tumor-secreting insulin. However, they are confined to the pancreas, and when all are enucleated or excised (distal pancreatectomy), the syndrome is cured and recurrences appear to be rare. Octreotide may be useful to palliate symptoms resulting from VIPoma, gastrinoma, glucagonoma, and carcinoid (316). Streptozocin plus doxorubicin achieved the best response in patients with unresectable, progressive malignant tumors (354). Symptomatic hepatic-dominant metastases can be palliated with surgical debulking or chemoembolization (355).

Prolactinoma should be treated with bromocriptine or other dopamine analogues first. Both prolactin level and tumor size will decrease in most patients. Transphenoidal hypophysectomy is reserved for patients who fail to respond to medical therapy, but surgery is the treatment of choice for GH-secreting adenoma. Octreotide reduces tumor size and circulating GH and somatomedin C levels in a significant portion of patients (349). Cushing's disease is best treated by transphenoidal hypophysectomy. Radiation, either limited sellar field or stereotaxic, can be used in patients who failed other modalities, but hormone level decreases very slowly, and hypopituitarism is common after conventional radiation (352).

Surgical resection is indicated for carcinoid tumors. Unfortunately, the thymic carcinoids have usually been too far advanced when detected to allow for total excision and have been the cause of death in those with this tumor. Periodic mediastinal and chest CT scans should be used routinely in the follow-up of MEN 1 patients.

MULTIPLE ENDOCRINE NEOPLASIA 2A, 2B, AND NON-MEN FAMILIAL MEDULLARY THYROID CARCINOMA

Epidemiology

All three syndromes have autosomal transmission patterns (Figure 102.10). Children of affected individuals have a 50% chance of inheriting the genetic abnormality with virtually 100% penetrance by biochemical screening, although only 60 to 70% manifest apparent clinical symptoms (282, 366). From the German *MTC* (Medullary Thyroid Cancer) registry, nearly 25% of patients have one of these familial syndromes. Two-thirds have MEN 2a , and the rest have non-MEN FMTC or MEN 2b (372). Five to twenty-three percent of all pheochromocytoma patients also have a familial disorder (327, 372), mostly either Von Hippel-Lindau disease or MEN 2. The syndromes have been described in virtually all ethnic groups throughout the world, and an appreciation of the genetic inheritance patterns has provided effective screening methods to direct early treatment to reduce morbidity and mortality in affected individuals (Figure 102.3).

Pathologic Characteristics

MEN 2a involves patients with virtually a 100% incidence of C-cell hyperplasia or medullary thyroid carcinoma (MTC), a 50% incidence of clinically significant, usually bilateral

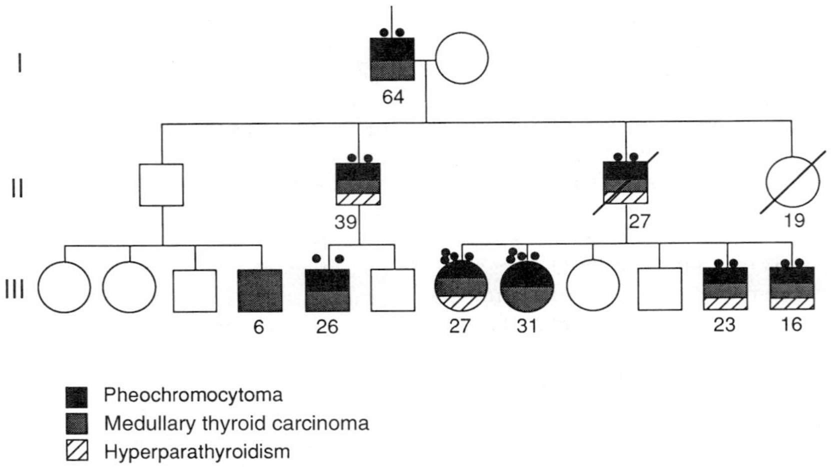

Figure 102.10. Pedigree of a typical kindred with MEN type 2a. Solid circles, number of pheochromocytomas found at surgery (courtesy of D. Pertsemlidis, Mount Sinai School of Medicine).

pheochromocytomas and 20 to 30% incidence of parathyroid adenomas with associated hyperparathyroidism. This syndrome always involves autosomal dominant transmission. A second syndrome, MEN 2b, as for MEN 2a, has 100% incidence of MTC and frequent pheochromocytomas. In addition, however, they have a characteristic physical appearance at birth or shortly after due to multiple neural defects including mucosal neuromas of the eyelids, lips, and tongue (135, 312). These patients also have a marfanoid habitus with hyperflexible joints but no lens or aortic abnormalities. The neural abnormalities also include widespread ganglioneuromatosis of the gastrointestinal tract leading to abnormal gut motility. Thus, even as infants or young children, patients with MEN 2b may have diarrhea, constipation, or may present with the clinical picture of megacolon. Patients with MEN 2b seldom have hyperparathyroidism.

The third and most recently defined form of genetic MTC is non-MEN MTC (72). Patients have MTC but no other associated endocrine or neural tissue involvement.

The major differences in the clinical pathology of MTC and pheochromocytomas in the MEN and familial syndromes, as compared to the sporadic forms of these tumors, involve the multifocality of the lesions, the presence of hyperplastic states as precursors to frank tumors, and the different clinical behavior of the tumors in each genetic disease.

Patients diagnosed as having genetic forms of MTC may manifest bilateral C-cell hyperplasia in the thyroid as the sole lesion or in association with frank MTC. Immunostaining of calcitonin is essential in making this diagnosis (Figure 102.3) since the hyperplasia may not be apparent on routine histologic examination. Patients diagnosed early may also have multifocal microscopic MTC diagnosed with such immunostaining. C-cell hyperplasia and microscopic MTC are the only stages of this cancer consistently curable by total thyroidectomy (20, 84). Similarly, patients with MEN 2a or 2b have a stage of adrenal hyperplasia that precedes development of pheochromocytomas. The clinical significance and management of this early condition is controversial.

Biological Characteristics

The biological properties of MTC, pheochromocytoma, and parathyroid neoplasms in the MEN syndromes are similar to those for each of the sporadic forms of these lesions described earlier. The gene for all three diseases has been identified to be RET proto-oncogene at the centromeric region of chromosome 10 (324, 328, 343, 344). RET proto-oncogene is a transmembrane tyrosine kinase. Its ligand and substrate have not been identified yet. MEN 2a and non-MEN FMTC have point mutations at one of the five cysteine residues in the extracellular domain. Eighty percent of MEN 2a and 50% of non-MEN FMTC have the mutation at codon 634 (370). MEN 2b has point mutation in the intracellular kinase catalytic domain, and most instances involve substitution of threonine for a methionine at codon 918 (328). All MEN 2a families studied so far have mutations at the RET proto-oncogene, but a few families with MEN 2b or non-MEN FMTC do not have such mutations (344, 374). Some sporadic MTC and, rarely, sporadic pheochromocytoma also have mutations at RET proto-oncogene (328, 344). Interestingly, mutations in the extracellular domain of this gene are found in Hirschsprung's disease. Therefore, RET proto-oncogene may be tightly associated with the growth regulation of neuroendocrine cells. Studies with transgenic mice do suggest RET proto-oncogene is involved in the embryologic development of the enteric nervous system. Both germ line (leukocyte) and tumors from patients with these syndromes contain a normal allele of RET gene. This suggests that the mutations at RET proto-oncogene act in a dominant fashion, which is contrary to the tumor-suppressive genes involved in MEN 1 and retinoblastoma. This is the first example of mutations at an oncogene causing a familial cancer syndrome (375). Besides RET proto-oncogene, loss of heterozygosity (LOH) at chromosome 1p, 22q, 17p, or 3p is commonly found in MTC and pheochromocytomas associated with MEN 2 and non-MEN FMTC (329, 332). Therefore, tumorigenesis in MEN 2 may also follow the model of multistage carcinogenesis established in colon cancer

(333). It is unknown why different families with the same point mutations can have different clinical manifestation. It may be possible that other genetic changes such as the deletions at chromosomes 1p, 22q, 17p, or 3p contribute to the difference.

Biochemical and Clinical Features

The biochemical features of MTC, pheochromocytomas, and parathyroid neoplasms in the genetic syndromes under discussion are similar to those for the sporadic forms of each of these disorders. There are no distinguishing markers that allow the genetic forms of each neoplasm to be separated from the non-inherited types.

Pheochromocytomas develop in 40 to 50% of MEN 2 patients and may arise bilaterally from medullary hyperplasia. Although the adrenal component usually develops at a later age than the thyroid disease, occasionally it may appear in childhood. The clinical course of pheochromocytomas in MEN 2a and 2b is typically that of benign tumors with peak incidence in the fourth and fifth decades. Malignant pheochromocytomas have been reported only rarely (131, 252, 291). The ratio of norepinephrine to epinephrine is generally lower in the genetic forms of pheochromocytoma than the sporadic form. In fact, epinephrine can actually be the dominant form in MEN 2a and 2b (35, 372). Most commonly these patients complain of palpitations, anxiety spells, or headache early in their disease. But many patients whose tumors were found by family screening have no symptoms. Hypertension may not be noted until a crisis is induced by an operation or delivery.

Familial MTC occurs at a younger age than sporadic MTC. The peak incidence is in the second and third decades for MEN 2a and non-MEN FMTC, whereas it is in the first and second decades for MEN 2b. But all ages can be affected. The clinical behavior of MTC differs for each of the genetic syndromes under discussion. In MEN 2a, the cancer, although it metastasizes early, often behaves in a relatively indolent fashion. Thus, the survival rates for patients with this syndrome are a bit longer than that for patients with the sporadic form of MTC (Figure 102.2). Aggressive malignant behavior of MTC occurs in a small subset of patients with MEN 2a. This fact emphasizes the need to excise all tumors at the very early stages of this disease to prevent the consequences of widely metastatic tumor. Cutaneous lichen amyloidosis, a pruritic lichenoid skin lesion of the upper back often appears before MTC in MEN 2a patients (372).

MTC in MEN 2b may be a more aggressive and lethal cancer (195, 244). Death from metastatic disease has been reported in young children with this disorder (130). When the physical stigmata of MEN 2b are recognized (e.g. mucosal neuromas), even in infants, surgical intervention for MTC should be undertaken as early as is feasible.

In non-MEN familial MTC, the thyroid neoplasm behaves in its least aggressive manner (72). The cancer generally appears in the fourth to fifth decade rather than in the second decade as in MEN 2a. Although local metastases may occur frequently, the disease usually follows an indolent course and virtually never results in death of the patient.

Diagnostic and Screening Tests

Patients with clinical MTC have elevated serum calcitonin. Pheochromocytoma can be diagnosed by urinary epinephrine or epinephrine/norepinephrine ratio and various imaging studies. Any patient with either MTC or pheochromocytoma should undergo investigation of the possibility of MEN 2. Their family members should be screened for both tumors. A negative family history is not reliable because 40% of MEN 2a gene carriers never develop apparent clinical disease. This has been demonstrated in a recently published study that 174 patients with MTC were screened for pheochromocytoma; in addition to five cases from known MEN 2 families, another five index cases were found, which led to discovery of five new MEN 2 families (364). Before the era of genetic screening, members of MEN 2a and non-MEN FMTC families began a yearly pentagastrin/calcium stimulation tests before age 5 and continued until age 40 if all tests were normal. The possibility of conversion to positive result after age 35 is less than 5% (372, 373). Urinary catecholamine measurement is done for MEN 2a and 2b families.

Patients with the earliest subclinical stages of MTC (premalignant C-cell hyperplasia and/or microscopic carcinoma) usually do not have elevated basal serum levels of calcitonin. However, even patients with C-cell hyperplasia increase calcitonin levels abnormally in response to the secretagogues calcium and/or pentagastrin. Although several regimens for stimulating calcitonin secretion are available, the combination test devised by Wells and colleagues consisting of a 50-second infusion of calcium gluconate (2 mg of elemental calcium/kg) followed by a 10-second bolus of pentagastrin (Peptavalon, Ayerst, 0.5 μg/kg) seems most reliable (307). This procedure results in less false negatives than tests performed with either of the two agents alone, is rapid, and has minimal side-effects consisting of only transient warmth, flushing, and nausea. Calcitonin levels, measured at 0, 2, 3.5, and 5 minutes of the test, generally peak at the 2- or 3.5-minute points. Several commercial diagnostic laboratories have standardized calcitonin results for this test in normal individuals. Although normal ranges vary somewhat for different calcitonin assays, in general, normal females do not have a provoked level higher than 29 pg/ml, and the limit for males is 106 pg/ml. It is critical that the physician screening patients for MTC be thoroughly familiar with the performance of a given calcitonin assay in detecting patients with early MTC. The provocative test becomes clearly abnormal at average age of 8 to 9 in the gene carriers of MEN 2a, and total thyroidectomy should be done. Patients operated at this stage typically have C-cell hyperplasia with/without microscopic MTC. Over 90% are cured. False positive results do occur in a small number of subjects with normal thyroid glands and in 5% of normal people who have C-cell hyperplasia (84, 369, 373).

Genetic screening with molecular linkage techniques can identify gene carriers with 95 to 99% accuracy. The identification of mutations at RET proto-oncogene has made the clinical calcium pentagastrin challenge technique almost obsolete. Four studies have confirmed that direct analysis of germ-line leukocyte DNA by polymerase chain reaction amplification, single strand conformation polymorphism

(SSCP), restriction enzyme digestion, or direct DNA sequencing can identify the index case of a new family and every gene carrier in any known family of MEN 2a with 100% accuracy (368, 370, 371, 376). Furthermore, all thyroid glands removed from gene carriers who have normal pentagastrin stimulation tests contain C-cell hyperplasia. Some even contain microscopic MTC (368, 376). The accuracy for MEN 2b and non-MEN FMTC might not be so good because a small number of families do not have the common mutations at the RET proto-oncogene. Because MTC, which is always malignant, has been the major cause of morbidity and mortality, preventive total thyroidectomy usually is done in MEN 2a as soon as gene carrier status is established by biochemical screening in the past. Morbidity from surgery is low, and hormone replacement is easy. The optimal timing for surgery is less certain now because gene carriers can be identified at birth by genetic screening. Probably surgery should not be later than age 6 because a metastatic MTC was reported to develop at this age. Family members of MEN 2a who are not gene carriers by genetic screening do not need to undergo biochemical testing. MTC in MEN 2b occurs in early age and can be more aggressive than in MEN 2a. Total thyroidectomy should be performed as soon as the typical phenotype is recognized, preferably before age 2, even before a calcitonin test is available. The accuracy of screening by direct analysis of RET proto-oncogene for non-MEN FMTC still needs to be confirmed.

Surgical Management

The primary management for the genetic forms of MTC is, as for sporadic disease, total thyroidectomy (Figure 102.3) (230). The effectiveness of surgical treatment is dependent on the stage at which the disease is first detected and treated. The object is to do surgery before there are any clinical signs of disease. C-cell hyperplasia and microscopic MTC are the only stages consistently curable by thyroidectomy (61, 307).

Patients with MEN 2 syndromes must be evaluated for possible pheochromocytomas before undergoing thyroidectomy for MCT. Operations for the adrenal disease component, if present, should always take precedence over any neck procedures to avoid a potential catastrophic hypertensive crisis following anesthesia induction.

Once the diagnosis of pheochromocytomas has been established by biochemical testing, noninvasive localization and surgical approaches are conducted as described previously for sporadic pheochromocytomas. MIBG scans are sensitive in detecting both medullary hyperplasia and small pheochromocytomas even when CT scans and biochemical screening have been considered normal. Conversely, an imaging study always reveals an abnormality when biochemical testing is abnormal (368), but CT and MIBG scans are not suitable screening modalities because of the radiation exposure. Although pheochromocytoma in an MEN 2 patient almost always occurs bilaterally (Figure 102.10), they often do not occur synchronously. In fact, the contralateral adrenal lesion can develop many years later. Pheochromocytoma is almost always benign in this situation. In addition, hormone replacement after bilateral adrenalectomy is more complicated than that after thyroidectomy. Addisonian crises do occur in these patients. Therefore, the treatment goal for pheochromocytoma should be different from MTC. Even though microscopic hyperplasia is common, surgery probably only needs to be done for patients who have demonstrated excess catecholamine secretion, tumors, or symptoms. Bilateral adrenalectomy should be performed for patients presenting with bilateral disease. But unilateral adrenalectomy can be considered for patients who present with unilateral disease. With yearly biochemical monitoring, the remaining adrenal gland can be removed if necessary before excess catecholamine causes symptoms. Actually, only one-third to one-half of the patients who had unilateral adrenalectomy for unilateral disease need second surgery for recurrent pheochromocytoma in the remaining adrenal gland. Another option instead of bilateral adrenalectomy is to perform a cortical sparing subtotal adrenalectomy (368).

Total thyroidectomy is essential in patients with the genetic forms of MTC because of the multifocal origins of the tumor in this setting. The operation must be extracapsular, leaving no thyroid tissue or rim of capsule. Embryologically, the C-cells are concentrated in the posterior portion of the upper two-thirds of the thyroid lobes. This is the area most frequently left by some surgeons in performing "near total" thyroidectomy. Any procedure less than a total thyroidectomy is an inadequate operation for this disease, since failrue to remove all thyroid tissue inevitably leads to recurrent disease (102, 230). This point cannot be over emphasized and is particularly important in children where the disease has an excellent chance of being cured. Some have even recommended ^{131}I scintiscanning following total thyroidectomy and ^{131}I ablation of any detected thyroid remnants. In addition to thyroidectomy, central compartment lymph nodes should be excised as described previously for sporadic MTC. In MEN 2 patients diagnosed by calcitonin testing, there are usually no palpable thyroid abnormalities, and perithyroidal lymph nodes are frequently free of disease. In performing both total thyroidectomy and central compartment lymph node dissection, it is imperative to identify and preserve all parathyroid glands until a decision has been made about which glands should be excised. In patients with involved central compartment lymph nodes, an ipsilateral or bilateral modified neck dissection should be considered. When a modified neck dissection has not been done and the postoperative calcitonin level remains elevated, we perform selective venous sampling for calcitonin. When elevated levels are detected from one or both sides of the neck, a modified neck dissection is then recommended.

Not infrequently, however, young adult patients have liver or bone metastases when initially diagnosed, preventing any curative operative attempts (195). The screening of first degree family members of those with newly discovered MTC, particularly when bilateral tumors and associated C-cell hyperplasia have been found, has led to earlier diagnosis and treatment of patients at risk during the past 15 years since calcitonin assays have been widely available (Figure 102.3). Calcitonin testing has been particularly valuable in MEN 2a family members who lack any of the characteristic features found in MEN 2b individuals. Genetic testing, when available, allows for recognition of MEN 2a family members with the trait in early infancy and eliminates the need for periodic childhood testing as currently done.

Clinical evidence of hyperparathyroidism is present in 20 to 30% of MEN 2a patients, whereas hypercalcemia rarely occurs in MEN 2b patients. Nevertheless, one or two parathyroid glands may be abnormal in MEN 2a patients even when they are normocalcemic preoperatively. The surgical treatment of MEN 2a parathyroid disease usually took place during total thyroidectomy for MTC in the past and does not differ from that of the MEN 1 disease. Subtotal parathyroidectomy or total parathyroidectomy and arm muscle autotransplant can be performed for patients who are hypercalcemic (369, 371). Recurrence, despite long term follow-up, rarely if ever occurs. Surgical treatment for normocalcemic patients has been controversial. More conservative surgery with removal of enlarged glands can be considered for patients whose family history reveals little hyperparathyroidism. Hyperparathyroidism is very rare after total thyroidectomy for C-cell hyperplasia discovered by screening, even though the parathyroid glands are left in place (371, 373).

Treatment of Recurrent or Metastatic Disease

The treatment of advanced MTC in a patient with a genetic syndrome is not distinguished from the approach used in sporadic disease. Locally recurrent disease in the neck may be amenable to further surgical management (288). There is little evidence supporting a role for radiation therapy (239), and in patients with progressive, symptomatic advanced disease, only anecdotal reports of combination chemotherapy have appeared (13, 212, 256). We have treated a patient from the MEN 2a kindred shown in Figure 102.10. This 26-year-old male with advanced MTC metastatic to lung and bones had little palliative benefit from radiation therapy to symptomatic lesions in the thoracic spine and pelvis. Following combination chemotherapy with cyclophosphamide, vincristine, and dacarbazine, the patient had a partial response with complete resolution of pulmonary metastases, improvement of bone pain, and markedly reduced serum calcitonin and CEA for 14 months (13). Subsequently, six sporadic MTC patients were treated with this regimen. Two had partial response and another one had stable disease. Response duration ranged from 9 to 29 months (335). Further improvement on this regimen and adjuvant treatment after total thyroidectomy for patients with gross MTC need to be explored.

References

1. Albright F. Case Records of the Massachusetts General Hospital: Case 27461. N Engl J Med 1941;225:789.
2. Alexander HR, Norton JA. Biology and management of medullary thyroid carcinoma of the parafollicular cells. In Thyroid Cancer: A Lethal Endocrine Neoplasm. Moderated by J. Robbins. Ann Intern Med 1991;115:133.
3. Allen JM, Yeats JC, Causon R, Brown MJ, Bloom SR. Neuropeptide Y and its flanking peptide in human endocrine tumors and plasma. J Clin Endocrinol Metab 1987;64: 1199.
4. Amara SG, Jonas V, Rosenfeld MF, Ong ES, Evans RM. Alternative RNA processing in calcitonin gene expression generates mRNAs encoding different polypeptide products. Nature 1982;298:240.
5. Amberson JB, Vaughan ED Jr, Gray GF, Naus J. Flow cytometric determination of nuclear DNA content in benign adrenal pheochromocytomas. Urology 1987;30.
6. Andersen GS, Toftdahl DB, Lund JO, Strandgaard S, Nielsen PE. The incidence rate of phaeochromocytoma and Conn's syndrome in Denmark, 1977–1981. J Hum Hypertens 1988;2:187.
7. Andrew A. The APUD concept: where has it led us? Br Med J 1982;38:221.
8. Arnaud CD. The parathyroid glands, hypercalcemia and hypocalcemia. In Cecil Textbook of Medicine. Edited by JB Wyngaarden, LH Smith Jr. Philadelphia: Saunders, 1988, p 1486.
9. Arnold A, Staunton CE, Kim GH, Gaz RD, Kronenberg HM. Monoclonality and abnormal parathyroid hormone genes in parathyroid adenomas. N Engl J Med 1988;318: 658.
10. Askanazy M. Ueber ostitis deformans ohne osteoides gewebe. Arb Geb Pathol Anat Inst Tubingen Leipez 1904;4:398.
11. Attie M. Treatment of hypercalcemia. Endocrinol Metab Clin North Am 1989;18:807.
12. Aurbach GD, Mallette LE, Patten BM, Heath DA, Doppman JL, Bilezikian JP. Hyperparathyroidism: recent studies. Ann Intern Med 1973;79:566.
13. Averbuch S, Wu L, Pertsemlidis D, Drakes T. Cyclophosphamide (C), vincristine (V), and dacarbazine (D) for advanced neuroendocrine carcinomas. Proc Am Soc Clin Oncol 1990;9:382.
14. Averbuch SD, Steakley CS, Young RC, Gelmann EP, Goldstein DS, Stull R, Keiser HR. Malignant pheochromocytoma: effective treatment with a combination of cyclophosphamide, vincristine, and dacarbazine. Ann Intern Med 1988;109:267.
14a. Averbuch SD. Unpublished observation.
15. Baba H, Kishihara M, Tohmon M, Fukase M, Kizaki T, Okada S, Matsuzuka F, Kobayashi A, Kuma K, Fujita T. Identification of parathyroid hormone messenger ribonucleic acid in an apparently nonfunctioning parathyroid carcinoma transformed from a parathyroid carcinoma with hyperparathyroidism. J Clin Endocrinol Metab 1986;62:247.
16. Bajorunas DR. Clinical manifestations of cancer-related hypercalcemia. Semin Oncol 1990;17(suppl 5):16.
17. Bale SJ, Bale AE, Stewart K, Dachowski L, McBride OW, Glaser T, Green JE, Mulvihill JJ, Brandi ML, Sakaguchi K, Aurbach GD, Marx SJ. Linkage analysis of multiple endocrine neoplasia type 1 with INT2 and other markers on chromosome 11. Genomics 1989;4:320.
18. Ballard HS, Frame B, Harstock RJ. Familial multiple endocrine adenoma-peptic ulcer complex. Medicine 1964;43:481.
19. Baylin SB. APUD cell fact and fiction. Trends Endocrinol Metab 1990;1:198.
20. Baylin SB, Mendelsohn G. Medullary thyroid carcinoma: a model for the study of human tumor progression and cell heterogeneity. In Tumor Cell Heterogeneity, Origins and Implications. Edited by AH Owens Jr, DS Coffey, SB Baylin. New York: Academic Press, 1982, p 9.
21. Beard CM, Sheps SG, Kurland LT. Occurrence of pheochromocytoma in Rochester, Minnesota, 1950 through 1979. Mayo Clin Proc 1983;58.
22. Benowitz NL. Pheochromocytoma. Adv Intern Med 1990;35:195.
23. Bergholm U, Adami HO, Auer G, Bergstrom R, Backdahl M, Grimelius L, Hansson G, Ljundberg O, Wilander E. Histopathologic characteristics and nuclear DNA content as prognostic factors in medullary thyroid carcinoma. A nationwide study in Sweden. The Swedish MTC Study Group. Cancer 1989;64:135.
24. Bergman SM, Sears HF, Javadpour N, Keiser HR. Postoperative management of patients with pheochromocytoma. J Urol 1978;120:109.
25. Berland Y, Olmer M, Lebreuil G, Grisoli J. Parathyroid carcinoma, adenoma and hyperplasia in a case of chronic renal insufficiency on dialysis. J Clin Nephrol 1982;18: 154.
26. Bierewaltes WH, Sisson JC, Shapiro B, Lloyd RV, Dmuchowski C, Rabbani R. Malignant potential of pheochromocytoma. Proc Am Assoc Cancer Res 1986;27:617.
27. Bilezikian JP. Etiologies and therapy of hypercalcemia. Endocrinol Metab Clin North Am 1989;18:389.
28. Bilezikian JP. Parathyroid hormone-related peptide in sickness and in health. N Engl J Med 1990;322:1151.
29. Black BK. Carcinoma of the parathyroid. Ann Surg 1954;139:355.
30. Blake GM, Lewington VJ, Fleming JS, Zivanovic MA, Ackery DM. Modification by nifedipine of ^{131}I-meta-iodobenzylguanidine kinetics in malignant phaeochromocytoma. Eur J Nucl Med 1988;14:345.
31. Blum R. Enalapril in pheochromocytoma (letter). Ann Intern Med 1987;106:326.
32. Bostwick DG, Null WE, Holmes D, Weber E, Barchas JD, Bensch KG. Expression of opioid peptides in tumors. N Engl J Med 1987;317:1439.
33. Brandi ML. Multiple endocrine neoplasia type I: general features and new insights into etiology. J Endocrinol Invest 1991;14:61.
34. Brandi ML, Aurbach GDA, Fitzpatrick LA, Quarto R, Spiegel A, Bliziotes MM, Norton JA, Doppman JL, Marx SJ. Parathyroid mitogenic activity in plasma from patients with familial multiple endocrine neoplasia type 1. N Engl J Med 1986;314:1287.
35. Bravo EL, Gifford RW Jr. Pheochromocytoma: diagnosis, localization, and management. N Engl J Med 1984;311:1298.
36. Bravo EL, Tarazi RC, Fouad FD. Clonidine suppression test: a useful aid in the diagnosis of pheochromocytoma. N Engl J Med 1981;305:623.
37. Brendel AJ, Jeandot R, Guyot M, Lambert B, Drouillard J. Radionuclide therapy of pheochromocytomas and neuroblastomas using iodine-131 metaiodobenzylguanidine (MIBG). Clin Nucl Med 1988;14:19.
38. Brennan MF, Keiser HR. Persistent and recurrent pheochromocytoma: the role of surgery. World J Surg 1982;6:397.
39. Broadus AE, Mangin M, Ikeda K, Insogna KL, Weir EC, Burtis WJ, Stewart AF. Humoral hypercalcemia of cancer. Identification of a novel parathyroid hormone-like peptide. N Engl J Med 1988;319:556.
40. Brogden RN, Heel RC, Speight TM. Alpha methyl-L-tyrosine: a review of its pharmacology and clinical use. Drugs 1981;21:81.
41. Budayr AA, Nissenson RA, Klein RF, Pun KK, Clark OH, Diep D, Arnaud CD, Strewler GJ. Increased serum levels of a parathyroid hormone-like protein in malignancy-associated hypercalcemia. Ann Intern Med 1989;111:807.
42. Bukowski RM, Sheeler L, Cunningham J, Esselstyn C. Successful combination chemotherapy for metastatic parathyroid carcinoma. Arch Intern Med 1984;144:399.
43. Bukowski RM, Vidt DG. Chemotherapy trials in malignant pheochromocytoma: report of two patients and review of the literature. J Surg Oncol 1984;27:89.
44. Burtis WJ, Brady TG, Orloff JJ, Ersbak JB, Warrell RP, Olson BR, Wu TL, Mitnick ME, Broadus WE, Stewart AF. Immunochemical characterization of circulating parathyroid hormone-related protein in patients with humoral hypercalcemia of cancer. N Engl J Med 1990;322:1106.
45. Bystrom C, Larsson C, Blomberg C, Sandelin K, Falkmer U, Skogseid B, Oberg K, Werner S, Nordenskjold M. Localization of the MEN 1 gene to a small region within

chromosome 11q13 by deletion mapping in tumors. Proc Natl Acad Sci USA 1990;87: 1968.

46. Cady B. Hyperparathyroidism. In Surgery of the Thyroid and Parathyroid Glands. Edited by CE Sedgwick, B Cady. Philadelphia: Saunders, 1980, p 206.
47. Calandra DB, Chejfec G, Foy BK, Lawrence AM, Paloyan E. Parathyroid carcinoma: biochemical and pathologic response to DTIC. Surgery 1984;96:1132.
48. Carney JA, Sizemore GW, Sheps SG. Adrenal medullary disease in multiple endocrine neoplasia, type 2: pheochromocytoma and its precursors. Am J Clin Pathol 1976;66:279.
49. Castleman B, Roth SI. Tumors of the parathyroid glands. In Atlas of Tumor Pathology. Edited by B Castleman, SI Roth. Wash. DC: Armed Forces Institute of Pathology, 1978, p 1.
50. Caty MG, Coran AG, Geagen M, Thompson NW. Current diagnosis and treatment of pheochromocytoma in children: experience with 22 consecutive tumors in 14 patients. Arch Surg 1990;125:978.
51. Chahinian AP, Holland JF, Nieburgs HE, Marinescu A, Geller SA, Kirschner PA. Metastatic nonfunctioning parathyroid carcinoma: ultrastructural evidence of secretory granules and response to chemotherapy. Am J Med Sci 1981;282:80.
52. Charbonnel B, Chatal JF, Brendel AJ, Lanehche B, Lumbroso J, Marchandise X, Mornex R, Schlumberger M, Wemeau JL. Le Traitement des phéochromocytomes malins par la 131-I-métaiodobenzylguanidine. Ann Endocrinol (Paris) 1988;49:344.
53. Cheung PS, Borgstrom A, Thompson NW. Strategy in reoperative surgery for hyperparathyroidism. Arch Surg 1989;124:676.
54. Clerkin EP. Hyperparathyroidism. In Surgery of the Thyroid and Parathyroid Glands. Edited by B Cady, RL Rossi. Philadelphia: Saunders, 1991, p 243.
55. Conlon MJ, McGregor GP, Gröndal S, Grimelius L. Synthesis of α- and β-calcitonin gene-related peptide by a human pheochromocytoma. Peptides 1989;10:327.
56. Cox TM, Fagan EA, Hillyard CJ, Allison DJ, Chadwick VS. Role of calcitonin in diarrhea associated with medullary carcinoma of the thyroid. Gut 1979;20:629.
57. Curley IR, Wheeler MH, Thompson NW, Grant CS. The challenge of the middle mediastinal parathyroid. World J Surg 1988;12:818.
58. Cushman P Jr. Familial endocrine tumors. Report of two unrelated kindreds affected with pheochromocytoma, one also with multiple thyroid carcinomas. Am J Med 1962;32:352.
59. de Asis DN, Ali MK, Soto A, Samaan NA. Acute cardiac toxicity of antineoplastic agents as the first manifestation of pheochromocytoma. Cancer 1978;42:2005.

59a. de Bustros, Baylin S. Personal observation.

60. Deftos LJ, Woloszczuk W, Krisch I, Horvat G, Ulrich W, Neuhold N, Braun O, Reiner A, Srikanta S, Krisch K. Medullary thyroid carcinomas express chromogranin A and a novel neuroendocrine protein recognized by monoclonal antibody HISL-19. Am J Med 1988;85:780.
61. Delius RE, Thompson NW. Early total thyroidectomy in patients with multiple endocrine neoplasia IIb syndrome. Surg Gynecol Obstet 1989;169:442.
62. Dhom G, Hohbach C. Case 12. Ultrastruct Pathol 1980;1:141.
63. Dinnen JS, Greenwood RH, Jones JH, Walker DA, Williams ED. Parathyroid carcinoma in familial hyperparathyroidism. J Clin Pathol 1977;30:366.
64. Drasin H. Treatment of malignant pheochromocytoma. West J Med 1978;128:106.
65. Duncan MW, Compton P, Lazarus L, Smythe GA. Measurement of norepinephrine and 3, 4-dihydroxyphenylglycol in urine and plasma for the diagnosis of pheochromocytoma. N Engl J Med 1988;319:136.
66. Eberle F, Grun R. Multiple endocrine neoplasia type I (MEN I). Ergeb Inn Med Kinderheilkd 1981;46:76.
67. Egglin TK, Hahn PF, Stark DD. MRI of the adrenal glands. Semin Roentgenol 1988;23: 280.
68. Ellison GT, Mansberger JA, Mansberger AR Jr. Malignant recurrent pheochromocytoma during pregnancy: case report and review of the literature. Surgery 1988;103: 484.
69. Erdheim J. Zur normalen und pathologischen histologie der glandula thyreoidea, parathyreoidea und hypophysis. Beitr Pathol Anat 1903;33:158.
70. Eriksson B, Skogseid B, Lundqvist G, Wide L, Wilander E, Oberg K. Medical treatment and long-term survival in a prospective study of 84 patients with endocrine pancreatic tumors. Cancer 1990;65:1883.
71. Farhangi M, Taylor J, Havey A, O'Dorisio T. Neuroendocrine (carcinoid) tumor of the lung and type 1 multiple endocrine neoplasia. South Med J 1987;80:1459.
72. Farndon JR, Leight GS, Dilley WG, Baylin SB, Smallridge RC, Harrison TS, Wells SAJ. Familial medullary thyroid carcinoma without associated endocrinopathies: a distinct clinical entity. Br J Surg 1986;73:278.
73. Feldman JM. Treatment of metastatic pheochromocytoma with streptozocin. Arch Intern Med 1983;143:1799.
74. Fink IJ, Reinig JW, Dwyer AJ, Doppman JL, LInehan WM, Keiser HR. MR imaging of pheochromocytomas. J Comput Assist Tomogr 1985;9:454.
75. Finklestein JZ, Klemperer MR, Evans A, Bernstein I, Leikin S, McCreadie S, Grosfeld J, Hittle R, Weiner J, Sather H, Hammond D. Multiagent chemotherapy for children with metastatic neuroblastoma: a report from Childrens Cancer Study Group. Med Pediatr Oncol 1979;6:179.
76. Fiore JJ, Kelsen DP, Cheng E, Dukeman M. Phase II trial of VP-16 in apudomas. Proc Am Assoc Cancer Res 1984;15:174.
77. Flye MW, Brennan MF. Surgical resection of metastatic parathyroid carcinoma. Ann Surg 1981;193:425.
78. Frankel F. Ein fall von doppelseitigem, vollig latent verlaufenen nebennierentumor und gleichzeitiger nephritis mit veranderungen am circulationsapparat und retinitis. Virchows Arch Pathol Anat Physiol 1886;103:244.
79. Friedman E, Sakaguchi K, Bale AE, Falchetti A, Streeten E, Zimering MB, Weinstein LS, McBride WO, Nakamura Y, Brandi, ML, Norton JA, Aurbach GD, Speigel AM, Marx SJ. Clonality of parathyroid tumors in familial multiple endocrine neoplasia type 1. N Engl J Med 1989;321:213.
80. Friesen SR. The development of endocrinopathies in the prospective screening of two families with MEA-I. World J Surg 1979;3:753.
81. Friesen SR. Update on the diagnosis and treatment of rare neuroendocrine tumors. Surg Clinic North Am 1987;67:379.
82. Fritsche AE. Clinical utility of serum osteocalcin. Cancer Invest 1990;8:441.
83. Fujimoto Y, Obara T. How to recognize and treat parathyroid carcinoma. Endocrinol Metab Clin North Am 1989;67:343.
84. Gagel RF, Tashjian AH Jr, Cummings T, Papathanasopoulos N, Kaplan MM, DeLellis RA, Wolfe HJ, Reichlin S. The clinical outcome of prospective screening for multiple endocrine neoplasia type 2a. N Engl J Med 1988;318:478.
85. Gazdar AF, Helman L, Israel MA, Russell EK, Linnoila RL, Mulshine J, Schuller H, Park JG. Expression of neuroendocrine cell markers L-dopa decarboxylase, chromogranin A, and dense core granules in human tumors of endocrine and non-endocrine origin. Cancer Res 1988;48:4078.
86. Giraud P, Eiden LE, Audigier Y. ACTH a-MSH and β-endorphin in human pheochromocytoma. Neuropeptides 1981;1:236.
87. Glover D, Riley L, Carmichael K, Spar B, Glick J, Kligerman MM, Agus ZS, Slatopolsky E, Attie M, Goldfarb S. Hypocalcemia and inhibition of parathyroid hormone secretion after administration of WR-2721 (a radioprotective and chemoprotective agent). N Engl J Med 1983;309:1137.
88. Glowniak J, Shapiro B, Vinik AI, Glaser B, Thompson HW, Cho KJ. Percutaneous transhepatic venous sampling of gastrin: value in sporadic and familial islet-cell tumors of G-cell. N Engl J Med 1982;307:293.
89. Goldfarb DA, Novick AC, Bravo EL, Straffon RA, Montie JE, Kay R. Experience with extra-adrenal pheochromocytoma. J Urol 1989;142:931.
90. Goldstein DS, Stull R, Eisenhofer G, Session JC, Weder A, Averbuch SD, Keiser HR. Plasma 3, 4-dihydroxyphenylalanine (dopa) and catecholamines in neuroblastoma or pheochromocytoma. Ann Intern Med 1986;105:887.
91. Goncalves E, Ninane J, Wese F, Leonet J, Piret L, Cornu G, De Meyer R. Familial phaeochromocytoma: successful treatment with 131I-MIBG. Med Ped Oncol 1990;18:126.
92. Gordon P, Comi RJ, Maton PN, Go VLW. Somatostatin and somatostatin analogue (SMS 201-995) in treatment of hormone-secreting tumors of the pituitary and gastrointestinal tract and non-neoplastic diseases of the gut. Ann Intern Med 1989;110: 35.
93. Gottlieb JA, Hill CS Jr. Adriamycin (NSC-123127) therapy in thyroid carcinoma. Cancer Chemother Rep (3). 1975;6:283.
94. Gough IR, Thompson NW. Phaeochromocytoma. Aust NZ J Surg 1988;58:365.
95. Grimelius L. A silver nitrate stain for alpha 2 cells in human pancreatic islets. Acta Soc Med Upsala 1968;73:243.
96. Grossman E, Goldstein DS, Hoffman A, Keiser HA. Glucagon and clonidine testing in the diagnosis of pheochromocytoma. Hypertension 1991;17:733.
97. Grouzmann E, Comoy E, Bohoun C. Plasma neuropeptide Y concentrations in patients with neuroendocrine tumors. J Endocrinol Metab 1989;64:808.
98. Grouzmann E, Gicquel C, Plouin PF, Schlumberger M, Comoy E, Bohoun C. Neuropeptide Y and neuron-specific enolase levels in benign and malignant pheochromocytomas. Cancer 1990;66:1833.
99. Guo JZ, Gong LS, Chen SX, Luo BY, Xu MY. Malignant pheochromocytoma: diagnosis and treatment in fifteen cases. J Hypertens 1989;7:261.
100. Hall EM, Chaffin L. Malignant tumors of the parathyroid glands. West J Surg Obstet Gynecol 1934;42:578.
101. Hamilton BPM, Cheikh IE, Rivera LE. Attempted treatment of inoperable pheochromocytoma with streptozocin. Arch Intern Med 1977;137:762.
102. Harness JK, Fung L, Thompson NW, Burney RE, McLeod MK. Total thyroidectomy: complications and technique. World J Surg 1986;10:781.
103. Harper MA, Murnaghan GA, Kennedy L, Hadden DR, Atkinson AB. Phaeochromocytoma in pregnancy: five cases and a review of the literature. Br J Obstet Gynaecol 1989;96:594.
104. Harrison M, James N, Broadley K, Bloom SR, Armour R, Wimalawansa S, Heath D, Waxman J. Somatostatin analogue treatment for malignant hypercalcaemia. Br Med J 1990;300:1313.
105. Hazard JB, Hawk WA, Crile G Jr. Medullary (solid) carcinoma of the thyroid—A clinicopathologic entity. J Clin Endocrinol Metab 1959;19:152.
106. Heath DA. Primary hyperparathyroidism: clinical presentation and factors influencing clinical management. Endocrinol Metab Clin North Am 1989;18:631.
107. Heath H III, Hodgson SF, Kennedy MA. Primary hyperparathyroidism: incidence, morbidity, and potential economic impact in a community. N Engl J Med 1980;302: 189.
108. Helman LJ, Cohen PS, Averbuch SD, Cooper MJ, Keiser HR, Israel MA. Neuropeptide Y expression distinguishes malignant from benign pheochromocytoma. J Clin Oncol 1989;7:1720.
109. Helman LJ, Gazdar AF, Park J, Cohen PS, Cotelingam JD, Israel MA. Chromogranin A expression in normal and malignant human tissues. J Clin Invest 1988;82:686.
110. Hirschel-Scholz S, Jung A, Fischer JA, Trechsel U, Bonjour JP. Suppression of parathyroid secretion after administration of WR-2721 in a patient with parathyroid carcinoma. Clin Endocrinol 1985;23:313.
111. Hoefnagel CA, Voute PA, deKraker J. Radionuclide diagnosis and therapy of neural crest tumors using iodine-131 metaiodobenzylguanidine. J Nucl Med 1987;28:308.
112. Holmes EC, Morton DL, Ketcham AS. Parathyroid carcinoma: a collective review. Ann Surg 1969;169:631.
113. Horton WA, Wong V, Eldridge R. Von Hippel-Lindau disease: clinical and pathological manifestations in nine families with 50 affected members. Arch Intern Med 1976;136:769.
114. Hosaka Y, Rainwater LM, Grant CS, Farrow GM, van Heerden JA, Lieber MM. Pheochromocytoma: nuclear deoxyribonucleic acid patterns studied by fluorocytometry. Surgery 1986;100:1003.
115. Hoskin PJ, Harmer C. Chemotherapy for thyroid cancer. Radiother Oncol 1987;10: 187.
116. Howard TJ, Passaro EJ. Gastrinoma: new medical and surgical approaches. Surg Clin North Am 1989;69:667.
117. Hull CJ. Phaeochromocytoma. Diagnosis, preoperative preparation and anaesthetic management. Br J Anaesth 1986;58:1453.
118. Husain M, Alsever RN, Lock JP, George WF, Katz FH. Failure of medullary carcinoma of the thyroid to respond to doxorubicin therapy. Hormone Res 1978;9:22.
119. Hussain S, Belldegrun A, Seltzer SE, Richie JP, Gittes RF, Abrams HL. Differentiation of malignant from benign adrenal masses: predictive indices on computed tomography. Am J Roentgenol 1985;14:61.
120. Insogna KL. Humoral hypercalcemia of malignancy: the role of parathyroid hormone-related protein. Endocrinol Metab Clin North Am 1989;18:779.
121. Ireland JP, Fleming SJ, Levison DA, Cattell WR, Baker LRI. Parathyroid carcinoma associated with chronic renal failure and previous radiotherapy to the neck. J Clin Pathol 1985;38:1114.

122. Javadpour N, Woltering E, Brennan MF. Adrenal neoplasms. Curr Probl Surg 1980;17:1.
123. Jodrell DI, Smith IE. Carboplatin in the treatment of metastatic carcinoid tumours and paraganglioma: a phase II study. Cancer Chemother Pharmacol 1990;26:62.
124. Kameda Y, Shigemoto H, Ikeda A. Development and cytodifferentiation of C-cell complexes in dog fetal thyroids. Cell Tissue Res 1980;206:403.
125. Kameya T, Bessho T, Tsumuraya M, Yamaguchi K, Abe K, Shimosato Y, Yanaihara N. Production of gastrin-releasing peptide by medullary carcinoma of the thyroid. Virchows Arch Pathol Anat Physiol Klin Med 1983;401:99.
126. Karlberg BE, Hedman L, Lennquist S. The value of the clonidine suppression test in the diagnosis of pheochromocytoma. World J Surg 1986;10:753.
127. Käser H. Clinical and diagnostic findings in patients with chromaffin tumors: pheochromocytomas, pheochromoblastomas. Journal 1990;97.
128. Kastan DJ, Kottamasu SR, Frame B, Greenwald K. Carcinoma in a mediastinal fifth parathyroid gland. JAMA 1987;257:1218.
129. Katz A, Braunstein GD. Clinical, biochemical, and pathologic features of radiation-associated hyperparathyroidism. Arch Intern Med 1983;143:79.
130. Kaufman FR, Roe TF, Isaacs H Jr, Weitzmann JJ. Metastatic medullary thyroid carcinoma in young children with mucosal neuroma syndrome. Pediatrics 1982;70:263.
131. Keiser HR, Doppman JL, Robertson CN, Linehan WM, Averbuch SD. Diagnosis, localization, and management of pheochromocytoma. In Pathology of the Adrenal Glands. Edited by EE Lack. New York: Churchill Livingstone, 1990, p 237.
132. Keiser HR, Goldstein DS, Wade JL, Douglas FL, Averbuch SD. Treatment of malignant pheochromocytoma with combination chemotherapy. Hypertension 1985;7(suppl I):18.
133. Kessinger A, Foley JF, Lemon HM. Therapy of malignant APUD cell tumors. Cancer 1983;51:790.
134. Khafagi FA, Shapiro B, Fig LM, Mallette S, Sisson JC. Labetalol reduces iodine-131 MIBG uptake by pheochromocytoma and normal tissues. J Nucl Med 1989;30:481.
135. Khairi MRA, Dexter RN, Burzynski NJ, Johnston CC Jr. Mucosal neuroma, pheochromocytoma, and medullary thyroid carcinoma. MEN type III. Medicine 1975;54:89.
136. Klein FA, Kay S, Ratliff JE, White FKH, Newsome HH. Flow cytometric determinations of ploidy and proliferation patterns of adrenal neoplasms: an adjunct to histological classification. J Urol 1985;134:862.
137. Koral KF, Wang X, Sisson JC, Botti J, Meyer L, Mallette S, Glazer GM, Adler RS. Calculating radiation absorbed dose for pheochromocytoma tumors in 131-I MIBG therapy. Int J Rad Oncol Biol Phys 1989;17:211.
138. Krisch K, Krisch I, Horvat G, Neuhold N, Ulrich W. The value of immunohistochemistry in medullary thyroid carcinoma: a systematic study of 30 cases. Histopathology 1985;9:1077.
139. Krubsack AJ, Wilson SD, Lawson TL, Kneeland JB, Thorsen MK, Collier BD, Hellman RS, Isitman AT. Prospective comparison of radionuclide, computed tomographic, sonographic, and magnetic resonance localization of parathyroid tumors. Surgery 1989;106:639.
140. Kvols LK, Buck M. Chemotherapy of endocrine malignancies: a review. Semin Oncol 1987;14:343.
141. Lack EE. Adrenal medullary hyperplasia and pheochromocytoma. In Pathology of the Adrenal Glands. Edited by EE Lack. New York: Churchill Livingstone, 1990, p 173.
142. Lack EE, Cubilla AL, Woodruff JM, Lieberman PH. Extra-adrenal paragangliomas of the retroperitoneum. Am J Surg Pathol 1980;4:109.
143. Lack EE, Kozakewich HPW. Embryology, developmental anatomy, and selected aspects of non-neoplastic pathology. In Pathology of the Adrenal Glands. Edited by EE Lack. New York: Churchill Livingstone, 1990, p 1.
144. Lafferty FW. Primary hyperparathyroidism: changing clinical spectrum, prevalence of hypertension and discriminant analysis of laboratory tests. Arch Intern Med 1981;141:1761.
145. Lairmore TC, Howe JR, Korte JA, Dilley WG, Aine L, Aine E, Wells SA Jr, Donis-Keller H. Familial medullary thyroid carcinoma and multiple endocrine neoplasia type 2B map to the same region of chromosome 10 as multiple endocrine neoplasia type 2A. Genomics 1991;9:181.
146. Lamers CB, Buis JT, Van Tongeren JH. Secretin-stimulated serum gastrin levels in hyperparathyroid patients from families with multiple endocrine adenomatosis-type I. Ann Intern Med 1977;86:719.
147. Lamers CB, Rotter JI, Jansen JB. Gastrin cell function in familial multiple endocrine neoplasia type 1. Gut 1988;29:1358.
148. Landsvater RM, Mathew CG, Smith BA, Marcus EM, te Meerman GJ, Lips CJ, Geerdink RA, Nakamura Y, Ponder BA, Buys CH. Development of multiple endocrine neoplasia type 2A does not involve substantial deletions of chromosome 10. Genomics 1989;4:246.
149. Larsson C, Skogseid B, Oberg K, Nakamura Y, Nordenskjold M. Multiple endocrine neoplasia type I gene maps to chromosome 11 and is lost in insulinoma. Nature 1988;332:85.
150. Law WL Jr, Heath H III. Familial benign hypercalcemia (hypocalciuric hypercalcemia): clinical and pathogenetic studies in 21 families. Ann Intern Med 1985;102:511.
151. Le Douarin NM. Developmental relationships between the neural crest and the polypeptide-hormone-secreting cells. In The Neural Crest. Edited by NML Douarin. London: Cambridge University Press, 1982, p 91.
152. Levinson PD, Hamilton BP, Mersey JH, Kowarski AA. Plasma norepinephrine and epinephrine responses to glucagon in patients with suspected pheochromocytomas. Metabolism 1983;32:998.
153. Lewi HJE, Reid R, Mucci B, Davidson JK, Kyle KF, MacPhersron SG, Semple P, Kaye S. Malignant pheochromocytoma. Br J Urol 1985;57:394.
154. Lewis PD. A cytophotometric study of benign and malignant pheochromocytomas. Virchows Arch 9:371, 1971.
155. Linnoila RI, Lack EE, Steinberg SM, Keiser HR. Decreased expression of neuropeptides in malignant paragangliomas: an immunohistochemical study. Hum Pathol 1988;19:41.
156. Lippman SM, Mendelsohn G, Trump DL, Wells SA Jr, Baylin SB. The prognostic and biological significance of cellular heterogeneity in medullary thyroid carcinoma: a study of calcitonin, L-dopa decarboxylase and histaminase. J Clin Endocrinol Metab 1982;54:233.
157. Lips KJM, Veer JVDS, Struyvenberg A. Bilateral occurrence of pheochromocytoma in patients with multiple endocrine neoplasia syndrome type 2a (Sipple's syndrome). Am J Med 1981;70:1051.
158. Lloyd RV, Shapiro B, Sisson JC. An immunohistochemical study of pheochromocytomas. Arch Pathol Lab Med 1984;108:541.
159. Loughlin KR, Gittes RF. Urological management of patients with von Hippel-Lindau's disease. J Urol 1986;136:789.
160. Lynn MD, Braunstein EM, Wahl RL, Shapiro B, Gross MD, Rabbani R. Bone metastases in pheochromocytoma: comparative studies of efficacy of imaging. Radiology 1986;160:701.
161. Mahler C, Verhelst J, De Longueville M, Harris A. Long-term treatment of metastatic medullary thyroid carcinoma with the somatostatin analogue octreotide. Clin Endocrinol 1990;33:261.
162. Mahoney EM, Harrison JH. Malignant pheochromocytoma: clinical course and treatment. J Urol 1977;118:225.
163. Malagelada JR, Edis AJ, Adsonl MA, van Heerden JA, Go VL. Medical and surgical options in the management of patients with gastrinoma. Gastroenterology 1983;84:1524.
164. Mangner TJ, Tobes MC, Wieland DW. Metabolism of iodine-131 metaiodobenzylquanidine in patients with metastatic pheochromocytoma. J Nucl Med 1986;27:37.
165. Manger WM, Gifford RW Jr. Pheochromocytoma. In Hypertension: Pathophysiology, Diagnosis, and Management. Edited by JH Laragh, BM Brenner. New York: Raven Press, 1990, p 1639.
166. Manger WM, Gifford RW, Hoffman BB. Pheochromocytoma: a clinical and experimental overview. Curr Probl Cancer 1985;9:1.
167. Mannelli M, DeFeo ML, Maggi M, Geppetti P, Baldi E, Pupilli C, Serio M. Effect of verapamil on catecholamine secretion by human pheochromocytoma. Hypertension 1986;8:813.
168. Manning PC Jr, Molnar GD, Black BM, Priestley JT, Woolner LB. Pheochromocytoma, hyperparathyroidism, and thyroid carcinoma occurring coincidentally. N Engl J Med 1963;268:68.
169. Marx SJ, Sakaguchi K, Green JI, Aurbach GD, Brandi ML. Multiple endocrine neoplasia type I: assessment of laboratory tests to screen for the gene in a large kindred. Medicine 1986;65:226.
170. Mason RT, Shulkes A, Zajac JD, Fletcher AE, Hardy KJ, Martin TJ. Basal and stimulated release of calcitonin gene-related peptide (CGRP) in patients with medullary thyroid carcinoma. Clin Endocrinol 1986;25:675.
171. Mathew CGP, Chin KS, Easton DF, Thorpe K, Carter C, Liou GI, Fong SL, Bridges CDB, Haak H. Nieuwenhuijzen Kruseman AC, Schifter S, Hansen HH, Telenius H, Telenius-Berg M, Ponder BAJ. A linked genetic marker for multiple endocrine neoplasia type 2A on chromosome 10. Nature 1987;328:527.
172. Mathew CGP, Smith BA, Thorpe K, Wong Z, Royle NJ, Jeffreys AJ, Ponder BAJ. Deletion of genes on chromosome 1 in endocrine neoplasia. Nature 1987;328:524.
173. Maton PN, Gardner JD, Jensen RT. The incidence and etiology of Cushing's syndrome in patients with Zollinger-Ellison syndrome. N Engl J Med 1986;315:1.
174. Maton PN, Gardner JD, Jensen RT. Diagnosis and management of Zollinger-Ellison Syndrome. Endocrinol Metab Clinics North Am 1989;18:519.
175. Mayo CH. Paroxysmal hypertension with tumor of retroperitoneal nerve: report of a case. JAMA 1927;89:1047.
176. McAuley P, Asa SL, Chiu B, Henderson J, Goltzman D, Drucker DJ. Parathyroid hormone-like peptide in normal and neoplastic mesothelial cells. Cancer 1990;66:1975.
177. McCance DR, Kenny BD, Sloan JM, Russell CJF, Hassen DR. Parathyroid carcinoma: a review. J Roy Soc Med 1987;80:505.
178. Medeiros LJ, Wolf BC, Balogh K, Federman M. Adrenal pheochromocytoma: a clinicopathologic review of 60 cases. Hum Pathol 1985;16:580.
179. Melicow MM. One hundred cases of pheochromocytoma (107 tumors) at the Columbia-Presbyterian Medical Center, 1926–1976: a clinicopathological analysis. Cancer 1977;40:1987.
180. Melvin KEW, Tashjian AH Jr, Cassidy CE, Givens JE. Cushing's syndrome caused by ACTH- and calcitonin-secreting medullary carcinoma of the thyroid. Metabolism 1970;19:831.
181. Mendelsohn G, Baylin SB. Medullary thyroid carcinoma: diagnostic and clinical features. Lab Management 1983;21:21.
182. Mendelsohn G, Bigner SH, Eggleston JC, Baylin SB, Wells SA Jr. Anaplastic variants of medullary thyroid carcinoma: a light microscopic and immunohistochemical study. Am J Surg Pathol 1980;4:333.
183. Modigliani E, Guliana JM, Maroni M, Guillausseau MP, Chabrier G, Dupont JL, Caron J, Roger P. Bentata Pessayre M, Jacob C. Effets de l'administration sous cutané de la sandostatine (SMS 201.995) en sous cutané dans 18 cas de cancer médullaire du corps thyroïde. Ann Endocrinol (Paris) 1989;50:483.
184. Modlin IM, Farndon JR, Shepard A, Johnston IDA, Kennedy TL, Montgomery DAD, Welbourn RB. Pheochromocytoma in 72 patients: clinical and diagnostic features, treatment and long term results. Br J Surg 1979;66:456.
185. Mundy GR. Hypercalcemia of malignancy revisited. J Clin Invest 1988;82:1.
186. Murphy MN, Glennon PG, Diocee MS, Wick MR, Cavers DJ. Nonsecretory parathyroid carcinoma of the mediastinum: light microscopic, immunocytochemical, and ultrastructural features of a case, and review of the literature. Cancer 1986;58:2468.
187. Nakagawara A, Ikeda K, Tsuneyoshi M. Malignant pheochromocytoma with ganglioneuroblastomatous elements in a patient with von Recklinghausen's disease. Cancer 1985;55:2794.
188. Narod SA, Sobol H, Nakamura Y, Calmettes C, Baulieu J, Bigorgne J, Chabrier G, Couette J, de Gennes J, Duprey J, Gardet P, Guillausseau P, Guilloteau D, Houdent C, Lefebvre J, Modigliani E, Parmentier C, Pugeat M, Siame C, Tourniaire J, Vandroux J, Vinot J, Lenoir GM. Linkage analysis of hereditary thyroid carcinoma with and without pheochromocytoma. Hum Genet 1989;83:353.
189. Nathaniels EK, Nathaniels AM, Wang C. Mediastinal parathyroid tumors: a clinical and pathological study of 84 cases. Ann Surg 1970;171:165.
190. Navaratnarajah M, White DC. Labetalol and phaeochromocytoma. Br J Anaesth 1984;56:10.
191. Nelkin BD, de Bustros AC, Mabry M, Baylin SB. The molecular biology of medullary thyroid carcinoma. JAMA 1989;261:3130.
192. Nelkin BD, Nakamura Y, White RW, de Bustros AC, Herman J, Wells SA Jr, Baylin SB. Low incidence of loss of chromosome 10 in sporadic and hereditary human medullary thyroid carcinoma. Cancer Res 1989;49:4114.
193. Nicholson JP, Vaughn ED, Pickering TG. Phaeochromocytoma and prazosin. Ann Intern Med 1983;99:477.
194. Norton JA, Doppman JL, Collen MJ, Harmon JW, Maton PN, Gardner JD, Jensen RT.

Prospective study of gastrinoma localization and resection in patients with Zollinger-Ellison syndrome. Ann Surg 1986;204:468.

195. Norton JA, Froome LJ, Farell RE, Wells SA Jr. Multiple endocrine neoplasia type IIb: the most aggressive form of medullary thyroid cancer. Surg Clin North Am 1979;59: 109.
196. Nourok DS. Familial pheochromocytoma and thyroid carcinoma. Ann Intern Med 1964;60:1028.
197. Nussbaum SR, Gaz RD, Arnold A. Hypercalcemia and ectopic secretion of parathyroid hormone by an ovarian carcinoma with rearrangement of the gene for parathyroid hormone. N Engl J Med 1990;323:1324.
198. O'Connor DT, Bernstein KN. Radioimmunoassay of chromogranin A in plasma as a measure of exocytic sympathoadrenal activity in normal subjects and patients with pheochromocytoma. N Engl J Med 1984;311:764.
199. O'Connor DT, Burton D, Deflos LJ. Immunoreactive human chromogranin A in diverse polypeptide hormone producing human tumors and normal endocrine tissue. J Clin Endocrinol Metab 1983;57:1084.
200. O'Connor DT, Deftos LJ. Secretion of chromogranin A by peptide producing endocrine neoplasms. N Engl J Med 1986;314:1145.
201. O'Hare MMT, Schwartz TW. Expression and precursor processing of neuropeptide Y in human pheochromocytoma and neuroblastoma tumors. Cancer Res 1989;49: 7015.
202. Obara T, Fujimoto Y, Hirayama A, Kanaji Y, Ito Y, Kodama T, Ogata T. Flow cytometric DNA analysis of parathyroid tumors with special reference to its diagnostic and prognostic value in parathyroid carcinoma. Cancer 1990;65:1789.
203. Obara T, Fujimoto Y, Kanaji Y, Okamoto T, Hirayama A, Ito Y, Kodama T. Flow cytometric DNA analysis of parathyroid tumors. Implication of aneuploidy for pathologic and biologic classification. Cancer 1990;66:1555.
204. Oberg K, Eriksson B. Medical treatment of neuroendocrine gut and pancreatic tumors. Acta Oncol 1989;28:425.
205. Oberg K, Skogseid B, Eriksson B. Multiple endocrine neoplasia type 1 (MEN-1): clinical, biochemical and genetical investigations. Acta Oncol 1989;28:383.
206. Padberg BC, Garbe E, Achilles E, Dralle H, Bressel M, Schroder, S. DNA cytophotometric findings in pheochromocytoma. Henry Ford Hosp Med J 1989;37:185.
207. Padberg CA, Garbe E, Achilles E, Dralle H, Bressel M, Schroder S. Adrenomedullary hyperplasia and phaeochromocytoma: DNA cytophotometric findings in 47 cases. Virchows Archiv A Pathol Anat 1990;416:443.
208. Palmer M, Ljunghall S, Akerstrom G, Adami HO, Berstrom R, Grimelius L, Rudberg C, Johansson H. Patients with primary hyperparathyroidism operated on over a 24 year period: temporal trends of clinical and laboratory findings. J Chronic Dis 1987;40: 121.
209. Pearse AGE. Common cytochemical and ultrastructural characteristics of cells producing polypeptide hormones (the APUD) series and their relevance to thyroid and ultimobranchial C-cells and calcitonin. Proc R Soc Lond (Biol) 1968;170:71.
210. Pearse AGE. The diffuse neuroendocrine system and the APUD concept: related endocrine peptides in brain, intestine, pituitary, placenta, and anuran cutaneous glands. Med Biol 1977;55:115.
211. Pearse AGE, Polack JM. Endocrine tumors of neural crest origin: neurolymphomas, apudomas and the APUD concept. Med Biol 1974;52:3.
212. Petursson SR. Metastatic medullary thyroid carcinoma: complete response to combination chemotherapy with dacarbazine and 5-fluorouracil. Cancer 1988;62:1899.
213. Pipeleers-Marichal M, Somers G, Willems G, Foulis A, Imrie C, Bishop AE, Polak JM, Hacki WH, Stamm B, Heitz PU, Kloppel G. Gastrinomas in the duodenums of patients with multiple endocrine neoplasia type 1 and Zollinger-Ellison syndrome. N Engl J Med 1990;332:723.
214. Plouin PF, Dudos JM, Menard J. Biochemical tests for diagnosis of phaeochromocytoma: urinary versus plasma determinations. Br Med J 1981;282.
215. Ponder B. Gene losses in human tumours. Nature 1988;335:400.
216. Ponder BA, Ponder MA, Coffey R, Pembrey ME, Gagel RF, Telenius-Berg M, Semple P, Easton DF. Risk estimation and screening in families of patients with medullary thyroid carcinoma. Lancet 1988;1:397.
217. Powell GJ, Southby J, Danks JA, Stillwell RG, Hayman JA, Henderson MA, Bennett RC, Martin TM. Localization of parathyroid hormone-related protein in breast cancer metastases: increased incidence in bone compared with other sites. Cancer Res 1991;51:3059.
218. Prinz RA, Gamvros OI, Sellu D. Subtotal parathyroidectomy for primary chief cell hyperplasia of the multiple endocrine neoplasia type 1 syndrome. Ann Surg 1981;193: 26.
219. Pritchard J, Kiely E, Rogers DW, Spitz L, Shafford EA, Brereton R, Muller C, Wright VM. Long-term survival after advanced neuroblastoma (letter). N Engl J Med 1987;317:1026.
220. Proye C, Fossati P, Fontaine P. Dopamine-secreting pheochromocytoma: an unrecognized entity? Classification of pheochromocytomas according to their type of secretion. Surgery 1986;100:1154.
221. Proye C, Thevenin D, Cecat P, Petillot P, Carnaille B, Verin P, Sautier M, Racadot N. Exclusive use of calcium channel blockers in preoperative and intraoperative control of pheochromocytomas: hemodynamics and free catecholamine assays in ten consecutive patients. Surgery 1989;106:1149.
222. Ralston SH, Alzais AA, Gardner MD, Boyle IT. A treatment of cancer associated hypercalcaemia with combined aminohydroxypropylidene diphosphonate and calcitonin. Br Med J 1986;292:1549.
223. Reinig JW, Doppman JL, Dwyer AJ, Johnson AR, Knop RH. Adrenal masses differentiated by MR. Radiology 1986;158:81.
224. Remine WH, Chong GC, van Heerden JA, Sheps SG, Harrison EG Jr. Current management of pheochromocytoma. Ann Surg 1974;179:740.
225. Ritch PS. Treatment of cancer-related hypercalcemia. Semin Oncol 1990;17(suppl 5):26.
226. Roos BA, Lindall AW, Ells J, Elde R, Lambert PW, Birnbaum RS. Increased plasma and tumor somatostatin-like immunoreactivity in medullary thyroid carcinoma and small cell lung cancer. J Clin Endocrinol Metab 1981;52:187.
227. Roth KA, Wilson DM, Eberwine J. Acromegaly and pheochromocytoma: a multiple endocrine syndrome caused by a plurihormonal adrenal medullary tumor. J Clin Endocrinol Metab 1986;63:1421.
228. Rougier P, Calmettes C, Laplanche A, Travagli JP, Lefevre M, Parmentier C, Milhaud G, Tubiana M. The value of calcitonin and carcinoembryonic antigen in the treatment and management of nonfamilial medullary thyroid carcinoma. Cancer 1983;51:855.
229. Rougier P, Parmentier C, Laplanche A, Lefevre M, Travagli JP, Caillou B, Schlumberger M, Lacour J, Tubiana M. Medullary thyroid carcinoma: prognostic factors and treatment. Int J Radiat Oncol Biol Phys 1983;9:161.
230. Russell CF, van Heerden JA, Sizemore GW, Edis AJ, Taylor WF, ReMine WH, Carney JA. The surgical management of medullary thyroid carcinoma. Ann Surg 1983;197: 42.
231. Saad MF, Fritsche HA, Samaan NA. Diagnostic and prognostic value of carcinoembryonic antigen in medullary carcinoma of the thyroid. J Clin Endocrinol Metab 1984;58:889.
232. Saad MF, Ordonez NG, Guido JJ, Samaan NA. The prognostic value of calcitonin immunostaining in medullary carcinoma of the thyroid. J Clin Endocrinol Metab 1984;59: 850.
233. Saad MF, Ordonez NG, Rashid RK, Guido JJ, Hill CS Jr, Hickey RC, Samaan NA. Medullary carcinoma of the thyroid: a study of the clinical features and prognostic factors in 161 patients. Medicine 1984;63:319.
234. Sager R. Tumor suppressor genes: the puzzle and the promise. Science 1989;246: 1406.
235. Saller B, Jacob K, Markl A, Zwiebel FM, Engelhardt D, Mann K. Rezidivierende Hochdruckkrisen und Dyspnoe nach einseitiger Adrenalektomie wegen Phäochromozytom bei einer 44 jährigen patientin. Internist 1990;31:78.
236. Samaan NA. Parathyroid carcinoma. In Cancer Medicine, 2nd ed. Edited by JF Holland, IE Frei. Philadelphia: Lea & Febiger, 1982, p 1692.
237. Samaan NA, Hickey RC, Shutts PE. Diagnosis, localization, and management of pheochromocytoma: pitfalls and follow-up in 41 patients. Cancer 1988;62:2451.
238. Samaan NA, Ouais S, Ordonez NG, Choksi UA, Sellin RV, Hickey RC. Multiple endocrine syndrome type 1. Clinical, laboratory findings, and management in five families. Cancer 1989;64:741.
239. Samaan NA, Schultz PN, Hickey RC. Medullary thyroid carcinoma: prognosis of familial versus sporadic disease and the role of radiotherapy. J Clin Endocrinol Metab 1988;67:801.
240. Sano T, Saito H, Inaba H, Hizawa K, Saito S, Yamanoi A, Mizunuma Y, Matsumura M, Yuasa M, Hiraishi K. Immunoreactive somatostatin and vasoactive intestinal polypeptide in adrenal pheochromocytoma: an immunochemical and ultrastructural study. Cancer 1983;52:282.
241. Sardesai SH, Mourant AJ, Sivathandon Y, Farrow R, Gibbons DO. Phaeochromocytoma and catecholamine induced cardiomyopathy presenting as heart failure. Br Heart J 1990;63:234.
242. Sasaki A, Yumita S, Kimura S, Miura Y, Yoshinaga K. Immunoreactive corticotropin-releasing hormone, growth hormone-releasing hormone, somatostatin, and peptide histidine methionine are present in adrenal pheochromocytomas, but not in extra-adrenal pheochromocytoma. J Clin Endocrinol Metab 1990;70:996.
243. Schifter S. Calcitonin gene-related peptide and calcitonin as tumour markers in MEN 2 family screening. Clin Endocrinol 1989;30:263.
244. Schimke RN. Multiple endocrine neoplasia: how many syndromes? Am J Med Genet 1990;37:375.
245. Schimke RN, Hartmann WH, Prout TE, Rimoin DL. Syndrome of bilateral pheochromocytoma, medullary thyroid carcinoma, and multiple neuromas. N Engl J Med 1968;279:1.
246. Schmedtje JF, Sax S, Pool JL, Goldfarb RA, Nelson EB. Localization of ectopic pheochromocytomas by magnetic resonance imaging. Am J Med 1987;83:770.
247. Scott HW, Halter SA. Oncologic aspects of pheochromocytoma: the importance of follow-up. Surgery 1984;96:1061.
248. Scott HW Jr, Reynolds V, Green N, Page D, Oates JA, Robertson D, Roberts S. Clinical experience with malignant pheochromocytomas. Surg Gynecol Obstet 1982;154: 801.
249. Shane E, Bilezikian JP. Parathyroid carcinoma: a review of 62 patients. Endocrinol Rev 1982;3:218.
250. Shane E, Bilezikian JP. Parathyroid carcinoma. In Textbook of Uncommon Cancer. Edited CJ Williams, JG Krikorian, MR Green, D Raghavan. Chichester: Wiley, 1988, p 763.
251. Shane E, Jacobs TP, Siris ES, Steinberg SF, Stoddart K, Canfield RE, Bilezikian JP. Therapy of hypercalcemia due to parathyroid carcinoma with intravenous dichloromethylene diphosphonate. Am J Med 1982;72:939.
252. Shapiro B, Fig LM. Management of pheochromocytoma. Endocrinol Metab Clin North Am 1989;18:443.
253. Shapiro B, Fig LM, Gross MD, Khafagi F. Contributions of nuclear endocrinology to the diagnosis of adrenal tumors. In Recent Results in Cancer Research: Hormone-related Malignant Tumors. Edited by L Beck, E Grundmann, R Ackermann, HD Roher. New York: Springer Verlag, 1990, p 113.
254. Shapiro B, Sisson JC, Eyre P, Copp JE, Dmuchowski C, Beierwaltes WH. 131I-MIBG—A new agent in diagnosis and treatment of pheochromocytoma. Cardiology 1985;72:(suppl 1):137.
255. Shapiro B, Sisson JC, Lloyd R, Nakajo M, Satterlee W, Beierwalters WH. Malignant pheochromocytoma: clinical, biochemical and scintigraphic characterization. Clin Endocrinol 1984;20:189.
256. Shimaoka K, Schoenfeld DA, DeWys W, Creech RH, DeConti R. A randomized trial of doxorubicin versus doxorubicin plus cisplatin in patients with advanced thyroid carcinoma. Cancer 1984;56:2155.
257. Siddiqui MZ, Von Eyben FE, Spanos G. High-voltage irradiation and combination chemotherapy for malignant pheochromocytoma. Cancer 1988;62:686.
258. Sikri KL, Varndell IM, Hamid QA, Wilson BS, Kameya T, Ponder BA, Lloyd RV, Bloom SR, Polack JM. Medullary carcinoma of the thyroid. An immunocytochemical and histochemical study of 25 cases using eight separate markers. Cancer 1985;56:2481.
259. Silverman ML. Pathology of thyroid and parathyroid glands. In Surgery of the Thyroid and Parathyroid Glands. Edited by B Cady, RL Rossi. Philadelphia: Saunders, 1991, p 31.
260. Simpson EL, Mundy GR, D'Souza SM, Ibbotson KJ, Bockman R, Jacobs JW. Absence of parathyroid hormone messenger RNA in nonparathyroid tumors associated with hypercalcemia. N Engl J Med 1983;309:325.
261. Simpson NE, Kidd KK. The mapping of the locus for multiple endocrine neoplasia type 2A by linkage with chromosome 10 markers. Horm Metab Res Suppl 1989;21:5.
262. Simpson NE, Kidd KK, Goodfellow PJ, McDermid H, Myers S, Kedd JR, Jackson CE, Duncan AMV, Farrer LA, Brasch K, Castiglione C, Genel M, Gertner J, Greenberg CR, Gusella JF, Holden JJA, White BN. Assignment of multiple endocrine neoplasia type 2A to chromosome 10 by linkage. Nature 1987;328:528.

263. Simpson WJ, Palmer JA, Rosen IB, Mustard RA. Management of medullary carcinoma of the thyroid. Am J Surg 1982;144:420.
264. Singer FR. Role of the bisphosphonate etidronate in the therapy of cancer-related hypercalcemia. Semin Oncol 1990;17(suppl 5):34.
265. Sipple JH. The association of pheochromocytoma with carcinoma of the thyroid gland. Am J Med 1961;31:163.
266. Sisson JC, Frager MS, Valk TW, Gros MD, Swanson DP, Wieland DM, Tobes MC, Beierwaltes WH, Thompson NW. Scintigraphic localization of pheochromocytoma. N Engl J Med 1981;305:12.
267. Snover DC, Foucar K. Mitotic activity in benign parathyroid disease. Am J Clin Pathol 1981;75:345.
268. Sobol H, Narod SA, Nakamura Y, Boneu A, Calmettes C, Chadenas D, Charpentier G, Chatal JF, Delepine N, Delisle MJ. Screening for multiple endocrine neoplasia type 2a with DNA-polymorphism analysis. N Engl J Med 1989;321:996.
269. Sobol RE, Memoli V, Deftos LJ. Hormone-negative, chromogranin A-positive endocrine tumors. N Engl J Med 1989;320:444.
270. Sofianides T, Chang, YS, Leary JS, Nichols FX. Localization of parathyroid adenomas by cervical esophagram. J Clin Endocrinol Metab 1978;46:587.
271. Sparagana M. Late recurrence of benign pheochromocytomas: the necessity for long term follow-up. J Surg Oncol 1988;37:140.
272. Sridhar KS, Holland JF, Brown JC, Cohen JM, Ohnuma T. Doxorubicin plus cisplatin in the treatment of apudomas. Cancer 1985;55:2634.
273. St. John Sutton MG, Sheps SG, Lie JT. Prevalence of clinically unsuspected pheochromocytoma: review of a 50-year autopsy series. Mayo Clin Proc 1981;56:354.
274. Stenstrom G, Haljamae H, Tisell LE. Influence of pre-operative treatment with phenoxybenzamine on the incidence of adverse cardiovascular reactions during anaesthesia and surgery for pheochromocytoma. Acta Anaesthesiol Scand 1985;29:797.
275. Stewart AF, Hoecker JL, Mallette LE, Segre GV, Amatruda TT Jr, Vignery A. Hypercalcemia in pheochromocytoma: evidence for a novel mechanism. Ann Intern Med 1985;102:776.
276. Stock JL, Weintraub BD, Rosen SW, Aurbach GD, Spiegel AM, Marx SJ. Human chorionic gonadotropin subunit measurement in primary hyperparathyroidism. J Clin Endocrinol Metab 1982;54:57.
277. Stokes KR. Invasive radiologic evaluation of hyperparathyroidism. In Surgery of the Thyroid and Parathyroid Glands. Edited by B Cady, RL Rossi. Philadelphia: Saunders, 1991, p 278.
278. Suva LJ, Winslow GA, Wettenhall EH, Hammonds RG, Moseley JM, Jasgger-Diefenback H, Rodda CP, Kemp BE, Rodriquez H, Chen EY, Hudson PJ, Martin TJ, Wood WI. A parathyroid hormone-related protein implicated in malignant hypercalcemia: cloning and expression. Science 1987;237:893.
279. Taub MA, Osburne RC, Georges LP, Sode J. Malignant pheochromocytoma. Severe clinical exacerbation and release of stored catecholamines during lymphoma chemotherapy. Cancer 1982;50:1739.
280. Taylor HC, Fallon MD, Velasco ME. Oncogenic osteomalacia and inappropriate antidiuretic hormone secretion due to oat-cell carcinoma. Ann Intern Med 1984;101:786.
281. Thakker RV, Bouloux P, Wooding C, Chotai K, Broad PM, Spurr NK, Besser GM, O'Riordan JLH. Association of parathyroid tumors in multiple endocrine neoplasia type 1 with loss of alleles on chromosome 11. N Engl J Med 1989;321:218.
282. Thakker RV, Ponder BAJ. Multiple endocrine neoplasia. Bailliere's Clin Endocrinol Metab 1988;2:1031.
283. Theilade K, Bak M, Olsen K, Nielsen SL, Christensen NJ. A case of malignant pheochromocytoma treated by 131 I metaiodobenzylguanidine. Acta Oncol 1988;27:296.
284. Thompson NW, Bondeson AG, Bondeson L, Vinik A. The surgical treatment of gastrinoma in MEN I syndrome patients. Surgery 1989;106:1081.
285. Thompson NW, Lloyd RV, Nishiyama RH, Vinik AI, Stroedel WE, Allo MD, Eckhauser FE, Talpos G, Mervak T. MEN I pancreas: a histological and immunohistochemical study. World J Surg 1984;8:561.
286. Thompson NW, Vinik AI, Eckhauser FE. Microgastrinomas of the duodenum: a cause of failed operations for the Zollinger-Ellison syndrome. Ann Surg 1989;209:396.
287. Tisell LE, Ahlman H, Jansson S, Grimelius L. Total pancreatectomy in the MEN-I syndrome. Br J Surg 1986;75:154.
288. Tisell LE, Hansson G, Jansson S, Salander H. Reoperation in the treatment of asymptomatic metastasizing medullary thyroid carcinoma. Surgery 1986;99:60.
289. Troncone L, Rufini V, Montemaggi P, Danza FM, Lasorella A, Mastrangelo R. The diagnostic and therapeutic utility of radioiodinated metaiodobenzylguanidine (MIBG). Eur J Nucl Med 1990;16:325.
290. Tsutsumi M, Yokota J, Kakizoe T, Koiso K, Sugimura T, Terada M. Loss of heterozygosity on chromosomes 1p and 11p in sporadic pheochromocytoma. JNCI 1989;81:367.
291. van Heerden JA, Roland CF, Carney A, Sheps SG, Grant CS. Long-term evaluation following resection of apparently benign pheochromocytoma(s)/paraganglioma(s). World J Surg 1990;14:325.
292. van Heerden JA, Sheps SG, Hamberger B, Sheedy PF, Poston JG, Remine WH. Pheochromocytoma: current status and changing trends. Surgery 1982;91:367.
293. van Heerden JA, Smith SL, Miller LJ. Management of the Zollinger-Ellison syndrome in patients with multiple endocrine neoplasia type I. Surgery 1986;110:971.
294. Velchik MG, Alavi A, Kressel HY, Engelman K. Localization of pheochromocytoma: MIBG, CT, and MRI correlation. J Nucl Med 1989;30:328.
295. Vetter H, Fischer M, Muller-Rensing R, Vetter W, Winterberg B. [^{131}I]-Meta-iodobenzylguanidine in treatment of malignant phaeochromocytomas. Lancet 1983;2(8341):107.
296. Viale G, Dell'Orto P, Moro E, Cozzaglio L, Coggi G. Vasoactive intestinal polypeptide-, somatostatin-, and calcitonin-producing adrenal pheochromocytoma associated with the watery diarrhea (WDHH) syndrome: first case report with immunohistochemical findings. Cancer 1985;55:1099.
297. Vinik AI, Shapiro B, Thompson NW. Plasma gut hormone levels in 37 patients with pheochromocytomas. World J Surg 1986;10:593.
298. Von Moll L, McEwan AJ, Shapiro B, Sisson JC, Gross MD, Lloyd R, Beals E, Beierwaltes WH, Thompson NW. Iodine-131 MIBG scintigraphy of neuroendocrine tumors other than pheochromocytoma and neuroblastoma. J Nucl Med 1987;28:979.
299. Voorhess ML. The catecholamines in tumor and urine from patients with neuroblastoma, ganglio-neuroblastoma and pheochromocytoma. J Pediatr Surg 1968;3:147.
300. Wang C. The anatomic basis of parathyroid surgery. Ann Surg 1976;183:271.
301. Wang C, Gaz RD. Natural history of parathyroid carcinoma: diagnosis, treatment and results. Am J Surg 1985;149:522.
302. Warrell RP, Israel R, Frisone M, Snyder T, Gaynor JJ, Bockman RS. Gallium nitrate for acute treatment of cancer-related hypercalcemia: a randomized, double-blind comparison to calcitonin. Ann Intern Med 1988;108:669.
303. Warrell RP, Issacs M, Alcock NW, Bockman RS. Gallium nitrate for treatment of refractory hypercalcemia from parathyroid carcinoma. Ann Intern Med 1987;107:683.
304. Warrell RPJ, Murphy WK, Schulman P, O'Dwyer PJ, Heller G. A randomized double-blind study of gallium nitrate compared with etidronate for acute control of cancer-related hypercalcemia. J Clin Oncol 1991;9:1467.
305. Weinstein RS, Ide LF. Immunoreactive calcitonin in pheochromocytomas. Proc Soc Exp Biol Med 1980;165:215.
306. Weiss RB. Failure of streptozotocin in rare hormonally active malignancies. Cancer Treat Rep 1978;62:847.
307. Wells SA, Dilley WG, Farndon JA, Leight GS, Baylin SB. Early diagnosis and treatment of medullary thyroid carcinoma. Arch Intern Med 1985;145:1248.
308. Wells SAJ, Gunnells DJ, Gutman RA, Shelbourne JD, Schneider AB, Sherwood LM. The successful transplantation of frozen parathyroid in man. Surgery 1977;81:86.
309. Wermer P. Genetic aspects of adenomatosis of endocrine glands. Am J Med 1954;16:363.
310. Williams ED. Histogenesis of medullary carcinoma of the thyroid. J Clin Pathol 1966;19:114.
311. Williams ED, Karin SMM, Sandler M. Prostaglandin secretion by medullary carcinoma of the thyroid: a possible cause of the associated diarrhea. Lancet 1968;1:22.
312. Williams ED, Pollock DJ. Multiple mucosal neuromata with endocrine tumours: a syndrome allied to Von Recklinghausen's disease. J Pathol Bacteriol 1966;91:71.
313. Williams SD, Birch R, Einhorn LH. Phase II evaluation of doxorubicin plus cisplatin in advanced thyroid cancer: a Southeastern Cancer Study Group trial. Cancer Treat Rep 1986;70:405.
314. Winzelberg GG. Parathyroid imaging. Ann Intern Med 1987;107:64.
315. Wolfe HJ, Melvin KEW, Cervi-Skinner SJ, Saadi AA, Juliar JF, Jackson CE, Tashjian AHJ. C-cell hyperplasia preceding medullary thyroid carcinoma. N Engl J Med 1973;289:437.
316. Woltering EA, Mozell EJ, O'Dorisio TM, Fletcher WS, Howe B. Suppression of primary and secondary peptides with somatostatin analog in the therapy of functional endocrine tumors. Surg Gynecol Obstet 1988;167:153.
317. Wynick D, Williams SJ, Bloom SR. Symptomatic secondary hormone syndromes in patients with established malignant pancreatic endocrine tumors. N Engl J Med 1988;319:605.
318. Zollinger RM, Ellison EH. Primary peptic ulcerations of the jejunum associated with islet cell tumor of the pancreas. Ann Surg 1955;142:709.
319. Zweifler AJ, Julius S. Increased platelet catecholamine content in pheochromocytoma: a diagnostic test in patients with elevated plasma catecholamines. N Engl J Med 1982;306:890.
320. Quint LE, Glazer GM. Pheochromocytoma and paraganglioma: comparison of MR imaging with CT and I-131 MIBG scintigraphy. Radiology 1987;165:89.
321. Bravo E, Fouad-Tarazi F, Rossi G. A reevaluation of the hemodynamics of pheochromocytoma. Hypertension 1990;15(suppl 1):128.
322. Bravo E, Tarazi R, Fouad F. Blood pressure regulation in pheochromocytoma. Hypertension 1982;4(suppl 2):193.
323. Bravo E. Pheochromocytoma: new concepts and future trends. Kidney Int 1991;40:544.
324. Donis-keller H, Dou S, Chi D. Mutations in the RET proto-oncogene are associated with MEN 2a and FMTC. Hum Mol Genet 1993;2:851.
325. Dralle H, Scheumann GF, Nashan B. Review: recent developments in adrenal surgery. Acta Chir Belg 1994;94:137.
326. Gifford RW, Manger WM, Bravo E. Pheochromocytoma. Endocronol Metab Clin North Am 1994;23:387.
327. Hartmut PH, Neumann MD, Dietmar P. Pheochromocytomas, multiple endocrine neoplasia type 2, and Von Hippel-Lindau disease. N Engl J Med 1994;329:1531.
328. Hofstra RM, Landsvater RM, Ceccherini I. A mutation in the RET proto-oncogene associated with multiple endocrine neoplasia type 2b and sporadic medullary thyroid carcinoma. Nature 1994;367:375.
329. Khosla S, Patel VM, Hay ID. Loss of heterozygosity suggests multiple genetic alterations in pheochromocytomas and medullary thyroid carcinomas. J Clin Invest 1991;87:1691.
330. Krempf M, Lumbroso J, Mornex R. Use of M -(131)iodobenzylguanidine in the treatment of malignant pheochromocytoma. J Clin Endocrinol Metab 1991;72:455.
331. Lee VM, Lui DM, Hall SJ. Unsuspected malignant pheochromocytoma: appearance on thallium and gallium scans. Am J Roentgenol 1993;161:1333.
332. Moley JF, Brother MB, Fong C-T. Consistent association of 1p loss of heterozygosity with pheochromocytomas from patients with multiple endocrine neoplasia type 2 syndromes. Cancer Res 1992;52:770.
333. Mulligan LM, Gardner E, Smith BA. Genetic events in tumor initiation and progression in multiple endocrine neoplasia type 2. Genes Chromosom Cancer 1993;6:166.
334. Reubi JC, Waser B, Khosla S. In vitro and in vivo detection of somatostatin receptors in pheochromocytomas and paraganglioma. J Clin Endocrinol Metab 1992;74:1082.
335. Wu L-T, Averbuch, SD. Treatment of advanced medullary thyroid carcinoma with a combination of cyclophosphamide, vincristine, and dacarbazine. Cancer 1994;73:432.
336. Sheps SG, Jiang N-S, Klee GG. Recent developments in the diagnosis and treatment of pheochromocytoma. Mayo Clin Proc 1990;65:88.
337. Shulkin BL, Wieland DM, Schwaiger M. PET scanning with hydroepinephrine: an approach to the localization of pheochromocytoma. J Nucl Med 1992;33:1125.
338. Stein PP, Black HR. A simplified diagnostic approach to pheochromocytoma: a review of the literature and report of one institution's experience. Medicine 1990;70:46.
339. Stimpel M, Reiss U, Volkmann H. The overnight clonidine suppression test. Hypertension 1993;21:560.
340. Unger P, Hoffman K, Pertsemlidis D. S-100 protein positive sustentacular cells in malignant and locally invasive adrenal pheochromocytoma. Arch Pathol Lab Med 1991;115:484.
341. Wu L-T, Dicpinigaitis P, Bruckner H, Manger W, Averbuch S. Hypertensive crises induced by treatment of malignant pheochromocytoma with a combination of cyclophosphamide, vincristine and dacarbazine. Med Pediatr Oncol 1994;22:389.
342. Boutros AR, Bravo E, Zanettin G. Perioperative management of 63 patients with pheochromocytoma. Cleve Clin J Med 1990;57:613.

343. Mulligan LM, Kwok JBJ. Germ-line mutations of the RET proto-oncogene in multiple endocrine neoplasia type 2a. Nature 1993;328:528.
344. Eng C, Smith DP. Point mutation within the tyrosine kinase domain of the RET proto-oncogene in multiple endocrine neoplasia type 2b and related sporadic tumors. Hum Mol Genet 1994;3:237.
345. Arnold A. Molecular mechanisms of parathyroid neoplasia. Endocrinol Metab Clin North Am 1994;23:93.
346. Benya RV, Metz DC. Zollinger-Ellison syndrome can be the initial endocrine manifestation in patients with multiple endocrine neoplasia-type 1. Am J Med1994;97:436.
347. Cadiot G, Laurent PP. Is the multiple endocrine neoplasia type 1 gene a suppressor for fundic argyrophil tumors in the Zollinger-Ellison syndrome? Gastroenterology 1993;105:579.
348. Doherty GM, Doppman JL. Results of a prospective strategy to diagnose, localize and resect insulinomas. Surgery 1991;110:989.
349. Ezzat S, Snyder PJ. Octreotide treatment of acromegaly. Ann Intern Med 1992;117:711.
350. Fraker DL, Norton JA. Controversies in surgical therapy for APUDomas. Semin Surg Oncol 1993;9:437.
351. Kvols LK, Reubi JC. Somatostatin-receptor imaging of carcinoid and islet cell tumors. Proc Am Soc Clin Oncol 1991;10:405.
352. McCutcheon IE. Management of individual tumor syndromes: Pituitary neoplasia. Endocrinol Metab Clin North Am 1994;23:37.
353. Melmed S. Pituitary neoplasia. Endocrinol Metab Clin North Am 1994;23: 81.
354. Moertel CG, Lefkopoulo M. Streptozocin-doxorubicin, streptozocin-fluorouracil or chlorozotocin in the treatment of advanced islet-cell carcinoma. N Engl J Med 1992;326:519.
355. Moertel CG, Johnson CM. The management of patients with advanced carcinoid tumors and islet cell carcinomas. Ann Intern Med 1994;120:302.
356. Norton JA, Doppman JL. Curative resection in Zollinger-Ellison syndrome. Results of a 10-year prospective study. Ann Surg 1992;215:8.
357. Rosch T, Lightdale CJ. Localization of pancreatic endocrine tumors by endoscopic ultrasonography. N Engl J Med 1992;326:1721.
358. Skogseid B, Eriksson B. Multiple endocrine neoplasia type 1: A 10-year prospective screening in four kindreds. J Clin Endocrinol Metab 1991;73:281.
359. Skogseid B, Rastad J. Multiple endocrine neoplasia type 1. Endocrinol Metab Clin North Am 1994;23:1.
360. Thakker RV. The role of molecular genetics in screening for multiple endocrine neoplasia type 1. Endocrinol Metab Clin North Am 1994;23:117.
361. Thom AK, Norton JA. Localization, incidence, and malignant potential of duodenal gastrinomas. Surgery 1992;110:1086.
362. Vassilopoulou R, Ajani J. Islet cell tumors of the pancreas. Endocrinol Metab Clin North Am 1994;23:53.
363. Wilkinson S, Teh BT. Cause of death in multiple endocrine neoplasia type 1. Arch Surg 1993;128:683.
364. Bonnin F, Schlumberger M. Screening for adrenal medullary disease in patients with medullary thyroid carcinoma. J Endocrinol Invest 1994;17:253.
365. Chi DD, Toshima K. Predictive testing for multiple endocrine neoplasia type 2a based on the detection of mutations in the RET protooncogene. Surgery 1994;116:124.
366. Easton DF, Ponder MA. The clinical and screening age-at-onset distribution for the MEN 2 syndrome. Am J Hum Genet 1989;44:208.
367. Evans DB, Lee JE. Adrenal medullary disease in multiple endocrine neoplasia type 2. Endocrinol Metab Clin North Am 1994;23:167.
368. Cornelis JM, Lips MD. Clinical screening as compared with DNA analysis in families with multiple endocrine neoplasia type 2a. N Engl J Med 1994;331:828.
369. Mallette LE. Management of hyperparathyroidism in the multiple endocrine neoplasia syndromes and other familial endocrinopathies. Endocrinol Metab Clin North Am 1994;23:19.
370. McMahon R, Mulligan LM. Direct, non-radioactive detection of mutations in multiple endocrine neoplasia type 2a families. Hum Mol Genet 1994;3:643.
371. O'Riordain DS, O'Brain T. Surgical management of primary hyperparathyroidism in multiple neoplasia type 1 and 2. Surgery 1993;114:1031.
372. Raue F, Frank-Raue K. Multiple endocrine neoplasia type 2: clinical features and screening. Endocrinol Metab Clin North Am 1994;23:137.
373. Snow KJ, Boyd AE III. Management of individual tumor syndromes, medullary thyroid carcinoma and hyperthyroidism. Endocrinol Metab Clin North Am 1994;23:157.
374. Tsai M-S, Ledger S. Identification of multiple endocrine neoplasia type 2 gene carriers using linkage analysis and analysis of the RET proto-oncogene. J Clin Endocrinol Metab 1994;78:1261.
375. Wells SA, Donis-Keller H. Current perspectives in the diagnosis and management of patients with multiple endocrine neoplasia type 2 syndromes. Endocrinol Metab Clin North Am 1994;23:215.
376. Wells SA, Chi DD. Predictive DNA testing and prophylactic thyroidectomy in patients at risk for multiple endocrine neoplasia type 2a. Ann Surg 1994;220:237.
377. Arnaud CD. The parathyroid glands, hypercalcemia and hypocalcemia. In Cecil Textbook of Medicine. 18th Edition. Edited by JB Wyngaarden, LH Smith Jr. Philadelphia: Saunders, 1988, p. 1486.
378. Arnold A, Staunton CE, Kim GH, Gaz RD, Kronenberg HM. Monoclonality and abnormal parathyroid hormone genes in parathyroid adenomas. N Engl J Med 1988;318:658.
379. Attie M. Treatment of hypercalcemia. Endocrinol Metab Clin North Am 1989;18:807.
380. Au WYW. Calcitonin treatment of hypercalcemia due to parathyroid carcinoma: synergistic effect of prednisone on long-term treatment of hypercalcemia. Arch Intern Med 1975;135:1594.
381. Aurbach GD, Mallette LE, Patten BM, Heath DA, Doppman JL, Bilezikian JP. Hyperparathyroidism: recent studies. Ann Intern Med 1973;79:566.
382. Baba H, Kishihara M, Tohmon M, Fukase M, Kizaki T, Okada S, Matsuzuka F, Kobayashi A, Kuma K, Fujita T. Identification of parathyroid hormone messenger ribonucleic acid in an apparently nonfunctioning parathyroid carcinoma transformed from a parathyroid carcinoma with hyperparathyroidism. J Clin Endocrinol Metab 1986;62:247.
383. Bajorunas DR. Clinical manifestations of cancer-related hypercalcemia. Semin Oncol 1990;17(suppl 5):16.
384. Berland Y, Olmer M, Lebreuil G, Grisoli J. Parathyroid carcinoma, adenoma and hyperplasia in a case of chronic renal insufficiency on dialysis. Clin Nephrol 1982;18:154.
385. Bilezikian JP. Management of acute hypercalcemia. N Engl J Med 1992;326:1196.
386. Bilezikian JP. Etiologies and therapy of hypercalcemia. Endocrinol Metab Clin North Am 1989;18:389.
387. Bilezikian JP. Parathyroid hormone-related peptide in sickness and in health. N Engl J Med 1990;332:1151 Editorial.
388. Black BK. Carcinoma of the parathyroid. Ann Surg 1954;139:355.
389. Bostwick DG, Null W, Holmes D, Weber E, Barchas JD, Bensch KG. Expression of opioid peptides in tumors. N Engl J Med 1987;317:1439.
390. Brandi ML, Aurbach GD, Fitzpatrick LA, Quarto R, Speigel AL, Bliziotes M, Norton JA, Doppman JL, Marx SJ. Parathyroid mitogenic activity in plasma from patients with familial multiple endocrine neoplasia type 1. N Engl J Med 1986;314:1287.
391. Broadus AE, Mangin M, Ikeda K, Insogna KL, Weir EC, Burtis WJ, Stewart AF. Humoral hypercalcemia of cancer: identification of a novel parathyroid hormone-like peptide. N Engl J Med 1988;319:556.
392. Budayr AA, Nissenson RA, Klein RF, Pun KK, Clark OH, Diep D, Arnaud CD, Strewler GJ. Increased serum levels of a parathyroid hormone-like protein in malignancy-associated hypercalcemia. Ann Intern Med 1989;111:807.
393. Bukowski RM, Sheeler L, Cunningham J, Esselstyn C. Successful combination chemotherapy for metastatic parathyroid carcinoma. Arch Intern Med 1984;144:399.
394. Burtis WJ, Brady TG, Orloff JJ, Ersbak JB, Warrell, Olson BR, Wu TL, Mitnick ME, Broadus AE, Stewart AF. Immunochemical characterization of circulating parathyroid hormone-related protein in patients with humoral hypercalcemia of cancer. N Engl J Med 1990;322:1106.
395. Cady B. Hyperparathyroidism. In Surgery of the Thyroid and Parathyroid Glands, 2nd Edition. Edited by CE Sedgwick and B Cady. Philadelphia: Saunders, 1980, p. 206.
396. Cai Q, Hodgson SF, Kao PC, Lennon VA, Klee GG, Zinsmiester AR, Kumar R. Brief report: Inhibition of renal phosphate transport by a tumor product in a patient with oncogenic osteomalacia. N Engl J Med 1994;330:1645.
397. Calandra DB, Chejfec G, Foy BK, Lawrence AM, Paloyan E. Parathyroid carcinoma: Biochemical and pathologic response to DTIC. Surgery 1984;96:1132.
398. Case records of the Massachusetts General Hospital: Case 27461. N Engl J Med 1941;225:789.
399. Castleman B, Roth SI. Tumors of the parathyroid glands. In Atlas of Tumor Pathology, Second Series, Fascicle 14. Washington, D.C.: Armed Forces Institute of Pathology, 1978.
400. Chahinian AP, Holland JF, Nieburgs HE, Marinescu A, Geller SA, Kirschner PA. Metastatic nonfunctioning parathyroid carcinoma: Ultrastructural evidence of secretory granules and response to chemotherapy. Am J Med Sci 1981;282:80.
401. Clerkin EP. Hyperparathyroidism. In Surgery of the Thyroid and Parathyroid Glands, 3rd Edition. Edited by B Cady, RL Rossi. Philadelphia: Saunders, 1991, p. 243.
402. Cryns VL, Thor A, Xu H-J, Hu S-X, Wierman ME, Vickery AL Jr, Benedict WF, Arnold A. Loss of the retinoblastoma tumor-suppressor gene in parathyroid carcinoma. N Engl J Med 1994;330:757.
403. Dhom G, Hohbach C. Case 12. Ultrastruct Pathol 1980;1:141.
404. Dinnen JS, Greenwood RH, Jones JH, Walker DA, Williams ED. Parathyroid carcinoma in familial hyperparathyroidism. J Clin Pathol 1977;30:366.
405. Flye MW, Brennan MF. Surgical resection of metastatic parathyroid carcinoma. Ann Surg 1981;193:425.
406. Friedman E, Sakaguchi K, Bale AE, Falghetti A, Streeten E, Zimering MB, Weinstein LS, McBride WO, Nakamura Y, Brandi ML, Norton JA, Aurbach GD, Spiegel AM, Marx S. Clonality of parathyroid tumors in familial multiple endocrine neoplasia type I. N Engl J Med 1989;321:213.
407. Fritsche AE. Clinical utility of serum osteocalcin. Cancer Invest 1990;8:441.
408. Fujimoto Y, Obara T. How to recognize and treat parathyroid carcinoma. Endocrinol Metab Clin North Am 1989;67:343.
409. Glover D, Riley L, Carmichael K, Spar B, Glick J, Kligerman MM, Agus ZS, Slatopolsky E, Attie M, Goldfarb S. Hypocalcemia and inhibition of parathyroid hormone secretion after administration of WR-2721 (a radioprotective and chemoprotective agent). N Engl J Med 1983;309:1137.
410. Heath DA. Primary hyperparathyroidism: Clinical presentation and factors influencing clinical management. Endocrinol Metab Clin North Am 1989;18:631.
411. Heath H III, Hodgson SF, Kennedy MA. Primary hyperparathyroidism: Incidence, morbidity, and potential economic impact in a community. N Engl J Med 1980;302:189.
412. Hirschel-Scholz S, Jung A, Fischer JA, Trechsel U, Bonjour JP. Suppression of parathyroid secretion after administration of WR-2721 in a patient with parathyroid carcinoma. Clin Endocrinol 1985;23:313.
413. Hodge MB. Thyroid and parathyroid disease during pregnancy. In Surgery of the Thyroid and Parathyroid Glands, 3rd Edition. Edited by B Cady, RL Rossi. Philadelphia: Saunders, 1991, p. 313.
414. Holmes EC, Morton DL, Ketcham AS. Parathyroid carcinoma: A collective review. Ann Surg 1969;169:631.
415. Insogna KL. Humoral hypercalcemia of malignancy: The role of parathyroid hormone-related protein. Endocrinol Metab Clin North Am 1989;18:779.
416. Ireland JP, Fleming SJ, Levison DA, Cattell WR, Baker LRI. Parathyroid carcinoma associated with chronic renal failure and previous radiotherapy to the neck. J Clin Pathol 1985:38:1114.
417. Kastan DJ, Kottamasu SR, Frame B, Greenwald K. Carcinoma in a mediastinal fifth parathyroid gland. JAMA 1987;257:1218.
418. Katz A, Braunstein GD. Clinical, biochemical, and pathologic features of radiation-associated hyperparathyroidism. Arch Intern Med 1983;143:79.
419. Krubsack AJ, Wilson SD, Lawson TL, Kneeland JB, Thorsen K, Collier BD, Hellman RS, Isitman AT. Prospective comparison of radionuclide, computed tomographic, sonographic, and magnetic resonance localization of parathyroid tumors. Surgery 1989;106:639.
420. Lafferty FW. Primary hyperparathyroidism: Changing clinical spectrum, prevalence of hypertension and discriminant analysis of laboratory tests. Arch Intern Med 1981;141:1761.
421. Law WL Jr, Heath H III. Familial benign hypercalcemia (hypocalciuric hypercalcemia): Clinical and pathogenetic studies in 21 families. Ann Intern Med 1985;102:511.
422. McAuley P, Asa SL, Chiu B, Henderson J, Goltzman D, Drucker DJ. Parathyroid hormone-like peptide in normal and neoplastic mesothelial cells. Cancer 1990;66:1975.
423. McCance DR, Kenny BD, Sloan JM, Russell CJF, Hassen DR. Parathyroid carinoma: A review. J Roy Soc Med 1987;80:505.

424. Mundy GR. Hypercalcemia of malignancy revisited. J Clin Invest 1988;82:1.
425. Murphy MN, Glennon PG, Diocee MS, Wick MR, Cavers DJ. Nonsecretory parathyroid carcinoma of the mediastinum: Light microscopic, immunocytochemical, and ultrastructural features of a case, and review of the literature. Cancer 1986;58:2468.
426. Nathaniels EK, Nathaniels AM, Wang C. Mediastinal parathyroid tumors: A clinical and pathological study of 84 cases. Ann Surg 1970;171:165.
427. Nussbaum SR, Gaz RD, Arnold A. Hypercalcemia and ectopic secretion of parathyroid hormone by an ovarian carcinoma with rearrangement of the gene for parathyroid hormone. N Engl J Med 1990;323:1324.
428. Obara T, Fujimoto Y, Hirayama A, Kanaji Y, Ito Y, Kodama T, Ogata T. Flow cytometric DNA analysis of parathyroid tumors with special reference to its diagnostic and prognostic value in parathyroid carcinoma. Cancer 1990;65:1789.
429. Obara T, Fujimoto Y, Kanaji Y, Okamoto T, Hirayama A, Ito Y, Kodama T. Flow cytometric DNA analysis of parathyroid tumors: Implication of aneuploidy for pathologic and biologic classification. Cancer 1990;66:1555.
430. O'Connor DT, Deftos LJ. Secretion of chromogranin A by peptide-producing endocrine neoplasms. N Engl J Med 1986;314:1145.
431. Palmer M, Ljunghall S, Akerstrom G, Adami HO, Berstrom R, Grimelius L, Rudberg C, Johansson H. Patients with primary hyperparathyroidism operated on over a 24 year period: Temporal trends of clinical and laboratory findings. J Chronic Dis 1987;40:121.
432. Parham GP, Orr JW. Hyperparathyroidism secondary to parathyroid carcinoma in pregnancy: A case report. J Reprod Med 1987;32:123.
433. Ponder B. Gene losses in human tumours. Nature 1988;335:400.
434. Ralston SH, Alzais AA, Gardner MD, Boyle IT. A treatment of cancer associated hypercalcaemia with combined aminohydroxypropylidene diphosphonate and calcitoni. Br Med J 1986;292:1549.
435. Ringenberg QS, Doll D. Endocrine tumors and miscellaneous cancers in pregnancy. Semin Oncol 1989;16:445.
436. Ritch PS. Treatment of cancer-related hypercalcemia. Semin Oncol 1990;17(suppl 5):26.
437. Rosenblatt M. Peptide hormone antagonists that are effective in vivo: Lessons from parathyroid hormone. N Engl J Med 1986;315:1004.
438. Sager R. Tumor suppressor genes: The puzzle and the promise. Science. 1989;246:1406.
439. Samaan NA. Parathyroid carcinoma. In Cancer Medicine, 2nd Edition. Edited by JF Holland, E Frei III. Philadelphia: Lea & Febiger, 1982, p. 1692.
440. Schantz A, Castleman B. Parathyroid carcinoma: A study of 70 cases. Cancer 1973;31:600.
441. Shane E, Bilezikian JP. Parathyroid carcinoma: A review of 62 patients. Endocrinol Rev 1982;3:218.
442. Shane E, Bilezikian JP. Parathyroid carcinoma. In *Textbook of Uncommon Cancer.* Edited by CJ Williams, JG Krikorian, MR Green, D Raghavan. Chichester: Wiley, 1988, p. 763.
443. Shane E, Jacobs TP, Siris ES, Steinberg SF, Stoddart K, Canfield RE, Bilezikian JP. Therapy of hypercalcemia due to parathyroid carcinoma with intravenous dichloromethylene diphosphonate. Am J Med 1982;72:939.
444. Silverman ML. Pathology of thyroid and parathyroid glands. In Surgery of the Thyroid and Parathyroid Glands, 3rd edition. Edited by B Cady, RL Rossi. Philadelphia: Saunders, 1991, p. 31.
445. Simpson EL, Mundy GR, D'Souza, SM, Ibbotson JK. Brockman R, Jacobs JW. Absence of parathyroid hormone messenger RNA in nonparathyroid tumors associated with hypercalcemia. N Engl J Med 1983;309:325.
446. Singer FR. Role of the bisphosphonate etidronate in the therapy of cancer-related hypercalcemia. Semin Oncol 1990;17(suppl 5):34.
447. Snover DC, Foucar K. Mitotic activity in benign parathyroid disease. Am J Clin Pathol 1981;75:345.
448. Sofianides T, Chang Y-S, Leary JS, Nichols FX. Localization of parathyroid adenomas by cervical esophagram. J Clin Endocrinol Metab 1978;46:587.
449. Stewart AF, Hoecker JL, Mallette LE, Segre GV, Amatruda TT Jr, Vignery A. Hypercalcemia in pheochromocytoma: Evidence for a novel mechanism. Ann Intern Med 1985;102:776.
450. Stock JL, Weintraub BD, Rosen SW, Aurbach GD, Spiegel AM, Marx SJ. Human chroionic gonadotropin subunit measurement in primary hyperparathryoidism. J Clin Endocrinol Metab 1982;54:57.
451. Stokes KR. Invasive radiologic evaluation of hyperparathyroidism. In Surgery of the Thyroid and Parathyroid Glands, 3rd Edition. Edited by B Cady, RL Rossi. Philadelphia: Saunders, 1991, p. 278.
452. Suva LJ, Winslow GA, Wettenhall EH, Hammonds RG, Moseley JM, Jasgger-Diefenback H, Rodda CP, Kemp BE, Rodriquez H, Chen EY, Hudson PJ, Martin TJ, Wood WI. A parathyroid hormone-related protein implicated in malignant hypercalcemia: Cloning and expression. Science 1987;237:893.
453. Taylor HC, Fallon MD, Velasco ME. Oncogenic osteomalacia and inappropriate antidiuretic hormone secretion due to oat-cell carcinoma. Ann Intern Med 1984;101:786.
454. Thakker RV, Bouloux P, Wooding C, Chotal K, Broad PM, Spurr NK, Besser GM, O'Riordan JLH. Association of parathyroid tumors in multiple endocrine neoplasia type 1 with loss of alleles on chromosome 11. N Engl J Med 1989;321:218.
455. Thompson GB, Mullan BP, Grant CS, Gorman CA, Van Heerden JA, O'Connor MK, Goellner JR, Ilstrup DM. Parathyroid imaging with technecium-99m-sestamibi: An initial institutional experience. Surgery 1994;116:966.
456. Wang C. The anatomic basis of parathyroid surgery. Ann Surg 1976;183:271.
457. Wang C, Gaz RD. Natural history of parathyroid carcinoma: Diagnosis, treatment and results. Am J Surg 1985;149:522.
458. Warrell RP, Israel R, Frisone M, Snyser T, Gaynor JJ, Bockman RS. Gallium nitrate for acute treatment of cancer-related hypercalcemia. A randomized, double-blind comparison to calcitonin. Ann Intern Med 1988;108:669.
459. Warrell RP, Issacs M, Alcock NW, Bockman RS. Gallium nitrate for treatment of refractory hypercalcemia from parathyroid carcinoma. Ann Intern Med 1987;107:683.
460. Winzelberg GG. Parathyroid imaging. Ann Intern Med 1987;107:64.

CHAPTER 103

Neoplasms of the Gastroenteropancreatic Endocrine System

AARON I. VINIK AND ROGER R. PERRY

Introduction

Endocrine tumors of the gastroenteropancreatic (GEP) axis consist of cells that are capable of amine precursor uptake and decarboxylation and therefore have been named apudomas (1). The morphologic similarity of the Apud cells suggested a common embryologic origin, which was believed to be the neural crest but was later revised to include the neuroectoderm or, in the case of endocrine cells, the dorsal placoderm. Various studies have cast doubt on this hypothesis, however, and most workers agree that these tumors should be classified according to their secretory products (i.e., gastrinoma, somatostatinoma, glucagonoma, and pancreatic polypeptide [PPoma]) (2–4). The generally held belief that the neuronal characteristics of these cells indicate an ectodermal origin during mammalian embryogenesis largely has been abandoned.

Developmental Origin of Islets during Pancreatic Embryogenesis

The developing pancreas appears as a protrusion from the dorsal surface of the embryonic gut (5). The different islet-cell types appear sequentially during development in vivo. Therefore, it seems reasonable to propose that coordinated growth depends on the specificity of growth factors.

Rosenberg and Vinik (6) used a model for new islet formation (i.e., nesidioblastosis) and showed that pancreatic ductal cells are capable of differentiating on stimulation into adult endocrine cells that are capable of secreting insulin in a fully regulated manner. This has led to the notion that endocrine tumors derive from a totipotential stem cell in the gut that is capable of differentiating into any one of a variety of cells that may be responsible for the clinical syndrome (Fig. 103.1).

A great deal of interest now is being focused on the factors responsible for the initiation of growth, growth proliferation, differentiation into adult endocrine cells, and in neuronal systems, for growth cessation and cell maintenance. Several models of pancreatic regeneration and tumor formation have been established (7–17).

Growth Factors

Multiple growth factors and receptors are frequently expressed in GEP tumors. These growth factors may include insulin-like growth factor-1, platelet-derived growth factor, transforming growth factors-α and -β, basic fibroblast growth factors, and nerve growth factor (18, 19). The frequent coexpression of TGF-α and its corresponding receptor, the epidermal growth factor receptor, suggests the presence of autocrine regulatory mechanisms in these tumors (19). TGF-β has been implicated in the desmoplastic reaction associated with carcinoid tumors (19, 20). Overall, the precise role of these growth factors and their importance in the growth and progression of GEP tumors is unknown.

Recently, apoptosis (i.e., programmed cell death) has been shown to be an important process that may occur under normal physiologic conditions, including embryonic growth and development, the differentiation of B-cell populations, and the involution of cells deprived of necessary growth factors (21). Apoptosis may be induced by a variety of chemotherapeutic drugs and cytokines (22). Several growth factors and substances that are secreted by neuroendocrine tumors, including TGF-β_1 (23), glucocorticoids (24), and somatostatin (25), have been shown in other model systems to induce apoptosis. The importance of apoptosis in the normal growth and differentiation of neuroendocrine tissues, however, and the importance of apoptosis in the response of GEP tumors to chemotherapy, remain unknown.

The multiple endocrine neoplasia type 1 syndrome (MEN-1) (i.e., combined occurrence of tumors of the pituitary, pancreas, and parathyroid glands) is associated with the loss of alleles on chromosome 11q13, which appears to be a tumor-suppressor gene (26, 27). This is the same chromosome on which the insulin gene has been located (28); and along with the finding of parathyroid mitogenic activity in the plasma of patients with MEN-1 (29, 30), and nesidioblastosis in certain families, suggests a genetic predisposition to tumor formation based on elaboration of a growth factor. Data from cell lineage analysis of pancreatic islets suggest that progenitor cells, which contain catecholamines, are present in pancreatic ducts and give rise to the glucagon and insulin cells of adult islets (31); and they can be stimulated to grow by plasma from patients with MEN-1. The findings that patients

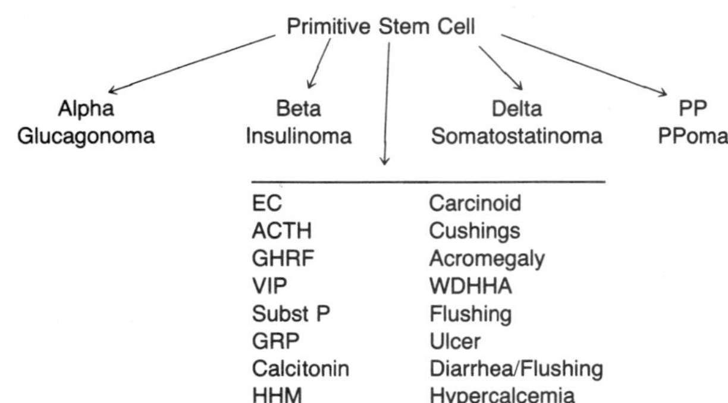

Figure 103.1. Gastroenteropancreatic tumors. ACTH, corticotropin; EC, enterochromaffin; GHRF, growth hormone-releasing factor; GRP, gastrin-releasing peptide; HHM, humoral hypercalcemia of malignancy; PP, pancreatic polypeptide; Subst P, substance P; VIP, vasoactive intestinal peptide; WDHHA, watery diarrhea hypokalemia, hypochlorhydria, and acidosis.

Table 103.1. Characteristics of Neuroendocrine Tumors

Rare
Usually small, <1 cm
Slow growing, months to years, "cancer in slow motion"
Usually metastasize before becoming symptomatic, often when tumor is >2 cm
Expression is episodic, may be silent for years
Symptoms mimic commonplace conditions and often are misdiagnosed
Complex diagnosis, rarely made clinically, requiring sophisticated laboratory and scanning techniques

with MEN-1 also might elaborate into their plasma mitogenic factors for pancreatic islet cells led McLeod and colleagues to postulate a genetically determined, circulating growth factor in the initiation of GEP tumor growth (Table 103.1) (32). It has been suggested, but not proven, that allelic loses in the MEN-I tumor-suppressor gene located in the 11q13 region also might be responsible for sporadic parathyroid, pituitary, and pancreaticoduodenal tumors (33). The few cases of carcinoid tumors studied have not shown losses in this region.

In addition, MEN-2a (34, 35), MEN-2b (36, 37), and familial medullary thyroid carcinoma (35) are associated with mutations of the *RET* proto-oncogene, which is a conventional dominant oncogene located on 10q11.2. Although mutations in this region have been associated with sporadic medullary thyroid carcinoma (37), the role, if any, of this gene in sporadic GEP tumors is unknown.

Neuroendocrine Characteristics

A number of peptides originally isolated from gut endocrine tissues have been shown to occur in nerves. These include gastrin, cholecystokinin, vasoactive intestinal polypeptide (VIP), and substance P (SP). As a corollary, peptides that have been found primarily in nervous tissues have now been identified in gut endocrine cells and include somatostatin (SRIF), enkephalins, SP, neurotensin, and thyrotropin-releasing hormone (TRH) (38–40) Because many of these peptides occur both in endocrine cells and nerves, "endocrine" tumors of the gut may in fact be endocrine or neurocrine. Unique to the GEP axis is the ability of the endocrine cell to secrete a variety of peptides and amines. Hormonal peptides not only have been found within the same cell (e.g., motilin and serotonin in the enterochromaffin [EC] cell), they have been localized to the same secretory granule. Whether these act within the secretory granule in a paracrine manner or are coregulated in some way is not clear. At any one point in time, several hormones and amines are cosecreted; in individual instances, the symptom complex derives from one or more of the peptides and amines produced and cannot simply be ascribed to a single factor. Thus, a tumor may secrete one peptide, recur, and secrete yet another, and its metastases may secrete still other peptides. In the British National Supra-Regional Survey of National Health Service Hospitals, 58% of 353 patients with neuroendocrine tumors had increased serum levels of two or more hormones at diagnosis. Nine percent of patients had clinical symptoms related to different hormones, and four patients developed new symptoms from secretion of a second hormone after diagnosis (41).

Anatomic Distribution

More than 50% of neuroendocrine tumors in clinical practice are of the so-called carcinoid variety and are found incidentally at operation, after metastasis has occurred, in the small intestine (especially the appendix). The remaining fraction comprises approximately 50% gastrinomas, 30% insulinomas, 13% vipomas, 5 to 10% glucagonomas, and rarely, less than 5% neurotensinomas, somatostatinomas, and etopic hormone-secreting tumors. Nonsecretory tumors were thought to make up the bulk of pancreatic tumors, but with better immunohistochemical stains for endocrine cells, especially for neuron-specific enclose (NSE), chromogranin, synaptophysin, and receptors for somatostatin (42), there is increasing recognition that tumors masquerading as carcinomas of liver, small cell carcinoma of the lung, and the like are endocrine tumors (Table 103.2). Most of these "nonsecretory" tumors actually store and secrete pancreatic polypeptide (PP), but because it has so little in the way of biologic activity, the tumor remains silent.

Approximately 60% of pancreatic gastrinomas are concentrated in Pasarro's Triangle, an area subtended by the head of pancreas, gastric antrum, and first portion of the duodenum. Other neuroendocrine tumors may be distributed more evenly across the pancreas or in ectopic sites such as the adrenal medulla, whereas carcinoid tumors most frequently occur in the appendix and small intestine.

The tumors are proliferative in nature and may take the form of hyperplasia or neoplasia (adenoma, adenomatous hyperplasia, microadenomatosis, nesidioblastosis, or carcinoma). Hyperplasia is relatively uncommon in benign sporadic tumors, but it is the rule in MEN-1 syndrome and often is present in the area of the pancreas surrounding a benign tumor.

Table 103.2. The Clinical Syndromes

Clinical syndrome	Tumor type	Site	Hormone(s)
Flushing/diarrhea/wheezing	Carcinoid	Mid foregut Pancreas/foregut Adrenal medulla	Serotonin, substance P NKA, TCT, PP, CGRP, VIP
Ulcer disease	Gastrinoma	Pancreas (85%) Duodenum (15%)	Gastrin
Hypoglycemia	Insulinoma Sarcomas Hepatoma	Pancreas/uterus Retroperitoneal Liver	Insulin/TNF IGF/BP
Dermatitis/dementia Diabetes/DVT	Glucagonoma	Pancreas	Glucagon
Diabetes/steatorrhea	Somatostatinoma	Pancreas	Somatostatin
Cholelithiasis/neurofibromatosis	Somatostatinoma	Duodenum	Somatostatin
Silent/liver mets	PPoma	Pancreas	PP
Acromegaly	GEP	Pancreas	GH (GHRH)
Cushings	GEP	Pancreas	ACTH/CRF
Hypercalcemia	VIPoma GEP	Pancreas Pancreas	VIP PTHrP
Pigmentation	GEP	Pancreas	MSH

ACTH—Adrenol corticotropic hormone, corticotropin; BP—binding protein; CGRP—calcitonin gene-related peptide; CRF—corticotropin releasing factor; DVT—deep venous thrombosis; GEP—gastroenteropancreatic; GH—growth hormone, somatotropin; GHRH—growth hormone-releasing hormone; IGF—insulin-like growth factor; MSH—melanocyte stimulating hormone; NKA—neurokinin A; PP—pancreatic polypeptide; PTHrP—parathyroid hormone related peptide; TCT—thyrocalcitonin; TNF—tumor necrosis factor; VIP—vasoactive intestinal peptide

The tumors may be further subdivided into (*a*) orthoendocrine, when they secrete the normal product of the cell type (e.g., α-cell glucagon), and (*b*) paraendocrine, when they secrete a peptide or amine that is foreign to the organ or cell of origin. Paraendocrine tumors are found in the adrenal medulla, kidney, lymph nodes, or liver and as a part of MEN-1 when a variety of peptides or amines are secreted.

When tumors metastasize, they do so to local lymph nodes, liver, peritoneum, and rarely, to bone. Metastases are notoriously highly vascular, which is a telltale sign of a GEP tumor and augurs well for the patient. Even with extensive liver metastasis, tumors can regress with treatment.

The occurrence of MEN-1 syndrome may be as frequent as one third of the cases of GEP tumors, depending on the endemic area. In high-risk areas, measurements of ionized Ca^{2+}, prolactin, and PP are important.

The sections that follow focus on the specific syndromes that are ascribed to GEP hyperfunction.

Carcinoid Tumors

Carcinoid tumors are the most commonly occurring gut endocrine tumors. The incidence is estimated to be approximately 1.5 cases per 100,000 of the general population (i.e., approximately 2,500 cases/year in the United States). Nonetheless, they account for 13 to 34% of all tumors of the small bowel and 17 to 46% of all malignant tumors of the small bowel (43). They derive from a primitive stem cell and generally are found in the gut wall. Carcinoids may, however, occur in the pancreas, rectum, ovary, lung, and elsewhere. The tumors grow slowly and often are clinically silent for many years before becoming manifest, usually when metastases have occurred. They frequently metastasize to the regional lymph nodes, liver, and less commonly, to bone. The likelihood of metastases relates to tumor size. The incidence of metastases is less than 2% with a carcinoid tumor smaller than 1 cm but rises to 100% with tumors larger than 2 cm. These tumors may be symptomatic only episodically, and their existence may go unrecognized for many years. The average time from onset of symptoms attributable to the tumor and diagnosis is a little over 9 years, and diagnosis usually is made only when the carcinoid syndrome occurs. The carcinoid syndrome occurs, however, in less than 10% of patients with carcinoid tumors (44). It is especially common in tumors of the ileum and jejunum but also occurs with bronchial, ovarian, and other carcinoids (45). This section discusses the incidence, natural history, clinical presentation, diagnosis, and management of carcinoid tumors.

One of the more clinically useful classifications of carcinoid tumors is according to the division of the primitive gut from which the tumor cells arise. There are two types of foregut carcinoid tumors: (*a*) sporadic primary, and (*b*) tumors secondary to achlorhydria. Sporadic primary foregut tumors include carcinoids of the bronchus, stomach, first portion of the duodenum, and pancreas. Midgut carcinoid tumors derive from the second portion of the duodenum, the jejunum, the ileum, and the right colon. Hindgut carcinoid tumors include those of the transverse colon, left colon, and rectum. This distinction assists in distinguishing a number of important biochemical and clinical differences between carcinoid tumors, because the presentation, histochemistry, and secretory products are quite different (Table 103.2).

Foregut carcinoids are argentaffin negative. They have a low content of serotonin (5-hydroxytryptamine [5-HT]). They often secrete the serotonin precursor 5-hydroxytryptophan (5-HTP), histamine, and a multitude of polypeptide hormones. Their functional manifestations include atypical carcinoid syndrome, gastrinoma syndrome, acromegaly, Cushing's disease, and a number of other endocrine disorders. Furthermore, they are unusual in that the flush tends to be of protracted duration, is often of a purplish or violaceous hue rather than the usual pink-red, and frequently leaves permanent telangiectasia and hypertrophy of the skin of the face and upper neck. The face assumes a leonine characteristic after repeated episodes. It is not unusual for these tumors to metastasize to bone.

Midgut carcinoids, in contrast, are argentaffin positive, have a high 5-HT content, rarely secrete 5-HTP, and often produce a number of other vasoactive compounds, such as kinins, prostaglandins, and SP. The clinical syndrome that derives is the classic carcinoid. These tumors may produce ACTH, albeit rarely, and very infrequently metastasize to bone.

Hindgut carcinoids are argentaffin negative, rarely contain 5-HT, rarely secrete 5-HTP or other peptides, and usually are silent in their presentation. However, they may metastasize to bone.

A further point of interest is that if a carcinoid tumor coexists with MEN-I, more than two thirds of the time in males the tumor is in the thymus, whereas in females, it is in the lung over 75% of the time.

Although carcinoids classically are tumors of enterochromaffin and argentaffin cells of the digestive tract, the term *carcinoid tumor* can be expanded to cover gut tumors of paracrine- and endocrine-like cells of unknown function (46, 47). It now is established that these tumors are of neuroendocrine origin and derive from a primitive stem cell. They may differentiate into any one of a variety of adult endocrine secreting cells: B cell and insulinoma; A cell and glucagonoma; D cell and somatostatinoma; and the PP cell and PPoma, or cells capable of producing ACTH, growth hormone-releasing hormone, VIP, SP, gastrin-releasing factor, calcitonin, and the enterochromaffin (EC) cell with its ability to cosecrete amines such as serotonin and the peptide motilin (Fig. 103.2). At any one point in time, these cells may secrete one humor, whereas at others, the peptide or amine secreted may differ and yield an entirely different clinical syndrome. Indeed, metastases are known to secrete hormones that differ from the parent tumor, and different metastases may secrete different hormones. Symptoms may derive from secretion of one or more of the hormones secreted.

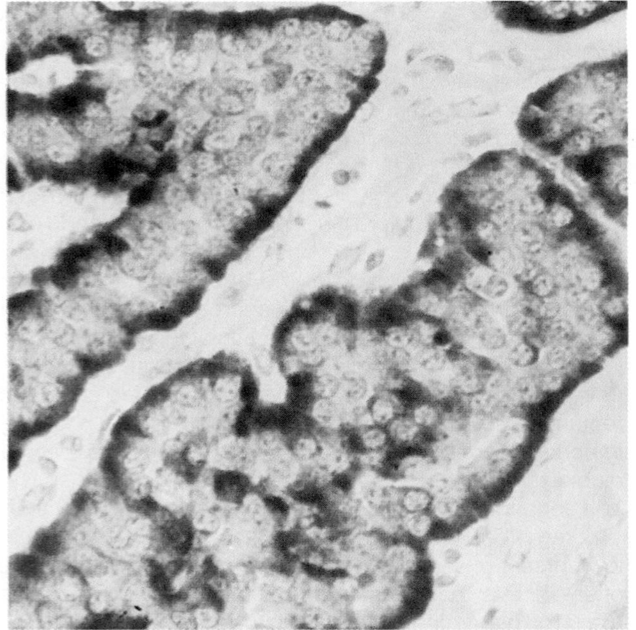

Figure 103.2. Ovarian carcinoid tumor stained positive for substance P.

AGE DISTRIBUTION

The distribution of carcinoids is gaussian in nature. The peak incidence occurs in the sixth and seventh decade of life, but patients as young as 10 years of age and people in their ninth decade are also seen.

NATURAL HISTORY

Carcinoid tumors are slow growing and may be present for years without overt symptoms, thus escaping attention. During the early stages, vague abdominal pain goes undiagnosed and invariably is ascribed to irritable bowel or spastic colon. Fully one third of patients with carcinoid tumors present with years of intermittent abdominal pain. Carcinoid tumors can present in a variety of ways. For example, duodenal tumors are known to produce gastrin and may present with the gastrinoma syndrome.

An interesting association between pernicious anemia, atrophic gastritis, chronic thyroiditis, and gastric carcinoid tumors has been described (48). These tumors arise from the gastric enterochromaffin-like (ECL) cell and usually are small and multiple. Development of these tumors is believed to be secondary to long-standing basal hypergastrinemia, resulting in stimulation of ECL cells and the development of hyperplasia, nodularity, and eventually, carcinoid tumors (49, 41). The association between hypergastrinemia and the development of gastric carcinoids supports the hypothesis that growth factors are important in the genesis of endocrine tumors. Patients with carcinoid tumors of the thymus most often manifest hyperparathyroidism or ectopic Cushing's syndrome. Bronchial carcinoids are associated with MEN-1.

The major clinical manifestations of carcinoid tumors include cutaneous flushing, which occurs in 84% of patients, gastrointestinal (GI) hypermotility with diarrhea (70%), heart disease (37%), bronchial constriction (17%), myopathy (7%), and an abnormal increase in skin pigmentation (5%) (49). When coexistence of the major symptoms of flushing and diarrhea are sought, it emerges that flushing and diarrhea occur simultaneously in 58%, diarrhea without flushing in 15%, flushing without diarrhea in 5%, and neither flushing nor diarrhea as a symptom complex in 22%.

With metastases to the liver, the correct diagnosis generally is arrived at, but with a delay of many years. Even then, mistaken identity is not uncommon, and unless biopsy material is examined for the neuronal glycolytic enzyme NE, or the secretory peptide chromogranin (50) of synaptophysin (51), tumors may be labeled erroneously as adenocarcinomas, with a negative impact on attitudes toward management and an underestimate of survival.

DIAGNOSIS

The diagnosis of carcinoid tumors rests on a strong clinical suspicion in patients who present with flushing, diarrhea, wheezing, myopathy, and right heart disease, and it includes appropriate biochemical and localization studies.

BIOCHEMICAL STUDIES

The rate-limiting step in carcinoid tumors for the synthesis of serotonin is the conversion of tryptophan into 5-HTP, catalyzed by the enzyme tryptophan hydroxylase. In midgut tumors, 5-HTP is rapidly converted to 5-HT by the enzyme aromatic amino acid decarboxylase (dopa-decarboxylase). 5-HT is either stored in the neurosecretory granules or may be secreted directly into the vascular compartment. Most of the secreted 5-HT is taken up by platelets and stored in their secretory granules. The rest remains free in the plasma, and circulating 5-HT then is largely converted into the urinary metabolite 5-hydroxyindoleacetic acid (5-HIAA) by the enzyme monoamine oxidase and by aldehyde dehydrogenase. These enzymes are abundant in the kidney, and the urine typically contains large amounts of 5-HIAA.

In patients with foregut tumors, the urine contains relatively little 5-HIAA but large amounts of 5-HTP. It is presumed that these tumors are deficient in dopa-decarboxylase, which therefore impairs the conversion of 5-HTP into 5-HT, leading to 5-HTP secretion into the vascular compartment. Some 5-HTP, however, is converted to 5-HT and 5-HIAA, thus the modest increase in these metabolites. The normal range for 5-HIAA secretion is 2 to 8 mg per 24 hours, and the quantitation of serotonin and all its metabolites usually permits the detection of 84% of patients with carcinoid tumors. No single measurement detects all cases of carcinoid syndrome, although the urine 5-HIAA appears to be the best screening procedure. Other peptides involved include SP, neuropeptide K, PP, and chromogranin A. In carcinoid tumors, neurotensin is elevated in 43%, SP in 32%, motilin in 14%, somatostatin in 5%, and VIP rarely (52). In miscellaneous illnesses, there may be elevation of the following hormones: neurotensin, SP, and motilin in 35, 7, and 5%, respectively. Up to one third of people with idiopathic flushing who do not have carcinoid syndrome, however, have elevated levels of a number of neuropeptides (5). Furthermore, we have examined the relationship between the products of the preprotachykinin gene, SP, and neurokinin A in healthy subjects and in patients with carcinoid tumors. SP was elevated 80% of the time in patients with carcinoid tumors, whereas neurokinin A was raised in all patients. Why there should be a discrepancy in these two peptides that derive from a common precursor gene product remains unclear. Measurement of circulating levels enhances the ability to identify more patients with carcinoid tumors.

Localization Studies

A number of techniques have been used to identify the primary site of the tumor and to evaluate the extent of the disease and presence of metastases. Chest radiography or computed tomography (CT) suffices to detect bronchial carcinoid. In contrast, carcinoids of the cecum, right colon, and hindgut carcinoids usually are demonstrable by endoscopy or barium enema examination. The greatest problems encountered are in localizing small bowel carcinoids, which may be small, and carcinoids in extraintestinal sites. These tumors usually are not identified by upper or GI roentgenographic studies. Abdominal CT scans and ultrasound usually are not helpful, because the primary tumors are below the resolution capacity of even the most sophisticated scanning apparatus. Superior mesenteric angiography, however, may be of help.

Several diagnostic methods have been evaluated for the diagnosis of carcinoid tumors, including barium examinations, CT, ^{131}I-metaiodobenzylguanidine (MIBG) scanning, octreotide scanning, angiography, and venous sampling with radioimmunoassay of hormones. Barium examinations rarely are diagnostic, but they may demonstrate fixation, separation, thickening, and angulation of the bowel loops. CT is the primary diagnostic procedure for tumor staging; it allows assessment of the extent of tumor spread to the mesentery and bowel wall as well as metastases to the lymph nodes and liver. The typical appearance of mesenteric invasion by carcinoid tumor on CT is a mesenteric mass with radiating linear densities representing thickened neurovascular bundles. Liver metastases appear as focal, hypodense lesions on nonenhanced CT scanning (53). The advantage of CT is its ability to localize the tumors precisely in relation to the adjacent structure. CT also remains the most useful roentgenographic method for localization of metastatic carcinoid tumors and evaluation of the response of metastatic carcinoid tumors to therapy. Magnetic resonance imaging (MRI) is a very sensitive technique for the detection of liver metastases, but it appears to be less sensitive for the diagnosis of extrahepatic disease. MRI needs further evaluation, however, before it is used as primary modality for the diagnosis and staging of carcinoid tumor (54), but overall, it appears to have little advantage over CT.

The role of angiography in the diagnosis of carcinoid tumor has been decreased by the availability of the newer imaging methods. Diagnostic angiography generally is employed when noninvasive imaging studies are equivocal and surgery is contemplated (Fig. 103.3). Liver metastases from carcinoid tumors vary in size and usually are vascular, with abundant neovascularity demonstrable on angiography. Percutaneous transhepatic portal and systemic venous sampling with hormone assay is not a very useful technique for the localization of carcinoid tumors. Positron-emission tomography (PET) has been used to image neuroendocrine gastrointestinal tumors, but experience thus far is very limited. Most patients who have been studied had classical midgut tumors and the carcinoid syndrome. Both tryptophan and 5-HTP have been used as tracer substances, but initial studies showed that only ^{11}C-5-HTP was taken up in serotonin-producing tumors (55). PET has been shown to be capable of identifying midgut carcinoid tumors that have metastasized to a variety of sites, and it may be of value in monitoring the effects of treatment (56).

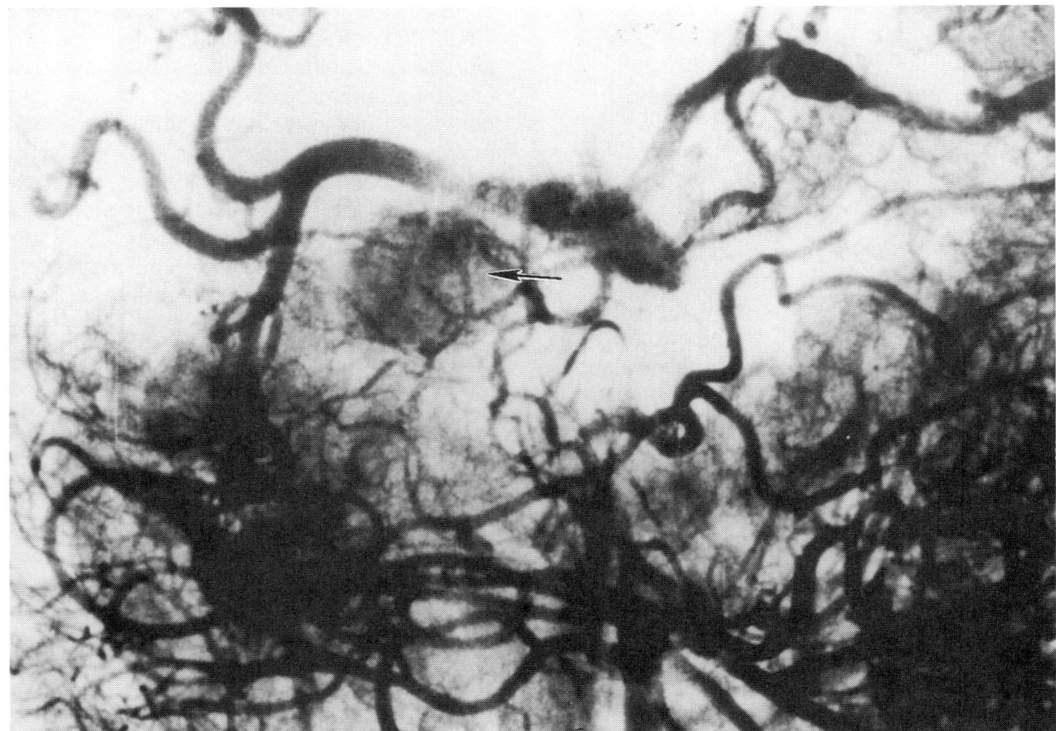

Figure 103.3. Celiac-axis angiogram (Subtraction films) showing tumor in the head of the pancreas (*arrow*).

Scintigraphic Detection with MIBG or Octreotide Scanning

The first report of ^{131}I-MIBG for the imaging of a carcinoid tumor was that of Fischer and colleagues in 1984, in which hepatic metastases that were seen as photopenic areas on a ^{99m}Tc-phytate liver scan concentrated ^{131}I-MIBG (57). Since this initial description, there have been a number of reports of successful imaging of carcinoid tumors using ^{131}I-MIBG. The number studied are far less than those reported for pheochromocytoma or neuroblastoma, however, but it probably is fair to say that the sensitivity is significantly lower (58–62). The overall sensitivity is calculated to be 55%. Because MIBG is taken up by a wide variety of neuroendocrine tumors (58–60, 62), specificity depends on the certainty of the clinical and biochemical diagnosis. In the correct clinical context, this is well over 95% for pheochromocytoma (29, 59, 60, 63) and neuroblastoma (60, 64–66), but it might well be less true for carcinoid tumors. Recently, somatostatin receptors have been identified on most endocrine tumors, including carcinoid tumors, which generally express a high density of the receptors. Five human somatostatin receptor subtypes have been cloned so far, and the binding affinity of octreotide may depend on the subtype(s) expressed (67). Several different imaging agents that bind to the receptor have been studied. ^{123}I-Tyr^3-octreotide was the agent initially used, but it has several disadvantages, including a short half-life, biliary excretion obscuring potential tumor sites, and difficulties with conjugation (68). The development of ^{111}In-DTPA octreotide, with a half-life of 3 days and renal excretion, has obviated many of these difficulties (69).

A recent analysis of the combined European experience showed that sensitivity of ^{111}In-DTPA octreotide scintigraphy for the detection of both primary and metastatic GEP tumors approaches 80 to 90% (70). The technique appears to be much less sensitive, however, in detecting tumors less than 1 cm in diameter (71). Another recent study showed that the sensitivity of this test only approaches 50% in primary or metastatic gastrinomas previously localized by other methods (72). Even those investigators who have shown good results with this technique admit the difficulty in imaging liver metastases, particularly when they are small; therefore, other modalities such as ultrasound or CT are recommended to investigate the liver (73).

Thus, octreotide scintigraphy, although useful, likely has limited benefit in identifying small primary tumors and liver metastases. This imaging technique may prove to be most valuable in identifying metastatic disease to extra-abdominal sites (Fig. 103.4) (71). In addition to tumor imaging, octreotide scanning may be useful in predicting responses to octreotide. One recent study showed that 22 of 27 patients with carcinoid tumor and positive scans responded to octreotide, whereas all three patients with negative scans failed to respond (74). Other investigators have shown similar results (75).

In the remaining cases, in whom the tumor has not been identified by the above techniques, total-body venous sampling with measurement of a peptide hormone that is produced may be considered. Measurements of serotonin may be misleading, but those of SP may well direct attention to the source of overproduction of the peptide. This has proved useful in SP-producing tumors (76).

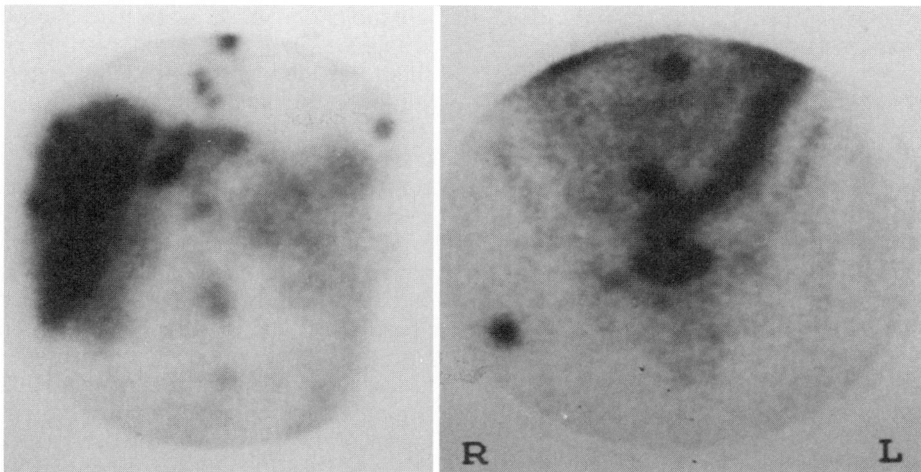

Figure 103.4. Octreotide scan at 24 hours showing liver and pelvic metastases in a patient with malignant carcinoid tumor.

Carcinoid Syndrome

Carcinoid syndrome occurs in less than 10% of patients with carcinoid tumors. Principal features include flushing, sweating, wheezing, diarrhea, abdominal pain, cardiac fibrosis, and pellagra dermatosis. Diarrhea is found in 83% of cases, flushing in 49%, dyspnea in 20%, and bronchospasm in 6% (77). The relationship between diarrhea and flushing is variable. One can occur without the other and there may be no temporal relationship between the two. The specific etiologic agent or agents for each of the protean manifestations of the carcinoid tumors are not known. Serotonin (78, 79), prostaglandins (80), 5-HTP (81–83), SP (76, 84), kallikrein (85), histamine (83), dopamine (86), and neuropeptide K (87) are thought to be involved in the clinical manifestations of carcinoid tumors. In addition, symptoms may relate to overproduction of peptides in the pro-opiomelanocortin family (e.g., endorphin and enkephalin). Pancreatic polypeptide and motilin levels often are raised (88), may be important markers of tumor activity, and may provide a means of monitoring tumor growth and response to therapy rather than contributing to specific symptomatology.

Feldman and O'Dorisio (89) examined the proportion of 43 patients with carcinoid tumor having increased levels of serotonin and various other vasoactive peptides (90). Serotonin, measured either as its urinary metabolite 5-HIAA (91) or whole-blood serotonin (92–94), was raised in 84% of patients with carcinoid tumors and within normal limits in patients having other tumors and miscellaneous illnesses. Urinary 5-HIAA alone had a 73% sensitivity and 100% specificity. Seven of these patients had normal urinary 5-HIAA levels but other elevated indices of serotonin production. Neurotensin and SP were raised in 43 and 32% of patients and had specificity values of 60 and 85%, respectively. False-positive results occurred in 23 and 26%, respectively, of patients with conditions other than carcinoid tumors. Motilin and somatostatin were raised in 14 and 50%, respectively.

These humors may prove useful as an aid in the localization of ostensibly occult carcinoid tumors. Whole-body venous sampling with measurements of plasma serotonin erroneously localized the tumor to the neck, for which a negative exploration was carried out; however, SP levels correctly localized certain of these tumors (76).

Diarrhea

The diarrhea syndrome that occurs with carcinoid tumors usually is of a secretory nature. Diarrhea persists with fasting or fails to disappear when feeding has been curtailed and sustenance given by the intravenous route. There are, however, a number of other causes of secretory diarrhea, but virtually all endocrine diarrheas are secretory in nature.

A history of improvement in the diarrhea with administration of H_2- receptor antagonists is strongly suggestive of the gastrinoma syndrome. Hypercalcemia is frequent with VIP-secreting tumors and steatorrhea and, for all intents and purposes, occurs only with the Zollinger-Ellison syndrome. Marked metabolic acidosis with bicarbonate wasting usually is only a characteristic of VIP-secreting tumors. The villous adenoma of the rectum causing secretory diarrhea is notoriously rare, and although it is referred to in many texts, most physicians have yet to see a case. A disturbing cause that may be very difficult to differentiate is laxative abuse, and in all circumstances, a KOH stool preparation to detect laxatives is mandatory. Measurement of intestinal secretion by passing a multilumen tube and quantifying electrolytes and water transport, in addition to the measurement of stool electrolytes, which should account for the total osmolarity, will help to exclude laxative abuse.

Flushing

Flushing in carcinoid syndrome is of two varieties. First, with midgut carcinoid, the flush usually is of a faint pink to red color and involves the face and upper trunk as far as the nipple line. The flush is initially provoked by alcohol and food containing tyramines, e.g., blue cheese, chocolate, red sausage, and red wine. With time, the flush may occur spontaneously and without provocation. It usually is ephemeral, lasting only a few minutes, may occur many times per day, but generally does not leave permanent discoloration.

In contrast, the second type, the flush of foregut tumors often is more intense, of protracted duration (lasting hours), purplish in hue, frequently followed by telangiectasia, and involves not only the upper trunk but also the limbs. The limbs may become acrocyanotic, and the nose resembles that of rhinophyma. The skin of the face often thickens, with the appearance of a leonine facies resembling that seen in leprosy and acromegaly.

Flushing cannot always be attributed to carcinoid syndrome. The differential diagnosis of flushing includes the postmenopausal state, simultaneous ingestion of chlorpropamide and alcohol, panic attacks, medullary carcinoma of the thyroid, autonomic epilepsy, autonomic neuropathy and mastocytosis.

Flushing in carcinoid syndrome has been ascribed to prostaglandins, kinins, and serotonin (5-HT). With the advent of sophisticated radioimmunoassay methods and region-specific antisera, a number of neurohumors now are thought to be secreted by carcinoid tumors, including serotonin (78), dopamine (86), histamine, and 5-HIAA (83), kallikrein (82), SP (81), neurotensin (89), motilin (76, 89), SRIF (89), VIP (95), prostaglandins (80), neuropeptide K (87), and gastrin-releasing peptide (GRP) (89).

Feldman and O'Dorisio have previously reported the incidence of elevated levels of plasma neuropeptides concentrations (89). Despite the elevated basal concentrations of SP and neurotensin, these authors were able to document further increases in these neuropeptides during ethanol-induced facial flushing. We support this contention and hasten to add that neuropeptide abnormalities frequently occur in patients with all forms of flushing and may be of pathogenetic significance (96).

Several new provocative tests have been developed for carcinoid syndrome. Ahlman and colleagues (97) reported the results of pentagastrin (PG) provocation in 16 patients with midgut carcinoid tumors and hepatic metastases. All patients tested had elevated urinary 5-HIAA levels, and 12 had profuse diarrhea requiring medication. PG uniformly induced facial flushing and GI symptoms in patients with liver metastases, but it had no effect in healthy control patients. All patients with PG-induced GI symptoms demonstrated elevated serotonin levels in peripheral blood. Administration of a serotonin-receptor antagonist had no effect on serotonin release but completely aborted the GI symptoms. The authors emphasized the improved reliability of PG compared with calcium infusion, another provocative test popularized by Kaplan and colleagues (98), and pointed out that PG provocation occasionally can be falsely negative in patients with subclinical disease. Our own experience is that PG uniformly induced flushing in 11 patients with gastric carcinoid tumors that was associated with a rise in circulating levels of SP in 80% (49). Thus, SP is one neurohumor that may be involved in the flushing of carcinoid syndrome.

Substance P has been found in tumor extracts and plasma from patients with carcinoid tumors and, in one reported case, was useful for tumor localization (76). Neurokinin A, its amino-terminally extended form, neuropeptide K, and SP are a group of peptides (i.e., tachykinins) with common biologic properties (99, 100). Norheim and colleagues (100) measured peptide responses to PG or ingestion of food or alcohol in 16 patients with metastatic carcinoid tumors and demonstrated twofold or greater increases in neurokinin A and neuropeptide K in 75% of patients, as well as variable increases in SP in approximately 20% of patients (101).

Conlon and colleagues (99) used region-specific antisera to SP and neurokinin A to measure circulating tachykinins during a meal-induced flush in 10 patients with metastatic carcinoid tumors. Five patients had undetectable levels of neurokinin A and SP after stimulation, thus suggesting that elevated tachykinin concentrations are not a constant feature of such patients. The authors also studied the effect of a somatostatin-analogue administration on meal-induced tachykinin responses in three patients with carcinoid tumors. Flushing was aborted in two patients, but tachykinin levels were only partially suppressed, indicating that these peptides cannot be solely responsible for the carcinoid flush.

PROGNOSIS

The general prognosis in carcinoid tumor is excellent compared with that of other visceral cancers. Based on a world literature of some 2,837 cases, the median 5-year survival rate for all cases is 82% (102). If, however, the tumor is localized, then the 5-year survival is 94%, decreasing to 64% with regional lymph node involvement and 18% with distant metastases. Davis and colleagues (45) reported a mean survival of 38 months from the first episode of flushing, with 25% of patients living for more than 6 years. With regional lymph node involvement, the figure falls to approximately 14 months (103), and with urinary 5-HIAA in excess of 150 mg per 24 hours or inoperable tumors, median survival is only 11 months (102).

Surgical removal of the primary tumor is the treatment of choice for small and localized tumors as well as for the alleviation of any obstructive symptoms, but surgical cure of carcinoid tumor is almost impossible in the presence of intra-abdominal and hepatic metastases. Different chemotherapeutic agents (104) and surgery or arterial embolization (105) have been used with variable success, but eventual relapse with increasing resistance to the drugs is encountered (102). Because the carcinoid is a slow-growing tumor, even patients with extensive metastatic disease can enjoy a normal quality of life so long as the endocrine syndrome is quiescent. Different chemical agents such as methysergide, cyproheptadene, heparin, phenothiazines, α-adrenergic antagonists, corticosteroids, H_1 and H_2 antihistamine blockers, symptomatic treatment of diarrhea with opioids, and codeine have been tried with variable results (102). Because somatostatin has very broad inhibitory effects, somatostatin-14 has been used successfully to suppress diarrhea and flushing in patients with carcinoid tumors (106), but its clinical use is limited by its short half-life (107) and the resulting need for continuous intravenous infusion. With the advent of the long-acting somatostatin analogue octreotide (SMS 201–995) (108), it has been used in the treatment of different neuroendocrine tumors, including carcinoid.

THERAPY

Various chemotherapeutic agents, including parachlorophenylalanine, cyproheptadene, methotrimeprazine, corticosteroids, aprotinin, phenoxybenzamine, and numerous antineoplastic agents have been used in carcinoid syndrome with variable success (77, 95). These medications either inhibit serotonin synthesis, act as systemic antagonists of serotonin, or block kallikrein release. Most recently, somatostatin 14 and its long-acting analogue, octreotide, have been used successfully to control the symptoms of diarrhea and flushing (46, 106, 109, 110) in the carcinoid syndrome. We have had variable experiences with carcinoid syndrome and report here factors that determine responsiveness.

Responses to Octreotide

The responses to therapy may be divided into four groups: (*a*) responders were those with a more than 75% improvement (i.e., a 75% drop in the frequency or intensity of a symptom or 75% drop in the level of a biochemical marker), (*b*) partial responders were those with a 25 to 75% improvement, (*c*) nonresponders were those with a less than 25% improvement, and (*d*) worsening was judged to occur if the clinical and/or biochemical values increased by more than 25% of their initial estimation.

Flushing

Our patients were a heterogeneous group with advanced carcinoid tumors refractory to conventional chemotherapeutic agents who were tried on the somatostatin analogue with variable clinical and biochemical responses. We have previously reported a dramatic response of flushing as a symptom during treatment with somatostatin (46). Frolich and colleagues (111) also reported on the value of native somatostatin given by continuous infusion to reverse the PG-induced flushing in patients with carcinoid tumors. We, however, were unable to show that PG was a reliable means to provoke flushing in our patients. Kvols and colleagues (112) found that 19 of 24 patients with carcinoid tumors had a 50% reduction in flushing, three had a minor response, and the octreotide failed in two patients. Richter and colleagues (113) showed that six of eight patients had improved symptoms.

Our more recent experience is that 64% of our patients presented with flushing as their major symptom. In all instances, the symptom complex improved, with a clear decrease in the frequency of symptoms using doses of octreotide in the range of 6 to 20 μg/kg/d. In no instance was there resistance to the drug. Tachyphylaxis did not occur, and withdrawal of the drug (or substitution with distilled water) was always followed by recurrence of the symptom complex. In contrast to another report (113), relapse of flushing did not occur with continued treatment once it was under control. However, in contrast to the reduction in a number of episodes, the severity in certain patients decreased only slightly, and the duration of each episode was essentially unchanged.

The extreme example of flushing is the carcinoid crisis with a profound fall in blood pressure. It is deemed unwise to submit a patient to anesthesia or operation without premedication using a combination of adrenergic blockade, steroids, thorazine, and aspirin. Preoperative use of octreotide also may help to prevent carcinoid crisis. Kvols and colleagues (109) presented data on one such patient, who soon after the induction of anesthesia had a fall in blood pressure that was unresponsive to intravenous fluid, calcium, Neo-Synephrine, or epinephrine administration. Within 1 minute of 100 μg of octreotide given intravenously, blood pressure rose, and the patient made an uneventful recovery.

Thus, while the mechanism of action by octreotide and the factors mediating flushing and vasodilatation is unclear, octreotide no doubt is a potent antidote to the vasoactive humors participating in the flush and hypotension. The drug may prove to be a useful adjunct in the preparation of patients for operative procedures and as a standby for the management of carcinoid crisis.

Diarrhea

Diarrhea occurred in 86% of our patients and responded variably to octreotide. Acute administration of octreotide normalized the water and electrolyte transport across the proximal intestine, as has been shown in patients with the watery diarrhea hypokalemia hypochlorhydria and acidosis (WDHHA) syndrome (110, 114). The acute reduction in electrolyte secretion did not, however, predict the long-term response of diarrhea to octreotide therapy, but this needs to be further examined in a larger number of patients. Only 58% of our patients with diarrhea had complete remission, which differs from the improvement in 19 of 25 patients (76%) reported by Kvols and colleagues (112). This could result from the fact that diarrhea in patients with carcinoid tumors has multiple etiologies (i.e., secretory, increased motility, malabsorption, partial luminal lymphatic obstruction, bacterial overgrowth, and short bowel syndrome because of surgical resection). The diarrhea may even seem to worsen with the appearance of steatorrhea, and the physician not infrequently is faced with the confounding situation of not knowing to what to attribute the symptom. However, although octreotide does inhibit exocrine pancreatic secretion (115), addition of pancreatic enzyme supplementation has not uniformly decreased octreotide-induced steatorrhea (116). We did not find any consistent changes in frequency or consistency of bowel movements in response to pancreatic supplements in those patients with steatorrhea before treatment or the bowel habits after therapy with octreotide, which is compatible with the notion that the steatorrhea has a complex pathogenesis and may be contributed to by alterations in bile flow, the direct effects of octreotide on nutrient absorption, and intestinal motility (117).

Effects of Octreotide on Pulmonary Function

All three of our patients with wheezing had clinical improvement, and spirometric improvement was documented. Pulmonary function did not improve further after 3 months of treatment, indicating an irreversible component or small airway disease secondary to long-standing smoking (118).

Effects of Octreotide on Myopathy

One patient in our series presented with severe proximal muscle weakness, with normal muscle enzymes and nerve conduction studies but electromyographic features of a proximal myopathy. Although a neurologic deficit secondary to metastatic carcinoid has been reported (119), metabolic-induced neuromuscular disease is very rare (120–122). Although our patient had a history of hypokalemia, his potassium was normal at the time of admission, with no biochemical evidence of thyrotoxicosis, ectopic ACTH production, or osteomalacia. We believe that his severe myopathy was caused by his carcinoid tumor, although it might have been aggravated by severe diarrhea, weight loss, and poor nutrition. Histologic changes can be induced in the skeletal muscle of mice by intraperitoneal injection of 5-HT (123), and 3 months after octreotide therapy, the patient had no clinical evidence of myopathy, with improvement in electromyographic features (118).

Biochemical Responses

Reports conflict regarding the biochemical responses of patients with carcinoid tumors to octreotide. Richter and colleagues reported a significant drop in 5-HT levels in eight patients treated with 150 μg/d of octreotide but no changes in urinary 5-HIAA; others have found a drop in urinary 5-HIAA (41, 113). In prolonging their treatment of four patients to 15 to 30 weeks, blood serotonin remained unchanged (116).

In our patients, urinary 5-HIAA dropped in almost all patients and normalized in one third, and four of eight patients normalized their 24-hour 5-HIAA. Although few of our patients had a fall in their blood serotonin level, the overall postoctreotide values were not significantly lower than the pretreatment values.

There were no clinical correlations between the clinical responses and either urinary 5-HIAA or the blood serotonin level. In contrast, for patients in whom urinary 5-HIAA fell, there was clinical improvement in one or more of the symptoms. This may reflect that multiple etiologic factors are involved in the symptomatology of carcinoid tumors. In our patients, those who responded clinically required no more than 500 μg/d of octreotide to control their symptoms, although we have examined the response to higher doses in certain instances.

Responses of Tumor Growth and Metastases to Octreotide

Because of the slow growth of carcinoid tumors, it is difficult to assess the effect of octreotide on tumor growth or regression. Shrinkage of liver metastases in patients with carcinoid (110, 112) and other functioning pancreatic neuroendocrine tumors (124) has been reported. We have had variable experiences. The relationship between tumor size and growth and the biochemistry is not a simple one. In one patient, the tumor clearly shrank, but ACTH levels rose to the 2,000 to 3,000 pg/mL range. On molecular sieve chromatography, the ACTH coeluted with native ACTH, but the patient has no clinical features of Cushing's syndrome, is gaining weight, and has no diarrhea or flushing. Another patient had progression of tumor growth after 18 months of octreotide therapy, yet there was a dramatic fall in blood serotonin values and the patient is entirely asymptomatic. The opposite also is not unusual, wherein there is no change in tumor size, a very well patient, and hormonal levels that are unaffected by octreotide even at doses as high as 1,000 μg/d (84).

We have follow-up CT data for 14 patients. Two showed some tumor regression, and in one case, the tumor infarcted. Five cases showed progression and seven cases no changes on the CT scan when followed for up to 2 to 5 years. It appears that the cessation or reversal of growth occurs in about two thirds of patients with carcinoid tumors who are treated with octreotide.

Short of an effective curative or palliative agent, octreotide can control flushing and wheezing in most, and diarrhea in some, patients with carcinoid tumors, with improvement in their general condition. The effects of octreotide on tumor growth need to be evaluated further in relation to the slow progression and indolent nature of these tumors. Octreotide increases the median survival of patients with metastatic carcinoid tumor from 11 to 33 months. Higher doses of octreotide may yield even better outcomes. A recent phase II study of apudomas showed no major tumor regressions but a 50% disease stabilization rate (125). A study of 14 patients with neuroendocrine tumor who received doses of octreotide of up to 9,000 μg/d showed partial responses in four patients (31%) and disease stabilization in two patients (16%) (126). Radiographic evidence of tumor necrosis was seen in five patients, but this did not correlate with response. A larger study of 55 patients showed an objective response rate of 37% (127). Because little effective therapy is available and much may be harmful, it seems not unreasonable to offer octreotide for control of symptoms and palliation at this point in time. The limits of safe and effective dosage need to be established, and long-term follow-up is a prerequisite to defining the ultimate role of this peptide therapy in the carcinoid syndrome.

When, however, there is clear evidence that tumor growth is not contained by octreotide, alternative forms of treatment should be considered (128). There also are experimental techniques that should be considered.

Internal Radiotherapy Delivered by MIBG

There is the potential to deliver therapeutic doses of radiation to those tumors in which there is intense and prolonged tumor uptake of tracer doses of MIBG. Target-to-background ratios with tracer doses that achieve diagnostic imaging may not, however, always permit the delivery of therapeutic radiation when large doses of activity are administered (129–131).

At present, therapy for carcinoid tumor with MIBG is considered to be highly experimental. Possible guidelines for its employment based on the experience with other neuroendocrine tumors would include: (*a*) lesions not readily treatable by alternative modalities, (*b*) patients with life expectancies sufficient to permit beneficial effects to become apparent (e.g., > 6 months or 1 year), and (*c*) undertaking dosimetric studies for whole-body and blood-absorbed radiation dose using tracer doses to guide the size of therapeutic administrations (129–131). The bone marrow and, especially, the platelets appear to be the dose-limiting tissues for MIBG therapy. Typical doses to date have been in the range of 100 to 250 mCi per administration, with cumulative doses sometimes exceeding 600 mCi (129–131). In addition, if at all possible, the absorbed radiation dose to one or more representative tumors should be determined from serial scintigraphic images. From these, the initial uptake and biologic reaction time of retention can be determined; the use of conjugate view technique with the inclusion of standard sources may be especially helpful (52). Tumor volume also must be determined by CT or another modality, and with the other parameters, this can be used with Medical Internal Radiation Dose formulas to calculate the radiation-absorbed dose (129–132).

The ability of somatostatin analogues to bind to GEP tumors has suggested other novel therapeutic approaches. Conjugating somatostatin with high energy β-emitters, short-acting α-particle emitters, or tumoricidal toxins such as ricin or modified diphtheria toxin has been proposed (133, 134). Although similar strategies have been used to deliver tumoricidal agents to other types of tumors, there are little data thus far on the therapeutic effectiveness of such an approach in GEP tumors.

Dearterialization

Today, angiography frequently is used for therapeutic purposes. Hepatic artery embolization has proved to be a relatively safe procedure for the palliation of carcinoid syndrome related to an excessive hormone production from hepatic carcinoid metastases (135). This method usually is beneficial to the patients whose hepatic metastases have failed to respond to chemotherapy and other pharmacologic therapy (87%). Gelfoam powder (particle sizes, 80–200 μM) and Ivalon particles (sizes, 149–250 μM) are the frequently used agents for devascularization of the hepatic metastases.

Several authors have described their experience with hepatic artery ligation or embolization in patients with malignant carcinoid tumors (136–138). In one study, the former procedure resulted in objective tumor responses in 9 of 19 patients, stable disease in 5 of 19 patients, and progressive disease in 4 of 19 patients when they were assessed 6 and 12 months after the procedure (138). Two patients died 1 and 3 months postoperatively from complications including liver abscesses, and the remainder of patients experienced mild abdominal pain, fever, and fatigue that was self-limiting. Hepatic artery gelfoam embolization performed in eight patients resulted in three objective responses and five with stable disease. Toxicity from this procedure included fever, abdominal pain, nausea, and elevation of serum hepatic enzymes, which returned to normal within 12 days. Overall, the duration of palliation tends to be short-lived (139). Hepatic arterial occlusion combined with sequential chemotherapy has resulted in an 80% response rate, with a median duration of 18 months (140). Although hepatic artery occlusion may produce subjective and objective responses in the majority of highly selected patients, the toxicity and duration of responses resulting from this therapy generally do not support its routine use (139).

Radiation Therapy

No available data support the use of radiation therapy in patients with metastatic carcinoid unless they have symptomatic bone metastases or spinal cord compression, which is amenable to this modality.

Chemotherapy

In malignant carcinoid tumor, chemotherapy has not been shown to be effective for most patients, and this approach should still be considered investigational. The single agent most studied in carcinoid tumor is 5-fluorouracil, which accounted for observed response rates of 26 and 18% in single institution and multi-institutional trials, respectively (141, 142) (Table 103.10). Melia and colleagues (137) reported a high complication rate with little benefit when 5-fluorouracil was administered by intra-arterial, portal, or peripheral intravenous routes. Few responses were observed following intravenous doxorubicin, 60 mg/m^2, every 3 to 4 weeks (102, 139, 143). Despite well-established activity in other GEP cancers, streptozotocin has not demonstrated significant efficacy in patients with carcinoid tumor (43, 102). Among other single agents, there have been anecdotal reports of objective responses to dacarbazine and dactinomycin (143, 144); however, a study of 32 patients demonstrated that dactinomycin or dacarbazine had little activity against metastatic carcinoid tumor (141). A larger, more recent study confirmed the ineffectiveness of dacarbazine in carcinoid tumor (145). Phase II studies in evaluable patients with carcinoid tumor have shown rare objective responses to either cisplatin or etoposide (141, 146, 147). No responses to carboplatinum were seen in a series of 20 patients.

Initial experience with combination chemotherapy suggested that this modality might be effective against malignant carcinoid tumor. Early, nonrandomized studies of combinations of cyclophosphamide plus methotrexate, streptozotocin plus 5-fluorouracil, or weekly streptozotocin plus doxorubicin reported response rates in excess of 50%; however, rigid criteria for response were not always employed and complete responses were not seen (43, 102, 142, 146, 148). Based on these observations, the Eastern Cooperative Oncology Group conducted a series of multi-institutional, randomized trials of combinations that all contained streptozotocin, despite the low activity of this drug when used alone. In two studies of 170 evaluable patients, the response rates ranged from 23 to 33%, and there was no evidence for any difference between streptozotocin administered every 6 weeks or every 10 weeks plus 5-fluorouracil versus streptozotocin plus cyclophosphamide versus single-agent doxorubicin (102, 142, 149). In a prospective trial, the Southwest Oncology Group reported similar response rates of brief duration following a combination of 5-fluorouracil, cyclophosphamide, and streptozotocin with or without doxorubicin (150). Only 10% of 31 patients had objective response following streptozotocin and 5-fluorouracil in another prospective clinical trial reported by Oberg and colleagues (151).

Feldman (152) suggested that streptozotocin alone or in combination with 5-fluorouracil may be beneficial for patients with foregut carcinoid tumors, in contrast to patients with midgut carcinoid tumors. This contrasts with the Eastern Cooperative Oncology Group experience (142), however, and it remains unsubstantiated. Thus, in the absence of randomized trials that contain a no-treatment arm, there is no persuasive evidence that single-agent or combination chemotherapy provide any significant impact on disease progression or on survival in patients with malignant carcinoid tumor.

Biologics

Several studies have used interferon against malignant carcinoid tumor. In the first, 17 of 36 patients (47%) with metastatic carcinoid tumor who were treated with human leukocyte interferon, 3 to 6 million units per day subcutaneously, had objective hormonal responses for a median duration of 34 months (153). Four patients had significant tumor regression, and two complete responses were noted. A second study randomized 20 patients to treatment with either a combination of streptozotocin and 5-fluorouracil or human leukocyte interferon, 6 million units five times per week (154). After 6 months, 50% of the patients treated with interferon had an objective hormonal response, and no patients treated with chemotherapy responded. Finally, Oberg and colleagues (151) conducted a study in 20 patients with malignant carcinoid tumor that suggested recombinant human interferon-α_{2b}, 5×10^6 U/m^2 three times a week subcutaneously for 6 months, was as active as leukocyte interferon, and that the two agents may not be cross-resistant. In this study, the development of neutralizing interferon antibodies correlated with lack of response to interferon in three patients.

Additional positive outcomes using recombinant human interferon-α_{2b} have been reported by several additional groups after small prospective trials (155, 156). Hanssen and colleagues (155) also gave interferon following hepatic artery embolization, and they observed five of seven patients with objective tumor and hormonal responses after 12 months. A recent review by Oberg (157) of 300 patients with carcinoid tumor treated with interferon-α for a median of 2.5 years concluded that this agent has significant antitumor effects in 70 to 80% of patients, as manifested by biochemical control and inhibition of tumor growth. Tumor progression generally occurred within 3 to 9 months after cessation of the drug.

These encouraging results with interferon must be interpreted with caution, however, considering the results from another prospective study using interferon reported by Moertel and colleagues (158). In this study, 27 previously treated patients with malignant carcinoid tumors were treated with recombinant human interferon-α_{2a}, $12–24 \times 10^6$ U/m^2 subcutaneously three times weekly for 8 weeks. Nine of 23 patients (39%) with elevated 5-HIAA had objective responses for a median of 40 weeks (range, 23–127 weeks), and 4 of 20 patients (20%) had objective tumor responses for a median of 7 weeks (range, 4–26 weeks). The flu-like syndrome and fatigue side effects from interferon were common in this study, requiring dose reduction in 10 patients and causing deterioration of performance status in 50% of all patients. In addition to differences in dose and observed toxicities, the variable response rates found in these reported studies may relate to the use of different recombinant interferon subtypes (alpha-2a vs. alpha-2b) and the subsequent development of neutralizing antibodies (159). The role for the combination of recombinant human interferon-α_{2a} and doxorubicin in patients with advanced pancreatic endocrine or carcinoid tumors currently is under investigation (160). A series of 19 patients treated with interferon-α combined with octreotide showed a 92% median biochemical response rate for a period of 10 months (127).

Adjuvant Therapy

Combined modality therapy, such as the use of adjuvant chemotherapy either before or following surgery, remains undefined for metastatic carcinoid. In the absence of well-established activity for chemotherapy in this disease, there is no rationale to support the use of adjuvant chemotherapy. In contrast, preliminary results of the prospective experience of sequential hepatic artery occlusion and alternating combination chemotherapy at the Mayo Clinic is of some interest (139, 143, 161). Following hepatic artery occlusion by surgical ligation or percutaneous embolization, 21 patients were treated with dacarbazine, 250 mg/m^2 daily for 5 days, plus doxorubicin, 60 mg/m^2, alternating every 4 to 5 weeks with 5-fluorouracil, 400 mg/m^2 daily for 5 days, plus streptozotocin, 500 mg/m^2 daily for 5 days until maximum response was observed. Using this combined-modality approach, Moertel (139) reported a hormonal response rate of 86%, with a median duration of response of 2 years. The toxicity of this approach notwithstanding and pending publication of the Mayo Clinic experience or other confirmatory experience, sequential hepatic artery occlusion and combination chemotherapy may be considered for selective patients with symptomatic metastatic carcinoid refractory to somatostatin therapy.

Gastrinoma Syndrome

The gastrinoma syndrome is characterized by a severe ulcer diathesis and persistent basal gastric acid hypersecretion because of hypergastrinemia (Table 103.3). It has been increasingly recognized that this syndrome can exist in multiple forms: benign sporadic, malignant metastatic, and as part of the MEN-1 syndrome. The gastrinoma syndrome needs to be distinguished from the G-cell hyperplasia syndrome and from those rare cases in which acid hypersecretion cannot be ascribed to gastrin (88, 162). From various series, it appears that approximately 66% of gastrinomas are sporadic (163). Most sporadic tumors in the pancreas are solitary and have been malignant in approximately 60 to 85% of cases. These usually are found in older subjects. Sporadic tumors generally occur in the pancreas, although primary tumors also may occur in the body of the stomach, duodenum, and jejunum, accounting for up to 23% of tumors found at operation (163). Less than 40% of these are malignant. Ec-

Table 103.3. Clinical Manifestations Suggestive of Gastrinoma

Multiple upper gastrointestinal ulcers
Peptic ulcers in unusual locations (e.g., postbulbar)
Ulcers resistant to medical therapy
Frequent and recurrent ulcers after cessation of therapy
Postoperative ulcer recurrence
Basal hyperchlorhydria
Prolonged unexplained diarrhea or steatorrhea
Symptoms of hypercalcemia, renal stones, pituitary tumors
Radiographic evidence of increased gastric or duodenal folds
Family history of pituitary, pancreas, or parathyroid tumors or kidney stones

topic tumors also have been identified in peripancreatic lymph nodes (163–169) in the splenic hilum, root of the mesentery, omentum, liver, gallbladder, and in the ovary (163, 170). Solitary tumors in these sites are less likely to be malignant, and the overall cure rate is higher than that reported for pancreatic tumors (169). In the past, the likelihood of a surgeon finding the tumor in these sites, however, has been less than 50%, but there still are difficulties finding tumors in these locations, leading to operative failures (167, 168, 171).

Because of the pioneering work of Debas and colleagues (172) as well as Thompson and colleagues (173) and others, the duodenum has been increasingly recognized as a site for gastrinomas. In several recent series, gastrinomas were located in extrapancreatic sites, including the duodenal wall, in 43 to 77% of patients (173–175).

Approximately 33% of gastrinomas are associated with the MEN-1 syndrome (171, 176–180). The problems attending gastrinoma in the MEN-1 syndrome are quite different from those associated with the sporadic variety, however. If patients with hyperparathyroidism are scrutinized carefully, up to 38% are found to have gastrinomas (178, 181). Whereas 50 to 60% of patients with MEN-1 develop gastrinoma, over 90% have hyperparathyroidism. Refined testing is indicated to detect the presence of gastrinoma in patients with ulcer and hyperparathyroidism (182). Tumors in the MEN-1 syndrome usually are multiple, often small or undetectable, and less frequently (7–12%), malignant (176, 177, 179, 183). Most cases, however, are discovered at a younger age than in the sporadic cases, and the frequency of malignancy may indeed be considerably higher. Both the multiplicity of the tumors and their small size may make it difficult to find the specific tumors that are secreting gastrin, and the likelihood of recurrence or persistence after excision militates against laparotomy without first identifying a specific site or sites of origin for the hypergastrinemia.

The G-cell hyperplasia syndrome has been considered by some to be part of the gastrinoma syndrome, but in general, the distinction from a tumor can be made based on equivocal responses to secretin and an exaggerated response to food ingestion, thus directing attention to the appropriate site of gastrin overproduction (184). There seldom is a need to pursue localization procedures.

Metastases from gastrinoma predominantly are located in the liver. The presence of gastrinoma in peripancreatic lymph glands should not be taken to indicate incurability (167, 168, 184–186), because it does not preclude removal of nodes and the primary tumor for possible cure. Some have advocated resection or a debulking procedure (169, 185–187) or even gastrectomy, which has been reported to cause regression of the primary tumor (165, 188). Nonetheless, it is vitally important to identify metastases, because tumor-related mortality can be as high as 79% (167). High serum levels of gastrin-17 compared with gastrin-34 may be of value (189, 190) or, if available, measurement of the NH_2 to COOH-terminal gastrin ratio (191, 192). Elevated circulating hCG subunits strongly favor the presence of metastases (193); in such cases, curative surgical attempts are unlikely to succeed.

DIAGNOSIS

The possibility of gastrinoma syndrome should be entertained in all patients with ulcer disease and in those with unexplained secretory diarrhea. Before development of the radioimmunoassay, 80% of patients with gastrinoma presented with a severe ulcer diathesis, bleeding, intestinal obstruction, or perforation. Two thirds had had at least one operation. Although this may seem extravagant, it can be calculated that one unnecessary operation costs at least 1,000 gastrin assays; thus, if the success rate is 1:1,000, it should more than compensate for the cost of the assay. Since 1970, only 20% of patients with the Zollinger-Ellison syndrome have presented with serious ulcer complications (ulcer diabetes because of gastrinoma), and only one third have had prior surgery (194). Today, the diagnosis of gastrinoma should be made even without ulcers, based on diarrhea or mild duodenitis.

Before carrying out an extensive work-up of hypergastrinemia, however, a careful family history inquiring for features of MEN-1 syndrome should be conducted. If this is positive or suspicious, then in most patients with MEN-1, hypercalcemia has developed before age 30. If present, this indicates autosomal dominant inheritance of the *MEN-1* gene (29). Measurement of serum calcium corrected for albumin will suffice, because esophagogastric duodenoscopy allows the examination of gastric juice for pH and visually identifies superficial ectopic lesions that are missed by barium studies. A urine testing tape is also useful, because in the absence of antisecretory drugs, a pH of 3.0 or higher excludes Zollinger-Ellison syndrome.

Studies of gastric acid secretion should include measurements of volume as well as basal and PG-stimulated acid secretion. The diagnosis is confirmed if: (*a*) the volume of gastric secretion is large (typically >10 L per 24 hours); (*b*) the basal acid output is over 15 mmol/h or, after vagotomy or gastrectomy, over 3 mmol/h (values in the 10–15 range are borderline, and <10 mmol/h excludes Zollinger-Ellison syndrome; and (*c*) the ratio of the basal acid output to the maximum response to pentagastrin is greater than 0.6, because the gastrinoma cells are maximally stimulating acid secretion and pentagastrin can cause no further rise. Of great importance is the need to stop H_2 blockers, K+/H+ ATPase inhibitors, and octreotide at least 24 hours before the study, because false-negative results may occur through iatrogenic inhibition of acid secretion.

Table 103.4. Causes of Hypergastrinemia

With increased acid	With decreased acid
Gastrinoma	Atrophic gastritis
G-cell hyperfunction	Pernicious anemia
Gastric outlet obstruction	Vagotomy
Short bowel syndrome	Gastric carcinoma
Retained antrum	Renal disease
Hypercalcemia	Rheumatoid arthritis
Hyperparathyroidism	Vitiligo
MEN-1	Diabetic pseudo ZE syndrome

MEN-1—Multiple endocrine neoplasia type 1; ZE—Zollinger-Ellison.

Serum gastrin levels are usually greater than 150 pg/mL in patients with Zollinger-Ellison syndrome, except for the small proportion who secrete a biologically active variant not recognized by the antiserum used (191). Gastrin levels may be raised for other reasons.

As Table 103.4 shows, it is apparent that only during conditions in which there is increased acid should Zollinger-Ellison syndrome be considered. The most sensitive and accurate test remains the secretin stimulation test for gastrin secretion. Secretin, 2 u/kg, is given intravenously and blood samples for gastrin drawn at 2, 5, 10, 20, and 30 minutes. A rise of more than 100 pg/mL is strongly suggestive of Zollinger-Ellison syndrome. No new test has emerged with a greater sensitivity or specificity. While false-positive results do occur, they are rare and usually found in hypochlorhydric states (88). The presence of normal hyperfunctioning antrum usually can be identified by a gastrin response to a meal greater than that to secretin.

GASTRINOMA LOCALIZATION

Tumor localization is needed to make the best treatment decisions in individual patients; the sensitivity and specificity of various localization procedures is given in Table 103.5. Selective angiography achieves visualization of the tumor in a minority of patients (195–197), although it often is useful for the demonstration of hepatic metastases. CT (198) and ultrasound (163, 198), even with the use of contrast, have proven to be of limited value, because the density of these tumors is within the limits of the surrounding pancreatic tissue or, as occurs not infrequently, the tumors are below the resolution capacity of the technique. Furthermore, the presence of small tumors in extrapancreatic sites, and even within the body of the liver, may go undetected by these means (168, 184, 186, 199). A technique using intraoperative ultrasound of the exposed pancreas (200–202) has been modestly successful, suggesting that this technique may be able to eliminate some of the artifacts created by external ultrasound. MRI was greeted with some enthusiasm, but apart from an enhanced capacity to visualize blood vessels, it generally has not been superior to previous techniques (203). A recent study of 11 patients with islet cell tumors showed that MRI combined with dynamic gadolinium scanning may be superior to CT (204).

On occasion, a combination of techniques may be useful. Although both CT and selective visceral angiography were found to be effective in identifying nearly all patients with metastatic disease to the liver and, in some cases, to retroperitoneal lymph nodes, these studies failed to identify primary tumors in more than 50% of the patients seen with biochemical proof of gastrinoma syndrome. Recently, selective intra-arterial injection of secretin has been used to help localize gastrinomas either by enhancing tumor/background differences in gastrin levels or by causing a tumor blush on angiography (172, 205). This technique has the advantage that it can be performed simultaneously with angiography with the addition of a catheter in a hepatic and a peripheral vein to sample gastrin levels. When secretin is injected into a vessel that supplies the gastrinoma, the hepatic vein levels of gastrin greatly exceed the peripheral levels. This technique may have a higher accuracy than percutaneous transhepatic venous sampling (PTHVS) alone (205).

The use of percutaneous transhepatic portal, pancreatic, and hepatic venous gastrin sampling (PTHVS) by Ingemansson and colleagues (206) in 1977, Burcharth and colleagues (207) in 1979, and subsequently by others (208–210) suggested that this new technique was of value in those patients with gastrinoma syndrome without liver metastases or those with a primary gastrinoma that was not detected by conventional imaging methods. Our initial studies were undertaken in 1978 (184, 209, 210). It soon became apparent that not only was a skilled angiographer imperative, but also expert technique, a detailed understanding of the variable venous anatomy, a sound and reliable assay method for gastrin, and thoughtful interpretation of the data in each case (184, 209, 210). The technique is both costly and time consuming (191). Gradients were determined by simultaneous measurements of gastrin in peripancreatic veins and central arterial samples to avoid the misinterpretations that the rapid changes in secretory rate often associated with gastrinomas can cause. Placement of cannulae without obstruction of the vessel and streaming of blood in the portal vessel had to be considered. Awareness of the peculiarities of the peripancreatic venous drainage was a prerequisite to avoid erroneous localization of tumors. Furthermore, hepatic venous sampling also was considered to be essential to detect occult liver metastases or the rare primary gastrinoma within the liver. In our experience, it has been possible to predict the presence or absence of liver metastases and, in two patients, to identify solitary resectable primary liver gastrinomas. Our results in 46 patients with gastrin hypersecretion indicate that the technique may be uniquely valuable in sporadic or ectopic gastrinomas (184, 209, 210), but false-negative results also have been reported (211).

The most recent analysis of a 10-year experience supports PTHVS as a useful method to regionalize a tumor. Early results suggested that the technique was of limited value in patients with MEN-1 who were much less likely to benefit from localization and excision of the tumor (179, 184). The results are based on the demonstration of tumors in the pancreas and in ectopic sites. Clearly, however, the surgeon would have found at least 50% of the tumors without the aid of PTHVS. Our approach has been aggressive: if there has been a gradient (by criteria that differ from those of others),

Table 103.5. Success of Tumor Localization in Gastrinoma

Factor	Ultrasound	Infusion	Computed tomography	Selective angiography		PTHVS	
						Local	Regional
Sensitivity	21	40	31	60	29	35	94
Specificity	92	100	66	100	100	89	97
Positive predictive value	80	100	83	100	100	—	94
Negative predictive value	40	50	15	60	100	89	—

PTHVS—Percutaneous transhepatic portal, pancreatic, and hepatic venous gastrin sampling.
Data from Norton and colleagues (211) as well as Vinik and colleagues (210, 328, 184).

the surgeon has pursued mobilization of the head of the pancreas and duodenotomy. These procedures have not been pursued by many other surgeons because of the relatively benign course of those patients in whom no tumor is found at standard laparotomy.

In experienced hands, endoscopic ultrasound may increase the ability to detect pancreatic gastrinomas, and localization rates of 80 to 100% have been reported (212, 213). The ability of this technique to detect lesions less then 5 mm in size or occult duodenal lesions, however, is uncertain. A typical instrument consists of a side-viewing endoscope combined with a 7.5- and 12.0-MHz ultrasonic transducer distal to the side-viewing optics, giving an ultrasonic section of 360° perpendicular to the shaft axis of the scope (213). The pancreatic head is examined with the scanner positioned in the duodenum. The body and tail of the pancreas are studied with the scanner in the stomach. A special saline-filled balloon at the tip of the instrument and instillation of approximately 400 mL of saline into the stomach are used to provide an interface between the ultrasonic unit and the GI wall (212, 213).

With the aggressive approach, at least 30% of patients with sporadic gastrinoma syndrome can be cured by tumor resection. With recent advances in localization methods and operative techniques, the percentage of patients cured likely will increase. Thus, in appropriate cases, an aggressive approach is distinctly advantageous in the localization and selection of operative treatment. Failure to find a tumor carries a good prognosis, and no patient has died in an 8.5-year follow-up (179). This must be contrasted with the 29% perioperative morbidity and mortality rate resulting from explorations of the head of the pancreas reported by some (167, 177, 187, 199, 210), although one group has reported 37% (214). The ultimate answer to the vexing question of whether to explore the head of the pancreas will no doubt be determined by longer follow-up; the approach will be dictated by the available expertise and experience of those involved.

TREATMENT

Treatment of the gastrinoma syndrome has undergone significant changes since the first case was described in 1955 (169). Until the development of drugs to control the excessive acid production (215–218), the purpose of operative intervention was to excise the acid-secreting stomach, which was the major cause of morbidity and mortality (from massive hemorrhage or perforation). These operations most frequently were done as emergency procedures under adverse conditions, and they were associated with a significant increase in mortality compared with elective partial or total gastrectomies. It soon was learned that partial gastrectomy with or without vagotomy usually was ineffective and total gastrectomy became the standard operation in patients with an established diagnosis of gastrinoma (163, 167, 169, 176). As experience accumulated, it became apparent that approximately 60% of patients with gastrinoma syndrome had malignant tumors, which although relatively slow-growing, became the major contributing factor to mortality after longer follow-up (163). Occasional cases were reported, however, in which the syndrome had been cured by tumor excision only, particularly when the primary neoplasm was in the duodenum and no metastases were found in either lymph nodes or the liver (167, 199, 219–221). In most of these cases, a total gastrectomy also was performed, because the surgeon was rightfully concerned that occult metastases might be present and remain a cause of continued hypersecretion of gastrin.

Most authorities now recommend a combined medical and surgical approach to the management of these tumors. If patients with MEN-1 syndrome are excluded, the cure rate for excision of a gastrinoma is approximately 14% (168, 179, 181, 222–225). These studies did not, however, define the nature of the primary disease. When only extrapancreatic tumors are examined, as many as 50% may be cured by excision of the tumor (163, 167, 168, 219), especially those in the duodenum. Even excision of tumors in lymph nodes may result in cure (199, 219, 222). For the most part, unfortunately, various reports have grouped their patients together and not identified the subgroups defined earlier. Surgical exploration should include mobilization of the pancreas along its entire length, allowing careful bimanual palpation if regionalization has not been achieved preoperatively. A variety of intraoperative methods are helpful to the surgeon in identifying gastrinomas. Intraoperative ultrasound has been shown by some investigators to detect nonpalpable lesions, identify the relationship of the lesion to major structures such as the main pancreatic duct, and detect signs suggesting malignancy (226, 227). The ability of this technique to detect duodenal lesions, however, is poor. Intraoperative endoscopy with transillumination of the duodenum has been shown to be capable of locating duodenal wall gastrinomas (228), but the most accurate method of detecting duodenal gastrinomas appears to be duodenotomy with careful palpation. Because the duodenum and extrapancreatic locations have been recognized increasingly as sites of gastrinomas (171, 179, 184, 214, 219), most experienced teams routinely employ duodenotomy during surgical exploration for gastrinoma (173, 175). Such an aggressive approach has increased significantly the number of positive explorations, with one group increasing the percentage of positive explorations from 64 to over 90%, primarily through the identification and resection of duodenal wall gastrinomas (174, 175).

The current treatment of the patient with MEN-1 and gastrinoma remains controversial (176, 180, 229). The total number of patients with the MEN-1 and gastrinoma syndromes who have been carefully evaluated for possible palliative or curative pancreatic operations based on selective venous sampling has been so limited that a definitive statement about optimal management cannot be made at present. In these patients, both the functional (i.e., hypergastrinemia) and malignant potential of the disease should be considered in the individual case. When there is no evidence of metastatic disease and venous sampling demonstrates an anatomically localized source of gastrin, enucleation (i.e., pancreatic head) or resection (i.e., body or tail) may offer excellent palliation, if not cure. The low incidence of malignancy in the patients with MEN-1 should not dictate a more cavalier approach than in sporadic cases without evidence of MEN-1.

Accurate estimates for chemotherapeutic activity in metastatic gastrinoma are difficult to ascertain, because most published series have studied chemotherapy for all histologic subtypes of pancreatic endocrine cancers pooled together. With respect to single-agent chemotherapy, streptozotocin probably is the most active antineoplastic drug in patients with metastatic gastrinomas (230–233). From their review, Maton and colleagues suggested that the drug appears to cause an objective response rate of 50% in patients with this disease. There is no evidence for improved outcomes when streptozotocin is used in combination with 5-fluorouracil with or without doxorubicin (234, 235). Inconsistencies in the reported dose and schedule of administration of streptozotocin as well as in the criteria used for reported objective tumor responses preclude reliable recommendations for chemotherapy with this agent in patients with metastatic gastrinoma. Among six patients with advanced gastrinoma that received dacarbazine, none had an objective response (234, 236).

Similarly, there has been little experience in the use of adjuvant chemotherapy following surgical resection. In one report of four patients who underwent complete resection of locally advanced gastrinoma followed by chemotherapy with streptozotocin, doxorubicin, and 5-fluorouracil, two patients remained free of disease at 14- and 32-month follow-up evaluations (237). The small number of patients and relatively short follow-up period is insufficient to recommend that this approach be generally adopted, however, although it may be appropriate to consider it for selected patients.

As discussed later for other pancreatic endocrine tumors, there appears to be a role for interferon in management (151). The number of reported patients with gastrinoma treated with interferon, however, is too few to reach any firm conclusions regarding its effectiveness in this specific disease.

Insulinomas

A firmly established diagnosis of an insulin-secreting lesion of the pancreas is essential to successful management. Therefore, it is critically important to rule out other causes of hypoglycemia associated with fasting (238). A detailed differential diagnosis may be found in Table 103.6. Nonislet cell neoplasms associated with hypoglycemia are given in Table 103.7.

An accurate diagnosis of organic hyperinsulinism can be established with near certainty in all cases (238). The specific causes of hyperinsulinism (Table 103.7) usually can be made before exploration. There are syndromes of autoimmunity that may lead to hypoglycemia which must be considered.

Antireceptor antibodies usually occur in the presence of other autoimmune disease, with antireceptor antibodies mimicking the effect of insulin and reducing insulin clearance. Therefore, insulin levels may be normal or high, but C-peptide levels are low. This is because islet cells are suppressed. Titres fall with time, leading to remission, although corticosteroids have been used. Autoimmune hypoglycemic disease syndrome usually occurs in the presence of other autoimmune disorders (e.g., Grave's disease, rheumatoid arthritis, lupus) and generally produces reactive hypoglycemia from prolongation of the half-life of circulating

Table 103.6. Classification of Hypoglycemia

Fasting hypoglycemia

- Hyperinsulinemia
  - Islet cell adenoma, carcinoma, hyperplasia, nesidioblastosis
- Autoimmune with insulin antibodies
- Counterregulatory hormone deficiency
  - Anterior pituitary insufficiency—GH, ACTH
  - Adrenocortical insufficiency
  - Hypothyroidism (severe)
- Large nonislet tumor
- Impaired hepatic function
  - Hepatocellular insufficiency
  - Ethanol/malnutrition
  - Sepsis
  - Specific enzymatic defects (childhood)
- Impaired renal function
- Substrate deficiency
  - Fanconi syndrome (renal loss)
  - Nursing
  - Severe inanition
  - Severe exercise
- Drug induced

Reactive Hypoglycemia

- Alimentary
- "Pre-diabetes"
- Endocrine
- Idiopathic

Factitious

- Surreptitious insulin administration
- Surreptitious sulfonylurea administration
- Leukemoid reaction polycythemia

ACTH—corticotropin; GH—growth hormone.

Table 103.7. Nonislet Cell Neoplasms Associated with Hypoglycemia

Mesenchymal
Mesothelioma
Fibrosarcoma
Rhabdomyosarcoma
Leiomyosarcoma
Hemangiopericytoma
Carcinoma
Hepatic: hepatoma, biliary carcinoma
Adrenocortical carcinoma
Genitourinary: hypernephroma, Wilms', prostate
Reproductive: cervical or breast carcinoma
Neurologic/neuroendocrine
Pheochromocytoma
Carcinoid
Neurofibroma
Hematologic
Leukemia
Lymphoma
Myeloma

insulin. Insulin levels generally are extremely elevated, which may result from interference by antibodies with the particular insulin assay or, if C peptide also is increased, increased insulin secretion by the pancreas to compensate for inactivation of insulin by circulating antibodies. Glucose tolerance testing reveals that plasma glucose is elevated early and reduced late because of the buffering effect of antibodies on the action of secreted insulin. The disease usually is self-limited, and it may be precipitated in some patients by exposure to drugs containing sulfhydryl groups that react with SH groups on insulin and render it immunogenic.

DIAGNOSIS

The blood glucose level alone is not diagnostic of insulinoma, nor in general is the absolute insulin level elevated in all cases of organic hyperinsulinism. The standard test remains a 72-hour fast while the patient is closely observed (238, 239). More than 95% of cases can be diagnosed based on responses to a 72-hour fast. Serial glucose and insulin levels are obtained over the 72 hours until the patient becomes symptomatic. Because the absolute insulin level is not elevated in all patients with insulinomas, a normal level does not rule out the disease; however, a fasting insulin level of greater than 24 μU/mL is found in approximately 50% of patients with insulinoma. This is strong evidence in favor of the diagnosis. Values of insulin greater than 7 μU/mL after a more prolonged fast in the presence of a blood glucose less than 40 mg/dL also are highly suggestive. A refinement in the interpretation of glucose and insulin levels has been established by determining the ratio of insulin levels in μU/mL to the concomitant glucose level in mg/dL. An insulin/glucose ratio of greater than 0.3 has been found in virtually all patients proven to have an insulinoma or other islet cell disease causing organic hyperinsulinism. The accuracy of the test can be increased by calculating the amended insulin/glucose ratio as follows:

$$\text{amended ratio} = \text{insulin } (\mu\text{U/mL})/\text{glucose (mg/dL)} - 30$$

If the value is greater than 50, then organic hyperinsulinism is certain (238). Measurements of proinsulin and C peptide also have proven to be valuable in patients suspected of having organic hypoglycemia (181). Normally, the circulating proinsulin concentration accounts for less than 22% of the insulin immunoreactivity, but it is greater than 24% in over 90% of individuals with insulinomas. Furthermore, when the proinsulin level is greater than 40%, a malignant islet cell tumor should be strongly suspected (187, 238, 240). The C-peptide level is useful in ruling out factitious hypoglycemia from self-administration of insulin. Commercial insulin preparations contain no C peptide, and combined with high insulin levels, low C-peptide levels confirm the diagnosis of self-administration of insulin. High-performance liquid chromatography to characterize the insulin species found in the blood was useful before the advent of recombinant human insulin, which has provided the malingerer with a more powerful tool to test the resourcefulness of the physician. Patients who take sulfonylureas surreptitiously may have raised insulin and C-peptide values soon after ingestion, but chronic use will result in hypoglycemia without raised insulin or C-peptide levels. Only an index of suspicion and measurement of urine sulfonylureas will lead to the correct diagnosis. A variety of insulin stimulation and suppression tests were once used when precise and accurate insulin measurements were not available. Each had its limitations, and all are currently considered to be obsolete (88, 238). The insulin response to secretin stimulation (2 μ/kg intravenously; peak response in 1–5 minutes) is a valuable measure to differentiate multiple adenomas from nesidioblastosis and single adenomas (241). The normal maximal increment is 74 μU/mL, whereas in single adenomas, the rise is only 17 μU/mL, in nesidioblastosis 10 μU/mL, and in two patients with multiple B-cell adenomas and hyperplasia, 214 and 497 μU/mL. Patients with single adenomas and nesidioblastosis do not respond to secretin, whereas those with multiple adenomas or hyperplasia have an excessive insulin response to the administration of secretin.

LOCALIZATION

Once the diagnosis of suspected hyperinsulinism is confirmed, every effort should be made to localize the source of excessive insulin production. Preoperative localization is important, because approximately 30% of insulinomas are less than 1 cm in diameter, 10% are multiple, 10 to 15% are malignant, and 10% will have either islet cell hyperplasia or nesidioblastosis and no tumor at all (Fig. 103.5) (88, 184, 219, 238, 239, 242–246). Because of their small size, the techniques most commonly used to demonstrate tumors in the upper abdomen, including ultrasound, CT, MRI, contrast studies of the upper GI tract, and endoscopic retrograde pancreatography, are of little value. Until the past decade, the only study considered to be of proven value in the localization of insulinomas was selective pancreatic angiography (239, 242, 245, 247). Highly selective injections of contrast,

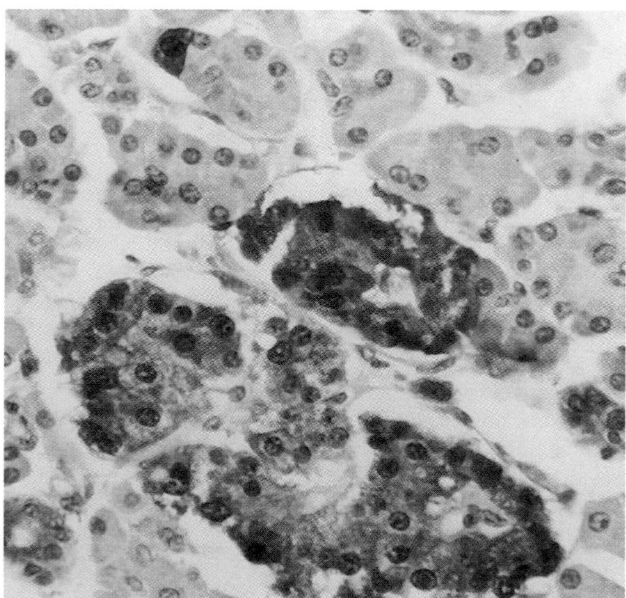

Figure 103.5. Nesidioblastosis showing islet hyperplasia, with immunoperoxidase evidence for insulin staining.

subtraction procedures, and magnification increase the number of insulinomas identified by this technique (Fig. 103.3). In one large series, 90% of insulinomas were reported to be localized by angiography alone (239); however, most groups report less satisfactory results (247). A summary of all reports in the literature found that approximately 60% of insulinomas have been detected by this method (184). Selective intra-arterial injection of calcium with sampling of hepatic vein insulin appears to improve the ability to detect insulinomas (71, 248), similar to the results seen with intra-arterial secretin in gastrinoma.

Percutaneous transhepatic venous sampling of insulin from pancreatic veins has been used successfully in localizing occult sources of hyperinsulinism (242, 249–252). We now believe that the combination of a secretin test to determine the nature of the hyperinsulinism (e.g., distinction of hyperplasia from adenoma or multiple adenomatosis) with PTHVS to localize provides the best means of establishing the specific cause of organic hyperinsulinism with near certainty. A skilled angiographer and careful analysis of the hormonal data in relationship to the venous anatomy in the individual case are required.

If PTHVS is not available and preoperative localization by angiography or other techniques has been negative, the surgeon may use intraoperative ultrasound if a careful exploration fails to detect a tumor. Some who have used this technique routinely have reported excellent results. Ultrasound does not identify hyperplasia or nesidioblastosis, however, and it appears to be operator dependent in its sensitivity.

TREATMENT OF ISLET β-CELL DISEASE WITH HYPERINSULINISM

The treatment of pancreatic islet β-cell disease usually is surgical; in the great majority of cases, it provides a complete cure. It should be performed only when the diagnosis is certain, however, and only by a surgeon who is skilled in pancreatic surgery. The surgical approach to insulinoma is straightforward when the tumor is localized. Precise localization obviates blind pancreatic resection (253). The results of PTHVS are very useful in helping to plan the surgical approach, even in the absence of finding a tumor during careful surgical exploration. In patients who have been unresponsive to medical therapy and in whom PTHVS suggests diffuse or multiple sources, such as adenomatosis, nesidioblastosis, or hyperplasia, a resection of at least 80% of the pancreas is indicated after a frozen-section specimen of the pancreatic tail confirms the diagnosis. When hypoglycemia can be controlled with diet alone or with small, well-tolerated doses of diazoxide, and/or when the medical condition of the patient may increase the hazard of surgery sufficiently, medical management alone may be considered. Patients with diffuse hyperinsulinism for whom an operation is planned first should have a trial of treatment with diazoxide and a natriuretic benzothiadiazine. Medical treatment is required for the great majority of malignant insulinomas, because only occasionally are they cured by operation. Medical treatment for benign insulinomas is a change in meals to include "lente carbohydrate" or unrefined carbohydrate given as frequently as required to prevent hypoglycemia. Antihormonal therapy may be useful if diet is insufficient. The management of malignant insulinoma is antihormonal and antitumor therapy.

MEDICAL MANAGEMENT OF BENIGN DISEASE

Diet

The cornerstone of medical management of insulinoma and other forms of hyperinsulinism is the diet. Not uncommonly, patients may avoid symptoms of hypoglycemia for variable periods of time by shortening the number of hours between feedings. For some, the inclusion of a bedtime (11:00 PM) feeding is sufficient; for others a midmorning, midafternoon, and/or a 3:00 snack are necessary. Although the tumor may be stimulated occasionally to secrete insulin by the ingestion of carbohydrates, it is inadvisable to restrict the intake of carbohydrate. More slowly absorbable forms of carbohydrates (e.g., starches, bread, potatoes, rice) generally are preferred. During hypoglycemic episodes, rapidly absorbable forms (e.g., fruit juices with added glucose or sucrose) are indicated. In patients with severe refractory hypoglycemia, use of a continuous intravenous infusion of glucose, coupled with increased dietary intake of carbohydrate, frequently alleviates hypoglycemia long enough to institute additional therapy.

Diazoxide and Natriuretic Benzothiadiazines

Diazoxide (Proglycem) owes its potent hyperglycemic properties to two effects (254, 255). it directly inhibits the release of insulin by B cells through stimulation of α-adrenergic receptors, and it has an extrapancreatic hyperglycemic effect, probably by inhibiting cyclic AMP phosphodiesterase, resulting in higher plasma levels of cyclic AMP and enhanced glycogenolysis. Because diazoxide induces the retention of sodium, edema is troublesome at higher dosages. The addition of a diuretic benzothiadiazine (e.g., trichlormethiazide) not only corrects or prevents edema but synergizes the hyperglycemic effect of diazoxide. At the doses needed to counteract the higher doses of diazoxide (e.g., 450–600 mg/d), natriuretic benzothiadiazines frequently induce hypokalemia. Nausea is an additional complication at higher dosages of diazoxide, and hypertrichosis may complicate long-term treatment. These compounds have been useful to elevate blood levels of glucose into the euglycemic range if operation must be delayed for weeks or months. Patients with benign insulinomas have been managed successfully for up to 16 years with diazoxide in doses of 150 to 450 mg/d in combination with trichlormethiazide in doses of 2 to 8 mg/d. If they can be tolerated, higher doses may be used in patients with malignant insulinomas.

Calcium Channel Blockers

Theoretically, calcium channel blockers are capable of inhibiting insulin secretion. Verapamil has been used successfully to alleviate the hypoglycemia caused by an insulin-secreting pancreatic tumor in a 94-year old woman (256). Verapamil and diltiazem have been used with variable results in other patients with organic hyperinsulinism.

Propranolol

β-Adrenergic-receptor blocking drugs inhibit insulin secretion and therefore may be of value in treating organic hyperinsulin. Only a few reports of the use of propranolol have appeared (257–259). Its use has been associated with the reduction of plasma insulin levels and with the relief of hypoglycemic attacks in patients with benign or malignant insulinoma. In a patient with a benign insulinoma, 80 mg of propranolol a day was sufficient, while a patient with malignant insulinoma, in whom streptozotocin was no longer effective, required 640 mg of propranolol orally per day (259). Because these changes can mask the adrenergic symptoms of hyperglycemia and inhibit muscle glycogenolysis, however, there is a risk of aggravating the clinical syndrome. The drug should be used with extreme caution and careful monitoring.

Dilantin

The anticonvulsive diphenylhydantoin (Dilantin) has been shown to inhibit the in vitro release of insulin from both the labile and storage B-cell pools. It has been used successfully to control refractory hypoglycemia, as evidenced by normal overnight fasting glucose levels and absence of hypoglycemia during total fasting of up to 24 hours (260, 261). In only one third or less of patients with benign insulinoma, however, is the hyperglycemic effect of Dilantin of any clinical significance. Furthermore, with the dosage required, ataxia, nystagmus, hypertrophic gums, and megaloblastic anemia may be side effects. Maintenance doses range from 300 to 600 mg/d. The concurrent administration of diazoxide lowers measurable blood levels of dilantin, and their concurrent use is not recommended.

Long-acting Somatostatin Analogue

We initially reported the successful use of octreotide (Sandostatin) in prolonging the ability to fast in a patient with a benign insulinoma (262), and a similar experience was reported by Osei and O'dorisio (263) in a patient with a malignant tumor. Our more recent experience has shown a variety of responses not easily predictable by the clinical or biochemical profile. We have examined the effects of a long-acting octreotide analogue in seven patients with endogenous hyperinsulinism, five with proven single adenomas, one with multiple adenomas, and one with organic hyperinsulinism associated with MEN-1 (245). In two patients, and possibly a third, octreotide prolonged the ability to fast without hypoglycemia, with variable decreases in plasma insulin concentrations. A trial of long-term administration of octreotide in one of these patients gave only short-term relief of hypoglycemia. Octreotide did not improve, or actually worsened, plasma glucose levels on fasting in the other four patients. In contrast, oral administration of diazoxide to four of these patients was effective in raising plasma glucose levels. A child treated for nesidioblastosis did well initially but subsequently required pancreatectomy and also grew at only the third percentile. It is unlikely that octreotide will be a useful addition to the therapeutic armamentarium for treatment of organic hyperinsulinism, except in familial forms of nesidioblastosis.

Glucocorticoids

The use of glucocorticoids, which increase gluconeogenesis and cause insulin resistance, also can help to stabilize blood glucose at an acceptable level. Pharmacologic doses (prednisone, approximately 1 mg/kg) must be used.

Glucagon

Glucagon may help to raise blood glucose concentrations, but it may simultaneously directly stimulate the release of insulin.

Vasoactive Intestinal Peptide Tumor (VIPoma)

In 1958, Verner and Morrison (264) first described refractory watery diarrhea and hypokalemia associated with non-insulin-secreting tumors of the pancreatic islets. The absence of gastric hypersecretion and even achlorhydria were documented in patients with this tumor syndrome (264–266), later termed *pancreatic cholera* because the observed severe diarrhea resembled *Vibrio cholerae* disease (267). The acronym *WDHA* (*w*atery *d*iarrhea [100%], *h*ypokalemia [100%], *A*chlorhydria) (268) was proposed, although a more appropriate acronym might be *WDHHA*, for *w*atery *d*iarrhea *h*ypokalemia, *h*ypochlorhydria, and *a*cidosis, because of bicarbonate wasting. Several reported series have confirmed the association between certain pancreatic tumors and watery diarrhea syndrome (257, 269, 270).

In a review of 55 patients with the diarrhea and hypokalemia syndrome, other features were sometimes ob-

Table 103.8. Differentiation of Gastrinoma and WDHHA Syndrome

Feature	Gastrinoma	WDHHA
Diarrhea	Acid	Alkaline (HCO_3 loss)
Gastric acid	Increased	Decreased
Gastric volume	Increased	Normal or decreased
Nasogastric suction	Diarrhea improves	Diarrhea unchanged
Motility	Increased[a]	Increased slightly[b]
Abdominal pain	Marked	Rare (initially)
Stool K^+ loss	Slight	Marked
Metabolic acidosis	No (alkalosis with gastric suction)	Yes
Lesion location	Primary pancreas (also liver, wall of stomach, and duodenum)	Primary pancreas Ganglioneuroblastoma
Mediator	Gastrin	VIP/other

[a] Motility enhanced secondary to gastric acid stimulation.
[b] Motility may be slightly increased secondary to direct effects of either intra-arterial or intraluminal VIP.
VIP—Vasoactive intestinal peptide; WDHHA—watery diarrhea, hypokalemia, hypochlorhydria, and acidosis.

served: alkalosis in mild cases but acidosis in severe diarrhea from bicarbonate wasting, flushing, hypercalcemia, tetany (perhaps from magnesium depletion), abnormal glucose tolerance, and dilation of the gallbladder (270). The most prominent symptom in most patients is profuse cholera-like diarrhea, which often is present for 3 or 4 years before diagnosis, with volumes usually exceeding 6 to 8 L of stool every 24 hours. Stool has the appearance of dilute tea and is rich in electrolytes, with an average secretion of 300 mmol of potassium per 24 hours. The diarrhea always is secretory in nature, will not disappear with fasting for 48 hours, and demonstrates an increased net secretion of electrolytes in the stool. This symptom may be confused with the diarrhea found in the Zollinger-Ellison syndrome; the distinguishing features are shown in Table 103.8.

Diarrhea that is not secretory always results from causes other than endocrine tumors. Laxative abuse may be very difficult to exclude, however, and the measurement of stool electrolytes and osmolarity may be required. Stool electrolytes should account for the osmolarity if the condition results from an endocrine tumor. An osmolarity exceeding that expected from the concentration of electrolytes invariably reflects laxative abuse, which must be carefully excluded.

The episodic and fulminating, secretory diarrhea associated with VIPomas results in profound hypokalemia, hypochlorhydria (rarely achlorhydria), bicarbonate wasting, and hyperchloremic metabolic acidosis. The more commonly observed hypochlorhydria results from the direct gastric acid inhibitory effect of VIP, a biologic property that is shared with other members of the secretin-glucagon family: secretin, glucagon, gastric inhibitory peptide (GIP), and polypeptide histidine and isoleucine (271). In the early stage of tumor growth, the predominant symptoms of diarrhea are episodic and intermittent. It generally is accepted that as the VIP tumor enlarges, the diarrhea becomes continuous and the ensuing electrolyte abnormalities life-threatening (257, 269). Increased intestinal motility as well as secretion may contribute to the diarrhea (132).

The clinical features of VIPomas are consistent with the known actions of VIP, which include: stimulation of intestinal secretion, facial flushing, inhibition of gastric acid secretion, stimulation of glycogenolysis, and hypercalcemia (272–275, 269, 276, 277, 270). The structural homology between VIP and secretin, glucagon, gastric inhibitory polypeptide (GIP) and peptide histidine and isoleucine (276) may account for enhanced secretion of pancreatic juice and inhibition of gastric acid secretion. VIP also has been reported to cause gallbladder relaxation; a large distended gallbladder often is found in patients with the VIPoma syndrome. Hypercalcemia has been noted in nearly 50% of patients with the syndrome. The cause is not clear, but it may relate to dehydration, electrolyte disturbances secondary to diarrhea, coincidental MEN accompanied by hyperparathyroidism, or secretion by the tumor of a calcitrophic peptide. Tetany has been reported in several patients and may result from hypomagnesemia secondary to the diarrhea. Nearly 8% of patients demonstrate facial flushing. The cause of this patchy erythematous and, sometimes, urticarial flushing is not clear, but it has been attributed to VIP or prostaglandins, which may be present in the tumor. The hyperglycemia often noted in patients with the watery diarrhea syndrome probably is secondary to the profound glycogenolytic effect of high portal vein VIP on the liver (275).

Sites of Tumors Secreting VIP

Tumors secreting VIP usually originate in the pancreas or along the sympathetic chain. In a series of 62 patients, 52 (84%) had pancreatic tumors, and 10 (16%) had ganglioneuroblastomas (278). Of the 10 patients with ganglioneuroblastomas, seven were children.

There have been 18 other case reports of elevated plasma levels of VIP that have been associated with neurogenic tumors, including ganglioneuroblastoma, ganglioneuromas, neurofibroma, and pheochromocytoma (279–288). Primary VIPomas now have been reported in other sites as well, including colon, lung, esophagus, jejunum, and liver, and we have reported the eventual emergence of tumors masquerading as hypernephroma and cutaneous mastocytomas (289). Most neurogenic tumors associated with the VIPoma syndrome have been found in children, but priapism has occurred, presumable resulting from a VIP-induced increase in blood flow to the corpora cavernosa. Catecholamines frequently are elevated; in patients with excess catecholamine secretion, flushing, increased sweating, and hypertension may occur. Hyperglycemia and hypercalcemia have not been noted in children. Plasma levels of PP are normal and have not been detected in VIP-producing ganglioneuroblastomas. Plasma PP levels nearly always are elevated if the tumor is in the pancreas. Thus, it was hoped that PP levels would distinguish pancreatic and nonpancreatic sources of VIP; however, three adults with neurogenic tumors and a 64-year-old woman with a VIPoma of the lower left kidney had high serum levels of PP (290). Excessive quantities of immunoreactive VIP and PP were found in the renal tumor tissue.

Biochemical Diagnosis and Experience

VIP is synthesized as the 170 amino acid precursor pre-proVIP, which posttranslationally is modified to yield the 28 amino acid VIP itself as well as peptide histidine and methionine (PHM) as well as other fragments (291). By definition, VIP levels are elevated in all patients with the VIPoma syndrome. Some of the non-VIP products of the precursor are secreted at higher levels than VIP itself, but unfortunately, assays for these products are not commercially available and their clinical usefulness not established. False-positive elevations of VIP can be observed in patients with small bowel ischemia or severe low-flow states caused by diarrhea and secondary dehydration not associated with VIP-producing tumors (274, 292, 293).

However, VIP is not the only agent implicated in the diarrhea syndrome. Gastrin, secretin, glucagon, enteroglucagon, gastric inhibitory polypeptide, PP, VIP, thyrocalcitonin (TCT), prostaglandins, and peptide fragments of pre-proVIP or any one of a number of combinations have been implicated as possible etiologic agents of the diarrhea syndrome (294). Bloom and colleagues reported 1,000 patients with various forms of diarrhea (79, 292, 295). Thirty-nine patients (3.9%) had greatly elevated levels of VIP, and in each case, a tumor was found. In more than 50% of these patients, the tumor was successfully removed, the symptoms remitted, and the plasma levels of VIP returned to normal. Twelve patients had diarrhea secondary to TCT-producing tumors of the thyroid, 13 had carcinoma of the lung, four had a villous adenoma of the rectum, and 24 had carcinoid tumors. All 53 of these patients had normal plasma VIP levels. Eleven additional patients had classic clinical features of the VIPoma syndrome in whom VIP levels were normal and no tumor was found; they probably were secreting an unidentified humoral substance with the biologic properties of VIP.

Biochemical detection of VIP-secreting tumors necessitates a highly sensitive and specific VIP radioimmunoassay. The range of normal VIP concentration is 0 to 170 pg/mL, which is similar to that (0–190 pg/mL) found by others (273, 281, 296).

Information gained from a single plasma VIP level may be misleading. The diagnosis of VIPoma in a patient with a good clinical history should not be excluded based on a single normal VIP because of vagaries in the assay. In addition between periods of watery diarrhea, the VIPoma, unlike many endocrine tumors of the gut (e.g., insulinoma, gastrinoma) may not be actively secreting VIP; thus, a normal level creates a false sense of security and may delay a more vigorous search for the cause.

Treatment

The first step in the treatment of these patients is prompt replacement of fluid and electrolyte losses. Symptoms of severe electrolyte imbalance include cardiac arrhythmias, neuromuscular deficits, profound shock, and cardiovascular collapse. The fluid of choice is an isotonic electrolyte solution containing adequate sodium, potassium, and base. In the series of 52 pancreatic cases reported by Long and colleagues (278), most of the solitary tumors were 8 cm or greater in diameter. Most of these tumors are demonstrable using ultrasound or CT, but occasionally, angiography or PTHVS are required (136). Somatostatin-receptor scintigraphy may be useful in identifying extrapancreatic VIPomas, particularly those in the sympathetic chain, or metastases (69).

If a tumor has been identified, complete surgical excision is the primary form of treatment. If the tumor cannot be removed completely, surgical debulking may have palliative benefit. In one series, surgical excision of the primary pancreatic tumor relieved all symptoms in 17 patients (27%) (177). Surgical removal of a ganglioneuroblastoma was successful in seven of 10 patients.

We do not advocate blind total pancreatectomy in patients who have diarrhea and in whom no tumor is demonstrable by angiography, CT, ultrasound, or PTHVS. Steroids have provided some symptomatic relief. A trial of prostaglandin synthesis inhibitors (e.g., indomethacin), phenothiazines, and lithium may be warranted (297). Octreotide has been used successfully in managing the diarrhea of VIPoma syndrome as well as that from the GEP tumors. Long-term octreotide treatment not only controls the diarrhea in these patients but also may cause arrest or regression of the tumor. Furthermore, we have seen spontaneous remission of watery diarrhea syndrome without establishing a cause, but we also have seen the eventual emergence of tumors in unusual sites, including the kidney and skin, only disclosed after careful follow-up for several years.

In summary, when confronted with severe chronic diarrhea, it must be established that the diarrhea is secretory in nature by fasting the patient for 48 hours and measuring stool volume. If diarrhea persists with fasting, VIP-producing tumors of the pancreas frequently are found, and plasma samples should be analyzed for VIP in these patients. If the VIP level is elevated, a VIP-secreting tumor (VIPoma) should be strongly suspected. In addition, a serum pancreatic polypeptide level should be determined simultaneously. If the tumor is located in the pancreas, this peptide almost invariably will be elevated. In children, catecholamine levels also should be obtained. If VIP levels are normal, screening for other causative agents, including gastrin, SP, somatostatin, PP, TCT, serotonin, glucagon, neuropeptide K, neurokinin A, peptide fragments of pre-pro VIP, and prostaglandins of the E series should be performed. Tumor localization should include CT, celiac, superior mesenteric, and renal angiography; and finally, PTHVS. Octreotide scanning may be useful, especially if metastases are being sought but may not be quite as helpful in small primary lesions. If a tumor is found, it should be excised. In the absence of finding a tumor, symptomatic therapy, not empiric surgery, is warranted. With malignant tumors, treatment with Sandostatin or chemotherapy must be considered.

Glucagonoma Syndrome

CLINICAL FEATURES

In 1966, McGavran and colleagues (298) called attention to a syndrome that included acquired diabetes and glucagon-producing tumors. It became apparent only later that these tumors usually were accompanied by a very characteristic skin rash (299, 300). The main features of the glucagonoma syndrome include a characteristic rash termed *necrolytic migratory erythema* (NME) (82% of patients) (Fig. 103.6), painful glossitis, angular stomatitis, normochromic normocytic anemia (61%), weight loss (90%), mild diabetes mellitus (80%), hypoaminoacidemia, deep vein thrombosis (50%) and depression (50%). The syndrome also goes by the acronym *4D syndrome*, which stands for *d*ermatosis, *d*iarrhea, *d*eep vein thromboses, and *d*epression.

The frequency of islet cell tumors has been estimated in autopsy series to be between 0.0 and 1.4% of all cases studied. In a very thorough study of 1,366 consecutive adult autopsies, Grimelius and Wilander (301) found a tumor frequency of 0.8%. All tumors were adenomas, and all contained histochemically defined glucagon cells. None of the tumors had been suspected during life. Although these adenomas contained glucagon, it is not known whether they were overproducing or even secreting glucagon. The incidence in vivo probably is 1% of all neuroendocrine tumors.

The NME rash of the glucagonoma syndrome has a characteristic distribution. It usually is widespread, but major sites of involvement are the perioral and perigenital regions along with the fingers, legs, and feet. It also may occur in areas of cutaneous trauma. The basic process in the skin seems to be one of superficial epidermal necrosis, fragile blister formation, crusting, and healing with hyperpigmentation. Skin biopsies usually show small bullae containing acantholytic epidermal cells as well as neutrophils and lymphocytes (299). The adjacent epidermis usually is intact, and the dermis contains a lymphocytic perivascular infiltrate. Different stages of the cutaneous lesions may be present simultaneously. Biopsy examination of a fresh skin lesion may be the most valuable aid in suggesting the diagnosis of glucagonoma syndrome, but repeated biopsy samples may be necessary to raise this possibility. A painful glossitis manifested by an erythematous, mildly atrophic tongue has been associated with the cutaneous lesions.

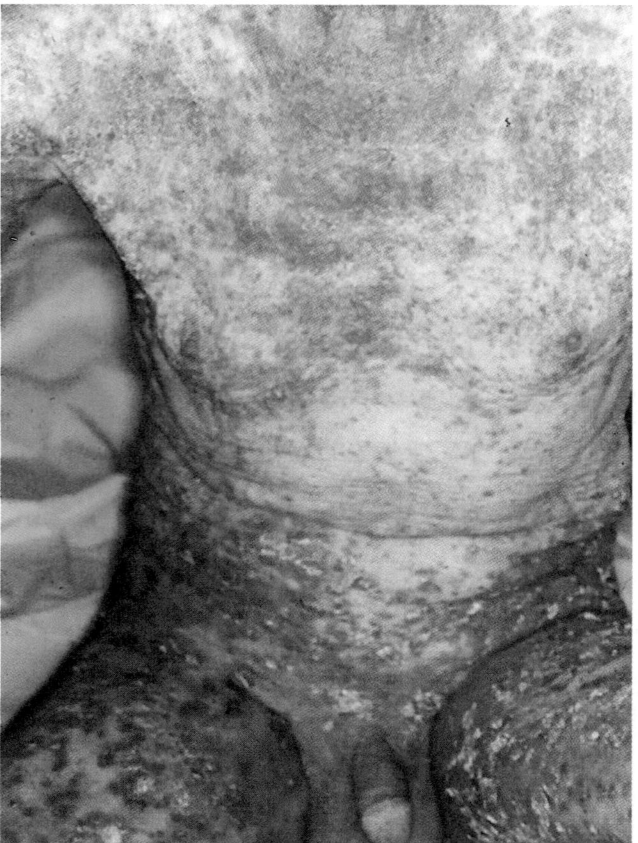

Figure 103.6. Migratory necrolytic erythema of glucagonoma syndrome.

Two other features of the syndrome are noteworthy. First, an alarmingly high rate of thromboembolic complications occurs in patients with glucagonomas, and many patients succumb to pulmonary embolism. Unexplained thromboembolic disease should alert one to the possibility of glucagonoma. Second, depression and other psychiatric disturbances including depression are common, but these may relate in part to the chronic dermatosis (292, 302).

Several metabolic disorders are associated with cutaneous lesions closely resembling the NME of the glucagonoma syndrome. These include acrodermatitis enteropathica, zinc deficiency induced by hyperalimentation, essential fatty acid deficiency, the dermatosis of protein calorie malnutrition of kwashiorkor, and pellagra resulting from niacin deficiency (297, 303–305). Cutaneous manifestations associated with malabsorptive states often are nonspecific, affecting approximately 20% of patients with steatorrhea. Improvement in the rash associated with the glucagonoma syndrome has been reported with amino acid repletion as well as administration of carbohydrate. The skin rash also has been shown to improve with the administration of zinc (306). Almost invariably, the dermatosis resolves after successful removal of a glucagon-producing tumor, even if the rash has been present for several years (307, 308). In addition, in those patients who do not undergo curative resection but are treated with chemotherapeutic agents, dermatitis improves as the glucagon levels decrease (85, 308, 309).

Glucose intolerance in the glucagonoma syndrome may relate to tumor size. Fasting plasma glucagon levels tend to be higher in patients with large hepatic metastases than in those without hepatic metastases (307), and all patients with large hepatic metastases had glucose intolerance. Massive hepatic metastases may decrease the ability of the liver to metabolize splanchnic glucagon, thus increasing peripheral plasma glucagon levels. Glucagon may not directly induce hyperglycemia, however, unless metabolism of glucose by the liver is directly compromised. Another factor may be variation in the molecular species of glucagon that is present in each case and its biological potency (310).

In previously reported cases of glucagonoma in which plasma glucagon concentrations were measured by radioimmunoassay, fasting plasma glucagon concentrations were 2,100 $\pm$ 334 pg/mL. These levels are markedly higher than those reported in normal, fasting subjects (i.e., $<$150 pg/mL) or in those with other disorders causing hyperglucagonemia, including diabetes mellitus, burn injury, acute trauma, bacteremia, cirrhosis, renal failure, or Cushing's syndrome, where fasting plasma glucagon concentrations often are elevated but less than 500 pg/mL.

As with other islet cell neoplasms, glucagonomas may overproduce multiple hormones. Insulin is the most common second hormone secreted by these tumors. Others include ACTH, pancreatic polypeptide, parathyroid hormone or substances with parathyroid hormone-like activity, gastrin, serotonin, VIP, and MSH in that order of frequency.

TREATMENT

All reported glucagonomas with the cutaneous syndrome originated from single pancreatic tumors of considerable size (diameter, 1.5–35 cm) (303, 311). All tumors occurred in the tail or body of the pancreas, where A cells normally are abundant, deriving from the dorsal anlage of the pancreas. At the time of diagnosis, 62% of the tumors had metastases. Glucagonomas not associated with the syndrome but characterized by morphologic and/or chemical criteria are diagnosed in various ways. First, the tumor may appear as a malignant pancreatic tumor, discovered because of local growth, with or without metastases. Second, the tumor may be associated with an insulinoma, gastrinoma, or as part of the MEN-1 syndrome. Glucagonoma also may occur as a single microadenoma found incidentally at autopsy in elderly patients (302).

If the diagnosis is made while the tumor still is localized, surgical resection can be curative (305, 312, 313). As in other islet cell tumors, even when malignant these tumors tend to be extremely slow-growing. Like others, we have been impressed with the dramatic response in these patients to both curative and major palliative resections (307). Preoperative preparation may require a period of total parenteral nutrition because of the severe weight loss induced by the catabolic effects of glucagon. Antibiotics, steroids, and both amino acid and zinc supplementation may improve the skin rash when it is severe, but cure of the rash is achieved only with the return of glucagon levels to normal. Octreotide also is useful in helping to improve the perioperative condition of these patients. Prophylactic measures to prevent venous thrombosis, including low-dose subcutaneous heparin or intermittent pneumatic compression stockings, are mandatory for all patients during the perioperative period. In patients for whom surgery is not feasible, streptozotocin with or without 5-fluorouracil should be considered (as described later).

Somatostatinoma

Somatostatin (somatotropin-release inhibiting factor [SRIF]) is a tetradecapeptide that inhibits numerous endocrine and exocrine secretory functions. Almost all gut hormones that have been studied are inhibited by SRIF, including insulin, PP, glucagon, gastrin, secretin, GIP, and motilin (314). In addition to inhibition of the endocrine secretions, SRIF has direct effects on a number of target organs (315). For example, it is a potent inhibitor of basal and PG-stimulated gastric acid secretion. It also has marked effects on GI transit time, intestinal motility, and absorption of nutrients from the small intestine. The major effect in the small intestine appears to be a delay in the absorption of fat and reduced absorption of calcium.

The salient features of the somatostatinoma syndrome are diabetes, diarrhea/steatorrhea, gallbladder disease, hypochlorhydria, and weight loss (316–318). The first cases of the somatostatinoma syndrome were reported in 1977 by Ganda and colleagues (316). We have examined the cases reported since 1977 and describe here the features now recognized to be a part of the syndrome. For convenience, we have divided the cases into those arising from the pancreas, the intestine, and extrapancreatic tumors. It appears that the syndrome differs among tumors arising from the pancreas and the intestine or extrapancreatic sites. Therefore, these will be considered separately.

CLINICAL FEATURES

Most patients were between 40 and 60 years of age. There is a 2:1 ratio of female to male patients, which contrasts with the equal sex incidence for other islet cell tumors (319).

Plasma Somatostatin-Like Immunoreactivity (SLI)

The mean SLI concentration in patients with pancreatic somatostatinoma was 50 times higher than normal (range, 1–250 times). Intestinal somatostatinomas, however, had only slightly elevated or normal SLI concentrations.

Diabetes Mellitus and Hypoglycemia

Seventy-five percent of patients with pancreatic tumors had diabetes mellitus. In contrast, diabetes occurred only in 11% of patients with intestinal tumors. In all instances, the diabetes was relatively mild and could be controlled with diet and/or oral hypoglycemic agents or with small doses of insulin. It is not clear, however, whether the differential inhibition of insulin and diabetogenic hormones can explain the usually mild degree of diabetes and the rarity of ketoacidosis in patients with somatostatinoma. Replacement of functional islet cell tissue by pancreatic tumor may be another reason for the development of diabetes in most patients with pancreatic somatostatinoma, contrasting with the low incidence in patients with intestinal tumors. These tumors usually are large and therefore destroy substantial portions of the pancreas.

Gallbladder Disease

Fifty-nine percent of patients with pancreatic tumors and 27% of patients with intestinal tumors had gallbladder disease. The high incidence of gallbladder disease in patients with somatostatinoma and the absence of such an association in any other islet cell tumor suggest a causal relationship between gallbladder disease and somatostatinoma. Infusion of somatostatin into normal human subjects has been shown to inhibit gallbladder emptying (315, 320), suggesting that somatostatin-mediated inhibition of gallbladder emptying may cause the observed high rate of gallbladder disease in patients with somatostatinoma. This thesis is supported by the observation of massively dilated gallbladders without stones or other pathology (321, 322) in patients with somatostatin-secreting tumors.

Diarrhea and Steatorrhea

Diarrhea consisting of 3 to 10 frequently foul-smelling stools per day and/or steatorrhea from 20 to 76 g of fat per 24 hours is common in patients with pancreatic somatostatinoma. This could result from the effects of high levels of somatostatin within the pancreas, serving as a paracrine mediator to inhibit exocrine secretion, or alternatively, from the somatostatinoma's causing duct obstruction. In some cases, the severity of diarrhea and steatorrhea parallels the course of the disease, worsening as the tumor advances and metastatic disease spreads, and improving after tumor resection. Somatostatin has been shown to inhibit the pancreatic secretion of proteolytic enzymes, water, bicarbonate (323), and gallbladder motility (324). In addition, it inhibits the absorption of lipids (325). All but one patient with diarrhea and steatorrhea have had high plasma somatostatin concentrations. The rarity of diarrhea and/or steatorrhea in patients with intestinal somatostatinomas may result from the lower SLI levels.

Hypochlorhydria

Infusion of somatostatin has been shown to inhibit gastric acid secretion in human subjects (326). Thus, hypochlorhydria in patients with somatostatinoma in the absence of gastric mucosal abnormalities likely results from elevated somatostatin concentrations. Basal and stimulated acid secretion was inhibited in 87% of patients with pancreatic tumors tested but in only 12% of patients with intestinal tumors.

Weight Loss

Weight loss ranging from 9 to 21 kg over several months occurred in one third of patients with pancreatic tumors and one fifth of patients with intestinal tumors. The weight loss may relate to malabsorption and diarrhea, but in small intestinal tumors, anorexia, abdominal pain and yet unexplained reasons may be relevant.

Associated Endocrine Disorders

Of great interest is the presence of café-au-lait spots, neurofibromatosis, and paroxysmal hypertension in patients with intestinal tumors. Thus, approximately 50% of all patients have other endocrinopathies in addition to their somatostatinoma. Occurrence of multiple endocrine tumors (MEN-1) has been recognized in patients with islet cell tumors, and MEN-2 or -3 syndromes are present in association with pheochromocytomas and neurofibromatosis, respectively. It seems that an additional dimension of the duct associated tumors is MEN-2. Secretion of different hormones by the same islet cell tumor, sometimes resulting in two distinct clinical disorders, now is being recognized with increasing frequency (327). These possibilities should be considered during endocrine work-ups of patients with islet cell tumors and their relatives.

TUMOR LOCATION

Of the reported primary tumors, 60% were found in the pancreas and 40% in the duodenum or jejunum. Of the pancreatic tumors, 50% were located in the head, 25% in the tail, and the remaining tumors either infiltrated the whole pancreas or were found in the body. Regarding extrapancreatic locations, approximately 50% originate in the duodenum, approximately 50% originate in the ampulla, and rarely, one is found in the jejunum. Thus, approximately 60% of somatostatinomas originate in the upper intestinal tract, which probably is a consequence of the relatively large number of D cells in this region.

TUMOR SIZE

Somatostatinomas tend to be large, similar to glucagonomas (329), but unlike insulinomas and gastrinomas, which as a rule are small (330, 331). Within the intestine, tumors have tended to be smaller. Symptoms associated with somatostatinomas and glucagonomas are less pronounced and probably do not develop until very high blood levels of the respective hormones have been attained. As a result, somatostatinomas and glucagonomas are likely to be diagnosed later.

INCIDENCE OF MALIGNANCY

Eighty percent of patients with pancreatic somatostatinomas were metastatic at diagnosis, and 50% with intestinal tumors had evidence of metastatic disease. Metastasis to the liver is most frequent, and regional lymph node involvement and metastases to bone are less so. Thus, in approximately 70% of cases, metatastic disease is present at diagnosis. This is similar to the high incidence of malignancy in glucagonoma (329) and in gastrinoma (330), but it is distinctly different from the low incidence of malignant insulinoma (331). The high prevalence of metastatic disease in somatostatinoma also may be a consequence of late diagnosis but apparently is not dependent on the tissue of origin.

MICROSCOPIC APPEARANCE

On light microscopy, most tumors appear to be well-differentiated islet cell or carcinoid-type tumors. Some show a mixed picture, consisting of separate zones of differentiated and anaplastic cells. In the differentiated areas, cells are arranged in lobular or acinar patterns that are separated by fibrovascular stroma. Less well-differentiated areas consist of sheets of cells interrupted by fibrous septa.

Diffuse positive immunoreactivity for somatostatin usually is found, which contrasts with the rarity of somatostatin-positive cells in gastrinomas and other tumors. There is a unique occurrence of psammoma bodies in somatostatinomas localized within the duodenum. In addition, there is abundant immunologic evidence for the presence of cells containing insulin, calcitonin, gastrin and VIP, ACTH, prostaglandin E_2, and SP. In tumors with multiple hormones, however, SLI-containing cells represent the large majority of all cells containing hormones detected by immunopathology.

SOMATOSTATIN-CONTAINING TUMORS OUTSIDE THE GI TRACT

Somatostatin has been found in many tissues outside the GI tract. Prominent among those are the hypothalamic and extrahypothalamic regions of the brain, the peripheral nervous system (including the sympathetic adrenergic ganglia), and the C cells of the thyroid gland. Not surprisingly, therefore, high concentrations of somatostatin have been found in tumors originating from these tissues. Sano and colleagues (333) as well as Saito and colleagues (332) reported seven patients with medullary carcinoma of the thyroid (MTC) who had high basal plasma SLI concentrations and high tumor SLI concentrations (332, 333). Roos and colleagues (334) reported elevated plasma SLI concentrations in three of seven patients with MTC and high tissue SLI concentrations in three of five MTC tumors. Some, but not all, of these patients exhibited the clinical somatostatinoma syndrome.

Elevated plasma SLI concentrations also have been reported in patients with small cell lung cancer (334). One case of metastatic bronchial oat cell carcinoma caused Cushing's syndrome, diabetes, diarrhea, steatorrhea, anemia and weight loss, and had a plasma SLI concentration 20 times greater than normal (335). We reported a patient with a bronchogenic carcinoma presenting with diabetic ketoacidosis and high levels of SLI (>5,000 pg/mL) (336). Pheochromocytomas (327, 337) and catecholamine-producing extra-adrenal paragangliomas (334) are other examples of endocrine tumors producing and secreting somatostatin in addition to other hormonally active substances. One-fourth of 37 patients with pheochromocytomas had elevated SLI levels (327).

DIAGNOSIS

In the reported series cited, somatostatinomas often were found more or less accidentally. In most cases, the tumors were found either during exploratory laparotomy or upper GI radiographic studies, CT, or ultrasound, or endoscopy performed because of various symptoms, including unexplained abdominal pain, melena, hematemesis, persistent diarrhea, or in search of insulinomas or ACTH-secreting tumors. Once found, the tumors were identified as somatostatinoma by the demonstration of elevated tissue concentrations of SLI and/or prevalence of D cells by immunocytochemistry or demonstration of elevated plasma SLI concentrations. Thus, events leading to the diagnosis of somatostatinoma usually occur in reverse order. In other islet cell tumors, the clinical symptoms and signs usually suggest the diagnosis, which then is established by demonstration of diagnostically elevated blood hormone levels, following which efforts are undertaken to localize the tumors. It can be expected that the same sequence of diagnostic procedures will be followed in the future for the diagnosis of somatostatinoma, mainly for two reasons: (*a*) the increasing familiarity of physicians with the clinical somatostatinoma syndrome (this symptom complex, while not pathognomonic, is nevertheless sufficiently characteristic of somatostatinoma to suggest the correct diagnosis), and (*b*) the greater availability of reliable radioimmunoassays for the determination of SLI in blood has increased the yield. Presently, these assays are complicated by the need for cumbersome extraction procedures and are not readily available. It should be recognized, however, that the syndrome is rare. Of 1,199 cases screened for somatostatinoma at the University of Michigan between 1982 and 1986, only 8 cases had diagnostic serum levels.

The diagnosis of somatostatinoma at a time when blood SLI concentrations are normal or only marginally elevated, however, requires reliable provocative tests. Increased plasma SLI concentrations have been reported after intravenous infusion of tolbutamide and arginine, and decreased SLI concentrations have been observed after intravenous infusion of diazoxide. Arginine is a well-established stimulant for normal D cells and thus is unlikely to differentiate between normal and supranormal somatostatin secretion. The same may be true for diazoxide, which has been shown to decrease SLI secretion from normal dog pancreas as well as in patients with somatostatinoma (338). Tolbutamide stimulates SLI release from normal dog and rat pancreas (323, 324, 338), but no change was found in the circulating SLI concentrations of three normal human subjects after intravenous injection of 1 g of tolbutamide (339). Therefore, at present, tolbutamide appears to be a candidate for a provocative agent in the diagnosis of somatostatinoma, but its reliability must be established in a greater number of patients and controls. Until then, it may be necessary to measure plasma SLI concentrations during routine work-ups for postprandial dyspepsia and gallbladder disorders (317), for diabetes in patients without a family history, and for unexplained steatorrhea as these findings can be early signs of somatostatinomas.

TREATMENT OF SOMATOSTATINOMAS

Forty percent of patients with somatostatinomas died at intervals ranging from 1 week to 14 months after diagnosis, while 60% of patients were alive from 6 months to 5 years after diagnosis. Thus, the syndrome is associated with a high malignant potential, and it is important to be aggressive in management and to attempt to remove all tumor tissue in benign cases. For patients in whom metastases already have occurred at diagnosis, bulk reduction may be justified, if feasible. The optimal form of chemotherapy remains to be determined.

Pancreatic Polypeptide (PP) PPoma

Pancreatic polypeptide was discovered by serendipity. In 1972, working in separate laboratories, Chance and Jones (340), as well as Kimmel and colleagues (341) independently purified a single major protein from a crude insulin preparation. The protein was named *pancreatic polypeptide* (PP) (340). In mammals, 93% of the cells producing PP are located in the pancreas.

There are very dramatic effects from meal ingestion, cerebral stimulation, and hormone administration on circulating levels of PP. A biologic role for PP has not been established, however (208, 342–344). The only physiologic effects that are recognized in humans are the inhibition of gallbladder contraction and pancreatic enzyme secretion (344). Thus, a tumor deriving from PP cells is predicted to be clinically silent, although this is not always the case.

Tomita and colleagues (345) reported two patients, one of whom had persistent watery diarrhea and the other high levels of circulating PP and PP-cell hyperplasia. A patient with chronic duodenal ulcer and a PP tumor also has been reported (346). A tumor that invaded the bile ducts, producing biliary obstruction was a PPoma (347). It has been suggested that the watery diarrhea syndrome, which is seen in GEP endocrine tumors, may have its origin in PP overproduction (348). The picture is complicated by the fact that mixed tumors, PP-cell hyperplasia in association with other functioning islet cell tumors, ductal hyperplasia of PP cells, nesidioblastosis, and multiple islet tumors producing PP also have been described, either alone or as part of the MEN-1 syndrome (349, 350). Basal concentrations of PP in plasma may be raised above 1,000 pg/mL in 22 to 77% of all endocrine secreting tumors and in 29 to 50% of patients with carcinoid syndrome, even if the carcinoid is located outside the pancreas. Among 53 patients with adenocarcinomas of the pancreas, however, no instance of an elevated basal concentration of PP was found (129, 178). The diagnostic accuracy of elevated basal PP concentrations as a marker for endocrine-secreting tumors can be marginally increased to around 50 to 60% by determining the response of PP to secretin administration (90, 351). A response of greater than 5,000 pg/min/mL (i.e., integrated response) is more than two standard deviations above that observed in healthy subjects. It appears, however, that many cases of so-called nonfunctional GEP endocrine tumors are indeed PPomas, because it is our experience that 50 to 75% of these have raised basal PP levels and in 67% the response to secretin is exaggerated. Thus, in the absence of factors, such as chronic renal failure, that are known to cause marked elevation of PP levels, a markedly elevated PP level in an older, healthy patient occasionally may indicate a nonfunctioning pancreatic endocrine tumor. Differentiation of a high basal concentration in a healthy subject from that appearing in patients with tumor has been difficult. Schwartz (325) suggested that administration of atropine would suppress concentrations in healthy subjects and would fail to do so in patients with tumors, but this has not been subjected to extensive examination.

Increased PP cells are found in 20 to 67% of functioning and nonfunctioning tumors of the pancreas (352). There does not appear to be a relationship between the number of cells and their function, because islet tumors containing subnormal, normal, or supernormal concentrations of PP compared with that in the normal pancreas may be associated with normal or high levels of circulating PP. There now are at least 21 patients in the literature with PPomas. Their age ranges from 20 to 74 years, with a mean of 51 years and an equal sex incidence.

Diabetes was found in only two cases. Diarrhea, which formerly was thought to be a part of the syndrome (348), occurred in only one third of cases. Steatorrhea was found in 100% of patients in whom it was sought. Decreased acid secretion was documented only in two of six people studied. Fifty-seven percent presented with weight loss. The PPoma syndrome is silent, and these tumors often are found unsuspectedly in the course of working up patients with hepatomegaly, abdominal pain, metastases to the liver, jaundice from obstruction of the common bile duct, or hematochezia. Upper GI bleeding may occur because of invasion of the wall of the duodenum or thrombosis of the splenic or portal vein, with consequent development of varices. Not infrequently, PPomas are recognized by the radiologist as highly vascular tumors with metastases to the liver. Six of the reported cases had PPomas as part of the MEN-1 syndrome.

It is our contention (88, 90, 184, 351, 352) that not every patient with raised PP levels has a tumor. If a tumor can be identified and localized, it should be removed. Raised PP levels occur as part of the MEN-1 syndrome and may reflect nesidioblastosis of PP cells or multiple adenomata not amenable to resection. The frequency of malignancy of these tumors is not established, and resection should be reserved for those patients with clearly identified solitary lesions.

It has been suggested that every patient with a markedly elevated level of PP should undergo exploratory laparotomy and careful inspection of the pancreas, even if the tumor cannot be diagnosed (353). This has not been our experience. Malignant PPomas are best treated with streptozotocin. PPomas rarely may occur outside the pancreas and can present a real dilemma, because these may occur in the chest and elsewhere. Laparotomy is not advised. We contend that percutaneous transhepatic portal venous sampling, and if necessary, total-body venous sampling, should be performed to localize the source of PP overproduction. If such a locus is found, the abdominal or other exploration should be performed. In patients who have metastatic tumors and those refractory to other forms of treatment, use of the somatostatin analogue octreotide (Sandoz) has proved to be useful and worthy of trial.

Neurotensinomas

Neurotensin (NT) is a 13 amino acid polypeptide first extracted from bovine brain by Carraway and Leeman (354). It subsequently was isolated from the human GI tract and found to have the same amino acid sequence (355). Neurotensin has a number of interesting pharmacologic effects that include hypotension, tachycardia and cyanosis (58, 356), and stimulation of secretion from the small intestine (357). It also has been reported to inhibit the interdigestive myoelectric complex and stimulate insulin release (358). Neurotensin also increases venous vascular permeability, raises blood glucose (152, 359, 360) and lowers blood pressure (354, 356).

High concentrations of neurotensin-like immunoreactivity (NTLI) are present in the ileal mucosa, where it is localized to a specific "N" cell (361). Plasma concentrations rise after food ingestion (191), and high circulating levels (362) have been found after surgery for duodenal ulcer and jejunoileal bypass for obesity (363). No clear physiologic role has been established for the peptide. High circulating levels also have been found in patients with VIPomas (39, 364–369).

In 1981, based on the pharmacologic actions of neurotensin, it was predicted (351) that a syndrome of excess would emerge, presenting with features that are consonant with the pharmacologic actions of the peptide: diabetes, hypotension, vasodilatation, cyanosis, and edema. In addition to these features, investigation would reveal net secretion of fluid and electrolytes, inhibition of gastric acid secretion, infrequent interdigestive myoelectric complexes, and prolonged biologic reaction of gastric emptying. The prediction that diabetes would occur was based on the predominant stimulation of adrenomedullary secretions despite stimulation of insulin secretion (370). The clinical features of reported cases include diarrhea, hypotension, hypokalemia, edema, weight loss, and occasionally, diabetes (90, 351).

Apart from these reported cases, Blackburn and colleagues (39) examined plasma neurotensin levels in 326 fasting patients with tumors in a variety of sites. Of these patients, 180 had tumors of the pancreas, including glucagonomas (339), gastrinomas (334), insulinomas (317), nonsecretory tumors (319), and VIPomas (326). Plasma NTLI levels were raised in only six patients with VIPomas and none with the other tumors. Twenty-one of the tumors containing VIP were removed surgically, and six were found to contain NTLI. The clinical features of these six patients did not appear to differ from those of the remaining 15 patients.

With so few cases, it is difficult to generalize on the clinical picture. Fifty percent of the cases were cured by resection of tumors in the pancreas (311) or lung (371), and the remainder have responded well to streptozotocin. The syndrome appears to comprise diarrhea, diabetes, and weight loss; as such, it may not be readily distinguishable from the VIPoma syndrome. Neurotensinomas probably are best characterized as yet another tumor that is capable of causing the WDHHA (watery diarrhea, hypokalemia, hypochlorhydria, and acidosis) syndrome. Edema, hypotension, and flushing should increase the suspicion of a neurotensinoma.

Octreotide in Treatment of Malignant Neuroendocrine Tumors

Somatostatin, a tetradecapeptide, inhibits the secretion and action of a number of peptide hormones, neurotransmitters, and exocrine secretions of the GEP axis. Its clinical use is limited because of its short half-life of 1 to 2 minutes. Development of its potent, long-acting octapeptide analogue (Sandostatin, octreotide acetate) with a half-life of over 100 minutes was a breakthrough for clinical application. Other analogues such as somatuline (BIM 23014 C) are being investigated (126). Thus far, their effectiveness and toxicity rates appear to be similar to those of octreotide. Several aspects of treatment of GEP neoplasms, including symptom reduction, hormone suppression, tumor growth, and survival, are discussed here.

SYMPTOM CONTROL

Octreotide has a potent action in reducing symptoms in certain neuroendocrine tumors. Detection of somatostatin receptors by octreotide scintigraphy correlates well with the predicted response to treatment with octreotide (74). In carcinoid tumor, flushing is reduced in all (118) or most patients (112, 113, 372). The acute effects on water and electrolyte transport is a reversal from a secretory to an absorptive state, thus normalizing transport across the proximal intestine (110). Long-term responses of diarrhea, however, differ in different reports: 9 of 14 of our patients with endocrine diarrhea responded to treatment (118), in contrast to 19 of 25 reported by Kvols and colleagues (112). Diarrhea in VIPoma improves 95% of the time (372). This difference might result from the involvement of different peptides causing diarrhea and different mechanisms. In five of our patients with gastrinoma, the presenting symptom was diarrhea, which improved, as did 65% of 26 reported cases (372). Diarrhea in 16 patients with glucagonomas also improved uniformly (372, 373). Diarrhea also improves in all patients with gastrinoma syndrome, and abdominal pain can be relieved in most patients (34). There is, however, the possibility of a rebound in symptoms and/or hormonal values during therapy. The mechanism of this is not clear, but it might involve accelerated enzymatic breakdown of octreotide and/or ligand-induced changes of somatostatin receptors on the target cell, preventing internalization of the hormone receptor complexes or a gradual adaptation of the target cell to the octreotide effect, as proposed by Koelz and colleagues (374).

Wheezing, as one of the symptoms in carcinoid syndrome, can be reversed by octroetide, and we have documented spirometric improvement in lung function (118). In one patient who had severe proximal myopathic muscle weakness, clinical and electromyographic improvement occurred with octreotide treatment (118). The arthropathy of carcinoid, which may be SP mediated, also improves (370). Hypoglycemia with insulinoma responds erratically because of unpredictable effects on food absorption, suppression of glucagon, and insulin (110). Of 15 patients, 50% improved, and 30% got worse (372). The necrolytic migratory erythema of glucagonoma clears in only 50% of the cases (198).

HORMONE SUPPRESSION AND BIOCHEMICAL FEATURES

Octreotide inhibits hormone secretion in some malignant GEP tumors. The most sensitive of these seems to be VIPoma, where lowering of VIP circulating levels parallels relief of symptoms (110, 114). Gastrin levels, however, are not equivalently lowered with octreotide. One recent study of eight patients with gastrinoma showed that octreotide decreased gastrin levels in five patients by a mean of 76% of baseline (34). We showed that in patients with metastatic disease whose basal gastrin levels were extremely high, there was no effect of lowering plasma gastrin levels. In worldwide pooled data (n = 26), 70% of patients are reported to respond. Furthermore, ACTH overproduction heralds unresponsiveness to the drug. Glucagon levels seldom decrease (372). The overall 5-HIAA level is significantly lower after octreotide treatment, whereas blood serotonin level does not differ significantly (113, 375). There is an overall reduction of 5-HIAA in 58% of patients (372).

PERIOPERATIVE MANAGEMENT

Carcinoid and other GEP tumors can be a major therapeutic problem perioperatively, when vast quantities of active peptides are released into the circulation from manipulation of the tumors. Octreotide is an effective suppressor of release and action of peptide hormones during surgery (262). Profound refractory hypotension in carcinoid syndrome can be rapidly reversed by octreotide (109), as can gastric acid secretion and fistula drainage (262).

TUMOR GROWTH

Because GEP tumors grow slowly, it is hard to assess the effect of treatment on tumor growth. Long-term CT monitoring, however, has shown shrinkage of liver metastasis in certain patients with carcinoid and other GEP tumors (112, 124). In 85 carcinoid tumors, no change was found with doses under 50 mg/d, but Kvols and colleagues (112) reported a 17% decrease in size using higher doses (1,500 mg/d). VIPoma,

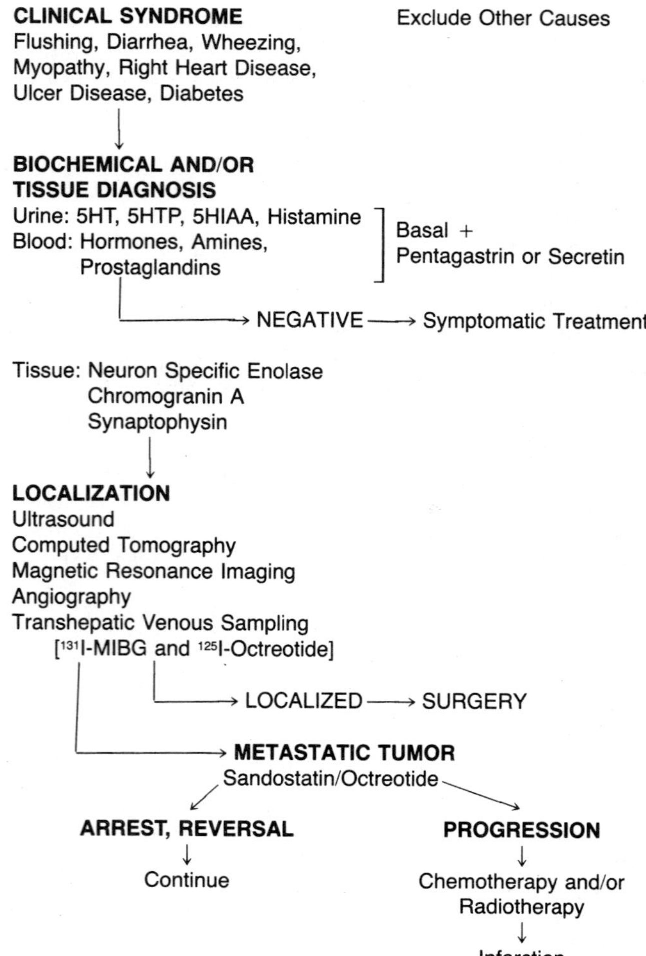

Figure 103.7. Suggested management of suspect neuroendocrine tumors.

glucagonoma, and gastrinoma generally do not change in size (372), although a tumor infarction has occurred in VIPoma (262). Tumor metastases to bone may occur despite apparent control of the primary tumor or liver metastases (110, 376).

CONCLUSION

The role of octreotide in the treatment of GEP tumors still is not well established. Because of the clear evidence of symptomatic relief (e.g., flushing, wheezing, diarrhea), it has established a place in treatment of such tumors both pre- and postoperatively. Perioperative use can prevent fatal episodes of rapid, extreme increases of hormones in the circulation. There is enough evidence for the control of tumor growth that primary treatment of select metastatic tumors, with proper monitoring of tumor growth, is recommended (Fig. 103.7).

Chemotherapy for Metastatic Islet Cell Carcinomas

Ajani and colleagues (377) performed repetitive hepatic artery embolization with polyvinyl alcohol particles in 22 patients with metastatic pancreatic endocrine tumors, and they achieved partial remission of measurable hepatic tumor in 12 of 20 evaluable patients. From this experience, the authors suggested this modality for prolonged palliation in selected patients. Recently, Marlink and colleagues (378) reported partial responses in all six patients with metastatic islet cell tumors following selective hepatic artery embolization; however, the duration of responses was not reported.

Because of the relative rarity of GEP neoplasms, chemotherapy trials frequently have combined several islet cell tumor subtypes within the same study. The experience from these studies suggests that while similar responses may be expected from chemotherapy for several tumor subtypes, there may be differences in the response of others. For example, streptozotocin alone or in combination with 5-fluorouracil is extremely effective against most VIPomas (136) and is moderately effective against gastrinomas and most other islet cell tumors. In contrast, streptozotocin has little activity against glucagonomas, whereas dacarbazine appears to have significant activity (144).

Streptozotocin is a drug that is selectively cytotoxic for pancreatic islet cells. Because of this property, the drug has been used to establish animal models for diabetes and islet cell hypofunction (379). This selective cytotoxicity also provided a rationale for using streptozotocin in neoplastic disorders of pancreatic endocrine cells. In several studies using intravenous and, less commonly, intra-arterial administration, streptozotocin was shown to be active against several pancreatic endocrine cancers, with nearly 40% tumor responses and over 50% hormonal responses reported (181, 230, 232, 380, 381). More frequent use of this agent is limited by its significant emetogenic and renal toxicities. In the case of symptomatic hepatic metastases from glucagonoma and somatostatinoma, Friesen (183) claims that use of intra-arterial administration of streptozotocin is effective, with reduced incidence of nephrotoxicity, but this has not been confirmed.

Other drugs that have single-agent activity in islet cell carcinoma are chlorozotocin and doxorubicin. At a dose of 100 to 200 mg/m^2, chlorozotocin resulted in a 53% objective response rate in 13 previously untreated patients (382). In 20 previously treated patients, doxorubicin, 60 mg/m^2 every 3 to 4 weeks, resulted in four (20%) objective responses (233).

Several authors have reported that dacarbazine is a highly effective agent for the treatment of pancreatic islet cell tumors, especially glucagon-secreting tumors (144). Using either 1,250 mg/m^2 in divided doses over 5 days or a single dose of 650 mg/m^2, Kessinger and colleagues (144) reported two complete responses and two partial responses of elevated serum glucagon in four patients with glucagonomas. Three of four additional patients with malignant islet cell carcinoma associated with glucagonoma syndrome were cited in this report as having responded to dacarbazine alone. In a recently reported prospective study of 48 evaluable patients with advanced islet cell carcinoma, Hahn and colleagues (383) reported 13 patients (27%) with objective responses (including three complete responses) following dacarbazine, 850 mg/m^2 given every 4 weeks. Severe or lethal toxicity was experienced by 15 patients. The median survival in all patients was 19 months, and the authors concluded that dacarbazine clearly had beneficial activity in patients with advanced islet cell carcinoma.

None of six evaluable patients with islet cell carcinoma responded to etoposide in a phase II study (146). Only 2 of 41 patients with a variety of advanced apudomas responded to carboplatinum (384). No other conventional chemotherapy agents are reported to have activity in this disease.

In a multi-institutional study, streptozotocin combined with 5-fluorouracil was shown to be effective against malignant pancreatic endocrine tumors, with an objective response rate of 63% for a duration of 17.4 months (143, 151, 232). Furthermore, this combination produced a 37% complete response rate and a more prolonged median survival than streptozotocin alone; however, the combination also was associated with a high prevalence of moderately severe GI, hematopoietic, and renal toxicity (232). A smaller, nonrandomized series of patients receiving the same combination chemotherapy regimen produced similar results, and this study also suggested that the response rate in patients with nonfunctional tumors (50%) may be less than that in those with functional tumors (68%) (151). Although the regimen of streptozotocin and fluorouracil is not considered to be the most active for malignant glucagonoma, responses to the combination have been reported (302).

In a randomized trial by the Eastern Cooperative Oncology Group, streptozotocin plus 5-fluorouracil was compared to a combination of streptozotocin plus doxorubicin or to chlorozotocin (143). Although the results have not been published, it is expected that this study will provide an important contribution toward further defining the optimal chemotherapeutic approach for malignant pancreatic endocrine tumors. A phase II study of the combination of streptozotocin and doxorubicin in patients with advanced miscellaneous neuroendocrine tumors (apudomas) was conducted by Frame and colleagues (385), who reported 6 of 31 (19%) objective tumor responses for a median duration of 7 months. This relatively low response rate might be improved by a higher dose intensity, but this approach is untested to date. Several other multicenter chemotherapeutic regimens have now been tried (Table 103.9) but in general, their activity is no better than that with single-agent therapy. There has been no prospective investigation of adjuvant chemotherapy in patients with islet cell carcinoma.

Finally, the interferons have been reported to be active in GEP endocrine neoplasms as well. As reviewed by Oberg and colleagues (151), an objective hormonal response of 73% was observed in patients with malignant pancreatic endocrine tumors treated with human leukocyte interferon, 3 to 6 million units per day subcutaneously. Among their first 22

Table 103.9. Systemic Anticancer Therapy for Neoplasms of the Gastroenteropancreatic System

Drug	Islet cell neoplasm(s)	Patients (n)	Objective biochemical or tumor response (%)	Reference
Single agents				
Streptozotocin	Gastrinomas	24	50	230, 232, 233, 235
	Unspecified	125	50	230, 320, 349, 380, 91
Dacarbazine	Gastrinoma	6	0	367, 17
	Glucagonoma	10	90	318, 345
	Unspecified	48	27	284
Carboplatin	Unspecified	12	50	6
	Unspecified	41	5	384
Chlorozotocin	Unspecified	13	53	186
		33	30	389
Doxorubicin	Unspecified	20	20	370
Etoposide	Unspecified	6	0	307
Interferon	Unspecified	32	73	219, 154
	Unspecified	67	51	387
	Gastrinoma	13	8	390
	Unspecified	372	44	388
Octreotide acetate	VIPoma	25	75	372, 128, 151, 88
	Glucagonoma	16	55	
	Gastrinoma	36	65	
	Insulinoma	15	50	
	GRFoma	4	75	
	Unspecified	19	31	287
	Insulinoma	7	71	391
	Unspecified	34	50	125
	Gastrinoma	9	62	34
	Unspecified	68	54	392
Somatuline	Unspecified	13	31	126
Combination agents				
Streptozotocin + 5-fluorouracil	Unspecified	40	63	367
		19	58	154
	Unspecified	31	54	287
		33	42	389
Streptozotocin + doxorubicin	Unspecified	31	19	380
		25	36	154
Streptozotocin + 5-fluorouracil + doxorubicin	Gastrinoma	10	40	235
5-flurouracil + leucovorin + interferon	Unspecified	3	33	393
Etoposide + cisplatinum	Unspecified	14	14	394

Table 103.10. Systemic Anticancer Therapy for Malignant Carcinoid

Drug	Patients (n)	Objective biochemical or tumor response (%)	Reference
Single agents			
5-Fluorouracil	19	26	102, 142
Doxorubicin	33	21	144, 143, 102
Streptozotocin	23	30	43, 102
Dacarbazine	15	13	141
	56	16	145
Dactinomycin	17	6	141
Etoposide	17	0	146
Cisplatin	15	6	147
Carboplatin	20	0	384
Interferon	99	≤50	155, 154, 151, 13
	27	39	158
	22	58	395
Octreotide acetate	85	71	372, 128, 151, 88
	14	31	126
	55	37	127
Combination agents			
Streptozotocin + 5-fluorouracil	154	≤33	45, 102, 142, 151
Streptozotocin + doxorubicin	47	26	102, 142
Streptozotocin + 5-fluorouracil + doxorubicin	20	35	150
Etoposide + cisplatin	13	0	394
Streptozotocin + doxorubicin + interferon	11	0	396
Octreotide + interferon	19	72	127

responders, six patients (27%) had a 50% reduction in tumor mass, and two patients (9%) had a complete response (386). The median duration of response was 9.5 months. Since 1986, this group has been using recombinant interferon-α_{2b}, 5 million units three times per week subcutaneously or intravenously. An update of their results in 57 patients showed objective responses in 29 patients (51%), with biochemical responses in 27 (47%) and radiologic responses in 7 (12%) (387). The median duration of response was 20 months (range, 2–96 months), and response rates were higher in patients with VIPomas (10 of 12 patients) than in those with other tumors. A review of 372 patients treated with interferon from various institutions showed an overall objective response rate of 44% (388). Interferon was well tolerated despite frequent occurrence of a flu-like syndrome, weight loss, and mild myelosuppression. A summary of these studies appears in Tables 103.9 and 103.10.

Conclusions

New approaches to the diagnosis and localization of GEP tumors have been stressed, including the importance of circulating hormone levels and sophisticated immunohistochemistry, tracer scanning, and the role of peptide therapy in the management of the symptom complex as well as the tumor. There is, however, much that remains unsolved, requiring diligent research and evaluation if we are ultimately to include neuroendocrine tumors among the curable cancers. An outline of the current approach to management of the patient suspected of harboring a GEP tumor is given in Figure 103.7.

Acknowledgments

The authors thank Lu-Ann Caron-Leslie, Deborah Bellingham, and Dr. Kerry Burnstein for editorial assistance and Tobi Schwartzman for manuscript preparation. The studies by A. I. Vinik reported here were supported by National Institutes of Health Grant 1-ROC1CA54641-01.

References

1. Pearse AGE. Common cytochemical and ultrastructural characteristics of cells producing polypeptide hormones (the APUD series) and their relevance to thyroid and ultimobronchial C cells and calcitonin. Proc R Soc Lond (Biol) 1968;170:71.
2. Andrew A. An experimental investigation into the possible neural crest origin of pancreatic APUD (islet) cells. J Embryol Exp Morphol 1976;35:577.
3. Le Douarin NM, Teillet MA. The migration of neural crest cells to the wall of the digestive tract in avian embryo. J Embryol Exp Morphol 1973;30:31.
4. Pictet RL, Rall LB, Phelps P, Rutter WJ. The neural crest and the origin of the insulin-producing and other gastrointestinal hormone-producing cells. Science 1967;191:191.
5. Pictet R, Rutter WJ. Development of the embryonic endocrine pancreas. In Handbook of Physiology. Session 7. Edited by J Field. Bethesda: American Physiological Society, 1972, p 25.
6. Rosenberg L, Vinik AI. Regulation of pancreatic islet growth and differentiation: evidence for paracrine and/or autocrine growth factor(s). Clin Res 1990;38:271A.
7. Brockenbrough JS, Weir GC, Bonner-Weir S. Discordance of exocrine and endocrine growth after 90% pancreatectomy in rats. Diabetes 1988;37:232–236.
8. Miyaura C, Chen L, Appel M, et al. Expression of *reg*/PSP, a pancreatic exocrine gene: relationship to changes in islet B-cell mass. Mol Endocrinol 1991;5:226–234.
9. Pour P, Mohr U, Cardesa A, Althoff J, Kruger FW. Pancreatic neoplasms in an animal model: morphological, biological and comparative studies. Cancer 1975;36:379.
10. Rosenberg L, Duguid WP, Brown RA, Vinik AI. Induction of neuroblastosis will reverse diabetes in the Syrian golden hamster. Diabetes 1988;37:334.
11. Rosenberg L, Duguid WP, Vinik AI. Cell proliferation in the pancreas of the Syrian golden hamster. Dig Dis Sci 1987;32:1185.
12. Sarvetnick N. Islet cell destruction and regeneration in IFN-g transgenic mice (abstract). J Cell Biochem 1991;CBO19:49.
13. Smith DB, Scarffe JH, Wagstaff J, Johnston RJ. Phase II trial of rDNA alfa 2b interferon in patients with malignant carcinoid tumor. Cancer Treat Rep 1987;71:1265.
14. Takasawa S, Yamamoto K, Terazono K, Okamoto H. Novel gene activated in rat insulinoma. Diabetes 1986;35:1178.
15. Terazono I, Uchiyama I, Ide M, Watanabe T, Yonekura H, Yamamoto H, Okamoto H. Expression of reg protein in rat regenerating islets and its co-localization with insulin in beta cell secretory granules. Diabetologia 1990;33:1.
16. Terazono K, Yamamoto H, Takasawa S, Shiga K, Yonemura Y, Tochino Y, Okamoto H. A novel gene activated in regenerating islets. J Biol Chem 1988;262:2111.
17. Watanabe T, Yonekura H, Terazono K, Yamamoto H, Okamoto H. Complete nucleotide sequence of human reg gene and its expression in normal and tumoral tissues. J Biol Chem 1990;265:7432.

18. Vinik AI, Pittenger GL, Pavlic-Renar I. Role of growth factors in pancreatic endocrine cells. Endocrinol Metab Clin North Am 1993;22:875.
19. Ahlman H, Wangberg B, Nilsson O. Growth regulation in carcinoid tumors. Endocrinol Metab Clin North Am 1993;22:889.
20. Chaudhry A, Funa K, Oberg K. Expression of growth peptides and their receptors in neuroendocrince tumors of the digestive system. Acta Oncol 1993;32:107.
21. Kerr JFR, Wyllie AH, Currie AR. Apoptosis: a basic biological phenomenon with wide ranging implications in tissue kinetics. Br J Cancer 1972;26:239.
22. Perry RR, Kang Y, Greaves B. Effects of tamoxifen on growth and apoptosis of estrogen-dependent and -independent human breast cancer cells. Ann Surg Oncol 1995.
23. Rotello RJ, Lieberman RC, Purchio AF, Gerscgebson LE. Coordinated regulation of apoptosis and cell proliferation by transforming growth factor β_1 in cultured uterine epithelial cells. Proc Natl Acad Sci USA 1991;88:3412.
24. Schwartzman RA, Cidlowski JA. Mechanism of tissue-specific induction of internucleosomal deoxyribonucleic acid cleavage activity and apoptosis by glucocorticoids. Endocrinology 1993;133:591.
25. Szende B, Zalatnai A, Schally AV. Programmed cell death (apoptosis) in pancreatic cancers of hamsters after treatment with analogs of both luteinizing hormone-releasing hormone and somatostatin. Proc Natl Acad Sci USA 1989;86:1643.
26. Larsson C, Skogseid B, Oberg K, Nakamura Y, Nordenskjold M. Multiple endocrine neoplasia type 1 gene maps to chromosome 11 and is lost in insulinoma. Nature 1988;332:85.
27. Thakker RV, Bouloux P, Wooding C, Chotai K, Broad PM, Spurr NK, Besser GM, O'Riordan JL. Association of parathyroid tumors in multiple endocrine neoplasia type 1 with loss of alleles on chromosome 11. N Engl J Med 1989;321:218.
28. Brandi ML, Aurbach GD, Fitzpatrick LA, Quarto R, Spiegel AM, Bliziotes MM, Norton JA, Doppman JL, Marx SJ. Parathyroid mitogenic activity in plasma from patients with familial multiple endocrine neoplasia type 1. N Engl J Med 1986;314:1287–1293.
29. Marx SJ, Vinik AI, Santen RJ, Floyd JC Jr, Mills J, Green J III. Multiple endocrine neoplasia type 1: assessment of laboratory tests to screen for the gene in a large kindred. Medicine 1986 65:226.
30. Owerbach D, Bell GI, Rutter WJ, Brown JA, Shows TB. The insulin gene is activated on the short arm of chromosome 11 in humans. Diabetes 1981;30:267.
31. Eisenbarth GS. Expression of receptors for tetanus toxin and monoclonal antibody A^2B_2 by pancreatic islet cells. Proc Natl Acad Sci USA 1982;77:5066.
32. McLeod MK, Fukuuchi A, Warnock M, Tutera A, Vinik AI. Mechanisms of stimulatory and inhibitory effects of somatostatin on cell proliferation in rat insulinoma (RIN m5F) cell line (abstract). 1991.
33. Larsson C, Weber G, Teh BT, Lagercrantz J. Genetics of multiple endocrine neoplasia type 1a. Ann N Y Acad Sci 1994;733:453.
34. Mozell EJ, Cramer AJ, O'Dorisio TM , Woltering EA. Long-term efficacy of octreotide in the treatment of Zollinger-Ellison syndrome. Arch Surg 1992;127:1019.
35. Donis-Keller H, Dou S, Chi D, et al. Mutations in the RET protooncogene are associated with MEN 2A and FMTC. Hum Mol Genet 1993;2:851.
36. Carlson KM, Dou S, Chi D, et al. A single missense mutation in the tyrosine kinase catalytic domain of the RET proto-oncogene is associated with multiple endocrine neoplasia type 2B. Proc Natl Acad Sci USA 1994;91:1579.
37. Hofstra RMW, Landsvater RM, Ceccherini I, et al. A mutation in RET proto-oncogene associated with multiple endocrine neoplasia type 2B and sporadic medullary thyroid carcinoma. Nature 1994;367:375.
38. Bissette G, Manberg P, Nemeroff CB, Jr Prange AJ. Neurotensin; a biologically active peptide. Life Sci 1978;23:2173.
39. Blackburn AM, Bryant MG, Adrian TE, Bloom SR, Christofides ND, Long RG, Fitzpatrick NR, Baron JH. Pancreatic tumours produce neurotensin. J Clin Endocrinol Metab 1981;52:820.
40. Sundler F, Alumets J, Hakanson R. Peptides in the gut with dual distribution in nerves and endocrine cells. In Gut Hormones. Edited by SR Bloom. Edinburgh: Churchill Livingstone, 1978, p 406.
41. Wynick D, Williams SJ, Bloom RS. Symptomatic secondary hormone syndromes in patients with established malignant pancreatic endocrine tumors. N Engl J Med 1988;319:605–605.
42. Reubi JC. Use of receptor autoradiography for the visualization of somatostatin receptors in human pituitary adenomas and other neuroendocrine tumors (abstract). J Endocrinol Invest 1989;12:18.
43. Buchanan KD, Johnston CF, O'Hare MMT, et al. Neuroendocrine tumors. A European view. Am J Med 1986;81(Suppl 6b):14.
44. Biorck G, Axen O, Throsen A. Unusual cyanosis in a boy with congenital pulmonary stenosis and tricuspid insufficiency. Am Heart J 1952;44:143.
45. Davis Z, Moertel CG, McLirath DC. The malignant carcinoid syndrome. Surg Gynecol Obstet 1973;137:637.
46. Solcia E, Capella C, Buffa R, Frigerio B, Usellini L, Fiocca R. Morphological and functional classification of endocrine cells and related growths in the gastrointestinal tract. In Gastrointestinal Hormones. Edited by GBJ Glass. New York: Raven, 1980, p 1.
47. Weil C. Gastroenteropancreatic endocrine tumors. Klin Wochenschr 1985;63:433.
48. Carney JA, Go VLW, Fairbanks VF, Moore SB, Alport EC, Nora FE. The syndrome of gastric argyrophil carcinoid tumors and nonantral gastric atrophy. Ann Intern Med 1983;99:761.
49. Eckhauser FE, Lloyd RV, Thompson NW, Raper SE, Vinik AI. Antrectomy for multicentric, argyrophil gastric carcinoids: a preliminary report. Surgery 1988;104:1046.
50. Cameron SJ, Doig A. Cerebellar tumours presenting with clinical features of phaeochromocytoma. Lancet 1970;1:492.
51. Weidenmann B, Franke WW, Kuhn C, Moll R, Gould VE. Synaptophysin: a marker protein for neuroendocrine cells and neoplasms. Proc Natl Acad Sci USA 1986;83:3500.
52. Simpson S, Vinik AI, Marangos PJ, Lloyd RV. Immunohistochemical localization of neuron-specific enolase in gastroentero-pancreatic neuroendocrine tumors. Correlation with tissue and serum levels of neuron-specific enolase. Cancer 1984;54:1364.
53. Gould M, Johnson RJ. Computed tomography of abdominal carcinoid tumor. Br J Radiol 1986;59:881.
54. Kressel HY. Strategies for magnetic resonance imaging of focal liver disease. Radiol Clin North Am 1988;26:607.
55. Eriksson B, Bergstrom M, Lilja A, Ahlstrom H, Langstrom B, Oberg K. Positron emission tomography (PET) in neuroendocrine gastrointestinal tumors. Acta Oncol 1993;32:189.
56. Eriksson B, Lilja A, Ahlstrom H, Bjurling P, Bergstrom M, Lindner KJ, Langstrom B, Oberg K. Positron-emission tomography as a radiological technique in neuroendocrine gastrointestinal tumors. Ann N Y Acad Sci 1994;733:446.
57. Fischer M, Kamanabroo D, Sonderkamp H, Proske T. Scintigraphic imaging of carcinoid tumors with I-131-metaiodobenzylguanidine. Lancet 1984;2:165.
58. Hammer RA, Leeman SE. Neurotensin: properties and actions. In Gut Hormones, vol 2. Edited by SR Bloom, JM Polak. Edinburgh: Churchill Livingstone, 1981, p 290.
59. Shapiro B. MIBG in the diagnosis and therapy of neuroblastoma and pheo-chromocytoma. In Proceedings of the International Symposium on Recent Advances in Nuclear Medicine. Edited by E Cattaruzi, E Englaro, O Geatti. Udine: Surin Biomedica, 1987, p 11.
60. Shapiro B. MIBG in the management of neuroendocrine tumors. Presented at the International Congress on Advances in Management of Malignancies, Ascoli Piceno, Italy, 1988, p 129.
61. Sinzinger H, Renner F, Granegger S. Unsuccessful I-131-MIBG imaging of carcinoids and apudomas. J Nucl Med 1986;27:1221.
62. von Moll L, McEwan AJ, Shapiro B, Sisson JC, Gross MD, Lloyd R, Beals F, Beierwaltes WH, Thompson NW. Iodine-131-MIBG scintigraphy of neuroendocrine tumors other than pheochromocytoma and neuroblastoma. J Nucl Med 1987;28:979.
63. Shapiro, B, Sisson JC. Sympatho-adrenal imaging with radioiodinated metaiodobenzylguanidine. In Atlas of Nuclear Medicine. Edited by D Von Nostrand, S Baum. Philadelphia: Lippincott, 1988, p 72.
64. Geatti O, Shapiro B, Sisson JC, Hutchinson RJ, Mallette S, Eyre P, Beierwaites WH. I-131-metaiodobenzylguanidine (I-131-MIBG) scintigraphy for the location of neuroblastoma: preliminary experience in 10 cases. J Nucl Med 1985;26:736.
65. Lumbroso J, Guermazi F, Hartmann O, Coonaert S, Rabarison Y, Lemerle J, Parmentier C. Sensitivity and specificity of metaiodoenzylguanidine (MIBG) scintigraphy in the evaluation of neuroblastoma: analysis of 115 cases. Bull Cancer 1988;75:97.
66. Treuner J, Feine U, Niethammer D, Muller-Schaumburg W, Meinke J, Elbach E, Dopfer R, Klingebliel T, Grumbach S. Scintigraphic imaging of neuroblastoma with I-131-MIBG. Lancet 1984;1:333.
67. Kubota A, Yamada Y, Kagimoto S, Shimatsu A, Imamura M, Tsuda K, Imura H, Seino S, Seino Y. Identification of somatostatin receptor subtypes and an implication for the efficacy of somatostatin analogue SMS 201–995 in treatment of human endocrine tumors. J Clin Invest 1994;93:1321.
68. Lamberts SW, Chayvialle JA, Krenning EP. The visualization of gastroenteropancreatic endocrine tumors. Metabolism 1992;41:111.
69. Krenning EP, Bakker WH, Kooij PP, Breeman WA, Oei HY, De Jong M, Reubi JC, Visser TJ, Bruns C, Kwekkeboom DJ. Somatostatin receptor scintigraphy with indium-111-DPTA-D-Phe-1-octreotide in man: metabolism, dosimetry and comparison with iodine-123-Tyr-3-octreotide. J Nucl Med 1992;33:652.
70. Krenning EP, Kwekkeboom DJ, Oel HY, de Jong RJB, Dop FJ, Reubi JC, Lamberts SWJ. Somatostatin-receptor scintigraphy in gastroenteropancreatic tumors. Ann N Y Acad Sci 1994;733:416.
71. Hammond PJ, Jackson JA, Bloom SR. Localization of pancreatic endocrine tumors. Clin Endocrinol 1994;40:3.
72. LeGuludes D, De Kervile E, Cadiot G, Lehbati P, Sobhatis I, Farragi M, Mignon M. Somatostatin receptor scintigraphy with In-111 octreotide: localization of gastrinomas and metastases in Zollinger-Ellison Syndrome. J Nucl Med 1993;34S:98.
73. Lamberts SWJ, Krenning EP, Klikn JG, Reubi JC. Validation of somatostatin receptor scintigraphy in the localization of neuroendocrine tumors. Acta Oncol 1993;32:167.
74. Janson ET, Westlin JE, Eriksson B, Ahlstrom H, Nilsson S, Oberg K. [111In-DTPA-D-Phe1] octreotide scintigraphy in patients with carcinoid tumors: the predictive value for somatostatin analogue treatment. Eur J Endocrinol 1994;131:577.
75. Kvols LK, Reubi JC, Horisberger U, Moertel CG, Rubin J, Carboneau JW. The presence of somatostatin receptors in malignant neuroendocrine tumor tissue predicts responsiveness to octreotide. Yale J Biol Med 1992;65:505.
76. Strodel WE, Vinik AI, Jaffe BM, Eckhauser F, Thompson NW. Substance P in localization of carcinoid tumors. J Surg Oncol 1984;27:106.
77. Strodel WE, Vinik AI, Thompson NW, Eckhauser FE, Talpos GB. Small bowel carcinoid tumors and the carcinoid syndrome. In Endocrine Surgery Update. Edited by NW Thompson, AI Vinik. New York: Grune & Stratton, 1983, p 293.
78. Feldman JM. Urinary serotonin in the diagnosis of carcinoid tumor. Clin Chem 1986;32:840.
79. Melmon KL, Sjoerdsma A, Oates JA, Laster L. Treatment of malabsorption and diarrhea of carcinoid syndrome with methysergide. Gastroenterology 1965;48:18.
80. Sandler M, Karim SM, Williams ED. Prostaglandin in amine-peptide-secreting tumors. Lancet 1968;2:1053.
81. Alumets J, Hakanson R, Ingemannson S, Sundler F. Substance P and 5-HT in granules isolated from an intestinal argentaffin carcinoid. Histochemistry 1977;52:217.
82. Oates JA, Pettinger WA, Doctor RB. Evidence for the release of bradykinin in the carcinoid syndrome. J Clin Invest 1966;45:173.
83. Pernow B, Waldenstrom J. Determination of 5-hydroxytryptamine, 5-hydroxyindoleacetic acid and histamine in 33 cases of carcinoid argentaffinoma. Am J Med 1957;53:16.
84. Wilander E, Grimelius L, Portela-Gomes G, Lundquist G, Skoog V, Westerwark P. Substance P and enteroglucagon-like immunoreactivity in argentaffin and argyrophil mid-gut carcinoid tumors. Scand J Gastroenterol 1979;53:19.
85. Lucas KJ, Feldman JM. Flushing in the carcinoid syndrome and plasma kallikrein. Cancer 1986;58:2290.
86. Feldman JM. Increased dopamine production in patients with carcinoid tumors. Metabolism 1985;34:255–260.
87. Theodrosson-Norheim E, Norheim KO, Brodin E, Lundberg JM, Tatemoto K, Lindgren PG. Neuropeptide K: a major tachykinin in plasma and tumor tissues from carcinoid patients. Biochem Biophys Res Commun 1985;131:77.
88. Vinik AI, Strodel WE, O'Dorisio TM. Endocrine tumors of the gastroenteropancreatic axis. In Diagnosis and Management of Endocrine-Related Tumors. Edited by RJ Santen, A Manni. Boston: Martinus Nijhoff, 1984, p 305.
89. Feldman JM, O'Dorisio TM. Role of neuropeptides and serotonin in the diagnosis of carcinoid tumors. Am J Med 1986;81:41–48.
90. Vinik AI, Achem-Karam S, Owyang C. Gastrointestinal hormones in clinical medicine. In Special Topics in Endocrinology and Metabolism, vol. 4. Edited by MP Cohen, PP Foa. New York: Alan R. Liss, 1983.
91. Udenfriend S, Titus E, Weissbach H. The identification of 5-hydroxy-3-indoleacetic acid in normal urine and a method for its assay. J Biol Chem 1955;216:499.
92. Das ML. A rapid sensitive method for direct estimation of serotonin in whole blood. Biochem Med 1972;6:299.
93. Davis RB. The concentration of serotonin in normal human serum as determined by an improved method. J Lab Clin Med 1973;24:177.

94. Walker TP. The determination of serotonin (5-hydroxytryptamine) in human blood. J Lab Clin Med 1959;55:824.
95. Modlin IM. Carcinoid syndrome. J Clin Gastroenterol 1980;2:349.
96. Aldrich LB, Moattari AR, Vinik AI. Distinguishing features of idiopathic flushing and carcinoid syndrome. Arch Intern Med 1988;148:2614–2618.
97. Ahlman H, Dahlstrom A, Gronstad K, et al. The pentagastrin test in the diagnosis of the carcinoid syndrome. Blockade of gastrointestinal symptoms by ketanserin. Ann Surg 1985;201:81–86.
98. Kaplan EL, Jaffe BM, Peskin GW. A new provocative test for the diagnosis of carcinoid syndrome. Am J Surg 1972;123:173.
99. Conlon JM, Deacon CF, Richter G, Stockman F, Creutzfeldt W. Circulating tachykinins (substance P, neurokinin A and neuropeptide K) and the carcinoid flush. Scand J Gastroenterol 1987;22:97.
100. Norheim I, Theodorsson-Norheim E, Brodin E, Oberg K. Tachykinins in carcinoid tumors: their use as a tumor marker and possible role in the carcinoid flush. J Clin Endocrinol Metab 1986;63:605.
101. Hoefnagel CA, Marcuse HR, DeKraker J, Voute PA. Detection of neuroblastoma with I-131-meta-iodobenzylguanidine. Clin Biol Res 1979;137:142.
102. Moertel CG. Treatment of the carcinoid tumor and the malignant carcinoid syndrome. J Clin Oncol 1983;1:727–740.
103. Godwin JD. Carcinoid treatment: an analysis of 2,837 cases. Cancer 1975;36:560.
104. Kvols LK. Metastatic carcinoid tumors and the carcinoid syndrome. A selective review of chemotherapy and hormonal therapy. Am J Med 1986;81:49–55.
105. Maton PN, Camilleri M, Griffin G, Hodgson H, Allison DJ, Chadwick VS. The role of hepatic arterial embolization in the carcinoid syndrome. Br Med J 1983;287:932.
106. Gyr NE, Kayasseh L, Keller U. Somatostatin as a therapeutic agent. In Gut Hormones, vol. 2. Edited by SR Bloom, JM Polak. Edinburgh: Churchill Livingstone, 1981, p 581.
107. Sheppard M, Shapiro B, Primstone B, Kronhein S, Berelowitz M, Gregory MJ. Metabolic clearance and plasma half disappearance time of exogenous somatostatin in man. Clin Endocrinol Metab 1979;48:50.
108. Bauer W, Briner U, Doepfner W, Waller R, Huguenin R, Marbach P, Fletcher TJ, Pless T. SMS 201-995: a very potent and selective octapeptide analogue of somatostatin with prolonged action. Life Sci 1982;31:1133.
109. Kvols LK, Martin K, Marsh HM, Moertel CG. Rapid reversal of carcinoid crisis with a somatostatin analogue (letter). N Engl J Med 1985;313:1229–1230.
110. Vinik AI, Tsai S, Moattari AR, Cheung P, Eckhauser F, Cho K. Somatostatin analogue (SMS 20–995) in the management of gastroenteropancreatic tumors and diarrhea syndromes. Am J Med 1986;81:23.
111. Frolich JC, Bloomgarden ZT, Oates J, McGuigan JE, Rabinowitz D. The carcinoid flush provocation by pentagastrin and inhibition by somatostatin. N Engl J Med 1978;299:1055.
112. Kvols LK, Moertel CG, O'Connell MJ, Schutt AJ, Rubin J, Hahn R. Treatment of the malignant carcinoid syndrome. Evaluation of a long-acting somatostatin analogue. N Engl J Med 1986;315:663–666.
113. Richter G, Stockman F, Lembeke B, Conlon JM, Creutzfeldt W. Short-term administration of somatostatin analogue SMS 201–995 in patients with carcinoid tumors. Scand J Gastroenterol 1986;21:193.
114. Santangelo WC, O'Dorisio TM, Kim JG, Severino G, Krejs GJ. Pancreatic cholera syndrome-effect of a synthetic somatostatin analogue on intestinal water and ion transport. Ann Intern Med 1985;103:363.
115. Arnold R, Lankisch PG. Somatostatin and the gastrointestinal tract. Clin Gastroenterol 1980;9:733.
116. Stockmann F, Richter G, Lembecke B, Conlon JM, Creutzfeldt W. Long-term treatment of patients with endocrine gastrointestinal tumors with the somatostatin analogue SMS 201–995. Scand J Gastroenterol 1986;21:230.
117. Hengl G, Prager J, Pointner H. The influence of somatostatin on the absorption of triglycerides in partially gastrectomized subjects. Acta Hepato-Gastroenterol 1979;26:392.
118. Vinik AI, Moattari AR. Use of somatostatin analogue in the management of carcinoid syndrome. Dig Dis Sci 1989;34:14S.
119. Poole CJM. Myelopathy secondary to metastatic carcinoid tumors. J Neurol Neurosurg Psychiatry 1984;47:1359.
120. Berry EM, Maunder C, Wilson M. Carcinoid myopathy and treatment with cyproheptadine (Periactin). Gut 1974;15:34.
121. Green D, Joynt RJ, Van Allen MW. Neuromyopathy associated with a malignant carcinoid tumor. Arch Intern Med 1964;114:494.
122. Wroe SJ, Ardon M, Bouden AR. Myasthenia gravis associated with a hormone producing malignant carcinoid tumor. J Neurol Neurosurg Psychiatry 1985;48:719.
123. O'Stern WK, Barnard JL Jr, Yates RD. Morphologic changes in skeletal muscle induced by serotonin treatment: a light and electron microscopy study. Exp Mol Pathol 1967;7:145.
124. Kraenzlin ME, Ching KC, Wood SM, Carr DH, Bloom SR. Long-term treatment of a VIPoma with somatostatin analogue resulting in remission of symptoms and possible shrinkage of metastases. Gastroenterology 1985;88:185.
125. Saltz L, Trochanowski B, Buckley M, Heffernan B, Niedziecki D, Tao Y, Kelsen D. Octreotide as an antineoplastic agent in the treatment of functional and nonfunctional neuroendocrine tumors. Cancer 1993;72:244.
126. Anthony L, Johnson D, Hande K, Shaff M, Winn S, Krozley M, Oates J. Somatostatin analogue phase I trials in neuroendocrine neoplasms. Acta Oncol 1993;32:217.
127. Janson ET, Oberg K. Long-term management of the carcinoid syndrome. Treatment with octreotide alone and in combination with a-interferon. Acta Oncol 1993;304:547.
128. Kvols LK. Therapy of the malignant carcinoid syndrome. Endocrinol Metab Clin North Am 1989;18:557–568.
129. McEwan AJ, Shapiro B, Sisson JC, Beierwaltes WH, Akery DM. Radioiodo-benzylgûanidine for the scintigraphic location and therapy of adrenergic tumors. Semin Nucl Med 1985;15:132.
130. Sisson JC, Shapiro B, Beierwaltes WH, et al. Radiopharmaceutical treatment of malignant pheochromocytoma. J Nucl Med 1984;25:197.
131. Sisson JC, Shapiro B, Beierwaltes WH, Nakajo M, Glowniak J, Mangner T, Carey JE, Swanson DP, Copp J, Satterlee W, Wieland DM. Treatment of malignant pheochromocytoma with a new radiopharmaceutical. Trans Assoc Am Physicians 1983;96:209.
132. Snisky CA, Wolfe MM, Martin JL, et al. Myoelectric effects of vasoactive intestinal peptide of rabbit small intestine. Am J Physiol 1983;244:G46.
133. Lamberts SWJ, Krenning EP, Klikn JG, Reubi JC. The clinical use of somatostatin analogues in the treatment of cancer. Baillieres Clin Endocrinol Metab 1990;4:29.
134. Schubert ML. In vivo samatostatin receptor imaging in the detection and treatment of gastrointestinal cancer. Gastroenterology 1991;100:1143.
135. Carrasco CH, Charnsangavej C, Ajani J, Samaan NA, Richli W, Wallace S. The carcinoid syndrome: palliation by hepatic artery embolization. Am J Roentgenol 1986;147:149.
136. Mekhjian HS, O'Dorisio TM. VIPoma syndrome. Semin Oncol 1987;14:282.
137. Melia WM, Nunnerley HB, Johnson PJ, Williams R. Use of arterial devascularization and cytotoxic drugs in 30 patients with the carcinoid syndrome. Br J Cancer 1982;46:331.
138. Nobin A, Mansson B, Lunderquist A. Evaluation of temporary liver dearterialization and embolization in patients with metastatic carcinoid tumour. Acta Oncol 1989;28:419.
139. Moertel CG. An odyssey in the land of small tumors. J Clin Oncol 1987;5:1502.
140. Moertel CG, Johnson CM, McKusick MA, Martin JK, Nagorney DM, Kvols LK, Rubin J, Kunselman S. The management of patients with advanced carcinoid tumors and islet cell carcinomas. Ann Intern Med 1994;120:302.
141. van Hazel GA, Moertel CG. Treatment of metastatic carcinoid tumor with dactinomycin or dacarbazine. Cancer Treat Rep 1983;67:583–585.
142. Moertel CG, Hanley JA. Combination chemotherapy trials in metastatic carcinoid tumor and the malignant carcinoid syndrome. Cancer Clin Trials 1979;2:327.
143. Kvols LK, Buck M. Chemotherapy of endocrine malignancies: a review. Semin Oncol 1987;14:343.
144. Kessinger A, Foley JF, Lemon HM. Therapy of malignant APUD cell tumors. Effectiveness of DTIC. Cancer 1983;51:790.
145. Bukowski RM, Tangen CM, Peterson RF, et al. Phase II trial of dimethyltriazenoimidazole carboxamide in patients with metastatic carcinoid. A Southwest Oncology Group Study. Cancer 1994;73:1505.
146. Kelsen D, Fiore J, Heelan R, Cheng E, Magill G. Phase II trial of etoposide in APUD tumors. Cancer Treat Rep 1987;71:305.
147. Moertel CG, Rubin J, O'Connell MJ. A phase II study of cisplatin therapy in patients with metastatic carcinoid tumor and the malignant carcinoid syndrome. Cancer Treat Rep 1986;70:1459.
148. Mengel CE, Shaffer RD. The carcinoid syndrome. In Cancer Medicine. Edited by JF Holland, E Frei. Philadelphia: Lea & Febiger, 1973, p 1584.
149. Engstrom PF, Lavin PT, Moertel CG, Folsch E, Douglass HO Jr. Streptozocin plus fluorouracil versus doxorubicin therapy for metastatic carcinoid tumor. J Clin Oncol 1984;2:1255–1259.
150. Bukowski RM, Johnson KG, Peterson RF, Stephens RL, Rivkin SE, Neilan B, Costanzi JH. A phase II trial of combination chemotherapy in patients with metastatic carcinoid tumors. Cancer 1987;60:2891.
151. Oberg K, Alm G, Magnusson A, et al. Treatment of malignant carcinoid tumors with recombinant interferon alfa-2b: development of neutralizing interferon antibodies and possible loss of antitumor activity. JNCI 1989;81:531–535.
152. Feldman JM. Carcinoid tumors and the carcinoid syndrome. Curr Probl Surg 1989;26:829.
153. Oberg K, Alm G, Norheim, et al. Treatment of malignant carcinoid tumors: a randomized controlled tachykinin production by carcinoid tumours in culture. Evidence for binding of gastrin toigandin, a cell cytosol protein. Clinical features, diagnosis, and localization of carcinoid tumors and their management. Gastroenterol Clin North Am 1989;1865–1896.
154. Oberg K, Eriksson B. Medical treatment of neuroendocrine gut and pancreatic tumors. Acta Oncol 1989;28:425.
155. Hanssen LE, Schrumpf E, Kolbenstvedt AN, Tausjo J, Dolva LO. Treatment of malignant metastatic midgut carcinoid tumours with recombinant human alfa-2b interferon with or without hepatic artery embolization. Scand J Gastroenterol 1989;24:787.
156. Sisson JC, Hutchinson R, Johnson J, Mallette S, Carey JE, Shapiro B, Beierwaltes WH. Acute toxicity of therapeutic I-131-MIBG relates more to whole body than to blood radiation dosimetry. J Nucl Med 1987;23:618.
157. Oberg K. The action of interferon alpha on human carcinoid tumours. Semin Cancer Biol 1992;3:35.
158. Moertel CG, Rubin J, Kvols LK. Therapy of metastatic carcinoid tumor and the malignant carcinoid syndrome with recombinant leukocyte A interferon. J Clin Oncol 1989;7:865–868.
159. Grander D, Oberg K, Lundqvist M, Janson ET, Eriksson B, Einhorn S. Interferon-induced enhancement of 2′,5′-oligoadenylate-synthetase in mid-gut carcinoid tumours. Lancet 1990;36:337.
160. Ajani JA, Carrasco CH, Charnsangavej C, Samann NA, Levin B, Wallace S. Islet cell tumors metastatic to the liver: effective palliation by sequential hepatic artery embolization. Ann Intern Med 1989;108:340.
161. Moertel CG, May GR, Martin JK, Rubin J, Schutt AJ. Sequential hepatic artery occlusion (HAO) and chemotherapy for metastatic carcinoid tumor and islet cell carcinoma (ICC). Proc Am Soc Clin Oncol 1985;4:80.
162. Vinik AI, Strodel WM, Lloyd RV, Thompson NW. Unusual gastroenteropancreatic tumors and their hormones. In Endocrine Surgery Update. Edited by NW Thompson, AI Vinik. New York: Grune & Stratton, 1983, pp 293–293.
163. McCarthy DM, Jensen RT. Zollinger-Ellison syndrome: current issues. In Hormone Producing Tumors of the Gastrointestinal Tract. Edited by S Cohen, R Soloway. New York: Churchill Livingstone, 1985, p 25.
164. Fox PS, Hofmann JW, DeCosse JJ, Wilson SD. The influence of total gastrectomy on survival in malignant Zollinger-Ellison tumors. Ann Surg 1974;180:558.
165. Friesen SR, Bolinger RE, A. Pearse GE, McGuigan JE. Serum gastrin levels in malignant Zollinger-Ellison syndrome after total gastrectomy and hypophysectomy. Ann Surg 1970;172:504.
166. Sircus W. Vagotomy in Z-E syndrome. Gastroenterology 1979;79:607.
167. Stabile BE, Passoro E Jr. Benign and malignant gastrinoma. Am J Surg 1985;148:144.
168. Wolfe MM, Alexander RW, McGuigan JE. Extrapancreatic, extraintestinal gastrinoma. N Engl J Med 1982;306:1533.
169. Zollinger RM. Gastrinoma: factors influencing prognosis. Surgery 1985;97:49.
170. Bhagavan BS, Slavin RE, Goldberg J, Rao RN. Ectopic gastrinoma and Zollinger-Ellison syndrome. Hum Pathol 1986;17:584–592.
171. Thompson NW, Lloyd RV, Nishiyama RH, et al. MEN 1 pancreas: a histological and immunohistochemical study. World J Surg 1984;8:561.
172. Debas HT, Soon-Shiong P, McKenzie AD, et al. Use of secretin in the roentgenologic and biochemical diagnosis of duodenal gastrinoma. Am J Surg 1983;145:408.

173. Thompson NW, Vinik AI, Eckhauser FE. Microgastrinomas of the duodenum. A cause of failed operations for the Zollinger-Ellison syndrome. Ann Surg 1989;209:396–404.
174. Norton JA, Doppman JL, Jensen RT. Curative resection in Zollinger-Ellison syndrome. Ann Surg 1992;215:8.
175. Sugg SL, Norton JA, Fraker DL, et al. A prospective study of intraoperative methods to diagnose and resect duodenal gastrinomas. Ann Surg 1993;218:138.
176. Deveney CW, Deveney KS, Stark D, Moss A, Stein S, Way LW. Resection of gastrinomas. Ann Surg 1983;198:546.
177. Friesen SR. The development of endocrinopathies in the prospective screening of two families with MEA-I. World J Surg 1979;3:753.
178. Lamers CB, Buis JT, Van Tongeren JH. Secretin-stimulated serum gastrin levels in hyperparathyroid patients from families with multiple endocrine adenomatosis-type 1. Ann Intern Med 1977;86:719.
179. Malagelada JR, Edis AJ, Adson MA, van Heerden JA, Go VL. Medical and surgical options in the management of patients with gastrinoma. Gastroenterology 1983;84:1524.
180. Mignon M, Ruszniewski P, Haffar S, Rigaud D, Rene E, Bonfils S. Current approach to the management of tumoral process in patients with gastrinoma. World J Surg 1986;10:703.
181. Friesen SR. Treatment of Zollinger-Ellison syndrome: a 25-year assessment. Am J Surg 1982;143:331.
182. Betts JB, O'Malley BP, Rosenthal FD. Hyperparathyroidism: a prerequisite for Zollinger-Ellison syndrome in MEA-I: report of a further family and a review of the literature. Q J Med 1980;49:69.
183. Friesen SR. Update on the diagnosis and treatment of rare neuroendocrine tumors. Surg Clin North Am 1987;67:379.
184. Vinik AI, Strodel WE, Cho KJ, Eckhauser FE, Thompson NW. Localization of hormonally active gastrointestinal tumors. In Endocrine Surgery Update. Edited by NW Thompson, AI Vinik. New York: Grune & Stratton, 1983.
185. Landor JH. Control of the Zollinger-Ellison syndrome by excision of primary and metastatic tumor. Am J Surg 1984;147:406.
186. Stabile BE, Morrow DJ, Passaro Jr E. The gastrinoma triangle: operative implications. Am J Surg 1984;147:25.
187. Thompson NW, Eckhauser FE. Malignant islet-cell tumors of the pancreas. World J Surg 1984;8:940.
188. Morowitz DA, Levine AE. Malignant Zollinger-Ellison syndrome: remission of primary and metastatic pancreatic tumor after gastrectomy: report of a case and review of the literature. Am J Gastroenterol 1986;81:471.
189. Fabri PJ, Johnson JA, Ellison EC. Prediction of progressive disease in Zollinger-Ellison syndrome—comparison of available preoperative tests. J Surg Res 1981;31:93.
190. Johnson JA, Fabri PJ, Lott JA. Serum gastrins in Zollinger-Ellison syndrome—identification of localized disease. Clin Chem 1980;26:867.
191. kothary pc, fabri pj, gower w, o'dorisio tm, ellis j, vinik ai. evaluation of nh_2-terminus gastrins in gastrinoma syndrome. J Clin Endocrinol Metab 1986;62:970–974.
192. Pauwels S, Desmond H, Dimaline R, Dockray GJ. Identification of progastrin in gastrinomas, antrum, and duodenum by a novel radioimmunoassay. J Clin Invest 1986;77:376.
193. McCarthy DM, Weintraub B, Rosen S. Subunits of human chorionic gonadotropin in the Zollinger-Ellison syndrome. Gastroenterology 1979;76:1198.
194. Ellison EC, Carey LC, Sparks J, et al. Early surgical treatment of gastrinoma. Am J Med 1987;82:17.
195. Giacobazzi P, Passaro E. Preoperative angiography in the Zollinger-Ellison syndrome. Ann Surg 1973;126:74.
196. Mills SR, Doppman JL, Dunnick NR, McCarthy DM. Evaluation of angiography in Zollinger-Ellison syndrome. Radiology 1979;131:317.
197. Wank SA, Doppman JL, Miller DL, Maton PN, Vinayek R, Slaff JI, Norton JA, Gardner JD, Jensen RT. Prospective study of the ability of computed axial tomography to localize gastrinomas in patients with Zollinger-Ellison syndrome. Gastroenterology 1987;92:905.
198. Dunnick NR, Doppman JL, Mills S, McCarthy DM. Computed tomographic appearance of non-beta (or non-insulin producing) pancreatic islet cell tumors. Radiology 1980;135:117.
199. Thompson NW, Vinik AI, Eckhauser FE, Strodel WE. Extrapancreatic gastrinomas. Surgery 1985;98:1113.
200. Hancke S. Localization of hormone-producing gastrointestinal tumors by ultrasonic scanning. Scand J Gastroenterol 1979;14(suppl 53):115.
201. Rueckert KF, Klotter HJ, Kummerle F. Intraoperative ultrasonic localization of endocrine tumors of the pancreas. Surgery 1984;96:1045.
202. Sigel B, Coelho JC, Nyhus LM, Velasco JM, Donahue PE, Wood DK, Spigos DG. Detection of pancreatic tumors by ultrasound during surgery. Arch Surg 1982;117:1058.
203. Cho KJ, Vinik AI, Thompson NW, Shields JJ, Porter DJ, Brady TM, Cadavid G, Fajans SS. Localization of the source of hyperinsulinism: Percutaneous transhepatic portal and pancreatic vein catheterization with hormone assay. AJR 1982;139:237–245.
204. Semelka RC, Cumming MJ, Shoenut JP, et al. Islet cell tumors: comparison of dynamic contrast-enhanced CT and MR-imaging with dynamic gadolinuium enhancement and fat suppression. Radiology 1993;186:799.
205. Thom AK, Norton JA, Doppman JL, Miller DL, Chang R, Jensen RT. Prospective study of the use of intraarterial secretin injection and portal venous sampling to localize duodenal gastrinomas. Surgery 1992;112:1002.
206. Ingemansson S, Larsson LI, Stadil F. Pancreatic vein catheterization with gastrin assay in normal patients and patients with Zollinger-Ellison syndrome. Am J Surg 1977;134:558.
207. Burcharth F, Stage JG, Stadil F, Jensen LI, Fischermann K. Localization of gastrinomas by transhepatic portal catheterization and gastrin assay. Gastroenterology 1979;77:444.
208. Glaser B, Vinik AI, Sive AA, Floyd JC Jr, Fajans SS, Pek S. Evidence for extravagal cholinergic dependence of pancreatic polypeptide responses to beef ingestion in man (abstract). Diabetes 1979;28:414.
209. Passaro E Jr. Localization of pancreatic endocrine tumors by selective portal vein catheterization and radioimmunoassay. Gastroenterology 1979;77:806.
210. Vinik AI, Glowniak J, Glaser B, et al. Localization of gastroenteropancreatic (GEP) tumors. In Surgery 2. Endocrine Surgery. Edited by IDA Johnston, NW Thompson. London: Butterworth's International Medical Reviews, 1983, p 76.
211. Norton JA, Doppman JL, Collen MJ, et al. Prospective study of gastrinoma localization and resection in patients with Zollinger-Ellison syndrome. Ann Surg 1986;204:468.
212. Rosch T, Lightdale CJ, Botet JF, et al. Localization of pancreatic endocrine tumors by endoscopic ultrasonography. N Engl J Med 1992;326:1721.
213. Zimmer T, Ziegler K, Liehr RM, Stolzel U, Riechen EO, Wiedenman B. Endosonography of neuroendocrine tumors of the stomach, duodenum, and pancreas. Ann N Y Acad Sci 1994;733:425.
214. Roche A, Raissonnier A, Gillon-Savouret MC. Pancreatic venous sampling and arteriography in the localising insulinomas and gastrinomas: procedure and results in 55 cases. Radiology 1982;145:621.
215. Deveney C, Steins S, Way LW. Cimetidine in the treatment of Zollinger-Ellison syndrome. Am J Surg 1983;146:116.
216. Maton PN, Vinayek R, Frucht H, McArthur RA, Miller LS, Saced ZA, Gardner JD, Jensen RT. Long-term efficacy and safety of one prazole in patients with Zollinger-Ellison syndrome. Gastroenterology 1989;97:827.
217. McCarthy DM. Report on the U.S. experience with cimetidine in Zollinger-Ellison syndrome and other hypersecretory states. Gastroenterology 1978;74:453.
218. Mignon M, Vallot T, Hervoir P, et al. Ranitidine versus cimetidine in the management of Zollinger-Ellison syndrome. In Proceedings of an International Symposium, World Congress of Enterology. Edited by AJ Riley, PR Salmon. Amsterdam: Excerpta Medica, 1982, p 169.
219. Glowniak JV, Shapiro B, Vinik AI, Glaser B, Thompson NW, Cho KJ. Percutaneous transhepatic venous sampling of gastrin: value in sporadic and familial islet-cell tumors of G-cell. N Engl J Med 1982;307:293–297.
220. Miyata M, Nakao K, Sakamoto T, et al. Removal of mesenteric gastrinoma: a case report. Surgery 1986;99:245.
221. Oberheiman HA. Excisional therapy for ulcerogenic tumors of the duodenum—long-term results. Arch Surg 1972;104:447.
222. Barreras RF, Mack E, Goodfriend T, Damm M. Resection of gastrinoma in the Zollinger-Ellison syndrome. Gastroenterology 1981;82:953.
223. Deveney CW, Deveney KS, Way LW. The Zollinger-Ellison syndrome—23 years later. Ann Surg 1978;188:384.
224. Stage JG, Stadil F. The clinical diagnosis of Zollinger-Ellison syndrome. Scand J Gastroenterol 1979;53:79.
225. Thompson JC, Lewis BG, Weiner I, Townsend CM Jr. The role of surgery in the Zollinger-Ellison syndrome. Ann Surg 1983;197:594.
226. Norton JA, Sigel B, Baker AR, et al. Localization of an occult insulinoma by intraoperative ultrasonography. Surgery 1985;97:381.
227. Norton JA, Cromack DT, Shawker TH, et al. Intraoperative ultrasonographic localization of islet cell tumors. Ann Surg 1988;207:160.
228. Frucht H, Norton JA, London JF, et al. Detection of duodenal gastrinomas by operative endoscopic transillumination: a prospective study. Gastroenterology 1990;99:1622.
229. van Heerden JA, Smith SL, Miller LJ. The management of Zollinger-Ellison syndrome in patients with multiple endocrine neoplasm Type 1. Presented at the Seventh Annual Meeting, American Association of Endocrine Surgeons, April 15, 1986. Surgery 1986;100:971–977.
230. Broder LE, Carter SK. Pancreatic islet cell carcinoma: II. Results of therapy with streptozotocin in 52 patients. Ann Intern Med 1973;70:108.
231. Friesen SR. Tumors of the endocrine pancreas. N Engl J Med 1982;306:580.
232. Moertel CG, Hanley JA, Johnson LA. Streptozotocin alone compared with streptoxocin plus fluorouracil in the treatment of advanced islet-cell carcinoma. N Engl J Med 1980;303:1189.
233. Moertel CG, Lavin PT, Hahn RG. Phase II trial of doxorubicin therapy for advanced islet cell carcinoma. Cancer Treat Rep 1982;66:1567.
234. Maton PN, Gardner JD, Jensen RT. Diagnosis and management of Zollinger-Ellison syndrome. Endocrinol Metab Clin North Am 1989;18:519.
235. von Schrenck T, Howard JM, Doppman JL, et al. Prospective study of chemotherapy in patients with metastatic gastrinoma. Gastroenterology 1988;94:1326.
236. Altimari AF, Badrinath K, Reisel HJ, Prinz RA. DTIC therapy in patients with malignant intra-abdominal neuroendocrine tumors. Surgery 1987;102:1009.
237. Norton JA, Sugarbaker PH, Doppman JL, et al. Aggressive resection of metastatic disease in selected patients with malignant gastrinoma. Ann Surg 1986;203:352.
238. Fajans SS, Vinik AI. Diagnosis and treatment of insulinoma. In Diagnosis and management of endocrine-related tumors. Edited by RJ Santen, A Manni. Boston: Martinus Nijhoff, 1984, p 235.
239. Edis AJ, McIlrath DC, van Heerden JA, et al. Insulinoma—current diagnosis and surgical management. Curr Probl Surg 1976;13:1.
240. Thompson NW. The surgical treatment of islet cell tumors of the pancreas. In Pancreatic Disease. Edited by TL Dent. New York: Grune & Stratton, 1981, p 461.
241. Glaser B, Shapiro B, Fajans SS, Vinik AI. Effects of secretin on the normal and pathological beta cell. J Clin Endocrinol Metab 1988;66:1138.
242. Kaplan E, Lee CH. Recent advances in the diagnosis and treatment of insulinomas. Surg Clin North Am 1979;59:119.
243. Le Quesne LP, Nabarro JD, Kurtz A, Zweig S. The management of insulin tumors of the pancreas. Br J Surg 1979;66:373.
244. Modlin IM. Endocrine tumors of the pancreas. Surg Gynecol Obstet 1979;149:751.
245. Stefanini P, Carboni W, Patrassi N, Basoli A. Beta-islet cell tumors of the pancreas: results of a study of 1,067 cases. Surgery 1974;75:597.
246. Stefanini P, Carboni W, Patrassi N, Benedetti-Valentini FJ. Surgical treatment and prognosis of insulinoma. Clin Gastroenterol 1974;3:697.
247. Robins JM, Bookstein JJ, Oberman HA, Fajans SS. Selective angiography in localizing islet cell tumors of the pancreas: a further appraisal. Radiology 1973;106:525.
248. Doppman JL, Miller DL, Chang R, Shawker TH, Gordon P, Norton JA. Insulinomas: localization with selective intraarterial injection of calcium. Radiology 1991;178:237.
249. Cho KJ, Vinik AI, Thompson NW, et al. Localization of the source of hyperinsulinism by percutaneous transhepatic portal and pancreatic vein catheterization with hormone assay. Am J Roentgenol 1982;139:237–245.
250. Ingemansson S, Kuhl C, Larsson L, Lunderquist A, Lunderquist I. Localization of insulinomas and islet cell hyperplasia by pancreatic vein catheterization and insulin assay. Surg Gynecol Obstet 1978;146:725.
251. Katz LB, Aufses AH, Rayfield E, Mitty H. Preoperative localization and intraoperative monitoring in the management of patients with pancreatic insulinoma. Surg Gynecol Obstet 1986;163:509.
252. Vinik AI, Thompson N. Controversies in the management of Zollinger-Ellison syndrome. Ann Intern Med 1986;105:956–959.
253. Pasieka JL, McLeod MK, Thompson NW, Burney RE. Surgical approach to insulinomas. Arch Surg 1992;127:442.

254. Fajans SS, Floyd JC Jr, Knopf RF, Rull J, Guntsche EM, Conn JW. Benzothiadiazine suppression of insulin release from normal and abnormal islet cell tissue in man. J Clin Invest 1986;45:481.
255. Fajans SS, Floyd JC Jr, Thiffault CA, Knopf RF, Harrison TS, Conn JW. Further studies on diazoxide suppression of insulin release from abnormal and normal islet tissue in man. Ann NY Acad Sci 1968;150:261.
256. Ulbrecht JS, Schmeltz R, Aarons JH, Greene DA. Insulinoma in a 94 year old woman: long-term therapy with verapamil. Diabetes Care 1986;9:196.
257. Blum I, Doron M, Laron Z, Atsmon A, Tigva P. Prevention of hypoglycemic attacks by propranol suffereing from insulinoma. Diabetes 1975;24:535.
258. Neri V, Bartorelli A, Faglia G. Effect of propranolol on the blood sugar, immunoreactive blood insulin in a patient with insulinoma. Acta Diabetol Lat 1969;6:809.
259. Schusdziarra V, Zyznar E, Rouiller D, et al. Splanchnic somatostatin: a hormonal regulator of nutrient homeostasis. Science 1980;207:530.
260. Brodows RG, Campbel RG. Control of refractory fasting hypoglycemia in a patient with suspected insulinoma with diphenylhydantoin. J Clin Endocrinol Metab 1974;38: 159.
261. Hofeldt FD, Dippe SE, Levin SR, Karam JH, Blum MR, Forsham PH. Effects of diphenylhydantoin upon glucose-induced insulin secretion in three patients with insulinoma. Diabetes 1973;23:192.
262. Tsai ST, Eckhauser FE, Thompson NW, Stroedel WE, Vinik AI. Perioperative use of long-acting somatostatin analogue (SMS 201–995) in patients with endocrine tumors of the gastroenteropancreatic axis. Surgery 1986;100:788.
263. Osei K, O'Dorisio TM. Malignant insulinoma: effects of a somatostatin analogue (compound 201–995) on serum glucose, growth and gastro-entero-pancreatic hormones. Ann Intern Med 1985;103:223.
264. Verner JV, Morrison AB. Islet cell tumor and a syndrome of refractory watery diarrhea and hypokalemia. Am J Med 1958;25:374.
265. Murray JS, Paton RR, Pope CE. Pancreatic tumor associated with flushing and diarrhea. Report of a case. N Engl J Med 1961;264:436.
266. Priest WM, Alexander MK. Islet-cell tumor of the pancreas with peptic ulceration, diarrhea, and hypokalemia. Lancet 1957;2:1145.
267. Matsumoto KD, Peter JB, Schultze RG, Hakin AA, Frank PT. Watery diarrhea and hypokalemia associated with pancreatic islet cell adenoma. Gastroenterology 1967;52: 965.
268. Marks IN, Bank S, Louw JH. Islet cell tumor of the pancreas with reversible watery diarrhea and achlorhydria. Gastroenterology 1967;52:695.
269. Kraft AR, Tompkins RK, Zollinger R. Recognition and management of the diarrheal syndrome caused by non-beta cell tumors of the pancreas. Am J Surg 1970;119:163.
270. Verner JV, Morrison AB. Endocrine pancreatic islet disease with diarrhea: report on a case due to diffuse hyperplasia of nonbeta islet tissue with a review of 54 additional cases. Arch Intern Med 1958;25:374.
271. Tatemoto K, Mutt V. Isolation of two novel candidate hormones using chemical method for finding naturally occurring polypeptide. Nature 1980;285:417.
272. Barbezat GO, Grossman M. Intestinal secretion: stimulation by peptides. Science 1971;174:422.
273. Bloom SR, Polak JM. VIP measurement in distinguishing Verner-Morrison syndrome and pseudo-Verner-Morrison syndrome. Clin Endocrinol (Oxf) 1976;5:223S.
274. Bloom SR, Polak JM. VIPomas. In Vasoactive Intestinal Peptides. Edited by SI Said. New York: Raven, 1982.
275. Go VLW, Korinik JK. Effect of vasoactive intestinal polypeptide on hepatic glucose release. In Vasoactive Intestinal Peptide. Edited by SI Said. New York: Raven, 1982.
276. Rambaud JC, Modiglioni R, Matuchansky C, et al. Pancreatic cholera: studies on tumoral secretions and pathophysiology of diarrhea. Gastroenterology 1975;69:110.
277. Said SI, Mutt V. Isolation from porcine intestinal wall of a vasoactive ocatcospeptide related to secretin and to glucagon. Eur J Biochem 1972;28:129.
278. Long RG, Byrant MG, Mitchell SJ, Adrian TE, Polak JM, Bloom SR. Clinicopathological study of pancreatic and ganglioneuroblastoma tumours secreting vasoactive intestinal polypeptide (vipomas). Br Med J 1981;282:1767.
279. Blair AW, Ahmed S. Presacral vipoma in a 16-month old child. Acta Paediatr Belg 1981;34:89.
280. Carson DJ, Glasgow J, Ardill FTJ. Watery diarrhea and elevated vasoactive intestinal polypeptide associated with a massive neurofibroma in early childhood. J R Soc Med 1980;73:69.
281. Ebeid AM, Murray PD, Fisher JE. Vasoactive intestinal peptide and the watery diarrhea syndrome. Ann Surg 1978;187:411.
282. Iida Y, Nose O, Kai H, et al. Watery diarrhea with a vasoactive intestinal peptide-producing ganglioneuroblastoma. Arch Dis Child 1980;55:929.
283. Kaplan SJ, Holbrook CT, McDaniel HG, Buntain WL, Crist WM. Vasoactive intestinal peptide secreting tumors of childhood. Am J Dis Child 1980;134:21.
284. Kudo K, Kitajima S, Munakata H, Yagihashi S. WDHA syndrome caused by VIP-producing ganglioneuroblastoma. J Pediatr Surg 1982;17:426.
285. Modlin IM, Bloom SR. VIPomas and the watery diarrhea syndrome. S Afr Med J 1978;54:53.
286. Tiedemann K, Long RG, Pritchard J, Bloom SR. Plasma vasoactive intestinal polypeptide and other regulaory peptides in children with neurogenic tumours. Eur J Pediatr 1981;137:147.
287. Tiedemann K, Pritchard J, Long R, Bloom SR. Intractable diarrhoea in a patient with vasoactive intestinal peptide-secreting neuroblastoma. Eur J Pediatr 1981;137:217.
288. Yamaguchi K, Abe K, Adachi I, et al. Clinical and hormonal aspects of the watery diarrhea-hypokalemia-achlorhydria (WGHA) syndrome due to vasoactive intestinal polypeptide (VIP)-producing tumor. Endocrinol Jpn 1980;27:79.
289. Wesley JR, Vinik AI, O'Dorisio TM, Glaser B, Fink A. A new syndrome ofsymptomatic cutaneous mastocytoma producing vasoactive intestinal polypeptide. Gastroenterology 1982;82:963.
290. Hamilton I, Reis L, Bilimoria S, Lang RG. A renal vipoma. Br Med J 1980;281:1323.
291. Itoh N, Obato K, Yanaihara N, Okamoto H. Human preprovasoactive intestinal polypeptide contains a novel PHI 27-like peptide PHM-27. Nature 1993;304:547.
292. Bloom SR, Polak JM. Glucagonomas, VIPomas and somatostatinomas. Baillieres Clin Endocrinol Metab 1980;9:285.
293. Modlin IM, Bloom SR, Mitchell SJ. Plasma vasoactive intestinal polypeptide (VIP) levels and intestinal ischemia. Experientia 1978;34:535.
294. Modlin IM, Mitchell SJ, Bloom SR. The systemic release and pharmacokinetics of VIP. In Gut Hormones. Edited by SR Bloom. Edinburgh: Churchill Livingstone, 1978.
295. Bloom SR, Polak JM. Hormone profiles. In Gut Hormones. Edited by SR Bloom, JM Polak. New York: Churchill Livingstone, 1981.
296. Said SI. Vasoactive intestinal polypeptide: elevated plasma and tissue levels in the watery-diarrhea syndrome due to pancreatic and other tumors. Trans Assoc Am Physicians 1975;88:87–93..
297. Binnick AN, Spencer SK, Dennison WL Jr. Glucagonoma syndrome. Arch Dermatol 1977;113:749.
298. McGavran MH, Unger RH, Recant L, Polk HC, Kilo C, Levin ME. A glucagon-secreting alpha-cell carcinoma of the pancreas. N Engl J Med 1966;274:1408.
299. Sweet RD. A dermatosis specifically associated with a tumour of pancreatic alpha cells. Br J Dermatol 1974;90:301.
300. Wilkinson DS. Necrolytic migratory erythema with carcinoma of the pancreas. Trans St Johns Hosp Dermatol Soc 1973;59:244.
301. Grimelius L, Wilander E. Silver stains in the study of endocrine cells of the gut and pancreas. Invest Cell Pathol 1980;3:3.
302. Khandekar JD, Oyer D, Miller HJ, Vick NA. Neurologic involvement in glucagonoma syndrome. Response to combination chemotherapy with 5-fluorouracil and streptozotocin. Cancer 1979;44:2014.
303. Holst JJ. Possible entries to the diagnosis of a glucagon-producing tumour. Scand J Gastroenterol 1979;53(suppl):53.
304. Norton JA, Kahn CR, Schiebinger R, Gorschboth C, Brennan MF. Acid deficiency and the skin rash associated with glucagonoma. Ann Intern Med 1979;91:213.
305. Unger RH, Orci L. Glucagon and the A cell. Physiology and pathophysiology. N Engl J Med 1981;304:1575.
306. Hoitsma HF, Cuesta MA, Starink TM, Uttendorfsky-Vander, Putten HJ, Vander Veen EA. Zinc deficiency syndrome versus glucagonoma syndrome. Arch Chir Neerlandicum 1979;13:131.
307. Montenegro F, Lawrence GD, Macon W, Pass C. Metastatic glucagonoma. Improvement after surgical debulking. Am J Surg 1980;139:424.
308. von Schenck H, Thorell JI, Berg J, Bojs G, Dymling JF, Hallengren B, Liungberg O, Tibblin S. Metabolic studies and glucagon gel filtation pattern before and after surgery in a case of glucagonoma syndrome. Acta Med Scand 1979;205:155–162.
309. Marynick SP, Fagadau WR, Duncan LA. Malignant glucagonoma syndrome: response to chemotherapy. Ann Intern Med 1980;93:453.
310. Conlon JM. The glucagon-like polypeptides—order out of chaos? Diabetologia 1980;18:85.
311. Zollinger RM, Ellison EH. Primary peptic ulcerations of the jejunum associated with islet cell tumors of the pancreas. Ann Surg 1955;39:231.
312. Higgins GA, Recant L, Fischman AB. The glucagonoma syndrome: surgical curable diabetes. Am J Surg 1979;137:142.
313. Villar HV, Johnson DG, Lynch PJ, Pond GD, Smith PH. Pattern of immunoreactive glucagon in portal, arterial and peripheral plasma before and after removal of glucagonoma. Am J Surg 1981;141:48.
314. Vale W, Rivier C, Brown B. Regulatory peptides of the hypothalamus. Annu Rev Physiol 1977;39:473.
315. Creutzfeldt W, Arnold R. Somatostatin and the stomach: exocrine and endocrine aspects. First International Somatostatin Symposium, Freiberg, Germany. Metabolism 1978;27(suppl):1309.
316. Ganda PO, Weir GC, Soeldner JS, et al. Somatostatinoma: a somatostatin-containing tumor of the endocrine pancreas. N Engl J Med 1977;296:963.
317. Krejs GJ, Orci L, Conlon M, et al. Somatostatinoma syndrome (biochemical, morphological, and clinical features). N Engl J Med 1979;301:285.
318. Larsson LI, Hirsch MA, Holst J, et al. Pancreatic somatostatinoma clinical features and physiologic implications. Lancet 1977;1:666.
319. Crain EL Jr, Thorn GW. Functioning pancreatic islet cell adenomas. Medicine 1949;28:427.
320. Fisher RS, Rock E, Levin G, Malmud L. Effects of somatostatin on gallbladder emptying. Gastroenterology 1983;92:885.
321. Axelrod L, Bush MA, Hirsch HJ. Malignant somatostatinoma: clinical features and metabolic studies. J Clin Endocrinol Metab 1981;52:886.
322. Penman E, Wass J, Besser AU, Rees LU. Somatostatin secretion by lung and thymic tumors. Clin Endocrinol (Oxf) 1980;13:613.
323. Boden G, Baile CA, McLaughlin CL, Matschinsky FM. Effects of starvation and obesity on somatostatin, insulin and glucagon release from an isolated perfused organ system. Am J Physiol 1981;241:E215.
324. Creutzfeldt W, Lankisch PG, Folsch UR. Hemmung der Secretin und Cholezystokinin-Pankreozymin-induzierten Saft und Enzymsecretion des Pancreas und der Gallenblasen-Kontraktion beim Menschen durch Somatostatin. Dtsch Med Wochenschr 1975;100:1135.
325. Schwartz TW. Atropine suppression test for pancreatic polypeptide. Lancet 1978;2: 43.
326. Bloom SR, Mortimer CH, Thorner MO, et al. Inhibition of gastrin and gastric-acid secretion by growth-hormone-release-inhibiting hormone. Lancet 1974;2:1106.
327. Vinik AI, Shapiro B, Thompson NW. Plasma gut hormone levels in 37 patient with pheochromocytomas. World J Surg 1985;10:593.
328. Vinik AI, Delbridge L, Moattari R, Cho K, Thompson N. Transhepatic portal vein catheterization for localization of insulinomas: A ten-year experience. Surgery 1991;109:1–11.
329. Bhathena SJ, Higgins GA, Recant L. Glucagonoma and glucagonoma syndrome. In Glucagon. Edited by RH Unger, L Orci. New York: Elsevier/North Holland, 1981, p 413.
330. Jensen RT, Gardner JD, Raufman JP, Pandol SJ, Doppman JL. Zollinger-Ellison syndrome: current concepts and management. Ann Intern Med 1983;98:59.
331. Vinik AI, Levitt NS, Pirnstone BL, Wagner L. Peripheral plasma somatostatin-like immunoreactive responses to insulin hypoglycemia and mixed meal in healthy subjects in non-insulin-dependent maturity-onset diabetes. J Clin Endocrinol Metab 1980;52: 330.
332. Saito S, Saito H, Matsumura M, Sano T. Molecular heterogeneity and biological activity of immunoreactive somatostatin in medullary carcinoma of the thyroid. J Clin Endocrinol Metab 1981;53:1117.
333. Sano T, Kagawa N, Hizawa K, et al. Demonstration of somatostatin production in medullary carcinoma of the thyroid. Jpn J Clin Oncol 1980;10:221.
334. Roos BA, Lindall AW, Ells J, Elde R, Lambert PN, Birnbaum RS. Increased plasma and tumor somatostatin-like immunoreactivity in medullary thyroid carcinoma and small cell lung cancer. J Clin Endocrinol Metab 1981;52:187.
335. Ghose RR, Gupta SK. Oat cell carcinoma of bronchus presenting with somatostatinoma syndrome. Thorax 1981;36:550.

336. Jackson J, Raju U, Janakivamon N, et al. Metastatic pulmonary somatostatin present with diabetic ketoacidosis: clinical biochemical and morphologic characterization. Clin Res 1986;34:196A.
337. Berelowitz M, Szabo M, Barowsky HW, Arbel GR, Frohman LA. Somatostatin-like immunoactivity and biological activity is present in a human pheochromocytoma. J Clin Endocrinol Metab 1983;56:134.
338. Samols E, Weir GC, Ramseur R, Day JA, Patel YC. Modulation of pancreatic somatostatin by adrenergic and cholinergic agonism and by hyper- and hypoglycemic sulfonamides. Metabolism 1978;24:1219.
339. Pipeleers D, Couturier E, Gepts W, Reynders J, Somers G. Five cases of somatostatinoma: clinical heterogeneity and diagnostic usefulness of basal and tolbutamide-induced hypersomatostatinemia. J Clin Endocrinol Metab 1983;56:1236.
340. Chance RE, Jones WE. Polypeptides from bovine, ovine, human, and porcine pancreas. US Patent Office 1974;842:63.
341. Kimmel J, Pollack H, Hazelwood R. Isolation and characterization of chicken insulin. Endocrinology 1968;83:1323.
342. Floyd JC Jr, Vinik AI, Glaser B, et al. Pancreatic polypeptide. In Proceedings of the 10th Congress of the International Diabetes Federation. Edited by W. Waldhusi. Amsterdam: Excerpta Medica, 1979, p 490.
343. Glaser B, Vinik AI, Sive AA, Floyd JJ. Plasma human pancreatic polypeptide responses to administered secretin: effects of surgical vagotomy, cholinergic blockage, and chronic pancreatitis. J Clin Endocrinol Metab 1980;50:1094–1099.
344. Greenberg GR, McCloy RF, Adrian TE, Chadwick VS, Baron JH, Bloom SR. Inhibition of pancreas and gallbladder by pancreatic polypeptide. Lancet 1978;2:1280.
345. Tomita T, Friesen SR, Kimmel JR. Pancreatic polypeptide cell hyperplasia with and without watery diarrhea syndrome. J Surg Oncol 1980;14:11.
346. Bordi C, Togni R, Baetens M, Malaisse-Lagae F, Orci L. Human islet cell tumor storing pancreatic polypeptide: a light and electronic microscopic study. J Clin Endocrinol Metab 1978;46:215.
347. Strodel WE, Vinik AI, Lloyd RV, Glaser B, Eckhauser FE, Fiddian-Green RG, Turcotte JG, Thompson NW. Pancreatic polypeptide-reproducing tumors. Silent lesions of the pancreas. Arch Surg 1984;119:508–514.
348. Larsson LI, Schwartz T, Lundquist G, et al. Pancreatic polypeptide in pancreatic endocrine tumors, possible implication in watery diarrhea syndrome. Am J Pathol 1976;85:675.
349. Larsson LI. Two distinct types of islet abnormalities associated with endocrine pancreatic tumors. Virchows Arch (Pathol Anat) 1977;376:209.
350. Polak JM, Bloom SR, Adrian TE, Heitz P, Bryant MG, Pearse AGE. Pancreatic polypeptide in insulinomas, gastrinomas, vipomas, and glucagonomas. Lancet 1976;1:328.
351. Vinik AI, Glaser B. Pancreatic endocrine tumors. In Pancreatic Disease. Diagnosis and Therapy. Edited by TL Dent. New York: Grune & Stratton, 1981, p 427.
352. O'Dorisio TM, Vinik AI. Pancreatic polypeptide and mixed peptide-producing tumors of the gastrointestinal tract. In Contemporary Issues in Gastroenterology. Edited by S Cohen, RD Soloway. New York: Churchill-Livingstone, 1985, p 117.
353. Friesen SR, Kimmel JR, Tomita T. Pancreatic polypeptide as screening for pancreatic polypeptide apudomas in multiple endocrinopathies. Am J Surg 1980;139:61.
354. Carraway R, Leeman SE. The isolation of a new hypotensive peptide, neurotensin, from bovine hypothalami. J Biol Chem 1973;248:6854.
355. Hammer RA, Leeman SE, Carraway R, Williams R. Isolation of human intestinal neurotensin. J Biol Chem 1980;255:2476.
356. Mitchenere P, Adrian TE, Kirk RM, Bloom SR. Effect of gut regulatory peptides on intestinal luminal fluid in the rat. Life Sci 1981;29:1563.
357. Andersson S, Rosell S, Hjelmquist U, Change D, Folkers K. Inhibition of gastric intestinal motor activity in dogs by (Gln^4)-neurotensin. Acta Physiol Scand 1977;100: 231.
358. Blackburn AM, Fletcher DR, Bloom SR. Effect of neurotensin on gastric function in man. Lancet 1980;1:987.
359. Carraway R, Demers LM, Leeman SE. Hyperglycemic effect of neurotensin, a hypothalamic peptide. Endocrinology 1976;99:1452.
360. Nagai, K, Frohman LA. Hyperglycemia and hyperglucagonemia following neurotensin administration. Life Sci 1976;19:273.
361. Polak JM, Sullivan SN, Bloom SR, Buchan AM, Facer P, Brown MR, Pearse AG. Specific localization of neurotensin to the N cell in human intestine by radioimmunoassay and immunocytochemistry. Nature 1977;270:183.
362. Blackburn AM, Bloom SR. A radioimmunoassay for neurotensin in human plasma. Life Sci 1979;83:175.
363. Besterman HS, Bloom SR, Sarson DL, Blackburn AM, Johnston DI, Patel HR, Stewart JS, Modigliani R, Guerin S, Mallinson CN. Gut hormone profile in coeliac disease. Lancet 1978;1:785.
364. Bloom SR, Lee YC, Lacroute JM, Abbass A, Sondag D, Baumann R, Weill JP. Two patients with pancreatic apudomas secreting neurotensin and VIP. Gut 1983;24:448.
365. Feurle GE, Helmstaeder V, Tischbirek K, Carraway R, Forssmann WG, Grube D, Rohe HD. A multihormonal tumor of the pancreas producing neurotensin. Dig Dis Sci 1981;26:1125.
366. Gutniak M, Rosenqvist U, Grimelius L, Lundberg JM, Hokfelt T, Rokaeus A, Lundquist G, Frahrenkrug J, Sunbad R, Gutniak E. Report on a patient with watery diarrhea syndrome caused by a pancreatic tumour containing neurotensin, enkephalin and calcitonin. Acta Med Scand 1980;208:95.
367. Maier W, Schumacher A, Etzrodt H, Arlart I. A neurotensinoma of the head of the pancreas: demonstration by ultrasound and computed tomography. Eur J Radiol 1982;2: 125.
368. Shulkes A, Boden R, Cook I, Gallagher N, Furness JB. Characterization of a pancreatic tumor containing vasoactive intestinal peptide, neurotensin and pancreatic polypeptide. J Clin Endocrinol Metab 1984;58:41.
369. Wood JR, Wood SM, Lee YC, Bloom SR. Neurotensin-secreting carcinoma of the bronchus. Postgrad Med J 1983;59:46.
370. Brown M, Vale W. Effects of neurotensin and substance P on plasma insulin, glucagon and glucose levels. Endocrinology 1976;98:819.
371. Yallow RS, Berson SA. Immunoassay of endogenous plasma insulin in man. J Clin Invest 1960;39:1157.
372. Dunne MJ, Elton R, Fletcher T, Hofker P, Shul J. Sandostatin and gastroenteropancreatic tumors—therapeutic Characteristics. In Sandostatin in the Treatment of GEP Endocrine Tumors. Edited by TM O'Dorisio. Berlin: Springer Verlag, 1987, p 93.
373. Moattari AR, Cho K, Vinik AI. Sandostatin in treatment of co-existing glucagonoma and pancreatic pseudocyst dissociation of responses. Surgery 1990;108:581.
374. Koelz A, Kraenzlin M, Gyr K, Meier V, Bloom SR, Heitz P, Stalder H. Escape of the response to a long-acting somatostatin analogue (Sandostatin) in patients with VIPoma. Gastroenterology 1987;92:527.
375. Vinik AI, Thompson N, Eckhauser F, Moattari AR. Clinical features of carcinoid syndrome and the use of somatostatin analogue in its management. Acta Oncol 1989;28: 389–402.
376. Vinik AI, Tsai ST, Moattari AR, Cheung P. Somatostatin analogue (SMS 201–995) in patients with gastrinomas. Surgery 1988;104:834.
377. Ajani JA, Kavanaugh J, Patt Y, Levin B, Edwards C, Gutterman J. Roferon and doxorubicin combination active against advanced islet cell or carcinoid tumors. Proc Am Assoc Cancer Res 1989;30:293.
378. Marlink RG, Lokich JJ, Robins JR, Clouse ME. Hepatic arterial embolization for metastatic hormone-secreting tumors. Cancer 1990;65:2227.
379. Rakieten N, Rakieten ML, Nadkani MV. Studies of the diabetogenic action of streptozotocin (NSC-37917). Cancer Chemother Rep 1969;29:91.
380. Murray-Lyon IM, Eddleston AL, Williams R, Brown M, Hogbin BM, Bennett A, Edwards JC, Taylor KW. Treatment of multiple hormone producing malignant islet cell tumour with streptozotocin. Lancet 1968;2:895.
381. Schein PS, Kahn R, Gorden P, Wells S, DeVita VT. Streptozotocin for malignant insulinomas and carcinoid tumors. Arch Intern Med 1973;132:555.
382. Bukowski RM, McCracken JD, Balcerzak SP, Fabian CJ. Phase II study of chlorozotocin in islet cell carcinoma. A Southwest Oncology Group Study. Cancer Chemother Pharmacol 1983;11:48.
383. Hahn RG, Caan A, Kessinger A, Foley JF, Doyal Y, Petrelli N, Tormey D, Smith T. A phase II study of DTIC in the treatment of nonresectable islet cell carcinoma: an ECOG treatment protocol. Proceedings of Annual Meeting, American Society of Clinical Oncology. Proc Am Soc Clin Oncol 1990;9:A417.
384. Saltz L, Lauwers G, Wiseberg J, Kelsen D. A phase II trial of carboplatin in patients with advanced APUD tumors. Cancer 1993;72:619.
385. Frame J, Kelsen D, Kemeny N, Cheng E, Niedzwiecki D, Heelan R, Lippemann R. A phase II trial of streptozotocin and adriamycin in advanced APUD tumors. Am J Clin Oncol 1988;11:490.
386. Eriksson B, Oberg K, Alm G, et al. Treatment of malignant endocrine pancreatic tumors with human leukocyte interferon. Lancet 1986;2:1307.
387. Eriksson B, Oberg K. An update of the medical treatment of malignant endocrine pancreatic tumors. Acta Oncol 1993;32:203.
388. Oberg K, Eriksson B, Janson ET. The clinical use of interferons in the management of neuroendocrine gastroenteropancreatic tumors. Ann N Y Acad Sci 1994;733:471.
389. Moertel CG, Lefkopoula M, Lipsitz M. Streptozocin-Doxorubicin, Streptozocin-Fluorouracil or Chlorozotocin in the treatment of advanced islet-cell carcinoma. N Engl J Med, 1992;326(8):519.
390. Pisegna JR, Slimak GG, Doppman JL, Strader DB, Metz DC, Benya RV, Orbuch M, Fishbeyn VA, Fraker DL, Norton JA, Maton PN, Jensen RT. An evaluation of human recombinant α interferon in patients with metastatic gastrinoma. Gastroenterology, 1993;105:1179.
391. von Eyben FE, Grodum E, Giessing HJ, Hagen C, Nielsen H. Metabolic remission with octreotide in patients with insulinoma. J Intern Med 1994;235(3):245.
392. Arnold R, Benning R, Neuhaus C, Rolwage M, Trautmann ME. Gastroenteropancreatic endocrine tumors: effect of Sandostatin on tumor growth. The German Sandostatin Study Group. Digestion 54 Suppl 1:72, 1993.
393. Seymour MT, Johnson PW, Hall MR, Wrigley PF, Slevin ML. Double modulation of 5-fluorouracil with interferon alpha 2a and high-dose leucovorin: a phase I and II study. Br J Cancer 1994;70(4):719.
394. Moertel CG, Kvols LK, O'Connell MJ, et al. Treatment of neuroendocrine carcinomas with combined Etoposide and Cisplatin. Evidence of major therapeutic activity in the anaplastic variants of these neoplasms. Cancer, 1991;68:227.
395. DiBartolomeo M, Bajetta E, Zilembo N, de Braud F, Di Leo A, Verusio C, D'Aprile M, Scanni A, Barduagni M, et al. Treatment of carcinoid syndrome with recombinant interferon α-2a. Acta Oncol 1993;32(2):235.
396. Tiensuu Janson E, Rönnblom L, Ahlström H, et al. Treatment with alpha-interferon versus alpha-interferon in combination with streptozocin and doxorubicin in patients with malignant carcinoid tumors: A randomized trial. Ann Oncol 1992;3:635.

CHAPTER 104

Pass through to the Gonads

JAMES F. HOLLAND, EMIL FREI, III, ROBERT C. BAST, JR., DONALD W. KUFE, DONALD L. MORTON, AND RALPH R. WEICHSELBAUM

Carcinomas of the ovary and of the testis are not commonly associated with exaggerated endocrine function. Many different carcinomas, sarcomas, and teratomas arise from the gonads, which display their malignant neoplastic character in ways other than endocrine dysfunction. Neoplasms of the gonads are therefore considered with their respective genitourinary organs systems (see Chapters 128 and 133).

SECTION XXIX

NEOPLASMS OF THE HEAD AND NECK

CHAPTER 105

Head and Neck Cancer

GARY L. CLAYMAN, SCOTT M. LIPPMAN, GEORGE E. LARAMORE, AND WAUN KI HONG

Introduction

The National Cancer Institute (NCI) predicted that in 1995 approximately 40,000 new cases of head and neck cancer would be diagnosed in the United States (28,150 with oral cavity and pharyngeal cancer and 11,600 with laryngeal cancer). The same grim reckoning projected more than 12,000 American deaths in 1995 from this class of cancers (62). These diagnosis and mortality figures correspond to over 4% of all new cancer cases and 2% of all cancer deaths in the United States annually. Nearly identical percentages are reported from Britain, but head and neck cancers have a much greater impact in certain other parts of the world and are the leading causes of cancer mortality worldwide (164, 657). Despite improvements in diagnosis and local management, long-term survival rates in head and neck cancer have not increased significantly over the past 30 years and are among the lowest worldwide of the major cancers. For American blacks, survival rates have decreased. Oropharyngeal cancer, the largest subgroup of head and neck cancers, has a 5-year relative survival rate of only 55% for United States whites and 34% for blacks (767). Although early-stage head and neck cancers (especially laryngeal and oral cavity) have high cure rates, over 60% of head and neck cancer patients present with advanced disease. Cure rates decrease, of course, in locally advanced cases, whose probability of cure is inversely related to tumor size and even moreso to the extent of regional node involvement.

Treatment advances have been undermined by the significant percentage of patients initially cured of head and neck squamous cell carcinoma (HNSCC) who go on to develop second primary tumors (427, 715). Second primaries are the major threat to long-term survival after successful therapy of early-stage HNSCC. Their high incidence probably results from the same carcinogenic exposure responsible for the initial primary—a process called field cancerization (see "Biology" below). The clinical significance of second primary tumors is that a patient who presents with HNSCC, even in its earliest stage, is a patient for life.

In addition to the problem of long-term survival in the face of second primary risk, HNSCC patients also can face tremendous reductions in their quality of life after definitive surgical therapy. Despite marked advances in reconstructive surgery and rehabilitation, patients who have undergone laryngectomy, glossectomy, or composite resection can have significant residual cosmetic and functional debilities. These compelling problems are responsible for the emerging importance of primary chemotherapy and chemoprevention of HNSCC.

New strategies for the management of cancers of the mucous membranes of the upper aerodigestive tract (UADT) are badly needed. A team concept is required. Already the role of each treatment modality is becoming more clearly defined. New combined-modality approaches (e.g., sequential and synchronous chemoradiotherapy) and advances in organ preservation and chemoprevention are beginning to offer realistic hopes for improvements in HNSCC patients' survival rates and quality of life. HNSCC research, both clinical and basic, is becoming a model for research into other epithelial cancers. This chapter reviews both the current status of and future investigative directions for the epidemiology, biology, chemoprevention, diagnosis, and therapy of head and neck cancer.

Etiology and Epidemiology

OVERVIEW

The complex process of head and neck carcinogenesis involves dynamic interactions among many factors (27, 91, 164, 464, 590). Approximately 90% of head and neck cancers occur after exposure to known UADT carcinogens. Chief among HNSCC-related carcinogens are tobacco and tobaccolike substances, such as betel leaf. Alcohol use is closely linked to tobacco in this regard and is part of a group of agents that can potentiate tobacco-related carcinogenesis. Other important etiologic factors are viruses, genetic predisposition, occupation, radiation exposure, and diet.

The incidence of HNSCC increases with age, and HNSCC patients typically are older than 50 (105, 177). Several retrospective series report a worse prognosis in younger patients (30 years of age or younger). Other data suggest, however, that the natural history of HNSCC is the same in stage-matched patients regardless of age (114, 441, 607, 633). Confounding factors in younger patients include genetic susceptibility and immunologic profile (580).

Complicating the issues of HNSCC etiology and epidemiology are carcinomas of the salivary gland and nasopharynx. Both cancers are distinct from head and neck cancers at other sites and, therefore, will be considered separately after a general discussion of etiologic factors in head and neck cancer.

TOBACCO AND ALCOHOL EXPOSURE

Tobacco initiates a linear dose–response carcinogenic effect in which duration is more important than the intensity of exposure. The major carcinogenic activity of cigarette smoke resides in the particulate (tar) fraction, which contains a complex mixture of interacting cancer initiators, promoters, and cocarcinogens. Although the risk of bronchogenic carcinoma appears to be less for cigar and pipe smokers, these forms of tobacco use are clearly associated with carcinogenesis of the UADT. The pooling of saliva containing carcinogens in gravity-dependent regions may account for the frequent location of oral SCC along the lateral and ventral surfaces of the tongue and in the floor of the mouth (489). Pipe smokers who have a habitual constant position for the pipe stem may develop carcinoma of the lip at that site, which initiates speculation that physical and thermal trauma may be contributing factors. In heavy smokers, approximately 15 years must pass before the risk is approximately back to the level of people who never smoked (91).

Tobacco is smoked and chewed in daunting quantities. Estimated 1986 world figures for smoking and smokeless tobacco use were 1 billion and 600 million people, respectively Smoking rates are rising by 2% per year in developing countries, offsetting a 1.5% annual decrease in developed nations. Smokeless tobacco use is a growing international problem in many parts of the world, including Asia and Africa. Although overall United States rates have not changed in 30 years, dramatic increases in smokeless tobacco use have occurred among younger people, which may account for the recent excess of oral cancer mortality rates in this group (105, 151, 169, 177, 657, 768).

Striking variations in head and neck cancer sites and incidence are seen among different regions, cultures, and demographic groups, due in large part to differing patterns of tobacco and other substance abuse (59, 169, 177, 657). SCC of the oral cavity and hypopharynx accounts for only 3% of all cancers in the United States, where smokers outnumber chewers, but for 50% of all cancers in Bombay, where "pan" (betel leaf, lime, catechu, and areca nut) is commonly chewed (657). SCC of the hard palate is endemic in other parts of Asia, where reverse chutta (homemade cigar) smoking—burning end held in the mouth—is common. Oral cancer incidence is highest in Southeast Asia, lip cancer in Newfoundland, and nasopharyngeal cancer in southern China. The male-to-female ratios of HNSCC incidence run the gamut from 12:1 in France to 1:1 in Bangalore, India. In the United States, this ratio has changed from about 4:1 40 years ago to about 2:1 today. The United States rates of head and neck cancer have changed over time as tobacco-use habits have shifted. Among American women and nonwhite men, HNSCC incidence and mortality rates have increased over the last 50 years—with the trends most striking for oral cancer (sevenfold increase in women) (177). Increased United States tobacco use among women, adolescents, and children portends increasing national death rates from head and neck cancer in the next several decades (151). In addition to causing head and neck cancer, smoking has also been shown to adversely affect radiotherapy (74).

Although primary, tobacco is not the only factor in the complex causality equation for these cancers. Alcohol is an important promoter of carcinogenesis and is a contributive factor in at least 75% of UADT cancers (59). It has only a modest independent effect, however (653). Studies attempting to correlate types of alcoholic beverages with specific cancer risks have been conflicting. Most investigators believe that ethanol itself is the important factor (363). The major clinical significance of alcohol consumption is that it potentiates the carcinogenic effect of tobacco at every level of tobacco use, and the causative effect is most striking at the highest levels of exposure to both. The magnitude of the effect is midway between additive and multiplicative.

Smoking marijuana appears to confer an even greater risk for HNSCC (but not for lung cancer) than does cigarette smoking (92, 189). Marijuana smoke has a four times higher tar burden and 50% higher concentrations of benzpyrene and aromatic hydrocarbons than are present in tobacco smoke.

VIRUSES

Viruses have been implicated in the pathogenesis of oral, laryngeal, and nasopharyngeal carcinoma (NPC) (69, 222, 316).

Seroepidemiologic studies in oral SCC suggest that herpes simplex virus 1 (HSV-1) may act as a mutagen in the development of this cancer. These studies have shown that patients with oral SCC have increased levels of HSV-1 IgA and IgM antibodies that are of prognostic significance (614). Recent laboratory work, however, has raised questions about the importance of HSV-1 in oral carcinogenesis, since HSV-1 gene products appear in oral SCC tissue only in isolated cases (615). If not critical by itself, HSV-1 still may be a cofactor with other viral or chemical agents in causing oral carcinogenesis.

More recently, an association between head and neck cancer and human papilloma viruses (HPVs) has been hotly pursued (69, 70, 167, 438, 604, 667). HPVs are a family of at least 65 viral subtypes that have been best studied in cervical carcinogenesis and recently linked to other epithelial cancers. Early studies suggested that the HPV-to-verrucous carcinoma relationship is stronger than that between HPV and other types of oral SCC, but they have not been confirmed. Immunohistochemical analysis of HPV capsid antigen and in situ hybridization and polymerase chain reaction studies of HPV DNA suggested the association of HPVs (numbers 6, 11, 16, and 18) with oral carcinogenesis (167, 438, 667). These uncontrolled small studies generated conflicting results, however, and suggested marked overlap between viral expression in oral SCC and in normal oral mucosa. Laryngeal papillomatosis is associated with HPVs 6 and 11, whereas laryngeal SCC is associated with HPVs 16 and 18. HPV DNA is not limited to lesion sites, but is present also in clinically and histologically normal UADT epithelium.

New work using polymerase chain reaction (PCR) probes in controlled studies, coupled with standard epidemiologic analysis data, should provide major insights into the role of HPVs in head-and-neck carcinogenesis.

GENETIC LINKS

Levels of aryl hydrocarbon hydroxylase, the enzyme that activates polycyclic aromatic hydrocarbons (the major carcinogens in cigarette smoke) are greater in laryngeal cancer patients than in controls. An association between the development of HNSCC in patients and specific human leukocyte antigens has also been reported. Recent data from several groups suggest that HNSCC patients have increased sensitivity to clastogen-induced chromosome damage when compared with case controls. A multiplicative risk of HNSCC has been reported when analyzing mutagen-induced chromosome damage and carcinogenic exposure (652). Along with environmental factors, genetic factors may become useful components of quantitative risk-assessment models (434, 583).

OCCUPATION

Although occupational exposures probably play a minor role overall in the development of HNSCC, they are major risk factors for adenocarcinoma of the sinonasal region (37, 91). The most important exposures occur in the environments of nickel refining, woodworking, and leather working. Additionally, thoratrast contrast ingestion has also been related historically to paranasal sinus malignancies. Asbestos exposure may be associated with certain UADT cancers, most notably in the larynx (101).

RADIATION

A strong association no longer exists between exposure to ionizing radiation and the development of squamous carcinoma of the head and neck. Other than in lip cancer, which, like skin cancer, is associated with ultraviolet-B exposure, only two associations are known to exist between radiation and UADT cancers—paranasal sinus cancers related to radium watch dial painting (really mesothorium) and thorotrast ingestion, and thyroid cancers related to radiotherapy (274). Therapeutic irradiation of HNSCC does not appear to induce second primary tumors in the aerodigestive tract. Patients with histories of head and neck irradiation in childhood, however, may have an increased incidence of head and neck sarcomas as adults.

DIET

Considerable epidemiologic evidence suggests that vitamin A and beta-carotene play a protective role in epithelial neoplasia (466). Deficiencies of carotenoids appear to be a risk factor for squamous UADT and lung cancers. It is not known, however, which of the more than 500 carotenoids are protective, what chemical interactions may occur, or what protective role other micronutrients in carotenoid-rich foods may play. Several groups specifically studied the association between dietary vitamin A and/or beta-carotene and risk for oral cancer. Winn and colleagues found that the risk of oral SCC in women was inversely related to the consumption of fresh fruits and vegetables (769). Diets are complex and difficult to assess and validate; in particular, there are often inaccuracies in translating foods into constituent nutrients. Further studies are needed to define sharply the relationship between dietary intake and serum levels of the various carotenoid components. Even in positive studies, it is impossible to determine which of the vast array of compounds is most beneficial, and controlling for other dietary variables and confounding risk factors has remained a difficult methodologic problem. Further confounding this situation, smoking has been associated with reduced dietary intake and serum levels of carotenoids.

Despite their many problems, prospective and retrospective nutritional (serum and dietary) epidemiologic studies, along with basic science research, have provided important clues to the development and prevention of specific cancers. Several large-scale clinical chemoprevention trials of beta-carotene and/or retinol in epithelial neoplasia have been designed on the basis of data from these studies.

SALIVARY GLAND AND NASOPHARYNGEAL CARCINOMA

As stated in the overview, nasopharyngeal and salivary carcinomas, each accounting for 0.2% of all United States cancers, are distinct from those in other head and neck sites (177). Neither has been strongly linked etiologically to tobacco and neither demonstrates the multiple-primary or second-primary patterns of the other head and neck cancer sites (307). Salivary gland cancer incidence has been stable for the past 25 years in the United States. These tumors are similar to nonmelanoma skin cancers and lip cancer in their epidemiologic association with ultraviolet-B and ionizing radiation exposure (44, 535, 618, 654). There may also be an association between breast carcinomas and salivary gland malignancies.

Nasopharyngeal carcinoma (NPC) presents in a younger population than other head and neck cancer sites. Its incidence increases with age, and plateaus at 50 to 60 years. In all races, NPC is twofold to threefold more common in males. It is 20 times more common in Asia than in North America, although in the latter it has an increased frequency among Alaskan natives. This carcinoma's pattern shows decreasing incidence in a gradient from southern to northern regions of China (30 to 50 per 100,000 person-years down to two or three per 100,000). Among Chinese in Hong Kong and Singapore, this is the most common cancer in people 15 to 34 years old (106, 220). Immigrant studies indicate that incidence differences seemingly associated with ethnicity are really largely associated with environment. Americans with Chinese ancestry have an incidence halfway between those of native Chinese and American whites. These are but a few of the wide variations in NPC incidence produced by geographic, ethnic, and cultural differences (106, 220, 307).

Two major, independent risk factors for NPC are salted fish as a diet standard and the Epstein-Barr virus (EBV) (785). Seven studies have used case-control methodology to look at whether eating salted fish correlates with NPC incidence (506). These studies were variously performed in high- and low-risk areas of China. All seven identified salted fish as an independent risk factor (attributable risk of 50%).

Even stronger than that of salted fish is the epidemiologic link between EBV and NPC (132, 220, 221). Regardless of histopathologic subtype (WHO I–III), geographic or ethnic setting, sporadic or endemic pattern, premalignant or malignant status, NPC is an EBV-associated malignancy. Types II and III NPC cells have EBV nuclear antigen (EBNA), DNA, and transmissible virus (104.132). The association between EBV and well-differentiated (WHO type I) NPC was recognized only recently with the detection of EBV genome in type I lesions by recombinant DNA technology (546). NPC may be the best example of a virus-related epithelial carcinoma and has served as a model for the study of virus-induced carcinogenesis elsewhere in the body. The fundamental and early role of EBV in the pathogenesis of NPC is suggested by the recent finding of EBV DNA in premalignant nasopharyngeal lesions. The transformation rate of these lesions, however, only 20%, indicates the importance of additional events in nasopharyngeal tumorigenesis.

Several serologic associations exist between EBV and types II and III NPC (104, 562, 788). Elevated IgG response to EBV capsid antigen (EBVCA) is most sensitive, seen in nearly 100% of types II and III NPC, but is the least NPC specific. The IgA EBVCA serologic measure is more specific but less sensitive. The most specific but least sensitive of current serologic tests is IgA response in a diffuse pattern to EBV early antigen (EBVEA)—positive in 40 to 60% of NPC patients and in fewer than 2% of other HNSCC patients and controls (788). These data illustrate that IgA response to both EBVCA and EBVEA is useful for recognizing occult disease in treated patients and for screening high-risk groups. Recent investigations have proposed PCR screening of metastatic unknown primary carcinomas to the neck for EBV capsid DNA as a molecular marker of NPC in the absence of biopsy-confirmed NPC in any primary site (221). In this regard, the management of unknown primary carcinomas may be altered by contemporary scientific advances.

ETIOLOGIC AND EPIDEMIOLOGIC GOALS

The ultimate goals of epidemiology and etiology are disease prevention and early detection. Studying incidence patterns and risk factors facilitates research and intervention strategies designed ultimately to reduce cancer mortality. Cancers of the head and neck are a devastating group of diseases for which many etiologic factors are known. The strong relationship of NPC with EBV has important diagnostic and therapeutic implications (221), and offers the unique opportunity to develop effective screening for early detection with viral markers in high-risk areas and vaccines for disease prevention (213). Significant efforts should be made toward eliminating, or at least diminishing, the effects of the major known causes of head and neck cancer (225). For example, given the double-barreled multiplicative effect of tobacco and alcohol, substantially reducing the use of either could dramatically reduce rates of HNSCC. Unfortunately, both smoking and drinking have proved so far to be highly resistant to primary-prevention (use-reduction) approaches (127). Some success has been achieved in getting patients to quit smoking after treatment of primary HNSCC: fear of recurrent disease disposes them to heed the physician's advice. Effective tobacco- and alcohol-cessation programs are prerequisite to the control and prevention of HNSCC.

Biology

CARCINOGENESIS (FIELD CANCERIZATION)

Slaughter's classic 1953 report (625) on oral cancer proposed that UADT carcinogenesis is a process of "field cancerization"—the repeated exposure of a region's entire tissue area to carcinogenic insult (e.g., tobacco and alcohol), which increases the tissue's risk for developing multiple independent premalignant and malignant foci (426, 427, 664, 747). This concept (also called field carcinogenesis or condemned-mucosa syndrome) may explain the clinical occurrence of multiple primary and second primary tumors in HNSCC. The data indicate that second primaries, whether synchronous or metachronous, generally are of squamous histology, develop at a constant rate (4 to 7% of treated patients per year), are not treatment related, and occur in the aerodigestive field at risk, that is, the head and neck, the upper two thirds of the esophagus, and the lung (426, 427,715). These characteristics of second primaries support the field cancerization hypothesis. Recent data on p53 mutations provide strong molecular support for the field carcinogenesis concept (109, 616, 632). Despite epidemiologic studies having long associated tobacco and alcohol use with the development of squamous cell carcinoma of the head and neck, the molecular targets of these agents remain to be identified. In recent investigations by Brennan et al. (71) significant tobacco and alcohol use was associated with a high frequency of p53 mutations. Their preliminary results suggest these p53 mutations occur at nonendogenous mutation sites. These findings suggest a role for tobacco in the molecular progression and field carcinogenesis process in head and neck cancer.

Despite intensive study, much of the complex fundamental biology of HNSCC remains poorly understood. Like other epithelial neoplasms, UADT carcinogenesis appears to evolve through a complex multistep process involving certain biomolecular changes that precede premalignant lesions, which in turn precede invasive cancer (63, 64, 197).

On the basis of animal studies, epithelial carcinogenesis has been divided into three phases: initiation, promotion, and progression. Although human neoplasia does not fit neatly into this tripartite framework, the framework serves as a useful model for understanding pharmacologic interventions. Pharmacologic interventions at each phase have attendant advantages and disadvantages. Chemoprevention's greatest potential is in the promotion and progression phases of carcinogenesis.

Occurring within the three-phase model described above, multiple subtle steps of UADT carcinogenesis involve genetic alterations, dysregulated epithelial differentiation, abnormal proliferation, and altered regulatory effects. Although the earliest genetic changes precede the relatively simultaneous occurrences of altered differentiation and proliferation, evolving genetic changes occur as carcinogenesis progresses. One important focus of combined clinical and basic research is to establish specific probes and markers for these carcinogenic steps. These probes would help identify individuals at highest risk of UADT cancer and would act as intermediate–end-point markers for early evaluations of the efficacy of chemopreventive agents (431).

Genetic Alterations. (See also "Molecular Biology")

The degree of genetic damage reflects a composite of carcinogen exposure and inherent tissue sensitivity. Genomic changes accumulate, presumably in the entire carcinogen-exposed tissue. Clonal malignant foci develop only in specific sites, however, where tumorigenesis is possible. Nonspecific (random) genomic alterations indicated by micronuclei, sister-chromatid exchanges, and aneuploidy can occur in normal, premalignant, and malignant aerodigestive tract tissue (50, 190, 409, 563). Although the fundamental genetic events associated with UADT cancers have not yet been established, several nonrandom chromosomal alterations (e.g., alterations in chromosomes 1, 3, 5, 7, 8, 9, 10, 11, 13, and 17) have been detected in HNSCC (fresh-tissue and cell-line studies) (50, 409, 417, 735, 760). Short-term cultures of oral premalignant cells may reveal early nonrandom cytogenetic changes.

Carcinogenesis is thought to be regulated fundamentally by the cellular balance between oncogenes and tumor-suppressor genes. This dynamic relationship is under intensive study in HNSCC (428, 430). Aberrant expressions (amplifications or mutations) of specific families of cellular oncogenes such as *myc*, *ras*, *neu*, *bcl*, *int*, *ems*-1, cyclin D_1 and hst–are associated with ADT carcinogenesis (45, 223, 249, 574, 638). Up to one-third of cases of primary HNSCC demonstrate amplification of either the *int*-2 or *hst*-1 gene (both members of the fibroblast growth-factor gene family) on chromosome 11q13 (45, 631, 696). Little is known, however, about when these events take place during the multistep process or what role their gene products play in regulating growth and differentiation. The families of *ras*, *neu*, and n-*myc* oncogenes are amplified in the more advanced stages of oral SCC, and activated oncogenes of these families in vitro alter the response to differentiation agents and promote uncontrolled cellular growth, aneuploidy, and tumorigenicity (223, 638).

Differentiation Alterations

Dysregulation of differentiation is another hallmark of multistep carcinogenesis. Human oral and esophageal epithelium is stratified squamous in type. Oral mucosa is noncornified except, for the mucosa on the gingiva and dorsal surface of the tongue, which undergo keratinization. Cytokeratins, a family of at least 19 intermediate-sized filaments that range from 40 to 68 kDa, are expressed in different complex patterns that correlate with distinct types of epithelial differentiation and with carcinogenic progression (133, 501, 783).

The spatial distribution of several cytokeratins, involucrin, transglutaminase I, and other differentiation antigens is also altered in dysplasia and carcinoma (93, 133, 154, 429).

Proliferation Alterations

The third major phase of multistep carcinogenesis is dysregulated proliferation. The transition from normal epithelium to hyperplasia and dysplasia is associated with an increased growth fraction and cells proliferating beyond the basal layer. Older histologic assays have correlated this process with increased frequencies of mitotic figures; more recently, DNA flow cytometry and monoclonal-antibody probes to nuclear antigens (e.g., Ki-67 and proliferating-cell nuclear antigen, PCNA) have revealed some strong positive correlations in UADT epithelium between abnormal suprabasal proliferation and later carcinogenic stages (severe dysplasia) (126, 431, 617).

Altered Regulatory Effects

Epithelial carcinogenesis is associated also with the abnormal expression of cellular factors that regulate growth and development. The importance of these factors is inferred from their differential expression in normal and malignant tissues. For example, high expression of epidermal growth factor receptor (EGF-R) is found in a significant fraction of experimental and human SCCs of the UADT (199, 778). EGF-R gene activation occurs early in experimental oral carcinogenesis, and foci of cells expressing EGF-R can be found in human premalignant lesions. Similarly, high expression of transforming growth factor-alpha (TGF-α) has been associated with malignant transformation of a variety of tumors (including oral cancers), and is frequently accompanied by elevated levels of EGF-R in SCC (276, 690). The relationship between high TGF-α and high EGF-R suggests that an autocrine loop mechanism drives the dysregulation of proliferation.

MOLECULAR BIOLOGY

As advances in molecular biology and biotechnology continue at a rapid pace, our understanding of the initiation and progression of carcinogenic processes will follow. The most frequent molecular abnormalities in these cancers, to date, are mutations in the tumor suppressor gene, p53, which occur at a rate of approximately 40 to 70% (69, 637). Mutations of p53 are present in premalignant areas, including carcinoma in situ or moderate to severe dysplasia, in approximately 20% of cases (67). No other oncogene or tumor suppressor gene has been found to be mutated as frequently as p53 in head and neck tumor specimens. Other genes have been investigated in these cancers, including the tumor suppressor gene Rb, and several oncogenes, such as *ras*, *myc*, *int*-2, *bcl*-1, cyclin D_1 and C-*erb*/*neu*; despite these studies, predictors of response to therapy, phenotypic behavior (478), and survival remain elusive (223, 478).

Biotechnology and scientific advances have also allowed identification of areas of frequent chromosomal loss, termed loss of heterozygosity (LOH). In head and neck cancer, LOH is frequent among chromosomes 3p, 17p, 13q, 11q, 6p, 9p, and 14q (705). These studies may lead to the identification of putative tumor suppressor genes in these malignancies as well as an understanding of the progression to malignancy.

The concepts of multistep carcinogenesis and field carcinogenesis have now been formulated in molecular biologic terms. The carcinogen-containing environment that initiated tumorigenesis has also affected the nontransformed surrounding tissues. Chromosome labeling and LOH studies have shown that LOH at 9p and abnormalities in chromosome 11 are present in histologically normal mucosa adjacent to tumors, supporting the field hypothesis (705).

Once a head and neck cancer has developed, its phenotypic behavior (the ability to invade, metastasize, respond to radiotherapy, and recur) is dependent on complex microenvironmental and biologic systems. Invasive and metastatic capabilities of a tumor depend on degradative enzymes, including collagenases, plasminogen activators (including urokinase), and cathepsin, as well as angiogenic factors, growth factors, cytokines, receptors, cell-surface properties, and motility factors. The tumor milieu is also influenced by nerve fibers, stromal cells, and tumor-associated and tumor-infiltrating lymphocytes. All of these characteristics provide attractive targets for new and more specific therapeutic approaches.

IMMUNOLOGY

A variety of immunologic abnormalities occur in HNSCC, but precise cause-and-effect relationships between abnormalities and cancer remain unclear (372). Both cellular and humoral immunity have important implications for HNSCC prognosis and therapy.

Cell-mediated immunity may be involved in tumor control (579). Defective cell-mediated immunity as determined by NK activity, skin tests, and other measures correlates with advanced disease, early recurrence, and poor survival. Large variations in tumor-infiltrating lymphocyte (TIL) levels in HNSCC have been reported. TILs in HNSCC are primarily CD3+ T cells (NK cells are rare), and 30 to 50% of TILs express HLA-DR–activation antigens. The prognostic significance of tumor-infiltrating cell subsets is unclear (310, 774).

Most recent work in HNSCC immunology has focused on humoral immune status. A large body of growing evidence suggests that humoral immunity plays a negative role in HNSCC (663). Increased serum levels of IgA, IgM, and immune complexes are associated with advanced disease and poor prognosis (498). Increased IgA can block many aspects of the host cell–mediated immune response, including cytotoxic effects of sensitized lymphocytes, NK cells, and macrophages, and IgG-mediated antibody-dependent cell-mediated cytotoxicity (ADCC). In contrast, increased IgE is associated with a good prognosis in HNSCC. The ratio of IgA to IgE, therefore, may be more predictive of prognosis than either IgA or IgE is individually. Posttreatment patterns of IgA and immune complexes differ: immune complex levels more accurately reflect tumor burden.

Although multiple and prominent immunologic deficits occur in HNSCC, immunologic therapeutic approaches (IFN-α, interleukin-2 [IL-2], plasmapheresis) have yielded only modest response rates and short response durations (see "Immunobiologic Therapy" below).

BIOLOGIC GOALS

Several nonrandom chromosomal alterations, activated oncogenes, and loss of heterozygosity sites likely for tumor-suppressor genes are being actively investigated to develop informative biologic and predictive markers for HNSCC. The recent development of antibody probes for key gene products and molecular probes for gene transcripts should allow future study to identify the timing and sequence of gene alterations during multistep UADT carcinogenesis.

The mechanisms of HNSCC invasion and metastasis are not well established. Recent studies have identified specific membrane proteins, degradative enzymes, and binding sites required for SCC invasion and metastasis (in animal models) and associated with early recurrence (in clinical studies) (93). This work opens the way to novel therapeutic approaches for future use of directed monoclonal antibodies/inhibitors to block key binding sites, thus preventing tumor invasion and metastasis.

Advances in molecular biology and biotechnology are also expanding our concept of the capabilities for molecular (or gene) therapy (117, 435). Novel gene intervention strategies may be applicable for augmenting immune response, delivering a toxic gene or metabolite, alternating chemo or radiation sensitivity, or inducing cell cycle control or cell death. Further studies that demarcate critical molecular events in the HNSCC progression model may be essential for gene therapy prevention strategies.

Chemoprevention Approaches

OVERVIEW

The control and management of HNSCC are hindered tremendously by poor overall survival rates and the high risk of second primary tumors in early-stage cases. Compounding these issues are severe disfigurements and debilities resulting from definitive local therapy of head and neck tumors. Although tobacco and alcohol cessation is of primary importance, cessation approaches have not succeeded in significantly reducing exposure to these carcinogens (127). Consequently, chemoprevention very recently has come to the forefront of head and neck cancer research efforts (323–325, 424–428, 434, 440).

In the mid-1970s, Michael Sporn of the NCI coined the term "chemoprevention"—the pharmacologic inhibition of carcinogenesis or its reversal in premalignant stages (655). Current HNSCC chemopreventive strategy focuses strongly on retinoids in oral premalignancy and in the adjuvant prevention of second primary tumors. The term "retinoid" was coined in 1976, also by Dr. Sporn (656). Ultimately, this study hopes to find effective agents or dietary manipulations with little or no toxicity for use in largely healthy subjects at risk (56, 162). (See Chapters 27, 28, and 29.) Another major focus of this work is on potential biologic markers of intermediate endpoints (431).

Anatomy

OVERVIEW

The term "cancer of the head and neck" describes a diverse collection of cancers of varying histologies arising from a variety of anatomic sites that make up the UADT (142). The UADT consists of a complex mucosa-covered conduit for food and air that extends from the vermilion surface of the lips to the cervical esophagus. In common usage, this terminology has been applied primarily to those cancers arising from the mucosal surfaces of the lips, oral cavity, pharynx, larynx, and cervical esophagus. Included in this designation, however, are other important sites, such as the nose and paranasal sinuses, salivary glands (major and minor), thyroid and parathyroid, and melanoma and nonmelanoma skin cancers. Some cancers arising in this region are typically excluded from the generic designation of "head and neck cancer." Examples are tumors of the central nervous system, ocular neoplasms, primary tumors of lymphatic origin, and neural and endocrine malignancies.

Because of the diversity of sites and tissues of origin, the biology of tumor growth, patterns of metastases, natural boundaries for tumor extension, and signs and symptoms of disease are quite varied. The anatomy of the region has also dictated that optimal evaluation, diagnosis, and treatment require specific multidisciplinary expertise that frequently crosses traditional training backgrounds to include neurosurgery, otolaryngology, head and neck surgery, oral surgery, cosmetic and reconstructive disciplines, and specialized radiology, pathology, radiation therapy, and chemotherapy. The clinical manifestations of disease are varied and have a significant impact on the cosmetic and functional integrity of the head and neck region. Although the anatomic structures are only millimeters apart, the low metastatic potential and high curability of vocal cord cancers stand in extreme contrast to the early dissemination and grim prognosis of stage-matched pyriform sinus cancers (39, 204, 235, 545, 584, 704). Clinical differences between cancers in different sites are not explained solely by anatomic factors but by major biologic differences. Regrettable, the relatively small number of head and neck cancer patients (in the United States, 40,000 annual diagnoses of HNSCC) often requires grouping many different types in each HNSCC therapy trial (767). Associated morbidities of disease and treatment involve all of the special senses to varying degrees, notably speech, swallowing, smelling, breathing, and mastication—functions critically important for social interaction, a good quality of life, and survival.

ORAL CAVITY

The oral cavity includes the lips, buccal mucosa, anterior tongue, floor of the mouth, hard palate, upper gingiva, and lower gingiva. The tongue occupies a major portion of the oral cavity and is contiguous with the floor of the mouth. The gingival mucosa overlying the mandibular and maxillary alveolar ridges is closely adherent to the underlying periosteum. The hard palate forms the roof of the oral cavity and consists of mucosa overlying the palatine portion of the maxilla extending from the superior alveolar ridge to the junction with the soft palate.

PHARYNX

The pharynx is a musculomembranous tube extending from the skull base to the level of the sixth cervical vertebra, supported by overlapping constrictor muscles (superior, middle, and inferior) and other muscles arising from the styloid process and skull base.

The region of the oropharynx consists of a complex three-dimensional musculomembranous conduit communicating with the oral cavity anteriorly, the nasopharynx superiorly, and the hypopharynx/larynx inferiorly. It is divided into four sites of clinical importance (*a*) the tonsillar area, which makes up the major portion of the lateral pharyngeal wall and blends with the tongue base, palate, and retromolar trigone; (*b*) the tongue base; (*c*) the soft palate; and (*d*) the posterior pharyngeal wall. Innervation of the pharynx is via the pharyngeal plexus with contributions from the glossopharyngeal (sensory) and vagus nerves (motor and sensory).

The hypopharynx is divided into three distinct regions: the pyriform sinuses, the posterior surface of the larynx (postcricoid area), and the inferior, posterior, and lateral pharyngeal walls. The pyriform sinus (a recess) is a paired mucosal cul-de-sac lying lateral to each side of the larynx, bounded superiorly by the pharyngoepiglottic folds and inferiorly by the cricoid cartilage.

LARYNX

The larynx consists of a mucosally covered cartilaginous framework (thyroid and cricoid cartilages) attached above to the hyoid bone by the thyrohyoid membrane and below to the trachea. The opening to the larynx is continuous with the pharyngeal airway. Unlike the rest of the pharynx, the mucosa of the larynx consists largely of columnar ciliated respiratory-type epithelium, although stratified squamous epithelium is found on the upper posterior epiglottis, aryepiglottic folds, and true vocal cords. Submucosal lymphatics in the upper larynx are extensive whereas they are sparse in the true vocal cords.

The larynx is divided into three anatomic regions: the supraglottic larynx, the glottic larynx, and the subglottic larynx. The supraglottic larynx includes the epiglottis, aryepiglottic folds, laryngeal surface of the arytenoids, false vocal cords, and ventricles. The glottic larynx is derived from the tracheobronchial anlage and consists of both true vocal cords and the mucosa of the anterior and posterior commissures extending 1 cm below the free edge of the vocal folds. The subglottic larynx consists of the region bounded by the vocal cords above and the inferior border of the cricoid cartilage. Lymphatic supply to the subglottic larynx is extensive and bilateral. The infraglottic lymphatics drain to the cervical nodes through the cricothyroid membrane, while supraglottic lymphatics drain through the thyrohyoid membrane.

NECK

Anatomic considerations in the treatment of cancers of the head and neck must include a thorough understanding of the neural, vascular, and lymphatic structures of the neck. Detailed anatomic studies have described the organization of the lymphatic drainage of the upper aerodigestive tract. Specific regions of the head and neck and the tumors that arise there have lymphatic drainage, which is consistent and predictable. There are 10 major groups of lymph nodes in the head and neck (Fig. 105.1). Primary and secondary echelons of lymph node drainage have been derived for each major region of the head and neck mucosa. The lip, cheek, and anterior gingiva drain to submandibular and submental lymph node groups. In addition, the cheek and upper lip also drain to inferior parotid nodes, while the posterior gingiva and palate drain to the internal jugular chain and lateral retropharyngeal groups. Lymphatic drainage for the tongue can be crossed and drains to the internal jugular, subdigastric, omohyoid, submandibular, and submental nodal groups. Although metastases to the lower neck nodes are infrequent from the oral cavity, generally the more anterior the tumor location in the tongue, the more likely it is that metastases also will spread to lower jugular nodes. The floor-of-mouth drainage is similar to that of the tongue. The upper portion of the pharynx drains directly to the upper cervical lymph nodes along the internal jugular chain. The oropharynx and tonsil drain through the peripharyngeal space to the midjugular region, particularly to the jugulodigastric nodes. The regions of the hypopharynx and larynx drain primarily along the routes of their vascular supply to either the deep cervical nodes along the midjugular (upper pharynx, larynx) or the deep nodes along the lower jugular and peritracheal region (lower pharynx, larynx).

For the purposes of local treatment, the various lymph node groups of the neck have been divided into five levels (Fig. 105.2). Level I includes the submental group of nodes located within the triangle bounded by the anterior belly of the digastric muscles and the hyoid bone and the submandibular group bounded by the digastric muscle and the body of the mandible. Level II nodes consist of the upper jugular lymph nodes located in proximity to the upper third of the internal jugular vein and extending from the skull base to the level of the bifurcation of the carotid artery. The anterior and posterior boundaries are the lateral border of the sternohyoid muscle and the posterior border of the sternocleidomastoid muscle, respectively. Level III nodes include those nodes located adjacent to the middle third of the internal jugular vein from the carotid bifurcation to the omohyoid muscle (level of the cricothyroid notch). Anterior and posterior boundaries are the same as level II. Level IV nodes include the lower jugular group extending from omohyoid muscle to the clavicle below. Level V nodes are those located along the lower half of the spinal accessory nerve and transverse cervical artery. This level is bounded by the anterior border of the trapezius muscle, the posterior border of the sternocleidomastoid muscle, and the clavicle below.

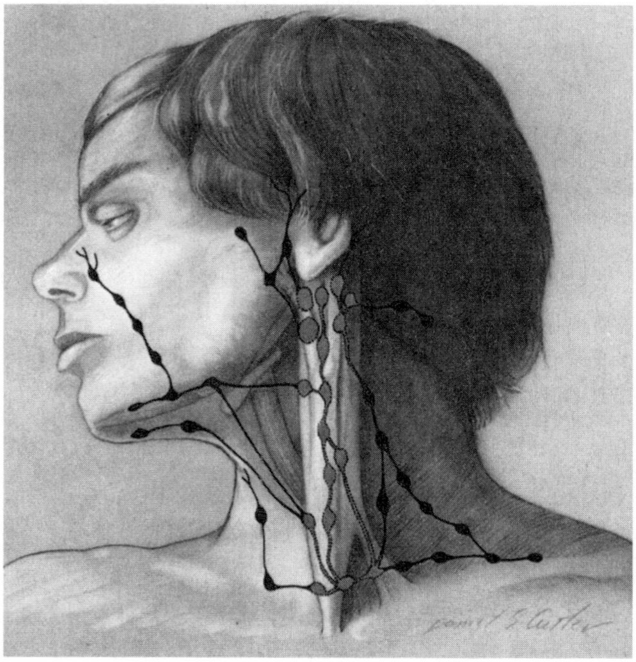

Figure 105.1. Major lymph node groups in the head and neck. These include occipital, mastoid, parotid, submandibular, facial, submental, sublingual, retropharyngeal, anterior cervical, and lateral cervical lymph node groups.

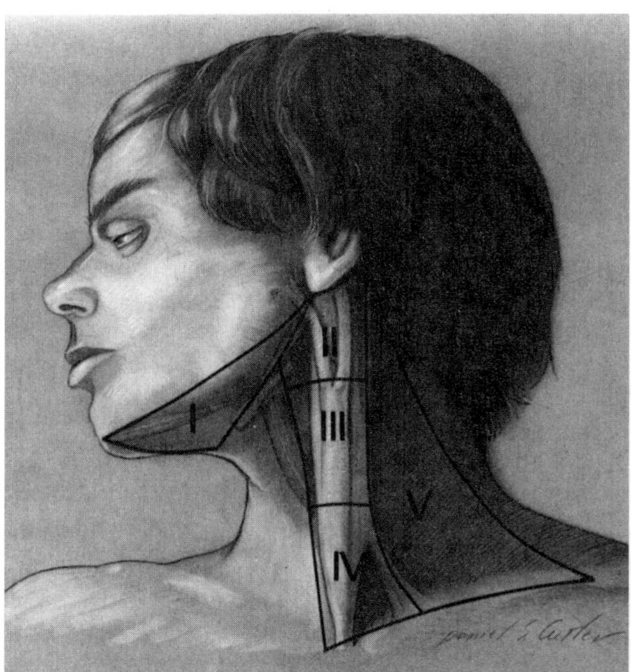

Figure 105.2. Division of lymph nodes by level. A system of five levels of lymph node groups in the lateral neck is used clinically to describe lymph node location. Level I includes submental and submandibular groups. Level II is upper jugular lymph nodes. Level III is middle jugular lymph nodes. Level IV is lower jugular lymph nodes. Level V is posterior cervical lymph nodes. A variably used designation is level VI, for lymph nodes of the anterior cervical compartment.

Pathology

HISTOLOGY AND PROGNOSIS

More than 90% of head and neck cancers of the upper aerodigestive tract are squamous carcinomas (40). Additional information usually reported by the pathologist includes tumor grade or differentiation. Traditionally, tumor grading has been based on criteria developed over 50 years ago by Broder (73, 145). Unfortunately, differentiation grade has not been consistently accurate in reflecting the biologic aggressiveness of squamous carcinomas (145). The difficulty in predicting the behavior of individual tumors, however, is well recognized. Prognosis is influenced by many factors other than grade (627, 773). These include tumor size, site, vascularity, lymphatic drainage, and host immune response; the patient's age, sex, nutritional status, and performance status; and other, as yet unrecognized variables.

The comprehensive histologic evaluation of squamous carcinomas includes characteristics of tumor–host interactions. Their incorporation into the determination of tumor grade was pioneered by Jakobsson and colleagues (354). Characteristics considered include degree of keratinization, nuclear grade, mitotic rate, inflammatory response, vascular-stromal response, vascular invasion, and pattern of invasion. These characteristics have variably correlated with biologic behavior. Keratinization is the major determinant of Broder grade. Better-differentiated tumors that produce more keratin are thought to be less likely to metastasize. Nuclear grade assesses nuclear pleomorphism. Enlarged, hyperchromatic nuclei are associated with less-differentiated tumors. Nuclear grade accurately predicts the behavior of advanced laryngeal cancers (776). Enlarged nuclear size and staining presumably reflect chromosomal abnormalities and increased DNA content. Numerous studies of DNA content have demonstrated high rates of aneuploidy in squamous cancers that range from 50 to 70%. Aneuploidy has been associated with poor prognosis (212, 392). Mitotic rate and labeling index have also been used to reflect proliferative activity, but large-scale studies of head and neck cancers have been lacking.

Features reflecting aggressive disease include lymphatic invasion, perineural invasion, lymph node metastases, and penetration of the tumor through the capsule of involved lymph nodes (extracapsular spread). The presence of regional lymph node metastases is the most important determinant of prognosis in head and neck cancer and is associated with a 50% decrease in survival rates as compared with patients without regional metastases.

More recently, the histologic pattern of invasion of these cancers was systematically studied. Tumors that invade with thin, fingerlike projections or single disassociated cells behave more aggressively regardless of differentiation grade and tend to be associated with vascular and neural invasion (354). The presence of extracapsular spread of tumor in the neck has been directly associated with high rates of distant metastases. These various histologic features play an important role in therapeutic decision making.

MOLECULAR PATHOLOGY

The head-and-neck surgical oncologist relies heavily on the histopathologic assessment of surgical margins to ensure total excision of the tumor in patients with head and neck cancer. Currently, surgeons depend on frozen-section analysis of margins to assess these issues. Recently, Sidransky et al. proposed using contemporary molecular techniques to determine whether clonal populations of infiltrating tumor cells harboring mutations of the p53 gene could be detected in histopathologically negative surgical margins and cervical lymph nodes of patients with squamous cell carcinoma of the head and neck (72). They found that 38% (5 of 13) of patients had molecular positive margins and approximately 50% had molecular identification of p53 mutations in histopathologically negative lymph nodes. Patients with these molecular positive margins had an increased risk of local recurrence. Although advances in molecular techniques are likely to augment enormously what is now considered standard histopathologic assessment, critical studies will be required to determine the meaning and impact of this new pathologic information and appropriate management steps that result.

Diagnosis

The identification and appropriate management of premalignant mucosal lesions in the head and neck are important aspects of patient management that have major impact on overall survival rates. Since stage (extent) of disease at the time of diagnosis is the most important prognostic factor in the treatment of HNSCC, the identification and early treatment of small cancers correlate with excellent survival statistics. Most early premalignant changes or in situ carcinomas of the oral mucosa occur as red (erythroplasia) or white (leukoplakia) patches that should be readily apparent on visual examination. In areas less easily visualized directly, such as the larynx and hypopharynx, early lesions cause such symptoms as chronic hoarseness, chronic sore throat, referred otalgia, or dysphagia. These symptoms demand visualization of the involved structures by direct or indirect laryngoscopy.

Appropriate management of leukoplakia and erythroplasia lesions includes a high index of suspicion, particularly in high-risk individuals. Although both lesions are considered premalignant, erythroplasia lesions are of greater clinical concern since approximately half of these lesions contain carcinoma in situ (CIS) or invasive cancer. Additionally, often erythroplasia and leukoplakia may coexist (63, 64). Erythroplasia mandates biopsy to rule out invasive cancer. The management of erythroplasia and leukoplakia depends on the location, extent, and histology. The diffuse field effect and multifocal nature of the epithelial carcinogenic process support the need for effective chemoprevention (see Chapter 29). White lesions can be confused with mucositis; lichen planus; local tissue irritation from mechanical, thermal, or chemical trauma; histoplasmosis; candidiasis; and other infectious processes. Lesions that persist despite the removal of local irritating factors, or that are associated with ulceration, vertical growth, induration, a recent change in size, or pain, should be biopsied. Topical supravital staining with toluidine blue of suspicious lesions can be helpful in identifying areas to biopsy and in screening high-risk populations.

Dysphagia, odynophagia, otalgia (referred), hoarseness, mucosal irregularities and ulceration, pain, weight loss, and the presence of an unexplained neck mass are the common presenting complaints of HNSCC. The predominant symptoms vary with the site: chronic dysphagia or odynophagia (for 6 weeks or even less) demands thorough visualization of the oropharynx, hypopharynx, and esophagus; chronic hoarseness demands visualization of the larynx; chronic, unilateral serous otitis media in an adult is a result of cancer of the nasopharynx until proved otherwise; and unilateral nasal polyps, nasal obstruction, or epistaxis is a common presenting sign of nasal cavity or paranasal sinus neoplasm. A firm or hard unilateral neck mass represents cancer until proved otherwise. More than 80% of the time, such a mass represents neoplasm, and 80% of these neoplasms are due to metastatic spread from an UADT primary.

In patients presenting with a suspicious neck mass, a complete head and neck examination usually reveals the primary malignant tumor. If it does not, a thorough search for occult primary cancers both above and below the clavicles is warranted. Technologic advances in fiberoptics and in flexible and rigid endoscopes now provide excellent upper airway visualization that previously required special skills in indirect mirror examination. Endoscopic evaluation should include the nasopharynx, oropharynx, hypopharynx, larynx, and esophagus. Endoscopic evaluation should be preceded by a barium swallow and chest radiograph. Most commonly, occult primaries responsible for neck metastases occur in the nasopharynx, tongue base, tonsil or hypopharynx. In the absence of an identifiable mass, directed biopsies of these sites are indicated during endoscopic evaluation. Metastasis to a solitary left supraclavicular lymph node (Virchow's node) is occasionally seen with intra-abdominal cancer. Generally, metastatic supraclavicular masses derive from breast, lung or infradiaphragmatic neoplasms. Nevertheless, thyroid malignancies may also metastasize to this area. Three-dimensional imaging with computer tomography (CT) and magnetic resonance imaging (MRI) is frequently used to supplement the clinical evaluation and staging of the primary tumor and regional lymph nodes.

Only after a thorough search for a primary tumor has been completed should a neck mass undergo biopsy. We recommend fine-needle aspiration biopsy when this is feasible. If an excisional biopsy is required for the biopsy of a neck mass, the surgeon and patient should be prepared for definitive neck dissection if the mass should prove to be metastatic squamous carcinoma. The introduction of fine-needle aspiration of neck masses has gained wide acceptance in the early evaluation of such masses and frequently supplements the diagnostic workup (221). The potential ramifications of false-negative results are inherently obvious. Accuracy of the cytologic interpretation of the aspirate is directly dependent on the skill and experience of the pathologist.

STAGING

Staging criteria for cancers arising in the upper aerodigestive tract, paranasal sinuses, and salivary glands have been developed by the American Joint Committee on Cancer (AJCC). The criteria undergo regular reevaluation and modification. The stage groupings utilized for head and neck cancer are based on T (primary tumor), N (regional node), and M (distant metastasis) designations. Because of variations in the growth, behavior, and prognosis of head and neck cancers according to site of origin and extent, differences exist in the staging criteria for each anatomic site and region in the head and neck. Despite the variations in primary tumor staging parameters, the characteristics used for staging regional nodes and distant metastases are uniform for all sites (Tables 105.1 and 105.2).

Careful documentation of tumor extent and accurate staging classification are also important for the comparison of the results of different treatment regimens. Accurate evaluation of the results of a given treatment or the efficacy of new treatment strategies requires comparisons with patient groups with tumors of similar extent and behavior. Restaging after treatment, or for recurrent cancers, must be clearly designated and separate from the primary staging of previously untreated cancers. Postsurgical, or pathologic, staging is gaining importance in the primary treatment of head and neck cancers because of the increasing use of postop-

Table 105.1. Clinical Tumor Stage and Groupings for Head and Neck Cancer

Stage 0	Tis	N0	M0
Stage 1	T1	N0	M0
Stage 2	T2	N0	M0
Stage 3	T3	N0	M0
	T1	N1	M0
	T2	N1	M0
	T3	N1	M0
Stage 4	T4	Any N	M0
	Any T	N2, 3	M0
	Any T	Any N	M1

Table 105.2. Clinical Tumor Staging Characteristics for Regional Lymph Nodes and Distant Metastases

Regional Lymph Nodes (N)	
Nx	Regional lymph nodes cannot be assessed
N0	No regional lymph node metastases
N1	Metastasis in a single ipsilateral lymph node, 3 cm or less in greatest dimension
N2a	Metastasis in a single ipsilateral lymph node, more than 3 cm, but not more than 6 cm in greatest dimension
N2b	Metastasis in multiple ipsilateral lymph nodes, none greater than 6 cm in greatest dimension
N2c	Metastasis in bilateral or contralateral lymph nodes, none greater than 6 cm in greatest dimension
N3	Metastasis in a lymph node greater than 6 cm in greatest dimension
Distant Metastases (M)	
Mx	Presence of distant metastasis cannot be assessed
M0	No distant metastasis
M1	Distant metastasis

erative radiation therapy and/or adjuvant chemotherapy for patients with specific tumor characteristics, such as histologically proved lymph node metastases, close surgical margins, or extracapsular spread into the soft tissues of the neck (360).

Treatment

GENERAL PRINCIPLES

After a histologic diagnosis has been established and tumor extent determined, the selection of appropriate treatment for a specific cancer depends on a complex array of variables, including tumor site, respective morbidity of various treatments, patient performance and nutritional status, concomitant health problems, social and logistic factors, therapy anticipated for potential recurrences or second primaries, and patient preference. These variables are each considered with respect to the established effectiveness of various treatment regimens available (Table 105.3).

Several generalizations are useful in therapeutic decision making, but variations on these themes are numerous. Surgical resection and radiation therapy are the mainstays of treatment for most head and neck cancers. For small primary cancers without regional metastases (stage I or II), wide surgical excision alone or curative radiation therapy alone is used. Functional and cosmetic results are usually better following radiotherapy. Local tumor control rates are generally better with primary surgical resection, but if local recurrences occur after primary radiation therapy, they can often be successfully treated with salvage surgery, resulting in similar overall survival rates. Surgical complication rates are generally increased following radiation. Salvage of surgical recurrences by radiation therapy is less effective than is surgical salvage of radiation failures.

For more extensive primary tumors or regional metastases (stage III or IV), planned combinations of pre- or postoperative radiation and complete surgical excision are generally used (258). For selected patients with advanced cancers of specific sites, such as the larynx, treatment approaches with

Table 105.3. Therapeutic Approaches in Head and Neck Cancer

Established
Definitive surgery (S)
Definitive radiation therapy (RT)
Surgery and planned preoperative or postoperative RT
Definitive RT with surgery reserved for salvage of recurrence
Palliative radiation therapy
Palliative chemotherapy
Investigational
Induction chemotherapy and S or RT
Induction chemotherapy with curative RT (organ preservation)
Concomitant chemoradiotherapy
S or RT and adjuvant chemotherapy
RT and adjunctive hyperthermia or radio-sensitizers
Altered fractionation RT
Immunobiologic therapy
Chemoprevention

radiation alone, with surgery held in reserve for salvage of recurrences, have been utilized in attempts to preserve structure and function. Although these organ-preserving techniques have been successful in many patients, they were generally associated with lower overall survival rates (158, 172, 374, 396, 517, 534).

The overall management goals in treating patients with head and neck cancer are to achieve the highest cure rates at the lowest cost in terms of functional and cosmetic morbidity. These goals include early diagnosis, effective rehabilitation, and appropriate palliation when cancers are incurable. The achievement of these goals requires the close interaction and cooperation of a multidisciplinary team of practitioners representing surgery, radiation, chemotherapy, prosthodontics, dentistry, social services, dietetics, physical medicine, pathology, nursing, and sometimes psychiatry.

Effective rehabilitation is an important part of the overall treatment of head and neck cancers. Modern advances in surgical reconstruction, microvascular free-tissue transfer, and prosthodontics have significantly improved functional performance (30). Rehabilitation concerns must be addressed at initial treatment planning and carefully integrated with the various treatment modalities used (see Chapter 89). Pretreatment dental evaluations and speech and swallowing assessments are routine. Needed dental care and/or extractions should be planned prior to chemotherapy or radiation to reduce dental-associated sepsis, mucositis, and osteoradionecrosis. The overall impact of treatment and rehabilitation decisions on a patient's quality of life is an important issue that may require utilization of specialized social or psychiatric support systems for the patient and family. Finally, the prolonged nature of treatment for advanced disease, which may extend over many months, requires consideration of the social and financial effect of treatment decisions on the patient, the family, and the patient's employer.

Biopsies of primary tumors should not be excisional unless the biopsy procedure is sufficient for definitive treatment and the surgeon performing the excision is responsible for providing curative treatment. Oncologic principles of surgical resection must not be compromised by ill-conceived reconstructive efforts or attempts at modifying the necessary resection in order to minimize functional or cosmetic morbidity. Head and neck cancers are serious threats to life. Temporary preservation of function at the cost of high morbidity and death from recurrent cancer is a poor bargain. Positive surgical margins after tumor resection or gross residual cancer portends inevitable treatment failure. Molecular pathologic staging may identify other patients earlier, where additional therapy may be essential to achieve cure (72). Appropriate management must also include the utilization of precise modern techniques of conservative surgical resection (e.g., partial laryngectomy and functional neck dissection) that, in selected patients, have cure rates similar to those of more radical techniques (408).

RADIOTHERAPY

General

Radiation therapy is an effective modality in treating local/regional disease. For early (T1 and T2) lesions, it gives results comparable to those achieved by surgery. For certain tumor sites, such as the larynx, it is preferred over surgery in the treatment of early tumors because it maintains organ function. When lesions are intermediate in size, it is used adjuvantly (following surgical excision) to improve local/regional control. Vikram and colleagues found that the rates of local/regional tumor recurrence were markedly higher if there was a greater than 6-week delay between surgery and postoperative radiotherapy (719). For advanced, inoperable lesions, and for lesions arising in certain sites, such as the nasopharynx, radiation therapy may be the only modality that offers a potential for cure. Its therapeutic effectiveness has now been enhanced by the concomitant use of chemotherapy.

Ionizing radiation (high-energy photons, electrons, neutrons, charged particles) interacts with matter in subtle ways (292). Tumors can vary dramatically in their ability to repair the DNA damage inflicted by radiation. Hyperthermia and concomitant chemotherapy are methods of reducing this repair ability. HNSCCs are generally characterized as moderately radioresponsive, meaning that fairly large dosages of radiation are required to achieve high probabilities of tumor control. Fortunately, the required dosages are within the tolerance of the various critical structures of the head and neck.

The effectiveness of a given quantity of radiation depends on the manner in which it is given (292). Many different radiation treatment schedules are in use, or under investigation in controlled clinical trials. Over the past 20 years in the United States, however, a regimen of 180 to 200 cGy once a day for 5 days a week has become standard for most head and neck cancer patients. This schema evolved empirically to allow the regeneration of normal tissues during the course of radiotherapy. Radiation kills the stem cells in the basal layer, and several weeks later, the cells in the superficial layers are not replaced when they are lost through normal physiologic processes. This denudes the epithelium, giving rise to the mucositis reaction that can greatly inhibit a patient's ability to swallow liquids and solids. Patients must be monitored closely during radiotherapy to ensure that this problem is minimized. It is important to note that this reaction does not occur immediately but develops after several weeks of treatment. A similar process takes place in skin layers exposed to therapeutic radiation, giving rise to a sunburnlike desquamation. Certain chemotherapeutic agents (5-fluorouracil, actinomycin D, doxorubicin, methotrexate, and mitomycin C) can potentiate these reactions.

Although mucositis can delay the delivery and increase the overall treatment time, the major limiting factors for final dose determination are the long-term effects of radiation on normal tissues. The late effects of head and neck irradiation can include thickening or fibrosis of the subcutaneous tissues or fibrosis in the temporomandibular joint (which can cause trismus). In contrast to acute reactions, the magnitude of the late effects is determined more by the total dose given than by the daily fraction size. Salivary gland function and taste perception are altered by radiation (494–496). The loss of saliva is significant after about 1,000 cGy is given to the glands; this decreased salivary output may persist for years. Approximately 4,000 to 5,000 cGy causes permanent loss of salivary gland function. Recent data suggest that xerostomia in this setting may be treated effectively with oral pilocarpine (361). Taste loss is significant after 4,000 to 4,500 cGy to the oral cavity.

The decrease in saliva and changes in its chemical composition cause alterations in the microorganisms inhabiting the mouth, which in turn can cause a marked increase in the number of caries. Aggressive dental prophylaxis can reduce this problem, and workup by a dentist with expertise in these problems is mandatory before radiotherapy is initiated. The incidence of osteoradionecrosis can be considerably reduced if the necessary repairs and/or extractions are done pretreatment rather than waiting until problems occur in a heavily irradiated field (43, 499, 538). A delay of 2 to 3 weeks is required between extractions and the initiation of radiotherapy to allow adequate healing.

Technological Advances

Advances in radiotherapy have been tied to advances in technology. Modern radiotherapy departments use linear accelerators rather than cobalt 60 units, producing sharper field edges and higher dose rates. Megavoltage electron beams are used to treat the posterior neck nodes to tumoricidal dosages without risk of spinal cord damage. Custom blocking techniques reduce the radiation dosage to normal tissues and thus reduce treatment-related morbidity. Computed tomography and MRI are used to localize tumors for radiation therapy treatment planning. Figure 105.3 shows a reconstructed CT scan with a large tumor of the maxillary, ethmoid, and frontal sinuses outlined on anterior and lateral projections. Information from such scans is inputted into treatment-planning computers to design individualized optimal treatment plans. Figure 105.4 shows the isodose distribution from a treatment plan for the tumor shown in Figure 105.3. Two levels are shown. Note how the radiation dose distribution lies deeper in the region of the maxillary and ethmoid sinuses but is "pulled" anteriorly at a level through the frontal sinus, thus sparing the frontal lobe. Noncoplanar field configurations, often using vertex presentations, are now fairly standard techniques in many radiotherapy centers. Treatment field arrangements are verified immediately using a fluoroscopic simulator. With such techniques, there should be many fewer marginal misses than in the past.

Curative Radiotherapy

HNSCCs respond to radiation injury through a loss of reproductive capability, resulting in a clonogenic cell death. This cell-killing ability is essentially an exponential function of the radiation dosage (within the context of a given radiation fractionation schema), and so the dosage required for a given level of tumor control is approximately proportional to the number of clonogenic cells in the tumor (292). Subclinical microscopic disease requires a dosage of approximately 5,000 cGy, a 1-cm (3) tumor requires approximately 6,500 cGy, and large (T3 or T4) tumors require dosages in the range of 7,000 to 7,500 cGy to maximize the chances of achieving tumor control (227, 401). (see Chapter 48.) Patients with head and neck tumors are generally treated with

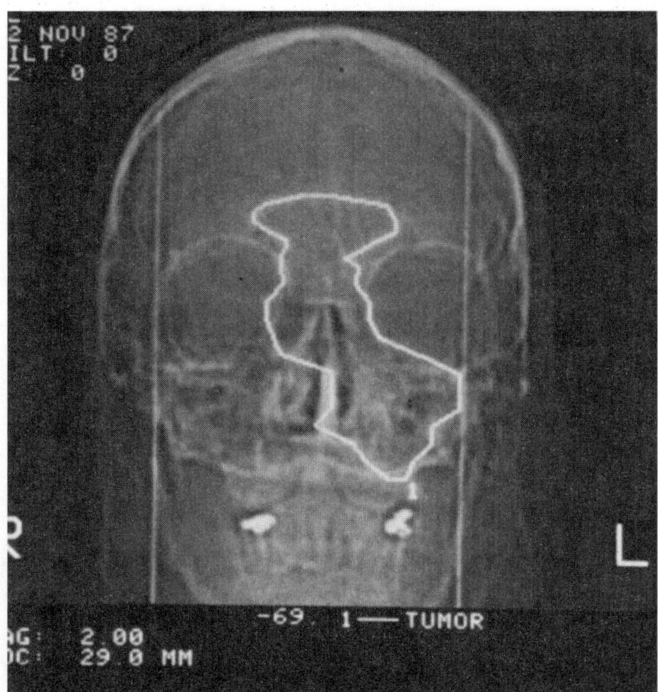

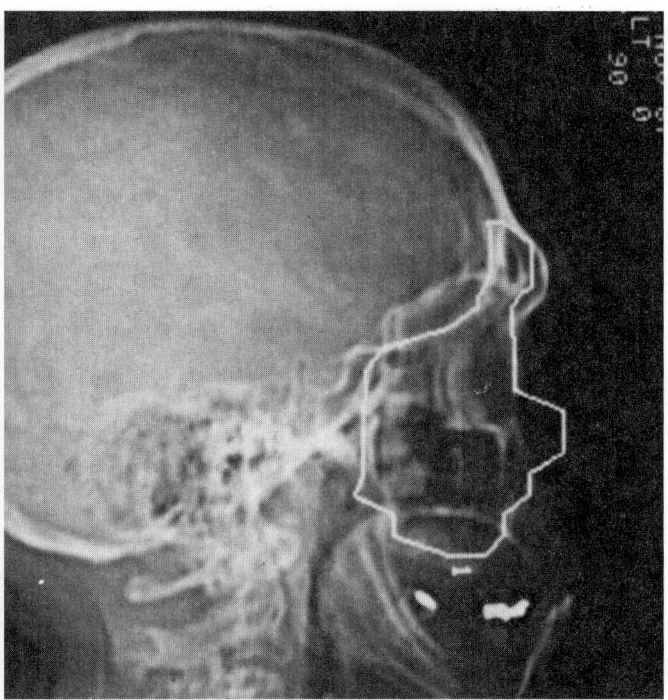

Figure 105.3. A large tumor of the maxillary, ethmoid, and frontal sinuses outlined on a CT scan reconstruction showing the patient in anterior and lateral views. This information is used to design radiation therapy treatment fields.

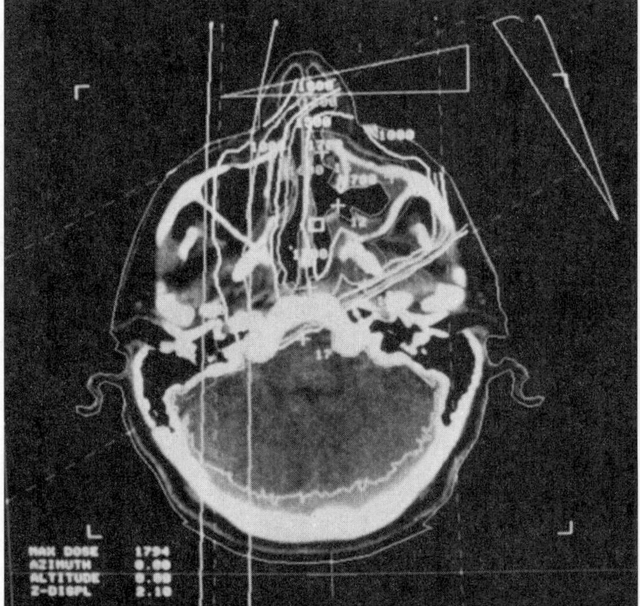

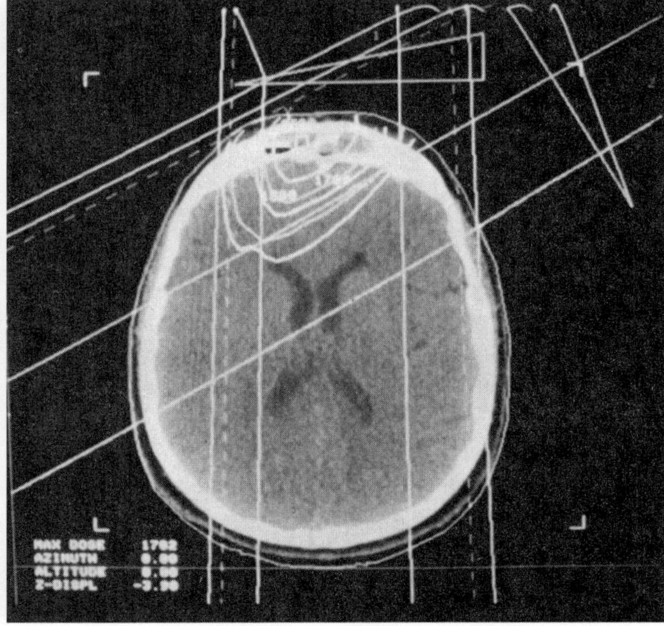

Figure 105.4. Radiation isodose distributions overlying transverse CT scan images at two different levels for the tumor shown in Figure 105.3. Note how the radiation isodoses extend posteriorly to cover the tumor in the maxillary and ethmoid sinus regions but are pulled anteriorly at the superior level, thus sparing the normal brain tissue at this level while adequately treating the frontal sinuses.

shrinking-field techniques, wherein the various regions at risk receive dosages commensurate with the tumor mass they are thought to contain. A typical head and neck treatment regimen involves at least three separate alterations in radiation field geometry. Dosages greater than 7,500 cGy may be achieved using interstitial radioactive implants, which allow the delivery of ultrahigh dosages to small volumes with the dose levels to critical normal tissues kept within safe limits. Table 105.4 shows representative local control rates and survival data for patients with SCCs of com-

Table 105.4. Representative Local Control Rates and Survival for Patients with Squamous Cell Carcinoma of Common Head and Neck Sites Treated with Definitive Radiotherapy

Stage by Site	Local Control (%)	Survival* (%)
Oral cavity		
Oral tongue		
T1	80–90	75–80
T2	60–85	40–60
T3	30–50	20–30
T4	25–45	10–15
Floor of mouth		
T1	75–85	70–85
T2	60–80	50–60
T3	30–50	15–40
T4	5–30	5–20
Oropharynx		
Base of tongue		
T1	80–95	65–85
T2	60–75	40–55
T3	40–65	15–20
T4	30–50	5–20
Tonsil/tonsillar fossa		
T1	75–95	65–85
T2	60–80	55–60
T3	35–70	20–40
T4	20–30	10–15
Soft palate		
T1	90–100	90–95
T2	75–85	65–75
T3	60–70	30–40
T4	25–35	10–15
Nasopharynx		
T1	70–85	60–75
T2	50–60	50–65
T3	20–45	25–50
T4	15–35	5–30
Hypopharynx		
Pyriform sinus		
T1	60–70	30–50
T2	40–50	20–45
T3	30–40	15–25
T4	10–25	5–20
Larynx		
Supraglottic		
T1	80–90	65–90
T2	60–80	50–65
T3	35–70	35–55
T4	30–60	15–40
Glottis		
T1	85–95	80–95
T2	65–75	60–85
T3	20–35	35–60
T4	15–30	10–30

* Adapted from Laramore (401). Local control is for radiation alone. Survival data include surgical salvage for radiation failures. Overlap in the two sets of figures is due to data coming from different patient series, which are a heterogeneous mix of nodal stages, Karnofsky scores, tumor differentiation.

mon head and neck sites treated with definitive radiotherapy (401). While the local/regional control rates are excellent for the small lesions, there is obviously a need for improvement regarding definitive radiation therapy for larger lesions (280).

The choice between radiotherapy and surgery as definitive primary treatment is dependent on the interplay among many factors (481). For early lesions of the larynx and the tip of the tongue, the two modalities yield equivalent local/regional control and survival. However, the functional result is better with radiotherapy, and so it is the treatment of choice. For early lesions of the lip or skin cancers of the nose or eyelid, the ultimate cosmetic result is better with radiotherapy. For sites, such as the nasopharynx, that are surgically unapproachable, radiotherapy is the only tenable form of definitive treatment. For early lesions of the tonsil and tongue (base and lateral aspect), the results are equivalent to those of surgery and informed patient choice should guide the treatment decision. Radiotherapy is also given following diagnosis of SCC metastatic to the cervical lymph nodes from an unknown primary site. The treatment fields encompass the probable sites of tumor origin: nasopharynx, tonsillar fossa, base of tongue, and hypopharynx. The patient survival at 2 to 3 years ranges from 30 to 60% (289).

Accelerated and Hyperfractionated Radiotherapy

An area of current clinical interest in radiotherapy is the use of nonstandard fractionation patterns in radiotherapy in an attempt to improve the therapeutic response ratio (330, 507). Late radiation effects limit the total amount of radiation that can be safely given in the standard treatment schema. The slowly proliferating normal tissues are the dose-limiting structures for these late effects. Such tissues tend to have large shoulders on their cell survival curves, which indicates an increased ability to repair sublethal radiation damage as compared with that of rapidly proliferating normal tissues (292). Hence, a logical approach would be to give smaller radiation treatment fractions so as not to exceed the shoulder on the late-effects tissue cell survival curves and then to go to a higher total dose. The assumption is implicit that the tumor will behave like the rapidly proliferating normal tissues in that it will not have a large shoulder on its radiation cell survival curve and so a therapeutic gain will result. To avoid inordinately prolonging the overall treatment time and allowing tumor repopulation kinetics to become the dominant effect, multiple daily fractions must be given (292, 685). A sufficient time interval (generally more than 6 hours) must be allowed between treatments to allow for adequate repair of sublethal and potentially lethal damage.

Hyperfractionation refers to giving multiple daily doses such that the overall treatment time is about the same as for a course of conventionally fractionated once-a-day radiotherapy (573). The Radiation Therapy Oncology Group (RTOG) has been systematically exploring this approach using twice-daily treatments of 120 cGy. Initially, a trial was performed that randomized this treatment to a total dose of 6,000 cGy versus delivery by conventional fractionation (449). Of 210 patients entered on the study, no differences arose in either local/regional control or survival. The acute effects were well tolerated; since the daily dose rate determines the acute effects, it should be possible on radiobiologic grounds to use a total dose considerably above 6,000 cGy. Currently, the RTOG is conducting a phase II randomized trial to determine the maximum total hyperfractionated dose that can safely be given to the head and neck region. A preliminary report on this work suggests improved local control at 2 years with increasing radiation dose on the three lower-dose arms: 25% for 6,720 cGy, 37% for 7,200 cGy, and 42% for 7,680 cGy (P = .08) (138). No survival differences were noted. The incidence of grade 4 necrosis was 10.0% on the 6,720-cGy arm, 5.1% on the 7,200-cGy arm, and 13.9% on the 7,680-cGy arm. Data on an 8,160-cGy arm are not yet available. The European Organization for Research and Treatment of Cancer (EORTC) has investigated three daily fractions of 160 cGY each for 10 days, a 3-week break in treatment, followed by a boost to 6,720 cGy with or without misonidazole (a hypoxic cell radiosensitizer), compared with a third arm of standard fraction radiotherapy alone in a total of 523 patients. No significant differences in local or regional control or survival have been reported among the three arms (702).

Early mucosal reactions were more severe on the hyperfractionation arms but late effects were equivalent. The EORTC subsequently conducted a phase III clinical trial for patients with oropharyngeal cancer (329). This study compared twice-daily treatments of 115 cGy to a total dose of 8,050 cGy versus a conventional fractionation schema of 200 cGy once a day to a total dose of 7,000 cGy. Eligible patients had stage T1–2, N0–1 tumors, with base-of-tongue primaries being excluded. A total of 356 patients were entered between 1980 to 1987. At the 5-year end point, local control was 59% on the hyperfractionation arm as compared with 40% on the conventional fractionation arm (P = .02). Subset analysis showed that the improved benefit was confined to patients with T3 tumors, since equivalent results were noted for patients with the smaller T2 lesions. The overall survival difference at 5-years (40 versus 31%; P = .08) did not achieve statistical significance. Late normal tissue toxicity was equivalent on the two treatment arms.

Accelerated fractionation refers to giving multiple daily doses of such a size that the overall treatment time is shortened relative to that of conventional radiotherapy. The fraction size and the total dose given are generally slightly less than that of conventional radiotherapy. C.C. Wang has developed a twice-daily schema utilizing 160-cGy fractions (742, 744). The total daily dose is thus 320 cGy, which is too high for the rapidly proliferating normal tissues (e.g., mucosa) to tolerate without a planned interruption in treatment to allow for recovery and repopulation. No randomized trial has been carried out to evaluate it, but historic comparison suggests a possible benefit to its use.

Other accelerated fractionation schemes have been utilized in various pilot studies, but no randomized trials have taken place (277, 473, 482, 504). Another version of accelerated fractionation that attempts to limit the normal tissue acute reaction is the concomitant "boost" regimen proposed by Ang et al. (21). In this approach, the accelerated portion of the radiation therapy is delivered only during the last phase of treatment when the proliferation rates of both tumor and normal tissues have been accelerated. The volume of tissue that receives the twice-daily treatment is limited to the primary target volume; there are no planned breaks in treatment. The RTOG currently is using this approach as one arm of a randomized trial for patients with inoperable head and neck cancer. Because of the acute toxicity with these regimens, a controlled trial is warranted before its acceptance into standard practice.

COMBINED SURGERY AND RADIOTHERAPY

Very few well-designed randomized trials have compared surgery alone with combined therapy in any disease site. When treatment is surgery or radiotherapy alone, local/regional control rates for stages I and II lesions are in the range of 75 to 90% (depending on disease site). The local/regional control rates with single-modality therapy are much less satisfactory in stages III and IV lesions, for which standard medical practice employs both modalities.

Radiotherapy can be given either preoperatively or postoperatively. The aims of preoperative radiotherapy are to sterilize microscopic disease outside the resection field and to shrink the tumor bulk, thus making the surgery easier to perform. Theoretically, preoperative radiotherapy should also reduce the risk of disseminating viable tumor cells at surgery. A dosage of 5,000 cGy over 5 to 5.5 weeks is usually given (229). No significant problems with delayed wound healing occur at this dosage.

When radiotherapy is postoperative, the surgical resection bed has a disrupted blood supply. Conventional wisdom says that higher dosages of radiation are needed because of the increased likelihood of hypoxic tumor cells, which are less radiosensitive. Generally, one delivers 5,500 to 6,000 cGy in 180- to 200-cGy fractions in a postoperative setting. Higher dosages are used if the surgical margins are compromised or if there is a high likelihood of the presence of macroscopic residual disease. Postoperative radiotherapy has the advantage of being given to only those patients thought to be at a significant risk for local/regional tumor recurrence based on a thorough review of the pathologic data. It has the further advantage of not delaying the surgical procedure, which for patients with operable disease is the most important treatment modality.

Preoperative radiotherapy and postoperative radiotherapy were compared in a randomized clinical trial by the RTOG. A total of 277 patients with tumors of the oral cavity, oropharynx, supraglottic larynx, or hypopharynx were entered into the study (396). Patients in the preoperative arm received 5,000 cGy followed by surgery in 4 to 6 weeks, whereas patients in the postoperative arm received 6,000 cGy starting 2 to 4 weeks after the surgical resection. A higher percentage of patients in the postoperative arm completed the combined course of therapy within protocol guidelines (74 versus 56%). The 4-year competing-risk local/regional tumor control was 65% in the postoperative arm versus 48% in the preoperative arm (P = .04). For the subgroup of 194 patients who completed overall treatment within protocol guidelines, the local/regional control rates were 74% in the postoperative arm and 56% in the preoperative arm. There were no significant differences between the two study arms in complication or survival rates.

Although it is generally felt that there is little role for debulking surgery in the treatment of head and neck cancers, there may be situations where a gross total resection followed by high-dose radiotherapy is preferable to treatment with radiation alone. A recent analysis by the Head and Neck Intergroup Study IG 0034 showed that the patients who were excluded because of positive surgical margins exhibited improved local/regional control of tumor as compared with a matched set of patients from the RTOG databases treated with radiotherapy alone (396, 406). At 4 years, respective local/regional controls were 44 versus 24% ($P = .007$). However, there was no difference in survival. This was not a randomized trial and no analysis was made of quality of life with either treatment. The authors argue for testing the concept in a controlled clinical trial rather than changing traditional resectability criteria.

Chemotherapy—General

Chemotherapeutic strategies for HNSCC are reviewed in detail under "Chemotherapy Approaches" below. Systemic approaches to salivary gland tumors, nasopharyngeal carcinoma, advanced skin cancer, esthesioneuroblastoma, and other nonsquamous cancers are distinct from head and neck cancers at other sites and, therefore, are discussed separately.

NATURAL HISTORY AND TREATMENT BY SITE

Oral Cavity

Both tumor growth and treatment significantly compromise speech and deglutition, particularly for those patients in whom cancer involves the tongue, the floor of mouth, or the mandible. Furthermore, the diversity of potential sites of cancer development in the oral cavity and variations of lymphatic drainage and rates of node metastases lend added complexity to treatment planning (364, 703, 732). Despite the fact that this region is readily amenable to visual examination and bimanual palpation, more than 50% of patients are diagnosed in advanced stages. The current T staging of oral cavity primaries is presented in Table 105.5.

SCCs of the lip are the most common oral cavity cancer. Over 90% occur on the lower lip, usually on the exposed vermilion border, midway between the midline and the oral commissure. Upper lip cancers most commonly are basal cell carcinomas (458). Well-differentiated and verrucous cancers rarely metastasize. Poorly differentiated and spindle cell varieties tend to grow aggressively and metastasize commonly. Perineural infiltration of large nerves is indicative of aggressive disease.

Lip

The treatment of lip cancers must consider adequate removal of tissue to encompass the disease, and yet provide the patient with a lip that functions in speech, chewing, and oral competence, and affords adequate cosmesis (28, 745). These goals are achieved equally well with either primary radiation or surgery when the tumors are less than 2 cm in size or are very superficial. Larger lesions are best treated with surgical resection and reconstruction, where there is greater accuracy in evaluating the extent of tumor and nerve or cervical lymphatic involvement (357, 586). Frequently, adjacent precancerous changes are present that can be treated with surgery (lip shaving and advancement) to prevent recurrences or the development of second primary tumors (470, 766). For large lesions, primary reconstruction with local and regional flaps avoids defects that result from tissue loss with radiotherapy, provides for future reconstructive and treatment options, and eliminates the risk of osteoradionecrosis of the mandible. Lesions demonstrating extensive infiltration, bone involvement, or lymphatic metastases are increasingly managed with combined surgery and postoperative radiation.

Radiation therapy techniques for management of lip cancers include external irradiation, interstitial implants (usually radium needles or iridium 192), and combinations of both. Local tumor control rates with irradiation exceed 80% (362, 446, 532), with determinant survival at 5 years, including surgical salvage, in excess of 95%. Similar tumor control and survival rates are reported with primary surgical excision (29). Confirmed regional metastases decrease the survival rates to 36 to 55% (149, 362). Five-year survival rates for patients with carcinomas of the upper lip are lower than for lower lip lesions and range from 40 to 60% (488, 592). Involvement of both lips or the lateral commissure is uncommon. The prognosis for commissure lesions is not as good as for cancers of other areas of the lip. Cross and colleagues report a 5-year survival rate of 34% for patients with oral commissure carcinoma (Table 105.6) (149).

Tongue

Tongue cancers account for 25% of oral cavity SCC and most commonly arise in the oral portion or anterior two thirds

Table 105.5. Primary Tumor Staging Characteristics for Oral Cavity Carcinoma

Tx	Primary tumor cannot be assessed
T0	No evidence of primary tumor
Tis	Carcinoma in situ
T1	Tumor 2 cm or less in greatest dimension
T2	Tumor more than 2 cm, but less than 4 cm in greatest dimension
T3	Tumor more than 4 cm in greatest dimension
T4	(lip) Tumor invades adjacent structures, e.g., through cortical bone, tongue, skin of neck
T4	(oral cavity) Tumor invades adjacent structures, e.g., cortical bone, deep tissues (extrinsic muscle of tongue, maxillary sinus, skin)

Table 105.6. Five-Year Survival Rates for Patients with Carcinoma of the Lip

Investigator	Number of patients	5-Year survival (%)	
		Determinant	Absolute
Burkell[82]	534	89	80
Gladstone[263]	519	82	65
Schreiner[592]	636	74	59
Wookey[780]	1,128	85	58
Molnar[488]	2,066	86	76
Cross[149]	563	58	50
Jorgensen[362]	869	97	84
MacKay and Sellers[446]	3,166	89	65

of the tongue on the lateral edge or ventral surface. Infiltration of the underlying tongue musculature occurs early. The intrinsic tongue muscles are loosely arranged, interdigitating and endowed with a rich vascular and lymphatic supply, which may explain the early high rate of regional metastases.

Most patients present with T2 or greater lesions. Prognosis is directly related to the degree of infiltration and the presence of regional metastases. The biologic aggressiveness of small (less than 4 cm) tongue cancers is noteworthy and is reflected in higher rates of occult regional metastases than similarly staged lesions arising from other oral sites (Table 105.7). Occult node metastases are present in 30 to 40% of early lesions (166, 187, 217, 646). Approximately 40% of patients have clinical evidence of node metastases at diagnosis (645). Primary-echelon node drainage is to the upper deep cervical lymphatics. Involvement of middle and lower neck nodes (levels III and IV) is not uncommon. Bilateral nodal involvement may be present with cancers of the tip of the tongue or those involving the midline of the tongue. Local-regional recurrence in patients with tongue cancer accounts for 60 to 70% of cancer deaths (87, 710, 736). Distant metastases account for 15% of deaths and second primaries for 20 to 40%.

The management of carcinomas of the tongue has been significantly influenced by a better appreciation of the aggressiveness of small, deeply infiltrative lesions; the high rate of occult lymph node metastases; and an interest in improving treatment without compromising oral function. Although surgical excision has been the mainstay of treatment, combined surgery and adjuvant radiation therapy to include the primary site and regional nodes is commonly used for most advanced (stages III and IV) cancers and is being used increasingly for small stage II cancers that exhibit pathologic indicators of lymph node metastasis or perineural invasion.

For stage I cancers, surgical excision is effective and expeditious with good preservation of function. For stage II lesions that are infiltrative, hemiglossectomy achieves excellent tumor control rates and can be combined with modified dissection of neck nodes (supraomohyoid dissections) to provide accurate staging information and determination of the need for adjuvant radiation. Hemiglossectomy may result in some functional morbidity in terms of articulation and deglutition. Because of this, radiation therapy may be used in selected cases. Nevertheless, surgery should remain the mainstay of treatment in oral tongue malignancies. For radiation to be as effective as surgery in controlling these cancers, interstitial brachytherapy combined with external radiation is essential. Radiation doses of 80 to 85 Gy are generally given via external megavoltage radiation or in combination with brachytherapy. Interstitial treatment requires precise placement and spacing of implants. Accurate dosimetry is enhanced by using afterloading techniques in which the radioactive source is inserted into previously placed hollow tubes. Tracheostomy at the time of implant should be considered because of the potential development of tongue edema after implantation. Occult or apparent neck disease is usually treated using external radiation or radiation combined with neck dissection (166). The long-term ramifications of radiation therapy for oral cavity malignancies must also be considered, including radiation fibrosis with impaired function of the oral structures (including the tongue), dry mouth, and osteoradionecrosis.

Extension of cancer to the floor of the mouth or the mandible may necessitate partial mandibulectomy or segmental mandibular resection. Modern reconstructive techniques with vascularized composite bone and soft tissue free flaps, titanium metal prostheses, pedicled myocutaneous regional flaps, and free bone grafts have improved the functional and cosmetic results of major mandibular resections. If the neck must be surgically entered to accomplish adequate resection of the primary tumor, a neck dissection should be simultaneously performed. When tumors grossly involve bone, radiation therapy is less effective in these poorly vascularized osseous tissues and requires high doses that are associated with osteoradionecrosis. After local failure of interstitial implants, complication rates for salvage surgical resections are extremely high and are associated with significant morbidity from fistulization, radionecrosis, and failure of primary reconstructive efforts. In many cases, control fistulas and delayed reconstruction with well-vascularized flaps are advantageous. Although the surgical salvage of radiation failures is often successful in early lesions, success drops to less than 50% in advanced lesions.

For more advanced primary lesions (stages III and IV), surgery and external radiation are generally used. Radiation has been administered as either planned preoperative or postoperative therapy, although currently we advocate postoperative treatment in most instances. Although no prospective controlled trials have proved the superiority of combined therapy over surgery alone, many studies indicate improved local/regional control rates (230, 413, 414, 715, 720). These improvements have generally been offset, in part, by an increased frequency of distant metastases and second primaries. Surgical management generally consists of partial glossectomy and neck dissection, with the mandibular apparatus spared unless directly involved. In instances with limited periosteal invasion, coronal and other partial mandibular resections can be performed that spare mandibular continuity and maximize function. Where tumors extend to the midline or involve the tongue base, subtotal or total glossectomy may be necessary. Modern reconstructive techniques have improved the functional results of these aggressive resections. Provision for temporary tracheostomy

Table 105.7. Occult Lymph Node Metastases for Oral Cavity Carcinoma by Level*

Level (# positive/total)	Tongue (18/58) %	Floor of mouth (15/57) %	Gingiva (20/52) %	Retromolar trigone (7/16) %	Buccal (5/9) %
I	14	16	27	19	44
II	19	12	21	12	11
III	16	7	6	6	0
IV	3	2	4	6	0
V	0	0	2	0	0

* Modified from Shah et al. (600).

and prolonged enteral nutrition should be made. Total glossectomy or sacrifice of both hypoglossal nerves frequently necessitates permanent feeding gastrostomy or jejunostomy. Current experience indicates that total glossectomy can often be accomplished without the need for laryngectomy (52).

Tumor resection is more difficult after preoperative radiation therapy unless precise tattooing of intended resection margins is accomplished prior to therapy. Likewise, the rates of surgical complications, fistulization, exposed bone, and radionecrosis may be increased with preoperative radiation, although studies have been conflicting. Because of this, most centers have adopted a policy of postoperative radiation. With postoperative radiation, higher doses can be delivered, the extent of disease is precisely defined, the histologic status of the lymph nodes is known, and high-risk areas of close margins or residual cancer can be treated to a high dose. Both ipsilateral and contralateral necks are irradiated, with the dosage determined by the extent of disease. Postoperative radiation should begin within 3 to 6 weeks of resection. Interstitial implants are not used. Close surgical margins require high doses (70 Gy) because of the difficulty in eradicating even small amounts of tumor in the tongue after glossectomy (34). Curative radiation alone with surgical salvage has been shown to be inferior to combined therapy in control of local/regional disease, and in the complication rate, even though survival rates are similar with these approaches (395, 396). Even with combined therapy, estimated 2-year disease-free and overall survival rates for advanced disease are only 51 and 53%, respectively (775). The 5-year survival rates range from 50 to 70% for stages I and II to 15 to 30% for stages III and IV (Table 105.8) (87).

The management of the neck is of particular interest in patients with tongue cancer because of the high rate of occult node metastases. For lesions T2 or greater in size, rates of occult metastases exceed 40% and some form of neck treatment is generally indicated. When the primary tumor can be adequately excised via a transoral technique, unilateral or bilateral neck dissections should be performed based on the location of the primary disease. Radiotherapy should be used postoperatively if pathologic indicators are recognized. When radiation alone is selected for the treatment of primary tumors with neck node metastases, this treatment is often combined with therapeutic neck dissection (166).

Table 105.8. Overall Five-Year Survival Rates (%) for Patients with Squamous Carcinoma of the Tongue

Investigator	N	Stage I	Stage II	Stage III	Stage IV
Callery[87]	252	75	60	40	20
Decroix[166]	602	59	45	25	13
Wallner[736]	424	68	50	33	20
Ildstad[342]	122	48	48	18	26
O'Brien[510]	97	73*	62*	—	—
Average	(N = 1,497)	65	53	29	20

* Disease-free survival

Floor of Mouth

Floor-of-mouth cancers occur with a frequency similar to that for tongue cancer. Early spread to adjacent areas (gingiva and periosteum of the mandible) is common. The periosteum is a natural barrier to spread. Fixation of the tongue is a sign of deep invasion. The tumor may extend to or through the myohyoid muscle, which serves as a natural barrier to direct spread below the hyoid bone. Lymph node metastases at presentation are seen in approximately 40% of patients and an additional 20% have occult lymphatic metastases (187). The occult metastatic rate increases with the T stage of the primary: T2 tumors have a 40% and T3 tumors a 70% occult metastasis rate.

First-echelon nodes of lymphatic drainage include the submandibular and jugulodigastric lymph nodes (levels I and II). Submental node involvement is unusual. Evaluation for early mandibular involvement is facilitated by palpation since fixation to the mandible indicates periosteal involvement and direct bone invasion is present in 50 to 60% of such tumors.

Small cancers (T1, T2) are generally treated effectively by wide resection or radiation therapy. Little morbidity results from surgical resection of superficial lesions. Lateral floor-of-mouth tumors can often be resected transorally and the resection defect closed with the advancement of adjacent mucosa, skin grafts, or secondary intention. Early cancers involving the mandible are best treated surgically because bone involvement compromises radiation efficacy. Surgery remains the mainstay of treatment for early floor-of-mouth malignancies, achieving excellent functional and curative results.

Radiation therapy for small floor-of-mouth cancers usually involves combinations of external radiation and brachytherapy. Decision making concerning primary therapy takes into consideration the expected functional result, the management of the neck nodes, and the risk of osteoradionecrosis. Radiotherapy for moderate-size (T2) anterior floor-of-mouth lesions and small or deeply invasive cancers must also include treating bilateral first-echelon lymph nodes. Rates of occult nodal metastases range from 30 to 40%.

More advanced floor-of-mouth cancers (T3, T4) are generally treated with resection combined with postoperative radiation of the primary and regional nodes. These resections require a transcervical approach and are combined with neck dissection and mandibular resections as needed. Again, mandibular continuity-sparing procedures with cortectomies can often be employed. In these instances, we have found the radial free forearm (fasciocutaneous) flap to offer excellent floor-of-mouth and tongue reconstructive potential. Large surgical defects are reconstructed with skin grafts, local flaps, myocutaneous pedicled regional flaps, and frequently free-tissue transfers. Mandibular reconstruction for segmental defects is performed primarily with composite free-tissue transfers.

Doses of radiation therapy for local/regional tumor control are based on actual tumor volume rather than T stage (472). Interstitial doses of 65 to 75 Gy are recommended for early lesions (1 to 3 cm) if brachytherapy alone is used, or external

Table 105.9. Overall Five-Year Survival Rates (%) in Patients with Squamous Carcinoma of the Floor of Mouth

Investigator	N	Stage I	Stage II	Stage II	Stage IV
Harrold[295]	634	69	49	25	7
Panje[517]	103	57	60	43	19
Trible[693]	56	100	65	37	11
Nason[502]	198	69	64	46	26
Shaha[606]	320	88	80	66	32
Fu[245]	153	83	71	43	10
Average	(N = 1,464)	78	65	43	18

beam radiation of 50 Gy combined with 25 to 30 Gy of interstitial radiation. Postoperative doses are given by external radiation only at doses of 65 Gy over 6 to 7 weeks, or preoperative doses of 50 Gy over 6 weeks. No significant differences in overall survival rates have been shown when comparing preoperative and postoperative radiation regimens (396).

Treatment results are influenced by the size of the primary tumor, presence of lymph node metastases, degree of mandibular involvement, and adequacy of resection. The 5-year survival rates for localized stages I and II carcinomas of the floor of mouth range from 60 to 80% (Table 105.9). Cancers that cross the midline or involve the tongue, or the mandible are associated with 5-year survival rates of 50 to 60% (517). Survival rates for more advanced lesions (stages III and IV) are less than 50%. Lymph node metastases decrease survival rates to approximately 25%. The major advantage of combined treatment (radiation and surgery) in these patients is improved control of ipsilateral and contralateral neck disease. Because rates of occult nodal disease are high in advanced primary lesions, elective treatment of the neck with radiation or bilateral neck dissections is indicated. Recurrence in the untreated, clinically negative neck is the most frequent site of failure in patients treated only with surgery (606).

The debate over performing elective neck dissection versus irradiation remains unresolved. If adequate primary tumor margins are uncertain or if multiple histologically positive lymph node metastases are detected, postoperative radiation to the ipsilateral and contralateral neck is administered. The development of second primary cancers is a major cause of morbidity and death. Fu and colleagues reported that 55 of 153 (36%) patients developed second primaries, of whom 30 died of their second cancer (245). Distant metastases occur in 10 to 15% of patients (245, 606).

Gingiva and Buccal Mucosa

Gingival cancers occur most commonly (80%) in the lower gingiva posterior to the bicuspid teeth (86). For both sites, trismus is an ominous sign. Clinical staging criteria are similar to those for other oral sites. Overall, regional metastases occur in approximately 15% of gingival cancers and are rarely associated with buccal cancers (58). Occult metastases occur in 10 to 20% of patients. Exophytic tumors tend to be papillary or verrucous in appearance and can be confused with benign hyperkeratosis.

Small, superficial gingival cancers can be effectively treated with surgical resection or radiation therapy with excellent preservation of function (84). Generally, the amount of bone resected for small lesions is minimal and resection can be accomplished transorally. Even larger lesions requiring partial maxillectomy or alveolectomy can be resected without external incision. External beam irradiation is not as effective in local tumor control once gross bone involvement has occurred. The intermediate (T2 or larger) lesions are best handled surgically; the risk of osteoradionecrosis is thereby avoided. For large lesions (T3 and T4), segmental mandibulectomy or maxillectomy is required and adjuvant radiation is frequently recommended. Elective neck dissection is not indicated unless the en bloc resection of a large primary tumor requires neck exposure. For patients in whom no neck dissection is performed, elective neck irradiation should be considered. Clinically positive neck nodes warrant neck dissection combined with resection of the primary tumor.

Buccal carcinomas of early stage (I or II) can be treated equally well with surgery or radiation. Radiation therapy offers the advantage of including the draining lymphatics in the treatment fields, but also risks posttreatment fibrosis and trismus. Large primary tumors or tumors with regional metastases are managed surgically, with the need for adjuvant radiation determined by the adequacy of resection and risk of suspected residual disease. Neck dissection is recommended only in cases of clinically positive lymph nodes with buccal cancers, unless neck access is required for surgical excision of the primary.

Overall survival rates for gingival and buccal cancers depend on tumor size, bone involvement, and node metastases. The 5-year survival rates for lower gingival lesions do not differ from those for the upper gingiva and range from 78% for stage I to 15% for stage IV disease (444). Surgical results are clearly superior to those of radiation when bone involvement is present. Survival rates (5-year) for stages I and II buccal carcinomas range from 65 to 75%. Determinant survival for stages III and IV disease varies from 20 to 30% (58). For both gingival and buccal mucosal cancers, overall survival rates have improved over recent years as surgical management has replaced radiation therapy as the primary treatment.

Retromolar Trigone

Cancers arising in the retromolar trigone (the narrow band of mucosa that lies behind the mandibular molar teeth and covers the ascending ramus) are rarely confined to that gingiva, but involve adjacent buccal mucosa, anterior tonsillar pillar, the floor of the mouth, or posterior gingiva. Thus, retromolar trigone cancers that involve the anterior tonsillar pillar behave more like oropharyngeal cancers than like oral cavity primaries. The risk of clinically positive and occult lymph node metastases is higher than with other gingival cancers. The frequent involvement of periosteum mandates partial (rim or marginal) mandibulectomy as part of the surgical management, even for small lesions. Primary radiation therapy is reserved for superficial lesions that cover a large surface area, such as extension to the soft palate or buccal mucosa, and remain mobile. Moderately advanced or deeply invasive lesions are best treated with surgical resection (mandibulectomy and neck dissection), followed by radiation therapy if pathologically indicated, unless the functional or cosmetic result would be unacceptable to the patient.

Oropharynx

The clinical staging of oropharyngeal cancers depends primarily on tumor size and is similar to the staging of oral cavity cancers (Table 105.10). Although tumors may arise from any site in the oropharynx, most commonly they arise from the tonsillar area and palatine arch. The most common presenting symptom is chronic sore throat (often unilateral) and referred otalgia. Change in voice, dysphagia, and trismus are late signs. Regional lymphatic metastases occur frequently and are related to the depth of tumor invasion and tumor size. Upper cervical nodes are generally first involved, but lower nodes can become clinically involved with skipping of the upper first-echelon nodes. Bilateral lymphatic metastases can occur, particularly with cancers of the soft palate, tongue base, and midline pharyngeal wall.

Tonsil

These cancers tend to be superficial, better differentiated, and of an earlier stage than other oropharyngeal tumors. The treatment of early tonsillar neoplasms (stages I and II) is usually radiation therapy alone. Transoral wide local excision of small, superficial lesions may be effective, but does not address the potential of subclinical lymph node metastasis. Deeply invasive cancers require extensive resections of the pharyngeal wall or mandible (529, 551).

Radiation for early cancers offers the advantage of treating upper-echelon lymph nodes. Treatment is usually unilateral unless extension to the tongue base or midline soft palate is present that warrants treatment of contralateral lymphatics. Ipsilateral treatment portals allow sparing of the contralateral mucosa and salivary glands. Because much of the tumor may be hidden from external beam photons by the mandible, deeper dose calculation with electron beam therapy is used, which can be combined with a small interstitial implant if invasion of adjacent tongue is present. Early cancers of the tonsillar pillar are less effectively treated with radiation alone than are cancers confined to the tonsillar fossa (487).

Radical radiotherapy to lymph nodes controls approximately 90% of limited nodal disease (N1) if the primary tumor is controlled, but nodal failure increases to more than 20% if failure occurs at the primary tumor site. Overall 5-year survival rates for patients with advanced primary tumors or regional metastases are generally less than 25% with single-modality therapy (110, 253, 487, 684). Combinations of surgery and radiation therapy offer improved rates of local and regional tumor control, which, in some studies, has translated into improved survival (158, 487, 619). Similar tumor-control and survival rates have been reported for stage III (T3N0) patients without nodal metastases who are treated with radiation alone or combined surgery and radiation or surgery alone (Table 105.11) (17, 525). In general, preoperative or postoperative radiation for advanced (stage III or IV) cancers of the tonsillar fossa is recommended, combined with resection to include the tonsillar fossa and regional nodes. In some instances, advances in surgical approaches may allow for sparing of the mandible, but composite resection of the pharynx, mandible, and neck remains a frequent surgical approach. Postoperative rather than preoperative radiation is currently preferred because it allows more accurate assessment of surgical margins, local extent of disease, and degree of lymphatic involvement, and is associated with lower rates of surgical complications.

Table 105.10. Primary Tumor Staging Characteristics for Cancer of the Oropharynx

Tx	Primary tumor cannot be assessed
T0	No evidence of primary tumor
Tis	Carcinoma in situ
T1	Tumor <2 cm in greatest dimension
T2	Tumor >2 cm, but not more than 4 cm in greatest dimension
T3	Tumor >4 cm in greatest dimension
T4	Tumor invades adjacent structures, e.g., through cortical bone, soft tissue of neck, deep muscle of tongue

Tongue Base

Base-of-the-tongue cancer poses a more difficult therapeutic problem than do tonsillar carcinomas. The 5-year survival rates are lower, metastases are more common, early diagnosis is less common, and treatment morbidity is greater. Because of the functional difficulties from wide local excision, even of small tongue-base cancers, most early (T1,T2) tumors are treated with definitive radiation. Three quarters of patients are first seen with stage III or IV disease, primarily because of the early development of regional metastases, even with T1 or T2 tumors. Understaging of the primary tumor is frequent because these cancers tend to be diffusely infiltrative beyond their clinical appearance. This may account for similarities in local tumor control rates for both "early" and advanced lesions. The poor outcome is largely attributable to late diagnosis (560).

The staging of tongue-base carcinomas is principally dependent on primary tumor size and the extent of regional metastases. Lymph node involvement is present in approximately 60% of patients with small (T1, T2) primaries (752) and is the major determinant of prognosis. Overall 5-year survival rates range from 11 to 45% (36, 749). The 5-year survival rates decrease from over 60% for N0 patients to less than 30% for N1 patients (36, 38, 752).

The results of radiation therapy alone as definitive treatment for small primary tumors (T1, T2) are better for exophytic than for deeply invasive tumors (752). Radiation alone is generally reserved for those patients without clinical node metastases, but can be combined with salvage neck dissection for patients with clinically positive nodes that persist

Table 105.11. Three-Year and Five-Year Survival Rates (%) in Patients with Squamous Carcinoma of the Tonsil

Investigator	N	Stage I	Stage II	Stage III	Stage IV	Duration
Perez[525]	218	76	40	42	25	3-year
Spiro[644]	117	89	83	58	49	3-year
Dasmahapatra[158]	174	83	72	23	15	5-year
Amornarn[17]	185	100	73	52	21	5-year
Mizono[487]	171	92	77	56	29	5-year determinant
Givens[262]	104	93	57	27	17	5-year determinant

Table 105.12. Overall Survival Rates (%) in Patients with Squamous Carcinoma of the Tongue Base According to T Class and Tumor Stage

Investigator	N	T class				Stage				Rate
		T1	T2	T3	T4	I	II	III	IV	
Thawley[686]	101	57	72	30	22	50	44	45	28	5-year
Weber[752]	173	100	58	38	20	100	72	50	30	5-year
Barrs[36]	119	63	56	31	—	68	55	55	11	3-year

after the completion of radiation. Local recurrence is more frequent after radiation alone in most series (36, 568, 752), and salvage of local failure with subsequent surgery is poor. In selected patients, interstitial radiation therapy has been used to treat residual palpable disease after external beam radiation in anticipation of better local control. The use of brachytherapy is associated with high rates of soft tissue necrosis and osteoradionecrosis, however (252, 314). The results of supplemental interstitial therapy appear to be highly dependent on the dose and technique, with the best results reported with extensive percutaneous lateral cervical loop implants to include treatment of the lateral oropharyngeal wall and pharyngoepiglottic fold (270). The acute morbidity with implantation techniques is severe and results in massive tongue edema that necessitates tracheostomy in all patients. The role of radiation therapy alone seems best reserved for small, exophytic primary tumors without node metastases.

Surgical management of small primary tongue-base tumors (T1) achieves results similar to those from radiation alone. In most cases, primary tumors are moderately advanced and require transcervical resection via mandibulotomy or lateral pharyngotomy approaches, combined with elective or therapeutic neck dissection. Local tumor control rates are superior to those with radiation alone (36, 752), but regional control is poor if clinically positive nodes are present. Elective neck dissection can serve an important role as a staging procedure, thereby providing a rationale for adjuvant radiation therapy. To date, no prospective randomized trial data are available that compare surgery alone with combined surgery with either pre- or postoperative radiation. Survival rates do not differ substantially by stage of disease for patients with tongue-base cancers, except for those with stage IV disease (Table 105.12).

Soft Palate and Pharyngeal Wall

These cancers are less common than other oropharyngeal neoplasms. Most soft palate cancers occur on the anterior surface of the palate and tend to be superficial. Regional metastases are uncommon, although lateral extension to the tonsillar area results in an increased rate of lymph node involvement and lesions close to the midline result in bilateral or contralateral neck metastases in 15% of patients. Occult node metastases are estimated to occur in 16% of patients (423). Posterior wall lesions tend to be superficial with less tumor bulk than similarly staged lesions elsewhere in the oropharynx. Tumor extension to the tongue base decreases survival and increases the rate of metastases, which are often bilateral. Advanced lesions with deep invasion have ready access to the prevertebral space, infratemporal fossa, and skull base, and can be associated with extensive submucosal spread with clinical "skip" areas.

Radiation alone as curative treatment is preferred in most cases, even for T3 or T4 primary tumors (228). Resection of all but the smallest soft palate lesions is associated with significant functional disability. The rates of occult regional metastases are difficult to determine because elective irradiation of bilateral nodal groups is included as part of primary treatment and must include the retropharyngeal lymphatics. Clinically positive lymph nodes at presentation occur in 30% of patients. Small primary tumors with positive nodes can be effectively treated with definitive radiation to the primary tumor and neck. Neck dissections should be initiated if disease in the neck persists for 6 weeks following the completion of external beam therapy. Extensive pharyngeal wall cancers or palate cancers with extension to the tonsil and those cases with advanced regional metastases are usually treated with combined surgical resection and postoperative radiation. Overall 5-year survival rates for soft palate and faucial pillar cancers are 60 to 70% and range from 80 to 90% for T1 or T2 lesions to 30 to 60% for stages III and IV lesions (752). Local/regional recurrence is the most frequent cause of failure (754).

HYPOPHARYNX

The hypopharynx represents one of the most lethal sites of SCC. Lymph node metastases are clinically evident at time of diagnosis in 70 to 80% of patients (39, 204, 480) and are indicative of advanced disease. Bilateral and contralateral lymph node metastases occur in 10 to 20% of cases, particularly if tumors cross the midline of the hypopharynx. Primary tumor extension beyond the hypopharynx is common (94, 534). Hypopharyngeal cancers are characterized by a propensity to spread submucosally to involve the oropharynx or esophagus. Ulcerated, deep infiltration and "skip areas" are common. This leads to difficulties in adequately assessing the margins of the tumor and contributes to poor local tumor control, even with the addition of adjuvant radiation (198). The majority (over 75%) of hypopharyngeal cancers arise in the pyriform sinus, while 20% occur in the posterior pharyngeal wall. Postcricoid cancers are rare (less than 5%). Posterior pharyngeal wall cancers tend to grow superficially and only involve the prevertebral fascia in advanced lesions. Pyriform cancers spread early to other contiguous structures, such as the larynx, postcricoid area, thyroid gland, and thyroid and cricoid cartilages. Most pyriform sinus cancers arise along the medial wall followed by the lateral wall of the sinus. The postcricoid mucosa is contiguous with the apex of the pyriform and tumor can spread circumferentially to involve the entire lower hypopharynx. Because of the locale of hypopharyngeal cancers and their growth patterns and proximity to the larynx, surgical management generally entails partial or total pharyngectomy combined with laryngectomy (584).

The staging of hypopharyngeal cancer is based primarily on the subsite of the pharynx involved, the presence of vocal cord fixation, and the extent of lymph node metastases (Table 105.13). Distant metastases at the time of diagnosis are rare. Staging evaluation is critical for treatment planning and must include endoscopic evaluation to determine precisely the tumor margins, extent of invasion of adjacent structures, and presence of second primary tumors or "skip areas" (461). Determination of the precise site of origin and inferior extent of a tumor can be difficult with large tumors or with those obstructing the esophageal inlet.

Because of the necessity to remove the larynx as part of the surgical treatment of most hypopharyngeal cancers, radiation therapy alone as treatment has been extensively investigated (484). Retrospective analyses have consistently demonstrated that survival rates are lower and local/regional failure rates higher with radiation alone as compared with surgery or surgery and radiotherapy (94, 196, 198, 204, 534, 550). However, for small (T1) cancers of the hypopharynx, and, in particular, for superficial posterior pharyngeal wall lesions, radiation therapy alone has been used effectively, with surgery reserved for salvage (548, 650). Radiation therapy offers the advantage of treating bilateral occult lymph node disease, including retropharyngeal nodes, which are frequently involved when cancer arises from the posterior pharyngeal wall (33). Small cancers of the hypopharynx can be treated equally effectively with surgical resection, often with sparing of the larynx for posterior wall lesions or with supraglottic laryngectomy for superficial cancers of the medial or lateral pyriform when the apex mucosa is tumor-free. Most patients, however, present with advanced primary tumors (T2–T4) and positive lymph nodes. In such patients, local control rates with radiation alone decrease to 50% and salvage surgery is rarely successful. Thus, surgical management has become the mainstay of treatment for most hypopharyngeal cancers. Resections may entail partial pharyngectomy, pharyngolaryngectomy, or total pharyngectomy combined with neck dissection.

Table 105.13. Primary Tumor Staging Characteristics for Carcinoma of the Hypopharynx

Tx	Primary tumor cannot be assessed
T0	No evidence of primary tumor
Tis	Carcinoma in situ
T1	Tumor limited to one subsite of the hypopharynx
T2	Tumor invades more than one subsite of the hypopharynx
T3	Tumor invades more than one subsite of the hypopharynx or adjacent site, with fixation of hemilarynx
T4	Tumor invades adjacent structures, e.g., cartilage or soft tissue of neck

Tumors arising in the lower laryngopharynx or postcricoid mucosa often spread to involve the esophagus. Distal submucosal spread in the esophagus can be extensive and require partial or total esophagectomy. Reconstruction with transposition of the stomach (gastric pullup) or jejunal free graft is currently recommended (293, 311, 585). Following the advent of total laryngopharyngectomy and postoperative radiation therapy, disease recurrence more commonly occurs in distant sites (i.e., the lung). Treatment approaches with combined preoperative or postoperative radiation have improved the control of lymph node disease, but survival rates have not improved substantially over those with surgery alone because of the increased rates of distant metastases. Postoperative radiation is currently preferred to preoperative radiation because of its lower local recurrence rates, fewer complications, and less difficulty in accurately assessing tumor margins (198). The clear superiority of combined surgery and radiation over surgery alone has not been established (94, 198, 704, 784). Although several studies demonstrate improved survival with combined therapy (196, 204), direct comparisons with surgery alone are difficult because of differences in patient selection factors, tumor extent, and degree of lymph node involvement. Well-designed, randomized trials to compare surgery alone with combined therapy have not been performed.

The presence of lymph node metastases, extracapsular lymph node involvement, and direct extension of the primary tumor into the soft tissues of the neck are major negative prognostic factors. Overall 5-year survival rates range from 10 to 30% for posterior pharyngeal wall cancers (78, 155, 548, 650, 738), and from 20 to 40% for pyriform sinus cancers (Table 105.14) (39, 196, 204, 534, 550, 704). Local/regional recurrence continues to account for the greatest number of deaths from disease (346, 704).

Distant metastases are rarely evident at the time of presentation. The development of distant metastases may appear many years after primary therapy and seems to correlate with extent of regional lymph node involvement (204, 353). The rates of distant metastases range from 20 to 50% (204, 704) and increase with the extent of lymph node metastatic disease. In a recent study by the EORTC, induction chemotherapy and radiation therapy were utilized for stages II and III hypopharyngeal cancers. In these randomized trials, which compared laryngeal preservation with combination chemotherapy and radiation therapy with surgery with postoperative radiation therapy, survival (including surgical salvage) remained equal. Approximately 30% of patients with stage III disease can preserve their larynx. The functional analysis of these patients regarding speech and swallowing remain unreported to date, however (411).

Larynx

Because of the prominent role the larynx plays in speech communication, swallowing, respiration, and protection of the lower airway, the treatment of cancer of the larynx presents formidable functional consequences in addition to the intrinsic threat to life posed by these cancers. Unique to this particular site of head and neck cancer, quality-of-life issues have been incorporated into treatment decision making more extensively than for other cancer sites (468). Cancer of the larynx is generally diagnosed at an earlier stage of development than are other head and neck sites, primarily owing to the early manifestation of symptoms. As a result, cure rates are generally higher than for other sites.

The three laryngeal subdivisions (see "Anatomy" above) form the basis for classifying cancers arising at the different sites within the larynx and have clinical importance in the embryologic development, vascular and lymphatic anatomy and the patterns of tumor growth in the larynx and in the frequency of metastases. The characteristics used in the clinical staging of primary tumors arising in each of these major subdivisions differ (Table 105.15).

Considerable attention has been devoted to anatomic studies of the vascular and lymphatic compartments of the larynx (242, 385, 544, 756). These studies have formed the basis for defining natural anatomic barriers to cancer spread within the larynx and have contributed to the development of precise surgical techniques for partial laryngeal resections for small cancers.

The true vocal cords present an effective apparent boundary between supraglottic and subglottic lymphatic spread within the larynx. This separation breaks down with tumors involving the anterior or posterior commissures and with deep invasive tumors that extend vertically across the true and false vocal cords (transglottic cancers). Normally, the internal perichondrium of the thyroid cartilage also presents an effective barrier to cancer spread. However, cancer involvement of the anterior commissure or transglottic extension is associated with invasion of the thyroid cartilage in 40 to 60% of cases (384, 399).

Early diagnosis is critical for achieving high survival rates and larynx preservation (171). Most cancers that are diagnosed at an early stage of development arise in the glottic larynx. This is so because minimal changes in the mass of the vibrating vocal cord due to tumor growth result in changes in its vibrating characteristics evident as dysphonia or hoarseness. Supraglottic cancers are usually more advanced than glottic cancers at the time of diagnosis because they do not generally produce early symptoms of hoarseness. Rather, the earliest symptoms of a supraglottic cancer are usually sore throat, dysphagia, referred otalgia, or the development of a neck mass representing regional metastasis. Airway compromise may be an early symptom with subglottic cancer.

Modern clinical evaluation of laryngeal cancers includes indirect mirror-assisted or fiberoptic laryngoscopy, direct laryngoscopy, CT, and MRI scanning of the larynx and neck, as well as videostroboscopic analysis. These radiologic assessments are of value in assessing direct extension to the preepiglottic and paraglottic spaces of the larynx, detecting

Table 105.14. Overall Five-Year Survival Rate (%) in Patients with Squamous Carcinoma of the Hypopharynx

Investigator	(n)	Stage I	Stage II	Stage III	Stage IV	Overall
Dubois[196]	(457)	60	47	23	8	16
Bataini[39]	(384)	36	33	24	10	19
Razack[550]	(120)	77	63	25	5	28
Carpenter[94]	(162)	100	66	51	0	47
Pingree[534]	(1,208)		35*		23*	25

* Stages I and II combined; III and IV combined

Table 105.15. Primary Tumor Staging Characteristics for Carcinoma of the Larynx

Supraglottis	
T1	Tumor limited to one subsite, normal vocal cord mobility
T2	Tumor invades more than one subsite, normal vocal cord mobility
T3	Tumor limited to larynx with vocal cord fixation and/or invades postcricoid area, medial wall of pyriform sinus or pre-epiglottic tissues
T4	Tumor invades thyroid cartilage and/or extends to tissues beyond larynx, e.g., oropharynx, soft tissue of neck
Glottis	
T1	Tumor limited to vocal cord(s) with normal mobility
T2	Tumor extends to supraglottis and/or subglottis and/or impaired vocal cord mobility
T3	Tumor limited to larynx with vocal cord fixation
T4	Tumor invades thyroid cartilage and/or extends to tissues beyond the larynx
Subglottis	
T1	Tumor limited to the subglottis
T2	Tumor extends to vocal cord(s) with normal or impaired mobility
T3	Tumor limited to larynx with vocal cord fixation
T4	Tumor invades cricoid or thyroid cartilage and/or extends to tissues beyond the larynx

cartilage invasion, and evaluating the soft tissues and lymph nodes of the neck. These studies have replaced conventional tomography and contrast laryngograms. The precise evaluation of tumor extent demands direct laryngoscopy under anesthesia. With large obstructive tumors, this may necessitate prior tracheostomy. In some patients with large obstructive lesions, debulking the tumor mass at the time of direct laryngoscopy can obviate the need for tracheostomy and thereby reduce the potential risk of tumor seeding of the tracheostomy site. Even with precise clinical evaluation, inaccurate estimation of tumor extent (usually underestimation) occurs in 30 to 40% of cases (533). Most often this involves failure to identify invasion of the laryngeal cartilage framework. Nevertheless, with clinical examination confirming normal vocal cord function and the absence of anterior commissure involvement, there is no clear role for radiologic imaging of the larynx.

Supraglottic primary tumors account for 25 to 50% of all laryngeal cancers (173, 176). A knowledge of the laryngeal compartments aids in understanding the spread and staging of supraglottic and glottic cancers. The staging of supraglottic cancers is based on the subsite or region of the supraglottis involved in the cancer. Subsites include the false vocal cords, arytenoids, lingual and laryngeal surfaces of the epiglottis, and aryepiglottic folds. The epiglottis itself is also subdivided into the region extending above the plane of the hyoid and that below the hyoid. Suprahyoid epiglottic tumors tend to have a better prognosis than infrahyoid cancers with the exception of those invading the aryepiglottic fold (marginal area) to involve the pyriform sinus. Early cancers (T1 and T2) involve one or more subsites, but have normal vocal cord motion. Those cancers that cause fixation of the vocal cord or involve the postcricoid region, medial wall of the pyriform sinus, or preepiglottic space are staged T3. Those that extend beyond the larynx or invade thyroid cartilage are staged T4.

Glottic carcinomas are also staged according to the subsites involved. Cancers limited to the true vocal cords are T1 (T1a—one vocal cord involved; T1b—both vocal cords involved) and those with extension to the false cord above or the subglottis below are staged T2. Vocal cord fixations are classified T3 whereas those with cartilage involvement or extension outside the larynx are T4.

Subglottic cancers that are limited to the subglottic region (T1) or to the subglottis and true vocal cords (T2) are early cancers. Fixation of the vocal cord (T3) and cartilage invasion or extension outside the larynx (T4) are associated with a worse prognosis. The nodal classification for staging is the same as for other HNSCC sites.

Curative radiotherapy is generally the treatment of choice for early-stage laryngeal lesions. It is for the moderately advanced lesions that one must consider the trade-offs between definitive radiotherapy with salvage surgery held in reserve and a surgical approach. The patient must be brought into the decision-making process when the various treatment options are being formulated.

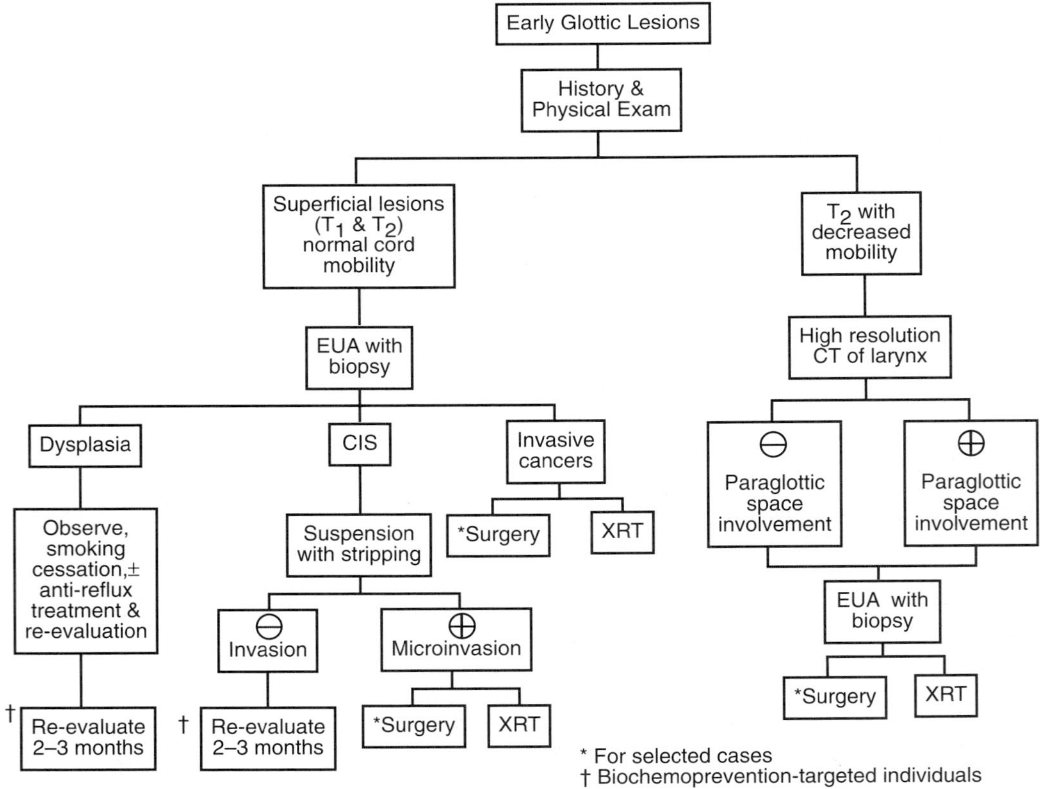

Figure 105.5. Algorithm for management of early glottic lesions. EUA, examination under anesthesia.

A treatment algorithm for premalignant and early glottic malignancies is shown in Figure 105.5. Obviously, examination under anesthesia and biopsy is the gold standard in the assessment of early lesions, with radiographic imaging reserved for assessment of the paraglottic space when decreased cord mobility is noted and thyroid cartilage if an infiltrative lesion of the anterior commissure is noted. Certainly, radiation therapy remains the management of choice in early glottic cancers. Nevertheless, in some instances, patients may choose conservative laryngeal surgery, including endoscopic laser excision of localized lesions, or partial laryngeal surgery; both require frozen-section analysis of margins if the patient and tumor factors support such an approach. Additionally, in some instances, conservative laryngeal surgical salvage may be attempted in those 10 to 20% of cases where external beam therapy has been unsuccessful in stages I and II cancers.

The design of the radiation portals must be tailored to the individual patient, but some general comments can be made. In general, supraglottic tumors have access to a richer lymphatic drainage than do tumors of the glottic larynx and so radiation fields tend to be larger in order to treat the larger volume at risk for metastatic disease (453). Typically, one treats the primary tumor volume and regions at risk for subclinical metastatic disease to 5,000 cGy, and then reduces the field size to areas of gross disease and delivers an additional 2,000 to 2,400 cGy. The spinal cord is shielded at 4,500 cGy and megavoltage electron beams are used to treat the posterior cervical nodes to higher doses as required. Because of the V shape of the anterior neck, wedge-compensating filters are often required to ensure uniform radiation dose distributions. If the anterior supraclavicular fossa is at risk for micrometastatic disease, it is treated to 5,000 cGy using an anterior field suitably matched to the upper neck fields. Early-stage (T1–2N0) glottic lesions are generally treated with relatively small fields localized to the primary tumor. Tumors of the subglottic larynx can spread to the upper paratracheal nodes, as well as to the nodes in the cervical chain, and radiation fields for this disease must, therefore, include the upper mediastinum (231).

The treatment of more advanced laryngeal cancers (T3 and T4) has historically included surgery with or without radiation therapy. Prospective randomized studies have shown convincingly that chemotherapy and radiation therapy (including surgical salvage) are equally effective in the long-term survival of patients with T3 laryngeal cancers as compared with surgery with or without radiation therapy. It is important to note that approximately 60% of patients may preserve their larynx, and thus quality of life has significantly improved (468,717) Unfortunately, success with laryngeal preservation attempts for T4 lesions that invade the thyroid cartilage are fraught with poor local control and chondronecrosis of the larynx. Therefore, these advanced lesions still require surgery, and frequently postoperative radiation therapy, if subglottic extension or peritracheal or other lymph node metastases are noted. A treatment algorithm for advanced glottic cancers is shown in Figure 105.6.

Many surgical procedures for laryngeal carcinoma involve the creation of a tracheal stoma. This area is sometimes at significant risk for tumor recurrence, which is most likely associated with peritracheal metastases that erode into the peristomal area. For this reason, bilateral peritracheal dissections should be performed in T4 glottic cancers and radiation therapy provided postoperatively if metastases to

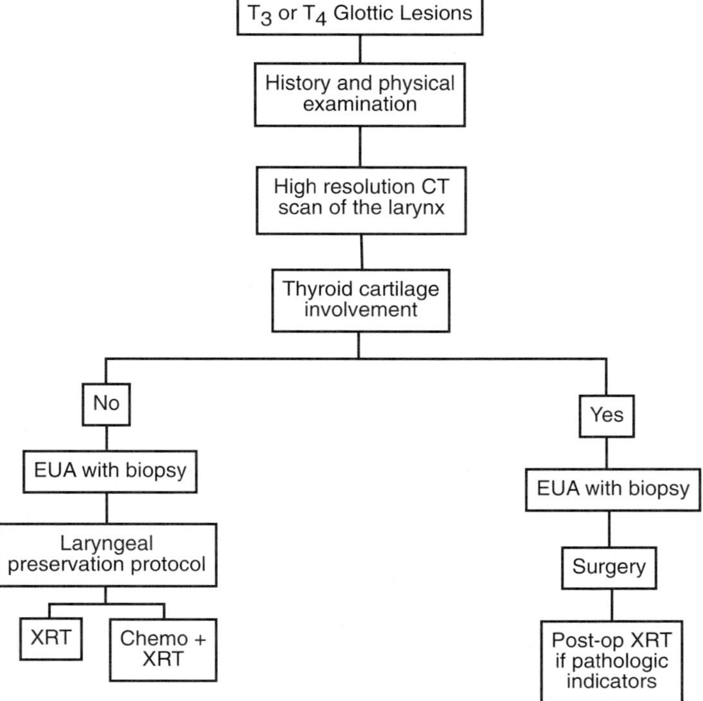

Figure 105.6. Algorithm for management of advanced glottic lesions. EUA, examination under anesthesia.

this echelon of nodes are found pathologically. Once a stomal recurrence has developed, the prognosis is very grave regardless of whether it is treated with surgery or radiotherapy. Sisson and colleagues report on a series of 28 patients with stomal recurrences treated with one or more surgical resections (623). The 5-year survival was only 17%. Schneider and colleagues report on patients with tracheal recurrences treated with radiotherapy; good palliation of local pain and/or bleeding was achieved, but the 2-year survival was only 6% (588). Given the poor results with salvage therapy, it is clearly better to prevent stomal recurrence in the first place. If risk factors for stomal recurrence are present (Table 105.16), then the tracheal stoma should be irradiated as part of the initial management.

Table 105.16. Risk Factors for Tracheal Stomal Recurrence

Extensive primary lesion (T_3 or T_4)
Subglottic tumor extension
Preliminary emergency tracheostomy for airway obstruction
Inadequate tumor margins on the pathologic specimen
Tumor involvement of the paratracheal lymphatics
Large, fixed nodes or multiple involved cervical nodes
Perineural or venous invasion by tumor

Supraglottic

Important factors in selecting therapy for supraglottic cancers are tumor location and preepiglottic extension. Tumors limited to the suprahyoid epiglottis are amenable to radiation with fields that encompass neck regions at risk for lymphatic metastases. Additionally, some proponents of limited surgical interventions recommend endoscopic laser excision with observation of the neck for N1 disease. An algorithm for early supraglottic cancers is shown in Figure 105.7. Tumors involving the aryepiglottic folds, pyriform sinuses, or infrahyoid epiglottis tend to be more aggressive, are deeply infiltrative, and frequently involve the preepiglottic space. Radiation alone is less effective than surgery, resulting in more frequent local recurrences that require surgical salvage. Often these recurrences are difficult to detect early enough to allow salvage by laryngeal conservation surgery and, therefore, require salvage total laryngectomy. Persistent postradiation edema of the supraglottic larynx is not uncommon and contributes to difficulty in detecting recurrence, which occurs in 40 to 50% (247, 739, 746).

Preepiglottic extension of cancer carries a poor prognosis. However, these situations can be managed effectively with horizontal supraglottic laryngectomy, which allows preservation of the voice. Indeed, even advanced tumors

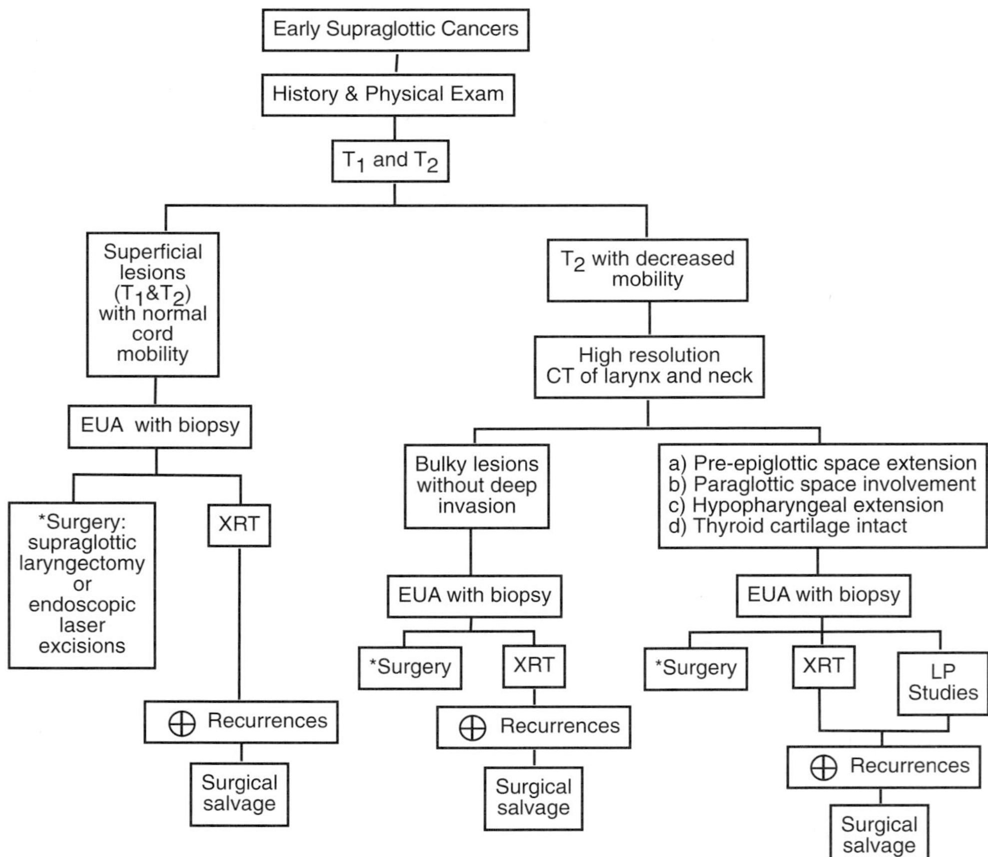

Figure 105.7. Algorithm for management of early supraglottic cancers. EUA, examination under anesthesia; LP, laryngeal preservation.

with extension of cancer to the valleculae and tongue base can often be treated by supraglottic laryngectomy with results equal to those of total laryngectomy. Very superficial tumors of the suprahyoid epiglottis can also be treated with simple epiglottectomy. Because supraglottic laryngectomy is associated with variable degrees of postoperative aspiration, adequate pulmonary status is a prerequisite for this surgery, as is intact mobility of the true vocal cords.

In every patient undergoing supraglottic laryngectomy, preoperative permission must be obtained for total laryngectomy in case the surgical findings dictate that more extensive surgery is needed to extirpate the cancer. Approximately 20% of patients require prolonged tracheostomy, and this is usually related to edema secondary to postoperative radiation. The rates of persistent swallowing difficulties are low, however, and the need for completion laryngectomy for persistent aspiration ranges only from 0 to 5% (61, 410, 445).

The frequency of neck node metastases is high with T2 or greater tumors. Treatment of the clinically negative neck may be accomplished with surgery or radiation. Surgical approaches should include removal of bilateral primary nodal groups at risk (levels II, III, IV) for occult disease. For N0 disease, most authors advocate elective modified radical dissection or selective dissection of nodal groups (60, 79, 175). Others argue that neck dissection can be delayed until clinically evident metastases occur (500, 602). For T1 and T2 lesions, most authors demonstrate overall cure rates of 68 to 73% (79, 119, 386) with determinate 3-year survival rates of 80 to 85% (60, 173, 418) when elective neck dissection is included. Most recurrences occur in the neck and this argues for prophylactic neck treatment.

Radiation is also effective for early lesions. Local control rates for patients with supraglottic tumors treated with radiation alone range from 68 to 94% and survival rates from 50 to 89%. The latter set of survival figures are comparable to those for planned surgery and adjuvant radiotherapy, which range from 46 to 90%. While the figures are comparable for T1 and T2 lesions, there is a trend favoring the combined approach for larger lesions. Nonrandomized series from different institutions are not strictly comparable since unstated patient-selection factors are generally involved. For example, the excellent local control results by Goepfert and colleagues for T3 and T4 lesions are for a selected set of tumors that were exophytic in nature (266). Survival rates tend to run lower than local control rates for supraglottic tumors because of deaths from second primaries and other intercurrent diseases. Cure rates range from 73 to 75% (297, 709, 740) and increase to 80 to 85% with the addition of surgical salvage (345, 471, 640). Most recurrences are local and preservation of voice is successful in 65 to 70% of patients when salvage surgery is included (443, 640).

The treatment of more advanced supraglottic cancers (T3, T4) remains controversial. Laryngeal preservation remains a focus on this population as well, however. A patient management algorithm is shown in Figure 105.8. In cases with clinically evident regional metastases, combined surgery and postoperative radiation are usually recommended since this treatment approach is associated with better local control rates (629) and better control rates for neck disease in both the ipsilateral and contralateral neck (244). Approximately 50% of patients have clinically palpable lymph nodes at the time of diagnosis and 20 to 25% have bilateral nodal

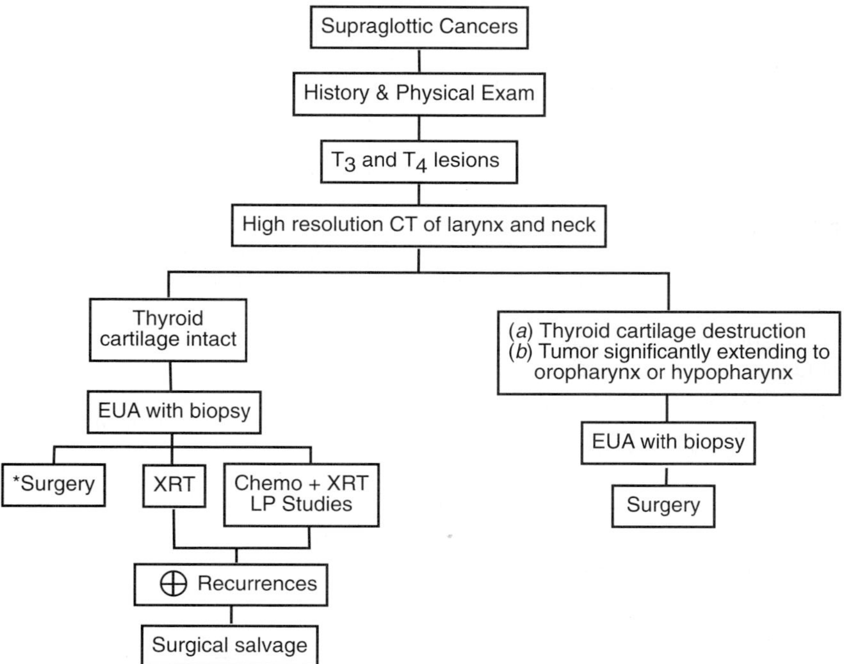

Figure 105.8. Algorithm for management of advanced supraglottic cancers. EUA, examination under anesthesia; LP, laryngeal preservation. * Selected cases.

Table 105.17. Overall Five-Year Survival Rates (%) for Patients with Squamous Carcinoma of the Supraglottic Larynx

Investigator	N	Stage I	Stage II	Stage III	Stage IV
Flynn[232]	234	93	49	50	33
Fu[244]	173	64	80	35	10
Shah and Tollefsen[603]	290	83	72	42	0*
Coates[119]	212	69	73	51	—
DeSanto[174]**	236	80	65	62	52
Goepfert[266]	241	100	68	59	32

* 3 patients
** Determinant survival, 2–13 yr. follow-up

involvement. In the clinically negative neck, elective neck dissection shows cancer metastases in 15 to 30% of patients. Failure to control disease in the neck is a major cause of mortality in advanced supraglottic cancers. In most reports, radiation alone for the control of supraglottic cancers with N2 or N3 nodes is clearly inferior to combined therapy. Therefore, in instances where T1–T3 lesions of the supraglottis are associated with N2 or N3 disease, neck dissection should be performed when the primaries are treated by radiation therapy. Although the issue of optimal initial management for the patient with N0 disease has not been settled, an individualized approach has been recommended in which bilateral selective node dissections are performed. Postoperative radiation is reserved for patients with proven regional metastases (410, 634).

Overall 5-year survival rates for supraglottic cancers range from 40 to 50% (Table 105.17) (454, 640). Local failures occur in approximately 10% of patients and regional failures in 15 to 20%. Rates of distant metastases range from 11 to 18% (259, 442, 453, 640), with rates approaching 30% in patients with stage IV disease (640). Second primaries (20 to 25% of failures) are a major cause of death (454, 640). Intercurrent illness accounts for up to 20% of deaths (454, 701).

Glottic

The treatment of glottic cancer is greatly influenced by the secondary goal of voice preservation. Mobility of the vocal cords is a critical factor in selecting treatment. For small cancers (T1, T2) with mobile vocal cords, radiation therapy alone for cure achieves excellent local control rates (T1, 85 to 95%, T2, 65 to 75%) and overall survival rates similar to those for surgical resection (301, 369). Voice quality, although often impaired by radiation, is generally better than that following surgical resection (370, 503). Local control rates are 10 to 15% better with primary surgery, but local recurrences after definitive radiation can often be salvaged by subsequent surgery, and this combined approach results in overall survival figures comparable to those with primary surgery. Tumor involvement of the anterior commissure or arytenoids may be associated with higher local recurrence rates with radiation alone, but this may historically have been related to understaging. As with supraglottic cancers, careful clinical tumor staging is necessary since underestimation of tumor extent is common. The "irradiate and watch" treatment strategy is predicated on close follow-up in order to detect recurrences when they are still salvageable by surgery. Delay in the diagnosis of recurrent glottic cancers after radiation is more frequent than with supraglottic cancers (175) and often requires total laryngectomy for cure. Thus, unreliable patients, or patients who are difficult to examine, may be more suitable for primary surgical treatment.

Survival figures in radiotherapy series are comparable to local control figures, reflecting the effectiveness of surgical salvage and the fact that few patients with early-stage glottic cancer die of their disease. The 5-year survival rates for T1 lesions range from 80 to 95% with either primary surgery or radiation (Table 105.18). Rates for T2 lesions are generally in the range of 70 to 80%, but these rates are decreased 10 to 15% (local control rates drop 20 to 25%) when the mobility of the vocal cords is impaired (300) or transglottic spread is present (485). Lesions with impairment due to invasion of muscle behave more like T3 cancers and have a poorer response to radiation alone (299, 367, 379, 700, 701). Transglottic cancers and those with subglottic extension have higher rates of regional metastases and often require total laryngectomy for cure. In selected patients with these more advanced lesions or impaired vocal cord mobility, extended hemilaryngectomy, or more extensive subtotal laryngectomy with resection of a major portion of the cricoid cartilage, can achieve excellent cure rates (51, 521). Voice quality is diminished with these extensive procedures, and chronic aspiration or permanent tracheostomy may result. Additionally, these procedures are technically challenging and experience dependent. However, if proper patient selection is accomplished, these procedures can be well tolerated. Although further study is required, hemilaryngectomy with postoperative radiation therapy has been advocated for some patients with close or involved surgical margins (267).

Management of advanced T3 glottic cancers had historically consisted of total laryngectomy with or without postoperative radiation therapy. Local control rates with radiotherapy alone for T3 and T4 lesions run between 20 and 35%, with survival rates between 36 and 57% for T3 lesions and 10% or less for T4 lesions. In patients without regional metastases, local tumor control rates with surgery alone are excellent. Significant increases in local control with the addition of radiation therapy have not been clearly demonstrated. However, in patients with regional metastases, overall prognosis

Table 105.18. Overall Five-Year Survival Rates (%) for Patients with Squamous Carcinoma of the Glottic Larynx

Investigator	N	Stage I	Stage II	Stage III	Stage IV
Mainpang[448]	143	93	83	—	—
Kelly[379]†	148	82	79	—	—
Hendrickson[308]‡	525	82	68	61	37*
Kaplan[367]	283	96	88	65	57*
Yuen[786]	192	—	—	80	63
Skolnick[624]	264	82	70	53	20

* <10 patients
† 3-year rates
‡ 4-year disease-free rates.

is poor and recurrence in the neck is a major problem when surgery is used alone. Better regional tumor control rates are achieved with the addition of adjuvant radiation therapy, and this justifies its use in these advanced cases (266). Because rates of occult regional metastases approach 30% in patients with advanced glottic (T3, T4) cancers, elective modified or selective node dissections for staging purposes are recommended when surgery is performed for primary disease. Demonstration of histologically positive nodal metastases has been used as an indication for postoperative radiation. Surgery alone is curative in 50 to 80% of patients without nodal metastases (172, 367, 416, 709, 786), and decreases to less than 40% if metastases are present (148, 485, 624).

Considerable controversy surrounds the use of definitive radiation with surgical salvage in patients with advanced (T3N0, T4N0) but localized glottic cancers (172, 298, 402). A very large, long-term British study demonstrated that salvage laryngectomy was possible in less than 50% of patients who suffered tumor recurrence after definitive radiation (764). The radiation-alone concept, however, presumes equal overall survivorship as compared with primary laryngectomy, with associated low complication rates. Overall survival rates range from 50 to 55% (148, 298, 374) with larynx preservation in 60 to 70% of these patients (148, 298, 485). High complication rates, however, have been reported with late surgical salvage of radiation failures (148). The overall patterns are confusing and based entirely on retrospective series. The resolution of this controversy in management will require carefully designed prospective studies that include assessments not only of survival, but also of voice and quality-of-life issues and complication rates.

A subset of laryngeal cancers that warrant special consideration are those that involve both the glottic and supraglottic regions (transglottic). These cancers are usually advanced and are associated with a high incidence (30 to 50%) of regional metastases (465, 485), extralaryngeal spread, and vocal cord fixation. Although clinical understaging is common, occasionally these cancers are quite superficial and amenable to conservation surgical techniques. Most patients, however, require total laryngectomy. In a careful review of 152 cases of transglottic carcinomas, Mittal reported a 55% cure rate with combined therapy as compared with a 5-year survival of 8% with radiation alone (485).

Subglottic

Primary subglottic carcinomas account for less than 5% of laryngeal cancers. Limited data may support the use of primary radiotherapy for early-stage (T1, T2) lesions. However, these lesions are usually advanced at diagnosis and require surgery (laryngectomy) and bilateral peritracheal lymph node dissections since regional metastases occur in about 20% of these patients (605). Many reported series contain glottic primaries with subglottic extension and confuse these analyses. Surgical treatment generally requires total laryngectomy combined with resection of adjacent soft tissues (thyroid gland, strap muscles, peritracheal lymph nodes). Five-year survival rates of 36% for radiation therapy and 42% for surgery (720) have been reported. Also, cure rates as high as 70% have been reported in a small number of patients treated with combined therapy (605). The addition of adjuvant radiation offers the advantage of improved regional control rates and treatment of peritracheal and upper mediastinal lymph nodes. Histologically positive lymph nodes can be found in 65% of cases. The risk of stomal recurrence increases substantially with cancers that involve the subglottic larynx, particularly if prior tracheostomy was necessary for impending airway obstruction (378). Early aggressive treatment (often within 24 hours) has been recommended for patients requiring tracheostomy for subglottic extension of laryngeal cancers (159).

Patterns of failure for glottic carcinoma differ somewhat from other laryngeal sites. Local failures are uncommon with primary surgical therapy and account for fewer than 10% of recurrences. However, after primary radiation therapy for local glottic primaries, recurrences account for 10 to 50% of failures (374, 764). Regional nodal recurrences are seen in 15 to 30% of patients with advanced disease who are treated with surgery alone (786). This contrasts to supraglottic cancers where regional recurrences are a major site of failure.

It previously was thought that distant metastases from laryngeal cancers were uncommon, accounting for less than 10% of failures. Distant spread is approximately four times more common with supraglottic than with glottic cancers (545). Rates of distant metastases associated with glottic cancer have increased, however, with the use of combined therapy and have been reported in approximately 20% of patients with advanced disease (374). Rates appear to be directly related to the extent of nodal disease, with reported rates as high as 40 to 50% of failures attributed to distant metastases in patients with N2 or N3 disease.

Carcinoma in Situ

A special issue relates to the treatment of carcinoma in situ of the vocal cords (144, 261). This disease often can be managed with vocal cord stripping, but if enough serial sections are examined, foci of invasive carcinoma are often found. Pane and Fletcher report on a series of 79 patients with carcinoma in situ and seven patients with leukoplakia/atypical hyperplasia who were treated with radiotherapy (522). Patients were staged as either T1 or T2 using the same criteria as for invasive tumors. Local control rates were the same as for invasive lesions—89% for T1 and 74% for T2. However, only 2 of 12 failures were on the initially involved cord, suggesting that most were not true recurrences but rather new disease developing in dysplastic epithelium. Furthermore, it took about 5 years for 80% of the failures to develop, which further suggests a second process. Most of the failures after primary radiotherapy tend to be invasive whereas failures after vocal cord stripping tend to be equally divided between carcinoma in situ and invasive disease.

Very superficial cancers limited to the free edge of the vocal cord or carcinoma in situ can be effectively treated by limited excision by conventional means, or with laser excision, with excellent voice preservation (513, 761). More extensive disease requires cordectomy or vertical hemilaryngectomy (508). Numerous methods have been devised for reconstructing the vocal cords after conservation surgery, although, in fact, they are probably not necessary if proper patient selection is pursued. Voice results, in general, are inferior to that with radiation therapy alone for early lesions. The patient with carcinoma in situ, however, by inference has diffuse premalignant mucosal findings and certainly should be targeted for novel prevention strategies due to the likelihood of later developing invasive disease.

PARANASAL SINUS AND NASAL CAVITY

Paranasal sinus and nasal cavity tumors represent 0.2% of all human cancers. Roughly two thirds occur in the maxillary sinus and one-third in the ethmoid sinus. Frontal and sphenoid sinus cancers are rare—0.3% of sinus tumors. These cancers are associated epidemiologically with occupational exposures (woodworking, nickel refining), inhaling noxious fumes (dioxane, nitrosamine), and tobacco (see "Epidemiology" above). Although 80% of paranasal sinus cancers are squamous cell, a variety of other cell types exist and are increasing in frequency relative to squamous cell carcinomas (40).

These tumors notoriously present at a late stage; over 80% have bony involvement at diagnosis by radiographic or clinical examination. This fact relates to their vague and often protean symptoms: sinusitis is the most common. The natural history is characterized by local invasion into adjacent structures—base of the skull and orbit. While nodal and distant metastases are staged according to the AJCC criteria for the HNSCC, a staging system for primary tumors exists only for the maxillary sinus.

The complex anatomy of the paranasal sinuses and nasal cavity and their proximity to the orbit and skull base pose major problems in staging and treatment planning. The maxillary sinus can be visualized as a pyramidal chamber, which is bordered inferiorly by the alveolar ridge and palate, medially by the nasal cavity, and laterally by the cheek. This tumor can invade superiorly to the orbit, inferiorly into the alveolar ridge impinging on the superior alveolar nerve, and posteriorly involving the trunk of the maxillary branch of the trigeminal nerve and extending into the skull base. Invasion superiorly into the orbit may frequently compromise ocular integrity.

The ethmoid sinus is a complex of air cells between the medial walls of the orbits. The sphenoid sinus is a deep midline structure. Lateral wall invasion commonly results in an abducens paralysis, but can also cause facial paresthesias and numbness in the first and second divisions of the trigeminal nerve, as well as ocular palsies. Invasion superiorly into the cribriform plate often occurs.

The treatment of tumors of the paranasal and nasal cavity has traditionally been linked to advances in surgical excision along with muscle preservation or reconstitution for effective prosthesis. Early reports indicated poor results with 5-year survivors of 20 to 40%. With the advance of craniofacial resections and improved diagnostic imaging over the last 2 decades, some improved success has been experienced in the treatment of extensive sinus malignancies (55). Traditional surgical therapy of paranasal/nasal sinus tumors consists of resection with free surgical margins for low-grade lesions. High-grade malignancies frequently require combined surgery and radiation therapy. The total maxillectomy involves transection of the malar bone from the zygomatic process of the frontal bone, transection of the hard palate, and separation of the maxilla from the pterygoid plates. Reconstruction requires skin grafting and maxillofacial prosthetic obturation.

Single-modality therapy is effective in early-stage disease. Radiation of the cervical or retropharyngeal lymph nodes is limited to the presence of positive nodes, advanced lesions, or perineurally invasive malignancies. Results of pre- versus postsurgical radiation are mixed. Wang found a 58% 3-year disease-free survival with preoperative radiation versus a 36% 3-year disease-free survival with postoperative radiotherapy (740). However, Jesse found no difference between the two groups (356). A recent series suggests that in patients with resectable tumors, survival rates are better in patients treated with surgery and postoperative radiotherapy (343). Radiotherapy data are mixed, with 5-year survivals ranging from 0 to 50%.

In maxillary sinus tumors without bone invasion, surgery or radiation is equally effective. Once bone invasion has occurred, however, combination radiation and surgery is the suggested therapy. An exception is seen in a study that achieved a 3-year disease-free survival of 40% and a 5-year disease-free survival of 35%, in a group of 20 patients of whom 18 had T4 lesions, using megavoltage beams, meticulous technique, and effective doses (3, 15). Additionally, the Japanese experience with chemotherapy and radiation therapy in conjunction with necrotomy and debridement also suggests that advances in organ preservation may be possible in this arena.

SCC of the nasal vestibule, a distinct type of skin cancer, is related more to tobacco usage than to sunlight exposure and presents a difficult management problem. Nasal vestibule cancers have a distinctly more aggressive natural history with a worse prognosis than skin cancers of other sites and, therefore, require more immediate evaluation and treatment (265). Unexpected deep extension may occur in the nasal vestibule itself, upper lip, and other midface regions (516). Radiation is now the favored approach for patients without regional node disease because recurrence rates and survival data appear equivalent to those seen with surgery, the cosmetic outcome is much better than with surgery, and the morbidity is low (107). Furthermore, many of the radiation failures can be salvaged surgically. In patients without clinical neck node involvement, either surgery or radiotherapy yields 10 to 20% recurrence overall and only a 3% recurrence rate after primary single-modality therapy of lesions smaller than 2 cm (777). Large lesions, or those infiltrating the upper lip, may be treated with external beam radiation combined with radioactive implants or paired wedged beam radiation. Regional neck node involvement is uncommon (6%) at presentation and confers a poor prognosis with a high (over 50%) recurrence rate despite aggressive local therapy (surgery and radiotherapy).

SALIVARY GLAND

Anatomy

Tumors can arise not only in the major glands, but also in the small foci of salivary gland tissue scattered throughout the upper respiratory and digestive tracts. The most common sites of minor salivary gland tumors are the palate, the base of the tongue, and the buccal mucosa (207, 284, 651). The majority of salivary gland tumors arise in the parotid glands, and about 80% of these are benign. Tumors arising in the submandibular, submaxillary, or minor salivary glands are much more likely to be malignant.

The largest salivary glands are the parotids, which lie anterior to the external auditory canals. The facial nerve passes through the parotid and divides it into superficial and deep lobes. About 80% of the parotid gland lies in the superficial lobe and 20% lies within the deep lobe. The internal carotid artery, the internal jugular vein, the cervical sympathetic chain, and cranial nerves IX, X, XI, and XII are in close proximity to the deep lobe of the parotid. The parotid's lymphatic drainage is to the parotid and upper jugular nodes. These nodal groups then drain into the nodes at the angle of the mandible, the subdigastric nodes, or the upper portion of the posterior cervical chain. Depending on histology, these nodes may be involved. Certain histologies, such as adenoid cystic carcinoma, tend to invade major nerve sheaths—the facial nerve and the auricular-temporal branch of cranial nerve V. In general, the presence of a parotid mass warrants surgical excision since progression of even benign neoplasms may place the facial nerve at risk. Fine-needle aspiration may, however, be utilized when inflammatory or infectious etiologies are strongly considered.

The second largest glands are the submaxillary (submandibular) glands, located in the submaxillary triangle of the neck, which lies just anterior, and inferior, to the angle of the mandible. Certain tumors of the submandibular glands may invade along nerve sheaths or perineural lymphatics to spread to the mandible or the base of the skull. The sublingual glands are the smallest of the major salivary glands and are located deep in the floor of the mouth.

Histopathology

Benign lesions account for about 80% of tumors arising in the parotid glands, 50% in the submandibular glands, and 25% in minor salivary glands. A list of such tumors is given in Table 105.19.

The basic histologic classification of malignant salivary tumors was developed by Foote and Frazell (Table 105.20) (234). Mucoepidermoid carcinomas constitute about 26%, 21%, and 10%, respectively, of malignant salivary gland tumors of the palatal, parotid, and sublingual glands (467).

Table 105.19. Benign Tumors of the Salivary Glands

Adenomas
Pleomorphic adenoma
Monomorphic adenoma
Warthin's tumor (adenolymphoma)
Sebaceous lymphadenoma
Oncocytoma
Myoepithelioma
Vascular tumors
Hemangiomas
Lymphangiomas

Table 105.20. Malignant Tumors of the Salivary Glands

Mucoepidermoid carcinoma
Low grade
High grade
Acinic cell carcinoma
Adenoid cystic carcinoma
Adenocarcinoma
Malignant mixed tumors (carcinoma ex-pleomorphic adenoma)
Squamous cell carcinoma

They are the most common malignant tumor of the parotid (358). Well-differentiated tumors are characterized by a slow growth rate, a low recurrence rate after complete surgical excision (about 15%), and rare metastatic potential. High-grade tumors are more aggressive; the local recurrence rate after surgery alone approaches 60% (467). About 50% of patients with high-grade mucoepidermoid carcinoma present with regional metastasis, and 30% develop distant metastasis (647).

Acinic cell carcinomas are usually well differentiated and account for about 13% of the cancers arising in the parotid glands. Lymph node metastasis occurs in about 15% of cases (467). Local recurrences and distant metastases may occur many years after treatment (40, 648).

Adenoid cystic carcinomas (cylindromas) account for approximately 10% of parotid gland cancers and approximately 60% of malignant neoplasms arising in the submandibular or minor salivary glands (129, 208, 467, 649). An outstanding feature of this neoplasm is its propensity to invade major nerves and to spread along the perineural sheath. This must be taken into account in designing treatment. Although these tumors often follow an indolent course, as many as 40% of patients ultimately develop regional and/or distant metastasis (400, 721).

Adenocarcinomas account for 10% of parotid gland cancers but they are common tumors of the minor salivary glands. The majority of them are high grade. About 36% of patients either present with or subsequently develop regional lymph nodes and therefore the draining lymphatics need to be addressed in treatment strategies for adenocarcinomas (647). Distant metastases (bone and lungs) are common.

Carcinomas, expleomorphic adenoma, arise from preexisting benign pleomorphic adenomas. The risk of malignant transformation increases with time—1.6% for adenomas of less than 5 years' duration and 9.4% for adenomas present for more than 15 years (54). True malignant mixed tumors are very rare, constituting about 2 to 5% of all malignant salivary gland tumors, and are aggressive tumors: the neck nodes become involved in about 25% of patients.

Primary SCC of the salivary gland is rare, accounting for less than 3% of all parotid neoplasms. However, given the rich lymphatic network that permeates the parotids, SCCs of the skin of the forehead, temple, or ear may metastasize to this region. Such primary sites must be excluded before the diagnosis of primary SCC of the parotid can be made. About 50% of patients with primary SCC of the parotid ultimately develop positive regional nodes, and again, the draining lymphatics should be addressed by surgery and usually postoperative radiation therapy.

The presentation of malignant salivary gland tumors is variable, depending on site and histology. Facial nerve paralysis is uncommon and generally indicates a malignant lesion. Tumors of the deep lobe of the parotid may produce dysphagia, otalgia or trismus. When the parapharyngeal space is invaded, there may be cranial nerve IX, X, XI, or XII involvement. The usual presentation of a submandibular gland tumor is painless swelling below the mandible.

Staging

Recently, the AJCC and the UICC agreed to changes in the staging system for salivary gland tumors to bring the two schema into agreement. T-stage criteria are reproduced in Table 105.21, along with stage groupings. The N- and M-stage criteria are the same as for the more common HN-SCCs.

Treatment

The treatment of benign salivary gland tumors is primarily surgical. However, there may be a role for postoperative radiation in high-risk situations. If microscopic disease remains overlying the facial nerve or a recurrence has developed, postoperative radiation may be effective in preventing subsequent recurrences (161, 748). These tumors must be followed for extended periods because of the late recurrence and spontaneous transformation (40).

Surgery is the primary form of treatment for patients with resectable salivary gland cancer. Early-stage (T1/T1), low-grade mucoepidermoid cancers should be treated with local excision with free surgical margins. Such tumors arising in the parotid are treated with parotidectomy with preservation of the facial nerve. Early-stage, high-grade tumors of all other histologies are treated with surgical resection plus dissection of the regional lymph nodes. Such tumors arising in the parotid require parotidectomy with facial nerve preservation unless the nerve is clinically involved with disease. Patients with clinically positive neck nodes should have a neck dissection on the involved side. For many years, salivary gland tumors were thought to be resistant to conventional photon irradiation, but now it is recognized that this treatment can be highly effective when given in a postoperative setting to eradicate subclinical disease. Postoperative radiotherapy is indicated (676) when (*a*) the tumor is high grade (any histology, except low-grade mucoepidermoid carcinoma or acinic cell carcinomas) or is metastatic SCC, regardless of the surgical margins; (*b*) the surgical margins are close or microscopically positive (which often may include tumors involving the deep lobe of the parotid gland), regardless of the grade; (*c*) resection has been performed for recurrent disease, regardless of the histology or margin status; (*d*) the tumor has invaded skin, bone, nerve, or extraparotid tissue; (*e*) regional nodes are confirmed as positive on neck dissection; or (*f*) there is gross residual or unresectable disease.

Table 105.21. Staging of Salivary Gland Primary Tumors According AJCC, 1988

T Stage

Tx	Primary tumor cannot be assessed
T0	No evidence of primary tumor
T1	Tumor less than or equal to 2 cm in greatest diameter
T2	Greatest diameter of tumor more than 2 cm but less than 4 cm
T3	Greatest diameter of tumor more than 4 cm but less than 6 cm
T4	Tumor more than 6 cm in greatest diameter

Subdivisions

The above categories are subdivided into (a) no local extension or (b) local extension. Local extension is defined as clinical or macroscopic evidence of tumor invading the skin, soft tissues of the neck, bone, or nerve.

Stage Grouping

Stage I	T1a	N0	M0	
	T2a	N0	M0	
Stage II	T1b	N0	M0	
	T2b	N0	M0	
	T3a	N0	M0	
Stage III	T3b	N0	M0	
	T4a	N0	M0	
	any T	N1	M0	(excluding T4b)

In the past, patients with T3 or T4 parotid disease required radical parotidectomy with sacrifice of the facial nerve. Now, unless the facial nerve is circumferentially encompassed by tumor, nerve-sparing surgery may be used followed by radiotherapy. Dosages given to the primary resection site are in the range of 5,500 to 6,500 cGy, depending on the post-surgical tumor status. In the case of low-grade mucoepidermoid carcinomas and acinic cell carcinomas, it is generally not necessary to treat the neck nodes in the N0 neck. For other histologies, the neck nodal drainage is generally treated to dosages in the range of 5,000 cGy. In the case of adenoid cystic carcinomas, the radiation fields must include the courses of the adjacent cranial nerves because perineural spread is common.

The results of treatment depend on both histology and site. In a series from M. D. Anderson Cancer Center, 5-year survivals were 100% for 11 patients with acinic cell carcinoma, 95% for 20 patients with adenoid cystic carcinoma, 90% for 10 patients with low-grade mucoepidermoid carcinoma, 82% for 20 patients with high-grade mucoepidermoid carcinoma, 70% for 30 patients with adenocarcinoma, and 59% for 16 patients with malignant mixed tumor. In a retrospective review of 407 patients treated at Princess Margaret Hospital, primary parotid disease was controlled by surgery alone in 24% cases and by surgery and radiotherapy in 74% of cases (226). In a surgical series of submandibular tumors (130), 8 of 17 patients with adenoid cystic histology were free of disease after 5 years compared with only 3 of 17 with mucoepidermoid histology. Minor salivary gland tumors arising in the paranasal sinuses often present in an advanced stage. Goepfert and colleagues found a 2-year local control rate of 47% (9 of 19) in patients treated with surgery alone compared with 76% (26 of 34) in patients treated with surgery and postoperative radiotherapy (268).

For patients with large, inoperable salivary gland cancers, fast-neutron radiotherapy is an alternative. A randomized clinical trial was performed comparing neutron irradiation and photon irradiation in patients with large, inoperable lesions (281). After only 32 patients had been entered, the trial was closed early for ethical reasons. The tumor clearance rate at the primary site was 85% for the neutron group versus 33% for the photon group ($P = .01$); the clearance rate in the neck for patients with clinically positive nodes was 86% for neutrons versus 25% for photons. Actuarial projections showed the 2-year survival at 62% for the neutron group, compared with 25% for the photon group ($P = .10$). Ten-year data on this study continue to show improved local/regional control on the neutron arm (56% versus 17%, $P = .009$) but no difference in survival (395). This appears to be due to distant metastases, which ultimately became of greater importance on the neutron arm owing to a reduction in deaths attributable to local disease. A review of the published data on nonrandomized trials shows a local control rate of 67% for 309 patients treated with neutrons as compared with 26% for 298 patients treated with conventional photon radiation (404). Fast neutron radiotherapy is of particular interest in situations where the surgical alternative would entail sacrifice of the facial nerve.

An analysis of the University of Washington experience by Buchholz et al. (80) showed no difference in either local/regional control or survival for patients treated postoperatively with neutrons after surgery that left behind gross residual disease versus a comparable group of patients treated with neutron radiotherapy alone. Neutron radiotherapy also appears to be an effective treatment for large, multiply recurrent pleomorphic adenomas, although the follow-up period is too short to make a definitive statement in this regard (81).

Control of local/regional disease is only a part of the problem. Table 105.22 shows the incidence of distant metastasis from a series of parotid tumors as a function of histology (359). This ranges from a low of 8% for mucoepidermoid tumors to a high of 42% for adenoid cystic tumors.

Although early-stage, low-grade tumors have high cure rates with surgery/radiotherapy, standard local therapy is not so successful in locally or regionally advanced metastatic or high-grade disease. Therefore, a moderate amount of phase II chemotherapeutic study has been conducted in search of effective systemic therapy for these difficult cases (552).

Whereas adenoid cystic carcinoma is a slow-growing neoplasm, the mucoepidermoid subtype appears to grow faster and more closely resemble HNSCC in its biologic and clinical behavior. The single-agent response patterns reflect these differences. Paralleling results in HNSCC, methotrexate has yielded a 36% response rate in mucoepidermoid cancer. In salivary gland cancers of other histologies, however, methotrexate has produced only a 6% response rate. In contrast to methotrexate, doxorubicin is relatively inactive in mucoepidermoid carcinoma and HNSCC but active in other salivary gland histologic subtypes (708). These suggestions must be interpreted with great caution, since they are based in large part on retrospective data and very small patient numbers. Furthermore, response rates do not correlate well with survival, with the more chemoresistant but slow-growing adenoid cystic subtype having the longest survival.

Several single-agent studies have been conducted in salivary gland cancers. Promising results have been achieved with cisplatin, methotrexate, doxorubicin, and 5-fluorouracil. Tannock and colleagues conducted a single-institution review of results with noncisplatin single agents in adenoid cystic cancer (673). Although achieving one of the lowest response rates (29%), compared with other single-agent or combination trials, it also revealed the longest median survival rate (nearly 2 years). More recently, regimens including cisplatin have been tested. Cisplatin alone or in combination has been evaluated in over 130 patients and has yielded response rates in the range of 17 to 100%. Studies have evaluated single-agent cisplatin, mainly in adenoid cystic carcinomas, and yielded conflicting results (Table 105.23). The combination of cyclophosphamide, doxorubicin (Adriamycin), and cisplatin (CAP) is the most extensively studied regimen (7). A recent study with a dose-intensive cisplatin-based regimen combining all four drugs active in this disease produced high toxicity without an improvement in response or survival over single-agent cisplatin or other combinations (183). Hormonal therapy (based on supportive preclinical work) appears to have limited activity (181). The taxanes are the most promising new agents under study in salivary gland tumors.

Table 105.22. Distant Metastasis Rates in Parotid Carcinomas by Histology

Histologic type	No. with metastases/total (%)
Mucoepidermoid	14/184 (8%)
Acinic cell	2/14 (14%)
Acenoid cystic	22/53 (42%)
Malignant mixed tumor	3/14 (21%)
Adenocarcinoma	25/91 (27%)
Squamous cell	2/13 (15%)

From Johns and Kaplan[359]

Table 105.23. Phase II Chemotherapy Results in Salivary Gland Cancers*

Author	No. of patients	Histology	Agent(s)	Objective response rate (%)	Median survival (mo)**
Tannock[673]	17	AC	Mult	29	21
Alberts[7]	5	Mult	CDP	100	8
Schramm[591]	10	AC	P	70	7–18
Posner[540]	13	Mult	CD	38	8
	3	Mucd	PBM	66	6
Suen[665]	14	AC	P	64	—
Sessions[599]	14	AC	P	50	—
Creagan[140]	34	Mult	P-based	38	15
Eisenberger[200]	4	Mult	CDP	100	11+
Dreyfuss[193]	13	Mult	CDP	46	—
Triozzi[694]	21	AC	COF	25	—
Venook[707]	17	Mult	PDF	35	15
Licitra[422]	23	Mult	P	17	—
Dimery[183]	16	Mult	FACP	50	18

Abbreviations: AC, adenoid cystic carcinoma; Mucd, mucoepidermoid carcinoma; Mult, multiple; D, doxorubicin; B, bleomycin; C, cyclophosphamide; F, 5-fluorouracil; M, methotrexate; O, vincristine; P, cisplatin; V, vinblastine; —, no data
* Excluding isolated case reports
** From diagnosis

NASOPHARYNGEAL CARCINOMA

In the United States, nasopharyngeal carcinoma (NPC) accounts for 2% of all HNSCCs (see "Epidemiology" above). Its unusual epidemiologic and natural history features include a remarkable tendency toward early regional and distant dissemination. NPC also is extremely sensitive to radiotherapy and cytotoxic chemotherapy.

Natural History

In the adult, the nasopharynx is a chamber that is approximately cuboidal in shape and 4 cm on an edge. Anteriorly it is bounded by the choana of the nasal cavity, superiorly by the base of the skull, and inferiorly by the soft palate, and its posterior wall is the mucosa that overlies the superior constrictor muscles of the pharynx and the C1 and C2 vertebral bodies. The lateral walls contain the eustachian tube orifices. The epithelium of the superior lateral walls contains pseudostratified columnar cells and occasional goblet cells while the inferior lateral and posterior walls are stratified squamous in nature. The region is richly endowed with lymphatics that drain to the retropharyngeal and deep cervical nodes.

Malignant neoplasms of the nasopharynx are primarily epithelial, with the presence of keratin associated with a poorer prognosis. The World Health Organization (WHO) recognizes three histopathologic types of NPC: type 1, differentiated SCC (of varying degrees); type 2, nonkeratinizing carcinoma; and type 3, undifferentiated or lymphoepithelial carcinoma (526). Mixed patterns are common. About 75% of nasopharyngeal carcinomas are type 1 or 2 (or predominantly one or both of these types). The term "lymphoepithelial carcinoma" (type 3) is used when numerous infiltrating lymphocytes are seen.

About one-third of patients present with a neck mass without other complaints and about 70 to 75% of patients have enlarged neck nodes at presentation. Other common complaints are epistaxis, nasal stuffiness, headache, or hearing loss (generally unilateral). The tumor can spread laterally and superiorly to cause bony destruction of the base of the skull. Frequently, there are cranial nerve findings, with the sixth nerve being most commonly involved (106). There are two principal cranial nerve syndromes associated with NPC: the retroparotidian syndrome, involving the 9th, 10th, 11th, and 12th cranial nerves, and the petrosphenoidal syndrome, involving the third, fourth, fifth, and sixth cranial nerves (and occasionally the second cranial nerve via extension through the foramen lacerum into the middle cranial fossa). Evaluation of the nasopharynx should consist of direct visualization with either a mirror or a fiberoptic scope. A CT and/or MRI scan is important in evaluating base-of-skull involvement and the possible presence of occult involved lymph nodes.

Staging

The staging for nodal disease is the same as for other head and neck cancers. The staging for the primary site is based on regions of tumor involvement rather than on size of the lesion as follows: Tis, carcinoma in situ; T1, tumor confined to one site of the nasopharynx or no tumor visible (positive biopsy only); T2, tumor involving two sites of the nasopharynx; T3, tumor extends into nasal cavity or oropharynx; and T4, tumor invades the base of the skull and/or involves the cranial nerve.

Treatment

Standard treatment for NPC is radiotherapy for early and locally advanced disease. Surgical resection even for early-stage disease is technically difficult because of the anatomic location of the primary tumor and the frequent bilateral cervical and retropharyngeal node involvement. The role of the surgeon is limited to obtaining tissue for diagnosis and occasionally to resecting residual adenopathy after definitive radiotherapy. Fortunately, these tumors tend to be fairly radiosensitive and even large lymph nodes often respond to moderate doses of radiotherapy (403). Prior to initiating therapy, a dental consultation is advised since it is necessary to irradiate the parotid glands bilaterally and the resulting xerostomia predisposes to serious oral problems.

The initial radiation fields encompass the adjacent base of the skull, as well as the nasopharynx itself. The fields are bilaterally directed and include the retropharyngeal drainage and the anterior and posterior cervical chains. A dose of 4,500 cGy is given using megavoltage photons, and then the fields are reduced to spare the spinal cord and an additional 500 cGy given. Megavoltage electrons are used to bring the posterior cervical nodes to this same dose. The fields are then reduced in size and an additional 2,000 to 2,200 cGy given to the nasopharyngeal primary. Regions of positive cervical adenopathy are also boosted with megavoltage photons and/or electrons to total doses of 6,500 to 7,500 cGy depending on the original size of the node and its response to the first phase of therapy (279). In selected patients, the boost dose to the nasopharynx itself can be given with an intracavitary implant (743). Critical normal structures in the treatment region include the cervical cord, the brain stem, the optic nerves, and orbital contents. Proper shielding and limiting the delivered dose to these structures are necessary to avoid untoward complications. An anterior supraclavicular field is generally matched to the initial large lateral fields and approximately 5,000 cGy given to treat submicroscopic disease in this area.

Treatment results are related to both stage and histopathology, but many series do not adequately document outcome as a function of these variables. Huang combines the above-listed T1, T2, and T3 stages into his T1/T2 categories (336). For a clinically negative neck, he reports a 5-year survival of 65%. For groups corresponding to T4N0–N2 and T4N3, he finds respective 5-year survivals of 41.3% and 23%. Vikram and colleagues note a 5-year local/regional control rate for early T-stage N0 patients of 65% (718). Scanlon and colleagues show a clear worsening of prognosis with increasing cervical adenopathy with 5-year survivals of 67%, 24%, and 14% when the patient has no clinical adenopathy, unilateral adenopathy, or bilateral adenopathy (576). It is important to note that these series were treated prior to routine CT/MRI scanning, which would have the tendency to increase the clinical stage of the neck disease.

A clear correlation exists between the degree of cervical

adenopathy and the subsequent development of distant metastases, with patients with bilateral adenopathy having a 5-year actuarial risk of approximately 80% of developing distant metastases. Common sites of distant metastases are the lung, bone, and liver. In selected cases, a failure at the primary site alone can be salvaged using a combination of external beam radiotherapy and an intracavitary implant (741). However, the morbidity associated with this may be substantial.

Although effective in early stages, standard radiotherapy (despite achieving high complete response rates) produces 5-year survivals in stage III disease of only 10 to 45% and in stage IV disease of 0 to 30% (322, 527). Despite major differences between NPC and other HNSCCs, many chemotherapy studies have included NPC patients, which confounds study results. Chemotherapeutic strategies in NPC now treat this disease as a distinct entity. With the exception of parts of China, the problem of small patient numbers is obviously even greater in NPC trials than in many other HNSCC trials.

Early United States reports of chemotherapy in NPC were single-institution retrospective surveys of recurrent or metastatic NPC patients treated over a many-year period with a variety of agents. Active single agents include cisplatin, bleomycin, methotrexate, 5-fluorouracil, doxorubicin, and Vinca alkaloids. Interferon has very limited activity, with response rates of less than 10%. Retrospective surveys from the early 1980s reported 40 to 70% response rates (less than 20% complete responses) with a variety of cisplatin- and non–cisplatin-based combination regimens in recurrent disease. More recent series with intensive cisplatin-based regimens in recurrent disease have reported higher and more durable complete response rates (26).

The use of combined-modality treatments (sequential chemotherapy and radiotherapy) is under active study in advanced NPC (322). Neoadjuvant series have reported 70 to 90% response rates (20 –40% complete) with cisplatin- and non–cisplatin-based regimens. Results of a large series from Taiwan treating 1,206 patients with a variety of chemotherapeutic agents given with split-course radiotherapy suggested that the combined-modality approach was more effective than radiotherapy alone in historic controls (337).

At least seven small, single-arm sequential-therapy studies have been reported, all but one with cisplatin-based regimens (24, 322, 382, 635, 672). Tannock and colleagues reported the largest series of 49 consecutive patients treated with methotrexate, cisplatin, and 3-day continuous-infusion bleomycin followed by radiotherapy (672). The overall response rate was high, but complete response was low—22% (8 of 36) in patients with measurable nodal disease. After radiotherapy, the complete response rate jumped to 82%. This group compared its results with 140 stage-matched historic controls and reported no differences in disease-free or overall survival. Furthermore, there was no apparent reduction in distant metastases in the chemotherapy group. This study was not confirmed by three similar series (113, 185, 526). Although complete-response rates were equivalent in the combined-modality and radiotherapy groups, the disease-free and median survivals of the combined-modality group were higher.

The need for effective systemic therapy in NPC is indicated by the high recurrence rate despite high initial complete response rates with primary therapy. Two phase III trials comparing neoadjuvant chemotherapy with radiotherapy alone (both in N2–3, undifferentiated NPC) have been reported and produced conflicting results. An international trial tested neoadjuvant epirubicin, cisplatin, and bleomycin for three cycles in 399 patients. Compared with standard radiotherapy, this trial showed a significant increase in the 3-year disease-free survival rate (31% versus 4%, $P < .02$), and a nonsignificant increase in overall survival at a median follow-up of 24 months (153).

A second phase III trial from Hong Kong included three cycles of neoadjuvant (cisplatin and 5-fluorouracil) followed by radiation and four cycles of adjuvant cisplatin and 5-fluorouracil in 77 patients (100). At a median follow-up of 29 months, the 2-year overall survival rates for the chemoradiotherapy arm and radiotherapy control arm were 80% and 81%, respectively. The respective figures for disease-free survival were 68% and 72%. In addition, there were no differences in local, regional, or distant treatment failure rates between the two arms.

A third recent phase III NPC trial from Taiwan compared sequential (neoadjuvant) and concomitant cisplatin-5-fluorouracil–radiation (781). In this trial of 68 patients, actuarial disease-free survival at 5 years favored the concomitant arm (65% versus 41%). The difference in disease-free survival reflected the much higher relapse rate at distant sites in the neoadjuvant arm. These data are consistent with the results in other head and neck sites, indicating that concomitant chemoradiotherapy is more effective than are sequential approaches.

ADVANCED SKIN CANCER

Although the skin of the head and neck accounts for less than 10% of the body's surface area, 70 to 80% of cutaneous malignancies occur in this region. As a result of greater sun exposure in occupational and recreational activities, and the depleted ozone layer (with increased ultraviolet-B exposure), the incidence of skin cancer seems to be increasing, and the initial age at presentation to be decreasing (see Chapter 137) (753). About 3,000 yearly deaths are attributable to nonmelanoma cutaneous malignancies; morbidity occurs in a manyfold greater number of people, however, in terms of medical costs, cosmetic deformity, and loss of function. About 850,000 new nonmelanoma skin cancers are projected annually in the United States. Treatment is protracted because of the recurrent nature of the disease, the need for repeated reconstructive efforts, and the propensity of second primary skin cancers to occur. Most early lesions are successfully controlled on the first attempt with conservative local therapy. But advanced skin cancer of the head and neck is not controlled easily, and its frequently devastating physical consequences can have tremendous influence on a patient's psychological well-being.

The only phase II study of systemic therapy in advanced SCC of the skin tested isotretinoin plus interferon-alpha (INF-α). The overall major response rate was 68%, primarily limited to advanced local and regional disease (432, 433).

Three smaller series of cytotoxic chemotherapy combinations in similar patient populations report overall response rates in the 60 to 70% range (287, 317, 547).

Melanoma of the head and neck region is considered in Chapter 138.

SARCOMAS

Sarcomas arising from bone or extraskeletal soft tissues of the head and neck are rare. The most commonly encountered include osteogenic sarcoma (see Chapter 139), malignant fibrous histiocytoma, rhabdomyosarcoma, fibrosarcoma, synovial sarcoma, angiosarcoma. and chondrosarcoma (see Chapter 140). Complete excision is the mainstay of treatment, with radiation or chemotherapy playing a less well-defined role in most head and neck sarcomas, with the exception of rhabdomyosarcoma (see Chapter 169) (463).

Osteogenic sarcoma is the most common malignant neoplasm of bone, although it is rare in the oral and facial bones. Less than 10% of all osteogenic sarcomas occur in the skull, with most of them in the mandible or maxilla. Among American children, osteogenic sarcoma is the most frequent primary malignant tumor of the jaw. Craniofacial osteogenic sarcomas tend to have a better prognosis than those arising in long bones, with the best survival seen for tumors of the maxilla. Overall 5-year survival approximates 35% (see Chapter 139) (254).

Approximately 10% of chondrosarcomas occur in head and neck sites (83), the most common of which are the jaws, paranasal sinuses, and larynx. Chondrosarcomas of the larynx deserve special note because they tend to be low-grade, well-differentiated sarcomas with low metastatic capability. Successful management usually consists of complete surgical excision, which can often spare functional and cosmetic structures. With advances in craniofacial surgery, complete surgical excision of skull-base and maxillary chondrosarcomas should ultimately improve overall tumor control rates. Survival rates for chondrosarcoma are directly related to resectability, site, and tumor grade. The 5-year survival rate for low-grade, completely resected tumors ranges from 70 to 90% and overall survival rates range from 0 to 50% for unresectable or high-grade tumors (see Chapter 129) (83, 216, 462).

Rhabdomyosarcoma is the most common soft tissue sarcoma in children, and in the head and neck it presents most frequently in the orbit, sometimes by invasion from the adjacent nasal cavity or pterygoid musculature. Other sites of involvement include the nasopharynx, ear, paranasal sinuses, and soft tissues of the oral cavity and neck. Histologically, the embryonal variety is the most common. Of prognostic importance in rhabdomyosarcomas of the head and neck is the site of origin. Orbital sites have the most favorable and parameningeal sites have the least favorable prognosis. Five-year survival rates for these sites of childhood rhabdomyosarcoma are 89%, 55%, and 47%, respectively (463).

The parameningeal group consists of sites at high risk for meningeal spread of tumor and includes the infratemporal fossa, ear, nasopharynx, nasal cavity, and paranasal sinuses. Prior to the mid-1960s, surgical excision was the mainstay of therapy, with survival rates of less than 20% and with more than 80% of patients developing metastatic disease within 1 year of diagnosis (666). Chemotherapy and radiation had achieved 5-year survival rates of 83% for localized, completely resected disease; 70% for grossly resected disease with microscopic residual; and 52% for patients with gross residual disease (481). Based on these results, chemotherapy and radiation therapy have emerged as the preferred therapy for rhabdomyosarcoma of the head and neck with surgery reserved for residual or recurrent disease (see Chapter 169).

Malignant fibrous histiocytoma is the most common soft tissue sarcoma in adults, but only 3 to 10% are found in the head and neck (35). The paranasal sinuses are the most common head and neck site of origin, followed by craniofacial bones, larynx, soft tissues of the neck, and oral cavity. Those tumors arising in the sinonasal tract or facial bones tend to be very aggressive, with high rates of local recurrence and distant metastases (25 to 30%). Regional node metastases are rare. The 2-year survival rates range from 30 to 40% (see Chapters 139 and 140) (35).

Lymphomas can arise in any structure in the head and neck region, and they must enter into the differential diagnosis of every neoplasm (see Chapters 150 and 170).

SMALL CELL UNDIFFERENTIATED CANCER

A variety of small cell neoplasms that occur in the head and neck pose particular diagnostic problems for the pathologist. They probably derive from cells of embryonic neuroectodermal or neuroendocrine origin. In general, these tumors tend to behave aggressively. Some are unique to the head and neck, such as esthesioneuroblastoma, but others, such as neuroendocrine carcinoma, carcinoids, and Merkel cell carcinoma, have counterparts that occur at sites outside the head and neck. Differentiation of distinct entities frequently requires electron microscopy, special stains (PAS, Grimelius), or immunohistochemical stains for keratin, neuron-specific enolase, and polypeptide hormones, such as calcitonin, somatostatin, or ACTH. Some tumors may have a mixed histologic appearance with evidence of squamous or glandular differentiation (see Chapters 102 and 103).

ESTHESIONEUROBLASTOMA

Esthesioneuroblastoma (olfactory neuroblastoma) is an uncommon tumor (3% of nasal tumors) arising from the olfactory epithelium of the superior nasal cavity and cribriform plate (206, 601, 695). A bimodal age distribution exists and the etiology is not known (see Chapter 167). Intracranial spread through the natural foramina of the cribriform plate is common. The type and extent of primary therapy depend on the tumor size and location. Generally, early-stage disease is treated with a single-modality approach, such as complete surgical excision, usually with craniofacial resection techniques that encompass the entire cribriform plate and ethmoid complex. Adjuvant radiation is used for extensive tumors or when microscopic residual disease is suspected.

Despite aggressive local therapy, this tumor has a high propensity for multiple local recurrences. The distant metastasis rate is 10 to 20%. Overall survival correlates with stage with a 3-year survival of 50% in stage C (Kadish system) after surgery and radiotherapy. Chemotherapy has been increasingly integrated into the management of stage C disease and in recurrent/metastatic disease. Although the data are limited, drug response patterns are similar to those for the lung and other small cell cancers; cyclophosphamide, Vinca alkaloids, doxorubicin, cisplatin, and epipodophyllotoxins appear to be active (271). The most frequently reported regimen, cyclophosphamide/vincristine (with or without doxorubicin), produces overall response rates of 50 to 70%. A retrospective series recently reported significantly improved survival with multimodality therapy (including primary chemotherapy) over local therapy alone for stage C disease (639). No improvement in disease-free survival was noted, however, despite multiagent chemotherapy and craniofacial resection. In an attempt to increase disease-free survival, high-dose chemotherapy and autologous bone marrow transplant were investigated (661). The series included eight heavily pretreated patients, five with esthesioneuroblastoma and three with sinonasal undifferentiated carcinoma. Prolonged disease-free survival (17+ to 60 months) was reported in four patients.

NEUROENDOCRINE CARCINOMA

The most common sites of origin for neuroendocrine carcinoma in the head and neck are the larynx and paranasal sinuses, although similar cancers have been reported in the trachea and parotid gland (see Chapter 102) (41, 759). Although biochemical evidence of hormone production is common, paraneoplastic syndromes are rare. The prognosis is directly related to the site of origin and degree of histologic differentiation. Five-year survival rates of 70% for paranasal sinus sites have been reported as compared with less than 20% for laryngeal neuroendocrine tumors (41). Biologic behavior also varies according to histologic spectrum, from low-grade, well-differentiated "carcinoid type" tumors to intermediate-grade or moderately differentiated neuroendocrine carcinoma to highly aggressive undifferentiated carcinomas.

A particularly virulent entity of undifferentiated carcinoma has been described in the sinonasal tract (419). The management of low-grade tumors consists of conservative resection, often combined with radiation. Because of the rapid occurrence of distant metastases with small cell carcinomas or undifferentiated tumors, chemotherapy combined with radiation therapy or surgery is under study.

MERKEL CELL CARCINOMA

Merkel cell carcinomas arise from Merkel cells located in the basal layer of the epidermis and occur most commonly as a primary neuroendocrine carcinoma of the skin. Merkel cells are tactile cells of neuroectodermal origin and histologically show ultrastructural neurosecretory granules and immunohistochemical staining for neuron-specific enolase. The skin of the head and neck is a common site of origin. These tumors generally are seen in elderly patients. Although previously viewed as fairly indolent cancers of the skin, these adnexal malignancies are biologically aggressive, with an 80% rate of regional metastases and 50% rate of distant dissemination (269). Overall 5-year survival rates are less than 20%. Wide local excision and regional node dissections are effective in controlling localized disease, often in conjunction with radiation therapy. Adjuvant radiation is indicated for large tumors, tumors with close surgical margins, or lymphatic invasion. Because of the propensity for distant metastases and evidence that these cancers are quite sensitive to chemotherapy (150, 257, 782), this modality may be explored.

Chemotherapy Approaches in HNSCC

OVERVIEW

Chemotherapy is investigational in primary (advanced untreated)HNSCC (9, 20, 22, 48, 49, 95, 272, 288, 302, 320, 346, 622, 628, 641, 660, 692, 770). Data from the many different single- and combined-agent trials do not indicate that chemotherapy currently is able to improve survival prospects over those of local therapy with surgery and/or irradiation alone. Chemotherapy does play a role in the palliation of recurrent disease and recently has proved effective in primary-therapy trials of organ preservation.

Research into breast, lung, prostate, and colon cancers benefits from large, relatively homogeneous study groups (767). HNSCC research, on the other hand, suffers from great disease heterogeneity and a low incidence in the United States, factors contributing to confusion and conflicting reports regarding chemotherapy outcome (response and survival) and underscoring the importance of large multicenter randomized chemotherapy trials. A large-scale study of laryngeal cancer by the Veterans Affairs group is contributing important data on organ preservation (see "Primary Chemotherapy" below) and demonstrating the importance of multicenter studies of specific HNSCC sites (699). Single-arm trials should be limited to feasibility testing of new drugs and innovative study designs.

PROGNOSTIC FACTORS

Prognostic factors for chemotherapy response generally accepted as standard include performance status, nutritional status, degree of tumor differentiation, tumor burden (size of primary tumor, resectability, and extent of regional nodal metastases), disease stage, and primary cancer site (112, 124, 146, 392, 628, 775). In head and neck cancer, however, correlative results are conflicting, and it is difficult in most cases to say which of these standard factors has significant effects on response. One clear exception relates to site: undifferentiated nasopharyngeal cancer is the most responsive and adenoid cystic salivary gland cancer the least responsive to chemotherapy.

Recent work looking for additional prognostic factors in HNSCC has focused on immunologic studies, tumor DNA content, and p53 (134, 346). Clq-binding macromolecules and circulating immune complexes are the best-studied immunologic factors; both appear to be inversely correlated with the response of previously untreated patients to cisplatin-based chemotherapy (581, 582). DNA content studies report a direct correlation between aneuploidy and complete response rate to cisplatin-based regimens (212). p53 mutations have been associated with resistance to chemotherapy and radiotherapy. However promising such studies of biologic factors are, further data are required.

Chemotherapy Response

Comparing the results of HNSCC chemotherapy trials can be difficult because of inconsistent standards for response determination (628). Confusion regarding tumor measurements can arise as a result of superinfection from ulcerative lesions or, in studies in recurrent disease, from scarring after local therapy. The timing of response determination also varies. Clinical response determinations 4 to 6 weeks after therapy often describe persistent nonmalignant abnormalities (e.g., fibrosis, edema) that resolve after longer follow-up. This is a problem with bulky tumors treated with chemoradiotherapy. These responses may be variably reported as complete or partial.

All investigators agree that a complete response to chemotherapy is of overwhelming importance to a patient's survival outlook. The current direction of response reporting in primary HNSCC trials is to differentiate between responses at primary sites and those at regional sites. Pathologic documentation of primary-site clinical complete response is critical, and the number and depth of biopsies must be rigorously defined. There is disagreement, however, as to the comparative importance of histologic and clinical complete responses (8, 214, 509). Much of the discrepancy in this area of research may relate to a lack of thoroughness in clinical staging and a lack of uniform specifications for the number and depth of postchemotherapy biopsies. Although critical in screening for new drug activity, partial responses generally do not increase survival in primary or recurrent disease.

Toxicities

Chemotherapy-related toxicities frequently encountered in HNSCC are reviewed briefly in the following discussions of each agent. They are classic toxicities seen with the use of these agents in other cancers (99). Toxicities that are not well established or that are unique to drugs not currently in common use are not mentioned here but only in the applicable discussion of each drug.

The most frequent and dose-limiting toxicities with current chemotherapeutic approaches in HNSCC fall into three areas: myelosuppression, mucositis, and the legendary toxicities associated with cisplatin. Myelosuppression is a well-known side effect of chemotherapy of great importance in UADT neoplasms. Its mitigation by hematopoietic growth factors is important in other tumors and intuitively should be of great value in UADT tumors although few studies have been reported. (see Chapter 82).

Mucositis is becoming the limiting acute toxicity in the chemotherapy of HNSCC (see Chapter 185). Two of the most promising new approaches for controlling advanced HNSCC—concomitant chemoradiotherapy and chemical/pharmacologic modulation of 5-fluorouracil—are severely limited by this toxic effect. How best to mitigate mucositis is not clear. Several strategies to limit therapy-induced mucositis in HNSCC are under study, but no proved standard approach currently exists (46, 251, 278, 286, 483, 530, 643). In a randomized study, sucralfate rinses decreased mucositis associated with cisplatin and 5-fluorouracil (530). Antimicrobial mouthwashes containing amphotericin B, polymyxin B, and tobramycin have been reported to limit radiation-induced oral mucositis by selectively decreasing colonization of the oral cavity by fungi and aerobic gram-negative bacteria (643). A novel approach for reducing drug-induced mucositis is the use of circadian infusion schedules of anticancer therapy (286). Two other approaches that have yielded promising results include the use of filgrastin (G-CSF) and cryotherapy.

Problems with cisplatin toxicities (renal, otologic, neurologic, and gastrointestinal) may be solved largely by substituting carboplatin, a platinum analogue (90). Nevertheless, cisplatin will remain a leading agent against HNSCC when management is hampered by myelosuppression. The recent availability of specific serotonin receptor antagonists (e.g., ondansetron and gramsetron) greatly enhance control of the major acute problem of cisplatin-induced nausea and vomiting (see Chapter 174). Cisplatin's relative lack of mucositis also contributes to its continued utility because of the association of mucositis with some of the newer strategies, especially concomitant chemoradiotherapy.

Preclinical data and suggestive results of single-arm clinical trials have pointed to other ways to control cisplatin toxicity. One such new strategy is the use of a heterogeneous group of agents called chemoprotectors, a group that includes thiol-containing compounds (e.g., sodium diethyldithiocarbamate, sodium thiosulfate, and amifostine, or WR-2721) and probenecid (47, 518).

Preclinical Screening

Preclinical drug screening for active new agents and combinations is of highest priority. Many groups are developing panels of HNSCC cell lines for this research, and these lines are as heterogeneous as the diseases themselves. The establishment of panels of site-specific HNSCC cell lines may be important for future chemosensitivity studies. However, different cell lines from the same HNSCC may have different chemosensitivity patterns (393).

In addition to drug screening, the in vitro work has allowed the study of chemical modulation of active drugs. This work has shown that leucovorin, hydroxyurea,alfa-interferon and methotrexate potentiate 5-fluorouracil cytotoxicity. In vitro interactions between chemotherapy (e.g., hydroxyurea, 5-fluorouracil) and irradiation and between chemotherapy (cisplatin, 5-fluorouracil) and hyperthermia have also led to clinical trials. In vivo (xenograft) work has identified promising new drugs, such as gemcitabine (68, 706).

CHEMOTHERAPY OF RECURRENT HNSCC

The majority of patients included in the following discussion have recurrent disease and constitute the principal study group; a minority have metastatic or advanced unresectable disease. We refer to this patient group generically as "recurrent," although many studies discussed under this rubric include the minority cases also.

The exclusive arena for testing new chemotherapeutic single agents and the principal arena for trials of new combinations of agents in HNSCC is in recurrent disease. So far, chemotherapy has had no impact on overall survival in recurrent HNSCC. The purely clinical, noninvestigational goal of chemotherapy in recurrent disease has been to achieve palliation, unlike the goal of primary chemotherapy trials, which is to cure locally advanced, untreated cancer. The overall prognosis in recurrent HNSCC is dismal (median survival of 5 to 6 months).

Lumped diagnostically under HNSCC is a diverse group of cancers with markedly variable natural histories (fully discussed in the "Biology" section above) and, therefore, markedly variable responses to chemotherapy. Important diversities also occur in HNSCC relapse patterns: at the primary site, in regional nodes, and at distant sites after definitive local therapy. These and many other diversities make it extremely difficult to interpret results of chemotherapy trials in cancers of this region.

Many chemotherapy studies encompass all guises of recurrent HNSCC. They run the gamut from minimal, resectable disease seen locally after radiation therapy to bulky regional and distant disease occurring after surgery, radiotherapy, and even primary and/or salvage chemotherapy. Often these last salvage patients are excluded from further chemotherapy trials because of their extremely high risk. Other poor-risk patients, such as those with unresectable disease resistant to neoadjuvant chemotherapy or with short disease-free intervals or persistent disease after primary therapy, are included in many trials. Although patients with advanced resectable disease should be included in trials of primary therapy (112, 772), the varying definition of resectable among different head and neck surgeons can place these patients in "recurrent" trials.

Single-Agent Trials

Response rates of different trials with the same agent have varied markedly due to HNSCC's great heterogeneity and because of differences in trial designs. Pooled results indicate that eight drugs show single-agent response rates of 15% or higher and remission durations of 3 to 5 months (Table 105.24).

Methotrexate, according to many oncologists, is the standard palliative therapy for recurrent or metastatic HNSCC (320, 415). The standard dose and schedule for palliation are 40 mg/m^2/w intravenously or intramuscularly (89), with dose escalations to 60 mg/m^2/w until mild toxicity or any tumor response is achieved. This methotrexate dose and schedule are relatively nontoxic, inexpensive, and convenient, features that are critical to palliative therapy.

Preclinical work and early single-arm HNSCC clinical studies suggested a dose–response effect with high-dose methotrexate plus delayed leucovorin. However, five randomized trials of standard-dose methotrexate versus high-dose (up to 100-fold increases) methotrexate plus delayed leucovorin failed to show superiority. Pooled response rates for the two arms (high dose versus low dose) from all of the five randomized studies are nearly identical (Table 105.25).

The issue of high-dose methotrexate has been revived, however. A randomized, placebo-controlled trial of standard-dose methotrexate with leucovorin or without it revealed that even delayed leucovorin (given 24 hours after high-dose methotrexate) suppressed not only toxicity, but also antitumor activity (75). This study indicates the need for

Table 105.24. Single-Agent Activiity in Recurrent Head and Neck Cancer*

Agent	N	Response (%)
Methotrexate	998	31
Bleomycin	347	21
Cisplatin	288	28
Carboplatin	115	26
5-Fluorouracil	118	15
Cyclophosphamide	86	36

* See text

Table 105.25. Randomized Trials of Weekly Standard-Doses vs. High-Dose Methotrexate in HNSCC

Author	Standard dose		High-dose		
	Dose[a]	Response (%)	Dose[a]	Response (%)	Leucovorin (mg)
Levitt[420]	80–240	7/16 (44)	240–1,080	15/25 (60)	40/m^2 IV then 25/m^2 every 6 hr × 4 at 36 hr
Vogler[724]	60	12/44 (27) 19/61 (31)[b]	500	11/49 (22)	5 every 6 hr × 6 at 36 hr
Woods[779]	50	7/27 (26)[c] 6/23 (26)	500–5,000	10/22 (46) 7/27 (26)	15 every 6 hr × 2 at 24 hr
DeConti[165]	40–60	21/81 (26)	120[d] (2 wks)	19/90 (21)	25 every 6 hr × 8 at 42 hr
Taylor[680]	40	4/18 (22)	1,500	6/19 (32)	25 × 2 then 10 every 6 hr at 30 hr
Total	40–240	76/270 (28)	120–5,000	68/232 (29)	

[a] mg/m^2 per week
[b] Standard dose used in two different schedules; both were compared to a single high-dose regimen
[c] Three dose levels tested; middle dose (500 mg) was used at high dose vs. 50 mg, and as standard dose vs. 5,000 mg
[d] 240 mg/m^2 per 2 week

further work in optimizing methotrexate/leucovorin doses and schedules.

Cisplatin is perhaps the most important chemotherapeutic drug for HNSCC (95, 770, 771). Most studies have given cisplatin in an intermittent standard-dose bolus schedule (80 to 120 mg/m^2 every 3 to 4 weeks). Altered drug schedules designed to enhance therapeutic index in HNSCC have been tested. A small randomized comparison of schedules showed no difference in activity between bolus cisplatin at 120 mg/m^2/d and the less-toxic schedule of 20 mg/m^2/d for 5 days (572). Cisplatin given as a continuous infusion in HNSCC has pharmacokinetic advantages and activity equivalent to those at the same dose given in boluses (237, 347).

The dose–response relationship between cisplatin and HNSCC has been studied by several groups but remains unproved. Single-arm studies of regional and high-dose (150 to 200 mg/m^2) systemic cisplatin have produced single-agent response rates of over 70% and definite objective responses in patients failing standard-dose cisplatin (305, 491). The only randomized HNSCC trial, however, tested a lower "high-dose" regimen and failed to confirm cisplatin's dose–response effect (712). This trial, which directly compared 120 mg/m^2 with 60 mg/m^2 via intravenous bolus, was stopped early because of very similar response rates between the two arms (16.1% and 17.8%, respectively) and identical median survivals (34 weeks).

Bleomycin has been studied extensively as a single agent and in combinations in HNSCC. Its spectrum of toxicity is distinctive. Dose intensity is directly associated with mucositis, and total cumulative dosage is directly associated with skin toxicity and with the most feared side effect, pulmonary fibrosis. Bleomycin's lack of myelosuppression, even with prolonged continuous infusion, promotes its use in combinations. Continuous-infusion regimens produce less pulmonary toxicity but are not clearly more active clinically than intermittent-bolus schedules in HNSCC (523, 539, 620).

5-Fluorouracil has limited single-agent activity in HNSCC (Table 105.24). It has been given in varying doses as an intravenous bolus daily (for 5 days), weekly or every 3 or 4 weeks. The dose-limiting toxicity of bolus administration is myelosuppression; prolonged administration is limited by mucositis, diarrhea, and cutaneous erythema (554). Schedule dependency of 5-fluorouracil treatment has received little study in HNSCC, although long-term continuous low-dose infusion (e.g., 6 weeks) is effective palliation for recurrent disease (218, 674). Continuous-infusion regimens were designed initially to reduce myelosuppression and seem to have enhanced activity (10).

Despite 5-fluorouracil's modest single-agent activity in HNSCC, preclinical studies indicating its synergistic interaction with radiation and its enhanced cytotoxicity with chemical modulators (e.g., leucovorin) have led to active recent study of this agent in HNSCC (256).

Randomized trials have compared different single agents in recurrent HNSCC. Two phase III studies have directly compared cisplatin and methotrexate (randomized, two-arm design). In the first of these studies, Hong and colleagues gave cisplatin at 50 mg/m^2 on days 1 and 8 every month versus methotrexate at 40 to 60 mg/m^2 per week (326). Both arms produced similar response rates, 28.6% and 23.5%, respectively. Similar findings were observed in the second phase III trial (282).

New drug development in HNSCC is following five major avenues: high-dose therapy; altered schedules (e.g., continuous infusion); chemical/pharmacologic modulation of activity and/or toxicity of currently active drugs (primarily 5-fluorouracil); structurally and mechanistically new drugs; and new analogues of known active drugs with increased therapeutic indices. The first four avenues of study are discussed elsewhere. Work along the last approach, analogue development, is discussed here.

The methotrexate analogues trimetrexate, piritrexim, and edatrexate have been studied in HNSCC and may have pharmacologic advantages and less renal toxicity (99, 397, 564, 589, 697). In preclinical studies, some lack of cross-resistance between these analogues and methotrexate has been observed. The dose-limiting toxicity of piritrexim is myelosuppression and mucositis is the major problem with edatrexate. Recent clinical data, including multicenter phase II and phase III trials of edatrexate, have been disappointing (589).

Driven by the major activity and legendary toxicities of cisplatin, analogue development has moved faster with this drug than with other drugs. Carboplatin is a second-generation platinum complex with activity equivalent to and toxicity less than those of cisplatin (1, 90). Bolus carboplatin has pharmacokinetic and toxicity profiles similar to those of continuous-infusion cisplatin and has significantly less renal, otologic, neurologic, and gastrointestinal (nausea/vomiting) toxicity than bolus cisplatin. Reversible myelosuppression (primarily thrombocytopenia) is the dose-limiting toxicity for carboplatin.

Single-agent studies of carboplatin given monthly in bolus (400 mg/m^2) or fractionated (80 mg/m^2/d for 5 days) schedules produced objective response rates of 20 to 30% in recurrent and metastatic HNSCC (141, 163, 201, 203, 332). These single-arm data were confirmed in a cooperative group randomized phase II trial of two second-generation platinum complexes: carboplatin (response rate 24%) and iproplatin (response 12%) (11). In contrast to the proved activity of carboplatin, this and other trials of iproplatin in recurrent HNSCC have been uniformly disappointing, with overall response rates of less than 10% and major toxicity (myelosuppression, nausea/vomiting).

In an attempt to increase platinum dose intensity in a number of solid tumors, researchers have studied the combined use of carboplatin and cisplatin. This approach may allow higher serum platinum levels by varying the types and thereby lowering the intensities of platinum toxicities. Two recent single-arm studies in advanced and recurrent disease, however, did not show increased response (17% in one, 33% in the other) (186, 543).

Bleomycin and 5-fluorouracil analogues, used systemically, in HNSCC, have shown no therapeutic advantages over the parent compounds (10, 505).

Several new agents that have recently shown activity in recurrent head and neck cancer are ifosfamide, topotecan, gemcitabine, Taxol, and Taxotere. Ifosfamide has been tested in a wide range of doses (from 5 to 17 g/m^2/cycle) and fractionation schedules, producing an overall major response rate of 32% in a total of over 200 patients reported from several series (338, 713). Topotecan (565) and gemcitabine (97) have produced promising early results, with phase II response rates of 29% (5 of 17) and 13% (7 of 54), respectively.

The taxanes are the newest class of established active agents in head and neck cancer (98, 195, 239, 248, 571, 687, 714). The best study is a recently completed ECOG phase II trial of pacitaxol (Taxol) at a dose of 250 mg/m^2 over 24 hours with G-CSF in 28 patients (239). This study reported an impressive 40% major response rate and 9.2-month median survival, which are even more noteworthy coming from a cooperative group study. The major toxicity was neutropenia that lasted a mean duration of only 2 days. To date, one other study of Taxol and three studies of Taxotere have reported major activity in the 15 to 35% range.

General classes of drugs with limited single-agent activity include the anthracyclines, Vinca alkaloids, mitomycin (and analogues), and nitrosoureas (260). The major role for anthracyclines in head and neck cancer appears to be in the therapy of nonsquamous cancers (salivary gland cancer, naso-pharyngeal carcinoma, small cell carcinoma, sarcoma, and esthesioneuroblastoma). Following is a partial list of drugs that are inactive in recurrent HNSCC or do not appear to have advantages over parent compounds in single-agent trials: PCNU, bisantrene, hexamethylmelamine, mitoguazone, m-AMSA, aclacinomycin, doxorubicin, epirubicin, mitoxantrone, tallysomycin S10b, vindesine, dibromodulcitol, triazinate, gallium nitrate, 6-thioguanine, triazofurin, homoharringtonine, porfiromycin, mitozolomide, lomustine, and hydroxyurea (9, 120, 147, 283, 320, 407, 520).

Multiagent Trials

Nearly all possible combinations and combination doses/schedules of methotrexate, cisplatin, bleomycin, and 5-fluorouracil and other agents listed in Table 105.24 have been tried in numerous single-arm studies in recurrent HNSCC. Results have covered a wide range of response rates, including generally low complete response rates, in heterogeneous subsets of patients. In the late 1970s, work focused on cisplatin–bleomycin combinations, which appeared from single-arm studies to be more active than noncisplatin combinations (264, 320, 770, 772). The highest complete response rate to a high-dose cisplatin–bleomycin combination strategy in recurrent disease was 24% (291).

The cisplatin/5-fluorouracil regimen in HNSCC was an important advance launched by preclinical studies indicating synergy between these drugs and by concern over bleomycin's pulmonary toxicity. Pioneering clinical work by the Wayne State group in the early 1980s yielded major objective response rates of 78% (27% complete responses) in recurrent disease (390, 751). Lower response rates have been reported by other centers, however, including disappointing phase II response rates of 11%, on an every-28-day schedule; 25% using the identical regimen (drugs, doses, schedules, and cycle number) in patients with recurrent (chemotherapy-naive) disease; and less than 10% in patients failing prior chemotherapy (9, 157, 474). Enthusiasm for this combination in recurrent disease is further diminished by the negative long-term results (727) and recent results of randomized trials comparing cisplatin-5-fluorouracil with other combinations and even single agents (Tables 105.26 and 105.27). Several phase II and III trials (over 300 reported patients) of the less-toxic carboplatin/5-fluorouracil regimen report response rates equivalent to cisplatin/5-fluorouracil (203, 309, 457).

Based on preclinical synergy and activity in other human tumors, the cisplatin etoposide and cisplatin cytarabine combinations have been studied in HNSCC. Cisplatin etoposide produced activity and toxicity equivalent to single-agent cisplatin in a phase III trial (451). Despite four negative phase II trials (139, 452, 542), cisplatin cytarabine produced

Table 105.26. Randomized Trials of Chemotherapy in Recurrent Head and Neck Cancer: Single Agents Versus Multiple Agents

Author	Agents	No. patients	% Response (complete)	Median survival (mo)
Davis[160]	*P* v PBM	*30* v 27	*13(3)* v 11(0)	*4.2* v 5.2[e]
DeConti[165]	*MIMI* v MICA	*81/80* v 76	*26(−) 24(−)* v 18(−)	*5.0/4.4* v 3.2
Drelichman[192]	*M* v POB	*24* v 27	*33(8)* v 41(11)	*5.5* v 3.2
Jacobs[351]	*P* v PM	*40* v 39	*18(8)* v 33(15)	*6.2* v 6.9
Vogl[723]	*M* v PBM	*83* v 80	*35(8)* v 48(16)[b]	*5.6* v 5.6
Morton[492]	*PIB* v PB	*31/22* v 38	*13(3)/14(0)* v 24(5)	*3.7/2.8* v 3.8
Williams[765]	*M* v PVB	*98* v 92	*16(0)* v 24(1)	*7.3* v 6.8
Jacobs[349]	*PIF* v PF	*83/83* v 79	*17(4)/13(2)* v 32(6)[d]	*5.0/6.1* v 5.5
Eisenberger[202]	*M* v CpM	*20* v 20	*25(5)* v 25(0)	*6* v 6
Forastiere[238]	*M* v CpF/PF	*88/87* v 87	*11(1)* v 18(2)/30(5)[e]	*5.6* v 5.2/6.6
Liverpool[436]	*PIM* v PF/PM	*50/50* v 50/50	*29(2)/12(0)* v 24(6);22(0)	*2.7/8.7* v 5.3/6.7[f]
Total (Median Response—*Single Agent* v Multiagent)			*16(3)* v 24(5)	*5.5* v 5.5

Abbreviations: P, cisplatin; Cp. carboplatin; F, 5-fluorouracil; M, methotrexate; B, bleomycin; C, cyclophosphamide; O. vincristine; V, vinblastine; A, cytarabine; I, leucovorin; −, not available; v, versus. *Italic* = single agents

[a] Median partial response duration

[b] Initial report significant (P = .04, 1-sided T-test); final report (P = .07, 1-sided T-test)

[c] Four-arm study with a no treatment (supportive care) control arm. Single arm cisplatin associated with a significantly increased median survival *v* control arm

[d] PF *v* P, P = .035; PF *v* F, P = .005

[e] Response rate significant PF *v* M, P = .02

[f] Taken from interim report, not available in final report.

Table 105.27. Randomized Trials of Cisplatin/5-Fluorouracil vs Other Agent(s)

Author	No.	Agents	% Response (complete)	Survival
Neoadjuvant				
Clark[111]	56	*PF* v PBMI (2 cycles)	*77(19)* v 70(19)	P = NS
Gonzales[273]	36	*PF* v PA (3 cycles)	*83(16)* v 89(35)[a]	P = NS
Recurrent				
Kish[389]	40	*PF* v PF (bolus)	*72(22)* v 20(10)[b]	P = NS
Clavel[116]	382	*PF* v PBMO	*31(2)* v 34(10)	P = NS
Jacobs[349]	104	*PF* v P/F	*32(6)* v 17(4)/13(2)[c]	P = NS
Forastiere[238]	262	*PF* v CpF/M	*30(5)* v 18(2)/11(1)	P = NS
Amrein[18,19]	55	*PF* v PFBMI	*46(0)* v 63(7)	P = NS
Liverpool[436]	200	*PF* v P/M/PM	*24(6)* v 29(2)/12(0)/22(0)	P = NS

Abbreviations: P, cisplatin; Cp, carboplatin; F, 5-fluorouracil; B, bleomycin; M, methotrexate; A, cytarabine; O, vincristine; I, leucovorin; NS, not statistically significant ($P > 0.05$)
[a] Significant difference complete response ($P < .05$)
[b] Significant difference ($P < .01$)
[c] PF v P, P = .035; PF v F, P = .005

significantly higher response rates as compared with cisplatin/5-fluorouracil in a small randomized trial (273).

RANDOMIZED STUDIES

Only two of the 12 trials comparing multiagent and single-agent (methotrexate in seven trials and cisplatin in five) therapies produced significant differences in response, and the overall single-agent and multiagent median survivals are similar at 5 to 6 months (Table 105.26).

Jacobs and colleagues reported a three-arm comparative trial of cisplatin and 5-fluorouracil as single agents and in combination (349). Although no major survival differences occurred, the response rate was highest in the cisplatin/infusional 5-fluorouracil combination (Table 105.26).

The Southwest Oncology Group (SWOG) reported a three-arm randomized phase III study comparing cisplatin/5-fluorouracil, carboplatin (300 mg/m^2)/5-fluorouracil and single-agent methotrexate in recurrent HNSCC (238). The response rate and toxicity of cisplatin/5-fluorouracil were significantly greater than they were in the methotrexate arm. The carboplatin/5-fluorouracil arm did not differ significantly from the two other arms in response or toxicity. Median survival was poor and not significantly different among the three groups. Interpretation of these results is clouded by atypical toxicity patterns. Moderate to severe myelosuppression (leukopenia) was significantly more frequent in the cisplatin arm, suggesting suboptimal dosing of carboplatin.

Five studies compared single-agent cisplatin with cisplatin combinations. Despite promising single-arm studies, cisplatin combinations have not performed better than cisplatin alone in phase III trials (Table 105.26). Multiagent survival rates are equivalent to those with single-agent cisplatin (88, 436, 492).

Two phase III trials compared cisplatin-based combinations and similar regimens without cisplatin (2, 115). These trials reported significant increases in response rates with the cisplatin regimen but no survival differences.

A randomized trial designed to test the schedule dependency of 5-fluorouracil in the cisplatin 5-fluorouracil combination compared cisplatin (100 mg/m^2) bolus plus 5-fluorouracil given by continuous infusion (1,000 mg/m^2/d for 4 days) with the same bolus dose of cisplatin plus 5-fluorouracil as a bolus (600 mg/m^2 on day 1 and day 8) (389). The continuous-infusion regimen produced a higher response rate of 72% (22% complete) compared with the bolus-group response rate of 20% (10% complete) ($P < .01$). Despite the lower total dose, the bolus arm was associated with greater toxicity (myelosuppression). The interpretation of this study is clouded by the bolus 5-fluorouracil arm's unusual day 1 and 8 schedule, and more than fourfold lower total dose of 5-fluorouracil. Furthermore, single-arm trials of different schedules (e.g., cisplatin and 5-fluourouracil given as daily intravenous bolus for 5 days) (380, 477) or different sequences (381), produced response rates comparable to those, in similar-risk patients, of the standard regimen of cisplatin plus continuous-infusion 5-fluorouracil.

Single-arm clinical trials of methotrexate pretreatment and 5-fluorouracil in advanced and recurrent HNSCC yielded mixed results: response rates ranging from 16 to 94% (537, 561). However, three randomized studies differing somewhat in design and results clearly indicate that the methotrexate/5-fluorouracil sequence, predicted by preclinical studies to be active, does not produce a response or survival advantage over simultaneous administration or the reverse sequence (Table 105.28) (76, 77, 118).

CONCLUSIONS

All these data for recurrent, unresectable, and metastatic disease fail to show that multiagent therapy is more effective than single-agent therapy. Although combination chemotherapy for recurrent or metastatic HNSCC may produce higher response rates than single agents, none of the 12 randomized combination trials (including those comparing cisplatin/5-fluorouracil) produced improved survival over single-agent treatment (Tables 105.26 and 105.27).

Single-agent and combination chemotherapy can provide effective palliation for these patients. Because of its documented activity, acceptable toxicity, convenience of administration, and low cost, methotrexate remains a single-agent standard of comparison, but other agents are active, e.g., platinums, 5FU, and taxanes. Indeed, cisplatin is at least comparable to methotrexate in response and survival rates,

Table 105.28. Randomized Trials of Sequential Methotrexate-5-Fluorouracil

Author	No.	Chemotherapy	% Response (complete)	Median survival (mo.)
Browman[76,77]	79	*M-F*[a] *v* MF[b]	*38(5)* *v* 62(12)	*19* *v* 18
Coates[118]	70	*M-F*[a] *v* F-M	*51(11)* *v* 40(6)[c]	*13.3* *v* 13.0
			65(12) *v* 39(4)[d]	*13.3* *v* not reached
Browman[75]	113	*M-F*[f] *v* MF[b]	*47(5)* *v* 45(10)	*34* *v* 33

[a] 1-hour sequential methotrexate-5-fluorouracil
[b] Simultaneous
[c] All patients (advanced plus recurrent)
[d] Advanced untreated only
[e] Mostly advanced (11% recurrent). Toxicity (mucositis) increased in sequential arm ($p < .05$)
[f] 18-hour sequential methotrexate-5-fluorouracil

albeit with increased toxicity. Single-agent carboplatin is active against HNSCC, but has not been compared adequately with cisplatin in this setting (90). Nevertheless, carboplatin may be preferred as palliation for selected patients due to its favorable toxicity profile.

The current standard chemotherapy options for recurrent HNSCC are all palliative. The development of new, more active drugs and combinations must assume high priority. Although the combination of cisplatin and infusion 5-fluorouracil had generally been the regimen of choice for palliation in patients able to tolerate the increased toxicity, the results of large series with long follow-up (727) and of recent phase III trials indicate no advantage over other combinations (in response or survival) or over less toxic single-agent therapy (in survival). The choice of regimen depends on the important balance between efficacy and toxicity (quality of life), which must be considered on a case-by-case basis.

REGIONAL CYTOTOXIC THERAPY

Preclinical data support regional therapy in HNSCC, as do the predominantly local-regional tumor spread and a relatively selective access to tumor blood supply (see Chapter 55) (31, 125, 182, 439, 493, 497, 556, 598, 675, 762). High total-body clearance and low regional exchange rates are the major pharmacokinetic factors that allow optimization of regional drug delivery. Total-body clearance for drugs active in HNSCC is highest for floxuridine (FUDR) and lowest for methotrexate, with cisplatin at the low end (598). Although not ideal for regional therapy from a pharmacokinetic perspective, cisplatin is active and achieves an estimated fourfold greater intratumoral drug concentration when given intra-arterially (i.e., regionally) rather than intravenously. Single-arm clinical and pharmacokinetic studies of regional therapy in HNSCC have reported low regional exchange rates, increased intratumoral drug levels, enhanced toxicity in the infused area (mucositis, alopecia), reduced systemic toxicity, and modest increases in response rates (complete and partial) without apparent survival benefit over the systemic route (236).

Although the future of regional drug therapy in HNSCC is uncertain, newer microcatheters and catheter placement techniques that have reduced morbidity have led to a renewed interest in intra-arterial therapy. A phase I study using a highly selective intra-arterial infusion of high-dose cisplatin with concurrent intravenous thiosulfate (used to neutralize systemic cisplatin) in locally advanced and recurrent disease was recently reported (566). The MTD was 150 mg/m^2/w and the overall response rates were 86% (complete, 41%) in 22 stage III or IV disease patients and 62% (complete, 25%) in 16 recurrent-disease patients. This encouraging phase I work led to a phase II trial integrating this regimen with concurrent radiotherapy in 25 patients with locally advanced disease (567). Although only 18 of the 25 patients were evaluable, all evaluable patients achieved a complete response and 13 were alive and disease-free at a median follow-up of 16 months. These results appear superior to historic results with systemic therapy and previous intra-arterial therapy trials. Future phase III trials will be required to determine whether this approach is superior in terms of survival to systemic chemotherapy.

IMMUNOBIOLOGIC THERAPY

Immunotherapeutic approaches to head and neck cancer have been disappointing. Early clinical trials adding nonspecific immunoadjuvants to chemotherapy were negative. Despite limited encouraging results (682), most of the nine phase III adjuvant trials with bacilli Calmette-Guérin (BCG), thymosin, *Corynebacterium parvum*, and levamisole were negative (16, 42, 152, 366, 512, 668, 737).

Cytokines, differentiation agents, and plasma exchange have received limited study in HNSCC (6, 180, 224, 310, 373, 429, 430, 559, 578, 596). Studies using recombinant interferon-alpha have reported response rates in the 10% range (224, 469, 486, 671, 722, 734).

Two factors led to the study of interferons in NPC: (*a*) these patients have increased antibody-dependent cytotoxicity and a selective deficit in anti-EBV T-cell activity, and (*b*) interferons have antiviral activity against EBV and are immunomodulators. Although early study of interferon alfa (IFN-α) produced a response rate of 16% (25 treated patients), more recent data indicate single-agent response rates of 10% or less (65, 131, 132, 430).

The study of biologic therapy is now focusing on the best ways to combine cytokines, differentiation agents, cytotoxic agents, and irradiation. Several biologic agents (e.g., IFN-α, IL-2, retinoic acid) used systemically have produced objective tumor regression in HNSCC patients. Overall, however, response rates have been low and remissions incomplete and of short duration. Preclinical mechanistic data provide a basis for clinical dosing and scheduling decisions, although major differences and complex dose–response relationships occur in humans. Based on preclinical data, type I interferons are under phase I/II clinical study as radiosensitizers (102, 318). Small series of regional cytokine therapy (IFN-α and IL-2) and of adoptive cellular therapy have reported objective responses in advanced HNSCC (341, 344, 597).

The integration of biologic agents into cytotoxic regimens as primary therapy is more complex. Early results suggest that IFN-α may enhance both the activity and toxicity of 5-fluorouracil (see Chapters 61 and 80) (99, 726). It is not yet clear if the therapeutic index of the IFN-α/5-fluorouracil regimen is greater than that of high-dose, single-agent 5-fluorouracil. The possible contribution of additional antitumor activity by IFN-α immune modulation in vivo is under study. In recurrent HNSCC, adding IFN-α or IL-2 (184) to the cisplatin/5-fluorouracil regimen was associated with significant toxicity and relatively low response rates (30% and 35%). A new area of specific immunologic therapy in HNSCC is the use of monoclonal antibodies (593, 789).

As a rule, immunobiologic therapy is more effective when tumor volume is low, well differentiated, or only partially transformed (premalignant). Carefully controlled trials monitoring clinical response and markers of biologic activity will be required to clearly define the roles of these agents—alone and in combination—as primary, adjuvant, and chemopreventive therapy.

PRIMARY CHEMOTHERAPY

Although chemotherapy has not improved the short survival of patients with recurrent or metastatic HNSCC, promising results are beginning to emerge from the intense study of chemotherapy as an adjunct to standard primary treatment (surgery and/or radiotherapy) of advanced local disease. A patient's prognosis and treatment depend on the primary tumor site and TNM stage. Primary chemotherapy is not called for in early-stage (T1–2N0M0) disease, usually cured through standard treatment. After cure, early-stage patients require chemoprevention, however, because of their high risk of second primary tumors (427).

Chemotherapy can play a role in the primary treatment of more than 60% of all HNSCC patients, or those who are diagnosed with advanced or extensive (T3–4N2–3M0) local-regional disease. This is so because advanced HNSCC is both a local-regional and a systemic phenomenon. Although optimal surgery or radiotherapy has improved local or regional control, it has not improved survival. Two years after standard treatment, clinical evaluations indicate that less than 40% of these patients will be disease-free: local invasion and regional lymph node metastases are diagnosed in 60% and distant metastases in 15 to 25% (595). The rate of distant metastases is actually far greater. Autopsy series show that occult distant metastases are present in up to 50% of HNSCC fatalities (94, 168, 275, 333, 394, 510, 787).

Severe morbidities after surgery, high mortality rates, and the poor outcome of chemotherapy for recurrent tumors led to clinical investigations of many therapeutic variations of primary chemotherapy. These approaches fall into three main categories: (*a*) neoadjuvant or induction, chemotherapy (before standard surgery and/or radiotherapy); (*b*) maintenance, or true adjuvant, chemotherapy (following definitive standard primary therapy); and (*c*) concomitant chemotherapy (in combination with radiotherapy, usually in unresectable HNSCC). The principal goals of primary chemotherapy in HNSCC are to enhance local-regional control (relapse prevention, organ preservation, and primary curative treatment), decrease distant metastases, and improve overall survival.

Many reports have used the terminology of primary chemotherapy loosely. Some authors refer to adjuvant chemotherapy as any and all primary chemotherapy (346, 628, 660). They intend this phrase merely to distinguish it from the treatment of recurrent disease. However, we distinguish among neoadjuvant, adjuvant, and concomitant chemotherapy. We use the term "adjuvant chemotherapy" only to refer to prevention of relapse after standard therapy. "Neoadjuvant chemotherapy" refers specifically to tumor reduction prior to definitive therapy, and "concomitant chemotherapy" applies to chemotherapy given concomitantly with radiotherapy intended to achieve definitive control of local, regional, and micrometastatic disease.

Although many phase II studies of chemotherapy in HNSCC have been conducted, the great heterogeneity of head and neck disease and patient populations mandates controlled trials to establish the role of chemotherapy. Innovative single-arm phase I and II trials are important, however, for testing promising new agents and combinations before phase III study.

The following discussion focuses primarily on results from randomized phase III chemotherapy trials in primary HNSCC. The problem of small trial populations and heterogeneous tumors creates the need for multicenter cooperative studies in HNSCC.

NEOADJUVANT

Neoadjuvant (induction) therapy prior to surgery is sometimes referred to as sequential chemoradiotherapy when chemotherapy is followed by definitive radiotherapy. This latter approach specifically excludes or limits the extent of surgery, except in treatment failures, and is growing in importance as an "organ preservation" approach for locally advanced resectable disease (322). The neoadjuvant concept has been expanded to include novel studies of neoadjuvant chemotherapy followed by concomitant chemoradiotherapy (14).

The use of chemotherapy as induction treatment prior to local therapy for advanced HNSCC has been evaluated for over 15 years (123, 156, 170, 179, 199, 205, 319, 320, 322, 327, 348, 387, 628, 733, 770, 772). The strong rationale for this approach comes from mathematical models of cell kinetics and acquired drug resistance and from preclinical in vivo data (577). The principal objectives of induction are as follows: to promote regression and thereby enhance subsequent local-regional therapy; to identify patients with responding lesions that might be controlled by more conservative local treatment (organ preservation) rather than by extensive surgical procedures; to use chemotherapy before tumor and normal vasculature was altered by surgery or radiation; to identify responding tumors that may benefit from adjuvant chemotherapy following surgery or radiotherapy (214); and to provide early treatment for micrometastatic disease.

Early nonrandomized neoadjuvant trials based their selections of agents on trials in recurrent disease. Single agent early trials achieved response rates of 30 to 40% (320, 770). Gradually, neoadjuvant studies expanded to include multiagent therapy (320). The first major advance of chemotherapy in this area came in the late 1970s when Randolph and colleagues reported a 71% objective response rate (20% complete responses) in 21 HNSCC patients receiving cisplatin and continuous-infusion bleomycin (549, 772). Single-arm studies that followed and confirmed Randolph's initial report achieved overall response rates in advanced untreated HNSCC ranging from 37 to 87%, including complete-response rates of approximately 20% (291, 319–321, 327, 524, 611). The addition of other drugs to cisplatin/bleomycin to create three- and four-drug regimens produced significant increases in toxicity without improving response or survival rates (770, 772).

The next advance occurred in the early 1980s when Wayne State investigators reported a neoadjuvant trial of cisplatin infusional 5-fluorouracil, which produced a response rate of 88% (complete, 54%). The unprecedented complete-response rate of greater than 50% was perhaps the most important finding because of the significant impact complete responses have on survival. Wayne State data suggested that 5-fluorouracil was better given for 5 days than for 4 days, and that three cycles were significantly more active than were two; their complete-response rates doubled between the second and third cycles (9, 569, 750). Recent study suggests that complete response rates continue to increase from cycle 3 to 5. Subsequent studies used a variety of doses and schedules of cisplatin and 5-fluorouracil, and confirmed the activity of this combination, although generally at lower objective (mean, 77%; range, 38 to 100%) and complete (mean, 34%; range, 13 to 54%) response rates (9, 10, 628). The RTOG used the Wayne State regimen and corroborated its activity by achieving a 38% complete-response rate.

More recently, many uncontrolled trials have attempted to further enhance the activity of cisplatin/5-fluorouracil. They have given high-dose cisplatin with fixed-dose 5-fluorouracil; high-dose 5-fluorouracil with fixed-dose cisplatin; cisplatin intra-arterially rather than intravenously; other cytotoxic drugs, such as bleomycin, methotrexate, cyclophosphamide, mitoguazone, or Vinca alkaloids; and dose-intensive multicourse alternating regimens (9, 10, 211, 278, 388, 698). These trials have produced increased toxicity and no consistent improvements in response or survival. Phase II and phase III trials of carboplatin/5-fluorouracil yielded response rates of 70 to 80% (complete in 30 to 40%)—results comparable to those of cisplatin/5-fluorouracil (203, 457).

Noncisplatin combinations are under development because of cisplatin's relatively high toxicity. Alternative foundations used most commonly are 5-fluorouracil, cyclophosphamide, bleomycin, and methotrexate, with or without Vinca alkaloids. Response rates have ranged from 11 to 69%. One of the best studied of these regimens is Price and Hill's schedule A developed over 10 years ago, a complex combination of vincristine, bleomycin, methotrexate/leucovorin, 5-fluorouracil, hydrocortisone, and doxorubicin based on stem-cell kinetics and cell-cycle specificity (312, 313). Doxorubicin was later excluded.

Randomized trials of neoadjuvant therapy versus standard local therapy have been conducted with single-agent and multiagent regimens (Table 105.29). Eight of these trials using single-agent neoadjuvant treatment have been reported. All used methotrexate (standard or high dose with leucovorin). The only trial reporting significantly improved survival used methotrexate intra-arterially in SCC of the oral cavity, oropharynx, and maxillary antrum (23).

Twenty-nine randomized multiagent trials of neoadjuvant therapy without (21 trials) or with (eight trials) adjuvant chemotherapy compared with local therapy control groups have been reported to date. Although none has shown that neoadjuvant therapy significantly improves survival, many of these trials had major design limitations, including suboptimal patient numbers, relatively inactive induction regimens (median complete-response rate under 20%), variations in local-regional therapies (surgery alone, surgery and radiotherapy, radiotherapy alone) and heterogeneous study populations with multiple primary sites, and resectable and unresectable cases (Table 105.29). None of the neoadjuvant regimens produced a complete-response rate of over 50%. Twenty-one of the 29 randomized studies had such small study numbers (fewer than 75 patients per arm) that they could not detect significant survival differences below 25%.

Organ preservation is second to improving survival as a goal of primary chemotherapy. Those patients fortunate enough to survive their cancer often face a lifetime of significant morbidity because of cosmetic and functional debilities from surgical resection. Despite marked advances in reconstructive surgery and rehabilitation, patients who have undergone laryngectomy, glossectomy, or composite resection still have major debility. Unfortunately, the importance of organ and function preservation often is ignored. Many opt to receive the less effective therapy of radiation alone to avoid curative surgery (468). They risk shorter survival rather than face increased survival with severe surgical morbidity. An active area of HNSCC research involves chemoradiotherapy (sequential or concomitant) to facilitate organ-preserving approaches for advanced disease (322). This research is designed to preserve anatomic structures without compromising survival. In such studies, extensive surgery is reserved to salvage patients who fail to respond to initial therapy or who recur.

Laryngeal preservation is the most advanced application of organ-preservation chemotherapy. In advanced laryngeal SCC (T3 or T4,and/ or nodal metastasis), total laryngectomy improves survival at the price of impaired speech, and upfront irradiation preserves the voice at the price of a decreased chance of survival. Survival remains low with strate-

Table 105.29. Randomized Trials of Neoadjuvant (Induction) Multiagent Chemotherapy for Head and Neck Cancer

Author	N	Induction therapy		Local therapy	% Disease-free survival (yr)[a]		% Survival (yr)[a]	
		Regimen (no. cycles)	% Response (complete)		Control	Chemotherapy	Control	Chemotherapy
Petrovich[528]	23	MLO (2) (ia)	25 (0)	R	—	—	9 (2)	17
Richard[555]	225 (oc,op)	OB (12d)	—	S ± R	—	—	— (3)[b]	—
Shetty[612]	42 (tb)	OBMFMc (2)	—	R	50 (0.54)	50 (0.58)	—	—
Stolwijk[662]	68	VBMCF (2)	21 (0)	S ± R	—	—	77 (1)	58
Kun[398]	83	CMBF (2)	67 (5)	R ± S	64 (2)	59	43 (2)	31
Szpirglas[669]	114	DOBP (3)	53 (11)	R	3 (3+)	5	5 (3+)	11
Toohill[691]	60	PF (3)	85 (19)	R + S	70 (2)	70	70 (2)	56
Schuller[594]	158	PMBO (3)	70 (18)	S + R	23 (5)	23	28 (5)	28
Martin[460]	107 (oc,op)	PFBML (3)	48 (6)	S + R; R	42 (2)	49[f]	—	—
Carugati[96]	120	PB +/− M (1)	44–59 (—)	—	25 (5)	33	18 (5)	38
Jaulerry[355]	100	PBVdMc (2)	50 (10)–p	R	38 (2)	44	45 (2)	34
VACSP[699]	332 (lc)	PF (2)	85 (31)	R	—	—	56 (3)	53
Martin[456,459]	75	PF (3)	68 (46)	S + R; R	61 (1)	73	—	—
Paccagnella[514,515]	221	PF (4)	70 (29)	S + R	58	62	—	—
Martin[455]	218 (op)	CpF (3)	81 (34)	S + R; R	21 (2)	22	60 (2)	65

Abbreviations: P, cisplatin; Cp, carboplatin; F, 5-fluorouracil; M, methotrexate; L, leukovorin; B, bleomycin; O, vincristine; Vd, Videsine; Mc, mitomycin-C; R, radiotherapy; S, surgery; p, primary site; oc, oral cavity; op, oropharynx; tb, tongue base; lc, laryngeal cancer; ia, intraarterial

[a] Published values or estimated from published data/survival curves

[b] Reduction in local-regional recurrence ($P < .05$) in chemotherapy arm

[c] Freedom from local-regional recurrence (53 *v* 35%, $P = .06$)

[d] Reduced distant metastasis rate in chemotherapy arm ($P < .05$)

[e] Low-dose cisplatin (50 mg/m^2/cycle; distant metastases lower (49% *v* 28%, $P = .07$) in chemotherapy arm

[f] Disease-free survival favored control arm at 1 year (70 *v* 54%, $P = .01$)

[g] 3-arm study—2 chemotherapy arms combined for analysis

Table 105.30. The Veterans Affairs Cooperative Studies Program Trial in Laryngeal Cancer: Patterns of First-Site Failure

Failure site/type	Surgery + radiotherapy	Chemotherapy + radiotherapy
Local recurrence	4	20
Regional recurrence	9	14
Distant metastasis	29	18
Second primary tumor	10	3
Total	52 (31%)	55 (33%)

From VACSP[699]

gies to combine radiotherapy and surgery because of the high frequency of local-regional and distant recurrence.

Loss of natural speech, of course, is the chief forfeit of surgery for laryngeal cancer. Laryngectomy also can result in the need of a neck stoma (for breathing), an inability to smell or sneeze, a diminished sense of taste, and problems with swallowing. Cosmetic and psychologic consequences can be great.

Although preservation of the voice long has been an important goal of the treatment of these patients, interest in the issue has heightened over recent years. A trend of decreasing use of radical surgery so as to preserve normal function and improve quality of life is developing in a variety of other solid tumor settings as well. Two examples are limb preservation in osteosarcoma and breast preservation in breast cancer.

Based on promising pilot data (210, 322, 348, 371) in 1985, the Veterans Affairs Cooperative Studies Program (VACSP) initiated a multi-institutional randomized prospective trial that attempted laryngeal preservation in previously untreated patients with locally advanced resectable laryngeal cancer (Fig. 105.9). Patterns of treatment failure differed (Table 105.30). At a median follow-up of 8 years, an increased local-regional recurrence rate and a decreased distant metastasis rate were seen in the sequential chemoradiotherapy group in comparison with the surgery-radiotherapy group. The findings also indicated that delay of definitive local therapy in chemotherapy nonresponders was not detrimental. Chemotherapy responders and nonresponders in the experimental arm had about the same rate of survival. Eight-year rates were similar (approximately 30%) in the two study arms, and laryngeal preservation was achieved in over 60% of the chemotherapy recipients. Sequential chemoradiotherapy was least effective in advanced local (T4) and regional disease (N2,N3), over 50% of these patient subgroups required salvage laryngectomy (699).

These long-term results from the large VACSP trial indicate that sequential induction chemotherapy and definitive radiotherapy can be an effective strategy for achieving laryngeal preservation in a high percentage of patients without compromising overall survival. The trial's success argues strongly for adoption of this new treatment strategy in order to spare patients the functional, psychologic, and cosmetic deformities resulting from total laryngectomy.

While the VACSP study shows that induction chemotherapy plus radiotherapy is as effective as the previous standard treatment of surgery and postoperative radiotherapy, the question of "what role chemotherapy actually plays" has been raised. Does it add efficacy or is it merely predictive? For certain laryngeal cancer subsets such as T3N0 glottic

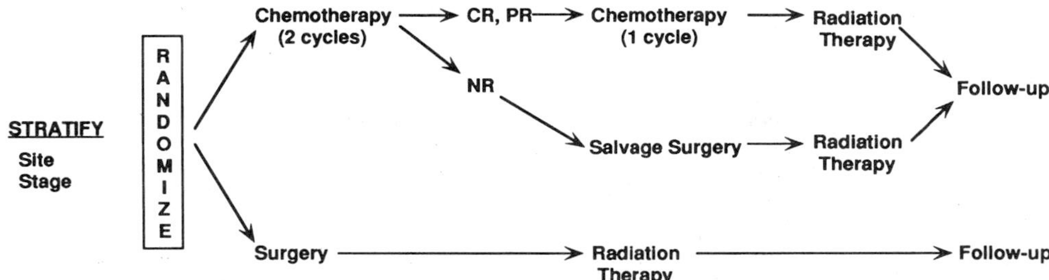

Figure 105.9. Veterans Affairs Laryngeal Cancer Study Group trial schema: induction chemotherapy plus radiation compared with surgery plus radiation in patients with advanced laryngeal cancer (see text).

tumors, it appears that definitive radiotherapy alone with surgery held in reserve as a salvage gives essentially the same results as either arm of the VACSP study and is much more cost effective (394). Considerations of cost are becoming important in an increasingly "managed care" environment. There is currently a Head and Neck Intergroup randomized trial for stage T2–3N0–3 tumors of the supraglottic and glottic larynx that compares radiotherapy alone versus concomitant radiotherapy and cisplatin versus the VACSP cisplatin 5-fluorouracil radiotherapy experimental arm that addresses this question.

Two recent European phase III trials add further support to this organ-preservation approach. A French trial had a design similar to the VA trial, except that it used carboplatin instead of cisplatin and included all head and neck cancer subsites. The local-regional therapy was surgery and/or radiotherapy, determined by the treating physician. Patients were assigned randomly to chemotherapy followed by standard local therapy (in 152 patients) or standard local therapy alone (154 patients). The neoadjuvant carboplatin plus 5-fluorouracil produced overall and complete response rates of 57% and 31% respectively. The chemotherapy-radiotherapy arm produced an increased 4-year survival rate (49% versus 38%, $P = .053$) and organ-preservation rate (48% versus 20%, $P = .001$), compared with the standard local therapy arm (455).

The EORTC reported the most recent phase III trial. This trial randomized 197 patients with locally advanced hypopharyngeal cancer: 100 patients were randomized to chemo-radiotherapy with cisplatin/5-fluorouracil and 97 to standard local therapy of total laryngectomy, partial pharyngectomy, and radical neck dissection and postoperative radiotherapy. In this study, patients in the neoadjuvant arm who achieved less than a complete response after two cycles of cisplatin/5-fluorouracil underwent immediate surgical therapy as outlined in the standard arm. At a follow-up of 3 years, survival rates were similar in the two arms and 28% of patients in the neoadjuvant arm were alive, disease-free, and had preserved their larynxes (411).

Future trials aimed at laryngeal preservation will need to establish chemotherapy regimens that achieve higher complete response rates, investigate innovative fractionated-radiation schemes, and assess concomitant chemoradiation programs (approaches detailed elsewhere in this chapter).

Promising new combinations are being tried to overcome the major disappointment of neoadjuvant chemotherapeutic approaches; that is, despite achieving high response rates of 70 to 90% (20 to 40% complete) in advanced untreated patients, neoadjuvant chemotherapy has not translated into improved survival (327, 524, 594, 688). Data suggest that neoadjuvant regimens capable of significantly improving survival must be able to produce reproducible complete response rates of over 50%. So far, complete-response rates in phase II trials have appeared to be inflated and always drop in phase III trials. Although developed most often in recurrent disease, promising new dose-intensive regimens are designed for later integration into primary chemotherapy. The following discussion includes trials of new combinations in both the recurrent-disease and neoadjuvant settings.

Preclinical data suggested a promising new line of work to potentiate 5-fluorouracil cytotoxicity (726, 728–730). Laboratory studies indicate that 5-fluorouracil resistance can be overcome by adding reduced folates (e.g., leucovorin) before 5-fluorouracil exposure due to enhanced stability of the active ternary complex with thymidylate synthase. Although still in development, combined leucovorin with cisplatin and 5-fluorouracil (PFL regimen) has already produced the highest complete-response rates reported in locally advanced HNSCC.

Vokes and colleagues were among the first to test this concept clinically in HNSCC (729). Using a variation of the PFL regimen in untreated advanced disease, investigators from the Dana-Farber Cancer Institute gave high-dose leucovorin (500 mg/m^2/d for 6 days), cisplatin (25 mg/m^2/d for 5 days), and 5-fluorouracil (800 mg/m^2/d for 5 days), all by continuous infusion, starting the 5-fluorouracil 24 hours after the cisplatin and leucovorin (194). Preclinical data suggested that prior exposure to cisplatin and leucovorin enhanced the cytotoxicity of 5-fluorouracil. The striking finding in this phase II study was an apparent shift in the degree of response. The 80% objective response rate is in line with cisplatin/5-fluorouracil and other cisplatin-based regimens; however, the overall clinical complete-response rate was 66%, the highest complete-response rate reported to date with any chemotherapy regimen in advanced HNSCC. The clinical complete-response rate at the primary site was 77%, and 74% of these patients had a pathologic complete response. The clinical complete response in the regional (neck) nodes was 67% (83% in N2 and 46% in N3 disease). Toxicities were notable, including moderate to severe mucositis in 94% of patients, nausea and vomiting in 37%, and diarrhea in 17%, necessitating dose reductions after the first cycle in 31% of patients. Rash developed in 26% but significant myelosuppression was uncommon (less than 10%). As with the cisplatin/5-fluorouracil regimen, three cycles were critical in PFL administration—the complete response rate jumped from 26% to 66% with the third cycle.

PFL has now been studied extensively over the past 6 years with conflicting results. A recent phase II study of 22 patients from the Memorial Sloan-Kettering Cancer Center did not confirm the initial promising PFL results: compared with prior experience with cisplatin/5-fluorouracil, this study found no increase in complete or overall response rates but greatly increased the toxicity (531). More than 10 phase II studies of various PFL regimens have now been reported, producing an overall median complete-response rate of approximately 40%, which appears to represent a modest improvement over the 30% complete-response rate generally observed with other cisplatin-based regimens, including cisplatin/5-fluorouracil. To date, only one randomized trial involving PFL has been reported. This small study (55 patients) from Argentina compared cisplatin/5-fluorouracil with PFL and reported no difference in complete and overall response rates or survival (412). The overall (and complete) response rates for cisplatin/5-fluorouracil were 65% (15%) compared with respective figures for PFL of 68% (13%). Toxicity was substantially increased, however, in the PFL arm.

The addition of INF-α to cisplatin/5-fluorouracil (PFI) in various doses and schedules of all three agents has been tested in five uncontrolled trials. Although not having major clinical activity in advanced disease by itself, INF-α has been shown in vitro to potentiate the activity of both fluorouracil and cisplatin in some systems. The phase II results in recurrent disease overall indicate response rates and survivals similar to those of cisplatin/5-fluorouracil (339).

Vokes et al. have extended this approach to add INF-α to PFL (726). Although producing a high rate of severe toxicity, recent results in a series of 71 mostly stage IV patients are impressive, with an overall response rate of 100%, and a complete-response rate of 51%.

CONCOMITANT CHEMORADIOTHERAPY

Concomitant chemoradiotherapy is the most promising primary chemotherapy approach to prolonging the survival of patients with locally advanced resectable and unresectable disease. It is the only systemic approach consistently shown to improve local-regional control and survival in randomized trials. Schedules of concomitant chemoradiotherapy can be synchronous, with both modalities administered close together, or alternating, with both administered in a nonoverlapping fashion. Both of these schedules offer distinct therapeutic advantages over regimens of strictly sequential treatment.

Radiotherapy and chemotherapy given concomitantly is a dose-intensive approach that exploits the independent complementary activity of radiotherapy locally and chemotherapy distantly (spacial cooperation) and the potentially enhanced local activity (within the radiotherapy field) (241, 243, 730). Chemoradiotherapy approaches must attempt to incorporate full doses of both modalities. Suboptimal doses and/or schedules of either (e.g., low-dose cisplatin or split-course radiotherapy) compromise dose intensity and, ultimately, survival. Dose intensities possible with concomitant chemoradiotherapy are higher in 2 to 3 months than those allowed by sequential chemoradiotherapy given over twice the time. Even if no direct drug-radiation synergy occurs, concomitant therapy should produce additive effects and avoid critical delays of either therapy. Unfortunately, the concomitant approach incurs severe toxicity (primarily mucositis), which is difficult to balance effectively with desired activity (421, 677, 678, 716, 730).

Concomitant single-agent chemoradiotherapy has been under investigation in head and neck cancer for over 3 decades. Numerous phase II trials have reported encouraging but inconclusive results. All cytotoxic drugs with major activity in this disease have been studied (243, 730). Frequently, these have been administered in low doses during full-course conventional radiotherapy. The phase III trials are listed in Table 105.31.

Bleomycin, an active single agent and radiosensitizer, has been included in numerous single-arm trials. Nine randomized studies of this drug alone with concomitant radiotherapy have been published. Of the four trials with relatively large study cohorts (exceeding 100 patients), two reported significant long-term survival improvements in the concomitant arm (246, 609). A key feature of one positive trial was the use of very-low-dose bleomycin, suggesting that the subtherapeutic dose of bleomycin enhanced radiosensitivity of the tumor (246).

5-Fluorouracil, a radioenhancer in vitro (85) and active also in head and neck cancer, has been tested in four randomized trials. All four trials observed improvements in disease-free and overall survival, which were statistically significant in three and two trials, respectively. The most recent phase III trial was a Canadian-NCI–sponsored trial of 5-fluorouracil in 175 patients (66). Patients with stage III disease were randomly assigned to radiotherapy either with 5-fluorouracil (1.2 g/m^2/d) or saline (placebo) as a 72-hour infusion given in weeks 1 and 3 of radiotherapy. The complete-response rate was higher in the 5-fluorouracil than in the placebo group (68% versus 56%, $P = .04$). With minimum and median study follow-up times of 2 and 3.5 years, the median overall ($P = .08$) and progression-free ($P = .06$) survival rates favored the 5-fluourouracil group. Toxicity was also significantly greater in the 5-fluorouracil arm but did not interfere with radiation delivery.

Methotrexate, a drug that produces severe mucositis at full doses (especially when combined with radiotherapy) (391), was evaluated in two randomized trials. The largest concomitant trial (285) gave only two doses (100 mg/m^2 on days 0 and 14 with leucovorin rescue in selected patients with elevated methotrexate serum levels) along with nonstandard radiotherapy (40 to 55 Gy radiotherapy in 15 to 16 fractions over 3 weeks). At a median follow-up of 32 months, relapse-free ($P < .016$) and overall survivals ($P = .075$) were better in the methotrexate arm. The improvements in local control ($P = .002$) and survival ($P = .009$) were most striking in the oropharyngeal subset. The need for salvage surgery also was reduced in the methotrexate arm. Furthermore, toxicity was equivalent in the two treatment arms.

Hydroxyurea is a ribonucleotide reductase inhibitor with S-phase–specific cytotoxicity (99, 730) and single-agent activity in HNSCC (Table 105.24). Stefani and colleagues con-

TABLE 105.31. Phase III Studies of Concomitant Single Agent Chemotherapy (CT) and Radiotherapy (RT) in Head and Neck Cancer

Drug Author	N	% Complete response rate		% Disease-free survival (yr)[a]		% Survival (yr)[a]	
		RT	RT + CT	RT	RT + CT	RT	RT + CT
Bleomycin							
Scandolaro[575]	30	43	50			50(2)	50
Kapstad[368]	29	14[b]	27[b]	64(2+)	87	—	—
Shanta[609]	157 (oc)	19	79*	17(5)	72*	24(5)	66*
Morita[490]	45 (t)	61 (or)	64	65(2)	73	—	—
Shetty[612]	38 (tb)	—	—	50(0.54)	50(0.29)	—	—
Vermund[711]	222	58	63	58(5)	53	42(5)	38
Fu[246]	104	45	67	26(5)	64*	14(5)	28
Eschwege[215]	199	69	65	—	—	22(6)	24
Parvinen[519]	46	35	38	—	—	38(5)	35
5-Fluorouracil							
Shigematsu[613]	63 (ia;ci;ma)	—	—	18(2)	40*	61(2)	68
Lo[437]	136 (oc,op,tb)	32	44	18(2)	49*	13(5)	32*,[d]
Methotrexate							
Condit[128]	40	60	45	—	—	—	—[e]
Gupta[285]	313	—	—	48(5)	60*	27(5)	42[f]
Hydroxyurea							
Richards[557,558]	40	20	65*	—	—	35(5)	50
Stefani[658]	126	47	42	31(2)	22	51(2)	29
Hussey[340]	40	56	67	38(2)	38	27(2)	30
Mitomycin C							
Weissberg[755]	117	—	—	49(5)	75[g]	40(5)	48
Cisplatin							
Haselow[304]	319	30	34[h]	—	—	—	—

Abbreviations: RT, radiotherapy; CT, chemotherapy, —, not available; ci, continuous infusion; ia, intra-arterial; oc, oral cavity; t, tongue; ma, maxillary antrum; op, oropharynx; tb, tongue base, or, overall response rate

*$P < 0.05$

[a] Published or estimated from data/survival curves

[b] Histologic CR

[c] Histologic CR increased in RT + CT ($P < .05$)

[d] Even greater significance in tonsil and intraoral

[e] Only 25 completed therapy and no survival data reported

[f] Overall survival ($P = 0.075$)—oropharyngeal ($P < .002$)

[g] $P < .07$

[h] Overall response greater in CT + RT ($P < .05$)

ducted the largest randomized placebo-controlled trial of concomitant hydroxyurea and radiotherapy and found no increase in response or survival with this combination. Toxicity and distant metastases were increased in the concomitant arm.

Mitomycin C, a bioreductive alkylating agent, is differentially metabolized, is selectively toxic to hypoxic (radiotherapy-resistant) cells, and produces little mucositis, which provides a favorable toxicity profile for chemoradiotherapy studies. Weissberg and colleagues reported a randomized comparison in HNSCC of radiotherapy alone versus radiotherapy plus mitomycin (755). Mitomycin was given at a dose of 15 mg/m^2 on the fifth day of radiotherapy, and in some cases on a second occasion 6 weeks later. Despite limited single-agent activity in HNSCC, at a median follow-up exceeding 5 years, the actuarial disease-free ($P = .07$) and local-regional disease-free (87% versus 66%, $P = .02$) survivals were higher in patients treated with mitomycin. The addition of dicoumarol to mitomycin C did not improve survival over mitomycin alone (both with concurrent radiotherapy) in a recent phase III trial (290).

Cisplatin is ideal for concomitant chemoradiotherapy in HNSCC. It has established single-agent activity and synergistic interaction in vitro and nonoverlapping toxicities (no mucositis) in vivo with radiotherapy (137, 178). Cisplatin recently received extensive clinical evaluation in concomitance with radiotherapy. Despite high complete local control rates from phase II trials (Table 105.32), study follow-ups are short and the impact on disease-free and overall survival is unclear. Only one phase III study of this approach in locally advanced disease has been completed (304). This randomized study compared cisplatin (20 mg/m^2 weekly) during radiation with conventional radiotherapy in patients with inoperable HNSCC. Results indicate that concomitant therapy increased overall response but not complete-response, disease-free, or overall survival rates. Concomitant therapy's complete-response rate of only 34% in this phase III trial stands in marked contrast to the 84% complete-response rate achieved with the same dose and schedule in a pilot trial (303).

The optimal dose, schedule, and sequence of cisplatin with radiotherapy have undergone extensive evaluation (25, 137, 191, 240, 365). Preclinical (in vitro and in vivo) and clinical chemoradiotherapy data suggest that cisplatin used predominantly as a cytotoxic agent (large and infrequent doses) is more active than cisplatin used predominantly as a radiosensitizer (small and frequent weekly or daily doses). The clinical data are more difficult to sort out, inasmuch as

Table 105.32. Synchronous Single-Agent Platinum Chemo-Radiotherapy Trials

Author	Dose (mg/m^2) and schedule	Radiotherapy	N	Response (complete %)
Cisplatin				
Haselow[303]	10–30 (weekly)	Conventional	32	27 (84)
Bloom[57]	20 (5 d every 3 wk)	Conventional	34	18 (53)
Miller[479]	80 (d 1, 23, 43)	Conventional	22	10 (45)
Slotman[626]	20 (d1–4, 21–24)	Conventional	18	13 (72)
Snyderman[630]	15 (d 1–5, 21–25)	Conventional	29	9 (31)
Crispino[143]	20 (weekly)	Conventional	19	10 (53)
Tobias[689]	10[c] ×6 weeks	Conventional	16	9 (56)
Chang[103]	20 (d 1–4) × 3 cycles	Conventional	22	18 (82)
Choi[108]	5–7 CI (2–3 wk) × 2 courses	Conventional/Hyperfraction	23	16 (70)
Cognetti[121,122]	100 (d 1, 21, 43)	Conventional	30[d]	13[d](44)
Wheeler[763]	40 (5 d every 4–5 wk) × 3 cycles	Conventional	18	17 (94)
Gasparini[255]	80 (d 1, 21, 42)	Conventional	18	11 (61)
Al-Sarraf[12]	100 (d 1, 21, 42)	Conventional	27 (npc)	24 (89)
Fontanesi[233]	100 (d 1, 22, 42)	Hyperfraction	20	16 (80)
Harrison[294]	100 (d 1, 22)	Conventional/Hyperfraction	22	14 (64)
Haselow[304]	20 (weekly)	Conventional	159	54 (34)
Marcial[450]	100 (d 1, 21, 42)	Conventional	124	88 (71)
Shankar[608]	100 (d 1, 28, 56)	Accelerated	19	14 (68)
Carboplatin				
Sinibaldi[621]	60–100 weekly	Conventional	29	15 (52)
Schnabel[587]	70 (d 1–5, 29–33)	Conventional	54	36 (67)
Volling[731]	20–60 (4 d wk 1, 2, 5; 2 d/wk 6)	Accelerated	23	13 (57)
Total			500	346 (69%)

Abbreviations: d, day; wk, week; CI, continuous infusion; npc, nasopharyngeal carcinoma
[a] From randomized trial
[b] Split-course radiotherapy
[c] Total dose per day
[d] Percentage accurate; numbers estimated from abstract

they are based on comparisons of dose and schedule from many uncontrolled single-institution trials of heterogeneous and small patient groups and multiple variables (different doses, schedules, and routes of cisplatin administration; differing schedules, fractionation programs, and total doses of radiotherapy) (Table 105.32). The many dose-schedule clinical trials of cisplatin with irradiation suggest that cisplatin at 100 mg/m^2 on days 1, 22, and 43 of radiation treatment is most promising, mostly based on a large cooperative-group phase II trial with long-term follow-up (450). Fifty-eight percent of the patients received adequate radiotherapy (more than 64.5 Gy) and the full three cycles of cisplatin. The complete response rate was 71% and the 3-year absolute survival was 43%—results superior to those in historic controls (radiotherapy only). Acute and chronic toxicities were acceptable.

The activity of intermittent standard or high-dose cisplatin regimens is further supported by evidence that it can salvage patients who fail to respond to induction therapy with cisplatin and infusion 5-fluorouracil (209). Some recent single-arm work suggests that local control rates may be further improved with regional or higher-dose cisplatin and hyperfractionated or accelerated radiotherapy schedules. Randomized trials in HNSCC of this cisplatin dose and schedule are currently in progress (121, 122).

Carboplatin has not yet received adequate clinical evaluation in concomitance with radiotherapy (137). Preliminary data limited to five phase I/II trials with differing doses and schedules of carboplatin and of radiotherapy in unresectable disease have produced complete responses in the range of 50 to 70%. These carboplatin trials included patients with more advanced primary and nodal stage disease (621) than many concomitant cisplatin trials (450). Further study to establish optimal doses and schedules is needed.

The same RTOG concomitant cisplatin radiotherapy regimen (450) has been tested in 27 locally advanced NPC patients (26 stage IV). The complete-response rate was 89%; disease-free and overall survival rates were higher, and distant metastasis rates lower than those of historic controls (radiotherapy alone) from the RTOG database (12).

Pure radiosensitizer trials (i.e., drugs without independent activity in HNSCC) have been generally negative (32, 702). Misonidazole, the best-studied agent in this class, has achieved no improvement in survival in several randomized trials in a total of over 1,000 HNSCC patients (702). A recent double-blind, randomized Italian study of lonidamine with or without hyperfractionated radiotherapy reported improvements in complete response, response duration, and local control (447). The estimated 2-year disease-free survival was 51% in the lonidamine arm versus 25% without the drug.

Concomitant multiagent chemoradiotherapy began as a result of positive studies with concomitant single-agent chemotherapy and radiotherapy. The primary goal of these combined-agent trials was to reduce distant failures, which seem to be resistant to single-agent chemoradiotherapy; the secondary goal is to further enhance already excellent local control rates with concomitant approaches. Due to acute toxicity (mucositis), many trials used split-course radiotherapy, in which a period (or cycle) of concurrent chemoradiotherapy is followed by a planned interruption in all therapy to allow time for normal tissue recovery. Much of this work has been done in phase I/II feasibility trials designed to sort out issues of maximized dose intensity and minimized normal tissue toxicity. A popular variant of, or hybrid between, synchronous and sequential combined-agent chemoradiotherapy is the alternating approach (511, 716). Its rationale is based in part on preclinical in vivo work (murine model) indicating that the approach reduces normal-tissue toxicity and, therefore, represents a compromise between synchronous and sequential chemoradiotherapy.

A distinct advantage of single-agent over combined-agent concomitant trials is the simplicity of study design and more effective (continuous, uninterrupted) conventional or hyperfractionated radiotherapy. The split-course radiotherapy necessary with combined agents is inferior to uninterrupted radiotherapy. The rationale for pursuing combined-agent trials is based on the assumption that combined agents are better than single agents—an assumption that has not been proved in HNSCC. Survival rates with single-agent cisplatin are equivalent to those of any combination chemotherapy. Combined-modality approaches requiring reduced dose intensities of cisplatin may produce results inferior to cisplatin alone at high doses.

Cisplatin-based concomitant multiagent regimens have been studied in several recent phase II trials. An increasing trend toward employing combinations of cisplatin and 5-fluorouracil with conventional or hyperfractionated split-course radiotherapy has been reported (3, 135, 136, 377, 475, 476, 678, 681). Preclinical studies have demonstrated synergistic interactions between any two of these three treatments. Doses and schedules of cisplatin, 5-fluorouracil, and radiotherapy have varied considerably. The modulation of 5-fluorouracil by leucovorin and hydroxyurea as part of concomitant chemoradiotherapy regimens is under study (296, 729, 757, 758).

Taylor and colleagues administered a regimen of concomitant cisplatin (60 mg/m^2) and 5-fluorouracil (800 mg/m^2 for 5 days) with conventionally fractionated (total 70 Gy) radiation given every other week for seven cycles (678, 681). Results from 53 unresectable patients indicate a high rate of clinical complete (55%) and partial (43%) responses, and a median failure-free survival of 51 months (range, 12 to 83). The overall median survival was 37 months. Further, survival of patients with a partial response to therapy was remarkably high and not significantly different from that of patients achieving a complete response.

However promising they may be, studies of concomitant cisplatin, 5-fluorouracil (with or without modulators of 5-fluorouracil), and radiotherapy must be interpreted with caution in light of their radical designs and markedly increased normal-tissue toxicity. One study of alternating cisplatin/5-fluorouracil and hyperfractionated radiotherapy was terminated early because of excessive toxicity (135). Moreover, potential therapeutic gains with the concomitant regimen may be compromised by a significant decrease in the dose intensity of radiotherapy. Despite these potential drawbacks, the preliminary experience with concomitant cisplatin, 5-fluorouracil, and radiotherapy is promising and deserves future comparisons with conventional and hyperfractionated radiotherapy. These innovative concomitant approaches await confirmation of their efficacy in randomized trials.

To date, there have been 10 phase III trials that have compared concomitant combination chemoradiotherapy with radiotherapy alone (in four trials) (49, 376, 377, 475) or with sequential chemoradiotherapy (in six trials) (4, 476, 536, 636, 677, 781). Of the four trials with radiotherapy-alone control arms, one reported significant improvement in progression-free and overall survival. This positive randomized trial compared rapidly alternating cisplatin/5-fluorouracil chemotherapy and radiation therapy with continuous radiation therapy alone in 157 patients with locally advanced unresectable disease (475). The study was stopped early (planned sample size of 180) because of the major difference in complete-response rates (42% versus 22%, $P = .037$), causing investigator reluctance to randomize patients to radiotherapy only. Compared with radiation, the chemoradiotherapy arm had a significant increase in 3-year progression-free (25% versus 7%) and overall (41% versus 23%) survival. The rate of severe mucositis was similar in the chemotherapy and radiotherapy arms (19% and 18%). This study has been criticized because the survival rate in the radiotherapy control arm was lower than that observed in several other studies.

Of the six randomized trials comparing concomitant with sequential chemoradiotherapy, four reported significant improvements in disease-free or progression-free survival and two reported significant improvements in overall survival. The most recently published trial compared sequential and concomitant cisplatin/5-fluorouracil in 214 patients (677). This trial's major finding was a significant improvement in progression-free survival ($P = .03$) in the concomitant arm due mostly to a reduction in the local-regional failure rate (55% versus 39%). There were no significant differences in distant failure rates (only 7% and 10% in the concomitant and sequential arms, respectively) or in overall survival.

Recently, several groups developed more intensive combination chemoradiotherapy approaches (250, 725). Early results from these nonrandomized studies indicate that the severe toxicity may be balanced by improved survival results. Vokes et al. have studied the administration of 5-fluorouracil plus hydroxyurea given synchronously with radiotherapy (FHX) (383, 642, 725). FHX produced 23 complete responses in 24 stages II and III patients and a 2-year survival rate of 87%. Vokes has also applied this approach to stage IV disease. In a recent study, 71 patients were treated with FHX after PFLI (cisplatin, fluorouracil, leukovorin, interferon) induction. With a median follow-up time of 37 months, the 3-year disease-free and overall survival rates of 69% and 60% are far superior to historic figures for stage IV patients. However, toxicity was substantial: severe life-threatening mucositis and myelosuppression developed in 54% and 60%, respectively, and there were five treatment-related deaths.

Table 105.33. Randomized Trials of Adjuvant Chemotherapy for Head and Neck Cancer

Author	N	Adjuvant chemotherapy	% Disease-free survival (yr)[a]		% Survival (yr)[a]	
			Control	Chemotherapy	Control	Chemotherapy
Szpirglas[668]	95 (at,fom)	M1B (3-arm)	47 (2)	52	58 (4)	58
Bitter[53]	33 (oc)	MBO	24 (3)	68[b]	29 (3)	65[b]
Huang[334,335]	126	MBVL	58 (—)	72[c]	—	—
Rossi[570]	229 (npc)	ODC	56 (4)	58	67 (4)	59
Domenge[188]	287 (ecs)	PBM	— (3)	—	— (3)[d]	—
Intergroup[405]	448	PF	—[f]	—	—[f]	—

Abbreviations: at, anterior tongue; fom, floor of mouth; oc, oral cavity; npc, nasopharyngeal carcinoma; ecs, extracapsular spread; LF, 5-Fluorouracil; M, methotrexate; B, bleomycin; O, vincristine, V, vinblastine, L, lomustine; D, doxorubicin; C, cyclophosphamide; P, cisplatin; I, leucovorin; —, not available.
[a] published values or estimated from published data/survival curves
[b] statistically significant
[c] significant only for patients receiving more than 2 cycles
[d] statistically significant favoring control
[e] significant reduction in incidence of distant metastasis in chemotherapy arm (P = 0.05)
[f] no significant differences in median disease-free or overall survival rates

Adjuvant

Adjuvant (maintenance) chemotherapy to eradicate micrometastases following local therapy (adjuvant therapy in the strict sense) has not been studied extensively in HNSCC (219). The principal objectives of adjuvant trials have been to control subclinical persistent disease after surgery or radiotherapy and to decrease the rates of local-regional and distant relapse. The ideal study design would include enrollment of (high-risk) patients with resectable advanced disease, early administration after local therapy to avoid drug resistance, and an effective regimen. Although no study has met all these criteria, promising leads for future studies have emerged.

Seven randomized studies have evaluated the impact of adjuvant multiagent chemotherapy with no clear survival impact: significant differences occurred in two trials (Table 105.33), one small positive trial (53) and one large negative trial of delayed adjuvant therapy (188).

The most recent phase III trial was a Japanese multicenter study of uracil plus tegafur for one year in 398 patients with resectable advanced head and neck cancer (331). The minimum study follow-up was 36 months at the time of the report. Although no significant differences in overall or disease-free survival occurred, this study did report a significant systemic effect of adjuvant therapy (compared with the control group) as indicated by a reduction in the rate of distant metastases (7.9% versus 14.6%, $P = .03$).

Neoadjuvant (or Concomitant) Plus Adjuvant Chemotherapy

This is perhaps the most important primary-therapy study design (Table 105.34). The largest of these is an NCI-sponsored multi-institutional trial, begun in 1978, called the Head and Neck Contracts Program (306, 350). Over 400 patients with resectable stage III or IV disease were randomized to (*a*) induction chemotherapy (one cycle of cisplatin and bleomycin) followed by standard therapy (surgery and radiotherapy in all study arms); (*b*) induction chemotherapy followed by standard therapy followed by six cycles of adjuvant monthly cisplatin (80 mg/m^2) by 24-hour continuous infusion; or (*c*) standard local therapy only. At a median follow-up of more than 5 years, the disease-free and overall survivals were not significantly different among the three arms. This study has been criticized because of its one cycle of induction chemotherapy, considered suboptimal (3% complete response, 34% objective response), and a striking noncompliance rate in the adjuvant-therapy arm (47% never received any maintenance therapy). Subset analyses of this study suggested improved disease-free and/or overall survival in three subgroups: oral cavity, T1–2 primary lesions, and N1–2 regional disease (350).

An important aspect of the planned design of one study, the administration of adjuvant therapy to only those who responded to the chemotherapy, reported a definite disease-free survival improvement in the adjuvant arm (214). These promising results are not definitive in light of the extremely small sample size, but they do justify future large-scale study of this strategy.

SUMMARY AND FUTURE DIRECTIONS

Advanced local disease is the focus of primary chemotherapy investigation in HNSCC. Advanced local HNSCC is not controlled adequately by standard surgery and/or radiotherapy alone: 2-year disease-free survival after standard therapy is less than 40%. Preclinical work strongly supports the early integration of chemotherapy into the primary management of advanced HNSCC (99, 577).

Primary chemotherapy in HNSCC falls into three main treatment categories: (*a*) neoadjuvant chemotherapy, designed to reduce tumor burden prior to definitive local control; (*b*) concomitant chemoradiotherapy, designed to be a third definitive treatment (in addition to surgery and radiotherapy) for controlling advanced local HNSCC; and (*c*) adjuvant chemotherapy, designed to maintain, or prevent recurrence in, patients after definitive local control.

Major goals of the first treatment category, neoadjuvant chemotherapy, are to prolong disease-free and overall survivals and to improve the quality of life for surviving patients by providing effective organ-preservation approaches for

Table 105.34. Randomized Trials of Induction Plus Adjuvant Chemotherapy for Head and Neck Cancer

Author	N	Induction (schedule)	% Response (complete)	Local therapy	Adjuvant (cycles)	% Disease-free survival (yr)[a]		% Survival (yr)[a]	
						Control	Chemotherapy	Control	Chemotherapy
Tejada[683]	82	PM (—)	66 (4)	S ± R	PM (—)	576[b]	530[b]		
Stell[659]	86	BOFML CMp (2 cycles)	—	R	BOFML/CMp (12 cycles)	—	—	18 (8)	16
Taylor[679]	82	M (d 1,5,9)	40 (6)	S ± R	M (1 yr) or PD (4 cycles)	37 (3)	50	41 (3)	41
Kun[398]	83	BCMF (2 cycles)	67 (5)	S + R; R	BCMF[c] (2 cycles)	64 (2)	59[d]	43 (2)	31
Ervin[214]	114	PBML (2 cycles)	78 (26)	S + R; R	PBM (3 cycles)	61 (2)	84[e]	—	—
HNCP[306]	462 (see text)	PB (1 cycle)	37 (3)	S + R	P (6 cycles)	55 (5)	49-I 64-Ad	35 (5)	37-I 45-Ad
Rentschler[553]	60	M (4 doses)	73 (5)—p 60 (7)—r	S + R	M (12 weekly)	59 (3)	66	55 (3)	55

Abbreviations: M, methotrexate; P, cisplatin; d, doxorubicin; C, cyclophosphamide; F, fluorouracil; O, vincristine (oncovin); V, vinblastine; Mp, 6-mercaptopurine; L, leucovorin; Vds, vindesine; MMC, mitomycin-C; A, cytosine arabinoside (ara-C), S, surgery; R, radiotherapy; I, induction only; Ad, adjuvant; p, primary site, r, regional disease
[a] Published values or estimated from published data/survival curves
[b] Mean disease-free survival in days
[c] Adjuvant therapy stopped early in trial becuase of non-compliance
[d] Local-regional free survival significantly different $P < .02$
[e] Only 46 patients randomized to the adjuvant trial—benefit greatest for partial responders ($P = 0.14$ overall)

the control of advanced HNSCC. Data from the numerous phase I and II neoadjuvant studies reveal many positive features of this approach: multiagent response rates of 70 to 90% (complete in 20 to 50%), with 30 to 70% of clinically complete responders having complete pathologic tumor regression in biopsies or surgical specimens. Initial tumor stage or extent—whether defined by overall stage, T stage, N stage, or resectability—is predictive of response to chemotherapy and survival. Response to chemotherapy is predictive of response to radiotherapy. Further, chemotherapy responders have a better prognosis than do nonresponders (123, 524, 647), but whether this is a benefit of chemotherapy or a result of unknown factors in the responding subset of patients is not clear. Local-regional control is adequate with surgery or radiotherapy alone in selected patients who respond completely to induction. Induction chemotherapy does not significantly increase the toxicity of subsequent radiotherapy, surgery, or chemotherapy (541). Major concerns about the neoadjuvant approach are the possibilities of delaying and compromising definitive local therapy and the risk that responding patients may refuse definitive local therapy. Furthermore, neoadjuvant chemotherapy definitely prolongs the treatment course, is expensive, and compromises later palliative chemotherapy in recurring patients. Of the over 40 phase III trials incorporating neoadjuvant chemotherapy, only one (using single-agent regional chemotherapy) reported significantly improved survival over that of patients receiving standard local therapy (23). These trials were flawed in many aspects, including study size, heterogeneous patient populations/disease sites/local therapies, and ineffective chemotherapy (median complete-response rate of ≤ 10% in trials).

One randomized neoadjuvant trial, the VACSP, did have a large sample size, a relatively homogeneous patient population (advanced operable laryngeal cancer patients), and a relatively effective regimen of chemotherapy (cisplatin and infusion 5-fluorouracil at full doses). Although this trial produced a respectable complete-response rate, it did not increase survival. Still, neoadjuvant chemotherapy could not be evaluated as an independent variable because the local-regional treatments in the two study arms were not identical. Even so, this study achieved the positive results of laryngeal preservation in 60% of patients and a significant decrease in distant relapse rate in the neoadjuvant arm.

Phase I and phase II trials must continue to translate the preclinical study data into trials of new, more active regimens. Regimens deserving further study include combined cisplatin/5-fluorouracil/leucovorin and other combinations with such agents as IFN-α and hydroxyurea that enhance 5-fluorouracil cytotoxicity. Neoadjuvant trials also should investigate the issue of optimal numbers of chemotherapy cycles on response (clinical/histologic) and on survival. Future work should study the integration of biologic response modifiers, differentiation agents, other cytotoxic drugs (e.g., taxanes, ifosfamide), and irradiation into primary therapy (5, 315, 571).

The second major category of primary chemotherapy is that of regimens designed to achieve definitive local and distant control. So far, concomitant chemoradiotherapy is the only approach in this category that has shown potential by increasing survival in randomized testing. This survival benefit has appeared in trials in both resectable and unresectable HNSCC. Although early trials have used suboptimal intensities, concomitant chemoradiotherapy is designed ultimately to maximize dose intensities of both treatment modalities. All the positive single-agent concomitant trials used suboptimal doses of active drugs (e.g., bleomycin and methotrexate) and full doses of relatively inactive drugs (e.g., mitomycin C). This indicates that chemotherapy enhances radiotherapy. Recent data from numerous phase II trials now support the promise of concomitant cisplatin/radiotherapy. The lack of overlapping toxicities allows the optimal administration of both modalities. Randomized trials are required, however.

Concomitant multiagent chemoradiotherapy (which includes synchronous therapy with split-course radiotherapy and alternating chemoradiotherapy) greatly increases acute toxicity and so requires creative study designs to make this approach feasible (375). The major problem with multiagent regimens is the need to lower radiotherapy's dose intensity, which compromises local control rates. Paradoxically, "aggressive" multiagent chemoradiotherapy programs ultimately may be of decreased rather than increased dose intensity. Nevertheless, early results from all 10 randomized trials are encouraging, with survival favoring the experimental (concomitant) arm in most of these studies. Six trials had no standard local-therapy-only arms. These studies have been criticized for comparing only two experimental arms. Although faulty, this study design has a silver lining: it has provided the best support for concomitant chemoradiotherapy (4, 136, 476, 636). Before accepting concomitant chemoradiotherapy as standard, the results of these and other planned randomized trials (especially those with standard-therapy control arms) will need to mature with more patients, longer follow-ups, and more careful assessments of toxicity and quality of life.

Concomitant therapy does not appear significantly to increase surgical complications, and clearly it has altered the natural history of locally advanced unresectable HNSCC. It has produced lower local-regional failure rates, which suggests that a direct chemotherapy–radiotherapy interaction occurs at primary sites. The lack of impact on distant relapse rates, however, suggests that concomitant chemoradiotherapy should be followed by adjuvant therapy, and support for this approach comes from randomized trials.

No survival benefit is evident in trials of adjuvant chemotherapy, the third major treatment category. The adjuvant approach in HNSCC has not been adequately tested, however. Regimens, cycle number, and timing may not have been optimal; study size and stratification (by site and stage, for example) have not been adequate to allow for this disease's heterogeneity; postoperative delays in initiating adjuvant therapy have compromised results; and toxicity and noncompliance rates have been uniformly high. In the HNCP study, nearly 50% of the patients randomized to adjuvant therapy did not receive any chemotherapy after surgery, and only 8% of all the patients in the adjuvant arm completed the full six cycles (306). Still, this series produced a significant reduction in distant relapse rate, notwithstanding the inclusion of all the many untreated patients in the analysis of this effect. This result underscores the potential value of adjuvant chemotherapy.

The collective data suggest that adjuvant chemotherapy may be useful in the management of selected head and neck cancer patients: those with disease in specific primary sites (e.g., the oral cavity), those with small-volume disease, and those with response who retain a high risk of relapse (Tables 105.33 and 105.34). The data indicate further that trials should incorporate active regimens of chemotherapy in the immediate postoperative period, either before or concomitant with radiotherapy. It also seems evident that large-scale studies designed to detect modest but clinically important survival differences will be required to test the role of adjuvant chemotherapy in HNSCC.

The timing of therapy may be crucial. A novel strategy to circumvent the toxicity of adjuvant chemotherapy given after radiotherapy is adjuvant chemotherapy sandwiched between standard local therapies. This interposition of chemotherapy between surgery and radiotherapy is a carefully conceived strategy (13, 352). Initiating chemotherapy after surgery means that tumor margins are not obscured by prior chemotherapy responses (nor in this protocol are they obscured by responses to prior radiotherapy). It eliminates the problem of patients who refuse surgery because they have responded to chemotherapy, and it allows chemotherapy to attempt its effect in an already debulked tumor. Drug delivery before radiotherapy is through an intact vascular supply. Furthermore, this approach avoids the expected toxicity of postirradiation chemotherapy.

Ultimately, the optimum control of advanced HNSCC certainly may require primary chemotherapy in all three of its strategic roles (i.e., as neoadjuvant, concomitant, and adjuvant therapy). Meta-analysis, or analysis of pooled data from all randomized trials, reveals that concomitant chemotherapy has produced a significant reduction in local-regional failure (660).

Unfortunately, the greatest hope for primary chemotherapy—that it would eradicate systemic disease—has not been fulfilled. This is so even though elegant mathematical and preclinical models support the early use of chemotherapy to eradicate micrometastases, and, thus, to prevent distant relapse. Heterogeneous cancer cell populations and relatively low growth fractions may be the major hurdles to developing effective chemotherapy for this disease. Significant decreases (13, 306, 405, 669, 699) and increases (16, 658, 660, 711) in distant relapse rates have been reported from the more than 50 phase III trials incorporating primary chemotherapy (Tables 105.29, 105.31, 105.33, 105.34, and 105.35). All types of analyses, including meta-analysis of the more than 50 trials, indicate that neither single-agent nor multiagent regimens have consistently diminished distant relapse rates.

Although overall results show no improvement, well-designed, large-scale, cooperative group trials achieved significantly reduced distant relapse rates (13, 306, 328, 405, 699). Through their large patient bases, these trials were able to show statistically significant, small improvements and, therefore, to suggest that currently available platinum-based chemotherapy may have clinically important, albeit modest, activity in micrometastatic disease. Future work should build on these findings, and must continue to search for more effective programs in the systemic control of advanced HNSCC.

References

1. Abele R, Clavel M, Rossi A, Bruntsch U, Pinedo HM. Iproplatin (CHIP, JM-9) in advanced squamous cell carcinoma of the head and neck. A phase II study of the EORTC early clinical trials group (abstract 575). Proc Am Soc Clin Oncol 1986;5:147.
2. Abele R, Honegger HP, Grossenbacher R, Mermillod B, Kaplan E, Gervasi A, Wolfensbeager M, Lehmann W, Cavalli F. A randomized study of methotrexate, bleomycin, hydroxyurea with versus without cisplatin in patients with previously untreated and recurrent squamous cell carcinoma of the head and neck. Eur J Cancer Clin Oncol 1987;23:47.
3. Adelstein DL, Kalish LA, Adams GL, Wagner H, Oken MM, Remick SC, Mansour E. G, Haselow RE. Concurrent radiation therapy and chemotherapy for locally unresectable squamous cell head and neck cancer. J Clin Oncol 1993;11:2136.
4. Adelstein DJ, Sharan VM, Earle AS, Shah AC, Vlastou C, Haria CD, Damm D, Carter SG, Hines JD. Simultaneous versus sequential combined technique therapy for squamous cell head and neck cancer. Cancer 1990;65:1685.
5. Afridi N, Taghian A, Nogueira C, et al. Interferon-α2a/13cis-retinoic acid enhance the radiation sensitivity of squamous cell carcinoma of the head and neck in vitro. Proc Am Soc Clin Oncol 1995;14:295.
6. Vlock D, Anderson J, Whiteside T, Herbeman R, Kirkwood J, Adams G. Immunologic correlates in patients (PTS) with head and neck cancer (SCCHN) treated with interferon alpha (IFN): association between natural killer cell (NK) activity and prolonged survival (abstract 900). Proc Am Soc Clin Oncol 1994;13:280.
7. Alberts DS, Manning MR, Coulthard SW, Koopmann CF Jr, Herman TS. Adriamycin/*cis*-platinum/cyclophosphamide combination chemotherapy for advanced carcinoma of the parotid gland. Cancer 1981;47:645.
8. Al-Kourainy K, Kish J, Ensley J, Tapazoglou E, Jacobs J, Weaver A, Crissman J, Cunnings G, Al-Sarraf M. Achievement of superior survival for histologically negative versus histologically positive clinically complete responders to cisplatin combination in patients with locally advanced head and neck cancer. Cancer 1987;59:233.
9. Al-Sarraf M, Hussein M. Head and neck cancer: present status and future prospects of adjuvant chemotherapy. Cancer Invest 1995;13:41–53.
10. Al-Sarraf M. Clinical trials with fluorinated pyrimidines in patients with head and neck cancer. Invest New Drugs 1989;7:71.
11. Al-Sarraf M, Metch B, Kish J, Ensley J, Rinehart JJ, Schuller DE, Coltman CA Jr. Platinum analogs in recurrent and advanced head and neck cancer: a Southwest Oncology Group and Wayne State University study. Cancer Treat Rep 1987;71:723.
12. Al-Sarraf M, Pajak TF, Cooper JS, Mohiuddin M, Herskovic A, Ager PJ. Chemo-radiotherapy in patients with locally advanced nasopharyngeal carcinoma: A radiation therapy oncology group study. J Clin Oncol 1990;8:1342.
13. Al-Sarraf M, Scott CB, Ahmad R, Schwade JG, Schuller D, Laramore GE, Jacobs J. Phase III study comparing sequential chemotherapy (CT) and radiotherapy (RT) to RT for resected and negative margins squamous cell carcinoma of the head and neck: intergroup study #0034. Proc Am Soc Clin Oncol 1992;11.
14. Al-Sarraf M, Tapazoglou F, Ensley JF, Ahmad K, Jacobs JR, Suchowski C, Kish JA. Significant loco-regional control of advanced head and neck cancer (HN-CA) with concurrent cisplatin and radiotherapy (RT) after initial response to induction chemotherapy (CT) (abstract 670). Proc Am Soc Clin Oncol 1990;9:173.
15. Amendola BE, Eisert D, Hazra TA, King ER. Carcinoma of the maxillary antrum: surgery or radiation therapy? Int J Radiat Oncol Biol Phys 1981;7:743.
16. Amiel JL, Sancho-Garnier H, Vandenbrouck C, Eschwege F, Droz JP, Schwaab G, Wibault P, Stromboni M, Rey A. First results of a randomized trial on immunotherapy of head and neck tumors. Recent results. Cancer Res 1978;68:318.
17. Amornarn R, Prempre T, Jaiwatana J, Wixwnberg MJ. Radiation management of carcinoma of the tonsillar region. Cancer 1984;54:1293.
18. Amrein PC. Cisplatin and 5-fluorouracil vs.the same plus bleomycin and methotrexate in recurrent squamous cell carcinoma of the head and neck (SCC H+N) (abstract 676). Proc Am Soc Clin Oncol 1990;9:175.
19. Amrein PC, Fabian RL. Treatment of recurrent head and neck cancer with cisplatin and 5-fluorouracil vs. the same plus bleomycin and methotrexate. Laryngoscope 1992;102:901–906.
20. Amrein PC, Fingert H, Weitzman SA. Cisplatin-vincristine-bleomycin therapy in squamous cell carcinoma of the head and neck. J Clin Oncol 1983;1:421.
21. Ang KK, Peters LJ, Weber RS, Maio MH, Morrison WH, Wendt CD, Brown BW. Concomitant boost radiotherapy schedules in the treatment of carcinoma of the oropharynx and nasopharynx. Int J Radiat Oncol Biol Phys 1990;19:1339.
22. Ansfield FJ, Ramirez G, Davis HL Jr, Korbitz BC, Vermund H, Gollin FF. Treatment of advanced cancer of the head and neck. Cancer 1970;25:78.
23. Arcangeli G, Nervi C, Righini R, Creton G, Mirri MA, Guerra A. Combined radiation and drugs: the effect of intra-arterial chemotherapy followed by radiotherapy in head and neck cancer. Radiother Oncol 1983;1:101.
24. Atichartakarn V, Kraiphibul P, Clongsusuek P, Pochanugool L, Kulapaditharom B, Ratantharathorn V. Nasopharyngeal carcinoma Result of treatment with *cis*-diamminedichloroplatinum II, 5 fluorouracil, and radiation therapy. Int J Radiat Oncol Biol Phys 1988;14:461.
25. Bachaud JM, David JM, Boussin G, et al. Combined postoperative radiotherapy and weekly cisplatin infusion for locally advanced squamous cell carcinoma of the head and neck: preliminary report of a randomized trial. Int J Radiat Oncol Biol Phys 2 1991;0:243-246.
26. Bachouchi M, Cvitkovic E, Azli N, Gasmi J, Cortes-Funes H, Boussen H, Rahal M, Kalifa C, Schwaab G, Eschwege, F. High complete response in advanced nasopharyngeal carcinoma with bleomycin, epirubicin, and cisplatin before radiotherapy. JNCI 1990;82:616.
27. Baden E. Prevention of cancer of the oral cavity and pharynx. CA 1987;37:49.
28. Bailey BJ. Management of carcinoma of the lip. Laryngoscope 1977;87:250.
29. Baker SR, Krause CJ. Carcinoma of the lip. Laryngoscope 1980;90:19.
30. Baker SR, Sullivan MJ. Osteocutaneous free scapular flap for one-stage mandibular reconstruction. Arch Otolaryngol 1988;114:267.
31. Baker SR, Wheeler RH. Intraarterial chemotherapy for head and neck cancer, Part I: theoretical considerations and drug delivery systems. Head Neck Surg 1983;6:664.
32. Bakowski MT, MacDonald E, Mould RF, Cawte P, Sloggem J, Barrett A, Dalley V, Newton KA, Westbury G, James SE, Hellman K. Double blind controlled clinical trial of radiation plus razoxane (ICRF 159) versus radiation plus placebo in the treatment of head and neck cancer. Int J Radiat Oncol Biol Phys 1978;4:115.
33. Ballantyne AJ. Methods of repair after surgery for cancer of the pharyngeal wall, postcricoid area and cervical esophagus. Am J Surg 1971;122:482.
34. Bamberg M, Schulz U, Scherer E. Postoperative split course radiotherapy of squamous cell carcinoma of the oral tongue. Int J Radiat Oncol Biol Phys 1979;5:515.
35. Barnes L, Kanbour A. Malignant fibrous histiocytoma of the head and neck. Arch Otolaryngol Head Neck Surg 1988;114:1149.
36. Barrs DM, DeSanto LW, O'Fallon WM. Squamous cell carcinoma at the tonsil and tongue-base regions. Arch Otolaryngol 1979;105:479.
37. Barton RT, Hogetveit AC. Nickel-related cancers of the respiratory tract. Cancer 1980;45:3061.
38. Bataini P, Bernier J, Jaulerry C, Brunin F, Pontvert D. Impact of cervical disease and its definitive radiotherapeutic management on survival: experience in 2013 patients with squamous cell carcinoma of the oropharynx and pharyngolarynx. Laryngoscope 1990;100:716.
39. Bataini P, Brugere J, Bernier J, Jaulerry CH, Picot C, Ghossein NA. Results of radical radiotherapeutic treatment of carcinoma of the pyriform sinus: experience of the Institute Curie. Int J Radiat Oncol Biol Phys 1982;8:1277.
40. Batsakis JG. Tumors of the head and neck. In Clinical and Pathological Considerations. Edited by JG Batsakis. Baltimore: Williams & Wilkins, 1974.
41. Baugh RF, Wolf GT, McClatchey KD. Small cell carcinoma of the head and neck. Head Neck Surg 1986;8:343.
42. Beatty JD, Terz JJ, Brown PW, Lawrence W Jr, Schuller GB, Kaplan AM. Adjuvant intralesional and systemic *Corynebacterium parvum* immunotherapy for surgically treated head and neck cancer. Surg Forum 1978;29:155.
43. Bedwinek JM, Shukovsky LJ, Fletcher GH, Daly TE. Osteonecrosis in patients treated with definitive radiotherapy for squamous cell carcinomas of the oral cavity and naso- and oropharynx. Radiology 1976;119:665.
44. Belsky JL, Tachikawa C, Cihak RW, Yamamoto T. Salivary gland tumors in the atomic bomb survivors. Hiroshima-Nagasaki 1957 to 1970. JAMA 1972;219:864.
45. Berenson JR, Yang J, Koga H, Slamon D, Mickel RA. bcl-1 and Int-2 coamplification in squamous cell carcinomas of the head and neck and lung (abstract 1749). Proc Am Assoc Cancer Res 1989;30:440.
46. Berger AM, Bartoshuk LM, Duffy VB, Nadoolman W. Capsaicin for the treatment of oral mucositis pain. Prin Pract Oncol Updates 1995;9(1):1–11.
47. Berry M, Jacobs C, Sikic B, Halsey J, Borch RF. Modification of cisplatin toxicity with diethyldithiocarbamate. J Clin Oncol 1990;8:1585.
48. Bertino JR, Boston B, Capizzi RL. The role of chemotherapy in the management of cancer of the head and neck: a review. Cancer 1975;36:752.
49. Bezwoda WR, de Moor NG, Deman DP. Treatment of advanced head and neck cancer by means of radiation therapy plus chemotherapy: a randomized trial. Med Pediatr Oncol 1979;6:353.
50. Bijman JT, Wagener D, van Rennes H, Wessels JM, van den Brock P. Flow cytometric evaluation of cell dispersion from human head and neck tumors. Cytometry 1985;6:334.
51. Biller HF, Lawson W. Partial laryngectomy for vocal cord cancer with marked limitations or fixation of the vocal cord. Laryngoscope 1986;96:61.
52. Biller HF, Lawson W, Baek SM. Total glossectomy. A technique of reconstruction eliminating laryngectomy. Arch Otolaryngol 1983;109:69.
53. Bitter K. Postoperative chemotherapy versus postoperative cobalt 60 radiation in patients with advanced oral carcinoma: Report on a randomized study (abstract). Head Neck Surg 1981;3:264.
54. Bjorkland A, Eneroth CM. Management of parotid gland neoplasms. Am J Otolaryngol 1980;1:155.
55. Blacklock JB, Weber RS, Lee YY, Goepfert H. Transcranial resection of tumors of the paranasal sinuses and nasal cavity. J Neurosurg 1989;71:10.
56. Blomhoff R, Green MH, Berg T, Norum KR. Transport and storage of vitamin A. Science 1990;250:399.
57. Bloom EJ, Green MD, Cooper JS, Cohen N, Muggia FM. Concomitant use of *cis*-platinum (CDDP) chemotherapy and radiation therapy (RT) in the treatment of advanced head and neck cancer. (abstract C-533) Proc Am Soc Clin Oncol 1985;4:137.
58. Bloom ND, Spiro RH. Carcinoma of the cheek mucosa: A retrospective analysis. Am J Surg 1980;140:556.
59. Blot WJ, McLaughlin JK, Winn DM, Austin DF, Grumbers RS, Preston-Martin S, Bernstein L, Schoenberg JB, Stemhagen A, Fraumeni JF Jr. Smoking and drinking in relation to oral and pharyngeal cancer. Cancer Res 1988;48:3282.
60. Bocca E. Supraglottic cancer. Laryngoscope 1975;85:1318.
61. Bocca E, Pignataro O, Oldini C. Supraglottic laryngectomy: 30 years of experience. Ann Otol Rhinol Laryngol 1983;92:14.
62. Boring CC, Squires TS, Tong T. Cancer statistics 1993. CA 1993;43:7.
63. Bouquot JE, Kurland LT, Weiland LH. Carcinoma in situ of the upper aerodigestive tract. Incidence, time trends, and follow-up in Rochester, Minnesota 1935–1984. Cancer 1988;61:1691.
64. Bouquot JE, Weiland LH, Kurland LT. Leukoplakia and carcinoma in situ synchronously associated with invasive oral/oropharyngeal carcinoma in Rochester, Minn 1935–1984. Oral Surg Oral Med Oral Pathol 1988;65:199.
65. Boussen H, Khalfallah S, Mezlini A, et al. Phase II trial of alpha-2 interferon (IFN) in metastatic (MTS) nasopharyngeal carcinoma (NPC) (abstract 878). Proc Am Soc Clin Oncol 1995;4:303.
66. Bowman GP, Cripps C, Hodson DI, et al. Placebo-controlled randomized trial of infusional fluorouracil during standard radiotherapy in locally advanced head and neck cancer. J Clin Oncol 1994;12:2648–2653.
67. Boyle JO, Hakin J, Koch W, et al. The incidence of p53 mutations increases with progression of head and neck cancer. Cancer Res 1993;53:4477–4480.
68. Braakhuis BJM, van Dongen GAMS, Vermorken JB, Snow GB. Preclinical in vivo activity of 2′, 2′-difluorodeoxycytidine (Gemcitabine) against human head and neck cancer. Cancer Res 1991;51:211.
69. Brachman DG, Graves D, Vokes E, Beckett M, Haraf D, Motag A, Dunphy E, Mick R, Yandell D, Weichselbaum RR. Occurrence of p53 gene deletions and human papilloma virus infection in human head and neck cancer. Cancer Res 1992;52:4832.
70. Brandsma JL, Abramson AL. Association of papillomavirus with cancer of the head and neck. Arch Otolaryngol Head Neck Surg 1989;115:621.
71. Brennan JA, Boyle JO, Koch WM, Goodman SN, Hruban RH, Eby YJ, Couch MJ, Forastiere AA, Sidransky D. Association between cigarette smoking and mutation of

the p53 gene in squamous-cell carcinoma of the head and neck. N Engl J Med 1995;332(11):712–717.

72. Brennan JA, Mao L, Hruban RH, Boyle JO, Eby YJ, Koch WM, Goodman SN, Sidransky D. Molecular assessment of histopathological staging in squamous-cell carcinoma of the head and neck. N Engl J Med 1995;332(7):429–35.
73. Broders AC. The microscopic grading of cancer. Surg Clin North Am 1941;21:947.
74. Browman GP, Wong G, Hodson I, Sathya J, Russell R, McAlpine L, Skingley P, Levine MN. Influence of cigarette smoking on the efficacy of radiation therapy in head and neck cancer. N Engl J Med 1993;328:159.
75. Browman GP, Goodyear MD, Levine MN, Russell R, Archibald SD, Young JE. Modulation of the antitumor effect of methotrexate by low-dose leucovorin in squamous cell head and neck cancer: A randomized placebo-controlled clinical trial. J Clin Oncol 1990;8:203.
76. Browman GP, Levine MN, Goodyear MD, Russell R, Archibald SD, Jackson BS, Young JE, Basrur V, Johanson C. Methotrexate/fluorouracil scheduling influences normal tissue toxicity but not antitumor effects in patients with squamous cell head and neck cancer: results from a randomized trial. J Clin Oncol 1988;6:963.
77. Browman GP, Levine MN, Russell R, Young JE, Archibald SD. Survival results from a phase III study of simultaneous versus 1-hour sequential methotrexate-5-fluorouracil chemotherapy in head and neck cancer. Head Neck Surg 1986;8:146.
78. Bryce D. The conventional surgical management of carcinoma of the hypopharynx. J Laryngol Otol 1971;85:1221.
79. Bryce DP. The management of laryngeal cancer. J Otolaryngol 1979;8:105.
80. Buchholz TA, Laramore GE, Griffin BR, Koh WJ, Griffin TW. The role of fast neutron radiation therapy in the management of advanced salivary gland malignant neoplasms. Cancer 1992;69:2779.
81. Buchholz TA, Laramore GE, Griffin TW. Fast neutron irradiation of recurrent pleomorphic adenomas of the parotid gland. Am J Clin Oncol 1992;15:441.
82. Burkell CC. Cancer of the lip. Can Med Assoc J 1950;62:28.
83. Burkey BB, Hoffman HT, Baker SR, Thornton AF, McClatchey KD. Chondrosarcoma of the head and neck. Laryngoscope 1990;100:1301.
84. Byers RM, Newman R, Russell N, Yue A. Results of treatment of squamous carcinoma of the lower gum. Cancer 1981;47:236.
85. Byfield JE, Calabro-Jones P, Klisak I, Kulhanian F. Pharmacologic requirements for obtaining sensitization of human tumor cells in vitro to combined 5-fluorouracil or ftorafur and x-rays. Int J Radiat Oncol Biol Phys 1982;8:1923.
86. Cady B, Catlin D. Epidermoid carcinoma of the gum. Cancer 1969;23:551.
87. Callery CD, Spiro RH, Strong EW. Changing trends in the management of squamous carcinoma of the tongue. Am J Surg 1984;148:449.
88. Campbell JB, Dorman EB, McCormick M, Miles J, Morton KP, Rugman F, Stell PM, Stoney PJ, Vaughn ED, Wilson JA. A randomized phase III trial of cisplatinum, methotrexate, cisplatinum + methotrexate, and cisplatinum + 5-fluorouracil in end-stage head and neck cancer. Acta Otolaryngol 1987;103:519.
89. Campbell MA, Perrier DG, Dorr RT, Alberts DS, Finley PR. Methotrexate bioavailability and pharmokinetics. Cancer Treat 1985;69:833.
90. Canetta R, Bragman K, Smaldone L, Rozencweig MI. Carboplatin: current status and future prospects. Cancer Treat Rev 1988;15(suppl B):17.
91. Cann CI, Fried MP, Rothman KJ. Epidemiology of squamous cell cancer of the head and neck. Otolaryngol Clin North Am 1985;18:367.
92. Caplan GA, Brigham BA. Marijuana smoking and carcinoma of the tongue. Is there an association? Cancer 1990;66:1005.
93. Carey TE, Wolf GT, Hsu S, Poore J, Peterson K, McClatchey KD. Expression of A9 antigen and loss of blood group antigens as determinants of survival in patients with head and neck squamous carcinoma. Otolaryngol Head Neck Surg 1987;91:221.
94. Carpenter RJ, DeSanto LW, Devine KD, Taylor WF. Cancer of the hypopharynx: analysis of treatment and results in 162 patients. Arch Otolaryngol 1976;102:716.
95. Carter SK, Livingston RB. The chemotherapy of head and neck cancer. In Principles of Cancer Treatment. Edited by SK Carter, E Glatstein, RB Livingston. New York: McGraw-Hill, 1982.
96. Carugati A, Pradier R, de la Torre A. Combination chemotherapy (CT) pre radical treatment of head and neck squamous cell carcinoma (SCC) (abstract 589). Proc Amer Soc Clin Oncol 1988;7:152.
97. Catimel G, Vermorken JB, Clavel M, et al. A phase II study of gemcitabine (LY188011) in patients with advanced squamous cell carcinoma of the head and neck. Ann Oncol 1994;5:543–547.
98. Catimel G, Verweij J, Mattijssen V, et al. Docetaxel (Taxotere): an active drug for the treatment of patients with advanced squamous cell carcinoma of the head and neck. Ann Oncol 1994;5:533–537.
99. Chabner BA, Collins JM. Cancer Chemotherapy: Principles and Practice. Philadelphia: Lippincott 1990.
100. Chan ATC, Teo PML, Leung WT, et al. Chemotherapy adjunctive to definitive radiotherapy in locoregionally advanced nasopharyngeal carcinoma (NPC): results of a prospective randomized trial using cisplatin and 5-fluorouracil (5-FU) (abstract 863). Proc Am Soc Clin Oncol 1995;14:299.
101. Chan CK, Gee JBL. Asbestos exposure and laryngeal cancers: an analysis of the epidemiologic evidence. J Occup Med 1988;30:23.
102. Chang AY, Keng PC. Potentiation of radiation cytotoxicity by recombinant interferons, a phenomenon associated with increased blockage at the G2-M phase of the cell cycle. Cancer Res 1987;47:4338.
103. Chang H, Leone L, Tefft M, Nigri PT. Simultaneous *cis*-platinum and radiotherapy as an induction therapy for advanced head and neck squamous cell carcinoma (abstract 579). Proc Am Soc Clin Oncol 1988;8:150.
104. Chen JY, Chen CJ, Liu MY, Cho SM, Hsu MM, Lynn TC, Shieh T, Tu SM, Beasley RP, Hwang LY. Antibody to Epstein-Barr virus specific DNase as a marker for field survey of patients with nasopharyngeal carcinoma in Taiwan. J Med Virol 1989;27:269.
105. Chen K, Katz RV, Krutchkoff DJ. Intraoral squamous cell carcinoma: epidemiologic patterns in Connecticut from 1935 to 1985. Cancer 1990;66:1288.
106. Chiang TC, Griem ML. Nasopharyngeal cancer. Surg Clin North Am 1973;53:121.
107. Chobe R, McNeese M, Weber R, Fletcher GH. Radiation therapy for carcinoma of the nasal vestibule. Otolaryngol Head Neck Surg 1988;98:67.
108. Choi K, Aziz H, Stark R, Sohn C, Rosenthal J, Braverman A, Khil S, Isaacson S, Marti J, Rotman M. Concomitant radiation and infusion *cis*-platinum in advanced cancers of the head and neck: Influence of radiation fractionation (abstract 607). Proc Am Soc Clin Oncol 1988;8:157.
109. Chung KY, Mukhopadhyay T, Kim J, Casson A, Ro JY, Goepfert H, Hong WK, Roth JA. Discordant p53 gene mutations in primary head and neck cancers and corresponding second primary cancers of the upper aerodigestive tract. Cancer Res 1993;53:1676.
110. Chung TS, Stefani S. Distant metastases of carcinoma of tonsillar region: A study of 475 patients. J Surg Oncol 1980;14:5.
111. Clark J, Fallon B, Norris C, Miller D, Fabian R, Weichselbaum R, Anderson R, Chaffey J, Ervin T, Frei E. A randomized trial of two induction regimens for advanced squamous cell carcinoma of the head and neck (SCCHN): preliminary results (abstract 515). Proc Am Soc Clin Oncol 1986;5:132.
112. Clark J Fallon B, Weichselbaum R, Miller D, Norris C, Frei E, Ervin T. The influence of resectability on response to induction chemotherapy and survival in advanced squamous cell carcinoma of the head and neck (SCCHN) (abstract C-542). Proc Am Soc Clin Oncol 1985;4:139.
113. Clark JR, Norris CM Jr, Dreyfuss AI, Fallon BG, Balogh K, Anderson RF Jr, Chaffey JT, Anderson JW, Miller D. Nasopharyngeal carcinoma. The Dana-Farber Cancer Institute experience with 24 patients treated with induction chemotherapy and radiotherapy. Ann Otol Rhinol Laryngol 1987;96:608.
114. Clark RM, Rosen IB, Laperriere NJ. Malignant tumors of the head and neck in a young population. Am J Surg 1982;144:459.
115. Clavel M, Cognetti F, Dodion P, Wildiers J, Rosso R, Rossi A, Gignoux B, Van Rymenart M, Cortez-Funes H, Dalesio O. Combination chemotherapy with methotrexate, bleomycin, and vincristine with or without cisplatin in advanced squamous cell carcinoma of the head and neck. Cancer 1987;60:1173.
116. Clavel M, Vermorken JB, Cognetti F, et al. Randomized comparison of cisplatin, methotrexate, bleomycin and vincristine (CABO) versus cisplatin and 5-fluorouracil (CF) versus cisplatin (C) in recurrent or metastatic squamous cell carcinoma of the head and neck. Ann Oncol 1994;5:521–526.
117. Clayman GL, El-Naggar AK, Roth JA, et al. In vivo therapy with p53 adenovirus for microscopic residual head and neck squamous carcinoma. Cancer Res 1995;55:1–6.
118. Coates AS, Tattersall MH, Swanson C, Hedley D, Fox RM, Raghavan D. Combination therapy with methotrexate and 5-fluorouracil: A prospective randomized clinical trial of order of administration. J Clin Oncol 1984;2:756.
119. Coates HL, DeSanto LW, Devine KD, Elveback LR. Carcinoma of the supraglottic larynx. A review of 221 cases. Arch Otolaryngol 1976;102:686.
120. Cobleigh MA, Hill JH, Lad TE, Shevrin DE, Applebaum EL. Phase II study of etoposide in previously untreated squamous cell carcinoma of the head and neck. Cancer Treat Rep 1987;71:321.
121. Cognetti F, Carlini P, Pinnaro P. Prospective randomized trial of neoadjuvant cisplatin and 5-FU followed by radiotherapy versus concurrent cisplatin and radiotherapy in locally advanced head and neck squamous cell cancer: preliminary results. Proceedings Second International Conference on Head and Neck Cancer. Boston: July 31–August 5, 1988.
122. Cognetti F, Carlini P, Pinnaro P, Ruggeri EM, Perrino A, Del Vecchio MR, Ambesi Impiombato F, Calabresi F. Preliminary results of a randomized trial of sequential versus simultaneous chemo and radiotherapy (CT-xRT) in patient (pts) with locally advanced unresectable squamous cell carcinoma of the head and neck (SCCHN) (abstract 661). Proc Am Soc Clin Oncol 1989;8:170.
123. Cognetti F, Pinnaro P, Carlini P, Ruggeri EM. Neoadjuvant chemotherapy in previously untreated patients with advanced head and neck squamous cell cancer. Cancer 1988;62:251.
124. Cognetti F, Pinnaro P, Ruggeri EM, Carlini P, Perrino A, Impiobato FA, Calabresi F, Chilelli MG, Giannarelli D. Prognostic factors for chemotherapy response and survival using combination chemotherapy as initial treatment of advanced head and neck squamous cell cancer. J Clin Oncol 1989;7:829.
125. Collins JM. Pharmacologic rationale for regional drug delivery. J Clin Oncol 1984;2:498.
126. Coltrera MD, Zarbo RJ, Gown AM, et al. Comparison of two putative markers of premalignant change in the oral cavity: Suprabasal expression of CK-19 and proliferating cell nuclear antigen (PCNA). Proceedings, Third International Head and Neck Oncology Research Conference. Las Vegas, 1990.
127. COMMIT Research Group Community intervention trial for smoking cessation (COMMIT): I. Cohort results from a four-year community intervention. Am J Pub Health 1995;85:183–192.
128. Condit PT. Treatment of carcinoma with radiation therapy and methotrexate. Mo Med 1968;65:832.
129. Conley J, Dingman DK. Adenoid cystic carcinoma in the head and neck (cylindroma). Arch Otolaryngol 1974;100:81.
130. Conley J, Myers E, Cole R. Analysis of 115 patients with tumors of the submandibular gland. Ann Otol Rhinol Laryngol 1972;81:323.
131. Connors JM, Andiman WA, Howarth CB, Liu E, Merigam TC, Savage ME, Jacobs C. Treatment of nasopharyngeal carcinoma with human leukocyte interferon. J Clin Oncol 1985;3:813.
132. Connors JM, Jacobs C. Nasopharyngeal carcinoma: Relationship to Epstein-Barr virus and treatment with interferon. In Cancers of the Head and Neck. Edited by C Jacobs. Boston: Martinus Nijhoff, 1987, pp 167–175.
133. Conti CJ. Markers of keratinocyte differentiation in preneoplastic and neoplastic lesions. In Immunocytochemistry in Tumor Diagnosis. Edited by J Russo. Proceedings of the Workshop on Immunocytochemistry in Tumor Diagnosis, Detroit, Michigan. Boston: Martinus Nijhoff, 1984, pp 59–71.
134. Cooke LD, Cooke TG, Bootz F, Forster G, Helliwell TR, Spiller D, Stell PM. Ploidy as a prognostic indicator in end stage squamous cell carcinoma of the head and neck region treated with cisplatinum. Br J Cancer 1990;61:759.
135. Corvo R, Merlano M, Looney WB, Benasso M, Bacigalupo A, Margarino G. Integration of chemotherapy in an MFD-radiotherapy plan for advanced inoperable squamous cell carcinoma of the head and neck. Head Neck 1990;12:60.
136. Corvo R, Merlano M, Scarpati D, Grimaldi A, Benasso M, Franzone P, Santelli A, Scasso F, Rosso R, Vitale V. Sequential or alternate chemo-radiotherapy in the treatment of advanced head and neck tumors. Results of a randomized study. Radiol Med 1988;75:653.
137. Coughlin CT, Richmond RC. Biologic and clinical developments of cisplatin combined with radiation: Concepts, utility, projections for new trials, and the emergence of carboplatin. Sem Oncol 1989;16:31.
138. Cox JD, Pajak TF, Marcial VA, Hanks GE, Mohiuddin M, Fu KK, Byhard RW, Rubin P.

Dose response for local control with hyperfractionated radiation therapy in advanced carcinomas of the upper aerodigestive tracts: preliminary report of Radiation Therapy Oncology Group protocol 83–13. Int J Radiat Oncol Biol Phys 1990;18:515.
139. Craig JB, Powell BL, Jackson DV, Atkins JN, Smith LR, White DR, Richards F, Capizzi RL. Phase II trial of high-dose cytarabine and cisplatin in locoregional previously untreated squamous carcinoma of the head and neck. A Piedmont Oncology Association study. Cancer Treat Rep 1987;71:151.
140. Creagan ET, Woods JE, Schutt AJ, O'Fallon JR. Cyclophosphamide, Adriamycin and *cis*-diamminedichloroplatinum (II) in the treatment of advanced nonsquamous cell head and neck cancer. Cancer 1983;52:2007.
141. Creekmore SP, Micetich KC, Vogelzang N, Canzoneri C, Choudhurg A, Fisher RI. Low toxicity and significant tumor responses in phase II trials of carboplatin (CBDCA) in head and neck, non-small cell lung, urothelial, and ovarian cancers. (abstract C-562) Proc Am Soc Clin Oncol 1985;4:144.
142. Crile G. Excision of cancer of the head and neck. JAMA 1906;258:1780.
143. Crispino O, Tancini O, Barni S, Colombo A, Paolorossi F, Frigerio F, Lissoni P, Buratti C, Ferri L. Simultaneous cisplatinum (CDDP) and radiotherapy in patients with locally advanced head and neck cancer (abstract 482). Proc Am Soc Clin Oncol 1987;6: 123.
144. Crissman JD. Laryngeal keratosis and subsequent carcinoma. Head Neck Surg 1979;1:386.
145. Crissman JD, Liu WY, Gluckman JL, Cummings G. Prognostic value of histopathologic parameters in squamous cell carcinoma of the oropharynx. Cancer 1984;54: 2995.
146. Crissman JD, Pajak TF, Zarbo RJ, Marcial VA, Al-Sarraf M. Improved response and survival to combined cisplatin and radiation in non-keratinizing squamous cell carcinomas of the head and neck. An RTOG study of 114 advanced stage tumors. Cancer 1987;59:1391.
147. Crivellari D, Veronesi A, Magri MD, Tirelli U, Comoretto R, Barzan L, Caruso G, Carbone A, Grigoletto E. Phase II trial of oral VP 16–213 (etoposide) in patients with advanced head and neck cancer. Tumori 1985;71:499.
148. Croll GA, Gerritsen GJ, Tiwari RM, Snow GB. Primary radiotherapy with surgery in reserve for advanced laryngeal carcinoma: results and complications. Eur J Surg Oncol 1989;15:350.
149. Cross JE. Carcinoma of the lip: a review of 563 case records of carcinoma of the lip at the Pondville Hospital. Surg Gynecol Obstet 1948;87:153.
150. Crown J, Lipzstein R, Cohen S, Goldsmith M, Wisch N, Pacincci PA, Silverman L, Weiner M, Jaffrey I, Norton L, Holland JF. Chemotherapy of metastatic Merkel cell cancer. Cancer Invest 1991;9:129–132.
151. Cullen JW, Blot W. Henning Field J, Boyd G, Mecklenberg R, Massey MM. The health consequences of using smokeless tobacco. Summary of the Advisory Committee's Report to the Surgeon General. Pub Health Rep 1986;101:355.
152. Cunningham TJ, Antemann R, Paonessa D, Sponzo RW, Steiner D. Adjuvant immuno- and/or chemotherapy with neuraminidase-treated autogenous tumor vaccine and bacillus Calmette-Guerin for head and neck cancers. Ann NY Acad Sci 1976;277: 339.
153. Cvitkovic E. Neoadjuvant chemotherapy (NACT) with epirubicin (EPI), cisplatin (CDDP), bleomycin (BLEO) (BEC) in undifferentiated nasopharyngeal cancer (UCNT) Preliminary results of an international. (int) phase (PH) III trial. Proc Am Soc Clin Oncol 1994;14:283.
154. Dabelsteen E, Vedtofte P, Hakomori S, Young WW Jr. Accumulation of a blood group antigen precursor in oral premalignant lesions. Cancer Res 1983;43:1451.
155. Dalley VM. Cancer of the laryngopharynx. J Laryngol Otol 1968;20:1859.
156. Dalley D, Beller E, Aroney R, et al. The value of chemotherapy (CT) prior to definitive local therapy (DLT) in patients with locally advanced squamous cell carcinoma (SCC) of the head and neck (HN) (abstract 856). Proc Am Soc Clin Oncol 1995;14:297.
157. Dasmahapatra KS, Citrin P, Hill GJ, Yee R, Mohit-Tabatabai MA, Rush BF Jr. A prospective evaluation of 5-fluorouracil plus cisplatin in advanced squamous cell cancer of the head and neck. J Clin Oncol 1985;3:1486.
158. Dasmahapatra KS, Mohit-Tabatabai MA, Rush BF Jr, Hill GJ, Feuerman M, Ohanian M. Cancer of the tonsil: improved survival with combination therapy. Cancer 1986;57: 451.
159. Davis RK, Shapshay SM. Peristomal recurrence Pathophysiology, prevention and treatment. Otolaryngol Clin North Am 1980;13:499.
160. Davis S, Kessler W. Randomized comparison of *cis*-diamminedichloroplatinum versus cis-diamminedichloroplatinum, methotrexate, and bleomycin in recurrent squamous cell carcinoma of the head and neck. Cancer Chemother Pharmacol 1979;3:57.
161. Dawson AK, Orr JA. Long term results of local excision and radiotherapy in pleomorphic adenoma of the parotid. Int J Radiat Oncol Biol Phys 1985;11:451.
162. Dawson MI, Okamura WH. Chemistry and Biology of Synthetic Retinoids. Boca Raton, FL: CRC, 1990.
163. De Andres Basauri L. Lopez Pousa A, Alba E, Sanpedro F. Carboplatin, an active drug in advanced head and neck cancer. Cancer Treat Rep 1986;70:1173.
164. Decker J, Goldstein JC. Risk factors in head and neck cancer. N Engl J Med 1982;306:1151.
165. DeConti RC, Schoenfeld D. A randomized prospective comparison of intermittent methotrexate, methotrexate with leucovorin, and a methotrexate combination in head and neck cancer. Cancer 1981;48:1061.
166. Decroix Y, Ghossein NA. Experience of the Curie Institute in treatment of cancer of the mobile tongue I: treatment policies and results. Cancer 1981;47:496.
167. De Villiers EM, Weidauer H, Otto H, zur Hausen M. Papillomavirus DNA in human tongue carcinomas. Int J Cancer 1985;36:575.
168. Dennington ML, Carter DR, Meyers AD. Distant metastases in head and neck epidermoid carcinoma. Laryngoscope 1980;90:196.
169. Depue RH. Rising mortality from cancer of the tongue in young white males (letter). N Engl J Med 1986;315:647.
170. Demard F, Chauvel P, Santini J, Vallicioni J, Thyss A, Schneider M. Response to chemotherapy as justification for modification of the therapeutic strategy for pharyngolaryngeal carcinomas. Head Neck Surg 1990;12:225.
171. DeSanto LW. The options in early laryngeal carcinoma. N Engl J Med 1982;306:910.
172. DeSanto LW. T3 glottic cancer: options and consequences of the options. Laryngoscope 1984;94:1311.
173. DeSanto LW. Cancer of the supraglottic larynx: a review of 260 patients. Otolaryngol. Head Neck Surg 1985;93:705.
174. DeSanto LW. Early supraglottic cancer. Ann Otol Rhinol Laryngol 1990;99:593.
175. DeSanto LW, Lillie JC, Devine KD. Surgical salvage after radiation for laryngeal cancer. Laryngoscope 1976;87:649.
176. DeSanto LW, Lillie JC, Devine KD. Cancer of the larynx: supraglottic cancer. Surg Clin North Am 1977;57:505.
177. Devesa SS, Blot WJ, Stone BJ, Miller BA, Tarone RE, Fraumeni JF. Recent cancer trends in the United States. JNCI 1995;87:175–182.
178. Dewit L. Combined treatment of radiation and cisdiamminedichloroplatiunum (II): a review of experimental and clinical data. Int J Radiat Oncol Biol Phys 1987;13:403.
179. Di Blasio B, Barbien W, Bozzetti A, et al. A prospective randomized trial in resectable head and neck carcinoma: locoregional treatment with and without neoadjuvant chemotherapy (abstract 899.) Proc Am Soc Clin Oncol 1994;13:279.
180. Dimery IW, Jacobs C, Tseng A Jr, Saks S, Pearson G, Hons WK, Gutterman JU. Recombinant interferon-gamma in the treatment of recurrent nasopharyngeal carcinoma. J Biol Response Mod 1989;8:221.
181. Dimery IW, Jones LA, Verjan RP, Raymond AK, Goepfert H, Hong WK. Estrogen receptors in normal salivary gland and salivary gland carcinoma. Arch Otolaryngol Head Neck Surg 1987;113:1082.
182. Dimery I, Lee YY, VanTassel P, Goepfert H, Byers R, Guillamondegui O, McCarthy K, Hong WK. Combined intra-arterial (I.A.) and systemic chemotherapy (CT) for paranasal sinus carcinoma (PNSC). Proc Am Soc Clin Oncol 1988;7:150.
183. Dimery IW, Legha SS, Shirinian M, Hong WK. Fluorouracil, doxorubicin, cyclophosphamide, and cisplatin combination chemotherapy in advanced or recurrent salivary gland carcinoma. J Clin Oncol 1990;8:1056.
184. Dimery IW, Martin T, Bradley E, Kramer A, Hong W. Phase I trial of interleukin-2 (rIL-2) plus cisplatin (CDDP) and 5-fluorouracil (5-FU) in recurrent or advanced squamous cell carcinoma of the head and neck. Proc Am Soc Clin Oncol 1989;8:170.
185. Dimery IW, Peters L, Goepfert H, Atkinson EN, McCarthy K, Bennett L, Byers R, Weber R, Hong WK. Long-term survival in advanced stage IV nasopharyngeal carcinoma after combination chemotherapy and radiotherapy. In Adjuvant Therapy of Cancer VI. Edited by SE Jones and SE Salmon. Orlando, FL; Grune and Stratton, 1990, pp 82–91.
186. Dimery IW, Brooks BJ, Winn R, Martin T, Shirinian M, Hong WK. Phase II trial of carboplatin plus cisplatin in recurrent and advanced squamous cell carcinoma of the head and neck. J Clin Oncol 1991;9:1939.
187. DiTroia JF. Nodal metastases and prognosis in carcinoma of the oral cavity. Otolaryngol Clin North Am 1972;5:333.
188. Domenge C, Marandas P, Vignond J, et al. Postsurgical adjuvant chemotherapy in extracapsular spread invaded lymph node of epidermoid carcinoma of the head and neck: a randomized multicentric trial (abstract 108). Proceedings, second International Conference on Head and Neck Cancer:Combined Therapy, Boston: July 31–August 5, 1988, p 74.
189. Donald PJ. Marijuana smoking—possible cause of head and neck carcinoma in young patients. Otolaryngol Head Neck Surg 1986;94:517.
190. Doseva D, Christov K, Kristeva K. DNA content in reactive hyperphasia, precancerosis, and carcinomas of the oral cavity. Acta Histochem 1984;75:113.
191. Douple EB. Platinum-radiation interactions, NCI Monogr 1988;6:315.
192. Drelichman A, Cunnings G, Al-Sarraf M. A randomized trial of *cis*-platinum, oncovin and bleomycin (COB) versus methotrexate in patients with advanced squamous cell carcinoma of the head and neck. Cancer 1983;52:399.
193. Dreyfuss AI, Clark JR, Fallon BG, Posner MR, Norris CM Jr, Miller D. Cyclophosphamide, doxorubicin, and cisplatin combination chemotherapy for advanced carcinomas of salivary gland origin. Cancer 1987;60:2869.
194. Dreyfuss AI, Clark JR, Wright JE, Norris CM Jr, Busse PM, Lucarini JW, Fallon BG, Casey D, Andersen JW, Klein R. Continuous infusion high-dose leucovorin with 5-fluorouracil and cisplatin for untreated stage IV carcinoma of the head and neck. Ann Intern Med 1990;112:167.
195. Dreyfuss A, Posner M, Clark J, et al. Docetaxel (TXTR): an active drug against squamous cell carcinoma of the head and neck (SCCHN) (abstract 875). Proc Am Soc Clin Oncol 1995;14:302.
196. Dubois JB, Guerrier B, DiRuggiero JM, Pourquier H. Cancer of the pyriform sinus: treatment by radiation therapy alone and with surgery. Radiology 1986;160:831.
197. Einhorn J, Wersall J. Incidence of oral carcinoma in patients with leukoplakia of the oral mucosa. Cancer 1967;20:2189.
198. Eisbach KJ, Krause CJ. Carcinoma of the pyriform sinus: A comparison of treatment modalities. Laryngoscope 1977;87:1904.
199. Eisbruch A, Blick M, Lee JS, Sacks PG, Gutterman J. Analysis of the epidermal growth factor receptor gene in fresh human head and neck tumors. Cancer Res 1987;47:3603.
200. Eisenberger MA. Supporting evidence for an active treatment program for advanced salivary gland carcinomas. Cancer Treat Rep 1985;69:319.
201. Eisenberger M, Hornedo J, Silva H, Donehower R, Spaulding M, Van Echo D. Carboplatin (NSC-241-240): An active platinum analog for the treatment of squamous-cell carcinoma of the head and neck. J Clin Oncol 1986;4:1506.
202. Eisenberger M, Krasnow S, Ellenberg S, Silva H, Abrams J, Sinibaldi V, Van Echo D, Aisner J. A comparison of carboplatin plus methotrexate versus methotrexate alone in patients with recurrent and metastatic head and neck cancer. J Clin Oncol 1989;7: 1341.
203. Eisenberger M, Van Echo D, Aisner J. Carboplatin: the experience in head and neck cancer. Sem Oncol 1989;16(suppl 5):34.
204. El Badawi SA, Goepfert H, Fletcher GH, Herson J, Oswald MJ. Squamous cell carcinoma of the pyriform sinus. Laryngoscope 1982;92:357.
205. Elias EG, Chretien PB, Monnard E, Kahn T, Bouchelle WH, Wiernik PH, Lipson SD, Mande KR, Zentai T. Chemotherapy prior to local therapy in advanced squamous cell carcinoma of the head and neck: Preliminary assessment of an intensive drug regimen. Cancer 1979;43:1025.
206. Elkon D, Hightower SI, Lim ML, Cantrell RW, Constable WC. Esthesioneuroblastoma. Cancer 1979;44:1087.
207. Eneroth CM. Salivary gland tumors in the parotid gland, submandibular gland and the palate region. Cancer 1971;27:1418.
208. Eneroth CM, Hamberger CA. Principles of treatment of different types of parotid tumors. Laryngoscope 1974;84:1732.
209. Ensley JF, Ahmed K, Kish JA. Salvage of patients with advanced squamous cell can-

cers of the head and neck (SCCHN) following induction chemotherapy failure using radiation and concurrent cisplatinum (CACP). In Adjuvant Therapy of Cancer IV. Edited by SE Jones and SE Salmon. Orlando, FL; Grune and Stratton,1990 pp. 92–100.

210. Ensley JF, Jacobs JR, Weaver A, Kinzie J, Crissman J, Kish JA, Cummings G, Al Sarraf M. Correlation between response to cisplatinum-combination chemotherapy and subsequent radiotherapy in previously untreated patients with advanced squamous cell cancers of the head and neck. Cancer 1984;54:811.
211. Ensley J, Kish J, Tapazoglou E, Jacobs J, Weaver A, Atkinson D, Ahmed K, Mathog R, Al Sarraf M. An intensive, five course, alternating combination chemotherapy induction regimen used in patients with advanced, unresectable head and neck cancer. J Clin Oncol 1988;6:1147.
212. Ensley JF, Maciorowski Z, Pietraszkiewicz H, deBaud F, Sakr W, Kish J Al Sarraf M, Tapazoglou E. Clinical applications of cellular DNA content parameters determined by flow cytometry in squamous cell cancers of the head and neck. In Adjuvant Therapy of Cancer VI. Edited by SE Jones and SE Salmon. Orlando, FL; Grune and Stratton, 1990, pp 101–108.
213. Epstein MA. Vaccination against Epstein-Barr virus Current progress and future strategies. Lancet 1986;1:1425.
214. Ervin TJ, Clark JR, Weichselbaum RR, Fallon BG, Miller D, Fabian RL, Posner MR, Norris CM Jr, Tuttle SA, Schoenfeld DA. An analysis of induction and adjuvant chemotherapy in the multidisciplinary treatment of squamous-cell carcinoma of the head and neck. J Clin Oncol 1987;5:10.
215. Eschwege F, Sancho-Garnier H, Gerard JP, Madelain M, DeSaulty A, Jortay A, Cachin Y. Ten-year results of randomized trial comparing radiotherapy and concomitant bleomycin to radiotherapy alone in epidermoid carcinomas of the oropharynx: Experience of the European Organization for Research and Treatment of Cancer. NCI Monographs 1988;6:275.
216. Evans HL, Ayala AG, Romsdahl MM. Prognostic factors in chondrosarcoma of bone. A clincopathologic analysis with emphasis on histologic grading. Cancer 1977;40: 818.
217. Fakih AR, Rao RS, Borges AM, Patel AR. Elective versus therapeutic neck dissection in early carcinoma of the oral tongue. Am J Surg 1989;158:309.
218. Fandi A, Taamma A, Bachouchi M, Azli N, Yanes B, Cvitkovic E, Armand JP. Palliative treatment by low dose 5-fluorouracil (5FU) continuous infusion (FUCI) in recurrent and/or metastatic (REC/MTS) undifferentiated nasopharyngeal carcinoma type (UCNT). (abstract 946). Proc Am Soc Clin Oncol 1994;13:291.
219. Fazekas JT, Sommer C, Kramer S. Adjuvant intravenous methotrexate or definitive radiotherapy alone for advanced squamous cancers of the oral cavity, oropharynx, supraglottic larynx or hypopharynx. Int J Radiat Oncol Biol Phys 1980;6:533.
220. Fedder M, Gonzalez MF. Nasopharyngeal carcinoma: brief review. Am J Med 1985;79:365.
221. Feinmesser R, Miyazaki I, Cheung R, Freeman JL, Noyek AM, Dosch HM. Diagnosis of nasopharyngeal carcinoma by DNA amplification of tissue obtained by fine-needle aspiration. N Engl J Med 1992;326:17.
222. Fey SJ, Larsen PM. DNA viruses and human cancer. Cancer Lett 1988;41:1.
223. Field JK, Spandidos DA, Stell PM, Vaughan ED, Evan GI, Moore JP. Elevated expression of the c-*myc* oncoprotein correlates with poor prognosis in head and neck squamous cell carcinoma. Oncogene 1989;4:1463.
224. Fierro R, Johnson J, Myers E, Colao D, Pelch K, Rust D, Wagner R, Whiteside J, Vlock D. Phase II trial of non-recombinant interferon alpha (INF) in recurrent squamous cell carcinoma of the head and neck (SCCHN) (abstract 605). Proc Am Soc Clin Oncol 1988;7:156.
225. Fiore MC, Pierce JP, Remington PL, Fiore BJ. Cigarette smoking: the clinician's role in cessation, prevention, and public health. Dis Mon 1990;36:181.
226. Fitzpatrick PJ, Therialut C. Malignant salivary gland tumors. Int J Radiat Oncol Biol Phys 1986;12:1743.
227. Fletcher GH. Clinical dose-response curves of human malignant epithelial tumors. Br J Radiol 1973;46:1.
228. Fletcher GH. Squamous cell carcinomas of the oropharynx. Int J Radiol Oncol Biol Phys 1979;5:2073.
229. Fletcher GH. Lucy Wortham James Lecture: subclinical disease. Cancer 1984;53: 1274.
230. Fletcher GH, Jesse RH. The contribution of supervoltage roentgen therapy to the integration of radiation and surgery in head and neck squamous cell carcinoma. Cancer 1962;15:566.
231. Fletcher GH, Lindberg RD, Hamberger A, Horiot JC. Reasons for irradiation failure in squamous cell carcinoma of the larynx. Laryngoscope 1975;85:987.
232. Flynn MB, Jesse RH, Lindberg RD. Surgery and irradiation in the treatment of squamous cell cancer of the supraglottic larynx. Am J Surg 1972;124:477.
233. Fontanesi J, Kun LE, Beckford N, Babin R, Kavanagh K, Lester E, Pao WJ, Tai D, Eddy T. Hyperfractionated irradiation and concomitant cisplatin for advanced squamous cell carcinoma of the head and neck: Early experience. Presented at Third International Head and Neck Oncology Research Conference, Las Vegas, 1990.
234. Foote FW Jr, Frazell EL. Tumors of the major salivary glands. Cancer 1953;6:1065.
235. Foote RL, Buskirk SJ, Stanley RJ, Grambsh PM, Olsen KD, De Santo LW, Earle JD, Weiland LH. Patterns of failure after total laryngectomy for glottic carcinoma. Cancer 1989;64:143.
236. Forastiere AA, Baker SR, Wheeler R, Medvec BR. Intra-arterial cisplatin and FUDR in advanced malignancies confined to the head and neck. J Clin Oncol 1987;5:1601.
237. Forastiere AA, Belliveau JF, Goren MP, Vogel WC, Posner MR, O'Leary GP Jr. Pharmacokinetic and toxicity evaluation of five-day continuous infusion versus intermittent bolus *cis*-diamminedichloroplatinum(II) in head and neck cancer patients. Cancer Res 1988;48:3869.
238. Forastiere AA, Metch B, Schuller DE, Ensley JF, Hutchins LF, Triozzi P, Kish JA, McClure S, VonFeldt E, Williamson SK, Von Hoff DD. Randomized comparison of cisplatin plus fluorouracil and carboplatin plus fluorouracil versus methotrexate in advanced squamous-cell carcinoma of the head and neck: a Southwest Oncology Group study. J Clin Oncol 1992;10:1245.
239. Forastiere AA, Neuberg D, Taylor IV SG, et al. Phase II evaluation of taxol in advanced head and neck cancer: an Eastern Cooperative Oncology Group trial. Proc Amer Soc Clin Oncol 1993;12:277.
240. Forastiere AA, Koch W, Lee DJ, Eisele D, Cummings C. Cisplatin and carboplatin combined with radiation to preserve organ function in patients with cancer of the oral cavity, oropharynx and hypopharynx (abstract 69). Proc Head Neck Res Workshop 1994:491.
241. Franchin G, Gobitti C, Minatel E, Barzan L, De Paoli A, Boz G, Mascarin M, Lamon S, Trovo MG. Simultaneous radiochemotherapy in the treatment of inoperable, locally advanced head and neck cancers. Cancer 1995;75:1025–1029.
242. Freeland AP, Van Nostrand AW, Jahn AF. Metastasis to the larynx. J Otolaryngol 1979;8:448.
243. Fu KK. Biological basis for the interaction of chemotherapeutic agents and radiation therapy. Cancer 1985;55:2123.
244. Fu KK, Eisenberg L, Dedo HH, Phillips TL. Results of integrated management of supraglottic carcinoma. Cancer 1977;40:2874.
245. Fu KK, Lichter A, Galante M. Carcinoma of the floor of mouth: an analysis of treatment results and the sites and causes and failures. Int J Radiol Oncol Biol Phys 1976;1:829.
246. Fu KK, Phillips TL, Silverberg IJ, Jacobs C, Goffinet DR, Chun C, Friedman MA, Kohler M, McWhirter K, Carter SK. Combined radiotherapy and chemotherapy with bleomycin and methotrexate for advanced inoperable head and neck cancer: Update of a Northern California Oncology Group randomized trial. J Clin Oncol 1987;5: 1410.
247. Fu KK, Woodhouse RJ, Quivey JM, Phillips TL, Dedo HH. The significance of laryngeal edema following radiotherapy of carcinoma of the vocal cord. Cancer 1982;49: 655.
248. Fujii H, Sasaki Y, Ebihara S, et al. An early phase I study of docetaxel in patients with head and neck cancer. Proc Am Soc Clin Oncol 1995;14:298.
249. Gallick GE, Sacks PG, Maxwell SA, Steck PA, Gutterman JU. Head and neck squamous cell carcinoma cell lines as a model system for the study of oncogene expression during tumor progression and metastasis. Prog Clin Biol Res 1986;212:97.
250. Gandia D, Wibault P, Guillot T, et al. Simultaneous chemoradiotherapy as salvage treatment in locoregional recurrences of squamous head and neck cancer. Head Neck 1993;15:8–15.
251. Garbrilove JL, Jakubowski A, Scher H, Sternberg C, Wong G, Grovs J, Yagoda A, Fain K, Moore MA, Clarkson B. Effect of granulocyte colony-stimulating factor on neutropenia and associated morbidity due to chemotherapy for transitional-cell carcinoma of the urothelium. N Engl J Med 1988;318:1414.
252. Gardner KE, Parsons JT, Mendenhall WM, Million RR, Cassisi NJ. Time dose relationships for local tumor control and complications following irradiation of squamous cell carcinoma of the base of tongue. Int J Radiol Oncol Biol Phys 1987;13:507.
253. Garrett PG, Beale FA, Cummins BJ, Harwood AR, Keane TJ, Payne DG, Rider WD. Cancer of the tonsil: results of radical radiation therapy with surgery in reserve. Am J Surg 1983;146:432.
254. Garrington GE, Scotfield HH, Coryn J, Hooker SP. Osteosarcoma of the jaws. Analysis of 56 cases. Cancer 1967;20:377.
255. Gasparini G, Recher G, Favretto S, Visona A, Bevilacqua P, Del Fior S. Simultaneous *cis*-platinum (CDDP) and radiotherapy (RT) in inoperable or advanced squamous cell carcinoma of the head and neck (H&N) (abstract 663). Proc Am Soc Clin Oncol 1989;8:170.
256. Gebbia V, Gebbia N, Russo A, Testa A, Valenza R, Zerillo G, Ingria F, Spadafora G, Rausa L. Hydroxyurea modulates 5-fluorouracil antineoplastic activity in advanced head and neck carcinoma pretreated with chemotherapy. Anti-Cancer Drugs 1992;3: 347–349.
257. George TK, Sant Agnese AD, Bennett JM. Chemotherapy for metastatic Merkel cell carcinoma. Cancer 1985;56:1034.
258. Ghossein NA, Bataini JP. The role of radiotherapy in the treatment of neck metastases from head and neck cancer. In Head and Neck Cancer. Edited by GT Wolf. Boston: Martinus Nijhoff, 1984, pp 169–199.
259. Ghossein NA, Bataini JP, Ennuyen A, Stacey P, Krishnaswamy V. Local control and site of failure in radially irradiated supraglottic laryngeal cancer. Radiology 1974;112: 187.
260. Giaccone G, Bagatella M, Donadio M, Calciati A. Phase II study of divided-dose vinblastine in advanced cancer patients. Tumori 1989;75:248.
261. Gillis TM, Incze J, Strong MS, Vaughan CW, Simpson GT. Natural history and management of keratosis, atypia carcinoma-in situ, and microinvasive cancer of the larynx. Am J Surg 1983;146:512.
262. Givens CD, Johns ME, Cantrell RW. Carcinoma of the tonsil: analysis of 162 cases. Arch Otolaryngol 1981;107:730.
263. Gladstone WS, Kerr HO. Epidermiod carcinoma of the lower lip: results of radiation therapy of the local lesions. Am J Roentgenol 1958;79:101.
264. Glick JH, Marcial V, Richter M, Velez-Garcia E. The adjuvant treatment of inoperable stage III and IV epidermoid carcinoma of the head and neck with platinum and bleomycin infusions prior to definitive radiotherapy: An RTOG pilot study. Cancer 1980;46:1919.
265. Goepfert H, Guillamondegui OM, Jesse RH, Lindberg RD. Squamous cell carcinoma of nasal vestibule. Arch Otolaryngol Head Neck Surg 1974;100:8.
266. Goepfert H, Jesse RH, Fletcher GH, Hamberger A. Optimal treatment for technically resectable squamous cell carcinoma of the supraglottic larynx. Laryngoscope 1975;85:14.
267. Goepfert H, Lindberg RD, Jesse RH. Combined laryngeal conservation surgery and irradiation: Can we expand on the indications for conservative therapy? Otolaryngol Head Neck Surg 1981;89:974.
268. Goepfert H, Luna M, Lindberg R, White A. Malignant salivary gland tumors of the paranasal sinuses and nasal cavity. Arch Otolaryngol 1983;109:662.
269. Goepfert H, Remmler D, Silva E, Wheeler B. Merkel cell carcinoma (endocrine carcinoma of the skin) of the head and neck. Arch Otolaryngol 1984;110:707.
270. Goffinet DR, Fee WE, Wells J, Austin-Seymour M, Clarke D, Mariscal JM, Goode RL. 192Ir pharyngoepiglottic fold interstitial implants: The key to successful treatment of base of tongue carcinoma by radiation therapy. Cancer 1985;55:941.
271. Goldsweig HG, Sundaresan N. Chemotherapy of recurrent esthesioneuroblastoma. Am J Clin Oncol 1990;13:139.
272. Gollin FF, Ansfield FJ, Brandenburg JH, Ramirez G, Vermund H. Combined therapy in advanced head and neck cancer: a randomized study. Am J Roentgenol Radium Ther Nucl Med 1972;114:83.
273. Gonzalez MF, Valdivieso JG, Sartiano GP, Hollman JM, Worster CF. Comparative study with two platinum containing combinations in locally advanced head and neck squamous cell carcinoma (HNSCC) (abstract 572). Proc Am Soc Clin Oncol 1986;5: 146.
274. Goolden AWG. Radiation cancer. A review with special reference to radiation tumours in the pharynx, larynx, and thyroid. Br J Radiol 1957;30:626.

275. Gowan GF, deSuto-Nagy G. The incidence and sites of distant metastases in head and neck carcinoma. Surg Gynecol Obstet 1953;116:603.
276. Grandis JR, Tweardy DJ. Elevated levels of transforming growth factor alpha and epidermal growth factor receptor messenger RNA are early markers of carcinogenesis in head and neck cancer. Cancer Res 1993;53:3579.
277. Gray AJ. Treatment of advanced head and neck cancer with accelerated fractionation. Int J Radiat Oncol Biol Phys 1986;12:9.
278. Greenberg B, Ahmann F, Garewal H, Koopmann C, Coulthard S, Berzes M, Alberts D, Shimm D, Slymen D. Neoadjuvant therapy for advanced head and neck cancer with allopurinol-modulated high dose 5-fluorouracil and cisplatin. A phase I–II study. Cancer 1987;59:1860.
279. Griem ML, Chiang DTC. Nasopharynx. In Radiation Therapy of Head and Neck Cancer. Edited by GE Laramore. Berlin: Springer-Verlag, 1989.
280. Griffin TW, Pajak TF, Gillespie BW, Davis LW, Brady LW, Rubin P, Marcial VA. Predicting the response of head and neck cancers to radiation therapy with a multivariate modelling system: an analysis of the RTOG head and neck registry. Int J Radiat Oncol Biol Phys 1984;10:481.
281. Griffin TW, Pajak TF, Laramore GE, Duncan W, Richter MP, Hendrickson FR, Maor MH. Neutron vs photon irradiation of inoperable salivary gland tumors: Results of an RTOG-MRC cooperative randomized study. Int J Radiat Oncol Biol Phys 1988;15:1085.
282. Grose WE, Lehane DE, Dixon DO, Fletcher WS, Stuckey WJ. Comparison of methotrexate and cisplatin for patients with advanced squamous cell carcinoma of the head and neck region: a Southwest Oncology Group study. Cancer Treat Rep 1985;69:577.
283. Grunberg SM, Felman IE, Gala KV, Johnson KB, Owens JC. Phase II study of etoposide (VP-16) in the treatment of advanced head and neck cancer. Am J Clin Oncol 1985;8:393.
284. Guillamondegui OM, Byers RM, Tapley N du V. Malignant tumors of the salivary gland. In Textbook of Radiotherapy, 3rd ed. Edited by GH Fletcher. Philadelphia: Lea & Febiger, 1980.
285. Gupta NK, Pointon RC, Wilkinson PM. A randomized clinical trial to contrast radiotherapy with radiotherapy and methotrexate given synchronously in head and neck cancer. Clin Radiol 1987;38:575.
286. Guthrie TH, Brubaker LH, Porubsky ES, Isaacs JH, Erwin SA, Roberts WH. Circadian cisplatin (C), bleomycin (B) and 5-fluorouracil (F) in advanced squamous cell carcinoma of the head and neck (SCCH) (abstract 689). Proc Am Soc Clin Oncol 1990;9:178.
287. Guthrie TH, Jr., Porubsky ES, Luxenberg MN, Shah KJ, Wurtz KL, Watson PR. Cisplatin-based chemotherapy in advanced basal and squamous cell carcinoma of the skin: results in 28 patients including 13 patients receiving multimodality therapy. J Clin Oncol 1990;8:342.
288. Haas C, Anderson T, Byhardt R, Cox J, Duncavage J, Grossman T, Haas J, Libnoch J, Malin T, Ritch P, Toohill R. Randomized neo-adjuvant study of 5-fluorouracil (FU) and *cis*-platinum (DDP) for patients (PTS) with advanced resectable head and neck squamous carcinoma (ARHSC) (abstract 735). Proc Am Assoc Cancer Res 1986;27:185.
289. Haas JS, Cox JD. Cervical nodal metastasis from an unknown primary carcinoma. In Radiation Therapy of Head and Neck Cancer. Edited by GE Laramore. Berlin: Springer-Verlag, 1988.
290. Haffty B, Papac R, Son Y, et al. Mitomycin C (MC) with dicoumarol (D) as an adjuvant to radiation therapy (RT) in squamous cell carcinoma (SCC) of the head & Neck: Results of a randomized clinical trial (abstract 884). Proc Am Soc Clin Oncol 1995;14:304.
291. Haines I, Bosl G, Pfister D, Spiro R, Gerold F, Sessions R, Shah J, Strong E, Vikram B, Harrison L. Very-high-dose cisplatin with bleomycin infusion as initial treatment of advanced head and neck cancer. J Clin Oncol 1987;5:1594.
292. Hall EJ. Radiobiology for the Radiologist, 3rd ed. Hagerstown, MD: Harper & Row 1988.
293. Harrison DFN. Surgical management of hypopharyngeal cancer. Arch Otolaryngol Head Neck Surg 1979;105:149.
294. Harrison L, Bosl G, Fass D, Armstrong J, Pfister DG, Motzer R, Weisen S, Teeple C, Sessions R, Shah J, Spiro R, Strong E. A new chemo-radiation program for advanced, unresectable head and neck cancer. Presented at Third International Head and Neck Oncology Research Conference, Las Vegas, 1990.
295. Harrold CC. Management of cancer of the floor of mouth. Am J Surg 1971;122:487.
296. Hartenstein R, Wendt TG, Kastenbauer ER. 5-Fluorouracil/folinic acid/cisplatin-combination and accelerated split-course radiotherapy in advanced head and neck cancer. Adv Exp Med Biol 1988;244:275.
297. Harwood AR, Beale FA, Cummings BJ, Keane TJ, Payne DG, Rider WD, Rawlinson E, Elhakim T. Supraglottic laryngeal carcinoma: An analysis of dose-time-volume factors in 410 patients. Int J Radiat Oncol Biol Phys 1983;9:311.
298. Harwood AR, Bryce DP, Rider WD. Management of T3 glottic cancer. Arch Otolaryngol 1980;106:697.
299. Harwood AR, DeBoer G. Prognostic factors in T2 glottic cancer. Cancer 1980;45:991.
300. Harwood AR, Hawkins NV, Keane T, Cummings B, Beale FA, Rider WD, Bryce DP. Radiotherapy in early glottic cancer. Laryngoscope. 1980;90:465.
301. Harwood AR, Hawkins NV, Rider WD, Bryce DP. Radiation therapy of early glottic cancer I. Int J Radiat Oncol Biol Phys 1979;5:473.
302. Hasegawa Y, Matsuura H, Fukushima M, et al. A randomized trial of neoadjuvant chemotherapy with cisplatin and 5FU in advanced head and neck cancer (abstract 926). Proc Am Soc Clin Oncol 1994;13:286.
303. Haselow RE, Adams GS, Oken MM. Simultaneous *cis*-platinum (DDP) and radiation therapy (RT) for locally advanced unresectable head and neck cancer (abstract C-780). Proc Am Soc Clin Oncol 1983;2:160.
304. Haselow RE, Warshaw MG, Oken MM. Radiation alone versus radiation with weekly low dose *cis*-platinum in unresectable cancer of the head and neck. In Head and Neck Cancer, vol II. Edited by WE Fee Jr, H Goepfert, ME Johns, EW Strong, PH Ward Jr. Philadelphia: Decker, 1990, pp 279–281.
305. Havlin KA, Kuhn JG, Myers JW, Ozols RF, Mattox DE, Clark GM, von Hoff DD. High-dose cisplatin for locally advanced or metastatic head and neck cancer: a phase II pilot study. Cancer 1989;63:423.
306. Head and Neck Contracts Program: Adjuvant chemotherapy for advanced head and neck squamous carcinoma. Final report of the Head and Neck Contracts ProgrAm Cancer 1987;60:301.
307. Henderson BE, Louie E, SooHoo Jing J, Buell P, Gardner MB. Risk factors associated with nasopharyngeal carcinoma. N Engl J Med 1977;295:1101.
308. Hendrickson FR. Radiation therapy treatment of larynx cancers. Cancer 1985;55:2058.
309. Henriquez I, Martin Algarra S, Bilbao I, Calvo FA. Continuous intra-arterial (ia) infusion of carboplatin (CBDCA) and 5-fluorouracil (5FU) in unresectable locally advanced (stage III–IV) head and neck cancer (abstract 684). Proc Am Soc Clin Oncol 1989;8:176.
310. Heo DS, Whiteside TL, Johnson JT, Chen KN, Barnes EL, Herberman RB. Long term interleukin 2 dependent growth and cytotoxic activity of tumor-infiltrating lymphocytes from human squamous cell carcinomas of the head and neck. Cancer Res 1987;47:6353.
311. Hester TR, McConnel FM, Nahal F, Juriewicz MJ, Brown RG. Reconstruction of the cervical esophagus, hypopharynx and oral cavity using free jejunal transfer. Am J Surg 1980;140:487.
312. Hill BT, Price LA. Long term survival advantage in patients with advanced oropharyngeal squamous cell carcinoma receiving two courses of initial schedule a non-cisplatin containing combination chemotherapy before definitive local therapy (abstract 685). Proc Am Soc Clin Oncol 1990;9:177.
313. Hill BT, Price LA, MacRae K. Importance of primary site in assessing chemotherapy response and 7-year survival data in advanced squamous-cell carcinomas of the head and neck treated with initial combination chemotherapy without cisplatin. J Clin Oncol 1986;4:1340.
314. Hintz BL, Kagan R, Wollin M, Rao AR, Ryoo MC, Nussbaum H, Rowland J. Treatment selection for base of tongue carcinoma. J Surg Oncol 1989;41:165.
315. Hoffmann W, Kley J, Schiller U, et al. Retinoids and interferon-alpha enhance the antiproliferative effect of radiation in cultured human squamous cell carcinoma cell lines (abstract 1683). Proc Am Soc Clin Oncol 1995;14:513.
316. Hollingshead AC, Lee O, Chretien PB, Tarpley JL, Rawls WE, Adam E. Antibodies to herpesvirus nonvirion antigens in squamous carcinomas. Science 1973;182:713.
317. Holoye PY, Byers RM, Gard DA, Goepfert H, Guillamondegui OM, Jesse RH. Combination chemotherapy of head and neck cancer. Cancer 1978;42:1661.
318. Holsti LR, Mattson K, Niiranen A, Standertskiold-Nordenstam CG, Stenman S, Sovijarvi A, Cantell K. Enhancement of radiation effects by alpha interferon in the treatment of small cell carcinoma of the lung. Int J Radiat Oncol Biol Phys 1987;13:1161.
319. Hong WK, Bhutani R, Shapshay SM, Strong MS. Induction chemotherapy in advanced previously untreated squamous cell head and neck cancer with cisplatin and bleomycin. In Cisplatin: Current Status and New Developments. Edited by AW Prestayki, ST Crooke, SK Carter. New York: Academic, 1980, pp 431–444.
320. Hong WK, Bromer R. Chemotherapy in head and neck cancer. Current concepts. N Engl J Med 1983;308:75.
321. Hong WK, Bromer RH, Amato DA, Shapshay S, Vincent M, Vaughan C, Willett B, Katz A, Welch J, Fofonoff S, Strong MS. Patterns of relapse in locally advanced head and neck cancer patients who achieved complete remission after combined modality therapy. Cancer 1985;56:1242.
322. Hong WK, Choksi A, Dimery IW. Sequential induction chemotherapy and radiotherapy for advanced head and neck cancer: potential impact of treatment in advanced laryngeal and nasopharyngeal carcinomas. In Head and Neck Cancer: Proceedings of the International Conference, Volume 2. Toronto: Decker, 1989, pp 282–285.
323. Hong WK, Endicott J, Itri LM, Doos W, Batsakis JG, Bell R, Fofonoff S, Byers R, Atkinson EN, Vaughan C. 13-*cis*-retinoic acid in the treatment of oral leukoplakia. N Engl J Med 1986;315:1501.
324. Hong WK, Lippman SM, Hittelman WN, Lotan R. Retinoid chemoprevention of aerodigestive cancer: basic to clinic. Clin Cancer Res 1995;1:677.
325. Hong WK, Lippman SM, Itri LM, Karp DD, Lee JS, Byers RM, Schantz SP, Kramer AM, Lotan R, Peters LJ, Dimery IW, Brown BW, Goepfert H. Prevention of second primary tumors with isotretinoin in squamous cell carcinoma of the head and neck. N Engl J Med 1990;323:795.
326. Hong WK, Schaefer S, Issell B, Cummings C, Luedke D, Bromer R, Fofonoff S, D'Aoust J, Shapshay S, Welch J, Levin E, Vincent M, Vaughan C, Strong S. A prospective randomized trial of methotrexate versus cisplatin in the treatment of recurrent squamous cell carcinoma of the head and neck. Cancer 1983;52:206.
327. Hong WK, Shapshay SM, Bhutani R, Craft ML, Ucmakli A, Yamaguchi KT, Vaughan CW, Strong MS. Induction chemotherapy in advanced squamous head and neck carcinoma with high-dose *cis*-platinum and bleomycin infusion. Cancer 1979;44:19.
328. Hong WK, Lippman SM, Wolf GT. Recent advances in head and neck cancer—larynx preservation and cancer chemoprevention. The 17th Annual Richard and Hinda Rosenthal Foundation Award Lecture. Cancer Res 1993;53:5113.
329. Horiot JC, LeFur R, N'Guyen T, Chenal C, Schraub S, Alfonsi G, Gardani G. Van Den Bogaert W, Danczak S, Bolla M, Van Glabbeke M, De Pauw M. Hyperfractionation versus conventional fractionation in oropharyngeal carcinoma: final analysis of a randomized trial of the EORTC Cooperative Group of Radiotherapy. Radiother Oncol 1992;25:231.
330. Horiot JC, van den Bogaert W, Ang KK, van der Schueren E, Bartelink H, Gonzales D, de Pauw M, van Glabbeke M. European Organization for Research on Treatment of Cancer trials using radiotherapy with multiple fractions per day: a 1978–1987 survey. Front Radiat Ther Oncol 1988;22:149.
331. Horiuchi M, Inuyama Y, Miyake H. Efficacy of surgical adjuvant with tegarfor and uracil (UFT) in resectable head and neck cancer: a prospective randomized study. Proc Am Soc Clin Oncol 1994;13:284.
332. Hornedo-Muguiro J, So M, Spaulding MB, Van Echo DA, Donehouser R, Ettinger D, Aisner J. Phase II trial of carboplatin (CBDCA) in aerodigestive malignancies (abstract C-530). Proc Am Soc Clin Oncol 1985;4:136.
333. Hoye RC, Herrold KM, Smith R. A clincopathological study of epidermoid carcinoma of the head and neck. Cancer 1962;15:741.
334. Huang AT, Cole TB, Fishburn R, Jelovsek SB. Adjuvant chemotherapy after surgery and radiation for stage III and IV head and neck cancer. Ann Surg 1984;200:195.
335. Huang AT, Fisher SR, Cole TB. A study of postoperative and/or postradiation adjuvant chemotherapy (abstract). Proceedings, second International Head and Neck Oncology Research Conference, Arlington, VA: September 10–13, 1987.
336. Huang SC. Nasopharyngeal cancer. A review of 1605 patients treated radically with cobalt 60. Int J Radiat Oncol Biol Phys 1980;6:401.
337. Huang SC, Lui LT, Lynn TC. Nasopharyngeal cancer: Study III. A review of 1206 patients treated with combined modalities. Int J Radiat Oncol Biol Phys 1985;11:1789.
338. Huber MH, Lippman SM, Benner SE, et al. A phase II study of ifosfamide in recurrent

squamous cell carcinoma of the head and neck. Am J Clin Oncol (in press).

339. Huber MH, Shirinian M, Lippman SM, et al. Phase I/II study of cisplatin, 5-fluorouracil and α-interferon for recurrent carcinoma of the head and neck. Invest New Drugs 1994;12:223–229.
340. Hussey DH, Abrams JP. Combined therapy in advanced head and neck cancer: Hydroxyurea and radiotherapy. Prog Clin Cancer 1975;6:79.
341. Ikic D, Padovan I, Brodarec I, Knezevic M, Soos E. Application of human leucocyte interferon in patients with tumours of the head and neck. Lancet 1981;1:1025.
342. Ildstad ST, Bigelow ME, Remensnyder JP. Squamous cell carcinoma of the tongue: A comparison of the anterior two thirds of the tongue with its base. Am J Surg 1983;146:456.
343. Isaacs JH, Mooney S, Mendenhall WM, Parsons JT. Cancer of the maxillary sinus treated with surgery and/or radiation therapy. Am Surg 1990;56:327.
344. Ishikawa T, Ikawa T, Eura M, Fukiage T, Masuyama K. Adoptive immunotherapy for head and neck cancer with killer cells induced by stimulation with autologous or allogeneic tumour cells and recombinant interleukin-2. Acta Otolaryngol 1989;107:346.
345. Issa PY. Cancer of the supraglottic larynx treated by radiotherapy exclusively. Int J Radiat Oncol Biol Phys 1985;15:843.
346. Jacobs C. Adjuvant chemotherapy for head and neck cancer. J Clin Oncol 1989;7:823.
347. Jacobs C, Bertino JR, Goffinet DR, Fu WE, Good RL. 24-Hour infusion of *cis*-platinum in head and neck cancers. Cancer 1978;42:2135.
348. Jacobs C, Goffinet DR, Goffinet L, Kohler M, Fee WE. Chemotherapy as a substitute for surgery in the treatment of advanced resectable head and neck cancer: A report from the Northern California Oncology Group. Cancer 1987;60:1178.
349. Jacobs C, Lyman G, Velez-Garcia E, Sridhar KS, Knight W, Hochster H, Goodnough LT, Mortimer JE, Einhorn LH, Schacter L, Cherng N, Dalton T, Burroughs J, Rozencweig M. A phase III randomized study comparing cisplatin and fluorouracil as single agents and in combination for advanced squamous cell carcinoma of the head and neck. J Clin Oncol 1992;10:257.
350. Jacobs C, Makuch R. Efficacy of adjuvant chemotherapy for patients with resectable head and neck cancer: a subset analysis of the Head and Neck Contracts Program. J Clin Oncol 1990;8:838.
351. Jacobs C, Meyers F, Hendrickson C, Kohler M, Carter S. A randomized phase III study of cisplatin with or without methotrexate for recurrent squamous cell carcinoma of the head and neck. A Northern California Oncology Group study. Cancer 1983;52:1563.
352. Jacobs JR, Pajak TF, Al-Sarraf M, Kinzie J, Stetz J, Davis LW, Leibel S, Laramore GE. Chemotherapy following surgery for head and neck cancer. A Radiation Therapy Oncology Group study. Am J Clin Oncol 1989;12:185.
353. Jacobs JR, Sessions DG, Ogura JH. Recurrent carcinoma of the larynx and the hypopharynx. Otolaryngol Head Neck Surg 1980;88:425.
354. Jakobsson PA, Eneroth DM, Killander D, Moberger G, Martensson B. Histologic classification and grading of malignancy in carcinoma of the larynx. Acta Radiol Ther Phys Biol 1973;12:1.
355. Jaulerry C, Rodriquez J, Brunin F, Jouve M, Mosseri V, Point D, Pontvert D, Validire P, Zafrani B, Blaszka B, Asselain B, Pouillact P, Brugere J. Induction chemotherapy in advanced head and neck tumors: Results of two randomized trials. Int J Radiat Oncol Biol Phys 1992;23:483.
356. Jesse RH. Radiation in the treatment of squamous carcinoma of paranasal sinus. Am J Surg 1965;110:552.
357. Jesse RH. Extensive cancer of the lip. Surgical therapy. Arch Surg 1967;94:509.
358. Johns ME, Goldsmith MM. Incidence, diagnosis, and classification of salivary gland tumors. Oncology 1989;3:47.
359. Johns ME, Kaplan MJ. Malignant neoplasms. In Otolaryngology Head and Neck Surgery, vol. II. Edited by CW Cummings, JM Fredreickson, LA Harker, CJ Krause, DE Schuller. St. Louis: Mosby, 1986, p 1049.
360. Johnson JT, Myers EN, Bedetti CD, Barnes EL, Schramm VL Jr, Thearle PB. Cervical lymph node metastases. Incidence and implications of extracapsular carcinoma. Arch Otolaryngol 1985;111:534.
361. Johnson JT, Ferretti GA, Nethery WJ, Valdez IH, Fox PC, Ng, D., Muscoplat CC, Gallagher SC. Oral pilocarpine for post-irradiation xerostomia in patients with head and neck cancer. N Engl J Med 1993;329:390.
362. Jorgensen K, Elbrond O, Anderson AP. Carcinoma of the lip. A series of 869 cases. Acta Radiol Ther Phys Biol 1973;12:177.
363. Kabat GC, Wynder EL. Type of alcoholic beverage and oral cancer. Int J Cancer 1989;43:190.
364. Kalnins IK, Leonard AG, Sako K, Razack MS, Shedd DP. Correlation between prognosis and degree of lymph node involvement in carcinoma of the oral cavity. Am J Surg 1977;134:540.
365. Kamioner D, Haddad,E., Dana M, Coscas Y, Vuillemin E, Daoui S. Carboplatin-radiotherapy versus cisplatin-radiotherapy according to a concurrent schedule in advanced head and neck cancer: Preliminary results of a randomized study (abstract 606). Ann Oncol 1992;3(5):158.
366. Kaplan BH, Schoenfeld D, Vogl SE. Treatment of recurrent (REC) or metastatic (MET) squamous cancer of the head and neck (SCH&N) with methotrexate (M), M plus *Corynebacterium parvum* (CP) or M plus bleomycin (B) plus diamminedichloroplatinum (D): a prospective randomized trial of the Eastern Cooperative Oncology Group (abstract C-780). Proc Am Assoc Cancer Res 1981;22:532.
367. Kaplan MJ, Johns ME, Clark DA, Cantrell RW. Glottic carcinoma: The role of surgery and irradiation. Cancer 1984;53:2641.
368. Kapstad B, Bang G, Rennaes S, Dahler A. Combined preoperative treatment with cobalt and bleomycin in patients with head and neck carcinoma: A controlled clinical study. Int J Radiat Oncol Biol Phys 1978;4:85.
369. Karim ABMF, Snow GB, Hasman A, Chang SC, Kelhotz A, Hoekstra F. Dose response in radiotherapy for glottic carcinoma. Cancer 1978;41:1728.
370. Karim AB, Snow GB, Siek HT, Njo KH. The quality of voice in patient irradiated for laryngeal carcinoma. Cancer 1983;51:47.
371. Karp D, Vaughan C, Carter R, Willett B, Heeren T, Calarese P, Zeitels S, Strong MS, Hong W. Voice preservation using induction chemotherapy (CT) plus radiation therapy (RT) as an alternative to laryngectomy in advanced head and neck cancer: Long term follow up. Am J Clin Oncol 1991;14:273.
372. Katz AE. Immunobiologic staging of patients with carcinoma of the head and neck. Laryngoscope 1983;93:445.
373. Katz DE, Seder RH, Keggins JJ. Plasmapheresis in patients with advanced carcinoma of the head and neck. In Head and Neck Oncology Research. Edited by GT Wolf, TE Carey. Amsterdam: Kugler & Ghedini, 1988, pp 151–157.
374. Kazem I, van den Broek P. Planned preoperative radiation therapy vs definitive radiotherapy for advanced laryngeal carcinoma. Laryngoscope 1984;94:1355.
375. Keane TJ, Harwood AR, Beale FA, Cummings BJ, Payne DG, Elhakim T, Rawlingson E. A pilot study of mitomycin-C/5-fluorouracil infusion combined with split course radiation therapy for carcinomas of the larynx and hypopharynx. J Otolaryngol 1986;15:286.
376. Keane TJ, Harwood AR, Danjoux C. Results of a randomized trial of radiation compared to radiation and chemotherapy for advanced laryngeal and hypopharyngeal squamous carcinoma (abstract 55). Proceedings second International Conference on Head and Neck Cancer, Boston: July 31–August, 5, 1988.
377. Keegan P, Pillsbury HC, Weissler M, Rosenman J, Varia M, Tepper J. Hyperfractionated radiotherapy with or without simultaneous cisplatin and fluorouracil (5-FU) in the treatment of advanced head and neck cancer (abstract 667). Proc Am Soc Clin Oncol 1990;9:172.
378. Keim WF, Shapiro MJ, Rosin HD. Study of post laryngectomy stomal recurrence. Arch Otolaryngol 1965;81:183.
379. Kelly MD, Hahn SS, Spaulding CA, Kersh CR, Constable WC, Cantrell RW. Definitive radiotherapy in the management of stage I and II carcinomas of the glottis. Laryngoscope 1989;98:235.
380. Kerpel-Fronius S, Mechl Z, Csetenyi J, Nagykalnai T, Gyergyay F, Jassem J, Vuletic L, Kolaric K, Eckhardt S. Pharmacokinetic and response rate of 5-fluorouracil (5-FU) given in daily 4 H infusion combined with cisplatin (CDDP) in head and neck cancer (H&N CA): phase I-II. A South-East European Oncology Group (SEEOG) study (abstract 581). Proc Am Soc Clin Oncol 1988;8:150.
381. Khojasteh A, Reynolds R, Ruble K, Garcia A, Coleman J, Gohel M. A phase III, comparison of sequence-dependent schedules of cisplatin (DDP) and 5-fluorouracil (5FU) in carcinoma of head and neck (H&N Ca). An up date report (abstract 611). Proc Am Soc Clin Oncol 1988;8:158.
382. Khoury GG, Paterson IC. Nasopharyngeal carcinoma. A review of cases treated by radiotherapy and chemotherapy. Clin Radiol 1987;38:17.
383. Kies M, Haraf D, Mick R, et al. Cisplatin, 5FU, leucovorin, and interferon α-2B (PFL-α) followed by concurrent 5FU-hydroxyurea (HU) and radiation (FHX) for stage IV squamous cell cancer of the head and neck (abstract 913). Proc Am Soc Clin Oncol 1994;13:283.
384. Kirchner JA. Two hundred laryngeal cancers: Patterns of growth and spread as seen in serial sections. Laryngoscope 1977;87:474.
385. Kirchner JA, Cornog JL, Holmes RE. Transglottic cancer Its growth and spread within the larynx. Arch Otolaryngol 1974;99:247.
386. Kirchner JA, Som ML. Clinical and histologic observation on supraglottic cancer. Ann Otol Rhinol Laryngol 1971;80:638.
387. Kirkwood JM, Miller D, Weichselbaum R, Pitman S. Predefinitive and postdefinitive chemotherapy for locally advanced squamous cell carcinoma of the head and neck. Laryngoscope 1979;89:573.
388. Kish JA, Ensley JF, Jacobs JR, Binns P, Al Sarraf M. Evaluation of high-dose cisplatin and 5-FU infusion as initial therapy in advanced head and neck cancer. Am J Clin Oncol 1988;11:553.
389. Kish JA, Ensley JF, Jacobs J, Weaver A, Cummings G, Al Sarraf M. A randomized trial of cisplatin (CACP) + 5-fluorouracil (5-FU) infusion and CACP + 5-FU bolus for recurrent and advanced squamous cell carcinoma of the head and neck. Cancer 1985;56:2740.
390. Kish JA, Weaver A, Jacobs J, Cummings G, Al Sarraf M. Cisplatin and 5-fluorouracil infusion in patients with recurrent and disseminated epidermoid cancer of the head and neck. Cancer 1984;53:1819.
391. Knowlton AH, Percarpio B, Bobrow S, Fischer JJ. Methotrexate and radiation therapy in the treatment of advanced head and neck tumors. Radiology 1975;116:709.
392. Kokal WA, Gardive RL, Sheibani K, Zak IW, Beatty JD, Riihimaki DU, Wagman LD, Terz JJ. Tumor DNA content as a prognostic indication in squamous cell carcinoma of the head and neck region. Am J Surg 1988;156:276.
393. Komiyara S, Matsui K, Kudoh S, Nogae I, Kuratoma Y, Saburi Y, Asoh K, Kohno K, Kuwano M. Establishment of tumor cell lines from a patient with head and neck cancer and their different sensitivities to anti-cancer agents. Cancer 1989;63:675.
394. Kotwall C, Sako K, Razack MS, Rao U, Bakamjian V, Shedd DP. Metastatic patterns in squamous cell cancer of the head and neck. Am J Surg 1987;154:439.
395. Kramer S. Methotrexate and radiation therapy in the treatment of advanced squamous cell carcinoma of the oral cavity, oropharynx, supraglottic larynx, and hypopharynx: (Preliminary report of a controlled clinical trial of the Radiation Therapy Oncology Group). Can J Otolaryngol 1975;4:213.
396. Kramer S, Gleber RD, Snow JB, Marcial VA, Lowry LD, Davis LW, Chandler R. Combined radiation therapy and surgery in the management of advanced head and neck cancer: Final report of the study 73–03 of the Radiation Therapy Oncology Group. Head Neck Surg 1987;10:19.
397. Kuebler JP, Benedetti J, Schuller DE, et al. Phase II study of edatrexate in advanced head and neck cancer. Invest New Drugs 1994;12:341–344.
398. Kun LE, Toohill RJ, Holoye PY, Duncavage JA, Byhardt RW, Ritch PS, Grossman TW, Hoffmann RG, Cox JD, Malin T. A randomized study of adjuvant chemotherapy for cancer of the upper aerodigestive tract. Int J Radiat Oncol Biol Phys 1986;12:173.
399. Laccourreye H, Brasnu DF, Beutter P. Carcinoma of the laryngeal margin. Head Neck Surg 1983;5:500.
400. Lampe I, Zatzkin H. Pulmonary metastases of pseudoadenomatous basal cell carcinoma (mucous and salivary gland tumor). Radiology 1949;53:379.
401. Laramore GE. Radiation Therapy of Head and Neck Cancer. Berlin: Springer-Verlag, 1988.
402. Laramore GE. T3NOMO glottic cancer: Are more treatment modalities necessarily better? Int J Radiat Oncol Biol Phys 1995;31:423.
403. Laramore GE, Clubb B, Quick C, Amer MH, Ali M, Greer W, Mahboubi E, El-Senoussi M, Schultz H, El-Akkad SM. Nasopharyngeal carcinoma in Saudi Arabia: A retrospective study of 166 cases treated with curative intent. Int J Radiat Oncol Biol Phys 1988;15:1119.
404. Laramore GE, Krall JM, Griffin TW, Duncan W. Richter MP, Saroja KR, Maor MH, Davis LW. Neutron versus photon irradiation for unresectable salivary gland tumors: Final

report of an RTOG-MRC randomized clinical trial. Int J Radiat Oncol Biol Phys 1993;27:235.
405. Laramore GE, Scott CB, al-Sarraf M, Haselow RE, Ervin TJ, Wheeler R, Jacobs JR, Schuller DE, Gahbauer RA, Schwade JG, Campbell BH. Adjuvant chemotherapy for resectable squamous cell carcinomas of the head and neck: Report on Intergroup Study 0034. Int J Radiat Oncol Biol Phys 1992;23:705.
406. Laramore GE, Scott CB, Schuller DE, Haselow RE, Ervin TJ, Wheeler R, Al-Sarraf M, Gahbauer RA, Jacobs JR, Schwade JG, Campbell BH. Is a surgical resection leaving positive margins of benefit to the patient with locally advanced squamous cell carcinoma of the head and neck? A comparative study using the Intergroup Study 0034 and the Radiation Therapy Oncology Group database. Int J Radiat Oncol Biol Phys 1993;27:1011.
407. Lee G, Pitman SW, Bertino JR. Weekly hydroxyurea in squamous head and neck cancer (abstract C-572). Proc Am Soc Clin Oncol 1985;4:147.
408. Lee JG, Krause CJ. Radical neck dissection: elective, therapeutic and secondary. Arch Otolaryngol 1975;101:656.
409. Lee JS, Kim SY, Hong WK, Lippman SM, et al. Detection of chromosomal polysomy in oral leukoplakia, a premalignant lesion. JNCI 1993;85:1951.
410. Lee NK, Goepfert H, Wendt CD. Supraglottic laryngectomy for intermediate-stage cancer: UT MD Anderson Cancer Center experience with combined therapy. Laryngoscope 1990;100:831.
411. Lefebvre JL, Chevalier D, Luboinski B, Kirkpatrick A, Collette L, Sahmoud T. Larynx preservation in pyriform sinus cancer: preliminary results of an EORTC Phase III trial. J Natl Cancer Inst (in press).
412. Lehmann OA, Santos RL, Batagelj E, et al. Cisplatin and fluorouracil vs cisplatin, fluorouracil and leucovorin in advanced head and neck cancer (abstract 927). Proc Am Soc Clin Oncol 1994;13:286.
413. Leipzig B, Cummings CW, Chung CT, Johnson JT, Sagerman RH. Carcinoma of the anterior tongue. Ann Otol Rhinol Laryngol 1982;91:94.
414. Leonard JR, Litton WB, Latourette HB, McCube BF. Combined radiation and surgical therapy: Tongue, tonsil and floor of mouth. Ann Otol Rhinol Laryngol 1968;77:514.
415. Leone LA, Albala MM, Rege VB. Treatment of carcinoma of the head and neck with intravenous methotrexate. Cancer 1968;21:828.
416. Leroux RJ. A statistical study of 620 laryngeal carcinomas of the glottic region personally operated upon more than 5 years ago. Laryngoscope 1985;85:1440.
417. Lester EP, Tharapel SA. Chromosome abnormalities in squamous carcinoma cell lines of head and neck origin. Presented at Third International Head and Neck Oncology Research Conference, Las Vegas, 1990.
418. Levendag P, Sessions R, Vikran B, Strong EW, Shah JP, Spiro R, Gerold F. The problem of neck relapse in early stage supraglottic larynx cancer. Cancer 1989;63:345.
419. Levine PA, Frierson HF, Stewart FM, Mills SE, Fechner RE, Cantrell RW. A distinctive and highly aggressive neoplasm. Laryngoscope 1987;97:905.
420. Levitt M, Mosher MB, DeConti RC, Farber LR, Skeel RT, Marsh JC, Mitchell MS, Papac RJ, Thomas ED, Bertino JR. Improved therapeutic index of methotrexate with "leucovorin rescue." Cancer Res 1973;33:1729.
421. Leyvraz S, Pasche P, Bauer J, Bernasconi S, Monnier P. Rapidly alternating chemotherapy and hyperfractionated radiotherapy in the management of locally advanced head and neck carcinoma: Four-year results of a phase I/II study. J Clin Oncol 1994;12:1876–1885.
422. Licitra L, Marchini S, Spinazze S, De Braud F, Rossi A, Salvatori P, Bonadonna G. Phase II study with cisplatin (DDP) for advanced carcinoma of salivary gland origin (abstract 584). Proc Amer Soc Clin Oncol 1988;8:151.
423. Lindberg RD, Barkley HT, Jesse RH, Fletcher GH. Evolution of the clinically negative neck in patients with squamous cell carcinoma of the faucial Arch Am J Roentgenol 1971;111:60.
424. Lippman SM, Batasakis JF, Toth BB, Weber RS, Lee JJ, Martin JW, Hays GL, Goepfert H, Hong WK. Comparison of low-dose isotretinoin with beta carotene to prevent oral carcinogenesis. N Engl J Med 1993;328:15.
425. Lippman SM, Benner SE, Hong WK. Cancer chemoprevention. J Clin Oncol 1994;12: 851–73.
426. Lippman SM, Benner SE, Hong WK. The chemoprevention of cancer. In Cancer Prevention and Control. Edited by P Greenwald, RS Kramer, DL Weed. New York: Marcel Dekker, 1995, pp 329–352.
427. Lippman SM, Hong WK. Retinoid chemoprevention of upper aerodigestive tract carcinogenesis. In Important Advances in Oncology. Edited by VT DeVita, S Hellman, SA Rosenberg. Philadelphia: Lippincott, 1992, pp 93–109.
428. Lippman SM, Shin DM, Lee JJ, Batsakis JG, Lotan R, Tainsky MA, Hittelman WN, Hong WK. p53 and retinoid chemoprevention of oral carcinogenesis. Cancer Res 1995;55:16–19.
429. Lippman SM, Kessler JF, Al-Sarraf M, Alberts DS, Itri LM, Mattox D, Von Hoff DD, Loescher L, Meyskens FL. Treatment of advanced squamous cell carcinoma of the head and neck with isotretinoin: a phase II randomized trial. Invest New Drugs 1988;6:51.
430. Lippman SM, Hong WK. Chemotherapy and chemoprevention. In Cancer of the Head and Neck, 3rd ed. Edited by E Myers, JY Suen. Philadelphia: Saunders, 1995.
431. Lippman SM, Lee JS, Lotan R, Hittelman W, Wargovich MJ, Hong WK. Biomarkers as intermediate endpoints in chemoprevention trials. JNCI 1990;82:555.
432. Lippman SM, Meyskens FL. Treatment of advanced squamous cell carcinoma of the skin with isotretinoin. Ann Intern Med 1987;107:499.
433. Lippman SM, Parkinson DR, Itri LM, Weber RS, Schantz SP, Ota DM, Schusterman MA, Krakoff IH, Gutterman JU, Hong WK. 13-*cis*-retinoic acid and interferon α-2a Effective combination therapy for advanced squamous cell carcinoma of the skin. JNCI 1992;84:235.
434. Lippman SM, Spitz MR, Trizna Z, et al. Epidemiology, biology and chemoprevention of aerodigestive cancer. Cancer 1994;74:2719–2725.
435. Liu TJ, El-Naggar AK, McDonnell TJ, Steck KD, Wang M, Taylor DL, Clayman GC. Apoptosis induction mediated by wild-type p53 adenovirus gene transfer in squamous cell carcinoma of the head and neck. Cancer Res 1995;55:3117–3122.
436. Liverpool Head and Neck Oncology Group. A phase II randomized trial of cisplatinum, methotrexate, cisplatinum + methotrexate and cisplatinum + 5-FU in end stage squamous cell carcinoma of the head and neck. Liverpool Head and Neck Oncology Group. Br J Cancer 1990;61:311.
437. Lo TC, Wiley AL Jr, Ansfield FJ, Brandenburg JH, Davis ML Jr, Gollin FF, Johnson RO, Ramirez G, Vermund H. Combined radiation therapy and 5-fluorouracil for advanced squamous cell carcinoma of the oral cavity and oropharynx: A randomized study. Am J Roentgenol 1976;126:229.
438. Loning T, Ikenberg H, Becker J, Gissman L, Hoepfer I, zur Hausen M. Analysis of oral papillomas, leukoplakias, and invasive carcinomas of human papillomavirus type related DNA. J Invest Dermatol 1985;84:417.
439. LoRusso P, Tapazoglou E, Kish JA, Ensley JF, Cummings G, Kelly J, Al-Sarraf M. Chemotherapy for paranasal sinus carcinoma. A 10-year experience at Wayne State University. Cancer 1988;62:1.
440. Lotan R, Xu C, Lippman SM, et al. Suppression of retinoic acid receptor β in oral premalignant lesions and its upregulation by isotretinoin. N Engl J Med 1995;332: 1405–1410.
441. Lund VJ, Howard DJ. Head and neck cancer in the young: a prognostic conundrum? J Laryngol Otol 1990;104:544.
442. Lustig RA, DeMare PA, Kramer S. Adjuvant methotrexate in the radio-therapeutic management of advanced tumors of the head and neck. Cancer 1976;37:2703.
443. Lutz CK, Johnson JT, Wagner RL, Myer EN. Supraglottic carcinoma Patterns of recurrence. Ann Otol Rhinol Laryngol 1990;99:12.
444. MacComb WS, Fletcher GH. Cancer of the Head and Neck. Baltimore: Williams & Wilkins, 1967.
445. Maceri DR, Laupe HB, Makielski KH, Passamani PP, Krause CJ. Conservation laryngeal surgery. A critical analysis. Arch Otolaryngol 1985;111:361.
446. Mackay EN, Sellers AH. A statistical review of carcinoma of the lip. Can Med Assoc J 1964;90:670.
447. Magno L, Terraneo F, Bertino F, Tordiglione M, Bardelli D, Rosignoli MT, Ciottoli GB. Double-blind randomized study of lonidamine and radiotherapy in head and neck cancer. Int J Radiat Oncol Biol Phys 1994;29:45–55.
448. Mainpang T, Razack MS, Sako K, Chen TY. Surgical salvage for recurrent "early" glottic cancers. J Surg Oncol 1989;40:32.
449. Marcial VA, Pajak TF, Chang C, Tupchong L, Stetz J. Hyperfractionated photon radiation therapy in the treatment of advanced squamous cell carcinoma of the oral cavity, pharynx, larynx, and sinuses, using radiation therapy as the only planned modality: (Preliminary report) by the Radiation Therapy Oncology Group (RTOG). Int J Radiat Oncol Biol Phys 1987;13:41.
450. Marcial VA, Pajak TF, Mohiuddin M, Cooper J S. Al Sarraf M, Mowry PA, Curran W, Crissman J, Rodriguez M, Velez-Garcia E. Concomitant cisplatin chemotherapy and radiotherapy in advanced mucosal squamous cell carcinoma of the head and neck. Cancer 1990;66:1861.
451. Marechal F, Nasca S, Morel M, Jezekova D, Coninx P, Legros M, Nguyen TD, Cattan A. A phase III of cisplatinum versus cisplatinum-etoposide for previously untreated squamous cell carcinoma of the head and neck. Anticancer Res 1987;7:455.
452. Margolin K, Doroshow J, Leong L, Akman S, Carr BI, Odujinrin O, Flanagin B. Combination chemotherapy with cytosine arabinoside (Ara-C) and *cis*-diamminedichloroplatinum (CDDP) for squamous cancers of the upper aerodigestive tract. Am J Clin Oncol 1989;12(6):494.
453. Marks JE, Breaux S, Smith PG, Thawley SE, Spector GG, Sessions DG. The need for elective irradiation of occult lymphatic metastases from cancer of the larynx and piriform sinus. Head Neck Surg 1985;8:3.
454. Marks JE, Freeman RB, Lee F, Ogua JH. Carcinoma of the supraglottic larynx. Am J Roentgenol 1979;132:255.
455. Martin M, Gehanno P, Depondt J, et al. A phase III study: Induction carboplatin and 5-fluorouracil before locoregional treatment versus locoregional treatment alone in head and neck carcinomas. Proc Am Soc Clin Oncol 1994;13:281.
456. Martin M, Hazan A, Vergnes L, Peytral C, Lelievre G, Senechaut JP, Mazeron JP, Peynegre R. Randomized study of 5 fluorouracil (5.F.U.) and *cis* platinum (D.D.P) as neoadjuvant therapy in head and neck cancer. A preliminary report (abstract 680). Proc Am Soc Clin Oncol 1989;8:175.
457. Martin M, Lelievre G, Gehanno P, Depondt J, Guerrier B, Peytral C, Hazan A, Dubreuil P, Margotton A, Pellae-Cosser B. Induction carboplatin (CBDCA) and 5 fluorouracil (5FU) treatment versus no chemotherapy before locoregional treatment for oro and pharyngolaryngeal cancers: preliminary results of a randomized study. Proc Am Soc Clin Oncol 1992:11.
458. Martin H, MacComb WS, Blady JV. Cancer of the lip. Ann Surg 1941;114:226.
459. Martin M, Malaurie E, Langlet PM, et al. A randomized prospective study of CDDP and 5FU as neoadjuvant chemotherapy in head and neck cancer: a final report. Proc Am Soc Clin Oncol 1995;14:294.
460. Martin M, Mazeron JJ, Brun B, Vergnes L, Lelievre G, Feuillade F, Juvanon JM, Haddad E, Delacour IS, Peynegre R, Pierquin B. Neo-adjuvant polychemotherapy of head and neck cancer: results of a randomized study (abstract 590). Proc Am Soc Clin Oncol 1988;7:152.
461. Martin SA, Marks JE, Lee JY, Bauer WC, Ogura JH. Carcinoma of the pyriform sinus: predictors of TNM relapse and survival. Cancer 1980;46:1974.
462. Marwood AR, Krajbich JI, Fornasier VL. Radiotherapy of chondrosarcoma of bone. Cancer 1980;45:2769.
463. Mauer HM, Beltangady M, Gehan EA, Christ W, Hammond D, Hays DM, Heyn R, Lawrence W, Newton W, Ortega J. The intergroup rhabdomyosarcoma study—I: a final report. Cancer 1985;61:209.
464. McCoy GD, Hecht SS, Wynder EL. The roles of tobacco, alcohol, and diet in the etiology of upper alimentary and respiratory tract cancers. Prev Med 1980;9:622.
465. McGovern MH, Bauer WC, Ogura JH. The incidence of cervical lymph node metastases from epidermoid carcinoma of the larynx and their relationship to certain characteristics of the primary tumor. Cancer 1961;14:55.
466. McLaughlin JK, Gridley G, Block G, Winn DM, Preston-Martin S, Schoenberg JB, Greenberg RS, Stemhagen A, Austin DF, Ershow AG. Dietary factors in oral and pharyngeal cancer. JNCI 1988;80:1237.
467. McNeese MD, Fletcher GH. Tumors of the major and minor salivary glands. In Radiation Therapy of Head and Neck Cancer. Edited by GE Laramore. Berlin: Springer-Verlag, 1988.
468. McNeil BJ, Weichselbaum R, Parker SG. Speech and survival: Tradeoffs between quality and quantity of life in laryngeal cancer. N Engl J Med 1981;305:982.
469. Medenica RN, Slack N. Clinical results of leukocyte interferon-induced tumor regression in resistant human metastatic cancer resistent to chemotherapy and/or radiotherapy-pulse therapy schedule. Cancer Drug Deliv 1985;2:53.
470. Mehregan DA, Roenigk RK. Management of superficial squamous cell carcinoma of

the lip with Mohs micrographic surgery. Cancer 1990;66:463.

471. Mendenhall WM, Parsons JT, Stringer SP, Cassisi NJ, Million RR. Carcinoma of the supraglottic larynx: A basis for comparing the results of radiotherapy and surgery. Head Neck 1990;12:204.
472. Mendenhall WM, VanCise WS, Bova FJ, Million RR. Analysis of time-dose factors in squamous cell carcinoma of the oral tongue and floor of mouth treated with radiation therapy alone. Int J Radiol Oncol Biol Phys 1981;7:1005.
473. Meoz RT, Fletcher GH, Peters LJ, Barkley HT, Thames HD. Twice daily fractionation schemes for advanced head and neck cancer. Int J Radiat Oncol Biol Phys 1984;10:831.
474. Merlano M, Conte PF, Tatarek R, Scarsi P, Barbieri A, Benedetti G, Rosso R. Ineffectiveness of 5-fluorouracil and cisplatin as a second line chemotherapy in head and neck cancer. Tumori 1984;70:267.
475. Merlano M, Vitale V, Rosso R, Benasso M, Corvo R, Cavallari M, Sanguineti G, Bacigalupo F, Margarino G, Brema F, Pastorino G, Marziano C, Grimaldi A, Scasso F, Sperati G, Pallestrini E, Garaventa G, Accomando E, Cordone G, Comella G, Daponte A, Rubagotti A, Bruzzi P, Santi L. Treatment of advanced squamous-cell carcinoma of the head and neck with alternating chemotherapy and radiotherapy. N Engl J Med 1992;327:1115.
476. Merlano M, Carvé R, Margarino G, et al. Combined chemotherapy and radiation therapy in advanced inoperable squamous cell carcinoma of the head and neck: The final report of a randomized trial. Cancer 1991;67:915–921.
477. Merlano M, Tatarek R, Grimaldi A, Margarino G, Rosso R. Phase I–II trial with cisplatin and 5-FU in recurrent head and neck cancer: An effective outpatient schedule. Cancer Treat Rep 1985;69:961.
478. Michalides R, van Veelen N, Hart A, Loftus B, Wientjens E, Balm A. Overexpression of cyclin D1 correlates with recurrence in a group of forty-seven operable squamous cell carcinomas of the head and neck. Cancer Res 1995;55(5):975–978.
479. Miller B, Yu A, Tefft M, Leone L. Improved response rate in patients with advanced unresectable cancer of the head and neck (abstract C-552). Proc Am Soc Clin Oncol 1985;4:142.
480. Million RR, Cassisi NJ. Radical irradiation for carcinoma of the pyriform sinus. Laryngoscope 1981;91:439.
481. Million RR, Cassisi NJ, Wittes RE. Cancer in the head and neck. In Cancer—Principles and Practice of Oncology. Edited by VT Devita, S Hellman, SA Rosenberg. Philadelphia: Lippincott, 1982 pp 301–395.
482. Million RR, Parsons JT, Cassisi NJ. Twice a day irradiation technique for squamous cell carcinoma of the head and neck. Cancer 1985;55:2096.
483. Mills EE. The modifying effect of beta-carotene on radiation and chemotherapy induced oral mucositis. Br J Cancer 1988;57:416.
484. Mirimanoff RO, Wang CC, Doppke KP. Combined surgery and postoperative radiotherapy for advanced laryngeal and hypopharyngeal tumors. Int J Radiat Oncol Biol Phys 1985;11:499.
485. Mittal B, Marks JE, Ogura JH. Transglottic carcinoma. Cancer 1984;53:151.
486. Miyake H, Horiuchi M, Togawa K, Kawamoto K, Kaneko T, Iruyama Y, Hondo Y, Baba S, Matsunaga T, Ishikawa T. Recombinant interferon alpha 2 (sch 30500) in patients with head and neck cancer. Gan To Kagaku Ryoho 1985;12:1651.
487. Mizono GS, Diaz RF, Fu KK, Boles R. Carcinoma of the tonsillar region. Laryngoscope 1986;96:240.
488. Molnar L, Ronay P, Tapolcsanyi L. Carcinoma of the lip: analysis of the material of 25 years. Oncology 1974;29:101.
489. Moore C, Catlin D. Anatomic origins and locations of oral cancer. Am J Surg 1967;114:510.
490. Morita K. Clinical significance of radiation therapy combined with chemotherapy. Strahlentherapie 1980;156:228.
491. Mortimer JE, Taylor ME, Schulman S, Cummings C, Weymuller E Jr, Laramore G. Feasibility and efficacy of weekly intraarterial cisplatin in locally advanced (stage III and IV) head and neck cancers. J Clin Oncol 1988;6:969.
492. Morton RP, Rugman F, Dorman EB, Stoney PJ, Wilson JA, McCormick M, Veevers A, Stell PM. Cisplatinum and bleomycin in the treatment of advanced or recurrent squamous cell carcinoma of the head and neck: a randomized factorial phase III controlled trial. Sonderb-Strahlenther Oncol 1987;81:141.
493. Moseley HS, Thomas LR, Everts EC, Stevens KR, Ireland KM. Advanced squamous cell carcinoma of the maxillary sinus: results of combined regional infusion chemotherapy, radiation therapy and surgery. Am J Surg 1981;141:522.
494. Mossman KL. Quantitative radiation dose response relationships for normal tissues in man. II. Response of the salivary glands during radiotherapy. Radiat Res 1983;95:392.
495. Mossman KL, Chencharick JD, Scheer AC, Walker WP, Ornitz RD, Rogers CC, Hendin RI. Radiation induced changes in gustatory function: comparison of effects of neutron and photon irradiation. Int J Radiat Oncol Biol Phys 1979;5:521.
496. Mossman KL, Shatzman AR, Chencharick JD. Effects of radiotherapy on human parotid saliva. Radiat Res 1981;88:403.
497. Muggia FM, Wolf GT. Intra-arterial chemotherapy of head and neck cancer: worth another look? Cancer Clin Trials 1980;3:375.
498. Mukhopadhyaya R, Rao RS, Fakih AR, Gangal SG. Detection of circulating immune complexes in patients with squamous cell carcinoma of the oral cavity. J Clin Lab Immunol 1986;21:189.
499. Murray CG, Herson J, Daly TE, Zimmerman SO. Radiation necrosis of the mandible: A 10 year study. Part I: Factors influencing the onset of necrosis. Int J Radiat Oncol Phys 1980;6:543.
500. Nadol JB Jr. Treatment of carcinoma of the epiglottis. Ann Otol Rhinol Laryngol 1981;90:442.
501. Nagle RB, Moll R, Weidauer H, Nemetschek H, Franke WW. Different patterns of cytokeratin expression in the normal epithelia of the upper respiratory tract. Differentiation 1985;30:130.
502. Nason RW, Sako K, Beecroft WA, Razack MS, Bakamjian VY, Shedd DP. Surgical management of squamous cell carcinoma of the floor of mouth. Am J Surg 1989;158:292.
503. Nass JM, Brady LW, Glassburn JR, Prasasvinichai S, Schatanoff D. Radiation therapy of glottic carcinoma. Int J Radiat Oncol Biol Phys 1976;1:867.
504. Nguyen TD, Demange L, Froissart D, Panis X, Liorette M. Rapid hyperfractionated radiotherapy. Clinical results in 178 advanced squamous cell carcinomas of the head and neck. Cancer 1985;56:16.
505. Nicaise C, Hong WK, Dimery W, Usakewicz J, Rozencweig M, Krakoff I. Phase II study of tallysomycin S10b in patients with advanced head and neck cancer. Invest New Drugs 1990;8:325.
506. Ning JP, Yu MC, Wang QS, Henderson BE. Consumption of salted fish and other risk factors for nasopharyngeal carcinoma (NPC) in Tianjin, a low-risk region for NPC in the People's Republic of China. JNCI 1990;82:291.
507. Nissenbaum M, Browde S, Bezwoda WR, de Moor NG, Derman DP. Treatment of advanced head and neck cancer: Multiple daily dose fractionated radiation therapy and sequential multimodal treatment approach. Med Pediatr Oncol 1984;12:204.
508. Norris CM. Laryngectomy and neck dissection. Otolaryngol Clin North Am 1969;69:667.
509. Norris CM Jr, Clark JR, Frei E, Ervin TJ, Fallon B, Tuttle SA, Fabian RL, Miller P. Pathology of surgery after induction chemotherapy: An analysis of resectability and locoregional control. Laryngoscope 1986;96:292.
510. O'Brien PH, Carlson R, Steubber EA. Distant metastases in head and neck epidermoid carcinoma. Laryngoscope 1980;90:196.
511. O'Connor D, Clifford P, Edwards WG, Dallen VM, Durden-Smith J, Hollis BA, Calman FM. Long-term results of VBM and radiotherapy in advanced head and neck cancer. Int J Radiat Oncol Biol Phys 1982;8:1525.
512. Olivari AJ, Glait HM, Guardo A, Califano L, Pradier R. Levamisole in squamous cell carcinoma of the head and neck. Cancer Treat Rep 1979;63:983.
513. Ossoff RH, Shapshay SM, Sisson GA. Endoscopic management of selected early vocal cord carcinoma. Ann Otol Rhinol Laryngol 1985;94:560.
514. Paccagnella A, Cavaniglia G, Zorat PL, Pappagallo GL, Orlando A, Balli M, Bononi A, Puccetti C, Fila G, Vinante O, Sala O, Calzavara F, Fiorentino MV. Chemotherapy (CT) before loco-regional treatment (LRT) in stage III+IV head and neck cancer: Intermediate results of an ongoing randomized phase III trial. A GSTTC study (abstract 669). Proc Amer Soc Clin Oncol 1990;9:173.
515. Paccagnella A, Orlando A, Marchiori C, et al. Phase III trial of initial chemotherapy in stage III or IV head and neck cancers: A study by the Gruppo di Studio sui Tumori Della Testa e del Collo. JNCI 1994;86:265–272.
516. Panje WR, Ceilley RI. The influence of embryology of the mid-face on the spread of epithelial malignancies. Laryngoscope 1979;89:1914.
517. Panje WR, Smith B, McCabe BF. Epidermoid carcinomas of the floor of mouth. Surgical therapy vs combined therapy vs radiation therapy. Otolaryngol Head Neck Surg 1980;88:714.
518. Paredes J, Hong WK, Felder T, Dimery IW, Choksi AJ, Newman RA, Castellanos AM, Robbins KT, McCarthy K, Atkinson N. Prospective randomized trial of high-dose cisplatin and 5-FU infusion with or without sodium diethyldithiocarbamate (DDT) in recurrent and/or metastatic squamous cell carcinoma of the head and neck. J Clin Oncol 1988;6:955.
519. Parvinen LM, Parvinen M, Nordman E, Kortekangas AE. Combined bleomycin treatment and radiation therapy in squamous cell carcinoma of the head and neck region. Acta Radiol Oncol 1985;24:487.
520. Peacock N, Kuhn J, Hardy J, Burris H, Shaffer D, Thurman A, Von Hoff D, Rodriguez G. A phase I trial of hydoxyurea in patients with head and neck cancer (abstract 924). Proc Am Soc Clin Oncol 1993;12:285.
521. Pearson BW, Woods RD II, Hartman DE. Extended hemilaryngectomy of T3 glottic carcinoma with preservation of speech and swallowing. Laryngoscope 1980;90:1950.
522. Pene F, Fletcher GH. Results in irradiation of the in situ carcinomas of the vocal cord. Cancer 1976;37:2586.
523. Peng YM, Alberts DS, Chen HS, Mason N, Moon TE. Antitumor activity and plasma kinetics of bleomycin by continuous and intermittent administration. Br J Cancer 1980;41:644.
524. Pennacchio JL, Hong WK, Shapshay S, Gillis T, Vaughan C, Bhutani P, Ucmakli A, Katz AE, Bromer R, Willet B, Strong SM. Combination of *cis*-platin and bleomycin prior to surgery and/or radiotherapy compared with radiotherapy alone for the treatment of advanced squamous cell carcinoma of the head and neck. Cancer 1982;50:2795.
525. Perez CA, Purdy JA, Breaux SR, Ogura JH, von Essen S. Carcinoma of the tonsillar fossa. Cancer 1982;50:2314.
526. Peters LJ, Batsakis JG, Goepfert H, Hong WK. The diagnosis and management of nasopharyngeal cancer in caucasians. In Textbook of Uncommon Cancer. Edited by CJ Williams, JG Krikorian, MR Green, D Raghaven. Chichester, England: Wiley, 1988, pp 975–1006.
527. Peters LJ, Harrison ML, Dimery IW, Fields R, Goepfert M, Oswald MJ. Acute and late toxicity associated with sequential bleomycin-containing chemotherapy regimens and radiation therapy in the treatment of carcinoma of the nasopharynx. Int J Radiat Oncol Biol Phys 1988;14:623.
528. Petrovich Z, Block J, Kuisk H, Mackintosh R, Casciato D, Jose L, Berton R. A randomized comparison of radiotherapy with radiotherapy-chemotherapy combination in stage IV carcinoma of the head and neck. Cancer 1986;47:2259.
529. Petrovich Z, Kuisk H, Jose L, Barton R, Rice D. Advanced carcinoma of the tonsil. Treatment results. Acta Radiol Oncol 1980;19:425.
530. Pfeiffer P, Madsen EL, Hansen O, May O. Effect of prophylactic sucralfate suspension on stomatitis induced by cancer chemotherapy. A randomized, double-blind cross-over study. Acta Oncol 1990;29:171.
531. Pfister DG, Bajorin D, Motzer R, et al. Cisplatin, fluorouracil and leucovorin. Increased toxicity without improved response in squamous cell head and neck cancer. Arch Otolaryngol Head Neck Surg 1994;120:89–95.
532. Pigneux J, Richaud PM, Lagarde C. The place of interstitial therapy using 192 Indium in the management of carcinoma of the lip. Cancer 1979;43:1073.
533. Pillsbury HR, Kirchner JA. Clinical vs histopathologic staging in laryngeal cancer. Arch Otolaryngol 1979;105:157.
534. Pingree TF, Davis RK, Reichman O, Derrick L. Treatment of hypopharyngeal carcinoma: A 10 year review of 1362 cases. Laryngoscope 1987;97:901.
535. Pinkston JA, Wakabuyashi T, Yamamoto T, Asano M, Harada Y, Kumagami H, Takeuchi, M Cancer of the head and neck in atomic bomb survivors: Hiroshima and Nagasaki, 1957–1976. Cancer 1981;48:2172.
536. Pinnaro P, Cercato MC, Giannarelli D, et al. A randomized phase II study comparing sequential versus simultaneous chemo-radiotherapy in patients with unresectable locally advanced squamous cell cancer of the head and neck. Ann Oncol 1994;5:513–519.
537. Pitman SW, Kowal CD, Bertino JR. Methotrexate and 5-fluorouracil in sequence in squamous head and neck cancer. Semin Oncol 1983;10(suppl 2):15.

538. Pomp J, Levendag PC, van Putten L. Reirradiation of recurrent tumors in the head and neck. Am J Clin Oncol 1988;11:543.
539. Popkin JD, Hong WK, Bromer RH, Moffer SM, Doos WG, Willett BL, Katz AE, Vaughn CW, Strong MS. Induction bleomycin infusion in head and neck cancer. Am J Clin Oncol (CCT) 1984;7:199.
540. Posner MR, Ervin TJ, Weichselbaum RR, Fabian RL, Miller D. Chemotherapy of advanced salivary gland neoplasms. Cancer 1982;50:2261.
541. Posner MR, Weichselbaum RR, Fitzgerald TJ, Clark JR, Rose C, Fabian RL, Norris CM Jr, Miller D, Tuttle SA, Ervin TJ. Treatment complications after sequential combination chemotherapy and radiotherapy with or without surgery in previously untreated squamous cell carcinoma of the head and neck. Int J Radiat Oncol Biol Phys 1985;11:1887.
542. Powell BL, Craig JB, Muss HB, Zekan PJ, Cooper MR, Schnell FM, Hampton JW, White DR, Smith LR, Capizzi RL. Phade II trial of high-dose cytosine arabinoside and cisplatin in recurrent squamous carcinoma of the head and neck. Am J Clin Oncol 1988;11:550.
543. Powell BL, Stanley V, Brockschmidt J, White D, Muss H, Livesay L, McNeill J, Schifeling D, Jackson D, Baker A, Caldwell D, O'Rourke M, Paschal B, Brodkin R, Pavy M. Combination carboplatin (CBDCA) and cisplatin (CDDP) for advanced squamous carcinoma of the head and neck (SCHN) (abstract 693). Proc Am Soc Clin Oncol 1990;9:179.
544. Pressman JJ, Dowdy A, Libby M. Further studies upon the submucosal compartments and lymphatics of the larynx by the injection of dye and radioisotopes. Ann Otol Rhinol Laryngol 1956;65:963.
545. Probert JC, Thompson RW, Bagshaw MA. Patterns of spread of distant metastases in head and neck cancer. Cancer 1974;33:127.
546. Raab-Traub N, Flynn K, Pearson G, Huang A, Levine P, Lanier A, Pagano J. The differentiated form of nasopharyngeal carcinoma contains Epstein-Barr virus DNA. Int J Cancer 1987;39:25.
547. Rahal M, Sadek H, Azli M, Cvitkovic E, Djemma A, Wendling JL, Filali T, Avril MF, Armand JP. Advanced loco-regional skin carcinoma. Primary chemotherapy with cisplatin (CDDP), bleomycin (BLM) and 5-JP: fluorouracil (5 FU) (abstract 1142). Proc Am Soc Clin Oncol 1989;8:293.
548. Raine CH, Stell PM, Dalby J. Squamous cell carcinoma of the posterior wall of the hypopharynx. J Laryngol Otol 1982;96:997.
549. Randolph VL, Vallejo A, Spiro RH, Shah J, Strong EW, Huvos AG, Wittes RE. Combination therapy of advanced head and neck cancer: Induction of remissions with diamminedichloroplatinum (II) bleomycin and radiation therapy. Cancer 1978;41:460.
550. Razack MS, Sako K, Marchetta FC, Calamel P, Bakamjian V, Shedd DP. Carcinoma of the hypopharynx: Success and failure. Am J Surg 1977;134:489.
551. Remmier D, Medina JE, Byers RM, Meoz R, Pfalzgraf K. Treatment of choice for squamous carcinoma of the tonsillar fossa. Head Neck Surg 1985;7:206.
552. Rentschler R, Burgess MA, Byers R. Chemotherapy of malignant major salivary gland neoplasms: a 25-year review of M. D. Anderson Hospital experience. Cancer 1977;40:619.
553. Rentschler RE, Wilbur DW, Petti GH, Chonkich GD, Hilliard DA, Camacho ES, Thorpe RB. Adjuvant methotrexate escalated to toxicity for resectable stage III and IV squamous head and neck carcinomas—A prospective, randomized study. J Clin Oncol 1987;5:278.
554. Rezkalla S, Ensley J, Turi Z, Kloner RA, Kish J, Tapazoglou E, Bhasin S, Revels S, Olivienstein A, Wynne J, Al-Sarraf M. 5-fluorouracil (5FU) cardiotoxicity A controlled, prospective investigation of ischemic changes during 5-FU infusions (abstract 580). Proc Am Soc Clin Oncol 1988;8:150.
555. Richard J, Molinari R, Sancho-Garnier H, et al. A randomized trial comparing surgery preceded or not by intra-arterial chemotherapy in squamous cell carcinomas of the head and neck. Proceedings, International Conference on Head and Neck Cancer. Baltimore, 1984, p 113.
556. Richard JM, Sancho H, Lepintre Y, Rodary J, Pierquin B. Intra-arterial methotrexate chemotherapy and telecobalt therapy in cancer of the oral cavity and oropharynx. Cancer 1974;34:491.
557. Richards GJ Jr, Chambers RG. Hydroxyurea. A radiosensitizer in the treatment of neoplasms of the head and neck. Am J Roentgenol Radium Ther Nucl Med 1969;105:555.
558. Richards GJ Jr, Chambers RG. Hydroxyurea in the treatment of neoplasms of the head and neck: a resurvey. Am J Surg 1973;126:513.
559. Richtsmeier WJ. Interferon gamma induced oncolysis: an effect of head and neck squamous carcinoma cultures. Arch Otolaryngol Head Neck Surg 1988;114:432.
560. Riley RW, Fee WE Jr, Goffinet D, Cox R, Goode RL. Squamous cell carcinoma of the base of the tongue. Otolaryngol Head Neck Surg 1983;91:143.
561. Ringborg U, Ewert G, Kinnman J, Lundgvist PG, Strander H. Sequential methotrexate-5-fluorouracil treatment of squamous cell carcinoma of the head and neck. Cancer 1983;52:971.
562. Ringborg U, Henle W, Henle G, Ingimarson S, Klein G, Silfversward C, Strander H. Epstein-Barr virus—specific serodiagnostic tests in carcinomas of the head and neck. Cancer 1983;52:1237.
563. Roa RA, Carey TE, Passamani PP, Greenwood JH, Hsu S, Ridings EO, Schwartz DR, Wolf GT, Hudson JL. DNA content of human squamous cell carcinoma cell lines. Analysis by flow entometry and chromosome enumeration. Arch Otolaryngol 1985;111:565.
564. Robert F. Trimetrexate as a single agent in patients with advanced head and neck cancer. Sem Oncol 1988;15(suppl 2):22.
565. Robert F, Wheeler RH, Molthrop DC, et al. Phase II study of topotecan in advanced head and neck cancer: Identification of an active new agent. Proc Am Soc Clin Oncol 1994;13:281.
566. Robbins KT, Storniolo AM, Kerber C, et al. Phase I study of highly selective supradose cisplatin infusions for advanced head and neck cancer. J Clin Oncol 1994;12:2113–2120.
567. Robbins KT, Howell SB. Head and Neck Study Groups: Concurrent regional supradose cisplatin infusions and radiotherapy for advanced head and neck cancer. Head Neck 1995;498:103.
568. Rollo J, Rozenbom CV, Thawley S, Korba A, Ogura J, Perez CA, Powers WE, Bauer WC. Squamous carcinoma of the base of the tongue: A clinicopathologic study of 81 cases. Cancer 1981;47:333.
569. Rooney M, Kish J, Jacobs J, Kinzie J, Weaver A, Crissman J, Al-Sarraf M. Improved complete response rate and survival in advanced head and neck cancer after three-course induction therapy with 120-hour 5-FU infusion and cisplatin. Cancer 1985;55:1123.
570. Rossi A, Molinari R, Boracchi P, Del Vecchio M, Marubini E, Nava M, Morandi L, Zucali R, Pilotti S, Grandi C. Adjuvant chemotherapy with vincristine, cyclophosphamide, and doxorubicin after radiotherapy in local-regional nasopharyngeal cancer: results of a 4-year multicenter randomized study. J Clin Oncol 1988;6:1401.
571. Rowinsky EK, Donehower RC. Paclitaxel (Taxol). N Engl J Med 1995;332:1004–1014.
572. Sako K, Razack MS, Kalnins I. Chemotherapy for advanced and recurrent squamous cell carcinoma of the head and neck with high and low dose *cis*-diamminedichloroplatinum. Am J Surg 1978;136:529.
573. Sanchiz F, Milla A, Torner J, Bonet F, Artola N, Carreno L, Moya LM, Riera D, Ripol S, Cirera L. Single fraction per day versus two fractions per day versus radiotherapy in the treatment of head and neck cancer. Int J Radiat Oncol Biol Phys 1990;19:1347.
574. Saranath D, Panchal RG, Nair R, Mehta AR, Sanghavi V, Sumegi J, Klein G, Deo MG. Oncogene amplification in squamous cell carcinoma of the oral cavity. Jpn J Cancer Res 1989;80:430.
575. Scandolaro L, Bertoni F. Tolleranza cutanea e mucosa e risposte cliniche a breve termine nella associazione tra radioterapia e bleomycina per tumori del distretto cervico-cefalico. Acta Otorhinol Ital 1982;2:213.
576. Scanlon PW, Rhodes RE, Woolner LB, Devine KD, McBean JB. Cancer of the nasopharynx. One hundred forty-two patients treated in the 11-year period 1950–1960. Am J Roentgenol 1967;99:313.
577. Schabel FM Jr. Concepts for treatment of micrometastases developed in murine systems. Am J Roentgenol 1976;126:500.
578. Schantz SP, Dimery I, Lippman SM, et al. A phase II study of interleukin-2 and interferon-alpha in head and neck cancer. Invest New Drugs 1992;10:217–223.
579. Schantz SP, Guillamondegui OM. Developing perspectives in head and neck tumor immunology. Prob Gen Surg 1988;5:99.
580. Schantz SP, Hsu TC, Ainslie N, Moser RP. Young adults with head and neck cancer express increased susceptibility to mutagen-induced chromosome damage. JAMA 1989;262:3313.
581. Schantz SP, Savage HE, Brown BW, Reuben JM, Hong WK, Rossen RD. Association of levels of Clq binding macromolecules with induction chemotherapy response in head and neck cancer patients. Cancer Res 1988;48:5868.
582. Schantz SP, Savage HE, Race T, Liu FJ, Brown BW, Rossen RD, Hong WK. Immunologic determinants of head and neck cancer response to induction chemotherapy. J Clin Oncol 1989;7:857.
583. Schantz SP, Spitz MR, Hsu TC. Mutagen sensitivity in patients with head and neck cancers: A biologic marker for risk of multiple primary malignancies. JNCI 1990;82:1773.
584. Schechter GL, Kalafsky JT. Cancer of the hypopharynx and cervical esophagus: management concepts. Oncology 1988;2:17, 34.
585. Schechter GL, Baker JW, El-Mahdi AM, Bumata JT. Combined treatment of advanced cancer of the laryngopharynx and cervical esophagus. Laryngoscope 1982;92:11.
586. Schmidseder R, Dick H. Spread of epidermoid carcinoma of the lip along the inferior alveolar nerve. Oral Surg Oral Med Oral Pathol 1977;43:517.
587. Schnabel T, Zamboglou N, Pape H, Achterrath W, Lenaz L, Schmitt G, Preusser P. Phase II trial with carboplatin and simultaneous radiation in previously untreated advanced squamous cell carcinoma of the head and neck (SCCHN) (abstract 680). Proc Am Soc Clin Oncol 1990;9:176.
588. Schneider JJ, Lindberg RD, Jesse RH. Prevention of tracheal stoma recurrences after total laryngectomy by postoperative irradiation. J Surg Oncol 1975;7:187.
589. Schornagel JH, Verweij J, de Mulder PHM, Cognetti F, Vermorken JB, Cappelaere P, Armand JP, Wildiers J, de Graeff A, Clavel M, Sahmoud T, Kirkpatrick A, Lefebvre JL. Randomized phase III trial of edatrexate versus methotrexate in patients with metastatic and/or recurrent squamous cell carcinoma of the head and neck: a European Organization for the Research and Treatment of Head and Neck Cancer Cooperative Group study. J Clin Oncol 1995;13:1649–1655.
590. Schottenfeld D. Epidemiology, etiology, and pathogenesis of head and neck cancer. In Head and Neck Cancer. Edited by PB Chretien, ME John, DP Shedd. New York: Dekker, 1985, pp 6–18.
591. Schramm VL Jr, Srodes C, Myers EN. Cisplatin therapy for adenoid cystic carcinoma. Arch Otolaryngol 1981;107:739.
592. Schreiner BF, Christy CJ. Results of irradiation treatment of cancer of the lip: analysis of 636 cases from 1926–1936. Radiol 1942;39:293.
593. Schrijvers AH, Quak JJ, Uyterlinde AM, van Walsum M, Meijer CJ, Snow GB, van-Dogen GA. MAb U36, a novel monoclonal antibody successful in immunotargeting of squamous cell carcinoma of the head and neck. Cancer Res 1993;53:4383.
594. Schuller DE, Metch B, Stein DW, Mattox D, McCracken JD. Preoperative chemotherapy in advanced resectable head and neck cancer: final report of the Southwest Oncology Group. Laryngoscope 1988;98:1205.
595. Schuller DE, Stein DW, Metch B. Analysis of treatment failure patterns. A Southwest Oncology Group study. Arch Otolaryngol Head Neck Surg 1989;115:834.
596. Seder RH, Vaughan CW, Oh SK, Keegins JJ, Hayes JA, Blanchard GC, Vincent ME, Katz AE. Tumor repression and temporary restoration of immune response after plasmapheresis in patients with recurrent oral cancer. Cancer 1987;60:318.
597. Selvaggi KJ, Vlock DR, Johnson JT, Snyderman CH, Rubin J, Kirkwood J, Haselow R, Letessier E, Whiteside T, Prescott K. Phase Ib trial of peritumoral and intranodal injections of IL-2 in patients with advanced squamous cell carcinoma of the head and neck (SCCHN)—preliminary results (abstract 691). Proc Am Soc Clin Oncol 1990;9:178.
598. Sessions RB, Lehane DE, Bryan RN, Horowitz BL. Intra-arterial cisplatin in the treatment of aerodigestive squamous carcinoma and nasopharyngeal carcinoma. In Head and Neck Cancer. Edited by PB Chretian, ME Johns, DP Shedd, EW Strong, PH Ward. Philadelphia: Dekker, 1985, pp 451–455.
599. Sessions RB, Lehane DE, Smith RJ, Bryan RN, Suen JY. Intra-arterial cisplatin treatment of adenoid cystic carcinoma. Arch Otolaryngol 1982;108:221.
600. Shah JP, Caudela FC, Poddar AK. The patterns of cervical lymph node metastases from squamous carcinoma of the oral cavity. Cancer 1990;66:109.
601. Shah JP, Feghali J. Esthesioneuroblastoma. Am J Surg 1981;142:456.
602. Shah JP, Anderson PE. The impact of patterns of nodal metastasis on modifications of neck dissection. Ann Surg Oncol 1994;1(6):521–532.
603. Shah JP, Tolletsen HR. Epidermoid carcinoma of the supraglottic larynx. Role of neck dissection in initial surgical treatment. Am J Surg 1974;128:494.

604. Shah KV. Papillomavirus infections of the respiratory tract, the conjunctiva, and the oral cavity. In Papillomaviruses and Human Cancer. Edited by H Pfister. 1990, pp 73–261.
605. Shaha AR, Shah JP. Carcinoma of the subglottic larynx. Am J Surg 1982;144:456.
606. Shaha A, Spiro R, Shah J, Strong EW. Squamous carcinomas of the floor of mouth. Am J Surg 1984;148:455.
607. Sham JS, Poon YF, Wei WI, Choy D. Nasopharyngeal carcinoma in young patients. Cancer 1990;65:2606.
608. Shankar PG, Taylor SA, Gemer LS. Accelerated fractionation radiation therapy and concurrent *cis*-platin chemotherapy for advanced head and neck cancer (abstract 696). Proc Am Soc Clin Oncol 1990;9:180.
609. Shanta V, Krishnamurthi S. Combined bleomycin and radiotherapy in oral cancer. Clin Radiol 1980;31:617.
610. Shapira A, Virolainen E, Jameson JJ, Ossakow SJ, Carey TE. Growth inhibition of laryngeal UM-SCC cell lines by tamoxifen: comparison with effects on the MCF-7 breast cancer cell line. Arch Otolaryngol Head Neck Surg 1986;112:1151.
611. Shapshay SM, Hong WK, Incze JS, Sismanis A, Bhutani R, Vaughn CW, Strong MS. Prognostic indicators in induction *cis*-platinum bleomycin chemotherapy for advanced head and neck cancer. Am J Surg 1980;140:543.
612. Shetty P, Mehta A, Shinde S, Mazumdar A, Hingorani C. Controlled study in squamous cell carcinoma of base of tongue using conventional radiation, radiation with single drug and radiation with multiple drug chemotherapy (abstract C-595). Proc Am Soc Clin Oncol 1985;4:152.
613. Shigematsu Y, Sakai S, Fuchihata H. Recent trials in the treatment of maxillary sinus carcinoma with special reference to the chemical potentiation of radiation therapy. Acta Otolaryngol 1971;71:63.
614. Shillitoe EJ, Greenspan D, Greenspan JS, Silverman S Jr. Five-year survival of patients with oral cancer and its association with antibody to herpes simplex virus. Cancer 1986;58:2256.
615. Shillitoe EJ, Hwang CB, Silverman S Jr, Greenspan JS. Examination of oral cancer tissue for the presence of the proteins ICP4, ICP5, ICP6, ICP8, and gB of herpes simplex virus type 1. JNCI 1986;76:371.
616. Shin DM, Kim J, Ro JY, Hittelman J, Roth JA, Hong WK, Hittelman WN. Activation of p53 gene expression in premalignant lesions during head and neck tumorigenesis. Cancer Res 1994;54:321–326.
617. Shin DM, Voravud N, Ro JY, Lee JS, Hong WK, Hittleman WN. Sequential increases in proliferating cell nuclear antigen expression in head and neck tumorigenesis: A potential biomarker. JNCI 1993;85:971.
618. Shore-Friedman E, Abrahams C, Recant W, Schneider AB. Neurilemonas and salivary gland tumors of the head and neck following childhood irradiation. Cancer 1983;51:2159.
619. Shresbury D, Adams GL, Duvall AJ III, Maisel RH, Haselow RE. Carcinoma of the tonsillar region: A comparison of radiation therapy with combined preoperative radiation and surgery. Otolaryngol Head Neck Surg 1981;89:979.
620. Sikic BT, Collins JM, Mimnaugh EG, Gram TE. Improved therapeutic index of bleomycin when administered by continuous infusion in mice. Cancer Treat Rep 1978;62:2011.
621. Sinibaldi V, Eisenberger M, Jacobs M. Treatment of advanced unresectable stage IV squamous cell carcinoma of the head and neck (SCCHN) with combined carboplatin (CBDCA) and radiotherapy (RT) (abstract 659). Proc Am Soc Clin Oncol 1989;8:169.
622. Siodlak MZ, Dalby JE, Bradley PJ, Campbell JB, Strickland P, Fraser JG, Willatt DJ, Flood LM, Stell PM. Induction VBM plus radiotherapy, versus radiotherapy alone for advanced head and neck cancer: Long-term results. Clin Otolaryngol 1989;14:17.
623. Sisson GA, Bytell DE, Edison BD, Yeh S. Transsternal radical neck dissection for control of stomal recurrences—end results. Laryngoscope 1975;85:1504.
624. Skolnick EM, Yee KF, Wheatley MA, Martin LO. Carcinoma of the laryngeal glottis therapy and end results. Laryngoscope 1975;85:1453.
625. Slaughter DP, Southwick HW, Smejkal W. "Field cancerization" in oral stratified squamous epithelium: Clinical implications of multicentric origin. Cancer 1953;6:963.
626. Slotman GJ, Cummings FJ, Glicksman AR, Doolittle CL, Leone LA. Preoperative simultaneously-administered *cis*-platinum plus radiation therapy for advanced squamous cell carcinoma of the head and neck. Head Neck Surg 1986;8:159.
627. Snow GB, Annyas AA, van Slooten EA, Bartelink H, Hart AA. Prognostic factors of neck node metastases. Clin Otolaryngol 1982;7:185.
628. Snow GB, Vermorken JB, Pinedo HM. Adjuvant chemotherapy: The EORTC trials. In Head and Neck Oncology. Edited by HJG Bloom, et al. New York: Raven, 1986, pp 83–92.
629. Snow JB, Gelber RD, Kramer S, Davis LW, Marcial VA, Lowry LD. Comparison of preoperative and postoperative radiation therapy for patients with carcinoma of the head and neck. Interim Report Act Otolaryngol 1981;91:611.
630. Snyderman NL, Wetmore SJ, Suen JY. Cisplatin sensitization to radiotherapy in stage IV squamous cell carcinoma of the head and neck. A follow-up report. Arch Otolaryngol Head Neck Surg 1986;112:1147.
631. Somers KD, Cartwright SL, Schechter GL. Coamplification of int-2 and HST-1 genes in squamous cell carcinoma of the head and neck. Presented at Third International Head and Neck Oncology Research Conference, Las Vegas, 1990.
632. Somers KD, Merrick MA, Lopez ME, Incognito LS, Schecter GL, Casey G. Frequent p53 mutations in head and neck cancer. Cancer Res 1992;52:5996–6000.
633. Son YH, Kapp DS. Oral cavity and oropharyngeal cancer in a younger population: Review of literature and experience at Yale. Cancer 1985;55:441.
634. Soo KC, Shah JP, Gopinath KS, Gerold FP, Jaques DP, Strong EW. Analysis of prognostic variables and results after supraglottic partial laryngectomy. Am J Surg 1988;156:301.
635. Souhami L, Rabinowits M. Combined treatment in carcinoma of the nasopharynx. Laryngoscope 1988;98:881.
636. South East Cooperative Oncology Group: A randomized trial of combined multidrug chemotherapy and radiotherapy in advanced squamous cell carcinoma of the head and neck. Eur J Surg Oncol 1986;12:289.
637. Sozzi G, Miozzo M, Donghi R, Pilotti S, Cariani CT, Pastorino U, Porta GD, Pierotti MA. Deletions of 17p and p53 mutations in preneoplastic lesions of the lung. Cancer Res 1992;52:1.
638. Spandidos PA, Lamothe A, Field JK. Multiple transcriptional activation of cellular oncogenes in human head and neck solid tumors. Anticancer Res 1985;5:221.
639. Spaulding CA, Kranyak MS, Constable WC, Stewart FM. Esthesioneuroblastoma: A comparison of two treatment eras. Int J Rad Oncol Biol Phys 1988;15:581.
640. Spaulding CA, Krochak RJ, Hahn SS, Constable WC. Radiotherapeutic management of cancer of the supraglottis. Cancer 1986;57:1292.
641. Spaulding MB, Lore JM, Sundquist N. Long-term follow-up of chemotherapy in advanced head and neck cancer. Arch Otolaryngol Head Neck Surg 1989;115:68.
642. Spencer S, Wheeler R, Peters G, et al. Concomitant chemotherapy and re-irradiation as managment for recurrent cancer of the head and neck (abstract 104). Head Neck, Sept/Oct 1994:498.
643. Spijkervet F, Vermey A, Panders AV, Saene H, Mehta D. Prevention of irradiation mucositis in head-neck cancer patients (abstract 673). Proc Am Soc Clin Oncol 1990;9: 174.
644. Spiro JD, Spiro RH. Carcinoma of the tonsillar fossa: An update. Arch Otolaryngol Head Neck Surg 1989;115:1186.
645. Spiro RH. Squamous cancer of the tongue. Cancer 1985;35:252.
646. Spiro RH, Alfonso AE, Farr HW, Strong EW. Cervical node metastases from epidermoid carcinoma of the oral cavity and oropharynx. A critical assessment of current staging. Am J Surg 1974;128:562.
647. Spiro RH, Huvos AG, Strong EW. Cancer of the parotid gland: A clinicopathologic study of 288 primary cases. Am J Surg 1975;130:452.
648. Spiro RH, Huvos AG, Strong EW. Acinic cell carcinoma of salivary origin: A clinicopathologic study of 67 cases. Cancer 1978;41:924.
649. Spiro RH, Huvos AG, Strong EW. Adenoid cystic carcinoma: Factors influencing survival. Am J Surg 1979;138:579.
650. Spiro RH, Kelly J, Vega AL, Harrison LB, Strong EW. Squamous carcinoma of the posterior pharyngeal wall. Am J Surg 1990;160:420.
651. Spiro RH, Koss LG, Hajdu SI, Strong EW. Tumors of minor salivary gland origin a clinicopathologic study of 492 cases. Cancer 1973;31:117.
652. Spitz MR, Fueger JJ, Beddingfield NA, Annegers JF, Hsu TC, Newell GR, Schantz SP. Chromosome sensitivity to bleomycin-induced mutagenesis: An independent risk factor for upper aerodigestive tract cancers. Cancer Res 1989;49:4626.
653. Spitz MR, Fueger JJ, Geopfert H, Hong WK, Newell GR. Squamous cell carcinoma of the upper aerodigestive tract: a case comparison analysis. Cancer 1988;61:203.
654. Spitz MR, Sider JG, Newell GR, Batsakis JG. Incidence of salivary gland cancer in the United States relative to ultraviolet radiation exposure. Head Neck Surg 1988;10:305.
655. Sporn MB. Approaches to prevention of epithelial cancer during the preneoplastic period. Cancer Res 1976;36:2699.
656. Sporn MB, Dunlop NM, Newton DL, Smith JM. Prevention of chemical carcinogenesis by vitamin A and its synthetic analogs (retinoids). Fed Proc 1976;35:1332.
657. Squier CA. Smokeless tobacco and oral cancer: a cause for concern? CA 1984;34: 242.
658. Stefani A, Chung TS. Hydroxyurea and radiotherapy in head and neck cancer—long term results of a double blind randomised prospective study. Radiat Oncol Biol Phys 1980;6:1398.
659. Stell PM, Dalby JE, Strickland P, Fraser JG, Bradley PJ, Flood LM. Sequential chemotherapy and radiotherapy in advanced head and neck cancer. Clin Radiol 1983;34:463.
660. Stell PM, Rawson NS. Adjuvant chemotherapy in head and neck cancer. Br J Cancer 1990;61:779.
661. Stewart FM, Lazarus HM, Levine PA, Stewart KA, Tabbara IA, Spaulding CA. High-dose chemotherapy and autologous marrow transplantation for esthesioneuroblastoma and sinonasal undifferentiated carcinoma. Am J Clin Oncol 1989;12:217.
662. Stolwijk C, Wagener DJ, van den Broek Levendaj PC, Kazem I, Bruaset I, DeMulder PH. Randomized adjuvant chemotherapy trial for advanced head and neck cancer. Neo-Neth J Med 1985;28:347.
663. Strome M, Clark J, Fried M, Rodliff S, Blazar BA. Prognostic implications of defining natural killer cell function and T-cell sub-sets in patients with squamous cell carcinoma. In Head and Neck. Edited by W Fee, W Goepfert, ME Johns, EW Strong, PH Ward. Philadelphia: Dekker, 1990, pp 89–93.
664. Strong MS, Incze J, Vaughan CW. Field cancerization in the aerodigestive tract—Its etiology, manifestation, and significance. J Otolaryngol 1984;13:1.
665. Suen JY, Johns ME. Chemotherapy for salivary gland cancer. Laryngoscope 1982;92:235.
666. Sutow WW, Sullivan MP, Reid HL, Taylor MG, Griffith KM. Prognosis in childhood rhabdomyosarcoma. Cancer 1970;25:1238.
667. Syrjanen SM, Syrjanen KJ, Happonen RP. Human papillomavirus (HPV) DNA sequences in oral precancerous lesions and squamous cell carcinoma demonstrated by in situ hybridization. J Oral Pathol 1988;17:273.
668. Szpirglas H, Chastang C, Bertrand JC. Adjuvant treatment of tongue and floor of the mouth cancers. Rec Results Cancer Res 1978;68:309.
669. Szpirglas H, Nizri D, Marneur M, et al. Neo-adjuvant chemotherapy. A randomized trial before radiotherapy in oral and oro-pharyngeal carcinomas: end results. Head and Neck Oncology Research Proceedings, Second International, Head and Neck Oncology Research Conference, Arlington VA, Sep 1987, pp 261–264.
670. Taguchi T. Clinical studies of recombinant interferon alfa-2a (Roferon-A) in cancer patients. Cancer 1986;57:1705.
671. Takaku F. Clinical trials and cancer risk in Japan. JNCI 1984;73:1483.
672. Tannock I, Payne D, Cummings B, Hewitt K, Panzarella T. Sequential chemotherapy and radiation for nasopharyngeal cancer: Absence of long-term benefit despite a high rate of tumor response to chemotherapy. J Clin Oncol 1987;5:629.
673. Tannock IF, Sutherland DJ. Chemotherapy for adenocystic carcinoma. Cancer 1980;46:452.
674. Tapazoglou E, Kish J, Ensley J, Al-Sarraf M. The activity of a single-agent 5-fluorouracil infusion in advanced and recurrent head and neck. Cancer 1986;57:1105.
675. Tapazoglou E, Lorusso P, Kish J, Ensley J, Al-Sarraf M. The management of paranasal sinus cancer. Proceedings, Second International Head and Neck Oncology Research Conference, 1987, pp 357–364.
676. Tapley N-du V. Irradiation treatment of malignant tumors of the salivary glands. Ear Nose Throat J 1977;56:110.
677. Taylor SG, Murthy AK, Vannetzel JM, et al. Randomized comparison of neoadjuvant cisplatin and fluorouracil infusion followed by radiation versus concomitant treatment in advanced head and neck cancer. J Clin Oncol 1994;12:385–395.
678. Taylor SG IV. Combined chemotherapy and radiation for unresectable head and neck

cancer. In Carcinomas of the Head and Neck: Evaluation and Management. Edited by C Jacobs. Boston: Kluwer, 1990, pp 195–208.

679. Taylor SG IV, Applebaum E, Showel JL, Norusis M, Holinger LD, Hutchinson JL Jr, Murthy AK, Caldarelli DD. A randomized trial of adjuvant chemotherapy in head and neck cancer. J Clin Oncol 1985;3:672.
680. Taylor SG IV, McGuire WP, Hauck WW, Showel JL, Lad TE. A randomized comparison of high-dose infusion methotrexate versus standard-dose weekly therapy in head and neck squamous cancer. J Clin Oncol 1984;2:1006.
681. Taylor SG IV, Murthy AK, Caldarelli DD, Showel JL, Kiel K, Griem KL, Mittal BB, Kies M, Hutchinson JC Jr, Molinger LD. Combined simultaneous cisplatin/fluorouracil chemotherapy and split course radiation in head and neck cancer. J Clin Oncol 1989;7:846.
682. Taylor SG, Sisson GA, Bytell DE, Raynor WJ. A randomized trial of adjuvant BCG immunotherapy in head and neck cancer. Arch Otolaryngol 1983;109:544.
683. Tejada F, Chandler JR. Combined therapy for stage III and IV head and neck cancer (H&N) (abstract C-774). Proc Am Soc Clin Oncol 1982;1:199.
684. Terz JJ, Farr HW. Carcinoma of the tonsillar fossa. Surg Gynecol Obstet 1967;125: 581.
685. Thames HD, Peters LJ, Withers HR, Fletcher GH. Accelerated fractionation vs hyperfractionation: rationales for several treatments per day. Int J Radiat Oncol Biol Phys 1983;9:127.
686. Thawley SE, Simpson JR, Marks JE, Perez CA, Ogura JH. Preoperative irradiation and surgery for carcinoma of the base of the tongue. Ann Otol Rhinol Laryngol 1983;92: 485.
687. Thornton D, Singh K, Putz B, et al. A phase II trial of taxol in squamous cell carcinoma of the head and neck (abstract 933). Proc Am Soc Clin Oncol 1994;13:288.
688. Tobias JS. Has chemotherapy proved itself in head and neck cancer? Br J Cancer 1990;61:649.
689. Tobias JS, Smith BJ, Blackman G, Finn G. Concurrent daily cisplatin and radiotherapy in locally advanced squamous carcinoma of the head and neck and bronchus. Radiother Oncol 1987;9:263.
690. Todd R, Donoff BR, Gertz R, Chang AL, Chow P, Matossian K, McBride J, Chiang T, Gallager GT, Wong DT. TGF-alpha and EGF-receptor mRNAS in human oral cancer. Carcinogenesis 1989;10:1553.
691. Toohill RJ, Anderson T, Byhardt RW, Cox JD, Duncavage JA, Grossman TW, Haas CD, Haas JS, Hartz AJ, Libroch JA. Cisplatin and fluorouracil as neoadjuvant therapy in head and neck cancer. A preliminary report. Arch Otolaryngol Head Neck Surg 1987;113:758.
692. Toohill RJ, Duncavage JA, Malin TC, Wilson JF, Haas JS, Anderson T, Ritch PS, Libnoch J, Grossmam TW, Teplin RW, Byhardt RW, Cox JD, Holoye PY, Haas CD, Hoffmann RG. The effects of delay in standard treatment due to induction chemotherapy in two randomized prospective studies. Laryngoscope 1987;97:407.
693. Trible WM. Cancer of the oral cavity: Five year end results in 237 patients. Ann Otol Rhinol Laryngol 1969;78:716.
694. Triozzi PL, Brantley A, Fisher S, Cole TB, Crocker I, Huang AT. 5-Fluorouracil, cyclophosphamide, and vincristine for adenoid cystic carcinoma of the head and neck. Cancer 1987;59:887.
695. Trojanowski JQ, Lee V, Pillsbury N, Lee S. Neuronal origin of human esthesioneuroblastoma demonstrated with antineurofilament monoclonal antibodies. N Engl J Med 1982;307:159.
696. Tsuda T, Tahara E, Kajiyama G, Sakamoto M, Tejada M, Sugimura T. High incidence of coamplification of hst-1 and int-2 genes in human esophageal carcinomas. Cancer Res 1989;49:5505.
697. Uen W, Huang AT, Mennel R, Jones SE, Spaulding MB, Killion K, Havlin K, Keegan P, Clendeninn NJ. A phase II study of piritrexim in patients with advanced squamous head and neck cancer. Cancer 1992;69:1008.
698. Urba S, Forastiere AA, Wolf GT, Sullivan M, Thronton A, Husted S. Induction chemotherapy (CT) with intensive continuous infusion high dose cisplatin (CDDP), 5-fluorouracil (5FU) and mitoguazone (MGBG) for advanced head and neck cancer (H&N CA) (abstract 663). Proc Am Soc Clin Oncol 1990;9:171.
699. VA Laryngeal Cancer Study Group. Induction chemotherapy plus radiation compared with surgery plus radiation in patients with advanced laryngeal cancer. N Engl J Med 1991;324:1685.
700. Van den Bogaert W, Ostyn F, Van der Schueren E. The significance of extension and impaired mobility in cancer of the vocal cord. Int J Radiat Oncol Biol Phys 1983;9:181.
701. Van den Bogaert W, Ostyn F, Van der Schueren E. The differential clinical presentation, behaviour and prognosis of carcinomas originating in the epilarynx and the lower supraglottic. Radiother Oncol 1983;1:117.
702. Van den Bogaert W, Van der Schueren E, Horiot JC, Chaplin G, Devilhena M, Rapso S, Leonor J, Schraub S, Chenal C, Barthelme E, Daban A, Eschwege F, Gonzales D, Leer JW, Hamers H, Svoboda V, Rigon A, Arcangeli G, Sack H, de Pauw M, van Glabbeke M. Early results of the EORTC randomized clinical trial on multiple fractions per day (MFD) and misonidazole in advanced head and neck cancer. Int J Radiat Oncol Biol Phys 1986;12:587.
703. Van den Brouck C, Sancho-Garnier H, Chassagne D, Saravane D, Chachin Y, Micheau C. Elective versus therapeutic radical neck dissection in epidermoid carcinoma of the oral cavity: Results of a randomized clinical trial. Cancer 1980;46:386.
704. Van den Brouck C, Eschwege F, De La Rochefordiere A, Sicot H, Mamelle G, Le Ridant AM, Bosq J, Domenge C. Squamous cell carcinoma of the pyriform sinus: Retrospective study of 351 cases treated at the Institute Gustave-Roussy. Head Neck Surg 1987;10:4.
705. Van der Riet P, Nawroz H, Hruban RH, Corio R, Tokino K, Koch W, Sidransky D. Frequent loss of chromosome 9 p21–22 early in head and neck cancer progression. Cancer Res 1994;54:1156–1158.
706. van Dongen G, Braakhuis BJ, Bagnay M, Leyva A, Snow GB. Activity of differentiation-inducing agents and conventional drugs in head and neck cancer xenografts. Acta Otolaryngol 1988;105:488.
707. Venook AP, Tseng A Jr, Meyers FJ, Silverberg I, Boles R, Fu KK, Jacobs CD. Cisplatin, doxorubicin, and 5 fluorouracil chemotherapy for salivary gland malignancies: A pilot study of the Northern California Oncology Group. J Clin Oncol 1987;5:951.
708. Vermeer RJ, Pinedo HM. Partial remission of advanced adenoid cystic carcinoma obtained with Adriamycin: a case report with a review of the literature. Cancer 1979;43: 1604.
709. Vermund H. Role of radiotherapy in cancer of the larynx as related to the TNM system of staging. Cancer 1970;25:485.
710. Vermund H, Brennhovd I, Kaalhus O, Poppe E. Incidence and control of occult neck node metastases from squamous cell carcinoma of the anterior two-thirds of the tongue. Int J Radiol Oncol Biol Phys 1984;10:2025.
711. Vermund H, Kaalhus O, Winther F, Trausj J, Thorud E, Marang R. Bleomycin and radiation therapy in squamous cell carcinoma of the upper aero-digestive tract: A phase III clinical trial. Int J Radiat Oncol Biol Phys 1985;11:1877.
712. Veronesi A, Zagonel V, Trielli U, Galligioni E, Tumolo S, Barzan L, Lorenzini M, Comoretto R, Grigoletto E. High-dose versus low-dose cisplatin in advanced head and neck squamous carcinoma: a randomized study. J Clin Oncol 1985;3:1105.
713. Verweij J, Alexieva-Figusch J, de Boer MF, Reichquelt B, Stoter G. Ifosfamide in advanced head and neck cancer. A phase II study of the Rotterdam Cooperative Head and Neck Cancer Study Group. Eur J Cancer Clin Oncol 1988;24:795.
714. Verweij J, Clavel M, Chevalier B. Paclitaxel (Taxol) and docetaxel (Taxotere): not simply two of a kind. Ann Oncol 1994;5:495–505.
715. Vikram B. Changing patterns of failure in advanced head and neck cancer. Arch Otolaryngol 1984;110:564.
716. Vikram B. Cisplatin-based chemotherapy rapidly alternating with accelerated radiation therapy for carcinomas of the hypopharynx and upper esophagus. Presented at Third International Head and Neck Oncology Research Conference, Las Vegas, 1990.
717. Vikram B, Bosl GJ, Pfister D, Assad W, Strong EW, Spiro RH, Sessions RB, Gerold FP, Shah JP. New strategies for avoiding total laryngectomy in patients with head and neck cancer. NCI Monogr 1988;6:361.
718. Vikram B, Mishra UB, Strong EW, Manolatos S. Patterns of failure in carcinoma of the nasopharynx I: failure at the primary site. Int J Radiat Oncol Biol Phys 1985;11:1455.
719. Vikram B, Strong EW, Shah J, Spiro RH. Elective postoperative irradiation in stages III and IV epidermoid carcinoma of the head and neck. Am J Surg 1980;140:580.
720. Vikram B, Strong EW, Shah JP, Spiro R. Failure at the primary site following multimodality treatment in advanced head and neck cancer. Head Neck Surg 1984;6:720.
721. Vikram B, Strong EW, Shah JP, Spiro RH. Radiation therapy in adenoid-cystic carcinoma. Int J Radiat Oncol Biol Phys 1984;10:221.
722. Vlock D, Kalish L, Crouse C, Dutcher J, Adams G. Phase II trial of interferon alpha (IFN) and chemotherapy in locally recurrent or metastatic head and néck cancer (SC-CHN). Preliminary results of ECOG trial EST 1390 (abstract 918). Proc Am Soc Clin Oncol 1993;12:284.
723. Vogl SE, Schoenfeld DA, Kaplan BH, Lerner HJ, Engstrom PF, Horton J. A randomized prospective comparison of methotrexate with a combination of methotrexate, bleomycin, and cisplatin in head and neck cancer. Cancer 1985;56:432.
724. Vogler WR, Jacobs J, Moffitt S, et al. Methotrexate therapy with or without citrovorum factor in carcinoma of the head and neck, breast, and colon. Cancer Clin Trials 1979;2:227.
725. Vokes EE, Haraf DJ, Mick R, et al. Intensified concomitant chemoradiotherapy with and without filgrastim for poor-prognosis head and neck cancer. J Clin Oncol 1994;12:2351–2359.
726. Vokes EE, Ratain MJ, Mich R, McEvilly JM, Haraf D, Kozloff M, Hamasaki V, Weichselbaum RR, Panje WR, Wenig B, Berezin F. Cisplatin, fluorouracil, and leucovorin augmented by interferon alfa-2b in head and neck cancer: A clinical and pharamcologic analysis. J Clin Oncol 1993;11:360.
727. Vokes EE, Mick R, Lester EP, Panje WR, Weichselbaum RR. Cisplatin and fluorouracil chemotherapy does not yield long-term benefit in locally advanced head and neck cancer: results from a single institution. J Clin Oncol 1992;9:1376.
728. Vokes EE, Weichselbaum RR, Mick R, McEvilly JM, Haraf DJ, Panje WR. Favorable long-term survival following induction chemotherapy for locally advanced head and neck cancer. JNCI 1992;84:877.
729. Vokes EE, Schilsky RL, Weichselbaum RR, Kozloff MF, Parje WR. Induction chemotherapy with cisplatin, fluorouracil, and high-dose leucovorin for locally advanced head and neck cancer: a clinical and pharmacologic analysis. J Clin Oncol 1990;8:241.
730. Vokes EE, Weichselbaum RR, Lippman SM, Hong WK. Head and neck cancer. N Engl J Med 1993;328:184.
731. Volling P, Mueller RP, Staar S, Schroeder M, Achterrath W, Lenaz L. Pilot study with carboplatin (CBDCA) and simultaneous accelerated radiation (RT) in advanced squamous cell carcinoma of the head and neck (SCCHN) (abstract 681). Proc Am Soc Clin Oncol 1990;9:176.
732. Volterrani F, Chiesa F, Molinari R. Argument in favor of precautional treatment of cervical nodes in clinically no oral cancer. Tumori 1982;68:241.
733. Von Essen CP, Joseph LB, Simon GT, Singh AD, Singh SP. Sequential chemotherapy and radiation therapy of buccal mucosa carcinoma in South India. Methods and preliminary results. Am J Roentgenol Radium Ther Nucl Med 1968;102:530.
734. Voravud N, Lippman SM, Weber RS, et al. Phase-II study of 13-*cis*-retinoic acid plus interferon-α in recurrent head and neck cancer. Invest New Drugs 1993;11:57–60.
735. Voravud N, Shin DM, Ro JY, Lee JS, Hong WK, Hittelman WN. Increased polysomies of chromosomes 7 and 17 during head neck multistage tumorigenesis. Cancer Res 1993;53:2874.
736. Wallner PE, Hanks GE, Kramer S, McLean CJ. Patterns of care study: Analysis of outcome survey data—anterior two thirds of tongue and floor of mouth. Am J Clin Oncol 1986;9:50.
737. Wanebo HJ, Hilal EY, Strong EW, Pinsky CM, Mike V, Oettgen HF. Adjuvant trial of levamisole in patients with squamous cancer of the head and neck: A preliminary report. Rec Results Cancer Res 1978;68:324.
738. Wang CC. Radiotherapeutic management of carcinoma of the posterior pharyngeal wall. Cancer 1971;27:894.
739. Wang CC. Megavoltage radiation therapy for supraglottic carcinoma: Results of treatment. Radiology 1973;109:183.
740. Wang CC. Radiation Therapy for Head and Neck Neoplasms: Indications, Techniques and Results. Boston: John Wright, 1983.
741. Wang CC. Re-irradiation of recurrent nasopharyngeal carcinoma—treatment techniques and results. Int J Radiat Oncol Biol Phys 1987;13:952.
742. Wang CC. Local control of oropharyngeal carcinoma after two accelerated hyperfractionation radiation therapy schemes. Int J Radiat Oncol Biol Phys 1988;14:1143.
743. Wang CC, Busse J, Gitterman M. A simple afterloading application for intracavitary irradiation of the nasopharynx. Radiology 1975;115:737.

744. Wang CC, Suit HD, Blitzer PH. Twice a day radiation therapy for supraglottic carcinoma. Int J Radiat Oncol Biol Phys 1986;12:3.
745. Ward GE, Hendrick JW. Results of treatment of carcinoma of the lip. Surgery 1950;27: 321.
746. Ward PH, Calcaterra TC, Kagan AR. The regimen of postradiation edema and recurrent or residual carcinoma of the larynx. Laryngoscope 1975;85:522.
747. Warren S, Gates O. Multiple primary malignant tumors: a survey of the literature and statistical study. Am J Cancer 1932;51:1358.
748. Watson TA. Irradiation in the management of tumors of the head and neck. Am J Surg 1965;110:542.
749. Wawro NW, Babcock A, Ellison L. Cancer of the tongue: experience at the Hartford Hospital from 1931–1963. Am J Surg 1970;119:455.
750. Weaver A, Fleming S, Ensley J, Kish JA, Jacobs J, Kinzie J, Crissman J, Al-Sarraf M. Superior clinical response and survival rates with initial bolus of cisplatin and 120 hour infusion of 5-fluorouracil before definitive therapy for locally advanced head and neck cancer. Am J Surg 1984;148:525.
751. Weaver A, Flemming S, Kish J, Vandenberg M, Jacob J, Crissman J. *cis*-Platinum and 5-fluorouracil as induction therapy for advanced head and neck cancer. Am J Surg 1982;144:445.
752. Weber RS, Gidley P, Morrison WH, Peters LJ, Hankins P, Wolf P, Guillamondegui O. Treatment selection for carcinoma of the base of the tongue. Am J Surg 1990;160: 415.
753. Weber RS, Lippman SM, McNeese MD. Advanced basal and squamous cell carcinoma of the head and neck. In Carcinomas of the Head and Neck. Edited by C Jacobs. Norwell, MA: Kluwer, 1990, pp 61–81.
754. Weber RS, Peters LJ, Wolf PS, Guillamondegui O. Squamous cell carcinoma of the soft palate, uvula and anterior faucial pillar. Otolaryngol Head Neck Surg 1988;99:16.
755. Weissberg JB, Son YH, Papac RJ, Sasaki C, Fischer DB, Lawrence R, Rockwell S, Sartorelli AC, Fischer JJ. Randomized clinical trial of mitomycin C as an adjunct to radiotherapy in head and neck cancer. Int J Radiat Oncol Biol Phys 1989;17:3.
756. Welsh LW, Welsh JJ, Rizzo TA Jr. Laryngol spaces and lymphatics: current anatomic concepts. Ann Otol Rhinol Laryngol 1983;105(suppl):19.
757. Wendt TG, Hartenstein RC, Wustrow TP. 4-Years-update of simultaneous chemo-radiotherapy with 5-FU/folinic acid (FA)/cisplatin (DDP) and accelerated radiation in inoperable head and neck cancer (HNC) (abstract 658). Proc Am Soc Clin Oncol 1989;8:169.
758. Wendt TG, Hartenstein RC, Wustrow TP, Lissner J. Cisplatin, fluorouracil with leucovorin calcium enhancement, and synchronous accelerated radiotherapy in the management of locally advanced head and neck cancer: A phase II study. J Clin Oncol 1989;7:471.
759. Wenig BM, Hyam VJ, Heffner DK. Moderately differentiated neuroendocrine carcinoma of the larynx. Cancer 1988;62:2658.
760. Wennerberg J, Heim S, Jin Y, et al. Rearrangements involving chromosome bands 1p22 and 11q13 in squamous cell carcinomas of the head and neck. Presented at Third International Head and Neck Oncology Research Conference, Las Vegas, 1990.
761. Wetmore SJ, Key MJ, Suen JY. Laser therapy for T1 glottic carcinoma of the larynx. Arch Otolaryngol Head Neck Surg 1986;112:853.
762. Wheeler RH, Baker SR, Medvec BR. Single-agent and combination-drug regional chemotherapy for head and neck cancer using an implantable infusion pump. Cancer 1984;54:1504.
763. Wheeler R, Salter M, Stephens S, Hardy I, Peters G, Urist M, Maddox W. Simultaneous therapy with high-dose cisplatin and radiation for unresectable squamous cell cancer of the head and neck: A phase I–II study. NCI Monogr 1988;6:339.
764. Wiernik G, Bates TD, Bleehen MN, Brindle JM, Bullimore J, Fowler JF, Haybittle JL, Howard N, Laing AH, Lindup R. Final report of the general clinical result of the British Institute of Radiology fractionation study of the 3F wk versus 5F wk in radiotherapy of carcinoma of the laryngo-pharynx. Br J Radiol 1990;63:169.
765. Williams SD, Velez-Garcia E, Essessee I, Ratkin G, Birch R, Einhorn LH. Chemotherapy for head and neck cancer: Comparison of cisplatin + vinblastine + bleomycin versus methotrexate. Cancer 1986;57:18.
766. Wilson JS, Walker EP. Reconstruction of the lower lip. Head Neck Surg 1981;4:29.
767. Wingo PA, Tong T, Bolden S. Cancer statistics 1995. CA 1995;45:1, 8–30.
768. Winn DM, Blot WJ, Shy CM, Pickle LW, Toledo A, Fraumeni JF Jr. Snuff dipping and oral cancer among women in the southern United States. N Engl J Med 1981;304:745.
769. Winn DM, Ziegler RG, Pickle LW, Gridley G, Blot WJ, Hoover RN. Diet in the etiology of oral and pharyngeal cancer among women from the southern United States. Cancer Res 1984;44:1216.
770. Wittes RE. Chemotherapy of head and neck cancer. Otolaryngol Clin North Am 1980;13:515.
771. Wittes RE, Cvitkovic E, Shah J, Gerold FP, Strong WE. *cis*-Dichlorodiammineplatinum (II) in the treatment of epidermoid carcinoma of the head and neck. Cancer Treat Rep 1977;61:359.
772. Wittes R, Heller K, Randolph V, Howard J, Vallejo A, Farr H, Harrold C, Gerold F, Shah J, Shapiro R, Strong E. *cis*-Dichlorodiammineplatinum(II)-based chemotherapy as initial treatment of advanced head and neck cancer. Cancer Treat Rep 1979;63:1533.
773. Wolf GT, Carey TE, Schmaltz SP, McClatchey KD, Poore J, Glaser L, Hayashida DJ, Hsu S. Altered antigen expression predicts outcome in squamous cell carcinoma of the head and neck. JNCI 1990;82:1566.
774. Wolf GT, Hudson JL, Peterson KA, Miller HL, McClatchey D. Lymphocyte subpopulation infiltrating squamous carcinomas of the head and neck: correlations with extent of tumor and prognosis. Otolaryngol Head Neck Surg 1986;95:142.
775. Wolf GT, Makuch RW, Baker SR. Predictive factors for tumor response to pre-operative chemotherapy in patients with squamous carcinoma. The Head and Neck Contracts Group. Cancer 1984;54:2869.
776. Wolf GT, Truelson JM, Beals T, Fisher S. Nuclear area and adjusted DNA index: A new correlate of prognosis in squamous carcinoma of the larynx. Proc Am Assoc Cancer Res 1990;31:189.
777. Wong CS, Cummings BJ. The place of radiation therapy in the treatment of squamous cell carcinoma of nasal vestibule: a review. Acta Oncol 1988;27:203.
778. Wong DT. Amplification of the c-erb B1 oncogene in chemically-induced oral carcinomas. Carcinogenesis 1987;8:1963.
779. Woods RL, Fox RM, Tattersall MH. Methotrexate treatment of squamous-cell head and neck cancers: dose-response evaluation. Br Med J (Clin Res) 1981;282:600.
780. Wookey H, Ash C, Welsh WK, Mustard RA. The treatment of oral cancer by a combination of radiotherapy and surgery. Ann Surg 1951;134:529.
781. Wu C-J, Su C-C, Hsu W-L, Jen Y-M. Locally advanced nasopharyngeal carcinoma treated with radiotherapy plus chemotherapy: analysis of patterns of failure in different treatment arms (abstract 72). Proc Head Neck Res Workshop 1994;490.
782. Wynne CJ, Kearsley JH. Merkel cell tumor: a chemosensitive skin cancer. Cancer 1988;62:28.
783. Xu X-C, Lee JS, Lippman SM, Hong WK, Lotan R. Increased expression of cytokeratins CK8 and CK19 are associated with premalignancy in head and neck tumorigenesis. Cancer Epidemiol Biomarkers Prev 1995;4:871.
784. Yates A, Crumley RL. Surgical treatment of pyriform sinus cancer: a retrospective study. Laryngoscope 1984;94:1586.
785. Yu MC. Diet and nasopharyngeal carcinoma. Prog Clin Biol Res 1990;346:93.
786. Yuen A, Medina JE, Goepfert H, Fletcher G. Management of stage T3 and T4 glottic carcinoma. Am J Surg 1984;148:467.
787. Zbaeren P, Lehmann W. Frequency and sites of distant metastases in head and neck squamous cell carcinoma. Arch Otolaryngol Head Neck Surg 1987;113:762.
788. Zeng Y. Seroepidemiological studies on nasopharyngeal carcinoma in China. Adv Cancer Res 1985;44:121.
789. Zenner HP. Selective killing of laryngeal carcinoma cells by a monoclonal immunotoxin. Ann Otol Rhinol Laryngol 1986;95:115.

CHAPTER 106

Odontogenic Tumors

GEORGE T. GALLAGHER AND GERALD SHKLAR

Introduction

Odontogenic tumors comprise an unusual group of lesions of the jaws, derived from primordial tooth-forming tissues, and presenting in a large number of histologic patterns. Some of these lesions, particularly the odontomas, are now interpreted as developmental malformations or hamartomatous lesions rather than true neoplasms. Other lesions, such as ameloblastoma, are accepted as true neoplasms and must be diagnosed and treated as such. The true odontogenic tumors are essentially benign lesions but infiltrate the adjacent bone between the spicules of the medulla. This form of bony infiltration, common to all benign tumors of bone, such as giant cell tumors, is not the true invasiveness of malignant tumors but represents a clinical problem, in that the tumor can recur after surgical therapy if the bony margins still contain some of the tumor infiltration.

In general terms, odontogenic tumors tend to be more common in younger patients, but can occur at any age (9a, 29). They originate in the jaws and usually are found in the tooth-bearing sites. The odontomas are often associated with impacted or missing teeth. Since the odontomas represent maldevelopment of a tooth bud, that tooth will not develop. The common sites for odontogenic tumors are the mandibular molar region and the maxillary cuspid region. The odontogenic tumors are slowly growing and asymptomatic. Pain is not a feature of benign tumors of the jaws but is a common symptom of malignant tumors of the jaws. The odontogenic tumors are expansile lesions and may expand the bony cortex, but will not invade or perforate it. Radiographically, the odontomas will present as mixed radiolucent and radiopaque lesions. Among true neoplasms, the radiographic appearance may vary from entirely radiolucent to mixed.

The odontomas usually occur in cyst-like cavities with a connective tissue lining. They can be removed surgically by simple enucleation and will not recur since they are not true neoplasms and do not infiltrate the contiguous bone. Neoplasms such as ameloblastoma are benign tumors and treated by conservative surgical removal. Simple enucleation rarely offers a permanent cure for ameloblastoma since recurrence of the tumor will eventually occur from the infiltrative foci at the tumor margin. A block resection is favored, leaving the cortical lower border of the mandible intact. These benign tumors are relatively unaffected by radiation, and the risks of radiation in stimulating the development of a malignant tumor or of radiation necrosis is unwarranted for a benign tumor.

Over the years, very extensive and complicated classifications have been used for the odontogenic tumors and related lesions. A simple classification will suffice, based upon the derivation of the lesions and the degree of cellular differentiation involved (Table 106.1).

Other lesions, which probably are different from odontogenic lesions, but which are frequently included in this general topic are: Periapical Cemental Dysplasia and Gigantiform Cementoma; Peripheral Odontogenic Fibroma and Odontogenic Epithelial Hamartoma of Gingiva; Craniopharyngioma; Adamantinoma of Long Bones; and Teratoma.

Odontogenic lesions share two major characteristics: 1) they arise from tissue with the potential for differentiation into tooth or periodontal ligament structures, and 2) they are found predominantly to arise at tooth-bearing sites. Variable, but distinctive features of odontogenic lesions include: 1) formation of tooth-related extracellular substance, some of which may calcify and be visible on radiographs, and 2) epithelial-mesenchymal interactions ("induction").

Odontogenic lesions vary widely in their degree of differentiation, and there is a rough correlation between the degree of differentiation and the biologic behavior associated with any given lesion. True malignant transformation of benign odontogenic lesions or the development of malignancy de novo from odontogenic tissues have both been reported, but such occurrences are extremely rare. In general, the less-differentiated odontogenic lesions (the immature ones) are more likely to have indistinct radiographic borders, invasive growth patterns, and relatively aggressive clinical behavior, while the mature or well-differentiated entities are more likely to produce recognizable extracellular product, to be well circumscribed, and to be self-limiting in terms of growth.

Although odontogenic lesions may be discovered at any age, certain lesions are typically found in patients of particular age groups and at certain sites; knowledge of these patterns, plus careful radiographic interpretation, enables the astute clinician to make an accurate clinical diagnosis of odontogenic lesions fairly frequently.

Clinical, Radiographic, Histologic Features

EPITHELIAL ODONTOGENIC LESIONS

Enamel pearl is a developmental defect whereby enamel is deposited on the root surface of a tooth separate from the

Table 106.1. Classification of Odontogenic Tumors

	Epithelial	Mixed	Mesenchymal
Immature	Ameloblastoma	Ameloblastic fibroma	Myxoma
Intermediate	Calcifying odontogenic cyst (Gorlin lesion) Calcifying epithelial odontogenic tumor	Ameloblastic fibro-odontoma	Cementoblastoma (true cementoma)
Mature	Adenomatoid odontogenic tumor Squamous odontogenic tumor Enamel pearl?	Odontoma	Odontogenic fibroma (central ossifying/cementifying fibroma)

coronal enamel. Such defects are most commonly found in the furcation region of maxillary molars. On the radiograph, enamel pearls appear as rounded, well-circumscribed densities associated with tooth roots. These nodules are of little clinical significance, except that they may be complicating factors in periodontal disease, and they may contain cores of dentin and projections of dental pulp that could complicate their removal.

Squamous Odontogenic Tumor (S.O.T.)

S.O.T. is a well-differentiated odontogenic tumor composed of islands or sheets of squamous epithelium that lack recognizable features of enamel organ differentiation (16, 28). The typical clinical presentation is of a slowly growing, well-circumscribed radiolucent lesion in a young adult, which is associated with the cervical portion of a tooth root. No site is really typical, but maxillary anterior and mandibular posterior regions have been most frequently affected. Multifocal lesions have been reported more frequently than in the case of other odontogenic tumors. This is an uncommon lesion, so it should not be high on the differential diagnostic list when considering radiolucent jaw lesions; if the clinical situation fits, however, and at exploration one discovers that a solid fleshy lesion is associated with a vital tooth root, then the S.O.T. becomes more likely.

Microscopically, the lesion consists of bland nests of squamous cells. No palisading or polarization of peripheral cells should be demonstrable.

Aggressive behavior or recurrences seem to be rare in S.O.T., but care must be taken to differentiate the lesion histologically from acanthomatous ameloblastoma, odontogenic carcinoma, and central mucoepidermoid carcinoma, all of which are more serious.

Nests of squamous epithelium may be found in the walls of odontogenic cysts or in small gingival nodules that resemble the S.O.T. microscopically; these may be called odontogenic epithelial hamartomas if they seem to lack the characteristics of a true tumor.

Adenomatoid Odontogenic Tumor (A.O.T.)

A.O.T. is a well-circumscribed odontogenic tumor composed of sheets and nests of spindle-shaped epithelial cells resembling somewhat the stellate reticulum of the enamel organ, along with palisaded, polarized ameloblast-like cells, which frequently produce extracellular product (1, 8, 15). The typical clinical presentation is that of a well-circumscribed radiolucency (sometimes with small foci of calcification) associated with an unerupted tooth in the anterior maxilla of a young female patient. In general, affected patients are likely to be in the second and third decade of life, females are more frequently affected than males, the maxilla is more frequently affected than the mandible, the anterior regions are more frequently affected than the posterior, and most A.O.T.s are associated with unerupted tooth crowns (that is, they are in a dentigerous relationship to a tooth). No other odontogenic lesion has this clinical pattern.

A.O.T. is not common, but many may have been misdiagnosed in the past as ameloblastomas; true incidence is difficult to know. A.O.T. should be considered in the differential diagnosis of a radiolucent lesion about the crown of an impacted maxillary canine, especially.

Microscopically, the main cell type consists of basophilic spindle-shaped epithelial cells in sheets and whorls. Focally, one finds columnar cells in duct-like array or forming rosettes, and frequent deposits of eosinophilic, hyaline material are seen. Dystrophic calcifications are not uncommon, and these are usually found within the epithelium. Pleomorphism and mitotic activity are not expected.

A.O.T. is differentiated from ameloblastoma microscopically by the absence of polarized or palisaded cells at the periphery of the epithelial aggregates and by the production of extracellular product and calcifications. A.O.T. is distinguished from C.E.O.T. (see below) by the predominantly spindle-cell morphology it exhibits and its failure to produce amyloid.

Clinical behavior is generally that of a slow-growing, expansile lesion that seldom, if ever, would be expected to recur after conservative removal.

Calcifying Epithelial Odontogenic Tumor (C.E.O.T.)

C.E.O.T. is a moderately differentiated odontogenic tumor composed of somewhat pleomorphic and polyhedral epithelial cells in sheets and nests, along with extracellular material that has the characteristics of amyloid. Calcifications are quite commonly found, associated both with the epithelial cells and with the amyloid material. This lesion is also sometimes called Pindborg Tumor, after the pathologist who first described it as distinct from ameloblastoma (11, 19, 27, 31). The typical clinical presentation is similar in most respects to that of ameloblastoma, in that there is a predominance of cases in adults, in the mandible, and in the posterior region. The lesion exhibits radiolucency, sometimes with small focal opacities, and may be associated with a tooth (Fig. 106.1).

The histologic appearance is quite characteristic; the growth pattern is usually that of a solid lesion with amorphous amphophilic extracellular material mixed with islands or sheets of polyhedral epithelial cells, some of which may undergo degeneration. The nuclei of the cells may be large and basophilic, but mitotic activity is absent. Special stains for amyloid are positive when applied to the extracellular material. Calcifications are frequently spherical and lamellar (Fig. 106.2).

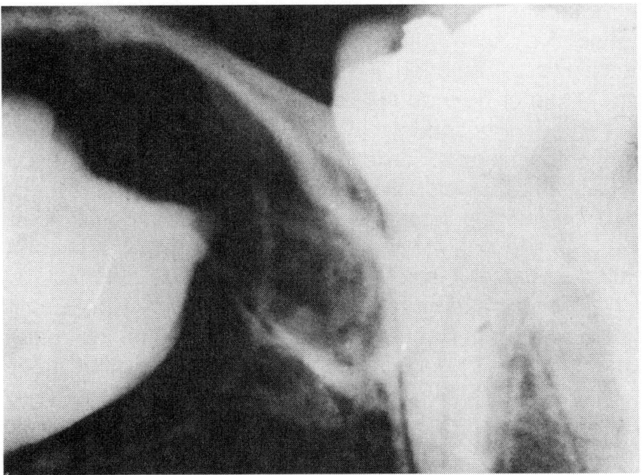

Figure 106.1. Calcifying epithelial odontogenic tumor with impacted third molar tooth.

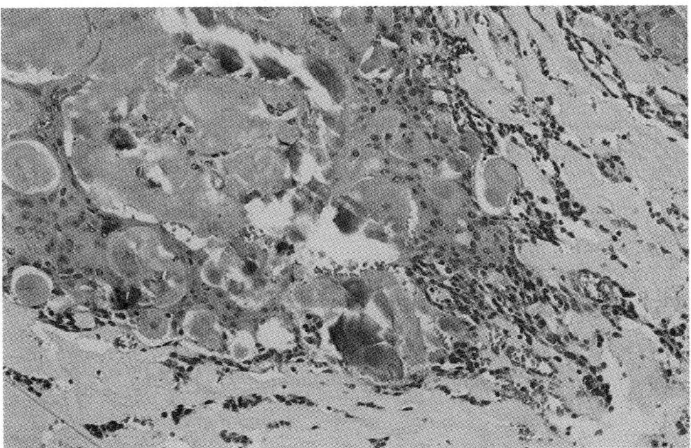

Figure 106.2. Microscopic appearance of calcifying epithelial odontogenic tumor showing clusters of epithelial cells, calcifications, and amyloid material. 200x.

No ameloblastic differentiation is noted in the epithelial islands, and the cohesive nature of the epithelial cell nests, along with the absence of mitotic activity, militates against a malignant interpretation.

This lesion, while uncommon, should be considered in the differential diagnosis of posterior jaw radiolucencies in the adult, especially if there are foci of radiopacity within the lesion. The clinical course is usually that of slow growth and uncommon recurrence, but radiographic evidence of poorly circumscribed borders should suggest the need for removal of bone to ensure tumor-free margins.

Calcifying Odontogenic Cyst (C.O.C.)

This term is applied to a heterogeneous group of lesions, which have in common the histologic finding of ghost-cell keratinization (22). Many lesions, histologically designated as C.O.C. (or Gorlin cyst), are probably best viewed as simple odontogenic cysts that happen to contain ghost cells, as nothing about that alteration per se seems to predispose to altered biologic behavior. Often, the lesions demonstrate radiopaque foci, and this usually designates a moderately well-differentiated odontogenic lesion. Many C.O.C.s are associated with either impacted teeth or odontomas.

Histologically, ghost cells are squamous epithelial cells that lose their nuclei as they keratinize, leaving empty space in the cytoplasm where the nuclei had been. Frequently, foci of keratinizing cells escape into the connective tissue, whereupon a foreign-body reaction with inflammation and giant cells supervenes. Calcium may deposit in the foci of keratinization, but no tooth-related matrix is generally produced. In one rare variant form, designated the type *II* ghost cell lesion, a tumor-like proliferation of epithelium with ghost cells is noted, along with production (perhaps by mesenchyme) of an osteoid or dentin-like extracellular substance.

The clinical course of most ghost-cell lesions is similar to that of a dentigerous cyst, with relatively easy removal and a low frequency of recurrence. A few of the rare variants may behave more aggressively.

Ameloblastoma

This immature benign odontogenic lesion replicates the histologic appearance of the early enamel organ, with palisaded, polarized ameloblast-like cells at the border between epithelium and connective tissue, and stellate reticulum-like cells centrally (24, 35, 37). No extracellular product is produced.

The typical clinical presentation is that of a slowly growing, radiolucent, destructive lesion in the mandibular molar-ramus region of a young adult (over 50% are first discovered between the ages of 20 and 40 years) (2, 18, 24). The radiolucency usually has well-circumscribed borders. Early lesions usually appear unilocular (Fig. 106.3) (30), while established ones are generally multilocular (Figs. 106.4 and 106.5). Calcifications within the lesion are never found. Approximately 20% of ameloblastomas appear in the dentiger-

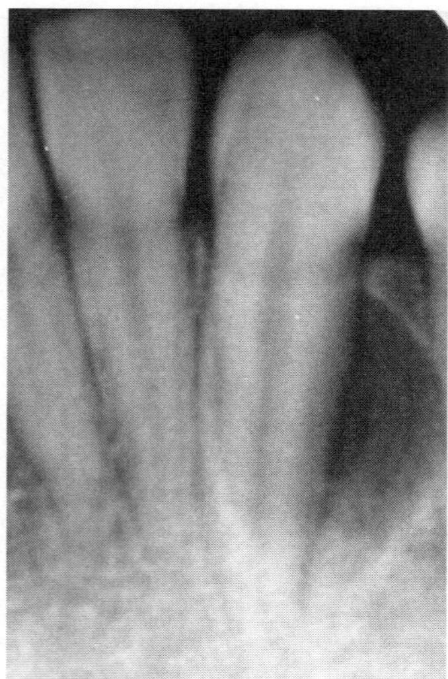

Figure 106.3. Unilocular ameloblastoma between mandibular cuspid and bicuspid teeth.

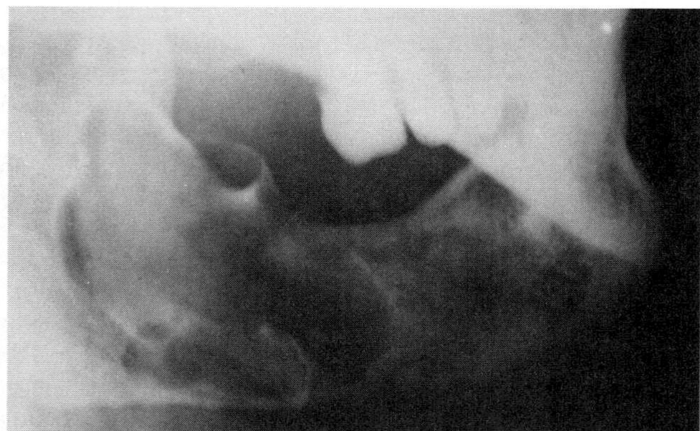

Figure 106.4. Large cystic ameloblastoma in posterior mandible.

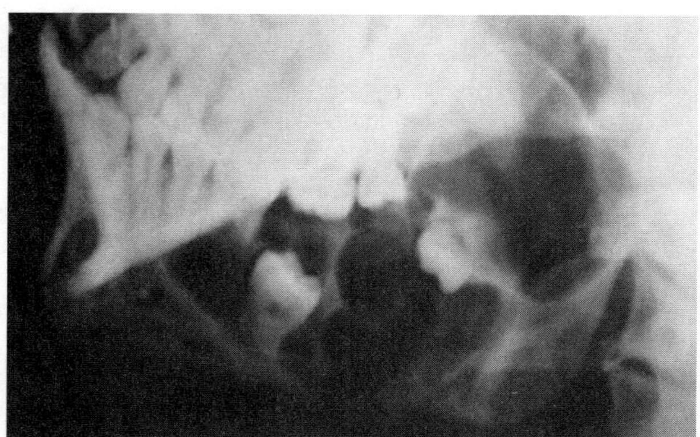

Figure 106.5. Large multilocular ameloblastoma of mandible with two impacted teeth. The entire body and ramus of the mandible are involved.

ous relationship to unerupted teeth, and these usually are noted before the age of 30. Some ameloblastoma-like lesions may arise from cyst lining (23, 32) and proliferate entirely *within* the cyst lumen; if there is no invasive component, such lesions are termed *unicystic ameloblastoma,* and probably behave as cysts, with little potential for recurrence. "Mural" ameloblastomas are those that arise in cyst linings and proliferate *away* from the cyst lumen, invading bone; these lesions behave as conventional ameloblastomas, with a high recurrence potential.

Microscopically, in ameloblastoma one sees proliferating epithelial islands and strands, a mature collagenous stroma, and an invasive pattern of growth (Fig. 106.6). The identification of mature collagen fibers in the stroma is very important for distinguishing the ameloblastoma from ameloblastic fibroma, a mixed odontogenic tumor. The tumor cells exhibit both palisading (alignment of the cell nuclei at one level in the cells) and polarization (migration of the nuclei to one end of the cell). Of great importance, also, is the nature of the polarization; in ameloblasts, secretion of matrix occurs toward connective tissue, with the nuclei polarized *away* from connective tissue, an orientation that is almost unique to this cell type. Little or no inductive effect occurs in ameloblastoma, so we see no mesenchymal differentiation and no matrix production by the tumor cells. (In *normal* tooth formation, we do not speak of "ameloblast" until actual enamel matrix formation is initiated; columnar cells with palisaded, polarized nuclei that are not yet producing matrix are most properly called "preameloblasts.")

Histologic patterns of ameloblastoma have led to classification of subgroups such as acanthomatous ameloblastoma (3) with development of keratin-like substance within the epithelial islands or plexiform ameloblastoma (13), with an extensive network of strands with a loose inner reticulum. These histologic variants do not appear to relate to different clinical behavior of the lesions.

The stellate reticulum within the nests and cords of columnar epithelium tends to undergo degeneration, forming mi-

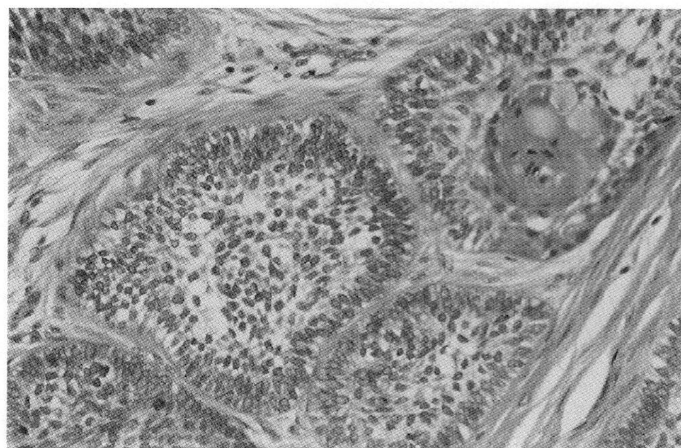

Figure 106.6. Microscopic appearance of ameloblastoma showing cords and nests of ameloblastic cells with a central stellate reticulum. The ameloblastic structures are surrounded by a fibrous connective tissue matrix. 200x.

croscopic cysts (Fig. 106.7) (20). The microcysts then expand to form large cystic spaces within the tumor and give the ameloblastoma its multicystic gross and radiologic appearance (Fig. 106.8). No calcifications are found in ameloblastomas, not even dystrophic calcification.

Ameloblastoma is a slowly growing lesion (mitoses are hardly ever seen), but, unlike its better-differentiated epithelial relatives, it displays a marked propensity for invasive growth, spreading between trabeculae of medullary bone for a moderate distance beyond its apparent radiographic or surgical margins. Seldom, however, does the tumor penetrate the cortical plate of bone, although expansion of bony cortex is sometimes seen in longstanding lesions.

The clinical behavior of the tumor relates mainly to the difficulty at surgery of establishing tumor-free margins; recurrence is predictable unless 1 to 2 cm of clinically uninvolved bone is resected in addition to that which is obviously infiltrated by tumor. Curettage is inadequate treatment; recommended approaches involve en bloc excision, usually with preservation of the inferior border of the mandible. Maxillary lesions, although less frequently encountered (5, 36), are more dangerous than mandibular ones due to the tendency for the lesion to spread more extensively in the more porous maxillary bone and the possibility of the involvement of the cranial base. Patients who have been treated for ameloblastoma should be followed carefully with radiographs to recognize recurrence early.

Craniopharyngioma is a tumor that occurs within the skull with palisading and polarizing nuclei, in the region around the pituitary gland, and it is said to arise from remnants of the stomadeal ectoderm that invaginates to form Rathke's pouch. Fusion of Rathke's pouch with a process of the forebrain produces the anterior and posterior pituitary in the adult. Although epithelial remnants of the craniopharyngeal duct are said to be quite common, craniopharyngioma develops infrequently, accounting for fewer than 5% of all C.N.S. tumors (see XXIV) (6).

Clinical features of craniopharyngioma relate to destruction of the pituitary (diabetes insipidus) or compression of nearby cranial nerves; radiographically, a suprasellar mass,

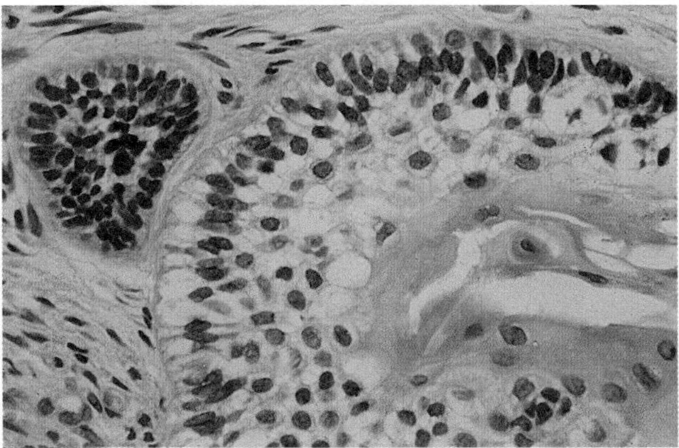

Figure 106.7. High power view showing rystic degeneration of stellate reticulum. The ameloblastic cells are columnar with Polarizing and Palisading nuclei. 400x.

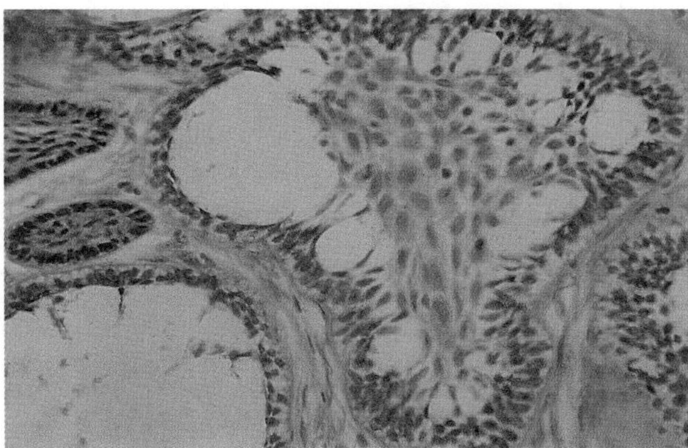

Figure 106.8. Cystic development within the islands of an ameloblastoma. 400x.

often with calcifications (75% of cases), is the usual finding. Although the most common presenting age is in the second and third decades, any age may be affected.

Microscopic findings are quite variable; lesions in children seem to be rather invasive, with epithelium in islands or sheets, often showing ghost cell keratinization, calcification, and foreign-body reactions similar to that which is seen in the C.O.C. (see above). Adult lesions may be more squamous in their morphology without calcifications or necrosis. The resemblance of those lesions to ameloblastoma, although frequently cited, is usually not great.

Prognosis in craniopharyngioma must be guarded, since complete excision is difficult and damage to vital structures is a risk. Subtotal removal followed by radiation results in outcomes at least as favorable as treatment by total removal alone (38) and superior to surgery alone (39).

Adamantinoma is a tumor of long bones with a striking predilection for occurrence in the tibial diaphysis (79% of reported cases) (26). Its name implies a relationship to enamel organ, given originally because odontogenic lesions are the only other primary tumors in which epithelial elements are seen to arise within bone. Although recent studies show that the cells in adamantinoma are probably, in fact, epithelial (the cells have desmosomes and produce keratin), there is no good explanation of the origin of the lesion. No enamel organ differentiation is found in these lesions, nor is toothy product produced.

The clinical course is quite variable, with some lesions behaving quite aggressively and sometimes metastasizing. Histologic features cannot be used to predict clinical behavior.

MIXED ODONTOGENIC LESIONS

Odontoma

This is a term applied to odontogenic proliferations in which enamel, dentin, and pulp are present within the lesion; this represents terminally differentiated odontogenic tissue. Although toothy tissues are present, the structures formed are arranged either as collections of small, morphologically atypical teeth ("compound" odontoma) or as a disorderly mass of dental tissues that lack recognizable tooth form altogether ("complex" odontoma).

The typical clinical presentation of odontoma is that of a well-circumscribed radiopacity, usually located either in the anterior maxilla (compound type), or posterior mandible (complex type), which may be associated with an unerupted tooth but which is otherwise asymptomatic. An important finding is the presence of toothy structures or a radiodensity indicative of the presence of enamel (Fig. 106.9). Generally, a radiolucent rim is noted between the opaque area and the surrounding bone. The common presenting age is during the second decade, but since the growth of the lesion is self-limiting, it may persist and be discovered during later life. In occasional cases, a dentigerous cyst may develop in association with an odontoma, and this would appear as a larger surrounding radiolucency.

Microscopically, one sees mixtures of odontogenic epithelium and mesenchyme, with recognizable enamel matrix, dentin, pulp, and periodontal ligament. Two major subgroups of odontomas are recognized. In a compound composite odontoma, all dental tissues are present and are arranged in the form of numerous miniature teeth. In a complex composite odontoma, the dental tissues are arranged in a haphazard pattern and do not resemble tooth-like structures

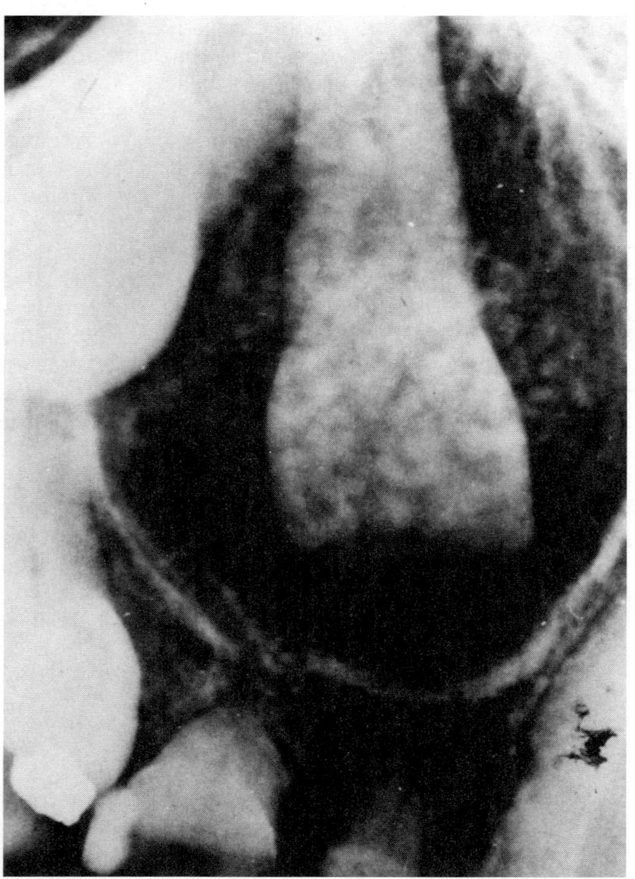

Figure 106.9. Radiograph of complex composite odontoma with impacted maxillary central incisor tooth. The calcified materials within the odontoma appear as opaque granules.

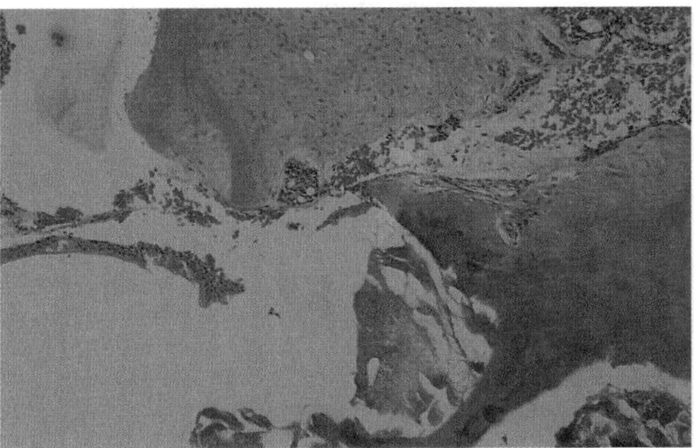

Figure 106.10. Microscopic features of complex composite odontoma showing enamel matrix, dentin, odontogenic epithelial rests, reduced enamel epithelium, and fibroblastic connective tissue. 100x.

(Fig. 106.10). No proliferations of immature odontogenic tissues should be found in the uncomplicated odontoma; rare cases of ghost-cell lesion or ameloblastoma in association with odontomas have been reported, but these lesions' behavior is usually dominated by the epithelial proliferation and may be more aggressive.

The clinical behavior of odontomas is more in keeping with the view that they are developmental disorders of the odonotogenic apparatus rather than true neoplasms. They are usually surgically removed so that normal alignment of teeth is not jeopardized by pressure of the odontoma. The surgical procedure is usually quite straightforward. Complications are rare, and recurrences are not expected.

Ameloblastic Fibro-odontoma

This name is applied to an odontogenic lesion that exhibits mixed epithelial-mesenchymal proliferation and both mature and immature areas (33). There has been a controversy as to whether, with the passage of time, such lesions would become completely mature odontomas. At present, the prevailing opinion is that at least some ameloblastic fibro-odontomas would never be expected to progress to maturity.

The usual clinical presentation of ameloblastic fibro-odontoma is somewhat similar to that described in connection with an odontoma developing in a dentigerous cyst; there is an expansile lesion that is mostly radiolucent and well circumscribed but that contains foci of radiopacity that may resemble teeth. Teenagers and young adults are most commonly affected.

The microscopic appearance is that of a combination of ameloblastic fibroma and odontoma, frequently with fairly well-formed teeth. Since tooth-like structures are frequently removed from soft tissues before histologic processing, the diagnosis might be missed on the basis of the soft-tissue specimen alone.

Clinical behavior of this lesion seems to be similar to that of the ameloblastic fibroma. There are reported instances in which lesions have behaved rather aggressively following multiple attempted excisions and recurrences.

Ameloblastic Fibroma

This is an immature mixed odontogenic neoplasm within which is commonly observed a very slight inductive effect, but in which no extracellular matrix is elaborated (33, 40). The usual clinical presentation is that of a radiolucent, expansile lesion in the posterior mandible of a young person. The radiographic appearance is indistinguishable from ameloblastoma (no calcified foci are present), but the lesion occurs usually in children or teenagers rather than in adults. A dentigerous relationship to an unerupted tooth seems to be relatively uncommon, but the lesion may present as if it were a primordial cyst (a radiolucency replacing a tooth).

Microscopically, the lesion exhibits proliferating odontogenic epithelium, which may resemble dental lamina (cords of cuboidal cells) or enamel organ (like ameloblastoma). In addition, there is invariably a substantial amount of immature mesenchymal tissue, consisting of spindle-shaped or stellate fibroblastic cells that are widely separated by myxoid-appearing extracellular material. No mature collagen fibers are seen. The mesenchymal tissue resembles dental papilla, and a hyalinized basement membrane-like product is frequently observed at the interface between mesenchyme and epithelium ("inductive" effect). No calcified material is present. Mitotic activity should be absent.

The expected clinical course is that of a slowly growing noninvasive lesion; although the ameloblastic fibroma may become quite large and produce substantial clinical deformity, it is usually easily excised. Recurrence may occur if tumor is left behind, however, and there are reports of lesions that seemed to have evolved into mesenchymal malignancies when subjected to multiple incomplete surgical attempts. Hypercellularity and mitotic activity among the mesenchymal components are worrisome pathologic findings in this regard. Probably, a valid approach to the ameloblastic fibroma involves an initial attempt at conservative removal by curettage; those lesions that recur should probably be treated at the second attempt by a more aggressive, en bloc type excision. Radiation treatment would seem to be contraindicated, as in most benign conditions.

MESENCHYMAL ODONTOGENIC LESIONS

Odontogenic Fibroma

This name is applied to lesions of the jaws that behave as though they are neoplastic, and that show a propensity for production of extracellular mesenchymal matrix substances that are associated with periodontal ligament.

The clinical presentation is of an expansile central lesion, which begins as a radiolucency (12), but which develops progressive diffuse radiopacity with the passage of time. The molar region of the mandible is the most common site, and the lesion usually appears spherical, displacing the cortical plate of bone as it expands but without penetration or periosteal reactive bone formation. No connection with tooth roots is generally observed, nor is there pain. A radiolucent rim separates the lesion from surrounding bone. Young adults are most commonly affected (9).

Microscopically, the lesion consists of mature fibroblastic elements, with varying amounts of collagen, osteoid, or cementum in a manner reminiscent of periodontal ligament (Fig. 106.11). "Cementifying fibroma" or "cemento-ossifying fibroma" are names that have been applied to these lesions, according to the amounts and types of products observed, but distinctions of this sort have little, if any, clinical relevance. Just as epithelial nests may be observed in periodontal ligament, some odontogenic fibromas possess epithelial elements; these are most frequently sparsely distributed, rudimentary epithelial nests, without apparent inductive influence.

The expected clinical behavior is that of a slow-growing benign neoplasm. Excision is usually relatively easy, and recurrence is uncommon. Lesions that present as described here seem to have little malignant potential.

Peripheral Odontogenic Fibroma

This is a lesion of gingival soft tissue that may resemble the central lesion histologically but that usually behaves as a self-limiting reactive nodule. The presence of odontogenic epithelial nests and/or calcified product has led to the suggestion that these might be neoplasms of odontogenic tissues, but in the absence of unlimited growth potential, this hypothesis is hard to support. Epithelial nests are common in gingiva (dental lamina rests of Serres), and gingival fibroblasts seem to readily express potential for calcified matrix production; although the occasional true neoplasm of gingival mesenchyme probably does occur, the vast majority of gingival "fibromas" are unlikely to be neoplastic.

Cementoblastoma

This is a distinctive odontogenic lesion that is always attached to the root of a tooth and that exhibits robust cementum production. The usual clinical presentation is associated with pain and tenderness in a mandibular posterior tooth of a teenager or young adult. Radiographically, there is a radiolucency with localized disruption of the periodontal ligament space and lamina dura, usually involving a single root. The tooth possesses a vital pulp (confusion with periapical

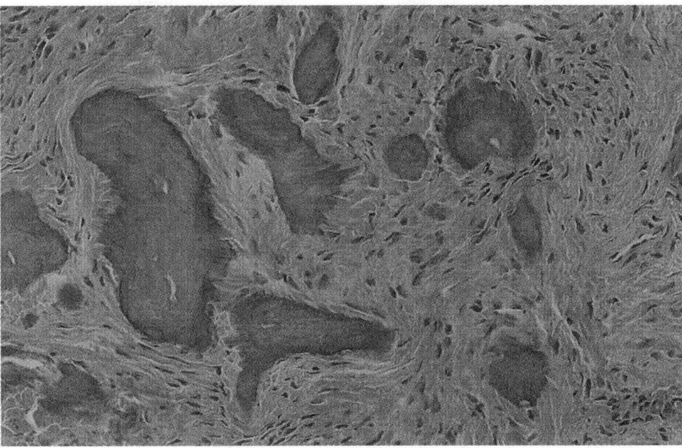

Figure 106.11. Microscopic appearance of odontogenic fibroma with some cementum forming. 80×.

cyst or granuloma may occur if the tooth happens to be carious, but the cemental lesion, per se, is not associated with pulpal pathosis). As the lesion enlarges, radiopacity develops, first in the central portions, and, in the well-developed lesion, the opacity is connected to the cementum of the root, with a peripheral radiolucent rim.

The microscopic appearance may be somewhat alarming, with large numbers of hyperchromatic, basophilic cells depositing cementum matrix, which may resemble osteoid in some cases. Actual cellular atypia is absent, and if the clinical information is available, the microscopic interpretation is not too difficult. Mitotic activity is not prominent.

The clinical course is of unlimited expansile growth; if the tooth is extracted without curettage of the lesion, the cementoblastoma continues to grow. In times past, the affected tooth was always sacrificed; recently, there have been reports of attempts to treat the lesion via apicoectomy, with salvage of the tooth and later endodontic therapy. Malignant transformation is not reported.

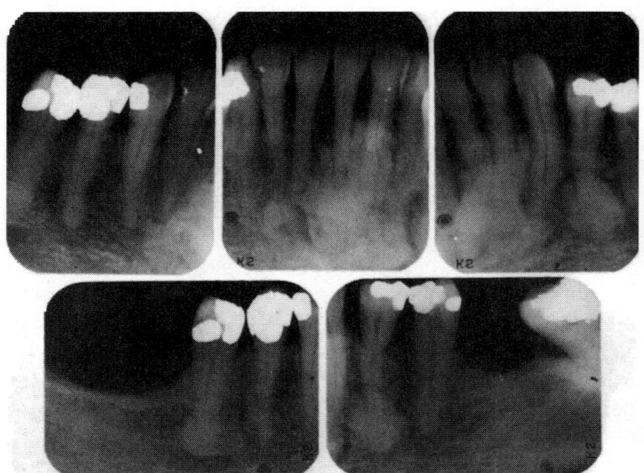

Figure 106.12. Multiple cementomas of the mandible at the apices of the teeth (periapical cemental dysplasia).

Osteoblastoma and Osteoid Osteoma

These are lesions of bone with a histologic resemblance to one another and to cementoblastoma. They are not associated with the roots of teeth, and they occur in bone generally, not being confined to occurrence within the jaws. These lesions are best considered as benign tumors of bone and so will not be further treated here.

Cementoma

This is a term used with respect to a cemental lesion that is probably not neoplastic, but that is of great clinical importance. Cementoblastoma is sometimes called "true cementoma" to distinguish it from this other condition, which would be better termed *periapical cemental dysplasia.* The clinical presentation of periapical cemental dysplasia is that of asymptomatic periapical radiolucencies involving, usually, mandibular anterior teeth. The patients are frequently young adult black females. The teeth possess vital pulps. The lesion(s) may be single or multiple, and the lesion evolves radiographically in a predictable fashion: the radiolucencies may be observed to enlarge to a certain size, after which the lesions stop growing and begin to opacify. Finally, the lesions opacify completely and seem to become confluent with the tooth and the surrounding bone (Fig. 106.12). If there is no clinical intervention, no adverse sequelae result.

The microscopic appearance varies depending upon the stage at which biopsy is performed, but the lesion is indistinguishable from fibro-osseous lesions or odontogenic fibroma.

The importance of the lesion lies in the fact that needless extraction or endodontic therapy may be carried out if the lesion is not recognized by the clinician. Periodic follow-up is the only management required.

Gigantiform Cementoma

This is another lesion with a marked predilection for black females, and this is characterized by diffuse patchy radiopacities throughout the jaws. There is a histologic resemblance to other osteoid or cementum-forming jaw lesions, but the true nature of the condition is still unknown. It seems unlikely to be a neoplastic disorder but rather to represent a florid development of periapical cemental dysplasia. The relationship of the lesion to infection or other inflammatory influences has been postulated but is unproven. Management is conservative, but the condition may be associated with pain, and the clinical problems may become complex. As with periapical cemental dysplasia, the diagnosis is usually made on clinical and radiographic grounds, and biopsy should be *avoided* whenever possible.

Myxoma

Myxoma refers to a proliferation of fibroblastic elements that do not produce mature extracellular product. Although soft-tissue myxomatous tumors have been reported throughout the body, myxomas of bone seem to occur only in the jaws and are presumed, therefore, to arise from odontogenic tissues. The usual clinical presentation is that of an expansile, ill-defined radiolucency of the jaw in a young adult. Symptoms are variable, and growth is usually slow.

Myxoma is relatively invasive, and at surgery a gelatinous consistency may be noted. The microscopic appearance is that of bony replacement by a myxoid mass without mature collagen formation. No giant cells, adipocytes, or neurogenic elements should be noted. Mitoses should not be found. The tissue somewhat resembles dental papilla.

The clinical course is unpredictable, since complete excision by conservative approaches is often very difficult. Persistent destructive growth is frequently encountered, and wide margins may be required for definitive treatment. Although mitotic activity, hypercellularity, and more rapid growth may characterize some lesions, metastatic spread seems distinctly uncommon.

MALIGNANT ODONTOGENIC TUMORS

The odontogenic tumors and tumor-like lesions are to be considered benign and managed as such. Malignant odontogenic tumors have been described but are *exceedingly* rare. They are either an ameloblastic sarcoma (7, 21), in which an ameloblastoma-like component is seen within a fibrosarcoma, or a carcinoma (34) arising from ameloblastic cells, either within an ameloblastoma or de novo from ameloblastic cells within the mandible. As in all malignant tumors, they are characterized microscopically by hypercellularity, pleomorphism, and abnormal and increased mitotic activity. Pain and paresthesia are clinical features of all malignant tumors of the jaws. The prognosis and management of *ameloblastic* sarcoma is similar to fibrosarcoma of the jaws (9b). The carcinomas arising in the jaws are undifferentiated and aggressive with a poor prognosis.

Management

The treatment of odontogenic tumors is surgical, conservative, and based on proper microscopic and clinical evaluation (14). The odontomas are well circumscribed, non-infiltrative, and usually surrounded with a connective tissue membrane. They can be enucleated, and the healing is uneventful. The ameloblastoma is an infiltrative tumor of bone, and simple enucleation will not remove finger-like projections of tumor into medullary bone at the margins of the lesion. This explains the recurrence of ameloblastoma following incomplete surgical removal. A block-resection is favored, leaving the lower border of the mandible intact. The cortex is rarely infiltrated. The block-resection may involve the sacrifice of adjacent teeth.

Radiation therapy is not indicated for odontogenic tumors, although some recent reports have reconsidered the question, using current techniques (4). The ameloblastoma is relatively resistent to radiation, and the risks of radiation are unwarranted for the management of a benign lesion where access is relatively easy and total surgical removal can be effected without significant complications.

References

1. Abrams AM, Melrose RJ, Howell FJ. Adenoameloblastoma. A clinical pathological study of ten new cases. Cancer 1968;22:175.
2. Adekeye EO. Ameloblastoma of the jaws: a survey of 109 Nigerian patients. J Oral Surg 1980;38:36.
3. Anneroth G, Heindahl A, Wersall J. Acanthomatous ameloblastoma. Int J Oral Surg 1980;9:231.
4. Atkinson CH, Harwood AR, Cummings BJ. Ameloblastoma of the jaw: a reappraisal of the role of megavoltage irradiation. Cancer 1984;53:869.
5. Batsakis JG, McClatchey KD. Ameloblastoma of the maxilla and peripheral ameloblastoma. Ann Otol Rhinol Laryngol 1983;92:532.
6. Bernstein M, Buchino J. The histologic similarity between craniopharyngioma and odontogenic lesions: a reappraisal. Oral Surg 1983;56:501.
7. Cataldo E, Nathanson N, Shklar G. Ameloblastic sarcoma of the mandible. Oral Surg 1963;16:953.
8. Courtney RM, Kerr DA. The odontogenic adenomatoid tumor. Oral Surg 1975;39:424.
9. Dahl E, Wolfson S, Haugen J. Central odontogenic fibroma. J Oral Surg 1981;39:120.
9a. Daley TD, Wysocki GP, Bringle GA. Relative incidence of odontogenic tumors and oral jaw cysts in a Canadian population. Oral Surg Oral Med Oral Pathol 1994;77:276–280.
9b. Dallera P, Bertoni F, Marchetti C, Bacchini P, Campobassi A. Ameloblastic fibrosarcoma of the jaw: report of five cases. J Cranio Maxillofac Surg 1994;22:349–354.
10. Eversole LR, Tomich CE, Cherrick HM. Histogenesis of odontogenic tumors. Oral Surg 1971;32:569.
11. Franklin CD, Pindborg JJ. The calcifying epithelial odontogenic tumor. Oral Surg 1976;42:753.
12. Gardner DG. The central odontogenic fibroma: an attempt at clarification. Oral Surg 1980;50:425.
13. Gardner DG, Corio RL. Plexiform unicystic ameloblastoma: a variant of ameloblastoma with a low-recurrence rate after enucleation. Cancer 1984;53:1730.
14. Gardner DG, Pecak AMJ. The treatment of ameloblastoma based on pathologic and anatomic principles. Cancer 1980;46:2514.
15. Giansanti JS, Someren A, Waldron CA. Odontogenic adenomatoid tumor (adenoameloblastoma). Oral Surg 1970;30:69.
16. Goldblatt LI, Brannon RB, Ellis GL. Squamous odontogenic tumor: report of five cases and review of the literature. Oral Surg 1982;54:187.
17. Gorlin RJ, Chaudhry AP, Pindborg JJ. Odontogenic tumors, classification, histopathology and clinical behavior in man and domestic animals. Cancer 1961;14:73.
18. Kahn MA. Ameloblastoma in young persons: a clinicopathologic analysis and etiologic investigation. Oral Surg 1989;67:706.
19. Krolls SO, Pindborg JJ. Calcifying epithelial odontogenic tumor. A survey of 23 cases and discussion of histomorphologic variations. Arch Pathol 1974;98:206.
20. Leider A, Eversole L, Barkin M. Cystic ameloblastoma. Oral Surg 1985;60:624.
21. Leider AS, Nelson JF, Trodahl JN. Ameloblastic fibrosarcoma of the jaws. Oral Surg 1972;33:559.
22. McGowan RH, Browne RM. The calcifying odontogenic cyst: a problem of preoperative diagnosis. Br J Oral Surg 1982;20:203.
23. McMillan MD, Smillie AC. Ameloblastomas associated with dentigerous cysts. Oral Surg 1981;51:489.
24. Mehlisch DR, Dahlin DC, Masson JK. Ameloblastoma. A clinicopathologic report. J Oral Surg 1972;30:9.
25. Minderjahn A. Incidence and clinical differentiation of odontogenic tumors. J Maxillofac Surg 1979;7:142.
26. Perez-Atayde A, Kozakewich H, Vawter G. Adamantinoma of the tibia. Cancer 1985;55:1015.
27. Pindborg JJ, Kramer IRH, Torloni H. Histologic typing of odontogenic tumors, jaw cysts, and allied lesions. International Histological Classification of Tumors, No. 5, Geneva: World Health Organization, 1971.
28. Pullon PA, Shafer WG, Elzay RP, Kerr DA, Corio RL. Squamous odontogenic tumor: report of six cases of a previously undescribed lesion. Oral Surg 1975;40:616.
29. Regezi JA, Kerr DA, Courtney RM. Odontogenic tumors: an analysis of 706 cases. J Oral Surg 1978;36:771.
30. Robinson L, Martinez MG. Unicystic ameloblastoma. A prognostically distinct entity. Cancer 1977;40:2278.
31. Sadeghi EM, Hopper TL. Calcifying epithelial odontogenic tumor. J Oral Surg 1982;40: 225.
32. Shteyer A, Lustmann J, Lewin-Epstein J. The mural ameloblastoma: review of literature. J Oral Surg 1978;36:866.
33. Slootweg PJ. An analysis of the interrelationship of the mixed odontogenic tumor–ameloblastic fibroma, ameloblastic fibro-odontoma, and the odontomas. Oral Surg 1981;51:266.
34. Slootweg PJ, Muller H. Malignant ameloblastoma or ameloblastic carcinoma. Oral Surg 1984;57:168.
35. Small IA, Waldron CA. Ameloblastomas of the jaws. Oral Surg 1955;8:281.
36. Tsaknis PJ, Nelson JF. The maxillary ameloblastoma: an analysis of 24 cases. J Oral Surg 1980;38:336.
37. Waldron C, El-Mofty S. A histopathologic study of 116 ameloblastomas with special reference to the desmoplastic variant. Oral Surg 1987;63:441.
38. Weiss M, Sutton L, Marcial V, Fowble B, Packer R, Zimmerman R, Shut L, Bruce D, D'Angio G. The role of radiation therapy in the management of childhood craniopharyngioma. Int J Radiat Oncol Biology Phys 1989;17:1313.
39. Wen BC, Hussey DH, Staples J, Hitchon PW, Jani SK, Vigliotti AP, Doornbos JF. A comparison of the roles of surgery and radiation therapy in the management of craniopharyngiomas. Int J Radiat Oncol Biol Phys 1989;16:17.
40. Zallen RD, Preskar MH, McClary SA. Ameloblastic fibroma. J Oral Surg 1982;40: 513.

INDEX

Page numbers in *italics* denote figures; those followed by "t" denote tables.